KU-262-278

Applied Therapeutics:
THE CLINICAL USE OF DRUGS
Eighth Edition

Edited By

Mary Anne Koda-Kimble, PharmD
Professor and Dean
TJ Long Chair in Chain Pharmacy Practice
School of Pharmacy
University of California, San Francisco
San Francisco, California

Lloyd Yee Young, PharmD
Professor and Chair
TA Oliver Chair in Clinical Pharmacy
School of Pharmacy
University of California, San Francisco
San Francisco, California

Wayne A. Kradjan, PharmD, BCPS
Professor and Dean
College of Pharmacy
Oregon State University
Oregon Health & Science University
Corvallis, Oregon

B. Joseph Guglielmo, PharmD
Professor and Vice Chair
Department of Clinical Pharmacy
School of Pharmacy
University of California, San Francisco
San Francisco, California

Assistant Editors

Brian K. Alldredge, PharmD
Professor of Clinical Pharmacy
Clinical Professor of Neurology
Departments of Clinical Pharmacy and Neurology
University of California, San Francisco
San Francisco, California

Robin L. Corelli, PharmD
Associate Professor of Clinical Pharmacy
Department of Clinical Pharmacy
University of California, San Francisco
San Francisco, California

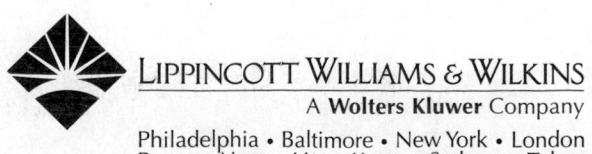

LIPPINCOTT WILLIAMS & WILKINS
A **Wolters Kluwer** Company

Philadelphia • Baltimore • New York • London
Buenos Aires • Hong Kong • Sydney • Tokyo

Editor: David Troy
Managing Editor: Matthew J. Hauber
Marketing Manager: Sam Smith
Senior Project Editor: Paula C. Williams
Designer: Risa Clow
Compositor: Graphic World, Inc.
Printer: Quebecor World—Versailles

Copyright © 2005 Lippincott Williams & Wilkins

351 West Camden Street
Baltimore, Maryland 21201-2436 USA

530 Walnut Street
Philadelphia, Pennsylvania 19106-3621 USA

All rights reserved. This book is protected by copyright. No part of this book may be reproduced in any form or by any means, including photocopying, or utilized by any information storage and retrieval system without written permission from the copyright owner.

The publisher is not responsible (as a matter of product liability, negligence, or otherwise) for any injury resulting from any material contained herein. This publication contains information relating to general principles of medical care, which should not be construed as specific instructions for individual patients. Manufacturers' product information and package inserts should be reviewed for current information, including contraindications, dosages, and precautions.

Printed in the United States of America

Library of Congress Cataloging-in-Publication Data

Applied therapeutics : the clinical use of drugs / edited by Mary Anne Koda-Kimble . . . [et al.] ; assistant editors, Brian K. Alldredge, Robin L. Corelli.—8th ed.
    p. ; cm.
Includes bibliographical references and index.
ISBN 0-7817-4845-3
1. Chemotherapy. 2. Pharmacology. I. Koda-Kimble, Mary Anne.
[DNLM: 1. Drug Therapy. WB 330 A651 2004]
RM262.A65 2004
615.5′8—dc22

The publishers have made every effort to trace the copyright holders for borrowed material. If they have inadvertently overlooked any, they will be pleased to make the necessary arrangements at the first opportunity.

To purchase additional copies of this book call our customer service department at **(800) 638-3030** or fax orders to **(301) 824-7390**. International customers should call **(301) 714-2324**.

Visit Lippincott Williams & Wilkins on the Internet: **http://www.lww.com**. Lippincott Williams & Wilkins customer service representatives are available from 8:30 am to 6:00 pm, EST, Monday through Friday, for telephone access.

04 05 06
1 2 3 4 5 6 7 8 9 10

PREFACE TO THE EIGHTH EDITION

It has been nearly 30 years since the first edition of Applied Therapeutics: The Clinical Use of Drugs was published. The use of case studies and problem solving integrated with timely clinical information served as a founding principle for this innovative text; this format remains integral to the current edition. The editors and authors strive to provide current treatment recommendations in an ever-changing health care environment. Human immunodeficiency virus was unheard of in 1975, but now the dynamics of this disease and new strategies involved in its treatment, are drivers, among others, stimulating the need to publish updated editions in rapid succession. In this edition are new chapters (Culturally Competent Care, End of Life, Smoking Cessation), renewed emphases on complementary and alternative medical therapies, and significant new therapies in all chapters.

It is critical that health care providers make informed decisions regarding the clinical use of drugs. As our population ages, more people carry the burden of multiple chronic diseases. New knowledge about pathophysiology and drug targets have expanded our approaches to drug therapy, and in many cases, polypharmacy has become the standard of care. This, in turn, increases patient exposure to adverse medica-

tion events. Furthermore, the latest statistics show that health care spending in the United States topped $1.6 trillion dollars in 2002. Spending for prescription drugs exceeded $160 billion, the fastest growing component of health care spending and under ever increasing scrutiny. Landmark legislation providing prescription drug benefits for Medicare recipients will increase further the demand for prescription drugs and the accompanying economic burden. We hope our readers can more rationally care for their patients and make decisions that will assure the most cost effective use of limited time and resources.

As in previous editions, our authors present patient cases that stimulate the reader to integrate and apply therapeutic principles in the context of specific clinical situations. We also strive to provide students and practitioners with a glimpse into the minds of clinicians who are assessing and solving therapeutic problems so that they too can develop and refine their own problem-solving skills. *Although the authors have been careful to recommend therapies that are in agreement with current standards and responsible literature, we recommend that our readers consult several appropriate information sources when dealing with new and unfamiliar drugs.*

PREFACE TO THE SEVENTH EDITION

The last chapter for the seventh edition of Applied Therapeutics, Inc. (ATI) has been delivered to the publisher and we celebrate its completion. The dedication of our authors, editors, reviewers, and publisher has been remarkable and very much appreciated. Although the work on this edition now comes to a gradual close, we see much work awaiting all of us as we observe a health care system under considerable stress. Shortages of nurses, pharmacists, and other health care providers interface with remarkable new technologies, increased costs, and decreased access to care. The roles of the disadvantaged and the underserved continue to increase at a time of remarkable economic growth over the past decade. Meanwhile, health care strives to find better approaches to manage escalating costs, to enhance the quality of care provided, and to meet and exceed rising customer expectations. Systems to guarantee safety and freedom from errors (including medication errors) are urgently needed as our rapidly growing elderly populations increasingly access health care.

The future of health care ultimately resides in the next generation of practitioners. We need to recruit the best and the brightest to health care and we need to prepare them to meet the challenges of tomorrow. Our understanding of diseases has improved, new drugs are available, and we eagerly await the result of continuing research in fields such as neurochemical biology, genetics, genomics, medicine, and public health. We hope this edition shares sufficient thought processes to assist students in the formulation of the problem-solving skills needed to integrate present and future knowledge about its appropriate drug use.

All chapters in this edition have been revised and updated to reflect our changing knowledge of drugs and the application of this knowledge to the therapy of patients. As in previous editions, we have encouraged our authors to present patient cases that stimulate the reader to integrate and apply therapeutic principles to the specific patient. In this text, we have striven to provide students and practitioners with a glimpse into the minds of clinicians who are assessing and solving therapeutic problems so that they too can begin to develop their own set of problem-solving skills.

The authors have drawn much information from their clinical experiences. *It remains the responsibility of every practitioner to evaluate the appropriateness of a particular opinion in the context of the actual clinical situation and with due consideration of any new developments in the field. Although the authors have been careful to recommend therapies that are in agreement with current standards and responsible literature, we recommend the student or practitioner consult several appropriate information sources when dealing with new and unfamiliar drugs.*

B. Joseph Guglielmo
Mary Anne Koda-Kimble
Wayne A. Kradjan
Lloyd Yee Young

October 2000

PREFACE TO THE FIRST EDITION

In the past decade, new roles for the pharmacist have emerged. More and more frequently the pharmacist is placed in increasingly responsible positions within the health care delivery system. In this capacity (s)he is able to have a significant influence on the quality of health care delivered to the patient. M. Silverman and P. Lee have skillfully assessed the current and future role of the pharmacist in *Pills, Profits and Politics.*[1]

". . . It is the pharmacist who can play a vital role in assisting physicians to prescribe rationally, who can help see to it that the right drug is ordered for the right patient at the right time, in the right amounts and with due consideration of costs and that the patient knows how, when and why to use both prescription and non-prescription products.

It is the pharmacist who has been most highly trained as an expert in drug products, who has the best opportunity to keep up-to-date on developments in this field and who can serve both physician and patient as a knowledgeable advisor. It is the pharmacist who can take a key part in preventing drug misuse, drug abuse and irrational prescribing."

Many schools of pharmacy have made substantial curriculum changes to prepare their graduates for these responsibilities. Although traditional pharmacy courses have imparted factual information about drugs, they have not enabled the students to apply these facts to the drug therapy of patients. Similarly, traditional pharmacology and medical textbooks do not provide the professional with sufficient information to make a judgment regarding the selection and dosing of a particular product for a specific patient. To arrive at this decision, the clinician must consider a number of patient factors, including age, renal and hepatic function, concurrent disease states and medications and allergies. (S)he must also consider drug product factors, including bioavailability, pharmacokinetics, efficacy, toxicity, risk to benefit ratio, and cost.

We have found that students have most difficulty in *integrating* and *applying* the multiple components of their education to formulate the safest, most rational drug regimen for a given patient. We have also observed that although the student is able to enumerate the adverse effects on a drug, (s)he is unable to recognize or monitor for these effects should they occur in his/her patient.

This text is an outgrowth of the clinical pharmacy courses taught at the University of California and at Washington State University. The major objective of these courses is to enable the student to practice effectively in the clinical setting. Lectures on the pathophysiology and medical management of disease states are supplemented with conferences where students are challenged with drug therapy questions frequently asked by physicians and by case histories, which require drug therapy assessment and the selection of appropriate alternatives. The objective of these conferences and this text is to enable the student to identify relevant factors in drug treatment, such as the probability of whether or not a specific drug is responsible for a patient's symptoms; the clinical significance of a drug interaction; why a specific drug is not achieving therapeutic blood levels; the dose for a patient with multiple disease states.

The success of the conference portion of our courses was a major determinant of the format used for this text; case histories that simulate the actual practice situations and frequently asked therapeutic questions are followed by well-referenced responses.

The authors have drawn much information from their clinical experiences. *It remains the responsibility of every practitioner to evaluate the appropriateness of a particular opinion in the context of the actual clinical situation and with due considerations of any new developments in the field.* Although the authors have been careful to recommend dosages that are in agreement with current standards and responsible literature, we suggest the student or practitioner consult several appropriate information sources when dealing with new and unfamiliar drugs.

ACKNOWLEDGMENTS TO EIGHTH EDITION

We are deeply indebted to the many dedicated people who have given of themselves to complete the eighth edition of this book. As always, we are most grateful to our contributing authors who are attentive to meeting our stringent time deadlines and unique writing format. We especially thank the following section editors for their truly remarkable support as they edited chapters, assisted authors, and worked with our publishers at Lippincott Williams & Wilkins (LWW): Ann Bolinger-Churukian (Pediatrics), Thomas J. Comstock (Renal Disorders), Allan J. Ellsworth (Dermatologic Disorders), Beverly J. Holcombe (Nutrition), Celeste M. Lindley (Neoplastic Disorders), Mark D. Watanabe and Patrick R. Finley (Psychiatric Disorders), and Bradley R. Williams (Geriatric Therapy).

We also wish to acknowledge our colleagues David Troy, Matt Hauber, Loftin (Paul) Montgomery, and Paula Williams at LWW for their diligence in reviewing our work, helping us all to stay on task, and for their attention to detail. Above all, we are especially grateful for the understanding and long-suffering patience of our spouses (Carolyn, Kimberly, Tom, Deter, Don, and Linda), respectively, during those nights and weekends we spent writing or editing; our children (both young and old); and now our grandchildren.

Finally, we dedicate our work to the patients we have cared for. They have taught us over and over again how critical it is to tailor our knowledge to their specific circumstances; to listen well; and to welcome them as true partners in their care.

WAYNE A. KRADJAN
BRIAN K. ALLDREDGE
ROBIN L. CORELLI
B. JOSEPH GUGLIELMO
MARY ANNE KODA-KIMBLE
LLOYD YEE YOUNG

COMPANION CD-ROM AND INSTRUCTOR WEB SITE

New to the Eighth Edition of *Applied Therapeutics*—
- *LWWBookView CD-ROM,* containing the full text of the Eighth Edition in an indexed, page-view format. Also includes a series of pathophysiology animations for self-study.

- *LWW Connection web site,* available at http://connection.lww.com. Site features quarterly updated drug information provided by Facts and Comparisons and sourced from A to Z DrugFacts.

See inside back cover for details.

NOTICE TO READER

Drug therapy information is constantly evolving. Our ever-changing knowledge and experience with drugs and the continual development of new drugs necessitates changes in treatment and drug therapy. The editors, authors, and publisher of this work have made every effort to ensure the information provided herein was accurate at the time of publication. *It remains the responsibility of every practitioner to evaluate the appropriateness of a particular opinion or therapy in the context of the actual clinical situation and with due consideration of any new developments in the field.* Although the authors have been careful to recommend dosages that are in agreement with current standards and responsible literature, the student or practitioner should consult several appropriate information sources when dealing with new and unfamiliar drugs.

Steven R. Abel, PharmD
Professor and Head
Department of Pharmacy Practice
Purdue University School of Pharmacy
and Pharmacal Sciences
Indianapolis, Indiana

Brian K. Alldredge, PharmD
Professor of Clinical Pharmacy
Clinical Professor of Neurology
Departments of Clinical Pharmacy and Neurology
Northern California Comprehensive Epilepsy Center
University of California, San Francisco
San Francisco, California

Judith Ann Alsop, PharmD
Associate Clinical Professor of Pharmacy
Department of Clinical Pharmacy
University of California, San Francisco
San Francisco, California

J. V. Anandan, PharmD, BCPS
Adjunct Associate Professor
Eugene Applebaum College of Pharmacy and Health Sciences
Wayne State University
Pharmacy Specialist, Department of Pharmacy, Henry Ford
    Hospital
Detroit, Michigan

Edgar R. Arriola, PharmD
Coordinator, Drug Information Center
UCLA Medical Center
Department of Pharmaceutical Services
Los Angeles, California

Sara Grimsley Augustin, PharmD, BCPP
Assistant Professor
Clinical and Administrative Sciences
Mercer University Southern School of Pharmacy
Atlanta, Georgia

Francesca T. Aweeka, PharmD
Professor, Director of Drug Research Unit
Department of Clinical Pharmacy
University of California, San Francisco
San Francisco, California

Omar Badawi, PharmD
Assistant Clinical Professor
Department of Pharmacy Practice and Science, University of
    Maryland
Clinical Pharmacist, Cardiac Intensive Care Unit
University of Maryland Medical Center
Baltimore, Maryland

Andrew D. Barnes, PharmD
Clinical Pharmacist
Cardiothoracic Surgery, Department of Pharmacy, University of
    Washington Medical Center
Clinical Assistant Professor, School of Pharmacy
University of Washington
Seattle, Washington

David T. Bearden, PharmD
Clinical Assistant Professor
Department of Pharmacy Practice
College of Pharmacy
Oregon State University
Portland, Oregon

Sandra Benavides, PharmD
Assistant Professor
University of Texas, Pan American
Edinburg, Texas

William H. Benefield Jr., PharmD, BCPP, FASCP
Clinical Assistant Professor
Department of Pharmacotherapy, University of Texas, Health
    Sciences Center at San Antonio
Consultant, Pharmerica
San Antonio, Texas

Paul M. Beringer, PharmD
Associate Professor
USC School of Pharmacy
Los Angeles, California

Daniel Bestul, PharmD
Oncology Pharmacy Specialist
Pharmacy Department, University of Colorado Hospital
Department of Clinical Pharmacy
Univesity of Colorado School of Pharmacy
Denver, Colorado

Nicholas Ronald Blanchard, PharmD, Med
Associate Professor
Pharmacy Practice
Wingate University
Wingate, North Carolina

Ann M. Bolinger, PharmD
Associate Professor of Clinical Pharmacy
Department of Clinical Pharmacy
School of Pharmacy
University of California, San Francisco
San Francisco, California

Thomas C. Bookwalter, PharmD
Assistant Clinical Professor
Department of Clinical Pharmacy, School of Pharmacy
Clinical Pharmacist, Department of Clinical Pharmacy,
    Long-Moffit Hospital
University of California, San Francisco
San Francisco, California

Mary C. Borovicka, PharmD, BCPP
Assistant Professor
Department of Pharmacy Practice, University of Toledo
Clinical Pharmacy Specialist, Pharmacy Department,
Louis Stokes VA Medical Center
Toledo, Ohio

Tina Penick Brock, PharmD
Clinical Associate Professor
Department of Pharmacy, University of North Carolina at Chapel Hill
Clinical Specialist, Pharmacy Department ,
UNC Hospitals
Chapel Hill, North Carolina

Donald F. Brophy, PharmD, BCPS
Associate Professor
Departments of Pharmacy Practice and Internal Medicine
School of Pharmacy
Virginia Commonwealth University
Richmond, Virginia

Glen R. Brown, PharmD
Clinical Coordinator
Pharmacy Department
St. Paul's Hospital
Vancouver, British Columbia, Canada

Jill S. Burkiewicz, PharmD
Assistant Professor
Director, Primary Care Residency Program Midwestern Univesity
Midwestern University Chicago College of Pharmacy
Clinical Pharmacisi, Advocate Health Centers
Downer's Grove, Illinois

Betsy A. Carlisle, PharmD, CDF
Clinical Coordinator
Department of Pharmacy
Seton Medical Center
Austin, Texas

Barry L Carter, PharmD, FCCP, BCPS, FAHA
Professor and Head
Division of Clinical and Administrative Pharmacy
College of Pharmacy and Department of Family Medicine
University of Iowa
Iowa City, Iowa

Pauline Ann Cawley, PharmD
Clinical Assistant Professor
Clinical Pharmacy, University of Utah
Clinical Pharmacist Specialist, Critical Care
LDS Hospital
Salt Lake City, Utah

Jennifer C. Y. Chan, PharmD
Clinical Assistant Professor
College of Pharmacy, The University of Texas at Austin
Clinical Associate Professor of Pediatrics and Clinical Assistant Professor of Pharmacology
The University of Texas Health Science Center
San Antonio, Texas

Stanley W. Chapman, MD
Director, Division of Infectious Diseases
Professor of Medicine, Department of Medicine
University of Mississippi Medical Center
Jackson, Mississippi

Steven W. Chen, PharmD, FASHP, CDM
Assistant Professor of Clinical Pharmacy
University of Southern California
Los Angeles, California

Michael F. Chicella, PharmD
Clinical Specialist, Pediatrics
Children's Hospital of the King's Daughters
Norfolk, Virginia

Moses S. S. Chow, PharmD, FCP, FCCP
Professor and Director
School of Pharmacy
Faculty of Medicine
The Chinese University of Hong Kong
Shatin, Hong Kong

Tom B. Christian, RPh, BCPS
Staff Pharmacist
Pharmacy Department, Southwest Washington Medical Center
Vancouver, Washington

John D. Cleary, PharmD
Professor,
School of Pharmacy, Department of Clinical Pharmacy Practice
School of Pharmacy
Department of Clinical Pharmacy Practice
Associate Professor of Infectious Diseases
University of Mississippi Medical Center
Jackson, Mississippi

Lenore Coleman, PharmD
Research Fellow
School of Pharmacy
Howard Univesity
Washington, DC

Thomas J. Comstock, PharmD
Associate Professor
Department of Pharmacy
Virginia Commonwealth University
Richmond, Virginia

Michelle Condren, PharmD
Assistant Professor
Departmnet of Pharmacy Practice
Texas Tech University Health Science Center School of Pharmacy
Amarillo, Texas

Andrea Cooper, PharmD, BCPS
Assistant Professor of Clinical Pharmacy
Pharmacy Department
University of Southern California School of Pharmacy
Los Angeles, California

Robin L. Corelli, PharmD
Associate Professor of Clinical Pharmacy
Department of Clinical Pharmacy
University of California, San Francisco
San Francisco, California

Larry H. Danziger, PharmD
Professor of Pharmacy Practice
Department of Pharmacy Practice
University of Illinois at Chicago
Chicago, Illinois

Lisa E. Davis, PharmD, FCCP, BCPS, BCOP
Associate Professor of Clinical Pharmacy
Philadelphia College of Pharmacy
University of the Sciences in Philadelphia
Philadelphia, Pennsylvania

Suzanne D. Day, PharmD, BCOP
Clinical Pharmacy Associates, Inc.
Atlanta, Georgia

Cathi Dennehy, PharmD
Associate Clinical Professor
Department of Clinical Pharmacy
University of California, San Francisco
San Francisco, California

Betty Jean Dong, PharmD
Professor of Clinical Pharmacy
Departments of Clinical Pharmacy and Family and Community
    Medicine
University of California, San Francisco
San Francisco, California

Andrew J. Donnelly, PharmD, MBA
Director, Hospital Pharmacy Services
University of Illinois Medical Center at Chicago
Clinical Professor Department of Pharmacy Practice
University of Illinois Medical Center at Chicago
Chicago, Illinois

Julie Ann Dopheide, PharmD, BCPP
Associate Professor of Clinical Pharmacy,
Psychiatry and the Behavioral Sciences
USC Schools of Pharmacy and Medicine
University of Southern California
Los Angeles, California

Richard Drew, PharmD, BCPS
Associate Professor
Duke School of Medicine,
Campbell University School of Pharmacy
Clinical Pharmacist, Infectious Diseases, Duke Medical Center
Durham, North Carolina

Vicky Dudas, PharmD
Assistant Clinical Professor of Pharmacy
Department of Clinical Pharmacy, School of Pharmacy
University of California at San Francisco
San Francisco, California

Robert E. Dupuis, PharmD, BCPS
Clinical Associate Professor
School of Pharmacy
Division of Pharmacotherapy
University of North Carolina at Chapel Hill
Chapel Hill, North Carolina

Sandra B. Earle, PharmD, BCPS
Assistant Professor of Pharmacy Practice
Department of Pharmacy Practice, College of Pharmacy
Oregon State University
Portland, Oregon

Allan Ellsworth, PharmD, BCPS, PA-C
Professor of Pharmacy and Family Medicine
Schools of Pharmacy and Medicine, Departments of Pharmacy and
    Family Medicine
Clinical Pharmacist/Physician Assist, Department of Family
    Medicine
University of Washington
Seattle, Washington

Michael E. Ernst, PharmD
Assistant Professor (Clinical)
Division of Clinical and Administrative Pharmacy
Assistant Professor (Clinical)
Department of Family Medicine
The University of Iowa Hospitals and Clinic
University of Iowa College of Pharmacy
Iowa City, Iowa

Martha P. Fankhauser, MS Pharm, FASHP, BCPP
Clinical Associate Professor
Department of Pharmacy Practice and Science
University of Arizona College of Pharmacy
Tucson, Arizona

Patrick R. Finley, PharmD, BCPP
Associate Clinical Professor
Department of Clinical Pharmacy,
University of California, San Francisco
San Francisco, California

Douglas N. Fish, PharmD, BCPS
Associate Professor of Pharmacy
Department of Pharmacy Practice,
University of Colorado School of Pharmacy
Clinical Pharmacist
Medical/Surgical Intensive Care Units, Department of Pharmacy
University of Colorado Hospital
Denver, Colorado

Mark W. Garrison, PharmD
Associate Professor
Department of Pharmacotherapy
Washington State University, Spokane
Spokane, Washington

Steven P. Gelone, PharmD
Associate Professor of Pharmacy
Pharmacy Practice Department
School of Pharmacy
Assistant Professor of Medicine
Section of Infectious Diseases
Department of Medicine, School of Medicine
Clinical Pharmacist in Infectious Diseases
Temple University Health System
Temple University
Philadelphia, Pennsylvania

Jane Maria Gervasio, PharmD,BCNSP
Nutrition Support Pharmacist
Clinical Pharmacy
Clarian Health at Methodist Hospital
Indianapolis, Indiana

Barry E. Gidal, PharmD
Assistant Professor
University of Wisconsin
School of Pharmacy and Department of Neurology
Division of Neurology
Madison, Wisconsin

Jeffery A. Goad, PharmD, BCPS
Assistant Professor of Clinical Pharmacy
Pharmacy Department
University of Southern California School of Pharmacy
Los Angeles, Californa

Julie A. Golembiewski, PharmD
Clinical Associate Professor
Department of Pharmacy Practice, College of Pharmacy, University
   of Illinois at Chicago, University of Illinois Medical Center at
   Chicago
Phamacotherapist, Pharmacy Services - Anesthesiology
University of Illinois Medical Center
Chicago, Illinois

William C. Gong, PharmD, FASHP
Associate Professor of Clinical Pharmacy
Director, Residency and Fellowship Training
University of Southern California, School of Pharmacy
Los Angeles, California

Susan Goodin, PharmD, BCPS, BCOP
Associate Professor of Medicine
Division of Medical Oncology
UMDNJ/Robert Wood Johnson Medical School
Director, Division of Pharmaceutical Sciences
The Cancer Institute of New Jersey
New Brunswick, New Jersey

B. Joseph Guglielmo, PharmD
Professor and Vice Chair
Department of Clinical Pharmacy
School of Pharmacy
University of California, San Francisco
San Francisco, California

Mark R. Haase, PharmD
Assistant Professor of Pharmacy Practice
Department of Pharmacy Practice
Texas Tech University School of Pharmacy
Amarillo, Texas

Emily B. Hak, PharmD
Associate Professor, Pharmacy and Pediatrics
University of Tennessee Health Sciences Center
Clinical Pharmacist, Pharmacy Department, Le Bonheur Children's
   Medical Cen
Memphis, Tennessee

Raymond W. Hammond, PharmD, FCCP, BCPS
Associate Dean for Practice Programs
Clinical Associate Professor
College of Pharmacy
University of Houston
Houston, Texas

Jennifer L. Hardman, PharmD
Clinical Assistant Professor
Department of Pharmacy Practice and Obstetrics and Gynecology,
   University of Illinois at Chicago
Clinical Pharmacist, Department of Pharmacy Practice
University of Illinois Medical Center
Chicago, Illinois

R. Donald Harvey,III, PharmD, BCPS, BCOP
Division of Pharmacoterapy
University of North Carolina
Senior Clinical Specialist, Department of Pharmacy
University of North Carolina Hospitals
Chapel Hill, North Carolina

Fotini K. Hatzopoulos, PharmD
Clinical Associate Professor
Pharmacy Practice
Assistant Director, Clinical Services, Hospital Pharmacy Services
University of Illinois at Chicago Medical Center
Chicago, Illinois

David W. Henry, M.S., B.C.O.P., FASHP
Associate Professor, Pharmacy Practice
Pharmacy Specialist in Pediatric Hematology/Oncology
University of Kansas Medical Center
Kansas City, Kansas

Beverly J. Holcombe, PharmD, BCNSP
Clinical Professor
Division of Pharmacotherapy, School of Pharmacy
Clinical Specialist, Department of Pharmacy, University of North
   Carolina Health Care
University of North Carolina at Chapel Hill
Chapel Hill, North Carolina

Mark T. Holdsworth, PharmD, BCOP
Associate Professor of Pharmacy and Pediatrics
College of Pharmacy
University of New Mexico
Albuquerque, New Mexico

Curtis D. Holt, PharmD
Associate Clinical Professor
Department of Surgery
UCLA Medical Center
Los Angeles, California

Yvonne Huckleberry, PharmD
Clinical Assistant Professor
Department of Pharmacotherapy
College of Pharmacy
Washington State University
Pullman, Washington

Karen Suchanek Hudmon, Dr. P. H.
Assistant Clinical Professor
Department of Clinical Pharmacy
University of California, San Francisco
San Francisco, California

Joanna Q. Hudson, PharmD, BCPS
Assistant Professor
Departments of Clinical Pharmacy and Medicine (Nephrology)
Clinical Pharmacist, Pharmacy Department, UT Bowld Hospital
University of Tennessee, Memphis
Memphis, Tennessee

Gail S. Itokazu, PharmD
Clinical Assistant Professor
Department of Pharmacy Practice
University of Illinois at Chicago
Clinical Pharmacist, Department of Medicine, Division of
    Infectious Diseases
Cook County Hospital
John H. Stroger, Jr. Hospital of Cook County
Chicago, Illinois

Timothy J Ives, PharmD, MPH, FCCP, BCPS
Associate Professor of Pharmacy
School of Pharmacy and Medicine
University of North Carolina at Chapel Hill
Chapel Hill, North Carolina

Curtis A. Johnson, PharmD
Professor
School of Pharmacy
University of Wisconsin-Madison
Madison, Wisconsin

Paul W. Jungnickel, PhD
Professor and
Associate Dean for Academic and Student Affairs
Harrison School of Pharmacy
Auburn University
Auburn, Alabama

Angela Kashuba, PharmD
Associate Professor of Pharmacy
Division of Pharmacotherapy, School of Pharmacy
University of North Carolina at Chapel Hill
Chapel Hill, North Carolina

Michael B. Kays, PharmD, BCPS, FCCP
Associate Professor of Pharmacy Practice
Department of Pharmacy Practice
Perdue University School of Pharmacy
Indianapolis, Indiana

Jiwon W. Kim, PharmD
Assistant Professor
Department of Pharmacy, Univesity of Southern California
Clinical Pharmacist, Department of Pharmacy,
University of Southern California University Hospital
Los Angeles, California

Mary Anne Koda-Kimble, PharmD
Professor and Dean
TJ Long Chair in Chain Pharmacy Practice
School of Pharmacy
University of California, San Francisco
San Francisco, California

Peter J.S. Koo, PharmD
Pharmacist Specialist, Pain Management
Associate Clinical Professor of Pharmacy,
Department of Clinical Pharmacy
University of California, San Francisco
San Francisco, California

Wayne A. Kradjan, PharmD
Dean and Professor
College of Pharmacy
Oregon State University
Oregon Health and Science University
Corvallis, Oregon

Donna M. Kraus, PharmD
Pediatric Clinical Pharmacist
Associate Professor of Pharmacy Practice
Departments of Pharmacy Practice and Pediatrics
Colleges of Pharmacy and Medicine
University of Illinois at Chicago
Chicago, Illinois

Lisa Kroon, PharmD, CDE
Associate Clinical Professor
Department of Clinical Pharmacy
University of California, San Francisco
San Francisco, California

Jonathan Lacro, PharmD, BCPS, BCPP
Associate Clinical Professor
Psychiatry Department, University of California, San Diego
VA San Diego Healthcare System, Clinical Pharmacist, Pharmacy
    Service
University of California San Diego
San Diego, California

Alan H. Lau, PharmD, FCCP
Professor
Department of Pharmacy Practice
College of Pharmacy
University of Illinois at Chicago
Chicago, Illinois

Kelly C. Lee, PharmD
Assistant Professor of Pharmacy Practice
Clinical Pharmacy
Loma Linda University School of Pharmacy
Loma Linda, California

Susan H. Lee, PharmD
Clinical Pharmacist
Department of Pharmacy Services
University of Washington
Clinical Care Pharmacist
Department of Pharmacy Services
Harborview Medical Center
Seattle, Washington

Celeste Lindley, PharmD, FCCP, FASHP, BCOP
Associate Professor of Pharmacy
Clinical Associate Professor of Medicine
University of North Carolina at Chapel Hill
Chapel Hill, North Carolina

Rex S. Lott, PharmD
Associate Professor
Department of Pharmacy Practice & Administrative Science
College of Pharmacy
Idaho State University
Clinical Pharmacist, Psychiatric Department
Boise Veterans Affairs Medical Center
Boise, Idaho

Raymond C. Love, PharmD, BCPP, FASHP
Professor
Department of Pharmacy Practice & Science
School of Pharmacy
University of Maryland
Baltimore, Maryland

Andrew D. Luber, PharmD
Executive Director
Pacific Oaks Research
Clinical Pharmacy Specialist—HIV/Infectious Diseases
Pacific Oaks Medical Group
Beverly Hills, California

Sherry Luedtke, PharmD
Associate Professor
Pharmacy Practice
Associate Dean for Professional Affairs
Texas Tech University Health Science Center School of Pharmacy
Amarillo, Texas

James W. McAuley, PhD
Associate Professor
College of Pharmacy
The Ohio State University
Columbus, Ohio

James P. McCormack, PharmD
Associate Professor
Faculty of Pharmaceutical Sciences
University of British Columbia
Vancouver, British Columbia, Canada

Jeannine McCune, PharmD
Assistant Professor
University of Washington
Seattle, Washington

James M. McKenney, PharmD
Professor Emeritus
Virginia Commonwealth University
President and CEO, National Clinical Research
Richmond, Virginia

Robert J. Michocki, PharmD
Professor
Pharmacy Practice and Science
School of Pharmacy
University of Maryland
Baltimore, Maryland

Robert Keith Middleton, PharmD
Clinical Coordinator
Department of Pharmacy,
Beebe Medical Center
Lewes, Delaware

Milap C. Nahata, PharmD
Professor and Chair
College of Pharmacy
The Ohio State University
Columbus, Ohio

Jean M. Nappi, PharmD, FCCP, BCPS
Professor of Pharmacy
Department of Pharmacy Practice
Medical University of South Carolina
Charleston, South Carolina

Paul G. Nolan Jr., PharmD, FCCP, FASHP
Professor
Department of Pharmacy Practice and Science
University of Arizona
Tucson, Arizona

Cindy Lea O'Bryant, PharmD, BCOP
Assistant Professor
Department of Clinical Pharamacy University of Colorado School
  of Pharmacy
University of Colorado Health Sciences Center
Denver, Colorado

Judith A. O'Donnell, PharmD
Associate Professor of Medicine and Public Health
Division of Infectious Diseases,
Drexel University College of Medicine
Attending Physician - Hospital Epidemiologist, Division of
  Infectious Diseases
Medical College of Pennsylvania Hospital
Philadelphia, Pennsylvania

Ali J. Olyaei, PharmD, BCPS
Assistant Professor of Medicine
School of Medicine
Oregon Health & Science University
Portland, Oregon

Neeta Bahal O'Mara, PharmD, BCPS
Clinical Pharmacist
Dialysis Clinics, Inc.
North Brunswick, New Jersey

Robert Lee Page, PharmD
Assistant Professor
Department of Clinical Pharmacy
UCHSC School of Pharmacy
Clinical Specialist, Cardiology/Heart Failure
Department of Pharmacy
University of Colorado
Denver, Colorado

Louise Parent-Stevens, PharmD, BCPS
Clinical Assistant Professor
Department of Pharmacy Practice
College of Pharmacy
Pharmacotherapist, Department of Family Medicine
University of Illinois at Chicago
Chicago, Illinois

Jennifer Tran Pham, PharmD, BCPS
Clinical Assistant Professor
Department of Pharmacy Practice
University of Illinois at Chicago
Neonatal Clinical Pharmacist, Pharmacy Department
University of Illinois Medical Center at Chicago
Chicago, Illinois

David J. Quan, PharmD
Associate Clinical Professor
Department of Clinical Pharmacy
Clinical Pharmacist, Pharmaceutical Services, UCSF Medical
    Center
University of California San Francisco
San Francisco, California

Carrie Quigley, PharmD
Assistant Professor
Pharmacy Practice, Midwestern University
Chicago College of Pharmacy
Clinical Pharmacist, Pharmacy Department, North Chicago VA
    Medical Center
Downers Grove, Illinois

Ralph H. Raasch, PharmD
Associate Professor
Division of Pharmacotherapy
School of Pharmacy
Clinical Specialist, Pharmacy Department, University of North
    Carolina Hospitals
University of North Carolina at Chapel Hill
Chapel Hill, North Carolina

Lori Reisner, PharmD
Palo Alto Medical Foundation
Palo Alto, California

Marjorie D. Robinson, PharmD
Antiviral Global Project Team, GPRD
Abbott Laboratories
Fort Lauderdale, Florida

Carol J. Rollins, RD, PharmD, BCNSP
Clinical Associate Professor
College of Pharmacy, Department of Pharmacy Practice and
    Science
Clinical Specialist, Pharmacy Department, University Medical
    Center
University of Arizona
Tucson, Arizona

Tricia M. Russell, PharmD, BCPS
Assistant Professor
Department of Pharmacy Practice,
Wilkes Univesity Nesbitt School of Pharmacy
Geisinger Health System, Clinical Pharmacist, Lipid Management
    Clinic, Geisinger Medical Group - Lake Scranton
Wilkes-Barre, Pennsylvania

Rosalie Sagraves, PharmD
Dean and Profesor of Pharmacy Practice
College of Pharmacy
University of Illinois at Chicago
Chicago, Illinois

Joseph J. Saseen, PharmD, BCPS
Associate Professor
Departments of Pharmacy and Family Medicine
University of Colorado Health Sciences Center
Denver, Colorado

Larry D. Sasich, PharmD, MPH
Pharmacist
Public Citizen's Health Research Group
Washington, District of Columbia

Terry L. Seaton, PharmD, FCCP, BCPS
Associate Professor
Division of Pharmacy Practice
Clinical Pharmacist Faculty, Mercy Family Medicine, St. John's
    Mercy Medical Center
St. Louis College of Pharmacy
St. Louis, Missouri

Timothy H. Self, PharmD
Professor, Department of Pharmacy
Director, Internal Medicine
Pharmacy Practice Residency Program
UT Bowld Hospital
University of Tennessee
Memphis, Tennessee

John Siepler, PharmD, BCNSP
Clinical Professor
Department of Clinical Pharmacy, School of Pharmacy, University
    of California San Francisco
Nutrition Support Specialty Pharmacist, Department of Pharmacy
University of California Davis Medical Center
Davis, California

Robert K. Smith, PharmD
Professor and Head
Department of Pharmacy Practice
Auburn University, Harrison School of Pharmacy
Auburn University, Alabama

Jessica Song, PharmD
Assistant Professor, Pharmacy Practice
University of the Pacific School of Pharmacy
San Jose Clerkship Coordinator
Department of Pharmacy Services
Santa Clara Valley Medical Center
University of the Pacific School of Pharmacy
San Jose, California

Suellyn J. Sorensen, PharmD, BCPS
Clinical Pharmacy Manager
Pharmacy Manager
Indiana University Hospital of Clarian Health Partners
Indianapolis, Indiana

Anne P. Spencer, PharmD, BCPS
Assistant Professor of Pharmacy Practice
College of Pharmacy
Clinical Specialist, Department of Pharmacy Services, Medical
    University of South Carolina Medical Center
Medical University of South Carolina
Charleston, South Carolina

Renee Spencer, PhD
Assistant Clinical Professor
School of Pharmacy, University of California San Francisco
Drug Information Coordinator and Clinical Pharmacist, Child,
    Youth and Family Services
San Francisco Community Mental Health Service
San Francisco, California

Glen L. Stimmel, PharmD
Professor of Clinical Pharmacy and Psychiatry
University of Southern California
School of Pharmacy
Los Angeles, Californa

Sana Sukkari, B Sc Phm, M. Phil
Oncology Palliative Care Pharmacist
Pharmacy Department
Joseph Brant Memorial Hospital
Burlington, Ontario, Canada

David Taber, PharmD
Clinical Assistant Professor
College of Pharmacy
Clinical Specialist, Pharmacy Department
Medical University of South Carolina
Charleston, South Carolina

Daniel J.G. Thirion, M.Sc, PharmD, BCPS
Clinical Assistant Professor
Faculte de Pharmacie,
Universite de Montreal
Clinical Pharmacist- Internal Medicine Teaching Unit, Pharmacy
    Department, Hospital Sacre-Coueu de Montreal
Montreal, Quebec, Canada

John F. Thompson, PharmD, FCP
Adjunct Associate Professor of Pharmacy Practice
University of Southern California
Los Angeles, California

Toby C. Trujillo, PharmD, BCPS
Adjunct Assistant Professor
Department of Pharmacy Practice, Massachusetts College of
    harmacy and Health Sciences
Clinical Coordinator - Cardiovascular Specialist, Pharmacy
    Department
Boston Medical Center
Boston, Massachusetts

Candy Tsourounis, PharmD
Associate Clinical Professor
Department of Clinical Pharmcy
School of Pharmacy
University of California, San Francisco
San Francisco, California

John Valgus, PharmD, BCOP
Clinical Assistant Professor
Division of Pharmacotherapy, UNC School of Pharmacy
Clinical Hematology/Oncology Specialist, Department of
    Pharmacy
University of North Carolina Hospitals and Clinics
Chapel Hill, North Carolina

Geoffrey Wall, PharmD, BCPS
Assistant Professor
Department of Pharmacy Practice,
College of Pharmacy, Drake University
Internal Medicine Clinical Pharmacist, Department of Pharmacy
Iowa Methodist Medical Center
Des Moines, Iowa

Mark D. Watanabe, PharmD, PhD, BCPP
Assistant Clinical Specialist, Pharmacy Practice
Northeastern University
Boston, Massachusetts

Charles Wayne Weart, PharmD, BCPS, FASHP
Professor
Department of Pharmacy Practice, College of Pharmacy
Medical University of South Carolina
Charleston, South Carolina

Timothy Edward Welty, PharmD, FCCP, BCPS
Associate Professor of Pharmacy Practice
McWhorter School of Pharmacy
Samford University
Adjunct Associate Research Professor,
Department of Neurology
University of Alabama, Birmingham
Birmingham, Alabama

C. Michael White, PharmD
Associate Professor of Pharmacy Practice
University of Connecticut School of Pharmacy
Co-Director, Arrhythmia and Cardiovascular Pharmacology
    Research, Pharmacy Department
Hartford Hospital Drug Information Center
Storrs, Connecticut

Bradley R. Williams, PharmD
Associate Professor
Clinical Pharmacy and Clinical Gerontology
Schools of Pharmacy and Gerontology
University of Southern California
Los Angeles, California

Dennis M. Williams, PharmD
Associate Professor
Division of Pharmacotherapy
Senior Clinical Specialist, Pharmacy Department, UNC Hospitals
University of North Carolina
Chapel Hill, North Carolina

Laura Winter, PharmD
Clinical Assistant Professor
Department of Pharmacy, Univesity of Washington School of
    Pharmacy
Clinical Pharmacist, Hematology/Oncology and HCT, Pharmacy
    Department
Children's Hospital and Regional Medical Center
Seattle, Washington

Ann K. Wittkowsky, PharmD, CACP
Clinical Professor
University of Washington School of Pharmacy
Director of Anticoagulation Services
University of Washington Medical Center
Seattle, Washington

Annie Wong-Beringer, PharmD
Associate Professor of Pharmacy Practice
University of Southern California, School of Pharmacy
Los Angeles, California

Lloyd Y. Young, PharmD
Professor and Chair
Department of Clinical Pharmacy
TA Oliver Endowed Chair in Clinical Pharmacy, School of
    Pharmacy
University of California, San Francisco
San Francisco, California

Veronica S.L. Young, PharmD
Clinical Assistant Professor
College of Pharmacy
University of Texas at Austin
Assistant Director, Drug Information Service
University of Texas Health Science Center
University of Texas Health Science Center at San Antonio
San Antonio, Texas

Wendy Zerngast, MD, PharmD
Resident Physician
Department of Anesthesiology
University of Washington Medical Centers
University of Washington
Seattle, Washington

Paolo V. Zizzo, DO
Assistant Clinical Professor
Department of Medicine, UCSD School of Medicine
Clinical Internist, Mobile Physician Services
San Diego, California

Wendy Zizzo, PharmD
Adjunct Professor of Behavioral Sciences
Alcohol and Other Drugs Study Program, San Diego City College
Assistant Clinical Professor of Pharmacy, Division of Clinical
    Pharmacy, School of Pharmacy
University of California, San Francisco
San Francisco, California

Margaret M. Pearson, PharmD, MS
Division of Epidemiology
Mississippi State Department of Health
Jackson, Mississippi

TABLE OF CONTENTS

Assessment of Therapy and Pharmaceutical Care

Robin L. Corelli, Wayne A. Kradjan, Mary Anne Koda-Kimble, Lloyd Y. Young,
B. Joseph Guglielmo, Brian K. Alldredge

This chapter presents several approaches to assessing drug therapy and providing basic pharmaceutical care. The illustrations used in this chapter primarily focus on the pharmacist; however, the principles used to assess patients' response to drug therapy are of value to all who have responsibility for the health and well-being of the patients they serve.

Pharmaceutical care has been described as "the responsible provision of drug therapy to achieve definite outcomes that are intended to improve a patient's quality of life."[1-3] Several key concepts form the basis of pharmaceutical care. The first is a belief and commitment by the practitioner that he or she shares *equal responsibility* with the patient and prescriber for optimal drug therapy outcomes and is willing to make this belief the driving force of practice. Second, the practitioner must be able to establish a trusting *professional–*

patient relationship. This allows him or her to gather the essential medical and social history needed to identify therapeutic problems, assess the patient's knowledge about drug therapy, and establish and evaluate therapeutic outcomes. This information is essential to the design and implementation of a pharmaceutical care plan that is specific to an individual patient's needs. The provision of such ongoing, individualized pharmaceutical care also encourages patients to use the pharmacist as a resource for drug therapy dilemmas. The third critical component of pharmaceutical care is *formal documentation,* not only of the pharmaceutical care plan, but also of all clinical interventions and therapeutic outcomes. These records enhance the continuity of care and can be used to facilitate communication with other providers involved in the patient's care.

ESTABLISHING THE PATIENT RECORD

The patient record provides readily available information that is needed to identify and assess medical problems. It is necessary for designing patient-specific care plans and documenting pharmaceutical care.

Pharmaceutical care has not progressed as readily in the community setting as it has in the institutional setting for several reasons. One explanation for this slow progress is attributed to the inaccessibility of patient "data" and the lack of easy communication between community practitioners and the other providers of care to their patients. Ideally, all practitioners providing care to a patient would have access to and communicate through a common patient record. Although computer technology is making patient records more readily available to all practitioners who are responsible for the care of a patient, practitioners within each practice site currently establish and maintain their own patient records. Therefore, community pharmacists must do the same. The development of a patient database by community pharmacists primarily entails gleaning a detailed history from the patient and supplementing this history with direct observations (e.g., physical appearance, mental acuity, insulin-injection technique), physical examination (e.g., blood pressure [BP], pulse), and laboratory tests (e.g., blood glucose or cholesterol levels).

Knowledge

To establish an accurate patient record, the practitioner must have a good understanding of the pathophysiology and clinical presentation of commonly encountered medical conditions so that he or she can correlate certain signs and symptoms with diseases. Pharmacists and other providers also must have a clear understanding of the appropriate use of drugs that are prescribed commonly to manage these diseases, including a thorough knowledge of pharmacology, how drugs are used to treat disease, and most important, the expected outcome of the therapy. The remaining chapters throughout this textbook provide knowledge for disease-specific interventions. This chapter provides a framework for the application of knowledge in various patient care settings.

Sources of Patient Information

Successful patient assessment and monitoring requires the gathering and organizing of all relevant information.[2,3] The patient (or a family member or other representative) is always the primary source of information. The primary care provider asks the patient a series of questions to obtain subjective information that is helpful in making a diagnosis or evaluating ongoing therapy. Likewise, pharmacists, home care nurses, and other providers without direct access to patient data also must obtain subjective data or measure objective physical data to guide recommendations for therapy and to monitor previously prescribed therapy.

Data-Rich Environment

In a "data-rich environment," such as a hospital or long-term care facility, a wealth of information is available to practitioners from the medical chart, pharmacy profile, and nursing medication administration record. In these settings, physicians, nurses, and patients are readily available. This facilitates timely, effective communication among those involved in the drug therapy decision-making process. Objective data (e.g., diagnosis, physical examination, laboratory and other test results, vital signs, weight, medications, intravenous [IV] flow rates, and fluid balance) are readily available. Likewise, the cases presented throughout this text usually provide considerable data on which to make more thorough assessments and therapeutic decisions.

Data-Poor Environment

In reality, many clinicians often are required to make assessments with limited information. Even in a relatively "data-poor environment," such as a community pharmacy, two valuable sources of information are still available: the medication profile and the patient. In addition, it usually is possible to consult with the prescriber (or the prescriber's office staff); however, contact with the prescriber may be delayed, and in some cases, requests for information may be met with resistance owing to time constraints or other factors. As illustrated later in this chapter, the successful practitioner can make assessments and intervene on the patient's behalf even in the absence of all the available information.

Interviewing the Patient

An ability to use effective communication principles (e.g., active listening, body language, voice intonation) and history-taking skills is crucial to a successful patient interaction.[2,3] Ideally, the initial patient interaction should occur by appointment in a private, professional, and unhurried environment; however, the ideal often is not an option. The process may be expedited by asking the patient to complete a written self-assessment history form (current medical conditions and medications) before obtaining a verbal history. Figure 1-1 presents a sample form.[3]

To the extent possible, the practitioner should ask open-ended questions so that the patient is encouraged to explain and elaborate. Skilled use of these questions puts the practitioner in the role of observer, listener, recorder, and prompter, and the patient in the role of storyteller. This technique also allows the practitioner to assess quickly the patient's depth of knowledge and understanding of his or her medications and health situation. Closed-ended questions (e.g., those that can be simply answered "yes" or "no") can be used to prompt patients who know little about their health situation and to systematically minimize inadvertent omissions. For example, many practitioners use a "head-to-toe" organ systems approach at the conclusion of the interview: "Just to be sure we haven't missed anything important, can you tell me if you have ever had any problems with your head? eyes? heart? lungs? gastrointestinal (GI) tract? liver? kidney? urinary tract? legs?" These questions are asked one at a time with a pause in between each to allow the patient to answer. All "yes" responses should be followed with additional questions such as, "Please explain what you experienced." As the practitioner gains experience and becomes more sophisticated in interviewing patients, subtle clues (e.g. unusual information, observation, body language) can be used to pursue a line of questioning that could elucidate an unexpected problem or clarify an existing problem. Finally, an important principle is to pay close attention to what the patient is saying and tailor

Name: _____   Date: _____

Mailing Address: _____
                      street   city   state   zip

Social Security Number: _____   Phone: (H) _____ (W) _____

DOB: _____   Height: _____   Weight: _____   HR: _____   BP: _____

Gender: _____   Pregnancy Status: _____

Allergies: _____   Reactions: _____

_____   _____

Devises/Alerts: _____

PRESCRIPTION MEDICATION HISTORY

Name/Strength	Directions	Start Date	Stop Date	Physician	Purpose	Effectiveness

OTC USE: Check conditions for which you have used a non-prescription medication.

_____ headache   _____ drowsiness   _____ heartburn/GI upset/gas
_____ eye/ear problems _____ weight loss   _____ vitamins
_____ cold/flu   _____ diarrhea   _____ herbal products
_____ allergies   _____ hemorrhoids   _____ organic products
_____ sinus   _____ muscle/joint pain   _____ other: _____
_____ cough   _____ rash/itching/dry skin
_____ sleeplessness

OVER-THE-COUNTER MEDICATION HISTORY

Name/Strength	Directions	Purpose	How Often	Effectiveness

FIGURE 1-1 Patient history form. (Reprinted with permission from Patient history form. A Practical Guide to Pharmaceutical Care, pp. 36–37, 2003, by the American Pharmaceutical Association.)

responses to his or her comments. The patient should be encouraged to do most of the talking, while the interviewer carefully listens and observes.

In all interactions, the health care provider must treat the patient with respect and must make every effort to ask questions and receive information in a nonjudgmental way (e.g., "Please tell me how you take your medications," as opposed to, "Do you take your medications exactly as prescribed?"). Practitioners who provide pharmaceutical care also must keep in mind that patients hold them in trust and often share intimate details of their medical and social histories. Thus, practitioners must maintain the confidentiality of that information

MEDICAL PROBLEMS: Have you experienced, or do you have: (circle Y or N)

known kidney problems?	Y	N	sores on legs or feet?	Y	N
frequent urinary infections?	Y	N	known blood clot problems?	Y	N
difficulty with urination?	Y	N	leg pain or swelling?	Y	N
frequent urination at night?	Y	N	unusual bleeding or bruising?	Y	N
known liver problems/hepatitis?	Y	N	anemia?	Y	N
trouble eating certain foods?	Y	N	thyroid problems?	Y	N
nausea or vomiting?	Y	N	known hormone problems?	Y	N
constipation or diarrhea?	Y	N	arthritis or joint problems?	Y	N
bloody or black bowel movements?	Y	N	muscle cramps or weakness?	Y	N
abdominal pain or cramps?	Y	N	memory problems?	Y	N
frequent heartburn/indigestion?	Y	N	dizziness?	Y	N
stomach ulcers in the past?	Y	N	hearing or visual problems?	Y	N
shortness of breath?	Y	N	frequent headaches?	Y	N
coughing up phlegm or blood?	Y	N	rash or hives?	Y	N
chest pain or tightness?	Y	N	change in appetite/taste?	Y	N
fainting spells or passing out?	Y	N	walking/balance problems?	Y	N
thumping or racing heart?	Y	N	other problems? _____	Y	N

MEDICAL HISTORY: Have you or any blood relative had: (mark all that apply)

	self	relative		self	relative
high blood pressure	___	___	heart disease	___	___
asthma	___	___	stroke	___	___
cancer	___	___	kidney disease	___	___
depression	___	___	mental illness	___	___
lung disease	___	___	substance abuse	___	
diabetes	___	___	other _____		

SOCIAL HISTORY: Please indicate your tobacco, alcohol, caffeine and dietary habits.

Nicotine Use
_____ never smoked
_____ packs per day for _____ years
_____ stopped _____ year(s) ago

Caffeine Intake
_____ never consumed
_____ drinks per day
_____ stopped _____ year(s) ago

Alcohol Consumption
_____ never consumed
_____ drinks per day/week
_____ stopped _____ year(s) ago

Diet Restrictions/Patterns
_____ number of meals per day
_____ food restrictions: _____
_____

OTHER INFORMATION/COMMENTS:

_____
Pharmacist Signature   Date

FIGURE 1-1 *(continued)*

and share it only with those providers who need this information to provide patient care. Additionally, clinicians must adhere to the regulations set forth by the Health Insurance Portability and Accountability Act (HIPAA) of 1996, which provides standards to protect the security and confidentiality of individually identifiable protected health information (PHI). PHI includes information created during the provision of patient care that can be linked with a specific patient. Examples of PHI include the patient's name, home address, date of birth, medical record number, medical diagnoses, treatment records, prescriptions, and laboratory and test results. Further discussion of the HIPAA regulations is beyond the scope of this chapter; consult the United States Department of Health and Human Services website (http://www.hhs.gov/ocr/hipaa/) for additional information. The process of interviewing the patient, how to set the stage for the interview, and the essential information to be gleaned from the interview are outlined in Table 1-1.

Table 1-1 Interviewing the Patient

Importance of Interviewing the Patient
Establishes professional relationship with the patient to:
- Obtain subjective data on medical problems
- Obtain patient-specific information on drug efficacy and toxicity
- Assess patient's knowledge about, attitudes toward, and pattern of medication use
- Formulate problem list
- Formulate plans for medication teaching and pharmaceutical care

How to Set the Stage for the Interview
- Have the patient complete a written health and medication questionnaire if available
- Introduce yourself
- Make the setting as private as possible
- Do not allow friends or relatives without permission of the patient
- Do not appear rushed
- Be polite
- Be attentive
- Maintain eye contact
- Listen more than you talk
- Be nonjudgmental
- Encourage the patient to be descriptive
- Clarify by restatement or patient demonstration (e.g., of a technique)

General Interview Rules
- Read chart or patient profile first
- Ask for patient's permission or make an appointment
- Begin with open-ended questions
- Move to close-ended questions
- Document interaction

Information to be Obtained
- History of allergies
- History of adverse drug reactions
- Weight and height
- Drugs: dose, route, frequency, and reason for use
- Perceived efficacy of each drug
- Perceived side effects
- Adherence to prescribed drug regimen
- Nonprescription medication use (including complementary and alternative medications)
- Possibility of pregnancy in women of childbearing age
- Family or other support systems

Adapted from work by Teresa O'Sullivan, PharmD, University of Washington.

ORGANIZING THE PATIENT RECORD

Those who provide pharmaceutical care should develop standardized forms to record patient information. Standardization facilitates quick retrieval of information, minimizes the inadvertent omission of data, and enhances the ability of other practitioners to use shared records.[2,3]

For convenience, the patient record can be divided into sections such as the history (the medical history, the drug history, and the social history), assessment, and plan (including expected outcomes). In some situations, these histories can be supplemented by the generation of flowchart diagrams to monitor changes in specific parameters (e.g., blood glucose concentrations, weight) over time. Several software packages have been developed to expedite record keeping (Table 1-2). Most allow a convenient Windows-based interface between the patient history, monitoring forms, and the prescription dispensing system.

Medical History

The medical history is essential to the provision of pharmaceutical care. It can be as extensive as the medical records that are maintained in an institution or in a physician's office, or it can be a simple patient profile that is maintained in a community pharmacy. The purpose of the medical history is to identify significant past medical conditions or procedures; identify, characterize, and assess current acute and chronic medical conditions and symptoms; and gather all relevant health information that could influence drug selection or dosing (e.g., function of major organs such as the GI tract, liver, and kidney that are involved in the absorption and elimination of drugs; height and weight, including recent changes in either; age and gender; pregnancy and lactation status; and special nutritional needs).

1. P.J., a 45-year-old woman of normal height and weight, states that she has diabetes. What questions might the practitioner ask of P.J. to determine whether type 1 or type 2 disease should be documented in her medical history?

Patients usually can enumerate their medical problems in a general way, but the practitioner often will have to probe more specifically to refine the diagnosis and assess the severity of the condition. Diabetes mellitus is used to illustrate the types of questions that can be used to gather important health information and assess drug therapy. The following questions should generate information that will help determine whether P.J. has type 1 or type 2 diabetes mellitus.

- **How old were you when you were told you had diabetes?**
- **Do any of your relatives have diabetes mellitus? What do you know of their diabetes?**
- **Do you remember your symptoms? Please describe them to me.**
- **What medications have you used to treat your diabetes?**

When questions such as these are combined with knowledge of the pathophysiology of diabetes, appreciation of the typical presenting signs and symptoms of the disease, and understanding of the drugs generally used to treat both forms of diabetes, meaningful pharmaceutical care can be provided. Even simple assessments such as the observation of a patient's body size can provide information useful for therapeutic

Table 1-2 Application Software for Case Management and Documentation

Company	Web Site	Telephone Number
AlphaCare by HealthCare Computer Corp (HCC)	http://www.hcc-care.com/	888-727-5422
Apothecare by Etreby Computer Co.	http://www.etreby.com/	800-292-5590
Guardian by CarePoint Inc.	http://www.carepoint.com/	800-296-1825
Encounter by jASCorp	http://www.jascorp.com/	800-444-4498
QARx by Cygnus Systems	http://www.qarx.com	816-525-6141
QS/1 by QS/1 Data Systems	http://www.qs1.com	800-845-7558

Data compiled by Bill G. Felkey, Harrison School of Pharmacy, Auburn University. For more information, visit his website at http://pharmacy.auburn.edu/pcs/review/manage.htm

interventions. For example, a person with type 2 diabetes is more likely to be an overweight adult (See Chapter 50, Diabetes Mellitus).

Drug History

After the initial visit, patients often present themselves to community pharmacists in one of three ways: (1) with a self-diagnosed condition for which nonprescription drug therapy is sought, (2) with a newly diagnosed condition for which a drug has been prescribed, or (3) with a chronic condition that requires refill of a previously prescribed drug or the initiation of a new drug. In the first and second situations, the practitioner must confirm the diagnosis using disease-specific questions as illustrated in Question 1. In the third situation, the practitioner uses the same type of questioning as in the first two situations; however, this time the practitioner needs to evaluate whether the desired therapeutic outcomes have been achieved. The practitioner must evaluate the information gleaned during follow-up visits in the context of the history and incorporate it into his or her assessment and pharmaceutical care plan. The goals of the therapeutic history are to obtain and assess the following information: the specific prescription and nonprescription drugs the patient is taking (the latter includes over-the-counter [OTC] medications, botanicals, dietary supplements, recreational drugs, alcohol, tobacco, and home remedies); the intended purpose or indications for each of these medications; how (e.g., route, ingestion in relation to meals), how much, and how often these medications are used; how long these agents have been taken or used (start and stop dates); whether the patient believes any of these agents are providing therapeutic benefit; whether the patient is experiencing or has experienced any adverse effects that could be caused by each of these agents (idiosyncratic reactions, toxic effects, adverse effects); and allergic reactions and any history of hypersensitivity or other severe reactions to drugs. This information should be as specific as possible, including a description of the reaction, the treatment, and the date of its occurrence.

2. P.J. has indicated that she is injecting insulin to treat her diabetes. What questions might be asked to evaluate P.J.'s use of, and response to, insulin?

The following types of questions when asked of P.J. should provide the practitioner with information on P.J.'s understanding about the use of and response to insulin.

Drug Identification and Use
- What type of insulin do you use?
- How many units of insulin do you use?
- When do you inject your insulin in relationship to meals?
- Where do you inject your insulin? (Rather than the more judgmental question, "Do you rotate your injection sites?")
- Please show me how you usually prepare your insulin for injection. (This request of the patient requires the patient to demonstrate a skill.)

Assessment of Therapeutic Response
- How do you know if your insulin is working?
- What blood glucose levels are you aiming for?
- How often and when during the day do you test your blood glucose concentration?
- Do you have any blood glucose records that you could share with me?
- Would you show me how you test your blood glucose concentration?
- What is your understanding of the hemoglobin A_{1c} blood test?
- When was the last time you had this test done?
- What were the results of the last hemoglobin A_{1c} test?

Assessment of Adverse Effects
- Do you ever experience reactions from low blood sugar?
- What symptoms warn you of such a reaction?
- When do these typically occur during the day?
- How often do they occur?
- What circumstances seem to make them occur more frequently?
- Examine injection sites.

The patient's responses to these questions on drug use, therapeutic response, and adverse effects will allow a quick assessment of the patient's knowledge of insulin and whether she is using it in a way that is likely to result in blood glucose concentrations that are neither too high nor too low. The responses to these questions also should provide the practitioner with insight about the extent to which the patient has been involved in establishing and monitoring therapeutic outcomes. Based on this information the practitioner can begin to formulate the patient's educational needs.

Social History

The social history is used to determine the patient's occupation and lifestyle; important family relationships or other support systems; any particular circumstances (e.g., a disability) or stresses in her life that could influence the pharmaceutical care plan; and attitudes, values, and feelings about health, illness, and treatments.

3. A patient's occupation, lifestyle, and attitudes often can determine the success or failure of drug therapy. Therefore, P.J.'s nutritional history, her level of activity or exercise in a typical day or week, the family dynamics, and any particular stresses that may affect glucose control need to be documented and assessed. What questions might be asked of P.J. to gain this information?

Work
- Describe a typical work day and a typical weekend day.

Exercise
- Describe your exercise habits. How often, how long, and when during the day do you exercise? Describe how you change your meals or insulin when you exercise?

Diet
- How many times per day do you usually eat? Describe your usual meal times.
- What do you usually eat for each of your main meals and snacks?
- Are you able to eat at the same time each day?
- What do you do if a meal is delayed or missed?
- Who cooks the meals at home? Does this person understand your dietary needs?
- How often do you eat meals in a restaurant?
- How do you order meals in a restaurant to maintain a proper diet for your diabetes?

Support Systems
- Who else lives with you? What do they know about diabetes? How do they respond to the fact that you have diabetes? How do they help you with your diabetes management? Does it ever strain your relationship? What are the issues that seem to be most troublesome? (*Note:* These questions apply equally to the workplace or school setting. Often, the biggest barrier to multiple daily injections is refusal of the patient to inject insulin while at work or school.)

Attitude
- How do you feel about having diabetes?
- What worries or bothers you the most about having diabetes? (*Note:* The patient's demeanor and response to this and other questions will cue the history taker to the issues the patient considers most important. By addressing these concerns first, the patient is encouraged to actively participate in his or her own care. This approach is likely to enhance the patient-provider relationship, which should translate into improved care.)

SYSTEMATIC APPROACHES TO PATIENT THERAPY ASSESSMENT

Patient therapy assessment is the process whereby a practitioner integrates general diagnostic and therapeutic knowledge with medical and social information obtained from an individual to develop an optimal patient-specific therapeutic plan. At first, the process seems overwhelming because of the multiple steps involved and the difficulty in transcending from generalities to specifics. Abnormal *laboratory values* must be placed into perspective regarding what is clinically relevant and what is considered normal variation. When *dosages* are recommended, they must be patient-specific and not generalities based on the package insert, the Physicians Desk Reference (PDR),[4] or Facts and Comparisons.[5] Terms such as *frequent monitoring* must be translated to specific time points such as hourly, daily, weekly, or annually based on the severity of the patient's problem.

When faced with multiple treatment options, the practitioner must decide which option is preferred. When a treatment regimen has been prescribed that the practitioner does not consider optimal, he or she must decide to either accept the plan or advocate for a change on the patient's behalf. With time and practice, the process of assessing patient therapy and prioritizing the need to make an intervention becomes second nature and does not require a concerted effort to mentally check off each step after it has been performed. Recall of prior clinical experience helps make assessments easier. Time constraints and the amount of patient information available in certain practice environments may dictate the level of assessment that can be undertaken and the need to prioritize certain patient situations over others, but the need to intervene on the patient's behalf should never be abdicated. At one extreme, simply accepting all difference of opinion without an intervention because of time constraints or fear of angering the prescriber is not acceptable. On the other hand, frequent questioning of another practitioner is an inefficient use of time and may lead to a strained professional relationship.

Implementing pharmaceutical care entails integrating, assessing, and applying the information from the patient's record or database to the identification and solution of therapeutic problems. This requires an organized thought process for evaluating information. Therefore, a systematic approach is needed for analyzing a case history, setting priorities about which patients require more in-depth intervention, monitoring drug therapy, and communicating information to other health care providers in an organized and concise format.

Problem-Oriented Medical Record Approach

Organizing information according to medical problems (e.g., diseases) helps break down a complex situation (e.g., a patient with multiple medical problems requiring multiple drugs) into its individual parts.[1-3] The medical community has long used a *problem-oriented medical record (POMR)* or *SOAP note* to record information in the medical record or chart using a standardized format (Table 1-3). Each medical problem is identified, listed sequentially, and assigned a number. *Subjective* data and *objective* data in support of each problem are delineated, an *assessment* is made, and a *plan* of action identified. The first letter of the four key words (subjective, objective, assessment, and plan) serve as the basis for the SOAP acronym.

Problem List

Problems are listed in order of importance and supported by the subjective and objective evidence gathered during the patient encounter. Each individual problem in the list can then be given an identifying number. All subsequent references to

Table 1-3 Elements of the Problem-Oriented Medical Record[a]

Problem name: Each "problem" is listed separately and given an identifying number. Problems may be a patient complaint (e.g., headache), a laboratory abnormality (e.g., hypokalemia), or a specific disease name if prior diagnosis is known. When monitoring previously described drug therapy, more than one drug-related problem may be considered (e.g., nonadherence, a suspected adverse drug reaction or drug interaction, or an inappropriate dose). Under each problem name, the following information is identified:

Subjective	Information that explains or delineates the reason for the encounter. Information that the patient reports concerning symptoms, previous treatments, medications used, and adverse effects encountered. These are considered nonreproducible data because the information is based on the patient's interpretation and recall of past events.
Objective	Information from physical examination, laboratory results, diagnostic tests, pill counts, and pharmacy patient profile information. Objective data are measurable and reproducible.
Assessment	A brief but complete description of the problem, including a conclusion or diagnosis that is supported logically by the above subjective and objective data. The assessment should not include a problem/diagnosis that is not defined above.
Plan	A detailed description of recommended or intended further workup (laboratory, radiology, consultation), treatment (e.g., continued observation, physiotherapy, diet, medications, surgery), patient education (self-care, goals of therapy, medication use and monitoring), monitoring, and follow-up relative to the above assessment.

[a]Sometimes referred to as the *SOAP* (subjective, objective, assessment, plan) note.

a specific problem can be identified or referenced by that number (e.g., "problem 1" or simply "1"). These generally are thought of in terms of a diagnosed disease, but they also may be a symptom complex that is being evaluated, a preventive measure (e.g., immunization, contraception), or a cognitive problem (e.g., nonadherence). Problems should be identified based on the practitioner's level of understanding. For example, the symptoms of "difficulty breathing at night" or "two-pillow orthopnea" are consistent with the symptom complex of heart failure (HF); however, these symptoms could be assessed as individual problems if the student or practitioner is unaware of the association of these symptoms with HF. Any condition that requires a unique management plan should be identified as a problem to serve as a reminder to the practitioner that treatment is needed for that problem.

Medical problems can be *drug-related* including prescribing errors, dosing errors, adverse drug effects, adherence issues, and the need for medication counseling. Drug-related problems may be definite (i.e., there is no question that the problem exists) or possible (i.e., further investigation is required to establish whether the problem really exists). The most commonly encountered types of drug-related problems are listed in Table 1-4.[2,3]

The distinction between medical problems and drug-related problems sometimes is unclear, and considerable overlap exists. For example, a medical problem (i.e., a disease, syndrome, symptom, or health condition such as pregnancy) can be prevented, cured, alleviated, or exacerbated by medications. When assessing drug therapy, several situations could exist: treatment is appropriate, and therapeutic outcomes have

Table 1-4 Drug-Related Problems

Drug Needed (also referred to as no drug)
Drug indicated but not prescribed; a medical problem has been diagnosed, but there is no indication that treatment has been initiated (maybe it is not needed)
Correct drug prescribed but not taken (nonadherence)

Wrong/Inappropriate Drug
No apparent medical problem justifying the use of the drug
Drug not indicated for the medical problem for which it has been prescribed
Medical problem no longer exists
Duplication of other therapy
Less expensive alternative available
Drug not covered by formulary
Failure to account for pregnancy status, age of patient, other contraindications
Incorrect non-prescription medication self-prescribed by the patient
Recreational drug use

Wrong Dose
Prescribed dose too high (includes adjustments for renal and hepatic function, age, body size)
Correct prescribed dose, but overuse by patient (overadherence)
Prescribed dose too low (includes adjustments for age, body size)
Correct prescribed dose, but underuse by patient (underadherence)
Incorrect, inconvenient, or less-than-optimal dosing interval (consider use of sustained-release dosage forms)

Adverse Drug Reaction
Hypersensitivity reaction
Idiosyncratic reaction
Drug-induced disease
Drug-induced laboratory change

Drug Interaction
Drug–drug interaction
Drug–food interaction
Drug–laboratory test interaction

been achieved; drugs that have been selected are ineffective, or therapeutic outcomes are partially achieved; dosages are subtherapeutic or medication is taken improperly; an inappropriate drug for the medical condition being treated has been prescribed or is being used; or the condition is not being treated.

Likewise, a drug-related problem can cause or aggravate a medical problem. Such drug-related problems could include hypersensitivity reactions; idiosyncratic reactions; toxic reactions secondary to excessive doses; adverse reactions (e.g., insulin-induced hypoglycemia or weight gain); or drug–drug, drug–disease, drug–laboratory test, and drug–lifestyle interactions.

Subjective and Objective Data

Subjective and objective data in support of a problem are important because assessment of patients and therapies requires the gathering of specific information to verify that a problem continues to exist or that therapeutic objectives are being achieved. Subjective data refer to information provided by the patient or another person which cannot be confirmed independently. Objective data refer to information observed or measured by the practitioner (e.g., laboratory tests, BP measurements). Sometimes, the distinction between subjective and objective is unclear. For example, the subjective assessment by a practitioner that the "patient appears to be in pain" could be considered objective if the assessment is confirmed independently by another individual.

4. P.N., a 28-year-old man, has a BP of 140/100 mm Hg. What is the primary problem? What subjective and objective data support the problem, and what additional subjective and objective data are not provided, but usually are needed to define this particular problem?

The primary problem is hypertension. No subjective data are given. The objective data are the patient's age, gender, and BP of 140/100 mm Hg. Each of these is important in designing a patient-specific therapy plan. Because hypertension often is an asymptomatic disease (See Chapter 14, Essential Hypertension), subjective complaints such as headache, tiredness or anxiety, shortness of breath (SOB), chest pain, and visual changes usually are absent. If long-term complications such as rupturing of blood vessels in the eye, glomerular damage, or encephalopathy were present, subjective complaints might be blurring or loss of vision, fatigue, or confusion. Objective data would include a report by the physician on the findings of the chest examination (abnormal heart or lung sounds if secondary HF has developed), an ocular examination (e.g., presence of retinal hemorrhages), and laboratory data on renal function (blood urea nitrogen [BUN], creatinine, or creatinine clearance). To place these complications in better perspective, the rate of change should be stated. For example, the serum creatinine has increased from a level of 1 mg/dL 6 months ago to a value of 3 mg/dL today. Vague descriptions such as "eye changes" or "kidney damage" are of little value because progressive damage to these end organs results from uncontrolled high BP and disease progression needs to be monitored more precisely.

5. D.L., a 36-year-old construction worker, tripped on a board at the construction site 2 days ago, sustaining an abrasion of his left shin. He presents to the emergency department (ED) with pain, redness, and swelling in the area of the injury. He is diagnosed as having cellulitis. What is the primary problem? What subjective and objective data support the problem? What additional subjective and objective data are not provided, but usually are needed to define this particular problem?

The primary problem is cellulitis of the left leg. Useful pieces of subjective information are D.L.'s description of how he injured his shin during his work as a construction worker and his current complaints of pain, redness, and swelling. The fact that he was at a construction site is indirect evidence of a possible dirty wound. Further information must be obtained about how he cleaned the wound after the injury and whether he has received a booster dose of tetanus toxoid within the past 10 years. Objectively, the wound is on the left shin. No other objective data are given. Additional data to obtain would be to document the intensity of the redness on a one-to-four-plus scale, the size of the inflamed area as described by an area of demarcation, the circumference of his left shin compared with his right shin, the presence or absence of pus and any lymphatic involvement, his temperature, and white blood cell (WBC) count with differential.

6. C.S., a 58-year-old woman, has had complaints of fatigue, ankle swelling, and SOB, especially when lying down, for the past week. Physical examination shows distended neck veins, bilateral rales, an S₃ gallop rhythm, and lower extremity edema. A chest radiograph shows an enlarged heart. She is diagnosed as having HF and is being treated with furosemide and digoxin. What is/are the primary problem(s)? What subjective and objective data support the problem(s)? What additional subjective and objective data are not provided but usually are needed to define this (these) particular problem(s)?

The primary problem is systolic HF. Subjectively, C.S. claims to be experiencing fatigue, ankle swelling, and SOB, especially when lying down. She claims to have been taking furosemide and digoxin. An expanded description of these symptoms and of her medication use would be helpful. The findings on physical examination and the enlarged heart on chest radiograph are objective data in support of the primary problem of HF. In addition, other objective findings that would help in her assessment would be the pulse rate, BP, serum creatinine, serum potassium concentration, digoxin blood level, and a more thorough description of the rales on lung examination, extent of neck vein distension, and degree of leg edema. Pharmacy records could be screened to determine current dosages and refill patterns of the medications.

In this case, a second primary problem may be present. Current recommendations for the management of HF include use of an angiotensin-converting enzyme (ACE) inhibitor before or concurrent with digoxin therapy. Thus, a possible drug-related problem is the inappropriate choice of drug therapy ("wrong drug"). The patient and/or prescriber should be consulted to ascertain whether an ACE inhibitor has been used previously, if any contraindications exist, or if possible adverse effects were encountered.

Assessment

After the subjective and objective data have been gathered in support of specific listed problems, the practitioner should assess the acuity, severity, and importance of these problems. He or she should then identify all factors that could be causing or contributing to the problem. The assessment of the severity and acuity is important because the patient expects relief from the symptoms that are of particular concern at this time. During the initial encounter with a patient, it might be discovered that the medical problem is only a symptom complex and that a diagnosis is needed to more accurately identify the problem and further define its severity.

Plan

After the problem list is generated, subjective and objective data are reviewed, and the severity and acuity of the problems are assessed, the next step in the problem-oriented (i.e., the SOAP) approach is to create a plan. The plan, at the minimum, should consist of a diagnostic plan and a pharmaceutical care plan that includes patient education.

DIAGNOSTIC PLAN

The diagnostic plan could include further diagnostic tests, evaluation of drug-induced problems, or referral to another health care provider. The extent of the diagnostic plan, of course, would differ with different specialists. For example, primary care providers would have a more general diagnostic plan, medical subspecialists would have a more narrowly focused diagnostic plan, and pharmacists would have a more drug-focused component to their diagnostic plan and would likely defer to the diagnostic plan of other practitioners.

PHARMACEUTICAL CARE PLAN
Therapeutic Objectives

The pharmaceutical care plan describes desired clinical outcomes or therapeutic objectives. Well-conceived targets of desired clinical outcomes must be patient specific and should be established in collaboration with the patient and other members of the health care team. These clinical outcomes also must be clearly defined and either measurable (e.g., laboratory test) or observable (e.g., task performance) by the patient and the practitioner within a specified time so that both know whether progress is being made toward the targeted objective. The therapeutic objectives should be realistic (i.e., what can be accomplished reasonably) and should begin with interventions that are essential to the patient's acute well-being or those that the patient perceives to be most important. Examples of clinical outcomes or therapeutic objectives are as follows: curing a disease (e.g., treatment of an infection), eliminating or reducing a patient's symptoms (e.g., pain control), arresting or slowing the disease process (e.g., lowering a patient's cholesterol or BP to reduce the risk of coronary heart disease), preventing an unwanted condition or disease (e.g., contraception, immunizations, prophylactic antibiotics, avoiding the complications of diabetes or hypertension), or improving the quality of life.

In a patient with multiple medical problems, the practitioner must consider the therapeutic objective for each problem separately and in the aggregate. Ideally, a single treatment that achieves the targeted clinical outcome of more than one problem concomitantly is desirable. Conversely, care must be taken to ensure that the therapy given for one problem does not worsen another problem or create a new problem. Furthermore, more than one therapeutic objective may be needed for each of the patient's problems; recognizing the ideal clinical outcome may have to be achieved through a se-

ries of intermediate step-wise goals. In some situations, an intermediate goal may be that which is realistic within the context of the patient's situation. For example, with peptic ulcer disease the short-term goal is symptomatic relief, an intermediate goal is healing the ulcer, and a long-term goal is preventing recurrence of the disease.

These examples all relate to achieving a positive outcome (i.e., ensuring that the therapy is effective). However, there are other concurrent goals related to drug therapy: avoidance of adverse effects, convenience (to improve adherence), and cost-effectiveness. Although these latter three elements of the therapeutic goal may not always be articulated, they are part of every desired clinical outcome and must be considered when evaluating a pharmaceutical care plan. The potential benefits always should be balanced against the potential risks of therapy. As an example, higher-than-average dosages may be acceptable if the patient is not responding to "usual dosages" and has not been experiencing side effects. The interventions necessary to achieve the specified clinical outcomes also are integral to the pharmaceutical care plan. The following are examples of interventions in a pharmaceutical care plan: reinstituting correct use of a prescription medication when it is being taken or used improperly; educating and working with the patient to self-diagnose, evaluate, and solve therapeutic problems; initiating nonprescription drugs, non-drug therapies, administration aids, or monitoring tools; recommending or prescribing prescription medications; reinforcing continuation of already prescribed medications; alerting physicians to potential drug-related problems that can be solved only through an alteration of the original prescription (these include discontinuing the medication, prescribing an alternative drug, altering the dosage or route of the current medications, and adding other medications); and referring the patient back to his or her primary care provider.

7. In Question 4, the subjective and objective data were considered for P.N., who has a BP of 140/100 mm Hg. What would be some therapeutic objectives or desired clinical outcomes of P.N.'s treatment?

Eradicating or curing the disease is not a realistic goal for hypertension (see Chapter 14, Essential Hypertension). Symptomatic control also is not relevant because BP often is an asymptomatic disease. To simply state that the therapeutic objective is to control BP technically is correct, but it is not specific enough to define how attainment of this therapeutic objective will be measured. Thus, a starting therapeutic objective may be to "achieve a diastolic BP of 85 mm Hg within the next 3 months." This objective clearly is measurable, has a time line, and hopefully is realistic. It also addresses both efficacy and, to a lesser extent, a side effect (i.e., avoidance of hypotension). Another short-term objective for this patient is for him "to be able to explain the long-term risks of untreated hypertension" and "the importance of adherence to the prescribed treatment plan."

The clinician's interventions in the effort to attain these therapeutic objectives would be to educate the patient about both of these issues. The clinician also would assess medication refill patterns and measure the patient's BP to determine whether these short-term therapeutic objectives have been met within the established time line. A long-term therapeutic objective is to "prevent the long-term complications of hypertension such as kidney damage, loss of eyesight, and the development of HF or other cardiovascular complications." This latter objective is better defined than simply stating that the goal is to "prevent complications of his disease." As always, unstated objectives are to avoid side effects and to make the treatment regimen as simple and cost-effective as possible.

8. **D.L. (see Question 5) presented to the ED with subjective and objective data sufficient to support a diagnosis of cellulitis. What would be some therapeutic objectives or desired clinical outcomes of his treatment?**

Unlike the hypertension case presented earlier, a simple statement of objective such as "to cure his infection" technically is correct, but in terms of specifics, it leaves much to be desired. In this case, the therapeutic objectives or desired clinical outcomes are to provide symptomatic relief, eradicate the infection, and prevent spread of the infection to adjacent tissues (See Chapter 67, Traumatic Skin and Soft Tissue Infections). When faced with an infectious disease case and the need to choose or evaluate antibiotic options, the practitioner must know the usual causative organisms for a particular site or type of infection, the bacterial coverage of available antibiotics, and the patient's drug allergy history (See Chapter 56, Principles of Infectious Diseases). The practitioner should formulate treatment decisions based on the results from culture and sensitivity testing when available. The most likely causative organisms for cellulitis are streptococci or staphylococci. Thus, a therapeutic objective could be "to eradicate a probable streptococcal or staphylococcal cellulitis, prevent bacteremia, and reduce pain and swelling" within a specific time. In this case, the inclusion of the type of infection and probable organisms helps define the antibiotic of choice (e.g., penicillinase-resistant penicillin or a first-generation cephalosporin). Culture and sensitivity data would not be available at the time of initial treatment, and a Gram's stain of the involved tissue seldom provides accurate data for this type of skin infection. The practitioner should ask D.L. about possible allergies to antibiotics including penicillins or cephalosporins. As always, other implied therapeutic objectives are to avoid side effects and to prescribe a regimen that is convenient and cost-effective. The education of the patient is an intervention that usually helps patients and practitioners achieve their mutually developed therapeutic objectives.

9. **C.S. (see Question 6) presented with subjective and objective data sufficient to support a diagnosis of HF and is being treated with furosemide and digoxin. What would be the therapeutic objective in this case?**

Short of a heart transplant, cure or eradication of the disease is impossible. A narrow therapeutic objective might be "to increase cardiac output." Obviously, there is more to treating HF than increasing cardiac output (See Chapter 19, Heart Failure). Also, this stated objective implies that invasive procedures can be performed to actually measure cardiac output. This would be beyond the scope of most practitioners. A more realistic statement of a therapeutic objective is "to provide symptomatic relief of HF, including increased exercise capacity, decreased SOB, and reduced ankle swelling." A long-range objective is to prolong the patient's survival. The physician's objectives may be more specific and include reducing neck vein distension, eliminating the S_3 gallop rhythm, and

minimizing pulmonary and ankle edema. The specificity of the goal is determined by the practitioner's knowledge of the pathophysiology, signs, and symptoms of HF and by prior experience in treating such patients. Once again, other goals are to minimize toxicity and strive for a convenient, cost-effective regimen. Finally, it must be decided whether an ACE inhibitor is indicated, and if so, which drug and at what dosage.

Patient Education

Educating patients to better understand their medical problem(s) and treatment also is an implied goal of all treatment plans. This process is categorized as the development of a *patient education plan*. The level of teaching has to be tailored to the patient's educational background, willingness to learn, and general state of health and mind. The patient should be taught the knowledge and skills needed to achieve and evaluate his or her therapeutic outcome. An important component of the patient education plan emphasizes the need for patients to follow prescribed treatment regimens.

Illustration of SOAP

10. **Based on the data presented in Questions 1 to 3, the practitioner believes that P.J. is experiencing frequent hypoglycemic reactions. What SOAP note could be developed for P.J.?**

The following example of a SOAP note illustrates the importance of integrating the patient's medical, therapeutic, and social history into the design of a pharmaceutical care plan (also see Chapter 50, Diabetes Mellitus).

Problem 1
Patient has been experiencing frequent hypoglycemia reactions.

SUBJECTIVE
Patient reports episodes characterized by severe hunger, tremors, and profuse sweating that are relieved by drinking orange juice. Episodes occur twice weekly, generally in the late afternoon. Patient often skips lunch to exercise. Patient states that she uses 30 U of NPH insulin every morning mixed with 30 U of regular insulin. She claims to never miss a dose and takes her insulin at 8 AM each day.

OBJECTIVE
Occasional blood glucose values of 30 to 60 mg/dL in the late afternoon, often followed by values >300 mg/dL before dinner and at bedtime.

ASSESSMENT
Total daily dose of insulin is high (1.2 U/kg). Morning dose of NPH insulin may be excessive. May require multiple daily injections of insulin. Carbohydrate intake and exercise patterns erratic.

PLAN
Therapeutic Objectives
- Initially, fasting blood glucose <140 mg/dL, postprandial blood glucose <180 mg/dL, all blood glucose concentrations >70 mg/dL.
- No symptoms of hypoglycemia such as those noted above under "Subjective."
- Patient to eat more regularly and carbohydrate intake to be distributed appropriately throughout the day.
- Patient to be able to predict time of peak NPH insulin activity and the relationship between carbohydrate intake and insulin dosage.

- Patient and family members can describe symptoms of hypoglycemia and its treatment.
- Patient can make appropriate insulin and dietary adjustments for exercise.
- Patient can demonstrate correct blood glucose testing procedure; bring in records of blood glucose test results that reflect appropriate testing frequency.

Education Plan

- Teach patient and key family members about dangers of hypoglycemia, symptoms of hypoglycemia, relationship between insulin action and food intake (insulin pharmacodynamics), and treatment of hypoglycemia.
- Ask patient to demonstrate blood glucose testing technique. Correct as necessary. Institute more frequent glucose testing (before meals and at bedtime) to document patterns of glucose response to insulin therapy. Instruct patient to perform additional tests when she experiences symptoms of hypoglycemia to verify reaction.
- Educate patient about effect of exercise on blood glucose.
- Refer to dietitian. Objective is to emphasize importance of eating regularly and spreading out carbohydrate content of meals.
- Review and evaluate patient glucose records, signs, symptoms, and dietary and exercise history weekly. Help patient interpret and adjust insulin dosages accordingly until target is achieved. Then evaluate quarterly.
- Contact primary care provider regarding hypoglycemic reactions and insulin dosage and regimen.
- Recommend adjustment of doses based on glucose test results.

This SOAP note demonstrates that pharmaceutical care is an iterative process with the potential for a high level of sophistication and complexity. Each time the practitioner interacts with the patient, he or she monitors and evaluates the patient's progress toward the designated therapeutic outcome or target. This, along with any new information, is used to redefine or refine the problem list, clarify the assessment, or modify the therapeutic targets or plan. Thus, a continuous readjustment occurs with the overall goal of improving therapeutic outcomes and the patient's quality of life.

Pharmacist's Workup of Drug Therapy

The pharmacist's workup of drug therapy (PWDT) is an alternative to the SOAP approach for solving clinical problems in that it focuses specifically on the identification of drug-related problems.[2] The PWDT uses the following six interrelated steps: (1) establishing a comprehensive patient-specific database; (2) identifying patient-specific, drug-related problems; (3) describing desired therapeutic outcomes; (4) listing all therapeutic alternatives that might produce the desired outcomes; (5) selecting the drug recommendation(s) that most likely will result in the desired outcomes; and (6) establishing a plan for therapeutic drug monitoring that documents that desired effects occur and undesired effects are minimized.

The key to both the PWDT and the SOAP techniques is a *systematic approach to assessing and monitoring drug therapy.* Although the PWDT is preferred by some pharmacists for monitoring continuing drug therapy, the SOAP approach should be used when communicating in writing with other health care providers (e.g., chart notes, formal letters) because it is recognized universally by physicians, nurses, and other health care professionals. Regardless of whether the PWDT or the SOAP technique is used, in the final analysis, it is more important to develop an organized thought process for identifying and solving clinical problems than to make every situation fit a specific mnemonic.

Drug Therapy Assessment

A responsibility of the practitioner is to monitor the response of patients to prescribed therapeutic regimens. This responsibility is shared by nurses, pharmacists, physicians, physician assistants, and other health care practitioners. For the pharmacist, this includes dispensing or refilling prescriptions in the community pharmacy, assessing a patient's therapy on the medical ward during hospitalization, or as part of routine monthly evaluations of patients residing in long-term care facilities. Many states have enacted legislation allowing pharmacists to develop collaborative drug therapy agreements with physicians for disease state management of common disorders such as asthma, diabetes, dyslipidemia, and hypertension. Additional services commonly provided by pharmacists through collaborative drug therapy agreements include anticoagulation monitoring, emergency contraception, and immunizations.[6] The individual patient's need (this should be the primary consideration), time constraints, the working environment (a determinant of the amount of patient information that is available), and the individual practitioner's skill level govern the extent of monitoring. Similarly, the exact steps used to monitor therapy and the order in which they are executed need to be adapted to a practitioner's personal style. Thus, the examples given in this chapter should be used by the reader as a guide, rather than as a recipe in a cookbook.

The purpose of drug therapy monitoring is to identify and solve drug-related problems and to ensure that all therapeutic objectives are being achieved. Unless proven otherwise, the medical diagnosis should be assumed to be correct. On occasion, the diagnosis may not be readily apparent, or a drug-induced problem may have been diagnosed incorrectly as being a disease entity.

Previously Prescribed Drug Therapy
Community Pharmacy Setting

11. T.M. has requested a refill of a previously dispensed prescription from her community pharmacy. This particular pharmacy has a computerized patient profile system that can display all drugs that the patient has taken in the past 2 years, including the date and quantity of each drug refill. What should the pharmacist be expected to do before dispensing this medication for T.M.?

The problem-oriented medical record approach (i.e., SOAP) begins the process of problem solving with the development of a problem list. In reality, the medical record generally begins with demographic data (e.g., age, address) followed by a history of present illness, significant past medical history, physical examination findings, and the results of laboratory tests. In essence, problem solving must begin first with the accumulation of a database. Because the community pharmacist seldom has access to such data, the pharmacist also must *upgrade and update the patient's database* (i.e., the patient profile). The community pharmacist could begin by carefully reviewing the patient profile for all drugs currently being taken by the patient; for drugs that have been taken previously, but are now discontinued; and for the apparent refill frequency rates for regularly scheduled, routine medications as well as for those medications with the potential for abuse.

The pharmacist should now be ready to generate a problem list by *identifying patient-specific, drug-related problems*. The pharmacist should prioritize the problems listed, with the most important problem or the patient's current complaint (chief complaint) being ranked first, followed in an order based on the pharmacist's personal assessment of the severity of the problems. The order of the pharmacist's problem list may be greatly different from that of the physician or nurse because each has a different perspective when evaluating a patient. In some cases, an abbreviated problem list that includes only the currently active problems or even a single problem that is being given priority (e.g., specific suspected adverse drug effect) can be developed. The risk of an abbreviated problem list is that confounding variables from other problems may be overlooked, thus affecting the practitioner's ability to assess the current problem accurately.

Although the community pharmacist in this scenario is not likely to have access to the patient's medical records, the pharmacist can formulate a problem list predicated on the most likely indications for the drugs that the patient is taking. When in doubt, the most valuable source of information can be accessed (i.e., the patient can be interviewed). In a tactful way, the practitioner can ask the patient about current medical problems or why medical help was sought. One example is to say, "I see that you are taking digoxin. What did your physician tell you this medication was for?" or "Are you taking this to help regulate your heartbeat or for heart failure?" The exact phrasing of these sample questions needs to be adapted to the patient and the professional "style" of the pharmacist. Questions also should be asked to determine how well the patient thinks the drug is working and whether the patient has experienced any problems. At the same time, the pharmacist can ask the patient about medications that are obtained from another pharmacy, nonprescription medications being used, and any previous drug allergy experiences. Gathering of information may be expedited by using written history forms for the patient to complete, but the importance of talking directly with the patient at the time of the initial filling of a prescription or when the patient is obtaining refills cannot be overemphasized. Note that at this point, the practitioner is gathering *subjective data* (i.e., information gleaned from the patient) while preparing a problem list for the patient.

A helpful intermediate step in gathering *objective data* is to link the patient's drugs to one or more of his or her medical problems (Table 1-5). This process aids in identifying drugs that may have been prescribed for more than one indication or drugs that are inappropriate (i.e., have no apparent indication). Drugs with multiple indications should be listed separately under each relevant problem. Some medications, such as vitamins, analgesics, sedatives, antacids, and laxatives, may be difficult to categorize. These nonprescription medications can be grouped under a general category such as "general care," but these should not be ignored because overuse or side effects can occur with these drugs as well. Alternatively,

Table 1-5	Example Problem List
Problem[a]	*Drugs Prescribed*
Medical problem 1 (usually the chief complaint)	Drug A
Medical problem 2	Drug B
	Drug C
Medical problem 3	Drug B
	Drug D
	Drug E
Medical problem 4	No drug therapy
Drug-related problem 1	
Drug-related problem 2	

[a]Identify problem name.

medication issues can be used as a generic term for issues such as adherence, need for medication counseling, and other possible drug-related problems.

If a *drug-related problem* is suspected, objective data (e.g., physical findings, laboratory tests) are often needed to confirm this suspicion. To start, it is helpful to ask the patient whether he or she has knowledge of these clinical or laboratory test results. It is also appropriate for the pharmacist to perform minor physical assessments, such as monitoring pulse rate (e.g., digoxin, by slowing conduction through the AV node, should decrease pulse rate), measuring BP (e.g., to check the effectiveness of antihypertensives), or observing the patient for obvious dermatologic conditions (e.g., skin color, rashes, presence of edema, insulin injection sites). Further referral to a specialist may be necessary for a more thorough evaluation.

Pharmacists also can perform simple laboratory tests (e.g., measure lipid or glucose serum concentrations). Alternatively, the physician's office can be called (to find out the values or suggest laboratory tests that may be needed). With the advent of collaborative drug therapy agreements and changes in state pharmacy practice acts, some pharmacists can initiate orders for laboratory tests.[6]

Monitoring the patient's drug list for drug-related problems can be facilitated by a series of questions, as elaborated here. These questions are summarized in Table 1-6 and in a series of algorithms in Figure 1-2.[7]

- Is the treatment working? If this question identifies a possible drug-related problem (i.e., the therapeutic objective is not being achieved), the problem list must be expanded accordingly. Relative to the drug-related problems in Table 1-3, this could provide a clue to one of several problems: an adherence problem exists (medication not being taken), an ineffective drug has been prescribed (wrong drug), the prescribed dosage is too low, or a drug interaction has led to lower-than-desired blood levels of the drug.
- Is there evidence of actual or potential side effects, drug interactions, or duplications within the same therapeutic category? If this question identifies a possible drug-related problem, the problem should be labeled and added to the problem list until the problem is either confirmed or ruled out.

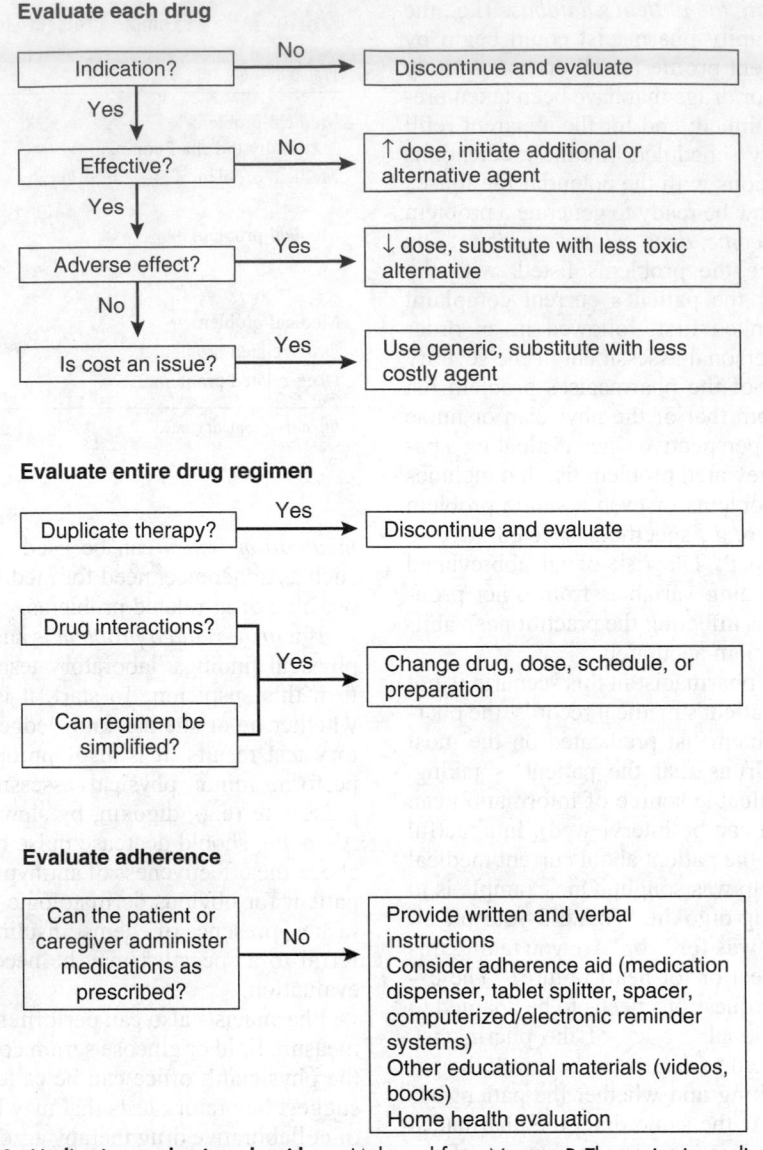

FIGURE 1-2 Medication evaluation algorithms. (Adapted from Newton P. The geriatric medication algorithm. A pilot study. J Gen Int Med 1994;9:164–167.)

- Are there any contraindications that need to be considered? If the profile indicates prior allergies, the current regimen should be screened for possible cross-reacting drugs. For women of childbearing age, the practitioner must consider the possibility of pregnancy and review the profile to see whether contraceptives are being taken. When possible teratogenic drugs are prescribed, the practitioner should ask women whether they are pregnant or considering pregnancy and counsel them about the risks of becoming pregnant.
- Are the dosages correct? For all drugs that a patient is taking, the provider should evaluate the appropriateness of the dosage, schedule, and the dosage form considering ease of use, reliability of the drug product, the patient's renal and hepatic function, the patient's age (especially pediatric and geriatric patients), body size, and possible interactions with food or other drugs that are being taken. If this question identifies one or more possible drug-related problems, the practitioner should add them to the problem list and deter-

mine a possible cause (e.g., high cost, inconvenient dosage schedule, patient misunderstanding of directions, or an adverse effect).
- Is the patient taking the medications as prescribed (i.e., is there evidence of poor technique, nonadherence, underuse, or overuse)? If this question identifies a possible drug-related problem, the clinician should add it to the problem list.
- Are more cost-effective alternatives available for any of the treatments? If this question identifies a possible drug-related problem, the problem list should be expanded.
- Are there any drugs prescribed for the patient with no apparent indication (i.e., when constructing the problem list, there is a prescribed drug that does not match with any of the medical diagnoses)? If the answer is "yes," one of the patient's problems may have been overlooked, an unusual use of a drug specific to this patient's needs has been missed, or the drug has been prescribed inappropriately.

Table 1-6   Monitoring Questions

1. Is the treatment working? (i.e., is the therapeutic objective being achieved?)

2. Is there evidence of actual or potential side effects?

3. How adherent is the patient to the prescribed therapy?

4. Is there evidence of actual or potential drug interactions or duplications within the same therapeutic category?

5. Are there any contraindications or allergies that need to be considered?

6. Is the patient pregnant?

7. Are the doses, dosage regimens, and dosage forms correct?

8. Have adjustments been made for renal function, hepatic function, age, and body size?

9. Could a less expensive or more convenient dosage form be used?

10. Are there any drugs prescribed for the patient with no apparent indication?

11. Are there any medical problems (diagnoses) listed for which no drug therapy has been prescribed? Could any of the medical problems or abnormal laboratory values be drug induced?

The clinician should investigate each of these possibilities and modify the problem list accordingly. This may involve adding a new medical problem to the list, linking the drug to an existing problem, or adding a new drug-related problem (wrong drug, inappropriate use) to the list.

- Are there any medical problems (diagnoses) listed for which no drug therapy has been prescribed? If the answer is "yes," it may be appropriate (e.g., a patient with a medical history of hypertension who has achieved acceptable BP control with weight loss alone). Other possible explanations include that (1) the pharmacist failed to identify a drug that was prescribed for the patient, (2) the patient is getting a drug from another pharmacy, (3) a drug is being given for one problem and the pharmacist thought it was being used for something else, or (4) the prescriber has inadvertently forgotten to order something for that patient. The pharmacist should investigate each of these possibilities further and modify the problem list accordingly.

- Could any of the medical problems or abnormal laboratory values be drug induced? If so, the pharmacist should add a new drug-related problem to the list.

- Are there any other obvious drug-related problems of the types listed in Table 1-4?

These questions will identify suspected drug-related problems that might need to be substantiated by additional data. The challenge at this stage is to *clarify the problem.* Although this task may sound simple, it is the most difficult component of patient assessment. In some cases, the signs and symptoms of diseases or adverse drug effects are similar to those found in textbooks; more often, some of the classic signs may be absent, or the patient may have unusual symptoms that require further observation. Generally, more data need to be obtained, but time is limited. With experience and continual expansion of one's own knowledge base, this process becomes easier.

The problem list for both medical and drug-related problems now has been finalized, and considerable subjective and objective data have been reviewed. After the listed problems have been assessed for severity and acuity, *a plan can be developed.* As previously presented, the plan should include both therapeutic objectives and an educational component for each of the defined medical or drug-related problems. The immediate emphasis may be on short-term therapeutic objectives, but the clinician also should formulate intermediate and long-term objectives from the beginning.

The therapeutic objectives, of course, include the correction of possible drug-related problems. After *considering all potential corrective actions,* the clinician ultimately must choose the one option that is best for the patient. The process of merely identifying several possible solutions to a problem without being able to prioritize and select what seems to be the best option does not benefit the patient. If a change in therapy is necessary or if there is sufficient concern to warrant contacting the prescriber, the recommended solution to the problem must be clearly defined and include a specific alternative drug, route of administration, dose, and frequency of administration. Furthermore, the pharmacist must be prepared to justify the reasoning behind his or her recommendations (i.e., provide supporting evidence). If more cost-effective alternatives are available, the pharmacist will need to work with both the patient and the prescriber to change the therapy.

A plan for ongoing monitoring also needs to be established for the patient. The ongoing plan should contain specifics about what parameters will continue to be monitored for efficacy, side effects, appropriateness of dosage, and adherence to treatment. The clinician will have to decide how often monitoring for these parameters will be necessary. It also is helpful to anticipate possible future complications (e.g., changes in disease control, future complications of the disease) that may necessitate a change in the dosage or drug of choice. For example, if a diabetic patient develops decreased visual acuity and worsening renal function, the therapeutic plan may have to be altered by using larger print on labels, recommending a magnifying attachment for the patient's insulin syringes, and adjustment of the dosage of one or more of the patient's drugs. Finally, issues for future counseling also need to be considered, taking into consideration the level of sophistication of the individual patient (i.e., education plan).

Inpatient Pharmacy Setting

12. **W.G. has just been hospitalized in a large medical center where the pharmacist has access to the medical chart, nursing record, medication administration record, and a computer that directly links to the clinical laboratory. The pharmacists at this facility assess the patients' drug therapy and routinely provide clinical pharmacokinetic monitoring. How would the pharmacist approach W.G. differently in this clinical setting compared with the pharmacist in Question 11 who worked in a community pharmacy?**

The process of monitoring drug therapy is similar in both situations, and the same SOAP or PWDT formats should be used. In the medical center setting, a problem list can be generated more easily because objective data (i.e., diagnoses, laboratory tests) are readily available. On the other hand, a hospitalized patient usually has acute medical problems that often are superimposed on previous chronic problems. As a result, new therapies are being added and home medications may or may not be continued. For this reason, the problem list development step needs to be modified. Instead of making a two-column matrix of medical diagnoses and drug therapy as previously described, a multiple-column matrix is created. For each medical problem, drugs previously taken at home are compared with those prescribed while in the hospital. Later, an additional column can be added, listing discharge medications. If the lists are not the same, the pharmacist should seek an explanation. Many times, the reasons are obvious (e.g., if a patient is changed from oral to parenteral therapy or if a side effect of one of the home medications was the cause for the admission). At other times, this process helps identify a home medication that the prescriber has forgotten to reorder. Medication counseling at discharge is more effective when the pharmacist can differentiate between drugs that are new for the patient and those that are continuations of prior therapy. This also makes it easier to alert the patient to changes in dosage and give instructions about medications at home that should be discarded.

Assessing the appropriateness of drug dosages requires knowledge of basic pharmacokinetic parameters (e.g., route of elimination) and the patient's weight and height. For hospitalized patients or those in long-term care facilities, the clinician should review the patient's renal function (BUN and serum creatinine) and liver function (hepatic aminotransferases, bilirubin, and albumin). If either of these organs is compromised, the clinician must review the prescribed drugs to determine whether dosage adjustment should be considered. Drug level monitoring may be necessary for certain agents (e.g., aminoglycosides, digoxen, phenytoin). Appropriate timing and frequency of obtaining drug levels also should be suggested. If serum levels have been reported previously, they should be reviewed for validity. Pharmacokinetic assessments should use actual patient data, rather than theoretical models, when possible. If a serum drug concentration seems unusually high or low, the clinician must consider all the various factors that might influence the serum concentration of the drug in that particular patient (e.g., assess patient adherence and the timing of the sample collection relative to the last dose). When the reason for an abnormal serum drug concentration is not apparent, the test should be repeated before considering a dosage change that may cause toxic or subtherapeutic concentrations because of spurious data. For some drugs (e.g., anticonvulsants) dosage alterations are made on the basis of clinical response rather than solely because of an abnormal serum concentration value.

Initiating Over-the-Counter Treatment in the Community Pharmacy Setting

13. S.F., a woman who appears to be about 25 years of age, asks her community pharmacist whether Vagistat-1 Cream is better than Monistat-7 vaginal suppositories. How does the workup of drug therapy principles presented in this chapter apply to S.F.?

First, it is important to identify the real question being asked. Superficially, the question relates to choosing one type of vaginal antifungal product versus another. S.F.'s question is

confusing because two different agents are involved (tioconazole versus miconazole) and the dosage forms are different (a cream versus suppository). There are also differences in how long each drug is to be used (1 day for tioconazole and 7 days for this particular form of miconazole). S.F. may be asking the question because she simply is curious, but more likely, she is indirectly asking the pharmacist to diagnose a problem and to recommend a therapy. Moreover, the treatment may be for her, or it may be for someone else. The pharmacist should ask several questions and mentally develop a problem list before recommending therapy.

The only approved indication for nonprescription vaginal antifungal products is the treatment of a recurrent candidal vaginal infection. Therefore, the pharmacist needs to gather subjective and objective data to verify the existence of this problem in S.F. or in whomever will be using the product. As a minimum, the pharmacist should inquire about symptoms (e.g., vaginal itching or burning, inflammation, a cottage-cheese–like discharge) and confirm that previous symptoms were diagnosed by a physician. Possible questions to ask are: "Will you be using this product or will someone else?" "What symptoms are you having?" "Describe the discharge." "Have you been treated for this problem before?" "How were you treated before?" "Have you ever used either of these two products?" "Was the drug effective last time?"

At least two other important questions should be asked: "What other medications are you taking?" and "Is it possible that you are pregnant?" The answer to the first question will help identify other possible medical problems to add to the problem list as well as possible drugs that could be the cause of her infection (e.g., antibiotics or oral contraceptives). If she is pregnant, referral to her obstetric provider is indicated.

14. At this point, an initial assessment can be made about whether S.F. has a recurrent vaginal yeast infection. Assume for the moment that the diagnosis is confirmed and S.F. is not taking any other medications and has no other medical problems. What is the therapeutic goal of her treatment, and what is the next step for the pharmacist to take?

The two interrelated primary goals are to relieve S.F.'s symptoms and to eliminate the current vaginal yeast infection. A secondary goal is to prevent or minimize future infections. S.F. must be educated about how to use the medication properly to treat the current infection and counseled on techniques to avoid future infections.

Next, the pharmacist must consider all therapeutic options. Possibilities include referral to a physician for prescription therapy, use of nondrug therapies (e.g., avoidance of occlusive clothing, daily ingestion of cultured yogurt), and one of several nonprescription drugs (butoconazole, clotrimazole, miconazole, or tioconazole). If a nonprescription product is chosen, the pharmacist must consider evidence for relative efficacy of 1-, 3-, and 7-day products. Note that this list of options is for illustrative purposes only and is not meant to be an exhaustive review of treatment modalities (Also see Chapter 48, Gynecological and Women's Health Disorders, and Chapter 71, Fungal Infections).

From these options, the pharmacist will make one or more specific recommendations to the patient. Tioconazole and miconazole (as well as butoconazole and clotrimazole) generally are considered equally effective; therefore, the selection of one drug over the other can be based on cost and convenience. The choice of a cream versus a suppository will be based on whether there is external vaginal involvement, patient convenience, and patient preference. The one-dose product (tioconazole) is obviously more convenient than 7 days of treatment with miconazole. However, 3-day miconazole dosage forms are available. Counseling about how to apply the medication, how long to use it, and hygienic precautions to avoid future infections also should be part of the plan.

The recommendations obviously will be different if the pharmacist determines that the patient does not have a vaginal yeast infection (e.g., the discharge is more characteristic of bacterial vaginosis), the patient has not had a previous diagnosis of a yeast infection, she has a drug-induced cause, or she is pregnant. Discussion of treatment options for each of these possibilities is beyond the scope of this chapter.

Establishing Priorities

15. How are priorities decided regarding which patients should be monitored and when the pharmacist should intervene?

Ideally, all patients should be monitored closely and interventions made in every instance that an actual or potential problem is identified. For the pharmacist working in a specialized unit (e.g., a bone marrow transplant unit), it may be feasible to monitor all patients with the same level of intensity because the number of patients may be relatively small and the underlying problem is similar for all the patients. On the other hand, pharmacists practicing on a general medicine ward, at a nursing home, or in a busy community pharmacy have a greater diversity and larger volume of patients, making universal monitoring impractical. Thus, criteria need to be established to determine which patients need to be monitored more extensively. Although there are no absolute rules on how to set priorities, the following guidelines might be helpful.

Age and Gender
The dosages of medications should be reviewed for children younger than 12 years of age and adults older than 65 because of smaller body size and possible impaired drug clearance or enhanced sensitivity to drug effects. Women of childbearing age should be evaluated more closely if possible teratogenic drugs are prescribed.

Number of Medications Prescribed or Number of Doses Per Day
People receiving multiple medications should be monitored more closely for duplication of therapy, potential adverse drug effects, and possible drug interactions. Complicated drug regimens should be evaluated for the possibility of using sustained-release preparations or combination products to improve adherence.

Drugs With a High Risk for Adverse Drug Effects or Drug Interactions
Pharmacists should develop a list of key drugs within their practice that trigger a more in-depth review when they are encountered. This list could include drugs such as anticoagulants, digoxin, metered-dose inhalers, oral corticosteroids, insulin or oral hypoglycemics, aminoglycosides, and anticonvulsants. Drugs with a high potential for triggering drug interactions include enzyme inhibitors and inducers, anticonvulsants, cimetidine, macrolide antibiotics, fluoroquinolones, and serotonin reuptake inhibitors.

Target Diseases
As with the drug examples just listed, drug therapy of some patient populations needs to be monitored more closely. This will have to be tailored to an individual's specific practice site and may change over time. For example, one may wish to develop a specialty interest in patients with asthma, diabetes, hypertension, or dyslipidemia. For 6 months or a year, a pharmacist could target all patients with asthma using more than one canister of a metered-dose β-agonist inhaler per month to receive special counseling and intervention. In some cases, disease state management protocols (collaborative drug therapy agreements) can be developed with local prescribers to help the target population treat their condition more effectively.[6] During the following year, different screening criteria could be established, such as all patients with hypertension who fail to refill their prescriptions within 2 weeks of their next scheduled refill.

High-Cost Drugs
The most cost-effective therapy always should be considered. Pharmacists practicing in acute care settings may closely screen and monitor orders for high-cost agents (e.g., hematopoietic growth factors, intravenous immune globulin, and intravenous antifungal agents) to ensure usage is consistent with criteria developed by the institution. In the community setting, pharmacists might target prescriptions for brand name drugs when therapeutically equivalent generic alternatives are available. Additionally, patients filling separate prescriptions for high-cost agents available in combination formulations may realize significant cost savings by switching to the combination product. For example, an asthmatic patient whose condition is well controlled with fluticasone (Flovent) 88 μg BID and salmeterol (Serevent) 50 μg BID will reduce drug costs and simplify the regimen (2 versus 6 puffs per day) by switching to the combination fluticasone/salmeterol formulation (Advair 100/50).

Altered Drug Clearance
In practice settings where laboratory values are available for monitoring, all patients with an elevated serum creatinine should be assessed for renally eliminated drugs that may need dosage adjustment. For patients with evidence of hepatic insufficiency (elevated bilirubin and hepatic aminotransferase concentrations, reduced albumin) dosage adjustments are more complicated because these endogenous biomarkers are not reliable in predicting alterations in hepatic drug clearance.[8] However, derangements in these tests suggest the possibility of liver dysfunction and should place the clinician on alert for more closely monitoring drugs that rely on the liver for elimination or are potentially hepatotoxic. Similarly, patients taking drugs with well-established pharmacokinetic monitoring parameters, such as aminoglycosides, carbamazepine, digoxin, phenytoin, and vancomycin, should be monitored closely.

Allergy
Patients whose drug profile indicates a drug allergy should be screened to make sure that no cross-reacting drugs have been

ordered. If possible, the patient should be consulted to ascertain the nature of the allergy and a notation made in his or her medical or pharmacy record regarding the clinical presentation of the allergy.

Prescriber Contact

The next level of priority setting is to determine when to contact a prescriber. This requires establishing a balance between patient safety, convenience, and the time available for both the pharmacist and prescriber. Any situation that represents potential harm to the patient (e.g., a newly identified adverse drug effect, a well-documented drug interaction, a dosing error) must be acted on immediately. Switching to less costly drugs or more convenient regimens also should have a high priority, but sometimes can be postponed until a more convenient time. If the pharmacist practices in the patient care area, it is easier to sense when the prescriber is stressed and, thus, postpone an intervention until a more convenient time. The pharmacist should not confront the prescriber in front of his or her peers, so it is prudent that he or she make an intervention during a private one-on-one consultation as opposed to during rounds or in a crowded room. If the same prescriber has several potential problem patients, it may be best to intervene on the most pressing issues and leave the others to another time. When a good working relationship has been established with the prescriber, it may be possible to schedule a time to review all of his or her patients in a collegial fashion. Interventions over the telephone are less desirable because it is difficult to judge how busy the individual is at the time of the phone call. Nonurgent communication to inform the physician of an intervention or to make suggestions for change can be made by notes sent by a fax machine, written in the chart, or by formal letters.

Example of the PWDT

16. M.B. practices in the outpatient pharmacy of a community hospital. V.C., a 30-year-old woman, comes to the pharmacy with a prescription for nitrofurantoin sustained-release (Macrobid) 100 mg BID for 7 days. The computer profile shows that the only other medicine V.C. is taking is metronidazole (Flagyl) 500 mg BID for 7 days, which she received 7 days prior. Both of the prescriptions were written by the same general practitioner in the hospital's medical clinic. No other information is available at this time. Based on the information given, what medical problems does V.C. have? Develop a tentative problem list with corresponding drug therapy.

The data given are insufficient to definitively state the diagnoses at this time. The most likely use for the nitrofurantoin is a urinary tract infection, probably cystitis or urethritis. The metronidazole could have been prescribed for a trichomonal infection, for bacterial vaginosis, or as an adjunct for anaerobic bacterial coverage. Given the dosage prescribed and the general circumstances, the most likely indication is bacterial vaginosis. Upon questioning V.C., these conclusions are confirmed. She claims good adherence to the metronidazole (she will take her last dose tonight), notes no side effects, and states that her vaginal itching and discharge are decreased, but now she has some burning on urination. Thus the problem list is as follows:

Problem	Drugs
1. New-onset urinary tract infection	Nitrofurantoin 100 mg BID
2. Bacterial vaginosis	Metronidazole 500 mg BID

17. **Are there any drug-related problems illustrated by V.C.?**

No. The indications and dosages are appropriate. It is too early to determine whether the therapy is effective. V.C. claims to not be experiencing any adverse effects, and there is no evidence of an adherence problem. There also are no obvious drug interactions. V.C. should be counseled about the GI effects of the nitrofurantoin.

18. **Four days later, V.C. presents to the ED with a chief complaint of nausea and vomiting of mixed coffee-ground–appearing material and bright red blood. She states that she was in her usual state of health until 2 days ago, when the nausea and vomiting began soon after dinner. Blood appeared in the vomitus after the first several episodes and she has continued to vomit intermittently since then to the point where she has vomited "more times than she can count." V.C. also states that her stools turned black this morning and appear to be tarry. She has had no oral intake since the vomiting began and now has some dizziness. She denies fever, chills, abdominal pain, or diarrhea. Her urinary tract infection symptoms have subsided. Her medical history includes a "nervous stomach" since childhood, occasional heartburn when lying down after a large meal, and endometriosis diagnosed 2 years ago. She has no history of ulcer disease. Her only current medication is the nitrofurantoin identified previously. She completed her metronidazole treatment course 4 nights ago. V.C. reports occasional alcohol use; she did not ingest any alcohol while taking the metronidazole per her pharmacist's directions, but she drank 2 glasses of wine with dinner the night her vomiting began. She denies use of aspirin or nonsteroidal agents.**

Physical examination shows temperature, 37.3(C; respiratory rate, 20 breaths/min; BP, 114/74 mm Hg, without a postural drop; and pulse, 64 beats/min lying down, increasing to 100 beats/min on standing. The findings of the rest of the examination are unremarkable, except for dry oral mucous membranes. Bowel sounds are normal.

Laboratory results show sodium (Na), 140 mEq/L (normal, 135 to 147 mEq/L); potassium (K), 3.3 mEq/L (normal, 3.5 to 5.0 mEq/L); chloride (Cl), 109 mEq/L (normal, 95 to 105 mEq/L); total carbon dioxide (CO_2), 24 mEq/L (normal, 22 to 28 mEq/L); glucose, 94 mg/dL (normal, 70 to 110 mg/dL); BUN, 22 mg/dL (normal, 8 to 18 mg/dL); creatinine, 0.9 mg/dL (normal, 0.5 to 1.5 mg/dL); hematocrit (Hct), 36% (normal, 33% to 43%); WBC count, 9,600 cells/mm³ (normal, 3,200 to 9,800 cells/mm³); platelets, 249,000/mm³ (normal, 150,000 to 350,000/mm³); prothrombin time, 11.6 seconds; and International Normalized Ratio (INR), 0.9. Urine and blood cultures are pending. Nasogastric aspirate is now negative for blood, but the stool sample is hemoccult positive. The physician's assessment is GI bleeding, volume depletion, and hypokalemia. Admission orders are for ranitidine 50 mg IV Q 8 hr, prochlorperazine 5 to 10 mg IV Q 4 to 6 hr PRN nausea, nitrofurantoin SR 100 mg BID, and 1 L of dextrose 5% in 0.45% normal saline with 40 mEq KCl at 125 mL/hr. Based on this information, develop an updated medical problem list.

[SI units: Na, 140 mmol/L; K, 3.3 mmol/L; Cl, 109 mmol/L; total CO_2, 24 mmol/L; glucose, 5.2 mmol/L; BUN, 5.35 mmol/L; creatinine, 68.6 μmol/L; Hct, 0.36; WBC count, 9,600 × 10^9 cells/L; platelets, 249 × 10^9/L]

Problem	Drugs
1. Nausea, vomiting, GI bleeding	Ranitidine, prochlorperazine
2. Volume depletion, hypokalemia	D_5½NS, KCl
3. Resolving urinary tract infection	Nitrofurantoin 100 mg BID
4. Bacterial vaginosis (resolved)	None
5. History of endometriosis	None

It is possible that V.C. also has underlying gastro-esophageal reflux disease (GERD). This is not listed as a separate problem, although it may contribute to her primary problem.

19. Are any drug-related problems present that should be added to this list? Make an assessment regarding the likelihood of any of the problems that could be drug induced.

There is a distinct possibility that V.C.'s GI distress and bleeding may be drug related. The most common side effect of nitrofurantoin is nausea and abdominal distress. She took the drug for several days without difficulty, but this could represent a cumulative effect or a combined effect with the factors that follow. Metronidazole generally is well tolerated, but when taken with alcohol it can cause a disulfiram-like reaction with severe nausea, vomiting, and flushing. V.C. drank alcohol 2 days after taking her last evening dose of metronidazole. Although this may raise a suspicion that she is having a disulfiram-like reaction, the possibility is less likely considering the half-life of metronidazole (6 to 8 hours) and the fact that most of the drug would have been eliminated by the time she ingested the alcohol (48 hours later). Finally, alcohol is a GI irritant itself, but she has continued to have symptoms for several days despite no further alcohol ingestion. Any of these factors could help explain the initial GI distress, but frank ulceration and bleeding as a result of taking her drugs are not as easy to explain. Of the three drugs, the one most likely to cause bleeding would be the alcohol, but only with chronic ingestion. She denies alcohol abuse. Of course, other factors, such as coincident viral gastroenteritis, cannot be ruled out. As a final assessment, it cannot be said with certainty that any of her drugs played a direct role in her admission. Nonetheless, she should be cautioned about future combinations of alcohol with metronidazole and the importance of taking nitrofurantoin with food.

An endoscopic examination the following day showed gastritis and an esophageal tear (Mallory-Weiss tear) from retching. The actual cause of the gastroenteritis remains unknown. She was discharged home with omeprazole 20 mg PO QD ×14 days (for acid suppression) and prochlorperazine 10 mg PO Q 6 hr as needed for nausea and vomiting. This case illustrates how a possible incorrect assessment (e.g., metronidazole–alcohol interaction with a disulfiram-like effect) could be made if one does not consider all facts known about the patient's history and the drug's pharmacokinetic properties. A second principle is that it is often difficult to definitely differentiate a drug-induced problem from a primary medical problem unrelated to current medications.

Evaluating a Possible Adverse Drug Effect

20. D.G. is a 63-year-old woman presenting to the ED with a chief complaint of fatigue and blurred vision, which has caused her to remain in bed for the past 2 days. This morning, D.G. became dizzy and fell in the shower, sustaining a head injury. Her past medical history is significant for stage III colon cancer (underwent surgical resection 4 months ago; now receiving adjuvant chemotherapy); seizure disorder (generalized tonic-clonic) since childhood, but has not had a seizure in more than 25 years; hypertension; and a recent diagnosis of depression. Her medication history includes phenytoin (Dilantin) 300 mg PO Q HS; hydrochlorothiazide 25 mg PO Q am; prochlorperazine 10 mg PO Q 6 hr PRN nausea; and fluoxetine (Prozac) 20 mg PO Q am which was started 1 week ago. Her chemotherapy consists of fluorouracil (5-FU) 700 mg IV daily in combination with leucovorin 35 mg IV daily for 5 consecutive days each month. D.G. has tolerated the treatment well, with only mild nausea. She completed the fourth of six cycles of chemotherapy 3 days ago. She has no known allergies. Family history and social history are noncontributory. When asked, D.G. states she has been taking all medications as prescribed and has taken no extra doses. She denies recent nausea or vomiting, but she has been taking the prochlorperazine prophylactically Q 6 hr because during the first cycle of chemotherapy she experienced nausea and vomiting.

Physical examination reveals weight, 58 kg; BP, 136/85 mm Hg; pulse, 78 beats/min; respiratory rate, 16 breaths/min; and temperature, 37°C. On neurologic exam she appears to be somnolent with bilateral nystagmus and ataxic gait. She has a bruise on the left side of the forehead and mild gingival hyperplasia. Admission laboratory results are unremarkable with normal electrolytes, liver function tests, renal function tests, and complete blood count. A STAT phenytoin concentration is 39.6 μg/mL; albumin is 4.4 g/dL. A repeat phenytoin level drawn 2 hours later was found to be 39.4 μg/mL. Of note, a phenytoin concentration measured 6 months ago was 10.5 μg/mL. The tentative diagnosis is phenytoin toxicity. Based on this information, develop a medical problem list and corresponding drug therapies.

Problem	Drugs
1. Possible phenytoin toxicity (ataxic gait, blurred vision)	Phenytoin (causative)
2. Head injury (bruise, fall, and dizziness probably secondary to no. 1)	Phenytoin and/or prochlorperazine (?causative)
3. Stage III colon cancer	Fluorouracil, leucovorin
4. Nausea and vomiting	Prochlorperazine
5. Depression	Fluoxetine
6. Hypertension	Hydrochlorothiazide
7. Seizure disorder	Phenytoin
8. Gingival hyperplasia	Phenytoin (causative)

The order of this problem list is prioritized based on the pharmacist's primary interest; therefore, possible phenytoin toxicity is listed as the first problem. The patient's oncologist may have listed colon cancer as the number one problem, and other practitioners may have different priorities. If the diagnosis of phenytoin toxicity had not been established, the problem list would have included ataxia and blurred vision as separate medical problems or as a complex of symptoms that needed further assessment. A practitioner evaluating these symptoms in a patient receiving anticonvulsant therapy would have to be suspicious of possible phenytoin toxicity.

21. **Which of the problems on the list require further intervention or consideration?**

The pharmacist should further explore the predisposing factors to the possible phenytoin toxicity. DG is receiving adjuvant chemotherapy to prevent recurrence of colon cancer following surgical resection. This appears to be a stable problem not requiring any urgent intervention. The therapeutic objective for the cancer may be either cure or palliation. Not enough information is provided to assess the current status of this problem, but for the moment, it does not appear to be the problem requiring the most immediate attention. The nausea and vomiting are not bothering D.G. at this time, and the prochlorperazine should be discontinued to prevent further worsening of her mental status. D.G. recently started fluoxetine for depression; thus, it is too early to assess her response to therapy. However, the period between initiation of the antidepressant therapy (1 week ago) and the recent change in her neurologic and mental status suggests a temporal relationship that merits further investigation. Her seizure disorder and hypertension appear to be well controlled and there is no need for an intervention at the present time. The gingival hyperplasia may be an unavoidable consequence of her phenytoin therapy. The tentative diagnosis is phenytoin toxicity; however, additional data are needed to confirm the diagnosis of this drug-related problem.

Subjective and Objective Data

22. **What subjective and objective data are given to help verify the diagnosis of phenytoin toxicity in D.G.? What other information is needed? Do you agree with the assessment?**

Subjectively, D.G.'s complaints are classic for phenytoin toxicity (e.g., fatigue, blurred vision, staggering when walking, dizziness). The latter problem led to her fall. Objectively, she appears somnolent; she has nystagmus, ataxia, and an obvious supratherapeutic phenytoin serum concentration of 39.6 µg/mL, which was verified by a repeat measurement. A free (unbound) serum phenytoin concentration could be measured, but this is not necessary because her albumin level is normal. The gingival hyperplasia is a side effect of chronic phenytoin therapy but is not relevant to her current problem. The assessment of phenytoin toxicity is appropriate.

23. **Which of the drug-related problem types in Table 1-4 does D.G.'s case illustrate? What factors could have contributed to the problem?**

This is an example of a patient getting too much of the correct drug. In other words, phenytoin is an appropriate drug for D.G.'s seizure disorder and, for a long time, has provided the desired therapeutic objective of good seizure control. Possible causes for the new onset of toxicity include an inappropriately prescribed dosage, overadherence, possible purposeful overdose (e.g., suicidal gesture), changes in drug metabolism, or a possible drug interaction. A laboratory error can be ruled out because a subsequent phenytoin serum concentration also was high and D.G.'s clinical complaints are compatible with phenytoin toxicity. Finally, it is possible that the symptoms are

related to another cause (e.g., a cerebrovascular accident, brain metastases from her cancer). None of these latter possibilities can be ruled out absolutely with the present data.

Assessment

24. **Which of the preceding factors are the most likely explanation for D.G.'s problem?**

D.G. claims good adherence and says she has not taken any extra doses. It is possible that she is an unreliable historian, but she has taken the drug at the same dosage for many years without previous complications. Colon cancer commonly metastasizes to the liver, raising the suspicion of hepatic involvement and possibly impaired phenytoin metabolism, but her liver function tests are all normal and she has no evidence of jaundice. There are no reported drug–drug interactions between phenytoin and fluorouracil or leucovorin and she has tolerated three previous cycles of chemotherapy with only mild nausea, so it is unlikely that the recent course of chemotherapy is causing the elevated phenytoin level. Phenothiazines (including prochlorperazine) have been reported to increase and in some cases decrease serum phenytoin levels by an unknown mechanism,[9] and it is possible that the prophylactic antiemetic therapy may have a causal role. However, a prochlorperazine–phenytoin interaction seems less likely considering D.G. did not experience these symptoms during the previous two cycles. D.G.'s symptoms began 5 days after starting fluoxetine, suggesting the possibility of a drug–drug interaction. Indeed, there have been numerous case reports of phenytoin toxicity observed in previously stable patients following the initiation of fluoxetine.[9,10] This interaction is thought to be caused by fluoxetine-mediated inhibition of cytochrome P450 2C9 (CYP2C9), a key hepatic microsomal enzyme involved in the metabolism of phenytoin. The time course between the initiation of antidepressant therapy and the development of symptoms strongly suggests a fluoxetine–phenytoin interaction as the cause of D.G.'s altered mental status and worsening neurologic function. D.G.'s other drug hydrochlorothiazide should not be contributing to the phenytoin toxicity because she has taken it for many years without problems.

Therapeutic Goals

25. **What is the desired therapeutic outcome relative to D.G.'s phenytoin toxicity?**

The short-term goal is to provide symptomatic relief with cessation of ataxia, dizziness, and blurred vision. The long-term goal is continued seizure control and avoidance of future phenytoin toxicity.

26. **Identify the therapeutic alternatives to help solve this potential problem.**

For the short term, phenytoin should be discontinued until the plasma level returns to the therapeutic range. No definitive therapy or antidotes are needed. Long-term alternatives include (1) restarting phenytoin at a lower dosage, (2) deleting phenytoin with the substitution of an alternative anticonvulsant such as carbamazepine or valproate, (3) discontinuing anticonvulsant therapy altogether considering she has been seizure-free for more than 25 years, or (4) deleting fluoxetine with the substitution of an alternative antidepressant that does not impair the metabolism of phenytoin.

Plan

27. **Which of the alternatives listed should be recommended?**

There is no one right answer to this question. Factors to consider are efficacy, risk for side effects, patient acceptance, and cost. Recommendations must be specific, including drug name, dosing, and timing of monitoring. Contingency plans need to be available in case the primary plan fails.

It is not the purpose of this example to exhaustively examine the rationale for the best recommendations. For illustrative purposes, assume that the recommendation was to discontinue fluoxetine and to restart phenytoin when the serum concentration of phenytoin had decreased to 10 to 12 μg/mL. It may take days to weeks for the serum concentration of phenytoin to decrease to this range because of its nonlinear pharmacokinetics. These recommendations would be reasonable because phenytoin has been effective in D.G. and her phenytoin toxicity is likely caused by inhibition of hepatic metabolism by fluoxetine. She will need to be counseled extensively and further questioned to make sure that she, in fact, did not take extra doses. The issue of starting an alternative antidepressant is

complicated in D.G. because some antidepressant drugs can lower the seizure threshold and precipitate seizures in patients with epilepsy. Agents to consider for use in D.G. include those less likely to decrease the seizure threshold and those without inhibitory effects on the CYP2C9 metabolic pathway such as citalopram, mirtazapine, and venlafaxine. Additionally, although not likely to be considered in the ED, is the issue of withdrawing anticonvulsant drug therapy altogether considering that D.G. has been seizure-free for more than 25 years. Given D.G.'s age, she is at increased risk for complications associated with phenytoin therapy including folate deficient anemia, osteopenia, and peripheral neuropathy. She already has gingival hyperplasia, which increases her risk for periodontal disease. D.G. should be evaluated further to determine if gradual tapering and withdrawal of anticonvulsant therapy is appropriate. If a decision is made to continue anticonvulsant drug therapy in D.G., changing to an alternate drug such as carbamazepine or valproate should be undertaken with caution. Phenytoin has controlled her seizures for many years and, although carbamazepine and valproate are also effective for generalized tonic-clonic seizures, there is no guarantee that these agents would offer similar protection. In addition, carbamazepine and valproate have been reported to interact with fluoxetine.

Table 1-7 Sample Chart Note

9/13; 5 PM

Problem 1: Possible phenytoin toxicity

S 63-year-old female admitted with head injury resulting from fall secondary to dizziness. Pt reports a 2-day history of fatigue and blurred vision. PMH significant for stage III colon cancer, seizure disorder since childhood (seizure free for 25 years), hypertension, and recently diagnosed depression. Patient taking Dilantin (phenytoin) 300 mg Q HS; hydrochlorothiazide 25 mg Q am; Prozac (fluoxetine) 20 mg Q am (started 1 week ago); and prochlorperazine 10 mg Q 6 hr PRN nausea. Has not taken any extra doses. Denies use of any OTC medications or other non-prescribed drugs. Completed fourth cycle of chemotherapy (5-FU and leucovorin) 3 days ago.

O *Weight:* 58 kg; NKDA

PE: Bruise on left side of forehead; mild gingival hyperplasia; bilateral nystagmus and ataxic gait, otherwise nonfocal neurologic examination; remaining examination WNL

Labs: Admission phenytoin concentration = 39.6 μg/mL (therapeutic: 10–20 μg/mL); repeat level 2 hours later 39.4 μg/mL; previous phenytoin concentration on 3/16 was 10.5 μg/mL with an albumin of 4.4 g/dL

A Pt with supratherapeutic phenytoin levels and symptoms consistent with phenytoin toxicity. The temporal relationship between initiation of fluoxetine for depression and the new onset CNS symptoms suggests a possible drug–drug interaction. Fluoxetine is a known inhibitor of cytochrome P450 2C9 (a key hepatic enzyme involved in the metabolism of phenytoin) and cases of phenytoin toxicity have been reported in previously stable patients following the initiation of fluoxetine. Patient reports taking medications as prescribed and denies intentional overdose. Other medications in the regimen (hydrochlorothiazide, prochlorperazine, 5-FU, leucovorin) are unlikely to be contributing as she has tolerated these agents in the past without problems.

R Consider temporarily discontinuing phenytoin and monitoring for further seizure activity. Suggest measuring serum phenytoin every 2–7 days until the concentration falls below 15 mg/mL, then reinstate phenytoin at 300 mg PO Q HS. Monitor for dizziness, blurred vision, ataxia, and nystagmus. Suggest discontinuing fluoxetine as this agent is likely causing the elevated phenytoin level. Consider citalopram, mirtazapine, or venlafaxine for the treatment of depression as these agents are unlikely to inhibit the metabolism of phenytoin or lower the seizure threshold.

Although not appropriate acutely, given her long seizure-free period, D.G. may be a candidate for withdrawal of anticonvulsant therapy. Given her age, she is at increased risk for phenytoin-induced folate deficient anemia, osteopenia, and peripheral neuropathy. Consider further evaluation to determine if gradual tapering and withdrawal of anticonvulsant therapy is appropriate. Please call for further questions. Will follow. Thank you for the consult.

Signature, Pharm.D.

A, assessment; CNS, central nervous system; NKDA, no known drug allergies; O, objective; OTC, over the counter; PE, physical examination; PMH, past medical history; Pt, patient; R, recommendation; S, subjective; WNL, within normal limits.

28. What follow-up monitoring is required?

After phenytoin is restarted, a follow-up serum concentration should be obtained 1 week later. D.G. should be observed for further signs of toxicity (ataxia, nystagmus, dizziness) and for seizure control. Weekly monitoring of phenytoin serum concentrations may be needed for the next month until a steady state is achieved. If seizures recur, the dosage should be increased or another therapy started. D.G. will require follow up to assess her response to antidepressant therapy and counseled that the beneficial effects of treatment may not be realized for up to 4 to 6 weeks after initiating therapy.

WRITING A CONSULT NOTE

Practitioners must be able to communicate patient information effectively both verbally and in writing.[2,3] Written consults may take the form of faxed communications, notes in the patient's medical record, or a formal letter of correspondence through the mail. Brevity and clarity are important; recommendations should be complete and specific. Elements to include in the consult are a brief overview of patient data necessary to show the thought process and assessment of the problem. Recommendations for drugs should include the specific dose for the patient, the route, and the dosage frequency. The practitioner should include parameters that he or she would recommend for monitoring to ensure efficacy of the treatment regimen, prevention of toxicity, and the assessment of adherence. The practitioner should also be sure to include how often it is recommended that the parameters be monitored. The SOAP format is desirable for the medical record, although the P (plan) may be changed to R (recommend) if it seems more logical.

29. Using D.G.'s case, how would you formulate your consult note for D.G.'s medical record?

At the top of the note, the current date, time, and name of the problem being addressed should be included. The body of the note should be in the SOAP format, and the practitioner should sign his or her name at the end. Common abbreviations and incomplete sentences often are used to keep the length of the note manageable. A formal consult written as a letter may be more formal, including full sentences and fewer abbreviations. See Table 1-7 for the note written in D.G.'s chart.

REFERENCES

1. Hepler CD, Strand LM. Opportunities and responsibilities in pharmaceutical care. Am J Hosp Pharm 1990;47:533.
2. Cipolle R et al, eds. Pharmaceutical Care Practice. New York: McGraw-Hill, 1998.
3. Rovers JP et al, eds. A Practical Guide to Pharmaceutical Care. 2nd Ed. Washington, DC: American Pharmaceutical Association, 2003.
4. Physicians' Desk Reference. 58th Ed. Montvale, NJ: Medical Economics 2004.
5. Drug Facts and Comparisons. St. Louis, MO: Wolters Kluwer Health, 2004.
6. Ferro LA et al. Collaborative practice agreements between pharmacists and physicians. J Am Pharm Assoc 1998;38:655.
7. Newton PF et al. The geriatric medication algorithm: a pilot study. J Gen Intern Med 1994;9:164.
8. Verbeeck RK, Horsmans Y. Effect of hepatic insufficiency on pharmacokinetics and drug dosing. Pharm World Sci 1998;20:183.
9. Drug Interaction Facts. St. Louis, MO: Wolters Kluwer Health, 2004.
10. Spina E, Perucca E. Clinical significance of pharmacokinetic interactions between antiepileptic and psychotropic drugs. Epilepsia 2002;43:37.

CHAPTER 2

Interpretation of Clinical Laboratory Tests

Mark W. Garrison, Lloyd Y. Young

This chapter introduces the reader to some of the most commonly encountered laboratory tests used in clinical medicine. Specialized laboratory tests that commonly are used to monitor specific disease states or specific drug therapy are integrated into the case histories, questions, and answers in subsequent chapters of this book rather than in this introductory chapter.

Students will find Kathleen and Timothy Pagana's *Diagnostic and Laboratory Test Reference* (6th ed., Mosby), Frances Fischbach's *A Manual of Laboratory and Diagnostic Tests* (7th ed., Lippincott Williams & Wilkins), or Scott L. Traub's *Basic Skills in Interpreting Laboratory Data* (American Society of Health-System Pharmacists) essential in the clinical setting. If a more comprehensive review of clinical laboratory tests is needed, the reader is referred to the most recent edition of *Clinical Diagnosis and Management by Laboratory Methods* (W.B. Saunders). The major pharmaco-

kinetic and pharmacodynamic principles governing the clinical use of specific drugs are reviewed critically in *Applied Pharmacokinetics: Principles of Therapeutic Drug Monitoring* (Lippincott Williams & Wilkins). In addition, Michael E. Winter's *Basic Clinical Pharmacokinetics* (4th ed., Lippincott Williams & Wilkins) and the companion handbook, *Basic Clinical Pharmacokinetic Handbook* (Lippincott Williams and Wilkins), by White and Garrison cover the clinical aspects of pharmacokinetically monitored drugs.

GENERAL PRINCIPLES

The serum, urine, and other fluids of patients are analyzed routinely; however, the economic cost of obtaining these data always must be balanced by benefits to patient outcomes. Generally, laboratory tests should be ordered only if the results of the test will affect decisions about the therapeutic management of the patient. There is little justification for frequent multiorgan baseline studies in the absence of a suspected problem or diagnosis.

Normal Values

Clinical laboratory test results that appear within a predetermined range of values are termed *normal,* and those outside this range are called *abnormal.* Abnormal laboratory values are not always of diagnostic significance (see Question 1); in addition, normal values sometimes can be interpreted as being abnormal in some diseases (see Question 2). Various factors (e.g., age, gender, weight, height, time since last meal, drugs) can affect the range of normal values for a given test.

Clinical laboratories may analyze sample specimens by different laboratory methods; therefore, each laboratory has its own set of normal values. When a laboratory department changes its analytic procedures or equipment, normal values also will change accordingly. Consequently, clinicians should use the normal values listed by their own clinical laboratory facility when interpreting laboratory test results in preference to those published in reference texts.

Laboratory Error

The clinician must always consider the possibility of laboratory error when laboratory results do not correlate with clinical expectations. Common sources of laboratory error are as follows.

Spoiled Specimen

Improper handling, improper preservation, or undue delay in analyzing the specimen may invalidate test results. For example, if a blood sample is allowed to hemolyze, a spurious hyperkalemia may be noted because potassium concentrations are higher within erythrocytes than in plasma.

Specimen Taken at Wrong Time

The concentrations of some substances in biologic fluids can be influenced by the time of day and the relationship to meals, as well as other factors. Thus, specimens obtained at improper times can yield misleading test results.

Incomplete Specimen

Studies requiring 24-hour collections (e.g., urine) can be a source of error because of the difficulty inherent in the collection of every sample specimen throughout the 24-hour collection period.

Faulty Reagents

Reagents that are prepared improperly or those that have deteriorated may produce erroneous results. This is more often seen with infrequently ordered laboratory tests.

Technical Errors

Laboratory personnel may make an error in reading an instrument or making a calculation. Patient names and samples might be interchanged, or results can be transcribed incorrectly.

Diagnostic and Therapeutic Procedures

Some diagnostic and therapeutic procedures can alter laboratory test results. For example, digital examination of the prostate can increase the serum concentration of acid phosphatase, and electrocardioversion can increase the serum concentration of creatine kinase (CK).

Diet

Certain foods contain substances that can appear in biologic fluids and interfere with various laboratory tests.

Medication

Drugs can alter laboratory results in the following ways:

- *By interfering with the testing procedure.* For example, spironolactone can interfere with some digoxin assays, resulting in false increases in the serum concentration of digoxin. Digoxin assays using sheep antibodies may be less likely to be affected by spironolactone than digoxin assays using rabbit antibodies.[1]
- *By altering laboratory values by virtue of their pharmacologic or toxicologic properties.* For example, thiazide diuretics can increase uric acid serum concentrations by inhibiting the tubular secretion of urate.

Units of Measure

The Système International (SI) units of measure is a method of reporting clinical laboratory values in a standard metric format. The basic unit of mass for the SI system is the mole, which is not influenced by the added weight of salt or ester formulations. It is technically and pharmacologically more meaningful than the gram because each physiologic reaction occurs on a molecular level.

When substances are expressed in mass concentration units (e.g., milligrams), the amount of the substance relative to others in the body is unclear. For example, a substance of a high molecular weight can react with a substance of low molecular weight on a molar-to-molar basis, yet the number of moles of these substances relative to each other is not readily apparent to most clinicians. The use of SI units makes it possible to better appreciate the influence of albumin concentrations on the binding of drugs. The SI system is based on fundamental units for measuring quantity from which derivations are made (Table 2-1).

Table 2-1   SI Units and Symbols

Physical Quantity Measured	Unit	Symbol
Length	Meter	m
Mass	Kilogram	kg
Time	Second	s
Amount of substance	Mole	mol
Temperature	Kelvin	K
Electric current	Ampere	A
Luminous intensity	Candela	cd
Area	Square meter	m^2
Volume	Cubic meter	m^3
Force	Newton	N
Pressure	Pascal	Pa
Work energy	Joule	J
Density	Kilogram per cubic meter	kg/m^3
Frequency	Hertz	Hz

Efforts to implement the SI system internationally began in the 1970s and resulted in the adoption of full SI transition policies by several major medical and pharmaceutical journals in the late 1980s.[2,3] However, acceptance of this system has met resistance among many American clinicians. In January 1992, in recognition of this resistance, two major medical journals announced adjustments to their former policies and compromised by reporting both the SI units and conventional U.S. units or a method for conversion between the two.[4,5] The most appropriate method to report clinical laboratory values remains controversial. Proponents of further implementation of the SI system argue that its adoption by the United States would enhance international collaboration in the medical field. Proponents of continuing the use of conventional units claim that conversion to SI units offers little benefit in daily use and its adoption would require learning unfamiliar reference ranges, with the possibility for errors. For an effective conversion to the SI reporting system in the United States, there must be a concerted effort within the medical community to implement the change. Most journals in the United States continue to use the conventional U.S. units and supplement these with SI units or conversion factors.

In this chapter, laboratory values are expressed in traditional units and the comparable SI units are included at the end of a question. Table 2-1 lists the units and corresponding SI symbols. Conversion factors for changing common individual laboratory values from the traditional units to SI units can be found in Table 2-2 (Blood Chemistry Reference Values), Table 2-4 (Hematologic Laboratory Values), and Table 2-7 (Therapeutic Drug Concentrations). Comprehensive conversion tables and guides are available.[6,7]

ELECTROLYTES

Sodium

Sodium (135 to 147 mEq/L or mmol/L) is the predominant cation of the extracellular fluid (ECF). Along with chloride, potassium, and water, sodium is important in establishing osmotic pressure relationships between intracellular fluid (ICF) and ECF. An increase in the serum sodium concentration may signify impaired sodium excretion or volume contraction. Conversely, a decrease in the serum sodium concentration to less-than-normal values may reflect hypervolemia, abnormal sodium losses, or sodium starvation. Healthy individuals are able to maintain their sodium balance without difficulty; however, patients with kidney failure, heart failure, or pulmonary disease often have problems with sodium and water balance. In adults, changes in serum sodium concentrations most often represent water imbalances and not salt imbalances. Hence, the serum sodium concentration often is a reliable indicator of a patient's fluid status rather than sodium balance.

Hyponatremia

Hyponatremia may be related to dilution of serum sodium or to total body depletion of sodium. Because water moves freely across cell membranes in response to oncotic pressures, hyponatremia simply means that sodium is diluted throughout all body fluids. Dilutional hyponatremia occurs when the ECF compartment expands without an equivalent increase in sodium. Clinical conditions such as cirrhosis, heart failure (HF), and nephrosis or the administration of osmotically active solutes such as albumin or mannitol commonly are associated with dilutional hyponatremia.

Hyponatremia that results from sodium depletion presents as a low serum sodium concentration in the absence of edema. Sodium depletion hyponatremia might be caused by mineralocorticoid deficiencies, sodium-wasting renal disease, or replacement of sodium-containing fluid losses with nonsaline solutions.

Hypernatremia

Hypernatremia represents a state of relative water deficiency and hence excessive concentrations of sodium in all body fluids (hypertonicity). Therefore, hypernatremia can be caused by the loss of free water, loss of hypotonic fluid, or excessive sodium intake. Free water loss is uncommon except in the presence of diabetes insipidus. Fluid loss that occurs with gastroenteritis is the most common cause of hypotonic fluid loss in infants and the elderly (the "nursing home prune syndrome"). Excessive salt intoxication usually is accidental or iatrogenic, resulting from intravenous administration of hypertonic salt solutions. In addition, some β-lactam antibiotics (e.g., ticarcillin) contain a modest sodium load and can cause fluid overload when high dosages are administered.

The primary defense against hypertonicity is thirst and subsequent fluid intake. Therefore, hypernatremic syndromes usually occur in patients who are unable to drink sufficient fluids. Infants who cannot demand fluid or patients who are vomiting, comatose, or not allowed oral fluids are at greatest risk for the development of hypernatremia.

1. T.T., a 75-year-old woman, was hospitalized with a chief complaint of increasing shortness of breath (SOB) and orthopnea over the past week. She had been treated previously for HF but has not taken any medication over the past 2 weeks. T.T. was noted to have severe (4+) pedal edema and to be in respiratory distress. An SMA-6 was ordered and revealed the following blood chemistries: sodium (Na), 123 mEq/L (normal, 135 to 147); potassium (K), 4.1 mEq/L (normal, 3.5 to 5.0); chloride (Cl), 90 mEq/L (normal, 95 to 105); carbon dioxide (CO_2), 28 mEq/L (normal, 22 to 28); blood urea nitrogen (BUN), 30 mg/dL (normal, 8 to 18); and glucose, 100 mg/dL (normal, 70 to 110). Why should T.T., with a serum sodium concentration of 123 mEq/L, not be given sodium chloride to return her serum sodium concentration to normal values?

[SI units: Na, 123 mmol/L; K, 4.1 mmol/L; Cl, 90 mmol/L; CO_2, 28 mmol/L; BUN, 10.7 mmol/L urea; glucose, 5.5 mmol/L]

All body fluids are in osmotic equilibrium, and changes in serum sodium concentration are associated with shifts of water into and out of cells. The serum sodium concentration should not be used as an index of sodium need because cell membranes are freely permeable to water. The serum sodium concentration does not reflect total body sodium content. The serum sodium concentration, however, does detect water balance disturbances because the serum sodium concentration is a significant component of body osmolality.

In T.T., who has 4+ pedal edema and HF, the serum concentration of sodium probably is low because the plasma volume is increased relative to sodium. The usual treatment of this type of hyponatremia is salt and water restriction plus diuretics. (See Chapter 17, Ischemic Heart Disease: Anginal Syndromes, and Chapter 12, Fluid and Electrolyte Disorders, for further discussion.)

Table 2-2 Blood Chemistry Reference Values

Laboratory Test	Normal Reference Values		Conversion Factor	Comments
	Conventional Units	SI Units		
ALT (SGPT)	0–35 U/L	0–0.58 μkat/L[a]	0.01667	From heart, liver, muscle, kidney, pancreas. ↑ negligible unless parenchymal liver disease. More liver-specific than AST.
Albumin	4–6 g/dL	40–60 g/L	10	Produced in liver; important for intravascular osmotic pressure. ↓ in liver disease, malnutrition, ascites, hemorrhage, protein-wasting nephropathy. May influence highly protein-bound drugs.
Alk Phos	30–120 U/L	0.5–2.0 μkat/L	0.01667	Large amounts in bile ducts, placenta, bone. ↑ in bile duct obstruction, obstructive liver disease, rapid bone growth (e.g., Paget's), pregnancy.
Amylase	35–120 U/L	0.58–2.0 μkat/L	0.01667	Pancreatic enzyme; ↑ in pancreatitis or duct obstruction.
AST (SGOT)	0–35 U/L	0–0.58 μkat/L	0.01667	Large amounts in heart and liver; moderate amounts in muscle, kidney, and pancreas. ↑ with myocardial infarction and liver injury. Less liver-specific than ALT.
Bilirubin				Breakdown product of hemoglobin, bound to albumin, conjugated (direct) in liver. ↑ with hemolysis, cholestasis, liver injury.
Total	0.1–1 mg/dL	1.7–17.1 μmol/L	17.1	
Direct	0–0.2 mg/dL	0–3.4 μmol/L	17.1	
BUN	8–18 mg/dL	3–6.5 mmol/L	0.357	End product of protein metabolism, produced by liver, transported in blood, excreted renally. ↑ in renal dysfunction, high protein intake, upper GI bleeding, volume contraction.
Calcium				
Total	8.8–10.2 mg/dL	2.20–2.55 mmol/L	0.250	Regulated by body skeleton redistribution, parathyroid hormone, vitamin D, calcitonin. Plasma level affected by changes in albumin concentration (40% bound to albumin). ↓ by hypothyroidism, loop diuretics and vit D deficiency; ↑ malignancy and hyperthyroidism.
Unbound	4.6–5.2 mg/dL	1.15–1.3 mmol/L	0.250	Physiologically active form. Unbound "free" calcium remains unchanged as albumin fluctuates. Total calcium ↓ when albumin ↓.
CO_2 content	22–28 mEq/L	22–28 mmol/L	1	Sum of HCO_3 and dissolved CO_2. Reflects acid-base balance and compensatory pulmonary (CO_2) and renal (HCO_3) mechanisms. Primarily reflects HCO_3.
Chloride	95–105 mEq/L	95–105 mmol/L	1	Important for acid-base balance. ↓ by GI loss of chloride-rich fluid (vomiting, diarrhea, GI suction, intestinal fistulas, overdiuresis).
Cholesterol				Desirable = Total <200; LDL <130; HDL >45 mg/dL; ↑ LDL or ↓ HDL are risk factors for cardiovascular disease. High in hypothyroid, nephrotic syndrome, systemic lupus erythematosus, multiple myeloma, obstructive liver disease.
Total	<200 mg/dL	<5.2 mmol/L	0.02586	
LDL	<130 mg/dL	<3.36 mmol/L	0.02586	
HDL	>45 mg/dL	>1.16 mmol/L	0.02586	
CK	0–150 U/L	0–2.5 μkat/L	0.01667	In tissues that use high energy (skeletal muscle, myocardium, brain). ↑ by IM injections, myocardial infarction, acute psychotic episodes. Isoenzyme CK-MM in skeletal muscle; CK-MB in myocardium; CK-BB in brain. MB fraction >5–6% suggests acute MI.
CK-MB	0–12 U/L	0–0.2 μkat/L	0.01667	

Continued

Table 2-2   Blood Chemistry Reference Values *(continued)*

Laboratory Test	Normal Reference Values		Conversion Factor	Comments
	Conventional Units	SI Units		
Creatinine	0.6–1.2 mg/dL	50–110 μmol/L	88.4	Major constituent of muscle; rate of formation constant; affected by muscle mass (lower with aging); excreted renally. ↑ in renal dysfunction. Used as a primary marker for renal function.
Cl$_{Cr}$	75–125 mL/min	1.24–2.08 mL/s	0.01667	Reflects glomerular filtration rate; ↓ in renal dysfunction.
GGT	0–70 U/L	0–1.17 μkat/L	0.01667	Sensitive test reflecting hepatocellular injury; not helpful in differentiating liver disorders. Usually high in chronic alcoholics.
Globulin	2.3–3.5 g/dL	23–35 g/L	10	Active role in immunologic mechanisms. Immunoglobulins ↑ in chronic infection, rheumatoid arthritis, multiple myeloma.
Glucose (fasting)	70–110 mg/dL	3.9–6.1 mmol/L	0.05551	↑ in diabetes or by adrenal corticosteroids. Important to obtain fasting glucose level.
LD (LDH)	100–190 U/L	1.67–3.17 μkat/L	0.01667	High in heart, kidney, liver, and skeletal muscle. 5 isoenzymes— LD$_1$ and LD$_2$ mostly in heart, LD$_5$ mostly in liver and skeletal muscle. ↑ in malignancy, extensive burns, PE and renal disease.
Lipase	0–160 U/L	0–2.67 μkat/L	0.01667	Pancreatic enzyme, ↑ acute pancreatitis, elevated for longer period than amylase.
Magnesium	1.6–2.4 mEq/L or 1.8–3.0 mg/dL	0.8–1.20 mmol/L 0.8–1.20 mmol/L	0.5 1 0.5 1	↓ in malabsorption, severe diarrhea, alcoholism, pancreatitis, diuretics, hyperaldosteronism (symptoms of weakness, depression, agitation, seizures, hypokalemia, and arrhythmias). ↑ in renal failure hypothyroidism and Mg containing antacids.
Phosphate^b	2.5–5 mg/dL	0.8–1.60 mmol/L	0.323	↑ with renal dysfunction, hypervitaminosis D, hypocalcemia and hypoparathyroidism. ↓ with excess aluminum antacids, malabsorption, renal losses, hypercalcemia and re-feeding syndrome.
Potassium	3.5–5 mEq/L	3.5–5 mmol/L	1	↑ by renal dysfunction, acidosis, K-sparing diuretics, hemolysis, burns, crush injuries. ↓ by diuretics, alkalosis, severe vomiting and diarrhea, heavy NG suctioning.
Prealbumin	15–36 mg/dL	150–360 g/L	10	Indicates acute changes in nutritional status, useful for monitoring TPN.
Sodium	135–147 mEq/L	135–147 mmol/L	1	Low sodium usually due to excess water (e.g., excess serum antidiuretic hormone) and is treated with water restriction. ↑ in severe dehydration, diabetes insipidus significant renal and GI losses.
Triglycerides (fasting)	<160 mg/dL	<1.80 mmol/L	0.0113	↑ by alcohol, saturated fats, drugs (propranolol, diuretics, oral contraceptives). Obtain fasting level.
Troponin cTnI cTnT	<0.03 ng/ml <0.2 ng/ml	<0.03 μg/L <0.2 μg/L	1 1	More specific than CK-MB for myocardial damage, elevated sooner and remains elevated longer than CK-MB. cTnI > 2.0 suggests acute myocardial injury.
Uric acid	2–7 mg/dL	120–420 μmol/L	59.48	↑ in gout, neoplastic, or myeloproliferative disorders, and drugs (diuretics, niacin, low-dose salicylate, cyclosporine).

^{a}Enzyme activity can be reported as U/L, where 1 unit equals the amount of enzyme generating 1 μmol of product per minute, or as a katal (kat) unit, which reports product formation in moles per second. One μkat = 60 U.
^{b}Phosphate as inorganic phosphorus.
Alk Phos, alkaline phosphatase; ALT, alanine aminotransferase; AST, aspartate aminotransferase; BUN, blood urea nitrogen; CO$_2$, carbon dioxide; CK, creatine kinase, formerly known as creatine phosphokinase (CPK); Cl$_{Cr}$, creatinine clearance; GGT, gamma-glutamyl transferase; HDL, high density lipoprotein; LD, lactate dehydrogenase, formerly known as LDH; LDL, low-density lipoprotein; MI, myocardial infarction; SGOT, serum glutamate oxaloacetic transaminase; SGPT, serum glutamate pyruvate transaminase; cTnI, cardiac troponin I; cTnT, cardiac troponin T; TPN, total parenteral nutrition; PE, pulmonary embolism.

Potassium

The major intracellular cation in the body is potassium (3.5 to 5.0 mEq/L or mmol/L); approximately 3,500 mEq of potassium is contained in the body of a 70-kg person. Only about 10% of this total body concentration of potassium is extracellular, and only about 50 mEq is in the ECF. The potassium ion is filtered freely at the glomerulus of the kidney, reabsorbed in the proximal tubule, and secreted into the distal segments of the renal nephron.

The serum potassium concentration is not a good measure of total body potassium because most of the potassium is sequestered within cells. Intracellular potassium, however, cannot be measured easily. Fortunately, the clinical manifestations of potassium deficiency (fatigue, drowsiness, dizziness, confusion, electrocardiographic changes, muscle weakness, and pain) correlate well with serum concentrations.

The serum potassium concentration is buffered and may be within normal limits despite abnormalities in total body potassium. During potassium depletion, potassium moves from the ICF into the ECF to maintain the serum concentration. There is a total body potassium deficit of approximately 100 mEq when the serum concentration decreases by only 0.3 mEq/L. Consequently, serum potassium concentrations may be misleading, and no assumptions may be made as to the status of total body potassium concentrations.

Hypokalemia

The renal system is responsible for about 90% of daily potassium losses (about 40 to 90 mEq/day). The gastrointestinal (GI) system and sweating account for the remainder of potassium losses.

The kidney has a limited ability to conserve potassium. Even when potassium intake is reduced to zero, the urine will contain at least 5 to 20 mEq of potassium per 24 hours. Therefore, prolonged intravenous therapy with potassium-free solutions in a patient who is unable to eat can result in hypokalemia. Hypokalemia also can be induced by osmotic diuretics (e.g., mannitol) or by substantial glucosuria. Thiazide or loop diuretics commonly cause hypokalemia, as does excessive mineralocorticoid activity.

Protracted vomiting is another common cause of potassium depletion. Although the fluid secreted along most of the upper GI tract contains only 5 to 20 mEq/L of potassium, vomiting of this fluid in conjunction with decreased food intake, loss of acid, loss of sodium, and the development of alkalosis all combine to produce hypokalemia. Severe diarrhea especially leads to potassium depletion because of the loss of large volumes of colonic fluid containing 30 to 40 mEq/L of potassium. Insulin and stimulation of β_2-adrenergic receptors are other causes of hypokalemia resulting from increased movement of potassium intracellularly.

Hyperkalemia

Hyperkalemia most often results from decreased renal excretion of potassium, excessive exogenous potassium administration, or excessive cellular breakdown (e.g., hemolysis, burns, crush injuries, surgery, infections). In addition, metabolic acidosis can induce hyperkalemia as hydrogen ions move into the cell in exchange for potassium and sodium.

Potassium excesses or deficits primarily affect the excitability of nerve and muscle tissue. As a result, cardiac function can be affected adversely. Potassium also affects certain enzyme systems, acid–base balance, and carbohydrate and protein metabolism.

2. K.C., a 27-year-old man with type 1 diabetes mellitus, was hospitalized for ketoacidosis. His blood glucose was 918 mg/dL (normal, 70 to 110), his urine output was 135 mL/hr (normal, 50), and his urine was positive (4+) for glucose and ketones. K.C.'s blood pH was 7.1, and his serum potassium concentration was 4.1 mEq/L. Why should the clinician monitoring K.C. be concerned that the potassium serum concentration appears "normal"?

[SI units: glucose, 51.0 mmol/L (normal, 3.9 to 6.1); K, 4.1 mmol/L]

Treatment of K.C.'s diabetic ketoacidosis without supplemental potassium could result in life-threatening hypokalemia. When the pH of the blood is acidic, potassium shifts out of cells in response to increased concentrations of intracellular hydrogen ion. K.C.'s total body potassium concentration is decreased as a result of glycosuria and polyuria. However, the serum potassium concentration appears "normal" because the acidotic state results in a shift of potassium from intracellular storage sites into the circulating plasma volume. When the acidosis and hyperglycemia are corrected and the potassium re-equilibrates back into the intracellular storage sites, the serum potassium concentration will decrease dramatically if potassium supplementation is not provided. As a very general guideline, every decrease in pH by 0.1 unit from 7.4 will falsely elevate the serum potassium concentration by about 0.6 mEq/L. Because K.C.'s pH is 7.1 (i.e., 0.3 units <7.4), his serum potassium concentration will be about 2.3 mEq/L when the acidosis is corrected and potassium returns intracellularly (i.e., three 0.1-units × 0.6 mEq/L = 1.8 mEq/L; 4.1 mEq/L − 1.8 mEq/L = 2.3 mEq/L). (See Chapter 12 for a thorough presentation on the treatment of fluid and electrolyte disorders.)

Carbon Dioxide Content

The CO_2 content (22 to 28 mEq/L or mmol/L) in the serum represents the sum of the bicarbonate concentration and the concentration of dissolved CO_2 in the serum. Although there are several buffer systems in the body (including hemoglobin, phosphate, and protein), the carbonic acid–sodium bicarbonate system is the most important in regulating pH within physiologic limits. From a clinical standpoint, most disturbances of acid–base balance can be considered in terms of imbalances in this system.

Combinations of weak acids and strong bases are called *buffer systems* because they resist changes in hydrogen ion concentration by binding and releasing H+. For example, the bicarbonate ions bind hydrogen ions to form carbonic acid as follows:

$$HCO_3^- + H^+ \rightleftharpoons H_2CO_3 \rightleftharpoons H_2O + CO_2 \qquad \textbf{2-1}$$

Normally, a ratio of 1 part carbonic acid to 20 parts bicarbonate is present in the ECF. This ratio is uniquely important and can be appreciated best when viewed in the context of the Henderson-Hasselbalch equation:

$$pH = pKa + \log \frac{[Salt]}{[Acid]}$$

$$= pKa + \log \frac{HCO_3^-}{H_2CO_3} \qquad \textbf{2-2}$$

$$= 6.1 + \log \frac{20}{1}$$

$$= 7.4$$

This equation unequivocally states that it is the *ratio* of HCO_3 to H_2CO_3 (or PCO_2), and *not* the absolute value of either one, that defines the pH or acid–base status of the patient. To assess the acid–base status of the patient accurately, the clinician must know two of the three variables (pH, PCO_2, bicarbonate). The clinician cannot use either the bicarbonate concentration or the pH by itself to determine a patient's acid–base balance.

Decreases in blood pH (acidosis) may be compensated for by either "blowing off" CO_2 from the lungs or by excreting H^+ in the urine. Increases in pH (alkalosis) result in compensatory retention of CO_2 by the lungs.

In clinical practice, the serum bicarbonate concentration is measured because the acid–base balance can be inferred if a patient has normal pulmonary function based on past medical history and present bedside evaluation. For example, if a clinician reasonably can conclude that a patient's PCO_2 would not be greatly altered because of normal pulmonary function, an increase in measured serum bicarbonate concentration most likely would indicate alkalosis based on the Henderson-Hasselbalch equation. (See Chapter 11, Acid–Base Disorders, for additional clinical examples.)

Chloride

Hyperchloremia and Hypochloremia

Chloride (95 to 105 mEq/L or mmol/L) is the principal inorganic anion of the ECF and is important in maintaining acid–base balance. A decreased serum chloride concentration often accompanies metabolic alkalosis, whereas an increased serum chloride concentration may be indicative of a hyperchloremic metabolic acidosis. The serum chloride level, however, also may be slightly decreased in acidosis if organic acids or other acids are the primary cause of the acidosis. Clinically, hyperchloremia in the absence of metabolic acidosis seldom is encountered because chloride retention usually is accompanied by sodium and water retention. Hypochloremia may result from excessive GI loss of chloride-rich fluid (e.g., vomiting, diarrhea, gastric suctioning, intestinal fistulas). Because chloride ions are excreted renally with cations, hypochloremia also may result from significant diuresis.

Generally, alteration in the serum concentration of chloride seldom is the primary indicator of a major medical problem. The serum chloride level per se has no real diagnostic significance. In fact, the only real reason for measuring the serum chloride is to validate the serum sodium concentration. The relationship between serum concentrations of sodium, bicarbonate, and chloride can be described by Equation 2-3, as follows (where R is the anion gap):

$$Cl^- + HCO_3^- + R = Na^+ \qquad \textbf{2-3}$$

Anion Gap

The R factor (or anion gap) represents the contribution of unmeasured acids. Although it may vary widely under different clinical conditions, it normally has a value of 10. If the anion gap is established for a given patient by measuring the serum concentrations of chloride, bicarbonate, and sodium at the same time, subsequent electrolyte measurements can be checked against each other because the anion gap should remain fairly constant or at least change in a predictable manner.

An elevated anion gap may result from metabolic acidosis (e.g., caused by lactic acids, ketoacids, salicylic acids, methanol, ethylene glycol), sodium salts of strong acids with "unmeasured anions" (e.g., sodium citrate, sodium acetate), or high dosages of certain antibiotics (e.g., carbenicillin). A low anion gap may be the result of reduced concentrations of unmeasured anions (e.g., hypoalbuminemia) or from systematic underestimation of serum sodium (e.g., hyperviscosity of myeloma). (See Chapter 11 for a discussion of the clinical use of the anion gap.)

3. The electrolyte values for K.C. (the patient in Question 2) were as follows: Na, 130 mEq/L; Cl, 100 mEq/L; and HCO₃, 20 mEq/L. The following evening's laboratory results were as follows: Na, 140 mEq/L; Cl, 100 mEq/L; and HCO₃, 20 mEq/L. Why is this second set of laboratory results suspicious?

[SI units: Na, 130 and 140 mmol/L; Cl, 100 mmol/L; and HCO₃, 20 mmol/L]

K.C.'s R fraction has increased from 10 to 20, and the R fraction should be fairly constant. There is either a laboratory error in reporting these electrolyte values, or organic acids and/or other acids are accumulating in K.C. In this case, the possibility of ketoacidosis should be considered because K.C. is diabetic. Otherwise, one would have to question the validity of these electrolyte values.

Osmolality

The osmolality (280 to 300 mOsm/kg or mmol/kg) of a solution is a measure of the osmotic strength, or number of osmotically active ions (i.e., particles present) per unit of solution. It is the total number of particles in the solution, not the weight of the particle or the nature of the particle, that determines osmolality. Because one mole of a substance contains 6×10^{23} molecules, equimolar concentrations of all substances in the undissociated state exert the same osmotic pressure. A mole of an ionized compound such as NaCl contributes twice as many particles in solution as one mole of an undissociated compound such as glucose.

The principal determinants of serum osmolality in most situations are sodium (and its accompanying anions), glucose, and urea. If one corrects for the concentrations of glucose and urea, the serum concentration of sodium closely mirrors the serum osmolality.

The serum osmolality can be calculated as follows:

$$\text{Osmolality*} = 1.86\,[\text{Na}^+] + \frac{[\text{Glucose}]}{18} + \frac{[\text{BUN}]}{2.8} \qquad \textbf{2-4}$$

*Osmolality is measured in mOsm/kg H$_2$O

Under normal physiologic conditions, only about 93% of sodium chloride dissociates in plasma; hence, the osmolality for sodium chloride in plasma is $1.86 \times$ molality. The glucose and BUN concentrations are divided by 18 and 2.8, respectively, to convert the units from mg/dL to mmol/L. A more simplified formula useful for rule-of-thumb calculations is as follows:

$$\text{Osmolality*} = 2\,[\text{Na}^+] + \frac{[\text{Glucose}]}{20} + \frac{[\text{BUN}]}{3} \qquad \textbf{2-5}$$

*Osmolality is measured in mOsm/kg H$_2$O

If the measured serum osmolality exceeds the calculated serum osmolality by more than 10 mOsm/kg H$_2$O, the clinician must consider the possibility of decreased water content in the serum because of hyperlipidemia or hypoproteinemia, the presence of substantial amounts of low-molecular-weight substances (e.g., ethanol, methanol, isopropyl alcohol, acetone, paraldehyde, ethyl ether, ethylene glycol), or laboratory error. The difference between the measured serum osmolality and the calculated serum osmolality commonly is referred to as the *osmol gap.*

Although the serum osmolality commonly is measured to evaluate hyponatremia, it is of limited usefulness in this disorder. Tonicity is more important than osmolality in the clinical assessment of hydration because tonicity measures the movement of water across a semipermeable membrane. Some solutes, such as urea and alcohol, freely enter cells and thereby can increase the measured osmolality without affecting tonicity. These solutes do not shift water out of cells and, therefore, do not affect water balance or the serum sodium concentration. However, impermeable solutes, such as sodium or mannitol, in the ECF increase tonicity and pull water out of cells. As a result, measurement of serum osmolality is unnecessary for the evaluation of hyponatremia unless the diagnosis of hyperlipidemia or hypoproteinemia is a consideration.[8]

Osmolality also can be used in the evaluation of renal function by comparing the ratio of urine to plasma (or serum) osmolality (U/P osmol ratio). The ratio of urine to serum osmolality ranges from 1:1 to 3:1. This ratio validates the clinical finding that urine usually is more concentrated than plasma. If the kidney loses its ability to concentrate urine, the U/P ratio cannot increase beyond a ratio of 1.2:1. For example, in acute and chronic renal dysfunction, the urine sodium is >20 mEq/L and the U/P ratio is 1.2:1. In cases of prerenal azotemia, the U/P ratio is >1.2:1 and urinary sodium is <20 mEq/L.[9,10]

In summary, measurement of serum osmolality assists in the determination of whether there are large deviations in water content and also whether low-molecular-weight substances are present in substantial amounts in the plasma.

4. **Q.P., a 35-year-old man, was seen in the emergency department (ED) after complaining of a peculiar whiteness to his vision, like a "snow field." He also reported being restless and short of breath with mild exertion. He had been watching television and drinking alcohol. He was afebrile, his blood pressure (BP) was 170/105 mm Hg, his pulse was 110 beats/min, and his respiration rate was 30 breaths/min. Physical examination was unremarkable, including a thorough eye examination. Routine laboratory studies showed the following: Na, 135 mEq/L; K, 4.7 mEq/L; Cl, 107 mEq/L; HCO$_3$, 9 mEq/L; pH, 7.10; PCO$_2$, 11 mm Hg; blood glucose, 100 mg/dL; BUN, 12 mg/dL; and serum osmolality, 335 mOsm/kg H$_2$O. Blood ethanol level was 100 mg/dL, and blood methanol was 50 mg/dL. Calculate the serum osmol gap and explain why it is high. Why was the osmolality measured?**

[SI units: Na, 135 mmol/L; K, 4.7 mmol/L; Cl, 107 mmol/L; HCO$_3$, 9 mmol/L; PCO$_2$, 1.5 kPa; glucose, 5.5 mmol/L; BUN, 4.3 mmol/L urea; osmolality, 335 mmol/kg; ethanol, 21.7 mmol/L; methanol, 15.6 mmol/L]

Patients presenting to an ED with a recent history of alcohol consumption complaining of whitish vision concurrent with restlessness and shortness of breath are highly suspect for methanol ingestion. The patient's calculated osmolality is determined from Equation 2-5 to be 279 mOsm/kg H$_2$O ($2 \times 135 + 100/20 + 12/3$). The osmol gap is $335 - 279$ or 56 mOsm/kg H$_2$O. An osmol gap >10 suggests the presence of osmotically active substances in addition to the normal contributors to osmolality. Methanol, as indicated by a level of 50 mg/dL, is the osmotically active substance in this case that caused the osmol gap.[11]

BLOOD CHEMISTRY

SMA-6, SMA-12, and Chem Profile-20

5. **What are the advantages and disadvantages of biochemical profiles such as the Chem Profile-20, SMA-12, or the SMA-6 ordered for T.T. (from Question 1)?**

The SMA-6, SMA-12, and Chem Profile-20 are compilations of 6, 12, or 20 biochemical tests that analyze blood chemistries on large-volume, automated instruments. Such tests have become increasingly routine procedures because they quickly provide basic information concerning organ function at relatively low cost. If abnormal values are noted, additional tests can be ordered to further investigate specific organ function. Nevertheless, the routine use of biochemical profiles is controversial. When biochemical profiles are ordered without regard to the clinical evidence in an individual patient (i.e., routine testing is done on all patients upon admission to a hospital), there is no evidence that such batteries of tests have improved patient care, lessened hospital costs, or shortened lengths of stay.

The SMA-6 blood chemistry panel typically analyzes the sodium, potassium, chloride, CO$_2$, BUN, and glucose concentrations. This particular blood chemistry panel rapidly provides insights into the nature of T.T.'s serum electrolytes, acid–base status, renal function, and metabolic state. If an SMA-12 is ordered instead of the SMA-6 panel, six additional blood chemistry tests are performed. These six additional tests usually include a determination of the serum concentrations of albumin, total protein, bilirubin, alkaline phosphatase, calcium, and creatinine. The creatinine provides a more specific evaluation of renal function than the BUN, and some of the other added tests provide an evaluation of liver function.

An abbreviated method to report the SMA-6 and serum creatinine that is used commonly by clinicians is shown in the following figure.

A Chem Profile-20 provides an additional eight tests: phosphorus, cholesterol, triglycerides, uric acid, iron, lactic dehydrogenase (LD), aspartate aminotransferase (AST), and alanine aminotransferase (ALT). These eight tests provide additional information for a general evaluation of metabolism, cardiovascular risk factors, and liver function, which are not provided by some SMA-6 or SMA-12 automated biochemical profiles. The cost of a Chem Profile-20 seldom is much greater than that of an SMA-6 or SMA-12 because of the automated nature of these tests. Costs and the particular grouping of tests into an SMA-6, SMA-12, or Chem Profile-20 panel vary with different clinical laboratories.

Although additional automated blood chemistry tests are relatively inexpensive, the probability of obtaining a false "abnormal" test result increases with the number of tests. For example, an estimated 65% of patients would have at least one abnormal test result if 20 tests were performed. When faced with an unexpected abnormal test result, the clinician has the choice of ignoring it, repeating the test, or obtaining further tests for confirmation. The induced costs, inconvenience, and potential risk of further investigations may more than offset the initial benefits ascribed to profile testing. Although clinicians often state that they should follow up on the unexpected abnormality, in practice most often they do not.[12] Therefore, laboratory abnormalities based on routine biochemical profiles should be interpreted with appropriate caution.

Calcium

The total calcium (8.8 to 10.2 mg/dL or 2.20 to 2.55 mmol/L) content of normal adult humans is 20 to 25 g/kg of fat-free tissue, and about 44% of this calcium is in the body skeleton. About 1% of the skeletal calcium is freely exchangeable with that in the ECF. This reservoir of calcium in bones maintains the concentration of calcium in the plasma constant despite pronounced changes in the external balance of calcium. If the homeostatic factors (i.e., parathyroid hormone, vitamin D, calcitonin) that regulate the calcium content of body fluid are intact, a patient may lose 25% to 30% of total body calcium without a change in the concentration of calcium ion in the plasma.

About 40% of the calcium in the ECF is bound to plasma proteins (especially with albumin); 5% to 15% is complexed with phosphate and citrate; and about 45% to 55% is in the unbound, ionized form. Most laboratories measure the total calcium concentration, although it is the free, ionized calcium level that is important physiologically and the form that is regulated closely.

Hypocalcemia

A reduced calcium concentration, or hypocalcemia, usually implies a deficiency in either the production or response to parathyroid hormone or vitamin D. The abnormality in the parathyroid hormone system may result from hypoparathy-

roidism, pseudohypoparathyroidism, or hypomagnesemia. The abnormality in the vitamin D system may be caused by decreased nutritional intake; decreased absorption of vitamin D because of gastrectomy, chronic pancreatitis, or small bowel disease; decreased production of 25-hydroxycholecalciferol because of liver disease; increased metabolism of 25-hydroxycholecalciferol because of enzyme-stimulating drugs (e.g., phenobarbital, phenytoin, rifampin); or decreased production of 1,25-dihydroxycholecalciferol because of chronic renal disease.

Hypercalcemia

An elevated calcium concentration commonly is associated with malignancy or metastatic diseases. Other causes of hypercalcemia include hyperparathyroidism, Paget's disease, milk-alkali syndrome, granulomatous disorders, thiazide diuretics, and vitamin D intoxication.

6. V.C., a 38-year-old man, was hospitalized because of obtundation, somnolence, and severe alcohol intoxication. Laboratory tests revealed the following: albumin, 2.0 g/dL (normal, 4 to 6); Ca, 6.8 mg/dL (normal, 8.8 to 10.2); total bilirubin, 10.8 mg/dL (normal, 0.1 to 1.0); serum AST, 280 U/L (normal, 0 to 35 U/L); and alkaline phosphatase 240 U/L (normal, 30 to 120 U/L). Why should V.C. not be treated with calcium despite his apparently low serum concentration of calcium?

[SI units: albumin, 20 g/L; Ca, 1.7 mmol/L; total bilirubin, 184.6 μmol/L; AST, 4.67 μkat/L; alkaline phosphatase, 4 μkat/L]

This case presentation provides insufficient patient data to make a conclusion concerning treatment. Clinicians must not become so engrossed in the patient's "numbers" that the patient as a person is overlooked. Always remember to *treat* the patient and *observe* laboratory tests; it is not appropriate to treat laboratory values. Furthermore, remember that serum calcium is partially bound to plasma proteins and the serum concentration depends on the concentration of these plasma proteins, particularly albumin. If the concentration of plasma proteins is low, the reported serum calcium generally will be less than the lower limit of normal. Although it would be best to measure ionized calcium, available instrumentation and methodology make such measurement difficult on a routine basis. In the absence of a direct measurement of ionized calcium, a useful method to estimate a corrected value for serum calcium in the presence of a low serum albumin is to use the following rule: the total serum calcium will decrease by 0.8 mg/dL for each decrease of 1.0 g/dL in serum albumin concentration. V.C.'s serum albumin concentration is about 3.0 mg/dL less than "normal" (5.0 mg/dL − 2.0 mg/dL = 3.0 mg/dL). Therefore, the amount of available ionized calcium in V.C. is comparable to that available if his serum calcium were 9.2 mg/dL (i.e., calculated ionized calcium = 3.0 × 0.8 = 2.4 mg/dL; "corrected" serum calcium = 2.4 + 6.8 = 9.2 mg/dL). The "corrected" serum calcium concentration is within the normal range; therefore, V.C. should not be treated with calcium based on the available data.

Phosphate

The extracellular concentration of phosphate, as inorganic phosphorus (2.5 to 5.0 mg/dL or 0.80 to 1.60 mmol/L), is the prime determinant of the intracellular concentration, which in turn is the source of phosphate for adenosine triphosphate

(ATP) and phospholipid synthesis. Intracellular phosphate also is important in the regulation of nucleotide degradation.

Hyperphosphatemia and Hypophosphatemia

The ECF concentration of phosphate is influenced by parathyroid hormone, intestinal absorption, renal function, bone metabolism, and nutrition. Hyperphosphatemia most commonly is caused by renal insufficiency, although hypervitaminosis D and hypoparathyroidism also are significant causes. Moderate hypophosphatemia appears in malnourished patients, especially when anabolism is induced; in patients with excessive use of aluminum-containing antacids that bind phosphorus in the GI tract; in chronic alcoholics; and in septic patients. Clinical consequences of severe hypophosphatemia involve nervous system dysfunction, muscle weakness, rhabdomyolysis, cardiac irregularities, and dysfunction of leukocytes and erythrocytes.

Glucose

The glucose (70 to 110 mg/dL or 3.9 to 6.1 mmol/L) concentration in the ECF is regulated closely by homeostatic mechanisms to provide body tissues with a ready source of energy. The plasma glucose concentration usually is measured in either the fasting or postprandial state, depending on the type of information desired. Generally, normal glucose values refer to the plasma glucose concentration in the fasting state. The specific laboratory assay of blood sugar determinations also must be considered because different assay methods vary in their specificity and sensitivity to glucose.

Hyperglycemia and Hypoglycemia

Hyperglycemia and hypoglycemia are nonspecific signs of abnormal glucose metabolism. Diabetes mellitus is the most common cause of hyperglycemia, and insufficient carbohydrate intake because of a missed meal in a patient receiving insulin or another hypoglycemic medication is the most common cause of hypoglycemia. (See Chapter 50, Diabetes Mellitus, for an in-depth presentation of the laboratory tests associated with abnormal glucose metabolism.)

Uric Acid

Uric acid (2.0 to 7.0 mg/dL or 0.12 to 0.42 mmol/L) is an endproduct of nucleoprotein metabolism. It serves no biologic function, is not metabolized, and must be excreted renally. Gout usually is associated with increased serum concentrations of uric acid and deposits of monosodium urates.

Increased serum uric acid concentrations can result from either a decrease in renal urate excretion or excessive urate production (e.g., from the nucleoprotein turnover that accompanies neoplastic or myeloproliferative disorders). Low serum uric acid concentrations are inconsequential and usually are reflective of drugs that have hypouricemic activity (e.g., high dosages of salicylates). The determinants of the serum concentration of uric acid, the clinical implications of hyperuricemia, and the therapeutic management of uric acid disorders are presented in Chapter 42, Gout and Hyperuricemia.

Blood Urea Nitrogen

Urea nitrogen (8 to 18 mg/dL or 3.0 to 6.5 mmol/L) is an endproduct of protein metabolism. It is produced solely by the liver, is transported in the blood, and is excreted by the kidneys. The concentration of BUN reflects renal function because the urea nitrogen in blood is filtered completely at the glomerulus of the kidney, then reabsorbed and tubularly secreted within nephrons. Acute or chronic renal failure is the most common cause of an elevated BUN. Although the BUN is an excellent screening test for renal dysfunction, it is not sufficiently selective for quantifying the extent of renal disease. A number of factors other than renal function can affect the serum BUN concentration. For example, unusually high protein intake or conditions that increase protein catabolism tend to increase the BUN. Upper GI bleeding or esophageal varices can increase the BUN because blood is converted by bacteria in the bowel to ammonia and urea nitrogen. The hydrational status of a patient may either increase or decrease the BUN because a water deficit tends to concentrate the urea nitrogen and a water excess dilutes the urea nitrogen. Finally, the BUN may be decreased in the terminal stages of liver disease because of the inability of the liver to form urea.

7. **Why is the BUN abnormal for T.T. (from Question 1)?**

The BUN serum concentration in T.T. is somewhat increased, perhaps because of inadequate renal perfusion secondary to her heart failure. Her renal function also could be more severely compromised than one would anticipate from her slightly increased BUN value because of dilution by increased ECF volume. Therefore, T.T.'s renal status should be evaluated.

Creatinine

Creatinine (0.6 to 1.2 mg/dL or 50 to 110 mmol/L) is derived from creatine and phosphocreatine, a major constituent of muscle. Its rate of formation for a given individual is remarkably constant and is determined primarily by an individual's muscle mass or lean body weight. Therefore, the serum creatinine concentration is slightly higher in muscular subjects, but unlike the BUN, it is less affected by exogenous factors. Once creatinine is released from muscle into plasma, it is excreted renally almost exclusively by glomerular filtration. A decrease in the glomerular filtration rate results in an increase in the serum creatinine concentration. Thus, careful interpretation of the serum creatinine concentration is used widely in the clinical evaluation of patients with suspected renal disease.

A doubling of the serum creatinine (SrCr) level roughly corresponds to a 50% reduction in the glomerular filtration rate. This general rule of thumb only holds for steady-state creatinine levels.[13]

8. **T.T. was given digoxin 0.25 mg/day, and an SrCr was ordered to further assess her renal function. The clinical laboratory determined that her SrCr was 1.2 mg/dL. Because this laboratory test result is within normal limits, does it indicate normal renal function for T.T.?**

[SI unit: SrCr, 106 mmol/L]

A serum creatinine of 1.2 mg/dL in T.T. does not necessarily reflect normal renal function. As patients become older, muscle mass represents a smaller proportion of total weight and creatinine production is decreased. Furthermore, the serum creatinine concentration in female patients generally is 0.2 to 0.4 mg/dL (85% to 90%) less than for males because females have relatively smaller kidneys. Because T.T. is a 75-year-old woman, a creatinine clearance determination would reflect more accurately her renal function status.

Creatinine Clearance

The clearance of any substance that is filtered freely at the glomerulus and is not absorbed, secreted, synthesized, or metabolized by the kidney is equal to the glomerular filtration rate. Creatinine meets these criteria; therefore, creatinine clearance (Cl_{Cr}) reflects the glomerular filtration rate.

An accurate estimation of Cl_{Cr} is crucial to administering appropriate drug therapy because many drugs are partially or totally eliminated by the kidney. Cl_{Cr} is a specific measurement of renal function that requires a 24-hour urine collection. It more accurately reflects renal function than the serum creatinine; however, 24-hour urine collections often are unreliable. An incomplete urine collection could result in a substantial underestimation of renal function. Urine should be collected over a 24-hour period rather than over a shorter time interval because of the possibility of a daily cyclical pattern in the clearance of creatinine. Nevertheless, in critically ill, trauma, or postsurgical patients, the 24-hour creatinine clearance can be estimated from an 8-hour urine collection if a deviation of up to 20% from the 24-hour value is clinically acceptable.[14] No significant cyclical variation in creatinine excretion was found over the 24-hour period of this latter study.

Urine collections are time-consuming and expensive. As a result, several nomograms and formulas have been developed to provide estimates of creatinine clearances by using measured serum creatinine values. The following formula created by Jelliffe is used commonly[15]:

$$\begin{array}{c} Cl_{Cr} \\ \text{for Males} \\ (\text{mL/min/1.73 m}^2) \end{array} = \frac{98 - [(0.8)(\text{Age} - 20)]}{SrCr_{ss}} \qquad \textbf{2-6}$$

This Jelliffe formula must be multiplied by 90% to calculate creatinine clearances for females.

An evaluation of various formulas that estimate creatinine clearance noted that all methods of calculation appeared to be equally reliable for patients with a serum creatinine in the range of 1.5 to 5.0 mg/dL.[16] Equation 2-6 by Jelliffe, however, substantially underestimated the creatinine clearance in patients with a serum creatinine of <1.5 mg/dL. The following Cockcroft and Gault[17] formula uses age, body weight, and serum creatinine and has the highest correlation and the greatest accuracy in patients with serum creatinine concentrations <1.5 mg/dL[18]:

$$\begin{array}{c} Cl_{Cr} \\ \text{for Males} \\ (\text{mL/min}) \end{array} = \frac{(140 - \text{Age})(\text{Body weight in kg})}{(SrCr)(72)} \qquad \textbf{2-7}$$

The Cockcroft and Gault formula must be multiplied by 85% to calculate creatinine clearance for females.

For patients with liver dysfunction, all methods of calculating creatinine clearance from a serum creatinine value are associated with significant overprediction of creatinine clearance.[16] Thus, methods for predicting creatinine clearance should not be used in patients with liver disease as a basis for the adjustment of drug dosages.

9. A 24-hour Cl_{Cr} determination was ordered for B.J., a 44-year-old, 50-kg man. The following data were returned from the clinical laboratory: total collection time, 24 hours; urine volume, 1,200 mL; urine creatinine concentration, 42 mg/dL; SrCr,

1.5 mg/dL; and Cl_{Cr}, 23 mL/min (uncorrected) and 30 mL/min (corrected). Why should B.J.'s reported Cl_{Cr} be viewed with considerable suspicion?

[SI units: SrCr, 132.6 mmol/L; Cl_{Cr}, 0.38 and 0.50 mL/s, respectively]

When creatinine clearance determinations are reported, clinicians always should verify the reliability of the test result before altering drug dosing schedules. First of all, it would be appropriate to determine whether the urine collection was complete. The total amount of creatinine actually collected in the 24-hour period should be compared with the calculated amount of creatinine that is expected to be produced.

$$\begin{array}{l} \begin{array}{c} \text{Creatinine} \\ \text{Excreted} \end{array} = (\text{Urine Volume/24 hr}) \left(\begin{array}{c} \text{Urine Creatinine} \\ \text{Concentration} \end{array} \right) \\ \qquad = (1200 \text{ mL/24 hr})(42 \text{ mg/100 mL}) \qquad \textbf{2-8} \\ \qquad = 504 \text{ mg Creatinine/24 hr} \end{array}$$

The total amount of creatinine excreted per 24 hours can be divided by the patient's body weight to determine the apparent creatinine production per day.

$$\begin{array}{c} \text{Apparent Rate} \\ \text{of Creatinine} \\ \text{Production} \\ \text{per Day} \end{array} = \frac{\text{Amount of Creatinine Excreted}}{\text{Patient's Weight}}$$

$$\qquad = \frac{504 \text{ mg Creatinine/24 hr}}{50 \text{ kg}} \qquad \textbf{2-9}$$

$$\qquad = 10.08 \text{ mg/mg/day}$$

This apparent rate of creatinine production of approximately 10 mg/kg per day is considerably less than the expected 20 mg/kg per day creatinine production for a 44-year-old man (Table 2-3). Therefore, this collection of urine for B.J. probably was incomplete, and the reported creatinine clearance probably is much less than his actual creatinine clearance. However, if B.J. has a very small muscle mass because of atrophy, cachexia, or age, the urine collection could be adequate and the reported creatinine clearance accurate.

As shown in B.J.'s laboratory test results, both uncorrected and corrected creatinine clearance values are reported by clinical laboratories. The uncorrected value usually represents the patient's actual creatinine clearance and the corrected value predicts what the patient's creatinine clearance would be if he or she were 1.73 m² or 70 kg.[12] (See Chapter 31, Acute Renal Failure, for a more thorough description of renal function assessments.)

Table 2-3	Expected Daily Creatinine Production for Males
Age (yr)	Daily Creatinine Production (mg/kg/day)
20–29	24
30–39	22
40–49	20
50–59	19
60–69	17
70–79	14
80–89	12
90–99	9

Reprinted with permission of reference 13.

Lactate Dehydrogenase

The glycolytic enzyme LD (100 to 190 units/L or U/L) catalyzes the interconversion of lactate and pyruvate and is present in most tissues. It is present in especially high concentrations in the heart, kidney, liver, and skeletal muscle, although it also is abundantly present in erythrocytes and lung tissue. Because increased serum concentrations of LD can be associated with diseases in many different organs and tissues, the diagnostic usefulness of an LD determination is somewhat limited. However, there are five isoenzymes of LD, and there are striking differences in the isoenzyme content of different tissues. Most tissues contain all five isoenzymes, but LD_1 and to a lesser extent LD_2 predominate in the heart. Skeletal muscle and the liver have mostly LD_5. Red blood cells, kidneys, brain, stomach, and pancreas are other important sources of LD_1. Consequently, chemical or electrophoretic separation of these isoenzymes can increase the diagnostic usefulness of serum LD determinations. For example, the elevated serum LD associated with myocardial infarction (MI) consists mostly of LD_1 and LD_2, whereas with acute liver disease there is a greater proportion of LD_4 and LD_5. Unfortunately, these isoenzyme patterns are not necessarily typical of all myocardial or liver diseases.

The LD isoenzymes are removed from the serum at different rates. The biologic half-life of LD_5 is 8 to 10 hours, whereas the biologic half-life of LD_1 is estimated to be 48 to 113 hours. The liver will liberate LD quickly when damaged by physical trauma, infection, or ischemia. If the insult is an isolated event and not an ongoing process, the released LD will be cleared from the serum within a day.

Creatine Kinase

The CK (0 to 150 units/L or U/L) enzyme (formerly known as creatine phosphokinase) catalyzes the transfer of high-energy phosphate groups in tissues that consume large amounts of energy (e.g., skeletal muscle, myocardium, brain). Therefore, total CK can be increased by strenuous exercise, intramuscular injections of drugs that are irritating to tissue (e.g., diazepam, phenytoin), acute psychotic episodes, or myocardial injury.

CK is composed of M and B subunits, which are further divided into three isoenzymes: MM, BB, and MB. The CK-MM isoenzyme is found predominantly in skeletal muscle, the CK-BB in the brain, and the CK-MB in the myocardium. Myocardial CK activity consists of 80% to 85% CK-MM and 15% to 20% CK-MB. Noncardiac tissues that contain large amounts of CK have either CK-MM or CK-BB. The MB fraction is either absent or present only in trace amounts in tissues other than the myocardium.

After an MI, the CK-MB fraction accounts for about 5% or more of the total CK.[19] Myocardial damage appears to correlate with the amount of CK-MB released into the serum (i.e., the higher the amount of CK-MB, the more extensive the myocardial injury). Although CK-MB levels >25 U/L usually are associated with MI,[20] the absolute amount may vary depending on the assay technique used. Generally, if the amount of CK-MB exceeds 6% of the total, myocardial injury presumably has occurred. Analysis of CK-MB provides a rapid, sensitive, specific, cost-effective, and definitive means of detecting MI.[21]

10. O.D., a 55-year-old man, presents to the ED with sudden onset of acute chest pain, diaphoresis, and nausea that began about 1 hour ago. He describes his pain as severe and not relieved by position change, antacids, or nitroglycerin. An electrocardiogram (ECG) reveals changes consistent with an acute evolving MI. The total CK serum concentration is 118 U/L and the CK-MB is 5 U/L. O.D. was admitted to the coronary care unit to rule out an acute MI. Why are the total CK and CK-MB serum concentrations within the normal range in O.D., who presents with strong evidence of an MI?

[SI units: CK, 1.97 μkat/L; CK-MB, 0.08 μkat/L]

The total CK and CK-MB are both within the normal range for O.D.; however, an MI cannot be excluded. CK serum concentrations usually do not rise above normal values until 4 to 8 hours after myocardial injury and usually peak in about 12 to 24 hours. Therefore, it is important to measure CK and CK-MB serum concentrations 12 to 24 hours after the initial determination to be sure that subsequent increases in the serum concentrations of these myocardial enzymes will be detected. About 10% of patients with suspected MIs fail to demonstrate an increase in the total CK, although serial CK-MB fractions will be increased. Therefore, when CK-MB is >6% of total CK, an MI probably has occurred even if the total CK is not elevated.[19]

Troponin

11. How can myocardial enzymes be detected earlier than 4 to 8 hours after myocardial injury?

Troponins T, I, and C are a complex of proteins that mediate the calcium-mediated interaction of actin and myosin within muscles. Whereas troponin T is present in cardiac and skeletal muscle cells, troponin I is present only in cardiac muscle. Troponin C is present in two distinct isoforms that are present in both skeletal and cardiac muscle.[22,23] Compared with the detection of CK-MB, the detection of the presence of troponin T and I is a more specific and sensitive indicator of myocardial damage.[24] Furthermore, the concentration of troponin increases within 2 to 4 hours of an acute MI, enabling clinicians to initiate appropriate therapy very quickly following presentation to the ED. Troponin also remains elevated for 10 to 14 days compared to the 2- to 3-day elevation typically observed with CK-MB. Levels of troponin I >2.0 ng/mL are suggestive of acute myocardial tissue injury. The use of troponin as a primary diagnostic test for acute MI is becoming widely accepted as a standard.[24] (See Chapter 18, Myocardial Infarction, for a thorough discussion regarding the appropriate initial therapy of acute MI.)

Albumin

Albumin (4.0 to 6.0 g/dL or 40 to 60 g/L) is produced by the liver and contributes approximately 80% of serum colloid osmotic pressure. Therefore, hypoalbuminemic states commonly are associated with edema and transudation of ECF. A lack of essential amino acids from malnutrition or malabsorption or impaired synthesis by the liver can result in decreased serum albumin concentrations. Most forms of hepatic insufficiency are associated with decreased synthesis of albumin. Albumin can be lost directly from the blood because of hemorrhage, burns, or exudates, or it may be lost directly into the urine because of nephrosis. Serum albumin concentrations seldom increase, but increases may be noted in volume depletion or shock or immediately after the administration of large amounts of intravenous albumin. In addition to its diagnostic value, the serum albumin concentration is an important consideration in the therapeutic monitoring of drugs and electrolytes that are highly protein bound (e.g., phenytoin, digoxin, calcium). In cases of severe hypoalbuminemia, determination of the "free" or unbound concentration of these entities may be required for an accurate assessment of drug therapy.

Prealbumin

Prealbumin (15 to 36 mg/dL or 150 to 360 mg/L) is one of the primary proteins but accounts for a relatively small percentage of circulating proteins. It is also referred to as thyroxine-binding prealbumin (TBA) due to its role as a transport mechanism for triiodothyronine (T_3) and thyroxine (T_4). However, prealbumin is most frequently used in the assessment of a patient's nutritional status. Compared to the relatively long half-life of albumin (roughly 3 weeks), the half-life of prealbumin is only 1 to 2 days. This shorter half-life provides a more accurate reflection of acute changes in protein synthesis and catabolism and is an effective and useful marker in patients receiving total parenteral nutrition. Similar to albumin, hepatic disease and malnutrition are associated with decreases in prealbumin. Hodgkin's disease, pregnancy, chronic renal disease, and steroid use may increase prealbumin levels.

Globulin

The plasma proteins primarily consist of albumin, globulin (2.3 to 3.5 g/dL or 23 to 35 g/L), and fibrinogen fractions. Whereas albumin principally functions to maintain serum oncotic pressure, globulins play an active role in some immunologic processes. The globulins can be separated into several subgroups (e.g., α, β, γ). The γ-globulins can be separated further into various immunoglobulins (e.g., IgA, IgM, IgG). Chronic infection or rheumatoid arthritis can increase immunoglobulin levels, and fractionation of immunoglobulins can provide useful information in the evaluation of immune disorders. When the immunoglobulins are separated by electrophoresis, elevations of one or several of the immunoglobulins in a specific pattern can suggest a diagnosis of multiple myeloma, a plasma cell malignancy.

Because globulin is not manufactured solely by the liver, the ratio of albumin to globulin (the A/G ratio) is changed in patients with liver disease. Changes in this ratio result from decreased albumin concentration and a compensatory increase in globulin concentration.

Aspartate Aminotransferase

The AST enzyme (0 to 35 units/L or U/L), formerly called serum glutamic oxaloacetic transaminase (SGOT), is abundant in heart and liver tissue and moderately present in skeletal muscle, the kidney, and the pancreas. In cases of acute cellular injury to the heart or liver, the enzyme is released into the blood from the damaged cells and presumably is metabolized within the body. In clinical practice, AST determinations are used to evaluate myocardial injury and to diagnose and assess the prognosis of liver disease resulting from hepatocellular injury.

The serum concentration of AST activity is increased in about 96% to 98% of patients after an MI. However, the serum concentrations do not become abnormal until 4 to 6 hours after the onset of myocardial injury. The AST activity in serum peaks after 24 to 36 hours, and the activity returns to the normal range in about 4 to 5 days. The peak values of AST approximate the extent of myocardial damage (see Chapter 18).

Serum AST values are elevated significantly in patients with acute hepatic necrosis, whether caused by viral hepatitis (see Chapter 73, Viral Hepatitis) or a hepatotoxin such as carbon tetrachloride. In these situations, the serum concentrations of both AST and ALT (see the following section) will be increased, even before the appearance of clinical symptoms (e.g., jaundice). The AST and ALT serum concentrations may be increased by as much as 100 times greater than the usual upper limits of normal in the presence of parenchymal liver disease. Patients with intrahepatic cholestasis, posthepatic jaundice, or cirrhosis usually experience more moderate elevations of AST, depending on the extent of cell necrosis. The AST serum concentration usually is higher than that of ALT in patients with cirrhosis, and the AST increase usually is about four to five times greater than the upper limit of normal.

Alanine Aminotransferase

The enzyme ALT (0 to 35 units/L or U/L), formerly called serum glutamic pyruvic transaminase (SGPT), is found in essentially the same tissues that have high concentrations of AST. In liver diseases, serum ALT elevations parallel those of AST, although slightly more acute hepatocellular parenchymal damage must occur to produce abnormal values. The ALT is relatively more abundant in hepatic tissue versus cardiac tissue than AST; however, the liver still contains 3.5 times more AST than ALT. Although serum concentrations of both AST and ALT increase when disease processes affect liver cell structure, the ALT is the more liver-specific enzyme. ALT serum concentrations rarely are increased except in parenchymal liver disease. The ALT activity is increased only marginally by an MI because the ALT activity in heart muscle is only a small fraction of the quantity of AST present. Furthermore, elevations of ALT persist longer than those of AST.

Alkaline Phosphatase

The alkaline phosphatases (30 to 120 units/L or U/L) constitute a large group of isoenzymes that play important roles in the transport of sugar and phosphate. These isoenzymes of alkaline phosphatase have different physiochemical properties and originate from different tissues (e.g., liver, bone, placenta, intestine).

In normal adults, the circulating alkaline phosphatase is derived primarily from liver and bone. Although only small amounts of alkaline phosphatase are present in the liver, this enzyme is secreted into the bile, and its serum concentration increases substantially with mild intrahepatic or extrahepatic biliary obstruction. Thus, the presence of early bile duct abnormalities can result in alkaline phosphatase elevations before increases in the serum bilirubin are observed. Drug-induced cholestatic jaundice (e.g., chlorpromazine or sulfonamides) can increase the serum concentration of alkaline phosphate. The serial evaluation of serum concentrations of alkaline phosphatase is not particularly useful in assessing the degree of hepatic impairment. In mild cases of acute liver cell damage, the alkaline phosphatase level seldom is elevated, and even in cirrhosis, the alkaline phosphatase serum concentration is variable and depends upon the degree of hepatic decompensation and obstruction. The serum alkaline phosphatase concentration is an excellent indicator of space-occupying lesions in the liver, primarily because of disruption of biliary canaliculi within the liver.[25]

The osteoblasts in bone produce large amounts of alkaline phosphatase. Thus, alkaline phosphatase concentrations in serum are increased markedly in Paget's disease, hyperparathyroidism, osteogenic sarcoma, osteoblastic cancer metastatic to bone, and other conditions of pronounced osteoblastic activity. The serum alkaline phosphatase is increased during periods of rapid bone growth (e.g., infancy, early childhood, healing bone fractures) and during pregnancy because of the contributions of the placenta and fetal bones.

Gamma-Glutamyl Transferase

Although the enzyme gamma-glutamyl transferase (GGT) (0 to 70 units/L or U/L) is found in the kidney, liver, and pancreas, its major clinical value is in the evaluation of hepatobiliary disease. An increase in the serum concentration of GGT parallels the increase of alkaline phosphatase in obstructive jaundice and infiltrative disease of the liver. Because GGT is a hepatic microsomal enzyme, tissue concentrations increase in response to microsomal enzyme induction by alcohol and other drugs (e.g., phenobarbital, phenytoin). As a result, GGT is a sensitive indicator of recent alcohol exposure.

Bilirubin

Bilirubin (0.1 to 1.0 mg/dL or 1.7 to 17 μmol/L for total bilirubin; 0 to 0.2 mg/dL or 0 to 3.4 μmol/L for direct conjugated bilirubin) primarily is a breakdown product of hemoglobin and is formed in the reticuloendothelial system (step 1 of Fig. 2-1). It is transferred then into the blood (step 2), where it is almost completely bound to serum albumin (step 3). When the bilirubin arrives at the sinusoidal surface of the liver cells, the free fraction rapidly is taken up into the cell (step 4) and converted primarily to bilirubin diglucuronide (step 5). A monoglucuronide also is formed that is metabolized predominantly to the diglucuronide. The conjugated bilirubin diglucuronide then is excreted into the bile (step 6) and appears in the intestine, where bacteria convert most of it to urobilinogen (step 7). Most of the urobilinogen is destroyed or excreted in the feces (step 13), but some is reabsorbed into the blood (step 8). A portion of this small amount of urobilinogen in the blood is then reabsorbed into the liver (step 9) and subsequently excreted into the bile (step 12); the other portion is excreted into the urine (step 10). The mechanism by which conjugated bilirubin in the liver cell is transferred to the blood (step 14) is not well understood. However, in many types of liver disease, the conjugated form of bilirubin (direct-acting) is present in increased concentrations in the blood. When this concentration exceeds 0.2 to 0.4 mg/dL, bilirubin will begin to appear in the urine (step 11). Unconjugated bilirubin (indirect-acting) is water insoluble and is highly bound to serum albumin; both of these factors account for its lack of excretion in the urine.[26]

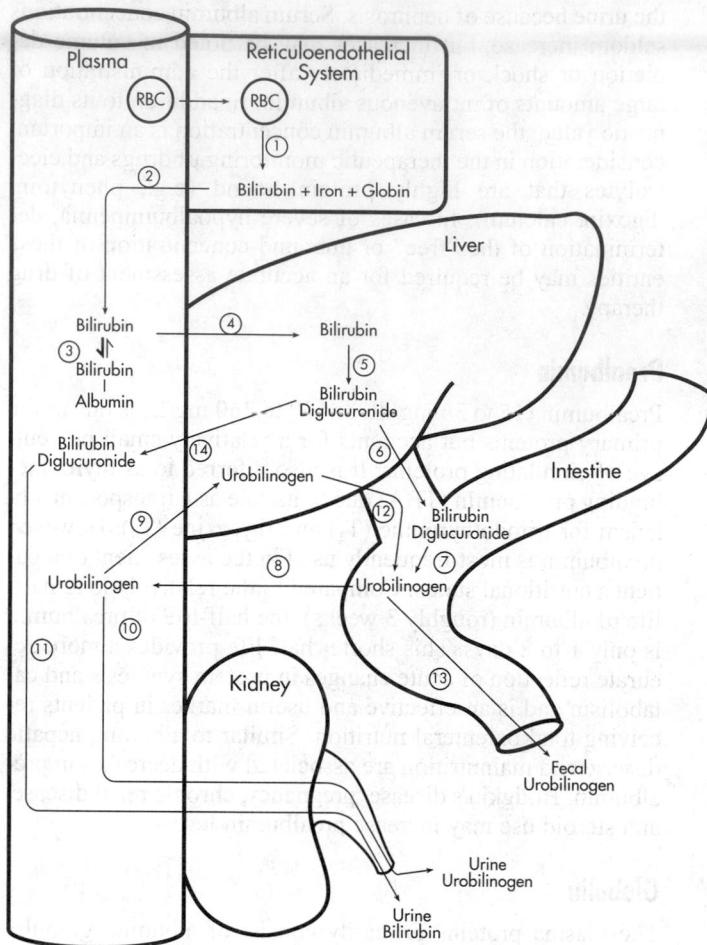

FIGURE 2-1. Bilirubin metabolism.

Causes of Increased Bilirubin

12. A.R., a 42-year-old man with a 2-year history of hypertension controlled with hydrochlorothiazide and 1-year history of Parkinson's controlled by levodopa, is hospitalized after an episode of orthostatic hypotension. Admitting laboratory results show a hematocrit (Hct) of 27%. Because A.R. had a long history of alcoholism, additional laboratory tests were obtained. His results were as follows: bilirubin (total), 3.5 mg/dL; bilirubin (direct), 0.5 mg/dL; alkaline phosphatase, 40 U/L; AST, 32 U/L; and ALT, 27 U/L. Based on this information and Figure 2-1, what are three major causes of increased bilirubin in adults, and what might be the most logical cause of increased bilirubin in A.R.?

[SI units: Hct, 0.27; bilirubin, 59.8 and 8.6 μmol/L, respectively; alkaline phosphatase, 0.67 μkat/L; AST, 0.53 μkat/L; ALT, 0.45 μkat/L]

HEPATOCELLULAR DAMAGE

When the liver is unable to conjugate bilirubin, the serum concentration of total bilirubin will increase out of proportion to the direct bilirubin (i.e., the indirect bilirubin will be increased). A.R.'s normal AST and ALT values, however, indicate that hepatocellular damage is not likely. Therefore, in this situation, a diagnosis of hepatocellular damage cannot be confirmed by the serum bilirubin concentrations alone.

CHOLESTASIS (POSTHEPATIC)

When bile flow is obstructed in the absence of severe liver impairment, the increase in the total bilirubin serum concentration can be attributed primarily to an increase in the direct or conjugated bilirubin. A determination of the alkaline phosphatase serum concentration is useful in differentiating cholestasis from other forms of jaundice. In this case, the normal serum concentrations of alkaline phosphatase and direct bilirubin indicate that there is not a cholestatic component to A.R.'s problem.

HEMOLYSIS (PREHEPATIC)

When erythrocytes are hemolyzed rapidly, the serum concentration of indirect bilirubin increases. If the liver is conjugating and eliminating bilirubin normally, the total bilirubin will increase out of proportion to the direct bilirubin. This is evident in the previous case. Thus, A.R.'s increased indirect bilirubin concentration probably is caused by hemolysis.

Prostate-Specific Antigen

Prostate-specific antigen (PSA) is a protease glycoprotein produced almost exclusively by prostate epithelial cells. Serum concentrations of PSA are increased when the normal prostate glandular structure is disrupted by benign or malignant tumor or inflammation. In fact, the serum concentration of PSA is elevated in 55% to 83% of men with benign prostatic hyperplasia. Nevertheless, the PSA is most useful for the staging of cancer and for monitoring the progression and response to therapy of prostate cancer.[27]

PSA serum concentrations increase after prostatic manipulation such as digital rectal examination (DRE), transrectal ultrasound, cystoscopy, or biopsy of the prostate. Although elevated serum concentrations of PSA can occur in men with benign prostatic hyperplasia, these concentrations are higher and encountered more often in men with cancer. As a result, the American Cancer Society[28] and the American Urological Association[29] currently recommend that health care providers offer a PSA blood test and DRE yearly to men over 50 years of age. For men considered to be at high risk (family history or African American men), testing at age 45 years is suggested. After reviewing the test results of >6,300 men, a U.S. Food and Drug Administration (FDA) panel noted that PSA blood testing when combined with a DRE was much more effective in detecting prostate cancer than either a DRE or a PSA test alone. Subsequently, the FDA approved Hybritech Corporation's PSA assay for early diagnosis of prostate cancer.

The serum half-life of PSA is 2 to 3 days, but serum PSA concentrations can remain high for several weeks after manipulation of the prostate. When PSA levels from blood samples of men in the Physician's Health Study (an ongoing, randomized trial that enrolled 22,071 men 40 to 84 years of age in 1982) were analyzed, high sensitivities and specificities for the entire 10-year follow-up were detected.[30] This group concluded that "PSA has the highest validity of any circulating cancer screening marker discovered thus far, and that intensive efforts to identify cost-effective screening strategies incorporating PSA testing are warranted."[30] Therefore, the optimal cutoff serum PSA concentrations for delineation of aggressive cancers versus nonaggressive cancers, the estimated relative risks of prostate cancer within given ranges of PSA, and the predictive value of PSA screening relative to costs and benefits will be clarified in the near future. An aggressive approach to localize prostate cancer for men with life expectancies more than 10 years is now favored.[27,31] (Prostate cancer and its treatment are presented in Chapter 91, Solid Tumors.)

Amylase and Lipase

Amylase (35 to 120 U/L or 0.58 to 2.0 μkat/L) and lipase (0 to 160 U/L or 0 to 2.67 μkat/L) are enzymes produced in the pancreas and secreted into the duodenum to assist in the digestive process. Amylase is responsible for breaking down complex carbohydrates into simple sugars and is also found in the saliva. Significant elevations in serum amylase are observed in patients with acute pancreatitis or pancreatic duct obstruction. Amylase levels tend to rise 6 to 48 hours after onset of the disease and usually return to normal 3 days after the acute event. In chronic pancreatitis or obstruction, amylase levels may remain elevated for longer periods. Other nonpancreatic conditions such as bowel perforation, biliary disease, perforated peptic ulcer, ectopic pregnancy, and parotitis (mumps) can be associated with elevated serum amylase levels. Lipase is responsible for breaking down triglycerides into fatty acids. Elevated serum lipase levels are also suggestive of pancreatic disease and tend to be more specific for pancreatic disease than amylase. The onset of lipase elevation is similar to amylase; however, lipase typically remains elevated for 5 to 7 days and can be useful in diagnosing patients in later stages of pancreatic disease. Narcotics such as morphine may constrict the sphincter of Oddi and cause elevations in amylase and lipase.

HEMATOLOGY

Complete Blood Count

The complete blood count (CBC) is one of the most commonly ordered clinical laboratory tests. A CBC measures the hemoglobin (Hgb), hematocrit (Hct), total white blood cells (WBCs), red blood cells (RBCs), mean cell volume (MCV), and mean cell hemoglobin concentration (MCHC). Depending on the laboratory, an order for a CBC may or may not include a platelet count, reticulocyte count, or leukocyte differential count. For a list of hematologic laboratory values, see Table 2-4.

Red Blood Cells (Erythrocytes)

RBCs (4.3 to 5.9 $\times$ 10^6/mm^3 or 4.3 to 5.9 $\times$ 10^{12}/L for males and 3.5 to 5.0 $\times$ 10^6/mm^3 or 3.5 to 5.0 $\times$ 10^{12}/L for females) or erythrocytes are produced in the bone marrow, released into the peripheral blood, circulate for approximately 120 days, and are cleared by the reticuloendothelial system. The primary function of RBCs is to transport oxygen to tissues.

The concentration of RBCs in the blood can be measured to detect anemia, calculate RBC indices, or calculate the Hct. For monitoring quantitative changes in RBCs, the hematocrit and hemoglobin concentration generally are used.

Hematocrit

The Hct (packed cell volume [39% to 49% or 0.39 to 0.49 for males; 33% to 43% or 0.33 to 0.43 for females]) is determined by centrifuging a capillary tube of whole blood and

Table 2-4   Hematologic Laboratory Values[a]

| Laboratory Test | Normal Reference Values | | Comments |
	Conventional Units	SI Units	
ESR	0–20 mm/hr	0–20 mm/hr	Nonspecific; ↑ with inflammation, infection, neoplasms, connective tissue disorders, pregnancy, nephritis. Useful monitor of temporal arteritis and polymyalgia rheumatica.
Male	0–30 mm/hr	0–30 mm/hr	
Female			
Hct			↓ with anemias, bleeding, hemolysis. ↑ with polycythemia, chronic hypoxia.
Male	39–49%	0.39–0.49 I[a]	
Female	33–43%	0.33–0.43 I[a]	
Hgb			Similar to hematocrit.
Male	14–18 g/dL	140–180 g/L	
Female	12–16 g/dL	120–160 g/L	
Iron			
Male	80–180 μg/dL	14–32 μmol/L	Body stores ⅔ in hemoglobin; ⅓ in bone marrow, spleen, liver; only small amount present in plasma. Blood loss major cause of deficiency.
Female	60–160 μg/dL	11–29 μmol/L	↑ needs in pregnancy and lactation.
TIBC	250–460 μg/dL	45–82 μmol/L	↑ capacity to bind iron with iron deficiency.
MCH	27–33 pg/cell	27–33 pg/cell	Measures average weight of Hgb in RBC.
MCHC	33–37 g/dL	330–370 g/L	More reliable index of red cell hemoglobin than MCH. Measures average concentration of Hgb in RBC. Concentration will not change with weight or size of RBC.
MCV	76–100 μm³	76–100 fL[b]	Describes average RBC size; ↑ MCV = macrocytic, ↓ MCV = microcytic.
Platelets	130–400 × 10³/mm³	130–140 × 10⁹/L	<100 × 10³/mm³ = thrombocytopenia; <20 × 10³/mm³ = ↑ risk for severe bleeding.
RBC count			
Male	4.3–5.9 × 10⁶/mm³	4.3–5.9 × 10¹²/L	
Female	3.5–5.0 × 10⁶/mm³	3.5–5.0 × 10¹²/L	
Reticulocyte count (adults)	0.1–2.4%	0.001–0.024 I[a]	Indicator of RBC production; ↑ suggests ↑ number of immature erythrocytes released in response to stimulus (e.g., iron in iron deficiency anemia).
WBC count	3.2–9.8 × 10³/mm³	3.2–9.8 × 10⁹/L	Consists of neutrophils, lymphocytes, monocytes, eosinophils, and basophils; ↑ in infection and stress.
Neutrophils	54–62%	0.54–0.62 I[a]	An ↑ in neutrophils suggests bacterial or fungal infection. ↑ in bands suggests bacterial infection.
Bands	3–5%	0.03–0.05 I[a]	
Lymphocytes	25–33%	0.25–0.33 I[a]	ANC = (% neutrophils + % bands) × WBC; if
Monocytes	3–7%	0.03–0.07 I[a]	<500 = ↑ risk infection, if >1,000 = ↓ risk infection.
Eosinophils	1–3%	0.01–0.03 I[a]	Eosinophils ↑ with allergies and parasitic infections.
Basophils	<1%	<0.01 I[a]	

[a]With the SI, the concept of number fraction replaces %. Thus, for mass fraction, volume fraction, and relative quantities, the unit "I" is used to replace former units.
[b]fL, femtoliter; femto, 10^{-15}; pico, 10^{-12}; nano, 10^{-9}; micro, 10^{-6}; milli, 10^{-3}.
ESR, erythrocyte sedimentation rate; MCH, mean corpuscular hemoglobin; MCHC, mean cell hemoglobin concentration; MCV, mean cell volume; RBC, red blood cell; WBC, white blood cell; ANC, absolute neutrophil count; Hgb, hemoglobin; Hct, hematocrit; TIBC, total iron-binding capacity.

comparing the height of the settled red cells to the height of the column of whole blood. The percentage of red cells to the blood volume is the Hct.

A decrease in Hct may result from bleeding, bone marrow suppressant effects of drugs, chronic diseases, genetic alterations in red cell morphology (sickle cell anemia), or hemolysis. An increase in Hct may result from hemoconcentration, polycythemia vera, or polycythemia secondary to chronic hypoxia.

Hemoglobin

Hgb (14.0 to 18.0 g/dL or 140 to 180 g/L for males; 12.0 to 16.0 g/dL or 120 to 160 g/L for females) is the oxygen-carrying compound contained in RBCs. Therefore, the total Hgb concentration primarily depends on the number of red cells in the blood sample, although it also is slightly influenced by the amount of Hgb in each red cell. The same medical conditions that increase or decrease the Hct or the number of RBCs affect the Hgb concentration in a similar fashion.

A Hgb determination is preferable to an RBC determination because it more directly reflects the oxygen transport capability of blood; however, the Hct most commonly is used clinically because it is technically simpler to perform.[32]

Red Blood Cell Indices (Wintrobe Indices)

RBC indices are useful in the classification of anemias. These indices include the MCV, the mean cell hemoglobin (MCH), and the MCHC. These indices are calculated as follows:

$$MCV = \frac{Hct \times 1,000}{RBC \text{ (in millions/}\mu L)} = 76 - 100 \text{ (in } \mu m^3 \text{ or fL)} \quad \textbf{2-10}$$

$$MCH = \frac{Hgb \text{ (in g/dL} \times 10)}{RBC \text{ (in millions/}\mu L)} = 27 - 33 \text{ (in pg)} \quad \textbf{2-11}$$

$$MCHC = \frac{Hgb \text{ (in g/dL)}}{Hct} = 33 - 37 \text{ (in g/dL)} \quad \textbf{2-12}$$

MEAN CELL VOLUME

The MCV detects changes in cell size. Therefore, descriptive terms such as *macrocytosis* or *microcytosis* can be used for abnormal MCV values. For example, a decreased MCV suggests a microcytic cell, which can result from iron deficiency anemia. A large MCV suggests a macrocytic cell, which can be caused by a vitamin B_{12} or folic acid deficiency. The MCV can be normal in a patient with a "mixed" (microcytic and macrocytic) anemia. RBC indices cannot take the place of direct observation of a blood smear.

An increased MCV has been correlated with many disease states (e.g., alcoholism, habitual alcohol ingestion, chronic liver disease, anorexia nervosa, hypothyroidism, reticulocytosis, and hematologic disorders).[33] Although one could speculate as to whether the macrocytosis or increased MCV noted in these disorders represents preclinical folate or B_{12} deficiencies, an increased MCV may indicate an underlying disorder, and an MCV determination might be useful as a screening tool for occult disease.[33]

MEAN CELL HEMOGLOBIN CONCENTRATION

The MCHC is a more reliable index of red cell hemoglobin than the MCH. The former measures the concentration of Hgb, whereas the latter measures the weight of Hgb in the average red cell. In normochromic anemias, changes in the size of RBCs (MCV) are associated with corresponding changes in the weight of Hgb (MCH), but the concentration of Hgb (MCHC) remains normal.[9]

Changes in the Hgb content of red cells alter the color of these cells. Thus, the terms *hypochromic* and *normochromic* indicate decreased or normal amounts of Hgb in cells, respectively. Hypochromic red cells are characteristic of an iron deficiency anemia. Hyperchromic cells are rare.[14]

13. C.U., a 58-year-old chronic alcoholic, was hospitalized after a barroom brawl. A CBC was ordered, and the following RBC indices were noted: MCV, 108 μm^3; MCH, 38 pg; and MCHC, 34 g/dL. How should these indices be interpreted in C.U.?

[SI units: MCV, 108 fL; MCH, 38 pg; MCHC, 340 g/L]

Usually, the MCH and MCV are both increased and the MCHC is normal in macrocytic anemias associated with vitamin B_{12} or folic acid deficiency. The MCH is increased because the RBCs have increased in size; however, the concentration of Hgb (MCHC) has not changed. This characteristic picture is illustrated in the alcoholic patient, C.U., who is likely to have a dietary folic acid deficiency. If C.U.'s indices were normal (normocytic, normochromic) and if anemia was present (decreased Hgb or Hct), acute blood loss from injuries he sustained in the brawl should be considered. If the anemia seems to be more chronic in nature, alcohol-induced bone marrow suppression should be considered (see Chapter 29, Alcoholic Cirrhosis, and Chapter 84, Alcohol Abuse).

Reticulocytes

Reticulocytes (0.1% to 2.4% of red cells or 0.001 to 0.024 I) are young, immature erythrocytes. The reticulocyte count measures the percentage of these new corpuscles in the circulating blood. An increase in the number of reticulocytes suggests that an increased number of erythrocytes are being released into the blood in response to a stimulus. Because erythrocytes regenerate rapidly, reticulocytosis can be noted within 3 to 5 days after hemolysis (e.g., sickle cell anemia) or after a hemorrhagic episode. The reticulocyte count can be as high as 40% during rapid erythrocyte regeneration. Appropriate treatment of anemias caused by iron, vitamin B_{12}, or folic acid deficiencies should result in an increased reticulocyte count as well. If a properly functioning bone marrow is present and the reticulocyte count does not increase in response to replacement therapy, the diagnosis or the treatment should be re-evaluated. Furthermore, caution must be exercised in the interpretation of reticulocyte counts. Changes in the number of RBCs will result in proportional changes in the reticulocyte count because the reticulocyte count is reported as a percentage of the number of RBCs.

Erythrocyte Sedimentation Rate

The erythrocyte sedimentation rate (ESR) (0 to 20 mm/hour for males and 0 to 30 mm/hour for females) is the rate at which erythrocytes settle to the bottom of a test tube through the forces of gravity. The ESR is nonspecific and seldom is the sole clue to disease in asymptomatic persons.

The ESR is increased abnormally in acute and chronic inflammatory processes, acute and chronic infections, neoplasms, infarction, tissue necrosis, rheumatoid-collagen disease, dysproteinemias, nephritis, and pregnancy. On the other hand, it sometimes is normal in diseases in which it usually is abnormal, and laboratory technique can affect the sedimentation rate substantially.[25] Because many factors can enhance the settling rate of RBCs, moderate to marked elevation of the ESR merely indicates a disease state. An increased ESR in the setting of a normal physical examination usually is transitory and rarely is the harbinger of serious occult disease.[34]

The ESR is useful in the diagnosis and monitoring of temporal arteritis and polymyalgia rheumatica. When patients with rheumatoid arthritis are being monitored, the ESR principally is used to help resolve conflicting clinical evidence and to evaluate response to therapy.[34] The ESR has been correlated with the severity of illness in patients with chronic HF; however, the test is of limited value in the clinical management of HF because of its lack of discriminatory specificity.[35] The ESR also has been identified as one of the most important pretherapy prognostic factors in patients with early-stage Hodgkin's disease.[36] The ESR may also be useful in differentiating organic diseases from those of psychosomatic origin in symptomatic patients.

White Blood Cells (Leukocytes)

WBCs (3.2 to $9.8 \times 10^3/mm^3$ or 3.2 to $9.8 \times 10^9/L$), unlike RBCs and platelets, perform no physiologic function within the vascular system. The blood merely serves as a transportation network that allows white cells to move from their site of origin, the bone marrow, into various body tissues and cavities.

Neutrophils are the most abundant of the circulating WBCs, followed in order of frequency by lymphocytes, monocytes, eosinophils, and basophils. The neutrophils, eosinophils, basophils, and monocytes are formed from stem cells in the bone marrow. Some lymphocytes are formed in the bone marrow, but most are formed in the lymph nodes, thymus, and spleen. Also in the bone marrow, another type of leukocyte, the plasma cell, is observed. The entire system of WBCs contributes to the host defense mechanisms; however, each of these types of cells has unique functions. Therefore, it is best to think of these cell types as individual types of cells rather than collectively as "leukocytes."[37] A convenient mnemonic for remembering the various types of white blood cells is "Never Let Monkeys Eat Bananas" (N = neutrophils; L = lymphocytes; M = monocytes; E = eosinophils; and B = basophils).

NEUTROPHILS

The terms *polys, segs, PMNs,* and *granulocytes* are synonymous with the term *neutrophil* in clinical practice. The normal maturation sequence of the neutrophil in the bone marrow is as follows: the stem cell gives rise to the myeloblast, which then matures progressively into a promyelocyte, myelocyte, metamyelocyte, band neutrophil, and finally into a polymorphonuclear segmented neutrophil. Segmented neutrophils constitute 54% to 62% of circulating leukocytes, and band neutrophils usually represent about 3% to 5%. Normally, about 35% of the polymorphonuclear segmented neutrophils have two lobes, 41% have three lobes, and 20% have four or more lobes. At one time, the maturation of neutrophils was depicted with the more immature neutrophils on the left and the more mature forms on the right. Therefore, a "shift to the left" occurred when band neutrophils and other immature neutrophils increased and a lower average number of lobes of segmented neutrophils appeared in the blood.[9]

The number of neutrophils commonly is increased during bacterial or fungal infections because these cells are essential in killing invading microorganisms. As the bone marrow increases production of new leukocytes, there is an increase in the number of circulating immature neutrophils or bands, frequently referred to as a shift to the left, indicating a bacterial infection. However, neutrophils also are important in the pathogenesis of tissue damage in some noninfectious diseases.[38]

The same processes that are so important to the destruction of organisms also can induce tissue injury in diseases such as rheumatoid arthritis, inflammatory bowel disease, asthma, or myocardial infarction (Table 2-5). Neutrophilia also can be encountered during metabolic toxic states (e.g., diabetic ketoacidosis, uremia, eclampsia) and during physiologic response to stress (e.g., physical exercise, childbirth). Drugs (e.g., epinephrine, corticosteroids) also can cause significant neutrophilia, primarily by demargination from blood vessel walls.

Table 2-5 Diseases in Which Tissue Injury or Symptoms May Be Mediated by Neutrophils[38]

Adult respiratory distress syndrome
Asthma
Emphysema
Glomerulonephritis
Gout
Immune vasculitis
Inflammatory bowel disease
Malignant neoplasms at sites of chronic inflammation
Myocardial infarction
Neutrophil dermatoses
Rheumatoid arthritis
Thermal injury-associated hemolysis

Agranulocytosis and Absolute Neutrophil Count. Decreased neutrophils, or neutropenia, is defined as a neutrophil count of $<2,000$ cells/mm^3; agranulocytosis refers to severe neutropenia. The degree of neutropenia often is expressed by the absolute neutrophil count (ANC). The ANC is defined as the total number of granulocytes (polymorphonuclear leukocytes and band forms) present in the circulating pool of WBCs and can be calculated as WBC × (%neutrophils + % bands)/100. Generally, the risk of infection is low when the ANC exceeds 1,000/mm^3; however, the risk of infection increases significantly when the ANC is <500/mm^3. The risk of developing bacteremia is increased further as the ANC decreases to <100/mm^3, a condition commonly referred to as profound neutropenia (see Chapter 68, Prevention and Treatment of Infections in Neutropenic Cancer Patients). The most common causes of neutropenia are metastatic carcinoma, lymphoma, and chemotherapeutic agents.

LYMPHOCYTES

Lymphocytes constitute the second most common white cell in circulating blood. These leukocytes respond to foreign antigens by initiating the immune defense system. The vast majority of the lymphocytes are located in the spleen, lymph nodes, and other organized lymphatic tissue. The lymphocytes circulating in blood represent $<5\%$ of the total amount in the body.

There are two major types of lymphocytes. *T lymphocytes* (thymic dependent) participate in cell-mediated immune responses, and *B lymphocytes* (bone marrow derived) are responsible for humoral antibody responses. Therefore, diseases affecting lymphocytes primarily manifest themselves as immune deficiency disorders that render the patient unable to defend against normal pathogens (see Chapter 69, Pharmacotherapy of Human Immunodeficiency Virus Infection) or as autoimmune diseases in which immune responses are directed against the body's own cells.[37]

Increased numbers of lymphocytes on a white count differential sometimes accompany viral infections such as infectious mononucleosis, mumps, and rubella. A relative lymphocytosis sometimes is encountered when the total lymphocytes have remained constant despite a decline in the total neutrophils.

MONOCYTES

The precursors to macrophages are the monocytes, which are formed in the bone marrow and transported by the blood to tissues, where they mature.[39] Monocytosis may be observed in subacute bacterial endocarditis, malaria, and tuberculosis, as well as during the recovery phase of some infections.

EOSINOPHILS

Because eosinophils have surface receptors that bind IgG and IgE, they can modify reactions associated with IgG- and IgE-mediated degranulation of mast cells. These receptors are responsible for damaging larval-tissue states of some helminth parasites, especially *Schistosoma mansoni*.[40] Primary lysosomal granules, small dense granules, and specific or secondary granules are the three types of granules found within eosinophils. The specific granules account for most of the biologic activity of eosinophils and consist of three basic polypeptides: major basic protein (MBP), eosinophil cationic protein (ECP), and eosinophil-derived neurotoxin (EDN). These basic polypeptides are toxic to parasites, tumor cells, and some epithelial cells.[41]

Investigations have focused on this WBC because of the fatalities associated with tryptophan-induced eosinophilic-myalgia syndrome[42]; however, little is known about the natural function of eosinophils. Eosinophils have phagocytic activity, catalyze the oxidation of many substances, facilitate killing of microorganisms, initiate mast cell secretion, protect against various parasites, and play some role in host defense. Eosinophilia probably is associated most commonly with allergic reactions to drugs, allergic disorders (e.g., hay fever, asthma, eczema), invasive parasitic infections (e.g., hookworm, schistosomiasis, trichinosis), collagen vascular diseases (e.g., rheumatoid arthritis, eosinophilic fasciitis, eosinophilic-myalgia syndrome), and malignancies (e.g., Hodgkin's disease).[40,43]

BASOPHILS

An increase in basophils commonly accompanies chronic myeloid leukemia, myelofibrosis, and polycythemia vera. A decrease in the number of basophils generally is not readily apparent because of the paucity of these cells in the blood.[37]

14. R.L., a 45-year-old man, is hospitalized with a sustained high fever of 39.4°C, SOB, and pleurisy. His cough is productive of rusty sputum, and he appears to be in acute distress. The results of the CBC and leukocyte differential are as follows: total WBC count, 18,000/mm³; neutrophils ("polys"), 76%; bands, 13%; lymphocytes, 10%; monocytes, 0; eosinophils, 1%; and basophils, 0. On the basis of this laboratory report and other findings, a diagnosis of pneumococcal pneumonia is suspected. How is R.L.'s laboratory report consistent with bacterial infection?

[SI units: WBC, 1.8 × 10⁹/L; neutrophils, 0.76; bands, 0.13; lymphocytes, 0.10; eosinophils, 0.01]

WBCs are the host's chief defense system, and the neutrophil is the main component of that system. During bacterial infections, the leukocyte count and the neutrophils generally are increased and a shift to the left may be noticeable. The percentage of other types of white cells is decreased proportionately because the number of neutrophils is increased.

As the infection progresses, the percentage of band cells may decrease as a result of an increase in the number of neutrophils that have a longer half-life. This decrease in bands does not necessarily indicate improvement. A decrease in the percentage of neutrophils with a decrease in the total WBC count is characteristic of effective antibiotic therapy.

15. S.Q., a 35-year-old woman, was treated for 7 days with dicloxacillin for a cellulitis of the left leg. On the eighth day, an allergic urticarial rash developed. The CBC showed a total leukocyte count of 10,000/mm³ with 6% eosinophils. What is the significance of this eosinophil count?

[SI units: WBC, 1.0 × 10⁹/L; eosinophils, 0.06]

Eosinophils usually are increased in allergic reactions; therefore, a drug-induced hypersensitivity reaction is a strong probability in S.Q. with 600 eosinophils/mm³ (i.e., 6% of 10,000 leukocytes). The clinician should be suspicious of an allergic drug reaction when the absolute eosinophil count exceeds 300 cells/mm³. Eosinophils may increase before, after, or concurrent with other evidence of allergy (e.g., rash). Eosinophilia without evidence of allergy is not sufficient cause to discontinue a suspected medication unless the eosinophilia is massive (i.e., >2,000 cells). In addition, the lack of eosinophilia in a patient with an apparent allergic drug reaction does not exclude that diagnosis.

Coagulation Studies

The control of bleeding depends on the formation of a platelet plug and the formation of a stable fibrin clot. The formation of this clot, the complex interactions of plasma proteins and clotting factors, and the clinical application of laboratory tests of coagulation are described in Chapter 16, Thrombosis. The prothrombin time (PT), international normalized ratio (INR), and activated partial thromboplastin time (aPTT) are commonly used laboratory tests of coagulation to assist clinicians in localizing the specific factor or factors responsible for a coagulation abnormality. These tests are described briefly in this chapter with the understanding that the reader will need to refer to Chapter 16 to gain the appropriate perspective on the clinical applicability of these tests.

Activated Partial Thromboplastin Time

The aPTT measures the intrinsic clotting system, which depends on factors VIII, IX, XI, and XII and the factors involved in the final common pathway of the clotting cascade (factors II, X, and V). The aPTT is a modified PTT and is a more sensitive test than the PTT. The typical control ranges from 35 to 45 seconds. The aPTT commonly is used to monitor unfractionated heparin therapy.

Prothrombin Time

Prothrombin is synthesized in the liver and is converted to thrombin during the blood clotting process. Thrombin formation is the critical event in the hemostatic process because thrombin creates fibrin monomers that ultimately assemble into a clot, and thrombin stimulates platelet activation. The PT test directly measures the activity of clotting factors VII, X, prothrombin (factor II), and fibrinogen. Automated laboratory instruments measure and record the time required for the blood to clot (i.e., the PT) after tissue thromboplastin has been added to the patient's blood sample. The reference range depends on the specific laboratory but usually is between 10 and 12 seconds when rabbit brain thromboplastin is used. Previously, the PT ratio (patient's PT divided by the laboratory's control PT) was used to monitor warfarin therapy; however, the INR has replaced the use of the PT ratio.

International Normalized Ratio

In the United States, the laboratory testing procedures of the PT commonly use rabbit brain thromboplastin; however, rabbit thromboplastins from different manufacturers vary in their sensitivity and precision. In an effort to standardize the interpretation of the PT, the use of the INR is recommended. The INR is the PT ratio that would result if the World Health Organization's international reference thromboplastin was used to test the patient's blood sample.

Although the INR is the recommended method to accurately monitor oral anticoagulant therapy, several potential problems have been identified with the INR system. Because of the variable sensitivity of thromboplastin reagents to decreases in specific clotting factors, there may be a lack of reliability of the INR system when it is used at the onset of warfarin therapy and for screening for a coagulopathy. Despite these potential problems with the INR system, the American College of Chest Physicians unanimously recommends that the INR system of reporting be used during the initiation and maintenance of oral anticoagulant therapy.[44] However, despite these attempts at standardizing laboratory reporting, clinicians must be cautious when interpreting PTs that have been obtained for a patient by more than one clinical laboratory because the INR and PTs are specific to each institution.

The INR is calculated using Equation 2-13, where the prothrombin ratio (PTR) is the ratio between the patient's PT and the laboratory's control PT, and the ISI is the international sensitivity index. The commercial manufacturer of the thromboplastin reagent calculates the ISI and includes it in the product package insert. The ISI is specific for each lot.

$$\text{INR} = \left\{ \frac{\text{PT}_{\text{(Patient)}}}{\text{PT}_{\text{(Control)}}} \right\}^{\text{ISI}} = \text{PTR}^{\text{ISI}} \qquad \textbf{2-13}$$

For a thorough review on the monitoring of anticoagulant therapy, see Chapter 16.

URINALYSIS

A standard urinalysis begins with simple observation of the color and the gross general appearance of the urine specimen. The urine pH and specific gravity then are recorded. Formed elements in the urine are examined microscopically, and the urine is searched routinely for pathologically significant substances that normally are not present (e.g., glucose, blood, ketones, and bile pigments).

Gross Appearance of the Specimen

The concentrated, first-morning urine specimen usually is analyzed to eliminate effects of undue dilution as a result of water intake. The color should be slightly yellow depending on the degree of dilution, and the appearance should be clear. The appearance of the urine may reveal clouds of crystals, bilirubin, blood, porphyrins, proteins, food or drug colorings, or melanin.

Discolored urine is abnormal. A red coloration of the urine may be imparted by blood, porphyria, or ingestion of phenolphthalein. A brown urine color may be caused by the acid hematin of blood or from melanin pigments. The excessive excretion of urobilinogen or the effects of drugs such as rifampin or phenazopyridine may cause a dark orange urine color. A blue to blue-green color of the urine may result from the systemic administration of methylene blue.

Specimen pH

When freshly produced, urine normally is acidic (pH 4.6 to 8). Alkaline urine may indicate an aged specimen, systemic alkalosis, failure of renal acidifying mechanisms, or infection in the urinary tract.

Specific Gravity

A normal morning urine specimen should have a specific gravity of 1.020 to 1.025. The upper end of this range is close to the maximal concentrating ability of the kidney. Glomerular filtrate has a specific gravity of 1.010, and a urine of such a low specific gravity, under conditions of restricted water intake, would suggest failure of renal concentrating mechanisms. When water intake is not restricted, specific gravity readings are difficult to interpret.

Protein

A positive test for urine protein is common (e.g., 1%) and often is a transient and insignificant laboratory finding. Proteinuria, however, is a classic sign of renal injury and a matter of concern. If proteinuria is found during the evaluation of a patient with a nonrenal illness, it suggests that the disease also may involve the kidneys (i.e., hypertension, diabetes).[45] A healthy adult generally excretes 30 to 130 mg/day of protein into the urine.

The protein in a urine sample generally is tested qualitatively on a random urine sample by a dipstick method and usually is reported on a scale of 0 (<30 mg/dL), 1+ (30 to 100 mg/dL), 2+ (100 to 300 mg/dL), 3+ (300 to 1,000 mg/dL), and 4+ (>1,000 mg/dL). A positive qualitative test for urine protein should be repeated after a few days because transient proteinuria can accompany various physiologic and pathologic states even when kidney function is normal. Therefore, patients with HF, seizures, or febrile illnesses and normal renal function need not undergo invasive renal function tests if the proteinuria is modest and likely to be transient. Another qualitative evaluation of proteinuria can be performed in about 2 weeks to confirm the diagnosis of transient proteinuria.[46] If subsequent qualitative test results are positive, a 24-hour urine sample should be collected to quantitatively test for protein and creatinine. In patients with a normal 24-hour urinary protein concentration, previous positive qualitative test results probably represent either false-positive results or a transient phenomenon.[45] This approach should minimize unwarranted risks and costs without overlooking serious and treatable conditions.

Microscopic Examination

The urine sediment is examined for red cells, white cells, casts, yeast, crystals, and epithelial cells. RBCs should be absent in normal urine, although one or two RBCs per high-power field (HPF) still would be considered in the normal range. Bleeding or clotting disorders, some collagen diseases, and various bladder, urethral, and prostatic conditions may cause microscopic hematuria. In females, vaginal blood occasionally contaminates the urine specimen, but the presence of numerous squamous epithelial cells should be sufficient to alert clinicians to this artifact. WBCs should be virtually absent in normal urine, although up to five WBCs/HPF still would be in the normal range. The presence of white cells in the urine usually suggests an acute infection in the urinary tract (see Chapter 64, Urinary Tract Infections). Some noninfectious inflammatory diseases of the kidney, ureter, or bladder may also contribute white cells to the urine sediment. Casts are composed of proteinaceous or fatty material that outlines the shape of the renal tubules where they were deposited. The presence of casts in the urine must be interpreted in light of other factors related to the kidney and its function; however, fatty casts, RBC casts, and WBC casts always are significant. Red cell casts usually suggest glomerular injury, and white cell casts suggest tubular or interstitial injury. Lipid casts with proteinuria are characteristic findings in patients with the nephrotic syndrome.[47] The finding of hyaline casts alone in the presence of proteinuria suggests a renal origin for the protein. Hyaline or granular casts alone, however, only suggest some defect in factors that affect cast formation, and are therefore difficult to interpret. Crystals originally may appear as a cloud in the urine. Their formation is pH dependent, and they often appear only as the urine cools to room temperature or in concentrated urine. In acid urine, crystals may be uric acid or calcium oxalate; in alkaline urine, they may be phosphates. Crystals per se are not highly significant, although they may reflect a tendency toward the formation of renal calculi (see Chapter 31, Acute Renal Failure).

16. R.C. is a 23-year-old man who was diagnosed with type 1 diabetes mellitus about 10 years ago; up until now, his diabetes has been well controlled with an aggressive insulin regimen. His sister brings him to the ED with a 3-day history of fever, chills, dysuria, malaise, and some confusion. He also complains of nausea and vomiting and a poor appetite. Because he has not been able to keep any food down for about 48 hours, he has not taken his insulin. A fingerstick blood glucose is 545 mg/dL, and a stat midstream urinalysis and Gram's stain indicate the following: pH 5.2; appearance cloudy; specific gravity 1.033; urine protein 3+; urine glucose 4+; urine ketones positive; urine bacteria 4+; urine WBC, too numerous to count (TNTC); squamous epithelial, few per HPF; urine nitrite positive; and Gram's stain, numerous Gram-negative rods. What objective data from the urinalysis indicate that R.C. is critically ill?

[SI unit: glucose, 30.3 mmol/L]

The cloudy appearance of R.C.'s urine indicates the presence of bacteria, protein, and WBCs, which is substantiated by the data (4+ bacteria, 3+ protein, and TNTC WBCs). The lack of a significant amount of squamous epithelial cells, the presence of a significant amount of nitrite-producing bacteria, and the Gram's stain indicate a clean-catch urine specimen and a urinary tract infection (UTI) from Gram-negative organisms. Because the renal threshold of glucose is typically 180 mg/dL, the presence of 4+ glucose in the urine indicates that the blood glucose concentration significantly exceeds this figure (substantiated by blood glucose of 545 mg/dL). Acidification of the urine and ketonuria occur after the release of ketone bodies into the bloodstream after the breakdown of fatty acids for energy utilization. It is likely that R.C. has a severe UTI and probably diabetic ketoacidosis. (See Chapters 50, Diabetes Mellitus, and Chapter 64 for thorough discussions of diabetes, diabetic ketoacidosis, and UTIs.)

Urine Drug Screening

With one exception, urine drug screening is the preferred method to screen for an unknown drug. The exception is ethyl alcohol, which is more reliably detected in the blood. Drugs that were taken days to weeks before the test may be detectable because drug concentrations are higher in the urine and drug metabolites are excreted for a longer period through urine (Tables 2-6 and 2-7). There are several indications for toxicology screening, such as confirming the clinical diagnosis and contributing diagnoses and testing for drug abuse/use in the workplace or as a pre-employment screen. It is important to recognize the psychological, social, and legal implications of urine drug screening.[48] (See Chapter 83, Drug Abuse.)

Table 2-6   Approximate Detection Times in Urine with Enzyme Multiplied Immunoassay Technique (EMIT) Methods[48]

Drug	Detection Time in Urine
Amphetamines	Within 24–48 hr after ingestion. Oral decongestants (ephedrine, pseudoephedrine, or phenyl propanolamine) may give positive results.
Barbiturates	1 dose of 250 mg phenobarbital detectable for up to 9 days. Others detectable for up to 1–3 days.
Benzodiazepines	1 dose usually not detectable. Therapeutic doses for 3 days. Up to 5–7 days in chronic users.
Cocaine	Up to 48 hr after a single dose. 1–4 days for chronic users.
Codeine	1 dose of 120 mg detectable for up to 48 hr. Excreted and detected as morphine.
Heroin (morphine)	1 dose of 10 mg detectable for up to 24 hr. 4–5 days for chronic users.
Marijuana	Dependent on use; 3 days for single use; 5 days for moderate use (4 times/week); and 21–27 days for chronic, heavy users.
Methadone	≈ 3 days. Possible interference from high levels of chlorpromazine, promethazine, and dextromethorphan.
Methamphetamines	Same as amphetamines.
Methaqualone	Typical dose 5–7 days.
Morphine	1 dose of 10 mg detectable for 24–48 hr.
Phencyclidine	1 dose detectable for up to 8 days; 14 days in chronic users.
Propoxyphene	Up to 48 hr after a single dose.

Table 2-7   Therapeutic Drug Concentrations[a]

Laboratory Test	Normal Reference Values		Conversion Factor
	Conventional Units	SI Units	
Acetaminophen	15–20 μg/mL	100–130 μmol/L	6.62
Toxic levels	>120 μg/mL	>795 μmol/L	
Amitriptyline	120–250 ng/mL	433–900 nmol/L	3.61
Carbamazepine	4–12 μg/mL	17–51 μmol/L	4.23
Desipramine	150–300 ng/mL	562–1125 nmol/L	3.75
Diazepam	100–1000 ng/mL	0.35–3.5 μmol/L	0.0035
Digoxin	0.5–2 ng/mL	0.6–2.6 nmol/L	1.28
Disopyramide	2–6 μg/L	6–18 μmol/L	2.95
Ethosuximide	40–110 μg/mL	280–780 μmol/L	7.08
Imipramine	150–250 ng/mL	535–892 nmol/L	3.57
Lidocaine	1–5 μg/mL	4.3–21.4 μmol/L	4.27
Lithium	0.5–1.5 mEq/L	0.5–1.5 mmol/L	1
Phenobarbital	15–50 μg/mL	65–215 μmol/L	4.34
Phenytoin	5–20 μg/mL	20–80 μmol/L[b]	3.96
Procainamide	4–10 μg/mL	17–42 μmol/L	4.25
Quinidine	2–5 μg/mL	6.2–15.4 μmol/L	3.08
Salicylate	150–300 μg/mL	1.0–2.1 μmol/L	0.007
Toxic levels	>300 μg/mL	>2.1 μmol/L	
Theophylline	10–20 μg/mL	56–110 μmol/L	5.55
Valproic acid	50–100 μg/mL	346–693 μmol/L	6.93

[a]Drug concentrations of antibiotics are presented in the Infectious Disorders chapters.
[b]Unbound phenytoin = 0.5–2 μg/mL = 2–8 μmol/L.

REFERENCES

1. Hansten PD, Horn JR. Drug Interactions. Baltimore: Lippincott Williams & Wilkins, 1999.
2. Evans PC, Cleary JD. SI units—are we leaders or followers? [Editorial] Ann Pharmacother 1993; 27:97.
3. Vaughan LM. SI units: is it pass the mass but hold the mole? [Editorial] Ann Pharmacother 1993;29:99.
4. Making it easier [Editorial]. Ann Intern Med 1992; 117:87.
5. Campion EW. A retreat from SI units [Editorial]. N Engl J Med 1992;327:49.
6. The New England Journal of Medicine SI Unit Conversion Guide. Waltham, MA: Massachusetts Medical Society, 1992:56.
7. Kratz A, Lewandrowski KB. Case records of Massachusetts General Hospital normal reference laboratory values. N Engl J Med 1998;339:1063.
8. Gennari FJ. Serum osmolality—use and limitations. N Engl J Med 1984;310:102.
9. Henry JB, ed. Clinical Diagnosis and Management by Laboratory Methods. 20th Ed. Philadelphia: WB Saunders, 2001.
10. Kassirer J. Clinical evaluation of kidney function-glomerular function. N Engl J Med 1971;285:385.
11. Becker CE. Methanol poisoning. J Emerg Med 1983;1:51.
12. Cebul RD, Beck JR. Biochemical profiles. Ann Intern Med 1987;106:403.
13. Winter ME et al. Basic Clinical Pharmacokinetics. 4th Ed. Baltimore: Williams & Wilkins, 2004.
14. Baumann TJ et al. Minimum urine collection periods for accurate determination of creatinine clearance in critically ill patients. Clin Pharm 1987;6:393.
15. Jelliffe RW. Creatinine clearance: bedside estimate. Ann Intern Med 1973;79:604.
16. Hull JH et al. Influence of range of renal function and liver disease on predictability of creatinine clearance. Clin Pharmacol Ther 1981;29:516.
17. Cockcroft DW, Gault MH. Prediction of creatinine clearance from serum creatinine. Nephron 1976; 16:31.

18. Rhodes PJ et al. Evaluation of eight methods for estimating creatinine clearance in men. Clin Pharm 1987;6:399.
19. Lee TH, Goldman L. Serum enzyme assays on the diagnosis of acute myocardial infarction. Ann Intern Med 1986;105:221.
20. White RD et al. Diagnostic and prognostic significance of minimally elevated creatine kinase-MB in suspected acute myocardial infarction. Am J Cardiol 1985;55:1478.
21. Roberts R. Where, oh where has the MB gone? N Engl J Med 1985;313:1081.
22. Hamm CW. New serum markers for acute myocardial infarction. N Engl J Med 1994;331:607.
23. Chapelle JP. Cardiac troponin I and troponin T: recent players in the field of myocardial markers. Clin Chem Lab Med 1999;37(1):11-20.
24. Malasky BR, Alpert JS. Diagnosis of myocardial injury by biochemical markers: problems and promises. Cardiol Rev 2002;10:306.
25. Ravel R. Clinical Laboratory Medicine: Clinical Application of Laboratory Data. 6th Ed. St. Louis: Mosby, 1995.
26. Schmid R. Bilirubin metabolism in man. N Engl J Med 1972;285:703.
27. Barry MJ. Prostate-specific-antigen testing for early diagnosis of prostate cancer. N Engl J Med 2001;344:1373.
28. Smith RA et al. American Cancer Society guidelines for the early detection of cancer: update of the early detection guidelines for prostate, colorectal, and endometrial cancers. CA Cancer J Clin 2001;51:38.
29. American Urological Association. Prostate-specific-antigen (PSA) best practice policy. Oncology (Huntingt) 2000;14:267.
30. Gan PH et al. Prospective evaluation of plasma prostate-specific antigen for detection of prostate cancer. JAMA 1995;273:289.
31. Lange PH. New information about prostate-specific antigen and the paradoxes of prostate cancer. JAMA 1995;273:336.

32. Hillman RS, Finch CA. Red Cell Manual. 7th Ed. Philadelphia: FA Davis, 1996.
33. Keenan WF. Macrocytosis as an indicator of human disease. J Am Board Fam Pract 1989;2:252.
34. Sox HC, Liang MH. The erythrocyte sedimentation rate. Ann Intern Med 1986;104:515.
35. Haber HL et al. The erythrocyte sedimentation rate in congestive heart failure. N Engl J Med 1991;324:353.
36. Henry-Amar M et al. Erythrocyte sedimentation rate predicts early relapse and survival in early-stage Hodgkin disease. Ann Intern Med 1991;114:361.
37. Winkelstein A, Kaplan SS, Boggs DR. White Cell Manual. 5th Ed. Philadelphia: FA Davis, 1998.
38. Malech HL, Gallin JI. Neutrophils in human diseases. N Engl J Med 1987;317:687.
39. Cline MG et al. Monocytes and macrophages: functions and diseases. Ann Intern Med 1978;88:78.
40. Butterworth AE, David JR. Eosinophil function. N Engl J Med 1981;304:154.
41. Beeson PB. Cancer and eosinophilia. N Engl J Med 1983;309:792.
42. Clauw DJ et al. Tryptophan-associated eosinophilic connective-tissue disease. JAMA 1990;263:1502.
43. Dombrowicz D, Capron M. Eosinophils, allergy and parasites. Curr Opin Immunol 2001;13:716.
44. Fifth ACCP Consensus Conference on Antithrombotic Therapy. Chest 1998;114(Suppl):445S.
45. Abuelo JG. Proteinuria: diagnostic principles and procedures. Ann Intern Med 1983;98:186.
46. Reuben DB et al. Transient proteinuria in emergency medical admissions. N Engl J Med 1982;306:1031.
47. Morrin PAF. Urinary sediment in the interpretation of proteinuria. Ann Intern Med 1983;98:254.
48. Council on Scientific Affairs. Scientific issues in drug testing. JAMA 1987;257:3110.

Table 3-1   Summary of Herbal Products and Nutritional Supplements Reviewed—cont'd

Herbal/ Nutritional Supplement	Proposed Indication(s)	Authors' Interpretation of Level of Evidence for Use in a Clinical Setting[a]	Dosing
Saw palmetto *Serenoa repens*	Benign prostatic hyperplasia	Promising	Lipophilic extract standardized to contain 85–95% fatty acids and sterols; 160 mg 2 times daily
Panax ginseng	Adaptogen	Unknown	*P. ginseng* extract standardized to contain at least 7% ginsenosides; 1–2 g of the crude root or its equivalent (1 g of crude root is equivalent to 200 mg of the extract)
	Ergogenic	Unknown	
	Immune modulation	Investigational	
	Anticancer/antitumor	Investigational	
	Diabetes/hypoglycemia	Unknown	
	Hyperlipidemia	Unknown	
	Hypertension/cardiovascular	Unknown	
	Hepatoprotectant	Unknown	
	Erectile dysfunction/infertility	Investigational	
Dehydroepian-drosterone (DHEA)	Weight loss	Doubtful	*Replacement dosing:* men 50–100 mg daily; women 25–50 mg daily
	Anticancer	Unknown	*Systemic lupus erythematosus:* 50–200 mg daily
	Antioxidant effects	Investigational	*Hyperlipidemia:* 1,600 mg daily in divided doses
	Hormone replacement therapy	Doubtful	*HIV:* 750–2,250 mg in 3 divided doses
	Aging	Doubtful	
	Alzheimer's disease	Doubtful	
	Cardiovascular protection	Investigational	
	Hyperlipidemia	Doubtful	
	HIV	Doubtful	
	Systemic lupus erythematosus	Promising	
	Diabetes	Doubtful	
	Depression	Promising	
Glucosamine	Osteoarthritis	Promising	500–1,000 mg 3 times daily
	Wound healing	Doubtful	
	Antioxidant	Investigational	
Shark cartilage	Anticancer	Doubtful	1 g/kg/day or 80–100 g/day given in 3 divided doses
	Antimicrobial	Doubtful	*ZGG:* 13.3 mg Q 2 hr while awake
Zinc	Common cold	Promising	*ZG:* 23 mg Q 2 hr while awake
	Allergic rhinitis	Investigational	*ZA:* 10 mg Q 2 hr while awake
Melatonin	Jet lag	Promising	*Jet lag:* 5–8 mg IR the evening of departure and for 3–5 days after
	Insomnia	Promising	*Insomnia:* 0.3–5 mg once nightly for sleep onset
	Reproduction	Investigational	Higher dosages may be required for sleep maintenance
	Antioxidant	Investigational	
	Immune modulation	Investigational	
	Anticancer	Investigational	
	Aging	Doubtful	
	Depression	Doubtful	

[a]Promising: A sufficient number of double-blind, placebo-controlled studies have been conducted that indicate an effect may exist.
Investigational: Studies have indicated promising results in animal models or in epidemiologic studies. Small trials in humans may currently be underway.
Unknown: There is an equivalent amount of scientific evidence, which shows both positive and negative results of studies that have been conducted and indicate positive findings but were generally of poor study design, or there is a relative lack of trials that have been performed for this indication.
Doubtful: Studies that have been conducted have generally shown no effect.
HIV, Human immunodeficiency virus; IR, immediate release; ZA, zinc acetate; ZG, zinc gluconate; ZGG, zinc gluconate-glycine.

that one of the first groups to examine the safety and efficacy of herbal products was established in Germany. In 1978, the German Commission E, an expert panel composed of physicians, toxicologists, pharmacists, pharmacologists, biostatisticians, and others, was assembled by the German Federal Health Agency.[6] Its purpose was to review the available clinical information on herbs and to determine which ones achieved "reasonable certainty of efficacy and absolute safety."[7] More than 300 herbs and herbal combinations were reviewed by the German Commission E, and its findings were published in the German Bundesanzeiger, which is similar to the U.S. Federal Register.[7] Only recently was this information translated and published in English by the American Botanical Council. Practitioners in the United States can now use these monographs as a source of information regarding herbal remedies.

Dietary Supplement Health and Education Act

In 1994, the U.S. Congress passed a bill that revolutionized nonprescription drugs. The Dietary Supplement Health and Education Act (DSHEA) of 1994 was created to regulate dietary supplements: botanicals, vitamins, minerals, tissue extracts, and amino acids.[8] DSHEA has special provisions that regulate dietary supplements as foods, removing them from regulation as pharmaceuticals. Manufacturers of dietary supplements can make labeling claims without submitting evidence to the FDA, but they are responsible for the truthfulness of those claims. The FDA cannot remove a product from the market unless the product is proven to pose a serious or unreasonable risk to consumers. In contrast, pharmaceuticals must demonstrate a significant degree of safety and efficacy before they are approved for marketing. These differences have led to the rapid growth of the dietary supplement industry.

The terms used in this chapter to refer to dietary supplements differ from the FDA definition. Herbal remedy (botanical) is used to refer to any product derived from a plant source. Nutritional supplement is used to refer to hormones, vitamins, minerals, cofactors, enzymes, amino acids, and others. Despite the legal classifications and variations in nomenclature, any product that alters the structure and function of the body or endogenous process for the treatment or prevention of disease is considered a drug.

Product Labeling

Product labeling refers to both the label of the actual product and any accompanying written information. The labeling on a product must conform to the provisions in the Code of Federal Regulations (CFR) for foods,[8] which states that the principal display panel (PDP) must contain the name of the product and the contents in net weight. Other information about the product is located on the information panel, usually found to the right of the PDP. Currently, not all supplements on the market conform to these regulations, especially if they are imported from other countries. As of March 23, 1999, specific labeling requirements were required for all products sold as dietary supplements. The rules require manufacturers to include the term dietary supplement as part of the name of the product. For example, vitamin C is sold as "Vitamin C Dietary Supplement." Ingredient requirements also changed. Products are required to include a "Supplement Facts" panel similar to the "Nutrition Facts" panels used for many processed foods. The labels contain information on as many as 14 ingredients when present in "significant amounts." Examples include sodium, calcium, iron, ascorbic acid, and other vitamins and minerals. If the product was derived from a plant, the product identifies the part of the plant used and the Latin binomial. Similarly, for nonherbal dietary supplements, the source of the substance is listed: animal, human, and synthetic. When the ingredients exceed 100% of the dietary reference intake (DRI) for that vitamin or mineral, the product is referred to as high potency. DRI is a general term for nutrient requirements in a population. The DRI differs from the recommended dietary allowance (RDA) in that the RDA is based on individual nutrient requirements rather than population requirements.

The most significant labeling change requires each ingredient listed on a dietary supplement label to provide the "% Daily Value." The "% Daily Value" is based on the RDA; a supplement containing 60 mg vitamin C is considered to provide 100% of the daily value for adults. However, the problem is that the RDAs are based on 1968 nutrition recommendations. For example, the recommended calcium intake based on the RDA is too low for most adults, including postmenopausal women. For postmenopausal women, the National Institutes of Health recommends 1,200 mg of calcium daily, whereas the RDA for adults is 800 mg. In this example, an 800-mg dose represents 100% of the daily value for calcium. However, based on the new calcium requirements, the value is closer to 67%. The National Academy of Sciences is updating the human nutrient requirements for vitamins, minerals, and antioxidant dietary supplements. New recommendations are anticipated by 2005. Substances such as choline, betaine, glutamic acid, inositol, and botanicals are considered nonessential for health. These products are added to supplements and are easily identified on a product label that states that the "% Daily Value" has not been established.

Structure-Function Claims

Manufacturers of dietary supplements can make only "structure-function" claims, which may include a statement on the supplement's role in a person's well-being. Under DSHEA, manufacturers who make structure-function claims on product labels must also include the following disclaimer, "This statement has not been evaluated by the Food and Drug Administration. This product is not intended to diagnose, treat, cure or prevent any disease." Consequently, a product can claim that it "enhances memory," but it cannot claim that it "treats dementia." Manufacturers who wish to use a structure-function claim must inform the FDA no later than 30 days after the product is marketed. The manufacturer must be able to substantiate the claim, but is not required to submit supporting evidence to the FDA or make the evidence publicly available.

Fraudulent claims are common in the dietary supplement field. Phrases such as miracle cure suggest that the product is a cure for a disease, whereas terms such as detoxify and purify are vague and misleading. The most troubling labeling claims suggest that these products are free of side effects. If a dietary supplement is potent enough to cause a beneficial effect, it will likely be potent enough to cause a side effect.

Supplement Labeling

Consumers may receive informational leaflets on a particular supplement at the time of purchase. The informational leaflets might consist of an article, a newsletter, a summary, or other written document. The quality of the information provided is not reviewed by FDA, an expert panel, or other authority. DSHEA specifies that dietary supplement labeling excludes accompanying written information from regulation when the information (1) is not false or misleading, (2) does not promote a particular manufacturer or brand, (3) is physically separate from the dietary supplement, and (4) does not have other information appended to it.[8] It is difficult to enforce these provisions. Consequently, the information distributed to consumers may be false, biased, inaccurate, or misleading.

Product Formulations

Herbal remedies come in a variety of formulations, some of which include teas, extracts, oil macerations, and fresh expressed juice or tinctures.[9]

Teas: Infusions, Decoctions, and Cold Maceration

Teas are prepared by drying the herb, which is then marketed in its coarse cut form or in tea bags. In general, tea formulations have not been studied in a randomized, controlled fashion because they are difficult to mask.[7]

Thus, empirical data have been used to establish indications for use.[7] Teas can be prepared by infusion, decoction, or cold maceration. The most common preparation, infusion, involves steeping the herb in boiling hot water for up to 10 minutes and then straining.[9] To prepare a decoction, the herb is placed in cold water and the combination is heated to a boil, steeped for up to 10 minutes, and then strained.[9] Macerations are prepared by letting the herb stand in water at room temperature for many hours before straining.[9]

Extracts

The term extraction is used when a portion of the herb or the entire herb is processed for the purpose of concentration. Extractions are formulated as fluids, powders, solids, and volatile oils. Extraction of the dried herb with ethanol, water, or both is used to make fluid extracts.[7] Fluid extracts, which use alcohol as a solvent, are further classified as tinctures. Evaporation of the solvent is used to prepare solid and powder extracts.[7] Either distillation or lipophilic extraction can be used to prepare volatile oils.[7]

Oil Maceration and Fresh Pressed Juice or Tincture

Oil macerates can be prepared with fresh or dried herbs. In either case, similar to tea macerations, the herb is allowed to stand in oil macerate (e.g., vegetable oil) at room temperature for many hours before straining. Fresh pressed juice is prepared by macerating the herb in water and then squeezing the juice from it.[7] Fresh herbal tinctures also can be prepared by using an alcohol-based solvent.

Good Manufacturing Practices

In the United States, pharmaceutical manufacturers are required by law to conform to strict standards. Good manufacturing practices (GMP) were designed to protect consumers from contamination and improper conditions during manufacturing. Dietary supplements are not required by law to conform to the same level of GMPs as pharmaceutical manufactures. Under DSHEA, dietary supplements are subject to current good manufacturing practice in production, packing, or holding human food.[8] These guidelines include maintenance of buildings and facilities, food handler requirements, and safety standards. Products imported from other countries are more difficult to regulate. Consequently, problems related to product purity, potency, and contamination have been documented in the scientific literature.[10] Often, neither the distributor nor the consumer have any assurance that product content matches the labeling claims. Adulteration, whether intentional or accidental, is dangerous and puts the public health in jeopardy. In an attempt to begin addressing this issue, the United States Pharmacopeia (USP) established a program called the Dietary Supplement Verification Program (DSVP). This program helps establish ingredient quality and other standards unique to herbs and dietary supplements. Participation in the program is voluntary. Manufacturers who meet the DSVP criteria will be allowed to carry the USP cer-

tified seal on their labels. This will help consumers distinguish a particular manufacturer's product as having the highest quality standards for content. Other organizations have established similar programs including Consumer Lab and the National Science Foundation. Importantly, none of these programs address issues of pharmacologic safety or efficacy.

As the demand for dietary supplements increases, unscrupulous companies may attempt to cut costs through product adulteration. This is especially true of herbs that are expensive to acquire or that take years to cultivate. As a consequence of adulteration, the product could fail to have the desired effect, could cause serious side effects, or could interact with other drugs.

Herbal Hazards

Consumers sometimes believe that "natural" products available without a prescription also must be safe.[11] Often, this is not the case because hazards can be introduced during the collection and manufacturing process or, unknowingly, by the patient. Other hazards can result from toxic components within the herb.

Manufacturing Hazards (Adulteration)

In some cases, substances that do not appear on the package labeling may be introduced into a product, either deliberately or by accident. For example, plant misidentification resulted in renal failure in up to 100 women who ingested a Chinese herbal diet aid. In this case, *Stephania tetrandra* was replaced with a nephrotoxic herb, *Aristolochia fangchi*.[12] Similar cases of misidentification have resulted in digitalis poisoning.[13]

High levels of heavy metals (e.g., lead, mercury, and arsenic) have been observed in some traditional Chinese and Ayurvedic (Indian) herbal remedies.[14,15] A recent survey of 260 Asian products distributed in the United States revealed that high levels of heavy metals or adulterants were present in 83 products (32%).[10] In these cases, the amounts exceeded the recommended maximum amounts set by the U.S. Pharmacopeia (USP). Heavy metal toxicity has resulted in cases of anemia, hepatitis, and death.[14,15]

There are many reports of toxicity caused by adulterated products. In the United States, an outbreak of eosinophilic-myalgia syndrome (EMS) occurred in patients using the nutritional supplement L-tryptophan.[16] An aniline-derived contaminant was later found to be the cause. Cases of digitalis poisoning prompted the chemical analysis of an herbal product advocated for bowel cleansing. *Digitalis lanata* was isolated from the plantain (plantago) portion of the product.[12] Adulteration of herbal remedies with prescription drugs such as diazepam, nonsteroidal anti-inflammatory drugs (NSAIDs), hydrochlorothiazide, and steroids has been observed as well.[17]

Direct Hazards: Products to Avoid or Use Cautiously

Products associated with severe adverse reactions are listed in Table 3-2. Herbs containing pyrrolizidine alkaloids generally should be avoided because they are metabolized to pyrroles, which are hepatotoxic. Ephedrine and ephedrine-containing products can increase the risk of stroke, myocardial infarction, and seizures. Many cases of adverse events, including fatalities in otherwise healthy adults, have prompted several countries and individual states to ban the sale of ephedra-containing products. Currently, ephedra-containing products

Table 3-2 Hazards Associated with Some Nutritional Supplements

Supplement/Latin Binomial	References	Associated Clinical Use[a]	Toxicity	Recommendation
Comfrey rhizome, roots, leaves *Symphytum* spp.	6, 11, 19, 20	Internal digestive aid External wound healing	Pyrrolizidine alkaloids—hepato-toxicity	Avoid ingestion External application only. Limit use to 4–6 wk Do not use on unbroken skin
Coltsfoot flower, leaves *Tussilago farfara*	6, 11, 19	Upper respiratory tract infections	Pyrrolizidine alkaloids—hepatotoxicity	Avoid herb, root, or flower products. Leaf can be used as an external anti-inflammatory agent. Limit use to 4–6 wk
Germander leaves, tops *Teucrium chamaedrys*	11, 19, 21	Diet aid	Hepatotoxicity	Avoid
Borage leaves, tops *Borago officinalis*	6, 11, 19	Anti-inflammatory, diuresis	Pyrrolizidine alkaloids—hepatotoxicity	Avoid
Chaparrel leaves, twigs *Larrea tridentata*	11, 19, 22	Anti-infective, antioxidant, anticancer	Hepatotoxicity	Avoid
Sassafras root bark *Sassafras albidum*	19	Tonic, blood thinner	Safrole oil—hepatocarcinogen in animal studies	Avoid
Aconite (found in some Chinese herbal remedies) *Aconitum* spp.	23	Analgesic	Alkaloids—cardiac and central nervous system toxicity	Avoid
Kava *Piper methysticum*	24	Anxiety	Hepatotoxicity	Avoid
Pennyroyal Extract from *Mentha pulegium* or *Hedeoma pulegoides*	11, 25	Digestive aid, induction of menstrual flow, abortifacient	Pulegone and its metabolite—hepatic and renal failure	Avoid
Life root, whole plant *Senecio aureus*	19	Induction of menstrual flow	Pyrrolizidine alkaloids—hepatotoxicity	Avoid
Poke root, root of plant *Phytolacca americana*	19	Antirheumatic	Hemorrhagic gastritis	Avoid
Jin Bu Huan (a Chinese herbal remedy)	26	Analgesic, sedative	Hepatotoxicity—mechanism unknown, but levotetrahydropalmatine is structurally similar to pyrrolizidine alkaloids	Avoid
Aristolochic acid *Aristolochia* spp.	26	Weight loss	End-stage renal failure	Avoid
Ephedra *Ma huang, Ephedra* spp.	18	Weight loss, stimulant, bronchodilation	Extension of pharmacologic effects	Avoid use in patients in whom stimulant effects could be harmful (e.g., hypertension, diabetes, heart disease, anxiety, hyperthyroidism)
Royal jelly from the honeybee (*Apis mellifera*)	27	Tonic	IgE-mediated bronchospasm, and anaphylaxis in patients with atopy or asthma	Avoid use in patients with history of asthma, atopy, or allergies
Guar gum *Cyamopsis psorabides* or *tetragonolobus*	11, 28	Weight loss, diabetes, hypercholesterolemia	Esophageal, small-bowel obstruction	Avoid

[a]Associated clinical use is based on patient report at time of event or reported use in listed references.

Table 3-3 Guidelines for Selecting or Recommending on Herbal Remedy or Dietary Supplement Product

- Read all labels carefully
- Never share these products with others
- Avoid using in children
- Avoid if you are pregnant or nursing or trying to become pregnant
- Never take more than the recommended amount listed on the label
- Do not select a product that does not have dosing recommendations on the label
- Avoid products that do not carry a lot number or expiration date
- Discard products 1 year from the date of purchase with no other expiration date present
- Select products that list the manufacture's name, address, and telephone number
- Avoid purchasing these products from mail-order companies; instead purchase from pharmacies and large outlet nutrition stores
- Speak to your health care professional if you are trying to treat a life-threatening condition, such as cancer, HIV, and others
- If you are taking a prescription medicine, do not take an herbal remedy or dietary supplement for the same condition
- Avoid taking multiple-ingredient preparations; select single-ingredient products that list the strength per dose
- Do not store these products in a medicine cabinet or glove compartment; store them in a dry environment out of direct sunlight and humidity
- The term *natural* does not mean safe; be diligent and report any unusual experiences to your doctor or pharmacist
- Store products away from young children and pets
- Always inform your health care provider of the products you are taking; keep a list if necessary or bring them with you to your appointment
- Do not take these products with alcohol until you know it is safe to do so or are familiar with the effects
- Check with your health care provider if you are taking "blood thinning" drugs; some products may interact
- Never use these products in place of proper rest and nutrition; eat a balanced diet
- Do not expect a cure or unrealistic results; these agents are not "cure-alls"
- If it sounds too good to be true, it probably is; use discretion when evaluating claims

carry a warning indicating the risks in people with certain health conditions.[18]

Hazards Introduced by the Consumer

Consumers should not exceed the doses recommended on the package label because overuse may lead to toxicity. Indirect toxicity can occur if consumers attempt to self-treat serious disorders. In general, dietary supplements should not be used to treat cancer or serious infection if more effective therapies exist. However, if the patient is terminally ill and the supplement provides relief, use may be justified. Use during pregnancy, during lactation, or in children also should be avoided because the products have not been adequately studied for safety in these vulnerable patient populations.

Patient Recommendations

General recommendations regarding the use of herbal products are outlined in Table 3-3. These may be used when counseling patients on product selection and appropriate use. Many of the recommendations are conservative because data on quality, safety, and efficacy of these products, specifically in special patient populations, are unavailable. These recommendations are not intended to promote use, but rather to educate patients and practitioners. Each decision should be made on an individual basis with the best interest of the patient in mind.

GARLIC (ALLIUM SATIVUM)
Garlic Formulations

1. **M.J., a 65-year-old obese man, is concerned about his cholesterol and wants to start taking garlic. What types of commercial preparations are available and how is garlic standardized? Which formulations are preferred?**

Preparations of Garlic and Active Constituents

A variety of organosulfur compounds in garlic have been reported to have therapeutic effects. Fresh bulbs contain all of these compounds, but their potency varies depending on how the plant was grown, harvested, and stored. The type and amount of organosulfur compounds in commercial preparations also may vary based on the manufacturing process.[29]

Di-allyl-disulfide-oxide, or allicin, is responsible for the characteristic odor of garlic and many of the reported therapeutic effects. When bulb garlic is crushed, chewed, or chopped, the odorless precursor, S-allyl-l-cysteine sulfoxide, or alliin, is exposed to the enzyme allinase, and allicin and other thiosulfinates are formed.[30] Allinase is a very unstable enzyme and can be destroyed by heat and stomach acid.[31] Allicin is water-soluble and highly volatile and is easily converted into diallylsulfides, vinyl dithiins, and ajoenes.[29]

The instability of allicin and allinase causes commercial preparations to vary in product content. Oil-based preparations that have been steam-distilled predominantly contain diallylsulfides.[29] Macerated oil preparations, which are made without heating, contain diallylsulfides, vinyl dithiins, and ajoenes.[29] Fermented or aged garlic extracts, which are odor free, are less likely to contain active constituents due to degradation with prolonged storage.[7,29]

If processed appropriately, alliin and allinase activity can be preserved when dried sliced garlic is manufactured into powdered preparations.[7,29] Therefore, the amount of allicin and other thiosulfinates generated upon ingestion may be comparable to homogenated fresh pickled or store-bought garlic.[7,29] For this reason, powdered formulations are generally preferable to oil formulations.[7] Drying also concentrates the active organosulfur compounds, minimizing the need to ingest large quantities of fresh garlic.[7] Enteric-coating of powdered formulations prevents allinase degradation in the stomach and releases allicin in the small intestine, minimizing the odor.[30] Consumers should look for preparations that are standardized by their alliin or allicin content. Powdered formulations used in clinical trials were most commonly standardized to 1.3% alliin or 0.6% allicin (based on allicin-releasing ability).[6]

Antihyperlipidemic Effects

2. M.J. weighs 105 kg and is 6′ tall. He rarely exercises and eats a diet high in fat; his medication profile indicates that he has been taking benazepril (Lotensin) 10 mg PO QD for 2 years. M.J.'s doctor has recommended a diet and exercise program. Upon questioning, he recalls his cholesterol values from last month: total cholesterol, 290 mg/dL; high-density lipoprotein cholesterol (HDL-C), 30 mg/dL; low-density lipoprotein cholesterol (LDL-C), 230 mg/dL; and triglycerides (TG), 150 mg/dL. Can garlic significantly improve M.J.'s lipid profile?

Many studies have examined the lipid-lowering effects of garlic,[31–40] but only a few have included sample sizes of more than 100 subjects.[33,34] Because a study of at least 1,000 individuals would be necessary to support or refute the combined results of previously published studies,[33] the antihyperlipidemic properties of garlic are largely based on published meta-analyses.[41–44]

Two initial meta-analyses concluded that 600 to 900 mg of powdered garlic per day significantly reduced levels of total cholesterol by 9% to 12%, reduced TG by 13%, and had little effect on HDL-C.[41,42] Both the 600- and 900-mg doses were equally effective in reducing total cholesterol by 1 month, and benefits extended up to 6 months. Nonpowder preparations appeared to have a greater effect, but formulations varied considerably, which may have skewed results.[42]

A more recent meta-analysis and systematic review suggests a small but favorable effect of garlic on hyperlipidemia, lowering total cholesterol by 4% to 6%. In the presence of dietary controls, however, this effect became insignificant.[43,44] The results of recent studies on the antihyperlipidemic effects of garlic have been mixed and are summarized in Table 3-4. It is hypothesized that variations in efficacy seen in more recent trials may be related to the poor allicin releasing ability of some powdered formulations marketed after 1993.[30]

Mechanism of Action

In vitro, inhibition of hepatic 3-hydroxy-3methylglutaryl coenzyme A (HMG-CoA) reductase has been observed and is considered the primary mechanism for garlic's antihyperlipidemic action.[45] Inhibition of later steps in cholesterol synthesis also has been observed, but this effect requires garlic concentrations exceeding those achieved with normal or long-term human consumption.[45] Whether these mechanisms apply in humans remains uncertain because no significant differences in serum levels of mevalonate (the end-product of the HMG-CoA reductase reaction) and lanosterol (a cholesterol precursor) were observed in 25 individuals after 12 weeks of treatment with steamed garlic oil.[36]

3. Is M.J. a candidate for garlic?

M.J. should be advised that dietary modification and exercise are the best ways to reduce cholesterol without pharmacotherapy. His high total cholesterol and LDL-C and low HDL-C are not likely to be normalized by the limited effect, if any, of garlic. As already noted, the benefits of garlic remain

Table 3-4 Clinical Trials: Garlic and Hyperlipidemia

Author, Year	Number Total	Formulation and Dose	Duration (wk)	Design	Results
Neil, 1996	106[a,b]	Powder, 900 mg/day	24	R, DB, P, PD	NS—TC, H, L, TG
Breithaupt-Grogler, 1997	202	Powder, ≥300 mg/day; mean, 460 mg/day	≥2 yr; mean, 7 yr	Observational cross-sectional, matched pairs	NS—TC, L, H, TG, BP
Bordia, 1998	60[c]	Oil equivalent of 1 clove/day	12	P, PD Not randomized or blinded	Significant differences from baseline, not placebo TC ↓ 12.8%[e] H ↑ 22.3%[e] TG ↓ 15.2%[e]
Berthold, 1998	25[a,b]	Steamed oil, 10 mg/day Powder, 900 mg/day	12	R, DB, P, C	NS—TC, L, H, TG
Isaacsohn, 1998	50[a,b]	Powder, 900 mg/day	12	R, DB, P, PD	NS—TC, L, H, TG, BP
Superko, 2000	50[a,b]	Powder, 500 mg/day, 1000 mg/day	20	R, DB, P, PD	NS—TC, L. H, TG
Gardner, 2001	51[a,b]	Powder, 880 mg/day	12	R, DB, P, PD	NS—TC, L, H, TG, BP
Kannar, 2001	45[a,b]	Powder, 880 mg/day	12	R, DB, P, PD	TC ↓ 4.2%[d] L ↓ 6.6%[d] NS—H, TG

[a]Patients with baseline elevated cholesterol.
[b]Dietary compliance assessed.
[c]Patients with baseline coronary artery disease.
[d]Significant reduction compared to placebo, unless otherwise noted.
BP, blood pressure; C, crossover design; DB, double blind; H, HDL cholesterol; L, LDL cholesterol; NS, not significant; P, placebo controlled; PD, parallel design; R, randomized; TC, total cholesterol; TG, triglycerides.

questionable because only small numbers of patients have been evaluated. Furthermore, its benefit in people who are already modifying their diets may be insignificant.

Hypotensive Activity

4. M.J. decides to purchase garlic and tells you that he also will begin the diet and exercise plan his doctor recommended. M.J. is taking benazepril (Lotensin) for hypertension. Do you have any additional questions or concerns?

Although there have been no drug–drug interactions reported for garlic and benazepril, M.J. should be aware that garlic may lower blood pressure (BP). M.J. should watch for symptoms of hypotension (e.g., dizziness) and monitor his BP after initiating therapy to ensure against a possible hypotensive event.

Fifteen studies published between 1986 and 1995 evaluated the effect of 600 to 900 mg/day of powdered garlic on BP. Twelve studies noted reductions in both systolic blood pressure (SBP) and diastolic blood pressure (DBP), ranging from 2% to 27%.[7] Reductions were deemed significant in seven of the studies. A review of 30 randomized controlled trials measuring BP outcomes concluded that although several trials reported significant reductions in BP with at least 4 weeks of use, statistical significance was only achieved in three studies. Among these three studies the SBP was reduced by approximately 3% and the DBP by 2% to 7%.[44] The long-term effects of garlic on BP remain unknown. Stimulation of nitric oxide (NO) synthesis (a potent vasodilator), inhibition of angiotensin converting enzyme, and reductions in intracellular calcium have all been observed in vitro and may be responsible for this effect.[46-48]

Antiatherosclerotic Effects

5. T.L. is a 70-year-old man with a history of coronary artery disease (CAD) and peripheral vascular disease (PVD). He began taking warfarin (Coumadin) after a stroke 2 months ago. His other medications include metoprolol (Lopressor) 50 mg PO QD, simvastatin (Zocor) 20 mg PO QD, and isosorbide dinitrate (Isordil) 20 mg PO TID. T.L.'s friend told him that garlic might help his heart condition. Is there any evidence that garlic is beneficial in treating CAD?

The antiatherosclerotic effects of garlic are largely based on its potential to reduce coronary risk factors of hyperlipidemia, hypertension, platelet aggregation, LDL-oxidation, and fibrin formation (see Question 6). Reductions in atherosclerotic lesions, atherosclerotic cell proliferation, aortic collagen accumulation, and vascular damage caused by oxidized LDL have been observed in vitro and in garlic-treated animals fed a cholesterol-rich diet.[48,49]

Only a few clinical trials have evaluated the effect of garlic in patients with CAD.[48,49] A double-blind, placebo-controlled trial randomized patients with advanced atherosclerotic plaques and at least one risk factor for CAD to receive 900 mg/day of powdered garlic or placebo. At 2 years, plaque volume in the carotid and femoral arteries was significantly reduced by 5% to 18% in the treatment group.[50] In a much smaller trial, blood serum atherogenicity was significantly reduced in patients with CAD who received 4 weeks of powdered garlic compared with placebo controls. The authors suggest that a reduction in LDL-oxidation may have been responsible.[48] In healthy subjects, an epidemiologic, cross-sectional, matched-pairs study found that aortic stiffness was significantly lower in older patients who consumed ≥300 mg/day of powdered garlic (mean, 460 mg/day) for ≥2 years (mean, 7.1 years).[34] Aortic stiffness has been correlated with progression of atherosclerosis in animals.[34]

Antiplatelet and Thrombolytic Effects

6. You inform T.L. that garlic may reduce coronary risk factors for CAD, but that its effectiveness in treating CAD has not been adequately studied in humans. Nevertheless, T.L. wishes to take garlic. Do you have any concerns about T.L.'s use of garlic given his current medication profile?

Some studies evaluating the effects of garlic on platelets have observed a decrease in platelet aggregation,[35,44] whereas others observed no effect.[44] Significant fibrinolytic effects also have been associated with chronic ingestion of garlic for ≥14 days.[35,44] Small sample size, use of variable garlic preparations, and variable study duration have made drawing definitive conclusions from these studies difficult.

A few studies using larger sample sizes (60 to 80 people) have observed substantial reductions in spontaneous platelet aggregation and plasma viscosity.[51,52] All these studies used 800 mg/day of garlic powder for 4 to 12 weeks. One study was conducted in patients with stage 2 peripheral arterial occlusive disease and another in patients at increased risk for ischemic attack.[51,52]

Mechanism of Action

Allicin and adenosine have antiplatelet effects in vitro.[53,54] However, because both of these compounds are metabolized in vivo, antiplatelet effects have been attributed to diallylsulfides, particularly diallyl trisulfide, and ajoene,[53,54] although ajoene is unlikely to play a role when fresh or powdered preparations are used.[53] These metabolites may inhibit thromboxane (TXB_2) formation and platelet aggregation in response to various activating factors such as collagen, adenosine diphosphate (ADP), and epinephrine.[35,54] Stimulation of NO synthesis also may play a role because NO is a potent inhibitor of platelet aggregation and adhesion.[46]

In summary, T.L. should be told that garlic might increase his risk for bleeding. He should be advised not to initiate garlic because he is currently taking warfarin. Two cases of increased international normalized ratio have been reported in patients stabilized on warfarin who initiated garlic. If T.L. still wishes to try garlic, he should watch for signs and symptoms of bleeding and have frequent INR testing.

Other Effects of Garlic

Anticarcinogenic/Antitumor Effects

Epidemiologic studies in China and Italy reported a reduced incidence of stomach cancer in patients who consumed high amounts of garlic,[55] but other studies failed to show a similar effect. In one of the largest studies, 120,852 Netherlanders, ages 55 to 69, were followed for 3.3 years for the development of cancer. Overall, there was no association between garlic supplement use and a lower risk of lung, breast, or colorectal cancer.[56] A recent meta-analysis, however, seems to support a protective effect of raw or cooked garlic on reducing the relative risk of colorectal and stomach cancers to 0.69 and 0.53, respectively.[56]

In vivo animal studies looking at the anticarcinogenic properties of garlic have focused on the water soluble constituent, S-allylcysteine (SAC), and the lipid soluble diallyl-sulfide constituents, particularly diallylsulfide (DAS) and allyl methyl disulfides and trisulfides.[55,57] Water and oil constituents of garlic inhibited pro-carcinogens for colon, esophageal, lung, breast, and stomach cancers in animal models.[55] Garlic constituents also enhanced glutathione and glutathione-S-transferase activity, a step in the detoxification of carcinogens, and decreased cytochrome P450 2E1 activity, a step in the activation of carcinogens.[55,57] In vitro garlic also inhibited the growth of *Helicobacter pylori,* a known risk factor in the development of stomach cancer.[56,57]

In vitro, the growth of established tumors has been inhibited by the oil, but not the water soluble, constituents of garlic.[57,58] A review of studies involving the antiproliferative effects of garlic in animals speculated that usefulness in humans would be limited based on the difficulty in controlling the growth of established tumors and the small numbers of cells that could be inhibited.[58] Whether the concentrations of garlic constituents used to inhibit tumor growth in vitro could be achieved or tolerated in vivo also is of concern.

Anti-Infective Effects

Garlic has antibacterial, antifungal, antiprotozoal, and antiviral properties in vitro.[59,60] Allicin has been identified as the primary anti-infective component.[59] Today, the availability of potent antimicrobials limits the use of garlic as an anti-infective in industrialized countries.

Antidiabetic/Hypoglycemic Effects

Some studies have reported that garlic has a hypoglycemic effect.[44] However, others, including two trials in patients with type 2 diabetes mellitus, failed to find an effect.[44] Until further research confirms a consistent effect on blood glucose, garlic should not be used to treat diabetes. Furthermore, patients with diabetes who take garlic need not monitor their blood sugar more frequently than normal.

Adverse Drug Reactions/Drug Interactions

An observational study of 1997 patients taking 900 mg/day of garlic for 16 weeks found the following incidence of side effects: 6% nausea, 1.3% hypotension, and 1.1% allergy.[7] A dose-ranging study of the odiferous effects of enteric-coated garlic found that 14 days of garlic, 1,200 mg, resulted in a 50% incidence of perceived odor. Doses of 300 to 900 mg were associated with a 20% to 40% incidence of perceived odor.[7]

Contact dermatitis has been reported most often in people who frequently handle raw garlic (e.g., cooks, farmers).[61] The reaction is preceded by an eczematous rash followed by the potential for desquamation and hyperkeratosis of the palms.[61] A case report of anaphylaxis has been described in a patient who ingested young garlic and who also had a prior allergic history to pollen and dried fruit.[62]

The antiplatelet effects of garlic have been cited as a risk factor for postoperative bleeding.[63,64] A case report of a spinal epidural hematoma in a previously healthy patient suggested that the patient's use of four cloves/day of raw garlic may have been the cause.[64] Patients should be advised to avoid garlic 7 to 10 days before and after surgery.

There have been few reported drug–drug interactions between garlic and other medications. As already noted, patients taking anticoagulants and BP medications should be monitored closely. A 50% reduction in the bioavailability of saquinavir also has been reported.[65] Ritonavir, however, was not similarly affected.[66]

Pharmacokinetics and Dosing

Pharmacokinetic studies evaluating the bioavailability, half-life, and absorption of garlic are needed. Breakdown products have been found in the urine of patients who ingested 200 mg of garlic extract.[67]

Patients wishing to reduce the possibility of garlic odor should purchase an enteric-coated formulation. A daily dosage of 600 to 900 mg of powdered garlic in two to three divided doses is recommended.[7] This is equivalent to 1.8 to 2.7 g, or 0.5 to 1 clove of fresh garlic, per day.[41] Products should be standardized for alliin or allicin content. The recommended standard is an alliin concentration of 1.3% or an allicin content of 0.6%.[43]

GINKGO (GINKGO BILOBA)

Neuroprotection

7. E.B., a 22-year-old woman, comes to the pharmacy to purchase ginkgo biloba for her 80-year-old grandmother. E.B.'s grandmother has difficulty recalling past events and often becomes disoriented and anxious. Her grandmother was recently diagnosed as having cerebral insufficiency (CI) secondary to early Alzheimer's disease (AD), but the neurologist suggested waiting before initiating donepezil (Aricept) because she has a history of low BP and dizziness when standing. E.B. heard that ginkgo biloba may be helpful for patients with AD. Her grandmother's medications include aspirin 325 mg PO QD and buspirone (BuSpar) 2.5 mg PO TID. Are there any clinical data demonstrating ginkgo biloba efficacy in the treatment of AD?

CI includes a variety of clinical symptoms, some of which can include confusion, poor concentration and memory, forgetfulness, fatigue, depression, anxiety, vertigo, tinnitus, and hearing loss.[68] Many of these symptoms are said to be relieved by ginkgo biloba extract (GBE). Studies using GBE for CI conducted before 1991 assessed efficacy based on improvements in clinical symptoms and tests designed to assess cognitive improvement.[7] In 1991, the German Commission E developed new criteria for evaluation of nootropic (i.e., cognition enhancing) therapies. It recommended that clinical improvement be based on three distinct levels of observation involving (1) patients' and families' impression of effect on daily living, (2) objective testing of cognitive performance, and (3) clinicians' impressions of symptomatic improvement.[7] GBE was recommended only for patients with AD or vascular or mixed-type degenerative dementia.[7]

A few published studies evaluating the efficacy of GBE have used these new criteria.[69,70] A meta-analysis of 40 studies published before 1992 evaluating the benefits of GBE for CI determined that only eight met the criteria for quality study design.[68] The analysis included 434 patients who received GBE 112 to 160 mg/day for 6 to 12 weeks and 415 patients who received placebo. All eight studies showed positive effects on cognitive testing or symptoms.

Larger studies using three levels of observation extended treatment duration to better assess effects on daily life. A 1-year randomized, double-blind, placebo-controlled trial evaluated the effects of 120 mg/day GBE in 309 patients with mild to moderately severe dementia.[69] Only 44% of patients completed the study, but the data from early withdrawals were carried over to the study endpoint. Significant improvements in the cognition and daily living scales were observed in patients receiving GBE. However, there was no difference in the clinician global impression scale. Twenty-seven percent of GBE-treated patients showed a 4-point improvement in the Alzheimer's Disease Assessment Scale for Cognition (ADAS-Cog), which may correlate with a 6-month decrease in disease progression. However, the results could have been influenced by the high patient dropout rate and the inclusion of data from the point of patient withdrawal for analysis, because the disease worsens over time. The clinical relevance of these findings is also tempered by the lack of perceived improvement by clinicians.

In another large-scale, randomized, double-blind trial, 216 patients with mild to moderate dementia received 240 mg/day of GBE or placebo for 6 months.[70] At the study endpoint, GBE-placebo differences were significant for the cognition scale (20%) and the clinician global impression scale (15%). An insignificant trend in favor of GBE was observed for the daily living scale.

These trials, as well as recent systematic reviews and a meta-analysis, indicate a small but significant benefit of GBE on cognitive function.[71–73] Using the ADAS-Cog, an effect size of 3% has been estimated when GBE 120 to 240 mg is used for 3 to 6 months.[71]

8. Is E.B.'s grandmother a candidate for GBE? If so, how long should therapy be continued?

E.B.'s grandmother has been diagnosed with AD of mild severity. Clinical studies suggest that GBE may be of some benefit for dementia of mild to moderate severity, but further research should be conducted to firmly establish efficacy. One researcher concluded that the magnitude of clinical response after 6 months of GBE administration was only slightly less potent than the highest dose of the prescription drug, tacrine (Cognex) or donepezil (Aricept) 10 mg/day.[74] However, because of methodologic shortcomings in some GBE studies, this comparison may be premature. GBE is an option for E.B.'s grandmother, but her primary care provider should be informed if she initiates therapy. The optimal dosage and duration of therapy is unknown, but no significant adverse events have been noted in studies that have treated subjects with GBE for 6 to 12 months.[69,70]

Mechanism of Action

9. What are the proposed mechanisms of action for ginkgo biloba's neuroprotective effects?

Cerebral ischemia, oxidative stress, and neuronal degeneration are thought to be involved in the pathogenesis of dementia and dementia of the Alzheimer's type.[68] The mechanism of ginkgo biloba's action as a neuroprotective agent has

been examined in many in vitro and some in vivo studies. Potential mechanisms include improved blood flow, antioxidant effects, antagonism of platelet-activating factor (PAF), alterations in neurotransmitter concentrations and binding sites, and inhibition of amyloid-beta (Abeta) fibrils.[75–80]

Patients with AD have higher levels of cerebral oxidation and inflammation and modified neurotransmission. Reductions in acetylcholine, serotonin, gamma-aminobutyric acid (GABA), somatostatin, and norepinephrine have been reported, as well as reductions in receptors for serotonin, glutamate, and somatostatin.[81] If GBE can decrease inflammation and improve blood flow through PAF antagonism, decrease oxidation through its antioxidant and radical scavenging properties, affect neurotransmission in humans as it does in animals, and inhibit the aggregation and toxicity of Abeta fibrils, it may be clinically meaningful for patients like E.B.'s grandmother who have AD.

Preparations and Active Constituents

10. E.B.'s grandmother loves tea. Will a tea formulation of ginkgo biloba be beneficial?

Ginkgo biloba is prepared from the leaves of the Ginkgo tree.[6] The active constituents include a flavonoid fraction (kaempferol, quercetin, and isorhamnetin) and a terpene fraction (ginkgolides A, B, C, J, and M and bilobalide).[75] These compounds require concentration for optimal potency. The German Commission E recommends an herb:extract ratio of 50:1, which means that 50 parts of ginkgo leaf are used to generate one part extract.[7] Extracts should be standardized to contain 22% to 27% flavone glycosides and 5% to 7% terpene lactones.[7] Although crude leaf teas are available, they are unlikely to be beneficial because of their low potency. Standardization for flavones and terpenes should be indicated on the package labeling.

Stress and Anxiety

11. E.B.'s grandmother is taking buspirone (BuSpar). Can GBE be used as a substitute for buspirone to treat her anxiety?

GBE has exhibited physiologic stress-relieving properties in rodent models that differ from those of classic anxiolytics and antidepressants.[79] In rats, an 8-day treatment of GBE reduced corticosterone synthesis by reducing adrenal peripheral-type benzodiazepine receptor (PBR) expression. This receptor has been linked to the stress response through enhanced steroid production.[79] In humans, exposure to physiologic or psychologic stress can result in steroid production. GBE may control the stress response by minimizing this elevation in steroids and promoting a more "normal" circulating corticosteroid level. GBE may improve cognitive deficiency, and anxiety is considered one of many symptoms associated with cognitive deficiency.[68] However, there are no trials in humans that have assessed improvements in anxiety or stress. Therefore, GBE should not be used as a substitute for buspirone in E.B.'s grandmother. The potency and effectiveness of GBE as an antianxiety or antistress agent need to be studied further before it can be recommended for this indication.

Intermittent Claudication

12. E.B.'s grandmother has always had a problem with "poor circulation" in her legs, which limits her ability to walk. Will gingko biloba help this problem?

Although GBE may improve vascular insufficiency through enhanced blood flow, there is less literature that supports its use for complications of peripheral arterial occlusive disease (PAOD) than there is for dementia.[7,68] One recent meta-analysis of eight randomized, double-blind, placebo-controlled trials evaluated GBE for intermittent claudication, a painful symptom of PAOD. It concluded that GBE was more effective than placebo at improving pain-free walking distance.[82] Among the eight trials, seven favored ginkgo but only four met statistical significance. The weighted mean improvement in walking distance for GBE versus placebo was 34 meters. Effective dosing ranged from 120 to 160 mg/day for 24 weeks.

The largest trial of GBE for intermittent claudication involved 111 patients who received 120 mg/day of GBE or placebo for 6 months.[83] Walking distance increased by 45.1 meters or 41% with GBE treatment compared with 20.9 meters or 20% with placebo treatment. GBE-treated patients were able to walk twice as far as the placebo group, which met the definition of clinical relevance (20% to 30% difference) used by the German Society of Angiology. The clinical effect of GBE has been compared with the prescription drug, pentoxifylline (Trental). One meta-analysis suggested the improvement in pain-free walking distance was comparable, with an increase of 45% for GBE and 57% for pentoxyfylline.[84] However, this analysis is disputed by a more recent one in which GBE improved pain-free walking distance by 32 meters versus 138 meters for pentoxyfylline.[85] In summary, GBE may enhance E.B.'s grandmother's ability to walk longer distances.

Pharmacokinetics, Dosing, and Onset

13. What are the pharmacokinetic characteristics of GBE? What dose should be recommended for E.B.'s grandmother? When can beneficial effects be expected?

Pharmacokinetic parameters have been reported for the flavonoid fraction of ginkgo, ginkgolides A and B, and bilobalide.[68,86] Kinetics for the ginkgolides and bilobalide were determined following a single 80-mg oral dose of GBE.[68] Single-dose kinetics for the flavonoid fraction were determined following the oral administration of equivalent doses of GBE (dose not stated) in capsules, drops, or tablets.[86] All the GBE constituents studied were well absorbed (>60%) and reached peak concentrations within 1 to 3 hours. Half-life ranged from 2 to 6 hours for all constituents. Studies in animals identified many routes of clearance: 38% appeared in expired air, 22% in urine, and 29% in feces.[68]

The recommended dosage of GBE is 120 to 240 mg/day taken orally in two to three divided doses.[7] GBE is available as 40-, 60-, and 120-mg capsules or tablets. Studies in patients with CI suggest that clinical benefits may not be observed for 4 to 6 weeks.

Adverse Drug Reactions/Drug Interactions

14. Should E.B. be warned of any adverse effects or drug interactions with GBE?

Adverse effects associated with GBE are minimal. An evaluation of >10,000 individuals who took GBE for at least 3 months found that only 183 patients (1.69%) reported adverse events.[7] All reported side effects occurred with a frequency of >0.5%; ranked in order from the most to the least common, they included nausea, headache, stomach upset, diarrhea, allergy, anxiety, and insomnia.[7]

Case reports suggest an association between GBE use and the development of hemorrhage, especially when used in combination with aspirin or warfarin (Coumadin).[87,88] Patients should be monitored for bleeding when taking antiplatelet or anticoagulant medications based on these case reports and discontinue ginkgo at least 7 to 10 days before or after surgery. E.B.'s grandmother should not use ginkgo in combination with aspirin. Ginkgo also should be avoided in patients with a history of epilepsy or seizures. Case reports of seizures associated with ginkgo are likely due to product contamination with ginkgo seeds, which are known to contain an epileptogenic neurotoxin.[89] Coma has occurred following the use of ginkgo in combination with trazodone (Desyrel).[90]

Short-Term Memory

15. C.S. is a college student and has a big test in 4 days. Can GBE improve her memory?

A number of randomized, double-blind, placebo-controlled studies in healthy young (ages 20 to 30) and older (ages > 50) adults have looked at the effect of GBE on memory.[91–94] In general, improvements were undetectable, inconsistent, and limited to a small fraction of cognitive tests.[91,92] Some argue that beneficial effects, even though limited, seem more likely to occur following acute administration of very high doses of GBE (e.g., one 600-mg dose) or chronic administration of lower doses (e.g., 120 mg for 30 days). The only study that included a global measure that assessed effects on daily living in addition to objective cognitive tests found no benefit in healthy older adults.[91] A recent review of the literature concluded that GBE cannot be recommended for memory enhancement.[94]

Because the benefits of GBE in young and healthy patients is not well established, it should not be recommended to C.S. as a means to improve her memory for her upcoming examination.

Other Indications

16. What other conditions might be improved by the use of GBE?

GBE has been used for several other conditions, but in most cases, only a few studies have been conducted or results have been conflicting. The use of GBE for tinnitus has been studied with conflicting results.[95] A review of five randomized trials (four placebo-controlled) for this indication generally reported significant improvement in audiometry or the severity score.[95] Variations in GBE dosage, duration of therapy, etiology or hearing loss, duration of tinnitus, and study methodology, however, limited these researchers from drawing a firm conclusion about efficacy.

Beneficial effects of GBE have been reported for stroke infarct volume, acute mountain sickness, erectile dysfunction, antidepressant-induced sexual dysfunction, and age-associated macular degeneration.[96–99] GBE cannot be recommended for these indications until more definitive clinical studies are completed.

ST. JOHN'S WORT (HYPERICUM PERFORATUM)

Depression

17. G.C., a 47-year-old man, heard that St. John's Wort can be used to treat depression. He is tired of the side effects associated with prescription antidepressants and would like to try this herb. G.C. was diagnosed with major depression of moderate severity 2 years ago and was treated with fluoxetine (Prozac) 40 mg PO QD, which he discontinued after 2 months because it caused sexual dysfunction. G.C. never returned to the physician because he believed that his symptoms had improved. However, for the past few months, he has noted recurrent symptoms of lethargy, insomnia, poor appetite, a feeling of hopelessness, and a general disinterest in pleasurable activities. Assuming that G.C.'s depression is moderate in severity, is there any evidence that hypericum is a safe and effective alternative to prescription antidepressants for this indication?

Systematic reviews and meta-analyses evaluating the efficacy of hypericum in the treatment of depression have been published.[100–103] The Hamilton Depression Scale (HAMD) was the primary tool used to assess response in a majority of these studies.[100–103] The HAMD score is based on a 17- to 21-item survey of the patient's somatic symptoms in which a score of 18 to 24 is indicative of modest depression.[101] Treatment response in these studies was typically defined as a HAMD score of <10 or a 50% drop in the HAMD score by the study endpoint.[101]

The most recent systematic review and meta-analysis included 22 randomized, double-blind, controlled trials published from 1989 to 2001.[100] Most patients were defined as having mild to moderate depression and were treated with 900 mg/day of hypericum (range, 300 to 1800 mg/day) for 4 to 8 weeks. Meta-analysis of all studies showed hypericum to be more effective than placebo (relative risk [RR], 1.98) and to be comparable in efficacy to prescription antidepressants (RR, 1.0). A subanalysis of six placebo-controlled and four antidepressant controlled trials that employed stricter methodology (e.g., intention-to-treat analysis and adherence to predefined inclusion and exclusion criteria) revealed similar RRs of 1.77 and 1.04, respectively. Unfortunately, only one of the nine antidepressant controlled trials employed a placebo arm, and only two compared hypericum to the more commonly used selective serotonin reuptake inhibitors (SSRIs).

Other reviews support the superiority of hypericum over placebo and an efficacy similar to or slightly less than tricyclic antidepressants (TCAs) in the treatment of mild to moderate depression.[101–103] Adverse effects were consistently more likely to occur with prescription antidepressants than with hypericum.

A number of newly released randomized, double-blind trials comparing hypericum to SSRIs exist. All these show hypericum to be equivalent in efficacy.[104–106] The dose of fluoxetine used in these trials was 20 mg/day, while sertraline dosing ranged from 50 to 100 mg/day. Study durations extended 6 to 12 weeks. All these trials failed to include a placebo-control arm.

Trials assessing the effects of hypericum in patients with moderate to severe depression have generally met with negative findings.[107,108] One of these included treatment arms for hypericum, an SSRI, and placebo. Patients (N = 340) with a HAMD score of 20 or higher received 900 to 1500 mg/day hypericum, 50 to 100 mg/day sertraline, or placebo for 8 weeks. Neither hypericum nor sertraline produced a significant improvement in the HAMD score versus placebo. The clinician's global impression of improvement (CGI-I), however, was significantly better for sertraline.

The only other trial to include three treatment arms compared hypericum, imipramine, and placebo. In this trial, 263 patients with mild to moderate depression were randomized to receive 100 mg imipramine, 1,050 mg hypericum, or placebo in a double-blind fashion. At 8 weeks, HAMD scores were reduced by 14.2 (±7.3), 15.4 (±8.1), and 12.1 (±7.4), respectively. Although the response rate for hypericum was superior to placebo and similar to imipramine, the large standard deviation in HAMD scores, the use of a low to moderate dosage of imipramine, and the use of a relatively high dosage of hypericum make these results less convincing.[109]

In summary, hypericum is effective and has a more tolerable side effect profile than prescription antidepressants. It may be an alternative for patients, such as G.C., with mild to moderate depression who are unwilling or unable to tolerate the side effects of prescription antidepressants. Current evidence suggests that hypericum should not be used in severely depressed patients.[107,108] In addition, hypericum should not be recommended for patients who have experienced suicidal ideation, therapy resistance, or complicated depressive courses.[102]

Mechanism of Action

18. What is the mechanism of action for St. John's Wort in depression?

In vitro and animal studies have been conducted to evaluate the antidepressant mechanism for St. John's Wort.[110] Originally, the hypericin constituent was reported to have monoamine oxidase inhibitor (MAOI) qualities based on in vitro data, but this has not been affirmed.[110] Recent attention has focused on hyperforin and its structural analog, adhyperforin, as the primary antidepressant constituents in the extract.[122] In vitro, hyperforin equally inhibits the reuptake of serotonin, dopamine, norepinephrine, gamma-amino butyric acid (GABA), and L-glutamate.[110] Unlike other antidepressants, hyperforin does not act as a competitive antagonist at transmitter binding sites to decrease reuptake; instead, it attenuates the sodium gradient to alter neurotransmitter transport. This could also explain why its effects on neurotransmitters are less specific than with other antidepressants. Hypericum can also affect the density of neurotransmitter binding sites. In rats, chronic administration of hypericum results in a significant downregulation of cortical β-receptors and an upregulation of serotonin 5HT$_2$ receptors.[110] Many prescription antidepressants also downregulate cortical β-receptors, and electroconvulsive treatment, a highly effective antidepressant treatment, upregulates 5HT$_2$ receptors.[110]

19. **How should G.C. be advised regarding his request for St. John's Wort?**

G.C. should be advised against self-treatment of his depressive symptoms without first consulting his physician. Although G.C. did not tolerate fluoxetine, he did report temporary relief of symptoms, indicating that a reduction in dosage may be an option. In addition, there are a variety of other atypical antidepressants (e.g., bupropion [Wellbutrin], nefazodone [Serzone]) that G.C. may be able to tolerate. It is unclear what level of depression G.C. is currently experiencing. Although he was diagnosed as being moderately depressed 2 years ago, his relapse of symptoms is concerning, warranting re-evaluation of his depressive state. The long-term benefits of treatment with hypericum remain unknown because study durations typically lasted 8 to 12 weeks.[100–103]

Adverse Drug Reactions/Drug Interactions

20. **One month later, G.C.'s physician indicates that he has improved on a lower dosage of fluoxetine 20 mg PO QD. However, G.C. still has complaints consistent with depression and wants to try St. John's Wort. Is it safe to use St. John's Wort in combination with a prescription antidepressant? Are there any adverse effects that G.C. should watch for?**

There have been no clinical studies evaluating the combined use of prescription antidepressants and hypericum. Because the mechanism of action for hypericum is still unclear, it would be wise to avoid its combined use with agents that could enhance adrenergic or serotonergic neurotransmission (e.g., amphetamines, phenylephrine or phenylpropanolamine, antidepressants). There have been case reports of possible "serotonergic syndrome" in patients who began taking hypericum 600 to 900 mg/day in combination with prescription antidepressants or buspirone (BuSpar).[111,112] All these patients reported symptoms such as nausea, vomiting, dizziness, headache, restlessness/anxiety, and confusion within 2 to 4 days of initiating hypericum. All symptoms resolved with discontinuation of hypericum, and in two cases cyproheptadine, a serotonin antagonist, was administered. In another case report, a patient developed sedative hypnotic symptoms when hypericum was used in combination with paroxetine (Paxil).[112] The latter is an unexpected reaction given the proposed mechanism for these agents.

Mania, hypomania, anxiety, autonomic arousal, and psychotic relapse have been reported in patients taking hypericum.[12,113,114] In most cases, patients had a history of psychiatric illness (e.g., panic disorder, post-traumatic stress disorder, mania, schizophrenia, severe depression) but were not taking psychiatric medications. One woman had initiated hypericum within 1 week of discontinuing sertraline, so an additive effect may have occurred.

Hypericum induces multiple cytochrome P450 isoenzymes (e.g., 3A4, 2D6, 2C9)[115] as well as the activity of the P-glycoprotein drug transporter, which is responsible for drug excretion from cells. There are multiple case reports of patients who experienced a reduction in efficacy or serum drug concentration of digoxin, theophylline, cyclosporine, warfarin, indinavir, nevirapine, amitriptyline, midazolam, simvastatin, tacrolimus, oral contraceptives, and other medications after beginning hypericum therapy.[12,112] Patients using these medications or medications that are essential to their health should avoid hypericum or initiate therapy under the direction of a physician.

Few side effects have been reported in people taking 900 mg/day of hypericum. In comparative trials with prescription antidepressants, the most common side effects were gastrointestinal (GI) disturbances (8.5%), dizziness/confusion (4.5%), tiredness/sedation (4.3%), dry mouth (4%), restlessness (2.6%), and headache (1.7%).[116] As previously noted, side effects occur less commonly with hypericum than with prescription antidepressants.[100–103] Other adverse effects that have been observed in at least one case report and may have been caused by hypericum include hypertension and hypertensive crisis, sexual dysfunction, elevated thyrotropin levels, withdrawal symptoms after one month of use, cardiovascular collapse during anesthesia, and delayed emergence from anesthesia.[112,117,118] Photosensitization is a rare side effect caused by the hypericin constituent in St. John's Wort.[116] The effect has been observed more commonly in animals who ingest large amounts of the plant and can include symptoms such as blisters, burns, restlessness, seizures, and death.[116] In humans, phototoxic reactions are rare at recommended doses up to 1800 mg/day; they occur more often in patients with HIV who are receiving parenteral hypericin or taking the extract while undergoing laser treatment.[119–121] Hypericin enhances the oxidation of lens proteins in the eye, which could lead to the formation of cataracts.[122] Sunglass protection is therefore advisable. If high doses of hypericum are ingested acutely (e.g., in a suicide attempt), sun exposure should be avoided for several days because of hypericin's long half-life.[7]

Case reports of possible "serotonin syndrome" when St. John's Wort was used in combination with other prescription antidepressants should be brought to the physician's attention. If he still wishes to proceed with St. John's Wort therapy, G.C. should monitor himself for symptoms of GI upset, headache, anxiety/restlessness, sedation, and dizziness/confusion. He should also wear sunscreen, sunglasses, and protective clothing and avoid prolonged sun exposure. Warning patients to avoid tyramine-containing foods when taking hypericum is unnecessary based on in vitro data showing low levels of MAO inhibition.

Preparations and Active Constituents

21. **What factors should G.C. consider when selecting a product? What type of product would you recommend?**

St. John's Wort is prepared from the dried above-ground parts of the plant.[6] A variety of constituents have been isolated, including flavonoids biflavonoids, tannins and proanthocyanidins, xanthones, phloroglucinols (e.g., hyperforin, pseudohyperforin), phenolic acid, volatile oils, napthodianthrones (e.g., hypericin, pseudohypericin), sterols, vitamins, and choline.[6] Products are typically standardized by the hypericin content, even though it is unlikely to be the active constituent.[110] Hyperforin, which represents 2% to 4% of the crude herbal drug, could be the primary antidepressant constituent,[110] although a combination of chemicals is likely involved.

A dried alcoholic extract can be prepared by extraction with ethanol or methanol and is the formulation most commonly used in the treatment of depression.[7] Alcoholic extracts are formulated with an herb:extract ratio of 4:1 to 7:1 and should contain no less than 0.3% hypericin or 2% to 5% hyperforin.[7,110] Tea formulations are less concentrated and generally contain approximately 300 mg or one-third of the recommended antidepressant dose.[7] An oil formulation, prepared by steeping the crushed leaves of the flower in olive oil, is not recommended for treating depression but has been used historically as a topical agent for wound healing.[7]

G.C. should be told that alcoholic extracts have been used most often in clinical studies reporting antidepressant efficacy.[7] In addition, although the active constituents are unknown, total hypericin and hyperforin content are still considered markers of pharmaceutical quality and should be indicated on the package labeling.[7]

Pharmacokinetics and Dosing

22. What is known about the pharmacokinetics of hypericin and hyperforin? What dosage should be recommended, and when can G.C. expect to see a reduction in his symptoms for depression?

Pharmacokinetic parameters have been determined for the hypericin, pseudohypericin, and hyperforin constituents of hypericum.[123-125] Results after single- and multiple-dose oral kinetics indicate an apparent linear relationship for hypericin and pseudohypericin with doses up to 3.6 g of hypericum.[123] Both hypericin and pseudohypericin are poorly bioavailable (14% and 21%, respectively).[124] There is a 2-hour lag time in the onset of action for hypericin compared with 30 minutes for psuedohypericin.[124] Time to peak levels also are delayed for hypericin compared with pseudohypericin (6.0 to 7.1 hours versus 3.2 to 3.5 hours).[123] At steady state, the half-life of hypericin is increased substantially from its single-dose value of 27.5 to 29.1 hours to 41.7 hours.[123] The half-life of pseudohypericin is less affected and increased from 16.1 to 19.4 hours to 22.8 hours.[123] Hypericin and pseudohypericin appear to be completely cleared by the liver because neither the primary compounds nor their glucuronide or sulfate metabolites have been detected in urine.[124]

Hyperforin demonstrates linear pharmacokinetics after single doses of up to 600 mg of hypericum.[125] Larger doses of up to 1,200 mg resulted in serum concentrations that were less than what would have been expected with linear extrapolation. Pharmacokinetic parameters for hyperforin after a single dose of 300, 600, and 1,200 mg of hypericum (enriched to 5% hyperforin) revealed a lag time in the onset of action of 1 hour, a 9-hour half-life, and a time to peak of 3 hours. Half-life increased to 16 hours with multiple dosing of 900 mg of the extract for 8 days, but no accumulation occurred.

Hypericum extract 900 mg/day was the dosage most commonly used in clinical studies of mild to moderate depression.[100-103] Each tablet is formulated to contain 300 mg hypericum with 0.3% hypericin or 2% to 5% hyperforin and is administered three times daily.[100-103] Although hyperforin is now considered the primary antidepressant constituent, most commercial preparations do not always bear this standardized marker. Patients should be told that 2 to 4 weeks is required for onset of effect.[100-103]

Other Indications

23. What other conditions have been treated with hypericum?

In the past, hypericum was used as a topical agent for wound healing, an effect that was thought to be mediated by the astringent properties of the tannin constituents.[7] The hyperforin constituent also inhibits the growth of various Gram-positive bacteria in vitro.[126] Despite these properties, the use of hypericum oil for wound healing is now considered obsolete.[7]

In vitro, hypericin and pseudohypericin have demonstrated antiviral properties against HIV-1, human cytomegalovirus, and herpes simplex virus; in vivo, murine retrovirus was inhibited.[124] The antiviral effect of St. John's Wort is dose dependent and enhanced by exposure to light.[124] The mechanism may involve the generation of singlet oxygen radicals and damage to the viral envelope.[124] Antiviral efficacy has been assessed in patients with AIDS, but the dosages required for antiretroviral activity were generally high.[119] An intravenous (IV) formulation of the isolated hypericin constituent was used and caused phototoxicity in most patients.[119] Until more research is conducted, hypericin and hypericum extract cannot be recommended for the treatment of AIDS.

In vitro studies indicate that hypericin inhibits the growth of a variety of cancer cell types.[127] Photoactivation is required to enhance its antiproliferative effects.[127] Phase I trials in humans are currently under way. Hypericum extract has also been studied in the treatment of seasonal affective disorder (SAD), depression with somatic symptoms, reactive depression, premenstrual syndrome, and neuropathy. Additional research is required before hypericum can be recommended for these indications.[6,7,128]

ECHINACEA (ECHINACEA PURPUREA)
Preparations and Active Constituents

Many different factors have contributed to the variability in marketed echinacea products, including product content (e.g., parts used, addition of other non-*Echinacea* plant species), method of extraction, and the formulation most likely to trigger biologic activity.[129] Three species of echinacea have been evaluated in clinical studies for their immune stimulating effects: *Echinacea purpurea, E. angustifolia,* and *E. pallida.* Chemical studies conducted before 1990 often confused the botanical identity of these different species, especially *E. pallida* and *E. angustifolia,* making interpretation of therapeutic properties among individual species more difficult.[7] Furthermore, *E. angustifolia* and *E. pallida* have been the predominant species evaluated in chemical analysis, whereas *E. purpurea* was most often used for testing in clinical trials.[129]

In 1992, the German Commission E approved the root of *E. pallida* and the above-ground parts of *E. purpurea* for clinical use.[6] The Commission recommends that the root of *E. pallida* be manufactured as a water-alcohol extract (1:5 tincture, 50% ethanol), whereas the above-ground parts of

E. purpurea must be manufactured as a fresh pressed juice in 22% ethanol by volume as a preservative (e.g., *Echinacin, Echinaguard*).[6] *Echinacea* may stimulate the lymph tissue in the mouth.[7] Although this mechanism of action remains to be proven, such an assumption would indicate preference for a liquid versus a tablet formulation.[7]

Although chemically distinct, *E. purpurea, E. pallida,* and *E. angustifolia* share some common fractions; however, these common fractions can still vary in concentration and individual chemical components based on the plant parts used, the species being studied, and the type of formulation. All three species contain a lipophilic fraction (e.g., alkamides, polyacetylenes), water-soluble polysaccharides, caffeol conjugates (e.g., echinacoside, chicoric acid, caffeic acid), and flavonoids.[130] The alkamides, chicoric acid, and the polysaccharides have been recognized most often for possible immune-modulating effects.[130] Various constituents have also been studied for possible anti-infective, antioxidant and anti-inflammatory properties.[129–132]

Cold Treatment

24. A.T. is an otherwise healthy 32-year-old man who wants to purchase echinacea. Over the past 2 days, A.T. has had symptoms consistent with a new onset cold: a sore throat, stuffy nose, and general body aches. He is not taking any other over-the-counter or prescription medications and asks you if echinacea will shorten the duration of his cold symptoms.

Clinical trials evaluating the efficacy of echinacea in the relief of respiratory infections have been complicated by methodologic shortcomings, among them poor study design, use of heterogeneous echinacea preparations, and failure to ensure adequate blinding. Placebo control is also complicated by the distinctive flavor of liquid formulations of echinacea.

Recent trials involving Echinacea monopreparations prepared from the above-ground portions of the plant have typically noted significant improvements in cold symptoms when taken at the onset of a cold for 7 to 10 days.[133–135] All these trials were randomized, double-blind, and placebo-controlled. In the largest trial, 246 patients with upper respiratory infection (URI) symptoms received either a dried ethanolic extract of *E. purpurea* (95% herb, 5% root) known as Echinaforce, a highly concentrated version of Echinaforce (approximately seven times stronger), or a crude extract of *E. purpurea* root or placebo.[133] A complaint index of 12 common symptoms was used as the primary endpoint. Both preparations of Echinaforce significantly reduced the complaint index compared with placebo. However, the concentrated formulation was no more effective than the standard concentration. The root formulation of *E. purpurea* did not improve symptoms. The latter may have been the result of differences in chemical composition between the root and the above-ground portions of the *E. purpurea* plant. The method of manufacture can also influence the presence of pharmacologically active constituents (e.g., ethanolic extracts contain minimal amounts of polysaccharides).[130]

In another trial, 120 patients with initial URI symptoms received either *E. purpurea* fresh pressed juice preserved in ethanol (i.e., Echinaguard) or placebo (identical in color and ethanol concentration).[134] Treatment was continued for up to 10 days or until symptoms resolved. Forty percent of patients taking echinacea developed a "real" cold compared with 60%

of patients taking placebo. Time to symptom improvement in the subgroup of patients who developed a cold was significantly shortened from 8 to 4 days in the echinacea group.

The most recent trial evaluating Echinacea for cold treatment used a tablet formulation of an unrefined mixture of *E. purpurea* herb (25%), *E. purpurea* root (25%), and *E. angustifolia* root (50%).[136] Use of this product for a maximum of 10 days did not result in a significant improvement in severity or duration of cold symptoms compared to placebo. A limitation, however, could have been the formulation used, as the roots of *E. purpurea* and *E. angustifolia* are not currently approved by the German Commission E.[6]

A.T. should be informed that the use of echinacea in the treatment of cold symptoms is still under investigation. However, the evidence to date is positive when the above-ground parts of the *E. purpurea* plant are used. Cold symptoms and duration may be reduced by 10% to 50% when echinacea is taken early in the course of illness.[129] Echinacea is not a cure for the common cold. Adequate hydration, proper nutrition, and rest also are important during this period.

Mechanism of Action

25. What is *Echinacea's* purported mechanism of action in the abatement of cold symptoms?

Both in vitro and in vivo studies suggest that echinacea has an immune-modulating effect. In vitro studies have been conducted using murine and human macrophages. Using a purified polysaccharide fraction of *E. purpurea,* significant increases in polymorphonuclear (PMN) cell activation; macrophage activation; macrophage cytotoxicity against tumor and bacterial target cells; and macrophage secretion of IL-1, IL-6, tumor necrosis factor-α (TNF-α), and reactive oxygen intermediates were observed.[129,137] In vivo, the polysaccharide fraction enhanced immune activation in mice against fungal and bacterial pathogens.[129] In healthy volunteers, IV administration of the polysaccharide fraction enhanced PMN activity, macrophage activity, and migration of cells from bone marrow to peripheral blood.[137] However, the mechanisms described for the parenterally administered polysaccharide fraction of *E. purpurea* may not be applicable to the oral formulation used commercially.

Few studies have evaluated the mechanism of action of echinacea in its commercially available form. One in vitro study showed a significant increase in the production of IL-1, IL-6, IL-10, and TNF-α by human phagocytes in the presence of *E. purpurea* juice.[138] In vitro, natural killer (NK) cell and antibody-dependent cell cytotoxicity was also enhanced by *E. purpurea* extract in both healthy and immunocompromised patients.[139] However, in vivo, only enhancement of phagocytic activity has been noted.[140] Specifically, 4 weeks of an orally administered echinacea extract combination product failed to influence IL-1, IL-2, IL-6, TNF-α, or IFN-γ levels in 23 postsurgical tumor patients.[140] In contrast, 24 subjects given *E. purpurea* juice or placebo for 5 days had significantly enhanced neutrophil phagocytic activity.[129] A more recent study failed to find an effect of an orally administered *E. purpurea* juice on either cytokine expression or phagocytosis in 40 healthy volunteers who took the product for 14 days as compared to placebo.[141]

Echinacea's mechanism of action remains uncertain. Immune modulation or stimulation may play a role, but to date, only enhancement of phagocytic activity has been observed in humans. Future studies using the orally administered commercial formulations are required to determine if cytokine activity is enhanced in vivo as it is in vitro for humans.

Pharmacokinetics and Dosing

26. What is known about the pharmacokinetics of echinacea? What dose should be recommended for A.T.?

The pharmacokinetic parameters of echinacea have not been studied. Echinacea dosing for the supportive treatment of colds or URI is 6 to 9 mL/day of fresh pressed juice preserved in ethanol prepared from the above-ground parts of *E. purpurea* (e.g., Echinaguard) or 900 mg/day of *E. pallida* root (1:5 tincture, 50% ethanol).[7] Both preparations are administered in divided doses (e.g., 15 to 30 drops of *E. purpurea* juice, equivalent to 0.75 to 1.5 mL, two to five times daily). Appropriate dosing should be indicated on the package labeling. The German Commission E recommends that neither preparation be used for longer than 8 weeks because the mechanism for reported immune modulation is unclear.[6] However, studies as long as 12 weeks have been conducted without serious adverse effects.[129] External preparations should contain no less than 15% *E. purpurea* fresh pressed juice.[6]

Adverse Drug Reactions/Drug Interactions

27. Should A.T. be warned of any adverse effects caused by echinacea?

Toxic effects were not observed in animals given supratherapeutic parenteral and oral formulations of *E. purpurea* juice.[142] In vitro mutagenicity and carcinogenicity studies were also negative.[142] In humans, flu-like symptoms (e.g., fever, shivering, headache, vomiting) have been reported infrequently after parenteral administration.[143] This reaction may be caused by stimulation of phagocytes, cytokine production, or by a transient decrease in lymphocyte counts immediately after parenteral administration.[143] Few adverse effects have been associated with oral dosing. Unpleasant taste and upset stomach have occurred in 1.7% and 0.48% of patients, respectively, using *E. purpurea* lozenges for 4 to 6 weeks.[143] Hypersensitivity reactions have been commonly reported in patients with pre-existing atopy, which predisposes individuals to IgE-mediated allergic reactions.[144]

There are no reported drug–drug interactions for *E. purpurea* or *E. pallida*.[6] Theoretically, however, echinacea should be avoided in patients taking immunosuppressive medications (e.g., cyclosporin, steroids). Because of the high alcohol content of certain preparations, patients taking drugs known to cause an Antabuse-like reaction (e.g., metronidazole [Flagyl], griseofulvin [Fulvicin], chlorpropamide [Diabinese]) should be warned of this effect.

Cold Prophylaxis

28. A.T. purchases a product called Echinaguard, a fresh pressed juice formulation preserved in alcohol made from the above-ground parts of *E. purpurea*. Two days later, he indicates

that his partner, who has had HIV for 6 years, wants to use echinacea to protect himself from A.T.'s cold. His partner's most recent CD4+ lymphocyte count was 300 cells/mm³, and his viral load is undetectable. How would you advise A.T.?

Randomized, double-blind, placebo-controlled trials have failed to observe a prophylactic benefit of echinacea in reducing the frequency of the common cold.[145–147] In one trial, echinacea root extracts from the *E. purpurea* and *E. angustifolia* plants were compared with placebo in 289 patients who had experienced three or more colds in the past year. Twelve weeks of treatment failed to produce any significant differences in the frequency of URI infections or the time to first occurrence.[145] In another trial, 109 patients with three or more colds in the preceding year received 8 mL/day of Echinacin, a fresh pressed juice prepared from the above-ground portions of the plant, or placebo. After 8 weeks, there were no differences between groups in the frequency, duration, or severity of URI infections.[146] The most recent trial used an experimental cold model by injecting patients with rhinovirus. Patients received 14 days of an *E. purpurea, E. angustifolia* alcohol extract, 900 mg, before the injection and 5 days of the extract after the injection. There were no significant differences in infection rates between the treatment and placebo groups.[147]

A.T.'s partner should be informed that the prophylactic benefit of echinacea has not been established. Instead, he should be advised to wash his hands frequently and avoid close contact with A.T. while he is symptomatic.

States of Immune Deficiency

29. Could echinacea have other beneficial or harmful effects on A.T.'s partner who is HIV positive? What are the contraindications to *Echinacea's* use?

Because the immune modulating effects of echinacea are still being evaluated, it is unclear how this herb will affect the immune status of patients with HIV infection. On the one hand, echinacea may enhance immune function and this could be viewed as beneficial. In vitro analysis using cells from patients with AIDS showed enhancement of NK-cell activity by *E. purpurea* extract.[139] NK cells, in turn, can have a cidal effect on HIV-infected cells.[139] On the other hand, replication of HIV also may be stimulated by other effects of echinacea: enhancement of TNF-α levels and T-lymphocyte activation.[129] Therefore, until the effects of echinacea are clearly defined, it should not be used by patients who have HIV.

Additional disorders have been cited by the German Commission E as contraindications to echinacea use. Many of these disorders could be activated by immunostimulation, such as multiple sclerosis, tuberculosis, leukosis, collagen disorders (i.e., rheumatoid arthritis), and other autoimmune disorders.[5] As further clinical research is conducted, these contraindications may be removed.

Other Indications

30. What other conditions have been treated with echinacea?

Echinacea has been used to enhance hematologic recovery after chemotherapy, but this use is investigational. Two studies used intramuscular *E. purpurea* juice in combination with thymostimulin (an immune-enhancing thymic hormone) after low-dose cyclophosphamide (Cytoxan) therapy.[148,149] In both studies, patients had advanced stage hepatocellular or colorectal cancer, and sample sizes were small. Although certain immune parameters were significantly increased, it was unclear whether thymostimulin or echinacea was predominantly responsible. A pilot study investigated the effect of *E. purpurea* polysaccharides on leukocyte counts before and during chemotherapy. Patients had advanced gastric cancers, and no benefits were observed from the intervention.[150]

The German Commission E recommends *E. purpurea* but not *E. pallida* for the "supportive treatment of lower *urinary tract infections*"[6]. This indication is largely based on (1) studies performed in the 1950s using parenteral echinacea preparations and (2) unpublished studies performed by the manufacturer (Madaus) using echinacea lozenges in patients with respiratory and urinary tract infections (UTIs).[143] Despite support by the German Commission E, the use of echinacea for UTIs requires further clinical study. To date, most clinical trials have used injectable, not commercially available, formulations of echinacea and have lacked high-quality study design.[143]

Echinacea has also been evaluated for the treatment of recurrent vaginal candidiasis and recurrent genital herpes. In a nonrandomized, open-label study involving 203 women with recurrent vaginal candidiasis, patients received 6 days of topical econazole (Spectazole) with or without a 10-week course of subcutaneous, IV, intramuscular, or oral fresh pressed juice of *E. purpurea*.[129,143] Recurrence rates in patients receiving echinacea versus econazole alone were significantly lower, 5% to 16.7% versus 60%, respectively. The other trial was randomized and double-blinded and evaluated 50 patients with recurrent genital herpes. Patients received 6 months of an *E. purpurea* extract (Echinaforce) or placebo, but no benefits were observed at the end of the study.[151]

Historically, echinacea has been used for wound healing by Native Americans.[7] The German Commission E has approved *E. purpurea* for the topical treatment of "poorly healing wounds and ulcerations."[6] In vitro, echinacea has many effects that are compatible with a variety of possible anti-inflammatory effects. These include inhibition of enzymes involved in the inflammatory process (e.g., cyclooxygenase, 5-lipooxygenase, hyaluronidase) and a reduction in free radical formation.[129,131] In animals, echinacea reduces skin inflammation in response to chemical irritants.[129,131] Although topical anti-inflammatory effects have been demonstrated, there are no well-designed published trials in humans supporting this indication.[129] Thus, the use of echinacea for wound healing requires further research.

SAW PALMETTO (SERENOA REPENS)
Background

Prostate growth is largely dependent on the enzymatic conversion of testosterone to dihydrotestosterone (DHT) by 5α-reductase. Elevated DHT levels have been observed in patients with benign prostatic hyperplasia (BPH).[152] Prostatic growth factors, focal inflammation, and upregulation of androgen receptors also may be involved in the hyperplasia of prostatic stroma.[152] Prostatic enlargement can lead to physical obstruction of the urethra and symptoms of urinary hesitancy,

dribbling, incomplete bladder emptying, straining, and decreased urinary flow.[153] In addition, α-mediated adrenergic innervation of the prostate smooth muscle and bladder neck can lead to vasoconstriction and further compression of the urethra.[153] This dynamic component of BPH can account for up to 40% of the prostatic tone exerted on the urethra and can contribute to urinary symptoms.[153] Disease progression may lead to UTIs, urinary retention, hematuria, renal insufficiency, and bladder dysfunction from poor detrusor contractility or instability.[152,153]

The American Urological Association (AUA) Symptom Index is the standard scale for prostate symptom assessment.[154] Using this validated symptom scale, seven questions are scored from 0 to 5 and the total sum is used to classify disease progression as mild (0 to 7), moderate (8 to 18), or severe (19 to 35).[154] The International Prostate Symptom Score (I-PSS) is the European equivalent of the AUA Index and is also used to assess BPH.[155] Prostatic enlargement may often be detected by digital rectal examination (DRE); a prostate size >20 g is considered abnormal.[153] Urinary flow rate is the most frequent objective test used to assess bladder outlet obstruction.[154] Although peak flow rate can vary with age or voided volume, a guideline for classification of prostatism is mild (15 to 20 mL/sec), moderate (10 to 14 mL/sec), and severe (<10 mL/sec).[154] Prostate-specific antigen (PSA) values, produced by both benign and malignant prostate cells, can be used to detect prostate abnormalities.[153] Normal PSA values range between 0 and 4 ng/mL. However, PSA values may also be within normal limits in patients with BPH or prostate cancer; therefore, they are not a truly specific marker for either disease.[153] The reader is refereed to Chapter 101, Geriatric Urologic Disorders for more information.

31. B.F. is a 70-year-old man who presents to the ambulatory care clinic for a follow-up visit with his primary care provider. B.F. was recently referred to the urology clinic for symptoms of frequent urination, urgency, dysuria, and decreased urinary flow. Additional objective tests performed by the urologist included a urinalysis and a peak urinary flow rate. Prostate cancer was ruled out on rectal examination. Results of B.F.'s examination included the following: AUA score, 12 out of 35; PSA, 3.2 ng/mL; estimated prostate weight, 32 g; peak urinary flow, 12 mL/sec; normal urinalysis; BP, 110/60 mm Hg; HR, 70 beats/min; and normal renal function. B.F. has no other medical problems and is not taking any other prescription medications. How would you rate the severity of B.F.'s BPH? What objective parameters contribute to this rating?

Based on B.F.'s AUA score, his disease is of moderate severity. Objective parameters include his increased prostate size of 32 g and a restricted urinary flow of 12 mL/sec. Subjective symptoms of dysuria, urgency, and frequent urination should not be used as tools to assess disease severity because both obstructive and irritative symptoms of BPH often wax and wane.[153]

Treatment Options for Benign Prostatic Hyperplasia

32. B.F. is extremely bothered by his symptoms and wants to know the treatment options available besides the minimally invasive procedures and surgical procedures described by his urologist. What are these options?

Because B.F. has moderate disease, a number of treatment options are available. Generally, patients with mild to moderate disease are afforded the "watchful waiting" option, which means that the patient's symptoms are monitored for disease progression.[153] This option is recommended for mild prostatism because over a 5-year period, 45% of patients will have no deterioration, 40% will improve, and 15% will deteriorate.[154] The dynamic nature of BPH also has been noted in placebo studies of 2 to 24 weeks' duration in which 42% of patients improved, 46% had no change, and 12% had worsening of symptoms.[154] Patients like B.F. who are significantly bothered by their symptoms and are requesting nonsurgical treatments are candidates for prescription medications such as α_1-adrenergic antagonists (e.g., prazosin [Minipress], terazosin [Hytrin], doxazosin [Cardura], tamsulosin [Flomax]) and 5α-reductase inhibitors (e.g., finasteride [Proscar]).[154] Saw palmetto, a phytotherapeutic agent, also has been advocated for the treatment of BPH by many physicians in Europe.[152]

Finasteride is most effective in patients with prostate volumes >40 mL and may be no more effective than placebo in patients with prostate volumes <30 mL.[156] B.F.'s prostate volume of 32 mL makes him a poor candidate for finasteride. His BP of 110/60 mm Hg is also a concern if α-blockers are prescribed because they reduce BP in both hypertensive and nonhypertensive patients.[154] If α-blockers were initiated, B.F.'s BP would have to be monitored closely. Tamsulosin is 10 to 12 times more specific for the α-receptor subtype located on the prostate versus the vasculature and may be less problematic for B.F.[157] If B.F. is initiated on α-blockers, he should be counseled about first-dose syncope and monitoring his BP when beginning therapy. B.F. should arise slowly from the sitting or lying position, especially when getting out of bed in the morning.

33. B.F. begins the titration schedule for prazosin, but returns to the clinic 1 week later complaining of intolerable dizziness. The primary care physician is considering switching B.F.'s prescription to tamsulosin. Given B.F.'s lack of insurance coverage and financial constraints, he is considering saw palmetto. What are the active ingredients and mechanism of action of saw palmetto?

Preparations and Active Constituents

Saw palmetto berry is composed of many constituents; the active ingredients, however, are as yet unknown.[155] Permixon, the brand most commonly used in Europe, contains 90% free and 7% esterified fatty acids.[155] Phytosterols (i.e., β-sitosterol, campesterol, stigmasterol, cycloartenol, lupeol, lupenone, and methylcycloartenol), aliphatic alcohols, polyprenic compounds, and flavonoids also are present.[155,158,159] Reported pharmacologic activity may reside in the lipophilic fraction.[152] Saw palmetto is commercially formulated as a concentrated fat-soluble extract that is standardized to contain 85% to 95% fatty acids and sterols.[159]

Mechanism of Action

Preliminary in vitro studies suggested that saw palmetto has antiandrogenic properties. In human foreskin fibroblasts and rat prostate cell lines, saw palmetto competitively inhibited DHT binding to cytosolic and nuclear receptors.[152] Unlike finasteride, which inhibits 5α-reductase type-2, saw palmetto inhibited type-1 and, in some cases, both isoforms of the enzyme in vitro.[152] This could be beneficial because the type-1 isoenzyme is also expressed in normal and pathologic prostate glands to some degree.[160] Another study failed to confirm an effect on DHT production or 5α-reductase inhibition and suggested that supraphysiologic dosing had been used in initial studies.[152] Additional mechanisms that have been observed in vitro include inhibition of prostatic growth factors and inflammatory mediators produced by the 5-lipooxygenase pathway (e.g., leukotrienes) and α_1-adrenoreceptor antagonism.[152]

In vivo, saw palmetto reduced estrogen- and androgen-stimulated prostate growth in rats.[161] However, in healthy males, 1 week of treatment failed to influence 5α-reductase activity, DHT levels, and testosterone levels when compared with finasteride.[152] Eight days of treatment also had no effect on α_1-adrenoreceptor antagonism in healthy men.[162] In men with BPH, saw palmetto failed to influence plasma levels of testosterone, follicle stimulating hormone, and luteinizing hormone after 1 month of treatment.[152] PSA levels were also unaffected by saw palmetto after 6 months of treatment, suggesting a lack of 5α-reductase activity.[155] Contrary to these reports, some studies in men with BPH report significant reductions in epidermal growth factor, DHT production, and antiestrogenic activity with 3 months of treatment.[160,163] These reductions were comparable with that observed with 3 months of finasteride.[160] In summary, the mechanism of action of saw palmetto on the prostate remains unclear, but it is likely to involve a number of different processes. More clinical research is required to confirm previously published reports.

34. B.F.'s primary care physician is still unsure whether to initiate tamsulosin or saw palmetto. Are there any clinical trials that have evaluated the efficacy of saw palmetto in the treatment of BPH? How does the effect of saw palmetto compare with the α-blockers? Would it benefit B.F.? If so, what dosage should be used?

In a number of uncontrolled studies, 320 mg/day of saw palmetto for 3 to 6 months improved BPH symptoms, urinary flow rate, and postvoid residual volume.[158,164] However, as previously described, BPH is a dynamic disease and clinical benefits have also been observed in placebo-treated patients for up to 2 years.[154] Therefore, studies that lack blinding, placebo control, or a placebo run-in phase offer only weak support for clinical efficacy.

A meta-analysis looked at 21 randomized controlled trials conducted between 1966 and 2002 involving saw palmetto for BPH.[165] There were more than 3000 participants: 1408 in trials of saw palmetto versus placebo and 1701 in trials of saw palmetto versus another treatment medication. Urinary symptom scale scores were reported in 13 studies and revealed an absolute improvement of 28% for saw palmetto versus placebo. The weighted risk ratio (RR) for patient and physician rated symptomatic improvement were 1.76 and 1.72, respectively. The weighted mean difference (WMD) for nocturia and peak urine flow between saw palmetto and placebo were -0.76 times/evening and 1.86 mL/sec. Saw palmetto and finasteride showed similar absolute improvements in urinary peak flow and I-PSS scores. Saw palmetto was typically administered at a dose of 320 mg/day for a mean of 13 weeks.

Small comparative trials of saw palmetto versus prazosin and alfuzosin have been conducted in patients with mild to moderate BPH.[166,167] The prazosin study was not analyzed statistically, but both treatment groups noted symptomatic improvements at 3 months. Improvements were slightly greater for prazosin 2 mg orally twice a day versus saw palmetto 320 mg/day in the 41 patients studied.[166] A shorter 3-week trial compared saw palmetto 320 mg/day with alfuzosin 2.5 mg orally three times daily in 63 patients.[167] A standardized scale, the Boyarsky rating scale, was used for symptomatic assessment. Improvements in symptom score (38.8% versus 26.9%), obstructive score (37.8% versus 23.1%), and peak urinary flow (71.8% versus 48.4%) all favored alfuzosin over saw palmetto.

A large comparative trial of saw palmetto and tamsulosin also exists.[168] This 1-year trial compared 320 mg/day of saw palmetto to 0.4 mg/day of tamsulosin among 811 men with moderate BPH. The primary endpoints were the I-PSS score and maximal urinary flow. All outcomes were significantly improved in both groups to a similar degree. Approximately 80% of those treated had an improvement in I-PSS scores.

A large comparative trial of saw palmetto 320 mg/day and finasteride 5 mg/day was conducted in 1,098 patients.[155] The 6-month trial used the I-PSS rating scale to evaluate BPH symptoms in patients with mild to moderate disease. Objective parameters included peak urinary flow, prostate volume, and PSA levels. Quality of life and sexual dysfunction also were assessed. Both treatment groups had significant improvements in I-PSS score, quality of life, and peak urinary flow upon study completion. PSA was reduced by 41% by finasteride but was unaffected by saw palmetto. Finasteride significantly reduced prostate volume (18%) compared with saw palmetto (6%). Sexual dysfunction was significantly more frequent with finasteride (+9%) than with saw palmetto (−6%).

Although impressive in size, the latter trial had methodologic shortcomings. There was no placebo control and the study lasted only 6 months. Because clinical improvement with finasteride continues for 6 to 12 months into treatment, a longer follow-up period of 1 year may have revealed a significant difference between treatment groups.[169] In addition, enrollment in this comparative study required a prostate volume >25 mL. As previously noted, finasteride generally is reserved for patients with a prostate volume >40 mL and may be no more effective than placebo in patients with a prostate volume <30 mL.[156] Therefore, without a placebo arm, the clinical response observed in both treatment groups may be no greater than placebo. Saw palmetto had a lower incidence of sexual dysfunction, which was significant but not of substantial magnitude. Absolute percentages for side effects of erectile dysfunction and decreased libido, respectively, were 2.8% and 3.0% for finasteride and 1.5% and 2.2% for saw palmetto.

In summary, saw palmetto improves overall urinary tract symptoms by approximately 28% compared with placebo.[165] In comparative trials, saw palmetto demonstrated similar efficacy to finasteride at 6 months, tamsulosin at 1 year, and a slightly reduced efficacy versus other α-blockers at 1 and 3 months.[155,166–169] The benefits of saw palmetto extending beyond 1 year remain uncertain because of short study dura-

tions. B.F. may benefit from saw palmetto because it has a quick onset of action (4 weeks) that is similar to α-blockers (4 to 6 weeks) but shorter than finasteride (6 months).[154,158] B.F.'s low BP and financial constraints also make saw palmetto a reasonable choice. The dose of saw palmetto used most often in trials of patients with BPH was 320 mg/day, taken as 160 mg orally twice a day. The German Commission E recommends 1 to 2 g of saw palmetto berry or 320 mg of lipophilic extract.[6] The lipophilic extract is available as 80- and 160-mg tablets and capsules.

If B.F. does not achieve any symptomatic relief by 6 weeks, another therapy should be instituted. Saw palmetto is not indicated for severe BPH or prostate cancer. B.F. should continue to schedule regular follow-up visits with his primary care physician to continuously assess the need for saw palmetto.

Adverse Drug Reactions/Drug Interactions

35. **B.F. begins saw palmetto therapy. Two days later, he complains of stomach upset after ingesting the herb. What adverse effects and drug interactions are associated with saw palmetto? Is stomach upset a common reaction, and is there anything that can be done to minimize it?**

To date, no drug–drug interactions have been reported for saw palmetto, but a small number of side effects have been observed in clinical trials. In the comparative study involving 1,098 patients, saw palmetto–associated side effects occurring with an incidence of 1% to 3% included hypertension, decreased libido, abdominal pain, erectile dysfunction, back pain, urinary retention, and headache.[155] Additional complaints that occurred with an incidence of <1% were diarrhea, flulike symptoms, nausea, constipation, and dysuria.[155] In another trial involving 500 men, side effects were reported with an incidence of 2%. The most commonly reported side effect was GI upset, which resolved when saw palmetto was taken with food.[158]

B.F. should be assured that this type of reaction has occurred before in patients taking saw palmetto. To minimize stomach upset, B.F. can try taking the herb with food. If his stomach upset does not resolve, he should inform his primary care physician so that another treatment can be considered.

Pharmacokinetics

36. **What is known about the pharmacokinetics of saw palmetto? Will administration with food affect the absorption or the overall efficacy of the herb?**

Few pharmacokinetic trials have been performed with saw palmetto. Single-dose kinetics were evaluated in 12 fasting men who ingested 320 mg of the herb. Peak plasma levels were reached in 1.5 hours and the elimination half-life was 1.9 hours.[152] No trials have been conducted evaluating the effect of food on bioavailability or efficacy. Tissue distribution of saw palmetto has been studied in rats.[152] Saw palmetto supplemented with oleic acid, lauric acid, or β-sitosterol revealed tissue concentrations that were greater in the prostate than other genital organs or the liver.

GINSENG (PANAX SPP.)
Preparations and Active Constituents

37. A.J., an overweight 55-year-old man with type 2 diabetes mellitus, hypercholesterolemia, and hypertension, has come to the pharmacy to purchase a dietary supplement to boost his energy. His current medications include simvastatin (Zocor) 10 mg PO QD, metformin (Glucophage) 750 mg PO BID, and benazepril (Lotensin) 10 mg PO QD. His current laboratory values are as follows: total cholesterol, 225 mg/dL; LDL-C, 185 mg/dL; HDL-C, 30 mg/dL; TG, 110 mg/dL; and BP 150/80 mm Hg. There have been no changes to A.J.'s medication regimen in the past year. A.J. has no family history of coronary heart disease. He states that he has been under a lot of stress lately and has not been feeling as energetic as he normally does. He selects two herbal products, both of which claim to enhance energy. The first is a combination herbal product containing ephedra as the primary ingredient; the other is labeled "Siberian ginseng." There are so many ginseng products that A.J. asks you if there is any difference between his current selection and the other bottles labeled "Panax."

There are a variety of species of ginseng, many of which are distinguished by their country of origin. Some of these include *Panax ginseng* C.A. Meyer (Chinese or Korean variety), *P. quinquefolius* (American variety), *P. japonicus* C.A. Meyer (Japanese variety), and *P. notoginseng* (Sanchi variety).[170] Twenty-eight different triterpenoid saponin glycosides known as *ginsenosides* have been isolated from ginseng. Additional constituents include polysaccharides, flavonoids, daucosterin, mucilaginous substances, amino acids, bitter substances, vitamins, choline, pectin, fatty oil, and ethereal oil.[171] Composition may vary between different species or within the same species when cultivated at different locations. The ginsenosides are thought to be responsible for many of the reported effects and can be subdivided into three main categories based on their chemical structure: oleanolic acid, panaxadiol, and panaxatriol types.[171] Individual saponins have been further classified and are chemically designated by the letter "R" followed by a subscript letter, number, or both.[7] It is generally the root of the plant that is used for commercial manufacturing, although the flower buds, leaves, and root stock also contain ginsenosides.[171] The length of time required for maturation of ginseng root and optimal ginsenoside levels is 5 to 6 years.[171] For this reason, commercial supply can be scarce, leading to higher prices and a greater risk of plant substitution or suboptimal ginsenoside content.[172] Rg_1 is used as a marker to assess ginsenoside content in *P. ginseng roots;* 1.5% is considered standard.[6] Both *P. ginseng* extract and crude herb formulations are recommended by the German Commission E.[6] Ginseng extract should be standardized to contain at least 4% ginsenosides.[6] Crude herb products are available as fresh ginseng (younger than 4 years of age), peeled and dried white ginseng (4 to 6 years of age), or steamed and dried red ginseng (older than 6 years of age).[170] The latter products may be further processed into powder, extract, or tea formulations.

Other plants that have been reported to have similar clinical effects to ginseng but are not of the *Panax species* include *Eleutherococcus senticosus* (Siberian ginseng) and *Pfaffia paniculata* (Brazilian ginseng).[173] Both of these species lack the characteristic ginsenosides of the Panax species but contain eleutherosides and pfaffosides, respectively.[173] Siberian ginseng was developed as a substitute for the Panax species by the former Soviet Union. Many of the clinical studies for Siberian ginseng have been published in the Russian language, making them less available to the scientific community.[174] Both the *Panax* species and *Eleutherococcus* are approved by the German Commission E as "a tonic to counteract weakness and fatigue, as a restorative for declining stamina and impaired concentration, and as an aid to convalescence."[6]

Therefore, A.J. should be informed that Siberian ginseng is not part of the Panax species and contains no ginsenosides. However, both preparations are approved for the treatment of similar conditions in Europe. In general, *P. ginseng* C.A. Meyer may be a superior choice because it has been studied more thoroughly by the scientific community and carries a marker of standardization based on its ginsenoside content.

38. Given A.J.'s clinical presentation, what concerns would you have before recommending a ginseng product?

A.J.'s fatigue may be a symptom of poor glucose control. Thus, his recent blood glucose measurements should be reviewed, and his glycosylated hemoglobin (A1c) level should be checked. In addition, A.J. should be asked about other symptoms that can cause a loss of energy such as depression (e.g., appetite, quality of sleep), a cold (e.g., congestion, runny nose, sore throat), or hypothyroidism (e.g., constipation, cold intolerance, weight gain).

39. A.J. states that his most recent A1c was 8% (normal, 4% to 6%). He performs fingerstick blood glucose measurements twice daily and values range between 130 and 160 mg/dL. He has no other symptoms suggestive of hyperglycemia or other conditions associated with fatigue. A.J. asks for your assistance in choosing between the supplements he has selected. What claims are made for each of these supplements, and how does the proposed mechanism of action for each of these agents affect your recommendation?

Mechanism of Action

A.J. has selected a combination product that includes ephedra (abbreviation for ephedrine), a sympathomimetic. Sympathomimetics act as central nervous system (CNS) stimulants to boost energy; they also constrict blood vessels and raise glucose levels. Because these effects could worsen A.J.'s hypertension and diabetes, he should avoid the use of this combination supplement.

Ginseng has been labeled as an "adaptogen," which refers to the body's ability to normalize itself when exposed to stressful or noxious stimuli. Adaptogenic properties that have been reported for ginseng include stress relief, improved mood and cognitive function, enhanced physical performance, immune modulation, improved cardiovascular function, antidiabetic activity, anticancer effects, and protection against liver damage.[6] The postulated mechanism of action in humans is based on the results of in vitro and animal studies. This extrapolation may be premature because many studies used formulations (e.g., individual ginsenosides or polysaccharides) and routes of administration (e.g., parenteral) that differ from commercially available formulations. Some of the mechanisms reported for ginseng are listed in Table 3-5. Based on these mechanisms, A.J. has no contraindications to ginseng and may or may not benefit from its reported homeostatic effects on glucose control and BP. Of the two supplemental products A.J. has selected, *P. ginseng* would be the preferred agent.

Ergogenic and Nootropic Effects

40. A.J. agrees to avoid the ephedra-containing supplement but wants to know what types of benefits he can expect once he initiates ginseng.

The effects of ginseng on physical (ergogenic) and mental (mood, nootropic) performance have been inconsistent. In 83 healthy patients, 200 to 400 mg/day of *P. ginseng* extract (Ginsana, G115) or placebo for 8 weeks failed to show a significant benefit on positive affect, negative affect, or total mood disturbance.[183] A larger 9-week, double-blind study in 127 healthy patients using 400 mg/day of standardized *P. ginseng* extract (Gerimax) failed to show consistent enhancement of cognitive function.[184] A series of tests were used to assess psychomotor function, attention and concentration, learning and memory, and abstraction. Significant improvements occurred for the abstraction test and the Auditive Reaction Test (one of three tests designed to assess psychomotor function).

Many human studies evaluating the ergogenic effects (i.e., parameters of muscular oxygen utilization and work load) of ginseng have been criticized for their poor methodology.[185] Well-designed trials involving small numbers of healthy patients (8 to 38) have been performed. *P. ginseng* extract (Ginsana, G115) at dosages of 200 to 400 mg/day or 8 to 16

mg/day of *P. quinquefolius* extract for 1 to 8 weeks failed to improve parameters of oxygen consumption, blood lactic acid concentration, or respiration under conditions of submaximal or maximal exercise.[186–188] Many studies reporting positive ergogenic effects were not placebo controlled.[185] Those that were blinded and reported benefit were of small sample size (12 to 30 patients) and conducted in athletes; significant improvements in oxygen uptake, recovery heart rate, and endurance were noted.[185]

Combination products of *P. ginseng* extract (G115) complexed with vitamins, minerals, and trace elements also have been used to assess adaptogenic properties.[189–192] The dosage of ginseng extract used in these studies ranged from 40 to 80 mg/day for up to 12 weeks. Unfortunately, only one study used a control group, which accounted for the effects of vitamins, minerals, and trace elements.[192] Without such a control, the effects of ginseng cannot be distinguished from the other nutritional elements in the product. Ergogenic benefits were observed in one of these studies.[190] In two other studies, quality of life was assessed.[189,192] In 390 patients, 80 mg/day of extract significantly improved one of three scales used to assess quality of life.[189] A subgroup analysis revealed that patients with the lowest quality of life scores had the greatest benefit. In contrast, 80 mg/day of extract in 49 sick and geriatric patients failed to influence cognitive function or somatic symptoms.[191] The only study that used an appropriate control group was conducted in 625 patients, 501 of whom completed the trial. Ginseng extract (40 mg/day) significantly improved quality of life based on an 11-item questionnaire.[192]

A.J. should be told that the reported adaptogenic benefits of ginseng have not occurred with any consistency. Some studies reported significant effects, whereas others demon-

References	Mechanism	Adaptogenic Quality
	Table 3-5 Adaptogenic Mechanisms Reported for Ginseng and Its Constituents Based on In Vitro and Animal Studies	
175	↓ adrenal catecholamine release	Antistress
176	↑ adrenocorticotropin hormone (ACTH) and corticosterone release, agonist at glucocorticoid receptor	Antistress
175	Centrally mediated enhancement of GABA$_A$ and opioid systems, inhibition of substance P	↓ psychologic and pain-mediated stress
175	↑ central levels of acetylcholine	Nootropic
175	Possible dopamine antagonism or reversal of immunodepressant effects of narcotics	↓ narcotic tolerance and dependence
177	Anti-inflammatory, possibly mediated through anticomplement activity	↓ acute and chronic inflammation
178	Antioxidant	↓ cellular damage in states of hypoxia
175	Calcium channel blockade	Vasoregulatory, effect may vary depending on dose and target tissue
176, 179	↑ nitric oxide and/or prostacyclin release	Vasoregulatory effect
180, 181	↓ platelet aggregation by ↓ effect of activating triggers: collagen, thrombin, thromboxane (TXA$_2$), and platelet-activating factor (PAF); increase effect of aggregation inhibitors; cGMP, cAMP	Antiplatelet activity
176	↑ insulin release and number of insulin receptors	Improved glucose homeostasis
182	Induced mRNA expression for IL-2, IL-1α, IFN-γ, and GM-CSF; activated T cells, NK cells, and macrophages	Immunomodulation
175	↓ tumor angiogenesis, ↑ tumor cell apoptosis (death)	↓ tumor metastasis

GM-CSF, granulocyte-macrophage colony-stimulating factor; IFN-γ, interferon-γ; IL, interleukin; NK, natural killer.

strated no effect. When benefits were observed, they typically occurred after 6 to 12 weeks of treatment. Dosages of *P. ginseng* extract ranged from 40 to 400 mg/day. Improvements, when noted, included enhanced quality of life, cognition, alertness, and physical performance with exertion.

Glucose Homeostasis

41. To what degree will A.J.'s diabetes, hypertension, and hyperlipidemia be affected by ginseng?

Few studies have assessed the role of ginseng in the treatment of diabetes.[193,194] In 36 patients with type 2 diabetes mellitus, 100- and 200-mg doses of ginseng extract (species not indicated) were compared with placebo.[194] At 8 weeks, both ginseng groups had significant reductions in fasting blood glucose (FBG); A1c was significantly reduced only in the 200 mg group. Absolute changes in FBG and A1c from baseline were not reported. A more recent trial evaluated an American ginseng product, *Panax quinquefolius* L, for its effect on postprandial blood sugar levels.[193] Both nondiabetic subjects and subjects with type 2 diabetes mellitus had significant drops in postprandial blood sugar values when 3 g of ginseng was taken 40 minutes before a meal, compared with placebo. A significant drop also was observed in patients with diabetes, but not in healthy subjects, when ginseng was taken at the time of the meal. Overall, this evidence suggests that ginseng use could reduce the blood glucose, but more clinical studies are needed. A.J. should continue to check his blood glucose regularly and report any changes to his doctor.

Cardiac and Lipid Homeostasis

Some studies suggest that ginseng may have a beneficial effect on BP and lipid profiles, but results are inconclusive.[194–196] For example, 7 days of powdered *P. ginseng* 4.5 g (equivalent to 900 mg/day of extract) significantly increased HDL-C and reduced TGs in 11 patients.[196] In contrast, *P. ginseng* had no effect on lipids in 36 patients with type 2 diabetes mellitus.[194]

Vasodilatory effects of *P. ginseng* have been observed in animal models.[175,176] In young healthy adults, reductions in SBP and DBP as well as platelet aggregation were reported for a ginkgo/ginseng combination product.[195] The contribution of ginseng to this response is unclear. In contrast, a rise in BP was reported after chronic ingestion (for >1 month) of ginseng and Siberian ginseng products.[197] Patients developing hypertension typically consumed an average of 3 g of ginseng root per day,[197] but many of these patients also consumed caffeinated beverages, which may have contributed to the hypertension. Furthermore, no chemical analysis was performed for product content. Additional studies have evaluated the cardiovascular effects of ginseng in patients with congestive heart failure, essential and white coat hypertension, and in subjects undergoing coronary bypass for mitral valve replacement. Although low in patient numbers (<30 patients), these studies reported improvements in cardiac performance and BP.[179,198,199]

A.J. should be informed that hypotensive and antihyperlipidemic effects of ginseng have not been clearly demonstrated. A.J.'s current BP and lipid values are elevated despite prescription therapy and he has several other cardiovascular risk factors, including his age, diabetes, hypertension, and low HDL-C. A.J.'s dosages of simvastatin and benazepril should be increased, and he should monitor his BP more frequently after initiating ginseng. Any episodes of hypotension or hypertension should be discussed with his physician.

Immune Modulation

42. A.J. has received his flu shot already. Will taking ginseng further decrease his risk of catching the flu this season?

Ginseng is under investigation as an immune modulator. In vitro, ginseng appeared to have a greater effect on stimulating lymphocyte proliferation in elderly versus young patients.[200] A lack of effect on leukocyte and lymphocyte counts was also observed in vivo when 300 mg/day of *P. ginseng* extract was studied for 8 weeks in young and healthy adults.[201] However, other research has shown significant enhancement of immune function in healthy patients.[202] Eight weeks of aqueous or standardized *P. ginseng* extract significantly increased PMN cell chemotaxis, phagocytosis fraction and index, intracellular killing, total lymphocytes (T3), T helper (T4) subset, suppressor cells (T8), and NK cell activity.[202] Both time to effect and degree of immune stimulation were superior in the standardized versus the aqueous extract group.[202] The largest study to date was performed in 227 patients. Influenza vaccine was administered with and without 100 mg/day of *P. ginseng* extract (Ginsana). Forty-two cases of influenza were reported in the vaccination-only group versus 15 in the vaccination and ginseng group at 12 weeks. Antibody titers and NK-cell activity also were significantly enhanced at 8 and 12 weeks in the ginseng group.[203] A more recent study examined the effect of ginseng plus amoxicillin/clavulanic acid [Augmentin] versus antibiotics alone in the clearance of infection in patients with chronic bronchitis.[204] Clearance over 10 days was significantly accelerated with the combination versus antibiotics alone. Thus, ginseng may indeed decrease A.J.'s risk for catching the flu this season.

43. J.L. is a 32-year-old woman with a history of multiple sclerosis who last had an exacerbation 6 months ago. She would like to initiate ginseng to improve her athletic performance in an upcoming race. How would you advise J.L.?

Multiple sclerosis is an autoimmune disorder, and ginseng may enhance cytokine expression and stimulate the immune system. Although the German Commission E does not contraindicate the use of ginseng in patients with autoimmune disorders, it is reasonable to avoid ginseng in patients with multiple sclerosis and other immune system disorders (AIDS, collagen vascular disease, and others) given the possibility of immune activation. More extensive clinical research is needed to substantiate the effects of ginseng on the immune system.

Anticarcinogenic/Antitumor Effects

44. R.B. is a 32-year-old woman who has a strong family history of stomach cancer. She has heard that ginseng can prevent cancer. Is there any evidence for this effect?

Animal studies have demonstrated anticarcinogenic properties for ginseng. In long-term experiments, ranging in duration from 28 to 56 weeks, ginseng significantly reduced procarcinogen-induced lung adenoma and hepatoma in mice.[170] The incidence and proliferation of tumors also was reduced.[170]

In humans, two large-scale epidemiologic trials observed reductions in the incidence of cancer in patients consuming ginseng.[170] Evaluation of 921 cancer patients and 605 controls on an oncology service in Korea found a direct correlation between ginseng intake and the risk for cancer development.[170] The odds ratio with no ginseng intake was 1.0. This was reduced to 0.6 in patients who consumed ginseng one to three times per year, and to 0.36 if consumption was increased to once per month or more. Duration of ginseng use also correlated to cancer development. At 1, 3, and 5 years of use, the odds ratio for cancer development was 0.64, 0.36, and 0.31, respectively. Fresh ginseng juice or slices and white ginseng tea had no influence on cancer risk, but fresh and white ginseng extract, white ginseng powder, and red ginseng did. Types of cancers that were reduced included oral, pharyngeal, esophageal, gastric, colorectal, hepatic, pancreatic, laryngeal, pulmonary, and ovarian. There were no reductions in breast, cervical, bladder, or thyroid cancer.

A larger prospective study of 4,634 patients compared quantity of ginseng ingested to future cancer development.[170] The relative risk (RR) of cancer development was significantly lower in individuals who consumed ginseng more often. The RR for consumption once per month or more was 0.34. Stomach and lung cancers were significantly reduced.

In both epidemiologic studies, other patient-specific variables could have influenced cancer development. Although smoking was taken into account, diet, environmental carcinogen exposure, and sexual behavior were not.

In summary, R.B. can be told that ginseng extract or powder may reduce her risk of developing stomach cancer. However, it should not be considered a cure for cancer. The greatest benefit is associated with frequent consumption (once or more per month) and long duration of use. If a fresh formulation is used, it should be manufactured as an extract, as other formulations showed no benefit.

45. B.J. is a 45-year-old man with a history of mild alcohol-induced liver dysfunction, bipolar disorder, and recent intermittent episodes of erectile dysfunction. B.J. has been alcohol-free for 2 years and clinically his bipolar disorder has been stabilized with lithium (Lithobid) for 10 years. He has never been evaluated for sexual dysfunction. His current laboratory values include the following: lithium, 1.0 mEq/L; AST, 80 U/L (normal, 5 to 40 U/L); ALT, 60 U/L (normal, 7 to 35 U/L); alkaline phosphatase, 100 U/L (normal, 30 to 120 U/L); albumin, 3.0 g/dL (normal, 4 to 6 g/dL); and an International Normalized Ratio (INR) of 1.3. B.J. read that ginseng can improve liver function and alleviate sexual dysfunction; he wishes to purchase a bottle. How would you instruct this patient?

Liver Function

There have been only a few studies of small sample size (14 to 24 patients) that have evaluated the hepatic effects of ginseng in humans. A large dose of *P. ginseng* extract, 3 g, significantly accelerated blood alcohol clearance after acute alcohol ingestion,[205] but ginseng's effects on alcohol and drug-induced chronic liver disease have not been clearly demonstrated.[206] In elderly patients with hepatotoxin-induced chronic liver disease (>80 g/day of alcohol and/or medicines known to cause chronic liver damage), a combination ginseng

product containing *P. ginseng* with vitamins, minerals, and trace elements was compared with a control group without ginseng. Twelve weeks of ginseng extract 80 mg/day failed to affect AST, ALT, or bilirubin. Other measures of liver function, including gamma-glutamyl transpeptidase, postprandial bile salts, and bromsulfophthalein, were significantly reduced from baseline but not compared with placebo.

Erectile Dysfunction, Fertility, and Sex Hormones in Men

Ginseng may enhance fertility and erectile dysfunction in men. In one study, 46 patients with oligoasthenospermia and 20 controls were treated with *P. ginseng* extract.[207] Sperm number and motility were significantly enhanced, and testosterone, dihydrotestosterone, follicle-stimulating hormone (FSH), and luteinizing hormone levels were increased compared with controls. In another study of 45 men, 2,700 mg of red *P. ginseng* extract significantly enhanced parameters of erectile dysfunction compared with placebo (60% versus 20%, respectively) after 8 weeks of treatment.[208] Nitrogen oxide release has been suggested as a possible mechanism of action.[179]

In summary, B.J. should be advised not to initiate ginseng for his history of alcoholic liver dysfunction because there is insufficient evidence to support this claim. Instead, he should continue to refrain from alcohol use and have his liver function evaluated periodically by his doctor. Furthermore, although preliminary studies suggest that ginseng might improve fertility and erectile dysfunction, more research is needed. Because B.J.'s erectile dysfunction is of recent onset, he should be evaluated by his physician before initiating any treatment. If ginseng is initiated for sexual dysfunction, patients should be informed that efficacy cannot be assured.

Adverse Drug Reactions/Drug Interactions

46. B.J.'s physician was unable to find any physical abnormalities to explain B.J.'s temporary erectile dysfunction. Therefore, B.J. would like to try ginseng to alleviate his symptoms. What are the side effects and drug–drug interactions that have been associated with ginseng? Are any of these of concern in B.J.?

CNS stimulation, insomnia, hypertension, and nervousness have been reported in patients using ginseng and Siberian ginseng products.[197] Additional case reports of irritability, sleeplessness, and manic behavior have been observed in patients with a history of psychiatric illness taking ginseng in combination with other psychiatric medications (i.e., lithium, neuroleptics, phenelzine [Nardil]).[205] In all of these cases, product analysis was not performed, and adulteration could have occurred. However, in animal studies ginseng has altered corticosterone release, neurotransmitter function, and pain modulation (see Table 3-5). Because B.J. has a history of bipolar disorder, he and his physician should be informed of these reports. If B.J. initiates ginseng, he should be alert for changes in mood and discuss these with his physician if they occur.

Additional drug–drug interactions that have been reported include a case report of diuretic resistance in a patient using a germanium-containing ginseng product.[205] Germanium, which has been associated with renal dysfunction, was considered to be the cause.[205] Elevated digoxin levels were observed in a patient consuming Siberian ginseng.[209] This may have been the result of contamination of Siberian ginseng products with *Periploca sepium* (silk vine), which contains cardiac glycosides.[210] In another case report, ginseng was associated with a probable reduction in warfarin efficacy,[205] and in animals, antiplatelet properties have been observed (see Table 3-5). Antiplatelet properties could increase bleeding risk in patients taking other antiplatelet or anticoagulant medications, so this combination should be avoided. Preoperative and postoperative patients should also be advised to discontinue ginseng 7 to 10 days before and after surgery. Finally, reports of Stevens-Johnson syndrome and cerebral arteritis have occurred after standard and supratherapeutic (25 g fresh root) ginseng doses, respectively.[205]

The German Commission E lists no drug–drug interactions, contraindications, or adverse events associated with the use of *P. ginseng*.[6] However, high BP has been listed as a contraindication to the use of Siberian but not *P. ginseng*.[6] Adulteration cannot be ruled out in most adverse events and drug interactions that have been reported. Product analyses were not performed.

Sex Hormones in Women

47. **Does ginseng have any "hormonal effects" in women?**

In women, ginseng has been reported to have weak estrogenic activity.[205] In vitro, *P. quinquefolius* demonstrated a possible protective role against breast cancer.[211] In vivo, case reports of vaginal bleeding and mastalgia have occurred after the acute or chronic use of ginseng products.[205] In one of these cases, rechallenge with the ginseng product resulted in a return of the bleeding and a reduced plasma FSH level.[205] Neonatal androgenization was reported after a mother's use of Siberian ginseng.[212] This was later discredited when product analysis revealed the presence of *P. sepium* (silk vine) as a contaminant.[212]

Pharmacokinetics and Dosing

48. **What is known about the pharmacokinetics of ginseng? What doses are generally recommended?**

After oral dosing of red, white, and *P. ginseng* extract, urinary excretion of 20(S)-protopanaxadiol and 20(S)-protopanaxatriol ginsengosides was >2%.[214] Elimination half-life ranged between 13.5 and 17.0 hours based on urinary excretion data.[214] After single-dose administration, a linear relationship was observed between the amount of ginseng ingested and the rate of ginsenoside excretion. Steady-state excretion of ginsenosides after multiple daily doses was achieved in 5 days.[214] These data provide some information regarding the absorption and excretion of ginsenosides in humans, but the primary route of metabolism and excretion of ginsenosides requires further investigation.

The dose of *P. ginseng* recommended by the German Commission E is 1 to 2 g of the crude root or its equivalent; 1 g of crude root is equivalent to 200 mg of the extract.[187,188] Ginsana is a standardized extract of *P. ginseng* that has been used in some clinical trials and can be found in the United States. Dosing for Siberian ginseng is 2 to 3 g of crude root or its equivalent. The Commission recommends limiting the continuous use of these agents to 3 months.[6]

DEHYDROEPIANDROSTERONE AND WILD YAMS (DIOSCOREA EXTRACTS)
Background

Dehydroepiandrosterone (DHEA) is a precursor hormone secreted by the adrenal cortex and to a lesser extent, by the CNS.[215] It is the most abundant adrenal steroid and is rapidly converted to the sulfate ester, dehydroepiandrosterone-sulfate (DHEAS). Although no specific function has been attributed to DHEAS, endogenous levels have correlated with a variety of disease states. DHEA may be involved in the aging process, enhancing the immune system,[216] improving cardiovascular risk factors,[217] promoting weight loss,[218] and preventing certain types of cancers.[219] Research is under way to assess the effects of exogenous DHEA supplementation on these conditions.

Before DSHEA was enacted, DHEA was marketed as a product that could stimulate weight loss, improve longevity, and enhance libido, but these claims were never proven in clinical trials and the hormone was never assessed for safety. In 1985, the FDA prohibited manufacturers from marketing DHEA as a drug product. Today, DHEA is widely available as a dietary supplement through health and nutrition stores, pharmacies, and other places where drug products are sold. DHEA is commonly compounded to specific strengths for research purposes and for individual use. It also is widely available at high doses from "buyers groups" for its affect on HIV. Currently, DHEA has orphan drug status for the treatment of burns, autologous skin grafting, and systemic lupus erythematosus (SLE).

Regulation and Release

The secretion of DHEA is regulated by the hypothalamic-pituitary axis. Adrenocorticotropin hormone (ACTH) is largely responsible for the release of DHEA from the pituitary. However, unlike glucocorticoids, DHEA and DHEAS do not exert negative feedback effects on the production of ACTH from the pituitary.[220] The responsiveness to ACTH stimulation decreases with age. Therefore, levels of DHEA and the conjugated sulfate, DHEAS, decline with age. Peak DHEA levels occur at age 25 to 30 years and decline progressively by 25% per decade of life until age 70. See Table 3-6.[221,222] DHEA levels in males are higher than those in females in every decade of life until age 65.[223] Most studies evaluating endogenous levels have measured DHEAS because DHEA levels have a large diurnal variation.[224] DHEA is primarily produced in the morning hours, when levels are highest; levels then decline rapidly throughout the day. In contrast, DHEAS levels remain stable throughout the day because DHEAS is cleared slowly.

Because DHEA is a precursor hormone, it is ultimately converted to either estrogen or testosterone. A theoretical model for DHEA conversion has been described and is the basis for DHEA administration in a variety of disease states (Table 3-7).[225] In men, DHEA is predominantly converted to estrogen with negligible amounts converted to testosterone. Premenopausal women, who have abundant estrogen and low testosterone levels, convert DHEA predominantly to testosterone. In postmenopausal women, who have low levels of estrogen and testosterone, DHEA is converted to both hormones. This model also serves to explain many of the observed and theoretical DHEA side effects. Many doses and

Table 3-6   Age-Related DHEAS Levels for Women and Men

	Age (yr)	DHEAS Levels (ng/mL)
Males	15–39	1,500–5,500
	40–49	1,000–4,000
	50–59	600–3,000
	≥60	300–2,000
Females	15–29	1,000–5,000
	30–39	600–3,500
	40–49	400–2,500
	≥50	200–1,500

formulations of DHEA are available in the United States, including tablets, capsules, sublingual tablets, and sublingual sprays. The doses available include but are not limited to 5, 10, 25, 30, 50, and 100 mg. Patients should be instructed to read the labels carefully. See Table 3-8 for general recommendations.

Pharmacokinetics

After DHEA administration, approximately 50% of the dosage is absorbed.[226] DHEA undergoes first-pass metabolism and has an elimination half-life of 15 to 30 minutes. DHEA metabolism involves hepatic phase one and phase two reactions through esterification into fatty acids, transportation by lipoproteins,[227] and peripheral conversion in target tissues to estrogens and androgens. DHEA is weakly bound to sex hormone–binding globulin and albumin with negligible renal reabsorption; however, DHEAS is strongly bound to albumin and undergoes renal tubule reabsorption. Renal tubule reabsorption contributes to the high interindividual variation

in DHEAS levels[228] (see Table 3-6). DHEAS has an elimination half-life between 8 and 10 hours and, unlike other hormones, does not have a circadian pattern of production or release.[223]

Weight Loss

49. C.K., a 66-year-old male smoker with chronic stable angina, wants to take DHEA to lose weight. He is 5`6" tall and currently weighs 95.5 kg. C.K. has tried many diets but states that he cannot follow the dietary restrictions. His diet primarily consists of fast-food burgers and beer. C.K. does not exercise regularly, but he walks one to two times per week to catch the bus. His medications include enteric-coated aspirin 325 mg QD and atenolol (Tenormin) 50 mg QD. C.K. would like to know if DHEA is effective when used for weight loss.

Few studies have assessed the effects of DHEA on body fat in humans.[218,229,230] Each of these had an extremely small sample size (<10 subjects), used varying fat calibration techniques, and only one included obese men.[218] All patients received a total daily DHEA dose of 1,600 mg for 4 weeks. The greatest loss in body fat occurred in patients who were already lean at study entry; four of the five patients studied had a 31% decrease in body fat.[229] In normal men, DHEA had no effect on body mass or body fat.[230] However, in obese men, the results are less clear. Only two obese men displayed a reduction in weight, three had no change, and one patient had a slight increase in body weight.[218] Based on these studies, DHEA cannot be recommended for weight loss. C.K. is considered obese because his body mass index (BMI) is 34 (normal, 20 to 25) and he is >30% above his ideal body weight (IBW) (actual body weight, 95.5 kg; IBW, 63.8 kg). Therefore, until more information is available, C.K. should avoid using DHEA for

Table 3-7   Theoretical Basis of the Effects of DHEA[288]

Patients	Hormonal Environment		Effect of DHEA		Potential Outcome
	Estrogens	Androgens	Estrogenic	Androgenic	
Premenopausal women	High	Low	Decreases estradiol effect by binding competitively to estrogen receptor	Enhances androgenic effect on fat distribution and CVD, which are balanced by high estrogens	If DHEA is low, breast cancer risk is increased because estradiol effect is unopposed
Postmenopausal women	Low	Low	Binds to unoccupied estrogen receptors and enhances estradiol effects	Enhanced androgenic effect on fat distribution and CVD, which are less well balanced by low estrogen levels	If DHEA is high, both pathways are active with androgenic predominance: 1. Androgenic effects (central obesity, insulin resistance, risk for CVD) 2. Estradiol-like effect (increased risk for breast cancer)
Men	Low	High	Binds to unoccupied estrogen receptors and enhances estradiol effects	Negligible additional androgenic effect	If DHEA is high, estrogenic effect may offer protection against CVD

Reprinted with permission from Ebeling P, Koivisto VA. Physiological importance of dehydroepiandrosterone. Lancet 1994;343:1479. © The Lancet Ltd.
CVD, cardiovascular disease.

Table 3-8 DHEA: General Recommendations

- Because DHEA is a precursor hormone, women should avoid using DHEA during pregnancy and lactation

- Replacement doses are associated with few adverse effects but may depend on gender and menopausal status; if patients decide to replace low DHEA levels, they should start with the lowest tolerable DHEA dosage

- Patients should be informed that the hormonal protective effects of DHEA have not been clearly defined and have not been compared to standard pharmaceuticals

- The long-term safety and efficacy of DHEA has not been systematically studied; with long-term supplementation, endogenous regulation of DHEA may be adjusted to account for the excess hormone

- DHEA is not released from wild yam extracts

- The antioxidant properties of DHEA have not been applied in a clinical setting; it is unknown whether DHEA improves longevity or well-being

- The role of DHEA in diabetes has not been defined; patients should not use DHEA to help regulate their insulin or blood glucose levels

- There is no evidence to prove DHEA supplementation reverses age-related diseases, including cancer, cardiovascular disease, and Alzheimer's disease

- DHEA may have a role in improving the quality of life of patients with systemic lupus erythematosus, but side effects may limit routine use

- DHEA is not effective in preventing HIV disease progression

- DHEA drug interactions have not been formally studied

weight loss. He should try to increase his physical activity by walking daily and setting reasonable and attainable dietary goals. He also should meet with a dietician to learn how he can lower the fat and alcohol content in his diet.

DHEA Levels, Dose, and Side Effects

50. **P.R. is a 63-year-old man who recently discovered that his DHEAS level was lower than normal for his gender and age. He has heard that low levels are associated with accelerated aging, so he would like to take a DHEA supplement. However, a friend told him that large doses cause "female-like" side effects. P.R. has a 40 pack-year smoking history and currently smokes one pack a day. Given his smoking history, what dose of DHEA (if any) should P.R. use to replace his endogenous levels? How do replacement doses differ from pharmacologic doses with regard to their conversion to hormones in men and women? What are their side effects?**

Besides hereditary and gender differences, DHEA levels can be altered by smoking.[217] Although higher-than-normal DHEAS levels have been seen in young smokers, lower DHEAS levels occur in older smokers like P.R. Because DHEA and DHEAS levels decline with age, there is a popular belief that supplementing with DHEA may slow or reverse aging. DHEA has been used to augment normal endogenous levels at replacement doses and also has been used in much higher pharmacologic doses. Only a few studies have assessed

the effects of DHEA dose in men and women. Dose, study duration, patient population studied, and outcome parameters have varied greatly.

Replacement Dosing

Replacement doses, sufficient to replace the age-related decline, vary between men and women. Studies assessing the effects of replacement doses have used 25 to 50 mg administered once daily as lactose-based capsules or a micronized wax vegetable oil matrix.[216,231–233] One study used 40-mg sublingual tablets to avoid first-pass effects by the liver.[218] In general, women require 25 to 50 mg/day, whereas males require 25 to 100 mg/day to supplement endogenous levels for their respective age groups (see Table 3-6). Side effects associated with replacement doses are uncommon. Replacement doses of DHEA have been associated with an improved sense of well-being, which appear upon DHEA initiation and dissipate with continued use. A similar effect is commonly reported with corticosteroid (prednisone) administration.

Pharmacologic Dosing

Pharmacologic doses are much higher than replacement doses (1,600 mg versus 25 to 100 mg/day) and produce elevated levels of hormones that vary by gender and menopausal state. Men who took 1,600 mg of DHEA daily for 4 weeks had significant elevations of DHEA(S) levels, whereas other androgens were unaffected.[218,226,229,230] However, similar doses in postmenopausal women significantly elevated DHEA(S) levels as well as those of androstenedione, testosterone, and dihydrotestosterone.[226] Elevations in estrone and estradiol also increased. Because greater conversion to androgens and estrogens occurs, there is a greater risk for adverse effects. Adverse effects largely depend on gender and menopausal status (see Table 3-7).[234] Most often DHEA is converted to the hormone in deficit. Thus, women typically complain of masculinizing effects such as hirsutism, acne, and deepening of voice because androgens are produced. However, men may experience gynecomastia and breast tenderness. The effects of chronic pharmacologic dosing are unknown because they may induce effects not normally seen at physiologic levels.[231]

P.R.'s DHEA level of 250 ng/mL is lower than the normal for his gender and age (see Table 3-6), but he should be told that DHEAS levels vary greatly, that the level may have been depressed by smoking, and that his level may not necessarily mean he is at greater risk for accelerated aging. If P.R. still wishes to supplement his DHEAS levels, a dosage of 50 to 100 mg/day would be adequate. This replacement dose should not produce "female-like" effects associated with higher pharmacologic dosages.

Benign Prostatic Hyperplasia

51. **P.R. has an enlarged prostate. He has only mild symptoms of urinary hesitancy and is not taking any medications. Should he be concerned about prostate enlargement or prostate cancer while taking DHEA supplements?**

The role of DHEA replacement in BPH or prostate cancer has not been established, but there is some concern that DHEA may worsen BPH or prostate cancer. This is because prostate enlargement is caused by testosterone produced by the testicles and, to a lesser extent, by the adrenal glands. Because DHEA is a precursor hormone for both estrogen and testosterone, it may increase adrenal testosterone production. Previous studies found that in men, DHEA is preferentially converted to estrogen, with negligible conversion to testosterone.[218,229,230,231] More recent evidence suggests that replacement doses of DHEA in men result in a 10% increase in mean free testosterone levels 3 months into treatment.[235,236] It is unknown whether this elevation persists or whether a compensatory mechanism adjusts for this increase with continued DHEA treatment.

The effects of DHEA supplementation have not been studied in patients like P.R. with prostate enlargement. DHEA conversion to testosterone may contribute to prostate cell growth. Therefore, P.R. should avoid using DHEA. If he still feels strongly about using DHEA, P.R. should be informed of the risks and urged to undergo yearly digital rectal examinations and periodic PSA level measurements. These should be checked before initiating DHEA therapy and every 3 to 6 months thereafter. If P.R. develops symptoms suggestive of prostatic hypertrophy (urinary hesitancy, frequency, low urine volume, hematuria), he should discontinue DHEA and seek medical attention promptly.

Cancer

52. Will DHEA prevent certain types of cancers?

Advanced age and body weight have been associated with an increased risk of certain cancers, and because corresponding endogenous DHEAS levels are lower in these patient populations, some believe they can be used as a predictor for certain cancers. The relationship between endogenous DHEA levels and the development of prostate, bladder, gastric, and ovarian cancers is under study. DHEA levels were lower in patients who went on to develop bladder and gastric cancers.[237,238] In contrast, the risk for developing breast cancer was greater in postmenopausal women with elevated DHEA and DHEAS levels than in those with normal levels.[239] The opposite has been seen in premenopausal women in whom low serum DHEAS levels have been associated with increased risk of breast cancer.[240] One case–control study reported a greater risk for developing ovarian cancer in women with higher DHEAS levels.[241] Because the effects of DHEA supplementation on cancer risk have not been fully studied, patients who have been diagnosed with any type of cancer should avoid using DHEA until more information is known.

Wild Yams (Mexican Yams)

53. R.D. is a 48-year-old woman with Graves' hyperthyroidism that was treated with radioactive iodine (RAI) 8 years ago. She has been euthyroid on levothyroxine (Synthroid) 100 mcg daily for several years as evidenced by normal levels of thyroid-stimulating hormone (TSH) and FT₄. R.D.'s physical examination is normal and she has an intact uterus. She takes conjugated estrogens (Premarin) 0.625 mg QD and medroxyprogesterone (Provera) 2.5 mg QD continuously. The clerk at her local health food store told her that taking wild yams is a natural way to replace hormones because they are converted to DHEA "naturally." Are wild yams effective for hormone replacement therapy?

Wild yam extracts have been marketed as a natural way to supplement endogenous female hormones. Wild yams or Mexican yams are members of the *Dioscorea* species. The yam with the most abundant source of steroids is a Mexican yam derived from *Dioscorea floribunda*. Diosgenin, one of many steroid sapogenins that has been isolated from the Mexican yam, has been used to produce cortisone, estrogen, and progesterone derivatives commercially. Because *Dioscorea* is a steroid precursor, the endogenous conversion to DHEA in humans was measured. One study measured DHEAS levels in seven adults (six postmenopausal women, one man) ages 65 to 82 years after administration of *Dioscorea* extracts and DHEA.[242] Over the course of 9 weeks, patients sequentially received *Dioscorea* extracts (2, 4, and 8 pills daily), placebo, then 85 mg DHEA once daily. *Dioscorea* extracts (at all doses) had no effect on serum DHEAS levels, whereas DHEA supplements increased DHEAS levels significantly. Despite this finding, Dioscorea appeared to have hormonal effects because both DHEA and *Dioscorea* extracts reduced triglyceride and increased HDL-C levels to a statistically significant extent. Although DHEA increased HDL-C levels in this study, other studies have shown statistically significant decreases in HDL-C levels.[243] This is concerning because a decrease in HDL-C can contribute to heart disease in postmenopausal women.

There is some evidence that replacing DHEA (300 mg) 60 minutes before sexual activity may improve sexual arousal in postmenopausal women.[244] Although more research is needed, the mechanism of action may be related to small increases in testosterone, which may enhance libido and improve vaginal blood flow and lubrication. Wild yam extracts, however, have not been studied for this purpose.

In summary, there is no evidence supporting the claim that "natural" hormonal replacement with wild yam extracts is better than prescription versions of estrogen and progesterone. R.D. should be advised that there are no clinical studies on the long-term safety of these products, nor are there studies that have assessed the rate and amount of hormones generated from yam precursors. This is important because DHEAS levels apparently do not correspond to *Dioscorea* hormonal activity. Furthermore, natural products do not undergo the standardization and purification processes required of pharmaceutical grade products. Therefore, it is difficult to assess the amount of hormones released. The amount of protection afforded against osteoporosis also is unknown because dose-response relationships have not been established. Specifically, DHEA's effects on HDL-C levels are undesirable in postmenopausal women because low HDL-C levels can contribute to heart disease. Single dose DHEA shows some promise in helping improve sexual arousal before intercourse; however, long-term use in postmenopausal women should be discouraged.

Hormone Replacement

54. If R.D. decides to take wild yam extracts for "natural" hormone replacement, what side effects should she expect?

Five of seven patients who used high-dose *Dioscorea* extracts (8 pills/day) reported side effects, including headache, xerostomia, nausea, vomiting, and sleep difficulties.[242] However, patients who took lower doses (2 to 4 pills/day) reported no side effects. Because the dose of *Dioscorea* extracts has not been established, it is difficult to predict which side effects R.D. will experience. For example, *Dioscorea* extracts may not provide the same controlled amount of progesterone that R.D. was receiving with medroxyprogesterone. Therefore, because R.D. is still undergoing the climacteric, she should expect some breakthrough bleeding, especially because she was receiving continuous combined hormone replacement therapy. R.D. should be warned to look for headache, dry mouth, nausea, vomiting, and perhaps insomnia. If these side effects become bothersome, she should discontinue taking the product and schedule a follow-up visit with her primary care provider. R.D. also should be advised to increase her dietary intake of calcium through low-fat dairy products to prevent osteoporosis. If she cannot meet the dietary requirements, she should consider taking a calcium supplement that provides 1,200 mg of elemental calcium daily.

Antioxidant Properties

55. R.D. has heard that yams can also help her "live longer" because they are "antioxidants." Do wild yams (*Dioscorea* extracts) and DHEA have antioxidant properties? Are they equivalent?

Both DHEA and yam extracts have been evaluated for their antioxidant properties. In one study, DHEA and *Dioscorea* extracts reduced lipid peroxidation after 3 weeks, compared with placebo.[242] However, DHEA was significantly more effective than *Dioscorea* extracts. Antioxidants are promoted for longevity because free radical lipid peroxidation has been associated with aging, atherosclerosis, and various cancers. Endogenous antioxidants and free radical scavengers inhibit the formation of free radicals, but whether taking supplemental antioxidants will prevent tissue damage from free radicals is unclear. Thus, although wild yam extracts may have antioxidant effects, the beneficial effects on R.D.'s health, well-being, or longevity are not known.

Thyroid Effects

56. Could DHEA interfere with R.D.'s thyroid function?

Two studies have assessed the effect of DHEA supplementation on endogenous thyroid hormone levels,[226,230] and both used pharmacologic doses (1,600 mg once daily) for 4 weeks. Six postmenopausal women and eight men were enrolled. In men, no significant changes in TT_3 or TT_4 were observed, but a statistically significant decrease in thyroid-binding globulin (TBG) was seen in all six women studied, as was a slight decrease in TT_4. No patients reported clinical signs or symptoms of hypothyroidism or hyperthyroidism. These findings suggest that postmenopausal women are more susceptible to androgen-induced fluctuations in protein binding, specifically TBG capacity. Although the binding capacity of TBG decreased, free thyroid hormone levels did not change. Because these changes in TBG binding are transient and appear as laboratory interference, a change in R.D.'s levothyroxine dose is not necessary. Compensatory increases in levothyroxine clearance usually occur before clinical signs and symptoms of hyperthyroidism develop. In postmenopausal women, it is unlikely these effects will result in clinical or subclinical

hyperthyroidism. However, TSH and FT_4 should be checked once yearly during DHEA supplementation.

If R.D. decides to take DHEA supplements as hormone replacement therapy, she should be counseled on the signs and symptoms of hyperthyroidism, especially during DHEA therapy initiation. These include palpitations, chest pain, and heat intolerance, which are more likely to be prevalent at night or during exercise. She should see her primary care provider once yearly to measure TSH and FT_4 levels. R.D. also should inform her primary care provider that she is taking DHEA because she will need to discontinue the prescription estrogen and progesterone.

Aging

Alzheimer's Disease

57. E.B. is a 73-year-old woman complaining of increased memory problems over the past 2 years. She writes notes to herself but now forgets to look at them. She denies changes in sleep or eating habits, suicidal ideation, hallucinations, delusional thoughts, or symptoms of anxiety. She has no neurologic deficits and maintains the capacity for independent living; her Mini-Mental State Exam (MMSE) score is 26 (normal, >25). E.B.'s mother had Alzheimer's disease (AD) and lived 8 years after the diagnosis. She would like to try DHEA for her memory problems. Is there evidence that DHEA improves symptoms of or slows the progression of AD?

Aging is associated with physiologic changes that include increased body fat, decreased lean body mass, and reduced protein synthesis. Because DHEA and DHEAS levels decline with age,[221] some have promoted DHEA supplementation to reverse these age-related effects.

The role of DHEA in the progression of AD is controversial. The majority of research suggests low endogenous levels of DHEA and DHEAS correlate with dementia and AD.[245] The Rancho Bernardo study, one of the best designed trials, found no relationship between DHEAS levels and cognitive function in elderly patients.[246] Another well-designed study assessed the effects of aging on DHEAS levels in otherwise healthy elderly patients.[223] In men, there was a direct relationship between low DHEAS levels and self-appreciated poor health. In women, low levels were associated with symptoms of depression, dyspnea, and level of independence. Overall, age, gender, and poor subjective health were correlated with low DHEAS levels to a statistically significant degree. However, no associations were found between dementia and DHEAS levels in men or women. After 4 years, no statistically significant correlations were found between DHEAS levels and death from any cause in either men or women.

The research thus far does not support a correlation between DHEA synthesis or metabolism and AD. Furthermore, there is no evidence to prove DHEA supplementation improves symptoms or slows the progression of AD. Because E.B. is in the early stages of the disease, treatment with donepezil (Aricept) should be considered. Donepezil is a reversible acetylcholinesterase inhibitor indicated for patients with mild disease as defined by an MMSE score of 10 to 26. E.B. also should be evaluated for reversible causes of dementia and told about drugs that can induce or contribute to dementia.

Cardiovascular Effects

Background

DHEA may affect the synthesis of cholesterol and other lipids involved in atherogenesis. It is a noncompetitive inhibitor of glucose-6-phosphate dehydrogenase (G6PDH),[247] which is the rate-limiting enzyme in the production of nicotinamide adenine dinucleotide phosphate (NADPH). NADPH is a coenzyme involved in the synthesis of cholesterol, aldosterone, cortisol, and fatty acids. Based on these actions, exogenous DHEA supplementation has been advocated in both men and women to reduce the risk(s) for developing cardiovascular disease. No studies have evaluated the effect of exogenous DHEA supplementation in reducing the risks for cardiovascular disease.

Both high[248] and low[217] serum DHEAS levels have been associated with an increased risk of cardiovascular morbidity in men. In postmenopausal women, DHEAS levels are poor predictors of cardiovascular disease.[249] However, in postmenopausal women with diabetes, low DHEAS levels predicted ischemic heart disease–associated mortality.[250] Based on the current literature, DHEAS levels are poor predictors of cardiovascular morbidity or mortality in both men and women.

Lipids

58. A.B. is 38-year-old man who presents to the lipid clinic for a follow-up appointment. Three months ago, A.B.'s laboratory results were as follows: total cholesterol, 245 mg/dL (normal, <200 mg/dL); LDL-C, 169 mg/dL (normal, <130 mg/dL); and HDL-C, 23 mg/dL (normal, ≥60 mg/dL). Since this time, he has been following the National Cholesterol Education Program (NCEP) Step 1 diet, but he rarely exercises. A.B. denies smoking or using drugs of abuse. His mother is alive and well, and his 62-year-old father has had two acute myocardial infarctions, one 5 years ago and another last year. His father is currently awaiting coronary artery bypass surgery. A.B.'s BP is 138/88 mm Hg and his heart rate is 100 beats/min and regular. A.B.'s current fasting cholesterol values are as follows: total cholesterol, 216 mg/dL; LDL-C, 162 mg/dL; and HDL-C, 24 mg/dL. Currently, he takes no medications. A.B. read in the newspaper that DHEA could lower cholesterol. What should he know about DHEA and cholesterol?

The effects of DHEA on blood cholesterol levels are modest and variable.[218,226,229–233] Pharmacologic doses of DHEA in women seem to have the best results,[226] whereas some effects have been seen with lower replacement doses.[231–233] However, in men, the results are less clear. Only one study has evaluated the effects of replacement doses in men,[231] and there were no changes in lipid markers at 3 months. However, in one small study, pharmacologic doses resulted in statistically significant decreases in cholesterol values.[229] After 4 weeks, the five patients enrolled displayed a 7.1% reduction in total cholesterol and a 7.5% reduction in LDL-C. Other investigators using similar doses have failed to find similar reductions.[218,230] Variations in study design and patient population limit the clinical application of these results. Many of the studies had a small sample size (usually ≤17 patients) and subjects with other cardiovascular risk factors, such as family history of premature coronary heart disease (CHD), history of cigarette smoking, or evidence of hypertension, were not included or assessed at study entry.

Based on A.B.'s previous laboratory results, it appears that the dietary modifications have worked to lower his total cholesterol and LDL-C levels. Although A.B. has a family history of heart disease, he has only one risk factor for CHD, a low HDL-C. Because A.B.'s LDL-C has decreased from 169 to 162 mg/dL, drug therapy is not indicated at this time. Dietary modifications should be continued. He should begin some form of regular physical activity (See Chapter 13, Dyslipidemias, Atherosclerosis, and Coronary Heart Disease).

In summary, the role of DHEA in treating hypercholesterolemia is not defined. Based on the available studies in men, it appears that DHEA does not alter cholesterol regulation or synthesis. DHEA may have a role in decreasing total cholesterol in postmenopausal women. However, decreases in HDL-C make DHEA undesirable.

HIV

59. S.D., a 29-year-old man, was diagnosed with HIV 2 years ago, at which time his CD4+ cell count was 520 cells/mm³ (>1,200 cells/ mm³) with a viral load of 25,000 copies/mL (normal, undetectable). One year ago, his CD4+ cell count was 480 cells/mm³, with a viral load of 25,000 copies/mL. Today, his CD4+ cell count remains at 480 cells/mm³, and his viral load is undetectable. S.D. began a three-drug regimen last year consisting of lamivudine (Epivir) 150 mg BID, zidovudine (Retrovir) 200 mg TID, and ritonavir (Norvir) 600 mg BID. He states he adheres to his medication regimens. S.D. is asymptomatic and denies weight loss, but he read on the Internet that taking DHEA stabilizes CD4+ cell counts. What should S.D. know about the role of DHEA in HIV disease?

Animal studies suggest that DHEA supplementation affords protection against experimentally induced viral illness.[251] Other research demonstrates effects on T lymphocytes by improving IL-2 production and decreasing IL-4, IL-5, and IL-6 release.[252] These findings led investigators to examine the relationship between DHEA and the immune system. Low plasma DHEAS levels have been seen in patients with HIV and in those with AIDS.[253] Two studies in patients with HIV have demonstrated a relationship between declining DHEA levels and the progression to AIDS.[254,255] One study found that DHEA levels <180 ng/mL were an independent predictor for the progression to AIDS. This relationship persisted after correcting for age, hematocrit, and CD4+ cell counts.[254] Viral load measurements were not assessed or available at the time. However, DHEAS levels were not similarly predictive.

One open-label study evaluated DHEA tolerance in patients with HIV (CD4+ cell counts 250 to 600 cells/mm³). Patients were assigned to receive one of three DHEA regimens for 16 weeks: 250 mg three times daily, 500 mg three times daily, and 750 mg three times daily.[256] All patients reported adverse effects unrelated to dose. Some of these effects may have been related to HIV infection, DHEA exposure, or concomitant medications. The most common adverse effects reported were nasal congestion (39%), headache (35%), fatigue (29%), and nausea (26%). One patient receiving 2,250 mg DHEA reported insomnia that resolved on drug discontinuation and recurred on rechallenge. The 2,250-mg DHEA regimen was associated with a slower decline in CD4+ cell count than the 250-mg regimen; this effect was not statistically significant. A statistically significant improvement in lymphocyte response to cytomegalovirus antigen was observed at 8 weeks in patients receiving the 2,250-mg regimen. Although the study duration was short and sample size small, the authors concluded that low DHEA levels are associated with HIV disease progression. None of these studies assessed viral load measurements as a marker for disease progression.

The effects of DHEA on mood, fatigue, and depression have been studied in 32 HIV-positive patients.[257] After 12 weeks, oral mircronized DHEA (100 to 500 mg daily) improved mood by 50% as measured by the HAMD rating scale. Measures of fatigue and libido also improved in a majority of patients. Although this study had a high dropout rate and a high placebo response rate, the use of DHEA in improving mood and libido appears promising.

In summary, the studies evaluating DHEA supplementation on HIV progression have many limitations. The initial studies were small, enrolled only male patients, and did not use viral load measures to assess disease progression. Based on these limitations, it is difficult to assess the benefits of DHEA on CD4+ cell counts.

DHEA appears to have a positive effect in improving mood and possibly libido. Although there is limited evidence that DHEA is effective in HIV, it should not be excluded as an option. S.D. should discuss the benefits and risks of DHEA therapy with his primary care provider. Currently, there is no information regarding drug interactions between DHEA and protease inhibitors or the nucleoside analogs. Therefore, S.D. should be warned that DHEA therapy has not been systematically studied in clinical trials for its potential to cause nucleoside analog failure or inactivate protease inhibitors. He should be reminded that DHEA does not eradicate HIV. Because S.D.'s CD4+ cell count is stable and his viral load remains undetectable, DHEA therapy is not likely to improve the effect of his current antiviral regimen.

Dosing

60. Which DHEA dose is associated with the best improvement in CD4+ cell counts?

Only one study has assessed the effect of DHEA dose on HIV disease progression.[256] Daily doses of 750, 1,500, and 2,250 mg (in three divided doses) were used. The highest dosages, 750 mg three times daily, were associated with the lowest drop in CD4+ cell count, but none of the doses prevented disease progression. S.D. may respond better to this high-dose regimen than to the lower dosages. Recent studies have evaluated the effects of replacement doses (50 mg given once daily for 4 to 6 months) in both women and men with HIV.[258,259] Women reported improvements in energy, cognitive and physical functioning, emotional well-being, and health perception.[259] A modest increase in body weight and increased CD4+ cell counts also were seen in these women, but no one had a statistically significant decline in viral load. Although males reported improvements in well-being, no changes in CD4+ cell counts were observed. Because the optimal dosage of DHEA has not been determined, S.D. should be informed of the side effects associated with high-dose DHEA in

males such as gynecomastia, breast tenderness, nasal congestion, headache, fatigue, nausea, and insomnia. S.D. should continue taking all his medications and should keep all his follow-up appointments.

Drug Interactions

61. Will DHEA interact with S.D.'s other medications?

It is unknown whether DHEA interacts with protease inhibitors, nucleoside analogs, or other medications. There is evidence that DHEA does not interact with indinavir, nelfinavir, ritonavir, or saquinavir soft gels; however, pharmacokinetic studies have not been conducted.[257] Zidovudine may increase endogenous DHEA concentrations in patients with HIV, but the clinical implications of this effect relative to exogenous DHEA are unknown.[260] S.D. should monitor himself for symptoms of disease progression if he takes DHEA; if symptoms develop, he should stop taking DHEA and contact his primary care provider.

Systemic Lupus Erythematosus

62. T.M., a 28-year-old woman with systemic lupus erythematosus (SLE), is managed with prednisone 60 mg QD. Will DHEA supplementation improve her condition and decrease her reliance on corticosteroids?

Perhaps. DHEA supplementation has been used in patients with SLE, a condition associated with abnormal T-cell function and B-cell hyperactivity that leads to the production of autoantibodies. SLE also results in abnormal estrogen metabolism and decreased androgen, DHEA, and DHEAS levels.[261] The production of IL-2 from T lymphocytes is decreased and may be associated with symptoms of disease. These findings led investigators to assess the effects of DHEA on the SLE disease process. In vitro and in vivo data have shown that DHEA restores T-cell IL-2 production.[262,263] Studies in female patients with SLE have found lower DHEA and DHEAS levels for each patient in their respective age groups.[263] One study evaluated the effects of supplemental DHEA in 28 females with mild to moderate SLE.[264] After 3 months of therapy (200 mg/day), patients receiving placebo had significantly more frequent lupus flares as assessed by medical record reviews. Patients receiving DHEA were able to decrease their prednisone requirements but did not differ statistically from the placebo group. In an open-label study using similar DHEA dosing in patients with SLE of the same duration and severity, DHEA significantly reduced mean daily corticosteroid requirements.[265] Side effects included acneiform dermatitis, hirsutism, decreased menstrual blood flow, emotional changes, and weight gain.[264,265] The most recent study evaluated DHEA (200 mg/day) or placebo over 24 weeks in 119 women with SLE..[266] DHEA resulted in significantly fewer SLE flares and a greater improvement in overall symptoms. The most common side effects of DHEA included an increased incidence of acne and increased testosterone levels. Currently, DHEA is considered an orphan drug for the treatment of SLE in the United States. Various multicenter studies are underway to further define the role of DHEA in SLE therapy.

Diabetes

63. C.N., a 52-year-old man with a 20-year history of type 2 diabetes, presents to the outpatient clinic for a follow-up appointment. He developed peripheral neuropathy 5 years ago when he was not taking his medications but states that he is now very compliant. C.N. is currently taking metformin (Glucophage) 850 mg orally three times daily, amitriptyline (Elavil) 25 mg orally once nightly, and benazepril (Lotensin) 5 mg once daily. His home blood glucose readings have been between 160 and 180 mg/dL. Today his A1c is 5.2% (normal, 4 to 6%) and his fasting blood glucose is 140 mg/dL (normal, <126 mg/dL). C.N. read that DHEA helps regulate insulin levels, so eventually, he will not need to use metformin. Does DHEA alter insulin levels?

Many studies have assessed the relationship between insulin and endogenous DHEA(S) levels, but there are no consistent patterns. Both positive and negative relationships have been observed between insulin levels and DHEA(S) levels in obese and nonobese men and premenopausal women.[271] More research is needed to better define the relationship between insulin levels and endogenous production of DHEA(S).

DHEA Supplementation and Insulin Levels

Replacement doses (50 mg/day) and high dosages (1,600 mg/day) of DHEA may cause or contribute to insulin resistance in postmenopausal women, especially those with type 2 diabetes.[226] It is unknown if similar effects would be observed in men. The effects of DHEA on blood glucose levels require further study. Although C.N. should not expect DHEA to alter his blood glucose levels, he should continue to monitor his blood glucose as usual. His A1c is within normal limits, indicating good blood glucose control. DHEA has not been shown to decrease insulin or metformin requirements. Furthermore, the effects of DHEA supplementation on insulin response were seen only in postmenopausal women. C.N. should continue metformin therapy as indicated. More research is needed to assess the effects of exogenous DHEA on blood glucose control in male and female patients with type 2 diabetes mellitus. Currently, it cannot be recommended for blood glucose regulation.

GLUCOSAMINE

Background

Glucosamine has been promoted for use alone and in combination with chondroitin to treat and prevent osteoarthritis (OA). Glucosamine and chondroitin have been used in veterinary medicine for years. Glucosamine is said to increase cartilage formation, and chondroitin is commonly advocated as a product that decreases cartilage breakdown. Both products have been studied clinically as a way to prevent cartilage breakdown.

Human Cartilage

Human cartilage is a connective tissue composed of cartilage cells (chondrocytes) and the extracellular matrix. The extracellular matrix accounts for nearly 90% of articular cartilage[275] and is predominantly avascular. Chondrocyte nutrients and waste products are transported by diffusion through the blood supply of trabecular bone, blood, synovial fluid, and the perichondrium.[276] Chondrocyte nutrients help build the extracellular matrix.

The extracellular matrix of cartilage serves as the anchor for chondrocytes and imparts structural stability. Fibronectin, produced by fibroblasts, also is found within the extracellular matrix and is responsible for many cell repair processes. The extracellular matrix is a mesh of connective tissue that is composed of collagen, hyaluronic acid, and proteoglycans (PGs).

PGs are macromolecules composed of a protein core covalently linked to sulfated glucosaminoglycan (GAG) side chains. The PG structure resembles a "bottle brush" appearance. In articular cartilage, two types of GAGs are linked to the protein core: chondroitin sulfate and keratan sulfate. Hyaluronate serves as a link protein, which is bound to the PG subunit ionically (Fig. 3-1). The strength of articular cartilage largely depends on collagen, hyaluronate, and the GAGs of the PG aggregates (mostly chondroitin). Chondroitin imparts tensile strength, whereas PGs impart compressive strength. During cartilage synthesis, cations and water are bound to PG. This forms a viscous layer, which cushions and lubricates the joint.

Pharmacology

Glucosamine is an amino monosaccharide and is a product of glucose metabolism via the hexosamine pathway. Glucosamine is found in many human tissues and is a substrate for PG synthesis. Glucosamine is the rate-limiting step in GAG synthesis (Fig. 3-2). Based on in vitro data, glucosamine increases sulfate uptake and increases production of PG synthesis.[277] Exogenous glucosamine sulfate is taken into cells and enters the extracellular matrix through diffusion where it is incorporated into cartilage.[276] The sulfate salt component, as well as glucosamine, is necessary for the production of PG. Although the exact mechanism of glucosamine uptake has not been determined, PG channels have been suggested as a way of entry into the synovial fluid and chondrocytes.[276]

Osteoarthritis

Osteoarthritis (OA) is characterized by a loss of PGs and GAGs and an increase in cartilage degradation, leading to joint stiffness and decreased elasticity.[278] In early OA, GAG

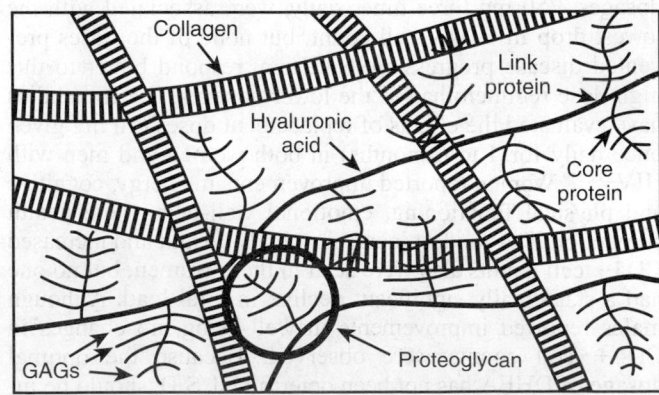

FIGURE 3-1 GAG and PG structures in human cartilage.

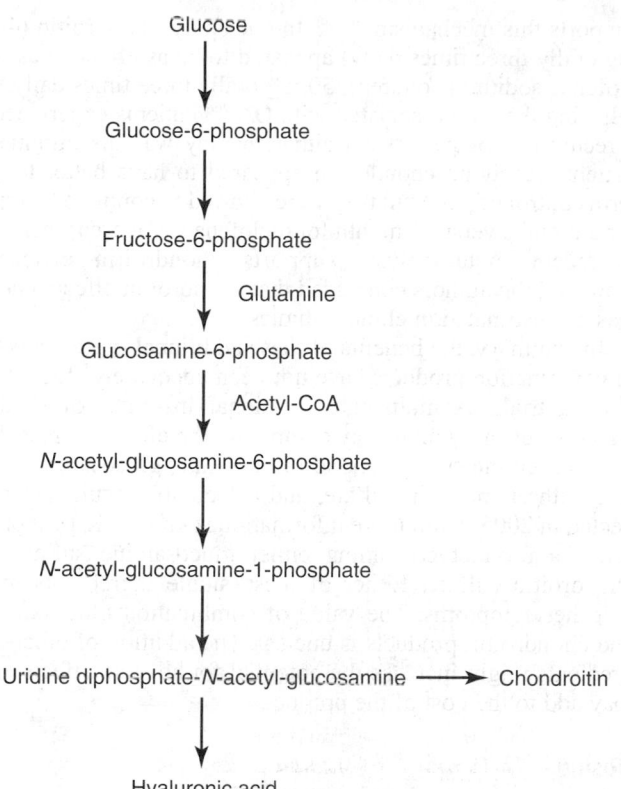

FIGURE 3-2 Biosynthesis of glucosamine, chondroitin, and hyaluronic acid.

synthesis increases.[279] PG aggregates, consisting of noncovalently linked PGs to a single monomer of hyaluronic acid, tend to be smaller and contain a lower proportion of PGs than that found in patients without OA.[280]

Pharmacokinetics

Approximately 26% of oral glucosamine is absorbed after first-pass metabolism.[281] It is distributed into tissues (kidneys, liver, articular cartilage) and incorporated into plasma proteins and other structures. The volume of distribution approaches 71 mL/kg after IV administration.[281] Unmetabolized and unbound glucosamine is predominantly eliminated in the urine. Unabsorbed glucosamine is largely eliminated by the fecal route. Although the exact amount has not been quantified, glucosamine is also metabolized to carbon dioxide and excreted through the lungs as expired air.[281]

64. K.E. is a 66-year-old obese woman with type 2 diabetes (managed with diet) who has had OA of the left knee for 10 years. She is 5'4" and weighs 95 kg (IBW, 55 kg). Five years ago, her knee pain responded to maximum doses of acetaminophen (Tylenol), but it has progressively worsened over the past 2 years. Radiographic examination of the left knee reveals osteophyte formation and articular space narrowing. K.E. is currently taking ibuprofen 400 mg TID, which provides only moderate relief of her pain. She would like to try glucosamine because a friend told her that it would help alleviate knee pain and increase her mobility. What is the clinical evidence for using glucosamine in osteoarthritis?

Glucosamine is commonly marketed as a cure for OA. Many poorly designed studies evaluating the safety and effi-

cacy of glucosamine for OA[282–291] have observed improved joint mobility. A recent meta-analysis found similar results but also noted that studies overestimated the beneficial effects.[292] Two well-designed, randomized, double-blind, placebo-controlled trials have shown improvements in symptom scores and pain after 2 to 3 months of glucosamine administration.[289,290] Both trials used once daily dosing of 1,500 mg glucosamine sulfate for 3 years. The Lequesne index, a tool used to measure pain, minimum walking distance, and movement limitation in activities of daily living, was used to measure efficacy. The Western Ontario and McMaster Universities knee osteoarthritis index (WOMAC) was used to assess severity of joint pain, stiffness, and physical function. Patients enrolled had similar baseline OA disease; mild to moderate severity as measured by radiograph and the Lequesne and WOMAC rating scales. Statistically significant improvements in symptoms and joint space narrowing were observed for patients receiving glucosamine sulfate. Improvements in joint space narrowing were observed at 1 year and continued to improve at 3 years. The patients receiving placebo experienced a progression of joint space narrowing and a worsening of symptom scores. In both studies, the use of rescue medications (e.g., acetaminophen, NSAIDs) was variable and inconsistent between the glucosamine and placebo groups. Interestingly, there was little correlation between structural joint improvements (as seen on radiograph) and symptom improvement. This finding is commonly accepted in the treatment of osteoarthritis; symptom relief can occur independently of structural changes. One comparative study assessed the effects of glucosamine against ibuprofen.[291] Patients were treated for unilateral OA of the knee for 8 weeks. Pain scores were significantly lower for those patients receiving ibuprofen at week 1; by week 8, glucosamine resulted in statistically improved pain scores as compared with ibuprofen. Ibuprofen resulted in fast-onset pain relief; glucosamine had a slower onset of action but maintained efficacy longer. Although these studies had design limitations, glucosamine may alleviate subjective pain and improve symptoms.

Therefore, K.E. should be advised that oral glucosamine may help to prevent the breakdown of cartilage and alleviate some of her pain long-term, but it will not cure OA. Glucosamine may take longer to work than ibuprofen, but the duration of pain relief may last longer. Weight loss and physical therapy should also improve her joint mobility.

Nonsteroidal Anti-Inflammatory Drug Combination Therapy

65. Can glucosamine be used in conjunction with NSAIDs to treat OA pain?

Combined glucosamine and NSAID therapy has not been studied, but due to the significant side effects associated with NSAIDs in elderly patients like K.E., the decision to use them should be based on her risks for GI bleeding or ulceration, renal function, and pain severity. Because the analgesic effects of glucosamine are not seen immediately,[289] combined use with ibuprofen may help alleviate acute pain. After 7 to 21 days, K.E. may consider discontinuing NSAID therapy while continuing glucosamine monotherapy. In any case, she should review her treatment decision with her primary care provider.

Product Selection

66. K.E. is determined to try glucosamine but is confused about which product to select because the ingredients vary. Which glucosamine product should K.E. use?

In the United States, glucosamine is widely available in grocery stores, health food stores, and pharmacies as an over-the-counter dietary supplement. Although glucosamine is predominantly derived from chitin, which is found in yeast, fungi, and marine invertebrates, it also is prepared synthetically. K.E. should use a synthetic product that lists the source of glucosamine on the label. People with shellfish allergies may wish to avoid products derived from chitin; there are no reports of cross-allergenicity with glucosamine sulfate. Many salts of glucosamine are available, including glucosamine sulfate, glucosamine hydrochloride, and glucosamine hydroiodide. Glucosamine sulfate is the preferred product because the sulfate salt is required for GAG synthesis and is the most widely studied.[277] The formulations of glucosamine sulfate that have been used in clinical trials are Dona, Viartril-S, or Xicil, all of which are manufactured by Rottapharm in Italy. Dona can be purchased directly from the manufacturer's Internet site. Glucosamine hydroiodide may be problematic in patients with undiagnosed thyroid disease or in those taking thioamides and therefore should be avoided. Glucosamine hydrochloride has been studied for OA knee pain for 3 months and was found to be ineffective in improving mobility and joint function as compared with placebo.[293] The only statistically significant improvements noted were in subjective pain relief and objective knee improvements on radiographic examination. Therefore, the value of glucosamine hydrochloride remains unknown. Many oral preparations also contain N-acetyl-glucosamine (NAG), which is a GAG intermediate. However, exogenous NAG is poorly used by cells and is thought to be a poor substrate for kinase phosphorylation, which is needed for GAG synthesis.[294] The role of NAG in preventing OA has not been determined.

Other ingredients added to glucosamine products include herbs, amino acids, sodium, selenium and potassium salts, zinc, copper, manganese, and vitamins. Some of these ingredients are added to make the product more attractive to consumers. Others are added because they are essential cofactors for GAG synthesis. For example, manganese is added because nutritional deficiencies have been associated with bone and joint malformations. Ascorbic acid is added because it is an essential cofactor for collagen synthesis and to ensure that collagen synthesis occurs at an effective rate.[295] There is no evidence, however, that these added ingredients are necessary in patients who eat a balanced diet. Sodium and potassium are added to increase glucosamine stability.

Chondroitin Sulfate

Dietary supplement manufacturers often combine chondroitin sulfate with glucosamine because it is thought to inhibit cartilage-destroying enzymes. Chondroitin sulfate is the most abundant GAG in articular cartilage and consists of repeating units of glucosamine and aminosugars. Whether chondroitin is absorbed intact from the GI tract remains controversial. Chondroitin is likely broken down into individual glucosamine monomers and absorbed via the GI tract. Clinical evidence

supports this mechanism.[296–298] In one study, chondroitin (400 mg orally three times daily) appeared to be as effective as diclofenac sodium (Voltaren), 50 mg orally three times daily, in relieving the pain associated with OA.[296] Patients experienced a recurrence of pain when either therapy was discontinued. Patients receiving chondroitin appeared to have better long-term control of pain, but they were allowed to continue therapy for 3 months versus 1 month for diclofenac (Voltaren) therapy. A recent meta-analysis supports chondroitin efficacy. However, the authors concluded that chondroitin effectiveness was overestimated in clinical studies.

In summary, the benefits of these additional ingredients or of combination products have not been adequately studied in clinical trials. A multicenter, National Institutes of Health study is currently underway comparing the effects of placebo to glucosamine sulfate, chondroitin sulfate, glucosamine sulfate with chondroitin sulfate, and celecoxib. Results are expected in 2005. Until more information is known, K.E. should select a product containing either glucosamine sulfate or chondroitin sulfate. Either of these single ingredients may help her symptoms. The value of combination glucosamine and chondroitin products is unclear. The addition of other ingredients might increase the potential for adverse effects and may add to the cost of the product.

Dosing

67. What is the most effective dose for glucosamine?

Dose-response studies have not been conducted. In clinical trials, glucosamine has been administered as either 500 mg given three times daily or 1500 mg given once daily with or without meals. If compliance is a concern, K.E. should consider taking 1500 mg once daily.

Adverse Drug Effects/Drug Interactions

68. K.E. has been experiencing stomach upset while taking ibuprofen. Will glucosamine cause stomach upset as well or other serious side effects? Are there any known drug interactions with glucosamine?

Although adverse effects of glucosamine have not been systematically studied, information can be gleaned from patient reports in four clinical trials[283,289–291] and one uncontrolled study.[285] Overall, glucosamine appears to be well tolerated and better tolerated than NSAIDs. The most commonly reported adverse symptoms involve the GI tract and include constipation, epigastric pain, tenderness, heartburn, diarrhea, and nausea.[283,284,289–291] Therefore, K.E. should be told that glucosamine is well tolerated compared with NSAIDs, but it also may produce symptoms of GI irritation. Taking glucosamine with food may prevent GI irritation. Because K.E. already is complaining of stomach upset while taking ibuprofen and is at high risk for GI bleeding secondary to NSAID use, she should be referred to her primary care provider for further evaluation before she adds glucosamine to her regimen.

It is unknown whether glucosamine administration can affect blood sugar. Animal studies suggest glucosamine increases blood glucose[299] and insulin resistance.[300] A recent human study in patients without diabetes suggests that glucosamine, when administered orally at regular doses (500 mg three times daily), increases fasting insulin levels.[301] In this study, blood glucose levels did not change. Glucosamine acts intracellularly and not extracellularly, which may explain why blood glucose levels were unaffected. In healthy volunteers, intravenous administration of glucosamine was not associated with insulin resistance.[302,303] The long-term effects of glucosamine sulfate on insulin resistance have not been adequately studied. Because K.E. has type 2 diabetes, it is possible that over time glucosamine may contribute to insulin resistance and worsen her blood glucose control. Until more information is available, patients like K.E. with diabetes mellitus or glucose intolerance who use glucosamine should monitor their blood sugar regularly. Although drug–drug interactions have not been formally evaluated, none have been reported to date.

SHARK CARTILAGE

Background

Shark cartilage has been advocated for many disorders, including cancer, psoriasis, diabetic retinopathy, neurovascular glaucoma, inflammation, Kaposi's sarcoma, and arthritic pain. It has also been said to have antimicrobial properties[304] and antioxidant effects,[305] neither of which is well studied. Shark cartilage is derived from the elastic cartilage found in the endoskeleton of sharks. The spiny dogfish shark (*Aqualus acanthias*) is the primary source of commercial shark cartilage products in the United States. Native shark cartilage contains three components: chondrocytes (cartilage cells), water, and an extracellular matrix. Shark cartilage dietary supplements contain various proteins including collagen, proteoglycans (PG), phospholipids, sterols, and a variety of minerals (calcium, phosphorus, sodium, magnesium, potassium, zinc, iron). Chondroitin-6-sulfate appears to be one of the primary PGs found in shark cartilage, although it is not known whether this is the active ingredient. Various angiogenesis inhibitors have been identified and extracted from native shark cartilage. It is unknown if these are present or active in commercially available shark cartilage supplements. The proposed antineoplastic activity of shark cartilage or its glycoprotein extracts is based on its ability to inhibit the proliferation of various animal and human cell types and to inhibit angiogenesis in vitro or in animal models. However, results have been inconsistent.[306–315] Angiogenesis, or the development of new blood vessels, is an important process in wound healing, building of the corpus luteum, embryonic development, and solid tumor growth and metastases.[316,317]

69. S.N., a 51-year-old woman, was recently diagnosed with stage III colon cancer. She has had two previous adenomatous polyps removed, and her recent colonoscopy revealed adenocarcinoma of the colon. S.N. recently watched a television news program that claimed shark cartilage is a cure for cancer. She is currently awaiting surgery and will be receiving adjuvant chemotherapy, fluorouracil (Adrucil), and levamisole (Ergamisol). She would like to start taking shark cartilage. Is shark cartilage effective as an anticancer agent?

There is limited information on the effectiveness of shark cartilage or its extracts in the prevention or cure of cancer. Shark cartilage is available in liquid, powder, tablets, and a variety of unique capsule formulations. Each formulation of shark cartilage requires unique processing. Two common methods of processing shark cartilage involve creating an aqueous extract or a dry powder formulation. Among the commercially available shark cartilage dietary supplements, little information is provided to consumers about the type of extract or the extent of the processing. This is important since dosing recommendations vary among the various formulations and limited data exist regarding an effective dose. One aqueous extract derived from shark cartilage (Neovastat AE-941) has been studied in a Phase II renal cell carcinoma study.[318] In this study, Neovastat was given to 22 patients as a twice daily oral preparation. The study began using 60 mL/day; subsequently, some patients received a higher dose, 240 mL/day, based on tolerability. The only responders included two patients receiving 240 mL/day who survived 14 months compared with 7 months for those taking 60 mL/day. Although this study suggests Neovastat had a favorable effect, the degree of improvement was minimal. Furthermore, the open label design makes these findings difficult to interpret. In one preliminary 16-week study in Cuba, only 3 of 29 patients with cancer responded to shark cartilage supplements. Although the findings were not published, the National Cancer Institute reviewed the data and concluded that the results were "incomplete and unimpressive."[319] One unpublished clinical trial evaluated the effect of 80 to 100 g of shark cartilage powder self-administered orally or rectally daily in 70 subjects with cancer (type of cancer and other concomitant therapy unspecified). After 8 weeks, 10 of 20 patients who had been evaluated reported an improvement in quality of life, pain, and appetite; 4 showed partial or complete responses to therapy.[319]

Another study described the use of shark cartilage in 60 adult patients with advanced cancers (16 breast, 16 colon, 14 lung, 8 prostate, 3 lymphoma, 1 brain, 2 unknown) that were resistant to conventional therapies and had objective measurable disease.[320] Life expectancy was greater than or equal to 12 weeks and none of the patients had received recent or concomitant cancer chemotherapy. All patients received shark cartilage 1 g/kg per day given in three divided doses. After 12 weeks, 47 patients were evaluated for efficacy and toxicity. Five patients dropped out because of GI side effects. Quality-of-life scores did not improve after 12 weeks of therapy, and no complete or partial responses were noted. Based on these findings, shark cartilage did not alter disease progression.

The current scientific literature does not support the use of commercially available shark cartilage for the treatment of any type of cancer, including colon cancer. If S.N. decides to use shark cartilage in combination with her chemotherapy, she should be told that it is not a cancer cure. Furthermore, the effect of shark cartilage on the activity of any other drugs she may be taking or the course of her disease is unknown.

Product Selection, Dosage, and Administration

70. If S.N. chooses to use shark cartilage, what type of product should she use and how should she be advised to take it?

There is no evidence that one formulation or source of shark cartilage is superior to another. However, the product selected should not have been exposed to excessive heat during the manufacturing process because this may denature any active proteins.[321,322] This information can be obtained only by contacting the manufacturer directly, since dietary supplement labels often do not disclose the specific formulation type.

Clinically, shark cartilage has been administered orally and rectally. The most commonly recommended oral dose is 1 g/kg per day.[320,321] The GI absorption of shark cartilage has not been studied, and skeptics suggest that substantial oral absorption of its macromolecular constituents (40% proteins; 5% to 20% GAGs) is unlikely because they will be destroyed by GI enzymes. However, others argue that the active ingredient is unknown and one GAG, chondroitin, has been shown to undergo significant intestinal absorption.[323] For these reasons, some advocate using products that have been pulverized to the finest particle size.[321] To avert enzymatic degradation, maximize absorption, and minimize GI irritation, shark cartilage also has been administered as a retention enema for 25 minutes. The recommended mixture is 20 g of bulk shark cartilage powder diluted in 20 mL of tepid water. In the lay press, "colonic cleansing" has been recommended before the retention enema to clear the bowel of fecal material and to enhance absorption. This practice is dangerous, can cause dehydration, and should not be used.

Adverse Effects

71. Are there any adverse effects associated with this product? Does S.N. have any contraindications to its use?

S.N. should be warned to watch for GI upset, the most common dose-limiting side effect of shark cartilage.[321] Shark cartilage may also contain calcium; therefore, patients taking calcium supplements along with shark cartilage may need to adjust their calcium supplementation. Two cases of hepatitis also have been reported.[324] In one case, the patient was also taking oral comfrey, which is known to be hepatotoxic. Use of other hepatotoxic agents, including alcohol and prescription medications, were not described. While taking shark cartilage, S.N. should report any changes in stool or urine color, flu-like symptoms, and fatigue. Because the cause of these effects is unknown, S.N. should discontinue use and discard any product that has changed in color, odor, or consistency.

S.N. does not have any contraindications to the use of this product. These include situations in which neovascularization is crucial for tissue growth and repair, such as fetal development (pregnancy), wound healing, and normal growth (infants and children). Drug interactions with shark cartilage have not been identified or reported. Shark cartilage should be used cautiously in patients receiving anticoagulants because certain proteins isolated from shark cartilage resemble the structure of heparin and other endogenous human proteins that enhance the effects of tissue plasminogen activator.[325]

ZINC

Background

Zinc is a trace element that serves as an enzymatic cofactor and protects cell membranes from lysis through complement activation and toxin release.[326] Many salt forms of zinc are available, including acetate, gluconate, gluconate-glycine, ascorbate, aspartate, orotate, sulfate, and chloride. Each of these formulations varies in solubility, palatability, and zinc

ion (Zn^{2+}) release characteristics. Zn^{2+} in zinc acetate (ZA), zinc gluconate (ZG), and zinc gluconate-glycine (ZGG) has been studied clinically for its role in treating the common cold.

Mechanism of Action

The mechanism of action of Zn^{2+} ions is controversial but may involve a combination of several actions. In vitro studies have shown that Zn^{2+} ions interfere with the formation of rhinoviral capsid proteins, preventing viral replication.[327–329] Zn^{2+} ions also block binding of human rhinovirus to intracellular adhesion molecule-1 (ICAM-I), which subsequently interferes with the inflammatory process.[330] ICAM-1, an immunoglobulin present on the surface of endothelial and epithelial cells, serves as a receptor for the human rhinovirus. However, Zn^{2+} ions do not seem to affect mature rhinoviruses.[328] Other research suggests that Zn^{2+} induces interferon-γ production in human white blood cell cultures[331]. At physiologic serum concentrations, zinc has been shown to inhibit histamine release from mast cells and basophils.[332] An astringent or drying effect on mucus-producing goblet cells may contribute to the efficacy of Zn^{2+} in treating the common cold.[333] Finally, Zn^{2+} ions have been shown to inhibit depolarization and impulse transmission in the trigeminal and facial nerves, leading to cold symptom relief in as rapidly as 1 to 3 minutes.[334]

The role for zinc lozenges in the symptomatic relief of the common cold is based on Zn^{2+} release characteristics. Once released into the oral and nasal passages, Zn^{2+} ions are at supraphysiologic concentrations, causing an osmotic gradient.[330] This gradient is thought to cause the transfer of Zn^{2+} ions from the mouth to the nasal and mucosal passages, sometimes referred to as a biologic closed electric circuit (BCEC), where they prevent rhinoviral binding and activation.[330,335] The Zn^{2+} cation appears to be the most effective form of zinc for the common cold because it may interact with the electronegative cell surfaces in the oropharyngeal cavity. The administration of zinc products that release neutral or negatively charged Zn^{2+} has been associated with a worsening of symptoms.[336,337] Neutral zinc may decrease transport through the BCEC, and negatively charged zinc may be repelled by mucosal cell surfaces.

Common Cold

The discovery that zinc may help treat the common cold occurred in 1979. A 3-year-old girl with acute lymphocytic leukemia suffering from a cold was taking ZG tablets to help stimulate lymphocyte responses after chemotherapy. Instead of swallowing the tablet whole, she let it dissolve in her mouth. The next day, her cold symptoms were gone.[338] This finding led researchers to begin studying ZG for the treatment and prevention of the common cold.[339,340]

Many studies have been conducted on the effects of zinc and the common cold (Table 3-9). These studies have generated controversy and have received a great deal of scrutiny. In addition to study design flaws, much of the criticism involves limitations in the nature of common cold. Study design flaws include poor placebo matching (blinding), lack of randomization information and power analysis, small sample size, variations in dosage, frequency of administration, time of first

Table 3-9 Summary of Clinical Trials: Zinc and the Common Cold

Reference/Study Design	Sample Size	Patient Population	Duration of Symptoms	Dose/Excipient(s)	Initiation/Duration of Treatment	Outcome
Eby 1984[339] R*, DB, PC	n = 65 ZG = 37 P = 28	Community acquired (autumn)	≤3 days	Adults: 46 mg initially, then 23 mg Q 2 hr while awake Max: 276 mg/day Children (≤27 kg): 11.5 mg Q 2 hr while awake Max: 69 mg/day	Within 3 days/until symptom free for 6 hr	At 7 days, 86% zinc-treated patients reported no symptoms vs. 46% of the placebo-treated patients Differences were significant Average duration of cold symptoms, 3.9 days for zinc group vs. 10.8 days for the placebo group
Al-Nakib 1987[340] R*, DB, PC	PS n = 57 ZG = 29 P = 28 TS n = 12 ZG = 6 P = 6	HRV-2 inoculation	Not applicable	PS: Adults: 23 mg Q 2 hr while awake Max: 276 mg/day TS: Adults: 23 mg Q 2 hr while awake Max: 276 mg/day	PS: 24 hr before inoculation; continued for 3.5 days after inoculation TS: 6 days	PS: ZG = 6/29 developed colds P = 8/28 developed colds Not statistically significant TS: ZG = 6/12 developed colds P = 6/12 developed colds Zinc reduced mean daily symptom scores compared with placebo; statistically significant on days 4 and 5
Farr 1987[336] R*, DB, PC	T1: n = 32 ZG = 16 P = 16 T2: n = 41 ZG = 21 P = 20	T1: RV-39 inoculation T2: RV-13 inoculation	Not applicable	T1:Adults: 46 mg initially, then 23 mg Q 2 hr while awake Max: 184 mg/day (Citric acid) T2:Adults: 23 mg Q 2 hr while awake Max: 184 mg/day (Citric acid)	T1: 36 hr after inoculation; continued for 5 days T2: 2 hr after inoculation; continued for 7 days	T1: No statistically significant differences in viral shedding T2: No statistically significant differences in frequency, severity, and duration of symptoms
Douglas 1987[337] R*, DB, PC	n = 55 ZA = 35 P = 35	Community acquired (season not stated)	Two symptoms for 1 day or one symptom for 2 days	Adults: 10 mg Q 2 hr while awake Max: 60–80 mg/day (Tartaric acid)	Duration 3–6 days	No reduction in symptoms
Smith 1989[344a] R*, DB, PC	n = 110 ZG = 57 P = 53	Community acquired (spring)	Not stated	Adults: 4 lozenges (11.5 mg each) initially then 2 Q 2 hr while awake (Mannitol/sorbitol)	Duration 7 days or 24 hr after symptom disappearance	No statistically significant differences in duration of symptoms; days 4 and 7 showed statistically significant improvements in subjective symptoms with ZA, small change in clinical significance
Weisman 1990[44] R, DB, PC	n = 130 ZG = 61 P = 69	Community acquired (spring and winter)	At symptom onset	Adults: 1 lozenge (4.5 mg) Q 1–1.5 hr while awake Max: 45 mg/day	Duration of cold up to 10 days	No statistically significant differences in symptom duration or severity

Table 3-9 Summary of Clinical Trials: Zinc and the Common Cold—cont'd

Reference Study Design	Sample Size	Patient Population	Duration of Symptoms	Dose/Excipient(s)	Initiation/Duration of Treatment	Outcome
Godfrey 1992[335] R*, DB, PC	n = 73 ZGG = 35 P = 38	Community acquired (season not stated)	≤2 days	Adults: One 23.7-mg lozenge Q 2 hr while awake Max: 189.6 mg/day	Duration of cold/complete elimination of symptoms	ZGG resulted in significant reduction of symptom severity compared to placebo by day 7 Average duration of cold symptoms was significantly less; 1.27 days less than normal with ZGG than placebo ZGG started after day 1 of symptoms resulted in a shorter duration and significantly lessened severity of symptoms than if started on day 2
Mossad 1996[348] R, DB, PC	n = 99 ZGG = 49 P = 50	Community acquired (autumn)	≤24 hr	Adults: 13.3 mg Q 2 hr while awake	Duration of cold symptoms	Median time to symptom resolution was 7.6 days in the placebo group compared with 4.4 days for the ZGG group; differences were significant ZGG-treated patients had statistically significant improvements in any nasal symptom
Macknin 1998[358] R, DB, PC	n = 249 ZGG = 117 P = 122	Community acquired (winter)	≤24 hr	Children (grades 1–6): 10 mg 5 times per day Children (grades 7–12): 10 mg 6 times per day	Symptom resolution for 6 hr	Time to any or all symptom resolution did not differ between groups
Prasad 2000[341] R, DB, PC	n = 48 ZA = 25 P = 23	Community acquired (year-round)	≤24 hr	Adults: 12.8 mg every 2–3 hours while awake	Duration of cold symptoms	Mean time to symptom resolution was 8.1 days in the placebo group compared to 4.5 days for the ZA group Mean duration of cough and nasal discharge was significantly shorter for ZA than placebo
Turner 2000[342] R, DB, PC	Study 1: n = 281 ZG = 68 ZA = 72 ZA = 68	Community acquired (year-round)	≤36 hr	Adults: ZG: 13.3 mg ZA: 5 mg ZA: 11.5 mg Every 2–3 hr while awake Max: 6/day	Until symptoms resolved up to 14 days	No difference in the duration of illness for any group No difference in severity of cold symptoms for any group
	Study 2: n = 273 ZG = 69 ZA = 66 ZA = 70 P = 71	Inoculated with RV-39	24 hr after challenge if symptoms present	Adults: ZG: 13.3 mg ZA: 5 mg ZA: 11.5 mg Every 2–3 hr while awake Max: 6/day		Duration of illness for zinc gluconate was 2.5 days compared to 3.5 days for placebo No difference in the duration of illness for zinc acetate doses None of the zinc groups had any effect on symptom severity

CO, crossover; DB, double-blind; HRV-2, human rhinovirus 2; P, placebo; PC, placebo-controlled; PS, prophylactic study; R, random allocation; R*, random allocation and selection; TS, therapeutic study; ZA, zinc acetate; ZG, zinc gluconate; ZGG, zinc gluconate-glycine; T1, treatment group 1; T2, treatment group 2.

dose, varying patient populations, lack of patient follow-up, and disparity in excipients or flavoring agents used. Other drawbacks that limit the applicability of the results involve a lack in documentation of rhinovirus infection, variations in the time of year studied, variations in location of study, differences in inoculum, and concomitant medication use.

Meta-Analysis Review

Two meta-analyses reviewed the clinical trials using zinc lozenges for the common cold.[343] The studies considered for review in the first meta-analysis included those listed in Table 3-9. After excluding the two studies evaluating experimentally induced colds,[336,340] the overall odds ratio for the incidence of any cold symptom at 1 week was 0.50. Patients taking zinc lozenges were 50% less likely to have any cold symptoms at 1 week compared with placebo. One study[344] used a smaller zinc dose of 4.5 mg. When this study was excluded from the analysis, the odds ratio decreased to 0.37, indicating a 37% chance of any cold symptom at 1 week with ZG administration. The authors then excluded studies that used excipients or formulations that prevent Zn^{2+} ion release (citric acid, tartaric acid, mannitol, and sorbitol). The odds ratio after exclusion and reanalysis decreased to 0.32, indicating a 32% chance of having any cold symptom with zinc lozenges at week 1. When this meta-analysis was reanalyzed using better methodology, a similar result was found, an odds ratio of 0.52.[343] These similar findings demonstrate the significant study design and formulation variability in the clinical trials. There are many variables that can affect zinc efficacy. Among these, patients should be counseled about variations in dose and zinc lozenge formulations.

72. C.D. is a 32-year-old woman suffering from a "cold." She complains of a sore throat, runny nose, and nasal stuffiness that began yesterday and has worsened since. Today, she developed watery eyes and sneezing. She is taking pseudoephedrine tablets (30 mg Q 8 hr PRN) for her nasal stuffiness. She is not immunocompromised and states that she does not have any other medical problems. She denies headaches, nausea, vomiting, cough, or myalgias and fever. An oral temperature taken at home is 98.0°F (37°C). She would like to try zinc lozenges for her cold symptoms. Are zinc lozenges appropriate for this patient?

Although many viruses are associated with the common cold, rhinovirus is involved in 30% to 50% of community-acquired colds.[345,346] C.D.'s symptoms began yesterday and have worsened today. The rapid onset is consistent with rhinovirus infections because the majority of viral replication is complete 1 day before symptom onset.[347] Peak symptoms usually appear 2 to 3 days after infection. C.D. is not complaining of headache, sinus pain, fever, fatigue, or myalgias, symptoms that are typically associated with influenza or respiratory syncytial virus. These symptoms usually develop more slowly over the course of ≥5 days. C.D. should see an improvement in her symptoms within 1 to 2 weeks because the common cold is self-limiting. C.D.'s symptoms began yesterday, so she is still a candidate for zinc therapy. In studies that have documented efficacy, improvements in cold symptoms have been seen when zinc therapy is started within 1 to 2 days from the start of symptoms.[335,339,348] C.D. states she wants rapid relief of her cold symptoms. Zinc may help relieve these symptoms,

but the onset of relief varies. In clinical trials, zinc therapy appeared to shorten the subjective duration of respiratory symptoms by 1 to 2 days. Remind C.D. that zinc lozenges are not a cure for the common cold. They also do not replace rest, proper nutrition, and hydration.

Product Selection and Dosing

73. C.D. now would like to know which product to select. Many formulations of zinc are available. What should C.D. know about zinc dosing and administration for the common cold?

Various zinc formulations have been used to deliver Zn^{2+} including zinc lozenges and nasal gels delivered as nasal sprays.

Clinical trials have used oral ZA, ZG, and ZGG, but adequate study blinding has been a problem because zinc lozenges have a characteristic taste that is difficult to mask. Various excipients and fillers have been used to overcome the flavor: citrate, tartaric acid, and mannitol–sorbitol mixtures. These products resulted in a tightly bound zinc complex, as measured by high stability constants, preventing the release of Zn^{2+}.[330] Based on its theoretical Zn^{2+} release characteristics, ZGG was studied. Some research suggests ZGG releases approximately 90% to 93% of the available Zn^{2+} in the mouth,[349] whereas other investigators have found that ZGG does not release any Zn^{2+} in the mouth at physiologic pH as measured by zinc ion availability (ZIA).[350] The ZIA method was developed to measure the amount of Zn^{2+} released under physiologic conditions in the mouth and oropharyngeal areas.[350] Based on this principle, the ZIA values were estimated for each of the formulations used in clinical trials. ZIA values varied based on rate of lozenge dissolution, dosage, and excipients used. ZIA values do not correspond to statistically significant treatment outcomes or to statistically significant changes in the duration of common colds. The clinical relevance of this method is controversial and is currently being evaluated.

Four randomized, double-blind, placebo-controlled trials have examined the effects of zinc gluconate nasal gel on the duration and severity of common cold symptoms.[351–354] Three studies have used the same formulation called Zicam. One study inoculated healthy volunteers with the rhinovirus,[353] and the other two studies evaluated efficacy in naturally acquired colds. All patients were instructed to begin using the spray within 24 to 48 hours of the onset of cold symptoms. They were further instructed to spray one dose into each nostril every 4 hours for as long as they experienced cold symptoms. In all but one study, zinc nasal gel significantly reduced the duration of cold symptoms. The average symptom duration was 2 to 4 days in the zinc group versus 6 to 9 days in the placebo. Side effects were reported equally in the zinc and placebo groups and included a slight tingling or burning sensation. Other side effects included nasal tenderness, dry nose, dry mouth, dysgeusia, and epistaxis.

Another similar trial used a nasal spray containing 0.12% zinc (as zinc sulfate heptahydrate).[354] Patients were instructed to administer two inhalations into each nostril four times daily until the symptoms resolved up to a maximum of 14 days. After the treatment period, there were no differences in the time to symptom resolution or cold duration; however, the zinc group did have a lower symptom score compared to placebo. The efficacy of zinc nasal spray appears similar to oral zinc lozenges, although zinc lozenges have been studied to a greater extent than zinc nasal spray. More research is needed to determine the best zinc formulation and method of administration in the common cold. Currently, both oral lozenges and nasal spray appear equally effective.

In summary, C.D. should select a zinc formulation that has been shown to release Zn^{2+} readily in the mouth and oropharyngeal areas, but it is currently unclear which of the zinc products can best accomplish this. Oral ZGG, ZG, and ZA as well as nasal sprays seem to be somewhat effective. C.D. should select a product that she finds the most palatable, convenient, and affordable.

Dosage

The commercially available zinc nasal spray (Zicam) has been administered as one spray in each nostril four times daily while awake. All zinc lozenges studied have been administered every 2 hours while awake. Although the most effective ZGG oral dose has not been established, 13.3-mg lozenges were used in clinical trials. C.D. may benefit from taking one 13.3-mg ZGG lozenge every 2 hours while awake. A higher ZGG dosage may be used, but may be associated with poor palatability. If C.D. chooses to take a ZA formulation, she should select a product with at least 10 mg of ZA per lozenge. If she prefers to take a ZG formulation, each lozenge should contain at least 23 mg of elemental zinc. For any zinc product selected, C.D. should let the lozenges dissolve completely in her mouth without chewing or swallowing them. C.D. should continue taking the lozenges every 2 hours while awake for the duration of her cold symptoms. Most clinical studies have continued Zicam for up to 10 days and zinc lozenge therapy from 5 to 10 days or until symptoms have completely resolved. C.D. should be reminded that neither zinc nasal spray nor zinc lozenges are a cure for the common cold. If she does not see an improvement in her symptoms after 10 days or if she develops a fever, purulent sputum, vomiting, or diarrhea, she should stop taking the zinc product and seek medical care.

Adverse Effects

74. What are the side effects of zinc lozenges? What should C.D. expect?

The most common side effects associated with zinc lozenges are related to poor palatability, often resulting in poor adherence and sometimes discontinuation. Other common side effects include nausea, taste disturbances, and mouth irritation. Vomiting, diarrhea, mouth sores, and stomach distress have also been reported. These symptoms are more likely to occur with higher doses of zinc (23 mg every 2 hours).[336,337,339] One acute overdose of ZG resulted in nausea and vomiting and an elevated serum zinc level.[355] Despite a total ingestion of 4.2 g, no caustic effects were observed. If C.D. develops nausea, she should try taking the lozenges after a meal.

Long-Term Safety

75. C.D. returns to the pharmacy 1 month later. She would like to take zinc lozenges again to treat another cold. Is it safe for C.D. to reinitiate zinc lozenges? What are the long-term concerns associated with zinc?

In clinical trials, the average duration of therapy for zinc lozenges has varied between 5 and 10 days or until symptom resolution. Zinc lozenges should be used only for colds of short duration. Currently, there is no information documenting the degree of systemic absorption, resistance to treatment, or the cumulative effects of zinc lozenges. Because the amount of elemental zinc absorbed from zinc lozenges has not been measured, the consequences of long-term use are unclear. Studies of elemental zinc supplementation at oral dosages of 150 mg twice daily for 6 weeks did not have adverse consequences.[356] However, with chronic use, oral zinc has resulted in copper and other nutrient imbalances because zinc is an effective copper chelator.[357] C.D. may begin another course of zinc therapy if she follows the same treatment recommendations mentioned earlier and does not exceed the dosing recommendations.

Pregnancy and Lactation

76. The following year C.D. wants to know if she can safely take zinc lozenges for her cold if she is pregnant. What should C.D. know about the safety of zinc lozenges during pregnancy or lactation?

Women who are pregnant or nursing should avoid zinc lozenges because subjects who were pregnant or lactating were excluded from study enrollment. C.D. should attempt to manage her cold symptoms without medications if possible. A humidifier may help her congestion and adequate hydration is especially important.

Efficacy in Children

77. L.P. is a 5-year-old girl who has caught a cold from her brother. L.P.'s mother wants to give her child zinc lozenges. Has the efficacy of zinc lozenges been evaluated in children?

Only two studies to date have assessed the value of zinc lozenges in children.[339,358] Dosing in these trials was estimated based on the empiric adult dose. For children weighing <27 kg, a dose of 11.5 mg (as ZG) was given every 2 hours while awake.[339] ZGG doses were estimated based on average body surface area and corresponding year in school (at the expected age). Children in school grades one to six received 10 mg ZGG five times per day. Children in school grades 7 to 12 received 10 mg six times per day.[358] Unfortunately, variations in both the formulation and the dose produced conflicting results. The 11.5-mg ZG lozenge, although higher in dose, resulted in a higher incidence of withdrawals because of taste disturbances and poor mucosal tolerability. The ZGG lozenges were better tolerated but did not shorten the duration of cold symptoms in children. In children, lozenge flavor is especially important in ensuring medication adherence. Macknin and colleagues attempted to characterize the amount of time missed from school because of colds.[358] Although children taking zinc lozenges returned to school sooner than those taking placebo, this difference was not statistically significant. Because a dose-response relationship in children has not been established, dosing of zinc lozenges in children is empiric; adverse effects are similar for both children and adults.

Various formulations of zinc specifically marketed to children are now available. These formulations include zinc gluconate bubble gum, zinc lollipops and sugar-free zinc lozenges. None of these formulations have been specifically studied in children for the relief of the common cold and should not be recommended. L.P.'s mother should be advised to ensure that L.P. gets adequate hydration and nutrition and to monitor her temperature. She may achieve symptomatic relief with pediatric over-the-counter cough and cold preparations.

Zinc Deficiency

78. Can zinc lozenges be used to supplement the normal dietary intake of zinc?

Zinc is an essential component in hundreds of cellular and enzymatic processes. The recommended dietary allowance for adult males is 15 mg.[359] Some researchers suspect that zinc lozenges correct an underlying zinc deficiency and therefore strengthen the immune response. In developing countries, zinc deficiencies have been documented in both children and adults.[360] In the United States, zinc deficiencies have been described in the elderly and in premenopausal women.[361,362] Many of the clinical manifestations of zinc deficiency (growth retardation, poor appetite, mental lethargy, delayed wound healing, susceptibility to infection) are reversible after supplementation. Therapeutic zinc supplementation at dosages of 150 mg/day for 1 to 3 months reverses these effects. The amount of elemental zinc delivered in a 7-day course of zinc lozenges given at the maximum recommended dose is about 1.9 g, but because it is unknown how much of the dose is absorbed systemically, they should not be used to correct nutritional deficiencies. The average U.S. diet provides 10 to 15 mg of zinc.[363] Patients should eat a balanced diet containing foods rich in zinc: red meats, eggs, whole grains, legumes, oysters, and other shellfish.[364] Otherwise, a multiple vitamin with minerals should be adequate to prevent zinc deficiency.

Allergic Rhinitis

79. S.L. is a 38-year-old man who read on the Internet that zinc lozenges alleviate the symptoms of allergic rhinitis. S.L. knows that zinc has been studied for the common cold to relieve nasal congestion and rhinitis. Currently, he is taking loratadine (Claritin) 10 mg PO QD. Should S.L. take zinc lozenges for his allergic rhinitis symptoms?

Some patients enrolled in the clinical trials for the common cold experienced "antiallergic effects" after zinc lozenge administration,[334,335] but there are no studies that have evaluated this effect in people with allergic rhinitis. However, some literature suggests that Zn^{2+} interferes with the inflammatory process by inhibiting leukocyte migration. The expression of ICAM-1, an adhesion molecule, is increased during an allergic response, and its expression has been correlated with an increased migration of neutrophils and eosinophils.[334] Because Zn^{2+} can prevent ICAM-1 expression, it may therefore inhibit the inflammatory process; Zn^{2+} also may have antihistaminic effects.[332] If S.L. decides to take zinc lozenges for his allergic rhinitis, he should be told that Zn^{2+} has antihistaminic properties. Although the degree of systemic antihistaminic effects has not been measured clinically, S.L. should be made aware of possible additive effects with his antihistamine.[334] Symptoms to look for include excessive dryness and irritation of the oral and nasal passages and headache. Because there is no clinical information on the use of zinc lozenges for allergic rhinitis, it cannot be recommended.

MELATONIN

Background

Melatonin is an endogenous hormone that is secreted by the pineal gland, located at the base of the brain. Melatonin secretion is primarily controlled by daylight and darkness and corresponds to typical sleep–wake hours. Darkness stimulates melatonin release. Secretion increases progressively after the onset of darkness, usually between 9 PM and 4 AM; peak melatonin levels occur between 2 AM and 4 AM.

Melatonin has received orphan drug status to regulate the sleep cycle in blind patients who have no light perception.[365] In the United States, it is sold as a dietary supplement as 0.1-, 0.3-, 1-, 5-, and 10-mg oral tablets or capsules in immediate and various sustained-release formulations. Synthetic formulations of melatonin are available and should be used exclusively. Animal-derived or human-derived products carry a risk for viral transmission, contamination, and variable potency. Melatonin has been used for jet lag, insomnia, aging, depression, reproduction, HIV, and a variety of cancers. Other uses include cluster headache prophylaxis, use in night-shift workers, and in children. Melatonin is currently being investigated for use in children undergoing computed tomography (CT) scans and in children with developmental disorders. Many studies evaluating the effects of melatonin are limited by small sample size, incomplete information, and inadequate laboratory monitoring. In addition, short treatment duration and variable dosing schedules make treatment recommendations difficult. Many treatment recommendations are based on pharmacologic principles, rather than clinical evidence.

Pharmacokinetics

The effects of several medications on melatonin levels have been studied, as have the pharmacokinetics of endogenous and exogenous melatonin (Table 3-10 and Table 3-11). After administration of an 80 mg oral dose, melatonin levels peaked between 60 and 150 minutes and returned to normal in 8 to 19 hours. Melatonin disposition is characterized by a rapid distribution phase followed by an elimination phase. The initial half-life is estimated to be 2 minutes, and the elimination half-life is 20 to 50 minutes.[366] Other research has shown that doses of 0.05, 0.5, and 5 mg have mean elimination half-lives of 65, 43, and 70 minutes, respectively.[367,368]

Endogenous melatonin is metabolized in the liver to 6-hydroxy-melatonin and excreted as sulfate and glucuronide conjugates.[366] In 22 patients with liver cirrhosis, endogenous melatonin serum levels were significantly elevated compared with age-matched controls.[369] A positive correlation between total bilirubin and daytime melatonin level was also seen.[369] As expected, the elimination half-life of exogenous melatonin increased from 44 to 97 minutes, on average, in people with liver cirrhosis.[370] Competition with bilirubin for elimination, decreased liver blood flow, or decreased activity of the enzyme 6-β-hydroxylase may contribute to these observations as well.[369] Other research has suggested that the endogenous production rate of melatonin appears to be reduced in patients with liver cirrhosis.[370]

Table 3-10 The Effect of Various Drugs on Endogenous Melatonin secretion

Drug Name	Reference	Direction of Change
NSAIDs	Murphy et al.[a]	↓
Fluvoxamine	Skene et al.[b]	↑
Desipramine	Farney et al.[c] Skene et al.[c]	↑
Fluoxetine	Childs et al.[d]	↓
Tryptophan	Namboodiri et al.[e]	↑
Corticotropin-releasing hormone (CRH)	Kellner[f]	↓
Sodium valproate	Childs et al.[d]	↓
Clonidine	Kennedy et al.[g]	—
Yohimbine	Kennedy et al.[g]	—
Atenolol	Cowen et al.[h]	↓
Propranolol	Rommel and Demisch[i] Vaughan et al.[j]	↓
Scopolamine	Vaughan et al.[j]	↓
Isoproterenol	Vaughan et al.[j]	↓
Zolpidem	Copinschi et al.[k]	—
Pyridoxine	Luboshitzky et al.[l]	—

[a]Murphy PJ et al. Nonsteroidal anti-inflammatory drugs alter body temperature and suppress melatonin in humans. Physiol Beh 1996; 59:133.
[b]Skene DJ et al. Comparison of the effects of acute fluvoxamine and desipramine administration on melatonin and cortisol production in humans. Br J Clin Pharmacol 1994;37:181.
[c]Farney C et al. Acute treatment with desipramine stimulates melatonin and 6-suphatoxy melatonin production in man. Br J Clin Pharmacol 1986;22:73.
[d]Childs PA et al. Effect of fluoxetine on melatonin in patients with seasonal affective disorder and matched controls. Br J Psychiatry 1995;166:196.
[e]Namboodiri MA et al. 5-hydroxyptophan elevates serum melatonin. Science 1983;221:659.
[f]Kellner M et al. Corticotropin-releasing hormone inhibits melatonin secretion in healthy volunteers: a potential link to low-melatonin syndrome in depression? Neuroendocrinology 1997;65:284.
[g]Kennedy SH et al. Melatonin responses to clonidine and yohimbine challenges. J Psychiatry Neurosci 1995;20:297.
[h]Cowen PJ et al. Atenolol reduces plasma melatonin concentration in man. Br J Clin Pharmacol 1983;15:579.
[i]Rommel T, Demisch L. Influence on chronic beta-adrenoreceptor blocker treatment on melatonin secretion and sleep quality in patients with essential hypertension. J Neural Transm Gen Sect 1994;95:39.
[j]Vaughan GM et al. Nocturnal elevation of plasma melatonin and urinary 5-hydroxyindoleacetic acid in young men: attempts at modification by brief changes in environment lighting and sleep and by autonomic drugs. J Clin Endocrinol Metab 1976;42:752.
[k]Copinschi G et al. Effects of bedtime administration of zolpidem on circadian and sleep-related hormonal profiles in normal women. Sleep 1995;18:417.
[l]Luboshitzky R et al. The effect of pyridoxine administration on melatonin secretion in normal men. Neuroendocrinol Lett 2002;23:213.

Table 3-11 Mean Nocturnal Levels of Circulating Melatonin

Age	Mean Melatonin Levels
First 6 mo of life	27.3 pg/mL (0.12 nmol/L)
1–3 yr	329.5 pg/mL (1.43 nmol/L)
15–20 yr	62.5 pg/mL (0.27 nmol/L)
70–90 yr	29.2 pg/mL (0.13 nmol/L)

The oral bioavailability of melatonin ranges between 40% and 70% for dosages that vary from 2.5 to 100 mg. Food may enhance the absorption somewhat, resulting in higher mean plasma levels compared with those achieved when taken in the fasting state.[370]

Jet Lag (Rapid Time Zone Change)

Transmeridian air travel results in dysregulation of the sleep–wake cycle until the circadian secretion of melatonin adjusts to the new time zone (2 to 14 days). Adaptation is generally more difficult or slower for older patients when traveling eastward and when multiple time zones are crossed. The most common symptoms of jet lag include GI disturbances and insomnia, particularly daytime sleepiness and frequent awakenings during the night. Maximizing exposure to daylight can enhance symptom recovery.[371]

80. **S.T., a 33-year-old female flight attendant, complains of sleep disturbances, loss of mental alertness, and daytime drowsiness. Every 2 weeks, she travels from Los Angeles, California, to London, England, and on to Auckland, New Zealand. A friend recommended melatonin. How should S.T. manage her symptoms? Can melatonin help?**

S.T. is experiencing the classic symptoms of rapid and multiple time zone changes, which have caused an abrupt shift in her sleep–wake cycle. Usually, time to adjust to the new time zone and proper sleep hygiene is the only treatment necessary. However, because S.T. is a flight attendant and has to repeat this schedule on a regular basis, her body has little time to adapt and she is likely to suffer from jet lag symptoms on a more long-term basis.

Clinical trials have evaluated 5 to 8 mg of immediate-release (IR) melatonin for jet lag.[372–376] Although these studies included a small number of participants, patients reported subjective improvements in symptoms, including decreased daytime fatigue, normal sleep patterns, energy, alertness, and mood. Subjects who took 5 mg IR melatonin up to 3 days before departure seemed to have a worse recovery of jet lag symptoms (decreased energy and alertness) than those who began taking the medication on arrival in the new time zone. This difference was not statistically significant. The largest study assessed the effects of melatonin in 257 patients traveling across six time zones.[377] Subjects were randomized to receive placebo or one of three melatonin regimens. Melatonin was administered as a 0.5 mg at bedtime, 5 mg at bedtime, or 0.5 mg on a "shifting schedule." The shifting schedule was designed to mimic the circadian release of melatonin throughout the sleep–wake cycle; one dose was taken on the evening of departure and then at 1 hour earlier each night for 6 days. By day 6, the melatonin dose corresponded to the natural melatonin peak time. No differences were observed at all time points among patients receiving any melatonin dosage or placebo. No statistical differences were observed in total sleep time, napping, sleep onset, or other symptoms. Melatonin possesses some hypnotic effects, which may help S.T. However, improvement in jet lag symptoms seems to be more closely related to resynchronization by regular light–dark stimuli. Therefore, S.T. should also maximize her exposure to daylight and implement proper sleep hygiene techniques, which include going to bed at the same time each night and avoiding caffeine and daytime naps.

The optimal dose and timing of melatonin administration have not been determined, but S.T. may benefit from 5 mg of the IR formulation beginning on the evening of departure and then for the next 1 to 3 days after arrival at the destination.

Although melatonin is relatively well tolerated, she should be advised to watch for daytime drowsiness, tachycardia, dysthymia, and headache.[372–375,378] One case of acute psychosis, one case of retrograde amnesia, and two cases of melatonin-induced erythematous plaques have been reported.[379–381] Because melatonin can cause drowsiness, S.T. should use caution when performing tasks that require full alertness 30 minutes to 2 hours after a dose and she should avoid alcohol or other CNS depressants. The long-term effects of melatonin administration have not been studied.

81. **S.T. is trying to become pregnant. Is it safe for her to continue taking melatonin now or when she becomes pregnant? Should S.T. take melatonin while breast-feeding?**

Melatonin has been shown to inhibit ovulation when administered in combination with a progestin. Therefore, S.T. should avoid taking melatonin while trying to conceive because high dosages (75 to 300 mg/day) may inhibit ovulation.[382] Although it is unknown whether lower dosages (0.5 to 5 mg daily) can alter conception or pose a threat to the fetus, she should avoid taking any drugs while trying to become pregnant and during her pregnancy. Instead, she should try to control her jet lag symptoms through sleep hygiene.

S.T. also should avoid taking melatonin while breast-feeding because it may suppress prolactin secretion and diminish the production of breast milk.[383]

Insomnia

82. **T.X. is a 75-year-old woman who complains of insomnia and daytime fatigue. On further questioning, it becomes clear that T.X. falls asleep early (around 9 PM) and wakes up at about the same time each morning (6 AM). However, she wakes up two to three times each night and has difficulty getting back to sleep. Will melatonin help?**

Insomnia is a subjective awareness of inappropriate sleep. Patients may complain of difficulty falling asleep (sleep onset), staying asleep, sleep maintenance (as in T.X.'s case), or arising too early (early morning awakening). Melatonin has been studied in the treatment of various sleep disorders, including delayed sleep-phase syndrome (DSPS) and insomnia. Many studies have documented the hypnotic effect of melatonin[384] in improving sleep onset, duration, and quality when administered to healthy volunteers.[384–387] Increases in rapid eye movement (REM) sleep also have been documented.[384] One study demonstrated that peak hypnotic effects vary based on the time of day melatonin is ingested, suggesting that light is an important factor for efficacy. Melatonin 5 mg orally caused peak hypnotic effects within 3 hours when taken at noontime compared to 1 hour when taken at 9 PM.[384]

Five clinical studies have assessed the effect of oral melatonin in patients with insomnia or DSPS (Table 3-12). Improvements in the quality of sleep,[385,388] both in sleep onset and duration,[368,389,390] have been seen. However, these studies are limited by small sample size, inadequate monitoring, and poor study design. Dosing, patient age, timing of drug administration, randomization, study duration, and type of monitoring have varied greatly. Many of the clinical studies failed to establish a relationship between low endogenous melatonin levels and insomnia at study onset.[385,388–390] In addition, the cause of the sleep disorder is not often defined,[388–390] is not stated,[385] or is confounded by other disease states. Some patients with DSPS, for example, also had a diagnosis of depression,[389] and sleep disturbances often subside in the population once antidepressant therapy is initiated.[391] Larger studies are needed to determine the effect of patient age, dosage, duration of therapy, and sleep disorder etiology on melatonin efficacy.

Insomnia in the Elderly

As illustrated by T.X., sleep maintenance is the most prevalent sleep-related disorder in patients older than 65 years of age,[368] occurring in approximately 30% of the elderly population. Sleep-onset insomnia is less common (19%), followed by early morning awakening (18.8%).[368] Because melatonin serum levels can be low in elderly patients who suffer from insomnia, some have theorized that use of a sustained-release formulation will correct the low levels and prevent sleep maintenance insomnia. Although elderly patients taking either 0.5-mg sustained-release or IR products experienced significant improvements in sleep onset, the sustained-release formulation did not improve total sleep time. In fact, the effectiveness of melatonin administration on improving total sleep time (sleep maintenance) has been inconsistent. Therefore, it is unlikely that either formulation of melatonin can improve sleep maintenance insomnia. Despite this evidence and because there are few risks associated with its use, T.X. can try the lowest dose of melatonin at bedtime to see if it will maintain her sleep. The dosage can be gradually escalated to 5 mg.

83. **R.R. is a 28-year-old male medical student who has been having trouble falling asleep for the past week. He attributes his insomnia to stress because he has to take his medical licensing examination in 2 weeks. He wants to know if melatonin will help him get to sleep without feeling "hung-over" the next day. Will melatonin help?**

Melatonin has not been systematically studied in people with insomnia caused by stress, even though it is a common etiology. R.R. wants to achieve adequate rest but also wants to avoid the "hang-over" effects associated with antihistamines contained in over-the-counter sleep medications or prescription sedative-hypnotics. R.R. will likely benefit from melatonin because it has been shown to improve sleep onset. Because he does not experience early morning awakenings, an IR formulation of melatonin should be sufficient. IR melatonin has a short half-life and has not been associated with significant daytime drowsiness or a "hang-over" effect. R.R. should start with the lowest effective dose, 0.3 mg, if possible. If he has no response in 30 to 60 minutes, he may take a repeat dose as needed. Although melatonin is considered relatively safe with few dose-related side effects, using the minimal effective dose is best. Melatonin should only be used 30 minutes before the desired bedtime. There is some evidence, however, that up to 6 months of continuous melatonin use may decrease semen quality in otherwise healthy males. If R.R. is planning to start a family, he may wish to avoid using

Table 3-12 Select Studies Evaluating Oral Melatonin Supplementation on Insomnia or Delayed-Sleep Phase Syndrome

Author/Study Design	Sample Size	Sleep Disorder	Mean Age of Patients (yr)	Dose	Time of Administration	Duration	Outcome
Dahlitz et al.[a] R*, DB, PC	n = 8	DSPS	35	5 mg	22:00	4 wk	Improved sleep onset; Earlier wake-up time
Oldani et al.[b] NR, OL	n = 6	DSPS	31	5 mg	17:00–19:00	1 mo	Improved sleep onset; Earlier wake-up time
Wurtman and Zhdanova[c] R*, PC	n = 9	Insomnia	51–78 range	0.3 mg	30 min before bedtime	3 days	Improved sleep onset; Reduced nightly awakenings; Improved subjective sleep quality; No increase in morning sleepiness
Haimov[d] R*, DB, PC	n = 26	Insomnia	73	2 mg IR; 2 mg SR	2 hr before bedtime	1 wk to 2 mo (variable)	Improved sleep onset with IR; Improved quality and duration of sleep with SR form
Garfinkel et al.[e] R*, CO	n = 12	Insomnia	76	2 mg SR	Nightly	3 wk	Improved quality of sleep; No improvement in total sleep time
James et al.[f] R, DB, PC, CO	n = 10	Insomnia	33	1 mg IR; 5 mg IR	Nightly	3 wk	Improved perceived quality of sleep
Hughes et al.[g] DB, PC, CO	n = 14	Insomnia	57–79 range	0.5 mg IR; placebo; 0.5 mg SR; placebo; placebo; 0.5 mg IR; placebo; placebo	Bedtime; 4 hr later; Bedtime; 4 hr later; Bedtime; 4 hr later; Bedtime; 4 hr later	2 wk with each treatment	Melatonin in all treatment groups shortened sleep latency (sleep onset) and increased the average sleep period time; Total sleep time and wake time was not statistically improved with melatonin
Serfaty et al.[h] R*, DB, PC, CO	n = 44	Dementia with sleep disturbance	>65	6 mg SR	At bedtime	2 wk	No effect of total sleep time, number of awakenings, sleep efficiency
Zhdanova et al.[i] R, DB, PC	n = 15	Insomnia	>50	0.1 mg; 0.3 mg; 3 mg	30 min before bedtime	1 wk	0.1 mg and 0.3 mg dose restored sleep efficiency; 3 mg dose restored sleep efficiency and maintained high melatonin levels throughout the day
Kayumov et al.[j] R, DB, PC, CO	n = 22	DSPS	30–35	5 mg	19:00–21:00	4 wk	Improved sleep onset; No change in total sleep time

[a]Dahlitz M et al. Delayed phase syndrome response to melatonin. Lancet 1991;337:1121.
[b]Oldani A et al. Melatonin and delayed sleep phase syndrome; ambulatory polygraphic evaluation. Sleep Rhythms 1994;6:132.
[c]Wurtman RJ, Zhdanova I. Improvement of sleep quality by melatonin. Lancet 1995;346:1491.
[d]Haimov I et al. Melatonin replacement therapy of elderly insomniacs. Sleep 1995;18:598.
[e]Garfinkel D et al. Improvement of sleep quality in elderly people by controlled-release melatonin. Lancet 1995;346:541.
[f]James SP et al. Melatonin administration in insomnia. Neuropsychopharmacology 1990;3:19.
[g]Hughes RJ et al. The role of melatonin and circadian phase in age-related sleep-maintenance insomnia: assessment in a clinical trial of melatonin replacement. Sleep 1998;21:52.
[h]Serfaty M et al. Double blind randomized placebo controlled trial of low dose melatonin for sleep disorders in dementia. Int J Geriatr Psychiatry 2002;17:1120.
[i]Zhdanova IV et al. Melatonin treatment for age-related insomnia. J Clin Endocrino/Metab 2001;86:4727.
[j]Kayumov L et al. A randomized, double blind, placebo-controlled crossover study of the effect of exogenous melatonin on delayed sleep phase syndrome. Psychosom Med 2001;63:40.
CO, crossover; DB, double blind; DSPS, delayed sleep phase syndrome; IR, immediate-release formulation; NR, non-randomized; OL, open label; PC, placebo controlled; R, random selection and random allocation to treatment group; R*, random allocation; SR, sustained-release formulation.

melatonin. Rather, R.R. should try to follow proper sleep hygiene techniques. For example, he should avoid staying up all night studying, and he should try to maximize his exposure to daylight while awake.

84. P.B. is a 35-year-old man with AIDS. He is currently taking zidovudine (Retrovir), indinavir (Crixivan), and lamivudine (Epivir). His CD4+ cell counts have been between 300 and 400 cells/mm³, and his viral load is undetectable. P.B. would like to know if melatonin can augment his current three-drug regimen. What are melatonin's effects on the immune system, if any?

The lay press is replete with information suggesting that melatonin has beneficial effects in people with HIV. These effects include enhancement of the immune system and protection against AZT toxicity and the AIDS-related wasting syndrome. None of these claims are supported by clinical trials in healthy subjects or subjects who are HIV-positive, but in vitro and animal studies suggest that melatonin may affect the immune response.[392–394] For example, melatonin may stimulate the production of IL-4 from bone marrow T-helper cells and granulocyte-macrophage colony-stimulating factor from stromal cells.[392,393] IL-4 is partly responsible for inducing proliferation of T and B lymphocytes. Thus, it is not known whether melatonin will alter the course of P.B.'s HIV infection or prolong his life, and at this point, it would be difficult to evaluate because his viral load is undetectable. However, there are no data showing that melatonin interferes with any of P.B.'s medications. Therefore, if he feels strongly about taking melatonin, he may do so, provided he continues his follow-up care and continues to take his other medications as prescribed. Empiric melatonin doses that have been recommended for patients with AIDS range from 20 to 30 mg once nightly.[395]

Patients who are HIV-positive but who have not developed AIDS have taken 10 to 20 mg once nightly.

Anticancer Effects

85. J.T. is a 47-year-old woman who currently is taking tamoxifen for breast cancer. She recently read that melatonin may have antitumor effects. What evidence exists for this claim? Would melatonin be effective in her case?

The antitumor effects of melatonin have been studied in vitro[396–398] and in small clinical trials involving patients with metastatic breast cancer, malignant melanoma, and glioblastoma.[399–402] In all these cancers, some beneficial effect has been observed, which may be related to melatonin's immune modulating or antioxidant effects. With regard to breast cancer, in vitro studies have shown that melatonin decreases estrogen-binding capacity and the expression of estrogen receptors in the MCF-7 breast cancer cell line[396]; it also inhibits the growth of epithelial breast cancer cells.[403] In a clinical trial, patients with metastatic breast cancer refractory to tamoxifen displayed a slower progression of disease when given melatonin than patients receiving tamoxifen alone, regardless of estrogen-receptor status.[400] Melatonin also may lessen the cytotoxicity associated with chemotherapy or radiation therapy.[402] Nonetheless, more study is needed to better define the effects of melatonin based on the severity and type of cancer as well as on duration of disease. Thus, melatonin may have some beneficial effects in J.T.'s case, but she should add this therapy only in consultation with her oncologist, who is in the best position to evaluate its effects on her disease progression. Dosages of 20 to 40 mg/day have been used.

REFERENCES

1. Eisenberg DM et al. Trends in alternative medicine use in the United States, 1990–1997. JAMA 1998;280:569.
2. Balluz LS et al. Vitamin and mineral supplement use in the United States: results from the third national health and nutrition examination survey. Arch Fam Med 2000;9:258.
3. Blendon RJ et al. American's views on the use and regulation of dietary supplements. Arch Intern Med 2001;161:805.
4. Kaufman DW et al. Recent patterns of medication use in the ambulatory adult population of the United States: the Sloan survey. JAMA 2002;287:337.
5. Astin JA. Why patients use alternative medicine: results of a national study. JAMA 1998;279:1548.
6. Blumenthal et al, eds. Herbal Medicine: Expanded German Commission E Monographs. Integrative Medicine Communications, 2000.
7. Schulz V et al. Rational phytotherapy: a physician's guide to herbal medicine. Berlin, NY: Springer-Verlag, 2001.
8. Dietary Supplement Health and Education Act of 1994. 103rd Congress, 2nd session report 103-410, January 25, 1994.
9. Wichtl M. General part. In: Bisset NG, ed. Herbal Drugs and Phytopharmaceuticals: A Handbook for Practice on a Scientific Basis. Stuttgart: Medpharm Scientific Publishers; Boca Raton, FL: CRC Press, 1994:11.
10. Marcus DM, Grollman AP. Botanical medicines – the need for new regulations. N Engl J Med 2002;347:2073.
11. Ernst E. Harmless herbs? A review of the recent literature. Am J Med 1998;104:170.
12. De Smet PAGM. Herbal remedies. N Engl J Med 2002;347:2046.
13. Brustbauer R, Wenisch C. Bradycardic atrial fibrillation after consuming herbal tea. Dtsch Med Wochenschr 1997;122(30):930.
14. Ernst E, Coon JT. Heavy metals in traditional Chinese medicines: a systematic review. Clin Pharmacol Ther 2001;70(6):497.
15. Ernst E. Heavy metals in traditional Indian remedies. Eur J Clin Pharmacol 2002;57:891.
16. Blackburn WD Jr. Eosinophilia myalgia syndrome. Semin Arthritis Rheum 1997;26(6):781.
17. Ernst E. Adulteration of Chinese herbal medicines with synthetic drugs: a systematic review. J Int Med 2002;252:107.
18. Bent S et al. The relative safety of ephedra compared with other herbal products. Ann Intern Med 2003;138(6):468.
19. Tyler VE. What pharmacists should know about herbal remedies. J Am Pharm Assoc 1996;NS36(1):29.
20. Rode D. Comfrey toxicity revisited. Trends Pharmacol Sci 2002;23(11):497.
21. Polymeros D et al. Acute cholestatic hepatitis caused by Teucrium polium (golden germander) with transient appearance of antimitochondrial antibody. J Clin Gastroenterol 2002;34(1):100.
22. Shad JA et al. Acute hepatitis after ingestion of herbs. S Med J 1999;92(11);1095.
23. Chan TY. Incidence of herb-induced aconite poisoning in Hong Kong: impact of publicity measures to promote awareness among the herbalists and the public. Drug Saf 2002;25(11):823.
24. Russmann S et al. Kava hepatotoxicity. Ann Intern Med 2001;135(1):68.
25. Anderson IB et al. Pennyroyal toxicity: measurement of toxic metabolite levels in two cases and review of the literature. Ann Intern Med 1996;124:726.
26. McRae CA et al. Hepatitis associated with Chinese herbs. Eur J Gastroenterol Hepatol 2002;14:559.
27. Leung R et al. Royal Jelly consumption and hypersensitivity in the community. Clin Exp Allergy 1997;27(3):333.
28. Lewis J. Esophageal and small bowel obstruction from guar gum-containing "diet pills": analysis of 26 cases reported to the Food and Drug Administration. Am J Gastroenterol 1992;87(10):1424.
29. Amagase H et al. Intake of garlic and it's bioactive components. J Nutr 2001;131:955S.
30. Lawson LD, Wang ZJ. Low allicin release from garlic supplements: a major problem due to the sensitivities of allinase activity. J Agric Food Chem 2001;49(5):2592.
31. Harenberg J et al. Effect of dried garlic on blood coagulation, fibrinolysis, platelet aggregation and serum cholesterol levels in patients with hyperlipoproteinemia. Atherosclerosis 1988;74:247.
32. Kiesewetter H et al. Effect of garlic on thrombocyte aggregation, microcirculation, and other risk factors. Int J Clin Pharmacol Ther Toxicol 1991;29(4):151.
33. Neil HAW et al. Garlic powder in the treatment of moderate hyperlipidemia: a controlled trial and meta-analysis. J R Coll Physicians Lond 1996;30(4):329.
34. Breithaupt-Grogler K et al. Protective effect of chronic garlic intake on elastic properties of aorta in the elderly. Circulation 1997;96:2649.
35. Bordia A et al. Effect of garlic (Allium sativum) on blood lipids, blood sugar, fibrinogen, and fibrinolytic activity in patients with coronary artery

disease. Prostaglandins Leukot Essent Fatty Acids 1998;58(4):257.

36. Berthold HK et al. Effect of a garlic oil preparation on serum lipoproteins and cholesterol metabolism. JAMA 1998;279(23):1900.

37. Isaacsohn JL et al. Garlic powder and plasma lipids and lipoproteins: a multicenter, randomized, placebo-controlled trial. Arch Intern Med 1998;158:1189.

38. Superko RH, Krauss RM. Garlic powder, effect on plasma lipids, postprandial lipemia, low-density lipoprotein particle size, high-density lipoprotein sub-class distribution and lipoprotein(a). J Am Coll Cardiol 2000;35:321.

39. Gardner CD et al. The effect of a garlic preparation on plasma lipid levels in moderately hypercholesterolemic adults. Atherosclerosis 2001;154:213.

40. Kannar D et al. Hypercholesterolemic effect of an enteric-coated garlic supplement. J Am Coll Nutr 2001;20(3):255.

41. Warshafsky S et al. Effect of garlic on total serum cholesterol: meta-analysis. Ann Intern Med 1993; 119:599.

42. Neil HAW, Silagy C. Garlic as a lipid lowering agent: a meta-analysis. J R Coll Physicians Lond 1994;28(1):39.

43. Stevinson C et al. Garlic for treating hypercholesterolemia: a meta-analysis of randomized clinical trials. Ann Intern Med 2000;133:420.

44. Ackermann RT et al. Garlic shows promise for improving some cardiovascular risk factors. Ann Intern Med 2001;161:813.

45. Liu L, Yeh YY. S-alk(en)yl cysteines of garlic inhibit cholesterol synthesis by deactivating HMG-CoA reductase in cultured rat hepatocytes. J Nutr 2002;132:1129.

46. Ku DD et al. Garlic and it's active metabolite allicin produce endothelium and nitric oxide dependent relaxation in rat pulmonary arteries. Clin Exp Pharmacol Physiol 2002;29(1–2):84.

47. Suetsuna K. Isolation and characterization of angiotensin I-converting enzyme inhibitor dipeptides derived from Allium sativum (garlic). J Nutr Biochem 1998;9:415.

48. Orekhov AN, Grunwald J. Effects of garlic on atherosclerosis. Nutrition 1997;13:656.

49. Berthold HK, Sudhop T. Prevention of atherosclerosis. Curr Opin Lipidol 1998;9:565.

50. Koscielny J et al. The antiatherosclerotic effect of Allium sativum. Atherosclerosis 1999;144:237.

51. Kiesewetter H et al. Effect of garlic on platelet aggregation in patients with increased risk of juvenile ischemic attack. Eur J Clin Pharmacol 1993;45:333.

52. Jepson RG et al. Garlic for peripheral arterial occlusive disease (Cochrane review). In: The Cochrane Library, Issue 4, 2000. Oxford: Update Software.

53. Lawson LD et al. Inhibition of whole blood platelet-aggregation by compounds in garlic clove extracts and commercial garlic products. Thromb Res 1992;65:141.

54. Makheja AN, Bailey JM. Antiplatelet constituents of garlic and onion. Agents Actions 1990;29(3/4):360.

55. Wargovich MJ et al. Allium vegetables: their role in the prevention of cancer. Biochem Soc Trans 1996;24(3):811.

56. Fleischauer AT et al. Garlic consumption and cancer prevention: meta-analysis of colorectal and stomach cancers. Am J Clin Nutr 2000;72:1047.

57. Thomson M, Ali M. Garlic (Allium sativum): a review of it's potential use as an anti-cancer agent. Curr Cancer Drug Targets 2003;3(1):67.

58. Lau BHS et al. Allium sativum (garlic) and cancer prevention. Nutr Res 1990;10:937.

59. Ankri S, Mirelman D. Antimicrobial properties of allicin from garlic. Microbes Infection 1999;2:125.

60. Harris JC et al. Antimicrobial properties of Allium sativum (garlic). Appl Microbiol Biotechnol 2001; 57:282.

61. Jappe U et al. Garlic-related dermatoses: case report and review of the literature. Am J Contact Dermatol 1999;10(1):37.

62. Perez-Pimiento AJ et al. Anaphylactic reaction to young garlic. Allergy 1999;54:626.

63. Petry JJ. Garlic and postoperative bleeding. Plast Reconstr Surg 1995;96(2):483.

64. Rose KD et al. Spontaneous spinal epidural hematoma with associated platelet dysfunction from excessive garlic ingestion: a case report. Neurosurgery 1990;26(5):880.

65. Piscitelli SC et al. The effect of garlic supplements on the pharmacokinetics of saquinavir. Clin Infect Dis 2002;34(2):234.

66. Gallicano K et al. Effect of short-term administration of garlic supplements on single-dose ritonavir pharmacokinetics in healthy volunteers. Br J Clin Pharmacol 2003;55:199.

67. De Rooij BM et al. Urinary excretion of N-acetyl-S-allyl-L-cysteine upon garlic consumption by human volunteers. Arch Toxicol 1996;70:635.

68. Kleijnen J, Knipschild P. Ginkgo biloba. Lancet 1992;340:1136.

69. Le Bars PL et al. A placebo-controlled, double-blind, randomized trial of an extract of Ginkgo biloba for dementia. JAMA 1997;278(16):1327.

70. Kanowski S et al. Proof of efficacy of the Ginkgo biloba special extract EGb 761 in outpatients suffering from mild to moderate primary degenerative dementia of the Alzheimer type or multi-infarct dementia. Pharmacopsychiatry 1996;29:47.

71. Oken BS et al. The efficacy of Ginkgo biloba on cognitive function in Alzheimer's disease. Arch Neurol 1998;55:1409.

72. Ernst E, Pittler MH. Ginkgo biloba for dementia: a systematic review of double-blind, placebo-controlled trials. Clin Drug Invest 1999;17(4):301.

73. Birks J et al. Ginkgo biloba for cognitive impairment and dementia (Cochrane review). In: The Cochrane Library, Issue 4, 2002. Oxford: Update Software.

74. Le Bars PL et al. A 26-week analysis of a double-blind, placebo-controlled trial of Ginkgo biloba extract Egb 761 in dementia. Dement Geriatr Cogn Disord 2000;11:230.

75. Maclennan KM et al. The CNS effects of Ginkgo biloba extracts and ginkgolide B. Progr Neurol 2002;67:235.

76. Mehlsen J et al. Effects of a Ginkgo biloba extract on forearm haemodynamics in healthy volunteers. Clin Physiol Funct Imaging 2002;22:375.

77. Diamond BJ et al. Ginkgo biloba extract: mechanisms and clinical indications. Arch Phys Med Rehabil 2000;81:668.

78. Pietri S et al. Ginkgo biloba extract (EGb 761) pretreatment limits free radical-induced oxidative stress in patients undergoing bypass surgery. Cardiovasc Drugs Ther 1997;11:121.

79. Amri H et al. Transcriptional suppression of the adrenal cortical peripheral-type benzodiazepine receptor gene and inhibition of steroid synthesis by ginkgolide B. Biochem Pharmacol 2003;65: 717.

80. Bastianetto S, Quirion R. Egb 761 is a neuroprotective agent against B-amyloid toxicity. Cell Mol Biol 2002;48(6):693.

81. Cummings JL et al. Alzheimer's disease: etiologies, pathophysiology, cognitive reserve and treatment opportunities. Neurology 1998;51(Suppl 1):S2.

82. Pittler MH, Ernst E. Ginkgo biloba extract for the treatment of intermittent claudication: a meta-analysis of randomized trials. Am J Med 2000; 108:276.

83. Peters H. Demonstration of the efficacy of Gingko biloba special extract EGb 761 on intermittent claudication: a placebo-controlled, double-blind multicenter trial. Vasa 1998;27:106.

84. Letzel H, Schoop E. Gingko biloba extract EGb 761 and pentoxifylline in intermittent claudication. Vasa 1992;21:403.

85. Moher D et al. Pharmacological management of intermittent claudication: a meta-analysis of randomized trials. Drugs 2000;59(5):1057.

86. Wojcicki J et al. Comparative pharmacokinetics and bioavailability of flavonoid glycosides of Ginkgo biloba after a single oral administration of three formulations to healthy volunteers. Meter Med Pol 1995;27(4):141.

87. Hauser D et al. Bleeding complications precipitated by unrecognized Ginkgo biloba use after liver transplantation. Transpl Int 2002;15:377.

88. Vaes LP, Chyka PA. Interactions of warfarin with garlic, ginger, gingko, or ginseng: nature of the evidence. Ann Pharmacother 2000;34(12):1478.

89. Kajiyama Y et al. Ginkgo seed poisoning. Pediatrics 2002;109:325.

90. Galluzzi S et al. Coma in a patient with Alzheimer's disease taking low dose trazodone and ginkgo biloba. J Neurol Neurosurg Psych 2000;68:679.

91. Solomon PR et al. Ginkgo for memory enhancement: a randomized controlled trial. JAMA 2002;288:835.

92. Mix JA, Crews WD Jr. A double-blind, placebo-controlled, randomized trial of Ginkgo biloba extract Egb 761 in a sample of cognitively intact older adults: neuropsychological findings. Hum Psychopharmacol 2002;17:267.

93. Nathan PJ et al. The acute nootropic effects of Ginkgo biloba in healthy older subjects: a preliminary investigation. Hum Psychopharmacol 2002;17:45.

94. Canter PH, Ernst E. Ginkgo biloba: a smart drug? A systematic review of controlled trials of the cognitive effects of Ginkgo biloba extracts in healthy people. Psychopharmacol Bull 2002; 36(3):108.

95. Ernst E, Stevinson C. Ginkgo biloba for tinnitus: a review. Clin Otolaryngol 1999;24:164.

96. Clark WM et al. Therapeutic efficacy of Ginkgo biloba in transient focal ischemia. Neurology 2000;54(Suppl 3):A67.

97. Evans JR. Ginkgo biloba extract for age-related macular degeneration (Cochrane review). In: The Cochrane Library, Issue 3, 2000. Oxford: Update Software.

98. Cohen AJ, Bartlik B. Ginkgo biloba for antidepressant induced sexual dysfunction. J Sex Marital Ther 1998;24:139.

99. Gertsch JH et al. Ginkgo biloba for the prevention of severe acute mountain sickness (AMS). High Alt Med Biol 2002;3(1):29.

100. Whiskey E et al. A systematic review and meta-analysis of Hypericum perforatum in depression: a comprehensive clinical review. Int Clin Psychopharmacol 2001;16:239.

101. Linde K, Mulrow CD. St John's wort for depression (Cochrane review). In: The Cochrane Library, Issue 4, 2000. Oxford: Update Software.

102. Williams JW et al. A systematic review of newer pharmacotherapies for depression in adults: evidence report summary. Ann Int Med 2000; 132(9):743.

103. Gaster B, Holroyd J. St John's wort for depression: a systematic review. Arch Intern Med 2000;160:152.

104. Van Gurp G et al. St John's wort or sertraline? Randomized controlled trial in primary care. Can Fam Physician 2002;48:905.

105. Behnke K et al. Hypericum perforatum versus fluoxetine in the treatment of mild to moderate depression. Adv Ther 2002;19(1):43.

106. Schrader E. Equivalence of St. John's Wort extract (Ze 117) and fluoxetine: a randomized, controlled study in mild-moderate depression. Int Clin Psychopharmacol 2000;15:61.

107. Shelton RC et al. Effectiveness of St John's wort in major depression: a randomized, controlled trial. JAMA 2001;285(15):1978.

108. Hypericum Depression Trial Study Group. Effect of hypericum perforatum (St John's wort) in major depressive disorder: a randomized controlled trial. JAMA 2002;287:1807.

109. Philipp M et al. Hypericum extract versus imipramine or placebo in patients with moderate depression: randomized multicenter study of treatment for eight weeks. Br Med J 1999;319:1534.

110. Muller WE. Current St John's wort research from mode of action to clinical efficacy. Pharmacol Res 2003;47:101.

111. Dannawi M. Possible serotonin syndrome after combination of buspirone and St John's wort. J Psychopharmacol 2002;16(4):401.

112. Izzo AA, Ernst E. Interactions between herbal medicines and prescribed drugs: a systematic review. Drugs 2001;61(15):2163.

113. Moses EL, Mallinger AG. St John's wort: three cases of possible mania induction. J Clin Psychopharmacol 2000:20(1):115.

114. Brown TM. Acute St John's wort toxicity. Am J Emerg Med 2000;18(2):532.

115. Obach RS. Inhibition of human cytochrome P450 enzymes by constituents of St John's wort, an herbal preparation used in the treatment of depression. J Pharmacol Exp Ther 2000:249:88.

116. Ernst E et al. Adverse effects profile of the herbal supplement St. John's Wort (*Hypericum perforatum* L.). Eur J Clin Pharmacol 1998;54:589.

117. Bhopal JS. St John's wort induced sexual dysfunction. Can J Psych 2001;46(5):456.

118. Dean AJ et al. Suspected withdrawal syndrome after cessation of St John's wort. Ann Pharmacother 2003;37:150.

119. Gulick RM et al. Phase I studies of hypericin, the active compound in St. John's Wort, as an antiretroviral agent in HIV-infected adults. Ann Intern Med 1999;130(6):510.

120. Schempp CM et al. Effect of oral administration of Hypericum perforatum extract (St John's wort) on skin erythema and pigmentation induced by UVB, UVA, visible light and solar simulated radiation. Phytother Res 2003;17:141.

121. Cotterill JA. Severe phototoxic reaction to laser treatment in a patient taking St John's wort. J Cosmet Laser Ther 2001;3(3):159.

122. Schey KL et al. Photooxidation of lens α-crystallin by hypericin (active ingredient in St John's wort). Photochem Photobiol 2000;72:200.

123. Brockmoller J et al. Hypericin and pseudohypericin: pharmacokinetics and effects on photosensitivity in humans. Pharmacopsychiatry 1997; 30(Suppl 2):94.

124. Kerb R et al. Single-dose and steady-state pharmacokinetics of hypericin and pseudohypericin. Antimicrob Agents Chemother 1996;40(9):2087.

125. Biber A et al. Oral bioavailability of hyperforin from hypericum extracts in rats and human volunteers. Pharmacopsychiatry 1998;31:36.

126. Schempp CM et al. Antibacterial activity of hyperforin from St John's wort, against multiresistant Staphylococcus aureus and gram positive bacteria. Lancet 1999;353:2129.

127. Agostinis P et al. Hypericin in cancer treatment: more light on the way. Int J Biochem Cell Biol 2002;34(3):221.

128. Stevinson C, Ernst E. A pilot study of Hypericum perforatum for the treatment of premenstrual syndrome. Br J Obstet Gynecol 2000;107:870.

129. Barrett B. Medicinal properties of echinacea: a critical review. Phytomed 2003;10:66.

130. Bone K. Echinacea: what makes it work? Alt Med Rev 1997;2(2):87.

131. Raso GM et al. In-vivo and In-vitro anti-inflammatory effect of Echinacea purpurea and Hypericum perforatum. J Pharm Pharmacol 2002;54:1379.

132. Sloley BD et al. Comparison of chemical components and anti-oxidant capacity of different Echinacea species. J Pharm Pharmacol 2001; 53:849.

133. Brinkeborn RM et al. Echinaforce and other Echinacea fresh plant preparations in the treatment of the common cold. Phytomed 1998;6(1):1.

134. Hoheisel O et al. Echinaguard treatment shortens the course of the common cold: a double-blind, placebo-controlled clinical trial. Eur J Clin Res 1997;9:261.

135. Schulten B et al. Efficacy of Echinacea purpurea in patients with a common cold: a placebo-controlled, randomized, double-blind, clinical trial. Arzneim-Forsch/Drug Res 2001;51:563.

136. Barrett BP et al. Treatment of the common cold with unrefined echinacea: a randomized, double-blind, placebo-controlled trial. Ann Intern Med 2002;137:939.

137. Roesler J et al. Application of purified polysaccharides from cell cultures of the plant Echinacea purpurea to test subjects mediates activation of the phagocyte system. Int J Immunopharmacol 1991;13(7):931.

138. Burger R et al. Echinacea induced cytokine production by human macrophages. Int J Immunopharmacol 1997;19(7):371.

139. See DM et al. In vitro effects of echinacea and ginseng on natural killer and antibody-dependent cell cytotoxicity in healthy subjects and chronic fatigue syndrome or acquired immunodeficiency syndrome patients. Immunopharmacol 1997; 35:229.

140. Elsasser-Beile U et al. Cytokine production in leukocyte cultures during therapy with echinacea extract. J Clin Lab Anal 1996;10:441.

141. Schwarz E et al. Oral administration of freshly expressed juice of Echinacea purpurea herbs fail to stimulate the nonspecific immune response in healthy young men: results of a double-blind, placebo-controlled, crossover study. J Immunother 2002;25(5):413.

142. Mengs U et al. Toxicity of Echinacea purpurea. Acute, subacute and genotoxicity studies. Arzneimittelforschung 1991;41(10):1076.

143. Parnam MJ. Benefit-risk assessment of the squeezed sap of the purple coneflower (Echinacea purpurea) for long term oral immunostimulation. Phytomed 1996;3(1):95.

144. Mullins RJ, Heddle R. Adverse reactions associated with echinacea: the Australian experience. Ann Allergy Immunol 2002;88:42.

145. Melchart D et al. Echinacea root extracts for the prevention of upper respiratory tract infections. Arch Fam Med 1998;7:541.

146. Grimm W, Muller HH. A randomized controlled trial of the effect of fluid extract of Echinacea purpurea on the incidence and severity of colds and respiratory infections. Am J Med 1999;106:138.

147. Turner RB et al. Ineffectiveness of echinacea for prevention of experimental rhinovirus colds. Antimicrob Agents Chemother 2000;44(6):1708.

148. Lersch C et al. Stimulation of the immune response in outpatients with hepatocellular carcinomas by low doses of cyclophosphamide (LDCY), Echinacea pupurea extracts (Echinacin) and thymostimulin. Arch fur Geschwulstforschung 1990,60(5):379.

149. Lersch C et al. Nonspecific immunostimulation with low doses of cyclophosphamide (LDCY), thymostimulin, and Echinacea purpurea extracts (Echinacin) in patients with far advanced colorectal cancers: preliminary results. Cancer Invest 1992;10(5):343.

150. Melchart D et al. Polysaccharides isolated from Echinacea purpurea herbal cell cultures to counteract undesired effects of chemotherapy: a pilot study. Phytother Res 2002;16:138.

151. Vonau B et al. Does the extract of the plant Echinacea purpurea influence the clinical course of recurrent genital herpes? Int J STD AIDS 2001;12:154.

152. Koch E. Effects from fruits of saw palmetto (Sabal serrulata) and roots of stinging nettle (Urtica dioica): viable alternatives in the medical treatment of benign prostatic hyperplasia and associated lower urinary tract symptoms. Planta Med 2001;67:489.

153. Thorpe A, Neal D. Benign prostatic hypertrophy. Lancet 2003;361:1359.

154. Oesterling JE. Benign prostatic hyperplasia. Drug Ther 1995;332(2):99.

155. Carraro JC et al. Comparison of phytotherapy (Permixon) with finasteride in the treatment of benign prostate hyperplasia: a randomized international study of 1,098 patients. Prostate 1996; 29:231.

156. Holtgrewe HL. Current trends in management of men with lower urinary tract symptoms and benign prostatic hyperplasia. Urology 1998; 51(Suppl 4A):1.

157. Narayan P, Tewari A. Overview of alpha-blocker therapy for benign prostatic hyperplasia. Urology 1998;51(Suppl 4A):38.

158. Plosker GL, Brogden RN. Serenoa repens (Permixon): a review of its pharmacology and therapeutic efficacy in benign prostatic hyperplasia. Drugs Aging 1996;9(5):379.

159. Lowe FC, Ku JC. Phytotherapy in treatment of benign prostatic hyperplasia: a critical review. Urology 1996;48(1):12.

160. Di Silverio et al. Effects of long-term treatment with Serenoa repens (Permixon) on the concentrations and regional distribution of androgens and epidermal growth factor in benign prostatic hyperplasia. Prostate 1998;37:77.

161. Paubert-Braquet M et al. Effect of the lipidosterolic extract of Serenoa repens (Permixon) and its major components on basic fibroblast growth factor induced proliferation of cultures of human prostate biopsies. Eur Urol 1998;33:340.

162. Goepel M et al. Do saw palmetto extracts block human alpha-1 adrenoceptor subtypes in vivo? Prostate 2001;46:226.

163. Di Silverio et al. Response of tissue androgen and epidermal growth factor concentration to the administration of finasteride, flutamide and Serenoa repens in patients with benign prostatic hyperplasia (BPH). Eur Urol 1996;30(Suppl 2):96.

164. Gerber GS et al. Saw palmetto (Serenoa repens) in men with lower urinary tract symptoms: effects on urodynamic parameters and voiding symptoms. Urology 1998;51(6):1003.

165. Wilt T et al. Serenoa repens for benign prostatic hyperplasia (Cochrane review). In: The Cochrane Library, Issue 4, 2002. Oxford: Update Software.

166. Semino AM et al. Symptomatic treatment of benign hypertrophy of the prostate. Comparative study of prazosin and Serenoa repens. Arch Exp Urol 1992;45:211.

167. Grasso M et al. Comparative effects of alfuzosin versus Serenoa repens in the treatment of symptomatic benign prostatic hyperplasia. Arch Exp Urol 1995;48:97.

168. Debruyne F et al. Comparison of a phytotherapeutic agent (Permixon) with an alpha-blocker (tamsulosin) in the treatment of benign prostatic hyperplasia: a one year randomized international study. Eur Urol 2002;41:497.

169. Denis LJ. Editorial review of "Comparison of phytotherapy (Permixon) with finasteride in the treatment of benign prostatic hyperplasia: a randomized international study of 1098 patients." Prostate 1996;29:241.

170. Yun T-K. Panax ginseng: a non-organ specific cancer preventative. Lancet Oncol 2001;2:49.

171. Liu C-X, Xiao P-G. Recent advances on ginseng research in China. J Ethnopharmacol 1992; 36:27.

172. Cui J et al. What do commercial ginseng products contain? Lancet 1994;344:134.

173. Vignano C, Ceppi E. What is in ginseng? Lancet 1994;344:619.

174. Bucci LR. Selected herbals and human exercise performance. Am J Clin Nutr 2000;72:624S.

175. Attele AS et al. Ginseng pharmacology: multiple constituents and multiple actions. Biochem Pharmacol 1999;58:1685.

176. Nocerino E et al. The aphrodisiac and adaptogenic properties of ginseng. Fitoterapia 2000;71:S1.

177. Kim DS et al. Anticomplementary activity of ginseng saponins and their degradation products. Phytochemistry 1998;47(3):397.

178. Maffei-Facino R et al. Panax ginseng administration in the rat prevents myocardial ischemia-reperfusion damage induced by hyperbaric oxygen: evidence for an antioxidant intervention. Planta Med 1999;65:614.

179. Gillis NC. Panax ginseng pharmacology: a nitric oxide link. Biochem Pharmacol 1997;54:1.

180. Park HJ et al. Effects of dietary supplementation of lipophilic fraction from Panax ginseng on cGMP and cAMP in rat platelets and on blood coagulation. Biol Pharm Bull 1996;19(11):1434.

181. Jung KY et al. Platelet activating factor antagonist activity of ginsenosides. Biol Pharm Bull 1998; 21(1):79.

182. Kim K-H et al. Acidic polysaccharide from Panax ginseng, Ginsan, induces Th1 cell and macrophage cytokines and generates LAK cells in synergy with IL-2. Planta Med 1998;64:110.

183. Cardinal BJ, Engels HJ. Ginseng does not enhance psychological well being in healthy, young adults. Results of a double-blind, placebo-controlled, randomized clinical trial. J Am Dietetic Assoc 2001:101:655.

184. Sorenson H, Sonne J. A double-masked study of the effects of ginseng on cognitive functions. Curr Ther Res 1996;57(12):959.

185. Bahrke MS, Morgan WR. Evaluation of the ergogenic properties of ginseng: an update. Sports Med 2000;29:113.

186. Allen JD et al. Ginseng supplementation does not enhance healthy young adults' peak aerobic exercise performance. J Am Coll Nutr 1998;17(5):462.

187. Vogler BK et al. The efficacy of ginseng. A systematic review of randomized clinical trials. Eur J Clin Pharmacol 1999;55:567.

188. Engels HJ. Effects of ginseng on secretory IgA performance and recovery from interval exercise. Med Sci Sports Exerc 2003;35:690.

189. Wiklund I et al. A double-blind comparison of the effect on quality of life of a combination of vital substances including standardized ginseng G115 and placebo. Curr Ther Res 1994;55(1):32.

190. Pieralisi G et al. Effects of a standardized ginseng extract combined with dimethylaminoethanol bitartrate, vitamins, minerals, and trace elements on physical performance during exercise. Clin Ther 1991;13(3):373.

191. Thommessen B, Laake K. No identifiable effect of ginseng (Gericomplex) as an adjuvant in the treatment of geriatric patients. Aging Clin Exp Res 1996;8:417.

192. Caso Marasco A et al. Double-blind study of a multivitamin complex supplemented with ginseng extract. Drugs Exp Clin Res 1996;22(6):323.

193. Vuksan V et al. American ginseng (Panax quinquefolius L) reduces postprandial glycemia in non-diabetic subjects and subjects with type 2 diabetes mellitus. Arch Intern Med 2000;160:1009.

194. Sotaniemi EA et al. Ginseng therapy in non-insulin dependent diabetic patients. Diabetes Care 1995;18(10):1373.

195. Kiesewetter H et al. Hemorrheological and circulatory effects of Gincosan. Int J Clin Pharmacol 1992;30(3):97.

196. Yamamoto M et al. Serum HDL-cholesterol-increasing and fatty liver-improving actions of Panax ginseng in high cholesterol diet-fed rats with clinical effect on hyperlipidemia in man. Am J Chin Med 1983;11(1-4):96.

197. Siegel RK. Ginseng abuse syndrome. JAMA 1979;241(15):1614.

198. Han KH et al. Effect of red ginseng on blood pressure in patients with essential hypertension and white coat hypertension. Am J Chin Med 1998;26:199.

199. Cheng TO. Ginseng: is there a use in clinical medicine [Letter]? Postgrad Med J 1989;64:427.

200. Liu J et al. Stimulatory effect of saponin from Panax ginseng on immune function of lymphocytes in the elderly. Mech Ageing Dev 1995;83:43.

201. Srisurapanon S et al. The effect of standardized ginseng extract on peripheral blood leukocytes and lymphocyte subsets: preliminary study in young healthy adults. J Med Assoc Thai 1997; 80(Suppl 1):S81.

202. Scaglione F et al. Immunomodulatory effects of two extracts of Panax ginseng C.A. Meyer. Drugs Exp Clin Res 1990;16(10):537.

203. Scaglione F et al. Efficacy and safety of a standardized ginseng extract G115 for potentiating vaccination against the influenza syndrome and protection against the common cold. Drugs Exp Clin Res 1996;22(2):65.

204. Scaglione F et al. Effects of the standardized ginseng extract G115 in patients with chronic bronchitis. Clin Drug Invest 2001;21:41.

205. Coon J, Ernst E. Panax ginseng: a systematic review of adverse effects and drug interactions. Drug Safety 2002;25:323.

206. Zuin M et al. Effects of a preparation containing a standardized ginseng extract combined with trace element and multivitamins against hepatotoxin-induced chronic liver disease in the elderly. J Intern Med Res 1987;15:276.

207. Salvatti G et al. Effects of Panax ginseng C.A. Meyer on male fertility. Panminerva Medica 1996;38(4):249.

208. Hong B et al. A double-blind, crossover study evaluating the efficacy of Korean red ginseng in patients with erectile dysfunction: a preliminary report. J Urol 2002;168:2070.

209. McRae S. Elevated digoxin levels in a patient taking digoxin and Siberian ginseng. Can Med Assoc J 1996;155(3):293.

210. Awang DVC. Siberian ginseng toxicity may be case of mistaken identity [Letter]. Can Med Assoc J 1996;155(9):1237.

211. Duda RB et al. American ginseng and breast cancer therapeutic agents synergistically inhibit MCF-7 breast cancer cell growth. J Surg Oncol 1999;72:230.

212. Koren G et al. Maternal ginseng use associated with neonatal androgenization [Letter]. JAMA 1990;264(22):1828.

213. Awang DVC. Maternal use of ginseng and neonatal androgenization [Letter]. Can Med Assoc J 1991;266(3):363.

214. Cui JF et al. Gas chromatographic-mass spectrometric determination of 20(S)-protopanaxadiol and 20(S)-protopanaxatriol for study on human urinary excretion of ginsenosides after ingestion of ginseng preparations. J Chromatogr B Biomed Sci Appl 1997;689:349.

215. Baulieu EE. Neurosteroids: of the nervous system, by the nervous system, for the nervous system. Recent Prog Horm Res 1997;52:1.

216. Casson PR et al. Oral dehydroepiandrosterone in physiologic doses modulates immune function in postmenopausal women. Am J Obstet Gynecol 1993;169:1536.

217. Barrett-Connor E et al. A prospective study of dehydroepiandrosterone sulfate, mortality and cardiovascular disease. N Engl J Med 1986;315:1519.

218. Vogiatzi MG et al. Dehydroepiandrosterone in morbidly obese adolescents: effects on weight, body composition, lipids and insulin resistance. Metabolism 1996;45:1011.

219. Brownsey B et al. Plasma dehydroepiandrosterone sulfate levels in patients with benign and malignant breast disease. Eur J Cancer 1972;8:131.

220. Ziegler TR et al. Effects of growth hormone on dehydroepiandrosterone sulfate, androstenedione, testosterone and cortisol metabolism during nutritional repletion. Clin Endocrinol 1991;34:281.

221. Orentreich N et al. Age changes and sex differences in serum dehydroepiandrosterone sulfate concentrations throughout adulthood. J Endocrinol Metab 1984;59:551.

222. Belanger A et al. Changes in serum concentrations of conjugated and unconjugated steroids in 40- to 80-year-old men. J Clin Endocrinol Metab 1994;79: 1086.

223. Berr C et al. Relationships of dehydroepiandrosterone sulfate in the elderly with functional, psychological and mental status, and short-term mortality: a French community-based study. Proc Natl Acad Sci USA 1996;93:13410.

224. Nieschlag E et al. The secretion of dehydroepiandrosterone and dehydroepiandrosterone sulfate in man. J Endocrinol 1973;57:123.

225. Ebeling P, Koivisto VA. Physiological importance of dehydroepiandrosterone. Lancet 1994;343: 1479.

226. Mortola JF, Yen SSC. The effects of oral dehydroepiandrosterone on endocrine-metabolic parameters in postmenopausal women. J Clin Endocrinol Metab 1990;71:696.

227. Provencher PH et al. Pregnolone fatty acid esters incorporated into lipoproteins: substrates in adrenal steroidogenesis. Endocrinology 1992;130: 2717.

228. Dehennin L et al. Oral administration of dehydroepiandrosterone to healthy men: alteration of the urinary androgen profile and consequences for the detection of abuse in sport by gas chromatography-mass spectrometry. Steroids 1998;63:80.

229. Nestler JE et al. Dehydroepiandrosterone reduces serum low density lipoprotein levels and body fat but does not alter insulin sensitivity in normal men. J Clin Endocrinol Metab 1988;66:57.

230. Welle S et al. Failure of DHEA to influence energy and protein metabolism in humans. J Clin Endocrinol Metab 1990;71:1259.

231. Morales AJ et al. Effects of replacement dose of dehydroepiandrosterone in men and women of advancing age. J Clin Endocrinol Metab 1994;78: 1360.

232. Casson PR et al. Replacement of dehydroepiandrosterone enhances T-lymphocyte insulin binding in postmenopausal women. Fertil Steril 1995;63:1027.

233. Casson PR et al. Postmenopausal dehydroepiandrosterone administration increases free insulin-like growth factor-1 and decreases high-density lipoprotein: a six month trial. Fertil Steril 1998;70:107.

234. Ebeling P, Koivisto VA. Physiological importance of dehydroepiandrosterone. Lancet 1994;343:1479.

235. Reiter WJ et al. Dehydroepiandrosterone in the treatment of erectile dysfunction: a prospective, double-blind, randomized, placebo-controlled study. Urology 1999;53:590.

236. Flynn MA et al. Dehydroepiandrosterone replacement in aging humans. J Clin Endocrinol Metab 1999;84:1527.

237. Gordon GB et al. Serum levels of dehydroepiandrosterone and its sulfate and the risk of developing bladder cancer. Cancer Res 1991;51:1366.

238. Gordon GB et al. Serum levels of dehydroepiandrosterone and dehydroepiandrosterone sulfate and the risk of developing gastric cancer. Cancer Epidemiol Biomarkers Prev 1993;2:33.

239. Gordon GB et al. Relationship of serum levels of dehydroepiandrosterone and dehydroepiandrosterone sulfate to the risk of developing postmenopausal breast cancer. Cancer Res 1990;50: 3859.

240. Helzlsouer KJ et al. Relationship of prediagnostic serum levels of DHEA and DS to the risk of developing premenopausal breast cancer. Cancer Res 1992;52:1.

241. Helzlsouer KJ et al. Serum gonadotropins and steroid hormones and the development of ovarian cancer. JAMA 1995;274:1926.

242. Araghinknam M et al. Antioxidant activity of Dioscorea and dehydroepiandrosterone (DHEA) in older humans. Life Sci 1996;59:PL147.

243. Casson PR et al. Postmenopausal dehydroepiandrosterone administration increases free insulin-like growth factor-I and decreases high-density lipoprotein: a six-month trial. Fertil Steril 1998;70:107.

244. Hackbert L et al. Acute dehydroepiandrosterone (DHEA) effects on sexual arousal in postmenopausal women. J Womens Health Gen Based Med 2002;11:155.

245. Nasman B et al. Serum dehydroepiandrosterone sulfate in Alzheimer's disease and in multi-infarct dementia. Biol Psychiatry 1991;30:684.

246. Barrett-Connor E, Edelstein SL. A prospective study of dehydroepiandrosterone sulfate and cognitive function in an older population: the Rancho Bernardo Study. J Am Geriatr Soc 1994;42:420.

247. Beitner R, Naor Z. The effect of adenine nucleotides and dehydroepiandrosterone on the isoenzymes of NADP% and NAD% glucose-6-phosphate dehydrogenase from rat adipose tissue. Biochim Biophys Acta 1972;3:437.

248. Hautanen A et al. Adrenal androgens and testosterone as coronary risk factors in the Helsinki Heart Study. Atherosclerosis 1994;105:191.

249. Barrett-Connor E, Goodman-Gruen D. Dehydroepiandrosterone sulfate does not predict cardiovascular death in post-menopausal women: the Rancho Bernardo Study. Circulation 1995;91: 1757.

250. Haffner SM et al. Sex hormones and DHEA-SO4 in relation to ischemic heart disease mortality in diabetic subjects: the Wisconsin Epidemiologic

Study of Diabetic Retinopathy. Diabetes Care 1996;19:1045.

251. Loria RM et al. Protection against lethal viral infections with the native steroid dehydroepiandrosterone (DHEA). J Med Virol 1988;26:301.

252. Daynes RA, Araneo BA. Natural regulators of T-cell lymphokine production in vivo. J Immunother 1992;12:174.

253. Laudat A et al. Changes in systemic gonadal and adrenal steroids in asymptomatic human immunodeficiency virus-infected men: relationship with the CD4 cell counts. Eur J Endocrinol 1995;133:418.

254. Jacobson MA et al. Decreased serum dehydroepiandrosterone is associated with an increased progression of human immunodeficiency virus infection in men with CD4% cell counts of 200. J Infect Dis 1991;164:864.

255. Mulder JW et al. Dehydroepiandrosterone as predictor for progression to AIDS in symptomatic human immunodeficiency virus-infected men. J Infect Dis 1992;165:413.

256. Dyner TS et al. An open-label dose escalation trial of oral dehydroepiandrosterone tolerance and pharmacokinetics in patients with HIV disease. J AIDS 1993;6:459.

257. Rabkin JG et al. DHEA treatment of HIV+ patients: effects on mood, androgenic and anabolic parameters. Psychoneuroendrocrinology 2000;25:53.

258. Piketty C et al. Double blind placebo controlled trial of oral dehydroepiandrosterone (DHEA) in advanced HIV-infected patients. Abstract 42326. 12th World AIDS Conference, Geneva Switzerland June 28–July 3, 1998.

259. Umar S et al. Effect of dehydroepiandrosterone (DHEA) on clinical and laboratory parameters in female patients with AIDS (FPWA). Abstract 42373. 12th World AIDS Conference, Geneva Switzerland June 28–July 3, 1998.

260. Mulder JW et al. Dehydroepiandrosterone (DHEA) as a surrogate marker for monitoring zidovudine treatment [Abstract]. International Conference on AIDS: Amsterdam, Netherlands, July 19–24, 1992;127(2):B169.

261. Jungers P et al. Low plasma androgens in women with active or quiescent systemic lupus erythematosus. Arthritis Rheum 1982;25:454.

262. Suzuki T et al. Dehydroepiandrosterone enhances IL-2 production and cytotoxic effector function of human T cells. Clin Immunol Immunopathol 1991;61(2 Pt 1):202.

263. Suzuki T et al. Low serum levels of dehydroepiandrosterone may cause deficient IL-2 production by lymphocytes in patients with systemic lupus erythematosus (SLE). Clin Exp Immunol 1995;99:251.

264. Van Vollenhoven RF et al. Dehydroepiandrosterone in systemic lupus erythematosus. Arthritis Rheum 1995;38:1826.

265. Van Vollenhoven RF et al. An open study of dehydroepiandrosterone in systemic lupus erythematosus. Arthritis Rheum 1994;37:1305.

266. Chang DM et al. Dehydroepiandrosterone tretment of women with mild to moderate systemic lupus erythematosus. Arthritis Rheum 2002; 46:2924.

267. Haffner SM et al. Decreased testosterone and dehydroepiandrosterone concentrations are associated with increased insulin and glucose concentrations in non-diabetic men. Metabolism 1994;43:599.

268. Diamond MP et al. Effect of acute physiological evaluation of insulin on circulating androgen levels in non-obese women. J Clin Endocrinol Metab 1991;72:884.

269. Elkind-Hirsch K et al. Androgen responses to acutely increased endogenous insulin levels in hyperandrogenic and normal cycling women. Fertil Steril 1991;55:486.

270. Khaw KT, Barrett-Connor E. Fasting glucose and endogenous androgens in nondiabetic postmenopausal women. Clin Sci 1991;81:199.

271. Leenen R et al. Visceral fat accumulation in relation to sex hormones in obese men and women in relation to sex hormones in obese men and women undergoing weight loss therapy. J Clin Endocrinol Metab 1994;78:1515.

272. Nafziger AN et al. Dehydroepiandrosterone and dehydroepiandrosterone sulfate: their relation to cardiovascular disease. Epidemiol Rev 1991;13:267.

273. De Pergola G et al. Low dehydroepiandrosterone circulating levels in premenopausal obese women with very high body mass index. Metabolism 1991;40:187.

274. Yamauchi A et al. Depression of dehydroepiandrosterone in Japanese diabetic men: comparison between non-insulin-dependent diabetes mellitus and impaired glucose tolerance. Eur J Endorinol 1996;135:101.

275. Howell DS et al. Biochemical changes in cartilage relevant to the cause and management of osteoarthritis. Rheumatology 1982;7:29.

276. Cumming GJ et al. Permeability of composite chondrocyte-culture millipore membranes to solutes of varying size and shape. Biochem J 1979;181:257.

277. Bassleer C et al. In-vitro evaluation of drugs proposed as chondroprotective agents. Int J Tissue React 1992;14:231.

278. Kempson GE et al. Patterns of cartilage stiffness on normal and degenerate human femoral heads. J Biomech 1971;4:597.

279. Mankin HJ et al. Biochemical and metabolic abnormalities in articular cartilage from osteoarthritic human hips. II. Correlation of morphology with biochemical and metabolic data. J Bone Joint Surg 1971;53A:523.

280. Tenenbaum J et al. Biochemical and biomechanical properties of osteoarthritic dog cartilage. Arthritis Rheum 1979;22:666.

281. Setnikar I et al. Pharmacokinetics of glucosamine in man. Arzneimittelforschung 1993;43:1109.

282. Rovati LC. Clinical research in osteoarthritis: design and results of short-term and long-term trials with disease-modifying drugs. Int J Tissue React 1992;14:243.

283. Vajranetra P. Clinical trial of glucosamine compounds for osteoarthritis of knee joints. J Med Assoc Thai 1984;67:409.

284. Tapadinhas MJ et al. Oral glucosamine sulphate in the management of arthrosis: report on a multi-centre open investigation in Portugal. Pharmathera peutica 1982;3:157.

285. Pujalte IM et al. Double blind clinical evaluation of oral glucosamine sulphate in the basic treatment of osteoarthritis. Curr Med Res Opin 1980;7:110.

286. Crolle G, D'Este E. Glucosamine sulphate for the management of arthrosis; a controlled clinical investigation. Curr Med Res Opin 1980;7:110.

287. D'Ambrosio E et al. Glucosamine sulphate: a controlled clinical investigation in arthrosis. Pharmatherapeutica 1981;2:504.

288. Vajaradul Y. Double-blind clinical evaluation of intra-articular glucosamine in outpatients with gonarthrosis. Clin Ther 1981;3:336.

289. Reginster JY et al. Long-term effects of glucosamine sulphate on osteoarthritis progression: a randomized, placebo-controlled tiral. Lancet 2001;357:251.

290. Pavelka K et al. Glucosamine sulfate use and delay of progression of knee osteoarthritis. Arch Intern Med 2002;162:2113.

291. Vaz AL. Double-blind clinical evaluation of the relative efficacy of ibuprofen and glucosamine sulphate in the management of osteoarthrosis of the knee in out-patients. Curr Med Res Opin 1982;8:145.

292. McAlindon TE et al. Glucosamine and chondroitin for treatment of osteoarthritis: a systematic quality assessment and meta-analysis. JAMA 2000;283:1469.

293. Houpt JB et al. Effect of glucosamine hydrochloride in the treatment of pain of osteoarthritis of the knee. J Rheumatol 1999;26:2423.

294. Karzel K, Domenjoz R. Effects of hexosamine derivatives and uronic acid derivative on glycosaminoglycan metabolism of fibroblast cultures. Pharmacology 1971;5:337.

295. Leach RM. Role of manganese in mucopolysaccharide metabolism. Fed Proc 1971;30:991.

296. Morreale P et al. Comparison of the antiinflammatory efficacy of chondroitin sulfate and diclofenac sodium in patients with knee osteoarthritis. J Rheumatol 1996;23:1385.

297. Palmieri L et al. Metabolic fate of exogenous chondroitin sulphate in the experimental animal. Arzneimittelforschung 1990;40:319.

298. Conte A et al. Biochemical and pharmacokinetic aspects of oral treatment with chondroitin sulfate. Arzneimittelforschung 1995;45:925.

299. Miles PDG et al. Troglitazone prevents hyperglycemia-induced but not glucosamine-induced insulin resistance. Diabetes 1998;47:395.

300. Baron AD et al. Glucosamine induces insulin resistance in vivo by affecting GLUC4 translocation in skeletal muscle. J Clin Invest 1995;96:2792.

301. Almada AL et al. Effect of chronic oral glucosamine sulfate upon fasting insulin resistance index (FIRI) in nondiabetic individuals [Abstract]. Exp Biol 2000 meeting.

302. Monauni T et al. Effects of glucosamine infusion on insulin secretion and insulin action in humans. Diabetes 2000;49:926.

303. Pouwels MJ et al. Short-term glucosamine infusion does not affect insulin sensitivity in humans. J Clin Endocrinol Metab 2001;86:2099.

304. Moore KS et al. Squalamine: an aminosterol antibiotic from the shark. Proc Natl Acad Sci USA 1993;90:1354.

305. Gomes EM et al. Shark-cartilage containing preparation protects cells against hydrogen peroxide induced damage and mutagenesis. Mutat Res 1996;367:203.

306. Lee A, Langer R. Shark cartilage contains inhibitors of tumor angiogenesis. Science 1983; 221:1185.

307. Pettit GR, Ode RH. Antineoplastic agents L: isolation and characterization of sphyrnastatins 1 and 2 from the hammerhead shark Sphyrna lewini. J Pharm Sci 1977;66:757.

308. McGuire TR et al. Antiproliferative activity of shark cartilage with and without tumor necrosis factor-alpha in human umbilical vein endothelium. Pharmacotherapy 1996;16:237.

309. Eisenstein R et al. The resistance of certain tissue to invasion. III. Cartilage extracts inhibit the growth of fibroblasts and endothelial cells in culture. Am J Pathol 1975;81:337.

310. Pauli BU et al. Regulator of tumor invasion by cartilage-derived anti-invasion factor in vitro. J Natl Cancer Inst 1981;67:65.

311. Moses MA et al. Isolation and characterization of an inhibitor of neovascularization from scapular chondrocytes. J Cell Biol 1992;119:475.

312. Moses MA et al. Identification of an inhibitor of neovascularization from cartilage. Science 1990; 248:1408.

313. Cataldi JM, Osbourne DL. Effects of shark cartilage on mammary neovascularization in-vivo and cell proliferation in-vitro. FASEB J 1995;9:A135.

314. Langer R et al. Control of tumor growth in animals by infusion of an angiogenesis inhibitor. Proc Natl Acad Sci USA 1980;77:4331.

315. Sipos EP et al. Inhibition of tumor angiogenesis. Ann NY Acad Sci 1994;732:263.

316. Folkman J, Klagsbrun M. Angiogenic factors. Science 1987;235:442.

317. Folkman J et al. Control of angiogenesis with synthetic heparin substitutes. Science 1989;243 (4897):1490.

318. Batist G et al. Neovastat (AE 941) in refractory renal cell carcinoma patients: report of a phase II trial with two dose levels. Ann Oncol 2002;13:1259.

319. Mathews J. Media feeds frenzy over shark cartilage as cancer treatment. J Natl Cancer Inst 1993;85: 1190.

320. Miller DR et al. Phase I/II trial of the safety and efficacy of shark cartilage in the treatment of advanced cancers. J Clin Oncol 1998;16:3649.

321. Lane IW, Comac L. Sharks Don't Get Cancer: How Shark Cartilage Can Save Your Life. Garden City, NY: Avery Publishing Group, 1992.

322. Markman M. Shark cartilage: the Laetrile of the 1990s. Cleve Clinic J Med 1996;63:179.

323. Volpi N. Physico-chemical properties and the structure of dermatan sulfate fractions purified from plasma after oral administration in healthy

human volunteers. Thromb Haemost 1996; 75:491.

324. Ashar B, Vargo E. Shark cartilage induced hepatitis. Ann Intern Med 1996;125:780.

325. Neame PJ et al. Primary structure of a protein isolated from reef shark (Carcharhinus springeri) cartilage that is similar to the mammalian C-type lectin homolog, tetranectin. Protein Sci 1992;1:161.

326. Pasternak A. A novel form of host defense: a membrane protection by Ca^{++} and $Zn++$. Biosci Rep 1987;7:81.

327. Geist FC et al. In vitro activity of zinc salts against human rhinoviruses. Antimicrob Agents Chemother 1987;31:622.

328. Korant BD et al. Zinc ions inhibit replication of rhinoviruses. Nature 1974;248:588.

329. Korant BD, ButterWorth BE. Inhibition by zinc of rhinovirus protein cleavage: interaction of zinc with capsid proteins. J Virol 1976;18:298.

330. Novick SG et al. How does zinc modify the common cold? Clinical observations and implications regarding mechanisms or action. Med Hypotheses 1996;46:295.

331. Salas M, Kirchner H. Induction of interferon-gamma in human leukocyte cultures stimulated by $Zn++$. Clin Immunol Immunopath 1987;45:139.

332. Marone G et al. Physiological concentrations of zinc inhibit the release of histamine from human basophils and lung mast cells. Agents Actions 1986;18:103.

333. Eby GA. Handbook for Curing the Common Cold: The Zinc Lozenge Story. Austin: George Eby Research, 1994.

334. Novick SG et al. Zinc-induced suppression of inflammation in the respiratory tract, caused by infection with human rhinovirus and other irritants. Med Hypotheses 1997;49:347.

335. Godfrey JC et al. Zinc gluconate and the common cold: a controlled clinical study. J Int Med Res 1992;20:234.

336. Farr BM et al. Two randomized controlled trials of zinc gluconate lozenge therapy of experimentally induced rhinovirus colds. Antimicrob Agents Chemother 1987;31:1183.

337. Douglas RM et al. Failure of effervescent zinc acetate lozenges to alter the course of upper respiratory tract infection in Australian adults. Antimicrob Agents Chemother 1987;31:1263.

338. Eby GA. Zinc lozenges as cure for common colds. Ann Pharmacother 1996;30:1336.

339. Eby GA et al. Reduction in duration of common colds by zinc gluconate lozenges in a double-blind study. Antimicrob Agents Chemother 1984;25:20.

340. Al-Nakib W et al. Prophylaxis and treatment of rhinovirus colds with zinc gluconate lozenges. J Antimicrob Chemother 1987;20:893.

341. Prasad AS et al. Duration of symptoms and plasma cytokine levels in patients with the common cold treated with zinc acetate: a randomized, double-blind, placebo-controlled trial. Ann Intern Med 2000;133(4):245.

342. Turner RB et al. Effect of treatment with zinc gluconate or zince acetate on experimental and natural colds. Clin Infect Dis 2000;31:1202.

343. Jackson JL et al. Zinc and the common cold: a meta-analysis revisited. J Nutr 2000;130:1512S.

344. Weismann K et al. Zinc gluconate lozenges for common cold: a double blind clinical trial. Dan Med Bull 1990;37:279.

344a. Smith DS et al. Failure of zinc gluconate in treatment of acute upper respiratory tract infections. Antimicrob Agents Chemother 1989;33:646.

345. Jennings LC, Dick EC. Transmission and control of rhinovirus colds. Eur J Epidemiol 1987;3:327.

346. Makela MJ et al. Viruses and bacteria in the etiology of the common cold. J Clin Microbiol 1998;36:539.

347. Gwaltney JM. Rhinovirus. In: Mandell GL et al., eds. Principles and Practice of Infectious Diseases. New York: Churchill Livingstone, 1995:1656.

348. Mossad SB et al. Zinc gluconate lozenges for treating the common cold: a randomized, double-blind, placebo-controlled study. Ann Intern Med 1996;125:81.

349. Hirt M et al. Zinc nasal gel for the treatment of common cold symptoms: a double-blind, placebo controlled trial. Ear Nose Throat J 2000;79:778.

350. Mossad SB. Effect of zincum gluconicum nasal gel on the duration and symptom severity of the common cold in otherwise healthy adults. Q J Med 2003;96:35.

351. Turner RB. Ineffectiveness of intranasal zinc gluconate for prevention of experimental rhinovirus colds. Clin Infect Dis 2001;33:1865.

352. Belongia EA et al. A randomized trial of zinc nasal spray for the treatment of upper respiratory illness in adults. Am J Med 2001;111:103.

353. Zarembo JE et al. Zinc (II) in saliva: determination of concentrations produced by different formulations of zinc gluconate lozenges containing common excipients. J Pharm Sci 1992;81:128.

354. Eby GA. Zinc ion availability: the determinant of efficacy in zinc lozenge treatment of common colds. J Antimicrob Chemother 1997;40:483.

355. Lewis MR, Kokan L. Zinc gluconate: acute ingestion. J Toxicol Clin Toxicol 1998;36:99.

356. Chandra RK. Excessive intake of zinc impairs immune responses. JAMA 1984;252:1443.

357. Pfeiffer CC et al. Effect of chronic zinc intoxication on copper levels, blood formation and polyamines. Orthomol Psychiatry 1980;9:79.

358. Macknin ML et al. Zinc gluconate lozenges for treating the common cold in children: a randomized controlled trial. JAMA 1998;279:1962.

359. Committee on Dietary Allowances, Food and Nutrition Board: Recommended Dietary Allowances. Washington, DC: National Academy of Sciences, 1980.

360. Prasad AS. Zinc: the biology and therapeutics of an ion. Ann Intern Med 1996;125:142.

361. Prasad AS. Zinc: an overview. Nutrition 1995; 11:93.

362. Yokoi K et al. Iron and zinc nutriture of premenopausal women: associations of diet with serum ferritin and plasma zinc disappearance and of serum ferritin with plasma zinc and plasma zinc disappearance. J Lab Clin Med 1994;124:852.

363. Sandstead HH. Zinc nutrition in the United States. Am J Clin Nutr 1973;26:1251.

364. Mineral elements. In: Howe PS, ed. Basic Nutrition in Health and Disease: Including Selection and Care of Good. 7th Ed. Philadelphia: Saunders, 1981:107.

365. Kastrup H, ed. Facts and Comparisons. St. Louis: Facts and Comparisons.

366. Waldhauser F et al. Bioavailability of oral melatonin in humans. Neuroendocrinology 1984;39:307.

367. Deacon S, Arendt J. Melatonin-induced temperature suppression and its acute phase-shifting effects correlate in dose-dependent manner in humans. Brain Res 1995;688:77.

368. Hughes RJ et al. The role of melatonin and circadian phase in age-related sleep-maintenance insomnia: assessment in a clinical trial of melatonin replacement. Sleep 1998;21:52.

369. Iguchi H et al. Melatonin serum levels and metabolic clearance rate in patients with liver cirrhosis. J Clin Endocrinol Metab 1982;54:1025.

370. Lane EA, Moss HB. Pharmacokinetics of melatonin in man: first pass hepatic metabolism. J Clin Endocrinol Metab 1985;61:1214.

371. Daan S, Lewy AJ. Scheduled exposure to daylight: a potential strategy to reduce "jet lag" following transmeridian flight. Psychopharmacol Bull 1984;20:566.

372. Petrie K et al. Effect of melatonin on jet lag long haul flights. Br Med J 1989;298:705.

373. Claustrat B et al. Melatonin and jet lag: confirmatory result using a simplified protocol. Biol Psychiatry 1992;32:705.

374. Arendt J et al. Alleviation of jet lag by melatonin: preliminary results of a controlled double blind study. Br Med J 1986;292:1170.

375. Petrie K et al. A double-blind trial of melatonin as a treatment for jet lag in international cabin crew. Biol Psychiatry 1993;33:526.

376. Edwards BJ et al. Use of melatonin in recovery from jet-lag following an eastward flight across 10 time-zones. Ergonomics 2000;43:1501.

377. Spitzer RL et al. Jet lag: clinical features, validation of a new syndrome-specific scale, and lack of response to melatonin in a randomized, double-blind trial. Am J Psychiatry 1999;156:1392.

378. Arendt J et al. Some effects of jet lag and their alleviation by melatonin. Ergonomics 1987;30:1379.

379. Force RW et al. Psychotic episode after melatonin. Ann Pharmacother 1997;31:1408.

380. Bardazzi F et al. Fixed drug eruption due to melatonin. Acta Derm Venereol 1997;78:69.

381. Badia P et al. Effects of exogenous melatonin on memory, sleepiness and performance after a 4-hour nap. J Sleep Res 1996;5:11.

382. Voordouw BCG et al. Melatonin and melatonin-progestin combinations alter pituitary-ovarian function in women and can inhibit ovulation. J Clin Endocrinol Metab 1992;74:108.

383. Arendt J et al. Chronic, timed, low-dose melatonin (MT) treatment in man: effects on sleep, fatigue, mood and hormone rhythms. EPSG Newslet 1984;(Suppl)5:51.

384. Tzischinsky O, Lavie P. Melatonin possesses time-dependent hypnotic effects. Sleep 1994;17:638.

385. Wurtman RJ, Zhdanova I. Improvement of sleep quality by melatonin. Lancet 1995;346:1491.

386. Dollins AB et al. Effect of inducing nocturnal serum melatonin concentrations in daytime on sleep, body temperature and performance. Proc Natl Acad Sci USA 1994;91:1824.

387. James SP et al. The effect of melatonin on normal sleep. Neuropsychopharmacology 1987;1:41.

388. Garfinkel D et al. Improvement of sleep quality in elderly people by controlled-release melatonin. Lancet 1995;346:541.

389. Dahlitz M et al. Delayed sleep phase syndrome response to melatonin. Lancet 1991;337:1121.

390. Haimov I et al. Melatonin replacement therapy of elderly insomniacs. Sleep 1995;18:598.

391. Farney RJ, Walker JM. Office management of common sleep-wake disorders. Med Clin North Am 1995;79:391.

392. Maestroni GJM et al. Colony stimulating activity and hematopoietic rescue from cancer chemotherapy compounds are induced by melatonin via endogenous interleukin 4. Cancer Res 1994;54:4740.

393. Maestroni GJM et al. A hematopoietic rescue via T-cell-dependant, endogenous granulocyte-macrophage colony-stimulating factor induced by the pineal neurohormone melatonin in tumor-bearing mice. Cancer Res 1994;54:2429.

394. Gonzales-Haba MG et al. High-affinity binding of melatonin by human circulating T lymphocytes (CD4%). FASEB J 1995;9:1331.

395. Reiter RJ, Robinson J. Your Body's Natural Wonder Drug: Melatonin. New York: Bantam Books, 1995.

396. Molis TM et al. Modulation of estrogen receptor mRNA expression by melatonin in MCF-7 human breast cancer cells. Mol Endocrinol 1994;8:1681.

397. Hill SM, Blask DE. Effects of the pineal hormone melatonin on the proliferation and morphological characteristics of human breast cancer cells (MCF-7) in culture. Cancer Res 1988;48:6121.

398. Ying SW et al. Human malignant melanoma cells express high-affinity receptors for melatonin: antiproliferative effects of melatonin and 6-chloromelatonin. Eur J Pharmacol 1993;246:89.

399. Lissoni P et al. Increased survival time in brain glioblastomas by a radioneuroendocrine strategy with radiotherapy plus melatonin compared to radiotherapy alone. Oncology 1996;53:43.

400. Lissoni P et al. Modulation of cancer endocrine therapy by melatonin: a phase II study of tamoxifen alone. Br J Cancer 1995;71:854.

401. Gonzalez R et al. Melatonin therapy of advanced human malignant melanoma. Melanoma Res 1991;1:237.

402. Lissoni P et al. A randomized study with the pineal hormone melatonin versus supportive care alone in patients with brain metastases due to solid neoplasms. Cancer 1994;73:699.

403. Panzer A et al. Melatonin has no effect on the growth, morphology or cell cycle of human breast cancer (MCF-7), cervical cancer (HeLa), osteosarcoma (MG-63) or lymphoblastoid (TK6) cells. Cancer Lett 1998;122:17.

CHAPTER 4

Anaphylaxis and Drug Allergies

Robert K. Middleton and Paul M. Beringer

Allergic drug reactions account for 5% to 20% of all observed adverse drug reactions.[1-3] Adverse drug reactions have been reported to occur in as many as 30% of hospitalized patients, and 3% of all hospitalizations are a result of adverse drug reactions.[4] In a computerized surveillance study of >36,000 hospitalized patients, 731 adverse events were identified. Of those, 1% were categorized as severe, life-threatening, and allergic in nature.[5] The potential morbidity and mortality associated with allergic drug reactions is potentially great, although they occur infrequently.

Definition

To appropriately diagnose and treat a patient experiencing an allergic reaction, it is necessary to be able to differentiate allergic reactions from other closely related adverse drug reactions. One method of classification divides adverse reactions into those that are "predictable, usually dose dependent, and related to the pharmacologic actions of the drug" and those that are "unpredictable, often dose independent, and are related to the individual's immunologic response or to genetic differences in susceptible patients."[1] Under this classification scheme, drug allergy or drug hypersensitivity is an unpredictable adverse drug reaction that is immunologically mediated.[1,2,6]

Predisposing Factors

Factors known to affect the incidence of allergic reactions can be categorized as being drug or patient related.[7]

Age and Gender

Children are less likely to become sensitized than adults, presumably because younger age is likely to be associated with less cumulative drug exposure.[6-9] A concurrent evaluation of >15,000 patients revealed a significantly higher incidence (35%) of cutaneous reactions in females than in males.[10]

Genetic Factors

Patients with histories of allergic rhinitis, asthma, or atopic dermatitis who develop a systemic drug reaction tend to react more severely than others.[7,8,11] A patient's ability to metabolize a drug is influenced by his or her genetic makeup and may affect the incidence of allergic reactions. *Pharmacogenetics* is the study of genetically determined variability to drug response and is a rapidly growing area of research. The pharmacogenetics of drug-metabolizing enzymes is a major focus in this field because many drugs are metabolized by enzymes that are encoded by variations in DNA sequences or genetic polymorphisms.[12]

For example, patients who are slow acetylators are more likely to develop antinuclear antibodies (ANAs) and symptoms of systemic lupus erythematosus (SLE) when treated with procainamide or hydralazine. (Drug-induced lupus reactions may be considered allergic in nature because they are associated with an immune response, as evidenced by an increase in ANAs.) Acetylator phenotype (e.g., fast acetylator or slow acetylator) is genetically determined, and several variations in the gene encoding for *N*-acetyltransferase (NAT) are recognized.[12] The slow acetylator phenotype is an autosomal reces-

Table 4-1   Immunopathologic Classification of Allergic Drug Reactions

Immunologic Class	Antibody	Mechanism	Common Clinical Manifestations
Type I (anaphylactic)	IgE	Drug-hapten reacts with IgE antibody on the surface of mast cells and basophils, resulting in the release of mediators	Anaphylaxis
Type II (cytotoxic)	IgG	*Hapten–Cell Reaction:* Drug interacts with cell surfaces, resulting in the formation of an immunogenic complex and the production of antibodies	Hemolytic anemia
	IgM	*Immune Complex Reaction:* Drug reacts with antibody in circulation, forming a complex that with complement binds to the cell, resulting in injury (hematologic reactions only)	Granulocytopenia
		Autoimmune Reaction: Drug induces autoantibody production against red blood cells	Thrombocytopenia
Type III (immune complex)	IgG	Same as type II immune complex reactions (nonhematologic reactions)	Serum sickness
Type IV (cell mediated)		Interaction of sensitized T lymphocytes with drug antigen	Contact dermatitis

Adapted from reference 6.

sive trait. Slow acetylators are also at risk for sulfonamide hypersensitivity, as are patients with a deficiency of glutathione-s-transferase.[13] Anticonvulsant hypersensitivity syndrome, characterized by fever, generalized rash, and lymphadenopathy, is more common in patients with a heritable deficiency in epoxide hydrolase.[14] A genetic defect in the metabolism of cefaclor may be responsible for the serum sickness-like reaction seen with this antibiotic.[14] Numerous polymorphisms are known for the CYP isoenzyme family that catalyzes the oxidative metabolism of hundreds of drugs. The best studied of these are variations in genes that encode for CYP2D6, CYP2C9, CYP2C19, and CYP3A4. Examples of the phenotypic expression of these variations include poor metabolizers (who possess nonfunctional alleles and have reduced metabolic activity) and ultrarapid metabolizers (who have multiple copies of functional genes and have enhanced metabolic activity).[12] Genetic differences in CYP metabolizing enzymes may help to explain predisposition to drug allergy and hypersensitivity, as well as other forms of drug toxicity and drug response. In addition, a link between certain histocompatibility types and a few allergic reactions has been identified.[7] Examples include drug eruptions to gold, penicillamine, and allopurinol and the potentially life-threatening hypersensitivity syndrome seen with the antiretroviral agent abacavir.[13–16] In the future, it will be possible to identify those genes that are involved in life-threatening hypersensitivity reactions such as anaphylaxis, hepatotoxicity, blood dyscrasias, and dermatologic reactions such as Stevens-Johnson syndrome or toxic epidermal necrolysis.

Associated Illness
The incidence of maculopapular rash with ampicillin therapy is significantly higher in patients with Epstein-Barr virus infections (e.g., infectious mononucleosis), lymphocytic leukemia, or gout.[2,7] About 64% of patients with AIDS affected by *Pneumocystis carinii* pneumonia develop adverse reactions to medications (e.g., skin rash to sulfonamides). In addi-tion, a higher incidence of skin eruptions with amoxicillin-clavulanate therapy has been found in HIV-positive patients with CD4+ cell counts <200 cells/mm³ compared with those with higher counts (62% versus 11%). One explanation for this increased susceptibility is thought to be impaired T-cell regulation of IgE production.[7]

Previous Drug Administration
A previous history of allergic reaction to a drug being considered for treatment, or one that is immunochemically similar, is the most reliable risk factor for development of a subsequent allergic reaction.[6,7] A commonly encountered example is the patient with a history of penicillin allergy, in whom all structurally related penicillin compounds should be avoided, and in whom the possibility of a reaction when using other β-lactam antibiotics should be considered.[7]

Drug-Related Factors
The dose, frequency of exposure, and route of administration influence the incidence of drug allergy. For example, penicillin-induced hemolytic anemia requires high and sustained drug concentrations.[9] In β-lactam antibiotic IgE sensitivity, frequent intermittent courses rather than continuous therapy are more likely to result in drug sensitization.[12] The route of administration is important both in terms of the risk of sensitization and the risk of allergic reaction in a previously sensitized person. Topical administration carries the greatest risk of sensitization, while the oral route is the least sensitizing. Intramuscular administration is more sensitizing than the intravenous (IV) route. In a patient who is already sensitized to a specific medication, the risk of an allergic reaction to that medication is greatest when it is given intravenously and least when given orally. This is thought to be a function of the rate of drug delivery.[7]

Pathogenesis

The immunopathologic mechanisms that lead to an allergic drug reaction occur in two phases: initial sensitization and subsequent elicitation.[17] Sensitization occurs as a result of binding of a drug or a metabolite to a carrier protein in a process referred to as haptenization.[2,3,6,11,17] This drug–protein (or drug metabolite–protein) complex induces the production of drug-specific T or B lymphocytes and IgM, IgG, and IgE. Upon re-exposure to the drug, the patient is likely to present with allergic symptoms.[12]

Drugs as Allergens and Immunologic Classification

Allergic drug reactions can be classified into one of four types (Table 4-1).[6,7]

TYPE I: ANAPHYLACTIC REACTIONS

Anaphylactic reactions are acute generalized reactions that occur when a previously sensitized person is re-exposed to a particular antigen. Reactions range in severity from pruritus and urticaria to bronchospasm, respiratory distress, laryngeal edema, circulatory collapse, and death. Anaphylactic reactions to antibiotics and radiographic contrast media reportedly occur in 1 in every 5,000 exposures, 10% of which are fatal.[18] Initial exposure to an antigen results in production of specific IgE antibodies. Upon re-exposure, antigen interacts with antibodies bound to the surface of mast cells or basophils, causing the release of histamine and other mediators.[17] A period of several weeks is required after initial exposure and sensitization before an anaphylactic reaction can be elicited; once sensitized, however, an anaphylactic response can be elicited within minutes as a result of existing antibodies. In addition, an anaphylactic response can occur upon re-exposure to small amounts of drug administered by any route.[17–20] Reactions that clinically resemble anaphylaxis, but do not involve immunologic mediators (antibodies), are termed *anaphylactoid reactions.*

TYPE II: CYTOTOXIC REACTIONS

Cytotoxic reactions involve the interaction of IgG or IgM and can occur by three different mechanisms (see Table 4-1). Common clinical manifestations of cytotoxic reactions include hemolytic anemia, thrombocytopenia, and granulocytopenia. Penicillin-induced hemolytic anemia is the best-known example of a cytotoxic drug reaction. This reaction typically appears after 7 days of high-dose therapy.[9,21,22]

TYPE III: IMMUNE COMPLEX–MEDIATED REACTIONS

Immune complex–mediated reactions result from the formation of drug–antibody complexes in serum, which often deposit in blood vessel walls, resulting in activation of complement and endothelial cell injury.[18] Also referred to as *serum sickness,* these reactions typically manifest as fever, urticaria, arthralgia, and lymphadenopathy 7 to 21 days after exposure.[9,23]

TYPE IV: CELL-MEDIATED (DELAYED) REACTIONS

In cell-mediated (delayed) reactions, antigen binds with sensitized T lymphocytes. Contact dermatitis is the most common manifestation of cell-mediated reactions, although systemic reactions can occur.

An understanding of the immunologic mechanism can be helpful in the diagnosis and treatment of an allergic reaction; however, the exact immunologic mechanism is unknown for many allergic reactions to drugs. In addition, patients often present with several symptoms characteristic of more than one of the reactions described above. The use of many drugs concurrently in hospitalized patients also makes it difficult to identify the drug responsible for the reaction. Therefore, a careful drug history and diagnostic tests (e.g., wheal and flare, in vitro detection of drug-specific IgE antibodies) often are necessary to appropriately diagnose and treat a patient.

Diagnosis

Distinctive Features of Allergic Reactions

The first step in the diagnosis of an allergic drug reaction is to recognize and differentiate it from other adverse drug reactions. This can be accomplished by having a good understanding of the distinctive features of allergic drug reactions (Table 4-2).[2,6]

1. J.A., a 73-year-old woman, is admitted from a nursing home with an infected decubitus ulcer. Cultures reveal *Staphylococcus aureus,* which is sensitive to oxacillin, cefazolin, and vancomycin. Upon questioning, J.A. reports having experienced a rash to penicillin in the past. Her current medications include docusate 100 mg PO BID, enalapril 5 mg PO Q am, prednisone 20 mg PO QD, and ibuprofen 800 mg PO TID. What information should be obtained to determine whether J.A.'s rash represents an allergic drug reaction?

The single most informative diagnostic procedure for allergic drug reactions is a detailed drug history (Table 4-3), which is helpful in obtaining the information necessary to determine whether a reaction represents a drug allergy and in

---

Table 4-2   Clinical Features of Allergic Drug Reactions

- Have no correlation with known pharmacologic properties of the drug
- Require an induction period on primary exposure but not on readministration
- Can occur with doses far below therapeutic range
- Often include a rash, angioedema, serum sickness syndrome, anaphylaxis, and asthma
- Occur in a small proportion of the population
- Disappear on cessation of therapy and reappear after readministration of a small dose of the suspected drug(s) of similar chemical structure
- Desensitization may be possible

Reprinted from Assem E-SK. Drug allergy and tests for its detection. In: Davies DM, ed. Textbook of Adverse Drug Reactions. 3rd Ed. New York: Oxford University Press, 1985:689, by permission of Oxford University Press.

Table 4-3   Detailed Drug History

- Prior allergic and medication encounters
- Nature and severity of reaction
- Temporal relationships between drugs and reaction (dose, date initiated, duration)
- Prior exposure to the same or structurally related medications subsequent to the reaction
- Effect of drug discontinuation
- Response to treatment
- Prior diagnostic testing or rechallenge
- Route of administration (e.g., preservatives in formulations)
- Other medical problems (if any)

From references 3 and 19.

identifying the culprit drug. Inquiring about prior allergic and medication encounters is important to document the drugs to which the patient has or has not previously reacted. This can sometimes alert the clinician about certain types of compounds to which the patient is likely to react. In addition, the acquired information allows the clinician to characterize the drug reaction and to appreciate how such a reaction might be manifested in the patient upon exposure to the same, or an immunologically similar, compound in the future.

The temporal relationship between drugs and reactions often is the strongest piece of evidence implicating an allergic reaction to a particular agent. Drugs that the patient has received for long continuous periods before the onset of a reaction are less likely to be implicated than drugs that have been recently initiated or restarted.[24] Equally important is to determine when an adverse reaction occurred. Many compounds have been reformulated over the years, resulting in removal of sensitizing impurities (e.g., penicillin, vancomycin). Therefore, it is possible that re-exposure to the agent will not result in an adverse event. Inquiring about whether the patient has received the drug since the first episode by asking the patient about other brands or names of other drugs in the same class (e.g., amoxicillin, ampicillin) will assist in determining whether the patient is likely to react to the drug upon re-exposure. It usually is helpful to chart all the drugs the patient is currently taking, their dose, and start and stop dates of use. This can be compared with the onset and disappearance of the reaction.

2. **Upon further questioning, J.A. reports having experienced an urticarial rash in the past when given ampicillin for a kidney infection approximately 2 years ago. The rash developed over her entire body less than a day after starting the antibiotic and disappeared 2 days after discontinuation. Her treatment course was completed with ciprofloxacin. She denies having had a viral infection at the time of the rash to ampicillin. She does not recall having experienced any adverse effects when she received penicillin before this reaction. No other recent changes in her treatment regimen were made before the occurrence of the rash. Why is it likely that J.A. is allergic to penicillin?**

Several useful pieces of information were gleaned from the drug history obtained from J.A. that can be used to determine the likelihood of an allergic reaction to penicillin. Because J.A.'s rash appeared less than a day after initiation of ampicillin and no other recent changes in her treatment regimen had been made, it is likely that the rash is caused by ampicillin.

Another important method of identifying a potential drug-induced allergic reaction is to examine the patient's medication list to determine whether the patient is receiving an agent that commonly is implicated in causing the exhibited allergic manifestation. In an evaluation of drug-induced cutaneous reactions, amoxicillin and ampicillin were identified as two of the top three drugs implicated in drug rash.[10]

J.A. received penicillin in the past without any adverse effects until an urticarial rash (a relatively common allergic manifestation) developed upon subsequent exposure. This sequence of events follows the typical pattern of an allergic reaction. Allergic reactions require an induction period to sensitize the person to the antigen; however, once sensitized, allergic symptoms typically occur immediately upon re-exposure.[24] Therefore, any history of prior exposures to the same or structurally related compounds needs to be documented.

Finally, it is important to evaluate other medical problems that may elicit or mimic a reaction resembling drug allergy. Rashes to ampicillin occur in 69% to 100% of patients with concurrent Epstein-Barr virus infection.[16] Because J.A. denies having a viral infection during her rash, it further strengthens her reaction as being a true allergic reaction.

Skin Testing

3. **Why would skin testing for penicillin allergy be appropriate for J.A.?**

Based on J.A.'s elicited medication history, allergy to penicillin is highly suggestive. However, skin testing and drug rechallenge are the most definitive methods of diagnosing drug allergy. Although skin testing procedures have been described for local anesthetics, penicillin, β-lactams, and sulfamethoxazole, skin test antigens are currently available commercially for penicillin only.[9] Metabolism of penicillin results in the production of penicilloyl, penicillate, and penicillate derivatives of benzylpenicillin. The penicilloyl derivative is the primary metabolite and thus is referred to as the major determinant. The other derivatives, including the parent compound (penicillin), are referred to as minor determinants. When combined with proteins, penicillin and its metabolites become antigenic and can precipitate a hypersensitivity reaction in a patient upon re-exposure.

The terms "major determinant" and "minor determinant" refer to the frequency of antibody formation to these antigenic penicillin metabolite–protein complexes. These terms do *not* describe the severity of the allergic reaction. Indeed, the major determinant is thought to be responsible for accelerated reactions, but not anaphylaxis. The minor determinants are responsible for anaphylaxis and immediate systemic reactions.

Penicillin skin testing is a safe and effective procedure (Table 4-4), with <1% of positive responders developing systemic reactions.[22] In those in whom a false-negative response occurred, reactions were mild and in most cases did not require drug discontinuation.[21,22] Administration of the penicilloyl derivative, benzylpenicillin-polylysine (Pre-Pen), identifies 80% of patients allergic to penicillin. When the penicilloyl derivative is supplemented with skin tests for the minor determinants of penicillin,[21] 99.5% of penicillin-allergic patients can be identified. The minor determinants are found not only in vivo but also in the penicillin G solutions formulated for IV administration. Therefore, some investigators have recommended using the penicilloyl-polylysine (Pre-Pen) product to test for the major determinants and penicillin G to test for the minor determinants. The results from penicillin skin testing are highly predictive of potential adverse outcomes due to allergic reactions. A series of 38 patients with skin test negative results were followed prospectively during subsequent hospitalizations to determine antibiotic use and potential allergic reactions. There were 48 readmissions, of which 35 required antibiotics (86% β-lactams). No allergic drug reactions during any of the admissions were noted.[25]

In patients with a history of penicillin hypersensitivity, skin test reactivity is affected by the length of time since the allergic reaction and by the nature of the past reaction. Skin test positivity is greatest 6 to 12 months after a reaction and

Table 4-4   Penicillin Skin Testing Procedure

Agent	Procedure	Interpretation
Penicilloyl penicillin (Pre-Pen)	Scratch test 1 drop of full-strength solution (6×10^{-5} mol/L)[a]	*No wheal or erythema after 10 min:* proceed with intradermal test.
Major determinant		*Wheal or erythema within 10 min:* choose alternative agent, desensitization if no other alternatives exist
Penicilloyl penicillin (Pre-Pen)	*Intradermal test:* 0.01–0.02 mL PPL (Pre-Pen)[a] *Saline:* negative control *Histamine:* positive control (optional; useful if it is suspected that patient may be anergic)	*Negative response:* induration size similar or less than saline control *Positive response:* induration 14 mm or more greater than saline control with or without erythema: choose alternative agent, desensitization if no other alternatives exist
Penicillin G potassium (>1 wk old) most important of the minor determinants	Scratch test 1 drop of 10,000 U/mL solution	Same as scratch test with PPL (see above)
Penicillin G potassium	*Intradermal test:* 0.002 mL 10,000 U/mL solution *Serial testing* with 10, 100, or 1,000 U/mL solutions can be performed in those with strong history/serious reactions	Same as intradermal test with PPL (see above)

[a]The penicilloyl derivative of penicillin conjugated to polylysine (PPL) is administered initially as a scratch test. If no wheal or erythema develops, then intradermal testing is performed.
From Schwarz Pharma, Kremers Urban Company, Milwaukee, WI.

decreases with time. Skin test positivity in one study was found to be only 40% of patients with a history of anaphylaxis, 17% with urticaria, and 7% for maculopapular rashes.[21] Skin testing should not be performed in patients receiving antihistamines because they block the response to the antigen and result in misinterpretation. In patients receiving antihistamines (i.e., H_1- or H_2-receptor antagonists) or when skin testing is not possible because of severe skin disease, in vitro assays to detect drug-specific IgE antibodies have been developed for major and minor determinants of penicillin and sulfamethoxazole.

To determine whether skin testing is appropriate for J.A., the risks and benefits must be weighed. Because the time of the last reaction was approximately 2 years ago, J.A. may still retain some skin test positivity if the previous reaction was truly an allergic reaction to ampicillin (skin test positivity is greatest 6 to 12 months after a reaction). Testing with PPL (major determinant) and penicillin (minor determinant) could be useful in determining whether J.A. is likely to develop an urticarial or anaphylactic reaction to penicillin or its derivatives. The fact that J.A. is currently receiving prednisone should not alter the interpretation of the skin test results because the corticosteroids minimally affect the IgE-mediated immediate hypersensitivity reactions. The risks of developing serious systemic reactions to penicillin skin testing are minimal. The benefit of penicillin skin testing for J.A., however, is questionable because she could be treated with an antibiotic other than a penicillin. The most practical approach to penicillin-allergic patients is simply to avoid the drug. Therefore, the patient's drug history should always be evaluated carefully. In the unlikely situation in which treatment with a penicillin is essential, penicillin skin testing would be useful.

Cross-Reactivity

4. J.A. received a scratch test with PPL, which was negative; however, an intradermal test was positive. What treatment options are available to J.A. for her infection?

Because J.A. exhibited a positive skin test reaction, all penicillin derivatives should be avoided. Because the specific antigenic determinants for allergy to cephalosporins and other β-lactams are unknown, skin tests currently are not commercially available for these other β-lactam antibiotics. Some have recommended performing skin testing (prick followed by intradermal) using 0.01 mL of a concentration of 2 mg/mL of the cephalosporins in normal saline; however, there are no prospective studies evaluating this approach.[26] Therefore, the clinician must rely primarily on data on cross-reactivity to determine whether a cephalosporin or other nonpenicillin β-lactam antibiotic can be used for J.A. In one study, about 50% of patients with a history of penicillin allergy exhibited hypersensitivity reactions to the β-lactam carbapenem antibiotic imipenem (Primaxin).[21] Cross-reactivity (i.e., cross-antigenicity) occurs between penicillin and cephalosporins in 5% to 15% of patients;[21,22] however, the true incidence of cross-reactivity may be considerably less because these percentages are based on the patient's recollection of an allergic history rather than by objective skin tests. The cross-reactivity between penicillins and cephalosporins was thought to be primarily related to common nuclear determinants (i.e., β-lactam ring); however, side chain-specific reactions are now recognized to account for a significant portion of allergic reactions within and between the penicillin and cephalosporins families.[26–29] In a study of 30 patients with immediate allergic reactions to cephalosporins, <20% reacted to penicillin determinants (skin test positivity, RAST positivity, or both).[28]

The reported cross-reactivity is significantly less than earlier reports (up to 50%); however, this may be due to the greater use of third- rather than first-generation cephalosporins, which share more structural similarities with the penicillins. Additional support for side chain-specific reactions to β-lactams comes from observational data noting that 30% of patients with immediate reactions to penicillins were selective for amoxicillin.[29] These data suggest there is a relatively low rate of cross-reactivity between penicillins and third-generation cephalosporins. In fact, some have considered the risk of a serious allergic reaction with the use of an advanced-generation cephalosporin in a penicillin-allergic patient to be no greater then the risk to any alternative antibiotic.[27] Some patients also have multiple drug allergies and may manifest an allergic reaction to these drugs (and others that are not β-lactams) in a manner similar to their penicillin reaction.[21]

Desensitization with an appropriate cephalosporin is a potential option for J.A.; however, her infection is not life-threatening, and the organism is probably sensitive to other antimicrobial agents. In this case, it would be more prudent to treat J.A. with a non–β-lactam antibiotic. If J.A.'s skin tests had been negative, she may have been able to receive a cephalosporin or other β-lactam despite her positive history. Nevertheless, it would be prudent in this situation to use a small (i.e., "test") initial dose.[21]

GENERALIZED REACTIONS

Drug allergies can be grouped into three categories: generalized reactions, organ-specific reactions, and pseudoallergic reactions. Generalized reactions involve multiple organ systems and variable clinical manifestations. Anaphylactic reactions, serum sickness reactions, drug-induced fever, drug-induced vasculitis, and autoimmune drug reactions are the generalized drug reactions presented in this chapter.

Anaphylaxis

5. **L.P., a 43-year-old man, is brought to the emergency department (ED) with a chief complaint of a hand wound received while defending himself during an attempted robbery. Physical examination reveals a man in moderate distress with a 3.5-inch laceration on the palm of his right hand, requiring sutures. L.P.'s history is notable for migraine headaches, which are managed with atenolol 25 mg QD; adult-onset diabetes, controlled with diet; and multiple scars from wounds obtained during a barroom brawl 2 years before admission. He has no known allergies. The wound is cleansed and 1% lidocaine is infiltrated around the laceration in preparation for suturing. Four minutes after the lidocaine injections, L.P. notes tingling and pruritus of both his hands and feet, and appears flushed. Three minutes later he complains of light-headedness, difficulty breathing, and a lump in his throat. His vital signs at this time are blood pressure (BP) 80/40 mm Hg (normal, 130/85); heart rate 75 beats/min (normal, 60); and respiratory rate 27 breaths/min (normal, 12). Chest auscultation reveals restricted airflow and stridor. A diagnosis of anaphylaxis is made and emergency treatment is started. What subjective and objective evidence support the diagnosis of anaphylaxis in L.P.?**

Anaphylaxis is an acute, clinical syndrome that results from the rapid release of immunologic mediators from tissue mast cells and peripheral blood basophils. The symptoms of anaphylaxis vary widely, depending on the route of exposure, rate of exposure, and dose of allergen.[18,19,30,31] Symptoms usually begin within minutes of exposure, as in L.P., and most reactions occur within 1 hour; however, anaphylaxis can appear several hours after exposure on rare occasions. In general, the severity of the anaphylaxis is directly proportional to the speed of onset. L.P. displays symptoms in many of the organs commonly involved in anaphylaxis. Although almost any organ system can be affected, the cutaneous, gastrointestinal (GI), respiratory, and cardiovascular systems are involved most frequently, either singly or in combination.[18,19,30,31] Not surprisingly, these "shock organs" contain the largest number of mast cells and thus are the most highly affected.

L.P. exhibits erythema (flushed appearance) and complains of pruritus of his hands and feet, both common initial symptoms of anaphylaxis: the groin also is commonly affected. These symptoms may progress to urticaria and angioedema, especially of the palms, soles, periorbital tissue, and mucous membranes. L.P. describes the early manifestations of angioedema (laryngeal edema) with complaints of a lump in his throat; this also may be described as throat tightness or constriction by some patients.

The upper and/or lower respiratory tracts also can be involved during an anaphylactic event. L.P. exhibits stridor, indicating upper airway involvement. Hoarseness is another sign of upper respiratory tract involvement. In addition, L.P. is tachypneic with poor airflow, suggesting his lower airway also is affected. Although L.P. does not display wheezing and acute emphysema, these are further clues to lower airway involvement. Respiratory symptoms can lead to suffocation and death.[30] The principal event in 25% of the cases in one autopsy series was laryngeal edema, and in another 25% of cases acute emphysema was the cause of death.[32] Cardiovascular symptoms also are ominous. Cardiovascular collapse and hypotensive shock (anaphylactic shock) are caused by peripheral vasodilation, enhanced vascular permeability, leakage of plasma, low cardiac output, and intravascular volume depletion. Thus, hypotension, as seen with L.P., is a common cardiac manifestation. Tachycardia also is commonly seen in patients with cardiac complications of anaphylaxis. L.P. does not show a significant increase in heart rate, however, because he is taking the β-blocker atenolol. Other cardiac manifestations include a direct cardiodepressant effect and various electrocardiographic changes, including arrhythmias and ischemia.

Last, although not demonstrated by L.P., common GI manifestations such as abdominal cramping, diarrhea (which can be bloody), nausea, and vomiting also are manifested during an anaphylactic reaction.[18,19,30] In summary, L.P.'s rapid onset and progression of symptoms involving multiple organ systems (i.e., cutaneous, respiratory, and cardiovascular systems) are consistent with an anaphylactic reaction. L.P.'s anaphylaxis is a severe reaction given its speed of onset, the number of organ systems involved, and the degree of involvement. In particular, his respiratory and cardiovascular symptoms indicate a potentially life-threatening reaction.

6. **What is the likely cause of L.P.'s anaphylactic event?**

Anaphylaxis occurs through one of three mechanisms.[18] In the first type of reaction, exposure to a foreign protein, either in its native state or as a hapten conjugated to a carrier protein, causes IgE-antibody formation. The IgE antibodies then bind to receptors on mast cells and basophils. Upon re-exposure, the antigen stimulates cellular degranulation through antigen-IgE antibody formation and cross-linking. This causes massive release of preformed immunologic mediators from the mast cells and basophils. Histamine is the major mediator of anaphylaxis and the primary preformed cellular constituent. Histamine has multiple effects and is likely responsible for vasodilation, urticaria, angioedema, hypotension, vomiting, abdominal cramping, and changes in coronary flow.[19] Leukotrienes (e.g., leukotrienes C$_4$ and D, also known as slow-reacting substance of anaphylaxis [SRS-A]), platelet activating factor, and prostaglandins are generated rapidly as a result of cellular degranulation, and other mediators of anaphylaxis (e.g., tryptase, chymase, heparin, and chondroitin sulfate) are released as well.[18,30] Anaphylactic reactions to *Hymenoptera* venom (e.g., bee stings), insulin, streptokinase, penicillins, cephalosporins, local anesthetics, and sulfonamides occur through this IgE-mediated mechanism.

Anaphylaxis also can occur via a second mechanism. This involves the formation of immune complexes that activate the complement system and the subsequent formation of anaphylatoxins C3a, C4a, and C5a. Such anaphylatoxins can directly stimulate mast cell and basophil degranulation and mediator release. The third mechanism by which substances, such as radiocontrast media and other hyperosmolar agents, can cause anaphylaxis is by the direct stimulation of mediator release (primarily histamine). The pathway by which this occurs is as yet unknown, but it is independent of IgE and complement. Last, anaphylaxis can occur in situations where no distinct mechanism is identified; such cases are described as idiopathic recurrent anaphylaxis.[18,31]

Most likely, L.P.'s anaphylactic episode is related to the first mechanism (i.e., IgE-antibody formation). Specifically, L.P. probably received lidocaine when the wounds he sustained 2 years ago were sutured. Exposure to lidocaine at that time probably stimulated IgE-antibody formation. Following re-exposure to lidocaine during this admission, antibody–antigen complexes were formed, resulting in cellular degranulation and anaphylaxis. The temporal relationship of L.P.'s anaphylactic reaction to the administration of lidocaine also strongly implicates lidocaine as the precipitating agent. Furthermore, L.P. was not exposed to agents known to cause anaphylaxis by one of the other known mechanisms.

7. **Given L.P.'s signs and symptoms and the presumed cause of his anaphylactic reaction, how should he be treated?**

Effective management of anaphylaxis requires quick recognition and aggressive therapeutic intervention because of the immediate life-threatening nature of the reaction, as illustrated by L.P. The severity of the anaphylactic reaction must be assessed quickly, the probable causative agent determined, the administration of the offending substance discontinued, and the absorption of the offending agent minimized. All of these interventions must be undertaken promptly and the clinical status of the patient closely monitored. Vital signs, cardiac and pulmonary function, oxygenation, cardiac output, and tissue perfusion in particular must be immediately and continuously assessed.[18,30] Because lidocaine infiltrated around the wound is the probable cause of L.P.'s reaction, attempts should be made to prevent its further systemic absorption. Thus, the wound should be thoroughly flushed with normal saline.

L.P. is showing signs of anaphylactic shock and peripheral vasodilation, which must be managed immediately. Epinephrine is the drug of choice for the pharmacologic management of anaphylaxis and for all major or severe allergic reactions. It also can be used for the symptomatic relief of minor adverse allergic reactions. The α-adrenergic effects of epinephrine increase systemic vascular resistance and increase blood pressure. These actions counter the vasodilating and hypotensive effects of histamine and the other mediators of anaphylaxis. In addition, the β-adrenergic effects of epinephrine promote bronchodilation and increase cardiac rate and contractility. Epinephrine also inhibits the release of mediators from basophils and mast cells.

The route of epinephrine administration is important. In anaphylactic shock, epinephrine should be administered intravenously because the low cardiac output and intravascular volume depletion from shock decrease tissue perfusion and possibly the absorption of subcutaneously administered epinephrine. When shock is not present, subcutaneous epinephrine is acceptable. In L.P.'s case, an IV line should be placed rapidly and 5 mL of 1:10,000 epinephrine administered over 5 minutes. At the same time, another IV line should be established and 1 L of normal saline infused at a rate sufficient to maintain perfusion to vital organs (e.g., every 30 minutes until his BP is stabilized). Cerebral perfusion, as evidenced by adequate mentation, must always take precedence over BP readings when managing shock.

The effect of L.P.'s atenolol also must be anticipated. If L.P.'s BP and heart rate do not substantially improve shortly after the initial dose of epinephrine, IV glucagon, which can stimulate heart rate and cardiac contractility independent of β-adrenergic blockade, should be given as outlined in Table 4-5. Medications commonly used to augment the actions of epinephrine include H$_1$- and H$_2$-receptor antagonists, inhaled β-agonists, corticosteroids, and aminophylline. In light of L.P.'s severe pulmonary reaction, he should receive oxygen as well as a nebulized β-agonist, such as albuterol. Nebulized ipratropium bromide also may be a useful bronchodilator, although its use in anaphylaxis has not been documented. If L.P.'s respiratory status fails to improve after pharmacologic intervention, intubation must be considered. Atenolol would not be expected to diminish the effect of albuterol because atenolol is a β1 cardioselective β-blocker and the dose is low. Because histamine is the primary mediator of anaphylaxis, IV administration of an antihistamine such as diphenhydramine, 50 mg every 6 hours until the reaction resolves, is warranted. Similarly, giving an H$_2$-receptor antagonist is reasonable. Because L.P. is not receiving any drugs known to interact with cimetidine and because he has no diseases that require dose adjustment, cimetidine may be given as outlined in Table 4-5.

Last, given the severity of his reaction and his pulmonary involvement, L.P. is a candidate for IV corticosteroids. Methylprednisolone, 125 mg every 6 hours for four doses, may be beneficial and is associated with minimal risk. The effect of methylprednisolone on L.P.'s diabetes should be considered, but because L.P.'s clinical status is severe, diabetes certainly does not preclude its administration. Once stabilized, L.P. should be transferred to a critical care setting and

Table 4-5   Drug Therapy of Anaphylaxis

Drug	Indication	Adult Dosage	Complications
Initial Therapy			
Epinephrine	Hypotension, bronchospasm, laryngeal edema, urticaria, angioedema	0.3–0.5 mL of 1:1,000 SC or IM Q 10–20 min PRN. 3–5 mL of 1:10,000 IV over 5 min Q 10–20 min PRN. 1 mL of 1:1,000 in 500 mL of dextrose 5% IV at a rate of 0.5–5 μg/min. 3–5 mL of 1:10,000 intratracheally Q 10–20 min PRN	Arrhythmias, hypertension, nervousness, tremor
Oxygen	Hypoxemia	40–100%	None
Metaproterenol	Bronchospasm	0.3 mL of 5% solution in 2.5 mL of saline via nebulizer (i.e., 15 mg)	Arrhythmias, hypertension, nervousness, tremor
Or			
Albuterol		0.5 mL of 0.5% solution in 2.5 mL of saline via nebulizer (i.e., 2.5 mg)	
Or			
Isoetharine		0.5 mL of 1% solution in 2 mL of saline via nebulizer (i.e., 5 mg)	
IV fluids	Hypotension	1 L of crystalloid or colloid Q 20–30 min PRN	Pulmonary edema, CHF
Secondary Therapy[a]			
Antihistamines H₁-receptor Antagonists	Hypotension, urticaria	Diphenhydramine or hydroxyzine 25–50 mg IV/IM/PO Q 6–8 hr PRN	Drowsiness, dry mouth, urinary retention; may obscure symptoms of continuing reaction
H₂-receptor Antagonists		Cimetidine 300 mg IV over 3–5 min or PO Q 6–8 hr PRN *or* Ranitidine 50 mg IV over 3–5 min Q 8 hr PRN or 150 mg PO BID PRN	
Corticosteroids	Bronchospasm; patients undergoing prolonged resuscitation or severe reaction	Hydrocortisone sodium succinate 100 mg IM/IV Q 3–6 hr for 2–4 doses *or* Methylprednisolone sodium succinate 40–125 mg IV Q 6 hr for 2–4 doses	Hyperglycemia, fluid retention
Aminophylline	Bronchospasm	6 mg/kg loading dose (if necessary) IV over 30 min followed by 0.3–0.9 mg/kg/hr as a maintenance dose[b]	Arrhythmias, nausea, vomiting, nervousness, seizures
Norepinephrine	Hypotension	4 mg in 1 L dextrose 5% IV at a rate of 2–12 μg/min	Arrhythmias, hypertension, nervousness, tremor
Glucagon[c]	Refractory hypotension	1 mg in 1 L of dextrose 5% IV at a rate of 5–15 μg/min	

[a]Although not effective during acute anaphylaxis, these agents may reduce or prevent recurrent or prolonged reactions.
[b]Doses are for aminophylline; to convert to theophylline, multiply by 0.8. Lower rates may be required in elderly patients, those taking medications that reduce aminophylline metabolism, those with hepatic dysfunction, and those with HF. Higher doses may be required in younger patients or cigarette smokers.
[c]Glucagon may be particularly useful in patients taking β-adrenergic blockers, because it can increase both cardiac rate and contractility regardless of β-adrenergic blockade.
Adapted from references 18, 30, and 31. Choice of agent and starting doses should be patient-specific, weighing safety and efficacy.
HF, heart failure; IM, intramuscularly; IV, intravenously; PO, orally; PRN, as needed; SC, subcutaneously.

Table 4-6   Hypersensitivity Reactions to Drugs: Serum Sickness

Clinical Manifestations	Fever, cutaneous eruptions (95% of cases), lymphadenopathy, and joint systems (10–50%).[33–36] Onset 1–2 weeks after exposure, 2–4 days in sensitized individuals. Laboratory data relatively nonspecific: elevated ESR and circulating immune complexes. Complements C3 and C4 are often low, while activation products C3a and C3a des-arginine are elevated. RF sometimes present. UA may reveal proteinuria, hematuria, or an occasional cast.[33–36]
Prognosis	Usually mild and self-limiting. Most resolve within a few days to weeks after withdrawal of inciting agent.
Treatment	Aspirin and antihistamines can relieve arthralgias and pruritus. Corticosteroids may be required for severe cases and tapered over 10–14 days.[33–36]

From references 33–36.
ESR, erythrocyte sedimentation rate; RF, rheumatoid factor; UA, urinalysis.

monitored for a minimum of 24 hours because relapses of the anaphylactic reaction may occur.[18,19,30,31]

Serum Sickness

Serum sickness is a type III hypersensitivity reaction that results from the production of antibodies directed against heterologous protein or drug haptens with subsequent tissue deposition. The typical presentation of serum sickness (Table 4-6) includes fever, cutaneous eruptions (95%), lymphadenopathy, and joint symptoms (10% to 50%).[33–36] Symptoms usually occur 1 to 2 weeks after exposure, but accelerated reactions may occur within 2 to 4 days in previously sensitized persons. Laboratory data are relatively nonspecific and are of little diagnostic value. The erythrocyte sedimentation rate (ESR) is usually slightly elevated. The serum concentration of circulating immune complexes usually is increased. Complements C3 and C4 are often low, while activation products C3a and C3a des-arginine are elevated. Occasionally rheumatoid factor is present. Urinalysis may reveal proteinuria, hematuria, or an occasional cast.[33–36]

In most cases, serum sickness reactions are mild and self-limiting and resolve within a few days to weeks after withdrawal of the inciting agent. Antihistamines and aspirin can be used to relieve pruritus and arthralgias. In severe cases, corticosteroids may be required and can be tapered over 10 to 14 days.[33–36] Serum sickness reactions are rare because of the infrequent use of foreign serum today;[36] however, reactions to specific agents continue to be reported (Table 4-7).

Drug Fever

8. M.M. is a 47-year-old ill-appearing woman admitted to the hospital with a 3-day history of difficulty breathing, left-sided chest pain on inspiration, fever, chills, and a productive cough. Her medical history is significant only for hypertension, well controlled on hydrochlorothiazide; she has no known drug allergies. M.M.'s physical findings on admission are temperature 38°C; respirations 20 breaths/min; left-sided crackles heard on auscultation; oxygen saturation 85% on room air; and heart rate 85 beats/min. A chest radiograph reveals an infiltrate in her left lower lobe. Her WBC count is 17,500 cells/mm³ (normal, 5,000 to 10,000) with the following differential: polymorphonuclear neutrophil leukocytes (PMNs), 83% (normal, 45% to 79%); bands, 12% (normal, 0% to 5%); lymphocytes, 10% (normal, 16% to 47%); basophils, 0% (normal, 0% to 1%); and eosinophils, 1%

(normal, 1% to 2%). A diagnosis of community-acquired pneumonia is made, and M.M. is empirically started on ceftriaxone 1 g IV QD and oxygen at 2 L/min. Other medications include acetaminophen 325 mg PO Q 4 to 6 hr PRN for temperature >38°C, famotidine 20 mg PO BID, and hydrochlorothiazide 12.5 mg PO QD. Seventy-two hours later, M.M. is breathing without pain at a respiratory rate of 12 breaths/min, her lungs are clear to auscultation, and her oxygen saturation is 98% on room air. She appears much better and offers no new complaints. However, her temperature over the previous 48 hours has ranged from 38.6° to 40°C, her pulse has ranged from 90 to 100 beats/min, and her white blood cell (WBC) count is 22,000 with the following differential: PMNs, 89%; bands, 5%; lymphocytes, 12%; basophils, 0%; and eosinophils, 7%. Drug-induced fever is considered. What evidence supports this diagnosis? What is the mechanism for drug fever?

Drug fever is described as a febrile reaction to a drug without cutaneous symptoms and is estimated to occur in 3% to 5% of inpatients.[66] Drug fever can be challenging to identify and can be misinterpreted as a new infectious process or failure of an existing infection to respond to treatment. Such failure to recognize a drug fever can lead to prolonged hospitalization and unnecessary tests or medications. Table 4-8 lists the characteristics of hypersensitivity drug-induced fever. The most important finding in the case of M.M. is her clinical improvement with respect to her pulmonary status despite a high-grade fever and persistent leukocytosis; she also appears healthier than expected if she had an untreated infection. Whereas a drop in her WBC count would be anticipated given her improving respiratory function, her WBC count remains elevated, consistent with hypersensitivity drug fever. Notably, her eosinophil count is increased, a frequent sign of hypersensitivity reactions. Despite her high-grade fever, she has a relative bradycardia; that is, her heart rate is not as elevated as expected if an infectious process were ongoing. Further, the timing of the symptoms favors a drug-induced fever (i.e., within days of starting a new medication). However, a definitive diagnosis can be made only by stopping the suspected offending agent, since fever generally resolves within 48 to 72 hours if a rash is not present. When a rash is present, however, the fever may persist for several days after stopping the implicated drug.

Drug fever may be caused by various mechanisms, although it is ascribed most commonly to a hypersensitivity re-

Table 4-7   Allergic Reactions to Drugs

Serum Sickness[36–57]

6-Mercaptopurine	Furazolidone	Minocycline
Antithymocyte globulin	Haemophilus B vaccine	Pentoxifylline
Carbamazepine	Indomethacin	Phenytoin
Cefaclor	Intravenous immune globulin	Rabies vaccine
Ciprofloxacin	Iron dextran	
Fluoxetine	Itraconazole	

Drug Fever[58–69]

Allopurinol	Digoxin	Nitrofurantoin
Aminoglycosides	Epinephrine	Oral contraceptives
Amphetamine	Folate	Para-aminosalicylate
Amphotericin B	Griseofulvin	Penicillins
Anesthetics, inhaled	Heparin	Phenytoin
Antacids	Hydralazine	Procainamide
Anticholinergics	Hydroxyurea	Propylthiouracil
Antihistamines	Ibuprofen	Quinidine
Antilymphocyte globulin	Imipenem	Quinine
Antineoplastics	Insulin	Ranitidine
Azathioprine	Interferon	Rifampin
Barbiturates	Iodides	Salicylates
Bleomycin	Isoniazid	Streptokinase
Carbamazepine	Iron dextran	Streptomycin
Cephalosporins	Macrolide antibiotics	Sulfonamides
Chloramphenicol	Mebendazole	Sulindac
Cimetidine	Metoclopramide	Tacrolimus
Clofibrate	Methyldopa	Tetracyclines
Cocaine	Monamine oxidase inhibitors	Tolmetin
Corticosteroids	Muromonab-CD3	Triamterene
Cyclosporine	Neuroleptics	Trimethoprim
Diazoxide	Nifedipine	Vancomycin
		Vitamins

Drug-Induced Vasculitis[70–103]

Allopurinol	Mefloquine	Ritodrine
Azathioprine	Methotrexate	Sotalol
Carbamazepine	Naproxen	Sulfadiazine
Cephalosporins	Nizatidine	Terbutaline
Cimetidine	Ofloxacin	Torsemide
Ciprofloxacin	Penicillin	Trimethadione
Clarithromycin	Phenytoin	Valproate
Furosemide	Phenylbutazone	Vitamins
Hydralazine	Pneumococcal vaccine	Warfarin
Hydrochlorothiazide	Procainamide	Zidovudine
L-Tryptophan	Propylthiouracil	

Autoimmune Drug Reactions[104–149]

Anticonvulsants	Interferon	Procainamide
β-Blockers	Isoniazid	Quinidine
Chlorpromazine	Methyldopa	Sulfasalazine
Estrogen	Minocycline	Terbinafine
Hydralazine	Penicillamine	Zafirlukast

action. Other mechanisms include the pharmacologic action of the drug (e.g., cell destruction from antineoplastic agents releases endogenous pyrogens); altered thermoregulatory function (e.g., increased metabolic rate from thyroid hormone; decreased sweating from drugs, such as atropine, tricyclic antidepressants, or phenothiazines, with anticholinergic properties); administration-related fever (e.g., from amphotericin B or bleomycin); and idiosyncratic reactions (e.g., neuroleptic malignant syndrome from haloperidol, malignant hyperthermia from inhaled anesthetics).[61,66]

9. **What agent is the most likely cause of drug fever in M.M.?**

Most of the information available on drug fever is based on case reports or small case series, and the only critical appraisal of the literature[63] is not consistent with information found in other reports. Furthermore, the literature is inconsistent with regard to the frequency of drug fever (e.g., very common, common, uncommon), and such descriptions are not supported by good clinical data. Nevertheless, some drugs do stand out as being more commonly associated with drug fever than others. These include anti-infectives as a class (especially β-lactam antibiotics), antiepileptics (especially barbiturates and phenytoin), and antineoplastics. Other causes of drug fever include amphotericin B; antihistamines (except diphenhydramine); anticholinergics and drugs with anticholinergic properties (e.g., tricyclic antidepressants, phenothiazines); asparaginase; bleomycin; hydralazine; interferon; methyldopa; muromonab CD-3; para-aminosalicylic acid; procainamide; quinidine; quinine; and drugs containing a sulfonamide moiety (including antibiotics, stool softeners, and diuretics).[38-68] A more complete listing of drugs associated with fever is presented in Table 4-7.

In M.M.'s case, ceftriaxone is the most likely cause of her ongoing fever, given the timing of the reaction relative to beginning ceftriaxone and the frequency of febrile reactions attributed to β-lactam antibiotics. Febrile reactions have not been associated with acetaminophen, and famotidine is rarely a cause of fever without other symptoms of an allergic reaction. Although diuretics such as hydrochlorothiazide can cause fever, M.M. was taking this medication before admission without any ill effects, making this drug an unlikely culprit.

10. **How should M.M.'s drug fever be managed? Can M.M. receive cephalosporins in the future?**

Because M.M. has responded clinically, ceftriaxone should be discontinued and her fever curve, WBC count, heart rate, and respiratory status followed. An oral antibiotic from another drug class (e.g., a fluoroquinolone) should be started to complete a 7- to 10-day course of antibiotics. Acetaminophen and other antipyretics should be avoided unless M.M. becomes uncomfortable from the fever because they may mask the response to withdrawing ceftriaxone.

As with any hypersensitivity reaction, rechallenge with the offending drug can cause a similar, or sometimes greater, response. In M.M.'s case, re-exposure to ceftriaxone or another β-lactam antibiotic may cause a febrile reaction. It is unclear, however, how large the risk of re-exposure truly is. Although drug fever sometimes precedes more serious hypersensitivity reactions, evidence suggests there may be little risk to re-exposure. Should M.M. require ceftriaxone or another β-lactam antibiotic in the future, it would be prudent to administer the drug in a setting where M.M. can be monitored, at least initially, to ensure prompt treatment if an immediate hypersensitivity reaction develops.

Hypersensitivity Vasculitis

11. **M.G. is a 26-year-old woman with cystic fibrosis who is admitted for treatment of pneumonia. Sputum cultures obtained before admission reveal *Alcaligenes xylosoxidans* sensitive only to minocycline and chloramphenicol. M.G. is initiated on appropriate doses of these two antibiotics for a 2-week course. On day 8 of therapy M.G. begins to complain of a rash on her legs. Physical examination reveals palpable purpura and a maculopapular rash on both lower extremities. Laboratory data reveal an elevated ESR and leukocytosis. What is the likely cause of M.G.'s rash and laboratory abnormalities?**

M.G.'s presentation is suggestive of a diagnosis of hypersensitivity vasculitis. Hypersensitivity vasculitis is characterized by inflammation of the small blood vessel walls. These reactions occur when immune complex deposition within the small veins and arterioles activates complement, causing the release of chemotactic factors. These factors attract polymorphonuclear cells that cause vessel damage.[78,150,151]

Table 4-8	Hypersensitivity Reactions to Drugs: Drug-Induced Fever[58-65]
Frequency	True frequency is unknown because fever is a common manifestation and almost any drug may cause fever. However, it has been estimated that 3–5% of hospitalized patients experiencing adverse drug reaction suffer from drug fever alone or as part of multiple symptoms.
Clinical Manifestations	Temperatures may be 38°C or higher and do not follow a consistent pattern. Although patients may have high fevers with shaking chills, patients generally have few symptoms or serious systemic illness. Skin rash (18%), eosinophilia (22%), chills (53%), headache (16%), myalgias (25%), and bradycardia (11%) may occur in patients with drug fever. Onset of fever after exposure to the offending agent is highly variable, ranging from an average of 6 days for antineoplastics to 45 days for cardiovascular agents. Occurrence of fever is independent of the dose of the offending agent.
Treatment	Although drug fever may be treated symptomatically (e.g., with antipyretics, cooling blankets), stopping the offending agent is the only therapy that will eliminate fevers. Patients generally defervesce within 48–72 hr of stopping the suspect drug.
Prognosis	Drug fever is usually benign, although one review found a mean increased length of hospitalization of 9 days per episode of drug fever. Rechallenge with the offending drug usually results in rapid return of the fever. Although re-exposure to the suspect drug was previously thought to be potentially hazardous, there is little risk of serious sequelae.

Drug-Induced Vasculitis

Vasculitis secondary to drug use occurs infrequently. Among 10,000 cases of vasculitis, 8.8% were identified as drug related.[150] Table 4-7 lists implicated drugs. The diagnosis of hypersensitivity vasculitis is based on five clinical criteria (Table 4-9), three of which must be present.[77] M.G. meets three of the five criteria, including age >16 years, palpable purpura, and a maculopapular rash. In addition, minocycline, a medication that she was taking at the onset of the rash, has been associated with serum sickness and vasculitic-type reactions. Onset of symptoms typically occurs 7 to 10 days after initiation of drug therapy but can occur sooner upon re-exposure. Purpuric papules and macular eruptions, the most commonly observed findings, are usually symmetrical and occur on the extremities (Table 4-10).[150] Hypersensitivity vasculitis often involves multiple organ systems. Renal damage, ranging from microscopic hematuria to nephrotic syndrome and acute renal failure, is common in patients with disseminated disease.[150] An enlarged liver with elevated enzymes is indicative of hepatocellular involvement. Although the lungs and ears can be involved as well, clinical manifestations are usually mild.[150] Arthralgia also is commonly observed. Laboratory examinations usually show nonspecific abnormalities of inflammation such as an elevated ESR and leukocytosis. In patients with cystic fibrosis experiencing acute pneumonia, these laboratory abnormalities may be present already and therefore will not be helpful in establishing the diagnosis of hypersensitivity vasculitis in M.G.

12. What additional workup could be performed to confirm the diagnosis of drug-induced vasculitis in M.G.?

Table 4-9 1990 Criteria for the Classification of Hypersensitivity Vasculitis

Criteria[a]	Definition
Age at disease onset >16 yr	Development of symptoms after age 16
Medication at disease onset	Medication was taken at the onset of symptoms that may have been a precipitating factor
Palpable purpura	Slightly elevated purpuric rash over one or more areas of the skin; does not blanch with pressure and not related to thrombocytopenia
Maculopapular rash	Flat and raised lesions of various sizes over one or more areas of the skin
Biopsy including arteriole and venule	Histologic changes showing granulocytes in a perivascular or extravascular location

[a]The diagnosis of hypersensitivity vasculitis can be made if a patient exhibits at least 3 of these criteria.
Adapted with permission from Calabrese LH et al. The American College of Rheumatology 1990 criteria for the classification of hypersensitivity vasculitis. Clin Neuropharmacol 1993;16:19.

Table 4-10 Hypersensitivity Reactions to Drugs: Clinical Manifestations of Drug-Induced Vasculitis

- Palpable purpura and maculopapular rash occurring symmetrically on the extremities
- Multiple organ systems may be involved:
  Renal: microscopic hematuria to nephrotic syndrome and acute renal failure
  Liver: enlarged liver, elevated enzymes, and arthralgias
- Laboratory data usually show nonspecific abnormalities of inflammation: elevated erythrocyte sedimentation rate and leukocytosis. Peripheral eosinophilia may be present and serum complement concentrations can be low. Histologic findings upon biopsy reveal granulocytes in venule or arteriole walls
- Onset typically 7–10 days after initiation of therapy

From references 33, 51, 140, and 141.

In addition to the previous workup, other laboratory and diagnostic procedures can be performed. Peripheral eosinophilia sometimes is present, and serum complement concentrations can be low. The most definitive source of diagnostic information is a biopsy, which typically reveals granulocytes in the wall of a venule or arteriole and eosinophils at any location.[77]

13. How should M.G.'s hypersensitivity vasculitis be managed?

The first step is to discontinue the minocycline therapy. Drug-induced vasculitic reactions typically resolve on their own without additional interventions. If the reaction is severe, corticosteroids can be used.

Autoimmune Drug Reactions

14. R.F., a 24-year-old Caucasian male medical student, comes to the clinic for a routine follow-up visit following initiation of isoniazid therapy 5 months ago because of a positive skin test for tuberculosis demonstrated during a recent annual health screening. R.F. complains of new-onset myalgias and arthralgias. Laboratory values obtained the morning of the visit are within normal limits except for a positive ANA titer and elevated ESR. What is the likely cause of R.F.'s symptoms and laboratory abnormalities?

Some drugs may produce a state of autoimmunity characterized by the presence of autoantibodies and, in some instances, clinical features of an autoimmune disorder. A syndrome resembling SLE has been associated with several drugs (see Table 4-7). As described in Table 4-11, drug-induced lupus is characterized by myalgias, arthralgias, positive ANA titers, and an elevated ESR. All of these are observed in R.F. Drug-induced SLE was first recognized over 40 years ago in a group of patients taking hydralazine for antihypertensive therapy.[115] Subsequent reports of drug-induced lupus have implicated hydralazine and procainamide most frequently. Other drugs causing drug-induced lupus include isoniazid, chlorpromazine, anticonvulsants, β-adrenergic blockers, quinidine, methyldopa, penicillamine, and sulfasalazine.[111,116,137,153] The exact incidence of drug-induced lupus is difficult to ascertain because of the changing pattern of drug usage and the emergence of new lupus-inducing drugs.

15. How can the diagnosis of drug-induced lupus be differentiated from SLE in R.F.?

In contrast to idiopathic SLE, drug-induced lupus is less likely to affect females and Blacks.[116] Persons with a slow acetylator phenotype have a greater tendency to develop drug-induced lupus, and ANAs following exposure to lupus-inducing drugs also appear more rapidly.[117,154] In general, drug-induced lupus is a milder disease than idiopathic SLE. However, many patients with drug-induced lupus would fulfill the diagnostic criteria for SLE according to the American Rheumatism Association.[155] Arthralgias or myalgias accompanied by a positive ANA test may be the only clinical features for some patients with drug-induced lupus. Symptoms usually appear abruptly after several months to years of continuous therapy with the offending drug. Common complaints include fever, malaise, arthralgias, myalgias, pleurisy, and slight weight loss. Mild splenomegaly and lymphadenopathy have been reported occasionally. The classic butterfly malar rash, discoid lesions, oral mucosal ulcers, Raynaud's phenomenon, and alopecia are unusual features in drug-induced lupus in contrast to idiopathic SLE. In addition, the central nervous system and kidneys rarely are affected.[116] Laboratory abnormalities commonly include anemia and an elevated ESR. Thus, the evidence supporting a diagnosis of drug-induced lupus in this case includes Caucasian male predominance, the abrupt onset and relatively mild symptomatology, and lack of the classic butterfly malar rash. More definitive tests include determining whether antibodies to single-stranded (indicative of drug-induced lupus) or double-stranded DNA (indicative of SLE) are present.

16. Should R.F. have had frequent monitoring of ANAs to detect drug-induced lupus at an earlier stage?

No. Although all patients with symptomatic drug-induced lupus test positive for ANAs (which consist predominantly of single-stranded DNA and antihistone antibodies),[116] many patients taking lupus-inducing drugs become ANA positive without going on to develop lupus. In patients treated with procainamide, about 50% to 75% are positive for ANAs after 12 months and 90% after 2 years or more of continuous therapy; only 10% to 20% of those patients actually develop lupus symptoms.[156-158] Similarly, up to 44% of patients are ANA positive after 3 years of hydralazine therapy, but drug-induced lupus occurs in only 6.7% of patients after 3 years of treatment.[159] It is not necessary to discontinue therapy in asymptomatic patients with positive ANAs because most of them will never develop clinical symptoms.[116]

17. How should R.F.'s drug-induced lupus be managed?

Musculoskeletal complaints can be managed with aspirin or nonsteroidal anti-inflammatory drugs (NSAIDs). More severe symptoms from pleuropulmonary or pericardial involvement may require the use of corticosteroids.[137] Clinical features of drug-induced lupus usually subside and disappear in days to weeks with discontinuation of the offending drug. Occasionally, these symptoms linger or recur over a course of several months before eventually disappearing. Serologic tests tend to resolve more slowly; ANAs may persist for a year or longer.[116,160] Drug-induced lupus does not predispose patients to the subsequent development of idiopathic SLE.[146] In most instances, lupus-inducing drugs do not increase the risk of exacerbation of idiopathic SLE;[112] however, long-term treatment with isoniazid may worsen pre-existing SLE.[147] Because R.F. has not yet completed his 6-month course of isoniazid therapy, he should receive an additional month's therapy with an alternative agent.

ORGAN-SPECIFIC REACTIONS

The drug allergies in this chapter are grouped into categories of generalized reactions, organ-specific reactions, and pseudoallergic reactions. The organ-specific hypersensitivity drug reactions affecting the blood, liver, lung, kidney, and skin are described next.

Table 4-11   Hypersensitivity Reactions to Drugs: Autoimmune Drug-Induced Lupus

Frequency	Less likely to affect females and Blacks than idiopathic SLE. Drug-induced lupus is more common in individuals with slow acetylator phenotype.
Clinical Manifestations	Milder disease than idiopathic SLE. Arthralgias, myalgias, fever, malaise, pleurisy, and slight weight loss. Mild splenomegaly and lymphadenopathy. *Onset:* usually abrupt, occurring several months to years after continuous therapy with the offending drug. Classic butterfly malar rash, discoid lesions, oral mucosal ulcers, Raynaud's phenomenon, and alopecia are unusual features with drug-induced lupus as opposed to idiopathic SLE. *Laboratory studies:* positive ANA (predominantly single-stranded DNA and antihistone antibodies), anemia, and elevated erythrocyte sedimentation rate. Many patients demonstrate ANAs *without* development of lupus disease. It is, therefore, not necessary to discontinue therapy in asymptomatic patients with positive ANAs.
Treatment	Clinical features subside and disappear days to weeks after discontinuation of the offending drug. Serologic tests resolve more slowly. ANAs may persist for a year or longer.
Prognosis	Drug-induced lupus does not predispose to development of idiopathic SLE. Lupus-inducing drugs do not appear to increase the risk of exacerbation of idiopathic SLE. However, long-term treatment with interferon-γ may worsen pre-existing SLE.

From references 111, 112, 115–117, 137, 146, and 152–160.
ANA, antinuclear antibody; SLE, systemic lupus erythematosus.

Blood: Immune Cytopenias

Drug-induced immune cytopenias such as granulocytopenia, thrombocytopenia, and hemolytic anemia result from type II–mediated allergic reactions (see Table 4-1). A drug or drug metabolite binds to the surface of blood elements such as granulocytes, platelets, and red blood cells. IgG or IgM antibodies are formed and are directed against the drug/drug metabolite bound to the cell (i.e., hapten-cell reaction).[9] The immune complex and autoimmune mechanisms for hemolytic anemia are presented in Chapter 87, Drug-Induced Blood Disorders. Typical symptoms associated with immune thrombocytopenia include chills, fever, petechiae, and mucous membrane bleeding. Granulocytopenia manifests with chills, fever, arthralgias, and a precipitous drop in the leukocyte count. Symptoms of hemolytic anemia can be subacute or acute and may be sufficiently severe to cause renal failure in some instances. Coombs' test is useful in identifying antibodies bound to red cells or circulating immune complexes directed against red cells. Antibiotics are the most commonly implicated class of drugs causing either neutropenia or hemolytic anemia (see Chapter 87 for a more complete description of the immune cytopenias).

Liver

Hypersensitivity reactions involving the liver can be classified as cholestatic or cytotoxic. Jaundice is usually the first sign of a cholestatic reaction, in addition to pruritus, pale stools, and dark urine. Cholestatic reactions usually are reversible upon discontinuation of the offending agent.

Cytotoxic reactions can involve hepatocellular necrosis or steatosis and may result in irreversible damage if not recognized early. (See Chapter 30, Adverse Effects of Drugs on the Liver, for a discussion of hypersensitivity reactions involving the liver.)

Lung

Pulmonary manifestations of drug hypersensitivity include asthma and infiltrative reactions. Asthma typically occurs as part of a generalized systemic reaction. Most reactions to drugs that involve asthma alone represent a pharmacologic side effect rather than a true allergic reaction.

Infiltrative reactions typically develop 2 to 10 days after exposure and manifest with cough, dyspnea, fever, chills, and malaise.[6] Infiltrative reactions vary in presentation from eosinophilic pneumonitis to acute pulmonary edema. (See Chapter 26, Drug-Induced Pulmonary Disorders, for a discussion of hypersensitivity reactions to specific drugs.)

Kidney

The most common hypersensitivity reaction involving the kidney is interstitial nephritis. Typical findings include fever, rash, and eosinophilia. Methicillin is the drug most frequently implicated as a causative agent. Other agents that have been identified include other penicillins, sulfonamides, and cimetidine.[6,9] (See Chapter 31, Acute Renal Failure, for an analysis of hypersensitivity reactions to specific drugs that adversely affect the kidney.)

Skin

Adverse reactions involving the skin are the most common clinical manifestation of drug allergy. Although several different types of cutaneous reactions are possible, most drug-induced skin eruptions can be classified as erythematous, morbilliform, or maculopapular in nature.[9] A surveillance study of drug-induced skin reactions identified amoxicillin as the most common cause, followed by trimethoprim-sulfamethoxazole and ampicillin. Overall, allergic skin reactions were identified in 2% of hospitalized patients.[10]

Treatment of skin reactions includes discontinuation of the offending drug and general supportive care. (See Chapter 38, Dermatotherapy, for a discussion of causative agents and specific treatments of various cutaneous reactions.)

PSEUDOALLERGIC REACTIONS

18. C.C., a 37-year-old man with no known allergies, is hospitalized for treatment of methicillin-resistant *S. aureus* (MRSA) bacteremia associated with an infected central line. His medical history is significant for short-bowel syndrome requiring parenteral nutrition and one previous episode of MRSA line infection successfully treated with vancomycin. Similar to his last admission, vancomycin 750 mg IV over 60 min Q 12 hr is begun. A trough level taken after the fifth dose, however, is 5 mg/L and the vancomycin dose is doubled to 1,500 mg IV Q 12 hr, to be administered at the same rate. Fifteen minutes after the new dose of vancomycin is begun, C.C. experienced hypotension (100/70 mm Hg), tachycardia (85 beats/min), generalized pruritus, and facial flushing. C.C. is diagnosed as having a pseudoallergic reaction to vancomycin. What subjective and objective data in C.C. are important in differentiating vancomycin pseudoallergic reaction from a true allergic reaction?

Pseudoallergic reactions are drug reactions that exhibit clinical signs and symptoms of an allergic response but are not immunologically mediated.[161] They may manifest as relatively benign symptoms or as severe, life-threatening events indistinguishable from anaphylaxis (Table 4-12).[161] The latter response is described as an anaphylactoid reaction because it resembles true anaphylaxis but does not involve IgE-antibody formation.[9,161] The risk of such potentially severe reactions needs to be considered when prescribing agents known to be associated with anaphylactoid reactions. In particular, the prophylactic use of antibiotics such as ciprofloxacin to prevent meningococcal infections during an outbreak was associated with a relatively high rate (1:1,000) of serious anaphylactoid reactions.[162] This would be of potentially greater importance in the setting of a mass prophylaxis program to combat exposure to anthrax. Unlike true allergic reactions, which require an induction period during which a patient becomes sensitized to an antigen, pseudoallergic reactions can occur on the first exposure to a drug. The development of pseudoallergic reactions may be dose related, manifesting when large doses of the drug are administered, when the dose is increased, or when the rate of IV administration is increased.[6] C.C. has experienced a common pseudoallergic reaction to vancomycin, usually referred to as the "red man syndrome" or "red neck syndrome," which primarily occurs when large doses of vancomycin are administered rapidly. Differentiating between a

---

Table 4-12 Hypersensitivity Reactions to Drugs: Pseudoallergic Reactions

Frequency	Highly variable, depending on the agent involved. For example, up to 30% of patients taking aspirin develop a cutaneous pseudoallergic response. On the other hand, pseudoallergic reactions to other agents, such as phytonadione and thiamine, are rare.
Clinical Manifestations	Range from benign reactions (e.g., pruritus and flushing) to a life-threatening clinical syndrome in distinguishable from anaphylaxis
Treatment	Pseudoallergic reactions are treated the same as true allergic reactions (i.e., according to the clinical presentations of the patient). Thus, some reactions simply may require removal of the suspect agent, while some anaphylactoid reactions may require aggressive therapy (e.g., epinephrine, antihistamines, corticosteroids).
Prognosis	As with true allergic reactions, patients who have experienced a pseudoallergic drug reaction may have a similar reaction upon re-exposure. However, the severity of response may lessen with repeated administration. Furthermore, for some drugs, the frequency and severity of the reaction also may be influenced by the dose and/or rate of IV administration. Pretreatment regimens to reduce the frequency and the severity of responses have been developed for some drugs well known to cause pseudoallergic reactions (e.g., radiocontrast media).

From references 5, 9, and 161–174

true allergic response and a pseudoallergic response can be difficult because the signs and symptoms can be indistinguishable. For example, each of the symptoms experienced by C.C. (flushing, tachycardia, pruritus, and hypotension) is caused by histamine release and can occur during an anaphylactic episode. To conclusively determine the cause of the reaction would require immunologic testing for antibodies to the suspect drug or agent, which is not always possible or practical. In this case, C.C. had uneventfully received vancomycin previously and has tolerated five doses during this hospitalization; therefore, it is unlikely that the reaction is immunologically mediated (i.e., a true allergic reaction). Furthermore, the reaction occurred after an increase in his vancomycin dose, which further supports the diagnosis of a pseudoallergic reaction.

19. Why did vancomycin cause a pseudoallergic reaction in C.C.?

Two general mechanisms have been proposed for pseudoallergic reactions: complement activation and direct histamine release.[18] Complement activation is secondary to immune complex formation, leading to the production of C3a, C4a, and C5a. These anaphylatoxins directly stimulate tissue mast cell and basophil degranulation and the subsequent release of neurochemical mediators. Radiocontrast media, whole blood and blood products, and protamine cause pseudoallergic reactions via this mechanism of complement activation.[161] Pseudoallergic reactions from direct drug-induced histamine release occur through an as yet unknown pathway. Direct drug-induced release of histamine does not involve complement activation or IgE-antibody formation. Several drugs are known to directly stimulate histamine release: vancomycin, protamine, radiocontrast media, opiates, pentamidine, phytonadione, and deferoxamine.[6,161] Some drugs (e.g., radiocontrast media and protamine) cause pseudoallergic reactions via both mechanisms. Furthermore, some drugs (e.g., vancomycin, quaternary ammonium muscle relaxants, and ciprofloxacin) can cause both true allergic reactions and pseudoallergic reactions.[3]

20. How should C.C.'s pseudoallergic reaction be managed? Does treatment of pseudoallergic reactions differ from that of true allergic reactions?

The first step in treating C.C.'s reaction is to eliminate the underlying cause. Thus, his vancomycin infusion should be held until the reaction resolves. Because the reaction is histamine mediated, administration of an antihistamine such as diphenhydramine 50 mg IV is warranted. Observation of his BP and heart rate is mandatory. IV fluids should be administered if his BP continues to fall or fails to stabilize. Patients with allergic reactions should be treated based on their clinical signs and symptoms, regardless of the mechanism behind the reaction. Thus, for all intents and purposes, pseudoallergic reactions are treated in the same manner as true allergic reactions.

21. Can C.C. continue to receive vancomycin? How can future reactions be prevented?

It is not necessary to discontinue vancomycin therapy in C.C. This reaction can be prevented by administering smaller doses of the drug more frequently (e.g., 1,000 mg Q 8 hr rather than 1,500 mg Q 12 hr) and/or infusing the dose over a longer interval, typically 2 hours. Alternatively, pretreatment with an antihistamine 1 hour before vancomycin administration is effective. In addition, tachyphylaxis to vancomycin-induced red man syndrome is independent of pretreatment with antihistamine and is another characteristic that differentiates a pseudoallergic reaction from a true allergic reaction. Pretreatment regimens to prevent pseudoallergic reactions to various other drugs, in particular radiocontrast media, also are well described and can be effective.

22. What other drugs are commonly associated with pseudoallergic reactions?

Many other agents have been associated with pseudoallergic reactions, as shown in Table 4-13. Some of the agents more commonly associated with pseudoallergic reactions are described next.

Table 4-13 Pseudoallergic Reactions

Acetylcysteine[171]	Immune globulin[161]	Polyoxyethylated castor oil (Cremophor EL, a solubilizing agent
ACE inhibitors[166]	Iron dextran[198]	used in parenteral drugs such as cyclosporine, paclitaxel)[205,206]
Angiotensin II–receptor	Iron sucrose injection[197]	Protamine[9]
blocking agents[175–190]	Methotrexate[191]	Pyrethrin with piperonyl butoxide[163]
Aspirin[167,170]	Minocycline[192]	Quaternary ammonium muscle relaxants[5,161]
β-Adrenergic blockers[161]	Narcotic analgesics[161]	Radiocontrast media[165]
Ciprofloxacin[5,168,172,173]	NSAIDs[167,175]	Reserpine[161]
Cisplatin[194]	Ondansetron[169,174]	Sodium ferric gluconate[199]
Corticosteroids[203,204]	Paclitaxel[193]	Thiamine[175]
COX-2 inhibitors[176]	Pentamidine[161]	Vancomycin[9,164]
Deferoxamine[161]	Phytonadione[161]	

Aspirin/NSAIDs

After penicillins, aspirin is the drug most commonly reported as causing "allergic" reactions. Reactions to aspirin may be divided into three broad categories: respiratory reactions, cutaneous manifestations, and anaphylaxis. None of these reactions has been consistently associated with IgE.[175]

The prevalence of bronchospasm with rhinoconjunctivitis is 0% to 28% in children with aspirin sensitivity. In adult asthmatics, the prevalence of aspirin sensitivity ranges from 5% to 20%. The prevalence of aspirin sensitivity during aspirin challenge in adult asthmatics with a prior history of aspirin-induced respiratory reaction ranges from 66% to 97%.[167,170] Symptoms usually occur within 30 minutes to 3 hours of ingestion. The triad seen in many sensitive patients is aspirin sensitivity, nasal polyps, and asthma. All potent inhibitors of cyclooxygenase may cause respiratory symptoms in aspirin-sensitive patients. Thus, patients who react to aspirin should be considered sensitive to NSAIDs, and vice versa. Weak cyclooxygenase inhibitors, such as acetaminophen, choline magnesium salicylate, propoxyphene, salicylamide, salsalate, and sodium salicylate, are generally well tolerated in patients with aspirin sensitivity.[175]

The prevalence of cutaneous reactions to aspirin depends on the type of reaction and the population studied. For example, urticaria-angioedema occurs in 0.5% of children, 3.8% of the general adult population, and in 21% to 30% of patients with a history of chronic urticaria. Disease activity at the time of aspirin challenge plays an important role in the latter group, however. In one study, 70% of patients whose urticaria was active at the time of challenge reacted to aspirin, compared with only 6.6% of patients whose urticaria was not active at the time of challenge. Furthermore, aspirin or NSAIDs may aggravate preexisting urticaria.[167,170,175] Other dermatologic reactions to aspirin occur with less frequency; for example, eczema, purpura, and erythema multiforme occur in 2.4%, 1.5%, and 1% of the population, respectively.

The true prevalence of aspirin or NSAID-induced anaphylaxis is unknown but may range from 0.07% of the general population to 10% of patients with anaphylactic symptoms. As noted before, IgE is not consistently associated with aspirin/NSAID-related reactions, including anaphylaxis. However, aspirin/NSAID-induced anaphylaxis shares three characteristics with immune-mediated anaphylaxis that point to IgE as an etiology: (1) the reaction occurs after two or more exposures to the offending agent, suggesting that preformed IgE antibodies are responsible; (2) patients do not have underlying nasal polyposis, asthma, or urticaria; and (3) the patient who reacts to aspirin or a single NSAID can tolerate a chemically unrelated NSAID, suggesting that a drug-specific IgE antibody has been formed.[175,176]

Since 1998, NSAIDs selectively inhibiting cyclooxygenase-2 (COX-2) while sparing cyclooxygenase-1 (COX-1) have been marketed. These agents, referred to as COX-2 inhibitors or "coxibs," include celecoxib, rofecoxib, and valdecoxib. Selective inhibition of COX-2 provides anti-inflammatory effects while minimizing the renal effects, GI toxicity, and antiplatelet effects seen with inhibition of COX-1. Aspirin and older NSAIDs are nonselective inhibitors of cyclooxygenase, inhibiting both COX-1 and COX-2. Anaphylactoid/hypersensitivity reactions have been reported with each of the marketed COX-2 inhibitors, and it appears that the rate of hypersensitivity is comparable to that of traditional NSAIDs.[176] Notably, prescribing information for all COX-2 inhibitors states that as with any NSAID, use is contraindicated in patients who have experienced asthma, urticaria, or allergic-type reactions after taking aspirin or other NSAIDs. However, there are several reports that describe successful administration of both rofecoxib and celecoxib to patients with aspirin-sensitive asthma or a history of hypersensitivity reactions to traditional NSAIDs, and evidence suggests that inhibition of COX-1 rather than COX-2 is key to initiating these events.[177–180] Nevertheless, COX-2 selective agents may still elicit allergic responses by other means, such as IgE-mediated hypersensitivity. Thus, appropriate precautions and monitoring should be followed when initiating therapy in any patient with a history of allergic reactions to aspirin or other NSAIDs.

Angiotensin-Converting Enzyme Inhibitors and Angiotensin II–Receptor Blockers

23. K.J. is a 48-year-old woman with a history of hypertension, atrial fibrillation, and a new diagnosis of hypercholesterolemia (plasma cholesterol 290 mg/dL). Although her BP had been well controlled on hydrochlorothiazide, her diuretic was stopped because of its effect on cholesterol, and enalapril 5 mg QD, was started. K.J. also takes a multivitamin (1 tablet QD) and warfarin (5 mg QD). Three weeks after starting enalapril, K.J. developed red, swollen lips and tongue and puffy eyes. Although still able to swallow, her speech is impaired. She is evaluated at an urgent care center with the following vital signs: BP 130/87 mm Hg; heart rate 70 beats/min; lungs clear to auscultation and percussion; respirations 12 breaths/min; skin without rash or urticaria. A diagnosis of angioedema secondary to enalapril is made. What is angioedema, and what evidence supports this diagnosis? What is the mechanism behind angioedema?

Angioneurotic edema (angioedema) is an anaphylactoid reaction to angiotensin-converting enzyme (ACE) inhibitors that occurs in 0.1% to 0.2% of recipients. It is not dose related and occurs with all ACE inhibitors. Symptoms consist of local erythematous edema frequently involving the tongue, lips, and eyelids as well as mucous membranes of the mouth, nose, and throat. K.J. presents with classic symptoms of angioedema and does not have symptoms of a true anaphylactic reaction, further strengthening the diagnosis of angioedema. Symptoms of angioedema usually occur within the first week of starting therapy, although they may occur at any time. Thus, although the reaction developed many weeks after K.J. began the drug, the temporal relationship is not unreasonable.

The precise mechanism of angioedema remains unclear. However, studies suggest that increased concentrations of bradykinin, elevated levels of complement 1-esterase inactivator (an enzyme that inhibits complement activation), histamine-mediated reactions, and/or deficiencies in carboxypeptidase N, α_1-antitrypsin, and complement C4 may be involved.[166,175,190,191] (Also see Chapter 20, Heart Failure.)

24. How should K.J. be treated? Would an angiotensin receptor blocker (ARB) be an appropriate substitute for an ACE inhibitor?

Although angioedema can be life-threatening, symptoms are usually mild and resolve within hours to days of stopping the offending drug. More severe reactions can progress to laryngospasm, laryngeal swelling, and obstruction and must be treated emergently with appropriate measures to maintain airway patency. Because K.J. does not have any respiratory compromise or swallowing difficulty, she does not require hospitalization. Although little evidence supports their use, antihistamines and/or corticosteroids are commonly prescribed. K.J. should be observed at the urgent care center to ensure that the reaction does not worsen. After this is established, she can be sent home with a prescription for diphenhydramine 25 mg orally Q 6 hr for 24 hours, with instructions to seek emergent help if her breathing or swallowing becomes difficult. She should be instructed to follow up with her primary physician as soon as possible. Last, she should be told to discontinue her enalapril and to inform her community pharmacist of the reaction so that it is noted on her drug profile. As stated above, angioedema occurs with all ACE inhibitors, so K.J. must avoid all drugs in this class.

Angioedema with ARBs also has been reported,[182–189] although with less frequency than with ACE inhibitors. Clinical experience with these agents lags far behind that of the ACE inhibitors, however, which may explain the relatively few cases of angioedema reported to date. Many of the cases of ARB-induced angioedema involved patients with a history of

ACE inhibitor-induced angioedema, but this is not consistently the case. Similar to the ACE inhibitors, angioedema to ARBs may occur at any time during treatment. In K.J.'s case, it would be best to avoid ARBs and ACE inhibitors. Instead, other antihypertensive agents that have little effect on cholesterol, such as the calcium channel blockers, should be used.

25. Are there other pseudoallergic reactions that occur with ACE inhibitors and ARBs?

Besides angioedema, cough is a pseudoallergic reaction caused by ACE inhibitors. It may occur in up to 39% of patients after 1 week to 6 months of therapy. Interestingly, it is more common in nonsmokers than in smokers; the incidence does not increase in patients with chronic airway disease or asthma. Cough is more common in women than men, is not dose related, and, like angioedema, occurs with all ACE inhibitors.[166,175,190,194] Several mechanisms appear to be responsible, including inhibition of the breakdown of bradykinin in the lung and increases in local mediators of inflammation such as prostaglandins and substance P. Although many approaches to the management of ACE-induced cough have been proposed,[190] angiotensin II–receptor blocking agents are the most promising alternative. Cough can occur with ARBs, but the frequency appears to be no more than that of placebo. Furthermore, most direct comparative trials between ARBs and ACE inhibitors demonstrate that the frequency of cough with ARBs is much lower than with ACE inhibitors.[190]

Radiocontrast Media

Radiocontrast media are widely used diagnostic agents, exceeding 10 million administrations annually.[175] Reactions include nausea, flushing, BP changes, bronchospasm, urticaria, angioedema, cardiac arrhythmias, convulsions, angina, and symptoms indistinguishable from true anaphylaxis. The cause of radiocontrast media reactions remains unknown, although histamine release, complement activation, and direct toxic effects on end-organs may all play a role. Little evidence supports IgE mediation of these reactions; thus, they are classified as pseudoallergic. The overall incidence of reaction to radiocontrast media is 0.7% to 13%, depending on the type of agent selected and whether the patient was pretreated before administration.[165] Conventional, ionic, high-osmolality contrast media produce reactions in 4% to 13% of recipients, while the newer, nonionic, low-osmolality agents produce fewer reactions (0.7% to 3.1%). The mortality rate for all contrast media varies widely, from 1:15,000 to 1:117,000.[165,175]

Patients with a history of allergic reaction to contrast media are at increased risk for future reactions with repeat exposure. Several pretreatment regimens have been developed to minimize such occurrences. For example, 32 mg of oral methylprednisolone given 12 and 2 hours before a procedure involving a high-osmolality contrast medium can reduce the reaction rate by up to 45% in some patients.[165] Another pretreatment regimen uses oral prednisone 50 mg taken 13 hours, 7 hours, and 1 hour before the procedure, plus diphenhydramine 50 mg orally or intramuscularly 1 hour before the examination.[207] This regimen lowers the occurrence of pseudoallergic reactions to high-osmolality contrast media, even in high-risk patients (i.e., those with a prior history of severe anaphylactoid reactions).

Narcotic Analgesics

Some opiates can stimulate histamine release, causing hypotension, tachycardia, facial flushing, increased sweating, or pruritus. Fortunately, severe reactions are uncommon. In many cases, the opiate can be continued with administration of an antihistamine to treat the symptoms. If the reaction is significant, a nonnarcotic analgesic may be considered, or an opiate that does not cause histamine release can be substituted. In vitro and in vivo studies show that morphine and meperidine cause the greatest histamine release; codeine, hydromorphone, oxycodone, and butorphanol less commonly stimulate histamine release; and levorphanol, fentanyl, sufentanil, methadone, and oxymorphone have little to no effect on histamine levels. One of the more frequent reactions to epidurally or intrathecally administered opiates is pruritus. Interestingly, pruritus from spinal opiates does not appear to be mediated by histamine because narcotics that do not release histamine (e.g., fentanyl, sufentanil) still cause pruritus after spinal administration. Furthermore, the pruritus tends to develop several hours after the opiate has been administered, when serum levels of histamine are insignificant. The cause of pruritus from spinal opiates remains unclear. However, the reaction can be managed with antihistamines and low-dose naloxone or nalbuphine, while continuing with the spinal narcotic.[161]

Protamine

Protamine sulfate is a low-molecular-weight protein that is a component of some insulin preparations and is used extensively to neutralize heparin during cardiac procedures. One study found that 11% of patients receiving protamine during cardiac surgery experienced an adverse reaction, including angioedema, wheezing, erythema, and urticaria. Severe hypotension and shock leading to death have also been reported. The mechanism of these severe reactions is unknown but may be pseudoallergic as well as IgE mediated.[9,175]

Iron Dextran Injection

Iron dextran injection is a solution of ferric hydroxide complexed with low-molecular-weight dextran. Iron dextran is used in the treatment of iron deficiency when oral iron preparations cannot be used or are ineffective. This is most commonly seen in patients with anemia of chronic renal failure, particularly those treated with epoetin alfa and receiving hemodialysis (see Chapter 32, Chronic Kidney Disease). Iron dextran injection is associated with a wide spectrum of adverse events, including chest pain, hypotension, hypertension, abdominal pain, nausea, vomiting, weakness, syncope, backache, arthralgias, myalgias, and hypersensitivity reactions. Hypersensitivity reactions can manifest as urticaria, sweating, dyspnea, rash, fever, and anaphylactoid reactions, which can be fatal. Consistent with a nonimmunologic mechanism, hypersensitivity reactions to iron dextran are not dose related and can occur with the first drug exposure.[195] Serious life-threatening anaphylactoid reactions occur in 0.6% to 0.7% of patients treated with iron dextran; serious reactions that prevent further administration occur in 2.47% of recipients.[196] The cause of the hypersensitivity reactions from iron dextran is unclear but is thought to be due to the dextran component; anaphylaxis from dextran when used as a volume expander has been reported.[196] Because of the frequency of serious adverse reactions to iron dextran, a test dose is required to assess tolerance prior to administration of the full dose. However, hypersensitivity reactions have been reported despite successful tolerance to a test dose, rendering this practice unreliable.

Until 1999, the only parenteral iron preparation available in the United States was iron dextran injection. Since that time, two other parenteral iron products have been marketed: sodium ferric gluconate complex in sucrose for injection (Ferrlecit) and iron sucrose injection, also known as iron saccharate (Venofer). Both agents appear to have a better safety profile than iron dextran. In the two trials that formed the basis for FDA approval of sodium ferric gluconate, no fatal hypersensitivity reactions occurred after multiple doses in 126 patients. Three patients (3.4%) experienced a nonfatal hypersensitivity reaction that lead to study discontinuation.[197] In a review of the safety of sodium ferric gluconate, no deaths were reported from 1976 to 1996 in Europe, compared to 31 deaths from iron dextran in United States over the same time period. This same study reported 3.3 allergy episodes per million doses of sodium ferric gluconate per year compared to 8.7 allergy episodes per million doses of iron dextran injection per year.[198] In a postmarketing trial of sodium ferric gluconate, 0.4% of patients experienced drug intolerance (defined as a serious reaction that prevented re-exposure to the drug), compared to 0.1% of placebo-treated patients.[196] One patient (0.04%) experienced a life-threatening reaction, compared to no placebo-treated patients. These results were compared to historical iron dextran controls that showed an incidence of 0.61% and 2.47% for life-threatening reactions and drug intolerance, respectively. It is significant that the study protocol did not include a sodium ferric gluconate test dose. Based upon these findings, the FDA no longer requires a test dose prior to sodium ferric gluconate administration and removed the warning for rare potentially life-threatening hypersensitivity reactions from the product package insert. The same investigators performed a subset analysis of 144 iron dextran-sensitive patients, comparing their tolerance to sodium ferric gluconate to that of the iron dextran-tolerant subjects.[199] Three iron dextran-sensitive patients (2.1%) experienced a suspected allergic reaction to sodium ferric gluconate, compared to 0.4% of the iron dextran-tolerant patients. While this difference was statistically significant, regression analysis did not identify a history of iron dextran sensitivity as being predictive of a reaction to sodium ferric gluconate. This suggests that the reaction is not drug related or immunologically mediated. Instead, idiosyncratic patient factors may play an important role.

Based upon the three trials that formed the basis for approval of iron sucrose injection, none of the 231 patients enrolled (each receiving up to a total of 1,000 mg of elemental iron over 10 dialysis sessions) experienced a serious or life-threatening anaphylactoid reaction. Nonserious hypersensitivity reactions included "several" patients with pruritus and one patient with a facial rash.[200] There were no reports of generalized rashes or urticaria. A test dose was not required in two of these trials (but could be administered at the physician's discretion), and one trial administered a one-time 50-mg test dose. Tolerance to iron sucrose injection in 22 hemodialysis patients with a history of iron dextran sensitivity was investigated.[201] Reactions to iron dextran ranged from mild (rash, urticaria, GI complaints, back/flank pain, pruritus, hypotension) to severe (hypotension with dyspnea or arrest, bronchospasm, cough, and dyspnea). All patients received iron sucrose without a prior test dose by IV infusion or IV push in 10 consecutive doses of 100 mg each during consecutive dialysis sessions. There were no serious adverse reactions reported and no episodes of anaphylactoid reactions. Three mild adverse events that might have been related to iron sucrose were observed. However, no patient withdrew from the trial or was forced to stop the drug because of adverse events. Despite these encouraging results, postmarketing safety surveillance of iron sucrose has resulted in 27 reports of anaphylactoid reactions (out of an estimated 450,000 patient exposures), 8 of which were life-threatening.[200]

Both sodium ferric gluconate and iron sucrose cause fewer hypersensitivity reactions, including anaphylactoid reactions, and appear to be safer than iron dextran. The decision to give patients who are to receive parenteral iron preparation a test dose will depend on the product used. All patients receiving iron dextran should receive a test dose to assess tolerance. Neither sodium ferric gluconate nor iron sucrose requires a test dose per their prescribing information. However, the National Kidney Foundation-Dialysis Outcomes Quality Initiative 2000 guidelines recommended a one-time test dose for both iron dextran and sodium ferric gluconate, while making no statement regarding iron sucrose.[202] These guidelines do not reflect data that became available since their publication; future updates may provide different recommendations. It appears iron dextran-tolerant patients have little risk of experiencing a serious hypersensitivity or anaphylactoid reaction to sodium ferric gluconate or iron sucrose injection and can safely be given one of these products without a prior test dose. Similarly, patients who have never received any parenteral iron product can be administered sodium ferric gluconate or iron sucrose for injection without a prior test dose. While studies support the safety of both sodium ferric gluconate and iron sucrose for injection in iron dextran-sensitive patients, such patients may be at increased risk for an anaphylactoid reaction or other serious hypersensitivity response, and test dosing in this population may be reasonable. Regardless of whether a test dose is administered for any of the parenteral iron products, close monitoring of the patient following drug administration is necessary.

LATEX ALLERGY

Natural latex is a milky fluid consisting of extremely small particles of rubber obtained from the rubber tree. Natural rubber includes all products made from, or containing, natural latex.[208] Many products commonly used in health care are made wholly or in part of latex, such as gloves, BP cuffs, catheters, injection ports, and the rubber stoppers of many medication vials. Over the past few years, the significance of latex allergy has become clear as cases of allergic reactions, some life-threatening, have been reported.[208] Although not a drug allergy, health professionals must recognize the types of reactions latex may cause and must know how to minimize patient exposure to latex. Also, preparing parenteral drugs for latex-allergic patients can be difficult because of the number of materials involved that may contain latex. Last, health profes-

sionals are one of the groups at greatest risk for developing latex allergy because of their frequent exposure to latex products. Other groups at risk for developing latex allergy are workers in businesses that manufacture latex products, patients with spina bifida; and people with allergies to certain foods, including avocado, potato, banana, tomato, chestnuts, kiwi fruit, and papaya.[208]

Three types of reactions to latex have been described: irritant contact dermatitis, allergic contact dermatitis (chemical sensitivity dermatitis), and immediate hypersensitivity.[208,209] Irritant contact dermatitis is the most common form of reaction to latex and manifests as dry, itchy, irritated areas of the skin. This is not a true allergic reaction to latex.[208] Allergic contact dermatitis is a delayed hypersensitivity reaction and is caused by exposure to chemicals added during the processing and manufacturing of latex. A rash, similar to that seen with poison ivy, usually begins 24 to 48 hours after exposure and may progress to oozing blisters.[208] Last, immediate hypersensitivity is an IgE-mediated allergic response to proteins in the latex. The reaction may begin within minutes of exposure to latex but can occur hours later. Symptoms vary from mild skin redness, hives, and itching to respiratory involvement (runny nose, sneezing, itchy eyes, trouble breathing, asthma). Rare cases of anaphylactic shock have been described.[208] Reports of the prevalence of latex allergy vary from 1% to 6% of the general population and 8% to 12% of health care workers. Latex allergy is diagnosed by obtaining an accurate description of the reaction and establishing a temporal relationship to latex exposure. Diagnostic kits are available to detect latex antibodies as well as aid in the diagnosis of allergic contact dermatitis.[208,209]

Pharmacists, particularly those in settings in which IV or intramuscular medications are administered, may be faced with preparing parenteral products for a latex-allergic patient. This often poses a challenge because latex is in many of the materials used to prepare parenteral products, such as the rubber stoppers on medication vials, the injection ports on IV bags, rubber plungers for syringes, and IV transfer sets.[208,209] Many manufacturers are now preparing products in a latex-free form, which simplifies drug preparation. Furthermore, manufacturers of medical devices are now required to identify on their labels which products have natural latex and which have dry natural rubber.[210] Last, many institutions have instituted policies on how to prepare parenteral products for the "latex-sensitive" person. Readers are referred to these references for a detailed discussion of these procedures.[209,211–214]

PREVENTION AND MANAGEMENT OF ALLERGIC REACTIONS

26. A.M., a 40-year-old woman, is hospitalized with a diagnosis of community-acquired pneumonia. Her medical history is noncontributory except for an uneventful course of ampicillin 6 months before admission for an ear infection. A.M. is empirically treated with cefuroxime 0.75 g IV Q 8 hr. On day 2 of therapy, she develops a raised pruritic maculopapular rash on her back, abdomen, and upper extremities. Antacid, docusate sodium, albuterol by metered-dose inhaler, and multivitamins were initiated on the same day as the cefuroxime. How should A.M.'s allergic reaction be managed? How might her allergic reaction have been prevented?

When examining methods to prevent allergic reactions, three possibilities exist: (1) the patient has unknowingly been sensitized to a drug and experiences an allergic reaction upon receiving the same or a similar drug again; (2) the patient has a history of an allergic reaction to a medication and mistakenly receives the same or a similar medication a second time and again develops an allergic reaction; and (3) the patient has a history of an allergic reaction to a medication and intentionally receives the same or similar medication again. As in the first situation, A.M.'s allergic reaction was unpredictable and, therefore, could not be prevented. However, to prevent future allergic reactions (i.e., the second situation), A.M.'s reaction should be well documented in the medical chart and pharmacy records. In addition, all patients should undergo a thorough drug history upon hospitalization. Careful attention should be paid to differentiating drug intolerance (e.g., stomach upset) from true allergic reactions, and any allergic reactions elicited during an interview should be documented appropriately. Adequate communication of allergic reactions is the single most important method of preventing their occurrence.

As described earlier, the first step in managing an allergic reaction is to determine its cause. Given A.M.'s history of exposure to ampicillin, the timing of the reaction, and the low frequency of allergic reactions to her other medications, cefuroxime is the most likely candidate. Second, a decision regarding whether to stop the suspect drug should be made. This decision must be based on the severity of the reaction, the condition being treated, and the availability of suitable alternatives. When possible, an equally effective alternative drug should be substituted for the suspect agent, preferably one that is immunologically distinct to avoid cross-sensitivity (see Question 4 for a discussion of cross-reactivity).[215] If a suitable alternative exists, the offending agent should be stopped and the reaction treated symptomatically if necessary. In the case of A.M., another antimicrobial such as trimethoprim-sulfamethoxazole could be substituted for cefuroxime (see Chapter 60, Respiratory Tract Infections) and her symptoms treated with an oral or parenteral antihistamine, as well as a low-potency topical corticosteroid if necessary.

Last, some cases are described by the third situation: a patient develops an allergic reaction (or has a well-documented history of drug allergy), and it is inappropriate or not possible to change to an alternative drug. If the sensitivity reaction is severe or life-threatening, desensitization should be considered (see Questions 27 to 30); premedication to prevent or minimize anaphylaxis is not effective.[3] If the reaction is minor (e.g., pruritus, rash, or GI symptoms), premedication or management of the reaction with antiallergy medications (e.g., antihistamines) may be sufficient to allow completion of therapy. It is rare in such cases for the reaction to progress to more serious allergic symptoms such as anaphylaxis;[215] however, suppression of allergic symptoms should be undertaken cautiously because many immunologic reactions are not IgE mediated and may progress to serious reactions, despite treatment. In general, allergy suppression should be reserved for prevention of mild reactions that are known or strongly suspected to be IgE mediated.[3,215]

Desensitization

β-Lactams

27. K.A. is a 24-year-old primigravida in her eighth week of pregnancy with a history of angioedema secondary to penicillin. Her initial pregnancy screening revealed a positive Venereal Disease Research Laboratory (VDRL) reaction and a fluorescent treponemal antibody absorption (FTA-Abs) titer of 1:64. K.A. denies a history of genital lesions, currently does not exhibit clinical signs or symptoms of syphilis, and denies previous treatment for syphilis. Based on the serologic evidence and her history, a diagnosis of early latent syphilis is made. Current treatment guidelines indicate that penicillin is the drug of choice for K.A. How can a possible reaction to penicillin be prevented in K.A.? Is premedication an alternative to preventing a reaction?

Acute desensitization (or hyposensitization) is the process of administering gradually increasing doses of a drug over hours or days in an effort to develop clinical tolerance.[1,3,6,22,215] This process has been used successfully to reintroduce drugs to patients with known allergic reactions in situations in which no alternatives exist. It is most commonly used in patients with IgE-mediated hypersensitivity and is well described for penicillin-allergic patients. Desensitization, however, is not useful in preventing late penicillin reactions and should not be attempted in patients who have experienced severe dermatologic reactions such as exfoliative dermatitis.[22] Because K.A.'s reaction to penicillin may be potentially severe, premedication is not an option and desensitization to penicillin should be started. (See Chapter 65, Sexually Transmitted Diseases, for a discussion of alternative therapy.)

28. How should K.A. be desensitized? Why should she be skin tested before desensitization?

Before desensitization is begun, K.A. should be skin tested (see Questions 3 and 4) to confirm her penicillin allergy.[3,22,215] Patients who have a positive history of penicillin allergy, but whose skin tests are negative, can receive full therapeutic doses without desensitization with little risk of developing an allergic reaction. One author, for example, reported only one case of acute anaphylaxis in a skin test–negative patient given full therapeutic doses of penicillin in >1,500 skin tests; similar results have been reported by other investigators.[22,215] If K.A.'s skin test is positive, desensitization should be initiated. Acute oral desensitization to penicillin and other β-lactam antibiotics is well established; one such protocol is outlined in Table 4-14, although others have been used successfully.[216–219]

The oral route for β-lactam desensitization is preferred to the parenteral route because: (1) exposure by the oral route is less likely to cause a systemic allergic reaction than parenteral exposure; (2) fatal anaphylaxis from oral β-lactam drug therapy is rare; (3) preformed polymers and conjugates of penicillin major and minor determinants to penicillium proteins are not well absorbed after oral administration; (4) blood levels rise gradually, favoring univalent haptenation (appearance of multivalent hapten–carrier conjugates, on the other hand, is gradual); and (5) fatal or life-endangering reactions have not occurred using current methods. In addition, oral desensitization can be accomplished over several hours.[3] If oral desensitization is not possible (e.g., if oral absorption is question-

Table 4-14 β-Lactam Oral Desensitization Protocol

Stock Drug Concentration (mg/mL)[a]	Dose No.	Amount (mL)	Drug Dose (mg)	Cumulative Drug (mg)
0.5	1[b]	0.05	0.025	0.025
	2	0.10	0.05	0.075
	3	0.20	0.10	0.175
	4	0.40	0.20	0.375
	5	0.80	0.40	0.775
5.0	6	0.15	0.75	1.525
	7	0.30	1.50	3.025
	8	0.60	3.00	6.025
	9	1.20	6.00	12.025
	10	2.40	12.00	24.025
50	11	0.50	25.00	49.025
	12	1.20	60.00	109.025
	13	2.50	125.00	234.025
	14	5.00	250.00	484.025

[a]Dilutions using 250 mg/5 mL of pediatric suspension.
[b]Oral dose doubled approximately every 15–30 minutes.
Adapted from references 216 and 218. Dosing for the oral protocol is arbitrary and should be adjusted for individual patients based on the clinical sensitivity and the desired drug dose end point.

able), parenteral desensitization can be instituted. Although the subcutaneous and intramuscular routes have been used, the IV route is quicker and allows better control over the rate and concentration of drug administered, and any untoward reaction can be detected promptly and treated rapidly.[3,6,9] Table 4-15 outlines an IV β-lactam desensitization protocol. Unfortunately, oral and parenteral desensitization methods have not been compared formally. Patients should not be premedicated before desensitization, because this may prevent detection of minor allergic responses that may precede more serious reactions. In addition, desensitization should be performed in a setting where emergency resuscitative equipment and personnel are readily available.[215] Thus, K.A. should undergo oral desensitization as outlined in Table 4-14 if her skin test is positive.

29. Is K.A. at risk for an allergic reaction during desensitization? If desensitization is successful, is she at risk for a reaction during full-dose penicillin therapy?

Acute β-lactam desensitization, regardless of the route or protocol chosen, is not without risk. Approximately 5% of patients experience mild cutaneous reactions during desensitization, although one study reported reactions in 20% of patients during oral desensitization.[3,219] If a reaction occurs during the desensitization procedure itself, the reaction may be treated and desensitization continued using lower doses, increased intervals between doses, or both, after the reaction has abated. Severe, fatal reactions during desensitization are rare.[3]

Uneventful β-lactam desensitization, however, does not guarantee patients will be without reaction during full-dose therapy. Approximately 25% to 30% of patients experience a mild reaction during therapy, while 5% experience more severe reactions, including drug-induced serum sickness, hemolytic anemia, or nephritis.[3] Reaction rates are no different

in severely ill or pregnant patients compared with stable or nonpregnant patients, although those with cystic fibrosis may be more difficult to desensitize because of their high frequency of allergic reactions.[3,219–221] Despite the occurrence of reactions, full-dose therapy is possible for most desensitizations, but suppression of the reaction (e.g., by diphenhydramine) may be required.[3]

30. If K.A. requires penicillin at a later date, will she need to undergo desensitization again? What is chronic desensitization?

The desensitized state, once achieved, will persist for approximately 48 hours after the last full dose of antibiotic; after this time, drug sensitivity will return.[3] Thus, if K.A. requires future courses of penicillin, she will need to undergo desensitization once again. In some cases, those requiring long-term antibiotic therapy (e.g., for endocarditis), those who may require β-lactams at a future date (e.g., those with cystic fibrosis), or those who have occupational exposure to β-lactams, maintenance of the desensitized state can be considered. Chronic twice-daily dosing of oral penicillin has safely resulted in "chronic desensitization." However, similar to acute desensitization, once therapy is interrupted, the allergic state returns.[3,9]

Other Drugs

31. Have patients allergic to drugs besides β-lactams been desensitized successfully?

Although most experience with desensitization is with penicillin and other β-lactams, desensitization also has been accomplished with various other drugs, including rifampin,[221] isoniazid,[221] acyclovir,[222] sulfasalazine,[223–228] aminoglycosides,[220] vancomycin,[229,230] and several others.[231–244] Interest-

Table 4-15 β-Lactam Intravenous Desensitization Protocol

Stock Drug Concentration (mg/mL)[a]	Dose No.[b]	Amount per 50 mL (mg/mL)[c]	Cumulative Drug (mg)
0.005	1	0.0001	0.005
0.025	2	0.0005	0.030
0.125	3	0.0025	0.155
0.625	4	0.0125	0.780
3.125	5	0.0625	3.905
15.625	6	0.3125	19.530
31.25	7	0.625	50.780
62.50	8	1.25	113.280
125.00	9	2.5	238.280
250.00	10[d]	5.0	488.280

[a]Stock drug solutions are prepared using serial dilutions of the desired goal (e.g., 500 mg of β-lactam). Doses 1–5 represent fivefold dilutions; doses 6–10 represent twofold dilutions.
[b]Interval between doses is 15–30 minutes. If desensitization is interrupted for >2 half-lives of the β-lactam, desensitization should be repeated.
[c]Mix 1 mL of stock drug solution in 50 mL 5% dextrose/0.225 normal saline or other compatible solution. Infuse each dose over 20–45 minutes. Dilution volume may vary with patient age and weight.
[d]If all 10 doses are administered and tolerated, the remainder of a full therapeutic dose of the β-lactam should be administered.
Adapted from reference 255. Dosing for the IV protocol is arbitrary and should be adjusted for individual patients based on the clinical sensitivity and the desired drug dose end point.

Table 4-16 Oral Trimethoprim-Sulfamethoxazole Desensitization Protocol

Hour	Trimethoprim Component (Concentration or Tablet)	Volume	Dose of TMP-SMZ
0	0.0008 mg/mL	5 mL	0.004/0.02 mg
1	0.008 mg/mL	5 mL	0.04/0.2 mg
2	0.08 mg/mL	5 mL	0.4/2 mg
3	0.8 mg/mL	5 mL	4/20 mg
4	8 mg/mL	5 mL	40/200 mg
5	160 mg	1 tablet	160/800 mg

Stock solution of trimethoprim-sulfamethoxazole (TMP-SMZ) may be prepared by appropriate dilutions of the commercially available suspension (8 mg trimethoprim/40 mg sulfamethoxazole per mL) with simple syrup or distilled water.
Adapted with permission from Gluckstein D, Ruskin J. Rapid oral desensitization to trimethoprim-sulfamethoxazole use in prophylaxis for *Pneumocystis carinii* in patients with AIDS who were previously intolerant to TMP-SMZ. Clin Infect Dis 1995;20:849. This protocol should serve as a guide only. Obtaining informed consent from the patient before initiating desensitization is advisable.

ingly, not all of these cases represent IgE-mediated hypersensitivity reactions. Acute desensitization, which has until recently been used to manage only IgE-mediated reactions, appears to be effective in other forms of immunopathology.[3] For example, reactions to trimethoprim-sulfamethoxazole commonly occur in HIV-infected patients and may not be IgE mediated. Yet, successful desensitization to trimethoprim-sulfamethoxazole is increasingly common, given its role in treating and preventing *P. carinii* pneumonia.[3]

One procedure for trimethoprim-sulfamethoxazole desensitization[245] is outlined in Table 4-16, although several other protocols have been used successfully.[9,246-255] Although mild to moderate reactions may occur (e.g., fever, mild skin rash), patients may complete desensitization successfully by suppressing the reaction with antihistamines, reducing the dose to the highest level previously taken without a reaction until the reaction subsides, or both.[246,248,249] As with the β-lactams, before desensitization for any medication is undertaken, alternative therapies should be sought and used if possible. Furthermore, desensitization is contraindicated if the reaction is a serious dermatologic response such as toxic epidermal necrolysis or Stevens-Johnson syndrome. Last, desensitization should be undertaken only in an appropriate setting by experienced personnel, because severe reactions can develop.[256]

REFERENCES

1. DeSwarte RD. Drug allergy: problems and strategies. J Allergy Clin Immunol 1984;74(Pt 1):209.
2. Assem E-SK. Drug allergy and tests for its detection. In: Davies DM, ed. Textbook of Adverse Drug Reactions. 3rd Ed. New York: Oxford University Press, 1985:689.
3. Sullivan TJ. Drug allergy. In: Middleton E Jr et al, eds. Allergy. Principles and Practices. 4th Ed. St. Louis: Mosby, 1993:1726.
4. Jick H. Adverse drug reactions: the magnitude of the problem. J Allergy Clin Immunol 1984;74:555.
5. Classen DC et al. Computerized surveillance of adverse drug events in hospital patients. JAMA 1991;266:2847.
6. Van Arsdel PP Jr. Drug hypersensitivity. In: Bierman CW, Pearlman DS, eds. Allergic Diseases from Infancy to Adulthood. 2nd Ed. Philadelphia: WB Saunders, 1988:684.
7. Van Arsdel PP Jr. Classification and risk factors for drug allergy. Immunol Allergy Clin North Am 1991;11:475.
8. Adkinson NF Jr. Risk factors for drug allergy. J Allergy Clin Immunol 1984;74:567.
9. Anderson JA. Allergic reactions to drugs and biological agents. JAMA 1992;268:2845.
10. Bigby M et al. Drug-induced cutaneous reactions. JAMA 1986;256:3358.
11. Parker CW. Drug allergy. N Engl J Med 1975; 292(Pt 1–3):511,732,957.
12. Ma MK et al. Genetic basis of drug metabolism. Am J Health-Syst Pharm 2002;59:2061.
13. Breathnach SM. Mechanisms of drug eruptions: Part I. Australas J Dermatol 1995;36:121.
14. Svensson CK et al. Cutaneous drug reactions. Pharmacol Rev 2000;53:357.
15. Evans WE, McLeod HL. Pharmacogenomics: drug disposition, drug targets, and side effects. N Engl J Med 2003;348:538.
16. Mallal S et al. Association between presence of HLA-B*5701, HLA-DR7, and HLA-DQ3 and hypersensitivity to HIV-1 reverse-transcriptase inhibitor abacavir. Lancet 2002;359:722.
17. de Weck AL. Pharmacological and immunochemical mechanisms of drug hypersensitivity. Immunol Allergy Clin North Am 1991;11:461.

18. Bochner BS, Lichtenstein LM. Anaphylaxis. N Engl J Med 1991;324:1785.
19. Marquardt DL, Wasserman SI. Anaphylaxis. In: Middleton E Jr et al, eds. Allergy. Principles and Practices. 4th Ed. St. Louis: Mosby, 1993:1365.
20. Yunginger JW. Anaphylaxis. Ann Allergy 1992;69:87.
21. Shepherd GM. Allergy to β-lactam antibiotics. Immunol Allergy Clin North Am 1991;11:611.
22. Lin RY. A perspective on penicillin allergy. Arch Intern Med 1992;152:930.
23. Gruchalla RS, Sullivan TJ. In vivo and in vitro diagnosis of drug allergy. Immunol Allergy Clin North Am 1991; 11:595.
24. Weiss ME. Drug allergy. Med Clin North Am 1992;76:857.
25. Perencevich EN et al. Benefits of negative penicillin test results persist during subsequent hospital admissions. Clin Infect Dis 2001;32(2):317.
26. Romano A et al. Immediate hypersensitivity to cephalosporins. Allergy 2002;57(Suppl 72):52.
27. Robinson JL et al. Practical aspects of choosing an antibiotic for patients with a reported allergy to an antibiotic. Clin Infect Dis 2002;35:261.
28. Romano A et al. Immediate allergic reactions to cephalosporins: cross-reactivity and selective responses. J Allergy Clin Immunol 2000;106:1177.
29. Blanca M et al. Side-chain-specific reactions to beta-lactams: 14 years later. Clin Exp All 2002;32:192.
30. Fath JJ, Cerra FB. The therapy of anaphylactic shock. Drug Intell Clin Pharm 1984;18:14.
31. Atkinson TP, Kaliner MA. Anaphylaxis. Med Clin North Am 1992;76:841.
32. Delage C, Irey NA. Anaphylactic deaths: a clinicopathologic study of 43 cases. J Forensic Sci 1972;17:525.
33. Buhner D, Grant JA. Serum sickness. Dermatol Clin 1985;3:107.
34. Lin RY. Serum sickness syndrome. Am Fam Physician 1986;33:157.
35. Erffmeyer JE. Serum sickness. Ann Allergy 1986;56:105.
36. Lawley TJ et al. A study of human serum sickness. J Invest Dermatol 1985;85(Suppl):129S.

37. Andersen JM, Tiede JJ. Serum sickness associated with 6-mercaptopurine in a patient with Crohn's disease. Pharmacotherapy 1997;17:173.
38. Wolfe MS, Moede AL. Serum sickness with furazolidone. Am J Trop Med Hyg 1978;27:762.
39. Dukes MNG, ed. Meylers Side Effects of Drugs. 12th Ed. Amsterdam: Elsevier Science Publishers, 1992.
40. Cunningham E et al. Acute serum sickness with glomerulonephritis induced by antithymocyte globulin. Transplantation 1987;43:309.
41. Bielory L et al. Human serum sickness: a prospective analysis of 35 patients treated with equine antithymocyte globulin for bone marrow failure. Medicine 1988;67:40.
42. Bielory L et al. Cutaneous manifestations of serum sickness in patients receiving antithymocyte globulin. J Am Acad Dermatol 1985;13:411.
43. Calabrese LH et al. The American College of Rheumatology 1990 criteria for the classification of hypersensitivity vasculitis. Arthritis Rheum 1990;33:1108.
44. Panwalker AP et al. Serum sickness associated with cefoxitin and pentoxifylline therapy. Drug Intell Clin Pharm 1986;20:953.
45. Igarashi M et al. An immunodominant haptenic epitope of carbamazepine detected in serum from patients given long-term treatment with carbamazepine without allergic reaction. J Clin Immunol 1992;12:335.
46. Ferraccioli G et al. Indomethacin-related serum sickness-like illness with IgM lambda cryoparaprotein. Acta Haematol 1985;73:45.
47. Haruda F. Phenytoin hypersensitivity. Neurology 1979;29:1480.
48. Josephs SH et al. Phenytoin hypersensitivity. J Allergy Clin Immunol 1980;66:166.
49. Tomsick RS. The phenytoin syndrome. Cutis 1983;32:535.
50. Reynolds RD. Cefaclor and serum sickness-like reaction. JAMA 1996;276:950.
51. Comenzo RL et al. Immune hemolysis, disseminated intravascular coagulation, and serum sickness after large doses of immune globulin given intravenously for Kawasaki disease. J Pediatr 1992;120:926.

52. Tomas S et al. Ciprofloxacin and immunocomplex-mediated disease. J Intern Med 1991;230:550.
53. Slama TG. Serum sickness-like illness associated with ciprofloxacin. Antimicrob Agents Chemother 1990;34:904.
54. Bielory L. Serum sickness from iron-dextran administration. Acta Haematol 1990;83:166.
55. Vincent A et al. Serum sickness induced by fluoxetine. Am J Psychiatry 1991;148:1602.
56. Miller LG et al. A case of fluoxetine-induced serum sickness. Am J Psychiatry 1989;146:1616.
57. Park H, Knowles S, Shear NH. Serum sickness-like reaction to itraconazole. Pharmacotherapy 1998;32:1249.
58. Young EJ et al. Drug-induced fever: cases seen in the evaluation of unexplained fever in a general hospital population. Rev Infect Dis 1982;4:69.
59. Lipsky BA, Hirschmann JV. Drug fever. JAMA 1981;245:851.
60. Kumar KL, Reuler JB. Drug fever. West J Med 1986;144:753.
61. Tabor PA. Drug-induced fever. Drug Intell Clin Pharm 1986;20:413.
62. Cunha BA. Drug fever. Postgrad Med 1986;80:123.
63. Mackowiak PA, LeMaistre CF. Drug fever: a critical appraisal of conventional concepts. Ann Intern Med 1987;106:728.
64. Hofland SL. Drug fever: is your patient's fever drug-related? Crit Care Nurse 1985;5:29.
65. Hiraide A et al. IgE-mediated drug fever due to histamine H₂-receptor blockers. Drug Safe 1990;5:455.
66. Johnson DH, Cunha BA. Drug fever. Infect Dis Clin North Am 1996;10:85.
67. Cunha BA, Shea KW. Fever in the intensive care unit. Infect Dis Clin North Am 1996;10:185.
68. Fischer SA, Trenholme GM, Levin S. Fever in the solid organ transplant patient. Infect Dis Clin North Am 1996;10:167.
69. Lossos IS, Matzner Y. Hydroxyurea-induced fever: case report and review of the literature. Ann Pharmacother 1995;29:132.
70. Arellano F, Sacristan JA. Allopurinol hypersensitivity syndrome. Ann Pharmacother 1993;27:337.
71. Steinmetz JC et al. Hypersensitivity vasculitis associated with 2-deoxycoformycin and allopurinol therapy. Am J Med 1989;86:499.
72. Scerri L, Pace JL. Mefloquine-associated cutaneous vasculitis. Int J Dermatol 1993;32:517.
73. Enat R et al. Hypersensitivity vasculitis induced by terbutaline sulfate. Ann Allergy 1988;61:275.
74. Bergman SM et al. Azathioprine and hypersensitivity vasculitis. Ann Intern Med 1988;109:83.
75. Simonart T et al. Cutaneous necrotizing vasculitis after low-dose methotrexate therapy for rheumatoid arthritis: a possible manifestation of methotrexate hypersensitivity. Clin Rheumatol 1997;16:623.
76. Rustmann WC et al. Leukocytoclastic vasculitis associated with sotalol therapy. J Am Acad Dermatol 1998;38:111.
77. Drory VE, Korczyn AD. Hypersensitivity vasculitis and systemic lupus erythematosus induced by anticonvulsants. Clin Neuropharmacol 1993;16:19.
78. Singhal PC et al. Hypersensitivity angiitis associated with naproxen. Ann Allergy 1989;63:107.
79. Bear RA et al. Vasculitis and vitamin abuse. Arch Pathol Lab Med 1982;106:48.
80. Martinez-Taboada VM et al. Clinical features and outcome of 95 patients with hypersensitivity vasculitis. Am J Med 1997;102:186.
81. Suh JG, Oleksowicz L, Dutcher JP. Leukocytoclastic vasculitis associated with nizatidine therapy. Am J Med 1997;102:216.
82. Grunwald MH et al. Allergic vasculitis induced by hydrochlorothiazide: confirmation by mast cell degranulation test. Isr J Med Sci 1989;25:572.
83. Mitchell GG et al. Cimetidine-induced cutaneous vasculitis. Am J Med 1983;75:875.
84. Huminer D et al. Hypersensitivity vasculitis due to ofloxacin. Br Med J 1989;299:303.
85. Jungst G, Mohr R. Side effects of ofloxacin in clinical trials and in postmarketing surveillance. Drugs 1987;34(Suppl 1):144.

86. Palop-Larea V et al. Vasculitis with acute kidney failure and torsemide. Lancet 1998;352:1909.
87. Kanuga J et al. Ciprofloxacin-induced leukocytoclastic vasculitis with cryoglobulinemia [Abstract]. Ann Allergy 1991;66:76.
88. Choe U et al. Ciprofloxacin-induced vasculitis. N Engl J Med 1989;320:257.
89. Stubbings J et al. Cutaneous vasculitis due to ciprofloxacin. Br Med J 1992;305:29.
90. Hannedouche T, Fillastre JP. Penicillin-induced hypersensitivity vasculitides. J Antimicrob Chemother 1987;20:3.
91. Gavura SR, Nusinowitz S. Leukocytoclastic vasculitis associated with clarithromycin. Ann Pharmacother 1998;32:543.
92. Kamper AM et al. Cutaneous vasculitis induced by sodium valproate. Lancet 1991;337:497.
93. Lin RY. Unusual autoimmune manifestations in furosemide-associated hypersensitivity angiitis. NY State J Med 1988;88:439.
94. Leung AC et al. Phenylbutazone-induced systemic vasculitis with crescentic glomerulonephritis. Arch Intern Med 1985;145:685.
95. Reynolds NJ et al. Hydralazine predisposes to acute cutaneous vasculitis following urography with iopamidol. Br J Dermatol 1993;129:82.
96. Fox BC, Peterson A. Leukocytoclastic vasculitis after pneumococcal vaccination. Am J Infection Control 1998;26:365.
97. Tanay A et al. Dermal vasculitis due to Coumadin hypersensitivity. Dermatologica 1982;165:178.
98. Knox JP et al. Procainamide-induced urticarial vasculitis. Cutis 1988;42:469.
99. Torres RA et al. Zidovudine-induced leukocytoclastic vasculitis. Arch Intern Med 1992;152:850.
100. Travis WD et al. Hypersensitivity pneumonitis and pulmonary vasculitis with eosinophilia in a patient taking an L-tryptophan preparation. Ann Intern Med 1990;112:301.
101. Stankus SJ, Johnson NT. Propylthiouracil-induced hypersensitivity vasculitis presenting as respiratory failure. Chest 1992;102:1595.
102. Wolf D et al. Nodular vasculitis associated with propylthiouracil. Cutis 1992;49:253.
103. Carrasco MD et al. Cutaneous vasculitis associated with propylthiouracil therapy. Arch Intern Med 1987;147:1677.
104. Alarcon-Segovia D et al. Antinuclear antibodies in patients on anticonvulsant therapy. Clin Exp Immunol 1972;12:39.
105. Jacobs JC. Systemic lupus erythematosus in childhood. Report of 35 cases, with discussion of 7 apparently induced by anticonvulsant medication, and of prognosis and treatment. Pediatrics 1963;32:257.
106. Bleck TP, Smith MC. Possible induction of systemic lupus erythematosus syndrome by valproate. Epilepsia 1990;31:343.
107. Ahuja GK, Schumacher GA. Drug-induced SLE: primidone as a possible cause. JAMA 1966;198:201.
108. Drory VE et al. Carbamazepine-induced systemic lupus erythematosus. Clin Neuropharmacol 1989;12:115.
109. Livingston S et al. Carbamazepine in epilepsy. Nine-year follow-up with special emphasis on untoward reactions. Dis Nerv Syst 1974;35:103.
110. Livingston S et al. Systemic lupus erythematosus. Occurrence in association with ethosuximide therapy. JAMA 1968;204:185.
111. Wandl UB et al. Lupus-like autoimmune disease induced by interferon therapy for myeloproliferative disorders. Clin Immunol Immunopathol 1992;65:70.
112. Machold KP, Smolen JS. Interferon-gamma induced exacerbation of systemic lupus erythematosus. J Rheumatol 1990;17:831.
113. Ronnblom LE et al. Possible induction of systemic lupus erythematosus by interferon-alpha treatment in a patient with a malignant carcinoid tumour. J Intern Med 1990;227:207.
114. Schilling PJ et al. Development of systemic lupus erythematosus after interferon therapy for chronic myelogenous leukemia. Cancer 1991;68:1536.

115. Gilliland BC. Drug-induced autoimmune and hematologic disorders. Drug Allergy 1991;11:525.
116. Skaer TL. Medication-induced systemic lupus erythematosus. Clin Ther 1992;14:496.
117. Woosley RL et al. Effect of acetylator phenotype on the rate at which procainamide induces antinuclear antibodies and the lupus syndrome. N Engl J Med 1978;298:1157.
118. Lahita R et al. Antibodies to nuclear antigens in patients treated with procainamide or acetylprocainamide. N Engl J Med 1979;301:1382.
119. Roden DM et al. Antiarrhythmic efficacy, pharmacokinetics and safety of N-acetylprocainamide in human subjects: comparison with procainamide. Am J Cardiol 1980;46:463.
120. Stec GP et al. Remission of procainamide-induced lupus erythematosus with N-acetylprocainamide therapy. Ann Intern Med 1979;90:799.
121. Booth RJ et al. Beta-adrenergic-receptor blockers and antinuclear antibodies in hypertension. Clin Pharmacol Ther 1982;31:555.
122. Greenberg JH, Lutcher CL. Drug-induced systemic lupus erythematosus. JAMA 1972;222:191.
123. Lee SL, Chase PH. Drug-induced systemic lupus erythematosus. A critical review. Semin Arthritis Rheum 1975;6:83.
124. Perry HM. Late toxicity to hydralazine resembling systemic lupus erythematosus or rheumatoid arthritis. Am J Med 1973;54:58.
125. Kendall MJ, Hawkins CF. Quinidine-induced systemic lupus erythematosus. Postgrad Med J 1970;46:729.
126. Cohen MG et al. Two distinct quinidine-induced rheumatic syndromes. Ann Intern Med 1988;108:369.
127. West SG et al. Quinidine-induced lupus erythematosus. Ann Intern Med 1984;100:840.
128. Burlingame RW, Rubin RL. Anti-histone antibody induction by drugs implicates autoimmunization with nucleohistone [Abstract]. Arthritis Rheum 1980;32(Suppl 4):S22.
129. Dubois EL et al. Chlorpromazine-induced systemic lupus erythematosus. JAMA 1972;221:595.
130. Fabius AJM, Faulhofer WK. Systemic lupus erythematosus induced by psychotropic drugs. Acta Rheumatol Scand 1971;17:137.
131. Goldman LS et al. Lupus-like illness associated with chlorpromazine. Am J Psychiatry 1980;137:1613.
132. Quismorio FP et al. Antinuclear antibodies in chronic psychotic patients treated with chlorpromazine. Am J Psychiatry 1975;132:1204.
133. Harrington TM, Davis DE. Systemic lupus-like syndrome induced by methyldopa therapy. Chest 1981;79:696.
134. Dupont A, Six R. Lupus-like syndrome induced by methyldopa. Br Med J 1982;285:693.
135. Perry HM Jr et al. Immunologic findings in patients receiving methyldopa: a prospective study. J Lab Clin Med 1971;78:905.
136. Nordstrom DM et al. Methyldopa-induced systemic lupus erythematosus. Arthritis Rheum 1989;32:205.
137. Vyse T, So AKL. Sulphasalazine-induced autoimmune syndrome. Br J Rheumatol 1992;31:115.
138. Griffiths ID, Kane SP. Sulphasalazine-induced lupus syndrome in ulcerative colitis. Br Med J 1977;2:1188.
139. Crisp AJ, Hoffbrand BI. Sulphasalazine-induced systemic lupus erythematosus in a patient with Sjogren's syndrome. J R Soc Med 1980;73:60.
140. Carr-Locke D. Sulfasalazine-induced lupus syndrome in a patient with Crohn's disease. Am J Gastroenterol 1982;77:614.
141. Clementz GL, Doli BJ. Sulfasalazine-induced lupus erythematosus. Am J Med 1988;84:535.
142. Rafferty P et al. Sulphasalazine-induced cerebral lupus erythematosus. Postgrad Med J 1982;58:98.
143. Meier CR et al. Postmenopausal estrogen replacement therapy and risk of developing systemic lupus erythematosus or discoid lupus. J Rheumatol 1998;25:1515.
144. Elkayam O, Yaron M, Caspi D. Minocycline-induced autoimmune syndromes: an overview. Semin Arthritis Rheum 1999;28:392.

145. Holmes S, Kemmett D. Exacerbation of systemic lupus erythematosus induced by terbinafine. Br J Dermatol 1998;139:1133.

146. Solinger AM. Drug-related lupus. Clinical and etiologic considerations. Rheum Dis Clin North Am 1988;14:187.

147. Alarcon-Segovia D et al. Clinical and experimental studies on the hydralazine syndrome and its relation to SLE. Medicine 1967;46:1.

148. Chalmer A et al. Systemic lupus erythematosus during penicillamine therapy for rheumatoid arthritis. Ann Intern Med 1982;97:659.

149. Finekl TH et al. Drug-induced lupus in a child after treatment with zafirlukast (Accolate). J Allergy Clin Immunol 1999;103:533.

150. Calabrese LH. Differential diagnosis of hypersensitivity vasculitis. Cleve Clin J Med 1990;57:506.

151. Semble EL et al. Vasculitis: a practical approach to management. Postgrad Med 1991;90:161.

152. Morrow JD et al. Studies on the control of hypertension by hyphex. II. Toxic reactions and side effects. Circulation 1953;8:829.

153. Perry HJ et al. Relationship of acetyltransferase activity to antinuclear antibodies and toxic symptoms in hypertensive patients treated with hydralazine. J Lab Clin Med 1970;76:114.

154. Tan EM et al. The 1982 revised criteria for the classification of systemic lupus erythematosus. Arthritis Rheum 1982;25:1271.

155. Blomgren SE et al. Antinuclear antibody induced by procainamide. N Engl J Med 1969;281:64.

156. Henningsen NC et al. Effects of long-term treatment with procainamide. Acta Med Scand 1975;198:475.

157. Kowsowsky BC et al. Long-term use of procainamide following acute myocardial infarction. Circulation 1973;47:1204.

158. Cameron HA, Ramsay LE. The lupus syndrome induced by hydralazine: a common complication with low-dose treatment. Br Med J 1984;189:410.

159. Anderson JA, Adkinson NF Jr. Allergic reactions to drugs and biologic agents. JAMA 1987;258:2891.

160. Blombgren SE et al. Procainamide-induced lupus erythematosus: clinical and laboratory observations. Am J Med 1972;52:338.

161. Van Arsdel PP Jr. Pseudoallergic drug reactions. Introduction and general review. Immunol Allergy Clin North Am 1991;11:635.

162. Burke P, Burne SR. Allergy associated with ciprofloxacin. Br Med J 2000;320:679.

163. Culver CA. Probable anaphylactoid reaction to a pyrethrin pediculicide shampoo. Clin Pharm 1988;7:846.

164. Polk RE. Anaphylactoid reactions to glycopeptide antibiotics. J Antimicrob Chemother 1991; 27(Suppl B):17.

165. Lasser EC. Pseudoallergic drug reactions. Radiographic contrast media. Immunol Allergy Clin North Am 1991;11:645.

166. Israili ZH, Hall WD. Cough and angioneurotic edema associated with angiotensin-converting enzyme inhibitor therapy. A review of the literature and pathophysiology. Ann Intern Med 1992; 117:234.

167. Manning ME, Stevenson DD. Pseudoallergic drug reactions. Aspirin, nonsteroidal anti-inflammatory drugs, dyes, additives, and preservatives. Immunol Allergy Clin North Am 1991;11:659.

168. Davis H et al. Anaphylactoid reactions reported after treatment with ciprofloxacin. Ann Intern Med 1989;111:1041.

169. Chen M et al. Anaphylactoid-anaphylactic reactions associated with ondansetron [Letter]. Ann Intern Med 1993;119:862.

170. Stevenson DD, Simon RA. Sensitivity to aspirin and nonsteroidal anti-inflammatory drugs. In: Middleton E Jr et al, eds. Allergy. Principles and Practices. 4th Ed. St. Louis: Mosby, 1993: 1747.

171. Bonfiglio MF et al. Anaphylactoid reaction to intravenous acetylcysteine associated with electrocardiographic abnormalities. Ann Pharmacother 1992;26:22.

172. Deamer RL et al. Hypersensitivity and anaphylactoid reactions to ciprofloxacin. Ann Pharmacother 1992;26:1081.

173. Soetikno RM et al. Ciprofloxacin-induced anaphylactoid reaction in a patient with AIDS [Letter]. Ann Pharmacother 1993;27:1404.

174. Kossey JL, Kwok KK. Anaphylactoid reactions associated with ondansetron. Ann Pharmacother 1994;28:1029.

175. deShazo RD, Kemp SF. Allergic reactions to drugs. JAMA 1997;278:1895.

176. Berkes EA. Anaphylactic and anaphylactoid reactions to aspirin and other NSAIDs. Clin Rev Allergy Immunol 2003;24:137.

177. Woessner KM et al. The safety of celecoxib in patients with aspirin-sensitive asthma. Arthritis Rheum 2002;46:2201.

178. Szczeklik A et al. Safety of a specific COX-2 inhibitor in aspirin-induced asthma. Clin Exp Allergy 2001;31:219.

179. Pacor ML et al. Safety of rofecoxib in subjects with a history of adverse cutaneous reactions to aspirin and/or non-steroidal anti-inflammatory drugs. Clin Exp Allergy 2002;32:397.

180. Quiralte J et al. Safety of selective cyclooxygenase-2 inhibitor rofecoxib in patients with NSAID-induced cutaneous reactions. Ann Allergy Asthma Immunol 2002;89:63.

181. Alderman CP. Adverse effects of the angiotensin-converting enzyme inhibitors. Ann Pharmacother 1996;30:55.

182. Cha YJ, Pearson VE. Angioedema due to losartan. Ann Pharmacother 1999;33:936.

183. Rivera JO. Losartan-induced angioedema. Ann Pharmacother 1999;33:933.

184. Rupprecht R et al. Angioedema due to losartan. Allergy 1999;4:81.

185. van Rijnsoever EW, Kwee-Zuiderwijk WJ, Feenstra J. Angioneurotic edema attributed to the use of losartan. Arch Intern Med 1998;158:2063.

186. Frye CB, Pettigrew TJ. Angioedema and photosensitive rash induced by valsartan. Pharmacotherapy 1998;18:866.

187. Sharma PK, Yium JJ. Angioedema associated with angiotensin II receptor antagonist losartan. South Med J 1997;90:552.

188. Boxer M. Accupril- and Cozaar-induced angioedema in the same patient. J Allergy Clin Immunol 1996;98:471.

189. Acker CG et al. Angioedema induced by the angiotensin II blocker losartan. N Engl J Med 1995;333:1572.

190. Pylypchuk GB. ACE-inhibitor- versus angiotensin II blocker-induced cough and angioedema. Ann Pharmacother 1998;32:1060.

191. Alkins SA et al. Anaphylactoid reactions to methotrexate. Cancer 1996;77:2123.

192. Okano M, Imai S. Anaphylactoid symptoms due to oral minocycline. Acta Derm Venerol 1996;76:164.

193. Essayan DM et al. Successful parenteral desensitization to paclitaxel. J Allergy Clin Immunol 1996;97(1 Pt 1):42.

194. Hebert ME et al. Anaphylactoid reactions with intraperitoneal cisplatin. Ann Pharmacother 1995;29:260.

195. Fishbane S, Ungureanu V, Maesaka J, et al. The safety of intravenous iron dextran in hemodialysis patients. Am J Kidney Dis 1996;25:529.

196. Michael B, Coyne DW, Fishbane S, et al. Sodium ferric gluconate complex in hemodialysis patients: adverse reactions compared to placebo and iron dextran. Kidney Int 2002;61:1830.

197. Ferrlecit (sodium ferric gluconate complex in sucrose injection) prescribing information. Watson Pharma, Inc. November 2001.

198. Faich G, Strobos J. Sodium ferric gluconate complex in sucrose: safer intravenous iron therapy than iron dextrans. Am J Kidney Dis 1999;33:464.

199. Coyne DW, Adkinson Jr. NF, Nissenson AR, et al. Sodium ferric gluconate complex in hemodialysis patents. II. Adverse reactions in iron dextran-sensitive and dextran-tolerant patients. Kidney Int 2003;63:217.

200. Venofer injection (iron sucrose injection) prescribing information. American Regent Laboratories, Inc. December 2000.

201. Van Wyck DB, Cavallo G, Spinowitz BS, et al. Safety and efficacy of iron sucrose in patients sensitive to iron dextran: North American clinical trial. Am J Kidney Dis 2000;36:88.

202. National Kidney Foundation-Dialysis Outcomes Quality Initiative 2000. Guidelines for anemia of chronic kidney disease. Available at http://www.kidney.org/professionals/doqi/guidelines/doqi_up toc.html#an. Accessed April 26, 2003.

203. Valdivieso R et al. Pseudo-allergic reactions to corticosteroids: diagnosis and alternatives. J Invest Clin Immunol 1995;5:171.

204. Kamm GL, Hagmeyer KO. Allergic-type reactions to corticosteroids. Ann Pharmacother 1999;33:451.

205. Liau-Chu M, Theis JG, Koren G. Mechanism of anaphylactoid reactions: improper preparation of high-dose cyclosporine leads to a bolus infusion of Cremophor EL and cyclosporine. Ann Pharmacother 1997;31:1287.

206. Volcheck GW, Dellen RG. Anaphylaxis to intravenous cyclosporine and tolerance to oral cyclosporine: case report and review. Ann Allergy Asthma Immunol 1998;80:159.

207. Greenberger PA et al. Two pretreatment regimens for high-risk patients receiving radiographic contrast media. J Allergy Clin Immunol 1984;74:540.

208. DHHS (NIOSH) Publication No. 97-135: Preventing allergic reactions to natural rubber latex in the workplace. June 1997.

209. Senst BL, Johnson RA. Latex allergy. Am J Health-Syst Pharm 1997;54:1071.

210. Thompson CA. Medical devices with latex to become easier to identify. Am J Health-Syst Pharm 1998;55:2059.

211. Kim KT et al. Implementation recommendations for making health care facilities latex safe. AORN J 1998;67:615.

212. Rice SP, Gutfeld MB. Preparation of latex-safe sterile products. Am J Health-Syst Pharm 1998;55:1466.

213. Au AL, Sloskey GE, Knisely V. Important points to note when preparing nutritional admixtures for latex-sensitive patients. Am J Health-Syst Pharm 1997;54:2128.

214. McDermott JS, Gura KM. Procedures for preparing injectable medications for latex-sensitive patients. Am J Health-Syst Pharm 1997;54:2516.

215. Wedner HJ. Drug allergy prevention and treatment. Immunol Allergy Clin North Am 1991;11:679.

216. Sullivan TJ et al. Desensitization of patients allergic to penicillin using orally administered β-lactam antibiotics. J Allergy Clin Immunol 1982;69:275.

217. Sullivan TJ. Antigen-specific desensitization of patients allergic to penicillin. J Allergy Clin Immunol 1982;69:500.

218. Wendel GD Jr et al. Penicillin allergy and desensitization in serious infections during pregnancy. N Engl J Med 1985;312:1229.

219. Stark BJ et al. Acute and chronic desensitization of penicillin-allergic patients using oral penicillin. J Allergy Clin Immunol 1987;79:523.

220. Earl HS, Sullivan TJ. Acute desensitization of a patient with cystic fibrosis allergic to both beta-lactam and aminoglycoside antibiotics. J Allergy Clin Immunol 1987;79:477.

221. Holland CL et al. Rapid oral desensitization to isoniazid and rifampin. Chest 1990;98:1518.

222. Henry RE et al. Successful oral acyclovir desensitization. Ann Allergy 1993;70:386.

223. Farr M et al. Sulphasalazine desensitization in rheumatoid arthritis [Letter]. Br Med J 1982; 284:118.

224. Bax DE, Amos RS. Sulphasalazine in rheumatoid arthritis: desensitizing the patient with a skin rash. Ann Rheum Dis 1986;45:139.

225. Purdy BH et al. Desensitization for sulfasalazine skin rash. Ann Intern Med 1984;100:512.

226. Toila V. Sulfasalazine desensitization in children and adolescents with chronic inflammatory bowel disease. Am J Gastroenterol 1992;87:1029.

227. Taffet SL, Das KM. Desensitization of patients with inflammatory bowel disease to sulfasalazine. Am J Med 1982;73:520.
228. Holdsworth CD. Sulfasalazine desensitization [Letter]. Br Med J 1982;282:110.
229. Lerner A, Dwyer JM. Desensitization to vancomycin [Letter]. Ann Intern Med 1984;100:157.
230. Lin RY. Desensitization in the management of vancomycin hypersensitivity. Arch Intern Med 1990;150:2197.
231. Bell ET et al. Sulphadiazine desensitization in AIDS patients [Letter]. Lancet 1985;1:163.
232. Tenant-Flowers M et al. Sulphadiazine desensitization in patients with AIDS and cerebral toxoplasmosis. AIDS 1991;5:311.
233. de la Hoz Caballer B et al. Management of sulfadiazine allergy in patients with acquired immunodeficiency syndrome. J Allergy Clin Immunol 1991;88:137.
234. Greenberger PA, Patterson R. Management of drug allergy in patients with acquired immunodeficiency syndrome. J Allergy Clin Immunol 1987;79:484.
235. Walz-LeBlanc BAE et al. Allopurinol sensitivity in a patient with chronic tophaceous gout: success of intravenous desensitization after failure of oral desensitization. Arthritis Rheum 1991;34:1329.
236. Fasm AG et al. Desensitization to allopurinol in patients with gout and cutaneous reactions. Am J Med 1992;93:299.
237. Pleskow WW et al. Aspirin desensitization in aspirin-sensitive asthmatic patients: clinical manifestations and characterization of the refractory period. J Allergy Clin Immunol 1982;69:11.
238. Knight A. Desensitization to aspirin in aspirin-sensitive patients with rhino-sinusitis and asthma: a review. J Otolaryngol 1989;18:165.

239. Lumry WR et al. Aspirin-sensitive asthma and rhinosinusitis: current concepts and recent advances. Ear Nose Throat J 1984;63:102.
240. Smith H, Newton R. Adverse reactions to carbamazepine managed by desensitization [Letter]. Lancet 1985;1:753.
241. Carr A et al. Allergy and desensitization to zidovudine in patients with acquired immunodeficiency syndrome. J Allergy Clin Immunol 1993;91:683.
242. Kurohara ML et al. Metronidazole hypersensitivity and oral desensitization. J Allergy Clin Immunol 1991;88:279.
243. Rassiga AL et al. Cytarabine-induced anaphylaxis. Demonstration of antibody and successful desensitization. Arch Intern Med 1980;140:425.
244. Thompson DM, Ronco JJ. Prolonged desensitization required for treatment of generalized allergy to human insulin [Letter]. Diabetes Care 1993;16:957.
245. Gluckstein D, Rushkin J. Rapid oral desensitization to trimethoprim-sulfamethoxazole (TMP-SMZ) use in prophylaxis for *Pneumocystis carinii* pneumonia in patients with AIDS who were previously intolerant to TMP-SMZ. Clin Infect Dis 1995;20:849.
246. Smith RM et al. Trimethoprim-sulfamethoxazole desensitization in the acquired immunodeficiency syndrome [Letter]. Ann Intern Med 1987;106:335.
247. Hughes TE et al. Co-trimoxazole desensitization in bone marrow transplant [Letter]. Ann Intern Med 1986;105:148.
248. Torgovnick J, Arsura E. Desensitization to sulfonamides in patients with HIV infection [Letter]. Am J Med 1990;88:548.
249. Kletzel M et al. Trimethoprim-sulfamethoxazole oral desensitization in hemophiliacs infected with

human immunodeficiency virus with a history of hypersensitivity reactions. Am J Dis Child 1991;145:1428.
250. Finegold I. Oral desensitization to trimethoprim-sulfamethoxazole in a patient with acquired immunodeficiency syndrome. J Allergy Clin Immunol 1986;78:905.
251. White MV et al. Desensitization to trimethoprim sulfamethoxazole in patients with acquired immune deficiency syndrome and *Pneumocystis carinii* pneumonia. Ann Allergy 1989;62:177.
252. Gluckstein D, Ruskin J. Trimethoprim-sulfamethoxazole desensitization permits long-term Pneumocystis prophylaxis in AIDS patients with prior TS intolerance. Interscience Conference on Antimicrobial Agents and Chemotherapy. Los Angeles, 1992. Abstract 1475.
253. Rich JD et al. Successful oral desensitization to TMP/SMX in persons with HIV infection and prior hypersensitive reactions. Int Conf AIDS. Boston, 1993. Abstract PO-810-1482.
254. Moreno JN, Maggio CM. Oral desensitization to sulfadiazine and trimethoprim-sulfamethoxazole (TMP-SMZ) in 4 patients with acquired immunodeficiency syndrome. Int Conf AIDS. Miami, 1989. Abstract T.B.P. 320.
255. Borish L et al. Intravenous desensitization to beta-lactam antibiotics. J Allergy Clin Immunol 1987;80:314.
256. Sher MR et al. Anaphylactic shock induced by oral desensitization to trimethoprim/sulfamethoxazole (TMP-SMZ) [Abstract]. J Allergy Clin Immunol 1986;77:133.

Managing Acute Drug Toxicity

Judith A. Alsop

This chapter reviews and presents examples of the most common strategies used to evaluate and manage drug overdoses and poisonings. For detailed information about how to manage specific drug overdoses, the reader is referred to other toxicologic references or to a poison control center.

Epidemiologic Data
American Association of Poison Control Centers and Drug Abuse Warning Network
Toxicity secondary to drug and chemical exposure is one of the most common types of injury, especially in children.[1] The incidence of drug or chemical exposure, the agents involved, and the severity of the outcome varies based on the population studied (Table 5-1). The number of reported toxic exposures in the United States in 2002 was approximately 2.38 million according to the American Association of Poison Control Centers (AAPCC) Toxic Exposure Surveillance System (TESS).[2] In most cases, little or no toxicity was associated with the exposure. About 22% received treatment at a health care facility, 5.3% had moderate or severe symptoms, and 1,153 deaths were reported. The number of drug dependence and intentional overdose cases treated in U.S. emergency rooms was about 670,000 in the year 2002 according to the Drug Abuse Warning Network (DAWN).[3]

These disparate statistics from two national sources underscore the difficulty in determining the true incidence of poisoning and overdoses.[4] Nevertheless, epidemiologic data are useful in identifying trends and in instigating public health interventions. For example, from 2001 to 2002, the number of inhalant abuse cases reported by DAWN increased 187%, identifying the need for additional education about inhalant abuse toxicity.[3]

Age-Specific Data
Stratifying patients by age can be useful in assessing the likelihood of severe toxicity from an exposure. For example, most unintentional ingestions by patients 1 to 6 years of age occur because children are curious, become more mobile, and begin exploring their surroundings. Often, these children put objects or substances into their mouths, resulting in poisonings. According to AAPCC TESS data, about 52% of all reported poisonings occur in children under 6 years of age.[2] Fortunately, exposures usually involve the ingestion of relatively small amounts of a single substance. Only 10.5% of pediatric poisoning cases are treated in a health care facility; the remainder is managed at home.[2] Therefore, severe toxicity in young children are relatively uncommon despite the child's small body size.

In children older than 6 years, the reasons for exposure become less clear. Although suicide attempts are unlikely, the potential should not be ignored entirely in older-aged children. Adolescent children have poor knowledge of the potential toxicity of various nonprescription medications and may, therefore, overdose themselves unintentionally.[5] However, in adolescents and adults, potentially toxic exposures most commonly represent suicide attempts or intentional substance abuse. These intentional overdoses commonly involve mixed exposures to illicit drugs, prescribed medications, or ethanol, and they produce more severe toxicity and death than unintentional poisonings.

In geriatric patients, overdoses tend to have a greater potential for severe adverse effects compared with overdoses in other age groups because the elderly are more likely to have underlying cardiovascular or pulmonary disease and more often have access to a variety of potentially dangerous prescription medications.

Information Resources
Computerized Databases
A vast number of different substances can be involved in a poisoning or overdose, and reliable data about the contents of products, toxicities of substances, and treatment approaches need to be readily accessible. *Poisindex,* a computerized CD-ROM database[6] that is updated quarterly, is a primary resource for poison control centers. *Poisindex* lists hundreds of thousands of products, including brand name, generic, street, and foreign drugs, chemicals, pesticides, household products, personal care items, cleaning products, insects, snakes, plants,

Table 5-1 Substances Most Frequently Involved in Poisoning Exposures[a]

All Ages	Children Under 6 Years	Adults Over 19 Years	Fatalities
Analgesics	Cosmetics and personal care products	Analgesics	Analgesics
Cleaning substances	Cleaning substances	Sedative/hypnotics/antipsychotics	Sedative/hypnotics/antipsychotics
Cosmetics and personal care products	Analgesics	Cleaning substances	Antidepressants
Foreign bodies	Foreign bodies	Antidepressants	Stimulants and street drugs
Sedative/hypnotics/antipsychotics	Topical products	Bites, envenomations	Cardiovascular drugs
Topical products	Plants	Food poisoning	Alcohols
Cough and cold preparations	Cough and cold preparations	Alcohols	Chemicals
Antidepressants	Pesticides	Cosmetics and personal care products	Anticonvulsants
Bites, envenomations	Vitamins	Cardiovascular drugs	Fumes/gases/vapors
Pesticides	GI preparations	Pesticides	Antihistamines
Plants	Antimicrobials	Chemicals	Muscle relaxants
Food poisoning	Antihistamines	Hydrocarbons	Hormones and hormone antagonists
Alcohols	Arts, crafts, office supplies	Fumes/gases/vapors	Cleaning substances
Antihistamines	Hormones and hormone antagonists	Anticonvulsants	Automotive products
Antimicrobials	Hydrocarbons	Antihistamines	Cough and cold preparations

[a]Despite a high frequency of involvement, these substances are not necessarily the most toxic, but may reflect ready access.
Adapted from reference 2. These poisoning exposures are listed in order of frequency encountered.

and over 1,000 management protocols. Yearly subscriptions to *Poisindex* are expensive (several thousand dollars per year) and are generally available only in health care facilities.[7]

Printed Publications
Textbooks and manuals also provide useful clinical information about the presentation, assessment, and treatment of toxicities. *Goldfrank's Toxicologic Emergencies*[8] and the pocket-sized *Poisoning & Drug Overdose*[9] are valuable, inexpensive alternatives to computerized database programs. However, books are less useful than computerized databases because information must be condensed and cannot be updated as frequently. In addition, discussion of the treatment of acute toxicity is inadequate or inappropriate in drug package inserts.[10]

Poison Control Centers
Poison control centers provide the most accurate specific information for both the general public and health care providers. They also provide cost-effective care.[11,12] Poison centers are usually staffed by trained specialists in poison information who come from a pharmacy, nursing, or medical background. In addition, ancillary support poison information personnel, who often have a paramedic or pharmacy technician background, are used in some poison centers. Physician backup is provided 24 hours a day by board-certified medical toxicologists. Pharmacists, nurses, and nonphysician clinical toxicologists can become certified as specialists in poison information by the AAPCC or become board certified as clinical toxicologists by the American Board of Applied Toxicology.

A poison control center's most important function is to provide event specific toxicity information to the public and health care providers. The poison information specialist must be able to accurately and efficiently assess the toxicity and communicate, usually by telephone, without the benefit of direct observation of the patient. This assessment and communication needs to be conducted quickly, accurately, and professionally in a reassuring manner. Subsequent to the telephone consultation, the poison control center staff should initiate follow-up calls to determine the effectiveness of the recommended treatment, the need for additional evaluation or treatment, and the outcome.[24] The poison control center also should be able to coordinate treatment, which may include facilitating transportation to a health care facility that has appropriately trained personnel, equipment (e.g., hemodialysis, hyperbaric oxygen), and an analytic toxicology laboratory.[13]

Effective Communication
Effective communication is essential to the assessment of potential poisonings.[22] In most situations, the person seeking guidance on the management of a potentially toxic exposure is the parent of a small child who may have ingested a substance. The caller usually is anxious about the child and may feel guilty about the exposure. To calm the caller, the health care provider should quickly reassure the parent that telephoning for assistance was appropriate and that the best assistance possible will be provided. If English is not the first language of the caller or if there are other communication barriers, solutions must be found to enhance outcomes. Most poison centers subscribe to translation services to serve the needs of diverse populations.

Once calm, effective communication is established, the health care provider should first determine whether the patient is conscious and breathing and has a pulse. If life-threatening symptoms have occurred, the caller should call for emergency services. If the health care provider does not have the knowledge or resources to provide poison information, he or she should refer the caller to the closest poison control center. Information on the location and phone number of the nearest poison control center can be found on the Internet at www.aapcc.org or by calling 1-800-222-1222. The call is automatically transferred to the poison center that serves their area in the United States.

GENERAL MANAGEMENT
Supportive Care and "ABCs"
Management of poisoned or overdosed patients is primarily based on symptomatic and supportive care. Specific antidotes exist only for a small percentage of the thousands of potential drugs and chemicals that could be ingested. The first aspect of patient management should always be basic support of airway, breathing, and circulation (the "ABCs"). The assessment and treatment of the potentially poisoned patient can be separated into seven primary functions: (1) gathering history of exposure; (2) evaluating clinical presentation (i.e., toxidromes); (3) evaluating clinical laboratory patient data; (4) removing the toxic source (e.g., gastrointestinal [GI] decontamination); (5) considering antidotes and specific treatment; (6) enhancing systemic clearance, and (7) monitoring outcome.[23,24]

Gathering History of Exposure
Comprehensive historical information about the toxic exposure should be gathered from as many different sources as possible (e.g., patient, family, friends, prehospital health care providers). This information should be compared for consistency and evaluated relative to clinical findings and laboratory results. The patient's history of the exposure is often inaccurate and should be confirmed with objective findings.[23,25] For example, a patient who presents at the emergency department (ED) with a supposed hydrocodone and carisoprodol overdose is expected to be lethargic. If the patient arrives wide awake with tachycardia and agitation, the caregiver should suspect other drugs. This would be the case whenever the patient's symptoms are not consistent with the history presented.

Specific information should be sought concerning the patient's state of consciousness, present symptoms, probable intoxicant(s), maximum amount and dosage form(s) of substance ingested, as well as when the exposure occurred. Medications, allergies, and prior medical problems also should be ascertained (e.g., a history of renal failure may indicate the need for hemodialysis to compensate for decreased renal drug clearance).[22,26]

Evaluating Clinical Presentation and Toxidromes
A thorough physical examination should be performed to characterize the signs and symptoms of overdose. Physical examinations should be conducted serially to determine the evolution or resolution of the patient's intoxication. An evaluation of the presenting signs and symptoms can provide clues on the drug class causing the toxicity, confirm the historical data surrounding the toxic exposure, and suggest

initial treatment.[27,28] The patient may be asymptomatic upon presentation even though a potentially severe exposure has occurred if absorption of the drug or toxic substance is not complete or if the substance is metabolized to a toxic substance.[29]

Characteristic *toxidromes* (i.e., a constellation of signs and symptoms consistent with a syndrome) can be associated with some specific classes of drugs.[23,28] The most common toxidromes are those associated with anticholinergic activity, increased sympathetic activity, and central nervous system (CNS) stimulation or depression. The anticholinergic effects of drugs can increase heart rate, increase body temperature, decrease GI motility, dilate pupils, and produce drowsiness or delirium. Sympathomimetic drugs can increase CNS activity, heart rate, body temperature, and blood pressure (BP). Opioids, sedatives, hypnotics, and antidepressants can depress the CNS, but the specific class of CNS depressant often cannot be easily identified by a specific constellation of symptoms. Classic findings may not be present for all drugs within a therapeutic class. For example, opioids generally induce miosis, but meperidine can produce mydriasis. Also, the association of symptoms with a particular class of toxic substances is difficult when more than one substance has been ingested. Clinicians should not focus on specific clinical findings associated with a toxidrome; rather, they should consider all subjective and objective data gleaned from the patient history, physical examination, and laboratory findings.

Interpretation of Laboratory Data
DRUG SCREENS

A urine drug screen can be useful in identifying the presence of drugs and their metabolites in selected patients. Although a urine drug screen is not indicated in all cases of drug overdose, it may be useful in a patient with coma of unknown etiology, when the presented history is inconsistent with clinical findings, or when more than one drug might have been ingested.[30]

PHARMACOKINETIC CONSIDERATIONS

The absorption, distribution, metabolism, and elimination of drugs in the overdosed patient can be quite different compared to when the drug is taken in therapeutic doses.[32] The pharmacodynamic and pharmacokinetic behavior of drugs can be substantially altered by large drug overdoses, especially with drugs that exhibit dose-dependent pharmacokinetics. The rate of drug absorption generally is slowed by large overdoses, and the time to reach peak serum drug concentrations can be delayed. The volume of distribution can be increased, and when usual metabolic pathways become saturated, secondary clearance pathways can become important. For example, large overdoses of acetaminophen saturate glutathione mechanisms of metabolism, resulting in hepatotoxicity.

The altered pharmacokinetic parameters of an overdosed drug suggest that measurements of serial plasma concentrations are necessary to better define the absorption, distribution, and clearance phases of the ingested substance. Pharmacokinetic parameters that have been derived from therapeutic doses should not be used to predict whether absorption is complete or to predict the expected duration of intoxication caused by large overdoses.[33] Furthermore, the pharmacokinetics of an ingested substance can be significantly affected by other drugs that could have been ingested concurrently. The pharmacokinetic behavior of drugs and other substances in the setting of clinical intoxications is referred to as toxicokinetics.[32,33]

Decontamination

After the airway and the cardiopulmonary system are supported, efforts should be directed toward removing the toxic substance from the patient (i.e., decontamination). Decontamination presumes that both the dose and the duration of toxin exposure are important in determining the extent of toxicity and that preventing continued exposure will decrease the toxicity. This intuitive concept is clearly relevant to ocular, dermal, and respiratory exposures, when local tissue damage is the primary problem. Respiratory decontamination involves removing the patient from the toxic environment and providing fresh air or oxygen to the patient. Decontamination of skin and eyes involves flushing the affected area with large volumes of fluid to physically remove the toxic substance from the surface. Decontamination does not include neutralizing the substance because the chemical reaction of neutralization can produce heat that could further damage the exposed tissue.[34]

GASTROINTESTINAL DECONTAMINATION

Since most poisonings and overdoses result from oral ingestions, measures to decrease or prevent continued GI absorption commonly have been used to limit the extent of exposure.[23,24,35] GI decontamination should be considered if the ingestion is potentially large enough to produce clinically significant toxicity or if the potential severity of the ingestion is unknown. The following methods can be used: (1) evacuate gastric contents by emesis or lavage; (2) administer activated charcoal as an adsorbent to bind the toxic substance remaining in the GI tract; (3) use cathartics or whole bowel irrigation to increase the rectal elimination of unabsorbed drug; or (4) combine any of the above methods. When there is potential for severe toxicity, more aggressive GI decontamination methods should be undertaken. A history of spontaneous emesis before treatment does not negate the need to institute GI decontamination. GI decontamination should also be considered when patients have abused drugs intravenously or by inhalation because concurrent oral ingestion is possible.

The efficacy of GI decontamination varies depending on when the process is initiated relative to the time of ingestion, dose ingested, and other factors. The effectiveness of GI decontamination ranges from 0% to 70%.[15,35] In a meticulous review of the literature,[15–21] ipecac-induced emesis, gastric lavage, cathartics, and activated charcoal were not directly associated with improved patient outcomes. However, individualization of GI decontamination methods perhaps will enhance outcomes.

The most appropriate method for GI tract decontamination is unclear because sound comparative data for different methods of GI decontamination are unavailable. Clinical research in healthy subjects, by necessity, must use nontoxic doses of drugs. Because alterations in GI absorption can occur with large doses, studies using nontoxic doses cannot be applied to the overdose situation. Furthermore, low-dose studies generally rely on pharmacokinetic endpoints such as peak plasma concentrations, area under the plasma concentration-time curve, or quantity of drug recovered from the urine.[36,36a,37] In contrast, clinical studies of GI decontamination methods in patients who have ingested toxic doses of a substance use clinical outcomes or a directional change in serum drug concentrations (i.e., effective decontamination should prevent further increase in serum concentrations).[38,39] These latter trials are not standardized with respect to the dose ingested or to the time interval between drug ingestion and GI decontamination.

Ipecac-Induced Emesis

Ipecac-induced emesis and gastric lavage primarily remove substances from the stomach; and their efficacy is affected significantly by the time the ingested substance remains in the stomach. Gastric lavage or ipecac-induced emesis is most effective when implemented within 1 hour of the ingestion (i.e., before the substance moves past the stomach into the small or large intestine).[15–17] Unfortunately, most patients arrive in the ED more than an hour after ingestion of the substance, when absorption of the toxic substance from the stomach has most likely already occurred. As a result, the efficacy of these procedures in most overdose situations is minimal.

Established Guidelines

The American College of Emergency Physicians (ACEP) has published guidelines for the initial evaluation, diagnosis, stabilization, and management of patients who present with acute toxic ingestions; and the American Academy of Clinical Toxicology (AACT) along with the European Association of Poisons Centres and Clinical Toxicologists (EAPCCT) and other organizations, have published position papers on GI decontamination.[14,15,21] These evidence-based clinical guidelines also identify areas where additional research is needed. Guidelines also are available from ACEP for the management of dermal or inhalation exposures.

The AACT and EAPCCT clinical guidelines state that ipecac syrup and gastric lavage should not be routinely used.[15–17] In addition, the American Academy of Pediatrics no longer supports the use of ipecac syrup routinely as a home treatment of poisoning and advocates that ipecac syrup already in the home should be discarded safely.[40] As a result, the use of ipecac to induce vomiting in both the home and health care setting is likely to be curtailed significantly. Triage of common pediatric ingestions is now leaning toward keeping at home individuals who have had less-than-toxic exposures without recommendations for the use of ipecac. More serious exposures are treated in a health care facility where the individual can be monitored properly.

Whole bowel irrigation (WBI) with a polyethylene glycol–balanced electrolyte solution (e.g., Colyte, GoLYTELY) can remove substances from the entire GI tract by the ingestion of large volumes of fluid over several hours. This method of GI decontamination, however, takes much longer to complete than ipecac-induced emesis or gastric lavage and is associated with poor compliance of patients to the regimen. Whole bowel irrigation is effective with substances that disintegrate and dissolve very slowly (e.g., sustained-release dosage forms).[20,39] WBI is also used in circumstances in which the toxic agent is not adsorbed by activated charcoal (e.g., body-packer packets, lithium, or iron). According to AACT and EAPCCT clinical guidelines, the role of whole bowel irrigation in the treatment of poisoning cases is unclear.[15,20,39]

Activated Charcoal

Currently, activated charcoal is the preferred method of GI decontamination.[18,35,41] The adsorption of substances to charcoal prevents their absorption, and the charcoal-substance complex is excreted in stool. In the past, sorbitol (a cathartic) often was administered concurrently with the activated charcoal to enhance passage of the charcoal-substance complex through the intestinal tract. However, decreased transit time through the bowel has not been proven to decrease absorption.[19,41] Sorbitol is also associated with an increased incidence of vomiting and other potential complications (e.g., aspiration).[19] Currently, most EDs use aqueous activated charcoal mixtures rather than charcoal-sorbitol combinations. Cathartics are not effective as GI decontaminants and are rarely used alone or in combination with activated charcoal.[15,19]

The effectiveness of GI decontamination varies with the amount of the toxic substance ingested and its location in the GI tract. Since the absorption rates from various toxic doses of drugs generally are not known, the time from ingestion until initiation of GI decontamination treatment is not a good guide for determining the potential efficacy of this procedure. Nevertheless, this time estimate is one of the main determinants in the decision regarding whether GI decontamination should be used. The efficacy of decontamination of the GI tract needs to be studied further to provide guidelines for its clinical use. Meanwhile, the effectiveness of GI decontamination must be inferred based on symptoms of toxicity and their association with serial plasma drug concentrations.[35]

Antidotes and Specific Treatments

An antidote is a drug that antagonizes the toxicity of another substance in a specific manner. Antidotes can be useful if they do not produce other effects that could pose even greater hazards for the patient. Antidotes can displace a drug from receptor sites (e.g., naloxone for opioids, flumazenil for benzodiazepines) or inhibit the formation of toxic metabolites (e.g., N-acetylcysteine for acetaminophen, fomepizole for methanol). Antidotes also can be used as selective diagnostic aids.

Some treatments are highly effective for the management of individual drug overdoses, but they do not meet the definition of an antidote. For example, sodium bicarbonate is used to treat the cardiotoxicity arising from tricyclic antidepressant overdoses, and benzodiazepines are used to treat CNS toxicity associated with cocaine and amphetamine overdoses.[23,42]

Enhancing Systemic Clearance

Hemodialysis, hemoperfusion, and manipulation of urine pH can enhance the clearance of substances.[43] Generally, these interventions do not increase the total systemic clearance of the toxic substance enough to shorten the course of a drug overdose. Nevertheless, hemodialysis or hemoperfusion can successfully treat some specific intoxications (e.g., methanol, ethylene glycol, aspirin, lithium) and should be considered for patients with renal dysfunction.[24,44]

Monitoring Outcome

Selecting the appropriate parameters and length of time to monitor a patient who has been exposed to a toxic agent requires knowledge of toxic effects and the time course of the intoxication. Most patients who are at risk for moderate or severe toxicity should be monitored in an intensive care unit

(ICU) with careful assessments of cardiac, pulmonary, and CNS function.[45]

ASSESSMENT OF SALICYLATE INGESTION
Gathering a History

1. M.O., the mother of a 4-year-old child, states that her daughter D.O., has ingested some aspirin tablets. What additional information should be obtained from or given to M.O. at this time?

Requests for information should be evaluated more closely to determine whether an exposure to a toxic substance has occurred. Obtaining an initial assessment of the patient's status is essential. The caller's telephone number should be obtained in the event that the call is disconnected, initial recommendations need to be modified, or subsequent follow-up is needed. The health care provider should ask for patient-specific information with questions that are nonthreatening and nonjudgmental. For example, the caller could be asked to provide information about the ingestion with an explanation that better assistance could be provided as a result.

Evaluating Clinical Presentation

2. On further questioning, M.O. states that her daughter is crying and complaining of a stomachache. Otherwise, the child appears to be normal. The daughter was found sitting on the bathroom floor with an aspirin bottle in her hand and some partially chewed tablets on the floor next to her. The child had the same look on her face that she does when she eats things that she does not like. M.O. reports that she can see white tablet material gummed on the child's teeth. The mother was gone no more than 5 minutes and had asked her 5- and 6-year-old sons to watch their sister. What additional information is needed to correctly assess the potential for toxicity?

To determine the potential toxicity for an unintentional ingestion, it is important to assess the presence of symptoms and to identify the substance ingested. Begin with open-ended questions to determine the facts that the caller is certain of versus what may have been assumed. The answers usually point to more specific information that is needed to accurately assess the exposure.

D.O.'s symptoms presently are not life-threatening. Her stomachache and crying are usual behaviors for a child who is frightened. Instead, these behaviors are consistent with a response to the mother's anxiety when she discovered the ingestion. Once it has been established that the child does not need immediate lifesaving treatment, the caller generally is more willing and able to answer additional questions.

Because M.O. already has provided information about the child's symptoms, information is needed to ascertain the substance involved in the unintentional ingestion: the maximum potential dose and the time of ingestion. Additional information that is needed includes the brand of aspirin (to ensure that the product is not an aspirin-combination formulation), the dosage form, the number of dosage units in a full container, and the number of remaining dosage units. The actual number of remaining dosage units should be counted rather than estimated. Furthermore, the parent should be careful to look for tablets under beds, rugs, or other locations out of sight (e.g.,

wastepaper baskets, toilets, pet food dishes, pockets). The dosage forms in the container should all be identical in appearance, and the contents should be what are stated on the label. Information concerning the child's weight and health status, and whether the child is taking other medications is also important. The child's weight can be used to determine the precise maximum mg/kg dose of aspirin that was ingested. Other medications and health conditions that could increase aspirin toxicity should be considered as well.

If the ingested substance is a liquid, it can be more difficult to determine the amount ingested because the liquid is frequently spilled on or around the child. The caller may have witnessed the child actually drinking the liquid and be able to provide an estimate of how many swallows were ingested. In the average 2-year-old child, each swallow of liquid contains about 5 mL.[46]

When more than one child is present during an ingestion incident, the caller should be questioned as to whether an additional child also could have participated in the ingestion. Most poison information specialists have experienced drug ingestion incidents involving multiple children. In this situation, all the children may have shared equally in the missing dosage units of drug; all the drug may have been fed to one child (usually the youngest); or all the dosage units may have been ingested by the oldest or most aggressive child. When it is unclear how many missing dosage units of a substance may have been ingested among a group of children, each child should be evaluated and managed as if he or she may have ingested the total missing quantity.

Triage of Call

3. The caller, M.O., has now determined that a total of five tablets each containing 325 mg/tablet of aspirin are missing from the bottle. Because M.O. recalls having taken two aspirin tablets from this bottle, it is not likely that her daughter took more than three tablets. Does M.O. have to provide any treatment to her child?

The maximum dose of aspirin ingested by this child is likely to be much less than the minimum dose required to produce significant symptoms based on an assumption that this 4-year-old girl is of average weight for her age (i.e., 36 pounds or ~16 kg). A dose of 150 mg/kg of aspirin is the smallest dose at which treatment or assessment at a health care facility is necessary.[47] D.O. is likely to have ingested 975 mg of aspirin (i.e., three 325-mg tablets), which is about 60 mg/kg (975 mg divided by 16 kg). Providing this information to the mother will be reassuring and is likely to foster her continued cooperation with further questioning.

If this child is healthy, takes no medications, and is not allergic to aspirin, the mother does not need to induce vomiting. The child has not taken a toxic dose of aspirin and need not undergo any treatment. The mother should be instructed to continue to observe her daughter for any changes that she would consider abnormal. With this history of ingestion, adverse effects would not be expected, except possibly some mild nausea.

For many years, aspirin was the most common cause of unintentional poisoning and poisoning deaths among children. However, safety closure packaging and reduction of the total aspirin content in a full bottle of children's aspirin to approximately 3 g has steadily reduced the frequency of aspirin poisoning and deaths.[48] Although acute aspirin poisoning remains a problem, the largest percentage of life-threatening intoxications now results from therapeutic overdose.[49] Therapeutic overdoses occur when a dose is given too frequently, when both parents unknowingly dose the child with the drug, or when too large a dose is given. Therapeutic overdoses are especially a problem if the situation continues for a period of time and the drug is able to accumulate.

Aspirin is found less often in most households now because acetaminophen or ibuprofen are more commonly used for the relief of pain and fever. Salicylates are also found in less obvious places (e.g., bismuth subsalicylate in Pepto-Bismol, methyl salicylate [oil of wintergreen] in topical liniments or as peppermint flavoring for homemade candy).

Outcome

Follow-up of telephone consultations on toxic ingestions is important to identify children who unexpectedly develop symptoms that might need to be treated. A telephone call to this mother 6 to 24 hours after her initial call would be appropriate to follow up on the child.[22,26] On a call back to M.O., the parent stated she gave D.O. lunch at the appropriate time. D.O. then watched cartoons, took her usual nap, and remained asymptomatic.

Acute and Chronic Salicylism
Signs and Symptoms

4. V.K., a 65-year-old, 55-kg woman with a history of chronic headaches has taken 10 to 12 aspirin tablets a day for several months. On the evening of admission, she became lethargic, disoriented, and combative. Additional history revealed that she ingested up to 100 aspirin tablets on the morning of admission in a suicide attempt. She complained of ringing in her ears, nausea, and three episodes of vomiting. Vital signs were BP 140/90 mm Hg, pulse 110 beats/min, respirations 36 breaths/min, and temperature 102.5°F. V.K.'s laboratory data obtained on admission were as follows: serum sodium (Na), 148 mEq/L (normal, 135 to 153); potassium (K), 3.0 mEq/L (normal, 3.5 to 5.5); chloride (Cl), 105 mEq/L (normal, 95 to 105); bicarbonate, 12 mEq/L (normal, 24 to 31); glucose, 60 mg/dL (normal, 70 to 110); blood urea nitrogen (BUN), 35 mg/dL (normal, 5 to 25); and creatinine, 2.1 mg/dL (normal, 0.5 to 1.4). Arterial blood gas (ABG) values (room air) were as follows: pH, 7.25; PCO2, 20 mm Hg; and PO2, 95 mm Hg. A serum salicylate concentration measured approximately 12 hours after the acute ingestion was 80 mg/dL. Her hemoglobin was 9.6 g/dL (normal, 12 to 16 g/dL for females) with a hematocrit of 28.9% (normal, 37% to 47% for females) and a prothrombin time (PT) of 16.4 seconds (normal, 10 to 13 seconds). Describe the pathophysiology and clinical features of acute and chronic salicylism.

The symptoms and severity of salicylate intoxication depend on the dose consumed; the patient's age; and whether the ingestion was acute, chronic, or a combination of the two. This case illustrates an acute ingestion in someone who has also chronically ingested aspirin. Acute ingestion of 150 to 300 mg/kg of aspirin is likely to produce mild to moderate intoxication; >300 mg/kg implies severe poisoning; and >500

mg/kg is potentially lethal.[49,50] V.K., who ingested approximately 600 mg/kg, has taken a potentially lethal dose. Chronic salicylate intoxication usually is associated with ingestion of >100 mg/kg per day for >2 to 3 days.[49,50] V.K. has been taking 70 mg/kg per day for her headaches in addition to her acute ingestion.

Toxic doses of salicylate directly stimulate the medullary respiratory center (note V.K.'s increased respiratory rate) and influence several key metabolic pathways. Direct stimulation of the respiratory drive increases the rate and depth of ventilation, which can result in primary respiratory alkalosis. The respiratory alkalosis, in turn, causes increased renal excretion of bicarbonate resulting in diminution of buffering capacity. The patient usually presents clinically with a partially compensated respiratory alkalosis.

Hypokalemia can result from increased GI and renal losses as well as systemic alkalosis. Tinnitus is common when the salicylate concentration exceeds 25 to 30 mg/dL. It is essential to note the units of measurement on any salicylate serum concentration because different laboratories report concentrations in different units (e.g., mg/dL, μg/mL, mmol/L). An incorrect interpretation of the salicylate unit of measurement can result in overestimates or underestimates of the severity of salicylate exposure. Although marked metabolic and neurologic abnormalities are most commonly observed in young children with advanced salicylate intoxication, adolescents or adults acutely poisoned with a sufficiently large dose can develop these symptoms as well, as demonstrated by V.K.

Acute salicylism in a young child often takes a more severe course than that typically seen in adults. After acute ingestion, children quickly pass through the phase of pure respiratory alkalosis. Renal bicarbonate loss secondary to respiratory alkalosis reduces the buffering capacity more profoundly in a child and facilitates the development of metabolic acidosis.[51]

Salicylates also have toxic effects on several biochemical pathways that contribute to metabolic acidosis and other symptoms.[52] Mitochondrial oxidative phosphorylation is uncoupled and results in an impaired ability to generate high-energy phosphates, increased oxygen use and carbon dioxide production, increased heat production and hyperpyrexia, increased tissue glycolysis, and increased peripheral demand for glucose. Salicylates also inhibit key dehydrogenase enzymes within the Krebs cycle, resulting in increased levels of pyruvate and lactate. The increased demand for peripheral glucose causes increased glycogenolysis, gluconeogenesis, lipolysis, and free fatty acid metabolism. The latter results in enhanced formation of ketoacids and ketoacidosis.[51,52]

The patient may become severely volume depleted through several mechanisms. Hyperthermia and hyperventilation produce increased insensible water loss, vomiting may promote GI fluid losses, and the solute load caused by altered glucose metabolism results in an osmotic diuresis. Large amounts of sodium and potassium also may be lost through these mechanisms. However, depending on the patient's acid–base balance and net fluid and electrolyte intake and output, serum sodium and potassium concentrations may be normal, elevated, or decreased. Hypernatremia and hypokalemia are most common.[51,52]

Blood glucose concentration is usually normal or slightly elevated, although hypoglycemia may accompany chronic salicylism (e.g., as illustrated by V.K.) or occur late in acute intoxication.[48] CNS glucose levels can be markedly reduced in the presence of normal blood glucose concentrations[53] because increased CNS glucose utilization to generate high-energy phosphate exceeds the rate at which glucose can be supplied.

Other manifestations of severe acute salicylism include a variety of neurologic signs and symptoms: disorientation, irritability, hallucinations, lethargy, stupor, coma, and seizures. Hyperthermia may be marked and can result in the inappropriate administration of aspirin as an antipyretic. Coagulopathy can occur because of impaired platelet function, hypoprothrombinemia, reduced factor VII production, and increased capillary fragility, especially when taken chronically.[52] Pulmonary edema and acute renal failure also can occur, but the former occurs more commonly after chronic intoxication.[53,54]

In both adults and children, the principal manifestations of chronic salicylism are a partially compensated metabolic acidosis, increased anion gap, ketosis, dehydration, electrolyte loss, and encephalopathy.[48,52] Unless the history of salicylate intake is specifically sought, the problem may not be immediately apparent, especially in the elderly in whom such findings are likely to be attributed to other causes (e.g., encephalitis, meningitis, diabetic ketoacidosis, myocardial infarction).[55] Delay in diagnosis has been associated with increased mortality.[56] Unfortunately, plasma salicylate concentrations do not correlate well with the degree of poisoning in chronically intoxicated patients.[53]

Death in patients with salicylism, whether acute or chronic, results from CNS dysfunction, severe dehydration and electrolyte loss, or pulmonary edema.[52] The severity of CNS manifestations is related to the cerebrospinal fluid (CSF) salicylate concentration. This may increase in the presence of systemic acidosis because a greater fraction of salicylate is unionized and can cross the blood-brain barrier.[57] Thus, metabolic acidosis is especially dangerous in a salicylate-intoxicated patient. Maintaining a blood pH of 7.4 should be attempted.[9]

Assessment of Toxicity

5. Explain V.K.'s signs, symptoms, and laboratory values.

V.K. demonstrates many of the findings typical of severe acute salicylism. Hyperventilation has resulted from the direct respiratory stimulant effects of salicylate and as compensation for her metabolic acidosis (PCO_2, 20 mm Hg; pH, 7.25; serum bicarbonate, 12 mEq/L; respiratory rate, 36 breaths/minute). Hypokalemia (3.0 mEq/L) in the presence of metabolic acidosis represents severe potassium depletion because of increased renal and possibly GI losses. Hyperpyrexia caused by salicylate is present in V.K., although an infectious cause also must be considered. Last, her neurologic symptoms of lethargy, disorientation, and combativeness, as well as tinnitus, nausea, and vomiting are commonly seen in severe salicylate intoxication. In addition, being elderly and taking a lethal amount of aspirin bodes ill for this patient's outcome.

Laboratory Evaluation

6. What parameters should be measured to assess a patient with salicylate intoxication?

V.K.'s workup illustrates a thorough initial patient evaluation. Laboratory evaluation should include ABG values, serum electrolytes, blood glucose, and a complete blood count. Prothrombin, INR, and partial thromboplastin times are useful in severe acute or chronic intoxication to assess the presence of salicylate-induced coagulopathy. Physical examination should include an evaluation of cardiopulmonary and neurologic function and a measurement of urine output.

Measurement of serum salicylate concentration, when interpreted with the assistance of a published nomogram,[57] can be used along with other clinical data to assess acute salicylate ingestion. However, clinical symptoms and other laboratory findings are more useful than a nomogram to identify the degree of acute intoxication, assess patient prognosis, and guide therapy. In case of chronic ingestions, the nomogram is not useful, and other parameters such as acid–base and electrolyte balance should be used instead to determine severity of the case.

After acute ingestions, serum concentrations obtained less than 6 hours after ingestion are difficult to interpret and can result in an underestimation of the eventual degree of intoxication. This is because the salicylate concentration can continue to rise over approximately 24 hours if a large amount has been taken or enteric-coated tablets have been ingested.[53] Enteric-coated tablets can clump together forming a bezoar that slowly releases drug into the gut. Therefore, it is necessary to repeat a serum salicylate measurement every 4 to 6 hours to verify that the original concentration represented a peak level and that the salicylate level is decreasing rather than increasing.

Management

7. Outline a management plan for V.K.

Management of salicylate intoxication depends on the character and magnitude of acid–base and electrolyte disturbances that exist. V.K.'s initial management should include administration of activated charcoal. Gastric lavage may be considered even with the long period of time since ingestion because aspirin can be very slowly absorbed and the outcome of this overdose is potentially life threatening. In V.K., hypokalemia, acidosis, and hypoglycemia must be corrected. This generally is accomplished through the administration of intravenous hypotonic saline-dextrose solutions combined with potassium supplementation. This solution is administered at a rate that replaces the patient's deficits and keeps pace with continued losses. Care should be taken to avoid overzealous fluid therapy, which can predispose the patient to cerebral or pulmonary edema.[53] Because V.K. is hypoglycemic (60 mg/dL), administration of an IV dextrose bolus is also indicated.

SODIUM BICARBONATE

It is important to correct V.K.'s acidosis because acidosis will increase CSF salicylate concentrations. Correction of acidosis can be accomplished by administering an IV bolus of sodium bicarbonate or by adding sodium bicarbonate to each liter of IV fluids; occasionally, very large doses of sodium bicarbonate are necessary.[53] V.K.'s serum sodium concentration should be monitored closely. It is essential to provide adequate ventilation to prevent respiratory alkalosis. With a respiratory rate of 36 breaths per minute, placing the patient on a ventilator to assist with breathing might be considered. However, forced mechanical ventilation can interfere with the patient's need to compensate to maintain the serum pH.[9] Patients on ventilators can become severely acidotic, which can result in death because of an inability to compensate adequately.

SEIZURES

Seizures are not evident in V.K. but can be encountered in cases of severe salicylate poisoning. Seizures generally carry a poor prognosis and are indicative of a severe poisoning that requires hemodialysis.[51,53] Other treatable causes of seizures (e.g., marked alkalosis, hypoglycemia, hyponatremia), can be present in individuals such as V.K. and should be ruled out.

COAGULOPATHY

Coagulopathy generally responds to vitamin K[1], which should be given if the PT is prolonged.[52] Fresh frozen plasma will be required if there is evidence of GI bleeding or other hemorrhage. Hyperthermia usually does not require therapy, but cooling fans and mist may be required for extremely elevated temperatures.

ALKALINE DIURESIS

8. **What measures will enhance salicylate elimination? Which of these may be indicated in V.K.?**

Forced alkaline diuresis, hemodialysis, and hemoperfusion have been used to enhance salicylate excretion in overdose situations.[51] Of these, the use of alkaline diuresis is most debated. Although large doses of sodium bicarbonate together with forced fluids enhance the renal elimination of this weak acid and shorten its half-life, it does not favorably influence the morbidity or mortality of patients with salicylism. Alkaline diuresis may place the patient at risk for sodium and fluid retention as well as pulmonary edema. Furthermore, whether the urine can be adequately alkalinized (pH >7) in severely intoxicated pediatric patients has been questioned because of the large acid load that is excreted.[56] In these patients, sodium bicarbonate is nevertheless recommended to reduce the arterial pH with the goal of minimizing salicylate transport into the CNS. Potassium replacement in patients receiving alkaline diuresis is essential. These patients may require large amounts of potassium supplementation due to renal wasting of potassium. In adult patients such as V.K., who is severely intoxicated, urine alkalinization with sodium bicarbonate along with supplemental potassium should be attempted. The risk for pulmonary edema can be minimized if this is done without forcing fluids.

Hemodialysis or hemoperfusion should be considered in patients who show progression of severe salicylate intoxication and seizure activity, renal failure, or plasma salicylate concentrations in the potentially fatal range (note: check the units of measurement of salicylate levels). Peritoneal dialysis is much less effective than hemodialysis or hemoperfusion, and hemodialysis is preferred to hemoperfusion because it also can be used to correct fluid and electrolyte imbalances concurrently.[53] Patients with salicylate levels greater than 60 mg/dL after chronic exposure, with acidosis, CNS symptoms and who are elderly or ill are high-risk patients who should be considered for early dialysis.[9]

Outcome

V.K. received 50 g of activated charcoal via nasogastric tube. A repeat salicylate level 6 hours later (18 hours after ingestion) had increased to 93 mg/dL. Her chemistry panel revealed serum sodium (Na), 134 mEq/L (normal, 135 to153); potassium (K), 2.1 mEq/L (normal, 3.5 to 5.5); chloride (Cl), 100 mEq/L (normal, 95 to 105); bicarbonate, 11 mEq/L (normal 24 to 31); glucose, 78 mg/dL (normal, 70 to 110); creatinine, 4.8 mg/dL (normal, 0.5 to 1.4), BUN, 42 mg/dL (normal, 5 to 25). Her hemoglobin was now 8.5 g/dL (normal, 12 to 16 for females) with a hematocrit of 23% (normal, 37% to 47% for females) and a PT of 16.6 seconds (normal, 10 to 13 seconds). V.K.'s pH on blood gases remained in the 7.2 to 7.3 range.

Urinary alkalinization was attempted with high-dose IV sodium bicarbonate infusion in an attempt to reach a urine pH of 7.5. However, her urine pH never increased above 5.6. V.K. became fluid overloaded and developed dyspnea. She was placed on a ventilator with worsening of her symptoms. A chest radiograph showed pulmonary edema. V.K. became confused and agitated, pulling at her IV lines and trying to get out of bed. Nephrology was consulted to provide emergent hemodialysis to correct the acidosis, electrolyte abnormalities, and fluid overload. As the catheter was being placed, the patient had a tonic-clonic seizure. Diazepam 10 mg IV was administered and the seizure stopped. At this time, the patient was unresponsive. The nasogastric tube revealed the presence of copious amounts of bright red blood. She was rushed to surgery for an emergency laparotomy. On the way to the operating room, she had another seizure and coded and could not be resuscitated.

ASSESSMENT OF IRON INGESTION
Gathering History and Communications

9. The grandmother of F.E., a 20-month-old boy, calls the poison control center because her grandson is vomiting and appears to have been playing with some red tablets. The child was left alone in his room for about 15 minutes to take a nap. Why might the consultation with this grandmother be expected to be more difficult than the consultation in Question 1?

Phone calls to a poison control center from individuals other than the parent usually are more difficult to manage. The caller may not be able to provide all of the patient-specific information needed (e.g., patient weight, chronic medications) to accurately assess the drug ingestion. Supplemental information often is needed from a parent. Furthermore, nonparent callers tend to be more upset over an unintentional ingestion and may have more difficulty than a parent in taking decisive action.

Triage of Call

10. Despite additional questioning, the grandmother cannot identify the tablets and cannot find any labeling or empty medicine containers that could help in the tablet identification. F.E. is still vomiting, and some of the vomitus is red like the tablets. There are three children in the household and two adults who take medications for various chronic illnesses. According to the grandmother, F.E. is healthy and no one else in the household currently has the "flu" or other GI illness. The child's mother gave birth 3 weeks ago and is now at her obstetrician's office for a postnatal visit. What recommendations could be provided to this grandmother at this time?

With this history, the clinician should consider whether the information presented by F.E.'s grandmother is consistent with a classic drug ingestion and whether this incident is likely to be associated with a significant adverse outcome. Most 1.5- to 2-year-old children experience limited toxicity with unintentional drug ingestions because only a relatively small amount of substance usually is ingested. Nevertheless, some substances (e.g., methanol, ethanol, ethylene glycol, nicotine, clonidine, diphenoxylate-atropine, caustic substances, oral hypoglycemic agents, calcium channel blockers, tricyclic antidepressants, iron) can produce significant toxicity when only small amounts are ingested. As little as one dosage unit of camphor, chloroquine, tricyclic antidepressants, phenothiazines, quinine, methyl salicylate, or theophylline can be fatal in a 10-kg child.[58] These compounds represented 42% of all childhood fatalities secondary to acute drug ingestions between 1983 and 1989.[59]

Although the history of the presumed drug ingestion in F.E. is vague, the description of a red tablet, the vomiting of red material, and the recent pregnancy of his mother suggests possible ingestion of prenatal iron tablets. Iron ingestions are of concern as 12 deaths in small children were attributed to iron by poison centers between the years 1993 and 1999, making iron supplements one of the most common drugs associated with unintentional drug overdose fatalities.[60–67] Because this exposure would be categorized as an unknown toxicity, with a realistic potential for severe toxicity if iron tablets were ingested, F.E. should be referred to an ED for evaluation.

Depending on the distance to the hospital and the anxiety-level of the grandmother, the grandmother may be instructed to call for emergency medical services transportation rather than relying on other means of transportation. She should be instructed to take the red tablets to the ED along with the child, so that the tablets can be identified. Other medications that are in the house also should be taken to the ED, and the mother should be contacted at the obstetrician's office.

Substance Identification

11. **F.E.'s mother has been contacted and has confirmed that the only red tablets in the house are her prenatal iron supplements. She is in close proximity to the hospital and will await the arrival of her son. Meanwhile, the poison control center telephoned the ED to prepare them for F.E.'s arrival. F.E. arrived 20 minutes later along with one red tablet and an empty prescription container that was found by his older brother. F.E. is still vomiting but is awake and alert with a heart rate of 125 beats/min, a respiratory rate of 28-breaths/min, a temperature of 99.1°F, and pulse oximetry of 99%. How can the maximum potential severity of this ingestion be estimated at this time?**

F.E.'s vital signs, when corrected for age, are normal. Attention now should focus on identifying the ingested substance and the maximum potential severity of the ingestion. Although this case was referred to the ED as an unknown intoxication with the potential for being a severe iron intoxication, the ingestion of iron has not been verified. Therefore,

F.E. must be carefully assessed and the ingestion history reaffirmed.

All solid dosage prescription drugs are required by the U.S. Food and Drug Administration to have identification markings. Reference books (e.g., *Facts and Comparisons*),[68] computerized databases (e.g., *Identidex*),[69] and the proprietary manufacturers can assist in identifying solid dosage forms. The markings on the red tablet brought to the ED with F.E., the empty medication container, and the mother's assistance should be sufficient to correctly identify the tablet. Because most childhood ingestions usually involve only one substance, the identification of this red tablet will most likely establish the toxicity potential. Once the tablet has been identified, the maximum number of tablets ingested should be estimated. The label on the empty medication container should provide information on the identity and number of tablets dispensed. If the medication container is unlabeled, the date the prescription was obtained, the number of estimated doses taken, and the number currently remaining in the medication container can be used to approximate the maximum number of tablets that were ingested.

F.E.'s vital signs and symptoms should be monitored at frequent intervals to evaluate whether his clinical status is consistent with expectations based on the suspected ingestion. Nausea, vomiting, diarrhea, and abdominal pain are commonly encountered early in the course of iron intoxication. The caustic effects of iron may explain the presence of blood in the vomitus or stool. CNS effects (e.g., lethargy, seizures) or cardiovascular symptoms (e.g., hypotension, tachycardia) are suggestive of severe iron toxicity.[70] However, the absence of symptoms should not be interpreted as an indication that a poisoning has not occurred, especially if the patient is being evaluated within a short time after the presumed ingestion.

Evaluating Severity of Toxicity

12. **F.E. weighs 22 pounds, appears to be in no apparent distress, and has stopped vomiting. About 30 mL of dark red vomitus was recovered, but no tablets are seen, and testing demonstrates that no blood is present in the vomitus. A maximum of 11 tablets were ingested based on the bottle label and the mother's recall. What degree of toxicity should be expected in F.E.?**

The potential severity of ingestion can be estimated for commonly ingested drugs such as acetaminophen, salicylates, iron, and tricyclic antidepressants because of well-established dose–toxicity relationships.[49,70,71] Acute elemental iron ingestions of <20 mg/kg usually are nontoxic, 20 to 60 mg/kg doses result in mild to moderate toxicity, and >60 mg/kg doses are severe and potentially fatal ingestions.[72,73]

The label on the prescription medication container, as well as independent verification of the tablet by F.E.'s mother and the tablet imprint, indicate that each tablet contained 300 mg of ferrous sulfate in an enteric-coated formulation. Because the dose–toxicity relationship of iron is based on the amount of elemental iron ingested,[70] knowledge of the specific iron salt is important in calculating the ingested dose. Ferrous sulfate contains 20% elemental iron, ferrous gluconate contains 12%, and ferrous fumarate contains 33%. Therefore, each 300-mg ferrous sulfate tablet contains 60 mg of elemental iron. Because F.E. ingested a maximum of 11 enteric-coated ferrous sulfate 300-mg tablets and he weighs 22 pounds (10 kg), he is estimated to have ingested 66 mg/kg of iron, placing him at risk of severe toxicity. Although F.E.'s only symptom is vomiting at this time, absorption could be delayed because he ingested an enteric-coated formulation.

Abdominal Radiographs

13. Because F.E. is expected to experience potentially severe toxicity from his ingestion of iron, would an abdominal radiograph be useful to verify how many iron tablets actually were ingested?

Radiodense substances (e.g., iron, enteric-coated tablets, chloral hydrate, phenothiazines, heavy metals) can be visualized in the GI tract by an abdominal radiograph. However, the ability of a radiograph to demonstrate the presence of a radiodense substance depends on the dosage form, concentration, and the molecular weight of the substance. The intact dosage form can often be detected if the tablet has not already disintegrated or dissolved.[73]

Keep in mind that children are more likely than adults to chew tablets rather than swallow them whole, and false-negative results can occur even when whole tablets have not already started to disintegrate. If the tablets were chewed, an abdominal radiograph to verify the number of ingested iron tablets is not likely to be useful. However, an abdominal radiograph after the completion of GI decontamination can help assess whether additional decontamination is needed.

Gastrointestinal Decontamination

14. Why are activated charcoal and gastric lavage not indicated for the management of F.E.'s iron ingestion?

When selecting a GI decontamination method (lavage, charcoal), one should consider the substance ingested, maximum potential toxicity expected from drug dosage form, potential time course of toxicity, time elapsed between ingestion and the initiation of treatment, symptoms, and physical examination findings. Decontamination with activated charcoal is not indicated because F.E. has ingested iron tablets, which do not adsorb to activated charcoal,[35,75] and gastric lavage would not be effective in removing whole tablets of iron because the removal of large particles from the stomach is limited by the small internal diameter of the gastric lavage tube relative to the size of undissolved iron tablets.

Gastric Lavage

15. When is gastric lavage indicated and how should this process be implemented?

The commonly used adult gastric lavage tube (36F) has an internal diameter too small to allow recovery of large tablet or capsule fragments and an even smaller diameter lavage tube is used for children.[17,35] However, gastric lavage may be useful if the tablets were chewed or had already disintegrated.

Gastric lavage is generally used in patients who have ingested enough substance to produce severe toxicity and in patients who, because of a decreased level of consciousness, may be unable to protect their airway from aspiration. Because lavage can increase the risk of aspiration, these patients generally require intubation with a cuffed endotracheal tube before insertion of the lavage tube.[17,35] After the gastric tube is in place, the gastric contents are initially aspirated, and fluid is instilled into the stomach and then aspirated. This process is repeated until the gastric aspirate is clear. A total of several liters of fluid is usually instilled and aspirated. After gastric lavage, activated charcoal should be administered through the orogastric tube if the substance is adsorbed by charcoal.

Monitoring Effectiveness of Treatment

16. How should the effectiveness of GI decontamination be assessed in the ED?

The simplest method of assessing GI decontamination is to visually inspect the return fluid from lavage. Whole tablets can sometimes be seen, but one more often sees tablet fragments, which look like soft, crumbly white particles. However, it is not clear whether tablet fragments represent active drug or the inactive filler ingredients in the tablet dosage form.[76] Increasing serum iron concentrations, deteriorating clinical status, or evidence of radiodense tablets in the GI tract on abdominal radiograph would warrant more aggressive GI decontamination.

Whole Bowel Irrigation

17. What other method of GI decontamination should be considered for F.E.?

Whole bowel irrigation (WBI) with a polyethylene glycol electrolyte solution (PEG-ELS) can be considered in this case. WBI (PEG-ELS) is administered orally or infused by nasogastric tube at a rate of 1.5 to 2 L/hour for adults and at a rate of 25 mL/kg per hour for children.[20] Although the large volume of fluid to be ingested over a short period of time and the frequent association of the nausea and vomiting often result in poor patient compliance, F.E. is hospitalized and the fluid can be infused by nasogastric tube if needed. WBI should be continued until the rectal effluent is clear, which may take many hours.[20]

Serum Iron Concentrations

18. At this time, F.E. has no evidence of CNS, or cardiovascular symptoms that can occur with toxic iron ingestions. He did have one large dark-colored diarrheal stool that tested negative for blood. A serum iron concentration, obtained about 3 hours after the ingestion, was 470 µg/mL (normal, 60 to 160 µg/dL). What conclusions as to severity or likely clinical outcome can be derived from this serum concentration?

The higher than normal serum iron concentration confirms the suspicion that F.E. has ingested iron tablets despite both his current lack of serious symptoms and the absence of tablet evidence in the gastric fluid or abdominal radiograph. The serum iron concentration can also provide an indication as to whether more aggressive therapy is needed. This single value does not provide information as to whether the serum concentration will increase or decrease over the ensuing hours.

The time course of absorption is probably the most difficult pharmacokinetic parameter to evaluate with toxic ingestions. For example, serum phenytoin concentrations can continue to rise for 48 to 72 hours after an overdose with extended-release phenytoin despite continued GI decontamination.[77,78] This prolongation of absorption time is even further complicated when sustained-release or enteric-coated dosage forms have been ingested because the onset of symptoms is unpredictable.[79,80]

F.E.'s serum iron concentration of 470 μg/mL at this time suggests a serious ingestion because peak serum iron concentrations >500 μg/mL usually are predictive of significant toxicity.[70,72,74,80] This single serum iron concentration, however, does not provide information as to whether this serum concentration is rising or declining nor when the serum iron concentration will peak as a result of his iron ingestion. Samples for peak serum iron concentration should be obtained 2 to 6 hours after ingestion.[74] Because F.E.'s serum iron concentration was measured approximately 3 hours after ingestion, another serum iron measurement in 2 to 4 hours is indicated, particularly because he ingested an enteric-coated formulation.

Blood Glucose and White Blood Cell Count

19. F.E. had WBI (PEG-ELS) administered through the nasogastric tube for 4 hours until the rectal effluent was clear. At this time F.E. began to vomit numerous times and became drowsy and fussy. A second serum iron concentration was ordered (i.e., 6 hours after ingestion). What other laboratory tests could be helpful in assessing the potential toxicity of iron in F.E.?

Blood glucose concentrations and white blood cell (WBC) counts usually are increased when serum iron concentrations are >300 μg/mL. A WBC count >15,000/mm³ and a blood glucose concentration >150 mg/dL within 6 hours of an ingestion generally suggest a greater likelihood of severe iron intoxication.[70,74] These tests provide supplemental confirmation of iron intoxication, and are especially useful in medical facilities in which serum iron concentrations cannot be obtained immediately.

Asymptomatic Period and Stages of Toxicity

20. It is now 6 hours since F.E. ingested the iron tablets. His second serum iron concentration is not yet available. He continues to be fussy and drowsy but has missed his usual afternoon nap. He has several more episodes of vomiting. Why is F.E.'s relatively mild course at this time not particularly reassuring?

The time between the ingestion of an overdose of drugs and the development of severe toxicity often is delayed. It is unclear in some cases why there is an asymptomatic period, but it may be secondary to delayed absorption of the ingested drug, the time required for the drug to distribute to the sites of action, or the time needed to form a toxic metabolite. Consequently, F.E. may still develop further symptoms of severe toxicity. Four distinct stages of symptoms can be encountered with iron toxicity.[70,72,82,83]

Stage I
Stage I symptoms usually occur within 6 hours of ingestion. During this time, nausea, vomiting, diarrhea, and abdominal pain are encountered and probably are secondary to the erosive effects of iron on the GI mucosa. The caustic effects of free iron also may result in bleeding, with blood in the vomitus and stool. In more severe intoxications, CNS and cardiovascular toxicity may be present during Stage I.

Stage II
The second stage of iron toxicity is described as a period of decreasing symptoms with apparent improvement in the clinical condition. This stage may last for up to 12 to 24 hours after the ingestion and can be misinterpreted as resolving toxicity. The clinical course of iron intoxication may not be an accurate reflection of the severity of the toxicity during this stage. Although this stage can be the genuine beginning of complete recovery, it may progress to the more ominous stage III. It is unknown why this stage of apparent improvement occurs with iron toxicity. However, in most severe cases, there is no stage II and the patient's condition continues to progressively deteriorate.

Stage III
Stage III generally occurs 12 to 48 hours after iron ingestion and is characterized by CNS toxicity (e.g., lethargy, coma, seizures) and cardiovascular toxicity (e.g., hypotension, shock, pulmonary edema). Metabolic acidosis, hypoglycemia, hepatic necrosis, renal damage, and coagulopathy can be experienced at this stage.

Stage IV
The final stage is apparent 4 to 6 weeks after acute iron ingestion and consists of late-appearing GI tract sequelae that are secondary to the initial local toxicity. In this stage, prior tissue damage can progress to gastric scarring and strictures at the pylorus, with permanent abnormalities of function.

Deferoxamine Chelation

21. The clinical laboratory has reported that the second serum iron concentration that was obtained 6 hours after ingestion from F.E. has increased from 470 to 553 μg/mL. He has continued to vomit. F.E.'s mother states that the child looks "pale" to her. What criteria are most important in determining whether deferoxamine should be administered to F.E.?

[SI units: 84.18 and 99.04 μmol/L, respectively]

Deferoxamine (Desferal) chelates iron by binding ferric ions in plasma to form the iron complex ferrioxamine. Deferoxamine appears to have a greater affinity for iron than other chelating agents and probably also has additional mechanisms that decrease iron toxicity at the cellular level.[70,82] A relatively small amount of iron is bound (approximately 85 mg of iron to 1 g of deferoxamine). The iron–deferoxamine complex primarily is excreted renally as ferrioxamine. Renal elimination of the ferrioxamine usually results in a pinkish-orange colored urine, often described as "vin rose" in color.

Deferoxamine therapy should be initiated when serum iron concentrations exceed 500 μg/mL or when either >60 mg/kg of iron has been ingested or severe symptoms of iron toxicity (e.g., coma, shock, seizures) are present. F.E. is experiencing symptoms, he presumably ingested up to 66 mg/kg of elemental iron, and iron absorption appears to be ongoing based on the increase in his serum iron concentration. Therefore, F.E. should be treated with deferoxamine.

Deferoxamine Dose

22. What dose of deferoxamine should be prescribed for F.E., and how should it be administered?

The usual IM dose of deferoxamine for the treatment of acute iron intoxication is 90 mg/kg, not to exceed a maximum of 1 gram per dose. The dose can be repeated every 8 hours as needed; however, no more than 6 g of deferoxamine should be given to adults or children in a 24-hour period. Deferoxamine may be more effective when administered intravenously.[82,83] Pain at the injection site as well as induration is common after IM administration. Clinically, a slow IV infusion is preferred because the dose administered can be controlled more precisely. Many toxicologists prefer to use a constant intravenous infusion of deferoxamine at 15mg/kg per hour. In pediatric patients with severe iron poisoning, doses up to 35 mg/kg per hour have been infused with no adverse effects.[82] However, hypotension can result from administering IV boluses of deferoxamine too rapidly.[83] Because the adverse effects of deferoxamine are most likely related to rapid IV administration,[84] it should be administered to F.E. at a rate of about 10 mg/kg per hour, and his clinical status should be monitored closely.

Monitoring and Discontinuation

23. F.E. is admitted to the pediatric ICU 1 hour after the initiation of a deferoxamine infusion at 10 mg/kg per hour. How should deferoxamine therapy be monitored, and when should it be discontinued?

The rate of deferoxamine infusion should be increased if symptoms of severe iron toxicity develop, and the dosage should be decreased if adverse effects develop. The infusion of deferoxamine should be continued until the serum iron concentration is within the normal range and symptoms of iron toxicity are no longer present. The duration of deferoxamine infusion generally is about 6 to 12 hours. Chelation therapy that continues longer than necessary should be avoided because deferoxamine infusion of 15 mg/kg per hour for more than 24 hours has been associated with the development of acute respiratory distress syndrome (ARDS).[85]

Deferoxamine can interfere with some laboratory methods used to measure serum iron concentrations and cause falsely low values.[82] When deferoxamine is initiated, the clinical laboratory should be contacted to clarify whether deferoxamine will interfere with their serum iron tests. Disappearance of the "vin rose" color of urine also has been suggested as a way to determine the adequacy of deferoxamine therapy.

Outcome

F.E. was admitted to pediatric ICU overnight and treated with a constant infusion of deferoxamine at 10 mg/kg per hour for 7 hours. His GI symptoms stopped, he became more alert, and his vitals signs were stable. An analysis of a free iron blood sample the next morning revealed a serum iron level of 167 µg/mL. He was discharged home that afternoon.

[SI units: 34.39 µmol/L]

ASSESSMENT OF CENTRAL NERVOUS SYSTEM DEPRESSANT VERSUS ANTIDEPRESSANT INGESTION
Validation of Ingestion

24. T.C., a 30-year-old, unconscious woman, was found lying on the couch with a suicide note. The note stated that she had ingested 25 of her pills. Upon discovering T.C. unresponsive, T.C.'s 15-year-old daughter called paramedics. When the paramedics arrived, T.C.'s heart rate was 145 beats/min, BP was 110/70 mm Hg, and respirations were 12 breaths/min and shallow. T.C. had vomitus in her mouth. T.C. responded only to painful stimuli. The paramedics immediately started an IV line after completing their assessment of her airway, breathing, and circulation. Why does this drug overdose information from this suicidal patient need to be validated?

Assessing the accuracy of historical information in adult drug exposures is difficult, and many health care professionals question the validity of information, especially from suicidal patients.[23,25] The ingestion history could be inaccurate because the patient's altered mental status might prevent accurate recollection of what occurred. She may also try to intentionally deceive health care providers to minimize appropriate care. The supposition that the drug overdose history from a patient is unreliable is based on studies that demonstrate poor correlation between stated drug ingestions and urine drug tests.[25,86] However, these tests generally detect all recent drug and substance use, rather than just the overdosed drug. Every effort should be made to validate the history with information from other sources. In suicidal patients, one should consider all drugs that may have been available to the patient; the patient's presenting symptoms; laboratory tests; as well as information obtained from family members, police, paramedics, and other individuals who know the patient.

Interventions by Protocol

25. In addition to managing the ABCs of airway, breathing, circulation, and oxygenation, what pharmacologic interventions should be authorized for the paramedics to administer to T.C. in addition to the IV solution?

Glucose and Thiamine

Emergency medical service personnel often have protocols directing them to treat patients who are unconscious from an unknown cause. These protocols generally include administration of glucose, thiamine, and naloxone. If the paramedics cannot measure a blood glucose immediately, T.C. should be given 50 mL of 50% dextrose in water to treat possible hypoglycemia. The risks of hyperglycemia from this dose of glucose are negligible relative to the significant benefits if the patient is hypoglycemic. Thiamine should be given with glucose because glucose can precipitate the Wernicke-Korsakoff complex in thiamine-deficient patients (Chapter 29: Alcoholic Cirrhosis). Wernicke's encephalopathy is a reversible neurologic disturbance consisting of generalized confusion, ataxia, and ophthalmoplegia. Korsakoff's psychosis is believed to be irreversible and is associated with a more prolonged deficiency of thiamine.[87,88] The patient also should be evaluated for blood loss, hypoxia, and for evidence of head trauma from a possible fall.[23]

Naloxone

The pure opiate antagonist, naloxone is indicated for the treatment of respiratory depression induced by opioids,[88,90] but many emergency medical services protocols authorize paramedics to routinely administer naloxone to all patients with decreased mental status.[91] Although naloxone reportedly has reversed coma and acute respiratory depression in intoxicated patients who have no evidence of opiate use, its administration is not justified unless the use of opioids is suspected.[87,88] The response of these patients to naloxone might have been secondary to opioids that were not detected by the urine toxicology screens (e.g., oxycodone, fentanyl).

Drug-induced CNS depression usually waxes and wanes, and reports of naloxone success in patients who have not used opioids could also have been the result of responses to needle sticks, movement, or other stimuli rather than to naloxone. Although some patients might respond to naloxone, lack of consistent effectiveness, lack of clinical variables that can be used to predict when a patient should respond, and lack of well-controlled clinical studies minimize its clinical usefulness for nonopioid intoxications. Furthermore, violent and aggressive patient behavior can be precipitated when there is a sudden increased consciousness induced by naloxone. This can complicate emergency care in an emergency transport vehicle and put caregivers and patients at risk for trauma.[92]

Initial Treatment

26. The paramedics arrive at the ED with T.C. 30 minutes after her daughter called them. T.C.'s heart rate in the ED is 138 beats/min, BP is 90/55 mm Hg, and respirations have decreased from 12 breaths/min, spontaneous and shallow, to 7 breaths/min with assisted ventilation with a bag-valve mask. T.C. remains unresponsive. The paramedics were unable to find any prescriptions or other medications in the house. Her daughter thought that her mother was taking medication for depression, but she could not be more specific. The police will notify T.C.'s husband and try to obtain additional information about the ingested substance. What initial treatment should be provided for T.C. in the ED?

T.C. should be intubated and mechanically ventilated with 100% oxygen because of her shallow, slow respirations and the likelihood that vomitus has been aspirated into her lungs. The blood pressure taken by the paramedics was 110/70 mm Hg and now is 90/55 mm Hg. Because T.C.'s usual blood pressure is unknown at this time, the contribution of her hypotension to her mental status cannot be established. She should be given a bolus of IV fluids to determine whether increasing her intravascular fluid volume will increase her blood pressure and improve her mental status.

Antidotes

27. T.C.'s husband reports that T.C. is under the care of a psychiatrist for depression and two previous suicide attempts. He does not know the identity of her medication, but attempts are underway to contact T.C.'s psychiatrist. What antidotes can be administered in the ED for diagnostic purposes? Should flumazenil (Romazicon) be administered?

Theoretically, antidotes such as naloxone, flumazenil, deferoxamine, and antidigoxin FAB fragments could be administered in a hospitalized setting to identify an unknown toxin. However, the costs, time required for administration, and increased risks from these antidotes preclude their use for diagnostic purposes without some plausible suspicion of a particular drug ingestion. Although naloxone and flumazenil can reverse CNS depression caused by opioids and benzodiazepines, respectively, their use is not appropriate without historical, clinical, or toxicologic laboratory findings suggesting these drugs as a cause of T.C.'s intoxication.

Organ-System Evaluations

28. How can the initial physical assessment, using an organ-systems approach, be helpful in identifying the drugs ingested by T.C.?

The patient's airway, breathing, circulation, CNS, and cardiopulmonary function should be assessed with special attention to clinical manifestations that suggest ingestion of a specific class of drugs.[27] For example, T.C.'s history of depression suggests that antidepressants, antipsychotics, lithium, and/or benzodiazepines are candidates for ingestion in her case. An organ-system evaluation will help determine whether these (or other) drugs might have been ingested. Because adult drug ingestions usually involve more than one drug, nonprescription medications such as aspirin, acetaminophen, decongestants, and antihistamines, which are commonly available in most households, should also be considered.

Central Nervous System Function

Changes in CNS function are probably the single most common finding associated with drug intoxication. CNS depression or stimulation, seizures, delirium, pseudohallucinations, coma, or any combination of these can be manifested in intoxicated patients. CNS changes can be the direct result of an ingested drug or may be an additive to other underlying CNS processes or medical conditions. Many drug overdoses can produce different clinical manifestations at various times during the intoxication and different doses can produce different effects as well.

Drugs with anticholinergic properties can produce disorientation, confusion, delirium, and visual hallucinations early during the course of the intoxication; coma can become apparent as toxicity progresses. Generally, overdoses with anticholinergic drugs do not produce true hallucinations, but rather pseudohallucinations. When a patient with an intact sensorium presents with psychosis, paranoia, or visual hallucinations, CNS stimulants such as cocaine or amphetamines should be considered.[93] Drug intoxication–induced alterations in CNS function initially are difficult to distinguish from those caused by underlying psychiatric disorders, trauma, hypoxia, or metabolic disorders such as hepatic encephalopathy or hypoglycemia. However, with the passage of time, decreased CNS function secondary to drug toxicity is more likely to wax and wane in severity in contrast to the more constant CNS depression that occurs with significant trauma or metabolic disorders. Drug toxicity also rarely produces focal neurologic findings. Changes in pupil size, reflexes, and vital signs may provide insights into the pharmacologic class of drug involved in the intoxication.

CNS depression, seizures, disorientation, and other CNS changes that commonly are associated with drugs likely to be prescribed by psychiatrists should be evaluated carefully in T.C. For example, T.C.'s pupil size would most likely be dilated if she had ingested a tricyclic antidepressant because of the anticholinergic effects of these drugs. Tricyclic antidepressant intoxications also can cause myoclonic spasms. These spasms often are difficult to differentiate from seizure activity caused by tricyclic antidepressant overdoses, although the spasms often are asymmetrical and more persistent.[71]

Cardiovascular Function

Assessment of heart rate, rhythm, conduction, and measurements of hemodynamic function also can be used to help identify the type of drugs ingested. For example, overdoses of sympathomimetic drugs usually increase heart rate. Overdoses of cardiac glycosides or β-blockers may slow the heart rate. Although drugs can increase or decrease heart rate directly, indirect cardiac effects (e.g., reflex tachycardia in response to hypotension) also need to be considered. Abnormal heart rates produced by drug overdoses usually are not treated unless hypotension or severe dysrhythmias are precipitated.

Pulmonary Function

Evaluating the rate and depth of respiration and the effectiveness of gas exchange in an intoxicated patient also can help identify drugs that might have been ingested. For example, a decrease in respiratory rate is commonly associated with the ingestion of CNS depressants. An increased respiratory rate and depth generally is associated with CNS stimulant toxicity. An increase in respiratory rate also can be secondary to respiratory compensation for a drug-induced metabolic acidosis. Aspiration of gastric contents after vomiting is a common event in drug ingestions, and pneumonitis and pneumonia are the most common pulmonary abnormalities associated with significant intoxications.[112] Noncardiogenic acute pulmonary edema has been associated with drug overdoses of salicylates, especially with chronic intoxications, ethchlorvynol (Placidyl), tricyclic antidepressants, and the inhalation of drugs of abuse (e.g., cocaine).[94–97]

Temperature

Body temperature is an important and sometimes overlooked parameter when assessing potential intoxications. Decreased mental status often is associated with a loss of thermoregulation, and this results in a body temperature that falls toward the ambient temperature. Increased body temperature (hyperthermia) caused by overdoses of CNS stimulants (e.g., cocaine, amphetamines, ecstasy), salicylates, hallucinogens (e.g., phencyclidine), or anticholinergic drugs or plants (e.g., jimsonweed) can have serious consequences.[27] Body temperature should be measured rectally to obtain an accurate representation of core temperature.

Hyperthermia caused by drug overdoses is commonly encountered in hot, humid environments or when the intoxication is associated with physical exertion, increased muscle tone, or seizures. In these patients, it is important to obtain a serum creatine kinase (CK) measurement to determine whether rhabdomyolysis has occurred secondary to breakdown of muscle tissue. Patients with severe rhabdomyolysis can have CK levels in the tens of thousands range. These patients usually have significant increases in their BUN and serum creatinine measurements as well.

Gastrointestinal Function

The GI tract should be assessed for decreased motility because drug absorption can be delayed and prolonged. When this is the case, decontamination may be beneficial after an oral ingestion even when a long period of time has elapsed since the ingestion. The presence of blood in either emesis or stool may signal ingestion of a GI irritant or caustic substance.

Skin and Extremities

Examination of the skin and extremities can provide evidence of IV or subcutaneous drug injections. Fluid-filled bullae at gravity-dependent sites that have been in contact with hard surfaces for a long time suggest prolonged coma.[98] Muscle tone also should be assessed. Increased tone or myoclonic spasms can be caused by some drug overdoses (e.g., tricyclic antidepressants) and can produce rhabdomyolysis or hyperthermia.[71] Dry, hot, red skin may also be an indication of anticholinergic toxicity.

In summary, an organ system assessment in T.C. can provide useful insights into the identity of drugs that might have been ingested, the viability of organ function that might have been adversely affected, and the treatment that should be instituted.

Laboratory Tests

29. **What laboratory tests should be ordered for T.C.?**

The laboratory assessment of an intoxicated patient should be guided by the history of the events surrounding the ingestion, clinical presentation, and past medical history. The status of oxygenation, acid–base balance, and blood glucose concentration must be determined, especially in patients with altered mental status such as T.C. Oxygenation can be assessed initially by pulse oximetry, and acid–base status by arterial blood gases and serum electrolyte concentrations. T.C. was given oxygen and a bolus of IV fluid on her arrival at the ED. Paramedics administered a glucose load during her transportation to the ED.

A medical history of organ dysfunction or medical disorders (e.g., diabetes, hypertension) that can damage organs of elimination (e.g., kidney, liver) will also guide the need for laboratory tests. In this case, no medical history was obtained from T.C. Therefore, a serum creatinine concentration and liver function tests (e.g., aspartate aminotransferase [AST], alanine aminotransferase [ALT]) also should be ordered. Other more specific tests reflective of her past medical history can be ordered subsequent to dialogue with her psychiatrist, who already has been called. Until her medical records become available, a complete blood count (CBC), chemistry panel, and other baseline laboratory tests (e.g., electrocardiogram [ECG]) should be obtained.[99] Pregnancy tests should be considered in female patients of childbearing age because unwanted pregnancies are common causes of overdose.

A baseline ECG should be obtained when there is suspected exposure to a cardiotoxic drug or whenever the cardiovascular or hemodynamic status is altered. In these patients, continuous cardiac monitoring is appropriate. Because T.C. is likely to have ingested a psychotropic agent, possibly a tricyclic antidepressant, a 12-lead ECG and continuous cardiac monitoring should be ordered because of the significant cardiotoxicity associated with overdoses of these agents. Patients with severe tricyclic antidepressant overdoses frequently present with symptoms of coma, tachycardia with a prolonged QRS segment, seizures, and hypotension.

A chest radiograph is useful when the potential exists for either direct pulmonary toxicity or aspiration. Because T.C. had vomitus in her mouth, and tricyclic antidepressants are associated with the development of acute respiratory distress syndrome, a chest radiograph is indicated.

Qualitative Screening

30. Why should (or should not) T.C.'s urine, blood, or gastric fluid be screened to assist in identifying the ingested substance?

Toxicology laboratory testing can be used to identify the substances involved in a toxic exposure, to exclude substances, or to measure the concentration of substances in serum or other biologic fluids.[99,100] The identification and quantification of compounds should be considered as two distinct types of toxicologic testing. *Qualitative* screening is unique because it is intended to identify unknown substances. The test must be able to identify which substance, or class of substances, is involved in the toxic exposure. *Quantitative* testing is similar to therapeutic drug monitoring in that the presence of the substance usually is known, and the question being answered is how much is present.

Screening various biologic fluids suspected of having high concentrations of a parent drug and its metabolites can identify unknown substances. Urine is screened much more commonly than blood, while gastric fluid is rarely evaluated. A urine drug screen is preferred to a blood drug screen because urine generally contains a higher concentration of a drug and its metabolites than other body fluids.

When reviewing the results of urine screening panels for drugs and other substances, one must remember that the presence of a substance in urine is not necessarily related to a concurrent toxicity. A positive result on an urine-screening panel merely indicates that the patient has ingested or has been exposed to the substance, but it does not differentiate between toxic and nontoxic doses. If a drug and its metabolites are eliminated slowly into the urine over a prolonged period of time, and if the testing methodology detects small concentrations of the substance, urine drug screening may identify the presence of a substance many days, weeks, or even months subsequent to the exposure. Similarly, a negative toxicologic screening test does not necessarily rule out a drug overdose because the drug concentration may be undetectable or the substance may not be included in laboratory analyses. The sensitivity, specificity, and practicality of the test should be considered.

Sensitivity, Specificity, and Practicality
An understanding of the sensitivity, specificity, and practicality of analytic tests is crucial to their interpretation. The *sensitivity* of a test reflects the minimum concentration required to detect the substance. The *specificity* of a test reflects its ability to identify an unknown compound and to distinguish it from other substances. When compounds with similar chemical structures cross-react with an assay, the assay is deemed to have poor specificity. Cross-reactivity of compounds is ac-

ceptable in some instances. For example, the identity of a specific benzodiazepine is less important than knowing that a compound within the benzodiazepine pharmacologic class is present. On the other hand, taking pseudoephedrine for a cold may result in a false-positive screen for amphetamines. A positive drug screen on a work-mandated drug screen or a random drug screen for parolees may result in serious consequences.

The *practicality* of an assay is determined by its cost, availability, and turnaround time for test results. Practicality is probably the most important determinant of whether toxicology testing is useful to assess and manage drug intoxication.[99,102] For example, if the hospital laboratory sends out all of its methanol tests to a reference laboratory and results do not return for 3 days, this laboratory test cannot be used to determine the severity of the ingestion or the treatment of the patient in a timely manner.

Qualitative toxicology screening is most useful when these tests can confirm the absence of suspected toxic substances. These tests also can be useful in uncommon circumstances when results could alter the treatment plan.[100] It is appropriate when the history of a suspected toxic exposure is unavailable, inaccurate, or inconsistent with the clinical findings. A comprehensive qualitative urine drug screen should be ordered for T.C. because she is unable to provide information about the substances she ingested.

Quantitative Testing

31. Why should a quantitative toxicology laboratory test be ordered (or not ordered) for T.C. as well?

The qualitative screening of urine for drugs and other substances does not determine the amount of substance involved in an exposure; it only determines the presence or absence of the substance or its metabolite. Knowledge of the concentration of a substance in serum can help determine the severity of toxicity and the need for aggressive interventions.[101] Quantitative tests are especially useful when assessing the potential toxicity of drugs with delayed clinical toxicity or when the toxicity primarily is caused by metabolites (e.g., acetaminophen, methanol). Furthermore, the concentration of a drug in serum is sometimes much more predictive of end-organ damage than clinical findings (e.g., ethanol effects on CNS).[103]

Measuring the amount of drug in serum or plasma is useful when (1) there is a known correlation between the concentration of the substance and toxic effects; (2) the turnaround time for results is rapid; and (3) treatment can be guided by the serum concentration. For example, serum concentrations are commonly used to estimate the potential toxicity of acetaminophen, salicylates, theophylline, iron, lithium, digoxin, phenytoin, phenobarbital, methanol, ethanol, and ethylene glycol.[23,30,31]

When blood samples are collected to quantitate potentially intoxicating substances, as much information as possible should be obtained about the time course of events to determine whether absorption and distribution of the substance is complete. Serial samples collected at 3- to 6-hour intervals may be needed to determine whether significant absorption is still occurring and whether GI decontamination should be repeated or continued. In contrast to the interpretation of serum concentrations of chronically administered drugs, the serum concentration of a substance ingested in an overdose will not be at steady state.

Quantitative toxicologic testing will not benefit T.C. at this point in time because the identity of the ingested substance is unknown. However, because alcohol often is ingested concurrently in overdose situations, a serum ethanol concentration would be useful in T.C. Also, patients often do not consider acetaminophen a dangerous drug as it can be purchased over the counter. If an acetaminophen ingestion is missed, serious hepatotoxicity may occur at a time when it is too late to prevent damage. Because of that, many poison centers recommend obtaining a quantitative acetaminophen level on all intentional ingestions.

Assessment

32. T.C.'s clinical status has not changed over the last 10 minutes. A urine toxicology screen has been ordered along with a blood acetaminophen level and an ABG measurement. The 12-lead ECG has a prolonged QRS interval of 0.14 seconds (normal, <0.1 sec). No antidotes have been administered. T.C.'s physical examination did not detect any evidence of trauma to her head. Her pupils were dilated and slowly responsive to light, and her bowel sounds were hypoactive. What conclusions can be made at this time with regard to the likely substance ingested by T.C.?

Although the ingested substance still has not been specifically identified, the available data provide some clues as to the likely pharmacologic class of drug that was ingested. The presence of CNS depression (T.C. is unresponsive), slowed ventricular conduction (prolonged QRS on ECG), tachycardia (heart rate, 138 beats/minute), hypotension (BP, 90/55 mm Hg), decreased GI motility (hypoactive bowel sounds), and the history of a possible depressive illness (history from husband and daughter) are all consistent with a tricyclic antidepressant drug overdose. The antidepressant may have been ingested alone or with other agents concomitantly.

Antidepressant Toxicities

33. How would the different toxicities of the various available antidepressants affect the treatment of T.C.?

The major pharmacologic effects and toxicities of the antidepressants are similar for all drugs within the same class. When a specific drug within a therapeutic class has not yet been identified, the overdose should be managed as if the ingested drug can produce the most severe toxicity of any drug in the class. In this light, T.C.'s presumed antidepressant drug overdose should be evaluated and managed initially as a tricyclic antidepressant (e.g., amitriptyline) ingestion.[104] Antidepressants with different structures and actions (e.g., trazodone [Desyrel], fluoxetine [Prozac], sertraline [Zoloft]) generally do not produce toxicity as severe as that of the tricyclic antidepressants.[105]

Gastrointestinal Decontamination

34. If a tricyclic antidepressant ingestion is presumed, is GI decontamination appropriate at this time?

The longer GI decontamination is delayed relative to the time of ingestion, the less effective it is likely to be because absorption will already have occurred. Nevertheless, absorption generally is slowed and more erratic in the case of a toxic overdose. Therefore, T.C. should undergo some form of GI decontamination.

Activated Charcoal

35. What method of GI decontamination should be initiated for T.C.?

A combination of gastric lavage followed by activated charcoal could be used in T.C. She will require endotracheal intubation with a cuffed endotracheal tube before the lavage tube is inserted because passage of the lavage tube can stimulate emesis and place her at risk of aspiration. T.C. already is unresponsive and vulnerable to aspiration. Furthermore, tricyclic antidepressant overdoses can induce seizures. Although gastric lavage may not be effective and its role is controversial, >300 mg of antidepressants have been recovered from overdosed patients by gastric lavage.[106]

While gastric lavage may not remove significant amounts of drug in T.C., there is no contraindication. Also, once the gastric lavage tube is placed, activated charcoal will be easier to administer in this patient by simply instilling the charcoal slurry via the lavage tube.

The adsorption of tricyclic antidepressants to charcoal prevents absorption and the charcoal-drug complex can be excreted in the stool. A second dose of activated charcoal should be considered in patients with serious tricyclic antidepressant toxicity because of the possibility of desorption of the drug from the charcoal. Tricyclic antidepressants also undergo enterohepatic recirculation. Up to 15% of metabolized drug is excreted in bile and gastric secretions and then reabsorbed in the intestines. Because of the recirculation, multiple-dose charcoal might be of benefit. The combination of both gastric lavage and activated charcoal is indicated because of the potential for severe, life-threatening toxicity in T.C.

Monitoring Efficacy

36. How should the effectiveness of GI decontamination be monitored in T.C.?

Tricyclic antidepressants are commonly absorbed very slowly in an overdose situation.[71] Because of the anticholinergic nature of tricyclic antidepressants, GI transit time may be significantly increased.[107] As a result, GI decontamination should be monitored to determine whether additional decontamination would be beneficial. Activated charcoal can produce GI obstruction, especially when administered to patients who have ingested drugs with anticholinergic activity that slows GI motility.[108]

Sodium Bicarbonate and Hyperventilation

37. According to T.C.'s psychiatrist, he prescribed amitriptyline 100 mg at bedtime for her severe depression. How does this new information alter T.C.'s treatment plan?

This information confirms the assumptions made about a tricyclic antidepressant ingestion and specifically identifies the probable ingested drug. Moderate to severe toxicity is expected after the oral ingestion of 10 to 20 mg/kg of drugs in the tricyclic antidepressant class of drugs. T.C. ingested a total of 2,500 mg based on her suicide note that said she took 25 tablets. If she was truthful about the amount taken, she has clearly ingested a toxic amount.

Based on this information, T.C. should receive IV sodium bicarbonate because it counteracts the effects of amitriptyline on myocardial conduction and narrows the QRS. Because the suspicion of an antidepressant overdose was strong, sodium bicarbonate could have been administered empirically if her ECG demonstrated QRS prolongation, worsening myocardial conduction and if her BP continued to decline. The mechanism by which sodium bicarbonate decreases antidepressant-induced myocardial toxicity is unclear.[109] Hyperventilation via the ventilator setting to a pH of 7.5 also might decrease the cardiotoxicity of the antidepressants.

Monitoring Efficacy

38. **How should the sodium bicarbonate therapy in T.C. be monitored?**

Serial ECGs to measure the QRS interval can evaluate the efficacy of sodium bicarbonate. A prolonged QRS interval generally will narrow to normal after the systemic pH has been increased to about 7.5. Many patients intoxicated with tricyclic antidepressants present with severe acidosis. Numerous doses of sodium bicarbonate may be required to normalize the arterial pH. The toxicity of sodium bicarbonate administration can be evaluated by monitoring for systemic alkalosis. Acid–base status should be monitored using ABGs, especially if the patient is also being ventilated mechanically, because the combination of bicarbonate and mechanical ventilation is more likely to produce severe alkalosis.[110]

Seizures

39. **T.C. gradually developed more severely altered mental status and became comatose, not responding even to painful stimuli. She suddenly experienced a generalized tonic-clonic seizure, which lasted about 2 minutes and terminated spontaneously. Why should anticonvulsant therapy not be initiated for T.C. at this time?**

Drug overdose–induced seizures are most commonly single seizures that terminate before drug therapy can be administered.[111] Since this seizure episode terminated spontaneously, drug management of this event is not needed. However, if her seizures did not stop within 1 to 2 minutes, a benzodiazepine would have been administered parenterally. The onset of action of phenobarbital is too delayed for managing this acute seizure and phenytoin is usually ineffective in treating drug-toxicity related seizures. Chronic anticonvulsant therapy also should not be administered to T.C. because there is no evidence that she will have additional seizures. Furthermore, the potential for drug-induced seizures will decrease as the elimination of the antidepressant continues. Subsequent to a seizure, the patient may become more acidotic and hypotensive.

Interpretation of Urine Screens

40. **T.C.'s BP fell to 88/42 mm Hg and dopamine was started. Her pH on repeat arterial blood gases was 7.26. T.C.'s ECG normalized after the administration of 150 mL of sodium bicarbon-** ate by IV bolus. After dopamine, her BP increased to 102/68 mm Hg, and seizure activity ceased. The urine drug screen results were positive for amitriptyline and nortriptyline. Acetaminophen and alcohol were not detected in her blood. Does the presence of nortriptyline indicate that T.C. has ingested other drugs in addition to her combination of amitriptyline?

Nortriptyline is a metabolite of amitriptyline and therefore was identified on the urine drug screen. Metabolites often are identified on comprehensive urine drug screens as well as the parent compound.

Duration of Hospitalization

41. **How long should T.C. be monitored?**

T.C. should be admitted to the ICU from the ED and monitored until all evidence of CNS and cardiovascular toxicity has been reversed. As with all cases of tricyclic antidepressant overdoses, T.C. should be followed until at least 12 hours have elapsed without any evidence of toxicity and there is no further risk of continued GI absorption.[112] After the toxicity has completely resolved, T.C. should be evaluated by a psychiatrist to determine whether she should be admitted for inpatient treatment of her suicidal tendencies.

Outcome

T.C. had no further seizure activity. She remained on a dopamine infusion for 8 hours and required several more boluses of IV sodium bicarbonate. The next afternoon, she started to awake with her family at the bedside. She was tearful and expressed remorse that her suicide-attempt was unsuccessful. She repeatedly told her family that they would be better off without her. Her psychiatrist saw her and arrangements were made to transfer her to a psychiatric hospital once she was medically cleared.

ASSESSMENT OF ACETAMINOPHEN INGESTION
Complication of Pregnancy

42. **L.P., a 23-year-old woman who is about 32 weeks pregnant, presents to the ED 90 minutes after ingesting 50 acetaminophen 500-mg tablets. She is depressed and hoped to end her pregnancy by ingesting acetaminophen. Her pregnancy was unplanned, and she has received no prenatal care. L.P. has vomited spontaneously twice since the ingestion; her heart rate is 100 beats/min, BP is 100/70 mm Hg, and temperature is 97.5°F. L.P. does not have any chronic diseases, and the remainder of her medical history is unremarkable. How does L.P.'s pregnancy change the management of her acetaminophen ingestion?**

Pregnancy does not change the initial approach to the assessment or treatment of potentially toxic ingestions. Assessment should initially focus on the mother. Overdoses during pregnancy often are associated with attempted abortions or with depression.[113]

The exposure of the fetus to the toxic ingestion depends on the ability of the ingested substance or its toxic metabolites to cross the placenta into the fetal circulation. The ability of the fetus to produce the toxic acetaminophen metabolite and the ability of the N-acetylcysteine antidote to cross the placenta also must be considered. Fetal and neonatal hepatotoxicity and death have occurred after maternal acetaminophen intoxications.[114,115] The fetal liver begins to metabolize acetaminophen to its hepatotoxic metabolite some time during the second trimester, but it also may be less able to detoxify the metabolite by conjugation with glutathione.[116]

The effects of the intoxication on maintaining the pregnancy and organogenesis also should be considered. Data regarding the effect of maternal poisonings on fetal outcomes are sparse. In one series of 209 pregnant patients with acetaminophen overdoses, a higher rate of stillbirths, lower birth weights, and increased likelihood of CNS abnormalities were noted, but infant death rates, spontaneous abortions, or other congenital abnormalities were not observed.[117] In a later study, acetaminophen overdoses during pregnancy did not appear to increase the risk for birth defects or adverse pregnancy outcome unless the mother suffered severe toxicity.[119]

Mechanism of Hepatotoxicity

43. How do overdoses of acetaminophen cause hepatic necrosis?

At toxic serum concentrations, conjugation pathways for acetaminophen become saturated and a greater fraction of acetaminophen metabolism is dependent on the P450 pathway producing a potentially toxic metabolite. Normally this metabolite is detoxified by conjugation with glutathione. However, increase amounts of the toxic metabolite deplete hepatic glutathione stores. When glutathione stores decrease to approximately 30% of normal, the toxic metabolite binds to hepatocytes, resulting in the characteristic centrilobular hepatic necrosis seen in acetaminophen overdoses.[119]

Gastrointestinal Decontamination

44. What GI decontamination should be initiated for L.P.?

The use of GI decontamination for acetaminophen ingestions has been widely debated because N-acetylcysteine (Mucomyst), the antidote used to prevent hepatotoxicity, is administered orally. Although GI decontamination can be accomplished with activated charcoal, the activated charcoal may also inhibit the absorption of the N-acetylcysteine. While N-acetylcysteine serum concentrations in studies were decreased by activated charcoal,[120] the overall bioavailability of N-acetylcysteine was not decreased.[18] Therefore, activated charcoal is recommended in the management of acetaminophen overdose cases, but it should not be administered concurrently with N-acetylcysteine.[121] An interval of 1 to 2 hours between the administration of activated charcoal and N-acetylcysteine is preferred.

Activated charcoal 50 g should be administered to L.P. because her acetaminophen ingestion occurred 90 minutes ago. If N-acetylcysteine therapy is needed later, the activated charcoal will not impair its absorption. Furthermore, N-acetylcysteine therapy is not contraindicated in pregnant patients and might be helpful because it may cross the placenta, thereby protecting the fetus from hepatotoxicity.[115]

Alternatively, N-acetylcysteine can be given intravenously. Although not an FDA-approved route of administration because there is currently no sterile, pyrogen-free formulation of N-acetylcysteine in the United States, IV administration is often used. However, use of IV N-acetylcysteine is not completely risk free as there is a possibility of the patient developing bronchospasm or anaphylaxis during the first dose of the IV N-acetylcysteine, especially in asthmatic patients.[122] This reaction occurs rarely, but has resulted in death and must be carefully monitored when the IV route is being used.

Estimating Potential Toxicity

45. How should the potential toxicity of the acetaminophen ingestion be assessed in L.P.?

Acetaminophen toxicity is poorly correlated with the dose ingested. Serum acetaminophen concentrations are a better predictors of hepatotoxicity.[123,124] The Matthew-Rumack nomogram (Fig. 5-1) is used in the United States to assess the potential for hepatotoxicity from acute overdoses of acetaminophen. The serum acetaminophen concentration is plotted on a graph against the time of ingestion.[118] It is useful only for acute ingestions because it underestimates the potential for toxicity in instances of chronic acetaminophen over ingestion. This nomogram also can be used to guide therapy.

Acetaminophen Treatment Nomogram

46. A serum acetaminophen concentration is measured 4 hours after ingestion. Why was this analysis delayed for 4 hours even though L.P. arrived at the ED within 90 minutes after her ingestion?

Acetaminophen absorption generally is complete within 1.5 to 2.5 hours after ingestion of solid or liquid dosage forms.[125] The Matthews-Rumack nomogram is not applicable before 4 hours after ingestion because it is based on complete absorption. A report by the patient of an ingested dose is not as accurate as serum concentrations in predicting hepatotoxicity. Most clinical laboratories can complete their assays and report acetaminophen serum concentration results within 2 hours. The efficacy of N-acetylcysteine therapy is maximal if it is initiated during the first 8 hours after ingestion of the

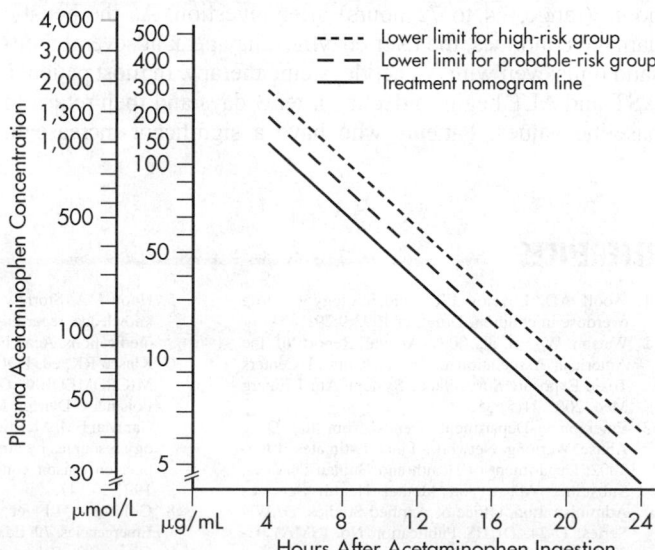

FIGURE 5-1 Nomogram for interpretation of severity of acetaminophen poisoning. (Copyright 2001 Massachusetts Medical Society. All rights reserved.)

toxic acetaminophen dose. Although it is less effective thereafter, late administration of *N*-acetylcysteine still diminishes hepatotoxicity compared with untreated historical controls.

N-Acetylcysteine Administration

47. The 4-hour acetaminophen concentration in L.P. was 245 μg/mL. How should *N*-acetylcysteine be administered, and what can be done if she vomits after *N*-acetylcysteine administration?

This concentration of acetaminophen at four hours is above the treatment line on Figure 5-1. The loading dose of *N*-acetylcysteine is 140 mg/kg orally. Oral *N*-acetylcysteine commonly causes nausea and vomiting, and as a result, it is diluted to a concentration of 5% using a carbonated beverage or fruit juice to mask the unpleasant taste and odor. Seventeen additional maintenance doses of 70 mg/kg of *N*-acetylcysteine are administered at 4-hour intervals after the initial dose for a total of 72 hours of therapy. Shorter *N*-acetylcysteine regimens are currently being used based on the efficacy of IV therapy.

If L.P. vomits within the first hour after her *N*-acetylcysteine dose, the dose should be repeated. If she experiences protracted vomiting, the use of antiemetic drugs (e.g., ondansetron, metoclopramide) or a duodenal feeding tube can improve GI tolerance.[126] Alternatively, the *N*-acetylcysteine can be administered intravenously.[127]

Monitoring Efficacy of *N*-Acetylcysteine

48. How should the efficacy and toxicity of *N*-acetylcysteine therapy be monitored in L.P.?

With the exception of vomiting, oral *N*-acetylcysteine does not produce other toxicity when administered orally. Patients should be monitored for allergic and anaphylactoid reactions when *N*-acetylcysteine is administered intravenously. The effectiveness of *N*-acetylcysteine intervention in L.P. should be monitored by daily assessment of her acetaminophen concentration (as long as it is still measurable), liver function tests, and PT.[126] The AST and ALT levels typically increase within 36 hours (range, 24 to 72 hours) after ingestion. As the hepatic damage continues, the liver enzymes may peak at several thousand units even with *N*-acetylcysteine therapy. In most patients, AST and ALT begin to decline after 3 days and then return to baseline values. Patients who have a significant increase in serum bilirubin concentration and PT and who develop encephalopathy have a decreased likelihood of survival.[118,127]

Liver transplantation is used as a last resort in patients with fulminant hepatic failure and encephalopathy. Each transplant institution has its own criteria for transplantation. In general, symptoms such as severe or persistent acidosis, coagulopathy, a significantly increased serum creatinine, and grade III to IV encephalopathy are consistent with fatal outcomes in patients with fulminant hepatic failure.[118]

Outcome

L.P. continued to have nausea and vomiting and had difficulty keeping the *N*-acetylcysteine down. She was treated with metoclopramide 30 minutes before the oral dose of *N*-acetylcysteine and was successful in keeping the *N*-acetylcysteine down afterward. An obstetrics consultation was requested to evaluate L.P.'s pregnancy. Fetal monitoring was instituted during her hospital admission. A sonogram was taken of the baby. Once L.P. saw her baby's picture from the sonogram, her depressed mood seemed to lift. Approximately 36 hours after ingestion, her acetaminophen level was no longer detectable, and her liver function tests showed a mild elevation of her AST at 134 units/L and an ALT of 88 units/L [normal AST and AST values, 8 to 45 units/L]. Her PT and total bilirubin values were normal at 11 seconds [normal PT time, 10 to 13 seconds] and 0.8 mg/dL [normal total bilirubin in adults: 0.3 to 1.0 mg/dL], respectively. L.P. was seen by a psychiatrist. She was scheduled for counseling and prenatal classes, which L.P. seemed eager to attend. She received all 17 maintenance doses of *N*-acetylcysteine in hopes of protecting the fetal liver as much as possible. Six weeks later, she had a normal delivery of a healthy 6-lb 1-oz baby girl.

SUMMARY

When challenged with a poisoning exposure, consult with a poison control center. By calling 1-800-222-1222, the call will be connected to the poison center nearest your location. Consultation is available 24 hours a day nationwide to provide toxicology assistance.

Acknowledgment
William Watson and Frank Paloucek contributed significantly to this chapter in a previous edition.

REFERENCES

1. Woolf AD, Lovejoy FR. Epidemiology of drug overdose in children. Drug Saf 1993;9:291.
2. Watson WA et al. 2002 Annual Report of the American Association of Poison Control Centers Toxic Exposure Surveillance System. Am J Emerg Med. 2003;21(5):353.
3. Emergency Department Trends from the Drug Abuse Warning Network, Final Estimates 1995-2002. Department of Health and Human Services, Substance Abuse and Mental Health Services Administration, Office of Applied Studies. DAWN Series: D-24, DHHS Publication No. (SMA) 03-3780, Rockville, Md, 2003.
4. Blanc PD et al. Surveillance of poisoning and overdose through hospital discharge coding, poison control center reporting, and the drug abuse warning network. Am J Emerg Med 1993;11:14.
5. Huott MA, Storrow AB. A survey of adolescents' knowledge regarding toxicity of over-the-counter medications. Acad Emerg Med 1997;4:214.
6. Klasco RK, ed. POISINDEX ® System. Thomson MICROMEDEX. Greenwood Village, Colorado. Poisindex. Denver: Micromedex.
7. Caravati EM, McElwee NE. Use of clinical toxicology resources by emergency physicians and its impact on poison control centers. Ann Emerg Med 1991;20:147.
8. Goldfrank LF et al. Goldfrank's Toxicologic Emergencies, 7th Ed. New York: McGraw-Hill, 2002.
9. Olson KR. Poisoning & Drug Overdose, 4th Ed. New York: McGraw-Hill, 2004.
10. Mullen WH et al. Incorrect overdose management advice in the Physicians Desk Reference. Ann Emerg Med 1997;29:255.
11. Harrison DL et al. Cost-effectiveness of regional poison control centers. Arch Intern Med 1996;156:2661.
12. Miller TR, Lestina DC. Costs of poisonings in the United States and savings from poison control centers: a benefit-cost analysis. Ann Emerg Med 1997;29:239.
13. Anon. Facility assessment guidelines for regional toxicology treatment centers. Clin Toxicol 1993; 31:211.
14. American College of Emergency Physicians. Clinical policy for the initial approach to patients presenting with acute toxic ingestion or dermal or inhalation exposure. Ann Emerg Med 1995;25:570.
15. Krenzelok EP, Vale JA. Position statements: gut decontamination. Clin Toxicol 1997;35:695.
16. Krenzelok EP, Vale JA. Position statement: ipecac syrup. Clin Toxicol 1997;35:699.

17. Vale JA. Position statement: gastric lavage. Clin Toxicol 1997;35:711.
18. Chyka PA, Seger D. Position statement: single-dose activated charcoal. Clin Toxicol 1997;35:721.
19. Barceloux GD, McGuigan M, Hartigan-Go K. Position statement: cathartics. Clin Toxicol 1997;35:743.
20. Tenebein M. Position statement: whole bowel irrigation. Clin Toxicol. 1997;35:753.
21. Vale JA, Krenzelok EP, Barceloux GD. Position statement and Practical Guidelines on the Use of Multi-dose Activated Charcoal in the Treatment of Acute Poisoning. Clin Toxicol 1999;37:731.
22. Manoguerra AS. The poison information telephone call. In: Haddad LM, Winchester JF, eds. Clinical Management of Poisoning and Drug Overdose, 2nd Ed. Philadelphia: WB Saunders, 1990:471.
23. Kulig K. Current concepts—initial management of ingestions of toxic substances. N Engl J Med 1992;326:1677.
24. Vale JA. Reviews in medicine—clinical toxicology. Postgrad Med J 1993;69:19.
25. Wright N. An assessment of the unreliability of the history given by self-poisoned patients. Clin Toxicol 1980;16:381.
26. Veltri JC. Regional poison control services. Hosp Forum 1982;17:1469.
27. Olson KR et al. Physical assessment and differential diagnosis of the poisoned patient. Med Toxicol 1987;2:52.
28. Nice A et al. Toxidrome recognition to improve efficiency of emergency urine drug screens. Ann Emerg Med 1988;17:676.
29. Spyker DA, Minocha A. Toxicodynamic approach to management of the poisoned patient. J Emerg Med 1988;6:117.
30. Mahoney JD et al. Quantitative serum toxic screening in the management of suspected drug overdose. Am J Emerg Med 1990;8:16.
31. Hepler BR et al. Role of the toxicology laboratory in the treatment of acute poisoning. Med Toxicol 1986;1:61.
32. Sue YJ, Shannon M. Pharmacokinetics of drugs in overdose. Clin Pharmacokinet 1992;23:93.
33. Watson WA. Toxicokinetics and management of the poisoned patient. US Pharm 1990;15:H1.
34. Knopp R. Caustic ingestions. J Am Coll Emerg Phys 1979;8:329.
35. Linden CH, Watson WA. Gastrointestinal decontamination. In: Harwood-Nuss A et al, eds. The Clinical Practice of Emergency Medicine. Philadelphia: JB Lippincott, 1991:438.
36. Dillon EC et al. Large surface area activated charcoal and the inhibition of aspirin absorption. Ann Emerg Med 1989;18:547.
36a. Krenzelok EP, Heller MB. Effectiveness of commercially available aqueous activated charcoal products. Ann Emerg Med 1987;16:1340.
37. Comstock EG et al. Assessment of the efficacy of activated charcoal following gastric lavage in acute drug emergencies. J Toxicol Clin Toxicol 1982;19:149.
38. Kulig K et al. Management of acutely poisoned patients without gastric emptying. Ann Emerg Med 1985;14:562.
39. Tenenbein M. Whole bowel irrigation as a gastrointestinal decontamination procedure after acute poisoning. Med Toxicol 1988;3:77.
40. Committee on Injury, Violence and Poison Prevention: American Academy of Pediatrics Policy Statement: Poison Treatment in the Home. Pediatrics 2003;112:1182.
41. Palatnick W, Tenenbein M. Activated charcoal in the treatment of drug overdose. Drug Saf 1992;7:3.
42. Goldfrank LR, Hoffman RS. The cardiovascular effects of cocaine. Ann Emerg Med 1991;20:165.
43. Garrettson LK, Geller RJ. Acid and alkaline diuresis: when are they of value in the treatment of poisoning. Drug Saf 1990;5:220.
44. Todd JW. Do measures to enhance drug removal save life? Lancet 1984;1:331.
45. Kulling P, Persson H. Role of the intensive care unit in the management of the poisoned patient. Med Toxicol 1986;1:375.
46. Watson WA et al. The volume of a swallow: correlation of deglutition with patient and container parameters. Am J Emerg Med 1983;1:278.
47. Temple AR. Acute and chronic effects of aspirin toxicity and their treatment. Arch Intern Med 1981;141:364.
48. Clarke A, Walton WW. Effect of safety packaging on aspirin ingestion by children. Pediatrics 1979;63:687.
49. Done AK. Aspirin overdosage: incidence, diagnosis, and management. Pediatrics 1978;62:890.
50. Done AK, Temple AR. Treatment of salicylate poisoning. Mod Treat 1971;8:528.
51. Temple AR. Pathophysiology of aspirin overdosage toxicity, with implications for management. Pediatrics 1978;62:873.
52. Yip L et al. Concepts and controversies in salicylate toxicity. Emerg Med Clin North Am 1994;12:351.
53. Heffner JE, Sahn SA. Salicylate-induced pulmonary edema. Clinical features and prognosis. Ann Intern Med 1976;85:745.
54. Paul BN. Salicylate poisoning in the elderly: diagnostic pitfalls. J Am Geriatr Soc 1972;20:387.
55. Anderson RJ et al. Unrecognized adult salicylate intoxication. Ann Intern Med 1976;85:745.
56. Hill JB. Experimental salicylate poisoning: observations on the effects of altering blood pH on tissue and plasma salicylate concentrations. Pediatrics 1971;47:658.
57. Done AK. Salicylate intoxication. Significance of measurements of salicylate in blood in cases of acute ingestion. Pediatrics 1960;26:800.
58. Koren G. Medications which can kill a toddler with one tablet or teaspoonful. Clin Toxicol 1993;31:407.
59. Litovitz T, Manoguerra A. Comparison of pediatric poisoning hazards: an analysis of 3.8 million exposure incidents: a report from the American Association of Poison Control Centers. Pediatrics 1992;89:999.
60. Schauben JL et al. Iron poisoning: report of three cases and a review of therapeutic intervention. J Emerg Med 1990;8:309.
61. Litovitz TL et al. 1993 Annual Report of the American Association of Poison Control Centers Toxic Exposure Surveillance System. Am J Emerg Med 1994;12(5):546.
62. Litovitz TL et al. 1994 Annual Report of the American Association of the Poison Control Centers Toxic Exposure Surveillance System. Am J Emerg Med 1995;13(5):551.
63. Litovitz TL et al. 1995 Annual Report of the American Association of Poison Control Centers Toxic Exposure Surveillance System. Am J Emerg Med 1996;14(5):487.
64. Litovitz TL et al. 1996 Annual Report of the American Association of Poison Control Centers Toxic Exposure Surveillance System. Am J Emerg Med 1997;15(5):447.
65. Litovitz TL et al. 1997 Annual Report of the American Association of Poison Control Centers Toxic Exposure Surveillance System. Am J Emerg Med 1998;16(5):443.
66. Litovitz TL et al. 1998 Annual Report of the American Association of Poison Control Centers Toxic Exposure Surveillance System. Am J Emerg Med 1999;17(5):435.
67. Litovitz TL et al. 1999 Annual Report of the American Association of Poison Control Centers Toxic Exposure Surveillance System. Am J Emerg Med 2000;18(5):517.
68. Cada DJ, ed. Drug Facts and Comparisons 2003. St. Louis: Wolters Kluwer, 2003.
69. IDENTIDEX® in MICROMEDEX®. In: Klasco RK, ed. POISINDEX ® System. Thomson MICROMEDEX. Greenwood Village, Colorado. Poisindex. Denver: Micromedex.
70. Mann KV et al. Management of acute iron overdose. Clin Pharm 1989;8:428.
71. Callaham M. Tricyclic antidepressant overdose. J Am Coll Emerg Phys 1979;8:413.
72. Engle JP et al. Acute iron intoxication: treatment controversies. Drug Intell Clin Pharm 1987;21:153.
73. Jaeger RW et al. Radiopacity of drugs and plants in vivo—limited usefulness. Vet Hum Toxicol 1981;23(suppl 1):2.
74. Lacouture PG et al. Emergency assessment of severity of iron overdose by clinical and laboratory methods. J Pediatr 1981;99:89.
75. Neuvonen PJ, Olkkola KT. Oral activated charcoal in the treatment of intoxications—role of single and repeated doses. Med Toxicol 1988;3:33.
76. Perrone J et al. Special considerations in gastrointestinal decontamination. Emerg Med Clin North Am 1994;12:285.
77. Albertson TE et al. A prolonged severe intoxication after ingestion of phenytoin and phenobarbital. West J Med 1981;135:418.
78. Dolgin JG et al. Pharmacokinetic modeling and simulation of the effect of multi-dose activated charcoal in phenytoin intoxication—report of two pediatric cases. DICP, Ann Pharmacother 1991;25:463.
79. Buckley NA et al. Controlled release drugs in overdose: clinical consideration. Drug Saf 1995;12:73.
80. Minocha A, Spyker DA. Acute overdose with sustained release drug formulations: perspectives in treatment. Med Toxicol 1986;1:300.
81. Ling LJ et al. Absorption of iron after experimental overdose of chewable vitamins. Am J Emerg Med 1991;9:24.
82. Lovejoy FH. Chelation therapy in iron poisoning. J Toxicol Clin Toxicol 1982;19:871.
83. Boehnert M et al: Massive iron overdose treated with high-dose deferoxamine infusion (abstract). Vet Human Toxicol 1985;28:291.
84. Pagliaro LA, Levin RH, eds: Problems in pediatric drug therapy. Hamilton, IL: Drug Intelligence Publications, 1979.
85. Tenenbein M et al: Pulmonary toxic effects of continuous desferrioxamine administration i acute iron poisoning. Lancet 1992;339:699.
86. Ingelfinger JA et al. Reliability of the toxic screen in drug overdose. Clin Pharmacol Ther 1981;29:570.
87. Watson AJS et al. Acute Wernicke's encephalopathy precipitated by glucose loading. Ir J Med Sci 1981;150:301.
88. Zubaran C et al. Wernicke-Korsakoff syndrome. Postgrad Med J 1997;73:27.
89. Handal KA et al. Naloxone. Ann Emerg Med 1983;12:438.
90. Hoffman RS, Goldfrank LR. The poisoned patients with altered consciousness. JAMA 1995;274:562.
91. Yealy DM et al. The safety of prehospital naloxone administration by paramedics. Ann Emerg Med 1990;19:902.
92. Gaddis GM, Watson WA. Naloxone-associated patient violence: an overlooked toxicity? Ann Pharmacother 1992;26:196.
93. Leikin JB et al. Clinical features and management of intoxication due to hallucinogenic drugs. Med Toxicol Adverse Drug Exp 1989;4:324.
94. Shannon M, Lovejoy FS. Pulmonary consequences of severe tricyclic antidepressant ingestion. Clin Toxicol 1987;25:443.
95. Heffner JE, Sahn SA. Salicylate-induced pulmonary edema. Ann Intern Med 1981;95:405.
96. Glauser FL et al. Ethchlorvynol (Placidyl)-induced pulmonary edema. Ann Intern Med 1976;84:46.
97. Ettinger NA, Albin RJ. A review of the respiratory effects of smoking cocaine. Am J Med 1989;87:664.
98. Parrish J, Arndt KA. Skin lesions in barbiturate poisoning. Lancet 1970;2:764.
99. Sohn D, Byers J. Cost effective drug screening in the laboratory. Clin Toxicol 1981;18:459.
100. Garriott JC. Interpretive toxicology. Clin Lab Med 1983;3:367.
101. Watson WA. Identifying the acetaminophen overdose (editorial). Ann Emerg Med 1989;18:1126.
102. Robinson MC et al. Analysis of cost benefit of toxicology laboratory determinations. Vet Hum Toxicol 1981;23(Suppl 1):26.
103. Starmer GA. Effects of low to moderate doses of ethanol on human driving-related performance. In: Crow KE, Batt RD, eds. Human Metabolism

of Alcohol, vol 1. Boca Raton, FL: CRC Press, 1989:101.

104. Cassidy S, Henry J. Fatal toxicity of antidepressant drugs in overdose. Br Med J 1987;295:1021.

105. Revicki DA et al. Acute medical costs of fluoxetine versus tricyclic antidepressants: a prospective multicentre study of antidepressant overdoses. Pharmacoeconomics 1997;11:48.

106. Watson WA et al. Recovery of cyclic antidepressants with gastric lavage. J Emerg Med 1989;7:373.

107. Harchelroad F et al. Gastrointestinal transit times of a charcoal/sorbitol slurry in overdose patients. Clin Toxicol 1989;27:91.

108. Watson WA et al. Gastrointestinal obstruction associated with multiple-dose activated charcoal. J Emerg Med 1986;4:401.

109. Wilens TE et al. Adverse cardiac effects of combined neuroleptic ingestion and tricyclic antidepressant overdose. J Clin Psychopharmacol 1990;10:51.

110. Wrenn K et al. Profound alkalemia during treatment of tricyclic antidepressant overdose. Am J Emerg Med 1992;10:553.

111. Olson KR et al. Seizures associated with poisoning and drug overdose. Am J Emerg Med 1993;11:565.

112. Callaham M, Kassel D. Epidemiology of fatal tricyclic antidepressant ingestion: implications of management. Ann Emerg Med 1985;14:1.

113. Lester D, Beck AT. Attempted suicide and pregnancy. Am J Obstet Gynecol 1988;158:1084.

114. Haiback H et al. Acetaminophen overdose with fetal demise. Am J Clin Pathol 1984;82:240.

115. Riggs BS et al. Acute acetaminophen overdose during pregnancy. Obstet Gynecol 1989;74:247.

116. Rollins DE et al. Acetaminophen: potentially toxic metabolite formed by human fetal and adult liver microsomes and isolated fetal liver cells. Science 1979;205:1414.

117. Czeizel A, Lendvay A. Attempted suicide and pregnancy. Am J Obstet Gynecol 1989;161:497. Letter.

118. POISINDEX® Editorial Staff: Acetaminophen (Management/Treatment Protocol). In: Klasco RK, ed. POISINDEX® System. Thomson MICROMEDEX, Greenwood Village, Colorado (edition expires 12/2003).

119. Lewis RK, Paloucek FP. Assessment and treatment of acetaminophen overdose. Clin Pharm 1991;10:765.

120. Watson WA, McKinney PE. Activated charcoal and acetylcysteine absorption: issues in interpret-

ing pharmacokinetic data. Ann Pharmacother 1991;25:1081.

121. Kozer E, Koren G. Management of paracetamol overdose. Current controversies (review). Drug Saf 2001;24:503.

122. Schmidt LE, Dalhoff K. Risk factors in the development of adverse reactions to N-acetylcysteine in patients with paracetamol poisoning. Br J Clin Pharmacol 2000;1:87.

123. Flanagan RJ. The role of acetylcysteine in clinical toxicology. Med Toxicol 1987;2:93.

124. Kumar S, Rex DK. Failure of physicians to recognize acetaminophen hepatotoxicity in chronic alcoholics. Arch Intern Med 1991;151:1189.

125. Anker AL, Smilkstein MJ. Acetaminophen: concepts and controversies. Emerg Med Clin North Am 1994;12:335.

126. Reed MD, Marx CM. Ondansetron for treating nausea and vomiting in the poisoned patient. Ann Pharmacother 1994;28:331.

127. Harrison PM et al. Serial prothrombin time as prognostic indicator in paracetamol induced fulminant hepatic failure. Br Med J 1990;301:964.

CHAPTER 6

Delivering Culturally Competent Care

Lenore T. Coleman

REASONS FOR HEALTH DISPARITIES

As far back as the early 20th century, a difference in diagnosis, treatment, and access to care for people of color has been noted. The reasons for health disparities are complex and difficult to understand. Some of the key indices are lack of access to health care, low socioeconomic status, discrimination, lack of available community resources, stressful lifestyle, poor nutrition, poor education, inadequate housing, low paying jobs, and lack of health insurance compounded by a lack of access to preventive health care services. In some situa-

tions, even when the access to care is equivalent, racial and ethnic minorities experience a lower quality of health services and are less likely to undergo routine medical procedures.

DEFINITION OF HEALTH DISPARITIES

The definition of health disparities related to the health care environment is defined as "racial or ethnic differences in the quality of healthcare that are not due to access related factors or clinical needs, preferences, and appropriateness of intervention."[1] Disparities can occur due to discrimination against the individual or at the patient-provider level or secondary to the operational systems within the health care organization. Discrimination within health care institutions is reflected in differences in care that result from biases, prejudices, stereotyping, and uncertainty in clinical communication and decision-making.

An example of disparities in health outcomes between minority and non-minority Americans can be demonstrated by the difference in life expectancy. In 1996, the average life expectancy of White males was 74 years compared with 66 years for African American males. These disparities become apparent when we observe the high mortality rates experienced by minority populations related to heart disease, cancer, cerebrovascular disease, and HIV/AIDS.

OVERVIEW OF RACIAL AND ETHNIC GROUPS IN THE UNITED STATES

African Americans[2]

Based on the year 2000 census data, the total population in the United States was 281.4 million. Of that total, 36.4 million reported themselves as Black or African American, representing 12.9% of the total U.S. population. Approximately 6% of the Black population were reported as foreign-born. The terms "Black" or "African American" refer to people having origins in any of the Black race groups of Africa. The rate of growth of the African American population is expected to slow over the next decade. According to the 2000 census, 54% of African Americans lived in the South, 19% lived in the Midwest, 18% lived in the Northeast, and 10% lived in the West. In cities where the population was 100,000 or more, New York and Chicago had the largest African American populations. Compared with Whites, African Americans are less likely to graduate from high school (79% versus 88.4%). African Americans have an increased prevalence of diabetes, cardiovascular disease, and HIV/AIDS.

Latino Americans[3]

In the 2000 census, 32.8 million Latinos lived in the United States, representing 12.0% of the total U.S. population. Latinos reported that their place of origin was Mexico, Puerto Rico, Cuba, Central America, or South America. The majority of Latino respondents were in the Mexican category (66%). Most Latinos (45%) live in the West, and 46.4% live in a central city within a metropolitan area. Latinos are twice as likely to die of diabetes than their White counterparts.

Native Americans/Alaska Natives[4]

In the 2000 census, there were 4.1 million Native Americans or Alaska Natives living in the United States. This represents 1.5% of the total population. The term Native American and Alaska Native refers to people having origins in any of the original peoples of North and South America (including Central America) and those who maintain tribal affiliations or community attachments. Forty-three percent of Native Americans live in the West, with more than 50% living in just 10 states (California, Oklahoma, Arizona, Texas, New Mexico, New York, Washington, North Carolina, Michigan, and Alaska). For Native Americans, the largest tribal groupings are Cherokee, Navajo, Latin American Indian, Choctaw, Sioux, and Chippewa. For

Alaska Natives the largest group is Eskimo, followed by Tlingit-Haida, Alaska Athabascan, and Aleut. Native Americans are more likely to die of diabetes, liver disease, and cirrhosis.

Asian Americans[5]

In the 2000 census, there were 11.9 million Asians representing 4.2% of the U.S. population. The term "Asian" refers to people having origins in the Far East, Southeast Asia, or Indian subcontinent (i.e., Cambodia, China, India, Japan, Korea, Malaysia, Pakistan, the Philippine Islands, Thailand, and Vietnam). The Chinese population is the largest Asian group in the United States. Forty-nine percent of the Asian population lives in the West, with more than 51% living in three states (California, New York, and Hawaii). The two cities with the largest Asian population are New York and Los Angeles. Asian Americans have high rates of stomach, liver, and cervical cancers.

INSTITUTE OF MEDICINE REPORT: UNEQUAL TREAMENT[6]

Overview

Over the years there have been many reports in the literature documenting differences in the level of care provided to minority populations in the United States. In 1999, Congress requested the Institute of Medicine (IOM) to study and assess the disparities in the kind and quality of health care received by U.S. racial and ethnic minorities and non-minorities. Specifically, Congress requested the IOM committee to:

- Assess the extent of racial and ethnic differences in health care that are not otherwise attributable to known factors such as access to care (ability to pay)
- Evaluate potential sources of racial and ethnic disparities in health care, including the role of bias, discrimination, and stereotyping at the individual (provider and patient), institutional, and health system levels
- Provide recommendations regarding interventions to eliminate health care disparities

The IOM committee performed a literature search that produced more than 600 citations regarding racial and ethnic differences in health care. The IOM reports on 100 studies that were published in peer-reviewed journals within the past 10 years.

There were several disease states and health categories that were covered in the report (Table 6-1).

Table 6-1 Disease States and Health Categories Addressed in the IOM Report on Unequal Treatment[6]

Cardiovascular
Cancer
Cerebrovascular disease
Renal transplantation
HIV/AIDS
Asthma
Diabetes
Pain management
Rehabilitative services
Maternal and child health
Children's health services
Mental health services

Findings of the IOM Report

The findings of the literature review support the hypothesis that patients' race and ethnicity significantly predict the quality and intensity of care they receive. The findings from the report are as follows:

- Racial and ethnic disparities in health care exist and, because they are associated with worse outcomes in many cases, are unacceptable
- Racial and ethnic disparities in health care occur in the context of broader historic and contemporary social and economic inequality, and there is evidence of persistent racial and ethnic discrimination in many sectors of American life
- Many sources—including health systems, health care providers, patients, and utilization managers—may contribute to racial and ethnic disparities in health care
- Bias, stereotyping, prejudice, and clinical uncertainty on the part of health care providers may contribute to racial and ethnic disparities in health care. Although indirect evidence from several lines of research supports this statement, a greater understanding of prevalence and influence of these processes is needed and should be sought through research
- A small number of studies suggest that racial and ethnic minority patients are more likely than White patients to refuse treatment. These studies find that differences in refusal rates are generally small and that minority patient refusal does not fully explain health care disparities

Strategies and Recommendations

Based on these findings, the IOM committee provided strategies and recommendations to help eliminate health disparities. The recommendations include the following:

- Increase awareness of racial and ethnic disparities in health care among the general public and key stakeholders within the health care system
- Increase health care providers' awareness of disparities through education.
- Avoid fragmentation of health care plans along socioeconomic lines
- Strengthen the stability of patient–provider relationships in publicly funded health care plans
- Increase the proportion of underrepresented U.S. racial and ethnic minorities among health professionals; this could be achieved through increased recruitment and retention of students from diverse communities
- Apply the same managed care protections to publicly funded HMO enrollees that apply to private HMO enrollees
- Provide greater resources to the U.S. DHHS Office for Civil Rights to strengthen and enforce civil rights laws
- Promote the consistency and equity of care through the use of evidence-based guidelines available on chronic disease management
- Structure payment systems designed to ensure an adequate supply of services to minority patients and limit provider incentives that may promote disparities

- Enhance patient-provider communication and trust by providing financial incentives for practices that reduce barriers and encourage evidence-based practice
- Support the use of interpretation services where community needs exist.
- Support the use of community health workers; implement multidisciplinary treatment and preventive care teams within health care systems
- Implement patient education programs to increase patients' knowledge of how to best access care and actively participate in treatment decisions
- Integrate cross-cultural education into the training of all current and future health care professionals
- Collect and report data on health care access and utilization by patients' race, ethnicity, socioeconomic status, and where possible, primary language
- Include measures of racial and ethnic disparities in performance measurement
- Monitor progress toward the elimination of health care disparities
- Report racial and ethnic data by Office of Management and Budget (OMB) categories, but use subpopulation groups when possible
- Conduct further research to identify sources of racial and ethnic disparities and assess promising intervention
- Conduct research on ethical issues and other barriers to eliminating disparities

In addition to the recommendations from the IOM report, Table 6-2 lists clinical and system-wide interventions that can be implemented to further reduce health disparities.

HEALTHY PEOPLE 2010[7]

Healthy People 2010 was developed from the ideas and expertise of 350 national organizations and 250 public health, mental health, substance abuse, and environmental agencies. The final report was developed by experts from key public agencies throughout the country. Healthy People 2010 had two major goals:

- Increase quality and years of healthy life of people living in the United States
- Eliminate health disparities among people of color

A complete listing of the Healthy People 2010 goals are found in Table 6-3. A partial listing of the Health People 2010 focus areas are described below.[7]

Access to Quality Health Services
Issues of Disparity
Minority populations have a wide array of barriers that affect their access to health care. These include:

- Financial barriers: no health insurance or limited health insurance coverage; Mexican Americans have the highest uninsured rates in the U.S. at 40%
- Personal barriers: cultural and language differences, disabilities due to environmental factors, lack of formal education, multiple co-morbid conditions, and spiritual beliefs that are not aligned with traditional medicine

Table 6-2 Clinical and System-Wide Interventions to Eliminate Health Disparities

Patient–Provider Interactions	System-Wide	Clinical
Minority patients feel: • Physicians do not listen to them • Physicians do not understand what they say due to language and cultural barriers 40% of Asian Americans did not have confidence in their doctors One in four patients did not follow the doctor's advice because they: • Disagreed • Could not afford the cost • Thought the advice was too complex • Felt it went against their personal beliefs	• On-site interpreters in health care systems where 15% of the population has limited English proficiency • Provide social services support to address issue of access and medical cost issues	Cross-cultural training of health care professionals on cultural, environmental, and social constructs that affect both diagnosis and treatment; professional training curriculum should be developed to include: • Racial and ethnic disparities in health • Importance of sociocultural factors on health beliefs and behaviors • Impact of race, ethnicity, culture, and class on clinical decision-making Professional workshop to: • Develop tools to assess the health beliefs and behaviors of populations being served • Develop human resource skills for cross-cultural assessment, communication, and negotiation
Minority populations feel: • They leave the medical encounter with unanswered questions on both diagnosis and treatment	• Design health education materials, signage, informed consent, and advance directives at the appropriate level of health literacy and language proficiency for the population being served	Health care professionals need to incorporate written and audiovisual aides in the education of patients related to chronic disease state management Visual aides that encourage patients to ask questions and clarify diagnostic and treatment recommendations need to be posted in waiting rooms and examination rooms
25% of African Americans and Latinos feel their doctors do not treat them with dignity and respect; cited reasons for the disrespect included their ability to pay, ability to speak English, or race/ethnicity	Large health care purchasers should require racial and ethnic data collection and interpreter services as part of the contract language JCAHO and the National Committee for Quality Assurance (NCQA) should incorporate standards for measuring systemic cultural competence Medicare and Medicaid should collect data on race, ethnicity, and language preference for all beneficiaries	Patient satisfaction surveys should be developed to include process and outcome measurements of culturally and linguistically appropriate care
Minorities receive less counseling on preventive measures like: • Smoking cessation • Healthy diet • Weight control • Mental health issues (i.e., depression, stress management) • Colon, prostate, breast cancer screening	Develop specific targeted programs on health promotion and disease prevention	Develop programs to help patients navigate the health care system, especially those related to preventive health services

Arthritis

Issues of Disparity

Arthritis affects more than 15% of the U.S. population (43 million people). It is one of the most common chronic conditions in the United States. Arthritis is the leading cause of activity limitation. African Americans and Whites have similar rates of arthritis but African Americans have more limitation of activity.[8] For Latinos and Native Americans/Alaska Natives, arthritis is the second most common chronic condition. In Asian Americans arthritis is the fourth most common chronic condition. The rate of arthritis and its disabilities is higher among persons with low education and low income.[8,9] African Americans have lower rates of total joint replacement.[10,11]

Cancer

Issues of Disparity in African Americans

African American men have a 20% higher incidence rate and a 40% higher death rate from all cancers combined than White men.[12] Cancer among African Americans is more frequently diagnosed after the cancer has metastasized and spread to regional or distant sites. African Americans tend to be diagnosed with more advanced stages of disease and have a lower survival rate. Reasons for the lower survival include unequal access to medical care, a higher prevalence of coexisting conditions, and differences in tumor biology. Approximately 132,700 new cancer cases are expected to be diagnosed among African Americans in 2003.[12] Prostate cancer is the most com-

Table 6-3   Healthy People 2010 Goals[7]

GOAL #1: Improve access to comprehensive, high quality health care services.

GOAL #2: Prevent illness and disability related to arthritis and other rheumatic conditions, osteoporosis, and chronic back conditions.

GOAL #3: Reduce the number of new cancer cases as well as the illness, disability and death caused by cancer.

GOAL #4: Reduce new cases of chronic kidney disease and its complications, disability, death, and economic costs.

GOAL #5: Through prevention programs, reduce the disease and economic burden of diabetes, and improve the quality of life for all persons who have or are at risk for diabetes.

GOAL #6: Promote the health of people with disabilities, prevent secondary conditions, and eliminate disparities between people with and without disabilities in the U.S. population.

GOAL #7: Increase the quality, availability, and effectiveness of educational and community-based programs designed to prevent disease and improve health and quality of life.

GOAL #8: Promote health for all through a healthy environment.

GOAL #9: Improve pregnancy planning and spacing and prevent unintended pregnancy.

GOAL #10: Reduce foodborne illnesses.

GOAL #11: Use communication strategically to improve health.

GOAL #12: Improve cardiovascular health and quality of life through the prevention, detection, and treatment of risk factors; early identification and treatment of heart attacks and strokes; and prevention of recurrent cardiovascular events.

GOAL #13: Prevent HIV infection and its related illness and death.

GOAL #14: Prevent disease, disability, and death from infectious diseases, including vaccine-preventable diseases.

GOAL #15: Reduce injuries, disabilities, and deaths due to unintentional injuries and violence.

GOAL #16: Improve the health and well-being of women, infant, children, and families.

GOAL #17: Ensure the safe and effective use of medical products.

GOAL #18: Improve mental health and ensure access to appropriate, quality mental health services.

GOAL #19: Promote health and reduce chronic disease associated with diet and weight.

GOAL #20: Promote the health and safety of people at work through prevention and early intervention.

GOAL #21: Prevent and control oral and craniofacial diseases, conditions, and injuries and improve access to related services.

GOAL #22: Improve health, fitness, and quality of life through daily physical activity.

GOAL #23: Ensure that Federal, Tribal, and State and local health agencies have the infrastructure to provide essential public health services effectively.

GOAL #24: Promote respiratory health through better prevention, detection, treatment, and education efforts.

GOAL #25: Promote responsible sexual behaviors, strengthen community capacity, and increase access to quality services to prevent sexually transmitted diseases (STD) and their complications.

GOAL #26: Reduce substance abuse to protect the health, safety, and quality of life for all, especially children.

GOAL #27: Reduce illness, disability, and death related to tobacco use and exposure to secondhand smoke.

GOAL #28: Improve the visual and hearing health of the Nation through prevention, early detection, treatment and rehabilitation.

mon cancer among African American men (39%), and breast cancer (31%) is the most common cancer among African American women. Approximately 63,100 African Americans are expected to die of cancer in 2003. It is estimated that 19,100 cases of lung cancer will occur in African Americans in 2003. Lung cancer is the second most common cancer in both African American men and women. The increased susceptibility may be due to more complete smoking of the cigarette, poor nutritional status, or genetic differences.[12]

When reviewing the various health disparities related to cancer, the following has been reported in the literature.[12]

- Cancer mortality rates among African American women are approximately 28% higher than in White women
- African Americans have the highest death rate from colon and rectal cancer of any racial or ethnic group in the United States

Issues of Disparities in Latinos
Although Latinos experience lower incidence and death rates for all cancers combined, they still have a higher rate of cer-

vical, esophageal, gallbladder, and stomach cancers compared with Whites. Cancer is the second leading single cause of death in the Latino population. In 2001, 54,100 new cases of cancer were diagnosed, with 21,000 persons dying of the disease. Latino women do not access the preventive health services available to screen and detect early signs of disease. They tend not to get pap tests, mammograms, and clinical breast examinations.[13–17]

When reviewing the various health disparities related to cancer, the following has been reported in the literature.[18]

- Lung cancer deaths are three times higher for Latino men compared with Whites
- The incidence of cervical cancer is three times higher in Mexican American and Puerto Rican women than in White women
- Latina women have the highest invasive cervical cancer incidence rates of any group other than Vietnamese women
- The rate of stomach cancer in Latino men is 30% to 90% higher than Whites living in the same geographic area

- Latina women have a two-fold higher incidence rate for cancer, with higher mortality rates

Issues of Disparity in Asians

Cancer is the leading cause of death for Asian Americans/Pacific Islanders. Breast cancer is the most common malignancy among Asian/Pacific Islanders. More breast cancer is being seen in Japanese women and is fast approaching that of White women.[19] When reviewing the various disparities in cancer rates:

- Cervical cancer is a significant health problem for Korean women and is five times more common among Vietnamese women compared with White women[20, 21]
- Vietnamese men have the highest rates of liver cancer for all racial/ethnic groups[21]
- Korean men experience the highest rate of stomach cancer of all racial/ethnic groups and a five-fold increased rate of stomach cancer compared with White men[21]
- Lung cancer rates among Southeast Asians are 18% higher than among Whites[22]
- Seventy-nine percent of Asian American women with breast cancer have tumors larger than 1 cm at diagnosis[23]
- Japanese women are more likely to undergo a mastectomy than White women[24]

Chronic Kidney Disease

Issues of Disparity

Kidney disease impacts certain racial and ethnic groups differently. African Americans have the highest overall risk of chronic kidney disease along with the one of the highest rates of treated end-stage renal disease in the world.[25] In 1999, the incidence of African Americans starting dialysis remained 311% higher than that for Whites.[26] This increased risk is not entirely explained by the higher number of African Americans with high blood pressure and diabetes.[27, 28] African Americans develop end-stage kidney failure at a younger age than Whites (55.8 years versus 62.2 years).[25]

Native Americans/Alaska Natives have a much higher risk of chronic kidney disease due to diabetes. The rate of new cases is 4 times higher in African Americans and Native Americans/Alaska Natives and 1.5 times higher in Asians than Whites.[7]

New data are emerging demonstrating an increased risk of chronic kidney failure in persons of Mexican ancestry.[29] Mexican Americans with diabetes are 4.5 to 6.6 times more likely to suffer end stage renal disease.[30]

Diabetes

Issues of Disparity

Approximately 13 million people in the United States have diabetes, with another 5.2 million undiagnosed.[30] The average life expectancy for people with diabetes is up to 15 years *less* than for people without diabetes. People of color are disproportionately affected by diabetes and its complications. When compared with Whites, the death rate from diabetes is 2 times greater in African Americans. There are 2.7 million African Americans in the United States with diabetes; 730,000 do not know they have the disease.[31] Diabetes affects African American men at a rate that is nearly 50% greater

than that for Whites, and for African American women the rate is 100% greater. Diabetes affects Latinos 1.9 times more often than non-Hispanic Whites, and Native Americans are 2.8 times more likely to have the disease than non-Hispanic Whites.[32]

Disability and Secondary Conditions

Issues of Disparity

People with disabilities tend to be overweight, less physically active, more stressed, and are less likely to undergo preventive screening tests (i.e., mammograms).[33]

Community Based Programs

Issues of Disparity

Communities with large numbers of racial and ethnic minorities tend to have fewer community based support programs. Effective prevention programs must be specific to the needs of the community and provide culturally and linguistically appropriate services. They should help families make better health choices and navigate the complex health care system.

Environmental Health

Issues of Disparity

Throughout the United States, there are more minority populations living in areas with poor air quality. Toxic air pollutants are suspected to cause cancer and birth defects. Lead poisoning is still present in minority populations living in substandard housing. Indoor allergens from dust mites, cockroaches, mold, and rodents can worsen symptoms of respiratory conditions such as asthma. Low-income populations have 3 to 5 times higher hospitalization and death rates from asthma. African American children are 4 to 6 times more likely to die of asthma than are White children.

Family Planning

Issues of Disparity

Women who are younger than 20 years of age, poor, or African American are more likely to become pregnant unintentionally.[34] Unintended pregnancies during contraceptive use are most common among African American and Latina females.[7]

Food Safety

Issues of Disparity

More than 30 million people in the United States are likely to be susceptible to foodborne disease.[35] The very young, elderly, and immunocompromised persons experience the most serious foodborne illnesses. At this time, there are very little data that address susceptibility of specific racial and ethnic groups.

Health Communication

Issues of Disparity

Many people in low-education and low-income groups receive no information or misinformation about health. Health literacy is key to the successful access of the health care system. A lack of cultural competency among health providers who do not appreciate differences in the ability to read and understand materials contributes to the problem. People with low health literacy are more likely to report poor health and have an incomplete understanding of their health problems and treatment. These patients are also at increased risk of hospitalization.[36] People with chronic conditions, such as diabetes, hypertension, and asthma, who also have low reading skills have been found to have less knowledge of their conditions than people with higher reading skills.[37]

Heart Disease and Stroke

Issues of Disparity

The strongest and most consistent evidence for the existence of racial and ethnic health disparities is found in studies of cardiovascular disease (CVD).

CVD is the no. 1 killer of African Americans, claiming more than 286,000 lives each year. An estimated 4 in every 10 African American adults have CVD. This includes diseases of the heart, stroke, high blood pressure, congestive heart failure, coronary heart disease (CHD), and congenital defects. Forty-one percent of African American men and 40% of African American women age ≥20 years old have CVD. In 2000, 48,708 African American males and 57,063 African American females died of CVD. In 2000, the relative risk for stroke was 4 times higher in African Americans between the ages of 35 and 54 when compared with Whites.[38] The rate of hypertension in African Americans is among the highest in the world. Racial and ethnic minorities tend to develop hypertension at a younger age and are less likely to undergo treatment or achieve target blood pressure goals. In the African American community, the characteristics that lead to hypertension include being middle aged, less educated, overweight, physically inactive, and having diabetes.

Latinos have a disproportionate burden of death and disability from CVD as well. Among Mexican Americans, about 29% of men and 27% of women have CVD. High blood pressure is seen more frequently in Mexican American women than men.

When reviewing the various health disparities related to CVD, the following have been reported in the literature. African Americans are:

- One-half to one-third less likely to receive cardiovascular procedures[39–41]; minorities are less likely to receive appropriate cardiac medications like thrombolytic therapy, aspirin, or β-blockers
- White patients were 50% more likely to receive thrombolytics than African American patients[42]
- African American men and women are up to 4 times less likely to undergo coronary artery bypass grafts (CABG) or angiography than Whites[43–45]

HIV

Issues of Disparity

In the year 2000, 55% of the reported AIDS cases occurred among African Americans and Latinos, although these populations only represent 13% and 12% of the U.S. population, respectively.[46] In 1997, AIDS remained the leading cause of death for all African Americans aged 25 to 44 years. It was the second leading cause of death among African American females and the leading cause among African American males.[47] In 2000, African American and Latina women accounted for 80% of reported cases in women. African Americans and Latinos with HIV/AIDS are more likely to have unmet social service needs. African Americans are less likely to receive appropriate HIV treatment and are more likely to experience delays in receiving appropriate treatment. The CDC estimates that 1 in 50 Black men and 1 in 160 Black women are infected with HIV. In other words, Blacks are 10 times more likely to be diagnosed with HIV and 10 times more likely to die of AIDS than Whites.[48] Socioeconomic problems that contribute to the increased prevalence of HIV/AIDS in the African American community include poverty, denial of the disease process, delays in treatment of HIV infection, substance abuse, and complicated social roles between genders.

Immunization and Infectious Disease

Issues of Disparity

African Americans and Latinos receive fewer vaccinations against pneumococcal infections and influenza. Increasing minority community participation, education, and partnership will help to improve these figures.

BARRIERS TO CULTURALLY COMPETENT CARE

Many ethnic minorities have limited access to health care as a result of their lower socioeconomic status. Compared with Whites, Latinos and African Americans are less likely to have graduated from high school (88%, 79%, and 57%, respectively) and are more likely to be living in poverty (8%, 21%, and 23%, respectively). They have lower median household incomes ($45,900, $33,400, and $30,439, respectively), are less likely to own a home, and are more likely to live in rental property that is substandard. Finally, compared with Whites, a greater proportion of Latinos and African Americans had no health insurance coverage (10%, 19%, and 32%) in the year 2000.[49] Many minority patients live in urban rather than rural areas. Studies have shown that for those people living in urban poverty zones, 67% are African Americans, 20% are Latino, and 12% are White.[50] All these circumstances—poverty, lack of insurance, low education, limited access to health care, lack of awareness of chronic disease risk factors and screening methods, lack of physician referrals, acculturation levels, language barriers, culture, and negative provider attitudes—play a part in the health disparities that occur in the health care system.

Minority populations tend to receive their care in urgent care and emergency departments and are also less likely to have a primary care provider. Latino children, working-age African American adults, and the African American and Latino elderly are at greater risk of being hospitalized for a preventable condition than Whites. This was after adjusting for socioeconomic status, insurance coverage, and availability of primary care.[51]

Language/Literacy Issues

Reading literacy is a major problem in the United States. Based on the 1992 National Adult Literacy Survey, 44 million adults scored in level 1. Someone with a level 1 score can read a little but not well enough to fill out a job application, read a food label, or read a simple children's book.[52] Accurate and linguistically appropriate oral and written communication between providers and patients is critical to the successful management of chronic diseases. Through the oral interview, the provider is able to assess the patient's medical and social history, health beliefs about illness, and medication adherence issues. Importantly, the interview can be critical to establishing a rapport and trusting relationship with the patient. Incomplete communication can lead to misunderstandings of the patient's concerns and to misdiagnosis. Miscommunication can result in poor adherence with the treatment regimen, inappropriate follow-up, missed appointments, and poor patient satisfaction.

Stereotypes and Health Care Disparities

Stereotyping can be defined as the process by which people use social categories (e.g., race, sex) in acquiring, processing, and recalling information about others. The beliefs (stereotypes) and general orientations (attitudes) that people bring to their interactions are important. Attitudes toward members of social groups based on race and ethnicity can shape interpersonal interactions with those groups. Stereotypes can shape interpretations, influence how information is recalled, and guide expectations. Negative stereotypes, held consciously or unconsciously by health care providers, can contribute to health care disparities. In one study, physicians believed African Americans were less likely to adhere to treatment and more likely to engage in destructive health behaviors (e.g., drug abuse). [53] In some cases, physicians may have the misconception that minority patients wish to avoid aggressive or new health care technologies. This may cause them to avoid these treatment strategies as a way to respect the patient's wishes.

MANAGEMENT ISSUES IN TREATING SELECTED CHRONIC DISEASES IN MINORITY POPULATIONS
Cancer—Asians
Evidence

1. R.W. is a 38-year-old Chinese woman who underwent a mammogram at a local health fair. Based on the results of the mammogram, R.W. was referred to her primary care provider. Review of the mammogram revealed a 2.4 cm mass in the upper, outer quadrant of her right breast. Biopsy of the mass revealed a moderately differentiated ductal carcinoma. Physical examination revealed some breast tenderness on palpation. All laboratory tests, including complete blood count (CBC) and liver function, were within normal limits, and the findings of a chest radiograph were negative. Her family history was significant in that her mother died at age 42 of breast cancer, and her 44-year-old sister had a breast tumor removed about 5 years ago. R.W. is married and has three children. Is there evidence of health disparities in the treatment of Chinese women with breast cancer?

Asian women are twice as likely to undergo mastectomy than White women.[54,55] Chinese women are more likely not to receive hormonal or radiation therapy after breast-conserving surgery.

Health Beliefs

2. What are the health beliefs of the Asian populations?

Asian cultures generally view illnesses as inevitable and unchangeable. Thus, they may avoid treatment and fail to seek medical care. Other cultural determinants include modesty, embarrassment, inconvenience of treatment on the family unit, and language barriers, all of which can lead to lack of understand regarding treatment options.[56]

Alternative Medicine

3. Describe the use of complementary (alternative) medicine in the treatment of breast cancer.

Approximately one in two Americans currently use alternative therapies and make 629 million visits to alternative medicine practitioners each year.[57] There are many traditional Chinese medicines (TCM), mostly botanical agents that have been used to prevent breast cancer. In one study, 22% of Chinese women used herbal remedies to treat their breast cancer.[58] A study in 460 women with benign breast lumps and increased breast density looked at the effect of Xiao He Ling on breast density. Complete disappearance of the lumps occurred in 24% of women and significant improvement was noted in 48%.[59] Some women used both Western medicines and TCM. In a study of 134 patients with early stage breast cancer, a combination of standard surgery, radiation, and chemotherapy with individualized Chinese herbal formula showed a 5-year survival rate of 82% compared with 67% with Chinese herbs alone.[60]

Diabetes—Latinos
Prevalence

4. S.S., a 42-year-old Mexican woman who recently moved from Mexico to the Los Angeles area, seeks medical care for symptoms she believes to be related to diabetes. A brother, mother, and grandmother have diabetes. Over the past 4 weeks S.S. has had symptoms of polyuria, polydipsia, and polyphagia and has lost 15 pounds. Her blood pressure was 120/74 mm Hg; she weighs 250 pounds; she is 5'3" tall; and her BMI is 44 kg/m². Laboratory values on the day of the clinic visit were fasting plasma glucose, 502 mg/dL (normal, <110 mg/dL) and A_{1C}, 13.4% (normal, 4% to 6%). S.S. was referred to a diabetes education class and given glyburide 20 mg/day. A return appointment was scheduled in 2 weeks.

S.S. has met the diagnostic criteria for type 2 diabetes (See Chapter 50, Diabetes Mellitus). Latinos and African Americans have an increased prevalence of diabetes. In the United States, 14% of Latinos and 12% of African Americans are affected by diabetes compared with 7% of Whites.[61]

Risk Factors

5. Do Latinos have risk factors that predispose them to diabetes?

A number of studies have found that Latinos are 2.5 times more likely than Whites to have risk factors for type 2 diabetes.[62] As illustrated by S.S., these include a positive family history of diabetes, obesity, and high blood pressure. Other risk factors include high cholesterol, stress associated with injury or illness, and a history of diabetes during pregnancy or delivery. Latinos with diabetes tend to have higher hemoglobin A_{1c} levels, fewer physician visits, greater insulin resistance, and problems with obesity. They also are less likely to self-monitor their blood glucose.[62]

Cultural Barriers

6. **What cultural barriers need to be addressed when educating S.S. about her diabetes?**

S.S. has been referred to a diabetes education class. Many minorities have a fatalistic view of diabetes and feel that its complications are inevitable.[63] One of the primary goals of culturally appropriate diabetes education programs is to provide patients with the knowledge that they have the power to delay and prevent many of the long-term complications. When designing an education program for minority populations, it is important that the program address the needs and preferences of the target community. All materials should be linguistically appropriate and at the correct reading level. For self-management education to be effective it must occur frequently and be combined with telephone follow-up and mail remainders for appointments. Minority populations tend to understand the complex concepts of diabetes self-management if educational materials provide visual images. It may be necessary to read questionnaires aloud and provide pictures and videotapes of pertinent information. Gagliardino and Etchegoyen demonstrated the effectiveness of a culturally specific diabetes education program implemented in 10 Latin American countries over a 12-month period for 446 adults with type 2 diabetes. The patients were able to achieve a decrease in weight, blood pressure, fasting blood sugar, and hemoglobin A_{1c}. There was a significant decrease in the percentage of patients taking oral antidiabetic, cholesterol, and antihypertensive agents. Drug costs were lowered by 34%.[64]

Social Networks

When educating Latino populations, the family unit should be incorporated as much as possible. Latino populations prefer intervention settings that are away from hospitals or clinics environments.[65] Many programs have found that soliciting social support from community and local church groups is beneficial. Because Mexican Americans and African Americans attend church on a regular basis,[65] programs delivered at these sites have been effective in both groups. Religious organizations offer the following advantages[66,67]:

1. Well-established social networks
2. Religious education programs and infrastructure
3. Facilities located in virtually every neighborhood in the United States
4. Clerical and other church leadership who are receptive to health programming
5. A history of volunteerism
6. Large membership rosters
7. Involvement of entire families

The risk for cardiac mortality in Latinos is 3 times higher than in the White population because of inadequate social support.[68] Thus, the use of volunteer community health workers who can provide ongoing educational support, interpretative services, and a linkage to the community at large is very beneficial in programs designed for Latinos.

Language/Literacy

S.S has recently moved from Mexico to Los Angeles and speaks very little English. For many Latinos, English is their second language. Several studies have evaluated the effect of language on health care outcomes. In a study in 74 Latino patients, those treated by a Spanish-speaking clinician reported greater satisfaction with the physician–patient encounter, better physical functioning, and better psychological well-being than those treated with a non-Spanish–speaking physician (60% versus 40%).[69]

When clinicians do not speak the patient's native language, it is important to use professional interpreters. Ad hoc interpretation by nonclinical employees, family, and friends is used much too often within health care systems. These nonprofessional interpreters lack the understanding of medical terminology and often misinterpret the questions being asked.[70] When using family members as interpreters, issues of patient privacy need to be considered, especially for chronic diseases that involve discussions surrounding sexual orientation or high risk behaviors.

Hypertension—Blacks

Increased Risk

7. **A.W. is a 47-year-old African American man referred to the community health clinic for evaluation of his blood pressure. A.W. has no complaints other than occasional headaches, which he attributes to his sinus condition. Over the past 5 years A.W. has put on 50 pounds due to a knee injury at his job. Past medical history is significant for osteoarthritis in his elbow for which he takes a nonsteroidal anti-inflammatory agent. A.W.'s father died of a myocardial infarction (MI) at age 60. His mother has diabetes and renal insufficiency.**

Physical examination reveals that he is overweight but in no acute distress. He is 6'2" and weighs 127 kg; his BMI is 36 kg/m² (normal, <25 kg/m²). Blood pressure readings are 170/102 mm Hg (left arm) and 168/100 mm Hg (right arm) while sitting. His pulse is 84 beats/min and regular.

A.W. smokes 0.5 pack of cigarettes daily and drinks no alcoholic beverages. Laboratory tests reveal BUN, 30 mg/dL; serum creatinine (Scr), 1.5 mg/dL; total cholesterol, 220 mg/dL; LDL cholesterol, 162 mg/dL; and HDL cholesterol, 40 mg/dL. An electrocardiogram (ECG) and echocardiogram reveal increased left ventricular wall thickness of 13 mm (normal, 6 to 11 mm) consistent with mild left ventricular hypertrophy. What are the data to support the increased risk for hypertension in African Americans?

According to the statistics of the American Heart Association, 36.7% of African American men and 36.6% of African American women have high blood pressure. Compared with Whites, African Americans develop high blood pressure earlier in life and their average blood pressures are much higher. Due to the higher pressures, African Americans have a 1.8 times greater rate of fatal stroke and a 4.2 times greater rate of end-stage kidney disease than the White population. In 2000, 4,670 African American males and 5,912 African American females died as a result of high blood pressure.[71] Even though the incidence of high blood pressure is increased in African Americans, 27% are unaware of their hypertension and 32% are receiving inadequate treatment.[72]

Hypertension in African Americans contributes to the development of left ventricular hypertrophy (LVH) and congestive heart failure (CHF). Both conditions contribute to the increased death rates in African Americans. In one study, 37% of total cardiac deaths were independently attributable to LVH. LVH in African Americans is a greater predictor of sudden death than three-vessel CVD or left ventricular dysfunction.[73]

Nephropathy

8. Is there a disparity in the incidence of nephropathy in African Americans?

End-stage renal disease (ESRD) occurs 4 times more frequently among African Americans when compared with their White counterparts; they suffer one of the highest rates of ESRD in the world.[25] The National Health and Nutrition Survey III (NHANES III) noted a prevalence of elevated serum creatinine that was nearly 3 times higher (>2.0 mg/dL) among African Americans than Whites.[74] It appears that African Americans are at an increased risk for rapid decline of their renal function and the development of ESRD. The reason for this propensity to renal disease is not totally understood but contributing factors include hypertension, poor glycemic and lipid control, obesity, genetics, low birth weight, and decreased access to health care.

Diabetic Nephropathy

9. Is the treatment of diabetic nephropathy different for minority populations?

Patients with diabetes and hypertension require tight control and aggressive management to minimize sequelae. A few small studies have looked at the response of African Americans with diabetic nephropathy to various antihypertensive regimens. Although clinical trials generally support a favorable effect of angiotensin-converting enzyme (ACE) inhibitors on proteinuria and progression of diabetic kidney disease,[75, 76] some have suggested that ACE inhibitors are not efficacious in African Americans. For example, a Collaborative Study Group showed a positive benefit of ACE inhibition in patients with serum creatinine levels >1.5 mg/dL. Crook and colleagues examined the effect of specific classes of antihypertensives in African Americans with advanced diabetic nephropathy. They found the ACE inhibitors had no effect on renal survival in the total cohort and in those patients with serum creatinine >4.0 mg/dL. Lack of effect of ACE inhibitors in this study may have been due to poor blood pressure control[77] (See Question 12).

Risk Factors for Hypertension

10. What risk factors for hypertension and CVD are present in A.W.? How should they be managed?

SMOKING

A.W. smokes cigarettes, which increases his risk for myocardial infarction and stroke. African Americans have the second-highest rate of smoking prevalence of all ethnic groups at 27.2%. Death rates from smoking in African Americans are 20% higher than in Whites, and many African Americans are unaware that smoking is associated with a worsening of their CVD. Recommendations for increased smoking cessation programs and a reduction in targeted marketing by tobacco companies to African American communities should be implemented. A.W. should be referred to a smoking cessation program and receive ongoing follow-up.

DYSLIPIDEMIA

A.W. has total cholesterol, 220 mg/dL (normal, <200 mg/dL); LDL cholesterol, 162 mg/dL (normal, <100 mg/dL); and HDL cholesterol, 40 mg/dL (normal, 40 mg/dL). African Americans have increased morbidity and mortality from CHD. Based on the NHANES III and CDC/NCHS data, the prevalence of hyperlipidemia (total cholesterol >200 mg/dL) is higher in both White men (52%) and women (49%) than in African American men (45%) and women (46%).[81] Nonetheless, in 2000, the overall death rate from CHD was 186.9 per 100,000 in Whites, while the death rate for African American men and women was 262.4 and 187.5, respectively. Due to the increased risk for heart attack and stroke in African Americans, aggressive management of hyperlipidemia is required, with a goal of less than 100 mg/dL for LDL cholesterol.

OBESITY

A.W. has gained 50 pounds over the past 5 years and has a BMI of 36 kg/m² (normal, <25). Obesity is considered the most prevalent and potentially controllable health problem in the U.S. today. Obesity has been linked to an increase in the incidence of diabetes, hypertension, coronary artery disease, and cancer. Currently, more than 60% of all adults in the United States are estimated to be overweight.[78] Obesity is common in both African American males and females. The NHANES III survey data demonstrated that 48.5% of African American females are overweight.[79] The reasons for persistent and pervasive obesity among African Americans are unclear but could include many factors such as dietary preferences, perception of ideal body size, lower levels of physical activity, less concern about obesity, less overall health knowledge, less likelihood of receiving health education, low income, and lower geographic mobility. The African American diet is generally high in saturated fat, salt, and simple sugars. High-fat diets are associated with an increased risk for a variety of cancers, CVD, and stroke.

NUTRITIONAL GOALS

There have been few randomized controlled studies looking at the effect of different diets in African Americans. The Dietary Approaches to Stop Hypertension (DASH) Trial was a randomized multi-center control trial that compared the effect of three dietary patterns on blood pressure among adults, aged 22 or older with diastolic pressures between 80 and 95 mm Hg and systolic blood pressures less than 160 mm Hg. The DASH diet (rich in fruits, vegetables, and low-fat dairy products) was compared against a control diet (low in fruits, vegetables, and dairy products with a fat content of 36%) versus a diet similar to the control diet except rich in just fruits and vegetables. Four hundred and fifty-nine adult patients were randomized and 373 (81%) completed the 11-week trial; 60% of the participants in the trial were African Americans. The DASH diet is composed of fruits, vegetables, fiber, and low-fat dairy foods. It includes both meat and poultry but has reduced amounts of saturated and total fats. In the African American cohort, the DASH diet reduced both the systolic (13.2 mm Hg) and diastolic (6.1 mm Hg) blood pressures significantly more than the other diets, without weight reduction or sodium restriction.[80] A.W. and all African American patients that are overweight or obese need to be encouraged to adhere to a healthy diet that decreases both salt and fat intake.

Clinical Characteristics

11. Characterize hypertension in African Americans. Is it different than that observed in Whites? What are the goals of therapy?

Hypertension in African Americans has been characterized by salt sensitivity, low renin levels, and the potential for reduced response to blood pressure lowering effects by some agents. The overall goal in the management of hypertension in African Americans is to reduce the cardiovascular and renal morbidity and mortality seen with elevated blood pressure. Table 6-4 shows blood pressures goals recommended by the Hypertension in African Americans Working Group (HAAW).[81]

There is a misconception that high blood pressure in African Americans is more difficult to control. Based on data from the Antihypertensive and Lipid-Lowering Treatment to Prevent Heart Attack Trial (ALLHAT) and African American Study of Kidney Disease and Hypertension (AASK) trial, that

thinking is unjustified. In the AASK trial, two to three drugs were required to reduce the mean arterial blood pressure to lower than 92 to 107 mm Hg in African Americans with hypertension and mild-to-moderate renal insufficiency. Previously, diastolic blood pressure has been used as an outcome measure for drug efficacy. A meta-analysis of pooled data from randomized controlled trials showed that an average reduction of 12 to 13 mm Hg in systolic blood pressure over 4 years was associated with a 21% reduction in CHD, 37% reduction in stroke, a 25% reduction in total cardiovascular mortality, and a 13% reduction in all-cause mortality. Based on this data, it is recommended that clinicians treat aggressively to achieve target goals for both diastolic and systolic blood pressure.[82]

Drug Effects

12. Are there differences in antihypertensive drug effects in African Americans?

Two hypertension trials had substantial representation of African Americans among their subjects. The ALLHAT was a 6-year, double blind, randomized controlled trial that studied 42,448 patients, 36% of which were African Americans. The target blood pressure in ALLHAT was <130/85 mm Hg with a primary outcome of a reduction in fatal and nonfatal cardiac endpoints. The agents used in the study were chlorthalidone versus amlodipine or lisinopril or doxazocin. The doxazocin arm of the study was discontinued in the year 2000 because patients had an increased rate of congestive heart failure.[83]

The AASK was a 4-year double blind, randomized controlled clinical trial of 1,094 patients. Two levels of target blood pressures were assessed with a primary outcome of decreasing the rate of decline in glomerular filtration rate. The effects of amlodipine versus ramipril versus metoprolol were evaluated.[81] Table 6-5 outlines recommendations for antihypertensive drug use based on the data from these two major studies.

Some of the differences in drug effects in African Americans are:[84]

- Thiazide diuretics and long-acting calcium channel blockers (CCB) appear to have greater blood pressure lowering effects than other classes of antihypertensive agents in African American patients

Table 6-4 Consensus Recommendations of the Hypertension in African Americans Working Group (HAAW)	
Disease State	Target Blood Pressure Goals
Diabetes	DBP < 80 mm Hg
Non-diabetics with hypertensive renal disease (proteinuria <1g/day)	BP <140/90 mm Hg
Non-diabetics with hypertensive renal disease (proteinuria >1 g/day)	BP <130/80 mm Hg
Patients with a history of cardio-vascular event, stroke, transient ischemic attacks, end organ damage, microalbuminuria, CHD, or high-risk CHD	BP <130/80 mm Hg

CHD, coronary heart disease; DBP, diastolic blood pressure.

Table 6-5 Consensus Recommendations of the Hypertension in African Americans Working Group (HAAW)	
Drug Class	Drug Use in African Americans
Diuretics Thiazides	Low-dose thiazides have well-established efficacy in African Americans; chlorthalidone provides cardiovascular benefits
Potassium-sparing diuretics	Recent data provide evidence for superior efficacy of eplerenone compared with losartan in Black patients[93]
β-Blockers	Not as efficacious as monotherapy
	Drugs of choice in post-myocardial infarction patients
α-Blockers	Doxazocin shown to cause increased congestive heart failure in the ALLHAT trial
Calcium channel blockers	Proven efficacy in African Americans
	May be beneficial in African Americans with renal failure
	Amlodipine found to be less renal protective in hypertensive patients with renal insufficiency than ramipril in the AASK trial
ACE inhibitors	Renal protective in African Americans (AASK trial)
	May be less effective in lowering blood pressure; therefore, generally used in combination therapy
	Increased incidence of angioedema and cough noted in African Americans compared with Whites
Angiotensin receptor blockers	Effective in lowering blood pressure especially when used in combination with diuretics

- ACE inhibitors have additional benefits in patients with diabetes and in patients with heart failure, and both ACE inhibitors and angiotensin II receptor blockers (ARB) have comparable benefits in patients with renal compromise
- β-blockers produce less blood pressure reduction in African Americans compared with Whites. Nevertheless, β-blocker therapy following a myocardial infarction has been proven to be beneficial in lowering mortality rate; therefore, they should be used by all patients who have had an MI, including African Americans
- Many clinicians perceive that they achieve greater reductions in blood pressure among African Americans treated with thiazide diuretics, but there are limited data to support this impression. A recent clinical trial has shown that African Americans have a polymorphism (allele of the gene encoding the β3-subunit of G proteins) linked to greater blood pressure response to thiazide diuretics. The disadvantage to thiazide diuretics in African Americans is decreased medication adherence due to frequent urination and erectile dysfunction noted in some male patients
- CCBs seem to be very effective in lowering blood pressure in African Americans. However, since CCBs do not provide the best protection against the progression of renal disease or reduce heart attack rates, they should not be used as monotherapy in African American patients with renal disease or heart failure
- ACE inhibitors effectively lower blood pressure in most African Americans, but higher doses may be required. In the AASK trial, ramipril was more beneficial in protecting renal function than amlodipine. Thus, ACE inhibitors should be used in combination with low-dose diuretics and other agents as necessary along with a sodium-reduced diet
- African Americans are at increased risk for ACE inhibitor–induced angioedema and cough. If these side effects occur, switching to an ARB may be beneficial
- ARBs are effective antihypertensive agents for African Americans when used in combination with other agents

Acquired Immune Deficiency Syndrome—Blacks

Prevalence

13. B.J. is a 24-year-old African American woman who has been HIV-positive for 2 years. She is a single parent with one child. B.J. has no symptoms of immunosuppression at this time, and her overall health status is good. Laboratory values show a CD4+ lymphocyte count of 600 cells/mm³ (normal, > 500 cells/mm³). What is the prevalence of HIV/AIDS in African American women?

African American women accounted for 64% of HIV cases reported in the United States in 2001.[85] Most of the HIV infections occurred among teenagers and young adults aged 25 years and younger. Of all the HIV cases reported since the epidemic began, African Americans account for 35%. AIDS is the leading cause of death among African American women ages 25 to 34.[86]

Health Disparities

14. Are there health disparities associated with African Americans with HIV/AIDS?

The literature suggests that African American women are:

- More likely to delay seeking treatment for their HIV infection for 6 months after learning they have it[87]
- Less likely than Whites to receive the newer combination treatments for HIV[88]
- Less likely to use condoms consistently; reasons for lack of consistent condom use include[89]:
  1. Sex may be used as an exchange for financial support of a male partner
  2. Implication that they may be sexually permissive
  3. Sex-ratio imbalance (Note: Among African Americans there are fewer marriageable men than women. Given this sex-ratio imbalance, African American women are more likely to tolerate objectionable behavior in men.)

African Americans are twice as likely to have a low knowledge level about the effectiveness of AIDS preventive measures relative to Whites.[90] When surveyed, African Americans had a low level of knowledge about the:

- Effectiveness of AIDS prevention; this could have an impact on their ability to use effective precautions
- Difference between infection with HIV and AIDS; this could create a false sense of safety from infection

AIDS Education

15. What are the components of a culturally competent AIDS education program?

Culture is composed of a vast structure of language, customs, knowledge, and patterns for interpreting reality. For instance, African American cultural values include a sense of appropriateness and excellence.[91] The values are combined with a profound sense of adaptability, respect, restraint, responsibility, reciprocity, cooperativeness, mutual aid, unconditional love, and interdependence. African Americans tend to be very humane and spiritual, which creates a very caring, sensitive, and concerned individual. Thus, when structuring an HIV/AIDS educational program it is important to incorporate the extended family and to stress individual survival and well-being. It is also important to ensure that educational efforts can be provided on a long-term basis. Programs should foster trust and respect, focus on both males and females, and mobilize the community.

Adherence

16. What are the factors that affect medication adherence in minority populations with HIV/AIDS?

Factors that affect medication adherence include drug side effects, complexity of the medication regimen, total number of medications, and complicated dosing schedules.

Graney and colleagues looked at medication adherence patterns among 57 inner city patients.[92] Eighty-two percent of the patients in this study were African American. Demographic factors such as age, education, household size, race, sex, and years since diagnosis were not associated with adherence. However, the number of doses per day, number of different medications, and total number of pills were inversely associated with adherence. All these variables showed statistical significance. Side effects were considered a barrier to adherence in 67% of the population studied, and privacy issues were considered an adherence problem by 42% of patients. Simply forgetting to take the medication was the most common problem mentioned as a barrier to adherence. The two most important factors that patients felt improved their adherence were the perceptions of the health care provider as a support person and educator and using written schedules for medication use.

Community outreach activities, including community-based screenings and lectures to local consumer groups, can begin to eradicate the misinformation and misconceptions of communities of color regarding drug therapy. All health care settings should aim to reflect the diverse population that they serve. A diverse staff can assist in communicating drug and health information to patients in a linguistically appropriate manner. Culturally and linguistically appropriate educational

materials on medication use and side effects should be available. Using technology and the media to reach out to minority populations is underutilized by the health care industry. Many minority patients are using the worldwide web to obtain information on medications and medical conditions. Using television, radio, and video teleconferencing are effective ways to communicate technical information to large numbers of people.

Through culturally appropriate educational strategies and commitment by all health care professionals to change minority health status, we can begin to reverse the ravages of chronic disease plaguing communities of color in the United States.

REFERENCES

1. Smedley BD et al., eds. Unequal Treatment: Confronting Racial and Ethnic Disparities in Health Care. National Academy Press, 2002.
2. Census 2000 briefs. The black population: 2000. Issued August 2001. www.census.gov/prod/www/abs/briefs.html
3. Therrien M, Ramirez RR. The Hispanic population in the United States: March 2000. Current Population Reports, P20-535. Washington, DC: U.S. Census Bureau, 2000.
4. Census 2000 briefs. The American Indian and Alaska Native population: 2000. Issued February 2002. www.census.gov/prod/www/abs/bricfs.html
5. Census 2000 briefs. The Asian population: 2000. Issued February 2002. www.census.gov/prod/www/abs/bricfs.html
6. Institute of Medicine, Haynes MA, Smedley BD, eds. The Unequal Burden of Cancer: An Assessment of NIH Research and Programs for Ethnic Minorities and the Medically Underserved. Washington, DC: National Academy Press, 1999.
7. Healthy People 2010. Conference edition in two volumes. Washington, DC: U.S. Department of Health and Human Services, January 2000.
8. Lawrence RC et al. Estimates of the prevalence of arthritis and selected musculoskeletal disorders in the United States. Arthritis Rheum 1998; 41(5):778.
9. CDC. Prevalence and impact of arthritis by race and ethnicity: United States, 1989-1991. MMWR 1996; 45(18):373.
10. Helmick CG et al. Arthritis and other rheumatic conditions: who is affected now, who will be affected later? National Arthritis Data Workgroup Arthritis Care and Research 1995;8:203.
11. Wilson MG et al. Racial differences in the use of total knee arthroplasty for osteoarthritis among older Americans: Ethnicity and Disease. 1994;4(1):57.
12. American Cancer Society. Cancer facts and figures for African Americans 2003-2004. Atlanta, GA: American Cancer Society; 2003.
13. American Cancer Society. Cancer facts and figures for Hispanics 2000-2001. Atlanta, GA: American Cancer Society; 2001.
14. U.S. Department of Health and Human Services. DATA 2010... the Healthy People 2010 database. August 6, 2002 edition.
15. Habbell FA et al. The influence of knowledge and attitudes about breast cancer on mammography use among Latinas and Anglo women. J Gen Intern Med 1997;12:505.
16. Zambrana RE et al. Use of cancer screening practices by Hispanic women: analysis by sub-group. Prev Med 1999;29:466.
17. Skaer TL et al. Breast cancer mortality declining by screening among subpopulations tags. Am J Public Health 1998;88:307.
18. Ramirez AG, Suarez L. The impact of cancer in Latino population. In: Aguirre-Molina M et al., eds. Latino Health Book. 2000 (in press).

19. Gotay CC, Wilson ME. Social support and cancer screening in African American, Hispanic and Native American women. Cancer Pract 1998;6:31.
20. Probst-Hensch NM et al. Ethnic differences in post-menopausal plasma oestrogen levels: high oestone levels in Japanese-American women despite low weight. Br J Cancer 2000;82(11):1867.
21. Lee MC. Knowledge, barriers, and motivators related to cervical cancer screening among Korean American women: a focus group approach. Cancer Nurs 2000;23(3):168.
22. Miller BA et al., eds. Racial/Ethnic Patterns of Cancer in the United States 1988-1992. Bethesda, MD: National Cancer Institute, 1996. NIH Publication No. 96-4104. Available from URL: http://wwwseer.ims.nci.nih.gov/Publications/REPoC/
23. Hedeen AN et al. Ethnicity and birthplace in relation to tumor size and stage in Asian American women with breast cancer. Am J Public Health 1999;89(8):1248.
24. Prehn AW et al. Differences in treatment patterns for localized breast carcinoma among Asian/Pacific Islander women. Cancer 2002;95:2268.
25. US Renal Data System. 2001 Annual Data Report: Atlas of End-Stage Renal Disease in the United States. Bethesda, MD: National Institutes of Health, National Institutes of Diabetes and Kidney Disease, 2001.
26. US Renal Data System. 1999 Annual Data Report: Atlas of End-Stage Renal Disease in the United States. Bethesda, MD: National Institutes of Health, National Institutes of Diabetes and Kidney Disease, 1999.
27. Whittle JC et al. Does racial variation in risk factors explain black-white differences in the incidence of hypertensive end-stage renal disease? Arch Intern Med 1991;151:1359.
28. Brancati FL et al. The excess incidence of diabetic end stage renal disease among blacks: a population based study of potential explanatory factors. JAMA 1992;268:3079.
29. Agodoa LYC et al. ESRD among Hispanics. J Am Soc Nephrol 1999;10:232A.
30. American Diabetes Association. www.diabetes.org.
31. Gavin JR. Management of diabetes: Issues for clinical success. Urban Cardiol 1999;6:13.
32. Harris MI et al. Prevalence of diabetes, impaired fasting glucose and impaired glucose intolerance in US Adults. The Third National Health and Nutrition Examination Survey 1988-1994. Diabetes Care 1998;21:518.
33. Office of Disease Prevention and Health Promotion (ODPHP). Healthy People 2000 Progress Review, People with Disabilities. Washington, DC: The Department of ODPHP, January 1997.
34. Brown SS, Eisenberg L. The Best Intentions: Unintended Pregnancy and the Well-Being of Children and Families. Washington, DC: National Academy Press,1995.

35. Council for Agricultural Science and Technology. Foodborne Pathogens: Risks and Consequences. Task Force Report No. 122. 1994.
36. Baker DW et al. The relationship of patients reading ability to self-reported health and use of health services. Am J Public Health 1997;87:1027.
37. Williams MV et al. Relationship of functional health literacy to patients' knowledge of their chronic disease: a study of patients with hypertension and diabetes. Arch Intern Med 1998;158;166.
38. MMWR 2000;49(4):
39. Gornick ME et al. Effects of race and income on mortality and use of services among Medicare beneficiaries. N Engl J Med 1996;335(11):791.
40. McBean AM, Gornick MD. Differences by race in the rates of procedures performed in hospitals for Medicare beneficiaries. Health Care Financ Rev 1994;15(4):77.
41. Escarce JJ et al. Racial differences in the elderly's use of medical procedures and diagnostic tests. Am J Public Health 1993;83(7):948.
42. Allison JJ et al. Racial differences in the medical treatment of elderly Medicare patients with acute myocardial infarction. J Gen Intern Med 1996; 11:736.
43. Ford et al. Coronary arteriography and coronary by-pass among whites and other racial groups relative to hospital-based incidence rates for coronary artery disease: findings from NHDS. Am J Public Health 1989;79(4):437.
44. Goldberg et al. Racial and community factors influencing coronary artery bypass graft surgery rates for all 1986 Medicare patients. JAMA 1992; 267:1473.
45. Carlisle et al. Underuse and overuse of diagnostic testing for coronary artery disease in patients presenting with new-onset chest pain. Am J Med 1999; 106(4):391.
46. US Census Bureau. Population profile on the United States: 2000. HIV/AIDS Surveillance Report, Midyear 2001 Edition. Atlanta, GA: Centers for Disease Control and Prevention, 2002.
47. National Center for Health Statistics. Health, United States, 1999, With Socioeconomic Status and Health Chartbook. Hyattsville, MD: National Center for Health Statistics, 2000.
48. CDC. Report on AIDS. MMWR 2001;50:429.
49. U.S. Census Bureau. Health Insurance Coverage: 2001. Table 3. http://www.census.gove/hhes/hlth-ins01/hi01t3.html. Accessed January 6, 2003.
50. Williams DR. African American health: the role of the social environment. J Urban Health 1998; 75:300.
51. Gaskin DJ, Hoffman C. Racial and ethnic differences in preventable hospitalizations across 10 states. Med Care Res Rev 2000;57(1):85.
52. National Adult Literacy Survey. www.nifl.gov.
53. van Ryn, M. Research on provide contribution to race/ethnicity disparities in medical care. Med Care 2002;40(Suppl):I-140.

54. Morris CR et al. Increasing trends in the use of breast-conserving surgery in California. Am J Public Health 2000;90:281.

55. Prehn AW et al. Differences in treatment patterns for localized breast carcinoma among Asian/Pacific Islander women. Cancer 2002;95:2268.

56. Prehn AW et al. Perceived risk and help-seeking behavior for breast cancer: a Chinese-American perspective. Cancer Nurs 2000;23:258.

57. Eisenberg DM et al. Trends in alternative medicine use in the United States, 1990-1997: Results of a follow-up national survey. JAMA 1998;280:1569.

58. Hedeen AN et al. Ethnicity and birthplace in relation to tumor size and stage in Asian American women with breast cancer. Am J Public Health 1999;89(8):1248.

59. Yin K. Observation on curative effect of Xiao He Ling applied to treat 460 patients with mastoplasia. Gansu J TCM 1995;8:30.

60. Cohen I et al. Traditional Chinese medicine in the treatment of breast cancer. Semin Oncol 2002;29(6):563.

61. Moss SE et al. Cause-specific mortality in a population-based study of diabetes. Am J Public Health 1991;81:1158.

62. Harris MI et al. Racial and ethnic differences in glycemic control for adults with type 2 diabetes. Diabetes Care 1999;22:403.

63. Egede LE, Bonadonna RJ. Diabetes self-management in African Americans: an exploration of the role of fatalism. Diabetes Educ 2003;29(1):105.

64. Gagliardino JJ, Etchegoyen G. A model education program for people with type 2 diabetes: a cooperative Latin American Implementation study (PEDNID-LA). Diabetes Care 2001;24:1001.

65. Brown SA, Reaching underserved populations and cultural competence in diabetes education. Curr Diabetes Rep 2002; 2(2):166.

66. Bertera EM. Psychosocial factors and ethnic disparities in diabetes diagnosis and treatment among older adults. Health Soc Work 2003;28(1):33.

67. Lasater TM. J Health Educ 1991;22(4):233.

68. Farmer IP et al. Higher levels of social support predict greater survival following acute myocardial infarction: the Corpus Christi Heart Project. Behav Med 22(2):59.

69. Perez-Stable et al. The effects of ethnicity and language on medical outcomes of patients with hypertension or diabetes. Med Care 1997;24:749.

70. Woloshin S et al. Language barriers in medicine in the United States. JAMA 1995;273(9):724.

71. American Heart Association. 2003 Heart and Stroke Statistical Update. Dallas: American Heart Association, 2003.

72. Hyman DJ, Pavlik VN. Characteristics of patients with uncontrolled hypertension in the United States. N Engl J Med 2001;345(7):479.

73. Sowers JR et al. Hypertension-related disease in African Americans. Postgrad Med 2002;112(4):24.

74. Jones CA et al. Serum creatinine levels in the US population: Third National Health and Nutrition Survey. Am J Kidney Dis 1998;32:992.

75. Lewis EF et al. The effect of angiotensin-converting enzyme inhibition on diabetic nephropathy: the Collaborative Study Group. N Engl J Med 1993;329:1456.

76. Kshirsagar AV et al. Effect of ACE inhibitors in diabetic and nondiabetic chronic renal disease: a systematic overview of randomized placebo-controlled trials. Am J Kidney Dis 2000;35:695.

77. Crook ED et al. End-stage renal disease due to diabetic nephropathy in Mississippi: an examination of factors influencing renal survival in a population prone to late referral. J Invest Med 2001;42:284.

78. Flegal K et al. Overweight and obesity in the United States: prevalence and trends, 1960-1994. Int J Obes Relat Metab Disord 1998; 22:39.

79. Kuczmarski R et al. Increasing prevalence of overweight among US adults: the National Health and Nutrition Examination Surveys, 1960 to 1991. JAMA 1994;272:205.

80. Appel LJ et al. for the DASH Collaborative Research Group. A clinical trial of the effects of dietary patterns on blood pressure. N Engl J Med. 1997;336:1117.

81. Wright JT Jr et al. Effect of blood pressure lowering and antihypertensive drug class on progression of hypertensive kidney disease: results from the AASK trial. JAMA 2002;288:2421.

82. Psaty BM et al. Health outcomes associated with antihypertensive therapies used as first-line agents:

a systematic review and meta-analysis. JAMA 1997;227:739.

83. ALLHAT Collaborative Research Group. Major cardiovascular events in hypertensive patients randomized to doxazosin vs. chlorthalidone: the Antihypertensive and Lipid-Lowering Treatment to Prevent Heart Attack Trial (ALLHAT). JAMA 2000;283:1967.

84. Douglas JG. Management of high blood pressure in African Americans. Arch Intern Med 2003; 163:525.

85. Lee L, Fleming P. Trends in HIV diagnoses among women in the United States. 1994-1998. JAMA 2001;56(3):94.

86. National Center for Health Statistics. National Vital Statistics Report. 2002:50(16).

87. Wohl AR et al. Sociodemographic and behavioral characteristics of African American Women with HIV and AIDS in Los Angeles. J Acquir Immune Defic Syndr and Human Retrovirology 1998;19:413.

88. McNaghten A et al. Inequities between gender and racial groups in prescription of highly active antiretroviral therapy. Abstract ThPeB5286. XIII International Conference on AIDS, Durban. Atlanta, GA : CDC, 2000.

89. Collins O et al. HIV/AIDS education and prevention among African Americans: a focus on culture. AIDS Educ Prev 1992;4(3):267.

90. Peruga A, Rivo M. Racial differences in AIDS knowledge among adults. AIDS Educ Prev 1992;4(1):52.

91. Nobles WW. Back to the roots: African culture as a basis for understanding black families. In: Nobles WW, ed. Africanity and the Black Family: The Development of a Theoretical Mode. Berkeley, CA: The Institute for the Advanced Study of Black Family Life and Culture.

92. Graney MJ et al. HIV/AIDS medication adherence factors: inner-city clinic patient's self-reports. Tenn Med 2003;96(2):73.

93. Flack JM et al. Efficacy and tolerability of eplerenone and losartan in hypertensive black and white patients. J Am Coll Cardiol 2003;41(7):1148.

CHAPTER 7

End-of-Life Care

Thomas C. Bookwalter

HOSPICE AND PALLIATIVE CARE

Hospice and palliative care are similar but distinct terms that share the concept that, *"the relief of suffering is a long standing, central, and fully legitimate aim of medicine."* "End-of-life care" incorporates both hospice care and palliative care. This philosophy of care strives to provide the best quality of life possible to the patient and his or her family in the last weeks and months of the patient's life; it extends beyond the end of the patient's life and into the family's bereavement period.

"Hospice," originally a place or way station for people making a pilgrimage, is considered both a philosophy of care and a place to deliver care. "Hospice care," therefore, can be delivered in a building designated as a hospice, in a skilled nursing facility, or at the patient's home. As a programmatic model for delivering palliative care, hospice care provides individualized management of a patient's symptoms (e.g., pain) as well as psychosocial, emotional, and spiritual support during the last months of life.[1] The National Hospice and Palliative Care Organization estimates that there are 3,200 hospice programs in the United States. Approximately 600,000 Americans died while under hospice care in 2000, and another 775,000 patients were admitted to hospice care in 2001. Hospices provide care for patients with various life-threatening illnesses, including those with chronic lung and heart disease, as well as those with acute illnesses such as HIV and cancer. Approximately 5,000 patients 24 years of age or younger were cared for by hospice in 2001.[1]

"Palliative care," which includes hospice care, takes a somewhat broader perspective, is introduced earlier in the disease progression, and includes all patients living with a life-threatening illness. The word "palliation," derived from the Latin word *pallium* (a cloak), has been defined as "treatment to reduce the violence of a disease."[2] The World Health Organization (WHO) defines palliative care as "an approach which improves the quality of life of patients and their families facing life-threatening illness, through the prevention and relief of suffering by means of early identification and impeccable assessment and treatment of pain and other physical, psychosocial and spiritual problems."[4] Palliative care:

- Provides relief from pain and other distressing symptoms

- Affirms life and regards dying as a normal process
- Intends neither to hasten nor postpone death
- Integrates the psychological and spiritual aspects of patient care
- Offers a support system to help patients live as actively as possible until death
- Offers a support system to help the family cope during the patient's illness and in their own bereavement
- Uses a team approach to address the needs of patients and their families, including bereavement counseling, if indicated
- Will enhance quality of life, and may also positively influence the course of illness
- Is applicable early in the course of illness, in conjunction with other therapies (e.g., chemotherapy, radiation therapy) that are intended to prolong life...and manage distressing clinical complications."[3]

Finally, the *Oxford Textbook of Palliative Care* defines palliative care as "the study and management of patients with active, progressive, far advanced disease for whom the prognosis is limited and the focus of care is the quality of life."[4] The provision of palliative care by interdependent health team members composed of physicians, nurses, pharmacists, social workers, and others has been successful in meeting the unique needs of patients with difficult or terminal illnesses.[5–11]

COMMUNICATION

Stages of Adjustment

1. K.D., a 26-year-old woman, has breast cancer with bony metastases. Her disease has failed to respond to all available treatment options. She has bravely endured hormonal therapy, lumpectomy with radiation, and combination chemotherapy. During a lengthy discussion with her oncologist, K.D. is informed that other treatment options are unlikely to be curative and that her prognosis is most likely terminal in weeks to months. After returning home she calls the infusion center where she receives regularly scheduled infusions of pamidronate to control elevated serum calcium concentrations and other medications to alleviate her symptoms of nausea, vomiting, and bone pain. This usually pleasant woman shouts angrily into the phone denouncing her oncologist, nurse, and pharmacist. She demands to know why there are no more options and wants to know how much longer she is likely to continue living with these symptoms. She asks for the reason she went through all the chemotherapy with its multiple side effects and the resultant deterioration in her quality of life. What may have prompted this behavior?

Reconciliation to one's own death is an extremely difficult task. Dr. Elisabeth Kubler-Ross in her landmark book, *On Death and Dying* identified five stages of adjustment that she observed in terminal patients.[12]

1. *Denial and Isolation.* During this stage, patients deny their diagnosis and tend to isolate themselves to further their denial. It is a time to prepare emotional defenses.
2. *Anger.* This stage can be described as a response to the "injustices" of the disease and often leads to the "dreaded questions." Patients ask: "Why me?" "Is there any hope?" "Are you going to let me die?" "Will you help me to die?"
3. *Bargaining.* This stage involves an attempt to postpone the unavoidable. "God, if you grant me a cure. . . ."
4. *Depression.* When the illness can no longer be denied, the patient may experience a great sense of loss, not only of life, but also of family, friends, finances, and other cherished things.
5. *Acceptance.* Not necessarily a "happy" phase, but the patient is able to face death without emotion (anger or denial) and with a quiet anticipation.[12]

These stages are rarely distinct and do not appear in a particular sequence. However, understanding these stages provides insight into the patient's needs and emotions during a difficult time in his or her life. The acceptance stage may be easier to achieve with good symptom management. K.D.'s behavior appears to be consistent with stage 2, and she likely would benefit from the understanding and support of family and caregivers as she progresses through the other stages before her death.

2. How should clinicians respond to K.D.'s questions of, "Why me?" "Why can't you tell me specifically how long I have?" or to other unasked questions (e.g., "Did I do something to cause this?" "Is there any hope?" "Are they just going to let me die?").

These questions are uncomfortable for clinicians because they are expressions that reflect the powerful emotions of patients, and sometimes these questions can trigger underlying emotions of clinicians (e.g., frustration with inability to do more, anger at being accused of incompetence or lack of sensitivity). These types of questions have no specific answer, but they merit a response. One possible approach is to first clarify ambiguity and then to respond as a person first and as a professional second by listening and offering empathy. For example, "*I wish* I could tell you more precisely how long you have, but each patient is different." Then the clinician can briefly discuss the prognostic uncertainty in these situations and follow with a question that focuses on the patient's specific underlying concerns (e.g., "Can you tell me more about what you were hoping that I could tell you?") Starting the reply with, "I wish..." provides an empathic response (not an answer) to K.D.'s concern. Some other helpful phrases to use in response to affective communications include, "I am sorry."

"How can I be most helpful?" and "What do you think?" Empathetic silence and touch can be appropriate.

Clinicians practicing palliative care may find that their personal experiences with death, and attitudes about death, can create barriers to communication, especially if the clinician is unaware that these experiences and attitudes are affecting communication. Practitioners must confront these experiences and attitudes to gain an understanding of how they can impinge on their relationships with dying patients and their families. This process has been called "confronting personal mortality"[13] and is difficult for several reasons. First, there is no established process or training to achieve this state of awareness. People have different experiences with death; and insights and self-awareness in the same person can be influenced by various stages of life.[14] It may be more useful to look at individual occurrences of vulnerability rather than abruptly "confronting mortality." Suppose the practitioner was unable to respond to K.D.'s questions because of feelings of inadequacy in addressing the "meaning of life"; or perhaps a family history of breast cancer makes this topic particularly painful. Reflecting on the encounter with K.D. may help the practitioner become more aware of his or her own vulnerabilities and enable coping with personalized feelings on death or feelings of inadequacy. Examining each episode of vulnerability in a similar manner can lead to increased self awareness. Self awareness is one way to define "confronting mortality."[14]

Goals

3. What are the goals of communication when caring for dying patients or their families?

In general, communications between clinicians and patients should focus on: 1) managing and monitoring medical problems and adverse events; 2) developing a caring professional relationship (i.e., "a therapeutic relationship"); and 3) providing instructions and guidance to the patient. The last two have particular relevance to end-of-life care. It is therapeutic for the patient and the family to disclose feelings, ventilate fears, and to assert as much control as possible. A therapeutic relationship can be developed by practicing active listening, respecting the patient's values, promoting partnership, and offering support. Since fear of abandonment is highly prevalent in patients with terminal illnesses, the promotion of a sense of partnership can be very important in allaying anxiety. "I'll be there for you," or a similar expression of nonabandonment is regarded as a central obligation of those caring for the terminally ill.[15]

Patients cannot make informed decisions without information that is factual and appropriate. In end-of-life care, it is important that the clinician knows what the patient already understands about the disease and associated symptoms so that education can proceed by building on the patient's current knowledge. It is supportive to give information in small amounts, to use understandable language, to reinforce information, and to check with the patient or family frequently to make sure that they understand what has been said. Clinicians should summarize what has been said and repeat mutual understandings before concluding a conversation.

It is important to recognize that despite our apprehensions, patients want to talk about death and dying.[16–19] The following seven-step approach for structuring end-of-life discussions has been useful to clinicians faced with situations such as "breaking bad news" or "advance care planning."[20] This approach also facilitates the establishment of treatment goals and provides a structure for these kinds of discussions. The steps are:

1. Prepare for the discussion
2. Establish what the patient (and family) knows
3. Determine how the information is to be handled (How is the information to be processed? How is the information to be shared? Do not assume that the patient's preferences follow any cultural, religious, or ethnic norm)
4. Deliver the information (be sensitive and straight forward)
5. Respond to emotions
6. Establish goals for care and treatment priorities
7. Establish a plan

PAIN MANAGEMENT

4. **After some time in hospice care, K.D.'s pain is successfully managed at home with extended release morphine tablets 100 mg PO TID and amitriptyline 50 mg PO Q HS. Morphine liquid 20 to 60 mg PO Q 3 hr PRN is prescribed to manage breakthrough pain. Her bowel regimen includes docusate 250 mg PO BID and senna 2 tablets HS. She is not complaining of any other symptoms. Her father asks whether his daughter has become addicted and if that is why she is drowsy all the time. In addition, he wants to know why K.D. is taking amitriptyline because she does not have a mental problem and the literature accompanying this medication indicated that it was a "psychotropic" used to treat depression. What might be some approaches for responding to these questions from K.D.'s father?**

Two important issues must be addressed before entering into a discussion with K.D.'s father. First, the hospice team must confirm that K.D. has provided approval for the sharing of her medical information with her father. Some patients do not wish to involve family members or others in their medical care, and the unapproved release of confidential medical information is a violation of federal statutes.

After confirming K.D.'s approval for release of this information, her father's understanding of her disease, prognosis, and care should be assessed before answering his specific questions. Her father's understanding may be elicited by using open-ended questions. Careful listening to his responses will facilitate the dialogue and help K.D.'s father and the hospice team to arrive at a common perception of the problems under discussion. In the course of this discussion, the practitioner should minimize the use of complex medical words (e.g., psychotropic), make empathic connections when possible, and try to determine whether the values and goals of K.D.'s father for the medical care of his daughter are consistent with those of his daughter.[13,21–25] After these issues have been assessed, the practitioner will be better prepared to answer the specific questions posed by him.

The response to his questions about addiction could begin with a discussion of the difference between physical dependence, tolerance, and addiction.[26,27] Physical dependence may be defined as the occurrence of withdrawal symptoms (e.g., anxiety, hyperactivity, shaking chills, abdominal cramps, nausea, vomiting, muscle spasms) after a drug is abruptly discontinued or when the dose of the opioid is decreased too rapidly. Tolerance can be described as the need for higher doses of a drug over time to produce the same effect, and addiction can be described as the psychological dependence on a drug for psychic effects (also see Chapter 83: Drug Abuse). Addicted patients will continue to use a drug despite social, psychological, economic, or legal harm.[8,28,29] Addiction should be distinguished from pseudoaddiction. Pseudoaddiction is a phenomenon noticed first in a leukemia patient who seemed to be exhibiting drug-seeking behavior, which ceased when the patient obtained adequate analgesia.[30–32] K.D.'s father needs to be reassured that the goal of analgesia is to relieve pain and to provide comfort to his daughter.

A description of the efficacy of amitriptyline in relieving the neuropathic component of pain would answer her father's specific question about the use of this "psychotropic" medication.[33] It would also be appropriate to mention that his daughter's symptom of drowsiness is one that is amenable to therapy and will be discussed with K.D. and with other team members.

5. **What are some possible solutions for K.D.'s drowsiness?**

The goals of pain management should be reviewed with K.D. If she is willing to accept her current level of sedation to obtain necessary pain relief, her opioid dose should not be decreased. If she is willing to accept more pain to be more alert and be better able to interact with her family and friends, then a dose reduction of her opioid should be attempted. Alternatively, another opioid, perhaps extended release oxycodone 80 mg PO TID or a fentanyl transdermal system 150 μg/hr, which can provide comparable pain relief with less sedation, could be selected. The sedating properties of amitriptyline also should be considered. Alternatives to amitriptyline include other less sedating tricyclic antidepressants with efficacy for neuropathic pain (e.g., imipramine, desipramine) or an anticonvulsant with similar properties (e.g., gabapentin, carbamazepine). If the neuropathic component of her pain is localized, topical lidocaine may be another alternative to amitriptyline.[33–36] The addition of a non-opioid analgesic can possibly reduce opioid requirements and thereby reduce K.D.'s sedation. Stimulants such as caffeine (100 to 200 mg/day), methylphenidate (5 to 10 mg/day), or dextroamphetamine (2.5 to 10 mg/day) also can be used to reduce the drowsiness caused by opioids.[33–39]

SYMPTOM MANAGEMENT

Patients living with a life-threatening illness or nearing the end-of-life can encounter as many as 53 symptoms.[40] In one study, patients (N = 176) experienced an average of 6.6 to 6.8 distressing symptoms during the last week of life.[41] In general, the prevalence of each symptom is difficult to measure and demonstrates a high degree of variability. The prevalence of pain (43% to 80%) varies with the primary site of advanced cancer.[41] Patients with terminal illnesses also experience nausea and vomiting (4% to 44%), dyspnea (15% to 79%), constipation (4% to 65%), insomnia (7% to 28%), delirium (4% to 85%), anorexia (6% to 74%), weight loss (58% to 77%), and fatigue (13% to 91%).[41–43] The disparity in symptom prevalence (Table 7-1) may be attributed to a host of variables

Table 7-1   Symptom Prevalence in Advanced Cancer

Symptom	Vainio[42] (%)	Curtis[59] (%)	Donnelly[43] (%)	Conill[41] (1st Evaluation) (%)	Conill[41] (2nd Evaluation) (%)
Pain	51	NR	64	52.3	30.1
Nausea/vomiting	21	32/25	36/23	26.1/18.8	23/10.2
Dyspnea	19	41	51	39.8	46.6
Constipation	23	40	51	49.4	55.1
Insomnia	9	NR	NR	34.7	28.4
Delirium	NR	NR	NR	NR	NR
Anorexia	30	55	74	68.2	80.1
Fatigue	NR	NR	NR	NR	NR
Weight loss	39	NR	NR	NR	NR
Weakness	51	NR	NR	76.7	81.8
Confusion	8	NR	NR	30.1	68.2
Dry mouth	NR	NR	NR	61.4	69.9
Dysphagia	NR	NR	NR	27.8	46.0
Anxiety	NR	20	23	50.6	45.5
Depression	NR	31	40	52.8	38.6
Diarrhea	NR	NR	NR	8.0	6.8

NR, not reported.

(e.g., study design, patient population, underlying disease, inconsistent definitions). The occurrence of symptoms, however, can vary significantly, even within the last week of life, and the need for frequent assessments of patients cannot be overemphasized.

6. A.S., a 79-year-old man with a 2-year history of multiple myeloma, presents to the emergency department after a fall with altered mental status, hallucinations, dizziness, and shortness of breath. Upon admission to the emergency department his systolic blood pressure was 117 mm Hg (supine) and 88 mm Hg (standing). His more recent medical history includes treatment with three cycles of melphalan and prednisone (complicated by neutropenia and thrombocytopenia), and his past medical history also includes gout, hypertension, coronary artery disease, and hyperlipidemia. His present medications include lisinopril 2.5 mg PO QD and isosorbide dinitrate 10 mg PO BID. Previously he had been taking dexamethasone, atenolol, ranitidine, and hydrocodone 5 mg/acetaminophen 500 mg. He lives at home with his wife and denies any alcohol or tobacco use. He has a daughter who lives outside his home, but she is involved in his care. After a discussion among the family and the medical team, conducted in the emergency department, it was decided for several reasons that the patient should have a do not resuscitate (DNR) order and that the goal of therapy should be to provide comfort to the patient and his family. His physical examination was pertinent for temperature, 101.1°F; blood pressure, 94/44 mm Hg; heart rate, 66 beat/min; respiratory rate, 20 breaths/min; oxygen saturation, 81% on room air, which improved to 93% with 3 liters O_2 by nasal cannula; and pain assessment, 0/10. He had coarse breath sounds at the right base but no egophony. A chest radiograph is consistent with pneumonia. His laboratory test results show Na, 135 mEq/L; K, 3.9 mEq/L; BUN, 30 mg/dL; Cr, 1.4 mg/dL; WBC, 5,900; HCT, 29.3; and platelets, 81,000. What symptoms are contributing to A.S.'s discomfort?

A.S. is dizzy, orthostatic, and has fallen down. In addition his blood pressure is low. His blood pressure medication will

be held and fluid repletion may help with these symptoms. His shortness of breath and fever are most likely secondary to his pneumonia. A course of antibiotics appropriate for community-acquired pneumonia should improve his shortness of breath, low oxygen saturation, and elevated temperature. His altered mental status and dizziness are the likely result of his low blood pressure and perhaps his pneumonia.

7. A.S. is admitted to the hospital; given IV fluids, ceftriaxone, doxycycline, and acetaminophen; and a physical therapist is consulted to provide an exercise program that will improve his strength. After several days of therapy A.S. can walk 40 feet with minimal assistance, and his oxygen saturation has improved to 93% on room air during rest. His blood pressure has stabilized at 130/70 mm Hg. Unfortunately, he is still confused and somewhat disoriented. His wife is unable to care for him at home at this time, and he is to be discharged to a skilled nursing facility on oral antibiotics, oxygen, and his current physical therapy program. During his stay at the nursing home, laboratory studies show a creatinine of 2.3 mg/dL and a hemoglobin of 7.8 g/dL. He has begun to complain of low back pain. A.S. no longer has skilled nursing needs and will be cared for by family members at home with the support of a local hospice. What services commonly are provided to terminal patients through hospice?

Eligibility for medical reimbursement for hospice services generally requires that the hospice patient be expected to live no longer than 6 months if the disease were to follow its normal course. A.S. is not eligible for further high-dose chemotherapy regimens or bone marrow transplant because of his medical condition and his age. His developing renal failure (creatinine, 2.3 mg/dL) and anemia (hemoglobin, 7.8 g/dL) make his prognosis quite poor. To participate in the Medicare hospice program, the hospice must provide physician's services for the direction of the patient's care; regular home visits by registered nurses and licensed practical nurses; home health aides and homemakers for services such as dressing and bathing; social work and counseling; medical equipment such as hospital beds; medical supplies such as bandages and catheters; drugs for symptom control and pain relief; volunteer support to assist patients and loved ones; and physical therapy, speech therapy, occupational therapy, and dietary counseling.

8. What medications may be prescribed to treat A.S.'s back pain?

Since A.S.'s back pain is most likely caused by osteolytic lesions secondary to his underlying disease, a nonsteroidal anti-inflammatory drug (NSAID) may be appropriate. A.S., however, has used hydrocodone/acetaminophen in the past with good results. Thus, it is reasonable to prescribe one or two tablets of hydrocodone 5 mg/acetaminophen 500 mg PO Q 4 to 6 hours as needed for his back pain. Although patients are usually cautioned to take no more than 8 tablets of this preparation daily, the usual 4gm/day limit on acetaminophen can be exceeded, when appropriate, in terminal patients. It is equally reasonable to prescribe an NSAID or an oral opioid without acetaminophen for A.S. because these may be safer despite his terminal illness. In the final analysis, it is difficult to make a strong case for any of these choices because his illness is terminal and it is difficult to argue against previous success with the combination of acetaminophen with hydrocodone.

9. What side effects can be expected with opioid administration?

Large doses of opioids are commonly associated with side effects such as constipation, nausea, vomiting, itching, and sedation. Just as frequent assessment of the patient is key to successful pain management, it also is key to the successful management of opioid side effects. The patient or his caregiver should be asked if A.S. is experiencing any side effects so that they may be managed appropriately. Patients may become tolerant to all opioid side effects except constipation. Usually, constipation may be managed with a stool softener (e.g., docusate) and a stimulant laxative (e.g., senna).

10. What other effective laxatives could be considered if A.S. were to develop refractory constipation?

If stool softeners and stimulant and saline laxatives are ineffective in resolving the opioid-induced constipation in A.S., a trial of lactulose 30 mL PO (10 g/15 mL) up to 4 times a day can be prescribed. The frequency of administration should be reduced if the patient has several bowel movements/day or develops diarrhea. When the injectable formulation of the opioid antagonist, naloxone, is administered orally, it can reverse opioid-induced constipation by antagonizing opioid effects within the gastrointestinal tract without antagonizing systemic analgesic effects because naloxone is poorly absorbed orally. The usual starting dose of naloxone for the management of opioid-induced constipation is 0.4 to 0.6 mg PO Q 6 hr. Naloxone doses of 2.4 mg PO Q 6 hr have been used, but the drug has caused withdrawal at higher doses.[44]

11. After 1 week of therapy it is clear that A.S requires 8 to 10 tablets of hydrocodone 5 mg/acetaminophen 500 mg daily for pain relief. The hospice nurse and the patient's wife often feel that pain control is suboptimal as they observe him grimacing and complaining of incomplete pain relief daily. A.S.'s wife understands "as needed for pain" to mean that she is not to give the medication until she sees signs of pain or discomfort or until A.S. asks her for it. What adjustments may be made to A.S.'s pain regimen?

A thorough assessment of A.S. should be completed before adjusting his pain medication regimen. The intensity and quality of his pain should be evaluated as well as the affective, behavioral, and cognitive dimensions of pain. The following types of questions could be used in this assessment. Is the pain causing A.S. to suffer, to be afraid, or to be angry? Is he demonstrating any behaviors associated with pain (e.g., his wife and nurse have observed him grimacing)? Does the pain have significant meaning for A.S.? Is it his "fault?" Pain should not be treated on an "as needed" basis when it is severe, moderately severe, or chronic. When a numeric rating scale from 0 to 10 is used to assess pain intensity (with zero being no pain and 10 the worst pain imaginable), ratings of 1 to 4 represent mild pain, 5 to 6 moderate pain, and 7 to 10 severe pain.[45] Patients with A.S.'s level of pain should receive pain medications on a regularly scheduled basis to provide basal control. Supplemental doses of pain medication also should be prescribed for use on an "as needed" basis to manage breakthrough pain. Long-acting opioid formulations (e.g., extended-release morphine, extended-release oxycodone) can be used to provide basal pain relief, and an immediate-release formulation of morphine can be used to manage intermittent breakthrough pain. Since the patient is requiring 40 to 50 mg hydrocodone/day, extended- release morphine 15 mg PO TID or extended-release oxycodone 10 mg PO TID would be an appropriate equianalgesic dose. The hydrocodone/acetaminophen product can be used to manage breakthrough pain. The plan and attainable goals for pain relief should be discussed with the patient, his family, and with all hospice team members. In addition, the principles of good pain management should be explained to A.S.'s wife to provide her with a better understanding of the rationale for the appropriate use of pain medications for her husband (See Chapter 9, Pain).

12. C.L. is a 63-year-old woman with a 6-year history of ovarian cancer treated with surgery, chemotherapy, and radiation. Subsequent metastases of the cancer to the head of the pancreas, liver, bone, and small bowel have resulted in several additional surgical procedures. She is currently in severe pain and, with the concurrence of her oncologists and family, has requested palliative care. She was given a morphine drip and currently requires morphine 1.4 g/hr to control her pain successfully. She has become increasingly agitated and has failed to respond to high doses of anxiolytics and neuroleptics. Would palliative sedation be appropriate for C.L. at this time?

In patients who are terminally ill, suffering may continue despite maximal palliative efforts. In this small number of patients, it may be desirable to reduce suffering by the thoughtful use of medications to induce sedation. It is not appropriate to increase opioid doses to achieve the desired sedated state. Medications used successfully to induce sedation for these patients include benzodiazepines, barbiturates, and phenothiazines. No drug or drug class is superior to any other for this use.[46]

A trial of palliative sedation with lorazepam could be initiated at a rate of 2 mg/hr and gradually increased if needed to as much as 6 mg/hr. Although palliative sedation has a small potential to shorten life, the need to relieve terminal agitation sometimes warrants this risk. Palliative sedation only should be initiated as a last resort in severe cases not responsive to other palliative measures and only after thorough discussion of the important clinical and ethical issues with the patient, family, and other clinical team members.

13. **What is the principle of "double effect?"**

"Double effect" is a moral principle that distinguishes between intended effects and effects that are merely foreseen. For example in the case above, the "intent" of controlled sedation was to relieve suffering, but we may foresee that this intervention has the potential to hasten C.L.'s death. The "bad" effect (death) must not be the means to the "good" effect (less suffering). Finally, proportionally the "good" effect must outweigh the risks of the "bad" effect.[47-49]

PHYSICIAN-ASSISTED SUICIDE

Whatever society ultimately decides about the legality and morality of physician-assisted suicide, practitioners might encounter requests by patients for the ending of their lives because of overwhelming suffering. According to the literature, most clinicians have significant aversion to this practice both ethically and legally.[50-56] State and national professional organizations have not been helpful in providing guidance for managing this ultimate end-of-life decision. Each clinician, therefore, must rely on his or her own conscience to decide whether to participate in facilitating a patient's death. Although substantial numbers of clinicians can imagine situations in which assisted suicide would be acceptable, few are willing to actively participate in response to the request of a patient for the ending of life.[57,58]

REFERENCES

1. NHPCO facts and figures. Available at www.nhpco.org. Accessed June 6, 2003.
2. Lamers W. Defining hospice and palliative care: some further thoughts. J Pain Palliat Care Pharmacother 2002;16:65.
3. Sepulveda C et al. Palliative care: the World Health Organization's global perspective. J Pain Sympt Man 2002;24:91.
4. Doyle D et al. Introduction. In: Doyle D et al., ed. The Oxford Textbook of Palliative Medicine. Oxford: Oxford University Press, 1993:3.
5. Lipman AG. Drug therapy in terminally ill patients. Am J Hosp Pharm 1975;32:270.
6. Berry JI et al. Pharmaceutical services in hospices. Am J Hosp Pharm 1981;38:1010.
7. Arter SG et al. Hospice care and the pharmacist. Am Pharm 1987;NS27:32.
8. Bonomi AE et al. Cancer pain management: barriers, trends, and the role of pharmacists. J Am Pharm Assoc (Wash) 1999;39:558.
9. Lucas C et al. Contribution of a liaison clinical pharmacist to an inpatient palliative care unit. Palliat Med 1997;11:209.
10. Hanif N. Role of the palliative care unit pharmacist. J Palliat Care 1991;7:35.
11. Wagner J, Goldstein E. Pharmacist's role in loss and grief. Am J Hosp Pharm 1977;34:490.
12. Kubler-Ross E et al. On death and dying. JAMA 1972;221:174.
13. Buckman R. Communication skills in palliative care: a practical guide. Neurol Clin 2001;19:989.
14. Warm E. Fast facts concepts #31: confronting personal mortality. Available at www.eperc.mcw.edu. Accessed June 6, 2003.
15. Quill TE, Cassel CK. Nonabandonment: a central obligation for physicians. Ann Intern Med 1995;122:368.
16. Matthews DA et al. Making "connexions": enhancing the therapeutic potential of patient-clinician relationships. Ann Intern Med 1993;118:973.
17. Schonwetter RS. Care of the terminally ill patient. Clin Geriatr Med 1996;12:xi.
18. Lo B et al. Patient attitudes to discussing life-sustaining treatment. Arch Intern Med 1986;146:1613.
19. Emanuel LL et al. Advance directives for medical care: a case for greater use. N Engl J Med 1991;324:889.
20. von Gunten CF et al. Ensuring competency in end-of-life care: communication and relational skills. JAMA 2000;284:3051.
21. Stolick M. Overcoming the tendency to lie to dying patients. Am J Hosp Palliat Care 2002;19:29.
22. Tattersall MH et al. Insights from cancer patient communication research. Hematol Oncol Clin North Am 2002;16:731.
23. DiBartola LM. Listening to patients and responding with care: a model for teaching communication skills. Jt Comm J Qual Improv 2001;27:315.
24. Cooley C. Communication skills in palliative care. Prof Nurse 2000;15:603.
25. Finlay IG et al. The assessment of communication skills in palliative medicine: a comparison of the scores of examiners and simulated patients. Med Educ 1995;29:424.
26. Porter J, Jick H. Addiction rare in patients treated with narcotics. N Engl J Med 1980;302:123.
27. Portenoy RK. Opioid therapy for chronic nonmalignant pain: a review of the critical issues. J Pain Sympt Man 1996;11:203.
28. Aronoff GM. Opioids in chronic pain management: is there a significant risk of addiction? Curr Rev Pain 2000;4:112.
29. Berry PE, Ward SE. Barriers to pain management in hospice: a study of family caregivers. Hosp J 1995;10:19.
30. Weissman DE, Haddox JD. Opioid pseudoaddiction: an iatrogenic syndrome. Pain 1989;36:363.
31. Breivik H. Opioids in cancer and chronic non-cancer pain therapy-indications and controversies. Acta Anaesthesiol Scand 2001;45:1059.
32. Kowal N. What is the issue?: pseudoaddiction or undertreatment of pain. Nurs Econ 1999;17:348.
33. Ramirez A et al. ABC of palliative care. The carers. BMJ 1998;316:208.
34. Chong MS, Bajwa ZH. Diagnosis and treatment of neuropathic pain. J Pain Sympt Man. 2003;25:S4.
35. Gammaitoni AR et al. Safety and tolerability of the lidocaine patch 5%, a targeted peripheral analgesic: a review of the literature. J Clin Pharmacol 2003;43:111.
36. Backonja M. Anticonvulsants for the treatment of neuropathic pain syndromes. Curr Pain Headache Rep 2003;7:39.
37. Manfredi PL, Gonzales GR. Symptomatic uses of caffeine in patients with cancer. J Palliat Care 2003;19:63.
38. Homsi J et al. Psychostimulants in supportive care. Support Care Cancer 2000;8:385.
39. Bruera E et al. Use of methylphenidate as an adjuvant to narcotic analgesics in patients with advanced cancer. J Pain Sympt Man. 1989;4:3.
40. Doyle D et al. Oxford Textbook of Palliative Medicine. 2nd Ed. Oxford: Oxford University Press, 1998:1283.
41. Conill C et al. Symptom prevalence in the last week of life. J Pain Sympt Man 1997;14:328.
42. Vainio A, Auvinen A. Prevalence of symptoms among patients with advanced cancer: an international collaborative study. Symptom Prevalence Group. J Pain Sympt Man 1996;12:3.
43. Donnelly S, Walsh D. The symptoms of advanced cancer. Semin Oncol 1995;22:67.
44. Meissner W et al. Oral naloxone reverses opioid-associated constipation. Pain 2000;84:105.
45. Serlin RC et al. When is cancer pain mild, moderate or severe? Grading pain severity by its interference with function. Pain 1995;61:277.
46. Cowan JD, Walsh D. Terminal sedation in palliative medicine: definition and review of the literature. Support Care Cancer 2001;9:403.
47. Twycross R. The 'principle', not 'doctrine' of double effect. Int J Palliat Nurs 2003;9:40.
48. Quill TE, Byock IR. Responding to intractable terminal suffering: the role of terminal sedation and voluntary refusal of food and fluids. ACP-ASIM End-of-Life Care Consensus Panel. American College of Physicians-American Society of Internal Medicine. Ann Intern Med 2000;132:408.
49. Quill TE et al. The rule of double effect: a critique of its role in end-of-life decision making. N Engl J Med 1997;337:1768.
50. Cato MA et al. Perspective on ASHP's assisted-suicide policy. Am J Health Syst Pharm 1999;56:1672.
51. ASHP statement on pharmacist decision-making on assisted suicide. Am J Health Syst Pharm 1999;56:1661.
52. Dixon KM, Kier KL. Longing for mercy, requesting death: pharmaceutical care and pharmaceutically assisted death. Am J Health Syst Pharm 1998;55:578.
53. Hamerly JP. Views on assisted suicide. Perspectives of the AMA and the NHO. Am J Health Syst Pharm 1998;55:543.
54. Rupp MT. Physician-assisted suicide and the issues it raises for pharmacists. Am J Health Syst Pharm 1995;52:1455.
55. Brock D. Death and dying. In: Vaeatch R ed. Medical Ethics. Boston: Jones and Bartlett, 1989:329.
56. Veatch RM. The pharmacist and assisted suicide. Am J Health Syst Pharm 1999;56:260.
57. Vivian J et al. Michigan pharmacists' attitudes about medically assisted suicide. J Mich Pharm 1993;31:490.
58. Rupp MT, Isenhower HL. Pharmacists' attitudes toward physician-assisted suicide. Am J Hosp Pharm 1994;51:69.
59. Curtis EB et al. Common symptoms in patients with advanced cancer. J Palliat Care 1991;7:259.

Nausea and Vomiting

Celeste Lindley

Nausea and vomiting are unpleasant consequences of many drugs and disorders (Table 8-1). The act of emesis is a protective mechanism designed to rid the body of ingested poisons and toxins before dangerous amounts can be absorbed. However, these symptoms may occur in situations in which they seem to be an inappropriate response. Nausea and vomiting are usually self-limiting events without serious sequelae. Severe and/or protracted nausea and vomiting, however, may result in serious medical complications such as dehydration, malnutrition, and metabolic disturbances. This is particularly true in infants and children. Recent data have confirmed that symptoms of nausea and vomiting significantly impact the quality of life and functional ability of sufferers.[1] Prevention is the goal of therapy in cases in which nausea and vomiting are predictable, such as surgical procedures, the administration of chemotherapy, and motion sickness. When prevention is unsuccessful or not feasible, treatment must be aimed at treating the underlying disorder, managing the symptoms, and correcting secondary complications.

PHYSIOLOGY

The act of vomiting may be divided into three phases: nausea, retching, and vomiting.[2,3] *Nausea,* which can persist for hours or days, represents an awareness of the urge to vomit. It is accompanied by loss of gastric tone and peristalsis with contraction of the duodenum and reflux of intestinal contents into the stomach. Additional symptoms such as increased perspiration, salivation, tachycardia, anorexia, and headache often occur simultaneously. *Retching* consists of rhythmic labored spasmodic movements, involving the diaphragm, chest wall, and abdominal muscles. Retching usually precedes or alternates with bouts of vomiting. *Vomiting,* or emesis, is the forceful expulsion of gastrointestinal (GI) contents through the mouth. It is associated with descent of the diaphragm, powerful sustained contractions of the abdominal muscles, and opening of the gastric cardia. Nausea is largely an autonomic response; however, vomiting is coordinated by the somatic nervous system. Although the act of vomiting typically combines nausea, retching, and vomiting, each of these physiologic processes can occur independently.

PATHOPHYSIOLOGY

Early researchers, recognizing the close integration of vomiting, respiration, salivation, and vasomotor control, determined that the vomiting center (VC) is located in the reticular formation of the medulla oblongata. Using surgical ablative techniques, researchers were able to more precisely locate the position of the VC in the dorsal portion of the lateral reticular formation in the medulla.[4,5] It represents the final common pathway that mediates vomiting from all causes. In numerous animal models, the VC coordinates the respiratory, GI, and abdominal musculature involved in vomiting. In addition, vomiting can be induced by electrical stimulation of the VC and the nearby nucleus tractus solitarius (NTS) (Fig. 8-1). It can also be indirectly induced by stimulation of the chemoreceptor trigger zone (CTZ), the GI tract, the vestibular apparatus, and higher brain centers. Stimulation of the VC from these remote locations is mediated by the release of neurotransmitters.

The CTZ, located in the area postrema on the floor of the fourth ventricle, is accessible to both blood and cerebrospinal fluid. For many years, the CTZ was believed to mediate emesis from all blood-borne drugs and toxins. This belief was based on studies demonstrating that surgical ablation of the area postrema afforded total protection against apomorphine-induced emesis. More recent studies have demonstrated that CTZ ablation does not prevent vomiting in response to pilocarpine or veratrum. This led researchers to propose the forebrain and a vagal nodose ganglion site, respectively, as the location of the CTZ.[6,7] Further studies demonstrated that the CTZ was not essential for vomiting induced by motion or by activation of vagal nerve afferents. Efficacy against acute chemotherapy-induced emesis by $5HT_3$ receptor antagonists and the identification of $5HT_3$ receptors in the GI tract prompted researchers to reappraise the relative involvement of the CTZ and the abdominal visceral afferents in the emetic reflex. Gut vagal afferent fibers were found to terminate directly underneath the CTZ in the NTS. Inadequate CTZ ablation techniques used in early studies may have damaged gut vagal afferents; hence, early reports designating the CTZ as the principal site of the emetic stimulus may have been based on erroneous microanatomy.[8] Proponents of the GI tract as the primary initiator of emesis cite the more rapid induction of emesis from ingested substances as opposed to systemic absorption of toxins for stimulation of the CTZ.

Table 8-1 Etiologies of Nausea and Vomiting

Fluid and electrolyte abnormalities
 Hypercalcemia
 Volume depletion
 Water intoxication
 Adrenocortical insufficiency
 Metabolic disturbances
Drug-induced
 Chemotherapy
 Opiates
 Antibiotics
 Cardiac glycosides
 Bronchodilators
Gastrointestinal obstruction
Increased intracranial pressure
Peritonitis
Metastasis
 Brain, meninges, hepatic
Uremia
Infections
Radiation therapy
Tube feeding
Anxiety

NEUROPHARMACOLOGY OF EMESIS

The CTZ and NTS contain several types of neurotransmitters and neuromodulators. Dopamine has received the most attention as a central mediator of emesis. However, opiate, serotonin, acetylcholine, and histamine receptors also are found in the CTZ. Histaminic, muscarinic, and serotonin receptors also are found in the NTS. Most recently, NK_1 (or Substance P) receptors have been identified in brain regions regulating eme-

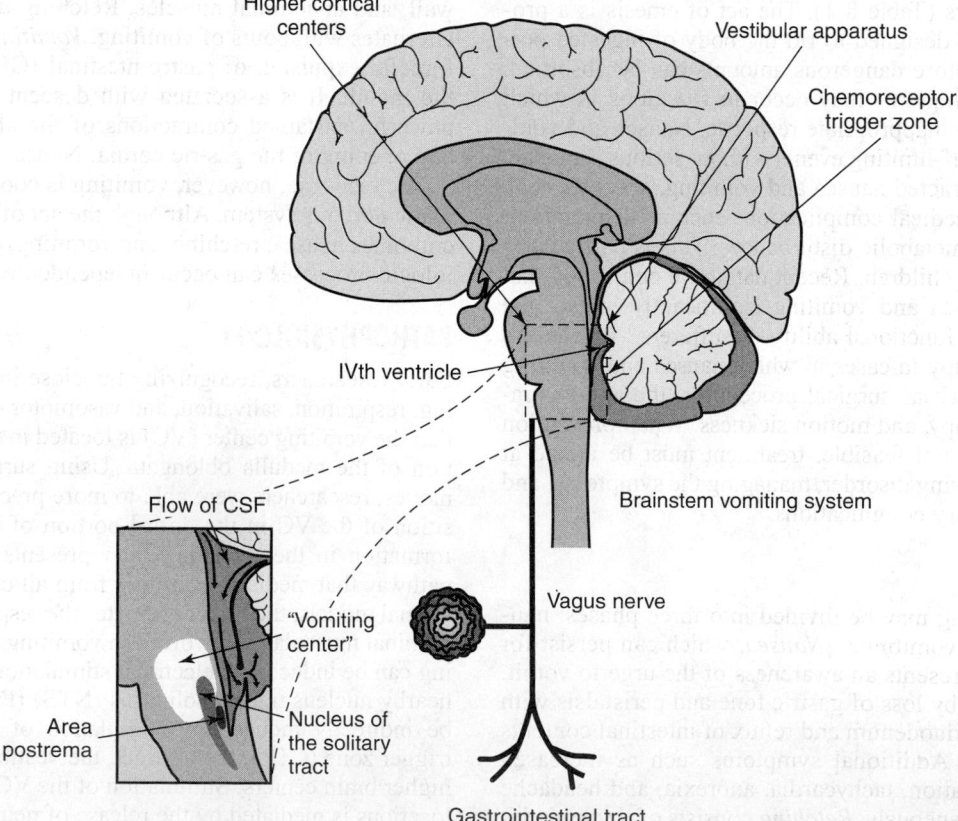

FIGURE 8-1 Vomiting center.

sis including the brain stem nuclei, the NTS, and area postrema regions. Blockade of these neurotransmitter receptors constitutes a major mechanism for antiemetic efficacy of various agents (Table 8-2). Inputs to the VC from higher cortical centers are the least understood of all pathways for initiating emesis. The existence of such signaling pathways is observed clinically in patients who experience nausea and emesis in response to emotional stimuli, such as terror. These connections also explain the conditioned response that occurs in cancer patients in whom cues, such as the sight of the hospital or thoughts of treatment, can trigger emesis.

Dopamine Receptors in the CTZ and Gastrointestinal Tract

As previously discussed, dopamine-2 receptors (D_2) located in the CTZ have long been recognized as a primary mediator of emesis caused by blood-borne drugs and toxins. Drugs that block dopamine receptors include the piperazine class of phenothiazines (prochlorperazine, thiethylperazine, and perphenazine) and the substituted benzamide, metoclopramide. Metoclopramide also blocks D_2 receptors located in the GI tract and in high doses has some blockade of serotonin receptors as well. Haloperidol and droperidol are also useful as antiemetics due to dopamine receptor blocking action. These agents are useful for nausea and vomiting resulting from a variety of emetogenic stimuli.

Serotonin Receptors in the Gastrointestinal Tract

More recently, serotonin and dopamine (D_2) receptors in the GI tract have been associated with the emetic syndrome. After cisplatin administration, increased urinary excretion of 5-hydroxyindolacetic acid (5-HIAA), the major breakdown product of serotonin, correlates with the onset and severity of nausea and vomiting.[9] This, coupled with efficacy of serotonin antagonists for preventing acute cisplatin-induced emesis, led researchers to conclude that serotonin is the major mediator of acute chemotherapy-induced nausea and vomiting (CINV). However, increased urinary excretion of 5-HIAA has not been observed in acute chemotherapy-induced emesis resulting from noncisplatin-based chemotherapy regimens. Increases in 5-HIAA also have not correlated with emesis re-

sulting from GI tract physical factors such as irritation, distention, motility disorders, or obstruction.[10] One cannot conclude from these data that all GI tract–associated etiologies of emesis will respond to blockade of serotonin receptors. Nausea and emesis associated with gastric distention and/or mechanical or autonomic dysfunction of the GI tract respond best to metoclopramide (10 to 40 mg three to four times daily), which has dopamine-receptor blocking activity at low dosages and prokinetic activity.

Neurokinin Stimulation

In the mid-1990s, animal studies demonstrated that a capsaicin analog was able to block the emetic response to emetic agents acting centrally (apomorphine) or peripherally (total body irradiation, intragastric copper sulfate).[12] It was proposed that the blockade was caused by the release and subsequent depletion of substance P in the NTS in the brainstem. The neurokinin-1 (NK_1) receptor is activated by substance P and closely related substances. Substance P is located primarily within the NTS in the central nervous system. A new class of compounds, the NK_1 receptor antagonists, have been investigated in animal models and found to block the emetic effect of apomorphine, morphine, nicotine, copper sulfate, ipecac, radiation, cyclophosphamide, cisplatin, motion, and anesthesia in the ferret, dog, cat, and house musk shrew.[13] Aprepitant (Emend) was approved by the FDA in 2003 for vomiting induced by highly emetogenic chemotherapy and is the first agent in this class to be marketed. Aprepitant, in combination with other antiemetic agents, is indicated for the prevention of acute and delayed nausea and vomiting associated with initial and repeat courses of highly emetogenic cancer chemotherapy, including high-dose cisplatin. The primary site of action of the NK_1 receptor antagonist appears to differ from the $5HT_3$ receptor antagonists. Unlike the latter, which appear to work primarily at a peripheral site, the NK_1 receptor antagonists require entry into the central nervous system to exert their antiemetic effect. Aprepitant, when added to standard therapy consisting of a $5HT_3$ receptor antagonist and dexamethasone on day 1 followed by dexamethasone alone on days 2 to 4, improves acute CINV by 10% to 15% and delayed CINV by 20%.[14] Receptor mapping studies have shown that the NK_1 receptor system is also expressed in brain regions

Table 8-2 Major Site of Action of Drugs Used to Control Chemotherapy-Induced Nausea and Vomiting

Class of Drug	Example	Receptor	Site of Action
Phenothiazines	Prochlorperazine	Dopamine	CTZ
Butyrophenones	Haloperidol	Dopamine	CTZ
Benzamides	Metoclopramide	Dopamine, serotonin[a]	GI, CTZ
Antihistamine	Diphenhydramine	Histamine	VA, NTS
Anticholinergic	Scopolamine	Acetylcholine	VA, NTS
Cannabinoids	Dronabinol	Unknown	CNS, NTS
Corticosteroids	Dexamethasone	Unknown	Unknown
Serotonin ($5HT_3$) antagonists	Ondansetron	Serotonin	NTS
NK_1-receptor antagonists	Aprepitant	NK_1	CNS, NTS
Anxiolytics	Lorazepam	Unknown	CNS

[a]At high dosages.
CNS, central nervous system; CTZ, chemoreceptor trigger zone; GI, gastrointestinal; NK1, neurokinin-1 receptor; NTS, nucleus tractus solitarius; VA, visceral vagal.
From references 2–5, 8, 9, 11, 13, 16.

involved in the regulation of affective disorders and the neurochemical response to stress.[15] Ongoing studies are assessing the role of NK$_1$ receptor antagonists in a variety of disorders.

Disturbances in Vestibular Function

Disturbances in vestibular function are believed to stimulate cranial nerve VIII, which in turn stimulates the VC. Motion sickness is the most common emetic syndrome elicited in response to a vestibular stimulus. Acetylcholine, muscarinic, and histamine receptors are thought to initiate the emetic cascade in this setting. Dopamine and serotonin do not appear to be involved in the development of motion sickness. Amphetamine and other agents that cause a release of norepinephrine are effective clinically in preventing motion sickness. The mechanism of action remains obscure, but it may be related to the role of the noradrenergic nervous system in central sensory information processing.[11]

PRINCIPLES OF PHARMACOTHERAPY OF EMESIS

It is important to emphasize that nausea and vomiting are common symptoms that occur in response to many drugs and disorders. Therefore, it is important to determine the potential causes before making a specific pharmacotherapeutic recommendation for prevention or treatment. Patients with acute onset emesis, who also have a viral infection or have recently ingested excessive amounts of food or alcohol, may not require antiemetic therapy. This is particularly true of acute viral gastroenteritis in children or in cases of food poisoning. Therefore, patient assessment should include the onset and duration of signs and symptoms; the nature of precipitating factors; a complete history of recent medication, food, and liquid ingestion; and current, chronic, or acute medical conditions. The presence of mild to moderate nausea and vomiting for <48 hours in the absence of more severe symptoms is best managed by close monitoring of hydration status. Over-the-counter products, such as phosphorated carbohydrate solution (Emetrol, Calm-X, Nausetrol) or Pepto-Bromol (Pepto-Bismol), may be helpful in these cases. Nausea and vomiting accompanied by blood in the vomitus, abdominal pain or distention, fever, severe headache, recent trauma, diabetes, or other medical conditions may affect nutritional intake or compliance with oral medications and require referral to a health care provider.

Specific pharmacotherapeutic interventions are often required to prevent and treat motion sickness, postoperative nausea and vomiting, and nausea and vomiting associated with administration of chemotherapy or radiation therapy. The cases that follow describe the pharmacotherapeutic principles and current treatment recommendations for these disorders. A variety of antiemetic regimens with specific mechanisms of action are available commercially. Current treatment recommendations reflect an attempt to link causes of emesis with mechanisms of action of antiemetics and rely extensively on published clinical trials. However, it is important to note that the etiology and pharmacology of emesis are not completely understood; therefore, continuous assessment and modification of a therapeutic plan for a specific patient is required.

THERAPEUTIC GUIDELINES

A number of multidisciplinary expert panels have developed evidence-based recommendations for the treatment of emesis associated with motion, postoperative nausea and vomiting, chemotherapy-induced emesis, and radiation-induced emesis.[16–20] The expert panel assigned a value to the evidence, ranging from 1 to 5, based on the quality of the source of information available. In addition, it graded the recommendations based on the type and level of evidence, as well as the consistency of findings. Table 8-3 indicates the areas addressed by the American Society of Health-Systems Pharmacists,[17]

Table 8-3 National and International Antiemetic Guidelines	
American Society of Clinical Oncology[18]	Acute and delayed CIE
	Anticipatory emesis
	Emesis in pediatric oncology
	High-dose chemotherapy
	Breakthrough emesis
	Radiation-induced emesis
American Society of Health-Systems Pharmacists[17]	Adult acute and delayed CIE
	Radiation-induced emesis
	PONV
	Pediatric CIE, radiation-induced emesis, PONV
Multinational Association of Supportive Care in Cancer[19]	Adult acute and delayed CIE
	Radiation-induced emesis
	High-dose chemotherapy
	Pediatric CIE
	Multiple day and rescue
National Comprehensive Cancer Center Network[20]	Acute and delayed CIE
	Radiation-induced emesis
	Anticipatory emesis
	Breakthrough emesis

CIE, chemotherapy-induced emesis; PONV, postoperative nausea and vomiting.

American Society of Clinical Oncology,[18] the Multinational Association of Supportive Care in Cancer,[19] and the National Comprehensive Cancer Center Network.[20] Specific references for each of these publications are included. These guidelines are incorporated into the recommendations for treatment of nausea and vomiting contained in this chapter.

MOTION SICKNESS

1. P.C. is a 27-year-old woman who has no significant medical history with the exception of moderate dysmenorrhea and motion sickness associated with travel by air. In the past, she has taken dimenhydrinate (Dramamine) before airplane trips with moderate success. She is engaged to be married, and she and her fiancé have decided on a Caribbean cruise for their honeymoon. P.C. is mildly concerned that dimenhydrinate may not control her symptoms, particularly in the event of rough weather at sea. What alternatives are available to prevent and treat P.C.'s motion sickness?

Motion sickness occurs when perceptions of motion by different proprioceptors (i.e., visual, vestibular, and sensory proprioreceptors) provide conflicting information.[16] Motion sickness occurs most commonly with boat travel, followed by air, car, and train travel, in descending order of frequency. Although the magnitude of the motion stimulus affects the likelihood of sickness, individuals vary in their propensity to experience this phenomenon as well. Some have stated that personal propensity to experience motion sickness remains stable throughout life; however, other evidence indicates that motion sickness in childhood is often diminished in later adolescence and adulthood. P.C.'s plan for an extended cruise, along with her history of motion sickness, suggest that dimenhydrinate, which typically is prescribed for moderate motion severity, may be inadequate to prevent motion sickness.

As indicated in Table 8-4, antihistamine agents, such as cyclizine, meclizine, and dimenhydrinate, are considered the agents of choice for mild to moderate motion sickness.[16,21] Promethazine is largely used in situations in which stimuli are severe and to treat established motion sickness. Several lines of evidence suggest that dextroamphetamine and related sympathomimetic agents also have significant efficacy in individuals experiencing motion sickness.[22,23] They often are used in conjunction with scopolamine or promethazine to increase efficacy and attenuate the adverse effects associated with these agents.[24–26] Scopolamine transdermal patch is as efficacious or more efficacious than dimenhydrinate.[27] This topical preparation is applied behind the ear at least 8 hours before the motion sickness stimulus is to begin. This formulation provides continuous systemic concentrations of scopolamine for 72 hours. Its convenience and long duration of action would make it particularly beneficial for P.C.'s protracted cruise. Commonly reported adverse effects associated with the scopolamine patch include dry mouth, drowsiness, blurred vision, and occasional confusional states and visual hallucinations, particularly in the elderly.

A scopolamine patch is the most appropriate drug product for P.C. in view of her high risk and prolonged exposure to motion. Promethazine (oral or rectal) may be prescribed for as-needed use. Table 8-5 outlines effective regimens for the

Table 8-4	Recommendations for Travelers

I.   Short-term exposure (≤6 hr)
   A.   Mild to moderate
      1.   Recommended
         a.   Dimenhydrinate
      2.   Alternatives
         a.   Meclizine
         b.   Promethazine
   B.   Intensive
      1.   Recommended
         a.   Promethazine plus amphetamine
      2.   Alternatives
         a.   Dimenhydrinate
         b.   Scopolamine patch
II.   Long-term exposure (>6 hr)
   A.   Mild
      1.   Recommended
         a.   Dimenhydrinate as needed
      2.   Alternatives
         a.   Scopolamine patch
         b.   Meclizine as needed
         c.   Promethazine as needed
   B.   Moderate to severe
      1.   Recommended
         a.   Scopolamine patch
      2.   Alternatives
         a.   Repeated doses of dimenhydrinate
         b.   Repeated doses of promethazine
         c.   Repeated doses of meclizine

Adapted from Committee to Advise on Tropical Medicine and Travel (CATMAT). Statement on motion sickness. Can Commun Dis Rep 1996:101.

prevention of motion sickness, and Table 8-6 recommends general measures for the prevention of motion sickness.

2. R.W. is a 50-year-old man who presents with the chief complaint of inability to ambulate because of severe nausea and vomiting. R.W. reports the recent onset of severe symptoms associated with any movement of his head. He also complains of sweating, headache, and dizziness. The diagnostic workup revealed lung cancer with central nervous system metastases that involved a large area of the cerebellum. What would you recommend as antiemetic therapy for this individual?

R.W.'s symptoms of motion sickness are stimulated by change in position of the head, presumably secondary to the presence of the tumor. Although neural mismatch between the vestibular, visual, and proprioceptive systems is the major factor contributing to motion sickness, motion sickness can be provoked by vestibular stimulation. Traditional treatment regimens for nausea and vomiting associated with vestibular disorders of any etiology include antihistamines and anticholinergic agents. Ideally, the primary problem affecting the vestibular apparatus should be corrected, which may be difficult to accomplish quickly in this patient. Treatment with promethazine should be initiated, and a short course of dextroamphetamine may be tried if symptoms are not adequately controlled with optimized doses of promethazine.

Little systematic research exists to assist in identifying agents beyond those traditionally used for motion sickness,

Table 8-5   Recommendations for Prevention of Motion Sickness

Drug	U.S. Availability	Oral Dose (mg)	Time to Efficacy (hr)	Dose Frequency (hr)	Use in Pregnancy	Use in Children
Amphetamine	Yes	5–10	1–2	Q 4–6	No	Not <3 yr
Cyclizine	Yes	50	1–2	Q 4–6	? No	Yes
Dimenhydrinate	Yes	50–100	1–2	Q 4–6	? No	Not <2 yr
Meclizine	Yes	25–50	2	Q 6–24	? No	Yes
Promethazine	Yes	25	1.5–2	Q 4–6	Yes	Not <2 yr
Scopolamine patch	Yes	Patch	8	Q 72	No	No

Adapted from Committee to Advise on Tropical Medicine and Travel (CATMAT). Statement on motion sickness. Can Commun Dis Rep 1996:101.

Table 8-6   General Measures for Prevention of Motion Sickness

Minimize exposure
Be located in the middle of the plane or boat where movement is least
Be in a semirecumbent position
Minimize head and body movements
Restrict visual activity
Fix vision on the horizon or some other stable external object
Avoid fixation on a moving object
Avoid reading
Close eyes if below deck or in an enclosed cabin
Improve ventilation and remove noxious stimuli
Reduce the magnitude of the motion stimulus
Avoid or minimize acceleration and deceleration and turning or moving of the vehicle
Engage in distracting activity
Be in control of the vehicle
Perform mental activity

but other classes of agents are under study. Conflicting information exists regarding the use of ginger as an antiemetic,[28–30] and preliminary studies exist for the antidepressant, doxepin, and the anticonvulsant, phenytoin.[31–33]

POSTOPERATIVE NAUSEA AND VOMITING

3. J.M. is a 4-year-old boy who is admitted to the ambulatory care operative center for placement of tympanostomy tubes. Balanced anesthesia consisting of propofol, fentanyl, and isoflurane is planned for this operative procedure. What is the incidence of postoperative nausea and vomiting (PONV)? What are the risk factors? Should J.M. receive prophylactic antiemetic medications?

Incidence and Risk Factors

Estimates of the incidence of PONV vomiting have ranged from 1% to 43%, with some of the highest rates reported in recent studies.[34] This variability, in part, reflects the anesthetic used as well as patient-specific and surgical factors that influence the likelihood of emesis. Whether J.M. should receive prophylactic antiemetic therapy will be determined by his risk factors for PONV. Women are two to four times more likely to experience PONV than men.[35,36] Various reports suggest that

the incidence of PONV range from 5% in infancy to as high as 50% in late childhood and adolescence[37,38]; the incidence decreases after puberty. Another significant patient characteristic is a history of PONV or motion sickness, which has been shown to increase the risk threefold to sixfold over patients without a similar history.[39] Before the 1960s, the use of the anesthetic agents such as ether and cyclopropane significantly contributed to the incidence of PONV.[40] Changing patterns of anesthetic use with the growth of ambulatory surgery and same-day admission surgery has altered the incidence of PONV.[41] Essentially, all surgical patients receive several drugs in the preoperative period (balanced anesthesia), but there is less use of narcotic and anticholinergic premedication. Often, midazolam is the only sedative used in some same-day surgery centers. Narcotics are no longer commonly used as premedication for surgery but they may be used for sedation, for analgesia, or as a component of general anesthesia. Several studies have shown that narcotics increase the risk of PONV.[42] Anesthetics also vary in their propensity toward promoting PONV. An area of current controversy relates to the use of newer agents, such as propofol, which are thought by some to be less emetogenic.[43] In addition, certain types of surgery carry a greater risk for PONV. In adults, high incidences are found following intra-abdominal surgery (70%),[44] major gynecologic surgery (58%),[45] laparoscopic surgery (40% to 77%),[46] and ear, nose, and throat (ENT) surgery (71%).[47] In children, the surgical procedures associated with the high incidences of PONV include strabismus surgery (up to 85%)[48] and tonsillectomy (35% to 75%).[49] Given his age and operative procedure that involves the ear, presurgical prophylaxis for PONV is warranted in this patient.

Prevention

4. What agents are available to prevent PONV?

The pathophysiology of PONV is multifactorial and incompletely understood. The high frequency of emesis associated with operative procedures that involve the ear, nose, and throat suggest a significant contribution of cranial nerve VIII. Similarly, high incidences of PONV in procedures that involve the abdomen suggest a prominent role of vagal afferents in stimulating the emetic center as well. Although many agents are being used successfully to prevent PONV, the best studied and most effective agents include droperidol and the $5HT_3$-receptor antagonists. Table 8-7 provides current recommended doses of droperidol and $5HT_3$-receptor antagonists for this indication.

Table 8-7   Antiemetics for Management of Postoperative Nausea and Vomiting in Adults and Pediatrics

Agents	Regimen	Route
Prophylaxis—adults		
Droperidol	0.625–1.25 mg 5 min before terminating anesthesia	IV
Ondansetron	4 mg immediately before induction of anesthesia	IV
	8 mg 1 hr before induction of anesthesia	PO
Dolasetron	12.5 mg intraoperatively	IV
	100 mg 1 hr before induction of anesthesia	PO
Metoclopramide	10 mg given near end of procedure (20 mg may be used)	IV
Promethazine	25 mg 1 hr before induction of anesthesia	PO
	12.5–25 mg immediately before induction of anesthesia	
Prochlorperazine	5–15 mg 1 hr before induction of anesthesia	PO
	5–10 mg 1–2 hr before induction of anesthesia; may repeat once in 30 min if needed	IM
	5–10 mg 15–30 min before induction of anesthesia; may repeat once as needed	IV
Treatment—adults		
Ondansetron	1–4 mg postoperatively	IV
Metoclopramide	10 mg may be given Q 4–6 hr as needed postoperatively	IV
Promethazine	10–25 mg Q 4–6 hr as needed postoperatively	PO
	12.5–25 mg Q 4 hr as needed postoperatively	IM/IV
Prochlorperazine	5–15 mg postoperatively	PO
	5–10 mg; may repeat once in 30 min as needed	IM
	5–10 mg; may repeat once as needed	IV
Droperidol	0.625–0.125 mg as needed	IV
Dolasetron	12.5 mg postoperatively	IV
Prophylaxis—pediatrics		
Dolasetron	>2 yr old; 1.8 mg/kg immediately before induction	IV
Ondansetron	0.05 mg/kg (range, 0.05–0.15 mg/kg) ⎤ when	IV
Droperidol	0.015–0.075 mg/kg/dose ⎦→	IV
Treatment—pediatrics		
Chlorpromazine	0.55 mg/kg	PO/IM
Droperidol	0.1 mg/kg/dose	IV
Ondansetron	0.05 mg/kg/dose	IV

IM, intramuscularly; IV, intravenously; PO, orally

Adapted from ASHP Therapeutic Guidelines on the Pharmacologic Management of Nausea and Vomiting in Adult and Pediatric Patients Receiving Chemotherapy, Radiation Therapy or Undergoing Surgery. Am J Health Syst Pharm 1999;56:729.

A number of randomized controlled trials have compared droperidol with ondansetron.[50–54] Most studies found no significant difference between the two agents with regard to efficacy or toxicity, although several studies did report better results with one or the other. Most experts consider droperidol and 5HT$_3$-receptor antagonists equivalent for the prevention of PONV. Costs and patient-specific factors may dictate the choice of one or the other, but given the low-risk profile associated with both agents and the lack of obvious contraindication to either agent, the decision ultimately depends on comparative costs. Traditionally, both 5HT$_3$ receptor antagonists and droperidol were considered to have low side effect and low risk profiles. Recently, however, a black-box warning has been added to droperidol's prescribing information, which describes droperidol's association with QT interval prolongation, cardiac arrhythmias, torsades de pointes, ventricular tachycardia, and cardiac arrest. Although these events are rare, they have diminished the use of droperidol in the postoperative setting. The lower dosages of serotonin antagonists used for PONV significantly diminish their cost relative to the use of high dosages in chemotherapy-induced emesis. Despite the reduced cost of the 5HT$_3$-receptor antagonists for PONV,

droperidol costs significantly less than 5HT$_3$-receptor antagonists at $0.50 per dose. Other medications that are considered alternatives to droperidol and 5HT$_3$-receptor antagonists include prochlorperazine, metoclopramide, and promethazine.

Treatment

5. J.M. received ondansetron 4 mg intravenously intraoperatively. His recovery was uneventful, and he was discharged home. Several hours after returning home, J.M.'s mother called to report that he had an episode of emesis associated with ingestion of a cup of juice. What advice would you give J.M.'s mother?

Although use of prophylactic antiemetics decreases the incidence and severity of PONV, these measures do not uniformly eliminate the symptoms. Most clinical trials show complete response rates of 30% to 70%, depending on the patient population and surgical procedures. It is not surprising or alarming that J.M. has experienced an episode of vomiting hours after discharge from the recovery room. Fortunately, most PONV resolves within 24 hours. J.M.'s mother should be reassured that the single episode of emesis is not particularly worrisome or unexpected. Maintaining hydration is important, particularly in the pediatric patient, and if emetic episodes continue, treatment is warranted. Droperidol is available only as an intravenous formulation, eliminating its use in the outpatient setting. Therefore, therapeutic options are limited to additional doses of ondansetron or promethazine. Prochlorperazine and metoclopramide, alternative agents for PONV, are usually avoided in pediatric populations because of the high incidence of extrapyramidal side effects associated with their use in this age group. J.M. has received an optimal dose of a $5HT_3$-receptor antagonist for prevention of PONV. If episodes of emesis persist in the initial 24-hour period, a drug from another pharmacologic class or a second dose of serotonin-receptor antagonist can be considered. Promethazine is an effective and commonly used antiemetic in children that is available in a suppository formulation, which may be necessary if emesis continues.

RADIATION-INDUCED EMESIS

Incidence and Risk Factors

6. **A.A. is a 32-year-old woman with acute nonlymphocytic leukemia who is undergoing preparation for receipt of an allogenic bone marrow transplant. The conditioning regimen includes administration of total body irradiation (TBI), which will be administered as 13.2 Gy in 11 fractions over 4 days. What is the frequency of and what are the risk factors for radiation-induced emesis (RIE)? Should A.A. receive prophylaxis against RIE?**

Frequency, severity, and onset of RIE relate both to the emetogenic potential of the therapy and to the emetogenic risk profile of the patient.[55] The site of radiation is the primary factor to consider when anticipating the risk, onset, peak, and duration of nausea and vomiting associated with radiation therapy. TBI is associated with the highest incidence of nausea and vomiting. Other radiation-related factors include dose, rate, and field size. Emesis occurs more often in patients receiving treatment to large fields, such as total body or hemibody irradiation in doses larger than 5 Gy.[56,57] Irradiation to the upper abdomen, in particular, is associated with a high incidence of RIE. Patient-related factors that influence the risk of RIE are less well identified. Some investigators report young age, female gender, and previous experience of emesis as risk factors.[55] Similar to chemotherapy, there is some evidence that high alcohol consumption has a preventive effect against radiation-induced illness.

The pathophysiology of emesis recurring after irradiation is complex, multifactorial, and incompletely understood. Two leading hypotheses include release of free radicals and chemical neurotransmitters from host and tumor cells. These mediators may induce emesis by stimulating the VC via the CTZ or the peripheral vagal afferent pathways. An increase in 5-HIAA urinary excretion after upper and mid hemibody irradiation has been reported, providing evidence that serotonin stimulates the VC via the vagal afferent fibers.[58]

Unfortunately, the prophylaxis and management of nausea and vomiting in patients receiving irradiation have not been studied extensively or rigorously. Many of the studies suffer from poor design, patient selection, irradiation treatment, and definition of successful outcome. Currently, the greatest body of evidence supports the use of $5HT_3$-receptor antagonists in patients like A.A. who are scheduled to receive TBI.[59–63] Trials with $5HT_3$ antagonists also have been conducted in patients receiving hemibody irradiation and radiation therapy to the upper abdomen.[64–66] Ondansetron and granisetron have been the most extensively studied of the $5HT_3$-receptor antagonists, and currently, these products have FDA-approved labeling for radiation-induced emesis. The recommended dose of ondansetron is 8 mg orally, three times a day, and for granisetron, 2 mg orally once a day or 1 mg twice a day. Although A.A. is scheduled to receive TBI for 4 days without chemotherapy, many TBI regimens combine radiation with the administration of chemotherapeutic agents. If A.A. has been scheduled to receive chemotherapy along with her TBI, recommendations for antiemetic prophylaxis would be based on the emetogenic potential of the chemotherapy.

A double-blind, randomized, paralleled group multicenter study compared the safety and efficacy of granisetron 2 mg and ondansetron 8 mg three times daily with a historical control group, who received conventional antiemetics administered before fractionated TBI. The percentage of patients with no emetic episodes over the 4-day study period was 33% in the granisetron group, 27% in the ondansetron, and 0% in historical controls.[66] These data suggest that 2 mg of granisetron administered once a day is equivalent to 8 mg of ondansetron administered three times a day in patients receiving TBI.[66] One published study reports similar response rates in patients receiving oral dolasetron for the control of emesis during fractionated TBI and high-dose cyclophosphamide.[67] To summarize, although no comparative studies exist and little systematic research has been conducted to determine the optimal dose of $5HT_3$-receptor antagonists, their use in patients receiving TBI is advocated by all experts in the field.[17–19]

Prophylaxis

7. **A.A. receives a prophylactic regimen of 8 mg of oral ondansetron TID for each day of TBI administration. On the second day, she complains of severe nausea (10 on a 10-point visual analog scale) and has experienced two episodes of emesis. What additional interventions are appropriate at this time?**

It is not surprising that A.A. is experiencing nausea and vomiting despite prophylaxis with a $5HT_3$-receptor antagonist. Complete response rates range from 20% to 80% among published reports. Unfortunately, there is very little scientific evidence to guide treatment in A.A.'s case. Anecdotal evidence supports maintaining a $5HT_3$ antagonist and adding medications with different mechanisms of action and side effect profiles to the regimen. Examples of medications that might improve A.A.'s control of RIE include prochlorperazine, metoclopramide, thiethylperazine, and dexamethasone.

In addition to TBI, $5HT_3$ antagonists are indicated to prevent emesis induced by other forms of radiation therapy. Their use is recommended for patients scheduled for single-fraction radiation therapy in doses of 5 to 10 Gy to the upper abdomen and hemibody irradiation, particularly when administered to the upper abdomen. The recent International Consensus on Antiemetic Therapy Conference of the Multinational Association of Supportive Care in Cancer (MASCC) recom-

Table 8-8   Radiation-Induced Emesis: Radiation Emetic Risk Categories

Risk Categories	Area Receiving Radiation	Antiemetic Guideline
ASCO[18]		
High risk	Total body irradiation	Before each fraction: 5HT$_3$ antagonist
Intermediate risk	Hemibody irradiation	Before each fraction: 5HT$_3$ antagonist or dopamine-receptor
	Upper irradiation	antagonist
	Abdominal–pelvic	
	Mantle	
	Cranium (radiosurgery)	
	Craniospinal	
Low risk	Cranium only	As-needed basis: dopamine receptor or 5HT$_3$ antagonist
	Breast	
	Head and neck	
	Extremities	
	Pelvis	
	Thorax	

Emetogenic^a Potential of Radiation Therapy	Risk Profile^b of the Patient	Antiemetic Prophylaxis
MASCC[19]		
Severe	Normal	5HT$_3$ antagonists (PO/IV) or
	High	5HT$_3$ antagonists + dexamethasone
Moderate	Normal	None
	High	Non-5HT$_3$ antagonists or 5HT$_3$ antagonists (PO)
Mild	Normal	None
	High	None

^{a}Severe, total body irradiation, upper half body irradiation, total nodal irradiation, abdominal bath; moderate, lower thorax region, upper abdominal region, pelvis, lower half body irradiation; low, head and neck, extremities.
^{b}Risk profile includes age <50, female gender, alcohol consumption, and prior experience with nausea and vomiting.

mends that patients receiving highly emetogenic radiotherapy *should* receive 5HT$_3$-receptor antagonist antiemetics to prevent RIE (consensus high, confidence high).[68] Dexamethasone should be administered with a 5HT$_3$ antagonist for antiemetic prophylaxis when the emetogenic potential of the radiation therapy is severe and the risk profile of the patient is normal to high (consensus moderate, confidence moderate). Table 8-8 lists the ASCO and MASCC guidelines for prevention of RIE.

Although some evidence supports the use of 5HT$_3$-receptor antagonists in conventional daily fractionated radiation therapy to the abdominal region, the benefit of prophylaxis with 5HT$_3$-receptor antagonists in this setting is far less clear. A recent study indicates that dexamethasone has efficacy similar to 5HT$_3$-antagonists when given to patients receiving radiotherapy to the upper abdomen.[113] Dexamethasone (2 mg tid) has been shown to be more effective than placebo in patients receiving radiotherapy to fields involving the upper abdomen.[114]

The patients for whom prophylactic 5HT$_3$-receptor antagonists are indicated constitute a relatively small proportion of the total number of cancer patients who receive radiation therapy. If a patient who has not received prophylaxis with a 5HT$_3$ receptor antagonist develops RIE, prochlorperazine, metoclopramide, or thiethylperazine is recommended. Limited data exist to support the use of 5HT$_3$-receptor antagonists for treatment of established RIE.

CHEMOTHERAPY-INDUCED EMESIS

8.   **H.M. is a 58-year-old man with newly diagnosed adenocarcinoma. He is scheduled to receive his first course of** chemotherapy with cisplatin 100 mg/m^2 on day 1 and fluorouracil 1 g/m^2 per day for 5 days by continuous infusion. He will be receiving concomitant radiation therapy during the chemotherapy and for the following 3 weeks. Outline a plan to prevent and treat acute chemotherapy-induced emesis in this patient.

Prevalence and Duration

Nausea and vomiting are common complications of chemotherapy administration. Patients have reported that nausea and vomiting are among their most important concerns while receiving treatment.[69,70] One study that examined the influence and duration of nausea and vomiting in an outpatient population receiving a broad range of chemotherapy regimens reported that nausea was present in 50% and vomiting in 27% of patients on the day of chemotherapy administration.[71] Three days after chemotherapy, nausea was reported by 22% and vomiting by 11% of patients. Nausea persisted for 5 days in 14% of patients, and vomiting persisted in 2.5% of patients. Although nausea and vomiting are most common and usually most severe in the 24-hour period following chemotherapy administration (acute phase), these complications can persist for up to 5 days in a significant proportion of patients.

Emetogenic Potential of Chemotherapy

The single most important factor influencing the frequency with which acute nausea and vomiting develops after treatment with antineoplastic chemotherapy agents is the emetogenic potential of the chemotherapy administered.[71–74] The emetogenic potential is determined by examining the number of patients who experience one or more episodes of emesis in the first 24 hours following chemotherapy administration. Agents classified as highly emetogenic (level 5) are those that produce one or more episodes of vomiting within the first 24 hours in ≥90% of patients who receive it. Agents classified as moderately high (level 4) have a 60% to 90% frequency of acute emesis; level 3, 30% to 60% incidence of acute emesis; level 2, 10% to 30% incidence of acute emesis; and level 1, <10% incidence of acute emesis.

To determine the incidence of emesis for an individual agent, single-agent therapy studies that reported the frequency of nausea and vomiting were evaluated. These methods of classifying the emetogenic potential of single chemotherapy agents are limited by the lack of consistency among the studies in the dose and regimen prescribed and the incomplete reporting of nausea and vomiting. Thus, there are often discrepancies between various classification schemas for the emetogenic potential of chemotherapeutic agents. Another limitation for determining the emetogenic potential of chemotherapy lies in the fact that little information exists to describe how combinations of chemotherapeutic agents affect the emetogenic potential of their individual components. Clearly, a combination chemotherapy regimen is at least as emetogenic as the most emetogenic single agent it contains, but the relative contribution of other agents in the regimen is less clear. A proposed classification schema for determining the acute emetogenicity of combination cancer chemotherapy has been proposed by Hesketh and colleagues (Fig. 8-2).[72] Using the Lindley schema as a starting point,[71] a group of antiemetic researchers sought to develop a more comprehensive classification system that would (1) take into account not only the chemotherapy dose, but also the rate and route of administration; (2) include new antineoplastic agents; (3) define an algorithm to predict the emetogenicity of combination chemotherapy regimens; and (4) reflect a consensus of a group of investigators active in the area of chemotherapy-induced emesis (CIE) and its treatment.

The emetogenic potential of single-agent chemotherapy developed by this group is found in Table 8-9. The algorithm to determine the emetogenicity of combination chemotherapy

regimens was designed by a consensus panel (Figure 8-2). The final algorithm was developed after a database of patients treated with combination chemotherapy on the placebo arm of four randomized antiemetic trials was analyzed. It is important to point out that the database consisted of female patients receiving adjuvant chemotherapy for breast cancer, a patient population that has been shown to have a higher incidence of emesis after chemotherapy than other cancer patient populations. Therefore, the rules for combining individual agents may overpredict the emetogenic potential of combination regimens.

This classification system for emetogenicity is quite important in that it is used as the basis for appropriate selection of antiemetic regimens. For example, the emetogenic potential of chemotherapy regimens and recommendations for appropriate therapy offered by the ASHP[17] and NCCN[20] use the Hesketh nomogram to determine the emetogenic potential of combination chemotherapy regimens. However, the ASCO and the MASCC define emetogenic potential somewhat differently. The ASCO classifies highly emetogenic (cisplatin and noncisplatin agents) as intermediate risk and low risk, respectively. The MASCC classifies chemotherapy as having high-risk, moderately high-risk, low- to moderate-risk, and low-risk emetogenic potentials. Neither group uses the Hesketh algorithm to determine the emetogenicity of combination chemotherapy regimens. Rather, their recommendations are based on the premise that the most emetogenic agent in the regimen dictates the appropriate antiemetic therapy.

Some of the differences in emetogenic classifications used by the various guidelines can be simplified by critically inspecting the agents included in the high-risk, moderately high-risk, and low- to moderate-risk categories (categories 5, 4, and 3). All guidelines recommend the use of a 5HT$_3$-receptor antagonist plus dexamethasone for regimens containing cisplatin, dacarbazine, mechlorethamine, cyclophosphamide, ifosfamide, doxorubicin, epirubicin, and idarubicin. Regimens that are typically classified as intermediate risk or low to moderate risk for emesis include docetaxel, etoposide, gemc-

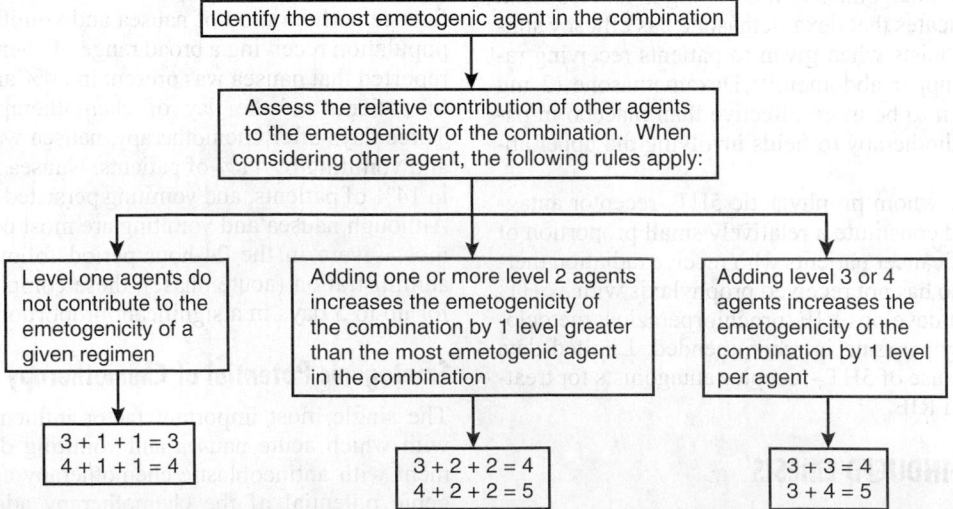

FIGURE 8-2 Algorithm for defining the emetogenicity of combination chemotherapy. (From Hesketh P et al. Proposal for classifying the acute emetogenicity of cancer chemotherapy. J Clin Oncol 1997;15:103.)

Table 8-9 Emetogenic Potential of Single Chemotherapy Agents

Hesketh[72]	ASCO[10]	MASCC[19]
Level 5	*High*	*High*
Carmustine (>250 mg/m²)	Cisplatin (>50 mg/m²)	Cisplatin
Cisplatin (>50 mg/m²)	Dacarbazine	Mechlorethamine
Cyclophosphamide	Actinomycin	Streptozocin
Dacarbazine (>500 mg/m²)	Mechlorethamine	Cyclophosphamide
Mechlorethamine	Carboplatin	Carmustine
Streptozocin	Cyclophosphamide (>1,500 mg/m²)	Dacarbazine
Level 4	Lomustine	*Moderate to High*
Carboplatin	Carmustine (>250 mg/m²)	Cisplatin
Carmustine (<250 mg/m²)	Daunorubicin	Cytarabine
Cisplatin (<50 mg/m²)	Doxorubicine	Carboplatin
Cyclophosphamide (>750–1,500 mg/m²)	Epirubicin	Ifosfamide
Cytarabine (>1 g/m²)	Idarubicin	Carmustine
Doxorubicin	Cytarabine (>1 g/m²)	Hexamethylmelamine
Methotrexate (>1,000 mg/m²)	Ifosfamide	Cyclophosphamide
Procarbazine (oral)	*Intermediate*	Anthracyclines
Level 3	Irinotecan	Topotecan
Cyclophosphamide (≤750 mg/m²)	Mitoxantrone	Cyclophosphamide (oral)
Cyclophosphamide (oral)	Paclitaxel	Procarbazine
Doxorubicin (20–60 mg/m²)	Docetaxel	Methotrexate
Epirubicin (≤90 mg/m²)	Mitomycin	Irinotecan
Hexamethylmelamine (oral)	Topotecan	Mitoxantrone
Idarubicin	Gemcitabine	*Low to Moderate*
Ifosfamide	Etoposide	Taxoids
Methotrexate (250–1,000 mg/m²)	Teniposide	Etoposide
Mitoxantrone (<15 mg/m²)	*Low*	Methotrexate
Level 2	Vinorelbine	Mitomycin
Docetaxel	Fluorouracil	Gemcitabine
Etoposide	Methotrexate (≤50 mg/m²)	Fluorouracil
5-Fluorouracil	Bleomycin	*Low*
Gemcitabine	Vinblastine	Bleomycin
Methotrexate (50 mg/m²; 250 mg/m²)	Vincristine	Busulfan
Mitomycin	Busulfan	Chlorambucil (oral)
Paclitaxel	Fludarabine	2-Chlorodeoxyadenosine
Level 1	Cladribine	Fludarabine
Bleomycin		Hydroxyurea
Busulfan (<4 mg/kg/day)		Methotrexate
Chlorambucil (oral)		L-phenylalanine mustard
2-Chlorodeoxyadenosine		6-Thioguanine (oral)
Fludarabine		Vinblastine
Hydroxyurea		Vincristine
Methotrexate (≤50 mg/m²)		Vinorelbine
L-phenylalanine mustard (oral)		
Thioguanine (oral)		
Vinblastine		
Vincristine		
Vinorelbine		

itabine, topotecan, mitomycin, and paclitaxel combination regimens. Although stratifying the dose of 5HT₃ antiemetic by emetogenic potential was once recommended, all guidelines now call for the maximally effective dose of 5HT₃ antagonist (combined with dexamethasone) that prevents acute (moderate or moderately high to high risk) CIE for level 3 to 5 regimens. For intermediate-risk or low- to moderate-risk regimens, a 5HT₃ antagonist, dexamethasone, or prochlorperazine is recommended. No prophylactic therapy is recommended for regimens containing agents with low emetogenic potential in any of the evidence-based guidelines published to date.

Other Risk Factors

Other factors that influence the incidence of acute CIE include gender and history of alcohol use. Women are at higher risk for CIE, and clinical trials with female subjects show a response rate that is about 20% lower than males. Past or current heavy use of alcohol (>12 drinks/week) confers a protective effect against CIE.[75] The influence of age is controversial. Although several other risk factors for CIE have been identified, selection of prophylactic therapy is based on the emetogenic potential of the chemotherapy and the patient's past response to chemotherapy and antiemetic therapy.

Table 8-10   Recommendations for Prevention of Acute Chemotherapy-Induced Emesis

Agent	Dose	Schedule[a]	Route
Adults			
Level 4–5 or moderate, moderately high, or high risk			
Ondansetron	8 mg	Single dose	IV
or	24 mg		PO
Granisetron	10 μg/kg	Single dose	IV
or	2 mg	Single dose	PO
Dolasetron	1.8 mg/kg or	Single dose	IV
or	100 mg	Single dose	PO
plus			
Dexamethasone	20 mg	Single dose	PO or IV
Level 3 or intermediate, low to moderate risk			
Ondansetron	8 mg	BID	PO
or			
Granisetron	2 mg	QD	PO
or			
Dolasetron	100 mg	QD	PO
or			
Palonosetron	0.25 mg	Single dose	IV
Dexamethasone	8 mg	BID	PO
Pediatrics			
Level 3–5			
Ondansetron	0.15 mg/kg/dose	4 hr × 3	IV
Granisetron	20–40 μg/kg	Single dose	IV
Dolasetron	1.8 mg/kg	Single dose	IV
plus			
Dexamethasone	5–10 mg/m^2	Single dose	PO or IV

[a]Single dose administered once 15–60 minutes before chemotherapy administration.
IV, intravenously; PO, orally.
Adapted from references 17–20 and product information.

Serotonin Receptor Antagonists

H.M. is receiving a combination chemotherapy regimen classified as highly emetogenic on day 1 and low emetogenicity on days 2 to 5. Therefore, the appropriate prophylactic antiemetic premedication should include a 5HT$_3$-receptor antagonist. Table 8-10 provides recommendations for specific 5HT$_3$ antagonists, doses, schedules, and route by level of emetogenicity, which are based on randomized controlled studies and FDA-approved labeling. A single dose administered before chemotherapy will produce optimal protection. This is consistent with the theory that serotonin release from enterochromaffin cells subsequently stimulates vagal afferent nerves to produce nausea. Thus, blockade of these receptors before chemotherapy is administered is the most critical determinant of their success. Repeated administration of 5HT$_3$ antagonists during the acute phase does not confer additional benefits.

Palonosetron is the newest 5HT$_3$-receptor antagonist to be marketed in the United States. Palonosetron differs from the other 5HT$_3$ antagonists in that they have higher receptor binding and a longer plasma elimination half-life of approximately 40 hours. Two studies in patients receiving moderately emetogenic chemotherapy regimens reported statistically superior delayed emesis control with a single palonosetron (0.25 mg IV) compared to a small dose of dolasetrol (100 mg IV) and ondansetron (32 mg IV).[110,111] A trial comparing palonosetron (0.25 and 0.75 mg IV) with ondansetron (32 mg IV) in patients receiving cisplatin based chemotherapy reported no significant difference in acute or delayed emesis control.[112] The improvement in delayed emesis control in patients receiving palonosetron for moderately emetogenic regimens likely reflects the prolonged half-life of palonosetron providing modest protection against emesis on days 2 and 3. It is reasonable to assume that repeat dosing of other 5HT$_3$ antagonists would have provided similar benefits.

Dose of 5HT$_3$ Antagonist

It is important to make one point regarding intravenous dose recommendations for level 4 and 5 emetogenic chemotherapy. There is controversy regarding the optimal intravenous dose of ondansetron for prevention of acute CIE. Based on a single U.S. study that showed 32 mg to be superior to 8 mg, 32 mg is the current FDA-approved dose in the United States.[76] In contrast, at least two European studies showed that 8 mg and 32 mg are equally efficacious; thus, the 8-mg dose of ondansetron is currently approved in Europe. One important difference between the European studies and the U.S. study was that the median dose of cisplatin in the U.S. study was higher than those used in the European studies. Guidelines for the prevention and treatment of CIE developed by professional organizations suggest 8-mg intravenous doses.[17–20]

The FDA-approved dose of dolasetron is 1.8 mg/kg or a 100-mg fixed dose. Dose ranging studies with this agent demonstrated that doses of 1.2 mg/kg and 2.4 mg/kg were

Table 8-11   Standard Doses of Non–5HT$_3$-Receptor Antagonist Antiemetics for Prevention and Management of Chemotherapy-Induced Emesis

Agents	Dose/Schedule[a]	Route
Phenothiazines		
Prochlorperazine	10–40 mg Q 6–8 hr	PO, IV, IM
	25 mg Q 6–8 hr	PR
Thiethylperazine	10 mg Q 8 hr	PO, IM, IV, PR
Perphenazine	4–5 mg Q 6 hr	PO, IV, IM
Butyrophenones		
Haloperidol	1–3 mg Q 2–8 hr	PO, IM, IV
Droperidol	5–15 mg × 1; 2-7.5 mg Q 2 hr	IV
Cannabinoids		
Marinol	5–10 mg/m² Q 3–4 hr	PO
Corticosteroids		
Dexamethasone	20 mg before chemotherapy	PO, IV
	4–8 mg Q 12 hr (delayed)	PO
Methylprednisolone	0.5–1 mg/kg before chemotherapy or Q 12 hr IV (maximum total 4 mg/kg/24 hr)	IM, PO
Substituted benzamides		
Metoclopramide	1–3 mg/kg Q 2 hr × 2–5 doses (maximum total, 12 mg/kg/24 hr)	IV
	0.5 mg/kg Q 2–6 hr (delayed)	PO
Benzodiazepines		
Lorazepam	1–2 mg before chemotherapy	IV, SL
	1 mg Q 6–12 hr	PO
Miscellaneous		
ACTH	1 mg Q 12 hr × 3	IM
Scopolamine	1 patch Q 72 hr	TD
NK$_1$ receptor antagonist Aprepitant	125 mg on day 1, then 80 mg on days 2 and 3	PO

[a]Dose and schedule pertain to use as antiemetics with chemotherapy only.
ACTH, adrenocorticotropin hormone; IM, intramuscularly; IV, intravenously; PO, orally; PR, per rectum; SL, sublingually; TD, transdermally.
Adapted from references 17–20 and product information.

both inferior to 1.8 mg/kg. Therefore, it may be advisable to restrict the use of the 100-mg fixed dose to patients weighing between approximately 50 and 70 kg.

Oral Versus Intravenous Route

For many years, it was believed that intravenous administration of serotonin antagonists was necessary to prevent acute CIE. Recognizing that the primary benefit of these agents is protection against emesis and not active treatment, studies have begun to investigate use of the oral route of administration. Currently, only granisetron and ondansetron have data to support a single oral dose before highly emetogenic chemotherapy.[77,78] Oral dolasetron is approved for use with moderately emetogenic chemotherapy regimens. Studies are currently being conducted to identify the optimal oral dose of dolasetron in the setting of highly emetogenic chemotherapy.

Efficacy

The percentage of patients who experience complete total control (defined as no nausea and no vomiting) for a 24-hour period following chemotherapy administration depends on the emetogenic potential of the chemotherapy. Approximately 40% to 60% of patients given single intravenous doses of 5HT$_3$ antagonists for highly emetogenic chemotherapy will have total control. This percentage of patients with total con-

trol increases as the emetogenic potential of the chemotherapy decreases.

NK$_1$ Receptor Antagonists

Efficacy and Dose

Aprepitant, a recently marketed NK$_1$ receptor antagonist, was studied in two multicenter, randomized, parallel, double-blind, controlled clinical trials. Relative to a combination of 5HT$_3$ receptor antagonists plus dexamethasone, complete control (no vomiting and no use of rescue medication) was improved by 11% and 15% in the first 24 hours following chemotherapy.[14] Relative to dexamethasone alone, aprepitant improved complete control of delayed emesis by 19% and 21% when added to conventional doses of dexamethasone. In both trials, cisplatin was administered at a dose >50 mg/m² (mean cisplatin dose was equal to 80.2 mg/m²). A total of 1,045 patients were represented in these two clinical trials. Aprepitant was administered as a 125 mg oral dose before chemotherapy on day 1 and 80 mg orally on days 2 and 3. This dose was selected because it was recognized early in phase II trials that aprepitant inhibits its own metabolism; therefore, 80 mg on days 2 and 3 produced the same systemic exposure as 125 mg administered on day 1.

Aprepitant is extensively metabolized by CYP3A4 and is a moderate inhibitor of CYP3A4 when administered acutely. With more prolonged administration (>14 days), aprepitant is a moderate to weak inducer of CYP3A4. For this reason, the dose of dexamethasone was reduced on day 1 to 12 mg followed by 8 mg once a day on days 2 and 3, as compared to the standard regimen that consisted of 20 mg once a day on day 1 and 8 mg twice a day on days 2, 3, and 4.

Drug Interactions

Because a number of antineoplastic agents are primarily metabolized by CYP3A4, the product information for aprepitant suggests that it be used cautiously in patients receiving certain drugs. Inhibition of CYP3A4 by aprepitant could result in elevated plasma concentrations of these agents. The effect of aprepitant on the pharmacokinetics of CYP3A4 substrates administered orally is expected to be greater than that when the same substrates are administered intravenously, because a major site of aprepitant's 3A4 inhibition is located in the GI tract. Despite these warnings, approximately 20% of the patients in the phase II trials were receiving antineoplastics metabolized by CYP3A4. No significant differences were observed in the adverse effect profiles of those in this group receiving aprepitant versus those receiving standard antiemetic therapy. However, these trials were not designed to assess the effect of aprepitant on concomitantly administered antineoplastic agents that are metabolized by CYP3A4; studies designed to address these questions are ongoing.

Separately, aprepitant was shown to reduce the metabolism of S-warfarin and tolbutamide, which are metabolized by CYP2C9. Therefore, coadministration of aprepitant with these drugs or other drugs that are known to be metabolized by CYP2C9, such as phenytoin, may result in lower plasma concentrations of these drugs. A single 125 mg dose of aprepitant was administered on day 1, 80 mg on days 2 and 3, to healthy subjects who were stabilized with chronic warfarin therapy. Although there was no effect of aprepitant on the plasma area under the curve (AUC) of R or S-warfarin on day 3, there was a 34% decrease in the S-warfarin trough concentration accompanied by a 14% decrease in the prothrombin time 5 days after aprepitant dosing was completed. Product information recommends that the international normalized ratio (INR) be monitored closely in the 2-week period following initiation of the 3-day regimen of aprepitant, particularly during posttreatment days 7 through 10. However, increasing the dose of warfarin at this point would be illogical because the induction effect of aprepitant on 2C9 would have recovered and an increase in INR would be expected in the absence of a dosage increase. The effect of aprepitant on warfarin is small and many patients would probably remain within the therapeutic range with a 14% reduction in INR. However, if patients are at the low end of the INR therapeutic range and are scheduled to receive aprepitant, it may be advisable to increase the dose before or concurrent with the initiation of aprepitant therapy. Unfortunately, none of this information has been published and the best source of data is the FDA website, which contains the data presented for regulatory approval.[14]

In summary, aprepitant works through a novel substance P pathway and has been shown to enhance control of cisplatin-induced acute and delayed CINV. Therefore, H.M. should receive the standard aprepitant regimen, 125 mg orally on day 1 followed by 80 mg orally on days 2 and 3 in addition to 5HT$_3$ receptor antagonists and dexamethasone. Aprepitant is not yet included in consensus guidelines for highly emetogenic chemotherapy only because they were established before its availability.

Dexamethasone

Dexamethasone is a highly effective antiemetic agent, which improves response rates of the serotonin-receptor antagonists by 15% to 30%. The optimal dose of dexamethasone to prevent acute CINV induced by cisplatin was recently identified as 20 mg administered intravenously as a single dose although this dose was not statistically superior to a 12 mg IV dose. The optimal dose of dexamethasone to prevent acute emesis in patients receiving moderately to highly emetogenic noncisplatin regimens was recently identified as 8 mg IV.[79] Dexamethasone may be administered either by the oral or the intravenous route because of its high bioavailability. The side effects associated with the single 20-mg dose of dexamethasone in this setting are few to none. Dexamethasone is also effective in the treatment of delayed nausea and vomiting, as discussed in question 9.

Lorazepam

Lorazepam in doses of 1 to 2 mg is often combined with serotonin-receptor antagonists and dexamethasone as premedication for administration of moderately high to highly emetogenic chemotherapy. Lorazepam was initially used to produce retrograde amnesia and to prevent the development of anticipatory nausea and vomiting, but it also mitigates the side effects associated with high-dose metoclopramide regimens. Although serotonin-receptor antagonists have replaced metoclopramide-based regimens, lorazepam still has a role as an antiemetic premedication. Clearly, administration of chemotherapy is an anxiety-provoking situation that may lead to anticipatory nausea and vomiting. Lorazepam's anxiolytic properties may reduce the incidence of anticipatory nausea and vomiting by providing a calming effect. Although lorazepam is not a recognized antiemetic agent, many patients feel that it is helpful for relieving delayed nausea and vomiting, as discussed further in question 9.

H.M. is a hospitalized patient who will receive highly emetogenic chemotherapy. There is no harm associated with sedation, and because he is likely to experience nausea and vomiting at some point during the course of therapy, lorazepam is indicated. In summary, he should receive a single dose of a 5HT$_3$ antagonist in conjunction with dexamethasone 12 mg and lorazepam 1 to 2 mg to decrease his likelihood of experiencing acute CINV. Aprepitant should be administered as described above to increase control of acute and delayed CINV. The dexamethasone dose should be reduced from the standard 20 mg to 12 mg because it will be administered with aprepitant.[19–21] The oral route of administration for all four agents is as efficacious as intravenous administration, is more convenient, and less expensive.

Delayed Chemotherapy-Induced Emesis

Prophylaxis: Cisplatin Regimens

9. H.M. was premedicated with a serotonin receptor antagonist and dexamethasone before cisplatin administration but did not receive aprepitant or prophylactic medication for delayed chemotherapy-induced emesis. He experienced no nausea and vomiting over the first 24 hours. However, a few hours thereafter, he began to complain of nausea and started retching. Assess H.M.'s case. Should he have received additional prophylactic antiemetic therapy? If he had not received cisplatin, would additional prophylaxis be recommended?

H.M. is experiencing delayed emesis, which has traditionally been defined as beginning ≥24 hours after chemotherapy. Observation of emesis patterns suggests that the syndrome can begin as early as 16 hours after cisplatin administration or beyond 24 hours with cyclophosphamide. The incidence and severity of delayed vomiting is greatest between 48 and 72 hours after cisplatin administration.[81-82] The period from 24 to 96 hours after chemotherapy is the time when rescue antiemetic treatment is most often required. Individuals who do not experience acute vomiting typically are less likely to experience delayed vomiting.[83]

H.M. should have received additional antiemetic prophylaxis for delayed emesis. Prophylaxis for delayed nausea and vomiting is clearly defined only for cisplatin-based regimens and has traditionally been initiated the morning following cisplatin administration. Recognizing the earlier onset of delayed emesis following cisplatin administration, many oncologists prefer to begin prophylactic antiemetics the evening or night of the day cisplatin will be given. Dexamethasone 4 to 8 mg twice daily plus metoclopramide 0.5 mg/kg orally four times daily or a $5HT_3$ antagonist twice daily are the currently recommended prevention regimens for delayed emesis,[84] although some use dexamethasone alone.[85,86] When a $5HT_3$-receptor antagonist is added to dexamethasone, the combination is more effective than the $5HT_3$-receptor antagonist alone,[87] but other studies have found that dexamethasone alone is as effective or more effective than a $5HT_3$-receptor antagonist alone, particularly in patients receiving less than highly emetogenic regimens.[88,89]

The pivotal phase III trials that led to the approval of aprepitant defined dexamethasone alone as the standard of care for prophylaxis of delayed nausea and vomiting. In this setting, the addition of aprepitant improved complete control in the delayed emesis phase by approximately 20% in patients receiving high-dose cisplatin.[14] There were some limitations to this study. Aprepitant should have been coadministered with a $5HT_3$ antagonist and dexamethasone on day 1 and with dexamethasone alone or, perhaps, a combination of dexamethasone and $5HT_3$ antagonist or metoclopramide on days 2, 3, and 4. The use of aprepitant plus dexamethasone (double therapy) compared to aprepitant, dexamethasone, and $5HT_3$ antagonists (triple therapy) in delayed cisplatin-induced emesis has not been evaluated. Similarly, the combination of aprepitant and dexamethasone has not been compared to standard two-drug delayed prophylaxis regimens consisting of dexamethasone combined with metoclopramide or a $5HT_3$ antagonist.

Prophylaxis: Noncisplatin Regimens

Although many patients experience delayed symptoms, it is unclear whether prophylactic therapy is indicated for patients receiving noncisplatin-containing regimens. For highly emetogenic noncisplatin chemotherapy, most guidelines support the use of combination therapy with dexamethasone and metoclopramide or a $5HT_3$ antagonist. Aprepitant is indicated for prophylaxis of acute and delayed CINV in patients receiving highly emetogenic chemotherapy. However, no studies have evaluated its use in noncisplatin regimens to date.

For moderately emetogenic chemotherapy regimens, oncologists often prescribe single-agent antiemetics to be taken on an as-needed basis in the delayed period, particularly after the first course of chemotherapy. Agents commonly prescribed include prochlorperazine, thiethylperazine, metoclopramide, dexamethasone, and ondansetron. Although lorazepam is technically not an antiemetic, many patients report that it helps control nausea. There is no clear evidence to support superior efficacy and lower toxicity for any single agent. However, dexamethasone is traditionally viewed as the most effective single agent for prevention and treatment of delayed emesis.

Breakthrough Emesis

10. C.L. is a 42 year-old woman receiving adjuvant chemotherapy for early stage breast cancer with cyclophosphamide and doxorubicin. She received a single oral dose of a $5HT_3$ antagonist plus dexamethasone before chemotherapy and a prescription for oral ondansetron (8 mg BID) and oral dexamethasone (8 mg BID) for the delayed emesis prophylaxis. It is now 36 hours after chemotherapy administration. Despite prophylaxis for acute CIE and oral ondansetron plus dexamethasone for delayed emesis, C.L. began to vomit 24 hours after chemotherapy administration. She has vomited four times in the last 12 hours and complains of severe nausea. What does this scenario represent and how should C.L. be managed at this time?

C.L. has breakthrough emesis, defined as symptoms that occur despite adequate prophylactic therapy. Not every episode of breakthrough emesis requires administration of rescue antiemetics. Many patients will experience one to two episodes of emesis despite adequate prophylaxis during the 2- to 5-day period following chemotherapy. If treatment is desirable, and in this case it clearly is, an agent with a different mechanism of action should be used. Most patients who receive moderate to highly emetogenic chemotherapy agents or regimens will have received dexamethasone and a serotonin antagonist; thus, a dopamine-receptor antagonist such as prochlorperazine or metoclopramide would be most appropriate for breakthrough symptoms. If C.L. had or does receive a dopamine-receptor antagonist and emesis persists, addition of dronabinol should be considered.

Patients who experience nausea and vomiting during the delayed phase should begin to take at least one antiemetic agent as described earlier. If emesis occurs despite the scheduled use of a single agent, the addition of a second agent with a different mechanism of action is recommended. Unfortunately, the use of aprepitant in a patient who is actually experiencing nausea and vomiting following chemotherapy has not been studied. However, a standard combination regimen for prevention of delayed emesis has failed in C.L., and the use of prophylactic aprepitant with the next cycle of chemotherapy is strongly advised.

Refractory Emesis

Refractory emesis can be defined as nausea and vomiting unresponsive to standard therapy (prophylaxis or treatment). It is commonly encountered in patients receiving high-dose chemotherapy with multiple alkylating agents and stem cell support. Antiemetic therapy in this population generally consists of a corticosteroid, serotonin antagonist, dopamine-receptor antagonist, and dexamethasone. However, some bone marrow transplantation programs prohibit the use of dexamethasone in patients receiving transplants for hematologic malignancies because of unfounded concerns of increased risk of infection. Other interventions used for refractory emesis include high-dose metoclopramide (2 mg/kg intravenous bolus, followed by 0.5 mg/kg per hour) or droperidol (5 to 15 mg intravenously, followed by 5 to 7.5 mg intravenously every 2 hours for 6 to 8 hours). Few, if any, trials have evaluated the optimal intervention for refractory emesis. The principle of combining active agents with different mechanisms of action is most likely to be successful. Similar to patients who experience breakthrough emesis despite prophylactic antiemetic therapy, the addition of serotonin antagonists, corticosteroids, dopamine-receptor antagonists, anxiolytics and dronabinol should be considered.

Pediatric Use

11. Are there special considerations for antiemetic use in pediatric patients receiving chemotherapy?

Few studies have attempted to describe the incidence, duration, and optimal management of CINV in the pediatric population. In the absence of information specific for pediatric patients, there are many variations in the indications and schedules of administration for 5HT$_3$-receptor antagonists and corticosteroids for this population.

Currently, the recommended ondansetron dosage is 0.15 mg/kg every 4 hours for three doses. The granisetron and dolasetron dosages recommended for pediatric patients are 10 μg/kg for granisetron and 1.8 mg/kg for dolasetron. These dosages translate into the currently approved, recommended single dose for granisetron and dolasetron. Although the use of single-dose 5HT$_3$-receptor antagonists in pediatric patients has not been studied, many centers have adopted this treatment approach. Similarly, oral dosing of 5HT$_3$ antagonists follows the same dosing guidelines in pediatric patients as in adults.[17–20]

A corticosteroid should be administered along with a 5HT$_3$ antagonist in pediatric patients who receive moderately to highly emetogenic chemotherapy regimens (Table 8-11). Both dexamethasone and methylprednisolone have been used. Dexamethasone (5 to 10 mg/m^2) and methylprednisolone (2 to 4 mg/kg) are administered as a single dose before chemotherapy or at intervals of 4 hours (methylprednisolone, maximum dose is 4 mg/kg per 24 hours) or 12 hours (dexamethasone, maximum dose is 20 mg/24 hours). These also can be administered by the oral route.

Most pediatric patients have a much greater risk of extrapyramidal symptoms (EPS) with dopamine-receptor antagonists than do adults. Thus, antiemetics with a high potential to produce EPS (e.g., metoclopramide, prochlorperazine, haloperidol) are not recommended for use in pediatric patients. This limits available choices for acute, delayed, and refractory emesis. Chlorpromazine has a lower potential for producing EPS and can be administered safely to children. However, evidence supporting the efficacy of this agent in the pediatric population is mixed.[89–91]

NONPHARMACOLOGIC THERAPIES FOR NAUSEA AND VOMITING

The precepts of traditional Chinese medicine are based on the belief that 14 major "life channels" interact to produce health and well-being. Alterations in these channels, charted on the body surface as meridians, result in disease and disorder. Stimulation of the meridian associated with symptoms of illness restores normal balance and relieves symptoms. The Neiguan point is located on the inner surface of the wrist below the tendon of the flexor carpi radialis and the palmaris longus, 3 to 5 cm proximal to the flexor grip. Several studies have suggested that acupuncture or acupressure stimulation of the Neiguan point is associated with significant relief from nausea and vomiting related to pregnancy, anesthesia, and chemotherapy.[93–95] Similar studies have documented suppression of nausea and vomiting by transcutaneous electrical nerve stimulation (TENS) over the Neiguan point.[96–97] Recently, a miniaturized wristband unit (ReliefBand) was developed and approved by the FDA to relieve symptoms of nausea and vomiting due to chemotherapy, motion sickness, pregnancy, and therapy related to AIDS. The ReliefBand is designated as neurostimulation therapy (NST). It differs from TENS in that it stimulates one location (i.e., the wrist) and produces a response in a remote location (i.e., the stomach). TENS devices use electrical stimulation to block nerve messages in close proximity to the point of application. For example, a TENS unit may be applied to a muscle in the back with the intent to relieve pain in that muscle. Another difference between NST and TENS is based on fundamental differences in the way each stimulates nerves. A TENS device uses faster, more powerful pulsing, which has the effect of jamming nerve communication, whereas NST devices provide slower, weaker electrical pulses, which may actually cause nerves to trigger rather than be blocked. Several studies have demonstrated positive results associated with the ReliefBand.[98,99,100] Additional work will be required to identify the optimal place for the use of this new commercially available device.

The National Institutes of Health Consensus Development Conference on Acupuncture, held in 1977, concluded that there is "clear evidence that needle acupuncture treatment is effective for postoperative and chemotherapy-induced nausea and vomiting, nausea, pregnancy, and postoperative dental pain."[101] The Panel issued their consensus statement after an extensive review of existing medical literature and a series of presentations by acupuncture research experts at a 3-day conference.

CANNABIS: INHALED VERSUS INGESTED

Natural and synthetic cannabinoids are known to be effective antiemetic agents.[102–105] Delta-9-terahydrocannabinol (THC) has been found to be superior to prochlorperazine.[106] Patients whose conditions are refractory to standard antiemetic agents have significant reduction in nausea and vomiting with oral THC.[105,107] There is little information on the efficacy of inhalation marijuana aside from anecdotal reports from patients who obtained the drug privately. A prospective pilot study of inhaled marijuana as an antiemetic for cancer chemotherapy was conducted in 57 patients who showed no improvement with standard antiemetic agents. Seventy-eight percent had a positive response to marijuana.[105] Younger age and prior marijuana exposure were factors that predicted positive response to treatment. Because of a lack of a randomized, placebo-control group, the precise role of inhaled marijuana is unknown. To date, only one trial reported in abstract form has directly compared THC and marijuana as chemotherapy antiemetics. The antiemetic efficacy and pharmacokinetics of ingested Delta-9-THC versus smoked marijuana were compared in 20 chemotherapy patients. A double-blind, double-dummy crossover design was used with the first and second consecutive identical courses of chemotherapy. Smoking was closely supervised to quantitatively follow an established technique. The mean age of patients was 54; 15 were male; 14 had bronchogenic carcinoma; and all received either two or three chemotherapy agents, including Adriamycin (17), cyclophosphamide (15), and cisplatin (12). Nine patients had no preference for either study drug; seven preferred THC; four preferred inhaled marijuana ($P > 0.1$). Seven had distortions of time perception or hallucinations (five with THC, three with marijuana, one with both).[108]

REFERENCES

1. Lindley CM et al. Quality of life consequences of chemotherapy-induced emesis. Qual Life Res 1992;1:331.
2. Andrews PLR, Davis CJ. The mechanism of emesis induced by anticancer therapies. In: Andrews PLR, Sanger GJ, eds. Emesis in Anticancer Therapy. London: Chapman and Hall Medical, 1993:113.
3. Borison HL, McCarthy LE. Neuropharmacology of chemotherapy-induced emesis. Drugs 1983;25(Suppl 1):8.
4. Borison HL, Wang SC. Functional localization of central coordinating mechanism for emesis in cat. J Neurophysiology 1949;12:305.
5. Borison HL, Wang SC. Physiology and pharmacology: vomiting. Pharmacol Rev 1953;5:193.
6. Borison HL et al. Central emetic action of pilocarpine in the cat. J Neuropathol Exp Neurol 1956;15:485.
7. Borison HL, Fairbanks VF. Mechanism of veratrum induced emesis in the cat. J Pharmacol Exp Ther 1952;104:398.
8. Andrews PLR et al. Neuropharmacology of emesis and its relevance to anti-emetic therapy. Supp Care Cancer 1998;6:197.
9. Cubeddu LX et al. Clinical evidence for the involvement of serotonin in acute cytotoxic-induced emesis. In: Reynolds J et al., eds. Serotonin and the scientific basis of antiemetic therapies. Oxford: Oxford Clinical Communications, 1995:142.
10. Cubeddu LX et al. Plasma chromogranin A marks emesis and serotonin release associated with dacarbazine and nitrogen mustard but not with cyclophosphamide-based chemotherapies. Br J Cancer 1995;72:1033.
11. Takeda N et al. Neurochemical mechanisms of motion sickness. Am J Otolaryngol 1989;10:351.
12. Andrews PLR, Bhandari PB. Resinferatoxin, an ultrapotent capsaicin analogue, has anti-emetic properties in the ferret. Neuropharmacology 1993;32:799.
13. Campos D et al. Prevention of cisplatin-induced emesis by the oral neurokinin-1 antagonist, MK-869, in combination with granisetron and dexamethasone or with dexamethasone alone. J Clin Oncol 2001;19:1759.
14. Aprepitant product information and FDA website www.FDS.gov/ohrms/dockets/ac/03/briefing/3928B1.
15. Hargreaves R. Imaging substance P receptors (NK1) in the living human brain using positron emission tomography. J Clin Psychiatry 2002;63(Suppl 11):18.
16. Committee to Advise on Tropical Medicine and Travel (CATMAT). Statement on motion sickness. Can Commun Dis Rep 1996:101–110.
17. ASHP Therapeutic Guidelines on the Pharmacologic Management of Nausea and Vomiting in Adult and Pediatric Patients Receiving Chemotherapy, Radiation Therapy or Undergoing Surgery. Am J Health Syst Pharm 1999;56:729.
18. Recommendations for the use of antiemetics: evidence-based clinical practice guidelines. J Clin Oncol 1999;17(9):297.
19. International (Perugia) consensus conference on antiemetic therapy. Supp Care Cancer 1998;6(3):195.
20. Antiemesis Practice Guidelines Panel (1997) NCCN Antiemesis Practice Guidelines (NCCN proceedings) Oncology 11:52-89.
21. Lucot JB. Pharmacology of motion sickness. J Vestibular Res 1998;8(1):61.
22. Kohl RL et al. Arousal and stability: the effects of five new sympathomimetic drugs suggest a new principle for the prevention of space motion sickness. Aviat Space Environ Med 1986;57:137.
23. Kohl RL, Macdonald S. New pharmacologic approaches to the prevention of space/motion sickness. J Clin Pharmacol 1991;31:934.
24. Wood CD et al. Therapeutic effects of antimotion sickness medications on the secondary symptoms of motion sickness. Aviat Space Environ Med 1990;61:157.
25. Wood CD et al. Side effects of antimotion sickness drugs. Aviat Space Environ Med 1984;55:113.
26. Wood CD et al. Effectiveness and duration of intramuscular antimotion sickness medications. J Clin Pharmacol 1992;32:1008.
27. Pyykko I et al. Transdermally administered scopolamine vs. dimenhydrinate: 1. Effect on nausea and vertigo in experimentally induced motion sickness. Acta Otolaryngol (Stockh) 1985;99:588.
28. Grontved A et al. Ginger root against seasickness: a controlled trial on the open sea. Acta Otolaryngol 1988;105:45.
29. Holtmann S et al. The anti-motion sickness mechanism of ginger: a comparative study with placebo and dimenhydrinate. Acta Otolaryngol 1989;108:168.
30. Mowrey DB, Clayson DE. Motion sickness, ginger, and psychophysics. Lancet 1982;1:655.
31. Kohl RL et al. Facilitation of adaptation and acute tolerance to stressful sensory input by doxepin and scopolamine plus amphetamine. J Clin Pharmacol 1993;33:1092.
32. Chelen W et al. Computerized task battery assessment of cognitive and performance effects of acute phenytoin motion sickness therapy. Aviat Space Environ Med 1993;64:201.
33. Woodard D et al. Phenytoin as a countermeasure for motion sickness in NASA maritime operations. Aviat Space Environ Med 1993;64:363.
34. Watcha MF, White PF. Postoperative nausea and vomiting: its etiology, treatment, and prevention. Anesthesiology 1992;77:162.
35. Cookson RF. Mechanisms and treatment of postoperative nausea and vomiting. In: Davis CJ et al., eds. Nausea and Vomiting: Mechanisms and Treatment. Berlin: Springer-Verlag, 1986:130.
36. Burtles R, Peckett BW. Postoperative vomiting. Br J Anaesth 1957;29:114.
37. Cohen MM et al. Pediatric anesthesia morbidity and mortality in the perioperative period. Anesth Analg 1990;70:160.
38. Vance JP et al. The incidence and aetiology of postoperative nausea and vomiting in a plastic surgical unit. Br J Plast Surg 1973;26:336.
39. Purkis IE. Factors that influence postoperative vomiting. Can Anaesthetists Soc J 1964;11:335.
40. Kenny GNC. Risk factors for postoperative nausea and vomiting. Anaesthesia 1994;49(Suppl):6.
41. Haynes GR, Bailey MK. Postoperative nausea and vomiting: review and clinical approaches. South Med J 1996;89(10):940.
42. Sung YF. Risk and benefits of drugs used in the management of postoperative nausea and vomiting. Drug Safety 1996;14(3):181.
43. Tramer M et al. Propofol anaesthesia and postoperative nausea and vomiting: quantitative systematic review of randomized controlled studies. Br J Anaesth 1997;78:247.
44. Dupeyron JP et al. The effect of oral ondansetron in the prevention of postoperative nausea and vomiting after major gynaecological surgery performed under general anaesthesia. Anaesthesia 1993;48:214.
45. Madej TH, Simpson KH. Comparison of the use of domperidone, droperidol and metoclopramide in the prevention of nausea and vomiting following gynaecological surgery in day cases. Br J Anaesth 1986;58:879.
46. Hovorka J et al. Nitrous oxide does not increase nausea and vomiting following gynaecological laparoscopy. Can J Anaesth 1989;36:145.
47. Grunwald Z et al. The pharmacokinetics of droperidol in anesthetized children. Anesth Analg 1993;76:1238.
48. Abramowitz MD et al. The antiemetic effect of droperidol following outpatient strabismus surgery in children. Anesthesiology 1983;59:579.
49. Dent S et al. Postoperative vomiting: incidence, analysis and therapeutic measures in 3000 patients. Anesthesiology 1955;16:564.
50. Alon E, Himmelseher S. Ondansetron in the treatment of postoperative vomiting: a randomized, double-blind comparison with droperidol and metoclopramide. Anesth Analg 1992;75:561.
51. Alon E et al. Ondansetron as prophylaxis for postoperative nausea and vomiting: a prospective randomized double-blind comparative trial with droperidol. Anaesthetist 1994;43:500.
52. Gan TJ et al. Double-blind comparison of ondansetron, droperidol and saline in the prevention of postoperative nausea and vomiting. Br J Anaesth 1994;72:544.
53. Heim C et al. Ondansetron versus droperidol: treatment of postoperative nausea and vomiting. Comparison of efficiency, side-effects and acceptance by gynaecological inpatients. Anaesthesist 1994;43:504.
54. Desilva PHDP et al. The efficacy of prophylactic ondansetron, droperidol, perphenazine, and metoclopramide in the prevention of nausea and vomiting after major gynecologic surgery. Anesth Analg 1995;81:139.
55. Feyer PC et al. Aetiology and prevention of emesis induced by radiotherapy. Supp Care Cancer 1998;6:253.
56. Westbrook C et al. Vomiting associated with whole body irradiation. Clin Radiol 1987;38:263.

57. Harding RK et al. Radiotherapy-induced emesis. In: Andrews PLR, Sanger GJ, eds. Emesis in Anticancer Therapy Mechanisms and Treatment. London: Chapman and Hall, 1993:163.

58. Scarantino CW et al. Radiation-induced emesis: effects of ondansetron. Semin Oncol 1992;6(Suppl 15):38.

59. Prentice GH et al. Granisetron in the prevention of irradiation-induced emesis. Bone Marrow Transplant 1995;15:445.

60. Belkacemi Y et al. Total body irradiation prior to bone marrow transplantation: efficacy and safety of granisetron in the prophylaxis and control of radiation-induced emesis. Int J Radiat Oncol Biol Phys 1996;36:77.

61. Huner AE et al. Granisetron, a selective 5HT₃ receptor antagonists for the prevention of radiation-induced emesis during total body irradiation. Bone Marrow Transplant 1991;7:439.

62. Tiley C et al. Results of a boule blind placebo controlled study of ondansetron as an antiemetic during total body irradiation in patients undergoing bone marrow transplantation. Leuk Lymphoma 1992; 7:317.

63. Schwella N et al. Ondansetron for efficient emesis control during total body irradiation. Bone Marrow Transplant 1994;13:169.

64. Roberts JT, Priestmann TJ. A review of ondansetron in the management of radiotherapy induced emesis. Oncology 1993;50:173.

65. Priestman TJ. Clinical studies with ondansetron in the control of radiation-induced emesis. Eur J Cancer Clin Oncol 1989;251:29.

66. Spitzer TR, Friedman CT, Bushnell W, Frankel SR, Raschko. Double-blind randomized, parallel group study of the efficacy and safety of oral granisetron and oral ondansetron in the prophylaxis of nausea and vomiting in patients receiving hyperfractionated total body irradiation. Bone Marrow Transplantation 2000;26:203–210.

67. Danjoux E et al. The acute radiation syndrome. Clin Radiol 1979;30:581.

68. Feyer PC et al. Aetiology and prevention of emesis induced by radiotherapy [Review]. Supp Care Cancer 1998;6(3).

69. Coates A et al. On the receiving end: patient perception of the side effects of cancer chemotherapy. Eur J Cancer 1983;19:203.

70. Griffin AM et al. On the receiving end V: patient perceptions of the side effects of cancer chemotherapy in 1993. Ann Oncol 1996;7:189.

71. Lindley CM et al. Incidence and duration of chemotherapy-induced nausea and vomiting in the outpatient oncology population. J Clin Oncol 1989; 7:1142.

72. Hesketh P et al. Proposal for classifying the acute emetogenicity of cancer chemotherapy. J Clin Oncol 1997;15:103.

73. Laszlo J. Treatment of nausea and vomiting caused by cancer chemotherapy. Cancer Treat Rev 1982; 9:3.

74. Craig JB, Powell BL. Review: the management of nausea and vomiting in clinical oncology. Am J Med Sci 1987;293:34.

75. D'Acquisto R et al. The influence of a chronic high alcohol intake on chemotherapy-induced nausea and vomiting [Abstract]. Proc Am Soc Clin Oncol 1986;5:257.

76. Beck TM et al. Stratified, randomized, double-blind comparison of intravenous ondansetron administered as a multiple-dose regimen versus two single-dose regimens in the prevention of cisplatin-induced nausea and vomiting. J Clin Oncol 1992; 10(12):1969.

77. Perez EA et al. Comparison of single-dose oral granisetron versus intravenous ondansetron in the prevention of nausea and vomiting induced by moderately emetogenic chemotherapy: a multicenter, double-blind, randomized parallel study. J Clin Oncol 1998;16:754.

78. Gralla RJ et al. Single-dose granisetron has equivalent antiemetic efficacy to intravenous ondansetron for highly emetogenic cisplatin-based chemotherapy. J Clin Oncol 1998;16:1568.

79. Double-blind, dose-finding study of four intravenous doses of dexamethasone in the prevention of cisplatin-induced acute emesis. Italian Group for Antiemetic Research J Clin Oncol 1998;16: 2937–2942.

80. Roila F, Basurto C, Bosnjak S, et al. Optimal dose of dexamethasone (DEX) in preventing acute emesis induced by highly-moderately emetogenic chemotherapy (HMECT): A randomized, double-blind, dose-finding study. Proc Am Soc Clin Oncol 2003;22:729 (abstr 2930).

81. Kris MG et al. Incidence, course, and severity of delayed nausea and vomiting following the administration of high-dose cisplatin. J Clin Oncol 1985;3:1379.

82. Fetting JH et al. The course of nausea and vomiting after high-dose cyclophosphamide. Cancer Treat Rep 1982;66:1487.

83. Italian Group for Antiemetic Research. Ondansetron versus metoclopramide, both combined with dexamethasone, in the prevention of cisplatin-induced delayed emesis. J Clin Oncol 1997;15:124.

84. Kris MG et al. Controlling delayed vomiting: double-blind, randomized trial comparing placebo, dexamethasone alone, and metoclopramide plus dexamethasone in patients receiving cisplatin. J Clin Oncol 1989;7:108.

85. Koo WH, Ang PT. Role of maintenance oral dexamethasone in prophylaxis of delayed emesis caused by moderately emetogenic chemotherapy. Ann Oncol 1996;7:71.

86. Jones AL et al. Comparison of dexamethasone and ondansetron in the prophylaxis of emesis induced by moderately emetogenic chemotherapy. Lancet 1991;338:483.

87. Moreno I et al. Comparison of three protracted antiemetic regimens for the control of delayed emesis in cisplatin-treated patients. Eur J Cancer (Am) 1992;28:1344.

88. Latreille J et al. Use of dexamethasone and granisetron in the control of delayed emesis for patients who receive highly emetogenic chemotherapy. J Clin Oncol 1998;16:1174.

89. Marshall G, et al. Antiemetic therapy for chemotherapy-induced vomiting: Metoclopramide, benztropine, dexamethasone, and lorazepam regimen compared with chlorpromazine along. J Pediatr 1989;115:156.

90. Graham-Pole J, et al. Antiemetics in children receiving cancer chemotherapy: A double-blind prospective randomized study of metoclopramide with chlorpromazine. J Clin Oncol 1986;4:1110.

91. Relling MV, et al. Chlorpromazine with and without lorazepam as antiemetic therapy in children receiving uniform chemotherapy. J Pediatr 1993; 123:811.

92. Not cited.

93. Vickers AJ. Can acupuncture have specific effects on health? A systematic review of acupuncture anti-emesis trials. J R Soc Med 1996;89(6):303.

94. Dundee JW et al. Acupuncture prophylaxis of cancer chemotherapy-induced sickness. J R Soc Med 1989;82:268.

95. Hu S et al. P-6 acupressure reduces symptoms of vection-induced motion sickness. Aviat Space Environ Med 1995;66(7):631.

96. Hu CM et al. Effect of P-6 acupressure on prevention of NV after epidural morphine for post-ccsarean section pain relief. Acta Anaesth Scand 1996;40(3):372.

97. Dundee JW et al. Non-invasive stimulation of the P-6 (Neiguan) antiemetic acupuncture point in cancer chemotherapy. R Soc Med 84:210.

98. Pearl ML et al. Transcutaneous electrical nerve stimulation as an adjunct for controlling chemotherapy induced nausea and vomiting in gynecologic patients. Cancer Nursing 1999 22(4) 307-311.

99. Evans T et al. Suppression of pregnancy-induced nausea and vomiting with sensory afferent stimulation. J Reprod Med 1993;28(8):603.

100. Bertolucci LE, DiDario B. Efficacy of a portable acustimulation device in controlling seasickness. Aviat Space Environ Med 1995;66(12):1155.

101. NIH Consensus Development Conference on Acupuncture http://consensus.nih.gov/cons/107/107

102. Laszlo J. Tetrahydrocannabinol: from pot to prescription. Ann Intern Med 1979;91:916.

103. Stack P. The pharmacologic profile of nabilone: a new antiemetic agent. Cancer Treat Rev 1982; 9(Suppl B):11.

104. Frytak S et al. Delta-9-tetrahydrocannabinol as an antiemetic for patients receiving cancer chemotherapy. Ann Intern Med 1979;91:825.

105. Vinciguerra V et al. Inhalation marijuana as an antiemetic for cancer chemotherapy. NY State Med J 1998;88(10):525.

106. Sallan SE et al. Antiemetics in patients receiving chemotherapy for cancer: a randomized comparison of delta-9-tetrahydrocannabinol and prochlorperazine. N Engl J Med 1980;302:135.

107. Lucas VS, Laszlo J. Delta-9-tetrahydrocannabinol for refractory vomiting induced by cancer chemotherapy. JAMA 1980;243:1241.

108. Levitt M et al. Randomized double-blind comparison of delta-9-tetrahydrocannabinol (THC) and marijuana as chemotherapy antiemetics. Proc Am Soc Clin Oncol 1984;3:91.

CHAPTER 9

Pain and Its Management

Lori Reisner, Peter J.S. Koo

Pain is an unpleasant sensation that can negatively affect all areas of a person's life, including comfort, thought, sleep, emotion, and normal daily activity. Chronic untreated pain can disturb quality of life and social functioning and disrupt employment. The pain sensation results from complex phenomena that involve physical perception as well as the emotional reaction to the perception. Physiologic variables such as tissue injury and psychological variables such as anxiety influence a person's reaction to pain. Ascending neural pathways transfer electrochemical pain signals from the periphery to the central cortex where perception occurs, whereas descending pathways may attenuate or modulate signaling back to the site where the pain is felt. The pain sensation is therefore the net effect of complicated interactions of ascending and descending neural pathways with biochemical and electrochemical processes.

Pain is categorized according to its cause, location, duration, and clinical features. The most simplistic categorization involves differentiating brief-duration (acute) pain from long-lasting (chronic) pain syndromes. Acute pain serves a useful purpose of alerting an individual to an injury and initiating a reflex withdrawal from a noxious or offensive stimulus. In contrast, persistent (chronic) pain serves no biologic protective purpose and can cause undue stress and suffering. Pain was formerly believed to be merely a symptom and not a diagnosis. However, recent advances in molecular biology and the understanding of neural mechanisms have demonstrated that chronic pain can lead to long-lasting changes in the nervous system, a phenomenon known as "neural plasticity." This concept is particularly important to the understanding of chronic pain because it helps explain difficulties observed in treating various painful conditions. Although initially considered static, pain processes are now realized to be plastic. Such changes therefore define a disease or process that induces physiologic change in the body. Regardless of its origin, however, pain requires a thorough evaluation to determine the underlying cause. By definition, pain is a subjective experience. Therefore, the patient is the only person who can best describe the intensity and character of pain. Pain is whatever the experiencing person says it is, existing wherever he or she says it does.

Because pain is a variable and personal experience, it is difficult to completely describe and measure objectively. The clinician must therefore guard against personal biases, which can interfere with treatment. One must also rely on tools such as pain scales to communicate with patients and understand the extent of their pain. Such tools allow clinicians to objectively measure the clinical results of their interventions. Most often with chronic painful conditions, total pain elimination is not a realistic goal, owing to the nervous system changes described above. Instead, a more attainable objective is reducing pain to a tolerable predetermined level as agreed on by consensus of the patient and clinician. A person with chronic pain should expect to achieve pain reduction with the ultimate objective of increasing daily function (e.g., activities of daily living) and minimizing suffering.

Mechanisms of Pain

Transduction, Transmission, Modulation, and Perception

Pain sensation involves a series of complex interactions between peripheral nerves and the central nervous system (CNS). This process is modulated by excitatory and inhibitory neurotransmitters released in response to stimuli. Such stimuli can be physical, psychological, or both. An example of a physical stimulus is a burn or cut to the skin. In a short time, local reactions occur in the damaged area that initiate the release of chemical mediators involved in inflammation. This is followed by sensitization of the nerve endings, which ultimately send signals to the sensory cortex of the brain. Nociception, or the sensation of pain, is composed of four basic processes: transduction, transmission, modulation, and perception (Fig. 9-1).[1]

Transduction is the process by which noxious stimuli are translated into electrical signals at peripheral receptor sites. This begins when nociceptors (free nerve endings located throughout the skin, muscle, and viscera) are exposed to a sufficient quantity of mechanical, chemical, or thermal noxious stimuli.[2,3] In addition, a variety of chemical compounds such as histamine, bradykinin, serotonin, prostaglandins and, substance P are released serially from damaged tissues and can activate or sensitize nociceptors.[2,3] Serotonin has the additional action of modulating the peripheral release of primary afferent neuropeptides that are responsible for neurogenic inflammation. These neuropeptides include substance P, calcitonin gene-related peptide and neurokinin A.[2,3]

Transmission involves the propagation of an electrical signal along neural membranes. Stimuli, such as prostaglandins and inflammatory mediators, change the permeability of the membrane, producing an influx of sodium and an efflux of potassium, thereby depolarizing neuronal membranes. Electrical impulses are transmitted to the spinal cord via two primary afferent nerve types: myelinated A-fibers and unmyelinated C-fibers. The A-delta fiber is responsible for rapidly conducting electrical impulses associated with thermal and mechanical stimuli to the dorsal horn of the spinal cord. A-delta fibers release excitatory amino acids, such as glutamate, which activate α-amino-3-hydroxy-5-methylisoxazole-4-propionic acid (AMPA) receptors located on dorsal horn neurons.[2,4] Transmission of signals along these fibers results in sharp or stabbing sensations that alert the subject to an injury or insult to tissue. CNS input rapidly produces reflex signals, such as musculoskeletal withdrawal, to prevent further injury.[5]

The smaller, unmyelinated C-fibers respond to mechanical, thermal, and chemical stimuli and conduct electrical impulses to the spinal cord at a much slower rate compared with myelinated A-delta fibers. C-fibers, which also terminate in the dorsal horn, release the excitatory amino acids, glutamate and aspartate. Unlike A-fibers, C-fibers also release peptides, such as substance P, neurokinin A, somatostatin, galanin, and calcitonin gene–related peptide (CGRP).[5] The role of these peptides is not completely understood. Substance P is known to activate neurokinin-1 receptors, which may play a role in increasing excitability of spinal cord neurons.[5,6] Transmission of electrical impulses via C-fibers results in pain that is dull, aching, burning, and poorly localized or diffuse. This type of pain is known as *second* pain because it is perceived after the first pain sensation.

Once dorsal horn receptors are activated, electrical signals are further propagated to the thalamus primarily via the spinothalamic tract. From the thalamus, signals are sent to the cortex and other regions of the brain for processing and interpretation.

Modulation of nociceptive information occurs quickly between descending inhibitory pathways from the thalamus and brain stem and interneurons in the dorsal horn. Neurons from the thalamus and brain stem release inhibitory neurotransmitters, such as norepinephrine, serotonin, gamma-aminobutyric acid (GABA), glycine, endorphins, and enkephalins, which block substance P and other excitatory neurotransmitter activity on primary afferent fibers.[7]

The conscious awareness, or *perception,* of pain is the end result of this complex cascade of actions. The perception of pain involves not only nociceptive processes, but also physiologic and emotional responses, which contribute significantly to the sensation that is ultimately experienced by the person.[7] The perception of pain may be influenced by abnormal gener-

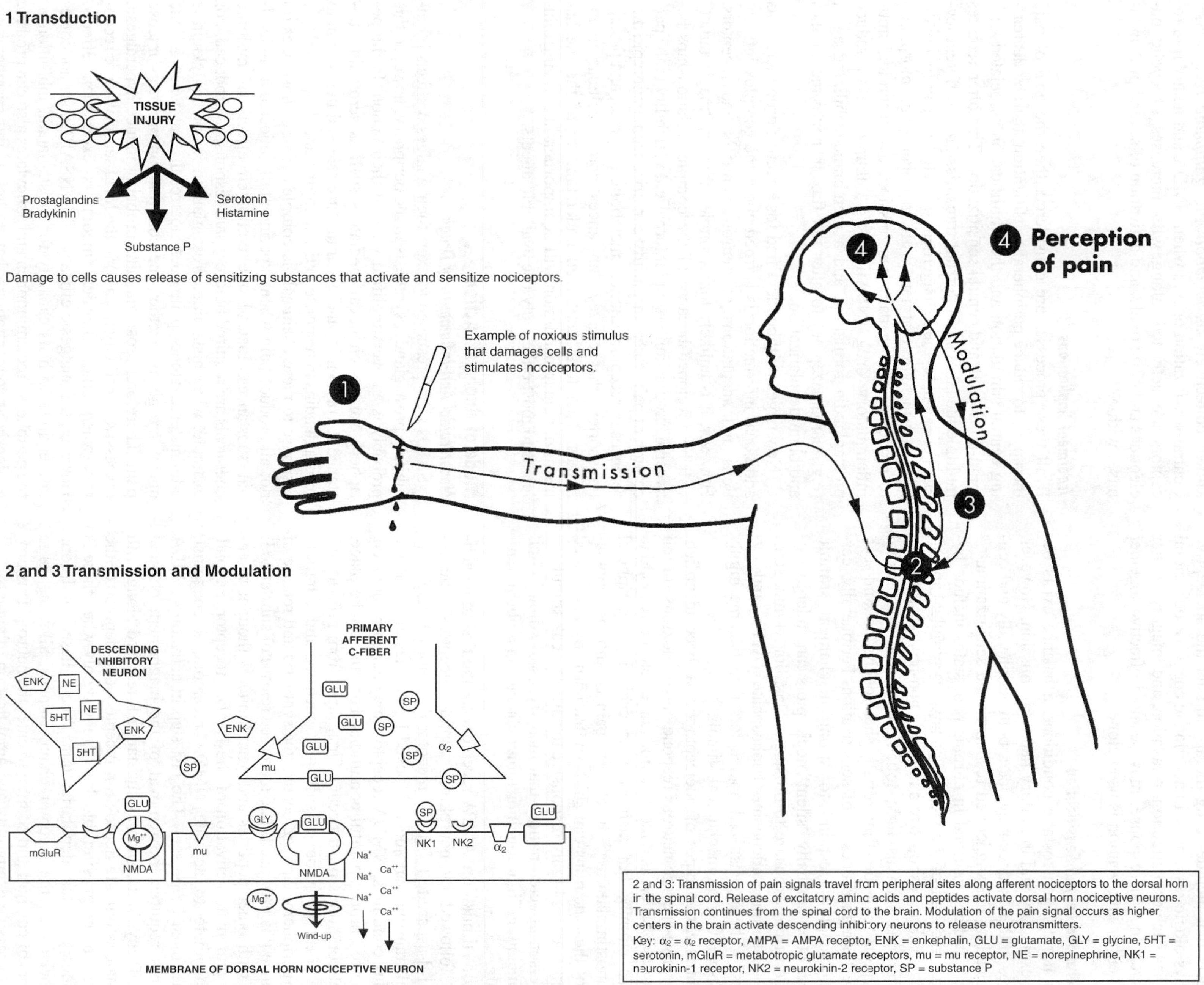

1 Transduction

TISSUE INJURY

Prostaglandins
Bradykinin

Substance P

Serotonin
Histamine

Damage to cells causes release of sensitizing substances that activate and sensitize nociceptors.

Example of noxious stimulus that damages cells and stimulates nociceptors.

Modulation

Transmission

4 Perception of pain

2 and 3 Transmission and Modulation

DESCENDING INHIBITORY NEURON

PRIMARY AFFERENT C-FIBER

MEMBRANE OF DORSAL HORN NOCICEPTIVE NEURON

2 and 3: Transmission of pain signals travel from peripheral sites along afferent nociceptors to the dorsal horn in the spinal cord. Release of excitatory amino acids and peptides activate dorsal horn nociceptive neurons. Transmission continues from the spinal cord to the brain. Modulation of the pain signal occurs as higher centers in the brain activate descending inhibitory neurons to release neurotransmitters.

Key: α_2 = α_2 receptor, AMPA = AMPA receptor, ENK = enkephalin, GLU = glutamate, GLY = glycine, 5HT = serotonin, mGluR = metabotropic glutamate receptors, mu = mu receptor, NE = norepinephrine, NK1 = neurokinin-1 receptor, NK2 = neurokinin-2 receptor, SP = substance P

FIGURE 9-1 Transduction, transmission, modulation, and perception of pain following a noxious stimulus. (Adapted from McCaffery M, Pasero C. Pain: Clinical Manual. St. Louis: Mosby, 1999.)

ation or processing of electrical pain signals and by the psychological framework created by the patient's temporal affective state or from previous painful experiences. Therefore, treatment that includes drug therapy to alter the nociceptive and physiologic responses, in addition to cognitive-behavioral strategies such as distraction, relaxation, and imagery to alter the psychological response, may be more effective together than if either intervention is used alone.[8]

Peripheral and Central Sensitization

Under normal homeostatic conditions, a balance exists between excitatory and inhibitory neurotransmission. However, changes in this balance may occur both peripherally and centrally, leading to exaggerated responses and sensitization.[8–10] Examples often observed in chronic pain states include hyperalgesia (enhanced pain to a given noxious stimulus) and allodynia (pain in response to a normally non-noxious mechanical stimulus such as light touch). Peripheral and central nociceptors can be functionally heterogeneous and can change through processes of sensitization. Peripherally, certain nociceptors respond to strong mechanical stimuli, whereas other normally "silent" nociceptors can undergo sensitization from exposure to prostaglandins, bradykinin, serotonin, histamine, adenosine triphosphate (ATP), and cytokines.[11] These sensitized nociceptors then become highly responsive to weak mechanical stimuli.[12]

Centrally, two types of nociceptors have been identified. Nociceptive-specific neurons respond only to noxious stimuli such as heat, whereas wide dynamic range neurons respond to noxious stimuli, but also may be excited by peripheral mechanostimulation.[9,12] In chronic pain conditions, populations of these neurons can shift, so that normally inactivated neurons become highly responsive to various weak stimuli.[2,12] The person affected notices that many types of stimuli elicit pain, including light touch or minor changes in ambient temperature.

Upon stimulation, AMPA receptors are the first to be activated, followed by neurokinin peptide receptors. The N-methyl-d-aspartate (NMDA) receptor does not participate in normal transmission and is blocked by magnesium.[5,13] If the stimulus continues, NMDA receptors may become activated, leading to chronic painful conditions. For this to take place, several conditions must occur.[5] First, input from primary afferent fibers must be of sufficient intensity and duration. When peripheral damage occurs, the synthesis and release of substance P is increased. The increased release of substance P, along with other peptides and neurokinins is thought to enhance glutamate activation of the NMDA receptor. Second, for glutamate to activate NMDA receptors, a coagonist, glycine, must be present. The last step in activating NMDA receptors requires the removal of the magnesium channel block. Tachykinins, such as substance P released along with glutamate, stimulate neurokinin receptors and depolarize the neuron. The magnesium block is removed only when there is sufficient repeated depolarization. When these conditions have been met, the receptor channel opens, allowing large amounts of calcium and sodium to enter the neuron. This produces excessive excitability and amplification of signals.

This initial activation of the NMDA receptor is known as *wind-up*. Wind-up progressively increases the number and response of nociceptive neurons in the dorsal horn without any change of input to the spinal cord.[5,13] In fact, this process can continue after peripheral input has stopped. With continued nociceptive input, spread occurs activating nearby receptors, known collectively as *metabotropic glutamate receptors*.[4,7] Central sensitization occurs when NMDA and neurokinin receptors are activated, along with increases of cyclic nucleotides and nitric oxide, and activation of several protein kinases within.[12]

Treatment Implications

If all these processes are considered, then the goal of pain therapy is to reduce peripheral sensitization, thereby decreasing central stimulation and the amplification associated with wind-up, spread, and central sensitization. This often requires multiple modalities to interrupt transmission at different levels. For example, the management of a chronic painful condition may include treatment with an opiate (e.g., morphine) to reduce ascending pain transmission, a nonsteroidal anti-inflammatory drug (NSAID) (e.g., ibuprofen) to reduce prostaglandin formation, and a membrane-stabilizing agent (e.g., carbamazepine) to alter ion flux in nerve membranes and blunt depolarization.

New targets will be identified for effective drug therapy as additional information is learned about the complex interactions and adaptations of neurotransmitters and receptors. However, it is unlikely that a single effective "magic bullet" will be developed because of the complex relationships between neurotransmitters and interpatient variability in the perception of pain. Such variability can arise from genotypic differences in receptor function, metabolic enzymes, and protein transporters that convey substances across cellular membranes. Therefore, continued understanding of the mechanisms of pain transmission will be important in allowing clinicians to most effectively use available agents.

Mode of Analgesic Action
Nonsteroidal Anti-Inflammatory Drugs

NSAIDs were presumed to exert their analgesic effects by inhibiting prostaglandin synthesis in the periphery; however, this probably is an oversimplified view of their action. In the periphery, various chemical mediators such as serotonin, substance P, bradykinin, and histamine are released in addition to prostaglandins in response to tissue injury, and the physiologic response to these chemicals is complex. These substances do not all produce pain when experimentally injected as individual substances. Instead, the combined effects of multiple chemicals are required before a pain response is produced. For example, when histamine, prostaglandin E_2, or bradykinin is administered alone, pain does not result; but when all the agents are given together, the combination produces intense pain. Therefore, prostaglandins probably induce hyperalgesia (excessive sensitivity to pain) in the local sensory nerve receptors when other chemical mediators exert their effects. However, the analgesic efficacy of an NSAID does not correlate entirely with its capacity for prostaglandin inhibition in the periphery. Acetaminophen and salicylates also can produce analgesia at concentrations that do not inhibit peripheral cyclooxygenase activity and prostaglandin formation. Therefore, the exact mechanism of NSAID analgesia has yet to be elucidated; however, the analgesic effect of NSAIDs is likely central in origin and involves substance-P receptors of the neurokinin-1 type and glutamate receptors of the NMDA type in addition to central prostaglandin inhibition. Because spinal NSAIDs reduce the hyperalgesia evoked by spinal substance P and NMDA, the action of the NSAIDs appears to be independent of peripheral inflammation. NSAID actions through GABAergic pathways, arachidonic acid byproducts, and AMPA receptors also are being studied. Aspirin, the prototypical NSAID, has demonstrated synergistic activity with endogenous opioids at opioid receptors as well as enhancing serotonin's effects in the central nervous system.[14,15]

Opiates

Opiates can attach to one or more of five opioid receptors: the μ-, δ-, ϵ-, κ-, and σ-receptors. These receptors can be differentiated further into subtypes (e.g., μ_1, μ_2, δ_1, δ_2, κ_1, κ_2, and κ_3). Animal models suggest that as many as seven subtypes of μ-receptors may exist, but it is not known how many of these can be found in humans. Stimulation of the μ_1-receptors may be responsible for the desired effects of supraspinal analgesia, and stimulation of μ_2-receptors may lead to unwanted consequences such as respiratory depression, euphoria, constipation, and physical dependence. Some κ-receptors, as well as δ- and ϵ-receptors, also mediate analgesic response, although the role of ϵ-receptors is not fully understood. Autonomic stimulation, dysphoria, and hallucinations may be caused by σ-receptors. These are not considered true opioid receptors, but may interact with some opioid-like agents.

The effect of opiates on these receptor subtypes is gradually being discovered. Morphine can stimulate μ_1-, μ_2-, and κ-receptors, and perhaps this capability to stimulate multiple receptors can account for morphine's mixed analgesic and side effect profile. Pure opiate antagonists (e.g., naloxone) occupy opiate receptors without eliciting a direct response and block the access of other opiate agonists such as morphine to these receptors. As a result, pure narcotic antagonists block both the desired and undesired opiate effects. Pentazocine and butorphanol (both mixed agonist/antagonists) produce analgesia through stimulation of κ-receptors, but cause unwanted dysphoria and hallucinations through their effect on σ-receptors. Pentazocine and butorphanol also block access of morphine to μ-receptors, leading to withdrawal symptoms in individuals who are physically dependent on morphine or its analogs.

In the spinal cord, the highest concentration of opioid receptors is located around the C-fiber terminal zones in the lamina 1 of the dorsal horn and the substantia gelatinosa. The μ-opioid receptors constitute approximately 70% of the total receptor population; δ- and κ-receptors account for 24% and 6% of the population, respectively. μ-Receptors also are located in the afferent terminals. Because morphine has a 50-fold higher affinity for the μ-receptor than the δ- or κ-receptors, it is a very effective analgesic. The pharmacologic action of opioids depends on the availability of opioid receptors, and the cutting of peripheral nerves leads to degeneration and loss of opioid receptors in the nerve itself. As a result, postamputation pain often is not relieved by morphine or other opioids.

Opioids produce analgesia by three main mechanisms[16]:

- Presynaptically, opioids reduce the release of inflammatory transmitters (e.g., tachykinin, excitatory amino acids, and peptides) from the terminals of afferent C-fiber neurons after activation of opioid receptors. This presynaptic action is achieved by the opening of potassium channels and closing of calcium channels, which reduce calcium influx into the C-fiber terminal. The μ- and δ-opioid receptors respond to the opening of potassium channels, and the κ-opioid receptors respond to the closing of calcium channels.
- Opioids also can reduce the activity of output neurons, interneurons, and dendrites in the neuronal pathways by means of postsynaptic hyperpolarization. The postsynaptic hyperpolarization is achieved by a mechanism similar to the opening of the potassium channels and closing of the calcium channels of the nerve terminal.
- Opioids also inhibit neuronal activity via GABA and enkephalin neurons in the substantia gelatinosa.

Analgesic Adjunctive Agents

Analgesic medications often are prescribed concurrently with other drugs to enhance analgesia or to treat pain exacerbations. These adjunctive medications are most often used in the management of chronic pain, particularly when the dose of the primary analgesic has been optimized or when the underlying condition has progressed and is no longer adequately controlled by the primary analgesic agent. Other adjuvant agents may be added to analgesic therapy to reduce side effects, such as excessive sedation, nausea and vomiting, or constipation. The most common drug classes used as adjunctive analgesic agents are corticosteroids, anticonvulsants, heterocyclic antidepressants, α_2- adrenergic agonists, NMDA receptor antagonists, local and oral anesthetics/antiarrhythmics, antihistamines and neuroleptics. Adjunct analgesic agents may be used as the primary analgesic agent in the treatment of neuropathic pain syndromes, where the usefulness of opioids is under debate. Neuropathic pain syndromes do not respond to NSAIDs.

Corticosteroids, such as dexamethasone, are useful in reducing pain associated with cerebral and spinal cord edema and in treating refractory neuropathic pain and bone pain, particularly metastatic bone pain. Corticosteroids may also provide other beneficial effects, such as mood elevation, antiemetic activity, and appetite stimulation.[17]

Antidepressants are commonly used to treat neuropathic pain (e.g., diabetic neuropathy, postherpetic neuralgia) and pain associated with insomnia or depression.[18] They are used to treat fibromyalgia, a syndrome characterized by diffuse muscle and joint pain, which is thought to result from central dysregulation. Their analgesic effect is independent of their antidepressant effect. Postulated mechanisms of action involve blockade of norepinephrine reuptake, antagonism of histamine and muscarinic cholinergic receptors, α-adrenergic blockade, or suppression of C-fiber–evoked activity in the spinal cord.[19]

Anticonvulsants; antiarrhythmics; α_2-adrenergic antagonists; and the NMDA receptor antagonists, ketamine and dextromethorphan, also have been used to manage neuropathic pain with varying degrees of success. Antihistamines, such as hydroxyzine and promethazine, are often prescribed postoperatively to augment the analgesic effects of opioid agents. Hydroxyzine may provide minimal analgesia, whereas there is little evidence to confirm analgesic action for promethazine.[20] The addition of phenothiazines and antihistamines may be useful in alleviating opioid-induced nausea and vomiting; however, these agents may potentiate orthostatic hypotension, respiratory depression, sedation, and extrapyramidal side effects.[21] Use of these agents should not be a substitute for appropriate doses of opioid analgesics.

Classification of Pain
Acute Pain
Pain immediately following an injury to the body is considered to be acute pain, whereas pain lasting beyond the expected healing time, or persistent pain that does not respond to usual pain control methods, is defined as chronic pain. Acute pain serves a useful purpose in minimizing the site of injury by causing an organism to recoil from a noxious or harmful stimulus. In most cases, the objective physical findings associated with acute pain can be localized directly to the site of injury. However, injury to nerves on visceral organ systems can present as diffuse, poorly differentiated, referred pain.

Acute pain is usually self-limiting and typically subsides when the injury heals. Untreated or inadequately treated pain can evoke physiologic hormonal responses that alter circulation and tissue metabolism; these can also produce tachypnea, tachycardia, widening of the pulse pressure, and increased sympathetic nervous system activity. Inadequately treated pain can produce significant psychological stress responses and compromise the body's immune system by provoking release of endogenous corticosteroids. Decreased range of motion, diminished vital pulmonary capacity, and a compromise in the overall well-being of a person secondary to poorly treated pain may delay recovery after surgery or trauma. Acute pain is often exacerbated by anxiety and secondary reflex musculoskeletal spasms.

Acute pain should always be aggressively managed, even before a definitive cause is known. In patients with traumatic head injury, medications should be withheld until a full neurologic workup can be performed because they may interfere with cognitive function. Patients with acute abdominal pain also may have pain medications withheld until a diagnosis is made; however, several studies support early pain management.[22,23] When pain is relieved, the patient is more comfortable and better able to cooperate with the history, physical examination, and diagnostic procedures. Unfortunately, postoperative and other acute pain syndromes often are ignored or inadequately treated. Part of the tendency to undertreat pain is the reluctance of caregivers to prescribe opiates for fear of causing addiction. However, addiction to opioids is essentially nonexistent when these drugs are prescribed for acute pain, and withholding appropriate pain treatment causes needless patient suffering.

Chronic Pain
The origins of chronic pain may be neurogenic, nociceptive, psychiatric, or idiopathic. As will be presented later, it is important to further differentiate chronic pain syndromes into those that are associated with malignancy from those that are not. However, all forms of chronic pain share some common characteristics. Unlike acute pain, which prompts the afflicted individual to avoid further injury or seek help, chronic pain usually serves no benefit to the individual. Chronic pain can

be episodic or continuous, or a combination of both. A patient may feel constant pain and also experience exacerbations of more intense pain at various times. Chronic pain may cause a person to feel "trapped" inside of his or her body, distinguished only by more painful and less painful days. Chronic pain often is destructive to the host by deteriorating quality of life, functional ability, spiritual and psychological well-being, interpersonal relationships, and financial status.[17] Chronic pain also can cause changes in appetite, psychomotor retardation, irritability, social withdrawal, sleep disturbances, and depression. The patient often cannot remember an existence free of pain and is convinced that the pain will be present until death. In short, chronic pain can become an all-consuming focus of the patient's life.

The key to successful chronic pain management rests on prevention and elimination of unnecessary suffering and despair. Chronic pain management should consider the applicability of cognitive interventions (relaxation technique, self-hypnosis, and/or psychiatric therapy) as well as physical manipulations (local application of heat, cold, massage, electrical nerve stimulation, acupuncture, and physical therapy). Pharmacologic agents (antidepressants, antiarrhythmics, anticonvulsants, major tranquilizers, and longer-acting opioids), regional anesthesia (local anesthetic blocks with or without corticosteroids or chemical neurolysis), surgical interventions (spinal decompression, release of nerve entrapment), and spinal analgesia (intraspinal opioids and/or local anesthetic agents) are also warranted.[24,25]

PAIN ASSOCIATED WITH MALIGNANCY (CHRONIC MALIGNANT PAIN)
Chronic malignant pain can have a combination of acute, intermittent, or constant components. Although the pain is chronic, it can have elements of acute pain when tissue damage continues from tumor infiltration. Nerve destruction, chemotherapy, radiation therapy, and surgery also contribute to malignant pain. Occasionally, chronic malignant pain has only minimal or no associated objective clinical physical findings, and may be erroneously dismissed by inexperienced clinicians.

Anticipation by the patient that malignant pain will be continuous leads to anxiety, depression, and insomnia.[26] These destructive feelings can accentuate the patient's perception of pain. Inadequately treated chronic malignant pain can become progressively more severe and cause relentless suffering. Persistent pain can accelerate the deterioration of the patient's physical and psychological condition more than the malignancy itself.

Some cancer patients, when confronted with a dreaded disease and the possibility of impending death, respond with fear not only for themselves, but for their loved ones as well, especially when young children are involved. Their anxiety is heightened by the fear of loss of social position, possible surgical mutilation, loss of self-control, and fear of uncontrollable pain. These fears and anxieties can be projected as resentment, anger, isolation, depression, and frustration. A full discussion of the psychological and emotional aspects of chronic malignant pain is beyond the scope of this chapter, but successful treatment of a large percentage of these patients requires a comprehensive multidisciplinary approach.[17,27–29]

The most important aspect of chronic malignant pain management is a logical and systematic approach with the goal of pain alleviation and prevention. A primary element of this approach is patient access to health care and pain management information. It is the duty of all health care providers to effectively assess their patients' pain management needs and to make the appropriate referrals or therapeutic changes.

CHRONIC NONMALIGNANT PAIN

Pain not associated with a malignant disease and lasting >6 months or beyond the healing period is considered to be chronic nonmalignant pain. Unfortunately, this pain also has been called *chronic benign pain,* an obvious misrepresentation because pain is never benign when it causes patient suffering. Chronic nonmalignant pain is recognized as a serious health problem that affects millions of people worldwide and carries far-reaching social implications.[30] The development of treatment guidelines is difficult because of the heterogeneity of causes. For most types of chronic pain, initial therapy is often conservative. Failure of conservative therapy may necessitate the use of more potent analgesics. The use of opiates in this patient population is controversial; however, increasing data support opiate use in psychologically healthy patients.[29,31–33] Since chronic pain affects many aspects of a patient's life, a multidisciplinary approach that addresses effective drug therapy and comprehensive rehabilitation often provides greater relief to the patient than drug therapy alone.

Much of the difficulty encountered in pain management arises when clinicians are not sufficiently educated or trained in dealing with the complex pharmacologic and psychosocial problems associated with chronic pain. Often the clinician fails to listen to the patient or fails to recognize clues to the subtle nature of his or her patient's pain complaints. Drug selection often is irrational and doses are frequently inadequate. However, the unfortunate tragedy occurs when clinicians occasionally withhold adequate analgesia because of a misunderstood fear of addiction, or when a patient refuses medications because of a similar fear of addiction.[34–36]

A BILL OF RIGHTS FOR PEOPLE WITH PAIN
1. I have the right to have my reports of pain accepted and acted on by health care professionals.
2. I have the right to have my pain controlled, no matter what its cause or how severe it may be.
3. I have the right to be treated with respect at all times. When I need medication for pain, I should not be treated like a drug abuser.

FIGURE 9-2 The rights of patients with pain. (From McCaffery M, Pasero C. Pain: Clinical Manual. St. Louis: Mosby, 1999:13.)

General Treatment Principles

Pain is one of the most common reasons for which patients seek medical attention; yet it remains significantly undertreated despite the availability of effective medications and other therapies.[37,38]

All patients deserve to have their pain managed in a timely and effective manner, yet many misconceptions, both from practitioners and patients, often preclude optimal pain care. To increase awareness about pain management, many states with pain initiatives have published a bill of rights for people with pain (Fig. 9-2).[39] In an attempt to address the undertreatment of pain and increase accountability for assessing and relieving pain, the Joint Commission on Accreditation of Healthcare Organizations (JCAHO) has developed standards that address pain assessment and management.[40] These standards help health care professionals assess their own pain management programs and improve the care they provide, make patients more aware of the right to receive adequate pain relief, and ultimately help dispel the many myths that interfere with effective pain control. Table 9-1 lists eight common causes of treatment failure when using analgesics.[41] In general, the reasons include a lack of understanding of pain management principles or the pharmacologic properties of the drugs; an overestimation of the risk of addiction by both patients and caregivers; or poor communication between the

Table 9-1   Common Causes of Analgesic Treatment Failure

Problem	Potential Impact on Pain Management	Example
1. Inappropriate or Unknown Diagnosis	Improper medication selection	Utilizing an NSAID for abdominal pain that may be related to a GI bleed
2. Misunderstanding of pharmacology or pharmacokinetics	Overestimating potency or half-life	Dosing an opioid less frequently than necessary to provide adequate relief
3. Inadequate management of adverse effects	Patient may discontinue therapy or misuse OTC remedies	Patient suffers constipation from antidepressants and uses daily bisacodyl
4. Fear of addiction	Physician or patient or caregiver may withhold medications	Evidence of tolerance after chronic use of opioids may be mistaken for addiction
5. Unrealistic goals for therapy	Patient will not be satisfied with pain management regimen and may seek other care	Patient states a desire to be "pain free" following significant nerve injury
6. Irrational polypharmacy	Over- or under-use of appropriate therapies	Patient with neuropathic pain using three different opioids without any adjuncts in the regimen
7. Patient barriers	Patient cannot understand appropriate medication use or other pain management modalities	• Language/comprehension deficits • Cognitive deficits - patient cannot remember regimen • Physical impediments to using medicines appropriately • Cultural barriers (e.g., stoicism)
8. Lack of understanding of pathophysiology of pain	Limitations of health care providers' ability to adequately relieve pain	Drugs that show benefit in animal models are not useful for human pain conditions

patient and medical personnel. A number of steps to overcome these barriers are described in the succeeding section.

Effective analgesic therapy begins with an accurate assessment of the patient. The Initial Pain Assessment Tool (Fig. 9-3) and the Brief Pain Inventory (Fig. 9-4) can help clinicians assess pain. When obtaining a pain history, it is important to gather details about the pattern, duration, location, and character of the pain. Pain intensity should be measured using

Date_____

Patient's name_____Age_____Room_____

Diagnosis_____Physician_____

Evaluator_____

1. LOCATION: Patient or clinician marks drawing.

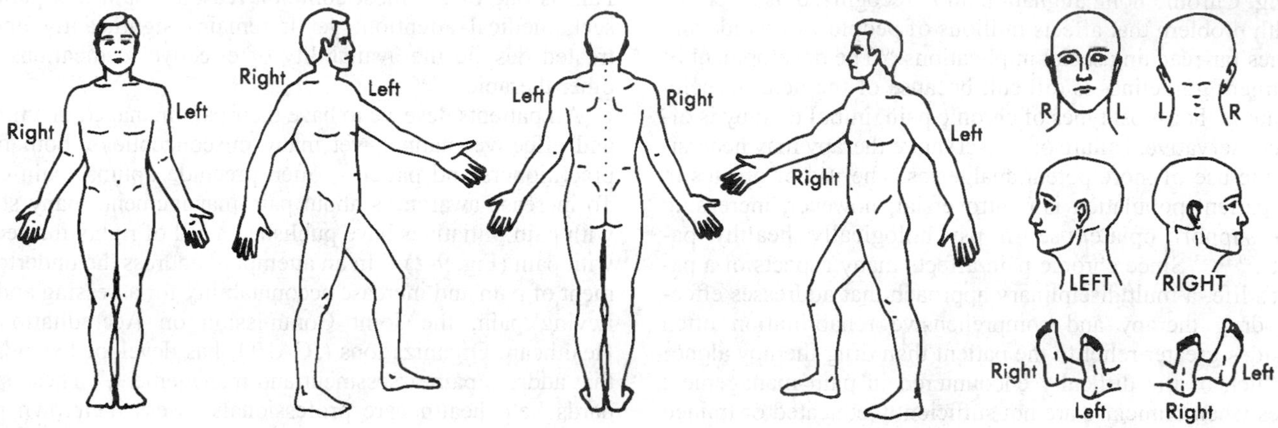

2. INTENSITY: Patient rates the pain. Scale used _____
    Present: _____
    Worst pain gets: _____
    Best pain gets: _____
    Acceptable level of pain: _____

3. QUALITY: (Use patient's own words, e.g., prick, ache, burn, throb, pull, sharp) _____

4. ONSET, DURATION, VARIATIONS, RHYTHMS: _____
    _____

5. MANNER OF EXPRESSING PAIN: _____
    _____
    _____

6. WHAT RELIEVES THE PAIN? _____
    _____
    _____

7. WHAT CAUSES OR INCREASES THE PAIN? _____
    _____

8. EFFECTS OF PAIN: (Note decreased function, decreased quality of life.)
    Accompanying symptoms (e.g., nausea) _____
    Sleep _____
    Appetite _____
    Physical activity: _____
    Relationship with others (e.g., irritability) _____
    Emotions (e.g., anger, suicidal, crying) _____
    Concentration _____
    Other _____

9. OTHER COMMENTS: _____
    _____

10. PLAN: _____
    _____

FIGURE 9-3 Initial pain assessment tool. (Modified from McCaffery M, Pasero C. Pain: Clinical Manual. St. Louis: Mosby, 1999:60.)

Date:____/____/____   Time:_____
Name:_____ _____ ____
                 Last   First   MI

1) Throughout our lives, most of us have had pain from time to time (such as minor headaches, sprains, and toothaches). Have you had pain other than these everyday kinds of pain today?
   1. Yes   2. No

2) On the diagram, shade in the areas where you feel pain. Put an X on the area that hurts the most.

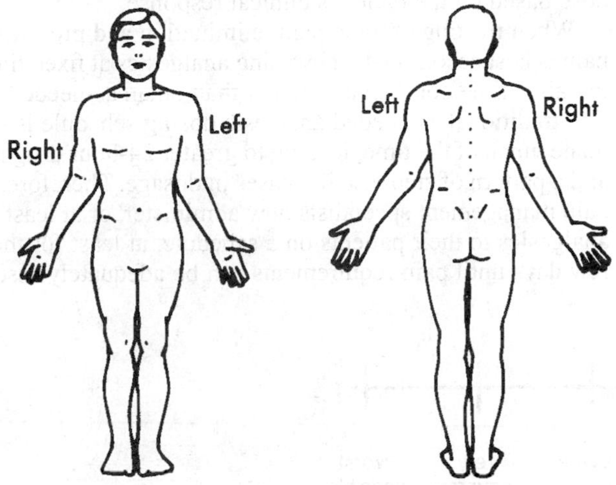

3) Please rate your pain by circling the one number that best describes you pain at its **worst** in the past 24 hours.

0	1	2	3	4	5	6	7	8	9	10
No pain										Pain as bad as you can imagine

4) Please rate your pain by circling the one number that best describes your pain at its **least** in the past 24 hours.

0	1	2	3	4	5	6	7	8	9	10
No pain										Pain as bad as you can imagine

5) Please rate your pain by circling the one number that best describes your pain on the **average.**

0	1	2	3	4	5	6	7	8	9	10
No pain										Pain as bad as you can imagine

6) Please rate your pain by circling the one number that tells how much pain you have **right now.**

0	1	2	3	4	5	6	7	8	9	10
No pain										Pain as bad as you can imagine

7) What treaments or medications are you receiving for your pain?
_____
_____

8) In the past 24 hours, how much relief have pain treatments or medications provided? Please circle the one percentage that most shows how much relief you have received?

0	1	2	3	4	5	6	7	8	9	10
No relief										Complete relief

9) Circle the one number that describes how, during the past 24 hours, pain has **interfered** with your:

A. General activity

0	1	2	3	4	5	6	7	8	9	10
Does not interfere										Completely interferes

B. Mood

0	1	2	3	4	5	6	7	8	9	10
Does not interfere										Completely interferes

C. Walking ability

0	1	2	3	4	5	6	7	8	9	10
Does not interfere										Completely interferes

D. Normal work (includes both work outside the home and housework)

0	1	2	3	4	5	6	7	8	9	10
Does not interfere										Completely interferes

E. Relations with other people

0	1	2	3	4	5	6	7	8	9	10
Does not interfere										Completely interferes

F. Sleep

0	1	2	3	4	5	6	7	8	9	10
Does not interfere										Completely interferes

G. Enjoyment of life

0	1	2	3	4	5	6	7	8	9	10
Does not interfere										Completely interferes

FIGURE 9-4 Brief Pain Inventory (Short Form). (From Agency for Health Care Policy and Research, Clinical Practice Guideline: Cancer Pain Management. Rockville: AHCPR Publication 94-0592; 1994.)

an appropriate pain scale (Figs. 9-5 and 9-6) according to the patient's ability to communicate.[17,24] Factors that exacerbate or relieve pain should be assessed. The names and amounts of all analgesics that the patient is taking should be documented as well as their effectiveness. In addition, other medical problems and medications should be documented, including over-the-counter and nonprescription remedies. A patient fearful of being accused of analgesic abuse might be reluctant to give an accurate drug use history unless a trusting relationship can be established.

Effective treatment considers the cause, duration, and intensity of pain and matches the appropriate intervention to the situation. The goal of therapy is to eliminate or reduce the pain to the lowest tolerable intensity and prevent it from recurring, rather than wait to treat the pain when it becomes unbearable. The patient should predetermine this lowest tolerable level with the health care provider based on a pain scale that is mutually understood. Guidelines from the World Health Organization, summarized in Table 9-2, can be useful when choosing initial therapy.[42] However, one also must consider the clinical situation when determining analgesic selection or whether the painful condition requires analgesic ther-

apy. For example, it would be irrational to treat the severe abdominal cramping pain of constipation with morphine, which may worsen the constipation. If pain is the result of a fracture, then stabilization and immobilization, in addition to appropriate analgesics, will reduce pain in the affected bone. Once a pain regimen is initiated, frequent reassessment will determine whether the goals of therapy are being met and whether they address any emerging side effects. Drug selection, doses, routes of administration, and dosing frequency should be adjusted as needed until the goals of therapy are met. In treating acute, severe postoperative pain, it may be necessary to begin with a potent opiate analgesic and then gradually reduce the dose based on the patient's clinical response.

When treating chronic pain, elimination and prevention of pain is best accomplished by using analgesics at fixed time intervals ("time-contingent") rather than on an as-needed basis. The traditional as-needed analgesic dosing schedule is inadequate much of the time, leading to greater 24-hour drug intake and a pattern of stepwise increases in dosage. Therefore, most pain management specialists now administer, or at least offer, analgesics to their patients on a schedule, at least for the first few days until pain requirements can be adequately assessed.

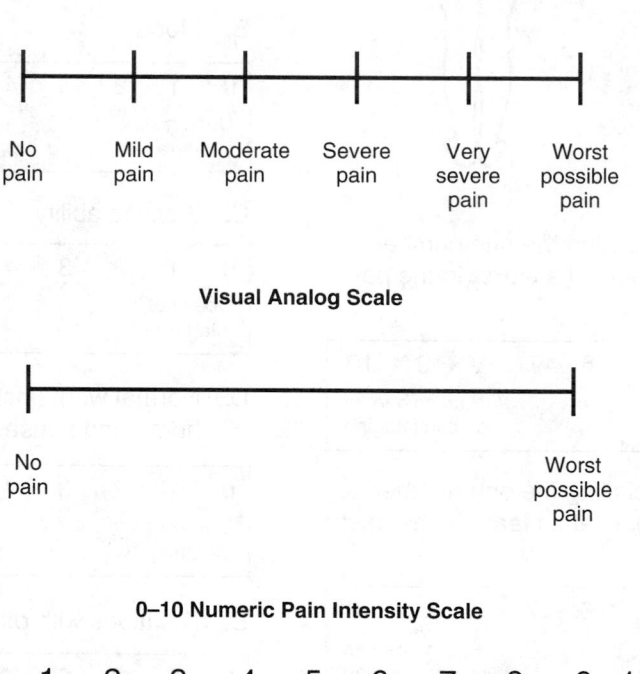

Visual Analog Scale

0–10 Numeric Pain Intensity Scale

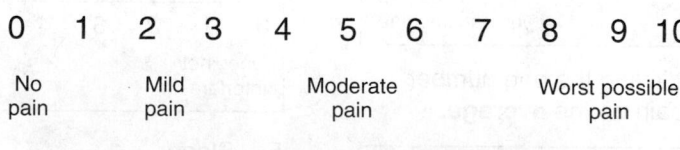

"Faces" Pain Scale

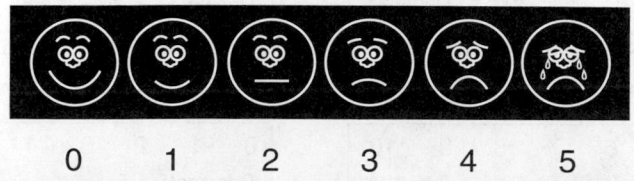

FIGURE 9-5 Pain intensity scales. (Adapted from Patt RB. Cancer Pain. Philadelphia: JB Lippincott, 1993; and Wong DL. Whaley and Wong's Essentials of Pediatric Nursing. St. Louis: Mosby, 1997.)

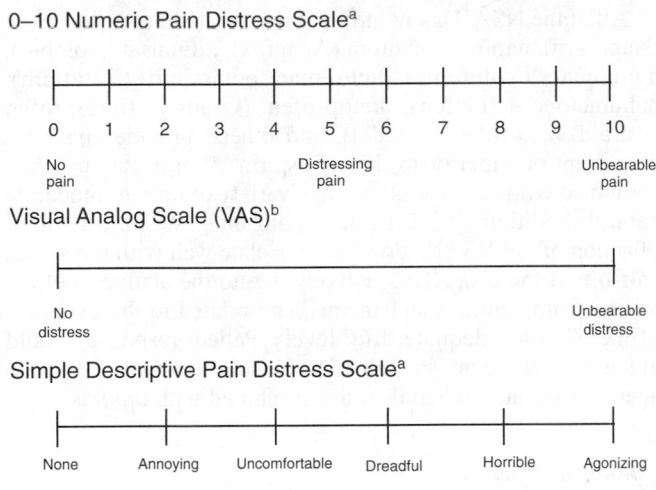

0–10 Numeric Pain Distress Scale[a]

| 0 | 1 | 2 | 3 | 4 | 5 | 6 | 7 | 8 | 9 | 10 |

No pain   Distressing pain   Unbearable pain

Visual Analog Scale (VAS)[b]

No distress   Unbearable distress

Simple Descriptive Pain Distress Scale[a]

None   Annoying   Uncomfortable   Dreadful   Horrible   Agonizing

[a]If used as a graphic rating scale, a 10-cm baseline is recommended.
[b]A 10-cm baseline is recommended for VAS scales.

FIGURE 9-6 Pain distress scales.

However, in patients with severe acute or malignant pain, scheduled analgesics alone may not be adequate without additional analgesics for breakthrough episodes. Until the dosage is stabilized, all patients who are receiving analgesics should be monitored closely for efficacy of analgesia as well as untoward side effects. Successful pain management may also include the use of nonpharmacologic measures, such as ensuring that the patient receives adequate rest and emotional support. Physical and occupational therapy may be useful to help improve strength or mobility and to ensure that there are no barriers at home or work that can interfere with the patient's activities of daily living.[29]

Anxiety and guilt often complicate the management of pain. Patients sometimes become anxious, fearing that their pain will become uncontrollable or that they will become addicted to opiates. Also, patients sometimes feel guilty about taking opioids for their pain because of the negative social connotations associated with these drugs. They may feel that they have failed their clinicians' expectations. Therefore, patient education about the rational use of analgesics is imperative. Pain can be managed best when there is trust and communication between the caregiver and the patient, known as a therapeutic alliance. Patients must feel comfortable telling caregivers whenever their pain needs arise, and caregivers must respond appropriately and in a timely fashion. Good communication between caregivers and patients can alleviate anxiety and guilt regarding patients' pain needs.

Analgesic Selection

The selection of the analgesic must be individualized for each patient, depending on the cause and chronicity of the pain as well as the patient's age and concomitant medical conditions that may alter drug response. Furthermore, the clinical response of the patient dictates the dose, route, or desired dosing interval. The selection of the most appropriate drug should be based on pharmacologic data as well as clinical experience. The selection of an opioid for the management of severe acute and chronic malignant pain must always include consideration of morphine or one of the other potent opioids; however, the role of NSAIDs should not be overlooked. Adjunctive analgesic medications such as antidepressants or anticonvulsants are often preferred because chronic nonmalignant pain often is associated with sympathetic dysfunction

Table 9-2   Example Initial Regimens for Different Pain Levels Based on Guidelines From the World Health Organization (WHO)

Pain Level Description	Typical Corresponding Numerical Rating (0 to 10 Scale)	WHO Therapeutic Recommendations	Example Medicines for Initial Therapy	Comments
"Mild" Pain	1–3/10	Nonopioid Analgesic: taken on a regular schedule, not prn	• Acetaminophen 650 mg Q 4 hr • Acetaminophen 1000 mg Q 6 hr • Ibuprofen 600 mg Q 6 hr	• Consider adding adjunct analgesic or using an alternate regimen if pain not reduced in 1–2 days • Consider step up if pain not relieved by ≥2 different regimens
"Moderate" Pain	4–6/10	Add opioid for moderate pain (e.g., moderate potency analgesic). Use on a schedule, not prn	• Acetaminophen 325 mg/ codeine 60 mg Q 4 hr • Acetaminophen 325 mg/ Oxycodone 5 mg Q 4 hr • Tramadol 50 mg Q 6 hr	• Consider adding adjunct analgesic or using an alternate regimen if pain not reduced in 1–2 days • Consider step up if pain not relieved by ≥2 different regimens
"Severe Pain"	7–10/10	Switch to a high potency (strong) opioid; administer on a regular schedule	• Morphine 15 mg Q 4 hr • Hydromorphone 4 mg Q 4 hr • Morphine controlled release 60 mg Q 8 hr	• Consider alternate regimen (e.g., different strong opioid) if pain not reduced in 1–2 days • Consider increased dose of strong opioid, or addition of nonopioid agents, if pain not adequately relieved by ≥2 regimens

Adapted from the World Health Organization, http://www.who.int/cancer/palliative/painladder/en/.

and neuropathies. The NSAIDs are the analgesic agents of choice in the management of mild to moderate pain involving the musculoskeletal tissues and also are extremely effective in the management of pain from bony neoplastic metastasis. Neurogenic pain often responds better to tricyclic antidepressants (TCAs) than to opioids. Neuropathic pain may not be relieved by opioids until the dose is large enough to cause significant side effects.

If the maintenance dose of an opioid analgesic is too high, the patient can become oversedated and less functional. In extreme cases, patients may become bedridden from excessive opiate use. When given the choice of eliminating the last trace of discomfort at the cost of some sensorial clouding, patients almost invariably select full alertness and the continued presence of some pain.[43,44] Patients who are receiving opioids also need to be monitored for deterioration in vital signs (pulse and respiratory rate), constipation, and urinary retention. Stool softeners and other prophylactic measures such as stimulant laxatives may be required. Similarly, a patient who is receiving NSAIDs or adjunctive analgesics also should be monitored for possible untoward side effects associated with such medications.

Orally or transdermally administered analgesics allow a patient a greater degree of independence and control over daily activities than parenteral administration by maximizing mobility. Similar advantages can be obtained with an intravenous (IV) infusion device, particularly a portable programmable infusion pump. Regular parenteral administration by other routes can be difficult and painful in cachectic patients.

Every patient has a right to expect his or her pain to be controlled, and clinicians should discuss pain management before surgical procedures or after an unexpected trauma or injury. The pain management team should be involved before surgery if severe pain is anticipated or if pain relief is less than satisfactory when treating an acute pain problem. It is important to convey realistic expectations in designing a pain management regimen, however. An expectation of pain control is not synonymous with the complete abolition of pain, particularly with chronic pain syndromes. It is important for the clinician, the patient, and the patient's caregivers or family to understand and agree with the treatment plan, and to design a systematic approach toward achieving the specified goals for pain relief as well as activities.

Low to Moderate Potency (Mild) Analgesics

The nonsteroidal anti-inflammatory analgesics have a relatively flat dose-response effect when contrasted with analgesics such as opioids, reaching maximum analgesia at low to moderate doses. Compared with opiate analgesics, higher doses do not produce greater analgesia. However, these drugs are frequently prescribed at doses in excess of the effective maximum analgesic dose because the duration of analgesia can increase with higher doses.. For example, ibuprofen given 600 mg every 6 hours produces a similar analgesic effect as 400 mg given every 4 hours. The total daily dose is the same, but side effects are experienced more often with larger doses. Although the NSAIDs have both analgesic and anti-inflammatory properties, it is often difficult to differentiate between these effects in published studies or during clinical use in patients, as the time courses of each effect overlap.

All of the NSAIDs, including ibuprofen (Motrin), naproxen (Naprosyn), naproxen sodium (Anaprox), diflunisal (Dolobid), diclofenac (Voltaren), diclofenac potassium (Cataflam), nabumetone (Relafen), ketoprofen (Orudis), flurbiprofen (Ansaid), ketorolac (Toradol), and others, provide analgesia equivalent or superior to that of aspirin[45,46] or acetaminophen combined with codeine 60 mg in a variety of mild to moderate painful conditions.[47–50] Like the opioid analgesics, the duration of action of the NSAID does not correlate well with the serum half-life of the drug. This is likely due to the analgesic effect arising from central mechanisms, and related to the exposure of the CNS to adequate drug levels. Patient response should guide the clinician in selecting dosing intervals of these agents, especially when they are combined with opioids.

Opioid Analgesics

In general, opioids are more potent than nonopioid analgesics such as NSAIDs, although the range of potencies is wide with this class of medicines. They are generally recommended for moderate to severe pain intensity and are used in chronic pain syndromes that are refractory to other classes of agents.

An intramuscular (IM) dose of 10 mg/70 kg of morphine sulfate provides significant analgesia in approximately 70% of patients with severe pain. The remaining 30% of patients require higher doses,[51] which not only increases the intensity and duration of analgesia, but also the incidence of side effects. Morphine dosage requirements also vary with the severity of pain, individual perceptions of pain, age, opioid tolerance or previous exposure, and the presence of concomitant diseases. Thus, single parenteral analgesic doses of morphine ranging from 4 to >20 mg are used to treat acute pain, and parenteral doses as high as 200 mg/hour have been required to treat end-stage malignant pain.

A 10-mg parenteral dose of morphine is the historical reference standard by which all other opioid analgesics are compared. Therefore, morphine equivalents are often used when calculating analgesic doses for other opioids. The duration of analgesia of an opioid correlates partially with its serum half-life, but also with the dose, route of administration, and the distribution characteristics of the drug.[52] For example, methadone has a very long serum half-life of 24 hours, but its duration of analgesia is only about 6 hours. However, single daily doses of methadone are retained on opiate receptors in the brain long enough to prevent abstinence symptoms in opiate abusers. When used for pain management, the long half-life of methadone may contribute to cumulative effects and drug toxicity such as QTc prolongation. When methadone is administered epidurally, its duration of analgesia is short because of its high lipophilicity that promotes rapid redistribution from the epidural space into systemic circulation, and consequently, clearance. Conversely, morphine has a relatively short duration of analgesia when administered parenterally, but when it is administered epidurally, it has a long duration of analgesia because of its low lipophilicity, which inhibits its redistribution from the epidural space.

The administration of opioid analgesics is frequently complicated by the need to convert between different routes of administration or different opioid formulations. The approximate equianalgesic doses of parenteral and oral opioid analgesics are listed in Table 9-3. The specific oral:parenteral ra-

Table 9-3 Properties of Opioid Analgesics

	Parenteral Dose (mg)	Oral Equivalent	Routes	Onset (min)	Duration (hr)	t½ (hr)	Notes
Opioid Agonists for Moderate to Severe Pain (mu Receptor Agonists)							
Phenanthrenes:							
Morphine (various)	10	30	PO, parenteral, PR	IV: 5, PO: 60	3–6	2–3	Sustained release PO preps available
Hydromorphone (Dilaudid)	1.5	7.5	PO, parenteral, PR	See morphine	3–6	2–4	
Levorphanol (Levo-Dromoran)	2	4	PO, SC, IM	30–90	4–6	4–16	Accumulates with chronic dosing
Oxymorphone (Numorphan)	1.5	N/A	Parenteral, PR	10–90	3–6	3–4	
Phenylpiperidines:							
Fentanyl (Sublimaze)	0.1	N/A	IV, spinal, buccal, patch	10	1–2	3–4	Nonlinear kinetics with repeat dosing
Sufentanil (Sufenta)	10 μg	N/A	Parenteral, spinal	10	2–4		Duration may be dose-related
Diphenylheptanes:							
Methadone (Dolophine)	10	5	PO, SC, IM	SC, IM = 60	6–8	21–25	Accumulates with chronic dosing
Opiods for Mild to Moderate Pain (mu Agonists)							
Phenanthrenes:							
Codeine (various)	120	200	PO, parenteral, PR	See morphine	3–6		
Hydrocodone (various)	N/A	30	PO	30–60	3–4		
Oxycodone (various)	N/A	20	PO	30–60	4–6		
Dihydrocodeine (various)	N/A	30	PO	30–60	4–6		
Phenylpiperidines:							
Meperidine (Demerol)	100	400	PO, parenteral	15–60	1–3	3–4	Normeperidine is a CNS irritant
Partial Agonists/Antagonists (mu and/or Kappa Agonists with or without mu Antagonism)							
Buprenorphine (Buprenex)	0.3	N/A	SC, IV, IM	15	4–6	2–3	Not naloxone reversible
Butorphanol (Stadol)	2	N/A	SC, IV, IM, intranasal	15–45	3–4		Dysphoric
Nalbuphine (Nubain)	10	N/A	SC, IV, IM	15	4–6	2–3	Respiratory ceiling
Opioid Antagonists							
Naloxone (Narcan)	0.4–0.8	N/A	IV	10	2–3	1–1.5	
Naltrexone (Trexan)	N/A	50	PO	30–60	24–72	9–17	Duration dose-dependent

NOTE: Most analgesic equivalents were derived from single dose studies
Adapted from Principles of Analgesic Use in the Treatment of Acute Pain and Cancer Pain, Fifth Edition. Glenview, IL: American Pain Society, 2003, pp14–17.

tios of these drugs also are listed in Table 9-3; however, the precision of these ratios is controversial, in part because of the methodologies used to infer these "equivalencies." For example, some investigators maintain that the oral:parenteral ratio for morphine is 6:1, but some hospice clinicians maintain that morphine's oral:parenteral ratio is closer to 2:1. Such confusion may result from differences in the design of single-dose versus multiple-dose clinical trials. First-pass hepatic metabolism may be greater in single-dose clinical studies than in multiple-dose studies because first-pass metabolic pathways can become saturated with repeated doses. Furthermore, the accumulation of the active metabolite morphine-6-glucuronide after chronic dosing may contribute to the clinically observed differences. When all factors are taken into account, the bioavailability of oral morphine varies from 17% to 70% of a dose; therefore, it is reasonable to expect individual patient response to be highly variable.[53,54] No matter which ratio the clinician uses, the dosing must be guided by the patient's clinical response and frequent clinical reassessment.

If an opioid analgesic is to be substituted with another opioid, the equivalent doses as listed in Table 9-3 can be used as an approximate guide to dosage conversions unless the patient has developed tolerance. Cross-tolerance between opioid analgesics exists, but is often not complete. Therefore, calculated doses may be reduced by as much as 50% when interchanging different opioids. This is especially true when switching to methadone from other opioids.[55] Patient comfort is the goal, and the response of the patient should always be the basis for dosage adjustments. Whenever a new opioid analgesic is initiated, the patient's response should be assessed within the first few hours because the initial dose of the new analgesic is only correctly estimated about half the time. Frequent reassessment of clinical responses should facilitate dosage adjustments and control the patient's pain more quickly.

The analgesic efficacy of propoxyphene and combinations of acetaminophen with propoxyphene 65 mg remains controversial. Most double-blind studies demonstrate no advantage of propoxyphene alone over aspirin, acetaminophen, or codeine in relieving various types of pain.[56,57] This lack of benefit conflicts with the observation that propoxyphene in combination with acetaminophen remains a commonly prescribed regimen in the United States. This may be partially explained by an additive or synergistic effect when opioids are combined with nonopioid analgesics. Another possible explanation is the tendency of many patients to take more than the prescribed doses. Because propoxyphene has a 13-hour half-life, repeated doses taken every 4 to 6 hours for several days can result in significant drug accumulation. Furthermore, analgesic assessments of propoxyphene efficacy have been based primarily on single-dose studies,[58] in spite of the fact that patients take as many as 10 to 12 tablets daily. Propoxyphene has significant CNS effects. At lower dosages, propoxyphene can produce mild CNS depressant effects. However, at higher dosages, it can have an amphetamine-like stimulant effect, and in overdoses, propoxyphene can produce seizures. Like other opioid analgesics, propoxyphene can produce physical dependence.

As with all opioid analgesics, patients taking propoxyphene need to be warned about the risks of concurrent alcohol use, the operation of equipment or machinery requiring mental acuity, and the potential for agitation and sleeplessness when the medication is discontinued abruptly after prolonged use. In addition to effects on the CNS, propoxyphene has been associated with hypoglycemia in patients with renal dysfunction.[59]

Differentiating Between Clinical Opioid Use and Drug Abuse

When using opiates to treat severe pain lasting more than a few days, several phenomena can occur. The terms used to describe these phenomena are *tolerance, physical dependence,* and *pseudoaddiction.* Clinicians must understand the differences and the context in which these phenomena occur to differentiate between expected developments and drug abuse. Much of the fear and reluctance to use opioid analgesics result from misunderstandings of these natural events by clinicians, patients, and caregivers.

Tolerance to the analgesic effects of opiates is a common physiologic finding that results from neuroadaptation by the body during chronic use.[60] It may be seen after several days of therapy and can be first recognized by a decrease in the duration of analgesia. Patients who develop tolerance require an increase in the opiate dose to achieve the same level of analgesia. Tolerance to opiates occurs fairly slowly, but should be anticipated in all patients requiring continuous opiate therapy, such as critical care patients or patients with chronic painful conditions. These types of patients should be informed that the need for increasing doses is an expected occurrence and does not indicate addiction.

Physical dependence is another natural physiologic process that occurs with chronic opioid administration.[60] Signs and symptoms of physical dependence are summarized

Table 9-4 Signs and Symptoms of Opiate Physical Dependence

1. Rhinorrhea—runny nose
2. Lacrimation—tearing
3. Hyperthermia, chills
4. Muscle aches (myalgia)
5. Emesis, diarrhea, GI cramping
6. Anxiety, agitation, hostility
7. Sleeplessness

Symptoms begin within 6 hours for short-acting opioids (e.g., morphine) and generally peak in approximately 36–48 hours. Symptoms of abstinence usually subside within 3–7 days (average = 5). With methadone, however, abstinence syndrome develops more slowly, and is less severe, but protracted. Opioid antagonists or mixed agonist-antagonist drugs can precipitate abstinence in some patients after chronic or subchronic opioid exposure.

in Table 9-4 and are seen only when opiates are stopped abruptly or the dose is markedly decreased. Physical dependence does not indicate addiction, and the difference should be made clear to patients and their caregivers. The symptoms of physical dependence may be observed in critical care patients who have their doses of opioid analgesics tapered too rapidly or in patients requiring chronic opioid therapy who are unable to obtain an adequate supply of medication or who are undertreated. Unintentional physical withdrawal can also occur if metabolic enzyme inducers, such as phenytoin, are added to a chronic pain regimen. Early symptoms of abstinence can include irritability and restlessness, and onset occurs within 6 to 24 hours of the time the last opioid dose was administered. Later, a person develops chills, sweating, joint and muscle pains, and gastrointestinal (GI) distress, including emesis and diarrhea with abdominal cramping. The time of onset is correlated to the drug's half-life, to the average doses required by an individual, and to the pattern and history of opioid dosing. For instance, abstinence induced by tolerance to hydrocodone (a drug with a short half-life) can be anticipated to develop in 4 to 6 hours after the last dose, whereas with methadone it may not occur for 24 to 48 hours after the last dose. Similarly, the abstinence syndrome can last longer when associated with long-acting agents. For short-acting agents such as hydrocodone or oxycodone, abstinence may resolve within 48 to 72 hours, whereas for drugs such as methadone, it may last as long as several days. Mood swings, myalgia, and arthralgia may persist for as long as several weeks after the last dose of an opioid.

Addiction to opioid analgesics is characterized by a dysfunctional pattern of use for purposes other than alleviation of pain. It may involve adverse consequences of opioid use, loss of control over their use, and preoccupation with obtaining opioids despite the presence of adequate analgesia. It is important to realize that tolerance and physical dependence may or may not be present in addiction and that the presence of tolerance and physical dependency does not imply addiction. *Pseudoaddiction* is an important type of behavior that clinicians must understand and recognize because it can easily be misinterpreted as addiction.[60] Pseudoaddictive behaviors may be seen in patients with severe, unrelieved pain. These behaviors may mimic those seen with addiction. Patients become preoccupied with obtaining opioids; however, their underlying focus is on finding relief for their pain. Their fear of not having an adequate amount of medication available to control their pain may result in medication hoarding. When patients with pseudoaddiction are provided adequate analgesia, the behaviors that mimic addiction resolve, the medications are used as prescribed, and the patient's daily functioning increases.[60]

If opioid misuse is suspected, pharmacists can help both patients and prescribers develop appropriate care plans by being vigilant for warning signs that the patient is not adhering to a care plan. These include prescriptions from multiple physicians or phone calls from unknown physicians; rapid or unsanctioned escalation of dosing requirements, particularly for nonmalignant pain syndromes; frequent excuses for running out of medication early or requests for "vacation" supplies; lack of requests for adjunct analgesic refills (e.g., antidepressants, anticonvulsants); extreme polypharmacy with multiple CNS depressants or multiple habituating substances; and injecting oral medicines or chewing matrix formulations.

Persons demonstrating these traits may require referral to an appropriate substance abuse program.[61]

ACUTE PAIN
Analgesic Goals

1. **E.T. is a 36-year-old woman recovering from the surgical repair of a left tibia fracture that resulted from a motor vehicle accident. She is otherwise healthy, with no other medical conditions. Her medication history reveals no drug allergies or history of recreational drug use, and occasional use of ibuprofen 400 mg PO Q 6 hr PRN for menstrual cramps. Postoperatively, E.T. received acetaminophen 325 mg with codeine 30 mg, two tablets PO Q 3 hr for pain; however, this analgesic regimen is inadequate for controlling her pain. After extensive complaints, E.T.'s analgesic medication was replaced with two tablets of hydrocodone 5 mg with acetaminophen 500 mg Q 4 hr. In spite of these changes, E.T. continues to complain of pain. Vital signs indicate the following: respiratory rate, 24 breaths/min; heart rate, 110 beats/min; blood pressure (BP), 140/85 mm Hg. She rates the intensity of her pain as 8 on a 10-point scale. What is your assessment of E.T.'s pain and what are reasonable analgesia goals for E.T.?**

The current analgesic regimen has not provided E.T. with adequate pain relief based on her pain evaluation rating of 8 on a 10-point scale. Physiologic responses to pain include autonomic findings, such as increased respirations, heart rate, and BP. The apparent analgesic failure in E.T. can be attributed to several factors. First, the choice of medication may not be effective for her level of pain, or she may simply require more analgesics than anticipated. Standard analgesic dosage recommendations are only conservative estimates of average initial doses. Ultimately, analgesic dosing must be tailored to the specific needs of the patient. Patients with compromised metabolic function may need smaller doses, whereas patients with extensive injuries may require larger doses. Acute pain always should be aggressively treated.

After an initial analgesic has been administered, the patient should be assessed frequently, and doses should be adjusted quickly in response to inadequate pain control or excessive sedation. The dose of an analgesic should be modified before a patient feels the need to express significant discomfort from pain. E.T.'s complaints of significant pain intensity may also be influenced by anxiety that commonly accompanies inadequate pain relief. E.T.'s possible anxiety over the current surgical outcome could intensify her pain because pain and anxiety are reinforcing phenomena. For most patients, pain is synonymous with injury. When an injury has been repaired and the patient continues to experience pain, the patient's anxiety and fear can intensify pain sensations. The use of Pain Distress Scales, as shown in Figure 9-6, may be more useful for evaluating pain in patients with significant anxiety.[24] The use of distraction or relaxation techniques can also help make E.T. more comfortable.

The goal for managing acute pain is to keep the patient as comfortable as possible while minimizing possible untoward adverse effects from the analgesic. It is important for the clinician to discuss the pain management plan with the patient, establishing goals of therapy, addressing patient concerns, and evaluating patient understanding. Use of pain rating scales, as shown in Figure 9-5, should be reviewed with the patient, and a pain rating goal that is acceptable to the patient should be determined. The importance of factual reporting should be emphasized to the patient. This helps eliminate behaviors of stoicism or exaggeration.[24] Appropriate goals for E.T. would be a pain rating of <4 out of 10, a return of vital signs toward her baseline values, and reduced anxiety. Only appropriate analgesic selection, careful follow-up evaluations, and rational analgesic dosage adjustments can accomplish these goals.

Combination Analgesics

2. **Is the choice of acetaminophen with hydrocodone appropriate for E.T.?**

Acetaminophen and opioid analgesics provide pain relief by different mechanisms of action and it is reasonable to use both for their additive or synergistic effects when managing pain. However, acetaminophen with hydrocodone is a fixed-dose combination, and these combination drug formulations decrease dosing flexibility and frequently lead to unintended toxic side effects. The combination of acetaminophen 500 mg and hydrocodone 5 mg given two tablets every 4 hours can result in the patient receiving 6 g of acetaminophen in a 24-hour period. Chronic administration of acetaminophen in doses exceeding 5 g/day has been associated with hepatic enzyme changes. Short-term use of 6 g of acetaminophen daily for a few days in patients without risk factors (e.g., alcoholism, malnutrition, concurrent administration of hepatic-enzyme inducers) is usually safe.[62] If patients need to use acetaminophen-containing combination analgesics frequently throughout the day, then one should consider products that contain lower amounts of acetaminophen. Several NSAIDs also have been associated with hepatotoxicity.[63] Acetaminophen and NSAIDs should be avoided in patients who have severe liver disease, as evidenced by elevated liver transaminases, a low serum albumin, or a prolonged prothrombin time. If acetaminophen is to be used at all in patients with impaired hepatic function, doses must be limited to <2 to 3 g/24 hours.

E.T. should have been initiated on more potent analgesics to control her pain. Analgesic combinations of acetaminophen with either codeine 30 mg or hydrocodone 5 mg are effective for mild to moderate pain (e.g., ≤5 on a 10-point scale), but these combinations are less than adequate for moderately severe to severe pain, unless the opioid dose is increased. Because E.T.'s pain has not been successfully controlled with either acetaminophen with codeine or acetaminophen with hydrocodone, it would be reasonable to start her on oral morphine 30 mg every 4 hours. If she is unable to tolerate oral medications following surgery, then morphine 4 mg IV every 2 to 3 hours can be used instead. Although the use of IM administration is often prescribed, many clinicians discourage the use of this route because of erratic or unpredictable absorption with some opiates and additional pain caused from the injection itself.

After initiation of morphine, E.T. should be evaluated for pain relief and adverse effects in a few hours. The dose or dosing interval should be adjusted if either is found to be inadequate. Sometimes, changing to an alternative opiate may be indicated if analgesia is still inadequate or unwanted side effects are experienced. Until an individual's response to a particular opioid is known, it is wise for the clinician to formulate a back-up plan with an alternative opiate regimen.

An NSAID such as ibuprofen or naproxen also may be used adjunctively for E.T.'s pain. Although NSAIDs alone usually are inadequate for controlling moderate to severe pain, they have additive analgesic effects when combined with opiates. In E.T., one also must consider the risk of bleeding after surgical intervention owing to the antiplatelet effect of NSAIDs. Newer cyclooxygenase-2 (COX-2) NSAIDs appear to have minimal antiplatelet effects, so may be considered if surgery or trauma presents a high risk of bleeding.

Equianalgesic Dosing of Opioid Analgesics

3. How should E.T.'s hydrocodone dose be converted to oral morphine?

Hydrocodone 20 mg orally is approximately equal to morphine 30 mg (see Table 9-3). Therefore, the 10 mg of hydrocodone as originally ordered for E.T. is equal to an oral morphine dose of approximately 15 mg, or 5 mg of morphine by injection. This dose of morphine would likely be inadequate for E.T. because her pain control is not controlled by this equivalent dose. Thus, E.T. should be started on oral morphine 30 mg every 4 hours around-the-clock for the first 24 hours, then changed to as-needed dosing afterward. Inflammation due to trauma often peaks around 48 to 72 hours following the inciting event, so pain is expected to decrease dramatically after this period.

Managing Side Effects of Opioid Analgesics

4. E.T. complains of itching after three doses of morphine, but shows no sign of rash. What can be done to alleviate the problem?

Opioid analgesics can cause pruritic rashes and other true allergic-type reactions. When administered parentally, they can stimulate local histamine release from mast cells and cause a local wheal, burning, itching, and erythema at the site of injection. In contrast, systemic release of histamine after both oral and parenteral administration of opioids can produce either localized or generalized flushing and itching. Although these latter reactions occur frequently and may be confused with an allergic reaction, true opioid allergies are infrequent. When they do occur, they are IgE-dependent.[64] Coadministration of diphenhydramine (Benadryl) or hydroxyzine (Vistaril) prevents histamine-induced itching and also provides antianxiety effects that may add to morphine's analgesic benefit.

Chemically, there are three distinct structural categories of opioids: the *phenanthrenes* (morphine, codeine, hydrocodone, hydromorphone, dihydrocodeine, oxycodone, oxymorphone, levorphanol, nalbuphine, butorphanol, dezocine, and dihydrocodeine), the *phenylpiperidines* (meperidine, fentanyl, alfentanil, sufentanil, and remifentanil), and the *phenylheptanones or diphenylheptanes* (methadone, levomethadyl, and the weak analgesic, propoxyphene). Allergic reactions may cross-manifest within the same chemical structural class, but are less likely between classes. Thus, in patients with true allergic reactions, treatment can be instituted

with a product from one of the other chemical groups. For example, if E.T. was allergic to morphine, she could be switched to fentanyl.

5. What other adverse effects from morphine should be monitored for in E.T.? What preventive measures should be considered?

The most common side effects reported with the use of opioid analgesics are nausea, vomiting, itching, and constipation. These are expected untoward opioid effects, and with some care they can be managed or minimized. These first three symptoms of nausea, vomiting, and itching can all be minimized by antihistamines, such as diphenhydramine or hydroxyzine 25 to 50 mg orally every 6 hours as needed. If drowsiness from the antihistamine is excessive when used in combination with the opioid, a nonsedating antihistamine such as fexofenadine can be substituted. Persistent and more problematic symptoms may require switching to an alternative opioid analgesic.

The best method for treating opioid-induced constipation is prevention. Postsurgical patients are especially prone to this effect because their GI motility is already slowed from decreased physical activity and from anesthetic agents received during surgery. Morphine and other opioids suppress the propulsive peristaltic action of the colon, increase colonic and anal sphincter tone, and reduce the reflex relaxation response to rectal distention. These actions, combined with decreased normal sensory stimuli for defecation because of their CNS-depressant actions, contribute to opioid-induced constipation. Stool softeners are effective in keeping the bowel contents moist, but do not stimulate bowel peristaltic propulsion. Only the stimulant laxatives and prokinetic agents can increase bowel propulsive activity. When opioid analgesics are initiated, a stimulating laxative plus stool softener should also be initiated. E.T. will be receiving morphine orally around the clock and probably would benefit from 1 senna tablet orally at bedtime in addition to docusate 250 mg orally twice daily. For more resistant constipation, one can use oral lactulose 30 mL every hour and/or sodium phosphate enemas.

Postoperative ileus frequently is exacerbated by opioid analgesics, but opioids rarely produce ileus or bowel obstruction alone without other underlying physiologic causes. Oral naloxone 0.4 to 12 mg every 6 hours has been used with some success in preventing opioid-induced constipation. Unlike parenteral naloxone, oral naloxone is poorly absorbed systemically (25%) and therefore will not interfere with analgesic effect unless doses are high.[65–71] An oral naloxone formulation is not yet commercially available, but the parenteral preparation can be administered orally if needed. The oral naloxone requirement rarely exceeds 2.4 mg every 6 hours. At higher dosages, systemic antagonist effects can occur, resulting in decreased analgesia in addition to the local intestinal effects.

6. On the third day of her morphine treatment, E.T. appears agitated. Could her agitation be attributed to her morphine?

Although opioids are CNS depressants, they can cause CNS excitation, especially if the patient receives large doses for a prolonged period. Anxiety, agitation, irritability, motor restlessness, tremors, involuntary twitching, and myoclonic seizures have been associated with meperidine, morphine, and hydromorphone, but not methadone, though methadone may rarely cause myoclonus. For meperidine and morphine, the CNS toxicity correlates to accumulation of their active metabolites, normeperidine and morphine-6-glucuronide, respectively. Because both of these metabolites are cleared renally, patients with renal insufficiency are at greatest risk, but toxicity can also occur when high doses are administered frequently even in patients with normal renal function.[71,72] With meperidine, the problem is compounded by the 17-hour half-life of normeperidine. In patients with normal renal function, avoiding doses in excess of 60 mg/hour of meperidine, 100 mg/hour of morphine, or 40 mg/hour of hydromorphone minimizes CNS toxicity.

The treatment of opioid-induced CNS irritability should include discontinuation of the opioid analgesic and treatment with a benzodiazepine. Myoclonic seizures resulting from meperidine administration are sometimes preceded by involuntary twitching in the extremities and can be averted by discontinuing the meperidine. Seizures induced by meperidine are resistant to naloxone, but respond to anticonvulsants such as phenytoin or diazepam. Because E.T. has normal renal function and her morphine dose is not excessive, it is unlikely that she is suffering from morphine-induced CNS effects. It is more likely that she is starting to recover from her surgery and is anxious from her environment. Nevertheless, it may be time to start reducing her morphine dose if her pain is well controlled.

Ketorolac

7. Could parenteral ketorolac (Toradol) be given to E.T. instead of the morphine?

Short-term opioids for acute pain, even at very large doses, do not cause dependency or abuse and therefore should not be withheld because of fear of addiction. E.T. will be receiving opioids only during the immediate postoperative period, and opioids can be rapidly tapered after the more severe acute pain has subsided. The acute clinical use of opioids in hospitalized patients does not cause drug addiction in an otherwise psychologically healthy individual. For patients like E.T. with acute severe pain, an opioid such as oral or parenteral morphine or hydromorphone should be the first-line agent for pain management. However, as E.T.'s pain severity decreases, NSAIDs may be considered for treating mild to moderate pain.

Because it is the only available injectable NSAID in the United States, ketorolac is sometimes used as an alternative to opioids. Although ketorolac is indicated for the short-term management of moderate to severe pain, it should not be substituted for appropriate opioid analgesics for the management of acute postoperative pain.[73,74] Ketorolac is most beneficial in postoperative pain if it is used in combination with the opioids instead of as monotherapy. Parenteral formulations of NSAIDs are no more effective than oral formulations given in equivalent doses (e.g., ibuprofen 600 mg orally every 6 hours is equally as effective as 15 to 30 mg parenteral ketorolac).[75] Ketorolac also has been associated with several cases of serious postsurgical bleeding. Although ketorolac could be effective in relieving E.T.'s pain, it is no more effective than morphine. Patients receiving ketorolac should be monitored for typical NSAID side effects, especially postsurgical bleeding.

NSAIDs cause sodium retention and can also block prostaglandin-induced vasodilation in patients with compromised renal blood flow. Thus, NSAIDs should be used with caution in patients with congestive heart failure, hypovolemia, dehydration or any other conditions that compromise renal blood flow and increase the risk of developing renal toxicity.

Nonsteroidal Anti-Inflammatory Drug Selection

8. Two days later, E.T. is ready to be discharged from the hospital. Although her pain is much improved, she still has mild to moderate intermittent pain. The pain management team is planning to send her home with NSAIDs to treat her pain. Is any one NSAID analgesic superior to the others?

In all probability, all NSAIDs, not just those with an approved indication for the treatment of mild to moderate pain, have analgesic properties. The superiority of any particular NSAID for a particular patient cannot be predicted, and no one NSAID has been demonstrated to have superior analgesia over any other. Nevertheless, patients who fail to benefit from one NSAID can respond to a different NSAID. Therefore, an NSAID should be selected based on the patient's previous history of response, efficacy, safety, and cost. Ibuprofen and other proprionic acids have a long history of safety and are available as less costly generic products. (See Chapter 43, Rheumatic Disorders, for a more detailed discussion of the clinical use of NSAIDs.)

When selecting one of these agents, the clinician must be aware of the considerable risk of systemic side effects. Although GI side effects are the most common, NSAIDs have caused undesirable nervous system, otic, ocular, hematologic, renal, and hepatic adverse effects. Once an NSAID has been selected, the doses should be increased until pain has been relieved or the maximum tolerable dose has been achieved. Some investigators have used rather large doses with remarkable success. The use of the newer selective COX-2 NSAIDs should be limited to patients who have demonstrated GI intolerance to other NSAIDs (e.g., history of ulcer). COX-2 NSAIDs have fewer effects on the intestinal mucosa, but other side effects are similar, including fluid retention and effects on renal prostaglandins.

9. If E.T. had a history of asthma, would NSAIDs be safe to use?

Aspirin and essentially all other NSAIDs can induce bronchospasm and other allergic manifestations in patients with a history of asthma, allergic rhinitis, and nasal polyps. However, the asthma response is not an allergic reaction, but rather a pharmacologic effect associated with prostaglandin inhibition and unopposed leukotriene activity in the respiratory tract.

Acetaminophen does not induce bronchospasm and is safe to give to patients with an asthma history. The risk of using NSAIDs or aspirin in chronic bronchitis, emphysema, and asthmatics without nasal polyps or history of drug-induced bronchospasm is less clear. If E.T. had a history of asthma, then NSAIDs should be avoided or used cautiously.[76,77]

Analgesic Nephrotoxicity

10. What are the risks of analgesic nephropathy from NSAIDs in E.T.?

Analgesic overuse is a common cause of chronic interstitial nephritis (CIN) and may account for approximately 5% of the cases of chronic renal failure in the United States. Historically, aspirin and phenacetin in combination were thought to be the causative agent for most cases of CIN; however, acetaminophen, aspirin,[78] and the NSAIDs[79,80] also have been implicated. Acetaminophen-induced renal toxicity is almost always accompanied by concomitant serum hepatic transaminase changes and generally is associated with acute acetaminophen intoxication.[81] Most cases of interstitial nephritis seem to be related to both dose and duration of NSAID therapy.[82,83] (Also see Chapter 31, Acute Renal Failure.)

The NSAID's effect on renal function may be twofold. NSAIDs can directly damage renal tubules and can also reduce renal blood flow by inhibiting prostacyclin. Prostacyclin modifies renal function in response to the effects of endogenous vasoconstrictors (e.g., norepinephrine and angiotensin II), especially if the patient is volume depleted, has been taking diuretics, or is elderly. Renal insufficiency may occur in 20% of patients with one or more of these identifiable risks who also take NSAIDs.[84,85] Patients with cirrhosis and ascites[86] and patients with significantly altered hemodynamic status can experience as much as a 50% decrease in creatinine clearance (Cl_{Cr}) when treated with indomethacin (Indocin)[87,88] or ibuprofen (Motrin). Some subjects with normal renal function have experienced profound changes in glomerular filtration rate when taking indomethacin concurrent with triamterene (Dyrenium).[89]

For E.T., who is fairly young and healthy without risk factors, the potential for NSAID-induced renal toxicity is quite low. However, her renal function still should be monitored if she is to be placed on NSAIDs for more than a few days because she has recently undergone surgery and may have relative volume depletion.

NSAID Use in Renal Disease

11. If E.T. was currently exhibiting renal dysfunction, what NSAID could be used?

Sulindac (Clinoril) and nabumetone (Relafen) have been reported to cause less renal insufficiency because of the absence of active urinary nephrotoxic metabolites. These two NSAIDs can still decrease renal blood flow in patients at risk and can cause renal dysfunction via hypersensitivity reactions unrelated to their effects on renal blood flow. Although sulindac and nabumetone appear to be preferred over other NSAIDs in patients with renal dysfunction, clinical experience is not as great with these two drugs relative to other NSAIDs.

Possible drug-induced nephrotic syndrome has been reported with indomethacin (Indocin), ibuprofen (Motrin), naproxen (Naprosyn), phenylbutazone (Butazolidin), fenoprofen (Nalfon), sulindac (Clinoril), and tolmetin (Tolectin). In particular, fenoprofen has been implicated in 71% of 31 cases.[90] The prognosis for recovery of renal function is excellent, although some patients require treatment with corticosteroids.[91] It is unclear whether patients with pre-existing renal dysfunction are at any greater risk of developing further

drug-induced abnormalities, but most clinicians consider it a relative contraindication.

Opioids
Patient-Controlled Analgesia

12. T.J., a 52-year-old woman, has had posterior spinal fusion with instrumentation because of severe scoliosis that had compromised her respiratory function and quality of life. She has just been transferred to the ward from the postanesthetic recovery critical care unit. She is now crying and complaining of severe pain not relieved by meperidine 75 mg IM Q 3 hr. T.J. has no known drug allergies. She has a history of taking acetaminophen 500 mg with hydrocodone 7.5 mg two tablets Q 3 hr before admission. Why would a patient-controlled analgesia (PCA) device be useful for T.J.?

PCA is a technique whereby patients self-administer narcotics by using a preprogrammed mechanical infusion device attached to tubing that delivers the drug to the patient through an IV or subcutaneous needle or catheter. Basically, the patient depresses a button to activate the PCA controller to deliver a preset dose of opiate medication. This prevents the need to call a nurse or other caregiver when pain arises and also obviates the problem of drug doses that are not ordered frequently enough. The controller is preprogrammed to establish "lock-out" periods that prevent the pump from delivering a dose if the patient presses the button too often. Safeguards against accidental overdose are instituted by adjusting the concentration of drug in the controller and/or the duration of the lock-out period. Either of these variables can be adjusted to fit the patient's analgesic needs. Caution must be taken to instruct parents of children or adolescents appropriately on the use of the PCA device, lest they inadvertently administer an excess amount of medication. In general, family members should not act as "surrogates" in helping patients control their pain with a PCA device.

Numerous programmable PCA devices are available, most of which have the capability of providing intermittent self-boluses of drug with or without continuous infusion. Some systems use syringe pump technology and others an IV pump system. Compact devices are convenient for ambulatory use. T.J.'s pain can be managed with a PCA device for as long as she is able to comprehend the operation of the device. Most postoperative patients require a basal continuous infusion of opioid in addition to intermittent boluses during the first 24-hour period. The need for continuous basal infusion usually diminishes after 24 to 48 hours. PCA is most useful in the first 3 to 5 postoperative days when the patient has the most severe pain. After this initial critical period, the pain can readily be managed with oral analgesic doses. The PCA allows T.J. to have control over her pain. She will determine how often and when the opioid analgesic is delivered, and she can titrate the dose to a level of comfort or side effects that is acceptable to her.

OPIOID SELECTION FOR USE IN PCA

13. What opioid analgesics could be used in T.J.'s PCA device?

Most of the commonly prescribed parenteral opioids can be used in a PCA, but fentanyl, hydromorphone, and mor-

Table 9-5   Recommended Doses of Opioid Analgesics

Initial Doses	Adult Oral Dose (mg)	Child Oral Dose (mg/kg)
Opioid Agonists for Moderate to Severe Pain (mu Receptor Agonists)		
Morphine(various)	15–30	0.30
Hydromorphone (Dilaudid)	4–8	0.06
Levorphanol (Levo-Dromoran)	2–4	0.04
Methadone (Dolophine)	5–10	0.20
Opioids for Mild to Moderate Pain (mu Agonists)		
Codeine (various)	30–60	0.5–1
Hydrocodone (various)	5–10	N/A
Oxycodone (various)	5	0.1
Tramadol (Ultram)	50–100	NR
Meperidine (Demerol)	Not Recommended (NR)	

Patient Controlled Analgesia (Parenteral)

	Usual Initial Dose (mg)	Dose Range (mg)	Interval Range (minutes)
Morphine	1.0	0.5–2.0	6 (5–10)
Hydromorphone	0.2	0.04–0.4	6 (5–10)
Fentanyl	0.01 (10 μg)	0.01–0.05	6 (5–10)

Example: A morphine PCA with a 1.0 mg initial dose that allows a patient to self-administer an additional 1 mg every 6 minutes provides a dosing range of 1.0–11 mg per hour available medication.

Adapted from Principles of Analgesic Use in the Treatment of Acute Pain and Cancer Pain, Fifth Edition. Glenview, IL: American Pain Society, 2003, pp14–17, 20.

phine are used most frequently. Meperidine is used less frequently due to the problems with the normeperidine metabolite discussed earlier. (See Table 9-5 for dosing guidelines.) Morphine usually is recommended first, followed by hydromorphone, fentanyl, and meperidine. If the patient has a history of morphine intolerance (e.g., itching or nausea), alternative agents such as hydromorphone should be initiated. Most of the opioids used for PCA have a broad range of acceptable doses with the exception of meperidine, which has a narrow dosing range because the active normeperidine metabolite can accumulate, even at normal therapeutic doses. Meperidine also has only a 3-hour half-life and perhaps an even shorter duration of action as an analgesic.[92] Therefore, meperidine is unsuitable for treatment of acute severe pain when the analgesic requirement is exceedingly high or when patients have impaired renal function. Fentanyl can be a safer alternative to meperidine.

PCA is used most commonly for administering opioids IV, and on rare occasions, subcutaneously. Subcutaneous opioid administration is limited by the fluid volume needed to deliver the drug. A subcutaneous infusion of 1 mL/hour is universally accepted; however, slightly larger volumes can be acceptable in some patients. Highly concentrated morphine solutions (e.g., 60 mg/mL) must be compounded to permit maximal doses for these patients. Alternatively, hydromorphone (Dilaudid HP) at concentrations of 10 mg/mL can be used. When necessary, hydromorphone powder can be purchased and higher concentrations can be prepared (maximum concentration of 40 mg/mL can be achieved), but it is unknown

whether concentrations that exceed those of commercial products increase local tissue irritation or other untoward effects.[93,94] Because no contraindications exist, T.J. should be started on IV morphine in her PCA pump.

PCA PRESCRIPTIONS

14. **How should T.J.'s PCA prescriptions be ordered?**

A basic PCA prescription for opioid analgesics must include the name of the drug, solution concentration, dose for self-bolus, lock-out period, continuous basal dose (if used), and hourly maximum dose limit. In addition, a "rescue dose" and frequency also should be ordered for breakthrough pain. Monitoring parameters such as respiratory rate, blood pressure, mental status, and frequency of assessment also should be included on the order. It is of utmost importance to have the name and telephone or pager number of the person responsible for pain management on the prescription. For example, the IV PCA order for morphine for T.J. would include the following:

Morphine sulfate	1 mg/mL
Self-dose	1 mg (1 mL) IV
Lock-out time	6 minutes
Basal dose	1 mg/hr (1 mL/hr) IV for 24 hr
Rescue	1 mg IV every 20 minutes as needed for pain
1-hr Limit Total	12 mg IV

Hold PCA for respiratory rate <10 breaths/minute or systolic BP <90 mm Hg.

T.J. should be reevaluated 2 hours after starting the PCA, and doses should be adjusted at that time if necessary.

PCA SELECTION CRITERIA

15. **What general criteria can one use in selecting a PCA device?**

A PCA device must be easy to use. If the operation of a device is too complicated, patients and caregivers can easily become confused, especially patients who are recovering from anesthetics and other medications administered during surgery. Patients generally are not interested in learning all the capabilities of a particular device. Most just want to learn the specifics of administering the analgesic. The device selected must have enough programming capability to allow the health care providers to increase or decrease the continuous infusion rate as well as the size of the self-bolus dose and lock-out interval. Most PCA devices allow programming of the dosage of analgesics in milliliters as well as in micrograms and milligrams. PCA devices that are capable of administering doses only in milligrams increase the risk of medication calculation errors and should be avoided. For ambulatory patients, the PCA pump also must be easily portable. Unlike the devices used for general inpatient postoperative care, the ambulatory PCA devices generally do not have extensive restrictions to patient access. If a patient is unreliable and a locked, tamper-proof PCA device is needed, the patient is probably unsuitable for PCA.

Subcutaneous or epidural PCAs can be an alternative for acute and chronic administration of analgesics[95–97] but are more costly than oral analgesics. PCA use does not replace the need to assess patient response. For example, it is not appropriate to assume that pain is automatically controlled when a patient is on a PCA. An institutionally acceptable measuring tool should be used to assess the patient's pain and appropriate documentation made in the patient's medical record. "Patient on PCA" is not adequate documentation for pain assessment. When assessing pain, the clinician should always use either a numeric or visual analog scale as a guide for adjusting therapy (see Fig. 9-5).

DOSE CONVERSION BETWEEN OPIOID ANALGESICS

16. **T.J. has requested another analgesic agent because of excessive sedation. She currently needs 10 mg of morphine per hour from her PCA. How should T.J. be converted to another PCA opioid analgesic?**

The IV equivalent of morphine 10 mg/hour is approximately equal to hydromorphone 2 mg/hour, meperidine 100 mg/hour, or fentanyl 100 μg/hour (see Table 9-3). Meperidine is not a viable alternative for T.J. because the equivalent meperidine dose of 100 mg/hour exceeds the maximum recommended dose of 60 mg/hour. The remaining options are either hydromorphone or fentanyl PCA. Example prescriptions for these two drugs are as follows:

Fentanyl	10 μg/mL
Self-dose	10 μg (1 mL) IV
Lock-out time	6 minutes
Basal dose	10 μg/hr (1 mL/hr) IV
Rescue	10 μg IV every 20 minutes as needed for pain
1-hr Limit Total	120 μg IV

Hold PCA for respiratory rate <10 breaths/minute or systolic BP <90 mm Hg.
Naloxone 0.4 mg 2 ampules by bedside.

OR

Hydromorphone	0.2 mg/mL
Self-dose	0.2 mg (1 mL) IV
Lock-out time	6 minutes
Basal dose	0.2 mg/hr (1 mL/hr) IV
Rescue	0.2 mg IV every 20 minutes as needed for pain
1-hr Limit Total	2.4 mg IV

Hold PCA for respiratory rate <10 breaths/minute or systolic BP <90 mm Hg.
Naloxone 0.4 mg 2 ampules by bedside.

As always, T.J. should be re-evaluated in 2 hours after changing the PCA, and doses should be adjusted at that time.

CONVERSION FROM PCA TO ORAL OPIOIDS

17. **Forty-eight hours later, T.J.'s requirement for hydromorphone has decreased significantly. Her requirement has averaged 0.5 mg hydromorphone/hr in the last 12 hours. How should T.J. be converted to oral opioid analgesics?**

PCA is rarely used beyond 72 hours postoperatively,[98] and continuous basal infusions frequently are discontinued after the first 24 hours. Transition to oral opioid analgesics from PCA should occur as soon as the patient is able to tolerate oral intake of solids. Oral opioid analgesia usually is given every 3 to 4 hours for convenience, as well as allowing time for drug absorption. Conversion to oral from parenteral opioids is best achieved based on the total opioid requirement of the previous 24-hour period. For T.J., the total 24-hour IV hydromorphone (0.5 mg/hour) required was 12 mg, which is roughly equivalent to IV morphine 60 mg, methadone 18 mg, or levorphanol 12 mg. Alternatively, the oral equivalent doses are as follows: morphine 180 mg, methadone 18 mg, levorphanol 24 mg, or hydromorphone 48 mg. Levorphanol, with its long duration of action and a lower incidence of GI side effects, would be a good oral agent to use for T.J. The levorphanol dose for T.J. would be 4 mg every 4 hours. A period of 4 to 6 hours of PCA overlapping dosing of oral opioids is recommended to allow equilibration of the oral medicines, but the PCA's continuous basal infusion should be stopped as soon as the oral dose is given.

Tapering of Opioid Analgesics

18. **How should T.J.'s opioid analgesics be tapered?**

Most patients gradually decrease their activation of a PCA pump as soon as their acute pain begins to subside. In instances in which patients have not decreased their PCA pump use, the dose may safely be reduced by 15% to 20% each day without precipitating symptoms of abstinence. For T.J., the oral levorphanol regimen should be changed to an as-needed schedule once the pain has stabilized. For most patients, a scheduled opioid taper is not essential unless the total daily requirement is in excess of 160 mg of oral morphine (or its equivalent) or if opioid use is prolonged. T.J. should be able to be converted to acetaminophen 325 mg with codeine 30 mg (or an equivalent opioid preparation) once her oral levorphanol has been completely discontinued.

Pain Management in the Opioid-Dependent Patient

19. If T.J. had a history of heroin and cocaine abuse, how would her pain treatment be modified?

Pain management in an IV drug abuser is not difficult as long as the clinician does not judge the patient's behavior or interject personal values into the decision-making process. As with any patient, the goal is to provide as much comfort as possible. Concerns over opiate abuse or addiction are not relevant when treating acute pain, although the clinician must recognize the potential for physical tolerance of opioids and adjust medication doses accordingly.

The first step in the management of a patient with a history of substance abuse is to try to determine the amount of illicit drugs the patient has been using, being alert to the possible abuse of multiple drugs in varying quantities.[99] Patients who have a history of opiate (heroin) and stimulant (cocaine) use are likely to demonstrate a much greater tolerance to opiates than a patient who has been using opiates alone. There is some evidence that cross-tolerance can occur between cocaine and some opiates, but not to methadone.[100]

The primary goal is to control the patient's pain. A combination of methadone titrated to prevent withdrawal and to provide background analgesia plus a short-acting opioid analgesic dosed adequately to prevent breakthrough pain can be used. If T.J. had a history of substance abuse, she could start with methadone 20 to 40 mg/day in four equally divided doses depending on how much heroin had been used (see Chapter 83, Drug Abuse). The methadone would prevent heroin withdrawal and possibly provide additional analgesia. Because her actual pain requirements are unknown, she also would be placed on a PCA with an agent such as morphine or hydromorphone. One should always reassess the patient 1 to 2 hours after starting the analgesic regimen for signs of withdrawal, clinical response, and toxicity, and then titrate the doses of both the methadone and hydromorphone accordingly, although it is best to adjust one medication at a time.[101] The final amount required may be higher than doses typically used in opioid-naive patients. Conversely, some patients may exaggerate their history of prior drug use and will be quite sensitive to the prescribed therapy. Long-term management should include offering the patient appropriate referrals to drug treatment centers, but the final responsibility should rest with the patient.

Use of Opioids in Recovering Addicts

20. Should opioid analgesics be prescribed to recovering opiate addicts?

Acute opioid use in the hospitalized setting is unlikely to cause opioid addiction; the rate of addiction from clinical opioid use is much less than 1%. Unless it is the patient's choice not to use opioids, there is no rational reason to avoid them.

Often the patient's fear of addiction can be alleviated by thorough education. The clinician should have a therapeutic contract with the patient that includes pain management as well as opioid tapering upon the resolution of the acute pain (see Chapter 83, Drug Abuse).

Use of Opioids in Renal Disease

21. What adjustments in analgesic dosing would be required if T.J. had an estimated creatinine clearance of 30 mL/min?

Uremia can produce CNS changes, which can cause patients with renal disease to be more sensitive to the CNS depressant effects of opioids. As discussed in Question 11, some opioids have active metabolites that are renally excreted, and uremia or significant renal disease can lead to their accumulation. For example, the active metabolites of meperidine and morphine (normeperidine and morphine-6-glucuronide, respectively) are renally excreted. Both of these active metabolites can cause CNS excitation; in particular, normeperidine can precipitate tonic-clonic seizures. Therefore, meperidine should be avoided in uremic patients, but other opioids can be used as long as one is aware of the potential toxicities, the patient is closely monitored, and the dosage is properly titrated. For T.J., hydromorphone PCA could still be a reasonable choice for the management of her acute pain; however, a continuous basal infusion would be unnecessary in a patient with significant renal dysfunction. As with all patients receiving opioid analgesics, close monitoring and follow-up care are essential.

Obstetric Pain: Special Considerations for Opioid Analgesia
EPIDURALS

22. M.T., a 28-year-old woman who has been in labor for 10 hours, is experiencing strong, erratic contractions at 5- to 15-minute intervals. Her cervix is minimally dilated, suggesting that delivery is still several hours away. Her pain is severe and, if it continues, may compromise her ability to assist in the labor and delivery process. A single, 50 μg epidural dose of fentanyl is ordered for M.T. by anesthesia. What guidelines are necessary for the safe use of epidural opioids?

Fentanyl and morphine are frequently administered epidurally during labor and during lower extremity surgical procedures (e.g., cesarean delivery, total joint replacements) because they have limited systemic effects and long durations of analgesic action.[102] Epidural analgesia has also been used in thoracic surgery.[103] A single dose of 2 to 10 mg morphine given epidurally may provide analgesia for >12 hours.[104] Respiratory depression can occur 1 to 3 hours after the administration of epidural morphine and can be readily reversed by naloxone. Facial or generalized pruritus also can occur hours after the administration of epidural morphine. If pruritus does occur, it can be controlled with low doses of IM or IV naloxone 0.02 to 0.08 mg without reversing the analgesic effect of the epidural morphine. Frequent monitoring of vital signs is essential after the administration of epidural opioids. One should be vigilant for delayed signs of toxicity, because their onset occurs up to several hours after the administration of the opioid.

Besides morphine, fentanyl (Sublimaze), sufentanil (Sufenta), and buprenorphine (Buprenex) also have been used epidurally. The duration of analgesia of epidurally administered opioids depends less on the serum half-life of the opioid than on the lipid solubility of the drug. The more lipophilic the opioid, the shorter its duration because these agents rapidly diffuse out of the epidural space. In contrast, the more hydrophilic opioids remain in the epidural space longer. For example, methadone, which is highly lipophilic, has a very short duration of activity when administered epidurally despite a long serum half-life of 24 hours.[105,106] For M.T., fentanyl is a good choice because it has a fairly long duration of analgesia but will not produce significant systemic effects that might compromise the fetus through transplacental migration. Also, the duration of fentanyl is short enough that it will not unnecessarily delay maternal postpartum recovery. A single 50-μg dose of epidural fentanyl was given to M.T. through an epidural catheter and complete analgesia was achieved.

Spinal Analgesia in Opioid-Dependent Patients

23. Why would spinal opioid analgesia still be appropriate if M.T. is opioid dependent?

Previous opioid use has minimal influence on epidural doses. Opioid-dependent patients can achieve adequate analgesia from epidural opioids, but their physical opioid dependency will not be satisfied. In fact, in spite of adequate analgesia, the opioid-dependent patient may exhibit symptoms of opiate withdrawal. These include restlessness, insomnia, nervousness, irritability, sweating, and GI hypermotility (nausea, emesis, and diarrhea). If withdrawal symptoms occur, they can be treated effectively by systemic administration of morphine or other opioids. Without treatment, such symptoms may persist for a few days. The dose of the systemic opioids varies with the patient's previous level of opioid dependence, and doses will need to be adjusted accordingly. It would be appropriate to start M.T. on a short-acting opioid such as meperidine 10 mg IV every 15 to 20 minutes until the symptoms of withdrawal subside. This may be somewhat hazardous because the incidence of respiratory depression in the first 24 hours may be increased when opioids are administered by simultaneous epidural and systemic routes.[107] Therefore, longer-acting opioids such as methadone or levorphanol should be avoided. The respiratory depression can be treated with the opioid antagonist naloxone, but the dose must be limited to 0.1-mg increments given IV to avoid precipitation of an acute withdrawal syndrome and reversal of analgesia. The naloxone dose can be repeated and the dose titrated to the desired clinical response.

Clonidine for Opioid Withdrawal Symptoms

24. If M.T. was opioid dependent, what are alternatives in managing the symptoms of physical withdrawal while she is treated with epidural opioids?

Clonidine (Catapres) 0.2 to 1.2 mg/day can effectively suppress the signs and symptoms of opioid withdrawal without eliciting other opioid effects.[108–111] The specific dose must be individualized for each patient to avoid hypotension, dry mouth, or drowsiness.[112–115] Clonidine also can be given sublingually or transdermally in equivalent doses. Clonidine transdermal patches of 3.5, 7, and 10.5 cm^2 deliver 0.1, 0.2, and 0.3 mg of clonidine, respectively, over a 24-hour period. Approximately 24 hours must elapse before steady-state plasma concentrations of clonidine are attained from the patches.[116,117] Therefore, supplemental oral or sublingual[112] clonidine 0.1 mg every 6 to 12 hours must be administered during the first 24 hours of the application of the transdermal patches. Clonidine transdermal patches should be used to treat the signs of physical opioid withdrawal only when these symptoms are expected to be severe or prolonged. In addition, clonidine is available for epidural administration and has been used in combination with opioids alone or with opioids and local anesthetics for epidural analgesia. For M.T., who is in labor, clonidine should be avoided owing to the risk of hypotension and possible adverse effects on the fetus. A shorter-acting opioid should be used as in Question 23.

SYSTEMIC OPIOIDS DURING LABOR

25. Should M.T. be given a systemic analgesic rather than epidural analgesia?

If possible, CNS depressants should be avoided during labor because they can compromise fetal vital functions.[118–121] Nevertheless, if an analgesic is deemed necessary, then an agent that meets the following criteria should be chosen: (1) provides adequate pain relief; (2) has little effect on the course or duration of labor; and (3) affects fetal vital signs minimally during labor, delivery, and postpartum phases. Meperidine and fentanyl meet most of these criteria and are therefore frequently preferred over other opioids in obstetrics when given in small, frequent parenteral injections or through a PCA.[120–123] As with all opioid analgesic use, close monitoring of the patient for analgesia and untoward effects is essential.

Although meperidine and fentanyl seem to have only minimal residual effects on the neonate at analgesic doses, adverse effects such as respiratory depression can still occur.[124,125] According to an early neonatal neurobehavioral scale, meperidine broadly depressed most measured neonatal activities on the first and second days of life.[126] Nevertheless, if the contractions are very strong, erratic, and prolonged early in the course of labor (as with M.T.), a short-acting analgesic (e.g., meperidine) could be useful to blunt the labor pain and calm the mother, so that she can regain control over her contractions and conserve her energy for the actual delivery.

Butorphanol (Stadol) also has minimal effects on fetal and neonatal function and is a reasonable alternative to meperidine or fentanyl in this situation.[127] All potent analgesics should be administered IM or subcutaneously because IV administration is associated with more neonatal and fetal depression because of the high peak serum concentration achieved by this route.[128–130] Pentazocine has similar effects as butorphanol, but is seldom used because of local tissue reactions at the site of IM or subcutaneous injections. Pentazocine and butorphanol are mixed opiate-agonists/antagonists and can precipitate acute withdrawal reactions in some opiate-dependent individuals. As a result, these drugs need to be used cautiously, if at all, in the opiate-addicted population (see Question 27).

If neonatal respiratory difficulties are manifested as a result of opioid analgesics administered during labor, they can be reversed with naloxone (Narcan). For M.T., meperidine 50 mg IM was given with good clinical response. As with all opioid analgesics, the dose has to be adjusted after an evaluation of the patient's history and clinical findings. Analgesic doses always should be individualized for the specific patient.

Variability in Intramuscular Meperidine Absorption

26. M.T. achieved excellent analgesia from the first dose of meperidine 50 mg IM, but she started to complain that subsequent doses produced variable pain relief, and she accused the nurse of giving her placebos. What are some of the explanations for this problem?

The most common cause of variable clinical response after an IM meperidine injection is erratic bioavailability after repetitive injections at the same site. The absorption of meperidine from an injection may vary by as much as 30% to 50% after repeated IM administrations. Other considerations include tachyphylaxis, progression of an underlying disease (e.g., in patients with cancer), and the possibility of opioid diversion by the patient or someone else through dilution or removal of active drug from its container.

Special Consideration for Using Partial Agonist and Antagonist Opioid Analgesics

27. What are precautions for using partial agonist and antagonist opioids for analgesia in M.T.?

Pentazocine, butorphanol, dezocine, and nalbuphine are partial agonist/antagonist opioid analgesics. Besides exhibiting agonist analgesic effects, they all possess opiate antagonist properties as well. Generally, they act as agonists at κ-opiate receptors and as antagonists at μ-opiate receptors, which explains their ability to simultaneously produce analgesia and precipitate withdrawal symptoms. Pentazocine has an opioid antagonist effect equal to 1/50 of nalorphine; 80 mg has been known to precipitate abstinence in patients who have been given opioids for chronic pain. If a partial opiate agonist is instituted in a patient previously taking a pure agonist, the dose should be increased gradually, and the patient should be observed closely for symptoms of abstinence. If possible, the pure agonist opioid should be withdrawn gradually. If the agonist dose is fairly low and the patient has not been on the drug for >10 days, then the patient can be changed over to pentazocine. In this situation, the patient may experience mild diaphoresis, but should not have significant withdrawal symptoms. A drug-free period of 2 days before the institution of pentazocine also has been suggested but this is impractical for a patient in pain.

When partial agonist/antagonist opioid analgesics are being considered, the risk of unpleasant psychotomimetic side effects must be weighed against the benefits. For example, butorphanol-induced dysphoric responses are well documented.[131,132] A 2-mg dose of butorphanol was associated with an 18% incidence of psychic disturbance, and a 4-mg dose with a 33% incidence. Pentazocine (Talwin) also is associated with a higher incidence of psychotomimetic reactions than traditional opiate agonist analgesics. Hallucinations occurred in 24 of 65 patients (37%) who received 40 to 50 mg of IM pentazocine. In another trial, psychic changes occurred in 1.7% of patients receiving morphine versus 11.4% of pentazocine-treated patients. In comparison, nalbuphine (Nubain) and other analgesics induce much less psychotomimetic effect than butorphanol or pentazocine.[133–135] Therefore, a partial agonist/antagonist opioid analgesic should be used in M.T. only if she cannot tolerate the available shorter-acting opioid agonist analgesics.

Tramadol

28. What is the purported advantage of tramadol (Ultram) over other opioid analgesics and NSAIDs?

Tramadol, a centrally acting analgesic with weak opioid agonist properties, activates monoaminergic spinal inhibition of pain. The *O*-demethylated metabolite of tramadol has a higher affinity for opioid receptors than the parent drug; however, after a single oral dose, the binding of tramadol to the μ-opioid receptor is overshadowed by its nonopioid analgesic effects.[136] The tolerance and dependence potential of tramadol during treatment for up to 6 months appear to be low; however, the possibility of dependence with long-term use cannot be excluded entirely.[137] Tramadol is indicated for the treatment of moderate to severe pain, but analgesia is not superior to other opiate analgesics.[138–140] However, it has a lower incidence of respiratory depression or significant GI dysmotility than most traditional opioids.

Tramadol is well tolerated in short-term use. Doses range from 50 to 100 mg orally every 4 to 6 hours and should not exceed 400 mg/day.[141] Like other opiate agonists, the principal adverse effects are sedation, dizziness, nausea, vomiting, dry mouth, constipation, and sweating; however, the potential for respiratory depression is low. Seizures have occurred during therapy with recommended doses. Seizure risk increases with doses exceeding 500 mg/day and in patients taking concurrent selective serotonin-reuptake inhibitors (SSRIs), TCAs, and other opiate agonists.[142,143] Tramadol should be used cautiously in patients taking drugs known to lower the seizure threshold, such as monoamine-oxidase inhibitors or antipsychotic agents. In addition, patients with epilepsy, head trauma, metabolic disorders, alcohol or drug withdrawal, or CNS infections may be at increased risk for seizures with tramadol therapy.[141] Tramadol also has SSRI-like properties that can initially overshadow the opiate effect in some patients. Therefore, instead of sedation, patients may experience excitation. For more on drug interactions with tramadol, see Question 67.

CHRONIC MALIGNANT PAIN
Goal of Malignant Pain Management

29. A.J., a 68-year-old man, was diagnosed with metastatic prostate cancer 6 months ago. Now he is admitted for evaluation of possible accidental opioid overdose. A.J. was started on a fentanyl patch 100 μg/hr 24 hours ago by his physician because of spinal pain not adequately relieved by oral acetaminophen 325 mg and hydrocodone 5 mg Q 3 hr. The fentanyl patch was removed 6 hours ago, and A.J. is again complaining of his spinal pain radiating to his buttocks and left leg. A.J. is currently awake and alert and relates that his pain level is at 9 of 10 on the pain scale. What is the goal in managing A.J.'s pain?

The goal in treating pain of terminal illness is comfort and an acceptable (to the patient) level of consciousness. Opioids should not be withheld for fear of addiction or that the dose may be too high. Instead, the dose should be titrated based on the patient's clinical response. Ideally, the patient should be comfortable and voice no complaints when questioned about his or her level of activity and alertness. Under these conditions, any dosage reductions or changes in therapy serve no purpose, even if the patient is receiving doses several times those typically used to treat acute pain. To emphasize, clinicians should focus attention on their patients' clinical response rather than on an arbitrary list of doses or ideal number of medications. The immediate goal for A.J. is to break the cycle of pain and to rapidly achieve the greatest degree of comfort possible.

Indications for Use of Fentanyl Patches

30. **What special considerations are necessary for use of fentanyl transdermal patches in patients such as A.J.?**

Transdermal fentanyl can effectively manage chronic cancer pain. Because of the nature of the transdermal delivery system, the onset of analgesia may be delayed by 6 to 12 hours after placement of the patch.[144-146] On removal of the patch, the fentanyl deposited in the subcutaneous tissue continues to release active drug for approximately another 8 to 12 hours. These delays in onset upon application and in offset after removal of the transdermal patch discourage use of the patch except for patients who require a steady maintenance analgesic dose. The transdermal patches do not provide sufficient flexibility in dosing to manage rapidly changing analgesic needs. Even after stabilized on a given drug regimen, cancer pain patients always should be given an immediate-onset opioid analgesic (e.g., morphine elixir) to take as needed for management of breakthrough pain.[147] If the need for breakthrough drugs becomes frequent, the underlying dosage regimen should be reassessed and the doses increased as appropriate. Fentanyl absorption from the patches can be affected by body temperature, and unintentional overdoses can occur with hyperthermia.[148]

A patient given fentanyl patches must be instructed to dispose of used patches appropriately to prevent inadvertent access by children or household animals. Fentanyl patches were thought to be safe from diversion and abuse, but the drug enclosure membrane can be removed and active drug accessed.[149]

Morphine
Use of Oral Morphine

31. **What oral dose of morphine should be selected for A.J.?**

The usual initial dose for morphine is 30 mg orally every 3 hours (see Table 9-5), but A.J. has been receiving acetaminophen with oxycodone for an unknown length of time and likely has some degree of opioid tolerance. His response to morphine should be monitored carefully 1 to 2 hours after his initial dose and the dose adjusted appropriately. If A.J.'s clinical response indicates that the dose is too high, it should be decreased; however, if he is still uncomfortable after the 2 hours, an additional 30 mg should be given at once and subsequent doses increased by 10 mg to a total of 40 mg every 3 hours. A.J.'s response should be the primary criterion for determining the dose, and the pharmacokinetics of the drug

should determine the dosing interval. Frequent reassessment of A.J.'s pain status and level of consciousness is essential.

When the pain has been relieved, the dose of morphine often can be decreased. Ideally, only one clinician should assume responsibility for coordinating frequent monitoring of the patient's level of awareness and pain control. Once the pain has been controlled, single-day dosage adjustment should be sufficient. If the dose is changed, then it should be reassessed within the first 2 hours to prevent unnecessary exposure to pain or adverse effects. Most oral opioids reach maximum analgesic effect within the first 2 hours after administration, but for longer-acting opioid analgesics such as methadone, the patient should be monitored for several days because of potential drug accumulation.

Tolerance, Dependence, and Addiction

32. **Should tolerance, dependence, and addiction to morphine be an issue in A.J.?**

Tolerance and physical dependence should be anticipated and discussed openly in patients who are receiving chronic opioid analgesia. Tolerance occurs when a given dose no longer produces the same effect over time. For patients with a malignant disease, it is difficult to differentiate between tolerance and increased pain from disease progression. A.J. should be instructed to inform his clinicians when his pain regimen becomes ineffective. Escalating doses of opioid analgesics should be expected and should not deter the clinician from continuing with analgesic therapy. However, the need for increasing doses should serve as a warning that alternative analgesic or adjunct agents need to be considered.

Physical dependence should also be anticipated. It should be explained to A.J. that this is a natural adaptation process of the body that occurs with opiates. The signs and symptoms of dependence are seen when abrupt withdrawal or a marked decrease in opioid administration occurs. Therefore, it is important that A.J. receive an adequate supply of medication to prevent exacerbating withdrawal symptoms caused by difficulties in obtaining medication or missed doses. The potential for dependency to opioid analgesics should never prevent the clinical use of opioid analgesics in malignant disease.

Addiction is a compulsive behavior relating to drug procurement and use. Addiction from clinical opioid use for the treatment of pain is rare. Misunderstanding by clinicians and caregivers regarding the difference between tolerance, dependence, and addiction is not uncommon and often results in undertreatment of painful conditions.[150-162] Addiction is not an issue in patients requiring opiates for the treatment of chronic malignant pain. Tolerance and dependence should be expected and should in no way be misconstrued as evidence of addiction.

Use of Sustained-Release Morphine

33. **A.J.'s pain was controlled on 40 mg of morphine solution orally Q 3 hr, but he is now complaining of the frequency of the morphine dose. He wishes to have the therapy changed to allow fewer daily doses so that he may have longer periods of rest. What can be done about A.J.'s request?**

A.J.'s daily morphine requirement of 320 mg can be provided by use of a sustained-release (SR) dosage form given every 8 to 12 hours. However, direct conversion of doses from oral morphine solutions or other immediate-release dosage forms to SR tablets often leads to oversedation initially, and particularly during the first hours of the dosing period. Therefore, the SR dose should be reduced by 25% to 240 mg/day (320 mg × 75%) for A.J. This can be given as 90 mg every 8 hours or as 120 mg every 12 hours. SR morphine is available as 15-, 30-, 60-, 100-, and 200-mg tablets and 20-, 50-, and 100-mg capsules. When starting a patient on oral SR preparations, it often is desirable to try an every-8-hour regimen to prevent the initial sedation that often is associated with the larger individual doses of the 12-hour regimen. Likewise, when larger doses are needed, 8-hour dosing intervals usually cause less sedation than 12-hour intervals (i.e., during the first 2 hours of the dosing period). Some patients also may have more breakthrough pain at the end of the 12-hour dosing interval. Careful assessment of the patient's response and toxicity by the clinician is the most essential ingredient between success and failure with either product in managing the patient's pain.

Rectal Use of Morphine Suppositories and Sustained-Release Tablets

34. **Several weeks later, A.J. is no longer able to swallow his medication because of worsening of an existing esophageal stricture. What are alternatives for giving A.J. his required daily analgesic?**

In addition to the parenteral routes already presented, morphine can be administered as an oral solution or via a rectal suppository. The absorption of the rectal suppository is at least comparable to or better than that of the morphine solution.[153,154] If A.J. was stabilized on 240 mg/ day of SR morphine, the initial morphine suppository dose also should be 240 mg/day. The duration of action of morphine suppositories is similar to that of morphine solution and therefore must be administered every 3 to 4 hours. For A.J., the starting dose is 30 mg rectally every 3 hours. Other agents such as hydromorphone (Dilaudid) and codeine are also available as suppositories. The equianalgesic doses of these agents for A.J. (see Table 9-3) would be 6 and 10 mg, respectively. SR oral morphine tablets also can be used for rectal administration. The rectal absorption of SR tablets is comparable to the oral route of administration.[155–158] There is no maximum dose for opioid analgesics for the management of pain of a terminal disease, but there is a limit as to how many suppositories or tablets the patient can hold rectally.

Oral Infusion

35. **Because A.J. was unable to swallow, he agreed to have a gastrostomy feeding tube placed by a general surgeon. He is now being fed through the tube at a rate of 50 mL/hr. Morphine sulfate solution is added to each feeding bag to deliver 10 mg/hr. He also is receiving amitriptyline (Elavil) 150 mg at bedtime, naproxen suspension 250 mg QID, and lorazepam (Ativan) 4 mg TID via the feeding tube. A.J. is reasonably alert and is only slightly uncomfortable. Are there any problems associated with placing A.J.'s morphine in the feeding formula?**

There is no reason why morphine cannot be given in this manner. The obvious questions about drug stability, solubility, and binding to proteins in the feeding formula do not appear to present a problem because A.J. has been receiving morphine in this manner for the past several days. The dose of morphine (240 mg/day) is apparently not causing undesirable effects, and A.J. is quite comfortable. Administering morphine as a continuous oral infusion at night while he is sleeping is perhaps the best method to ensure restful, pain-free sleep.

Tricyclic Antidepressants

36. **What are the indications for amitriptyline in A.J.'s treatment regimen?**

TCAs have been used experimentally at low to moderate doses as an adjunct to analgesic pain control. These agents may alter psychological responses to pain, have intrinsic analgesic activity, and may potentiate opioid analgesics.[159] European investigations noted an 82% overall response rate to these agents.[160] Imipramine (Tofranil) relieved cancer and surgical pain in approximately 75% to 80% of patients, and doxepin (Sinequan) relieved pain completely in approximately half of 16 depressed, chronic-pain patients.[161] Tension headaches also were improved with 25 to 100 mg of doxepin.[162] Imipramine 50 to 200 mg/day or amitriptyline 10 to 40 mg/day alone or in combination with fluphenazine (Prolixin) have also been investigated for neuropathic pain.[163] However, neuroleptic agents have fallen out of general use for chronic pain syndromes because of their potential for extrapyramidal syndromes (EPS) and other long-term effects. TCAs and methadone combination also have been used successfully for the long-term management of chronic phantom limb pain (see Question 49).[164] For A.J., the choice of TCAs is limited, because of his inability to swallow. However, a few TCAs are available as oral suspensions (doxepin and nortriptyline). Therefore, it would be reasonable to continue A.J.'s present TCA therapy.

Methadone
Guidelines

37. **The decision has been made to use oral methadone to treat A.J.'s pain. What are guidelines for the safe use of methadone in treating cancer pain?**

Clinical experience with the use of methadone for cancer pain is favorable.[165] The patient's physical and mental condition should be monitored closely, and clinicians should be aware of the long elimination half-life of methadone. Repeated dosing with methadone requires decreasing the dose when comfort is achieved to prevent drug accumulation and overdose. Methadone is 85% bound to serum proteins, and its average plasma half-life is approximately 23 hours with a range of 13 to 47 hours. Therefore, the drug probably is tightly bound and only slowly released from its binding sites. Plasma levels of methadone may continue to rise for up to 10 days after an increase in dose.

Unfortunately, duration of analgesia does not correlate to the serum half-life, and multiple doses must be given each day. The absolute amount of methadone in plasma, although it undoubtedly affects sedation and respiratory depression, is not a factor in the magnitude of analgesic response. Nevertheless, analgesic effects are obtained only while methadone plasma levels are above a certain individualized concentration. Most patients can be maintained on doses of methadone every 6 or 8 hours after pain control is achieved, but the drug often must be given every 4 hours or administered with another short-acting opioid analgesic during the first day or two of therapy to control pain.[166] Alternatively, methadone loading with larger doses for the first few doses can accomplish rapid analgesia at the onset of methadone administration. Unfortunately, this carries a higher risk of rapid drug accumulation and excessive drowsiness. Thus, loading doses must be reduced after the first one to two doses.

The necessity for shorter dosing intervals during the initiation of methadone can cause clinicians who are unfamiliar with the long half-life of methadone to adjust doses too frequently or to then maintain a patient at an inappropriately high dose after initial pain control is achieved. This can threaten the patient with dangerous drug accumulation. A scenario that often is repeated is one in which analgesia and patient comfort are achieved after 2 or 3 days of gradually increasing doses, On days 4 and 5, the patient becomes increasingly sedated and on day 6 alarmingly so. The drug is then discontinued, or the opioid antagonist naloxone (Narcan) is administered. Suddenly, the patient is no longer sedated, but the pain has reappeared. This sudden reversal of sedation may be short lived. Because the half-life of methadone is much longer than that of naloxone, the patient can still slip back into sedation once the naloxone is cleared from the plasma in 1 to 2 hours.[167] Elderly and severely debilitated patients may require smaller doses of methadone for pain control; therefore, caution must be exercised when methadone is used in these patients.[168]

Dosing

38. **What dose of methadone should be prescribed to treat A.J.'s pain?**

To convert A.J.'s dose of morphine to an equivalent dose of methadone, one must use Table 9-3 as a standard reference for comparison. A.J.'s 10-mg-every-hour oral morphine sulfate solution dose is estimated to be approximately equivalent to 10 mg every 3 hours of morphine IM. On a single-dose basis, IM doses of methadone and morphine are equally potent; however, with repeated doses on a chronic basis, the duration of methadone activity is approximately four times longer than that of morphine. Therefore, the total daily parenteral methadone dose will only be one-fourth that of parenteral morphine. In this case, A.J. would require 20 mg/day of IM methadone. Because oral methadone is only 75% as effective as methadone IM,[169] A.J. should receive approximately 7.5 mg of methadone orally every 6 hours. Approximately 5 to 10 days will elapse before the full methadone effect is realized, unless loading doses equal to twice that of the maintenance analgesic dose are used for the first two doses. These two larger doses accelerate the process of reaching the steady-state concentration.

Continuous Intravenous Morphine Infusion

39. **Three months later, A.J. is again hospitalized because of a compression fracture of his spine. He is cachectic and weighs only 87 pounds. He has been receiving 20 mg of morphine IM Q 3 hr since his admission. His pain is bothersome and his loss of muscle mass is not conducive to IM injections. What would be a reasonable IV analgesic program for A.J.?**

Continuous IV infusions of morphine are superior to IM injections in maintaining a pain-free condition in cancer and surgical patients.[170–172] In one study, six of eight children with cancer experienced complete pain control with 0.025 to 2.6 mg/kg per hour of morphine for 1 to 16 days.

A.J. has been receiving 160 mg of morphine daily, which is approximately 7 mg/hour. His initial IV infusion dose of morphine should be increased to 8 mg/hour because his pain is still bothersome. When 500 mg of morphine sulfate is added to 500 mL of 5% dextrose in water, the resulting 1-mg/mL solution can be infused IV at 8 mL/hour to deliver the 8-mg/hour dose. In addition, an order should be written for a 4-mg IV bolus of morphine every hour as needed for signs of pain or discomfort.

The supplemental bolus doses of IV morphine will facilitate subsequent adjustments of the continuous infusion rate. At the end of a predetermined period of time, the number of milligrams of drug that were administered by constant infusion are added to 1.5 times the number of milligrams of drug used in supplemental bolus doses. This amount of drug is then divided by the elapsed interval of time, thereby calculating the new infusion rate. For example, if at the end of 6 hours A.J. has received five supplemental doses of 4 mg each, then (6 hours at 8 mg/hour) plus (1.5 × 5 doses of 4 mg) = 78 mg per 6 hours. The new infusion rate should then be 13 mg/hour, and the new supplemental doses should be 6 mg (approximately equal to the amount of drug normally infused in 30 minutes) every hour as needed. Continual assessment of the patient and hourly adjustments of dose are probably superior to the method outlined previously, but the aforementioned method may be more practical for the busy clinician.

Brompton's Mixture

40. **What is Brompton's mixture? Will heroin (diamorphine) be superior to morphine for managing A.J.'s malignant pain?**

An opioid mixture for oral administration in severe pain was formulated at the Brompton Chest Hospital in London in 1926 and was included in the British Pharmaceutical Codex by 1973. The mixture contained diamorphine (heroin) in variable doses, cocaine, alcohol, chloroform water, and syrup. Because clinicians in the United States were precluded from using heroin, they formulated their own versions of Brompton's mixture by substituting either morphine or methadone for the heroin, often adding a phenothiazine as well. Because the analgesic effectiveness of heroin and morphine are comparable, cancer pain was successfully treated in approximately 90% of patients using these Brompton's mixtures.[173–175]

Studies comparing standard Brompton's mixture containing morphine, cocaine, ethanol, syrup, and chloroform water with a flavored aqueous solution of morphine alone have shown no differences in pain relief, drowsiness, or other side effects between the two products.[176,177] Studies in cancer patients have demonstrated that the analgesia claimed to be obtained from heroin is most likely due to its metabolites, morphine and 6-acetyl-morphine. Oral morphine solution should be prescribed for A.J. because Brompton's mixture is not superior.

Pentazocine

41. Why should pentazocine (Talwin) not be used in treating cancer pain?

The use of agonist/antagonists also should be avoided because of poor oral efficacy and because of the particularly disturbing nature of the psychotomimetic side effects in patients who are already fearful and anxious. Furthermore, pentazocine is a "ceiling" drug; that is, doses cannot be greatly increased to treat increasing pain without greatly increasing the incidence or severity of side effects.

Hydroxyzine or Phenothiazine

42. Would coadministration of either hydroxyzine or phenothiazine be beneficial for A.J.'s pain?

The addition of hydroxyzine (Vistaril, Atarax) to an analgesic regimen is thought to potentiate the analgesia of the opioid analgesic.[20,178,179] Whether this is a true analgesic effect or a consequence of its sedating properties is unclear. Two additional benefits related to the antihistamine properties of hydroxyzine are prevention of opiate-induced nausea and itching.

Phenothiazines, like antihistamines, often are administered concomitantly with opioids to "enhance" analgesia. However, claims of enhanced analgesia are not supported by well-designed studies. Many of these studies lack double-blinding, cross-over of patients, placebo control, or appropriate instruments capable of evaluating pain. Another problem in the design of studies evaluating the combination of a phenothiazine or antihistamine with an opioid is the failure to differentiate between analgesia and sedation. Two excellent reviews summarize the studies that demonstrate analgesia with antihistamines and discuss the proposed mechanisms of action.[180,181]

All phenothiazines, except for methotrimeprazine, initially demonstrated antianalgesic effects in experimental pain studies. Clinicians now realize that experimental pain is not a completely valid model to assess the response of a patient in pain. These studies could not assess the anxiolytic properties of the phenothiazines and the effect a reduction in anxiety has on pain perception. Furthermore, cancer and chronic pain cause anxiety, and anxiety worsens pain perception and, consequently, pain severity. This reinforcement cannot be overestimated and helps explain the apparent benefit many patients obtain from the combination of hydroxyzine with an opioid.

Adrenal Corticosteroids

43. Why might corticosteroids be useful for A.J.'s spinal pain?

Patients who have spinal metastatic disease often obtain pain relief with corticosteroids. This is thought to be due to a combination of direct anti-inflammatory effects and a reduction of pressure from edema around affected nerves. A short course of dexamethasone at a dose of 10 mg orally or IV three times daily with rapid tapering should be considered for A.J. Corticosteroid response may decrease with repeated use, but a single short-course therapy often can produce a significantly prolonged effect. Dexamethasone is most often used because of its long duration of action and lack of mineralocorticoid effects. However, other corticosteroids may be substituted for the dexamethasone using a conversion table to calculate equivalent doses.

Nonsteroidal Anti-Inflammatory Drugs

44. Why should the use of an NSAID be considered for A.J.'s spinal pain?

Pain from tumor metastasis to bone is particularly distressing and difficult to treat. Although the most effective therapy for the relief of bone pain is radiation to the site of the pain,[182] prostaglandin inhibitors may be another reasonable alternative to increased doses of opioids. Osseous metastases induce the production of prostaglandins that may cause osteolysis, sensitize free nerve endings, and augment pain perception. The NSAIDs effectively decrease prostaglandin and endoperoxide production and may be useful in treating metastatic bone pain if administered on a scheduled basis. Usual analgesic doses of NSAIDs often are effective, but maximum therapeutic doses may be necessary. Some specialists in treating cancer pain advocate doses considerably larger than the manufacturers' recommendations. Sometime IV ketorolac is used for this purpose.[183] In extremely painful cases, ketorolac has been used as a continuous infusion for managing metastatic bone pain. Beside the NSAIDs, strontium, and radiopharmaceuticals such as phosphorus 32, strontium 89, samarium 153, rhenium 186, and tin 117m have been used to treat metastatic bone pain, but occasionally with limited benefit. Nevertheless, they can be considered for severe bony metastatic pain unresponsive to corticosteroids or NSAIDs.

CHRONIC NONMALIGNANT PAIN
Goal of Therapy

45. W.C., a 38-year-old man, has been disabled for the past 2 years because of an injury to his cervical spine sustained while operating a forklift at a warehouse. He is currently taking oxycodone 5 mg with acetaminophen 325 mg (Percocet) PO two tablets QID as needed for severe pain, codeine 30 mg with acetaminophen 325 mg (Tylenol #3) or hydrocodone 5 mg with acetaminophen 325 mg (Lorcet-5) two tablets PO QID as needed for less severe pain, and diazepam 10 mg PO TID for neck spasms. W.C. describes the pain as sharp and stabbing, and the spasms in his neck are his most troublesome problem. The spasms become severe if he stops taking the diazepam, and the pain starts to build 2 hours after taking the opioids. W.C. currently is seeing an internist and an orthopedic surgeon who prescribed his analgesics. W.C. also has undergone several cervical discectomies and vertebral fusion with minimal pain relief. What are the treatment goals in W.C.?

Opioid use for chronic nonmalignant pain remains the most controversial issue facing clinical pain management. Not only is opioid efficacy subject to debate, but, in addition, the potential for opioid dependency creates considerable hesitation on the part of many prescribers.[184,185] Although neuropathic pain may respond to opioids, high dosages are often needed.[186] Opioid analgesics should be considered only after the patient has received and failed adequate trials of NSAIDs or other analgesic agents. In addition, patients should be evaluated for physical interventions, such as muscle strengthening or conditioning exercises that may improve their clinical situation, before becoming over-reliant on opioids for pain management. As with any chronic pain management, time-contingent dosing (fixed dose and interval) is superior to as-needed dosing. If an opioid is used to manage chronic pain, a longer-acting agent (e.g., SR morphine, methadone, levorphanol) should be used to minimize fluctuations in serum concentrations. Patients should be monitored closely for both efficacy and toxicity.

Shorter-acting opioid analgesics often can complicate chronic nonmalignant pain management by exacerbating the pain perception because of fluctuating serum concentrations and the production of opioid withdrawal hyperalgesia when serum concentrations are low. Analogous withdrawal effects can occur with sedative-hypnotics and antispasmodics as well, particularly those with relatively short half-lives.

A written agreement, as shown in Figure 9-7 (including provisions for a single prescriber, monitoring of serum drug concentrations, urine or blood substance abuse screening, agreement to inform all current and future health care providers regarding pain management, and termination of service), must be agreed on between the primary caregiver and the patient before any therapeutic modality is initiated. There should be only one prescriber for all of W.C.'s medications, and all of his health care providers must be informed of the therapeutic plans. The immediate goal of pain management for W.C. is to consolidate his analgesic regimen to a time-contingent, longer-acting opioid. Longer-term goals should include withdrawal of diazepam and consideration of opioid withdrawal, whereas alternative analgesic adjuncts (antidepressants or membrane stabilizers) are instituted. Psychological evaluation and support should supplement pharmacologic therapy. The overall therapeutic goal for W.C. is pain control and pain reduction, but not total pain elimination. He should be able to conduct activities of daily life with minimal discomfort, and ideally be able to return to gainful employment in some capacity, even if his work duties are modified.

Analgesic Consolidation

46. W.C. relates that he has been taking up to 18 tablets of various opioid analgesics daily. How should his pain be managed?

Chronic opiate use can lead to dependence as well as tolerance. The immediate need is to stabilize W.C.'s pain, but a longer-term goal should include analgesic tapering if tolerated. There is evidence from pain studies in animal models, and in longitudinal studies of humans, that chronic opioid use may lead to changes in the central nervous system that result in hyperalgesia. It is not known if this effect is drug- and time-dependent.[187,188]

However, tapering is not likely to be achieved quickly. W.C. should be started on an opiate tapering regimen after his pain is stabilized, and this process should occur within 24 hours after the analgesic dose has stabilized. The first step in opiate analgesic tapering is opiate consolidation. As in this case, the patient often is receiving several analgesics unnecessarily. A longer-acting opioid analgesic should be used for W.C. to minimize the pain and analgesia fluctuations. One method is to sum his total opioid use per day during the past several weeks and then convert to an equivalent dose of either methadone or SR morphine. Alternatively, an arbitrary dose such as oral methadone 5 mg every 6 hours could be started, and all of his current analgesics could be discontinued. If this

dose is insufficient, a temporary dosage increase may be necessary. The long half-life of methadone will be beneficial when instituting opioid tapering.

Alternative analgesic adjuncts such as antidepressants or anticonvulsants should also be considered and introduced at this time. Opiate consolidation in W.C. would also serve to reduce his exposure to acetaminophen. He is currently taking three different acetaminophen-containing products. Although concern for opioid dosing emphasizes a balance between benefits and risks from the opioids, the risk of either short-term overdose or cumulative effects from acetaminophen (e.g., liver or renal toxicity) should not be neglected. W.C. should be instructed not to exceed 4 to 5 g/day of acetaminophen from all sources, including products he may be purchasing over the counter.

Opioid Tapering and Withdrawal

47. How rapidly can opiate analgesics be discontinued in a patient such as W.C. without precipitating withdrawal symptoms?

W.C. would benefit from long-term multidisciplinary pain management that includes behavioral therapy as well as medication adjustments. An acute pain opiate analgesic dose can be decreased in hospitalized patients by 20% daily without precipitating opiate withdrawal symptoms; but in a patient such as W.C., who has been taking opiate analgesics for an extended period of time, the decrease in analgesic dose will have to be much more gradual. In chronic opiate dependence, the opioid dose can be decreased by approximately 10% every 3 to 5 days without inducing withdrawal symptoms. The addition of clonidine can also improve the overall opioid tapering process, since it may impart analgesic effects while assisting in controlling abstinence symptoms.

Managing Opioid Overdose

48. W.C. accidentally received an excessive dose of methadone leading to a respiratory rate of 8 breaths/min and excessive sedation. How should he be managed?

Methadone can accumulate when converting from short-acting opioids to this longer-acting opioid unless careful attention is paid to the differences in pharmacokinetic properties. Because methadone has a long half-life, steady-state plasma levels may not be achieved for 5–10 days. In W.C., the challenge is to treat the respiratory depression induced by methadone without interfering with the desired analgesic effects and without precipitating narcotic withdrawal. Opioid toxicity is not life threatening if it is managed immediately. Naloxone reverses opioid-induced CNS sedation and respiratory depression after overdose of all opiates except buprenorphine. W.C. should be given naloxone 0.1 mg parenterally at 2- to 3-minute intervals until the desired effect (improved respiration rate and increased alertness) is achieved. Because methadone has a long half-life, the naloxone dose may need to be repeated every 15 to 20 minutes, sometimes for several hours, until the methadone toxicity dissipates. Overly aggressive dosing of naloxone can cause agitation and exaggerated responses to pain. The methadone dose will have to be adjusted accordingly if too much naloxone has been administered.

Name:
ID number:

Dr. _[Physician Name]_ is prescribing opioid medicine, sometimes called narcotic analgesics, because other treatments have not adequately helped my pain. The purpose of this Agreement is to prevent misunderstandings about certain medicines for pain management. I understand that this Agreement is essential to the trust and confidence necessary in a doctor/patient relationship and that my doctor undertakes to treat me based on this Agreement.

1. I am aware that the use of opioid medicine is associated with certain risks, including but not limited to: sleepiness or drowsiness, constipation, nausea, itching, vomiting, dizziness, allergic reaction, slowing of breathing rate, slowing of reflexes or reaction time and possibility that the medicine will not provide complete pain relief. I am also aware that these side effects can be increased or made worse by the use of other medicines, as well as other substances, such as alcohol.

2. I am aware of the possible risks and benefits of other types of treatments that do not involve the use of opioids. These treatments can also be considered in the future, if my condition warrants.

3. I will tell my doctor about all other medicines and treatments that I am receiving.

4. I will not be involved in any activity that may be dangerous to me or someone else if I feel drowsy or am not thinking clearly. I am aware that even if I do not notice it, my reflexes and reaction time might still be slowed. Such activities include, but are not limited to: using heavy equipment or a motor vehicle, working in unprotected heights or being responsible for another individual who is unable to care for himself or herself.

5. I am aware that certain other medicines such as nalbuphine, pentazocine, buprenorphine, or butorphanol, may reverse the action of the medicine I am using for pain control. Taking any of these other medicines while I am taking my pain medicines can cause symptoms of a withdrawal syndrome, such as nausea or vomiting. I agree not to take any of these medicines and to tell any other doctors that I am taking an opioid as my pain medicine and can't take any of the medicines listed above.

6. I am aware that addiction is defined as the use of a medicine or substance even if it causes harm, having cravings for a drug, feeling the need to use a drug and interferes with quality of life. I am aware that the chance of becoming addicted to my pain medicine is low, and that the development of addiction has been reported rarely in medical journals and is much more common in a person who has a family or personal history of addiction. I agree to tell my doctor my complete and honest personal drug history and that of my family to the best of my knowledge.

7. I understand that physical dependence is a normal, expected result of using these medicines for longer than a few days. I understand that physical dependence is not the same as addiction. I am aware physical dependence means that if my pain medicine use is markedly decreased, stopped, or reversed by some of the agents mentioned above, I will experience a withdrawal syndrome. This means I may have any or all of the following: runny nose, yawning, large pupils, goose bumps, abdominal pain and cramping, diarrhea, irritability, aches throughout my body and a flu-like feeling. I am aware that opioid withdrawal is uncomfortable but not life threatening.

8. I am aware that tolerance to analgesia means that I may require more medicine to get the same amount of pain relief. I am aware that tolerance to analgesia has been seen and may occur to me. If it occurs, increasing doses may not always help and may cause unacceptable side effects. Tolerance or failure to respond well to opioids may cause my doctor to choose another form of treatment.

9. I will communicate fully with my doctor about the character and intensity of my pain, the effect of the pain on my daily life, and how well the medicine is helping to relieve the pain.

10. I will not use any illegal controlled substances, including marijuana, cocaine, etc.

11. I will not share, sell or trade my medication with anyone. I will not attempt to obtain any controlled medicines from another person, such as a friend or family member.

12. I will not attempt to obtain any controlled medicines, including opioid pain medicines, controlled stimulants, or anti-anxiety medicines from ANY OTHER doctor.

13. I agree that I will use my medicine no more often than the prescribed rate and that use of my medicine at a greater rate will result in my being without medication for a period of time.

14. I will report all unused pain medicine to my doctor and will bring it to an office visit if required by my doctor. I will make every effort to come to each scheduled visit with my doctor. If for any reason, I cannot make these appointments, I will notify the doctor's office at least 24 hours in advance and reschedule an appointment as soon as one is available.

15. I agree that refills of my prescriptions for pain medicine will be made only at the time of an office visit or during regular office hours. *NO refills will be available during evenings or on weekends.*

16. I agree that I will submit to a blood or urine test if requested by my doctor to determine if I am following my pain control program.

17. I agree to use *** Pharmacy, located at *** in ***. Tel # ***, for filling prescriptions for all of my pain medicine.

18. I authorize the doctor and my pharmacy to cooperate fully with any city, state or federal law enforcement agency, including this state's Board of Pharmacy, in the investigation of any possible misuse, sale, or other diversion of my pain medicine. I authorize my doctor to provide a copy of this Agreement to my pharmacy. I agree to waive any applicable privilege or right of privacy or confidentiality with respect to these authorizations.

19. I will safeguard my pain medicine from loss or theft. ** Lost or stolen medicines will NOT be replaced under any circumstances. **

20. *I understand that if I do not comply with this Agreement, my doctor will stop prescribing these pain-control medicines.*
In this case, my doctor will taper off the medicine over a period of several days, as necessary, to avoid withdrawal symptoms. Also, a drug-dependence treatment program may be recommended.

I have read this form or have it read to me. I understand all of it. I have had a chance to have all of my questions regarding this treatment answered to my satisfaction. By signing this form voluntarily, I give my consent for the treatment of my pain with opioid pain medicines. I agree to follow these guidelines.

A copy of this document has been given to me.

Patient signature: _____ Date ____/____/____
[PATIENT NAME]

Physician signature: _____ Date ____/____/____
[PHYSICIAN NAME] MD

Witnessed by: _____

NOTE: Components of this informed consent/agreement form are recommended but can be adapted to the needs of the health care practitioner.

(Adapted from the American Academy of Pain Medicine, http://www.painmed.org/ and "Partners Against Pain", http://www.partnersagainstpain.com/)

FIGURE 9-7 Patient agreement for pain medications.

In the event of a massive overdose of opioid analgesics, naloxone can be given as a continuous infusion of 2.5 μg/kg per hour to 0.4 mg/hour. In light of the low incidence of side effects from naloxone, it might be reasonable to start with a loading dose of 0.8 mg and a higher infusion dose such as 0.4 mg/hour, followed by subsequent dosage adjustments, depending on clinical response. The required duration of naloxone infusion will vary, depending on the specific opioid and the amount involved.[189,190]

A longer-acting opiate antagonist, nalmefene (Revex), may provide an alternative to naloxone. Approved for the use of conscious sedation reversal and management of opioid overdose, nalmefene may be most beneficial in overdoses of methadone or propoxyphene where repeated administration of antagonists is necessary due to their long elimination half-lives.[191] Nalmefene has a long half-life (8 to 11 hours) compared with naloxone (1 to 1.5 hours). Although fewer doses of nalmefene may be needed to reverse opioid intoxication, studies have not shown any difference in efficacy between nalmefene and naloxone.[191,192]

NEUROPATHIC PAIN

49. **R.L., a 40-year-old, generally healthy woman, suffered a superficial laceration of her left arm at work from a broken glass window. The initial laceration has since healed without complications, but now she is referred for evaluation of pain management because of persistent intolerable pain in her left arm and hand. Physical examination reveals allodynia (pain resulting from a non-noxious stimulus to normal skin) in her left hand and arm. What caused R.L.'s condition, and how would you manage her pain pharmacologically?**

Hyperalgesia after a minor injury is well described, but the pathogenic basis of such pain is not understood. In these afflicted patients, the pain threshold is decreased and stimuli response in the affected region is increased. This persistent pain also may be associated with changes in regional cutaneous blood flow, osteoporosis, swelling, changes in regional temperature, and atrophic musculocutaneous changes in the affected region without demonstrable nerve injury. In the affected areas, pain is elicited by even the slightest mechanical or thermal stimuli. This painful hyperalgesic condition, known as, *reflex sympathetic dystrophy,* or *chronic regional pain syndrome (CRPS)* has been attributed to sympathetic excess and has been called sympathetically maintained pain (SMP) by some. It also can be the result of other central or peripheral mechanisms that are independent of the sympathetic nervous system. SMP may partially respond to pharmacologic agents that interfere with the α-adrenergic function; therefore, one would expect it to respond to clonidine, prazosin, phenoxybenzamine, or guanethidine. Some symptoms of these syndromes may respond to other classes of pharmacologic agents such as steroids and nonsteroidal anti-inflammatory agents, TCAs, anticonvulsants, antiarrhythmics, or local anesthetics.

α₂-Agonists

50. **R.L.'s CRPS will be managed by a sympathoplegic agent. What doses of clonidine or prazosin will be required for pain management in R.L.?**

α₂-Agonists (e.g., clonidine) are useful in the management of SMP. They act by reversing the excessive sympathetic adrenergic response at central and peripheral receptors and by reversing local vasoconstriction with improvement in blood flow. Clonidine has analgesic effects when administered either systemically or locally at the spinal level. The α₁-antagonist, prazosin, also has been used in the management of SMP. The dosages for clonidine and prazosin are 0.2 to 0.6 mg/day and 1 to 6 mg/day, respectively, in two to three equally divided doses. The major disadvantage of these agents is their side effects, especially hypotension and exacerbation of depression.[193] In addition, rapid development of tachyphylaxis has been noted. Clonidine 0.1 mg orally four times daily would be a good starting dose for R.L., but the final dose must be titrated based on the patient's clinical response or side effects.

Tricyclic Antidepressants

51. **What types of pain are most responsive to antidepressants? Is there any advantage of using one antidepressant over another for pain management in patients such as R.L.?**

The analgesic properties of TCAs are independent of their antidepressant properties. However, depression often accompanies chronic pain, and in turn depression often exacerbates a patient's response to pain and inability to cope with pain-induced lifestyle changes.[194,195] Thus, the antidepressant may interrupt this cycle of events. TCAs produce analgesia directly through modulation of the descending inhibitory nerve pathway by either altering serotonin or norepinephrine neurotransmission. They are also believed to reduce pain through local anesthetic (sodium-channel blocking) effects. Another secondary benefit of some TCAs is their sedative effect, which can help the patient sleep and reduce feelings of anxiety.

Antidepressants have been most widely studied in patients with diabetic neuropathy and postherpetic neuralgia.[196,197] However, they also have some value in deafferentation pain (central pain resulting from loss of spinal afferent nerve pathway), phantom limb pain, HIV neuropathy,[198] postsurgical pain,[199,200] fibromyalgia, and chronic pain associated with depression. They also have limited usefulness in the management of lower back pain, radiation neuropathy, and direct malignant nerve infiltration.

Clinical data for the management of pain is most extensive for amitriptyline, but other TCAs also have been used for this purpose.[191–203] Data on the use of SSRIs such as fluoxetine, paroxetine, and sertraline are limited.[204] The major disadvantage associated with the use of TCAs is their side effect profile, which includes sedation, anticholinergic effects, and cardiotoxicity (quinidine-like widening of QRS on electrocardiogram [ECG]) (see Question 36). Sedation and anticholinergic effects are less severe with the secondary amine TCAs (desipramine, nortriptyline) than with the tertiary amine TCAs such as amitriptyline and doxepin. Weight gain can be a limiting factor as well.[205–209] In patients such as R.L., who have no histories of cardiac problems, a TCA can be helpful in pain management. Whether TCAs should be used to treat pain in the elderly population remains controversial because these agents also can produce cognitive impairment and hypotension.[210]

Anticonvulsants and Antiarrhythmics

52. What other alternatives are there for the management of R.L.'s neuropathic pain?

Anticonvulsants have been used frequently in the management of neuropathic pain with varying success. In randomized-controlled studies, gabapentin has improved symptoms of diabetic neuropathy and postherpetic neuralgia.[211,212] In addition, gabapentin has demonstrated anecdotal benefit in other neuropathic pain syndromes. Doses of gabapentin up to 3,600 mg/day or greater may be required in some patients. The reported use of antiarrhythmics in the management of neuropathic pain is primarily derived from anecdotal reports or uncontrolled trials. These drugs function primarily by stabilizing sodium channels and decreasing neuronal activation.[213,214] Mexiletine has been used for diabetic neuropathy, HIV neuropathy, and other neuropathic pain syndromes.[215–219] The total daily dose is approximately 10 mg/kg in three to four equally divided doses, but GI adverse effects limit its tolerability. Other antiarrhythmics such as regional application of bretylium and tocainide have been tried, but clinical data are limited and these agents carry a higher risk of toxicity.[220]

HEAD INJURY AND OPIOID ANALGESIA

53. M.C., a 24-year-old hemophiliac man, is admitted to the emergency department (ED) with several minor lacerations, contusions, and painful hemarthrosis secondary to a bicycle accident. Meperidine 50 mg IV was ordered and he was transferred to the medical ward for further evaluation. There, M.C. was given antihemophilic factor. He also was given meperidine 50 to 75 mg intravenously Q 3 hr PRN for pain. What was the danger in administering an opioid to M.C. in the ED or shortly after he was admitted?

Opioid analgesics generally are avoided in patients with head injury for the following reasons: (1) opioid-induced pupillary changes, nausea, and general CNS clouding may mask or confuse the neurologic evaluation; (2) head injury potentiates the respiratory depressant effects of opioids; (3) opioids induce carbon dioxide retention, which in turn causes vasodilation of cerebral arteries and an increase in cerebrospinal fluid pressure that might already be elevated because of head injury[221–223]; (4) opioids in excessive doses can mask internal organ injury; and (5) morphine and meperidine can produce further hypotension in patients who have blood loss due to trauma. However, these potential complications should not preclude the use of a short-acting opioid such as fentanyl for pain control in emergency situations, especially when the patient's clinical condition and analgesic responses are monitored closely. If fentanyl is to be used, small but frequent IV doses are preferred over single, large boluses (see Table 9-5 for starting doses). The final dose is based on the patient's analgesic and toxic responses. It would be reasonable to start M.C. on fentanyl 25 to 50 μg IV every 30 to 60 minutes followed by analgesic titration.

MYOCARDIAL PAIN

54. C.P., a 65-year-old man with a history of angina pectoris, is brought to the ED with a suspected acute myocardial infarc-

tion (MI). Meperidine 25 mg IV is prescribed for pain control. Would another analgesic be preferred over pentazocine in C.P.?

This dose of meperidine might be effective for analgesia; however, meperidine has variable hemodynamic effects in patients with hemodynamic instability, whereas fentanyl and morphine's effects are more predictable. Butorphanol (Stadol) and pentazocine can increase pulmonary vascular resistance and pulmonary artery pressure.[224–226] Furthermore, pentazocine can produce idiosyncratic hypotensive episodes, which could be disastrous in these patients. Therefore, these agents should be avoided after MI.

Morphine does not increase myocardial wall tension or oxygen consumption and does not affect cardiac dimensions. Morphine also can decrease heart rate and induces only minimal orthostatic changes in blood pressures. However, in postsurgical patients who are volume depleted, the orthostatic effect of morphine can be quite dramatic. Sedative and emetic effects of morphine are comparable to methadone, but may be greater than those of meperidine or hydromorphone. Methadone, hydromorphone, buprenorphine, and nalbuphine affect the cardiovascular system in a manner similar to that of morphine.[226]

In summary, although all the aforementioned agents are effective analgesics, pentazocine and butorphanol cause greater cardiovascular effects and can exacerbate an acute MI by increasing the cardiac workload and oxygen consumption. Therefore, morphine remains the preferred agent. (See Chapter 18, Myocardial Infarction, for further discussion.)

COLIC PAIN
Biliary Colic

55. B.C., a 42-year-old man, is admitted for severe, intermittent right upper quadrant pain accompanied by nausea, vomiting, and clay-colored stools. The differential diagnosis is biliary colic versus acute pancreatitis. Two doses of meperidine 100 mg IM 3 hours apart fail to ease the pain. What other potent analgesics are preferred in this situation?

Opioid analgesics can induce smooth-muscle spasms in the sphincter of Oddi and thereby increase intrabiliary pressures.[227–231] The resulting intraductal back pressure can aggravate pain symptoms and increase the serum concentrations of amylase 5 to 10 times above the control value.[232] Although it often is claimed that meperidine is less likely than morphine to cause spasm of the sphincter of Oddi, there is no clear evidence of the superiority of one agent over the other.[233] Significant increases in intrabiliary pressures of patients receiving fentanyl (Sublimaze), morphine, meperidine, pentazocine (Talwin), butorphanol (Stadol), and oxycodone are documented.[234,235]

In one study,[236] buprenorphine (Buprenex) did not increase biliary pressure, but further controlled investigations are needed to substantiate this finding. Generally, biliary pressures increase and spasms begin within 5 minutes of parenteral opioid administration. These effects peak within 20 to 60 minutes, and values gradually return to normal over 1 to 2 hours.[237,238] Because the reported severity, intensity, and duration of the biliary hypertension vary greatly, it is unlikely that any agent presently available has a clear advantage over another.[233]

Opioid-induced biliary hypertension and sphincter of Oddi spasm can be reversed by parenteral glucagon or naloxone.[237–241] It is still unclear whether orally administered naloxone will have similar effects, although orally administered naloxone prevented opioid-induced constipation in one study.[70] It is unclear whether B.C. is having more pain because of an adverse drug effect or primary failure of meperidine. Because there is no consistent way to clinically measure intraductal pressure, it is recommended that he be given a longer-acting opioid such as methadone 10 mg IM every 6 hours for pain.

Renal Colic

56. M.J., a 36-year-old woman with a history of urolithiasis, comes to the ED because of severe flank pain along with microscopic hematuria. She is diagnosed with renal colic by the ED physician who wishes to treat her pain with meperidine 100 mg IM, but M.J. does not want to take opioids. What can you give to M.J. for her severe pain from her renal colic?

Renal colic is extremely painful, and patients often require parenteral opioid analgesics. There is no significant clinical difference between any of the opioids for this type of acute analgesic indication. Because M.J. does not want to receive opioids, the choice of analgesics is limited. The parenteral nonsteroidal analgesic ketorolac is likely to be the best alternative.[242] It would be appropriate to start M.J. on ketorolac 15 mg IV every 6 hours as an alternative to the opioids for acute analgesia.

LIVER DISEASE AND ANALGESIA

57. A.A., a 54-year-old man with alcoholic cirrhosis, severe ascites, and mild jaundice, has been hospitalized with severe right upper quadrant abdominal pain. His stools are guaiac positive, and he occasionally has bright red blood present at the rectum secondary to hemorrhoids. He was placed on oral lactulose 30 g QID when the protein content of his diet was increased. Although he has a history of hepatic encephalopathy, he is currently alert and receiving only spironolactone 200 mg/day and prophylactic lactulose. What problems can arise upon administration of opioid analgesics to patients such as A.A.?

Morphine can induce electroencephalogram (EEG) changes similar to those associated with impending hepatic encephalopathy when administered to patients with hepatic cirrhosis.[243] These morphine-induced EEG changes cannot be correlated with alkalosis, hypokalemia, or increased blood ammonia levels, and the mechanism is unknown.

Because most opioid analgesics are significantly metabolized in the liver, their serum levels may accumulate if dosing intervals are not adjusted in patients with decreased hepatic function.[244–249] The oral bioavailability of some of the opioids also may be increased because of a decreased hepatic first-pass effect.[250] The opioids with the greatest first-pass effect or a high extraction ratio have the greatest variability in bioavailability. For example, oral morphine and meperidine have a higher extraction ratio than methadone and therefore are more likely to be absorbed unpredictably in patients with severe liver disease. In these patients, methadone is most likely to be absorbed consistently when administered orally.

It would be reasonable to treat A.A.'s pain with a single, modest dose of parenteral morphine, but subsequent doses should await the reappearance of signs of pain to prevent the possible precipitation of hepatic encephalopathy. Careful monitoring of A.A. is essential to minimize risk while maximizing analgesia. The clinician should remember that any CNS depressant may trigger significant problems in a patient such as A.A. If an oral opioid is to be used, then methadone will be a good choice because of its more consistent bioavailability. Although methadone has a long half-life, it is still safer to use orally than morphine. All opioid analgesics should be given in small, frequent, on-demand doses in patients such as A.A. Time-contingent dosing of opioids should be avoided in patients with liver disease because of the risk of drug accumulation. A.A. can be given methadone 2.5 mg no more often than every 6 hours, as needed, accompanied by close monitoring.

RESPIRATORY DISEASE AND ANALGESIA

58. C.T., a 65-year-old man admitted with a hip fracture, has a history of chronic obstructive pulmonary disease (COPD). On admission, C.T. has a nonpurulent productive cough and wheezing. His medical history includes several episodes of pneumonia. Morphine sulfate 6 to 10 mg IM Q 3 hr is ordered for his severe hip pain. What risks are associated with using morphine in C.T.? Are there better alternative potent analgesics?

Systemic opioids remain the first-line agents in managing pain in COPD patients. However, careful monitoring orders also should be written along with the opioid orders. Morphine and all other opioid analgesics can depress respiration when given in therapeutic doses and should be used cautiously in patients with advanced respiratory disease and decreased respiratory function. Respiratory rate, tidal volume, and sensitivity to hypercapnia or hypoxemia are all decreased by opioid analgesics.[251] Although all opioids and agonists produce respiratory depression at therapeutic doses, there appears to be a ceiling effect to the respiratory depression caused by butorphanol (Stadol), nalbuphine (Nubain), and buprenorphine (Buprenex) at higher doses.[252–254] Increased doses of these compounds do not further depress respiration and still provide increased analgesia. The antagonist naloxone reverses the respiratory difficulty (and analgesia) produced by nalbuphine and butorphanol. Although respiratory depression caused by buprenorphine is uncommon, naloxone does not reverse buprenorphine's effects predictably.[255] Ventilatory support is the only treatment.

Because C.T. is in severe pain, a lower dosage of morphine should be used initially. Opioids do not always depress respiration when dosed correctly, and in some instances they actually may improve respiratory function in patients who have recently undergone thoracotomy. These patients often are afraid to breathe deeply because of the pain elicited by such activity. The analgesic phenothiazine, methotrimeprazine, nerve block, or epidural anesthetics also can be used with fewer respiratory effects than systemic morphine.[256–258] Alternatively, morphine PCA should be considered for C.T., because PCA will allow him to self-administer small, frequent doses, thereby reducing the possibility of opioid-induced respiratory depression.

OPIATES IN SPECIAL AGE GROUPS
Advanced Age

59. B.V., a 75-year-old woman, is seen in the office for a routine physical examination. She has a history of osteoarthritis in both knees, osteoporotic vertebral disease, and peptic ulcer disease. In addition to estrogen and calcium supplementation, B.V. takes acetaminophen 650 mg every 4 hours during the day for general discomfort and ibuprofen 400 mg every night to "help [her] sleep." What further information should be assessed before modifying B.V.'s drug therapy?

Chronic pain can have a significant impact on daily functioning and quality of life and should be recognized as a significant problem requiring prompt attention. Chronic pain is common in older adults and may easily go unrecognized and untreated. Painful conditions affecting bones and joints often develop as people age. These conditions provide a chronic source of pain and are often incurable. Approximately one in five older adults takes analgesic medications regularly and more than half of these patients have taken prescription analgesics for >6 months. Prevalence rates for chronic pain among community-dwelling older people have been estimated to be between 25% and 50%.[259] Studies of nursing home residents have documented similar rates for chronic nonmalignant pain and also have shown a consistent trend toward undertreatment with analgesics.[260,261]

Clinical practice guidelines have been developed for the management of chronic pain in older persons.[259] All older patients should be assessed for evidence of chronic pain as well as for acute pain that may indicate a new illness or exacerbation of a chronic condition. Older patients may be reluctant to report pain because they may fear the consequences of a diagnostic workup. Older adults may also perceive pain to be synonymous with serious disease or death.[259] When providing a history, they may not use the word "pain" to describe how they feel. Instead, they may describe their discomfort as "aching, soreness, burning, or tightness." Finally, patients with dementia or language deficits may not be able to communicate the presence of pain. In these individuals and others, grimacing or other unusual behavior may provide clues to the presence of pain.

B.V. should receive a comprehensive assessment that includes a complete medical history and physical examination to determine any new underlying causes of pain, sensory deficits, or neurologic abnormalities. Physical function and pain associated with activities of daily living should be assessed as well as her psychosocial function to evaluate her for depression and to understand her social network and support system. A thorough evaluation of current pain should be performed to characterize her pain and to determine the patterns of her analgesic use and their effectiveness. The medication history should be reviewed for potential drug side effects and interactions. B.V.'s use of ibuprofen should be further evaluated, because older patients who use NSAIDs chronically have a higher frequency of GI bleeding, especially if they have a previous history of this condition.[259]

60. When asked, B.V. states that her current pain level is a 7 on a 10-point scale, and that it can vary from 4 to 8 during the day. It is usually better after rest and worsens later in the day, especially after physical exertion. Although she takes acetaminophen and ibuprofen regularly, they do not effectively reduce her pain. B.V. realizes that her current medical condition will probably not allow her to be completely pain free and states that a pain level of 3 would be acceptable. Would opiate analgesics be appropriate to control B.V.'s pain?

The use of opioid analgesic for chronic nonmalignant pain is controversial. However, the usefulness of this class of drugs should not be overlooked and may provide fewer risks than long-term or high-dose NSAID therapy. The doses needed are often much smaller than those needed to treat chronic malignant pain. Older patients often experience greater pain relief from opioid analgesics than do younger patients probably because both the extent and duration of analgesia are enhanced in this group.[262–268] Older patients achieve higher-than-expected plasma opioid levels (compared with younger patients) after IM or IV administration. Physiologic changes associated with aging, such as decreases in lean body mass, renal function, plasma proteins, hepatic blood flow, and hepatic metabolism[266,267] may be responsible for the enhanced activity of opioids in older patients.[269]

When initiating opioid or adjunct analgesics in older patients, one should remember the phrase "start low and go slow." Because B.V. has underlying conditions that cause continuous pain, time-contingent dosing will be more beneficial. An appropriate initial regimen for B.V. using oxycodone HCl 2.5 mg and acetaminophen 325 mg would be 1 tablet orally every 6 hours, with 1 tablet every 4 hours as needed. This would provide continuous analgesic therapy throughout the day and allow B.V. flexibility to take an additional dose before activities that may exacerbate her pain. B.V. should be instructed to discontinue taking ibuprofen and to avoid other products containing acetaminophen. B.V. may also respond to tramadol 25 to 50 mg (i.e., 1/2 to 1 tablet) Q 8 hr for her pain, because it has shown efficacy equivalent to NSAIDs in osteoarthritis pain. This agent can be considered as an alternative to a high-potency analgesic, but still presents a risk of dizziness and drowsiness.

B.V. should be monitored closely for sedation that could affect her concentration and ability to perform her activities of daily living. Since older patients are more sensitive to the constipating side effects of opioids, a bowel regimen consisting of a stimulant laxative and stool softener should be started at the beginning of therapy. Patients also should be encouraged to maintain good fluid intake and to include fruits and vegetables that are high in fiber in their diet. B.V.'s therapy should be adjusted based on careful monitoring for efficacy and side effects.

Neonates and Children

61. M.M., a 2-day-old, 3-kg girl, has just had bowel surgery for congenital bowel atresia. How should pain management be approached for M.M.?

Many misconceptions exist about the management of pain in the pediatric population. Historically, infants and children have been undertreated for pain and painful procedures. This is due in part to difficulty in communicating with and evaluating pain in children, particularly those who are nonverbal. It was also believed that children did not experience pain in the same way as adults do. Significant advances have been made in the understanding of children's pain perception, and assessment tools designed for different stages of development and communication abilities are available.[270,271] Nevertheless, misconceptions still exist, ranging from the amount of pain a child should experience after a painful procedure to the fear of addiction. Inadequately treated pain can interfere with the healing process, increase heart and respiratory rates, reduce oxygen saturation, and induce hyperglycemia and metabolic acidosis. Increased morbidity and mortality associated with unrelieved pain has been documented in neonates undergoing cardiac surgery.[272] The reality is that infants and children experience pain just as adults do and should receive appropriate medication and doses to treat their pain.

62. What would be a rational pain management plan for M.M.?

Because M.M. has undergone significant GI surgery, severe pain should be anticipated and prevented. Therefore, use of opiates, such as morphine or fentanyl, would be appropriate in this situation. Children appear to mature very early with respect to morphine metabolism. Infants as young as 5 months old show very similar pharmacokinetic parameters as adults; however, morphine concentrations in patients younger than 2.4 months are five times higher than in older patients because of slower metabolic clearance and a lower central compartment volume of distribution.[273] The dosing of morphine in children is similar to adults on a milligram-per-kilogram basis, but children younger than 5 months old may require less frequent dosing. The use of opiates in infants and children does not lead to addiction. Critically ill children who are receiving opiates for long periods of time develop tolerance and physical dependence and exhibit signs and symptoms of withdrawal if opiates are weaned too quickly. However, this should not preclude pediatric patients from receiving opiates.

An appropriate initial dosing regimen for M.M. would be fentanyl 1 µg/kg IV every 4 hours with 1 µg/kg every 2 hours as needed for breakthrough pain. When using parenteral morphine preparations in infants, close attention should be given to the preparation used and the age of the infant. Parenteral morphine preparations are available with and without preservatives. Infants younger than 3 months of age are more susceptible to respiratory depression caused by an allergic reaction to the sulfites or to CNS irritation induced by benzyl alcohol. Thus, neonates and infants younger than 3 months of age should receive only preservative-free morphine. When choosing a route of administration, attention should be given to the patient's clinical condition. Although oral routes are preferred, they may not be appropriate immediately following surgery. Opiates are frequently administered IM. However, IM administration offers no advantage over IV and causes much more pain and distress. Children receiving repeated IM injections often deny the presence of pain to avoid the injection.[271] Therefore, IV administration is the preferred parenteral route in pediatric patients.

Assessment of pain and relief in M.M. is more challenging because she is unable to verbalize specific information. Careful attention to behavioral responses such as crying characteristics, crying duration, facial expressions, visual tracking, response to stimuli, and body movement will be most useful in assessing pain and relief in M.M.[270,271] Heart rate, respiratory rate, blood pressure, and presence of diaphoresis can provide useful clues to M.M.'s level of pain or comfort and can alert the clinician to potential side effects. Careful monitoring together with adjustments to the dose and frequency of administration provides optimal therapy.

MORPHINE-INDUCED NAUSEA AND VOMITING

63. J.J., a 48-year-old woman, has advanced inoperable cervical cancer. The physician has ordered 30 mg of oral morphine solution Q 4 hr for pain, but she has vomited after each dose despite apparently adequate doses of prochlorperazine. What can be done to relieve pain in J.J. who vomits after oral morphine?

Morphine and its derivatives induce nausea and vomiting by stimulating the chemoreceptor trigger zone (CTZ). Although the chemoreceptor trigger zone is stimulated initially, subsequent doses of morphine generally suppress the vomiting center. Because the incidence of nausea (40%) and vomiting (15%) increases in ambulatory patients, a vestibular component also is likely to be involved. If the vomiting is vestibular in origin, instructing J.J. to lie quietly, with as little head motion as possible for an hour or two, often will help. The nausea usually persists for 48 to 72 hours.[274]

Levorphanol (Levo-Dromoran) may cause less nausea and vomiting than other potent opioid analgesics at equianalgesic doses and might be an alternative to morphine if the aforementioned recommendations are ineffective in modifying J.J.'s nausea and vomiting. An equipotent dose of levorphanol for J.J. according to Table 9-3 would be 4 mg. The reported duration of action of levorphanol is 6 hours, longer than that of morphine.[275]

Adjunctive drugs such as droperidol, prochlorperazine, hydroxyzine, scopolamine, and diphenhydramine have been used successfully to control opioid-induced nausea and vomiting. Patients who are extremely sensitive to this opioid-induced effect have to be placed on concurrent or scheduled antiemetics; transdermal scopolamine can be used for this purpose. Although much more costly, agents such as ondansetron may also be useful in patients who have contraindications to the use of phenothiazines or butyrophenones.

USE OF CENTRAL NERVOUS SYSTEM STIMULANTS

64. D.H., a 34-year-old man, is diagnosed with acquired immunodeficiency syndrome (AIDS) and Kaposi's sarcoma. He was discharged from the hospital with a prescription for oral morphine solution, 30 mg Q 3 hr. He has been relatively pain free for about a month, but now returns to the clinic complaining of excessive morning sedation. He cannot reduce his morphine dose because the pain makes him too uncomfortable. What therapeutic intervention can be used to alleviate D.H.'s problem of excessive morning sedation?

Limited clinical data suggest that a morning dose of methylphenidate (Ritalin) or dextroamphetamine (Dexedrine) could relieve not only opioid-induced drowsiness, but could also potentiate analgesia.[276] Less sleepiness has been associated with these combinations than with opioid analgesics alone, and a 10-mg dose of amphetamine combined with the opioid analgesic improved pain tolerance more than the analgesic alone.[277,278] Although these studies involved only single doses, these agents should cause enough CNS stimulation to obviate morning drowsiness. D.H. should try a morning dextroamphetamine dose of 5 to 20 mg. A somewhat smaller dose may be added around noon if he desires increased alertness in the late afternoon and early evening hours. Another alternative would be to switch D.H. to an opioid analgesic that is less sedating. Drugs such as hydromorphone, levorphanol, methadone, and fentanyl often produce the desired clinical response in a patient like D.H.

IMPORTANT DRUG INTERACTIONS
Phenytoin and Methadone

65. B.D., a 32-year-old man, has an 18-year history of chronic pain in the right hip as a result of a motor vehicle accident. He has a long problem list that includes grand mal seizures and gastric ulcer disease. In the past, he has been treated with a variety of opioid analgesics on a PRN schedule, which resulted in escalating drug requirements and a complex regimen of multiple-ingredient drugs (e.g., Percocet, Tylenol #3, Vicodin). B.D.'s attending physician prescribed methadone 10 mg Q 6 hr several weeks ago. This switch was initially very successful, but B.D. now presents with symptoms suggestive of opioid withdrawal and poor pain control despite good compliance to his methadone regimen. A note in his chart indicates that B.D. saw a neurologist recently who started him on phenytoin therapy. What important drug–drug interactions might explain this rather complex case?

Phenytoin (Dilantin) induces cytochrome P450 (CYP) 3A4 isoenzymes that are responsible for the clearance of methadone, and can thereby decrease serum concentrations of methadone and precipitate symptoms of withdrawal.[279,280] The methadone dose should be increased to 20 mg every 6 hours, and a note should be made in the chart that the doses will need to be reduced if the phenytoin is discontinued for any reason. After his dose has been increased, B.D. should be watched closely for the next several days for drug-induced drowsiness since the long half-life of methadone can produce accumulation.

Cimetidine and Methadone

66. One week later, B.D.'s wife calls and says that he is very drowsy and that his speech has started to slur. On further questioning, his wife notes that B.D. restarted cimetidine 400 mg PO TID for symptoms of gastritis. She confirms that B.D. has been taking methadone 20 mg PO Q 6 hr. What may explain B.D.'s symptoms of apparent opioid toxicity?

Cimetidine (Tagamet) inhibits CYP 3A4 isoenzymes, thereby decreasing the metabolism of methadone and potentially subjecting patients to toxic levels. B.D. also could be reaching serum methadone steady-state levels at this time. He should be instructed to withhold the methadone until his mental status returns to baseline; then, the dose of methadone needs to be decreased to 10 mg every 6 hours. When adding cimetidine to existing methadone therapy, methadone doses need to be decreased; the doses should be increased again if cimetidine is subsequently withdrawn.[281]

Similar precautions need to be instituted for other CYP3A4 inhibitors, such as antiretroviral agents, ketoconazole or fluconazole, erythromycin, and other agents.

Codeine Interactions With CYP 2D6 Inhibitors
Tramadol and SSRIs

67. T.R. is a 42-year-old man who suffered a right tibial fracture requiring pinning and external fixation. He is now able to ambulate with crutches. Before discharge from the hospital, four acetaminophen 500 mg with hydrocodone 5-mg tablets throughout the day provided good pain control. At the time of discharge, T.R.'s pain regimen was changed to acetaminophen 325 mg with codeine 60 mg, 2 tablets PO Q 3 to 4 hr, owing to his pharmacy benefit limitations. T.R. calls your office because the acetaminophen with codeine is not controlling his pain even when he takes 2 tablets every 3 hours. T.R. also is taking paroxetine 20 mg PO Q am for his chronic depression. His physician is considering switching his medication to tramadol or acetaminophen with oxycodone. What changes in T.R.'s therapy can you recommend to provide better pain control?

Codeine is metabolized to morphine in the liver by CYP 2D6 isoenzymes. Concurrent administration of codeine with agents that inhibit the CYP 2D6 system, such as paroxetine, fluoxetine, amiodarone, and ritonavir, may reduce the conversion of codeine to morphine and influence drug response.[282] In addition, this isoenzyme shows genetic polymorphism and individuals may demonstrate ultrarapid, extensive, or poor metabolism. Recognition of these potential drug interactions is important because concurrent administration of CYP 2D6 inhibitors may make some patients appear to be poor metabolizers and less responsive to codeine, which, in fact, may not be true.

Oxycodone, hydrocodone, and tramadol are also substrates for the CYP 2D6 isoenzyme. Although a potential interaction exists between oxycodone and paroxetine, there is little evidence at this time to indicate that oxycodone requires conversion to an active metabolite via the 2D6 pathway to be an effective analgesic. However, tramadol is partially metabolized by CYP 2D6 and has an active metabolite. Concurrent administration with a CYP 2D6 inhibitor could potentially reduce analgesic activity.[282]

The coadministration of tramadol and paroxetine could potentially cause more serious problems in this patient. Tramadol has SSRI-like activity because it decreases the synaptic reuptake of norepinephrine and serotonin. Coadministration with SSRI agents, such as paroxetine, fluoxetine, fluvoxamine and citalopram, can put the patient at risk for serotonin syndrome.[283] Signs and symptoms associated with serotonin syndrome include diaphoresis, chest pain, tachycardia, hypertension, confusion, psychosis, agitation, and tremor. Neurotoxicity can be severe and may progress to seizures or coma. Therefore, tramadol is not a good choice for this patient.

Similarly, tramadol can interact with the antimigraine agents known as "triptans," because their mode of action includes enhancing serotonin activity centrally. Therefore, combinations of tramadol, SSRIs, and/or triptans are relatively contraindicated and require close and judicious monitoring.

It would be reasonable to consider either acetaminophen with oxycodone or hydrocodone for pain control in this patient, especially because he has experienced good pain control with the hydrocodone preparation in the past.

PRIMARY DYSMENORRHEA

68. **P.O., a 27-year-old woman, is seen in the primary care clinic because of severe abdominal pain secondary to her menstrual periods. She reports having pain-free menstrual periods only once or twice yearly. She has been diagnosed as having primary dysmenorrhea with no other gynecologic pathology being found. How should P.O.'s menstrual pain be treated?**

Primary dysmenorrhea is a common gynecologic disorder effecting 60% to 80% of women at sometime in their life.[284] Pain usually occurs 2 to 12 hours before the commencement of menstrual flow, but it may occur simultaneously with, or a few hours after, the beginning of menstruation. It reaches maximal intensity at 2 to 24 hours, then decreases over the next few days.[285] Primary dysmenorrhea is associated with increases in endometrial and circulatory prostaglandins. Thus, the NSAIDs, which alter the production of the prostaglandins, are frequently used to manage primary dysmenorrhea. The dosages required for the treatment of primary dysmenorrhea usually are higher than those used for analgesia, but frequently a single dose is sufficient to terminate the dysmenorrhea pain. On some occasions, frequent, high doses may be required.

The best time to initiate NSAIDs remains controversial. Some clinicians recommend beginning drug therapy a few days before the start of menses; others argue that the prostaglandins are not stored and therefore prefer to initiate drug therapy only after the start of menses. Pretreatment with NSAIDs carries the risk of fetal drug exposure during early pregnancy. Studies comparing pretreatment with dosing at the onset of menses show no difference in the analgesia between either of the regimens.[286,287] (Also see Chapter 48, Gynecologic and Other Disorders of Women.) P.O. should be instructed to take 600 to 800 mg of ibuprofen at the onset of menses or when discomfort begins. Repeat dosages of 400 to 600 mg may be taken every 4 to 6 hours as needed. If this regimen is ineffective, she can take the first dose 1 to 2 days before the first day of menses is expected.

HEADACHES

69. **M.K., a 32-year-old man, is complaining of severe headaches that occur at least once every 2 weeks. He takes two Excedrin extra-strength tablets (acetaminophen 250 mg, aspirin 250 mg, and caffeine 65 mg) Q 2 hr until the headache starts to ease and sometimes requires a cumulative dose of up to 16 tablets. Migraine and vascular headaches have been ruled out in M.K. Would one of the nonsalicylate NSAIDs be more efficacious for M.K.? Are there any other considerations in managing M.K.'s headache? Is caffeine an effective analgesic for headaches?**

Headaches are common, afflicting nearly everyone at some time during their life. The incidence of headache is higher in females and increases with age; 10% of headaches develop into chronic disabling conditions. For M.K., who self-medicates chronically with large doses of acetaminophen, one must be concerned with toxicity from the analgesics. Chronic use of both NSAID analgesics and caffeine (either as single agents or in combination) can possibly precipitate withdrawal ("rebound") headaches on discontinuation. Although NSAIDs are not considered habituating, there is accumulating evidence

that chronic intake of peripheral-acting analgesics may perpetuate the underlying pain syndrome. In the case of M.K., one must consider the possibility of caffeine withdrawal headache as well, because he is taking a caffeine-containing combination product. Other dietary sources of caffeine ingestion from coffee, tea, and other foods should be determined as well.

Caffeine is used in analgesic combination products because it has both a CNS stimulant and a vasoconstrictive effect, which may reverse some of the headache symptoms. The value of caffeine, especially in the small quantities found in most pain relievers, has been controversial. However, a meta-analysis and subsequent study conclude that caffeine does add to the analgesic effect of aspirin and acetaminophen.[288,289]

Acute headache can be managed with parenteral ketorolac, but it is not a viable alternative for chronic headache management.[290] M.K.'s headaches may resolve upon gradual withdrawal of NSAID analgesics and caffeine, but this process is slow and requires the clinician's as well as the patient's determination to stay with the treatment plan. (Also see Chapter 52, Headache.)

PROCEDURAL PAIN

70. **C.T., a 26-year-old woman, injured her left knee during a fall while skiing. After immobilizing her left knee and using ice therapy, most of her swelling has subsided. She is now seen in the outpatient surgical center for an arthroscopic evaluation of her knee. She is very concerned that the lidocaine that is to be used to anesthetize her knee is going to produce pain, because she had a bad experience with regional lidocaine injections in her past. What can you recommend to reduce the pain associated with lidocaine infiltration?**

Lidocaine injection is quite acidic and can produce local irritation and pain during the infiltration procedure before the anesthetic effect takes place. Because this is a common complaint, C.T.'s concerns should be taken seriously. A simple solution is to neutralize the lidocaine injection solution by adding 1 mL of 1 mEq/mL sodium bicarbonate to 9 mL of 1% to 2% lidocaine before injecting C.T.[291–294] Because lidocaine is stable over a wide range of pH values, the bicarbonate will not reduce its efficacy of local anesthetic blockade. However, this technique should not be used with other local anesthetics, which may be subject to rapid degradation by basic agents.

TOPICAL ANESTHETICS AND ANALGESICS

71. **J.G., a 6-year-old boy, is being treated for osteomyelitis of his foot as a result of a skate boarding accident. Because of the need for long-term antibiotic therapy, he requires occasional IV access replacement. He is very fearful of the procedure because of the associated pain. What can you offer J.G. to reduce his discomfort?**

Insertion of a venous catheter often produces significant discomfort and pain, but there is no reason C.T. has to endure it. Topical lidocaine/prilocaine cream (EMLA) can provide good pain relief during catheter insertion for minor surgical procedures such as circumcision and skin grafts.[295–299] The cream must be applied 30 to 60 minutes before the procedure with an occlusive dressing; the anesthetic effect lasts approximately 60 to 120 minutes.[300] A smaller-gauge catheter also may reduce the amount of pain associated with the venipuncture.[301]

REFERENCES

1. Fields HL. Pain. New York: McGraw-Hill, 1987: 364.
2. Heller PH et al. Peripheral neural contributions to inflammation. In: Fields HL, Liebeskind JC, eds. Pharmacological Approach to the Treatment of Chronic Pain. Progress in Pain Research and Management. Seattle: IASP Press, 1994:31.
3. Dickenson AH. The roles of transmitters and their receptors in systems related to pain and analgesia. In: Max M, ed. Pain 1999—an updated review. Seattle: IASP Press, 1999:381.
4. Wilcox GL. Pharmacology of pain and analgesia. In: Max M, ed. Pain 1999—an updated review. Seattle: IASP Press, 1999:573.
5. Dickenson AH, Rahman W. Mechanisms of chronic pain and the developing nervous system. In: McGrath PJ, Finley GA, eds. Chronic and Recurrent Pain in Children and Adolescents. Progress in Pain Research and Management. Seattle: IASP Press, 1999:5.
6. Besson JM. The neurobiology of pain. Lancet 1999;353(9164):1610.
7. Golianu B et al. Pediatric acute pain management. Pediatr Clin N Am 2000;47(3):559.
8. McCaffery M, Pasero C. Pain: Clinical Manual. St. Louis: Mosby, 1999:15.
9. Price DP et al. Central neural mechanisms of normal and abnormal pain state. In: Fields HL, Liebeskind JC, eds. Pharmacological Approach to the Treatment of Chronic Pain. Progress in Pain Research and Management. Seattle: IASP Press, 1994:61.
10. Woolf CJ et al. Neuropathic pain: aetiology, symptoms, mechanisms, and management. Lancet 1999;353(9168):1959.
11. McMahon SB, Koltzenburg M. Silent afferents and visceral pain. In: Fields HL, Liebeskind JC, eds. Pharmacological Approach to the Treatment of Chronic Pain. Progress in Pain Research and Management. Seattle: IASP Press, 1994:11.
12. Willis WD Jr. Introduction to the basic science of pain and headache for the clinician: physiological concepts. In: Max M, ed. Pain 1999—an updated review. Seattle: IASP Press, 1999:561.
13. Dickenson AH. NMDA receptor antagonists as analgesics. In: Fields HL, Liebeskind JC, eds. Pharmacological Approach to the Treatment of Chronic Pain. Progress in Pain Research and Management. Seattle: IASP Press, 1994:173.
14. Pini LA, Vitale G, Sandrini M. Serotonin and opiate involvement in the antinociceptive effect of acetylsalicylic acid. Pharmacology 1997 Feb; 54(2):84.
15. Sandrini M, Vitale G, Pini LA. Central antinociceptive activity of acetylsalicylic acid is modulated by brain serotonin receptor subtypes. Pharmacology 2002 Aug;65(4):1937.
16. Dickenson AH. Where and how do opioids act? Proceedings of the 7th World Congress on Pain. Prog Pain Res Manag 1994;2:525.
17. Clinical Practice Guideline, Cancer Pain Management. U.S. Department of Health and Human Services, Agency for Health Care Policy and Research. AHCPR Pub. Rockville, MD, 1994.
18. Porternoy RK. Opioids and adjuvant analgesics. In: Max M, ed. Pain 1999—an updated review. Seattle: IASP Press, 1999:3.
19. Max MB et al. Effects of desipramine, amitriptyline, and fluoxetine on pain in diabetic neuropathy. N Engl J Med 1992;326:1250.
20. Beaver WT, Feise G. Comparison of the analgesic effects of morphine, hydroxyzine, and their combination in patients with postoperative pain. In: Bonica JJ et al, eds. Advances in Pain Research and Therapy. New York: Raven Press, 1976:553.
21. American Pain Society. Principles of analgesic use in the treatment of acute and chronic cancer pain, 2nd Ed. Clin Pharm 1990;9:601.
22. LoVecchio F et al. The use of analgesics in patients with acute abdominal pain. J Emerg Med 1997; 15(6):775.

23. Pace S et al. Intravenous morphine for early pain relief in patients with acute abdominal pain. Acad Emerg Med 1996;3(12):1086.
24. Clinical Practice Guideline, Acute Pain Management. U.S. Department of Health and Human Services, Agency for Health Care Policy and Research. AHCPR Pub. No. 92-0032. Rockville, MD, 1992.
25. Krames ES. Intrathecal infusional therapies for intractable pain: patient management guidelines. J Pain Symptom Manage 1993;8:36.
26. Skevington SM. The relationship between pain and depression: a longitudinal study of early synovitis. Proceedings of the 7th World Congress on Pain. Prog Pain Res Manage 1994;2:201.
27. Stieg RL et al. Cost benefits of interdisciplinary chronic pain treatment. Clin J Pain 1985;1:189.
28. MacDonald N. Palliative care-an essential component of cancer control. Can Med Assoc J 1998;158:1709.
29. Ashburn MA et al. Management of chronic pain. Lancet 1999;353(9167):1865.
30. Gureje O et al. Persistent pain and well-being: a World Health Organization study in primary care. JAMA 1998;280:147.
31. Rose-Innes AP et al. Low back pain: an algorithmic approach to diagnosis and management. Geriatrics 1998;53(10):26.
32. Leland JY. Chronic pain: primary care treatment of the older patient. Geriatrics 1999;54(1):23.
33. Rowbotham MC et al. Oral opioid therapy for chronic peripheral and central neuropathic pain.N Engl J Med. 2003 Mar 27;348(13):1223.
34. Weissman DE. Doctors, opioids, and the law: the effect of controlled substances regulations on cancer pain management. Semin Oncol 1993;20(2 Suppl 1):53.
35. Portenoy RK. Cancer pain management. Semin Oncol 1993;20(2 Suppl 1):19.
36. Hill CS Jr. The barriers to adequate pain management with opioid analgesics. Semin Oncol 1993;20(2 Suppl 1):1.
37. Weinstein SM et al. Physicians' attitudes toward pain and the use of opioid analgesics: results of a survey from the Texas Cancer Pain Initiative. South Med J 2000;93(5):479.
38. Sloan PA et al.Cancer pain assessment and management by housestaff. Pain 1996;67(2-3):475.
39. McCaffery M, Pasero C. Pain: Clinical Manual. St. Louis: Mosby, 1999:15.
40. Joint Commission on Accreditation of Healthcare Organizations. Pain assessment and management standards. Available at: www.jcaho.org/standard/pm_mpfrm.html. Accessed April, 17, 2000.
41. Foley KM. The treatment of cancer pain. N Engl J Med 1985;313:84. World Health Organization. Cancer pain relief and palliative care. Report of a WHO expert committee [World Health Organization Technical Report Series, 804]. Geneva, Switzerland: World Health Organization, 1990.
42. World Health Organization guidelines at http://www.who.int/cancer/palliative/painladder/en/.
43. Claiborne R. A patient looks at pain and analgesia. Hosp Pract 1982;17:21.
44. Donovan BD. Patient attitudes to postoperative pain relief. Anesth Intensive Care 1983;11:125.
45. Cooper SA et al. Comparative analgesic potency of aspirin and ibuprofen. J Oral Surg 1977;35:898.
46. Winter L Jr et al. Analgesic activity of ibuprofen (Motrin) in postoperative oral surgical pain. Oral Surg Oral Med Oral Pathol 1978;45:159.
47. Heidrich G et al. Efficacy and quality of ibuprofen and acetaminophen plus codeine analgesia. Pain 1985;22:385.
48. Ouellette RD et al. Naproxen sodium vs acetaminophen plus codeine in postsurgical pain. Curr Ther Res 1986;39(5):839.
49. Vargas Busquets MA et al. Naproxen sodium versus acetaminophen-codeine for pain following plastic surgery. Curr Ther Res 1988;43(2):311.
50. Indelicato PA et al. Comparison of diflunisal and acetaminophen with codeine in the treatment of

mild to moderate pain due to strains and sprains. Clin Ther 1986;8(3):269.
51. Lasagna L. Analgesic methodology: a brief history and commentary. J Clin Pharmacol 1980;20(Pt. 2):373.
52. Levine J et al. Relationship of duration of analgesia to opioid pharmacokinetic variables. Brain Res 1983;289(1–2):391.
53. Hammack JE, Loprinzi CL. Use of orally administered opioids for cancer-related pain. Mayo Clin Proc 1994;69(4):384.
54. Davis T et al. Comparative morphine pharmacokinetics following sublingual, intramuscular, and oral administration in patients with cancer. Hospice 1993;9:85.
55. Crews JC et al. Clinical efficacy of methadone in patients refractory to other mu-opioid receptor agonist analgesics for management of terminal cancer pain. Case presentations and discussion of incomplete cross-tolerance among opioid agonist analgesics. Cancer 1993;72:2266.
56. Miller RR. Propoxyphene: a review. Am J Hosp Pharm 1977;34:413.
57. Li Wan Po A et al. Systematic overview of co-proxamol to assess analgesic effects in addition of dextropropoxyphene to paracetamol. Br Med J 1997;315(7122):1565.
58. Beaver WT. Analgesic efficacy of dextropropoxyphene and dextropropoxyphene-containing combinations: a review. Hum Toxicol 1984; 3(Suppl):191S.
59. Almirall J et al. Propoxyphene-induced hypoglycemia in a patient with chronic renal failure. Nephron 1989;53(3):273.
60. Savage SR. Chronic pain and the disease of addiction: the interfacing roles of pain medicine and addiction medicine. In: Max M, ed. Pain 1999—an updated review. Seattle: IASP Press, 1999:15.
61. Portenoy RK. Opioid therapy for chronic nonmalignant pain: a review of critical issues. J Pain Symptom Manage 1996;11(4):203.
62. Lewis JH. Hepatic toxicity of nonsteroidal anti-inflammatory drugs. Clin Pharm 1984;3:128.
63. Seeff LB et al. Acetaminophen hepatotoxicity in alcoholics. A therapeutic misadventure. Ann Intern Med 1986;104:399.
64. Baldo BA, Pham NH, Zhao Z. Chemistry of drug allergenicity. Curr Opin Allergy Clin Immunol. 2001;1(4):327.
65. Longo WE, Vernava AM, 3rd. Prokinetic agents for lower gastrointestinal motility disorders. Dis Colon Rectum 1993;36:696.
66. Culpepper-Morgan JA et al. Treatment of opioid-induced constipation with oral naloxone: a pilot study. Clin Pharmacol Ther 1992;52:90.
67. Portoghese PS, Edward E. Smissman-Bristol-Myers Squibb Award Address. The role of concepts in structure-activity relationship studies of opioid ligands. J Med Chem 1992;35:1927.
68. Bassotti G et al. Extensive investigation on colonic motility with pharmacological testing is useful for selecting surgical options in patients with inertia colica. Am J Gastroenterol 1992;87:143.
69. Robinson BA et al. Oral naloxone in opioid-associated constipation [Letter]. Lancet 1991;338:581.
70. Sykes NP. Oral naloxone in opioid-associated constipation [Letter]. Lancet 1991;337(8755):1475.
71. Laizure SC. Considerations in morphine therapy. Am J Hosp Pharm 1994;51(16):2042.
72. Clark RF. Meperidine: therapeutic use and toxicity. J Emerg Med 1995;13(6):797.
73. Catapano MS. The analgesic efficacy of ketorolac for acute pain. J Emerg Med 1996;14(1):67.
74. Neighbor ML et al. Intramuscular ketorolac vs oral ibuprofen in emergency department patients with acute pain. Acad Emerg Med 1998;5:118.
75. Tramer MR et al. Comparing analgesic efficacy of non-steroidal antiinflammatory drugs given by different routes in acute and chronic pain: a qualitative systematic review. Acta Anaesth Scand 1998; 42:71.

76. Hallen H et al. The nasal reactivity in patients with nasal polyps. ORL J Otorhinolaryngol Relat Spec 1994;56:276.

77. Kowalski ML et al. Nasal secretions in response to acetylsalicylic acid. J Allergy Clin Immunol 1993;91:580.

78. Muther RS et al. Aspirin-induced depression of glomerular filtration rate in normal humans: role of sodium balance. Ann Intern Med 1981;94:317.

79. Schoch PH et al. Acute renal failure in an elderly woman following intramuscular ketorolac administration. Ann Pharmacother 1992;26:1233.

80. Pearce CJ et al. Renal failure and hyperkalemia associated with ketorolac tromethamine. Arch Intern Med 1993;153:1000.

81. Epstein M. Renal prostaglandins and the control of renal function in liver disease. Am J Med 1986;80(Suppl 1A):46.

82. Zipser RD, Henrich WL. Implication of nonsteroidal anti-inflammatory drug therapy. Am J Med 1986;80(Suppl 1A):78.

83. Brater DC. Drug-drug and drug-disease interactions with nonsteroidal anti-inflammatory drugs. Am J Med 1986;80(Suppl 1A):62.

84. Dunn MJ, Zambraski EJ. Renal effects of drugs that inhibit prostaglandin synthesis. Kidney Int 1980;18:609.

85. Blackshear JL et al. NSAID-induced nephrotoxicity, avoidance, detection and treatment. Drug Ther Hosp 1983;(Nov.):41.

86. Zipser RD et al. Prostaglandins: modulators of renal function and pressor resistance in chronic liver disease. J Clin Endocrinol Metab 1979;48:895.

87. Donker AJ et al. The effect of indomethacin on kidney function and plasma renin activity in man. Nephron 1976;17:288.

88. Walsche JJ, Venuto RC. Acute oliguric renal failure induced by indomethacin. Possible mechanism. Ann Intern Med 1979;91:47.

89. Favre L et al. Reversible renal failure from combined triamterene and indomethacin. Ann Intern Med 1982;96:317.

90. Stillman MT et al. Adverse effects of nonsteroidal anti-inflammatory drugs on the kidney. Med Clin N Am 1982;68:371.

91. Finkelstein A et al. Fenoprofen nephropathy: lipoid nephrosis and interstitial nephritis. A possible T-lymphocyte disorder. Am J Med 1982;72:81.

92. Fung DL et al. A comparison of alphaprodine and meperidine pharmacokinetics. J Clin Pharmacol 1980;20:37.

93. Poniatowski BC. Continuous subcutaneous infusions for pain control. J Intraven Nurs 1991;14:30.

94. Lang AH et al. Treatment of severe cancer pain by continuous infusion of subcutaneous opioids. Recent Results Cancer Res 1991;121:51.

95. Swanson G et al. Patient-controlled analgesia for chronic cancer pain in the ambulatory setting: a report of 117 patients. J Clin Oncol 1989;7(12):1903.

96. Bruera E et al. Use of the subcutaneous route for the administration of narcotics in patients with cancer pain. Cancer 1988;15;62:407.

97. Marlowe S et al. Epidural patient-controlled analgesia (PCA): an alternative to continuous epidural infusions. Pain 1989;37:97.

98. Sawaki Y et al. Patient and nurse evaluation of patient-controlled analgesia delivery systems for postoperative pain management. J Pain Symptom Manage 1992;7:443.

99. Shaffer HJ, LaSalvia TA. Patterns of substance use among methadone maintenance patients. Indicators of outcome. J Subst Abuse Treat 1992;9:143.

100. Gossop M et al. Severity of dependence and route of administration of heroin, cocaine and amphetamines. Br J Addict 1992;87:1527.

101. Hoffman M et al. Pain management in the opioid-addicted patient with cancer. Cancer 1991;68:1121.

102. Rickford WJ, Reynolds F. Epidural analgesia in labour and maternal posture. Anaesthesia 1983;38:1169.

103. Conacher ID et al. Epidural analgesia following thoracic surgery. A review of two years' experience. Anaesthesia 1983;38:546.

104. Adu-Gymafi Y et al. High dose epidural morphine for surgical analgesia. Middle East J Anaesthesiol 1985;8:165.

105. Haynes SR et al. Comparison of epidural methadone with epidural diamorphine for analgesia following caesarean section. Acta Anaesthesiol Scand 1993;37:375.

106. Jacobson L et al. Intrathecal methadone: a dose-response study and comparison with intrathecal morphine 0.5 mg. Pain 1990;43:141.

107. Krames ES. Intrathecal infusional therapies for intractable pain: patient management guidelines. J Pain Symptom Manage 1993;8:36.

108. Uhde TW et al. Clonidine suppresses the opioid abstinence syndrome without clonidine-withdrawal symptoms: a blind inpatient study. Psychiatry Res 1980;2:37.

109. Hoder EL et al. Clonidine treatment of neonatal abstinence syndrome. Psychiatry Res 1984;13:243.

110. Fantozzi R et al. Clonidine and naloxone-induced opiate withdrawal: a comparison between clonidine and morphine in man. Subst Alcohol Actions Misuse 1980;1:369.

111. Bond WS. Psychiatric indications for clonidine: the neuropharmacologic and clinical basis. J Clin Psychopharmacol 1986;6:81.

112. Gold MS et al. Opiate withdrawal using clonidine. A safe, effective and rapid non-opiate treatment. JAMA 1980;243:343.

113. Cami J et al. Efficacy of clonidine and methadone in the rapid detoxification of patients dependent on heroin. Clin Pharmacol Ther 1985;38:336.

114. Charney DS et al. The clinical use of clonidine in abrupt withdrawal from methadone. Arch Gen Psychiatry 1982;38:1273.

115. MacGregor TR et al. Pharmacokinetics of transdermally delivered clonidine. Clin Pharmacol Ther 1985;38:278.

116. Arndts D, Arndts K. Pharmacokinetics and pharmacodynamics of transdermally administered clonidine. Eur J Clin Pharmacol 1984;26:78.

117. Clark HW, Longmuir N. Clonidine transdermal patches: a recovery oriented treatment of opiate withdrawal. Calif Society Treat Alcohol Other Drug Depend News 1986;13:1.

118. Kanto J, Erkkola R. Obstetric analgesia: pharmacokinetics and its relation to neonatal behavioral and adaptive functions. Biol Res Pregnancy Perinatol 1984;5:23.

119. Barrier G, Sureau C. Effects of anaesthetic and analgesic drugs on mother, fetus and neonate. Clin Obstet Gynaecol 1982;9:351.

120. Nation RL. Drug kinetics in childbirth. Clin Pharmacokinet 1980;5:340.

121. Mirkin BL. Perinatal pharmacology: placental transfer, fetal localization, and neonatal disposition of drugs. Anesthesiology 1975;43:156.

122. McIntosh DG, Rayburn WF. Patient-controlled analgesia in obstetrics and gynecology. Obstet Gynecol 1991;78:1129.

123. Jepson HA et al. The Apgar score: evolution, limitations, and scoring guidelines. Birth 1991;18:83.

124. Bardy AH et al. Objectively measured perinatal exposure to meperidine and benzodiazepines in Finland. Clin Pharmacol Ther 1994;55:471.

125. Nimmo WS et al. Narcotic analgesics and delayed gastric emptying during labour. Lancet 1975;1(7912):890.

126. Refstad SO et al. Ventilatory depressions of the newborn of women receiving pethidine or pentazocine. Br J Anaesth 1980;52:265.

127. Atkinson BD et al. Double-blind comparison of intravenous butorphanol (Stadol) and fentanyl (Sublimaze) for analgesia during labor. Am J Obstet Gynecol 1994;171:993.

128. Isenor L, Penny-MacGillivray T. Intravenous meperidine infusion for obstetric analgesia. J Obstet Gynecol Neonatal Nurs 1993;22:349.

129. Thorp JA et al. The effect of intrapartum epidural analgesia on nulliparous labor: a randomized, controlled, prospective trial. Am J Obstet Gynecol 1993;169:851.

130. Rosaeg OP et al. Maternal and fetal effects of intravenous patient-controlled fentanyl analgesia during labour in a thrombocytopenic patient. Can J Anaesth 1992;39:277.

131. Galloway FM et al. Comparison of analgesia by intravenous butorphanol and meperidine in patients with post-operative pain. Can Anaesth Soc J 1977;24:90.

132. Ameer B, Salter FJ. Drug therapy reviews: evaluation of butorphanol tartrate. Am J Hosp Pharm 1979;36:1683.

133. Sprigge JS, Otton PE. Nalbuphine versus meperidine for post-operative analgesia: a double-blind comparison using the patient controlled analgesic technique. Can Anaesth Soc J 1983;30:517.

134. Pallasch TJ, Gill CJ. Butorphanol and nalbuphine: a pharmacologic comparison. Oral Surg Oral Med Oral Pathol 1985;59:15.

135. Young RE. Double-blind placebo controlled oral analgesic comparison of butorphanol and pentazocine in patients with moderate to severe post-operative pain. J Int Med Res 1977;5:422.

136. Dayer P et al. The pharmacology of tramadol. Drugs 1994;47(Suppl 1):3.

137. Lee CR et al. Tramadol: a preliminary review of its pharmacodynamic and pharmacokinetic properties, and therapeutic potential in acute and chronic pain states. Drugs 1993;46:313.

138. Stubhaug A et al. Lack of analgesic effect of 50 and 100 mg oral tramadol after orthopaedic surgery: a randomized, double-blind, placebo and standard active drug comparison. Pain 1995;62(1):111.

139. Turturro MA et al. Tramadol versus hydrocodone-acetaminophen in acute musculoskeletal pain: a randomized, double-blind clinical trial. Ann Emerg Med 1998;32:139.

140. Moore PA et al. Tramadol hydrochloride: analgesic efficacy compared with codeine, aspirin with codeine, and placebo after dental extraction. J Clin Pharmacol 1998;38:554.

141. Ortho-McNeil Pharmaceuticals, Inc. Ultram package insert. Raritan, NJ: 1998 April.

142. Spiller HA et al. Prospective multicenter evaluation of tramadol exposure. J Toxicol 1997;35(4):361.

143. Tobias JD. Seizures after tramadol overdose. S Med J 1997;90(8):826.

144. Portenoy RK et al. Transdermal fentanyl for cancer pain. Repeated dose pharmacokinetics. Anesthesiology 1993;78:36.

145. Zech DF et al. Transdermal fentanyl and initial dose-finding with patient-controlled analgesia in cancer pain. A pilot study with 20 terminally ill cancer patients. Pain 1992;50:293.

146. Payne R. Transdermal fentanyl: suggested recommendations for clinical use. J Pain Symptom Manage 1992;7(3 Suppl):S40.

147. Calis KA et al. Transdermally administered fentanyl for pain management. Clin Pharm 1992;11:22.

148. Rose PG et al. Fentanyl transdermal system overdose secondary to cutaneous hyperthermia. Anesth Analg 1993;77:390.

149. DeSio JM et al. Intravenous abuse of transdermal fentanyl therapy in a chronic pain patient. Anesthesiology 1993;79:1139.

150. Cohen FL. Postsurgical pain relief: patients' status and nurses' medication choices. Pain 1980;9:265.

151. Whipple JK et al. Analysis of pain management in critically ill patients. Pharmacotherapy 1995;15(5):592.

152. Brunier G et al. What do nurses know and believe about patients with pain? Results of a hospital survey. J Pain Symptom Manage 1995;10(6):436.

153. Westerling D et al. Absorption and bioavailability of rectally administered morphine in women. Eur J Clin Pharmacol 1982;23:59.

154. Westerling D. Rectally administered morphine: plasma concentration in children premedicated with morphine in hydrogel and in solution. Acta Anaesthesiol Scand 1985;29:653.

155. Babul N et al. Pharmacokinetics of two novel rectal controlled-release morphine formulations. J Pain Symptom Manage 1992;7:400.

156. Kaiko RF et al. The bioavailability of morphine in controlled-release 30-mg tablets per rectum com-

pared with immediate-release 30-mg rectal suppositories and controlled-release 30-mg oral tablets. Pharmacother 1992;12:107.

157. Babul N, Darke AC. Disposition of morphine and its glucuronide metabolites after oral and rectal administration: evidence of route specificity. Clin Pharmacol Ther 1993;54:286.

158. Wilkinson TJ et al. Pharmacokinetics and efficacy of rectal versus oral sustained-release morphine in cancer patients. Cancer Chemother Pharmacol 1992;31:251.

159. Feinmann C. Pain relief by antidepressants: possible modes of action. Pain 1985;23:1.

160. Kocher R. The use of psychotropic drugs in the treatment of chronic, severe pain. Eur Neurol 1976;14:458.

161. Ward NG et al. The effectiveness of tricyclic antidepressants in the treatment of coexisting pain and depression. Pain 1979;7:331.

162. Morland TJ et al. Doxepin in the prophylactic treatment of mixed 'vascular' and tension headache. Headache 1979;19:382.

163. Adler RH. Psychotropic agents in the management of chronic pain. J Human Stress 1978;4:15.

164. Urban BJ et al. Long-term use of narcotic/antidepressant medication in the management of phantom limb pain. Pain 1986;24:191.

165. Fainsinger R et al. Methadone in the management of cancer pain: a review. Pain 1993;52:137.

166. Fainsinger R et al. Methadone in the management of cancer pain: a review. Pain 1993;52:137.

167. Berkowitz BA. The relationship of pharmacokinetics to pharmacological activity: morphine, methadone and naloxone. Clin Pharmacokinet 1976;1:219.

168. Symonds P. Methadone and the elderly. Br Med J 1977;1:512.

169. Goulay GK et al. A comparative study of the efficacy and pharmacokinetics of oral methadone and morphine in the treatment of severe pain in patients with cancer. Pain 1986;25:297.

170. Miser AW et al. Continuous intravenous infusion of morphine sulfate for control of severe pain in children with terminal malignancy. J Pediatr 1980;96:930.

171. Bryan-Brown CW et al. Decremental morphine infusion for postoperative pain. Crit Care Med 1980;8:233.

172. Church JJ. Continuous narcotic infusions for relief of postoperative pain. Br Med J 1979;1:977.

173. Weintraub M. Potentiation of narcotic analgesics with central stimulant: the use of modified Brompton's mixture. Clin Pharmacol Reports 1976;5:9.

174. Davis AJ. Brompton's cocktail: making goodbyes possible. Am J Nurs 1978;78:611.

175. Melzack R et al. The Brompton mixture: effects on pain in cancer patients. Can Med Assoc J 1976;155:125.

176. Melzack R et al. The Brompton solution versus morphine solution given orally: effects on pain. Can Med Assoc J 1979;120:435.

177. Twycross RG. The Brompton cocktail. Adv Pain Res Ther 1979;2:291.

178. Hupert C et al. Effect of hydroxyzine on morphine analgesia for the treatment of postoperative pain. Anesth Analg 1980;59:690.

179. Stambaugh JE Jr, Lane C. Analgesic efficacy and pharmacokinetic evaluation of meperidine and hydroxyzine, alone and in combination. Cancer Invest 1983;1:111.

180. Rumore MM, Schlichting DA. Clinical efficacy of antihistaminics as analgesics. Pain 1986;25:7.

181. Rumore MM, Schlichting DA. Analgesic effects of antihistaminics. Life Sci 1985;36:403.

182. Campa JA 3rd, Payne R. The management of intractable bone pain: a clinician's perspective. Semin Nucl Med 1992;22:3.

183. Miller LJ, Kramer MA. Pain management with intravenous ketorolac. Ann Pharmacother 1993;27:307.

184. Terman GW, Loeser JD. A case of opiate-insensitive pain: malignant treatment of benign pain. Clin J Pain 1992;8:255.

185. Goldman B. Use and abuse of opioid analgesics in chronic pain. Can Fam Physician 1993;39:571.

186. Bowsher D. Pain syndromes and their treatment. Curr Opin Neurol Neurosurg 1993;6:257.

187. Mercadante S et al. Hyperalgesia: an emerging iatrogenic syndrome. J Pain Symptom Manage. 2003;26(2):769.

188. Sjogren P et al. Hyperalgesia and myoclonus in terminal cancer patients treated with continuous intravenous morphine. Pain 1993;55(1):93.

189. Romac DR. Safety of prolonged, high-dose infusion of naloxone hydrochloride for severe methadone overdose. Clin Pharm 1986;5:251.

190. Lewis JM et al. Continuous naloxone infusion in pediatric narcotic overdose. Am J Dis Child 1984;138:944.

191. Wang DS et al. Nalmefene: a long-acting opioid antagonist. Clinical implications in emergency medicine. J Emerg Med 1998;16(3):471.

192. Kaplan JL et al. Double-blind, randomized study of nalmefene and naloxone in emergency department patients with suspected narcotic overdose. Ann Emerg Med 1999;34(1):42.

193. Quan DB et al. Clonidine in pain management. Ann Pharmacother 1993;27:313.

194. Sullivan MJ et al. The treatment of depression in chronic low back pain: review and recommendations. Pain 1992;50:5.

195. Herr KA et al. Depression and the experience of chronic back pain: a study of related variables and age differences. Clin J Pain 1993;9:104.

196. Gonzales GR. Postherpes simplex type 1 neuralgia simulating postherpetic neuralgia. J Pain Symptom Manage 1992;7:320.

197. Max MB et al. Effects of desipramine, amitriptyline, and fluoxetine on pain in diabetic neuropathy. N Engl J Med 1992;326:1250.

198. Penfold J, Clark AJ. Pain syndromes in HIV infection. Can J Anaesth 1992;39:724.

199. Kerrick JM et al. Low-dose amitriptyline as an adjunct to opioids for postoperative orthopedic pain: a placebo-controlled trial. Pain 1993;52:325.

200. Dillin W, Uppal GS. Analysis of medications used in the treatment of cervical disk degeneration. Orthop Clin N Am 1992;23:421.

201. Richardson PH et al. Meta-analysis of antidepressant induced analgesia in chronic pain [Letter]. Pain 1993;52:247.

202. McQuay HJ et al. Dose-response for analgesic effect of amitriptyline in chronic pain. Anaesthesia 1993;48:281.

203. Onghena P, Van Houdenhove B. Antidepressant-induced analgesia in chronic non-malignant pain: a meta-analysis of 39 placebo-controlled studies. Pain 1992;49:205.

204. Max MB et al. Effects of desipramine, amitriptyline, and fluoxetine on pain in diabetic neuropathy. N Engl J Med 1992;326:1250.

205. Acton J et al. Amitriptyline produces analgesia in the formalin pain test. Exp Neurol 1992;117:94.

206. Magni G. The use of antidepressants in the treatment of chronic pain. A review of the current evidence. Drugs 1991;42:730.

207. Sullivan MJ et al. The treatment of depression in chronic low back pain: review and recommendations. Pain 1992;50:5.

208. Max MB et al. Effects of desipramine, amitriptyline, and fluoxetine on pain in diabetic neuropathy. N Engl J Med 1992;326:1250.

209. Panerai AE et al. Antidepressants in cancer pain. J Palliat Care 1991;7:42.

210. Conn DK, Goldman Z. Pattern of use of antidepressants in long-term care facilities for the elderly. J Geriatr Psychiatry Neurol 1992;5:228.

211. Backonja M et al. Gabapentin for the symptomatic treatment of painful neuropathy in patients with diabetes mellitus. JAMA 1998;280:1831.

212. Rowbotham M et al. Gabapentin for the treatment of postherpetic neuralgia: a randomized controlled trial. JAMA 1998;280:1837.

213. Tanelian DL, Brose WG. Neuropathic pain can be relieved by drugs that are use-dependent sodium channel blockers: lidocaine, carbamazepine, and mexiletine. Anesthesiology 1991;74:949.

214. Welch SP, Dunlow LD. Antinociceptive activity of intrathecally administered potassium channel openers and opioid agonists: a common mechanism of action? J Pharmacol Exp Ther 1993;267:390.

215. Pfeifer MA et al. A highly successful and novel model for treatment of chronic painful diabetic peripheral neuropathy. Diabetes Care 1993;16:1103.

216. Stracke H et al. Mexiletine in the treatment of diabetic neuropathy. Diabetes Care 1992;15:1550.

217. Chabal C et al. The use of oral mexiletine for the treatment of pain after peripheral nerve injury. Anesthesiology 1992;76:513.

218. Awerbuch GI, Sandyk R. Mexiletine for thalamic pain syndrome. Int J Neurosci 1990;55:129.

219. Davis RW. Successful treatment for phantom pain. Orthopedics 1993;16:691.

220. Hord AH et al. Intravenous regional bretylium and lidocaine for treatment of reflex sympathetic dystrophy: a randomized, double-blind study. Anesth Analg 1992;74:818.

221. Smith AL, Wollman H. Cerebral blood flow and metabolism: effects of anesthetic drugs and techniques. Anesthesiology 1972;36:378.

222. Sperry RJ et al. Fentanyl and sufentanil increase intracranial pressure in head trauma patients. Anesthesiology 1992;77:416.

223. Albanese J et al. Sufentanil increases intracranial pressure in patients with head trauma. Anesthesiology 1993;79:493.

224. Vandam LD. Drug therapy: butorphanol. N Engl J Med 1980;302:381.

225. Rosenfeldt FL et al. Haemodynamic effects of buprenorphine after heart surgery. Br Med J 1978;2:1602.

226. Scott DH et al. Haemodynamic changes following buprenorphine and morphine. Anaesthesia 1980;35:957.

227. Gaensler EA et al. A comparative study of the action of Demerol and opium alkaloids in relation to biliary spasm. Surgery 1948;23:211.

228. Levy MH. Pain management in advanced cancer. Semin Oncol 1985;12:394.

229. Radnay PA et al. The effect of equi-analgesic doses of fentanyl, morphine, piperidine and pentazocine on common bile duct pressure. Anaesthesist 1980;29:26.

230. Nossell HL. The effect of morphine on the serum and urine amylase and the sphincter of Oddi. Gastroenterology 1955;29:409.

231. Chisholm RJ et al. Narcotics and spasm of the sphincter of Oddi. A retrospective study of operative cholangiograms. Anaesthesia 1983;38:689.

232. Radnay PA et al. Common bile duct pressure changes after fentanyl, morphine, meperidine, butorphanol, and naloxone. Anesth Analg 1984;63:441.

233. Radnay PA et al. The effect of equi-analgesic doses of fentanyl, morphine, meperidine and pentazocine on common bile duct pressure. Anaesthesist 1980;29:26.

234. Staritz M et al. Effect of modern analgesic drugs (tramadol, pentazocine, and buprenorphine) on the bile duct sphincter in man. Gut 1986;27:567.

235. Economou G et al. A cross-over comparison of the effect of morphine, pethidine, pentazocine, and phenazocine on biliary pressure. Gut 1971;12:216.

236. Hopton DS et al. Action of various new analgesic drugs on the human common bile duct. Gut 1967;8:296.

237. McCammon RL et al. Reversal of fentanyl induced spasm of the sphincter of Oddi. Surg Gynecol Obstet 1983;156:329.

238. McCammon RL et al. Naloxone reversal of choledochoduodenal sphincter spasm associated with narcotic administration. Anesthesiology 1978;48:437.

239. Takahashi T et al. Pathogenesis of acute cholecystitis after gastrectomy. Br J Surg 1990;77:536.

240. Jones RM et al. Narcotic-induced choledochoduodenal sphincter spasm reversed by glucagon. Anesth Analg 1980;59:946.

241. McLean ER Jr et al. Cholangiographic demonstration of relief of narcotic-induced spasm of the sphincter of Oddi. Am Surg 1982;48:134.

242. Larsen LS et al. The use of intravenous ketorolac for the treatment of renal colic in the emergency department. Am J Emerg Med 1993;11:197.

243. Hoyampa AM Jr et al. The disposition and effects of sedatives and analgesics in liver disease. Ann Rev Med 1978;29:205.

244. Klotz U et al. The effect of cirrhosis on the disposition and elimination of meperidine in man. Clin Pharmacol Ther 1974;16:667.

245. McHorse TS et al. Effect of acute viral hepatitis in man on the disposition and elimination of meperidine. Gastroenterology 1975;68:775.

246. Neal EA et al. Enhanced bioavailability and decreased clearance of analgesics in patients with cirrhosis. Gastroenterology 1979;77:96.

247. Pond SM et al. Bioavailability and clearance of meperidine in patients with chronic liver disease. Clin Pharmacol Ther 1979;25:242.

248. Barre J et al. Disease-induced modifications of drug pharmacokinetics. Int J Clin Pharmacol Res 1983;3:215.

249. Roberts RK et al. Drug prescribing in hepatobiliary disease. Drugs 1979;17:198.

250. Pond SM et al. Enhanced bioavailability of pethidine and pentazocine in patients with cirrhosis of the liver. Aust NZ J Med 1980;10:515.

251. Lehmann KA et al. CO_2-response curves as a measure of opiate-induced respiratory depression. Studies with fentanyl. Anaesthesist 1983;32:242.

252. Gal TJ et al. Analgesic and respiratory depressant activity of nalbuphine: a comparison with morphine. Anesthesiology 1982;57:367.

253. Harcus AW et al. Buprenorphine: experience in an elderly population of 975 patients during a year's monitored release. Br J Clin Pract 1980;34:144.

254. Nagashima H et al. Respiratory and circulatory effects of intravenous butorphanol and morphine. Clin Pharmacol Ther 1976;19:738.

255. Heel RC et al. Buprenorphine: a review of its pharmacological properties and therapeutic efficacy. Drugs 1979;17:81.

256. Bailey CJ et al. Epidural morphine infusion. Continuous pain relief. AORN J 1984;39:997.

257. Staren ED, Cullen ML. Epidural catheter analgesia for the management of postoperative pain. Surg Gynecol Obstet 1986;162:389.

258. Jones SF, White A. Analgesia following femoral neck surgery. Lateral cutaneous nerve block as an alternative to narcotics in the elderly. Anaesthesia 1985;40:682.

259. American Geriatrics Society Panel on Chronic Pain in Older Persons. Clinical practice guidelines: the management of chronic pain in older persons. J Am Geriatr Soc 1998;46:635.

260. Won A et al. Correlates and management of nonmalignant pain in the nursing home. J Am Geriatr Soc 1999;47:936.

261. Fox PL et al. Prevalence and treatment of pain in older adults in nursing homes and other long-term care institutions: a systematic review. Can Med Assoc J 1999;160(3):329.

262. Faherty BS, Grier MR. Analgesic medication for elderly people post-surgery. Nurs Res 1984;33:369.

263. Wall RT 3rd. Use of analgesics in the elderly. Clin Geriatr Med 1990;6:345.

264. Gerbino PP. Complications of alcohol use combined with drug therapy in the elderly. J Am Geriatr Soc 1982;30(11 Suppl):S88.

265. Sengstaken EA, King SA. The problems of pain and its detection among geriatric nursing home residents. J Am Geriatr Soc 1993;41:541.

266. Cohen JL. Pharmacokinetic changes in aging. Am J Med 1986;80:31.

267. Ouslander JG. Drug therapy in the elderly. Ann Intern Med 1981;95:711.

268. McCaffery M. Narcotic analgesia for the elderly. Am J Nurs 1985;85:296.

269. Harkins SW et al. Pain and the elderly. Adv Pain Res Ther 1984;7:103.

270. Beyer JE et al. The assessment of pain in children. Pediatr Clin N Am 1989;36(4):837.

271. LaFleur CJ et al. School-age child and adolescent perception of the pain intensity associated with three word descriptors. Pediatr Nurs 1999;25:45.

272. Anand KJS et al. Halothane-morphine compared with high-dose sufentanil for anesthesia and postoperative analgesia in neonatal cardiac surgery. N Engl J Med 1992;326:1.

273. Olkkola KT et al. Kinetics and dynamics of postoperative intravenous morphine in children. Clin Pharmacol Ther 1988;44:128.

274. Gutner LB et al. The effects of potent analgesics upon vestibular function. J Clin Invest 1952;31:259.

275. Dixon R et al. Levorphanol: pharmacokinetics and steady-state plasma concentrations in patients with pain. Res Commun Chem Pathol Pharmacol 1983;41:3.

276. Forrest WH et al. Dextroamphetamine with morphine for the treatment of postoperative pain. N Engl J Med 1977;296:712.

277. Twycross RG et al. Long-term use of morphine in advanced cancer. Adv Pain Res Ther 1976;1:653.

278. Webb SS et al. Toward the development of a potent, nonsedating, oral analgesic. Psychopharmacol 1978;60:25.

279. Tong TG et al. Phenytoin-induced methadone withdrawal. Ann Intern Med 1981;94:349.

280. Bernard SA, Bruera E. Drug interactions in palliative care. J Clin Oncol 2000;18:1780.

281. Sorkin EM, Ogawa GS. Cimetidine potentiation of narcotic action. Drug Intell Clin Pharm 1983;17:60.

282. Poulsen L et al. The hypoalgesic effect of tramadol in relation to CYP2D6. Clin Pharmacol Ther 1996;60:636.

283. Egberts AC, et al. Serotonin syndrome attributed to tramadol addition to paroxetine therapy. Int Clin Psychopharmacol 1997;12:181.

284. Caufriez A. Menstrual disorders in adolescence: pathophysiology and treatment. Hormone Research 1991;36(3–4):156.

285. Mackinnon GL, Partker WA. Current concepts—the management of primary dysmenorrhea. Can Pharm J 1982;1150:3.

286. Mehlisch DR. Double-blind crossover comparison of ketoprofen, naproxen, and placebo in patients with primary dysmenorrhea. Clin Ther 1990;12(5):398.

287. Shapiro SS, Diem K. The effect of ibuprofen in the treatment of dysmenorrhea. Curr Ther Res Clin Exp 1981;30:327.

288. Laska E et al. Caffeine as an analgesic adjuvant. JAMA 1984;251:1711.

289. Migliardi J et al. Caffeine as an analgesic adjuvant in tension headache. Clin Pharmacal Ther 1994;56:576.

290. Harden RN et al. Ketorolac in acute headache management. Headache 1991;31:463.

291. Roberts JE et al. Improved peribulbar anaesthesia with alkalinization and hyaluronidase. Can J Anaesth 1993;40:835.

292. Lugo-Janer G et al. Less painful alternatives for local anesthesia. J Dermatol Surg Oncol 1993;19:237.

293. Benzon HT et al. Onset, intensity of blockade and somatosensory evoked potential changes of the lumbosacral dermatomes after epidural anesthesia with alkalinized lidocaine. Anesth Analg 1993;76:328.

294. Smith SL et al. The importance of bicarbonate in large volume anesthetic preparations. Revisiting the tumescent formula. J Dermatol Surg Oncol 1992;18:973.

295. Benini F et al. Topical anesthesia during circumcision in newborn infants. JAMA 1993;270:850.

296. Kaddour HS. Myringoplasty under local anaesthesia: day case surgery. Clin Otolaryngol 1992;17:567.

297. Holm J et al. Pain control in the surgical debridement of leg ulcers by the use of a topical lidocaine-prilocaine cream, EMLA. Acta Derm Venereol Suppl (Stockh) 1990;70:132.

298. Buckley MM, Benfield P. Eutectic lidocaine/prilocaine cream. A review of the topical anaesthetic/analgesic efficacy of a eutectic mixture of local anaesthetics (EMLA). Drugs 1993;46:126.

299. Young SS et al. EMLA cream as a topical anesthetic before office phlebotomy in children. South Med J 1996;89(12):1184.

300. Farrington E. Lidocaine 2.5%/prilocaine 2.5% EMLA cream. Pediatr Nurs 1993;19:484.

301. Gershon RY et al. Intradermal anesthesia and comparison of intravenous catheter gauge. Anesth Analg 1991;73:469.

CHAPTER 10

Perioperative Care

Andrew J. Donnelly, Julie A. Golembiewski

The operating room (OR) is one of the most medication-intensive settings in a hospital. During the perioperative period (broadly defined as the preoperative, intraoperative, and postoperative periods), a patient may receive many medications. Most of these medications are used primarily in the OR setting and have limited application elsewhere in the institution. For those medications employed elsewhere, their use in the OR often may differ from that seen in other patient care areas. Furthermore, the OR is unique in that a significant number of the medications are administered as single doses. To ensure continuity of care of the surgical patient, health care providers from all settings (e.g., acute care, home health care, extended care) should have a basic understanding of perioperative drug therapy.

This chapter reviews seven major classes of medications used during the perioperative period: preoperative medications, intravenous (IV) anesthetic agents, volatile inhalation agents, neuromuscular blocking agents, local anesthetics, antiemetic agents, and analgesic agents. Cardioplegia solution is also discussed. Because all health care providers are under pressure to reduce costs while maintaining or improving the quality of patient care, the chapter concludes with a discussion of economic considerations associated with the use of anesthesia-related medications.

PREOPERATIVE MEDICATIONS

Administration of preoperative medications (premedicants) to patients can be thought of as the start of their operative course. Many different medications are used preoperatively and can be grouped into the following classes: benzodiazepines, opioids, anticholinergics, dissociative anesthetics, gastric motility stimulants, H_2-receptor antagonists, antacids, and α_2-agonists.

A key point concerning preoperative medication is that not all patients will require premedicants. A preoperative visit by the anesthesia provider ensures that the patient is medically prepared for surgery, allows the provider to discuss the most appropriate anesthetic and postoperative pain management options with the patient, and helps reassure the patient, which can reduce the patient's anxiety.[1] Preoperative assessment by an anesthesia provider is considered an important component of the patient's preparation for surgery.[2] In fact, if the preoperative assessment occurs earlier (e.g., 1 to 2 weeks before surgery) in an outpatient consultation area, rather than the night before surgery, the patient's anxiety level will be more effectively lowered.[3] Patients should be assessed individually regarding their need for pharmacologic premedication; if required, premedicants should be selected based on patient-specific needs. Administration of a standard preoperative regimen to all patients should be avoided. Furthermore, the anesthesia provider and the surgeon must determine if the patient should take his or her regularly scheduled medications the morning of surgery. These medications are often necessary to maintain the patient's physiologic condition. Antihypertensives, bronchodilators, tricyclic antidepressants, selective serotonin reuptake inhibitors, corticosteroids, thyroid preparations, anxiolytics, and anticonvulsants generally are continued up to and including the morning of surgery. Alternatively, medications that increase the risk for bleeding (e.g., aspirin,

nonsteroidal anti-inflammatory drugs [NSAIDs], warfarin, clopidogrel) may need to be discontinued up to 7 days or more before surgery. Finally, patients with suppression of the pituitary-adrenal axis (e.g., patients currently or recently taking corticosteroids) may not be able to respond to surgical stress. Hydrocortisone can be administered intravenously before surgery, with subsequent doses dependent on the estimated amount of surgical stress and the need for supraphysiologic steroid replacement in the postoperative period.

Goals of Premedication

A major goal of premedication is to decrease the patient's fear and anxiety about his or her upcoming surgery. In addition to reducing anxiety, premedication is used for a variety of other reasons. Medications can be used before surgery to produce sedation, provide analgesia, produce amnesia, facilitate a smooth anesthetic induction, reduce anesthetic requirements, prevent autonomic responses resulting in intraoperative hemodynamic stability, decrease salivation and secretions, reduce gastric fluid volume, increase gastric pH, and/or prevent or minimize allergic reactions.[4] Table 10-1 lists medications commonly used preoperatively and their major indications, routes of administration, and dosages.[4-8] Benzodiazepines have largely replaced barbiturates as premedicants. Midazolam is by far the most common sedative premedicant, followed by diazepam and lorazepam for adults and ketamine for children.[9]

Selection Criteria

Factors to consider when selecting a preoperative drug for a patient include his or her American Society of Anesthesiologists (ASA) physical status class, medical conditions, degree of anxiety, age, surgical procedure to be performed, length of procedure, postoperative admission status (e.g., inpatient versus outpatient), drug allergies, previous experience with medications, and concurrent drug therapy. The ASA physical status classification system classifies patients as I through V. ASA-I patients are healthy with little medical risk, whereas ASA-V patients have little chance of survival. Severe systemic disorders (e.g., uncontrolled diabetes mellitus, coronary artery disease) are present in ASA-III through ASA-V patients. Selection of preoperative medications in this group of patients will be more difficult. These patients generally have limited physiologic reserve; administration of a cardiovascular depressant agent, for example, may be harmful. Furthermore, these patients will be taking a significant number of medications; hence, chances for drug interactions are increased. The patient's other medical conditions are important to consider to prevent the administration of contraindicated medications. For example, the benzodiazepines are contraindicated in pregnancy.[6] A patient's age will play a role in the response seen with premedicant administration. The elderly often are more sensitive to preoperative opioids and benzodiazepines as well as the central nervous system (CNS) effects of anticholinergic agents.[10]

Familiarity with the surgery to be performed will aid in selecting appropriate premedicants. In surgical cases in which painful procedures (e.g., line insertion) will be performed on the patient, an analgesic premedicant may be warranted. The length and type of the procedure is important to consider

Table 10-1   Indications, Routes of Administration, and Doses of Preoperative Agents[a]

Agent	Indications	Routes of Administration	Doses[b]
Benzodiazepines			
Diazepam (Valium)	Anxiolysis, amnesia, sedation	PO	*Adults:* 5–10 mg
		IV	*Adults:* 2–10 mg (titrate dose)
Lorazepam (Ativan)	Anxiolysis, amnesia, sedation	PO	0.025–0.05 mg/kg (range, 1–4 mg for adults)
		IV	*Adults:* 0.025–0.04 mg/kg; *pediatrics:* 0.01–0.05 mg/kg (titrate dose)
Midazolam (Versed)	Anxiolysis, amnesia, sedation	PO	*Adults:* 20 mg; *pediatrics:* 0.5–0.75 mg/kg (max 20 mg)
		IM	*Adults:* 0.05–0.15 mg/kg (max 10 mg); *pediatrics:* 0.08–0.3 mg/kg (max 10 mg)
		IV	*Adults:* 1–2.5 mg (titrate dose); *pediatrics:* 0.025–0.1 mg/kg (titrate dose; max 10 mg)
		IN	*Pediatrics:* 0.2 mg/kg (max 15 mg)
Opioids			
Morphine	Analgesia, sedation	IM	*Adults:* 2–10 mg; *pediatrics:* 0.05–0.1 mg/kg
		IV	Titrate dose
Fentanyl (Sublimaze)	Analgesia, sedation	IV	*Adults:* 1–2 µg/kg (titrate dose)
Anticholinergics			
Atropine (A)	Antisialagogue (S > G > A), sedation (S > A)	IM/IV	*Adults:* 0.4–0.6 mg; *pediatrics:* 0.02 mg/kg IM, 0.01 mg/kg IV
Scopolamine (S)	Sedation, amnesia, antisialagogue	IM/IV	*Adults:* 0.2–0.4 mg; *pediatrics:* 0.02 mg/kg IM, 0.01 mg/kg IV
Glycopyrrolate (G) (Robinul)	Antisialagogue	IM/IV	*Adults:* 0.2–0.3 mg; *pediatrics:* 0.005–0.01 mg/kg
Dissociative Anesthetics			
Ketamine (Ketalar)[c]	Sedation, amnesia, analgesia	PO	*Pediatrics:* 6 mg/kg
		IM	*Adults:* 3–4 mg/kg; *pediatrics:* 3–4 mg/kg
		IV	*Adults:* 0.5–1 mg/kg
Gastric Motility Stimulants			
Metoclopramide (Reglan)	Reduce gastric volume, antiemetic	PO	*Adults:* 10 mg; *pediatrics:* 0.15 mg/kg
		IV	*Adults:* 0.1–0.2 mg/kg (10–20 mg); *pediatrics:* 0.1–0.15 mg/kg
H$_2$-Receptor Antagonists			
Cimetidine (Tagamet)	↑ gastric pH	PO	*Adults:* 300 mg; *pediatrics:* 7.5 mg/kg
		IV	*Adults:* 300 mg; *pediatrics:* 7.5 mg/kg
Ranitidine (Zantac)	↑ gastric pH	PO	*Adults:* 150 mg; *pediatrics:* 2 mg/kg
		IV	*Adults:* 50 mg; *pediatrics:* 0.5–1 mg/kg
Famotidine (Pepcid)	↑ gastric pH	PO	*Adults:* 40 mg; *pediatrics:* 0.5 mg/kg
		IV	*Adults:* 20 mg; *pediatrics:* 0.25 mg/kg
Nizatidine (Axid)	↑ gastric pH	PO	*Adults:* 150 mg
Nonparticulate Antacids			
Sodium citrate/citric acid (Bicitra)	↑ gastric pH	PO	*Adults:* 30 mL
α$_2$-Agonists			
Clonidine (Catapres)	Anxiolysis, potentiate action of anesthetic agents, sedation, analgesia	PO	*Adults:* 0.2 mg

[a]General dosage guidelines; doses must be individualized based on patient-specific parameters.
[b]Doses listed are for agents when used as sole premedicant; doses may need to be reduced if premedicants are administered in combination (e.g., opioids, benzodiazepines).
[c]The duration and depth of sedation from ketamine is determined by the dose and route of administration. Low dosages (0.025 to 0.075 mg/kg IV or 2 to 3 mg/kg IM) should produce light sedation for a short period. Higher dosages will produce deep sedation to the point of general anesthesia. In addition, airway reflexes are depressed, increasing the patient's risk for aspiration. An anesthesia care provider should be present and resuscitative/suction equipment should be readily available.
IM, intramuscular; IN, intranasal; IV, intravenous; PO, oral.
Adapted from references 4–8.

when selecting premedicants. For example, a patient undergoing emergency surgery who has not fasted is often administered a nonparticulate antacid because they are at risk for aspiration of gastric contents.[4] Likewise, in short-duration, outpatient surgery, agents with a long duration of action should be avoided because residual effects may prolong discharge time. Certain agents should not be administered to patients because of drug allergies. However, it is important to differentiate between true allergies and adverse reactions resulting from administration of premedicants. Patients often state allergies to opioids, for example, after having experienced nausea and vomiting, which are common adverse reactions of these agents. A patient's previous experience with premedicants can assist in agent selection. If an agent has caused trouble in the past, it should be avoided. Finally, it is important to review the patient's current drug therapy before selecting an agent to prevent potentially harmful drug interactions.

Timing and Routes of Administration

Almost as important as the choice of the agent is its timing and route of administration. For optimal results, the agent's peak effects should occur before the patient arrives in the OR suite. This will require the agent to be administered at varying times before surgery depending on the route of administration. Preoperative agents are administered by several routes: IV, intramuscular (IM), oral (PO), and intranasal (IN). As a general rule, agents administered by the IV route produce the fastest onset of action and often are given after the patient arrives in the OR, whereas medications administered via the IM route usually are administered 30 to 60 minutes before the patient arrives in the OR. If possible, the IM route should be avoided as it is painful and undesirable for the patient. Onset of peak effect is the slowest with PO administration of agents, which should be administered 60 to 90 minutes before the patient's scheduled arrival in the OR.[4]

Drug Interactions

Preoperative medications can interact with one another as well as with drugs the patient is receiving currently or will receive in the OR. These drug interactions may be advantageous and intentionally produced, or they may be problematic. For example, patients must be closely monitored when they concurrently receive a benzodiazepine and an opioid for premedication due to synergistic respiratory and cardiovascular adverse effects.[4] The α_2-agonists, on the other hand, can reduce the requirements for inhalational anesthetics and opioids.[7]

Administration of a Premedicant

1. D.W., a 21-year-old man, is scheduled to undergo a laparoscopic hernia repair on an outpatient basis under general anesthesia. This is the first time D.W. has undergone surgery and he is highly anxious in the preoperative area. Should D.W. receive premedication and, if so, what medication(s) should be administered?

The administration of a preoperative sedative to a patient undergoing outpatient surgery is controversial. However, with midazolam, the delayed recovery and discharge that had been associated with agents used in the past (e.g., lorazepam, triazolam, and temazepam) is less of a concern. Midazolam should be titrated to the desired effect (in increments of 0.5 to 1 mg), with the average adult generally requiring 2 mg. Elderly patients who receive as little as 0.5 mg midazolam intravenously can experience decreased oxygen saturation in the preoperative period as well as prolonged postanesthesia care unit (PACU) stays following surgery of a short duration.[11] Midazolam premedication produces sedation and provides anterograde amnesia and anxiolysis,[11,12] which can be problematic if these effects continue into the postoperative period when outpatients are provided with discharge instructions. Regarding children, premedication with oral midazolam can reduce both the child and the parents' anxiety during the preoperative period,[12] the likelihood of a child's distress at induction of anesthesia,[13] and the manifestation of negative behavioral changes in the child during the first 7 postoperative days.[14] However, the use of oral midazolam premedication in children who are undergoing outpatient surgery can result in delayed discharge.[13] Therefore, nonpharmacologic approaches to reduce anxiety must be optimized. If explanation of upcoming events and reassurance by the anesthesia provider have not sufficiently allayed D.W.'s anxiety, small titrated doses of IV midazolam may be administered.

Aspiration Pneumonitis Prophylaxis

Definition

Aspiration pneumonitis, although uncommon, is a potentially fatal condition that occurs as a result of regurgitation and aspiration of gastric contents. Aspiration of undigested or semi-digested gastric contents into the respiratory tract can cause obstruction and an inflammatory response. An acute chemical pneumonitis can result from aspiration of acidic gastric secretions resulting in damage to the alveolar and capillary endothelium with progression to adult respiratory distress syndrome.[15] The acidity and volume of the gastric contents appear to influence the morbidity seen if aspiration occurs. Historically, a gastric pH of ≤ 2.5 and a gastric volume >25 mL (0.4 mL/kg) have been accepted as the cutoff values that place the patient at greater risk for severe pneumonitis should aspiration occur. However, it has been suggested that these values be changed to a gastric pH <3.5 and gastric volume >50 mL, with pH appearing to be a greater determinant of morbidity than volume.[16]

Risk Factors

Patients at risk for regurgitation and aspiration include those who have had previous surgery on the upper gastrointestinal (GI) tract, those who are under stress, those who are in pain, and those with an abnormal airway. Pregnant patients, obese patients, and trauma patients, as well as patients with a hiatal hernia, gastroesophageal reflux, esophageal motility disorders, hyperchlorhydria, peptic ulcer disease, or diabetes mellitus, are also at risk.[17–19] In addition to having delayed gastric emptying, obese patients often will present with increased abdominal pressure and an abnormal airway; both factors predispose these individuals to aspiration. Hormonal changes in pregnant patients account for delayed gastric emptying as well as relaxation of the lower esophageal sphincter. An increase in intra-abdominal pressure also is seen in pregnant patients.

Labor may increase gastrin levels, increasing gastric volume and acidity as well as delaying gastric emptying. Patients undergoing emergency surgery frequently have full stomachs because they have not had time to fast appropriately. Administration of drugs may delay gastric emptying (e.g., opioids) or decrease lower esophageal sphincter pressure (e.g., anticholinergics, thiopental, benzodiazepines, calcium channel blockers).[18]

Although pharmacologic prophylaxis is considered prudent in patients at risk, no study has shown that administration of these agents is cost-effective or reduces morbidity or mortality in healthy patients undergoing elective surgery. Rapid sequence induction, effective application of cricoid pressure, maintaining a patent upper airway, avoiding inflation of the stomach with anesthetic gases, inserting a large-bore gastric tube once the airway has been secured, as well as the use of regional anesthesia when possible, are probably the most important measures the anesthesia provider can take to reduce the patient's risk of aspiration.[17,19]

Agents

Many medications are used to reduce the risk of pneumonitis should aspiration occur; they can be grouped into the following categories: antacids, gastric motility stimulants, and H$_2$-receptor antagonists. These agents, with the possible exception of metoclopramide, are relatively free of adverse effects and have a favorable risk-benefit profile.

ANTACIDS

Antacids are effective in raising gastric pH to >3.5.[4] They should be given as a single dose (30 mL) approximately 15 to 30 minutes before induction of anesthesia. Nonparticulate antacids (e.g., sodium citrate/citric acid [Bicitra]) are the agents of choice because the suspension particles in particulate antacids can act as foci for an inflammatory reaction if aspirated and increase the risk of pulmonary damage.[20] Antacids have two major advantages when used for aspiration pneumonitis prophylaxis: there is no "lag time" with regard to onset of activity, and antacids are effective on the fluid already in the stomach. Their major disadvantages are (1) a short-acting buffering effect that is not likely to last as long as the surgical procedure (sodium citrate must be administered no more than 1 hour before induction of anesthesia, with its duration possibly dependent on gastric emptying); (2) the potential for emesis (due to their lack of palatability); (3) the possibility of incomplete mixing in the stomach; and (4) their administration adds fluid volume to the stomach.[18,21,22]

GASTRIC MOTILITY STIMULANTS

The gastric motility stimulant metoclopramide (Reglan) has no effect on gastric pH or acid secretion. This agent is used to reduce gastric volume in predisposed patients (e.g., parturients, obese patients) by promoting gastric emptying. Preoperative metoclopramide increases lower esophageal sphincter pressure and reduces gastric volume.[6,23] Metoclopramide should be administered 60 minutes before induction of anesthesia when given orally; when given by the IV route, metoclopramide should be administered 15 to 30 minutes before induction of anesthesia. Variable effects have been seen with metoclopramide; gastric emptying is not always seen after its administration, especially when used with other agents. The concomitant administration of anticholinergics (e.g., glycopyrrolate, atropine) or prior administration of opioids, for example, can reduce lower esophageal sphincter pressure which can offset metoclopramide's effects on the upper GI tract.[24]

H$_2$-RECEPTOR ANTAGONISTS

H$_2$-receptor antagonists reduce gastric acidity and volume by inhibiting gastric secretion. Unlike antacids, the H$_2$-receptor antagonists do not produce immediate effects. Onset time for these agents when administered orally is 1 to 3 hours; good effects will be seen in 30 to 60 minutes when administered intravenously.[18,21] Oral doses of the H$_2$-receptor antagonists should not be crushed and given via a nasogastric tube at the time of surgery. As already mentioned, onset of action is not immediate. Furthermore, administration of tablets introduces particulate matter into the stomach, which can be detrimental if aspirated. Duration of action of H$_2$-receptor antagonists also is important, because the risk of aspiration pneumonitis extends through emergence from anesthesia. After IV administration, the cimetidine (Tagamet) dose should be repeated in 6 hours if necessary, whereas therapeutic concentrations of ranitidine (Zantac) and famotidine (Pepcid) persist for 8 and 12 hours, respectively.[6] Although cimetidine is associated with more adverse reactions than famotidine or ranitidine, this probably is not clinically significant because only one or two doses of the agent are given.[4]

PROTON PUMP INHIBITORS

Proton pump inhibitors (PPIs) (omeprazole, rabeprazole, lansoprazole, esomeprazole, and pantoprazole) are effective in suppressing gastric acid secretion. However, oral PPIs most effectively reduce gastric volume and increase gastric pH when a dose is administered the night before surgery and the morning of surgery. In addition, one dose of ranitidine is as efficacious as these two consecutive oral doses of a PPI.[24] Therefore, there is no need to use the more expensive oral PPIs in patients at risk for pulmonary aspiration. There also is no clinical rationale for the administration of an IV PPI for aspiration prophylaxis before surgery.

Choice of Agent

2. D.W., a 5'4", 95-kg, 38-year-old woman, ASA-II, is scheduled to undergo a laparoscopic cholecystectomy under general anesthesia. D.W. has type 2 diabetes. Physical examination is normal except for an abnormal airway, which is anticipated to complicate intubation. Her medications include glipizide and an antacid for dyspepsia. The procedure is scheduled as a same-day surgery. What factors predispose D.W. to aspiration and what premedication, if any, should D.W. receive for aspiration prophylaxis?

D.W. has several factors that place her at risk for aspiration. She is obese with an abnormal airway and has diabetes. She also reports symptoms of dyspepsia that are relieved by antacids. These conditions will predispose D.W. to increased abdominal pressure, delayed gastric emptying, and increased risk of regurgitation. Her abnormal airway may delay intubation, increasing the amount of time D.W. is susceptible to aspiration. Therefore, aspiration prophylaxis with medications that buffer gastric acid and reduce gastric volume is prudent for D.W. Because D.W.'s surgery is scheduled as a same-day surgery, D.W. will arrive at the hospital or Surgicenter approximately 90 minutes before the start of surgery. Although oral agents, in general, are less expensive than their parenteral counterparts, cimetidine 300 mg (Tagamet), famotidine 40 mg (Pepcid), or ranitidine 150 mg (Zantac) should be administered approximately 1 to 2 hours before induction of anesthesia to effectively decrease gastric acidity. Hence, due to time constraints, cimetidine 300 mg, famotidine 20 mg, or ranitidine 50 mg should be administered intravenously 30 to 60 minutes before induction of anesthesia in D.W. Since obese and diabetic patients tend to have larger gastric fluid volumes secondary to delayed gastric emptying, metoclopramide 10 mg IV can be added to D.W.'s regimen to reduce her gastric volume. Finally, a nonparticulate antacid such as sodium citrate/citric acid solution (Bicitra) 30 mL orally may be administered to D.W. immediately before entering the OR rather than, or in addition to, an H_2-receptor antagonist.

3. C.T., a 28-year-old woman, ASA-I, is admitted for an emergency cesarean section under general anesthesia. She is otherwise healthy and currently taking no medications. Why is C.T. susceptible to aspiration pneumonitis and what preoperative medications would be appropriate to help prevent this adverse effect from occurring in C.T.?

C.T. is at an increased risk for aspiration and the possible development of pneumonitis because she is pregnant and about to undergo emergency surgery. An appropriate regimen for C.T. would be sodium citrate/citric acid solution (Bicitra) 30 mL orally, famotidine 20 mg intravenously (or whichever H_2-receptor antagonist is on the institution's formulary), and metoclopramide 10 mg intravenously. There is not sufficient time to administer famotidine and metoclopramide orally because of their slower onsets of action when administered by this route. Sodium citrate/citric acid solution provides immediate protection by raising gastric pH; metoclopramide will help reduce the increased gastric volume commonly seen in pregnant patients; and famotidine will provide sustained coverage throughout the surgery. These agents have not been shown to have detrimental effects on the fetus.[25]

INTRAVENOUS ANESTHETIC AGENTS

General Anesthesia

IV anesthetic agents commonly are used to induce general anesthesia. The general anesthetic state consists of the following components: unconsciousness, amnesia, analgesia, immobility, and attenuation of autonomic responses to noxious stimuli.[26] The induction of this state and subsequent endotracheal intubation can result in undesirable changes in cardiovascular dynamics, the magnitude of which can be affected by resting sympathetic tone and level of preoperative anxiety; preoperative ventilatory status; vascular volume; preexisting cardiovascular disease; chronic medications such as angiotensin-converting enzyme inhibitors and angiotensin-receptor antagonists; and premedicants such as opioids or benzodiazepines.

Anesthetic induction agents should produce unconsciousness rapidly and smoothly while minimizing any cardiovascular changes. A list of additional desirable, as well as undesirable, characteristics of an IV induction agent is found in Table 10-2. Although currently available IV induction agents possess many of the desirable characteristics, no agent lacks one or more of the undesirable effects. As mentioned, the administration of an IV induction agent is the most common method for initiation of general anesthesia and generally affords the highest patient acceptance and predictability of response over IM, inhalation, or rectal routes of drug administration.[27] Drugs commonly used for IV induction include ultrashort-acting barbiturates (thiopental, methohexital), etomidate, and propofol. The synthetic opioids (fentanyl, sufentanil, alfentanil, and remifentanil), benzodiazepines (primarily midazolam), and ketamine are less frequently used. The IV induction agents blunt the stress response to laryngoscopy and intubation; these perioperative events often result in maximal patient stimulation that is even greater than that seen with the initial surgical incision.[28] Propofol can also be used to maintain general anesthesia; drugs that do not accumulate during repeat or continuous dosing are ideal choices for maintenance therapy. When used at dosages lower than those necessary for unconsciousness, some of the IV anesthetic agents can be used to produce sedation for monitored anesthesia care or regional anesthesia or in the medical procedure units and intensive care units (ICUs). Table 10-3 lists common clinical uses for IV anesthetic agents.

Mechanisms of Action

Most IV anesthetic agents produce CNS depression by action on the gamma-aminobutyric acid (GABA)-benzodiazepine-chloride ion channel receptor. GABA is the principal inhibitory neurotransmitter in the CNS. The barbiturates bind to a receptor site on the GABA-receptor complex, reducing the rate of dissociation of GABA from its receptor. This results in increased chloride conductance through the ion channel, nerve cell hyperpolarization, and inhibition of nerve impulse transmission. At higher dosages, the barbiturates can directly activate the chloride channels, without the presence of GABA.[29,30] Benzodiazepines also bind to this GABA-receptor complex and their subsequent potentiation of the inhibitory action of GABA is well described.[31] The site of action of eto-

Table 10-2	Characteristics of an Intravenous Induction Agent	
Desirable Characteristics	*Undesirable Characteristics*
Water soluble	Histamine release
Stable in solution	Hypersensitivity reaction
Small volume required for dose	Local toxicity at injection site
	Pain on injection
Rapid, smooth onset of action	Adverse CNS effects
	Adverse cardiovascular effects
Predictable effect	Active metabolites
High therapeutic index	
Analgesic	
Amnestic	
Short duration to awakening	
Rapid full recovery	
Availability of reversal agent	

CNS, central nervous system.

Table 10-3 Common Clinical Uses of Intravenous Anesthetic Agents

Etomidate (Amidate)	**Midazolam (Versed)**
IV induction	Anxiolysis
Ketamine (Ketalar)[a]	Amnesia
Analgesia	Sedation
Sedation	**Propofol (Diprivan)**[a]
IV induction	Sedation
IM induction	IV induction
Methohexital (Brevital)[a]	Maintenance of general anesthesia
IV induction	**Thiopental**
Sedation	IV induction

[a]Dose-dependent effects; sedation at lower doses, anesthesia at higher doses.
IM, intramuscular; IV, intravenous.

midate (Amidate) and propofol (Diprivan) is thought to be at the GABA receptor, although the mechanisms by which they produce their effects are not fully elucidated. Ketamine (Ketalar) acts at a different site than other induction agents. It produces a dissociation between the cortex and thalamus within the limbic system, resulting in a dissociative state; the patient appears to be detached from his or her surroundings. Unlike anesthesia produced by other agents (e.g., thiopental for induction followed by isoflurane/nitrous oxide/oxygen for maintenance) where the patient's eyes are closed resembling normal sleep, a ketamine-anesthetized patient's eyes are often open and move from side to side. A patient receiving ketamine will have analgesia, amnesia, and often, lacrimation, salivation, and purposeless movements.[30] There is evidence that ketamine suppresses spinal cord-to-brain nerve transmission in specific cord lamina to reduce the emotional component of pain transmission, occupies opioid receptors in the brain and spinal cord, and is a noncompetitive antagonist of the N-methyl-d-aspartate (NMDA) receptor.[31,32] These actions of ketamine may be responsible for its analgesic and general anesthetic effects.[31]

Pharmacokinetics

The onset and duration of effect are the most important pharmacokinetic properties of IV anesthetic agents when used for induction of anesthesia. In general, the commonly used IV in-

duction agents have a rapid onset of action and short clinical duration, with the short clinical duration resulting from redistribution of the drug from the brain to other tissue sites. Using the barbiturates as an example, thiopental and methohexital undergo maximal brain uptake within 30 seconds of injection as a result of their high lipophilicity and high rate of blood flow to the brain. This is followed by a decline over the next 5 minutes to half of the initial peak brain concentration, predominately through drug redistribution. As a result, patients awaken in <10 minutes after a single induction dose of thiopental despite a half-life of approximately 11 hours.[30] The initial redistribution is most prominent in the skeletal muscle,[33] with equilibrium in this tissue reached within 15 minutes of injection. Fat concentrations slowly accumulate, continuing to rise 30 minutes after injection[33]; this slow initial uptake is due to relatively poor perfusion of adipose tissue. Because cumulative effects can be seen after repeat or continuous dosing of barbiturates due to fat deposition and storage, these drugs make poor choices for maintenance of general anesthesia. The degree to which metabolism plays a role in the clinical duration of IV induction agents is variable; rapid metabolism may be a significant factor in the relatively shorter duration to full recovery of propofol.[27] Table 10-4 provides a comparison of the pharmacokinetic properties of IV anesthetic agents.[29–31]

Adverse and Beneficial Effects

IV anesthetic agents can produce a variety of adverse and beneficial effects other than loss of consciousness. These effects include cardiovascular depression or stimulation, pain on injection, nausea and vomiting, respiratory depression or stimulation, CNS cerebroprotection or excitation, and adrenocorticoid suppression. Table 10-5 compares the relative significance of these effects among available agents.[29–31] Most troublesome are usually cardiovascular effects or CNS excitation reactions. Contribution to postoperative nausea and vomiting (PONV) and "hangover" can be significant and may delay full recovery and patient discharge from the PACU. This is particularly a concern in the ambulatory surgery setting because the patient will be discharged home. CNS effects can include hiccups, myoclonus, seizure activity, euphoria, hallucinations, and emergence delirium. The cerebroprotective effect produced by barbiturates, etomidate, and propofol results from a reduction in cerebral blood flow secondary to cerebral vasoconstriction. As a result, cerebral metabolic rate, cerebral

Table 10-4 Pharmacokinetic Comparison of Common Intravenous Anesthetic Agents

Drug	Half-Life (hr)	Onset (sec)	Clinical Duration (min)[a]	Hangover Effect[b]
Etomidate (Amidate)	2–5	≤30	3–12	+
Ketamine (Ketalar)	1–3	30–40	10–15	+ + − + + +[c]
Methohexital (Brevital)	4	≤30	4–8	+
Midazolam (Versed)	1–4	30–60	17–20	+ + +[d]
Propofol (Diprivan)	0.5–7	≤30	4–10	0 − +
Thiopental (Pentothal)	11	≤30	5–8	+ +

[a]Time from injection of agent to return to conscious state.
[b]Residual psychomotor impairment after awakening.
[c]When ketamine is administered as an induction agent (e.g., 5–10 mg/kg IM).
[d]When midazolam is administered as the induction agent (e.g., 0.15 mg/kg).
Adapted from references 29–31.

Table 10-5   Adverse Effects and Costs of IV Induction Agents

Adverse Effect	Etomidate (Amidate)	Ketamine (Ketalar)	Methohexital (Brevital)	Midazolam (Versed)	Propofol (Diprivan)	Thiopental (Pentothal)
Adrenocorticoid suppression	+[a]	−	−	−	−	−
Cerebral protection	+	−	+	+	+	+
Cardiovascular depression	−	−	++	+	++	++
Emergence delirium or euphoria	−	++	−	−	+	−
Myoclonus	+++	+	++	−	+	+
Nausea/vomiting	+++	++	++	+	−	++
Pain on injection	++	−	+	−	++	+
Respiratory depression	++	−	++	+/++	++	++
Relative cost	+++	++	+++	+	++++	+

[a]Not shown to be clinically significant in single dose.
+ to ++++, likelihood of adverse effect relative to other agents (or increasing cost for cost comparison); −, no effect; IV, intravenous.
Adapted from references 29–31.

blood flow, and intracranial pressure are reduced.[29–31] This effect is useful if these drugs are available in therapeutic concentrations at a time of potential cerebral ischemia. Thiopental, for example, has been given during deep hypothermic circulatory arrest to minimize the possibility of ischemic events.

Agent Selection

The selection of an IV anesthetic agent should be determined based on patient characteristics, circumstances associated with surgery, and cost. Patient characteristics may include history of PONV, allergy profile, psychiatric history, or cardiovascular status. Circumstances associated with surgery that may influence choice of IV anesthetic include the postoperative admission status (inpatient versus outpatient), placement of an IV line, duration of surgery, and extubation status at the end of the procedure. The cost of induction agents varies widely, with older agents usually priced lower per single induction dose. Newer agents, especially if used for maintenance of anesthesia, are more expensive but may offer cost advantages in some situations by reduction in length of PACU stay, fewer postoperative complications, and improved patient well-being. The multidisciplinary development of evidence-based guidelines has been promoted as a means to ensure the appropriate, cost-effective use of IV anesthetic agents. Most guidelines have specifically addressed propofol use. For example, one institution's guidelines allow for the routine use of propofol in outpatients for monitored anesthesia care or regional anesthesia with sedation; for inpatient monitored anesthesia care or regional anesthesia cases, propofol is indicated only if PONV is a major concern. For induction of anesthesia in outpatient procedures, propofol use is limited to cases expected to last <2 hours, because the associated antiemetic effect does not last beyond this time. For induction of anesthesia in same-day admissions, 23-hour patients, and inpatients, propofol is indicated in those cases expected to last <2 hours when there is a documented history of PONV or when the type of surgery predisposes the patient to PONV. For maintenance of outpatient general anesthesia, propofol use should be minimized.[34]

Propofol Use in Ambulatory Surgery: Antiemetic Effect and Full Recovery Characteristics

4. K.T., a 15-year-old girl, ASA-I, is admitted to the ambulatory surgery center for strabismus surgery to correct misalignment of her extraocular muscles. She is otherwise healthy, and all laboratory values obtained before surgery are within normal limits. The duration of K.T.'s surgery is anticipated to be approximately 90 minutes. Which IV induction agent should be used?

Propofol (Diprivan) is a good choice here for several reasons. Strabismus surgery is considered highly emetogenic because operative manipulation of extraocular muscles triggers the release of dopamine, serotonin, and acetylcholine in the chemoreceptor trigger zone (CTZ) through the oculoemetic reflex.[35] Therefore, precautions should be taken to reduce the possibility of nausea and vomiting postoperatively. Propofol produces the lowest incidence of PONV when compared with other IV induction agents and the volatile inhalation agents; it has even been associated with a direct antiemetic effect.[36] This effect may not preclude the need for prophylactic antiemetic therapy, but may contribute to the avoidance of emesis in K.T. Furthermore, ambulatory surgery demands rapid, full recovery from general anesthesia. Propofol, etomidate, and methohexital produce less hangover than other IV induction agents; propofol, especially, is associated with a more rapid recovery of psychomotor function and a patient-perceived superior quality of recovery.[31] Although thiopental certainly could be used for induction at a reduced direct cost than propofol, it is associated with a higher degree of hangover effect and a greater incidence of PONV. Propofol also offers advantages for maintenance of anesthesia in this case, and it does not accumulate when administered as a continuous infusion.

Etomidate Use in Cardiovascular Disease

5. L.M., a 73-year-old man, ASA-IV, is in need of repair of an abdominal aortic aneurysm. During a preoperative evaluation a few days before surgery, his blood pressure (BP) was 160/102 mm Hg, and his medical records revealed hypertension that was poorly controlled by hydrochlorothiazide 50 mg daily and propranolol LA (Inderal) 160 mg daily. He also has angina that occasionally requires treatment with SL nitroglycerin (NTG). An exercise stress test showed electrocardiogram (ECG) changes at a moderate exercise load. Two days before the elective aneurysm repair was scheduled, L.M. presented to the emergency department (ED) with a 4-hour history of severe back pain. His surgeon believes that there is a high likelihood that the aneurysm is leaking or expanding and schedules surgery immediately. What is the best plan for L.M.'s anesthetic induction and maintenance?

L.M. has significant cardiovascular disease, and care should be taken to minimize any cardiovascular depression, tachycardia, or hypertension during induction and maintenance of anesthesia. Of the currently available induction agents, etomidate has the most stable cardiovascular profile[31] and is associated with minimal cardiovascular depression. Opioids generally produce minimal cardiovascular effects and could potentially be used for induction. Thiopental, propofol, and ketamine can cause hemodynamic changes and are best avoided in L.M. Etomidate would be an excellent choice for induction, followed by isoflurane (with low-dose opioids) to maintain anesthesia. Although opioid-based anesthetics provide cardiovascular stability, the doses required to maintain anesthesia can prolong the duration of respiratory depression, which may necessitate postoperative mechanical ventilation.[37]

Methohexital for Electroconvulsive Therapy

6. T.B., a 33-year-old woman, ASA-I, will undergo an electroconvulsive therapy (ECT) procedure for treatment of her severe, medication-resistant depression. T.B. is scheduled to go home within 1 to 2 hours after the procedure, which will be performed under general anesthesia. What IV induction agent should be used?

ECT procedures are an important method of treatment of severe and medication-resistant depression, mania, and other serious psychiatric conditions. During the ECT procedure, an electrical current is applied to the brain, resulting in an electroencephalographic (EEG) spike and wave activity, a generalized motor seizure, and acute cardiovascular response. For an optimal therapeutic (antidepressant) response, T.B.'s seizure activity should last from 25 to 50 seconds. Therefore, when selecting an IV induction agent, its effect on EEG seizure activity, its ability to blunt the hemodynamic response to ECT, and its recovery profile (e.g., short time to discharge, non-emetogenic) are important considerations. Midazolam, lorazepam, fentanyl, propofol, and thiopental will significantly reduce the seizure duration, thereby reducing the efficacy of the ECT, when compared with methohexital. Although etomidate does not adversely affect the seizure duration, the hemodynamic response to ECT is accentuated because etomidate is cardiovascularly stable and cannot blunt the cardiovascular response to ECT. In addition, it can cause nausea and vomiting, resulting in delayed recovery. Therefore, methohexital is the agent of choice because, in a dose of 0.75 to 1 mg/kg IV, it will not affect the seizure duration or prolong T.B.'s recovery time.[38]

Ketamine Use in Pediatrics

7. R.L., a 4-year-old boy, ASA-II, is scheduled for a painful debridement and dressing change that is anticipated to take approximately 15 minutes. He is brought to the procedure room near the OR with his parents and is in distress over parting from them. He currently has no IV line in place. How could sedation and analgesia be provided to R.L.?

Ideally, analgesia should be provided without the need to start an IV and, for children with a high level of separation anxiety, in the presence of a parent. Although ketamine can be given intramuscularly, administration by this route is painful and not optimal. However, it may be preferred to starting an IV in R.L. for a short, painful procedure. At relatively low doses, ketamine produces analgesia and a compliant patient who is not heavily sedated. Because it causes little or no respiratory depression, intubation is unnecessary. However, R.L.'s parents should be warned that ketamine produces a dissociative stare and nystagmus, random movements of the head and extremities, and tonic/clonic movements. An anticholinergic drug, such as atropine, may be given along with ketamine to counteract its sialagogue effect. Because of the quality of sedation and analgesia produced by ketamine and its short duration of action (<30 minutes), its use has expanded to the emergency department. This practice is acceptable as long as appropriate guidelines are followed.[32]

An unusual adverse effect of ketamine is delirium and hallucinations that occur in 10% to 30% of patients upon awakening from anesthesia. Emergence reactions (e.g., dreaming, illusions, sense of floating out of body) vary in severity, occur within hours after awakening from anesthesia, and occur more often in adults, females, frequent dreamers, patients with personality disorders, and in patients receiving high doses of ketamine (>2 mg/kg) by rapid IV administration. Reactions can be attenuated by prophylactic administration of benzodiazepines.[31,32] R.L. is at very low risk for an emergence reaction, based on age, sex, dose, and route of ketamine administration; therefore, benzodiazepines are not needed in R.L.

VOLATILE INHALATION AGENTS

Currently, five volatile inhalation agents are available for use in the United States: desflurane, sevoflurane, isoflurane, enflurane, and halothane, with desflurane, sevoflurane, and isoflurane being the most commonly used in clinical practice. The volatile inhalation agents are unique in that they can produce all the components of the anesthetic state, to varying degrees (e.g., minimal analgesia), with immobility to noxious stimuli and amnesia postulated to be the predominant effects produced by these agents. These agents differ from the IV anesthetic agents in that they are administered into the lungs via an anesthesia machine. Because of this route of administration, it is easy to increase or decrease drug levels in the body. Current technology provides the anesthesia provider with the ability to estimate the anesthetic partial pressure at its site of action (brain), which helps maintain an optimal depth of anesthesia.[39]

Although the volatile inhalation agents produce all the components of the anesthetic state, anesthesia is often provided by administering a combination of drugs intended to utilize the advantages of smaller doses of each drug while avoiding the disadvantages of high doses of individual agents. This practice is referred to as *balanced anesthesia*. For example, midazolam is used routinely to produce sedation and amnesia, whereas the administration of a barbiturate (e.g., thiopental) or other IV anesthetic agent (e.g., propofol) followed by a neuromuscular blocking agent (e.g., succinylcholine) provides a rapid loss of consciousness and muscle relaxation to facilitate endotracheal intubation. Volatile inhalation agents provide anesthesia, along with reflex suppression (lowering BP and heart rate) and some muscle relaxation. Opioids (e.g., fentanyl) provide analgesia with reflex suppression, thus lowering total anesthetic requirements. Subsequent doses of a nondepolarizing neuromuscular blocking agent may be necessary to provide adequate relaxation for surgery.[39]

Uses

The volatile inhalation agents are primarily used in clinical practice to maintain general anesthesia. Because of their low pungency, sevoflurane and halothane also can be used to induce general anesthesia via a face mask. Desflurane and sevoflurane, because of their low blood solubility, are ideally suited for maintenance of general anesthesia in ambulatory surgery patients and for inpatients when rapid wake-up is desired (e.g., neurosurgery procedures).

Site/Mechanism of Action

The goal of inhalation anesthesia is to develop and maintain a satisfactory (anesthetizing) partial pressure of anesthetic in the brain, which is the site of anesthetic action.[39] The mechanism of action of the volatile inhalation agents is not fully understood. It is believed that these agents disrupt neuronal transmission in discrete areas throughout the CNS. They may either block excitatory or enhance inhibitory transmission through axons or synapses, with both presynaptic and postsynaptic effects demonstrated. The ultimate action of the volatile inhalation agents is believed to be on neuronal membranes, where these agents bind to and perturb membrane lipids and proteins; it is not clear which of these actions is most important with respect to the anesthetic state.[40,41]

Anesthesia Machine and Circuit

To understand fully many of the concepts associated with the administration of volatile inhalation agents, a basic understanding of the anesthesia machine and circuit is required. Three parts of the anesthesia machine are critically important in terms of volatile agent administration. The flowmeters regulate the amount of nitrous oxide (an anesthetic gas), air, and oxygen delivered to the patient. The vaporizers regulate the concentration of volatile inhalation agent administered to the patient, while the carbon dioxide absorber, which contains either soda lime or Baralyme, removes carbon dioxide from exhaled air. The first step in the administration of a volatile inhalation agent to a patient is to begin the flow of background gases. Flow is measured in liters per minute. A mixture of nitrous oxide and oxygen is commonly used. This gas mixture flows to one of the vaporizers, where a portion of it enters the vaporizer and "picks up" the anesthetic vapor of the volatile inhalation agent. The concentration of volatile inhalation agent delivered by the vaporizer is proportional to the amount of the gas mixture passing through it, which is regulated by adjusting the vaporizer's concentration dial. The gas and anesthetic vapor mixture exits the vaporizer and continues through the anesthetic circuit, where it is ultimately delivered to the patient via an endotracheal tube or face mask. The exhaled air from the patient, which contains the volatile inhalation agent and carbon dioxide, is returned to the circuit. Depending on the type of circuit and breathing system in place, a carbon dioxide absorber may be used to remove carbon dioxide from the exhaled air. If a semiclosed circle breathing system is being used, rebreathing of the exhaled volatile agent can occur if the fresh gas flow rate is low enough (e.g., ≤2 L/min).[42]

Potency

Potency of the volatile inhalation agents is compared in terms of minimum alveolar concentration (MAC). MAC is the alveolar concentration of anesthetic at one atmosphere that prevents movement in 50% of subjects in response to a painful stimulus (e.g., surgical skin incision).[39] The lower an agent's MAC, the greater the anesthetic potency. A value of 1.3 MAC is required to produce immobility in 95% of patients, whereas 1.5 MAC is required to block the adrenergic response to noxious stimuli.[39] In addition, the inhalation agents are almost additive in their effects on MAC; the addition of a second agent reduces the required concentration of the first agent. For example, when desflurane, isoflurane, and sevoflurane are administered with 60% to 70% nitrous oxide, their MAC values decrease from 6%, 1.15%, and 1.71% to 2.38%, 0.56%, and 0.66%, respectively.[39] Of the volatile inhalation agents routinely used, halothane has the lowest MAC and desflurane the highest (Table 10-6).[39]

Chemical Stability

Desflurane, isoflurane, and halothane are very stable compounds and are not broken down by the moist soda lime or Baralyme contained in the carbon dioxide absorber of the anesthesia machine. Sevoflurane degrades in the presence of carbon dioxide absorbent to multiple byproducts, with compound A being most important. In rats, compound A has caused nephrotoxicity,[43] but no clinically significant changes in serum creatinine and blood urea nitrogen (BUN) have been demonstrated in human studies.[44-46] However, in some of these studies, albuminuria, glucosuria, and increased urinary α-glutathione-S-transferase (GST) and increased urinary π-GST were noted, which are reflective of transient dysfunction of the glomerulus, proximal tubule, and distal tubule, respectively.[45,46] These transient changes do not appear to be clinically significant. One of the major factors that increases compound A concentration is administration of sevoflurane at low flow rates. Because of the association between flow rate and compound A concentration, the U.S. Food and Drug Administration (FDA) has required a warning in sevoflurane's package insert, which currently states that sevoflurane exposure should not exceed 2 MAC hours at flow rates of 1 to <2 L/min, with flow rates <1 L/min not recommended.

However, desflurane, isoflurane, and enflurane can react with dry carbon dioxide absorbent to produce carbon monoxide. This does not occur with sevoflurane or halothane.[47] The

Table 10-6 Pharmacologic and Pharmacokinetic Properties of the Volatile Inhalation Agents

Property/Effect	Desflurane	Sevoflurane	Isoflurane	Halothane	Enflurane
MAC in O_2 (adults)	6.0	1.71	1.15	0.77	1.7
Blood/gas partition coefficient[a]	0.42	0.69	1.46	2.54	1.91
Brain:blood partition coefficient[b]	1.29	1.7	1.6	1.9	1.4
Muscle:blood partition coefficient[c]	2.02	3.13	2.9	3.4	1.7
Fat:blood partition coefficient[d]	27.2	47.5	45	51	36
Metabolism	0.02%	3%	0.2%	15–20%	2%
Molecular weight (g)	168	201	184.5	197.4	184.5
Liquid density[e]	1.45	1.505	1.496	1.87	1.517

[a]The greater the blood:gas partition coefficient, the greater the blood solubility.
[b]The greater the brain:blood partition coefficient, the greater the brain solubility.
[c]The greater the muscle:blood partition coefficient, the greater the muscle solubility.
[d]The greater the fat:blood partition coefficient, the greater the fat solubility.
[e]Density determined at 25°C for desflurane, isoflurane, and enflurane and at 20°C for sevoflurane and halothane.
MAC, minimum alveolar concentration to prevent movement in 50% of subjects.
Adapted from reference 39.

major factor leading to the production of carbon monoxide is the water content of the absorbent.[48] Carbon monoxide is produced when desflurane, isoflurane, or enflurane passes through dry absorbent; this is most likely to occur on a Monday morning in an anesthesia machine that has been idle during the weekend and has had a continuous flow of fresh gas through the absorbent. Carbon monoxide production can be prevented by ensuring that only fully hydrated absorbent is used.

The development of alkali hydroxide-free carbon dioxide absorbents containing calcium hydroxide (versus sodium or potassium hydroxide), for example, have the potential to make the chemical stability of volatile inhalation agents in the absorbent not a clinical concern. An in vitro study of a carbon dioxide absorbent composed of calcium hydroxide demonstrated that compound A levels were no higher than those found in sevoflurane itself when it was passed through the new absorbent at a low flow rate (1 L/min). Likewise, negligible carbon monoxide production was seen when desflurane, isoflurane, or enflurane was passed through an anhydrous form of this absorbent.[49]

Pharmacokinetics

A series of anesthetic partial pressure gradients beginning at the anesthesia machine serve to drive the volatile inhalation agent across barriers to the brain. These gradients are as follows: anesthesia machine > delivered > inspired > alveolar > arterial > brain. Because the alveolar, arterial, and brain partial pressures equilibrate rapidly, the alveolar partial pressure provides an indirect measurement of the anesthetic partial pressure in the brain.[39]

Factors that influence the uptake and distribution of a volatile inhalation agent include the inspired concentration of the agent, alveolar ventilation, solubility of the agent in the blood (blood/gas partition coefficient), blood flow through the lungs, distribution of blood to individual organs (levels rise most rapidly in highly perfused organs—brain, kidney, heart, liver), solubility of the agent in tissue (tissue/blood partition coefficient), and mass of tissue.[39] If all other factors are equal,

agents with low solubilities will equilibrate quickly and, as a result, have a faster wash-in (onset). Solubility also is a factor in the elimination of volatile inhalation agents, in addition to metabolism and extent of tissue equilibration. Low-solubility agents are more rapidly washed-out (eliminated) because more of the agent is removed from the blood in one passage through the lungs.[39] As can be seen in Table 10-6, desflurane has the lowest solubility of any of the volatile inhalation agents, with sevoflurane's solubility being lower than isoflurane's for blood and muscle. As a result of their low solubility, quicker responses to intraoperative concentration changes are seen with desflurane and sevoflurane as well as a faster emergence and awakening from anesthesia and a more rapid return to normal motor function and judgment when compared with isoflurane.[50–52] Because of desflurane's low fat/blood solubility, its use in longer cases may result in a faster wake-up because less of the drug will have accumulated in the fat.[53] Pharmacokinetically, the profiles of the low-solubility agents, desflurane and sevoflurane, administered at low flow rates are similar to the more soluble agents when administered at higher flow (e.g., isoflurane at 4 L/min).[54]

The metabolism of the volatile inhalation agents varies (Table 10-6). Desflurane is metabolized to the least extent, whereas halothane has the greatest degree of metabolism. An important point is that metabolism does not alter the rate of induction or maintenance of anesthesia as the amount of anesthetic administered to the patient greatly exceeds its uptake.[39] Metabolism depends on the activity of the cytochrome P450 system and the amount and duration of availability of the volatile inhalation agent to the liver.[39] Halothane's metabolites may contribute to the hepatitis seen with this agent, possibly as a result of an immune response with repeat exposure.[55] Metabolism of sevoflurane has resulted in peak inorganic fluoride levels >100 μmol/L.[45] Historically, a fluoride level of 50 μmol/L has been used as a cutoff for potential nephrotoxicity based on reports of methoxyflurane-associated nephrotoxicity at levels >50 μmol/L.[54] Despite this, sevoflurane has not been demonstrated to produce nephrotoxicity. Potential reasons for this include the fact that sevoflurane's low blood-gas solubility may limit the degree of its metabolism once the anesthetic is discontinued and that sevoflurane, unlike methoxyflurane, undergoes minimal renal defluorination.[56] In clinical studies examining the preanesthetic and postanesthetic serum creatinine and BUN values in patients receiving sevoflurane anesthesia, there have been no reports of clinically significant renal damage in patients with normal renal function nor evidence of worsening renal function in patients with stable renal insufficiency or in those undergoing hemodialysis.[57–60]

Pharmacologic Properties

All the volatile inhalation agents depress ventilation (with an elevation of $PaCO_2$) and dilate constricted bronchial musculature in a dose-dependent manner. As mentioned previously, sevoflurane and halothane can be used for mask induction of general anesthesia because they are not as pungent as desflurane, isoflurane, and enflurane. Administration of a pungent agent by mask for induction can cause coughing, breath-holding, laryngospasm, and salivation in the patient. All the volatile inhalation agents depress myocardial contractility and decrease arterial BP in a dose-dependent manner through vasodilation, decreased cardiac output, and decreased sympathetic nervous system tone. Halothane does not increase heart rate, unlike sevoflurane, which increases heart rate at concentrations >1.5 MAC. Desflurane, isoflurane, and enflurane increase heart rate, with the increase being dose-dependent for desflurane and enflurane. At clinically used concentrations (1 MAC), desflurane has minimal effects on heart rate.[39,54] Desflurane can produce sympathetic nervous system activation, resulting in a transient increase in BP and heart rate, when concentrations are rapidly increased, when increasing the inspired concentration of desflurane from 1 to 1.5 MAC, and with 1% increases in end-tidal desflurane concentration >6%.[61,62] The sympathetic nervous system activation may be due to stimulation of medullary centers via irritant receptors in the upper airway and lungs;[63] rapid adaptation of the airway receptors as well as the direct depressant effects of the higher desflurane concentration account for the transient nature of this effect. Halothane can sensitize the myocardium to the arrhythmogenic effects of exogenously administered epinephrine. The volatile inhalation agents decrease cerebral metabolic rate and produce cerebral vasodilation, resulting in increased cerebral blood flow and volume. All the volatile inhalation agents produce muscle relaxation and potentiate the actions of the neuromuscular blocking agents; halothane potentiation is the least compared with the other volatile inhalation agents. The volatile inhalation agents relax uterine smooth muscle, which can contribute to perinatal blood loss. All the volatile inhalation agents have been implicated as triggers of malignant hyperthermia and are contraindicated in malignant hyperthermia-susceptible patients. Finally, all volatile inhalation agents are associated with postoperative nausea, vomiting, and shivering.[39,54]

Drug Interactions

Opioids, benzodiazepines, α_2-agonists, and neuromuscular blocking agents potentiate the effects of the volatile inhalation agents. Therefore, their administration permits use of lower dosages of the volatile inhalents, thereby reducing their potential for adverse effects. Halothane, an inhibitor of the cytochrome P450 system,[39] acutely reduces the metabolism of ketamine, propranolol, diazepam, enflurane, and barbiturates. The other volatile inhalation agents do not inhibit drug metabolism as readily as does halothane.[39]

Economic Considerations

The following items must be considered when examining the costs associated with the administration of volatile inhalation agents from an institutional perspective: cost of the volatile inhalation agent (including waste), cost of the equipment necessary to administer the volatile inhalation agent, cost of adjuvants used to treat adverse effects of the volatile agent, and time spent in the OR and PACU.

The cost of a volatile agent depends on (1) the cost per milliliter of the liquid anesthetic, (2) the amount of vapor generated per milliliter, (3) the amount of volatile agent that must be delivered from the anesthesia machine to sustain the desired alveolar concentration, and (4) the flow rate of the background gases.[64] Items 1 and 2 are, for the most part, constant, with price increases or decreases occurring periodically. Because desflurane and sevoflurane are less soluble in blood and tissue than isoflurane, lower amounts of these agents will need to be delivered to the alveoli to attain the desired anesthetic depth.[64] The flow rate of background gases is a major determinant of the cost; as flow rate increases, the amount of anesthetic consumed per time increases.[65] The following formula is frequently used to calculate the cost of volatile inhalation agent used:

$$Cost\ used = (PFTMC)/(2412d)$$

where P is vaporizer concentration (%), F is fresh gas flow (L/min), T is time (min), M is molecular weight of the agent, C is the cost of the agent ($/mL), and d is the density of the agent.[66] The use of low flow rates can result in impressive reductions in the volatile anesthetic drug cost per case.[67] An important point to keep in mind when comparing only the cost of the volatile inhalation agents themselves (e.g., excluding any benefits in terms of cost reduction that may be realized by a quicker discharge from the recovery room) is that the low-solubility volatile agents have to be administered at low flow rates to prevent their cost from being substantially higher than that of the more traditional agents, such as isoflurane, when administered at rates of 2 to 3 L/min.

The cost of purchasing new vaporizers and upgrading or replacing agent analyzers that are used to administer and monitor volatile inhalation agents, respectively, can be significant, ranging from a few hundred dollars to as high as $10,000. These costs become a concern when a new agent is introduced onto the market.

Medications used to treat adverse effects associated with the volatile inhalation agents include β-blockers, opioids, benzodiazepines, vasopressors, and antiemetic agents. Antiemetic agents routinely are used to prevent and/or treat the PONV seen with the volatile inhalation agents; nausea and vomiting postoperatively occur in 43% to 51% and 22% to 25% of patients, respectively.[68] The cost of an antiemetic agent can range from <$1 for a single dose of a traditional agent, such as droperidol, to >$15 for a dose of ondansetron, thereby adding to the cost of the anesthetic. However, this is significantly less than the cost of an unanticipated admission to the hospital secondary to PONV.

Reducing the time patients spend in the OR and PACU by using the low-solubility volatile inhalation agents can significantly reduce the overall net cost of the surgical procedure. This concept is discussed at the end of this chapter.

On a more global basis, the use of volatile inhalation agents, especially desflurane and sevoflurane, should be considered in place of propofol to maintain general anesthesia when appropriate. Studies have demonstrated similar or better recovery characteristics for desflurane and sevoflurane when compared with propofol,[66,69,70] and their costs were approximately one-third to one-half that of propofol per hour.[66,69,70] The introduction of generic propofol onto the market has reduced this cost difference to some extent, but a meaningful difference still exists. Although a higher incidence of PONV and resultant antiemetic agent use was seen with the volatile inhalation agents in many of these studies, it did not result in a longer PACU stay. Prophylaxis with a traditional antiemetic agent when administering a volatile inhalation agent may reduce the incidence of PONV to a rate comparable with propofol while still keeping anesthetic drug cost low.[71] Sevoflurane also can be used in place of propofol to induce general anesthesia at a reduced cost.[72]

Desflurane Use for Maintenance of General Anesthesia

Sympathetic Nervous System Activation

8. C.K., a 26-year-old man, ASA-I, is scheduled to undergo a laparoscopic hernia repair on an outpatient basis. During his preoperative evaluation on the morning of surgery, his BP was 115/75 mm Hg and his heart rate was 70 beats/min. The surgery is expected to last <2 hours, so a propofol induction is planned followed by maintenance of general anesthesia with desflurane without nitrous oxide. After induction of anesthesia, the desflurane concentration on the vaporizer was rapidly increased to 8%. Within 1 minute of the concentration increase, C.K.'s BP increased to 148/110 mm Hg and his heart rate increased to 112 beats/min. What could be causing C.K.'s increased BP and heart rate, and how could it have been prevented?

Desflurane can produce sympathetic nervous system activation with a resultant increase in BP and heart rate under certain circumstances. One of these is the rapid increase of desflurane concentration to 1.1 MAC as seen with C.K. This hemodynamic response can be attenuated by the IV administration of fentanyl approximately 5 minutes before the increase in desflurane concentration; parenteral esmolol (90 seconds before desflurane concentration increase) and oral clonidine (90 minutes before desflurane concentration increase) also can be used.[73] Fentanyl is a good choice because it effectively blunts the increase in heart rate and BP while having minimal cardiovascular depressant and postoperative sedative effects. Alternatively, nitrous oxide can be administered with desflurane, thereby allowing the desflurane concentration to be maintained at <1 MAC (6%).

Factors That Increase or Decrease Minimum Alveolar Concentration

9. P.F., a 39-year-old man, ASA-II, is scheduled to undergo a laparoscopic cholecystectomy. He will be admitted postoperatively. General anesthesia will be induced with thiopental and

maintained with isoflurane and nitrous oxide. P.F.'s social history reveals longstanding ethanol abuse. During the surgery, the anesthesia provider has to use a higher concentration of isoflurane than he expected for P.F. What could be causing the need for a higher isoflurane concentration?

Various physiologic or pharmacologic factors can increase or decrease the anesthetic requirement. Hyperthermia, hypernatremia, chronic ethanol abuse, and increased central neurotransmitter levels can increase MAC. On the other hand, the following factors can decrease MAC: increasing age; metabolic acidosis; hypoxia; induced hypotension; decreased central neurotransmitter levels; anemia; hypothermia; hyponatremia; acute ethanol administration; pregnancy; hypoosmolality; and medications such as the α_2-agonists, lithium, ketamine, pancuronium, physostigmine (10 times clinical dose), neostigmine (10 times clinical dose), lidocaine, the opioids, the opioid agonist–antagonists, the barbiturates, chlorpromazine, diazepam, hydroxyzine, verapamil, and Δ-9-tetrahydrocannabinol.[39]

P.F.'s history of chronic ethanol abuse is consistent with his increased requirement for isoflurane during the procedure to maintain an adequate level of anesthesia.

NEUROMUSCULAR BLOCKING AGENTS

Uses

Neuromuscular blocking agents are one of the most commonly used classes of drugs in the OR. They are used primarily as an adjunct to general anesthesia to facilitate endotracheal intubation and to relax skeletal muscle during surgery under general anesthesia.[74] Skeletal muscle relaxation optimizes the surgical field for the surgeon and prevents patient movement as a reflex response to surgical stimulation. Neuromuscular blocking agents are also used in the ICU to paralyze mechanically ventilated patients.[75] An important point to remember is that neuromuscular blocking agents have no known effect on consciousness or pain threshold. Consequently, adequate sedation and analgesia must be ensured when neuromuscular blocking agents are administered to ICU patients.

Mechanism of Action

Two molecules of acetylcholine must bind to the acetylcholine subunits of the nicotinic cholinergic receptors located on the motor nerve endplate for normal neuromuscular transmission to occur.[76] Neuromuscular blocking agents produce muscle relaxation by binding to these subunits. Two classes of neuromuscular blocking agents exist based on their mechanism of action: depolarizing and nondepolarizing. Succinylcholine, the only depolarizing neuromuscular blocking agent in clinical use today, acts like acetylcholine to depolarize the membrane. Because succinylcholine is not metabolized at the neuromuscular junction, its action at the nicotinic receptor persists longer than acetylcholine. As a result, succinylcholine causes a persistent depolarization of the motor endplate, which results in sustained skeletal muscle paralysis. The paralysis produced by depolarizing agents is preceded initially by fasciculations (transient twitching of skeletal muscle). The nondepolarizing neuromuscular blocking agents act as competitive antagonists to acetylcholine at the acetylcholine subunits of the nicotinic cholinergic receptors, thereby preventing depolarization of the muscle membrane and subsequent muscle contraction.[74,76]

Monitoring Neuromuscular Blockade

In addition to clinical assessment (e.g., lack of movement) by the anesthesia provider and the surgeon, the degree of neuromuscular blockade produced by neuromuscular blocking agents is monitored by nerve stimulation with a peripheral nerve stimulator. Most commonly, the ulnar or facial nerve is electrically stimulated and the response of the innervated muscle (adductor pollicis in the thumb or orbicularis oculi around the eyelid) is visually assessed. Adequate neuromuscular blockade is present when the train-of-four (4 electrical stimulations of 2 Hz delivered every 0.5 seconds) count is 1/4 or 2/4 (one or two visible muscle twitches out of a possible 4 twitches).[75]

Classification

Neuromuscular blocking agents commonly are classified by the type of blockade produced (depolarizing versus nondepolarizing), chemical structure (steroidal compound, acetylcholine-like, benzyl isoquinolinium compound), or duration of action (ultrashort, short, intermediate, long) as listed in Table 10-7.[77]

Adverse Effects

The underlying mechanisms for the cardiovascular adverse effects of neuromuscular blocking agents are listed in Table 10-8 and include blockade of autonomic ganglia (hypotension), blockade of muscarinic receptors (tachycardia), and/or release of histamine from circulating mast cells (hypotension).[76-78] In general, the steroidal compounds exhibit varying degrees of vagolytic effect, whereas the benzyl isoquinolinium compounds are associated with varying degrees of histamine release. Although not reported as a problem when used short term in the OR, the use of neuromuscular blocking agents in ICU patients for extended periods can result in prolonged neuromuscular blockade or acute quadriplegic myopathy syndrome, albeit infrequently.[76] Of the currently available neuromuscular blocking agents, cisatracurium (Nimbex), vecuronium (Norcuron), and doxacurium (Nuromax) are virtually devoid of clinically significant cardiovascular effects and are the agents of choice for patients with unstable cardiovascular profiles.[74,76,77] Succinylcholine (Anectine, Quelicin) is associated with a significant number of adverse effects including hyperkalemia; arrhythmias; fasciculations; muscle pain; myoglobinuria; trismus; phase II block; and increased intraocular, intragastric, and intracranial pressures.[77,78] Succinylcholine, like inhalational anesthetics, can trigger malignant hyperthermia.[76] Of these adverse effects, bradycardia,

---

Table 10-7   Classification of Neuromuscular Blocking Agents

Agent	Type of Block	Clinical Duration of Action[a]	Structure
Atracurium (Tracrium)	−	Intermediate	Benzylisoquinolinium
Cisatracurium (Nimbex)	−	Intermediate	Benzylisoquinolinium
Doxacurium (Nuromax)	−	Long	Benzylisoquinolinium
Mivacurium (Mivacron)	−	Short	Benzylisoquinolinium
Pancuronium (Pavulon)	−	Long	Steroidal
Rocuronium (Zemuron)	−	Intermediate	Steroidal
Succinylcholine (Anectine, Quelicin)	+	Ultra-short	Acetylcholine-like
Vecuronium (Norcuron)	−	Intermediate	Steroidal

[a]Time from injection of agent to return to twitch height to 25% of control (time at which another dose of agent will need to be administered to maintain paralysis); in general, clinical duration of a standard intubating dose of ultra-short agents ranges from 3 to 5 minutes, short agents from 15 to 30 minutes, intermediate agents from 30 to 40 minutes, and long agents from 60 to 120 minutes.
+, depolarizing; −, nondepolarizing.
Adapted from reference 77.

Table 10-8   Causes of Cardiovascular Adverse Effects of Neuromuscular Blocking Agents

Agent	Histamine Release[a]	Autonomic Ganglia	Vagolytic Activity	Sympathetic Stimulation
Atracurium[a] (Tracrium)	++	−	−	−
Cisatracurium (Nimbex)	−	−	−	−
Doxacurium (Nuromax)	−	−	−	−
Mivacurium (Mivacron)	+	−	−	−
Pancuronium (Pavulon)	−	Weak block	++	++
Rocuronium[b] (Zemuron)	−	−	+	−
Succinylocholine (Anectine, Quelicin)	+	Stimulates	−	−
Vecuronium (Norcuron)	−	−	−	−

[a]Histamine release is dose and rate related; cardiovascular changes can be lessened by minimizing dose and injecting agent slowly.
[b]Produces an increase in heart rate of approximately 18% with intubating dose of 0.6 mg/kg; effect usually transient and resolves spontaneously.
+-++, likelihood of developing the cardiovascular adverse effect relative to the other agents; −, no effect.
Adapted from references 76–78.

hyperkalemia (which can trigger arrhythmias and cardiac arrest in patients at risk), and the triggering of a MH crisis are severe and potentially life-threatening reactions. Nevertheless, succinylcholine is still used today because of its rapid onset and ultrashort duration of action as well as its ability to be administered intramuscularly in children in an emergent situation when IV access has not been established.

Drug Interactions

Several drugs interact with neuromuscular blocking agents. The volatile inhalation agents potentiate the neuromuscular blockade produced by nondepolarizing agents, thereby allowing a lower dose of the latter to be used when administered concomitantly. Isoflurane, enflurane, sevoflurane, and desflurane potentiate the neuromuscular blockade to a greater extent than does halothane.[77,78] Other agents reported to potentiate the effects of neuromuscular blocking agents include the aminoglycosides, clindamycin, magnesium sulfate, quinidine, furosemide, lidocaine, amphotericin B, and dantrolene. Carbamazepine, phenytoin, corticosteroids (chronic administration), and theophylline antagonize the effects of neuromuscular blocking agents.[76,77] By appropriately monitoring the patient and dosing the neuromuscular blocking agent to effect, significant problems from drug interactions can be minimized.

Reversal of Neuromuscular Blockade

The action of neuromuscular blocking agents ceases spontaneously as plasma concentrations decline or by reversal with anticholinesterases (e.g., neostigmine, edrophonium, pyridostigmine). Anticholinesterases inhibit the enzyme acetylcholinesterase, which degrades acetylcholine, and are used to reverse paralysis produced by nondepolarizing agents. Anticholinergic agents are coadministered (in same syringe) with the anticholinesterases to minimize other cholinergic effects (e.g., bradycardia, bronchoconstriction, salivation, increased peristalsis, nausea, vomiting) caused by the increase in acetylcholine concentration. Atropine is routinely administered with edrophonium, and glycopyrrolate with neostigmine or pyridostigmine, to take advantage of similar onset times and durations of action.[74,75,77] Reversal of neuromuscular blockade, as a general rule, is not attempted until spontaneous recovery is well established. Before extubation, adequacy of reversal is assessed with the use of a peripheral nerve stimulator and by clinical assessment of the patient (e.g., ability to sustain head lift for 5 seconds).[77,78]

Pharmacokinetics and Pharmacodynamics

10. R.D., a 36-year-old man, ASA-I, is admitted through the ED for an emergency appendectomy. R.D. is otherwise healthy, has no drug allergies, and is currently taking no medications. All laboratory values are normal. Admission notes reveal that R.D. ate dinner approximately 60 minutes earlier. Because of this, the anesthesia provider plans to perform a rapid sequence induction using the Sellick maneuver. Which neuromuscular blocking agent would be most appropriate for R.D.?

Rapid sequence induction is indicated for patients at risk for aspiration of gastric contents should regurgitation occur. Patients with a full stomach or history of gastroesophageal re-

flux are at risk for aspiration, as is the case for R.D. The goal of rapid sequence induction is to minimize the time during which the airway is unprotected by intubating the patient as fast as possible (e.g., within 60 seconds). In this technique, the patient is preoxygenated, after which an IV induction agent is administered, followed immediately by a neuromuscular blocking agent. Manual ventilation of the patient is not attempted after administration of these agents. Apnea occurs as the neuromuscular blocking agent takes effect; therefore, a neuromuscular blocking agent with as rapid an onset as possible is required to produce adequate intubating conditions as quickly as possible. The Sellick maneuver often is used during rapid sequence induction. It is performed by placing downward pressure on the cricoid cartilage, which compresses and occludes the esophagus and helps prevent passive regurgitation of gastric contents into the trachea.[78]

Table 10-9 lists the onset times of normal intubating doses and other information pertaining to the use of neuromuscular blocking agents.[75–78] Succinylcholine has the fastest onset time, which makes it an attractive agent to use in rapid sequence induction.[79]

Because R.D. is an otherwise healthy man with no contraindications to the use of succinylcholine, this agent should be used.

Depolarizing Agent Contraindications

11. What would be your choice of a neuromuscular blocking agent if R.D. presents with a history of susceptibility to malignant hyperthermia, and why?

Succinylcholine is contraindicated in patients with skeletal muscle myopathies; after the acute phase of injury (i.e., 5 to 70 days after injury) following major burns, multiple trauma, extensive denervation of skeletal muscle, or upper motor neuron injury; in children and adolescents (except when used for emergency tracheal intubation or when the immediate securing of the airway is necessary); and in patients with a hypersensitivity to the drug.[74,77] Succinylcholine also can trigger malignant hyperthermia and is absolutely contraindicated in malignant hyperthermia-susceptible patients.[80]

The nondepolarizing neuromuscular blocking agents are safe to use in malignant hyperthermia-susceptible patients.[81] Rocuronium (Zemuron) has the fastest onset time of the nondepolarizing agents, although it is slightly slower than succinylcholine.[82] The onsets of the remaining intermediate- and long-duration agents can be shortened in two ways. Increasing the dose results in a faster onset of action, but also prolongs the duration of action. Rocuronium's onset, for example, can be reduced to 60 seconds with an initial dose of 0.9 mg/kg (versus a normal initial dose of 0.6 mg/kg).[83] The onset of action of nondepolarizing agents, with the exception of rocuronium, also can be shortened by the use of the priming principle. With this technique, approximately 10% of the intubating dose is administered 5 minutes before the standard intubating dose. For vecuronium, for example, a priming dose could shorten the onset time from 2 to 3 minutes to 90 seconds.[84] However, a low level of neuromuscular blockade is produced with the priming dose, which can result in patients complaining of heavy eyelids, blurred vision, and difficulty in swallowing. In certain patients (e.g., obese patients), measurable neuromuscular blockade can put the patient at risk for more serious consequences.[85]

Table 10-9 Pharmacokinetic and Pharmacodynamic Parameters of Action of Neuromuscular Blocking Agents

Agent	Cl (mL/kg/min)	Vd$_{ss}$ (L/kg)	Half-Life (min)	ED95 (mg/kg)	Intubating Dose[a,b] (mg/kg)	Onset[c] (min)	Clinical Duration of Action of Initial Dose (min)
Atracurium[d] (Tracrium)	5–7	0.2	20	0.2–0.25	0.4–0.5	2–3	25–30
Cisatracurium (Nimbex)	4.6	0.15	22	0.05	0.15–0.2	2–2.5	50–60
Doxacurium (Nuromax)	1–2.5	0.2	100–120	0.025–0.03	0.05–0.08	4–6	100–160
Mivacurium[d] (Mivacron)	50–100[e]	0.2	2[e]	0.08–0.09	0.15–0.25	1.5–3	12–20
Pancuronium (Pavulon)	1–2	0.3	80–120	0.07	0.04–0.1	3–5	80–100
Rocuronium[d] (Zemuron)	4.0	0.3	60–70	0.3	0.6–1.2	1–1.5	30–60
Succinylcholine[d] (Anectine, Quelicin)	Unknown	Unknown	Unknown	0.25	1.0–1.5	1	5–20
Vecuronium[d] (Norcuron)	4.5	0.4	50–70	0.05–0.06	0.1	2–3	25–30

[a]Dose when nitrous oxide-opioid technique is used.
[b]Intermittent maintenance doses to maintain paralysis, as a general rule, will be approximately 20% to 25% of the initial dose.
[c]Time to intubation.
[d]Also can be administered as a continuous infusion to maintain paralysis; suggested infusion ranges under balanced anesthesia are as follows: atracurium, 4 to 12 μg/kg per minute; cisatracurium, 1 to 2 μg/kg per minute; mivacurium, 3 to 12 μg/kg per minute (higher in children); rocuronium, 6 to 14 μg/kg per minute; succinylcholine, 50 to 100 μg/kg per minute; vecuronium, 0.8 to 2 μg/kg per minute.
[e]Values reflect contribution of trans-trans and cis-trans isomers only.
Cl, clearance; ED95, effective dose causing 95% muscle paralysis; Vd$_{ss}$, steady-state volume of distribution.
Adapted from references 75–78.

Rocuronium, with its rapid onset of action, would be a suitable alternative to succinylcholine in R.D.'s case. Its cost and slightly longer onset prevent it from being the first-line agent in individuals who have no contraindications to succinylcholine. Furthermore, its longer clinical duration of action could be a concern if the airway cannot be immediately secured or if the procedure is shorter than the duration of an intubating dose of rocuronium. Because this procedure will last longer than the duration of muscle relaxation provided by the intubating dose of rocuronium, this is not a concern.

Routes of Elimination

12. M.M., a 70-year-old woman, ASA-IV, is scheduled to undergo a 2-hour GI procedure. Pertinent laboratory findings are as follows: aspartate aminotransferase (AST), 272 U/L (normal, 5 to 45 U/L); alanine aminotransferase (ALT), 150 U/L (normal, 5 to 37 U/L); BUN, 40 mg/dL (normal, 8 to 21 mg/dL); serum creatinine (SrCr), 1.8 mg/dL (normal, 0.5 to 1.1 mg/dL); albumin, 2.6 g/dL (normal, 3.5 to 5.0 g/dL); and bilirubin, 0.74 mg/dL (normal, 2 to 18 mg/dL). Which neuromuscular blocking agent would you recommend for M.M.?

[SI units: AST, 4.5 μkat/L; ALT, 2.5 μkat/L; BUN, 14.28 mmol/L; SrCr, 159 μmol/L; albumin, 26 g/L; bilirubin, 12.7 mol/L]

When selecting a neuromuscular blocking agent, one of the factors that must be considered is the patient's renal and hepatic function. Neuromuscular blocking agents depend on the kidneys and liver for their metabolism and excretion to varying degrees as can be seen in Table 10-10.[74,75,78] They are metabolized by plasma cholinesterase (pseudocholinesterase), Hofmann elimination (a nonbiologic process that

Table 10-10 Elimination of Neuromuscular Blocking Agents

Agent	Renal	Hepatic	Biliary	Plasma
Atracurium (Tracrium)	<5%	—	—	Hofmann elimination, ester hydrolysis
Cisatracurium (Nimbex)	Some[a]	—	Some[a]	Hofmann elimination
Doxacurium (Nuromax)	80–100%[b]	—	Yes[b]	—
Mivacurium (Mivacron)	<10%	—	Minor	Plasma cholinesterase
Pancuronium (Pavulon)	60–80%	15–40%	5–10%	—
Rocuronium (Zemuron)	Up to 30%	—	50%	—
Succinylcholine (Anectine, Quelicin)	—	—	—	Plasma cholinesterase
Vecuronium (Norcuron)	10–20%	20–30%	40–75%	—

[a]<20% by renal and hepatic routes combined.
[b]Excreted unchanged.
Adapted from references 74, 75 and 78.

does not require renal, hepatic, or enzymatic function), nonspecific esterases, and via hepatic metabolic pathways.

Hofmann elimination is a pH- and temperature-dependent process unique to atracurium (Tracrium) and cisatracurium (Nimbex). One of the products produced by Hofmann elimination is laudanosine, a CNS stimulant in high concentrations. Laudanosine undergoes renal and hepatic elimination. Due to the short-term use of atracurium and cisatracurium in the OR, accumulation of laudanosine with resultant seizure activity is not a concern, even in patients with end-stage renal failure.[86,87]

Because plasma cholinesterase levels may be decreased in patients with renal or hepatic dysfunction, the duration of action of agents metabolized by this enzyme (e.g., succinylcholine, mivacurium) could be prolonged. The increased duration of action of succinylcholine in patients with low levels of normal plasma cholinesterase is not clinically significant; however, it can be significant with mivacurium. Hence, patients with renal disease should receive a lower dose of mivacurium; succinylcholine, on the other hand, is generally avoided in patients with renal dysfunction because acute hyperkalemia can result from its administration. For patients with severe hepatic disease, the dose of mivacurium should be reduced because of the significant reduction in plasma cholinesterase activity.[88] Finally, atypical plasma cholinesterase can increase the duration of action of succinylcholine and mivacurium (Mivacron) significantly.[89,90]

Unchanged neuromuscular blocking agents and their metabolites are excreted by the renal or biliary routes. The duration of action of renally eliminated agents (pancuronium, tubocurarine, doxacurium) will be increased in patients with renal failure. Vecuronium's duration of action can be increased in patients with liver disease, particularly when larger doses (0.2 mg/kg) are administered, reflecting impaired metabolism or excretion rather than termination of effect by redistribution.[91]

Because M.M. has evidence of both significant renal and hepatic impairment, cisatracurium or atracurium would be appropriate choices for a neuromuscular blocking agent because their properties are not altered significantly by renal and hepatic failure. Furthermore, because these agents have an intermediate duration of action, they can easily be used in a 2-hour procedure. The availability of generic atracurium makes this agent a more economic choice; however, atracurium's greater propensity to cause histamine release with resultant hypotension makes cisatracurium a better choice in this 70-year-old, ASA-IV patient.

LOCAL ANESTHETICS

Local and Regional Anesthesia

Some surgical procedures can be performed under regional anesthesia (anesthesia selective for the surgical site) rather than general anesthesia (total body anesthesia with the patient rendered unconscious). Epidural, spinal (intrathecal), IV regional, peripheral nerve block, topical, or local infiltration anesthesia can be chosen depending on the location of the surgical site, extent of the surgery, patient health and physical characteristics, coagulation status, duration of surgery, and the desires and cooperativeness of the patient. For epidural anesthesia, the local anesthetic is administered into the epidural space, which is located between the dura and the ligament covering the spinal vertebral bodies and disks. To provide spinal anesthesia, the local anesthetic is injected into the subarachnoid (intrathecal) space. By injecting a local anesthetic in the tissue near a specific nerve or nerve plexus, anesthesia can be provided for a carotid endarterectomy (cervical plexus), upper extremity surgery (brachial plexus), or hand surgery (ulnar, median and/or radial nerve). Regional anesthesia can be selected to reduce or avoid the likelihood of complications such as postoperative pain, nausea, vomiting, and laryngeal irritation or dental complications, all of which are associated with general anesthesia. Peripheral nerve block may be selected over general, spinal, or epidural anesthesia because it is not associated with bowel obstruction or urinary retention, and it provides postoperative analgesia (particularly when long-acting local anesthetics are used).[92] Potential advantages of spinal or epidural anesthesia include reduction of the stress response to surgery, improvement in cardiac function in patients with ischemic heart disease, fewer postoperative pulmonary complications, potentially favorable effects on coagulation (lower risk of venous thrombosis), and the ability to continue epidural analgesia into the postoperative period.[93] Disadvantages of spinal, epidural, or peripheral nerve block include the additional time and manipulations required to perform it, possible complications or pain from invasive catheter placements or injections, slow onset of effect, possible failure of technique, and toxicity from absorption of the drugs administered.

Uses of Local Anesthetic Agents

Local anesthetics are a mainstay of analgesia because they prevent the initiation or propagation of the electrical impulses required for peripheral and spinal nerve conduction. These agents can be administered by all routes previously discussed, depending on the drug chosen. Table 10-11 lists the common uses of currently available local anesthetics.[94–96] Local anesthetics often are given in combination with other agents, such as sodium bicarbonate (to increase the speed of onset and reduce pain on local infiltration), epinephrine (to prolong the duration of action and to delay vascular absorption of the local anesthetic, thereby minimizing plasma concentration and systemic toxicity), or opioids (to provide analgesia by a different mechanism of action).

Mechanism of Action

The two structural classes of local anesthetics are characterized by the linkage between the molecule's lipophilic aromatic group and hydrophilic amine group: amides and esters. Both the amide and ester classes provide anesthesia and analgesia by reversibly binding to and blocking the sodium channels in nerve membranes, thereby decreasing the rate of rise of the action potential such that threshold potential is not reached; propagation of the electrical impulses required for nerve conduction is prevented. The axonal membrane blockade that results is selective depending on the drug, the concentration and volume administered, and the depth of nerve penetration. C fibers (pain transmission and autonomic activity) appear to be the most easily blocked, followed by fibers responsible for touch and pressure sensation (A-α, A-β, and A-Δ), and finally, those responsible for motor function (A-α and A-β). At the most commonly used doses and concentrations, some

Table 10-11 Clinical Uses of Local Anesthetic Agents

Agent	Primary Clinical Use
Esters	
Chloroprocaine (Nesacaine)	Epidural
Cocaine	Topical
Procaine (Novocain)	Local infiltration, spinal
Tetracacine (Pontocaine)	Topical, spinal
Amides	
Bupivacaine (Marcaine, Sensorcaine)	Local infiltration, nerve block, epidural, spinal
Etidocaine (Duranest)	Local infiltration, nerve block, epidural
Levobupivacaine (Chirocaine)	Local infiltration, nerve block, epidural
Lidocaine (Xylocaine)	Local infiltration, nerve block, spinal, epidural, topical, IV regional
Mepivacaine (Carbocaine, Polocaine)	Local infiltration, nerve block, epidural
Ropivacaine (Naropin)	Local infiltration, nerve block, epidural

IV, intravenous.
Adapted from references 94–96.

non–pain transmitting-nerve fibers also are blocked. The blockade of sensory, motor, or autonomic (sympathetic, parasympathetic) fibers may result in adverse effects such as paresthesia, numbness and inability to move extremities, hypotension, and urinary retention. Systemic effects (such as seizures or cardiac arrhythmias) are related to the inherent cardiac and CNS safety margins of these drugs. They also are related to the site of injection, because the interaction between local blood flow and tissue binding can result in a high degree of systemic drug absorption from sites such as intercostal nerves; less absorption is seen with epidural, brachial plexus, or sciatic/femoral nerve drug administration.[94,95]

Ropivacaine is a homolog of mepivacaine and bupivacaine. Like bupivacaine, it has a long duration of action. Higher plasma concentrations of ropivacaine are required to produce mild CNS toxicity (lightheadedness, tinnitus, numbness of the tongue) in volunteers, when compared with bupivacaine. In animal studies, ropivacaine was found to be less cardiotoxic than bupivacaine. In addition, ropivacaine may produce less motor blockade than bupivacaine.[97] As a result, some anesthesia providers feel that ropivacaine is safer than bupivacaine. However, inadvertent intravascular administration of ropivacaine can produce significant CNS toxicity (seizures), emphasizing the importance of ensuring appropriate placement of the local anesthetic solution by the anesthesia provider. The true place of ropivacaine in clinical practice is currently ill defined.

Levobupivacaine, the S-enantiomer of bupivacaine, appears to have a similar onset, duration, and extent of sensory and motor block as bupivacaine. Volunteer studies have found less CNS depression and potential for arrhythmias with levobupivacaine when given in comparable doses to bupivacaine. Animal studies have demonstrated significantly less effect from levobupivacaine than bupivacaine on the corrected QT interval and QRS duration.[96] However, levobupivacaine is significantly more expensive than bupivacaine, which means that it should replace bupivacaine only when the risk for inadvertent intravascular injection is high (e.g., a large dose is being administered or the site of injection has a high vascular absorption).

Allergic Reaction

Most adverse reactions to local anesthetics are manifestations of excessive plasma concentration (systemic toxicity) of the local anesthetic. Allergic reactions to local anesthetics are rare. Ester-type local anesthetic agents (benzocaine, procaine, tetracaine) produce most of the allergic reactions, which is probably caused by their metabolite, para-aminobenzoic acid (PABA). True allergy to amide-type local anesthetics is extremely rare and may be due to the preservative (methylparaben or other substances that are structurally similar to PABA) or to accidental intravascular injection of an epinephrine-containing local anesthetic. Because amide-type local anesthetics do not undergo metabolism to a PABA metabolite, a patient with a known allergy to an ester-type local anesthetic can safely receive an amide-type agent. Furthermore, it is best to administer a preservative-free preparation to a patient with a known allergy to a local anesthetic.[94,95]

Toxicity

Factors that influence the toxicity of local anesthetics include the total amount of drug administered, presence or absence of epinephrine, vascularity of the injection site, type of local anesthetic used, rate of destruction of the drug, age and physical status of the patient, and interactions with other drugs. Elderly patients have a smaller volume of distribution and clearance, necessitating smaller, less-frequent doses after the initial dose.[98]

Toxic levels of local anesthetics are most often achieved by unintentional intravascular injection, which result in excessive plasma concentrations. Systemic toxicity of local anesthetics involves the CNS and cardiovascular system. Local anesthetics tend to have a continuum of symptoms of CNS toxicity. Patients initially may complain of tinnitus, lightheadedness, metallic taste in their mouth, tingling, numbness, and dizziness. These symptoms can be followed by tremors, seizures, unconsciousness, and respiratory arrest as plasma levels rise. Toxic plasma levels of local anesthetics can cause hypotension, prolongation of the Q-T interval, re-entrant arrhythmias, and even cardiac arrest.[94,98]

Physicochemical Properties Affecting Action

The potency of a local anesthetic is primarily determined by the degree of lipid solubility. Local anesthetics such as bupivacaine are highly lipid soluble and can be given in concentrations of 0.25% to 0.5%. Less lipid-soluble agents, such as lidocaine, require concentrations of 1% to 2% for many anesthetic techniques.

Amide-type local anesthetics are metabolized primarily by microsomal enzymes in the liver. The cytochrome P450 enzyme system is involved in the metabolism of lidocaine (CYP 3A4), levobupivacaine (CYP 3A4, CYP 1A2),[99] and ropivacaine (CYP3A2, CYP3A4, and CYP1A2). [97] Agents that induce or inhibit these enzymes could affect the metabolism, and therefore the plasma concentration, of these drugs. Ester-type local anesthetics are hydrolyzed by plasma cholinesterase and, to a lesser extent, cholinesterase in the liver.[94,95]

Differences in the clinical activity of local anesthetics are explained by other physicochemical properties such as protein binding and pK_a (the pH at which 50% of the drug is present in the un-ionized form and 50% in the ionized form). Agents that are highly protein bound typically have a longer duration of action. Agents with a lower pK_a typically have a faster onset of action.[95]

Choice of local anesthetic is based on the duration of the surgical procedure (e.g., the duration of analgesia required). Usually, a local anesthetic that will, at least minimally, outlast the duration of surgery with a single injection is chosen; a continuous infusion also can be administered for titration of effect with shorter-acting agents. Important physiochemical and pharmacokinetic properties of local anesthetics are shown in Table 10-12.[94,95]

Regional Anesthesia in High-Risk Patients

13. M.S., a 52-year-old, 5′9″, 105-kg African-American man, is undergoing an emergent minor hand repair procedure after a fall-related injury. His medical history is positive for type 1 diabetes mellitus for 41 years, angina, and hypertension. On OR admission, laboratory values of note are as follows: plasma glucose, 240 mg/dL; and BP, 145/92 mm Hg. His sister tells the anesthesia provider that he has been having increasing difficulty walk-

ing up stairs and, of late, is often short of breath. The anesthesia provider chooses to provide regional anesthesia via an axillary block; the anticipated duration of surgery is 2 hours. M.S. agrees with this plan. Why is this a good plan for M.S., and which local anesthetic should be chosen?

[SI unit: glucose, 13.3 mmol/L]

With his medical conditions of diabetes, angina, and hypertension, M.S. is at risk for complications from general or regional anesthesia. General anesthesia is not absolutely necessary in this localized surgery. Regional anesthesia would be beneficial in M.S. because it does not disrupt autonomic function. In addition, his diabetes and obesity, and possibly full stomach (emergency surgery, diabetic gastroparesis), place him at significant risk for aspiration during induction or emergence from general anesthesia. An axillary block with a local anesthetic could provide M.S. with adequate anesthesia and analgesia during and after his procedure.

The local anesthetic of choice is one with a duration at least that of the anticipated surgery and with a good safety profile should systemic absorption inadvertently occur. A local anesthetic containing epinephrine would increase the agent's duration of action and reduce the systemic absorption; however, such an agent is not indicated in M.S. because of his diabetes (peripheral vascular effects) and hypertension (added effect from catecholamine administration). Lidocaine as a single injection without epinephrine has a duration of action that may be too short for M.S.'s procedure. Mepivacaine, an intermediate-acting local anesthetic, or bupivacaine, a long-acting agent, would be good choices to use in M.S.

Topical Cocaine

14. C.J., a 21-year-old woman, is scheduled for rhinoplasty surgery under general anesthesia. The surgeon requests 4% cocaine solution for topical anesthesia. How is cocaine useful in C.J. and what are other alternatives?

Table 10-12 Physicochemical and Pharmacokinetic Properties of Local Anesthetic Agents

Agent	pKa	Potency	Toxicity	Onset	Duration[a]	Maximum Recommended Dose[b]	
						Plain (mg)	With Epinephrine (mg)
Esters							
Cocaine[c]	—	—	—	—	—	1.5 mg/kg	—
Chloroprocaine (Nesacaine)	9.1	Low	Very low	Very fast	Short	800	1,000
Procaine (Novocain)	8.9	Low	Low	Fast	Short	400	600
Tetracaine (Pontocaine)	8.4	High	Moderate	Slow	Very long	100 (topical)	200
Amides							
Bupivacaine (Marcaine, Sensorcaine)	8.1	High	High	Slow	Long	175	225
Etidocaine (Duranest)	7.9	High	Moderate	Fast	Very long	300	400
Levobupivacaine (Chirocaine)	8.1	High	Moderate	Slow	Long	150	—
Lidocaine (Xylocaine)	7.8	Moderate	Moderate	Fast	Moderate	300	500
Mepivacaine (Carbocaine, Polocaine)	7.7	Moderate	Moderate	Moderate	Moderate	300	500
Ropivacaine (Naropin)	8.1	High	Moderate	Slow	Long	300	

[a]Depends on factors such as injection site, dose and addition of epinephrine. In general, a short duration is <1 hour, a moderate duration is 1 to 3 hours, and a long/very long duration of action is 3 to 12 hours when the local anesthetic is administered without epinephrine.
[b]Maximum recommended single dose for infiltration or peripheral nerve block in 70-kg adults.
[c]Topical use only; concentrations >4% are not recommended due to increased risk for systemic adverse effects.
Adapted from references 94 and 95.

Cocaine is unique among local anesthetics in its ability to produce intense and prolonged vasoconstriction in addition to anesthesia. It is indicated only for topical anesthesia of the ear, nose, and throat due to its abuse potential as well as its potential to cause unexpected rapid and severe adverse reactions. When cocaine is applied to mucosal surfaces, systemic absorption occurs. Cocaine, as well as other topical nasal decongestants (phenylephrine, oxymetazoline), effectively constrict nasal blood vessels by their agonist effects at α-adrenergic receptors. These sympathomimetic effects are also responsible for adverse effects such as hypertension, tachycardia, and myocardial infarction (MI).[100] General anesthesia magnifies cocaine's sympathomimetic effects, leading to increased toxicity.[101] Alternatives to cocaine include topical mixtures of another local anesthetic (for anesthesia) and a sympathomimetic agent (for vasoconstriction), such as lidocaine/phenylephrine or tetracaine/oxymetazoline. Such combinations have resulted in effects indiscernible from cocaine itself.[102]

Alkalinization of Local Anesthetics

15. T.F., a 22-year-old man, is scheduled for a hernia repair. He has never undergone surgery and is very anxious. In the preoperative area, the anesthesiologist chooses to locally infiltrate 1% lidocaine to reduce the pain and discomfort from IV catheter placement. Can the speed of onset of local anesthetic be shortened?

The onset of action of local anesthetics depends on their pK_a. Drugs with pK_as closest to body pH (7.4) will have the fastest onset, because a high percentage of the local anesthetic molecules will be unionized and therefore able to cross the nerve membranes to their intracellular site of action. Local anesthetics are formulated in solutions with acidic pHs to optimize their shelf-lives. When sodium bicarbonate is added to local anesthetic solutions, the pH is increased, the percentage of unionized drug is increased, and the onset of local anesthetic action can be shortened considerably. The amount of bicarbonate added to the solution depends on the pH of the local anesthetic agent. Because too much sodium bicarbonate will precipitate the local anesthetic, a dose of 0.1 mEq (0.1 mL of a 1 mEq/mL concentration) of sodium bicarbonate is added to 10 mL of bupivacaine, whereas 1 mEq (1 mL of a 1 mEq/ml concentration) is added to 10 mL of lidocaine.[100,102] Furthermore, alkalinized lidocaine can be significantly less painful for subcutaneous injection before IV catheter placement when compared with lidocaine at pH 5 (its normal pH in a vial for storage).[103]

CARDIOPLEGIA SOLUTION

Use in Cardiac Surgery

Hypothermic, hyperkalemic cardioplegia solution was first used in open-heart surgery in the 1970s and enjoys widespread clinical use today. Cardioplegia solution is infused into the coronary vasculature to produce an elective diastolic cardiac arrest. Inducing cardiac arrest, or cardioplegia, helps protect the myocardium while providing the surgeon with a still, bloodless operative field and a flaccid heart on which to work. Cardioplegia solution is administered via the cardiopulmonary-bypass pump through specialized circuits.

During open-heart surgery, the heart is excluded from normal circulation by diverting venous blood away from the right atrium via gravity drainage and by clamping the aorta. Systemic circulation of blood is maintained through the use of the cardiopulmonary-bypass pump; a cannula is placed in the aorta distal to the clamp and carries oxygenated blood from the pump to the patient. The blood circulates through the body and is returned to the cardiopulmonary-bypass pump through cannulas inserted into the superior and inferior venae cava.

Delivery Methods

Cardioplegia solution is delivered to the coronary circulation by three approaches: antegrade, retrograde, or a combination antegrade/retrograde. With antegrade administration, the solution is administered via a cannula placed in the aortic root, whereas with retrograde administration, the cannula is placed in the coronary sinus.[104] The commonly used combination approach eliminates problems such as the nonhomogeneous distribution of cardioplegia solution, which can occur with the antegrade approach, while still ensuring a rapid arrest (arrest produced by retrograde administration is not as fast as antegrade).[105,106] This approach has significantly reduced patient morbidity when compared with antegrade administration, especially in high-risk patients requiring reoperation.[105]

Phases of Cardioplegia

Cardioplegia can be divided into three phases: induction of arrest, maintenance of arrest, and reperfusion (immediately before aortic unclamping). Cardioplegia solution is used routinely during the induction and maintenance phases, and reperfusion solution is used at the end of surgery before aortic unclamping. The solutions used in each phase may differ in composition and characteristics.

Goal of Treatment

Cardioplegia solution is used to prevent myocardial ischemic damage that can occur during the induction and maintenance of arrest, whereas reperfusion solution is used to help prevent and minimize the destructive phenomena that can occur during reperfusion. Myocardial ischemia can result in a number of detrimental changes to the heart, including rapid cellular conversion from aerobic to anaerobic metabolism, high-energy phosphate (e.g., adenosine triphosphate [ATP]) depletion, intracellular acidosis, calcium influx, and myocardial cell membrane disruption. Destructive changes that can occur during reperfusion include intracellular calcium accumulation, explosive cell swelling, and inability to use delivered oxygen.[107] Chemical components are added to cardioplegia solution to counteract the specific cellular effects of ischemia as well as the cellular events that can occur during reperfusion.

Cardioplegia Solution Vehicles

The chemical composition of a cardioplegia solution depends on the vehicle used: blood or crystalloid. Each has advantages and disadvantages as can be seen in Table 10-13.[104,105,108] Blood, because of its many advantages, is the vehicle most commonly used. Blood cardioplegia provides oxygen while the heart is arrested, proteins in blood maintain osmotic pressures closer to normal and are capable of serving as buffers, and endogenous oxygen free-radical scavengers are beneficial during reperfusion.[108] The disadvantages listed for blood have not been shown to occur during clinical use of blood-based cardioplegia solution. The patient's own hemodiluted blood from the extracorporeal circuit is used. Blood-based cardioplegia solution delivery systems deliver a fixed ratio of blood with a premixed crystalloid cardioplegia solution. Ratios of blood to crystalloid composition range from 1:1 to 8:1. The concentration of additives in the crystalloid solution must be tailored to the specific delivery ratio used to prevent accidental overdosage or underdosage. A commonly used ratio in clinical practice today is 4:1; in other words, the blood-based cardioplegia solution being delivered to the patient contains four parts blood to one part crystalloid solution. Therefore, the concentration of additives contained in the crystalloid solution is five times greater than that actually delivered to the patient due to the dilution of this solution with blood before it reaches the patient. Furthermore, with blood-based cardioplegia solution, there is a reduced need to place additives in the crystalloid component of the solution. For example, calcium and magnesium need not be added to the crystalloid component because sufficient quantities are contained in blood.

Common Characteristics

Most cardioplegia solutions have certain basic characteristics in common. Crystalloid cardioplegia solutions are made hyperosmolar to help minimize myocardial edema associated with cardiac arrest and usually are made slightly basic to compensate for the metabolic acidosis that accompanies myocardial ischemia. Cardioplegia solutions are traditionally chilled to a temperature of 4 to 8°C before being infused into the coronary circulation. Hypothermia decelerates the metabolic activity of the heart, reduces myocardial oxygen demand and the detrimental effects seen with myocardial ischemia, and helps maintain cardiac arrest.[109,110] However, hypothermia also can produce deleterious effects on the heart, which in-

clude impaired mitochondrial energy generation and substrate utilization; membrane destabilization; and the need for a longer period of reperfusion to rewarm the heart, which can increase the chances of reperfusion injury. In an effort to minimize the adverse consequences of hypothermia, the use of normothermic cardioplegia solution for induction of arrest (with cardioplegia maintained with a hypothermic solution) and the administration of a normothermic reperfusion solution before aortic cross clamp removal was demonstrated to improve myocardial metabolic and functional recovery in energy depleted hearts.[108] The benefits seen with this technique prompted investigators to study the use of intermittent, normothermic (37°C) cardioplegia. Positive results were reported with this technique and included a decreased incidence of perioperative MI and need for intra-aortic balloon pump (IABP) support, as well as a lower incidence of postoperative low cardiac output syndrome.[111,112] However, studies examining the use of normothermic cardioplegia solution have not consistently demonstrated a decrease in mortality or perioperative MI when compared with hypothermic cardioplegia solution. With normothermic cardioplegia, a major concern is that not as much protection from ischemia is provided during the time that cardioplegia solution is not being infused as that provided with the use of hypothermic solution. Furthermore, when compared with hypothermic cardioplegia solution, warm cardioplegia is associated with a greater use of crystalloid and α-agonists to maintain perfusion pressure, higher total volumes of cardioplegia, increased use of high potassium cardioplegia to stop periodic episodes of electrical activity, a higher incidence of systemic hyperkalemia, and lower systemic vascular resistance.[113] In an attempt to reduce problems seen with normothermic cardioplegia, the use of tepid (29°C) cardioplegia solution has been advocated. When compared with hypothermic techniques, tepid cardioplegia resulted in greater left and right ventricular stroke work indices (slightly less than normothermic cardioplegia) and a much faster recovery of

Table 10-13   Advantages and Disadvantages of Cardioplegia Solution Vehicles

Vehicle	Advantages	Disadvantages
Blood	Oxygen-carrying capacity	Possible sludging at low temperatures
	Active resuscitation	Possible unfavorable shift in oxyhemoglobin association curve
	Reduction in systemic hemodilution	Potential for poor distribution of solution beyond coronary stenoses
	Avoidance of reperfusion damage	Possible RBC crenation
	Provision of inherent buffering, oncotic, and rheologic effects	
	Provision of physiologic calcium concentration	
	Presence of endogenous oxygen-free radical scavengers	
Crystalloid	History of effectiveness	Minimal oxygen-carrying capacity
	Ease of solution preparation	Possible damage of coronary endothelium
	Low cost	Reduced efficacy (compared with blood) in preserving left ventricular function postoperatively
	Minimal potential for capillary obstruction	Systemic hemodilution
		Possible role in production of late myocardial fibrosis

RBC, red blood cell.
Adapted from references 104 and 105.

myocardial function.[114,115] Currently, a combination normothermic/hypothermic technique is still used more frequently in practice. Additional work is needed in this area.

Additives

Table 10-14 presents additives commonly used in cardioplegia and/or reperfusion solutions, the reason for their addition, and frequently used concentrations.[104,105] In addition to these additives, several other classes of agents continue to be examined for their usefulness in cardioplegia and/or reperfusion solutions.

Oxygen-Free Radical Scavengers

Oxygen-free radicals (e.g., superoxide anion, hydrogen peroxide, free hydroxyl radical) are released during the sudden reintroduction of oxygen to ischemic tissue during reperfusion. They have been implicated in myocyte death, reperfusion-induced arrhythmias, and prolonged left ventricular dysfunction after reperfusion.[107] The addition to reperfusion solution of drugs that inhibit oxygen-free radical production or degrade free radicals (e.g., mannitol, deferoxamine, allopurinol) has been demonstrated to reduce post-reperfusion myocardial injury and other free-radical induced surgical complications.[116–118] An advantage of using blood-based cardioplegia solution is that blood contains endogenous oxygen-free radical scavengers (e.g., catalase, superoxide dismutase, glutathione).[119]

Adenosine

Adenosine is an endogenous nucleoside that is released from the ischemic myocardium during the catabolism of ATP. It protects the heart from ischemic and reperfusion injury and may have a role in ischemic preconditioning. Adenosine produces the majority of its effects through interaction at the adenosine A1, A2, and A3 receptors. Stimulation of A1 receptors causes activation of the ATP-sensitive potassium channel (K-ATP), ultimately resulting in positive chronotropic and dromotropic effects, antiadrenergic effects, stimulation of glycogenolysis, and stimulation of neutrophil adherence. Stimulation of A2 receptors results in vasodilation, renin release, inhibition of neutrophil adherence to endothelium, and inhibition of superoxide generation. The physiologic effects of stimulation of A3 receptors include inhibition of neutrophil adherence to endothelium.[120] The cardioprotective effects during preconditioning are believed to be the result of K-ATP channel activation. Preliminary results of a phase II trial found that adenosine may improve postoperative hemodynamic function and possibly reduce morbidity and mortality when patients receive IV adenosine immediately before and after aortic cross-clamping in addition to cold blood cardioplegia containing 2 mM adenosine.[121] However, further multicenter studies are needed to identify patients who will benefit the most from adenosine and if adenosine will definitively reduce the incidence of myocardial infarction or death following open heart surgery.

Table 10-14 Commonly Used Cardioplegia Solution Additives

Additive	Frequently Used Concentration[a]	Function
Amino acid substrates (glutamate/aspartate[b])	11–12 mL/L[c]	Improves myocardial metabolism; improves metabolic and functional recovery in energy-depleted hearts
Calcium	At least trace amounts (0.1 mEq/L)	Maintains integrity of myocardial cell membrane; prevents "calcium paradox"[d]
Chloride	90–110 mEq/L	Establishes a solution similar in composition to extracellular fluid
CPD solution	12 mL/L[e] 45 mL/L[c]	Chelates calcium in blood-based cardioplegia solution to produce safe levels of hypocalcemia for rapid diastolic arrest; limits postischemic calcium accumulation and improves postischemic performance
Glucose	5–10 g/L safely used	Helps achieve desired osmolarity of solution; serves as a metabolic substrate for the heart
Magnesium	32 mEq/L	Reduces magnesium loss during ischemia; reduces calcium influx and potassium efflux during ischemia; has a weak arresting action on heart
Potassium	15–30 mEq/L[f]	Induces rapid diastolic arrest
Sodium	120–140 mEq/L	Necessary for protective action of potassium; establishes a solution similar in composition to extracellular fluid
Sodium bicarbonate or THAM	Variable; added until desired pH is obtained	Provides buffering capacity; helps maintain physiologically normal pH range; counters acidosis produced by ischemia

[a]Concentration delivered to patient; concentration dependent on other cardioplegia solution additives (concentration of any one additive may be changed by inclusion of other additives).
[b]Not commercially available in parenteral formulation; each mL of solution contains 178.4 mg monosodium L-glutamate and 163.4 mg monosodium L-aspartate (for preparation directions, see reference 104).
[c]Warm, blood-based induction and reperfusion solutions.
[d]Calcium paradox is a condition that results in rapid consumption of high-energy phosphates, extensive ultrastructural damage of myocardial cells, and myocardial contracture; it results from an influx of calcium into the myocardial cells, resulting from the introduction of a calcium-containing perfusate (i.e., blood) into the system during reperfusion after the use of a cardioplegia solution completely lacking in calcium.
[e]Cold, blood-based induction and maintenance solutions.
[f]Lower concentrations (5 to 10 mEq/L) used during maintenance phase.
CPD, citrate-phosphate-dextrose; THAM, trihydroxymethylaminomethane.
Adapted from references 104 and 105.

L-Arginine

Ischemia results in decreased formation of nitric oxide; nitric oxide helps prevent neutrophils from adhering to the vascular endothelial cells. Neutrophil adhesion to the coronary endothelium is a prerequisite for neutrophil activation and accumulation in the myocardium. Activated neutrophils may be a major source of oxygen-free radical production; they enhance degranulation and the release of proteases, which cause cellular damage; and they adhere to microvascular endothelium or embolize in the microcirculation. Nitric oxide–dependent vasodilation and inhibition of neutrophil activity are thought to play important roles in preventing reperfusion damage after ischemia.

L-arginine is a nitric oxide donor and may have a role as a supplement to cardioplegia and/or reperfusion solutions. Animal studies have demonstrated benefits (reduction in oxygen-free radical formation, restoration of endothelial function) from the addition of L-arginine to cardioplegia solutions.[122–124] Limited trials in patients undergoing coronary artery bypass grafting have demonstrated that the addition of L-arginine (7.5 g/500mL) to blood cardioplegia reduced the release of cardiac troponin T, a marker of myocardial ischemia.[125]

Potassium

16. W.D., a 64-year-old man, ASA-III, is scheduled to undergo a coronary artery bypass graft (CABG). W.D.'s serum potassium concentration is 4 mEq/L. A blood-based cardioplegia solution is ordered for the patient with the concentration of potassium in the crystalloid component to be 76 mEq/1,000 mL. Cold induction (e.g., chilled cardioplegia solution) using a delivery system of 4 parts blood to 1 part cardioplegia solution will be used. Upon administration of the solution to W.D., cardiac arrest was not achieved. A STAT chemical analysis of the crystalloid solution revealed that it contained no potassium. Why is this consistent with the findings in W.D.?

Failure to see immediate arrest within 1 to 2 minutes after the administration of cardioplegia solution can be due to several factors, including incomplete aortic clamping, aortic insufficiency, and failure to have a potassium concentration sufficient to produce arrest. Because W.D.'s cardioplegia solution contained no potassium, a direct cause-and-effect relationship can be made to the inability to achieve an arrest.

Potassium's major role in cardioplegia solution is to induce a rapid diastolic arrest by blocking the inward sodium current and initial phases of cellular depolarization. This results in cessation of electromechanical activity and helps preserve ATP and creatine phosphate stores for postischemic work. A delivered potassium concentration in the range of 15 to 20 mEq/L is used most commonly. This concentration consistently has produced asystole while minimizing adverse effects (e.g., tissue damage, systemic hyperkalemia). Potassium concentrations >40 mEq/L alter myocardial cell membranes, allow extracellular calcium to enter the cell, and raise energy demands.[126] In laboratory studies, high concentrations of potassium (>100 mEq/L) increase myocardial contracture and wall tension, a condition referred to as *stone heart syndrome*.[127] Varying concentrations of potassium are used in the cardioplegia solution depending on the phase of cardioplegia. As previously discussed, a high concentration of potassium is

required to induce arrest, whereas lower concentrations (e.g., 5 to 10 mEq/L) are sufficient to maintain arrest.[128] On first glance, the concentration of potassium ordered in W.D.'s blood-based cardioplegia solution appears excessive. However, the concentration delivered to the coronary circulation is slightly <20 mEq/L if one considers that the potassium contribution from the blood component of this blood-based cardioplegia solution is approximately 4 mEq/L and that from the crystalloid component is approximately 15 mEq/L (76 mEq/L ÷5). This highlights the importance of knowing the delivery ratio being used for the administration of blood-based cardioplegia solution.

Amino Acids: Normothermic, Blood-Based Cardioplegia Solution

17. T.E., a 55-year-old man, ASA-IV, is admitted to the hospital with a MI. He currently is in the coronary care unit and is scheduled for myocardial revascularization surgery. He has poor left ventricular function (cardiac output, 2.2 L/min [normal, 4 to 6 L/min]; pulmonary capillary wedge pressure, 25 mm Hg [normal, 5 to 12 mm Hg]; left ventricular ejection fraction, 25% [normal, >60%]), and is on an IABP for circulatory support. In addition to being on the IABP, he is receiving dopamine and milrinone. A diagnosis of cardiogenic shock is made. What type of cardioplegia solution should T.E. receive during his revascularization surgery?

Normothermic (37°C), blood-based cardioplegia and reperfusion solutions containing the amino acids, glutamate and aspartate, have been advocated for the induction and reperfusion phases of cardioplegia in patients with ischemic hearts (e.g., extending MI, cardiogenic shock, hemodynamic instability) or those with advanced left or right ventricular hypertrophy or dysfunction.[129–131] Glutamate and aspartate, Krebs' cycle precursors, are added to cardioplegia solution to counteract the depletion of Krebs' cycle intermediates during myocardial ischemia and to enhance energy production during reperfusion.[129,131,132] These agents enhance oxidative metabolism optimally at normothermia (37°C).[132]

With this technique, cardioplegia induction is accomplished with an infusion of the normothermic, blood-based cardioplegia solution over 5 minutes. Normothermia optimizes the rate of cellular repair, whereas glutamate and aspartate improve oxygen utilization capacity.[118] The normothermic solution is immediately followed by a 5-minute infusion of hypothermic, blood-based cardioplegia solution. Cardioplegia is maintained with hypothermic, blood-based solution. Normothermic reperfusion solution is administered for 3 to 5 minutes immediately before aortic unclamping (reperfusion). The administration of normothermic solution at the conclusion of surgery is referred to by some as a *hot shot* and is felt to result in early resumption of temperature-dependent mitochondrial enzymatic function and to allow energy supplies to be channeled into cellular recovery rather than electromechanical work. This results in improved hemodynamic and myocardial metabolic recovery.[132,133]

T.E., with his poor myocardial function, is a suitable candidate to receive amino acid–enriched, normothermic, blood-based cardioplegia solution and reperfusion solution during the induction and reperfusion phases of cardioplegia, respectively.

Antiemetic Agents and Postoperative Nausea and Vomiting

Impact of Postoperative Nausea and Vomiting

PONV is a relatively common (overall incidence, 25% to 30%) yet highly undesirable anesthetic and surgical outcome. Patients who develop PONV are greatly dissatisfied with their surgical experience and require additional resources such as nursing time and medical/surgical supplies. PONV typically lasts <24 hours; however, symptom distress can continue at home, thereby preventing the patient from resuming normal activities or returning to work.[134] It is important to remember that nausea is a separate subjective sensation and is not always followed by vomiting. Nausea can be as, or more, distressing to patients as vomiting.

Mechanisms of and Factors Affecting Postoperative Nausea and Vomiting

The vomiting center is reflex activated through the chemoreceptor trigger zone (CTZ). Input from other sources can also stimulate the vomiting center. Afferent impulses from the periphery (e.g., manipulation of the eye, oropharynx, gastroin-testinal tract), the cerebral cortex (e.g., unpleasant tastes, sights, smells, emotions), and the endocrine environment (e.g., female gender) can also stimulate the vomiting center. In addition, disturbances in vestibular function (e.g., movement after surgery, middle ear surgery) can stimulate the vomiting center via direct central pathways. Neurotransmitter receptors that play an important role in impulse transmission to the vomiting center include dopamine type 2 (D_2), serotonin ($5HT_3$), muscarinic cholinergic (M_1), and histamine type 1 (H_1) (Fig. 10-1).[135-140] The vestibular apparatus is rich in M_1 and H_1 receptors. Opioid analgesics can activate the CTZ, as well as the vestibular apparatus, to produce nausea and vomiting.[134-137]

PONV probably is not caused by a single event, entity, or mechanism; instead, the cause is likely to be multifactorial. Factors that place a patient at risk for developing PONV have been identified by a consensus panel based on the published evidence and expert opinion. Independent risk factors for developing PONV in adults include female gender, history of PONV or motion sickness, nonsmoking status, use of opioids, type of surgery, duration of surgery, and general anesthesia with inhalation anesthetic agents and/or nitrous oxide.[140] For children, risk factors are similar to adults; the risk increases with the age of the child, but there is no difference in risk

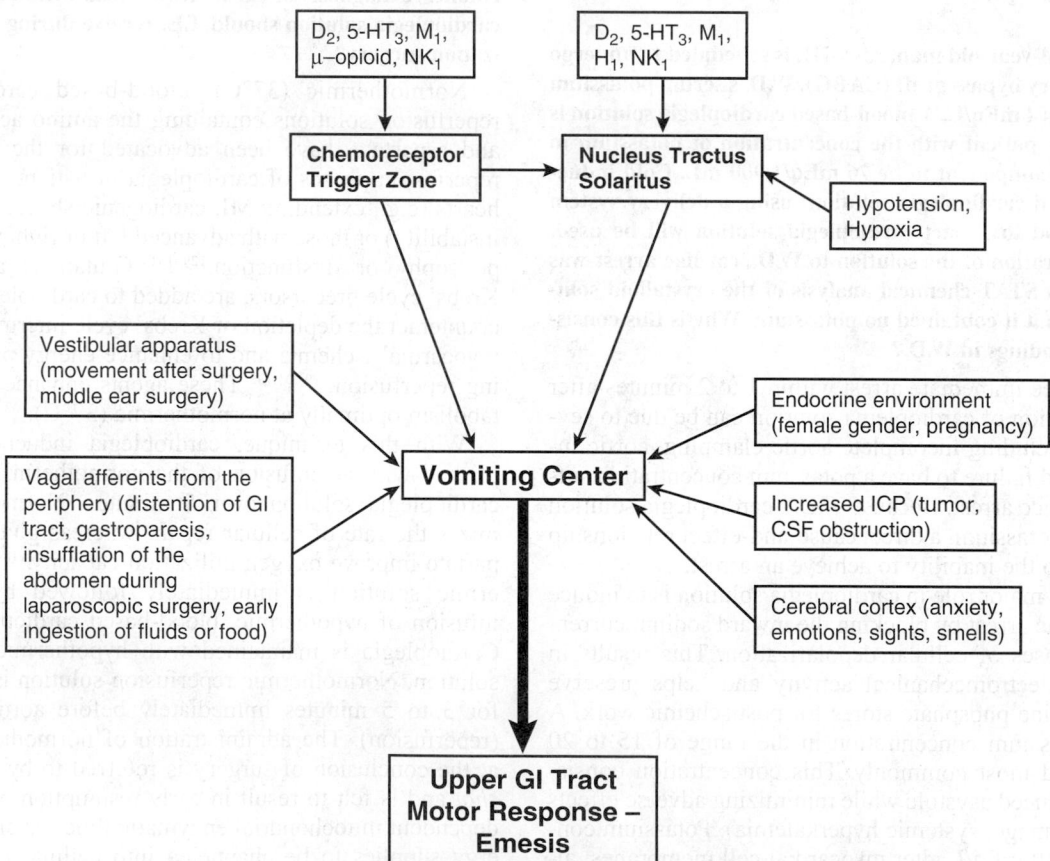

FIGURE 10-1 **Mechanisms and neurotransmitters of postoperative nausea and vomiting.** The chemoreceptor trigger zone (CTZ) is located in the area postrema of the midbrain. The vomiting center is also located in the midbrain, close to the nucleus tractus solaritus (NTS) and the area postrema. The CTZ, NTS, and area postrema are rich in $5-HT_3$, H_1, M_1, D_2, and μ-opioid receptors. Antiemetic agents used to manage postoperative nausea and vomiting block one or more of these receptors. $5HT_3$, serotonin type 3 receptor; H_1, histamine type 1 receptor; M_1, muscarinic cholinergic type 1 receptor; D_2, dopamine type 2 receptor; NK_1, substance P neurokinin type 1 receptor; GI, gastrointestinal; ICP, intracranial pressure; CSF, cerebral spinal fluid. (Adapted from references 135–139.)

based on gender. Unlike adults, nausea is not easily measured in children and hence not routinely assessed.

18. J.E., a 34-year-old, 55-kg woman, is scheduled to undergo a gynecologic laparoscopy under general anesthesia on an outpatient basis. She has had one previous surgery, has no known medication allergies, and is a nonsmoker. Upon questioning, she reports that she developed PONV following her first surgery. Her physical examination is unremarkable. Is J.E. a candidate for prophylactic antiemetic therapy?

J.E. has several risk factors that make her susceptible to developing PONV. Adult women are two to three times more likely than adult men to develop PONV. Previous PONV also increases the likelihood of developing PONV threefold. In addition, a nonsmoking status increases the risk of developing PONV. The type of procedure J.E. is undergoing (gynecologic laparoscopy) places her at a higher risk for developing PONV. Finally, J.E. is scheduled for general anesthesia, which is also associated with a greater risk of PONV when compared with regional anesthesia. Because of the presence of these risk factors, J.E. should be administered a prophylactic antiemetic agent. Patients undergoing surgery view PONV as a highly undesirable consequence, thereby reducing their overall level of satisfaction.

Prevention of Postoperative Nausea and Vomiting: Choice of Agent

19. Which antiemetic drug(s) would be most appropriate for J.E., and when should it (they) be administered?

Antiemetic drugs can be classified as antimuscarinics (scopolamine, promethazine, diphenhydramine, dimenhydrinate), serotonin antagonists (ondansetron, dolasetron, granisetron), benzamides (metoclopramide), butyrophenones (droperidol), phenothiazines (prochlorperazine), and miscellaneous agents. These drugs exert their antiemetic effects primarily by blocking one central neurotransmitter receptor. Dopamine antagonists include the benzamides, butyrophenones, and phenothiazines. Ondansetron, granisetron, and dolasetron block $5HT_3$ receptors of vagal afferent nerves in the GI tract and in the CTZ. Antimuscarinics likely exert their antiemetic effect by blocking acetylcholine in the vestibular apparatus, vomiting center, and CTZ, making these agents particularly useful for preventing and treating nausea and vomiting following procedures involving the vestibular apparatus (e.g., middle ear surgery).[134,136] The proposed site of action, usual adult dose, and select adverse effects of the commonly used antiemetic drugs for prevention and treatment of PONV are summarized in Table 10-15.[6,136,141,142]

Butyrophenones

Droperidol possesses significant antiemetic activity, with IV doses of 0.625 to 1.25 mg effectively preventing PONV. Droperidol is more effective for nausea than vomiting, even at a dose as low as 0.3 mg. Droperidol has an onset of action of 3 to 10 minutes, with peak effects seen at 30 minutes. Doses of 0.625 or 1.25 mg prevent PONV for up to 24 hours. The duration of action of a 0.3 mg dose, however, is short-lived, with repeated doses often necessary. Droperidol is most effective when administered near the end of surgery. Adverse

effects include sedation (especially at doses $\geq$2.5 mg), anxiety, hypotension, and rarely, restlessness or other extrapyramidal (EP) reactions.[143] Because of its effectiveness and cost, droperidol historically has been extensively used as a first-line agent. However, in December 2001, the FDA strengthened warnings regarding adverse cardiac events following droperidol administration. With the new warning to perform continuous 12-lead electrocardiographic monitoring before and for 2 to 3 hours following administration of droperidol, it became an issue, from both an expense and logistical viewpoint, to administer droperidol to an outpatient, patient in the postanesthesia care unit (recovery room), or a patient in an unmonitored bed. Many anesthesia providers challenged the decision of the FDA to issue this "black-box" warning.[144] Under the Freedom of Information Act, Habib and Gan[145] reviewed the FDA MedWatch forms submitted regarding serious cardiac adverse events or deaths associated with low-dose ($\leq$1.25 mg) droperidol. These authors concluded that there was no evidence of a cause-and-effect relationship in any of the 10 cases in which $\leq$1.25 mg of droperidol was administered.

Benzamides

Metoclopramide, in doses of 10 to 20 mg, has been used in the prevention and treatment of PONV. However, variable results have been seen with this agent.[146] For maximum benefit, metoclopramide must be administered near the end of surgery (secondary to its rapid redistribution after IV administration); 10 mg IV administered at the beginning of surgery is not effective.[146] Adverse effects of metoclopramide include drowsiness and EP reactions, such as anxiety and restlessness Metoclopramide should be administered by slow intravenous injection over at least 2 minutes to minimize the risk of EP reactions and cardiovascular effects such as hypotension, bradycardia, and supraventricular tachycardia.

Serotonin Antagonists

Ondansetron (4 mg intravenously) was the first $5HT_3$ antagonist to receive an indication for PONV. Dolasetron (12.5 mg intravenously) and granisetron (1 mg intravenously) are also approved for preventing and treating PONV. Serotonin antagonists are consistently more effective in reducing vomiting rather than nausea.[147] Ondansetron and dolasetron are equally efficacious in preventing[147] and treating[148] PONV, with dolasetron having been demonstrated to have a lower cost.[147] A single dose of ondansetron, dolasetron, or granisetron provides acute relief and can protect against nausea and vomiting for up to 24 hours after administration. For optimal efficacy, serotonin antagonists should be administered near the end of surgery. Adverse effects are minimal and include headache, constipation, and elevated liver enzymes.[141] Because of their good efficacy and adverse effect profile, serotonin antagonists are recommended as first-line therapy.[149]

Serotonin antagonists are significantly more expensive than the traditional antiemetic agents (prochlorperazine, promethazine, metoclopramide, droperidol). Serotonin antagonists should be used only in patients at moderate to high risk for PONV.

Dexamethasone

Dexamethasone is frequently used as an antiemetic in patients undergoing highly emetogenic chemotherapy. Its mechanism

Table 10-15 Classification, Proposed Site(s) of Action, Usual Dose, and Adverse Effects of Select Antiemetic Drugs

Antiemetic Drug	Proposed Receptor Site of Action	Usual Dose[a]	Duration of Action	Adverse Effects	Comments and Recommendations for Use
Butyrophenones Droperidol (Inapsine)	D_2	*Adult:* 0.625–1.25 mg IV *Pediatric:* 20–50 µg/kg IV	12–24 hr	Sedation, hypotension (especially in hypovolemic patients), EPS	Monitor ECG for QT prolongation/torsades de pointes
Phenothiazines Prochlorperazine (Compazine)	D_2	*Adult:* 5–10 mg IM or IV; 25 mg PR *Pediatric:*[b] 0.13 mg/kg IM, 0.1 mg/kg PO, 2.5 mg PR	2–6 hr (12 hr when given PR)	Sedation, hypotension (especially in hypovolemic patients), EPS	Effective first-line agent
Antimuscarinics Promethazine (Phenergan)	D_2, H_1, M_1	*Adult:* 6.25–25 mg IM, IV, or PR *Pediatric* (>2yr of age): 0.25–0.5 mg/kg IV, IM, PR[c]	4 hr	Sedation, hypotension (especially in hypovolemic patients), EPS	Good for patients with motion sickness or undergoing surgery affecting the vestibular apparatus
Diphenhydramine (Benadryl)	H_1, M_1	*Adult:* 12.5–50 mg IM or IV *Pediatric:* 1mg/kg IV, PO (max, 25 mg for <6 yr old)	4–6 hr	Sedation, dry mouth, blurred vision, urinary retention	Good for patients with motion sickness or undergoing surgery affecting the vestibular apparatus
Dimenhydrinate (Dramamine)	H_1, M_1	*Adult:* 50–100 mg IV, IM *Pediatric:* 1.25 mg/kg IV,IM[a]	6–8 hr	Sedation, dry mouth, blurred vision, urinary retention	Good for patients with motion sickness or undergoing surgery affecting the vestibular apparatus
Scopolamine (Transderm Scop)	M_1	*Adult:* 1.5 mg transdermal patch *Pediatric:* N/A	72 hr[a]	Sedation, dry mouth, visual disturbances, dysphoria, confusion, disorientation, hallucinations	Good for patients with motion sickness or undergoing surgery affecting the vestibular apparatus; therapeutic plasma levels are obtained 4 hr after patch is placed

Drug	Receptor	Dose[a]	Duration	Side effects	Comments
Benzamides					
Metoclopramide (Reglan)	D$_2$	Adult: 20 mg IV Pediatric: 0.25 mg/kg IV	6–8 hr	Sedation, hypotension, EPS	Good if N/V is due to gastric stasis; reduce dose to 5 mg in renal impairment; give slow IV push
Serotonin Antagonists					
Ondansetron (Zofran)	5-HT$_3$	Adult: 4 mg IV Pediatric: 0.05–0.1mg/kg IV	Up to 24 hr	Headache, lightheadedness	Much more effective for vomiting than nausea
Dolasetron (Anzemet)	5-HT$_3$	Adult: 12.5 mg IV Pediatric: 0.35 mg/kg IV	Up to 24 hr	Headache, lightheadedness	Much more effective for vomiting than nausea
Granisetron (Kytril)	5-HT$_3$	Adult: 1 mg IV Pediatric: Not known	Up to 24 hr	Headache, lightheadedness	Much more effective for vomiting than nausea
Other					
Trimethobenzamide (Tigan)	? (Probably M$_1$, D$_2$)	Adult: 200 mg IM or PR Pediatric: 5mg/kg PR	6–8 hr	Sedation, hypotension, blurred vision	Probably less effective than traditional agents
Dexamethasone (Decadron)	None	Adult: 4–8 mg IV Pediatric: 0.5–1mg/kg IV	Up to 24 hr	Watch blood sugar in diabetics; watch for fluid retention in cardiac patients	Well tolerated in healthy patients
Propofol (Diprivan)	None	Adult: 10–20 mg IV Pediatric: N/A	<10 min	Sedation	Very short acting

[a]Unless otherwise indicated, pediatric doses should not exceed adult doses.

[b]Children >10 kg or >2 years of age only. Change from IM to oral as soon as possible. When administering PR, the dosing interval varies from 8 to 24 hours depending on the child's weight.

[c]Maximum of 12.5 mg in children younger than 12 years of age.

[d]Children >2 years of age only. Do not exceed 75 mg/dose or 300 mg/day.

[e]Remove after 24 hours. Instruct patient to wash the site where the patch was, as well as their hands, thoroughly.

5-HT$_3$, serotonin type 3 receptor; D$_2$, dopamine type 2 receptor; ECG, electrocardiogram; EPS, extrapyramidal symptoms such as motor restlessness or acute dystonia; H$_1$, histamine type 1 receptor; IV, intravenous; IM, intramuscular; M$_1$, muscarinic cholinergic type 1; N/A, not applicable; N/V, nausea and/or vomiting; PO, per os (by mouth); PR, per rectum.

Adapted from references 6, 136, and 140–142.

of action as an antiemetic is not well understood, particularly in the surgical setting. When compared to placebo, a prophylactic dose of dexamethasone is antiemetic in high-risk patients. It is most effective in preventing late PONV (up to 24 hours). Adverse effects in otherwise healthy patients are minimal and include headache, dizziness, drowsiness, constipation, and muscle pain.[150] Because of dexamethasone's good efficacy and adverse effect profile (from a single dose), dexamethasone is also recommended as first-line therapy.[149] The optimal dose has not been established; doses less than 2.5mg do not appear to be effective.[151] Unlike droperidol and the serotonin antagonists, dexamethasone is most effective when administered at the beginning of surgery (immediately before induction).[152]

Phenothiazines

Prochlorperazine has been used successfully to prevent PONV. Prochlorperazine (10 mg intramuscularly) was found to have superior efficacy (less nausea and vomiting as well as need for rescue antiemetics) when compared with ondansetron for preventing PONV; cost savings were significant.[153] Prochlorperazine may cause sedation, EP reactions, and cardiovascular effects. Because it has a short duration of action, multiple doses may be necessary.

Antimuscarinics

Promethazine and dimenhydrate (contains equimolar proportions of diphenhydramine and chlorotheophylline) are useful for prevention and treatment of nausea, vomiting, and motion sickness. These agents primarily exert their antiemetic effects by blocking acetylcholine in the vestibular apparatus, as well as H_1 and M_1 receptors that activate the CTZ. For this reason, promethazine and dimenhydrate are particularly useful for preventing and treating vomiting following procedures involving the vestibular apparatus (e.g., middle ear surgery, ambulation after surgery). In a meta-analysis of 18 trials involving more than 3,000 patients, dimenhydrate was effective in preventing PONV when compared with placebo.[154] Excessive sedation is the primary concern that can limit the usefulness of these agents.

Scopolamine blocks afferent impulses at the vomiting center and blocks acetylcholine in the vestibular apparatus and CTZ. Like promethazine and dimenhydrate, transdermal scopolamine is useful for prevention of nausea, vomiting, and motion sickness. Compared with placebo, transdermal scopolamine effectively reduces the incidence of emetic symptoms.[155] Common side effects include dry mouth and visual disturbances. Patients can also have trouble correctly applying the patch. It is important to apply the patch before surgery because its onset of effect is 4 hours. Patients should also be instructed to wash their hands after applying the patch and how to dispose of the patch properly.

Combination of Agents

As discussed, droperidol, serotonin antagonists, dexamethasone, dimenhydrate, promethazine, and transdermal scopolamine effectively prevent PONV. However, these agents fail to prevent PONV in approximately 20% to 30% of patients. Most of the agents effectively block one receptor thought to be involved in the activation of the vomiting center. However, because the cause of PONV is likely multifactorial, a combi-

nation of antiemetic agents may be more efficacious for preventing PONV in a high-risk patient.

For prophylaxis of PONV, J.E. should receive dexamethasone 4 to 8 mg IV just before induction of anesthesia and dolasetron 12.5 mg IV 30 minutes before the end of surgery because she is at high risk for developing PONV. This combination can shorten the time in the ambulatory surgery center and improve the quality of recovery and patient satisfaction when compared with dolasetron alone.[156] Alternatively, if J.E. had a history of motion sickness, dexamethasone in combination with either promethazine 25 mg IV, transdermal scopolamine (applied at least 4 hours before the end of surgery), or dimenhydrate 50 to 100 mg IV would be appropriate first-line therapy.

Treatment of Postoperative Nausea and Vomiting

20. J.E. is taken to surgery. Anesthesia is induced with thiopental and maintained with isoflurane. Fentanyl is administered intraoperatively for analgesia. A prophylactic dose of dexamethasone is administered at the beginning of surgery, and dolasetron is administered near the end of surgery. Neuromuscular blockade produced by vecuronium is reversed with neostigmine and glycopyrrolate. In the recovery room, J.D. becomes nauseated and has several emetic episodes. What do you recommend?

Although dexamethasone and dolasetron are effective for both prevention and treatment of PONV, a rescue antiemetic is more efficacious if it works by a different mechanism of action.[157] Prophylactic dexamethasone and/or dolasetron should be effective for up to 24 hours. If nausea and emetic episodes occur in the recovery room, the prophylactic antiemetic agents were ineffective. Phenothiazines (prochlorperazine) and benzamides (metoclopramide) block dopaminergic stimulation of the CTZ, making these agents appropriate for J.E. Prochlorperazine may be preferred because metoclopramide's primary effect is in the gastrointestinal tract rather than the CTZ. Dimenhydrate, diphenhydramine, or promethazine, which block acetylcholine receptors in the vestibular apparatus, as well as histamine receptors that activate the CTZ, would also be appropriate choices for rescue for J.E. Because excessive sedation could delay J.E.'s discharge from the ambulatory surgery center, doses should not exceed 25 mg IV for promethazine, 50 mg IV for diphenhydramine, and 100 mg IV for dimenhydrate. In addition, it is important to assess J.E. for postoperative factors that could increase the likelihood of PONV. If postural hypotension is present, IV fluids and ephedrine would be appropriate therapy. Postoperative pain must also be assessed, because PONV is directly related to the degree of postoperative pain; a threefold higher frequency of PONV has been reported in ambulatory surgery patients with postoperative pain.[158]

Anesthetic Agents With a Low Incidence of Postoperative Nausea and Vomiting

21. How could J.E.'s anesthetic regimen have been modified to reduce the likelihood of PONV?

Several changes could be made in the anesthetic regimen to reduce the likelihood of PONV. Propofol has been postulated to have antiemetic properties, compared with the barbiturates (thiopental, methohexital), when used to induce anesthesia. However, it has been shown that propofol must be used for induction and maintenance of anesthesia to prevent PONV.[159] Patients receiving propofol for maintenance anesthesia have a significantly lower incidence of PONV than patients receiving inhalation anesthetic agents, regardless of the induction agent, presence or absence of nitrous oxide, choice of inhalation agent, age of the patient, or use of an opioid.[160] For females undergoing gynecological laparoscopic surgery, a 1-L IV fluid bolus preoperatively has been demonstrated to reduce the incidence of PONV from 51% to 17%.[161] Since perioperative administration of opioids is associated with PONV, the use of NSAIDs (oral agents preoperatively and postoperatively, parenteral ketorolac intraoperatively and postoperatively) , when appropriate, can reduce the need for postoperative opioids. In addition, surgical wound infiltration with a long-acting local anesthetic, such as bupivacaine, should also be used, when appropriate, to reduce postoperative incisional pain.

ANALGESIC AGENTS AND POSTOPERATIVE PAIN MANAGEMENT

Acute Pain

Surgery causes injury to the body, resulting in acute pain. Specifically, the tissue trauma from surgery directly stimulates nociceptors (receptors in the periphery that detect damaging or unpleasant stimuli, inflammation, pressure, and/or temperature). In addition, tissue injury causes the release of inflammatory mediators (e.g., prostaglandins, substance P) that sensitize and activate nociceptors. (Sensitized nociceptors amplify the pain impulse by generating nerve impulses more readily and more often; this is called peripheral sensitization.) The pain impulse propagates from the periphery to the dorsal horn of the spinal cord. From here, the pain impulse ascends to higher centers in the brain which results in the patient "feeling" the pain. Because both the cortical and limbic systems are involved and social and environmental influences are present, the same surgery can result in significant individual differences in pain perception. In postoperative pain, persistent bombardment of the dorsal horn with pain impulses from the periphery results in central sensitization ("wind-up"), where there is increased firing of dorsal horn neurons. Clinically, when this occurs, the patient will report spontaneous pain or an exaggerated response to a stimulus that does not generally cause pain (e.g., gentle touch) after healing has occurred.[162,163] The degree of pain usually depends on the magnitude of the surgery[164] and the patient's level of fear and anxiety. Patients vary in their response to pain (and interventions) as well as their personal preferences toward pain management. Acute pain usually resolves when the injury heals (hours to days). Unrelieved acute postoperative pain has detrimental physiologic and psychologic effects including impaired pulmonary function (leading to pulmonary complications); thromboembolism; tachycardia; hypertension and increased cardiac work; impairment of the immune system; nausea, vomiting, and ileus; chronic pain; and anxiety, fatigue, and fear.[163]

Adequate pain assessment and management are essential components of perioperative care. Education of patients and families about their roles, as well as the limitations and side effects of pain treatments, is critical to managing postoperative pain. Pain management must be planned for and integrated into the perioperative care of patients. Proactive planning includes obtaining a pain history based on the patient's own experiences with pain; determining the patient's pain goal; and anticipating preoperative, intraoperative, and postoperative pain therapies. The intensity and quality of pain as well as the patient's response to treatment and the degree to which pain interferes with normal activities should be monitored. Ideally, pain should be prevented by treating it adequately because once established, severe pain can be difficult to control. Based on our understanding of the mechanisms of postoperative pain, it makes sense to prevent the sensitization or stimulation of peripheral nociceptors.

Management Options

Effective postoperative pain management should provide subjective pain relief while minimizing analgesic-related adverse effects, allow early return to normal daily activities, and minimize the detrimental effects from unrelieved pain. The following techniques can be used to manage postoperative pain: (1) systemic administration of opioids, NSAIDs, and acetaminophen; (2) on-demand administration of IV opioids, also known as *patient-controlled analgesia* (PCA); (3) epidural analgesia (continuous and on-demand, usually with an opioid/local anesthetic mixture); (4) local nerve blockade such as local infiltration or peripheral nerve block; (5) cognitive-behavioral interventions such as relaxation or imagery to reduce anxiety and mild pain; and (6) application of heat or cold, guided imagery, music, or other nonpharmacologic intervention. Local anesthetics, opioids, acetaminophen, and NSAIDs can be used alone or in combination to create the optimal analgesic regimen for each patient based on factors such as efficacy of the agent to reduce pain to an acceptable level, type of surgery, underlying disease, adverse effects, and cost of therapy. For patients experiencing mild to moderate postoperative pain, local anesthetic wound infiltration or peripheral nerve blockade, or administration of a nonopioid analgesic such as a NSAID or acetaminophen are appropriate approaches to analgesia. For moderate postoperative pain, a less potent oral opioid, such as hydrocodone or codeine, is added. For moderate to severe pain following more invasive surgery, an IV opioid (e.g., morphine, hydromorphone), an epidural containing a local anesthetic and opioid, or a peripheral nerve block with local anesthetic is necessary. (For more information about general pain management, see Chapter 9, Pain.) Analgesia for acute pain in the perioperative setting is best achieved by using a multimodal (balanced) approach with a combination of two or more analgesic agents that have different mechanisms of action or that are administered by different techniques.[165] Wound infiltration with a local anesthetic not only blocks peripheral pain transmission but, more importantly, exerts a peripheral anti-inflammatory effect.[166] Peripheral nerve blocks significantly reduce or eliminate pain impulses from reaching the CNS (spinal cord), minimizing the effect of "wind-up." Finally, by minimizing the use of opioids and their related adverse effects, recovery can be improved.[167]

Patient-Controlled Analgesia
ADVANTAGES

22. J.A., a 60-year-old, 5'4", 50-kg woman, is immediately postoperative from a total abdominal hysterectomy for a neoplasm. Her laboratory values are remarkable for a SrCr of 1.3 mg/dL (normal, 0.6 to 1.0 mg/dL). She is allergic to penicillin. She will be admitted to the postsurgical floor for a planned stay of 2 to 3 days. What mode of pain management should be chosen for J.A.?

PCA is a popular method of administering analgesics and offers several advantages over traditional IM or IV opioid dosing. Patients treated with intermittent IM or IV dosing of opioids "as needed" can experience severe pain because the serum opioid concentration is allowed to fall to less than the minimum effective analgesic concentration (the concentration that provides approximately 90% pain relief). In addition, high peak plasma opioid concentrations can be seen with this administration method, often resulting in excessive nausea, vomiting, or sedation, as well as respiratory depression, which can lead to serious morbidity and/or mortality. Small, frequent opioid doses, as seen in PCA, minimize the peaks and valleys in serum concentrations seen with relatively larger intermittent IM or IV doses. This is helpful in avoiding adverse effects associated with high peak serum concentrations and inadequate pain relief caused by subtherapeutic serum concentrations. Small, frequent, patient-controlled dosing of opioids is efficacious because opioids have a steep sigmoidal dose–response curve for analgesia, resulting in the ability of a small opioid dose to move the plasma concentration from being subtherapeutic to above the minimum effective plasma concentration that will provide effective pain relief.[168] In terms of safety, analgesia occurs at lower opioid dosages than sedation, and sedation generally precedes respiratory depression.[169] Therefore, if a patient becomes sedated, self-administration of additional patient-controlled bolus doses will stop, allowing the serum opioid concentration to fall to a safe level.

Therapy can be individualized by using small doses of opioids at preset intervals (e.g., 1 mg morphine every 8 minutes), with the patient in control of his or her analgesic administration. An infusion pump with a programmed on-demand dose (the dose the patient can self-administer) and number of minutes between allowable doses (lock-out interval) is equipped with a button that the patient presses to receive a dose. IV bolus is the most common PCA route, with opioids being the drugs of choice to provide postoperative analgesia. The epidural route can also be used in select patients.

If the patient is educated to use PCA properly, it can be used to alleviate anticipated pain before movement or physical therapy in a preemptive fashion. J.A. has undergone a procedure for which moderate to severe pain is expected in the immediate postoperative period. J.A.'s pain requirement in the immediate postoperative period could be met with PCA opioid administration after first administering a bolus dose of opioid, which is titrated to achieve the appropriate level of analgesia. When her opioid requirements decline or when she can tolerate oral intake, she can then be switched to oral analgesics.

PATIENT SELECTION

23. J.A.'s surgeon decides to prescribe PCA for postoperative pain management. How should J.A. be evaluated for her ability to appropriately participate in her analgesic administration?

Patients receiving PCA therapy must be able to understand the concept behind PCA and to operate the drug administration button. J.A. must be alert and oriented before being put in control of her own pain management. She must be able to comprehend verbal and/or written instructions regarding the function and safety features of the infusion pump and how to titrate drug as needed for satisfactory analgesia. PCA has been used successfully in children, generally after ages 8 or 9 (adjusting doses appropriately) and in elderly patients. PCA is not indicated in patients who are expected to require parenteral opioids for analgesia for <24 hours, because these patients will generally be able to tolerate oral analgesics shortly after surgery.

PATIENT INSTRUCTIONS

24. J.A. is nervous about giving herself an overdose while using PCA. What instructions should be provided to her?

Patients often worry about the safety of PCA, which can lead to a reluctance to provide themselves with adequate pain relief. J.A. should be informed that when she administers a large amount of the prescribed opioid analgesic, she should fall asleep. Because she is asleep, she will not press the button. When this adverse effect of the opioid has worn off, she will wake up (plasma opioid level has fallen back into or below the therapeutic range). This is an important safety feature of PCA and is the reason why family members must not push the button for the patient. However, J.A. should also know that she may have to press the button several times (after the lock-out interval has passed) before her pain is relieved. She must also be informed that she may require a larger PCA dose, so it is important for J.A. to assess her pain relief from the "usual" dose most patients are initially started on following surgery. Accurate pain assessment following her prescribed dose is critical for ensuring that her dose is sufficient to provide the desired level of analgesia. She should also understand the possible adverse effects of her PCA medication and what can be done to prevent and treat these effects, as well as the advantages of providing herself with adequate analgesia (e.g., early ambulation). Finally, she should be told of the negligible risk of "narcotic" addiction from short-term PCA use and be given ample opportunity to ask questions.

CHOICE OF AGENT

25. Meperidine is ordered for J.A.'s PCA. Is this a reasonable drug choice for her?

Ideally, opioids for PCA administration have a rapid onset and intermediate duration of action (30 to 60 minutes), with no accumulation, ceiling effect, or adverse reactions. The physicians, nurses, and pharmacists involved with the care of the patient should be familiar with the drug selected for PCA. Morphine is by far the most common choice for PCA, although other opioids such as fentanyl and hydromorphone can be used. Drug choice is based on past patient experiences, allergies, adverse effects, and special considerations, such as renal function. Meperidine has a metabolite, normeperidine, which is renally excreted; has a long half-life; and can cause cerebral irritation and excitation. Symptoms of CNS toxicity from normeperidine include agitation, shaky feelings, delirium, twitching, tremors, and myoclonus/tonic-clonic seizures. These symptoms can be seen when meperidine is administered in higher doses and/or for a prolonged period.[170,171] The presence of renal insufficiency increases the risk of accumulation of normeperidine.[170] Unlike the other opioids, meperidine inhibits serotonin reuptake and has a high serotonergic potential. The risk of a patient developing the serotonin syndrome is greater when meperidine is coadministered with another drug that has moderate or high serotonergic potential (e.g., fluoxetine, fluvoxamine, paroxetine, venlafaxine).[172] For these reasons, meperidine is a poor choice for analgesia, particularly for J.A. who has diminished renal function. Morphine is conjugated with glucuronide in hepatic and extrahepatic sites (particularly the kidney) to its two major metabolites, morphine-3-glucuronide and morphine-6-glucuronide; both are excreted primarily in the urine. Morphine-6-glucuronide is an active metabolite that can accumulate in patients with renal failure, resulting in prolonged analgesia, sedation, and respiratory depression.[173] Because of J.A.'s diminished renal function, morphine should probably be avoided since other options exist. Hydromorphone and fentanyl are metabolized in the liver to inactive metabolites, thereby making these agents appropriate analgesic choices in patients with renal failure.[174] However, with repeat dosing or continuous infusion, fentanyl progressively accumulates in fat (due to its very high lipid solubility) and muscle. Fentanyl's serum concentration can then be slow to decline, resulting in prolonged effects. Therefore, hydromorphone would be the best analgesic choice for J.A. Table 10-16 lists common doses and lock-out intervals for drugs administered by PCA.[174–176]

DOSING

26. J.A. has not received any narcotics for several years. What dose of hydromorphone and what lock-out interval should be used for her initial PCA pump settings?

If J.A. is experiencing pain before PCA has been initiated, she should receive a loading dose of IV hydromorphone titrated to achieve baseline pain relief (usually, up to 1 mg). Demand doses of 0.1 mg with a lock-out interval of 8 minutes would be a good choice to maintain analgesia for this opioid-naive patient. If J.A.'s pain is not relieved after 1 hour, the demand dose can be increased to 0.2 mg.

USE OF A BASAL INFUSION

27. After the first postoperative evening, J.A. tells you that she had a terrible time sleeping. She describes waking up in pain frequently and wished that she did not have to press her PCA button while she was trying to sleep. During waking hours, she rates her pain relief as satisfactory. What can be done about this problem?

Many PCA infusion pumps offer a continuous infusion setting for a basal infusion during intermittent dosing. Use of a basal (continuous) infusion has not been shown to improve analgesia, and likely increases the risk of adverse effects (due to the potential of an opioid overdose in some patients). Therefore, routine basal (continuous) infusion of opioids cannot be recommended for acute pain management. A better approach is to increase the size of the bolus dose during nighttime hours. J.A.'s PCA hydromorphone dose could be increased at night to allow her to sleep for longer periods and returned to the previous amount during the day. Alternatively, a low, continuous (basal) infusion (0.1 mg/hr) of hydromorphone could be administered at night. The infusion should be discontinued when J.A. wakes up in the morning because she can then resume administering hydromorphone on demand.

ADVERSE EFFECTS

28. The next day, J.A. reports adequate pain relief with her PCA, but complains of feeling slightly groggy and nauseated. Bowel sounds are noted on physical examination, and J.A. plans to try to take clear liquids later that morning. What are the adverse effects of PCA opioids and how can J.A.'s complaints be addressed?

Opioids given by PCA can produce adverse effects similar to those given by other parenteral routes. Sedation, confusion, euphoria, nausea and vomiting, constipation, urinary retention, and pruritus can be experienced, and these can be managed by dose adjustments or pharmacologic intervention. Respiratory depression is extremely rare with PCA opioid administration.[175] However, elderly patients, patients with severe underlying systemic disease or pre-existing respiratory compromise, and those who are receiving other sedative-hypnotics concomitantly are predisposed to respiratory depression.[168] Technical problems also must be ruled out. The PCA pump should be checked to ensure that it is delivering the correct drug and dose, programming also should be checked for accuracy (e.g., drug concentration, dosing interval), and the opioid reversal agent naloxone must be readily

Table 10-16 Adult Analgesic Dosing Recommendations for IV Patient-Controlled Analgesia[a]

| Drug | Usual Concentration | Demand Dose (mg) | | Lock-Out Interval (min) |
		Usual	Range	
Fentanyl (as citrate) (Sublimaze)	10 µg/mL	0.01–0.015	0.01–0.05	3–10
Hydromorphone HCl (Dilaudid)	0.2 mg/mL	0.1–0.2	0.1–0.5	5–10
Morphine sulfate	1 mg/mL	1–2	0.5–3	5–10

[a]Analgesic doses are based on those required by a healthy 55- to 70-kg, opioid-naive adult. Analgesic requirements vary widely between patients. Doses may need to be adjusted because of age, condition of the patient, and prior opioid use.
HCl, hydrochloride; IV, intravenous.
Adapted from references 174–176.

available. Monitoring for efficacy and adverse effects of PCA therapy should include pain intensity and quality, response to treatment, number of on-demand requests, analgesic consumption, BP, heart rate, respiratory rate, and level of sedation, as well as other adverse effects of opioids.

J.A.'s PCA hydromorphone dose could be reduced to manage her sedation and nausea. However, her pain control must be carefully reassessed to ensure efficacy of the newly lowered dose. An order for an antiemetic could be provided as well. NSAIDs (ketorolac IM/IV or other NSAID orally) are not sedating and could be added to the analgesic regimen. However, because of her compromised renal function, NSAIDs should be administered with caution and in lower doses (e.g., 15 mg IM/IV ketorolac) to J.A. Before administering ketorolac, J.A.'s hydration status should be evaluated to ensure that she is not hypovolemic.[177] If J.A. is able to take fluids orally, PCA should be discontinued and oral analgesics administered as needed. As healing occurs, her pain intensity should lessen, and oral opioid/acetaminophen products should manage her pain adequately.

Epidural Analgesia

29. T.M., a 69-year old man, enters the surgical ICU after surgery for colorectal cancer (lower anterior resection, urethral stents, ileo-rectal pull-through). His pain is managed through a lumbar epidural catheter. What are the benefits and risks of epidural analgesia and why was this approach to postoperative analgesia chosen for T.M.?

ADVANTAGES AND DISADVANTAGES

Epidural analgesia can offer superior pain relief over traditional parenteral analgesia.[178] Continuous epidural infusions offer an advantage over intermittent epidural injections because peak and trough concentrations of drugs are avoided. Epidural catheter placement is an invasive procedure and can result in unintentional dural puncture resulting in postdural puncture headache, insertion site inflammation or infection, and rarely catheter migration during therapy and epidural hematoma.[175]

PATIENT SELECTION

Epidural analgesia should be chosen based on the need for good postoperative pain relief as well as reduced perioperative physiologic responses. Postoperative pain should be localized at an appropriate level for catheter placement in the lumbar or thoracic location of the epidural space. Patients undergoing abdominal, gynecologic, obstetric, colorectal, urologic, lower limb (e.g., major vascular or orthopedic), or thoracic surgery are excellent candidates for epidural pain management. Epidural analgesia with local anesthetics with or without low-dose opioids can reduce the incidence of pulmonary morbidity[179] and perioperative myocardial infarction.[178] Absolute contraindications to epidural analgesia include severe systemic infection or infection in the area of catheter insertion, known coagulopathy, significant thrombocytopenia, recent or anticipated thrombolytic therapy, full (therapeutic) anticoagulation, uncorrected hypovolemia, patient refusal, and anatomic abnormalities that make epidural catheter placement difficult or impossible.[180,181] T.M. is a good candidate for epidural analgesia based on the severity of pain associated with his surgery and the surgical procedure.

CHOICE OF AGENT AND MECHANISMS OF ACTION

30. What drug or drug combination can be used for T.M.'s epidural infusion? What are the mechanisms of action of the analgesics commonly administered in the epidural space?

Opioids and local anesthetics are administered alone or in combination in epidural infusions. Opioids in the epidural space are transported by passive diffusion and the vasculature to the spinal cord where they act at opioid receptors in the dorsal horn to inhibit the release of substance P and other neurotransmitters, thereby reducing the transmission of pain-related information (nociception). After epidural administration, opioids can reach brainstem sites by cephalad movement in the cerebrospinal fluid. Lipophilic opioids (fentanyl, sufentanil) are systemically absorbed and act in the brainstem, the brain, and the periphery to produce analgesia.[173,182] Opioids selectively block pain transmission and have no effect on nerve transmission responsible for motor, sensory, or autonomic function.[183] Local anesthetics, on the other hand, act on axonal nerve membranes crossing through the epidural space to produce analgesia by blocking nerve transmission. Depending on the drug, concentration, and depth of nerve penetration, local anesthetics also produce sensory, motor, or autonomic blockade (see Local Anesthetics). Table 10-17 describes the spinal actions, efficacy, and adverse effects of opioids and local anesthetics administered by the epidural route.[174,180,182,184]

Various opioids and local anesthetics have been used successfully in epidural drug preparations. Most often, opioids and local anesthetics are combined in the same solution because these two classes of drugs act synergistically at two different sites to produce analgesia, allowing the administration of lower doses of each drug to reduce the risk of adverse effects while providing effective analgesia. Table 10-18 lists the drugs, concentrations, and typical infusion rates for epidural administration.[175,176,182,183,185] Bupivacaine commonly is chosen as the local anesthetic agent because it can preferentially block sensory fibers (producing analgesia) without significantly blocking motor fibers.[175] The choice of opioid is based on pharmacokinetic differences among the available agents. Onset, duration, spread of agent in the spinal fluid (dermatomal spread), and systemic absorption are affected by the lipophilicity of the drug.[184] Highly lipophilic opioids such as fentanyl and sufentanil have a faster onset of action, a shorter duration of action (from a single dose), less dermatomal spread, and much greater systemic absorption. Morphine, which is relatively hydrophilic, has a slower onset of action, longer duration of action, greater dermatomal spread and migration to the brain, and less systemic absorption.[182,184] However, after several hours of epidural infusion, fentanyl's dermatomal (regional) effect is lost, and analgesia is achieved because of a therapeutic plasma concentration. Morphine, on the other hand, retains its spinal mechanism of action.[182] Hydromorphone's lipophilicity is intermediate between fentanyl and morphine. Clinically, hydromorphone has a faster onset and shorter duration than morphine. In terms of site of action, patients receiving IV hydromorphone following radical prostatectomy surgery required twice as much opioid as those who received epidural hydromorphone, suggesting a spinal mechanism of action.[186] A comparison of the pharmacokinetic properties important to epidural opioids is found in Table 10-19.[175,178,184,185] T.M should receive a combination of opioid and local anesthetic, such as fentanyl and bupivacaine, as an epidural infusion for postoperative pain management.

Table 10-17 A Comparison of the Spinal Actions, Efficacy, and Adverse Effects of Opioids and Local Anesthetics[a]

	Opioids	Local Anesthetics
Actions		
Site of action	Substantia gelatinosa of dorsal horn of spinal cord[b]	Spinal nerve roots
Modalities blocked	"Selective" block of pain conduction	Blockade of sympathetic pain fibers; can cause loss of sensation and motor function[c]
Efficacy		
Surgical pain	Partial relief	Complete relief possible
Labor pain	Partial relief	Complete relief
Postoperative pain	Fair/Good relief	Complete relief
Adverse Effects	Nausea, vomiting, sedation, confusion, pruritus, constipation/ileus, urinary retention, respiratory depression	Hypotension, urinary retention, loss of sensation, loss of motor function resulting in inability to ambulate

[a]Epidurally administered morphine and local anesthetics exert their effects mainly by a spinal mechanism of action; lipophilic opioids such as fentanyl and sufentanil achieve therapeutic plasma concentrations when administered epidurally.
[b]And/or other sites where opioid receptor-binding sites are present.
Adapted from references 174, 180, 182 and 184.

31. Fentanyl/bupivacaine is chosen for T.M. How should this be prepared and what infusion rate should be chosen?

Fentanyl and bupivacaine are commonly admixed in 0.9% sodium chloride (usual concentration ranges are found in Table 10-18). Concentrations are often institution specific and often depend on the rate of administration. Preservative-free preparations of each drug should be used because neurologic effects are possible with inadvertent subdural administration of large amounts of benzyl alcohol or other neurotoxic preservatives. Strict aseptic technique should be used when admixing and administering an epidural solution.

The rate of administration is chosen empirically based on the anticipated analgesic response, the concentration of opioid in the admixture, and the potential for adverse effects. Usually, a rate of 4 to 10 mL/hr is adequate; the epidural space can safely handle up to approximately 20 mL/hr of fluid. An initial infusion rate of 5 to 8 mL/hr would be reasonable for T.M., with titration based on efficacy and adverse effects.

Table 10-18 Adult Analgesic Dosing Recommendations for Epidural Infusion

Drug Combinations or Drug[a]	Infusion Concentration[b]	Usual Infusion Rate[b]
Morphine + bupivacaine	25–100 μg/mL (M) 0.5–1.25 mg/mL (B)	4–10 mL/hr
Hydromorphone + bupivacaine	3–50 μg/mL (H) 0.5–1.25 mg/mL (B)	4–10 mL/hr
Fentanyl + bupivacaine	2–10 μg/mL (F) 0.5–1.25 mg/mL (B)	4–10 mL/hr
Sufentanil + bupivacaine	1 μg/mL (S) 0.5–1.25 mg/mL (B)	4–10 mL/hr
Morphine	0.1 mg/mL	5–8 mL/hr
Hydromorphone	50 μg/mL	3–6 mL/hr
Fentanyl	10 μg/mL	3–8 mL/hr

[a]Use only preservative-free products and preservative-free 0.9% sodium chloride as the admixture solution.
[b]Exact concentrations and rates are institution-specific. Initial concentration and/or rate often depend on the age and general condition of the patient.
B, bupivacaine; F, fentanyl; H, hydromorphone; M, morphine; S, sufentanil.
Adapted from references 175,176,182, 183, and 185.

Table 10-19 Pharamacokinetic Comparison of Common Epidural Opioid Analgesics

Agent	Partition Coefficient[a]	Onset of Action of Bolus (min)	Duration of Action of Bolus (hr)	Dermatomal Spread
Fentanyl (Sublimaze)	955	5	3–6	Narrow
Hydromorphone (Dilaudid)	525	15	6–17	Intermediate-wide
Morphine Sulfate (Duramorph)	1	30	12–24	Wide
Sufentanil (Sufenta)	1,737	5	4–7	Narrow

[a]Octanol/water partition coefficient; used to assess lipophilicity; higher numbers indicate greater lipophilicity.
Adapted from references 175, 178, 184, and 185.

ADVERSE EFFECTS

32. Two hours after initiation of his fentanyl/bupivacaine epidural infusion, T.M. experiences discomfort in the form of an itchy feeling on his nose, torso, and limbs. Is this related to his epidural infusion?

Pruritus has been associated with almost all opioids, with a significantly greater frequency when the opioid is administered as an epidural infusion rather than by IV administration.[187] This effect is usually seen within 2 hours and is probably dose related. It generally subsides as the opioid effect wears off and can be more of a problem with continuous epidural administration of opioids or when opioids are administered via PCA. Although pruritus from opioids is probably μ-receptor mediated and not histamine-mediated,[188] antihistamines (e.g., diphenhydramine) can provide symptomatic relief. Alternatively, very small doses of opioid antagonists (e.g., naloxone 0.04 mg) can be used to effectively reverse opioid adverse effects, such as pruritus, but not analgesia. Due to naloxone's short duration of action, repeat doses or a continuous infusion may be necessary.

Other adverse effects possible with epidural opioids include nausea, vomiting, sedation, confusion, constipation, ileus, urinary retention, and respiratory depression. Although rare, respiratory depression from epidural opioids is the most dangerous adverse effect. Opioids depress respiratory drive by a direct action on the medullary respiratory center in a dose-dependent manner.[173] Opioids can reach this site in the brainstem after epidural administration either by systemic absorption and redistribution or by cephalad spread in the cerebrospinal fluid. Respiratory depression can occur as long as 12 to 24 hours after a single bolus of morphine[182,184] or within hours to 6 days after beginning a continuous infusion of fentanyl/bupivacaine.[189] Typically, regular assessments of sedation level and respiratory rate safely detect respiratory depression from opioids.[182] As with parenteral opioid administration, risk factors for opioid-related respiratory depression include severe underlying systemic disease or pre-existing respiratory compromise, concomitant use of other sedative-hypnotics (e.g., benzodiazepines, opioids administered by another route), and older age. As a result, reduced doses should be used in patients with these risk factors. Adverse effects of epidural local anesthetics include hypotension, urinary retention, lower limb paresthesias or numbness, and lower limb motor block. Depending on the degree of numbness and motor block, the patient may have difficulty ambulating. Monitoring for efficacy and adverse effects of epidural analgesia should include pain intensity and quality, response to treatment, number of on-demand requests (if PCA is being used), analgesic consumption, BP, heart rate, respiratory rate, level of sedation, and temperature.

ADJUNCTIVE KETOROLAC USE

33. On the second postoperative day, T.M. is able to rest comfortably when undisturbed, while receiving treatment with a lumbar epidural infusion of fentanyl 3 μg/mL and bupivacaine 1.25 mg/mL at a rate of 8 mL/hr. However, when he is moved at the change of each nursing shift, he complains of significant pain. Increasing the rate of his epidural infusion was tried, but caused unacceptable pruritus and sedation. How can T.M.'s intermittent pain needs be addressed?

The use of additional analgesics for breakthrough pain may be necessary in patients receiving continuous epidural infusion. T.M.'s intermittent pain could be managed by patient-controlled epidural analgesia. Like IV PCA, patient-activated epidural boluses can be administered to control pain during movement. Alternatively, ketorolac, an injectable NSAID, may be considered for T.M.; it does not contribute to respiratory depression, sedation, or pruritus and effectively treats moderate to severe pain. The analgesic effects of NSAIDs are additive with the opioids and can lower postoperative pain scores. Patient selection for ketorolac therapy should consider renal function, plasma volume and electrolyte status, GI disease, risk of bleeding, and concomitant drugs and therapies such as epidural analgesia.

ADJUNCTIVE ANTICOAGULANT ADMINISTRATION

34. The surgeon has determined that T.M. is at risk for developing postoperative venous thromboembolism. Enoxaparin 40 mg SC QD has been ordered postoperatively. What are the risks of enoxaparin in this situation? What are reasonable precautions?

Prolonged therapeutic anticoagulation appears to increase the risk of epidural and spinal hematoma formation, which can lead to long-term or permanent paralysis. Administration of antiplatelet or anticoagulant drugs in combination with low molecular weight heparin (LMWH) results in an even greater risk of perioperative hemorrhagic complications, including spinal hematoma.[190] These findings have led to concern for the safety of spinal and epidural anesthesia and analgesia in patients receiving LMWH. Important considerations for managing a patient being administered LMWH and receiving continuous epidural analgesia are: 1) the time of catheter placement and removal relative to the timing (and peak effect) of LMWH administration, 2) total daily dose of LMWH, and 3) the dosing schedule of LMWH.[181] For T.M., the epidural catheter is already in place and the LMWH is started postoperatively as a single daily dose. It is safe to leave the epidural catheter in place as long as the first dose of LMWH is administered 6 to 8 hours postoperatively. The second dose should be administered no sooner than 24 hours after the first dose. The timing of the catheter removal is of the utmost importance; it should be delayed for at least 10 to 12 hours after the last dose of LMWH, with subsequent dosing continued 2 or more hours after the catheter has been removed. There may be a greater risk of spinal hematoma when LMWH is administered twice a day. For that reason, if every 12 hour enoxaparin is required, the catheter should be removed and the first dose of LMWH administered 2 hours after catheter removal.[181] Since T.M. is receiving prophylactic daily enoxaparin, his catheter should be removed no earlier than 10 hours after his last dose of enoxaparin, with his next dose administered no earlier than 2 hours after catheter removal.

ANALGESIC LADDER FOR POSTOPERATIVE PAIN MANAGEMENT

35. W.W., a 16-year-old male, arrives at the ambulatory surgery center for arthroscopic knee surgery on his right knee (for removal of loose debris) under general anesthesia. His medical and surgical histories are unremarkable. He is not currently

taking any medication and reports no drug allergies. How should W.W.'s postoperative pain be managed?

In general, one would expect that the greater the magnitude of the surgical trauma, the greater the patient's postoperative pain.[164] For minor surgical procedures (e.g., laparoscopy, breast biopsy), there is minimal surgical trauma and the patient goes home shortly after surgery. For intermediate surgical procedures (e.g., hysterectomy, appendectomy), short-term hospitalization is often necessary to observe the patient's recovery and manage his or her pain. Patients undergoing major surgery (e.g., bowel resection, thoracotomy) experience a significant surgical stress response that can significantly increase postoperative morbidity. Effective pain management is essential.

The World Health Organization (WHO) has published recommendations for cancer pain management that include a three-step analgesic ladder based on pain intensity, with movement to the next step of the ladder occurring when pain relief is inadequate.[191] Step 1 is initiated with a nonopioid analgesic when pain is mild (e.g., acetaminophen ±NSAID). If pain is mild to moderate or persists, a low potency opioid analgesic (Step 2) is added to the nonopioid analgesic (e.g., acetaminophen + hydrocodone ±NSAID). When pain is moderate to severe (Step 3), a more potent opioid (e.g., morphine, oxycodone-CR) is necessary to supplement nonopioid analgesics. If a fixed combination of opioid and nonopioid is used, the total daily dose administered to the patient is limited by the maximum allowable daily dose of the nonopioid (e.g., acetaminophen, ibuprofen).

The WHO analgesic three-step ladder approach to pain management utilizes multimodal or "balanced" analgesia, which can also be applied to the postoperative setting. It is difficult to optimize postoperative pain relief, to the point of achieving normal function, by using one drug or route of administration. By using two or more agents that work at different points in the pain pathway, additive or synergistic analgesia can be achieved and adverse effects reduced because doses are lower and side effect profiles are different. Opioids are a mainstay of analgesic therapy for moderate to severe pain. However, opioids often are associated with intolerable adverse effects (e.g., nausea, vomiting, constipation, itching, sedation). Maximizing the use of nonopioid analgesics and nonpharmacologic techniques results in less need for opioids, particularly in patients undergoing minor procedures in the ambulatory surgery setting (Table 10-20).[164,165,192–194] For example, preoperative administration of 40 mg of IV parecoxib (the prodrug of the COX-2 inhibitor valdecoxib) followed by 40 mg of oral valdecoxib daily for 7 days at home to patients undergoing laparoscopic cholecystectomy resulted in less severe pain and less fentanyl and hydrocodone for postoperative analgesia when compared with placebo. In addition, patients who received parecoxib and valdecoxib returned to normal activities significantly sooner (i.e., at 24 and 48 hours) after surgery.[167]

Utilizing multimodal analgesia and the approach of the WHO three-step analgesic ladder (Fig. 10-2), Step 1 would be represented by mild pain that is anticipated following minor surgery. Nonopioid analgesics, such as local anesthetic infiltration or instillation and an oral NSAID/acetaminophen, should effectively manage this pain. A less-potent oral opioid such as hydromorphone or codeine in combination with acetaminophen can be intermittently added if needed. Step 2 would be applicable to mild-moderate pain that is anticipated following intermediate surgery. In addition to nonopioid analgesics, an IV or oral opioid should be prescribed to manage the anticipated pain of Step 2. Step 3 would be applicable to moderate to severe pain following major surgery. In addition to the nonopioid analgesics, IV opioids or epidural opioid plus local anesthetic would be necessary to manage the anticipated pain of Step 3. For all types of surgery, nonpharmacologic methods should be used in addition to pharmacologic agents.

Table 10-20 Commonly Used Analgesic Drugs and Nonpharmacologic Techniques for Postoperative Pain Management

Type of Agent	Examples	Potential Adverse Effects
Local anesthetics	Peripheral nerve block, tissue infiltration, wound instillation, topical	Tingling, numbness, residual motor weakness, hypotension, CNS and cardiac effects from systemic absorption
NSAIDs	Ketorolac (IV, IM, oral), ibuprofen (oral), naproxen (oral), celecoxib (oral), rofecoxib (oral)	GI upset, edema, hypertension, dizziness, drowsiness, GI bleeding, operative site bleeding (not celecoxib or rofecoxib)
Other nonopioids	Acetaminophen (oral, rectal)	GI upset, hepatotoxicity
	Clonidine (nerve block)	Sedation, hypotension
Nonpharmacologic	Transcutaneous electrical nerve stimulation, acupuncture	Skin irritation, discomfort
	Ice or cold therapy	Excessive vasoconstriction, skin irritation
	Distraction, music, deep breathing for relaxation	
Less potent opioids	Hydrocodone + acetaminophen or ibuprofen, codeine or oxycodone + acetaminophen, propoxyphene + acetaminophen	Nausea, vomiting, ileus, pruritus, constipation, rash, sedation, mental confusion, hallucinations, respiratory depression
More potent opioids	Morphine (IV, epidural), hydromorphone (IV, epidural), fentanyl (IV, epidural), oxycodone (oral)	Nausea, vomiting, ileus, pruritus, constipation, rash, sedation, mental confusion, hallucinations, respiratory depression

Adapted from references 192 and 194.
CNS, central nervous system; GI, gastrointestinal; IM, intramuscular; IV, intravenous.

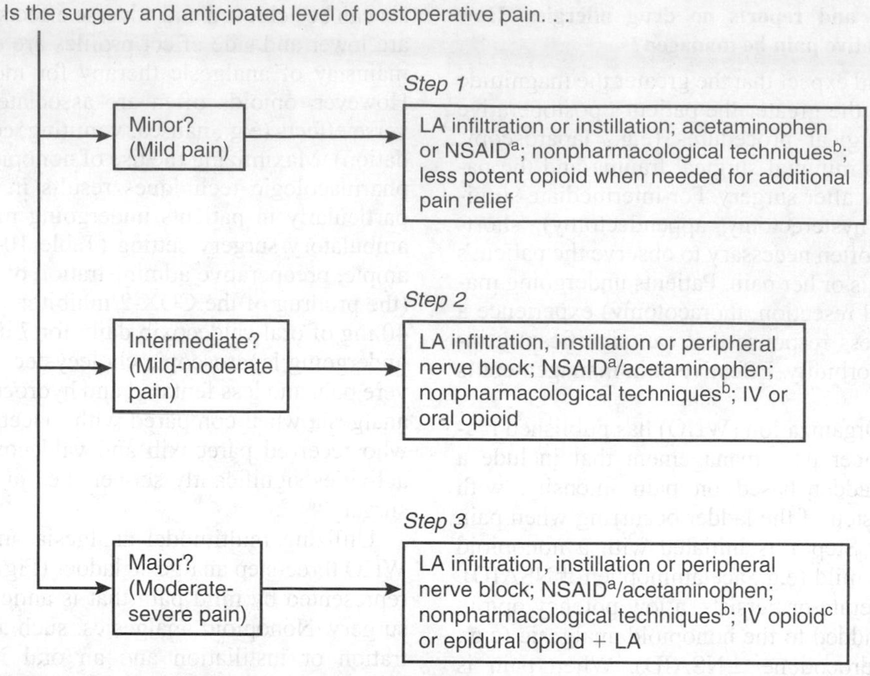

Is the surgery and anticipated level of postoperative pain. . .

```
                          ┌──────────────┐          ┌──────────────────────────────────────────┐
                          │              │  Step 1   │ LA infiltration or instillation; acetaminophen │
                  ┌──────▶│  Minor?      │─────────▶ │ or NSAIDᵃ; nonpharmacological techniquesᵇ; │
                  │       │  (Mild pain) │          │ less potent opioid when needed for additional │
                  │       └──────────────┘          │ pain relief                                  │
                  │                                  └──────────────────────────────────────────┘
                  │
                  │                                  Step 2
                  │       ┌──────────────┐          ┌──────────────────────────────────────────┐
                  │       │ Intermediate?│          │ LA infiltration, instillation or peripheral │
  ───────────────┼──────▶│ (Mild-moderate│────────▶ │ nerve block; NSAIDᵃ/acetaminophen;       │
                  │       │ pain)        │          │ nonpharmacological techniquesᵇ; IV or     │
                  │       └──────────────┘          │ oral opioid                                │
                  │                                  └──────────────────────────────────────────┘
                  │
                  │                                  Step 3
                  │       ┌──────────────┐          ┌──────────────────────────────────────────┐
                  │       │ Major?       │          │ LA infiltration, instillation or peripheral │
                  └──────▶│ (Moderate-   │────────▶ │ nerve block; NSAIDᵃ/acetaminophen;       │
                          │ severe pain) │          │ nonpharmacological techniquesᵇ; IV opioidᶜ │
                          └──────────────┘          │ or epidural opioid + LA                    │
                                                     └──────────────────────────────────────────┘
```

FIGURE 10-2 Analgesic ladder: management of postoperative pain.
[a]Nonspecific or COX-2 selective, depending on the patient history and risk for surgical bleeding.
[b]As appropriate for patient and surgical procedure.
[c]IV PCA is preferred to intermittent IV injections. When pain is anticipated to be severe and last more than a few days and surgery is being performed on an ambulatory (outpatient) basis, controlled release oxycodone can be used in place of IV opioids. An example of a type of surgery where controlled-release oxycodone is warranted is arthroscopic anterior cruciate reconstruction.
LA, local anesthetic; IV, intravenous; NSAID, nonsteroidal anti-inflammatory drug; COX-2, cyclooxygenase-2 enzyme.
(Adapted from references 164, 192, 193, and 195.)

For W.W., the anticipated surgical trauma is minor and recovery is anticipated to be faster than if there was ligament damage and surgical reconstruction. However, depending on the intra-articular structures of the knee that are involved, free nerve endings sensing painful stimuli can produce postoperative pain, and swelling can also occur. Good control of postoperative pain and swelling are important to allow successful rehabilitation of W.W.'s right knee, allowing return to his normal activities. A long-acting local anesthetic (bupivacaine) should be injected intra-articularly. For more extensive knee surgery, such as anterior cruciate ligament reconstruction, the addition of 5 mg of morphine intra-articularly provides additional analgesia because of the presence of peripheral opioid receptors.[195] In addition to intra-articular bupivacaine, W.W. should also receive acetaminophen or an NSAID. Because prostaglandins in the periphery are a significant cause of postoperative pain, NSAIDs may be more efficacious than acetaminophen in reducing the pain and swelling following many types of surgery. Ibuprofen 400 mg QID would be an appropriate choice for W.W. Analgesia from intra-articular bupivacaine would not be expected to last more than 8 hours, at which point W.W. will only be receiving analgesia from the ibuprofen. If he experiences pain, a less potent opioid (e.g., hydrocodone) combined with acetaminophen can be administered every 4 to 6 hours as needed for additional analgesia.

ECONOMIC ISSUES

Anesthesia-related medications account for an estimated 8% to 12% of a hospital's drug expenditures, with the 10 highest-expenditure medications accounting for >80% of all anesthesia medication expenditures.[67,196] Because of this, anesthesia-related medications are routinely targeted for cost-containment activities, which can include waste reduction,[34,197] development of appropriate guidelines for use,[34,198,199] formulary management, reduced access to select medications,[34,199] and financial incentives.[34,199] Large dollar savings can be realized from the systematic appropriate use of less expensive medications because thousands of patients are anesthetized per year in a hospital.

Value-Based Anesthesia Care

Cost containment should not be based on the use of the least expensive technology, piece of equipment, or drug because this strategy can lead to unacceptable patient outcomes and higher total costs. In responding to the need to consider both costs and outcomes, the anesthesiology profession has put forth the concept of value-based anesthesia care, which seeks the best patient outcomes at the most reasonable costs. The advantages and disadvantages of the technique or drug are balanced against all costs associated with the surgical experience.[200]

Total Costs of Surgical Stay

In one study, anesthesia costs, including medication use, accounted for 6% of the total costs for inpatient surgery, with approximately 50% being variable. Hence, modifying medication selection can impact, at most, 3% of the total costs associated with surgery. On the other hand, OR costs, including the costs of the PACU, accounted for 37% of the total costs of surgery, with approximately 44% being variable. Therefore, modifying practices that influence these costs can impact total cost by up to 16%.[201] In another study, labor costs were estimated to be two orders of magnitude greater than anesthesia maintenance costs for a 60-minute outpatient procedure; therefore,. a major component of cost-containment efforts should be directed at the reduction of labor costs by streamlining OR time and shortening PACU discharge time.[202] Methods to reduce a patient's PACU stay may allow personnel reductions and/or reassignment of staff during slow periods. These studies highlight the opportunity for cost reduction in the perioperative setting by focusing on nonmedication costs and support the concept of fast-track anesthesia.

Fast-Track Anesthesia

Fast-track anesthesia is defined as the acceleration of the movement of the patient through the perioperative experience (OR, PACU, and/or ICU). Fast-tracking has been promoted to improve patient satisfaction, to improve OR and PACU efficiency, and to lower the costs of the surgical experience. Several developments have facilitated the fast-track process and include the wide-scale use of less invasive surgical procedures (e.g., laparoscopy), the incorporation of new monitoring techniques to allow better titration of anesthesia, and the use of short-acting, fast-emergence anesthetic agents to reduce wake-up times and drug hangovers. A basic tenet of fast-track anesthesia is that medication costs will be higher compared with similar procedures not fast-tracked; however, fast-tracking can improve clinical and financial outcomes in both the inpatient and outpatient settings. Fast-tracking cardiac surgery patients has resulted in quicker extubation, reduced length of stay, reduced ICU readmission rate, and a 25% cost reduction.[203,204] Further, it has been demonstrated that fast-track cardiac surgery patients have a decreased

health care resource usage for at least 1 year following discharge.[205] In a landmark outpatient study, fast-tracking was implemented in five surgical centers and resulted in annual net savings from $50,000 to $160,000, with no significant differences in patient outcomes.[206,207] In this study, outpatients meeting a well-defined set of criteria were allowed to skip phase I recovery and proceed directly to phase II from the OR. Phase I recovery can be considered an ICU-type environment. Patients are taken here from the OR to recover hemodynamically and fully regain consciousness; this requires intensive nursing care (usually one nurse to two patients). Once patients are awake, hemodynamically stable, and able to sit upright, they are moved to phase II recovery to finish the recovery process. In this setting, the nurse:patient ratio is 1:3, or greater if nurse assistants are employed. The low-solubility, volatile inhalation agents (desflurane, sevoflurane) are ideally suited for fast-tracking in the outpatient setting.[208,209]

Monitoring Sedative and Hypnotic Effects of Anesthetic Agents

Finally, the introduction of devices that measure the hypnotic effects of anesthetic and sedative agents on the brain. Bispectral (BIS) Index Monitor and Patient State Analyzer (PSA 4000 monitor) have the potential to reduce the amount of anesthetic administered and facilitate recovery. The BIS index and the Patient State Index (PSI) are derived values from the EEG and are used as a quantifiable measure of the sedative and hypnotic effects of anesthetic drugs (e.g., level of consciousness).[210] Although decreased times to verbal responsiveness and a reduction in drug use have been noted when these devices were used,[209,211] other studies have not demonstrated similar results using these devices.[212,213] Further, these devices are not without costs (monitor, maintenance, disposable sensors), and their true place in practice still needs additional economic and outcome assessments.

Thus, the goal for the cost-effective use of medications in the perioperative setting is a net reduction in the cost of surgical procedures (either the result of a lower overall medication cost or process modifications such as fast-tracking) by taking advantage of the medications' properties and keeping in mind that patients' outcomes should not be negatively impacted and ideally should be improved.

REFERENCES

1. Klafta J, Roizen M. Current understanding of patients' attitudes toward and preparation for anesthesia: a review. Anesth Analg 1996;83:1314.
2. Matthey P et al. The attitude of the general public towards preoperative assessment and risks associated with general anesthesia. Can J Anaesth 2001;48:333.
3. Klopfenstein CE et al. Anesthetic assessment in an outpatient consultation clinic reduces preoperative anxiety. Can J Anaesth 2000;47:511.
4. Moyers JR, Vincent CM. Preoperative medication. In: Barash PG et al., eds. Clinical Anesthesia. Philadelphia: Lippincott Williams & Wilkins, 2001:551.
5. Rice LJ, Cravero J. Pediatric anesthesia. In: Barash PG et al., eds. Clinical Anesthesia. Philadelphia: Lippincott, Williams & Wilkins, 2001:1195.
6. Donnelly AJ et al. Anesthesiology and Critical Care Handbook. Hudson: Lexi-Comp, 2001.

7. Scholz J, Tonner PH. α_2-adrenoreceptor agonists in anaesthesia: a new paradigm. Curr Opin Anaesthesiol 2000;13:437.
8. Friedberg BL. Propofol ketamine anesthesia for cosmetic surgery in the office suite. Int Anesthiol Clin 2003;41:39.
9. Kain ZN et al. Premedication in the United States: a status report. Anesth Analg 1997;41:31.
10. Muravchick S. Anesthesia for the geriatric patient. In: Barash PG et al., eds. Clinical Anesthesia. Philadelphia: Lippincott-Raven, 1997:1125.
11. Fredman B et al. The effect of midazolam premedication on mental and psychomotor recovery in geriatric patients undergoing brief surgical procedures. Anesth Analg 1999;89:1161.
12. Kain ZN et al. Parental presence during induction of anesthesia versus sedative premedication. Which intervention is more effective? Anesthesiology 1998;89:1147.

13. Holm-Knudsen RJ et al. Distress at induction of anaesthesia in children: a survey of incidence, associated factors and recovery characteristics. Paediatr Anaesth 1998;8:383
14. Kain ZM et al. Postoperative behavioral outcomes in children: effects of sedative premedication. Anesthesiology 1999;90:758.
15. Knight PR et al. Pathogenesis of gastric particulate lung injury: a comparison and interaction with acidic pneumonitis. Anesth Analg 1993;77:754.
16. Rocke DA et al. At risk for aspiration: new critical values of volume and pH? Anesth Analg 1993; 76:666.
17. Rosenblatt WH. Airway management. In: Barash PG et al., eds. Clinical Anesthesia. Philadelphia: Lippincott, Williams & Wilkins, 2001:595.
18. Kallar SK, Everett LL. Potential risks and preventive measures for pulmonary aspiration: new con-

cepts in preoperative fasting guidelines. Anesth Analg 1993;77:171.

19. Minami H, McCallum RW. The physiology and pathophysiology of gastric emptying in humans. Gastroenterology 1984;86:1592.

20. Schneck H, Scheller M. Acid aspiration prophylaxis and caesarian section. Curr Opin Anaesthesiol 2000;13:261.

21. Lim SK, Elegbe EO. The use of single dose of sodium citrate as a prophylaxis against acid aspiration syndrome in obstetric patients undergoing caesarean section. Med J Malaysia 1991;46:349.

22. Schmidt JF et al. The effect of sodium citrate on the pH and the amount of gastric contents before general anesthesia. Acta Anaesthesiol Scand 1984;28:263.

23. American Society of Anesthesiologists. Practice guidelines for preoperative fasting and the use of pharmacologic agents to reduce the risk of pulmonary aspiration. Anesthesiology 1999;90:896.

24. Ng A, Smith G. Gastroesophageal reflux and aspiration of gastric contents in anesthetic practice. Anesth Analg 2001;93:494.

25. Stuart JC et al. Acid aspiration prophylaxis for emergency caesarean section. Anaesthesia 1996;51:415.

26. Evers AS. Cellular and molecular mechanisms of anesthesia. In: Barash PG et al., eds. Clinical Anesthesia. Philadelphia: Lippincott, Williams & Wilkins, 2001:121.

27. Murphy FL. Conduct of general anesthesia. In: Dripp RD et al., eds. Introduction to Anesthesia. Philadelphia: WB Saunders, 1997:159.

28. Forman SA et al. Administration of general anesthesia. In: Hurford WE et al., eds. Clinical Anesthesia Procedures of the Massachusetts General Hospital. Philadelphia: Lippincott-Raven, 2002;210.

29. Fragen RJ, Avram MJ. Barbiturates. In: Miller Rd, ed. Anesthesia. New York: Churchill Livingstone, 2000:209.

30. Stoelting RK. Pharmacology and Physiology in Anesthetic Practice. Philadelphia: Lippincott-Raven, 1999;113.

31. Reves JG et al. Nonbarbiturate intravenous anesthetics. In: Miller RD, ed. Anesthesia. New York: Churchill Livingstone, 2000:228.

32. Raeder J, Stenseth LB. Ketamine: a new look at an old drug. Curr Opin Anaesthesiol 2000;13:463.

33. Price HL et al. The uptake of thiopental by body tissues and its relation to the duration of narcosis. Clin Pharmacol Ther 1960;1:16.

34. Lubarsky DA et al. The successful implementation of pharmaceutical practice guidelines. Anesthesiology 1997;86:1145.

35. Greenwald MJ et al. Extraocular muscle surgery. In: Krupin T, Holker AE, eds. Complications of Ocular Surgery. St. Louis: Mosby, 1993.

36. Borgeat A et al. Subhypnotic doses of propofol possess direct antiemetic effects. Anesth Analg 1992;74:539.

37. Ellis JE et al. Anesthesia for vascular surgery. In: Barash PG et al., eds. Clinical Anesthesia. Philadelphia: Lippincott, Williams & Wilkins, 2001:929.

38. Ding Z, White PF. Anesthesia for electroconvulsive therapy. Anesth Analg 2002;94:1351.

39. Ebert TJ, Schmid PG III. Inhalation anesthesia. In: Barash PG et al., eds. Clinical Anesthesia. Philadelphia: Lippincott Williams & Wilkins, 2001:377.

40. Krasowski MD, Harrison NL. General anesthetic actions on ligand-gated ion channels. Cell Mol Life Sci 1999;55:1278.

41. Koblin DD. Mechanisms of action. In: Miller RD, ed. Anesthesia. Philadelphia: Churchill Livingstone, 2000:48.

42. Andrews JJ. Inhaled anesthetic delivery systems. In: Miller RD, ed. Anesthesia. Philadelphia: Churchill Livingstone, 2000:48.

43. Gonsowski CT et al. Toxicity of compound A in rats. Anesthesiology 1994;80:556.

44. Mazze RI et al. The effects of sevoflurane on serum creatinine and blood urea nitrogen concentrations: a retrospective, twenty-two-center, comparative evaluation of renal function in adult surgical patients. Anesth Analg 2000;90:683.

45. Eger II EI et al. Dose-related biochemical markers of renal injury after sevoflurane versus desflurane anesthesia in volunteers. Anesth Analg 1997;85:1154.

46. Karasch ED et al. Assessment of low-flow sevoflurane and isoflurane effects on renal function using sensitive markers of tubular toxicity. Anesthesiology 1997;86:1238.

47. Frink EJ et al. Production of carbon monoxide using dry Baralyme with desflurane, enflurane, isoflurane, halothane, or sevoflurane anesthesia in pigs. Anesthesiology 1996;85:A1018.

48. Fang ZX et al. Carbon monoxide production from degradation of desflurane, enflurane, isoflurane, halothane, and sevoflurane by soda lime and Baralyme. Anesth Analg 1995;80:1187.

49. Murray MM et al. Amsorb: a new carbon dioxide absorbent for use in anesthetic breathing systems. Anesthesiology 1999;91:1342.

50. Philip BK et al. A multicenter comparison of maintenance and recovery with sevoflurane or isoflurane for adult ambulatory anesthesia. Anesth Analg 1996;83:314.

51. Beaussier M et al. Comparative effects of desflurane and isoflurane on recovery after long lasting anesthesia. Can J Anaesth 1998;45:429.

52. Ebert TJ et al. Recovery from sevoflurane anesthesia: a comparison to isoflurane and propofol anesthesia. Anesthesiology 1998;89:1524.

53. Eger II EI et al. The effect of anesthetic duration on kinetic and recovery characteristics of desflurane versus sevoflurane, and on the kinetic characteristics of compound A, in volunteers. Anesth Analg 1998;86:414.

54. Stoelting RK. Pharmacology and Physiology in Anesthetic Practice. Philadelphia: Lippincott-Raven, 1999:36.

55. Njoku D et al. Biotransformation of halothane, enflurane, isoflurane, and desflurane to trifluoroacetylated liver proteins: association between protein acylation and hepatic injury. Anesth Analg 1997;84:173.

56. Karasch ED et al. Human kidney methoxyflurane and sevoflurane metabolism: intrarenal fluoride production as a possible mechanism of methoxyflurane nephrotoxicity. Anesthesiology 1995;82:689.

57. Conzen PF et al. Low-flow sevoflurane compared with low-flow isoflurane anesthesia in patients with stable renal insufficiency. Anesthesiology 2002;97:578.

58. Munday IT et al. Serum fluoride concentration and urine osmolality after enflurane and sevoflurane anesthesia in male volunteers. Anesth Analg 1995;81:353.

59. Higuchi H et al. Renal function in patients with high serum fluoride concentrations after prolonged sevoflurane anesthesia. Anesthesiology 1995;83:449.

60. Nishiyama T et al. Inorganic fluoride kinetics and renal tubular function after sevoflurane anesthesia in chronic renal failure patients receiving hemodialysis. Anesth Analg 1996;83:574.

61. Moore MA et al. Rapid 1% increase of end-tidal desflurane concentration to greater than 5% transiently increase heart rate and blood pressure in humans. Anesthesiology 1994;81:94.

62. Weiskopf RB et al. Rapid increase in desflurane concentration is associated with greater transient cardiovascular stimulation than rapid increase in isoflurane concentration in humans. Anesthesiology 1994;80:1035.

63. Muzi M et al. Site(s) mediating sympathetic activation with desflurane. Anesthesiology 1996;85:737.

64. Weiskopf RB, Eger EI. Comparing the costs of inhaled anesthetics. Anesthesiology 1993;79:1413.

65. Smith I. Cost considerations in the use of anesthetic drugs. Pharmacoeconomics 2001;19:469.

66. Rosenberg MK et al. Cost comparison: a desflurane-versus propofol-based general anesthetic technique. Anesth Analg 1994;79:852.

67. Szocik JF, Learned DW. Impact of a cost containment program on the use of volatile anesthetics and neuromuscular blocking drugs. J Clin Anesth 1994;6:378.

68. Ebert TJ et al. Recovery from sevoflurane anesthesia: a comparison to isoflurane and propofol anesthesia. Anesthesiology 1998;89:1524.

69. Kurpiers EMC et al. Cost-effective anesthesia: desflurane versus propofol in outpatient surgery. AANA J 1996;64:69.

70. Boldt J et al. Economic considerations of the use of new anesthetics: a comparison of propofol, sevoflurane, desflurane, and isoflurane. Anesth Analg 1998;86:504.

71. Tang J et al. Antiemetic prophylaxis with sevoflurane anesthesia: a comparison with propofol in the office setting. Anesth Analg 2000;90:519.

72. Thwaites A et al. Inhalation induction with sevoflurane: a double-blind comparison with propofol. Br J Anaesth 1997;78:356.

73. Weiskopf RB et al. Fentanyl, esmolol, and clonidine blunt the transient cardiovascular stimulation induced by desflurane in humans. Anesthesiology 1994;81:1350.

74. Bevan DR, Donati F. Muscle relaxants. In: Barash PG et al., eds. Clinical Anesthesia. Philadelphia: Lippincott, Williams & Wilkins, 2001:419.

75. McManus MC. Neuromuscular blockers in surgery and intensive care: part 2. Am J Health Syst Pharm 2001;58:2381.

76. McManus MC. Neuromuscular blockers in surgery and intensive care: part 1. Am J Health Syst Pharm 2001;58:2287.

77. Savarese JJ et al. Pharmacology of muscle relaxants and their antagonists. In: Miller RD, ed. Anesthesia. New York: Churchill Livingstone, 2000:412.

78. Campagna JA, Dunn PF. Neuromuscular blockade. In: Hurford WE et al., eds. Clinical Anesthesia Procedures of the Massachusetts General Hospital. Philadelphia: Lippincott-Raven, 2002:172.

79. Sparr HJ. Choice of muscle relaxant for rapid-sequence induction. Eur J Anaesth (Suppl) 2001;23:71.

80. Strazis KP, Fox AW. Malignant hyperthermia: a review of published cases. Anesth Analg 1993;77:297.

81. Sufit RL et al. Doxacurium and mivacurium do not trigger malignant hyperthermia in susceptible swine. Anesth Analg 1990;71:285.

82. Laurin EG et al. A comparison of succinylcholine and rocuronium for rapid-sequence intubation of emergency department patients. Acad Emerg Med 2000;7:1362.

83. Cheng CA et al. Comparison of rocuronium and suxamethonium for rapid tracheal intubation in children. Paediatr Anaesth 2002;12:140.

84. Schwarz S et al. Rapid tracheal intubation with vecuronium: the priming principle. Anesthesiology 1985;62:388.

85. Kopman AF et al. Precurarization and priming: a theoretical analysis of safety and timing. Anesth Analg 2001;93:1253.

86. Grigore AM et al. Laudanosine and atracurium concentrations in a patient receiving long-term atracurium infusion. Crit Care Med 1998;26:180.

87. Bryson HM, Faulds D. Cisatracurium besilate: a review of its pharmacology and clinical potential in anesthetic practice. Drugs 1997;53:848.

88. Jones RM. Mivacurium in special patient groups. Acta Anaesth Scand (Suppl) 1995;106:47.

89. Sockalingam I, Green DW. Mivacurium-induced prolonged neuromuscular block. Br J Anaesth 1995;74:234.

90. Viby-Mogenson J. Succinylcholine neuromuscular blockade in subjects homozygous for atypical plasma cholinesterase. Anesthesiology 1981;55:429.

91. Hunter JM et al. The use of different doses of vecuronium in patients with liver dysfunction. Br J Anaesth 1985;57:758.

92. Hartmannsgrube MWB, Atanassoff PG. Regional anesthesia versus general anesthesia: does it make a difference? Semin Anesth 1998;17:58.

93. Bode Jr RH, Lewis KP. Con: regional anesthesia is not better than general anesthesia for lower extremity revascularization. J Cardiothorac Vasc Anesth 1994;8:118.

94. Berde CB, Strichartz GR. Local anesthetics. In: Miller RD. Anesthesia. Philadelphia: Churchill Livingstone, 2000:491.

95. Haddad T, Min J. Local anesthetics. In: Hurford WE et al., eds. Clinical Anesthesia Procedures of the Massachusetts General Hospital. Philadelphia: Lippincott Williams & Wilkins, 2002:220.

96. McClellan KJ, Spencer CM. Levobupivacaine. Drugs 1998;56:355.

97. Markham A, Faulds D. Ropivacaine: a review of its pharmacology and therapeutic use in regional anesthesia. Drugs 1996;52:429.

98. Singh P, Lee JS. Cardiovascular and central nervous system toxicity of local anesthetics. Semin Anesthesia 1998;17:18.

99. Chirocaine Product Information. Norwalk, CT: Purdue Pharma L.P., 1999.

100. Kalyanaraman M et al. Cardiopulmonary compromise after use of topical and submucosal α-agonists: possible added complication by the use of β-blocker therapy. Otolaryngol Head Neck Surg 1997;117:56.

101. Fleming JA et al. Pharmacology and therapeutic applications of cocaine. Anesthesiology 1990;73:518.

102. Goodell JA et al. Reducing cocaine solution use by promoting the use of a lidocaine-phenylephrine solution. Am J Hosp Pharm 1988;45:2510.

103. Nuttall GA et al. Establishing intravenous access: a study of local anesthetic efficacy. Anesth Analg 1993;950.

104. Donnelly AJ, Djuric M. Cardioplegia solutions. Am J Hosp Pharm 1991;48:2444.

105. Golembiewski J, Bourtsos N. Cardioplegia solution. J Pharm Pract 1993;6:182.

106. Chitwood W et al. Complex valve operations: antegrade versus retrograde cardioplegia? Ann Thorac Surg 1995;60:815.

107. Loop FD et al. Myocardial protection during cardiac operations: decreased morbidity and lower cost with blood cardioplegia and coronary sinus perfusion. J Thorac Cardiovasc Surg 1992;104:608.

108. Buckberg GD. Myocardial protection: an overview. Semin Thorac Cardiovasc Surg 1993;5:98.

109. Griepp RB et al. The superiority of aortic cross-clamping with profound local hypothermia for myocardial protection during aorta-coronary bypass grafting. J Thorac Cardiovasc Surg 1975;70:995.

110. Barden C, Hansen M. Cold versus warm cardioplegia: recognizing hemodynamic variations. Dimensions Crit Care Nurs 1995;14:114.

111. Lichtenstein SV et al. Warm heart surgery. J Thorac Cardiovasc Surg 1991;101:269.

112. Naylor CD et al. Randomized trial of normothermic versus hypothermic coronary bypass surgery. Lancet 1994;343:559.

113. Christakis GT et al. A randomized study of the systemic effects of warm heart surgery. Ann Thorac Surg 1992;54:449.

114. Hayashida N et al. The optimal cardioplegic temperature. Ann Thorac Surg 1994;58:961.

115. Hayashida N et al. Tepid antegrade and retrograde cardioplegia. Ann Thorac Surg 1995;59:723.

116. Drossos G et al. Deferoxamine cardioplegia reduces superoxide radical production in human myocardium. Ann Thorac Surg 1995;59:169.

117. Ferreira R et al. Reduction of reperfusion injury with mannitol cardioplegia. Ann Thorac Surg 1989;48:77.

118. Bical O et al. Comparison of different types of cardioplegia and reperfusion on myocardial metabolism and free radical activity. Circulation 1991,84(5 Suppl):III-375.

119. Lapenna D et al. Blood cardioplegia reduces oxidant burden in the ischemic and reperfused human myocardium. Ann Thorac Surg 1994;57:1522.

120. Vinten-Johansen J et al. Broad-spectrum cardioprotection with adenosine. Ann Thorac Surg 1999;68:1942.

121. Mentzer R et al. Adenosine myocardial protection: preliminary results of a phase II clinical trial. Ann Surg 1999;229:643.

122. Engelman DT et al. Critical timing of nitric oxide supplementation in cardioplegic arrest and reperfusion. Circulation 1996:94(Suppl II):II-407.

123. Mizuno A et al. Endothelial stunning and myocyte recovery after reperfusion of jeopardized muscle: a role of l-arginine blood cardioplegia. J Thorac Cardiovasc Surg 1997;113:379.

124. Izhar U et al. Cardioprotective effect of L-arginine in myocardial ischemia and reperfusion in an isolated working rat heart model. J Cardiovasc Surg 1998;39:321.

125. Carrier M et al. Cardioplegic arrest with L-arginine improves myocardial protection: results of a prospective randomized clinical trial. Ann Thorac Surg 2002;73:837.

126. Tyers GFO. Cardioplegic additives: a critical review. In: Engleman RM, Levitsky S, eds. A Textbook of Clinical Cardioplegia. Mount Kisco, NY: Futura, 1982:139.

127. Rich TL, Brady AJ. Potassium contracture and utilization of high-energy phosphates in rabbit heart. Am J Physiol 1974;226:105.

128. O'Riordain DS et al. Low potassium cardioplegia: its effect on the incidence of complete heart block following cardiac surgery. Ir J Med Sci 1989;158:257.

129. Rosenkranz ER et al. Warm induction of cardioplegia with glutamate-enriched blood in coronary patients with cardiogenic shock who are dependent on inotropic drugs and intra-aortic balloon support. J Thorac Cardiovasc Surg 1983;86:507.

130. Pisarenki OI et al. Glutamate-blood cardioplegia improves ATP preservation in human myocardium. Biomed Biochem Acta 1987;46:499.

131. Teoh KH et al. The effect of lactate infusion on myocardial metabolism and ventricular function following ischemia and cardioplegia. Can J Cardiol 1990;6:38.

132. Buckberg GD. Strategies and logic of cardioplegic delivery to prevent, avoid, and reverse ischemic and reperfusion damage. J Thorac Cardiovasc Surg 1987;93:127.

133. Teoh KH et al. Accelerated myocardial metabolic recovery with terminal warm blood cardioplegia. J Thorac Cardiovasc Surg 1986;91:888.

134. Golembiewski JA, O'Brien D. A systematic approach to the management of postoperative nausea and vomiting. J Perianesth Nurs 2002;17:364.

135. ASHP therapeutic guidelines on the management of nausea and vomiting in adult and pediatric patients receiving chemotherapy or radiation therapy or undergoing surgery. Am J Health Syst Pharm 1999;56:729.

136. Kovac AL. Prevention and treatment of postoperative nausea and vomiting. Drugs 2000;59:213.

137. Watcha MF, White PF. Postoperative nausea and vomiting. Anesthesiology 1992;77:162.

138. Haynes GR, Bailey MK. Postoperative nausea and vomiting: review and clinical approaches. South Med J 1996;89:940.

139. Bailey PL et al. Intravenous opioid anesthetics. In: Miller RD. Anesthesia. Philadelphia: Churchill Livingstone, 2000:273.

140. Gan TJ et al. Consensus guidelines for managing postoperative nausea and vomiting. Anesth Analg 2003;97:62.

141. Tramr MR. A rational approach to the control of postoperative nausea and vomiting: evidence from systematic reviews. Part 1. Efficacy and harm of antiemetic interventions and methodological issues. Acta Anaesthesiol Scand 2001;45:4.

142. Taketomo CK et al. Pediatric Dosage Handbook. 9th Ed. Hudson: Lexi-Comp, 2002–2003.

143. Henzi I et al. Efficacy, dose-response, and adverse effects of droperidol for prevention of postoperative nausea and vomiting. Can J Anaesth 2000;47:537.

144. Gan TJ et al. FDA "Black-Box" warning regarding use of droperidol for postoperative nausea and vomiting: is it justified? Anesthesiology 2002;97:287.

145. Habib AS, Gan TJ. Food and Drug Administration black box warning on the perioperative use of droperidol: a review of the cases. Anesth Analg 2003;96:1377.

146. Domino KD et al. Comparative efficacy and safety of ondansetron, droperidol, and metoclopramide for preventing postoperative nausea and vomiting: a meta-analysis. Anesth Analg 1999;88:1370.

147. Zarate E et al. A comparison of the costs and efficacy of ondansetron versus dolasetron for antiemetic prophylaxis. Anesth Analg 2000;90:1352.

148. Roberson CR et al. IV dolasetron vs. ondansetron for the treatment of PONV in ambulatory surgery patients. Anesthesiology 1999;91:A4.

149. Gan TJ et al. Consensus guidelines for managing postoperative nausea and vomiting. Anesth Analg 2003;97:62.

150. Henzi I et al. Dexamethasone for the prevention of postoperative nausea and vomiting: a quantitative systematic review. Anesth Analg 2000;90:186.

151. Wang JJ et al. The use of dexamethasone for preventing postoperative nausea and vomiting in females undergoing thyroidectomy: a dose-finding study. Anesth Analg 2000;91:404.

152. Wand JJ et al. The effect of timing of dexamethasone administration on its efficacy as a prophylactic antiemetic for postoperative nausea and vomiting. Anesth Analg 2000;91:136.

153. Chen JJ et al. Efficacy of ondansetron and prochlorperazine for the prevention of postoperative nausea and vomiting after total hip replacement or total knee replacement procedures. Arch Intern Med 1998;158:2124.

154. Kranke P et al. Dimenhydrinate for prophylaxis of postoperative nausea and vomiting: a meta-analysis of randomized controlled trials. Acta Anaesthesiol Scand 2002;46:238.

155. Kranke P et al. The efficacy and safety of transdermal scopolamine for the prevention of postoperative nausea and vomiting: a quantitative systematic review. Anesth Analg 2002;95:133.

156. Coloma M et al. Dexamethasone in combination with dolasetron for prophylaxis in the ambulatory setting. Anesthesiology 2002;96:1346.

157. Kovac AL et al. Efficacy of repeat intravenous dosing of ondansetron in controlling postoperative nausea and vomiting: a randomized, double-blind, placebo-controlled multicenter trial. J Clin Anesth 1999;11:453.

158. Sinclair DR et al. Can postoperative nausea and vomiting be predicted? Anesthesiology 1999;91:109.

159. Gan TJ et al. Double-blind, randomized comparison of ondansetron and intraoperative propofol to prevent postoperative nausea and vomiting. Anesthesiology 1996;85:1036.

160. Sneyd JR et al. A meta-analysis of nausea and vomiting following maintenance of anaesthesia with propofol or inhalational agents. Eur J Anaesth 1998;15:433.

161. Monti S. Preoperative fluid bolus reduces risk of postoperative nausea and vomiting: a pilot study. Internet J Adv Nurs Prac 2000;4(2).

162. Reuben SS, Sklar J. Pain management in patients who undergo outpatient arthroscopic surgery of the knee. J Bone Joint Surg 2000;82A:1754.

163. Rowlingson JC. Acute pain management revisited. IARS Rev Course Lectures 2002.

164. Carpenter RL. Optimizing postoperative pain management. Am Fam Physician 1997;56:835.

165. Kehlet H, Wilmore D. Multimodal strategies to improve surgical outcome. Am J Surg 2002;183:630.

166. Hollmann MW, Durieux ME. Local anesthetics and the inflammatory response: a new therapeutic indication? Anesthesiology 2000;93:858.

167. Gan TJ et al. Postdischarge recovery experience after single presurgery dose of IV parecoxib sodium, a novel COX-2 inhibitor, followed by oral valdecoxib for pain after laparoscopic cholecystectomy. Anesthesiology 2002;96:A20.

168. Etches RC. Patient-controlled analgesia. Surg Clin North Am 1999;79:297.

169. Bennett RL et al. Patient-controlled analgesia: a new concept for postoperative pain relief. Ann Surg 1982;195:700.

170. Mernes ER, Hare BD. Meperidine neurotoxicity: three case reports and a review of the literature. J Pharmaceutic Care Pain Sympt Control 1993;1:5.

171. Kaiko RF et al. Central nervous system excitatory effects of meperidine in cancer patients. Ann Neurol 1983;13:180.

172. Mason PJ et al. Serotonin syndrome: presentation of 2 cases and a review of the literature. Medicine 2000;79:201.

173. Austrup ML, Korean G. Analgesic agents for the postoperative period. Surg Clin North Am 1999;79:253.

174. Lubenow TK et al. Management of acute postoperative pain. In: Barash PG et al., eds. Clinical Anesthesia. Philadelphia: Lippincott, Williams, & Wilkins, 2001:1403.

175. Ready LB. Acute perioperative pain. In: Miller RD ed. Anesthesia. Philadelphia: Churchill Livingstone, 2000:2323.

176. Peeters-Asdourian C. Acute pain management. In: Warfield CA, Fausett HJ eds. Manual of Pain Management. Philadelphia: Lippincott Williams & Wilkins, 2002:215.

177. Ketorolac tromethamine injection U.S.P. Bedford, OH: Bedford Laboratories, 1999.

178. Beattie WS et al. Epidural analgesia reduces postoperative myocardial infarction: a meta-analysis. Anesth Analg 2001;93:853.

179. Ballantyne JC et al. The comparative effects of postoperative analgesic therapies on pulmonary outcome: cumulative meta-analysis of randomized, controlled trials. Anesth Analg 1998;86:598.

180. Covino BG, Lambert DH. Epidural and spinal anesthesia. In: Barash PG et al., eds. Clinical Anesthesia. Philadelphia: Lippincott-Raven, 1997:1305.

181. Consensus statement. Regional anesthesia in the anticoagulated patient: defining the risks. American Society of Regional Anesthesia and Pain Medicine, 2002.

182. Cerda SE, Eisenach JC. Intrathecal and epidural opioids. Semin Anesth 1997;16:92.

183. Rawal N. Epidural and spinal opioids for postoperative analgesia. Surg Clin North Am 1999; 79:313.

184. Cousins MJ, Mather LE. Intrathecal and epidural administration of opioids. Anesthesiology 1984; 61:276.

185. DeLeon-Casasola OA, Lema MJ. Postoperative epidural opioid analgesia: what are the choices? Anesth Analg 1996;83:867.

186. Lui S et al. Intravenous versus epidural administration of hydromorphone: effects on analgesia and recovery after radical retropubic prostatectomy. Anesthesiology 1995;82:682.

187. Bromage PR et al. Nonrespiratory side effects of epidural morphine. Anesth Analg 1982;61:490.

188. Ko MC, Naughton NN. An experimental itch model in monkeys: characterization of intrathecal morphine-induced scratching and antinociception. Anesthesiology 2000;92:795

189. Scott DA et al. Postoperative analgesia using epidural infusions of fentanyl with bupivacaine. Anesthesiology 1995;83:727.

190. Vandermuelen EP et al. Anticoagulants and spinal-epidural anesthesia. Anesth Analg 1994;79:1165.

191. Cancer pain relief and palliative care. Geneva: World Health Organization, 1990.

192. White PF. The role of non-opioid analgesic techniques in the management of pain after ambulatory surgery. Anesth Analg 2002;94:577.

193. Crews JC. Multimodal pain management strategies for office-based and ambulatory procedures. JAMA 2002;288:629.

194. McCaffery M, Pasero C. Pain Clinical Manual. St. Louis: Mosby, 1999.

195. Reuben S, Sklar J. Pain management in patients who undergo outpatient arthroscopic surgery of the knee. J Bone Joint Surg 2000;82:1754.

196. Johnstone RE. Intraoperative strategies for cost containment in anesthesia. ASA Refresher Course Lecture, 1995.

197. Gillerman RB, Browning RA. Drug use inefficiency: a hidden source of wasted health care dollars. Anesth Analg 2000;91:921.

198. Bastron RD, Vallamaria FJ. Use of practice parameters to control drug costs. Anesthesiology 1995;83:A1059.

199. Freund PR et al. Cost-effective reduction of neuromuscular blocking drug expenditures: a two year follow-up. Anesth Analg 1997;84:537.

200. Orkin FK. Moving toward value-based anesthesia care. J Clin Ancsth 1993;5:91.

201. Macario A et al. Where are the costs in perioperative care? Analysis of hospital costs and charges for inpatient surgical care. Anesthesiology 1995;83:1138.

202. Lubarsky DA et al. A comparison of maintenance drug costs of isoflurane, desflurane, sevoflurane and propofol with OR and PACU labor costs during a 60 minute outpatient procedure. Anesthesiology 1995;83:A1035.

203. Cheng DCH et al. Early tracheal extubation after coronary artery bypass graft surgery reduces costs and improves resource use. Anesthesiology 1996;85:1300.

204. Cheng DCH et al. Morbidity outcome in early versus conventional tracheal extubation after coronary artery bypass graft surgery: a prospective randomized controlled trial. J Thorac Cardiovasc Surg 1996;112:755.

205. Cheng DCH et al. Randomized assessment of resource use in fast-track cardiac surgery 1 year after hospital discharge. Anesthesiology 2003;98:651.

206. Apfelbaum JL et al. Bypassing the PACU: a new paradigm in ambulatory surgery. Anesthesiology 1997;87:A32.

207. Apfelbaum JL et al. Eliminating intensive postoperative care in same-day surgery patients using short-acting anesthetics. Anesthesiology 2002; 97:66.

208. Song D et al. Fast-track eligibility after ambulatory anesthesia: a comparison of desflurane, sevoflurane, and propofol. Anesth Analg 1998; 86:267.

209. Song D et al. Titration of volatile anesthetics using bispectral index facilitates recovery after ambulatory anesthesia. Anesthesiology 1997;87:842.

210. Chan X et al. A comparison of patient state index and bispectral index values during the perioperative period. Anesth Analg 2002;95:1669.

211. Song D et al. The bispectral (BIS) index predicts fast-track eligibility after ambulatory anesthesia. Anesthesiology 1998;89:A16.

212. Pierce ET et al. Patient state index (PSI): optimization of delivery and recovery from propofol, alfentanil, and nitrous oxide. Anesthesiology 2001;95:A283.

213. Ahmad S et al. Impact of bispectral index monitoring on fast-tracking of gynecological patients undergoing laparoscopic surgery. Anesthesiology 2003;98:849.

Acid-Base Disorders

Raymond W. Hammond

To monitor drug therapy properly and recognize serious problems in patients, all clinicians need a basic knowledge of acid-base physiology, mechanisms that regulate acid-base balance, and interventions to correct problems occurring from an imbalance. Severe acid-base disorders may affect multiple organ systems: cardiovascular (e.g., impaired contractility, arrhythmias), pulmonary (e.g., impaired oxygen delivery, respiratory muscle fatigue, dyspnea), renal (e.g., hypokalemia, nephrolithiasis), or neurologic (e.g., decreased cerebral blood flow, seizures, coma).

ACID-BASE PHYSIOLOGY

To protect body proteins, acid-base balance must be tightly controlled in an attempt to maintain a normal extracellular pH of 7.35 to 7.45 and an intracellular pH of approximately 7.0 to 7.3.[1] This narrow range is maintained by complex buffer systems, ventilation to expel CO_2, and renal elimination of acids and reabsorption of HCO_3^-.[2] At rest, about 200 mL of CO_2, and even more during exercise, is transported from the tissues and excreted in the lungs.[3] While HCO_3^- is only responsible for about 36% of intracellular buffering, it provides about 86% of the buffering activity in extracellular fluid (ECF).[1] Extracellular fluid contains approximately 350 mEq HCO_3^-, which buffers generated H^+.

$$HCO_3^- + H^+ \Leftrightarrow H_2CO_3 \qquad (11\text{-}1)$$

Hydrogen ion (H^+) combines with HCO_3^- and shifts the equilibrium of Equation 11-1 to the right. In the proximal renal tubule lumen, carbonic anhydrase catalyzes the dehydration of H_2CO_3 to CO_2 and H_2O, which are absorbed into the tubule cell, as illustrated in Equation 11-2 and Figure 11-1. Within the tubule cell, H_2O dissociates into H^+ and OH^-. The H^+ is then secreted into the lumen by a Na^+-H^+ exchanger. Carbonic anhydrase then catalyzes the combination of OH^- and CO_2 to HCO_3^-, which is carried into the circulation by a $Na^+HCO_3^-$ cotransporter.[4]

$$HCO_3^- + H^+ \Leftrightarrow H_2CO_3 \overset{CA}{\Leftrightarrow} CO_2 \text{ (dissolved)} + H_2O \qquad (11\text{-}2)$$

To maintain acid-base balance, the kidney must reclaim and regenerate all the filtered HCO_3^-. The daily amount that must be reabsorbed can be calculated by the product of the glomerular filtration rate (GFR) and the HCO_3^- concentration in ECF (180 L/d GFR × 24 mEq/L HCO_3^- = 4,320 mEq/d).[1] The proximal tubule reabsorbs about 85% of the filtered HCO_3^-. The loop of Henle and the distal tubule reabsorb about 10%.[5] Salts of acids such as HPO_4^- (pK$_a$ of 6.8) that have a pK$_a$ greater than the pH of the urine (titratable acids) can accept a proton and be excreted as the acid, thus regenerating a HCO_3^- anion.[5] Sulfuric acid and other acids with a pK$_a$ <4.5 are not titratable. Protons from these acids must be combined with another buffer to be secreted. Glutamine deamination in proximal tubular cells forms NH_3 that accepts these protons. In the collecting tubule, the NH_4^+ produced is lipid-insoluble, trapping it in the lumen and causing its excretion, eliminating the proton, and allowing for regeneration of HCO_3^-.[4-6] Figure 11-2 is a simplified illustration of the buffering of these acids.

The daily metabolism of carbohydrates and fats generates about 15,000 mmol of CO_2. While CO_2 is not an acid, it reversibly combines with H_2O to form carbonic acid, (i.e.,

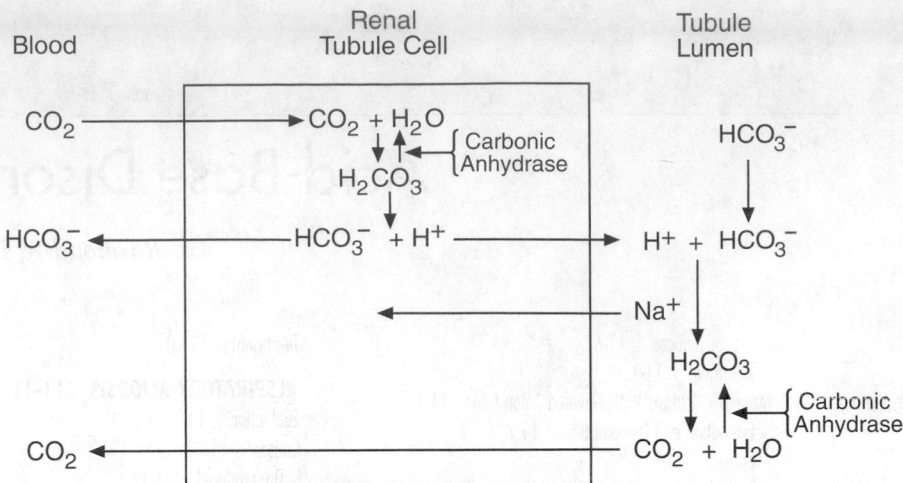

FIGURE 11-1 Renal tubular bicarbonate reabsorption.

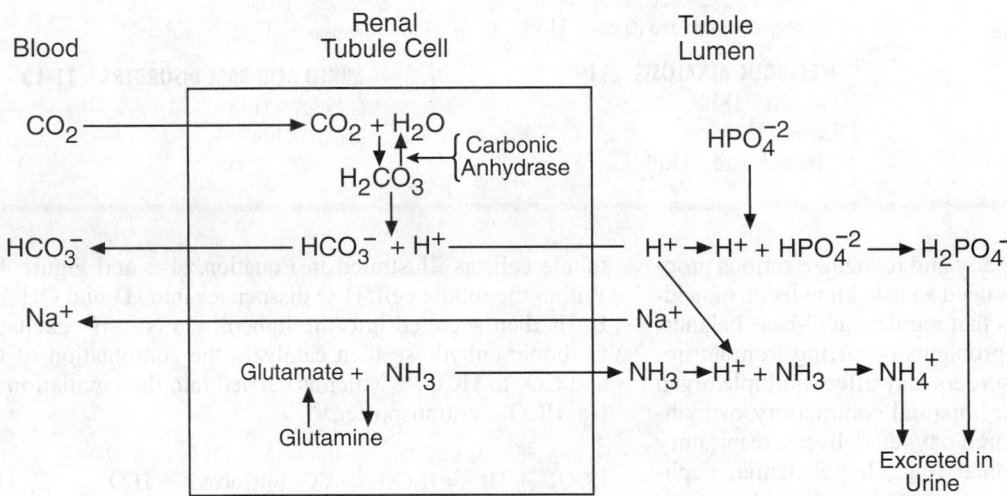

FIGURE 11-2 Renal tubular hydrogen ion excretion.

H_2CO_3). Respiration prevents the accumulation of volatile acid through the exhalation of CO_2. Metabolism of proteins and fats results in several fixed acids and bases. Amino acids like lysine and arginine have a net positive charge and serve as acids. Compounds, such as glutamate, aspartate, and citrate have a negative charge. In general, animal proteins contain more sulfur and phosphates, producing an acidic diet. Vegetarian diets consist of more organic anions, resulting in a more alkaline diet.[7] Normally, fatty acids are metabolized to HCO_3^-, but during starvation or diabetic ketoacidosis they may be incompletely oxidized to acetoacetate and β-hydroxybutyric acid.[6] The typical diet generates a net nonvolatile acid load of about 70 to 100 mEq of H^+ (1.0 to 1.5 mEq/Kg) per day.[1,8] Renal excretion of 70 mEq in 2 L of urine each day would require a pH of 1.5. Because the kidney cannot produce a pH less than 4.5, most of this fixed acid load must be buffered. The primary buffers for renal net acid excretion are NH_3-NH_4^+ and titratable buffers such as HPO_4^--$H_2PO_4^{2-}$, as mentioned above.[7] The correct assessment of acid-base disorders begins with an evaluation of appropriate laboratory data and an understanding of the physiologic mechanisms responsible for maintaining a normal pH.

Laboratory Assessment

Laboratory data used to evaluate acid-base status are arterial pH, arterial carbon dioxide tension ($PaCO_2$), and serum bicarbonate (HCO_3^-).[9–11] These values are obtained routinely with an arterial blood gas (ABG) determination. Acid-base abnormalities occur when the concentration of $PaCO_2$ (an acid) or HCO_3^- (a base) is altered. ABG measurements also include the arterial oxygen tension (PaO_2); however, this value does not directly influence decisions regarding acid-base abnormalities. Normal ABG values are listed in Table 11-1. When arterial pH is <7.35, the patient is considered acidemic, and the process that caused acid-base imbalance is called acidosis. Conversely, when the arterial pH is >7.45, the patient is considered alkalemic, and the causative process is alkalosis. The process is further defined as respiratory if there is an inappropriate elevation or depression of $Paco_2$ or metabolic if there is an inappropriate rise or fall in serum HCO_3^-.

Acid-base balance is normally maintained by the primary extracellular buffer system of HCO_3^--CO_2. Components of this buffer system are measured routinely to assess acid-base status. However, other extracellular buffers (e.g., serum proteins, inorganic phosphates) and intracellular buffers (e.g., hemoglobin, proteins, phosphates) also contribute significant buffering activity.[1,7–10] Serum electrolytes are obtained to calculate the anion gap, an estimate of the unmeasured cations and anions in serum. The anion gap helps determine the probable cause of a metabolic acidosis.[6,10,12–29] Urine pH, electrolytes, and osmolality help to further differentiate among the possible causes of metabolic acidosis.[10,30–34]:

Acid-Base Balance, Carbon Dioxide Tension, and Respiratory Regulation

In aqueous solution, carbonic acid [i.e., H_2CO_3) formed through the reaction described in Equation 11-1] reversibly dehydrates to form carbon dioxide (CO_2) and water (H_2O) as shown in equation 11-2.

The enzyme carbonic anhydrase (CA), present in red blood cells, renal tubular cells, and other tissues, catalyzes the interconversion of carbonic acid and carbon dioxide. Some of the carbon dioxide produced by dehydration of carbonic acid remains dissolved in plasma, but most exists as a volatile gas:

$$HCO_3^- + H^+ \Leftrightarrow H_2CO_3 \overset{CA}{\Leftrightarrow} CO_2 \text{ (dissolved)} + H_2O$$
$$\uparrow\downarrow$$
$$k \times CO_2 \text{ (gas)} \qquad \textbf{(11-3)}$$

In Equation 11-3, k is a solubility constant that has a value of approximately 0.03 in plasma at body temperature.[2,34] Virtually all the carbonic acid in body fluids is in the form of carbon dioxide. Therefore, the $Paco_2$, a measure of carbon dioxide gas, is directly proportional to the amount of carbonic acid in the HCO_3^-/H_2CO_3 buffer system. The normal range for $Paco_2$ is 35 to 45 mm Hg.

The lungs can rapidly exhale large quantities of carbon dioxide and thereby contribute significantly to the maintenance of a normal pH. Carbon dioxide formed through the reaction described in Equation 11-3 diffuses easily from tissues to capillary blood and from pulmonary capillary blood into the alveoli where it is exhaled from the body.[3] Pulmonary ventilation is regulated by peripheral chemoreceptors (located in the carotid arteries and the aorta) and central chemoreceptors (located in the medulla). The peripheral chemoreceptors are activated by arterial acidosis, hypercarbia (elevated $Paco_2$), and hypoxemia (decreased Pao_2). Central chemoreceptors are activated by cerebrospinal fluid (CSF) acidosis and by elevated carbon dioxide tension in the CSF.[3] Activation of these chemoreceptors stimulates the respiratory control center in the medulla to increase the rate and depth of ventilation, which results in increased exhalation of carbon dioxide.

Bicarbonate and Renal Control

As described in the Acid-Base Physiology section above, the kidneys are responsible for regulating the serum bicarbonate concentration. This is accomplished through two important and interrelated functions. First, they must reabsorb the bicarbonate that undergoes glomerular filtration and is present in the renal tubular fluid. Second, the kidneys must excrete hydrogen ions released from nonvolatile acids. Both functions are important in preventing systemic acidosis.

One mechanism of bicarbonate reabsorption in the proximal renal tubule is illustrated in Figure 11-1. Carbonic anhydrase catalyzes intracellular formation of carbonic acid (H_2CO_3) from carbon dioxide (CO_2) and water in the renal tubular cell. The carbonic acid then dissociates to form H^+ and HCO_3^-. The H^+ ion is secreted into the lumen of the tubule in exchange for a sodium ion (Na^+), and the bicarbonate from the renal tubule cell is reabsorbed into the capillary blood. Inside the lumen, carbonic acid is reformed from secreted H^+ and filtered HCO_3^-. Carbonic anhydrase present inside the lumen (on the brush border membrane of the cell) catalyzes conversion of carbonic acid to carbon dioxide that can readily diffuse back into the blood. Thus, the net result is reabsorption of sodium and bicarbonate. Although a hydrogen ion is secreted into the lumen in this process, no net excretion of acid occurs because of the reabsorption of carbon dioxide.[4–6] Figure 11-2 illustrates H^+ excretion by the kidney. This process was discussed in the physiology section above.

In clinical practice, the serum bicarbonate concentration usually is estimated from the total carbon dioxide content when the serum concentration of electrolytes are ordered on an electrolyte panel or calculated from the pH and $Paco_2$ on an ABG determination. These estimations of the serum bicarbonate concentration are more convenient than directly measuring serum bicarbonate. The total carbon dioxide content that is reported on serum electrolyte panels is determined by acidifying serum to convert all the bicarbonate to carbon dioxide and measuring the partial pressure of CO_2 gas. Approximately 95% of the total carbon dioxide content is bicarbonate. The serum bicarbonate concentration reported on ABG results is calculated from the patient's pH and $Paco_2$ using the Henderson-Hasselbalch equation (Equation 11-4). This calculated bicarbonate concentration should be within 2 mEq/L of the measured total carbon dioxide. The normal range of serum bicarbonate using these methods is 22 to 26 mEq/L.[10]

Bicarbonate:Carbonic Acid Ratio

The relationship between the pH and the concentrations of the acid-base pairs in buffer systems is described by the Henderson-Hasselbalch equation:

$$pH = pK + \log \frac{[base]}{[acid]} \qquad \textbf{(11-4)}$$

Table 11-1	Normal ABG Values
ABGs	Normal Range
pH	7.36–7.44
Pao_2	90–100 mm Hg
$Paco_2$	35–45 mm Hg
HCO_3^-	22–26 mEq/L

The pK is the negative logarithm of the equilibrium constant for the buffer reaction. The pK for the carbonic acid–bicarbonate buffer system is 6.1. Because most of the carbonic acid in plasma is in the form of carbon dioxide gas, the concentration of acid, [acid], can be estimated as $Paco_2$ multiplied by 0.03 (the solubility constant, k, in Equation 11-3). The concentration of base, [base], is equal to the serum bicarbonate concentration. Using these values, Equation 11-4 can be rewritten as follows:

$$pH = 6.1 + \log \frac{(HCO_3^-)}{(0.03)(P_{aco_2})} \quad (11\text{-}5)$$

As shown by Equation 11-5, the arterial pH will be 7.40 when the ratio of HCO_3^-:H_2CO_3 is approximately 20:1. Note that it is the *ratio* of bicarbonate to the carbon dioxide tension and not the absolute concentration of these factors that determines the arterial pH. Therefore, if the serum bicarbonate concentration and the carbon dioxide tension are increased or decreased proportionately, the ratio remains fixed and the pH is not affected.[33–36]

EVALUATION OF ACID-BASE DISORDERS

Acid-base disorders should be evaluated using a stepwise approach.[32,33]

1. Determine whether the pH is consistent with acidosis or alkalosis.
2. Check for laboratory validity. Using Equation 11-5, determine whether the CO_2 and HCO_3^- values are consistent with the pH.
3. Review the history to see if there are any clues to the cause of the disorder.

4. Determine whether the primary disorder is of respiratory or metabolic origin. The common laboratory findings of the four simple acid-base disorders are listed in Table 11-2.
5. Calculate the expected compensatory response and determine whether there is a mixed acid-base disorder. Normal compensatory changes for simple acid-base disorders have been identified and are outlined in Table 11-3.[5,8,32–34]
6. Calculate the anion gap to determine the probable cause of the disorder.
7. Consider other laboratory tests to further differentiate the cause of the disorder.
   a. If the anion gap is normal, consider calculating the urine anion gap.
   b. If the anion gap is high and a hypoxic origin is expected, obtain a serum lactate level.
   c. If the anion gap is high and a toxic ingestion is expected, calculate an osmolal gap.

METABOLIC ACIDOSIS

Metabolic acidosis is characterized by loss of bicarbonate from the body, decreased acid excretion by the kidney, or increased endogenous acid production. Two categories of simple metabolic acidosis are based on the calculated anion gap (AG) (Table 11-4).

The AG represents the concentration of unmeasured negatively charged substances (anions) in excess of the concentration of unmeasured positively charged substances (cations) in the extracellular fluid. The concentrations of total anions and cations in the body are equal because the body must remain electrically neutral. However, most clinical laboratories measure only a portion of these ions (i.e., sodium, chloride [Cl^-],

Table 11-2 Laboratory Values in Simple Acid-Base Disorders

Disorder	Arterial pH	Primary Change	Compensatory Change
Metabolic acidosis	↓	↓ HCO_3^-	↓ $Paco_2$
Respiratory acidosis	↓	↑ $Paco_2$	↑ HCO_3^-
Metabolic alkalosis	↑	↑ HCO_3^-	↑ $Paco_2$
Respiratory alkalosis	↑	↓ $Paco_2$	↓ HCO_3^-

Table 11-3 Normal Compensation in Simple Acid-Base Disorders

Disorder	Compensation[a]
Metabolic acidosis	↓ $Paco_2$ (mm Hg) = 1.0 − 1.2 × HCO_3^- (mEq/L)
Metabolic alkalosis	↑ $Paco_2$ (mm Hg) = 0.5 − 0.7 × ↑ HCO_3^- (mEq/L)
Respiratory acidosis	
Acute	↑ HCO_3^- (mEq/L) = 0.1 × ↑ $Paco_2$ (mm Hg)
Chronic	↑ HCO_3^- (mEq/L) = 0.4 × ↑ $Paco_2$ (mm Hg)
Respiratory alkalosis	
Acute	↓ HCO_3^- (mEq/L) = 0.2 × ↓ $Paco_2$ (mm Hg)
Chronic	↓ HCO_3^- (mEq/L) = 0.4 − 0.5 × ↓ $Paco_2$ (mm Hg)

[a]Based on change from normal $HCO_3^- = 24$ mEq/L and $Paco_2 = 40$ mm Hg.

and bicarbonate). The concentrations of other negatively and positively charged substances such as potassium (K^+), magnesium (Mg^{2+}), calcium (Ca^{2+}), phosphates, and albumin are measured less often. The concentration of unmeasured anions normally exceeds the concentration of unmeasured cations by 6 to 12 mEq/L and is calculated as follows:

$$Anion\ gap = Na^+ - (Cl^- + HCO_3^-) \quad (11\text{-}6)$$

Of the unmeasured anions, albumin is perhaps the most important. In critically ill patients with hypoalbuminemia, the calculated AG should be adjusted using the following formula: adjusted AG = AG + 2.5 × (normal albumin − measured albumin)g/dL, where a normal albumin concentration is assumed to be 4.4 g/dL.[19–22] For example, a hypoalbuminemic patient (serum albumin, 2.4 g/dL) with early sepsis and lactic acidosis may have a calculated AG of 11 mEq/L. After the calculation is corrected for the effect of abnormal serum albumin concentrations, the presence of elevated AG acidosis is more apparent (adjusted AG, 16 mEq/L).

Metabolic acidosis with a normal AG (hyperchloremic metabolic acidosis) usually is caused by loss of bicarbonate and can be further characterized as hypokalemic or hyperkalemic.[5,31,34,37–48] Diarrhea can result in severe bicarbonate loss and a hyperchloremic metabolic acidosis. Elevated AG metabolic acidosis usually is associated with overproduction of organic acids or with decreased renal elimination of nonvolatile acids.[34,49–51] Increased production of organic acids (e.g., formic, lactic acids) is buffered by extracellular bicarbonate with resultant consumption of bicarbonate and appearance of an unmeasured anion (e.g., formate, lactate).[32,49–50] The decrement in serum bicarbonate approximates the increment in the AG, the latter being a good estimate of the circulating anion level. Prolonged hypoxia results in lactic acidosis. Uncontrolled diabetes mellitus or excessive alcohol intake with starvation can cause ketoacidosis. In the case of renal failure, the capacity for H^+ secretion diminishes, resulting in

metabolic acidosis.[37] The accompanying increased AG results from decreased excretion of unmeasured anions such as sulfate and phosphate.[26]

Normal Anion Gap (Hyperchloremic) Metabolic Acidosis
Evaluation

1. A.B., a 27-year-old, 60-kg woman, is hospitalized for evaluation of weakness. She has a history of bipolar affective disorder and reports recent ingestion of lead-containing paint from the walls of her house. A.B.'s only current medication is lithium carbonate 300 mg TID. On admission, she appears weak and apathetic and complains of anorexia. Laboratory tests reveal the following: serum Na, 143 mEq/L (normal, 135 to 145 mEq/L); K, 3.0 mEq/L (normal, 3.5 to 5.0 mEq/L); Cl, 121 mEq/L (normal, 95 to 105 mEq/L); albumin, 4.4 g/dL (normal, 3.6 to 5.0 g/dL); pH, 7.28 (normal, 7.35 to 7.45); $Paco_2$, 26 mm Hg (normal, 35 to 45 mm Hg); HCO_3^-, 12 mEq/L (normal, 22 to 26 mEq/L); and urine pH, 5.5. A.B.'s urine pH following an ammonium chloride (NH_4Cl) 0.1 g/kg IV load is <5.1. A bicarbonate load of 1 mEq/kg infused IV over 1 hour induces bicarbonaturia (urinary pH, 7.0) and lowers the serum potassium to 2.0 mEq/L. Her blood pH only increased to 7.31. Assess A.B.'s acid-base status.

[SI units: Na, 143 mmol/L (normal, 135 to 145); K, 3.0 and 2.0 mmol/L, respectively (normal, 3.5 to 5.0); Cl, 121 mmol/L (normal, 95 to 105); albumin, 44 g/L (normal, 36 to 50); $Paco_2$, 3.5 kPa (normal, 4.7 to 6.0); HCO_3^-, 12 mmol/L (normal, 22 to 26)]

Using a stepwise approach, we see that A.B.'s low pH is consistent with acidosis, and here CO_2 and HCO_3^- are consistent with her pH as validated by Equation 11-5. A review of her history gives a clue that may lead to the cause for her acidosis. The next step is to determine whether the primary disorder is of respiratory or metabolic origin. As previously described, the serum bicarbonate concentration is regulated primarily by the kidneys, whereas the $Paco_2$ is controlled by the lungs. Alterations in pH resulting from a primary change in serum bicarbonate are metabolic acid-base disorders. Specifically, metabolic acidosis is associated with a decrease in serum HCO_3^- and decreased pH, whereas metabolic alkalosis is associated with an increase in serum HCO_3^- and increased pH. In respiratory disorders, the primary change occurs in the $Paco_2$. If A.B. had a decrease in pH and increase in $Paco_2$, a respiratory acidosis would be present. Because A.B. has a low $Paco_2$ and decreased serum HCO_3^-, she has a metabolic acidosis. The next step (i.e., Step 5 in the Evaluation of Acid-Base Disorders above) involves calculating the expected respiratory compensation to determine whether A.B. has a mixed acid-base disorder. In most cases of metabolic acidosis or alkalosis, the lungs compensate for the primary change in serum HCO_3^- concentration by increasing or decreasing ventilation. This respiratory compensation minimizes the change in the ratio of bicarbonate to the carbon dioxide tension and, thus, reduces the change in arterial pH (see Equation 11-5). The decrease in $Paco_2$ of 14 mm Hg for A.B. is consistent with respiratory compensation (see Table 11-3). A primary decrease in the serum bicarbonate to 12 mEq/L should result in a compensatory decrease in the $Paco_2$ by 12 to 17 mm Hg (see Table 11-3). A.B.'s $Paco_2$ has fallen by 14 mm Hg (normal, 40 mm Hg; current, 26 mm Hg), confirming that normal respira-

Table 11-4 Common Causes of Metabolic Acidosis

Normal AG	Elevated AG
Hypokalemic	Renal Failure
Diarrhea	Lactic Acidosis
Fistulous disease	(See Table 11-6)
Ureteral diversions	Ketoacidosis
Type 1 RTA	Starvation
Type 2 RTA	Ethanol
Carbonic anhydrase inhibitors	Diabetes mellitus
Hyperkalemic	Drug Intoxications
Hypoaldosteronism	Ethylene glycol
Hydrochloric acid or precursor	Methanol
Type 4 RTA	Salicylates
Potassium-sparing diuretics	
Amiloride	
Spironolactone	
Triamterene	

AG, anion gap; RTA, renal tubular acidosis.

tory compensation has occurred. When values for $Paco_2$ or serum HCO_3^- fall outside of normal compensatory ranges, either a mixed acid-base disorder, inadequate extent of compensation, or inadequate time for compensation should be suspected. Mixed acid-base disorders should also be suspected when the changes in serum HCO_3^- and $Paco_2$ occur in opposite directions.[5,33] For example, a patient with a pH of 6.92, decreased serum HCO_3^- concentration of 10 mEq/L, and increased $Paco_2$ of 50 mm Hg would have a mixed metabolic and respiratory acidosis. As this example illustrates, mixed acid-base disorders can result in profound alteration in arterial pH.

If A.B.'s $Paco_2$ was significantly lower than 23 mm Hg or higher than 28 mm Hg, a mixed disorder should be suspected (i.e., coexistent respiratory alkalosis or acidosis, respectively).

Causes

2. What are potential causes of metabolic acidosis in A.B.?

Steps 6 and 7 of the stepwise approach in the Evaluation of Acid Base Disorders (see above) are used to further determine the cause of the acid-base disorder. In patients with metabolic acidosis, calculation of the AG serves as a first stop in classifying the metabolic acidosis and provides additional information about the conditions that might be responsible for the acid-base disorder. A.B.'s calculated AG is 10 mEq/L (see Equation 11-6). Thus, A.B. has hyperchloremic metabolic acidosis with a normal AG.

The common causes of metabolic acidosis are presented in Table 11-4.[5,10,49] Normal AG metabolic acidosis usually is caused by gastrointestinal loss of bicarbonate (diarrhea, fistulous disease, ureteral diversions), exogenous sources of chloride (normal saline infusions), or altered excretion of hydrogen ions (renal tubular acidosis). A.B. reports a history of both lead ingestion and chronic use of lithium. These agents have been associated with the development of renal tubular acidosis.[31,52]

RENAL TUBULAR ACIDOSIS

3. How do the results of NH_4Cl and sodium bicarbonate ($NaHCO_3$) loading help identify the type of renal tubular acidosis in A.B.?

Renal tubular acidosis (RTA) is characterized by defective secretion of hydrogen ion in the renal tubule with essentially normal glomerular filtration rate. Many medical conditions and chemical substances have been associated with RTA (Table 11-5).[31,34] The recognized forms are type 1 (distal), type 2 (proximal), and type 4 (distal, hypoaldosterone). Type 1 RTA is caused by a defect in the distal tubule's ability to acidify the urine; type 2 by altered urinary bicarbonate reabsorption in the proximal tubule; and type 4 by hypoaldosteronism and impaired ammoniagenesis.[31,46]

Evaluation of bicarbonate reabsorption during bicarbonate loading and of response to acid loading by infusion of ammonium chloride is useful in distinguishing between the various types of RTA. In normal subjects, approximately 10% to 15% of the filtered bicarbonate escapes reabsorption in the proximal tubule but is reabsorbed in more distal segments of the nephron. Therefore, urine bicarbonate excretion is negligibly small, and urine pH is maintained between 5.5 and 6.5.

Table 11-5   Common Causes of Renal Tubular Acidosis

Type 1 (Distal)	*Type 2 (Proximal) (cont'd)*
Multiple myeloma	Medications/toxins
Sjögren's syndrome	Acetazolamide
Chronic pyelonephritis	Cadmium
Chronic renal transplant rejection	Copper
Medications/toxins	Lead
Amiloride	Ifosfamide
Amphotericin B	Outdated tetracycline
Foscarnet	Mercury
Lithium	Sulfamethoxazole
Toluene (glue sniffing)	
Triamterene	*Type 4 (Hypoaldosterone)*
	Adrenal insufficiency
Type 2 (Proximal)	Medications/toxins
Amyloidosis	Amiloride
Fanconi syndrome	Cyclosporine
Multiple myeloma	Spironolactone
Nephrotic syndrome	Trimethoprim

Type 2 (proximal) RTA is associated with a decrease in proximal tubular bicarbonate reabsorption. The distal tubular cells partially compensate for this defect by increasing bicarbonate reabsorption, but urinary bicarbonate excretion still is increased. As occurred with A.B., serum HCO_3^- concentration in patients with Type 2 RTA may acutely fall below a threshold of 15 but then stabilize around 15 mEq/L.[10,31] At this point, distal bicarbonate delivery no longer is excessive, allowing the distal nephron to acidify the urine appropriately and excrete acid in the form of titratable ammonia and phosphate.

In type 1 (distal) RTA, a defect in net hydrogen ion secretion results from a back-diffusion of H^+ from the tubule lumen to the tubule cell. Patients with type 1 RTA cannot reduce their urine pH below 5.5 even when systemic acidosis is severe.[46]

A.B.'s response to the acid (NH_4Cl) load demonstrates an ability to acidify the urine (i.e., pH <5.1), which helps rule out type 1 RTA. During bicarbonate loading in patients with type 2 RTA, serum bicarbonate concentration is increased and abnormally large amounts of bicarbonate are again delivered to the distal tubule. Its hydrogen secretory processes are overwhelmed, resulting in bicarbonaturia. Administration of bicarbonate to A.B. produced bicarbonaturia and an elevation in urine pH (7.0), with low blood pH (7.31). These findings indicate that the reabsorption of bicarbonate in the proximal tubule is impaired, which is characteristic of type 2 RTA. Type 4 (hypoaldosterone) RTA is unlikely given her initial serum potassium of 3.0 mEq/L.

LEAD-INDUCED

4. What is the cause of A.B.'s proximal RTA?

The most likely cause of A.B.'s proximal RTA is her exposure to lead (see Table 11-5). The pathogenesis of lead-induced type 2 RTA is unclear. Some studies suggest that carbonic anhydrase deficiency in the proximal tubule is the major factor, but these data are inconclusive.

5. **Why is A.B. hypokalemic?**

Bicarbonate wasting in proximal RTA is associated with sodium loss, extracellular fluid reduction, and activation of the renin-angiotensin-aldosterone axis. Aldosterone increases distal tubular sodium reabsorption and greatly augments potassium and hydrogen ion secretion. This results in potassium wasting, which explains A.B.'s hypokalemia.[53] When plasma bicarbonate achieves steady state, less bicarbonate reaches the distal tubule, and the stimulus for aldosterone release is removed. Therefore, A.B. experiences only a mild depletion of potassium body stores. When A.B. is exposed to bicarbonate loading, the renin-angiotensin-aldosterone axis is reactivated, and hypokalemia worsens. In addition, raising bicarbonate in the blood drives potassium intercellularly, contributing to the hypokalemia.

Treatment

6. **What treatment is indicated for A.B.?**

Although it is rare for patients with type 2 RTA to develop severe acidosis and potassium depletion chronically, it is not uncommon in an acute situation such as this. A.B. has a bicarbonate deficit; thus, she should be treated with alkali replacement, and the offending agent (lead) should be removed concurrently. Her serum potassium is also dangerously low and bicarbonate correction could further decrease it. A.B. needs potassium supplementation. The clinician should obtain hourly blood samples for electrolytes until her potassium is >3.5 mEq/L. In adults like A.B., chronic treatment often is not needed because acidosis is self-limited. However, A.B. should be treated with sodium bicarbonate until proximal RTA resolves. Very large doses of bicarbonate (6 to 10 mEq/kg per day) would be required to increase serum bicarbonate to the normal range.[10] In adults with proximal RTA, however, the goal is to increase serum bicarbonate to no more than 18 mEq/L.[31] Bicarbonate can be provided as sodium bicarbonate tablets (8 mEq/600-mg tablet) or Shohl's solution. Shohl's solution, USP, contains 334 mg citric acid and 500 mg sodium citrate per 5 mL. Sodium citrate is metabolized to sodium bicarbonate in the liver. Shohl's solution provides 1 mEq of sodium and 1 mEq of bicarbonate per mL of solution. Therapy for A.B. should be initiated with 1 mEq/kg per day . The clinician should monitor A.B.'s lithium levels while she is receiving alkali therapy. Sodium ingestion might increase renal lithium excretion and exacerbate her bipolar disorder. Because of severe hypokalemia resulting from alkali administration, supplemental potassium as chloride, bicarbonate, acetate, or citrate salts also should be administered.

Metabolic Acidosis With Elevated Anion Gap

Evaluation and Osmolal Gap

7. G.D., a 34-year-old, 60-kg man, is brought to the emergency department (ED) by the police in a semicomatose state. He was found lying on the floor of his hotel room 30 minutes ago. G.D. has a long history of alcohol abuse.

In the ED, supine blood pressure (BP) is 120/60 mm Hg, pulse is 100 beats/min, and respiratory rate is 40 breaths/min. G.D.'s pupils are reactive, and mild papilledema is noted. Laboratory tests reveal the following: serum Na, 140 mEq/L (normal, 135 to 145 mEq/L); K, 5.8 mEq/L (normal, 3.5 to 5.0 mEq/L); Cl, 103 mEq/L (normal, 95 to 105 mEq/L); blood urea nitrogen (BUN), 25 mg/dL (normal, 10 to 26 mg/dL); creatinine, 1.4 mg/dL (normal, 0.7 to 1.4 mg/dL); and fasting glucose, 150 mg/dL (normal, 70 to 105 mg/dL). ABGs include pH, 7.16 (normal, 7.35 to 7.45); $Paco_2$, 23 mm Hg (normal, 35 to 45); HCO_3^-, 8 mEq/L (normal, 22 to 26). His toxicology screen is negative for alcohol and his serum osmolality is 332 mOsm/kg (normal, 280 to 295).

What acid-base disturbance is present in G.D., and what are possible causes of the disorder?

[SI units: Na, 140 mmol/L; K, 5.8 mmol/L; Cl, 103 mmol/L; BUN, 8.9 mmol/L (normal, 3.57 to 9.28); creatinine, 124 mmol/L (normal, 62 to 124); fasting glucose, 8.3 mmol/L (normal, 2.8 to 5.8); $Paco_2$, 3.1 kPa; HCO_3^-, 8 mmol/L; osmolality, 332 mmol/kg (normal, 280 to 295)]

The stepwise approach reveals that GD has an acidosis, and the laboratory values are validated with the Henderson-Hasselbalch equation. His alcohol abuse may give a clue to the cause. G.D. has severe metabolic acidosis (pH, 7.16; HCO_3^-, 8 mEq/L) with a large AG (29 mEq/L). Respiratory compensation for a primary decrease in serum HCO_3^- to 8 mEq/L should result in a $Paco_2$ between 21 and 24 mm Hg (see Table 11-3). Therefore, G.D.'s laboratory findings on admission represent metabolic acidosis with normal respiratory compensation ($Paco_2$, 22 mm Hg). If his $Paco_2$ were significantly lower than 19 mm Hg or higher than 24 mm Hg, a mixed disorder should be suspected (i.e., coexistent respiratory alkalosis or acidosis, respectively).

An elevated AG metabolic acidosis often indicates lactic acidosis resulting from intoxications (e.g., salicylates, acetaminophen, methanol, ethylene glycol, paraldehyde, metformin) or ketoacidosis induced by diabetes mellitus, starvation, or alcohol.[14,29,33,37,50,54–59] The seventh step in the stepwise approach leads to the consideration of additional laboratory tests that may be helpful in the differential diagnosis of an elevated AG. These include serum ketones, glucose, lactate, BUN, creatinine, and plasma osmolal gap.[33] Osmolal gap is defined as the difference between measured serum osmolality (SO) and calculated SO using Equation 11-7.

$$\text{Calculated SO (mOsm/Kg)} = 2 \times Na^+ (mEq/L) + \frac{Glucose(mg/dL)}{18} + \frac{BUN(mg/dL)}{2.8} \quad \textbf{(11-7)}$$

When the difference between measured and calculated SO is greater than 10 mOsm/kg, the presence of an unmeasured osmotically active substance, such as ethanol, methanol, or ethylene glycol, should be considered.[33,59,60] G.D.'s calculated SO is 297 mOsm/kg, compared with the measured value of 332; therefore, his osmolal gap is 35 mOsm/kg. An increase in AG and osmolal gap without diabetic ketoacidosis and chronic renal failure suggests the possibility of metabolic acidosis resulting from a toxic ingestion.[33] On the basis of G.D.'s presentation (papilledema, history of alcohol abuse, increased osmolal gap, increased AG metabolic acidosis), methanol intoxication should be considered.

Causes
METHANOL-INDUCED

8. **How would G.D.'s methanol intake induce metabolic acidosis with an elevated AG?**

Methanol intoxication results in the formation of two organic acids, formic and lactic acid, that consume bicarbonate with production of an AG metabolic acidosis. Alcohol dehydrogenase in the liver metabolizes methanol to formaldehyde and then to formic acid. The formic acid contributes to the metabolic acidosis and also is responsible for the retinal edema and blindness associated with methanol intoxication.[33,34,59]

Serum lactic acid concentrations also are increased in patients with methanol intoxication.[33] Lactic acidosis classically has been divided into type A, which is associated with inadequate delivery of oxygen to the tissue, and type B, which is associated with defective oxygen utilization at the mitochondrial level (Table 11-6). Although great overlap usually exists within these distinctions, the lactic acidosis caused by methanol intoxication is most consistent with the type B variety.[63]

Treatment

9. **How should G.D.'s methanol intoxication be managed acutely?**

ANTIDOTES

Therapy is directed toward treatment of the underlying cause and may include additional supportive management. Ethanol and fomepizole (Antizol) compete with methanol for alcohol dehydrogenase binding sites.[34,59-63] Because ethanol and fomepizole have much greater affinity for alcohol dehydrogenase than methanol, these agents may reduce the conversion of methanol to its toxic metabolite, formic acid. The unmetabolized methanol then is excreted by the lungs and kidneys. Fomepizole may be given intravenously as a 15 mg/kg loading dose over 30 minutes, followed by bolus doses of 10 mg/kg Q 12 hr. Because of induction of metabolism of fomepizole, doses should be increased to 15 mg/kg every 12 hours if therapy is required beyond 2 days.[59] Fomepizole is usually continued until the serum methanol concentration is less than 20 mg/dL (6.2 mmol/L). Adverse effects of fomepizole are relatively mild, consisting of headache, nausea, dizziness, agitation, metallic taste, abnormal smell, and rash.

Because of its high cost and infrequent use, some small hospitals do not stock fomepizole. In such cases, ethanol is an alternative. Administration of intravenous (IV) ethanol as an antidote can be technically difficult and may produce central nervous system (CNS) depression.[59,61] For patients with methanol toxicity, an IV loading dose of 0.6 gm/kg ethanol solution may be administered over 30 minutes, followed by a continuous infusion of about 150 mg/kg/hr for drinkers and 70 mg/kg/hr for nondrinkers. Serum ethanol concentration should be maintained above 100 mg/dL.[34,63] Charcoal can be given orally to inhibit the absorption of methanol, but because of the small size of the methanol molecule, effectiveness will be limited. Charcoal may be more beneficial in binding other agents that may be co-ingested.[34,64] Charcoal could also inhibit the absorption of ethanol, if it were given orally.[34]

When other low-molecular-weight toxins such as ethanol or ethylene glycol are not present, the serum methanol level can be estimated by multiplying the patient's osmolal gap by a standardized conversion factor of 2.6. Using this methodology, G.D.'s osmolal gap of 35 mOsm/L may reflect a methanol level of approximately 91 mg/dL (35 mOsm/L × 2.6). When methanol blood levels are higher than 50 mg/dL, hemodialysis is indicated to rapidly reduce concentrations of methanol and its toxic metabolite. The dosage of fomepizole or ethanol should be increased in patients receiving hemodialysis to account for the increased elimination of these antidotes.[34,63] Ethylene glycol poisoning can also be treated by using fomepizole or ethanol.

BICARBONATE

Severe acidosis causes reduced myocardial contractility, impaired response to catecholamines, and impaired oxygen delivery to tissues as a result of 2,3-diphosphoglycerate depletion. For this reason, some clinicians have judiciously administered IV sodium bicarbonate to patients with metabolic acidosis in an attempt to raise the arterial pH to about 7.20.[65-67] If IV sodium bicarbonate is given, the amount required to correct serum HCO_3^- and arterial pH can be estimated using Equation 11-8 as follows:

$$\text{Bicarbonate dose (mEq)} = 0.5 \text{ (L/kg)} \times \text{Body Weight (kg)} \times \text{Desired increase in serum } HCO_3^- \text{ (mEq/L)} \quad \textbf{(11-8)}$$

Bicarbonate distributes to approximately 50% of total body weight (thus, the factor of 0.5 L/kg in Equation 11-8). To prevent overtreating, bicarbonate doses should only attempt to increase the bicarbonate concentration by 4 to 8 mEq/L (see Question 10).[66] For G.D., the dose required to raise serum bicarbonate from 8 to 12 mEq/L amounts to 120 mEq of bicarbonate (0.5 L/kg × 60 kg × 4 mEq/L; Equation 11-8). Clinical assessment of the effect of bicarbonate can be determined about 30 minutes after administration.[66] Arterial pH and serum bicarbonate concentrations should be obtained before any additional therapy.

Risks of Bicarbonate Therapy

10. **What are the risks of G.D.'s bicarbonate therapy?**

Table 11-6	**Common Causes of Lactic Acidosis**
Type A	*Type B*
Anemia	Diabetes mellitus
Carbon monoxide poisoning	Liver failure
Congestive heart failure	Renal failure
Shock	Seizure disorder
Sepsis	Leukemia
	Drugs
	Didanosine
	Ethanol
	Isoniazid
	Metformin
	Methanol
	Salicylates
	Zidovudine

Concerns about the risks of bicarbonate administration and studies failing to demonstrate significant short-term benefits have raised questions about the appropriateness of bicarbonate therapy in metabolic acidosis, particularly in ketoacidosis and lactic acidosis caused by cardiac arrest or other hypoxic events.[67–74] Bicarbonate administration may result in overalkalinization and a paradoxical transient intracellular acidosis. Whereas arterial pH can increase rapidly following bicarbonate administration, intracellular pH increases more slowly because of slow penetration of the negatively charged bicarbonate ion across cell membranes. The bicarbonate in plasma, however, is converted rapidly to carbonic acid, and the carbon dioxide tension increases as a result (see Equation 11-2). Because CO_2 diffuses into cells more rapidly than HCO_3^-, the intracellular $HCO_3^-:CO_2$ ratio decreases, resulting in a decrease in intracellular pH. This intracellular acidosis will persist as long as bicarbonate administration exceeds the CO_2 excretion; therefore, adequate tissue perfusion and ventilation must be provided in patients with diminished CO_2 excretion (e.g., cardiac or pulmonary failure).[69]

Overalkalinization also will cause a shift to the left in the oxygen-hemoglobin dissociation curve. This shift increases hemoglobin affinity for oxygen, decreases oxygen delivery to tissues, and potentially increases lactic acid production and accumulation.[34] Sodium bicarbonate administration also can cause hypernatremia, hyperosmolality, and volume overload; however, the excessive sodium and water retention usually can be avoided by the administration of loop diuretics.[34,60] Hypokalemia is another potential adverse effect of bicarbonate therapy. Acidosis stimulates movement of potassium from intracellular to extracellular fluid in exchange for hydrogen ions. When acidosis is corrected, potassium ions move intracellularly and hypokalemia can occur. This translocation of potassium tends to reduce serum potassium levels by approximately 0.4 to 0.6 mEq/L for each 0.1 unit increase in pH, although wide interpatient variability in this relationship exists.[5,8] In G.D. and other patients with organic acid intoxications, raising extracellular pH helps to provide a gradient to shift the toxin from the CNS and "trap" it into the blood and urine, enhancing elimination. To prevent the risks of bicarbonate therapy, G.D.'s mental status, serum sodium and potassium levels, and ABGs should be monitored.

ALTERNATIVE ALKALINIZING THERAPY

Although sodium bicarbonate is the most commonly used agent to raise arterial pH, alternative therapies are available. Sodium lactate and acetate have been used in select patients; however, these agents require metabolic conversion to bicarbonate, and are associated with many of the same risks as sodium bicarbonate (i.e., sodium and fluid overload, overalkalinization, carbon dioxide production).[37]

Tromethamine (THAM) acetate is a sodium-free organic amine with a pH of 8.6. THAM can combine with hydrogen ions from carbonic acid and lactic, pyruvic, or other metabolic acids. THAM is available commercially as a 0.3 M (36 mg/mL) solution for IV administration. The dose (in mmol) can be estimated by multiplying 0.3 × the base deficit (in mEq/L) × patient's weight (in kg). A loading dose of 25% to 50% of the calculated dose can be given over 5 to 10 minutes, and the remainder can be given over 1 hour. The rate of ad-

ministration should not exceed 5 mmol/kg in 1 hour. The maintenance dose can be adjusted according to creatinine clearance: Infusion rate (mmol/h) = 0.06 × Cl_{Cr} (mL/min) × Plasma THAM concentration. Dosage should be adjusted to maintain a serum concentration of ≤0.6 mmol/L. If used over several days, the 24-hour dosage should be limited to 15 mmol/kg.[75]

The role of THAM in the management of metabolic acidosis has not been clearly defined. THAM may produce hyperkalemia in patients with renal impairment and is contraindicated in anuric or uremic patients. Administration of THAM also has been associated with other serious side effects including respiratory depression, increased coagulation times, and hypoglycemia.[75–78] Carbicarb and dichloroacetate are investigational agents that have been studied in patients with metabolic acidosis.[37,63,79] Carbicarb and THAM are better than bicarbonate at improving extracellular pH and bicarbonate and intracellular pH, while not increasing CO_2; however, neither has yet resulted in better patient outcomes.[5,24,69]

METABOLIC ALKALOSIS

Metabolic alkalosis is associated with an increase in serum bicarbonate concentration and a compensatory increase in $PaCO_2$ (caused by hypoventilation). The two general classifications of metabolic alkalosis, saline-responsive and saline-resistant (Table 11-7), are usually distinguishable based on an assessment of the patient's volume status, BP, and urinary chloride concentration.

Saline-responsive metabolic alkalosis is associated with disorders that result in the loss of chloride-rich, bicarbonate-poor fluid from the body (e.g., vomiting, nasogastric suction, diuretic therapy, cystic fibrosis). Physical examination may reveal volume depletion (orthostatic hypotension, tachycardia, poor skin turgor), and the urinary chloride concentration often will be <10 to 20 mEq/L (although urine chloride levels >20 mEq/L may be seen in patients with recent diuretic use).[10,35,80]

Severe hypokalemia or excessive mineralocorticoid activity may result in a saline-resistant metabolic alkalosis, but this disorder is rare in comparison with saline-responsive metabolic alkalosis. Saline-resistant metabolic alkalosis should be suspected in alkalemic patients with evidence of increased extracellular fluid volume, hypertension, or high urinary chloride values (>20 mEq/L) without recent diuretic use.[10,80]

Table 11-7 Classification of Metabolic Alkalosis

Saline-Responsive	Saline-Resistant
Diuretic therapy	Normotensive
Extracellular volume contraction	Potassium depletion
Gastric acid loss	Hypercalcemia
Vomiting	Hypertensive
Nasogastric suction	Mineralocorticoids
Exogenous alkali administration	Hyperaldosteronism
Blood transfusions	Hyperreninism
	Licorice

Evaluation

11. K.E., a 60-year-old, 50-kg woman, was admitted to the hospital 4 days ago with peripheral edema and pulmonary congestion consistent with a congestive heart failure exacerbation. Since admission, she has been treated aggressively with furosemide 80 to 120 mg IV daily, which has generated approximately 3 L of urine output each day. Her chest radiograph and peripheral edema have improved considerably with diuresis; however, she now complains of dizziness when she gets out of bed to go to the bathroom. Physical examination reveals a tachycardic (heart rate [HR], 100 beats/min), thin elderly woman with poor skin turgor and slight muscle weakness. K.E.'s electrocardiogram shows flattened T waves and U waves. Laboratory tests reveal the following: serum Na, 138 mEq/L; K, 2.5 mEq/L; Cl, 92 mEq/L; creatinine, 0.9 mg/dL; BUN, 28 mg/dL; pH, 7.49; Paco₂, 46 mm Hg; and HCO₃⁻, 34 mEq/L. Urine Cl concentration is 60 mEq/L.

What acid-base disorder is present in K.E.?

[SI units: Na, 138 mmol/L; K, 2.5 mmol/L; Cl, 92 mmol/L; creatinine, 79.6 mmol/L; BUN, 10 mmol/L; Paco₂, 6.1 kPa; HCO₃⁻, 34 mmol/L; urine Cl, 60 mmol/L]

Using the stepwise approach, K.E.'s elevated pH is found to be consistent with alkalosis, and the laboratory values are validated. Furosemide-induced diuresis may be a clue to her acid-base disorder. The increased serum HCO_3^- and increased Paco₂ suggest primary metabolic alkalosis with respiratory compensation (see Table 11-2). A primary increase in bicarbonate concentration to 34 mEq/L should result in a compensatory increase in Paco₂ by 5 to 7 mm Hg (see Table 11-3). K.E.'s Paco₂ of 46 mm Hg suggests normal respiratory compensation for metabolic alkalosis. If her Paco₂ were significantly lower than 45 mm Hg or higher than 47 mm Hg, a mixed disorder should be suspected (i.e., coexistent respiratory alkalosis or acidosis, respectively).

Causes

Diuretic-Induced

12. What is the most likely cause of K.E.'s acid-base imbalance?

Common causes of metabolic alkalosis are listed in Table 11-7. The hypokalemic, hypochloremic, metabolic alkalosis in K.E. most likely is the result of diuretic-induced volume contraction. The incidence of this adverse effect is influenced by the type, dose, and dosing frequency of the diuretic.

Diuretics cause metabolic alkalosis (sometimes referred to as a "contraction alkalosis") by the following mechanisms. First, they enhance excretion of sodium chloride and water, resulting in extracellular volume contraction. Volume contraction alone will cause only a modest increase in plasma bicarbonate; however, volume contraction also stimulates aldosterone release. Aldosterone increases distal tubular sodium reabsorption and induces hydrogen ion and potassium secretion, resulting in alkalosis and hypokalemia. In addition, hypokalemia induced by diuretics will stimulate intracellular movement of hydrogen ions to replace cellular potassium, producing extracellular alkalosis. Hypochloremia also is important in sustaining metabolic alkalosis. In a hypochloremic state, sodium will be reabsorbed, accompanied by bicarbonate generated by secreted hydrogen (see Fig. 11-1).[80–82]

Treatment

13. How should K.E.'s acid-base imbalance be corrected and monitored?

Treatment of metabolic alkalosis depends on removing the cause. K.E.'s diuretic therapy should be temporarily discontinued until her volume status and electrolytes can be restored. The initial goal is to correct fluid deficits and replace chloride and potassium by infusing sodium and potassium chloride. As long as hypochloremia exists, renal bicarbonate excretion will not occur and the alkalosis will not be corrected.[81] The severity of alkalosis dictates how rapidly fluid and electrolytes should be administered. In patients with hepatic or renal failure or congestive heart failure, infusion of large volumes of sodium and potassium salts may produce fluid overload or hyperkalemia. Thus, fluid and electrolyte replacement should proceed cautiously and these patients should be monitored closely for these complications.

Potassium chloride should be administered to correct K.E.'s hypokalemia. The amount of potassium required to replace total body stores is difficult to determine accurately because 98% of the potassium in the body is intracellular. Although there is wide variation, for each 1 mEq/L decrease in K^+ from an ECF concentration of 4 mEq/L, the total body K^+ deficit is about 4 to 5 mEq/kg.[10] . K.E.'s serum potassium is 2.5 mEq/L, which correlates with a decrease of about 350 mEq in total body potassium stores. K.E. should be treated with the chloride salt to ensure potassium retention and correction of alkalosis. Potassium replacement can be achieved over several days with supplements of 100 to 150 mEq/day given either orally in divided doses or as a constant IV infusion. K.E.'s laboratory tests for BUN, creatinine, chloride, sodium, and potassium should be monitored during sodium and potassium chloride therapy. ABGs also should be measured to monitor adequacy of replacement therapy. Hypercapnia should disappear after correction of alkalemia.

14. What other agents are available for the management of K.E.'s alkalosis if fluid and electrolyte replacement does not correct the arterial pH?

Patients unresponsive to sodium and potassium chloride therapy or those at risk for complications with these agents may be treated with acetazolamide, hydrochloric acid (HCl), or a hydrochloric acid precursor. The most commonly used agent is acetazolamide, a carbonic anhydrase inhibitor that blocks hydrogen ion secretion in the renal tubule, resulting in increased excretion of sodium and bicarbonate. Although the serum bicarbonate concentration often improves with acetazolamide, metabolic alkalosis may not completely resolve. Other concerns with the use of acetazolamide include its ability to promote kaliuresis and its relative lack of effect in patients with renal dysfunction.[80,83,84]

A solution of 0.1 N HCl may be administered to patients who require rapid correction of alkalemia. The dose of HCl is based on the bicarbonate excess using Equation 11-9, where the factor $0.5 \times$ body weight (kg), represents the estimated bicarbonate space.[10,80,81,83]

$$\text{Dose of HCl (mEq)} = 0.5 \times \text{body weight (kg)} \times \\ (\text{plasma bicarbonate} - 24) \quad \text{(11-9)}$$

Parenteral hydrochloric acid is prepared extemporaneously by adding the appropriate amount of 1 N HCl through a 0.22-micron filter into a glass bottle containing 5% dextrose or normal saline. The dilute solution should be administered via central venous catheter in the superior vena cava to reduce the risk of extravasation and tissue damage. The infusion rate should not exceed 0.2 mEq/kg/hr.[83] ABGs should be monitored at least every 4 hours during the infusion. HCl should not be added to total nutrient solutions.[84]

Precursors of hydrochloric acid, such as ammonium and arginine hydrochloride, are not recommended.[80] The adverse effect profile of these agents has significantly limited their role.[83] Ammonium hydrochloride is metabolized to HCl and NH_3 in the liver. Severe ammonia intoxication with CNS depression can occur during rapid infusion of ammonium hydrochloride or in patients with liver disease.[80] Arginine may cause rapid shifts in potassium from the intracellular to extracellular space, resulting in dangerous hyperkalemia.[80]

RESPIRATORY ACIDOSIS

Respiratory acidosis occurs as a result of inadequate ventilation by the lungs. When the lungs do not excrete CO_2 effectively, the $Paco_2$ rises. This elevation in $Paco_2$ (a functional acid) causes a fall in pH (see Equations 11-3 and 11-5). Common causes of respiratory acidosis are listed in Table 11-8. They generally can be categorized into conditions of airway obstruction, reduced stimulus for respiration from the CNS, failure of the heart or lungs, and disorders of the peripheral nerves or skeletal muscles required for ventilation.[85]

Evaluation

15. B.B., a 56-year-old man, is admitted to the hospital for treatment of an exacerbation of chronic obstructive pulmonary disease (COPD). He complains of worsening shortness of breath and increased production of sputum for the past 3 days. He has also noted a mild headache, a flushed feeling, and drowsiness within the past 24 hours. He has a history of COPD, hypertension, coronary artery disease, and low back pain. Current medications are ipratropium (Atrovent) inhaler 2 puffs QID, salmeterol (Serevent) dry powder inhaler 1 inhalation BID, hydrochlorothiazide 25 mg daily, diltiazem (Cardizem LA) 240 mg daily, and diazepam (Valium) 5 mg TID PRN for back pain.

Vital signs include respiratory rate of 16 breaths/min and HR of 90 beats/min. Diffuse wheezes and rhonchi are heard on chest auscultation. ABGs are pH, 7.32; $Paco_2$, 58 mm Hg; Pao_2, 58 mm Hg; and HCO_3^-, 29 mEq/L. B.B's baseline ABG at the physician's office last month was pH, 7.35; $Paco_2$, 51 mm Hg; Pao_2, 62 mm Hg; and HCO_3^-, 28 mEq/L.

Which of B.B.'s signs and symptoms are consistent with the diagnosis of respiratory acidosis?

[SI units: $Paco_2$, 7.7 and 6.8 kPa; Pao_2, 7.7 and 8.3 kPa; HCO_3^-, 29 and 28 mmol/L]

A stepwise evaluation reveals an acidosis, with validated laboratory results. A history of COPD and physical findings of dyspnea, headache, drowsiness, and flushing give a clue that the disorder is probably of respiratory origin. Respiratory acidosis also can cause more severe symptoms, including CNS effects such as disorientation, confusion, delirium, hallucinations, and coma. These CNS abnormalities probably are in part caused by the direct effects of carbon dioxide. Hypoxemia (decreased Pao_2), which commonly accompanies respiratory acidosis, also contributes to these symptoms. Elevated $Paco_2$ causes cerebral vascular dilation, resulting in headache caused by increased blood flow and increased intracranial pressure. Cardiovascular effects typically include tachycardia, arrhythmias, and peripheral vasodilation.[86]

16. Is the compensatory response to the respiratory acidosis present in B.B. consistent with an acute or a chronic disorder?

After determining that B.B. has respiratory acidosis, his compensatory response is calculated. In respiratory acidosis, increased renal reabsorption of bicarbonate compensates for the increase in $Paco_2$; however, at least 48 to 72 hours are needed for this compensatory mechanism to become fully established.[10] In acute respiratory acidosis, the small increase in the serum bicarbonate concentration is caused by titration of acid by other buffers (e.g., hemoglobin) that generate bicarbonate. If B.B.'s $Paco_2$ increased acutely from a normal value of 40 to 58 mm Hg, one would expect an increase in the serum bicarbonate concentration of only 1.8 mEq/L (i.e., increased to 26 mEq/L from a normal of 24 mEq/L). Alternatively, a purely chronic respiratory acidosis with a $Paco_2$ of 58 mm Hg should be associated with a serum bicarbonate concentration of 31 mEq/L (see Table 11-3). B.B.'s bicarbonate concentration of 29 mEq/L falls somewhere between these two predicted values. This is most likely the result of a chronic respiratory acidosis (his baseline $Paco_2$ was 51 mm Hg) with an acute worsening to 58 mm Hg. Patients with COPD commonly present with an "acute-on-chronic" respiratory acidosis similar to B.B.

Table 11-8	Common Causes of Respiratory Acidosis
Airway Obstruction	**Cardiopulmonary**
Foreign body aspiration	Cardiac arrest
Asthma	Pulmonary edema or infiltration
COPD	Pulmonary embolism
β-Adrenergic blockers	Pulmonary fibrosis
CNS Disturbances	**Neuromuscular**
Cerebral vascular accident	Amyotrophic lateral sclerosis
Sleep apnea	Guillain-Barré syndrome
Tumor	Myasthenia gravis
CNS depressant drugs	Hypokalemia
Barbiturates	Hypophosphatemia
Benzodiazepines	**Drugs**
Opioids	Aminoglycosides
	Antiarrhythmics
	Lithium
	Phenytoin

CNS, central nervous system; COPD, chronic obstructive pulmonary disease.

Causes

17. What potential causes of respiratory acidosis are present in B.B.?

Respiratory acidosis often is caused by airway obstruction, as shown in Table 11-8.[85,86] Chronic obstructive airway disease is a common cause of both acute and chronic respiratory acidosis. Upper respiratory tract infections, such as acute bronchitis, can worsen airway obstruction and produce acute respiratory acidosis.

Drug-Induced

B.B.'s drug therapy also may be contributing to respiratory insufficiency. Many drugs (see Table 11-8) decrease ventilation, but usually these drugs only significantly affect patients who are predisposed to respiratory problems because of underlying diseases. Because B.B. has COPD, he may be more sensitive to drugs affecting respiration. The benzodiazepines, barbiturates, and opioids minimally decrease respiration in normal subjects and in most patients with COPD when given usual therapeutic doses. However, these drugs can cause significant respiratory insufficiency when administered either in large doses or in combination with other respiratory depressant drugs.[86] B.B.'s diazepam may be contributing to hypoventilation and respiratory acidosis and should be withdrawn from his regimen. β-adrenergic blocking drugs should be avoided in patients with COPD.

Treatment

18. How should B.B.'s respiratory acidosis be treated?

As with most cases of respiratory acidosis, treatment primarily involves correction of the underlying cause of respiratory insufficiency. In this case, treatment of acute bronchospasm with ipratropium or a β-adrenergic agent such as inhaled albuterol is warranted. The role of corticosteroids and antibiotic therapy in acute exacerbations of COPD is controversial. B.B's respiratory status should be monitored closely during his hospitalization. If the acidosis, hypercarbia, or associated hypoxemia progress, mechanical ventilation may be required.[66]

Treatment with IV sodium bicarbonate is not recommended in most cases of acute respiratory acidosis because of the risks associated with bicarbonate therapy (see Question 10) and because an absolute deficiency of bicarbonate is not present. When the excess CO_2 is excreted, arterial pH should return to normal. Hypercapnia should not be overcorrected, as hypocapnia results in decreased lung compliance, increases dysfunctional surfactant production, and shifts the oxyhemoglobin dissociation curve to the left, restricting the release of oxygen to tissues.[73,74,87]

RESPIRATORY ALKALOSIS

Respiratory alkalosis usually is not a severe disorder. Excessive rate or depth of respiration results in increased excretion of carbon dioxide, a fall in $PaCO_2$, and a rise in arterial pH. Common causes of respiratory alkalosis are presented in Table 11-9. Many conditions can cause respiratory alkalosis by stimulating respiratory drive in the CNS. In addition,

Table 11-9 Common Causes of Respiratory Alkalosis

CNS Disturbances	Pulmonary
Bacterial septicemia	Pneumonia
Cerebrovascular accident	Pulmonary edema
Fever	Pulmonary embolus
Hepatic cirrhosis	*Tissue Hypoxia*
Hyperventilation	High altitude
Anxiety-induced	Hypotension
Voluntary	CHF
Meningitis	*Other*
Pregnancy	Excessive mechanical ventilation
Trauma	Rapid correction of metabolic acidosis
Drugs	
Progesterone derivatives	
Respiratory stimulants	
Salicylate overdose	

CHF, congestive heart failure; CNS, central nervous system.

pulmonary diseases can stimulate receptors in the lung to increase ventilation, and conditions that decrease oxygen delivery to tissues also can stimulate ventilation, causing respiratory alkalosis.[88,89]

Evaluation

19. S.P., a 35-year-old, 60-kg woman, is admitted for treatment of presumed bacterial pneumonia. She was in good health until 24 hours before presentation when she noted a fever; onset of a productive cough with thick, yellowish sputum; and chest pain on deep inspiration. She has taken aspirin 650 mg Q 4 hr since the onset of fever, with mild relief. Since arriving in the ED, she has become anxious and lightheaded and has developed tingling in her hands, feet, and lips. Vital signs include the following: temperature, 38°C; respiratory rate, 24 breaths/min; HR, 110 beats/min; and BP, 135/70 mm Hg. Physical examination reveals dullness to percussion, rales, and decreased breath sounds over the left lower lung field.

Laboratory findings include the following: serum Na, 135 mEq/L; Cl, 105 mEq/L; pH, 7.49; $PaCO_2$, 30 mm Hg; PaO_2, 90 mm Hg; and HCO_3^-, 22 mEq/L. Gram's stain of sputum reveals 25 white blood cells (WBCs) per high-power field and many Gram-positive diplococci. WBC count is 15,400 cells/mm³ (normal, 3,500 to 10,500 cells/mm³) with a left shift. A left lower lobe infiltrate is seen on chest radiograph.

What acid-base disorder is present in S.P.?

[SI units: $PaCO_2$, 4.0 kPa; PaO_2, 12.0 kPa; HCO_3^- 22 mmol/L; other SI units are: Na, 135 mmol/L; Cl, 105 mmol/L]

Steps 1 to 4 in the evaluation of the ABG values reveal a respiratory alkalosis (increased pH, decreased $PaCO_2$) with history and physical findings of deep, rapid breathing and tingling sensations providing a clue to the cause. According to the criteria for renal compensation in Table 11-3, S.P. has an acute respiratory alkalosis (predicted decrease in HCO_3^- of 2 mEq/L) rather than chronic respiratory alkalosis (predicted decrease in HCO_3^- of 4 to 5 mEq/L). If her bicarbonate concentration were significantly lower than 19 mEq/L or higher than 22 mEq/L, a mixed acid-base disorder should be suspected (coexistent metabolic acidosis or alkalosis, respectively).[8]

20. Which of S.P.'s signs and symptoms are consistent with the diagnosis of acute respiratory alkalosis?

Respiratory alkalosis typically produces paresthesias of the extremities and perioral region, lightheadedness, confusion, decreased mental acuity, and tachycardia.[5,6,10] Increased rate and depth of respiration may be evident. Simple respiratory alkalosis rarely produces life-threatening abnormalities.

Causes

21. What is the cause of the acid-base disorder in S.P.?

Common causes of respiratory alkalosis are listed in Table 11-9.[5,6,10,88–90] Based on physical examination, laboratory findings, and chest radiograph, S.P. appears to have an acute bacterial pneumonia. Pneumonia and other pulmonary diseases can result in stimulation of ventilation and respiratory alkalosis, even with a normal PaO_2, as in this case. The anxiety S.P. is experiencing also may be contributing to respiratory alkalosis by producing the familiar anxiety-hyperventilation syndrome. Although salicylate intoxication is a potential cause of respiratory alkalosis because of the direct respiratory stimulant effect of salicylate,[90] S.P. displays few other symptoms of salicylate intoxication (e.g., nausea, vomiting, tinnitus, altered mental status, elevated AG metabolic acidosis). The total aspirin dose reportedly ingested (65 mg/kg over 24 hours) is not large enough to be associated with significant risk for toxicity.

Treatment

22. What is the appropriate treatment for S.P.'s respiratory alkalosis?

Similar to respiratory acidosis, treatment of respiratory alkalosis usually involves correcting the underlying disorder. Initiation of appropriate antibiotic therapy is indicated in this case. Simple respiratory alkalosis is unlikely to cause life-threatening symptoms, although mortality rates for critically ill patients with this disorder can be high.[86] The well-known remedy of rebreathing expired air from a paper bag for treatment of hyperventilation associated with anxiety appears to be effective for this cause of respiratory alkalosis and may be helpful for S.P.

MIXED ACID-BASE DISORDERS

Evaluation

23. B.L., a 58-year-old man, was transferred from a nursing home 2 days previously with disorientation and lethargy. He was doing well until 1 week before admission, when the staff noted that he was somnolent. He progressively became more lethargic and could no longer remember the names of other persons. B.L. has a history of alcoholic cirrhosis, non–insulin-dependent diabetes mellitus, and hypertension. Medications before admission were nadolol 80 mg QD, isosorbide mononitrate 20 mg BID, glyburide 10 mg QD, and spironolactone 50 mg BID. On admission, B.L. was disoriented to person, place, and time and was difficult to arouse. Vital signs include the following: temperature, 37°C; respirations, 16 breaths/min; HR, 70 beats/min; and BP, 154/92 mm Hg. Physical examination revealed asterixis and mild ascites. Laboratory studies included the following: Na, 133 mEq/L;

K, 4.3 mEq/L; Cl, 106 mEq/L; BUN, 5 mg/dL; creatinine, 0.7 mg/dL; fasting glucose, 150 mg/dL; albumin, 3.2 g/dL (normal, 3.6 to 5.0 g/dL); and ammonia, 120 μmol/L (normal, 19 to 43 μmol/L); ABGs: pH, 7.43; $PaCO_2$, 30 mm Hg; PaO_2, 90 mm Hg; and HCO_3^-, 19 mEq/L.

On admission, spironolactone was increased to 75 mg BID and lactulose 60 mL PO QID was started for treatment of hepatic encephalopathy. Within the first 24 hours of lactulose therapy, B.L. produced four loose, watery stools; however, his mental status worsened to the point of being unresponsive, his BP dropped to 100/60 mm Hg, and his breathing became labored and eventually required mechanical ventilation. At the time of intubation, his laboratory values were Na, 136 mEq/L; K, 4.5 mEq/L; Cl, 105 mEq/L; BUN, 10 mg/dL; creatinine, 1.2 mg/dL; arterial pH, 7.06; $PaCO_2$, 48 mm Hg; PaO_2, 58 mm Hg; and HCO_3^-, 13 mEq/L. Gram's stain of peritoneal fluid reveals many WBCs and Gram-negative rods; the diagnosis of spontaneous bacterial peritonitis with possible septicemia is made.

Describe B.L.'s acid-base status on admission and at the current time.

[SI units: Na, 133 and 136 mmol/L; K, 4.3 and 4.5 mmol/L; Cl, 106 and 105 mmol/L; BUN, 1.8 and 3.6 mmol/L; creatinine, 62 and 106 mmol/L; fasting glucose, 8.3 mmol/L; albumin, 32 g/L; $PaCO_2$, 4.0 and 6.4 kPa; PaO_2, 12.0 and 7.7 kPa; HCO_3^-, 19 and 13 mmol/L]

Steps 1 and 2 of the evaluation seem to indicate that initially there was no disorder in acid-base balance; however, a complete evaluation of B.L.'s ABGs reveals abnormal $PaCO_2$ and serum bicarbonate values, suggesting the existence of an underlying acid-base abnormality. The direction of change in his $PaCO_2$ and serum HCO_3^- is suspicious for either respiratory alkalosis with renal compensation or metabolic acidosis with respiratory compensation. Because the pH was trending toward the upper limit of normal (i.e., >7.40), respiratory alkalosis would be more likely. Examination of the ranges of expected compensation in Table 11-3 reveals that these values are indeed consistent with chronic respiratory alkalosis (serum HCO_3^- decreased by 0.5 mEq/L for each 1-mm Hg drop in $PaCO_2$). If B.L. had a metabolic acidosis, the primary decrease in HCO_3^- from 24 to 19 mEq/L would be expected to result in a $PaCO_2$ of about 34 or 35 mm Hg. B.L.'s history of alcohol-induced liver disease is consistent with the diagnosis of chronic respiratory alkalosis (see Table 11-9).[8,10]

The second set of ABGs reveals severe acidosis. B.L.'s serum bicarbonate has fallen from 19 to 13 mEq/L, and his $PaCO_2$ has increased acutely from 30 to 48 mm Hg. Because these values have changed in opposite directions, a mixed acid-base abnormality should be suspected.

The diagnosis of a mixed, metabolic and respiratory acidosis can be confirmed by applying the principles in Table 11-3. If the acidosis was purely metabolic in nature, a serum HCO_3^- of 13 mEq/L should result in hyperventilation and a $PaCO_2$ between 27 and 25 mm Hg. B.L.'s $PaCO_2$ of 48 mm Hg is significantly higher than the predicted compensatory range, which would be consistent with coexistent respiratory acidosis.

The same conclusion could be reached by looking at the respiratory acidosis first. Simple respiratory acidosis with a $PaCO_2$ of 48 mm Hg should be associated with a compensatory increase in serum HCO_3^- to either 25 mEq/L (acute) or 27 mEq/L (chronic). A serum HCO_3^- of 13 mEq/L is significantly lower than either of these predicted compensatory responses, leading once again to the diagnosis of a mixed, metabolic and respiratory acidosis. Clinically, the time frame in which B.L.'s $PaCO_2$ increased from 30 to 48 mm Hg would be more consistent with an acute respiratory acidosis. The order in which the metabolic and respiratory abnormalities occurred is not important, and each needs to be treated in a separate fashion.

Causes

24. **What are possible causes for the mixed acidosis in B.L.?**

The AG should be calculated in all patients with a metabolic acidosis. B.L.'s calculated AG has increased from 8 to 18 mEq/L (11 and 21 mEq/L, respectively, after adjusting for hypoalbuminemia), suggesting that an elevated AG acidosis is now present. Septicemia from bacterial peritonitis can produce profound hypotension, which leads to tissue hypoperfusion, generation of lactic acid, and a subsequent elevation in the AG. Other causes of elevated AG metabolic acidosis can be excluded with additional laboratory data (e.g., serum ketones, glucose, osmolal gap).

Although diarrhea and spironolactone should be considered in the differential diagnosis, these are usually associated with hyperchloremic, normal AG metabolic acidosis (see Table 11-4).[91] The coexisting respiratory acidosis is most likely the result of B.L.'s altered mental status and his diminished respiratory drive.

25. **Over the next 6 hours, B.L.'s hepatic encephalopathy, peritonitis, and acid-base disorders are aggressively treated with lactulose, antibiotics, sodium bicarbonate, and mechanical ventilation. His most recent ABG reveals the following: pH, 7.45; $PaCO_2$, 24 mm Hg; PaO_2, 90 mm Hg; and HCO_3^-, 16 mEq/L. Ventilator settings are assist-control mode at 16 breaths/min,** tidal volume 700 mL, and inspired oxygen concentration 40%. **B.L. is noted to be more awake, anxious, and initiating 25 to 30 breaths/min. Describe the current acid-base status and probable cause.**

[SI units: $PaCO_2$, 3.2 kPa; PaO_2, 12.0 kPa; HCO_3^-, 16 mmol/L]

Evaluation of the ABG reveals a pH at the upper limit of normal with significant decreases in both $PaCO_2$ and serum HCO_3^- concentration. This clinical scenario is most consistent with a mixed, acute respiratory alkalosis and ongoing metabolic acidosis. The time frame in which B.L.'s $PaCO_2$ decreased from 48 to 24 mm Hg is consistent with acute respiratory alkalosis; therefore, the diagnosis of coexistent metabolic acidosis should be confirmed by comparing B.L.'s serum HCO_3^- (16 mEq/L) with that predicted by the equation in Table 11-3 for acute respiratory alkalosis (21 mEq/L). B.L.'s serum HCO_3^- is significantly lower than expected, suggesting ongoing metabolic acidosis as a result of his septicemia. The metabolic acidosis should improve with time, given adequate antibiotic therapy and supportive measures that maintain BP and increase oxygen delivery to the tissues.

The acute respiratory alkalosis in this case is most likely caused by the mechanical ventilator and B.L.'s anxiety. In the assist-control mode, any inspiratory effort by B.L. results in delivery of a full assisted breath by the ventilator.[92] B.L.'s anxiety and resultant tachypnea are stimulating the ventilator to hyperventilate him, producing excessive CO_2 excretion and respiratory alkalosis. Appropriate changes in therapy include use of an anxiolytic agent, such as a benzodiazepine, changing the ventilator mode to intermittent mandatory ventilation, or both.

Acknowledgment
The author acknowledges S. Troy McMullin, the author of this chapter in the previous edition. Some of his work remains in this edition.

REFERENCES

1. Androgue HE, Androgue HJ. Acid-base physiology. Respir Care 2001;46:328.
2. Rose BD, Post TW. Acid-base physiology. In: Rose BD, Post TW, eds. Clinical Physiology of Acid-Base Disorders. 5th Ed. New York: McGraw-Hill, 2001:299.
3. Ganong WF. Review of Medical Physiology. 20th Ed. New York: McGraw-Hill, 2001.
4. Rose BD, Post TW. Regulation of acid-base balance. In: Rose BD, Post TW, eds. Clinical Physiology of Acid-Base Disorders. 5th Ed. New York: McGraw-Hill, 2001:325.
5. Bongard FS, Sue Dy. Fluids, electrolytes, & acid-base. In: Bongard FS, ed. Current Critical Care Diagnosis & Treatment. 2nd Ed. New York: McGraw Hill, 2003:14.
6. Gluck SL. Acid-base. Lancet. 1998;352:474.
7. Alpern RJ, Preisig PA. Renal acid-base transport. In: Schrier RW, ed. Diseases of the Kidney and Urinary Tract. Philadelphia: Lippincott Williams & Wilkins, 2001:203.
8. Rose BD, Post TW. Introduction to simple and mixed acid-base disorders. In: Rose BD, Post TW, eds. Clinical Physiology of Acid-Base Disorders. 5th Ed. New York: McGraw-Hill, 2001:535.
9. Ravel R. Clinical Laboratory Medicine: Clinical Application of Laboratory Data. 6th Ed. St. Louis: Mosby, 1995:393.
10. Fukagawa M et al. Fluid & electrolyte disorders. In: Tierney LM Jr, ed. Current Medical Diagnosis & Treatment. 42nd Ed. New York: McGraw-Hill, 2003:839.
11. Kelly AM et al. Venous pH can safely replace arterial pH in the initial evaluation of patients in the emergency department. Emerg Med J 2001;18:340.
12. Paulson WD et al. Wide variation in serum anion gap measurements by chemistry analyzers. Am J Clin Pathol 1998;110:735.
13. Story DA et al. Estimating unmeasured anions in critically ill patients: anion-gap, base-deficit, and strong-ion-gap. Anesthesia 2002;47:1102.
14. Balasubramanyan N et al. Unmeasured anions identified by the Fencl-Stewart method predict mortality better than base excess, anion gap, and lactate in patients in the pediatric intensive care unit. Crit Care Med 1999;27:1577.
15. Fencl V, Leith DE. Stewart's quantitative acid-base chemistry: applications in biology and medicine. Respir Physiol 1993;91:1.
16. Stewart PA. Modern quantitative acid-base chemistry. Can J Physiol Pharmacol 1983;61:1444.
17. Cusack RJ et al. The strong ion gap does not have prognostic value in critically ill patients in a mixed medical/surgical adult ICU. Intens Care Med 2002;28:864.
18. Wooten EW. Strong ion difference theory: more lessons from physical chemistry [Letter]. Kidney Int 1998;54:1769.
19. Salem MM, Mujais SK. Gaps in the anion gap. Arch Intern Med 1992;152:1625.
20. Fencl V. Reliability of the anion gap [Letter]. Crit Care Med 2000;28:1693.
21. Jurado RL et al. Low anion gap. South Med J 1998;91:624.
22. Carvounis CP, Feinfeld DA. A simple estimate of the effect of the serum albumin level on the anion gap. Am J Nephrol 2000;20:369.
23. Yaron T. Calculating the anion gap for patients with acidosis and hyperglycemia [Letter]. Ann Intern Med 1998;129:753.
24. Borawski J, Mysliwiec M. Hemoglobin level is an important determinant of acid-base status in hemodialysis patients. Nephron 2002;90:111.
25. Lorenz JM et al. Serum anion gap in the differential diagnosis of metabolic acidosis in critically ill newborns. J Pediatr 1999;135:751.
26. Oster JR et al. Metabolic acidosis with extreme elevation of anion gap: case report and literature review. Am J Med Sci 1999;317:38.
27. Matsumoto LC et al. Anion gap determination in preeclampsia. Obstet Gynecol 1998;91:379.
28. Kirschbaum B, Peng T. The anion gap associated with pregnancy-induced hypertension. Clin Nephrol 2000;53:264.
29. Chang CT et al. High anion gap metabolic acidosis in suicide: don't forget metformin intoxication-two patients' experiences. Renal Fail 2002;24:671.
30. Annerose H et al. Acid-base and endocrine effects of aldosterone and angiotensin II inhibition in metabolic acidosis in human patients. J Lab Clin Med 2000;136:379.
31. Smulders YM et al. Renal tubular acidosis: pathophysiology and diagnosis. Arch Intern Med 1996; 156:1629.

32. Fall PJ. A stepwise approach to acid-base disorders: practical patient evaluation for metabolic acidosis and other conditions. Postgrad Med 2000;107:249.
33. Kraut JA, Madias NE. Approach to patients with acid-base disorders. Respir Care 2001;46:392.
34. Rose BD, Post TW. Metabolic acidosis. In: Rose BD, Post TW, eds. Clinical Physiology of Acid-Base Disorders. 5th Ed. New York: McGraw-Hill, 2001:578.
35. Breen PH. Arterial blood gas and pH analysis: clinical approach and interpretation. Anesthesiol Clin North Am. 2001;19:835.
36. Sirker AA et al. Acid-base physiology: the 'traditional' and the 'modern' approaches. Anesthesia 2002;57:348.
37. Swenson ER. Metabolic acidosis. Respir Care 2001;46:342.
38. DuBose TD. Hyperkalemic metabolic acidosis. Am J Kidney Dis 1999;33:xlv.
39. Doberer D et al. Dilutional acidosis: an endless story of confusion [Letter]. Crit Care Med 2003;31:337.
40. Kellum JA. Dilutional acidosis: an endless story of confusion: the author replies [Author Reply]. Crit Care Med. 2003;31:338.
41. Stephens RCM, Mythen MG. Saline-based fluids can cause a significant acidosis that may be clinically relevant [Letter]. Crit Care Med 2000;28:3375.
42. Waters J. Saline-based fluids can cause a significant acidosis that may be clinically relevant [Letter]. Crit Care Med 2000;28:3376.
43. Waters JH et al. Cause of metabolic acidosis in prolonged surgery. Crit Care Med 1999;27:2142.
44. Izzedine H et al. Drug-induced Fanconi's syndrome. Am J Kidney Dis 2003;41:292.
45. Schoolwerth AC, DiGiovanni SR. Renal metabolism. In Schrier RW, ed. Diseases of the Kidney and Urinary Tract. 7th Ed. Philadelphia: Lippincott Williams & Wilkins, 2001:228.
46. Daphnis E et al. Isolated renal tubular disorders: molecular mechanisms and clinical expression of disease. In: Schrier RW, ed. Diseases of the Kidney and Urinary Tract. 7th Ed. Philadelphia: Lippincott Williams & Wilkins, 2001:620.
47. Verheist D et al. Fanconi syndrome and renal failure induced by tenofovir: a first case report. Am J Kidney Dis 2002;40:1331.
48. Kamel KS et al. A new classification for renal defects in net acid excretion. Am J Kidney Dis 1997;29:136.
49. Prough DS. Physiologic acid-base and electrolyte changes in acute and chronic renal failure patients. Anesthesiol Clin North Am 2000;18:809.
50. Luft FC. Lactic acidosis update for critical care clinicians. J Am Soc Nephrol 2001;12:S15.
51. Kellum JA. Metabolic acidosis in the critically ill: lessons from physical chemistry. Kidney Int 1998;43(Suppl 66);S81.
52. Boton R et al. Prevalence, pathogens, and treatment of a renal dysfunction associated with chronic lithium therapy. Am J Kidney Dis 1987;10:329.
53. Gill JR et al. Correction of renal sodium loss and secondary aldosteronism in renal tubular acidosis with bicarbonate loading. Clin Res 1961;9:201.
54. Bell AJ, Duggin G. Acute methyl salicylate toxicity complicating herbal skin treatment for psoriasis. Emerg Med 2002;14:188.
55. Koulouris Z et al. Metabolic acidosis and coma following a severe acetaminophen overdose. Ann Pharmacother 1999;33:1191.
56. Moyle GJ et al. Hyperlactatemia and lactic acidosis during antiretroviral therapy: relevance, reproducibility and possible risk factors. AIDS 2002;16:1341.
57. Reynolds HN et al. Hyperlactatemia, increased osmolar gap, and renal dysfunction during continuous lorazepam infusion. Crit Care Med 2000;28:1631.
58. Caravaca F et al. Metabolic acidosis in advanced renal failure: differences between diabetic and nondiabetic patients. Am J Kidney Dis 1999;33:892.
59. Brent J et al. Fomepizole for the treatment of methanol poisoning. N Engl J Med 2001;344:424.
60. Hanston P et al. Ethylene glycol poisoning treated by intravenous 4-methylpyrazole. Intens Care Med 1998;24:736.
61. Brent J et al. Fomepizole for the treatment of ethylene glycol poisoning. N Engl J Med 1999;340:832.
62. Poldelski V et al. Ethylene glycol-mediated tubular injury: identification of critical metabolites and injury pathways. Am J Kidney Dis 2001;38:339.
63. Halperin ML, Goldstein MB. Fluid, Electrolyte, and Acid-Base Physiology. 3rd Ed. Philadelphia: WB Saunders, 1999:73.
64. Rao RB, Hoffman RS. Acid-base disorders [Letter]. N Engl J Med 1998;338:1626.
65. Hood V, Tannen RL. Mechanisms of disease: protection of acid-base balance by regulation of acid production. N Engl J Med 1998;339:819.
66. Androgue HJ, Madias NE. Management of life-threatening acid-base disorders: first of two parts. N Engl J Med 1998;338:26
67. Androgue HJ, Madias NE. Acid-base disorders [Letter]. N Engl J Med 1998;338:1626.
68. Marik P, Varon J. Acid-base disorders [Letter]. N Engl J Med 1998;338;1626.
69. Kraut JA, Kurtz I. Use of bas in the treatment of severe acidemic states. Am J Kidney Dis 2001;38:703.
70. Laffey JG. Acid-base disorders in the critically ill. Anesthesia 2002;57:183.
71. Levy MM. Evidence-based critical care medicine. Crit Care Clin 1998;14:458.
72. Vukmir RB et al. Sodium bicarbonate in cardiac arrest: a reappraisal. Am J Emerg Med 1996;14:192.
73. Laffey JG, Kavanagh BP. Carbon dioxide and the critically ill: too little of a good thing? Lancet 1999;354:1283.
74. Laffey JG et al. Buffering hypercapnic acidosis worsens acute lung injury. Am J Respir Crit Care Med 2000;161:141.
75. Nahas GG et al. Guidelines for the treatment of acidaemia with THAM. Drugs 1998;55:191.
76. Kallet RH et al. The treatment of acidosis in acute lung injury with tris-hydroxymethyl aminomethane (THAM). Am J Respir Crit Care Med 2000;161:1149.
77. Nahas GG et al. More on acid-base disorders [Letter]. N Engl J Med 1998;339:1005.
78. Androgue HJ, Madias NE. More on acid-base disorders [Letter]. N Engl J Med 1998;339:1005.
79. Leung JM et al. Safety and efficacy of intravenous Carbicarb in patients undergoing surgery: comparison with sodium bicarbonate in the treatment of mild metabolic acidosis. Crit Care Med 1994;22:1540.
80. Rose BD, Post TW. Metabolic alkalosis. In: Rose BD, Post TW, eds. Clinical Physiology of Acid-Base Disorders. 5th Ed. New York: McGraw-Hill, 2001:551.
81. Galla JH. Metabolic alkalosis. J Am Soc Nephrol 2000;11:369.
82. Khanna A, Kurtzman AK. Metabolic alkalosis. Respir Care 2001;46:354.
83. Adrogue H, Madias NE. Management of life-threatening acid-base disorders. N Engl J Med 1998;338:107.
84. Bistrian BR et al. Acid-base disorders [Letter]. N Engl J Med 1998;338:1626.
85. Rose BD, Post TW. Respiratory acidosis. In: Rose BD, Post TW, eds. Clinical Physiology of Acid-Base Disorders. 5th Ed. New York: McGraw-Hill, 2001:647.
86. Epstein SK, Nirupam S. Respiratory acidosis. Respir Care 2001;46:366.
87. Laffey JG, Kavanagh BP. Medical progress: hypocapnia. N Engl J Med 2002;347:43.
88. Foster GT et al. Respiratory alkalosis. Respir Care 2001;46:384.
89. Brandon JOW et al. Hormone replacement therapy causes a respiratory alkalosis in normal postmenopausal women. J Clin Endocrinol Metab 1999;84:1997.
90. Rose BD, Post TW. Respiratory alkalosis. In: Rose BD, Post TW, eds. Clinical Physiology of Acid-Base Disorders. 5th Ed. New York: McGraw-Hill, 2001:673.
91. Milionis HJ, Elisaf MS. Acid-base abnormalities in a patient with hepatic cirrhosis. Nephrol Dial Transplant 1999;14:1599.
92. Tobin MJ. Current concepts: mechanical ventilation. N Engl J Med 1994;330:1056.

CHAPTER 12

Fluid and Electrolyte Disorders

Alan H. Lau

BASIC PRINCIPLES

Body Water Compartments and Electrolyte Composition

In newborns, approximately 75% to 85% of the body weight is water. After puberty, the percentage of water per kilogram of weight decreases as the amount of adipose tissue increases with age.[1-3] Body water constitutes 50% to 60% of the lean body weight (LBW) in adult men but only 45% to 55% in women because of their greater proportion of adipose tissue. The water content per kilogram of body weight further decreases with advanced age.

Two thirds of the total body water resides in the cells (intracellular water). The extracellular water can be divided into different compartments: the interstitial fluid (12% LBW) and the plasma (5% LBW) are the two major compartments. Other compartments of the extracellular fluid include the connective tissues and bone water, the transcellular fluids (e.g., glandular secretions), and other fluids in sequestered spaces, such as the cerebrospinal fluid.[1]

The electrolyte composition differs between the intracellular and extracellular compartments. Potassium (K), magnesium (Mg), and phosphate (PO_4) are the major ions in the intracellular compartment, whereas sodium (Na), chloride (Cl), and bicarbonate (HCO_3) are predominant in the extracellular space.[3] Water travels freely across cell membranes of most parts of the body. However, the cell membrane is only selectively permeable to solutes. The impermeable solutes are osmotically active and can exert an osmotic pressure that dictates the distribution of water between fluid compartments. Water moves across the cell membrane from a region of low osmolality to one of high osmolality. Net water movement ceases when osmotic equilibrium occurs. Each fluid compartment contains a major osmotically active solute: potassium in the intracellular space and sodium in the extracellular fluid. The volumes of the two compartments reflect the asymmetrically larger number of solute particles or osmoles inside the cells.[3,4]

The capillary wall separates the interstitial fluid from plasma. Since sodium moves freely across the capillary wall, its concentration is identical across both sides of the wall. Therefore, there is no osmotic gradient generated, and water distribution between these two spaces is not affected. Plasma proteins, which are confined in the vascular space, are the primary osmoles that affect water distribution between the interstitium and the plasma.[3] In contrast, urea, which traverses both the capillary walls and most cell membranes, is osmotically inactive.[3,4]

Plasma Osmolality

Osmolality is defined as the number of particles per kilogram of water (mOsm/kg). It is determined by the number of particles in solution and not by particle size or valence. Nondissociable solutes, such as glucose and albumin, generate 1 mOsm/mmol of particles; and dissociable salts, such as sodium chloride, which liberates two ions in solution, produce 2 mOsm/mmol of salt. The osmolality of body fluid is maintained between 280 and 295 mOsm/kg. Because all body fluid compartments are iso-osmotic, plasma osmolality reflects the osmolality of total body water. Plasma osmolality can be measured by the freezing point depression method, or estimated by the following equation, which takes into account the osmotic effect of sodium, glucose, and urea[3,4]:

$$P_{OSM} = 2(Na)(mmol/L) + \frac{Glucose\ (mg/dL)}{18} + \quad \textbf{12-1}$$

$$\frac{BUN\ (mg/dL)}{2.8}$$

This equation predicts the measured plasma osmolality within 5 to 10 mOsm/kg. Although urea contributes to the measured osmolality, it is an ineffective osmole because it readily traverses cell membranes and therefore does not cause significant fluid shift within the body. Hence, the effective plasma osmolality (synonymous with tonicity, the portion of total osmolality that has the potential to induce transmembrane water movement) can be estimated by the following equation:

$$P_{OSM} = 2(Na)(mmol/L) + \frac{Glucose\ (mg/dL)}{18} \quad \textbf{12-2}$$

An osmolal gap exists when the measured and calculated values differ by >10 mOsm/kg[5]; it signifies the presence of unidentified particles. When the individual solute has been identified, its contribution to the measured osmolality can be estimated by dividing its concentration (mg/dL) by one tenth of its molecular weight. Calculating the osmolal gap is used to detect the presence of substances such as ethanol, methanol, and ethylene glycol, which have high osmolality. Occasionally, the osmolal gap can also result from an artificial decrease in the serum sodium secondary to severe hyperlipidemia or hyperproteinemia.

1. **J.F., a 31-year-old man, is admitted to the inpatient medicine service for methanol (molecular weight, 32) intoxication. Routine laboratory analysis reveals the following: Na, 145 mEq/L (normal, 134 to 146); K, 3.4 mEq/L (normal, 3.5 to 5.1); Cl, 105 mEq/L (normal, 92 to 109); carbon dioxide (CO_2), 20 mEq/L (normal, 22 to 32); blood urea nitrogen (BUN),** 10 mg/dL (normal, 8 to 25); creatinine, 1.1 mg/dL (normal, 0.5 to 1.5); and glucose, 90 mg/dL (normal, 60 to 110). The blood methanol concentration was 108 mg/dL, and the measured plasma osmolality was 333 mOsm/kg. What is J.F.'s calculated osmolality? Are other unidentified osmoles present?**

[SI units: Na, 135 mmol/L; K, 3.4 mmol/L; Cl, 105 mmol/L; CO_2, 20 mmol/L; BUN, 3.57 mmol/L; creatinine, 97.4 µmol/L; glucose, 5.0 mmol/L; methanol, 33.7 mmol/L]

Using Equation 12-1, J.F.'s total calculated osmolality is as follows:

$$P_{OSM} = 2(145\ mEq/L) + \frac{90\ mg/dL}{18} + \frac{10\ mg/dL}{2.8} \quad \textbf{12-A}$$

$$= 290 + 5 + 3.6$$
$$= 299\ mOsm/kg$$

$$Osmolal\ gap = 333\ mOsm/kg - 299\ mOsm/kg \quad \textbf{12-B}$$
$$= 34\ mOsm/kg$$

In J.F., the entire osmolal gap can be accounted for by the presence of the methanol (because 108 mg/dL of methanol will provide 108/3.2 = 33.7 mOsm/kg). It is therefore unlikely that other unmeasured osmoles are present (e.g., ethylene glycol, isopropanol, and ethanol). The laboratory determination of osmolality measures the total number of osmotically active particles but not their permeability across the cell membrane. Methanol increases plasma osmolality but not tonicity because the cell membrane is permeable to methanol. Therefore, there is no net water shift between the intracellular and extracellular compartments. Conversely, mannitol, which is confined to the extracellular space, contributes to both plasma osmolality and tonicity.

Tubular Function of Nephron

The kidney plays an important role in maintaining a constant extracellular environment by regulating the excretion of water and various electrolytes. The volume and composition of fluid filtered across the glomerulus are modified as the fluid passes through the tubules of the nephron.

The renal tubule is composed of a series of segments with heterogeneous structures and functions: the proximal tubule, the medullary and cortical thick ascending limb of Henle's loop, the distal convoluted tubule, and the cortical and medullary collecting duct[3] (Fig. 12-1). The mechanism for sodium reabsorption is different for each nephron segment but is generally mediated by carrier proteins or channels located on the luminal membrane of the tubule cell.[3] Na^+-K^+-ATPase actively pumps sodium out of the renal tubule cell in exchange for potassium in a 3:2 ratio. Hence, the intracellular sodium concentration is kept at a low level. The potassium that is pumped into the cell leaks back out through potassium channels in the membrane, rendering the cell interior electronegative. The low intracellular sodium concentration and a negative intracellular potential produce a favorable gradient for passive sodium entry into the cell.[3] The Na^+-K^+-ATPase also indirectly provides the energy for active sodium transport and the reabsorption and secretion of other solutes across the luminal membrane of the renal tubule. The distal segments are mainly involved in the reabsorption of sodium and chloride ions and the secretion of hydrogen and potassium ions.[3]

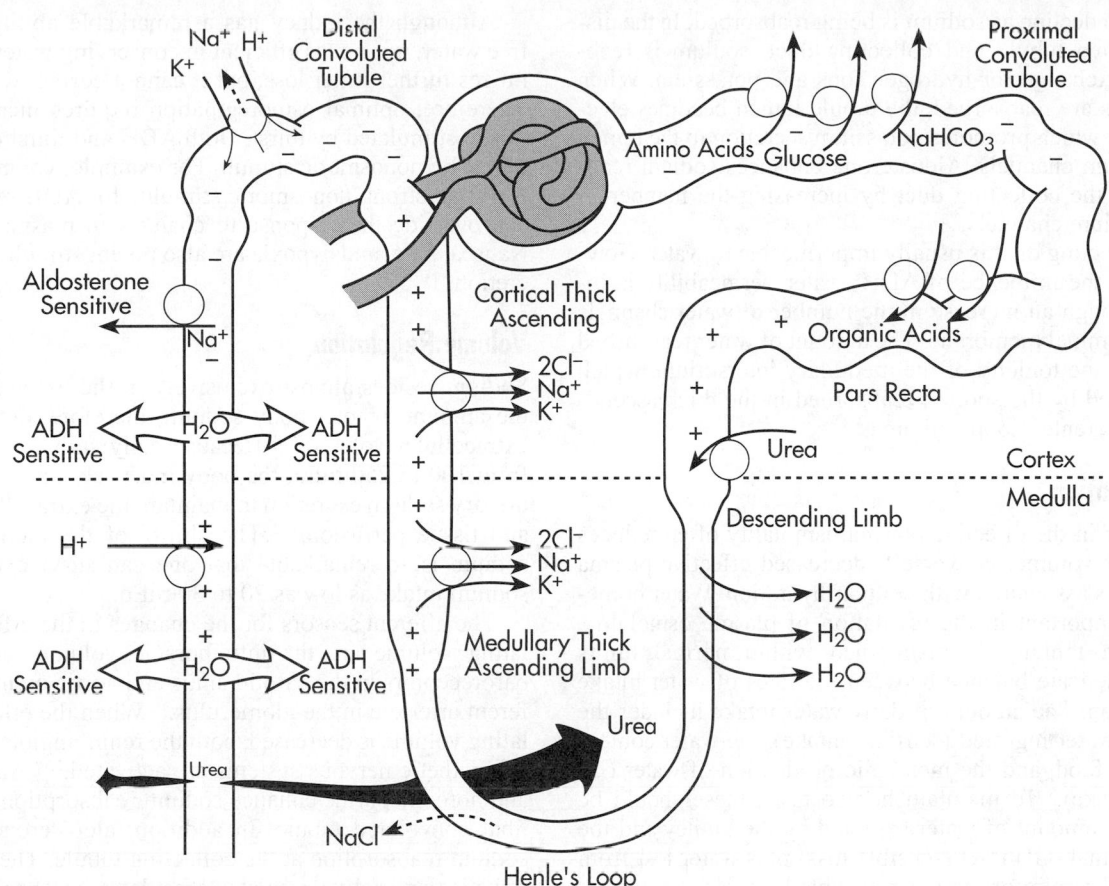

FIGURE 12-1 Sites of tubule salt and water absorption. Sodium is reabsorbed with inorganic anions, amino acids, and glucose in the proximal tubule against an electrical gradient that is lumen negative. In the late part of the proximal tubule (pars recta), sodium and water are reabsorbed to a lesser extent and organic acids (hippurate, urate) and urea are secreted into the urine. The electrical potential is lumen positive in the pars recta. Water, but not salt, is removed from tubule fluid in the thin descending limb of Henle's loop, but in the ascending portion salt is reabsorbed without water, rendering the tubule fluid hyposmotic with respect to the interstitium. Sodium, chloride, and potassium are reabsorbed by the medullary and cortical portions of the ascending limb; the lumen potential is positive. Sodium is reabsorbed and potassium and hydrogen ions are secreted in the distal tubule and collecting ducts. Water absorption in these segments is regulated by antidiuretic hormone (ADH). The electrical potential is lumen negative in the cortical sections and positive in the medullary segments. Urea is concentrated in the interstitium of the medulla and assists in the generation of maximally concentrated urine. (Reproduced with permission from reference 23.)

Iso-osmotic reabsorption of the glomerular filtrate occurs in the proximal tubule such that two thirds of the filtered sodium and water and 90% of the filtered bicarbonate are reabsorbed. The Na^+-H^+ antiporter (exchanger) in the luminal membrane is instrumental in the reabsorption of sodium chloride, sodium bicarbonate, and water. The reabsorption of most nonelectrolyte solutes such as glucose, amino acids, and phosphates are coupled to sodium transport.[3,6]

Both the thick ascending limb of Henle's loop and the distal convoluted tubule serve as the diluting segments of the nephron because they are impermeable to water. Sodium chloride is extracted from the filtrate without water. Sodium transport in both of these segments is flow dependent and varies with the amount of sodium ions delivered from the proximal segments of the nephron. Decreased sodium ions in the tubular fluid will limit sodium transport in the thick ascending limb of Henle's loop and the distal convoluted tubule.[3,7]

Reabsorption of sodium in the thick ascending limb of Henle's loop accounts for approximately 25% of the total sodium reabsorption. Sodium, chloride, and potassium are reabsorbed by the medullary and cortical portions of the ascending limb, but the leakage of reabsorbed potassium ions back into the tubular lumen, via potassium channels, makes the tubular lumen electropositive. This electrical gradient promotes the passive reabsorption of cations, such as sodium, calcium, and magnesium, in the distal convoluted tubules. Because the thick ascending limb of Henle's loop is impermeable to water, it contributes to the interstitial osmolality in the medulla. This high osmolality is key to the reabsorption of water by the medullary portion of the collecting duct under the influence of antidiuretic hormone (ADH, vasopressin). Therefore, the thick ascending limb of Henle's loop is important for both urinary concentration and dilution.[7]

Because, as noted previously, the distal convoluted tubule also is impermeable to water, the osmolality of the filtrate continues to decline as sodium is being reabsorbed. In the distal convoluted tubule and collecting duct, sodium is reabsorbed in exchange for hydrogen ions and potassium. When sodium ions are reabsorbed, the tubule lumen becomes electronegative, which promotes potassium secretion in the lumen via potassium channels. Aldosterone enhances sodium reabsorption in the collecting duct by increasing the number of opened sodium channels.[3,8]

The collecting duct is usually impermeable to water. However, under the influence of ADH, water permeability is increased through an increase in the number of water channels along the luminal membrane. The amount of water reabsorbed depends on the tonicity of the medullary interstitium, which is determined by the sodium reabsorbed in the thick ascending limb of Henle's loop and urea.[3,8,9]

Osmoregulation

An increase in the effective plasma osmolality often reduces intracellular volume; conversely, decreased effective plasma osmolality is associated with cellular hydration. Water homeostasis is important in the regulation of plasma osmolality, and plasma tonicity is maintained within normal limits through a delicate balance between the rates of water intake and excretion. The amount of daily water intake includes the volume of water ingested (sensible intake), the water content of ingested food, and the metabolic production of water (insensible intake).[3] To maintain homeostasis, these should be equal to the amount of water excreted by the kidney and the gastrointestinal (GI) tract (sensible loss) plus water lost from the skin and respiratory tract (insensible loss).[3,4]

Changes in plasma tonicity are detected by osmoreceptors in the hypothalamus, which also houses the thirst center and is the site for ADH synthesis.[10,11] When the plasma tonicity falls below 280 mOsm/kg as a result of water ingestion, ADH release is inhibited,[3] water is no longer reabsorbed in the collecting duct, and a large volume of dilute urine is excreted. Conversely, when the osmoreceptors in the hypothalamus sense an increased plasma osmolality, ADH is released to increase water reabsorption. A small volume of concentrated urine is then excreted. The threshold for ADH release is 280 mOsm/kg, and maximal ADH secretion occurs when the plasma osmolality is 295 mOsm/kg.[10] Thus, urine osmolality varies from 50 mOsm/kg in the absence of ADH to 1,200 mOsm/kg during maximum ADH release. The volume of urine produced depends on the solute load to be excreted, as well as the urine osmolality[3,4,10,11]:

$$\text{Urine volume (L)} = \left(\frac{\text{Solute load (mOsm)}}{\text{Urine osmolality (mOsm/kg)}} \right) \quad \textbf{12-3}$$

$$\left(\frac{1}{\text{Density of water (kg/L)}} \right)$$

Therefore, for a typical daily solute load of 600 mOsm:

Urine volume in the absence of ADH

$$= \left(\frac{600 \text{ mOsm}}{50 \text{ mOsm/kg}} \right)\left(\frac{1}{1 \text{ kg/L}} \right) = 12 \text{ L} \quad \textbf{12-C}$$

Urine volume with maximal ADH release

$$= \left(\frac{600 \text{ mOsm}}{1,200 \text{ mOsm/kg}} \right)\left(\frac{1}{1 \text{ kg/L}} \right) = 0.5 \text{ L} \quad \textbf{12-D}$$

Although the kidney has a remarkable ability to excrete free water, it is not as efficient in conserving water. ADH minimizes further water loss, but it cannot correct water deficits. Therefore, optimal osmoregulation requires increased water intake stimulated by thirst. Both ADH and thirst can be stimulated by nonosmotic stimuli. For example, volume depletion is such a strong nonosmotic stimulus for ADH release that it can override the response to changes in plasma osmolality. Nausea, pain, and hypoxia are also potent stimuli for ADH secretion.[11]

Volume Regulation

Sodium resides almost exclusively in the extracellular fluid; the amount of total body sodium, therefore, determines the extracellular volume.[3,12] Because daily sodium intake varies from 100 to 250 mEq, the body must rely on adjustments in urinary sodium excretion to maintain the extracellular volume and tissue perfusion.[3,12] The ability of the kidney to retain sodium is so remarkable that one can survive with a daily sodium intake as low as 20 to 30 mEq.

The afferent sensors for the changes in the effective circulating volume are the intrathoracic volume receptors, the baroreceptors in the carotid sinus and aortic arch, and the afferent arteriole in the glomerulus.[12] When the effective circulating volume is decreased, both the renin-angiotensin and the sympathetic nervous systems are activated.[3,12] Angiotensin II and norepinephrine enhance sodium reabsorption at the proximal convoluted tubule. In addition, aldosterone stimulates sodium reabsorption at the collecting tubule. The decrease in effective arterial volume also stimulates ADH release, which enhances water reabsorption at the collecting duct. Conversely, after a salt load, the increases in atrial pressure and renal perfusion pressure suppress the production of renin and, subsequently, angiotensin II and aldosterone. The release of atrial natriuretic peptide secondary to increased atrial filling pressure and intrarenal production of urodilation increase urinary excretion of the excess sodium.[13,14]

Although the kidney can excrete a 20-mL/kg water load in 4 hours, only 50% of the excess sodium is excreted in the first day.[3] Sodium excretion continues to increase until a new steady state is reached after 3 to 4 days, when intake equals output.[3,12] It is important to recognize that osmoregulation and volume regulation occur independently of each other.[3,4] The two homeostatic systems regulate different parameters and possess different sensors and effectors. However, both systems can be activated simultaneously.

DISORDERS IN VOLUME REGULATION

Sodium Depletion

2. A.B., a 17-year-old girl, presented to the emergency department (ED) with complaints of anorexia, nausea, vomiting, and generalized weakness for the past 3 days. She denied other medical problems and had not used any medications. Upon examination, her supine blood pressure (BP) was 105/70 mm Hg, with a pulse of 80 beats/min. Her standing BP was 85/60 mm Hg with a pulse of 100 beats/min, and she complained of feeling dizzy when she stood up. Her mucous membranes were dry but her skin turgor was normal. The jugular vein was flat, and peripheral or sacral edema was not present. Laboratory blood tests showed serum Na, 134 mEq/L (normal, 134 to 146); K, 3.5 mEq/L (normal, 3.5 to 5.1); Cl, 95 mEq/L (normal, 92 to 109); total CO_2 content, 35 mEq/L (normal, 22 to 32); BUN, 18 mg/dL (normal, 8 to 25); creatinine, 0.8 mg/dL (normal, 0.5 to 1.5); and glucose, 70 mg/dL (normal, 60 to 110). Random urinary Na was 40 mEq/L, K was 40 mEq/L, and Cl was <15 mEq/L. The hemoglobin (Hgb) was 14 g/dL (normal, 12 to 16), and white cell and platelet counts were normal. Why were the clinical and laboratory data in A.B. consistent with an assessment of volume depletion?

[SI units: serum Na, 134 mmol/L; K, 3.5 mmol/L; Cl, 95 mmol/L; CO_2, 35 mmol/L; BUN, 5.7 mmol/L; creatinine, 70.72 μmol/L; glucose, 3.9 mmol/L; urine Na, 40 mmol/L; K, 40 mmol/L; Cl, <15 mmol/L; Hgb, 140 g/L]

The signs and symptoms of A.B. were consistent with volume depletion. The loss of gastric fluid due to vomiting and decreased oral intake secondary to anorexia had led to moderate to severe volume depletion. There were orthostatic changes in both her BP (a drop in systolic BP of 20 mm Hg) and pulse (an increase of 20 beats/minute). The dry mucous membranes, the flat jugular vein, and the absence of edema support volume depletion as well, and dizziness on standing indicates extracellular volume depletion.[15] Her hypochloremic metabolic alkalosis was probably initiated by loss of acidic gastric contents through vomiting. Her volume depletion increased renal bicarbonate reabsorption, which perpetuated the metabolic alkalosis. The decreased renal perfusion brought about by volume depletion enhanced proximal tubular reabsorption of urea, resulting in an increased BUN-to-creatinine ratio (prerenal azotemia). When renal perfusion is decreased and the renin-angiotensin-aldosterone system is activated, the proximal reabsorption of sodium and chloride is increased. A.B.'s urinary sodium is therefore <10 mEq/L.[16] However, excretion of the poorly permeable bicarbonate ions results in obligatory urinary sodium loss in order to maintain luminal electroneutrality. A.B.'s urinary sodium was therefore elevated (40 mEq/L). In this situation, the urinary chloride remained low, and this is a better index of volume status.[16] However, both urinary sodium and chloride will be elevated in patients using diuretics, in those undergoing osmotic diuresis, and in those with underlying renal disease or hypoaldosteronism, even in the face of volume depletion. Physical examination should therefore be conducted as part of the volume status assessment. A.B.'s volume depletion increased the concentration of red blood cells, which could explain her slightly elevated Hgb concentration of 14 g/dL.

3. How should A.B.'s volume depletion be managed?

The etiology of A.B.'s vomiting should be sought and the cause removed. Because the patient is neither hypernatremic nor hyponatremic, normal saline should be administered intravenously to replenish the extracellular volume and improve tissue perfusion.[3,15] If the patient is hypernatremic (having a greater deficit of water than solute), half-isotonic saline (1/2NS) or dextrose solution, which contains more free water, should be administered. In contrast, hyponatremic hypovolemic patients have a greater deficit of solute than water; isotonic or hypertonic saline should then be given. The amount of volume deficit is often difficult to ascertain. Because A.B. was severely orthostatic, 1 or 2 L of fluid can be given over 2 to 4 hours. The subsequent rate of infusion will depend on A.B.'s response and the prevailing symptoms. The clinician should monitor her body weight, skin turgor, supine and upright BP, jugular venous pressure, urine output, and urine chloride concentration to assess the adequacy of volume repletion. Since the goal of treatment is to achieve a positive fluid balance, the rate of infusion should be 50 or 100 mL/hour in excess of the sum of urine output, insensible losses, and other losses, such as emesis and diarrhea.[3]

Sodium Excess

4. L.J., a 45-year-old man, presented to the clinic with complaints of swollen legs and puffy eyelids. He also noticed that his urine had been foamy recently. Upon examination, his BP was found to be 180/100 mm Hg and his pulse was 80 beats/min. There was bilateral periorbital edema and 2+ bilateral pitting edema up to the thigh. On auscultation, his heart was normal and his lungs had bilateral crackles. His jugular venous pressure was elevated at 10 cm H_2O. Laboratory tests revealed serum Na, 132 mEq/L (normal, 134 to 146); K, 3.8 mEq/L (normal, 3.5 to 5.1); Cl, 100 mEq/L (normal, 92 to 109); bicarbonate, 26 mEq/L (normal, 22 to 32); BUN, 40 mg/dL (normal, 8 to 25); creatinine, 2.5 mg/dL (normal, 0.5 to 1.5); glucose, 120 mg/dL (normal, 60 to 110); and albumin, 2 g/dL (normal, 3.4 to 5.4). The serum transaminases, alkaline phosphatase, and bilirubin were within normal limits. The serum cholesterol level was 280 mg/dL (normal, <200), and the triglyceride level was 300 mg/dL (normal, 30 to 200). Urinalysis showed specific gravity of 1.015 (normal, 1.002 to 1.030), pH 7.0 (normal, 4.6 to 7.9), protein >300 mg/dL, oval fat bodies, and fatty casts. The 24-hour urinary protein excretion was 6 g and the measured creatinine clearance (Cl_{Cr}) was 40 mL/min. L.J. was taking no medications and he denied illicit drug use. Hepatitis B serology and HIV antibody were negative. The impression was anasarca (total body edema) secondary to nephrotic syndrome. What is nephrotic syndrome? What could be the etiology of L.J.'s sodium excess state?

[SI units: Na, 132 mmol/L; K, 3.8 mmol/L; Cl, 100 mmol/L; bicarbonate, 26 mmol/L; BUN, 14.3 mmol/L; serum creatine (SrCr), 221 μmol/L; glucose, 6.7 mmol/L; albumin, 20 g/L; cholesterol, 7.24 mmol/L; triglyceride, 3.4 mmol/L; protein, 3 g/L, Cl_{Cr}, 0.67 mL/sec]

Nephrotic syndrome is characterized by hypoalbuminemia, urine protein excretion >3.5 g/day, hyperlipidemia, lipiduria, and edema.[17,18] The heavy proteinuria is a result of damage to the selective barrier of the glomerulus. The etiologies of nephrotic syndrome are multiple and diverse.[17] The cause of nephrotic syndrome can be idiopathic (primary glomerular disease) or secondary to chronic systemic diseases (e.g., diabetes mellitus, amyloidosis, sickle cell anemia,[19] lupus), cancer (e.g., multiple myeloma, Hodgkin's disease), infections (e.g., HIV,[20] hepatitis B, syphilis, malaria), intravenous (IV) drug abuse, and medications (e.g., gold, penicillamine, captopril, nonsteroidal anti-inflammatory drugs [NSAIDs][21]).

The heavy urinary protein loss results in various extrarenal complications.[17,18] Hypoalbuminemia reduces plasma oncotic pressure and contributes to the increased hepatic synthesis of both albumin and lipoproteins. This, coupled with the decreased catabolism of lipoproteins, resulted in L.J.'s hyperlipidemia.[17,22] Loss of inhibitors of coagulation in the urine predispose these patients to thromboembolism.[17] Specific therapy of nephrotic syndrome ranges from simple removal of the offending medication and treatment of the underlying infection, to the use of immunosuppressive agents in specific glomerular diseases.

The edematous state (L.J.'s anasarca) results from changes in both capillary hemodynamics and renal sodium and water retention.[23] The hypoalbuminemia (2 g/dL) and proteinuria (>300 mg/dL) produced an imbalance in the Starling forces across the capillary wall, namely the hydrostatic and oncotic pressures in the capillary and interstitial compartments. The reduced capillary oncotic pressure favors movement of fluid from the vascular space into the interstitium.[24] This leads to contraction of the effective arterial blood volume, which in turn activates humoral, neural, and hemodynamic mechanisms that signal the kidney to retain sodium and water.[25,26] However, this *underfill hypothesis* has been challenged by data suggesting that hypoalbuminemia plays a minor role in nephrotic edema[27,28] and the observation that patients with nephrotic syndrome can have increased, normal, or decreased plasma volumes.[24]

A defect in the intrarenal sodium handling mechanism that causes inappropriate sodium retention also contributes to nephrotic edema.[24,27] According to this *overflow hypothesis,* proteinuric renal disease leads to increased sodium reabsorption in the distal nephron. The mechanism is not well defined but may be related to cellular resistance to atrial natriuretic peptide.[24] Thus, a sodium excess state occurs and edema results. It is likely that the interaction between the "underfill" and "overflow" mechanisms results in the production of nephrotic edema.[29] Patients with severe hypoalbuminemia (i.e., serum albumin level <1.5 g/dL) who have a severe reduction in plasma oncotic pressure are most likely to exhibit evidence of the underfill phenomenon.[23]

5. How should L.J.'s sodium excess state be managed?

The etiology of L.J.'s nephrotic syndrome should be identified for specific treatment. Although L.J.'s serum sodium concentration of 132 mEq/L is low, it reflects dilution secondary to fluid excess. Salt restriction is therefore important to control L.J.'s generalized edema.[24] For most nephrotic patients, modest dietary sodium restriction to approximately 50 mEq/day may be sufficient to maintain neutral sodium balance.[23,24] However, for nephrotic patients who are very sodium avid (urine sodium concentration <10 mEq/L), sufficient restriction is difficult to achieve. Thus, slowing the rate of edema formation rather than hastening its resolution should be the goal of therapy for these patients.[24] Bed rest reduces orthostatic stimulation of the renin-angiotensin-aldosterone and sympathetic systems, thereby favoring the movement of interstitial fluid into the vascular space.[24] The central blood volume is thus increased and natriuresis and diuresis are facilitated. However, prolonged bed rest might predispose these hypercoagulable patients to thromboembolism.[17] Similarly, use of support stockings may reduce the stimulation for sodium retention by redistributing blood volume to the central circulation.[24,30]

Diuretics

Usually, loop diuretics are the mainstay of therapy in the management of nephrotic edema.[3,24] In most of these patients, the edema can be removed safely with rapid diuresis without compromising the systemic circulation, probably because of the rapid refilling of the plasma volume by interstitial fluid.[24] Nevertheless, as the edema resolves, the rate of fluid removal

and weight loss should be decreased to avoid compromising the effective circulating volume. The patient should be monitored for the development of orthostatic hypotension.

Infusions of albumin can expand the plasma volume. However, it is expensive, the relief is temporary, and it should therefore be used only for resistant edema.[31] In patients who are resistant to the aforementioned measures, extracorporeal fluid removal, namely ultrafiltration, may be necessary.[24,32]

L.J. was initially treated with IV furosemide 60 mg twice daily and placed on a low-sodium (50 mEq), low-fat, high–complex-carbohydrate diet that consisted of 0.8 g/kg protein of high biologic value with additional protein to match gram-per-gram of urinary protein loss. Fluid was restricted to 1,000 mL/day.[33] He had 5 L of diuresis in 2 days, with resolution of respiratory symptoms and improvement in the anasarca. Parenteral furosemide was discontinued on the fifth day of hospitalization and oral furosemide 120 mg twice daily was started. After a total weight loss of 12 kg, he was then discharged with instructions to maintain the diet and oral furosemide.

DISORDERS IN OSMOREGULATION

Hyponatremia

Serum sodium concentration reflects the ratio of total body sodium to total body water and is not an accurate indicator of total body sodium. Both hyponatremia and hypernatremia can occur in the presence of a low, normal, or high total body sodium.[34,35] Because the kidney can excrete >12 to 16 L of free water daily, hyponatremia does not occur unless the water intake overwhelms the kidney's ability to excrete free water (e.g., psychogenic polydipsia),[36,37] or free water excretion is impaired.[3,38]

Free water formation requires a normal glomerular filtration rate (GFR), the reabsorption of sodium chloride without water in the thick ascending limb of Henle's loop and the distal convoluting tubule, and the excretion of a dilute urine in the absence of ADH[38] (see Fig. 12-1). Therefore, hyponatremia can occur when the kidney's diluting ability is exceeded or impaired due to volume depletion and nonosmotic stimulation of ADH release or inappropriate stimulation of ADH production.[3,38]

Although plasma sodium is the primary determinant of plasma tonicity, hyponatremia does not always represent hypotonicity.[3,38] In patients with severe hyperlipidemia or hyperproteinemia (e.g., multiple myeloma), pseudohyponatremia may occur because the increased amounts of lipids and proteins displace plasma water, which sodium ions dissolve in, resulting in a lower concentration of sodium per unit volume of plasma.[35,38,39] Normally, water accounts for 93% of the plasma volume, and lipids and proteins make up the rest.[38] The increase in plasma lipid and protein contents expands plasma volume, displaces water, and increases the percentage of solids in plasma.[35,38] Because sodium is distributed only in the aqueous phase, the sodium content per liter of the newly recomposed plasma is thus decreased and the plasma sodium concentration is reduced.[35,38,39] However, the sodium concentration in plasma water remains the same. Because osmolality depends on the solute concentration in plasma water, serum osmolality remains unchanged.[35] Indeed, the measured osmolality is normal. Another example of isotonic hyponatremia can be found when a large volume of isotonic mannitol irrigant is used during prostate surgery.[35,38] Absorption of the irrigation solution can result in severe hyponatremia but normal osmolality. In contrast, use of large amounts of isotonic sorbitol and isotonic, or slightly hypotonic, glycine solutions during urologic surgery may cause the hypotonicity as a late complication.[35,38] Similar to mannitol, sorbitol and isotonic glycine initially distribute only in the extracellular space, resulting in hyponatremia without a change in osmolality.[38] Unlike mannitol, both sorbitol and glycine are later metabolized, leaving water behind to result in hypotonicity. The severe hypotonic hyponatremia, in conjunction with the neurotoxic effects of glycine and its metabolites, puts the patient at significant risk for severe neurologic symptoms (Table 12-1).[38,40]

6. T.T., a 23-year-old man with end-stage renal disease due to diabetic nephropathy, is receiving chronic ambulatory peritoneal dialysis. Because of dietary noncompliance, T.T. complained of shortness of breath (SOB) and his dialysis prescription was adjusted to include six cycles of 2.5% peritoneal dialysis solutions. Today, his laboratory values are Na, 128 mEq/L (normal, 134 to 146); K, 4 mEq/L (normal, 3.5 to 5.1); Cl, 98 mEq/L (normal, 92 to 109); total CO_2, 24 mmol/L (normal, 22 to 32); BUN, 50 mg/dL (normal, 8 to 25); creatinine, 6 mg/dL (normal, 0.5 to 1.5); and glucose, 600 mg/dL (normal, 60 to 110). Evaluate T.T.'s plasma osmolality. What is the etiology of T.T.'s hyponatremia?

[SI units: Na, 128 mmol/L; K, 4 mmol/L; Cl, 98 mmol/L; CO_2, 24 mmol/L; BUN, 17.85 mmol/L; creatinine, 530.4 μmol/L; glucose, 33.3 mmol/L]

T.T.'s effective plasma osmolality is calculated to be 289 mOsm/L, of which 33 mOsm/L is contributed by the hyperglycemia. The slow utilization of glucose, due to the lack of insulin, causes water to move from the intracellular compartment into the plasma space because of the increased tonicity, thereby lowering the plasma sodium concentration.[35,38] Despite the lowered plasma sodium concentration, the plasma osmolality is normal because of hyperglycemia. Hence, no symptoms attributable to hypo-osmolality are observed. Indeed, when serum glucose is normalized with insulin and hydration, the serum sodium level will increase to approximately 136 mEq/L. For each 100-mg/dL increment in serum glucose, serum sodium decreases by 1.3 to 1.6 mEq/L.[35,38] Use of hypertonic mannitol or glycine solutions in patients suffering from cerebral edema also results in a hyperosmolar hyponatremia.[35]

Hypotonic Hyponatremia With Decreased Extracellular Fluid

7. Q.B., a 30-year-old male athlete who has had multiple bouts of diarrhea over the last several days, has been drinking Gatorade to keep himself from getting dehydrated. His vital signs are supine BP, 145/80 mm Hg, and pulse, 70 beats/min; standing BP, 128/68 mm Hg, and pulse, 90 beats/min. Respiratory rate (RR) was 12 breaths/min, and he was afebrile. His skin turgor was mildly decreased and laboratory data were Na, 128 mEq/L (normal, 134 to 146); K, 3.0 mEq/L (normal, 3.5 to 5.1); Cl, 100 mEq/L (normal, 92 to 109); bicarbonate, 17 mEq/L (normal, 24 to 31); BUN, 27 mg/dL (normal, 8 to 25); and creatinine, 1.2 mg/dL (normal, 0.5 to 1.5). Urinary Na and Cl were

both <10 mEq/L. Assess Q.B.'s electrolyte and fluid status. What is the etiology of Q.B.'s hyponatremia?

[SI units: plasma Na, 128 mmol/L; K, 3 mmol/L; Cl, 100 mmol/L; bicarbonate, 17 mmol/L; BUN, 7.14 mmol/L; creatinine, 106.1 μmol/L; urinary Na, <10 mmol/L; Cl, <10 mmol/L]

Q.B. has true hypotonic hyponatremia with extracellular fluid depletion, suggesting that his total body sodium deficit is greater than that of total body water.[35] His poor skin turgor, orthostasis, prerenal azotemia, and low urinary sodium are consistent with volume depletion. The urinary sodium concentration helps distinguish between renal and nonrenal losses that result in the sodium and water deficits.[16,35,41] When the plasma volume is depleted, the urinary sodium concentration is <10 mEq/L, suggesting appropriate renal sodium conservation.[16] This is usually seen in patients such as Q.B. with GI fluid loss as in vomiting, diarrhea, or profuse sweating.[35,38,41] Other causes of hypotonic hyponatremia are less likely in Q.B. They include surreptitious cathartic abuse and "third spacing," or accumulation of extracellular fluid in the abdominal cavity during acute pancreatitis, ileus, or pseudomembranous colitis.[38,41] If the urinary sodium is >20 mEq/L in the face of volume depletion, renal salt wastage should be considered.[16,38,41] The potential causes of this latter problem include diuretic use,[42–44] adrenal insufficiency,[45] and salt-wasting nephropathy[36] (e.g., chronic interstitial nephritis, medullary cystic disease, polycystic kidney disease, obstructive uropathy, and cisplatin toxicity[45,46]). In patients with renal insufficiency, neither the urinary sodium nor chloride concentration is a reliable index of volume status.[16]

Volume depletion leads to increased reabsorption of sodium and water in the proximal tubule and, thus, decreased sodium delivery to the diluting segments for free water formation.[35,38,41] Decreased effective arterial volume is also a potent nonosmotic stimulus for ADH release.[10,11] These factors combine to dampen the ability of the kidney to form dilute urine and result in high urine osmolality despite a low serum sodium concentration.[35,38,41] Although the fluid lost in diarrhea is hypotonic, it is the replacement of fluid loss with an even more hypotonic fluid such as Gatorade or tap water that causes hyponatremia in patients like Q.B.[38,41]

Q.B.'s diarrhea probably caused loss of potassium and bicarbonate through the GI tract, resulting in hypokalemia and hyperchloremic metabolic acidosis. The potassium depletion can sensitize ADH secretion in response to hypovolemic stimuli, and the hypokalemia also can lead to hyponatremia.[38] The cellular efflux of potassium causes cellular uptake of sodium, further reducing the serum sodium concentration.

8. How should Q.B.'s hyponatremia be managed?

The treatment of hypovolemic hyponatremia involves sodium replacement to correct the deficit. The sodium deficit can be estimated by the following formula:

Na Deficit = Vd of Na × Patient Weight (Desired − Current Na concentration)   **12-4**

= (0.5 L/kg)(70 kg)(140 − 125 mEq/L)   **12-E**
= 525 mEq

Roughly one third of the deficit can be replaced over the first 12 hours at a rate of <0.5 mEq/L per hour. The remaining amounts can be administered over the next several days.

Table 12-1   Clinical Presentation and Treatment of Hyponatremia

Na⁺ and H₂O Status	Clinical Presentation/Cause	Treatment
Edematous, Fluid Overload **(Hypervolemic, Hypotonic)** $\uparrow$ Total Body Na⁺ $\uparrow\uparrow$ Total Body H₂O	*Cirrhosis/CHF/nephrotic syndrome:* A $\downarrow$in renal blood flow activates renin an- giotensin system. $\uparrow$ aldosterone leads to $\uparrow$ Na⁺, and $\uparrow$ ADH leads to free H₂O retention. Urine Na⁺ is low (0-20 mEq/L) and urine os- molality $\downarrow$. Diuretics can induce paradoxical effects on urine Na⁺ and osmolality. This form also can occur in patients with renal failure who drink excessive amounts of wa- ter. Patients have symptoms of fluid over- load (ascites, distended neck veins, edema).	Fluid and Na⁺ restriction. Correct underlying disorder (e.g., paracentesis for ascites). Di- urese cautiously; avoid $\downarrow$ ECF and accom- panying $\downarrow$ tissue perfusion. $\uparrow$ BUN may indicate overly rapid diuresis.
Nonedematous Hypovolemic **(Hypotonic with ECF Depletion)** $\downarrow\downarrow$ Total Body Na⁺ $\downarrow$ Total Body H₂O	Occurs in: *GI fluid loss (e.g., diarrhea) with hypotonic electrolyte-poor fluid replacement, overdiuresis, "third spacing," Addison's dis- ease, renal tubular acidosis, osmotic diure- sis.* Replacement of fluid losses with solute- free fluid predisposes these patients to hyponatremia. Kidneys concentrate urine to conserve fluid (urine Na⁺ <10 mEq/L). *Symptoms:* nonedematous; ECF depletion (collapsed neck veins, dehydration, orthosta- sis). *Neurologic symptoms:* (See Hypona- tremia: Symptoms in text).	Discontinue diuretics. Replace fluid and elec- trolyte (especially K⁺) losses. 0.9% saline preferred unless Na⁺ deficit severe, then use 3%-5% saline. See footnote *a* for method of estimating Na⁺ deficit.
Nonedematous, Normovolemic **(Normovolemic, Hypotonic)** $\downarrow$ Total Body Sodium $\uparrow$ Total Body H₂O	*SIADH[a]*: Hyponatremia, hypoosmolality, renal Na⁺ wasting (>40 mEq/L), absence of fluid depletion, $U_{osm} > P_{osm}$, normal renal and adrenal function. Free H₂O retained while Na⁺ lost. *Causes:* a) ADH production (infec- tious disease, vascular disease, cerebral neo- plasm, cancer of lung, pancreas, duodenum); b) exogenous ADH administration; c) drugs; d) psychogenic polydipsia.	*Chronic treatment:* Restrict fluids to less than urine loss. *Demeclocycline* (300-600 mg BID) induces reversible diabetes insipidus. *Emergency treatment* for unresponsive pa- tients includes *furosemide* diuresis to achieve negative H₂O balance with careful replacement of Na⁺ and K⁺ using hypertonic saline solutions.[b] See footnote *b* for method of calculating TBW excess and type of solu- tions to use.

ADH = Antidiuretic hormone; BUN = Blood urea nitrogen; CHF = Congestive heart failure; ECF = Extracellular fluid; GI = Gastrointestinal; NS = Normal saline (0.9% Na); SIADH = Syndrome of Inappropriate ADH.

[a]Estimate Na deficit: (mEq) = (0.5 L/kg × wt in kg) (Na desired − Na observed), where 0.5 L/kg is volume of distribution (Vd) of Na in the body. Rate of Na and fluid reple- tion used depends on severity. Mild: Replace with NS. 1st third over 6-12 hours at a rate of <0.5 mEq/L per hour, remaining 2/3 over 24-48 hr. Severe (e.g., seizures): Use 3%-5% saline, rate gauged by patient's ability to tolerate Na and volume load. Monitor CNS function, skin turgor, BP, urine Na, signs of Na/H₂O overload, especially in patients with cardiovascular, renal, and pulmonary disease.

[b]Total body water (TBW) = 0.5 L/kg × wt in kg.

$$\text{TBW excess} = \text{TBW} - \text{TBW}\ \frac{\text{(Observed serum Na)}}{\text{Desired serum Na)}}$$

Remove estimated excess free water with IV furosemide (1 mg/kg). Repeat as necessary. Since furosemide generates a urine that resembles 0.5% NaCl, urine losses of Na and K must be carefully measured and replaced hourly with hypertonic salt solutions. *Correction Rate:* 1-2 mEq Na/hr in symptomatic patients; 0.5 mEq/hr in asymptomatic patients.

The use of isotonic sodium chloride solution is ideal for the treatment of volume-depleted hyponatremia. As renal perfusion is restored, free water will be excreted with appropriate retention of sodium.[41] Because Q.B. suffered from only mild volume depletion, oral replacement fluids can be given. Oral solutions containing both electrolyte and glucose[47] or rice-based solutions[48] are ideal for the management of persistent fluid loss. Glucose not only provides calories but also promotes the intestinal absorption of ingested sodium.[49] Because the rice-based solution provides more glucose and amino acids, both of which can promote intestinal sodium absorption, it is more effective than glucose alone.[3,49]

In patients with renal salt wasting, the ongoing daily sodium loss also should be taken into consideration when estimating the amount of replacement. Potassium should be given to correct hypokalemia, thereby improving the hyponatremia as well. The serum sodium concentration may rise faster than expected because as tissue perfusion is restored, sodium delivery to the distal tubules will increase and ADH secretion will be suppressed appropriately.[35,38,41] In the absence of ADH, increased free water excretion will improve the serum sodium concentration faster than initially estimated.

Hypervolemic Hypotonic Hyponatremia

9. T.W., a 55-year-old man with a longstanding history of alcoholic liver cirrhosis, is admitted to the hospital for worsening SOB. His medical history includes portal hypertension, esophageal varices, and noncompliance with dietary restriction and medications. His BP is 120/60 mm Hg; pulse, 100 beats/ min; RR, 20 breaths/min. He is afebrile. Physical examination reveals a jaundiced man in respiratory distress. His jugular vein is flat and lung examination reveals bilateral basal rales. Abdominal examination shows tense ascites with hepatomegaly and spider angiomas (telangiectasias resembling a spider). He has 1+ pedal edema bilaterally. Laboratory data upon admission are Na, 127 mEq/L (normal, 134 to 146); K, 3.4 mEq/L (normal, 3.5 to 5.1); Cl, 95 mEq/L (normal, 92 to 109); total CO_2 content, 24 mEq/L (normal, 22 to 32); BUN, 10 mg/dL (normal, 8 to 25); SrCr, 1.2 mg/dL (normal, 0.5 to 1.5); and albumin, 2.5 g/dL (normal, 3.5 to 5.4). Urine Na was <10 mEq/L, and osmolality was 380 mOsm/L (normal, 250 to 1,000). Identify the possible causes of hyponatremia in T.W. and discuss its pathophysiology. How should he be managed?

[SI units: serum Na, 127 mmol/L; K, 3.4 mmol/L; Cl, 95 mmol/L; CO_2, 24 mmol/L; BUN, 3.57 mmol/L; SrCr, 106.1 μmol/L; albumin, 25 g/L; urine, Na <10 mmol/L]

T.W. had no history of vomiting or diarrhea and had stopped using diuretics before admission. The physical findings of ascites and bilateral edema are not consistent with volume depletion but indicate a sodium-excess state. Both sodium and water retention take place, but the disproportionate accumulation of ingested water relative to sodium leads to hyponatremia.[35,38,41]

Cirrhotic patients who are prone to develop hyponatremia have a decreased effective arterial blood volume.[25,38,47,48] The low urinary sodium concentration suggests that the effective arterial blood volume was decreased.[16] However, the high urinary osmolality in the face of hypotonic hyponatremia suggests that the release of ADH has been stimulated, impairing free water excretion. Peripheral vasodilation causes decreases

in systemic arterial BP despite a normal to high cardiac output. This, along with splanchnic venous pooling and decreased oncotic pressure secondary to hypoalbuminemia, decreases renal perfusion in patients like T.W. with cirrhosis.[23,29,47] Decreased renal perfusion activates the renin-angiotensin-aldosterone system, the sympathetic nervous system, and the release of ADH. Reabsorption of sodium and water in the proximal tubules is enhanced, diminishing sodium and water delivery to the distal segments of the nephron. The diluting capacity of the kidney is thus impaired. Increased secretion of antidiuretic hormone also promotes free water reabsorption at the collecting tubule and contributes to the hyperosmolality of urine and hyponatremia. The hypervolemic hyponatremia also is seen in patients with congestive heart failure (CHF) and nephrotic syndrome[25-29] and in patients with chronic renal disease who drink excessive amounts of water.[38,41] (See Chapter 19, Heart Failure, and also Question 2.) As the GFR decreases, distal delivery of sodium is reduced and the ability to generate free water is impaired. In addition, the capacity to conserve sodium is impaired in these patients.[16]

Most edematous, hyponatremic patients are asymptomatic, but the degree of hyponatremia probably reflects the severity of the underlying disease.[47,48,50] Unless there is an acute decrease in serum sodium, rapid therapeutic correction is not warranted.[38,41,47,48,51] Water restriction, the mainstay of therapy, is determined by the degree of hyponatremia and the severity of symptoms. Sodium restriction and judicious use of diuretics may help reduce the edematous state, but the patient must be monitored closely to avoid prerenal azotemia, which suggests overaggressive diuresis. Furthermore, diuretics can induce or worsen hyponatremia and volume depletion by impairing the diluting capacity of the kidney.[44-48]

T.W. underwent abdominal paracentesis to relieve respiratory discomfort with no sequelae. He was then prescribed a 1,000-mg sodium diet, and water was restricted to 500 mL/day. Diuretic therapy was resumed.

Normovolemic Hypotonic Hyponatremia

10. C.C., a 50-year-old man who was diagnosed recently with small-cell lung carcinoma, was brought to the ED by his family because he had become progressively lethargic and stuporous over the past week. Laboratory data revealed the following: serum Na, 110 mEq/L (normal, 134 to 146); K, 3.6 mEq/L (normal, 3.5 to 5.1); Cl, 78 mEq/L (normal, 92 to 109); bicarbonate, 22 mEq/L (normal, 24 to 31); BUN, 10 mg/dL (normal, 8 to 25); SrCr, 0.9 mg/dL (normal, 0.5 to 1.5); glucose, 90 mg/dL (normal, 60 to 110); serum osmolality, 230 mOsm/kg (normal, 274 to 296); urine osmolality, 616 mOsm/kg (normal, 250 to 1,000); and urine Na, 60 mEq/L. Arterial blood gas (ABG) examination at room air showed pH, 7.38 (normal, 7.35 to 7.42); P_{CO_2}, 38 mm Hg (normal, 35 to 45); and P_{O_2}, 80 mm Hg (normal, 80 to 100). Upon physical examination, C.C. was normotensive, appeared to be euvolemic, and had no edema detected. Review of his medical records showed normal adrenal and thyroid function. C.C. was currently not using any medications. Upon admission to the ward, C.C. weighed 60 kg and was given 1 L of normal saline, after which his serum sodium concentration was 108 mEq/L. Identify the etiology of hyponatremia in C.C. and describe its pathophysiology.

[SI units: serum Na, 110 mmol/L; K, 3.6 mmol/L; Cl, 78 mmol/L; bicarbonate, 22 mmol/L; BUN, 3.57 mmol/L; SrCr, 79.6 μmol/L; glucose, 5.0 mmol/L; serum osmolality, 230 mmol/kg; urine osmolality, 616 mmol/kg; urine Na, 60 mmol/L; Pco₂, 5.1 kPa; Po₂, 853.1 mmol/L; serum Na, 108 mmol/L]

In a patient with hypo-osmolar hyponatremia with a volume status that is apparently normal, the differential diagnosis[41] includes hypothyroidism,[52] cortisol deficiency,[53] a reset osmostat,[54] psychogenic polydipsia,[37,39] and the syndrome of inappropriate antidiuretic hormone secretion (SIADH),[55-57] which is a diagnosis of exclusion. C.C.'s normal thyroid and adrenal function tests exclude hypothyroidism and cortisol insufficiency as causes of his hyponatremia. The inappropriately elevated urine osmolality (>100 mOsm/kg) is inconsistent with psychogenic polydipsia or a reset osmostat, because free water excretion is usually not impaired in these disorders. These findings, in addition to a urine sodium concentration >40 mEq/L and a normal acid–base and potassium balance, are consistent with SIADH.[38,56,57]

In SIADH, the ADH secretion is considered inappropriate because of its persistence in the absence of appropriate osmotic and hemodynamic stimuli. Water ingestion is essential to the development of hyponatremia in SIADH because persistent ADH activity impairs water excretion, resulting in expansion of body fluids and hypo-osmolar hyponatremia. Edema rarely is apparent because only one third of the retained water resides in the extracellular space and the sodium homeostatic mechanisms are intact.[35,41] The extracellular fluid expansion activates volume receptors and results in natriuresis. At steady state, urinary sodium excretion reflects sodium intake and is usually >40 mEq/L, as in C.C.'s case. Nonetheless, if sodium intake is reduced severely, the urinary sodium concentration may become <40 mEq/L.[38]

The etiologies of SIADH are diverse and are shown in Table 12-1. Four different patterns of inappropriate ADH release have been identified.[38] However, no correlation has been found between these patterns and the underlying causes of SIADH. Mechanisms for drug-induced SIADH include ADH-like action on the collecting tubule, central stimulation of ADH release, and potentiation of the ADH effect.[38,58] Small-cell lung carcinoma is the most likely cause of C.C.'s SIADH.

11. Why was C.C.'s serum sodium concentration lower after the saline infusion?

Isotonic sodium chloride solution (154 mEq/L each of Na and Cl ions, or 308 mOsm/L) initially will increase the plasma sodium concentration because its osmolality is higher than C.C.'s.[59] However, C.C. has a relatively fixed urine osmolality of 616 mOsm/kg due to persistent ADH activity; thus, he must excrete an osmolar load of 616 mOsm in a volume of 1,000 mL of urine at steady state. Because a total of 1 L of fluid containing 308 mOsm was administered, all the solutes were excreted in 500 mL of urine output, and 500 mL of free water was retained to cause a further dilution of sodium and a reduction in serum sodium concentration.[38,59]

Neurologic Manifestations

12. Why are C.C.'s neurologic manifestations characteristic of hyponatremia?

As the plasma osmolality declines, the osmotic gradient created across the blood–brain barrier favors the movement of water into the brain and other cells.[38,41] Water movement from the cerebrospinal fluid into the cerebral interstitium results in cerebral edema. However, brain swelling is limited by the meninges and cranium, giving rise to increased intracranial pressure and neurologic symptoms. The degree of cerebral overhydration and the rapidity of its development appear to correlate with the severity of symptoms.[38,41]

When hyponatremia develops in less than 2 to 3 days or the rate of decline in serum sodium exceeds 0.5 mEq/L per hour, the situation is regarded as acute.[38,60,61] The patient often becomes symptomatic when serum sodium concentration falls to 125 mEq/L; early complaints include nausea, vomiting, and malaise.[38,62] Severe symptoms occur more commonly when the serum sodium falls to <120 mEq/L and the rate of decline exceeds 0.5 mEq/L per hour. The patient may present with headache, tremors, incoordination, delirium, lethargy, and obtundation. As the serum sodium drops below 110 to 115 mEq/L, seizure and coma may result.[38,62] On occasion, severe brain edema leads to transtentorial herniation and eventually death. Women, especially those who are premenopausal, apparently are more susceptible to the development of severe neurologic symptoms and irreversible neurologic damage than are men.[63,64]

In contrast to acute hyponatremia, patients who are chronically hyponatremic are usually asymptomatic.[38,60] If present, symptoms are usually vague and nonspecific and tend to occur at lower serum sodium concentrations than those associated with symptomatic acute hyponatremia.[38,60,62] The patient may experience anorexia, nausea, vomiting, muscle weakness, and cramps. Irritability, hostility, confusion, and personality changes also may be seen. At extremely low sodium levels, stupor and, rarely, seizures have been reported.

Brain Adaptation to Hyponatremia

The difference in symptoms between acute and chronic hyponatremia is related to cerebral adaptation to hypotonicity. Two adaptive mechanisms are important in minimizing cerebral edema.[38,41,65,66] First, *cerebral overhydration* increases the hydrostatic pressure in the cerebral interstitium, which results in the movement of fluid from the cerebral interstitial space to the cerebrospinal fluid. Second, the *extrusion of intracellular solutes* reduces cellular osmolality, which in turn enhances water movement out of the cells. Sodium and potassium ions are the initial solutes extruded, followed over a period of hours to days by osmolytes such as inositol, glutamine, glutamate, and taurine.[65] Therefore, when the serum sodium concentration falls faster than the onset of brain osmotic adaptation processes, serious and permanent neurologic damage can occur.[38,41,65,66] On the other hand, when hyponatremia develops over 2 to 3 days, symptoms are not usually seen unless the serum sodium concentration is reduced markedly.

It is often difficult to determine the acuity and chronicity of hyponatremia. Unless there is an obvious cause for acute hyponatremia, one should assume that the condition is chronic.[38,60,61,66] A rapid decline in serum sodium concentration usually suggests that hypotonic fluid was administered to a patient with a condition that overwhelms or impairs renal water excretion. These conditions include psychogenic polydipsia[36,37]; postoperative hyponatremia[63,64,67,68]; postprostatectomy syndrome[40]; and administration of thiazide diuretics,[42,43] parenteral cyclophosphamide,[69] oxytocin,[70] and arginine vasopressin or its analogs.[58] C.C.'s symptoms appear to have developed over 7 days and are consistent with chronic hyponatremia.

Rate of Correction of Hyponatremia

13. **How should C.C.'s hyponatremia be managed?**

C.C.'s water excess should be calculated to estimate the amount of water that should be removed to achieve the desired sodium concentration.

$$\text{Water excess} = \text{TBW} - \text{TBW} \left(\frac{\text{Observed serum Na}}{\text{Desired serum Na}} \right) \quad \textbf{12-5}$$

$$= 30 \text{ L} - 30 \text{ L} \left(\frac{110 \text{ mEq/L}}{120 \text{ mEq/L}} \right) \quad \textbf{12-F}$$

$$= 2.4 \text{ L}$$

$$\text{where TBW} = (0.5 \text{ L/kg})(60 \text{ kg}) = 30 \text{ L} \quad \textbf{12-G}$$

The treatment of hyponatremia has been controversial. Severe hyponatremia is associated with high rates of morbidity and mortality, but its treatment may also result in morbidity. The rate of correction has been implicated as the main cause of complications.[60–62,66,71–73]

It takes time for the brain to lose osmolytes to reduce cerebral swelling during hyponatremia; conversely, the rate of reaccumulation of these osmolytes must keep pace with the rise in serum sodium concentration to avoid brain dehydration and damage. Indeed, rapid correction of hyponatremia can cause a constellation of neurologic findings known as *osmotic demyelination syndrome* (ODS).[72,73] Clinical manifestations usually are delayed and occur 1 to several days after the treatment has been started. Neurologic findings include transient behavioral changes, seizures, akinetic mutism in mild cases, and features of a pontine disorder in severe cases (pseudobulbar palsy, quadriparesis, and coma). In some patients the damage is irreversible, and central pontine myelinolysis can be documented in fatal cases. Patients at greatest risk for osmotic demyelination are those with severe hyponatremia lasting >2 days and those in whom the rate of correction of hyponatremia is >12 mEq/L in any 24-hour period.[66,72,73] Hypokalemia, which was found in about 90% of patients with ODS associated with rapid hyponatremia correction, has been suspected as a predisposing factor in the development of ODS.[73] Since the etiology of this complication is unclear, it may be beneficial to correct the hypokalemia before correcting the severe hyponatremia.[73]

Retrospective reviews suggest that acute hyponatremia can be treated safely at a rate of 1 mEq/L per hour initially, until the serum sodium concentration reaches 120 mEq/L. Thereafter, the rate of correction should be reduced to ≤0.5 mEq/L per hour, such that an increment in sodium concentration does not exceed 12 mEq/L in the first 24 hours.[60,74] Slow correction is indicated for severe chronic hyponatremia. No neurologic complications were seen in patients with severe hyponatremia when the average rate of correction to serum sodium was <0.55 mEq/L per hour or when the increase in serum sodium was <12 mEq/L in 24 hours or <18 mEq/L in 48 hours.[74]

In C.C., the serum sodium concentration should be raised to approximately 120 mEq/L at a correction rate of approximately 0.5 mEq/L per hour, using hypertonic saline and furosemide. Serum sodium concentrations should be monitored closely because the equation for calculating water excess does not take into account insensible loss, which can increase the rate of sodium correction.

The use of normal saline is not useful in C.C. because he excretes salt normally (urine Na, 60 mEq/L). C.C.'s sodium deficit is as follows:

$$(0.5 \text{ L/kg})(60 \text{ kg})(120 - 110 \text{ mEq/L}) = 300 \text{ mEq} \quad \textbf{12-H}$$

Because 1 L of 3% sodium chloride solution contains 513 mEq of sodium, approximately 600 mL of 3% saline solution, which contains 308 mEq of sodium, will be required to correct the sodium deficit. The recommended serum sodium concentration correction rate is 0.5 mEq/L per hour; therefore, a minimum of 20 hours will be needed to raise the serum sodium concentration by 10 mEq/L (from 110 to 120 mEq/L). The amount of sodium replacement to safely increase the serum sodium concentration can be determined by the product of the rate of replacement (0.5 mEq/L per hour) and total body weight (TBW) (30 L, Equation 12-G)—that is, 15 mEq/hour. The maximum rate of infusion of 3% saline, which contains 0.513 mEq/mL of sodium, is therefore 29.2 mL/hour [15 mEq/hour]/[0.513 mEq/mL]). A rate of 25 mL/hour is therefore appropriate to safely replace C.C.'s sodium deficit.

Because calculations for water excess and sodium deficits are only approximations, the patient's serum osmolality, serum sodium, and clinical response must be monitored closely. Urinary losses can be replaced with 3% sodium chloride solution and appropriate amounts of potassium.

Chronic Management of the Syndrome of Inappropriate Antidiuretic Hormone Secretion

SIADH is usually transient if the underlying cause can be removed. However, chronic SIADH can occur, as illustrated by C.C. Water restriction sufficient to create a negative water balance is the primary therapy and should be attempted first.[38,41] In general, all fluids, not just water, should be included in the restriction. Salt intake, however, should not be reduced or solute depletion may occur. The extent of fluid restriction depends on urine output, the amount of insensible water loss, and urine osmolality. For a given amount of solute excretion, patients with a high urine osmolality require a smaller volume of urine (i.e., more water retained) than those with a lower urine osmolality (i.e., less water retained). Hence, more stringent water restriction is required in patients with a high urine osmolality. Commonly, several days of restriction are needed before a significant increase in plasma osmolality is observed.

When fluid restriction fails to reverse the hypo-osmolar state or when the patient is unwilling or unable to comply with the severe fluid restriction, drugs that antagonize the effect of ADH can be used.[38,41] These include loop diuretics,[75,76] demeclocycline,[77] and lithium.[78] Furosemide, 20 to 40 mg/day, reduces urine osmolality by blocking the concentrating ability of the kidney.[75] Demeclocycline and lithium directly impair the response to ADH at the collecting tubule, inducing nephrogenic diabetes insipidus.[77,78] Demeclocycline (300 to 600 mg twice daily) is usually better tolerated than lithium. Its effect on water excretion is delayed for a few days and it dissipates over a similar period of time after the drug is stopped. Nephrotoxicity has been reported with its use in patients with cirrhosis.[79] V_2 (vasopressin)-receptor antagonists, which directly block ADH action, may be useful in the treatment of SIADH and dilutional hyponatremia secondary to cirrhosis. However, the longer-term safety and efficacy of these drugs remain under investigation.[80-82] Limited data suggest that phenytoin may inhibit ADH secretion, but its effectiveness is questionable.[83] Urea can correct hypo-osmolality by increasing solute-free water excretion and reducing urinary sodium excretion.[84] It has been used effectively, at 30 to 60 g/day, both short and long term, to reduce the need for fluid restriction.[85] An IV formulation of urea is available commercially; however, for oral administration, 30 g of urea crystals can be dissolved in 10 mL of aluminum-magnesium antacid (Maalox) and 100 mL of water. Alternatively, orange juice or other strongly flavored liquids can be used to improve palatability.

Hypernatremia

Hypernatremia can occur under the following conditions: (1) normal total body sodium with pure water loss, (2) low total body sodium with hypotonic fluid loss, and (3) high total body sodium as a result of pure salt gain.[86] Therefore, as in hyponatremia, one should assess the volume status of the extracellular fluid when evaluating hypernatremia.

Pure water loss can result from the inability of the kidney to conserve water (diabetes insipidus) or from extrarenal water loss through the respiratory tract or the skin.[87] Usually, pure water loss does not cause hypernatremia unless the thirst center is damaged or access to free water is limited.[86]

Hypotonic fluid loss can occur renally as a result of osmotic diuresis, use of loop diuretics, postobstruction diuresis, or intrinsic renal disease. Extrarenally, hypotonic fluid loss may result from diarrhea, vomiting, burns, and excessive sweating.

Pure salt gain can result from the use of hypertonic saline during abortion, sodium bicarbonate administration during cardiopulmonary resuscitation, hypertonic feedings in infants, and, rarely, mineralocorticoid excess.

The management of hypernatremia includes correcting the underlying etiology of the hypertonic state, replacing the water deficits, and administering adequate water to match ongoing losses.[86] The pure water deficit can be estimated as follows:

$$\text{Water deficit} = \text{Normal TBW} - \text{Present TBW} \qquad \textbf{12-6}$$

$$= 0.6\left(\text{LBW}\right) - \left(\frac{\text{Normal Na concentration}}{\text{Present Na concentration}}\right)0.6\left(\text{LBW}\right) \qquad \textbf{12-I}$$

$$= 0.6\left(\text{LBW}\right)\left[1 - \left(\frac{\text{Normal Na concentration}}{\text{Present Na concentration}}\right)\right]$$

The rate at which hypernatremia should be corrected depends on the severity of symptoms and degree of hypertonicity. Too rapid correction may precipitate cerebral edema, seizures, and irreversible neurologic damage and can be fatal. For asymptomatic patients, the rate of correction probably should not exceed changes of 0.5 mEq/L in plasma sodium per hour. A rule of thumb is to replace half the calculated deficit with hypotonic solutions over 12 to 24 hours. Any ongoing water loss, including insensible loss, also should be replenished while carefully monitoring the patient's neurologic status. The remaining deficit can then be replaced over the ensuing 24 to 48 hours. Concomitant solute deficits and ongoing solute losses should also be replaced as appropriate. If hyperna-

tremia is caused only by pure water loss, free water can be administered as 5% dextrose in water. Half-normal or quarter-normal saline is used if a sodium deficit is also present. In patients with hypotension or shock, the effective arterial blood volume should be restored with normal saline or colloids before the plasma tonicity is corrected.

CLINICAL USE OF DIURETICS

Diuretics reduce sodium chloride reabsorption in the kidney tubules, thereby increasing urine volume. Enhanced solute and fluid excretion can be initiated through osmotic diuresis or inhibition of transport in the kidney tubules. Diuretics are categorized according to the sites within the kidney tubules where they inhibit sodium reabsorption. (See Chapter 14, Essential Hypertension, and Chapter 31, Chronic Renal Failure.)

Loop Diuretics

The loop diuretics furosemide, bumetanide, torsemide, and ethacrynic acid are the most potent diuretics available. They are also known as *high-ceiling diuretics* because they can inhibit the reabsorption of up to 20% to 25% of the filtered sodium load. The loop diuretics act in the medullary and cortical portion of the thick ascending limb of Henle's loop. Sodium and chloride transport through the Na^+-K^+-$2Cl^-$ carrier in the luminal membrane is inhibited. Reabsorption of calcium and magnesium is reduced secondary to the reduction in sodium chloride transport. The loop diuretics also possess a vasodilatory effect that can contribute to their diuretic activity.

Thiazide Diuretics

The thiazide diuretics are a group of structurally similar compounds that share a common mechanism of action. Several other sulfonamide diuretics that differ chemically, such as chlorthalidone, indapamide, and metolazone, also have diuretic effects similar to the thiazides. The primary site of action of these diuretics is at the proximal portion of the distal tubule. Sodium reabsorption via the Na^+-Cl^- cotransporter is blocked through competition with the Cl^- site of the transporter. Some of these agents, such as chlorothiazide, may also reduce sodium transport in the proximal tubule. However, the contribution of this effect toward net diuresis is negligible because the sodium ions that are not reabsorbed in the proximal tubule will subsequently be reabsorbed in Henle's loop. Thiazide diuretics can enhance the reabsorption of calcium ion through a direct action on the early distal tubule. Therefore, these agents are useful to reduce calciuria in patients with kidney stones. In contrast, magnesium excretion is increased by the thiazides, which may result in hypomagnesemia.

Potassium-Sparing Diuretics

Spironolactone, Triamterene, and Amiloride

Spironolactone, triamterene, and amiloride are potassium-sparing diuretics that inhibit sodium reabsorption in the cortical collecting tubules through different mechanisms. Spironolactone (Aldactone) is a competitive receptor-site antagonist of aldosterone in the distal segment of the renal tubule and is indicated especially for patients with hyperaldosteronism secondary to decreased renal perfusion. Patients with hyperaldosteronism can be identified by urinary electrolyte screening, which shows high urine potassium excretion with concomitant diminished or absent urine sodium excretion. By serving as an aldosterone antagonist, spironolactone inhibits sodium reabsorption and decreases the excretion of potassium and hydrogen ions. Dosages as high as 200 to 400 mg/day may be needed to induce natriuresis in patients with hyperaldosteronism.

In contrast to spironolactone, triamterene and amiloride reduce the passage of sodium ions through the luminal membrane, independent of aldosterone activity, by directly acting on sodium and potassium transport processes in the distal renal tubular cells. Triamterene and amiloride offer the advantage of a more rapid onset of action than spironolactone.

The initial effects of spironolactone are usually delayed for 2 or 3 days, and several additional days are needed to attain maximal diuretic effect. This delay is due partly to the formation of an active metabolite, canrenone, which accounts for approximately 70% of the antimineralocorticoid activity of spironolactone. The elimination half-life of canrenone is 13.5 to 24 hours in normal subjects and is prolonged in patients with chronic liver disease (59 hours [range, 32 to 105 hours]) or CHF (37 hours [range, 19 to 48 hours]).[88] Although the elimination half-life of canrenone is prolonged in these patients, plasma canrenone concentrations do not differ significantly from those in normal subjects because assay methods for canrenone are nonspecific and include measurement of both active and inactive metabolites.[89,90]

Triamterene (Dyrenium) is absorbed incompletely from the GI tract. The drug has a short half-life of 1.5 to 2.5 hours. The total body clearance is high because of rapid and extensive metabolism by the liver. Both the parent compound and the metabolite undergo biliary and renal excretion. As with spironolactone, the hepatic metabolism of triamterene can be altered in patients with cirrhosis.[91] The diuretic effect of triamterene begins within 2 to 3 hours of administration, with a maximum duration of 12 to 16 hours.

Amiloride (Midamor) does not undergo hepatic metabolism; approximately 50% of amiloride is excreted in the urine unchanged and the remainder is recovered in the stool as unabsorbed drug or through biliary excretion. Serum amiloride concentrations peak 3 hours after oral ingestion, and the half-life is 6 hours. Although commonly administered doses are in the range of 2.5 to 10 mg, diuresis increases over a much greater range. The onset of action is 2 hours, with maximal effects at 4 to 6 hours. Duration of action is dose dependent and ranges from 10 to 24 hours. Amiloride does not undergo hepatic metabolism, and the drug can accumulate in patients with renal insufficiency.

The maximum amount of filtered sodium that can be excreted through the action of potassium-sparing diuretics is approximately 1% to 2%. Their natriuretic activity is therefore relatively limited compared with the thiazide and loop diuretics. These agents are often used currently with thiazide and loop diuretics to reduce potassium loss. Spironolactone is especially useful in patients with liver cirrhosis and ascites, who are likely to have high levels of aldosterone.

Acetazolamide

Acetazolamide inhibits carbonic anhydrase, an enzyme that mediates the excretion of sodium, bicarbonate, and chloride ions in the proximal tubule. Use of the drug will increase urine pH due to the increased excretion of bicarbonate ion. The net diuretic and natriuretic effects are limited, similar to those of the potassium-sparing diuretics. Because of the drug's proximal site of action, the sodium ions that are not reabsorbed will subsequently be reclaimed in Henle's loop and the distal tubule. In addition, metabolic acidosis associated with the use of acetazolamide diminishes its diuretic effect.

Osmotic Diuretics

Osmotic diuretics are nonreabsorbable solutes in the kidney tubule. They act primarily in the proximal tubule, where the osmotic pressure they generate impedes the reabsorption of water and solutes. Unlike other diuretics, the amount of water loss exceeds the concurrent loss of sodium and potassium. Mannitol has been used in the early treatment of oliguric postischemic acute renal failure to increase urine output. Urea, another osmotic diuretic, and mannitol are used to reduce intracranial pressure through cellular dehydration.

Complications of Diuretic Therapy

Disturbances in fluid, electrolyte, and acid–base balance are common side effects associated with diuretic therapy. These side effects, including hypokalemia, are discussed in detail in Chapter 14, Essential Hypertension; Chapter 19, Heart Failure; and Chapter 42, Gout and Hyperuricemia. However, two complications, hyponatremia and metabolic alkalosis and acidosis, are discussed in the following section because of their specific relevance to fluid balance.

Hyponatremia

Thiazides induce diuresis by inhibiting sodium and water reabsorption in the kidney tubule. Because both sodium and water are lost, overdiuresis per se is not expected to cause hyponatremia. Instead, hyponatremia represents a dilution of plasma sodium by excess free water caused by volume depletion–induced ADH activity. The enhanced ADH secretion increases free water reabsorption, resulting in hyponatremia. Large doses of diuretic, excessive water drinking, and severe sodium intake restriction all will accentuate the hyponatremia. Elderly patients are prone to this diuretic-induced complication.

Metabolic Alkalosis and Acidosis

Metabolic alkalosis often occurs in conjunction with potassium depletion secondary to diuretic use. The diuretic-induced contraction of extracellular fluid volume stimulates the secretion of aldosterone, which promotes the absorption of sodium and the retention of hydrogen ions in the kidney tubule. The net urinary loss of hydrogen ions into the urine results in metabolic alkalosis. Generally, reducing the dose of the diuretic will restore the acid–base balance.

Acetazolamide causes metabolic acidosis by inhibiting carbonic anhydrase, which results in urinary excretion of sodium bicarbonate. Spironolactone, amiloride, and triamterene may cause hyperchloremic metabolic acidosis because of their ability to decrease potassium and hydrogen ion tubular secretion. Patients with renal dysfunction or those taking potassium supplements or angiotensin-converting enzyme inhibitors, which reduce aldosterone secretion, are at increased risk for developing hyperkalemia and metabolic acidosis.

POTASSIUM

Homeostasis

The total amount of potassium stored in the body is approximately 45 to 55 mEq/kg and varies with age, gender, and muscle mass. Lower total body potassium is found in older adults, females, and individuals with a low lean body mass-to-fat ratio. Potassium is distributed unevenly between the intracellular and extracellular compartments: 98% of the total body potassium resides in the intracellular compartment, predominantly the muscle, and only 2% is found in the extracellular space.[35,92,93] The disproportionate intracellular distribution of potassium is maintained by the Na^+-K^+-ATPase pump, which transports sodium out of the cell in exchange for potassium.[92–95] The cell membrane resting potential is determined by the ratio of intracellular to extracellular potassium concentrations. As this ratio increases, hyperpolarization of the cell membrane occurs. Conversely, cellular depolarization results when the ratio decreases. In both situations, generation of the action potential is impaired.

The plasma potassium concentration is maintained within a narrow range: 3.5 to 5.0 mEq/L. Although the plasma potassium concentration can be affected by the total body potassium store, one cannot accurately estimate total body potassium excess or deficit based solely on the plasma concentration. In fact, a normal plasma potassium concentration does not imply normal total body potassium because multiple factors affect the plasma potassium concentration independent of total body potassium.[92]

Potassium homeostasis is maintained by both renal and extrarenal processes. The renal process regulates total body potassium by matching potassium excretion to dietary intake (external balance),[96] whereas the extrarenal process regulates potassium distribution across cell membrane (internal potassium balance).[92,94]

The normal daily intake of potassium ranges between 50 and 100 mEq. Approximately 90% of the ingested potassium is eliminated by the kidneys and approximately 10% is eliminated via the GI tract.[96] Potassium is filtered freely through the glomerulus and then reabsorbed. By the time the filtrate reaches the distal convoluted tubule, >90% of filtered potassium has already been reabsorbed. The amount of potassium excreted is determined by distal tubular potassium secretion in the principal cells of the cortical collecting duct, which is under the influence of aldosterone. Hyperkalemia, increased potassium load, and angiotensin II can all stimulate aldosterone secretion.[92]

Factors that affect renal potassium excretion include tubular flow, sodium delivery to the distal segments of the nephron, the presence of poorly absorbable anions that increase luminal electronegativity, acid–base status, and aldosterone activity.[97] Potassium excretion increases during hyperkalemia and decreases during potassium depletion. Excretion of an acute potassium load is a slow process, with only half the potassium load excreted in the first 4 to 6 hours. Lethal hyperkalemia would ensue were it not for the extrarenal process that regulates intracellular–extracellular potassium distribution.[92]

The Na^+-K^+-ATPase pump, which extrudes sodium from the cell in exchange for potassium, is pivotal in maintaining internal potassium balance.[95] Different hormonal factors regulate the activity of the Na^+-K^+-ATPase pump, namely insulin, catecholamines, and aldosterone. Insulin, the most important regulator, enhances potassium uptake by muscle, liver, and adipose tissue by stimulating Na^+-K^+-ATPase.[98] Indeed, basal insulin secretion is essential for potassium homeostasis.[92] Whereas β_2-adrenergic agonists activate the Na^+-K^+-ATPase pump via cyclic adenosine monophosphate (cAMP) and cause hypokalemia, α-adrenergic stimulation promotes hepatic potassium release and causes hyperkalemia.[99] Epinephrine, an α- and β-agonist, causes a transient increase in plasma potassium (α-agonism) followed by a more sustained decrease in plasma potassium (β-agonism).[99,100] Besides its kaliuretic effect and enhanced potassium secretion in the colon, aldosterone also stimulates Na^+-K^+-ATPase.

Other factors that affect the transcellular distribution of potassium include systemic pH, plasma tonicity, and exercise.[92,95] The effect of *acid–base balance* on potassium distribution is not readily predictable and depends on both the nature and the direction of the underlying disorder. The concomitant effect of the acid–base disorder on renal potassium excretion further complicates the relationship between plasma potassium concentration and pH.[92,101] In acute inorganic acidosis, plasma potassium concentration increase by 0.2 to 1.7 mEq/L per 0.1-U decrease in pH. However, chronic inorganic metabolic acidosis usually is associated with hypokalemia because of urinary potassium loss associated with both proximal (type II) and distal (type I) renal tubular acidosis.[92,101] In contrast, organic acidosis commonly has no effect on potassium distribution.[102] However, other associated factors in the organic acidosis may affect cellular potassium distribution.[101] For example, hyperglycemia in diabetic ketoacidosis may increase the serum potassium concentration because of the hypertonic effect of glucose.[103] Hypertonicity causes cell shrinkage and increases the intracellular to extracellular fluid potassium gradient, favoring potassium egress. Acute metabolic alkalosis only modestly decreases the plasma potassium concentration: 0.3 mEq/L for each 0.1-U pH increment.[92,101] Like chronic metabolic acidosis, chronic metabolic alkalosis causes profound renal potassium wasting and is associated with hypokalemia. Respiratory acid–base disorders usually are associated with less significant changes in plasma potassium concentration than are metabolic acid–base disorders.[101] Exercise often causes an increase in the serum potassium concentration to a degree that varies with the intensity of the exercise.[104]

Hypokalemia

Etiology

14. **J.P., a 60-year-old woman, presents to the ED with complaints of malaise, generalized weakness, nausea, and vomiting for 3 days. Her medical history includes hypertension for 20 years. J.P.'s current medications include hydrochlorothiazide 25 mg/day and nifedipine XL 30 mg/day. However, she has not been able to take her medications in the past few days because of vomiting. J.P. denies recent diarrhea or use of laxatives. Her BP is 130/70 mm Hg with a pulse of 80 beats/min while sitting, and 120/70 mm Hg with a pulse of 95 beats/min on standing. Physical examination reveals a thin, older woman with poor skin turgor, dry mucous membranes, and a flat jugular vein. T-wave flattening is noted on the electrocardiogram (ECG). Laboratory**

tests show serum Na, 138 mEq/L (normal, 134 to 146); K, 2.1 mEq/L (normal, 3.5 to 5.1); Cl, 100 mEq/L (normal, 92 to 109); bicarbonate, 32 mEq/L (normal, 24 to 31); BUN, 30 mg/dL (normal, 18 to 25); creatinine, 1.2 mg/dL (normal, 0.5 to 1.5); and glucose, 100 mg/dL (normal, 60 to 110). ABG shows pH 7.50 (normal, 7.35 to 7.45); PCO_2, 45 mm Hg (normal, 35 to 45); and PO_2, 70 mm Hg (normal, 80 to 100) at room air. Urine electrolytes are Na, 30 mEq/L; K, 60 mEq/L; and Cl, <15 mEq/L. The patient's presentation is consistent with gastroenteritis. What are the etiologies for J.P.'s hypokalemia?

[SI units: serum Na, 138 mmol/L; K, 2.1 mmol/L; Cl, 100 mmol/L; bicarbonate, 32 mmol/L; BUN, 10.7 mmol/L; creatinine, 106.1 μmol/L; glucose, 5.55 mmol/L; PCO_2, 6.0 kPa; PO_2, 9.33 kPa; urine Na, 30 mmol/L; K, 60 mmol/L; Cl, <15 mmol/L]

When evaluating hypokalemia, the clinician should determine whether the hypokalemia is a result of low intake, increased cellular uptake of potassium, or excessive loss of potassium via the kidneys, GI tract, or skin.[35,105] History and physical evidence of potassium depletion; medication history (including use of over-the-counter medicines); and assessment of the patient's BP, extracellular volume, and concurrent acid–base status can provide clues to the etiologies of hypokalemia.[35,105]

Because J.P. has been unable to eat for the past few days, decreased oral intake may have contributed to her hypokalemia. However, because most foods are rich in potassium, inadequate intake rarely is the sole cause of potassium depletion unless there is inappropriate and continued renal or extrarenal losses, or potassium intake is severely restricted to <10 to 15 mEq/day.[105] Alkalosis,[101] insulin administration,[92] hypertonic solution administration, periodic paralysis,[106] β_2-agonists,[107] barium poisoning,[108] and treatment of megaloblastic anemia with vitamin B_{12}[109] all have been associated with increased cellular potassium uptake (Table 12-2). Although

the relationship between the degree of hypokalemia and increase in blood pH varies widely,[101] J.P.'s metabolic alkalosis probably enhances the cellular uptake of potassium. However, the transcellular shift of potassium should not result in total body potassium depletion.

The GI tract is an important site of potassium loss, particularly through vomiting and diarrhea. However, because the potassium content of gastric secretion (5 to 10 mEq/L) is much less than that of the intestinal secretion (up to 90 mEq/L),[105] loss of a large volume of gastric secretion is needed to produce substantial potassium depletion. However, potassium deficit induced by vomiting is commonly secondary to renal potassium loss, especially within the initial 24 to 48 hours.[110] The loss of hydrogen ion in gastric juice results in an elevated plasma bicarbonate concentration. The increased amount of bicarbonate ion, as a nonreabsorbable anion, increases water delivery to the distal nephron and enhances sodium reabsorption and potassium secretion, resulting in hypokalemia. The potassium wasting is often transient, as increased proximal reabsorption of sodium and bicarbonate will result in diminished bicarbonate delivery to the distal site. Reduced potassium excretion will ensue, commonly within 48 to 72 hours. Subsequent potassium loss will then be primarily consequent to gastric secretion removal.

The absence of diarrhea in J.P. excludes the GI tract as the source of potassium loss. Potassium loss through the skin also is unlikely in J.P. because the potassium concentration of sweat is <10 mEq/L. Therefore, profuse sweating, such as that induced by vigorous exercise in a hot, humid environment, or severe burns are needed to cause substantial loss.

J.P.'s inappropriately high urinary potassium concentration indicates that the kidney is the source of the potassium loss.[35,105] The urinary potassium concentration is a good marker for differentiating various hypokalemic syndromes. A

Table 12-2 Drugs That Most Commonly Induce Hypokalemia

Drug	Mechanism	Predisposing Factors
Acetazolamide	Marked ↑ in renal K^+ loss	Most profound with short-term therapy
Amphotericin	Renal K^+ loss (renal tubular acidosis)	Concurrent piperacillin, ticarcillin
β_2-agonists	Intracellular shift of K^+	—
Cisplatin	Renal K^+ loss secondary to renal tubular damage	May be dose related but can occur after a single 50 mg/m² dose
Corticosteroids	Renal K^+ loss. Enhanced Na^+ reabsorption at distal tubule and collecting ducts in exchange for K^+ and H^+	Supraphysiologic doses of agents with moderate to strong mineralocorticoid activity (e.g., prednisone, hydrocortisone)
Insulin with glucose	Intracellular shift of K^+	Predictable effect when insulin administered to patients with diabetic ketoacidosis. Combination used to treat hyperkalemia
Penicillins (piperacillin, ticarcillin)	High Na^+ load and nonreabsorbable anions can ↑ K^+ loss	Was more common with carbenicillin when it was available. Newer penicillins are used in lower doses. Less likely to produce hypokalemia
Thiazide and loop diuretics	Renal K^+ loss. ↑ Na^+ delivery to the late distal tubule, resulting in Na^+ resorption in exchange for K^+	Patients with hyperaldosteronism (e.g., cirrhosis, CHF) predisposed. May be dose related

CHF = Congestive heart failure.

urinary potassium excretion of <20 mEq/day suggests extrarenal potassium loss. However, renal potassium wastage cannot be excluded unless the low urinary potassium excretion is accompanied by a sodium intake of at least 100 mEq/day, because a low-sodium diet can reduce renal potassium excretion.[35] In J.P., the metabolic alkalosis and hypovolemia promote renal potassium wastage.[35,105] The distal delivery of a large sodium bicarbonate load and increased aldosterone activity (from hypovolemia) enhance potassium secretion and severely impair the kidney's ability to conserve potassium. The hydrochlorothiazide, which J.P. had been taking until 3 days before admission, could also have induced hypokalemia through volume depletion, hypochloremic metabolic alkalosis, and renal potassium wastage. However, the diuretic is unlikely to be the cause for J.P.'s hypokalemia because she has stopped taking the medication, and this is reflected by the low urinary chloride concentration.[16] Bartter's syndrome, which presents as normotension, hypokalemia, hypochloremic metabolic alkalosis, and renal potassium wastage, is characterized by impaired renal sodium and chloride reabsorption. The low urinary chloride concentration in J.P. can rule out Bartter's syndrome. Other causes of hypokalemia are listed in Table 12-2.

In an asymptomatic hypokalemic patient with no apparent causes for potassium depletion or transcellular redistribution, pseudohypokalemia should be excluded before pursuing an intensive evaluation.[105] Spurious hypokalemia can occur in leukemic patients whose leukocyte count ranges from 100,000 to 250,000 cells/μL.[111] The potassium in serum is taken up by the large number of leukemic cells when the blood specimen is allowed to stand at room temperature.

Clinical Manifestations

15. What clinical manifestations of hypokalemia are evident in J.P.?

The clinical presentation of hypokalemia depends on the severity of potassium depletion and is a result of changes in cell membrane polarization.[105] Patients are usually asymptomatic when the plasma potassium level is 3.0 to 3.5 mEq/L, but they may complain of malaise, weakness, fatigue, and myalgia. J.P.'s muscle weakness and ECG changes reflect the muscular and cardiac manifestations of hypokalemia, respectively.[112,113]

Potassium depletion can lead to hyperpolarization of myocardial cells and a prolonged refractory period. When serum potassium concentrations fall below 3 mEq/L, T-wave flattening, straight tubule segment depression, and prominent U waves are seen on the ECG.[113] Mild hypokalemia (potassium concentration of 3.0 to 3.5 mEq/L) is potentially arrhythmogenic in patients with underlying coronary artery disease. The incidence of ventricular arrhythmia increases with the degree of hypokalemia. Patients without underlying heart disease may be prone to these myocardial effects during exercise, especially if the patient's pre-exercise potassium concentration is <3.5 mEq/L, because the potassium concentration may drop below 3.0 mEq/L as a result of β_2-adrenergic receptor-mediated cellular potassium uptake.[105] Potassium depletion may also increase the BP,[105] which can be lowered with potassium supplementation.[114]

When the serum potassium concentration is <2.5 to 3.0 mEq/L, muscle weakness, cramps, general malaise, fatigue, restless leg syndrome, and paresthesia can occur, probably because potassium is necessary for vasodilation in skeletal muscle. In addition, severe potassium depletion (<2.5 mEq/L) may result in elevation of serum creatine phosphokinase, aldolase, and aspartate aminotransferase levels. Rhabdomyolysis can ensue when the serum potassium concentration falls below 2.0 mEq/L.[105,112]

Chronic potassium depletion can alter renal function and structure, which can manifest as decreased GFR and renal blood flow, disturbance in tubular sodium handling, impaired urinary concentrating ability with polydipsia, and ADH-resistant nephrogenic diabetes insipidus.[105,115] Reversible pathologic changes include renal hypertrophy and epithelial vacuolization of the proximal convoluted tubule. However, interstitial scarring and tubular atrophy have been reported with prolonged potassium depletion.[105]

Other effects of hypokalemia and potassium depletion include decreased insulin secretion resulting in carbohydrate intolerance,[115] metabolic alkalosis, and increased renal ammoniagenesis, which may play a role in the development of hepatic encephalopathy.[116]

Treatment

16. How should J.P.'s hypokalemia be managed?

J.P.'s protracted vomiting should be corrected, and fluids and electrolytes (sodium, potassium, and chloride) should be replaced to correct the volume deficit, hypokalemia, and hypochloremic metabolic alkalosis. Hydrochlorothiazide should continue to be withheld.

The amount of potassium deficit and the rate of continued potassium loss should be determined to guide replacement therapy. It has been estimated that a 1-mEq/L fall in serum potassium from 4 to 3 mEq/L represents a total body deficit of approximately 200 mEq. When the serum potassium falls below 3 mEq/L, the total body deficit increases by 200 to 400 mEq for each 1-mEq/L reduction in serum concentration. Other data suggest that even greater degrees of potassium loss may occur: a deficit of 100 mEq per 0.27-mEq/L fall in the serum potassium concentration.[92] However, transcellular redistribution of potassium may significantly alter the relationship between serum concentration and total body deficit.[105] Therefore, potassium repletion should be guided by close monitoring of serum concentrations and analysis of J.P.'s urine for potassium content to help assess the need for additional replacement.

The route of potassium administration depends on the acuity and severity of hypokalemia,[117] but oral supplementation is usually preferred. The parenteral route is indicated for patients who cannot tolerate high dosages of oral potassium supplements and for those with severe or symptomatic hypokalemia. J.P.'s potassium deficit is estimated to be 300 to 500 mEq, but because she is only moderately symptomatic, aggressive therapy is not indicated. Potassium chloride can be added to her IV fluid in a concentration of 40 mEq/L and infused at a rate that does not exceed 10 mEq/hour. For patients with life-threatening hypokalemia-induced arrhythmias or those with a serum potassium level <2.0 mEq/L, a more concentrated potassium solution (60 mEq/L) can be infused at a rate not exceeding 40 mEq/hour. A solution that is too concentrated or a rate of infusion that is too rapid would likely cause phlebitis in the peripheral veins and could cause arrhythmias, especially when administered through a central line. The potassium concentration should be monitored every 4 hours, more frequently in patients with severe potassium depletion or when a rapid infusion is given.[118] ECG monitoring is mandatory to identify life-threatening hyperkalemia.

Parenteral potassium can be given as chloride, acetate, or phosphate. The chloride salt is preferred in J.P., who has concurrent hypochloremic metabolic alkalosis. The acetate preparation is useful in cases of concomitant metabolic acidosis. Potassium phosphate is in order if hypophosphatemia coexists. In the latter condition, the serum calcium concentration should also be monitored because hypocalcemia may ensue. Glucose solution should be avoided as the vehicle because glucose-induced insulin secretion will promote intracellular potassium uptake.[119]

Once J.P.'s potassium levels are replenished and she can take medicine by mouth, oral potassium chloride can be started (see Chapters 14, Essential Hypertension, and 19, Heart Failure).

Hyperkalemia

Etiology

17. A.B., a 25-year-old woman with type 1 diabetes and hypertension, returns to the clinic for follow-up. Her BP is 170/90 mm Hg with a pulse of 80 beats/min, and her physical examination is remarkable for 2+ pedal edema. Laboratory tests show plasma Na, 135 mEq/L (normal, 134 to 146); K, 5.8 mEq/L (normal, 3.5 to 5.1); Cl, 108 mEq/L (normal, 92 to 109); total CO_2, 20 mEq/L (normal, 22 to 32); BUN, 28 mg/dL (normal, 8 to 25); creatinine, 2 mg/dL (normal, 0.5 to 1.5); and glucose, 200 mg/dL (normal, 60 to 110). Current medications include captopril 25 mg PO TID, Dyazide 1 capsule daily, human NPH insulin 30 U SC Q am, and ibuprofen 200 mg PRN for menstrual cramps. She uses a salt substitute occasionally. What is the etiology of her hyperkalemia?

[SI units: Na, 135 mmol/L; K, 5.8 mmol/L; Cl, 108 mmol/L; total CO_2, 20 mmol/L; BUN, 10 mmol/L; creatinine, 176.8 μmol/L; glucose, 11.1 mmol/L]

Before conducting any extensive evaluation to identify the etiology of hyperkalemia, the serum potassium concentration ought to be repeated to confirm the presence of hyperkalemia. Also to be ruled out are the different causes of spurious hyperkalemia, which may result from severe leukocytosis (>500,000/mm³),[120] thrombocytosis (>750,000/ mm³),[121] or hemolysis within the blood collection tube.[122] *Pseudohyperkalemia* is a test-tube phenomenon that occurs when potassium is released from leukocytes, platelets, or erythrocytes during blood coagulation. These disorders can be confirmed easily by comparing serum (clotted) and plasma (unclotted) potassium concentrations from the same blood sample. The two values should agree within 0.2 to 0.3 mEq/L. Improper tourniquet technique, causing strangulation of the patient's arm before blood sampling, may also result in spurious hyperkalemia.[123]

Identifying the etiology of hyperkalemia can be approached systematically by considering possible disturbances in internal and external potassium balance. The former involves transcellular flux of potassium from the intracellular to the extracellular space, whereas the latter involves either increased intake, including increased endogenous potassium load (e.g., rhabdomyolysis,[129] tumor lysis syndrome[125]), or decreased elimination. A thorough medication history is important to identify drugs associated with hyperkalemia.[126–128] (Also see Chapter 32, Chronic Kidney Disease, for additional information on hyperkalemia.)

A dietary history should ascertain whether A.B.'s consumption of potassium-rich foods, salt substitutes, or potassium supplements has increased. Dietary intake alone will *not* induce hyperkalemia unless renal excretion is impaired. Usually, the GFR must be <10 to 15 mL/minute, unless there is concurrent hypoaldosteronism or distal tubular potassium secretory defects.[129] A.B.'s renal insufficiency is mild, with an estimated Cl_{Cr} of 40 mL/minute.

Conditions associated with low renin and aldosterone, which usually present as hyperkalemia and hyperchloremic metabolic acidosis, decrease potassium excretion by the kidneys. These include diabetes (present in A.B.),[130] obstructive uropathy, sickle cell disease, lupus nephritis, and various tubulointerstitial diseases (e.g., gouty nephropathy, analgesic nephropathy). Adrenal insufficiency presents commonly with hyperkalemia because of mineralocorticoid deficiency.[132] A.B.'s poorly controlled hyperglycemia may cause movement of potassium-rich fluid from the intracellular space to the extracellular space because of the increased tonicity. Elevating the plasma tonicity by 15 to 20 mOsm/kg will increase the plasma potassium concentration by 0.8 mEq/L.[131] Patients with diabetes, mineralocorticoid deficiency, or end-stage renal failure, which commonly results in hyporeninemic hypoaldosteronism, are particularly susceptible.

A.B. is also taking several medications that may impair her ability to excrete potassium. Captopril indirectly decreases aldosterone secretion by decreasing the formation of angiotensin II.[133] Ibuprofen inhibits prostaglandin production as well as renin and aldosterone secretion.[134] Other drugs that cause hyperkalemia by impairing renin and aldosterone production include angiotensin II receptor antagonists,[135] β-adrenergic blockers,[136] lithium,[137] heparin,[138–140] and pentamidine.[141] Triamterene, the diuretic in Dyazide, inhibits tubular potassium secretion, as do amiloride, spironolactone, high-dose trimethoprim,[141,142] cyclosporine,[143] tacrolimus,[144] and digitalis preparations.[145] By inhibiting Na^+-K^+-ATPase, digitalis decreases tubular potassium secretion and reduces cellular potassium uptake. Arginine,[146] succinylcholine,[147] β-adrenergic blockers, α-adrenergic agonists, and hypertonic solutions also cause hyperkalemia by impairing transcellular potassium distribution into the intracellular space.

Clinical Manifestations

18. V.C., a 44-year-old woman with chronic renal failure, returns to the outpatient unit for routine hemodialysis with complaints of severe muscle weakness. Her vital signs are BP, 120/80 mm Hg; pulse, 90 beats/min; RR, 20 breaths/min; and temperature, 98°F. Laboratory data are serum K, 8.9 mEq/L (normal, 3.5 to 5.1); total CO_2, 15 mmol/L (normal, 22 to 32); BUN, 60 mg/dL (normal, 8 to 25); creatinine, 9 mg/dL (normal, 0.5 to 1.5); and glucose, 100 mg/dL (normal, 60 to 110). The ECG reveals an increased P-R interval and a widened QRS complex. What clinical manifestations of hyperkalemia are evident in V.C.?

[SI units: K, 8.9 mmol/L; total CO_2 15 mmol/L; BUN, 21.42 mmol/L; creatinine, 795.6 μmol/L; glucose, 5.55 mmol/L]

Hyperkalemia decreases the intracellular-to-extracellular potassium ratio. Hence, the resting membrane potential becomes less negative and moves closer to the threshold excitation potential. Muscle weakness and flaccid paralysis result when the resting membrane potential approaches the threshold potential, rendering the excitable cells unable to sustain an action potential.

The cardiac toxicity of hyperkalemia is a major cause of morbidity and mortality, with ECG findings paralleling the degree of hyperkalemia. When plasma potassium exceeds 5.5 to 6.0 mEq/L, narrow, peaked T waves and a shortened Q-T interval are seen. As the plasma potassium concentration increases further, the QRS complex widens and the P-wave amplitude decreases. As the level reaches 8 mEq/L, the P wave disappears and the QRS complex continues to widen and merge with the T wave to form a sine wave pattern. If these ECG changes are not recognized and no treatment is initiated, ventricular fibrillation and asystole will ensue. Hyponatremia, hypocalcemia, and hypomagnesemia all reduce the threshold potential, thereby increasing the patient's susceptibility to the cardiac effects of hypokalemia.[129] V.C.'s muscle weakness, ECG, chronic renal failure, and serum potassium concentration all are consistent with severe hyperkalemia.

Treatment

19. **How should V.C.'s hyperkalemia be treated?**

Hyperkalemia with ECG changes requires urgent treatment. Three therapeutic modalities are available: (1) agents that antagonize the cardiac effects of hyperkalemia, (2) agents that shift potassium from the extracellular into the intracellular space, and (3) agents that enhance potassium elimination. Considering V.C.'s severe ECG changes, calcium should be administered at a dose of 10 to 20 mL of 10% calcium gluconate IV over 1 to 3 minutes. Calcium counteracts the depolarizing effect of hyperkalemia by increasing the threshold potential, thus making it less negative and moving it away from the resting potential. The onset of action occurs in a few minutes, but the effect is short-lived, lasting approximately 15 to 60 minutes. The dose can be repeated in 5 minutes if ECG changes do not resolve and as needed afterward for recurrence. However, if there is no response after the second dose, additional attempts are not beneficial. When the hyperkalemia presents with a digitalis overdose, calcium should be used cautiously since it can worsen the cardiotoxic effects of digoxin.[129,148]

Since the serum potassium concentration is not affected by calcium administration, maneuvers should be employed to shift potassium from plasma into the cells. Three modalities are available: insulin and glucose, β$_2$-agonists, and sodium bicarbonate.

Insulin rapidly shifts potassium into the cell in a dose-dependent fashion. The maximum effect occurs at insulin concentrations exceeding 20 to 40 times the basal levels. Therefore, endogenous insulin secreted in response to dextrose administration is insufficient, and exogenous insulin must be administered.[92] Even though high concentrations of dextrose may worsen hyperkalemia, particularly in diabetic patients because intracellular potassium may be shifted to the

extracellular space due to the elevated plasma tonicity,[149] it is always administered with insulin to prevent hypoglycemia. Regular insulin (5 to 10 U) can be given with 50 mL of 50% dextrose as IV boluses, followed by a continuous infusion of 10% dextrose at 50 mL/hour to prevent late hypoglycemia.[93] In dialysis patients prone to developing fasting hyperkalemia, 20 U of insulin can be added to 1 L of 10% dextrose and administered at a rate of 50 mL/hour to prevent the hyperkalemia.[150] The insulin–dextrose combination lowers serum potassium by direct stimulation of cellular potassium uptake and potentiates the potassium-lowering effect of β-adrenergic stimulation.[150] The reduction in potassium is apparent 15 to 30 minutes after the start of the therapy and persists for 4 to 6 hours.[129] In a diabetic patient who is both hyperkalemic and hyperglycemic, insulin alone may be insufficient. If the patient has end-stage renal disease, the insulin–glucose combination is more predictable in lowering plasma potassium concentrations than epinephrine or sodium bicarbonate.[93,148,150]

β$_2$-Agonists, by binding with the β$_2$-adrenoreceptor to activate adenylyl cyclase, have an additive effect with the insulin–dextrose combination in decreasing serum potassium. When albuterol nebulization is used alone, the hypokalemic effect may be inconsistent.[151] Although side effects of albuterol nebulization are minimal, these agents can cause tachycardia and should be used cautiously in patients with underlying coronary artery disease.[152] Although not commercially available, has a faster onset of action (30 versus 90 minutes).[153] In contrast, nebulization is easier to set up and is less likely to be associated with tachycardia, but multiple doses are often necessary to attain an adequate response. In conjunction with the insulin–dextrose combination, albuterol (20 mg dissolved in 4 mL of saline) can be administered by nebulization and inhaled over 10 minutes to further decrease serum potassium if necessary.[154]

Although sodium bicarbonate has long been recommended for the acute treatment of hyperkalemia, its efficacy in this setting has been questioned.[93,148] The usual dose, 44 to 50 mEq, is infused slowly over 5 minutes and repeated in 30 minutes when necessary. Alternatively, it can be added to dextrose and saline solution to form an isotonic sodium bicarbonate infusion.[155] The hypokalemic effect is variable and may be delayed up to 4 hours, and it is reportedly ineffective in patients on maintenance hemodialysis. Although bicarbonate therapy is not a reliable option in the acute management of hyperkalemia, it may be beneficial in patients with severe metabolic acidosis (pH <7.20).[93] Potential complications of sodium bicarbonate therapy are volume overload and metabolic alkalosis.

The definitive treatment of hyperkalemia is removal of potassium from the body. Sodium polystyrene sulfonate (SPS) with sorbitol is an ion-exchange resin that binds potassium in the bowel and enhances its excretion in the stools.[156] Each gram of SPS exchanges 0.5 to 1.0 mmol of potassium for an equal amount of sodium. SPS can be administered orally or rectally; the latter route is preferred in the symptomatic hyperkalemic patient because intestinal potassium exchange occurs mainly in the ileum and colon. A dose of 50 g of SPS in sorbitol can be given as an enema, retained for at least 30 to 60 minutes, at 4- to 6-hour intervals. Alternatively, 15 to 60 g of SPS with sorbitol suspension can be given orally, which can be repeated as needed. The onset of action is ap-

Table 12-3 Treatment of Hyperkalemia

Drug	Mechanism	Dose	Comment
Ca gluconate	Reverse cardiotoxicity caused by K^+	10–20 mL 10% Ca gluconate IV over 1–3 min. May repeat once.	*Onset:* 1–3 min *Duration:* 30–60 min. $[K^+]$ remains unchanged
Insulin and glucose	Redistribution of K^+ intracellularly	5–10 U regular insulin with 50 ml 50% dextrose, then $D_{10}W$ infused at 50 mL/hr[a]	*Onset:* 15–30 min *Duration:* several hr Watch for hypoglycemia and hypokalemia. Does not ↓total body K^+
β_2-agonists (e.g., albuterol)	Redistribution of K^+ intracellularly	2 or 4 mg PO TID-QID. Inhalation: 20 mg in 4 mL saline via nebulizer	*Onset:* 30–60 min *Duration:* 2 hr
Sodium polystyrene sulfonate (SPS)	Cationic binding resin. 1 gm of resin binds 0.5–1 mEq K^+ in exchange for Na^+	*Oral:* 15–20 g with 20–100 mL 70% sorbitol Q 4–6 hr. PRN preferred *Retention enema:* 50 g in 50 mL (70% sorbitol and 150 mL H_2O). Retain 30 min and follow with nonsaline irrigation	*Onset:* Slow; 50 g will lower $[K^+]$ by 0.5–1 mEq/L over 4–6 hr. Watch for Na^+ overload (100 mg Na^+/1 g SPS).
$NaHCO_3$	Redistribution of K^+ intracellularly	50 mEq IV over 5 min. Repeat PRN.	*Onset:* variable, ≈30 min. May work best in acidosis. Watch for Na^+ overload and hyperosmolar state. No change in total body K^+
Dialysis	Removal of K^+	—	Use as last resort

[a]Glucose unnecessary in patients with high glucose concentrations.

proximately 1 to 2 hours after administration. The major side effects are GI intolerance, including diarrhea and sodium overload, and, rarely, intestinal necrosis.[157]

Hemodialysis is the most efficient way to remove potassium; potassium clearance by peritoneal dialysis is lower than for hemodialysis.[158] The hypokalemic effect is immediate and lasts for the duration of dialysis[148]; however, the amount of potassium removed is variable.[159] Dialysis with a glucose-free dialysate will remove 30% more potassium than one containing 200 mg/dL of glucose.[160]

Table 12-3 summarizes the treatment alternatives for hyperkalemia.

Although V.C. is receiving chronic maintenance hemodialysis, the severe cardiac effects of hyperkalemia she experienced warrant immediate institution of the aforementioned measures while awaiting preparation for dialysis. Loop diuretics, which enhance kaliuresis, are rarely useful in managing severe hyperkalemia, especially in patients with renal dysfunction.

After V.C.'s condition stabilized, she admitted to eating a lot of fruits in the past few days. Because noncompliance with dietary potassium restriction is the most common cause for acute and chronic hyperkalemia in a dialysis patient, V.C. should be counseled to consume potassium-rich foods in moderation. Medications that impair V.C.'s extrarenal potassium handling should be avoided. If V.C. remains chronically hyperkalemic, SPS will then be needed, probably three or four times weekly. However, if hyperkalemia is associated with

metabolic acidosis, an alkalinizing agent should be added to maintain a serum bicarbonate concentration of about 24 mEq/L.

CALCIUM

Homeostasis

In normal adults, there is approximately 1,400 g of calcium in the body, of which >99% is stored in bone. Nonetheless, the 0.1% of the total body calcium that is in the plasma and extravascular fluid plays a critical role in many physiologic and metabolic processes. Calcium is important in maintaining nerve tissue excitability and muscle contractility. It regulates the secretory activities of exocrine and endocrine glands and serves as a cofactor for enzyme systems and the coagulation cascade. It also is an essential component of bone metabolism.

Plasma calcium concentration is normally maintained within a relatively narrow range: 8.5 to 10.5 mg/dL. This is accomplished through a complex interaction between parathyroid hormone (PTH), vitamin D, and calcitonin, as well as the effect of these hormones on calcium metabolism in bone, the GI tract, and the kidneys.

Normally, about 40% of the plasma calcium is protein bound, primarily to albumin, and is nondiffusible.[109] Of the 60% that is diffusible, about 13% is complexed to various small ligands: phosphate, citrate, and sulfate. The remaining

47% is ionized, free, and physiologically active. Changes in serum protein concentration will alter the concentrations of both protein-bound and total calcium. Therefore, the serum albumin concentration needs to be monitored to adequately interpret the total serum calcium concentration. Each 1-g/dL increase in serum albumin concentration is expected to increase the protein-bound calcium by 0.8 mg/dL, thus increasing the total serum calcium concentration by the same amount. The total serum calcium therefore can be corrected by the following equation:

$$\text{Correct Ca} = \text{Observed Ca} + \qquad \textbf{12-7}$$
$$0.8 \, (\text{Normal albumin} - \text{Observed albumin})$$

Calcium is also bound to plasma globulins: 0.16 mg of calcium for each gram of globulin. When the total globulin concentration exceeds 6 g/dL (normal, 2.3 to 3.5 g/dL), moderate hypercalcemia may be seen. Changes in pH have an effect on calcium protein binding: acidosis decreases calcium binding, resulting in an increase in free calcium fraction, whereas an increase in pH reduces the amount of ionized calcium. Changes in serum phosphate and sulfate concentrations are expected to alter the fraction of ionized calcium due to the formation of calcium complexes with these anions. The presence of abnormal plasma proteins with a high affinity for calcium binding, as in patients with multiple myeloma, also affects the preceding equation for serum calcium concentration correction.[161]

Serum calcium concentration is regulated by the combined effect of GI absorption and secretion, renal reabsorption, and turnover of the skeletal calcium pool. Several hormones, such as PTH, 1,25-dihydroxyvitamin D_3, and calcitonin, have significant effects on these processes. Balanced diets generally contain 600 to 1,000 mg of calcium, although the minimum daily requirement is 400 to 500 mg. Calcium is primarily absorbed in the duodenum and jejunum via saturable and nonsaturable processes.[162] The nonsaturable process is diffusive in nature and varies with luminal calcium concentration. The saturable carrier-mediated component is stimulated by 1,25-dihydroxyvitamin D_3. Absorption of calcium is enhanced when the calcium intake is low and also when the demand is increased, such as in pregnancy and when total body calcium is depleted. Conversely, protein deficiency can reduce intestinal calcium absorption, presumably because of the reduced amount of specific calcium-binding protein.[163] Calcium also is secreted into the bowel lumen, which may account for the presence of a negative calcium balance when there is no oral calcium intake.[164]

The portion of plasma calcium that is not bound to protein is filtered by the glomerulus. Approximately 97% to 99.5% of the filtered calcium is reabsorbed: 60% in the proximal tubule, 20% in the ascending limb, 10% in the distal tubule, and 3% to 10% in the collecting duct. Approximately 20% of the calcium in the kidney tubule is ionized, whereas the remainder is bound to cations such as citrate, sulfate, phosphate, and gluconate. The extent of calcium resorption depends on the presence of specific cations and also on the urine pH, which affects the fraction of calcium bound to cations. Passive reabsorption at the proximal convoluted tubule is linked closely to sodium transport and is increased by extracellular fluid contraction and decreased by volume expansion. At the proximal straight tubule, the transport process is active and dissociable from sodium and water transport. PTH increases the calcium reabsorption at the distal tubule and also at the collecting duct independent of sodium reabsorption. Acidosis can also increase renal calcium excretion by inhibiting tubule reabsorption and by increasing the ultrafiltrable calcium through reduced binding of calcium to plasma proteins. Conversely, alkalosis promotes calcium protein binding, thus reducing the amount of ultrafiltrable calcium. It also induces hypocalciuria independent of PTH. Phosphorus administration reduces renal calcium excretion, whereas phosphorus depletion increases urinary calcium elimination. Normally, approximately 50 to 300 mg of calcium is excreted by the kidneys daily, but this can be increased to 600 mg/day.[165]

The other important factor regulating plasma calcium concentration is bone metabolism. The rate of bone turnover and calcium resorption is influenced by PTH, 1,25-dihydroxyvitamin D_3, and calcitonin.

Hypercalcemia

Etiology

20. A.C., a 62-year-old woman, is brought to the hospital by family members because she has become more lethargic and unresponsive over the past several days. Approximately 4 years ago, she underwent a radical mastectomy and node dissection followed by radiation and chemotherapy for breast carcinoma. Despite several courses of chemotherapy, she developed metastasis to the bone. About 1 week before this admission, A.C. complained of fatigue, muscle weakness, and anorexia. Since then, she has spent most of her time in bed and has had very limited oral intake. Medications taken before admission included hydrochlorothiazide, oral morphine sulfate, and tamoxifen. Physical examination reveals a dehydrated, cachectic woman responsive only to painful stimuli. Vital signs include BP, 100/60 mm Hg, and RR, 16 breaths/min. Pertinent laboratory values are Na, 138 mEq/L (normal, 134 to 146); K, 4.5 mEq/L (normal, 3.5 to 5.1); Cl, 99 mEq/L (normal, 92 to 109); CO_2, 33 mEq/L (normal, 22 to 32); BUN, 40 mg/dL (normal, 8 to 25); creatinine, 1.2 mg/dL (normal, 0.5 to 1.5); Ca, 19 mg/dL (normal, 8.0 to 10.4); P, 4.5 mg/dL (normal, 2.6 to 4.6); and albumin, 3.0 g/dL (normal, 3.5 to 5.4). The ECG revealed a shortened Q-T interval. What are the common causes of hypercalcemia? Which of these might be responsible for the hypercalcemia seen in A.C.?

[SI units: Na, 138 mmol/L; K, 4.5 mmol/L; Cl, 99 mmol/L; CO_2, 33 mmol/L; BUN, 14.3 mmol/L; creatinine, 106.1 μmol/L; Ca, 4.75 mmol/L; P, 1.45 mmol/L; albumin, 30 g/L]

MALIGNANCY

Malignancy and primary hyperparathyroidism are the most common causes for hypercalcemia. Hematologic malignancies, such as multiple myeloma, tend to be responsible for more hypercalcemia than solid tumors. Cancer of the breast, lung, head, and neck, as well as renal cell carcinoma, are solid tumors commonly associated with hypercalcemia. Malignancy may cause paraneoplastic hypercalcemia secondary to bone metastasis, which results in increased bone resorption. Alternatively, patients may develop hypercalcemia in the absence of bone metastasis due to the production of osteolytic humoral factors by the tumor. The mediators secreted may be PTH, PTH-like substances, prostaglandins, cytokines, transforming growth factor-α, and tumor necrosis factor.[166]

HYPERPARATHYROIDISM

Hyperparathyroidism is the other common cause of hypercalcemia. Although the etiology of primary hyperparathyroidism is unclear, women tend to develop the condition more frequently, especially in the fourth to sixth decades of life. Approximately 75% of patients have a single adenoma, whereas much smaller percentages of patients have multiglandular disease, hyperplasia, or carcinoma.[165] Other conditions that may result in hypercalcemia include postkidney transplantation, immobilization, vitamin A intoxication, hyperthyroidism, Addison's disease, and pheochromocytoma. Hypercalcemia may also occur secondary to increased intestinal calcium absorption because of vitamin D intoxication, sarcoidosis, and other granulomatous diseases. Use of thiazide diuretics, lithium, estrogens, and tamoxifen, as well as excessive calcium ingestion together with alkali (milk-alkali syndrome), may result in hypercalcemia.

A.C.'s breast cancer bone metastasis, volume contraction, and use of hydrochlorothiazide and tamoxifen may all contribute to her hypercalcemia.

Clinical Manifestations

21. How is hypercalcemia manifested in A.C.?

The clinical presentations of hypercalcemia vary substantially among patients, but the severity of the symptoms correlates well with free calcium concentrations.[167] The specific presentation depends on the rate of serum calcium concentration elevation, the presence of malignancy, the PTH concentration, and the patient's age. Concurrent electrolyte and metabolic abnormalities and underlying diseases also will have an effect. Because calcium is an important regulator of many cellular functions, hypercalcemia can produce abnormalities in the neurologic, cardiovascular, pulmonary, renal, GI, and musculoskeletal systems. As seen in A.C., the signs and symptoms can be nonspecific: fatigue, muscle weakness, anorexia, thirst, polyuria, dehydration, and a shortened Q-T interval on the ECG.

The effect of hypercalcemia on the central nervous system includes lethargy, somnolence, confusion, headache, seizures, cerebellar ataxia, altered personality, acute psychosis, depression, and memory impairment. The neuromuscular manifestations include weakness, myalgia, hyporeflexia or areflexia, and arthralgia.

Symptoms of impaired renal function include polyuria, nocturia, and polydipsia. These may reflect a defective concentrating ability, possibly due to resistance to the effects of ADH.[168] The GFR may be decreased because of afferent arteriolar vasoconstriction, and if hypercalcemia is prolonged, nephrolithiasis, nephrocalcinosis, chronic interstitial nephritis, and renal tubular acidosis may be present. Hypermagnesuria and metabolic alkalosis may also be observed.[165]

Calcium has a positive inotropic effect and reduces heart rate, similar to cardiac glycosides. ECG changes indicative of slow conduction, with prolonged P-R and QRS intervals and shortened Q-T intervals, are commonly seen. In severe hypercalcemia, increased Q-T intervals, widened T waves, and arrhythmia may be present.[165,169]

The GI symptoms of hypercalcemia are related primarily to the depressive action of calcium on smooth muscle and nerve conduction. Constipation, anorexia, nausea, and vomiting result from reduced GI motility and delayed gastric emptying. Duodenal ulcer may occur because of increased acid and gastrin secretion. Pancreatitis may occur during acute hypercalcemia due to the blockade of the pancreatic ducts caused by intraductal calcium deposits.[165] Proteolytic enzymes may also be activated by calcium to cause tissue damage. Both ulcer disease and pancreatitis are more common in hypercalcemia associated with primary hyperparathyroidism; they are less likely to be seen in patients with malignancy-induced hypercalcemia.[169]

Treatment

22. After vigorous fluid resuscitation with IV saline, combined saline and furosemide diuresis was instituted in A.C. Her serum calcium concentration declined very slowly, prompting the use of calcitonin. Despite initial success, the serum calcium concentration rose to pretreatment values within 24 hours. Higher dosages of calcitonin could have been attempted at this point; however, plicamycin was used instead. Her serum calcium concentration finally stabilized at 8 mg/dL (normal, 8.0 to 10.4) after several days of therapy. What was the rationale for each of these regimens? What other agents are available for hypercalcemia treatment?

Several therapeutic approaches are used to lower serum calcium concentration: increasing urinary calcium excretion, inhibiting release of calcium from bone, reducing intestinal calcium absorption, and enhancing calcium complex formation with chelating agents. The underlying disease that causes the hypercalcemia should also be treated if possible. The specific treatment used depends on the serum ionized calcium concentration, the presenting signs and symptoms, and the severity and duration of hypercalcemia. Immediate therapy was needed for A.C., who had symptoms consistent with severe hypercalcemia.

Specific interventions are described in the following paragraphs, but as an overview, hydration and diuresis with furosemide generally are the first steps in the acute treatment of hypercalcemia. If these measures fail to reduce the serum calcium concentration adequately, several other agents can be added. Calcitonin provides a rapid onset of hypocalcemic effect, but its duration of action is relatively short. Thus, one of the bisphosphonates could be used to elicit a longer hypocalcemic response. Gallium nitrate is an alternative to plicamycin without such toxic effects. Other agents, such as inorganic phosphates, glucocorticoids, and prostaglandin inhibitors, also have been used to treat hypercalcemia with varying success (Table 12-4).

HYDRATION AND DIURESIS

As noted previously, the first-line emergency treatment for hypercalcemia is hydration and volume expansion. Most patients with hypercalcemia are volume depleted due to the accompanying polyuria, nausea, and vomiting. One to two liters of normal saline is commonly given to correct the fluid deficit and to expand extracellular volume, which will increase urinary calcium excretion by increasing the GFR and inhibiting calcium reabsorption in the proximal tubule. Because both sodium and calcium are reabsorbed at the same site in the proximal tubule, saline hydration will reduce the reabsorption of both cations simultaneously. A.C. was hypotensive and ap-

Table 12-4   Treatment of Hypercalcemia

Intervention	Dose	Comment
Saline and furosemide	1–2 L NS. Then furosemide 80–100 mg Q 2–4 hr. Establish and maintain normovolemia. Other electrolytes as needed.	Saline diuresis and volume expansion depresses Ca^{++} reabsorption in tubules. Lowers $[Ca^{++}]$ within 24 hr. Treatment of choice in patients without CHF or renal failure.
Calcitonin	4 IU/kg SC or IM Q 12 hr. ↑ dose or use another therapy if unresponsive after 24 hr. (*Max*: 8 IU/kg Q 6 hr). Human calcitonin = 0.5 mg if allergic or resistant to salmon.	Inhibits osteoclast resorption and renal reabsorption of calcium. Calcimar (salmon-derived) is preferred over human-derived calcitonin because it is more potent and longer acting. Preferred 2nd-line agent because it has a rapid onset (6 hr) and is nontoxic. It can be used safely in CHF and renal failure. Nausea is the major adverse effect. Tolerance occurs in 24–72 hr. Concomitant plicamycin can lead to hypocalcemia.
Plicamycin	25 μg/kg/day IV over 4–6 hr. Repeat PRN in 48 hr. *Renal failure*: 12.5 μg/kg.	Inhibits osteoclast bone resorption. Onset 24–48 hr; duration 3–14 days. Common side effects: N/V, minimized by slow IV. Since the dose is 10% of an antineoplastic dose, cytotoxic effects less severe. Obtain baseline renal and hepatic function, platelet counts.
Biphosphonates (etidronate, pamidronate)	Etidronate: 7.5 mg/kg IV QD × 3 days over at least 2 hr. Maintenance: 20 mg/kg/day PO. Pamidronate: 60–90 mg IV over 4 hr × 1. Repeat in 7 days PRN.	Inhibits osteoclast reabsorption in malignancy state. Efficacy 75%–100%. Onset 48 hr. Duration, days. Concomitant hydration is imperative. Do not use in renal failure. Adverse effects: ↑ P, ↑ SrCr, N/V (oral).
Zoledronic acid	4 mg doses intravenous administration over 15 minutes	Potent effect on bone resorption. Preferred biphosphonate for hypercalcemia of malignancy. May have promising effects on skeletal complications secondary to bone metastasis.
Phosphate	IV PO_4^- not recommended. PO PO_4^- gradually titrate to 30–60 mmol/day (1–3 gm/day in divided doses)	Inhibits bone resorption; soft tissue calcification. IV onset 24 hr, but not drug of choice. Oral agents used for chronic therapy. Contraindicated in renal failure.
Corticosteroids	Prednisone 60–80 mg/day. Hydrocortisone 5 mg/kg/day IV × 2–3 days.	Impair GI absorption and bone resorption. Onset several days. Best in patients with multiple myeloma, vitamin D intoxication, granulomatous conditions. Can be used in CHF, renal failure.
Indomethacin	75–150 mg/day.	Reports of efficacy are mixed.

CHF, Congestive heart failure; GI, Gastrointestinal; IM, Intramuscular; IV, Intravenous; NS, Normal saline; N/V, Nausea and vomiting; SrCr, Serum creatinine.

peared dehydrated; therefore, saline hydration was used initially to treat the hypercalcemia. However, in patients who have renal failure or CHF, saline hydration and forced diuresis should be avoided.

After adequate volume repletion has been established, IV furosemide can be administered to augment calciuresis. Furosemide blocks the reabsorption of sodium, chloride, and calcium at the thick ascending limb of Henle's loop. Doses of 80 to 100 mg every 2 to 4 hours can be used until a sufficient decline of the serum calcium concentration is attained.[170] However, smaller doses (20 to 40 mg) commonly are given to avoid the significant loss of fluid and electrolytes caused by the more aggressive regimen. Adequate amounts of sodium, potassium, magnesium, and fluid should be used to replace any therapy-induced electrolyte abnormalities. Fluid balance as well as serum and urine concentrations of these electrolytes must be monitored closely. Urine flow must be maintained and the renal loss of sodium chloride must be replaced to preserve the calciuric effect of furosemide.[171] In A.C., the decline of serum calcium concentration was slow, possibly because of

inadequate restoration of plasma volume and/or replacement of renal sodium loss. More aggressive hydration with adequate sodium replacement will ensure that the efficacy of furosemide is not compromised.

CALCITONIN

Calcitonin can be used when saline hydration and furosemide diuresis fail to adequately lower serum calcium concentration or when their use is contraindicated. Calcitonin reduces serum calcium concentration by inhibiting osteoclastic bone resorption. It may also increase the renal excretion of calcium and phosphorus. Salmon-derived calcitonin is more potent and longer acting than human calcitonin. Salmon calcitonin is generally the preferred preparation because of its low cost and longer duration of action. Human calcitonin usually is used for patients with resistance or allergic reactions to the salmon calcitonin.[173]

The serum calcium concentration is often reduced several hours after calcitonin is administered, and the response may last approximately 6 to 8 hours. If used with plicamycin, the effect is additive and can lead to hypocalcemia. The drug is relatively nontoxic compared with agents such as plicamycin and organic phosphates and may be used in patients with dehydration, CHF, or renal failure.[171] Nausea, vomiting, diarrhea, and facial flushing are the more common side effects; soreness and inflammation at the injection site may also be seen.[165] Because of the potential for developing a hypersensitivity reaction to salmon calcitonin but not human calcitonin, the manufacturer recommends skin testing with 1 U of the salmon calcitonin before the first dose. As seen in A.C., tolerance to the hypocalcemic effect of calcitonin can develop after 24 to 72 hours of therapy. This "escape phenomenon" may be secondary to the altered responsiveness of the hormone receptors and might be prevented by concurrent use of corticosteroids.[174] After long-term therapy, antibodies may develop as well.[174]

The dosage of salmon calcitonin is 4 IU/kg given subcutaneously or intramuscularly every 12 hours; the maximum dosage is 8 IU/kg every 6 hours. The hypocalcemic response is often limited, and serum calcium concentration seldom drops to the normal range.[175] The starting dose for human calcitonin usually is 0.5 mg.[176]

PLICAMYCIN

Plicamycin (Mithramycin) is an antibiotic resembling actinomycin D, which was used to treat refractory testicular cancer. With the advent of cisplatin-based regimens, plicamycin is now used primarily to treat hypercalcemia. It inhibits RNA synthesis, which suppresses osteoclast-mediated calcium resorption from bone. The drug is effective for hypercalcemia associated with breast cancer, myelomas, lung, renal cell, or parathyroid carcinoma, and hypervitaminosis D.

The recommended dosage of plicamycin is 25 μg/kg infused over 4 to 6 hours. Generally, a response is seen within 24 to 48 hours, and most patients attain normocalcemia after a single dose.[175] The response lasts 3 to 14 days or longer in some patients. If an adequate response is not obtained, the dose may be repeated 48 hours later.

Many serious adverse effects are associated with plicamycin therapy. However, the drug is usually well tolerated at the lower doses used for hypercalcemia treatment, which is only one-tenth the antineoplastic dose.[175] Nausea and vomiting are common side effects that can be minimized by infusing the drug slowly and by using an antiemetic such as prochlorperazine. The drug is a vesicant and should be administered as a dilute solution to minimize the injury associated with extravasation. Other toxicities include impaired platelet function, proteinuria, azotemia, bone marrow suppression, and elevated hepatic transaminases.[177] Plicamycin may also cause hepatic toxicity, nephrotoxicity, and dose-related acute hemorrhagic syndrome. Because the drug is excreted primarily through the kidneys, impaired renal function may increase the risk for adverse effects.[165] Renal and hepatic function and platelet count should be assessed before and during therapy.

Plicamycin's side effect profile may potentiate the toxic effects of chemotherapeutic agents used to treat patients with malignancy-induced hypercalcemia. Thus, its use is limited to patients unresponsive to other antiresorptive agents. It also is used intermittently to take advantage of its relatively long duration of action. In addition, the drug should not be used in patients with severe hepatic or renal dysfunction, thrombocytopenia, or coagulopathies or those who are dehydrated or receiving myelosuppressive chemotherapy.[171]

BISPHOSPHONATES

Bisphosphonates are synthetic analogs of pyrophosphate that form stable bonds that are resistant to phosphatase degradation during osteoclast-mediated bone mineralization and resorption. The compounds adsorb to the hydroxyapatite crystals of the bone, inhibiting their growth and dissolution. In addition, the compounds may have a direct effect on the osteoclasts.

There are two distinct pharmacologic classes of bisphosphonates with different mechanisms of action. Etidronate, which does not contain any nitrogen atom, is metabolized to cytotoxic, nonhydrolyzable ATP analogs. In contrast, nitrogen-containing bisphosphonates, such as pamidronate and zoledronic acid, inhibit the prenylation of proteins and have potent inhibitory effects on osteoclast-mediated bone resorption.[178] In addition, they induce apoptosis of osteoclasts as well as certain tumor cells. Further antitumor activities may be mediated through their inhibitory effect on angiogenesis, stimulation of the γ-T-cell fraction in blood, and reduction of cancer cells' adherence to bone matrix. At present etidronate, pamidronate, and zoledronic acid are approved in the United States for the treatment of hypercalcemia secondary to malignancy.

Etidronate. Etidronate is administered in doses of 7.5 mg/kg for 3 consecutive days by IV infusion over 2 to 4 hours. Response may be seen after 1 to 2 days, and normocalcemia is expected to be attained in most patients, with response sustained for >10 days.[179] Because of the inconvenient dosing schedule as well as variability in its duration of action, other bisphosphonates are now preferred for the treatment of hypercalcemia of malignancy. In addition, etidronate may inhibit bone mineralization, a property not shared by other bisphosphonates.

Pamidronate. Pamidronate is more potent than etidronate as an inhibitor of bone resorption, but it has negligible effect on bone mineralization. For moderate hypercalcemia (albumin-corrected serum calcium concentration of 12.0 to 13.5 mg/dL), a single dose of 60 to 90 mg of pamidronate is commonly infused over 3 to 4 hours . For severe hypercalcemia (albumin-corrected serum calcium concentration >13.5 mg/dL), the dose is 90 mg. The advantages of pamidronate are that it requires only a single dose and produces a superior response compared with three doses of etidronate.[180]

If the hypercalcemia recurs, the etidronate or the pamidronate regimen may be repeated after an interval of ≥7 days. Etidronate (20 mg/kg per day by mouth) may be given to prolong the normocalcemic duration, but nausea and vomiting are common with the oral therapy. Long-term treatment may result in osteomalacia; however, the limited life expectancy of most patients may diminish the significance of this adverse effect.

Etidronate use has resulted in renal failure,[181] which probably is caused by the formation of biphosphonate–calcium complexes in the serum.[182] Because pamidronate requires a lower molar concentration to produce a comparable hypocalcemic effect, it is less likely to impair renal function. In fact, pamidronate has been given to a limited number of patients with end-stage renal disease without adverse consequence.[124]

Zoledronic Acid. Among the bisphosphonates approved for the treatment of hypercalcemia of malignancy, zoledronic acid has the most potent effect on bone resorption. It is superior to pamidronate with respect to the number of complete responses, time needed to attain calcium normalization, and duration of effect.[183] Since 8-mg doses were not superior to 4-mg, 4-mg doses are administered intravenously over 15 minutes.[184] The drug is well tolerated at 4-mg doses. Zolendroic acid's superior efficacy and convenience of administration make it the preferred biphosphonate for hypercalcemia of malignancy. Emerging studies show that zoledronic acid also may have promising effects in reducing skeletal complications secondary to bone metastasis associated with breast cancer, prostate cancer, non–small-cell lung cancer, and multiple myeloma.[184]

PHOSPHATE

Inorganic phosphates lower the serum calcium concentration by inhibiting bone resorption. They also promote the deposition of calcium salts ($CaHPO_4$) in the bone and soft tissue. If given orally, phosphate reduces intestinal calcium absorption by forming a poorly soluble complex in the bowel lumen and also by decreasing the formation of active vitamin D through enzyme inhibition.[189]

When given intravenously, phosphate is very effective, but renal failure and extensive extraskeletal calcifications are a concern. For these reasons, IV phosphate is not the agent of choice for acute treatment of hypercalcemia.

Oral phosphate (1 to 3 g/day in divided doses) may be used for long-term maintenance therapy, with the optimal dose determined by serum calcium concentrations. Nausea, vomiting, and diarrhea are common problems, especially when the daily dose exceeds 2 g. Soft tissue calcification is also a concern, and hyperphosphatemia and hypocalcemia may occur if the dose is not titrated appropriately. Phosphate therapy should not be given to patients with hyperphosphatemia or renal failure because it may cause further deterioration of renal function. Accumulation of the potassium and sodium salts in phosphate preparations may also present a therapeutic problem in certain patients.

CORTICOSTEROIDS

There are several possible mechanisms that may explain the hypocalcemic effect of corticosteroids. Vitamin D_3–mediated intestinal calcium absorption may be impaired[190] and the action of osteoclast-activating factor, which mediates bone resorption in malignancy, may be inhibited. Corticosteroids also may have a direct cytolytic effect on tumor cells and inhibit the synthesis of prostaglandins (see Prostaglandin Inhibitors). Prednisone (60 to 80 mg/day) is given initially, with subsequent dosage reduction based on the calcemic response. Alternatively, hydrocortisone (5 mg/kg per day for 2 to 3 days) may be given. The hypocalcemic effect will not be apparent for at least 1 to 2 days. Patients with hematologic malignancies and lymphomas tend to have a better response than those with solid tumors. Corticosteroids are also effective in treating hypercalcemia associated with vitamin D intoxication,[191] sarcoidosis,[192] and other granulomatous conditions. They are not generally used for long-term therapy because of their potential for serious adverse reactions.

PROSTAGLANDIN INHIBITORS

Because prostaglandins of the E series, especially PGE_2, may be responsible for hypercalcemia associated with some malignancies, NSAIDs may be useful for a select group of patients with hypercalcemia. For example, indomethacin is effective in lowering the serum calcium concentration in patients with renal cell carcinoma, but not in patients with other types of malignancy.[193] Indomethacin, 75 to 150 mg/day, can be tried in patients unresponsive to other therapy, especially when it is used as part of palliative treatment for cancer pain.

PHOSPHORUS

Homeostasis

Phosphorus is found primarily in bone (85%) and soft tissue (14%); <1% of the total body store resides in the extracellular fluid. Virtually all of the "free" or active phosphorus exists as phosphates in the plasma. However, most clinical laboratories measure and express the concentrations of elemental phosphorus contained in the phosphate molecules. One millimole of phosphate contains 1 mmol of phosphorus, but 1 mmol of phosphate is three times the weight of 1 mmol of phosphorus. Therefore, it is incorrect to equate a certain milligram weight of phosphorus as the same milligram weight of phosphate. Of the total plasma phosphorus, 70% exists as the organic form and 30% as the inorganic form. Organic phosphorus, primarily phospholipids and small amounts of esters, is bound to proteins. About 85% of inorganic phosphorus, or orthophosphate, is unbound or "free." The relative amounts of the two orthophosphate components, $H_2PO_4^-$ and HPO_4^{2-}, vary with the pH. At pH 7.40, the ratio of the two species is 1:4, giving rise to a composite valence of 1.8 for the orthophosphate. Serum phosphate concentrations reported by clinical laboratories reflect only the inorganic portion of the total plasma phosphate. To avoid confusion related to the pH effect on valence, phosphate concentrations are reported as mg/dL or mmol/dL rather than mEq/volume.

The normal range of serum phosphate concentration in healthy adults is 2.7 to 4.7 mg/dL. The value is higher in children, possibly because of the increased amount of growth hormone and the reduced amount of gonadal hormones.[194] In postmenopausal women, the range is slightly higher; however, it is lower in older men. The serum phosphate concentration is also affected by dietary intake. Phosphate-rich foods can transiently increase the serum phosphate concentration. In contrast, glucose decreases the serum phosphate concentration because of the flux of sugar and phosphate into cells and because of the phosphorylation of glucose. Similarly, administration of insulin and epinephrine decreases the serum phosphate concentration because of their effects on glucose. The serum concentration of phosphate is reduced in alkalosis and increased in acidosis.[199]

A balanced diet contains 800 to 1,500 mg/day of phosphorus. Both the organic and inorganic forms of phosphorus are present in food substances. Most of the phosphorus in milk is the organic form, whereas the phosphorus in meat, vegetable, and other nondairy sources represents organic forms bound to proteins, lipids, and sugars, which usually are hydrolyzed before absorption.[200] In general, 60% to 65% of the phosphorus ingested is absorbed, mostly in the duodenum and jejunum through an energy-dependent, saturable, active process.[201] Phosphorus absorption is linearly related to the dietary intake when the intake is 4 to 30 mg/kg per day.[141] The amount of phosphorus ingested probably is the most important factor in determining net absorption. Phosphorus absorption is also stimulated during periods of increased demand, such as active growth and pregnancy.[202] Increased intake of calcium and magnesium and concurrent use of aluminum hydroxide antacids may reduce phosphorus absorption due to formation of a nonabsorbable complex.[203] In addition, absorption is also affected by vitamin D, PTH, and calcitonin.[194]

Renal phosphorus excretion depends on the dietary phosphorus intake. Normally, >85% of the filtered phosphate load is reabsorbed; however, the fractional urinary excretion may vary from 0.2% to 20%.[144] Renal phosphate excretion is also affected by acid–base balance, extracellular fluid volume, and calcium and glucose concentrations.[194] In addition, PTH, thyroid hormone, thyrocalcitonin, vitamin D, insulin, glucocorticoid, and glucagon may also alter renal phosphate excretion.[194]

Hypophosphatemia

Etiology

23. M.R., a 72-year-old woman, was admitted to the hospital with a 1-week history of increasing malaise, confusion, and decreased activity. M.R. has a history of CHF, hypertension, type 2 diabetes, and peptic ulcer disease. She was receiving hydrochlorothiazide, Maalox, sucralfate, and insulin. She is febrile and in significant respiratory distress. ABG results at admission were pH 7.5 (normal, 7.36 to 7.44); Po_2, 42 mm Hg (normal, 80 to 90); and Pco_2, 20 mm Hg (normal, 34 to 46). Respiratory function continued to deteriorate, requiring intubation and mechanical ventilation. Serum electrolytes are Na, 128 mEq/L (normal, 134 to 146); K, 3.6 mEq/L (normal, 3.5 to 5.1); Cl, 96 mEq/L (normal, 92 to 109); CO_2, 23 mEq/L (normal, 22 to 32); glucose, 320 mg/dL (normal, 60 to 110); and phosphorus (P), 0.9 mg/dL (normal, 2.4 to 4.6). What may have contributed to the low serum phosphorus concentration in M.R.?

[SI units: Na, 128 mmol/L; K, 3.6 mmol/L; Cl, 96 mmol/L; CO_2, 23 mmol/L; glucose, 17.8 mmol/L; P, 0.29 mmol/L]

Hypophosphatemia may develop as the result of a phosphorus deficiency or secondary to a net flux of phosphorus out of the plasma compartment without a total body deficit. Moderate hypophosphatemia is defined as a serum phosphorus concentration of 1.0 to 2.5 mg/dL. A concentration of <1.0 mg/dL, as in M.R., is considered severe.[204] The extent of hypophosphatemia may not be assessed accurately by a single plasma phosphorus concentration determination because of diurnal variation.[205] Patients receiving large doses of mannitol may have pseudohypophosphatemia due to the binding of mannitol with molybdate, which is used in the calorimetric assay for phosphorus.[206]

Hypophosphatemia is commonly caused by conditions that impair intestinal absorption, increase renal elimination, or shift phosphorus from the extracellular to the intracellular compartments. Hypophosphatemia secondary to low dietary phosphorus is exceedingly rare because phosphorus is ubiquitous.[194] In addition, renal phosphorus excretion is reduced and intestinal phosphorus absorption is increased to prevent a deficiency state.[144,207] Starvation in itself does not result in severe hypophosphatemia because the phosphorus content in plasma and muscles is often normal. However, hypophosphatemia can develop during refeeding with a high-calorie diet low in phosphorus. Therefore, hyperalimentation without phosphorus supplementation is likely to cause severe hypophosphatemia.[208]

Impaired phosphorus absorption secondary to malabsorptive conditions, prolonged nasogastric suction, and protracted vomiting may also result in hypophosphatemia. In M.R., the use of aluminum- and magnesium-containing antacids may further reduce phosphorus absorption. The antacids bind with endogenous and exogenous phosphorus in the GI tract and cause severe hypophosphatemia in patients with or without renal failure.[209] In addition, M.R. was taking sucralfate, which can bind phosphorus in the GI tract.[210] Similarly, iron preparations can bind phosphorus.[211]

Hyperglycemia-induced osmotic diuresis and diuretic use may have increased the renal loss of phosphorus in M.R. Other conditions associated with renal phosphorus wasting include renal tubular acidosis, hyperparathyroidism, hypokalemia, hypomagnesemia, and extracellular volume expansion.[194] However, none of these situations was evident in M.R. Shifting of phosphorus into the intracellular compartment by glucose and/or insulin and profound respiratory alkalosis, especially during alcoholic withdrawal, may also have contributed to M.R.'s hypophosphatemic state.[212,213]

24. What other conditions are commonly associated with hypophosphatemia?

Diabetic ketoacidosis, chronic alcoholism, chronic obstructive airway disease, and extensive thermal burns are other conditions commonly associated with hypophosphatemia.[214,215] They are characterized by a combination of factors that result in phosphate loss and/or intracellular phosphate use and repletion. In patients with diabetic ketoacidosis, metabolic acidosis enhances the movement of phosphate from the intracellular compartment to plasma, whereas the concurrent osmotic diuresis secondary to hyperglycemia increases the renal elimination of extracellular phosphate.[216] The net result is a depletion of total body stores. Correction of the acidosis and administration of insulin then promotes the rapid uptake of phosphorus by tissues, and volume repletion dilutes the extracellular concentration. This sequence of events can ultimately lead to severe hypophosphatemia. The hypophosphatemia associated with chronic alcoholism and acute alcohol intoxication is also thought to be related to several factors, including reduced intestinal phosphorus absorption due to vomiting, diarrhea, and antacid use; repeated acidosis that results in increased urinary phosphate excretion; and a shift of phosphorus into cells because of respiratory alkalosis. Renal phosphorus wasting may also result from hypomagnesemia or as a direct effect of alcohol.[217]

Clinical Manifestations

25. What are the signs and symptoms associated with hypophosphatemia?

The clinical effects associated with chronic phosphorus depletion are often insidious and gradual in onset. In contrast, a rapid decline in plasma phosphorus concentrations results in sudden and serious organ dysfunction. Most of the effects can be attributed to impaired cellular energy stores and tissue hypoxia secondary to depletion of adenosine triphosphate (ATP) and/or erythrocyte 2,3-diphosphoglycerate (2,3-DPG).[218] Severe hypophosphatemia can result in generalized muscle weakness, confusion, paresthesias, seizures, and coma. In addition, reduced cardiac contractility, hypotension, respiratory failure, and rhabdomyolysis have been observed with acute severe hypophosphatemia.[194] Chronic phosphorus depletion has been associated with decreased mentation; muscle weakness; osteomalacia; rickets; anorexia; dysphagia; cardiomyopathy; tachypnea; reduced sensitivity to insulin; and dysfunction of red blood cells, white blood cells, and platelets. Renal function is altered, as manifested by hypophosphaturia, hypercalciuria, hypermagnesuria, bicarbonaturia, and glycosuria. M.R.'s decreased mentation, weakness, and respiratory failure are consistent with severe hypophosphatemia.

Treatment

26. How can phosphate depletion be assessed? Outline a treatment regimen that would effectively and safely correct the phosphorus deficit in M.R. How should her therapy be monitored?

Phosphorus resides primarily in the intracellular space; the amount in the extracellular fluid is only a small percentage of the total body store. Because the patient's pH, blood glucose concentration, and insulin availability may affect phosphorus distribution, it is difficult to determine the magnitude of the phosphorus deficit based on the serum concentration alone. As discussed previously, a patient may have hypophosphatemia secondary to a rapid shift of phosphorus into the intracellular space without a total body deficit. The duration of the hypophosphatemia is often limited because it may be corrected by renal phosphorus conservation and oral intake of phosphorus-containing foods. Aside from serum phosphorus concentrations, urinary phosphorus excretion may be used to further assess the phosphorus deficit. Typically, renal phosphorus excretion is severely limited in patients with significant deficits. A phosphorus excretion of <100 mg/day (fractional phosphorus excretion <10%) confirms appropriate renal phosphorus conservation when the serum phosphorus is <2 mg/dL. It also suggests a nonrenal etiology (e.g., impaired GI absorption) or some type of internal redistribution (e.g., respiratory alkalosis).[219]

Prophylactic supplementation should be used in situations that predictably increase the risk for developing hypophosphatemia. These include patients who are receiving total parenteral nutrition or large doses of antacids for an extended period, alcoholic patients, and those with diabetic ketoacidosis.

The specific treatment of hypophosphatemia depends on the presence of signs and symptoms, as well as the anticipated duration and severity of hypophosphatemia. In an asymptomatic patient with mild hypophosphatemia (1.5 to 2.5 mg/dL)

who has no evidence of phosphorus depletion, phosphorus supplementation is generally not necessary because the condition is usually self-limited.[194] In other patients with mild and moderate hypophosphatemia who have evidence of phosphorus deficit, oral supplementation is the safest and preferred mode of replacement. Skim or low-fat milk is a convenient source of phosphorus and calcium. Whole milk, because of its high fat content, may cause diarrhea if a large amount is consumed. Several oral phosphorus preparations can be used in patients who cannot tolerate milk products.

When hypophosphatemia is severe, as in M.R., or when the patient is vomiting or unable to take oral medication, parenteral phosphorus replacement is needed. Several empiric regimens have been evaluated. IV administration of 0.08 to 0.5 mmol of phosphorus per kilogram of body weight over 4 to 12 hours is safe and effective in restoring the serum phosphorus concentration.[220,221] Parenteral phosphorus replacement should be stopped once the serum phosphorus concentration reaches 2.0 mg/dL and also when oral supplementation is started. In general, no more than 32 mmol (1 g) of phosphorus should be administered IV in a 24-hour period. Regardless of the regimen used, serum phosphorus, calcium, and magnesium concentrations should be monitored closely because IV phosphorus administration can induce hyperphosphatemia quite rapidly, as well as hypocalcemia and hypomagnesemia. Monitoring of urine phosphorus concentration also helps determine the adequacy of therapy. Metastatic soft tissue calcification, hypotension, and, depending on the preparation used, potassium, sodium, or volume overload may occur. This could be significant in patients such as M.R. who have a history of CHF and hypertension. Therefore, renal function and volume status should be monitored during therapy. Diarrhea, a common dose-related side effect of oral phosphorus replacement, can be minimized by diluting the supplement and slowly titrating the dose. Large doses can also result in metabolic acidosis.[220]

Phosphorus can be administered orally in doses of 30 to 60 mmol/day using any commercially available oral supplement (e.g., Fleet or Neutra-Phos). Fleet Phospho-Soda (5 mL twice daily) delivers 40 mmol/day of phosphorus. Skim milk, the preferred agent for diluting the supplement, contains approximately 7 mmol of phosphorus/cup and provides calcium and potassium as well.

In M.R., oral supplementation was not feasible because she had intermittent diarrhea and vomiting. Potassium phosphate 15 mmol (providing 22 mEq of potassium) was therefore infused intravenously in 250 mL of 0.45% saline over 12 hours. The regimen was repeated once until the serum phosphorus concentration reached 2 mg/dL. Oral supplementation with Fleet Phospho-Soda then was begun by adding one teaspoonful twice daily to her enteral tube feeding.

MAGNESIUM

Homeostasis

Magnesium is an intracellular cation found primarily in bone (65%) and muscle (20%).[222] Only 2% of the total body store of 21 to 28 g (1,750 to 2,400 mEq) is located in the extracellular compartment. Serum magnesium concentrations, therefore, do not reflect the total magnesium body store accurately.

In healthy adults, the serum magnesium concentration is 1.40 to 1.75 mEq/L, with approximately 20% of the serum magnesium bound to proteins.

Magnesium plays an important role in different metabolic processes, particularly in energy transfer, storage, and utilization. Deficiency of the cation can impair many ATP-mediated energy-dependent cellular processes as well as the action of phosphatases.[223] Magnesium is necessary for many enzymes involved in the metabolism of carbohydrate, fat, and protein, as well as RNA aggregation, DNA transcription, and degradation. The normal operation of many sodium, proton, and calcium pumps and the regulation of potassium and calcium channels are all dependent on the availability of intracellular magnesium.[224,225] In addition, adequate magnesium stores are needed to maintain normal neuronal control, neuromuscular transmission, and cardiovascular tone.

The average diet in North America contains about 20 to 30 mEq of magnesium.[226] The daily requirement is approximately 18 to 33 mEq for young persons and 15 to 28 mEq for women.[227] Normally, 30% to 40% of the elemental magnesium is absorbed, primarily in the jejunum and ileum. However, absorption may be increased to 80% in deficiency states and reduced to 25% during high magnesium intake. In patients with uremia, GI absorption of magnesium is decreased; however, absorption in the jejunum can be normalized by physiologic doses of $1\alpha,25$-dihydroxyvitamin D_3.[228] In addition, PTH also modulates magnesium absorption.[229]

Magnesium is eliminated primarily by the kidneys; only 1% to 2% of the endogenous magnesium is eliminated by the fecal route.[164] The magnitude of renal removal is determined by GFR and tubular reabsorption. Approximately 20% to 30% of the tubular reabsorption takes place in the proximal tubule, whereas Henle's loop, primarily the thick ascending limb, is responsible for up to 65% of the total reabsorption.[230] Only about 5% to 6% of the filtered magnesium is generally eliminated in the urine. The extent of magnesium reabsorption changes in parallel with sodium reabsorption, which is affected by the extracellular fluid volume. The renal threshold for urinary magnesium excretion is 1.3 to 1.7 mEq/L, which is similar to the normal plasma magnesium concentration. Slight changes in plasma magnesium concentration may therefore substantially alter the amount of magnesium excreted in the urine.[231]

Urinary magnesium reabsorption is affected by many factors, including sodium balance; extracellular fluid volume; serum concentrations of magnesium, calcium, and phosphate; and metabolic acidosis and alkalosis.[232] Concurrent use of loop and osmotic diuretics will also modulate the reabsorption.[233,234] Hormones such as PTH and possibly calcitonin, glucagon, and mineralocorticoids may affect the routine maintenance of magnesium balance as well.[235–237]

Hypomagnesemia

Etiology

27. R.J., a 61-year-old man, is admitted to the hospital because of trauma to his forehead after falling at home. He has a long history of conditions related to his alcohol abuse: liver disease, ascites, seizures, pancreatitis, and malabsorption. R.J. complained of abdominal pain, nausea, vomiting, and diarrhea for the past several days. At admission, R.J. was confused, apprehensive, and combative, and he had marked tremors. He also had delirium, as evidenced by hallucinations, screaming, and delusions, and he was having multiple tonic-clonic seizures. The medical record revealed that R.J. had been taking furosemide for the last 2 months. Pertinent laboratory test results obtained at admission were K, 2.5 mEq/L (normal, 3.5 to 5.1); Mg, 0.8 mEq/L (normal, 1.6 to 2.8); and creatinine, 0.8 mg/dL (normal, 0.5 to 1.5). Phenytoin was administered for seizure control and R.J. was placed on nasogastric suction. Fluid restriction was instituted and furosemide therapy was continued to control his ascites. What are the circumstances that have contributed to R.J.'s hypomagnesemia?

[SI units: K, 2.5 mmol/L; Mg, 0.4 mmol/L; creatinine, 70.72 μmol/L]

Magnesium body stores are difficult to assess because magnesium is primarily an intracellular ion, and serum magnesium concentrations do not provide an accurate indication of the total body load. In fact, cellular magnesium depletion may be present with low, normal, or even high serum magnesium concentrations.[238,239] Conversely, hypomagnesemia may be seen without a net loss of body magnesium. Refeeding after starvation will result in increased trapping of magnesium by newly formed tissue, resulting in hypomagnesemia. Similarly, acute pancreatitis and parathyroidectomy may cause hypomagnesemia without a net loss of the cation.[240,241]

The prevalence of hypomagnesemia in ambulatory and hospitalized patients was found to be approximately 6% to 12%.[242] The incidence increased to 42% in patients who were hypokalemic[243] and to 60% to 65% in those under intensive care.[244] Multiple risk factors and clinical conditions can contribute to the high rate of hypomagnesemia in critically ill patients.

Magnesium depletion and hypomagnesemia can develop due to GI, renal, and endocrinologic causes. Depletion may occur in patients whose dietary magnesium intake is severely restricted[245] and in those who have protein calorie malnutrition.[246] Also at risk are patients who receive prolonged parenteral nutrition[247] and those who undergo prolonged nasogastric suction.[248] Hypomagnesemia may be present in patients who have increased magnesium requirements, such as pregnant women and infants.[249] Conditions associated with steatorrhea, such as nontropical sprue and short-bowel syndrome, may result in reduced GI magnesium absorption. Insoluble magnesium soaps may be formed in the GI tract due to the presence of unabsorbed fat.[250] Hypomagnesemia may also occur in patients with a bowel resection[251] and severe diarrhea.[252] A rare genetic disorder has also been reported in patients with defective GI magnesium absorption.[253] An impaired carrier-mediated magnesium transport system is believed to be responsible for the symptomatic deficiency, which requires high oral magnesium intake to overcome the defect.

Renal magnesium wasting may be caused by a primary defect or may be secondary to systemic factors. A rare form of renal magnesium wasting is congenital.[254] Various drugs can induce hypomagnesemia through increased renal loss: cisplatin,[255] aminoglycosides,[256] cyclosporine,[257] and amphotericin B.[258] Use of loop and thiazide diuretics may also result in hypomagnesemia, which can be reversed with the concurrent use of amiloride or triamterene.[185] Magnesium depletion may be associated with phosphate depletion,[259] calcium infusion,[260] and ketoacidosis.[261] Acute and chronic ingestion of alcohol will result in increased renal magnesium loss.[190,262] Various endocrinologic disorders, such as SIADH,[263] hyperthyroidism,[264] hyperaldosteronism,[237] and postparathyroidectomy,[265] are also associated with hypomagnesemia.

R.J. could be hypomagnesemic for many reasons. His long history of alcohol use, malnutrition, and malabsorption may all have contributed to his magnesium deficit. The vomiting and diarrhea that he experienced could have reduced GI magnesium absorption. Use of furosemide and nasogastric suction while in the hospital could also have exacerbated his magnesium depletion through renal and GI losses, respectively.

Clinical Manifestations

28. **What are the clinical manifestations of hypomagnesemia in R.J.?**

Magnesium depletion may result in abnormal function of the neurologic, neuromuscular, and cardiovascular systems. Hypomagnesemia lowers the threshold for nerve stimulation, resulting in increased irritability. Typical findings include Chvostek's and Trousseau's signs, muscle fasciculation, tremors, muscle spasticity, generalized convulsions, and possibly tetany. The patient may experience weakness, anorexia, nausea, and vomiting, as seen in R.J. Hypokalemia, hypocalcemia, and alkalosis may be present as well. In moderately depleted patients, changes in the ECG include widening of the QRS complex and a peaking T wave.[266] In severe depletion, a prolonged P-R interval and a diminished T wave may be seen. Ventricular arrhythmias also have been reported in some patients.[267]

Treatment

29. **Outline a regimen to replenish the body stores of magnesium for R.J., and develop a monitoring plan to assess efficacy and potential adverse effects.**

The specific regimen for magnesium replenishment depends on the clinical presentation of the patient. Symptomatic patients require more aggressive parenteral therapy, whereas oral replacement may suffice for asymptomatic hypomagnesemia. Patients with life-threatening symptoms, such as seizures and arrhythmias, need immediate magnesium infusion. Because serum magnesium concentrations do not reflect total body stores, symptoms are more important determinants of the urgency and aggressiveness of therapy.

The body stores of magnesium must be replenished slowly. Serum magnesium concentrations may return to the normal range within the first 24 hours, but total replenishment of body stores may take several days. Furthermore, approximately 50% of the administered IV dose of magnesium will be excreted in the urine.[195] Because the threshold for urinary magnesium excretion is low, the abrupt increase in serum magnesium after an IV dose will result in increased urinary magnesium excretion despite a total body magnesium deficit. Conversely, in patients with renal insufficiency, decreased excretion of magnesium will place the patient at risk for hypermagnesemia. A reduced rate of magnesium administration and frequent monitoring of serum magnesium concentrations are therefore necessary in patients with renal dysfunction.

Oral replacement of magnesium is indicated for asymptomatic patients with mild depletion. Magnesium-containing antacids, Milk of Magnesia, and magnesium oxide are effective choices for replacement. However, sustained-release preparations, such as Slow Mag (containing magnesium chloride) and Mag-Tab SR (containing magnesium lactate), are preferred. With 5 to 7 mEq (2.5 to 3.5 mmol or 60 to 84 mg) of magnesium per tablet, six to eight tablets should be given daily in divided doses for severe magnesium depletion. For mild and asymptomatic disease, two to four tablets per day may be sufficient.[196] A diet high in magnesium (cereals, nuts, meat, fruits, fish, legumes, and vegetables) also will help replenish body stores and prevent depletion.[197]

For patients with symptomatic hypomagnesemia, such as R.J., parenteral magnesium replacement is indicated. The magnesium deficit in patients with chronic alcoholism is estimated to be 1 to 2 mEq/kg.[198] Because up to half of the IV magnesium dose will be excreted in the urine during replacement, approximately 2 to 4 mEq/kg will be needed to replenish R.J.'s body store.[195] One milliequivalent per kilogram of magnesium, as magnesium sulfate 10% solution, should be administered intravenously in the first 24 hours. Half of this amount is given in the first 3 hours, and the remaining half is infused over the rest of the day. This dose may be repeated to keep the serum magnesium concentration >1.0 mg/dL.[196] Later on, 0.5 mEq/kg of magnesium may be replenished daily for up to 4 additional days.[195,268] Magnesium may be given intramuscularly as 50% solution, but the injections are painful and potentially sclerosing, and multiple administrations are needed. Therefore, the IV route is the preferred mode of parenteral administration. For patients with seizures or life-threatening arrhythmias, 16 to 32 mEq of magnesium sulfate may be administered as a short IV infusion over 2 to 4 minutes.[195]

After IV magnesium administration, the patient should remain in a supine position to avoid hypotension. He should be monitored carefully for marked suppression of deep tendon reflexes (Mg, 4 to 7 mEq/L); ECG, BP, and respiration changes; and high serum magnesium levels (see Question 24). Facial flushing, a sensation of warmth, and sweatiness may result from vasodilation secondary to a rapid magnesium infusion.[195] Particular caution is warranted in patients with renal impairment, in whom the rate of magnesium should be reduced. These patients should be monitored frequently to avoid toxicities related to hypermagnesemia. IV magnesium should also be administered cautiously in patients with severe atrioventricular heart block or bifascicular blocks because magnesium possesses pharmacologic properties similar to calcium channel blockers.[195,269]

In patients who develop hypomagnesemia secondary to a thiazide or loop diuretic, amiloride may be added to reduce renal magnesium loss by increasing reabsorption in the cortical collecting tubule.[196]

30. **Over the initial 2 days of hospitalization, R.J. received 3 mEq/kg of IV magnesium sulfate. However, his serum magnesium concentration remained <1.5 mEq/L (normal, 1.5 to 2.6). What might have contributed to the lack of favorable response to the magnesium therapy?**

The total amount of magnesium administered to R.J. over the past 2 days was higher than the usual recommended rate (4 to 5 days) of magnesium replenishment, leading to renal excretion of a large portion of the dose.[270] Furthermore, the use of nasogastric suction and furosemide have increased the magnesium loss during the replacement period, and hypokalemia may have reduced the effectiveness of magnesium replacement. In a patient whose serum magnesium concentration does not increase after appropriate magnesium therapy, a 24-hour urine collection to assess magnesium renal excretion can be helpful. A low urinary magnesium concentration is consistent with magnesium depletion, whereas high urinary magnesium excretion in the presence of hypomagnesemia suggests renal magnesium wasting.

Hypermagnesemia

Etiology

31. **J.O., a 63-year-old man with renal insufficiency, was admitted to the hospital because of increasing weakness over the past several days. J.O. began taking a magnesium–aluminum hydroxide antacid several times daily 2 weeks ago when he developed stomach upset. Physical examination reveals hypotension and depressed deep tendon reflexes. The ECG reveals prolonged P-R and QRS intervals. The serum magnesium concentration is 6.5 mEq/dL (normal, 1.6 to 2.8). What is the most likely cause of hypermagnesemia in J.O.?**

[SI unit: Mg, 3.25 mmol/L]

Because the kidney is the primary route of magnesium elimination, renal impairment is a virtual requisite for hypermagnesemia (see Chapter 32, Chronic Kidney Disease). A common cause of hypermagnesemia is the use of magnesium-containing medications, such as antacids and laxatives, by patients with impaired renal function, including older adults. When a renal failure patient, such as J.O., takes magnesium-containing medications, the serum magnesium concentration can increase substantially, resulting in toxicities. Hypermagnesemia may be seen when the creatinine clearance drops below 30 mL/minute; an inverse relationship is observed between the serum magnesium concentrations and the creatinine clearances.[271] Hypermagnesemia is also seen in patients with acute renal failure during the oliguric phase, but not the diuretic phase.[272] Other potential causes of hypermagnesemia include adrenal insufficiency,[223] hypothyroidism,[273] lithium,[273] magnesium citrate used as a cathartic for drug overdose,[274] and parenteral magnesium given for pre-eclampsia.[275]

Clinical Manifestations

32. **Describe the usual clinical presentation of a patient with hypermagnesemia.**

An elevated magnesium serum concentration alters the normal function of the neurologic, neuromuscular, and cardiovascular systems. When the serum magnesium concentration is >4 mEq/L, deep tendon reflexes are depressed; they are usually lost at >6 mEq/L. Flaccid quadriplegia may develop when the concentration is >8 to 10 mEq/L. Respiratory paralysis, hypotension, and difficulty in talking and swallowing may also be present.[276] Changes in the ECG may include a prolonged P-R interval and widening of the QRS complex. Complete heart block may be seen at concentrations of approximately 15 mEq/L. In mild hypomagnesemia, the patient may experience nausea and vomiting.

Drowsiness, lethargy, diaphoresis, and altered consciousness may be present at higher serum magnesium concentrations. J.O.'s increasing weakness, hypotension, depressed deep tendon reflexes, and ECG findings are consistent with hypermagnesemia.

Treatment

33. **How should J.O.'s hypermagnesemia be treated?**

If magnesium-containing medications are discontinued in patients with hypermagnesemia, the serum magnesium concentration will usually return to the normal range through renal elimination. However, when potentially life-threatening complications are present, as in J.O., 5 to 10 mEq of IV calcium should be administered to antagonize the respiratory and cardiac manifestations of magnesium.[275,276] The dose of the calcium may be repeated as necessary because its effect is short-lived. In patients with good renal function without life-threatening complications, IV furosemide, plus 0.45% sodium chloride to replace lost urine volume, will enhance urinary magnesium excretion while preventing volume depletion. Hemodialysis or peritoneal dialysis is indicated for patients with significant renal function impairment and possibly for those with severe hypermagnesemia.

REFERENCES

1. Fanestil DD. Compartmentation of body water. In: Narins RG, ed. Maxwell & Kleeman's Clinical Disorders of Fluid and Electrolyte Metabolism. 5th Ed. New York: McGraw-Hill, 1994:3.
2. Lesser GT et al. Body water compartments with human aging using fat-free mass as the reference standard. Am J Physiol 1979;236:R215.
3. Rose BD. Renal function and disorders of water and sodium balance. In: Rubenstein E, Federman DD, eds. Scientific American Medicine. New York: Scientific American Inc., 1994;Section 10(I):1.
4. Rose BD. Introduction to disorders of osmolality. In: Rose BD, Post TW, ed. Clinical Physiology of Acid-Base and Electrolyte Disorders. 5th Ed. New York: McGraw-Hill, 2001.
5. Oster JR, Singer I. Hyponatremia, hyposmolality, and hypotonicity: tables and fables. Arch Intern Med 1999;159:333.
6. Rose BD. Proximal tubule. In: Rose BD, Post TW, ed. Clinical Physiology of Acid-Base and Electrolyte Disorders. 5th Ed. New York: McGraw-Hill, 2001.

7. Rose BD. Loop of Henle and the countercurrent mechanism. In: Rose BD, Post TW, ed. Clinical Physiology of Acid-Base and Electrolyte Disorders. 5th Ed. New York: McGraw-Hill, 2001.
8. Rose BD. Functions of the distal nephron. In: Rose BD, Post TW, ed. Clinical Physiology of Acid-Base and Electrolyte Disorders. 5th Ed. New York: McGraw-Hill, 2001.
9. Sands JM et al. Vasopressin effects on urea and water transport in inner medullary collecting duct subsegments. Am J Physiol 1987;253:F823.
10. Gines P et al. Vasopressin in pathophysiological states. Semin Nephrol 1994;14:384.
11. Zerbe RL et al. Osmotic and nonosmotic regulation of thirst and vasopressin secretion. In: Narins RG, ed. Maxwell & Kleeman's Clinical Disorders of Fluid and Electrolyte Metabolism. New York: McGraw-Hill, 1994.
12. Rose BD. Regulation of the effective circulating volume. In: Rose BD, Post TW, ed. Clinical Physiology of Acid-Base and Electrolyte Disorders. 5th Ed. New York: McGraw-Hill, 2001.

13. Goetz KL. Renal natriuretic peptide (urodilatin?) and atriopeptin: evolving concepts. Am J Physiol 1991;261:F921.
14. Goetz K et al. Evidence that urodilatin, rather than ANP, regulates renal sodium excretion. J Am Soc Nephrol 1990;1:867.
15. Rose BD. Hypovolemic states. In: Rose BD, Post TW, ed. Clinical Physiology of Acid-Base and Electrolyte Disorders. 5th Ed. New York: McGraw-Hill, 2001.
16. Rose BD. Meaning and application of urine chemistries. In: Rose BD, Post TW, ed. Clinical Physiology of Acid-Base and Electrolyte Disorders. 5th Ed. New York: McGraw-Hill, 2001.
17. Kaysen GA. Proteinuria and the nephrotic syndrome. In: Schrier RW, ed. Renal and Electrolyte Disorders. 6th Ed. Philadelphia: Lippincott Williams & Wilkins, 2003.
18. Harris RE et al. Extrarenal complications of the nephrotic syndrome. Am J Kidney Dis 1994;23:477.
19. Saborio P, Scheinman JI. Sickle cell nephropathy. J Am Soc Nephrol 1999;10:187.

20. Klotman PE. HIV-associated nephropathy. Kidney Int 1999;56:1161.
21. Feinfeld DA et al. Nephrotic syndrome associated with the use of the nonsteroidal anti-inflammatory drugs: case report and review of the literature. Nephron 1984;37:174.
22. Kaysen GA et al. New insights into lipid metabolism in the nephrotic syndrome. Kidney Int 1999;56(Suppl. 71):S18.
23. Chonko AM, Grantham JJ. Treatment of edema states. In: Narins RG, ed. Maxwell & Kleeman's Clinical Disorders of Fluid and Electrolyte Metabolism. 5th Ed. New York: McGraw-Hill, 1994: 545.
24. Glassock RJ. Management of intractable edema in nephrotic syndrome. Kidney Int 1997;51(Suppl. 58):S75.
25. Schrier RW. Body fluid volume regulation in health and disease: a unifying hypothesis. Ann Intern Med 1990;113:155.
26. Schrier RW. An odyssey into the milieu? Interieur: pondering the enigmas. J Am Soc Nephrol 1992;2:1549.
27. Brown EA et al. Sodium retention in nephrotic syndrome is due to an intrarenal defect: evidence from steroid-induced remission. Nephron 1985;39:290.
28. Koomans HA et al. Renal function during recovery from minimal lesion nephrotic syndrome. Nephron 1987;47:173.
29. Schrier RW et al. A critique of the overfill hypothesis of sodium and water retention in the nephrotic syndrome. Kidney Int 1998;53:1111.
30. Bank N. External compression for the treatment of resistant edema. N Engl J Med 1980;302:969.
31. Davidson AM et al. Salt-poor human albumin in the management of nephrotic syndrome. Br Med J 1974;1:481.
32. Fancheld P et al. An evaluation of ultrafiltration as treatment of diuretic-resistant edema in nephrotic syndrome. Acta Med Scand 1985;17:127.
33. Yeun JY, Kaysen GA. The nephrotic syndrome: nutritional consequences and dietary management. In: Mitch WE, Klahr S, eds. Handbook of Nutrition and the Kidney. 4th Ed. Philadelphia: Lippincolt Williams & Wilkins, 2002.
34. Soupart A et al. Therapeutic recommendations for management of severe hyponatremia: current concepts on pathogenesis and prevention of neurologic complications. Clin Nephrol 1996;46:149.
35. Narins RG et al. Diagnostic strategies in disorders of fluid, electrolyte and acid-base homeostasis. Am J Med 1982;72:496.
36. Goldman MB et al. Mechanisms of altered water metabolism in psychotic patients with polydipsia and hyponatremia. N Engl J Med 1988;318:397.
37. Illowsky B et al. Polydipsia and hyponatremia in psychiatric patients. Am J Psychiatry 1988;145:6.
38. Sterns RH et al. Hyponatremia: pathophysiology, diagnosis, and therapy. In: Narins RG, ed. Maxwell & Kleeman's Clinical Disorders of Fluid and Electrolyte Metabolism. New York: McGraw-Hill, 1994.
39. Weisberg LS. Pseudohyponatremia: a reappraisal. Am J Med 1989;86:315.
40. Rothenberg DM et al. Isotonic hyponatremia following transurethral prostate resection. J Clin Anesth 1990;2:48.
41. Faber MD et al. Common fluid-electrolyte and acid-base problems in the intensive care unit: selected issues. Semin Nephrol 1994;14:8.
42. Ashraf N et al. Thiazide-induced hyponatremia associated with death or neurologic damage in outpatients. Am J Med 1981;70:1163.
43. Ashouri SD. Severe diuretic induced hyponatremias in the elderly. Arch Intern Med 1986;146:1355.
44. Shah PJ, Greenburg WM. Water intoxication precipitated by thiazide diuretics in polydipsic psychiatric patients. Am J Psychiatr 1991;48:1424.
45. Vassal G et al. Hyponatremia and renal sodium wasting in patients receiving cisplatinum. Pediatr Hematol Oncol 1987;4:337.
46. Hutchison FN et al. Renal sodium wasting in patients treated with cisplatin. Ann Intern Med 1988;108:21.

47. Vaamonde CA. Renal water handling in liver disease. In: Epstein M, ed. The Kidney in Liver Disease. Baltimore: Williams & Wilkins, 1988.
48. Papadakis MA et al. Hyponatremia in patients with cirrhosis. Q J Med 1990;76:675.
49. Carpenter CCJ et al. Oral rehydration therapy: the role of polymeric substrates. N Engl J Med 1988;319:1346.
50. Leier CV et al. Clinical relevance and management of the major electrolyte abnormalities in congestive heart failure: hyponatremia, hypokalemia, and hypomagnesemia. Am Heart J 1994;128:564.
51. Gore SM et al. Impact of rice-based oral rehydration solution on stool output and duration of diarrhea: meta-analysis of 13 clinical trials. Br Med J 1992;304:287.
52. Allon M et al. Renal sodium and water handling in hypothyroid patients: the role of renal insufficiency. J Am Soc Nephrol 1990;1:205.
53. Linas SL et al. Role of vasopressin in the impaired water excretion of glucocorticoid deficiency. Kidney Int 1980;18:58.
54. DeFronzo RA et al. Normal diluting capacity in hyponatremic patients: reset osmostat or variant of SIADH. Ann Intern Med 1975;82:811.
55. Schwartz WB et al. Syndrome of renal sodium loss and hyponatremia probably resulting from inappropriate secretion of antidiuretic hormone. Am J Med 1957;23:529.
56. Bartter FC et al. The syndrome of inappropriate secretion of antidiuretic hormone. Am J Med 1967;42:790.
57. Cooke RC et al. The syndrome of inappropriate antidiuretic hormone secretion (SIADH): pathophysiologic mechanisms in solute and volume regulation. Medicine 1979;58:240.
58. Marchioli CC, Graziano SL. Paraneoplastic syndromes associated with small cell lung cancer. Chest Surg Clin North Am 1997;7:65.
59. Rose BD. New approaches to disturbances in the plasma sodium concentration. Am J Med 1986;81:1033.
60. Cluitmans FHM et al. Management of severe hyponatremia: rapid or slow correction? Am J Med 1990;88:161.
61. Sterns RH. The treatment of hyponatremia: first, do no harm. Am J Med 1990;88:557.
62. Gross P. Treatment of severe hyponatremia. Kidney Int 2001;60:2417.
63. Arieff AI. Hyponatremia, convulsions, respiratory arrest, and permanent brain damage after elective surgery in healthy women. N Engl J Med 1986; 314:1529.
64. Ayus JC et al. Postoperative hyponatremic encephalopathy in menstruant women. Ann Intern Med 1992;117:891.
65. Lien Y et al. Study of brain electrolytes and organic osmolytes during correction of chronic hyponatremia: implications for the pathogenesis of central pontine myelinolysis. J Clin Invest 1991;88:303.
66. Berl T. Treating hyponatremia: damned if we do and damned if we don't. Kidney Int 1990;37:1006.
67. Chung HM et al. Post-operative hyponatremia. Arch Intern Med 1986;314:1529.
68. Cochrane JPS et al. Arginine vasopressin release following surgical operations. Br J Surg 1981;68:209.
69. DeFronzo RA et al. Water intoxication in man after cyclophosphamide therapy. Time course and relation to drug activation. Ann Intern Med 1973; 78:861.
70. Morgan DB et al. Water intoxication and oxytocin infusion. Br J Obstet Gynaecol 1977;84:6.
71. Cheng JC et al. Long-term neurologic outcome in psychogenic water drinkers with severe symptomatic hyponatremia: the effect of rapid correction. Am J Med 1990;88:561.
72. Laureno R et al. Pontine and extrapontine myelinolysis following rapid correction of hyponatremia. Lancet 1988;1(8600):1439.
73. Lohr JW. Osmotic demyelination syndrome following correction of hyponatremia: association with hypokalemia. Am J Med 1994;96:408.

74. Sterns RH et al. Neurologic sequelae after treatment of severe hyponatremia: a multicenter perspective. J Am Soc Nephrol 1994;4:1522.
75. Decaux G. Treatment of the syndrome of inappropriate secretion of antidiuretic hormone by long-loop diuretics. Nephron 1983;35:82.
76. Decaux G et al. Treatment of the syndrome of inappropriate secretion of antidiuretic hormone with furosemide. N Engl J Med 1981;304:329.
77. Cherill DA et al. Demeclocycline treatment in the syndrome of antidiuretic hormone secretion. Ann Intern Med 1975;83:654.
78. White MG et al. Treatment of the syndrome of inappropriate secretion of antidiuretic hormone with lithium carbonate. N Engl J Med 1975;292:390.
79. Miller PD et al. Plasma demeclocycline levels and nephrotoxicity: correlation in hyponatremic cirrhotic patients. JAMA 1980;243:2513.
80. Palm C, Gross P. V2-vasopressin receptor antagonists-mechanism of effect and clinical implication in hyponatraemia. Nephrol Dial Transplant 1999;14:2559.
81. Guyader D, Patat A, Ellis-Grosse EJ, Orczyk GP. Pharmacodynamic effects of a nonpeptide antidiuretic hormone V2 antagonist in cirrhotic patients with ascites. Hepatology 2002;36:1197.
82. Wong F, Blei AT, Blendis LM, Thuluvath PJ. A vasopressin receptor antagonist (VPA-985) improves serum sodium concentration in patients with hyponatremia: a multicenter, randomized, placebo-controlled trial. Hepatology 2003;37:182.
83. Decaux G et al. Lack of efficacy of phenytoin in the syndrome of inappropriate antidiuretic hormone secretion of neurological origin. Postgrad Med J 1989;65:456.
84. Decaux G et al. 5-year treatment of the chronic syndrome of inappropriate secretion of ADH with oral urea. Nephron 1993;63:468.
85. Decaux G et al. Hyponatremia in the syndrome of inappropriate secretion of antidiuretic hormone. Rapid correction with urea, sodium chloride, and water restriction. JAMA 1982;247:471.
86. Morrison G et al. Hyperosmolal states. In: Narins RG, ed. Maxwell & Kleeman's Clinical Disorders of Fluid and Electrolyte Metabolism. 5th Ed. New York: McGraw-Hill, 1994.
87. Snyder NA et al. Hypernatremia in elderly patients: a heterogeneous, morbid, and iatrogenic entity. Ann Intern Med 1987;107:309.
88. Beerman B, Groschinsky-Grind M. Clinical pharmacokinetics of diuretics. Clin Pharmacokinet 1980;5:221.
89. Merkus F. Is canrenone the major metabolite of spironolactone? Clin Pharm 1983;2:209.
90. Sklath H, Gums J. Spironolactone: a re-examination. DICP. Ann Pharmacother 1990;24:52.
91. Pruitt AW et al. Variations in the fate of triamterene. Clin Pharmacol Ther 1977;21:610.
92. Sterns RH et al. Internal potassium balance and the control of the plasma potassium concentration. Medicine 1981;60:339.
93. Allon M. Treatment and prevention of hyperkalemia in end-stage renal disease. Kidney Int 1993;43:1197.
94. Perrone RD, Alexander EA. Regulation of extrarenal potassium metabolism. In: Narins RG, ed. Maxwell & Kleeman's Clinical Disorders of Fluid and Electrolyte Metabolism. 5th Ed. New York: McGraw-Hill, 1994.
95. Salem MM et al. Extrarenal potassium tolerance in chronic renal failure: implications for the treatment of acute hyperkalemia. Am J Kidney Dis 1991;18:421.
96. Field MJ et al. Regulation of renal potassium metabolism. In: Narins RG, ed. Maxwell & Kleeman's Clinical Disorders of Fluid and Electrolyte Metabolism. 5th Ed. New York: McGraw-Hill, 1994:147.
97. Wright FS. Renal potassium handling. Semin Nephrol 1987;7:174.
98. Sterns RH et al. The disposition of intravenous potassium in normal man: the role of insulin. Clin Sci 1987;73:557.
99. Williams ME et al. Impairment of extrarenal potassium disposal by alpha-adrenergic stimulation. N Engl J Med 1984;311:345.

100. Rosa RM et al. Adrenergic modulation of extrarenal potassium disposal. N Engl J Med 1980;302:431.
101. Androgue HJ et al. Changes in plasma potassium concentration during acute acid-base disturbances. Am J Med 1981;71:456.
102. Oster JR et al. Plasma potassium response to acute metabolic acidosis induced by mineral and nonmineral acids. Miner Electrolyte Metab 1980;4:28.
103. Androgue HJ et al. Determinants of plasma potassium levels in diabetic ketoacidosis. Medicine 1986;65:163.
104. Hazeyama Y et al. A model of potassium efflux during exercise of skeletal muscle. Am J Physiol 1979;236:R83.
105. Krishna GG et al. Hypokalemic states. In: Narins RG, ed. Maxwell & Kleeman's Clinical Disorders of Fluid and Electrolyte Metabolism. 5th Ed. New York: McGraw-Hill, 1994.
106. Johnsen T. Familial periodic paralysis with hypokalemia. Dan Med Bull 1981;28(1):1.
107. Moravec MD et al. Hypokalemia associated with terbutaline administration in obstetrical patients. Anesth Analg 1980;59:917.
108. Kethersid TL et al. Dialysate potassium. Semin Dial 1991;4:46.
109. Moore EW. Ionized calcium in normal serum, ultrafiltrates and whole blood determined by ion-exchange electrode. J Clin Invest 1970;49:318.
110. Kassirer JP et al. The response of normal man to selective depletion of hydrochloric acid: factors in the genesis of persistent gastric alkalosis. Am J Med 1966;40:10.
111. Adams PC et al. Exaggerated hypokalemia in acute myeloid leukemia. Br Med J 1981;282:1034.
112. Knochel JP. Neuromuscular manifestations of electrolyte disorders. Am J Med 1982;75:521.
113. Surawicz B. Relationship between electrocardiogram and electrolytes. Am Heart J 1967;73:814.
114. Smith SR et al. Potassium chloride lowers blood pressure and causes natriuresis in older patients with hypertension. J Am Soc Nephrol 1992;2:1032.
115. Helderman JH et al. Prevention of the glucose intolerance of thiazide diuretics by maintenance of the body potassium. Diabetes 1983;32:106.
116. Tizianello A et al. Renal ammoniagenesis in humans with chronic potassium depletion. Kidney Int 1991;40:772.
117. Stanaszek WF et al. Current approaches to management of potassium deficiency. Drug Intell Clin Pharm 1985;19:176.
118. Kruse JA et al. Rapid correction of hypokalemia using concentrated intravenous potassium chloride infusions. Arch Intern Med 1990;150:613.
119. Kunin AS et al. Decrease in serum potassium concentration and appearance of cardiac arrhythmias during infusion of potassium with glucose in potassium-depleted patients. N Engl J Med 1962;266:228.
120. Bronson WR. et al. Pseudohyperkalemia due to release of potassium from white blood cells during clotting. N Engl J Med 1966;274:369.
121. Ingram RH Jr et al. Pseudohyperkalemia with thrombocytosis. N Engl J Med 1962;267:895.
122. Mather A et al. Effects of hemolysis on serum electrolyte values. Clin Chem 1960;6:223.
123. Romano AT et al. Mild forearm exercise during venipuncture and its effect on potassium determinations. Clin Chem 1977;2:303.
124. Morton AR. Bisphosphonates for the hypercalcemia of malignancy in end-stage renal disease. Semin Dialysis 1994;7:76.
125. Cohen LF et al. Acute tumor lysis syndrome. Am J Med 1980;68:486.
126. Perazella MA. Drug-induced hyperkalemia: old culprits and new offenders. Am J Med 2000;109:307.
127. Reston RA, et al. University of Miami Division of Clinical Pharmacology therapeutic rounds: drug-induced hyperkalemia. Am J Ther 1998;5:125.
128. Rimmer et al. Hyperkalemia as a complication of drug therapy. Arch Intern Med 1987;147:867.
129. DeFronzo RA et al. Clinical disorders of hyperkalemia. In: Narins RG, ed. Maxwell & Kleeman's Clinical Disorders of Fluid and Electrolyte Metabolism. 5th Ed. New York: McGraw-Hill, 1994:697.
130. DeFronzo RA. Hyperkalemia and hyporeninemic hypoaldosteronism. Kidney Int 1980;17:118.
131. Kurtzman NA et al. A patient with hyperkalemia and metabolic acidosis. Am J Kidney Dis 1990;15:333.
132. Fraser R. Disorders of the adrenal cortex: their effects on electrolyte metabolism. Clin Endocrinol Metab 1984;13:413.
133. Reardon LC, MacPherson DS. Hyperkalemia in outpatients using angiotensin-converting enzyme inhibitors: How much should we worry? Arch Intern Med 1998;158:26.
134. Schlondorff D. Renal complications of nonsteroidal anti-inflammatory drugs. Kidney Int 1993;44:643.
135. Bakris GL et al. ACE inhibition or angiotensin receptor blockade: impact on potassium in renal failure. VAL-K Study Group. Kidney Int 2000;58:2084.
136. Lundborg P. The effect of adrenergic blockade on potassium concentrations in different conditions. Acta Med Scand 1983;672(suppl):121.
137. Goggans FC. Acute hyperkalemia during lithium treatment of manic illness. Am J Psychiatry 1980;137:860.
138. Abdel-Raheem MM et al. Effect of low-molecular-weight heparin on potassium homeostasis. Pathophysiol Haemost Thromb 2002;32:107.
139. Oster JR et al. Heparin-induced aldosterone suppression and hyperkalemia. Am J Med 1995;98:575
140. Briceland LL, Bailie GR. Pentamidine-associated nephrotoxicity and hyperkalemia in patients with AIDS. DICP 1991;25:1171.
141. Velazquez H et al. Renal mechanisms of trimethoprim-induced hyperkalemia. Ann Intern Med 1993;119:296.
142. Alappan R et al. Trimethoprim-sulfamethoxazole therapy in outpatients: is hyperkalemia a significant problem? Am J Nephrol 1999;19:389.
143. Caliskan Y et al. Cyclosporine-associated hyperkalemia: report of four allogeneic blood stem-cell transplant cases. Transplantation 2003;75:1069.
144. Woo M et al. Toxicities of tacrolimus and cyclosporin A after allogeneic blood stem cell transplantation. Bone Marrow Transplant 1997;20;1095.
145. Bismuth C et al. Hyperkalemia in acute digitalis poisoning: prognostic significance and therapeutic implications. Clin Toxicol 1973;6:153.
146. Bushinsky DA et al. Life-threatening hyperkalemia induced by arginine. Ann Intern Med 1978;89:632.
147. Cooperman LH. Succinylcholine-induced hyperkalemia in neuromuscular disease. JAMA 1970;213:1867.
148. Blumberg A et al. Effect of various therapeutic approaches on plasma potassium and major regulating factors in terminal renal failure. Am J Med 1988;85:507.
149. Nicolis GL et al. Glucose-induced hyperkalemia in diabetic subjects. Arch Intern Med 1981;141:49.
150. Allon M et al. Effect of insulin-plus-glucose with or without epinephrine on fasting hyperkalemia. Kidney Int 1993;43:212.
151. Wong SL, Maltz HC. Albuterol for the treatment of hyperkalemia. Ann Pharmather 1999;33:103.
152. Allon M. Hyperkalemia in end stage renal disease: mechanism and management. J Am Soc Nephrol 1995;6:1134.
153. Liou HH et al. Hypokalemic effects of intravenous infusion or nebulization of salbutamol in patients with chronic renal failure: comparative study. Am J Kidney Dis 1994;23:266.
154. Allon M et al. Albuterol and insulin for treatment of hyperkalemia in hemodialysis patients. Kidney Int 1990;38:869.
155. Gutierrez R et al. Effect of hypertonic versus isotonic sodium bicarbonate on plasma potassium concentrations in patients with end-stage renal disease. Miner Electrolyte Metab 1991;17:291.
156. Scherr L et al. Management of hyperkalemia with a cation-exchange resin. N Engl J Med 1961;264:115.
157. Gestman BB et al. Intestinal necrosis associated with postoperative orally administered sodium polystyrene sulfonate in sorbitol. Am J Kidney Dis 1992;20:159.
158. Brown ST et al. Potassium removal with peritoneal dialysis. Kidney Int 1973;4:67.
159. Sherman RA et al. Variability in potassium removal by hemodialysis. Am J Nephrol 1986;6:284.
160. Ward RA et al. Hemodialysate composition and intradialytic metabolic acid-base and potassium changes. Kidney Int 1987;32:129.
161. Lindgarde F et al. Hypercalcemia and normal ionized serum calcium in a case of myelomatosis. Ann Intern Med 1973;78:396.
162. Favus MJ. Transport of calcium by intestinal mucosa. Semin Nephrol 1981;1:306.
163. LeRoith D et al. Bone metabolism and composition in the protein-deprived rat. Clin Sci 1973;44:305.
164. Bourdeau JE, Attie M. In: Narins RG, ed. Maxwell & Kleeman's Clinical Disorders of Fluid and Electrolyte Metabolism. 5th Ed. New York: McGraw-Hill, 1994:243.
165. Benabe JE et al. Disorders of calcium metabolism. In: Narins RG, ed. Maxwell & Kleeman's Disorders of Fluid and Electrolyte Metabolism. 5th Ed. New York: McGraw-Hill, 1994:1009.
166. Mundy GR. Pathophysiology of cancer-associated hypercalcemia. Semin Oncol 1990;17(Suppl. 5):10.
167. Ladenson JH et al. Relationship of free and total calcium in hypercalcemic conditions. J Clin Endocrinol Metab 1979;48:393.
168. Beck N et al. Pathogenetic role of cyclic AMP in the impairment of urinary concentrating ability in acute hypercalcemia. J Clin Invest 1974;54:1049.
169. Bajorunas DR. Clinical manifestations of cancer-related hypercalcemia. Semin Oncol 1990, 17(Suppl. 5):16.
170. Suki WN et al. Acute treatment of hypercalcemia with furosemide. N Engl J Med 1970;283:836.
171. Davidson TG. Conventional treatment of hypercalcemia of malignancy. Am J Health Syst Pharm 2001;58(Suppl 3):S8.
172. Ardaillou R et al. Renal excretion of phosphate, calcium and sodium during and after a prolonged thyrocalcitonin infusion in man. Proc Soc Exp Biol Med 1969;131:56.
173. Singer FR et al. An evaluation of antibodies and clinical resistance to salmon calcitonin. J Clin Invest 1972;51:2331.
174. Minstock ML et al. Effect of calcitonin and glucocorticoids in combination on the hypercalcemia of malignancy. Ann Intern Med 1980;93:269.
175. Ritch PS. Treatment of cancer-related hypercalcemia. Semin Oncol 1990;17(Suppl. 5):26.
176. Caro JF et al. Symptomatic hypocalcemia following combined calcitonin and mithramycin therapy for hypercalcemia due to malignancy. Cancer Treat Rep 1978;62:1561.
177. Green L et al. Hepatic toxicity of low doses of mithramycin in hypercalcemia. Cancer Treat Rep 1984;68:1379.
178. Major P. The use of zoledronic acid, a novel, highly potent bisphosphonate, for the treatment of hypercalcemia of malignancy. Oncologist 2002;7:481.
179. Ryzen E et al. Intravenous etidronate in the management of malignant hypercalcemia. Arch Intern Med 1985;145:449.
180. Gucalp R et al. Comparative study of pamidronate disodium and etidronate disodium in the treatment of cancer-related hypercalcemia. J Clin Oncol 1992;10:134.
181. Bounameaux HM et al. Renal failure associated with intravenous diphosphonates. Lancet 1983;1:471.
182. Francis MD et al. Acute intravenous infusions of disodium dihydrogen (1-hydroxy-ethylidene)

diphosphonate: mechanisms of cytotoxicity. J Pharm Sci 1983;73:1097.

183. Major P et al. Zoledronic acid is superior to pamidronate in the treatment of hypercalcemia of malignancy: a pooled analysis of two randomized, controlled clinical trials. J Clin Oncol 2001;19:558.

184. Brenson JR. Advances in the biology and treatment of myeloma bone disease. Am J Health-Syst Pharm 2001;58(Suppl 3):S16.

185. Widman L et al. Effect of Moduretic and Aldactone on electrolytes on skeletal muscle in patients on long-term diuretic therapy. Acta Med Scand 1982;661(Suppl.):33.

186. Todd PA, Fitton A. Gallium nitrate: a review of its pharmacological properties and therapeutic potential in cancer-related hypercalcemia. Drugs 1991; 42:261.

187. Warrell RP Jr. Clinical trials of gallium nitrate in patients with cancer-related hypercalcemia. Semin Oncol 1991;18(Suppl. 5):26.

188. Hughes TE et al. Gallium nitrate. Ann Pharmacother 1992;26:354.

189. Haussler MR et al. Basic and clinical concepts related to vitamin D metabolism and action. N Engl J Med 1977;297:974.

190. Kalbfleisch JM et al. Effects of ethanol administration on urinary excretion of magnesium and other electrolytes in alcoholic and normal subjects. J Clin Invest 1963;42:1471.

191. Streck WF et al. Glucocorticoid effects in vitamin D intoxication. Arch Intern Med 1979;139:974.

192. Baughman RP et al. Sarcoidosis. Lancet 2003;361:1111.

193. Smith BJ et al. Prostaglandins and cancer. Ann Clin Lab Sci. 1983;13:359.

194. Dennis VW. Phosphate disorders. In: Kokko JP, Tannen RL, eds. Fluids and Electrolytes. 3rd Ed. Philadelphia: WB Saunders, 1996:359.

195. Oster JR et al. Management of magnesium depletion. Am J Nephrol 1988;8:349.

196. Agus Z. Hypomagnesemia. J Am Soc Nephrol 1999;10:1616.

197. Alfrey AC. Normal and abnormal magnesium metabolism. In: Schrier RW, ed. Renal and Electrolyte Disorders. 6th Ed. Philadelphia: Lippincott Williams & Wilkins, 2003.

198. Flink EB. Magnesium deficiency in alcoholism. Alcoholism: clinical and experimental research. Alcohol Clin Exp Res 1986;10:590.

199. Harrison HE et al. The effect of acidosis upon renal tubular reabsorption of phosphate. Am J Physiol 1941;134:781.

200. Moog F et al. Phosphate absorption and alkaline phosphatase activity in the small intestine of the adult mouse and of the chick embryo and hatched chick. Comp Biochem Physiol 1972;42A:321.

201. Fox J et al. Stimulation of duodenal and head absorption of phosphate in the chick by low-calcium and low-phosphate diets. Calcif Tissue Int 1978;26:243.

202. Brommage R et al. Vitamin D-independent intestinal calcium and phosphorus absorption during reproduction. Am J Physiol 1990;259:G631.

203. Sheikh MS et al. Reduction of dietary phosphorus absorption by phosphorus binders. J Clin Invest 1989;83:66.

204. Levine BS et al. Hypophosphatemia and hyperphosphatemia: clinical and pathologic aspects. In: Narins RG, ed. Maxwell & Kleeman's Clinical Disorders of Fluid and Electrolyte Metabolism. 5th Ed. New York: McGraw-Hill, 1994:1045.

205. Portale AA et al. Dietary intake of phosphorus modulates the circadian rhythm in serum concentration of phosphorus: implications for the renal production of 1,25-dihyroxyvitamin D. J Clin Invest 1987;80:1147.

206. Eisenbrey AB et al. Mannitol interference in an automated serum phosphate assay. Clin Chem 1987;33:2308.

207. Lee DBN et al. Effect of phosphorus depletion on intestinal calcium and phosphorus absorption. Am J Physiol 1979;236:E451.

208. Crook MA et al. The importance of the refeeding syndrome. Nutrition 2001;17:632.

209. Lotz M et al. Evidence for phosphorus depletion syndrome in man. N Engl J Med 1968;278:409.

210. Roxe DM et al. Phosphate-binding effects of sucralfate in patients with chronic renal failure. Am J Kidney Dis 1989;13:194.

211. Cox GJ et al. The effects of high doses of aluminum and iron on phosphorus metabolism. J Biol Chem 1931;92:11.

212. Marwich TH et al. Severe hypophosphatemia induced by glucose-insulin-potassium therapy: a case report and proposal for altered protocol. Int J Cardiol 1988;18:327.

213. Stein JH et al. Hypophosphatemia in acute alcoholism. Am J Med 1996;252:78.

214. Fiaccadori E et al. Hypophosphatemia in course of chronic obstructive pulmonary disease: prevalence, mechanisms, and relationships with skeletal muscle phosphorus content. Chest 1990;97:857.

215. Lennquist S et al. Hypophosphatemia in severe burns. A prospective study. Acta Chir Scand 1979; 145:1.

216. Kebler R et al. Dynamic changes in serum phosphorus levels in diabetic ketoacidosis. Am J Med 1985;79:571.

217. Massry SG. The clinical syndrome of phosphate depletion. Adv Exp Med Biol 1978;103:301.

218. Lichtman MA et al. Reduced red cell glycolysis, 1,2-diphosphoglycerate and adenosine triphosphate concentration and increased hemoglobin-oxygen affinity caused by hypophosphatemia. Ann Intern Med 1971;74:562.

219. Narins RG et al. Diagnostic strategies in disorders of fluid, electrolyte and acid-base homeostasis. Am J Med 1982;72:496.

220. Subramanian R, Khardori R. Severe hypophosphatemia. Pathophysiologic implications, clinical presentations, and treatment. Medicine 2000;79:1.

221. Rubin MF, Narins RG. Hypophosphatemia: pathophysiological and practical aspects of its therapy. Semin Nephrol 1990;10:536.

222. Widdowson EM et al. Chemical composition of human body. Clin Sci 1951;10:113.

223. Wacker WEC, Parisi AF. Magnesium metabolism. N Engl J Med 1968;278:658.

224. Kurachi Y et al. Role of intracellular Mg^{2+} in the activation of muscarinic K^+ channel in cardiac atrial cell membrane. Pflugers Arch 1986;407:572.

225. White RE et al. Magnesium ions in cardiac function. Regulator of ion channels and second messengers. Biochem Pharmacol 1989;38:859.

226. Seelig MS. The magnesium requirement by the normal adult: summary and analysis of published data. Am J Clin Nutr 1964;14:212.

227. Jones JE et al. Magnesium requirements in adults. Am J Clin Nutr 1967;20:632.

228. Schmulen AC et al. Effect of 1,25-(OH)$_2$D$_3$ on jejunal absorption of magnesium in patients with chronic renal disease. Am J Physiol 1980;238:G349.

229. Heaton FW. The parathyroid glands and magnesium metabolism in the rat. Clin Sci 1965;28:543.

230. Quamme GA. Renal magnesium handling: new insights in understanding old problems. Kidney Int 1997;52.

231. Massry SG et al. Renal handling of magnesium in the dog. Am J Physiol 1969;216:1460.

232. Lennon EJ et al. A comparison of the effects of glucose ingestion and NH$_4$Cl acidosis on urinary calcium and magnesium excretion in man. J Clin Invest 1970;49:1458.

233. Quamme GA. Effect of furosemide on calcium and magnesium transport in the rat nephron. Am J Physiol 1981;241:F340.

234. Wong NLM et al. Effects of mannitol on water and electrolyte transport in the dog kidney. J Lab Clin Med 1979;94:683.

235. Morel F. Sites of hormone action in the mammalian nephron. Am J Physiol 1981;240:F159.

236. Massry SG et al. The hormonal and non-hormonal control of renal excretion of calcium and magnesium. Nephron 1973;10:66.

237. Horton R et al. Effect of aldosterone on the metabolism of magnesium. Clin Endocrinol Metab 1962;22:1187.

238. Lim P et al. Tissue magnesium levels in chronic diarrhea. J Lab Clin Med 1977;80:313.

239. Alfrey AC et al. Evaluation of body magnesium stores. J Lab Clin Med 1974;84:153.

240. Thoren L. Magnesium metabolism. Proc Surg 1971;9:131.

241. Potts JT et al. Clinical significance of magnesium deficiency and its relationship to parathyroid disease. Am J Med Sci 1958;235:205.

242. Jackson CE et al. Routine serum magnesium analysis: correlation with clinical state in 5100 patients. Ann Intern Med 1968;69:743.

243. Rasmussen HS et al. Intravenous magnesium in acute myocardial infarction. Lancet 1986;1:234.

244. Chernow B et al. Hypomagnesemia in patients in post-operative intensive care. Chest 1989;95:391.

245. Shils ME. Experimental human magnesium depletion. Medicine 1969;118:61.

246. Caddell JL et al. Studies in protein-calorie malnutrition. 1: Chemical evidence for magnesium deficiency. N Engl J Med 1967;276:533.

247. Flink EB et al. Magnesium deficiency after prolonged parenteral fluid administration and after chronic alcoholism, complicated by delirium tremens. J Lab Clin Med 1954;43:169.

248. Baron DN. Magnesium deficiency after gastrointestinal surgery and loss of excretions. Br J Surg 1960;48:344.

249. Coons CM et al. The retention of nitrogen, calcium, phosphorus and magnesium by pregnant women. J Biol Chem 1930;86:1.

250. Booth CC et al. Incidence of hypomagnesaemia in intestinal malabsorption. Br Med J 1963;2:141.

251. Hallberg DAG. Magnesium problems in gastroenterology. Acta Med Scand 1961:62.

252. Thoren L. Magnesium deficiency in gastrointestinal fluid loss. Acta Chir Scand 1963;306(Suppl.):1.

253. Milla PJ et al. Studies in primary hypomagnesemia: evidence for defective carrier-mediated small intestinal transport of magnesium. Gut 1979;20:1028.

254. Evans RA et al. The congenital magnesium-losing kidney: report of two patients. Q J Med 1981;197:39.

255. Lam M et al. Hypomagnesemia and renal magnesium wasting in patients treated with cisplatin. Am J Kidney Dis 1986;8:164.

256. Keating MJ et al. Hypocalcemia with hypoparathyroidism and renal tubular dysfunction associated with aminoglycoside therapy. Cancer 1977;39:1410.

257. Wong NLM et al. Cyclosporin-induced hypomagnesaemia and renal magnesium wasting in rats. Clin Sci 1988;75:505.

258. Barton CH et al. Renal magnesium wasting associated with amphotericin B therapy. Am J Med 1984;77:471.

259. Coburn JW et al. Changes in serum and urinary calcium during phosphate depletion. Studies on mechanisms. J Clin Invest 1970;49:1073.

260. Quamme GA, Dirks JH. Magnesium transport in the nephron. Am J Physiol 1980;8:393.

261. Butler AM et al. Metabolic studies in diabetic coma. Trans Assoc Am Phys 1947;60:102.

262. Flink EB et al. Magnesium deficiency after prolonged parenteral fluid administration and after chronic alcoholism, complicated by delirium tremens. J Lab Clin Med 1954;43:169.

263. Hellman ES et al. Abnormal water and electrolyte metabolism in acute intermittent porphyria: transient inappropriate secretion of antidiuretic hormone. Am J Med 1962;32:734.

264. Tapley DF. Magnesium balance in myxedematous patients treated with triiodothyronine. Johns Hopkins Med J 1955;96:274.

265. Heaton FW, Pyrah LN. Magnesium metabolism in patients with parathyroid disorders. Clin Sci Mol Med 1963;25:475.

266. Seelig MS. Magnesium deficiency and cardiac dysrhythmia. In: Seelig MS, ed. Magnesium Defi-

ciency in Pathogenesis of Disease. New York: Plenum, 1980:219.

267. Iseri LT. Magnesium and cardiac arrhythmias. Magnesium 1986;5:111.

268. Flink EB. Therapy of magnesium deficiency. Ann NY Acad Sci 1969;162:901.

269. Iseri LT, French JH. Magnesium: nature's physiologic calcium blocker. Am Heart J 1984;108:188.

270. Rude RK et al. Renal tubular maximum for magnesium in normal, hyperparathyroid, and hypoparathyroid man. J Clin Endocrinol Metab 1980;51:1425.

271. Coburn JW et al. The physicochemical state and renal handling of divalent ions in chronic renal failure. Arch Intern Med 1967;124:302.

272. Massry SG et al. Divalent ion metabolism in patients with acute renal failure: studies on the mechanisms of hypocalcemia. Kidney Int 1974;5:437.

273. Mordes JP, Wacker WEC. Excess magnesium. Pharmacol Rev 1978;29:273.

274. Jones J et al. Cathartic-induced magnesium toxicity during overdose management. Ann Emerg Med 1986;15:1214.

275. Pritchard JA. The use of magnesium ion in the management of eclamptogenic toxemias. Surg Gynecol Obstet 1955;100:131.

276. Alfrey AC et al. Hypermagnesemia after renal homotransplantation. Ann Intern Med 1970;73:367.

CARDIAC AND VASCULAR DISORDERS

Wayne A. Kradjan
SECTION EDITOR

CHAPTER 13

Dyslipidemias, Atherosclerosis, and Coronary Heart Disease

James M. McKenney

Dyslipidemias (one or more abnormalities of blood lipids) produce atherosclerosis, which in turn produces coronary heart (artery) disease (CHD, CAD). Successful management of dyslipidemias alters the natural course of atherosclerosis and prevents CHD. This is the simple but profound notion behind the modern approach to reducing the incidence of the nation's number-one killer. The challenge for the clinician is to know how to assess the patient's CHD risk, to understand lipid-modulating therapies, to match the intensity of treatment with the patient's risk, and to implement treatments that meet and maintain treatment goals. The principal focus of this chapter is on providing the information required to meet this challenge.

Lipid Metabolism and Drug Effects

The journey begins with acquiring an understanding of how lipids are formed, transported, and utilized; how these processes can go awry; and how our therapies alter these aberrant processes. At the center of these processes are cholesterol, triglycerides, and phospholipids. Of these three, cholesterol plays the central role in the pathogenesis of atherosclerosis. Cholesterol is a naturally occurring alcohol that is essential for life. It is the precursor molecule for the formation of bile acids (which are required for absorption of nutrients), the synthesis of steroid hormones (which provide important modulating effects in the body), and the formation of cell membranes.

In Vivo Cholesterol Synthesis

Cells derive cholesterol in two ways: by intracellular synthesis or by uptake from the systemic circulation. Within each cell, cholesterol is synthesized through a series of biochemical steps, many of which are catalyzed by enzymes[1] (Fig. 13-1). One important and early step in its synthesis is the conversion of hydroxymethylglutaryl-coenzyme A (HMG-CoA) to mevalonic acid. The enzyme HMG-CoA reductase catalyzes this step. One of the most effective therapies developed to date for managing dyslipidemias (i.e., HMG-CoA reductase inhibitors or statins) interferes with this enzyme and thereby reduces the cellular synthesis of cholesterol. Other catalytic enzymes involved in the biosynthesis of cholesterol, including HMG-CoA synthase and squalene synthase, have been targets in the search for therapies to reduce cholesterol synthesis. Unfortunately, drugs modifying these enzymes caused more, not less, atherosclerotic disease. For example, a drug released for cholesterol lowering in the 1950s, MER 29, interfered with a late step in cholesterol biosynthesis and effectively reduced cellular cholesterol production, but caused a toxic accumulation of desmosterol and other cholesterol precursors that resulted in the development of cataracts and myocardial ischemia.

Intracellular cholesterol is stored in an esterified form. Free cholesterol is converted to this ester form through the action of the enzyme acetyl CoA acetyl transferase (ACAT). ACAT also is required for the esterification and absorption of dietary cholesterol from the gut. In theory, inhibition of this enzyme should reduce the absorption of dietary cholesterol, the secretion of cholesterol by the liver, and even the uptake and storage of circulating cholesterol in artery beds. Several inhibitors of ACAT have been developed. These drugs generally produce only modest effects on plasma cholesterol levels, but studies are ongoing to determine if interference with the penetration of cholesterol into artery walls will alter the pathogenesis of atherosclerosis.

Lipoproteins

The second way cells obtain cholesterol is by extracting it from the systemic circulation. The source of this cholesterol is the liver, where it is synthesized and secreted into the systemic circulation. Because cholesterol and other fatty substances are insoluble in water, they are formed into complexes (particles) in the hepatocyte and gut before being secreted into the aqueous medium of the blood. These particles contain an oily inner lipid core made up of cholesterol esters and triglycerides (TGs) and an outer hydrophilic coat made up of phospholipids and unesterified cholesterol (Fig. 13-2). The outer coat also contains at least one protein, which provides the ligand for interaction with receptors on cell surfaces. The presence of a central lipid core and an outer protein gives rise to the name of these particles, *lipoproteins.*

The three major lipoproteins found in the blood of fasting patients are very-low-density lipoprotein (VLDL), low-density lipoprotein (LDL), and high-density lipoprotein (HDL).[2] These particles vary in size, composition, and accompanying proteins (Table 13-1).

VERY-LOW-DENSITY LIPOPROTEINS

VLDL particles are formed in the liver and to a lesser extent in the intestine (Fig. 13-3). They normally contain 15% to 20% of the total blood cholesterol concentration and most of the total blood TG concentration. The concentration of cholesterol in these particles is approximately one fifth of the total TG concentration; thus, if the total TG concentration is known, the VLDL-cholesterol (VLDL-C) level can be estimated by dividing total TG by 5. VLDL particles are large and appear to play only a small role in the pathogenesis of atherosclerosis.

VLDL REMNANTS

As VLDL particles flow through capillaries, some of their TG content is removed through the action of the enzyme lipoprotein lipase. Drugs that enhance the activity of lipoprotein lipase (i.e., fibrates) increase the delipidization process and lower blood TG levels. The removed TG is converted to fatty acids and stored as an energy source in adipose tissue. As TGs are removed, the VLDL particle becomes progressively smaller and relatively more cholesterol rich. The particles formed through this process include small VLDL particles (called remnant VLDL), intermediate-density lipoproteins (IDL), and LDL (see Fig. 13-3). Approximately 50% of the remnant VLDL and IDL particles are removed from the systemic circulation by receptors on the surface of the liver (receptors called LDL or B-E receptors); the other 50% are converted into LDL particles.

LOW-DENSITY LIPOPROTEINS

LDL particles carry 60% to 70% of the total blood cholesterol and make the greatest contribution to the development of atherosclerosis. This is why LDL-C is the primary target of cholesterol-lowering therapy. Approximately half of the LDL particles are removed from the systemic circulation by the liver; the other half may be taken up by peripheral cells or deposited in the intimal space of coronary, carotid, and other

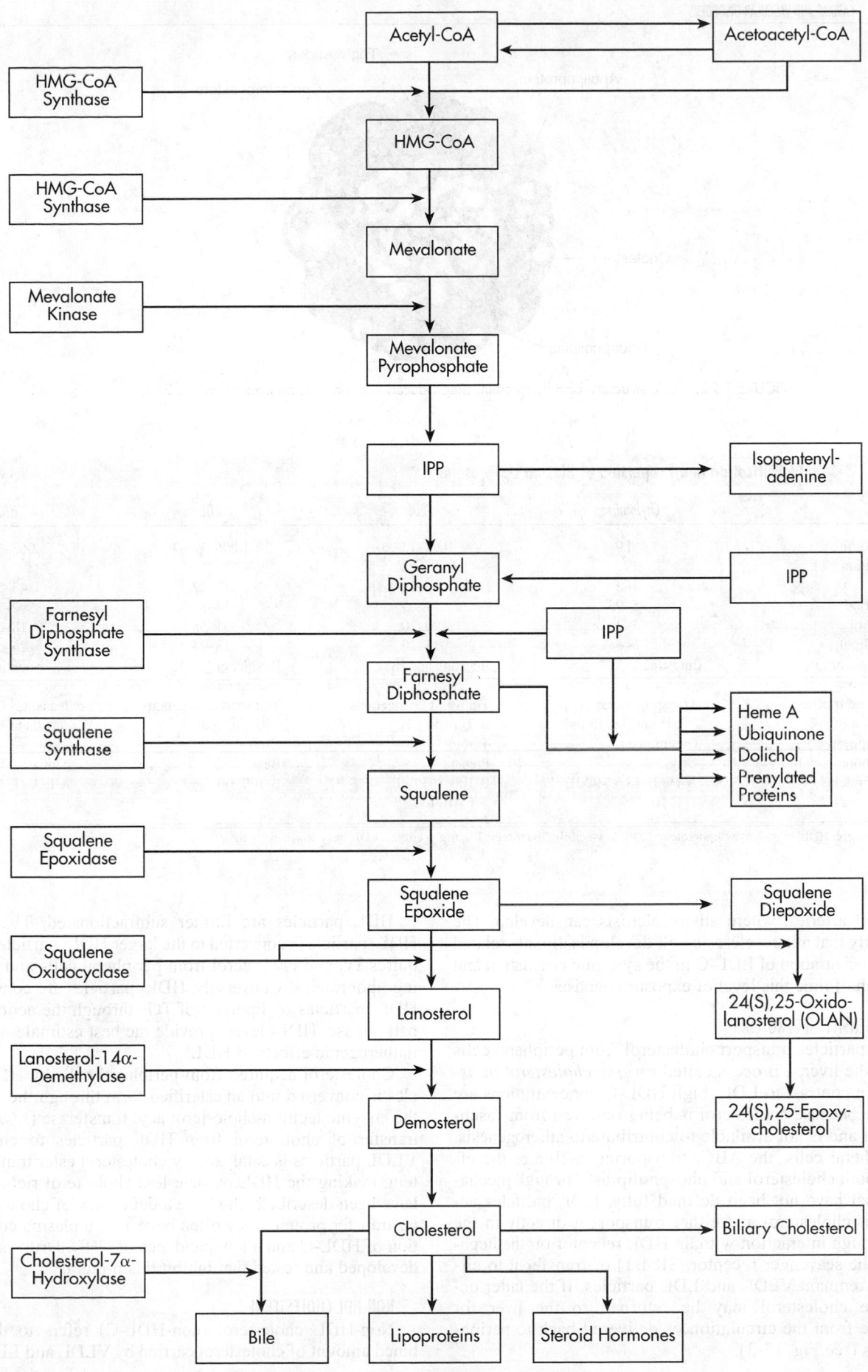

FIGURE 13-1. Biosynthetic pathway of cholesterol.

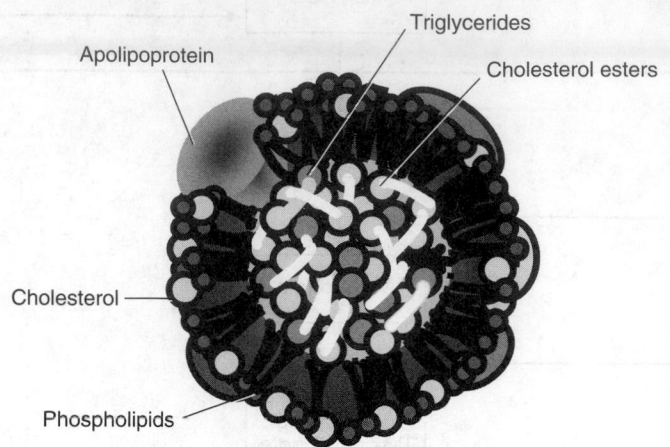

FIGURE 13-2. Basic structure of a lipoprotein. (Reproduced with permission from reference 273)

Table 13-1   Classification and Properties of Plasma Lipoproteins

	Chylomicron	*VLDL*	*LDL*	*HDL*
Density (g/mL)	<0.94	0.94–1.006	1.006–1.063	1.063–1.210
Composition (%)				
Protein	1–2	6–10	18–22	45–55
Triglyceride	85–95	50–65	4–8	2–7
Cholesterol	3–7	20–30	51–58	18–25
Phospholipid	3–6	15–20	18–24	26–32
Physiologic origin	Intestine	Intestine and liver	Product of VLDL catabolism	Liver and intestine
Physiologic function	Transport dietary CH and TG to liver	Transport endogenous TG and CH	Transport endogenous CH to cells	Transport CH from cells to liver
Plasma appearance	Cream layer	Turbid	Clear	Clear
Electrophoretic mobility	Origin	Prebeta	Beta	Alpha
Apolipoproteins	A-IV, B-48, C-IC-II, C-III	B-100, C-IC-III, C-III, E	B-100, (a)	A-I, A-II, A-IV

CH, cholesterol; HDL, high-density lipoprotein; LDL, low-density lipoprotein; TG, triglyceride; VLDL, very-low-density lipoprotein.

peripheral arteries, where atherosclerosis can develop. The probability that atherosclerosis will develop is directly related to the concentration of LDL-C in the systemic circulation and the length of time this level of exposure persists.

HIGH-DENSITY LIPOPROTEINS

HDL particles transport cholesterol from peripheral cells back to the liver, a process called *reverse cholesterol transport*.[3–5] In contrast to LDL, high HDL-C concentrations are desirable because cholesterol is being removed from vascular tissue and is not available to contribute to atherogenesis. In peripheral cells, the ABC_1 transporter facilitates the efflux of both cholesterol and phospholipids. Through mechanisms that have not been defined fully, HDL particles acquire this cholesterol and either transport it directly to the liver through interaction with an HDL receptor on the hepatocyte (the scavenger receptor, SR-B1) or transfer it to circulating remnant VLDL and LDL particles. If the latter occurs, the cholesterol may be returned to the liver for clearance from the circulation or delivered back to peripheral cells (see Fig. 13-3).

HDL particles are further subfractionated. The smaller HDL_3 particle is converted to the larger HDL_2 particle as it acquires TG and cholesterol from peripheral cells and circulating lipoproteins. Conversely, HDL_2 particles are converted to HDL_3 particles by lipolysis of TGs through the action of hepatic lipase. HDL_2 levels provide the best estimate of the antiatherogenic effects of HDL.

Cholesterol acquired from peripheral cells by HDL particles is converted into an esterified form through the action of the enzyme lecithin-cholesterol acyl transferase (LCAT). The transfer of cholesterol from HDL particles to circulating VLDL particles is catalyzed by cholesteryl ester transfer protein, making the HDL particle less cholesterol rich. Patients have been described who have a deficiency of cholesterol ester transfer protein; they often have a high plasma concentration of HDL-C and a low incidence of CHD. Drugs are being developed and tested that inhibit this protein.

NON-HDL CHOLESTEROL

Non-HDL cholesterol (non-HDL-C) refers to the combined amount of cholesterol carried by VLDL and LDL parti-

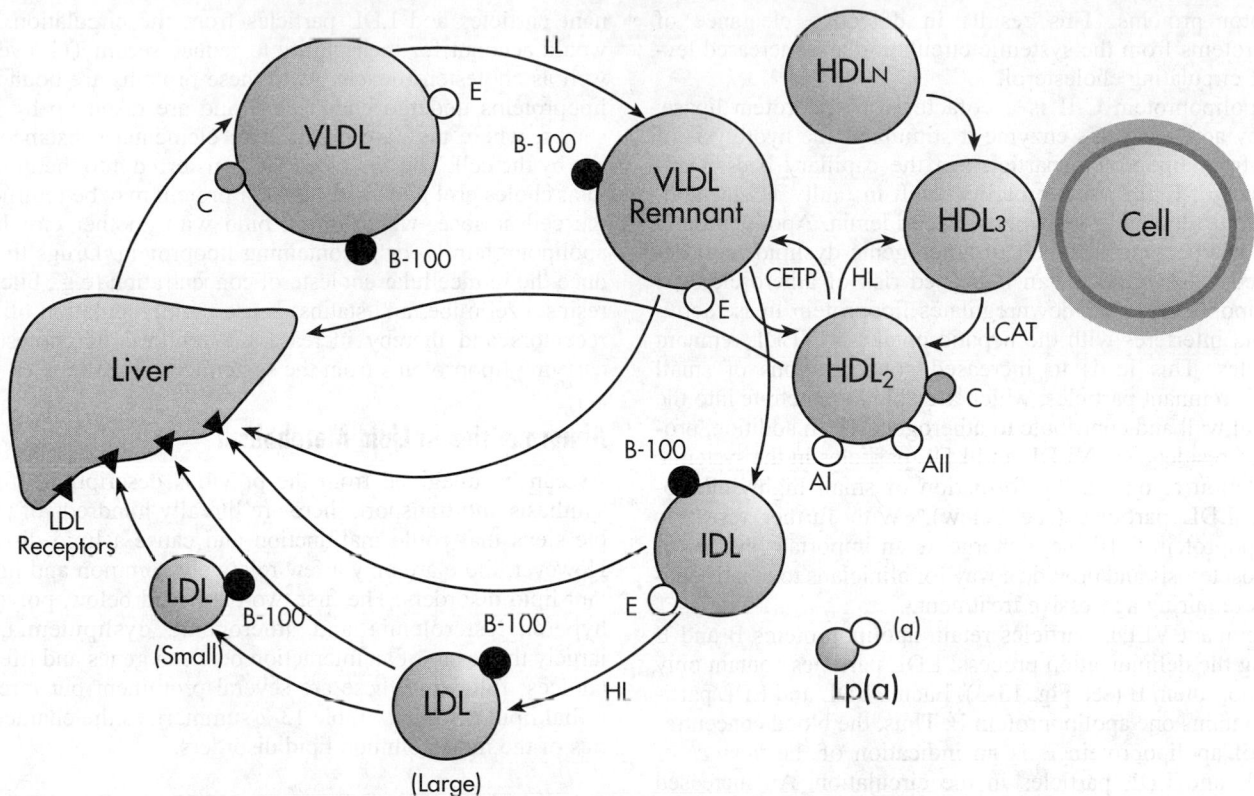

FIGURE 13-3. The lipoproteins, apolipoproteins, and enzymes involved in the transport of cholesterol and triglycerides. HDL, high-density lipoprotein; IDL, intermediate-density lipoprotein; LDL, low-density lipoprotein; VLDL, very-low-density lipoprotein.

cles (the cholesterol carried by IDL particles is reported as part of LDL cholesterol). As indicated, most often an elevated LDL-C is encountered, but in about 30% of cases, VLDL-C is also elevated. In these cases, it is helpful to know how much cholesterol is being carried by all of these particles. Non-HDL-C is determined by subtracting the HDL-cholesterol (HDL-C) level from the total cholesterol level.

CHYLOMICRONS

Unlike the lipoproteins that transport cholesterol from the liver to peripheral cells and back (endogenous system), chylomicrons transport fatty acids and cholesterol derived from the diet or synthesized in the intestines from the gut to the liver (exogenous system) (see Fig. 13-3 and Table 13-1). Chylomicrons are large, TG-rich lipoproteins. As they pass through capillary beds on the way to the liver, some of the TG content is removed through the action of lipoprotein lipase in a manner similar to that described for TG removal from VLDL particles. In the rare individual who has a lipoprotein lipase deficiency, this removal process is faulty and TG levels in the blood become very high (e.g., 1,000 to 5,000 mg/dL).

Following a fatty meal, the number of chylomicron particles (and therefore the concentration of TGs) is high. However, if the patient fasts for 10 to 12 hours, chylomicrons will have time to be removed from the blood. TG concentrations obtained during fasting reflect TG that is produced by the liver and carried in VLDL and other remnant particles (unless the patient has a rare chylomicron clearance disorder). This is

why patients are asked to fast before a lipoprotein profile is obtained. A blood sample that is rich in chylomicrons (and to a lesser extent VLDL particles) appears turbid; the higher the TG level, the more turbid the sample. If the sample from a patient with hyperchylomicronemia is refrigerated, chylomicrons will float to the top and form a frothy white layer, while smaller VLDLs stay suspended below.

Apolipoproteins

Each lipoprotein particle contains proteins on its outer surface called *apolipoproteins* (see Fig. 13-2 and Table 13-1). These proteins have three functions: (1) provide structure to the lipoprotein, (2) activate enzyme systems, and (3) bind with cell receptors.[2] Abnormal metabolism of apolipoproteins, even in the face of seemingly normal blood cholesterol levels, may result in faulty enzyme activity or cholesterol transport and an increased risk of atherosclerosis. Because of this, lipid specialists often assess blood levels of apolipoproteins to fully evaluate dyslipidemic patients, especially those who have a family history of premature CHD. The five most clinically relevant apolipoproteins are A-I, A-II, B-100, C, and E.

VLDL particles contain apolipoproteins B-100, E, and C (see Fig. 13-3). The B and E proteins are ligands for LDL receptors (also called *B-E receptors*) on the surface of hepatocytes and peripheral cells. Linkage allows the transfer of cholesterol from the circulating lipoprotein into the cell through absorptive endocytosis and cellular uptake of the particle. Defects in these proteins reduce their ability to bind with receptor proteins. This results in defective clearance of lipoproteins from the systemic circulation and increased levels of circulating cholesterol.

Apolipoprotein C-II is a cofactor for lipoprotein lipase, and by activating this enzyme it stimulates the hydrolysis of TGs from lipoprotein particles in the capillary beds. Deficiencies of C-II apolipoproteins result in faulty TG metabolism and ultimately in hypertriglyceridemia. Apolipoprotein C-III has become a marker of atherogenic dyslipidemia (described below) and for an increased risk of atherosclerosis. Apolipoprotein C-III downregulates lipoprotein lipase activity and interferes with the hepatic uptake of VLDL remnant particles. This leads to increased concentrations of small VLDL remnant particles, which are able to penetrate into the arterial wall and contribute to atherogenesis. In addition, prolonged residence of VLDL and LDL particles in the systemic circulation results in the formation of small highly atherogenic LDL particles (see below).[6] With further research, apolipoprotein C-III may emerge as an important marker of atherosclerosis and provide a way for clinicians to identify patients requiring aggressive treatment.

Remnant VLDL particles retain apolipoproteins B and E during the delipidization process; LDL particles contain only apolipoprotein B (see Fig. 13-3). Each VLDL and LDL particle contains one apolipoprotein B. Thus, the blood concentration of apolipoprotein B is an indication of the *number* of VLDL and LDL particles in the circulation. An increased number of lipoprotein particles (i.e., an increased apolipoprotein B concentration) is a strong predictor of CHD risk. The ratio of non–HDL-C (total cholesterol − HDL-C) to apoprotein B gives an estimate of the cholesterol contained in each VLDL and LDL particle. Some patients have high levels of apolipoprotein B (suggesting an increased number of VLDL and LDL particles in the circulation), even though their cholesterol level is in the desirable range. These patients have an increased risk of atherosclerosis.

HDL particles contain apolipoproteins A-I, A-II, and C. A-I protein activates LCAT, which catalyzes the esterification of free cholesterol in HDL particles. Levels of apolipoprotein A-I have a stronger inverse correlation with CHD risk than apolipoprotein A-II levels. HDL particles that contain only A-I apolipoproteins (LpA-I) are associated with a lower CHD risk than are HDL particles containing both A-I and A-II (LpA-I, A-II).[7]

LDL Receptor

The uptake of cholesterol into peripheral and hepatic cells is accomplished by the binding of apolipoproteins B and E on circulating lipoproteins to cell-surface LDL receptors (B-E receptors). The synthesis of LDL receptors is stimulated by a low intracellular cholesterol concentration.[7] Within the cell, the receptor protein travels from the mitochondria (where it is synthesized) to the cell surface (where it migrates to an area called the *coated pits*). Once in this position, it is capable of binding with lipoproteins that contain apolipoprotein E or B-100, including VLDL, remnant VLDL, IDL, and LDL. Because remnant VLDL and IDL particles contain both B and E proteins, they may have a higher affinity for LDL receptors than do LDL particles, which contain only the B protein. Furthermore, drugs that increase the synthesis of LDL receptors (e.g., statins) may increase the clearance of both VLDL rem-

nant particles and LDL particles from the circulation. This would account for their ability to reduce serum TG levels as well as cholesterol levels. After these proteins are bound, the lipoproteins undergo endocytosis and are taken up by lysosomes, where they are broken into elemental substances for use by the cell. The cholesterol is transferred into the intracellular cholesterol pool. The receptor protein may be returned to the cell surface, where it can bind with another circulating apolipoprotein E- or B-containing lipoprotein. Drugs that reduce the intracellular cholesterol concentration (e.g., bile acid resins, ezetimibe, and statins) cause the upregulation of LDL receptors and thereby increase the removal of cholesterol-carrying lipoproteins from the systemic circulation.

Abnormalities in Lipid Metabolism

As can be imagined from the previous description of lipid synthesis and transport, there are literally hundreds of possible steps that could malfunction and cause a lipid disorder. However, there are only a few relatively common and important lipid disorders. The first two described below, polygenic hypercholesterolemia and atherogenic dyslipidemia, are largely the result of an interaction between genes and lifestyle choices; following these are several prominent but rarer familial lipid disorders. Table 13-2 summarizes the characteristics of the most common lipid disorders.

Polygenic Hypercholesterolemia

Polygenic hypercholesterolemia, the most prevalent form of dyslipidemia, is found in more than 25% of the U.S. population and is caused by a combination of environmental (e.g., poor nutrition, sedentary lifestyle) and genetic factors (thus the term "polygenic"). Saturated fatty acids in the diet of these patients can reduce LDL receptor activity, thus reducing the clearance of LDL particles from the systemic circulation. As a result, patients with polygenic hypercholesterolemia have mild to moderate LDL-C elevations (usually in the range of 130 to 250 mg/dL). There are no unique physical findings. Family history of premature CHD is present in approximately 20% of cases. These patients are effectively managed with dietary restriction in saturated fats and cholesterol and by drugs that lower LDL-C levels (i.e., statins, bile acid sequestrants, niacin, and ezetimibe).

Atherogenic Dyslipidemia

Atherogenic dyslipidemia is found in about 25% of patients who have a lipid disorder. It is characterized by a moderate TG elevation (150 to 500 mg/dL; indicative of the increased presence of VLDL remnant particles), a low HDL-C level (<40 mg/dL), and a moderately high LDL-C level (including increased concentrations of small LDL particles.) Most commonly, these patients are either overweight or obese with increased waist circumference and/or diabetic and are said to have the *metabolic syndrome.*

Patients with obesity or diabetes have an increased mobilization of fatty acids from adipose cells to the systemic circulation, which leads to increased TG synthesis and secretion of VLDL particles by the liver. Often these particles contain apoprotein C-III, which interferes with the action of lipoprotein lipase, thus retarding lipolysis of TG from VLDL particles. This results in the formation of TG-rich VLDL remnant

Table 13-2   Characteristics of Common Lipid Disorders

Disorder	Metabolic Defect	Lipid Effect	Main Lipid Parameter	Diagnostic Features
Polygenic hyper-cholesterolemia	↓ LDL clearance	↑ LDL-C	LDL-C: 130–250 mg/dL TG: 150–500 mg/dL	None distinctive
Atherogenic dyslipidemia	↑ VLDL secretion, ↑ C-III synthesis, ↓ LPL activity, ↓ VLDL removal	↑ TG ↑ Remnant VLDL ↓ HDL ↑ Small dense LDL	HDL-C: <40 mg/dL	Frequently accompanied by central obesity or diabetes
Familial hyper-cholesterolemia (heterozygous)	Dysfunctional or absent LDL receptors	↑ LDL-C	LDL-C: 250–450 mg/dL	Family history of CHD, tendon xanthomas
Familial defective apoB-100	Defective apoB on LDL and VLDL	↑ LDL-C	LDL-C: 250–450 mg/dL	Family history of CHD, tendon xanthomas
Dysbetalipopro-teinemia (type III hyperlipidemia)	ApoE2:E2 phenotype, ↓ VLDL remnant clearance	↑ Remnant VLDL, ↑ IDL	LDL-C: 300–600 mg/dL TGs: 400–800 mg/dL	Palmar xanthomas, tuberoeruptive xanthomas
Familial combined hyperlipidemia	↑ ApoB and VLDL production	↑ CH, TGs, or both	LDL-C: 250–350 mg/dL TGs: 200–800 mg/dL	Family history, CHD Family history, Hyper-lipidemia
Familial hyperapo-betalipoproteinemia	↑ ApoB production	↑ ApoB	ApoB: >125 mg/dL	None distinctive
Hypoalphalipo-proteinemia	↑ HDL catabolism	↓ HDL-C	HDL-C: <40 mg/dL	None distinctive

ApoB, apolipoprotein B; apoE, apolipoprotein E; CH, cholesterol; CHD, coronary heart disease; IDL, intermediate-density lipoprotein; LDL, low-density lipoprotein; LDL-C, low-density lipoprotein cholesterol; TGs, triglycerides; VLDL, very-low-density lipoprotein.

particles. TG from these particles is exchanged with cholesterol esters from HDL under the influence of cholesterol ester transfer protein, which means the VLDL remnant particles become enriched with cholesterol while HDL particles lose cholesterol (and gain TG) (see Fig. 13-3). TG is also exchanged from VLDL remnant particles with cholesterol esters from LDL particles. Thus, VLDL remnants become even more cholesterol enriched and LDL becomes TG enriched. The cholesterol-enriched, small VLDL remnant particle is atherogenic. TG-rich LDL particles undergo lipolysis catalyzed by hepatic lipase to remove TG, leaving small, cholesterol ester–deficient LDL particles (called small dense LDL) that are highly atherogenic.[8]

Patients with atherogenic dyslipidemia can often be effectively managed with weight reduction and increased physical activity. If needed, drugs that enhance the removal of remnant VLDL and small dense LDL particles (i.e., statins) and that lower TG levels (i.e., niacin or fibrates) are effective in the management of these patients.

Familial Hypercholesterolemia

Familial hypercholesterolemia (FH) is the classic lipid disorder of defective clearance. This autosomal dominant disorder is found in 1 of 500 people in the United States and is strongly associated with premature CHD.[9,10] Heterozygotes of this disorder inherit one defective LDL receptor gene. Consequently, they possess approximately half the number of functioning LDL receptors and double the LDL-C level of unaffected patients (i.e., LDL-C of 250 to 450 mg/dL).[11,12] Clinically, heterozygous FH patients may deposit cholesterol in the iris, leading to arcus senilis. Cholesterol also deposits in tendons,

particularly the Achilles tendon and extensor tendons of the hands, leading to tendon xanthomas. The clinical diagnosis of FH is established by documenting a very high LDL-C level, a strong family history of premature CHD events, and the presence of tendon xanthomas. Untreated heterozygous FH patients have approximately a 5% chance of a myocardial infarction (MI) by age 30, a 50% chance by age 50, and an 85% chance by age 60. The mean age of death in untreated male heterozygotes is in the mid-50s; for untreated female heterozygotes, it is in the mid-60s.[13]

Homozygotes for this disorder inherit a defective LDL receptor gene from both parents and generally have LDL-C levels >500 mg/dL. This rare disorder results in CHD by age 10 to 20 years. Because these individuals have lost the ability to clear cholesterol-carrying lipoproteins from the circulation, apheresis (analogous to dialysis for the kidney patient) is required to help remove these atherogenic particles.

Familial defective apoprotein B-100 (FDB) is a genetic disorder clinically indistinguishable from heterozygous FH. These patients have normally functioning LDL receptors but a defective apolipoprotein B protein, which results in reduced binding to LDL receptors and reduced clearance of LDL particles from the systemic circulation.[14,15] Like FH, LDL-C levels are 250 to 450 mg/dL.[14,16,17] Presumably, the apoprotein E and half of the apoprotein B in heterozygous FDB patients function normally, providing mechanisms for removal of these lipoproteins from the systemic circulation. Clinical diagnosis of FDB, like FH, is based on a very high LDL-C level, a family history of premature CHD, and tendon xanthomas. The definitive diagnosis requires molecular screening techniques.

Familial Dysbetalipoproteinemia

Familial dysbetalipoproteinemia (also called *type III hyper-lipidemia* and *remnant disease*) is caused by poor clearance of VLDL and chylomicron particles from the systemic circulation.[18] Apolipoprotein E is necessary for the normal clearance of these particles. It is inherited as an E2, E3, or E4 isoform from each parent. The E2 isoform has a low binding affinity for the LDL receptor. Thus, individuals with an apoprotein E2:E2 phenotype have delayed clearance of VLDL remnant (and possibly chylomicron) particles from the circulation and a reduced conversion of IDL to LDL particles. However, a lipid disorder usually does not result unless triggered by other metabolic problems such as diabetes, hypothyroidism, or obesity. Clinically, these patients have high cholesterol (owing to an enrichment of cholesterol esters in VLDL remnant particles), high TGs (usually in the range of 400 to 800 mg/dL), and a VLDL-C:TG ratio >0.3.[19] Some patients have palmar xanthomas (yellow-orange discoloration in the creases of the palms and fingers) and tuberoeruptive xanthomas (small, raised lesions in areas of pressure, particularly the elbows and knees). A personal and family history of premature atherosclerotic vascular disease often is present. As noted above, these patients often have diabetes mellitus, hypertension, obesity, and hyperuricemia.

Familial Combined Hyperlipidemia

Familial combined hyperlipidemia (FCHL) is the classic example of a dyslipidemia caused by increased production of lipoproteins. For reasons that are not clear, FCHL patients overproduce apolipoprotein B-containing particles, VLDL, and LDL.[20–22] Many patients have an elevated apoprotein B level.[23] As the name implies, patients with this disorder may have hypercholesterolemia (usually in the range of 250 to 350 mg/dL), or hypertriglyceridemia (usually between 200 and 800 mg/dL) or a combination of both (usually with a low HDL-C level). First-degree relatives of these individuals frequently have a lipid disorder. A family history of premature CHD is often present as well. FCHL patients commonly are overweight and hypertensive and also may have diabetes or hyperuricemia. A diagnosis of FCHL is presumed in patients who have increased cholesterol and/or TG levels, a strong family history of premature CHD, and a family history of dyslipidemia.

Familial Hyperapobetalipoproteinemia

Familial hyperapobetalipoproteinemia (*hyperapoB* for short) is a variant of FCHL. This disorder is characterized by increased hepatic production of apolipoprotein B in the absence of other lipid abnormalities.[24,25] These patients have acceptable LDL-C and TG levels and a family history of CHD. Their apolipoprotein B concentration is usually >125 mg/dL, indicating an increase in the *number* of cholesterol-carrying lipoprotein particles. It is likely that FCHL and hyperapoB are related disorders, both resulting from excessive secretion of apolipoprotein B-containing lipoproteins.[26]

Hypoalphalipoproteinemia

Low HDL-C (<40 mg/dL; hypoalphalipoproteinemia) without an increase in TG level is fairly uncommon, but is associated with increased CHD risk.[27,28] Unfortunately, little is known about the precise molecular defect causing this problem, although genetic influences undoubtedly are involved.[29] Recently, Tangier disease, which is characterized by low HDL-C, orange tonsils, and hepatosplenomegaly, has been linked to a defect in the ABC_1 transporter responsible for the efflux of cholesterol from peripheral cells. The inherited tendency to have low HDL-C is accentuated by lifestyle factors such as obesity, smoking, and lack of exercise. Despite strong epidemiologic evidence showing an inverse relationship between HDL-C and CHD, clinical trials demonstrating a benefit of raising isolated low HDL-C with drugs are lacking. What has been shown is that lowering LDL-C in patients with low HDL-C reduces CHD risk.[30] It is anticipated that therapies to raise HDL-C will become available and can be tested to see if they reduce CHD risk also.

Rationale for Treating Dyslipidemia

Scientific data from animal studies, genetic studies, epidemiologic studies, and clinical trials support the link between cholesterol, atherosclerosis, and CHD. This collective body of knowledge resoundingly supports a critical role for cholesterol in the pathogenesis of atherosclerosis. Even more important, in clinical trials the lowering of blood cholesterol levels has been consistently associated with reduced CHD, whether the blood cholesterol was reduced by drug, diet, or surgical means. However, even the most vigorous cholesterol-lowering approach does not result in the complete amelioration of CHD, suggesting that there are other etiologies in play. Some of the significant literature on the pathogenesis of atherosclerosis and clinical trials establishing the link between blood cholesterol and CHD is summarized below.

Pathogenesis of Atherosclerosis

Circulating cholesterol has a central role in the pathogenesis of atherosclerosis. Even the name *atherosclerosis* depicts this (from the Latin *athero* ["porridge-like"] and *sclerosis* ["fibrous-like"]. Atherosclerotic lesions begin with the accumulation of cholesterol from LDL and VLDL remnant particles in the intimal space (Fig. 13-4). The reason this occurs is unknown, but in some way it appears directly related to the level of circulating cholesterol and the provocation by risk factors such as hypertension, smoking, diabetes, stress, and genetic predisposition. An important finding is that native LDL-C per se does not contribute to the development of atherosclerosis; instead, LDL-C must be modified (e.g., oxidized) before it becomes a factor in causing atherosclerosis.

Soon after taking up residence in the subendothelial space, LDL-C is modified primarily by oxidation. Simultaneously, monocyte adhesion molecules are released from endothelial cells on the surface of the lumen.[31,32] They cause circulating monocytes to attach to the intact endothelial surface, and then chemoattractants cause these monocytes to squeeze between endothelial cells into the intima (see Fig. 13-4).[33]

Once recruited, the monocytes are converted to activated macrophage cells, which begin to ingest modified LDL-C and remnant VLDL particles. These modified particles are taken up by special scavenger or acetyl-LDL receptors on the surface of macrophage cells.[34] Modified LDL serves as another chemoattractant for circulating monocytes, thus causing more monocytes from the systemic circulation to take up residence in the intima. It also inhibits the mobility of resident

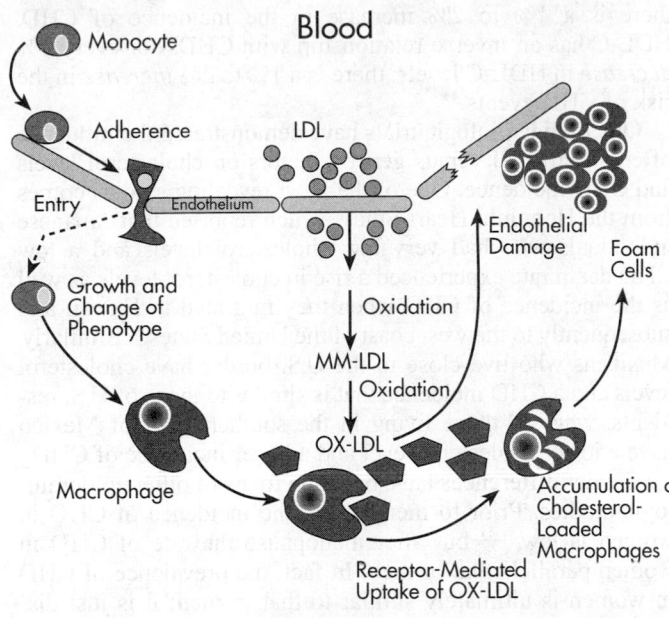

Blood

Monocyte

Adherence

LDL

Entry

Endothelium

Endothelial Damage

Foam Cells

Growth and Change of Phenotype

Oxidation

MM-LDL

Oxidation

OX-LDL

Macrophage

Accumulation of Cholesterol-Loaded Macrophages

Receptor-Mediated Uptake of OX-LDL

Artery Wall

FIGURE 13-4. Some of the steps involved in the development of the fatty streak. LDL, low-density lipoprotein.

macrophage cells (blocking the egress of these cells from the intima); macrophage cells become a cytotoxic agent (causing damage to the endothelium).[31] As the uptake of modified LDL-C into macrophage cells continues, the cells become laden with lipid, grow in size, and eventually become *foam cells* (Figs. 13-4 and 13-5).

Early in the process, the monocellular layer surrounding the lumen (the endothelium) becomes dysfunctional. Notably, the release of nitric oxide from these cells is impaired, which results in vasoconstriction and ischemic symptoms. Regulation of blood cholesterol levels and management of other risk factors restore endothelial function, nitrous oxide release, and the vasodilatory response.

The accumulation of foam cells in the intimal space eventually results in a raised lesion, the *fatty streak,* which is widely recognized as the precursor to atherosclerosis. Fatty streaks transform the once smooth endothelial surface of the artery into a lumpy, uneven surface. As this process continues, an atherosclerotic plaque is formed. In the initial stages, this plaque is characterized by a large lipid core made up of macrophage (foam) cells filled with cholesterol along the surface and at the shoulders of the lesion (see Fig 13-5).

During plaque growth, a number of cells (including macrophages, endothelial cells, platelets, and smooth muscle cells) secrete chemoattractant and growth factors, which cause smooth muscle cells from the media to migrate and proliferate near the luminal surface.[35] Collagen synthesis is increased. This leads to conversion of atherosclerotic lesions that initially are weak and unstable (because they contain a large lipid core surrounded by a thin fibrous cap) to become strong and hard (because they contain a small inner lipid core and much collagen, and matrix). At any given time, atherosclerosis at various stages of development can be found all along the arterial tree in susceptible patients (see Fig. 13-5).

As atherosclerotic lesions grow, the coronary artery remodels. Lesions initially grow away from the lumen toward the media, thus preserving the luminal opening and ensuring

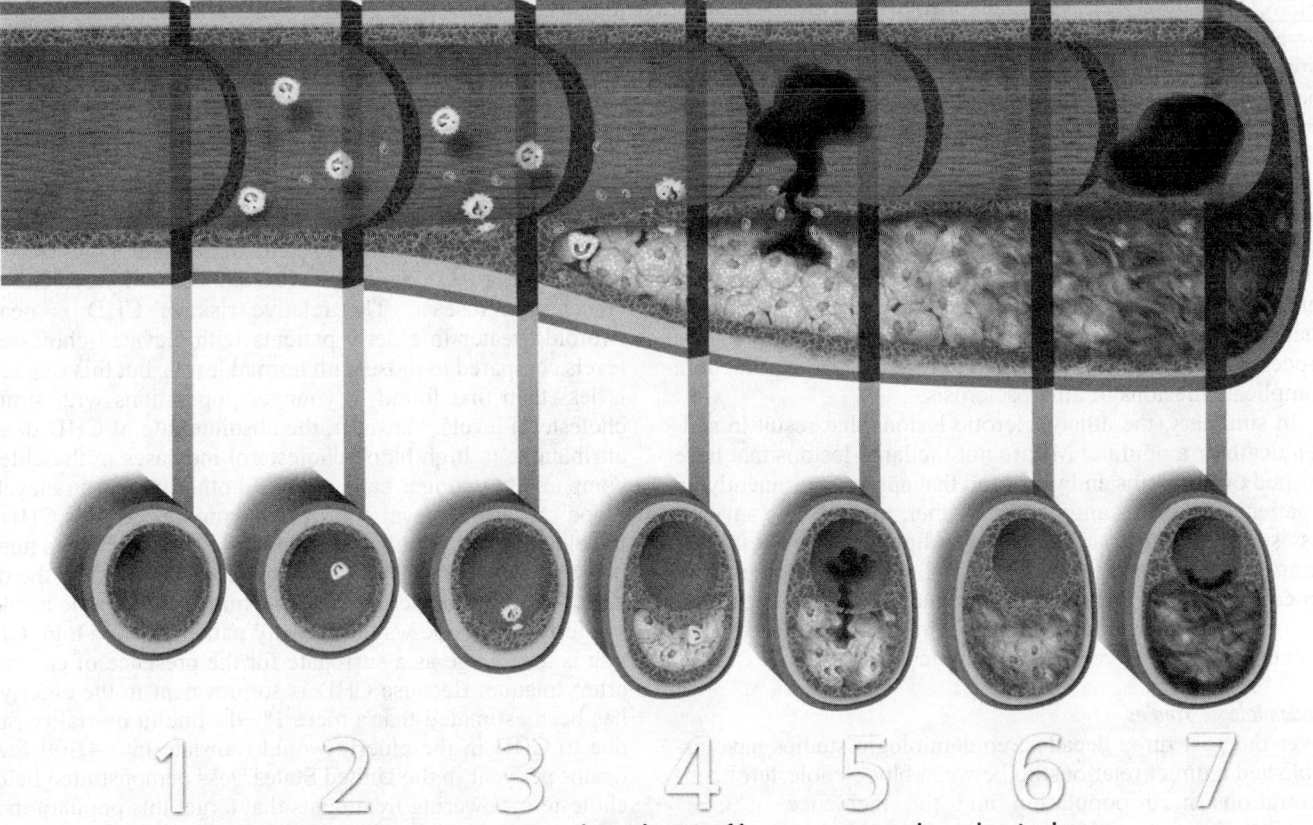

FIGURE 13-5. Initiation, progression, and complication of human coronary atherosclerotic plaque.

normal blood flow. However, late in the growth of the lesion, the luminal space is invaded and becomes progressively narrowed as the atherosclerotic lesion grows.

Similar to the stages of development, atherosclerotic lesions exist along a continuum from vulnerable lesions that can rupture and cause a thrombosis to older, rigid lesions that will not rupture. The younger lesions occupy only the intimal space, while the older lesions may protrude into the luminal space. As one examines the coronary angiogram of a patient, evidence of stenosis (narrowing of the lumen) indicates the presence of older, more advanced lesions. When these lesions are seen, other lesions distal to the narrowing are likely to be present. They are younger and more prone to erosion or rupture, which can cause a thrombosis. In fact, the culprit lesion that results in an MI is usually not at the site of the greatest stenosis, but distal to it.[36]

A number of processes cause younger lesions to become unstable; most of these are a part of an active inflammatory process. The uptake of cholesterol by activated macrophage cells is one of these processes. Chemoattractants such as monocyte chemoattractant protein-1 (MCP-1), adhesion molecules, and a family of T-cell substances participate in the migration of monocytes into the intima. Macrophage colony-stimulating factor (M-CSF) contributes to the differentiation of blood monocytes into macrophage cells. T-cells elaborate inflammatory cytokines that stimulate macrophages, endothelial cells, and smooth muscle cells. Activated macrophage cells produce proteolytic enzymes that degrade collagen and weaken the fibrous cap.[37] The release of metalloproteinase enzymes causes the destruction of connective tissue and renders the atherosclerotic lesion vulnerable to rupture. Apoptosis (cell death) of smooth muscle cells in the shoulders of the atherosclerotic cap further weakens the lesion.[38–43] These processes increase the chance that the atherosclerotic lesion will rupture or erode, especially at the shoulders of the lesion, and expose the underlying tissue to circulating blood elements.[44] With this exposure, platelets may adhere and microthrombi may form. The resultant clot can occlude blood flow entirely, causing an MI. More commonly, there is only partial occlusion of blood flow, causing transient ischemic symptoms and unstable angina. The clot creates a barrier between the underlying tissue and circulating blood and allows healing to take place. Subsequently, as the atherosclerotic plaque grows further and again ruptures, a new clot can form to mend the lesion. This process of fissuring and rehealing appears to lead to the more complicated lesions of atherosclerosis.

In summary, the atherosclerotic lesions that result in sudden death or a nonfatal MI are not the large lesions that have formed over months and years and that appear prominently on a patient's coronary angiogram. Rather, they are the smaller, less stable lesions that have a large lipid core and a thin fibrous cap.[45] When shear forces, blood pressure, or other toxic processes in the artery cause these plaques to fissure, erode, or rupture, a thrombosis may develop, leading to the occlusion of the affected vessel and a clinical event.

Epidemiologic Studies

Over the past three decades, epidemiologic studies have established a direct relationship between blood cholesterol concentrations in a population and the incidence of CHD events.[46–48] For every 1% increase in blood cholesterol levels, there is a 1% to 2% increase in the incidence of CHD. HDL-C has an inverse relationship with CHD. For every 1% *decrease* in HDL-C levels, there is a 1% to 2% *increase* in the risk of CHD events.[49]

Other epidemiologic trials have demonstrated the influence of environmental versus genetic factors on cholesterol levels and CHD incidence. One of the most revealing studies comes from the Honolulu Heart Study, which reported that Japanese individuals who had very low cholesterol levels and a low CHD death rate experienced a rise in cholesterol levels as well as the incidence of CHD when they migrated to Hawaii and subsequently to the west coast of the United States.[50] Similarly, Mexicans who live close to the U.S. border have cholesterol levels and a CHD incidence that is similar to those of U.S. residents, whereas those living in the southern part of Mexico have a lower cholesterol level and a lower incidence of CHD.

Gender differences have been the focus of other epidemiologic studies. Prior to menopause, the incidence of CHD in women is low,[51,52] but after menopause the rate of CHD in women parallels that of men. In fact, the prevalence of CHD in women is ultimately similar to that in men; it is just displaced by about 10 years.[48,53] Whereas men begin to experience CHD events in their 50s and 60s, women experience it in their 60s and 70s. Eventually, CHD causes nearly as many deaths in women as it does in men.[54] In fact, CHD is the cause of more deaths in women than all forms of cancer combined, including cancer of the breast, ovary, and cervix. Furthermore, the presence of diabetes in a woman with dyslipidemia negates whatever protection she may have had before menopause and is associated with a very high incidence of CHD events.[55,56] Conversely, a high HDL-C level may offer women more protection from CHD than a similar level offers a man.[49]

Finally, epidemiologic trials have taught us lessons about the influence of age on blood cholesterol levels and CHD. A direct relationship exists between blood cholesterol and CHD at all ages, to at least the mid-80s.[57] Because CHD risk increases with age, most CHD events occur among the elderly. In fact, CHD is the most common cause of death among the elderly.[58] Intravascular ultrasound studies that examine the inner walls of coronary arteries demonstrate that practically all patients older than 70 years have advanced and prevalent atherosclerotic disease. The relative risk of CHD is nearly twofold greater in elderly patients with elevated cholesterol levels compared to those with normal levels, but this risk level is less than that found in younger populations with similar cholesterol levels. However, the absolute rate of CHD deaths attributable to high blood cholesterol increases in the elderly compared to younger patients.[58,59] In other words, an elevated blood cholesterol level contributes to more cases of CHD in the older patient population than in the young, which is due in part to the sheer number of elderly people affected by the disease. Some authorities see age as a marker for plaque burden, suggesting that one way to identify patients with a high CHD risk is to use age as a surrogate for the presence of coronary artery plaque. Because CHD is so prevalent in the elderly, it has been estimated that a mere 1% decline in mortality rates due to CHD in the elderly would translate into 4,300 fewer deaths per year in the United States.[60] As demonstrated below, cholesterol-lowering treatments that target this population result in a substantial reduction in CHD, underscoring the importance of age in forecasting a high risk of future CHD events.

Clinical Trials

ANGIOGRAPHIC REGRESSION TRIALS

Based on animal, epidemiologic, and genetic studies, the direct relationship between blood cholesterol levels and CHD events was established. The critical hypothesis that remained to be proven before cholesterol-lowering therapies could be widely recommended was that lowering blood cholesterol levels would reduce CHD risk. The proof for this hypothesis was ultimately demonstrated in clinical trials. However, the initial test of this hypothesis involved angiographic trials that sought to demonstrate that by lowering blood cholesterol levels, coronary stenosis visualized on coronary angiography would regress.[61-78] Much to the surprise of investigators, this did not occur. In fact, more commonly, cholesterol lowering seemed only to slow lesion progression.

Despite these disappointing results, angiographic trials taught us many important lessons. They demonstrated that aggressive lipid lowering caused lesions to progress at a slower rate regardless of the vascular bed under study, including coronary,[62-70,73,74,76-78] carotid,[71,72,75] and femoral arteries.[67,75] They established that this effect was achieved regardless of the lipid-lowering therapy deployed: diet and other lifestyle modification,[64] lipid-lowering drugs,[6,30,38-43,62,63,66,68-78] or ileal bypass surgery.[61] They also suggested that the more aggressive the lipid lowering, especially if it resulted in >40% reduction in LDL-C, the greater the chance of plaque regression.[79]

The reason angiographic studies failed to demonstrate lesion regression was not because this process did not occur, but because the methodology could not detect it. Angiograms outline the lesion from the outside of the coronary artery. Since atherosclerotic lesions initially remodel outward away from the lumen, as explained above, the lumen would appear normal until the late stage of atherosclerosis plaque development.

Thus, lesions that were visible on a coronary angiogram were the older, more rigid lesions that were less likely to change with lipid-lowering therapy. However, younger lesions, which were not visualized in a coronary angiogram, may well have regressed. Recent investigations of the contour of the inner lining of the lumen using intravascular ultrasound report that lipid lowering does cause widespread plaque regression without any change in lumen size.[80]

Angiographic studies were the first to suggest that lipid-modifying therapy could alter the composition of plaque. As summarized earlier, plaques are initially characterized by a large lipid core and a thin fibrous cap; these lesions are more prone to rupture.[32,44] Additionally, these lesions are small; usually <50% the size of the lumen diameter. Angiographic studies revealed that the lesions that caused MI were not the large ones that caused substantial stenosis, but the smaller lesions. Subsequently, pathology studies performed during autopsies on patients who had died following MI showed that these smaller lesions were lipid-laden and had thin fibrous caps.

Even though angiographic trials were primarily designed to study coronary angiograms, they reported fewer CHD events in treated patients. Most of these observations did not reach statistical significance because of the small numbers of patients in the study and the relatively short (1 to 3 years) duration of observation. However, when these studies were combined, the message was clear: cholesterol lowering was associated with fewer CHD events.[45] These results set the stage for the larger clinical trials.

CHOLESTEROL-LOWERING CLINICAL TRIALS

The proof of whether LDL-C lowering reduces CHD events has been demonstrated by well-designed, large, placebo-controlled clinical trials. Since the early 1990s, the results of a dozen or more major clinical trials have conclusively demonstrated the value of lipid-modifying therapy to prevent CHD events (Table 13-3).

Table 13-3 Randomized Endpoint Trials With Cholesterol-Lowering Therapies

Trial	Intervention	LDL-C (Initial–On Rx)	LDL-C Changes	Placebo CHD Rate[a]	CHD Event Reduction
CHD and CHD Risk Equivalent Patients					
4S[82]	Simvastatin	188–117	↓ 35%	21.8%	↓ 34%
LIPID[84]	Pravastatin	150–112	↓ 25%	15.9%	↓ 24%
CARE[83]	Pravastatin	139–98	↓ 32%	13.2%	↓ 24%
Post-CABG[95]	Lovastatin/Resin	136–98	↓ 39%	13.5%	↓ 24%
HPS[86]	Simvastatin	131–89	↓ 32%	11.8%	↓ 24%
Acute Coronary Syndrome Patients					
MIRACL[92,93]	Atorvastatin	124–72	↓ 42%	—	↓ 26%[b]
AVERT[94]	Atorvastatin	145–77	↓ 42%	—	↓ 36%[b]
Patients Without Evidence of CHD					
LRC-CPPT[81]	Resin	205–175	↓ 15%	9.8%	↓ 19%
WOSCOPS[88]	Pravastatin	192–142	↓ 26%	14.9%	↓ 31%
Tex/AFCAPS[90]	Lovastatin	150–115	↓ 25%	3.0%	↓ 40%
ASCOT[89]	Atorvastatin	132–85	↓ 31%	4.7%	↓ 50%[c]

[a]Placebo CHD rate = nonfatal myocardial infarction and CHD death
[b]Ischemic events
[c]Estimated 5-year CHD risk reduction
CHD, coronary heart disease; LDL-C, low density lipoprotein cholesterol; Rx, drug therapy.

The first of these, the Lipid Research Clinics Coronary Primary Prevention Trial,[81] showed that a relatively modest 10% reduction in cholesterol levels with the bile acid sequestrant cholestyramine compared with placebo over a 5-year period reduced CHD deaths and nonfatal MIs by an impressive 19%. The results of this study launched the modern era of cholesterol management to reduce CHD risk.

Beginning in the mid-1990s, the results of clinical trials with the more potent cholesterol-lowering statins were reported. Three of these (4S,[80] CARE,[83] and LIPID[84]) were secondary prevention trials (i.e., they were conducted in patients with known CHD). In these trials, CHD death and nonfatal MIs occurred in 13% to 22% of placebo-treated patients over 5 years, compared to event rates of 10% to 14% with statin therapy. Total mortality was reduced significantly in two of these trials. Fewer revascularization procedures were required in patients receiving statin therapy; there were also 31% fewer strokes.[85] This important and unexpected finding suggests that the same mechanisms by which statins affect coronary atherosclerosis may be operable in extracranial carotid atherosclerosis. It also demonstrates that patients who have atherosclerosis in one vascular bed, such as the coronary vessels, are likely to have atherosclerosis in other vascular beds, and that cholesterol-lowering treatment can have beneficial effects throughout the vascular tree. Finally, these studies demonstrate that LDL-C–lowering therapy not only improves the quality of life (by preventing MIs, strokes, and revascularization procedures) but can also prolong life (by delaying deaths from any cause).

The Heart Protection Study (HPS) extended these results.[86] The HPS included 20,536 patients with a history of CHD or cerebrovascular disease (stroke or transient ischemic attacks), peripheral vascular disease, or diabetes. Of note, this grouping of patients is designated by the National Cholesterol Education Program's Adult Treatment Panel III (NCEP ATP-III) as being a "CHD equivalent population" because their risk of a CHD event is >20% in a 10-year period.[87] Statin therapy for 5 years lowered the future risk of a CHD event in each of these populations by about 24%. The CHD event rate exceeded 20% in each of the placebo-treated patient subgroups; statin therapy reduced this risk to <20% in all but the patients with peripheral vascular disease (and that group had a substantial risk reduction from 31% to 25%). The CHD event reduction was achieved equally in men and women; in all age groups, including those ages 75 to 85 years; and regardless of the baseline LDL-C, including those with initial levels <100 mg/dL. Patients in the upper tertile of LDL levels began with a mean LDL-C of 144 mg/dL that was reduced to a mean of 105 mg/dL on treatment; their corresponding CHD risk was reduced from approximately 27% to 22% in 5 years. Patients in the lower tertile of LDL levels began with a LDL-C of 105 mg/dL that was reduced to a mean of 70 mg/dL on statin treatment; their corresponding CHD risk was reduced from approximately 22% to 18% in 5 years. These data suggest that lowering LDL-C levels to at least 70 mg/dL is associated with the lowest level of risk in patients with CHD equivalent diseases. Further, these findings indicate that there is no LDL-C level in this population that is without risk.

Three trials with statin therapy have been reported in patients without evident CHD (i.e., primary prevention) but with multiple CHD risk factors. WOSCOPS, which included men who had two or more CHD risk factors, found that CHD events and revascularization procedures were reduced by 31% and 37%, respectively, in those receiving statin therapy for 5 years; total mortality was reduced 22% ($P < 0.051$).[88] The ASCOT trial, which included men and women with hypertension and an average of 3.7 other CHD risk factors, reported that CHD events were reduced by 36% and strokes by 27% after only 3.3 years of statin treatment.[89] The TexCAPS/AFCAPS trial was important because it included the lowest-risk population, with an estimated 10-year CHD risk of only 6%. Despite this relatively low CHD risk, the composite endpoint (i.e., fatal and nonfatal MIs, sudden cardiac death, and unstable angina) was reduced by 37%, fatal and nonfatal MIs were reduced by 40%, and unstable angina was reduced by 32%, with 5 years of statin treatment.[90] Significant reductions in CHD events were seen in women, older patients, and diabetic patients, emphasizing the value of treatment in these populations.

LDL-C lowering by other means also reduces CHD events.[61] For example, LDL-C lowering with ileal bypass surgery in the POSCH study resulted in a 40% reduction of CHD events compared with the groups not having this surgery.[61,88] These studies suggest that effective LDL-C lowering by any means can reduce CHD risk.

Trials carried out in patients with acute coronary syndromes have also demonstrated CHD risk reduction (see Table 13-3). The MIRACL study treated patients presenting to the hospital with unstable angina or non-Q-wave MI with statin therapy or placebo for 4 months. This resulted in a 24% reduction in symptomatic ischemia requiring emergency hospitalization and a 60% reduction in nonfatal strokes in those receiving the statin.[92,93] The AVERT study evaluated statin-based medical management versus revascularization and usual medical care in patients who had stable coronary artery disease and were candidates for a revascularization procedure. After 18 months of therapy, the statin-treated group had 36% fewer cases of ischemia requiring hospitalization compared with placebo-treated patients.[94] These studies show that intervention with a statin in patients with acute coronary syndromes can have important effects on ischemic symptoms in a relatively brief time after beginning therapy. The CHD risk reductions reported in the 5-year-long clinical trial were evident within the first 1 to 2 years of statin therapy and were significantly different from placebo after 5 years of treatment.

Taken together, these trials demonstrate that LDL-C lowering reduces the risk of a CHD event in patients at practically any level of risk. In the aggregate, common CHD events, including sudden CHD deaths and nonfatal MIs, were reduced by 25% to 40%. Revascularization procedures were reduced by 25% to 50%. Strokes were reduced by an average of 15% in primary prevention patients and 32% in secondary prevention patients.[85] In fact, practically any known adverse consequence of atherosclerosis has been reduced with lipid-lowering therapy. In some of these studies, especially those in patients at very high risk for CHD, total mortality was significantly reduced. These trials tell us that aggressive lipid lowering improves the quality of life as well as the length of life.

A key question for clinicians is, "what is the optimal LDL-C?" The clinical trials described above may help answer this question. Patients in the CARE[83] and HPS[86] studies achieved on-treatment LDL-C levels of 98 mg/dL and 89 mg/dL, respectively, and a significant reduction in CHD risk. Nonetheless, the 10-year CHD event rate was still 10% to 20% in patients who had received statin therapy for 5 years. Even the HPS patients with the lowest one third of LDL-C levels had a 10-year CHD event rate of about 17% despite an on-treatment LDL-C of 70 mg/dL.[86] It is likely that continued statin therapy for another 5 years would double the CHD risk reduction, which would mean that an event will still occur in 20% to 40% of treated patients. The two clinical trials in patients with an acute coronary syndrome reported statin-treatment LDL-C levels of 72 and 77 mg/dL and reductions in ischemic events of 26% and 36%, respectively.[92, 94]

The Post-CABG trial reported that aggressive statin–bile acid sequestrant combination therapy that lowered LDL-C from 154 to 93 mg/dL reduced revascularization procedures by 30% and cardiovascular endpoints (i.e., cardiovascular death, nonfatal MI, stroke, bypass surgery, or percutaneous transluminal coronary angioplasty) by 24% compared with patients receiving a less aggressive regimen that lowered LDL-C from 154 to 135 mg/dL.[78,95] Three other large trials are underway that will determine the benefit of lowering LDL-C to about 70 mg/dL versus about 100 mg/dL; the results of these trials should be available in the next several years. At present, clinical trials indicate that LDL-C levels well below 100 mg/dL provide substantial CHD risk reduction. In fact, plotting the CHD event rate and baseline and on-treatment LDL-C levels in the major statin clinical trials reveals a linear relationship and suggests that lower LDL-C levels are associated with the lowest levels of CHD events in both primary and secondary prevention populations (Fig. 13-6). This led the NCEP ATP III to define the "optimal" LDL-C level as <100 mg/dL and to recommend this as the goal of treatment for high-risk CHD patients.[87] These trials also indicate that LDL-C lowering alone is not likely to eliminate CHD events and that other, yet unidentified mechanisms and therapies are needed.

The above studies illustrate that the level of the patient's LDL-C predicts future events: the higher the level, the greater the chance of a future CHD event. For example, the 5-year CHD event rates in the placebo groups of 4S,[90] LIPID,[84] CARE,[83] and HPS[86] were 21.8%, 15.9%, 13.2%, and 11.8%, respectively, in patients who had a mean baseline LDL-C of 188, 150, 139, and 131 mg/dL (see Table 13-2). Treatment with a statin reduced the mean LDL-C in these studies to 117, 112, 98, and 89 mg/dL, respectively, with corresponding 5-year CHD event rates of 14.4%, 12.1%, 10.0%, and 9.0%.

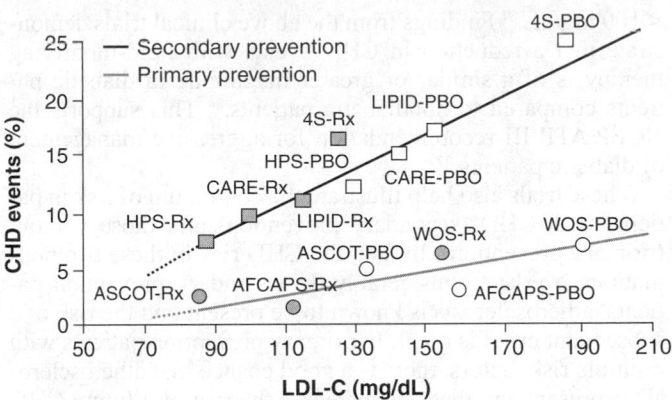

FIGURE 13-6. % CHD events by on-treatment LDL-C in major clinical trials.

A similar trend was observed in the primary prevention studies WOSCOPS,[88] AFCAPS,[90] and ASCOT.[89] In these studies, there was no baseline LDL-C level for which risk reduction was not demonstrated, suggesting that even patients with moderate CHD risk can benefit from treatment. Additionally, these studies support the current NCEP ATP III recommendation for aggressive lowering of LDL-C in patients with a high CHD risk.[87]

The statin trials further demonstrated that CHD risk reduction is achieved equally in older patients and younger patients[83,84,96] A meta-analysis of most of the major statin trials affirms this point[97] (Table 13-4). This has important implications in our treatment decisions. As noted, some specialists see age as a surrogate for plaque burden and thus more, not less, aggressive treatment is indicated as individuals age. HPS demonstrated that all patients, including those 75 to 85 years of age, benefited equally from statin therapy.[86]

Diabetic patients have a very high risk of macrovascular disease (i.e., CHD) as well as microvascular disease (e.g., retinopathy). Investigations have shown that diabetic patients with no history of CHD have the same risk of a future CHD event as do nondiabetic patients who have experienced an MI (approximately 20% risk in 7 years).[82,99] Close management of blood glucose levels appears to reduce microvascular disease, but not CHD.[100,101] Because of this, NCEP ATP III and the American Diabetic Association (ADA) considered patients with diabetes to be a CHD risk equivalent (>20% 10-year CHD risk) and recommended that these patients be treated with aggressive lipid-modifying therapy to an LDL-C goal of

Table 13-4   Overall Risk Reduction for CHD Events by Sex and Age

Group	Relative Risk Reduction (95% CI)	Absolute Risk Reduction/1,000 (95% CI)	Number Needed To Treat (95% CI)
Sex			
Women	29% (13–42)	33% (13–52)	31 (19–75)
Men	31% (26–35)	37% (29–44)	27 (23–34)
Age			
≥65 years	32% (23–39)	44% (30–58)	23 (17–33)
<65 years	31% (24–36)	32% (24–40)	31 (25–41)

CHD, coronary heart disease; CI, confidence interval.

<100 mg/dL.[87] Findings from the above clinical trials demonstrate that a reduction in CHD events with lipid-modifying therapy is of a similar or greater magnitude in diabetic patients compared to nondiabetic patients.[84] This supports the NCEP ATP III recommendation for aggressive management of diabetic patients.[87]

These trials also help illustrate the continuum of risk in patients with CHD (secondary prevention) and those without (primary prevention). In fact, the CHD risk in these two populations overlaps considerably. In secondary prevention patients, atherosclerosis is known to be present and the risk of a subsequent event is great. In primary prevention patients with multiple risk factors, there is a good chance that atherosclerosis is present and that this increases the risk of a future CHD event. In fact, some primary prevention patients have so many risk factors that they reach the level of a CHD risk equivalent (>20% CHD risk in 10 years). Others have only a few or no accompanying CHD risk factors and have a low to moderate future risk of a CHD event. Thus, the decision of how aggressively to treat patients begins with an assessment of their global CHD risk. The first step is to identify patients who have two or more risk factors and no CHD and CHD risk equivalent history (Table 13-5). The next step is to assess their global CHD risk with an instrument such as that illustrated in Figure 13-7 from the Framingham Heart Study.[87] (It is not necessary to conduct a global risk assessment of CHD patients, as their risk is known to be >20% in 10 years.) Patients with a very high risk of a future CHD event (e.g., diabetic patients and those with a global risk of >20% in 10 years) can be considered a CHD equivalent and given aggressive LDL-C–lowering treatment with the same LDL-C goal as applied to patients who have experienced a CHD event (i.e., an LDL-C treatment goal of <100 mg/dL).[102] Those with <20% risk of a CHD event in 10 years can be given lifestyle modification and drug therapy, if needed, to reach an intermediate LDL-C goal (<130 mg/dL). This approach of assessing a patient's CHD risk and matching the intensity of treatment is illustrated in the cases that follow.

TG-LOWERING CLINICAL TRIALS

Four clinical trials have tested TG-lowering therapies (fibrates and niacin) in randomized endpoint trials involving patients who generally had baseline TG levels of 150 to 500

Table 13-5	NCEP ATP III Major Risk Factors That Modify LDL-C Goals

Positive Risk Factors (↑ Risk)

Age: Male ≥45 yr
Female: ≥55 yr
Family history of a premature CHD (definite MI or sudden death before 55 yr in father or other male first-degree relative or before 65 yr in mother or other female first-degree relative)
Current cigarette smoking
Hypertension (≥140/90 mm Hg or on antihypertensive drugs)
Low HDL-C (<40 mg/dL)

Negative Risk Factor (↓ Risk, protective)

High HDL-C (≥60 mg/dL)

Expert Panel on Detection, Evaluation, and Treatment of High Blood Cholesterol in Adults, 2001.[87]
Note: Presence of diabetes mellitus is considered a CHD risk equivalent (see Table 13-8). It is not included in counting the number of risk factors because its presence automatically qualifies the patient for aggressive treatment whether or not true CHD is manifest.
CHD, coronary heart disease; HDL-C, high-density lipoprotein cholesterol; MI, myocardial infarction.

mg/dL and HDL-C <40 mg/dL (Table 13-6). The Helsinki Heart Study studied 4,081 men without CHD and found a 34% reduction in CHD death and nonfatal MI after 5 years of gemfibrozil therapy compared with placebo.[103] Post hoc analysis of this study showed that the group of patients with TG >200 mg/dL and an LDL/HDL ratio >5.0 (generally with LDL-C >194 mg/dL and HDL-C <40 mg/dL) accounted for 71% of the CHD reduction achieved in the entire study, even though the group represented only 10% of the total study population[104] (see Table 13-6). The VA-HIT (HDL Intervention Trial) studied 2,531 men with a history of CHD and low HDL-C levels (mean HDL-C level, 32 mg/dL) and reported a 22% reduction in CHD events with gemfibrozil therapy. The authors reported that approximately 25% of this risk reduction was due to the 6% increase in HDL-C. The Bezafibrate Infarction Prevention (BIP) trial studied CHD patients with a lipid profile similar to the patients in the

Table 13-6	Randomized Endpoint Trials With Triglyceride-Lowering Therapies				
Trial	Intervention	Lipids (Initial–On Rx)	Lipid Changes	Placebo CHD Rate	CHD Event Reduction
HHS[95]	Gemfibrozil	LDL: 189–170	↓ 10%		
		TG: 178–116	↓ 35%	4%	↓ 34%
		HDL: 47–52	↑ 11%		
VA-HIT[87]	Gemfibrozil	LDL: 111–113	0%		
		TG: 161–115	↓ 31%	22%	↓ 22%
		HDL: 32–34	↑ 6%		
BIP[106]	Bezafibrate	LDL: 148–138	↓ 7%		
		TG: 145–115	↓ 21%	15%	↓ 9.4%
		HDL: 35–41	↑ 18%		
CDP[81]	Niacin	TC: 250–235	↓ 10%	30%	↓ 13%
		TG: 480–354	↓ 26%		

CHD, coronary heart disease; HDL, high-density lipoprotein cholesterol; LDL-C, low-density lipoprotein cholesterol; Rx, drug therapy; TG, triglyceride.

Estimate of 10-Year Risk for Men

(Framingham Point Scores)

Age	Points
20-34	−9
35-39	−4
40-44	0
45-49	3
50-54	6
55-59	8
60-64	10
65-69	11
70-74	12
75-79	13

Total Cholesterol	Points				
	Age 20-39	Age 40-49	Age 50-59	Age 60-69	Age 70-79
<160	0	0	0	0	0
160-199	4	3	2	1	0
200-239	7	5	3	1	0
240-279	9	6	4	2	1
≥280	11	8	5	3	1

	Points				
	Age 20-39	Age 40-49	Age 50-59	Age 60-69	Age 70-79
Nonsmoker	0	0	0	0	0
Smoker	8	5	3	1	1

HDL (mg/dL)	Points
≥60	−1
50-59	0
40-49	1
<40	2

Systolic BP (mmHg)	If Untreated	If Treated
<120	0	0
120-129	0	1
130-139	1	2
140-159	1	2
≥160	2	3

Point Total	10-Year Risk %
<0	<1
0	1
1	1
2	1
3	1
4	1
5	2
6	2
7	3
8	4
9	5
10	6
11	8
12	10
13	12
14	16
15	20
16	25
≥17	≥30

10-Year risk _____ %

A

Estimate of 10-Year Risk for Women

(Framingham Point Scores)

Age	Points
20-34	−7
35-39	−3
40-44	0
45-49	3
50-54	6
55-59	8
60-64	10
65-69	12
70-74	14
75-79	16

Total Cholesterol	Points				
	Age 20-39	Age 40-49	Age 50-59	Age 60-69	Age 70-79
<160	0	0	0	0	0
160-199	4	3	2	1	1
200-239	8	6	4	2	1
240-279	11	8	5	3	2
≥280	13	10	7	4	2

	Points				
	Age 20-39	Age 40-49	Age 50-59	Age 60-69	Age 70-79
Nonsmoker	0	0	0	0	0
Smoker	9	7	4	2	1

HDL (mg/dL)	Points
≥60	1
50-59	0
40-49	1
<40	2

Systolic BP (mmHg)	If Untreated	If Treated
<120	0	0
120-129	1	3
130-139	2	4
140-159	3	5
≥160	4	6

Point Total	10-Year Risk %
<9	<1
9	1
10	1
11	1
12	1
13	2
14	2
15	3
16	4
17	5
18	6
19	8
20	11
21	14
22	17
23	22
24	27
≥25	≥30

10-Year risk _____ %

B

FIGURE 13-7. A: Estimate of 10-year risk for men. **B:** Estimate of 10-year risk for women.

Tex/AFCAPS trial (high LDL-C, low HDL-C, normal TG) and reported an insignificant 9% reduction in CHD events associated with an 18% increase in HDL-C and a 21% reduction in TGs.[106] A post hoc analysis of this trial found that patients who had TG levels of >175 and 200 mg/dL had significant CHD event reductions of 22% and 40%, respectively.

These studies, especially the post hoc analyses, suggest that patients with atherogenic dyslipidemia experience CHD risk reduction with fibrate therapy. The risk reduction may be similar to that achieved with statins, although there are no head-to-head trials to refute or affirm this. This presents a dilemma for the clinician; when presented with a patient who has atherogenic dyslipidemia, which is the drug of choice, a statin or fibrate? Some guidance to this question will be provided during the case discussions that follow.

Only one placebo-controlled endpoint study is available for niacin (see Table 13-6). The study was completed in men who had had a prior MI and mixed hyperlipidemia. After 5 years of niacin therapy, the CHD event rate was reduced by 13%.[107] Fifteen years after the start of the study, and 9 years after the study was terminated, the investigators reported that total mortality was 11% lower in the men in the niacin arm, suggesting that any period of lipid-modifying treatment may translate into a long-term benefit.[108] Combination therapy with niacin plus a statin has been studied in CHD patients with low HDL-C and normal LDL-C.[109] Compared with a mean 3.9% progression in coronary stenosis with placebo, niacin–simvastatin therapy was associated with a mean regression of 0.4% ($P < 0.001$). The authors posited that event reduction with this combination should be equivalent to the sum of the LDL-C reduction and the HDL-C increase. In the study LDL-C was reduced by 42% and HDL-C was increased by 26%, and the composite endpoint of death from coronary causes, MI, stroke, or revascularization for worsening ischemia was reduced 60% with the niacin–statin combination. ($P = 0.02$).

Niacin has long been an intriguing drug to lipid specialists. It is one of the few drugs that positively affects each component of the lipid profile (LDL-C, TG, and HDL-C). It is the best therapy available to raise HDL-C and one of the best at lowering TG. It is logical to expect that these effects would translate into substantial CHD risk reduction. It is especially interesting to speculate on how these effects may combine to offer better risk reduction, especially when combined with one of the statins. However, because niacin is an old therapy that is not as well tolerated as the newer statins and has no patent protection remaining, it is unlikely to be evaluated in a large randomized clinical trial for its ability to reduce CHD risk. This leaves the clinician with limited knowledge about the power of this therapy to reduce CHD risk. Guidance is provided in the cases as to how to integrate this therapy in the management of patients with a lipid disorder.

Mechanisms of CHD Risk Reduction

Given the consistent relationship between lowering blood cholesterol and reducing CHD events, the question arises, "what is the mechanism of this protection?" Scientists are offering many new and exciting answers to this question. At present, it appears that the reduction in CHD with lipid-altering therapy is mediated through, or at least tracked by, a reduction in cholesterol levels. However, in addition to lowering

blood cholesterol levels, statins and other lipid-altering therapies produce other, so-called pleiotropic, effects that may partly explain their CHD-reducing capability.

One way in which cholesterol lowering may reduce CHD is by changing atherosclerotic plaque from lesions with a large lipid core, thin fibrous cap, and many cholesterol-filled macrophage cells along the shoulders of the lesion to lesions with a small lipid core and much connective tissue and smooth muscle matrix throughout. The lesion does not appear to change much in size, or at least not in ways that can be visualized on an arteriogram. However, the harder lesion created with lipid lowering is much less likely to rupture or erode, thus reducing the risk of forming an occluding clot and producing CHD events.

Lipid lowering may also affect endothelial function. There is evidence that high LDL-C levels cause "endothelial dysfunction," as evidenced by a lowered ability of coronary arteries to dilate. Cholesterol lowering by practically any means restores endothelial function. Many studies have demonstrated improvement in brachial artery reactivity and coronary artery dilation when cholesterol levels are reduced.[110–115] Positron emission tomography (PET) scans demonstrate improved blood flow and reduced areas of ischemia throughout the myocardium in patients receiving lipid-altering therapy.[112,113] These effects may have important clinical benefits. In patients with coronary artery disease, cholesterol lowering reduces the number of ST-segment depressions recorded during a 48-hour electrocardiogram (ECG) Holter monitor study.[116,117] Therapy with a statin can also reduce ischemic events requiring acute management, a potential effect of restored endothelial function.[94]

Cholesterol lowering might also combat the inflammation that accompanies atherogenesis. Early in the development of plaques, monocyte-derived macrophages are recruited to engulf modified LDL particles, and in every stage of the disease, specific subtypes of T lymphocytes are present.[36,42] At various stages, cytokines, chemokines, and growth factors are released. Inflammatory processes may be especially active just before or after the plaque ruptures. Several investigators have attempted to identify markers of inflammation that may signal an increased risk of a CHD event. One promising marker is high-sensitivity C-reactive protein (hs-CRP). An elevated hs-CRP level predicts a high risk of future CHD events and appears to add to the risk predicted by LDL-C alone.[118] A subanalysis of the CARE trial reported that high levels of hs-CRP forecast CHD risk in placebo patients, but this was attenuated and nonsignificant in patients assigned to pravastatin, suggesting that statin treatment has an anti-inflammatory effect.[119] The American Heart Association has recently recommended that measurement of the hs-CRP level be considered in a patient with two or more risk factors as a way to further characterize the patient's future CHD risk.[120]

Cost-Effectiveness

Several cost-effectiveness analyses of lipid-lowering therapies have been conducted.[121–124] One variable used in these analyses is the cost per years of life saved (YOLS). Analyses of other prophylactic measures to reduce CHD risk, such as the use of aspirin in post-MI patients and the treatment of mild hypertension with antihypertensive drugs, indicate that it costs up to $50,000 per YOLS to treat these patients. Our society has accepted this level of expenditure as cost-effective. Analyses of cholesterol-lowering treatment in clinical trials have found that drug treatment of high-risk patients for secondary prevention costs approximately $12,000 per YOLS, while treatment of high-risk patients for primary prevention costs approximately $25,000 per YOLS. In the 4S study, the cost saved in reduced hospital days by treatment was so great that simvastatin was estimated to cost only $0.28 per day (an 88% savings).[125] In another analysis of the cost of treating patients to their NCEP goal in an office setting, atorvastatin was found to cost the least, approximately $1,064 per year, in combined expenses for drugs, office visits, and laboratory monitoring.[126] These analyses support aggressive (i.e., drug and lifestyle) treatment of CHD and high-risk patients with lipid-lowering therapy.

HYPERCHOLESTEROLEMIA

Evaluation of the Lipoprotein Profile

1. T.A., a 43-year-old premenopausal woman, is screened with a lipid profile during an annual medical evaluation. She has never taken cholesterol-lowering medication and currently takes only a multivitamin daily. She has had no symptoms of coronary, carotid, or peripheral vascular disease. She has a 20-pack/year history of smoking and exercises four times a week, without physical limitations. T.A. states that she follows a low-fat, low-cholesterol diet. Her father is alive and well at age 71, with a normal cholesterol level. Her mother had an MI at age 47 and died at age 57 from a second event. Her grandfather died of an MI at age 52; a sister has hypercholesterolemia and is taking simvastatin. Pertinent physical findings are weight, 125 lb; height, 63 in; BP, 120/82 mm Hg; pulse, 66 beats/min and regular; carotid pulses symmetric bilaterally without bruits; no neck masses; no abdominal bruit; and no evidence of tendon xanthomas. Pertinent laboratory findings, obtained after a 12-hour fast, show total cholesterol, 290 mg/dL; TGs, 55 mg/dL; HDL-C, 55 mg/dL; LDL-C, 224 mg/dL; non-HDL-C, 235; plasma glucose, 96 mg/dL (normal, 60 to 115); thyroid-stimulating hormone (TSH), 0.92 IU/mL (normal, 0.4 to 6.2); alanine aminotransferase (ALT), 11 U/L (normal, 6 to 34); aspartate aminotransferase (AST), 8 U/L (normal, 9 to 34); blood urea nitrogen (BUN), 12 mg/dL (normal, 4 to 24); creatinine, 1.0 mg/dL (normal, 0.4 to 1.1); and a negative urinalysis. What is your assessment of these results?

[SI units: total cholesterol, 7.5 mmol/L; TGs, 0.62 mmol/L; HDL-C, 1.42 mmol/L; LDL-C, 5.79 mmol/L; glucose, 5.33 mmol/L; TSH, <100 units; ALT, 0.18 μkat/L; AST, 0.13 μkat/L; BUN, 4.28 mmol/L urea; creatinine, 88.4 μmol/L]

T.A.'s LDL-C is considered "very high" (>190 mg/dl); NCEP defines the optimal LDL-C as <100 mg/dL.[87] Her HDL-C is right at the average HDL-C for a woman and her TG is normal (<150 mg/dL) (Table 13-7). In most cases, it is wise to repeat the lipid profile to be sure the first results are not atypical. However, T.A.'s LDL-C is so high a repeat test is not likely to change the assessment. Thus, in this case, a second test is optional.

In many labs, LDL-C is calculated. Total cholesterol, HDL-C, and TGs are measured directly and then the following formula is applied to calculate LDL-C:

Table 13-7 NCEP ATP III Classifications of Blood Lipids[87]

LDL-Cholesterol	
<100 mg/dL	Optimal
100–129 mg/dL	Near optimal or above optimal
130–159 mg/dL	Borderline high
160–189 mg/dL	High
≥190 mg/dL	Very high
Total Cholesterol	
<200 mg/dL	Desirable
200–239 mg/dL	Borderline high
≥240 mg/dL	High
HDL-Cholesterol	
<40 mg/dL	Low
≥60 mg/dL	High
Triglycerides	
<150 mg/dL	Normal
150–199 mg/dL	Borderline high
200–499 mg/dL	High
≥500 mg/dL	Very high

HDL, high-density lipoprotein; LDL, low-density lipoprotein.

$$LDL\text{-}C = \text{Total Cholesterol} - (HDL\text{-}C + VLDL\text{-}C)$$

Because the ratio of cholesterol to TG in LDL is 1:5, VLDL-C is estimated by dividing the total TG level by 5. Thus, the formula is rewritten as:

$$LDL\text{-}C = \text{Total Cholesterol} - (HDL\text{-}C + TG/5)$$

If the TG level is >400 mg/dL, the formula for estimating VLDL-C is not accurate and therefore LDL-C cannot be calculated. An accurate LDL-C measurement also requires that the patient fast for 10 to 12 hours. This provides sufficient time for exogenous TG, carried by chylomicrons, to be cleared from the systemic circulation (provided the patient does not have hyperchylomicronemia). Most labs can measure LDL-C directly and should be asked to do so when the TG is >400 mg/dL or the patient has not fasted. Applying the formula to T.A.'s lipid profile, the calculated LDL-C is 224 mg/dL.

$$\begin{aligned} LDL\text{-}C &= \text{Total Cholesterol} - (HDL\text{-}C + TG/5) \\ &= 290 - (55 + 55/5) \\ &= 224 \text{ mg/dL} \end{aligned}$$

Non-HDL-C is calculated by the following formula:

$$Non\text{-}HDL\text{-}C = \text{Total cholesterol} - HDL\text{-}C$$

For T.A.:

$$\begin{aligned} Non\text{-}HDL\text{-}C &= 290 \text{ mg/dL} - 55 \text{ mg/dL} \\ &= 235 \text{ mg/dL} \end{aligned}$$

Secondary Causes of High Blood Cholesterol

2. Is there any evidence that T.A.'s elevated LDL-C is secondary to other conditions or concurrent drug therapy?

As a routine, every new patient with hypercholesterolemia should be evaluated for four things in the following order: (1) secondary causes of the high cholesterol level, (2) familial disorders, (3) presence of CHD and CHD equivalents, and (4) CHD risk factors.

Conditions that may produce lipid abnormalities (i.e., secondary causes) include diabetes mellitus, hypothyroidism, nephrotic syndrome, and obstructive liver disease. Selected drugs may also produce lipid abnormalities (Table 13-8). When one of these secondary causes is identified, it should be managed first, as this may resolve the lipid abnormality.

In T.A.'s case, no secondary causes are evident. Her blood glucose level does not indicate the presence of diabetes; her TSH level does not indicate hypothyroidism; her ALT and AST levels are within acceptable levels, suggesting normal liver function; and her BUN, creatinine, and urinalysis are acceptable, signifying normal renal function. She is not taking any drugs that could have contributed to her cholesterol elevation.

Familial Forms of Hypercholesterolemia

3. Could T.A. have an inherited form of hyperlipidemia?

T.A.'s history is consistent with polygenic hypercholesterolemia, the form of hypercholesterolemia that affects 98% of patients with hypercholesterolemia. As described previously, polygenic hypercholesterolemia is suspected when the patient's LDL-C is 130 to 250 mg/dL and there is no evidence of tendon xanthomas (see Table 13-2). A family history of CHD is present in approximately 18% of these patients and is a strong finding in T.A.'s case. Polygenic hypercholesterolemia is caused by a combination of nutritional and genetic factors that reduce the clearance of LDL particles from the plasma. It is impossible to determine which of these factors are causing hypercholesterolemia in a given patient by simply examining the lipoprotein profile. However, if the patient's blood lipids normalize with a low-fat diet, one can assume that the diet is a major etiologic factor for that person. Conversely, if there is little or no change in blood cholesterol levels after dietary modification, genetics likely significantly influences the patient's elevated cholesterol. In most cases, a relatively equal contribution is made by genetic factors and environment on cholesterol elevations.

CHD and CHD Risk Equivalents

4. Does T.A. have evidence of CHD or a CHD risk equivalent?

Table 13-8 Drug-Induced Hyperlipidemia

	Effect on Plasma Lipids			Comments
	Cholesterol	*Triglycerides*	*HDL-C*	
Diuretics[255,256]				
Thiazides	↑ 5–7% initially ↑ 0–3% later	↑ 30–50%	↑ 1%	Effects transient; monitor for long-term effects
Loop	No change	No change	↓ to 15%	
Indapamide	No change	No change	No change	
Metolazone	No change	No change	No change	
Potassium-sparing	No change	No change	No change	
β-blockers[257–260]				
Nonselective	No change	↑ 20–50%	↓ 10–15%	Selective β-blockers have greater effects than nonselective; β-blockers with ISA or α-blocking effects are lipid neutral
Selective	No change	↑ 15–30%	↓ 5–10%	
α-Blocking	No change or ↓	No change	No change	
α-Agonists and antagonists (e.g., prazosin and clonidine)[261,262]	↓ 0–10%	↓ 0–20%	↑ 0 15%	In general, drugs that affect α-receptors ↓ cholesterol and ↑ HDL-C
ACE inhibitors[2633]	No change	No change	No change	
Calcium channel blockers	No change	No change	No change	
Oral contraceptives[264,265]				
Monophasics	↑ 5–20%	↑ 10–45%	↑ 15% to ↓ 15%	Effects due to reduced lipolytic activity and/or ↑ VLDL synthesis; mainly due to progestin component; estrogen alone protective
Triphasics	↑ 10–15%	↑ 10–15%	↑ 5–10%	
Glucocorticoids[266]	↑ 5–10%	↑ 15–20%		
Ethanol[267]	No change	↑ up to 50%	↑	Marked elevations can occur in hyper triglyceridemic patients
Isotretinoin[268]	↑ 5–20%	↑ 50–60%	↓ 10–15%	Changes may reverse 8 wk after stopping drug
Cyclosporine[269]	↑ 15–20%	No change	No change	

ACE, angiotensin-converting enzyme; HDL-C, high-density lipoprotein cholesterol; ISA, intrinsic sympathomimetic activity.

A search for CHD starts with a good medical history of symptomatic coronary artery disease but is quickly followed with a broader search for atherosclerotic disease in other artery beds, including the arteries of the limbs and carotid arteries[87] (Table 13-9). If detected in one site, atherosclerosis is likely to be present in all or most vessels, and it is associated with a five- to sevenfold higher risk of a major coronary event.[127–129]

The patient should be asked about a history of myocardial ischemia (exercise-induced angina), prior MI (i.e., severe angina with elevated cardiac creatine phosphokinase [CPK] and/or characteristic ECG changes), history of revascularizations (i.e., coronary artery bypass surgery, angioplasty with percutaneous transluminal coronary angioplasty or stent placement), or history of hospitalization due to unstable angina (see Table 13-9). The presence of any of these findings is associated with a very high (>20%) risk of a CHD death or nonfatal MI in the next 10 years; the risk approaches 40% if unstable angina and stroke are also considered. None of these signs are present in T.A.

The evaluation can stop here, but some would advocate continuing the search with noninvasive procedures, even if the patient has not experienced symptoms (Table 13-10). The case for pursuing these evaluations is more convincing in patients who have a high probability of atherosclerosis because of the presence of multiple risk factors or a strong family history of premature CHD events. One noninvasive evaluation is exercise testing with either ECG monitoring for signs of ischemia or pharmacologic perfusion imaging (e.g., exercise thallium). Because these tests are expensive and not widely available, they are reserved for selected use. Even if the results are found to be normal, atherosclerosis is not ruled out since both tests are designed to detect flow-limiting disease, and atherosclerosis can be present without causing obstructions in luminal blood flow.[87]

In recent years, electron beam computed tomography and spiral computed tomography have been used to detect calcium in coronary vessels. The presence of coronary calcium suggests the presence of old atherosclerotic plaque. If old disease is present, then it is likely that younger, more vulnerable plaques are also present. This test is simple, quick, and noninvasive, but it is relatively expensive and not widely available. High coronary calcium volume scores can add to the prediction of future coronary events based on traditional risk factor assessment.[87] Use of these tests is particularly helpful in modifying the assessment of risk in patients with multiple risk factors. In T.A.'s case, her strong family history could support obtaining an electron beam computed tomography evaluation. If she has a significantly positive calcium volume score, more aggressive medical therapy could be considered.

A good history should also probe for evidence of atherosclerotic vascular disease in peripheral vessels. Patients with flow-limiting atherosclerosis in peripheral vessels often describe claudication (pain and weakness in the limb muscles) after walking a distance (see Chapter 15, Peripheral Vascular Disorders). NCEP recommends that patients over age 50 be evaluated with an ankle:brachial index (ABI). This index is determined by measuring the systolic blood pressure of the brachial, posterior tibia, and dorsalis pedis arteries using a handheld Doppler device and dividing the higher of the two ankle systolic blood pressures by the higher of two systolic brachial pressures.[87] An ABI of ≤0.9 constitutes the diagnosis of peripheral vascular disease (PVD; also called peripheral arterial disease or PAD). Finding atherosclerosis in peripheral vessels probably means it is present in coronary arteries as

---

Table 13-9   NCEP APT III Definitions of CHD and CHD Risk Equivalents[87]

Clinical CHD
    Myocardial ischemia (angina)
    Myocardial infarction
    Coronary angioplasty and/or stent placement
    Coronary bypass graft
    Prior unstable angina

Carotid artery disease
    Stroke history
    Transient ischemic attack history
    Carotid stenosis >50%

Peripheral arterial disease
    Claudication
    ABI >0.9

Abdominal aortic aneurysm

Diabetes mellitus

Estimated global CHD risk >20% in 10 years for any of the factors above.
ABI, ankle:brachial blood pressure index; CHD, coronary heart disease.

Table 13-10   Emerging CHD Risk Factors[87]

Noninvasive Evaluations for Subclinical Atherosclerosis	Blood Tests
Exercise ECG	Lipoprotein (a)
Myocardial perfusion imaging	Small dense LDL
Stress echocardiography	Apolipoprotein B (particle concentration)
Carotid intimal-medial thickness (IMT)	High-sensitivity CRP (and other inflammatory markers)
Electron beam computed tomography (EBCT)	Homocysteine
	HDL subspecies
	Apolipoprotein A-1
	Apolipoprotein B:C-III
	Thrombogenic factors (e.g. fibrinogen, PAI-1, t-PA)

CRP, C-reactive protein; ECG, electrocardiogram; HDL, high-density lipoprotein cholesterol; LDL-C, low-density lipoprotein cholesterol; t-PA, tissue plasminogen activator.

well. In fact, most patients with PVD die of a CHD event. Further, most patients with PVD have a very high (>20%) risk of a CHD event in the next 10 years, and so are said to have a CHD risk equivalent.

The clinician should also evaluate the patient for atherosclerosis in the carotid vessels by asking about signs and symptoms of transient ischemic attacks (TIAs) and strokes (see Chapter 15, Peripheral Vascular Disorders). On the physical examination, the carotid vessels should be evaluated for the presence of a bruit (indicative of a space-occupying lesion in the carotid vessel). If a bruit is present, further evaluation with carotid duplex imaging is indicated to detect stenotic lesions. Some authorities recommend performing carotid sonography to measure the intimal-medial thickness. This test is safe and simple but relatively expensive and not widely available. Intimal-medial thickness results correlate with the severity of coronary atherosclerosis. Patients who have experienced a stroke or TIAs have more than a 20% 10-year risk of experiencing a CHD event and so are also considered a CHD risk equivalent. Patients found to have a stenosis of >50% in their carotid vessel, even if asymptomatic, have a >20% 10-year CHD risk and again can be considered a CHD risk equivalent. Patients found to have an increased intimal-medial thickness, suggesting the presence of subclinical atherosclerosis, may also have a high CHD risk and are therefore candidates for more aggressive medical therapy.[87]

Other conditions that confer a >20% risk of a CHD event in the next 10 years, and thus are considered by NCEP to be CHD risk equivalents, include abdominal aortic aneurysm and the diagnosis of diabetes. More will be said about diabetes below. T.A. does not have evidence of CHD or a CHD risk equivalent.

CHD Risk Factors

5. **Does T.A. have CHD risk factors, and what is her global CHD risk?**

Patients who are found to have CHD or CHD risk equivalent do not need a risk factor assessment to establish their LDL-C treatment goal; the presence of CHD or a CHD risk equivalent satisfies that. However, these patients should undergo an appraisal of risk factors so that risk factor modification can be incorporated in the overall treatment plan. For patients who do not have CHD or a CHD risk equivalent, risk factor counting and global risk assessment is important to establish treatment goals and approaches.

Begin this process by counting the number of risk factors present (see Table 13-5). Patients with either zero or one risk factor most likely have a low risk of a CHD event in the next 10 years and are assigned an LDL-C goal of <160 mg/dL. Patients with two or more risk factors have a moderate to high risk, depending on the number of risk factors present. These patients are assigned an LDL-C goal of <130 mg/dL. The presence of modifiable risk factors should become the target of any risk-reduction treatment program.

T.A. has two CHD risk factors: current cigarette smoking and a family history of premature CHD. She thus has an LDL-C treatment goal of <130 mg/dL (Table 13-11). NCEP recommends that patients who have two or more risk factors be further evaluated using the Framingham-based global risk assessment tool (see Fig. 13-7) to define the 10-year risk. T.A. is found to have a 5% 10-year CHD risk, which is several-fold greater than the average risk for women her age but below the threshold where aggressive drug treatment is indicated (i.e., >10% CHD risk in 10 years). If she were not a smoker, her 10-year CHD risk estimate would be 1%, illustrating the prominent influence that smoking has on her future risk of a CHD event.

Based on this assessment and assuming that the noninvasive assessments performed on her, if any, were negative, T.A. should be counseled on diet and exercise and strongly advised to stop smoking. Because of its strong effect on her risk, smoking cessation should be a primary focus of her risk-reduction program. If these measures fail to bring her LDL-C to her treatment goal of <130 mg/dL and her LDL-C remains >160 mg/dL, drug therapy should be considered (see Table 13-11). However, if she stopped smoking, she would have only one risk factor (family history), and her new LDL-C goal would be <160 mg/dL. In this case, drug therapy would be considered only if the LDL-C remains >190 mg/dL.

Therapy for Lowering Cholesterol Levels

Diet Therapy

6. **What dietary changes should be recommended to T.A.?**

The centerpiece of treatment for high blood cholesterol is a diet low in saturated fat and cholesterol. The therapeutic lifestyle change ("TLC") diet recommended by NCEP restricts total fat intake to 25% to 35% of calories, saturated fats to <7% of calories, and dietary cholesterol to 200 mg/day (Table 13-12).[87] The TLC diet is aggressive and requires in-

---

Table 13-11 NCEP ATP III LDL-C Goals and Cutpoints for Therapeutic Lifestyle Changes (TLC) and Drug Therapy[87]

Risk Category	LDL-C Goal	LDL-C at which to Initiate TLC	LDL-C at which to Consider Drug Therapy
CHD or CHD risk equivalents (10-year risk >20%)	<100 mg/dL	≥100 mg/dL	≥130 mg/dL (100–129 mg/dL, drug selection optional)[a]
≥2 risk factors (10-year risk ≤20%)	<130 mg/dL	≥130 mg/dL	With 10-year risk 10–20%: ≥130 mg/dL With 10-year risk ≤10%: ≥160 mg/dL
<2 risk factors	<160 mg/dL	≥160 mg/dL	190 mg/dL (160–189 mg/dL, LDL-C lowering drug therapy is optional)

[a]The clinician may select TLC, statin, niacin, or fibrate therapy to achieve the LDL-C goal of <100 mg/dL.
CHD, coronary heart disease; LDL-C, low-density lipoprotein cholesterol.

Table 13-12 **NCEP ATP III Therapeutic Lifestyle Change Diet**[87]

Nutrient	Recommended Intake
Total fat	25–35% of total calories
Saturated fat	<7% of total calories
Polyunsaturated fat	Up to 10% of total calories
Monounsaturated fat	Up to 20% of total calories
Carbohydrate	50–60% of total calories
Fiber	20–30 g/day
Cholesterol	<200 mg/d
Protein	Approx. 15% of total calories

struction by a dietitian, nurse, or other health professional well versed in nutrition counseling. The TLC diet is also flexible and allows for modification of carbohydrate and monounsaturated fat intake according to the individual patient's needs. The goals presented by the TLC diet are minimum goals, and some patients will want to exceed them, even to the point of following a "vegetarian" diet. This is permissible, as long as the diet is nutritionally balanced.

When saturated fat is removed from the diet, it is important to understand what should be given in replacement. In the overweight or obese patient, it may be appropriate to do nothing, because a reduction in saturated fat is a good way to lower calories and encourage weight loss.

In individuals who are close to their ideal weight, such as T.A., replacing saturated fats with carbohydrates may not be the best choice. Increased intake of sugar and highly refined starches, as found in the many low-fat, high-calorie snack foods, may actually increase weight and reduce HDL-C as well as LDL-C.[130] More importantly, a low-fat, high-carbohydrate diet has not been shown to reduce the risk of CHD. However, consumption of complex carbohydrates is recommended and could be a replacement for saturated fat calories in a TLC diet.

Replacing saturated fat with unsaturated fats, especially monounsaturated fats (e.g., canola, olive oil products) and omega-3 polyunsaturated fats (e.g., fish oil sources), is highly desirable.[131] This is the diet of the Mediterranean people, who have a low incidence of CHD, and has the advantage of lowering LDL-C without affecting HDL-C. In fact, in a major randomized clinical trial in which it was compared with a "prudent Western-type diet," the Mediterranean diet was associated with a ≥70% reduction in cardiovascular endpoints and total mortality, a result that exceeds that achieved by our best lipid-lowering drug trials.[132] This study alone illustrates how important it is to initiate a good diet in hyperlipidemic patients, even with the available of very potent, highly efficacious, and safe drugs to lower serum cholesterol levels.

In our society, diets high in protein and saturated fats and low in carbohydrates (e.g., Atkins Diet) promise quick weight loss and other health effects. While these diets are capable of reducing lipid levels and causing weight loss, they are not nutritionally sound and may even be unhealthy. Patients should be advised to avoid them.

T.A. is likely to need help in translating the dietary recommendations of a TLC diet into practical terms and concepts that she can easily implement in her everyday life. Two ap-

proaches can be used to achieve this: (1) teach her to count calories or (2) provide general guidance in the selection of low-fat foods.

The more sophisticated patient may want to count calories or grams of total and saturated fat per day. The first step in teaching a patient to do this is to determine his or her daily caloric requirements, adjusted for his or her level of activity. The average caloric requirement for women is 1,800 calories/day; for men it is 2,500 calories/day. Based on this, T.A. should be instructed to keep her total fat intake to 450 to 630 calories/day (25% to 35% of calories) and saturated fat to <126 calories/day (<7% of total calories). Converting fat calories to grams (i.e., dividing calories by 9 calories/g), T.A. should be instructed to restrict her total fat intake to <50 to 70 g/day and saturated fat to <14 g/day.

Once these calculations have been made, the next step is to teach T.A. how to determine the grams of saturated and unsaturated fat contained in the foods she eats by reading food labels and referring to reference charts or books that list the nutritional content of foods. A good source for this nutrition information is the National Institutes of Health website on Therapeutic Lifestyle Change (http://www.nhlbi.nih.gov under the Health Information icon). This site contains information on the TLC diet, a 10-year risk calculator, recipes, a virtual grocery store, a cyberkitchen, a fitness room, and a resource library. The American Heart Association sites (www.americanheart.org and www.deliciousdecisions.org) provide equally good information on risk assessment, a cholesterol tracker, low-fat recipes, and guidance for eating in restaurants, cooking, and fitness.

For patients who are not able or willing to count calories or grams, general instruction on how to select low-fat foods and control portion sizes of higher-fat foods would provide an alternative approach. Principles to teach include the following:

- Eat less high-fat food (especially food high in saturated fats).
- Replace saturated fats with monounsaturated fats and fish oils whenever possible.
- Eat less high-cholesterol food.
- Choose foods high in complex carbohydrates (starch and fiber).
- Attain and maintain an acceptable weight.

T.A. should be counseled to recognize and minimize the three main sources of saturated fats in her diet: meat products, dairy products, and oils used in processed foods and cooking.

All meat products, including beef, pork, and poultry, contain fat. Much of the fat is visible and should be trimmed off before consumption. The remaining fat is contained within the meat and can be limited by (1) selecting the leanest meat (e.g., lean beef, skinless chicken, fish), (2) limiting portion size to about the size of a deck of playing cards (no more than 6 oz/day), and (3) cooking the meat in a manner that allows the fat to drip away from the meat (i.e., broiling, grilling).

High-fat dairy products are made with whole milk; low-fat alternatives are made with skim or 1% milk (which contain all of the nutrient value of whole milk products). T.A. should be taught to substitute low-fat alternatives for high-fat products—for example, by choosing soft margarine (or no fatty spread at all) instead of stick butter (note that unsaturated fats exist normally in liquid form and saturated fats in solid form);

nonfat creams rather than whole milk creams; low-fat or non-fat soft cheese (e.g., cottage cheese) rather than natural or processed hard cheese (including cream cheese); skim milk rather than whole milk; light or nonfat sour cream rather than regular sour cream; and nonfat frozen yogurt rather than ice cream. She also should avoid or limit cream sauces on meats and vegetables and creamy soups.

Products prepared with coconut, palm, or palm kernel oils, as well as lard and bacon fat contain a high concentration of saturated fats, and intake should be restricted. In their place, products made with monounsaturated fats (e.g., olive oil, canola oils) or polyunsaturated fats (especially oils that contain omega-3 fatty acids) may be substituted. Monounsaturated fats have little or no effect on blood lipids, and polyunsaturated fats actually may help reduce total cholesterol. Although unsaturated fats do not elevate cholesterol levels, they are sources of dense calories and, therefore, may contribute to the development of obesity and hypertriglyceridemia. Also, when the "good" (unsaturated) oils are partially hydrogenated (i.e., saturated to make them solid, as in some margarine products), they take on the character of saturated oils and may raise cholesterol levels. These are called trans fatty acids. Major sources of saturated and trans fatty acids include cakes, pies, cookies, chips, and crackers. T.A. should be advised to avoid or limit not only saturated fats, but also trans fatty acids by reading food labels.

It is best not to give the patient a list of foods to avoid; this aversive approach is likely to fail. Rather, good instruction about a low-fat diet should teach the patient how to make good selections. Any food, even a high-fat food, is not prohibited as long as portion size and frequency of use are controlled.

Another dietary approach to lowering blood cholesterol is to use dietary adjuncts. For example, adding 5 to 10 g of viscous fiber (e.g., guar, pectin, oat gum, psyllium) or other dietary sources of fiber (e.g., vegetables, legumes, whole grains, fruits) to the diet daily will aid in lowering blood cholesterol levels about 5% on average. Also, plant stanol and sterol esters have been made available in margarine and salad dressing products (Benecol and Total Control) and can lower LDL-C 5% to 15% when the equivalent of one tablespoonful is ingested one to three times a day. They act by reducing the absorption of cholesterol in the intestine.

T.A. will need to follow a low-fat diet indefinitely to sustain its benefit. For this reason, it might be necessary to have T.A. work with a registered dietitian or other professional who understands low-fat, low-cholesterol diets and who can give her personalized instruction. Particularly important is instruction on how to shop for and prepare low-fat foods and how to select low-fat foods in restaurants.

EFFECT ON LDL-C

7. **What changes in T.A.'s LDL-C can be expected if she follows a TLC diet?**

Serum cholesterol is reported to be reduced by an average of 3% to 14% in males who restrict saturated fat to <10% of calories; a slightly smaller response is attained in women, perhaps because their intake of saturated fats is generally lower than that of men.[133–135] Patients who can restrict saturated fat intake to <7% of daily calories should experience an addi-

tional 3% to 7% average reduction. Most patients can attain at least a 5% reduction in cholesterol levels with a TLC diet, some patients much more. If dietary adjuncts are added, LDL-C may be lowered by an additional 5% to 15%.

Patients' response to a low-fat diet is variable. In some patients, blood cholesterol levels fall substantially, whereas in others practically no change occurs. Response to a low-fat diet depends on many factors, including the patient's dietary habits before implementing the low-fat diet, the patient's adherence with the diet, the degree to which the patient restricts fats and cholesterol, and the influence of genetic factors. The patient should not be discouraged if LDL-C levels do not change much or at all despite close adherence to the diet. The Mediterranean diet, for example, which is high in monounsaturated fats and fiber, has no appreciable effect on blood lipids, but can still reduce cardiovascular disease and mortality by 70%.[132] Patients who adhere to a low-fat diet might also respond to lower doses of lipid-lowering drugs.

Because T.A. is a woman and was following a low-fat diet before her diagnosis, a TLC diet is not likely to have a substantial effect on her blood cholesterol levels. It would be prudent to have her maintain a 3-day diary of everything she eats to allow a more objective view of her eating habits. If there are ways for her to improve her diet, this approach will reveal them.

Other Lifestyle Changes

8. **What other changes are prescribed in the TLC program?**

Weight reduction in the overweight patient can reduce LDL-C and is a key component to the TLC plan. A 5- to 10-lb weight loss, for example, can up to double the LDL-C reduction achieved with a low–saturated fat diet alone.[133] However, the predominant effect of weight loss is a reduction in serum TGs and a small increase in HDL-C.[136] In addition, weight reduction may offset the risk of developing hypertension and diabetes. The initial goal of a weight loss program is to reduce body weight by approximately 10% within about 6 months.[137] This is best achieved by restricting total daily energy consumption through a reduction in saturated and trans fatty acid intake and by increasing physical exercise. A normal weight is defined as a body mass index (BMI) between 18.5 and 24.9, and a desirable waist circumference is <40 inches for male patients and <35 inches for female patients.[137] Because T.A. has an acceptable weight, these considerations do not apply.

Smoking cessation substantially reduces the risk of CHD, pulmonary disease, and cancer and is a central component of a TLC program. This is an important consideration in T.A. The CHD risk she has from smoking is greater than the risk she has from her LDL-C elevation. By stopping smoking, T.A. will not only reduce her blood cholesterol levels slightly, but will also substantially alter her risk profile. Because most patients gain weight when they stop smoking and because weight gain may worsen lipid levels, plans to alter her diet and increase physical activity to counter these effects should be made.

Increasing physical activity should be a component of the management of any patient with high blood cholesterol. Regular physical exercise may reduce TG and VLDL-C levels, raise HDL-C levels slightly, promote weight loss or maintenance of desired weight, lower BP, and cause favorable changes in coronary blood flow.[138] Regular aerobic exercise such as brisk walking, jogging, swimming, bicycling, and tennis should be prescribed in terms of amount (e.g., walking 4 miles), intensity (e.g., walking 4 mph), and frequency (walking each day if possible, but at least three times a week). T.A. states that she is already physically active. The level of her activity should be documented and enhancements recommended if needed.

Goal of Therapy

9. **A lipid profile obtained 12 weeks after T.A. initiated a TLC diet and exercise program and had stopped smoking revealed an LDL-C level of 195 mg/dL; HDL-C and TG were not different from baseline values. What is your assessment of the need for additional lipid-modifying treatment?**

[SI units: LDL-C, 5.40, 5.43, and 5.17 mmol/L, respectively]

Based on her initial assessment, T.A.'s LDL-C goal is <130 mg/dL; drug therapy can be considered if her LDL-C is above 160 mg/dL (see Table 13-11). However, she has stopped smoking and now has a global CHD risk of 1% in the next 10 years. Thus, her LDL-C goal today is <160 mg/dL. While she is not currently smoking, it may take a year or more for the associated risk to fully dissipate. NCEP recommends that drugs be considered in patients with less than 2 risk factors if their LDL-C remains >160 mg/dL after implementing a TLC plan. Realistically, this is a therapeutic gray area where clinical judgment must be exercised. T.A. has a relatively low risk of CHD despite her current LDL-C level, supporting a decision to maximize TLC and withhold lipid-lowering drug therapy until her CHD risk rises to a high level. However, her strong family history suggests there is more to the story than LDL-C alone.

Emerging Risk Factors

10. **To help determine whether to initiate lipid-lowering drug therapy in T.A., is there value in ordering additional laboratory tests to identify possible emerging risk factors?**

As mentioned in question 4, noninvasive tests, such as ABI, carotid intimal-medial thickness, and electron beam computed tomography, can uncover evidence of subclinical atherosclerotic disease and help the clinician decide whether to pursue more aggressive therapy with lipid-lowering drugs. In addition, the clinician can measure several specialized laboratory tests of emerging risk factors to help with these decisions (see Table 13-10). In T.A.'s case, a global risk assessment indicating about a 1% risk of a CHD event in 10 years and her strong family history for premature CHD events present conflicting information. Measuring one or more of the emerging risk factors may help focus the treatment decision in one direction or another.

Lp(a) (pronounced "el, pea, little a") appears to be an independent risk factor for CHD, although this is not a universal finding.[139] This very small cholesterol-containing lipoprotein particle contains the apolipoprotein(a). Its structure suggests that it could be an important source of cholesterol for the formation of atherosclerosis as well as a stimulus for thrombogenic mechanisms. High Lp(a) levels suggest a high CHD risk and support a more aggressive approach to lowering LDL-C. Evidence has shown that lowering LDL-C aggressively can overcome the increased CHD risk predicted by an elevated Lp(a) level. The only drug that can lower Lp(a) is niacin, but there are no studies showing that giving niacin to these patients reduces CHD risk.

Apolipoprotein B is a marker for the number of atherogenic lipoproteins (VLDL and LDL) in the circulation. It is a strong predictor of CHD risk, at least as strong as LDL-C. It is a surrogate for LDL-C, but provides different information.[140] Some specialists prefer to use apolipoprotein B levels rather than, or in addition to, LDL-C in managing patients. Apolipoprotein B levels are usually disproportionately high in patients with high TGs, although they may also parallel LDL-C levels. There is a genetic dyslipidemia that is characterized by increased apolipoprotein B levels (increased particle number) and normal LDL-C levels. Based on this information, it appears reasonable to measure apolipoprotein B to gain additional information.

Severe elevations in homocysteine are positively correlated with CHD risk, especially in patients with inherited forms of hyperhomocysteinemia.[141] Several clinical trials are underway to determine whether treating moderate hyperhomocysteinemia will lower CHD events. High levels of homocysteine are easily treated with folic acid; the recent fortification of foods with folic acid is predicted to substantially reduce homocysteine levels. NCEP ATP III does not recommend homocysteine measurements in risk assessment to modify LDL-C goals because panel members were uncertain of the relationship between homocysteine levels and CHD risk.[87] However, it may be useful in patients such as T.A. when searching for causes of a strong family history of CHD.

Increasingly, it is recognized that atherosclerosis is a chronic inflammatory disease. Thus, markers of inflammation have been sought to measure arterial inflammation. The marker that has emerged from this search is high-sensitivity C-reactive protein (hs-CRP). Many observational studies have found that hs-CRP predicts a two- to fourfold increase in CHD risk over what is predicted by LDL-C alone.[118] Recently, the AHA has recommended that hs-CRP levels between 3 and 10 be considered suggestive evidence of a chronic inflammatory disease.[120] Levels >10 suggest the presence of an acute inflammation caused by infection, trauma, connective tissue disease or other causes; in this case, the hs-CRP measurement should be repeated after 6 weeks.

T.A. was found to have a slightly elevated apolipoprotein B level (135 mg/dL) (which is consistent with her elevated LDL-C level), normal Lp(a) and homocysteine levels, and an hs-CRP of 4.7 mg/dL. An hs-CRP >3.0 is consistent with the presence of a chronic inflammatory disease, possibly atherosclerosis. Some clinicians believe that these findings would support more aggressive LDL-C lowering therapy in T.A.

Drug Therapy

11. **L.W. is a 53-year-old man with a LDL-C of 200 mg/dL. He states that he follows a low–saturated fat diet and jogs 2 miles three times a week. He does not smoke and has no family history of premature CHD. His high BP is under marginal control with enalapril 10 mg/day (BP, 134/88 mm Hg). His glucose level is 80 mg/dL (normal). He does not have hypothyroidism. His total cholesterol is 261 mg/dL, HDL-C is 45 mg/dL (normal average**

Table 13-13   Drugs of Choice for Dyslipidemia

Lipid Disorder	Drug of Choice	Alternative Agents	Combination Therapy
Polygenic hypercholesterolemia	Statin	Resin, ezetimibe, niacin Combination	Statin-ezetimibe, Statin-resin, resin-niacin, statin-niacin
Familial hypercholesterolemia or severe polygenic hypercholesterolemia	Statin (high dose)		Statin-ezetimibe, statin-resin, resin-niacin, statin-niacin, statin-ezetimibe-niacin, statin-resin-niacin
Atherogenic dyslipidemia	Statin, niacin, fibrate	Statin, niacin, fibrate	Statin-niacin, statin-fenofibrate, niacin-resin, niacin-fibrate
Isolated low HDL	Statin	Niacin	Statin-niacin

[a]Use cautiously because there is an increased risk of myopathy.
HDL, high-density lipoprotein; HDL-C, high-density lipoprotein cholesterol; LDL-C, low-density lipoprotein cholesterol; TGs, triglycerides.

for a man), LDL-C is 200 mg/dL, and TG level is 80 mg/dL. No secondary or familial causes of his hypercholesterolemia are evident, and his physical exam is normal. Is L.W. a candidate for cholesterol-lowering drug therapy?

[SI unit: LDL-C, 5.17 mmol/L]

According to NCEP guidelines, L.W. has two CHD risk factors: male older than 45 and a diagnosis of hypertension; this makes his LDL-C goal <130 mg/dL (see Tables 13-5 and 13-7). Because he has two risk factors, his global risk was assessed (see Fig. 13-7A). L.W was found to have a 12% risk of a CHD event in the next 10 years. With two risk factors and an estimated 10-year risk assessment between 10% and 20%, he is a candidate for cholesterol-lowering drug therapy in addition to therapeutic lifestyle change (see Table 13-11).

BILE ACID RESINS AND CHOLESTEROL ABSORPTION INHIBITORS

12. The NCEP recognizes four drug categories for lowering LDL-C: bile acid resins, cholesterol absorption inhibitors, niacin, and the statins.[87] Which of these is preferred to treat L.W. (Table 13-13)?

Bile acid resins have appeal in the management of hypercholesterolemia because they have a strong safety record established from years of use, effectively lower LDL-C, and demonstrated the ability to reduce CHD events in the Coronary Primary Prevention Trial.[81,142] Resins are not absorbed from the gastrointestinal (GI) tract and thus lack systemic toxicity. They are available in powder and tablet forms. They reduce total and LDL cholesterol in a dose-dependent manner (Table 13-14). LDL-C is reduced approximately 15% with 5 g (1 packet) daily of colestipol (Colestid) powder (equivalent to 4 g of cholestyramine [Questran]), 23% with 10 g/day, and 27% with 15 g/day.[142] Therapy should be initiated with one packet, scoop, or tablet of resin daily (Table 13-15). The reduction achieved is inversely proportional to the baseline, untreated LDL-C level.[143] Thus, patients with a moderate cholesterol elevation (such as L.W.) will have a greater relative reduction than if the LDL-C were higher.

Unfortunately, the older resins are not well tolerated because of numerous GI side effects and the unpleasant granular texture of the powder. A new bile acid resin, colesevelam (WelChol), is available in 0.625-g tablets; the daily dose is six tablets (3.8 g) administered in one or two divided doses daily. Although the tablets are large and difficult for some patients to swallow, the product is much easier to administer and, due in part to a smaller total daily dose, less prone to cause GI side

effects than the older products. The standard daily dose reduces LDL-C by 15% to 18%.

Mechanism of Action. The resins are anion exchange agents that bind bile acids in the intestinal lumen and cause them to be eliminated in the stool.[144] By disrupting the normal enterohepatic recirculation of bile acids from the intestinal lumen to the

Table 13-14   Dose-Related LDL-C Lowering of Major Drugs

Drug	Daily Dosage	LDL-C Lowering
Bile acid resins (colestipol)[271]	5 g	−15%
	10 g	−23%
	15 g	−27%
Bile acid resin (Cosevelam)	3.8 g	−15%
	4.5 g	−18%
Ezetimibe[145]	10 mg	−18 to −22%
Niacin (crystalline)[152]	1,000 mg	−6%
	1,500 mg	−13%
	2,000 mg	−16%
	3,000 mg	−22%
Niaspan	1,000 mg	−9%
	1,500 mg	−14%
	2,000 mg	−17%
Atorvastatin[164]	10 mg	−39%
	20 mg	−43%
	40 mg	−50%
	80 mg	−60%
Fluvastatin[164]	20 mg	−22%
	40 mg	−24%
	80 mg	−34%
Lovastatin[164,271]	20 mg	−24%
	40 mg	−34%
	80 mg	−40%
Pravastatin[164,272]	10 mg	−22%
	20 mg	−32%
	40 mg	−34%
Rosuvastatin[274]	10 mg	−46%
	20 mg	−52%
	40 mg	−55%
Simvastatin[164]	5 mg	−26%
	10 mg	−30%
	20 mg	−38%
	40 mg	−41%
	80 mg	−47%

Table 13-15   Dosages of Selected Lipid-Modulating Drugs

Drug	Initial Dosage	Usual Dosage	Maximum Dosage	Comment
Cholestyramine	4 g before main meal	4 g BID before heaviest meals	8 g BID before heaviest meals	May prescribe 24 g/day, but few patients can tolerate.
Colestipol	5 g powder or 2 g tabs QD before main meal	5 g of powder or 4 g of tabs BID before heaviest meals	10 g powder or 8 g of tabs BID before heaviest meals	May prescribe 30 g of powder per day, but few patients can tolerate.
Colesevelam	6 × 0.63-g tablets per day	Same	7 × 0.63-g tablets per day	Less bulk is associated with less gastrointestinal intolerance.
Niacin	100–125 BID with food	750–1,000 mg BID	1,500 mg BID	Dosages up to 6 g/day have been used, but few can tolerate. Dosages may be increased 200–250 mg/ day every 3–7 days until desired dosage has been obtained.
Niaspan	500 mg q HS	1,000–2,000 mg q HS	2,000 mg q HS	Increase dose by 500 mg daily Q 4 wks.
Atorvastatin	10–40 mg QD	10–40 mg QD	80 mg QD	Administer any time of day.
Fluvastatin	20–40 mg QHS	20–40 mg QHS	40 mg BID 80 mg XL QD	Modified-release form (XL) has similar efficacy but has less bioavailability (and less risk of adverse effects).
Lovastatin	20 mg with dinner	20–40 mg with dinner	40 mg BID	Administration with food increases bioavailability. BID dosing provides greater LDL-C lowering efficacy than QD.
Pravastatin	10–40 mg QD	10–40 mg QD	40 mg QD	Administer with food to reduce dyspepsia.
Rosuvastatin	10–20 mg QD	10–20 mg QD	40 mg QD	Administer any time of the day.
Simvastatin	20–40 mg Q pm	20–40 mg Q pm	80 mg Q pm	Administer with food to reduce dyspepsia.
Gemfibrozil	600 mg BID	Same	Same	
Fenofibrate	67–201 mg QD	Same	200 mg QD	

liver, the liver is stimulated to convert hepatocellular cholesterol into bile acids. This in turn causes a reduction in the concentration of cholesterol in the hepatocyte, prompting the upregulation of LDL receptor synthesis. Finally, circulating LDL-C levels are lowered by binding to the newly formed LDL receptors on the liver surface.[57] This mechanism has appeal not only because it effectively lowers LDL-C but also because it is additive with other therapies to lower cholesterol. For example, combining a drug that reduces hepatocellular cholesterol biosynthesis (e.g., statins) with a resin that interferes with bile acid recycling can cause a substantial upregulation of LDL receptors and enhance removal of cholesterol from the blood.[9]

Adverse Effects. The disadvantage of the older resins (i.e., colestipol or cholestyramine) is their side effects. These resins often cause GI symptoms, including constipation, bloating, epigastric fullness, nausea, and flatulence[141] (Table 13-16). Colesevelam is associated with less GI intolerance. If one of the older resins is prescribed, the patient should be instructed to mix the resin powder in noncarbonated, pulpy juices; to swallow it without engulfing air (administering it through a straw may help avoid air entrapment); and to maintain an adequate intake of fluids and fiber in the diet.

The older resins also can *raise* TG levels by 3% to 10% or more, especially in patients with high TG levels; this ap-

pears to be less of a problem with colesevelam. Reduction in the absorption of fat-soluble vitamins and folic acid has been reported with high dosages of resins, but this is rarely a problem in otherwise healthy patients consuming a nutritionally balanced diet. The older resins also can reduce the absorption of digitoxin (but not digoxin), warfarin, thyroxine, thiazide diuretics, β-blockers, and presumably other anionic drugs. This interaction can be minimized by administering other drugs 1 hour before or 4 hours after the resin dose. Colesevelam appears to have a high specificity for binding with bile acids and not with other anionic drugs, including warfarin; thus, it may be safely administered with other drugs.

Based on this summary, there are no contraindications to the use of resin therapy in L.W. Colesevelam, which can safely be taken along with his BP medication and is less likely to cause intolerable symptoms, would be the preferred choice. However, it lowers LDL-C only about 20% on average, which is not likely to be sufficient to reduce L.W.'s LDL-C from 200 mg/dL to <130 mg/dL.

EZETIMIBE
Ezetimibe represents a new class of lipid-altering drugs called cholesterol absorption inhibitors. One advantage of this compound is its ability to reduce LDL-C by an action in the

Table 13-16   Monitoring Parameters, Adverse Effects, and Drug Interactions with Major Cholesterol-Lowering Drugs

Drug	Adverse Effects	Drug Interactions	Monitoring Parameters
Resin	Indigestion, bloating, nausea, constipation, abdominal pain, flatulence	GI binding and reduced absorption of anionic drugs (warfarin, β-blockers, digitoxin, thyroxine, thiazide diuretics); administer drugs 12 hr before or 4 hr after resin	Lipid profile Q 4–8 wk until stable dose; then Q 6–12 mo long term. Check TG level after stable dose achieved, then as needed.
Niacin	Flushing, itching, tingling, headache, nausea, gas, heartburn, fatigue, rash, worsening of peptic ulcer, elevation in serum glucose and uric acid, hepatitis, and elevation in hepatic transaminase levels	Hypotension with BP-lowering drugs such as α-blockers possible; diabetics taking insulin or oral agents may require dosage adjustment because of increase in serum glucose levels	Lipid profile after 1,000–1,500 mg/day and then after stable dosage achieved; then Q 6–12 mo long term. LFTs at baseline and Q 6–8 wk during dose titration; then as needed for symptoms. Uric acid and glucose at baseline and again after stable dose reached (or symptoms produced), more frequently in diabetic patients.
Statins	Headache, dyspepsia, myositis (myalgia, CPK >10 times normal), elevation in hepatic transaminase levels	Increased myositis risk with concurrent use of drugs that inhibit or compete for P450 3A4 system (e.g., cyclosporine, erythromycin, calcium blockers, fibrates, nefazodone, niacin, ketoconazole); risk greater with lovastatin and simvastatin; caution with concurrent fibrate or niacin use; lovastatin increases the pro-time with concurrent warfarin	Lipid profile 4–8 wk after dose change, then Q 6–12 mo long term. LFTs at baseline, in 3 months, and periodically thereafter. CPK at baseline and if the patient has symptoms of myalgia.

BP, blood pressure; CPK, creatinine phosphokinase; GI, gastrointestinal; LFTs, liver function tests; TC, total cholesterol; TG, triglyceride.

gut, with minimal systemic exposure. This suggests that the drug may be very safe, much like the resins. It is administered once a day as a 10-mg tablet.

Ezetimibe reduces LDL-C by 18% to 22% but has little effect on TG or HDL-C.[145] In combination with a statin, it demonstrates an additive effect, enhancing LDL-C lowering by an additional 10% to 20%. In fact, when added to a low dose of a statin, the net LDL-C reduction can be similar to the lowering achieved with the maximum dose of the statin.[146] When added to the maximum dose of a statin, it causes further LDL-C reduction, an effect important in patients with very high LDL-C levels requiring substantial reduction to achieve treatment goals.

Mechanism of Action.   Cholesterol that is ingested in the diet and circulated through the bile from the liver is actively reabsorbed in the intestines. Once transported across the intestinal lumen into the enterocyte, it is combined with TGs and apolipoprotein B48 to form chylomicron particles that transport the lipids through the lymphatic system to the hepatocyte. The TGs and cholesterol can then be packaged into VLDL particles and secreted into the systemic circulation.

Ezetimibe interferes with the active absorption of cholesterol from the intestinal lumen into the enterocyte. The exact mechanism that is inhibited is not yet identified but presumably is an active transport system located on the brush border along the enterocyte in the intestinal lumen. By interfering with the absorption of cholesterol, about 50% less cholesterol is transported from the intestines to the liver by the chylomicrons. This causes an upregulation in hepatic cholesterol synthesis, which is diverted to the intestines via the bile to replenish the cholesterol available for absorption processes. It also causes an upregulation of hepatic LDL receptors and increased clearance of circulating VLDL and LDL particles. The net effect of the inhibition of cholesterol absorption in the gut is approximately a 70% increase in GI sterol excretion, a 50% reduction in hepatic cholesterol concentration, a 90% increase in hepatic cholesterol synthesis, and approximately a 20% increase in LDL-C taken up from the systemic circulation via upregulated LDL receptors.[147] Ezetimibe also inhibits the absorption of sitosterol, a plant sterol, from the gut, resulting in about a 40% reduction in blood sitosterol levels. The occurrence of sitosterolemia is rare, but patients who have it have a high CHD risk. Ezetimibe provides one of the first effective treatments for this rare disorder.

Adverse Effects.   Ezetimibe's side effects include diarrhea, arthralgias, cough and fatigue. These occur no more frequently with ezetimibe than they do with placebo. Whether used alone or together with a statin, there have been no increases in liver function abnormalities and no reported cases of myopathy or rhabdomyolysis. As with resin therapy, ezetimibe can safely reduce the LDL-C by about 20%, which is not likely to be sufficient to reduce L.W.'s LDL-C to his goal of <130 mg/dL.

NIACIN
Clinical Use.   Niacin (or nicotinic acid) is a water-soluble B vitamin that can improve the levels of all serum lipids. Favorable attributes are low cost, a long history of use, and clinical

trial evidence that it can reduce CHD events.[107-109] Crystalline (immediate-release) niacin lowers LDL-C levels by 15% to 25% and TGs 30% to 60% and raises HDL-C levels 20% to 35%[107,148,149] (Tables 13-14 and 13-17). Reduction in LDL-C follows a linear relationship to dose: doses need to be increased to 2 to 3 g/day to reduce LDL-C levels by 20% to 25%. Conversely, the increase in HDL-C and reduction in TG follows a curvilinear relationship with dose: low to moderate doses (i.e., 1 to 2 g/day) can increase HDL-C by 25% and lower TG by 30% to 40%[148] (Table 13-14, Fig. 13-8). Crystalline niacin should be started at a low level (e.g., 250 mg in two or three divided doses daily) and slowly titrated as tolerated (e.g., daily doses increased by 250 mg every 3 to 7 days) to a maximum of 3,000 mg/day (see Table 13-15). Higher doses have been used but are associated with unpleasant side effects. Niacin is also the only drug that lowers Lp(a), with reductions being as great as 30%.[150] Its metabolite, nicotinamide, has no effect on cholesterol and should not be used as a substitute to lower side effects.

Sustained-release (timed-release) dosage forms of niacin were developed to reduce the flushing side effects associated with crystalline niacin. These products are sold over the counter ostensibly for treating niacin deficiency but are purchased by patients to treat high blood cholesterol. These products may have slightly greater LDL-C–lowering efficacy at each dose level and slightly less HDL-C and TG effects compared with crystalline niacin, but they cannot be recommended because of a substantially increased risk of liver toxicity at higher dosages (see Adverse Effects).

An extended-release dosage form of niacin, Niaspan, is available by prescription for the treatment of elevated cholesterol and TG levels and appears to be better tolerated than either the crystalline or sustained-release forms. Niaspan releases niacin over an 8- to 12-hour period, a feature that turns out to be important in improving its side effect profile, and has the efficacy pattern of crystalline niacin. It lowers LDL-C by 10% to 15% and TGs by 20% to 30%, and it raises HDL-C by 15% to 25% with daily doses between 1,000 and 2,000 mg. Daily doses of Niaspan should not exceed 2,000 mg/day to reduce the risk of liver side effects.

Mechanism of Action. Niacin inhibits the mobilization of free fatty acids from peripheral adipose tissue to the liver, which, either alone or together with other hepatic effects, results in reduced synthesis and secretion of VLDL particles by the liver.[151] This explains its effectiveness in lowering TG levels. Because LDL is a VLDL degradation product, reducing the secretion of VLDL particles secondarily lowers the LDL-C level. Niacin reduces the amount of apolipoprotein A-I ex-

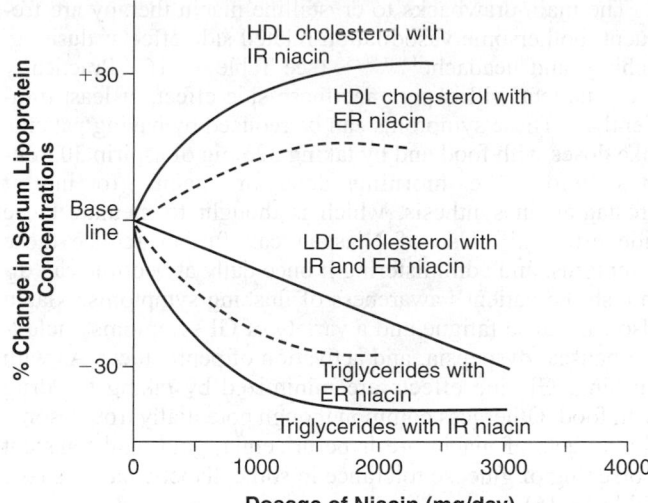

FIGURE 13-8. Dose-related effects of niacin on lipoproteins. (Reproduced with permission from reference 234)

tracted and catabolized from HDL during the hepatic uptake of cholesterol, thus preserving the structural and functional integrity of HDL particles.[152] As a result, cholesterol-deficient apolipoprotein A-I–containing HDL particles are recirculated from the liver to the peripheral cells, maintaining HDL levels and enhancing reverse cholesterol transport.[153]

Adverse Effects. The differences in release characteristics among various niacin products are important because they determine how the drug is metabolized, in turn influencing the side effect profile of the product. Niacin is metabolized through two separate metabolic pathways (Fig. 13-9).[154] The nicotinamide (NAM) pathway is a high-affinity, low-capacity pathway. Crystalline niacin quickly saturates this pathway and is predominately metabolized through the high-capacity conjugation pathway. The flushing effect with crystalline niacin results from prostaglandin-mediated vasodilation associated with the formation of nicotinuric acid (NUA) by the conjugation pathway. In contrast, sustained-release niacin is slowly absorbed and preferentially metabolized via the nicotinamide pathway. Because of this, sustained-release niacin rarely causes flushing, but it can cause serious, dose-related hepatotoxicity due to the formation of toxic metabolites of the nicotinamide pathway. Niaspan, with its intermediate absorption rate, has a more balanced metabolism between the two pathways. The result is less flushing and less risk of hepatotoxicity, at least with daily doses of ≤2 g.

Table 13-17 Average Effects of Selected Drugs on Lipoprotein Cholesterol and Triglycerides

Drug	LDL	HDL	TG
Resin	−15–30%	±3%	+3–10%
Ezetimibe	−18–22%	+0–2%	−0–5%
Niacin	−15–30%	+20–35%	−30–60%
Statin	−25–60%	+5–15%	−10–45%
Fibrates	±10–25%	+10–30%	−30–60%

HDL, high-density lipoprotein; LDL, low-density lipoprotein; TG, triglycerides.

FIGURE 13-9. Niacin metabolism. NAM, nicotinamide; NUA, nicotinuric acid. (Reproduced with permission from reference 154)

The main drawbacks to crystalline niacin therapy are frequent, bothersome vasodilation-related side effects: flushing, itching, and headache[148,149,155] (see Table 13-16). Practically every patient will experience these side effect, at least transiently.[156] These symptoms can be reduced by having patients take doses with food and by taking 325 mg of aspirin 30 minutes before the morning dose of niacin (to inhibit prostaglandin synthesis, which is thought to mediate these side effects).[157] Use of Niaspan can further reduce these symptoms, and administering it once daily at bedtime can diminish the patient's awareness of flushing symptoms. Niacin also can cause fatigue and a variety of GI symptoms, including nausea, dyspepsia, and activation of peptic ulcer. As with flushing, GI side effects are minimized by taking the drug with food. Other less common though potentially troublesome side effects of niacin are hyperuricemia, gout, and transient worsening of glucose tolerance in some diabetic patients (see Table 13-16).

The most worrisome side effect associated with niacin is hepatotoxicity, which is associated almost exclusively with the sustained-release forms of niacin.[148, 158–161] Hepatotoxicity is detected by an increase in liver transaminase enzymes exceeding three times the upper limit of normal; in severe cases, this may be accompanied by symptoms such as fatigue, anorexia, malaise, and nausea. This side effect occurs when daily doses of sustained-release niacin exceed 1,500 mg. Hepatotoxicity has been reported to occur in up to half of the patients titrated to daily doses of 3,000 mg of sustained-release niacin; many of these patients had symptoms, as well as laboratory findings, consistent with toxicity.[148] Conversely, <1% of patients titrated up to 2,000 mg/day of Niaspan have elevated liver function tests. Rare cases of fulminant hepatitis have been reported with sustained-release niacin. Niacin-induced hepatotoxicity appears to be completely reversible when the drug is discontinued.

Because of the hepatotoxic effects of sustained-release niacin and the flushing side effects of crystalline niacin, Niaspan is the preferred form of niacin for general use. It can be safely used in a daily dose up to 2,000 mg. An estimated 30% of patients experience flushing symptoms that will cause them to discontinue therapy.

There are no apparent contraindications to the use of niacin in L.W. However, niacin would not be expected to lower his LDL-C by the 35% required to reach his treatment goal of <130 mg/dL.

STATINS

Clinical Use. The group of drugs with the most potent cholesterol-lowering potential is the statins. They lower LDL-C by approximately 20% to 40% with initial doses and 35% to 60% with maximal doses[162-164] (see Table 13-14). Statins also reduce TG levels by 15% to 45% and increase HDL-C modestly (5% to 8%) (see Table 13-17). The LDL-C lowering achieved is dose dependent and log-linear. Low dosages produce substantial LDL-C–lowering effects, and with each doubling of the daily dose, LDL-C is lowered an additional 6% to 7% on average (see Table 13-14).

The currently available statins are atorvastatin (Lipitor), fluvastatin (Lescol), lovastatin (Mevacor), pravastatin (Pravachol), rosuvastatin (Crestor), and simvastatin (Zocor). Rosuvastatin provides the most substantial LDL-C lowering, followed by atorvastatin, simvastatin, lovastatin, pravastatin, and fluvastatin in descending order. With clinical trial evidence that lower LDL-C levels are associated with less CHD, higher initial doses of these statins are being advocated, thus blurring these LDL-C differences. The efficacy of many statins is greater if administered in the evening to coincide with the nighttime upturn in endogenous cholesterol biosynthesis; atorvastatin, and rosuvastatin with their longer half-lifes and more potent LDL-C lowering, may be administered without regard to time of day. The LDL-C–lowering efficacy of twice-daily administration of statins is slightly greater (by 2% to 4%) than once-daily evening doses, but this difference is rarely great enough to make a clinical difference. The bioavailability of lovastatin is improved by administration with food; thus, it is recommended for dosing with the evening meal. This, too, may not make much difference in the clinical setting.

The major statin trials described earlier in this chapter demonstrate that statins can significantly reduce CHD death and nonfatal MI, revascularization procedures, strokes, and total mortality. The mechanism for these beneficial outcomes is not fully known, but is at least partially associated with LDL-C reduction. Most authorities believe that the CHD event reduction with statins is a class effect and can be accomplished with any of the available statins. This, coupled with their favorable safety profile and their potency in lowering LDL-C, supports the NCEP ATP III recommendation that statins are the drugs of first choice to lower cholesterol and reduce CHD risk.[87,165]

Mechanism of Action. Statins competitively inhibit the enzyme responsible for converting HMG-CoA to mevalonate in an early, rate-limiting step in the biosynthetic pathway of cholesterol (see Fig. 13-1).[9] Reduction in hepatocellular cholesterol prompts an upregulation of LDL receptor proteins and thus increases the clearance of circulating LDL particles from the blood. The TG-lowering effects appear to be produced in two ways: by an increase in the clearance of VLDL and VLDL remnant particles from the systemic circulation (by the upregulation of LDL receptors) and by a reduced secretion of VLDL particles from the liver.[166–168] All statins have the ability to lower TG levels. However, their TG-lowering efficacy is related to their LDL-C–lowering effectiveness (thus, statins with greater LDL-C–lowering efficacy will have greater TG-lowering efficacy) and to the patient's baseline TG level (the higher the TG level, the greater the percentage of reduction produced by the statin).

Adverse Effects. Statins are well tolerated by most patients. Headache; myalgias (without CPK changes); and GI symptoms, including dyspepsia, flatus, constipation, and abdominal pain, occasionally are experienced[162,163,169,170] (see Table 13-16). These symptoms are usually mild and disappear with continued therapy. The statin side effects receiving the most attention include increases in liver function tests and myopathy. These two problems are described in detail below.

Statins can cause an elevation in transaminase enzyme levels of more than three times the upper limit of normal in 1% to 1.5% of patients in a dose-dependent manner.[162] The transaminase level may return to normal spontaneously even with continued statin therapy. Similarly, elevations in transaminase will return to normal if the statin is discontinued. Rechallenge with the same or a different statin after enzymes have returned to normal limits is acceptable. If the drug is tolerated upon rechallenge, it can be continued; recurrence of transaminase elevation warrants further evaluation of other potential causes. No cases of hepatic failure or liver transplant associated with statin therapy have been reported, leading many to conclude that transaminase elevations are relatively unimportant and not associated with worrisome adverse consequences.

The potential for muscle toxicity is a different matter. Myositis, defined as the presence of muscle symptoms, including aches, soreness, or weakness (i.e., myalgia), *and* an increase in serum CPK >10 times the upper limit of normal, occurs in approximately 0.1% to 1% of patients in a dose-dependent manner.[162] Routine monitoring of CPK levels is unnecessary; rather, unexplained symptoms of muscle aches, weakness, and/or soreness should prompt a CPK evaluation. If myositis is present, a careful history is necessary to rule out usual causes (i.e., trauma, increased physical activity). If no explanation is present for the findings and the CPK is elevated, the statin should be withdrawn until CPK levels return to normal. Occasionally, symptoms of myalgia are bothersome to the patient, even with a normal CPK, resulting in discontinuation of the statin. Once symptoms subside, statin therapy can be restarted, preferably with a different statin. Myositis is more likely to occur with high systemic concentrations of the statin and when there is a provocation for the event such as hypothyroidism, trauma, or flulike syndromes. Myositis has also been reported more often when a statin is combined with gemfibrozil or when a drug is given concurrently that can increase blood levels of the statin, such as a macrolide antibiotic (e.g., erythromycin). Cases of rhabdomyolysis, myoglobinuria, and acute tubular necrosis have been reported in patients receiving statin therapy. Most of these cases have occurred with high doses, in patients with impaired renal or hepatic function, in older individuals, or when statins are used in combination with interacting drugs.

Drug interactions with statins that result in higher blood levels of the statin or an active metabolite can increase the risk of myositis. Statins that depend on the P450 3A4 enzyme system to be metabolized are most vulnerable to this interaction (i.e., lovastatin, simvastatin, and to a lesser extent atorvastatin). Fluvastatin is metabolized by the P450 2C9 system and is therefore more vulnerable to interactions with drugs that directly inhibit 2C9 or act as competitive inhibitors (substrates) for this alternate system. Rosuvastatin is metabolized minimally (i.e., about 10%) by 2C9 to less active metabolites. Pravastatin is not metabolized at all. Some of the more commonly encountered drugs that inhibit the 3A4 enzyme system are macrolide antibiotics (clarithromycin and erythromycin), certain calcium channel blockers (diltiazem and verapamil), azole antifungals (itraconazole, ketoconazole, and miconazole), protease inhibitors (ritonavir), and antidepressants (nefazodone). Drugs that are substrates for the 3A4 system include alprazolam, midazolam, triazolam, calcium channel blockers (especially diltiazem), carbamazepine, cisapride, cyclosporine, estradiol, felodipine, loratadine, quinidine, and terfenadine. When these substrate drugs are used together with simvastatin or lovastatin (and to a lesser extent atorvastatin), systemic blood levels of the statin may be increased

due to competitive inhibition of the 3A4 enzymes, and this may increase the risk for myositis. Inhibitors of 2C9 isoenzymes include alprenolol, diclofenac, hexobarbital, tolbutamide, and warfarin.

It is preferable to avoid the combined use of interacting drugs with statins. If the patient requires a short course of therapy with a potentially interacting drug (e.g., erythromycin), the statin should be discontinued during this period and restarted when the course has been completed. If an interacting drug must be used long term (e.g., cyclosporine) with a statin, the lowest effective dose of the statin should be selected, with careful monitoring of muscle symptoms. If myositis occurs, it is quickly reversible when the statin is discontinued.

Caution should also be exercised when adding gemfibrozil with a statin to treat patients with high blood cholesterol and TGs. Gemfibrozil interferes with the glucuronidation of statins, thereby interfering with their renal clearance. This interaction results in two- to fourfold increases in systemic statin levels and has been demonstrated with all statins except fluvastatin. Because the interaction has not been reported to occur with fenofibrate, it is the preferred fibrate to add to a statin when treating patients with a mixed lipid disorder.

Hospitalizations and deaths due to rhabdomyolysis led to the withdrawal of one statin, cerivastatin, from the market, punctuating the importance of this potential side effect. Cerivastatin at its top dosage of 0.8 mg daily caused a significantly higher incidence of myotoxicity than other currently marketed statins. Additionally, when interacting drugs or gemfibrozil were added to this dose of cerivastatin, many cases of severe muscle toxicity and rhabdomyolysis occurred. The FDA subsequently observed that factors that appeared to raise the risk of severe muscle toxicity and rhabdomyolysis with cerivastatin included older individuals (especially females), small body frame, reduced renal function, multiple organ diseases, and use of multiple concurrent medications, particularly those known to interact with statins. Whenever these factors are present in a patient receiving a statin, it is advisable to use the lowest effective statin dose, to avoid or use with caution interacting drugs, and to monitor the patient carefully. It is also advisable not to unduly frighten the patient with dire warnings about the potential for this side effect: it occurs only rarely, especially when these drugs are used responsibly in the manner described.

Lovastatin and rosuvastatin may prolong the prothrombin time in patients receiving Coumarin anticoagulants concurrently; this effect is not caused by pravastatin.[183] Statins should not be used in patients with active liver disease or those who are or hope to become pregnant because of potential hazards to the fetus.

Based on this information, a statin would be the preferred drug for L.W. He is not receiving a potentially interacting drug and has no apparent contraindication to its use. Further, it is most likely to help him reach his LDL-C goal.

In selecting the specific statin for the patient, it is assumed, for reasons previously stated, that all statins are equally safe and have a similar potential to reduce CHD events. The characteristic that differentiates the statins is their ability to lower LDL-C (see Tables 13-14 and 13-17). Given the 35% reduction required to achieve L.W.'s LDL-C goal, it would be preferable to select the statin with the greatest LDL-

C–lowering potency, such as simvastatin, atorvastatin, or rosuvastatin. At 20 mg/d of simvastatin, 10 mg/d of atorvastatin, or 10 mg of rosuvastatin, LDL-C is reduced by an average of 39%, indicating that 50% of patients will experience at least this level of LDL-C reduction. Starting therapy with even higher doses (i.e., simvastatin 40 mg or atorvastatin 20 mg) will increase the chance of reaching L.W.'s treatment goal of <130 mg/dL.

Fiber

13. **What role can supplemental fiber play in the treatment of L.W.?**

Increasing fiber intake in the diet or adding supplemental fiber in the form of psyllium (Metamucil), oat bran, gums, or other products might temporarily aid in LDL-C reduction. When given to a patient who is following a low-fat diet, the LDL-C reduction is modest (usually about 5%). A dietary supplement of fiber would make little overall contribution to L.W.'s treatment, although appropriate fiber intake in the form of fresh fruits, beans, and vegetables is highly advisable. Overuse of fiber is associated with bothersome GI symptoms, including flatulence and bloating.

Fish Oils

14. **Is there a role for fish oil supplements in L.W.'s treatment?**

Fish oils predominantly contain polyunsaturated (omega-3) fatty acids, which lower TG levels significantly (30% to 60%) but have variable effects on cholesterol levels. They serve little value in achieving LDL-C reduction, as is needed by L.W. However, as noted under the discussion of diet, consumption of foods rich in omega-3 fatty acids (e.g., fish) several times a week has been associated with a reduced risk of heart disease, and they are recommended as part of a low-fat diet. Supplements of fish oils demonstrated a reduction in CHD events in several large clinical trials.[172] Commercial sources of fish oils vary in their content. The fish oil supplements used in the GISSI study, which demonstrated a CHD risk reduction, contained 850 mg of eicosapentaenoic acid (EPA) and docosahexanoic acid (DHA). Fish oils are most useful in the management of patients who have hypertriglyceridemia and who cannot achieve adequate control with conventional TG-lowering drugs (niacin and a fibrate) alone. The CHD risk reduction with fish oils appears to be due to an antiarrhythmic effect and not a change in atherosclerosis, since sudden CHD deaths are the outcome primarily affected by fish oil therapy.

Postmenopausal Drug Therapy

15. **C.M. is a 57-year-old woman whose last menses was 2 years ago. She follows a TLC diet and participates in an aerobic exercise program three times a week. She has a strong family history of CHD (her father died suddenly at age 59 and her 43-year-old brother has had a heart attack). Her mother is alive at age 78, but lives in a nursing home because of a hip fracture last year. C.M. does not have diabetes or hypertension; she smokes half a pack of cigarettes per day. Her mean BP for the last two visits is 142/88. She does not have hypothyroidism. Her lipid profile is total cholesterol, 260 mg/dL; LDL-C, 186 mg/dL; HDL-C, 58 mg/dL; and TGs, 78 mg/dL. C.M. has no evidence of secondary or familial**

dyslipidemia or atherosclerotic vascular disease on her physical examination. She has not had a hysterectomy. She complains of frequent daily hot flashes and night sweats. Does C.M. need cholesterol-lowering drug therapy, and if so, with which drug? Is she a candidate for estrogen replacement therapy?

[SI units: LDL-C, 5.17 mmol/L; HDL-C, 1.5 mmol/L; and TGs, 0.88 mmol/L]

Being postmenopausal, whether natural, surgical, or premature, is associated with an increased CHD risk. C.M. has three risk factors: postmenopausal status, smoking, and family history of premature CHD (see Table 13-5). Because she has two or more risk factors, her LDL-C goal is <130 mg/dL. An assessment of her global risk (see Fig. 13-7B) indicates that she has an 11% risk of a CHD event in the next 10 years. Because her mean LDL-C after diet is still 186 mg/dL, she will require a 30% reduction to achieve her goal. Until recently, C.M. would have been a candidate for estrogen therapy before (or instead of) other cholesterol-lowering drugs. Estrogen is known to improve lipid and lipoprotein profiles and was thought to provide cardioprotective effects as well as minimizing osteoporosis and menopausal symptoms. Today, with new data in hand, this approach has changed.

Estrogen Replacement Therapy

CONSIDERATIONS FOR USE IN HYPERCHOLESTEROLEMIA

16. **What are the considerations for using estrogen therapy in C.M. to reduce her CHD risk?**

Epidemiologic studies report up to 50% lower CHD rates in women who use estrogens compared with those who do not.[173–176] A meta-analysis of 31 case-control, cross-sectional, and cohort studies found an overall relative risk of 0.56—that is, a 44% lower rate of CHD in estrogen users compared with nonusers.[177] The difference in CHD rates between estrogen users and nonusers is even greater in women who have developed CHD.[175,178] Despite calls for caution,[179] the epidemiologic evidence of lower CHD risk was so impressive and consistent that many authorities supported the use of estrogen therapy as a first-line treatment to reduce CHD risk in dyslipidemic, postmenopausal women, especially if they were experiencing menopausal symptoms or were at risk from osteoporosis.

Following the reports of the Heart and Estrogen/Progestin Replacement Study (HERS) and the Women's Health Initiative (WHI), this position has changed. HERS evaluated 2,763 women with known CHD.[180] The active treatment group received conjugated equine estrogen 0.625 and medroxyprogesterone 2.5 mg/day (Prempro) for 5 years. Compared with placebo, the hormone replacement therapy (HRT) regimen lowered LDL-C by 11% and increased HDL-C by 10%. At the conclusion of the study, there was no difference between the groups with regard to CHD death and nonfatal MI (the primary study outcome measure) or total mortality. Of greatest concern, there was a 52% *increase* in CHD events during the first year of the study. By the fourth and fifth years of the study, HRT-treated women had 33% *fewer* CHD events, but this difference was not great enough to counter the first-year results. Venous thromboembolic events occurred in 0.6% of treated women compared with 0.2% in placebo-treated women; the incidence of gallbladder disease was 38% greater in HRT-treated than in placebo-treated patients. There were no significant differences between the groups with respect to breast cancer, endometrial cancer, or fracture. Study investigators searched for explanations of these surprising results but ultimately concluded that in this well-controlled study of estrogen therapy in CHD women, estrogen provided no benefit and may have caused harm.

Subsequently, the WHI reported the results of a 5.2-year, randomized, placebo-controlled study of the same estrogen/progestin product in 16,608 postmenopausal women who had no prior evidence of CHD.[181] The study was stopped before its planned 8.5-year duration because the rate of invasive breast cancer exceeded the stopping boundary. Investigators reported the following negative outcomes: a 29% increase in CHD events (nonfatal MI or CHD death), a 26% increase in breast cancer, a 41% increase in stroke, and a twofold increase in pulmonary embolism. Positive outcomes included a 37% reduction in colorectal cancer, a 17% reduction in endometrial cancer, a 34% reduction in hip fracture, and an 8% reduction in death due to non-CHD causes. These relative changes in risk camouflage a low overall absolute risk of harmful study events. That said, however, the absolute excess risk of adverse events during the study was 19 per 10,000 person-years, supporting an overall conclusion that the risks of estrogen/progestin (Prempro) therapy exceeded the benefits among healthy postmenopausal women. Since the whole purpose of healthy women taking a therapy is to preserve health and prevent disease, this study provides further strong evidence that women should not receive combination estrogen/progestin therapy for long-term use to prevent CHD. It should be noted that the WHI study arm with postmenopausal women taking estrogen alone was not stopped prematurely, suggesting that the adversities reported above were due to the progestin component of the combination and not to the estrogen. Nonetheless, until further data are available, long-term use of estrogen for lipid management is not recommended. Short-term (1 to 2 years) use for relief of C.M.'s menopausal symptoms is acceptable.

Alternative Lipid Therapy for Postmenopausal Women

17. If C.M. should not be started on estrogen/progestin therapy, what should she be given?

C.M.'s risk of dying of CHD is as great as it is for a male. Further, her risk rises after menopause in a log-linear manner parallel to men (although behind men by about 10 years). The Heart Protection Study and a meta-analysis of most of the major statin trials has shown strong evidence that postmenopausal women benefit from lipid-lowering treatment just as much as men[86, 97] (see Table 13-3). For all of these reasons, C.M. is a candidate for lipid-modifying therapy. Since she requires a 30% reduction to achieve her LDL-C goal of <130 mg/dL, a statin with sufficient LDL-C–lowering potency to achieve this target (i.e., simvastatin, atorvastatin, or rosuvastatin) would be the drug of choice. Even if the decision is made by her and her gynecologist to initiate short-term hormone replacement therapy to reduce vasomotor symptoms, a statin will still be needed to reduce her LDL-C to the goal level and to reduce her CHD risk.

Familial Hypercholesterolemia

18. D.E. is a 45-year-old man with no evidence of CHD. His father and grandfather both died suddenly from apparent heart attacks in their early 50s, but D.E. has no other CHD risk factors. He has no evidence of secondary causes of dyslipidemia. On physical examination, he is noted to have bilateral corneal arcus and bilateral Achilles tendon xanthomas; the rest of his examination is normal. Likewise, his laboratory test results are within normal limits, except for the following lipid profile: total cholesterol, 440 mg/dL; TGs, 55 mg/dL; HDL-C, 55 mg/dL; and LDL-C, 374 mg/dL. What form of hypercholesterolemia does D.E. most likely have? Is he a candidate for drug therapy at this time?

[SI units: total cholesterol, 11.38 mmol/L; TGs, 0.62 mmol/L; HDL-C, 1.42 mmol/L; LDL-C, 9.67 mmol/L]

The combination of a very high LDL-C, tendon xanthomas, and a strong family history of premature CHD is consistent with a diagnosis of familial hypercholesterolemia (FH) (see Table 13-2). The risk of a CHD event in the next 10 years associated with FH is very high, well in excess of 20%. Thus, it is not necessary to conduct a global risk assessment, since the diagnosis of the genetic disorder defines his risk. Although D.E. has bilateral tendon xanthomas, this finding would not necessarily be detected in all 45-year old patients because it takes time for xanthomas to develop. However, with a strong family history and a very high LDL-C level independent of the presence or absence of xanthomas, it is still presumed that the person has either FH or severe polygenic hypercholesterolemia. Thus, he deserves aggressive lipid management to reduce his high CHD risk. D.E. should be given therapy to lower his LDL-C to 130 mg/dL, lower if possible. To achieve this goal, D.E. will require a 65% LDL-C reduction, which almost assuredly will require combination drug therapy in addition to a low-fat diet. Because this is a genetically induced lipid abnormality, a low-fat diet alone will not correct the problem; in fact, diet may have little effect on his LDL-C.

Combination Drug Therapy

19. What cholesterol-lowering drugs should be combined to manage D.E.'s lipid disorder?

As stated previously, four drugs effectively reduce LDL-C: a statin, a resin, ezetimibe, and niacin (see Table 13-13). When two or more of these are combined, an additive LDL-C effect is achieved. Combinations of niacin and resin result in LDL-C reductions of 32% to 43%[62]; a statin and a resin lower LDL-C by 45% to 55%[63], and ezetimibe plus a statin reduces LDL-C by 46% to 61%.[146,182] LDL-C reductions of 50% to 60% are possible when the three-drug regimen of a statin plus resin plus niacin is used.[183–185]

The major limiting factor in combining drugs is side effects. Niacin and the older resins both cause bothersome side effects to the extent that 25% to 50% of patients cannot tolerate them. However, the use of Niaspan rather than crystalline niacin may reduce the vasodilatory side effects, and the use of colesevelam rather than one of the older resins should reduce GI intolerance.[186] The combination of a statin and niacin is said to be associated with an increased risk of myositis, although this risk appears to be very low.[171] The combination of a statin and ezetimibe is the best tolerated and offers the most convenient once-a-day dosing of the possible combinations. This is the combination that was selected for D.E.

INITIATING THERAPY

20. How should combined therapy with a statin and ezetimibe be initiated in D.E.?

Given the amount of LDL-C lowering needed to reach D.E.'s LDL-C goal, it is reasonable to select one of the more potent LDL-C–lowering statins (e.g., simvastatin, atorvastatin or rosuvastatin) and to start with a high daily dose (40 mg/d). Before therapy is initiated, baseline liver function tests and CPK levels should be obtained (see Table 13-16). Renal function should be assessed because impaired renal clearance of the statin or its active metabolite could result in increased systemic levels, which might increase the risk of myotoxicity. LDL-C levels should be evaluated in about 6 weeks, when the maximum effect of the statin is anticipated. If the LDL-C is within 6% of D.E.'s goal, the dosage of the statin may be advanced to 80 mg as this should be sufficient to achieve the goal. However, if the LDL-C is >6% below goal, ezetimibe 10 mg daily should be added to the regimen. This should add an additional 10% to 20% LDL-C–lowering effect.[182] D.E. should be seen in another 6 weeks for further LDL-C evaluation.

If D.E. does not achieve his goal with this two-drug combination, the addition of a third drug should be considered. Choices are to add a bile acid resin, such as colesevelam, or niacin. At the time of this writing, there is no study describing the efficacy of an ezetimibe, resin, and statin combination. Theoretically, the combination should be effective, but there may be a limit to how much hepatic LDL receptors can be up-regulated. Since each of the drugs (statins, ezetimibe, and resins) use this same mechanism, the combination of all three may not be as effective as a statin with either a resin or ezetimibe. Niacin has been successfully added as a third drug in a regimen and provides a 10% to 15% additional LDL-C–lowering effect when titrated to about 2,000 mg per day.

ADDING A THIRD LIPID-LOWERING DRUG TO THE REGIMEN

21. How should niacin be initiated in D.E., and what monitoring is required?

Before niacin therapy is started (and after its maximum dosage is reached), liver function tests should be evaluated (see Table 13-16). Patients with an active peptic ulcer or liver disease should not receive niacin. Niacin may increase glucose levels by 10% to 20% in some diabetic patients or patients with impaired fasting glucose levels, necessitating careful monitoring of glucose control. None of these issues is a factor in D.E.

The addition of niacin to D.E.'s statin and ezetimibe regimen should be initiated with low doses that are slowly titrated upward to allow tolerance to develop at each dosage level (see Table 13-15). D.E. should be given as much control over niacin administration as possible. Crystalline niacin can be started at 250 to 300 mg/day, administered in two or three divided doses. Thereafter, daily dosages may be increased every 3 to 7 days in the following sequence: 500, 1,000, 1,500, 2,000, and 3,000 mg. Niaspan is initiated at 500 mg at bedtime and increased every 7 days to 1,000 mg, 1,500 mg, and 2,000 mg daily as tolerated by the patient. The over-the-counter sustained-release niacin dosage form is not recommended due to its increased risk of causing hepatotoxicity.

D.E. should be warned about the vasodilatory symptoms associated with niacin use (facial flushing, itching, rash) and reassured that these symptoms are not dangerous and that tolerance should develop after several weeks of therapy. He should be advised to take 325 mg of aspirin or another prostaglandin-inhibiting drug 30 minutes before the morning dose of crystalline niacin or the bedtime dose of Niaspan to decrease these symptoms. Taking each dose with food will help to reduce flushing and GI symptoms. Instruction can also be provided to reduce doses if necessary to manage bothersome symptoms. He should be encouraged to call his clinician whenever troublesome symptoms occur.

Several weeks after the 1,500-mg/day dosage is reached (see Table 13-15), the patient should be evaluated for achievement of the LDL-C goal and side effects. If the LDL-C goal is not achieved with 1,500 mg/day, further increments can be made up to the maximum tolerated dose or a ceiling dose of 3,000 mg of crystalline niacin or 2,000 mg of Niaspan. In addition to a fasting lipid profile, laboratory tests of liver function, glucose, and uric acid may be indicated.

MIXED HYPERLIPIDEMIA

Assessing the Patient With Mixed Hyperlipidemia

22. B.C., a 56-year-old man, experienced acute chest pain 3 months ago and was admitted to the local hospital with a diagnosis of unstable angina. His only known medical problem was hypertension treated with enalapril 10 mg QD. His lipid profile on admission was total cholesterol, 235 mg/dL; HDL-C, 30 mg/dL; LDL-C, 165 mg/dL; and TG, 300 mg/dL. He underwent a cardiac catheterization, which revealed a 90% stenotic lesion in his left anterior ascending artery. A drug-coated stent was placed without difficulty. He was subsequently discharged on simvastatin 40 mg QD, ASA 325 mg QD, propranolol 40 mg BID, and enalapril 10 mg QD.

Today, he weighs 220 lb, is 6 feet tall (ideal body weight [IBW], 140 to 185 lb), and has a waist circumference of 42″. He has lost 10 lb since his MI by following a low-fat diet and an exercise program. He swims 1 mile three times a week without symptoms of cardiac ischemia, and he drinks two glasses of wine each evening with dinner. His father died at age 58 of an MI (lipids unknown). He has never smoked. Pertinent physical findings include BP 148/90 mm Hg; heart rate 60 regular; arcus senilis; carotid pulses equal without bruits; and chest clear to auscultation without cardiomegaly. Laboratory tests disclose normal thyroid-stimulating hormone levels, normal renal and liver function, and a fasting glucose level of 120 mg/dL. His urinalysis was normal. The lipid profile while taking the above regimen is total cholesterol, 175 mg/dL; TGs, 225 mg/dL; HDL-C, 32 mg/dL; and LDL-C, 98 mg/dL.

What is your assessment of B.C.'s lipids and lipoprotein cholesterol concentrations?

[SI units: glucose, 6.66 mmol/L; total cholesterol, 8.28 mmol/L; TGs, 3.39 mmol/L; HDL-C, 0.78 mmol/L; LDL-C, 5.95 mmol/L]

According to NCEP guidelines, B.C. has reached the LDL-C treatment goal (<100 mg/dL) for a patient with a history of CHD[87] (see Table 13-11). He has experienced a 40% LDL-C reduction since his hospitalization 3 months ago. The LDL-C should be confirmed with a second lipid profile (since there is biologic and analytical variability). According to NCEP guidelines, his TG level remains high (200 to 500 mg/dL) and his HDL-C is low (<40 mg/dL) (see Table 13-7). The lipid profile obtained during his hospitalization can be interpreted in a normal manner, since it was drawn within 24 hours of his acute coronary event. However, profiles drawn after 24 hours are generally lower than pre-event levels and remain so for several weeks.

Based on his recent CHD event, B.C. has a >20% chance of a recurrent CHD event in the next 10 years. He is therefore considered to be a high-risk, CHD risk equivalent patient. Post-MI patients in the placebo group of the LIPID study had an LDL-C level of 150 mg/dL and a 16% incidence of a non-fatal MI or CHD death in 5 years (or about a 32% risk of CHD events in 10 years).[84] Additionally, B.C. has several risk factors for CHD that add to his risk: family history, male older than 45, high BP, and low HDL-C. His fasting blood sugar is defined as impaired fasting glucose (i.e., a fasting value 110 to 126 mg/dL). Some clinicians would consider him to be diabetic, given how close he is to the definition of diabetes (fasting blood sugar >126 mg/dL). Evaluation of HgA1c and a glucose tolerance test are indicated to further define B.C.'s diabetes state.

B.C. was appropriately treated with a statin (as well as antiplatelet, angiotensin-converting enzyme [ACE] inhibitor, and beta-blocker therapy) and a TLC diet and exercise program to achieve an LDL-C <100 mg/dL. In such a high-risk patient, therapeutic interventions should not be delayed. Not only will the initiation of drug treatment in the hospital setting provide risk-reducing benefit, but the patient is more likely to relate this therapy to his acute event and adhere to it.[186]

Although B.C. has reached his LDL-C goal, the job of reducing his CHD risk is not complete. The next step is to evaluate the CHD risk associated with the high TG level and, if indicated, develop a plan to address it (Table 13-18).

Relation of Triglycerides to Coronary Heart Disease

23. Does the increased TG level in B.C. indicate an increased CHD risk?

The exact role that TGs play in the pathogenesis of CHD is under intense investigation. Most epidemiologic studies have found that a high TG level is an independent risk factor for CHD when evaluated with univariate analysis. However, when other lipid abnormalities such as increased LDL-C or low HDL-C are included in a multivariate analysis, TGs often lose their independent predictive power.[187] Part of the reason for this is the close interrelationship between lipids. Patients with high TG levels almost always have a low HDL-C, which also predicts CHD risk.[188,189] In addition, elevated TG levels are associated with increased levels of TG-rich lipoproteins (i.e., remnant VLDL particles) and small, dense LDL particles.[8,190] These particles are atherogenic and mediate a higher CHD risk than associated with an elevated LDL-C

alone.[191–194] When epidemiologic studies were combined, a meta-analysis found that TGs independently predicted CHD risk, even after adjustment for other lipid risk factors.[195] High TG levels are also found in certain familial disorders, including dysbetalipoproteinemia and familial combined hyperlipidemia, which carry increased CHD risk.[18,196] Additionally, hypertriglyceridemia is associated with a procoagulant state, which promotes coronary thrombosis.[190]

Paradoxically, very high TG levels (>500 mg/dL) are not commonly associated with an increased CHD risk, but do cause an increased risk of pancreatitis, especially when levels exceed 1,000 mg/dL. Often, a genetic defect in lipoprotein lipase is present in these cases that impairs the removal of TGs from TG-rich particles (VLDL and chylomicrons). These particles do not become enriched with cholesterol and, therefore, are not often atherogenic.[196,197] If the blood sample is stored in the refrigerator overnight, a thick creamy layer often appears on the surface, indicating the presence of chylomicrons. Although most patients with very high TGs remain free of CHD throughout their lives, some develop it.[187]

On the other hand, patients like B.C., with TGs in the borderline to high range (150 to 500 mg/dL), have an increased CHD risk because they likely have atherogenic TG-rich lipoproteins (see Table 13-7B). Characteristically, B.C. has a high TG level and a low HDL-C and is likely to also have elevated remnant VLDL-C and small dense LDL levels. This is the profile of atherogenic dyslipidemia described earlier in this chapter and is linked to a high CHD risk. This is exemplified by the placebo groups in the HIT and BIP trials, two studies that included patients with mixed hyperlipidemia. Untreated subjects had CHD event rates of 15% to 22% in 5 to 6 years, respectively.[105,106]

Atherogenic Dyslipidemia

24. Why does atherogenic dyslipidemia occur? How should the clinician assess and treat atherogenic dyslipidemia?

Patients like B.C. with borderline high or high TG levels (see Table 13-7) secrete large numbers of TG-enriched VLDL particles from the liver. One reason for this is increased levels of nonesterified fatty acids in the systemic circulation that come from adipose cells (especially in patients with central obesity). The liver clears these fatty acids and is stimulated to increase the synthesis of triglycerides.[198]

A second reason for the increased secretion of VLDL particles is an upregulation of the gene expression for microsomal triglyceride transfer protein (MTP) that is caused by the elevated insulin levels in these patients.[199] MTP is responsible for assembling VLDL particles in the hepatocyte. It brings together TG, cholesterol, and apolipoproteins to form the

Table 13-18 Treatment Targets for Patients Who Have Achieved Their LDL-C Goal and Have a Triglyceride Level ≥200 Mg/DL			
Patient Category	LDL-C Treatment Target	Non-HDL-C Treatment Target	Apolipoprotein B Treatment Target
CHD or CHD risk equivalent	<100 mg/dL	<130 mg/dL	<90 mg/dL
No CHD, ≥2 risk factors	<130 mg/dL	<60 mg/dL	<110 mg/dL
No CHD, <2 risk factors	<160 mg/dL	<190 mg/dL	<130 mg/dL

CHD, coronary heart disease; HDL, high-density lipoprotein cholesterol; LDL-C, low-density lipoprotein cholesterol.

VLDL particle. This mechanism suggests a molecular basis for the link between insulin resistance and increased VLDL secretion. One way of telling that there are increased numbers of lipoprotein particles in the systemic circulation is to measure apolipoprotein B. One apolipoprotein B is attached to each VLDL and LDL particle. An increased apolipoprotein B level indicates an increased number of particles. Patients with a high apolipoprotein B level have a high risk of CHD.

With the increase in VLDL particles, plasma levels of apolipoprotein C-III also increase. Apolipoprotein C-III has two detrimental effects. It interferes with the normal removal of TG from VLDL by reducing the action of lipoprotein lipase. This reduces lipolysis and increases the concentration of TGs in the VLDL particle. The second negative effect of apolipoprotein C-III is an interference with the normal removal of VLDL particles from the circulation via LDL receptors on the haptocyte.[198]

TG-rich VLDL particles interact with other circulating lipoproteins through the action of cholesterol ester transfer protein. Through this protein, a molecule of cholesterol ester is exchanged from circulating HDL and LDL particles for a molecule of TG from VLDL particles. With time, the HDL particles give up >50% of their cholesterol content and become enriched with TG. This results in low HDL-C levels. VLDL becomes more enriched with cholesterol and simultaneously smaller in size, close to the size of LDL, and thus more atherogenic (both because of its smaller size and its higher cholesterol content). LDL particles take on more TG than normal. Subsequently, under the influence of hepatic lipase, TG is removed from LDL particles, leaving a very small particle that is deficient in cholesterol and TG, but is present in great numbers. Because of their small size and concentration, small dense LDL particles are very atherogenic.

The net result of the above mechanisms is a high VLDL-C, low HDL-C, and increased small dense LDL, a lipid triad termed atherogenic dyslipidemia. How does the clinician measure this in the clinical setting? Unfortunately, VLDL-C and VLDL-TG levels are not available from most clinical laboratories. Several companies provide measurements of particle size, but these are not widely available and do not yet relate to a reference standard; particle size measurements are best reserved for research purposes at present. The clinician can measure apolipoprotein B as an indicator of the number of atherogenic particles; these levels are available from most clinical laboratories. However, a much easier, more accessible measure is non-HDL-C. Non-HDL-C is the product of VLDL-C and LDL-C and is determined by subtracting HDL-C from total cholesterol. NCEP recommends that non-HDL-C be determined in patients who have a TG >200 mg/dL after attaining their LDL-C goal.[87] Once the patient is at his or her LDL-C goal, any elevation in non-HDL-C will be due to an increase in VLDL-C. Since VLDL-C levels are normally <30 mg/dL, non-HDL-C treatment goals are set 30 mg/dL above LDL-C treatment goals (see Table 13-18). Included in the same table are alternative apolipoprotein B treatment goals that have been recommended by authorities.[200] Note that non-HDL-C levels can be determined from a nonfasting sample measuring only total cholesterol and HDL-C, thus making it very convenient for the clinician to make these measurements any time of the day without regard to food intake.

Secondary Causes of Hypertriglyceridemia

25. In addition to an assessment of B.C.'s lipid profile, what other evaluations should be made?

One of the questions that should be answered routinely when evaluating patients with lipid disorders is: Is there a secondary cause of the patient's lipid disorder? Secondary causes of hypertriglyceridemia include chronic renal failure; diabetes mellitus; alcohol use and abuse; a sedentary lifestyle; obesity; and the use of TG-raising drugs, including β-blockers, estrogens, and glucocorticoids (see Table 13-8). B.C. has a normal TSH level, normal liver and renal function tests, and a normal urinalysis. His blood glucose is elevated into the impaired fasting glucose range, which can be associated with impaired TG metabolism, as described earlier. In addition, he is overweight, with much of the weight distributed around his waist (i.e., a waist circumference >40 inches). Patients who have truncal obesity often overproduce TGs and oversecrete VLDL particles, thereby raising their TG level. The HDL-C is inversely reduced. This would appear to be an important factor affecting TG levels in B.C. A reduction in weight through an exercise program and a low-calorie, low–saturated fat, and low-carbohydrate diet would be one of the most effective ways to improve B.C.'s glucose level, raise his HDL-C, and lower his TG level.

Light to moderate alcohol intake, defined as up to two drinks per day (1 drink = 5 oz wine, 12 oz beer, or 1.5 oz 80-proof liquor), as is practiced by B.C., has been associated with lower CHD rates. The observed reduction in CHD among light to moderate alcohol drinkers is consistently on the order of 40% to 60% in epidemiologic trials.[201,202] Available epidemiologic evidence supports arguments of causality.[203,204] However, it is problematic to recommend alcohol consumption for CHD prevention. From a public health point of view, the adverse consequences of alcohol consumption are large and may outweigh the benefits gained. One known adverse consequence of alcohol consumption is hypertriglyceridemia, especially when alcohol is abused, but it may be seen with only moderate intake as well. Even though B.C.'s alcohol intake appears moderate, it may be contributing to his hypertriglyceridemia, so a period of abstinence is warranted to determine whether this is the case.

Use of a β-blocker could also raise TG levels (see Table 13-8) and might be a contributing factor in B.C.'s lipid profile. However, he already had a high TG level on admission to the hospital prior to starting propranolol therapy. In this case, the β-blocker is providing an important health benefit that probably outweighs the small risk posed by its effect of TG levels. More probably, B.C.'s weight and impaired glucose are the key factors contributing to his increased TG level and are the logical places to start when attempting to correct secondary causes of elevated TG levels.

Metabolic Syndrome

26. B.C. has a combination of obesity, impaired fasting glucose, and hypertension in addition to atherogenic dyslipidemia. What is the significance of this constellation of findings?

Not only does B.C. have CHD and a combination of lipid abnormalities that substantially raise his risk of CHD, but he also has a number of nonlipid risk factors that raise it as well.[205] These factors include obesity, impaired fasting glucose, and hypertension. Most of B.C.'s excess weight is concentrated around his waist. This central distribution of fat may reflect an excess of intra-abdominal fat, which in turn may influence the development of atherogenic dyslipidemia, as already described.[206] An increased outflow of fatty acids from intra-abdominal TG stores may provide the substrate for increased hepatic TG synthesis and VLDL secretion. This could explain B.C.'s elevated TG level.

Abdominal obesity also is strongly associated with insulin resistance.[198,207] Insulin resistance leads to mild hyperglycemia, and the pancreas responds by increasing insulin secretion; hyperinsulinemia results.[208,209] Some genetically predisposed patients are not able to secrete enough insulin to overcome this resistance and develop impaired glucose metabolism or diabetes. The presence of a blood sugar between 110 and 126 mg/dL in B.C. suggests impaired glucose metabolism (fasting) and probably insulin resistance (with hyperinsulinemia).[210]

B.C. has hypertension. The β-blocker and ACE inhibitor he is receiving to reduce his CHD risk also help lower his blood pressure. According to the most recent guidelines, B.C. still has stage 1 hypertension (systolic BP 140 to 159 mm Hg); his untreated BP may be higher.[211] Before one can conclude inadequate BP control, however, BP readings should be obtained on at least two other occasions and adherence to therapy documented. Abdominal obesity and insulin resistance also are commonly associated with high BP and could be a factor in B.C.[212,213] The exact mechanisms for this remain speculative.

What emerges from the preceding discussion is the strong possibility that B.C.'s risk factors are not independent, but rather represent a constellation of medical problems that have a common pathway. This pathway may be related to insulin resistance.[212,214] NCEP called this constellation the *metabolic syndrome*.[87] Other names given the same problem in the literature are *syndrome X, the deadly quadrangle, insulin resistance syndrome,* and *Reavan's syndrome*.[193,194,209,212,214,215] Metabolic syndrome is diagnosed when any three of the factors listed in Table 13-19 are present. The syndrome is associated with a substantial increase in CHD risk; the exact level of risk should be determined by using the risk-scoring charts in Figure 13-7. B.C. has the metabolic syndrome by having met all five criteria in Table 13-19. Weight loss, especially loss of visceral abdominal adiposity, will be the centerpiece of his nondrug treatment program. The goal is for weight reduction

Table 13-19 Clinical Identification of the Metabolic Syndrome

Presence of any three of the following:

• Waist Circumference	
○ Men	>40 inches
○ Women	>35 inches
• Triglycerides	≥150 mg/dL
• High-density lipoprotein cholesterol	
○ Men	<40 mg/dL
○ Women	<50 mg/dL
• Blood pressure (systolic/diastolic)	≥130/≥85
• Fasting glucose	>110 mg/dL

to correct, or at least substantially improve, his blood glucose, TG, and HDL-C levels and BP.

Hypertension Management With Atherogenic Dyslipidemia

27. **If B.C.'s BP elevation persists after lifestyle changes are made, how should he be managed?**

Consideration of antihypertensive therapy in a patient with dyslipidemia should take into account how BP-modifying drugs affect blood lipids. As noted above, the propranolol B.C. is receiving can elevate TG levels, but the benefit in post-MI prophylaxis warrants its continued use.[216] Substitution of a β-blocker with intrinsic sympathomimetic activity (e.g., pindolol) or a mixed α-β–blocker (e.g., labetalol) may have less effect on lipids (see Table 13-8), but their benefits for post-MI prophylaxis are unproven.

The ACE inhibitor B.C. currently is receiving for his hypertension has a neutral effect on serum lipids. However, his BP is not under good control, so an adjustment to his antihypertensive regimen is in order. One of the best drugs to reduce BP in patients receiving an ACE inhibitor is a thiazide diuretic.[211] Although thiazides may increase blood cholesterol levels (see Table 13-8), these effects usually are small, especially with long-term use. The thiazide dose should be kept low (i.e., 12.5 mg/d) to minimize the effect on his blood lipids. Calcium channel blockers, like ACE inhibitors, are lipid neutral and are possible alternatives to a thiazide.

Treatment of the Metabolic Syndrome
CHOLESTEROL LOWERING AND WEIGHT-LOSS DIET

28. **What nondrug therapies should be implemented to help B.C. achieve his treatment goals?**

B.C. needs to lose weight in addition to lowering his LDL-C and non-HDL-C levels. Effective weight loss and subsequent weight maintenance could substantially or fully correct his atherogenic dyslipidemia, lower his BP, reduce his waist circumference, and correct his blood glucose. He has already shown progress, having lost 10 pounds since his MI 3 months ago. He appears to be following a low-fat diet, which undoubtedly has helped him lose weight. However, he needs to lose more weight and needs to modify his lipids further. A more rigorous restriction of saturated fats might help him accomplish these goals. This will also substantially reduce total daily calories, since fats contain 9 calories/g. Restriction of saturated fat calories will encourage weight loss and will reduce TG levels; however, it may also reduce HDL-C levels. If saturated fat calories are replaced with polyunsaturated fats, HDL-C usually does not change and may increase. An increase in carbohydrate intake will increase TG and may cause weight gain. Therefore, in a weight-loss diet for the metabolic syndrome, saturated fats and carbohydrates should generally both be restricted. This level of complexity supports the involvement of a registered dietitian who can provide expert advice and practical meal planning.

DRUG THERAPY FOR THE METABOLIC SYNDROME

29. **If weight loss and an exercise program are insufficient to fully correct B.C.'s lipid disorder, it is appropriate to consider drug therapy. What lipid-modulating drugs should be considered?**

In patients with the metabolic syndrome and not at their non-HDL-C goal, three drugs are used: statins, niacin, or a fibrate. The statin given to B.C. has achieved his primary treatment goal, a LDL-C <100 mg/dL. It has also reduced his TG level about 25% and raised his HDL-C level modestly, both typical effects of statins. The effect of statins on TGs is dose dependent; the higher the statin dose, the greater the TG lowering. Also, the reduction of TG serum levels achieved with a statin is greatest in patients who have high baseline TG levels.[217] The reduction in non-HDL-C with each dose doubling of a statin is about 6%. Thus, an increase in the daily dose of simvastatin from 40 mg to 80 mg per day would be expected to reduce B.C.'s non-HDL-C level from 143 mg/dL to approximately 134 ng/dL, not likely to be enough to achieve his non-HDL-C goal of <130 mg/dL (see Table 13-18). Atorvastatin lowers LDL-C, non-HDL-C, and TGs more than the other statins and may achieve B.C.'s treatment goal with daily doses of 40 to 80 mg.

An alternative is to add other drugs to a moderate statin dose to achieve the non-HDL-C treatment goal. The advantages of doing this are to take advantage of the additive LDL-C–and non-HDL-C–lowering effects of these drugs, to take advantage of using two drugs with potentially different mechanisms of reducing CHD risk, and to avoid use of high doses of the statin and the accompanying increase in side effects (although this risk is quite small). Disadvantages include adding exposure to two drugs, both with their own side effect profile, adding complexity to the regimen, and adding cost. Choices of drugs to add to a statin include the bile acid resins, ezetimibe, niacin, or a fibrate.

The bile acid resins and ezetimibe will add 10% to 20% additional LDL-C lowering when added to a statin; non-HDL-C will be lowered nearly as much. However, much of the reduction in non-HDL-C will be from a reduction in LDL-C. VLDL-C and TG levels will not be lowered much with ezetimibe (over what is achieved with the statin) and may not change or may even increase with a bile acid resin. This effect of resins is most pronounced in patients like B.C. with hypertriglyceridemia. Thus, neither ezetimibe nor a resin appears to address the mechanisms causing the atherogenic dyslipidemia.

Niacin generally enhances VLDL-C and TG lowering (up to double the amount) and substantially increases HDL-C levels when added to a statin.[218] The effects on VLDL-C, TG, and HDL-C with niacin follow a curvilinear pattern such that substantial changes in these parameters can be achieved with modest daily doses of niacin (1 to 1.5 g/day) (see Fig. 13-8). Thus, when niacin is added to a statin, it need not be titrated to maximal doses, which might in turn increase patient tolerance of niacin. In one study, the addition of 750 mg/d of niacin to simvastatin extended the reduction in TG from 26% to 31% and in VLDL-C from 28% to 44%, while increasing HDL-C from 13% to 31%.[219] The principal concern with niacin in patients with the metabolic syndrome is its potential to worsen glucose metabolism. Several recent studies in subjects with and without diabetes have shown that niacin causes transient increases in fasting glucose and glycosylated hemoglobin levels in about a third of patients. These increases return to baseline levels in about 6 weeks, presumably because of adjustments made to the subject's diabetic therapy.[200,220] Investigators with the Coronary Drug Project reported that fasting and 1-hour postprandial blood glucose levels were increased in patients assigned to niacin, but this metabolic change did not adversely effect CHD risk reduction. In fact, nonfatal MI and all-cause death after 6 years of therapy was reduced by 29% and 12%, respectively, among study patients with a 1-hour postprandial glucose of <140 mg/dL compared with reductions of 42% and 20% among patients with a 1-hour postprandial glucose of ≥220 mg/dL.[221] Nonetheless, it is important to use appropriate doses of insulin or oral hypoglycemics in patient with inadequately controlled diabetes.

FIBRIC ACID DERIVATIVES

30. **What are the characteristics of gemfibrozil and fenofibrate that would qualify either drug for use in B.C.?**

Clinical Use. Gemfibrozil (Lopid) and fenofibrate (TriCor) (and the other fibric acid derivative available in the United States, clofibrate [Atromid S]) lower TG levels by 20% to 50% and in patients with hypertriglyceridemia, raise HDL-C by 10% to 15%[222–226] (see Table 13-17). Gemfibrozil generally lowers LDL-C by 10% to 15%, but in patients with both hypercholesterolemia and hypertriglyceridemia it may have no effect on or may actually increase LDL-C levels. Fenofibrate lowers LDL-C by 15% to 25%.[226–228] This effect is blunted in patients with combined hypercholesterolemia and hypertriglyceridemia, but an LDL-C reduction of 10% to 15% is still expected.[222,223,227,228]

Gemfibrozil and fenofibrate are both indicated for the reduction of TG levels in patients with hypertriglyceridemia.[218] In patients who have TG levels >1,000 mg/dL and are at risk for developing pancreatitis, fibrates, along with niacin, are the drugs of choice. Similarly, in patients with familial dysbetalipoproteinemia, fibric acid derivatives are highly effective and are considered the drugs of choice. Fibrates also have a place in the management of combined or mixed hyperlipidemia. Support for this comes primarily from the results of the Helsinki Heart Study and the HIT trials, in which gemfibrozil combined with diet therapy was associated with a reduction in CHD deaths and nonfatal MIs.[103,105] These positive outcomes are attributed to significant reductions in serum TGs (and, therefore, a reduction in TG-rich VLDL remnants and in small, dense LDLs) and an increase in HDL-C. Persons most likely to benefit are those with diabetes or the lipid triad found in patients with the metabolic syndrome.[229,230]

Mechanism of Action. Fibrates activate peroxisome proliferator-activated receptors (PPARα), which explains most of their effects on blood lipids.[231] PPARα receptors are located in the nucleus of cells and are ligand-dependent transcription factors that regulate target gene expression. Stimulation of PPARα suppresses the gene responsible for synthesis of apolipoprotein C-III and stimulates the gene responsible for LDL receptor synthesis.[232,233,234] As a result, lipolysis of TG from VLDL particles and the removal of these particles via hepatic LDL receptors is enhanced. Stimulation of PPARα also increases fatty acid oxidation, which reduces the synthesis of TG in the liver, and this in turn reduces the TG content of secreted VLDL particles.[233,235] Stimulation of PPARα may increase the synthesis of apolipoprotein A-1, the critical building block of nascent HDL, thereby enhancing reverse cholesterol transport. Research also suggests that fibrates stimulate the expression of ABC_1 transporters in macrophage cells, which are responsible for bringing cholesterol from within the cell to the cell surface, where it can be taken up by nascent HDL particles and removed from these cells.[231]

Adverse Effects. Gemfibrozil and fenofibrate are usually well tolerated. Gemfibrozil causes mild GI symptoms (nausea, dyspepsia, abdominal pain) in about one third of patients. Fenofibrate causes a rash in 2% to 4% of patients. Fibrate therapy may also cause muscle side effects, including myositis and rhabdomyolysis.[236] Most cases of muscle toxicity have been reported with gemfibrozil, especially when it is used in combination with a statin. Recent studies reveal that the area under the blood-concentration curve of most statins is increased two- to fourfold when given concurrently with gemfibrozil. These effects are not seen with fenofibrate. The mechanism causing this interaction appears to be related to an interference by gemfibrozil with the glucuronidation of statins and thereby a reduction in statin renal clearance from the systemic circulation.[237,238] This supports the preferential use of fenofibrate over gemfibrozil when a combination with a statin is indicated in managing patients such as B.C. with a mixed hyperlipidemia. Patients who receive gemfibrozil or fenofibrate therapy alone or in combination with a statin should be monitored for symptoms of muscle soreness and pain. If these symptoms emerge, a CPK level should be obtained. A CPK level >10 times the upper limit of normal along with muscle symptoms supports a diagnosis of myositis. The presence of myositis is an indication to withdraw fibrate therapy, provided other possible causes are not apparent, such as increased physical exercise or a recent trauma or fall.

Gemfibrozil increases biliary secretion of cholesterol, which increases the lithogenicity of bile and results in the development of cholesterol gallstones. Presumably the same effect occurs with all fibrates.

The results of two major primary prevention trials have raised questions about the safety of fibrates. In the World Health Organization trial, clofibrate reduced nonfatal MIs by 25% but caused an increase in total mortality.[239,240] As a result, its use has declined markedly in the United States. Some of these deaths may have been related to gallstone disease.[239] In the Helsinki Heart Study, gemfibrozil reduced fatal and nonfatal MIs by 37% but was associated with a slight increase in non-CHD mortality such that there was no net reduction in total mortality.[103] In a 3.5-year follow-up to this study, total mortality in gemfibrozil patients was increased due to an increase in non-CHD mortality.[241] Follow-up evaluations of non-gemfibrozil therapies were associated with continued event reduction.[107] In the HIT trial, death from CHD was significantly reduced by 22% with gemfibrozil, but total mortality was not.[105] Fenofibrate has not been tested in major clinical trials. Thus, there is little information about its effect on non-CHD events. Fenofibrate was evaluated against placebo in 418 patients with diabetes and at least one visible lesion on angiographic evaluation in the DAIS trial.[242] The trial was not powered to examine clinical endpoints, but there were fewer events, including deaths, in the fenofibrate group. Taken together, these data support a cautious and restricted use of gemfibrozil and perhaps other fibric acid derivatives.

DRUG SELECTION FOR MANAGING ATHEROGENIC DYSLIPIDEMIA

31. **Given these considerations, what drugs are indicated for B.C.?**

One approach would be to replace simvastatin with atorvastatin or rosuvastatin at 40 mg daily; atorvastatin may be to 80 mg daily if needed. This should attain both the LDL-C and non-HDL-C goals. Alternatively, consideration could be given to adding a TG-lowering (i.e., non-HDL-C lowering) drug such as niacin or fenofibrate. Gemfibrozil should be avoided, given its documented pharmacodynamic drug interaction with statins and the increased risk of muscle toxicity. Both niacin and fenofibrate effectively lower TGs by 30% to 50%; more importantly, they reduce VLDL-C and small dense LDLs and raise HDL-C (see Table 13-17). Both alter the mechanisms responsible for atherogenic dyslipidemia, although the effect of PPARα agonism has a broader and more fundamental effect on these mechanisms. Fibrate therapy is not likely to worsen B.C.'s impaired fasting glucose, whereas niacin might do so. Fenofibrate is certainly more tolerable than niacin: about 30% of niacin-treated patients cannot tolerate its vasodilatory side effects. Niacin is less expensive and has demonstrated CHD risk reduction alone or together with a statin in major clinical trials. Given these considerations, it is obvious that there is no one correct choice; the choice will be based on individual preferences.

INITIATING COMBINATION DRUG THERAPY FOR ATHEROGENIC DYSLIPIDEMIA

32. **How should combined therapy with a statin and fenofibrate be initiated in B.C.? What monitoring is required?**

Fenofibrate can be added as a 200-mg capsule once a day and the lipid profile rechecked in 6 to 8 weeks. A lower daily dose of 67 mg should be selected for patients with impaired renal function and in patients older than 65 (since creatine clearance declines with older age). As with all lipid-altering therapies, patients should be instructed on the purpose of the medication and its expected effects on blood lipids and on CHD risk reduction. They should be encouraged to remain adherent with the regimen to sustain its effects on serum lipids and, thereby, attain its CHD risk-reducing benefit. Withdrawal, even after a long period of consistent cholesterol control, will likely result in a return of blood lipids to pretreatment levels. Patients should be counseled to call a health professional if they experience any untoward symptoms, especially muscle soreness or discomfort or a rash. A CPK level should be obtained whenever a patient experiences symptoms of myositis (muscle soreness and aches).

LOW HDL-C

33. **J.M. is a 60-year-old man who has no history of CHD or a CHD risk equivalent. He has no known medical problems. He does not smoke. His mother had an ischemic episode at age 70 and subsequently had coronary artery bypass surgery. There is no other family history of CHD. J.M. eats a diet low in saturated fat and is sedentary. His physical examination is unremarkable: BP, 122/82 mm Hg, heart rate, 66 regular. He weighs 206 lb and is 6 feet tall (BMI 28). His laboratory values are fasting blood glucose, 80 mg/dL; total cholesterol, 137 mg/dL; LDL-C, 84**

mg/dL; TG, 120 mg/dL; HDL-C, 29 mg/dL. Should J.M. be treated for his low HDL-C?

J.M. has two CHD risk factors (age and low HDL) and a LDL-C goal of <130 mg/dL. His NCEP CHD risk is 10% in 10 years, mostly because of his age. His LDL-C is well within his treatment goal. His TGs are in the normal range. Epidemiologic studies clearly link low HDL-C with increased CHD events, especially in those over age 50. These studies show that a 1% decrease in HDL-C is associated with a 1% to 2% increase in CHD risk. Most commonly, low HDL-C is secondary to a number of lifestyle and medical conditions (Table 13-20). Of these conditions, overweight, physical inactivity, and a diet very low in fat may play a part in J.M.'s low HDL-C. Patients who substantially restrict saturated fats have lower HDL-C levels as well as LDL-C. A careful dietary history would be important to determine whether this is occurring with J.M. Vegetarians who have a low LDL-C and low BP have a low CHD risk in spite of having a low HDL-C. Increasing intake of monounsaturated fats and lowering carbohydrate intake is one maneuver to raise HDL-C. An obvious approach to improving J.M.'s HDL-C is to encourage him to increase his physical activity.

In addition to secondary causes, there are rare primary (genetic) causes of low HDL-C. Some are associated with increased CHD risk, while others are not. Tangier disease is associated with a reduction in the ABC_1 transporter that moves cholesterol out of peripheral cells. Patients with Tangier disease have characteristic orange tonsils as well as splenomegaly and neuropathy. Fish-eye disease is characterized by corneal opacification and an HDL deficiency. About a third of fish-eye patients develop CHD. Patients with apolipoprotein A-1$_{Milano}$ have very low HDL-C levels, but live well into their ninetieth decade, apparently because their reverse cholesterol transport is very efficient. J.M. does not appear to have any of these disorders. Importantly, he also does not have a family history of premature CHD. This suggests that his low HDL-C is not due to a genetic abnormality associated with an increased CHD risk.

What makes patients such as J.M. difficult to manage is that there is little clinical trial evidence that raising low levels of HDL-C with diet or drugs will reduce CHD risk. Part of the problem is that there are no effective drugs that substantially and specifically increase HDL-C. Niacin has the most substantial raising effect (mean increases of 25% to 35%). Fibrates also raise HDL-C by 10% to 20%, but they may also raise LDL-C in patients with hypertriglyceridemia. The available evidence indicates that aggressive LDL-C lowering is the most powerful way to reduce CHD risk in patients with low HDL-C. In fact, the lower the HDL-C level, the greater the CHD risk reduction with statin therapy.[243] Based on this evidence, NCEP recommended aggressive LDL-C lowering with a statin in patients with a low HDL-C.[87] In cases of isolated low HDL-C (without hypertriglyceridemia), NCEP recommended lifestyle modification with weight reduction and increased physical activity and the empiric use of HDL-C–raising drugs (niacin or a fibrate) if indicated to reduce CHD risk.[87]

It would be prudent to encourage J.M. to lose weight and especially to adopt a more physically active lifestyle. This will help his overall well-being. However, since he lacks a family history of premature CHD or associated CHD risk factors, his CHD risk would appear to be low and not supportive of an aggressive effort to raise his low HDL-C. If he did have a family history of premature CHD, a more aggressive approach, particularly with increased physical activity and possibly niacin therapy, would be advisable.

ANTIOXIDANT THERAPY

34. **Should antioxidants, such as vitamin E or β-carotene, be considered in the management of hyperlipidemic patients, especially patients who have developed CHD?**

Only oxidized (or otherwise modified) LDL is taken up by macrophage cells in the initial phase of atherogenesis. This observation has lead to the supposition that drugs that have antioxidant properties might reduce or block the development of atherosclerosis. Vitamins E, C, and β-carotene (the precursor of vitamin A) have antioxidant properties and have been variably recommended to prevent CHD.[244] Studies in hypercholesterolemic animals have demonstrated that antioxidants, such as probucol, can reduce the development of atherosclerosis.[244,245] In humans, oxidized LDL-C has been detected in atheromatous lesions, and circulating antibodies to oxidized LDL have also been detected.[246,247] In epidemiologic studies, people who frequently used β-carotene and vitamin E had 35% to 50% fewer CHD events.[248,249] However, when the hypothesis that antioxidant therapy will prevent CHD events was tested in well-controlled, randomized clinical trials, no benefit was observed. For example, vitamin E, whether administered in low, moderate, and high daily doses, either as monotherapy or combined with other antioxi-

Table 13-20 Factors Causing Low HDL-C

Secondary Causes
- Hypertriglyceridemia
- Obesity (visceral fat)
- Physical inactivity
- Type 2 diabetes
- Smoking
- Very-low-fat diet
- Drugs
  - β-blockers
  - Androgenic steroids
  - Androgenic progestins

Primary (Genetic) Causes
- Apo A-1
  - Apo A-1 mutations (e.g., ApoA-1$_{Milano}$)
- LCAT
  - Complete LCAT deficiency
  - Partial LCAT deficiency (fish-eye disease)
- ABC_1
  - Tangier disease
  - Familial hypoalphalipoproteinemia (some families)
- Unknown genetic etiology
  - Familial hypoalphalipoproteiniemia (most families)
  - Familial combined hyperlipidemia with low HDL-C
  - Metabolic syndrome

HDL-C, High-density lipoprotein cholesterol; LCAT, lecithin-cholesterol acyl transferase.

Table 13-21 Randomized Clinical Trials of Vitamin E Supplementation and CHD Events

Investigator	Number of Subjects	Vitamin E Dose (U)	Population	Follow-Up (yrs)	Relative Risk
Rapola[250]	29,133	50	Males, no CHD	4.7	0.9 (NS)
Stephens[252]	2,002	400 and 800	Males and females, with CHD	1.4	0.53
Vitamo[251]	27,271	50	Males, no CHD	6.1	0.98 (NS)
GISSI[172]	2,830	300	Males and females, with CHD	3.5	0.95 (NS)
HOPE[253]	9,541	400	Males and females, high risk	4.5	1.05 (NS)
HPS[254]	20,536	600 (+ vitamin C and β-carotene)	Males and females, with CHD	5.0	1.02 (NS)

CHD, coronary heart disease; NS, not significant.

dants, failed to demonstrate a CHD risk-reducing effect during clinical trials involving close to 100,000 patients (Table 13-21).[172,250–254] The latest, and one of the largest of these trials, the Heart Protection Study, prescribed vitamin E 600 U plus β-carotene or placebo daily for 5 years to 20,536 high-risk individuals. There was no demonstrable benefit, whether measured as CHD death, nonfatal MI, stroke, or revascularization procedures and whether or not the study population had a history of CHD, stroke, peripheral vascular disease, or diabetes. Further, there was no change in the incidence of cancer, another claim of potential benefit for antioxidant therapy.[254] These results effectively close the door on the use of antioxidant therapy for the prevention of CHD events. Future randomized clinical trials will have to demonstrate a benefit before these products can be recommended.

HYPERCHYLOMICRONEMIA

35. M.B., an asymptomatic woman, is screened with a lipoprotein profile during an annual physical evaluation by her primary care provider. She has non–insulin-dependent diabetes, which is treated with 60 U/day of NPII insulin. M.B. is approximately 20% overweight. Her fasting lipoprotein profile is total cholesterol, 234 mg/dL; TGs, 2,300 mg/dL; HDL-C, 24 mg/dL; and LDL-C (direct measured), 160 mg/dL. Fasting blood glucose is 290 mg/dL.

What is your assessment of M.B.'s CHD risk, and what treatment, if any, should she be given?

[SI units: total cholesterol, 6.05 mmol/L; TGs, 25.97 mmol/L; and HDL-C, 0.62 mmol/L]

Patients with fasting TGs >500 mg/dL have an increase in TG-rich chylomicron and VLDL particles. TG elevations of this magnitude typically increase the risk of pancreatitis, but usually not atherosclerosis and CHD. On the other hand, type II diabetic patients have a high CHD risk. Thus, it is possible that M.B. has two lipid disorders, one causing hyperchylomicronemia and a second causing the typical pattern of atherogenic dyslipidemia. There is no way of knowing whether M.B. has atherogenic dyslipidemia until her TG levels are lowered. Because of the life-threatening nature of TG levels of this magnitude, the priority in managing this patient is to first lower her TGs to as close to normal as possible, then assess her LDL.

Most likely, she has an inherited deficiency of lipoprotein lipase, as this is the most common cause of very high TG levels. TG levels this high can also be triggered by uncontrolled diabetes mellitus, alcohol abuse, obesity, or drugs, including estrogens, β-blockers, and steroids. Treatment of these patients should be aggressive. One of the first steps is to improve her diabetes control, because this alone may normalize lipid levels. A TG-lowering diet (severe carbohydrate restriction) and drug therapy (gemfibrozil or fenofibrate or niacin) should be initiated. If the patient has symptoms of pancreatitis, she should be managed in the hospital. In the absence of symptoms, outpatient management is possible, but frequent follow-up and aggressive therapy are indicated. Once the TG level is reduced to <400 mg/dL, a calculated LDL-C can be determined; if it is >100 mg/dL, therapy with a statin or other suitable lipid-modifying agent should be initiated to achieve a LDL-C level <100 mg/dL.

REFERENCES

1. Russell DW. Cholesterol biosynthesis and metabolism. Cardiovasc Drugs Ther 1992;6:103.
2. Eisenberg S. Metabolism of apolipoproteins and lipoproteins. Curr Opin Lipidol 1990;1:205.
3. Kwiterovich PO. The metabolic pathways of high-density lipoprotein, low-density lipoprotein, and triglycerides: A current review. Am J Cardiol 2000; 86(suppl):5L.
4. Barter P. High-density lipoproteins and reverse cholesterol transport. Curr Opin Lipidol 1993;4:210.
5. Brewer HB, Santamarina-Fofo S. New insights into the role of the adenosine triphosphate-binding cassette transporters in high-density lipoprotein metabolism and reverse cholesterol transport. Am J Cardiol 2003;91(suppl):3E.
6. Hoddis HN et al. Triglyceride-rich lipoproteins and the progression of coronary artery disease. Curr Opin Lipidol 1995;6:209.

7. Schmitz G, Williamson E. High-density lipoprotein metabolism, reverse cholesterol transport and membrane protection. Curr Opin Lipidol 1991;2:177.
8. Austin MA et al. Low-density lipoprotein subclass patterns and risk of myocardial infarction. JAMA 1988;260:1917.
9. Brown MS, Goldstein JL. A receptor-mediated pathway for cholesterol homeostasis. Science 1986;232:34.
10. Goldstein JL, Brown MS. Familial hypercholesterolemia. In: Scriver CR et al, eds. The Metabolic Basis of Inherited Disease. New York: McGraw-Hill, 1989:1215.
11. Hobbs HH et al. Molecular genetics of the LDL receptor gene in familial hypercholesterolemia. Hum Mutat 1992;1:445.
12. Hobbs HH et al. Deletion of the gene for the low-density-lipoprotein receptor in a majority of French

Canadians with familial hypercholesterolemia. N Engl J Med 1987;317:734.
13. Mabuchi H et al. Development of coronary heart disease in familial hypercholesterolemia. Circulation 1989;79:225.
14. Soria LF et al. Association between a specific apolipoprotein B mutation and familial defective apolipoprotein B-100. Proc Natl Acad Sci USA 1989;86:587.
15. Vega GL, Grundy SM. In vivo evidence for reduced binding of low-density lipoproteins to receptors as a cause of primary moderate hypercholesterolemia. J Clin Invest 1986;78:1410.
16. Innerarity TL et al. Familial defective apolipoprotein B-100: a mutation of apolipoprotein B that causes hypercholesterolemia. J Lipid Res 1990;31:1337.
17. Innerarity TL et al. Familial defective apolipoprotein B-100: low-density lipoproteins with abnormal

receptor binding. Proc Natl Acad Sci USA 1987;84:6919.

18. Mahley RW, Rall SC Jr. Type III hyperlipoproteinemia (dysbetalipoproteinemia): the role of apolipoprotein E in normal and abnormal lipoprotein metabolism. In: Scriver CR et al, eds. The Metabolic Basis of Inherited Disease. 6th Ed. New York: McGraw-Hill, 1991:1195.

19. Brewer HB Jr et al. Type III hyperlipoproteinemia: diagnosis, molecular defects, pathology, and treatment. Ann Intern Med 1983;98:623.

20. Kissebah AH et al. Integrated regulation of very low density lipoprotein triglyceride and apolipoprotein-B kinetics in man: normolipemic subjects, familial hypertriglyceridemia, and familial combined hyperlipidemia. Metabolism 1981;30:856.

21. Haffner SM et al. Metabolism of apolipoprotein B in members of a family with accelerated atherosclerosis: influence of apolipoprotein E-3/E-2 pattern. Metabolism 1992;41(3):241.

22. Cortner JA et al. Familial combined hyperlipidemia: use of stable isotopes to demonstrate overproduction of very low-density lipoprotein apolipoprotein B by the liver. J Inherit Metab Dis 1991;14(6):915.

23. Austin MA et al. Bimodality of plasma apolipoprotein B levels in familial combined hyperlipidemia. Atherosclerosis 1992;92:67.

24. Sniderman A, Cianftone K. Substrate delivery as a determinant of hepatic ApoB secretion. Arterioscler Thromb 1993;13:629.

25. Teng B et al. Composition and distribution of low-density lipoprotein fractions in hyperapobetalipoproteinemia, normolipidemia, and familial hypercholesterolemia. Proc Natl Acad Sci USA 1983;80:6662.

26. Sniderman A et al. From familial combined hyperlipidemia to hyperapoB: unraveling the overproduction of hepatic apolipoprotein B. Curr Opin Lipidol 1992;3:137.

27. Rifkind BM. High-density lipoprotein cholesterol and coronary artery disease: survey of the evidence. Am J Cardiol 1990;66:3A.

28. Miller M, Kwiterovich PO Jr. Isolated low HDL-cholesterol as an important risk factor for coronary heart disease. Eur Heart J 1990;11(Suppl H):9.

29. Genest JJ Jr et al. Prevalence of familial lipoprotein disorders in patients with premature coronary artery disease. Circulation 1992;85:2025.

30. Campeau L et al. Aggressive cholesterol lowering delays saphenous vein graft atherosclerosis in women, the elderly, and patients with associated risk factors. NHLBI Post Coronary Artery Bypass Graft Clinical Trial. Circulation 1999;99:3241.

31. Steinberg D et al. Beyond cholesterol: modification of low-density lipoprotein that increases its atherogenicity. N Engl J Med 1989;320:915.

32. Davies MJ et al. Atherosclerosis: inhibition or regression as therapeutic possibilities. Br Heart J 1991;65:302.

33. Faggiotto A et al. Studies of hypercholesterolemia in the nonhuman primate. I. Changes that lead to fatty streak formation. Arterioscler Thromb 1984; 4:323.

34. Witztum JL, Steinberg D. Role of oxidized low-density lipoprotein in atherogenesis. J Clin Invest 1991;88:1785.

35. Ross R, Agius L. The process of atherogenesis: cellular and molecular interaction: from experimental animal models to humans. Diabetologia 1992;35(Suppl 2):34.

36. Libby P. Current concepts of the pathogenesis of the acute coronary syndromes. Circulation 2001;104:365.

37. Libby P et al. Inflammation and atherosclerosis. Circulation. 2002;105:1135.

38. Henderson EL et al. Death of smooth muscle cells and expression of mediators of apoptosis by T-lymphocytes in human abdominal aortic aneurysms. Circulation 1999;99:96.

39. Galina K et al. Evidence for increased collagenolysis by interstitial collagenases-1 and -3 in vulnerable human atheromatous plaques. Circulation 1999;99:2503.

40. Libby P. Molecular basis of the acute coronary syndromes. Circulation 1995;91:2844.

41. Ridker PM. Inflammation, infection, and cardiovascular risk. How good is the clinical evidence? Circulation 1998;97:1671.

42. Ross R. Atherosclerosis: an inflammatory disease. N Engl J Med 1999;340:115.

43. Libby P et al. Novel inflammatory markers of coronary risk. Theory versus practice. Circulation 1999;100:1148.

44. Fuster V et al. The pathogenesis of coronary artery disease and acute coronary syndromes. N Engl J Med 1992;326:242.

45. Brown BG et al. Lipid lowering and plaque regression. New insights into prevention or plaque disruption and clinical events in coronary disease. Circulation 1993;87:1781.

46. Neaton JD et al. Serum cholesterol level and mortality findings for men screened in the Multiple Risk Factor Intervention Trial. Arch Intern Med 1992;152:1490.

47. Jacobs D et al. Report of the conference on low blood cholesterol: mortality associations. Circulation 1992;86:1046.

48. Castelli WP. Epidemiology of coronary heart disease: the Framingham Study. Am J Med 1984;76:4.

49. Gordon DJ et al. High-density lipoprotein cholesterol and cardiovascular disease: four prospective American studies. Circulation 1989;79:8.

50. Kagan A et al. Epidemiologic studies of coronary heart disease and stroke in Japanese men living in Japan, Hawaii and California: demographic, physical, dietary and biochemical characteristics. J Chronic Dis 1974;27:345.

51. Rosenberg L et al. Myocardial infarction in women under 50 years of age. JAMA 1983;250:2801.

52. Rosenberg L et al. Myocardial infarction and cigarette smoking in women younger than 50 years of age. JAMA 1985;253:2965.

53. Castelli WP et al. Cardiovascular risk factors in the elderly. Am J Cardiol 1989;63:12H.

54. Thom TJ. Cardiovascular disease mortality among United States women. In: Eaker ED et al, eds. Coronary Heart Disease in Women. New York: Haymarket Doyma, 1987.

55. Garg A, Grundy SM. Management of dyslipidemia in NIDDM. Diabetes Care 1990;13:153.

56. Kannel WB. Lipids, diabetes, and coronary heart disease: insights from the Framingham Study. Am Heart J 1985;110:1100.

57. Kannel WB, Gordon T. Evaluation of cardiovascular risk in the elderly. The Framingham Study. Bull NY Acad Med 1978;54:573.

58. Manolio TZ et al. Cholesterol and heart disease in older persons and women. Review of an NHLBI workshop. Ann Epidemiol 1992;2:161.

59. Malenka DJ, Baron JA. Cholesterol and coronary heart disease: the importance of patient-specific attributable risk. Arch Intern Med 1988;148:2247.

60. LaRosa JC et al. The cholesterol facts: a summary of the evidence relating dietary fats, serum cholesterol, and coronary heart disease. Circulation 1990; 81:1721.

61. Buchwald H et al. Effect of partial ileal bypass surgery on mortality and morbidity from coronary heart disease in patients with hypercholesterolemia: report of the Program on the Surgical Control of Hyperlipidemias (POSCH). N Engl J Med 1990; 323:946.

62. Blankenhorn DH et al. Beneficial effects of combined colestipol-niacin therapy on coronary atherosclerosis and coronary venous bypass grafts. JAMA 1987;257:3233.

63. Brown G et al. Regression of coronary artery disease as a result of intensive lipid-lowering therapy in men with high levels of apolipoprotein B. N Engl J Med 1990;323:1289.

64. Ornish D et al. Can lifestyle changes reverse coronary heart disease: the Lifestyle Heart Trial. Lancet 1990; 336:129.

65. Watts GF et al. Effects on coronary artery disease of lipid-lowering diet, or diet plus cholestyramine, in the St. Thomas' Atherosclerosis Regression Study (STARS). Lancet 1992;339:563.

66. Kane JP et al. Regression of coronary atherosclerosis during treatment of familial hypercholesterolemia with combined drug regimens. JAMA 1990; 264:3007.

67. Duffield RGM et al. Treatment of hyperlipidemia retards progression of symptomatic femoral atherosclerosis. A randomized controlled trial. Lancet 1983;ii:639.

68. MAAS Investigators. Effect of simvastatin on coronary atheroma: the Multicentre Anti-Atheroma Study (MAAS). Lancet 1994;344:633.

69. Waters D et al. Effects of monotherapy with an HMG-CoA reductase inhibitor on the progression of coronary atherosclerosis as assessed by serial quantitative arteriography. The Canadian Coronary Atherosclerosis Intervention Trial. Circulation 1994;89:959.

70. Haskell WL et al. Effects of intensive multiple risk factor reduction on coronary atherosclerosis and clinical cardiac events in men and women with coronary heart disease. The Stanford Coronary Risk Intervention Project (SCRIP). Circulation 1994;89:975.

71. Furberg CD et al. Pravastatin, lipids, and major coronary events. Am J Cardiol 1994;73:1133.

72. Furberg CD et al. Effect of lovastatin on early carotid atherosclerosis and cardiovascular events. Circulation 1994;90:1679.

73. Blankenhorn DH et al. Coronary angiographic changes with lovastatin therapy. The Monitored Atherosclerosis Regression Study (MARS). Ann Intern Med 1993;119:969.

74. Pitt B et al. Pravastatin limitation of atherosclerosis in the coronary arteries (PLACI): Reduction in atherosclerosis progression and clinical events. J Am Coll Cardiol 1995;26:1133.

75. Salonen R et al. Kuopio atherosclerosis prevention study (KAPS). A population-based primary prevention trial of the effect of LDL lowering on atherosclerotic progression in carotid and femoral arteries. Circulation 1995;92:1758.

76. Jukema JW et al. Effects of lipid lowering by pravastatin on progression and regression of coronary artery disease in symptomatic men with normal to moderately elevated serum cholesterol levels. The Regression Growth Evaluation Statin Study (REGRESS). Circulation 1995;91:2528.

77. Herd JA et al. Effects of fluvastatin on coronary atherosclerosis in patients with mild to moderate cholesterol elevations (Lipoprotein and Coronary Atherosclerosis Study [LCAS]). Am J Cardiol 1997;80:278.

78. The Post Coronary Artery Bypass Graft Trial Investigators. The effect of aggressive lowering of low-density lipoprotein cholesterol levels and low-dose anticoagulation on obstructive changes in saphenous-vein coronary-artery bypass grafts. N Engl J Med 1997;336:153.

79. Thompson GR. What targets should lipid-modulating therapy achieve to optimise the prevention of coronary heart disease? Atherosclerosis 1997;131:1.

80. Takagi T et al. Intravascular ultrasound analysis of reduction in progression of coronary narrowing by treatment with pravastatin. Am J Cardiol 1997;79:1673.

81. Lipid Research Clinics Program. The Lipid Research Clinics Coronary Primary Prevention Trial results; I: reduction in incidence of coronary heart disease. JAMA 1984;251:351.

82. Scandinavian Simvastatin Survival Study (4S) Group. Randomised trial of cholesterol lowering in 4444 patients with coronary heart disease. Lancet 1994;344:1383.

83. Sacks FM et al. The effect of pravastatin on coronary events after myocardial infarction in patients with average cholesterol levels. N Engl J Med 1996;335:1001.

84. The Long-Term Intervention With Pravastatin in Ischaemic Disease (LIPID) Study Group. Prevention of cardiovascular events and death with pravastatin in patients with coronary heart disease and a broad range of initial cholesterol levels. N Engl J Med 1998;339:1349.

85. Crouse JR III et al. Reductase inhibitor monotherapy and stroke prevention. Arch Intern Med 1997;157:1305.

86. Heart Protection Study Collaborative Group. MRC/BHF Heart Protection Study of cholesterol lowering with simvastatin in 20,536 high-risk individuals: a randomized placebo-controlled trial. Lancet 2002;360:7.

87. Expert Panel on Detection, Evaluation, and Treatment of High Blood Cholesterol in Adults. Third Report of the National Cholesterol Education Program (NCEP) Expert Panel on detection, evaluation, and treatment of high blood cholesterol in adults (Adult Treatment Panel III). Final Report. Circulation 2002;106:3143. Executive Summary in JAMA 2001:2486.

88. West of Scotland Coronary Prevention Study Group. Influence of pravastatin and plasma lipids on clinical events in the West of Scotland Coronary Prevention Study (WOSCOPS). Circulation 1998;97:1440.

89. Sever PS et al. Prevention of coronary and stroke events with atorvastatin in hypertensive patients who have average or lower-than-average cholesterol concentrations, in the Anglo-Scandivvian Cardiac Outcome Trial–Lipid Lowering Arm (AS-COT-LLA): A multicentre randomized controlled trial. Lancet 2003;361:1149.

90. Downs JR et al. Primary prevention of acute coronary events with lovastatin in men and women with average cholesterol levels. Results of AFCAPS/ TexCAPS. JAMA 1998;279:1615.

91. Buchwald H et al. Effective lipid modification by partial ileal bypass reduced long-term coronary heart disease mortality and morbidity: five-year posttrial follow-up report from the POSCH. Arch Intern Med 1998;158:1253.

92. Schwartz GG et al. Effects of atorvastatin on early recurrent ischemic events in acute coronary syndromes. The MIRACL study: A randomized controlled trial. JAMA 2001;285:1711.

93. Waters DD et al. Effects of atorvastatin on stroke in patients with unstable angina or non-Q-wave myocardial infarction. A Myocardial Ischemia Reduction With Aggressive Cholesterol Lowering (MIRACL) substudy. Circulation 2002;106:1690.

94. Pitt B et al. Aggressive lipid-lowering therapy compared with angioplasty in stable coronary artery disease. N Engl J Med 1999;341:70.

95. Knatterud GL et al. Long-term effects of clinical outcomes of aggressive lowering of low-density lipoprotein cholesterol levels and low-dose anticoagulation in the post coronary artery bypass graft trial. Circulation 2000;102:157.

96. Miettinen TA et al. Cholesterol-lowering therapy in women and elderly patients with myocardial infarction or angina pectoris. Findings from the Scandinavian Simvastatin Survival Study (4S). Circulation 1997;96:4211.

97. LaRosa JC et al. Effects of statins on risk of coronary disease. A meta-analysis of randomized controlled trials. JAMA 1999;282:2340.

98. Pyorala K et al. Cholesterol lowering with simvastatin improved prognosis of diabetic patients with coronary heart disease. A subgroup analysis of the Scandinavian Simvastatin Survival Study (4S). Diabetes Care 1997;20:614.

99. Haffner SM et al. Mortality from coronary heart disease in subjects with type 2 diabetes and in nondiabetic subjects with and without prior myocardial infarction. N Engl J Med 1998;339:229.

100. The Diabetes Control and Complications Trial Research Group. The effect of intensive treatment of diabetes on the development and progression of long-term complications in insulin-dependent diabetes mellitus. N Engl J Med 1993;329:977.

101. UK Prospective Diabetes Study (UKPDS) Group. Intensive blood-glucose control with sulphonylureas or insulin compared with conventional treatment and risk of complications in patients with type 2 diabetes (UKPDS 33). Lancet 1998;352:837.

102. Grundy SM. Primary prevention of coronary heart disease. Integrating risk assessment with intervention. Circulation 1999;100:988.

103. Frick MH et al. Helsinki Heart Study: primary-prevention trial with gemfibrozil in middle-aged men with dyslipidemia. Safety of treatment, changes in risk factors, and incidence of coronary heart disease. N Engl J Med 1987;317:1237.

104. Manninen V et al. Joint effects of serum triglyceride and LDL cholesterol and HDL cholesterol concentrations on coronary heart disease risk in the Helsinki Heart Study: implications for treatment. Circulation 1992;85:37.

105. Rubins HB et al. Gemfibrozil for the secondary prevention of coronary heart disease in men with low levels of high-density lipoprotein cholesterol. N Engl J Med 1999;341:410.

106. The BIP Study Group. Secondary prevention by raising HDL cholesterol and reducing triglycerides in patients with coronary heart disease. The Bezafibrate Infarction Prevention Study. Circulation 2000;102:21.

107. Coronary Drug Project Research Group. Clofibrate and niacin in coronary heart disease. JAMA 1975;231:360.

108. Canner PL et al. for the Coronary Drug Project Research Group. Fifteen-year mortality in coronary drug project patients: long-term benefit with niacin. J Am Coll Cardiol 1986;8:1245.

109. Brown BG et al. Simvastatin and niacin, antioxidant vitamins, or the combination for the prevention of coronary disease. N Engl J Med 2001;345:1583.

110. Vogel RA et al. Effect of a single high-fat meal on endothelial function in healthy subjects. Am J Cardiol 1997;79:350.

111. O'Driscoll G et al. Simvastatin, an HMG-coenzyme reductase inhibitor, improves endothelial function within 1 month. Circulation 1997;95:1126.

112. Gould KL et al. Short-term cholesterol lowering decreases size and severity of perfusion abnormalities by positron emission tomography after dipyridamole in patients with coronary artery disease. Circulation 1994;89:1530.

113. Baller D et al. Improvement in coronary flow reserve determined by positron emission tomography after 6 months of cholesterol-lowering therapy in patients with early stages of coronary atherosclerosis. Circulation 1999;99:2871.

114. Treasure CB et al. Beneficial effects of cholesterol-lowering therapy on coronary endothelium in patients with coronary artery disease. N Engl J Med 1995;332:481.

115. Anderson TJ et al. Effects of cholesterol-lowering and antioxidant therapy on endothelium-dependent coronary vasomotion. N Engl J Med 1995;332:488.

116. Andrews TC et al. Effect of cholesterol reduction on myocardial ischemia in patients with coronary disease. Circulation 1997;95:324.

117. Van Boven AJ et al. Reduction of transient myocardial ischemia with pravastatin in addition to the conventional treatment in patients with angina pectoris. Circulation 1996;94:1503.

118. Ridker PM. Clinical application of C-reactive protein for cardiovascular disease detection and prevention. Circulation 2003;107:363.

119. Ridker PM et al. Inflammation, pravastatin, and the risk of coronary events after myocardial infarction in patients with average cholesterol levels. Circulation 1998;98:839.

120. Pearson TA et al. Markers of inflammation and cardiovascular disease. Application to clinical and public health practice. A statement for healthcare professionals from the Centers for Disease Control and Prevention and the American Heart Association. 2003;107:499.

121. Schulman KA et al. Reducing high blood cholesterol level with drugs: cost-effectiveness of pharmacologic management. JAMA 1990;264:3025.

122. Goldman L et al. Cost-effectiveness of HMG-CoA reductase inhibition for primary and secondary prevention of coronary heart disease. JAMA 1991;265:1145.

123. Weinstein MC et al. Forecasting coronary heart disease, mortality, and cost: the coronary heart disease policy model. Am J Public Health 1987;77:1417.

124. Weissfeld JL et al. A mathematical representation of the expert panel's guidelines for high blood cholesterol case-finding and treatment. Med Decis Making 1990;10:135.

125. Pederson TR et al. Cholesterol lowering and the use of healthcare resources. Results of the Scandinavian Simvastatin Survival Study. Circulation 1996;93:1796.

126. Koren MJ et al. The cost of reaching National Cholesterol Education Program (NCEP) goals in hypercholesterolaemic patients. A comparison of atorvastatin, simvastatin, lovastatin, and fluvastatin. Pharmacoeconomics 1998;1:59.

127. Pekkanen J et al. Ten-year mortality from cardiovascular disease in relation to cholesterol level among men with and without preexisting cardiovascular disease. N Engl J Med 1990;322:1700.

128. Criqui MH et al. Mortality over a period of 10 years in patients with peripheral arterial disease. N Engl J Med 1992;326:381.

129. Salonen JT, Salonen R. Ultrasonographically assessed carotid morphology and the risk of coronary heart disease. Arterioscler Thromb 1991;11:1245.

130. Katan MB et al. Beyond low-fat diets. N Engl J Med 1997;337:563.

131. Leaf A. Dietary prevention of coronary heart disease. The Lyon Diet Heart Study. Circulation 1999;99:733.

132. de Lorgeril M et al. Mediterranean diet, traditional risk factors, and the rate of cardiovascular complications after myocardial infarction. Final Report of the Lyon Diet Heart Study. Circulation 1999;99:779.

133. Caggiula AW et al. The Multiple Risk Factor Intervention Trial (MRFIT), IV: intervention on blood lipids. Prev Med 1981;10:443.

134. Ramsay LE et al. Dietary reduction of serum cholesterol concentration: time to think again. Br Med J 1991;303:953.

135. Boyd NF et al. Quantitative changes in dietary fat intake and serum cholesterol in women: results from a randomized, controlled trial. Am J Clin Nutr 1990;52:470.

136. Wood PD et al. Changes in plasma lipids and lipoproteins in overweight men during weight loss through dieting as compared with exercise. N Engl J Med 1988;319:1173.

137. The Expert Panel. Executive summary of the clinical guidelines on the identification, evaluation, and treatment of overweight and obesity in adults. Arch Intern Med 1998;158:1855.

138. Wood PD et al. The effects of plasma lipoproteins of a prudent weight-reducing diet, with or without exercise, in overweight men and women. N Engl J Med 1991;325:461.

139. Danesh J et al. Lipoprotein (a) and coronary heart disease: meta-analysis of prospective studies. Circulation 2000;102:1082.

140. Bloch S et al. Apolipoprotein B and LDL cholesterol: which parameter(s) should be included in the assessment of cardiovascular risk? Ann Biol Clin 1998;68:539.

141. Malinow MR et al. Homocysteine, diet, and cardiovascular diseases: A statement for healthcare professionals for the Nutrition Committee, American Heart Association. Circulation 1999;99:178.

142. Lipid Research Clincs Program. The Lipid Research Clinics Coronary Primary Prevention Trial results; II: the relationship of reduction in incidence of coronary heart disease to cholesterol lowering. JAMA 1984;251:365.

143. Superko HR et al. Effectiveness of low-dose colestipol therapy in patients with moderate hypercholesterolemia. Am J Cardiol 1992;70:135.

144. Einarsson K et al. Bile acid sequestrants: mechanisms of action on bile acid and cholesterol metabolism. Eur J Clin Pharm 1991;40(Suppl 1):S53.

145. Bays HE et al. Ezetimibe Study Group. Effectiveness and tolerability of ezetimibe in patients with

primary hypercholesterolemia: pooled analysis of two phase II studies. Clin Ther 2001;23:1209.

146. Davidson MH et al. Ezetimibe co-administered with simvastatin in patients with primary hypercholesterolemia. J Am Coll Cardiol. 2002;40:2135.

147. Sudhop T et al. Inhibition of intestinal cholesterol absorption by ezetimibe in humans. Circulation 2002;106:1943.

148. McKenney JM et al. A comparison of the efficacy and toxic effects of sustained- vs. immediate-release niacin in hypercholesterolemic patients. JAMA 1994;271:672.

149. Drood JM et al. Nicotinic acid for the treatment of hyperlipoproteinemia. J Clin Pharmacol 1991;31:641.

150. Carlson LA et al. Pronounced lowering of serum levels of lipoprotein Lp(a) in hyperlipidemic subjects treated with nicotinic acid. J Intern Med 1989;226:271.

151. Grundy SM et al. Influence of nicotinic acid on metabolism of cholesterol and triglycerides in man. J Lipid Res 1981;22:24.

152. Sakai T et al. Niacin, but not gemfibrozil, selectively increases LP-A1, a cardioprotective subfraction of HDL, in patients with low HDL cholesterol. Arteriosclero Thromb Vasc Biol 2001;21:1783.

153. Jin FY et al. Niacin decreases removal of high-density lipoprotein apolipoprotein A-I but not cholesterol ester by Hep G2 cells: implication for reverse cholesterol transport. Arterioscler Thromb Vasc Biol 1997;17:2020.

154. Piepho RW. The pharmacokinetics and pharmacodynamics of agents proven to raise high-density lipoprotein cholesterol. Am J Cardiol 2000;86(suppl):35L.

155. Henkin Y et al. Niacin revisited: clinical observations on an important but underutilized drug. Am J Med 1991;91:239.

156. Knopp RH et al. Contrasting effects of unmodified and time-release forms of niacin on lipoproteins in hyperlipidemic subjects: clues to mechanism of action of niacin. Metabolism 1985;34:642.

157. Wilkin J et al. Aspirin blocks nicotinic acid-induced flushing. Clin Pharmacol Ther 1982;31:478.

158. Mullin GE et al. Fulminant hepatic failure after ingestion of sustained-release nicotinic acid. Ann Intern Med 1989;111:253.

159. Henkin Y et al. Rechallenge with crystalline niacin after drug-induced hepatitis from sustained-release niacin. JAMA 1990;264:241.

160. Etchason JA et al. Niacin-induced hepatitis: a potential side effect with low-dose time-release niacin. Mayo Clin Proc 1991;66:23.

161. Rader JI et al. Hepatic toxicity of unmodified and time-release preparations of niacin. Am J Med 1992;92:77.

162. Mevacor. Physician's Desk Reference. 56th Ed. Montvale, NJ: Medical Economics Company, 2002:2133.

163. Hunninghake DB et al. Efficacy and safety of pravastatin in patients with primary hypercholesterolemia; II: once-daily versus twice-daily dosing. Atherosclerosis 1990;85:219.

164. Jones P et al. Comparative dose efficacy study of atorvastatin versus simvastatin, pravastatin, lovastatin, and fluvastatin in patients with hypercholesterolemia (The Curves Study). Am J Cardiol 1998;81:582.

165. Grundy SM et al. Guide to primary prevention of cardiovascular diseases. A statement for healthcare professionals for the task force on risk reduction. Circulation 1997;95:2329.

166. Grundy SM et al. Influence of combined therapy with mevinolin and interruption of bile-acid reabsorption on low-density lipoproteins in heterozygous familial hypercholesterolemia. Ann Intern Med 1985;103:339.

167. Ginsberg HN et al. Suppression of apolipoprotein B production during treatment of cholesteryl ester storage disease with lovastatin: implications for regulation of apolipoprotein B synthesis. J Clin Invest 1987;80:1692.

168. Arad Y et al. Effects of lovastatin therapy on very-low-density lipoprotein triglyceride metabolism in subjects with combined hyperlipidemia: evidence for reduced assembly and secretion of triglyceride-rich lipoproteins. Metabolism 1992;41:487.

169. Hunninghake DB et al. Efficacy and safety of pravastatin in patients with primary hypercholesterolemia; I: a dose-response study. Atherosclerosis 1990;85:81.

170. Dujovne CA et al. Expanded Clinical Evaluation of Lovastatin (EXCEL) study results. IV. additional perspectives on the tolerability of lovastatin. Am J Med 1991;91(Suppl 1B):25S.

171. Tobert JA et al. Clinical experience with lovastatin. Am J Cardiol 1990;65:23F.

172. GISSI Prevenzione Investigators. Dietary supplementation with omega-3 polyunsaturated fatty acids and vitamin E after myocardial infarction: results of the GISSI-Prevenzione trial. Lancet 1999;354:447.

173. Stampfer MJ et al. Post-menopausal estrogen therapy and cardiovascular disease: ten-year follow-up from the Nurses Health Study. N Engl J Med 1991;325:756.

174. Barrett-Connor E, Bush TL. Estrogen and coronary heart disease in women. JAMA 1991;265:1861.

175. Grady D et al. Hormone therapy to prevent disease and prolong life in postmenopausal women. Ann Intern Med 1992;117:1016.

176. Grodstein F et al. Postmenopausal hormone therapy and mortality. N Engl J Med 1997;336:1769.

177. Stampfer MJ, Colditz GA. Estrogen replacement therapy and coronary heart disease: a quantitative assessment of the epidemiologic evidence. Prev Med 1991;20:47.

178. Gruchow HW et al. Postmenopausal use of estrogen and occlusion of arteries. Am Heart J 1988;115(5):88.

179. The Writing Group for the PEPI trial. Effects of estrogen or estrogen/progestin regimens on heart disease risk factors in postmenopausal women. The Postmenopausal Estrogen/Progestin Interventions (PEPI) trial. JAMA 1995;273:199.

180. Hulley S et al. Randomized trial of estrogen plus progestin for secondary prevention of coronary heart disease in postmenopausal women. JAMA 1998;280:605.

181. Writing Group for the Women's Health Initiative Investigators. Risks and benefits of estrogen plus progestin in healthy postmenopausal women. Principal results from the Women's Health Initiative randomized controlled trial. JAMA 2002;288:321.

182. Ballantyne CM et al. Effect of ezetimibe coadministered with atorvastatin in 628 patients with primary hypercholesterolemia: A prospective, randomized, double-blind trial. Circulation 2003;107:2409.

183. Illingworth DR. Clinical implications of new drugs for lowering plasma cholesterol concentrations. Drugs 1991;41:151.

184. Brown BG et al. Moderate dose, three-drug therapy with niacin, lovastatin, and colestipol to reduce low-density lipoprotein cholesterol <100 mg/dL in patients with hyperlipidemia and coronary artery disease. Am J Cardiol 1997;80:111.

185. Brown BG et al. Very intensive lipid therapy with lovastatin, niacin, and colestipol for prevention of death and myocardial infarction: a 10-year Familial Atherosclerosis Treatment Study (FATS) follow-up [abstract]. Circulation 1998;98:I-635.

186. Grundy SM et al. When to start cholesterol-lowering therapy in patients with coronary heart disease. A statement for healthcare professionals from the American Heart Association Task Force on Risk Reduction. Circulation 1997;95:1683.

187. NIH Consensus Development Panel on Triglyceride, High-Density Lipoprotein, and Coronary Heart Disease. Triglyceride, high-density lipoprotein, and coronary heart disease. JAMA 1993;269:505.

188. Gordon DJ, Rifkind BM. High-density lipoprotein—the clinical implications of recent studies. N Engl J Med 1989;321:1311.

189. Grundy SM et al. The place of HDL in cholesterol management. A perspective from the National Cholesterol Education Program. Arch Intern Med 1989;149:505.

190. Grundy SM, Vega GL. Two different views of the relationship of hypertriglyceridemia to coronary heart disease. Implications for treatment. Arch Intern Med 1992;152:28.

191. Reardon MF et al. Lipoprotein predictors of the severity of coronary artery disease in men and women. Circulation 1985;71:881.

192. Steiner G et al. The association of increased levels of intermediate-density lipoproteins with smoking and with coronary heart disease. Circulation 1987;75:124.

193. Grundy SM. Small LDL, atherogenic dyslipidemia, and the metabolic syndrome. Circulation 1997;95:1.

194. Grundy SM. Hypertriglyceridemia, atherogenic dyslipidemia, and the metabolic syndrome. Am J Cardiol 1998;81(4A):18B.

195. Austin MA et al. Hypertriglyceridemia as a cardiovascular risk factor. Am J Cardiol. 1998;81(4A):7B.

196. Brunzell JD et al. Plasma lipoproteins in familial combined hyperlipidemia and monogenic familial hypertriglyceridemia. J Lipid Res 1983;24:147.

197. Lamarche B et al. Small, dense low-density lipoprotein particles as a predictor of the risk of ischemic heart disease in men. Prospective results from the Quebec Cardiovascular Study. Circulation 1997;95:69.

198. Ginsberg HN. Insulin resistance and cardiovascular disease. J Clin Invest 2000;106:453

199. Sato R et al. Sterol regulatory element-binding protein negatively regulates microsomal triglyceride transfer protein gene transcription. J Biol Chem 1999;274:24714.

200. Grundy SM. Approach to lipoprotein management in 2001 National Cholesterol Guidelines. Am J Cardiol 2002;90 (8A):11i.

201. Marmot M, Brunner E. Alcohol and cardiovascular disease: the status of the U-shaped curve. Br Med J 1991;303:565.

202. Jackson R, Beaglehole R. The relationship between alcohol and coronary heart disease: is there a protective effect? Curr Opin Lipidol 1993;4:21.

203. Steinberg D et al. Davis conference, alcohol and atherosclerosis. Ann Intern Med 1991;114:967.

204. Klatsky AL et al. Alcohol and mortality: a ten-year Kaiser-Permanente experience. Ann Intern Med 1981;95:139.

205. Assmann G, Schulte H. Triglycerides and atherosclerosis: results from the Prospective Cardiovascular Munster Study. In: Gotto AM Jr, Paoletti R, eds. Atherosclerosis Reviews. Vol. 22. New York: Raven, 1991:51.

206. Fujioka S et al. Contribution of intra-abdominal fat accumulation to the impairment of glucose and lipid metabolism in human obesity. Metabolism 1987;36:54.

207. Barakat HA et al. Influence of obesity, impaired glucose tolerance, and NIDDM on LDL structure and composition. Possible link between hyperinsulinemia and atherosclerosis. Diabetes 1990;39:1527.

208. Bierman EL. Atherogenesis in diabetes. Arterioscler Thromb 1992;12:647.

209. DeFronzo RA, Ferrannini E. Insulin resistance. A multifaceted syndrome responsible for NIDDM, obesity, hypertension, dyslipidemia, and atherosclerotic cardiovascular disease. Diabetes Care 1991;14:173.

210. American Diabetes Association. Screening for type 2 diabetes. Diabetes Care 1998;21:S20.

211. Chobanian AV et al. The seventh report of the Joint National Committee on prevention, detection, evaluation, and treatment of high blood pressure. The JNC 7 Report. JAMA. 2003;289:2560.

212. Reaven GM. Insulin resistance and compensatory hyperinsulinemia: role in hypertension, dyslipidemia, and coronary heart disease. Am Heart J 1991;121:1283.

213. Gwynne J. Clinical features and pathophysiology of familial dyslipidemic hypertension syndrome. Curr Opin Lipidol 1992;3:215.

214. Reaven GM. Role of insulin resistance in human disease. Diabetes 1988;37:1595.

215. Kaplan NM. The deadly quartet: upper-body obesity, glucose intolerance, hypertriglyceridemia, and hypertension. Arch Intern Med 1989;149:1514.

216. Campos H et al. Low-density lipoprotein particle size and coronary artery disease. Arteriosclerosis 1992;12:187.

217. Stein EA et al. Comparison of statins in hypertriglyceridemia. Am J Cardiol 1998;81(4A):66B.

218. Gingsburg HN. Hypertriglyceridemia: New insights and new approaches to pharmacologic therapy. Am J Cardiol 2001;87:1174.

219. Stein EA et al. Efficacy and tolerability of low-dose simvastatin and niacin, alone and in combination, in patients with combined hyperlipidemia: a prospective trial. J Cardiovasc Pharmacol Ther 1996;1:107.

220. Elam MB et al. Effect of niacin on lipid and lipoprotein levels and glycemic control in patients with diabetes and peripheral arterial disease. The ADMIT study: a randomized trial. JAMA 2000;284:1263.

221. Canner PL et al. Niacin decreases myocardial infarction and total mortality in patients with impaired fasting glucose or glucose intolerance: results from the coronary drug project [abstract]. Circulation 2002;106(suppl II):II-636.

222. Hunninghake DB, Peters JR. Effect of fibric acid derivatives on blood lipid and lipoprotein levels. Am J Med 1987;83:44.

223. Manttari M et al. Effect of gemfibrozil on the concentration and composition of serum lipoproteins: a controlled study with special reference to initial triglyceride levels. Atherosclerosis 1990;81:11.

224. Rubins HB, Robins SJ. Effect of reduction of plasma triglycerides with gemfibrozil on high-density-lipoprotein-cholesterol concentrations. J Intern Med 1992;231:421.

225. Vega GL, Grundy SM. Comparison of lovastatin and gemfibrozil in normolipidemic patients with hypoalphalipoproteinemia. JAMA1989;262:3148.

226. Miller M et al. Effect of gemfibrozil in men with primary isolated low high-density lipoprotein cholesterol: a randomized, double-blind, placebo-controlled, crossover study. Am J Med 1993;94:7.

227. Manninen V et al. Relation between baseline lipid and lipoprotein values and the incidence of coronary heart disease in the Helsinki Heart Study. Am J Cardiol 1989;63:42H.

228. Brown WV et al. Effects of fenofibrate on plasma lipids. Double-blind, multicenter study in patients with type IIA or IIB hyperlipidemia. Arteriosclerosis 1986;6:670.

229. American Diabetic Association. Management of dyslipidemia in adults with diabetes. Diabetes Care 1998;21(Suppl 1):S36.

230. Grundy SM et al. Diabetes and cardiovascular disease. A statement for healthcare professionals from the American Heart Association. Circulation 1999;100:1134.

231. Berger J, Moller DE. The mechanisms of action of PPARα. Annu Rev Med. 2002;53:409.

232. Saku K et al. Mechanism of action of gemfibrozil on lipoprotein metabolism. J Clin Invest 1985;75:1702.

233. Grundy SM, Vega GL. Fibric acids: effects on lipids and lipoprotein metabolism. Am J Med 1987;83:9.

234. Knopp RH. Drug treatment of lipid disorders. N Engl J Med 1999;341:498.

235. Kesaniemi YA, Grundy SM. Influence of gemfibrozil and clofibrate on metabolism of cholesterol and plasma triglycerides in man. JAMA 1984;251:2241.

236. Pierce LR et al. Myopathy and rhabdomyolysis associated with lovastatin-gemfibrozil combination therapy. JAMA 1990;264:71.

237. Prueksaritanont T et al. Effects of fibrates on metabolism of statins in human hepatocytes. Drug Metab Dispos 2002;30:1280.

238. Prueksaritanont T et al. Mechanistic studies on metabolic interactions between gemfibrozil and statins. J Pharmacol Exp Ther 2002;301:1042.

239. Committee of Principal Investigators. World Health Organization. WHO cooperative trial on primary prevention of ischaemic heart disease using clofibrate to lower serum cholesterol: mortality follow-up. Lancet 1980;2:379.

240. Committee of Principal Investigators. A co-operative trial in the primary prevention of ischaemic heart disease using clofibrate. Br Heart J 1978;40:1069.

241. Lopid package insert, Pfizer Inc., New York, 1992.

242. Diabetes Atherosclerosis Intervention Study Investigators. Effect of fenofibrate on progression on coronary-artery disease in type 2 diabetes: the Diabetes Atherosclerosis Intervention Study, a randomised study. Lancet 2001;357:905.

243. Gotto AM et al. Relationship between baseline and on-treatment lipid parameters and first major coronary events in the Air Force/Texas Coronary Atherosclerosis Prevention Study (TexCAPS/AFCAPS). Circulation 2000;101:477.

244. Parthasarathy S et al. Probucol inhibits oxidative modification of low-density lipoprotein. J Clin Invest 1986;77:641.

245. Kita T et al. Probucol prevents the progression of atherosclerosis in Watanabe heritable hyperlipidemic rabbits, and animal models for familial hypercholesterolemia. Proc Natl Acad Sci USA 1987;84:5928.

246. Parums D et al. Serum antibodies to oxidized low-density lipoprotein and ceroid in chronic periaortitis. Arch Pathol Lab Med 1990;114:383.

247. Salonen JT et al. Autoantibody against oxidized LDL and progression of carotid atherosclerosis. Lancet 1992;339:883.

248. Gaziano JM et al. Beta-carotene therapy for chronic stable angina [abstract]. Circulation 1990;82:III-201.

249. Stampfer MJ et al. A prospective study of vitamin E supplementation and risk of coronary disease in women [abstract]. Circulation 1991;86:I-463.

250. Rapola JM et al. Effect of vitamin E and beta-carotene on the incidence of angina pectoris: a randomized, double-blind, controlled trial. JAMA 1996;275:693.

251. Virtamo J et al. Effect of vitamin E and beta carotene on the incidence of primary nonfatal myocardial infarction and fatal coronary heart disease. Arch Intern Med 1998;158:668.

252. Stephens NG et al. Randomised controlled trial of vitamin E in patients with coronary disease: Cambridge Heart Antioxidant Study. Lancet 1996;347:781.

253. The Heart Outcomes Prevention Evaluation (HOPE) Study Investigators. Vitamin E supplementation and cardiovascular events in high-risk patients. N Engl J Med 2000;342:154.

254. Heart Protection Study Collaborative Group. MRC/BHF Heart Protection Study of antioxidant vitamin supplementation in 20,536 high-risk individuals: A randomized placebo-controlled trial. Lancet 2002;360:233.

255. Grimm RH et al. Effects of thiazide diuretics on plasma lipids and lipoproteins in mildly hypertensive patients. Ann Intern Med 1981;84:7.

256. Ames RP. Metabolic disturbances increasing the risk of coronary heart disease during diuretic-based antihypertensive therapy: lipid alteration and glucose intolerance. Am Heart J 1983;106:1207.

257. Lasser NL et al. Effects of antihypertensive therapy on plasma lipids and lipoproteins in the multiple risk factor intervention trial. Am J Med 1984;76:52.

258. Day JL et al. Adrenergic mechanisms in the control of plasma lipids in man. Am J Med 1984;76:94.

259. Pagman A et al. Effects of labetalol on lipids and carbohydrate metabolism. Pharmacol Res Commun 1979;11:227.

260. Laren P et al. Antihypertensive drugs and blood lipids: the Oslo study. Br J Clin Pharmacol 1982;13:441S.

261. Lowenstein J. Effects of prazosin on serum lipids in patients with essential hypertension. Am J Cardiol 1984;53:21A.

262. Ames RP, Hill P. Antihypertensive therapy and the risk of coronary heart disease. J Cardiovasc Pharmacol 1982;5(Suppl 2):S206.

263. Weinberger MH. Comparison of captopril and hydrochlorothiazide alone and in combination in mild to moderate hypertension. Br J Clin Pharmacol 1982;14:127S.

264. Knopp RH et al. Oral contraceptive and post-menopausal estrogen effects on lipoprotein triglycerides and cholesterol in an adult female population: relationship to estrogen and progestin potency. J Clin Endocrinol Metab 1981;53:1123.

265. Wahl P et al. Effect of estrogen/progestin potency on lipid/lipoprotein cholesterol. N Engl J Med 1983;308:862.

266. Bagdade JD et al. Steroid-induced hyperlipemia: a complication of high-dose corticosteroid therapy. Arch Intern Med 1970;125:129.

267. Ginsburg H et al. Moderate ethanol ingestion and plasma triglyceride levels. Ann Intern Med 1974;80:143.

268. Bershad S et al. Changes in plasma lipids and lipoproteins during isotretinoin therapy for acne. N Engl J Med 1985;313:981.

269. Ballantyne CM et al. Effects of cyclosporine therapy on plasma lipoprotein levels. JAMA 1989;262:53.

270. Superko, HR. Effectiveness of low-dose colestipol therapy in patients with moderate hypercholesterolemia. Am J Cardiol 1992;70:135

271. Bradford RH et al. Expanded Clinical Evaluation of Lovastatin (EXCEL) study results I: efficacy in modifying plasma lipoproteins and adverse event profile in 8245 patients with moderate hypercholesterolemia. Arch Intern Med 1991;151:43.

272. Jones PH et al. Once-daily pravastatin in patients with primary hypercholesterolemia: A dose response study. Clin Cardiol 1991;14:146.

273. Harper C, Jacobsen T. New perspectives on the mangement of low levels of high-density lipoprotein cholesterol. Arch Intern Med 1999;159:1049.

274. Jones PH et al. Comparison of the efficacy and safety of rosuvastatin versus atorvastatin, simvastatin, and pravastatin across doses (STELLAR Trial). Am J Cardiol 2003;92:152–160.

CHAPTER 14

Essential Hypertension

Joseph J. Saseen, Barry L. Carter

Continues

INTRODUCTION

It is estimated that approximately 50 million Americans have hypertension.[1,2] Although the prevalence is much lower than in other European countries,[3] approximately 25% of the adult American population have this disease. Hypertension is the most frequently encountered chronic medical condition and is also one of the most significant risk factors for cardiovascular morbidity and mortality from coronary artery disease (ischemic heart disease, myocardial infarction [MI], sudden death), other forms of cardiac disease (left ventricular hypertrophy [LVH], heart failure [HF]), chronic kidney disease, stroke, and blindness. The etiology of essential hypertension is unknown and requires lifelong management.

In 1972, the National Institutes of Health (NIH) funded the development of the National High Blood Pressure Education Program (NHBPEP). This program was established to increase awareness among health care professionals and the public about the importance of treating hypertension. Although this effort has been partly successful, recent statistics suggest that awareness, treatment, and control of hypertension are not optimal. From 1976 to 1980, only 51% of hypertensive persons were aware they had elevated blood pressure (BP). This has increased to 70% between 1999 to 2000. Similarly, 59% of hypertensives are receiving some form of treatment (up from 31% between 1976 and 1980). Ultimately, the most disappointing statistic is that only 34% of hypertensive patients have controlled BP (liberally defined as both systolic BP <140 mm Hg and diastolic BP <90 mm Hg).[1] Improvement in the management of hypertension is desperately needed.

Blood Pressure

During systole the left ventricle contracts, ejecting blood into the vasculature to cause a sharp rise in BP. This is the systolic BP (SBP). The left ventricle relaxes during diastole, and BP decreases to a trough value as blood returns to the right heart from the venous system. This is the diastolic BP (DBP). When recording BP (e.g., 120/76 mm Hg), the numerator refers to SBP and the denominator refers to DBP. BP has a predictable diurnal rhythm with fluctuations throughout the day. Values are lowest during the nighttime, sharply rise starting in the early morning, and peak in the late-morning to early afternoon.[4] These fluctuations are less pronounced in the African American population and may be absent in patients with secondary hypertension.[5] Mean arterial pressure (MAP) is sometimes used to represent BP. It collectively reflects both SBP and DBP. MAP is calculated using the following equation:

$$MAP = (SBP - DBP)/3 + DBP$$

Hypertension

The Seventh Report of the Joint National Committee on Detection, Evaluation, and Treatment of High BP (JNC 7) classifies BP based on systolic and diastolic values (Table 14-1).[1] Hypertension is defined as an elevated SBP, DBP, or both. A clinical diagnosis of hypertension is based on the mean of two or more properly measured seated BP measurements taken on two or more occasions. This mean BP is also used to initially classify and stage hypertension. The JNC 7 classification includes normal BP, prehypertension, stage 1 hypertension, and stage 2 hypertension. The use of qualitative terms (e.g., mild, moderate, high-normal, severe) is not recommended. Initial therapy for hypertension is also listed in Table 14-1. A thiazide type diuretic is recommended under most circumstances. However, the presence of a compelling indication for a specific agent and the category of hypertension are also used to guide therapy. These issues are discussed later in this chapter.

Goals

The ultimate goal of treating hypertension is to reduce associated morbidity and mortality. These hypertension-related complications manifest as target-organ damage (Table 14-2), which includes cardiovascular disease, and are the primary causes of death in hypertensive patients. Several major risk factors have been identified. These risk factors increase the likelihood of developing target-organ damage, not hypertension.

CARDIOVASCULAR RISK AND BLOOD PRESSURE

Direct correlations between BP values and risk of cardiovascular disease have been established using epidemiologic data. These findings have been highlighted in the JNC 7 report.[1] Beginning at a benchmark BP of 115/75 mm Hg, the risk of cardiovascular disease doubles with every increment of 20/10 mm Hg. There is a significant increase in risk of cardiovascular events in patients with prehypertension versus normal BP, as depicted in Figure 14-1.[6] Differences in risk are also present within the prehypertension classification. Clinically, it is important to note that having elevated SBP (≥140 mm Hg) is a more reliable predictor of cardiovascular disease

Table 14-1   Classification and Management of BP for Adults[1,a]

Classification	SBP[a] (mm Hg)	DBP[a] (mm Hg)	Lifestyle Modifications	Initial Drug Therapy Without Compelling Indication	With Compelling Indication (Fig. 14-4)
Normal	<120	and <80	Encourage	—	—
Prehypertension	120–139	or 80–89	Yes	No antihypertensive drug indicated	Drug(s) for compelling indications[c]
Stage 1 hypertension	140–159	or 90–99	Yes	Thiazide-type diuretic for most; may consider ACE inhibitor, ARB, β-blocker, CCB, or combination	Drug(s) for compelling indications[c]; other antihypertensive drugs (diuretics, ACE inhibitor, ARB, β-blocker, CCB) as needed
Stage 2 hypertension	≥160	or ≥100	Yes	Two-drug combination for most (usually a thiazide-type diuretic and an ACE inhibitor or ARB or β-blocker or CCB)[b]	Drug(s) for compelling indications; antihypertensive drugs (diuretics, ACE Inhibitor, ARB, β-blocker, CCB) as needed

[a]Treatment determined based on highest BP category.
[b]Use initial combination therapy cautiously in those patients at risk for orthostatic hypotension.
[c]Treat patient with chronic kidney disease or diabetes to a BP goal of <130/80 mmHg.
ACE, angiotensin converting enzyme; ARB, angiotensin receptor blocker; BP, blood pressure; CCB, calcium channel blocker; DBP, diastolic blood pressure; SBP, systolic blood pressure.

Table 14-2   Hypertension-related Target Organ Damage and Major Cardiovascular Risk Factors[1]

Target Organ Damage
- Brain (stroke or transient ischemic attack)
- Eyes (retinopathy)
- Heart (left ventricular hypertrophy, angina, or prior myocardial infarction, prior coronary revascularization, heart failure)
- Kidney (chronic kidney disease)
- Peripheral vasculature (peripheral arterial disease)

Major Cardiovascular Risk Factors
- Age (>55 years for men, >65 years for women)
- Cigarette smoking
- Diabetes mellitus
- Dyslipidemia
- Family history of premature cardiovascular disease (men <55 years or women <65 years)
- Hypertension
- Kidney disease (microalbuminuria or estimated GFR <60 mL/min)
- Obesity (BMI ≥30 kg/m²)
- Physical inactivity

BMI, body mass index; GFR, glomerular infiltration rate.

---

than elevated DBP in people older than 50 years of age. Therefore, SBP is the primary target of evaluation and intervention for most patients.[1,7]

BLOOD PRESSURE VALUES

The surrogate goal in hypertension is to achieve target SBP and DBP values. Most patients with hypertension have a BP goal of <140/90 mm Hg. However, the BP goal is <130/80 mm Hg for patients with diabetes or chronic kidney disease (either an estimated glomerular filtration rate [GFR] <60 mL/min or albuminuria [>300 mg albumin in a 24-hour urine collection or 200 mg albumin/g creatinine on a spot urine measurement]).[1,8,9] A more aggressive BP goal is justified in these patients because they are at very high risk for target-organ damage, and lowering BP to this level has been shown to maximize risk reduction.[10,11] Although elevated SBP is more predictive of cardiovascular disease than DBP for the majority of patients,[1,7] goal achievement requires reduction of both SBP and DBP to target values. Control of SBP is imperative and this usually results in control of DBP. Clinicians should follow these recommendations and be appropriately aggressive with therapy despite the tendency to accept BP values that are close to, but not at, the goal.

White-Coat Hypertension

White-coat hypertension refers to patients without target-organ disease who have consistently elevated BP values measured in a clinical environment (e.g., physician's office) that are significantly higher than those obtained by either a manual reading outside this environment (e.g., home) or with 24-hour ambulatory monitoring.[12] This phenomenon was seen in 21 of 292 patients with untreated prehypertension who had normal ambulatory pressure readings.[13] Home BP monitoring and/or 24-hour ambulatory BP monitoring (ABPM) is warranted in patients suspected of having white-coat hypertension to differentiate this from true hypertension.[14]

Patients with white-coat hypertension are at risk for developing hypertension and need to be closely monitored with a device that can measure BP outside the clinic environment. This device should be checked regularly against the instru-

Women

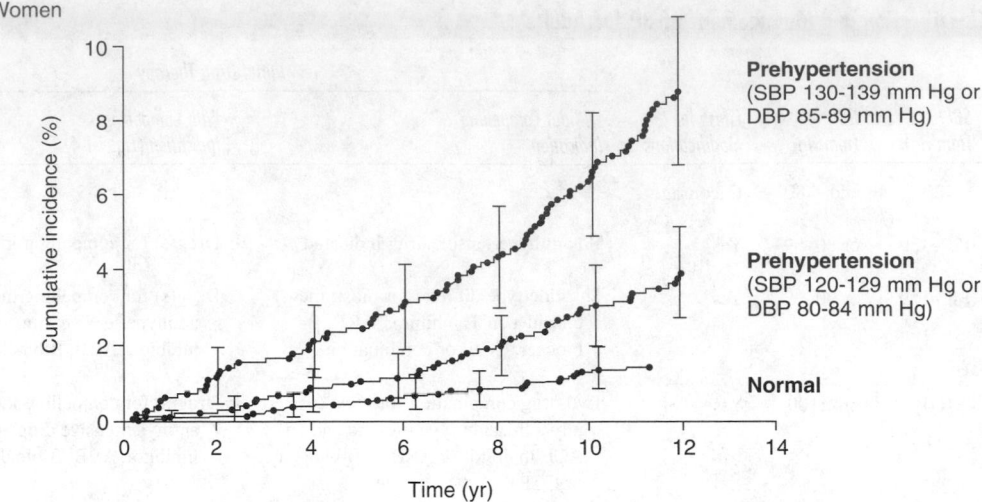

Men

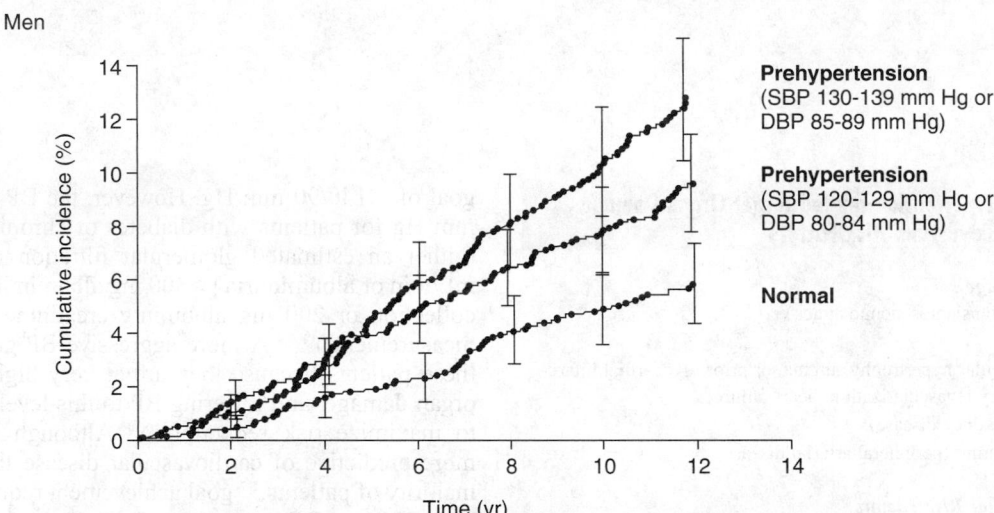

FIGURE 14-1 Cumulative incidence of cardiovascular events in women and men without hypertension according to baseline BP values. BP categories are assigned based on the JNC 7 classification.[1] (Adapted with permission from Vasan RS et al. Impact of high-normal blood pressure on the risk of cardiovascular disease. N Engl J Med 2001;345:1291. Copyright 2001 Massachusetts Medical Society. All rights reserved.)

ment used in the clinic environment to ensure accuracy. Data suggest that patients with white-coat hypertension are at a higher risk for cardiovascular disease than normotensive patients.[15] However, treating white-coat hypertension is controversial.

Hypertensive Crises

Hypertensive crises situations arise when measured BP values are excessively high, generally in the upper range of stage 2 hypertension (>180/110 mm Hg). They are further classified as either a *hypertensive emergency* (with acute or chronic end-organ damage) or *urgency* (without acute end-organ damage).[16] Hypertensive emergencies require hospitalization for immediate BP lowering using IV medications. Hypertensive urgencies do not require immediate BP lowering; instead, BP should be slowly reduced within 24 hours (but not generally

to goal BP so quickly) following drug therapy recommendations for stage 2 hypertension (See Chapter 21, Hypertensive Emergencies). However, the optimal rate of BP lowering in hypertensive emergencies and urgencies remains unclear.[17] Examples of acute end-organ damage include encephalopathy, MI, unstable angina, pulmonary edema, eclampsia, stroke, head trauma, life-threatening arterial bleeding, aortic dissection, severe retinopathy, or acute renal failure.

Blood Pressure Measurements

Auscultatory Method

BP measurement should be standardized to minimize variability in readings. The American Heart Association's technique for auscultatory BP measurement (described in Table 14-3) should be used.[1,18] Correct BP measurements require

Table 14-3 Recommended Technique for Auscultatory BP Measurement in Adults.[18]

1. Patient should be seated for 5 minutes with arm bared, unrestricted by clothing, and supported at heart level. Smoking or food ingestion should not have occurred within 30 minutes before the measurement.

2. An appropriately sized cuff should be chosen. The internal inflatable bladder width should be at least 40% and the bladder length at least 80% of the upper arm circumference. The cuff should be wrapped snugly around the arm with the center of the bladder over the brachial artery.

3. Measurements should be taken with a mercury sphygmomanometer, a recently calibrated aneroid manometer, or a validated electronic device.

4. The palpatory method should be used to estimate SBP. The cuff is inflated while simultaneously palpating the radial pulse on the cuffed arm and observing the manometer. The point at which the radial pulse is no longer palpable is the estimated SBP. The cuff is then deflated.

5. The BP should be measured with a stethoscope positioned over the brachial artery and the cuff rapidly inflated to 20 to 30 mm Hg above the estimated SBP from the palpatory method. The cuff is deflated at a rate of 2 mm Hg per second while listening for Phase 1 (the first appearance of sounds) and Phase 5 (the disappearance of sounds) Korotkoff sounds and observing the manometer. When 10 to 20 mm Hg below Phase 5, the cuff can be rapidly deflated.

6. The BP should be recorded. The Phase 1 (SBP) and Phase 5 (DBP) value should be recorded in even numbers (rounded up form an odd number) along with the patient's position, arm used, and cuff size documented.

7. A second measurement should be taken after 1 to 2 minutes in the same arm. If the readings differ by more than 5 mm Hg, additional measurements should be obtained. The mean of these two values should be used to make clinical decisions. BP should be taken in both arms at the initial visit with the BP taken in the arm with the higher reading at subsequent visits.

BP, blood pressure; DBP, diastolic blood pressure; SBP, systolic blood pressure.

that the clinician listen through a stethoscope that is placed over the brachial artery for the appearance of the five phases of the Korotkoff sounds. Each sound has distinct features, which are depicted in Figure 14-2.[18]

Pseudohypertension

The possibility of pseudohypertension should be considered when measuring BP in elderly patients. In pseudohypertension, blood vessels become stiff and thick because of calcification and resist compression from the bladder of the inflatable BP cuff. Greater pressure is then needed to occlude the artery, and this results in an inaccurate overestimation of SBP. Osler's maneuver is used to detect pseudohypertension. A BP cuff is inflated above the SBP while palpating the brachial and/or radial arteries to determine whether the pulseless artery is still palpable. If the artery is still palpable, the patient might have pseudohypertension. Pseudohypertension is thought to be relatively rare.

Blood Pressure Monitoring Outside the Office

Ambulatory blood pressure monitoring typically measures BP every 20 to 30 minutes throughout the day and is warranted in patients with suspected white-coat hypertension. It also may be helpful in patients with apparent drug resistance, hypotensive symptoms while receiving antihypertensive therapy, episodic hypertension, and autonomic dysfunction. ABPM values are usually lower than office-based measurements. Hypertensive patients have average values of >135/85 mm Hg while awake and >120/75 mm Hg while asleep. Therefore, the threshold for acceptable values are lower than those obtained during office-based measurements. Growing evidence indicates that ABPM recordings may be better predictors of target organ damage than office BP measurements in patients with treated hypertension.[19]

Self-measurement of BP can provide information on response to therapy and may help improve adherence to therapy and goal BP achievement.[1,20] Home measurement devices (e.g., electronic monitors, auscultatory monitors) need to be routinely checked for accuracy. As is the case with ambulatory monitoring, patients with average home BP values that are >135/85 mm Hg are considered hypertensive. Wrist or finger devices that measure BP are not accurate and should not be used.

BP values measured outside the office should be considered in the overall treatment of hypertensive patients, but definitive routine use cannot be recommended. The major clinical trials that have established that appropriate treatment of hypertension reduces morbidity and mortality rates used office-based BP measurements. Therefore, office-based BP measurements are still considered the gold standard values that guide antihypertensive drug therapy.

Etiology

The majority of hypertensive patients have essential hypertension (also known as primary hypertension), with no identifiable cause for their disorder. Patients with secondary hypertension have a specific identified cause for elevated BP (Table 14-4). Although only 5% to 10% of the hypertensive population has secondary hypertension, further diagnostic evaluation should occur if physical or laboratory findings are consistent with a secondary cause (Table 14-5). Secondary causes are potentially correctable. Further diagnostic workup also should be considered in patients who do not respond to increasing doses of antihypertensive medication or who have a sudden increase in BP or accelerated or malignant hypertension.[1] A thorough review of prescription medications, nonprescription medications, and herbal products should be conducted to rule out drug induced BP elevations.

Pathophysiology

Various neural and humoral factors are known to influence BP.[21] These include the adrenergic nervous system (controls α- and β-receptors), the renin-angiotensin-aldosterone system (regulates systemic and renal blood flow), renal function and renal blood flow (influences fluid and electrolyte balance),

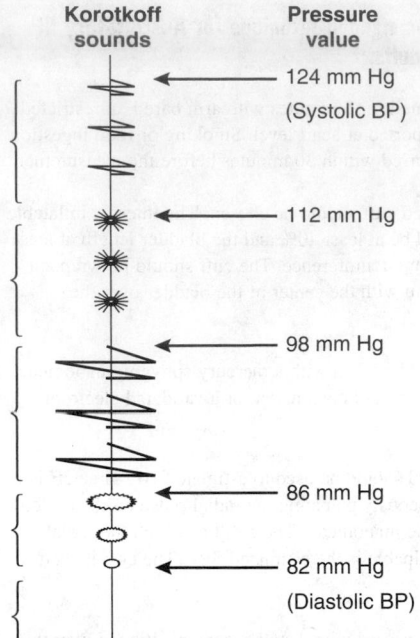

Phases

Phase 1: The pressure level at which the first faint clear tapping sounds are heard. These sounds gradually increase in intensity as the cuff deflates.

Phase 2: That time during cuff deflation when a murmur or swishing sounds are heard. They are softer and longer than in Phase 1.

Phase 3: The period during which sounds are crisp, loud and increase in intensity.

Phase 4: That time when sounds are less distinct, and change to a muffled and soft (or blowing) quality.

Phase 5: The pressure value when the last sound is heard and after which all sounds disappear.

Korotkoff sounds

Pressure value

124 mm Hg (Systolic BP)

112 mm Hg

98 mm Hg

86 mm Hg

82 mm Hg (Diastolic BP)

FIGURE 14-2 Phases of the Korotkoff sounds heard when indirectly measuring blood pressure.

Table 14-4 Secondary Causes of Hypertension[1]

Chronic Kidney Disease

Chronic Steroid Therapy and Cushing's Syndrome

Coarctation of the Aorta

Drug-Induced or Drug-Related
- Adrenal steroids
- Alcohol in excess
- Amphetamines/anorexiants (e.g., phentermine, sibutramine)
- Cocaine and other illicit drugs
- Cyclosporine and tacrolimus
- Erythropoietin
- Licorice (including some chewing tobacco)
- Nonsteroidal anti-inflammatory drugs/COX-2 Inhibitors
- Oral contraceptives
- Oral decongestants (e.g., pseudoephedrine)
- Some over-the-counter dietary supplements and medicines (e.g., ephedra, ma haung, bitter orange)

Pheochromocytoma

Primary Aldosteronism

Renovascular Disease

Sleep Apnea

Thyroid or Parathyroid Disease

several hormonal factors (adrenal cortical hormones, vasopressin, thyroid hormone, insulin), and the vascular endothelium (regulates release of nitric oxide, bradykinin, prostacyclin, endothelin). Knowledge of these mechanisms is important in understanding antihypertensive drug therapy. BP is normally regulated by compensatory mechanisms that respond to changes in cardiac demand. An increase in cardiac output (CO) normally results in a compensatory decrease in total peripheral resistance (TPR); likewise, an increase in TPR

results in a decrease in CO. These events occur to maintain MAP, as is evidenced by the following equation:

$$MAP = CO \times TPR$$

Adverse changes in BP can occur when these compensatory mechanisms are not functioning properly. It has been suggested that in hypertension an initial increase in fluid volume increases CO and arterial pressure. Eventually, with long-standing hypertension, it is believed that TPR increases so that CO returns to normal.

The kidney plays an important role in the regulation of arterial pressure, especially through the renin-angiotensin-aldosterone system. Decreases in BP and renal blood flow, volume depletion or decreased sodium concentration, and an activation of the sympathetic nervous system can all trigger an increased secretion of the enzyme renin from the cells of the juxtaglomerular apparatus in the kidney. Renin acts on angiotensinogen to catalyze the formation of angiotensin I. Angiotensin-converting enzyme (ACE) converts angiotensin I to angiotensin II (see Figs. 19-1 and 19-6 in Chapter 19, Heart Failure). Angiotensin II is a potent vasoconstrictor that acts directly on arteriolar smooth muscle and also stimulates the production of aldosterone by the adrenal glands. Aldosterone causes sodium and water retention and the excretion of potassium. Several factors influence renin release, especially those that alter renal perfusion. Lastly, the resultant increase in BP results in suppression of renin release through negative feedback.

Approximately 20% of patients with essential hypertension have lower-than-normal *plasma renin activity* (PRA), while approximately 15% have PRA concentrations that are higher than normal PRA. Those with normal to high PRA have decreased plasma volume and increased adrenergic activity and should theoretically be more responsive drug therapies that

Table 14-5 Clinical Findings Suggestive of Secondary Hypertension[1]

Causes	Historical Findings	Physical Examination Finding	Laboratory Finding
Sleep apnea	Daytime fatigue and somnolence; difficult concentration	Large neck circumference; overweight or obese	Abnormal sleep studies with frequent awakenings and anoxic episodes
Renovascular disease	Moderate or severe high BP before age 30 or after 55; rapidly progressive hypertension	Abdominal bruits with ↑ SBP and DBP; funduscopic hemorrhages	Suppressed or stimulated plasma renin activity; IVP (rapid sequence); digital subtraction angiography
Renoparenchymal disease	Dysuria, polyuria, nocturia; urinary tract infections; renal stones (or colic); family history of polycystic kidney disease; renal disease	Edema	Proteinuria; hematuria; bacteriuria
Coarctation of the aorta	Intermittent claudication	Diminished or absent femoral pulses compared to carotids; lower SBP in leg compared to arm	
Pheochromocytoma	Paroxysmal headaches, palpitations, sweating, dizziness, and pallor (in 30% of patients)	Nervousness, tremor, tachycardia, orthostatic hypotension	Clonidine suppression tests[a]; ↑ serum glucose; high urine metanephrine or vanillylmandelic acid
Primary aldosteronism	Weakness, polyuria, polydipsia, intermittent paralysis	Orthostatic hypotension	Hypokalemia
Cushing's syndrome	Menstrual irregularity	Moon face; truncal obesity; buffalo hump; hirsutism; violet striae	↑ serum glucose; ↑ plasma cortisol after suppression with dexamethasone

[a]Failure of plasma catecholamines to ↓ by 50% within 3 hr of administration of 0.3 mg clonidine highly suggests pheochromocytoma.
BP, blood pressure; DBP, diastolic blood pressure; IVP, intravenous pyelogram; SBP, systolic blood pressure.

target the renin-angiotensin-aldosterone system (e.g., ACE inhibitors or β-adrenergic blockers). Patients with low PRA have expanded fluid volume and may be more responsive to diuretic therapy. However, measuring PRA is problematic and is not advocated as a means for selection of drug therapy.

Arterial BP also is regulated by the *adrenergic nervous system,* which causes contraction and relaxation of vascular smooth muscle. Stimulation of α-adrenergic receptors in the central nervous system (CNS) results in a reflex decrease in sympathetic outflow causing a decrease in BP. Stimulation of postsynaptic α₁-receptors in the periphery causes vasoconstriction. α-Receptors are regulated by a negative feedback system; as norepinephrine is released into the synaptic cleft and stimulates presynaptic α₂-receptors, further norepinephrine release is inhibited. This negative feedback results in a balance between vasoconstriction and vasodilatation. Stimulation of postsynaptic β₁-receptors located in the myocardium causes an increase in heart rate and contractility, while stimulation of postsynaptic β₂-receptors in the arterioles and venules results in vasodilation.

A direct association between *sodium* and BP is supported by epidemiologic evidence and clinical trials.[22] Patients with a high dietary sodium intake have a greater prevalence of hypertension than those with a low sodium intake. The mechanism by which hypertension is caused by an increase in sodium intake is hypothesized to involve natriuretic hormone. This hormone is functionally and chemically different from atrial and brain natriuretic peptide. Natriuretic hormone is po-

tentially increased to facilitate sodium and water excretion in response to an increase in renal sodium retention and extracellular fluid volume. Natriuretic hormone might also cause an increase in intracellular sodium and calcium, resulting in increased vascular tone and hypertension. However, this hypothesis has not been definitively proven.

Epidemiologic evidence and clinical trials have demonstrated an inverse relationship between *calcium* and BP.[23] One proposed mechanism for this relationship involves an alteration in the balance between intracellular and extracellular calcium. Increased intracellular calcium concentrations can increase peripheral vascular resistance, resulting in increased BP.

A decrease in *potassium* has been associated with an increase in peripheral vascular resistance.[22] In theory, diuretic-induced hypokalemia could counteract some of the hypotensive effects of diuretic therapy, but this has not been well studied. It is important, however, that potassium concentrations be maintained within the normal range because hypokalemia increases the risk of cardiovascular events, such as sudden death.[24]

Insulin resistance and *hyperinsulinemia* also have been associated with hypertension.[25,26] Kaplan suggests that insulin resistance is responsible for the frequent coexistence of diabetes, dyslipidemia, hypertension, and abdominal obesity.[26] This is also referred to as the Metabolic Syndrome.[27] The exact role of insulin resistance in the development of hypertension is still evolving and is the subject of intense investigation.

The vascular epithelium is a dynamic system in which vascular tone is regulated by numerous substances. As noted previously, angiotensin II promotes vasoconstriction of the vascular epithelium. However, several other substances regulate vascular tone. Nitric oxide (NO) is produced in the endothelium and is a potent vasodilatory chemical that relaxes the vascular epithelium. The NO system has been firmly established as an important regulator of arterial BP. Hypothetically, hypertensive patients could have an intrinsic deficiency in NO release and inadequate vasodilation, which may contribute to hypertension and/or its vascular complications.[28]

Factors that regulate BP are well understood and continue to evolve. A decreased number of nephrons have also been associated with an increased incidence of essential hypertension in white patients.[29] However, the cause of essential hypertension is unknown. It is currently impossible to target therapy to specific abnormalities. Antihypertensive therapy should be based on outcome-based clinical data that demonstrate reductions in target organ damage.

CLINICAL EVALUATION
Patient Presentation

1. **D.C. is a 52-year-old African American man who complains of a throbbing headache in the morning for the past week. He was diagnosed with hypertension 6 years ago and was initially treated with lifestyle modifications, and then with antihypertensive medication (amlodipine). He took this medication for 2 years and then discontinued it because he did not think it was needed. Past medical history is unremarkable. D.C.'s father had hypertension and died of an MI at age 54. His mother had diabetes and hypertension and died of a stroke at age 68. D.C. smokes 1 pack per day of cigarettes (for 35 years) and thinks that his BP is high because of job-related stress. He does not believe that he has hypertension. D.C. states that he does not engage in any regular form of exercise and does not restrict his diet in any way.**

Physical examination shows he is 69" tall, weighs 108 kg (body mass index, 35.2 kg/m^2), BP is 148/88 mm Hg (left arm) and 150/86 mm Hg (right arm) while sitting, heart rate is 82 beats/min and regular. One month ago, his BP values were 152/88 mm Hg and 154/84 mm Hg. Funduscopic examination reveals mild arterial narrowing, arteriovenous nicking, with no exudates or hemorrhages. The remainder of the physical examination is essentially normal.

Laboratory examination reveals the following values: blood urea nitrogen (BUN), 24 mg/dL (normal, 7 to 20 mg/dL); serum creatinine (SrCr), 1.3 mg/dL (normal, 0.5 to 1.2 mg/dL); fasting glucose, 95 mg/dL (normal, 60 to 110 mg/dL); potassium (K), 4.0 mEq/L (normal, 3.5 to 5.2 mEq/L); uric acid, 8.0 mg/dL (normal, 2.0 to 8.0 mg/dL); low-density lipoprotein (LDL) cholesterol, 140 mg/dL (normal, <130 mg/dL); high-density lipoprotein (HDL) cholesterol, 35 mg/dL (normal, >40 mg/dL), and triglycerides 230 mg/dL (normal, <200 mg/dL). An electrocardiogram (ECG) and chest radiograph reveal mild LVH. What is the proper assessment of D.C.'s hypertension based on this information?

[SI units: BUN, 8.6 mmol/L (normal, 2.5 to 7.2 mmol/L); glucose, 5.3 mmol/L (normal, 3.3 to 6.1 mmol/L); K, 4.0 mmol/L (normal, 3.5 to 5.2 mmol/L); uric acid, 476 mmol/L (normal, 119 to 476 mmol/L); HDL, 0.96 mmol/L (normal, 1.09 to 1.64 mmol/L)]

D.C. has uncontrolled stage 1 hypertension that is above his BP goal of <140/90 mm Hg. His previous diagnosis alone should be enough to justify a diagnosis of hypertension, but D.C. fits the diagnostic criteria for hypertension because two or more of his BP measurements are elevated on separate days. SBP values are consistently stage 1, while DBP values are all in the prehypertension range. The higher of the two classifications is used to classify hypertension.[1] D.C.'s goal BP is <140/90 mm Hg since he does not have diabetes or chronic kidney disease. He has a pattern of hypertension that is common in the United States, in which SBP is ≥140 mm Hg (uncontrolled) with DBP <90 mm Hg (controlled).[30] Regardless of this discrepancy, D.C.'s hypertension is not at goal. Two BP measurements should always be obtained, with the average used to make clinical decisions (see BP measurements section and Table 14-3). The average of his most recent BP measurements is 149/87 mm Hg.

2. **Why does D.C. have hypertension?**

D.C.'s diagnosis is most likely essential hypertension, and the exact cause is not known. However, he has several characteristics (e.g., family history of hypertension, obesity) that may have increased his chance of developing hypertension. Race and gender also influence the prevalence of hypertension. Across all age groups, African Americans have a higher prevalence than whites and Mexican Americans.[2] The prevalence rates for men are 36.7%, 25.2%, and 24.2% for African Americans, whites, and Mexican Americans, respectively.[2] African Americans have a higher incidence of salt sensitivity, which might explain some of these trends. This appears to be caused by racially determined differences in renal handling of sodium. In addition, more men than women have hypertension. Similar to other forms of cardiovascular disease, hypertension is more severe, more likely to include target organ damage, and occurs at an earlier age in African American patients.

Patient Evaluation/Risk Assessment

Evaluation of patients with hypertension has multiple purposes.[1] First, the presence and absence of various forms of hypertension-related target organ damage should be assessed. Second, secondary causes of hypertension, if present, should be identified and managed accordingly. Third, major risk factors, concomitant disorders, and lifestyle habits should be evaluated so that they can be used to guide therapy and influence prognosis.

Target Organ Damage

3. **What hypertension-related complications might D.C. develop from his elevated BP?**

Avoiding the development of target organ damage is the primary purpose of treating hypertension. Hypertension adversely affects many organ systems throughout the body, including the heart, brain, kidneys, peripheral circulation, and eyes. These are summarized in Table 14-2. Damage to these systems (specified by terms such as coronary, myocardial, cerebrovascular, renal, or retinal disease) resulting from hypertension is termed target organ damage or cardiovascular disease (CVD). There are often misconceptions about the terms CVD and coronary artery disease (CAD). CVD encompasses the broad scope of all forms of *target organ damage.* CAD is simply a subset of CVD and refers specifically to disease related to the coronary vasculature, including ischemic heart disease and MI. Target organ damage and major risk factors for developing such complications should be assessed through a thorough patient history, a complete physical examination, and laboratory evaluation.

HEART

Hypertension can affect the heart either indirectly, by promoting atherosclerotic changes, or directly, via pressure-related effects. Hypertension can promote CVD and increase the risk for *ischemic events,* such as angina and MI. Antihypertensive therapy has been shown to reduce the risk of these coronary events.

Hypertension also promotes the development of LVH, which is a myocardial (cellular) change, not an arterial change. However, these two conditions often exist together. It is commonly believed that LVH is a compensatory mechanism of the heart in response to the increased resistance caused by elevated BP. LVH is a strong and independent risk factor for CAD, HF, and arrhythmias.[31] A finding of LVH does not necessarily indicate the presence of HF, but is a risk for progression to HF (See Chapter 19, Heart Failure).

A major cardiac outcome of hypertension is HF. This may be caused by repeated ischemia, excessive ventricular hypertrophy, and/or pressure overload. Ultimately, HF results in a decreased ability to contract (systolic dysfunction) or an inability of the heart to fill (diastolic dysfunction). Uncontrolled hypertension is one of the leading causes of HF.[2,32]

BRAIN

Hypertension is one of the most frequent causes of cerebrovascular disease.[2,33] Cerebrovascular signs can manifest as transient ischemic attacks, ischemic strokes, multiple cerebral infarcts, and hemorrhages. Residual functional deficits caused by stroke are among the most devastating forms of target organ damage. Clinical trials have demonstrated that antihypertensive therapy can significantly reduce the risk of both initial and recurrent stroke.[1,34] A sudden, prolonged increase in systemic BP also can cause hypertensive encephalopathy, which is classified as a hypertensive emergency. Hypertensive encephalopathy is now uncommon because effective antihypertensive therapy is available.

KIDNEY

The GFR is used to estimate kidney function. It declines with aging, but this rate of decline is greatly accelerated by hypertension.[35] Hypertension is associated with nephrosclerosis, which is caused by increased intraglomerular pressure. It is unknown whether a primary kidney lesion with ischemia causes systemic hypertension or whether systemic hypertension directly causes glomerular capillary damage by increasing intraglomerular pressure. Regardless, chronic kidney disease, whether mild or severe, can progresses to kidney failure (stage 5 chronic kidney disease) and the need for dialysis. Although studies have demonstrated that achieving aggressive BP control is the most important strategy to slow the rate of kidney decline,[35] it may not be entirely effective in slowing the progression of renal impairment in all patients.

Chronic kidney disease is staged based on estimated GFR values.[35] Moderate (stage 3) kidney disease is defined as a GFR <30 to 59 mL/min/1.73m^2, severe (stage 4) is 15 to 29 mL/min/1.73m^2, and kidney failure is <15 mL/min/1.73m^2 or the requirement of dialysis. In hypertension, moderate kidney disease or worse (estimated GFR <60 mL/min) identifies target organ damage. An estimated GFR <60 mL/min corresponds approximately to a creatinine of >1.5 mg/dL in an average man and >1.3 mg/dL in an average woman. This level of kidney compromise lowers an individual's BP goal to $<130/80$ mm Hg. The presence of albuminuria (>300 mg albumin in a 24-hour urine collection or 200 mg albumin/g creatinine on a spot urine measurement) also indicates chronic kidney disease. Achieving the more aggressive goal is a strategy to minimize the rate of progression to kidney failure. [Note: These definitions of the stages of kidney disease and albuminuria will be used throughout the remaining cases in this chapter.]

GFR can be estimated by calculating a patient's creatinine clearance. In adults, the MDRD study equation or the Cockcroft-Gault equation use the serum creatinine concentration and variables (e.g., age, sex, body size) to estimate GFR.[35,36] The Cockcroft-Gault equation is most universally accepted as an easy way to estimate GFR and requires knowledge of the patient's serum creatinine, ideal body weight, and gender.

PERIPHERAL ARTERIAL DISEASE

Peripheral arterial disease is another form of atherosclerotic vascular disease that is considered target organ damage. It is equivalent in risk to CAD.[1,27] Risk factor modifications, BP control, and antiplatelet agent(s) are needed to decrease progression. Complications of peripheral arterial disease can include infection and necrosis, which in some cases require revascularization procedures or extremity amputation.

EYE

Hypertension causes retinopathies that may progress to blindness. Retinopathy is evaluated according to the Keith, Wagener, and Barker funduscopic classification system. Grade 1 is characterized by narrowing of the arterial diameter, indicating vasoconstriction. Arteriovenous (AV) nicking is the hallmark of grade 2, indicating atherosclerosis. Longstanding untreated hypertension or accelerated hypertension also can cause cotton wool exudates and flame hemorrhages (grade 3). In severe cases, papilledema occurs, and this is classified as grade 4. Additional information on hypertensive retinopathy and pictures describing physical assessment findings can be found on the worldwide web (http://www. revoptom.com/handbook/SECT41b.HTM).

4. What forms of target organ damage are present in D.C.?

A complete physical examination to evaluate target organ damage includes examination of the optic fundi; auscultation for carotid, abdominal, and femoral bruits; palpation of the thyroid gland; heart and lung examination; abdominal examination for enlarged kidney, masses, and abnormal aortic pulsation; lower extremity palpation for edema and pulses; and neurologic assessment.[1] Routine laboratory assessment after diagnosis should include the following: electrocardiogram; urinalysis; fasting glucose; hematocrit; serum potassium, creatinine, and calcium; and a fasting lipid panel. Optional testing may include measurement of urinary albumin excretion or albumin/creatinine ratio, or additional tests specific for secondary causes if suspected.

D.C. has several signs of target organ damage. These have likely evolved from his longstanding, poorly controlled hypertension. D.C.'s electrocardiogram revealed LVH indicating cardiac damage. Although the gold standard for confirming LVH is with echocardiography, this confirmatory procedure is not usually necessary unless symptoms indicating LVH progression (i.e., HF) are present. His funduscopic examination reveals mild arterial narrowing and AV nicking, suggesting both early retinopathy and atherosclerosis. Finally, D.C.'s serum creatinine of 1.3 mg/dL is elevated. However, since his estimated GFR is >60 mL/min (approximately 64), he does not yet have chronic kidney disease. Additional testing for microalbuminuria is needed in D.C. to assure that he does not have chronic kidney disease. His complaint of headaches may or may not be related to hypertension. The presence or absence of headache is a poor indicator of hypertension, which is often an asymptomatic disease.

Major Risk Factors

5. Why is D.C. at high risk for hypertension-related complications?

Hypertension is one of nine major cardiovascular risk factors identified by the JNC 7. These are not necessarily risk factors for developing essential hypertension; rather, they increase the risk of target organ damage such as coronary heart disease (CHD) (see Table 14-2). Based on Framingham estimates, risk increases with higher SBP values.[27] Observational data in patients with untreated hypertension indicate an increased CHD risk related to the degree of BP elevation.[33,37,38] Even if BP is controlled with antihypertensive therapy, there is still an increased risk.

D.C. has many modifiable risk factors. He has a 35-pack-year history of cigarette smoking. This significantly increases the risk for CHD[27] and may reduce the efficacy of antihypertensive therapy.[39] Smoking cessation may not independently lower D.C.'s BP, but it will decrease his overall risk of CVD. D.C. is obese based on his body mass index. It is likely that this is influenced by his lack of physical activity and dietary patterns. A more focused patient interview on diet and exercise would be helpful to reinforce the assumption that he has a sedentary lifestyle.

D.C.'s elevated low-density lipoprotein (LDL) cholesterol and decreased high-density lipoprotein (HDL) cholesterol levels increase his risk of CHD.[27] Lipid-lowering therapy should be considered since intervention trials have repeatedly shown that treating dyslipidemia can decrease the risk of CHD and other forms of target organ damage[40–46] (See Chapter 13, Dyslipidemias, Atherosclerosis, and Coronary Heart Disease). Dyslipidemia in conjunction with hypertension and cigarette smoking has an additive effect for CHD risk.[37]

D.C. has no evidence of diabetes at this time based on his normal fasting glucose. However, if he did, his risk of CHD would be excessively high, especially if he had type 2 diabetes mellitus.[47] Patients with diabetes are predisposed to CVD for several reasons, although most relate to insulin resistance, the primary metabolic disturbance in type 2 diabetes. To address the high risk in this patient population, an aggressive BP goal

of <130/80 mm Hg is recommended to minimize the potential for heart and kidney complications.[1,8,9]

Advanced age, depending on gender, is considered a major risk factor in the JNC 7 report. Although CVD in the elderly age is not considered premature, increasing age increases the risk of hypertension-related complications. Premenopausal women are at low risk for CVD, presumably due to the production of endogenous estrogen. However, cardiovascular risk in women increases significantly after menopause, similar to the increased risk in men. Therefore, cut-off values for age as a risk factor in men and women are separated by 10 years (>55 years for men, >65 years for women). At age 52, D.C. does not yet have this risk factor. Premature CVD in first-degree relatives (i.e., parents and siblings) should be identified because it is a major risk factor for the development of CHD. D.C. has a significant family history of premature CHD because his father died of an MI before the age of 55.

PRINCIPLES OF TREATMENT

Goals of Therapy

6. What are the goals of treating D.C.?

Control of BP is currently the most feasible clinical end point used to guide therapy. It is considered a surrogate marker, or target of therapy.[48] In most patients, including D.C., the BP goal is <140/90 mm Hg. However, the ultimate goal of therapy is to lower hypertension-related morbidity and mortality. Pharmacotherapy principles to achieve these goals include selecting and designing a cost-effective treatment regimen with antihypertensive agent(s) that have been proven to reduce morbidity and mortality, complemented by appropriate lifestyle modifications. Provision of thorough patient education is needed to ensure that D.C. understands his disease and its complications.

Health Beliefs

7. D.C. has misconceptions regarding his hypertension. How can these be corrected?

Patients like D.C. often incorrectly explain BP elevation as stress related. A certain percentage of patients may have an increase in BP because of anxiety, as seen in those with white-coat hypertension. However, most patients with essential hypertension will have an elevated BP regardless of their stress level. Similarly, symptoms such as headache have little correlation to the presence or absence of hypertension. D.C. should be informed about the etiology of his disease and the lack of correlation between stress or symptoms and high BP. Most importantly, D.C. needs to realize that elevated BP, although most often asymptomatic, can cause serious long-term complications. It is essential that he understand the chronic nature of hypertension and the need for long-term therapy. Otherwise, as evidenced by his previous behavior, he may adhere to the prescribed treatment only when he "feels his BP is high" or during stressful events.

Some patients believe they can control their BP by stress management rather than with prescribed therapy (lifestyle modifications and antihypertensive agents). Stress management has not consistently been proven beneficial in controlled trials.[49] Attitudes regarding a chronic disease state can result not only in denial, but depression or perceived worsening of health status. It is important to determine the patient's health beliefs and attitudes and to educate him or her about the etiology and management of hypertension to promote BP control.

Another common myth patients believe is that treating hypertension leads to fatigue, lethargy, and sexual dysfunction. This misconception can be a limiting factor in appropriate management. Clinical trials have repeatedly reported that quality of life is better with active medication than placebo.[50–52] Data have indicated that as many as 27% of men with hypertension have erectile dysfunction.[53] Although many believe this to be a side effect of their medication, erectile dysfunction is likely caused by penile arterial changes (probably atherosclerosis) and could also be a result of the BP reduction itself.[53]

Patient Education

8. What information about hypertension, antihypertensive therapy, and methods of improving adherence should the clinician provide to D.C.?

Patient education for hypertensive patients should comprehensively include information on disease, treatment, adherence, and complications. Several approaches can be effective, but all methods should include direct communication between a clinician and the patient (Table 14-6).[54] Multidisciplinary approaches to disease state management in hypertension can effectively utilize a team of different clinicians. Clinicians can be physicians, nurse practitioners, physician assistants, pharmacists, dietitians, or exercise trainers. Providing education in a face-to-face manner is preferred, but the key components in patient education may be delivered via indirect interactions (i.e., on the telephone).

Recommendations should be tailored to the patient's specific needs, as not all patients respond to the same approach. For example, some patients are able to comprehend the importance of achieving controlled BP by reading written materials, whereas others understand this only after implementing self-BP monitoring. This patient education process must be continuous throughout the duration of therapy. Not all aspects need to be discussed during each clinical interaction. Careful selection of both written and verbal information is needed so that patients are not overwhelmed or frightened by too much information. It is important that clinicians review all materials provided to patients to identify the source of information, assess ease of reading, and identify omitted information or sources of confusion or anxiety (e.g., drug side effects). Patient needs can also change over time as their disease and/or circumstances change, and different strategies might be necessary to enhance education and adherence.

Benefits of Treatment

General Population

9. What are the data indicating that antihypertensive therapy will reduce hypertension-related complications?

Numerous landmark placebo-controlled studies have clearly demonstrated that treating hypertension reduces morbidity and mortality rates. The first large-scale trial was the

Table 14-6   Patient Education (Adapted From the JNC VI)[57]

Patient/Clinician Discussions

- Treatment is needed to reduce morbidity and mortality
- Establish the appropriate BP goal
- BP values cannot be determined based on patient symptoms
- Treatment will control, not cure hypertension
- Chronic treatment is usually necessary
- Treatment should not be discontinued without medical consultation
- Review potential adverse consequences of poor adherence to antihypertensive therapy and uncontrolled blood pressure
- Patients should be able to verbalize an understanding of their diagnosis
- Encourage open discussions or treatment and any problems or side effects

Clinician Responsibilities to Enhance Patient Education and Improve Adherence

- Ask open-ended questions
- Provide encouragement for achieving goals
- Involve patients' families or caregivers in the treatment process
- Encourage patients to self-monitor BP
- Provide alternative treatments and be willing to modify the patient's regimen
- Simplify treatment regimens to maximize compliance (QD regimens, combination products)
- Keep therapy inexpensive if possible
- Provide oral and written instructions and information on drug regimens and goals
- Provide assistance to noncompliant patients (i.e., pill boxes, frequent follow-up visits, mail and/or telephone refill reminders)
- Contact patients who fail to either refill medications or attend follow-up appointments
- Collaborate with other health care professionals (e.g., pharmacists, physicians, nurses)

BP, blood pressure.

Veterans Administration (VA) study in men with DBPs between 115 and 129 mm Hg.[55] This study was prematurely stopped because benefits of treatment were so dramatic that continuing the placebo arm would have been unethical. Antihypertensive therapy significantly reduced cerebral hemorrhage, MI, HF, retinopathy, and kidney disease. Other studies evaluating antihypertensive therapy in patients with less severe hypertension (DBP, 90 to 109 mm Hg) have shown a reduced risk of stroke, ischemic heart disease, HF, progression to more severe hypertension, and death.[38,54,56,57] Long-term placebo-control studies evaluating morbidity and mortality in hypertension are not only unnecessary, but are considered unethical because treatment is beneficial.

Older Population

In the past it was argued that data from these landmark placebo-controlled studies in younger patients did not apply to older patients with hypertension because of a potentially higher risk of drug-related adverse effects in the elderly compared to the benefits of BP lowering. Subsequently, several studies conducted specifically in older patients (ages 60 to 74) with elevated DBP have demonstrated significant reductions in stroke, CAD, HF, and CVD.[52,58-64]

Isolated Systolic Hypertension

Isolated systolic hypertension (ISH) is defined as an elevated SBP ($\geq$140 mm Hg) with a normal DBP (<90 mm Hg).[54,65] This pattern of hypertension is most common in patients older than 65. Although ISH incurs a significant risk for CVD, it was once thought that patients with ISH required high SBP to ensure normal perfusion of the heart and brain and that treating ISH would further lower DBP and worsen organ perfusion. Evidence has now clearly established that treating ISH reduces the risk of CVD.[52,64,66]

The JNC 7 report advocates that care of patients with ISH should follow the same general hypertension care principles that apply to all patients. These patients might require lower doses when starting therapy, but should be increased eventually to doses that are needed to achieve BP goals.[1]

10. **Will D.C.'s present hypertension-related complications improve with appropriate BP control?**

Most antihypertensive drugs (with the possible exception of direct vasodilators) reduce LVH through varying mechanisms.[31,67] It is logical that regression of LVH is desirable, but this remains unproven. Theoretically, myocardial function might be compromised when hypertrophied muscle regresses in size because of the increased ratio of collagen to muscle. Nonetheless, until proven otherwise, regression of LVH in D.C. is desirable.

Significant structural renal damage has already occurred once serum creatinine is elevated. D.C.'s serum creatinine is elevated, and his estimated GFR classifies him as having mild chronic kidney disease (stage 2), although he is at risk for progressing to moderate disease.[35] BP control may not stop the decline or reverse the change in D.C.'s renal function, but it might reduce the rate of decline.[8,35]

Reductions in BP can reverse many of the changes associated with D.C.'s retinopathy. In particular, studies have demonstrated that the risk of retinopathy in diabetic patients increases significantly when the DBP is higher than 70 mm Hg and that control of BP can slow this progression. D.C. does not have diabetes, but regardless, lowering BP is desirable for anticipated beneficial effects on his retinopathy.

Absence of a J-Curve Phenomenon

11. **What harm might occur if D.C.'s DBP decreased to <80 mm Hg?**

Data from observational studies generated concern that lowering BP too far may be harmful.[68,69] These data found that CAD events were decreased as expected when DBP was reduced to approximately 85 mm Hg.[70] However, below this level, the risk of events actually increased. This has been termed the *J-curve phenomenon.*[70]

Several limitations of this J-Curve phenomenon must be appreciated. The data used to establish this phenomenon are observations from retrospective evaluations and, therefore, cannot establish cause and effect. The J-curve has been asso-

ciated only with CAD events, not stroke or renal impairment. For stroke prevention and renal impairment, data consistently suggest that the lower the BP the better, unless BP reductions are too abrupt or are excessive. For example, a population-based cohort study in the Netherlands found that risk of stroke is increased in hypertensive elderly patients treated for hypertension even when DBP goes below 65 mm Hg, which is well below normal.[71] If the J-curve has any validity, it would occur when BP is reduced much lower than the therapeutic range. Furthermore, patients with very low BP may have other illnesses that predispose them to coronary events (e.g., autonomic dysfunction, volume depletion).

The Hypertension Optimal Treatment (HOT) trial was a prospective clinical trial designed to evaluate lower BP goals and CVD events (challenging the J-curve).[11] More than 18,700 patients were randomized to target DBP values of <90 mm Hg, <85 mm Hg, or <80 mm Hg. The risks for major CVD events were the lowest when treatment BP was $\leq$139/83 mm Hg. The risk for cerebrovascular events was lowest at a treatment BP of $\leq$142/80 mm Hg. Only in patients with ischemic heart disease and diabetes did the lowest risk occur at a DBP <80 mm Hg. A significant increase in events was not seen in patients with lower BP values. Therefore, the HOT trial does not support the concept of a J-curve.

With these factors in mind, D.C.'s goal should be to lower his BP to <140/90 mm Hg. Specifically, emphasis should be placed on lowering his SBP to <140 mm Hg. D.C.'s DBP may decrease to <80 mm Hg with treatment since he is already <90 mm Hg. His cardiovascular risk would benefit from lowering his DBP to <80 mm Hg if he had diabetes or chronic kidney disease (he is close to, but not at, a GFR <60 mL/min), but should not be harmed unless DBP becomes excessively low.

THERAPY FOR HYPERTENSION

Lifestyle Modifications

12. **Which non-drug therapies can effectively lower BP?**

Lifestyle modifications can be used to lower BP. Independent of BP lowering, cardiovascular risk may also be reduced. These therapies are encouraged in all persons, but are especially recommended in patients with prehypertension or hypertension (Table 14-1)[1] and are summarized in Table 14-7. Aside from lowering BP, the progression to hypertension in patients with prehypertension might be prevented or minimized with lifestyle modification. There may be an opportunity to decrease the number or dose of antihypertensive medication(s) in patients who adhere to lifestyle modification.[54] Patient education, encouragement, and continued reinforcement are essential to successful lifestyle modification implementation and adherence.

Weight Reduction

Weight loss as small as 5% to 10% of body weight in overweight individuals may significantly lower cardiovascular risk.[72] In overweight hypertensive patients, clinical data estimate that for every 1 kg of weight loss, SBP and DBP can be lowered as much as 2.5 and 1.5 mm Hg, respectively.[73] For most patients, an average weight loss of 10 kg can reduce SBP by 5 to 20 mm Hg.[74] Larger reductions in BP have been

Table 14-7   Lifestyle Modifications to Manage Hypertension[1]

Modification	Recommendation
Weight reduction	Maintain normal body weight (BMI, 18.5 to 24.9 kg/m²)
Adopt DASH eating plan	Consume a diet rich in fruits, vegetables, and low-fat dairy products with a reduced content of saturated and total fat
Dietary sodium restriction	Reduce daily dietary sodium intake to ≤100 mEq (2.4 g sodium or 6 g sodium chloride)
Physical activity	Engage in regular aerobic physical activity (at least 30 min/day, most days of the week)
Moderate alcohol consumption	Limit consumption to ≤2 drinks/day (1 oz or 30 mL ethanol [e.g., 24 oz beer, 10 oz wine, 3 oz 80-proof whiskey] in most men and ≤1 drink/day in women and lighter-weight persons)

BMI, body mass index; DASH, Dietary Approaches to Stop Hypertension; SBP, systolic blood pressure.

demonstrated in hypertensive versus nonhypertensive patients with similar degrees of weight loss.[75]

DASH Diet

The DASH (Dietary Approaches to Stop Hypertension) diet is rich in fruits, vegetables, and low-fat dairy foods, coupled with reduced saturated and total fat.[76] This diet can substantially reduce BP (8 to 14 mm Hg in SBP for most patients) and yield similar results to single drug therapy.[76–78] The low-fat component of this diet is important as weight loss is more readily achieved by a low-fat diet and it also reduces the risk of CVD by improving cholesterol.[27,72]

Dietary Sodium Restriction

The average American intake of sodium is >6 g/day. Epidemiologic data show a positive relationship between sodium intake and BP.[79] Therefore, restricting sodium seems reasonable for hypertensive patients. However, the efficacy of implementing sodium restriction in hypertensive patients may vary. Evidence from clinical trials have shown that SBP reductions of 2 to 8 mm Hg can be achieved with restricting sodium intake to ≤2.4 g daily.[77,78,80,81] Some populations (diabetics, African Americans, and elderly persons) respond better to sodium restriction than the general population, but all patients with hypertension should be instructed to reduce their sodium intake. They should be counseled to not add salt to foods, and to avoid or minimize ingestion of processed or packaged foods, foods with high sodium content, and nonprescription drugs containing sodium (See Chapter 19, Heart Failure).

Physical Activity

Regular physical activity can reduce SBP by 4 to 9 mm Hg in most patients.[82,83] Benefits include reducing the incidence of hypertension, promoting weight loss, and improving overall cardiovascular fitness. Most hypertensive patients can safely increase their aerobic activity. However, those with more severe forms of cardiac target organ damage (e.g., angina, previous MI) may need a medical evaluation before increasing their activity level. Physical activity should occur for at least 30 minutes, 3 to 5 days of the week.[1,72] Aerobic exercise such as walking, running, cycling, swimming, cross-country skiing, and calisthenics are examples of physical activity that can be recommended.

Moderate Alcohol Consumption

Explaining the need to limit alcohol consumption is complicated. Whereas data suggest that small daily doses of ethanol are associated with lower cardiovascular risk, excessive alcohol intake can elevate BP, decrease the effectiveness of antihypertensive medications, and increase the risk of stroke. Patients who consume three to four drinks a day experience a 3- to 4-mm Hg increase in SBP and a 1- to 2-mm Hg increase in DBP compared to those who do not drink. These increases are even higher in patients who consume more alcohol. Moderating alcohol consumption of two or fewer drinks daily in men and one or fewer drinks daily in women or lighter weight persons can decrease SBP approximately 2 to 4 mm Hg.[84] Patients should be instructed that one drink is equal to 1 oz of ethanol (3 oz 80-proof whiskey, 8 oz wine, 24 oz beer).

Smoking Cessation

Smoking cessation is the most important and significant modifiable major cardiovascular risk factor in hypertension. Cigarette smoking independently has been shown to increase cardiovascular and overall mortality, and cessation can decrease the incidence of CVD.[85] Although smoking may not chronically alter BP, it interferes with the response to certain antihypertensive medications (e.g., β-blockers).[39,86] Hypertensive smokers should be continually educated about the risks associated with cigarette smoking and directed to behavior modification programs that can assist smoking cessation efforts (See Chapter 85, Tobacco Use and Dependence).

Unnecessary Modifications

The role of electrolyte supplementation with potassium, calcium, and magnesium in hypertension is unclear. Higher concentrations of these electrolytes correlate with lower BP values based on observational data, but a limited number of intervention trials have not demonstrated reduced cardiovascular risk.[22,87] Efforts should be made to maintain the patient's potassium concentration within the normal range, especially for patients taking potassium-wasting diuretics. It should be noted that potassium and magnesium supplementation in hypertensive patients with chronic kidney disease may be harmful. Electrolyte supplementation in this population could increase the risk of hyperkalemia and hypermagnesemia, which can lead to significant cardiac toxicity.

Caffeine ingestion has been associated with an acute elevation in BP. However, these elevations appear to be transient. Limitations on caffeine intake are not recommended unless caffeine ingestion is detrimental for other medical reasons (e.g., cardiac arrhythmias, panic attacks).

13. **Which lifestyle modifications should be recommended for D.C.?**

Weight reduction with dietary modifications and physical activity, sodium restriction, and smoking cessation are the most apparent lifestyle modifications for D.C. A thorough patient interview includes a diet history to quantify his intake of total calories, sodium, fat, and cholesterol. A social history should also be obtained to determine alcohol consumption and to confirm cigarette use. Based on these interviews, customized recommendations can be made.

The DASH diet should be strongly encouraged in D.C. Patient information explaining this regimen has been developed by the NHBPEP. Publications such as Facts About the DASH Eating Plan, are readily available on the NHLBI website (http://www.nhlbi.nih.gov/guidelines/hypertension/index.htm) and are written in language easily understood by most patients. D.C.'s body mass index (BMI) of ≥30 kg/m² classifies him as obese. He needs greater than a 16-kg weight loss to lower his weight classification to overweight. However, as little as a 5% to 10% loss in weight (5 to 10 kg) will provide global health benefits. Strategies that increase his aerobic activity, in addition to diet, can augment weight loss.

Antihypertensive Agents

Diuretics

Diuretics have been extensively studied in large clinical trials for hypertension. They have historically been the most commonly prescribed antihypertensive agents in the United States. When initially started, they induce a natriuresis that decreases plasma volume. Diuresis usually decreases after chronic use with some of these agents, especially with thiazide diuretics. However, the long-term BP lowering effects are maintained because of a sustained decrease in peripheral vascular resistance (PVR).

Overwhelming evidence from large outcome-based clinical trials indicates that diuretic therapy reduces morbidity and mortality rates.[1] Diuretics are generally well tolerated, and most can be given once daily. They are especially effective in lowering BP in elderly and African American patients. Dose-related biochemical alterations (e.g., hypokalemia, hyperuricemia, hyperglycemia, hypercholesterolemia) can occur with diuretics. These effects were particularly problematic when high doses of older agents were used (e.g., HCTZ 100 to 200 mg/day). Adverse effects are drastically minimized by using lower doses that are now considered the standard of care (e.g., HCTZ 12.5 to 25 mg).[57,88] Other biochemical changes in glucose and cholesterol are minimal and mostly transient with low-dose therapy.[89,90]

β-Blockers

β-Blockers have several direct effects on the cardiovascular system. They can decrease cardiac contractility and output, lower heart rate, blunt sympathetic reflex with exercise, reduce central release of adrenergic substances, inhibit norepinephrine release peripherally, and decrease renin release from the kidney. All these contribute to their antihypertensive effects. Adverse biochemical effects include altered lipids and increased glucose concentrations. However, similar to diuretics, these changes are generally temporary and have minimal to no clinical significance.[89]

Angiotensin-Converting Enzyme Inhibitors

ACE inhibitors directly inhibit angiotensin-converting enzyme and, therefore, block the conversion of angiotensin I to angiotensin II. This action reduces angiotensin II mediated vasoconstriction and aldosterone secretion, and ultimately lowers BP. Because there are additional pathways for the formation of angiotensin II, ACE inhibitors do not completely block the production of angiotensin II. These agents generally do not cause metabolic effects. However, hyperkalemia is possible and potassium concentrations should be monitored. Patients with chronic kidney disease or volume depletion may be more prone to hyperkalemia or to further progression of renal dysfunction. Bradykinin accumulates in some patients since inhibiting ACE prevents the breakdown and inactivation of bradykinin. Although this may lead to additive vasodilation by releasing nitrous oxide, bradykinin can also cause a dry cough in some patients. Cough is the most frequent, yet harmless side effect of ACE inhibitor therapy.

Angiotensin II Receptor Blockers

Angiotensin II receptor blockers (ARBs) are the newest antihypertensive agents. They modulate the renin-angiotensin-aldosterone system by directly blocking the angiotensin II type 1 receptor site. Therefore, they block angiotensin II mediated vasoconstriction and aldosterone release. Overall, ARBs are very well tolerated. They do not affect bradykinin and, therefore, do not cause a dry cough like ACE inhibitors. Since aldosterone is blocked, monitoring of potassium is important to avoid hypokalemia. Because they are all relatively new, none are available generically.

Aldosterone Antagonists

Spironolactone and eplerenone are two aldosterone antagonists, also classified as potassium sparing diuretics. Potent blockade of the aldosterone receptor inhibits sodium and water retention, and inhibits vasoconstriction.[91] Hyperkalemia is a known dose-dependent effect with these agents that is more prominent in patients with chronic kidney disease and with eplerenone (compared with spironolactone) because eplerenone is a more specific aldosterone blocker. Gynecomastia is a side effect of spironolactone that does not occur with eplerenone.

Calcium Channel Blockers

Calcium channel blockers (CCBs) are pharmacologically complex. They reduce calcium entry into smooth muscles, cause coronary and peripheral vasodilation, and lower BP. All have been shown to decrease cardiac contractility (except amlodipine). Dihydropyridine CCBs are primarily vasodilators that can cause a reflex tachycardia. Non-dihydropyridine CCBs (verapamil and diltiazem) directly block the AV node, decrease heart rate, decrease cardiac contraction, and have some vasodilatory effects. Side effects depend on the individual CCB used, but can include flushing, peripheral edema, tachycardia, bradycardia or heart block, and constipation.

α-Blockers

α-Blockers (doxazosin, prazosin, terazosin) attach to peripheral $α_1$-receptors, inhibit the uptake of catecholamines in smooth muscle, and cause vasodilation. Although effective in lowering BP, they have more side effects than diuretics, β-blockers, ACE inhibitors, ARBs, or CCBs. The most prominent side effect is hypotension, which is most evident after the first dose and with postural changes (arising from a lying position to a standing position).

Central α₂-Agonists

Central α_2-agonists (e.g., clonidine, methyldopa) work in the vasomotor centers of the brain where they stimulate inhibitory neurons, and decrease sympathetic outflow from the CNS. The resultant decrease in PVR and cardiac output lowers BP. These agents commonly cause anticholinergic side effects (e.g., sedation, dizziness, dry mouth, fatigue) and possibly sexual dysfunction. Although α_2-agonists lower BP, they often cause fluid retention. This might compromise BP control, and ideally they should be used in combination with a diuretic.

Adrenergic Antagonists

Adrenergic antagonists (reserpine, guanadrel, guanethidine) are not frequently used to treat hypertension. Reserpine depletes catecholamines from storage granules to decreases BP. Potential advantages include low cost and it can be given once daily. High doses are associated with more side effects, but low-dose reserpine (0.05 to 0.1 mg/day), when used as third-line therapy has been shown to be well tolerated.[52] Due to the potential for fluid retention, reserpine generally requires concurrent diuretic therapy. Guanadrel and guanethidine have numerous significant adverse effects and should be avoided.

Arterial Vasodilators

Direct vasodilators (hydralazine, minoxidil) work on the arterial vasculature. They are considered last-line therapy, reserved for patients with specific indications or very difficult to control BP. Fluid retention and reflex tachycardia are frequent side effects. Concomitant therapy with both a diuretic and an agent that lowers heart rate (a β-blocker, diltiazem, or verapamil) are usually needed.

14. **Should D.C. start antihypertensive drug therapy, or should lifestyle modifications be his primary treatment?**

It is reasonable to assume that lifestyle modifications can partially help D.C. achieve his BP goal. Previous JNC guidelines recommended lifestyle modifications for 6 to 12 months before starting drug therapy in patients with few to no risk factors and no target organ damage.[54] D.C. not only has several major risk factors for developing hypertension-related complications, he has evidence of target organ damage. Although lifestyle modifications are germane to the appropriate treatment of hypertension, they have not been shown to prevent CVD in hypertensive patients.[65] The initiation of drug therapy should not be delayed unnecessarily, especially for patients with cardiovascular risk factors.[65] D.C. has stage 1 hypertension with risk factors and should start drug therapy (see Table 14-1) along with lifestyle modification.

SELECTING DRUG THERAPY

Evidence-Based Medicine in Hypertension

15. **Which treatment principles need to be considered when choosing an initial antihypertensive agent for D.C.?**

Selecting an antihypertensive is difficult considering the numerous choices. All antihypertensive agents can effectively lower BP. Depending on the dose used, pressure reductions are similar.[92] However, BP reduction is only a surrogate endpoint of therapy that does not necessarily reflect overall efficacy. Reducing hypertension-related complications (target organ damage) is the ultimate goal of treatment. Evidence-based medicine is the conscientious, explicit, and judicious use of current best-evidence in making decisions about the care of individual patients.[93] Practicing evidence-based medicine in hypertension requires a balance between weighing the findings from outcome-based studies showing reduced hypertension-related complications and considering specific drug therapies for each patient's individual situation.

The JNC 7 report outlines drug therapy recommendations that follow an evidence-based approach. These recommendations are based on the interpretation of clinical trials. A thiazide-type diuretic, either alone or in combination with another antihypertensive (depending on hypertension stage), is the initial drug choice recommendation of the JNC 7 for most patients, as depicted in Figure 14-3.[1] This recommendation is based on the propensity of data showing reduced morbidity and mortality with thiazide-type diuretics.[57] ACE inhibitors, ARBs, β-blocker, and CCBs also have been shown to reduce hypertension-related complications.[57,64,94–100] They are recommended in the treatment of hypertension, especially if there is a *compelling indication* for their use. This concept is discussed later in the Hypertension With Compelling Indications section.

Hypertension in Most Patients

Three older landmark placebo-controlled hypertension studies (the Systolic Hypertension in the Elderly Program [SHEP],[52] Swedish Trial of Old Patients with Hypertension [STOP-hypertension],[61] and Medical Research Council [MRC][62]) showed significant reductions in stroke (25% to 47%, $P < 0.05$), heart attacks (13% to 27%, $P < 0.05$), and all cause CVD (17% to 40%, $P < 0.05$) with thiazide-type diuretic-based therapy. Most importantly, these studies found improvement in survival. Several clinical trials evaluating newer agents (ACE inhibitors, ARBs, and CCBs) provide new evidence on cardiovascular event reduction.[11,64,66,94–96,98–112] In those studies in which newer antihypertensive agents were compared to thiazide-type diuretics, very similar effects were seen, with ACE inhibitors possibly showing better effects.[99,113] Most of these newer trials do not include a placebo group (since this is unethical) and use prospective open-label, blinded endpoint (PROBE) study methodology that is not double-blinded. Therefore, ability of these data to prove equivalence is somewhat limited.

16. **What recent evidence supports the use of thiazide-type diuretics to treat hypertension?**

The ALLHAT Study

The Antihypertensive and Lipid-Lowering Treatment to Prevent Heart Attack Trial (ALLHAT) was a prospective double-blind trial that randomized hypertensive patients to chlorthalidone, amlodipine, doxazosin or lisinopril for planned follow-up of approximately 4 to 8 years.[96] This was the largest hypertension trial ever conducted and included 42,418 patients. The primary objective was to compare combined endpoint of fatal CHD and nonfatal MI in patients randomized to these four therapies. Other hypertension-related complications were evaluated as secondary endpoints.

The doxazosin arm was terminated prematurely because of a significantly increased risk of HF.[114] However, the other arms were continued as scheduled for a mean of 4.9 years. At the end of the study, there were no significant differences in the

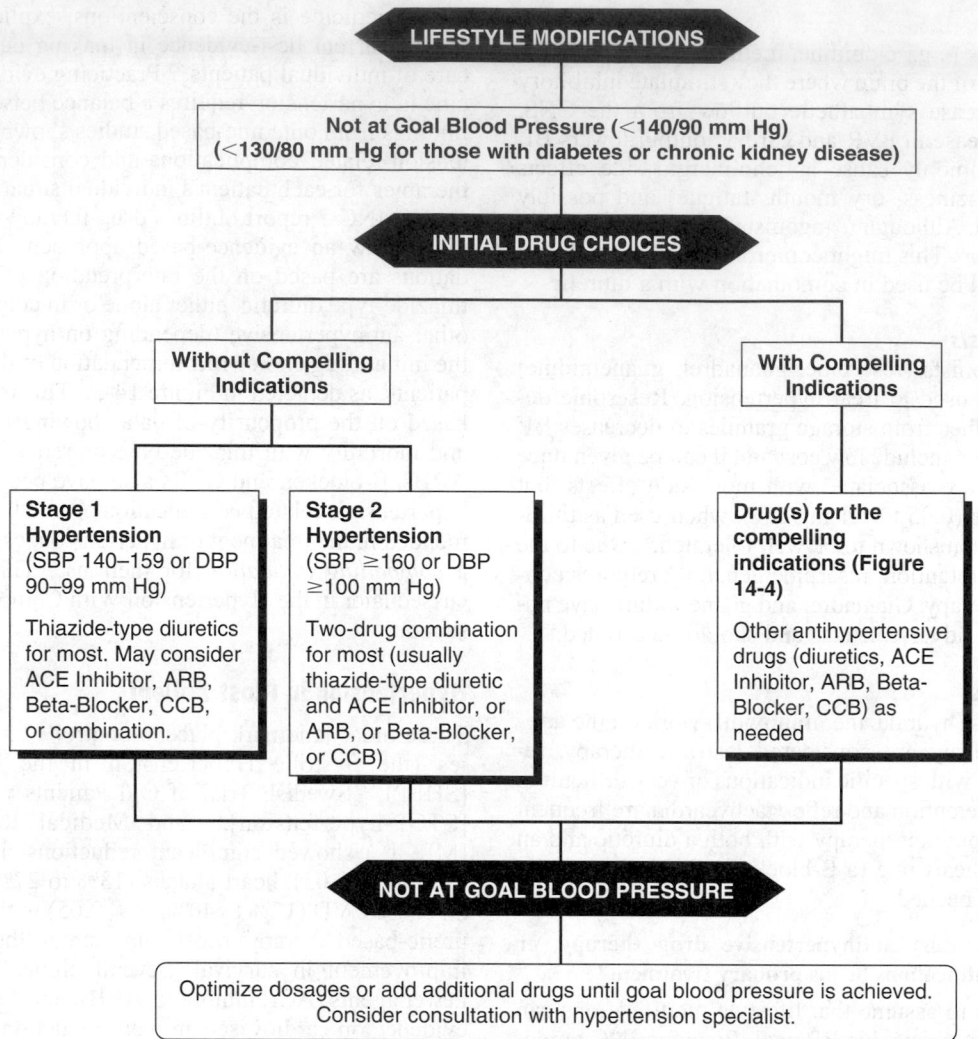

FIGURE 14-3 Algorithm for treatment of hypertension.[1]

primary endpoint between chlorthalidone and either lisinopril or amlodipine. However, secondary endpoints statistically favored the thiazide over both amlodipine (less HF) and lisinopril (less combined CVD, HF, and stroke). Investigators concluded that thiazide-type diuretics are superior in preventing one or more major forms of CVD and are less expensive.

The ALLHAT data is the primary justification for the thiazide-type diuretic recommendation by the JNC 7. Unlike other comparative studies, the ALLHAT was double-blinded and provided more scientific rigor to their results. However, not all agencies agree with this recommendation. The 2003 European Society of Hypertension-European Society of Cardiology guidelines for the management of arterial hypertension do not support thiazide diuretics as a superior drug class. Instead they advocate that target organ and survival benefits of therapy are a function of BP lowering that are largely independent of the specific drug(s) used.[65] They cite limitations of the ALLHAT as reasons to support BP control over recommending specific drug classes. These limitations include a high percentage of previously treated patients, differences (1 to 4 mm Hg) in BP values between regimens, racial diversity of the population, unreasonable add-on therapy (e.g., β-blockers, clonidine, reserpine), and excessive reliance on HF as an endpoint.

Often forgotten is that the ALLHAT was designed as a superiority study with the hypothesis that the newer agents (amlodipine, doxazosin, and lisinopril) would be better than chlorthalidone in reducing combined fatal CHD or nonfatal MI.[115] In the strictest sense of study interpretation, the ALLHAT did not prove this hypothesis since there were no statistical differences in the primary endpoint. Thiazide-type diuretics were unsurpassed in their ability to reduce hypertension-related complications before the ALLHAT and remain unsurpassed based on the findings of the ALLHAT. This has been reinforced by a 2003 meta-analysis of 42 clinical trials that found that low-dose diuretics were the most effective first-line treatment for preventing CVD and mortality.[57] Evidence supports the JNC 7 recommendation of using a thiazide-type diuretic, unless there are contraindications or if a compelling indication for another agent is present.

Hypertension With Compelling Indications

Throughout the remainder of this chapter the term *compelling indications* will be used frequently. The JNC 7 identifies certain compelling indications that are defined as diseases/situations for which antihypertensive classes may be specifically indicated based on evidence from clinical trials. Although these clinical trials may not have evaluated hypertension-related complications alone, they show significant benefits in reducing morbidity and/or mortality that warrant their use in a hypertensive patient with a given compelling indication (see Fig. 14-4). The drug therapy recommendation(s) for the compelling indication is/are recommended in addition to, or in place of, a thiazide-type diuretic. Each of the compelling indications is identified below.

Heart Failure

Systolic HF is a common complication of hypertension in which cardiac contractility is compromised.[32] Diuretics and ACE inhibitors have traditionally been recommended as the drugs of choice based on numerous outcome studies showing reduced morbidity and mortality rates.[116] Diuretics provide primarily symptomatic benefit, but as systolic HF progresses, loop diuretics are almost always needed. ACE inhibitors have been shown to modify HF by reducing morbidity and mortality and are a part of first-line systolic HF therapy.[117–119] However, β-blocker therapy has evolved as additional treatment that modifies HF by reducing morbidity and mortality and is an important component in managing these patients.[120–123]

Other antihypertensive agents reduce cardiovascular risk in this patient population. It was speculated that ARBs would be even better than ACE inhibitors in systolic HF,[124] but when compared head-to-head, ACE inhibitors were found to provide better outcomes.[125] However, data support the role of ARBs in HF as a very effective alternative for ACE-intolerant patients.[126] Aldosterone blockers such as spironolactone (in severe HF) and eplerenone (post-MI with left ventricular dysfunction) reduced morbidity and mortality rates in clinical trials.[127,128] These two agents should be considered in appropriate patients only after diuretics, ACE/ARBs, and β-blockers are utilized (See Chapter 19, Heart Failure).

Post-Myocardial Infarction

Many patients with hypertension experience an MI. The American College of Cardiology/American Heart Association guidelines recommend β-blocker and ACE inhibitor therapy in post-MI patients to prevent recurrent cardiovascular events.[129] β-Blockers (those without ISA) decrease the risk of a subsequent MI or sudden cardiac death by decreasing the adrenergic burden on the heart.[120,130] An ACE inhibitor promotes cardiac remodeling, improved cardiac function, and reduces cardiovascular events.[97,131] Eplerenone is the most recent drug shown to reduce morbidity and mortality in post-MI patients with symptoms of left ventricular dysfunction[128] (See Chapter 18, Myocardial Infarction).

High Coronary Disease Risk

Coronary disease presents as ischemic heart disease (chronic stable angina or MI). It is the most common form of target organ disease in hypertension. Patients with a history of stable angina pectoris should be managed first-line with a β-blocker to improve myocardial oxygen consumption and decrease demand.[1] A long acting CCB can be used as an alternative. Evolving information from the International Verapamil SR/Trandolapril (INVEST) study suggests there is no difference between β-blocker and CCB-based therapy in this population.[131a] For patients with acute coronary syndromes (non-ST segment elevation MI and unstable angina), BP should be managed first with a β-blocker and ACE inhibitor.[129] Diuretics can be added for BP if goal is not met with a first line agent (See Chapter 17, Ischemic Heart Disease: Anginal Syndromes).

Diabetes

Kidney disease (especially with type 1 diabetes) and CVD (especially with type 2 diabetes) are long-term complication of diabetes. Evidence shows many benefits of antihypertensive agents in diabetes: thiazide-type diuretics, β-blockers,

Compelling Indication	Diuretic	Beta-blocker	ACE inhibitor	ARB	CCB	Aldosterone antagonist
Heart failure	✓	✓	✓	✓		✓
Post-myocardial infarction		✓	✓			✓
High coronary disease risk	✓	✓	✓		✓	
Diabetes	✓	✓	✓	✓	✓	
Chronic kidney disease			✓	✓		
Recurrent stroke prevention	✓		✓			

FIGURE 14-4 Compelling indications for individual drug classes.[1] Compelling indications for antihypertensive drugs are based on benefits from outcome studies or existing clinical guidelines; the compelling indication should be managed in parallel with BP.

ACE, angiotensin converting enzyme; ARB, angiotensin receptor blocker; CCB, calcium channel blocker.

and ACE inhibitors reduce coronary events; β-blockers, ACE inhibitors, and ARBs reduce progression of kidney disease; and thiazide-type diuretics, β-blockers, ACE inhibitors, and CCBs (specifically dihydropyridine CCBs) reduce stoke.[8,9,96,107] When compared head-to-head, ACE inhibitors are superior to dihydropyridine CCBs at reducing cardiovascular events.[105,106] Subanalyses of larger clinical trials further support cardiovascular event reduction with ACE inhibitors and ARBs[132,133] (See Chapter 50, Diabetes Mellitus).

Patients with diabetes have an aggressive BP goal of <130/80 mm Hg. Numerous clinical trial have shown that tighter BP control in diabetes minimizes complications.[11,104,134] However, to get to these lower BP goals, two or more antihypertensive drugs are almost always needed.[8] ACE inhibitors (or alternatively an ARB) in combination with a diuretic are considered reasonable first-line agents when treating hypertension in patients with diabetes. This combination has consistently demonstrated cardiovascular risk reduction.

Chronic Kidney Disease
Chronic kidney disease initially presents as microalbuminuria (30 to 299 mg albumin in a 24-hour urine collection) that can progress to overt kidney failure.[35] Progression is expedited in both hypertension and diabetes. ACE inhibitors and ARBs reduce the progression of chronic kidney disease in type 1 diabetes,[135] in type 2 diabetes,[101,108–110] and in those without diabetes.[8,112,136] Patients with an estimated GFR <60 mL/min/m^2 or with albuminuria (see section on BP Values) have chronic kidney disease and an aggressive BP goal of <130/80 mm Hg.[1] At this point, risk of CVD and deterioration of kidney function increases. These patients typically require three or more antihypertensive agents which should include an ACE inhibitor or ARB with a diuretic and a third antihypertensive drug class (e.g., β-blocker or calcium channel blocker).[8,112]

Recurrent Stroke Prevention
Lowering BP to goal in patients with a history of stroke is beneficial once patients have stabilized after their acute event. Clinical trials data from the Perindopril protection against recurrent stroke study (PROGRESS) show that the combination of an ACE inhibitor with a thiazide-type diuretic reduces the incidence of recurrent stroke.[98] This event reduction was seen even in patients who were at goal BP values, which is consis-

tent with other studies using ACE inhibitor therapy in high-risk patients when at goal BP values.[97]

Other High-Risk Patients
Left Ventricular Hypertrophy
LVH independently increases the risk of CVD in patients with hypertension. As previously discussed, all antihypertensives along with appropriate BP control will help in regression of LVH. However, the clinical significance of this is unclear. One outcome-based study, the Losartan Intervention For Endpoint reduction in hypertension (LIFE) trial, prospectively evaluated losartan versus atenolol in patients with LVH and hypertension. Losartan was superior to atenolol in reducing the combined endpoint of stroke, MI, and death.[95] However, specific drug therapy recommendations for patients with LVH are not provided by the JNC 7.

Peripheral Arterial Disease
Patients with peripheral arterial disease have a risk for CHD that is equivalent to a patient with a history of MI.[27] Achievement of goal BP and aggressive management of risk factors (e.g., smoking cessation, dyslipidemia management) are important in the overall management of this population, but no specific antihypertensive class has been shown to be better than another in reducing morbidity or mortality. Antiplatelet therapy provides additional risk reduction to patients with peripheral arterial disease (See Chapter 15, Peripheral Vascular Disorders).

Additional Considerations
Potential Favorable/Unfavorable Effects
When looking beyond a thiazide-type diuretic, or when a compelling indication does not direct the clinician to one specific drug class, choices can be narrowed by selecting an agent that has potentially favorable effects (other than BP reduction) and/or by avoiding an agent that may elicit potentially unfavorable effects. These are summarized in Table 14-8. For example, consider a patient with hypertension, asthma, and benign prostatic hyperplasia (prostatism) who has uncontrolled BP while taking the maximum dose of a thiazide. Adding an α-blocker might have a favorable effect on benign prostatic hyperplasia, while a β-blocker could have an unfavorable ef-

Table 14-8 Additional Considerations in Antihypertensive Drug Choice[1] (in addition to compelling indications in Table 14-7)

Antihypertensive Agent	Potential Favorable Effects	Potential Unfavorable Effects[a]
Thiazide-type diuretics	Osteoporosis	Gout, hyponatremia
β-Blockers	Atrial tachyarrhythmias/fibrillation, migraine, thyrotoxicosis, essential tremor, preoperative hypertension	Asthma/reactive airways disease exacerbation, heart block
ACE inhibitors		Teratogenic effects, history of angioedema
Angiotensin II receptor blockers		Teratogenic effects
Aldosterone Antagonists		Hyperkalemia (as with other potassium-sparring diuretics)
Calcium channel blockers	Raynaud's syndrome, arrhythmias (verapamil and diltiazem only)	
α$_1$-Antagonists	Prostatism	

[a]May require special monitoring.

fect on asthma. Therefore, an α-blocker would be a reasonable choice. Other agents such as calcium channel blockers, ACE inhibitors, or ARBs could also be chosen, but they would not have the extra benefit of having a favorable effect on this patient's comorbid illness.

Cost

The costs of treating hypertension and related complications are substantial to patients and health systems. These include expenses for diagnostic laboratory evaluations, office visits, and medication. Selecting therapy should balance patient-specific information with documented evidence-based benefit on morbidity and mortality. Cost of a given regimen is another significant consideration and may be a deciding factor when two or more agents offer similar benefits. Whenever possible, inexpensive regimens that do not compromise efficacy should be designed. Generic products are usually much less expensive than brand-name products. ARBs are the only antihypertensives for which there is not a generic alternative within the given drug class.

Convenience

The frequency of administration of antihypertensive medications must be considered because it can influence patients' lifestyle and adherence to regimens. Once-daily administration maximizes compliance and is most desirable. Twice-daily administration may be acceptable but is less desirable. Studies have found that compliance is highest with once once-daily (86% to 87%), followed by twice-daily (78% to 81%), three-times-daily (58% to 77%), and four-times-daily (39% to 46%) dosing.[58,59,137,138] All major antihypertensive drug classes offer a once-daily product, so optimizing regimens is feasible.

Demographic Factors
AFRICAN AMERICAN PATIENTS

17. **D.C. is a middle-aged African American man. How does knowledge of this information influence the choice of therapy? What other factors should be considered?**

African American patients have a higher incidence of hypertension, hypertension-related complications, and an increased need for combination therapy to achieve and maintain BP goals.[1,2,139] It is well documented in this population that monotherapy with β-blockers, ACE inhibitors, or ARBs does not lower BP as much as it does in white patients. When these agents are used in combination, especially with a thiazide-type diuretic, BP lowering is greatly improved. Thiazide-type diuretics and CCBs are the most effective antihypertensives in lowering BP in African Americans.

The Hypertension in African American Working Group (HAAWG) of the International Society on Hypertension in Blacks recommendations are similar to the JNC 7 relative to lifestyle modifications and drug therapy selection (Figs. 14-3 and 14-4; Table 14-8).[1,139] However, they recommend combination therapy when SBP values are ≥15 mm Hg above goal (versus ≥20 mm Hg from the JNC 7). These more aggressive recommendations are reasonable strategies for optimal control. African American patients are also at higher risk of side effects with ACE inhibitors (both angioedema and cough) compared with whites.[96] The best antihypertensives for lowering D.C.'s BP are either a thiazide-type diuretic or a CCB. A

thiazide-type diuretic is recommended based on evidence and should be used to treat his hypertension.

ELDERLY PATIENTS

D.C. is only 52 years old. Older hypertensive patients (older than 65 years of age) have the lowest rates of BP control.[2,30] In the past, it was believed that elderly patients responded better to diuretics and CCBs and poorly to β-blockers and ACE inhibitors. However, numerous studies refute these generalities.[59,61,99,100] They should be viewed as medical myths rather than realities.

The elderly are at risk for ISH. In earlier JNC recommendations, BP goals for ISH and drug selection advocated slow introduction of medications that would cause gradual SBP reductions to minimize further decreases in DBP.[54] The use of thiazide-type diuretics and long-acting dihydropyridine CCBs were preferred based on the evidence of reduced hypertension-related complications.[52,54,64] The JNC 7 recommends that elderly patients be managed according to the same general treatment philosophies as for other patients with hypertension, as previously described.[1] Whereas lower starting doses may be needed to minimize the risk of side effects, elderly patients eventually need standard treatment doses and often require combination therapy to reach and maintain their BP goals.

Starting Drug Therapy
Monotherapy

Starting with one drug to treat hypertension is recommended when initial BP is close to goal values. The JNC 7 defines this as within 20 mm Hg of the SBP goal and within 10 mm Hg of the DBP goal. This would encompass patients with stage 1 hypertension and a BP goal <140/90 mm Hg (Fig. 14-3). However, other guidelines define a narrower range.[8,139] The HAAWG (for African Americans) and the National Kidney Foundation (for patients with diabetes) define close to goal (and a range at which starting a single agent is reasonable) as within 15 mm Hg of the SBP and within 10 mm Hg of the DBP.

STEPPED-CARE APPROACH

The stepped-care approach has traditionally been used when initiating therapy. A single agent is selected with the dose increased until BP is controlled, the maximum dose is reached, or dose-limiting toxicity occurs. If the goal BP is not achieved, a second drug from a different class is added. Theoretically, this process can be continued, if necessary, until three or even four drugs are used in combination.

18. **If D.C. started monotherapy using a stepped-care approach, how likely would it be that he would achieve his goal BP of <140/90 mm Hg?**

The Veterans Affairs (VA) Cooperative Studies Group on Antihypertensive Agents evaluated single-drug therapy (atenolol, captopril, clonidine, diltiazem, HCTZ, and prazosin) versus placebo in patients with stage 1 or 2 hypertension.[50] With single-agent therapy started and titrated to maximum doses (data combined for all drugs), 58.7% of patients reached a DBP <90 mm Hg. After 1 year of frequent medical follow-up, approximately 50% maintained a DBP of <90 mm

Hg. These results may overestimate what is seen in clinical practice because of the rigorous study design used. D.C. has stage 1 hypertension. Thiazide monotherapy could result in BP control, but close follow-up is essential because he has numerous risk factors and goal achievement is not guaranteed.

SEQUENTIAL THERAPY

The sequential therapy approach is similar to the stepped-care approach in that an agent is started and titrated to the maximum dose as needed. If goal BP is not achieved, an alternative agent is selected to replace the first. Combination drug therapy is reserved for patients who do not achieve goal BP values after the second agent. Sequential therapy seems most appropriate when the first drug is either poorly tolerated or results in minimal or no reduction in BP.

19. **If D.C. did not achieve his BP goal with a thiazide-type diuretic, how likely is it that he will get to goal with a second agent as monotherapy?**

The VA Cooperative Studies Group on Antihypertensive Agents evaluated sequential therapy in a follow-up to the single-drug therapy study.[140] Only an additional 49% of the nonresponders to the first agent achieved a DBP <90 mm Hg when switched to a second drug. Putting this into perspective, in patients requiring a moderate reduction in SBP (approximately 10 to 20 mm Hg), up to 80% of patients will have their hypertension controlled after a trial of two different agents. Although this appears good, in clinical practice, this high success rate is not likely to occur. If D.C. was not at goal with his first agent, a reasonable approach would be to add on a second agent, assuming that the first agent gave at least a partial effect and was well tolerated.

Combination Therapy

Starting therapy with a combination of two drugs is now strongly encouraged for certain patients. This approach is recommended for all patients with stage 2 hypertension or those who are far from their goal (e.g., ≥20 mm Hg from SBP goal or ≥10 mm Hg from DBP goal, according to JNC 7).[1] Initial combination therapy is also an option for patients in whom goal achievement may be difficult (i.e., diabetes, chronic kidney disease, African Americans) or in complex patients in whom there are multiple compelling indications for different antihypertensive agents. This is a significant change in the new guidelines. It is justified by the observation that most patients with hypertension do not have the condition controlled, and most patients require two or more agents.[1,8,30,65]

IDEAL COMBINATIONS

The JNC 7 recommends that the initial two-drug regimen should include a thiazide-type diuretic. Moreover, when selecting a second agent as add-on therapy for additional BP reduction, a diuretic should be added as the second drug if it was not the first drug added and if there are no contraindications. This does not always apply if the second drug is being added to treat a compelling indication, although most patients will respond to a two-drug regimen if it includes a diuretic.[1,65] By appropriately selecting combination regimens, many patients can achieve their BP goal with the combination of two drugs. However, patients with aggressive BP goals (diabetes and chronic renal disease) commonly require a third agent.[8]

ORTHOSTATIC HYPOTENSION

Orthostatic hypotension occurs when standing up results in a SBP decrease >10 mm Hg and is accompanied by dizziness or fainting.[1] This is a risk of aggressive BP lowering. Orthostatic hypotension is more frequent in older patients (especially those with ISH), diabetes, autonomic dysfunction, and in patients taking certain drugs (diuretics, nitrates, α-blockers, sildenafil, or psychotropic agents). Combination therapy can still be used in these patients, but close evaluation is needed. Dose titration should be gradual and caution applied to minimize the risk of hypotension and to avoid volume depletion.

Monitoring Therapy

When evaluating antihypertensive therapy, four aspects must always be considered: 1) BP response, 2) adherence, 3) progression of illness, and 4) toxicity. This includes determining whether the desired therapeutic goal has been achieved, whether the patient is complying with prescribed medications and lifestyle modifications, if new target organ damage has developed (or whether present damage has worsened), and if adverse reactions have occurred.

BP control should be evaluated 1 to 4 weeks after starting or modifying therapy for most patients. BP usually begins to fall within 1 to 2 weeks of starting an agent, but steady-state antihypertensive effects typically take up to 4 weeks. If patients have experienced a hypertensive crisis, evaluation should occur sooner. For example, hypertensive emergencies are triaged for hospitalized care, and BP response is evaluated with continuous monitoring. For patients with hypertensive urgency (BP values in the upper range of stage 2 hypertension without signs of acute target organ damage), BP response to treatment should be assessed within 3 to 7 days.

Two BP values should be measured to evaluate response, with the average of the two used to properly make an assessment. Ideally, BP measurements should be made in both the seated and standing positions to detect orthostatic changes, but if symptoms of dizziness are absent, this is not necessary. If home BP monitoring values are available, these should also be considered, but are expected to be slightly lower than clinic values.

All patients should be questioned in a nonthreatening manner regarding adherence to lifestyle modifications and drug therapy. This is especially important for complex regimens, when drug intolerance is likely, or when financial or insurance constraints hinder acquisition of medications. Medical evaluation to assess target organ damage and drug side effects is essential. The presence of new target organ damage may necessitate modification of therapy. Drug therapy may require changes based on the need to treat a compelling indication or target a new BP goal. The presence of drug-related side effects might similarly result in the need to modify therapy.

CLINICAL SCENARIOS

Diuretics

20. **B.A. is a 65-year-old white woman who presents to her family physician for hypertension management. She is postmenopausal, does not smoke, and never drinks alcohol. Since being diagnosed with hypertension, she has modified her diet, begun routine aerobic exercise, and has lost 10 kg over the past 18**

months. She now weighs 72 kg and is 65 inches tall. Her present BP is 152/94 mm Hg and has consistently remained near this value over the past year. Her BP when first diagnosed was 158/94 mm Hg. There is no evidence of LVH or retinopathy. Urinalysis is negative for protein. Other laboratory tests are normal, except for slightly elevated cholesterol. B.A. has no health insurance and is concerned about the cost of therapy. She takes over-the-counter calcium with vitamin D to strengthen her bones (she also has osteoporosis) and is to start a thiazide-type diuretic for hypertension. Why is a thiazide-type diuretic, but not a loop diuretic, appropriate for her?

Several types of diuretics are used to manage hypertension (Table 14-9). All lower BP, with the primary differences being duration of action, potency of diuresis, and potential for electrolyte abnormalities.

Thiazides
Thiazide-type diuretics are the diuretics of choice for hypertension. Goal BP values <140/90 mm Hg are achieved in 45% to 80% of patients who take these drugs.[50,140,141] Hydrochlorothiazide (HCTZ) and chlorthalidone have been used in several major outcome trials including the ALLHAT.[1,57,96,99] They are viewed as interchangeable with no reason to choose one over the other. HCTZ is most frequently used in the United States, is very inexpensive, and is dosed once daily. Chlorthalidone may be slightly more potent on a mg per mg basis, but this difference has questionable clinical relevance. The usual starting dose of HCTZ or chlorthalidone is a low-dose of 12.5 or 25 mg once daily. Maintenance doses of 25 mg once daily can lower SBP by 15 to 20 mm Hg and DBP by 8 to 15 mm Hg, with a low incidence of side effects.[50,57,92,140] The propensity of evidence showing benefit with thiazide-type diuretics is with low-dose therapy, considered to be the equivalent of HCTZ or chlorthalidone 12.5 mg to 25 mg daily.[57]

Loop Diuretics
Loop diuretics produce a more potent diuresis, a smaller decrease in PVR, and less vasodilation than thiazide-type diuretics. HCTZ is more effective at lowering BP than loop diuretics in most patients.[142,143] Furosemide, the most frequently used loop diuretic, has a short duration of effect and should be given two or three times daily when used in hypertension. Loop diuretics are the diuretics of choice for hypertensive patients with severe chronic kidney disease or failure (an estimated GFR <30 mL/min/1.73 m² or a serum creatinine of 2.5 to 3.0 mg/dL). Loop diuretics are also the preferred agent for patients with HF or severe edema that require diuresis.

Potassium-Sparing Diuretics
Potassium-sparing diuretics (especially amiloride and triamterene) are reserved for patients who develop hypokalemia while taking a diuretic. With low-dose thiazide-type diuretics, <25% of patients develop hypokalemia, and most cases are not severe. Several fixed-dose products are available that include HCTZ with a potassium-sparing agent. However, empirically starting all diuretic treated hypertensive patients on one of these fixed-dose combination products to avoid hypokalemia is not rational. Potassium-sparing diuretics have modest antihypertensive effects, compared with thiazide-type diuretics, when used as monotherapy.

Aldosterone Receptor Blockers
Spironolactone and eplerenone are considered aldosterone receptor blockers. Similar to potassium sparing diuretics, they can increase potassium and cause hyperkalemia. When used in hypertension, increases in potassium are small in most patients. However, this risk increases in patients with chronic kidney disease because they have a propensity to accumulate potassium.

Eplerenone is more specific than spironolactone in aldosterone blockade.[91,144] Compared to spironolactone, gyneco-

Table 14-9 Diuretics in Hypertension

Category	Selected Products	Usual Dosage Range (mg/day)[a]	Dosing Frequency
Thiazide	Chlorthalidone (Hygroton)	12.5–25	QD
	Hydrochlorothiazide (Esidrix, Hydrodiuril, Microzide)	12.5–50[b]	QD
	Indapamide (Lozol)[c]	1.25–5	QD
	Metolazone (Zaroxolyn)	2.5–10	QD
	Metolazone (Mykrox)	0.5–1.0	QD
Loop[b]	Bumetanide (Bumex)	0.5–4	BID
	Furosemide (Lasix)	20–80	BID
	Torsemide (Demadex)	2.5–10	QD
Potassium-sparing	Amiloride (Midamor)	5–10	QD to BID
	Triamterene (Dyrenium)	50–100	QD to BID
Aldosterone Receptor Blockers	Eplerenone (Inspra)	50–100	QD to BID
	Spironolactone (Aldactone)	25–50	QD to BID
Diuretic combinations	Triamterene/Hydrochlorothiazide (Maxide, Dyazide)	37.5–75/25–50	QD
	Spironolactone/Hydrochlorothiazide (Aldactazide)	25–50/25–50	QD
	Amiloride/Hydrochlorothiazide (Moduretic)	5–10/50–100	QD

[a]Geriatric patients may be more sensitive and require lower doses.
[b]25 mg/day is generally the maximum effective dose in hypertension.
[c]Metolazone and loop diuretics are no more effective than thiazides, except in patients with severe chronic kidney disease or failure (estimated GFR <30 ml/min/1.73 m²)

mastia is not a frequent side effect. However, the incidence of hyperkalemia is greater with eplerenone, thus it is contraindicated in populations at high risk for hyperkalemia. This includes type 2 diabetes with microalbuminuria, an estimated creatinine clearance <50 mL/min, or elevated serum creatinine (>1.8 mg/dL in women and >2.0 mg/dL in men). These agents are indicated for hypertension, but their greatest use may be in HF because of evidence showing reduced morbidity and mortality.[127,128] This evidence shows that spironolactone is beneficial in more severe HF patients who have experienced decompensation,[127] whereas eplerenone reduces mortality in patients with HF and LV dysfunction soon after MI.[128]

21. **How should a thiazide-type diuretic be started in B.A.?**

Monotherapy with a thiazide-type diuretic is best for B.A. She is stage 1 based on her BP, has no apparent additional risks for hypertension-related complications, no apparent target organ damage, and no compelling indications for other agents. Thiazide-type diuretics have evidence to support their use and are recommended as first-line treatment in most patients (Fig. 14-3), especially after lifestyle modifications. She has no contraindications to diuretic therapy (Table 14-10). Her cholesterol is moderately elevated, but thiazide-type diuretics are unlikely to have a clinically significant effect on

cholesterol when used in low doses.[89,90] B.A.'s osteoporosis may benefit from a thiazide (unlike a loop diuretic) because of retention of calcium and improved bone density (Table 14-8).

HCTZ is available generically at low cost. An appropriate starting dose for B.A. is 25 mg daily. Lifestyle modifications have reduced her BP, but she still requires >10 mm Hg reduction in SBP. It is unlikely that 12.5 mg daily will get her to goal. She has no additional risks for orthostatic hypotension, so starting at 25 mg daily is safe.

Patient Education

22. **B.A. is prescribed HCTZ 25 mg daily. How should she be counseled regarding this therapy?**

Several counseling points regarding hypertension need to be included when counseling B.A., as summarized in Table 14-6. She should be encouraged to continue these efforts to maximize her response to drug therapy. Some patients disregard lifestyle modifications when they start antihypertensive therapy. Education before starting and during drug therapy should focus on beneficial effects of lifestyle modification.

Drug-specific counseling for diuretics includes informing B.A. that diuretics effectively lower BP and that taking her daily dose at about the same time each morning is best to

Table 14-10 Side Effects and Contraindications of Antihypertensive Agents

	Side Effects		
	Innocuous but Sometimes Annoying	Harmful or Potentially Harmful	Contraindications
Oral Diuretics Thiazide type	↑ urination (onset of therapy), weakness, muscle cramps, hyperuricemia (sometimes with gout), GI disturbances	Hypokalemia,[a] hyponatremia,[b] hyperglycemia, hypercalcemia,[b] hypovolemia, azotemia[b] (↑ BUN), skin rash[b] (cross-reacts with sulfa drugs), photosensitivity,[b] purpura,[b] marrow depression,[b] lithium toxicity[b] (patients on lithium therapy), pancreatitis, hypercholesterolemia, hypertriglyceridemia	Persistent anuria/oliguria, advanced kidney failure
Loop diuretics	↑ urination (onset of therapy), weakness, muscle cramps, hyperuricemia (sometimes with gout), GI disturbances	Hypokalemia,[a] hyponatremia,[b] hyperglycemia, hypocalcemia,[b] hypovolemia, azotemia[b] (↑ BUN), skin rash[b] (cross-reacts with sulfa drugs), photosensitivity,[b] lithium toxicity[b] (patients on lithium therapy), pancreatitis, hypercholesterolemia, hypertriglyceridemia. Hearing loss with large IV doses	Not contraindicated in kidney failure
Aldosterone Antagonists	Hirsutism, menstrual irregularities,[c] gynecomastia,[c] GI disturbances	Hyperkalemia,[b] hyponatremia[b]	Kidney failure (eplerenone is contraindicated with CrCl <50 ml/min, Type 2 diabetes with proteinuria, and elevated serum creatinine [>1.8 in women, >2.0 in men]), hyperkalemia, hyponatremia

Table 14-10 Side Effects and Contraindications of Antihypertensive Agents—cont'd

	Side Effects		
	Innocuous but Sometimes Annoying	Harmful or Potentially Harmful	Contraindications
Beta Blockers	Bradycardia, weakness, lethargy, GI disturbances	Systolic heart failure (carvedolol, metoprolol approved for sysotic heart failure), bronchospasm[b] (patients with asthma), hypoglycemia (nonselectives can mask the symptoms of or potentiate hypoglycemia), hyperglycemia (nonselectives can ↓ insulin secretion in Type 2 diabetes patients), aggravation of peripheral arterial disease,[b] nightmares, insomnia,[b] impotence, hypertriglyceridemia, ↓ HDL	Asthma, 2nd or 3rd degree heart block, systolic heart failure exacerbation, "brittle" diabetes mellitus
ACE Inhibitors	Dizziness, faintness, lightheadedness (check orthostatic BP), cough, palpitation, taste changes[d]	Hypotension (more frequent in elderly), skin rash (disappears or discontinuation), proteinuria,[d] leukopenia[d]	Bilateral renal artery stenosis, volume depletion, hyponatremia, pregnancy
Angiotensin II Receptor Antagonist	Same as ACE inhibitors, except without cough	Same as ACE inhibitors	Same as ACE inhibitors
Calcium Channel Blockers			
Dihydropyridines	Dizziness, lightheadedness, headache, weakness, nausea	Peripheral edema, hypotension, tachycardia. Possibly angina, MI or stroke with high-dose immediate-release nifedipine	Severe hypotension
Verapamil and diltiazem	Dizziness, lightheadedness, headache, weakness, nausea, constipation[e]	AV block, bradycardia, systolic heart failure, digoxin interaction	Systolic heart failure, 2nd or 3rd degree AV block, sick sinus syndrome, severe hypotension
Alpha₁-Blockers	Headache, palpitation, dizziness	Sudden collapse and loss of consciousness related to orthostatic hypotension (usually after initial dose)	None
Alpha₂-Agonists			
Clonidine	Dry mouth, drowsiness/lethargy, constipation, skin rash with transderm	"Rebound hypertension,"[g] parotid pain	
Methyldopa	Drowsiness, lethargy, dry mouth, sexual difficulty, direct Coombs' test, nasal congestion	Abnormal liver function tests, hepatitis,[b] drug fever,[b] hemolytic anemia,[b] retroperitoneal fibrosis,[b] skin rash,[b] orthostatic hypotension, depression[b]	Coombs' positive hemolytic anemia, hepatic disease
Hydralazine	Tachycardia,[h] palpitation,[h] headache,[h] flushing,[h] nasal congestion, GI disturbances	Aggravation of angina,[b,h] drug-induced lupus,[b] drug fever,[b] skin rash[b]	Symptomatic angina (unless used with beta-blocker)
Minoxidil	Tachycardia,[h] hypertrichosis, initial rise in plasma rennin activity	Na and water retention (can lead to heart failure or pulmonary edema), pericardial effusion	Advanced kidney disease, limited to patients unresponsive to usual high BP therapy, pheochromocytoma
Reserpine	Drowsiness, nasal congestion	Depression,[b] activation of peptic ulcer,[b] parkinsonian state[b]	Depression (past or present), Parkinsonism, peptic ulcer disease

[a]Routine use of potassium supplements and/or concurrent potassium sparing diuretics should be discouraged unless hypokalemia is documented or the patient is taking digoxin.
[b]Usually requires cessation of therapy, at least temporarily.
[c]Noted with spironolactone, not eplerenone
[d]Skin rash, proteinuria, leukopenia, and taste change are minimized by using low doses of captopril or any of the other ACE inhibitors.
[e]Adverse reactions may be less frequent with diltiazem.
[f]Verapamil may ↑ digoxin levels.
[g]Rebound hypertension worse after doses >0.6 mg/day.
[h]These side effects are minimized or prevented by coadministration of a β-blocker.

minimize nocturia and provide consistent effects. Patients experience increased urination when starting this medicine, but this diminishes with time. Missed doses should be taken as soon as possible within the same day (as soon as she remembers), but doubling doses the next day is not recommended. B.A. should be informed of the potential for hypokalemia and the need for routine monitoring of serum potassium, but that this is easily identified and managed. She should be counseled on the signs and symptoms of electrolyte abnormalities (e.g., leg cramps, muscle weakness) and encouraged to report these to her physician if they occur. Increasing dietary intake of potassium-rich foods (i.e., bananas, orange juice) to minimize electrolyte depletion is an option to minimize potassium loss. This should be encouraged only with thiazide and loop diuretics, as a potassium enhanced diet could contribute to hyperkalemia with potassium-sparing agents.

Monitoring Therapy

23. After 4 weeks of HCTZ 25 mg daily, B.A. returns to the clinic for evaluation without complaints. She has not missed a dose of HCTZ, is still exercising, and is following the DASH diet. Her BP values are 142/90 (left arm) and 144/90 mm Hg (right arm). Her serum potassium is 3.8 mEq/L (normal, 3.5 to 5.2 mEq/L), uric acid is 7.3 mg/dL (normal, 2.0 to 7.5 mg/dL), fasting glucose is 100 mg/dL (normal, 60 to 110 mg/dL), and the other laboratory values are unchanged. One month ago, her potassium was 4.1 mEq/L, uric acid was 6.8 mg/dL, and fasting glucose was 95 mg/dL. What is your assessment from the data given regarding efficacy and toxicity?

[SI units: K, 3.8 mmol/L (normal, 3.5 to 5.2 mmol/L); uric acid, 432 mmol/L (normal, 119 to 476 mmol/L); and glucose, 5.6 mmol/L (normal, 3.3 to 6.1 mmol/L)]

B.A.'s goal BP of <140/90 mm Hg has not been met. Despite improvements, she still has stage 1 hypertension based on today's BP average of 143/90 mm Hg. B.A. had significant improvements with lifestyle modifications before starting HCTZ. She appears persistent and she should be encouraged to continue with her efforts. There are also no new signs of target organ damage present.

ADVERSE EFFECTS

Adverse reactions with low-dose thiazide-type diuretics are minimal compared with high-dose therapy. This has been shown in multiple long-term placebo-controlled treatment trials. The Treatment of Mild Hypertension Study (TOMHS) found that adverse reactions from a low-dose diuretic were no different from placebo.[92] The VA Cooperative group found that low-dose thiazide diuretics were better tolerated than a β-blocker, ACE inhibitor, CCB, α-blocker, or clonidine.[50]

B.A. should be questioned regarding increased urination. Increased urination usually subsides after the first few weeks of therapy with HCTZ or other thiazide-type diuretics. However, this is sometimes a cause for nonadherence, especially in elderly patients who fear incontinence. Signs and symptoms of metabolic changes such as hypokalemia, hyperglycemia, or hyperuricemia should be evaluated. Her serum potassium has dropped and uric acid has risen. These could be normal variations in laboratory measurements, but are consistent with thiazide-induced abnormalities. B.A. should be questioned about muscle cramps, weakness, or new joint pains.

Hypokalemia

24. Is B.A.'s decrease in potassium concerning? How should this be managed?

Thiazide and loop diuretics can reduce serum potassium concentrations, but clinically relevant hypokalemia is not common. Diuretic-induced hypokalemia is dose related and is most apparent within the first week of therapy. Most often thiazide diuretic-induced hypokalemia is mild with serum potassium concentrations reaching a nadir within the first month of therapy and generally remaining stable thereafter.[50,90] HCTZ in doses of 12.5, 25, and 50 mg daily can decrease serum potassium by an average of 0.21, 0.34, and 0.5 mEq/L, respectively.[89,90] With HCTZ ≤25 mg daily, only 10% to 15% of patients develop hypokalemia.

Most total body potassium is intracellular (approximately 98%). Decreases in serum potassium concentrations can be important, but the clinical significance of small decreases (≤0.5 mEq/L) when serum potassium concentrations are still in the normal range is unknown. B.A.'s potassium has dropped slightly but is still in the normal range. She is not taking other drugs that increase her risk of hypokalemia-associated cardiovascular toxicity (e.g., digoxin) and has no previous history of heart disease, so there is no cause for alarm.

A retrospective analysis of the Multiple Risk Factor Intervention Trial (MRFIT) showed that a subgroup of patients with baseline ECG abnormalities who were treated with a diuretic had an increased CAD mortality rate.[145] This finding created controversy suggesting that diuretic-induced hypokalemia may have been the cause. However, other similar placebo-controlled studies have failed to demonstrate this relationship.[52,61,146] Moreover, low-dose thiazide type diuretics have been identified as the most effective first-line agents for preventing the occurrence of CVD morbidity and mortality.[57]

25. When is potassium supplementation needed to manage diuretic-induced hypokalemia? What therapeutic options are available?

Diuretic-associated hypokalemia should be treated when serum concentrations are below normal or are less than 4.0 mEq/L in patients also taking digoxin regardless of whether symptoms of weakness and muscle cramps are present. Serum potassium should be measured at baseline and within 4 weeks of initiating therapy or with increasing diuretic therapy. Starting potassium supplementation and/or adding a potassium-sparing diuretic are therapeutic options. Other conditions such as chronic diarrhea, high-dose corticosteroid use, and hyperaldosteronism can contribute to hypokalemia.

Patients can be encouraged to increase consumption of potassium-rich foods to maintain normal potassium concentrations. Dried fruit, bananas, potatoes, and avocados are foods rich in potassium. Although potassium-rich foods may help prevent the development of hypokalemia in some patients, they cannot be used as sole therapy to correct severe hypokalemia (<3.0 mEq/L). For instance, one medium-size banana has 11.5 mEq of potassium. The usual replacement dose of prescribed potassium chloride is 20 to 40 mEq/day. Also, potassium-rich food may increase caloric intake and incur additional costs.

The dose of potassium needed to correct diuretic-induced hypokalemia is highly variable and can range from as little as 10 to more than 100 mEq/day. The average replacement dose is 20 to 60 mEq/day. Asymptomatic diuretic-induced hypokalemia can be corrected with oral potassium replacement products. Potassium chloride, bicarbonate, gluconate, acetate, and citrate salts are available as single ingredients and as components of combination products. However, chloride preparations are generally preferred. Oral potassium supplements are available in liquid, enteric-coated, and slow-release preparations. The slow-release tablets are preferred because they cause fewer gastrointestinal adverse effects (e.g., nausea, vomiting, abdominal discomfort, diarrhea) than the liquid and enteric-coated tablets. Small bowel ulcerations have been documented with enteric-coated tablets and these should be avoided (See Chapter 19, Heart Failure).

Potassium-sparing diuretics are prescribed frequently in combination with the thiazide-type diuretic. Unfortunately, the potassium-conserving capacity of these diuretics is difficult to quantify. They may be as effective as potassium supplementation in maintaining serum potassium concentrations within the normal range, but patients sometimes require both supplementation and a potassium-sparing diuretic to maintain normal serum concentrations.

B.A.'s potassium is still within the normal range. Potassium replacement is not indicated. She should be encouraged to continue a low-salt diet and to increase her dietary intake of potassium. Her potassium should be re-evaluated in 4 weeks at her next BP check.

Other Metabolic Abnormalities

26. B.A.'s glucose and uric acid both increased after starting HCTZ. Are these changes clinically significant? Should these adverse effects be treated?

Altered glucose metabolism is a recognized complication of diuretic therapy, but response is variable. Patients with diabetes and impaired glucose tolerance exhibit the most exaggerated glucose increases, but this effect has also been observed in patients without diabetes.[59] Serum glucose concentrations actually declined in patients who received long-term low-dose chlorthalidone in the TOMHS trial, compared to placebo.[92] However, different trends were seen in other long-term placebo-controlled studies in which fasting blood glucose values were increased 3.6 to 6.7 mg/dL in patients treated with HCTZ.[50,90] Small, but statistically significant, increases in glucose concentrations were seen with long-term low-dose chlorthalidone in the ALLHAT, compared to lisinopril and amlodipine.[96] It appears that these changes are not clinically relevant since morbidity and mortality are reduced despite these changes.

Diabetes is not a contraindication to the use of diuretics; rather, it is actually a compelling indication for a diuretic (Fig. 14-4). Decreases in morbidity and mortality have been consistently demonstrated in thiazide treated patients who have diabetes.[1,8,52,96] Altering diet or the dose of diabetes medications can manage hyperglycemia if it occurs.

The hyperglycemic effect of diuretics appears to parallel potassium loss. Patients with decreased serum potassium concentrations exhibit more impaired glucose tolerance,[59] and potassium supplementation can prevent thiazide-induced hyperglycemia. Maintaining normal serum potassium concentrations in patients with diabetes who are treated with diuretic therapy is essential. Hyperosmolar, non-ketotic coma has been reported with very high-dose HCTZ (100 mg/day).[147] This further reinforces using low-dose thiazide diuretics in hypertension.

B.A. does not have a strong family history of diabetes. If she did, she could be at an increased risk for hyperglycemia. Her baseline fasting glucose values should be documented and monitored at least once a year to detect any increases.

Thiazide-type and loop diuretics can increase serum uric acid concentrations in a dose-dependent fashion. It has been suggested that increased proximal tubular renal reabsorption, decreased tubular secretion, and/or increased postsecretory reabsorption of uric acid contribute to diuretic-induced hyperuricemia. Thiazide-induced hyperuricemia is minimal (≤ 0.5 mg/dL) in most patients.[89,90] If symptoms of gout (localized arthritic pain commonly in the great toe) are absent, treatment is rarely required. If acute gouty attacks are precipitated, then treatment or discontinuation of the diuretic should be considered. Very few patients have to discontinue a thiazide-type diuretic secondary to symptoms associated with gout.[148] If this happens, uric acid returns to pretreatment concentrations soon after the diuretic is discontinued. A history of gout is not a contraindication to diuretic therapy but is a potentially unfavorable effect. B.A.'s serum uric acid concentration is elevated, but switching to a different agent or lowering the dose of HCTZ is unnecessary since she is not symptomatic.

27. Can HCTZ alter B.A.'s cholesterol values?

Hypercholesterolemia and hypertriglyceridemia are potential side effects of diuretic therapy. Controversy exists over the significance of these effects. These alterations are characterized by increases in low-density lipoprotein cholesterol and total triglycerides.[149] Dietary fat restrictions help minimize, but do not necessarily prevent, these effects. Contrary to other biochemical disturbances, diuretic-induced changes in the lipid profile do not appear to be dose related.[150] Many clinical trials lasting more than 1 year have shown that hypercholesterolemia and hypertriglyceridemia with diuretic therapy is not sustained with prolonged use.[89,90,151] However, even if these changes are persistent, they do not appear to be clinically significance with low-dose thiazide-type diuretics (See Chapter 13, Dyslipidemias, Atherosclerosis, and Coronary Heart Disease).

Diuretic therapy should not be avoided in patients who have normal or borderline lipid profiles. Clinical judgment should be used in patients with significant dyslipidemia in whom the potential for a diuretic-induced rise in cholesterol or triglycerides would warrant lipid-lowering drug therapy. B.A. has no history of dyslipidemia and, therefore, is an excellent candidate for a diuretic.

28. What other metabolic abnormalities should be monitored as a result of B.A.'s diuretic therapy?

Thiazide diuretics decrease urinary calcium excretion and have been used to prevent stone formation in patients with calcium-related kidney stones. The resulting elevations in serum calcium concentrations are usually asymptomatic and of little clinical significance, but may be beneficial in postmenopausal patients like B.A. or in patients with osteoporosis. Contrary to thiazide-type diuretics, loop diuretics increase renal clearance of calcium and have been used for acute management of severe hypercalcemia. Baseline serum calcium concentrations should be obtained when diuretic therapy is started and then checked as needed during the course of therapy.

Hypomagnesemia is an often-overlooked metabolic complication of diuretic therapy. Thiazide and loop diuretics both increase urinary excretion of magnesium in a dose-dependent manner. Symptoms of significant magnesium deficiency include muscle weakness, muscle tremor or twitching, mental status changes, and cardiac arrhythmias (including torsades de pointes). Presence of these symptoms would necessitate magnesium supplementation. Hypomagnesemia frequently coexists with hypokalemia, further increasing the risk of cardiac conduction abnormalities. Until hypomagnesemia is corrected, attempts to replenish potassium in hypokalemia can be ineffective, even when high doses of potassium are given. After magnesium supplementation, hypokalemia is easier to correct.

Hyponatremia is a serious, yet infrequent adverse effect of diuretics. Changes in sodium concentrations are usually small, and patients are usually asymptomatic. Decreased renal excretion of free water, inappropriate antidiuretic hormone secretion, urinary sodium loss, and depletion of magnesium and potassium may all contribute to diuretic-induced hyponatremia. Severe hyponatremia (<120 mEq/L) rarely occurs with diuretic administration, but definitely requires discontinuation of the diuretic.

Reasons for Inadequate Blood Pressure Control

29. B.A.'s medications were not modified at her previous evaluation. She was instructed to purchase a home monitor, document her morning BP measurements each day, and bring her values back for evaluation in 4 weeks. Her BP values over the past 4 weeks have ranged from 138 to 146/88 to 94 mm Hg, with the average BP being 142/92 mm Hg. She has been taking HCTZ 25 mg daily for 8 weeks and has missed only three doses during that time. Her BP today is 144/92 mm Hg (142/90 mm Hg when repeated). Other than calcium and vitamin D, she uses no over-the-counter products or prescription drugs. Today her serum potassium concentration is 3.8 mEq/L, serum creatinine is 0.9 mg/dL, and uric acid is 7.2 mg/dL. Why is B.A.'s BP not at goal?

B.A. still has stage 1 hypertension. Although some of her home (self-monitoring) values are <140/90 mm Hg, her average is elevated and it is desirable to have home BP values consistently <135/85 mm Hg. The full antihypertensive effect of HCTZ has been achieved since it is well beyond 2 to 4 weeks. Potential reasons for inadequate response with an antihypertensive should be considered before choosing to modify her drug therapy regimen. These are displayed in Table 14-11. Evaluation requires a comprehensive medication history and medical evaluation to rule out identifiable causes. Based on the given information, her BP measurements appear accurate, as her clinic measurements are similar to her home values. She is taking a diuretic with good kidney function and without edema, so volume overload is unlikely. Lastly, no drug-induced or associated conditions are identified. It is reasonable to conclude that B.A. needs additional therapy to achieve her goal BP.

Table 14-11 Causes of Resistant Hypertension[1]
Improper Blood Pressure Measurement
Volume Overload and Pseudotolerance
• Excess sodium intake
• Volume retention from kidney disease
• Inadequate diuretic therapy
Drug-Induced Causes (See Table 14-4)
Other Drug-Related Causes
• Nonadherence
• Inadequate doses
• Inappropriate combinations
Associated Conditions (Obesity, Excess Alcohol Intake)
Identifiable Causes of Hypertension (See Table 14-4)

Modifying Therapy

B.A.'s present dose of HCTZ is considered low-dose. One option is to avoid adding a second drug by increasing the dose of HCTZ to the maximum recommended dose of 50 mg daily (considered high-dose diuretic therapy). Unfortunately, there is an increased risk of side effects and minimal to no additional BP lowering when increasing from low-dose to high-dose therapy.[57,88] B.A.'s potassium dropped to 3.8 mEq/L with low-dose HCTZ, and further dosage increases may produce significant hypokalemia (<3.5 mEq/L) requiring supplementation. She also has hyperuricemia that may be worsened. Increasing HCTZ is not desirable.

Discontinuing HCTZ and starting a different agent is another option, but is not ideal in B.A. for several reasons. HCTZ did lower her BP, it is known to reduce morbidity and mortality, is inexpensive, and may benefit her osteoporosis. In addition, other agents may not be completely effective for B.A. without a diuretic. Hypokalemia might lead some authorities to switch to another agent, but she is still within the normal range.

Two-Drug Regimens

The role of two-drug regimens as combination therapy in the treatment of hypertension is clear. With an increased emphasis on controlling BP and the realization that most patients require multiple agents for BP control, combination therapy is strongly recommended. Several guidelines now recommend two-drug regimens as initial therapy for patient far from their BP goal, in patients with multiple compelling indications, and in patients with uncontrolled BP.[1,8,139]

Adding a second agent to B.A.'s regimen is an ideal option. The overall goal of using combination antihypertensive therapy is to produce an additive response that targets goal BP achievement and/or treat a compelling indication with drug therapy that reduces morbidity and mortality. Ideally, a combination of two drugs with different mechanisms of action should be selected to produce a complimentary effect to lower BP. Various combinations are depicted in Figure 14-5, with the most rational combinations identified.

COMBINATIONS INCLUDING A DIURETIC

Diuretics, when combined with several agents (especially an ACE inhibitor or ARB), result in additive antihypertensive effects that are independent of reversing fluid retention.[152] Diuretics reduce BP initially by decreasing fluid volume, but

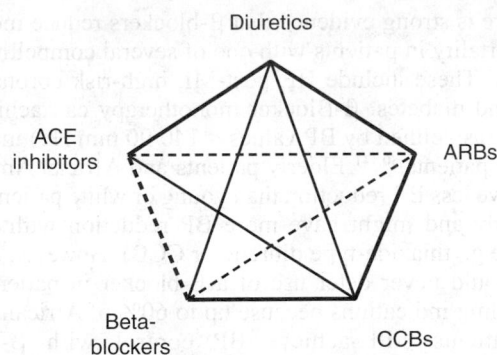

FIGURE 14-5 Possible combinations of different classes of antihypertensive agents. The most rational combinations are represented as thick lines. The combination of a CCB with a β-blocker is rational only if the CCB is a dihydropyridine. ACE, angiotensin-converting enzyme; ARB, angiotensin II receptor blocker; CCB, calcium channel blocker. (Adapted with permission from 2003 European Society of Hypertension-European Society of Cardiology guidelines for the management of arterial hypertension. J Hypertens 2003;21:1011–1053.)[6]

maintain their antihypertensive effects by lowering PVR. However, BP lowering can stimulate renin release from the kidney and activate the renin-angiotensin-aldosterone system. This compensatory mechanism is an in vivo attempt to neutralize BP changes and regulate fluid loss.

ACE inhibitors and ARBs block the renin-angiotensin-aldosterone systems, explaining why combinations of these agents with diuretics are additive. One mechanism by which β-blockers reduce BP is by suppressing renin release and activity. Thus, adding a diuretic to a β-blocker results in an ad-

ditive antihypertensive response. Even very low doses of HCTZ (6.25 mg daily) have additive effects when combined with bisoprolol.[153] Certain nondiuretic antihypertensive agents (i.e., reserpine, arterial vasodilators, and centrally acting agents) can eventually cause significant sodium retention and increased fluid volume. These agents should be given in combination with a diuretic to maximize BP lowering and provide maximal reductions on morbidity and mortality.

QUESTIONABLE COMBINATIONS

Several studies show little additive antihypertensive effect with the combination of an ACE inhibitor with a β-blocker. The primary mechanism of action of ACE inhibitors is to decrease angiotensin II production. Less angiotensin II is produced when PRA is suppressed by β-blockers. Therefore, if the angiotensin II–mediated BP effects are suppressed by a β-blocker, adding an ACE inhibitor might not result in an additive effect. Although this combination may not be additive, it is often used when multiple conditions or compelling indications require treatment with each of these individual agents (e.g., hypertension with CAD, diabetic nephropathy, HF).[1] ACE inhibitors/β-blocker combinations should be avoided if BP reduction is the only indication for combination therapy.

FIXED-DOSE COMBINATION PRODUCTS

The traditional approach with two-drug regimens has been to use two separate dosage forms. This allows for individual titration of each drug. However, there are several fixed-dose combinations of two antihypertensives available (Table 14-12). Although individual dose titration is not possible with fixed-dose combination products, their use can reduce the

Table 14-12   Combination Antihypertensive Agents

Combination Type	Fixed-Dose Combination	Unit strengths (mg/mg)
ACE inhibitor with diuretic	Benazepril/HCTZ (Lotensin HCT)	5/6.25, 10/12.5, 20/12.5, 20/25
	Captopril/HCTZ (Capozide)	25/15, 25/25, 50/15, 50/25
	Enalapril/HCTZ (Vaseretic)	5/12.5, 10/25
	Lisinopril/HCTZ (Prinzide, Zestoretic)	10/12.5, 20/12.5, 20/25
	Moexipril/HCTZ (Uniretic)	7.5/12.5, 15/25
	Quinapril/HCTZ (Accuretic)	10/12.5, 20/12.5, 20/25
ARB with diuretic	Candesartan/HCTZ (Atacand HCT)	16/12.5, 32/12.5
	Eprosartan/HCTZ (Teveten HCT)	600/12.5, 600/25
	Irbesartan/HCTZ (Avalide)	75/12.5, 150/12.5, 300/12.5
	Losartan/HCTZ (Hyzaar)	50/12.5, 100/25
	Olmesartan/HCTZ (Benicar HCT)	20/12.5, 40/12.5, 40/25
	Telmisartan/HCTZ (Micardis HCT)	40/12.5, 80/12.5
	Valsartan/HCTZ (Diovan HCT)	80/12.5, 160/12.5
β-Blocker with diuretic	Atenolol/Chlorthalidone (Tenoretic)	50/25, 100/25
	Bisoprolol/HCTZ (Ziac)	2.5/6.25, 5/6.25, 10/6.25
	Propranolol LA/ HCTZ (Inderide)	40/25, 80/25
	Metoprolol/HCTZ (Lopressor HCT)	50/25, 100/25
	Nadolol/Bendroflumethiazide (Corzide)	40/5, 80/5
	Timolol/HCTZ (Timolide)	10/25
Centrally acting agent with diuretic	Methyldopa/HCTZ (Aldoril)	250/15, 250/25, 500/30, 500/50
	Reserpine/Chlorothiazide (Diupres)	0.125/250, 0.25/500
	Reserpine/HCTZ (Hydropres)	0.125/25, 0.125/50
ACE inhibitor with CCB	Amlodipine/Benazepril (Lotrel)	2.5/10, 5/10, 10/20
	Enalapril/Felodipine (Lexxel)	5/5
	Trandolapril/Verapamil	2/180, 1/240, 2/240, 4/240

HCTZ, hydrochlorothiazide.

number of tablets/capsules taken by patients. This can benefit patients by promoting adherence, which may potentially increase the likelihood of achieving or maintaining goal BP values.

Most fixed-dose combinations include a thiazide-type diuretic. Many are available generically and are moderately priced or inexpensive. All commercially available ARBs are available in fixed-dose combinations with HCTZ, but only as relatively expensive brand-name products. Newer nondiuretic containing fixed-dose combination products combine a CCB with an ACE inhibitor. Use of fixed-dose combination products has increased, a prescribing trend that will likely grow further now that new hypertension guidelines recommend two-drug regimens under many circumstances. Clinicians are also comfortable with choosing a fixed-dose combination product in an attempt to simplify regimens and expedite goal achievement. Although many fixed-dose products are available generically, there may even be an economic advantage to using a brand-name product if it allows the patient to receive two drugs for one medication copayment.

B.A. is a candidate for a diuretic containing fixed-dose combination product. Cost should be taken into account since expense of therapy is a concern for B.A. No coexisting medical condition (i.e., a compelling indication) in B.A. requires a specific second antihypertensive drug class. The most attractive second agent for her is either an ACE inhibitor or a β-blocker. B.A. has no reason to avoid a β-blocker, and this would be an inexpensive second agent. However, an ACE inhibitor is particularly attractive because data have shown that it can blunt the potential for hypokalemia and hyperuricemia caused by diuretics. Although ACE inhibitors can potentially cause significant hypotension leading to acute renal insufficiency in volume-depleted patients (e.g., those who have been overdiuresed), there is no evidence that B.A. is volume depleted so this risk is very small. When this is a concern, one to two doses of the diuretic can be withheld before initiating the ACE inhibitor. Depending on the dose of ACE inhibitor used, it also might be necessary to lower the maintenance diuretic dosage.

Several ACE inhibitors are available generically or as a fixed-dose combination with a thiazide-type diuretic, and can be dosed once daily. The fixed-dose combination of enalapril/HCTZ at a dose of 10 mg/25 mg once daily can replace her current HCTZ 25 mg daily. This product is generically available, will likely lower her BP to goal, and may blunt B.A.'s decrease in potassium. Adherence should be maximized since this modification still requires her to take only one medication daily, yet should improve her overall antihypertensive response.

β-Blockers

30. E.K. is a 78-year-old African American man with a history of hypertension, who recently was hospitalized for an acute MI 2 months earlier. He has been treated with atenolol 25 mg daily and aspirin 325 mg daily since then. Today his BP readings are 148/92 and 146/90 mm Hg, and his heart rate is 80 beats/min. He denies any side effects with his medications. Since E.K. is African American and elderly, is a β-blocker an appropriate agent to treat his hypertension?

There is strong evidence that β-blockers reduce morbidity and mortality in patients with one of several compelling indications.[1] These include HF, post-MI, high-risk coronary disease, and diabetes. β-Blocker monotherapy can achieve BP control (as defined by BP values <140/90 mm Hg) in 35% to 70% of patients.[50,141] Elderly patients and African Americans may have less BP reduction than young or white patients. E.K. is elderly and might have more BP reduction with another agent (e.g., thiazide-type diuretic or CCB). However, age and race should never deter use of a β-blocker in patients with compelling indications because up to 60% of African American patients still achieve BP control with β-blocker theapy.[112,141,154] E.K.'s post-MI history requires the use of a β-blocker since he has no absolute contraindications to this therapy. Moreover, all β-blockers have similar activity with regard to BP lowering, and patients whose conditions fail to respond to one generally fail to respond to others.

β-Blockers are inexpensive with several generic products available. β-Blockers were combined with thiazide-type diuretics during some of the landmark trials that established BP reduction as a standard of care in hypertension. For these reasons, β-blockers were at one time the most widely prescribed agents for hypertension worldwide, but their use diminished after the introduction of ACE inhibitors and CCBs.[155] Despite these advantages, β-blockers are associated with adverse metabolic alterations and bothersome side effects that limit their universal use. However, the incidence of adverse reactions (e.g., sexual dysfunction, exercise intolerance, fatigue) is lower than popular medical myth suggests. Adverse reactions are dose-dependent and are minimized with low to moderate doses.

Pharmacologic Differences

31. What are some pharmacologic advantages of using atenolol, compared with other β-blockers, in treating E.K.'s hypertension?

Many different β-blockers are available (Table 14-13). Clinically important differences relate primarily to cardioselectivity, intrinsic sympathomimetic activity (ISA), relative lipid solubility, and benefit to risk in systolic HF. These differences might be useful when selecting an individual agent.

CARDIOSELECTIVITY

β_1-Adrenergic receptors are primarily located in the heart, and β_2-adrenergic receptors are in the lungs, kidneys, and peripheral arteriolar endothelium. Low-affinity β_1-receptors are also present in the lung, and low-affinity β_2-receptors are present in the heart. Some β-blockers demonstrate relative cardioselectivity with greater antagonism of cardiac β_1-receptors and less activity on β_2-receptors in the lung or bronchial tissue. However, selectivity is not absolute since it is dose-dependent. For instance, asthma has been precipitated even with cardioselective agents when they are used in higher doses, but not with low to moderate doses.[156]

Nonselective β-blockers potentially have the disadvantage of blunting the symptoms of hypoglycemia in patients with type 1 diabetes. β_2-Blockade from nonselective β-blockers can lead to unopposed α-induced peripheral vasoconstriction. This may worsen Raynaud's phenomenon, peripheral arterial disease, or hypertension caused by catecholamine-producing

Table 14-13   β-Blockers in Hypertension

Drug	Usual Dosage Range (mg/day)	Dosing Frequency	Relative β₁ Selectivity[b]	Intrinsic Sympatho-mimetic Activity[c]	Lipid Solubility[d]
Atenolol (Tenormin)	25–100	QD to BID	++	0	Low
Acebutolol (Sectral)	200–800	BID	++	+	Moderate
Bisoprolol (Zebeta)	2.5–10	QD	++	0	Low
Betaxolol (Kerlone)	5–20	QD	++	0	Low
Carteolol (Cartrol)	2.5–10	QD	0	++	Low
Carvedilol (Coreg)	12.5–50	BID	0	0	High
Labetalol (Trandate, Normodyne)	200–800	BID	0	0	Moderate
Metoprolol (Lopressor, Toprol XL[a])	50–100	QD[a] to BID	+	0	Moderate to high
Nadolol (Corgard)	40–120	QD	0	0	Low
Penbutolol (Levatol)	10–40	QD	0	+	High
Pindolol (Visken)	10–60	BID	0	+++	Moderate
Propranolol (Inderal, Inderal LA[a])	40–180	QD[a] to BID	0	0	High
Timolol (Blocadren)	20–40	BID	0	0	Low to moderate

[a]QD dosing for the extended release product only.
[b]None are entirely β₁ specific. Use cautiously in patients with asthma, COPD, or peripheral vascular insufficiency (e.g., Raynaud's).
[c]ISA = Intrinsic sympathomimetic activity. Whether ISA has a protective effect in patients predisposed to bradycardia, CHF, or vasospasm is controversial.
[d]Lipid solubility might predict other drug characteristics. Highly lipid-soluble agents have shortest t½, a greater percentage of hepatic metabolism, more variability in dose due to high presystemic (1st-pass) metabolism, and possibly more CNS side effects. Low lipid solubility drugs have longer t½, ↑ renal clearance, narrower dosage ranges, and possible ↓ CNS penetration.

tumors (pheochromocytoma). Despite these shortcomings, nonselective β-blockers are preferred in patients with noncardiovascular indications for β-blocker therapy such as migraine prophylaxis or essential tremor. Absent these indications, cardioselective β-blockers are preferred. E.K. is taking atenolol for cardiovascular indications (hypertension and post-MI). Atenolol, being a cardioselective agent, is appropriate therapy for E.K.

INTRINSIC SYMPATHOMIMETIC ACTIVITY

32. **Why are acebutolol, carteolol, penbutolol, and pindolol contraindicated in E.K.?**

Pure β-blockers occupy the β-receptor, inhibiting stimulatory catecholamine access while exerting no effect on their own. β-Blockers with ISA (acebutolol, carteolol, penbutolol, and pindolol) partially stimulate β-receptors while attached to this receptor, but much less than a pure agonist. When given to a patient with a slow resting heart rate, ISA β-blockers can increase the heart rate. Conversely, these agents can slow heart rate in patients with resting or exercise-induced tachycardia, because β-blocking properties predominate.

β-Blockers with ISA are theoretically less likely to cause bradycardia, bronchospasm, reduced cardiac output, peripheral vasoconstriction, and increased plasma lipids than nonselective β-blockers. Nonetheless, these agents still might worsen asthma or exacerbate HF or angina in patients with CAD. ISA β-blockers should be avoided in patients who have contraindications to or adverse reactions with non-ISA β-blockers. Perhaps the only role for ISA β-blockers is in patients who require a β-blocker, but experience severe bradycardia from non-ISA agents. They should never be used in patients with a history of MI because they may have detrimental effects as a result of their agonist properties. Since E.K. has a history of MI, a β-blocker with ISA (e.g., acebutolol) is contraindicated.

LIPID SOLUBILITY

Lipophilic β-blockers (e.g., propranolol) have a larger volume of distribution and undergo more extensive first-pass hepatic metabolism than hydrophilic β-blockers. Highly hydrophilic β-blockers (e.g., atenolol) are primarily excreted by the kidneys and may require lower doses in patients with moderate to severe chronic kidney disease.

Highly lipophilic agents theoretically penetrate the CNS more extensively and readily than hydrophilic β-blockers. It is possible that lipophilic agents are associated with increased side effects such as drowsiness, mental confusion, nightmares, or depression. However, comparative studies have not demonstrated significant differences between low to moderate doses of lipophilic and hydrophilic β-blockers.[157] Considering lipid solubility is most clinically relevant when selecting a β-blocker for a patient with renal or hepatic impairment. High lipid soluble drugs are hepatically cleared, while low lipid soluble drugs are excreted by the kidneys. Likewise, a high lipid soluble drug is desirable for migraine prophylaxis due to better CNS penetration.

Compelling Indications
HEART FAILURE

33. **Since β-blockers decrease cardiac contractility, how do they benefit patients with HF?**

β-Blockers lower heart rate, decrease cardiac contractility, and reduce cardiac output when first initiated. In patients with systolic HF, the primary physiologic abnormality is decreased contractility. Therefore, using a β-blocker seems pharmacologically flawed. However, extensive research has shown that slow introduction of certain β-blockers using doses much lower than what is used for BP lowering (i.e., carvedilol 3.125 mg twice daily and metoprolol 12.5 mg daily), followed by very slow and careful titration up to high dose, actually improves cardiac function (See Chapter 19, Heart Failure). Cardiac β-receptor upregulation occurs, and the detrimental compensatory tachycardia and excessive catecholamine release is halted. The end result is decreased morbidity and mortality.[116] Specifically, metoprolol and carvedilol are approved for systolic HF based on evidence showing reduced cardiovascular events and mortality.[120–122] When β-blockers are used in patients with both hypertension and systolic HF, only these two agents should be selected following dose recommendations as approved for HF (start with a low dose followed by gradual titration upward).

β-Blockers other than carvedilol and metoprolol should be avoided in systolic HF. This is not the case, however, for diastolic HF in which the primary physiologic abnormality is decreased left ventricular filling. β-Blockers lower heart rate and allow the heart more time to fill. Any β-blocker (e.g., atenolol) can be used for this type of HF, and antihypertensive doses can be used when starting therapy.

POST-MYOCARDIAL INFARCTION

Overwhelming evidence supports β-blocker therapy in acute MI and post-MI.[129] β-Blockers prolong survival and reduce the risk of recurrence.[120,130] These agents are often underutilized in this population because of perceived contraindications. However, patients with relative contraindications to β-blocker therapy (e.g., older patients, chronic pulmonary disease, non–Q-wave MI, diabetes) still benefit from β-blocker therapy.[158,159] All patients, even if they have controlled BP, should receive a β-blocker post-MI unless they have demonstrated intolerance or have an absolute contraindication (See Chapter 18, Myocardial Infarction).

HIGH-RISK CORONARY DISEASE

Hypertensive patients with chronic stable angina or acute coronary syndromes (non-ST segment elevation MI and unstable angina) have high coronary risk. These conditions can easily progress to more severe and sometimes fatal coronary events. β-Blocker therapy is recommended by the American College of Cardiology and American Heart Association as first-line therapy to treat these conditions.[129,160] In addition to lowering BP, these agents reduce heart rate, contractility, and myocardial oxygen demand. All these pharmacologic actions make β-blockers excellent and essential therapy in high-risk coronary disease (See Chapter 17, Ischemic Heart Disease: Anginal Syndromes).

DIABETES

34. Diabetes is a compelling indication for β-blocker therapy. Why is caution sometimes recommended when using these drugs in patients with diabetes?

β-Blockers reduce coronary events, progression of kidney disease, and stroke in patients with diabetes.[8,9,161,162] These drugs can inhibit insulin secretion and cause hyperglycemia, but the relatively low risk of this effect is usually outweighed by the potential reduction in hypertension-related complications. If blood glucose should rise, either the β-blocker dose can be reduced, or diabetes therapy can be adjusted.

All β-blockers can mask symptoms of impending hypoglycemia associated with epinephrine release (e.g., palpitations, tremor, hunger), but do not prevent hypoglycemia-related sweating. While they do not cause hypoglycemia, non-

selective β-blockers can worsen a hypoglycemic episode and may prolong recovery from hypoglycemia. The risk of masking and potentiating hypoglycemia is not an absolute contraindication. Although β-blockers are best avoided in insulin dependent type 1 diabetes, they can be used if other agents fail or if concurrent diseases are present that justify the use of a β-blocker. Because hypoglycemia is less common in patients with type 2 diabetes who do not require insulin, β-blockers are less likely to create adverse effects in this population.

All patients with diabetes who take β-blockers should be monitored carefully with regular glucose measurements and targeted patient education about how the signs and symptoms of hypoglycemia may change. Nonselective β-blockers should be avoided in tightly controlled patients with diabetes, especially those receiving insulin therapy. If a β-blocker is needed to control BP, or treat a compelling indication in diabetes, a cardioselective agent is preferred.

Other Considerations

β-Blockers have potential benefits in other conditions. They can slow the rate of cardiac conduction and may be useful in patients with paroxysmal supraventricular tachycardia or atrial fibrillation. They are also used in patients with tachycardia and/or anxiety from mitral valve prolapse, or preoperative hypertension. Finally, β-blockers are effective in treating other noncardiac conditions such as thyrotoxicosis, essential tremor, and migraine prophylaxis.

Nonselective β-blockers have been associated with increased serum triglycerides and reductions in HDL cholesterol. Agents with ISA have little or no effects on lipids, whereas cardioselective β-blockers have intermediate effects. Similar to diuretics, these changes are often not sustained with chronic therapy. β-Blockers have definitively been shown to lower morbidity and mortality, so their effects on cholesterol have little clinical significance. If a β-blocker is indicated in a patient with dyslipidemia, HDL cholesterol and fasting triglyceride values should be monitored closely.

35. How can monitoring heart rate optimize β-blocker therapy?

β-Blockers decrease conduction through both the SA and AV node. Lowering of the resting heart rate can be used as a marker of response. While receiving β-blocker therapy, heart rate should ideally be controlled to a resting pulse rate of no less than 60 beats/min to avoid heart block. First-degree heart block may be present when the heart rate is <60 beats/min, but normal conduction is maintained. β-Blocker therapy should, under most circumstances, be reduced if this occurs. Second- and third-degree heart block result in heart rates typically <55 and <40 beats/min, respectively, with abnormal cardiac conduction. β-Blocker therapy should be stopped if this occurs. Failure to achieve a lowered resting pulse could indicate inadequate dosage (i.e., need for a higher dose) or poor patient adherence to the prescribed regimen. However, if the BP target has been obtained, this is more important that pulse response.

36. Why should a β-blocker never be abruptly discontinued? What if a β-blocker needs to be stopped?

Chronic β-blocker therapy upregulates the expression of β-receptors. However, this does not result in rise of BP while β-blocker therapy is maintained to occupy the receptors. If β-blocker therapy is abruptly stopped, rebound hypertension can occur because more β-receptors are available to be activated, causing cardiac stimulation and vasoconstriction. Symptoms of rebound hypertension can include headache, tachycardia, and possibly anxiety. Patients with ischemic heart disease can have significant increases in angina frequency if β-blockers are abruptly stopped. If a β-blocker requires discontinuation, rebound hypertension or ischemia can be avoided by gradually tapering the dose by 50% for 3 days and then another 50% for 3 days. Replacing one β-blocker with another should not cause rebound hypertension.

Angiotensin-Converting Enzyme Inhibitors

37. A.R. is a 49-year-old African American woman with type 2 diabetes mellitus. She started lisinopril 10 mg daily 4 weeks ago when her BP values were consistently in the 140 to 150/85 to 90 mm Hg range. Since then she has come into the clinic weekly for BP measurements. They have ranged from 130 to 140/80 to 85 mm Hg despite strict adherence to her American Diabetes Association diet. Her BP today is 132/80 mm Hg (134/80 when repeated), and her heart rate is 78 beats/min. She is not a smoker, and her body mass index is 29 kg/m² (normal, <25 kg/m²). Her latest hemoglobin A1C was 8.5% (normal, 4% to 6%). All her laboratory test results, including renal function, are within normal limits, except that her spot urine albumin to creatinine ratio is 80 mg/g. How long should A.R. take lisinopril before her BP response is evaluated?

ACE inhibitors lower BP by causing peripheral arterial vasodilation without significant changes in cardiac output, heart rate, or GFR. The principal activity of ACE inhibitors is through inhibition of the renin-angiotensin-aldosterone system (see ACE Inhibitor section previously discussed). Additional mechanisms (vasodilatation from accumulation of bradykinin and prostaglandins, and direct local effects on arterioles of the systemic and renal vasculature) are also reported. ACE inhibitors are believed to provide unique cardiovascular benefits by improving endothelial function, promoting LVH regression and collateral vessel development, and improving insulin sensitivity.[31,163,164] The effects on renal blood flow and glomerular filtration are complex, depending on sodium balance and if renal artery stenosis is present (See Chapter 19, Heart Failure).

Pharmacologic Considerations

Several ACE inhibitors are currently marketed for the management of hypertension (Table 14-14). Some of these agents are primarily renally eliminated (benazepril, enalapril, lisinopril, quinapril, ramipril), and others have mixed hepatic and renal elimination (captopril, fosinopril, perindopril, trandolapril). Moexipril is the only ACE inhibitor that is almost completely hepatically eliminated. These characteristics may be important when selecting a product in patients with unstable organ function. Other differences such as a slower rate of elimination, a longer duration of action, prolonged onset of action with pro-drugs, and a slower dissociation from binding sites have been described. However, these differences have not been shown to have major clinical importance.

The time to reach steady-state BP conditions is similar to what is seen with other antihypertensive agents. Following the initiation of therapy, it may take several weeks before the full antihypertensive effects of these drugs are observed. Therefore, evaluating BP response 2 to 4 weeks after starting or changing the dose of an ACE inhibitor is appropriate. A.R. has been taking lisinopril for 4 weeks, and her present BP should be used to determine whether she has attained goal. Both her BP range over the past few weeks and today's average BP (133/80 mm Hg) are above her goal of <130/80 mm Hg (since she has diabetes).

ACE inhibitors can increase serum potassium, especially in patients with renal insufficiency, as a result of aldosterone reduction. ACE inhibitor therapy can also cause acute renal compromise (primarily in a small subset of patients with bilateral renal artery stenosis). Therefore, potassium and serum creatinine need to be monitored with ACE inhibitor therapy. One common mistake is to discontinue ACE inhibitors when there is a modest rise in serum creatinine. In these patients, the ACE inhibitor should be continued because they are more likely to benefit from the renal protective effects.[8]

DOSING

Most ACE inhibitors are dosed once daily in hypertension, but some require more frequent dosing, especially when higher doses are used as described in Table 14-14. Captopril was the first ACE inhibitor and is the only one for which at least twice daily dosing is needed. When first marketed, high doses (400 to 600 mg/day) were commonly used. These high

Drug	Starting Dose[a] (mg/day)	Usual Dosage Range (mg/day)	Dosing Frequency
Benazepril (Lotensin)	10	20–40	QD to BID
Captopril (Capoten)	25	50–100	BID to TID
Enalapril (Vasotec)	5	10–40	QD to BID
Fosinopril (Monopril)	10	20–40	QD
Lisinopril (Prinivil, Zestril)	10	20–40	QD
Moexipril (Univasc)	7.5	7.5–30	QD to BID
Perindopril (Aceon)	4	4–16	QD
Quinapril (Accupril)	10	20–80	QD to BID
Ramipril (Altace)	2.5	2.5–20	QD to BID
Trandolapril (Mavik)	1	2–4	QD

Table 14-14 Angiotensin-Converting Enzyme (ACE) Inhibitors in Hypertension

[a]Starting dose may be decreased 50% if patient is volume depleted, very elderly, or taking a diuretic.

dosages were associated with several adverse effects such as skin rash (5% to 10%), taste disturbances (5% to 10%), neutropenia (rare), and proteinuria (rare). Much lower dosages of captopril are now used, resulting in less frequent adverse effects. In general, most ACE inhibitors, if used in equivalent doses, are considered interchangeable.

TISSUE PENETRATION

Greater than 90% of ACE is localized in tissues and organs. Tissue penetration of individual ACE inhibitors varies. Ramipril, quinapril, and lisinopril have high penetration; captopril has low penetration.[165] Ramipril, an ACE inhibitor with high tissue penetration, provides cardiovascular event reduction in high-risk patients that may be largely independent of the degree of BP lowering.[97] Moreover, based on studies on endothelial function, ACE inhibitors with high tissue penetration may theoretically be superior to low penetration ACE inhibitors.[165] Despite this hypothesis, captopril, an ACE inhibitor with low tissue penetration, has been shown in numerous outcomes studies to reduce morbidity and mortality in a variety of high-risk CVD patients.[103,107,111,124,125,131,133] Therefore, evidence does not support the speculation that one ACE inhibitor is definitively better than another for cardiovascular protection based on tissue penetration.

RISK OF HYPOTENSION

38. **A.R.'s lisinopril dose is increased to 20 mg daily. Although A.R. did not experience hypotension when she first started lisinopril, will this doubling of her dose place her at risk for significant hypotension?**

Patients who are either volume depleted, hyponatremic, or have an exacerbation of HF may experience a significant first-dose response to an ACE inhibitor. This can manifest as orthostatic hypotension, dizziness, or possibly syncope. The increased pretreatment activity of the renin-angiotensin-aldosterone system coupled with acute blockade of this system by an ACE inhibitor explains this effect. These patients should initiate ACE inhibitor therapy at half the normal dose (see Table 14-14).

Concurrent diuretic therapy may predispose some patients to first-dose hypotension. When ACE inhibitors were first approved, dosing guidelines recommended starting at half the standard dose of the ACE inhibitor, decreasing the dose of the diuretic, or stopping the diuretic before initiating the ACE inhibitor. This was due to fear that BP would sharply and acutely drop. These recommendations are not necessary unless the patient is hemodynamically unstable (volume depleted, hyponatremic, or having a HF exacerbation), very elderly, or frail. A.R. did not exhibit these characteristics when she first started lisinopril; thus, she did not experience first-dose hypotension. Currently, she does not have these characteristics and can safely increase her dose of lisinopril without fear of significant hypotension.

AFRICAN AMERICAN PATIENTS

39. **Will an ACE inhibitor work in A.R. since she is African American?**

ACE inhibitor monotherapy is more effective at lowering BP in young white patients than in African American or elderly patients.[50] Elderly and African American patients are more likely to have low renin hypertension, which may partially explain some of the differences in response. Nevertheless, many of these patients still respond to ACE inhibitors as monotherapy. Several studies found that BP can be reduced to <140/90 mm Hg in 50% to 60% of elderly white patients and in approximately 50% of African American patients with an ACE inhibitor.[50,141,166] However, in the VA Cooperative trial, ACE inhibitors were effective as monotherapy in the following age and racial groups: 62% of young whites, 62% of elderly whites, 43% of young African American, and 33% of elderly African Americans.[50,167] These findings clearly show a trend of lower efficacy in African American patients, but not a complete lack of response.

Combination therapy, especially with a diuretic, can often overcome the race- or age-related differences in BP response to ACE inhibitors. In patients whose conditions do not adequately respond to an ACE inhibitor, the addition of a low-dose diuretic (e.g., HCTZ 12.5 mg) can achieve BP control in 80% to 90% of patients.[54] Diuretic use results in compensatory increases in renin. An ACE inhibitor in combination with a diuretic results in significant additive antihypertensive effects through complementary mechanisms.

When an antihypertensive agent is being selected for an African American patient with no other problems or disease states, an ACE inhibitor should generally not be chosen. A thiazide-type diuretic is preferred. However, if a compelling indication such as HF, diabetes, or chronic kidney disease is present, an ACE inhibitor is the drug of choice. Of note, African American patients have a two- to four-fold increased risk of angioedema and cough compared with whites.[96] While this does not preclude ACE inhibitor use in African Americans, it requires additional patient education regarding these potential side effects. A.R. has type 2 diabetes mellitus and microalbuminuria. Her goal BP is <130/80 mm Hg, and an ACE inhibitor is ideal treatment. Monotherapy is not expected to get her to goal, but nonetheless, she has had some BP reduction from lisinopril.

Compelling Indications

ACE inhibitors are useful for many patients with hypertension, including those who may not adequately respond to other therapies, or those who cannot take these agents due to contraindications or adverse reactions (e.g., patients with asthma, gout). Evidence has clearly demonstrated reduction in hypertension-related complications in patients with several medical conditions.

HEART FAILURE

ACE inhibitors reduce morbidity and mortality in patients with systolic HF and are standard therapy for these patients.[116–119] Although recent outcome-based studies have identified that several other antihypertensive agents can reduce morbidity and mortality in systolic HF (ARBs, aldosterone blockers, β-blockers),[121,126–128] ACE inhibitor therapy (with diuretics) is considered the standard regimen to which these other agents should be added. Therefore, ACE inhibitor therapy is the first-line intervention in hypertensive patients with systolic HF. The original trials evaluating ACE inhibitor therapy in HF primarily used captopril and enalapril. Since then, several other studies have been published using other

ACE inhibitors. In general, the beneficial effects are considered a class effect, and ACE inhibitors are used interchangeably at equivalent dosages in these patients.

POST-MYOCARDIAL INFARCTION

ACE inhibitor therapy is recommended indefinitely in all patients who are post-MI.[129,168] This is in addition to β-blockers. Evidence consistently shows reduced cardiovascular risk that is independent of LV function and BP in patients post-MI.[97,131]

HIGH CORONARY DISEASE RISK

ACE inhibitors have been evaluated in patients at risk for coronary disease, and similar to β-blockers, should be started early in patients with acute coronary syndromes (non-ST segment elevation MI and unstable angina).[129] In patients with chronic stable angina, ACE inhibitors can be added after β-blocker therapy (or a non-dihydropyridine CCB) as a strategy to either further lower BP or reduce risk of further CVD.[160]

DIABETES

ACE inhibitors are strongly recommended in the management of diabetes.[1,8,9] This recommendation is based on evidence showing reduced hypertension-related complications, including cardiac events, progression of kidney disease, and stroke.[162] ACE inhibitor therapy is likely the most important antihypertensive agent for patients with diabetes, independent of BP lowering.

The Heart Outcomes Prevention Evaluation (HOPE) study evaluated more than 9,000 patients, who were either at high risk for cardiovascular events or had diabetes, for 4 to 6 years.[97] They were randomized to ramipril (up to 10 mg daily) or placebo. Interestingly, these patients did not necessarily all have hypertension (the mean baseline BP was 139/77 mm Hg). Most of these high-risk patients had CAD (81%), hypercholesterolemia (66%), a previous MI (53%), or diabetes (38%, mostly type 2). The primary endpoint (a composite of MI, stroke, or death from cardiovascular causes) was reduced 32% with ramipril ($P < 0.001$). A substudy of the HOPE showed that in the 3,577 patients with diabetes, ramipril significantly reduced cardiovascular events and overt nephropathy.[101]

The United Kingdom Prospective Diabetes Study (UKPDS) group prospectively evaluated type 2 diabetes in several clinical trials. Consistent with findings from other trials, complications were reduced with lower levels of BP.[11,104,134] An added benefit of ACE inhibitors in diabetes is that they do not have biochemical adverse effects on glucose regulation like other agents may. Moreover, evidence suggests these ACE inhibitors are at least as good, if not better, than diuretics at reducing cardiovascular risk in diabetes.[133] Similarly, when ACE inhibitors were directly compared with CCBs, ACE inhibitors showed better reductions in cardiovascular events.[105,106]

CHRONIC KIDNEY DISEASE

ACE inhibitors protect the kidney from the unrelenting deterioration that occurs with chronic kidney disease, hypertension, and diabetes.[1,8] Chronic kidney disease is characterized by increased intraglomerular pressure and mesangial cell proliferation, which leads to proteinuria and a progressive decline in kidney function. Reductions in renal blood flow cause the kidneys to increase renin release, thus activating the angiotensin hormonal system locally. This local action constricts the efferent renal arteriole to preserve glomerular pressure, but may aggravate further renal impairment.

ACE inhibitors preferentially dilate the efferent arteriole, which relieves intraglomerular pressure. Data suggest that ACE inhibitors may have unique renal preservation properties, making chronic kidney disease a compelling indication for ACE inhibitor therapy. Some of the risk reduction is also related to systemic BP lowering. Control of BP, to a goal of <130/80 mm Hg, is a very important treatment goal in the management of chronic kidney disease.[35]

Patients with diabetes are at risk for nephropathy. This is especially true in type 1 diabetes. There is evidence that ACE inhibitor therapy reduces significant progression to severe chronic kidney disease and kidney failure in patients with type 1 diabetes and proteinuria.[135] ACE inhibitor therapy also reduces significant worsening of proteinuria in patients with type 2 diabetes and proteinuria,[8] but evidence showing progression to severe chronic kidney disease or failure is not available. Nonetheless, ACE inhibitor therapy is considered highly effective and is strongly recommended as a compelling indication in both type 1 and type 2 diabetes.

RECURRENT STROKE PREVENTION

The PROGRESS was a double-blind, placebo controlled evaluation of an ACE inhibitor in combination with a thiazide-type diuretic for 4 years in 6,105 patients with a history of stroke or transient ischemic attack.[98] Hypertensive and nonhypertensive patients were included. The incidence of stroke and total major vascular events were significantly reduced with combination regimen, and reductions were seen regardless of baseline BP or reduction in BP. These data justify the compelling indication to use an ACE inhibitor (in combination with a thiazide-type diuretic) to reduce recurrence in patients who have had a stroke.

Other Considerations

ACE inhibitors may not lower BP as well in elderly patients as in young patients. However, reductions in hypertension-related complications with ACE inhibitors in elderly patients are similar to those seen with diuretics and β-blockers. The Swedish Trial in Old Patients-2 (STOP-2) study was designed to prospectively evaluate elderly patients and compare reductions in complication with newer agents (ACE inhibitors and CCBs) versus older agents (diuretics and β-blockers).[100] The primary finding was that fatal cardiovascular events (stroke, MI, and other) were no different in the two groups. These data indicate that elderly patients receive cardiovascular protection with ACE inhibitors.

40. A.R. has microalbuminuria based on her spot urine. ACE inhibitor therapy may help preserve her kidney function. However, how can ACE inhibitors also cause acute renal dysfunction?

ACE inhibitors are effective in patients with hypertension-related renal artery disease. However, they are contraindicated in bilateral renal artery stenosis, pregnancy, and volume depletion (see Table 14-10). They should be used cautiously in patients who have suspected bilateral renal artery stenosis, or in those who have stenosis in a solitary kidney after nephrectomy. In these patients, high angiotensin concentrations maintain renal blood flow. Acute renal dysfunction can be precipitated when ACE inhibitors are started. Because it is often not known if a patient has bilateral renal artery stenosis, problems with ACE inhibitors can be minimized by starting with recommended doses and careful monitoring of serum creatinine within 4 weeks of starting therapy. Modest elevations in serum creatinine of ≤35% (for baseline creatinine values ≤3.0 mg/dL) or absolute increases ≤1.0 mg/dL, do not warrant changes.[8] These changes might even be expected in some patients. If larger increases occur, ACE inhibitor therapy should be stopped. Patients with elevated serum creatinine at baseline (up to 3.0 mg/dL) may particularly benefit from the vasodilatory effects of ACE inhibitors in the kidney, but definitely require close monitoring. A.R.'s renal function tests were normal after 4 weeks of lisinopril therapy. It appears as though she is not experiencing any kidney-related adverse effects from lisinopril.

41. What are the risks of using ACE inhibitors in women of childbearing age?

ACE inhibitors are teratogenic in the second and third trimester. Their use in pregnancy is contraindicated. Moreover, their use in women of child bearing potential is discouraged. If used in this population, patient education should be explicitly clear regarding risks to the fetus which include potentially fatal hypotension, anuria, renal failure, and developmental deformities. A highly effective form of contraception should be strongly recommended.

Angiotensin II Receptor Blockers

42. Four weeks after increasing lisinopril to 20 mg daily, A.R.'s BP is 126/78 mm Hg (128/76 mm Hg when repeated). Her serum potassium and creatinine are unchanged from previous values. However, her husband states that she has had a persistent dry cough for the past few months that sometimes keeps them both awake at night. She has no other signs of an upper respiratory infection or HF. Should A.R.'s lisinopril be replaced with an ARB?

The most well-known side effect of ACE inhibitors is a nonproductive and dry cough, which may occur in up to 15% of patients.[169] Patients may describe this as a tickling sensation in the back of the throat that commonly occurs late in the evening. This is distinctly different from the cough associated with HF, which is commonly associated with crackles and rales (on auscultation) and is wet and productive. ACE inhibitor–related

cough subsides with discontinuation. Many agents have been used to treat an ACE inhibitor cough with variable and poor results. The best treatment option for a patient with an intolerable ACE inhibitor cough is to switch agents.

ARBs are the newest antihypertensive class. There are seven of these agents commercially available as brand-name only products (Table 14-15). Fixed-dose combination products with HCTZ are also available (Table 14-12).

Pharmacology and Blood Pressure Lowering

Unlike ACE inhibitors, ARBs specifically bind to angiotensin II receptors in vascular smooth muscle, adrenal glands, and other tissues.[170] As a result, access of angiotensin II to its receptors is blocked and angiotensin II–mediated vasoconstriction and aldosterone release is prevented, resulting in BP reduction. Reduction in intraglomerular blood flow and pressure is mediated by angiotensin II actions in the efferent arteriole of the kidney. ARBs do not affect bradykinin. Therefore, there is no associated dry cough (See Chapter 19, Heart Failure).

Considerable investigation has focused on describing the pharmacologic differences between the angiotensin II type 1 and type 2 receptors.[171] Stimulation of the type 1 receptor causes vasoconstriction, salt and water retention, and vascular remodeling. Other deleterious effects from type 1 receptor stimulation include myocyte and smooth muscle hypertrophy, fibroblast hyperplasia, cytotoxic effects in the myocardium, altered gene expression, and possible increased concentrations of plasminogen activator inhibitor.[170] Stimulation of the type 2 receptor results in antiproliferative actions, cell differentiation, and tissue repair when stimulated.[170]

Theoretically, an ideal antihypertensive agent would block only type 1 and not type 2 receptor, as is the case with ARBs. Therefore, it is possible that an ARB would be superior to an ACE inhibitor in reducing hypertension-related complications because ACE inhibitors ultimately decrease stimulation of both type 1 and type 2 receptors by decreasing production of angiotensin II. This argument is purely speculative and is not supported by clinical trial data.

Another factor considered in the debate over relative BP lowering efficacy of ARBs versus ACE inhibitors is the role of bradykinin, a potent vasodilator normally metabolized by ACE. Because bradykinin serum concentrations rise with ACE inhibitors, but not with ARBs, it is suggested that ACE inhibitors may theoretically provide greater BP reductions

Table 14-15	Angiotensin II Receptor Blockers in Hypertension		
Drug	Starting Dose[a] (mg/day)	Usual Dosage Range (mg/day)	Dosing Frequency
Candesartan (Atacand)	16	8–32	QD to BID
Eprosartan (Teveten)	600	600–800	QD to BID
Irbesartan (Avapro)	150	150–300	QD
Losartan potassium (Cozaar)	50	50–100	QD to BID
Olmesartem (Benicar)	20	20–40	QD
Temisartan (Micardis)	20–40	20–80	QD
Valsartan (Diovan)	80–160	80–320	QD

[a]Starting dose may be decreased 50% if patient is volume depleted, very elderly, or taking a diuretic.

than ARBs.[172] However, these speculations are not substantiated with convincing evidence. ARBs are viewed as effective as other antihypertensive agents for BP lowering. Similar to ACE inhibitors, combinations with a thiazide-type diuretic are highly efficacious in lowering BP.

Differences Between Angiotensin II Receptor Blockers

The various ARBs have minor differences in their ability to antagonize the type 1 receptor site. Candesartan, irbesartan, and telmisartan have much stronger blockade than either losartan or valsartan.[173] The clinical significance of these effects is unclear. Most of these agents can be dosed once daily, except twice daily dosing may be needed when high doses of candesartan, eprosartan, or losartan are used. Similar to ACE inhibitors, initial doses may need to be lower in elderly patients and those who are taking a diuretic or are volume depleted.

There is debate regarding potential differences in BP lowering between individual ARBs. Some of the observed BP lowering differences may relate to comparisons that did not utilize equipotent doses. For instance, when comparing steady-state 24-hour BP reduction with recommended starting doses, olmesartan (20 mg daily) provides significantly better reductions when compared with losartan (50 mg daily) and valsartan (80 mg daily).[174] The magnitude of these differences is small (up to 4.5 mm Hg for SBP and up to 2.9 mm Hg for DBP) with debatable clinical relevance. However, steady-state BP reductions are similar with the starting doses of olmesartan (20 mg daily) and irbesartan (150 mg daily).[174] In general, it appears as though the starting doses of ARBs may not provide similar levels of BP lowering. However, difference may not to be present when using ARB doses above the starting dose.

Compelling Indications
HEART FAILURE

Pharmacologic blockade of the renin-angiotensin-aldosterone system in systolic HF is of paramount importance. It has been definitively proven that ACE inhibitor therapy reduces morbidity and mortality in this population.[116] Several studies have evaluated ARB therapy as alternatives to ACE inhibitors in the management of HF.[124–126] Overall, these two drug classes provide equal symptomatic improvement in HF, but ARBs are either similar or less efficacious in reducing mortality rates.[124,125] However, evidence from the VaLsartan in Heart Failure Trial (VaL-HeFT) indicates that patients with systolic HF given valsartan have less combined morbidity and mortality than patients taking placebo.[126] This benefit was less evident if patients were taking a combined regimen of an ACE inhibitor and valsartan (See Chapter 19, Heart Failure, for an expanded discussion of the VaL-HeFT trial).

ARBs are reasonable alternatives in patients with hypertension and HF who cannot tolerate ACE inhibitors (e.g., those who experience cough). The American College of Cardiology/American Heart Association HF guidelines also recommend an ARB in patients that have experienced angioedema from an ACE inhibitor[116] However, there are case reports of ARB induced angioedema (see Chapter 19, Heart Failure).

DIABETES
ARB-based treatment regimens have been shown in clinical trials to reduce the progression of diabetic nephropahy.[108–110] In type 2 diabetes with proteinuria, the incidence

of kidney disease progression (a composite end point of serum creatinine doubling, end-stage renal disease, or all cause mortality) improved more with irbesartan than with amlodipine.[109] Moreover, ARBs are the only antihypertensive agents for which evidence shows reduced kidney failure in patients with type 2 diabetes and nephropathy.[108] These benefits are independent of BP reduction, suggesting that improvements are due to inhibition of angiotensin II effects in the kidney. The American Diabetes Association recommends ARBs to decrease nephropathy in patients with hypertension, diabetes, and proteinuria.[9]

CHRONIC KIDNEY DISEASE

As discussed previously, ACE inhibitors protect the kidney from damage that occurs with chronic kidney disease.[8] Because of similar pharmacologic effects on the renal vasculature, ARBs share these same effects. Both ACE inhibitors and ARBs preferentially dilate the efferent arteriole, which relieves intraglomerular pressure. Thus, chronic kidney disease is a compelling indication for ARB therapy. However, for non–diabetic kidney disease, there is less evidence supporting ARB use, and they should be reserved as alternatives to ACE inhibitors.

ADDITIONAL POPULATIONS

Evidence shows decreased hypertension-related complications with ARBs compared to β-blocker therapy, as previously discussed.[95] The LIFE trial evaluated losartan versus atenolol in hypertensive patients with LVH. The incidence of primary cardiovascular events (including stroke, MI, and death) was statistically lower with losartan than with atenolol, primarily due to a significant reduction in stroke. The incidence of MI was similar with these two agents. The LIFE data were convincing enough that the Food and Drug Administration approved losartan for stroke reduction in hypertensive patients with LVH. Moreover, a subanalysis of the 1,195 patients with diabetes from the LIFE trial revealed statistically less cardiovascular morbidity and mortality with losartan in this subgroup.

Other Considerations
ARB VERSUS ACE INHIBITOR

Monitoring requirements, contraindications, and side effects (other than cough) are similar for ARBs and ACE inhibitors. Because of the potential hyperkalemia and acute renal dysfunction, serum creatinine and potassium should be monitored. ARBs are contraindicated in pregnancy and in patients with bilateral renal artery stenosis or volume depletion. Acute hypotension is possible when starting ARB therapy in patients with hyponatremia, volume depletion, or HF exacerbation.

There is an abundance of evidence in a wide range of patients showing benefits of ACE inhibitors on morbidity and mortality. Similar evidence demonstrating benefits with ARBs is growing. Head-to-head comparisons evaluating reductions in morbidity and mortality with ACE inhibitors versus ARBs are sparse. In HF, evidence indicates that ARB therapy is equal to or less effective than ACE inhibitor therapy in reducing complications.[111,125] In the Optimal Trial In Myocardial Infarction with Angiotensin II Antagonist Losartan (OPTIMAAL) trial, losartan was compared to captopril in 5,477 post-MI patients with HF. There were statistically fewer cardiovascular deaths with captopril and a trend showing reduced all cause mortality with captopril.

In summary, when examining cardiovascular outcomes, evidence supports ACE inhibitors being superior to ARBs. Data evaluating reductions in diabetic kidney disease are more difficult to evaluate since there are no comparative studies. ARBs have evidence showing reduced complications in type 2 diabetic nephropathy,[108,109] and ACE inhibitors have evidence showing reduced complications in type 1 diabetic nephropathy.[135]

A.R.'s BP has responded well to the lisinopril, and her cough appears to be drug induced. If her cough is caused by lisinopril, it should resolve over several days to 2 weeks after the drug is discontinued. One option is to lower the dose to that which she previously tolerated an add a second drug. Alternatively, switching to an ARB is warranted; it will likely control her BP and could minimize progression of her diabetic nephropathy. Other choices, such as CCBs, are potential alternatives to replace her ACE inhibitor for BP reduction, but they do not have a chronic kidney disease compelling indication.

Calcium Channel Blockers

43. **What are the pharmacologic actions of CCBs, and how do dihydropyridine CCBs differ from verapamil and diltiazem?**

Pharmacologic Actions

Vascular smooth muscle normally has low intracellular calcium. Smooth muscle contraction depends on an influx of extracellular calcium through calcium channels located on the cell membrane. The major hemodynamic alteration in most patients with hypertension is increased PVR caused in part by a direct effect of higher intracellular free calcium increasing arterial smooth muscle tone. CCBs prevent intracellular influx of calcium and promote vasodilation.

CCBs are very effective in lowering BP. Elderly and African Americans patients have greater BP reduction with CCBs than other agents (β-blockers, ACE inhibitors, ARBs).The addition of a diuretic to a CCB provides additive antihypertensive effects. CCBs do not alter serum lipids, glucose, uric acid, or electrolytes and they do not aggravate asthma or peripheral vascular disease.

CCBs are a heterogeneous drug class. All CCBs inhibit the movement of extracellular calcium, but there are two primary subtypes: dihydropyridines and nondihydropyridines (i.e., diltiazem and verapamil). Each has distinctly different pharmacologic effects that are summarized in Table 14-16.

Table 14-16 Pharmacologic Actions of Calcium Channel Blockers

	Verapamil	Diltiazem	Dihydropyridines
Peripheral vasodilation	↑	↑	↑↑
Heart rate	↓↓	↓	↑
Cardiac contractility	↓↓	↓	0/↓[a]
SA/AV nodal conduction	↓	↓	0
Coronary blood flow	↑	↑	↑↑

[a]No significant decreases are seen with amlodipine.
↑, increase; ↑↑, marked increase; ↓, decrease; ↓↓, marked decrease; 0, no change.

DIHYDROPYRIDINE CALCIUM CHANNEL BLOCKERS

Dihydropyridines are potent vasodilators of peripheral and coronary arteries. They do not block AV nodal conduction and do not effectively treat arrhythmias. Moreover, the potent vasodilation associated with most dihydropyridines can induce a reflex tachycardia. With the exception of amlodipine, dihydropyridines can decrease cardiac contractility and should be avoided in patients with systolic HF. Side effects of dihydropyridines are related to their potent vasodilatory effects, such as reflex tachycardia, headache, flushing, and peripheral edema.

NONDIHYDROPYRIDINE CALCIUM CHANNEL BLOCKERS

The nondihydropyridines, diltiazem and verapamil, are similar. Relative to dihydropyridines, they are only moderately potent vasodilators, but they directly decrease AV nodal conduction and have negative inotropic actions. The blockade of AV nodal conduction can slow heart rate and is the basis for their use in treating supraventricular arrhythmias (See Chapter 20, Cardiac Arrhythmias). Because vasodilation causes a reflex increase in heart rate, most patients only have a modest decrease in heart rate. However, first-, second-, or third-degree heart block are potential adverse effects with large doses.

Verapamil can cause bradycardia, heart block, and possible asystole when given via intravenous administration or when used in combination with a β-blocker. These reactions are rare with oral verapamil (due to differences in stereoselective metabolism) and oral diltiazem. Both are considered a safe and effective antihypertensives. Verapamil and diltiazem should be avoided in patients with second- or third-degree heart block. Under these circumstances a dihydropyridine can be used if a CCB is needed. Verapamil and diltiazem should also be avoided in patients with systolic HF because they can significantly reduce cardiac contractility. Diltiazem is slightly better tolerated than verapamil regarding potential side effects such as constipation.

Formulations

Several dihydropyridine and nondihydropyridine CCBs are available for the treatment of hypertension. They are listed in Table 14-17.

IMMEDIATE-RELEASE NIFEDIPINE

44. **A 68-year-old man has a new prescription for immediate-release nifedipine 10 mg three times daily for newly diagnosed hypertension. He has no contraindications to CCB therapy. Why should immediate-release nifedipine not be used to treat his hypertension?**

Most dihydropyridines, except amlodipine, are formulated as sustained-release products to provide 24-hour effects. Nifedipine has a very short half-life, and is available as an immediate-release capsule. It was once used to quickly reduce BP in hypertensive urgencies, but it should never be used for this indication. Immediate-release nifedipine, given sublingually or orally, has been associated with several adverse effects such as severe hypotension, cerebral ischemia, acute MI, fetal distress, conduction abnormalities, and even death.[175–177] The rapid and potent hypotensive effect can "steal" blood flow from coronary arteries, induce reflex tachycardia, and acutely decrease cardiac contractility (See Chapter 21, Hypertensive Emergencies).

Table 14-17   **Calcium Channel Blockers in Hypertension**[a]

Drug	Usual Dosage Range (mg/day)	Dosing Frequency
Nondihydropyridines[b]		
Diltiazem, sustained-release capsule (Cardizem SR, Tiamate)	120–360	BID
Diltiazem, sustained-release capsule (Cardizem CD, Cartia XT, Dilacor XR, Tiazac)	120–360	QD
Verapamil, sustained-release tablet (Calan SR, Isoptin SR)	180–480	QD to BID
Verapamil, sustained-release capsule (Verelan)	180–480	QD to BID
Verapamil, controlled-onset extended-release tablet (Covera HS)[c]	180–480	QHS
Verapamil, chronotherapeutic oral drug absorption system (Verelan HS)[c]	100–400	QHS
Dihydropyridines		
Amlodipine, immediate-release tablet (Norvasc)	2.5–10	QD
Felodipine, extended-release tablet (Plendil)	2.5–20	QD
Isradipine, controlled-release tablet (DynaCirc CR)	5–20	QD
Nicardipine, sustained-release capsule (Cardene SR)	60–120	BID
Nifedipine, sustained-release[d] tablet (Procardia XL, Adalat CC)	30–90	QD
Nisoldipine, extended-release tablet (Sular)	10–40	QD

[a]Immediate release (IR) diltiazem, nifedipine, and verapamil should be avoided in hypertension.
[b]Many sustained release (SR) products exist, but vary in release characteristics. Thus, they are not directly interchangeable using a mg-per-mg conversion.
[c]Covera HS (a "GITS" formulation) and Verelan HS (a beaded capsule) are "chronotherapeutic" agents. An outer coating delays initial release for 4 to 5 hours with both, followed by sustained release. They are taken at bedtime, but offer a peak response in the early AM when BP is often highest. Because they use different delivery systems, they are not interchangeable.
[d]Only sustained-release nifedipine is approved for hypertension. Immediate release should be avoided.

A link between immediate-release CCBs and MI was first reported in 1995.[176] This observational population-based analysis demonstrated that immediate-release CCBs were associated with a significantly higher risk of MI compared with thiazide-type diuretics (almost three-fold higher) and β-blocker therapy (almost two-fold higher). This risk was present with all three prototypical CCBs (nifedipine, diltiazem, and verapamil), but was strongest with nifedipine. Several other retrospective analyses have shown similar effects.

Immediate-release nifedipine has never been approved for the treatment of hypertension, and the Cardiorenal Advisory Panel of the Food and Drug Administration concluded that the use of immediate-release nifedipine is neither safe nor efficacious.[175] Immediate-release dihydropyridines, especially nifedipine, should be avoided. Even with verapamil and diltiazem, once daily sustained-release formulations are preferred for hypertension.

SUSTAINED-RELEASE FORMULATIONS

45. **C.F. is a 60-year-old man with a history of hypertension, asthma, and type 2 diabetes. His hypertension has been treated with HCTZ 25 mg daily, controlled-onset extended-release verapamil 240 mg daily (Covera HS), and ramipril 10 mg daily for the past 5 years. Today his BP is 124/74 mm Hg (128/72 mm Hg when repeated), and his heart rate is 64 beats/min. C.F. is interested in a generic alternative for his controlled-onset extended-release verapamil, such as sustained-release verapamil. What are the differences between these two verapamil products, and are they interchangeable?**

All CCBs have short half-lives, except amlodipine. Immediate-release forms require multiple daily doses to provide 24-hour effects. Sustained-released formulations are preferred when CCBs are used to treat hypertension. Various sustained-release delivery devices are available. Most of these are dosed once daily, except for Cardizem SR, verapamil SR, and Cardene SR. Sustained, extended, or controlled-release products all have unique biopharmaceutical delivery characteristics. Nifedipine is available as an osmotic pump (Procardia XL) that continually releases drug and as a core-coat release mechanism (Adalat CC) where two boluses of drug are released.

Serum drug concentrations differ between sustained-release CCBs, but the overall BP lowering effects are usually similar. Nonetheless, most of these products that include the same drug are not AB rated as equivalent (except Isoptin SR and Calan SR). Insurance formularies often require therapeutic substitution between these agents. However, therapeutic interchange with sustained-release diltiazem products or with chronotherapeutic verapamil are not equivalent using a mg-per-mg conversion. Therapeutic substitution between these products may result in variable BP lowering effects if not adjusted appropriately. BP and heart rate monitoring should occur within 2 weeks of interchanging sustained-release CCBs.

CHRONOTHERAPEUTIC VERAPAMIL

BP has a predictable circadian rhythm characterized by a sharp rises in pressure starting in the early morning, peaking in the mid to late morning, followed by a gradual decrease to lowest values during early to mid-nighttime.[4] Importantly, MI incidence also has a circadian rhythm in which events are most frequent during the time of the early morning BP surge. Chronopharmacology is the concept of recognizing circadian rhythms of disease and targeting drug delivery to blunt such rhythms. The prevailing assumption is that targeting BP reduction according to the circadian rhythm can maximally reduce the risk of cardiovascular events.

Two sustained-release verapamil products (Covera HS and Verelan PM) are chronotherapeutically designed to target the circadian BP rhythm. Covera HS uses an osmotic pump to provide a sustained release of verapamil with a once daily bedtime dose. The outer coating delays drug release by 4 to 5 hours. With evening dosing, drug is delivered during the morning BP surge with no delivery during the early evening. Verelan PM uses a different device that provides the same 4- to 5-hour delay but uses drug-loaded beads to control drug release. Covera HS and Verelan PM are not interchangeable using a mg-to-mg conversion, so therapeutic substitution between products must involve close monitoring.

The scientific rationale supporting chronotherapy in hypertension is logical. However, evidence from the Controlled Onset Verapamil Investigation of Cardiovascular Endpoints (CONVINCE) trial shows that chronotherapeutic verapamil is similar, but not better than, a thiazide-type diuretic/β-blocker based regimen in reducing hypertension-related complications.[94] C.F. has achieved his goal BP of <130/80 mm Hg with his present form of verapamil. Therefore, it may be ideal to continue using this product. However, if a switch must occur, his present controlled-onset extended release verapamil 240 mg daily should be changed to sustained-release generic verapamil 240 mg daily. This conversion requires BP and heart rate monitoring in 2 weeks to detect whether BP remains controlled after the switch, because these two products are not identical and are not AB rated as interchangeable.

Compelling Indications
HIGH CORONARY DISEASE RISK

46. **A.P. is a 71-year-old man with a BP of 168/96 mm Hg (170/100 mm Hg when repeated) and a heart rate of 88 beats/min. He has a history of angina, which is controlled with sublingual nitroglycerin as needed, and severe asthma that is poorly controlled. He currently has no chest pain, and his ECG shows no acute ischemia. Other lab results are within normal range, except his serum creatinine is 1.3 mg/dL (normal, 0.5 to 1.2 mg/dL). Is a CCB appropriate for A.P.? If yes, which type is preferred?**

β-Blocker therapy is first-line treatment for patients with a chronic stable angina pectoris, non-ST segment elevation MI, and unstable angina.[129,160] However, a CCB can be used as an alternative, especially when contraindications and/or intolerances to β-blockers are present. Sustained-release CCB formulations should be used for outpatient management of these patients. The INVEST study has recently found that verapamil-based therapy provides the same reductions in cardiovascular events as atenolol therapy in patients with chronic stable angina.[131a]

CCBs were first developed to treat ischemic heart disease and were later proven to be effective in hypertension. Nondihydropyridine CCBs decrease myocardial oxygen demand, improve myocardial blood flow, and have negative inotropic and chronotropic effects. All these can benefit high coronary risk patients (e.g., those with angina, ST-segment elevation MI, or acute coronary syndromes). Dihydropyridine CCBs are similar, but do not lower heart rate, and have less negative inotropic effects. They can be used in patients with chronic stable angina, but verapamil and diltiazem are preferred. Moreover, dihydropyridine CCBs are not particularly helpful in patients with ST-segment elevation MI or acute coronary syndromes.

CCB therapy is preferred in A.P., since β-blockers may worsen his severe asthma. If he had mild asthma, a cardioselective β-blocker would be a reasonable option.[156] Verapamil is an attractive agent for A.P. It will lower his elevated heart rate and BP as well as treat his angina. Sustained-release verapamil is available generically and is generally well tolerated. Constipation, which may be more prominent in an elderly patient, is the most frequent side effect. Of all the CCBs, constipation is most commonly associated with verapamil, but can be countered with dietary changes or bulk-forming laxatives. Similar to other antihypertensive agents, a low dose (120 to 180 mg daily) should be used initially and slowly titrated at 2- to 4-week intervals.

DIABETES

47. **Why is diabetes a compelling indication for a CCB?**

CCBs are recommended as options to treat hypertension in patients with diabetes.[1,8,9] They do not affect insulin sensitivity or glucose metabolism and would appear to be ideal antihypertensive drugs for patients with diabetes and hypertension. However, evidence showing reduced cardiovascular events with CCBs in patients with diabetes is not as convincing as that seen with other antihypertensive (thiazide-type diuretics, β-blockers, ACE inhibitors, and ARBs). Evidence suggests that the risk of stroke is significantly reduced with dihydropyridines in diabetes, but the effect on stroke is unknown with verapamil and diltiazem.[162] Evidence for reductions in coronary events with dihydropyridines in diabetes is controversial and is unknown with diltiazem and verapamil.[162] The results of the Fosinopril versus Amlodipine Cardiovascular Events randomized Trial (FACET) and Appropriate Blood pressure Control in Diabetes (ABCD) trials suggest that ACE inhibitors have more cardiovascular protection than CCBs.[105,106]

Data imply that nondihydropyridine CCBs (especially diltiazem) may slow the progression of chronic kidney disease, although evidence is not as extensive or definitive as it is with ACE inhibitors or ARBs.[8,108–110,112] The proposed mechanism is dilation of the afferent and efferent arterioles, which would decrease intraglomerular pressure. Dihydropyridines have unclear effects on progression of kidney disease. The prevailing opinion is that the renal protective effects of ACE inhibitors and ARBs are superior to CCBs.

CCBs do not appear to be harmful in persons with diabetes, and stroke reduction is a proven benefit. Nonetheless, CCBs are considered second-line agents after thiazide-type diuretics, β-blockers, ACE inhibitors, and ARBs. The BP goal in diabetes is <130/80 mm Hg. Because most patients with diabetes need three or more antihypertensives to achieve this goal, CCBs are useful agents in this population, especially in combination with other agents.

Additional Populations
ISOLATED SYSTOLIC HYPERTENSION

48. **T.C. is a 77-year-old woman with hypertension for the past 5 years. She was first treated with HCTZ 12.5 mg daily. It was stopped after she developed acute gout, which resolved shortly thereafter. Her hypertension has not been treated since this event. She now is being re-evaluated by a new physician. Her BP values are 164/76 mm Hg (168/78 mm Hg when repeated). She has no other cardiovascular risk factors, no evidence of target organ damage, and no compelling indications. Her laboratory**

values and ECG are all normal. What are the benefits of using a CCB to treat T.C.'s hypertension?

T.C. has isolated systolic hypertension. This should be managed according to the general patient care principles for hypertension. Thiazide-type diuretics should be used first, but this patient cannot use them. If another compelling indication is present, drug therapy recommended for that indication should predominate. If no compelling indication is present, a long-acting dihydropyridine CCB, as recommended in the previous JNC report, should be used.[54]

Thiazide-type diuretics and long-acting dihydropyridine CCBs reduce morbidity and mortality in patients with ISH. The SHEP trial proved that treating ISH in the elderly is beneficial and established thiazide diuretic-based regimens as first-line agents.[52] The Systolic hypertension in Europe (Syst-Eur) study was similar to the SHEP trial, but used a nitrendipine-based (a long-acting dihydropyridine CCB similar to long-acting nifedipine) regimen instead of a thiazide-type diuretic-based regimen.[64,178] Over a median of 2 years, there was a significant reduction in cardiovascular events (stroke, MI, and sudden cardiac death). Evidence suggests that long-acting (i.e., once daily) dihydropyridine CCBs reduce hypertension-related complications. Since T.C.'s gout was induced by HCTZ and she has no other compelling indications, a dihydropyridine CCB is her best option.

ADDITIONAL POPULATIONS

CCBs may also have potential benefits for other conditions. Diltiazem and verapamil can be used in atrial fibrillation, atrial flutter, and supraventricular arrhythmias. Verapamil is effective in migraine prophylaxis, but is second-line to β-blockers (e.g., propranolol) for this indication. Patients with Raynaud's syndrome can obtain symptomatic relief from the peripheral vasodilation associated with dihydropyridine CCBs. Lastly, CCBs are effective in treating cyclosporine-induced hypertension, but should be used cautiously because verapamil and diltiazem increase cyclosporine concentration.

Other Considerations
HEART FAILURE

49. What are the problems with using CCBs in HF?

CCBs decrease cardiac contractility due to negative inotropic effects. This is most pronounced with verapamil, but is also present with diltiazem and most dihydropyridines (see Table 14-16). In systolic HF, the primary physiologic problem is decreased cardiac contractility. Using a CCB in this population can exacerbate HF due to the direct negative inotropic effects. CCBs may also induce symptoms of HF in patients with no previous history of HF, but with underlying risk factors.

Some patients with systolic HF may require a CCB to treat another related condition (i.e., angina or uncontrolled hypertension). Amlodipine, a dihydropyridine with a long half-life, has been evaluated in patients with severe systolic HF. Available evidence indicates that amlodipine does not cause adverse cardiovascular effects in this population, but it does not protect against HF related mortality.[179] Amlodipine and felodipine are the only CCB that have been convincingly shown to be safe in systolic HF and may be used if needed for either angina or hypertension.

In diastolic HF, the primary physiologic problem is decreased cardiac filling time, not decreased contractility.

Therefore, verapamil and diltiazem can be helpful since they can decrease heart rate and allow more time for the LV to fill.

Dual Calcium Channel Blocker Therapy

50. If one CCB is not completely effective, is there any rationale for using two CCBs together?

It is rarely rational to combine two agents from the same therapeutic class in hypertension. Nevertheless, the three prototypical CCBs (i.e., nifedipine, diltiazem, and verapamil) each bind to different sites on the calcium channel. Combinations have been studied in hypertension and in refractory angina.[180,181] The combination of a dihydropyridine with a nondihydropyridine is more effective than each agent alone, especially when high-dose monotherapy is needed to control BP.

Dual CCB therapy is considered a last-line therapy, but may be needed in certain patients (those with chronic kidney disease or diabetes) to achieve aggressive BP goals or for severe angina.[8] If dual therapy is used, it should consist of a dihydropyridine with either diltiazem or verapamil.[8] The combination of a dihydropyridine with diltiazem may be more effective at lowering BP than a dihydropyridine with verapamil.[181] Diltiazem with verapamil should be avoided because of the potential for exaggerated AV nodal blocking and heart block.

Alternative Antihypertensive Agents

Several alternative agents are available to treat difficult-to-control hypertension, as listed in Table 14-18. None of these drugs should be used as monotherapy in the treatment of hypertension because they have not been shown to reduce hypertension-related complications. They should primarily be used as last-line agents in combination with better-tolerated antihypertensive agents that reduce morbidity and mortality (i.e., diuretics, β-blockers, ACE inhibitors, ARBs, or CCBs).

α-Blockers

51. J.L. is a 64-year-old man with hypertension. His BP is 138/82 mm Hg (138/84 mm Hg when repeated) while taking HCTZ 25 mg daily and amlodipine 10 mg daily. He also takes simvastatin 40 mg QD for dyslipidemia. J.L. is not completely compliant with lifestyle modifications, but he insists that this is the best he can do. He has been experiencing frequent nocturia, difficulty in starting urination, and a decrease in his urinary flow for the past several months. He is diagnosed with benign prostatic hyperplasia (BPH). J.L.'s physician is considering changing one of his antihypertensive agents to an α-blocker. How do α-blockers compare with other agents in reducing cardiovascular events?

The role of α-blockers as a first-line agent in the management of hypertension is discouraged. The ALLHAT, as discussed previously, originally included an α-blocker (doxazosin) treatment arm. Interim results after a mean follow-up of 3.3 years revealed that doxazosin had a statistically higher risk of combined CVD (RR = 1.25; $P < 0.001$) and HF (RR = 2.04; $P < 0.001$) than chlorthalidone.[114] Based on these findings, the doxazosin arm of the study was terminated early.

The ALLHAT data show that thiazide-type diuretic therapy is more protective against hypertension-related complications than α-blocker therapy. This study did not include a placebo group; therefore, to conclude that doxazosin is harmful is inaccurate. The average SBP of patients receiving chlorthali-

Table 14-18   Other Drugs Used in Hypertension

Drugs/Mechanism of Action	Usual Dosage Range (mg/day)	Dosing Frequency
α₁-Blockers		
Doxazosin (Cardura)	1–8	QD
Prazosin (Minipress)	2–20	BID to TID
Terazosin (Hytrin)	1–20	QD to BID
α₂-Agonists (Central)[a]		
Clonidine (Catapres)	0.1–0.8	BID
Clonidine Transdermal (Catapres TTS)[b]	0.1–0.3	Once weekly
Methyldopa (Aldomet)	250–100	BID
Arterial Vasodilators[a]		
Hydralazine (Apresoline)	25–100	BID
Minoxidil (Loniten)	2.5–800	QD to BID
Adrenergic Neuron Blockers[a]		
Reserpine (Serpasil)	0.5–0.25	QD

[a]May cause fluid retention and/or reflex tachycardia that requires concurrent diuretic and/or beta blocker therapy.
[b]Transdermal clonidine patch may ↓ incidence of side effects and ↑ compliance. Acceptability limited by skin rash.

done was approximately 2 to 3 mm Hg lower than those treated with doxazosin and may explain the difference in clinical outcomes. For J.L., discontinuing HCTZ to start an α-blocker is not prudent. However, it may be appropriate to use a combination of HCTZ and an α-blocker.

52. Do α-blockers reduce cardiovascular events in patients with hypertension? Is there any other potential benefit of using an α-blocker in J.L.?

α-Blockers are clearly last-line options in hypertension. Beneficial effects of reducing morbidity and mortality may be provided only if an α-blocker is used in combination with a proven effective agent. An α-blocker can potentially improve the symptoms of BPH by reducing urethral tone and alleviating the bladder outlet obstruction. Terazosin and doxazosin are both approved for the treatment of symptoms caused by BPH. Prazosin may be used, but requires more frequent dosing. Decreased symptoms of BPH with α-blockers are dose-related, and titration to high doses are often needed. This increases the risk of side effects with α-blockers. In J.L., an α-blocker will lower his BP and might also relieve his urinary symptoms.

53. How would J.L.'s dyslipidemia be affected by α-blocker therapy?

One theoretical advantage of the α-blockers is that they do not cause adverse metabolic effects. They have been shown to modestly lower total cholesterol, LDL cholesterol, and triglycerides and to increase HDL cholesterol. These effects are considered small and may not be clinically significant. An α-blocker should never be selected solely on the basis of these minor effects on plasma lipids.

54. J.L. prefers to try doxazosin rather than undergo surgery to relieve his symptoms of BPH. How should this agent be started?

For J.L., it would be best to add a low dose of an α-blocker to his present two-drug regimen. Based on his tolerance of the new drug and BP response, it can be titrated up. One of his other antihypertensive agents (preferably amlodipine since he does not have a compelling indication for a CCB) can be

stopped if he becomes hypotensive. The initial dose of doxazosin should not exceed 1 mg daily and it should be given at bedtime. This can minimize orthostatic hypotension (i.e., profound hypotension, dizziness, and possible fainting), which is the most frequent side effect of α-blockers. This complication is most pronounced with the first dose, but may persist in some patients. The dose can be increased to symptom control based on BP and tolerability.

55. What patient education should be provided to J.L. about the potential adverse effects of doxazosin?

α-Blockers are relatively well tolerated if dosed appropriately. J.L. could experience side effects such as drowsiness, headache, weakness, palpitations from reflex tachycardia, and nausea, but these do not occur in all patients. All α-blockers, especially prazosin due to its short half-life, can cause orthostatic hypotension. Patients starting an α-blocker should be instructed to take the initial dose at bedtime and to anticipate a first-dose effect, in which they may experience dizziness when changing their body posture. Specifically, patients should be counseled to rise more slowly from a seated or supine position. These side effects are most apparent when first starting therapy with prazosin, and are less frequent with chronic use.

Mixed α/β-Blockers

56. R.P. is a 68-year-old man with hypertension and a history of stroke (1 year ago). One month ago, his BP values were 164/94 mm Hg and 162/98 mm Hg, with a heart rate of 62 beats/min while on atenolol 50 mg daily. He started the fixed-dose combination of benazepril/HCTZ 10/12.5 mg daily and is being seen for follow-up. His BP today is 142/82 mm Hg (144/82 mm Hg when repeated). All his laboratory values are normal except his serum creatinine, which is 1.7 mg/dL (normal, 0.5 to 1.2 mg/dL). J.L. has implemented lifestyle modification to the best of his ability. Because R.P.'s BP is still not at goal, could his atenolol be replaced with an agent such as labetalol and carvedilol?

Labetalol and carvedilol are nonselective β-blockers that also have α₁-receptor blocking activity. Their hemodynamic properties are similar to a combination of a nonselective β-blocker (e.g., propranolol) with an α_1-antagonist (e.g., terazosin). Dosing recommendations are listed in Table 14-13.

These agents produce intense vasodilation and can cause more adverse reactions than β-blocker or α-blocker monotherapy. These reactions include postural dizziness, lightheadedness, and fatigue. The same precautions and typical contraindications relevant to β-blockers (e.g., patients with asthma) apply to these agents because they basically are nonselective β-blockers (see Table 14-10). However, unlike pure β-blockers, both carvedilol and labetalol may be safer to use in patients with peripheral arterial disease because unopposed peripheral α-constriction does not occur.

Carvedilol was first approved for the management of hypertension. In addition to its primary cardiovascular effects, it also has antioxidant properties that are of unknown relevance.[182] Carvedilol has been shown to reduce morbidity and mortality in a wide range of patients with systolic HF and is approved for this condition.[120,122,183] Carvedilol is not available generically. Since other less-expensive agents are equally effective in lowering BP, its use in hypertension is limited.

Labetalol and carvedilol have no clear advantage over other agents in the management of hypertension and have more side effects. If R.P. had the compelling indication of systolic HF, switching to carvedilol would be reasonable. His heart rate is between 60 and 70 beats/min, so this indicates he is adherent with atenolol. Increasing the atenolol dose to 100 mg daily is not wise since it may induce heart block. Atenolol is renally eliminated, so his present dose is probably causing more BP lowering than usual doses based on his chronic kidney disease. Increasing his ACE inhibitor will help to control both his BP and preserve his kidney function. This can be done without increasing his HCTZ by switching his fixed-dose combination product to benazepril/HCTZ 20/12.5 mg daily. This is the simplest option for R.P.

Central α_2-Agonists
CLONIDINE

57. T.M. is a 37-year-old male truck driver with a 5-year history of hypertension. Secondary causes have been ruled out previously. His regimen is losartan/HCTZ 100/25 mg daily and sustained-release diltiazem 240 mg daily. Other antihypertensive drugs have failed because of various side effects (captopril and lisinopril caused a dry cough, atenolol caused severe fatigue, nifedipine and amlodipine caused edema, and terazosin caused orthostasis). T.M. has been adherent to his present medications and lifestyle modification, but has been unable to quit smoking. His BP values have averaged 150/95 mm Hg for the past 3 months, based on clinic measures. Home values have been similar. The plan is to add clonidine 0.1 mg BID for BP control. How can it be that an α_2-agonist is effective in lowering BP when α_1-antagonists are also antihypertensive agents?

The antihypertensive effects of α_2-agonists (clonidine, guanabenz, guanfacine, methyldopa) are attributed to their central α_2-agonist activity. Stimulation of α_2-receptors in the CNS inhibits sympathetic outflow (via negative feedback) to the heart, kidneys, and peripheral vasculature, resulting in peripheral vasodilation. Although the α_2-agonists are effective as monotherapy, they are not considered first-line therapy for the treatment of hypertension because of their potential side

effects and a lack of evidence showing reductions in morbidity and mortality.

α_2-Agonists are most effective when used with a diuretic because they all can potentially cause fluid retention. They should ideally be used in combination with agents that have different mechanisms of action (e.g., diuretics, vasodilators) and with agents that do not affect other central adrenergic receptors (e.g., β-blockers).

Clonidine also has been used to attenuate withdrawal symptoms in people who are undergoing smoking cessation. Although response is variable, there may be an advantage to using clonidine in T.M. as an adjunct to a smoking cessation program. Clonidine can cause rebound hypertension when abruptly stopped. T.M.'s occupation may place him at risk for this complication if he misses doses due to unusual work hours and/or prolonged travel.

58. How should T.M.'s clonidine dose be titrated?

Clonidine should be started at a low dosage and gradually increased to achieve optimal BP lowering with minimal side effects. It is started as 0.1 mg twice daily, with 0.1 or 0.2 mg/day increases every few weeks until the desired response is achieved. Clonidine also is available as a transdermal patch, which releases the medication at a controlled rate over 7 days, and may have fewer side effects than the oral dosage form. The onset of initial BP effect may be delayed for 2 to 3 days after application; thus, rebound hypertension (which can occur with this drug class) might occur if the oral clonidine is switched to transdermal. To prevent this, an oral dose should be taken on the first day the transdermal patch is used. Anticholinergic side effects such as sedation and dry mouth are the most frequent and bothersome side effects of clonidine. These can be especially problematic in elderly patients. A patch may be preferred in T.M. as a strategy to avoid missing doses.

59. After several weeks, T.M.'s BP is 138/84 mm Hg with clonidine 0.2 mg twice daily. However, he wants to discontinue it because he is now experiencing daytime somnolence and dry mouth. What other α_2-agonists are available?

METHYLDOPA

Methyldopa, like clonidine, is an α_2-agonists. It has been extensively evaluated and is considered safe in pregnancy. Therefore, it is recommended as a first-line agent when hypertension is first diagnosed during pregnancy.[184] Beyond that, there is little role for methyldopa in the management of hypertension.

The usual initial dose is 250 mg administered twice daily up to 2,000 mg/day. Methyldopa causes side effects similar to those associated with clonidine including sedation, lethargy, postural hypotension, dizziness, dry mouth, headache, and rebound hypertension. These may decrease with continued use. Other significant side effects include hemolytic anemia and hepatitis. Although these are both rare, they necessitate discontinuing the medication.

OTHERS

Guanfacine and guanabenz are also α_2-agonists and have a high incidence of side effects. The adverse effects of guanfacine include dry mouth (occurring in up to 60% of patients), sedation, dizziness, orthostatic hypotension, insomnia, constipation, and impotence. Although complaints of sedation appear to be less common than with clonidine or guanabenz, the dose should be administered at bedtime if given once daily. Guanfacine has a long half-life (approximately 17 to 20 hours) that allows once daily administration and may have less rebound hypertension than other α₂-agonists with shorter half-lives. Guanabenz is similar, but has a shorter half-life and is dosed twice daily. Adverse effects include sedation (which may be more common than with methyldopa or clonidine), dizziness, and dry mouth.

The adverse effects of other α-agonists (methyldopa, guanfacine, and guanabenz) are nearly identical to that of clonidine. In general, patients who do not tolerate one α-agonist will not tolerate the others. An antihypertensive agent from a different class should be chosen for T.M.

Reserpine

60. **What is the role of reserpine in the contemporary management of hypertension?**

Reserpine is one of the oldest antihypertensive agents currently available. It is extremely effective in lowering BP when added to a diuretic.[185] Reserpine is inexpensive, and is dosed once daily. Several of the landmark trials that demonstrated reduced morbidity and mortality with BP lowering in hypertension used reserpine. More recently, the SHEP trial used reserpine as a second-step agent added to chlorthalidone in patients who could not take atenolol.[52] Reserpine is not commercially promoted since it has been available generically for more than 20 years.

Many clinicians avoid the use of reserpine because of the common impression that it can cause depression. This fear was generated from case reports in the 1950s. However, the doses used in those reports were much higher (0.5 to 1.0 mg/day) than what is needed to treat hypertension. Furthermore, many of the patients described in these cases would not meet modern criteria for depression; rather, they would be described as oversedated. When reserpine is limited to a maximum of 0.25 mg daily, depression is no more frequent than with other antihypertensive agents.

Low-dose reserpine (0.05 to 0.1 mg once daily) is effective at lowering BP and has significantly fewer side effects compared with high doses. The German Reserpine in Hypertension Study Group compared the combination of low-dose reserpine with a thiazide-type diuretic to a dihydropyridine CCB.[185] Antihypertensive effect was greater with the reserpine combination; there were fewer side effects and an increased quality of life with reserpine compared to the CCB.

Reserpine can cause nasal stuffiness in many patients. Gastrointestinal ulcerations have been reported, but are associated with either parenteral administration or very large doses. Although reserpine does not stimulate gastric acid secretion when doses ≤0.25 mg daily are used, it should be avoided in patients with a history of peptic ulcer disease. T.M. is a good candidate for low-dose reserpine. He is already taking HCTZ, which should always be used with reserpine, and his therapeutic options are limited. Of all the agents remaining for T.M., reserpine has the most favorable side effect profile.

Arterial Vasodilators
HYDRALAZINE

61. **C.M. is a 56-year-old woman with a history of hypertension and severe chronic kidney disease with an estimated GFR of 20 mL/min. Her antihypertensive regimen consists of furosemide 40 mg twice daily, captopril 100 mg twice daily, metoprolol 100 mg twice daily, and felodipine 20 mg daily. She started hydralazine 50 mg twice daily 4 weeks ago when her BP was 144/92 and 142/90 mm Hg. She has been very compliant, and her BP is now 136/86 mm Hg with a heart rate of 82 beats/min. Her lung fields are clear, with 1+ bilateral pitting edema. Serum electrolytes are within normal limits. Why was hydralazine used in this patient?**

Hydralazine causes direct relaxation of arteriolar smooth muscle with little effect on the venous circulation. Arterial vasodilators are infrequently used, except for patients with severe chronic kidney disease. In this population, hypertension is difficult to control and often requires four or five agents. Severe chronic kidney disease results in increased renin release and increased fluid retention. Potent vasodilation, in combination with diuresis, is often effective in lowering BP under these conditions.

Unfortunately, potent vasodilation stimulates the sympathetic nervous system and results in a reflex tachycardia, increased PRA, and additional fluid retention. Thus, the hypotensive effectiveness of direct arterial vasodilators can quickly diminish with time when used as monotherapy. To prevent this effect, arterial vasodilators should be used in combination with both a β-blocker to counteract reflex tachycardia and a diuretic to minimize fluid retention.

62. **After 18 months, C.M.'s hydralazine dose has been titrated up to 150 mg twice daily. She now complains of joint pain in both her right and left hands, which extends to the wrists, and generalized weakness with frequent fevers. What is a possible explanation for C.M.'s subjective complaints? What objective data can be obtained to confirm your suspicions?**

C.M.'s symptoms are consistent with drug-induced lupus (DIL). Hydralazine and procainamide are the most common agents reported to cause DIL. Musculoskeletal pains are the most frequent symptoms, but systemic symptoms (e.g., pericardial chest pain) and rash may also occur. Hydralazine doses as low as 100 mg/day of can cause DIL, and the risk significantly increases when >200 mg/day is used.

Laboratory tests are used to establish a diagnosis of DIL in patients taking hydralazine. A positive antinuclear antibody (ANA) is a common finding in 70% to 100% of those with long-term hydralazine exposure. However, only a small percentage of these patients will experience symptoms of DIL. A positive ANA test without symptoms of DIL does not warrant stopping hydralazine, so routine ANA testing is not necessary. The typical ANA pattern in DIL is diffuse and directed against single-stranded DNA (ss-DNA), not against double-stranded DNA (ds-DNA), as is the case with systemic lupus erythematosus (SLE). Other common laboratory findings include an elevated erythrocyte sedimentation rate (ESR), lupus erythematosus (LE) cells, and a false-positive serologic test for syphilis.

Patients with DIL from hydralazine rarely develop serious complications, which include blood dyscrasias such as leukopenia, and thrombocytopenia. Renal complications are not frequently associated with DIL. However, of all causative agents associated with DIL, hydralazine has the highest incidence of renal dysfunction. A serum creatinine should be obtained to identify any elevations, and a urinalysis should be conducted to monitor for signs of proteinuria and hematuria. In C.M. these tests may not be helpful since she suffers from severe chronic kidney disease.

63. Laboratory findings for C.M. showed a positive ANA (diffuse), a white blood cell count of 3,500/mm³, and an ESR of 45 mm/hr. DIL is diagnosed. How should this drug-induced toxicity be managed?

Hydralazine should be discontinued. Symptoms should begin to subside within days or weeks and complete resolution of symptoms can be expected; however, a positive ANA may persist for several months. Corticosteroids may be necessary to treat patients with persistent symptoms or more serious manifestations, such as nephritis.

MINOXIDIL

64. How should C.M.'s BP be managed?

C.M.'s BP responded to hydralazine, so she would likely benefit from another arterial vasodilator. Minoxidil, a potent arterial vasodilator, is similar to hydralazine with regard to causing reflex tachycardia, increased cardiac output, increased PRA, and fluid retention. Therefore, concomitant β-blocker and diuretic therapy is also required with this agent. Minoxidil therapy should be reserved for patients like C.M. who have severe chronic kidney disease or have refractory and difficult to control hypertension.

65. What instructions should C.R. receive concerning side effects with oral minoxidil administration?

Hypertrichosis is an adverse effect of oral minoxidil, occurring in 80% to 100% of patients. The hair growth is not associated with an endocrine abnormality and begins within the first few weeks. It commonly occurs on the temples, between the eyebrows, on the cheeks, and on the pinna of the ear. Hair growth can extend to the back of the legs, arms, and scalp with continued use. Shaving and use of depilatories can manage excessive growth. However, some patients, especially women, find the hypertrichosis so intolerable that they stop treatment.

Fluid retention with minoxidil is common, presenting as edema and weight gain. If adequate diuresis is not achieved during minoxidil therapy, HF may be precipitated or worsened. The compensatory reflex tachycardia with minoxidil also may precipitate angina in patients who have, or are at risk for, ischemic heart disease.

Step-Down Therapy

66. T.J., a 58-year-old white man who has a history of hypertension, systolic HF, and CAD (he had an MI 4 years ago). He has been treated with furosemide 20 mg daily, metoprolol XL 200 mg daily, spironolactone 25 mg daily, and lisinopril 20 mg daily for the past 2 years. T.J.'s BP has been stable since his last hospitalization for HF exacerbation 1 year ago. Today his BP readings are 118/68 and 116/70 mm Hg. He denies any problems, dizziness, or difficulties with his medications. Should his antihypertensive therapy be changed to reduce his medication doses and/or possibly discontinue some of his medications?

A small number of patients with long-standing hypertension can later have their BP medications slowly withdrawn, resulting in normal BP values for weeks or months following discontinuation of their medications. This is called step-down therapy. It should only be considered in a small subset of patients. Those with well-controlled BP for at least 1 year, who are at low cardiovascular risk, and have no compelling indications for antihypertensive therapy are eligible for a trial of step-down therapy. This consists of attempting to decrease the dosage and/or number of antihypertensive drugs without compromising BP control. Step-down therapy is most often successful in patients who have lost significant amounts of weight or have drastically changed their lifestyle. Any attempt at step-down therapy must be accompanied by scheduled follow-up evaluations because BP values can rise over months to years after drug discontinuation, especially if lifestyle modifications are not maintained.

Step-down therapy in T.J. is not an option. He has compelling indications for all of his drug therapies and is at very high risk for recurrent CVD based on his target organ damage. Although his BP is low, he does not have symptomatic hypotension, and his BP is considered normal.

REFERENCES

1. Chobanian AV et al. The seventh report of the Joint National Committee on Prevention, Detection, Evaluation, and Treatment of High Blood Pressure: the JNC 7 report. JAMA 2003;289:2560.
2. American Heart Association. Heart disease and stroke statistics: 2003 update. Dallas: American Heart Association, 2002.
3. Wolf-Maier K et al. Hypertension prevalence and blood pressure levels in 6 European countries, Canada, and the United States. JAMA 2003; 289:2363.
4. Smolensky MH. Chronobiology and chromotherapeutics: applications to cardiovascular medicine. Am J Hypertens 1996;9:11S.
5. Profant J, Dimsdale JE. Race and diurnal blood pressure patterns: a review and meta-analysis. Hypertension 1999;33:1099.

6. Vasan RS et al. Impact of high-normal blood pressure on the risk of cardiovascular disease. N Engl J Med 2001;345:1291.
7. Izzo JL Jr et al. Clinical advisory statement: importance of systolic blood pressure in older Americans. Hypertension 2000;35:1021.
8. Bakris GL et al. Preserving renal function in adults with hypertension and diabetes: a consensus approach. National Kidney Foundation Hypertension and Diabetes Executive Committees Working Group. Am J Kidney Dis 2000;36:646.
9. Arauz-Pacheco C, et al. Treatment of hypertension in adults with diabetes. Diabetes Care 2003; 26(Suppl 1):S80.
10. Lazarus JM et al. Achievement and safety of a low blood pressure goal in chronic renal disease. The

Modification of Diet in Renal Disease Study Group. Hypertension 1997;29:641.
11. Hansson L et al. Effects of intensive blood-pressure lowering and low-dose aspirin in patients with hypertension: principal results of the Hypertension Optimal Treatment (HOT) randomised trial. HOT Study Group. Lancet 1998;351:1755.
12. National High Blood Pressure Education Program Working Group report on ambulatory blood pressure monitoring. Arch Intern Med 1990;150:2270.
13. Pickering TG et al. How common is white coat hypertension? JAMA 1988;259:225.
14. Pickering T. Recommendations for the use of home (self) and ambulatory blood pressure monitoring. American Society of Hypertension Ad Hoc Panel. Am J Hypertens 1996;9:1.

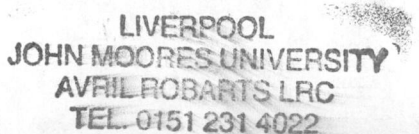
LIVERPOOL
JOHN MOORES UNIVERSITY
AVRIL ROBARTS LRC
TEL. 0151 231 4022

15. Glen SK et al. White-coat hypertension as a cause of cardiovascular dysfunction. Lancet 1996; 348:654.
16. Gifford RW Jr. Management of hypertensive crises. JAMA 1991;266:829.
17. Cherney D, Straus S. Management of patients with hypertensive urgencies and emergencies: a systematic review of the literature. J Gen Intern Med 2002;17:937.
18. American Heart Association. Human Blood Pressure Determination by Sphygmomanometry. Dallas: American Heart Association, 1994.
19. Clement DL et al. Prognostic value of ambulatory blood-pressure recordings in patients with treated hypertension. N Engl J Med 2003;348:2407.
20. Mehos BM et al. Effect of pharmacist intervention and initiation of home blood pressure monitoring in patients with uncontrolled hypertension. Pharmacotherapy 2000;20:1384.
21. Frohlich ED. Mechanisms contributing to high blood pressure. Ann Intern Med 1983;98:709.
22. Intersalt Cooperative Research Group. Intersalt: an international study of electrolyte excretion and blood pressure. Results for 24 hour urinary sodium and potassium excretion. BMJ 1988;297:319.
23. Cutler JA, Brittain E. Calcium and blood pressure: an epidemiologic perspective. Am J Hypertens 1990;3:137S.
24. Materson BJ. Diuretics, potassium, and ventricular ectopy. Am J Hypertens 1997;10:68S.
25. Reaven GM. Banting lecture 1988. Role of insulin resistance in human disease. Diabetes 1988;37:1595.
26. Kaplan NM. The deadly quartet. Upper-body obesity, glucose intolerance, hypertriglyceridemia, and hypertension. Arch Intern Med 1989;149:1514.
27. Executive Summary of The Third Report of The National Cholesterol Education Program (NCEP) Expert Panel on Detection, Evaluation, And Treatment of High Blood Cholesterol In Adults (Adult Treatment Panel III). JAMA 2001;285:2486.
28. Dominiczak AF, Bohr DF. Nitric oxide and its putative role in hypertension. Hypertension 1995;25:1202.
29. Keller G et al. Nephron number in patients with primary hypertension. N Engl J Med 2003;348:101.
30. Hyman DJ, Pavlik VN. Characteristics of patients with uncontrolled hypertension in the United States. N Engl J Med 2001;345:479.
31. Eselin JA, Carter BL. Hypertension and left ventricular hypertrophy: is drug therapy beneficial? Pharmacotherapy 1994;14:60.
32. Levy D, et al. The progression from hypertension to congestive heart failure. JAMA 1996;275:1557.
33. MacMahon S et al. Blood pressure, stroke, and coronary heart disease. Part 1: prolonged differences in blood pressure: prospective observational studies corrected for the regression dilution bias. Lancet 1990;335:765.
34. Tortorice KL, Carter BL. Stroke prophylaxis: hypertension management and antithrombotic therapy. Ann Pharmacother 1993;27:471.
35. K/DOQI clinical practice guidelines for chronic kidney disease: evaluation, classification, and stratification. Kidney Disease Outcome Quality Initiative. Am J Kidney Dis 2002;39:S1.
36. Calculators and modeling aids. GFR/1.73 M2 by MDR (+/-SUN and SAlb). Available at: http://www.hdcn.com/calcf/gfr.htm. Accessed June 1, 2003.
37. Kannel WB et al. Overall and coronary heart disease mortality rates in relation to major risk factors in 325,348 men screened for the MRFIT. Multiple Risk Factor Intervention Trial. Am Heart J 1986;112:825.
38. Collins R et al. Blood pressure, stroke, and coronary heart disease. Part 2: short-term reductions in blood pressure: overview of randomised drug trials in their epidemiological context. Lancet 1990; 335:827.
39. Materson BJ et al. Cigarette smoking interferes with treatment of hypertension. Arch Intern Med 1988;148:2116.
40. Shepherd J et al. Prevention of coronary heart disease with pravastatin in men with hypercholesterolemia. West of Scotland Coronary Prevention Study Group. N Engl J Med 1995;333:1301.
41. Downs JR et al. Primary prevention of acute coronary events with lovastatin in men and women with average cholesterol levels: results of AFCAPS/TexCAPS. Air Force/Texas Coronary Atherosclerosis Prevention Study. JAMA 1998;279:1615.
42. Randomised trial of cholesterol lowering in 4444 patients with coronary heart disease: the Scandinavian Simvastatin Survival Study (4S). Lancet 1994;344:1383.
43. The Long-Term Intervention with Pravastatin in Ischaemic Disease (LIPID) Study Group. Prevention of cardiovascular events and death with pravastatin in patients with coronary heart disease and a broad range of initial cholesterol levels. N Engl J Med 1998;339:1349.
44. Sacks FM et al. The effect of pravastatin on coronary events after myocardial infarction in patients with average cholesterol levels. Cholesterol and Recurrent Events Trial Investigators. N Engl J Med 1996;335:1001.
45. Heart Protection Study Collaborative Group. MRC/BHF Heart Protection Study of cholesterol lowering with simvastatin in 20,536 high-risk individuals: a randomised placebo-controlled trial. Lancet 2002;360:7.
46. Sever PS et al. Prevention of coronary and stroke events with atorvastatin in hypertensive patients who have average or lower-than-average cholesterol concentrations, in the Anglo-Scandinavian Cardiac Outcomes Trial-Lipid Lowering Arm (ASCOT-LLA): a multicentre randomised controlled trial. Lancet 2003;361:1149.
47. Turner RC et al. Risk factors for coronary artery disease in non-insulin dependent diabetes mellitus: United Kingdom Prospective Diabetes Study (UKPDS: 23). BMJ 1998;316:823.
48. Carter BL. Blood pressure as a surrogate end point for hypertension. Ann Pharmacother 2002;36:87.
49. The effects of nonpharmacologic interventions on blood pressure of persons with high normal levels. Results of the Trials of Hypertension Prevention, Phase I. JAMA 1992;267:1213.
50. Materson BJ et al. Single-drug therapy for hypertension in men: a comparison of six antihypertensive agents with placebo. The Department of Veterans Affairs Cooperative Study Group on Antihypertensive Agents. N Engl J Med 1993;328:914.
51. Grimm RH Jr et al. Relationships of quality-of-life measures to long-term lifestyle and drug treatment in the Treatment of Mild Hypertension Study. Arch Intern Med 1997;157:638.
52. SHEP Cooperative Research Group. Prevention of stroke by antihypertensive drug treatment in older persons with isolated systolic hypertension. Final results of the Systolic Hypertension in the Elderly Program (SHEP). JAMA 1991;265:3255.
53. Jensen J et al. The prevalence and etiology of impotence in 101 male hypertensive outpatients. Am J Hypertens 1999;12:271.
54. The sixth report of the Joint National Committee on prevention, detection, evaluation, and treatment of high blood pressure. Arch Intern Med 1997; 157:2413.
55. Veterans Administration Cooperative Study Group on Antihypertensive Agents. Effects of treatment on morbidity in hypertension: results in patients with diastolic blood pressures averaging 115 through 129 mm Hg. JAMA 1967;202:1028.
56. Hebert PR et al. Recent evidence on drug therapy of mild to moderate hypertension and decreased risk of coronary heart disease. Arch Intern Med 1993; 153:578.
57. Psaty BM et al. Health outcomes associated with various antihypertensive therapies used as first-line agents: a network meta-analysis. JAMA 2003;289:2534.
58. Treatment of mild hypertension in the elderly: a study initiated and administered by the National Heart Foundation of Australia. Med J Aust 1981;2:398.
59. Amery A et al. Glucose intolerance during diuretic therapy in elderly hypertensive patients. A second report from the European Working Party on high blood pressure in the elderly (EWPHE). Postgrad Med J 1986;62:919.
60. Coope J, Warrender TS. Randomised trial of treatment of hypertension in elderly patients in primary care. Br Med J (Clin Res Ed) 1986;293:1145.
61. Dahlof B et al. Morbidity and mortality in the Swedish Trial in Old Patients with Hypertension (STOP-Hypertension). Lancet 1991;338:1281.
62. MRC Working Party. Medical Research Council trial of treatment of hypertension in older adults: principal results. BMJ 1992;304:405.
63. Hypertension Detection and Follow-up Program Cooperative Group. Five-year findings of the hypertension detection and follow-up program. II. Mortality by race-sex and age. JAMA 1979;242:2572.
64. Staessen JA et al. Randomised double-blind comparison of placebo and active treatment for older patients with isolated systolic hypertension: the Systolic Hypertension in Europe (Syst-Eur) Trial Investigators. Lancet 1997;350:757.
65. 2003 European Society of Hypertension-European Society of Cardiology guidelines for the management of arterial hypertension. J Hypertens 2003;21:1011.
66. Wang JG et al. Chinese trial on isolated systolic hypertension in the elderly. Systolic Hypertension in China (Syst-China) Collaborative Group. Arch Intern Med 2000;160:211.
67. Dahlof B. Left ventricular hypertrophy and angiotensin II antagonists. Am J Hypertens 2001; 14:174.
68. Cruickshank JM et al. Benefits and potential harm of lowering high blood pressure. Lancet 1987;1:581.
69. Merlo J et al. Incidence of myocardial infarction in elderly men being treated with antihypertensive drugs: population based cohort study. BMJ 1996; 313:457.
70. Farnett L et al. The J-curve phenomenon and the treatment of hypertension: is there a point beyond which pressure reduction is dangerous? JAMA 1991;265:489.
71. Voko Z et al. J-shaped relation between blood pressure and stroke in treated hypertensives. Hypertension 1999;34:1181.
72. National Institutes of Health. Clinical guidelines on the identification, evaluation, and treatment of overweight and obesity in adults—the evidence report. Obes Res 1998;6(Suppl 2):51S.
73. Ramsay LE et al. Weight reduction in a blood pressure clinic. Br Med J 1978;2:244.
74. He J et al. Long-term effects of weight loss and dietary sodium reduction on incidence of hypertension. Hypertension 2000;35:544.
75. Schotte DE, Stunkard AJ. The effects of weight reduction on blood pressure in 301 obese patients. Arch Intern Med 1990;150:1701.
76. Appel LJ, et al. A clinical trial of the effects of dietary patterns on blood pressure. DASH Collaborative Research Group. N Engl J Med 1997; 336:1117.
77. Sacks FM, et al. Effects on blood pressure of reduced dietary sodium and the Dietary Approaches to Stop Hypertension (DASH) diet. DASH-Sodium Collaborative Research Group. N Engl J Med 2001;344:3.
78. Vollmer WM, et al. Effects of diet and sodium intake on blood pressure: subgroup analysis of the DASH-sodium trial. Ann Intern Med 2001;135:1019.
79. Gifford RW Jr. et al. Office evaluation of hypertension: a statement for health professionals by a writing group of the Council for High Blood Pressure Research, American Heart Association. Circulation 1989;79:721.
80. Midgley JP et al. Effect of reduced dietary sodium on blood pressure: a meta-analysis of randomized controlled trials. JAMA 1996;275:1590.
81. Chobanian AV, Hill M. National Heart, Lung, and Blood Institute Workshop on Sodium and Blood

Pressure : a critical review of current scientific evidence. Hypertension 2000;35:858.

82. Whelton SP et al. Effect of aerobic exercise on blood pressure: a meta-analysis of randomized, controlled trials. Ann Intern Med 2002;136:493.

83. Kelley GA, Kelley KS. Progressive resistance exercise and resting blood pressure: a meta-analysis of randomized controlled trials. Hypertension 2000;35:838.

84. Xin X et al. Effects of alcohol reduction on blood pressure: a meta-analysis of randomized controlled trials. Hypertension 2001;38:1112.

85. The Tobacco Use and Dependence Clinical Practice Guideline Panel, Staff, and Consortium Representatives. A clinical practice guideline for treating tobacco use and dependence: A US Public Health Service report. JAMA 2000;283:3244.

86. Buhler FR et al. Impact of smoking on heart attacks, strokes, blood pressure control, drug dose, and quality of life aspects in the International Prospective Primary Prevention Study in Hypertension. Am Heart J 1988;115:282.

87. Nonpharmacological approaches to the control of high blood pressure: final report of the Subcommittee on Nonpharmacological Therapy of the 1984 Joint National Committee on Detection, Evaluation, and Treatment of High Blood Pressure. Hypertension 1986;8:444.

88. Freis ED. The efficacy and safety of diuretics in treating hypertension. Ann Intern Med 1995; 122:223.

89. Lakshman MR et al. Diuretics and beta-blockers do not have adverse effects at 1 year on plasma lipid and lipoprotein profiles in men with hypertension. Department of Veterans Affairs Cooperative Study Group on Antihypertensive Agents. Arch Intern Med 1999;159:551.

90. Savage PJ et al. Influence of long term, low-dose, diuretic-based, antihypertensive therapy on glucose, lipid, uric acid, and potassium levels in older men and women with isolated systolic hypertension: the Systolic Hypertension in the Elderly Program. SHEP Cooperative Research Group. Arch Intern Med 1998;158:741.

91. Zillich AJ, Carter BL. Eplerenone: a novel selective aldosterone blocker. Ann Pharmacother 2002;36:1567.

92. Neaton JD et al. Treatment of Mild Hypertension Study. Final results. Treatment of Mild Hypertension Study Research Group. JAMA 1993;270:713.

93. Sackett DL et al. Evidence based medicine: what it is and what it isn't. BMJ 1996;312:71.

94. Black HR et al. Principal results of the Controlled Onset Verapamil Investigation of Cardiovascular End Points (CONVINCE) trial. JAMA 2003; 289:2073.

95. Dahlof B et al. Cardiovascular morbidity and mortality in the Losartan Intervention For Endpoint reduction in hypertension study (LIFE): a randomised trial against atenolol. Lancet 2002; 359:995.

96. ALLHAT Officers and Coordinators for the ALLHAT Collaborative Research Group. Major outcomes in high-risk hypertensive patients randomized to angiotensin-converting enzyme inhibitor or calcium channel blocker vs diuretic: the Antihypertensive and Lipid-Lowering Treatment to Prevent Heart Attack Trial (ALLHAT). JAMA 2002;288:2981.

97. Yusuf S et al. Effects of an angiotensin-converting-enzyme inhibitor, ramipril, on cardiovascular events in high-risk patients. The Heart Outcomes Prevention Evaluation Study Investigators. N Engl J Med 2000;342:145.

98. PROGRESS Collaborative Group. Randomised trial of a perindopril-based blood-pressure-lowering regimen among 6,105 individuals with previous stroke or transient ischaemic attack. Lancet 2001;358:1033.

99. Wing LM et al. A comparison of outcomes with angiotensin-converting–enzyme inhibitors and diuretics for hypertension in the elderly. N Engl J Med 2003;348:583.

100. Hansson L et al. Randomised trial of old and new antihypertensive drugs in elderly patients: cardiovascular mortality and morbidity the Swedish Trial in Old Patients with Hypertension-2 study. Lancet 1999;354:1751.

101. Heart Outcomes Prevention Evaluation Study Investigators. Effects of ramipril on cardiovascular and microvascular outcomes in people with diabetes mellitus: results of the HOPE study and MICRO-HOPE substudy. Lancet 2000; 355:253.

102. Hansson L, et al. Randomised trial of effects of calcium antagonists compared with diuretics and beta-blockers on cardiovascular morbidity and mortality in hypertension: the Nordic Diltiazem (NORDIL) study. Lancet 2000; 356:359.

103. Hansson L, et al. Effect of angiotensin-converting-enzyme inhibition compared with conventional therapy on cardiovascular morbidity and mortality in hypertension: the Captopril Prevention Project (CAPPP) randomised trial. Lancet 1999; 353:611.

104. Estacio RO, et al. Effect of blood pressure control on diabetic microvascular complications in patients with hypertension and type 2 diabetes. Diabetes Care 2000; 23 Suppl 2:B54.

105. Estacio RO, et al. The effect of nisoldipine as compared with enalapril on cardiovascular outcomes in patients with non-insulin-dependent diabetes and hypertension. N Engl J Med 1998; 338:645.

106. Tatti P, et al. Outcome results of the Fosinopril Versus Amlodipine Cardiovascular Events Randomized Trial (FACET) in patients with hypertension and NIDDM. Diabetes Care 1998; 21:597.

107. Efficacy of atenolol and captopril in reducing risk of macrovascular and microvascular complications in type 2 diabetes: UKPDS 39. UK Prospective Diabetes Study Group. BMJ 1998; 317:713.

108. Brenner BM, et al. Effects of losartan on renal and cardiovascular outcomes in patients with type 2 diabetes and nephropathy. N Engl J Med 2001; 345:861.

109. Lewis EJ, et al. Renoprotective effect of the angiotensin-receptor antagonist irbesartan in patients with nephropathy due to type 2 diabetes. N Engl J Med 2001; 345:851.

110. Parving HH, et al. The effect of irbesartan in patients with type 2 diabetes. N Engl J Med 2001; 345:870.

111. Dickstein K, Kjekshus J. Effects of losartan and captopril on mortality and morbidity in high-risk patients after acute myocardial infarction: the OPTIMAAL randomised trial. Optimal Trial in Myocardial Infarction with Angiotensin II Antagonist Losartan. Lancet 2002; 360:752.

112. Wright JT, Jr., et al. Effect of blood pressure lowering and antihypertensive drug class on progression of hypertensive kidney disease: results from the AASK trial. JAMA 2002; 288:2421.

113. Saseen JJ, et al. Treatment of uncomplicated hypertension: are ACE inhibitors and calcium channel blockers as effective as diuretics and beta-blockers? J Am Board Fam Pract 2003; 16:156.

114. ALLHAT Collaborative Research Group. Major cardiovascular events in hypertensive patients randomized to doxazosin vs chlorthalidone: the antihypertensive and lipid-lowering treatment to prevent heart attack trial (ALLHAT). JAMA 2000; 283:1967.

115. Davis BR, et al. Rationale and design for the Antihypertensive and Lipid Lowering Treatment to Prevent Heart Attack Trial (ALLHAT). ALLHAT Research Group. Am J Hypertens 1996; 9:342.

116. Hunt SA, et al. ACC/AHA guidelines for the evaluation and management of chronic heart failure in the adult: executive summary. A report of the American College of Cardiology/American Heart Association Task Force on Practice Guidelines (Committee to revise the 1995 Guidelines for the Evaluation and Management of Heart Failure). J Am Coll Cardiol 2001; 38:2101.

117. The SOLVD Investigators. Effect of enalapril on survival in patients with reduced left ventricular ejection fractions and congestive heart failure. N Engl J Med 1991; 325:293.

118. The Acute Infarction Ramipril Efficacy (AIRE) Study Investigators. Effect of ramipril on mortality and morbidity of survivors of acute myocardial infarction with clinical evidence of heart failure. Lancet 1993; 342:821.

119. Kober L, et al. A clinical trial of the angiotensin-converting-enzyme inhibitor trandolapril in patients with left ventricular dysfunction after myocardial infarction. Trandolapril Cardiac Evaluation (TRACE) Study Group. N Engl J Med 1995; 333:1670.

120. Dargie HJ. Effect of carvedilol on outcome after myocardial infarction in patients with left-ventricular dysfunction: the CAPRICORN randomised trial. Lancet 2001;357:1385.

121. Effect of metoprolol CR/XL in chronic heart failure: Metoprolol CR/XL Randomised Intervention Trial in Congestive Heart Failure (MERIT-HF). Lancet 1999;353:2001.

122. Packer M et al. Effect of carvedilol on survival in severe chronic heart failure. N Engl J Med 2001; 344:1651.

123. CIBIS Investigators and Committees. A randomized trial of beta-blockade in heart failure. The Cardiac Insufficiency Bisoprolol Study (CIBIS). Circulation 1994;90:1765.

124. Pitt B et al. Randomised trial of losartan versus captopril in patients over 65 with heart failure (Evaluation of Losartan in the Elderly Study, ELITE). Lancet 1997;349:747.

125. Pitt B et al. Effect of losartan compared with captopril on mortality in patients with symptomatic heart failure: randomised trial—the Losartan Heart Failure Survival Study ELITE II. Lancet 2000;355:1582.

126. Cohn JN, Tognoni G. A randomized trial of the angiotensin-receptor blocker valsartan in chronic heart failure. N Engl J Med 2001;345:1667.

127. Pitt B et al. The effect of spironolactone on morbidity and mortality in patients with severe heart failure. Randomized Aldactone Evaluation Study Investigators. N Engl J Med 1999;341:709.

128. Pitt B et al. Eplerenone, a selective aldosterone blocker, in patients with left ventricular dysfunction after myocardial infarction. N Engl J Med 2003;348:1309.

129. Braunwald E et al. ACC/AHA 2002 guideline update for the management of patients with unstable angina and non-ST-segment elevation myocardial infarction—summary article: a report of the American College of Cardiology/American Heart Association task force on practice guidelines (Committee on the Management of Patients With Unstable Angina). J Am Coll Cardiol 2002;40:1366.

130. A randomized trial of propranolol in patients with acute myocardial infarction. I. Mortality results. JAMA 1982;247:1707.

131. Pfeffer MA et al. Effect of captopril on mortality and morbidity in patients with left ventricular dysfunction after myocardial infarction. Results of the survival and ventricular enlargement trial. The SAVE Investigators. N Engl J Med 1992;327:669.

131a. Pepine CJ et al. A calcium-antagonist vs a non-calcium antagonist hypertension treatment strategy for patients with coronary artery disease: The International Verapamil-Trandolapril Study (INVEST): A randomized controlled trial. JAMA 2003;290:2805.

132. Lindholm LH, et al. Cardiovascular morbidity and mortality in patients with diabetes in the Losartan Intervention For Endpoint reduction in hypertension study (LIFE): a randomised trial against atenolol. Lancet 2002;359:1004.

133. Niskanen L et al. Reduced cardiovascular morbidity and mortality in hypertensive diabetic patients on first-line therapy with an ACE inhibitor compared with a diuretic/beta-blocker-based treatment regimen: a subanalysis of the Captopril Prevention Project. Diabetes Care 2001;24:2091.

134. UK Prospective Diabetes Study Group. Tight blood pressure control and risk of macrovascular

and microvascular complications in type 2 diabetes: UKPDS 38. BMJ 1998;317:703.

135. Lewis EJ et al. The effect of angiotensin-converting-enzyme inhibition on diabetic nephropathy. The Collaborative Study Group. N Engl J Med 1993; 329:1456.

136. The GISEN Group (Gruppo Italiano di Studi Epidemiologici in Nefrologia).Randomised placebo-controlled trial of effect of ramipril on decline in glomerular filtration rate and risk of terminal renal failure in proteinuric, non-diabetic nephropathy. Lancet 1997;349:1857.

137. Cramer JA et al. How often is medication taken as prescribed? A novel assessment technique. JAMA 1989;261:3273.

138. Eisen SA et al. The effect of prescribed daily dose frequency on patient medication compliance. Arch Intern Med 1990;150:1881.

139. Douglas JG et al. Management of high blood pressure in African Americans: consensus statement of the Hypertension in African Americans Working Group of the International Society on Hypertension in Blacks. Arch Intern Med 2003;163:525.

140. Materson BJ et al. Response to a second single antihypertensive agent used as monotherapy for hypertension after failure of the initial drug. Department of Veterans Affairs Cooperative Study Group on Antihypertensive Agents. Arch Intern Med 1995;155:1757.

141. Carter BL et al. Selected factors that influence responses to antihypertensives: choosing therapy for the uncomplicated patient. Arch Fam Med 1994; 3:528.

142. Finnerty FA Jr et al. Long-term effects of furosemide and hydrochlorothiazide in patients with essential hypertension a two-year comparison of efficacy and safety. Angiology 1977; 28:125.

143. Araoye MA et al. Furosemide compared with hydrochlorothiazide: long-term treatment of hypertension. JAMA 1978;240:1863.

144. Brown NJ. Eplerenone: cardiovascular protection. Circulation 2003;107:2512.

145. Multiple Risk Factor Intervention Trial Research Group. Baseline rest electrocardiographic abnormalities, antihypertensive treatment, and mortality in the Multiple Risk Factor Intervention Trial. Am J Cardiol 1985;55:1.

146. The Hypertension Detection and Follow-up Program Cooperative Research Group. The effect of antihypertensive drug treatment on mortality in the presence of resting electrocardiographic abnormalities at baseline: the HDFP experience. Circulation 1984;70:996.

147. Fonseca V, Phear DN. Hyperosmolar non-ketotic diabetic syndrome precipitated by treatment with diuretics. Br Med J (Clin Res Ed) 1982;284:36.

148. Langford HG et al. Is thiazide-produced uric acid elevation harmful? Analysis of data from the Hypertension Detection and Follow-up Program. Arch Intern Med 1987;147:645.

149. Ames RP. The effects of antihypertensive drugs on serum lipids and lipoproteins. I: Diuretics. Drugs 1986;32:260.

150. McKenney JM et al. The effect of low-dose hydrochlorothiazide on blood pressure, serum potassium, and lipoproteins. Pharmacotherapy 1986; 6:179.

151. Amery A et al. Influence of anti-hypertensive therapy on serum cholesterol in elderly hypertensive patients: results of trial by the European Working Party on High blood pressure in the Elderly (EWPHE). Acta Cardiol 1982;37:235.

152. Neutel JM et al. Combination therapy with diuretics: an evolution of understanding. Am J Med 1996;101:61S.

153. Frishman WH et al. A multifactorial trial design to assess combination therapy in hypertension: treatment with bisoprolol and hydrochlorothiazide. Arch Intern Med 1994;154:1461.

154. Saunders E et al. A comparison of the efficacy and safety of a beta-blocker, a calcium channel blocker, and a converting enzyme inhibitor in hypertensive blacks. Arch Intern Med 1990;150: 1707.

155. Manolio TA et al. Trends in pharmacologic management of hypertension in the United States. Arch Intern Med 1995;155:829.

156. Salpeter SR et al. Cardioselective beta-blockers in patients with reactive airway disease: a meta-analysis. Ann Intern Med 2002;137:715.

157. Gengo FM et al. The effect of beta-blockers on mental performance on older hypertensive patients. Arch Intern Med 1988;148:779.

158. Hennekens CH et al. Adjunctive drug therapy of acute myocardial infarction—evidence from clinical trials. N Engl J Med 1996;335:1660.

159. Smith SC Jr et al. AHA consensus panel statement. Preventing heart attack and death in patients with coronary disease. The Secondary Prevention Panel. J Am Coll Cardiol 1995;26:292.

160. Gibbons RJ et al. ACC/AHA/ACP-ASIM guidelines for the management of patients with chronic stable angina: executive summary and recommendations. A Report of the American College of Cardiology/American Heart Association Task Force on Practice Guidelines (Committee on Management of Patients with Chronic Stable Angina). Circulation 1999;99:2829.

161. Mooradian AD. Cardiovascular disease in type 2 diabetes mellitus: current management guidelines. Arch Intern Med 2003;163:33.

162. Arauz-Pacheco C et al. The treatment of hypertension in adult patients with diabetes. Diabetes Care 2002;25:134.

163. O'Keefe JH et al. Should an angiotensin-converting enzyme inhibitor be standard therapy for patients with atherosclerotic disease? J Am Coll Cardiol 2001;37:1.

164. Frohlich ED et al. The heart in hypertension. N Engl J Med 1992;327:998.

165. Dzau VJ et al. The relevance of tissue angiotensin-converting enzyme: manifestations in mechanistic and endpoint data. Am J Cardiol 2001;88:1L.

166. Cummings DM et al. The antihypertensive response to lisinopril: the effect of age in a predominantly black population. J Clin Pharmacol 1989; 29:25.

167. Materson BJ, Reda DJ. Correction: single-drug therapy for hypertension in men. N Engl J Med 1994;330:1689.

168. Smith SC Jr et al. AHA/ACC Scientific Statement: AHA/ACC guidelines for preventing heart attack and death in patients with atherosclerotic cardiovascular disease: 2001 update: a statement for healthcare professionals from the American Heart Association and the American College of Cardiology. Circulation 2001;104:1577.

169. Luque CA, Vazquez Ortiz M. Treatment of ACE inhibitor-induced cough. Pharmacotherapy 1999; 19:804.

170. Willenheimer R et al. AT1-receptor blockers in hypertension and heart failure: clinical experience and future directions. Eur Heart J 1999;20:997.

171. Horiuchi M et al. Recent progress in angiotensin II type 2 receptor research in the cardiovascular system. Hypertension 1999;33:613.

172. Gainer JV et al. Effect of bradykinin-receptor blockade on the response to angiotensin-converting-enzyme inhibitor in normotensive and hypertensive subjects. N Engl J Med 1998; 339:1285.

173. Oparil S. Newly emerging pharmacologic differences in angiotensin II receptor blockers. Am J Hypertens 2000;13:18S.

174. Oparil S et al. Comparative efficacy of olmesartan, losartan, valsartan, and irbesartan in the control of essential hypertension. J Clin Hypertens (Greenwich) 2001;3:283.

175. Grossman E et al. Should a moratorium be placed on sublingual nifedipine capsules given for hypertensive emergencies and pseudoemergencies? JAMA 1996;276:1328.

176. Psaty BM et al. The risk of myocardial infarction associated with antihypertensive drug therapies. JAMA 1995;274:620.

177. Borhani NO et al. Final outcome results of the Multicenter Isradipine Diuretic Atherosclerosis Study (MIDAS). A randomized controlled trial. JAMA 1996;276:785.

178. Staessen JA et al. Calcium channel blockade and cardiovascular prognosis in the European trial on isolated systolic hypertension. Hypertension 1998;32:410.

179. Packer M et al. Effect of amlodipine on morbidity and mortality in severe chronic heart failure. Prospective Randomized Amlodipine Survival Evaluation Study Group. N Engl J Med 1996;335: 1107.

180. Saseen JJ, Carter BL. Dual calcium-channel blocker therapy in the treatment of hypertension. Ann Pharmacother 1996;30:802.

181. Saseen JJ et al. Comparison of nifedipine alone and with diltiazem or verapamil in hypertension. Hypertension 1996;28:109.

182. Moser M, Frishman W. Results of therapy with carvedilol, a beta-blocker vasodilator with antioxidant properties, in hypertensive patients. Am J Hypertens 1998;11:15S.

183. Consensus recommendations for the management of chronic heart failure. On behalf of the membership of the advisory council to improve outcomes nationwide in heart failure. Am J Cardiol 1999; 83:1A.

184. National High Blood Pressure Education Program Working Group Report on High Blood Pressure in Pregnancy. Am J Obstet Gynecol 1990;163:1691.

185. Kronig B et al. Different concepts in first-line treatment of essential hypertension. Comparison of a low-dose reserpine-thiazide combination with nitrendipine monotherapy. German Reserpine in Hypertension Study Group. Hypertension 1997; 29:651.

CHAPTER 15

Peripheral Vascular Disorders

Anne P. Spencer, C. Wayne Weart

INTERMITTENT CLAUDICATION AND OCCLUSIVE PERIPHERAL ARTERIAL DISEASE

Intermittent claudication (IC) is a common and painful complication developing from atherosclerosis of the peripheral arteries of the legs. Some clinicians and patients have characterized claudication pain as "angina" of the legs. When one considers the risk factors and pathology of IC, the association with coronary disease becomes clear.

IC is described as aching, cramping, tightness, or weakness of the legs, which usually occurs during exertion. Claudication pain is relieved when the physical activity is discontinued. Numbness or continuous pain in the toes or foot may be present, indicating tissue ischemia, which can lead to ulceration. IC is a painful condition that can severely limit the patient's mobility and lead to tissue necrosis or amputation of the affected limb. Because symptoms of IC develop gradually, patients may not seek medical attention until the condition is advanced.

Epidemiology

Intermittent claudication is a relatively common condition that affects men and women equally, with a prevalence of 12%.[1] The annual incidence of IC increases dramatically with age (Table 15-1). In a population with only a 2% prevalence of IC symptoms, 11.7% of patients had detectable large vessel atherosclerosis of the lower extremities.[2] This indicates that the majority of patients with peripheral arterial disease (PAD) are largely asymptomatic, although their risk of developing symptoms of IC in the future is greatly increased. This disparity between IC symptoms and the presence of PAD contributes to the observation that 50% to 90% of patients with IC do not mention the symptoms to their physician. Patients attribute the symptoms of IC to normal walking difficulties

associated with aging, not a medical condition requiring treatment.[3]

Risk factors for developing occlusive PAD are similar to those for coronary artery disease. Longstanding diabetes is the most significant risk factor, with 30% of patients with diabetes affected by PAD.[4] PAD is five times more common in patients with diabetes than in patients without diabetes; in diabetics, it develops at a younger age and progresses more rapidly. Other risk factors include cigarette smoking, hypertension, dyslipidemia, and hyperhomocysteinemia.[5] Hypertriglyceridemia is a more significant risk factor for PAD than for coronary artery disease, and this may partially explain the increased prevalence of PAD in patients with diabetes.[6]

Cigarette smoking has a higher correlation with the development of IC pain than any other risk factor, and the risk increases dramatically with the number of cigarettes smoked per day and the duration of smoking history.[7] In patients with other cardiovascular risk factors, including hypertension or diabetes, smoking further increases the rate of claudication development. Smoking confers a sevenfold increase in risk for PAD compared to nonsmokers. In contrast, the risk of coronary artery disease is only increased twofold in smokers. Thus, the mechanism by which cigarette smoking causes damage may be different for these two vascular diseases.[8]

Epidemiologic studies show that IC is nonprogressive in 75% of patients over a period of 4 to 9 years. However, the other 25% of IC sufferers have worsening painful ischemic episodes over this period. Although rare, more serious complications can occur. Ischemic tissue changes, ulceration, and gangrene can accompany advanced peripheral atherosclerosis. Amputation of the affected limb may be necessary in up to 5% of patients with claudication.[9] The presence of two independent risk factors, such as diabetes and cigarette smok-

Table 15-1 Annual Incidence of Intermittent Claudication by Age[2]

Age Group	Annual Incidence
40 years	2%
50 years	4.2%
60 years	6.8%
70 years	9.2%

ing, has an additive affect on the risk for the development of progressive IC and serious limb complications (Table 15-2).

During a relatively short 2-year follow-up of a population with IC, 3.6% of patients died, while 22% experienced a nonfatal cardiovascular event (defined as any cardiac, cerebral, or peripheral vascular event). Furthermore, 26% experienced a decline in their walking capability during the same time frame.[10,11] While a relatively small fraction of patients died during the 2-year observation period, it is paramount to recognize that severe, short-term morbidity is highly likely in this patient population. IC clearly reflects generalized atherosclerosis and is associated with considerable morbidity.

Pathophysiology

Intermittent claudication is the predominant complication of occlusive PAD. The major cause of occlusive PAD is arteriosclerosis obliterans, defined as the development of atherosclerotic plaques in the peripheral vasculature. These plaques develop as a result of endothelial activation associated with conditions such as dyslipidemia, diabetes mellitus, hypertension, and tobacco use. Plaques result in the proliferation of vascular smooth muscle, with subsequent damage to the vascular structure. The damaged endothelium of the vasculature has impaired vasodilatory capabilities because secretion of nitric oxide, also known as endothelium-derived relaxing factor, is decreased and secretion of vasoconstrictive substances, such as endothelin, is increased. Both defects impede blood flow to the extremities. In addition, growth of the atherosclerotic lesions may physically limit blood flow. Exercise may induce IC symptoms in patients who have lesions with ≥50% stenosis, while patients with lesions of >80% stenosis can have pain at rest. The lesions themselves can be unstable and rupture, or adjacent smaller vessels experiencing high hemodynamic pressure caused by nearby plaques may rupture. Either situation can lead to acute vascular occlusion, analogous to unstable angina or acute myocardial infarction (MI) in affected coronary arteries.[12]

Figure 15-1 illustrates the distribution of the major peripheral arteries. Plaques that develop in central vessels (e.g., in the ilioaortic artery) are primarily associated with buttock

Table 15-2 Long-Term Incidence of Outcomes in Patients With Intermittent Claudication[9,10]

Patient Population	Abrupt Limb Ischemia	Amputation
All patients	23%	7%
Diabetics	31%	11%
Smokers	35%	21%

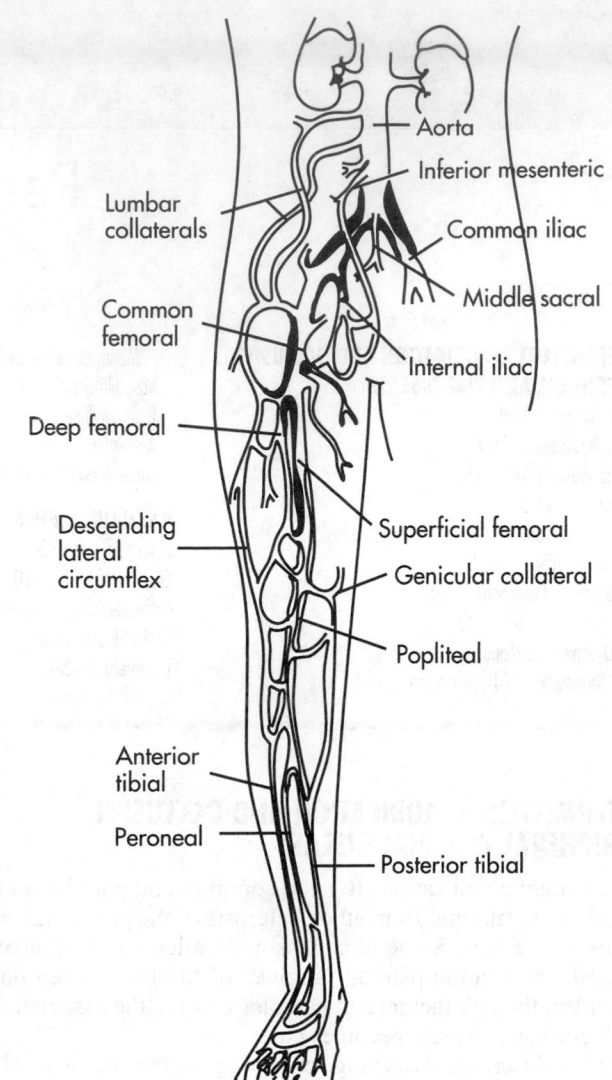

FIGURE 15-1 Common sites of atherosclerosis (shown in black) in the aorta and lower extremities. (Reproduced with permission from reference 12)

pain and erectile dysfunction. Those confined to the more distal femoropopliteal arteries characteristically cause thigh and calf pain. Occlusion of the tibial arteries will produce claudication pain in the foot. When more than one artery bed is affected by severe atherosclerosis, symptoms of IC will be diffuse. Symptoms of IC indicate an inadequate supply of arterial blood to peripheral muscles. Exercise, including walking, increases the metabolic demands of the muscles and can lead to claudication pain. Reduced blood supply to the muscles is due to changes in perfusion pressures and vascular tone caused by atherosclerosis.

Atherosclerosis can impair the microcirculation of the peripheral muscles by altering the pressure gradient needed for perfusion of the capillaries (Fig. 15-2). When obstruction develops, perfusion of tissue distal to the stenotic lesion relies on collateral blood flow. Collateral circulation consists of new blood vessels that develop to carry blood around the occluded area.

LEG ARTERY

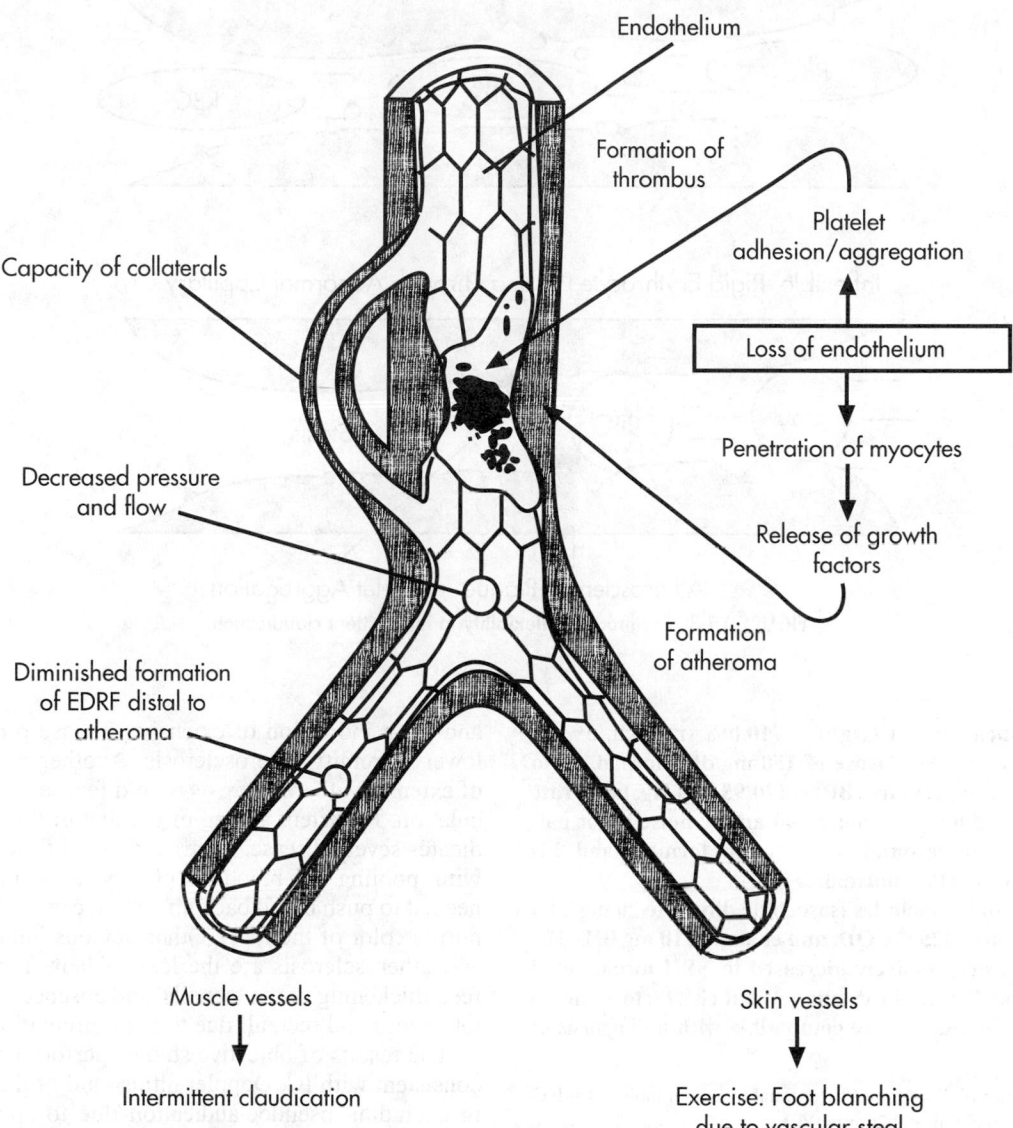

FIGURE 15-2 Consequences of occlusive atherosclerotic disease in the lower limbs. EDRF, endothelium-derived relaxing factor. (Reproduced with permission from reference 13)

Erythrocyte deformability is an important factor for in vitro capillary perfusion.[15,16] In areas free of compromised blood flow, normal red blood cells (RBCs) have the ability to deform when passing through a small capillary. By aligning themselves in a planar manner, the RBCs also reduce the viscosity of the blood suspension, enabling them to pass smoothly through the capillary. In many patients with IC, RBCs have a marked decrease in this intrinsic ability to deform, which results in increased blood viscosity. This defect is promoted by chronic tissue ischemia and hypoxia caused by increased intracapillary leukocyte adherence, platelet aggregation, and activation of complement and clotting factors.[12] The vascular responses to hypoxia are detrimental because this sequence of events further inhibits blood flow and oxygen delivery to the tissues (Fig. 15-3).

Clinical Presentation

1. J.S. is a 54-year-old, 100-kg man with a history of type 2, insulin-treated diabetes mellitus, angina, dyslipidemia, and tobacco use. His chief complaint today is right upper thigh pain while walking around the block. The pain has gradually increased over the past 12 months, but only recently has become intolerable. The pain is relieved within minutes after he stops walking. J.S. smokes 1.5 packs of cigarettes a day.

His most recent laboratory results are significant for total cholesterol, 290 mg/dL (optimal, <150 mg/dL); fasting triglycerides, 350 mg/dL (optimal, <200 mg/dL); LDL, 188 mg/dL (optimal, <100 mg/dL); and HDL, 32 mg/dL (optimal, >40 mg/dL). His serum creatinine (SCr) is 1.0 mg/dL (normal, 0.7 to 1.5 mg/dL), blood urea nitrogen (BUN) 15 mg/dL (normal, 8 to

Normal Erythrocyte Passing Through Capillary

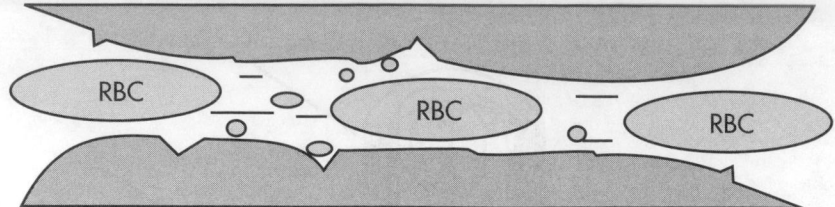

Inflexible, Rigid Erythrocyte Passing Through Abnormal Capillary

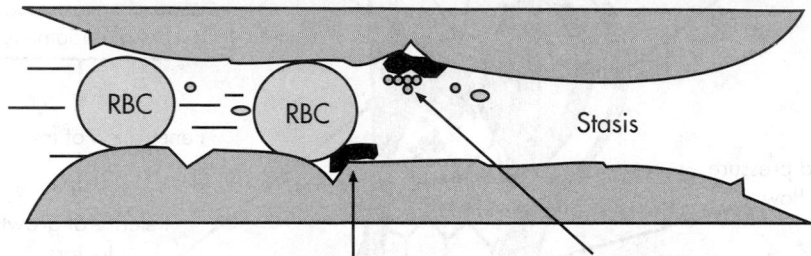

FIGURE 15-3 Erythrocyte inflexibility in intermittent claudication.

20 mg/dL), and hemoglobin (Hgb) A$_{1c}$ 10.0% (normal, 5% to 6%), and he has a fasting glucose of 150 mg/dL (normal, 70 to 115 mg/dL). His blood pressure (BP) is 170/95 mm Hg, heart rate (HR) is 89 bpm, and his posterior tibial artery pulse is not palpable. A Doppler ultrasound study is performed, and his ankle:brachial index is 0.7 (normal, >0.90).

J.S.'s medication list includes isosorbide dinitrate 20 mg TID (while awake), aspirin 325 mg QD, and enalapril 10 mg BID. His insulin doses have progressively increased to NPH insulin 40 U in the morning and 35 U in the evening. What risk factors and elements of J.S.'s presentation are compatible with a diagnosis of IC?

[SI units: total cholesterol, 7.49 mmol/L (optimal, <3.88 mmol/L); triglycerides, 3.95 mmol/L (optimal, <2.26 mmol/L); LDL, 4.86 mmol/L (normal, <2.58 mmol/L); HDL, 0.83 mmol/L (normal, >1.04 mmol/L); SCr, 60 mmol/L; BUN, 5.3 mmol/L; HgbA$_{1c}$, 0.1, glucose 8.3 mmol/L]

J.S.'s past medical history shows classic risk factors for vascular occlusion and IC, including dyslipidemia (specifically hypertriglyceridemia), diabetes, hypertension, and tobacco use. In particular, his diabetes is not adequately controlled based on elevated HgbA$_{1c}$ and fasting glucose levels, and he is obese. This constellation of disorders is known as the metabolic syndrome and is sometimes referred to as syndrome X or the "deadly quartet" (obesity, hypertension, diabetes mellitus, and dyslipidemia). These factors, along with smoking, commonly are seen together and have been linked with hyperinsulinemia and accelerated atherosclerosis (Fig. 15-4).[17,18] The presence of angina indicates coronary artery disease, so it is not surprising that he has peripheral vascular occlusion as well.

The classic pain of IC described by J.S. is associated with exercise of the affected muscle group(s) and subsides with a few minutes of rest and reperfusion. IC pain also can occur at rest; however, this type of claudication pain is less common

and is an indication of extensive disease progression due to lower extremity atherosclerosis. Another common symptom of extensive atherosclerosis is cold feet secondary to poor circulation. Persistent aching of the feet during rest or sleep indicates severe disease. Restricted blood flow to the feet along with pooling of blood secondary to inadequate pressure needed to push blood back up the leg can lead to rubor (red or purple color of the foot). Other obvious indicators of peripheral atherosclerosis are the loss of hair from the top of the feet, thickening of the toenails, and absence of sweating of the lower legs and feet, all due to poor circulation.[12]

The results of objective studies performed on J.S. also are consistent with IC. Doppler ultrasound of the spine is helpful in excluding pseudoclaudication due to spinal stenosis and other neurogenic or musculoskeletal causes of leg pain. Ul-

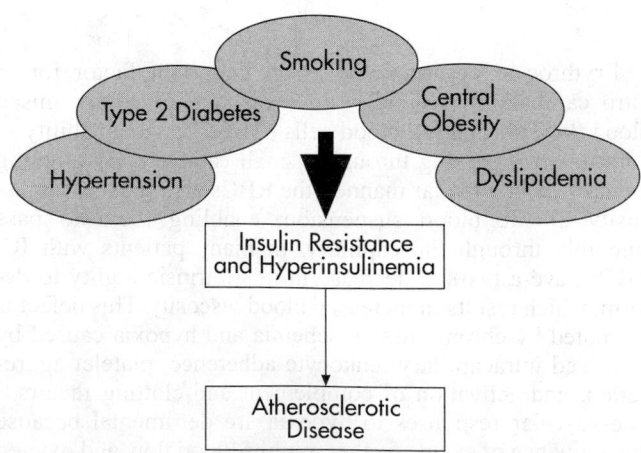

FIGURE 15-4 The metabolic syndrome in atherosclerosis.

Table 15-3 Severity of Arterial Obstruction As Assessed by Ankle:Brachial Index[29]

Severity	Ankle:Brachial Index
Normal	>0.90
Mild	0.70–0.89
Moderate	0.50–0.69
Severe	>0.50

Ankle:brachial index is the systolic blood pressure in the arm/systolic blood pressure in the ankle

trasound also is useful to measure BP of the lower extremities. An ankle:brachial index of 0.7 means that the ankle systolic BP reading is only 70% of the systolic pressure in the brachial artery supplying blood to the arm. In patients with IC, this is due to atherosclerotic obstruction of blood flow in the lower limbs and subsequent decreased perfusion pressures in the ankle compared to the arm (Table 15-3). The lower the ankle:brachial index, the more blood flow to the extremities is compromised and the greater the severity of symptoms. Also, loss of the posterior tibial pulse, as seen in J.S., is not uncommon in those with peripheral vascular occlusion; it is the single best criterion for the diagnosis of IC.

Treatment

Therapeutic Objectives and Nonpharmacologic Interventions

2. What is the therapeutic objective in treating J.S.? What interventions should be initiated to prevent claudication pain and arrest progression of the disease?

The specific treatment goals for J.S. are prevention of further claudication pain, arresting the progression of underlying disease, and decreasing his risk of any cardiovascular event. Achieving these goals will provide J.S. with the best chance of avoiding increased mobility impairment, amputation, and cardiovascular events such as stroke or MI. An important concept that should be stressed when explaining these treatment goals to J.S. is that all his diseases are closely interrelated, and that a beneficial intervention for one disease is beneficial for all. Interventions that can be initiated include proper diet and weight loss, control of his diabetes, hypertension therapy optimization, and dyslipidemia therapy. However, the two most important things that J.S. can do for his IC are summed up in five words: "Stop smoking and keep walking."[19]

SMOKING CESSATION

The importance of smoking cessation cannot be overemphasized to patients with IC. It is the most important modifiable factor in preventing the development of rest pain, prolonged limb ischemia, and amputation. Several studies have documented improved survival and decreased amputation rates in patients with IC who stopped smoking compared to patients who continue to smoke.[20,21] Other benefits, such as improved treadmill walking distance, decreased progression to symptoms, and decreased complications following vascular reconstructive surgery, have been shown in patients who are able to quit smoking compared to patients who continue to

smoke.[20,22–24] It also is the intervention that will decrease J.S.'s claudication pain most rapidly. If J.S. is able to stop smoking, his risk of developing rest pain or of requiring a limb amputation will be very low. He also will decrease his risk of MI and mortality by three- and fivefold, respectively. Table 15-4 summarizes the risk of cigarette smoking and the value of smoking cessation on cardiovascular complications.

Many pharmacologic products and strategies are available to aid patients like J.S. to stop smoking (see Chapter 85, Treatment of Tobacco Use and Dependence). Many are nicotine replacement products, which may be administered as a nasal spray, chewed as a gum, consumed as a lozenge, or absorbed through a transdermal patch. If these are needed to help him stop smoking, their use is warranted. However, nicotine itself has harmful effects on the vasculature via catecholamine release and vasoconstriction and may play a role in endothelial damage and atherosclerosis progression.[25] Medications that do not contain nicotine, such as bupropion (Zyban), and smoking cessation counseling or support groups should be used as necessary to help the patient stop smoking.

EXERCISE

An individualized exercise program has been endorsed for patients with IC and will benefit J.S.'s other risk factors as well.[26,27] The pain associated with IC results in decreased mobility, and because of deconditioning from lack of exercise, patients with IC may slowly become dependent on others for activities of daily living. An exercise program is the most effective way to not only preserve mobility, but also increase mobility. It is more effective than the best pharmacologic therapy currently available.[28] The ideal exercise program consists of walking for 30 to 60 minutes three to five times a week.[27] J.S. should walk as fast and far as he can until the pain becomes severe; he should then wait until the pain subsides, and then resume walking.[29] At first, J.S. may experience several painful episodes during each exercise session, but these should gradually decrease as the beneficial effects of exercise therapy begin to emerge. Studies have documented that this type of exercise program can more than double the pain-free distance a patient with IC is able to walk.[27] An exercise program should be supervised and individually designed, and the patient should understand the importance of exercise to his or her continued mobility.[28]

Rheologic abnormalities of increased blood viscosity, impaired RBC filterability, hyperaggregation, and polycythemia (elevated hematocrit) have been shown to return to normal in

Table 15-4 Patient Outcomes Based on Smoking Status After Intermittent Claudication Diagnosis[9,20]

Outcome	Length of Follow-up	Patient Population	
		Current Smokers	Past Smokers[a]
Rest pain	7 years	16%	0%
Myocardial infarction	10 years	53%	11%
Amputation	5 years	11%	0%
Mortality	10 years	54%	18%

[a]Quit after intermittent claudication diagnosis.

many patients with IC who participate in a regular exercise program.[30] Exercise may offset the need for pharmacologic intervention. The potential mechanisms by which exercise benefits patients with IC are listed in Table 15-5.

DYSLIPIDEMIA MANAGEMENT

3. **Is lipid-lowering therapy indicated for J.S.?**

Since IC is a consequence of atherosclerosis, arresting the progression of J.S.'s atherosclerotic disease is important (see Chapter 13, Dyslipidemias). The initiation of the nutritional and exercise recommendations outlined in the Therapeutic Lifestyle Changes (TLC) guidelines,[31] as well as cholesterol-lowering agents, are the cornerstones for attaining this goal. Considerable data suggest that aggressive dietary and pharmacologic management of dyslipidemia, particularly lowering LDL cholesterol, leads to regression of atherosclerotic lesions in the coronary and carotid vasculature.[32–34] In contrast, there are relatively few prospective data about the effect of successful lipid-lowering therapy on the regression or stabilization of peripheral lesions, or on clinical events in patients with PAD. However, a post hoc analysis of a large lipid-lowering study in subjects with known coronary artery disease treated with simvastatin demonstrated a significant decrease in new or worsening IC, suggesting that benefit is seen in the prevention of clinically symptomatic PAD in high-risk patients.[35] Another study randomized patients with known arterial disease of various types to simvastatin 40 mg daily or placebo. After 5 years, there was a 15% decrease in noncardiac revascularizations, including amputations, among the patients receiving simvastatin.[36]

A meta-analysis of 698 subjects from several small, randomized trials using a variety of lipid-lowering therapies in patients with PAD demonstrated reduced severity of claudication and decreased disease progression as measured by angiography. A decrease in mortality was also seen, but this did not reach statistical significance.[37] Limited data suggest high Lp(a) lipoprotein concentrations may be particularly important in the development of PAD.[5]

All patients with evidence of atherosclerotic disease and a LDL cholesterol >100 mg/dL (SI: 2.6 mmol/L) are candidates for a lipid-lowering regimen according to the National

Table 15-5 Primary Mechanisms of Symptom Improvement With Exercise Therapy in Intermittent Claudication[28]

Decrease of blood viscosity
Metabolic changes in the muscle
  Improved muscle metabolism
  Improved oxygen extraction
Improved endothelial function and microcirculation
Decreased occurrence of ischemia and inflammation
Atherosclerosis risk factors improved via:
  Weight loss
  Glycemic control
  Blood pressure control
  Increased HDL
  Decreased triglycerides
  Decreased thrombotic tendency

Cholesterol Education Program (NCEP).[31] J.S. has angina and lower extremity atherosclerosis, both of which indicate a need for aggressive lipid lowering. His LDL cholesterol is 180 mg/dL, so a reduction of almost 50% is desired. Lowering triglycerides and raising HDL cholesterol are secondary goals in J.S. and can be reassessed after his LDL goal has been reached and the effect of therapy on these parameters is measured. In addition to an aggressive dietary management program, an HMG-CoA reductase inhibitor agent should be prescribed as initial therapy for J.S. HMG-CoA reductase inhibitors, exercise, and the American Heart Association diet will all improve his LDL cholesterol level. They also have beneficial effects on triglycerides and HDL cholesterol, and the need for additional therapy can be assessed after the impact of these measures is determined. Niacin is the best alternative or additional agent if lipid goals are not met with statin therapy, or if the statin is not tolerated.[5]

MANAGEMENT OF HYPERTENSION

4. **J.S.'s blood pressure is elevated to 170/95 mm Hg despite enalapril therapy. Since he has angina, and his heart rate is 89, a β-adrenergic blocker is considered. Are there alternative antihypertensive therapies that might be preferable for J.S.?**

J.S.'s hypertension has likely contributed to the development of his atherosclerosis and PAD. Hypertension has been associated with deficiencies in the synthesis of vasodilating substances such as prostacyclin, bradykinin, and nitric oxide by the endothelial cells lining the vasculature. Hypertension also increases concentrations of vasoconstricting substances, such as angiotensin II. An increase in vascular tone can alter local hemodynamics, especially in the presence of a stenotic lesion. Hypertension is also a component of the metabolic syndrome, along with dyslipidemia, central obesity, and type 2 diabetes. While it has not been determined whether normalization of blood pressure has a positive effect on IC, it is well established that uncontrolled BP, as in J.S., results in vascular complications such as MI and stroke. In light of J.S.'s numerous risk factors for these complications, improved management of his hypertension is warranted.

β-Blockers are frequently cited as contraindicated in patients with IC due to the potential for unopposed α-adrenergic-mediated vasoconstriction during peripheral β-blockade. However, the evidence to document worsening IC by β-blockade is sparse. Calf blood flow and symptoms of claudication were not worsened by either metoprolol or propranolol in one study.[38] In contrast, another study documented decreased calf blood flow and walking distance with atenolol, labetalol, and pindolol.[39] These latter three β-blockers possess various ancillary properties that may have different effects on the symptoms of IC: β_1 selectivity (atenolol), combination α- and β-blockade (labetalol), and intrinsic sympathomimetic activity (pindolol). The mechanism of the observed detrimental effect with β-blockade in this study may be via attenuation of epinephrine-induced vasodilation during exercise and the blocking of peripheral β_2-adrenergic receptors.[40] Overall, controlled studies have been inconclusive; however, a meta-analysis of placebo-controlled trials and studies with control groups concluded that β-blockers did not worsen claudication.[41]

Thus, β-blockers should be used cautiously in patients with severe PAD. If used, a β-blocker should be started at a low dose and titrated slowly to reduce BP. Angiotensin-converting enzyme (ACE) inhibitors may preserve collateral blood supply compared to β-blockers and are an alternative for the treatment of hypertension in patients with IC.[39] Furthermore, the Heart Outcomes Prevention Evaluation (HOPE) study of the ACE inhibitor ramipril versus placebo included >4,000 patients with PAD, and this subgroup derived benefit in terms of decreased mortality, MI, and stroke.[42]

Because J.S. is hypertensive and has diabetes, his BP goal is <130/80.[43] He is already taking an ACE inhibitor, which is an excellent initial antihypertensive choice in a patient with diabetes. It definitely delays the development of nephropathy in patients with type 1 diabetes[44] and is thought to provide the same protection in patients with type 2 diabetes, based on data using surrogate markers. The dose of enalapril could be increased, or a low-dose diuretic, such as hydrochlorothiazide or chlorthalidone, could be added. This combination is synergistic and should be very effective in reducing J.S.'s BP.[45,46] Other options include a calcium channel blocker or a β-blocker, both of which are useful in patients such as J.S. with angina. If J.S. develops angina symptoms with exercise as a result of sympathetic stimulation, a β-blocker may be required to permit participation in an exercise program that could greatly benefit his IC. If β-blocker therapy is necessary, a β_1-selective agent should be chosen to minimize the peripheral blockade of β_2 receptors that could otherwise result in decreased perfusion.

MANAGEMENT OF DIABETES

5. Will improving J.S.'s diabetes control slow the progression of his PAD? What changes in his diabetes management do you recommend?

Patients with type 2 diabetes mellitus are able to minimize macrovascular and microvascular complications of their disease with aggressive pharmacologic glucose control.[47–49] Insulin, sulfonylurea, or metformin therapy has a beneficial effect on slowing the development of the microvascular complications of diabetes, such as retinopathy and nephropathy.[47] Metformin has specifically been shown to further reduce the occurrence of macrovascular complications such as stroke or myocardial infarction compared to therapy with insulin or sulfonylureas in obese patients with type 2 diabetes.[48]

J.S.'s diabetes is a significant risk factor for progression to further ischemic events (Table 15-6). He has a twofold greater risk of death and a seven-fold greater risk of amputation compared to a patient without diabetes. Although a specific benefit on IC has not been demonstrated, it seems prudent to initiate or continue aggressive diabetes management in patients with type 2 diabetes mellitus and IC. The addition of metformin to J.S.'s therapy could minimize his insulin requirement and decrease his risk of vascular complications. This agent will favorably affect hepatic glucose production and insulin sensitivity and could result in weight loss. The addition of a short-acting insulin before meals is another possible intervention. It is hoped that J.S. can reach his hemoglobin A_{1c} goal of <7% and a fasting blood glucose of 90 to 130 mg/dL with diet, exercise, and metformin therapy, in addition to his standing dose of insulin.[50] It would also be helpful to have J.S. check his blood glucose before meals, 1 to 2 hours after meals, and at bedtime and to keep a log of the results. This may help improve understanding of his medication and nutrition therapies and help guide future therapy changes.

J.S. also must take proper care of his feet to prevent ulcerative complications of IC. He should be encouraged to keep his feet warm and dry and to wear properly fitted shoes. He should seek medical attention immediately for minor trauma to his feet or legs.[3] These measures can reduce the incidence of amputation in patients with diabetes.

VASODILATORS

6. J.S. is already taking isosorbide dinitrate for his angina. Since IC is made worse by vasoconstriction, should another vasodilating agent be added to treat both his hypertension and IC?

The use of vasodilators for J.S. would at first appear to be a logical pharmacologic intervention to prevent claudication pain. Vasodilators, including isosorbide dinitrate, directly or indirectly relax blood vessel walls and increase both skin and muscle blood flow as long as cardiac output is maintained. However, with obstructive arterial disease, vessels may be so sclerotic that they are unable to dilate any further. With systemic vasodilation, BP distal to the occlusion may become lower than systemic BP, leading to decreased perfusion pressure of the tissues. Furthermore, systemic vasodilation may decrease blood flow provided by collateral blood vessels. This is because vasodilation in other areas of the body shunts blood away from the diseased areas that need perfusion the most. This is known as the steal phenomenon.

Numerous vasodilators (i.e., isoxsuprine, papaverine, ethaverine, cyclandelate, niacin derivatives, reserpine, guanethidine, methyldopa, tolazoline, nifedipine, buflomedil, L-carnitine) have been used to treat IC. However, none has convincingly or consistently improved exercise performance, despite earlier beliefs that they were effective.[51] Other vasodilators, such as ACE inhibitors, also have failed to demonstrate a clinical benefit. However, a recent small, but well-controlled study demonstrated improvement in walking distance with verapamil, a calcium channel blocker, compared to placebo in patients with IC.[52] Thus, although vasodilators have generally been eliminated from the treatment of IC and related obstructive vascular disorders,[12] verapamil may be a vasodilator that is useful in patients with IC.

Smoking cessation and the initiation of an exercise program are the two therapies that will improve J.S.'s IC to the largest degree. After these two measures have been implemented and the impact of the new BP regimen has been assessed, the addition of verapamil could be considered. Verapamil is initiated at 120 mg daily if further BP lowering is required to reach his goal of <130/80, or if angina symptoms are limiting his exercise capacity. Implementing verapamil at this time solely to increase walking distance is not likely to re-

Table 15-6 Effect of Diabetes Mellitus on Intermittent Claudication Outcomes After 5 Years[8]		
	Patients With Diabetes (%)	Patients Without Diabetes (%)
Mortality	49	23
Major amputation	21	3
Deterioration	35	19

liably yield clinically significant improvement, and well-proven measures therapies should be tried first. Since some improvement in walking distance may be obtained, verapamil is a good add-on therapy for BP or angina symptom control in patients with concomitant IC (see Chapter 17, Ischemic Heart Disease: Anginal Syndromes).

Pentoxifylline

7. **Has pentoxifylline been shown to be efficacious in patients like J.S.? How does this drug benefit patients with IC?**

Pentoxifylline, a methylxanthine derivative, is one of several agents currently approved by the FDA for the treatment of IC. The exact mechanism of action is unclear; however, it appears to decrease blood viscosity by decreasing fibrinogen, improving the deformability of both red and white blood cells, and eliciting antiplatelet effects.[53] While the theoretical and in vitro data on pentoxifylline are unique and positive, the data demonstrating clinical usefulness of this agent are controversial. Subjective measures of efficacy are limited to claudication distance and maximum walking distance. Claudication distance, the distance the patient can walk before pain begins, has been judged as the most clinically significant outcome measure for pentoxifylline treatment.[26] The maximum walking distance is the furthest the patient can walk with claudication pain and is considered a less reliable measure.

Some clinical trials of pentoxifylline at dosages of 600 to 1,200 mg/day have shown statistically significant improvements in these subjective measurements when compared to placebo, while others have found no benefit over placebo.[26,54] In general, the improvements in walking distances from study to study are unpredictable, and the clinical importance of the sometimes minimal increases in walking distances is not clear (e.g., pain-free walking of approximately 30 meters greater than with placebo).[55] Some experts assert that these potential benefits of questionable clinical significance are not worth the expense of drug therapy.[26] Furthermore, some patients taking pentoxifylline experience gastrointestinal side effects such as dyspepsia, nausea, or vomiting; others experience headache or dizziness.[56] Because the therapy is of questionable benefit, the expense and potential for side effects are rarely justified.

Pentoxifylline's role in IC therapy is limited. It may have a role in patients who are unable to engage in exercise therapy or in patients with markedly reduced walking distances, in whom any small increase in walking distance would greatly improve the patient's level of activity.[54] It also may be tried in patients who have not gained the desired benefit from smoking cessation and exercise therapy. A 2-month trial of pentoxifylline is adequate to determine if the patient will benefit from the therapy.[29]

J.S. is not severely debilitated, and the benefits of smoking cessation and exercise therapy have not been fully realized. Therefore, pentoxifylline therapy should be withheld until his response to these two well-proven therapies has been determined and the need for further improvement in walking distance is established.

Antiplatelet Therapy

8. **Is the aspirin that J.S. is taking beneficial for preventing IC? Would newer agents such as ticlopidine, clopidogrel, or cilostazol offer any advantages over aspirin?**

Aspirin is one of several antiplatelet agents that may be considered for indefinite use in patients like J.S. with IC. There has been a paucity of studies directly addressing the effects of antiplatelet agents on IC symptoms. Rather, most available data address the impact of antiplatelet agents on overall cardiovascular morbidity and mortality.

Aspirin exerts its antiplatelet effect by irreversibly inhibiting cyclooxygenase. This enzyme is essential for the production of thromboxane A_2, a stimulus for platelet aggregation. While aspirin has no direct effect on plaque regression, it does prevent and retard the role platelets play in the thrombogenic events that occur in the vicinity of atherosclerotic plaques.[57]

The antiplatelet mechanism of ticlopidine and clopidogrel, closely related thienopyridine derivatives, involves the blockade of adenosine $5'$-diphosphate (ADP) receptors on platelets. This blockade decreases platelet–fibrinogen binding.[58] Cilostazol is the newest antiplatelet agent that may be used for IC. It inhibits platelet aggregation via phosphodiesterase III inhibition. It also prevents calcium-induced contractions in the vasculature, providing additional vasodilatory properties.[59]

Aspirin is the overwhelming antiplatelet agent of choice in patients with vascular disease of any origin (this includes stroke, MI, PAD, and angina). At dosages of 80 to 325 mg per day, it decreased vascular death by approximately 15% and nonfatal vascular events by approximately 30% in secondary prevention trials.[60] In patients with PAD, aspirin will delay the progression of established lesions as assessed by angiography.[61] When used for primary prevention of cardiovascular disease in men, aspirin decreased the need for arterial reconstructive surgery due to PAD.[62] A subgroup analysis of a larger trial also indicated that aspirin decreases MI, stroke, and vascular death in patients with PAD.[60] However, whether aspirin has any beneficial effects on walking distance or claudication pain in patients with IC has not been studied.

In contrast, several small studies have shown that ticlopidine increases pain-free walking distance and absolute walking distance compared to placebo in patients with PAD.[63,64] Furthermore, ticlopidine (250 mg twice daily) decreases the risk of death from cardiovascular causes by approximately 30%[65] and the need for revascularization surgery over a 5-year treatment period in this patient population.[66] Most of the mortality benefits are derived from decreasing death due to ischemic heart disease.[65] However, side effects are 2.4 times more likely in patients receiving ticlopidine compared to placebo.[67] Diarrhea is a common complaint, with a prevalence in one trial of 21.7% compared to 8.8% of patients receiving placebo.[65] The most serious side effects are hematologic in nature (specifically neutropenia, occurring in approximately 1.6% of patients).[67,68] Ticlopidine also carries a black box warning concerning the rare but life-threatening development of thrombotic thrombocytopenic purpura (TTP).[69] Unfortunately, there are no data directly comparing ticlopidine to aspirin in this patient population, although the magnitude of mortality benefit in independent studies appears comparable.

Clopidogrel, an antiplatelet agent with the same mechanism of action as ticlopidine but with an improved safety profile, was compared to aspirin in patients with known atherosclerotic disease. Dosages of 75 mg daily significantly reduced cardiovascular endpoints by approximately 25% compared to aspirin in this patient population.[70] In fact, the treatment effect was most pronounced in the subgroup that had PAD, leading to the suggestion that clopidogrel may be preferable in the patient population with PAD. Unfortunately, there was no measure of clopidogrel's effect on walking distance or claudication pain.

Several studies have confirmed that cilostazol, the phosphodiesterase III inhibitor, increases walking distance by approximately 40% to 50%.[71–74] Discontinuation of cilostazol therapy worsened maximum walking distance in patients stabilized on therapy for 6 months.[75] However, while there was an overall benefit with cilostazol, only about half of the patients receiving cilostazol attained an improvement in walking distance.[76] One study incorporated quality-of-life measurements and found that cilostazol improved overall quality of life in these patients.[71] Despite all these positive findings with cilostazol, there are several drawbacks to its use. Cilostazol is contraindicated in patients with heart failure, because other phosphodiesterase inhibitors cause excess mortality in patients with heart failure, presumably due to increased arrhythmias.[77] Other common side effects include headache, loose stools or diarrhea, and dizziness.[72] Cilostazol is a cytochrome P450 3A4 substrate; therefore, any inhibitor of this enzyme system may substantially increase cilostazol levels. Most importantly, there are no data substantiating the long-term effects of cilostazol therapy on cardiovascular morbidity and mortality, nor is there any information about bleeding risks if used in combination with other antiplatelet agents except for aspirin.

Even though ticlopidine, clopidogrel, and cilostazol have been specifically studied for their effects on patients with PAD to a greater extent than aspirin, the latter remains the antiplatelet drug of choice for PAD. This is because such a large body of evidence documents aspirin's beneficial effect on mortality in patients with all types of cardiovascular diseases, and PAD rarely exists as the only manifestation of atherosclerotic disease. As discussed earlier, the presence of symptomatic atherosclerosis in the extremities is strongly associated with atherosclerosis in other vascular beds, such as the coronary arteries and the carotid arteries. Aspirin's unchallenged benefit in these disease processes, coupled with its limited but known benefits in PAD, makes it first-line antiplatelet therapy for J.S. However, some data suggest that hypertension should be controlled prior to the initiation of aspirin therapy to decrease the small increased incidence of cerebral hemorrhage associated with its use.[78] Clopidogrel is an option if aspirin is not tolerated or contraindicated; however, ticlopidine should be avoided due to its side effects. Cilostazol could be added to aspirin therapy in suitable patients as it is one of the few agents proven to improve walking distance. It cannot be considered a solo antiplatelet agent until a long-term benefit on mortality is proven.

9. What dose of aspirin should J.S. take?

Aspirin is an effective antithrombotic agent at dosages ranging from 50 to 1,500 mg daily. The minimum dosages proven to decrease cardiovascular events are 75 to 160 mg daily, with the higher dosage showing benefit in active processes such as acute ischemic stroke[79] and acute MI.[80] A dosage of 75 mg daily has demonstrated benefit in patients with hypertension[81] and stable angina.[82] There is no evidence that these "low doses" are any more or any less effective than dosages of 900 to 1,500 mg daily.[60]

Since all dosages of aspirin are similarly efficacious in decreasing cardiovascular events in this patient population, side effects determine the dose chosen. Although few studies have directly compared varying doses, side effects appear to be dose related. Thirty milligrams of aspirin daily results in less minor bleeding compared to approximately 300 mg daily,[83] and 300 mg daily results in less GI side effects compared to 1,200 mg daily.[84] Therefore, J.S. should take the lowest effective dose of aspirin; for convenience, 81 mg daily.

Other Therapeutic Alternatives

10. The sales clerk at a health food store told J.S. about several nutritional supplements and herbal products that would help his circulation so that he could walk better. Do any of these products really work?

Several herbs and vitamins have been used to treat IC, but most have not been rigorously studied. To complicate matters, many studies are published in foreign journals, making access and interpretation of the data challenging.

Ginkgo biloba is one of the few herbal therapies with double-blind placebo-controlled trials to support its use. A meta-analysis of eight trials representing data from 385 patients reported a mean increase in pain-free walking of 34 meters (a 47% increase) with a median dosage of 160 mg daily for 6 months.[85] This effect may be attributed to its antiplatelet properties.[86] Gingko is generally well tolerated with no major side effects, except for the increased risk of bleeding associated with any platelet inhibitor.[87] Occasionally, mild GI upset or headache has been reported.[88] While the treatment benefit is modest in size, there is a consistent trend in benefit and the side effects are minor.

Vitamin E has been advocated for the treatment of intermittent claudication for many years.[89] However, only a handful of very small, poorly controlled studies support its ability to improve blood flow and walking distance.[90,91] Vitamin E has not prevented cardiovascular events in patients with both established coronary artery disease and risk factors for cardiovascular disease.[91–93] Although it is generally not harmful at dosages of 400 to 800 IU/day, vitamin E is unlikely to offer any symptomatic relief or long-term protection from cardiovascular events to J.S.

Patients with IC have decreased intramuscular carnitine levels, and this impairs oxidative metabolism in the skeletal muscle.[94,95] Exogenous propionyl-L-carnitine, 1 to 2 g/day, improves energy production in ischemic muscles. Small studies have demonstrated beneficial effects on walking distances[96,97] and quality of life[98] in patients with IC. Although it is not approved by the FDA, similar agents, such as levocarnitine, are available in the United States. Limited data suggest its effects are less than those seen with propionyl-L-carnitine.[99]

J.S. should inform his doctors and pharmacist if he uses any of these agents to avoid potential drug interactions (e.g., ginkgo biloba plus antiplatelet drugs) and to allow appropriate assessment of other treatments.

11. What options are there for J.S. if nonpharmacologic and pharmacologic interventions fail?

Surgical intervention eventually may be necessary for persistent and complicated disease. Because success rates for preventing amputation and postsurgical complications vary from institution to institution, surgery should be considered only for severely ischemic limbs and should be performed in a hospital with a good history of success.[100] Arterial bypass grafting and percutaneous transluminal angioplasty of the femoral and/or iliac arteries, similar to cardiac revascularization, are two procedures that can be performed. Angioplasty is beneficial in patients with localized disease, especially in the iliac or superficial femoral arteries, and should be considered in patients who truly are incapacitated by their recreational, vocational, or personal exercise limitations.[101] Stent placement during angioplasty appears to improve postoperative patency and long-term outcomes.[102] Guidelines for patients who should have angioplasty were published in 1994.[101] Interestingly, angioplasty has not decreased the number of amputations, yet costs for revascularization procedures have doubled.[103] The more invasive reconstructive arterial (bypass) surgery can be employed if diffuse lesions preclude the use of localized angioplasty. The true benefits and pitfalls of these skilled interventions remain unclear.

Emergency surgical intervention may be required if acute, persistent ischemia develops. This is frequently due to a thrombosis associated with advanced atherosclerosis, although other causes, such as cardiac emboli, cannot be excluded.[54] Both surgical thrombectomy and localized thrombolytic administration[104] with tissue-plasminogen activator (t-PA) or urokinase have equal success in alleviating acute limb-threatening ischemia.[105,106]

RAYNAUD'S PHENOMENON

Raynaud's disease, first described by Maurice Raynaud in 1862,[107] remains largely a medical enigma today. This disorder is characterized by ischemia and vasospasm of the peripheral arteries. It is usually limited to the skin of the hands and fingers, but can also occur in the feet. Between attacks, the digits may appear cool and moist or normal. This abrupt and discomforting phenomenon can be brought on by exposure to cold or emotional stress, both likely mediated through an exaggerated sympathetic response to the precipitating stimuli. While both IC and Raynaud's phenomenon are disorders of the peripheral arterial circulation, they differ significantly in that IC results primarily from atherosclerotic obstruction, while Raynaud's is due to vasospasm.

Diagnosis

This disorder can be separated into primary Raynaud's phenomenon, indicating an idiopathic origin, and secondary Raynaud's.[108] Secondary Raynaud's consists of signs and symptoms of Raynaud's phenomenon in the presence of an associated disease or condition, most commonly a connective tissue disorder, such as scleroderma, rheumatoid arthritis, or systemic lupus erythematosus. Primary Raynaud's disease is diagnosed only when secondary causes have been excluded.[109] Common criteria for the diagnosis of primary Raynaud's phenomenon are listed in Table 15-7. The diagnosis is primarily a subjective one, consisting of clinical signs and symptoms, and simply reflects cold hands and/or feet without normal recovery following a cold stimulus or emotional stress.[110] In unaffected individuals, a cold provocation should result in some mottling and cyanotic changes in the hands, with recovery

Table 15-7   Diagnosis of Primary Raynaud's Phenomenon[114]

Vasospastic attacks caused by cold or emotional stress
Symmetrical attacks involving both hands
No evidence of digital ulcerations, pitting, or gangrene
Normal nailfold capillaries
No suggestion of a secondary cause
A negative antinuclear test
A normal sedimentation rate

once the stimuli is removed. However, in patients with Raynaud's phenomenon, the same cold provocation causes closure of the digital arteries, which produces a sharply demarcated pallor and cyanosis of the digits that persists despite removal of the stimulus.[110] The most reliable objective method to measure artery closure during an attack is the finger systolic BP;[111] however, the subjective diagnostic criteria are most commonly and easily employed to diagnose Raynaud's phenomenon.

Epidemiology

In general, the prevalence of Raynaud's phenomenon is about 3% to 4% across several ethnic groups;[112] however, it may be as high as 20% in some geographically defined populations.[113] It is more common in women than men, tends to affect young patients, and has a higher prevalence in patients with family members that also experience Raynaud's phenomenon. An onset in the teenage years suggests primary Raynaud's phenomenon, whereas an onset after 30 years of age suggests a secondary cause.[114] Secondary Raynaud's is usually associated with a connective tissue disorder, but several other conditions may predispose individuals to the development of Raynaud's phenomenon. These include occupational-related exposures to vibratory machinery (e.g., drills, grinders, chain saws), vinyl chloride, or hand trauma. It may also be associated with medications, including β-adrenergic blocking agents, ergots, and cytotoxic drugs, all of which can induce vasoconstriction.[115] While avoidance of β-adrenergic blocking agents in patients with Raynaud's phenomenon appears prudent, no discernible effect as measured by skin temperature and blood flow was found with the administration of both selective and nonselective β-blockers to patients with Raynaud's phenomenon.[116] The effect of smoking on Raynaud's phenomenon has yielded conflicting results. Overall, there appears to be a negligible effect of smoking on the prevalence of Raynaud's phenomenon, the incidence of attacks, and digital blood flow.[117,118]

Pathophysiology

The blood vessels of the digital skin have a prime role in the regulation of body temperature and are supplied with vast amounts of sympathetic vasoconstricting nerves.[109] Cold-induced vasospastic attacks in patients with primary Raynaud's phenomenon involve a heightened vasoconstriction of these digital arteries that is mediated by α_2-adrenergic receptors.[119] The cause of this exaggerated response to cold stimuli is unknown; however, there are several plausible mechanisms involving peripheral α_2-adrenoreceptors that could result in an intense vasoconstriction. These include an increased number of α_2-adrenoreceptors, increased temperature sensitivity of the α_2-adrenoreceptors, and increased activity of the α_2-adrenergic intracellular signal-transduction pathway.[112] The mechanism of secondary Raynaud's is also not known but is thought to be similar to primary Raynaud's. The α_2-adrenoreceptor aberrancy may be the result of arterial damage induced by an associated disease state, such as a connective tissue disorder.[112] It is also possible that serotonin receptors (S2) play a role in Raynaud's phenomenon. Serotonin agonists have caused decreased finger blood flow, and conversely antagonists have increased digital blood flow.[120]

Clinically, the patient with Raynaud's disease will present with a waxy pallor of one or more of the fingers after the sudden decrease of arterial blood flow. Hemoglobin desaturation occurs with static venous blood flow and causes the digit or digits to have a cyanotic appearance. The attack subsides over time, and the affected arteries vasodilate. As the skin temperature increases, classic rubor, or reddening of the afflicted area, will be seen. Many patients will be observed to have pallor only during the initial attack, in which the digits take on a white or yellow, sometimes patchy, appearance. In most cases, the ischemia produced by the phenomenon does not have important consequences; however, in severe cases, atrophy of the skin, irregular nail growth, and wasting of the tissue pads can occur.[109]

Clinical Presentation

12. F.K., a 39-year-old man, presents today with a 4-day history of left hand pain. He notes that the third digit of his left hand is "cold and somewhat blue," especially in the distal area. The other areas of his hand have recovered, but the distal portion of the digit remains cyanotic and numb. He has used acetaminophen and warm-water soaks without success. He is a construction worker who uses his hands "quite a bit" in his work.

He has a history of gastroesophageal reflux and has no allergies. His social history is significant for smoking 1.5 packs of cigarettes a day for 19 years. Upon physical examination, his extremities reveal appropriate sensation of the forearm and hand. There are some blue areas on the distal portion on the third phalanx, with no other signs and symptoms. When F.K.'s opposite hand was placed in cold water, several white splotches appeared and he experienced tingling in this hand as a result of the cold-water exposure. He is diagnosed as having Raynaud's phenomenon. Does F.K. present with primary or secondary Raynaud's phenomenon?

F.K. presents with what is most likely secondary Raynaud's phenomenon due to one of several potential underlying causes. His clinical presentation is classic for Raynaud's, with vasospasm, pallor, and a cyanotic overtone. The diagnosis is confirmed by the cold-water test, which indicates that the vasospastic attack is precipitated by cold exposure. He has a work history that may easily include hand trauma and the use of vibrating machinery. Due to Raynaud's association with connective tissue disorders, other laboratory tests such as an antinuclear antibody (ANA) and sedimentation rate should be checked.

Treatment

Nonpharmacologic Management

13. What conservative measures can be taken with F.K. to prevent or decrease the painful vasospasm of Raynaud's disease?

The majority of patients with both primary and secondary Raynaud's phenomenon will respond to conservative management. Avoiding cold stimuli is the primary treatment. F.K. should be instructed to protect his hands and fingers from exposure by using mittens and Styrofoam or foam rubber wrappers when handling cold drinks. While protecting his hands is important, he must also protect other parts of the body from cold exposure to prevent a sympathetic response, which may trigger symptomatic vasoconstriction in his hands. This includes layering his clothing when working outside in cold weather. He should avoid medications that can induce vasoconstriction, particularly sympathomimetics, clonidine, serotonin receptor agonists, and ergot preparations.[114] He should be encouraged to stop smoking, due to its overall health benefit and because it promotes vasoconstriction, although its impact on Raynaud's actually appears negligible.[117,118]

F.K. has new-onset and relatively mild Raynaud's phenomenon. For others who have more severe symptoms and manifestations, especially patients with underlying connective tissue disorders, it is important to immediately and aggressively manage any ulcers that develop on the digits and to be extremely vigilant in detecting infected digits. Antibiotic therapy should be initiated if necessary.[115]

Calcium Channel Blockers

14. Nifedipine extended-release 30 mg QD is ordered for F.K. What is the rationale for using a calcium channel blocker in this case?

Drugs may be used to treat primary and secondary Raynaud's phenomenon if it interferes with the patient's ability to work or perform daily activities or if digital lesions develop. Unfortunately, most proposed treatments for Raynaud's are variably effective, introduce the risk for significant side effects, and may be expensive. Drug therapy should always be in addition to nonpharmacologic measures.

Calcium channel blockers decrease calcium ion influx and prevent smooth muscle contraction, especially in vascular responses evoked by cold exposure. Nifedipine, a potent peripheral vasodilating calcium channel blocker, has become the drug of choice in patients with Raynaud's disease not controlled by conservative measures. In two thirds of patients with either primary or secondary Raynaud's disease, the frequency and severity of attacks decrease with nifedipine therapy, although patients with primary disease show the most improvement.[112,121,122] Doses of 10 to 30 mg three times daily of immediate-release nifedipine are beneficial. Most clinicians administer nifedipine in an extended-release formulation to increase convenience and decrease side effects such as dizziness, headache, facial flushing, and peripheral edema, which can occur in up to 50% of patients.[123] Several small studies have confirmed the efficacy of 30 to 120 mg/day of an extended-release nifedipine preparation.[124–126] Even the extended-release preparation of nifedipine can cause bothersome edema due to dilation of the precapillary bed. While less effective than nifedipine, other vasoselective calcium channel blockers such as amlodipine, felodipine, isradipine, and nisoldipine decrease the frequency and severity of ischemic attacks.[114,127–130]

Diltiazem, a less potent peripheral-dilating calcium channel blocker, also has beneficial effects in patients with primary and secondary Raynaud's disease at dosages of 90 to 360 mg/day.[131–133] The response rates are not as high as with nifedipine or the other dihydropyridine calcium channel blockers, and patients who have not responded to nifedipine probably will not gain any benefit with diltiazem. However, side effects, such as headache, dizziness, or peripheral edema, are less common than with nifedipine. Therefore, patients who are responding to dihydropyridine therapy, but cannot tolerate the side effects can be given a trial of diltiazem. Verapamil, another intermediate-potency, peripheral-vasodilating calcium channel blocker, was shown in one small study to be ineffective for Raynaud's phenomenon and should not be recommended.[134]

In summary, nifedipine is the current drug of choice for both primary and secondary Raynaud's disease. Patients who do not benefit from nifedipine likely will not benefit by switching to another calcium channel blocker. However, patients who cannot tolerate the side effects of nifedipine (such as ankle edema) might benefit by switching to another calcium channel blocker.

F.K. should be warned of the potential side effects with nifedipine therapy and should return to the clinic in 2 weeks for assessment. A 30-mg daily dose of extended-release nifedipine is a reasonable starting dose. He should be instructed to keep a diary documenting the number of attacks he experiences and details surrounding each attack, such as time course and precipitating factors. In addition to the usual side effects mentioned above, F.K. should be aware that his symptoms of gastroesophageal reflux could worsen with nifedipine therapy due to a decreased lower esophageal sphincter pressure. This side effect should be specifically assessed at his follow-up appointment in 2 weeks.

Other Therapeutic Agents

15. **What other drugs may be tried if F.K. cannot tolerate the calcium channel blocker?**

Other than calcium channel blockers, there is no proven therapy for Raynaud's phenomenon. However, many agents have been used based on minimal data and anecdotal reports. The α_1-adrenergic antagonists are one such class of drugs. Prazosin, 1 mg three times a day, yielded moderate benefit in two thirds of patients in two small studies.[135,136] Side effects of prazosin are significant at maximum doses and include dizziness, edema, fatigue, and orthostasis. The longer-acting α_1-adrenergic antagonist terazosin was evaluated in one small study and improved symptomatology as well as objective measures of blood flow.[137] However, there are not enough data with this class of drugs to routinely recommend their use in patients with Raynaud's phenomenon.

ACE inhibitors act as vasodilators and have been investigated in several small studies. Unfortunately, ACE inhibitors appear to have no beneficial effects in patients with Raynaud's phenomenon.[138] In contrast, one small study of losartan (an angiotensin-receptor blocker) in patients with secondary Raynaud's phenomenon due to scleroderma demonstrated benefit compared to nifedipine therapy.[139] Larger trials are needed to confirm this finding before recommending losartan therapy for Raynaud's phenomenon. Fluoxetine, a selective serotonin reuptake inhibitor, has also been shown in one study to improve the symptoms of Raynaud's phenomenon.[140] It is hypothesized to exert its effect by depleting platelet serotonin, rendering the platelet unable to release a significant amount of the vasoconstrictive serotonin during activation and aggregation.

The application of nitroglycerin (NTG) ointment to the hands of Raynaud's patients has been tried since the mid-1940s. High doses of NTG ointment (3.5 inches) three times a day applied to the hands for 6 weeks resulted in fewer and less severe attacks.[141] Transdermal nitroglycerin patches also provide some benefit, although headaches may be a limiting factor.[142] The potential for tolerance developing to the nitrates for this indication has not been studied. Because the data supporting nitrate use in the management of Raynaud's phenomenon are sparse, these agents should be discontinued after 2 to 3 weeks if no benefit is observed.[143]

Other vasodilators are not available in the United States but are used in Europe, often in combination with a calcium channel blocker, for the treatment of Raynaud's phenomenon. These include naftidrofuryl and ketanserin, serotonin receptor antagonists; inositol nicotinate, a direct vasodilator; and thymoxamine, an α_1-adrenergic antagonist.[144–149]

While currently not recommended for use in Raynaud's phenomenon, prostaglandins, most specifically the PGI2 analog iloprost, have shown promising results in studies[150] and were as efficacious as nifedipine in one study.[151] Iloprost requires intravenous administration and is not available in the United States. Intravenous epoprostenol is available, and while there are no data to support its use in acute Raynaud's phenomenon crises with severe digit ischemia, it has been used in this emergent setting.[114] Oral prostaglandin formulations such as misoprostol, iloprost, cicaprost, and beraprost have all failed to improve the symptoms associated with Raynaud's phenomenon.[152–154]

In the United States, there is no available medication other than calcium channel blockers with proven efficacy in Raynaud's phenomenon. All patients with Raynaud's phenomenon should be counseled regarding cold avoidance and other protective measures. A calcium channel blocker, nifedipine if tolerated, should be initiated if conservative measures are ineffective and titrated to the highest tolerated dose and symptom resolution. Combination therapies have not been investigated, but another agent, such as an α_1-adrenergic antagonist, may be considered in addition to the calcium channel blocker if symptom resolution is not satisfactory and side effects permit.

NOCTURNAL LEG MUSCLE CRAMPS

Nocturnal leg muscle cramps are idiopathic, involuntary contractions occurring at rest that cause a visible and palpable knot in the affected muscle. This type of muscle cramp usually afflicts middle-aged to elderly persons and is a distressing and painful condition. Its cause is unknown. The two primary hypotheses that attempt to explain the pathophysiology propose neurologic impairments. One involves a central nervous system impairment of γ-aminobutyric acid (GABA)[155] and the other, an impaired peripheral response to muscle lengthening.[156] While the incidence of nocturnal cramps is unknown, some data indicate it is very common. In a survey of veterans (95% men averaging 60 years of age), 56% complained of leg cramps, with 12% having cramping nearly every night;[157] 36% of these veterans were also attempting some type of drug treatment for their symptoms. A survey of a general population revealed that the prevalence of nocturnal leg cramps was 37% in people >50 years of age, and increased to 54% in people >80 years of age. The prevalence in men and women is equal.[158] Nocturnal leg cramps are associated with lower extremity atherosclerosis, coronary artery disease, and peripheral neurologic deficits.[158,159]

Clinical Presentation

16. E.A., a 62-year-old woman, complains of cramps in her left calf that began last night around 10 PM. The cramping occurred several times throughout the night and has resolved slowly since she arose this morning. These nighttime cramping episodes occur frequently, are very painful, and cause her calf muscle to become "knotted." She denies any trauma, fever, or chills, has no other medical problems, and takes no medications. The pain is not associated with walking. The physical examination is unremarkable and her vital signs are stable. An extended chemistry panel and thyroid function tests are within normal limits. E.A. works at an elementary school and walks up and down stairs throughout the day. Her physician associates the pain with nocturnal leg cramps. What characteristics differentiate E.A.'s nocturnal leg cramps from other pain syndromes?

Benign nocturnal leg cramps usually occur in the early hours of sleeping, are asymmetric, and are not exclusive to but primarily affect the calf muscle and small muscles of the foot. These cramps are not associated with exercise, specific electrolyte or laboratory abnormalities, or medication use. The nocturnal cramp occurs with the further contraction of a muscle already in its most shortened position. For example, sleeping in the supine position may place the calf and ventral foot muscles in their most shortened and vulnerable position, predisposing these muscles to contraction.[160]

For diagnosis and treatment, true muscle cramps first should be distinguished from other causes of muscle cramping, including drug-induced cramps (Table 15-8). The onset of cramps at rest is characteristic of ordinary leg cramps and is the primary symptom used for diagnosis. Clinical signs of sodium depletion, hyper- and hypothyroidism, tetany, and lower motor neuron disease should be evaluated. Laboratory measurements such as standard electrolytes and thyroid function tests can help rule out some of these other conditions.

Treatment

Therapeutic Objectives and Nonpharmacologic Interventions

17. What are the therapeutic objectives in treating E.A.? What nonpharmacologic recommendations can be made?

The primary treatment goal is prevention of this uncomfortable condition. Sufferers of leg cramps are commonly ad-

Table 15-8 Other Causes of Muscle Cramps[160,165]

Drug-Induced Cramps	Biochemical Causes	Other
Alcohol	Hyponatremia	Tetany
Antipsychotics (dystonia)	Dehydration	Contractures
β-agonists (e.g., albuterol, terbutaline, salbutamol)	Calcium deficiency	Lower motor neuron disease
	Magnesium deficiency	
	Hemodialysis	Peripheral vascular disease
Cimetidine		
Clofibrate		
Diuretics		
Lithium		
Narcotic analgesics		
Nicotinic acid		
Nifedipine		
Penicillamine		

vised to stretch out the afflicted muscle or perform dorsiflexion of the feet throughout the day and before bedtime, but this therapeutic modality has never been studied. Patients are also warned to avoid plantar flexion while sleeping by hanging the feet over the edge of the bed when sleeping on the stomach. Once a cramp occurs, the goal is to relieve the cramp as quickly as possible. Acute therapy consists of dorsiflexion (grasping the toes and pulling them upward in the opposite direction of the cramp). This can be accomplished with the hands, by walking, or by leaning toward a wall while standing 2 feet away from it, maintaining the feet flat on the floor.[160]

Quinine

18. After evaluating E.A., her physician prescribes quinine sulfate 260 mg (1 tablet) at bedtime for 2 weeks to see if E.A. achieves relief of further cramping. Has quinine been shown to be effective in preventing nocturnal leg cramps?

Before initiating quinine, prophylactic stretching and alteration of sleeping position should be initiated and evaluated. If these measures do not result in relief, therapy with quinine can be considered. Quinine is the most frequently prescribed medication for nocturnal leg cramps and was once a nonprescription product. In 1995, the FDA stated that quinine was not considered safe and effective for nocturnal leg cramps[161] and discontinued its over-the-counter status. Physicians may still prescribe quinine for the treatment of nocturnal leg cramps because it is commercially available and indicated for the treatment of malaria.

Quinine has been used to treat nocturnal leg cramps since the 1940s, when four patients suffering from leg cramps experienced marked improvement in symptoms after being treated with quinine.[162] When given placebo, their symptoms apparently worsened. Quinine may exert a beneficial effect by increasing the refractory period of skeletal muscle and by decreasing the excitability of the motor endplate. Despite its frequent use, there is significant controversy over its benefit. Only a few small controlled trials have been done, with mixed conclusions. A meta-analysis was published in 1998 that included both published and unpublished data addressing the efficacy of quinine in the treatment of leg cramps.[163] Pooled data from 659 patients indicated that quinine, at 200 to 325 mg/day, reduces the severity and average number of cramps experienced in a 4-week period from 17.1 to 13.5. Thus, the efficacy of quinine is proven; however, the magnitude of benefit is rather small, and the risks associated with quinine therapy for a benign condition must also be considered.

Precautions With Quinine

19. What side effect information should both the physician and E.A. know about prior to initiation of quinine therapy? How long should therapy be continued?

If quinine therapy is successful, E.A. should see a decrease in the severity and frequency of her cramping attacks. Quinine is available in the United States only as the sulfate salt in a number of generic doses and dosage forms. A 200- to 300-mg evening dose is commonly recommended, with an additional early-evening dose taken only if needed.

Cinchonism, a syndrome that includes nausea, vomiting, blurred vision, tinnitus, and deafness, is a dose-related side effect of quinine.[160] Tinnitus alone occurs in up to 3% of patients.[163] With overdose, central nervous system manifestations such as headache, confusion, and delirium can occur. Self-limiting rashes that resolve with drug discontinuation have been described.[160] The unpredictable and life-threatening side effect of thrombocytopenia was the impetus for the FDA to ban the over-the-counter status of this preparation. Thrombocytopenia has been estimated to occur in up to 1 in 1,000 patients taking quinine.[161] Since quinine is the optical isomer of quinidine, cross-reactivity of thrombocytopenia may occur between these agents. Care should also be taken with the use of quinine because its clearance is decreased in the elderly,[164] and several drugs decrease its clearance, such as cimetidine, verapamil, amiodarone, and alkalinizing agents.[165] Each of these could increase the risk of quinine dose-related side effects, specifically the central nervous system manifestations. Quinine can also produce toxic levels of digoxin, phenobarbital, and carbamazepine[165] and is contraindicated in patients with G6PD deficiency.

E.A. should be instructed to take the dose of quinine with food to minimize GI irritation. If a response is not seen within 2 weeks, it should be discontinued in light of the potentially serious side effects.[160] E.A. should be instructed to keep a diary documenting the frequency of the cramping episodes so that its efficacy can be objectively assessed.

Other Therapies

20. Are there other treatment options for E.A.?

Electrolyte replacement (e.g., sodium, potassium, calcium, magnesium) may be indicated if specific deficiencies are noted or if the onset of cramping is associated with a recent initiation or dosage increase of diuretic therapy. Prophylactic use of other pharmacologic agents has been attempted, but their use is mostly anecdotal. Diphenhydramine, riboflavin, carbamazepine, methocarbamol, and phenytoin have been used empirically,[160] but there are no data to support their use in nocturnal leg cramps. Vitamin E has been recommended, but one controlled study with 800 IU/day of vitamin E showed no benefit.[166] Verapamil has been shown in an open-label trial of eight elderly patients to relieve quinine-resistant cramps. A dose of 120 mg of verapamil at bedtime was used, and relief was seen after 6 days of treatment.[167] Similar results were reported from a similar small study using diltiazem.[168] A small study found benefit associated with vitamin B complex administration for nocturnal leg cramps, but no quantification of a decrease in the number of cramps was provided.[169] Two small crossover studies suggested that chronic magnesium administration is not effective for the treatment of nocturnal leg cramps.[170,171]

While nocturnal leg cramps are relatively benign, they do cause considerable discomfort. Nonpharmacologic measures should be maximized before drug therapy is contemplated. If drug therapy is warranted, quinine is the only agent with proven benefit, but the potential for side effects, especially in the elderly population, is very real. Careful patient selection, patient education, and vigilant monitoring for side effects should all be used to minimize the occurrence and progression of adverse effects from quinine.

REFERENCES

1. Criqui M et al. The prevalence of peripheral arterial disease in a defined population. Circulation 1985; 71:210.
2. Caspary L. Epidemiology of vascular disease. Dis Manage Health Outcomes 1997;2:9.
3. Boccalon H. Intermittent claudication in older patients. Drugs Aging 1999;14:247.
4. Kannel WB, McGee DL. Diabetes and cardiovascular disease: The Framingham Study. JAMA 1979; 241:2035.
5. Hiatt W. Medical treatment of peripheral arterial disease and claudication. N Engl J Med 2001; 334:1608.
6. MacGregor AS et al. Role of systolic blood pressure and plasma triglycerides in diabetic peripheral arterial disease. Diabetes Care 1999;22:453.
7. Kannel W, Shurtleff D. The Framingham Study: cigarettes and the development of intermittent claudication. Geriatrics 1973;28:61.
8. Price JF et al. Relationship between smoking and cardiovascular risk factors in the development of peripheral arterial disease and coronary artery disease. Eur Heart J 1999;20:344.
9. McDaniel CD, Cronenwett JL. Basic data related to the natural history of intermittent claudication. Ann Vasc Surg 1989;3:273.
10. Hertzer N. The natural history of peripheral vascular disease. Circulation 1991;83:I12.
11. Brevetti G et al. Intermittent claudication and risk of cardiovascular events. J Vasc Dis 1998; 49:843.
12. Rockson SG, Cooke JP. Peripheral arterial insufficiency: mechanisms, natural history, and therapeutic options. Adv Intern Med 1998;43:253.
13. Krajewski LP, Olin JW. Atherosclerosis of the aorta and lower-extremity arteries. In: Young JS et al, eds. Peripheral Vascular Diseases. St. Louis: Mosby, 1996:208.
14. Clement DL, Verhaeghe R. Atherosclerosis and other occlusive arterial diseases. In: Clement DL, Sherhert JF, eds. Vascular Diseases in the limbs. St. Louis: Mosby, 1993:71.
15. Weed RI. The importance of erythrocyte deformability. Am J Med 1970;49:147.
16. Braasch D. Red cell deformability and capillary blood flow. Physiol Rev 1971;51:679.
17. Kaplan NM. The deadly quartet. Upper body obesity, glucose intolerence, hypertriglyceridemia, and hypertension. Arch Intern Med 1989;149:1514.
18. Sowers JR. Insulin resistance, hyperinsulinemia, dyslipidemia, hypertension, and accelerated atherosclerosis. Clin Pharmacol 1992;32:529.
19. Housley E. Treating claudication with five words. Br Med J 1988;296:1483.
20. Jonason T, Bergstrom R. Cessation of smoking in patients with intermittent claudication: effects on the risk of peripheral vascular complications, myocardial infarction, and mortality. Acta Med Scand 1987;221:253.
21. Faulkner KW et al. The effect of cessation of smoking on the accumulative survival rates of patients with symptomatic peripheral vascular disease. Med J Aust 1983;1:217.
22. Wiseman S et al. Influence of smoking and plasma factors on patency of femoralpopliteal vein grafts. Br Med J 1989;299:643.
23. Quick CRG, Cotton LT. Measured effect of stopping smoking on intermittent claudication. Br J Surg 1982;69:524.

24. Hughson WG et al. Intermittent claudication: factors determining outcome. Br Med J 1978;1:1377.

25. Powell JT. Vascular damage from smoking: disease mechanisms at the arterial wall. Vasc Med 1998; 3:21.

26. Radack K, Wyderski RJ. Conservative management of intermittent claudication of the lower limbs. Ann Intern Med 1990;113:135.

27. Gardner AW, Poehlman ET. Exercise rehabilitation programs for the treatment of claudication pain. JAMA 1995;274:975.

28. Stewart K et al. Exercise training for claudication. N Engl J Med 2002;347:1941.

29. Gray BH, Sullivan TM. Vascular claudication: how to individualize treatment. Cleve Clin J Med 1997;64:492.

30. Ernst E, Matrai A. Intermittent claudication, exercise, and blood rheology. Circulation 1987;76:1110.

31. Summary of the third report of the National Cholesterol Education Program (NCEP) Expert Panel on Detection, Evaluation, and Treatment of High Blood Cholesterol in Adults (Adult Treatment Panel III). JAMA 2001;285:2486.

32. Brown G et al. Regression of coronary artery disease as a result of intensive lipid lowering therapy in men with high levels of lipoprotein b. N Engl J Med 1990;323:1289.

33. Blankenhorn DH et al. Beneficial effects of combined colestipol-niacin therapy on coronary atherosclerosis and coronary venous bypass grafts. JAMA 1987;257:3233 [published erratum appears in JAMA 1988 May 13;259(18):2698].

34. Blankenhorn DH et al. Coronary angiographic changes with lovastatin therapy. The Monitored Atherosclerosis Regression Study (MARS). The MARS Research Group. Ann Intern Med 1993; 119:969.

35. Pedersen TJ et al. Effect of simvastatin on ischemic signs and symptoms in the Scandinavian Simvastatin Survival Study (4S). Am J Cardiol 1998; 81:333.

36. MRC/BHF heart protection study of cholesterol lowering in 20,536 individuals: a randomised placebo-controlled trial. Lancet 2002;360:7.

37. Leng G et al. Lipid-lowering for lower limb atherosclerosis. Cochrane Database Syst Rev 2000; 2:CD000123.

38. Hiatt WR et al. Effect of beta-adrenergic blockers on the peripheral circulation in patients with peripheral vascular disease. Circulation 1985; 72:1226.

39. Roberts DH et al. Placebo-controlled comparison of captopril, atenolol, labetalol, and pindolol in hypertension complicated by intermittent claudication. Lancet 1987;2:650.

40. Houben H et al. Effect of low-dose epinephrine infusion on hemodynamics after selective and nonselective beta-blockade in hypertension. Clin Pharmacol Ther 1982;31:685.

41. Radack K, Deck C. Beta-adrenergic blocker therapy does not worsen intermittent claudication in subjects with peripheral arterial disease. A meta-analysis of randomized controlled trials. Arch Intern Med 1991;151:1769.

42. Investigators THOPES. Effects of an angiotensin converting enzyme inhibitor, ramipril, on cardiovascular events in high-risk patients. N Engl J Med 2000;342:145.

43. Chobanian A et al. The Seventh Report of the Joint National Committee on Prevention, Detection, Evaluation, and Treatment of High Blood Pressure. JAMA 2003;289: 2560.

44. Lewis EJ et al. The effect of angiotensin-converting-enzyme inhibition on diabetic nephropathy. N Engl J Med 1993;329:456.

45. Ismail N et al. Renal disease and hypertension in non-insulin-dependent diabetes mellitus. Kidney Int 1999;55:1.

46. Rodgers P. Combination drug therapy in hypertension: a rational approach for the pharmacist. J Am Pharm Assoc 1998;38:469.

47. Intensive blood-glucose control with sulphonylureas or insulin compared to conventional treatment and risk of complications in patients with type 2 diabetes (UKPDS 33). Lancet 1998;352:837.

48. Effect of intensive blood-glucose control with metformin on complications in overweight patients with type 2 diabetes (UKPDS 34). Lancet 1998; 352:854.

49. Goede P et al. Multifactorial intervention and cardiovascular disease in patients with type 2 diabetes. N Engl J Med 2003;348:383.

50. ADA. Standards of medical care for patients with diabetes mellitus. Diabetes Care 2003;26 (Suppl 1):S33.

51. Cameron HA et al. Drug treatment of intermittent claudication: a critical analysis of the methods and findings of published clinical trials, 1965–1985. Br J Clin Pharmacol 1988;26:569.

52. Bagger JP et al. Effect of verapamil in intermittent claudication. A randomized, double-blind, placebo controlled, cross-over study after individual dose-response assessment. Circulation 1997;95:411.

53. Samlaska C, Winfield E. Pentoxifylline. J Am Acad Dermatol 1994;30:603.

54. Jackson MR, Clagett GP. Antithrombotic therapy in peripheral arterial occlusive disease. Chest 1998; 114:666S.

55. Frampton JE, Brogden RN. Pentoxifylline. A review of its therapeutic efficacy in the management of peripheral vascular and cerebrovascular disorders. Drugs Aging 1995;7:480.

56. Ward A, Clissold SP. Pentoxifylline: a review of its pharmacokinetic and pharmacodynamic properties, and its therapeutic efficacy. Drugs 1987;34:50.

57. Patrono C et al. Platelet active drugs: the relationships among dose, effectiveness and side effects. Chest 1998;114:470S.

58. Sharis P et al. The antiplatelet effects of ticlopidine and clopidogrel. Ann Intern Med 1998;129:394.

59. Sorkin E, Markham A. Cilostazol. Drugs Aging 1999;14:63.

60. Collaborative overview of randomized trials of antiplatelet therapy: I. Prevention of death, myocardial infarction, and stroke by prolonged antiplatelet therapy in various categories of patients. Antiplatelet Trialists' Collaboration. Br Med J 1994;308:81.

61. Hess H et al. Drug-induced inhibition of platelet function delays progression of peripheral occlusive arterial disease. Lancet 1985;1:415.

62. Goldhaber S et al. Low-dose aspirin and subsequent peripheral arterial surgery in the physician's health study. Lancet 1992;340:143.

63. Arcan J, Panak E. Ticlopidine in the treatment of peripheral occlusive arterial disease. Sem Thromb Hemost 1989;15:167.

64. Balsano F et al. Ticlopidine in the treatment of intermittent claudication: a 21 month double-blind trial. J Lab Clin Med 1989;114:84.

65. Janzon L et al. Prevention of myocardial infarction and stroke in patients with intermittent claudication: effects of ticlopidine. Results from STIMS, the Swedish ticlopidine multicenter study. J Intern Med 1990;227:301.

66. Bergqvist D et al. Reduction of requirement for leg vascular surgery during long-term treatment of claudication patients with ticlopidine: results from the Swedish Ticlopidine Multicenter Study (STIMS). Eur J Vasc Endovasc Surg 1995;10:69.

67. Boissel J et al. Is it possible to reduce the risk of cardiovascualr events in subjects suffering from intermittent claudication of the lower limbs? Thromb Haemost 1989;62:681.

68. Love B et al. Adverse haematological effects of ticlopidine. Drug Safety 1998;19:89.

69. Chen D et al. Thrombotic thrombocytopenic purpura associated with ticlopidine use: a report of 3 cases and review of the literature. Arch Intern Med 1999;159:311.

70. A randomised, blinded, trial of clopidofrel versus aspirin in patients at risk of ischaemic events (CAPRIE). Lancet 1996;348:1329.

71. Beebe H et al. A new pharmacologic treatment for intermittent claudication: results of a randomized multicenter trial. Arch Intern Med 1999;159:2041.

72. Money S et al. Effect of cilostazol on walking distances in patients with intermittent claudication caused by peripheral vascular disease. J Vasc Surg 1998;27:267.

73. Dawson D et al. Cilostazol has beneficial effects in treatment of intermittent claudication. Circulation 1998;98:678

74. Dawson DL et al. A comparison of cilostazol and pentoxifylline for treating intermittent claudication. Am J Med 2000;109:523.

75. Dawson D et al. The effect of withdrawal of drugs treating intermittant claudication. Am J Surg 1999;178:141.

76. Dawson D. Cilostazol: a viewpoint. Drugs Aging 1999;41:72.

77. Cruickshank J. Phosphodiesterase III inhibitors: long-term risks and short-term benefits. Cardiovasc Drugs Ther 1993;7:655.

78. Meade T, Brennan P. Determination of who may derive most benefit from aspirin in primary prevention: subgroup results from a randomised controlled trial. Br Med J 2000;321:13.

79. CAST: randomised placebo-controlled trial of early aspirin use in 20,000 patients with acute ischemic stroke. Lancet 1997;349:1641.

80. Randomised trial of intravenous streptokinase, oral aspirin, both, or neither among 17,187 cases of suspected acute myocardial infarction: ISIS-2. Lancet 1988;2:349.

81. Hansson L et al. Effects of intensive blood-pressure lowering and low-dose aspirin in patients with hypertension: principle results of the Hypertension Optimal Treatment (HOT) randomised trial. Lancet 1998;351:1755.

82. Juul-Moller S et al. Double-blind trial of aspirin in primary prevention of myocardial infarction in patients with stable chronic angina pectoris. The Swedish Angina Pectoris Aspirin Trial (SAPAT) Group. Lancet 1992;340:1421.

83. The Dutch TIA trial study group. A comparison of two doses of aspirin (30mg vs. 283mg a day) in patients after a transient ischemic attack or minor ischemic stroke. N Engl J Med 1992;325:1261.

84. Farrell B et al. The United Kingdom transient ischemic attack (UK-TIA) aspirin trial: final results. J Neurol Neurosurg Psychiatry 1991;54:1044.

85. Pittler M, Ernst E. Ginkgo biloba extract for the treatment of intermittant claudication. a meta-analysis of randomized trials. Am J Med 2000; 108:276.

86. Campbell W, Halushka P. Lipid-derived autocoids, In: J Hardman, L Limbird, P Molinoff, R Ruddon, eds. Goodman and Gillman's the Pharmacological Basis of Therapeutics. New York: McGraw-Hill, 1996:601.

87. Kincheloe L. Gynecological and obstetric concerns regarding herbal medicinal use, In: L Miller, W Murray, eds. Herbal Medicines: A Clinician's Guide. New York: Pharmaceutical Product Press, 1998:279.

88. Newall C et al. Herbal Medicine: A Guide for Health Care Professionals. London: The Pharmaceutical Press, 1996:138.

89. Haeger K. Long-time treatment of intermittent claudication with vitamin E. Am J Clin Nutr 1974;27:1179.

90. Williams H et al. Alpha tocopherol in the treatment of intermittent claudication. Surg Gynecol Obstet 1971;132:662.

91. Stephens N et al. Randomised controlled trial of vitamin E in patients with coronary artery disease: Cambridge Heart Antioxidant Study (CHAOS). Lancet 1996;347:781.

92. Dietary supplementation with n-3 polyunsaturated fatty acids and vitamin E after myocardial infarction: results of the GISSI Prevenzione Trial. Lancet 1999;354:447.

93. Vitamin E supplementation and cardiovascular events in high-risk patients. N Engl J Med 2000;342:154.

94. Hiatt W et al. Skeletal muscle carnitine metabolism in patients with unilateral peripheral arterial disease. J Appl Physiol 1992;73:346.

95. Brevetti G, Angelini C et al. Muscle carnitine deficiency in patients with severe peripheral vascular disease. Circulation 1991;84:1490.

96. Brevetti G et al. Propionyl-L-carnitine in intermittent claudication: double-blind, placebo controlled, dose titration, multicenter study. J Am Coll Cardiol 1995;26:1441.

97. Brevetti G et al. European multicenter study on propionyl-L-carnitine in intermittent claudication. J Am Coll Cardiol 1999;34:1618.
98. Brevetti G et al. Effect of propionyl-L-carnitine on quality of life in intermittent claudication. Am J Cardiol 1997;79:777.
99. Brevetti G et al. Superiority of L-propionylcarnitine vs L-carnitine in improving walking capacity in patients with peripheral vascular disease: an acute, intravenous, double-blind, cross-over study. Eur Heart J 1992;13:251.
100. Coffman J. Intermittent claudication: be conservative. N Engl J Med 1991;325:577.
101. Pentecost M et al. Guidelines for peripheral percutaneous transluminal angioplasty of the abdominal aorta and lower extremity vessels: a statement for health professionals from a special writing group of the Councils on Cardiovascular Radiology, Arteriosclerosis, Cardiothoracic and Vascular Surgery, Clinical Cardiology, and Epidemiology and Prevention, the American Heart Association. Circulation 1994;89:511.
102. Bosch J, Hunink M. Meta-analysis of the results of percutaneous transluminal angioplasty and stent placement for aortoiliac occlusive disease. Radiology 1997;204:87.
103. Tunis S et al. The use of angioplasty, bypass surgery and amputation in the management of peripheral vascular disease. N Engl J Med 1991;325:556.
104. Thrombolysis in the management of lower limb peripheral arterial occlusion-a consensus document. Am J Cardiol 1998;81:207.
105. Nilsson L et al. Surgical treatment versus thrombolysis in acute arterial occlusion: a randomised controlled study. Eur J Vasc Surg 1992;6:189.
106. Ouriel K et al. A comparison of thrombolytic therapy with operative revascularization in the initial treatment of acute peripheral arterial ischemia. J Vasc Surg 1994;19:1021.
107. Raynaud M. On local asphyxia and symmetrical gangrene of the extremities, In: T Barlow,eds. Selected Monographs, 121. London: The Sydenham Society, 1888:1.
108. LeRoy E, Medsger T. Raynaud's phenomenon: a proposal for classification. Clin Exp Rheumatol 1992;10:485.
109. Shepard F, Shepard J. Primary Raynaud's disease, In: Vascular Diseases of the Limbs: Mechanisms and Principles of Treatment. St. Louis: Mosby Yearbook, 1993: 153.
110. Gasser P et al. Evaluation of reflex cold provocation by laser Doppler flowmetry in clinically healthy subjects with a history of cold hands. Angiology 1992;43:389.
111. Nielson S. Raynaud's phenomena and finger systolic blood pressure during cooling. Scand J Clin Lab Invest 1978;38:765.
112. Wigley F, Flavahan N. Raynaud's phenomenon. Rheum Dis Clin North Am 1996;22:765.
113. Maricq H et al. Geographic variation in the prevalence of Raynaud's phenomenon: a five region comparison. J Rheumatol 1997;24:879.
114. Wigley F. Raynaud's Phenomenon. N Engl J Med 2002;347:1001.
115. Belch J. Raynaud's phenomenon. Cardiovasc Res 1997;33:25.
116. Franssen C et al. The influence of different beta-blocking drugs on the peripheral circulation in Raynaud's phenomenon and in hypertension. J Clin Pharmacol 1992;32:652.
117. Goodfield M et al. The acute effects of cigarette smoking on cutaneous blood flow in smoking and nonsmoking subjects with and without Raynaud's phenomenon. Br J Rheumatol 1990;29:89.
118. Palesch Y et al. Association between cigarette and alcohol consumption and Raynaud's phenomenon. J Clin Epidemiol 1999;52:321.
119. Freedman R et al. Blockade of vasospastic attacks by alpha 2-adrenergic but not alpha1-adrenergic antagonists in idiopathic Raynaud's disease. Circulation 1995;92:1448.
120. Coffman J, Cohen R. Serotonergic vasoconstriction in human fingers during reflex sympathetic response to cooling. Am J Physiol 1988;254:H889.

121. Smith C, McKendry R. Controlled trial of nifedipine in the treatment of Raynaud's phenomenon. Lancet 1982;2:1299.
122. Rodeheffer R et al. Controlled double-blind trial of nifedipine in the treatment of Raynaud's phenomenon. N Engl J Med 1983;308:880.
123. Landry G et al. Current management of Raynaud's syndrome. Adv Surg 1996;30:333.
124. Finch M et al. A double-blind cross-over study of nifedipine retard in patients with Raynaud's phenomenon. Clin Rheumatol 1988;7:359.
125. Waller D et al. Clinical and rheological effects of nifedipine in Raynaud's phenomenon. Br J Clin Rheumatol 1986;22:449.
126. Comparison of sustained-release nifedipine and temperature biofeedback for treatment of primary Raynaud phenomenon. Results from a randomized clinical trial with 1-year follow-up. Arch Intern Med 2000;160:1101.
127. Leppert J et al. The effect of isradipine, a new calcium-channel antagonist, in patients with primary Raynaud's phenomenon: a single-blind dose-response study. Cardiovasc Drugs Ther 1989;3:397.
128. La Civita L et al. Amlodipine in the treatment of Raynaud's phenomenon. Br J Rheumatol 1993;32:524.
129. Kallenberg C et al. Once daily felodipine in patients with primary Raynaud's phenomenon. Eur J Clin Pharmacol 1991;40:313.
130. Schmidt J et al. The clinical effect of felodipine and nifedipine in Raynaud's phenomenon. Eur J Clin Pharmacol 1989;37:191.
131. Rhedda A et al. A double-blind placebo controlled crossover randomized trial of diltiazem in Raynaud's syndrome. J Rheumatol 1985;12:724.
132. Kahan A et al. A randomised double-blind trial of diltiazem in the treatment of Raynaud's phenomenon. Ann Rheum Dis 1985;44:30.
133. Matoba T, Chiba M. Effects of diltiazem on occupational Raynaud's syndrome. Angiology 1985;36:850.
134. Kinney E. The treatment of severe Raynaud's phenomenon with verapamil. J Clin Pharmacol 1982;22:74.
135. Wollersheim H, Thien T. Dose-response study of prazosin in Raynaud's phenomenon: clinical effectiveness versus side effects. J Clin Pharmacol 1988;28:1089.
136. Wollersheim H et al. Double-blind, placebo controlled study of prazosin in Raynaud's phenomenon. Clin Pharmacol Ther 1986;40:219.
137. Paterna S et al. Raynaud's phenomenon: effects of terazosin. Minerva Cardioangiol 1997;45:215.
138. Challenor V. Angiotensin converting enzyme inhibitors in Raynaud's phenomenon. Drugs 1994;48:864.
139. Dziadzio M et al. Losartan therapy for Raynaud's phenomenon and scleroderma: clinical and biochemical findings in a fifteen-week randomized, parallel-group, controlled trial. Arthritis Rheum 1999;42:2646.
140. Coleiro B et al. Treatment of Raynaud's phenomenon with the selective serotonin reuptake inhibitor fluoxetine. Rheumatology 2001;40:1038.
141. Franks A. Topical glyceryl trinitrate as adjunctive treatment in Raynaud's disease. Lancet 1982;1:76.
142. Teh L et al. Sustained-release transdermal glyceryl trinitrate patches as a treatment for primary and secondary Raynaud's phenomenon. Br J Rheumatol 1995;34:636.
143. Belch J, Ho M. Pharmacotherapy of Raynaud's phenomenon. Drugs 1996;52:682.
144. Davinroy M, Mosnier M. Double-blind clinical evaluation of naftidrofuryl in Raynaud's phenomenon. Sem Hop 1993;69:12.
145. Nilsen K. Effects of naftidrifuryl on microcirculatory cold sensitivity in Raynaud's phenomenon. Br Med J 1979;1:20.
146. Coffman J et al. International study of ketanserin in Raynaud's phenomenon. Am J Med 1989;87:264.
147. Murphy R. The effect of inositol nicotinate in patients with Raynaud's phenomenon. Clin Trials J 1985;22:521.

148. Sunderland J et al. A double blind randomised placebo controlled trial of hexopal in primary Raynaud's disease. Clin Rheumatol 1988;7:46.
149. Grigg M et al. The efficacy of thymoxamine in primary Raynaud's phenomenon. Eur J Vasc Surg 1989;3:309.
150. Wigley F et al. Intravenous iloprost infusion in patients with Raynaud's phenomenon secondary to systemic sclerosis. A multicenter, placebo-controlled, double-blind study. Ann Intern Med 1994;120:199.
151. Rademaker M et al. Comparison of intravenous infusion of iloprost and oral nifedipine in treatment of Raynaud's phenomenon in patients with systemic sclerosis: a double-blind randomised study. Br Med J 1989;298:561.
152. Wigley F et al. Oral iloprost treatment in patients with Raynaud's phenomenon secondary to systemic sclerosis: a multicenter, placebo-controlled, double-blind study. Arthritis and Rheum 1998;41:670.
153. Lau C et al. A randomised, double-blind study of cicaprost, an oral prostacyclin analogue, in the treatment of Raynaud's phenomenon secondary to systemic sclerosis. Clin Exp Rheumatol 1993;11:35.
154. Vayssairat M. Controlled multicenter double blind trial of an oral analog of prostacyclin in the treatment of primary Raynaud's phenomenon: French microcirculation society multicentre group for the study of vascular acrosyndromes. J Rheumatol 1996;23:1917.
155. Obi T et al. Muscle cramps as the result of impaired GABA function-an electrophysiological and pharmacological observation. Muscle Nerve 1993;16:1228.
156. Bertolasi L et al. The influence of muscle lengthening on cramps. Ann Neurol 1993;33:176.
157. Oboler S et al. Leg symptoms in outpatient veterans. West J Med 1991;155:256.
158. Naylor J, Young J. A general population survey of rest cramps. Age Ageing 1994;23:418.
159. Haskell S, Fiebach N. Clinical epidemiology of nocturnal leg cramps in male veterans. Am J Med Sci 1997;313:210.
160. Leclerc K, Landry F. Benign nocturnal leg cramps. Current controversies over use of quinine. Postgrad Med 1996;99:177.
161. Drug products for the treatment and/or prevention of nocturnal leg cramps for over-the-counter human use. Fed Reg 1994;59:43234.
162. Moss H, Herrmann L. Use of quinine for relief of "night cramps" in the extremities. JAMA 1940;115:1358.
163. Man-So-Hing M et al. Quinine for nocturnal leg cramps: a meta-analysis including unpublished data. J Gen Intern Med 1998;13:600.
164. Krishna S, White N. Pharmacokinetics of quinine, chloroquine, and amodiaquine: clinical implications. Clin Pharmacokinet 1996;30:263.
165. Brasic J. Should people with nocturnal leg cramps drink tonic water and bitter lemon? Psychol Report 1999;84:355.
166. Connolly P et al. Treatment of nocturnal leg cramps: a crossover trial of quinine vs vitamin E. Arch Intern Med 1992;152:1877.
167. Baltodano N et al. Verapamil vs quinine in recumbent nocturnal leg cramps in the elderly. Arch Intern Med 1988;148:1969.
168. Voon W, Sheu S. Diltiazem for nocturnal leg cramps. Age Ageing 2001;30:91.
169. Chan P et al. Randomized, double-blind, placebo-controlled study of the safety and efficacy of vitamin B complex in the treatment of nocturnal leg cramps in elderly patients with hypertension. J Clin Pharmacol 1998;38:1151.
170. Frusso R et al. Magnesium for the treatment of nocturnal leg cramps: a crossover randomized trial. J Fam Pract 1999;48:868.
171. Roffe C et al. Randomised, cross-over, placebo controlled trial of magnesium citrate in the treatment of chronic persistent leg cramps. Med Sci Monitor 2002;8:CR326.

CHAPTER 16

Thrombosis

Ann K. Wittkowsky

GENERAL PRINCIPLES

Thrombosis is the process involved in the formation of a fibrin blood clot. Both platelets and a series of coagulant proteins (clotting factors) contribute to clot formation. An *embolus* is a small part of a clot that breaks off and travels to another part of the vascular system. Damage is caused when the embolus becomes trapped in a small vessel, causing occlusion and leading to ischemia or infarction of the surrounding tissue. Normal clot formation maintains the integrity of the vasculature in response to injury, but pathologic clotting can occur in many clinical settings. Abnormal thrombotic events include deep venous thrombosis (DVT) and its primary complication, pulmonary embolism (PE), as well as stroke and other systemic manifestations of embolization of clots that form within the heart. Anticoagulant drug therapy is aimed at preventing pathologic clot formation in patients at risk and at preventing clot extension and/or embolization in patients who have developed thrombosis. The emphasis of this chapter is on arterial and venous thromboembolic disease and the use of heparin and warfarin as anticoagulants. Chapter 17, Ischemic Heart Disease; Chapter 18, Myocardial Infarction; and Chapter 55, Cerebrovascular Disorders, provide more in-depth discussions of thrombolytic agents and antiplatelet therapy.

Etiology of Thromboembolism

Three primary factors influence the formation of pathologic clots and are described in a model referred to as Virchow's triad (Fig. 16-1).[1] First, abnormalities of blood flow that cause venous stasis can result in DVT, which can progress to PE if embolization occurs. Intracardiac stasis also can result in clot formation, and embolization of intracardiac thrombi may lead to stroke or other systemic manifestations. Abnormalities of blood vessel walls, such as those that occur in injury or trauma to the vasculature, are a second source of thrombus formation. The presence of foreign material within the vasculature, including artificial heart valves and central venous catheters, is also thrombogenic and, like vascular injury, represents the presence of an abnormal surface in contact with blood. Finally, hypercoagulability resulting from alterations in the availability or the integrity of blood-clotting components or naturally occurring anticoagulants also represents a significant risk factor for thromboembolic disease.[2]

Clot Formation

The intact endothelial lining of blood vessels normally repels platelets and inhibits clot formation through secretion of numerous inhibitory substances. Damage to this endothelium leads to exposure of circulating blood to subendothelial substances, and this results in a complex series of events, including platelet adhesion, activation, and aggregation, followed by activation of the clotting cascade. These events result in formation of a fibrin clot.[3]

Platelet Adhesion, Activation, and Aggregation

Endothelial damage leads to exposure of blood to subendothelial collagen and phospholipids, resulting in platelet adhesion to the surface. Von Willebrand factor (vWF) serves as the binding ligand for platelet adhesion, via the glycoprotein I (GPI) receptor on the platelet surface. Adhered platelets become activated and release numerous compounds, including adenosine diphosphate (ADP) and thromboxane A_2 (TXA_2), which stimulate platelet aggregation. Fibrinogen serves as the binding ligand for platelet aggregation, via the GPIIb/IIIa receptor on the platelet surface.[4]

Clotting Cascade

Transformation of the relatively unstable platelet plug (i.e., the aggregated platelets) to a stable fibrin clot occurs as a result of an imbalance between other procoagulant and anticoagulant factors. In addition to stimulating the platelet response, endothelial damage results in activation of the clotting cascade (Fig. 16-2). The extrinsic pathway of the clotting cascade is activated by the release of thromboplastin (tissue factor) from endothelial cells. Tissue factor converts factor VII to factor VII_a, which mediates the activation of factor X. The intrinsic pathway of the clotting cascade is activated by exposure of factor XII to subendothelial components exposed during vessel injury. The intrinsic pathway mediates factor X activation via a chain of events initiated by factor XI. The distinction between these pathways is primarily an in vitro phenomenon; in vivo, the two pathways are activated simultaneously.

Once stimulated, both the extrinsic and intrinsic pathways activate the common pathway of the clotting cascade via factor X. Activated forms of factors V and VIII serve independently to accelerate this process. The final steps include conversion of factor II (prothrombin) to factor II_a (thrombin), with eventual formation of a stable fibrin clot.

Naturally occurring inhibitors of clotting factors play a role in localizing fibrin formation to the sites of injury and in

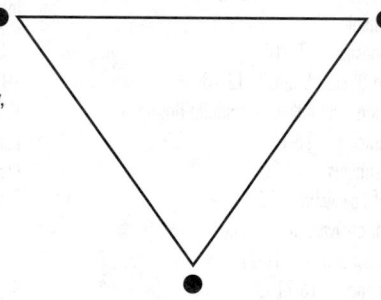

Abnormalities of Blood Flow
  Atrial fibrillation
  Left ventricular dysfunction from:
    ischemic/idiopathic cardiomyopathy,
    congestive heart failure, or
    myocardial infarction
  Bed rest/immobilization/paralysis
  Venous obstruction from
    tumor/obesity/pregnancy

Abnormalities of Surfaces in Contact With Blood
  Vascular injury/trauma
  Heart valve disease
  Heart valve replacement
  Atherosclerosis
  Acute myocardial infarction
  Indwelling catheters
  Previous DVT/PE
  Fractures
  Chemical irritation (potassium, hypertonic solutions,
    chemotherapy)
  Tumor invasion

Abnormalities of Clotting Components
  Protein C deficiency
  Protein S deficiency
  Antithrombin deficiency
  Factor V Leiden
  Prothrombin G20210A mutation
  Antiphospholipid antibody syndrome
    (lupus anticoagulant; anticardiolipin
    antibody)
  Estrogen therapy
  Pregnancy
  Malignancy
  Homocystenemia
  Dysfibrinogenemia
  Polycythemia
  Myloproliferative disorder
  Thrombocytosis

FIGURE 16-1 Risk factors for thromboembolism. DVT, deep venous thrombosis; PE, pulmonary embolism.

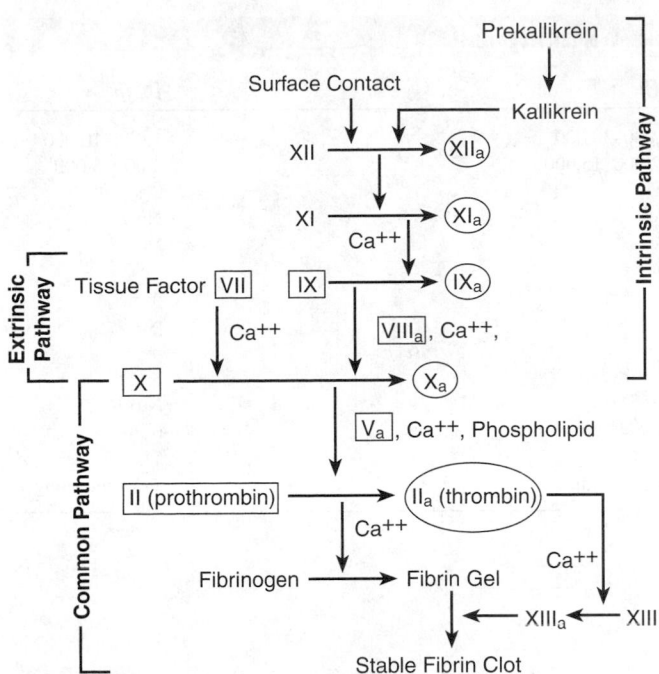

FIGURE 16-2 Simplified clotting cascade. Components in ovals are influenced by heparin; components in boxes are influenced by warfarin.

maintaining the fluidity of circulating blood. Table 16-1 outlines these clotting inhibitors and their primary actions. In addition, the fibrinolytic system is involved in degradation of fibrin clots. The actions of both clotting inhibitors and the fibrinolytic system prevent excessive coagulation. Thus, the process of clot formation is dynamic and involves various factors that can stimulate, inhibit, and dissolve a fibrin clot.

Pathologic Thrombi
Pathologic thrombi sometimes are classified according to location and composition. Arterial thrombi are composed primarily of platelets, although they also contain fibrin and occasional leukocytes. Arterial thrombi generally occur in areas of rapid blood flow (i.e., arteries). Venous thrombi are found primarily in the venous circulation and are composed almost entirely of fibrin and erythrocytes. Venous thrombi have a small platelet head and generally form in response to either venous stasis or vascular injury after surgery or trauma. The

Table 16-1   Inhibitors of Clotting Mechanisms

Inhibitor	Target
Antithrombin	Inhibits factors IIa, IXa, and Xa
Protein S	Cofactor for activation of protein C
Protein C	Inactivates factors Va and VIIIa
Tissue factor pathway inhibitor (TFPI)	Inhibits activity of factor VIIa
Plasminogen	Converted to plasmin via tissue plasminogen activator (t-PA)
Plasmin	Lyses fibrin into fibrin degradation products

areas of stasis prevent dilution of activated coagulation factors by blood flow.

The selection of an antithrombotic agent may be influenced by the type of thrombus to be treated. The anticoagulants heparin, low-molecular-weight heparins, and warfarin are used in the treatment and prevention of both arterial and venous thrombi. Drugs that alter platelet function (e.g., aspirin), alone and in combination with anticoagulants, are used in the prevention of arterial thrombi. Fibrinolytic agents are used for rapid dissolution of thromboemboli, most notably during myocardial infarction (MI).

Pharmacology of Antithrombotic Agents

Heparin
Heparin is a rapid-acting anticoagulant that is administered parenterally. Standard heparin (unfractionated heparin [UFH]) is a heterogeneous mixture of glycosaminoglycans of varying molecular weights obtained from bovine lung or porcine intestinal mucosa (Table 16-2). The action of heparin is facilitated by its binding to the naturally circulating anticoagulant antithrombin (AT), a serine protease also referred to as heparin cofactor. Binding of heparin to AT accelerates the anticoagulant effect of AT. The heparin–AT complex attaches to and irreversibly inactivates factor II_a (thrombin) and factor X_a as well as activated factors IX, XI, and XII (Fig. 16-3).[5] Approximately one third of the molecules present in UFH bind to AT and provide the anticoagulant properties of heparin. The remaining two thirds of the heparin molecules bind to plasma proteins and to endothelial cells, saturable processes that contribute to the dose-dependent pharmacokinetic profile of the drug and limit its bioavailability. In addition to its anticoagulant effects, heparin inhibits platelet function and increases vascular permeability; these properties contribute to the hemorrhagic effects of heparin.

In cases of acute DVT or PE, the clotting cascade has been activated, generating abnormal quantities of thrombin and fibrin. In these situations, thrombin must be inactivated directly, a process that may require relatively large doses of heparin. However, when the clotting cascade is in a normal balance, it is possible to indirectly inactivate thrombin with smaller heparin doses by complexing factor X_a. Because of the amplification effect of the clotting cascade, inactivation of relatively small amounts of factor X_a indirectly prevents the production of large quantities of thrombin. This phenomenon is the basis for low-dose heparin prophylaxis after surgery or in cases of prolonged bed rest or immobilization.

Heparin may be administered intravenously (IV) by continuous infusion, or subcutaneously (SC), although its bioavailability is significantly reduced by SC administration. Intramuscular administration should be avoided because of the potential for hematoma formation.

After IV administration, the anticoagulant effect of heparin is noted immediately. During active thromboembolism, the high concentration of clotting factors present necessitates a higher concentration of heparin to neutralize these clotting factors. This increased dosing requirement may also be related to continuing thrombin formation on the surface of the thrombus. Once endothelialization (localization and incorporation of the clot into the vascular endothelium) of the clot begins and the concentration of clotting factors decreases, dos-

Table 16-2   Comparison of Unfractionated Heparin and Low-Molecular-Weight Heparins[5]

Property	UFH	LMWH
Molecular weight range[a]	3,000–30,000	1,000–10,000
Average molecular weight[a]	12,000–15,000	4,000–5,000
Anti-X_a:anti-II_a activity	1:1	2:1–4:1
aPTT monitoring required	Yes	No
Inactivation by platelet factor 4	Yes	No
Capable of inactivation of platelet-bound factor X_a	No	Yes
Inhibition of platelet function	++++	++
Increases vascular permeability	Yes	No
Protein binding	++++	+
Endothelial cell binding	+++	–
Dose-dependent clearance	Yes	No
Primary route of elimination	1. Saturable binding processes 2. Renal	Renal
Elimination half-life	30–150 min	2–5 times longer

[a]Measured in daltons.
LMWH, low-molecular-weight heparin; UFH, unfractionated heparin.

ing requirements typically decrease. Considerable variability in dosing requirements among patients necessitates routine therapeutic monitoring to maintain an appropriate intensity of anticoagulation with heparin. The primary laboratory test for monitoring therapeutic heparinization is the activated partial thromboplastin time (aPTT) (see Tests Used to Monitor Antithrombotic Therapy).

The plasma half-life of heparin varies from 30 to 150 minutes, but the half-life increases with increasing doses. Heparin is cleared by extensive binding to plasma proteins and en-

dothelial cells, saturable processes that explain both its nonlinear kinetics and the variability in dosing requirements among patients. Additional clearance occurs by transfer to the reticuloendothelial system, with ultimate elimination controlled by the kidneys.

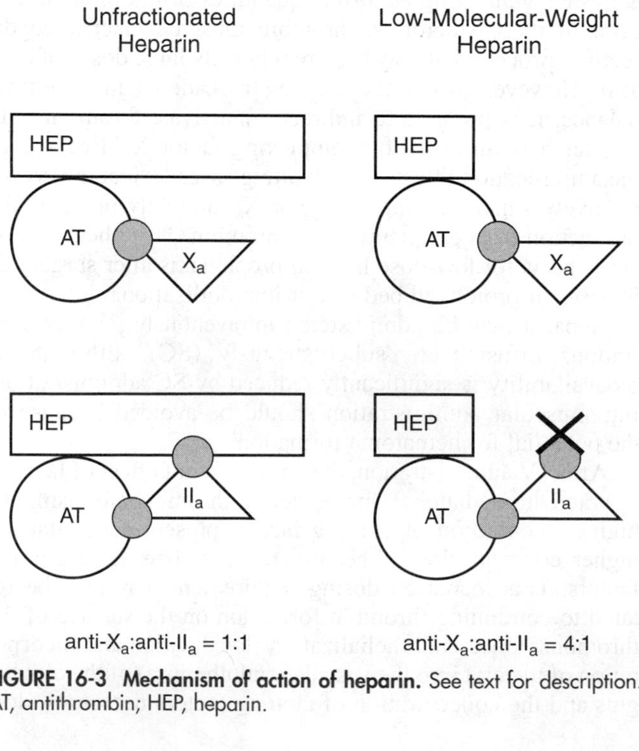

Low-Molecular-Weight Heparins

Using chemical or enzymatic depolymerization techniques, UFH can be separated into fragments based on molecular weight.[5] Low-molecular-weight heparin (LMWH) molecules have been isolated and commercially marketed as anticoagulants. These compounds differ substantially from UFH with respect to molecular weight, antithrombotic and pharmacokinetic properties, adverse effect profiles, and monitoring requirements (see Table 16-2).

To inactivate factor X_a, only the AT component of the heparin–AT complex is required to bind to factor X_a (see Fig. 16-3). Both the longer, high-molecular-weight fragments of UFH and the shorter, low-molecular-weight fragments of LMWHs are capable of inactivating factor X_a. However, to inactivate factor II_a (thrombin), both the heparin component and the AT component of the heparin–AT complex are required to bind to factor II_a. This binding requires heparin molecules of at least 18 saccharide units in length, which are less prevalent in LMWHs. Therefore, the anti-X_a properties of LMWHs are more significant than their anti-II_a properties. The resultant antithrombotic effect does not prolong the aPTT, meaning that these compounds do not require laboratory monitoring to ensure a therapeutic effect.

Additional advantages of LMWHs over UFH are explained by their reduced binding affinity for plasma proteins. These compounds display improved bioavailability after SC injection, predictable dose response, and longer pharmacodynamic effect compared with UFH. In general, these compounds are administered subcutaneously every 12 to 24 hours at fixed doses. Many LMWH products have been studied in the prevention and treatment of thromboembolic disease (Table 16-3). They

FIGURE 16-3 **Mechanism of action of heparin.** See text for description. AT, antithrombin; HEP, heparin.

Table 16-3 Selected Low-Molecular-Weight Heparin Products

Generic Name	Brand Name	Average Molecular Weight (range)[a]	Anti-Xa: Anti-IIa Activity
Dalteparin	Fragmin	5,000 (2,000–9,000)	2.0:1
Enoxaparin	Lovenox	4,500 (3,000–8,000)	2.7:1
Tinzaparin	Innohep	4,500 (3,000–6,000)	1.9:1

[a]Measured in daltons.

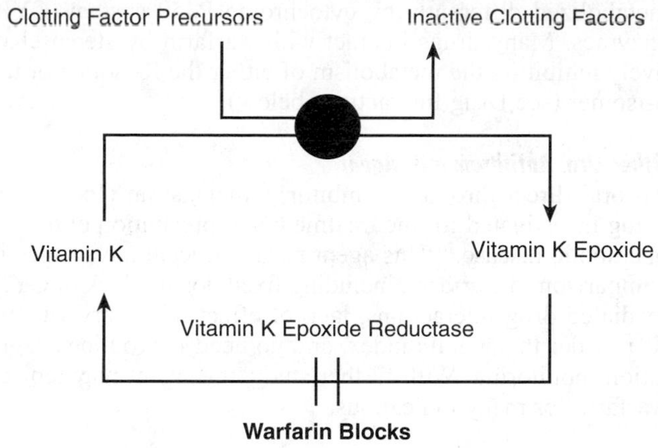

FIGURE 16-4 Mechanism of action of warfarin.

differ significantly in their molecular weight distributions, methods of preparation, and the ratio of anti-X_a:anti-II_a activities, as well as in their pharmacokinetic and pharmacodynamic characteristics. The LMWH products available in the United States are enoxaparin (Lovenox), dalteparin (Fragmin), and tinzaparin (Innohep). These products have replaced the use of UFH in many clinical situations.

Other Injectable Antithrombotic Agents

Several newer parenteral antithrombotic agents are available for limited indications. Fondaparinux (Arixtra) is a selective factor X_a inhibitor that is indicated for the prevention of venous thrombosis associated with orthopedic surgery.[6] This agent has a long elimination half-life, allowing for once-daily SC administration at a fixed dose without the need for routine coagulation monitoring. Argatroban and lepirudin (Refludan) are direct thrombin inhibitors that are used as alternative anticoagulants in patients with heparin-induced thrombocytopenia.[7] These agents are administered by continuous infusion and require aPTT monitoring for appropriate dosing adjustments. Finally, bivalirudin (Angiomax) is a direct thrombin inhibitor used in patients undergoing percutaneous coronary intervention. This agent appears to be associated with a lower rate of hemorrhagic complications than UFH and may reduce the need for concurrent therapy with glycoprotein IIb/IIIa receptor antagonists.[8]

Warfarin

Warfarin is an oral anticoagulant with a delayed onset of effect that acts as a vitamin K antagonist. Vitamin K is essential for the conversion (carboxylation) of precursors to clotting factors II, VII, IX, and X into inactive clotting factors and for the synthesis of protein C and protein S. During factor conversion, vitamin K is oxidized to inactive vitamin K epoxide (Fig. 16-4). In the non-anticoagulated patient, vitamin K epoxide is in reversible equilibrium with vitamin K, but this equilibrium is disrupted in patients taking oral anticoagulants. Warfarin (Coumadin) interferes with the hepatic recycling of vitamin K by inhibiting the reductase enzyme system that converts vitamin K epoxide to vitamin K.[9] The accumulation of vitamin K epoxide reduces the effective concentration of vitamin K and reduces the synthesis of coagulation factors.

Concentrations of clotting factors II, VII, IX, and X are diminished gradually at rates commensurate with their elimination half-lives (Table 16-4). Thus, the onset of the anticoagulant effect of warfarin is delayed. It takes approximately 5 to 7 days to reach a steady state of anticoagulation after warfarin therapy is initiated or after dosing changes. Protein C and its cofactor protein S are also vitamin K dependent, and these proteins are also depleted by warfarin at rates dependent on their elimination half-lives.

Warfarin is rapidly and completely absorbed in the upper gastrointestinal (GI) tract by passive diffusion, with nearly 100% bioavailability. Peak absorption of warfarin occurs in 60 to 120 minutes. It is approximately 99% bound to serum albumin. The volume of distribution (Vd) for warfarin is 12.5% of body weight. This small volume of distribution is consistent with the extensive binding of warfarin to albumin. The primary laboratory test for monitoring warfarin therapy is the prothrombin time (PT). No correlation appears to exist between PT and the dose of warfarin, the total warfarin concentration, or the free warfarin concentration among individuals, although in individual patients, an increasing dose of warfarin will increase the serum concentration (free and total) and the PT.

Warfarin is administered orally as a racemic mixture containing equal parts of the enantiomers R(+)-warfarin and S(−)-warfarin. The S-isomer is 2.7 to 3.8 times more potent as an anticoagulant than the R-isomer. These enantiomers are

Table 16-4 Elimination Half-Lives of Vitamin K–Dependent Clotting Factors

Clotting Factors	Half-Life (hrs)
II	42–72
VII	4–6
IX	21–30
X	27–48
Protein C	9
Protein S	60

metabolized differently by cytochrome P450 system (CYP) enzymes. Many drugs interact with warfarin by stereoselectively inhibiting the metabolism of either the R-isomer or the S-isomer (see Drug Interactions below).

Other Oral Antithrombotic Agent

An oral direct thrombin inhibitor, ximelagatran (Exanta), is being investigated for the treatment and prevention of thromboembolic disease.[10] This agent has significant advantages in comparison to warfarin, including fixed dosing, lack of CYP-mediated drug interactions, lack of effect of dietary vitamin K, a wider therapeutic index, and no need for routine coagulation monitoring. With further study, this agent may replace warfarin for many indications.

Tests Used to Monitor Antithrombotic Therapy

Before the initiation of antithrombotic therapy, an assessment of coagulation status is necessary. The clinician should obtain a baseline platelet count and hematocrit (Hct) and evaluate the baseline integrity of the extrinsic and intrinsic coagulation pathways with PT and aPTT.

Prothrombin Time/International Normalized Ratio

The PT is prolonged by deficiencies of clotting factors II, V, VII, and X, as well as by low levels of fibrinogen and very high levels of heparin. It reflects alterations in the extrinsic and common pathways of the clotting cascade, but not in the intrinsic system.[11] The PT is measured by adding calcium and tissue thromboplastin to a sample of plasma from which platelets have been removed by centrifugation. The time to clot formation is detected by automated instruments using light-scattering techniques that measure optical density. The mean normal PT, obtained by averaging a number of PT results from non-anticoagulated subjects, is approximately 12 seconds for most reagents.

The thromboplastins used in PT monitoring are extracted from various tissue sources by a number of techniques and prepared for commercial use as reagents. Unfortunately, thromboplastins are not standardized among manufacturers or among batches of reagent produced by the same manufacturer, leading to significant variability in PT results for anti-coagulated patients.[12] To standardize PT results, the World Health Organization developed a system by which all commercially available thromboplastins are compared with an international reference thromboplastin and then assigned an International Sensitivity Index (ISI). This value is used to mathematically convert PT to the International Normalized Ratio (INR) by exponentially multiplying the PT ratio to the power of the ISI of the thromboplastin being used in the laboratory to measure the test (INR = [PT patient/PT mean normal]^{ISI}). The ISI of the international reference thromboplastin is 1.0.

INR is the internationally recognized standard for monitoring warfarin therapy. Current recommendations for intensity of oral anticoagulation therapy for accepted clinical indications are summarized in Table 16-5. Regular-intensity therapy is defined as dosing warfarin to reach a goal INR of 2.5 (range, 2.0 to 3.0) and is appropriate for most settings that require the prevention and/or treatment of thromboembolic

disease. High-intensity therapy is used in mechanical valve replacement and certain situations of thromboembolic recurrence despite adequate anticoagulation and is defined as dosing warfarin to reach a goal INR of 3.0 (range, 2.5 to 3.5).

Activated Partial Thromboplastin Time

The aPTT reflects alterations in the intrinsic pathway of the clotting cascade and is used to monitor heparin therapy.[13] The test is performed by adding a surface-activating agent (kaolin; micronized silica), a partial thromboplastin reagent (phospholipid; platelet substitute), and calcium to the plasma sample. Mean normal values vary among reagents, but typically fall between 24 and 36 seconds.

Like PT, the aPTT is a highly variable test based on differences among commercially available partial thromboplastin reagents. However, a system equivalent to the INR has not been developed for standardization of aPTT results. Heparinization to prolong the aPTT to 1.5 to 2.5 times the mean normal value historically has been considered adequate to prevent propagation or extension of thrombus, but is not appropriate for all reagents and testing systems. Although not suitable for routine patient monitoring, the evaluation of heparin plasma levels by protamine titration has established a range of 0.2 to 0.4 U/mL that is correlated with clinical efficacy and safety. A reagent-specific therapeutic range in seconds is determined by measuring in vitro aPTT values (in seconds) for plasma samples containing known concentrations of heparin or by using protamine titration or anti-X_a activity to measure heparin concentrations in in vivo samples from heparinized patients. These concentrations are then correlated to aPTT values. The use of reagent-specific therapeutic ranges for monitoring heparin therapy is recommended for routine clinical practice. The therapeutic range for each aPTT reagent should be reported in seconds and calibrated to correspond with heparin serum levels of 0.2 to 0.4 U/mL by protamine titration or anti-X_a activity of 0.3 to 0.7 U/mL.[14]

Anti-X_a Activity

Although LMWHs do not require coagulation monitoring to ensure an appropriate antithrombotic effect or to adjust dosing, certain clinical situations may require evaluation of the anti-X_a activity of LMWHs.[15] Because these agents are eliminated renally, patients with severe renal failure may accumulate LMWHs, leading to an increased risk of hemorrhagic complications and necessitating evaluation of anti-X_a activity. LMWHs are dosed according to total body weight, but clinical trials have included only limited numbers of obese patients. Therefore, it may be appropriate to monitor anti-X_a activity in these patients. Anti-X_a activity also should be evaluated in patients who experience unexpected bleeding complications secondary to anticoagulation with LMWHs, and in pregnant patients in whom LMWHs are used for treatment or prevention of thrombosis..

Anti-X_a activity is measured using a chromogenic assay that is expensive and of limited availability. Peak activity levels should be obtained 3 to 4 hours after a SC dose of LMWH, with empiric dosing adjustments to maintain a level of roughly 0.5 to 1.0 U/mL.[16] Like other measures of hemostasis, results vary considerably, requiring both instrument- and method-specific determination of therapeutic ranges.

Table 16-5   Optimal Therapeutic Range and Duration of Warfarin Therapy

Indication	Target INR (range)	Duration	Comment
Atrial fibrillation (AF)			
No high or moderate risk factors	none	chronic	Use aspirin 325 mg QD alone
One moderate risk factor	2.5 (2.0–3.0)	chronic	Or aspirin 325 mg
(age 65–75, diabetes, CAD)			
Any high risk factor or >1 moderate risk factor	2.5 (2.0–3.0)	chronic	
(age >75; history of TIA/stroke/TE; HTN;			
poor LV function; rheumatic mitral valve disease;			
valve replacement)			
Precardioversion (atrial fib or flutter >48 hr)	2.5 (2.0–3.0)	3 weeks	
Postcardioversion (in NSR)	2.5 (2.0–3.0)	4 weeks	
Cardioembolic stroke			
With risk factors for stroke	2.5 (2.0–3.0)	chronic	
(AF, HF, LV dysfunction; mural thrombus,			
history of TIA/stroke/TE)			
Following embolic event despite anticoagulation	2.5 (2.0–3.0)	chronic	Add antiplatelet therapy
LV dysfunction			
Ejection fraction <30%	2.5 (2.0–3.0)	chronic	
Transient, following MI	2.5 (2.0–3.0)	3 months	
Following embolic event despite anticoagulation	2.5 (2.0–3.0)	chronic	Add antiplatelet therapy
MI			
Following anterior MI	2.5 (2.0–3.0)	3 months	
Following inferior MI with transient risk(s)	2.5 (2.0–3.0)	3 months	
[AF; HF, LV dysfunction, mural thrombus,			
history of TE]			
Following initial treatment with persistent risks	2.5 (2.0–3.0)	chronic	
Thromboembolism (DVT, PE)			
Treatment/prevention of recurrence			
Transient risk factors	2.5 (2.0–3.0)	3 months	
Idiopathic/first episode	2.5 (2.0–3.0)	6 months	
Idiopathic/recurrent	2.5 (2.0–3.0)	chronic	
Isolated calf vein	2.5 (2.0–3.0)	6–12 weeks	
Heterozygous factor V Leiden/first event	2.5 (2.0–3.0)	3 months	
Persistent risk factors	2.5 (2.0–3.0)	chronic	
[AT, protein C, protein S deficiencies;			
factor V Leiden; prothrombin gene mutation			
malignancy]			
Antiphospholipid antibody syndrome	3.0 (2.5–3.5)	chronic	Higher range may be required
Following recurrent DVT/PE	2.5 (2.0–3.0)	chronic	
Valvular disease			
Aortic valve disease	2.5 (2.0–3.0)	chronic	
With mobile atheroma or aortic plaque >4 mm,			
Mitral valve prolapse, regurgitation, or annular			
calcification			
With AF or history of systemic embolization	2.5 (2.0–3.0)	chronic	
With history of TIA despite ASA therapy	2.5 (2.0–3.0)	chronic	
Rheumatic mitral valve disease			
With AF, history of systemic embolization,			
LA>5.5cm	2.5 (2.0–3.0)	chronic	
Following embolic event despite anticoagulation	3.0 (2.5–3.5)	chronic	Or 2.0–3.0 plus aspirin 81 mg[a]
Valve replacement (bioprosthetic)			
Aortic or mitral	2.5 (2.0–3.0)	3 months	Followed by aspirin
With LA thrombus	2.5 (2.0–3.0)	>3 months	Followed by aspirin
With prior history systemic embolism	2.5 (2.0–3.0)	3–12 months	Followed by aspirin
With atrial fibrillation	2.5 (2.0–3.0)	chronic	
Following systemic embolism	2.5 (2.0–3.0)	chronic	Add aspirin

Continued

Table 16-5 Optimal Therapeutic Range and Duration of Warfarin Therapy *(continued)*

Valve replacement (mechanical)			
Aortic			
Bileaflet (or Medtronic Hall tilting disk)			
In NSR, normal EF, normal LA size	2.5 (2.0–3.0)	chronic	
All others	3.0 (2.5–3.5)	chronic	Or 2.0–3.0 plus aspirin 81 mg[a]
Tilting disk (all other brands)	3.0 (2.5–3.5)	chronic	Or 2.0–3.0 plus aspirin 81 mg[a]
Ball and cage	3.0 (2.5–3.5)	chronic	With aspirin 81 mg QD
Mitral			
Bileaflet	3.0 (2.5–3.5)	chronic	Or 2.0–3.0 plus aspirin 81 mg[a]
Tilting disk	3.0 (2.5–3.5)	chronic	Or 2.0–3.0 plus aspirin 81 mg[a]
Ball and cage/caged disk	3.0 (2.5–3.5)	chronic	With aspirin 81 mg QD
With additional risk factors or post-TE	3.0 (2.5–3.5)	chronic	Add aspirin 81 mg QD

[a]In patients with risks for hemorrhage.
ASA, acetylsalicylic acid; AT, antithrombin; CAD, coronary artery disease; EF, ejection fraction; HF, heart failure; HTN, hypertension; LA, left atrial; LV, left ventricular; NSR, normal sinus rhythm; TE, thromboembolism; TIA, transient ischemic attack.

DEEP VENOUS THROMBOSIS

Clinical Presentation

Signs and Symptoms

1. L.N., a 76-year-old, obese (92 kg, 6 ft tall) man, was admitted to the hospital 3 days ago for management of recurrent angina. He was started on a nitroglycerin drip and confined to bed rest with gradual increases in his oral antianginal medications. On the third day of hospitalization, he noted progressive swelling and soreness of the right calf. He denied shortness of breath (SOB), cough, or chest pain. His medical history includes coronary artery disease, MI at ages 55 and 67, and hypercholesterolemia. His medications are diltiazem CD (Cardizem CD) 360 mg/day PO, isosorbide mononitrate (Imdur) 120 mg/day PO, atenolol (Tenormin) 50 mg/day orally, aspirin 325 mg/day PO, and simvastatin (Zocor) 5 mg PO Q pm. Initial laboratory values include Hct, 36.5% (normal, 42% to 52%); PT, 10.8 sec (INR, 1.0); aPTT, 23.6 sec (normal, 24 to 36 sec); and platelet count, 255,000/mm³ (normal, 150,000 to 300,000/mm³). What signs and symptoms demonstrated by L.N. are consistent with DVT?

[SI units: Hct, 0.365 (normal, 0.42 to 0.52); platelet count, 255×10^9/L (normal, 150 to 300×10^9/L)]

One of the most reliable, although nonspecific, physical findings of DVT is unilateral leg swelling that often is accompanied by local tenderness or pain.[17] A tender, cordlike entity caused by venous obstruction sometimes can be palpated in the affected area. L.N. presented with the sudden onset of swelling along with soreness, but without evidence of a cord. Discoloration of the affected limb, including pallor from arterial spasm, cyanosis from venous obstruction, or a reddish color from perivascular inflammation, also may occur. The presence or absence of a positive Homans' sign (pain behind the knee or calf upon dorsiflexion of the foot) rarely is helpful in making the diagnosis because it is present in only about 30% of patients with DVT.

Risk Factors

2. What risk factors does L.N. exhibit that are associated with DVT?

The diagnosis of DVT depends not only on the presenting signs and symptoms, but also on the presence of risk factors. A summary of risk factors for thromboembolism is presented in Figure 16-1. L.N. has presented with obesity and immobilization (i.e., prolonged bed rest), two important risk factors for thromboembolism. It is common for more than one risk factor to be present in patients who develop DVT, and factors are cumulative in their effect.

Diagnosis

3. How should the final diagnosis of DVT be made in L.N.?

After evaluation of the signs and symptoms of DVT and consideration of risk factors for the development of thrombus, a definitive diagnosis should be made. The most common noninvasive test is duplex scanning, which combines B-mode imaging or color flow imaging with Doppler ultrasonography to visualize veins and thrombi while investigating flow patterns.[17] Other noninvasive testing options include ^{125}I-fibrinogen leg scanning (injection of radiolabeled fibrinogen followed by scanning to detect areas of accumulation corresponding to thrombosis), impedance plethysmography (use of pneumatic cuffs to detect leg blood volume changes associated with thrombosis), and Doppler ultrasonography alone (use of a transducer to audibly detect venous flow changes indicative of thrombosis). Each of these options differs with respect to sensitivity, specificity, and cost. Venography (radiographic visualization of the involved vessels with injection of radiocontrast material), an invasive diagnostic test, is the most sensitive and specific method for diagnosis of DVT, but exposes patients to the risks associated with contrast material.

Treatment

Baseline Information

4. What additional baseline data should be obtained before administering anticoagulants to L.N.?

In addition to assessing the integrity of the clotting process with platelet count, Hct, PT, and aPTT, the clinician should obtain a stool sample for occult blood. Generally, it is unnecessary to type and cross-match blood, but if this information is available, it should be recorded. Baseline values are used for comparison with the parameters that will be used in monitoring both the therapeutic and adverse effects of anticoagulant therapy.

Initiation of Therapy

5. Duplex scanning reveals clot formation in L.N.'s right calf extending to the right thigh. He does not exhibit signs of PE. What is the appropriate therapy for L.N., and how should it be initiated?

L.N.'s right leg was elevated and heat applied. Prompt and optimal anticoagulant therapy is indicated to minimize thrombus extension and its vascular complications, as well as to prevent PE. Options include UFH therapy initiated with a loading dose followed by a continuous infusion, or a LMWH, administered by SC injection. Because L.N. currently is hospitalized, UFH is selected for initial treatment of DVT.

Heparin
LOADING DOSE

6. L.N.'s medical resident ordered a heparin bolus dose of 5,000 U IV, to be followed by a continuous infusion of 1,000 U/hr. Is this heparin dosing regimen appropriate?

A loading dose of heparin is required for several reasons. Based on pharmacokinetic principles, a therapeutic serum level will be achieved more quickly; thus, pharmacodynamic and therapeutic responses to help prevent progression of clot will occur rapidly. Second, a relative resistance to anticoagulation exists during the active clotting process. Therefore, a larger initial dose generally is necessary to achieve a therapeutic effect.

Although many clinicians traditionally have turned to standardized doses for the initiation of heparin therapy (e.g., 5,000-U loading dose; 1,000-U/hour maintenance dose), this approach can result in significant delays in reaching a therapeutic intensity of anticoagulation. Body weight represents the most reliable predictor of heparin dosing requirement. Compared with standardized dosing, weight-based dosing (80-U/kg loading dose; 18-U/kg per hour initial infusion rate) increased both the number of patients whose first aPTT was within the therapeutic range (86% versus 32%) and the number of patients who were within the therapeutic range within the first 24 hours of therapy (97% versus 77%).[18]

Initial heparin loading doses of 70 to 100 U/kg followed by an infusion rate of 15 to 25 U/kg per hour commonly are recommended. Selection of the lower or upper dosage range is guided by the severity of the patient's symptoms and his or her potential sensitivity to adverse effects. For this 92-kg patient, a midrange loading dose of 7,400 U (92 kg × 80 U/kg) fol-

lowed by a continuous infusion of 1,700 U/hour (92 kg × 18 U/kg per hour) is recommended. Loading doses are typically rounded to the nearest 500 U and maintenance infusion rates to the nearest 100 U for convenience of administration.

DOSE ADJUSTMENTS

7. The orders for L.N. were rewritten by his attending physician. Based on the data that follow, explain the variability in laboratory results. (At this institution, aPTT values of 60 to 100 sec correspond with heparin serum concentrations of 0.2 to 0.4 U/mL.)

Time	APTT (sec)	Heparin Dosage Order
0800	31 (baseline)	7,400-U bolus followed by 1,700-U/hr infusion
0900	130	Hold infusion for 30 min, then ↓ to 1,500-U/hr
1500	40	Rebolus with 2,400 U, then ↑ to 1,700 U/hr
2100	85	Continue at 1,700 U/hr; recheck aPTT Q am

Although the aPTT drawn 1 hour after the initiation of the maintenance infusion (9 AM) demonstrates excessive prolongation of the aPTT (130 sec), this value most likely is explained by inappropriate timing of the test. When aPTT values are drawn too soon after a heparin bolus dose (i.e., before the maintenance infusion has achieved a steady-state concentration in serum), they are predictably very high, but are not associated with a bleeding risk and do not accurately reflect the anticipated level of anticoagulation in the patient. To ensure accuracy, the clinician should obtain aPTT values no sooner than 6 hours after a bolus dose or any change in infusion rate. Even results obtained at 6 hours may be excessively prolonged in some patients because of the dose-dependent pharmacokinetic characteristics of heparin.

L.N.'s heparin dose was decreased based on this prolonged, yet inappropriately timed, value. A repeat aPTT at 3 PM was only 40 seconds. The decrease in the dosage to 1,500 U/hour and the repeat aPTT of 40 seconds reflect near steady-state conditions because 6 hours have elapsed since the dosage change. Because the aPTT was subtherapeutic at 3 PM (40 seconds), administration of a smaller repeat bolus dose (2,400 U) and an increase in the maintenance infusion to 1,700 U/hour was the correct course of action. Subsequent aPTT values reflected therapeutic anticoagulation.

Dosing nomograms or protocols have been recommended for adjustment of heparin dosing based on aPTT results.[5,19] Nomogram-based dosing reduces the time to reach therapeutic range compared with empiric dosing.[19] After initiation based on patient weight, dosing adjustments may also be weight based or may simply be made in units per hour. A heparin dosing nomogram specific for a reagent with a therapeutic aPTT range of 60 to 100 seconds (and used in the adjustment of heparin doses for L.N.) is illustrated in Table 16-6.

Responses to changes in infusion rates of heparin are not always linear, and to some extent heparin doses are adjusted by trial and error. As the patient's condition improves after several days and endothelialization of the clot occurs, heparin dosing requirements may decrease.

Table 16-6 Heparin Protocol for Acute Thromboembolic Event[a]

1. Suggested loading dose
   Treatment: 80 U/kg (rounded to nearest 500 U)
   Prevention: 70 U/kg (rounded to nearest 500 U)
2. Suggested initial infusion
   Treatment: 18 U/kg/hr (rounded to nearest 100 U)
   Prevention 15 U/kg/hr (rounded to nearest 100 U)
3. First aPTT check: 6 hr after initiating therapy
4. Dosing adjustments: Per chart below (rounded to nearest 100 U)

aPTT[b] (sec)	Heparin Bolus	Infusion Hold Time	Infusion Rate Adjustment	Next aPTT
<40–49	4,000 U	0	↑ 200 U/hr	In 6 hr
50–59	2,000 U	0	↑ 100 U/hr	In 6 hr
60–100	0	0	None	Q am
101–110	0	0	↓ 100 U/hr	In 6 hr
111–120	0	0	↓ 200 U/hr	In 6 hr
>120	0	30 min	↓ 200 U/hr	In 6 hr

[a]University of Washington Medical Center.
[b]Based on aPTT reagent-specific therapeutic range of 60–100 sec corresponding to in vitro heparin concentrations of 0.2–0.4 U/mL.

THERAPEUTIC MONITORING

8. How should L.N.'s heparin therapy be monitored?

Once baseline clotting parameters have been established and a loading dose of heparin has been administered, the aPTT should be measured routinely to guide subsequent dosing adjustments. The aPTT should be evaluated no sooner than 6 hours after the loading dose or after any changes in infusion rate, as noted previously. If dosing is stable, the aPTT should be evaluated once daily (see Table 16-6).

Additional monitoring parameters for heparin therapy include evaluation for potential adverse reactions and possible therapeutic failure. Hct and platelet count should be checked every 1 to 2 days. L.N. should be examined for signs of bleeding as well as for signs and symptoms associated with thrombus extension and PE. Finally, if unusual or unexpected aPTT results are reported, the clinician should consider the possible influence of solution preparation errors, infusion pump failure, infusion interruption, and administration or charting errors in the assessment of L.N.'s heparin therapy.[20]

DURATION OF THERAPY

9. How long should heparin therapy be continued in L.N.?

Adherence of a thrombus to the vessel wall and subsequent endothelialization or resolution usually takes 7 to 10 days. However, anticoagulation generally must continue for 3 to 6 months to prevent recurrent thrombosis.[21] Warfarin is preferred for this long-term anticoagulation because it can be administered orally, and it is generally initiated on the same day as heparin. The long elimination half-life of warfarin and the long elimination half-lives of factors II and X necessitate a prolonged period of overlap between warfarin and heparin. Heparin is, therefore, continued for ≥5 days and until the INR has been therapeutic for 2 consecutive days. Heparin therapy should not be discontinued before 5 days even if the INR is therapeutic before then because of the time required for adequate elimination of factors II and X by warfarin. Shortening the duration of heparin is associated with an increased risk of recurrent thrombosis.

ADVERSE EFFECTS

10. On day 2 of heparin therapy, L.N.'s complete blood count (CBC) reveals a platelet count of 180,000/mm³, decreased from 255,000/mm³ at baseline. What is a reasonable explanation for this thrombocytopenia, and how should it be managed?

Thrombocytopenia. Thrombocytopenia induced by heparin has two distinct presentations.[22] Type I heparin-induced thrombocytopenia (HIT) occurs as a direct effect of heparin on platelet function, causing transient platelet sequestration and clumping with reductions in platelet count, but remaining above 100,000/ mm³. This reversible form of thrombocytopenia occurs within the first several days of heparin therapy. Patients remain asymptomatic and platelet counts return to normal even when heparin therapy is continued. L.N.'s reduction in platelet count is somewhat modest and likely represents type I HIT. His platelet count should be monitored daily, and heparin therapy should be continued.

Reductions in platelet count to <100,000/mm³ suggest the development of type II HIT, a more severe condition with a delay in onset of 5 to 14 days after the initiation of heparin therapy or with immediate onset in patients previously exposed to heparin. In this immune-mediated reaction, heparin binds to an IgG antibody to form a heparin–antibody complex that then binds to platelets, leading to significant platelet aggregation. In HIT, the observed thrombocytopenia is the result of drug-induced platelet aggregation as opposed to platelet destruction or bone marrow suppression. Laboratory analysis of the presence of the heparin-dependent platelet antibody can aid in differentiating type II HIT from other causes of thrombocytopenia.[23]

The overall incidence of type II HIT is <3%. It may occur somewhat more frequently with bovine lung heparin than with heparin derived from porcine gut mucosa. However, despite the low incidence, this is a life-threatening condition with high morbidity and mortality. Platelet aggregation secondary to type II HIT can lead to significant venous and arterial thrombosis, as well as thromboembolic stroke, acute MI, skin necrosis, and thrombosis of other major arteries. Amputation is necessary in up to 25% of patients, and mortality approaches 25% to 30% (see Chapter 87, Drug-Induced Blood Disorders).[22]

In patients who develop type II HIT, heparin therapy should be stopped immediately and treatment with an alternative anticoagulant should be initiated.[7] Although associated with a lower risk of type II HIT than UFH, LMWH products are contraindicated in patients with type II HIT because of a high incidence of immunologic cross-reactivity with heparin.[24] Preferred options include argatroban, a synthetic direct thrombin inhibitor, and lepirudin (Refludan), a recombinant form of the direct thrombin inhibitor hirudin. If necessary, an inferior vena cava filtration device such as the Greenfield filter can be implanted. These devices prevent pulmonary embolization by trapping embolic material originating from areas of the vasculature distal to their placement point.[25]

11. On day 3 of heparin therapy, L.N.'s Hct has dropped from a baseline of 36.5% to 29%, and blood is noted in his urine. Describe an approach to evaluate and interpret this event.

Hemorrhage. Bleeding is the most common adverse effect associated with heparin. A summary of eight inception cohort studies reporting heparin-associated bleeding found the absolute frequency of fatal, major, and all (major or minor) bleeding to be 0.4%, 6%, and 16%, respectively.[26] The corresponding average daily frequencies were 0.05% for fatal bleeding, 0.8% for major bleeding, and 2% for major or minor bleeding; cumulative risk increased with the duration of therapy. The most common sites for heparin-associated bleeding are soft tissues, the GI and urinary tracts, the nose, and the oral pharynx.

In addition to length of therapy, many factors influence the risk of bleeding during heparinization, including advanced age, serious comorbid illnesses (heart disease, renal insufficiency, hepatic dysfunction, cerebrovascular disease, malignancy, and severe anemia), and concomitant aspirin therapy.[27] Soft tissue bleeding commonly occurs at sites of recent surgery or trauma. Previously undiagnosed lesions, including malignancy, have been identified in a significant percentage of patients with GI or urinary tract bleeding associated with heparin therapy.

The influence of the intensity of heparinization on bleeding risk is controversial. Although an elevated aPTT historically has been considered a risk factor for bleeding complications, several investigators have been unable to substantiate a relationship between supratherapeutic aPTT values and hemorrhagic effects.[27] In addition, bleeding episodes can occur when coagulation test results are within the therapeutic range. These conflicting results may be explained in part by the influence of additional risk factors for bleeding and by the effect of heparin on platelet function and vascular permeability. These two factors, in addition to heparin's anticoagulant effect, influence hemorrhagic complications.

L.N. has developed hematuria despite an acceptable intensity of anticoagulation. He should be questioned and examined for the presence of nose bleeding (epistaxis), increased tendency to bruise (ecchymosis), bright red blood in the stool (hematochezia), black or tarry stool (melena), or coughing up of blood (hemoptysis). Blood pressure and pulse, both sitting and standing, should be obtained to determine whether orthostasis representing blood loss is present. A thorough evaluation of the urinary tract may reveal a previously unknown abnormality that will explain the bleeding episode.

12. What other side effects of heparin should be considered in L.N.?

Osteoporosis. The development of osteoporosis has been associated with administration of >20,000 U/day of heparin for 6 months or longer.[28] Various mechanisms have been suggested, but the underlying pathophysiology of this rare adverse effect remains unclear. Affected patients may present with bone pain and/or radiographic findings suggestive of fractures. The possibility of osteoporosis should be considered in patients receiving long-term, high-dose heparin therapy.

Hyperkalemia. Although rare, hyperkalemia has been attributed to heparin-induced inhibition of aldosterone synthesis. Hypoaldosteronism leading to hyperkalemia has been described with both high-dose and low-dose heparin therapy, may occur as quickly as within 7 days after initiation of heparin therapy, and appears to be reversible after discontinuation of heparin.[5] Patients with diabetes or renal failure may be at greatest risk.

Hypersensitivity Reactions. Other rarely occurring adverse effects associated with heparin include generalized hypersensitivity reactions, such as urticaria, rash, rhinitis, conjunctivitis, asthma, and angioedema, as well as a reversible temporal alopecia.[5]

ADJUSTED-DOSE SUBCUTANEOUS ADMINISTRATION

13. By day 4 of heparinization, IV access for L.N. has become difficult. What alternatives can be considered?

The most common strategy for treatment of venous thrombosis in hospitalized patients without IV access is the use of SC LMWH (see Question 15). Another alternative is SC administration of unfractionated heparin with adjustment of dosing to maintain a therapeutic aPTT.[29] Typically, SC heparin is administered at 12-hour intervals and aPTT is monitored at the mid-dosing interval (i.e., 6 hours after a dose).

For L.N., whose current heparin dosage is 1,700 U/hour, the initial SC heparin dose would be 20,500 U (1,700 U/hour × 12 hours and rounded to the nearest 500 U). Because a 20,000-U/mL preparation should be used to minimize the administration volume, the dose should be simplified to 20,000 U SC every 12 hours. L.N.'s aPTT should be checked 6 hours after the first dose, with adjustment of dosing as necessary. Because of the reduced bioavailability of SC heparin in comparison with IV administration, increased dosing may be required. A weight-based dosing nomogram, specific for a reagent with a therapeutic aPTT range of 60 to 100 seconds, is described in Table 16-7.

REVERSAL OF EFFECT

14. **P.B. is a 64-year-old woman with DVT. On day 4 of heparin therapy, she received 25,000 U of heparin during a 1-hour period as a result of an infusion pump malfunction. The infusion was stopped and within 30 minutes, she became diaphoretic and hypotensive. Bright red blood was evident upon rectal examination, and a large retroperitoneal mass was noted. How should the excessive heparin effect be reversed?**

P.B. has definite signs of hemorrhage from the GI tract, a site associated with considerable mortality. Heparin should be discontinued immediately, and treatment should include maintenance of fluid volume and replacement of clotting factors with whole blood, fresh frozen plasma, or clotting factor concentrates. If hemorrhage had not been present and the only manifestation of overdose had been a prolonged aPTT, administration of heparin simply could have been discontinued, permitting the effects to clear within a few hours.

Table 16-7 Heparin Protocol for Adjusted-Dose Subcutaneous Administration[a]

Initial Dosage

A. Initial therapy with adjusted-dose SC heparin
   1. Give SC heparin 240 U/kg × 1 STAT.
   2. Check first aPTT 6 hr after first dose.
   3. Adjust dosing per chart below.

B. Conversion from continuous infusion heparin to adjusted-dose SC heparin
   1. Calculate total 24-hr heparin requirement necessary to maintain therapeutic aPTT.
   2. Divide 24-hr heparin requirement by 2 to determine initial Q 12 hr SC dosing requirement.
   3. Discontinue IV heparin and administer initial Q 12 hr SC dose within 1 hr.
   4. Check first aPTT 6 hr after first dose.
   5. Adjust dosing per chart below.

C. Conversion from warfarin to adjusted-dose SC heparin
   1. Discontinue warfarin.
   2. Give 240 U/kg SC heparin within 24 hr.
   3. Check first aPTT 6 hr after first dose.
   4. Adjust dosing per chart below.

Dosing Adjustments

aPTT[b] (sec)	Dosing Adjustment[c]	Next aPTT
<40	↑ by 48 U/kg Q 12 hr	6 hr after dose
40–59	↑ by 24 U/kg Q 12 hr	6 hr after dose
60–100	No change	Q am
101–120	↓ by 12 U/kg Q 12 hr	6 hr after dose
121–140	↓ by 24 U/kg Q 12 hr	6 hr after dose
>140	↓ by 36 U/kg Q 12 hr	6 hr after dose

[a]University of Washington Medical Center.
[b]Based on aPTT reagent-specific therapeutic range of 60–100 sec corresponding to in vitro heparin concentrations of 0.2–0.4 U/mL.
[c]Rounded to nearest 500 U.
aPTT, activated partial thromboplastin time; IV, intravenous; SC, subcutaneous.

Protamine can be used to neutralize heparin by forming an inactive protamine–heparin complex.[30] Protamine has a rapid onset of action, with effects lasting about 2 hours. Protamine sulfate is infused as a 1% solution in a dose of 1 mg for each 100 U of heparin administered, but only if it is given within 30 minutes of heparin administration. If protamine therapy is delayed, dosing should be based on the estimated amount of heparin remaining, taking into consideration the elimination half-life of heparin. Response to protamine therapy can be assessed by a return of the aPTT to baseline. Adverse effects associated with protamine include systemic hypotension secondary to rapid administration; anaphylaxis characterized by edema, bronchospasm, and cardiovascular collapse; and catastrophic pulmonary vasoconstriction (see Chapter 4, Anaphylaxis and Drug Allergies).

LOW-MOLECULAR-WEIGHT HEPARIN

15. **H.K. is a 32-year-old woman who presents to the emergency department (ED) complaining of right calf pain of 1 day's duration. She denies trauma to the calf but reveals that she has just returned to the United States from Australia on a lengthy flight. She has no significant medical history, has no family history of clotting disorders, and takes no medications. A duplex ultrasound is positive for DVT, and immediate anticoagulation is indicated. What therapeutic alternative to hospitalization for UFH is available for this patient?**

Historically, UFH has been the initial treatment of choice for acute DVT. However, LMWHs have been shown to be as safe and effective as UFH, with many important practical advantages.[31] Weight-based, once- or twice-daily SC dosing of LMWHs provides a consistent anticoagulant effect that does not require aPTT monitoring. Based on these advantages, outpatient use of LMWH has become the most common approach to treatment of uncomplicated DVT. Home treatment is safe and effective and improves the overall physical and social functioning of patients being treated for DVT.[32,33] The drug costs associated with LMWH treatment are much higher than the costs of UFH, but overall costs to health care systems are significantly reduced when patients can be treated at home rather than in the hospital.[34]

For H.K. to be treated at home with LMWH, she or a family member must be willing and able to administer SC injections and she must be able to return for frequent follow-up visits, particularly during the first week while warfarin therapy is initiated. In addition, her health care insurance should cover the cost of the drug, or she must be able to pay out of pocket. Contraindications to home treatment of DVT include a pre-existing condition that requires hospitalization, symptoms of PE, recent or active bleeding, and severe renal impairment.

H.K. meets the eligibility requirements for home treatment and is interested in self-injection of LMWH at home, with support from her partner, for initial treatment of DVT. Most institutional formularies carry only a single LMWH product, with formulary decisions based on FDA-approved indications and clinical data supporting use for treatment and prevention of thromboembolism in various settings. In this case, enoxaparin is the LMWH available for use.

The usual dosing of enoxaparin for treatment of DVT is 1 mg/kg total body weight SC Q 12 hours, rounded to the nearest 10-mg increment. Once-daily dosing, at 1.5 mg/kg Q

24 hours is also an option, but this strategy is inferior to twice-daily dosing in patients with malignancy or obesity.[35] Because LMWHs are eliminated renally, patients with significant renal impairment require dosing adjustments. Some clinicians use enoxaparin 0.85 mg/kg Q 12 hours for patients with creatinine clearances of 30 to 60 mL/min, and 0.65 mg/kg Q 12 hours for patients with creatinine clearances of <30 mL/min.[36] Renal impairment is not a contraindication to the use of LMWH, but may preclude outpatient treatment and requires anti-X_a monitoring and dosing adjustments to avoid overanticoagulation and bleeding complications.[37]

16. **What systems must be in place for H.K.'s home treatment to be successful? What is the role of the pharmacist or other caregiver in her therapy?**

H.K. should be weighed to determine her dose of enoxaparin. Since she is not obese and does not have a malignancy, a 1.5-mg/kg dose once daily is acceptable. Dosing is typically rounded to the nearest 10 mg based on the availability of prefilled syringes. At 64 kg, H.K. will receive 100 mg SC Q 24 hours. Warfarin therapy is initiated concurrently to expedite the conversion to oral treatment.

H.K. must be taught to self-administer enoxaparin by SC injection. Patient education resources, including videotaped instructions and written materials, should supplement hands-on instruction. H.K. will administer the first dose of enoxaparin in the ED with the assistance of a pharmacist. She should also be given prescriptions for enoxaparin and warfarin that must be filled immediately at the pharmacy of her choice.

H.K. should be instructed regarding the potential adverse effects of LMWH therapy (bleeding, thrombocytopenia, pain and bruising at the injection site), required laboratory monitoring, and the expected duration of anticoagulation. At baseline, Hct, INR, and platelet count should be determined. Platelets will continue to be monitored at least every other day for the first two weeks of LMWH therapy. H.K. can expect to continue enoxaparin therapy for a minimum of 5 days. If by day 5 her INR has been therapeutic for 2 consecutive days, enoxaparin can be discontinued. Oral anticoagulation with warfarin will continue for 3 to 6 months.

To ensure the safety and efficacy of home treatment, H.K. should be provided with the names and telephone numbers of the health care providers who will assume responsibility for her care, including her primary physician and her anticoagulation management team. No patient should be sent home with LMWH without an adequate follow-up plan.

Prevention

17. **D.F., a 63-year-old obese woman, is to undergo elective abdominal surgery for treatment of diverticulitis. She has a medical history significant for mild hypertension, currently controlled by enalapril 10 mg QD (blood pressure, 135/85 mm Hg) and peripheral vascular disease. What therapeutic interventions might decrease the risk of DVT or PE in D.F.?**

Surgical procedures, particularly those involving the pelvis or lower extremities, represent a significant risk factor for DVT formation. All hospitalized patients, including both surgical and nonsurgical patients, should be stratified for risk of DVT based on the presence of various factors.[38] Risk stratification is used to select the most appropriate therapeutic interventions to prevent DVT, and thereby reduce the risk of fatal PE.[39,40] These interventions include both mechanical and pharmacologic strategies.

Nonpharmacologic Measures
Mechanical interventions aimed at preventing venous stasis and increasing venous return include the use of elastic compression stockings as well as leg elevation, leg exercises, and early postoperative ambulation. Intermittent pneumatic compression (IPC) of the leg muscles, using inflatable cuffs applied to the calf and thigh, represents another alternative for the prevention of DVT.

Pharmacologic Measures
Fixed, low-dose unfractionated heparin (LDUFH), administered as 5,000 U SC Q 8 to 12 hours depending on the indication, is an inexpensive and effective pharmacologic approach to DVT prevention in the setting of venous stasis or after surgical procedures. Because low-dose heparin inactivates factor X_a without a direct effect on factor II_a, the aPTT is not prolonged, and therefore aPTT monitoring is unnecessary. Bleeding complications are minimized using this dosing regimen.

Fixed-dose LMWH is an alternative approach for preventing DVT in most clinical situations. Enoxaparin 30 mg SC Q 12 hours or 40 mg SC once daily, and dalteparin 2,500 to 5,000 IU SC once daily are effective strategies, although enoxaparin has been studied for a larger number of indications. Current recommendations for prevention of venous thromboembolism based on risk stratification are presented in Table 16-8.[41]

D.F. is at high risk for DVT and PE, not only because of general surgery, but also because of her age (>60) and the presence of other risk factors for venous thromboembolism (obesity, peripheral vascular disease, and probable postoperative immobilization). Options for DVT prevention include SC heparin at 5,000 U Q 8 to 12 hours or enoxaparin 40 mg SC QD. The first dose should be administered several hours preoperatively, and dosing should continue postoperatively until she is fully ambulatory. If bleeding risk is of concern, IPC could alternatively be used.

PULMONARY EMBOLISM
Clinical Presentation
18. **D.J. is a 38-year-old, 90-kg man. Several days ago he developed a swollen left calf, which was painful and warm. This swelling gradually increased, affecting the entire left leg to the groin and prompting him to seek medical attention. In the ED, he also notes the recent onset of right-sided pleuritic chest pain without SOB or hemoptysis. His medical history includes a gastric ulcer 4 years ago, treated medically without recurrence. Physical examination reveals a pleasant, obese man with an enlarged left leg and mild to moderate tenderness in the entire leg. Chest examination reveals a loud, pulmonary heart sound (P_2). Vital signs include blood pressure, 150/85 mm Hg; heart rate, 100 beats/min; and respiratory rate, 28 breaths/min and regular. Laboratory data include Hct, 26.7% (normal, 45% to 52%); SCr 1.1 mg/dL (normal, 0.8 to 1.2 mg/dL); and arterial blood gases (on room air) Po_2, 72 mm Hg (normal, 75 to 100);**

Table 16-8 Prevention of Venous Thromboembolism

General surgery

Low risk	Early ambulation
Moderate risk	LDUH Q 12 hr, LMWH QD, IPC, or ES
High risk	LDUH Q 8–12 hr, LMWH QD, or IPC
Very high risk	LDUH Q 8–12 hr or LMWH QD + IPC

Gynecologic surgery

Brief procedures	Early ambulation
Major surgery	LDUH Q 12 hr, LMWH QD, or IPC
Major surgery for malignancy	LDUH Q 12 hr + IPC or ES; LDUH Q 8 hr; or LMWH QD

Urologic surgery

Low risk procedures	Early ambulation
Major open procedures	LDUH Q 12 hr, LMWH QD, IPC, or ES
Highest-risk patients	LDUH Q 12 hr or LMWH QD with IPC ± ES

Orthopedic surgery

Hip replacement	LMWH QD or BID or warfarin ± IPC
Knee replacement	LWMH BID, warfarin, or IPC
Hip fracture surgery	LMWH BID or warfarin
Trauma	LMWH BID
Acute spinal cord injury	LMWH BID ± IPC or ES
Neurosurgery	IPC ± ES; LDUH Q 12 hr or LMWH QD ± IPC or ES
Acutely medically ill	LDUH Q 8–12 hr or LMWH QD

LDUH, low-dose unfractionated heparin (5,000 U Q 8–12 h); LMWH, low-molecular-weight heparin (enoxaparin 40 mg QD or 30 mg Q 12 hr; dalteparin 2,500–5000 IU QD); ES, elastic stockings; IPC, intermittent pneumatic compression; VTE, venous thromboembolism.

Low risk: minor surgery, age <40, and no additional risk factors for VTE. Moderate risk: minor surgery and additional risk factors for VTE; nonmajor surgery, age 40–60, and no other risk factors for VTE; major surgery, age <40 and no other risk factors for VTE. High risk: nonmajor surgery with age >60 or additional risk factors for VTE; major surgery with age >40 or additional risk factors for VTE. Very high risk: multiple risk factors for VTE.

P_{CO_2}, 30 mm Hg (normal, 35 to 45); and pH 7.48 (normal, 7.35 to 7.45). The chest radiograph and lung scan (ventilation-perfusion [V/Q] scan) are highly suggestive of PE. An angiogram was not performed. The electrocardiogram (ECG) shows sinus tachycardia. The venogram is positive for defects in the ileofemoral vein. Coagulation test results include PT, 11.2 sec (INR, 1.0); aPTT, 28 sec; and platelet count, 248,000/mm³ (normal, 150,000 to 350,000). What subjective and objective evidence in D.J. is compatible with PE?

[SI units: Hct, 0.267 (normal, 0.45 to 0.52); platelets, 248 × 10⁹/L (normal, 150 to 300)]

Signs and Symptoms

The clinical diagnosis of PE often is difficult to make because of the nonspecificity of symptoms.[42] The most commonly observed subjective symptoms are dyspnea, pleuritic chest pain, apprehension (anxiety or a feeling of impending doom), and cough. Hemoptysis occurs occasionally. The objective signs most commonly observed are tachypnea at a rate of 20 breaths/min or more, tachycardia of 100 beats/min or more, accentuated pulmonary component of the second heart sound (P_2), and rales. DVT precedes PE in 80% or more of patients. A combination of these signs and symptoms provides further evidence for acute PE. D.J. has presented with pleuritic chest pain, tachycardia, tachypnea, loud P_2, and a decrease in Po_2; therefore, he may have developed PE.

Diagnosis

Because the clinical signs and symptoms of PE are difficult to distinguish from many other medical conditions, further evaluation is necessary. Chest radiograph, ECG, and arterial blood gas (alveolar-arterial oxygen gradient [A-a gradient]) abnormalities often are present in patients with PE, but like clinical signs and symptoms, they are somewhat nonspecific. V/Q lung scans and pulmonary angiograms are useful diagnostic procedures to document the presence of PE. Lung scans that incorporate an assessment of perfusion, or regional distribution of pulmonary blood flow, and ventilation are referred to as V/Q scans and involve both the injection and the inhalation of radiolabeled compounds. Test results are expressed as a high, intermediate, or low probability of PE. When ventilation (air movement) is normal over an area that shows abnormal perfusion (blood flow), a V/Q mismatch exists and PE is highly probable. If a matched defect is noted (abnormal ventilation over an area of abnormal perfusion), another disease state, such as chronic obstructive airway disease, is more likely.

A positive lung scan (D.J. had one highly suggestive of PE) or a positive pulmonary angiogram would confirm the presence of a PE. Nonetheless, when the diagnosis of PE is suspected, anticoagulation should be initiated immediately while awaiting results of more definitive diagnostic procedures. Mortality associated with PE has been documented to be as high as 17.5% over 3 months.[43]

Treatment

19. What anticoagulant strategy should be initiated for D.J.?

As with the treatment of DVT, there are two treatment options for initial management of PE. UFH therapy could be started in D.J. with a loading dose of 7,200 U (80 U/kg × 90 kg) followed by continuous infusion of 1,600 U/hr (18 U/kg/hr × 90 kg). Monitoring of the aPTT would be used to adjust dosing to maintain treatment within the therapeutic range.

The alternative to UFH for treatment of PE is the use of LMWH.[21] D.J. could receive fixed-dose enoxaparin 90 mg SC Q 12 hours (1mg/kg Q 12 hours × 90 kg). However, PE should not be treated on an outpatient basis. In this case, LMWH would be used during the complete hospital course.

Warfarin
TRANSITION FROM HEPARIN/LMWH THERAPY

20. When should warfarin be administered, and how should the transition be accomplished?

Either heparin or LMWH therapy should be continued for 5 days in the setting of PE and until warfarin therapy has been therapeutic for 2 consecutive days. Warfarin should be started

Table 16-9 Factors That Increase Sensitivity to Warfarin

Age >75	Clinical congestive heart failure
Malnutrition/NPO >3 days	Clinical hyperthyroidism
Elevated baseline INR	Malignancy
Fever	End-stage renal disease
Diarrhea	Concurrent use of drugs known to reduce warfarin dosing requirements

NPO, nothing by mouth.

on the first day of hospitalization and continued for 3 to 6 months. However, a delay in the initiation of warfarin may be acceptable in the setting of an anticipated extended hospitalization, recent or anticipated surgery or other invasive procedures, or a medical condition with the potential for uncontrolled bleeding.

There are several reasons to overlap heparin and warfarin therapy. The onset of warfarin activity depends not only on its inherent pharmacokinetic characteristics (half-life >36 hours), but also on the rate of elimination of circulating clotting factors. Although warfarin inhibits production of the vitamin K–dependent clotting factors, previously synthesized clotting factors must be eliminated at rates that correspond with their elimination half-lives (see Table 16-4). Approximately four half-lives are required for these factors to reach a new steady state after their production is inhibited, so the effect of warfarin can be delayed for several days. Initial increases in the INR reflect only reductions in factor VII activity, but full anticoagulation with warfarin requires adequate suppression of factors II and X, which have significantly longer elimination half-lives. By overlapping heparin with warfarin therapy, adequate anticoagulation can be continued with heparin until warfarin therapy reaches a therapeutic intensity.

In addition to suppressing the synthesis of the vitamin K–dependent clotting factors, warfarin also inhibits the formation of the naturally occurring anticoagulant protein C and its cofactor, protein S. In patients with congenital protein C or protein S deficiency, initial warfarin therapy can suppress these proteins to concentrations that may result in hypercoagulability with possible thrombus extension unless concurrent heparin therapy provides adequate anticoagulation.[44] To prevent these complications, heparin and warfarin therapy should overlap.

Heparin therapy has been observed to prolong the INR,[45] and warfarin can prolong the aPTT by several seconds.[46] Thus, interference with laboratory tests should be considered in the evaluation of the intensity of anticoagulation during the overlap of heparin and warfarin therapy.

INITIATION OF THERAPY

21. In an effort to discharge D.J. from the hospital as soon as possible, an initial dose of warfarin 10 mg PO Q pm for 3 days has been ordered. Is such a "loading dose" reasonable? What would be a more appropriate approach to initiating therapy?

Initiation of warfarin dosing is complex because dosing requirements vary significantly among individuals. Daily doses as low as 0.5 mg and as high as 20 mg or more may be re-

quired in individual patients to reach a therapeutic INR.[47] Two methods for initiation of warfarin therapy have been developed.[48] The average daily dosing method relies on an understanding that although dosing requirements for warfarin vary significantly among patients, an average dosing requirement of 4 to 5 mg/day of warfarin is necessary to maintain an INR of 2.0 to 3.0. When the average daily dosing method is used for initiation of warfarin therapy, patients are started at 4 to 5 mg daily, with dosing adjustments as necessary until the therapeutic goal is reached. However, patients who may be more sensitive to the effects of warfarin (Table 16-9) are expected to require lower dosages of warfarin. In these patients, therapy should be initiated at 1 to 3 mg daily, with subsequent dosing adjustments as necessary. Average daily dosing is often used to initiate therapy in ambulatory patients; in this case, the first INR should be evaluated within 3 to 5 days of initiation of warfarin therapy. In hospitalized patients, it is more common to evaluate the INR daily during initiation of therapy.

Flexible initiation of warfarin is an alternative approach for starting therapy that is based on evaluating the rate of increase in the INR and making daily dosing adjustments based on daily INR evaluation, with a goal of determining the eventual maintenance dosing requirement. A popular flexible initiation nomogram is presented in Table 16-10.[49,50] Using this nomogram, warfarin can be initiated with either a 10-mg or a 5-mg starting dose, with daily dosing adjustments based on the rate of increase in the INR. Flexible initiation does not necessarily shorten the time to reach the goal INR, and initiating therapy

Table 16-10 Flexible Initiation Dosing Protocol for Warfarin Dosing, Including 10- and 5-mg Starting Dose Options

Day	INR	10-mg Initiation Dose	5-mg Initiation Dose
1		10 mg	5 mg
2	<1.5	7.5–10 mg	5 mg
	1.5–1.9	2.5 mg	2.5 mg
	2.0–2.5	1.0–2.5 mg	1–2.5 mg
	>2.5	0	0
3	<1.5	5–10 mg	5–10 mg
	1.5–1.9	2.5–5 mg	2.5–5 mg
	2.0–2.5	0–2.5 mg	0–2.5 mg
	2.5–3.0	0–2.5 mg	0–2.5 mg
	>3.0	0	0
4	<1.5	10 mg	10 mg
	1.5–1.9	5–7.5 mg	5–7.5 mg
	2.0–3.0	0–5 mg	0–5 mg
	>3.0	0	0
5	<1.5	10 mg	10 mg
	1.5–1.9	7.5–10 mg	7.5–10 mg
	2.0–3.0	0–5 mg	0–5 mg
	>3.0	0	0
6	<1.5	7.5–12.5 mg	7.5–12.5 mg
	1.5–1.9	5–10 mg	5–10 mg
	2.0–3.0	0–7.5 mg	0–7.5 mg
	>3.0	0	0

Reprinted with permission from Crowther MA et al. Warfarin: less may be better. Ann Intern Med 1997;127:332.[49]

with a 10-mg dose as described in some protocols may be associated with an increased risk of early overanticoagulation in certain patients. Nonetheless, these methods offer a more individualized approach to initiation of therapy.

The baseline INR for D.J. was 1.0. Using the flexible initiation protocol presented in Table 16-10, the first dose of warfarin should be 10 mg administered in the evening on the first day of hospitalization. Subsequent INR values obtained daily will guide dosing requirements until a therapeutic INR is reached. The order for warfarin 10 mg orally every evening for three doses should be discontinued and replaced with daily orders for warfarin and INR monitoring.

INTENSITY OF THERAPY

22. **What is the goal INR for D.J., and how long should anticoagulation be administered?**

In patients with DVT or PE, warfarin therapy should be aimed at prolonging the PT to an INR of 2.0 to 3.0, defined as low-intensity therapy.[21] This therapeutic range is recommended to maximize the antithrombotic effect of warfarin while minimizing potential bleeding complications associated with excessive anticoagulation.

DURATION OF THERAPY

Once formed, clots adhere to the vessel wall. Thus, the first step in resolution of a thrombus involves covering the clot with a layer of endothelial cells to prevent additional platelet aggregation at the site of vessel injury. This endothelialization process generally takes 7 to 10 days to be completed. Initial anticoagulant treatment is used to prevent clot extension while allowing adequate endothelialization to occur. Continued anticoagulation is directed at the prevention of further clotting.

Patients with DVT and PE associated with transient risk factors should be anticoagulated with warfarin for 3 to 6 months.[21] A multicenter comparison of 4 weeks versus 3 months of oral anticoagulation following DVT or PE and a second comparison of 6 weeks versus 6 months of therapy confirmed the appropriateness of this duration of therapy.[51,52] In these trials, the incidences of both treatment failure, defined as persistent signs and symptoms or new thromboembolic events during treatment, and thromboembolic recurrence during 1 year of follow-up were significantly lower in patients treated for longer periods. In patients with idiopathic DVT/PE or persistent risk factors, including AT deficiency, protein C or protein S deficiency, factor V Leiden, prothrombin gene mutation, antiphospholipid antibody syndrome, or other hypercoagulable states, including malignancy, warfarin treatment should be continued indefinitely.[53] Similarly, prolonged anticoagulation in patients with recurrent venous thromboembolism was associated with a lower rate of recurrent DVT or PE than when 6 months of therapy was given.[54]

ADVERSE EFFECTS

23. **What possible adverse effects from warfarin therapy should be considered in D.J., and how should they be monitored?**

Hemorrhage. Bleeding is the most common adverse effect associated with warfarin. A summary of experimental and observational inception cohort studies determined that the average annual frequency of fatal, major, and all (major or minor) bleeding in patients treated with warfarin was 0.6%, 3%, and 9.6%, respectively.[26] However, wide variation in bleeding frequencies has been reported, probably because of differences in patient characteristics, treatment protocols, and the definition and assessment of bleeding among trials.

Warfarin-associated bleeding most commonly occurs in the nose, oral pharynx, and soft tissues, followed by the GI and urinary tracts. Hemarthrosis (bleeding into joint spaces) and retroperitoneal and intraocular bleeding represent less common hemorrhagic complications of warfarin therapy.[26,27] As with heparin, GI and urinary tract bleeding associated with warfarin often is caused by previously undiagnosed lesions.

Although it is uncommon, intracranial bleeding resulting in hemorrhagic stroke represents the most common cause of fatal bleeding associated with warfarin therapy. Rates of intracranial hemorrhage associated with anticoagulants have been estimated to range from 0.3% to 2%, and up to 60% are fatal.[55]

Many factors influence the risk of hemorrhagic complications associated with warfarin. The frequency of bleeding is higher in the first 3 months of therapy than during subsequent months.[56] Unlike heparin, the intensity of anticoagulation with warfarin directly influences the risk of bleeding, including intracranial hemorrhage.[57] Other patient-specific variables that influence the risk of warfarin-associated bleeding include a history of GI bleeding, serious comorbid disease (including malignancy), and concomitant therapy with aspirin or nonsteroidal anti-inflammatory drugs (NSAIDs).[26,27,56-59]

The influence of age on bleeding risk is controversial. Older patients are known to require lower dosages of warfarin than younger patients to reach a therapeutic intensity of anticoagulation.[60] Inherent vitamin K deficiency or age-related differences in stereoisomeric disposition of warfarin may explain why older patients are more sensitive to the effects of warfarin and, therefore, require lower dosages than younger patients. This increased sensitivity to the effect of warfarin is not the result of differences in pharmacokinetic characteristics of warfarin between older and young patients, including protein binding and metabolism. It is also not related to gender, weight, underlying medical conditions, or the presence of interacting drugs. Nonetheless, increased sensitivity to warfarin does not imply an increased bleeding risk if older patients are managed appropriately.

Some studies have reported that age is an independent risk factor for bleeding, while others have suggested that age alone does not increase bleeding risk.[61] However, in two studies in which comprehensive anticoagulation monitoring and follow-up were provided through anticoagulation management services, elderly patients did not experience an increased incidence of major bleeding.[62,63]

Hemorrhagic risk assessment can be used to predict bleeding risk during anticoagulant therapy. A popular bleeding index scoring system assigns level of risk based on the presence of age >65, history of GI bleeding, history of stroke, and one or more of four comorbid conditions: recent MI, anemia (Hct <30), renal insufficiency (Scr >1.5), and diabetes.[64] The cumulative risk of major bleeding at 48 months in low-, intermediate-, and high-risk patients was 3%, 12%, and 53%, respectively. The bleeding index can be useful in making decisions about management of drug interactions, overanticoagulation, bridge therapy for invasive procedures, and other issues that may present during anticoagulant therapy.

Bleeding complications in D.J. can be minimized by careful attention to the signs and symptoms of bleeding by the patient and his caregivers, maintenance of the INR within the therapeutic range, avoidance of therapy with concomitant drugs known to increase the risk of bleeding or to increase the INR, and routine outpatient follow-up for INR monitoring and clinical assessment.

24. S.G., a 34-year-old woman with no significant medical history, presents to the ED with an extremely painful, erythematous lesion on her right thigh. The lesion appeared 2 days ago, progressing in size and tenderness, and now includes a purplish-black discoloration at the center. All laboratory values are within the normal range with the exception of INR, which is elevated to 4.8, and a significant reduction in protein C activity to 20% (normal, 65% to 150%). Careful questioning reveals that several days before admission, S.G. experienced pain in her right calf after a period of prolonged immobility. At that time, she began to self-administer warfarin 5-mg tablets QD that had previously been prescribed for her brother for a similar incident. According to S.G., her brother developed a blood clot in his leg and was diagnosed as a "clotter." A duplex ultrasound is positive for DVT, and the additional diagnosis of warfarin-induced skin necrosis is made. What is the pathophysiology of this process?

Skin Necrosis. Warfarin-induced skin necrosis is a rare, but serious adverse effect of oral anticoagulation, occurring in approximately 0.01% to 0.1% of patients treated with warfarin.[65,66] Patients present within 3 to 6 days of the initiation of warfarin therapy with painful discoloration of the breast, buttocks, thigh, or penis. The lesions progress to frank necrosis with blackening and eschar. Skin necrosis appears to be the result of extensive microvascular thrombosis within subcutaneous fat and has been associated with hypercoagulable conditions, including protein C or protein S deficiency. In these patients, rapid depletion of protein C before depletion of vitamin K–dependent clotting factors during early warfarin therapy can result in an imbalance between procoagulant and anticoagulant activity, leading to initial hypercoagulability and thrombosis. Adequate heparinization during initiation of warfarin can prevent the development of early hypercoagulability.

25. How should S.G. be managed? Is further anticoagulation with warfarin contraindicated?

Warfarin therapy should be discontinued in patients who develop skin necrosis. However, subsequent warfarin therapy is not necessarily contraindicated if it is required for treatment or prevention of thromboembolic disease.[65] In patients with protein C or protein S deficiency and a history of skin necrosis, warfarin therapy can be restarted at low dosages as long as therapeutic heparinization has been achieved. Therapy is maintained until the INR has been within the therapeutic range for 72 hours. Supplementation of protein C through administration of fresh frozen plasma also may be indicated.

Purple Toe Syndrome. Purple toe syndrome is a rarely reported adverse effect that typically occurs 3 to 8 weeks after the initiation of warfarin therapy and is unrelated to intensity of anticoagulation.[66] Patients initially present with painful discoloration of the toes that blanches with pressure and fades with elevation. The pathophysiology of this syndrome has been related to cholesterol microembolization from atherosclerotic plaques, leading to arterial obstruction. Because cholesterol microembolization has been associated with renal failure and death, warfarin therapy should be discontinued in patients who develop purple toe syndrome.

PATIENT EDUCATION

26. B.H. is a 30-year-old woman newly diagnosed with idiopathic DVT. Before anticoagulation is initiated, appropriate laboratory tests are drawn to evaluate the possibility of a hypercoagulable state. She will be treated as an outpatient with enoxaparin 1.5 mg/kg SC QD and started on warfarin 4 mg PO QD using the average daily dosing method. Her primary care physician would like her to receive follow-up care in the medical center's pharmacist-managed anticoagulation clinic. What information should B.H. receive regarding the benefits of formal anticoagulation management services?

One of the keys to successful oral anticoagulant therapy is appropriate outpatient management. In comparison with routine medical care, management of warfarin therapy by anticoagulation clinics is associated with significant reductions in bleeding and thromboembolic complications, with reductions in the rates of warfarin-related hospital admissions and ED visits, and with outcome-based cost savings for health care organizations.[67] Pharmacist-managed anticoagulation clinics offer many benefits for the management of anticoagulation therapy, including improved dosing regulation, continuous patient education, early identification of risk factors for adverse events, and timely intervention to avoid or minimize complications. B.H.'s referral to a pharmacist-managed anticoagulation clinic is likely to improve her overall satisfaction with care and to improve her clinical outcomes.

27. At her initial visit to the anticoagulation clinic, B.H. will receive extensive education about her warfarin therapy. What information should be conveyed to her by her anticoagulation provider to ensure the safety and efficacy of warfarin therapy?

Successful warfarin therapy depends on the active participation of knowledgeable patients. The anticoagulant effect of warfarin is influenced by various factors, and fluctuations in the intensity of the anticoagulant effect of warfarin can increase the risk of both hemorrhagic complications and recurrent thromboembolism.[68] Pharmacists and other providers can improve adherence to the medication schedule and ensure the safety and efficacy of warfarin therapy by providing appropriate education to patients treated with this agent.

Key elements that form the basis of a thorough patient education program for warfarin therapy are listed in Table 16-11. This information may be conveyed through written teaching materials, videotaped instruction, individual or group discussion, or a combination of these approaches. Many useful educational tools are available from the manufacturers of warfarin.

B.H. should receive extensive education about warfarin therapy in an individual teaching session or an organized education program. A wallet card, medical bracelet, or alternative method of identifying her as a patient treated with war-

Table 16-11   Key Elements of Patient Education Regarding Warfarin

Identification of generic and brand names
Purpose of therapy
Expected duration of therapy
Dosing and administration
Visual recognition of drug and tablet strength
What to do if a dose is missed
Importance of prothrombin time/INR monitoring
Recognition of signs and symptoms of bleeding
Recognition of signs and symptoms of thromboembolism
What to do if bleeding or thromboembolism occurs
Recognition of signs and symptoms of disease states that influence warfarin dosing requirements
Potential for interactions with prescription and over-the-counter medications and natural/herbal products
Dietary considerations and use of alcohol
Avoidance of pregnancy
Significance of informing other health care providers that warfarin has been prescribed
When, where, and with whom follow-up will be provided

farin should be provided. The health care provider who assumes responsibility for her outpatient warfarin therapy will need to provide continuing reinforcement of the essential elements of medication information at each follow-up visit.

FACTORS INFLUENCING DOSING

28. **After receiving 6 days of enoxaparin therapy and six doses of warfarin 4 mg/day PO, B.H.'s INR is 2.4. Enoxaparin is discontinued, and B.H. is instructed to continue her current dosage of warfarin. She is scheduled to return to the anticoagulation clinic in 1 week for re-evaluation. At that time, her INR is 1.7. What factors might account for this change in the intensity of anticoagulation?**

Numerous factors influence warfarin dosing requirements in individual patients during both the initiation and maintenance phases of therapy. Changes in dietary vitamin K intake, alcohol use, underlying disease states, and concurrent medications can significantly change the intensity of therapy, resulting in the need for dosing adjustments to maintain the INR within the therapeutic range.

Dietary Vitamin K Intake.   The two primary sources of vitamin K in humans are the biosynthesis of vitamin K_2 (menaquinone) by intestinal bacteria and dietary intake of vitamin K_1 (phytonadione). The recommended daily allowance (U.S. RDA) for vitamin K is 70 to 140 mcg/day, and the typical Western diet provides approximately 300 to 500 mcg/day.[69] Vitamin K is found in high concentrations in certain foods, including beef liver and pork liver, green leafy vegetables (asparagus, broccoli, Brussels sprouts, cabbage, cauliflower, chick peas, collard greens, endive, kale, lettuce, parsley, spinach, and turnip greens), soy milk, certain oils, certain nutritional supplements, and multiple vitamin products. Green tea and chewing tobacco are other significant sources of vitamin K.

Diets high in vitamin K content have been associated with acquired warfarin resistance, defined as excessive warfarin dosing requirements to reach a therapeutic INR range.[70] Numerous cases have been reported in which patients previously stabilized with warfarin experienced elevations in INR with or without hemorrhagic complications when dietary sources of vitamin K were eliminated. Conversely, reductions in INR with or without thromboembolic complications have been reported in patients in whom dietary sources of vitamin K have been added.

These cases illustrate the potential clinical significance of dietary changes in patients taking warfarin. To minimize these potential effects, B.H. should be counseled to maintain a *consistent* intake of dietary vitamin K. Her final warfarin maintenance dose will be partially influenced by her typical diet. However, restriction of dietary vitamin K intake is unnecessary, except in cases of significant resistance to warfarin's anticoagulant effect. B.H. should be aware of the types of foods that contain large quantities of vitamin K and should be counseled to maintain a consistent diet, to avoid bingeing with foods high in vitamin K content, and to report significant dietary changes to her health care provider. Appropriate assessment and follow-up are essential to prevent hemorrhagic or thromboembolic complications that may arise from changes in INR resulting from dietary alterations.

Alcohol Ingestion.   Chronic alcohol ingestion has been associated with induction of the hepatic enzyme systems that metabolize warfarin. Therefore, warfarin dosing requirements are sometimes higher in alcoholic patients. Conversely, acute ingestion of large amounts of alcohol can inhibit warfarin metabolism, leading to elevations in INR and an increased risk of bleeding complications.[71] In general, however, moderate intake of alcoholic beverages is not associated with alterations in the metabolism or the therapeutic effect of warfarin as measured by INR. B.H. does not need to abstain from drinking alcoholic beverages in moderation, but she should be counseled to avoid the sporadic ingestion of large amounts of alcohol.

Underlying Disease States.   The presence or exacerbation of various medical conditions can also influence anticoagulation status.[72] Diarrhea-associated alterations in intestinal flora can reduce vitamin K absorption, resulting in elevations in INR. Fever enhances the catabolism of clotting factors and can increase INR. Heart failure, hepatic congestion, and liver disease can also cause significant elevations in INR because of a reduction in warfarin metabolism.

Thyroid function can influence warfarin therapy significantly. Hypothyroidism decreases the catabolism of certain clotting factors, increasing their availability and producing a relative refractoriness to warfarin therapy. This results in the need for increased dosages to reach a therapeutic INR. The addition of thyroid supplementation in these patients reverses the influence of hypothyroidism and can lead to significant elevations in INR unless the warfarin dose is reduced. Conversely, hyperthyroidism increases the catabolism of clotting factors, leading to an increased sensitivity to warfarin. Frequent monitoring of and adjustments in warfarin therapy are necessary in patients with changing thyroid function.

Other Factors That Influence Warfarin Dosing Requirements. Acute physical or psychological stress has been reported to increase INR.[73] Increased physical activity has also been reported to increase the warfarin dosing requirement.[74] Smoking can induce CYP1A2, which may increase warfarin metabolism in certain patients.[75]

29. **How should B.H. be assessed and evaluated at this clinic appointment?**

At each clinic visit, regardless of the INR result, all factors that may influence B.H.'s anticoagulation status should be evaluated carefully. A patient assessment nomogram (Fig. 16-5) is a helpful tool to assist with patient evaluation.

The accuracy and reliability of the INR test should be considered. B.H. should be assessed thoroughly for signs and symptoms of thromboembolism and hemorrhage. Detailed questions should be asked to determine whether any changes in diet, alcohol intake, underlying disease states, concurrent

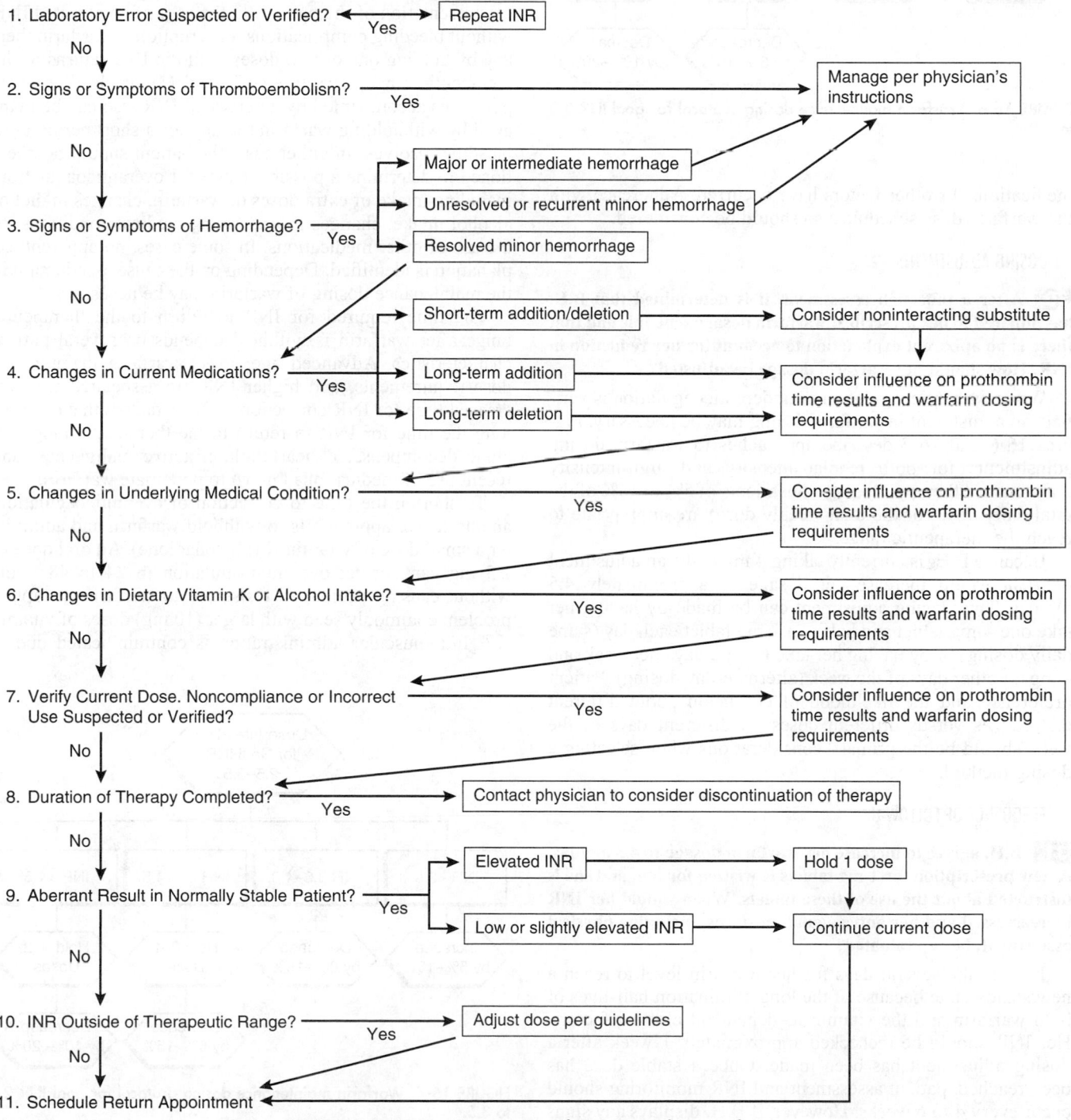

FIGURE 16-5 Assessment nomogram for patients taking warfarin.

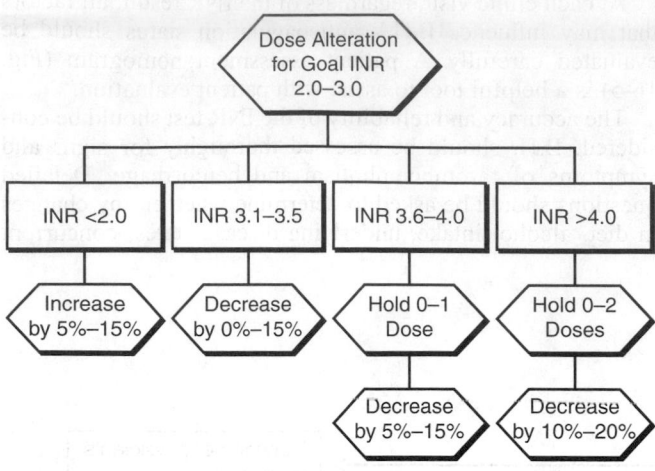

FIGURE 16-6 Warfarin maintenance dosing protocol for goal INR 2.0 to 3.0.

medications, or other factors have occurred. Adherence with the warfarin dose schedule also should be considered.

DOSING ADJUSTMENTS

30. After a thorough assessment, it is determined that B.H. has adhered to her prescribed warfarin dosage schedule and that there is no apparent explanation to account for her reduction in INR. How should her warfarin dosage be adjusted?

When overanticoagulation or underanticoagulation is verified, an adjustment in warfarin dosing may be necessary. Figures 16-6 and 16-7 describe approaches to warfarin dosing adjustments for both regular-intensity and high-intensity maintenance therapy. Dosing adjustments of 5% to 15% of the total daily dose (or the total weekly dose) are appropriate to reach the therapeutic range.

Because B.H. is currently taking 4 mg daily, an adjustment of 10% would increase her dosage to approximately 4.5 mg/day. This dosing adjustment can be made by having her take one 4-mg tablet and half of a 1-mg tablet each day (same daily dosing) or by having her take 6 mg 2 days per week and 4 mg all other days of the week (alternate-day dosing). Patient preference and the likelihood of confusion about different tablet sizes versus different doses on different days of the week should be the primary considerations when selecting a dosing method.[76]

FREQUENCY OF FOLLOW-UP

31. B.H. agrees to increase her warfarin dosage to 4.5 mg/day. A new prescription for 1-mg tablets is written for her, and she is instructed about the use of these tablets. When should her INR be reassessed and her anticoagulation status, including physical assessment, be re-evaluated?

It will take several days for her warfarin level to reach a new steady state because of the long elimination half-lives of both warfarin and the vitamin K–dependent clotting factors. Her INR should be rechecked approximately 1 week after a dosing adjustment has been made. Once a stable dose has been reached, patient assessment and INR monitoring should occur every 4 to 6 weeks. However, if B.H. displays any signs

of medical instability or nonadherence, a follow-up schedule of every 1 to 2 weeks is indicated (Table 16-12).

MANAGEMENT OF OVERANTICOAGULATION

32. E.M., who has been taking warfarin for 6 months with good laboratory control, noted a slight pink color to his urine. In the ED, an INR of 5.6 was reported. His Hct and hemoglobin (Hgb) were both within normal limits, as were his vital signs. A stool Hemoccult test was negative, but urinalysis revealed >50 red blood cells per high-power field. How should this adverse effect of warfarin be treated in E.M.?

Management of overanticoagulation depends on the clinical presentation of the patient. In the case of an elevated INR without bleeding complications, interruption of warfarin therapy by holding one or two doses until the INR returns to the therapeutic range usually is sufficient. Minor bleeding complications accompanied by an elevated INR also can be managed by withholding warfarin therapy for a short period until bleeding resolves. In either case, the patient should be questioned to determine a possible cause for overanticoagulation, including intake of extra doses of warfarin, changes in diet or alcohol intake, changes in underlying medical conditions, or the use of other medications. In some cases, no apparent explanation is identified. Depending on the cause, a reduction in the maintenance dosing of warfarin may be necessary.

The time required for INR to return to the therapeutic range after warfarin is withheld depends on several patient characteristics. Advanced age, lower warfarin maintenance dose requirements, and higher INR are associated with increased time for INR correction.[77] Other factors that can prolong the time for INR to return to the therapeutic range include decompensated heart failure, active malignancy, and recent use of medications known to potentiate warfarin.

To shorten the time to correction of overanticoagulation, an alternative approach is to withhold warfarin and administer a small dose of vitamin K (phytonadione). An oral dose of 2.5 mg can correct overanticoagulation in 24 to 48 hours without causing prolonged resistance to warfarin therapy, a problem commonly seen with larger (10 mg) doses of vitamin K.[78] Intramuscular administration is contraindicated due to

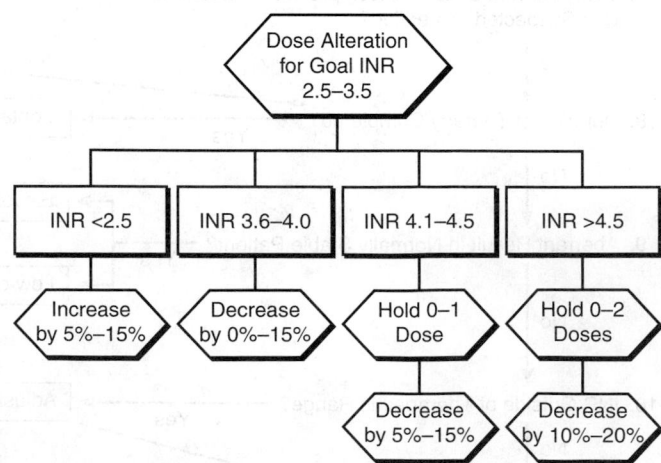

FIGURE 16-7 Warfarin maintenance dosing protocol for goal INR 2.5 to 3.5.

Table 16-12 Frequency of INR Monitoring and Patient Assessment During Warfarin Therapy

Initiation Therapy

Flexible initiation method	Daily through day 4, then within 3–5 days
Average daily dosing method	Within 3–5 days, then within 1 wk
After hospital discharge	If stable, within 3–5 days; If unstable, within 1–3 days
First month of therapy	Weekly

Maintenance Therapy

Dose held today	In 1–2 days
Dosage change today	Within 1–2 wk
Dosage change <2 wks ago	Within 2–4 wk
Routine follow-up of medically stable and reliable patients	Every 4–6 wk
Routine follow-up of medically unstable or unreliable patients	Every 1–2 wk

the risk of hematoma formation, and SC administration of vitamin K is not recommended because of variable absorption.[79]

IV doses of 0.5 to 1 mg of vitamin K can correct overanticoagulation within 24 hours.[80] This approach is also useful for reversal of therapeutic anticoagulation prior to invasive procedures and can be used to correct overanticoagulation in high-risk cases. IV vitamin K should be diluted and administered by slow infusion over 30 to 60 minutes to prevent flushing, hypotension, and cardiovascular collapse.[81] Although these symptoms resemble anaphylaxis, the mechanism of this adverse response is unclear: it is not known if it is caused by phytonadione or by the vehicle in which phytonadione is formulated. If this adverse reaction occurs, administration of epinephrine may be indicated, as well as other standard measures to support blood pressure and maintain the airway.

Rapid reversal of warfarin therapy is indicated in the setting of major, life-threatening bleeding. Fresh frozen plasma or factor concentrates to replace clotting factors will decrease the INR for 4 to 6 hours and should be administered as needed with careful monitoring of volume status. Supplementation with high-dose IV vitamin K (10 mg) also may be indicated. IV administration will reverse the effects of warfarin within 6 to 12 hours. However, if continued warfarin therapy is indicated when bleeding resolves, anticoagulation with heparin may be necessary for as long as 7 to 14 days until the effect of high-dose vitamin K is diminished and warfarin responsiveness returns.

Hematuria may be an early sign of more serious bleeding, but in many cases this condition is associated with only minor bleeding episodes. In a reliable patient, discontinuing warfarin until the INR returns to a therapeutic level usually suffices. A more rapid return to normal can be accomplished if low-dose vitamin K is administered. Because E.M. appears to be bleeding only into the urine and is hemodynamically stable, withholding warfarin and administering 2.5 mg of oral vi-

tamin K is appropriate. A thorough workup to evaluate the source of bleeding is indicated.

EFFECT ON MENSTRUATION

33. **J.Y., a 26-year-old woman, is taking warfarin. What instructions should be provided to J.Y. concerning the effect of warfarin on menstrual flow?**

Menstrual blood flow may be increased and prolonged in patients taking anticoagulants. This problem may be clinically significant if there is an underlying pathologic condition (ovarian cysts, uterine fibroids or polyps) resulting in abnormal vaginal bleeding. J.Y. should be advised to have her INR checked at least monthly. Should unusually heavy or excessively prolonged menstrual or breakthrough bleeding occur, gynecologic evaluation should be obtained because of the risk of an ovarian hemorrhage.

USE IN PREGNANCY

34. **E.S., a 30-year-old woman, has been taking warfarin for continuing therapy of a resolved PE. She has just learned she is pregnant. What effects might warfarin have on the fetus? Are UFH or LMWHs safer alternatives in this situation?**

Coumarin anticoagulants cross the placental barrier and may place the fetus at risk for hemorrhage and teratogenic effects.[82] Up to 30% of pregnancies that involve exposure to coumarins result in abnormal liveborn infants, and up to 30% in spontaneous abortion or stillbirth. Congenital abnormalities such as stippled calcifications and nasal cartilage hypoplasia primarily occurred in infants born to mothers receiving warfarin during the first trimester of pregnancy, with the highest risk during weeks 6 to 12. Other abnormalities, involving the central nervous system and eyes, are more likely to occur when the mother is taking warfarin later in the pregnancy. In addition, because warfarin crosses the placenta, fatal bleeding complications may occur.

Women of childbearing age who require anticoagulation should be counseled about options for contraception. Patients who become pregnant while receiving warfarin should be informed of the risks of continued anticoagulation to the fetus, as well as the risk to themselves of discontinuing anticoagulation.

Other options for pregnant women who require anticoagulation include UFH and LMWHs. Because these agents do not cross the placenta, they are preferred over warfarin for use in pregnancy.[83] UFH is typically recommended because it has been used extensively during pregnancy. However, many clinical trials have validated the safety and efficacy of LMWHs in the prevention and treatment of DVT and PE during pregnancy.[84] These agents represent an alternative to UFH, with advantages as previously described. When used at full doses for the treatment of venous thromboembolism during pregnancy, dosing must be adjusted throughout the pregnancy to account for the expected increase in the body weight of the mother and the reported increase in clearance of LMWH during pregnancy.[85]

In pregnant patients with mechanical heart valves, there is controversy regarding the use of LMHWs.[86] Several cases of valvular thrombosis and of maternal and fetal death have been reported. These cases may be the result of underdosing of

LMWH, and UFH.[87] Table 16-13 describes recommendations for anticoagulation during and after pregnancy for various conditions.

After being informed of the risks associated with warfarin, E.S. decided to continue her pregnancy and to begin anticoagulation with UFH. Warfarin therapy should be discontinued immediately and UFH initiated using SC treatment doses as previously described, or by continuous IV infusion. Dosing adjustments may be required throughout pregnancy as determined by aPTT monitoring. Potential adverse effects of UFH use, including hemorrhage, thrombocytopenia, and osteoporosis, should be monitored appropriately.

SC Heparin should be discontinued 24 hours before elective induction of labor and resumed as soon as bleeding from delivery has been controlled. IV heparin should be discontinued 6 hours before delivery. Warfarin therapy can then be safely reinitiated. If spontaneous labor occurs, protamine can be used to reverse the effect of UFH. Warfarin is not secreted in breast milk; therefore, E.S. can safely breast-feed.

PREVENTION OF CARDIOGENIC THROMBOEMBOLISM

Atrial Fibrillation

Anticoagulation Before Cardioversion

35. C.D., a 68-year-old woman with hypertension, presents to the cardiology clinic complaining of several days of fatigue and a "racing heart." On physical examination, her pulse is irregularly irregular and her heart rate is approximately 120 beats/min. Using ECG, a diagnosis of atrial fibrillation is made and cardioversion planned. Should C.D. be anticoagulated before cardioversion?

In atrial fibrillation, compromised atrial activity as well as atrial enlargement causes stasis of blood within the atria and the left atrial appendage, often resulting in atrial thrombus formation. Atrial thrombus formation increases the risk of systemic embolization; clinical manifestations include arterial embolization of the extremities or embolization of the splenic, renal, or abdominal arteries. However, the most prevalent site of embolization is the cerebral arterial system, resulting in either asymptomatic cerebral infarction or stroke with potentially devastating neurologic and functional impairment.[88]

Both direct current cardioversion and pharmacologic cardioversion using antiarrhythmic drugs expose patients with atrial fibrillation to an initial short-term increase in stroke risk from embolization secondary to resumption of normal atrial mechanical activity (see Chapter 20, Cardiac Arrhythmias). Data from a prospective cohort study of 437 patients noted a stroke incidence of 5.3% in patients with atrial fibrillation who were cardioverted without prior anticoagulation, but a significant reduction in stroke incidence to 0.8% was noted if patients who had received cardioversion were anticoagulated.[89] In addition to preventing the development of new atrial thrombi, anticoagulation allows any thrombus that may be present to endothelialize and adhere to the atrial wall so that the thromboembolic risk is minimized. Based on the as-

Table 16-13 Recommendations for Anticoagulation During Pregnancy

Clinical Situation	Peripartum Options	Postpartum
1. Prophylaxis		
Known hypercoagulable state with no prior history of VTE	• Surveillance • Minidose UFH • Prophylactic LMWH	Warfarin to INR 2–3 for 4–6 weeks with UFH/LMWH overlap until INR >2.0
Single prior episode of VTE associated with transient risk factors, not receiving long term anticoagulants	• Surveillance	Warfarin to INR 2–3 for 4–6 weeks with UFH/LMWH overlap until INR >2.0
Single prior episode of idiopathic or thrombophilia-related VTE, not receiving long-term anticoagulants	• Surveillance • Minidose UFH • Moderate-dose UFH • Prophylactic LMWH	Warfarin to INR 2–3 for 4–6 weeks with UFH/LMWH overlap until INR >2.0
Multiple prior episodes of VTE and/or receiving long term oral anticoagulants for VTE	• Adjusted-dose UFH • Prophylactic LMWH • Full-dose LMWH	Long-term warfarin to INR 2–3 with UFH/LMWH overlap until INR >2.0
Long-term oral anticoagulants for mechanical valve replacement	• Adjusted-dose UFH • Full-dose LMWH	Long-term warfarin to prior INR goal with UFH/LMWH overlap until INR above lower limit of therapeutic range
2. Treatment of VTE that occurs during pregnancy	• IV UFH for ≥5 days, followed by adjusted-dose UFH • Full-dose LMWH	Warfarin to INR 2–3 for a minimum of 6 wks with UFH/LMWH overlap until INR >2.0

VTE, venous thromboembolic disease; UFH, unfractionated heparin; LMWH, low-molecular-weight heparin; INR, International Normalized Ratio.
Minidose UFH: 5,000 U SQ Q 12 hr. Moderate-dose UFH: adjusted to 0.1–0.3 U/ml anti-X_a activity. Adjusted-dose UFH: adjusted to maintain therapeutic aPTT at mid-dosing interval. Prophylactic LMWH: enoxaparin 40 mg SQ QD or dalteparin 5,000 U SQ QD. Full-dose LMWH: enoxaparin 1 mg/kg SQ Q 12 hr or dalteparin 200 IU/kg and adjusted throughout pregnancy to maintain 4-hr-postinjection anti-X_a activity level of 0.5–1.2 U/mL (VTE) or approximately 1.0 U/mL (mechanical valves).

sumed time course of thrombus development, as well as the presumed time course of clot endothelialization, patients who have been in atrial fibrillation for >48 hours should receive 3 weeks of anticoagulation with warfarin to an INR of 2.0 to 3.0 before cardioversion is attempted.[88] Despite a lower risk of stroke than that associated with atrial fibrillation, patients with atrial flutter should be treated similarly.

Whether C.D. has been in atrial fibrillation for <48 hours is not known; therefore, she requires a 3-week course of therapeutic anticoagulation with a goal INR range of 2.0 to 3.0 before cardioversion is attempted. If C.D. cannot tolerate her heart symptoms despite control of the ventricular response rate, her medical team might consider immediate cardioversion without anticoagulation if transesophageal echocardiography (TEE) is used to rule out left atrial thrombi. Transthoracic echocardiography is not sensitive enough to visualize the left atrium and the left atrial appendage, but TEE is much more sensitive (although somewhat less than 100%).

In a clinical trial, 1222 patients with atrial fibrillation of more than 2 days' duration were randomly assigned to either treatment guided by TEE findings, or to conventional precardioversion anticoagulation.[90] Patients assigned to conventional treatment and patients in the TEE group in whom thrombus was detected received a 3-week course of warfarin prior to cardioversion. Patients without detectable thrombus by TEE were cardioverted without precardioversion anticoagulation. All patients received 4 weeks of postcardioversion anticoagulation. Thromboembolic rates were identical between patients who received conventional treatment and those whose treatment was guided by TEE (0.5% versus 0.8%, $P = 0.5$).

Anticoagulation After Cardioversion

36. After 3 weeks of regular-intensity warfarin therapy, C.D. is successfully cardioverted. Should warfarin be discontinued?

Despite normalization of atrial electrical activity, restoration of effective atrial mechanical activity after cardioversion of atrial fibrillation can be delayed for up to 3 weeks. In addition, a significant number of patients with atrial fibrillation who initially are cardioverted successfully revert to atrial fibrillation during the first month. Both of these factors contribute to the recognized delay in stroke presentation after cardioversion in patients with atrial fibrillation. For these reasons, anticoagulation with warfarin should be continued after successful cardioversion until normal sinus rhythm has been maintained for 4 weeks.

Anticoagulation for Chronic Atrial Fibrillation

37. Two weeks after successful cardioversion, C.D. presents to the ED with chest palpitations and light-headedness. An ECG is evaluated, and atrial fibrillation is diagnosed again. What decisions regarding anticoagulation need to be made?

ANTICOAGULATION IN VALVULAR ATRIAL FIBRILLATION

Atrial fibrillation secondary to valvular heart disease historically has been recognized as a significant risk factor for stroke. Patients with atrial fibrillation who have a history of rheumatic valvular disease have a 17-fold higher incidence of stroke than in matched controls. Patients with valvular atrial fibrillation require long-term, regular-intensity anticoagula-

tion to a goal INR of 2.0 to 3.0 to prevent thromboembolism and stroke.[88]

ANTICOAGULATION IN NONVALVULAR ATRIAL FIBRILLATION

Nonvalvular heart disease is the most common cause of atrial fibrillation and, like valvular heart disease, represents a significant risk for stroke in patients with atrial fibrillation. Five clinical trials have substantiated the role of warfarin in the primary prevention of systemic embolization and stroke in chronic, nonvalvular atrial fibrillation.[91] All five trials compared warfarin with a placebo and were terminated before completion because of the substantial benefit of warfarin. In comparison with a placebo, warfarin significantly reduced the risk of stroke from approximately 5% per year to approximately 2% per year, with an average relative risk reduction of 67%. Based on the results of these trials, long-term anticoagulation with warfarin to a goal INR of 2.5 (range, 2.0 to 3.0) is recommended in patients like C.D. who have atrial fibrillation secondary to nonvalvular heart disease.[88]

Several clinical trials have attempted to define the comparative efficacy of warfarin versus aspirin in the prevention of stroke associated with atrial fibrillation.[92] Compared with a placebo or control, aspirin decreases the risk of stroke in patients with atrial fibrillation. However, that reduction is not as substantial as the reduction seen with warfarin. In clinical trials comparing warfarin and aspirin, the risk reduction associated with warfarin is significantly larger than that of aspirin. However, aspirin may be appropriate in certain patients at low risk for stroke associated with atrial fibrillation (see Table 16-5).

The decision to continue long-term anticoagulation with warfarin in C.D. should be based on an evaluation of the likelihood that her atrial fibrillation will become chronic and not amenable to cardioversion, as well as an assessment of her risk of stroke compared with her risk of warfarin-associated bleeding complications. Because of her age and history of hypertension, the appropriate strategy should be long-term warfarin therapy with a goal INR of 2.5 (range, 2.0 to 3.0).

Cardiac Valve Replacement
Mechanical Prosthetic Valves

38. D.L., a 56-year-old woman with a history of rheumatic mitral valve disease, has undergone mitral valve replacement. A St. Jude (bileaflet mechanical) valve has been implanted, and heparin therapy is initiated postoperatively. Does D.L. require continued anticoagulation with warfarin?

Mechanical prosthetic valves confer a significant thromboembolic risk by providing a foreign surface in contact with blood components on which platelet aggregation and thrombus formation can occur. Valvular thrombosis can impair the integrity of valve function and can lead to embolization with systemic manifestations, including stroke.[93] The incidence of thromboembolic complications depends on the type of artificial valve (caged ball [Starr-Edwards] > tilting disk [Medtronic-Hall; Bjork-Shiley] > bileaflet [St. Jude]) as well as the anatomic position of the replacement (dual valve replacement > mitral > aortic).[94]

Long-term anticoagulation is required in patients with mechanical valve replacement because it significantly reduces the risk of stroke and other manifestations of systemic embolization. Trials comparing different intensities of oral anticoagulation with warfarin in mechanical valve replacement helped identify the intensity of anticoagulation that protects against thromboembolic risk while reducing the incidence of hemorrhagic complications.[94,95] Patients with mechanical valve replacement should receive long-term preventive anticoagulant therapy with warfarin to prolong the PT to an INR of 3.0 (range, 2.5 to 3.5).[93] Patients with bileaflet mechanical heart valves in the aortic position and who are in normal sinus rhythm with a normal ejection fraction and normal left atrial size are at reduced risk for valvular thrombosis and systemic embolization.[96] These patients can be anticoagulated to an INR of 2.5 (range, 2.0 to 3.0).

Bioprosthetic Valves

39. **E.K., an 86-year-old woman with a history of symptomatic aortic stenosis, has received a bioprosthetic (mammalian) aortic valve replacement. Is anticoagulant therapy required in E.K.?**

Prosthetic heart valves extracted from mammalian sources (porcine or bovine xenografts; homografts) are significantly less thrombogenic than mechanical prosthetic valves. The period of greatest thromboembolic risk appears to be during the first 3 months after implantation. Therefore, short-term, regular-intensity, preventive anticoagulation to an INR of 2.5 (range, 2.0 to 3.0) is recommended.[93] After this period, long-term aspirin therapy (minimum dose, 162 mg/day) is indicated. However, oral anticoagulation should be continued long term in patients with concurrent atrial fibrillation, a history of systemic embolism, or evidence of atrial thrombus at surgery.

Combined Anticoagulant/Antiplatelet Therapy

40. **W.W., a 69-year-old man, underwent mitral valve replacement 6 months ago with a mechanical valve prosthesis. Anticoagulation with warfarin resulted in stable INR values within the therapeutic range of 2.5 to 3.5. Despite adequate anticoagulation, he recently developed episodes of transient intermittent visual field and speech disturbances. Neurologic evaluation concluded that W.W. was having transient ischemic attacks (TIAs). Can antiplatelet therapy be added without increasing the risk of hemorrhagic complications?**

The primary approach to preventing valvular thrombosis and systemic thromboembolism associated with mechanical prosthetic valve replacement is anticoagulation with warfarin. If there is evidence of thromboembolism despite adequate anticoagulation, the addition of an antiplatelet agent is indicated.

In early studies, high-dose aspirin (500 mg/day) in combination with warfarin reduced the rate of systemic thromboembolism in patients with mechanical prosthetic valves, but was associated with an unacceptable risk of major bleeding. However, a trial comparing warfarin alone (adjusted to an INR of 3.0 to 4.5) and warfarin combined with low-dose aspirin (100 mg/day) in 370 patients with mechanical valve replacements or with tissue valve prostheses and underlying atrial fibrillation or a history of thromboembolism found a significant reduction in the incidence of systemic thromboembolism, as well as reduced mortality, in the combination therapy group.[97] Although the incidence of total bleeding was higher in patients receiving both warfarin and low-dose as-

pirin, this difference resulted entirely from differences in clinically insignificant minor bleeding. Major bleeding episodes were similar in both groups.

More recently, a clinical trial evaluated the efficacy and safety of very high-intensity oral anticoagulation (INR, 3.5 to 4.5) versus high-intensity oral anticoagulation (INR, 2.5 to 3.5) plus aspirin 100 mg/day in patients with mechanical valve prostheses.[98] In the group receiving combination therapy, the reported rate of thromboembolic events was 1.3% per year, similar to that of the group receiving very high-intensity therapy. The major bleeding rate was 1.1% per year, substantially lower than in the group receiving very high-intensity therapy.

Patients with mechanical prosthetic heart valves occasionally develop systemic thromboembolism despite adequate anticoagulation. In these patients, like W.W., the addition of an antiplatelet agent may be of benefit. Low-dose aspirin in combination with warfarin appears to offer an advantage in this setting while minimizing the potential for clinically significant major bleeding events.

Left Ventricular Thrombosis
In Dilated Cardiomyopathy

41. **Idiopathic cardiomyopathy has recently been diagnosed in M.F., a 39-year-old man with a left ventricular ejection fraction estimated at 18%. What is the risk of left ventricular thrombus formation in M.F.? Is preventive anticoagulation indicated?**

Left ventricular thrombus formation in dilated cardiomyopathy occurs as a result of intracavitary stasis because of systolic dysfunction. The resultant reduction in blood flow, often specifically in the apex of the left ventricle, represents a persistent risk for left ventricular thrombus formation and resultant systemic embolization, including stroke.[99]

The cause of dilated cardiomyopathy (i.e., ischemic or nonischemic) does not affect the risk of thromboembolism. The Vasodilators in Heart Failure (Ve-HeFT) trials substantiated an overall thromboembolic risk of 2.2% to 2.5% per year in patients with cardiomyopathy, regardless of the cause.[100,101] However, the degree of left ventricular dysfunction influences the risk of stroke. In a retrospective analysis of data from the Survival and Ventricular Enlargement (SAVE) trial (a placebo-controlled evaluation of angiotensin-converting enzyme [ACE] inhibitors after MI), the risk of stroke was found to increase as ejection fraction declined below 35%.[102] The overall risk of stroke was 1.5% per year of follow-up, and each 5% reduction in ejection fraction increased the cumulative risk of stroke by 18%. Anticoagulant therapy appeared to provide a protective effect in reducing the risk of stroke.

The role of anticoagulation in preventing thromboembolic events, including stroke, in patients with cardiomyopathy has not been evaluated in a randomized, placebo-controlled trial. However, data from other sources suggest a beneficial effect. In a cohort analysis of data from the Studies of Left Ventricular Dysfunction (SOLVD) trial (a placebo-controlled evaluation of ACE inhibitors in patients with an ejection fraction of <35%), warfarin therapy was associated with a significant reduction in overall mortality and in the risk of death or hospital admission for heart failure.[103]

Based on these data, it is suggested that patients with cardiomyopathy and an ejection fraction of <35%, like M.F., should receive long-term anticoagulation with warfarin to an

INR of 2.5 (range, 2.0 to 3.0).[104] If the patient-specific risk of bleeding is thought to be greater than the potential benefit of oral anticoagulation, aspirin should be considered as a substitute for warfarin therapy.

Following Myocardial Infarction

42. M.M, a 55-year-old woman with hypercholesterolemia and a 22-pack/year smoking history, recently sustained an anterior transmural MI. She was treated with thrombolytic therapy in the ED, and heparin was initiated. Is continued anticoagulation with warfarin indicated after her discharge from the hospital?

The primary role of anticoagulation in patients with MI is the prevention of coronary artery rethrombosis and reinfarction (see Chapter 18). The risk of venous thromboembolism (DVT, PE) also is substantial in this patient population because of prolonged immobilization during hospitalization and is reduced significantly by preventive anticoagulant therapy.[104] However, an additional source of thrombus formation is the infarcted myocardium. Abnormalities of intracardiac flow in areas of akinesis or dyskinesis, as well as the inflammatory changes at the endocardial surface of the infarcted myocardium, represent transient, additive risk factors for the development of left ventricular thrombi. These mural thrombi occur in up to 40% of patients following anterior MI and are associated with a risk of systemic embolization, including stroke. The risk of stroke following all MIs is 1% to 3%, and as high as 2% to 6% following anterior MI.

Anticoagulation with warfarin after an anterior MI significantly reduces the risk of systemic embolization and stroke and appears to be more effective than aspirin.[102,105] Based on the high incidence of left ventricular thrombus formation after anterior MI and the risk of stroke associated with mural thrombi, M.M. should be anticoagulated with warfarin for up to 3 months at a dosage sufficient to prolong the INR to 2.5 (range, 2.0 to 3.0).[104] An echocardiogram before hospital discharge will document the presence of mural thrombi, as well as determine left ventricular wall motion. The absence of mural thrombus on an initial echocardiogram does not preclude preventive anticoagulation because of the possibility of delayed clot formation. However, if left ventricular thrombus or significant wall motion abnormalities are evident on follow-up echocardiography at 3 months, continued anticoagulation is indicated.

BRIDGE THERAPY

Management of Anticoagulation Around Invasive Procedures

43. C.G. is a 43-year-old woman with a history of valvular heart disease associated with Marfan's syndrome. She has a St. Jude mitral valve replacement and is anticoagulated with warfarin 7.5 mg QD to a goal INR range of 2.5 to 3.5. Recently she has complained of episodic rectal bleeding despite adequate anticoagulation. She is scheduled for colonoscopy in several weeks. Her gastroenterologist calls you at the anticoagulation clinic to determine the most appropriate plan for reversal of her warfarin prior to the procedure. What are the options?

When an invasive procedure is planned, it is often necessary to reverse the effects of warfarin to minimize the risk of bleeding complications associated with the procedure, which can be worsened by the presence of an anticoagulant. It can take several days for the anticoagulant effect of warfarin to be reversed after discontinuation of the drug, but in that period of time, a patient may be at risk for thromboembolic complications associated with underanticoagulation. *Bridge therapy* is the term that refers to the use of a relatively short-acting injectable anticoagulant (UFH, LMWH) as a substitute for warfarin prior to and immediately following an invasive procedure.[106] Because UFH and LMWH have shorter elimination half-lives than warfarin, they can be stopped just prior to the invasive procedure without increasing the risk of bleeding associated with the procedure. In addition, because of their shorter onset of effect, they can be used while warfarin is restarted and until the INR reaches the therapeutic range.

Although bridge therapy has not been studied in randomized clinical trials, there are multiple options, many of which have been evaluated in case series.[107] The choice of a bridge therapy strategy depends on the risk of bleeding associated with continued anticoagulation for the surgery or procedure to be performed, and on the risk of thromboembolism associated with underanticoagulation in the patient in question. Individualized risk assessment and bridge therapy planning are necessary for each patient who may require temporary discontinuation of warfarin.

Since the use of IV UFH for bridge therapy requires hospitalization, there has been considerable interest in using LMWH on an outpatient basis for this purpose. Several case series have described successful use of LMWH in various populations, including patients with valve replacement.[108,109] As a bridge therapy strategy prior to colonoscopy, outpatient LWMH has been found to be considerably more cost-effective than inpatient UFH.[110] UFH, however, may be appropriate in patients with significant renal impairment, or in patients without third-party prescription coverage who cannot afford LMWH. A guideline for bridge therapy based on the risk of thromboembolism and on renal function is presented in Table 16-14.

Since C.G. has a mechanical valve replacement, her risk of thromboembolism associated with underanticoagulation is considered high. Therefore, warfarin should not simply be withheld; instead, she should receive bridge therapy with an injectable anticoagulant. Her renal function is normal, and her health care insurance covers injectable drugs. Therefore, her plan will include early discontinuation of warfarin 3 to 5 days prior to the procedure, and substitution with enoxaparin 1 mg/kg Q 12 hours when the INR falls below the lower limit of the therapeutic range. The last dose of enoxaparin should be given no later than 12 hours prior to the procedure to minimize the risk of bleeding at the time of the procedure. After the procedure, warfarin should be restarted at her usual dose and enoxaparin should be continued until the INR is >2.5.

Management of Anticoagulation Around Dental Procedures

44. A.V. is a 76-year-old man with a history of hypertension, hypercholesterolemia, adult-onset diabetes, and atrial fibrillation. He receives warfarin 2.5 mg on Monday, Wednesday, and Friday and 5 mg all other days for stroke prevention. He is scheduled to have a tooth removed, and his dentist has recommended that warfarin be withheld for 5 days prior to the procedure. He calls his anticoagulation provider for advice. What is your response?

Table 16-14 Bridge Therapy Guidelines for Invasive Procedures[a]

Thromboembolic Risk	Renal Function	Bridge Therapy
High • Atrial fibrillation (moderate to high stroke risk) • History of stroke/TIA • Hypercoagulable states • Mechanical valve • History of DVT/PE <3 mo ago	Cl_{cr} >30	• Last dose of warfarin on day −5 pre-procedure • Enoxaparin 1mg/kg Q 12 hr starting at 6 AM on day −3 • Vitamin K 2.5 mg PO on day −3 • Last dose of enoxaparin by 6 PM on day −1 • Resume enoxaparin or UFH 12–24 hr post-procedure and continue until INR > lower limit of therapeutic range • Resume warfarin 12–48 hr post-procedure using usual maintenance dose
	Cl_{cr} ≤30	• Last dose of warfarin on day −3 pre-procedure • Vitamin K 2.5 mg PO on day −2 • Admit on day −1 and begin IV UFH (70 U/kg bolus, 15 U/kg/hr and adjust per inpatient protocol) • If INR >1.5 on day −1, give vitamin K 1 mg IV • Stop IV UFH 6 hr pre-procedure • Resume UFH 12–24 hr post-procedure and continue until INR > lower limit of therapeutic range • Resume warfarin 12-48 hours post-procedure at usual maintenance dose
Low • Atrial fibrillation (low to moderate stroke risk) • Dilated cardiomyopathy with no history of thrombosis • History of DVT/PE >3 mo ago	all patients	• Last dose of warfarin on day −4 pre-procedure • Consider vitamin K 2.5 mg PO on day −2 if delayed reversal of oral anticoagulation is anticipated • Resume warfarin 12–48 hours post-procedure at usual maintenance dose

[a]University of Washington Medical Center Anticoagulation Clinics
DVT, deep vein thrombosis; PE, pulmonary embolism; UFH, unfractionated heparin; TIA, transient ischemic attack; IV, intravenous.

Based on his medical history, A.V. is considered at moderate to high risk for stroke. If his warfarin were to be discontinued for 5 days prior to this dental procedure, he would require bridge therapy with inpatient UFH or outpatient LMWH prior to the procedure, and afterward until his INR reached 2.0. However, for many dental procedures, it is often not necessary to withhold warfarin.[111] Oral bleeding can be prevented or controlled using a combination of local measures, including cold water rinse, local pressure (biting on gauze or tea bags [which release tannins, causing local vasoconstriction]), additional suturing, or electrocautery. Other options include packing the site with gelatin sponges (Gelfoam) or absorbable oxycellulose (Surgicel), or applying microcrystalline collagen (Avitene), topical thrombin, or a fibrin adhesive. A mouth rinse of 5% tranexamic acid or 5% aminocaproic acid can also be used to control oral bleeding.[112] Patients are instructed to hold 10 mL of the rinse in their mouths for 2 minutes, 30 minutes prior to the procedure, and then to repeat every 2 hours as needed afterward until bleeding is resolved. Table 16-15 describes guidelines for the management of warfarin around dental procedures based on the bleeding risk of the procedure.

The simple extraction planned for A.V. does not require discontinuation of his warfarin therapy. The anticoagulation clinic provider should call the dentist to offer suggestions regarding local prevention and control of oral bleeding. A.V. should be cautioned to avoid hot liquid, vigorous mouthwashes, hard foods, and NSAIDs and other antiplatelet agents during the first 24 to 48 hours after his tooth extraction.

DRUG INTERACTIONS
Interactions With Legend Drugs

45. D.G., a 72-year-old man, received a Bjork-Shiley tilting disk mitral valve prosthesis 5 years ago. He has been anticoagulated with warfarin 6 mg/day with good control. He is allergic to ampicillin and has gastric intolerance to tetracycline. Yesterday, he was seen in an acute-care clinic with symptoms of an acute prostatic infection and prescribed one double-strength tablet of trimethoprim-sulfamethoxazole (TMP-SMX) BID for 10 days. How will the combination of warfarin and TMP-SMX (Bactrim, Septra) affect D.G.'s anticoagulation control? Should his warfarin dosage be adjusted or another drug substituted for TMP-SMX?

Drug interactions with warfarin occur by a number of different mechanisms and can have a significant impact on the anticoagulant effect of warfarin.[113] Elevations or reductions in INR have been observed when interacting drugs are added to or discontinued from the medication regimens of patients taking warfarin or when used intermittently. Clinically significant hemorrhagic or thromboembolic complications can result. Careful selection of both prescription and nonprescription medications, appropriate INR monitoring, and detailed patient education regarding drug interactions are important interventions for pharmacists caring for patients taking warfarin. A summary of drugs that interact with warfarin, including mechanisms of interaction and effect on INR, is provided in Table 16-16.

Table 16-15   Suggestions for Anticoagulation Management Before and After Dental Procedures[a]

	Low Bleeding Risk	Moderate Bleeding Risk	High Bleeding Risk
Procedure	• Supragingival scaling • Simple restorations • Local anesthetic injections	• Subgingival scaling • Restorations with subgingival preparations • Standard root canal therapy • Simple extractions • Regional injection of local anesthetics	• Extensive surgery • Apicoectomy (root removal) • Alveolar surgery (bone removal) • Multiple extractions
Suggestions	• Do not interrupt warfarin treatment • Use local measures to prevent/control bleeding	• Interruption of warfarin treatment is not necessary • Use local measures to prevent or control bleeding *Consult with dentist to determine comfort with use of local measures to prevent bleeding when anticoagulation is not interrupted*	• May need to reduce INR or return to normal hemostasis • Follow bridge therapy guidelines for invasive procedures based on risk of thromboembolism

[a]University of Washington Medical Center Anticoagulation Clinics

Although warfarin is highly bound to protein, primarily to albumin, and can be displaced from protein-binding sites by a number of weakly acidic drugs, these interactions typically do not result in clinically significant elevations in PT/INR.[114] Warfarin displaced from protein-binding sites is readily available for elimination by hepatic metabolism, resulting in increased clearance without a significant change in the free drug concentration.

Other types of interactions with warfarin are much more significant. Pharmacodynamic interactions are those that alter the physiology of hemostasis, particularly interactions that influence the synthesis or degradation of clotting factors or that increase the risk of bleeding through inhibition of platelet aggregation. Pharmacokinetic interactions influence the absorption and metabolism of warfarin, and many clinically significant interactions with warfarin occur when warfarin metabolism is induced or inhibited. Interactions involving agents known to influence the hepatic microsomal enzyme systems responsible for the metabolism of the more potent (S)-warfarin (CYP2C9) are potentially more significant than those that influence the enzymes that metabolize (R)-warfarin (CYP1A2, CYP3A4).[115]

Sulfamethoxazole can increase the effect of warfarin significantly by stereoselectively inhibiting the metabolism of the more potent S-enantiomer of warfarin.[113] Potentiation of warfarin activity after inhibition of metabolism usually takes several days, and the effect may be slow to resolve once the offending agent is discontinued. In addition, fever associated with the infection for which TMP-SMX has been prescribed may enhance the catabolism of vitamin K–dependent clotting factors, resulting in an accentuated hypoprothrombinemic response. This effect will dissipate as the fever abates with antibiotic therapy.

For D.G., the best choice would be to discontinue TMP-SMX. Because ampicillin and tetracycline are contraindicated, either a first-generation cephalosporin or TMP alone may be used. Oral quinolones should be avoided because they also carry the risk of potentiating the anticoagulant effect of warfarin. Careful monitoring of the INR should continue because the introduction of any changes in treatment, as well as the acute illness, may alter the patient's response to warfarin therapy.

If these options are not appropriate, warfarin therapy is not an absolute contraindication to the use of TMP-SMX. TMP-SMX can be prescribed if D.G. is monitored frequently and carefully, with adjustment of warfarin dosages as necessary to maintain his INR within the therapeutic INR range of 2.5 to 3.5 and with attention to potential hemorrhagic complications. No initial change in the dosage of warfarin should be made, because it may take several days for the interaction to be apparent.

46. **D.R. is a 39-year-old woman recovering from unexplained ventricular fibrillation several weeks ago with significant, but improving, neurologic deficits. A defibrillator system has been implanted, with amiodarone 400 mg/day added for suppressive antiarrhythmic therapy. As a result of being immobile during her hospitalization, she developed a DVT and has been receiving heparin for 5 days. A full 3-month course of anticoagulation is indicated. How will amiodarone influence D.R.'s anticoagulation?**

Amiodarone appears to inhibit the hepatic metabolism of warfarin, resulting in 50% to 100% increases in INR in patients previously stabilized on warfarin therapy and in whom amiodarone is added.[116] Elevations in INR typically occur within 1 week and stabilize after approximately 1 month of combination therapy. These patients require frequent monitoring with downward adjustments in warfarin dosages.

In the case of D.R., warfarin is to be added to pre-existing amiodarone therapy. The use of a drug known to interact with warfarin is not an absolute contraindication to the addition of warfarin. Warfarin therapy should begin using a flexible initiation protocol or average daily dosing method, but with the expectation that D.R.'s INR likely will increase at a rate faster

Table 16-16 Clinically Significant Warfarin Drug Interactions

Mechanism	Effect on INR	Drugs/Drug Classes	
Increased synthesis of clotting factors	Decreased	• Estrogens	
		• Vitamin K (foods, green tea, chewing tobacco)	
Reduced catabolism of clotting factors	Decreased	• Methimazole	• Propylthiouracil
Induction of warfarin metabolism	Decreased	• Alcohol (chronic use)	• Nafcillin
		• Barbiturates[c]	• Phenytoin[a]
		• Bosentan[b,c]	• Primidone[c]
		• Carbamazepine[c]	• Rifabutin[c]
		• Dicloxacillin	• Rifampin[c]
		• Fosphenytoin[a]	• Ritonavir[c]
		• Griseofulvin	• Tobacco smoke[a]
Reduced absorption of warfarin	Decreased	• Cholestyramine	• Sucralfate
		• Colestipol	
Unexplained mechanisms	Decreased	• Azathioprine	• Mesalamine
		• Cyclophosphamide	• Raloxifene
		• Cyclosporin	
Increased catabolism of clotting factors	Increased	• Thyroid hormones	
Decreased synthesis of clotting factors	Increased	• Cefamandole	• Cefotetan
		• Cefmetazole	• Moxalactam
		• Cefoperazone	• Vitamin E
Impaired vitamin K production by GI flora	Increased	• Broad-spectrum antibiotics	
Inhibition of warfarin metabolism	Increased	• Acetaminophen	• Itraconazole[c]
		• Alcohol (acute use)	• Ketoconazole[c]
		• Allopurinol	• Lovastatin
		• Amiodarone[b,c,d]	• Metronidazole[b]
		• Azithromycin	• Miconazole[b,c]
		• Capecitabine[b]	• Nofloxacin[c,d]
		• Celecoxib[b]	• Omeprazole[e]
		• Citalopram	• Paroxetine
		• Cimetidine[c,d]	• Phenytoin[a]
		• Ciprofloxacin[c,d]	• Propafenone
		• Clarithromycin[c]	• Quetiapine[b,c]
		• Clotrimazole[c]	• Quinidine[c]
		• Disulfiram[b]	• Rofecoxib
		• Erythromycin[c]	• Saquinavir[c]
		• Fluconazole[b,c]	• Simvastatin
		• Fluoxetine[c,e]	• Sertraline
		• Fluoroquinolones[d]	• Sildenafil[b]
		• Fluorouracil[b]	• Sulfamethoxazole[b]
		• Fluvastatin	• Sulfasoxazole
		• Fluvoxamine[b,c,d,e]	• Tobacco smoke[a]
		• Gemfibrozil	• TCAs
		• Grapefruit juice[c,d]	• Zafirlukast[b]
		• Imatinib[c]	• Zileuton[d]
		• Isoniazid[c,e]	
Additive anticoagulant response	Increased	• Argatroban	• Lepirudin
		• Heparin	• Thrombolytic agents
		• Low-molecular-weight heparins	
Unexplained mechanisms		• Acarbose	• Corticosteroids[a]
		• Anabolic steroids	• Fenofibrate
		• Androgens	• Ifosfamide/mesna
		• Ascorbic acid	• Influenza vaccine
		• Clofibrate	• Tamoxifen
Increased bleeding risk	No effect	• Aspirin/acetylated salicylates	
		• Clopidogrel	
		• Cyclooxygenase 2 inhibitors	
		• Glycoprotein IIb/IIIa antagonists	
		• Nonsteroidal anti-inflammatory agents	
		• Ticlopidine	

[a]reported to both increase and decrease PT/INR
[b]via CYP2C9
[c]via CYP3A4
[d]via CYP1A2
[e]via CYP2C19
TCAs, tricyclic antidepressants.

than if she were not taking amiodarone and that her maintenance dosing likely will be significantly lower than if she were not taking amiodarone concurrently. Frequent monitoring will be required for D.R. to establish a maintenance dose because she may not yet have a steady-state amiodarone level.

If amiodarone therapy is discontinued while D.R. is anticoagulated, frequent monitoring also will be necessary. However, the effect of amiodarone on warfarin metabolism can continue for several months after amiodarone is discontinued because of its long elimination half-life and large volume of distribution. Gradual increases in warfarin dosing requirements over weeks to months have been observed after discontinuation of amiodarone.

47. M.G., a 67-year-old woman, was recently diagnosed with bursitis of the right shoulder. A course of anti-inflammatory medication is recommended by her doctor. M.G. is taking warfarin 12.5 mg/day for a history of chronic atrial fibrillation. What could be prescribed for M.G.'s shoulder pain that would not significantly interact with the warfarin she is taking?

This question illustrates one of the most difficult therapeutic dilemmas for a patient taking warfarin. All NSAIDs have the potential to cause gastric irritation by inhibiting cytoprotective prostaglandins, thereby providing a focus for GI bleeding. In addition, most NSAIDs inhibit platelet aggregation, which compromises effective clotting and can lead to bleeding complications.[117] Some NSAIDs (phenylbutazone, sulfinpyrazone, mefenamic acid) also may have specific pharmacokinetic interactions with warfarin that can increase the hypoprothrombinemic effect of warfarin.

These effects can increase the risk of hemorrhagic complications significantly in patients taking warfarin who are prescribed concurrent NSAID therapy. In a retrospective cohort study of patients aged 65 years or older, the risk of hospitalization for bleeding peptic ulcer disease was approximately three times higher for patients taking concurrent warfarin and an NSAID versus patients taking either drug alone, and almost 13 times higher than in patients taking neither warfarin nor an NSAID.[58] Warfarin therapy is considered a relative contraindication to NSAID use.

In patients like M.G. who require combination therapy, clinical experience suggests that ibuprofen (Motrin), naproxen (Naprosyn), or nabumetone (Relafen) are somewhat better tolerated than other NSAIDs with respect to additive hemorrhagic complications, particularly for short-term use. Alternative agents include the nonacetylated salicylates such as salsalate or choline salicylate. These agents have minimal effect on platelet aggregation compared with other salicylates. However, all patients requiring combined warfarin and NSAID therapy should be followed closely and observed routinely for signs and symptoms of bleeding, with frequent stool testing for GI bleeding. Patients should be counseled to avoid additional NSAID use, including use of aspirin, and to seek assistance from a pharmacist when selecting over-the-counter medications to prevent inadvertent NSAID use.

The cyclooxygenase-2 inhibitors celecoxib (Celebrex) and rofecoxib (Vioxx) represent potential alternatives to a nonspecific NSAID. These agents offer anti-inflammatory and analgesic properties with limited impact on platelet aggregation or gastric mucosa, and they are associated with significantly lower rates of GI bleeding, ulceration, or perforation than NSAIDs.[118] Further study is needed to determine their safety in combination with warfarin, since they have been associated with gastric hemorrhage, particularly in the elderly.[119]

The analgesic and antipyretic of choice in patients taking warfarin is acetaminophen, which has not been shown to increase the risk of bleeding. However, in a controversial case-control study of patients taking warfarin, acetaminophen use of >2,275 mg/week was an independent risk factor for developing an INR >6.0.[120] Controls were matched for age, gender, and race, but patients had a higher frequency of febrile illness and reduced oral intake, factors that may influence the INR independently as well as account for acetaminophen use. Acetaminophen may increase the INR by inhibition of CYP1A2 metabolism of (R)-warfarin, but this effect has not been reported consistently.[121] Appropriate monitoring and assessment of patients taking concurrent warfarin and acetaminophen, either routinely or as needed, is sufficient to detect any potential interaction.

Interactions With Natural Products/Dietary Supplements

48. A.B. is a 32-year-old woman who developed a left lower extremity DVT after sustaining a skiing injury 1 month ago. She has been taking warfarin 5 mg on Mondays, Wednesdays, and Fridays and 7.5 mg all other days of the week. She has maintained stable INRs between 2.0 and 3.0 for the last 2 weeks. She has no known medical problems and takes no other medications. However, she has felt increasingly lethargic since her accident and feels that she cannot participate fully in physical therapy because of fatigue. She is interested in taking an herbal supplement to increase her level of energy. How should she be counseled?

Dietary supplements, including herbal medicinals, amino acids, and other nonprescription products, are not tested before marketing for interactions with other medications, including warfarin.[122] Therefore little is known about their interactive properties, other than published case reports. In addition, dietary supplements are not required to meet *United States Pharmacopeia* (USP) standards for tablet content uniformity. Therefore, the actual ingredients and quantity of ingredients of a given product may change from batch to batch, and different products produced by different manufacturers may also differ substantially. These limitations influence the availability and reliability of information regarding potential interactions between warfarin and dietary supplements.

Table 16-17 lists herbal medicinals reported to influence INR or suspected to interact with warfarin based on known or implied properties.[115] In general, little is known about the actual risk of combining these and other dietary supplements with warfarin. Therefore, it is appropriate to counsel patients taking warfarin to avoid use of these products. However, up to 70% of patients may not report their use of dietary supplements to health care providers. Ongoing, detailed evaluation of all current medications is necessary to prevent potential adverse effects associated with interactions between warfarin and dietary supplements.

Table 16-17 Potential Warfarin Interactions With Dietary Supplements

Presumed Mechanism	Effect on INR	Case Reports	Potential Interactions	
Inhibition of CYP2C9	Increased	Chinese wolfberry		
Inhibition of CYP1A2/3A4	Increased	grapefruit juice		
Contains coumarin constituents	Increased	danshen (Salvia)	alfalfa	melilot
		dong quai (Angelica)	aniseed	licorice
		fenugreek	arnica	parsley
			artemisia	passionflower
			asa foetica	prickly ash
			bogbean	quassia
			bochu	red clover
			capsicum	sweet clover
			celery seed	sweet woodruff
			chamomile	tonka beans
			dandelion	wild carrot
			horse chestnut	wild lettuce
			horseradish	
Unknown	Increased	papain		
Contain vitamin K derivatives	Decreased	coenzyme Q$_{10}$		
Induction of CYP3A4	Decreased	St. John's wort		
Unknown	Decreased	ginseng		
Inhibition of platelet aggregation	↑ Risk of bleeding	garlic[a]	cassio	ginger
		ginkgo[a]	clove	onion
			feverfew	tumeric
Contains salicylate derivatives	↑ Risk of bleeding		agrimony	poplar
			meadowsweet	willow
Enhanced fibrinolysis	↑ Risk of bleeding		bromelains	ginseng
			capsicum	onion
			dihydroepiandrosterone (DHEA)	
			garlic	
Procoagulant activity	↑ Risk of thromboembolism		agrimony	
			goldenseal	
			yarrow	

[a] Case reports of bleeding when used alone.

DISSEMINATED INTRAVASCULAR COAGULATION

Pathophysiology

49. W.K., a 63-year-old woman, was admitted to the intensive care unit with respiratory failure secondary to acute pulmonary edema. She required ventilatory support until 48 hours ago, when she was extubated. At that time, aspiration was suspected, but no antibiotic coverage was prescribed. Within the last 24 hours, W.K. developed tachycardia (heart rate, 120 beats/min), tachypnea (respiratory rate, 30 breaths/ min), and a fever to 39°C. Sepsis was suspected, broad-spectrum antibiotic coverage was started, and W.K. was reintubated. Because of the sudden appearance of bright red blood per rectum and through her nasogastric tube, a coagulation screen was ordered. Until this time, all coagulation parameters had been within normal limits. Now the results show platelets, 43,000/mm³ (normal, 150,000 to 350,000); PT, 24 sec (mean normal, 12); aPTT, 76 sec (mean normal, 34); thrombin time, 48 sec (normal, 16 to 27); fibrinogen, 60 mg/dL (normal, 150 to 400); and fibrin degradation products, 580 ng/mL (normal, <250). The diagnosis of disseminated intravascular coagulation (DIC) is made. How does the pathophysiology of DIC explain these hematologic abnormalities?

[SI units: platelets, 43 × 10⁹/L (normal, 150 to 300), and fibrinogen, 0.6 g/L (normal, 1.5 to 4)]

Thrombosis in response to endothelial damage or the presence of an altered surface in contact with blood components is a localized phenomenon. Thrombus formation occurs at the site of injury or abnormality, where procoagulant and anticoagulant mechanisms, as well as fibrinolytic and antifibrinolytic mechanisms, are regulated. The term *localized extravascular coagulation* describes the site-specific nature of venous and arterial thrombosis.

In contrast, DIC is a diffuse response to systemic activation of the coagulation system (Fig. 16-8).[123] Circulating thrombin converts fibrinogen to fibrin, resulting in fibrin deposition within the microcirculation. Clinical manifestations of microvascular thrombosis are the result of tissue ischemia resulting from thrombotic occlusion of small and midsize vessels.

The presence of systemic circulating thrombin causes simultaneous systemic activation of the fibrinolytic system, resulting in circulating plasmin within the systemic circulation. Plasmin causes systemic lysis of fibrin to fibrin degradation products and results in hemorrhagic complications.

Bleeding manifestations of DIC occur not only as a result of systemic fibrinolysis, but also secondary to thrombocytopenia, clotting factor deficiency, and platelet dysfunction. Circulating thrombin promotes platelet aggregation, resulting in thrombocytopenia as platelet aggregates deposit in the microcirculation. Circulating plasmin degrades clotting factors as well as fibrin, and the presence of fibrinogen degradation products from fibrinolysis inhibits platelet function. Normal mechanisms of platelet and clotting factor synthesis are unable to compensate for this consumption. In essence, the patient shows paradoxical bleeding secondary to overactivation and eventual consumption of available clotting factors and platelets.

Clinical Presentation

50. What subjective and objective evidence in W.K. is consistent with the diagnosis of acute DIC?

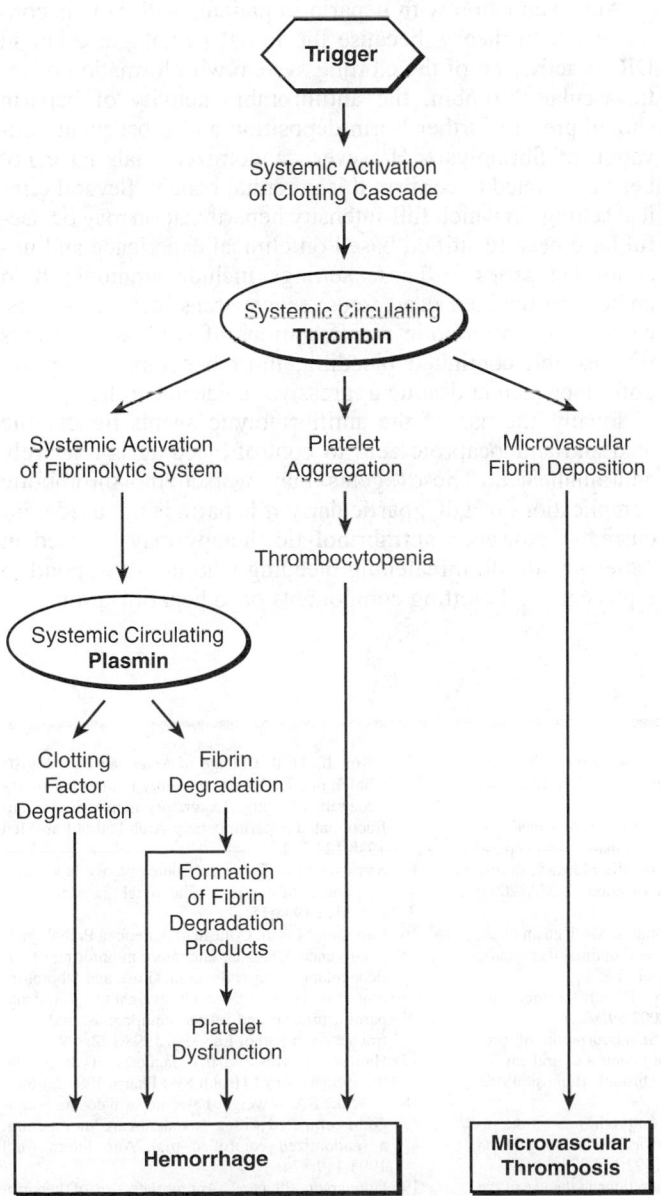

FIGURE 16-8 Pathophysiology of disseminated intravascular coagulation (DIC).

Laboratory Findings

Many coagulation laboratory abnormalities occur in DIC.[124] The PT/INR, aPTT, and thrombin time are increased because clotting factors are consumed more quickly than they can be replenished by hepatic synthesis. Platelet count is diminished secondary to thrombin-mediated platelet aggregation. Fibrinogen is reduced as a result of plasmin-mediated fibrinolysis, with an elevation in fibrinogen degradation products indicative of a fibrinolytic state. W.K.'s coagulation panel findings are consistent with the laboratory abnormalities seen in acute DIC. A peripheral smear will often show thrombocytopenia and red blood cells fragmented by exposure to microcirculatory fibrin (schistocytes).

Hemorrhagic Manifestations

As illustrated by W.K., hemorrhagic manifestations are the predominant clinical finding in DIC.[123] Bleeding can occur at sites of injury, including surgical incisions, venipuncture sites, nasogastric tubes, or gastric ulcers. However, spontaneous bleeding also occurs from intact sites or organ systems.

Spontaneous ecchymosis, petechiae, epistaxis, hemoptysis, hematuria, and GI bleeding commonly are encountered. Intracranial, intraperitoneal, and pericardial bleeding also may occur.

Thrombotic Manifestations

Thrombotic manifestations of DIC result in the obstruction of blood flow to multiple organ systems. The resultant ischemic damage to end organs, including the skin, kidneys, brain, lungs, liver, eyes, and GI tract, can result in multisystem failure. Despite the severity of hemorrhagic complications, microvascular thrombosis represents a significant cause of morbidity and mortality in patients with acute DIC.

Precipitating Events

51. What events may have precipitated the development of DIC in W.K.?

DIC is a pathologic syndrome triggered by disease states or conditions that activate coagulation systemically rather than locally.[123,124] The presence of thrombin within the systemic circulation can be triggered by systemic endothelial damage (e.g., bacterial endotoxin), by systemic contact activation of the clotting cascade (e.g., cardiopulmonary bypass), or by the release of procoagulants into the systemic circulation (e.g., malignancy). Table 16-18 presents an abbreviated list of disorders associated with the development of DIC. Although the most likely stimulus for DIC in W.K. is sepsis, both hypoxia and acidosis associated with respiratory compromise also may have contributed.

Treatment

52. Over the course of several hours, W.K. has developed more severe GI bleeding. Her Hct has fallen from 43% to 35%. What treatment course should be pursued? Should heparin be given?

The most important element of treatment in patients with DIC is alleviation of the underlying cause to eliminate the stimulus for continued thrombosis and hemorrhage.[123] For W.K., this involves appropriate antibiotic therapy as well as supportive measures to correct or prevent the hemodynamic,

Table 16-18 Clinical Conditions Associated with Disseminated Intravascular Coagulation

Obstetric States
Amnionic fluid embolism
Eclampsia
Retained dead fetus
Septic or saline abortion

Intravascular Hemolysis
Hemolytic transfusion reactions
Massive transfusions
Minor hemolysis

Tissue Injury
Burns
Crush injuries
Extensive surgery
Multiple trauma

Infectious Diseases
Bacterial infections
Gram-negative sepsis
Gram-positive sepsis
Viral infections
Cytomegalovirus
Hepatitis
Varicella
Fungal infections
Aspergillosis
Candidiasis
Histoplasmosis
Miscellaneous infections
Mycobacteria malaria
Mycoplasma
Psittacosis
Rocky Mountain spotted fever

Malignancy
Myeloproliferative diseases
Solid tumors

Vascular Disorders
Aortic aneurysm
Giant hemangioma

Miscellaneous
Acidosis
Anaphylaxis
ARDS
Cardiopulmonary bypass
Hematologic disorders
Heat stroke
Hepatic disease
Hypoperfusion
Hypovolemia
Severe allergic reaction
Snake bites
Transplant rejection

ARDS, adult respiratory distress syndrome.

respiratory, and metabolic manifestations of shock. Fluid replacement, maintenance of blood pressure and cardiac output, and adequate oxygenation are essential components of the treatment of patients with DIC.

The selection of other therapies aimed at correcting the hemorrhagic or thrombotic manifestations of DIC are controversial and to some extent depend on whether hemorrhagic manifestations or thrombotic complications predominate in the clinical presentation. Initial treatment in patients with hemorrhage involves replacement of components of clotting that have been consumed in DIC, guided by coagulation laboratory data.[125] Transfusion of platelets, fresh frozen plasma (containing all clotting factors), and/or cryoprecipitate (containing factor VIII and fibrinogen) may be necessary, with close monitoring of platelet count and fibrinogen level. Transfusion of AT concentrates, resulting in inhibition of coagulation processes, has been associated with reduced mortality in DIC.

Anticoagulation with heparin in patients with DIC is controversial. In theory, because the initial pathologic event in DIC is activation of the clotting system with formation of intravascular thrombin, the antithrombin activity of heparin should prevent further fibrin deposition and subsequent activation of fibrinolysis. However, randomized trials have not been conducted to confirm this potential benefit. Several clinical settings in which full-intensity heparinization may be useful have been identified based on clinical experience and uncontrolled series.[123] These settings include amnionic fluid embolism, retained dead fetus, severe transfusion reactions, evidence of thrombotic manifestations of DIC, and patients who exhibit continued bleeding, thrombocytopenia, or hypofibrinogenemia despite aggressive replacement therapy.

Finally, the use of the antifibrinolytic agents tranexamic acid and aminocaproic acid to control bleeding is relatively contraindicated. These agents may worsen the thrombotic complications of DIC, particularly if heparin is not used concurrently. However, antifibrinolytic therapy may be used in patients with life-threatening bleeding who fail to respond to replacement of clotting components or to heparinization.

REFERENCES

1. Haines ST, Bussey HI. Thrombosis and the pharmacology of antithrombotic agents. Ann Pharmacother 1997;29:892.
2. Federman DG, Kirsner DS. An update on hypercoagulable disorders. Arch Intern Med 2001; 161:1051.
3. Hirsh J, et al. Overview of thrombosis and its treatment. In: Coleman RW et al, eds. Hemostasis and Thrombosis. Basic Principles and Clinical Practice. 4th Ed. Philadelphia: Lippincott Williams and Wilkins, 2001.
4. Coleman RW et al. Overview of hemostasis. In: Coleman RW et al, eds. Hemostasis and Thrombosis. Basic Principles and Clinical Practice. 4th Ed. Philadelphia: Lippincott Williams and Wilkins, 2001.
5. Hirsh J et al. Heparin and low molecular weight heparin: mechanism of action, pharmacokinetics, dosing considerations, monitoring, efficacy and safety. Chest 2001;119(Suppl 1):64.
6. Turpie AGG et al. Fondaparinux vs enoxaparin for the prevention of venous thromboembolism in major orthopedic surgery. Arch Intern Med 2002; 162:1833.
7. Dager WE, White RH. Treatment of heparin-induced thrombocytopenia. Ann Pharmacother 2002;36:489.
8. Lincoff AM et al. Bivalirudin and provisional glycoprotein IIb/IIIa blockade compared with heparin and planned glycoprotein IIb/IIIa blockade during percutaneous coronary intervention. JAMA 2003; 289:853.
9. Hirsh J et al. Oral anticoagulants. Mechanism of action, clinical effectiveness, and optimal therapeutic range. Chest 2001;119(Suppl 1):8.
10. Kaplan KL, Francis CW. Direct thrombin inhibitors. Semin Hematol 2002;39:187.
11. Kitchen S, Preston FE. Standardization of prothrombin time for laboratory control of oral anticoagulant therapy. Semin Thromb Hemost 1999; 25:17.
12. Bussey HI et al. Reliance on prothrombin time ratios causes significant errors in anticoagulation therapy. Arch Intern Med 1992;152:278.
13. Nelson DE. Current considerations in the use of the aPTT in monitoring unfractionted heparin. Clin Lab Sci 1999;12:359.
14. Olson JD et al. College of American Pathologists Conference XXXI on laboratory monitoring of anticoagulant therapy. Laboratory monitoring of unfractionated heparin therapy. Arch Pathol Lab Med 1998;122:782.
15. Samama MM, Poller L. Contemporary laboratory monitoring of low-molecular-weight heparins. Clin Lab Med 1995;15:119.
16. Laposata M et al. College of American Pathologists Conference XXXI on laboratory monitoring of anticoagulant therapy: the clinical use and laboratory monitoring of low-molecular-weight heparin, danaparoid, hirudin and related compounds, and argatroban. Arch Pathol Lab Med 1998;122:799.
17. Haines ST, Bussey HI. Diagnosis of deep vein thrombosis. Am J Health Syst Pharm 1997;54:66.
18. Raschke RA. A weight-based heparin dosing nomogram compared with a "standard-care" nomogram: a randomized controlled trial. Ann Intern Med 1993;119:874.
19. Gunnarson PS et al. Appropriate use of heparin. Empiric vs. nomogram-based dosing. Arch Intern Med 1995;155:526.

20. Hylek E et al. Challenges in the effective use of unfractionated heparin in the hospitalized management of acute thrombosis. Arch Intern Med 2003; 163:621.

21. Hyers TM. Antithrombotic therapy for venous thromboembolic disease. Chest 2001;119(suppl 1):176.

22. Warkentin TE et al. Heparin induced thrombocytopenia: towards consensus. Thromb Haemost 1998;79:1.

23. Warkentin TE. Platelet count monitoring and laboratory testing for heparin-induced thrombocytopenia. Recommendations of the College of American Pathologists. Arch Pathol Lab Med 2002;126:1415.

24. Warkentin TE et al. Heparin-induced thrombocytopenia in patients treated with low-molecular-weight heparin or unfractionated heparin. N Engl J Med 1995;332:1330.

25. Whitehall TA. Caval interruption methods: comparison of options. Semin Vasc Surg 1996;9:59.

26. Landefeld CS, Beyth RJ. Anticoagulation-related bleeding: clinical epidemiology, prediction and prevention. Am J Med 1993;85:315.

27. Levine MN et al. Hemorrhagic complications of anticoagulant treatment. Chest 2001;119(Suppl 1):108.

28. Barbour LA et al. A prospective study of heparin-induced osteoporosis in pregnancy using bone densitometry. Am J Obstet Gynecol 1994;170:862.

29. Hommes DW et al. Subcutaneous heparin compared with continuous intravenous heparin administration in the initial treatment of deep vein thrombosis: a meta-analysis. Ann Intern Med 1992; 116:279.

30. D'Ambra M. Restoration of the normal coagulation process: advances in therapies to antagonize heparin. J Cardiovasc Pharmacol 1996;27(suppl 1):58

31. Gould MK et al. Low-molecular-weight heparins compared to with unfractionated heparin for treatment of acute deep vein thrombosis. A meta-analysis of randomized, controlled trials. Ann Intern Med 1999;130:800.

32. Levine M et al. A comparison of low molecular-weight heparin administered primarily at home with unfractionated heparin administered in the hospital for proximal deep vein thrombosis. N Engl J Med 1996;334:677.

33. Koopman MM et al. Treatment of venous thrombosis with intravenous unfractionated heparin administered in the hospital as compared with subcutaneous low-molecular-weight heparin administered at home. N Engl J Med 1996;334:682.

34. O'Brien B et al. Economic evaluation of outpatient treatment with low-molecular-weight heparin for proximal vein thrombosis. Arch Intern Med 1999;2298.

35. Merli G et al. Subcutaneous enoxaparin once or twice daily compared with intravenous unfractionated heparin for treatment of venous thromboembolic disease. Ann Intern Med 2001;134:191.

36. Collet JP et al. Enoxaparin in unstable angina patients with renal failure. Int J Cardiol 2001;80:81.

37. Nagge J, et al. Is impaired renal function a contraindication to the use of low-molecular-weight heparin? Arch Intern Med 2002;162:2605

38. Caprini JA et al. Effective risk stratification of surgical and nonsurgical patients for venous thromboembolic disease. Semin Hematol 2001;38(2 suppl 5):12.

39. Kaboli P et al. DVT prophylaxis and anticoagulation in the surgical patient. Med Clin North Am 2003;87:77.

40. Enders JM et al. Prevention of venous thromboembolism in acute medical illness. Pharmacotherapy 2002;22:1564.

41. Geerts WH et al. Prevention of venous thromboembolism. Chest 2001;119 (suppl 1):132.

42. Dalen JE. Pulmonary embolism: what have we learned since Virchow? Natural history, pathophysiology, and diagnosis. Chest 2002;122:1440.

43. Goldhaber SZ et al. International Cooperative Pulmonary Embolism Registry detects high mortality rate. Circulation 1997;96(Suppl 1):1.

44. D'Angelo A et al. Relationship between international normalized ratio values, vitamin K-dependent clotting factor levels and in vivo prothrombin activation during the early and steady phases of oral anticoagulant treatment. Hematologica 2002; 87:1074.

45. Leech BF, Carter CJ. Falsely elevated INR results due to the sensitivity of the thromboplastin reagent to heparin. Am J Clin Pathol 1998;109:764.

46. Kearon C et al. Effect of warfarin on activated partial thromboplastin time in patients receiving heparin. Arch Intern Med 1998;158:1140.

47. James AH, Britt RP, Raskind CL, Thompson SG. Factors affecting the maintenance dose of warfarin. J Clin Pathol 1992;45:704

48. Weiland K, Wittkowsky AK. Initiation of therapy and estimation of maintenance dose. In:Ansell J, Oertel L, Wittkowsky AK, eds. Managing Oral Anticoagulant Therapy. Clinical and Operational Guidelines. 2d Ed. Gaithersburg, MD: Aspen Publishers, 2002.

49. Crowther MA, Harrison L, Hirsh J. Warfarin: less may be better. Ann Intern Med 1997;127:332.

50. Crowther MA et al. A randomized trial comparing 5-mg and 10-mg warfarin loading doses. Arch Intern Med 1999;159:46.

51. Research Committee of the British Thoracic Society. Optimum duration of anticoagulation for deep vein thrombosis and pulmonary embolism. Lancet 1992;40:873.

52. Schulman S et al. A comparison of six weeks with six months of oral anticoagulant therapy after a first episode of venous thromboembolism. N Engl J Med 1995;332:1661.

53. Kearon C et al. A comparison of three months of anticoagulation with extended anticoagulation for a first episode of idiopathic venous thromboembolism. N Engl J Med 1999;340:901.

54. Schulman S et al. The duration of oral anticoagulant therapy after a second episode of venous thromboembolism. N Engl J Med 1997;336:393.

55. Hart RG et al. Oral anticoagulants and intracranial hemorrhage. Facts and hypotheses. Stroke 1995;26:1471.

56. Palareti G et al. Bleeding complications of oral anticoagulant treatment: an inception cohort, prospective collaborative study (ISCOAT). Lancet 1996;348:423.

57. Hyleck EM et al. Risk factors for intracranial hemorrhage in outpatients taking warfarin. Ann Intern Med 1994;120:897.

58. Shorr RI et al. Concurrent use of nonsteroidal anti-inflammatory drugs and oral anticoagulants places elderly persons at high risk for hemorrhagic peptic ulcer disease. Arch Intern Med 1993;153:1665.

59. Gitter MJ et al. Bleeding and thromboembolism during anticoagulant therapy: a population based study in Rochester Minnesota. Mayo Clin Prac 1995;70:725.

60. Henderson MC, White RH. Anticoagulation in the elderly. Curr Opin Pulm Med 2001;7:365.

61. Beyth RJ, Landefeld CS. Anticoagulants in older patients. A safety perspective. Drugs and Aging 1995;6:45.

62. Beyth RJ et al. A multicomponent intervention to prevent major bleeding complications in older patients receiving warfarin. Ann Intern Med 2000; 133:687.

63. Copland M et al. Oral anticoagulation and hemorrhagic complications in an elderly population with atrial fibrillation. Arch Intern Med 2001;161:2125.

64. Beyth RJ et al. Prospective evaluation of an index for predicting risk of major bleeding in outpatient treated with warfarin. Am J Med 1998;105:91.

65. Chan YC et al. Warfarin-induced skin necrosis. Br J Surg 2000;87:266.

66. Sallah S. Warfarin and heparin-induced skin necrosis and the purple toe syndrome: infrequent complications of anticoagulant treatment. Thromb Haemost 1997;78:785.

67. Chiquette E, Amato MG, Bussey HT. Comparison of an anticoagulation clinic with usual medical care. Arch Intern Med 1998;185:1641.

68. Fihn SD et al. Risk factors for complications of chronic warfarin therapy. A multicenter study. Ann Intern Med 1993;118:511.

69. Booth SL et al. Food sources and dietary intakes of vitamin K-1 (phylloquinone) in the American diet: data from the FDA Total Diet Study. J Am Diet Assoc 1996;96:149.

70. Booth SL et al. Vitamin K: a practical guide to the dietary management of patients on warfarin. Nutr Rev 1999;57(9 Pt 1):288.

71. Weathermon R, Crabb DW. Alcohol and medication interactions. Alcohol Res Health 1999;23:40.

72. Demirkan K et al. Response to warfarin and other oral anticoagulants: effects of disease states. South Med J 2000;93:448.

73. Hawk TL, Havrda DE. Effect of stress on International Normalized Ratio during warfarin therapy. Ann Pharmacotheraphy 2002;36:617.

74. Shibata Y et al. Influence of physical activity on warfarin therapy. Thromb Haemost 1998;80:203.

75. Zevin S, Benowitz NL. Drug interactions with tobacco smoking: an update. Clin Pharmacokinet 1999;36:425.

76. Wong W et al. Influence of warfarin regimen type on clinical and monitoring outcomes in stable patients in an anticoagulation management service. Pharmacotherapy 1999;19:1385.

77. Hylek EM et al. Clinical predictors of prolonged delay in return of the International Normalized Ratio to within the therapeutic range after excessive anticoagulation with warfarin. Ann Intern Med 2001;135:393.

78. Weibert RT et al. Correction of excessive anticoagulation with low-dose oral vitamin K_1. Ann Intern Med 1997;125:959.

79. Crowther MA et al. Oral vitamin K lowers the international normalized ratio more rapidly than subcutaneous vitamin K in the treatment of warfarin-associated coagulopathy. A randomized, controlled trial. Ann Intern Med 2002;137:251.

80. Hung A et al. A prospective randomized study to determine the optimal dose of intravenous vitamin K in reversal of over-warfarinization. Br J Haematol 2001;113:839.

81. Shields RC et al. Efficacy and safety of intravenous phytonadione (vitamin K1) in patients on long-term oral anticoagulant therapy. Mayo Clin Proc 2001;76:260.

82. Bates SM, Ginsberg JS. Anticoagulants in pregnancy:fetal effects. Baillieres Clin Obstet Gynaecol 1997;11:479.

83. Ginsberg JS, Hirsh J. Use of antithrombotic agents during pregnancy. Chest 2001;119(Suppl 1):122.

84. Laurent P et al. Low-molecular-weight heparins: a guide to their optimum use in pregnancy. Drugs 2002;62:463.

85. Casele HL et al. Changes in the pharmacokinetics of the low-molecular-weight heparin enoxaparin sodium during pregnancy. Am J Obstet Gynecol 1999;181:1113.

86. Shapira Y et al. Low-molecular-weight heparins for the treatment of patients with mechanical valves. Clin Cardiol 2002;25:323.

87. Chan WS et al. Anticoagulation of pregnant women with mechanical heart valves: a systematic review of the literature. Arch Intern Med 2000;160:191.

88. Albers GW et al. Antithrombotic therapy in atrial fibrillation. Chest 2001;119(Suppl 1):194.

89. Bjerkelund CJ et al. The efficacy of anticoagulant therapy in preventing embolism related to DC electrical conversion of atrial fibrillation. Am J Cardiol 1969;23:208.

90. Klein AL et al. Use of transesophageal echocardiography to guide cardioversion in patients with atrial fibrillation. New Engl J Med 2001;344:1411.

91. Atrial Fibrillation Investigators. Risk factors for stroke and efficacy of antithrombotic therapy in atrial fibrillation. Analysis of pooled data from five randomized controlled trials. Arch Intern Med 1994;154:1449.

92. Atrial Fibrillation Investigators. The efficacy of aspirin in patients with atrial fibrillation: analysis of pooled data from three randomized trials. Arch Intern Med 1997;157:1237.

93. Stein PD et al. Antithrombotic therapy in patients with mechanical and biologic prosthetic heart valves. Chest 2001;119(Suppl 1):220.

94. Cannegeiter SC et al. Optimal oral anticoagulant therapy in patients with mechanical heart valves. N Engl J Med 1995;333:11.

95. Saour JN et al. Trial of different intensities of anticoagulation in patients with prosthetic heart valves. N Engl J Med 1990;322:428.

96. Acar J et al. AREVA: multicenter randomized comparison of low-dose versus standard-dose anticoagulation in patients with mechanical prosthetic heart valves. Circulation 1996;94:2107.

97. Turpie AGG et al. A comparison of aspirin with placebo in patients treated with warfarin after heart-valve replacement. N Engl J Med 1993;329:524.

98. Meschengieser SS et al. Low-intensity oral anticoagulation plus low-dose aspirin versus high-intensity oral anticoagulation alone: a randomized trial in patients with mechanical prosthetic heart valves. J Thorac Cardiovasc Surg 1997;113:910.

99. Koniaris LS, Goldhaber SZ. Anticoagulation-indilated cardiomyopathy. J Am Coll Cardiol 1998; 31:745

100. Cohn JN et al. Effect of vasodilator therapy on mortality in chronic congestive heart failure. N Engl J Med 1986;314:1547.

101. Cohn JN et al. A comparison of enalapril with hydralazine-isosorbide dinitrate in the treatment of chronic congestive heart failure. N Engl J Med 1991;325:303.

102. Loh E et al. Ventricular dysfunction and the risk of stroke after myocardial infarction. N Engl J Med 1997;336:251.

103. Al-Khadra AS et al. Warfarin anticoagulation and survival: a cohort analysis from the studies of left ventricular dysfunction. J Am Coll Cardiol 1998;31:749.

104. Cairns JA et al. Antithrombotic therapy in coronary artery disease. Chest 2001;199(suppl 1):228.

105. Hurlen M et al. Warfarin, aspirin, or both after myocardial infarction. N Engl J Med 2002; 347:969.

106. Heit JA. Perioperative management of the chronically anticoagulated patient. J Thromb Thrombolysis 2002;12:81.

107. Ansell J et al. Managing oral anticoagulant therapy. Chest 2001;119(suppl 1):22.

108. Johnson J, Turpie AGG. Temporary discontinuation of oral anticoagulants: role of low-molecular-weight heparin. Thromb Haemost 1999;82 (suppl):62.

109. Montalsecot G et al. Low-molecular-weight heparin after mechanical valve replacement. Circulation 2000;101:1083.

103. Goldstein JL et al. Low-molecular-weight heparin versus unfractionated heparin in the colonoscopy peri-procedure period: a cost modeling study. Am J Gastroenterol 2001;96:2360.

111. Wahl MJ et al. Dental surgery in anticoagulated patients. Arch Intern Med 1998;158:1610.

112. Scully C, Wolff A. Oral surgery in patients on anticoagulant therapy. Oral Surg Oral Med Oral Pathol Oral Radiol Endod 2002;94:57.

113. Hansten PD, Wittkowsky AK. Warfarin drug interactions. In:Ansell J, Oertel L, Wittkowsky AK, eds. Managing Oral Anticoagulant Therapy: Clinical and Operational Guidelines. 2d Ed. Gaithersburg MD: Aspen Publishers, 2002.

114. Sands CD et al. Revisiting the significance of warfarin protein-binding displacement interactions. Ann Pharmacotherapy 2002;36:1642.

115. Wittkowsky AK. Drug interaction update: drugs, herbs and oral anticoagulation. J Thromb Thrombolysis 2001;12:67.

116. Kerin NZ et al. The incidence, magnitude and time course of the amiodarone–warfarin interaction. Arch Intern Med 1988;148:1779.

117. Chan TYK. Adverse interactions between warfarin and nonsteroidal antiinflammatory drugs: mechanisms, clinical significance, and avoidance. Ann Pharmacother 1995;29:1274.

118. Kaplan-Machlis B, Klostermeyer BS. The cyclooxygenase-2 inhibitors: safety and effectiveness. Ann Pharmacother 1999;33(9):979.

119. Mamdani M et al. Observational study of upper gastrointestinal hemorrhage in elderly patients given selective cyclooxygenase-2 inhibitors or conventional nonsteroidal antiinflammatory drugs. Br Med J 2002;325:624.

120. Hylek EM et al. Acetaminophen and other risk factors for excessive warfarin anticoagulation. JAMA 1998;279:657.

121. Kwan D, Bartle WR, Walker SE. The effects of acetaminophen on pharmacokinetics and pharmacodynamics of warfarin. J Clin Pharmacol 1999;39:68.

122. Heck AM et al. Potential interactions between alternative therapies and warfarin. Am J Health Syst Pharm 2000;57:1221.

123. Bick RL. Disseminated intravascular coagulation: a review of etiology, pathophysiology, diagnosis, and management: guidelines for care. Clin Appl Thromb Hemost 2002;8:1.

124. Levi M et al. The diagnosis of disseminated intravascular coagulation. Blood Rev 2002;16:217.

125. deJone E et al. Anticoagulant factor concentrates in disseminated intravascular coagulation: rationale for use and clinical experience. Semin Thromb Hemost 2001;27:667.

CHAPTER 17

Ischemic Heart Disease: Anginal Syndromes

Toby C. Trujillo, Paul E. Nolan

Angina pectoris is a symptom of myocardial ischemia that usually is secondary to atherosclerosis of the coronary arteries. This is part of the syndrome of coronary heart disease (CHD), also known as ischemic heart disease (IHD) or coronary artery disease (CAD). Other signs of CHD include acute coronary syndromes (ACS) such as unstable angina (USA) and acute myocardial infarction (MI), arrhythmias, heart failure (HF), and sudden cardiac death. Because angina is a marker for underlying heart disease, its management is of great importance.

Definitions

Angina pectoris is a "clinical syndrome characterized by discomfort in the chest, jaw, shoulder, back, or arm."[1] Although angina is typically brought on by exertion and relieved by nitroglycerin (NTG), its presentation is variable. At one extreme, angina occurs predictably with strenuous exercise; at the other, angina can develop unexpectedly with little or no exertion.

Patients who have a reproducible pattern of angina that is associated with a certain level of physical activity have *chronic stable angina* or exertional angina. In contrast, patients with unstable angina experience new-onset angina or a change in their angina intensity, frequency, or duration.[2] Both chronic stable angina and USA often reflect underlying atherosclerotic narrowing of coronary arteries. Classic Prinzmetal's variant angina, or vasospastic angina, occurs in patients without CHD and is due to a spasm of the coronary artery that decreases myocardial blood flow.[3,4] When coronary vasospasm occurs at the site of a fixed atherosclerotic plaque, mixed angina can result.[2]

Silent (asymptomatic) myocardial ischemia, which can result in transient changes in myocardial perfusion, function, or electrical activity, is detected on an electrocardiogram (ECG) in most angina patients.[2,5] However, the patient does not experience chest pain or other signs of angina (e.g., jaw pain, shortness of breath [SOB]) during these episodes. Silent myocardial ischemia also can occur in patients with no angina history (see Chapter 18, Myocardial Infarction).

Epidemiology

Cardiovascular disease (CVD) is the leading cause of death in the United States, and death due to CHD is responsible for approximately half of all deaths from CVD. Chronic stable angina is the first clinical sign of CHD in approximately 50% of patients.[2,6] CVD remains the leading cause of death in our society despite a decline in the death rate from CVD in the late 20th century. The incidence of angina is difficult to assess because it often is unrecognized by patients and physicians. However, in 1999, an estimated 12.6 million people were alive with a history of CHD.[6]

Although CHD accounts for 1 of every 5 deaths in the United States, individual mortality varies according to the patient's age, gender, cardiovascular risk profile, myocardial contractility, coronary anatomy, and specific anginal syndrome. The annual mortality rate increases as the number of coronary vessels with high-grade atherosclerotic lesions increases. Patients with left main CAD have an increased mortality rate compared with patients without left main coronary disease. Similarly, patients with diminished left ventricular (LV) function (ejection fraction [EF]<50%) have higher mortality rates compared with patients without impaired LV function.

In addition to the high morbidity and mortality associated with CHD, the economic cost to the U.S. health care system is substantial. Total direct and indirect costs associated with CHD were estimated to be $112 billion in 1999.[6]

Coronary Anatomy

Figure 17-1 illustrates the normal distribution of the major coronary arteries, although variation is common from individual to individual. The anterior and lateral portions of the left ventricle receive blood flow from the left coronary artery, usually the largest diameter and shortest of all coronary arteries. From its main stem, the left coronary artery divides into its two major branches: the left anterior descending (LAD) coronary artery and the circumflex. The LAD further subdivides into the first diagonal, the first septal, the right ventricular, the minor septals, the second diagonal, and the apical branches. Similarly, the circumflex also subdivides into four or five branches, the largest branch being the obtuse marginal.[7]

The right coronary artery (RCA) supplies blood flow to most of the right ventricle as well as the posterior part of the left ventricle. Like the LAD, the right coronary branches into major vessels, which supply blood flow to specific areas of the heart. In order of origin, the RCA divides into the conus branch, sinus node branch, right ventricular branches, atrial branch, acute marginal branch, atrioventricular (AV) node

branch, posterior descending, LV, and left atrial branches.[7] Because of wide variation in coronary artery distribution and the need to confirm the precise location of atherosclerotic plaques, most patients with angina undergo coronary arteriography. Patients with severe left main CAD are at higher risk because obstruction of this large coronary artery jeopardizes almost the entire left ventricle. Similarly, patients with three-vessel CAD are at higher risk than patients with single-vessel disease (see Chapter 18, Myocardial Infarction).

Pathophysiology

The myocardium must constantly generate a constrictive force (systolic contraction) and, unlike other muscle tissues, can function only in the presence of oxygen. Without oxygen, myocardial cells cease energy production, and if oxygen deprivation is widespread, the heart deteriorates and ceases to pump.

Angina pectoris typically occurs when myocardial oxygen demand exceeds myocardial oxygen supply (perfusion). The underlying pathologic condition of this mismatch invariably is the presence of atherosclerosis in one or more of the epicardial coronary arteries.[1,2] If the size of the atherosclerotic plaque obscures <50% of the diameter of the vessel, coronary blood flow during exertion usually is sufficient and the patient is pain free. In patients with chronic stable angina, most coronary artery stenoses are ≥70%. A linear decrease in coronary blood flow occurs as the plaque occupies more of the arterial lumen until high-grade (≥80%) obstruction develops. At this point, the decrease in blood flow is out of proportion to plaque size. The impaired blood flow with high-grade lesions can be affected by increased vasomotor tone, vasospasm, and thrombotic occlusion. Functionally, coronary blood flow is absent when lesions obstruct ≥95% of the vessel lumen.[8]

Collateral blood vessels (i.e., side branches of a coronary artery that join one of the three principal arteries or connect two points along the same artery) may offer protection against myocardial ischemia. The distribution and extent of collateral vessels are variable. These usually are very small and have no function in the normal heart. However, if blood flow is obstructed, collateral vessels assume more importance and can restore some myocardial blood flow. Unfortunately, when myocardial oxygen demand is increased excessively, collateral blood flow usually is insufficient, and angina or other myocardial ischemia syndromes develop.[2,9]

A thorough understanding of the determinants of myocardial oxygen supply and demand is needed to better comprehend the rationale for the use of various pharmacotherapeutic agents in the treatment of CHD.

Myocardial Oxygen Supply and Demand

The oxygen demand of the heart is determined by its work load. The major determinants of myocardial oxygen consumption are heart rate, contractility, and intramyocardial wall tension during systole (Fig. 17-2; also, see Chapter 19, Heart Failure). Intramyocardial wall tension is the force the heart is required to develop and sustain during contraction and is affected primarily by changes in ventricular chamber pressures and volume. Both enlargement of the ventricle and increased pressure within the ventricle increase the systolic wall force and consequently myocardial oxygen demand. Increases in contractility and heart rate also result in increased

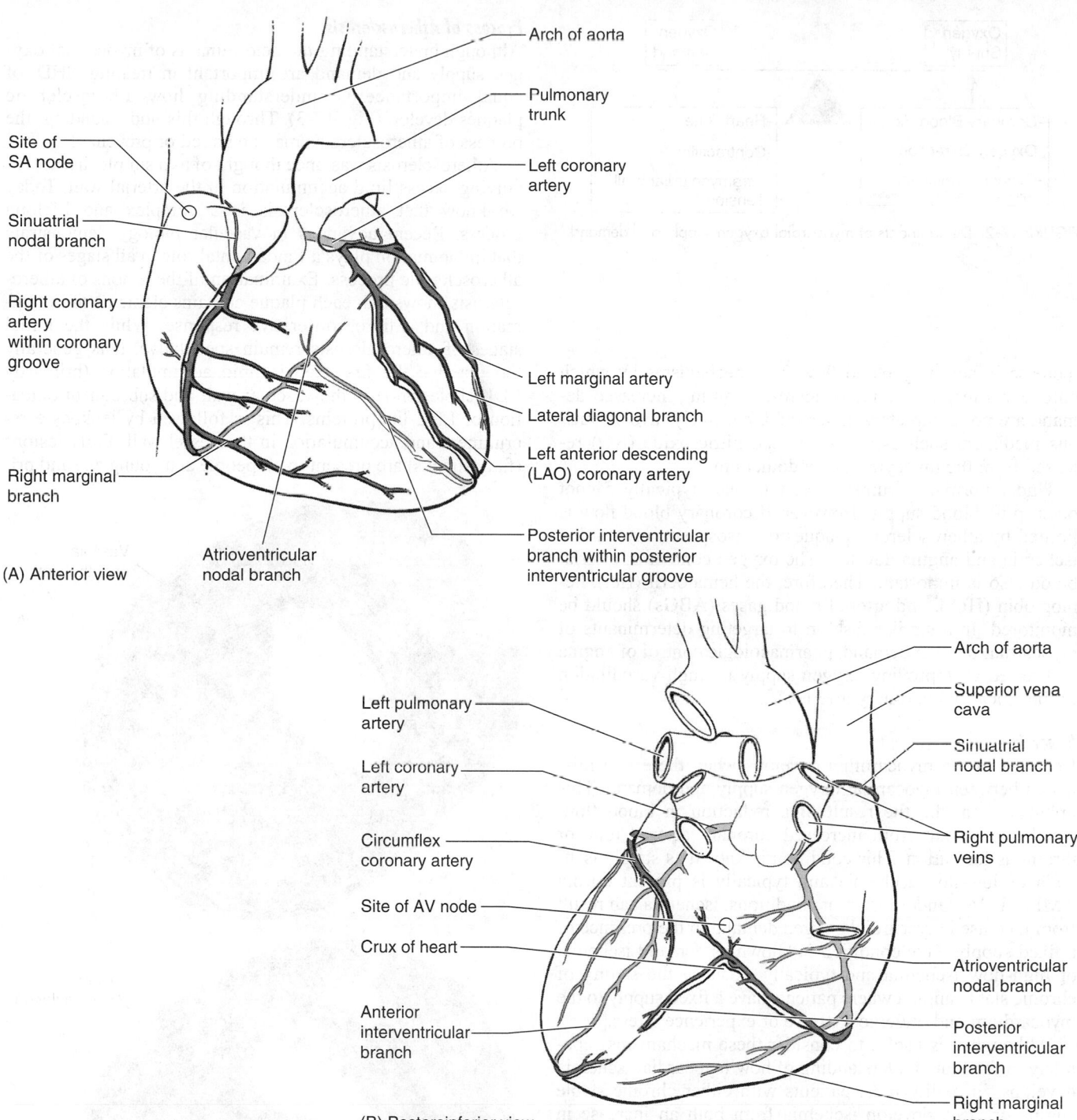

FIGURE 17-1. Coronary arteries. Observe that the right coronary artery (RCA) originates from the aorta and courses in the atrioventricular (coronary) groove to reach the posterior surface of the heart. Observe also that the left coronary artery splits into the circumflex branch that supplies blood to the lateral and posterior walls of the left ventricle, and a left anterior descending (LAD) branch, which supplies blood to the anterior wall of the left ventricle.

oxygen demand. Pharmacologic control of angina is, in part, directed toward decreasing the myocardial oxygen demand by decreasing heart rate, myocardial contractility, or ventricular volume and pressures.[8]

Of the many factors that affect oxygen supply to the heart (see Fig. 17-2), coronary blood flow and oxygen extraction are most important. Oxygen extraction by heart cells is high

(about 70% to 75%) even at rest. When extra demand is placed on the heart, myocardial oxygen extraction increases slightly and plateaus at approximately 80%. Because oxygen extraction is increased only modestly when the heart is heavily stressed, high oxygen demands must be met by increases in coronary blood flow. Sudden increases in oxygen demand lead to a rapid decrease in coronary vascular resistance and an

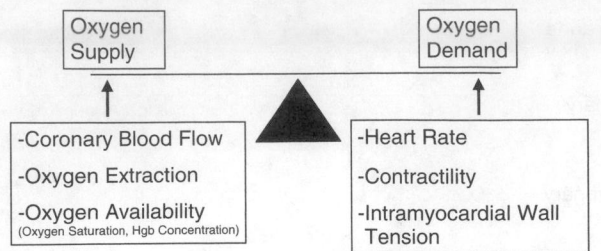

FIGURE 17-2. Determinants of myocardial oxygen supply and demand.

increase in coronary blood flow. The mechanisms by which coronary artery resistance is decreased during increased demand are not completely understood, but likely involve various mediators such as adenosine and nitric oxide (NO) released from the myocytes and endothelium.[8,10]

Under normal circumstances, the heart typically cannot outstrip its blood supply. However, if coronary blood flow is limited by atherosclerotic plaques or vasospasm, myocardial ischemia and angina develop. The oxygen content of arterial blood also is important. Therefore, the hematocrit (Hct), hemoglobin (Hgb), and arterial blood gases (ABGs) should be monitored. In a similar fashion to targeting determinants of myocardial oxygen demand, pharmacologic control of angina is directed at improving oxygen supply through vasodilation of the epicardial coronary arteries.

Ischemia

Ischemia in the myocardium develops when there is a mismatch between myocardial oxygen supply and demand. This imbalance can be the result of a reduction in blood flow, which may result from increased coronary arterial tone or thrombus formation. This condition is known as supply ischemia or low-flow ischemia and typically is present during AMI or USA. Under different conditions, ischemia can result from increased myocardial oxygen demand in the presence of a fixed supply. This condition is known as demand ischemia or high-flow ischemia and typically exists in the setting of chronic stable angina where patients have a fixed supply to the myocardium and undergo exercise or experience stress.[8]

Although it is useful to consider these mechanisms separately to facilitate understanding of how myocardial ischemia develops, in reality most patients with either chronic stable angina or USA develop ischemia from both an increase in oxygen demand and a reduction in oxygen supply. In diseased segments of the coronary arteries where atherosclerotic lesions have developed, vasomotor function (vasodilatory capacity) of the arterial wall is often abnormal secondary to endothelial dysfunction. This may lead to inappropriate vasoconstriction on top of a flow limiting atherosclerotic plaque, resulting in the precipitation or worsening of ongoing ischemia in patients with chronic stable angina.[8] In the setting of USA or AMI, coronary blood flow is often acutely decreased or completely interrupted secondary to the development of a pathologic thrombus superimposed on a flow limiting atherosclerotic plaque. Coronary vasoconstriction can be present in these acute coronary syndromes (ACS) as well.[11]

Process of Atherosclerosis

Although understanding the determinants of myocardial oxygen supply and demand are important in treating CHD, of equal importance is understanding how atherosclerotic plaques develop (Fig. 17-3). Through this understanding, the process of atherosclerosis may be halted or prevented.

Atherosclerosis was once thought of as a simple disease involving excess lipid accumulation in the arterial wall. Today we know that atherosclerosis is a complex and lifelong process. Recent advances in vascular biology demonstrate that inflammation plays a fundamental role in all stages of the atherosclerotic process. Examination of the lesions of atherosclerosis shows that each plaque contains elements of inflammation and a fibroproliferative response. While the initial stages of atherosclerosis remain speculative, it is generally thought that the first step is lipid accumulation (primarily LDL cholesterol) in the vascular wall and subsequent oxidation of LDL lipoproteins. This is followed by leukocyte recruitment and accumulation in the vessel wall. Early lesions (fatty streaks) are present in all people at a young age and pri-

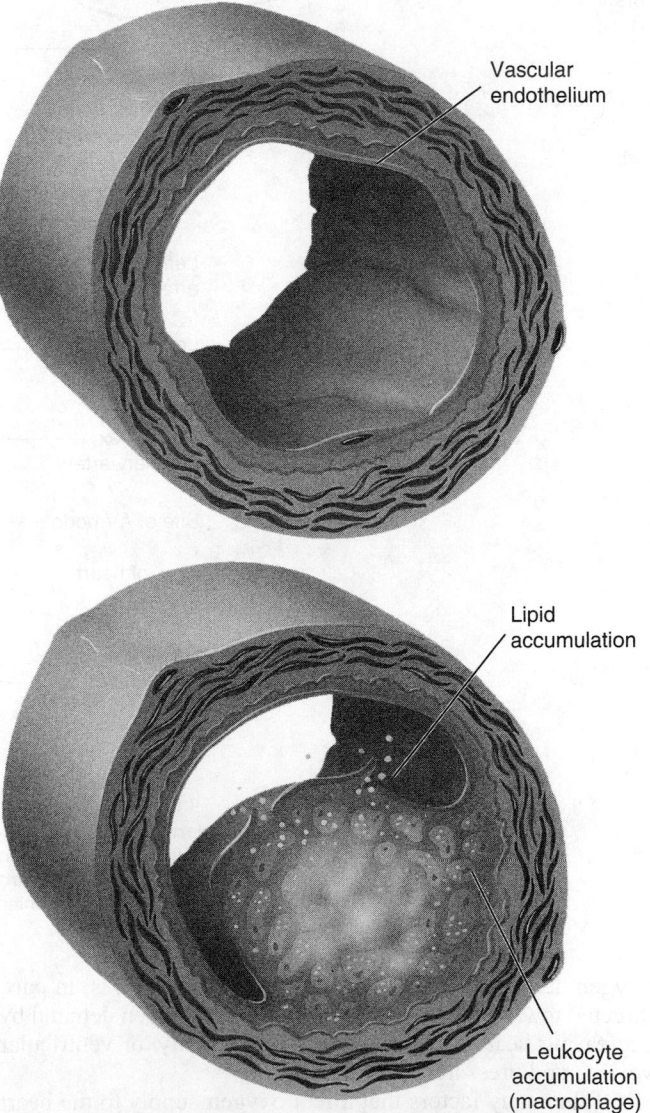

FIGURE 17-3. Cholesterol, consequence of high cholesterol, atherosclerosis. (Copyright Anatomical Chart Co.)

marily consist of activated macrophages and T lymphocytes. Once within the arterial wall, the leukocyte can take up oxidized cholesterol and become a lipid laden macrophage (foam cell). As lesions progress, smooth muscle cells (SMC) migrate, proliferate, and secrete large amounts of extracellular matrix (collagen). SMC migration and proliferation is promoted by the release of several pro-inflammatory cytokines by leukocytes. The end result is the presence of an elevated plaque, which occludes the vessel lumen. (Also see Chapter 13, Dyslipidemias, Atherosclerosis, and Coronary Heart Disease.) The inflammatory process is not only involved in the initiation and a development of atherosclerosis, but also is directly involved in the acute thrombotic complications of atherosclerosis, such as MI or USA. Cytokines produced by activated macrophages induce the production of proteolytic enzymes, which break down the extracellular matrix and render the plaque more prone to rupture.[12,13]

A key factor in plaque formation is the functional status of the vascular endothelium (Fig. 17-4) Historically, the endothelium was thought to act simply as the inner barrier of blood vessels. However, this single-cell layer has several functions, including the synthesis and secretion of many different substances and the regulation of the local vascular environment. One of the key substances synthesized is endothelium-derived relaxing factor (EDRF), identified as nitric oxide. Nitric oxide has vasodilatory, antithrombotic, anti-inflammatory, and growth-inhibiting properties. In the response to injury hypothesis, the endothelium is damaged and loses the ability to secrete nitric oxide and the ability to regulate the vascular environment. Without nitric oxide, the endothelium facilitates inflammation, thromboses, and extracellular growth. In this setting, atherosclerotic plaques can develop.[14,15] Assessment of endothelial function with non-invasive measures can independently predict patients at risk for ACS and may become a key component of estimating overall cardiovascular risk in the future.[16]

Several risk factors increase the risk of developing atherosclerosis (Table 17-1).[17,18] These risk factors promote endothelial dysfunction, which then promotes the development of CAD. Recently, primary prevention strategies have moved away from considering individual risk factors independently to identifying global cardiovascular risk in an individual. Those individuals considered to be at high risk for the development of cardiovascular disease (defined as a 20% risk of having a cardiovascular event over the next 10 years as determined by the Framingham risk table; see Chapter 13, Dyslipidemias, Atherosclerosis, and Coronary Heart Disease) should receive aggressive risk factor modification, regardless of the status of individual risk factors.[18,19] Elevated C-reactive protein (CRP) has been shown to predict major cardiovascular events in multiple prospective epidemiologic studies. As a marker of systemic inflammation, a single determination of CRP adds prognostic information on global cardiovascular risk at all levels of calculated Framingham risk. Despite the favorable potential for CRP, no guidelines exist for when and how often risk

Table 17-1 Risk Factors for Coronary Artery Disease	
Causative risk factors (directly associated with the development of CAD)	Smoking Hypertension High total and LDL cholesterol Low HDL cholesterol Type 1 and type 2 diabetes mellitus

Conditional risk factors (potentially associated with CAD, but evidence still accumulating)	High triglycerides
	Small LDL particles
	Lipoprotein(a)
	Homocysteine
	C-reactive protein
	Coagulation factors:
	    Plasminogen activator
	      inhibitor-1
	      Elevated fibrinogen

Predisposing risk factors (directly impact the development of causative risk factors)	Obesity/overweight Physical inactivity Male gender Family history of CAD Socioeconomic factors Insulin resistance

CAD, coronary artery disease; HDL, high-density lipoprotein; LDL, low-density lipoprotein.
Adapted from references 12, 18.

Endothelial Layer

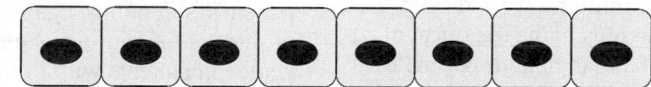

- Normal Function
  - Substances Produced
    - Nitric Oxide (NO)
    - Prosaglandin I_2 (PGI$_2$)
  - Main Actions
    - Anti-thrombotic
    - Anti-inflammatory
    - Extracellular Growth Inhibition

- Endothelial Dysfunction
  - Substances Produced
    - Angiotensin II
    - Endothelin
  - Main Actions
    - Pro-thrombotic
    - Pro-inflammatory
    - Extracellular Growth Facilitation

FIGURE 17-4. Endothelial function.

should be assessed in a given patient. A likely application for CRP will involve measuring it in patients who are determined to be at intermediate cardiovascular risk (calculated 10-year Framingham risk for a cardiovascular event between 5% and 20%). In circumstances in which CRP is elevated (level >3 mg/L) in patients at intermediate risk, physicians may opt for a more aggressive approach for risk factor modification. Likewise, if CRP is low (level <1 mg/L) in a patient at intermediate risk, a more conservative course of action may be warranted.[20,21] The targeting of risk factors is a critical strategy in the prevention and treatment of CHD and is discussed later.

Platelet Aggregation and the Formation of Thrombi

Although plaque rupture and the formation of a superimposing thrombus are commonly considered in the pathophysiology of acute coronary syndrome,[11] platelet activation and thrombus formation also are integral to the chronic atherosclerotic process. In response to arterial vessel wall injury (e.g., an atherosclerotic lesion), platelets aggregate and release granular contents.[12] These activities further enhance platelet aggregation, vasoconstriction (dynamic obstruction), and in many cases, thrombus formation. Although coronary atherosclerosis is the underlying mechanism for most patients with anginal syndromes, thrombotic factors commonly play a key role in the pathogenesis of myocardial ischemia. Both blood flow turbulence and stasis can cause intermittent platelet aggregation or intermittent coronary artery thrombosis. Thus, platelet-active agents are used in the treatment of chronic stable angina and USA, primary prevention of MI, secondary prevention of myocardial ischemia and acute MI, and in patients after coronary angioplasty or coronary artery bypass grafting (CABG).

Treatment Overview

The medical management of anginal syndromes always should be individualized. All patients should receive extensive education and counseling to help them reduce the risks of CHD. Risk factor modification is critical in the prevention and treatment of CHD. For most risk factors, national guidelines are available to assist in the formulation of a treatment plan. Table 17-2 lists risk factors and treatment guidelines. An assessment and treatment plan for each risk factor should be the first step in the overall treatment of patients with CHD.[1]

Six classes of drugs (nitrates, β-blockers, calcium channel blockers, antiplatelet drugs, oral anticoagulants, and angiotensin-converting enzyme [ACE] inhibitors) have been used either alone or in various combinations in the treatment of patients with CHD. Comparisons of antianginal drugs and treatment guidelines have been formulated to assist clinicians in the management of patients with chronic stable angina.[1]

The initial step in devising a treatment strategy for a particular patient should begin with an assessment of risk factors and should be followed by efforts to modify these risk factors. Although medications can treat symptoms and decrease mortality in patients with CHD, the value of risk factor modification and lifestyle changes in altering the progression of CHD should not be underestimated. A short-acting nitrate (either sublingual NTG tablets or lingual spray) should be prescribed for all patients to relieve or prevent an acute anginal episode. In the absence of any contraindications, all patients also should receive some form of antiplatelet therapy. Aspirin is

Table 17-2 Risk Factors and Associated Treatment Guidelines

Risk Factor	Treatment Guideline
Hypertension	JNC-VII[22]
Smoking	Assess tobacco use at every visit. Assist cessation with counseling and developing a plan to quit.
	Urge avoidance of second hand smoke[18,23]
Hyperlipidemia	NCEP-III[24]
	LDL <100 mg/dL
	HDL >40 mg/dL
	Triglycerides <150 mg/dL[18,24]
Type 1 and 2 diabetes mellitus	HgbA$_{1c}$ <7%[18,25]
Physical inactivity	Minimum 30 min exercise 3-4 times per week[18,26,27]
Obesity	Goal: BMI 18.5–24.9 Kg/m² [18,28]

BMI, body mass index; HDL, high-density lipoprotein; JNC, Joint National Committee; LDL, low-density lipoproteins.

the antiplatelet agent of choice, but clopidogrel is a viable alternative for patients with an allergy or intolerance to aspirin.[1] Furthermore, in patients who have recently experienced an acute coronary syndrome, optimal pharmacotherapy can include the combination of aspirin and clopidogrel for up to 1 year.[29,30] A long-acting nitrate, β-blocker, or calcium channel blocker also should be prescribed to prevent recurrent anginal syndromes. The selection of the optimal prophylactic antianginal medication should be based on the known effects of each medication on morbidity and mortality, the presence of concomitant diseases, and expected adverse reaction profiles. For example, a patient with both angina and moderately severe heart failure may benefit from either a long-acting nitrate or a cardioselective β-blocker (e.g. metoprolol), both of which can relieve the congestion symptoms of heart failure and also prevent angina. At the same time, specific calcium antagonists, such as verapamil, should be avoided in the same patient because verapamil can worsen HF.

Anginal episodes sometimes can be prevented with single-drug therapy (e.g., long-acting nitrate, β-blocker, calcium channel blocker). However, many patients require double- or triple-drug therapy. Combination drug therapy balances the patient's symptoms against the combined adverse reaction profiles of these drugs. Angina attacks can be completely prevented in patients with mild anginal syndromes. Patients with more severe disease continue to have angina attacks despite prophylactic drug therapy. Therefore, the goal of drug therapy in these patients is to decrease the frequency and intensity of attacks. The long-term goal of therapy is to prevent myocardial infarction and prolong life.

CHRONIC STABLE EXERTIONAL ANGINA

Signs and Symptoms

1. J.P., a 62-year-old retired dairy farmer, is hospitalized for evaluation of chest pain. About 3 weeks before admission, he noted substernal chest pain brought on by lifting heavy objects or walking uphill. He describes a crushing or viselike pain that never occurs at rest and is not associated with meals, emotional stress, or a particular time of day. When J.P. stops working, the pain subsides in about 5 minutes.

J.P.'s mother and brother died of a heart attack at ages 62 and 57, respectively; his father, who is alive at age 86, has survived one heart attack and one stroke. His family history is negative for diabetes mellitus. J.P. is 5'10" tall and weighs 235 lb; he drinks two or three beers per day and does not smoke or chew tobacco.

J.P.'s other medical problems include a 10-year history of hypertension, diabetes for 4 years, and traumatic amputation of the right hand. Until 3 weeks ago, J.P. could perform all his farm chores without difficulty, including heavy labor. He follows a no-added-salt diet, but consistently eats at fast-food establishments with his favorite meal consisting of two cheeseburgers and French fries.

J.P.'s medication history reveals the following: atenolol (Tenormin) 50 mg QD, glipizide (Glucotrol) 5 mg BID and losartan (Cozaar) 50 mg QD. He rarely uses over-the-counter medications. He has a history of an allergic reaction to sulfa drugs.

On admission to the cardiac ward, J.P. appears his stated age and is in no apparent distress. Resting vital signs include: supine blood pressure (BP), 164/98 mm Hg (normal, 120/80); regular pulse, 73 beats/min (normal, 65 to 75); and respiratory rate, 12 breaths/min (normal, 8 to 14). He has no peripheral edema or neck vein distention, and lung auscultation is within normal limits. Abdominal exam is unremarkable and he is alert and oriented ×3. Cardiac auscultation reveals a regular rate and rhythm with a normal S_1 and S_2; third or fourth heart sounds and murmurs are not noted. A 12-lead ECG reveals normal sinus rhythm at a rate of 75 without evidence of previous MI. All intervals are within normal limits.

Admitting laboratory values include the following: Hct, 43.5% (normal, 40% to 45%); white blood cell (WBC) count, 5,000/mm³ (normal, 5,000 to 10,000); sodium (Na), 140 mEq/L (normal, 136 to 144); potassium (K), 4.7 mEq/L (normal, 3.5 to 5.3); magnesium (Mg), 1.9 mEq/L (normal, 1.7 to 2.7); random blood glucose, 152 mg/dL (normal fasting, 65 to 110); blood urea nitrogen (BUN), 27 mg/dL (normal, 10 to 20); serum creatinine (SrCr), 1.4 mg/dL (normal, 0.5 to 1.2). Chest radiograph is within normal limits. What signs and symptoms of angina pectoris does J.P. exhibit? Can his symptoms be categorized on a measurement scale?

[SI units: Hct, 0.435 (normal, 0.40 to 0.45); WBC count, 5 ×10⁹/L (normal, 5 to 10×10⁹/L); Na, 140 mmol/L (normal, 136 to 144); K, 4.7 mmol/L (normal, 3.5 to 5.3); Mg, 0.95 mmol/L (normal, 0.85 to 1.35); random blood glucose, 6.16 mmol/L (normal, 3.6 to 6.1); BUN, 9.6 mmol/L of urea (normal, 3.57 to 7.14); SrCr, 124 μmol/L (normal, 44.2 to 106)]

J.P.'s description of his chest pain includes several common characteristics of angina pectoris (Table 17-3).[31] The substernal location of J.P.'s chest pain is typical, although some patients describe pain radiating down the left arm or pain that is referred to the shoulder area or jaw. J.P.'s pain is described as crushing or viselike in quality, which also is common: a fullness in the throat or jaw may occur simultaneously or in lieu of chest pain. In some cases, the patient may not consider these sensations as pain, describing them instead as a sense of pressure or heaviness. Many patients complain of SOB. J.P.'s symptoms are related to exercise and exertion—both known precipitating factors of angina. Most episodes of exertional angina last several minutes in duration and are relieved with

Table 17-3 Characteristics of Angina Pectoris[31]

Symptoms	Duration of Symptoms
• Sensation of pressure or heavy weight on chest alone or with pain	• 0.5–30 min
• Pain described variably as feeling of tightness, burning, crushing, squeezing, vice-like, aching, or "deep"	**ECG**
• Gradual ↑ in intensity followed by gradual fading away (distinguished from esophageal spasm)ᵃ	• ST-segment depression ≥2 mm
• SOBᵇ with feeling constriction about the larynx of upper trachea	• T-wave inversion
Location of Pain or Discomfort	**Precipitating Factors**
• Over the sternum or very near to it	• Mild, moderate, or heavy exercise, depending on patient
• Anywhere between epigastrium and pharynx	• Effort that involves use of arms above the head
• Occasionally limited to left shoulder and left arm	• Cold environment
• Rarely limited to left shoulder and left arm	• Walking against the wind
• Rarely limited to right arm	• Walking after a large meal
• Lower cervical or upper thoracic spine	• Emotions: fright, anger, or anxiety
• Left interscapular or suprascapular area	• Coitus
Radiation of Pain	**Nitroglycerin Relief**ᵃ
• Medial aspect of left arm	• Relief of pain occurring within 45 sec to 5 min of taking nitroglycerin
• Left shoulder	
• Jaw	
• Occasionally, right arm	

ᵃEsophageal spasm and other GI disorders occasionally mimic anginal pain and also can be relieved by nitroglycerin.
ᵇSOB, Shortness of breath.

rest. Because J.P. has never sought medical attention for his chest pain, his response to NTG cannot be determined.

After getting a detailed description of J.P.'s symptom complex, his physician can characterize his chest pain and make a global assessment. Initially, the chest pain should be classified as either typical angina, atypical angina, or noncardiac chest pain. Furthermore, angina should also be classified as either stable or unstable. This distinction is important because it indicates whether his short-term risk of an acute coronary event could be life-threatening. Unstable angina can also be subdivided by short term risk (Table 17-4). Patients at high or moderate risk should receive aggressive treatment to prevent adverse cardiovascular outcomes in the short term.[1] Attempts to categorize J.P.'s anginal symptoms on an objective measurement scale (e.g., Canadian Cardiovascular Society Grading Scale) can be misleading.[32] For example, a sedentary 65-year-old patient's class II symptoms may be tolerable, but the same symptoms could significantly disable an active 50-year-old patient.

J.P.'s chest pain is of a quality and duration characteristic of angina, provoked by exertion, and relieved by rest; therefore, J.P.'s constellation of symptoms can be classified as typical chest pain. However, J.P.'s symptoms do not occur at rest, so they can be classified as stable angina.[1]

2. **Assess J.P.'s physical examination. What signs and symptoms are relevant to the angina?**

The physical examination typically provides little information about the presence of CAD. The most useful findings pertain to the cardiovascular system where heart rate and BP can be increased during an acute anginal episode. J.P.'s physical examination is characteristic for a man of his age with angina.[2] He is obese and hypertensive, but his cardiac examination is normal. The presence of murmurs would have required further workup; the absence of a third heart sound suggests that the left ventricle may be functioning normally. (See Chapter 19, Heart Failure, for a description of third heart sounds.) The absence of a fourth heart sound in J.P. is indicative of a low probability of either CHD or a cardiac end-organ damage resulting from systemic hypertension. His chest radiograph, which is normal, does not present evidence of other complications commonly associated with myocardial ischemia (e.g., enlarged heart, heart failure).

J.P.'s physical examination should have evaluated the possibility of peripheral vascular disease and abdominal aortic aneurysm. The presence of xanthomas would suggest severe hypercholesterolemia, but these were not noted in J.P.

Risk Factors

3. **What independent risk factors for CAD are present in J.P.? Which of these may be altered?**

J.P. has several risk factors for CAD, some of which cannot be altered, such as middle age, male gender, and a strong family history of CAD. Risk factors such as hypertension, obesity, hypercholesterolemia, smoking, and possibly stress, can potentially be modified to decrease the likelihood of adverse sequelae for J.P. His hypertension should be controlled and his serum cholesterol concentration should be tested and fractionated for low-density lipoprotein (LDL), high-density lipoprotein (HDL), and triglycerides (TGs). (See Chapter 13, Dyslipidemias, Atherosclerosis, and Coronary Heart Disease.) A fasting hemoglobin A_1C should be drawn with a goal of less than 7%. (See Chapter 50, Diabetes Mellitus.) Dietary modification and weight reduction for J.P. are mandatory,

Table 17-4 Short-Term Risk of Death or Nonfatal MI in Patients With Unstable Angina

Feature	High Risk (At least one of the following must be present)	Intermediate Risk (No high-risk features, but must have one of the following)	Low Risk (No high- or intermediate-risk features, but may have any of the following)
History	Accelerating tempo of ischemic symptoms in preceding 48 hours	Prior MI, peripheral or cerebrovascular disease, or CABG, prior aspirin use	
Character of pain	Prolonged ongoing (>20 min), rest pain	Prolonged (>20 min) rest angina, now resolved, with moderate or high likelihood of CAD	New-onset angina[32] CCS class III or IV angina in the past 2 weeks without prolonged (>20 min) rest pain but with moderate or high likelihood of CAD
Clinical findings	• Pulmonary edema • New or worsening MR murmur • S_3 or new/worsening rales • Hypotension, bradycardia, tachycardia • Age >75 years		
ECG	• Angina at rest with transient ST-segment changes >0.05 mV • Bundle-branch block, new or presumed new	• T-wave inversions >0.2 mV • Pathologic Q waves	Normal or unchanged ECG during episode of chest discomfort
Cardiac markers	Markedly elevated (e.g., TnT or TnI >0.1 ng/ml)	Slightly elevated (e.g., TnT >0.01 but <0.1 ng/ml)	Normal

CABG, coronary artery bypass graft; CAD, coronary artery disease; CCS, Canadian Cardiovascular Society; ECG, electrocardiogram; MR, mitral regurgitation; S_3, third heart sound.
Adapted from reference 11.

since they positively influence several risk factors. Fortunately, J.P. does not smoke cigarettes, which would significantly increase his cardiovascular risk.[1] J.P.'s active lifestyle may influence his prognosis favorably.[33]

Diagnostic Procedures

4. **J.P.'s medical history and family history support the diagnosis of chronic stable angina. What other objective diagnostic procedures are helpful to confirm CHD and angina?**

A 12-lead ECG during an anginal episode would confirm CHD and angina if nonspecific ST-T changes, T-wave inversion, or ST-segment depression of ≥ 2 mm are noted (all are indicative of myocardial ischemia). Various arrhythmias can be detected on ECG, but generally are nonspecific for CHD. A normal ECG during chest pain would suggest a noncardiac cause for J.P.'s symptoms (e.g., esophagitis).[2]

Exercise Tolerance Test

An exercise tolerance test or treadmill test would be helpful in the diagnosis of CAD in J.P. Under controlled circumstances, J.P. would exercise to a preset level, and the test would be indicative of CAD upon the development of angina, ECG signs of ischemia, arrhythmias, abnormal heart rate, or abnormal BP response. The product of the heart rate and systolic BP (i.e., *the rate–pressure or double product*) correlates well with myocardial oxygen demand. The rate–pressure product normally rises progressively during exercise, with the peak value best describing the cardiovascular response to stress. Often, stable angina patients experience chest pain at a consistent rate–pressure product.[34]

Abnormal responses of either BP or heart rate may signal CAD. A normal BP response to exercise is a gradual rise in systolic BP with the diastolic BP remaining unchanged. A rise or fall of diastolic BP >10 mm Hg is considered abnormal. A fall in systemic BP during exercise is especially ominous because this indicates that the cardiac output cannot increase enough to overcome the vasodilation in the skeletal muscle vascular bed.

During exercise, the heart rate increases steadily until it reaches a plateau. The maximal heart rate depends on age, drug therapy, and cardiovascular fitness. Some patients can exhibit an abnormal slowing of heart rate, especially when taking β-blockers. Therefore, β-blockers should be tapered off (i.e., gradually discontinued) before treadmill testing when the test is being used for diagnosis or risk stratification. Similarly, digoxin can also interfere with the results of exercise testing, and other testing modalities are recommended if digoxin cannot be safely discontinued before treadmill testing. In patients with a history such as J.P.'s, the exercise tolerance test helps to confirm the presence of CAD and provides a risk stratification that may be helpful in determining whether he is a candidate for revascularization therapy.[34]

Myocardial Imaging

Stress imaging studies, either echocardiographic or nuclear, are preferred over the exercise tolerance test in patients with left bundle-branch block, electronically paced ventricular rhythm, prior revascularization (percutaneous coronary intervention or coronary artery bypass surgery), pre-excitation syndrome, greater than 1 mm ST-segment depression at rest, or other ECG conduction abnormalities. In addition, many patients are not able to develop an appropriate level of cardiac stress through exercise; pharmacologic stress testing is preferred in these patients.[1]

Pharmacologic stress may be achieved through the use of dipyridamole, adenosine, or dobutamine. Each of these agents is used to induce changes in the balance between myocardial oxygen supply and demand, similar to walking on a treadmill during the exercise stress test. Vasodilators (dipyridamole and adenosine) promote vasodilation in normal coronary segments, but have no effect in arteries affected by atherosclerosis. The net result is shunting of blood away from diseased coronary arteries and the development of ischemia that may be detected by changes in blood pressure, heart rate, or ECG changes. These agents are typically used in conjunction with myocardial perfusion scintigraphy. Stress thallium-201 myocardial perfusion imaging provides a dynamic picture of the heart. The radionuclide is injected at peak stress and an image is obtained within several minutes. A defect in myocardial uptake of the thallium indicates an area of ischemia or possible infarction.[1]

Dobutamine is a positive inotrope and typically is used with echocardiography. Administration of dobutamine leads to an increase in myocardial oxygen demand secondary to increases in heart rate and contractility. If demand exceeds available oxygen supply, ischemia develops. Subsequent to the infusion of dobutamine, defects or decreases in the wall motion or thickening of the left ventricle are indicative of ischemia.[1]

Cardiac Catheterization

5. **Should J.P. undergo cardiac catheterization? How will the results of this invasive procedure influence future therapy?**

CHD can be diagnosed definitively only by coronary catheterization and subsequent angiography. In addition, angiography is the most accurate means of identifying less common causes of chronic stable angina such as coronary artery spasm.[1,35] Cardiac catheterization is a procedure used to provide vascular access to the coronary arteries. Once access is gained with an intravascular catheter, a number of procedures (angiography, ventriculography, percutaneous coronary intervention) may be performed. Access to the vasculature is usually obtained percutaneously through the brachial or femoral arteries. From this point the catheter is advanced through the vasculature until the coronary arteries are accessible. After the tip of the catheter is advanced into the coronary arteries, radiocontrast dye is injected into the coronary arteries and the location and extent of atherosclerosis can be determined. Approximately 75% of patients with chronic stable angina such as J.P. are noted to have one-, two-, or three-vessel disease by this procedure (approximately equally divided).[2]

The results of angiography will be useful in determining the risk of death or MI in J.P. and, subsequently, the course of needed treatment. For example, patients who have a significant stenosis in the left main coronary artery are at high risk of death and should undergo coronary artery bypass grafting (CABG).[36]

Prognosis

6. **J.P. is found to have two-vessel CAD with lesions of 55% and 70%; the LAD coronary artery is not involved. What is his prognosis?**

J.P.'s history and physical examination suggest he does not have HF; poor LV function would be an ominous concurrent finding. J.P. also is fortunate not to have three-vessel disease or blockage of the LAD artery.[1] Overall, he probably will do well with medical therapy. His life expectancy depends on progression of the disease and development of other complications of CHD (e.g., heart failure, MI, sudden cardiac death). Although medical therapy is a reasonable treatment strategy for J.P., revascularization via percutaneous transluminal coronary angioplasty (PTCA) is an equally viable option. Although PTCA with or without stent placement would offer no mortality advantage over medical therapy at this time, it has been shown to decrease the incidence of recurrent symptoms.[1] Both strategies, including both pros and cons, should be offered to J.P. so that an informed decision can be made in accord with his wishes.

Presently, J.P. is not a candidate for CABG because the usual indications for surgical therapy include presence of left main CAD, presence of three-vessel disease (especially if LV function is impaired), or ineffectiveness of medical therapy.[36]

Overview of Medical Management

7. After consultation, J.P. and his cardiologist elect to control his angina medically. What are the goals of his therapy and how can they be achieved?

There are two major pharmacotherapeutic goals for treating all patients with angina. The first goal includes relief of symptoms and reduction of myocardial ischemia to improve quality of life. The second goal, and more important overall, is to prevent major complications of CAD such as AMI and death (increase quantity of life). Therapies that prevent death should receive priority. As with any chronic disease, education of the patient and his or her family are important objectives. The ultimate goal of patient education is a better quality of life through improved understanding of the disease and its therapy. Every effort should be made to reverse J.P.'s modifiable risk factors (i.e., his obesity, hypertension, and diabetes). He also could receive one or more of the following: nitrates, calcium channel blockers, β-adrenergic blockers, ACE inhibitors, or antiplatelet drugs.[1,37] J.P. should continue atenolol therapy because it will be helpful in treating both his hypertension and angina. Compliance to atenolol should be assessed because his BP was elevated upon admission. His BUN and creatinine are slightly elevated (probably as a consequence of his hypertension), and he developed angina symptoms despite use of the β-blocker. Reduction of precipitating factors may be difficult given J.P.'s work. However, he should be counseled to avoid sudden bursts of physical activity. Moderate exercise should be encouraged, such as a walking program. J.P.'s family members should be screened for smoking because passive (secondhand) smoke can aggravate angina.

NITRATES

Nitrates are almost always used in the treatment of all anginal syndromes. They are effective in treating all forms of angina because they decrease venous return to the heart and therefore decrease cardiac work load. Nitrates also promote coronary vasodilation, even in the presence of atherosclerosis. Nitrates generally are well tolerated, but to prevent loss of effect over

time must be scheduled to provide a nitrate-free interval of 10 to 12 hours. Therefore, nitrates should be combined with a β-blocker or a calcium channel blocker (e.g., verapamil, diltiazem). The individual nitrate products differ primarily in their onset and duration of action.

Mechanism of Action

8. During the first hospital day, J.P. decides to walk up three flights of stairs when returning to his room from the cafeteria instead of taking the elevator. Midway through the third flight of stairs J.P. develops chest pain. After quickly performing a 12-lead ECG, the physician instructs J.P. to place a 0.4-mg sublingual NTG tablet (Nitrostat) under his tongue. This relieves the pain. J.P.'s physician elects to continue atenolol and add both short- and long-acting nitrates. What is the mechanism by which nitroglycerin relieves angina? Why should J.P. continue his atenolol therapy?

The mechanism of action of NTG and the other nitrate esters is not completely understood, even though they have been used for >100 years. The overall benefits of nitrates result from a reduction in myocardial oxygen demand caused by venodilation and some arteriolar dilation.[1] Nitrates produce vasodilation by at least two mechanisms: stimulation of cyclic guanosine monophosphate (cGMP) production and inhibition of thromboxane synthetase. Organic nitrates are converted into nitric oxide. Nitric oxide is identical to endothelium-derived relaxation factor (EDRF), an endogenous vasodilator. Nitric oxide reacts with sulfhydryl groups in the vascular smooth muscle to produce S-nitrosothiols, which subsequently activate guanylate cyclase and increase the intracellular concentration of cGMP; cGMP controls the amount of vascular smooth muscle calcium available for muscle contraction by binding to calmodulin and phosphorylating myosin light chain kinase. The cGMP enhances calcium uptake into the sarcoplasmic reticulum, or inhibits its cellular influx. Because less calcium is available, dilation occurs.[38,39]

The peripheral effects of sublingual NTG in J.P. include dilation of both veins and arteries. Venous dilation is more pronounced because relaxation of arterial smooth muscle requires higher plasma NTG levels. By dilating the veins and reducing preload to the heart, filling pressures in the ventricles are reduced. This, in turn, reduces myocardial oxygen demand, thereby relieving J.P.'s angina.[38,39] (See Chapter 19, Heart Failure, for a more detailed discussion of preload.)

Nitrates also dilate epicardial coronary arteries.[38] Until recently, researchers assumed that arteries supplying ischemic areas already were maximally dilated and would not respond to nitrates. Angiographic studies show that coronary vessels that are not completely engulfed by the atherosclerotic lesions (eccentric lesions) will dilate further. Thus, nitrates will decrease J.P.'s coronary vasomotor tone.

Atenolol should be continued in J.P. because it both lowers BP and exerts antianginal effects. In addition, administration of nitrates must include a daily nitrate-free interval, and the atenolol will provide protection from ischemia during this time.[39] The addition of long-acting nitrates will provide J.P. additional protection against developing angina, and short-acting NTG will provide J.P. acute relief when an anginal attack occurs. Both short- and long-acting nitrates have well-documented effects and a low incidence of adverse reactions; they are reasonably priced.

Short-Acting Preparations

Sublingual Nitroglycerin
DOSING

9. How should J.P.'s dose of sublingual NTG be determined? Can NTG be used prophylactically?

Because sensitivity to NTG varies among patients, the dosage should be individualized (Table 17-5). However, most patients use a dose of 0.4 mg. An optimal dosage relieves pain and produces an objective hemodynamic response, such as a 10-mm Hg fall in systolic BP or a 10-beat/minute rise in heart rate. However, it should not cause intolerable orthostatic hypotension.[39]

The administration of sublingual NTG is also useful in patients who have a good understanding of what level of exertion produces their chest pain. Five to ten minutes before J.P. is about to undergo heavy exertion, he can take a sublingual NTG tablet to prevent angina.[1]

PATIENT INSTRUCTIONS

10. What instructions should J.P. receive with regard to the use and storage of sublingual NTG? How rapidly will sublingual NTG relieve J.P.'s chest pain?

When angina occurs, J.P. should sit down immediately and place the NTG tablet under his tongue; he should not swallow it. Many patients experience dizziness and lightheadedness, which is minimized by sitting. The onset of action is within 1 to 2 minutes, and pain usually is relieved within 3 to 5 minutes. If he needs more than one tablet, he can take a maximum of three tablets over 15 minutes. If the pain persists for >30 minutes, he should seek medical assistance because he may be having an MI.[39]

The tablets should be dispensed in the original, unopened manufacturer's container and stored in the original brown bottle. Because sublingual NTG tablets are degraded by heat, moisture, and light, they should be stored in a cool, dry place, but not refrigerated. The bottle should be closed tightly after each opening. Safety caps are not necessary, although patients should be cautioned to keep all medications out of the reach of children. The cotton plug sometimes is difficult to remove.

Table 17-5	Commonly Prescribed Organic Nitrates			
Nitrates	Dosage Form	Duration	Onset (min)	Usual Dosage
Short-acting				
NTG	SL	10–30 min	1–3	0.4–0.6 mg[a,b]
NTG	Translingual spray	10–30 min	2–4	0.4 mg/metered spray[a,b]
NTG	IV	3–5 min[c]	1–2	Initially 5 μg/min. ↑ Q 3–5 min until pain is relieved or hypotension occurs
Long-acting[d]				
NTG	SR capsule	4–8 hr	30	6.5–9 mg Q 8 hr
NTG	Topical ointment[e]	4–8 hr	30	½"–2" Q 4–6 hr[f] (Table 14-4)
NTG	Transdermal patch	4–8 hr	30	0.2–0.4 mg/hr[f]
NTG	Transmucosal	3–6 hr	2–5	1–3 mg Q 3–5 hr[f]
ISDN[g]	SL	2–4 hr	2–5	2.5–10 mg Q 2–4 hr[f]
	Chewable	2–4 hr	2–5	5–10 mg Q 2–4 hr[f]
	Oral	2–6 hr	15–40	10–60 mg Q 4–6 hr[f]
	SR	4–8 hr	15–40	40–80 mg Q 6–8 hr[f]
ISMN[h]	Tab (ISMO, Monoket)	7–8 hr	30–60	10–20 mg BID (a.m. and midday) to start. Titrate to 20–40 mg BID[f]
	SR tab (Imdur)	8–12 hr	30–60	60 mg QD to start. Titrate to 30–120 mg QD

[a]When using sublingual or translingual spray forms of nitroglycerin, patients should administer the dose while sitting to minimize tachycardia, hypotension, dizziness, headache, and flushing. The optimal dose relieves symptoms with ≤10–15 mm Hg drop in systolic BP or ≤10 beat/min rise in pulse. Pain relief is rapid (onset 1–2 min; relief in 3–5 min), but up to 3 doses at 5-min intervals may be given. After this, medical assistance should be summoned.
[b]Sublingual NTG tablets are degraded rapidly by heat, moisture, and light. They should be stored in a cool, dry place; do not leave the lid open or refrigerate. Tablets should be stored in the original manufacturer's container or a glass vial since the tablets volatilize and bind to many plastic vials and cotton. Previously, stinging of the tongue was an indicator of fresh tablets, but newer formulations only cause stinging in ~75% of patients.
[c]Duration after infusion discontinued.
[d]Longer-acting forms of nitrates are effective drugs, but one must understand their limitations to optimize effectiveness. Sublingual ISDN tablets display an onset and duration intermediate between that of sublingual NTG and oral ISDN. Because of high presystemic (1st-pass) metabolism of the oral forms of both NTG and ISDN, very large doses may be required compared to sublingual or chewable dosage forms. Small oral doses (2.5 mg NTG, 5 mg ISDN) are probably not effective; doses as large as 9 mg NTG and 60 mg ISDN are not uncommon. Despite claims for longer activity, ointments and oral forms are often only effective for 4-8 hr, even when given as sustained release (SR) preparations. Also, continued daily use leads to rapid development of tolerance (see f).
[e]Squeeze ½"–2" of ointment onto the calibrated paper enclosed in the package with tube. Carefully spread the ointment on chest in a thin layer ≈2" × 2" in size. Keep area covered with applicator paper. Wipe off previous dose before adding new dose or if hypotensive. If another person applies the ointment, avoid contact with fingers or eyes to prevent headache or hypotension.
[f]Dosage regimens should maintain a nitrate-free interval (e.g., bedtime) to ↓ tolerance development. Give last oral dose or remove ointment or transdermal patch at 7 p.m. Give last dose of SR ISDN in early afternoon.
[g]ISDN, Isosorbide dinitrate.
[h]ISMN, Isosorbide monohydrate = Major active metabolite of ISDN. 100% bioavailable; no first-pass metabolism, but tolerance may still occur. Rapid release (ISMO, Monoket) as 10- and 20-mg tablets. SR form (Imdur) as 60-mg tablets. OK to cut Indur in half, do not crush or chew.

Therefore, it should be discarded upon initial receipt of the prescription and should not be replaced. Use of cotton other than that supplied by the manufacturer should be discouraged because NTG tablets are volatile and are adsorbed by household cotton. This results in a significant loss in tablet effectiveness. Expiration dating should be monitored closely, and tablets should be replaced immediately if they are exposed to excessive light, heat, moisture, or air. Once a container is opened, the tablets should be used for only a limited time—usually from 6 months to 1 year.[39] A tablet left out of the bottle on a table will lose its effectiveness in just a few hours.

Nitroglycerin Lingual Spray

11. J.P. completes his evaluation and is maintained on atenolol 50 mg PO QD and sublingual NTG 0.4 mg PRN. His amputation makes opening of the sublingual NTG tablet bottle cumbersome. What other short-acting nitrate delivery system can be used? What are the possible side effects?

NTG lingual spray (Nitrolingual), available in a 0.4-mg metered-dose canister, is an attractive alternative for J.P.[40,41] Each canister dispenses 200 doses and has a shelf-life of 3 years.[41] He should bring the canister as close to his mouth as possible and spray a single dose of the NTG under or onto his tongue. The spray should not be inhaled. He should sit down and should not exceed the maximum recommended dose of three sprays over 15 minutes.

Adverse Effects

For practical purposes, side effects of all nitrates are limited to hypotension and headache.[39] Dizziness is a tolerable effect, but syncope (passing out, fainting) mandates a dosage reduction because severe hypotension and bradycardia have caused cardiac arrest in patients experiencing MI. Syncope is secondary to a NTG-induced vasovagal reaction and should be treated with leg elevation, atropine, and fluid infusion when necessary. Nitrates are converted in the body to nitrites, which can oxidize the ferrous ion in Hgb to the ferric state, thereby producing methemoglobinemia.[42] This adverse effect is of clinical importance only when large intravenous NTG doses are used.

Although headache is a common and expected side effect of the nitrates, patients usually develop a tolerance to this effect within several weeks of beginning therapy. Mild analgesics such as acetaminophen are helpful. Occasionally, patients experience continuing headaches causing them to discontinue nitrate therapy.

Long-Acting Nitrates

12. J.P. does well over the next several months, but he is still bothered by occasional angina episodes, ranging from one to four times per week. The attacks usually are precipitated by strenuous work and are relieved by rest and 2 or 3 NTG sprays (0.4 mg each). The quality and location of the pain are unchanged, although the duration has increased by 1 or 2 minutes. He follows a low cholesterol, no-added-salt diet.

Physical examination is unchanged except for a 20-lb weight loss. Vital signs include the following: supine BP, 119/76 mm Hg; heart rate, 65 beats/min; and respiratory rate, 12 breaths/min. J.P.'s cardiologist elected to start a long-acting prophylactic nitrate (isosorbide dinitrate) as well as continuing his β-blocker and angiotensin-receptor blocker therapy. What therapeutic end points should be used to evaluate the efficacy of long-acting nitrates? Could a calcium channel blocker have been used instead of the long-acting nitrate?

Long-acting nitrates occupy a key role in the prevention of angina of all types. Their mechanism of action is the same as that of short-acting NTG. The goals of therapy are to decrease the number, severity, and duration of J.P.'s anginal attacks.

A calcium channel blocker could be prescribed for J.P. instead of isosorbide dinitrate because he has no contraindications to this class of drugs. A calcium channel blocker would have been a good alternative if his BP had remained elevated, but for now, J.P.'s BP and pulse are within a desired range. Because sublingual nitrates were well tolerated by J.P., a long-acting nitrate would be acceptable. However, a calcium channel blocker (e.g., amlodipine) is an alternative as long as J.P.'s BP is not unduly decreased by this combination of drugs. Ultimately, the decision is based on the prescriber's personal choice and past experience, as well as the entire spectrum of the patient's disease complex.

Nitrate Tolerance

13. Will J.P. develop tolerance to the long-acting nitrate?

Early evidence for the development of nitrate tolerance and dependence came from the munitions industry. Workers in this industry were constantly exposed to NTG and ethylene glycol dinitrate, components of explosives.[43] Since 1898, the "Monday syndrome" has been recognized: workers developed mild to severe headaches late Sunday or Monday morning or during holidays. By rubbing NTG into their skin, wearing NTG impregnated headbands, or taking medicinal NTG, the workers avoided the Monday syndrome. In some workers without atherosclerosis, abrupt withdrawal from nitrates triggered coronary artery spasm.

Although tolerance to nitrate-induced headaches within several days of therapy commonly was observed, the clinical importance of this phenomenon in patients with CHD was not fully appreciated. Tolerance to both the headaches and the desired cardiovascular effect occur in tandem. However, tolerance can be limited by maintaining a nitrate-free interval of about 10 to 12 hours daily. Nitrate dosing schedules should be arranged to permit a nitrate-free interval during which time the patient may receive angina protection from β-adrenergic blockers or calcium channel blockers. Most often, this nitrate-free interval is arranged during the night because angina is more likely to occur during the work day. Patients with nocturnal angina should arrange their nitrate-free interval during the day.[44] Tolerance also is minimized by using the lowest effective nitrate dosage. Because long-acting nitrates must be dosed intermittently to avoid tolerance, atenolol therapy will provide J.P. with continuous protection, even during the nitrate-free interval. Even though J.P. uses a long-acting nitrate, he still will respond favorably to sublingual NTG. There is no evidence that use of long-acting nitrates leads to resistance or tolerance to the effects of sublingual NTG. He should clearly understand the differences between the indications for the two nitrate products.

MECHANISM OF ACTION

14. What is the mechanism of action for nitrate tolerance?

There are several proposed mechanisms of nitrate tolerance, including the depletion of sulfhydryl groups, which are necessary for the biotransformation of nitrate to nitric oxide, neurohormonal activation, plasma volume expansion, and abnormalities in NO signal transduction. A proposed unifying mechanism of these factors is that administration of nitroglycerin increases the production of superoxide anion (O_2^-), which reacts with NO to form peroxynitrite. Peroxynitrite further decreases production of NO by the endothelium, reduces clearance of O_2^-, increases activity of the sympathetic and renin-angiotensin-aldosterone (RAS) systems, and produces increased responsiveness of the endothelium to vasoconstrictors such angiotensin II (AT II). What is still unknown is the initial trigger of increased O_2^- production.[45,46]

One potential consequence of this current theory is that long-term administration of organic nitrates, by producing neurohormonal activation and endothelial dysfunction, may have long-term detrimental effects. Further research is needed to confirm this hypothesis for nitrate tolerance and it's long-term consequences on patient outcomes.

INTERMITTENT APPLICATION OF TRANSDERMAL NITROGLYCERIN

15. Are all nitrate delivery systems capable of inducing nitrate tolerance? How can tolerance be minimized?

All organic nitrates exhibit similar hemodynamic effects through a common pharmacologic mechanism; yet, the differing pharmacokinetic profiles of the nitrate delivery systems lead to a variation in the development of tolerance.[44] Short-acting formulations such as sublingual NTG, oral NTG spray, and sublingual isosorbide dinitrate are not likely to induce tolerance given their rapid onset of action and short duration of effect. Oral nitrates and transdermal products, both having an extended duration of action, are prone to induce tolerance.

Intermittent application of transdermal NTG can limit tolerance development in patients with both chronic stable angina and HF. The effects of continuous (24 hours/day) and intermittent (16 hours/day) transdermal NTG (10 mg/day) were compared in 12 men with chronic stable angina who also were being treated with β-blockers or calcium channel blockers.[47] Nitrate efficacy was maintained with intermittent treatment and an 8-hour nitrate-free interval. However, tolerance to the antianginal effects occurred with continuous transdermal NTG treatment. Twelve-hour intermittent patch therapy also prevents tolerance.[48] The minimum time necessary for a nitrate-free interval is unknown.

Intravenous NTG, a cornerstone therapy in management of patients with USA and severe HF, is associated with nitrate tolerance if it is administered as a sustained infusion. The immediate hemodynamic benefits observed with NTG infusions in patients with severe chronic heart failure were greatly reduced 24 to 48 hours after continuous IV therapy. The tolerance to IV NTG was prevented by infusing NTG for only 12 hours followed by a 12-hour nitrate-free interval.[49] Intermittent NTG infusions for patients with USA appear reasonable, but have not been fully evaluated.

Isosorbide Dinitrate

16. J.P. receives a prescription for oral isosorbide dinitrate (Isordil) 30 mg PO TID. How should he be instructed to take his medication so that he is nitrate free for 10 to 12 hours?

Despite the availability of nitrate preparations that can be dosed once or twice a day (isosorbide mononitrate), oral isosorbide dinitrate is still commonly used in the treatment of angina. J.P. should take his oral nitrate at 7 AM, noon, and 5 PM because his exercise-induced angina is likely to occur during daylight hours. He may need to adjust this schedule if he arises earlier than 7 AM because early-morning angina is common. Some physicians prescribe isosorbide dinitrate twice a day for patients with less severe anginal syndrome at 7 AM and noon.

Nitrate Pharmacodynamics

17. Is J.P.'s isosorbide dinitrate dose appropriate in light of nitrate pharmacokinetics and pharmacodynamics?

Understanding of the complex relationships between organic nitrate pharmacokinetics, vascular metabolism, and influence of first-pass effect have improved in recent years. After IV administration in man, both NTG and isosorbide dinitrate have high apparent volumes of distribution (3 to 4 L/kg), which reflect extensive distribution in the vascular and other peripheral tissues. NTG is cleared rapidly from plasma at about 50 L/minute, whereas isosorbide dinitrate is cleared at a rate of about 4 L/minute. 5-Isosorbide mononitrate is the active metabolite of isosorbide dinitrate. It has a small apparent volume of distribution (0.6 L/kg) and a low venous clearance (0.1 L/minute). Thus, its elimination half-life of about 275 minutes is much longer than that of NTG ($\beta t_{1/2} = 10$ minutes) and isosorbide dinitrate ($\beta t_{1/2} = 65$ minutes).[39] (Also see Question 22.) Nitrate pharmacokinetic parameters are influenced profoundly by the highly lipophilic and volatile properties of NTG. Enzyme systems in the gut, liver, skin, sublingual mucosa, and blood vessels contribute to NTG's metabolism,[50] and the influence of each metabolic site varies with the route of administration.

All nitrate dosages must be individualized (see Table 17-5). Because higher dosages contribute to nitrate tolerance, the smallest effective dosage should be used. Oral isosorbide dinitrate therapy usually is initiated with a single 10- or 20-mg dose and gradually titrated upward to a maximum dosage of 40 to 60 mg given two to three times a day. Titration also helps limit the occurrence of headaches. In many patients, maximal improvement in exercise tolerance is achieved with an isosorbide dinitrate oral dose of 15 to 30 mg given two to three times a day.[39] However, doses of 40 to 60 mg are common. J.P.'s starting dosage of 30 mg three times a day may increase his risk of headaches and could be lowered to 15 mg for the first few days to assess his tolerance.

Transdermal Ointment

18. J.P. has a friend who uses NTG ointment. Is this a reasonable alternative for him? How should he be instructed to apply the ointment if it is prescribed?

NTG ointment could be applied three times daily beginning in the early morning, but it should be removed around 7

PM so that a nitrate-free interval is maintained. The amount of ointment applied ranges between 1.5 and 2 inches (15 mg/inch).[38] The 2% ointment is squeezed from a tube onto a paper marked with a measuring scale. Using the paper, the ointment is spread in a thin layer over an area of about 2 by 3 inches on the skin of the anterior chest or upper limbs. Absorption can be markedly affected by administration technique.[51–53] J.P. should rotate application sites to avoid skin irritation; an ointment application system that uses an adhesive unit (TSAR, Rorer Laboratories) similar to a large bandage limits the variability and messiness of dosing. NTG ointment may be removed by first discarding the paper and then wiping off the application site with a tissue. However, the skin acts as a reservoir and NTG absorption continues for 10 to 20 minutes after the paste is removed. Because it can be removed rather easily, some critical care physicians prefer NTG ointment over other nitrate formulations. Nurses may wish to wear gloves when removing NTG ointment to avoid NTG-induced headaches. However, ambulatory patients may dislike the inconvenience of this dosage form. NTG ointment has a variable duration of action, but generally it is effective for 4 to 6 hours. The duration of action may be shorter with chronic use. The therapeutic efficacy of NTG ointment is acceptable if patients do not apply the ointment continuously (i.e., maintain a dosage-free interval).

Transdermal Patches

19. J.P. likes the idea of using topical nitrates, but does not want to work with the ointment, which he considers too messy. Are the transdermal patches a viable alternative? Is there any difference between products?

Transdermal NTG patches originally were designed to provide angina protection with once-daily application. The concept of a compact, easy-to-apply transdermal NTG patch prompted pharmaceutical manufacturers to design a number of products, which the U.S. Food and Drug Administration (FDA) subsequently approved based on plasma level data, not clinical efficacy studies (Table 17-6). Since the FDA approval of these products, the shortcomings of plasma level data have become apparent and prompted numerous clinical efficacy studies.

Transdermal NTG therapy has been shown to increase exercise duration and maintains an anti-ischemic effect for 12 hours after patch application. These beneficial responses remained consistent throughout 30 days of therapy. No significant nitrate tolerance or rebound was noted when the patch was applied for not more than 12 of 24 hours.[39]

Although the various patches use different pharmaceutical delivery systems, clear-cut advantages of one over another are not apparent. Despite variations in surface area and NTG content, the most important common denominator of the transdermal NTG systems is the amount of drug released per hour expressed as the release rate (e.g., 0.2 mg/hr). Each product label includes this information. Low dosages (0.2 to 0.4 mg/hr) may not produce sufficient plasma and tissue concentrations to produce a clinically significant effect.[2] However, it is still recommended to start with a low-dose patch and titrate upward as needed. Because the skin is the major factor influencing NTG absorption rate, product release characteristics do not favor one system over another. Contact dermatitis has been reported with the transdermal patches.[54] Patient instructions are included with the patches and should be reviewed with the patient, emphasizing the appropriate time for application and removal of the patch.

Table 17-6 Transdermal Nitroglycerin Systems[a]

Distributor/Product	Surface Area (cm²)	Total NTG Content (mg)
Schwarz Pharma		
Deponit 0.2 mg/hr (5 mg/24 hr)	16	16
Deponit 0.4 mg/hr (10 mg/24 hr)	32	32
Key Pharmaceuticals		
Nitro Dur 0.1 mg/hr (2.5 mg/24 hr)	5	20
Nitro Dur 0.2 mg/hr (5 mg/24 hr)	10	40
Nitro-Dur 0.3 mg/hr (7.5 mg/24 hr)	15	60
Nitro-Dur 0.4 mg/hr (10 mg/24 hr)	20	80
Nitro-Dur 0.6 mg/hr (15 mg/24 hr)	30	120
Nitro-Dur 0.8 mg/hr (20 mg/24 hr)	40	160
Novartis		
Transderm-Nitro 2.5 (0.1 mg/hr)	5	12.5
Transderm-Nitro 10 (0.4 mg/hr)	20	50
Transderm-Nitro 15 (0.6 mg/hr)	30	75
3M Pharm		
Minitran 0.1 mg/hr (2.5 mg/24 hr)	3.3	9
Minitran 0.2 mg/hr (5 mg/24 hr)	6.7	18
Minitran 0.4 mg/hr (10 mg/24 hr)	13.3	36
Minitran 0.6 mg/hr (15 mg/24 hr)	20	54

[a]Also generic in 0.2, 0.4, and 0.6 mg/hr.

Other Organic Nitrates

20. Do organic nitrates, other than oral isosorbide dinitrate or sublingual NTG, offer any significant advantages for J.P.?

Sublingual isosorbide dinitrate is available, but its onset of action is delayed when compared with sublingual NTG or the lingual spray; thus, it is used only for prophylaxis. Also, because the duration of action for sublingual isosorbide dinitrate is only 2 to 3 hours, it must be administered more frequently then oral or transdermal nitrates and this reduces compliance.[39] Chewable isosorbide dinitrate is prescribed occasionally, as are isosorbide dinitrate extended-release capsules and tablets: neither has undergone extensive clinical evaluation. Long-acting oral NTG capsules (e.g., Nitro-Bid) have questionable efficacy and may lead to tolerance. Larger doses (6.5 to 9 mg) of long-acting oral NTG may have physiologic effects persisting for 1 to 6 hours.[38]

21. Does isosorbide mononitrate offer any distinct advantages over other nitrate preparations for angina prophylaxis?

Isosorbide mononitrate (ISMO, Monoket, and Imdur) is the primary metabolite of isosorbide dinitrate. In fact, most of the clinical activity of isosorbide dinitrate is due to the mononitrate. Therefore, both drugs share a similar pharmacology. Isosorbide mononitrate does not undergo first-pass metabolism and has no active metabolites. Its oral bioavailability is almost 100%, and its overall elimination half-life is about 5 hours.[39] Maximum serum concentrations are observed 30 to 60 minutes after a dose. To minimize the potential development of nitrate tolerance, isosorbide mononitrate should be used in a twice-daily, asymmetric dosing regimen in which the first dose is taken upon awakening and the second dose about 7 hours later. Because of this unconventional dosing pattern and the availability of the sustained-release product, which can be taken once a day, most use of isosorbide mononitrate is in the form of the sustained-release preparation (Imdur).

General precautions and adverse reactions for isosorbide mononitrate are similar to those for the other nitrates. Potential advantages for the clinical use of isosorbide mononitrate are less dosage fluctuation because of the absence of presystemic clearance and an effective once- or twice-daily dosing schedule, which could perhaps lead to improved patient dosing adherence. Nevertheless, isosorbide dinitrate is effective clinically when administered two or three times a day and is a viable alternative.

β-ADRENERGIC BLOCKERS

Mechanism of Action

22. T.I. has a 5-year history of chronic stable angina. Cardiac catheterization 3 months ago showed two-vessel coronary disease with obstructions of 55% and 65% in the right coronary and circumflex coronary arteries, respectively. Despite appropriate use of sublingual NTG tablets (0.4 mg) and isosorbide dinitrate (40 mg PO at 6 AM, noon, and 5 PM), T.I. is having four to five angina attacks per week. His physician writes a prescription for atenolol (Tenormin) 50 mg QD. How do β-adrenergic blockers prevent angina?

β-Adrenergic blockers reduce myocardial oxygen demand by decreasing catecholamine-mediated increases in heart rate,

BP and, to some extent, myocardial contractility.[56] Traditionally, β-receptors are subdivided into two classes: β_1-receptors are found primarily in the myocardium, and β_2-receptors are distributed in the vascular and bronchial smooth muscle. Stimulation of the β_1-receptor accelerates heart rate, and β_2-stimulation relaxes or dilates peripheral vasculature and bronchial airways.

It was once believed that no β_2-receptors were located in the heart muscle. However, more recent evidence shows that β_2-receptors probably account for 10% to 40% of all β-receptors in the myocardium.[57] The functional role of myocardial β_2-receptors is not understood completely, but probably involves augmentation of contractility and perhaps heart rate. β-Blockers might also favorably affect myocardial metabolism, coronary microvasculature, collateral blood flow, myocardial blood flow, and oxygen-hemoglobin affinity.[56]

In patients with chronic angina, β-blockers generally should be administered before nitrates or calcium channel blockers when long-term therapy is indicated.[1] In a meta-analysis of clinical trials that compared the three classes of anti-ischemics, differences in long-term mortality were not noted. However, β-blockers were more effective in lowering the incidence of anginal episodes.[2] β-Blockers are generally considered the most effective class of agents at preventing silent myocardial ischemia.[2] In addition, β-blockers clearly lower morbidity and mortality in patients with hypertension,[22] acute MI,[59] and heart failure.[60] While calcium channel blockers have been shown to reduce cardiovascular outcomes in the treatment of hypertension,[22] the totality of evidence for improving prognosis in the treatment of various cardiovascular diseases is less than that seen with β-blockers. Nitrates do not have any supporting evidence for reducing cardiovascular outcomes. Although mortality benefits have not been demonstrated specifically in patients with chronic angina, the overwhelming body of literature suggests that all patients with angina should receive a β-blocker as initial therapy unless contraindicated. (See Chapter 14, Essential Hypertension, and Chapter 19, Heart Failure, for more in-depth information on β-blocker product availability, dosage forms, pharmacology, and dosing.)

Judging Therapeutic Endpoint

23. How can the efficacy of the atenolol be assessed?

All patients receiving antianginal drugs should be monitored for frequency of angina attacks and NTG consumption. Nevertheless, this provides only an estimate of therapeutic efficacy because the patient's exercise and stress levels change from day to day. Traditionally, clinicians have monitored the reduction in resting heart rate and have progressively increased the β-blocker dose until the resting heart rate was 55 or 60 beats/minute. Heart rates <50 beats/minute may be acceptable provided the patient is asymptomatic and heart block is not present. However, this approach does not take into account that although the initial β-blocker dose reduces heart rate, subsequent increases in dose may only slightly reduce the resting heart rate. Variations in resting heart rate are normal and subject to the influence of the endogenous sympathetic nervous system and other exogenous factors such as drugs, tobacco, and caffeine-containing beverages. β-Blockers with intrinsic sympathomimetic activity will not reduce the resting heart rate as much as β-blockers lacking this activity.[56,58]

Exercise testing is probably the most accurate, but least practical method of documenting the adequacy of β-blocker therapy. During an exercise tolerance test, atenolol should substantially increase the time T.I. walks before developing angina. There also may be a reduction in ST-segment depression during exercise indicating less myocardial ischemia. The heart rate–systolic BP product probably will be markedly lowered, reflecting a decrease in both heart rate and systolic wall tension.[58] β-Blocker dosages needed to achieve these effects are highly variable. Therefore, therapy should be initiated with the lowest possible effective dosage and titrated upward. Continuous assessment of T.I.'s exercise tolerance is advisable.

Dosing Frequency

24. Is once-daily dosing of atenolol sufficient to provide T.I. with 24-hour protection? How often should immediate-release propranolol be administered?

The pharmacodynamic effects of β-blockers are longer than their plasma half-lives, and β-blockers can be dosed once or twice a day for angina. The half-life of atenolol is about 10 hours during chronic dosing; however, clinical studies support a once-a-day dosing schedule.[56]

Propranolol has a relatively short plasma half-life of 2 to 3 hours, yet clinicians have observed that a single dose lowers the heart rate and BP for at least 12 hours. Subsequent studies have confirmed the efficacy of twice-daily dosing for propranolol in the treatment of angina (see Chapter 14, Essential Hypertension, for detailed pharmacokinetic and pharmacodynamic discussion of β-blockers).[56]

β-Blocker Cardioselectivity

Contraindications

25. R.O. is a 65-year-old man with a 40-pack-year smoking history and a 13-year history of insulin-dependent diabetes mellitus. His ability to walk is limited by peripheral vascular disease and claudication, as well as by exertional angina. A β-blocker is to be initiated for treatment of chronic angina. Which β-blocker would be preferable for this patient?

Although all β-blockers are equally effective in the treatment of angina, R.O.'s medical history poses several relative contraindications to the use of some β-blockers.[58] His smoking history may have caused some degree of chronic obstructive pulmonary disease (COPD) with a bronchospastic component despite the absence of medical history. His history of diabetes and peripheral vascular disease will influence the selection of a β-blocker for management of his angina. A cardioselective β-blocker offers several advantages in R.O.[61] Drugs such as acebutolol (Sectral), atenolol, and metoprolol (Lopressor) primarily inhibit β_1-receptors in the heart and produce less blockade of β_2-receptors in the bronchial and vascular smooth muscle. In patients with asthma and obstructive lung disease, β_2-receptors mediate airway responsiveness and blockade of β_2-receptors can cause severe bronchospasm and respiratory difficulty. In one meta-analysis, cardioselective β-blockers were not found to produce clinically signifi-

cant adverse respiratory effects in patients who had mild to moderate reactive airway disease.[62]

Cardioselective β-lockers also are less likely to inhibit β_2-mediated vasodilation in the peripheral arterioles. Therefore, cardioselective β-blockers are preferred over nonselective β-blockers for patients with peripheral vascular disease and Raynaud's disease. Blockade of the peripheral β_2-receptor would permit unopposed α-mediated vasoconstriction and could decrease R.O.'s walking tolerance markedly.

Although β-blockers may alter glucose metabolism and mask the symptoms of hypoglycemia, their use has clearly been demonstrated to lower overall mortality in diabetic patients after acute MI.[59] In addition, diabetic patients in general develop more severe CAD and overall have a worse prognosis than patients without diabetes. Because of the significant beneficial effects on mortality with β-blockers, diabetes should not be considered a contraindication to β-blocker therapy.

Adverse Effects

26. If R.O. receives a cardioselective β-blocker, could he still experience more difficulty breathing or walking?

Cardioselectivity is not an all-or-none response; instead, it is a dose-dependent phenomenon. As the dose is increased, cardioselectivity is lost. Unfortunately, the dose at which cardioselectivity will be lost in R.O. cannot be predicted; even a very small dose (e.g., metoprolol 37.5 mg) could cause wheezing.[56,58] Similarly, a cardioselective drug could worsen R.O.'s claudication. If R.O. experiences worsening control of COPD or peripheral vascular disease, a better alternative may be a calcium channel blocker either alone or with intermittent nitrate therapy.

β-Blockers With Intrinsic Sympathomimetic Activity

27. W.P. has a long cardiac history that includes three previous coronary artery bypass grafts, class III HF, and MI. He is experiencing angina that is unresponsive to maximally tolerated doses of isosorbide dinitrate. β-Blocker therapy is being considered, but there is concern that W.P.'s sinus bradycardia (resting heart rate, 45 to 52 beats/min) will be worsened. Would a β-blocker with intrinsic sympathomimetic activity (ISA) be safe to use for this patient?

Some β-blockers have ISA (i.e., a partial β-adrenergic agonist response). Because the β-blocking drugs with ISA have a chemical structure similar to, but not identical with, catecholamines, they can simultaneously block the receptor and attach to a small number of stimulating sites.[56] Theoretically, these drugs may produce less bradycardia, as well as less peripheral vasoconstriction and bronchial constriction, than pure β-adrenergic blockers. The clinical significance of ISA is actively debated. Overall, ISA appears to result in less derangement of lipid and glucose metabolism than pure β-blockers.[56] However, clinical studies have not yet definitively demonstrated advantages of ISA.

Because β-blockers with ISA do not decrease heart rate to the same extent as β-blockers without ISA, they theoretically would be less effective for the treatment of angina. Because of W.P.'s problems with a low resting heart rate, a β-blocker with ISA could be a consideration. However, a trial of a calcium channel blocker would be a more appropriate choice.

Central Nervous System Side Effects

28. C.G., a 43-year-old male executive who has received metoprolol 100 mg BID at 8 AM and 8 PM for 1 month, has new complaints of awakening five to six times during the night, nightmares, fatigue, and diminished libido. Would switching C.G.'s therapy to atenolol alleviate these troublesome side effects?

C.G. describes some common central nervous system (CNS) side effects of the β-adrenergic blockers: tiredness, fatigue, depression, sleep disturbances, psychomotor retardation, and sexual dysfunction.[56,58] Because patients may not associate these effects with their drug therapy, they often do not bring these complaints to their physician's attention. Therefore, all patients should be screened for these effects. Some investigators have suggested that these effects are related to the lipid solubility of the β-blockers; that is, the more lipophilic drugs can pass through the blood-brain barrier more easily and produce CNS disturbances more easily. On this basis, a hydrophilic drug such as atenolol may be better tolerated by C.G. This claim has not been substantiated by current clinical experience.[56] When administered in a larger single daily dose of >100 mg, atenolol therapy still may cause sedation.[63] Other investigators have reached opposite conclusions regarding lipophilics and CNS effects β-blockers (see Chapter 14, Essential Hypertension, for additional perspective).

β-Blockers in Acute Renal Failure

29. C.G. is severely injured in an automobile accident, becomes septic, and develops acute renal failure. He is to be started on hemodialysis. How will these events affect C.G.'s atenolol dose?

The β-blockers differ with regard to their pharmacokinetic profiles. The half-life of atenolol normally is about 9 hours, but dosages should be adjusted in renal failure because it primarily undergoes renal elimination. A dose of 12.5 or 25 mg can be used initially in C.G. and titrated upward as tolerated if atenolol is prescribed. Because atenolol also is removed by hemodialysis, patients generally receive 25 to 50 mg after each dialysis and are monitored closely for hypotension (see Chapter 14, Essential Hypertension).

Abrupt Withdrawal

30. J.F., a 76-year-old retiree with a long history of chronic stable angina controlled with oral isosorbide dinitrate 40 mg TID (7 AM, noon, 5 PM), and propranolol 80 mg BID (7 AM, 5 PM), stopped his propranolol 24 hours ago when he forgot to get his prescriptions refilled. He is transported to the hospital emergency department (ED) for treatment of angina unresponsive to five NTG tablets. How could J.F.'s situation have been avoided?

The β-blocker withdrawal syndrome places patients with severe atherosclerosis or USA at high risk for adverse cardiovascular events, which may include acute MI and sudden cardiac death. After J.F.'s angina has been controlled with medications during this particular hospitalization and before reinstitution of β-blocker therapy, he should be warned not to precipitously discontinue his β-blockers in the future. Failure

to renew prescriptions and financial hardship are common reasons for abrupt discontinuation, and clinicians need to have sufficient professional rapport with patients to understand when patients encounter difficulties in obtaining medications.

The β-blocker withdrawal syndrome is a rebound phenomenon resulting from heightened β-receptor density and sensitivity (i.e., upregulation) subsequent to receptor blockade. An "overshoot" in heart rate, as a consequence of sympathoadrenal activity from abrupt β-blocker withdrawal increases myocardial oxygen demand and platelet aggregation. Withdrawal syndromes may be less severe in patients taking β-blockers with partial agonist activity.[56,58]

If β-blockers are to be discontinued in the future, the propranolol withdrawal schedule illustrated below could be used for J.F. and modified to meet situational needs.[64]

Days	Dosage
1–4	40 mg BID
5–8	20 mg BID
9–12	10 mg BID
13–14	10 mg QD

Shorter periods for β-blocker withdrawal such as 2 to 3 days have also been proposed. The optimal strategy for discontinuation is not known. However, ensuring that β-blockers are tapered and that the patient is reasonably monitored for adverse events for the duration of the taper is imperative. Patients should limit physical activity throughout the β-blocker withdrawal period and seek prompt medical attention when angina symptoms become apparent.

Withdrawal Before Coronary Artery Surgery

31. V.T., a 67-year-old man, has been taking propranolol 160 mg BID for angina and hypertension for 10 years. He is scheduled to undergo CABG, and there is concern that propranolol will interact with general anesthesia to produce excessive myocardial depression. Should V.T. be tapered off propranolol before surgery? Could other drugs worsen V.T.'s angina?

V.T. should continue to receive propranolol because it will promote hemodynamic stability and protect him from intraoperative hypertension and tachycardia. Propranolol also will protect V.T. from postoperative supraventricular tachyarrhythmias, a common complication of open-heart surgery. He should receive 160 mg propranolol about 2 hours before surgery[64]; IV β-blockers may be needed during the surgery or in the immediate postoperative period. As soon as possible, oral therapy should be resumed (see Chapter 20, Cardiac Arrhythmias).

Most cases of drug-induced angina are related to withdrawal of antianginal drugs (e.g., abrupt discontinuation of propranolol). Any medication that lowers heart rate excessively (e.g., β-blocker therapy, verapamil/diltiazem therapy) potentially can precipitate angina when abruptly discontinued. Similarly, drugs that cause tachycardia (e.g., catecholamines, theophylline) may worsen angina by increasing workload on the heart. Drugs of abuse (e.g., cocaine, nicotine, ethanol) may cause ischemia and should be avoided by patients with ischemic heart disease.

CALCIUM CHANNEL BLOCKERS

The calcium channel blockers are a relatively recent addition to the family of drugs used to treat angina. Their clinical applicability extends to most cardiovascular diseases, although current FDA-approved indications are limited to angina, hypertension, and supraventricular arrhythmias. One calcium channel blocker, nimodipine (Nimotop), has FDA approval for treatment of cerebral spasm resulting from subarachnoid hemorrhage. Ongoing research suggests calcium channel blockers may be useful in the treatment of migraines, cerebral artery spasm, Raynaud's phenomenon, and pulmonary hypertension. (See Chapter 14, Essential Hypertension, for additional information on calcium channel blockers.)

Classification

Calcium channel blockers are highly diverse compounds. They differ markedly in chemical structure as well as specificity for cardiac and peripheral tissue. Using these character-

Table 17-7   Calcium Channel Blockers in Anginal Syndromes[a]

	FDA Approved[b]	Usual Dose for Chronic Stable Angina[c]	Product Availability[d]
Dihydropyridines			
Amlodipine (Norvasc)	Angina Hypertension	2.5–10 mg QD	2.5, 5, 10 mg tab
Felodipine (Plendil)	Hypertension	5–20 mg QD	5, 10 mg ER tab
Isradapine	Hypertension		
(DynaCirc)		2.5–10 mg BID	2.5, 5 mg IR cap
(DynaCirc CR)		5–10 mg QD	5, 10 mg CR tab
Nicardipine	Angina (IR only)		
(Cardene)	Hypertension	20–40 mg TID	20, 30 mg IR cap
(Cardene SR)		30–60 mg BID	30, 45, 60 mg SR cap
Nifedipine	Angina (not Adalat CC)		
(Adalat, Procardia, generic)	Hypertension (CC and XL only)	10–30 mg TID	10, 20 mg IR cap
(Adalat CC)		30–180 mg QD	30, 60, 90 mg ER tab
(Procardia XL)		30–180 mg QD	30, 60, 90 mg ER tab
Nisoldipine (Sular)	Hypertension	20–60 mg QD	10, 20, 30, 40 mg ER tab
Diphenylalkylamines			
Verapamil	Angina (IR and Covera		
(Calan, Isoptin, generic)	HS only)	30–120 mg TID/QID	40, 80, 120 mg IR tab
(Calan SR, Isoptin SR, generic)	Hypertension	120–240 mg BID	120, 180, 240 mg SR tab
(Covera HS)	SVT	120–480 mg Q HS	180, 240 mg DR, ER tab
(Verelan)		120–480 mg QD	120, 180, 240, 360 mg ER cap
(Verelan HS)		200–400 mg Q HS	100, 200, 300 mg DR, ER tab
Benzothiazepines			
Diltiazem	Angina		
(Cardizem, generic)	Hypertension	30–120 mg TID/QID	30, 60, 90, 120 mg IR tab
(Cardizem SR and generic)		60–180 mg BID	60, 90, 120, 180 mg SR cap
(Cardizem CD and generic)		120–360 mg QD	120, 180, 240, 300, 360 mg cap
(Dilacor XR)		120–480 mg QD	120, 180, 240 mg ER cap
Tiamate ER		120–480 mg QD	120, 180, 240 mg ER cap
Tiazac ER		120–480 mg QD	120, 180, 240, 300, 360, 420 mg ER cap
Bepridil (Vascor)	Refractory angina	200–400 mg QD	200, 300, 400 mg tab

Also see Tables 14-15 and 14-16 in Chapter 14: Essential Hypertension.
[a]Cap, capsules; CD, controlled diffusion; CR, controlled release; DR, delayed release; ER, extended release; FDA, Food and Drug Administration; HS, bedtime; IR, immediate release; SR, sustained release; SVT, supraventricular including atrial fibrillation, atrial flutter, and reentry; Tab, tablets; XL and XR, extended release.
[b]FDA-approved indications vary among IR and ER products. However, most all have been used clinically for both angina and hypertension. Avoid IR release products in hypertension.
[c]Because of short half-lives, most of these drugs are given TID if using IR tabs or caps. Amlodipine and bepridil have a long half-life and are given QD.
[d]Caution: Substituting one long-acting dosage form with another, even for the same drug, is not recommended. Cardizem SR capsules and verapamil SR tabs (Calan SR, Isoptin SR) still require BID dosing. Absorption of verapamil SR is more rapid and duration of action is shorter if taken on an empty stomach, further reducing its SR characteristics; generally it must be given Q 12 hours with food to maintain SR release, even though total bioavailability is reduced. Release characteristics of Verelan-beaded capsules have more reliable sustained-release characteristics allowing QD dosing, with or without food. Covera HS and Verelan HS are taken at bedtime to optimize AM release when blood pressure is often highest, but these two products are not interchangeable. Cardizem CD (copolymer-coated sustained-release beads) release 40% of the dose in the first 12 hours and 60% over the next 12 hours allowing QD dosing. Dilacor XR and Tiazac ER caps also given QD. Procardia XL uses the "GITS" technology and effectively releases the drug over 24 hours. Adalat CC also given QD but not GITS formulation. Some formularies allow therapeutic substitution of these two dosage forms.

istics, it is possible to classify calcium antagonists into several major types (Table 17-7).[65]

Both diltiazem and verapamil exert qualitatively similar effects on myocardial and peripheral tissue. They slow conduction and prolong the refractory period in the AV node. Ventricular refractory period is not affected. Therefore, the antiarrhythmic utility of these drugs is limited to controlling the ventricular rate in supraventricular tachyarrhythmias. Both agents can depress myocardial contractility and should be used with caution in patients with LV dysfunction. They are moderate peripheral vasodilators and potent coronary artery vasodilators.[65]

Nifedipine is the prototype compound of the dihydropyridine derivatives. Although amlodipine, felodipine, isradipine, and nicardipine are second-generation dihydropyridines, only nicardipine and amlodipine currently are approved for the treatment of chronic stable angina pectoris. In addition, amlodipine is indicated for vasospastic angina.[66] In contrast to diltiazem or verapamil, the dihydropyridines do not slow cardiac conduction and, therefore, have no antiarrhythmic action. However, they are more potent peripheral vasodilators and are associated with a reflex increase in the heart rate. All dihydropyridines have negative inotropic effects in vitro, but these effects, clinically, are overshadowed by the reflex sympathetic activation and decreased afterload. The net effect of these actions essentially results in no depression of myocardial function except in patients with evidence of heart failure (see Chapter 19, Heart Failure).[65] The dihydropyridines also can dilate coronary arteries, but vary in their potency.

Bepridil, unlike other calcium channel antagonists, blocks the fast sodium channel in the heart as well as the calcium channel. Therefore, it and related compounds are called *nonselective calcium channel antagonists*. They are potentially useful in a wide range of diseases, including supraventricular tachyarrhythmias, ventricular arrhythmias, and angina. However, the quinidine-like effect of these drugs raises concern about their deleterious arrhythmogenic effect, especially the induction of torsades de pointes. Currently, bepridil does not have a significant role in the treatment of angina and is indicated only for patients who have angina refractory to other drugs.[66]

Two distinct types of calcium channels have been isolated in the cardiovascular system and the agents discussed up to this point block the L-type receptor.[65] Mibefradil works by blocking the T-type calcium channel, resulting in vasodilation and lowering of heart rate. Although T-type channels are found in the sinoatrial (SA) node and conduction system, they are relatively absent in the myocardium and, therefore, negative inotropy is not a concern with mibefradil. Although mibefradil is an effective antianginal drug both alone and in combination with other agents, the drug is no longer available in the United States because of the large number of potential drug interactions that may result in life-threatening situations. The role of T-type calcium antagonists in the treatment of angina still remains to be defined.

Broad-based experience in the use of calcium channel blockers to treat angina is limited in the United States to the dihydropyridines, verapamil and diltiazem. During the mid- to late 1980s, oral nifedipine, verapamil, and diltiazem emerged as key agents in treating all types of angina. With the marketing of second-generation dihydropyridines, such as amlodipine and nicardipine, the clinician is faced with the difficult task of differentiating among calcium channel blockers.

Pharmacology

Calcium channel blockers decrease myocardial oxygen demand and increase myocardial blood supply.[65] By inhibiting smooth muscle contraction, the calcium channel blockers dilate blood vessels and decrease resistance to blood flow. Dilation of peripheral vessels reduces systemic vascular resistance and BP, thus decreasing the work load of the heart. Coronary artery dilation improves coronary blood flow. Diltiazem and verapamil also decrease the myocardial contractile force (negative inotropic effect). All these actions can reduce angina symptoms.

Potent arterial (peripheral) vasodilators, such as nifedipine, markedly reduce peripheral vascular resistance,[65] and reflexly stimulate sympathetic nervous system to cause a slight to moderate increase in heart rate and perhaps increase myocardial oxygen demand (see Table 17-7). The cardiodepressant effect of verapamil- and diltiazem-like drugs prevents reflex tachycardia. Verapamil and diltiazem are more likely to worsen ventricular function in patients with HF secondary to systolic dysfunction.[66] Two dihydropyridines, amlodipine and felodipine, have been studied in the setting of LV dysfunction and found to be relatively safer than other calcium blockers in heart failure, but have a negligible effect on mortality.[65] Therefore, these two drugs are available options in patients with HF who have other disease states that would benefit from calcium channel blocker therapy. Diltiazem, nifedipine, and verapamil should be avoided in heart failure. Individualization of calcium channel blocker therapy must consider the drug's overall pharmacologic effect and side effect profile.

Indications for Use

32. B.N., a 56-year-old man, has just undergone cardiac catheterization, which showed two-vessel CAD. He refuses to take nitrates because they cause severe headaches. His medical history includes asthma and hyperlipidemia. His physician begins antianginal therapy with nifedipine 10 mg PO TID. Are the calcium blockers indicated for all types of angina?

Calcium channel blockers are effective in both vasospastic and classic exertional angina. These drugs relieve vasospasm of the large coronary arteries and, as a result, are effective in treating Prinzmetal's variant angina. Their beneficial effect in chronic stable (effort-induced) angina is the result of multiple factors. Their vasodilatory effects in the coronary circulation increase myocardial oxygen supply, whereas dilation of the peripheral arterioles leads to a reduction in myocardial oxygen demand. Because coronary vasospasm can occur at the site of an atherosclerotic plaque, calcium channel blockers are particularly useful in patients who have a vasospastic component to their angina.

Although β-blockers are considered the drugs of choice when instituting antianginal therapy, B.N.'s asthma may be worsened by the addition of a β-blocker. While a cardioselective β-blocker could be tried to see if B.N. could tolerate it, a calcium channel blockers or long-acting nitrate are good alternatives to β-blockers for the treatment of angina in this situation. The choice of a calcium channel blocker as initial therapy in this patient is appropriate because of B.N.'s previous intolerance to nitrates and because nitrate therapy requires the scheduling of a nitrate-free period.[1]

Nifedipine

Adverse Effects

33. Two days after beginning nifedipine, B.N. calls his physician complaining of dizziness and a tripling of his angina attacks. He notices that his heart rate increases about 90 minutes after taking the nifedipine and shortly after that he develops chest pain. Could this be a side effect of nifedipine therapy?

Approximately 10% of all patients receiving nifedipine will experience worsening of their angina. B.N.'s complaints of dizziness probably are due to the powerful peripheral vasodilator effect of nifedipine that can precipitate an exaggerated reflex increase in the heart rate. Overall, nifedipine-induced hypotension and reflex increase in heart rate can increase myocardial oxygen demand. In extreme cases, nifedipine can precipitate an MI, and when used in the acute MI period, nifedipine has been demonstrated to increase mortality.[65]

Although the choice of a calcium channel blocker by B.N.'s physician was appropriate, the choice of immediate-release nifedipine was unwise because of the reasons stated earlier. Consequently, short-acting calcium antagonists such as nifedipine are no longer recommended in the treatment of any

disease state because of the potential for serious cardiac adverse effects.[1,65] Nifedipine, in an extended-release formulation to help minimize the reflex increase in sympathetic drive, would have been a more appropriate choice. Other appropriate options for B.N. are amlodipine or diltiazem if his LV function is normal.

Some side effects of calcium channel blockers reflect an extension of their hemodynamic and electrophysiologic profiles and therefore are predictable (Table 17-8). Dihydropyridine-induced hypotension and dizziness occurs in approximately 15% of patients. Patients also may complain of light-headedness, facial flushing, headache, and nausea. Swelling of the lower legs and ankles (peripheral edema) is related to the potent peripheral vasodilating effects of these agents.

Contraindications

34. Does B.N. have any contraindications to calcium channel blockers?

Contraindications to calcium channel blockers are based on pharmacologic actions of these agents (Table 17-9). Because B.N. has no apparent history of cardiac conduction disorders or heart failure, he is a suitable candidate for a trial of calcium blockers.

Table 17-8 Calcium Channel Blockers

	Dihydropyridine Derivatives[a]	Diltiazem	Verapamil	Bepridil
Peripheral vasodilation[b]	+++	++	++	++
Coronary vasodilation[b]	+++	+++	++	+++
Negative inotrope[c]	+/−	++	+++	++[f]
AV node suppression[c]	+/−	+	++	+[f]
Heart rate	↑ (reflex)	↓	↓	↓[f]
Pharmacokinetics[d]				
Dosing[e]				
Side Effects				
Nausea, vomiting	+ (most)	+/−	+/−	+/−
Constipation	Not observed	+/−	+	Not observed
Hypotension, dizziness[g]	++	+	+	+
Flushing, headache	++	+	+	+
Bradycardia, HF symptoms	+/−	+	++	+/−
Reflex tachycardia, angina	+[g]	Not observed	Not observed	++
Peripheral edema	+	+/−	+/−	Not observed
Drug Interactions[h]				Unknown

Also see Tables 14-15 and 14-16 in Chapter 14: Essential Hypertension.
[a]Dihydropyridine derivatives FDA approved for angina: Amlodipine (Norvasc), nicardipine (Cardene), and nifedipine (Adalat, Procardia). See Table 14-6 for others that are approved for hypertension but have been used clinically for angina. Investigational: nitrendipine (Baypress)
[b]Peripheral and coronary vasodilation helpful for angina, hypertension, and possibly HF, but peripheral dilation is the basis for side effects of flushing, headache, and hypotension.
[c]AV node suppression is helpful for controlling suproventricular arrhythmias, but this property plus the negative inotropic effect may worsen HF. Nifedipine has less negative inotropic effect than verapamil and diltiazem, but still may worsen HF. Amlodipine may have the least negative inotropic effect.
[d]All have poor bioavailability due to high 1st-pass metabolism and all are eliminated primarily by hepatic metabolism; intra- and interindividual variability in bioavailability and metabolism is extensive. Diltiazem, nifedipine, nicardipine, and verapamil have short t$\frac{1}{2}$ (<5 hr) requiring frequent dosing or use of SR products. Amlodipine, isradipine (8 hr), felodipine (10–20 hr), and bepridil (42 hr) have longer tt$\frac{1}{2}$. The long tt$\frac{1}{2}$ of bepridil makes dosage titration difficult.
[e]See Table 14-6 and Table 11-16 in Chapter 14: Essential Hypertension.
[f]Bepridil affects both sodium channels and calcium channels. Ventricular conduction can be depressed with prolonged QT interval on ECG. Ventricular toxicity including torsades de pointes has been reported. Hypokalemia and 2 cases of agranulocytosis also have been reported.
[g]Hypotension and reflex tachycardia most with immediate release nifedipine, occasional with immediate-release diltiazem and verapamil, minimal with sustained release products or intrinsically long-acting agents.
[h]Diltiazem and verapamil = weak CYP 3A4 inhibitors and strong p-glycoprotein inhibitors. ↑ cyclosporine and digoxin bioavailability via increased GI transport and possibly less gut metabolism. Case reports of cyclosporine renal toxicity with diltiazem. Bradycardia and heart failure risk with combined verapamil and digoxin via additive AV block and negative inotropic effects. Risk of interaction with drugs metabolized by CYP 3A4 not known.

Table 17-9 Contraindications to Calcium Channel Blockers*a*

Severe hypotension
Severe aortic stenosis
Extreme bradycardia
Moderate to severe heart failure
Cardiogenic shock
Sick sinus syndrome
Second- or third-degree AV block*b*
WPW syndrome with atrial fibrillation or flutter*b*

*a*Bepridil use requires extra precaution for potential drug-induced arrhythmias and agranulocytosis.
*b*Nifedipine and related dihydropyridines generally may be used safely as they do not depress sinoatrial or AV node conduction.
AV, atrioventricular; WPW, Wolff-Parkinson-White.

Diltiazem and Verapamil: Adverse Effects

35. **Diltiazem (Cardizem CD) 180 mg/day PO is prescribed for B.N. What side effects should be anticipated with diltiazem and other non–dihydropyridine calcium channel blockers?**

Verapamil and diltiazem have similar side effect profiles, although diltiazem appears to be better tolerated. The lower incidence of side effects reported with diltiazem, compared with verapamil, may reflect a true difference or, perhaps, less aggressive dosing regimens. Both drugs can cause sinus bradycardia and worsen already existing conduction defects and heart block.[65] Neither should be used in patients with sick sinus syndrome or advanced degrees of heart block unless a functioning ventricular pacemaker is present. Patients should be monitored for signs of worsening HF, such as SOB, weight gain, and peripheral edema. Verapamil-induced constipation can be particularly troublesome to the elderly. Rare instances of fecal impaction requiring surgery illustrate the need for the aggressive use of stool softening agents and, often, bulk-forming laxatives.

Generalized fatigue and nonspecific gastrointestinal (GI) complaints can occur with any of the calcium channel blockers. In rare instances, elevations of hepatic enzymes and acute hepatic injury have occurred with the calcium channel blockers. Appreciation for the individual side effect profiles helps determine preference for one calcium blocker over another. B.N. is not likely to experience major side effects with either verapamil or diltiazem.

36. **After several weeks' therapy with Cardizem CD 180 mg QD, B.N. still is having several angina attacks weekly. He has not experienced any side effects other than an occasional headache. What is the maximum diltiazem dose that can be used?**

All calcium channel blocker dosages are gradually titrated upward. Most patients start diltiazem therapy with 30 or 60 mg three or four times a day or, alternatively, an equivalent dosage of SR diltiazem. The dose can be increased every 1 or 2 days as needed or tolerated. Optimal daily diltiazem doses originally were thought to be 180 or 240 mg. However, in some patients, relief of angina occurred with divided doses of ≥240 mg/day. The maximum diltiazem dose is about 480 mg/day.[66] Careful monitoring for bradycardia and heart failure is imperative when large dosages are prescribed.

Verapamil: Risk-Benefit Assessment

37. **A.E., a 65-year-old man, has newly diagnosed angina pectoris. He refused cardiac catheterization; however, his coronary risk factors include a strong family history of cardiovascular disease and hyperlipoproteinemia. He experienced rheumatic fever at age 12; 5 years ago, his mitral valve was replaced. At that time, he had two-vessel CAD with 80% and 85% occlusion and an LV EF of 30% (normal, 55%). During this hospitalization, new-onset atrial fibrillation was observed with a ventricular response rate of 115 to 130/min. Current medications include warfarin (Coumadin) 5 mg for 5 days/wk and 2.5 mg for 2 days/wk; enalapril (Vasotec) 10 mg QD; digoxin (Lanoxin) 0.25 mg/day (serum digoxin concentration drawn 18 hours after the last dose is 1.0 ng/mL); and furosemide 40 mg/day. A.E.'s physician wishes to begin verapamil 60 mg PO QID. What is the risk versus benefit of adding verapamil to A.E.'s medical regimen?**

A.E. has a complicated history. Although a repeat cardiac catheterization would help confirm the progression of atherosclerosis, it is likely that he has significant CAD. Because calcium channel blockers are effective in all forms of angina, they are especially useful in patients with mixed angina syndromes or in patients in whom the diagnosis is not firmly established. Although A.E. has mild to moderate HF (as evidenced by his depressed EF), verapamil (or diltiazem) may be used for a short period of time in the treatment of his supraventricular arrhythmia. In A.E., verapamil (or diltiazem) should slow conduction through the AV node, thereby decreasing the ventricular response to his atrial fibrillation.[65] The long-term administration of verapamil (or diltiazem) would not be optimal given his LV dysfunction, but may be necessary if digoxin is not effective at controlling his ventricular rate over the long term. A β-blocker is another option at this point, as it is effective in angina and for slowing the ventricular rate in atrial fibrillation. However, the use of a β-blocker may not be feasible in the acute setting because the dosages needed to control A.E.'s ventricular rate may worsen his heart failure as well. The long-term administration of a β-blocker would be a better choice than verapamil or diltiazem because of the profound mortality benefits seen with β-blockers in patients with HF.[58] If a calcium channel blocker is needed for long-term treatment of angina, a dihydropyridine, such as amlodipine, would be a better choice.

Second-Generation Dihydropyridines

38. **A request has been made to add nicardipine and amlodipine to the hospital formulary. The current formulary includes verapamil, diltiazem, and nifedipine. What issues should be considered by the Pharmacy and Therapeutics (P&T) Committee?**

Nicardipine and amlodipine share many similar effects with the prototype dihydropyridine nifedipine.[65] Nicardipine is effective and reasonably well tolerated in the treatment of chronic stable angina pectoris. It appears to be as effective as nifedipine, propranolol, and atenolol in the treatment of chronic stable angina. Nicardipine also can be combined with β-adrenergic blockers and/or nitrates.

Adverse effects attributable to nicardipine generally are related to vasodilation and include flushing, headache, dizziness, and pedal or ankle edema.[65] Up to 10% of patients may require discontinuation of nicardipine because of intolerable adverse effects. Like nifedipine, nicardipine occasionally can precipitate an episode of angina pectoris, presumably secondary to reflex tachycardia or diminished coronary perfusion. However, nicardipine may impair ventricular systolic function to a lesser degree than nifedipine, and it may be used safely in patients with conduction deficits because it does not depress SA or AV node functions.[65]

Amlodipine is effective in the treatment of both chronic stable angina and vasospastic angina. It is as effective as verapamil and diltiazem in the treatment of chronic stable angina and safely can be used concomitantly with β-blockers.[65]

Like other dihydropyridines, the majority of amlodipine's adverse effects can be attributed to its vasodilating effects. Some of these, such as edema and flushing, may be dose related. Amlodipine appears to be tolerated as well as verapamil, diltiazem, and several β-blockers. Of all the calcium blockers, amlodipine (and perhaps felodipine) appears to be the safest in patients with heart failure.

Other second-generation dihydropyridines, such as felodipine and isradipine, currently are approved only for the treatment of hypertension. However, preliminary evidence suggests that these agents may be as effective as either β-adrenergic blockers or nifedipine in the management of chronic stable angina. Further clinical trials are needed to better assess the antianginal effects of these agents. In summary, the P&T Committee decision will be hampered by the lack of studies directly comparing the efficacy and safety of the various dihydropyridines in chronic stable angina. However, it is unlikely these drugs differ substantially in clinical effect. Therefore, the differences in acquisition cost may be a major factor in selecting agents for formulary inclusion. Amlodipine also may be added because of its potential safety in heart failure and because of its intrinsic long action (see Question 41).

Pharmacokinetics

39. Do any of the calcium channel blockers require dosage adjustment in patients with renal or hepatic disease?

Currently available calcium channel antagonists demonstrate similar pharmacokinetic properties.[65] With the exception of amlodipine and the SR formulations, all are absorbed rapidly after oral administration and generally reach peak concentrations within 1 to 2 hours. Peak concentrations for amlodipine usually are achieved within 6 to 9 hours after administration. Although calcium channel antagonists are well absorbed, bioavailability generally is low due largely to first-pass metabolism. In addition, calcium channel antagonists tend to have high metabolic clearances; their pharmacokinetic parameters are related to hepatic blood flow and intrinsic clearance, and they are metabolized almost exclusively by the liver. Furthermore, intraindividual and interindividual variations in bioavailability and total body clearance for most calcium channel antagonists are great. Therefore, dosage adjustment probably is necessary in patients with severe hepatic impairment, but not in those with renal disease.

Sustained-Release Calcium Channel Blockers

40. L.M., a 45-year-old female surgeon with a 3-year history of hypertension, recently was switched to SR verapamil 240 mg

BID. As a newly diagnosed chronic stable angina patient, she wonders if studies support the use of SR calcium channel blockers in angina.

Nifedipine, diltiazem, and verapamil all were originally introduced into the United States as immediate release preparations. As a consequence, dosing regimens called for TID or QID administration. SR calcium channel blockers are attractive alternatives to immediate-release products. The SR formulations of verapamil, diltiazem, and nifedipine offer promise in improving patient drug adherence and, thereby, better control of anginal episodes. L.M. uses the first SR calcium channel blocker marketed in the United States. SR verapamil is absorbed more slowly than immediate-release verapamil, thus providing more constant serum levels. The SR formulation, with a bioavailability of 0.9, extends the verapamil elimination half-life to 12 hours compared with about 6 hours observed with the immediate-release product.[67] Although some patients experience adequate control with once-daily SR verapamil, most patients require twice-daily dosing.[67] Another SR verapamil product (Verelan) uses beaded capsules and can be dosed reliably once a day. Therefore, SR verapamil and Verelan should not be interchanged.

The side effect profiles for immediate-release and SR verapamil are quite similar, with constipation being frequent. Diltiazem SR also exhibits slowed absorption and a prolonged half-life compared with immediate-release diltiazem. Like verapamil SR, twice-daily dosing of diltiazem SR is appropriate for most patients. A newer version of SR diltiazem (Cardizem CD available as 180, 240, and 300 mg capsules) may be given once daily. It is important that the Cardizem SR and Cardizem CD products are not confused. Another SR diltiazem product (Dilacor SR) uses yet another delivery system. Although verapamil SR and diltiazem SR and CD are FDA approved for treatment of hypertension only, many clinicians use these drugs to treat angina.

SR nifedipine (Procardia XL) uses a unique drug delivery system based on the osmotic pump principle. The GITS (GI system) nifedipine tablet consists of a semipermeable membrane that surrounds an active drug core. The core is composed of two layers: an active drug layer and an inert, but osmotically active push layer. Water entering the tablet from the GI tract activates the osmotic pump mechanism and pushes the active nifedipine out through a laser-drilled hole in the tablet's active layer. The inert components eventually are eliminated in the feces as a shell. The tablet should not be crushed, divided, or chewed. It should be taken at the same time each day and may be taken either with food or on an empty stomach.

The GITS nifedipine provides consistent (zero order rate), 24-hour serum nifedipine levels independent of pH or GI motility. Although this formulation decreases the vasodilatory effects observed with immediate-release nifedipine, dose-related edema is a common adverse experience occurring in 10% to 30% of patients. Headache is another common adverse effect. Limited experience suggests that patients switched from immediate-release nifedipine to GITS nifedipine will experience fewer angina episodes and side effects. Another form of extended-release tablets (Adalat CC) can be administered once daily and appears to be therapeutically equivalent to GITS nifedipine. Nevertheless, when patients are converted to any SR calcium channel blocker, reassessment of therapeutic efficacy is necessary. Because variations in SR products exist, they should not be substituted for one another without prior approval and patient counseling. The cost of the SR calcium channel blockers is similar to equivalent immediate-release doses. At one time, the use of generic immediate-release products was considered a cost-saving alternative, but now there are generic SR products marketed as well.

Any of the sustained release preparations of nifedipine, verapamil, or diltiazem are reasonable choices for patients with chronic stable angina. Immediate-release preparations of calcium channel blockers should be reserved for situations in which rapid titration of the dose is needed or desired, such as in patients with supraventricular arrhythmias. As stated previously, use of immediate-release nifedipine should be discouraged in any situation owing to the risk of reflex sympathetic drive and potential precipitation of myocardial ischemia. (See Chapter 14, Essential Hypertension, for further discussion of SR dosage forms of calcium channel blockers.)

COMBINATION THERAPY

41. E.R., a 62-year-old female with a long history of angina pectoris, has survived one out-of-hospital cardiac arrest and two MIs. She is not considered a surgical candidate for CABG because of severe COPD. Her current medications include isosorbide mononitrate 60 mg PO QD, metoprolol 50 mg PO BID, diltiazem CD 240 mg PO QD, fluticasone 2 puffs BID, albuterol 2 puffs PRN, NTG spray 0.4 mg PRN chest pain, and enteric-coated aspirin 325 mg/day. Is it rational for E.R. to receive a nitrate, β-blocker, and calcium channel blocker simultaneously?

E.R. is taking near maximal doses of all her medications. Using all three classes of drugs allows E.R.'s physician to titrate doses to maximize benefits and minimize troublesome side effects. E.R. probably cannot tolerate a higher β-blocker dosage because of her pulmonary disease. Disadvantages of triple-drug therapy include cost[68] and the potential for additive side effects, such as the possible worsening of heart failure by a combination of metoprolol and diltiazem. Excessive vasodilation and bradycardia are common side effects of triple-drug therapy, but these might be minimized by using a calcium channel blocker with less potent vasodilating properties.

As stated before, β-blockers should constitute initial therapy in patients with chronic angina. There are no formal recommendations regarding which class of agent to add next, and the choice should be made on a patient-by-patient basis.[1] Nitrates are preferred in patients who have coexisting LV dysfunction, whereas a calcium channel blocker would be preferred in patients who need additional BP control.

Simultaneous use of two calcium channel blockers is an alternative for patients who remain symptomatic despite maximal tolerated doses of single drugs and standard triple-drug therapy (nitrate + β-blocker + calcium blocker).[69] The combination of nifedipine with diltiazem or a verapamil-like calcium channel blocker will limit dizziness and effects on cardiac conduction and contractility. Addition of the second calcium channel blocker may permit use of a lower dosage of the other agent, thus minimizing the synergistic vasodilatory effects.

ANGIOTENSIN-CONVERTING ENZYME INHIBITORS

42. Would the addition of an ACE inhibitor be beneficial for E.R. at this time?

Historically, ACE inhibitors have not been thought of as having anti-ischemic properties. However, recent information indicates that ACE inhibitors have a prominent role in the overall treatment of patients with CAD.

ACE inhibitors have demonstrated significant benefits on morbidity and mortality in a number of patient groups such as HF, acute MI, and diabetes mellitus.[70] Interest in these agents for the treatment of chronic angina stems from results of studies investigating ACE inhibitors in patients with HF. Overall, ACE inhibitors decreased the risk of MI by approximately 23% in heart failure patients.[71,72] This set the stage for the investigation of ACE inhibitors in patients with CAD who do not have LV dysfunction or who are post-acute MI.

In a large, randomized, placebo-controlled trial in 9,297 patients with chronic CAD and no HF (the HOPE study), ramipril significantly decreased the incidence of death, MI, stroke, need for revascularization, and worsening angina. All patients were on appropriate medical therapy for angina, and the benefit appeared to be independent of any antihypertensive effect of ramipril in the treatment group.[37] Although the direct mechanism of action is unclear, it is thought that ACE inhibitors have a number of beneficial effects relative to the atherosclerosis process. These include antagonizing the growth mediating properties of angiotensin II on smooth muscle cells, preventing the rupture of atherosclerotic plaques by reducing inflammation, reducing LV hypertrophy, and improving endothelial function.[70]

An area of controversy after publication of the HOPE study was whether the results could be replicated with other ACE inhibitors. The issue stemmed mainly from cost, as ramipril is roughly 5 to 10 times more expensive than other ACE inhibitors, which are available in generic formulations (such as lisinopril and enalapril). The argument against a class effect is the variability in tissue binding (binding and inhibition of ACE in target organs such as the myocardium and endothelium) between various ACE inhibitors. Agents such as quinapril and ramipril are reported to have a high level of tissue binding, whereas as enalapril and fosinopril have a lower level of tissue binding. At issue is the ability to inhibit ACE not just in the circulation, but also at the tissue level as well and whether differences in the degree of tissue–ACE inhibition translate into differences in efficacy between ACE inhibitors.

Recently, the results of the European trial on reduction of cardiac events with perindopril in stable coronary artery disease (EUROPA) replicated the benefits seen in the HOPE study with the administration of perindopril in 12,218 patients with stable coronary heart disease and no apparent heart failure. Perindopril use (target dose 8 mg QD) for an average of 4.2 years resulted in a 20% relative risk reduction in the combined incidence of cardiovascular death, myocardial infarction, or cardiac arrest.[73]

While the results of the EUROPA trial confirmed the benefit of ACE inhibitors in patients with ischemic heart disease, it did not settle the question of tissue binding and whether agents with low tissue penetration will provide the same benefit. It is hoped that this issue will be further clarified when the results of the ongoing PEACE (trandolapril) trial become available.[74] These questions aside, the use of ACE inhibitors has become the standard of practice in the treatment of patients with chronic stable angina and other vascular diseases. Efforts should be directed at making sure patients with CAD receive these life saving medications.[1,75] In a patient such as E.R. who has maximized his antianginal therapy, the addition of an ACE inhibitor in the absence of any contraindication makes sense to improve his long-term outcome.

While in theory angiotensin-receptor blockers (ARBs) should produce the same beneficial effects as ACE inhibitors in patients with atherosclerosis, there are no clinical trials available documenting whether this is indeed true. However, given the similar results ARBs have shown to ACE inhibitors in patients with HF and post-MI, and the significant beneficial effects with ARBs seen in treating patients with hypertension and diabetes, the administration of an ARB in patients with CAD and intolerance to ACE inhibitors seems reasonable.[70,76]

ANTIPLATELET THERAPY

Aspirin

43. E.R. is taking enteric-coated aspirin every day. She wants your advice as to why she is getting this drug and if it is safe for her stomach. What is the most appropriate dose?

Platelet activation produces coronary occlusion either by formation of a platelet plug or through release of vasoactive compounds from the platelets. Two indices of platelet activity that have been studied intensely in patients with CAD are thromboxane A_2 and prostacyclin. Thromboxane A_2 is a cyclooxygenase-catalyzed product of arachidonic acid metabolism and a potent vasoconstrictor. Prostacyclin (PGI_2), another arachidonic acid metabolite produced under the influence of cyclooxygenase, counterbalances the effect of thromboxane A_2. It is a potent inhibitor of platelet aggregation and a vasodilator. Although PGI_2's production also is increased in USA and acute MI, the amount produced is insufficient to fully offset the effects of elevated thromboxane A_2 levels.[77]

The mechanism of action for aspirin's antiplatelet effect is inhibition of cyclooxygenase (see Chapter 16, Thrombosis). By acetylating the active site of cyclooxygenase, aspirin blocks the formation of prostaglandin endoperoxides from arachidonic acid. This inhibits the formation of both thromboxane and prostacyclin. Researchers have tested various aspirin doses in hopes of finding a dose that inhibits thromboxane synthesis but does not inhibit formation of prostacyclin. A single 100-mg aspirin dose virtually eliminates thromboxane A_2 production, whereas doses below 100 mg result in a dose-dependent reduction in thromboxane A_2 synthesis. Therapeutic benefit has been demonstrated with doses as low as 30 mg/day.[78]

Recent research has attempted to determine the effect of aspirin doses on the thromboxane A_2/prostacyclin (prostaglandin I_2) balance. Prostacyclin production recovers within hours of aspirin administration because the endothelial cell can resynthesize cyclooxygenase. In contrast, the inhibition of platelet cyclooxygenase is irreversible. Selective inhibition of platelet-generated thromboxane A_2 synthesis has been

shown with 75 mg of controlled-release aspirin daily.[77,78] This aspirin formulation undergoes extensive first-pass metabolism forming salicylic acid, a weak and reversible cyclooxygenase inhibitor. Theoretically, administration of 75 mg aspirin daily in a controlled-release formulation may selectively spare vascular endothelial prostacyclin production (preserving the vasodilator activity of prostacyclin), but at the same time still inhibit platelet cyclooxygenase. Unfortunately, controlled clinical trials on this proposed aspirin dosage regimen are lacking. Therefore, the proposed biochemical selectivity of aspirin on platelet function versus the vascular endothelium is difficult to achieve clinically.

Because of the lack of precise understanding of the pharmacodynamic effect of aspirin, it is not surprising that there is controversy regarding the optimal dose of aspirin to be used in patients with angina, as well as post-MI and as secondary prevention of stroke. In the past, it was believed that higher doses of aspirin would produce a higher level of efficacy than low doses. However, all available literature indicates that low dosages of aspirin (75 to 325 mg/day) are as effective as higher dosages (625 to 1,300 mg/day) in the treatment of patients with angina.[79] Conversely, as the aspirin dosage increases, the incidence of adverse effects, especially GI bleeding, increases as well. Therefore, current guidelines recommend a daily dosage of 75 to 325 mg orally for patients with CAD.[1,78,79] Aspirin at this dosage has been demonstrated to decrease the incidence of acute MI and death in patients with CAD, and it should be given to all patients barring any contraindications.[1]

Studies have also confirmed the protective effect of aspirin in patients with USA (see Question 57 for further discussion of USA). In these patients, aspirin reduces the incidence of MI and death from cardiac causes by 50% to 70%.[11]

Aspirin remains the most commonly prescribed antiplatelet agent for the treatment of cardiovascular disease. Essentially all patients with a history of angina or CAD, especially if they have also experienced an MI, should take aspirin daily. Further discussions of aspirin use in the secondary prevention of MI, combined therapy with thrombolytics in the treatment of acute MI, atrial fibrillation, prosthetic valves, and postoperative coronary artery bypass graft are discussed in Chapter 18, Myocardial Infarction, Chapter 16, Thrombosis, and Chapter 20, Cardiac Arrhythmias. Aspirin also is a key drug in treating cerebrovascular disease as presented in Chapter 55, Cerebrovascular Disorders.

Clopidogrel

44. As noted in question 41, ER was taking 325 mg per day of enteric-coated aspirin. This was later reduced to 75 mg per day based on the discussion above. Last week she was hospitalized for rapidly worsening angina, diagnosed as unstable angina. She is being discharged today with a new prescription for clopidogrel 75 mg PO QD, #60 with five refills. Is the combined use of aspirin and clopidogrel appropriate?

Clopidogrel (Plavix), a thienopyridine, inhibits platelet function in vivo. Its mechanism of action has not been identified, although it appears to be a noncompetitive antagonist of the platelet adenosine diphosphate (ADP) receptor. Stimulation of the ADP receptor produces platelet activation similar to thromboxane A_2. Clopidogrel at a dosage of 75 mg orally every day was demonstrated in one study to be slightly more effective than aspirin in the secondary prevention of MI and death in patients with various manifestations of atherosclerotic vascular disease.[77] However, the magnitude of difference in benefit seen with clopidogrel was quite small and not enough to justify its broad scale use in the treatment of CAD. Based on this study the role of clopidogrel historically was to serve as an alternative antiplatelet agent in patients with a true contraindication to aspirin and it is still used in this fashion.[1,77]

Recently, the combination of aspirin and clopidogrel was compared with aspirin alone in patients with acute coronary syndromes without ST-segment elevation in the CURE study. Patients received combination antiplatelet therapy acutely while in the hospital and continued it for an average of 9 months. The combination of aspirin and clopidogrel significantly reduced the occurrence of death from cardiovascular causes, nonfatal MI, or stroke.[29] The results of the CURE study were confirmed in the CREDO trial where patients with acute coronary syndromes who were treated with percutaneous coronary intervention with stent placement received aspirin plus clopidogrel acutely in hospital and then for 1 year. Patients receiving both aspirin and clopidogrel for 1 year had a lower incidence of death, MI and stroke in comparison to patients who only received aspirin.[30] Based on the results of these two studies, it appears appropriate for E.R. to receive the combination of aspirin and clopidogrel for up to 1 year after his recent episode of unstable angina. The occurrence of bleeding should be closely monitored because bleeding events were significantly increased in patients receiving combined antiplatelet therapy in both the CURE and CREDO study.[29,30] Dual therapy with aspirin and clopidogrel has not been investigated beyond 1 year; therefore, the combination should be limited to a duration of 1 year in patients who have experienced an acute coronary event.

Ticlopidine (Ticlid) is a related thienopyridine antiplatelet agent that is similar to clopidogrel in both structure and mechanism of action and is a potential alternative to aspirin for E.R. However, ticlopidine compares unfavorably with clopidogrel because of a lack of any data examining its use in ischemic heart disease (IHD) and its side effect profile. Of particular concern is a roughly 2% incidence of neutropenia, which may be life-threatening.[77] Because of these factors, ticlopidine should not be considered as a potential alternative to aspirin now that clopidogrel is available.

Oral anticoagulation with warfarin represents another alternative to aspirin in patients with angina. Although the efficacy of warfarin (International Normalized Ratio [INR] 2.0 to 3.0) appears to be similar to aspirin in the prevention of MI and death, the need for monitoring and the risk of bleeding relegate this mode of therapy as second line behind antiplatelet strategies.[79,80]

Primary Prevention

45. E.R. returns to your pharmacy 1 week later with her brother who wants to know if he should be taking an aspirin a day to prevent heart disease. His only medical history consists of hypertension for which he is taking hydrochlorothiazide 25 mg PO QD. Is primary prevention of CAD with aspirin appropriate for E.R.'s brother?

The question of whether aspirin is valuable in the primary prevention of cardiovascular events has been debated for over 20 years. In 2002, the U.S. Preventative Services Task Force developed guidelines for aspirin use in primary prevention based on the results of five large randomized studies.[81] Overall aspirin in this setting reduces the odds of having an MI by 28% (statistically significant), death from CHD by 13% (not statistically significant), and all-cause mortality by 7% (not statistically significant). Risk of stroke was not affected. The benefits of aspirin were not without risk because aspirin use increases the risk of hemorrhagic stroke and major gastrointestinal bleed.[82]

The net balance of risks versus benefits for any patient depends on the baseline risk of cardiovascular disease. In patients who have a high risk of developing cardiovascular disease ($>1.5\%$ per year), the benefits of aspirin in preventing cardiovascular events far outweighs the bleeding risks. In patients at low risk ($<0.6\%$/year), the risk of bleeding events negates any potential benefit in cardiovascular outcomes. Patients at intermediate risk (0.7% to 1.4% per year) derive some benefit in preventing cardiovascular events. However, the magnitude of benefit is not large enough to recommend routine administration of aspirin for primary prevention. In these circumstances patients should be informed about the risks and benefits of aspirin use in order to make an informed decision about whether they wish to take aspirin to prevent the occurrence of cardiovascular disease.[83]

For E.R.'s brother, the first step is to calculate what his risk of developing cardiovascular disease in the future. This can be done by using a validated risk assessment scoring system such as the Framingham risk score (see Chapter 13, Dyslipidemias, Atherosclerosis, and Coronary Heart Disease).[82] Once his risk is known, an appropriate recommendation can be made regarding his use of aspirin for primary prevention.

HORMONE REPLACEMENT THERAPY

46. E.R. returns to your pharmacy 4 months later to pick up refills of her isosorbide mononitrate, metoprolol, diltiazem, albuterol, lisinopril, and clopidogrel. She mentions to you that a few years back she remembers that her mother was put on estrogen by her doctor to help prevent heart disease and is wondering if she should be on estrogen replacement as well?

The increased popularity of hormone replacement therapy (estrogen alone or estrogen plus progesterone) to prevent adverse cardiovascular events stems from the results of many observational epidemiologic studies. These studies all suggested that postmenopausal women who use hormone replacement therapy (HRT) have a lower incidence of heart disease, bone fractures, and colorectal cancer; but also experience an increase the risk of breast cancer, endometrial cancer, stroke, and venous thromboembolism. Despite these risks, the use of hormone replacement therapy was attractive as heart disease is by far the number one cause of death for women in the U.S.[83]

Unfortunately, when put to the test of a randomized, placebo-controlled trial, the benefits of HRT on cardiovascular disease were not seen and potential harm was noted. The Women's Health Initiative (WHI) study sought to answer the question of whether administering estrogen alone (in women without a uterus) or estrogen plus progesterone (in women with a uterus) would prevent the development of CAD in healthy (without history of CAD) postmenopausal women. Unexpectedly, there was a 29% increase in the incidence of CAD in those women on estrogen plus progesterone compared with placebo after an average treatment duration of 5 years. No increase was noted in women on estrogen alone; that part of the trial is still ongoing.[84] Similar disappointing results were observed in the HERS study that evaluated the role of estrogen in secondary prevention of CAD. In women with documented cardiovascular disease, the use of estrogen plus progesterone had no effect on preventing recurrent cardiovascular events over an average of 4 years.[85] Based on the negative results of these two randomized trials of hormone replacement therapy, the American Heart Association released a specific recommendation in 2001 not to initiate HRT for prevention of cardiovascular disease.[86]

In the case of E.R., she should be educated regarding the current body of knowledge that does not support the use of HRT in the treatment of cardiovascular disease. Hormone replacement therapy still has a role in the treatment of menopausal symptoms and prevention of fractures.[83] E.R. should be directed to discuss these options with her physician if she feels that is warranted.

DIET AND ANTIOXIDANT THERAPY

47. **E.R. leaves your store a bit discouraged, but returns in 3 months to again pick up refills of her prescriptions. While she is paying for her medicines, she also has a bottle of vitamin E and a bottle of B complex vitamins to purchase. E.R. states she had heard that antioxidants such as vitamin E could benefit her along with a daily B vitamin. She also asks you whether there are other dietary changes she could make that would benefit her cardiovascular disease.**

Since oxidation of LDL in the arterial wall was identified as a key step in the atherosclerotic process, there has been considerable interest in the theory that supplementation with high doses of antioxidants such as vitamin E, vitamin C, and beta-carotene might mitigate this process and slow the progression of atherosclerosis. Early observational studies of dietary patterns high in these antioxidants seemed to confirm this theory. However, multiple large randomized studies have shown no positive effect from supplemental intake of antioxidants such as vitamin E on the incidence of cardiovascular outcomes such as MI or death. These findings were observed in both primary and secondary prevention of cardiovascular events. E.R. should be informed that beyond following a diet rich in fruits and vegetables (primary sources of antioxidants in the diet), supplemental intake of vitamin E will not have any positive or negative effect on her cardiovascular disease (see Chapter 13, Dyslipidemias, Atherosclerosis, and Coronary Heart Disease, for further discussion).[87]

Interest in the use of supplemental intake of folic acid and B vitamins stems from the relatively recent identification of elevated levels of homocysteine as a risk factor for cardiovascular disease.[88,89] Although elevated levels of homocysteine, a product of methionine metabolism, are associated with a higher rate of cardiovascular disease, it is unclear whether lowering levels of plasma homocysteine will have positive effects on the incidence of cardiovascular outcomes. Several large randomized trials are underway to determine whether supplemental administration of folic acid and other B vitamins decreases cardiovascular events by lowering homocysteine levels in patients with CHD.[90] Even though it is unknown whether supplemental intake of folic acid and B vitamins will have a positive effect, it may be reasonable for ER to use them, given the theoretical basis for benefit and a low risk for toxicity at usual doses. She should be instructed not to exceed 1 mg per day of folic acid.

Several dietary interventions have compelling evidence to support their implementation to prevent CHD. These include the substitution of nonhydrogenated saturated fats for saturated fats and trans-fats in the diet; consumption of omega-3 fatty acids (primary source is fish); and consumption of a diet high in fruits, vegetables, nuts, and whole grains.[91] When patients post-MI were randomized to a traditional Western diet or a Mediterranean diet high in fruits, vegetables, cereals, beans, nuts, and olive oil as the primary source of fat intake, there was a 50% to 70% lower risk of recurrent heart disease (which includes cardiac death and nonfatal MI).[92] These dietary alterations are in line with the current dietary guidelines from the American Heart Association.[93] In addition, the intake of 25 grams of soy protein per day (to replace protein from animal sources) can significantly decrease total and LDL cholesterol.[93] E.R. can make a number of dietary changes that can significantly benefit her cardiovascular disease, and she should be encouraged to do so. E.R. should be asked if she regularly consumes alcohol and counseled to limit her intake to one to two drinks per day if she does.[93]

VARIANT ANGINA (CORONARY ARTERY SPASM)

Clinical Presentation

48. **A.P., a 35-year-old woman, is hospitalized for evaluation of severe chest pain, which occurs almost daily at about 5 AM. A.P. ranks the severity of pain as 7 to 8 on a scale of 1 to 10. It is associated with diaphoresis and is not relieved by change in position. A.P. has no cardiovascular risk factors, and her hobbies include triathlon competition and rock climbing, neither of which has caused chest pain. She follows a strict vegetarian diet and takes no medications. Admission ECG reveals sinus bradycardia at 56 beats/min. Serum electrolytes, chemistry panel, and cardiac enzymes are all within normal limits.**

At 6 AM the next morning, A.P. is awakened abruptly by severe chest pain. Her vital signs include the following: heart rate, 55 beats/min; supine BP, 110/64 mm Hg; and respiratory rate, 12 breaths/min. A stat ECG shows sinus bradycardia with marked ST-segment elevation. The pain is relieved within 60 seconds by 1 NTG 0.4-mg sublingual tablet. During the day, she completes an exercise tolerance test without complication or evidence of CAD.

On the second day, A.P. undergoes cardiac catheterization, and no coronary atherosclerosis is visualized. An ergonovine provocation test is performed during cardiac catheterization. At 3-minute intervals, intravenous ergonovine maleate bolus doses are given: 0.05, 0.10, and 0.25 mg. After the 0.25-mg dose, A.P. develops severe chest pain associated with an ST-segment elevation of 0.3 mV. The cardiologist observes almost complete vasospasm of the RCA and immediately injects 200 μg NTG into

the coronary artery along with administering 2 lingual sprays of NTG. A.P.'s chest pain resolves within 60 seconds, and the ECG normalizes within 3 minutes. A.P. is diagnosed as having Prinzmetal's variant angina. Discharge medications include amlodopine 10 mg PO QD at 11 PM and NTG lingual spray 0.4 mg PRN chest pain. Is A.P.'s presentation typical for Prinzmetal's variant angina?

A.P. presents with a classic picture of variant (Prinzmetal's) angina, with transient total occlusion of a large epicardial coronary artery as a result of severe segmental spasm. Clinical manifestations include chest pain occurring at rest, often in the morning hours. Like A.P., patients with Prinzmetal's variant angina generally are younger than patients with chronic stable angina and do not carry a high-risk profile. Other vasospastic disorders, such as migraine attacks or Raynaud's phenomenon, may be present; smoking and alcohol ingestion may be important contributing factors. [2]

The hallmark of variant angina is ST-segment elevation on the ECG, which denotes rapid and complete occlusion of the coronary artery. Many patients also have asymptomatic episodes of ST-segment elevation. Transient arrhythmias and conduction disturbances may be observed during pain depending on the severity of the myocardial ischemia. In contrast to chronic stable angina in which the heart rate-BP product often is elevated with pain, no hemodynamic factors appear to contribute to Prinzmetal's variant angina. [2]

As documented by angiography, A.P. has vasospasm of the large RCA. This transient, reversible narrowing probably is caused by increased coronary vascular resistance. It can occur in the absence of atherosclerosis, as illustrated by A.P., or it may occur in the presence of CAD. One possible explanation for vasospasm occurring more commonly at night or during the early morning hours is increased vasomotor tone secondary to diurnal variations in catecholamines.

Ergonovine Stimulation Test

49. Why was the ergonovine test used? Was intracoronary NTG necessary to reverse the effects of ergonovine?

Because Prinzmetal's variant angina does not occur predictably, spasm must be induced under controlled circumstances. Ergonovine maleate, an ergot alkaloid that stimulates α-adrenergic and serotonergic receptors, exerts a direct vasoconstrictive effect on the vascular smooth muscle. [93] The ergonovine maleate provocation test is highly specific and sensitive, especially in patients with normal coronary arteries. The risks of the test, which often discourage some physicians from using ergonovine, include arrhythmias (heart blocks, ventricular tachycardia, ventricular fibrillation) and possible MI.

The vasospasm induced by ergonovine should be reversed promptly. Although sublingual NTG tablets or lingual spray may relieve the episode, the coronary vasospasm may be unresponsive to these agents. Direct injection of NTG into the coronary arteries immediately reverses the vasoconstrictor action of ergonovine. [94]

Therapy

50. Amlodopine 10 mg PO QD was ordered for A.P. Would long-acting nitrates or β-adrenergic blockers be alternatives to

verapamil for A.P.? Is one calcium channel blocker preferable to another for treatment of Prinzmetal's variant angina?

Because of their antispasmodic effects and low incidence of side effects, calcium channel blockers are generally selected over nitrates or β-blockers for nocturnal vasospastic angina. All calcium channel blockers appear equally effective in preventing Prinzmetal's variant angina. [66] However, intrinsically long-acting or SR forms are preferred, and some patients may respond better to one agent than to another.

In patients who continue to experience pain using maximal calcium channel blocker doses, combination therapy with nitrates should be tried. [2] Even though nitrates cause vasodilation by a different mechanism than calcium channel blockers, they are effective in treating Prinzmetal's variant angina. [2] To avoid tolerance, the nitrate-free interval for A.P. should be scheduled during the day so that the early morning hours are covered by NTG. For example, if needed, A.P. could apply a transdermal NTG patch at bedtime and remove it upon awakening. Aspirin therapy is indicated for A.P.

β-Blockers are likely to worsen A.P.'s angina because blockade of the β2-receptors that mediate vasodilation may allow unopposed α1-mediated vasoconstriction. A cardioselective β-blocker also could worsen Prinzmetal's variant angina. Therefore, calcium channel blockers or nitrates are preferable.

51. Will A.P. require treatment for the remainder of her life? [2]

During the first year of therapy, up to 50% of patients experience spontaneous remission by an unknown mechanism. This occurs most often in patients who have had a short duration of symptoms or have normal or mildly diseased coronary arteries (i.e., isolated vasospasm without atherosclerosis). If A.P. is pain free and not experiencing significant arrhythmias or silent ischemic episodes of Prinzmetal's angina after 1 year, the amlodopine could be tapered and discontinued. However, it is also possible that she will require treatment indefinitely. Modification of smoking and ethanol ingestion may promote remission of Prinzmetal's angina. [2]

52. Can variant angina lead to acute MI or death?

Variant angina, particularly in patients with multi-vessel coronary artery spasm, can lead to acute MI or death. In a study of 159 consecutive patients with variant angina in Japan who required hospitalization, 76% of patients experienced a cardiac event (acute MI in 19 patients, sudden death in 5 patients, and coronary artery bypass graft in 1 patient) within 1 month of onset of angina. [2] These patients had greatly improved outcomes if treated aggressively with calcium antagonists, nicorandil, and NTG infusion during the early stages. If variant angina persisted, revascularization of coronary arteries with underlying critical lesions was indicated.

MICROVASCULAR ISCHEMIA (SYNDROME X)

53. K.G., a 50-year-old female executive, has undergone an extensive cardiovascular workup for exertional angina associated with a 3-mm ST-segment depression. A recent cardiac catheterization did not reveal any atherosclerosis, and an ergonovine stimulation test did not produce observable coronary vasospasm. The cardiologists believe K.G. has microvascular ischemia. What drug therapy might be indicated for K.G.?

Syndrome X, increasingly known as *microvascular angina,* is the syndrome of angina or angina-like chest pain in the setting of a normal coronary arteriogram. There are several theories regarding the mechanism of pain production, including microvascular dysfunction producing ischemia or chest discomfort without ischemia in patients who may have an abnormal perception of pain. Microvascular dysfunction may be the result of either diminished responsiveness to vasodilating stimuli (e.g., endothelia relaxation factor[nitric oxide], kinins, atrial natriuretic peptide or prostaglandin I_2) or increased sensitivity to vasoconstricting stimuli (e.g., catecholamines, vasopressin, angiotensin II or thromboxane A_2). In patients who display a heightened perception of pain, there may be an awareness to pain in response to atrial stretch or changes in heart rate. Ischemia is not universally present in patients with syndrome X; therefore, different mechanisms may be responsible for symptoms in different patients.[2]

Microvascular angina differs substantially from variant angina. Although spasm-causing variant angina may be visible with coronary angiography, the microvascular coronary circulation is not visible. The changes in coronary artery tone are in the distal coronary arteries and perhaps the collateral vessels. Some patients with microvascular ischemia have other smooth muscle disorders, such as esophageal motility disorders. There is a definite link between coronary vasoconstriction and mental or psychological stress.[2]

By symptoms alone, K.G.'s presentation is not significantly different from that of a patient with exercise-induced angina secondary to atherosclerosis. However, with a 3-mm ST-segment depression as seen on ECG, one would expect to find severe CAD. The absence of these findings in K.G. confirms the diagnosis of syndrome X. Overall, the prognosis for patients with Syndrome X appears to be good. Long-term survival is no different from age-matched controls. However, most patients continue to experience symptoms and control of anginal pain is the main goal in therapy.[2]

Treatment with nitrates, calcium channel blockers and β-blockers all appear to offer some relief, but overall the response to therapy in these patients is poor. The choice of agent will likely depend on specific patient characteristics. Unfortunately, sublingual NTG is often ineffective at treating acute attacks although it should still be prescribed.

SILENT MYOCARDIAL ISCHEMIA

Definition

54. **Y.G., a 60-year-old man who has had his first complete physical examination in 12 years, is found to have Q waves on ECG, indicating a previous MI. Physical findings are normal except for borderline LV hypertrophy. Abnormal laboratory studies include a moderately elevated total serum cholesterol and TGs. His medical history is remarkable for hypertension controlled with hydrochlorothiazide 25 mg PO QD. Y.G. does not recall ever experiencing angina, nor has he ever been told he had a heart attack. What characteristic syndrome does Y.G. exhibit, and how does it differ from angina pectoris?**

Y.G. had a silent MI, often the first indicator of silent myocardial ischemia.[5] Silent myocardial ischemia is unrecognized by the patient because there are no symptoms of angina. It can occur in totally asymptomatic persons (type 1), in asymptomatic postinfarction patients (type 2), and in patients with angina (type 3).[5] The prevalence of silent myocardial ischemia is difficult to estimate because it often is undetected. An estimated 1 to 2 million totally asymptomatic men have silent myocardial ischemia, and approximately 50,000 new cases of postinfarction silent ischemia occur each year. Most patients with angina also appear to have episodes of silent ischemia, with the silent episodes occurring two to three times more often than the anginal episodes. The pathogenesis of silent ischemia is not fully defined. There may be an abnormality in pain threshold so that the anginal warning system is not triggered, or it may represent varying activation of coronary vasomotor tone or platelet activity.[2]

Prognosis

55. **What is Y.G.'s prognosis?**

Y.G.'s prognosis depends on the extent of his underlying CAD, ventricular function, and arrhythmia status. If Y.G. has multi-vessel disease, he is more likely to develop adverse cardiac events (reinfarction, USA, sudden death) than if he has single-vessel disease. Silent myocardial ischemia is especially ominous in patients with unstable angina.[5]

Diagnosis

56. **What diagnostic tests will be used to evaluate Y.G.'s total ischemic burden both before and after therapy is started?**

The total ischemic burden, the sum of painful and painless ischemic episodes that occur, is assessed with exercise testing and 24-hour ambulatory electrocardiographic (Holter) monitoring. Both tests measure ST-segment depression, the usual abnormal electrocardiographic response to ischemia. ST-segment depression >2 mm at low levels of exercise or ST-depression with hypotension or arrhythmias is a strong indicator of disease. Radionuclide procedures help confirm ECG responses.[5]

Management

57. **What management goals and techniques are likely to apply to Y.G.?**

Management of patients with silent myocardial ischemia is unresolved, but modification of risk factors is mandatory. Y.G.'s cholesterol and hypertension should be corrected and the aim of pharmacotherapy is to abolish all electrocardiographic evidence of ischemia. The same drugs used to treat angina (nitrates, β-blockers, calcium channel blockers, and aspirin) also prevents silent myocardial ischemia if used at high enough doses or in appropriate combinations. β-Blockers may be the most effective agents in decreasing the episodes of silent ischemia. Calcium antagonists are useful, but dihydropyridines are less efficacious than verapamil and diltiazem. Aspirin and nitrates also are key therapies in treating silent myocardial ischemia. Each patient requires careful titration to reduce both symptomatic and asymptomatic ischemic episodes. Even though many questions remain unanswered about silent myocardial ischemia, it is no longer acceptable to treat painful ischemic episodes only.[2,5]

REVASCULARIZATION

Percutaneous Coronary Intervention

58. T.T., a 54-year-old male, had a recent onset of angina that was precipitated by exertion. His current medications include isosorbide mononitrate 30 mg PO QD, atenolol 50 mg PO QD, NTG SL 0.4 mg PRN chest pain, and enteric-coated aspirin 81 mg/day. Would T.T be a candidate for revascularization therapy with either percutaneous coronary intervention (PCI) or coronary artery bypass (CABG), or should he be treated medically?

PCI, also known as angioplasty, involves the percutaneous insertion of a balloon catheter into the femoral artery in a similar fashion to angiography. The catheter is advanced up the aorta and into the coronary arteries at the coronary sinus. PCI, which was introduced in 1977, initially involved the inflation of a catheter-borne balloon that mechanically dilated a coronary artery obstruction through arterial intimal disruption, plaque fissuring, and stretching of the arterial wall. Balloon inflations are repeated until the plaque is compressed and coronary blood flow resumes. Since then, alternative devices have been developed including rotational blades designed to remove atheromatous material, lasers to ablate plaques, and intracoronary stents that are designed to maintain the patency of the vessel after it is re-opened.[1] It is estimated that more than 750,000 PCI procedures are performed in the United States each year. Approximately 70% of those procedures involve placement of a stent (Fig. 17-5). PCI is indicated in patients with single- or multi-vessel disease and who are either symptomatic or asymptomatic.[94]

Acute complications of PCI occur in approximately 2% to 21 % of patients, depending on patient risk factors and the procedure being performed. The incidence of Q-wave MI is 1.6% to 4.8% and in hospital mortality ranges anywhere from 0.7% to 2.5%. The overall success of any procedure is directly related to the experience of the operator, patient factors (such as LV function or number of vessels treated), and the equipment used. Repeat revascularization procedures (either repeat angioplasty or surgery) may be required in as many as 32% to 40% of first-time angioplasty patients because of the reoccurrence of plaque at the angioplasty site.[95] The process is known as *restenosis.*[96]

Many pharmacologic strategies have been studied in an attempt to reduce the risk of restenosis. The outcome with most methods has been disappointing. The only strategy that has been associated with a decrease in restenosis is the use of intraluminal stents.[97] Stents are essentially metal scaffolding that are deployed into the vessel wall after a balloon inflation has taken place. They provide a physical barrier to the reoccurrence of a significant stenosis at the site.[98] One of the early drawbacks of the use of stents was the need for complicated anticoagulation regimens including aspirin, heparin, dipyridamole, and warfarin to prevent in-stent thrombosis. However, it is now known that dual antiplatelet therapy is effective at reducing in-stent thrombosis. Currently, a combination of clopidogrel and aspirin is the recommended regimen of choice after stent placement. Clopidogrel is given for 2 to 4 weeks after stent placement and aspirin is continued for life.[99–101]

Recently, stents that elute antiproliferative agents such as sirolimus or paclitaxel have been demonstrated in clinical trails to reduce the incidence of restenosis compared with bare-metal stents. Although drug-eluting stents are attractive from the standpoint of reducing the rate of restenosis into single digits, their high cost likely limit their availability to patients who are at highest risk of developing restenosis or who have already experienced restenosis from a previous PCI. The duration of dual antiplatelet therapy (aspirin plus clopidogrel) to prevent in-stent thrombosis is at least 3 to 6 months when a drug-eluting stent is placed, compared with 2 to 4 weeks with bare-metal stents.[102]

Because of mechanical disruption of the atherosclerotic plaques and exposure of plaque contents to the bloodstream during PCI, potent antiplatelet and antithrombotic strategies are needed to prevent acute thrombotic events such as MI and death. Initially, strategies involved the use of high-dose unfractionated heparin and aspirin. With the development of the

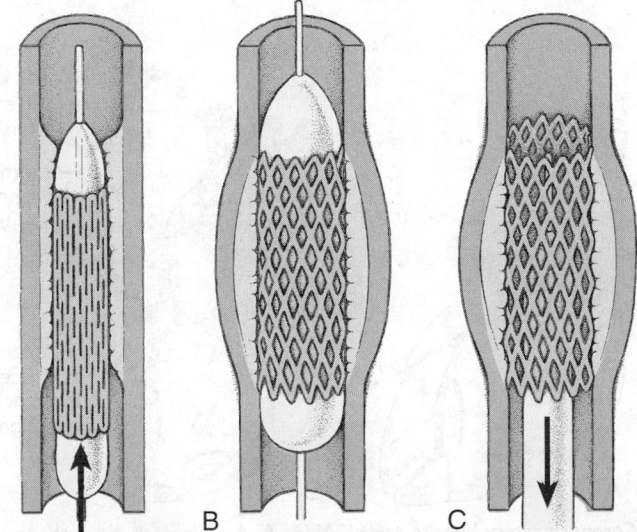

FIGURE 17-5. Vascular stent: **A,** a balloon catheter positions stent at site of arterial stenosis, **B,** inflation of balloon dilates artery and expands stent, **C,** balloon is collapsed and withdrawn, leaving expanded stent in position. (Illustration by Neil O. Hardy, Westpoint, Conn.)

Gp IIb/IIIa receptor antagonists, significant improvements were made in patient outcomes during and after PCI.[94] Currently, three agents are available in the United States (Table 17-10). Abciximab, a human-murine monoclonal antibody fragment, was the first agent available. Subsequently epitifibatide (cyclic heptapeptide) and tirofiban (nonpeptide mimetic) have become available.[103] All three agents, when administered intravenously during PCI and for 12 to 24 hours afterward, significantly decrease the risk of death, acute MI, or recurrent PCI. Major adverse effects include bleeding and thrombocytopenia. Therefore, Hct and platelet counts should be monitored appropriately. Clearance of both eptifibatide and tirofiban is renal, and dose adjustments should take place accordingly.[103]

In addition to appropriate use of the antiplatelet agents (aspirin, clopidogrel and Gp IIb/IIIa inhibitors), patients undergoing PCI should also receive adequate antithrombin therapy with unfractionated heparin (UFH) during the procedure. The intensity of anticoagulation in this setting is monitored via the activated clotting time (ACT) and the target range is 200 to 250 seconds in patients also receiving a Gp IIb/IIIa antagonist. Weight-based dosing strategies should be used with patients receiving a heparin bolus of 50 to 70 units/kg (in patients not receiving a Gp IIb/IIIa receptor antagonist, dose should be 70 to 100 units/kg). In patients who receive a Gp IIb/IIIa inhibitors during PCI, UFH should be discontinued at the end of the procedure.[95] There has been significant interest in using direct thrombin inhibitors such as bivalirudin in place of heparin during PCI. There have been some favorable results in clinical trials, but currently UFH is still considered the antithrombin of choice during PCI.[104]

Coronary Artery Bypass Graft Surgery

Coronary artery bypass graft (CABG) is a complicated surgical procedure during which an atherosclerotic vessel is "bypassed" using either a patient's saphenous vein or internal mammary artery (IMA; Fig. 17-6). The "graft" (i.e., the saphenous vein or IMA) then allows blood to flow past the obstruction in the native vessel. The goals of antianginal therapy,

Table 17-10	Indications and Dosing of Glycoprotein II_b/III_c Receptor Antagonists		
Indication	Abciximab (ReoPro)	Eptifibatide (Integrilin)	Tirofiban (Aggrestat)
Percutaneous transluminal coronary angioplasty (PCTA)	0.25 mg/kg IV bolus, then 0.125 µg/kg/min IV infusion × 12 hr	180 µg/kg IV bolus, then 2.0 µg/kg/min IV × 20–24 hr Repeat 180 µg/kg IV bolus 10 min after first bolus	Not approved use
Coronary stent placement	0.25 mg/kg IV bolus, then 0.125 µg/kg/min IV infusion × 12 hr	Same dose as for PCTA.	Not approved use
Acute coronary syndrome (unstable angina and non–Q-wave MI)	Not approved use	180 µg/kg IV bolus, then 2.0 µg/kg/min IV infusion × 72–96 hr	0.4 µg/kg/min IV load × 30 minutes, then 0.1 µg/kg/min IV infusion × 48–102 hr Reduce dose by 50% if CrCl <30 mL/min

CrCl, creatinine clearance; IV, intravenous.

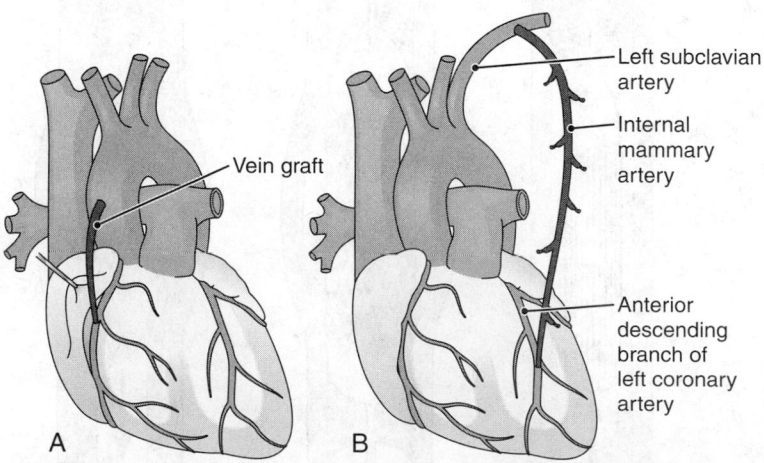

FIGURE 17-6. Coronary artery bypass graft (CABG). A. A segment of the saphenous vein carries blood from the aorta to a part of the right coronary artery that is distal to an occlusion. **B.** The mammary artery is used to bypass an obstruction in the left anterior descending (LAD) coronary artery. (From Cohen BJ. Medical Terminology, 4th Ed. Philadelphia. Lippincott Williams & Wilkins 2003.)

whether medical (pharmacologic) or revascularization, remain unchanged: (1) to prolong life, (2) to prevent MI, and (3) to improve the quality of life.

The choice of medical therapy or revascularization with CABG has been studied, and current guidelines are available.[36] Of interest to practitioners and patients are the relative effects of each treatment modality on mortality, occurrence of symptoms, and quality of life. Certain high-risk patient subgroups clearly have an improved outcome with CABG. These include (1) patients with significant left main coronary disease; (2) patients who have three-vessel disease, especially with LV dysfunction; (3) patients with two-vessel disease with a significant proximal LAD lesion; (4) patients who have survived sudden cardiac death; and (5) patients who are refractory to medical management. In patients who do not meet these criteria, medical management or PCI are viable options.[1,36] When compared with medical management in patients who would not be considered high risk, PCI in general offered no improvement in the long-term incidence of MI or cardiovascular death, but significantly improved symptoms.[1,94]

Whether T.T. undergoes either CABG or PCI depends on his coronary anatomy (one-, two-, or three-vessel disease along with location of lesions), associated patient-specific factors (LV function), and his preferences to undergo a surgical procedure versus managing his disease with medications.

ACUTE CORONARY SYNDROMES: UNSTABLE ANGINA AND NON–ST-SEGMENT ELEVATION MYOCARDIAL INFARCTION

59. F.G., a 54-year-old man, is brought to the ED by helicopter for management of severe, unrelenting chest pain of 2 hours' duration. He has no history of CAD, but cardiac risk factors include a strong positive family history of CAD, a 45-pack-year smoking history, and a 5-year history of hypertension. He is taking metoprolol 100 mg PO BID. Physical examination reveals a middle-aged man in obvious distress with the following vital signs: heart rate, 110 beats/min; BP, 176/108 mm Hg; respiratory rate, 18 breaths/min; and temperature, 37°C. Normal lung and heart sounds are heard with the exception of an S_4 gallop. Examination of F.G.'s abdomen and extremities is unremarkable, as is the funduscopic examination. F.G. has received 10 mg morphine sulfate IV and 3 sublingual 0.4 mg NTG tablets and is still experiencing severe pain that is associated with ST-segment depression. He is placed on oxygen (2 L by nasal prongs) and an NTG infusion (5 μg/min). Rapid upward titration of the NTG to 60 μg/min alleviates the chest pain. His admitting diagnosis is acute coronary syndrome. What general guidelines exist for the management of acute coronary syndromes?

Clinical Presentation

Acute coronary syndromes (ACS) include unstable angina (also known as *preinfarction angina, crescendo angina,* and *angina at rest*), non–ST-segment elevation myocardial infarction (NSTEMI) and ST segment elevation myocardial infarction (STEMI). On presentation, the ultimate diagnosis usually cannot be determined because the diagnosis of MI requires the presence of biomarkers such as creatinine kinase (CK) or troponin. Often these results are not available for the first 12 to 24

hours. Because of this delay in the determination of the final diagnosis, initial treatment must be driven by other factors. One critical factor during the acute presentation is the initial electrocardiogram (ECG) and, more specifically, whether ST-segment elevation is present on this initial ECG. Patients who have ST-segment elevation acute coronary syndromes (e.g., Acute MI) are candidates for immediate reperfusion therapy and are discussed in detail in Chapter 18, Myocardial Infarction. Treatment of patients who present with non–ST-segment elevation acute coronary syndromes (this includes patients presenting with ST-segment depression, T-wave inversions, or no ECG changes) is discussed briefly here.[11]

Unstable angina is a syndrome falling between chronic stable angina and MI. The prognosis of patients with USA is variable, and classification systems have been developed to determine whether a patient is at low, intermediate, or high risk for acute MI and death in the short term.[105] Patients at intermediate or high risk should be hospitalized for acute treatment and assessment of potential long-term treatment strategies. Patients at low risk may be managed without admission to the hospital. F.G. is a high-risk patient because he has ST-segment depression at rest or with pain.

Management

Coronary arteriographic studies of patients with USA usually reveal severe atherosclerotic disease complicated by the rupture of an atherosclerotic plaque with the formation of a superimposing thrombus.[11] Therefore, the pathophysiology of USA is closely related to that of MI, and similar treatment strategies are used in both disease states. The treatment of USA in recent years has evolved to include medical therapy as well as revascularization procedures. Typically, revascularization with PCI is reserved for patients who are considered intermediate to high risk for developing adverse cardiovascular outcomes in the next 30 days or who do not stabilize with medical therapy.[11]

The immediate challenge in the treatment of USA is relief of pain and control of all ischemic episodes. Hospitalization, bed rest, diagnosis, and treatment of underlying precipitating factors such as infection, anemia, hypertension, heart failure, and arrhythmias are essential. Pharmacologic therapy is targeted at relieving ischemia and at attenuating the thrombotic process.

As with patients experiencing an acute MI, β-blockers should be administered acutely because they have been demonstrated to prevent the progression to MI and death. Nitrates, both sublingually and then intravenously, are effective for relieving pain and acutely treating ischemia. Calcium channel blockers are effective for treating ischemia in patients with USA, but should be reserved for patients who have ischemia refractory to β-blockade.[11]

A 325-mg dose of chewable aspirin should be administered to all patients because it has been shown to prevent the progression to MI and death. In addition, the combined use of aspirin (81 to 325 mg daily) and clopidogrel (300 mg load, 75 mg PO QD) acutely and for up to 1 year in patients with USA/NSETMI has been shown to decrease the risk of cardiovascular death, MI, or stroke at 30 days and up to 1 year.[29,30] Based on these results from the CURE[29] and CREDO[30] studies, aspirin and clopidogrel should be administered to all patients with USA/NSTEMI who are unlikely to undergo PCI acutely. In patients who will undergo emergent PCI for treatment of USA/NSTEMI, clopidgrel administration may be delayed until after the procedure and then continued for 1 year.[11]

Historically UFH has been the primary antithrombin used in the treatment of ACS. The beneficial effects of UFH are additive to aspirin in the prevention of acute MI and death.[11] Several new antithrombotic strategies have become available, which may improve upon the results seen with aspirin and UFH. Several low-molecular-weight heparins (LMWH) have been investigated in the setting of USA and non–Q-wave MI and as a group are considered at least as effective as UFH at improving clinical outcomes.[106] However, results for individual agents have not been uniform. Trials comparing enoxaparin with UFH have consistently shown that enoxaparin is superior to UFH in preventing cardiovascular events. Trials investigating other LMWH's have only demonstrated equivalency to UFH. Based on these results from clinical trials, the current ACC/AHA guidelines specifically recommend enoxaparin at a dose of 1 mg/kg SC BID (an intravenous bolus dose of 30 mg may be used) as the preferred antithrombin agent for patients with USA or NSTEMI.[11]

The glycoprotein IIb/IIIa (Gp IIb/IIIa) receptor antagonists are relatively new antiplatelet agents that provide significantly improved outcomes in patients with USA/NSTEMI who are being treated medically or who undergo revascularization via PCI.[107] These agents have a unique mechanism of action in that they block the final common pathway in platelet aggregation. Platelets may be stimulated by a number of different agonists (e.g., epinephrine, serotonin, ADP, thromboxane A_2), some of which may be inhibited by aspirin (thromboxane A_2) or clopidogrel. Blockade of one or more of these agonists by aspirin or clopidogrel still leaves the platelet susceptible to stimulation via other agonists. Regardless of the initial stimulus, the end result is the expression of the Gp IIb/IIIa receptor. This receptor is critical because it binds and cross-links fibrin, which stabilizes the clot. This process is blocked with the receptor antagonists. Because of their mechanism of action, the Gp IIb/IIIa antagonists are significantly more potent in terms of their antiplatelet effects than aspirin or clopidogrel.

These agents, in addition to aspirin and UFH/LMWH, significantly decrease the composite risk of death, acute MI, and urgent revascularization in patients with USA/NSTEMI. The Gp IIb/IIIa receptor antagonists currently are recommended in patients with USA/NSTEMI: (1) in whom catheterization and PCI is planned; (2) who have continuing ischemia despite treatment with aspirin, UFH/LMWH, nitrates, β-blockers and clopidogrel; (3) who have other high risk features such as elevated troponin or ST-segment changes on the initial ECG.

REFERENCES

1. American College of Cardiology/American Heart Association Task Force on Practice Guidelines. ACC/AHA 2002 Guideline Update for the Management of Patients with Chronic Stable Angina. 2002. www.americanheart.org.
2. Gersh BJ et al. Chronic Coronary Artery Disease. In: Braunwald E, ed. Heart Disease: A Textbook of Cardiovascular Medicine, 6th Ed. Philadelphia: WB Saunders, 2001.
3. Sakata K et al. Assessment of regional sympathetic nerve activity in vasospastic angina: Analysis of iodine-123-labeled metaiodobenzylguanifdine scintigraphy. Am Heart J 1997;133:484.
4. Okumura et. al. Diffuse disorder of coronary artery vasomotility in patients with coronary spastic angina. Hyperreactivity to the constrictor effects of acetylcholine and the dilator effects of nitroglycerin. J Am Coll Cardiol 1996;27:45.
5. Cohn PF et al. Silent myocardial ischemia. Circulation 2003;108:1263.
6. American Heart Association. 2002 Heart and Stroke Statistical Update. Dallas, Tex.: American Heart Association, 2001.
7. Popma JJ, Bittl JA. Coronary Angiography and Intravascular Ultrasonography. In: Braunwald E, ed. Heart Disease: A Textbook of Cardiovascular Medicine, 6th Ed. Philadelphia: WB Saunders, 2001.
8. Ganz P, Ganz W. Coronary Blood Flow and Myocardial Ischemia. In: Braunwald E, ed. Heart Disease: A Textbook of Cardiovascular Medicine, 6th Ed. Philadelphia: WB Saunders, 2001.
9. Koerselman J et. al. Coronary collaterals: an important and underexposed aspect of coronary artery disease. Circulation 2003;107:2507.
10. Weber RT, Janicki JS. The metabolic demand and oxygen supply of the heart: physiologic and clinical considerations. Am J Cardiol 1974;44:722.
11. American College of Cardiology/American Heart Association Task Force on Practice Guidelines. ACC/AHA 2002 Guideline Update for the Management of Patients with Unstable Angina and Non-ST Segment Elevation Myocardial Infarction. 2002. www.americanheart.org.
12. Libby P. The Vascular Biology of Atherosclerosis. In: Braunwald E, ed. Heart Disease: A Textbook of Cardiovascular Medicine, 6th Ed. Philadelphia: WB Saunders, 2001.
13. Libby P, Ridker PM, Maseri A. Inflammation and atherosclerosis. Circulation 2002;105:1135.
14. Bonetti PO et al. Endothelial dysfunction. A marker of atherosclerotic risk. Arterioscler Thromb Vasc Biol 2003;23:168.
15. Laroia ST et al. Endothelium and lipid metabolism: the current understanding. Int J Cardiol 2003;88:1.
16. Halcox JPJ et al. Prognostic value of coronary vascular endothelial dysfunction. Circulation 2002;106:653.
17. AHA Conference Proceedings: Prevention Conference V, Beyond Secondary Prevention. Identifying the high-risk patient for primary prevention. Circulation 2000;101:111.
18. Pearson TA et al. AHA Guidelines for the Primary Prevention of Cardiovascular Disease and Stroke: 2002 Update. Circulation 2002;106:388.
19. Genest J, Pedersen TR. Prevention of cardiovascular ischemic events. High-risk and secondary prevention. Circulation 2003;107:2059.
20. Pearson TA et al. Markers of inflammation and cardiovascular disease. Application to Clinical and Public Health Practice. A statement for healthcare professionals from the centers for disease control and prevention and the American Heart Association. Circulation 2003;107:499.
21. Ridker PM. Clinical application of C-reactive protein for cardiovascular disease detection and prevention. Circulation 2003;107:363.
22. Chobanian AV et al. The Seventh Report of the Joint National Committee on Prevention, Detection, Evaluation, and Treatment of High Blood Pressure. The JNC 7 Report. JAMA 2003;289:2560.
23. Agency for Healthcare Policy and Research. Treating tobacco use and dependence. US Department of Health and Human Services Public Health Services Report. Washington, DC: US Government Printing Office; 2000
24. Expert Panel on Detection, Evaluation, and Treatment of High Blood Cholesterol in Adults. Executive Summary of the Third Report of the National Cholesterol Education Program (NCEP) Expert Panel on Detection, Evaluation, and Treatment of High Blood Cholesterol in Adults (Adult Treatment Panel III). JAMA 2001;285(19):2486.
25. American Diabetes Association. Standards of Medical Care for Patients with Diabetes Mellitus. Diabetes Care 2003;26:S33.
26. Thompson PD et al. Exercise and physical activity in the prevention and treatment of atherosclerotic cardiovascular disease: a statement from the council on clinical cardiology (subcommittee on exercise, rehabilitation, and prevention) and the council on nutrition, physical activity, and metabolism (subcommittee on physical activity). Circulation 2003;107:3109.
27. Polluck ML et al. AHA Scientific Advisory. Resistance exercise in individuals with and without cardiovascular disease: benefits, rationale, safety, and prescription: an advisory from the committee on Exercise Rehabilitation, and Prevention, Council on Clinical Cardiology, American Heart Association; Position paper endorsed by the American College of Sports Medicine. Circulation 2000;101:51S.
28. Clinical Guidelines on the identification, evaluation, and treatment of overweight and obesity in adults: the evidence report. National Institutes of Health. Obes Res 1998;6(suppl):51S.
29. The Clopidogrel in Unstable Angina to Prevent Recurrent Events Trial Investigators. Effects of clopidogrel in addition to aspirin in patients with acute coronary syndromes without ST-segment elevation. N Engl J Med 2001;345:494.
30. Steinhubl SR et al. Early and sustained dual oral antiplatelet therapy following percutaneous coronary intervention. JAMA 2002;288:2411.
31. Heifant RH, Banks VS. A clinical and angiographic approach to coronary heart disease. Philadelphia: F.A. Davis, 1978.
32. Cox J, Naylor CD. The Canadian cardiovascular society grading scale for angina pectoris: is it time for refinements? Ann Intern Med 1992;117:677.
33. Kannel WB et al. Epidemiological assessment of the role of physical activity and fitness in development of cardiovascular disease. Am Heart J 1985;109:876.
34. Gibbons RJ et al. ACC/AHA 2002 Guideline update for exercise testing: a report of the American College of Cardiology/American Heart Association

Task Force on Practice Guidelines (Committee of Exercise Testing). 2002. WWW.ACC.ORG.

35. ACC/AHA Guidelines for Coronary Angiography. A Report of the American College of Cardiology/American Heart Association Task Force on Practice Guidelines (Committee on Coronary Angiography). J Am Coll Cardiol 1999;33(6):1756.

36. ACC/AHA Guidelines for Coronary Artery Bypass Graft Surgery. A report of the American College of Cardiology/American Heart Association Task Force on Practice Guidelines (Committee to revise the 1991 guidelines for coronary artery bypass graft surgery). J Am Coll Cardiol 1999;34(4):1262.

37. The Heart Outcomes Prevention Evaluation Study Investigators. Effects of an angiotensin-converting enzyme inhibitor, ramipril, on cardiovascular events in high-risk patients. N Engl J Med 2000;342:145.

38. Parker JD, Parker JO. Nitrate therapy for stable angina pectoris. N Engl J Med 1998;338(8):520.

39. Abrams J, Frishman WH. The Organic Nitrates and Nitroprusside. In: Frishman WH, Sonnenblick EH, Sica DA, eds. Cardiovascular Pharmaceutics, 2nd Ed. New York: McGraw-Hill, 2003.

40. Abrams J. The role of nitrates in coronary artery disease. Arch Intern Med 1995;155:357.

41. Parker JO et al. Nitroglycerin lingual spray: clinical efficacy and dose-response relation. Am J Cardiol 1986;57:1.

42. Kaplan KJ et al. Association of methemoglobinemia and intravenous nitroglycerin administration. Am J Cardiol 1985;55:181.

43. Abrams J. Nitrate tolerance and dependence. Am Heart J 1980;99:113.

44. Shaw SV et al. Selection and dosing of nitrates to avoid tolerance during sustained antianginal therapy. Formulary 1999;34:590.

45. Gori T, Parker JD. The puzzle of nitrate tolerance: pieces smaller than we thought? Circulation 2002;106:2404.

46. Gori T, Parker JD. Nitrate Tolerance: a unifying hypothesis. Circulation 2002;106:2510.

47. Luke R et al. Transdermal nitroglycerin in angina pectoris: efficacy of intermittent application. J Am Col Cardiol 1987;10:642.

48. Cowan JC et al. Prevention of tolerance to nitroglycerin patches by overnight removal. Am J Cardiol 1987;60:271.

49. Packer M et al. Prevention and reversal of nitrate tolerance in patients with congestive heart failure. N Engl J Med 1987;317:799.

50. Noonan PK, Bennet LZ. Variable glyceryl dinitrate formation as a function of route of nitroglycerin administration. Clin Pharmacol Ther 1987;42:273.

51. Kirby JA, Woods SL. A study of variation in measurement of doses of nitroglycerin ointment. Heart Lung 1981;10:814.

52. Moe G, Armstrong PW. Influence of skin site on bioavailability of nitroglycerin ointment in congestive heart failure. Am J Med 1981;81:765.

53. Iafrate RP et al. Effect of dose and ointment application technique on nitroglycerin plasma concentrations. Pharmacotherapy 1983;3:118.

54. Rosenfeld AS, White WB. Allergic contact dermatitis secondary to transdermal nitroglycerin. Am Heart J 1984;108:1061.

55. DeBelder MA et al. Evaluation of the efficacy and duration of action of isosorbide mononitrate in angina pectoris. Am J Cardiol 1990;65:6J.

56. Goldstein S. Beta-blocking drugs and coronary heart disease. Cardiovasc Drug Ther 1997;11:219.

57. Bristow MR, Ginsburg R. Beta$_2$-receptors on myocardial cells in human ventricular myocardium. Am J Cardiol 1986;57:3F.

58. Alpha- and Beta-Adrenergic Blockings Drugs. In: Frishman WH, Sonnenblick EH, Sica DA, eds. Cardiovascular Pharmacotherapeutics, 2nd Ed. New York: McGraw-Hill, 2003.

59. Update: ACC/AHA Guidelines for the Management of Patients with Acute Myocardial Infarction. A report of the American College of Cardiology/American Heart Association Task Force on Practice Guidelines (Committee on Management of Acute Myocardial Infarction). J Am Coll Cardiol 1999;34(3):890.

60. Bonet S et al. Beta-adrenergic blocking agents in heart failure. Benefits of vasodilating and nonva-sodilating agents according to patients' characteristics: a meta-analysis of clinical trials. Arch Intern Med 2000;160:621.

61. Tafreshi MJ, Weinacker AB. Beta-adrenergic blocking agents in bronchospastic disease: a therapeutic dilemma. Pharmacotherapy 1999;19(8):974.

62. Salpeter S et al.. Cardioselective beta-blockers in patients with reactive airway disease: a meta-analysis. Ann Intern Med 2002;137:715.

63. Gengo FM et al. Lipid-soluble and water-soluble beta-blockers: comparison of the central nervous system depressant effect. Arch Intern Med 1987;146:39.

64. Feishman WH. Beta-adrenergic withdrawal. Am J Cardiol 1987;59:26F.

65. Frishman WH, Sica DA. Calcium Channel Blockers. In: Frishman WH, Sonnenblick EH, Sica DA, eds. Cardiovascular Pharmacotherapeutics, 2nd Ed. New York: McGraw-Hill, 2003.

66. Abernathy DR, Schwartz JB. Calcium antagonist drugs. N Engl J Med 1999;341(19):1447.

67. Davidson CL et al. Sustained-release calcium channel blockers. Hospital Therapy 1989 Nov; 35.

68. Crawford MH. The role of triple therapy in patients with chronic stable angina pectoris. Circulation 1987;75(II):V-122.

69. Prida XE et al. Comparison of diltiazem and nifedipine alone and in combination in patients with coronary artery spasm. J Am Coll Cardiol 1987;9:412.

70. Sica DA et al. The Renin-Angiotensin Axis: Angiotensin-Converting Enzyme Inhibitors and Angiotensin-Receptor Blockers. In: Frishman WH, Sonnenblick EH, Sica DA, eds Cardiovascular Pharmacotherapeutics, 2nd Ed. New York: McGraw-Hill, 2003.

71. Yusuf S et al. Effect of enalapril on myocardial infarction and unstable angina in patients with low ejection fractions. Lancet 1992;340:1173.

72. Pfeffer MA et al. Effect of captopril on mortality and morbidity in patients with left ventricular dysfunction after myocardial infarction: results of the Survival and Ventricular Enlargement Trial. N Engl J Med 1992;327:669.

73. The European trial on reduction of cardiac events with perindopril in stable coronary artery disease investigators. Efficacy of perindopril in reduction of cardiovascular events among patients with stable coronary artery disease: randomised, double-blind, placebo-controlled, multicentre trial (the EUROPA study). Lancet 2003;362:782.

74. Pfeffer MA et al. The continuation of the prevention of events with angiotensin-converting enzyme inhibition (PEACE) Trial. Am Heart J 2001; 142:375.

75. O'Keefe JH, et al. Should an angiotensin-converting enzyme inhibitor be standard therapy for patients with atherosclerotic disease? J Am Coll Cardiol 2001;37:1.

76. Jacoby DS, Rader DJ. Renin-angiotensin system and atherothrombotic disease. Arch Intern Med 2003;163:1155.

77. Frishman WH et al.. Antiplatelet and Antithrombotic Drugs. In: Frishman WH, Sonnenblick EH, Sica DA, eds. Cardiovascular Pharmacotherapeutics, 2nd Ed. New York: McGraw-Hill, 2003.

78. Awtry EH, Loscalzo J. Aspirin. Circulation 2000; 101:1206.

79. Cairns JA et al. Antithrombotic agents in coronary artery disease. Chest 2001;119:228S.

80. Anand SS, Yusuf S. Oral anticoagulant therapy in patients with coronary artery disease: a meta-analysis. JAMA 1999;282:2058.

81. U.S. Preventative Services Task Force. Aspirin for the primary prevention of cardiovascular events: recommendation and rationale. Ann Intern Med 2002;136:157.

82. Lauer MS. Aspirin for primary prevention of coronary events. N Engl J Med 2002;346:1468.

83. Michels KB, Manson JE. Postmenopausal hormone therapy. A reversal of fortune. Circulation 2003;107:1830.

84. Writing Group for the Women's Health Initiative Investigators. Risks and benefits of estrogen plus progestin in healthy postmenopausal women: principal results from the Women's Health Initiative Randomized Controlled Trial. JAMA 2002; 288:321.

85. Hulley S, Bush T et al. Randomized trial of estrogen plus progestin for secondary prevention of coronary heart disease in postmenopausal women. Heart and Estrogen/Progestin Replacement Study (HERS) Research Group. JAMA 1998;280:605.

86. Mosca L et al. American Heart Association. Hormone replacement therapy and cardiovascular disease: a statement for health care professionals from the American Heart Association. Circulation 2001;104:499.

87. Kritharides L, Stocker R. The use of antioxidant supplements in coronary heart disease. Atherosclerosis 2002;164:219.

88. Wald DS et al. Homocysteine and cardiovascular disease: evidence on causality from a meta-analysis. BMJ 2002;325:1202.

89. The Homocysteine Studies Collaboration. Homocysteine and risk of ischemic heart disease and stroke. JAMA 2002;288:2015.

90. Doshi SN et al. Lowering plasma homocysteine with folic acid in cardiovascular disease: what will trials tell us? Atherosclerosis 2002;165:1.

91. Hu FB, Willett WC. Optimal diets for the prevention of coronary heart disease. JAMA 2002;288:2569.

92. Kris-Etherton P et al. Lyon Diet Heart Study. Benefits of a Mediterranean-style, national cholesterol education program/American Heart Association step 1 dietary pattern on cardiovascular disease. Circulation 2001;103:1823.

93. Krauss RM et al. AHA Dietary Guidelines. Revision 2000: A statement for healthcare professionals from the nutrition committee of the American Heart Association. Circulation 2000;102:2284.

94. Hackett D et al. Induction of coronary artery spasm by a direct local action of ergonovine. Circulation 1987;75:577.

95. Smith SC Jr et al. ACC/AHA guidelines for percutaneous coronary intervention (revision of the 1993 PTCA guidelines). Executive Summary. A report of the American College of Cardiology/American Heart Association Task Force on Practice Guidelines endorsed by the Society for Cardiac Angiography and Interventions. Circulation 2001;103:3019.

96. Wurdeman RL et al. Restenosis. The Achilles' heel of coronary angioplasty. Pharmacotherapy 1998;18(5):1024.

97. Topol EJ, Serruys PW. Frontiers in Interventional Cardiology. Circulation 1998;98:1802.

98. Leon MB et al. A clinical trial comparing three antithrombotic drug regimens after coronary artery stenting. N Engl J Med 1998;339:1665.

99. Urban P et al. Randomized evaluation of anticoagulation versus antiplatelet therapy after coronary stent implantation in high-risk patients. Circulation 1998;98:2126.

100. Bertrand ME et al. Randomized multicenter comparison of conventional anticoagulation versus antiplatelet therapy in unplanned and elective coronary stenting. Circulation 1998;98:1597.

101. Moussa I et al. Effectiveness of clopidogrel and aspirin versus ticlopidine and aspirin in preventing stent thrombosis after coronary stent implantation. Circulation 1999;99:2364.

102. Levine GN et al. Management of patients undergoing percutaneous coronary revascularization. Ann Intern Med 2003;139:123.

103. Cheng JWM. Efficacy of glycoprotein IIb/IIIa-receptor inhibitors during percutaneous intervention. Am J Health Syst Pharm. 2002;59(suppl):S5.

104. Lincoff AM et al. Bivalirudin and provisional glycoprotein IIb/IIIa blockade compared with heparin and planned glycoprotein IIb/IIIa blockade during percutaneous coronary intervention. JAMA 2003;289:853.

105. Braunwald E. Unstable angina: a classification. Circulation 1989;80:410.

106. Zed PJ et al. Low-molecular-weight heparins in the management of acute coronary syndromes. Arch Intern Med 1999;159:1849.

107. Boersma E et al. Platelet glycoprotein IIb/IIIa inhibitors in acute coronary syndromes: a meta-analysis of all major randomised clinical trials. Lancet 2002;359:189.

CHAPTER 18

Myocardial Infarction

Jean M. Nappi, Robert L. Page II

Acute myocardial infarction (AMI), now referred to as ST segment elevation myocardial infarction (STEMI), is a manifestation of ischemic heart disease characterized by cellular death or necrosis occurring in the setting of severe or prolonged ischemia. STEMI is thought to be the result of complete occlusion in the coronary artery.

AMI is a medical emergency requiring immediate intervention. Until the 1980s, patients with AMI were treated symptomatically. Their pain was controlled; arrhythmic complications were treated; and bed rest, nitrates, and β-blockers minimized the amount of oxygen required by the heart. In 1980, an angiographic study by DeWood and colleagues found total occlusion in a coronary artery in 87% of patients who were examined by angiography within the first 4 hours of symptoms.[1] This study stimulated interest in using thrombolytics to interrupt the progression of myocardial necrosis. Thrombolytics and percutaneous transluminal coronary angioplasty are now considered first-line therapies unless a contraindication is present. A committee composed of representatives from the American College of Cardiology and the American Heart Association (ACC/AHA) periodically review the literature and publish practice guidelines to aid health care practitioners in selecting the most effective treatments for patients with AMI.[2]

Epidemiology

Approximately 540,000 Americans suffer an AMI annually.[3] Twenty to thirty percent of these patients die before reaching a hospital, presumably as a result of ventricular fibrillation.[3,4] Prompt recognition and treatment of AMI have dramatically reduced the mortality over the past two decades. In-hospital and 1-year postdischarge mortality rates have been estimated to be 9.9% and 7.1%, respectively. These rates are lower for patients <75 years of age, but greater for those >75.[5,6]

Pathophysiology

The majority of MIs result from occlusion of a coronary artery secondary to thrombus formation overlying a lipid-rich atheromatous plaque that has undergone fissuring or rupture.[4] Damage to the plaque results in blood being exposed to collagen and fatty acids; this in turn activates platelets, the first step in thrombosis and formation of a fibrin clot. Rarely, coronary artery spasm may cause an AMI in a patient with normal coronary arteries, particularly in the setting of cocaine abuse. More likely, spasm occurs before, during, or after the AMI and further compromises blood flow in an already stenotic artery.

Most infarctions are located in a specific region of the heart and are described as such (e.g., anterior, lateral, inferior).[4] Some patients develop permanent electrocardiographic (ECG) abnormalities (Q waves) following an AMI. In the past, patients with Q-wave infarctions generally were thought to have more extensive necrosis and a higher in-hospital mortality rate. Patients with a non–Q-wave infarct were thought to have a greater likelihood of experiencing postinfarction angina and early reinfarction. Recently, however, these distinctions have come into question.[7] Some cardiologists now believe there is no difference in prognosis. The terminology is changing: Q-wave MI is now called STEMI and non–Q-wave MI is now called non-ST segment elevation MI (NSTEMI) or the acute coronary syndrome. An anterior wall infarction carries a worse prognosis than an inferior or lateral wall infarction.

Clinical Presentation

It is important to make the diagnosis of AMI as quickly as possible so appropriate action may be taken. Patients may complain of prolonged substernal chest pain or pressure, shortness of breath, diaphoresis, nausea, and vomiting. In some patients, the symptoms may be confused with indigestion or other gastrointestinal complaints. The pain may be atypical in nature as well as location. The pain might be described as stabbing or knife-like, and it may occur in the arms, shoulder, neck, jaw, or back.[4] Some patients have a fever. However, not all AMIs are symptomatic: an estimated 20% of AMIs are "silent," and this presentation tends to occur more frequently in the elderly and people with diabetes. Elderly patients may present with hypotension or cerebrovascular symptoms rather than chest pain.

The physical examination is not particularly helpful in making the diagnosis of AMI, but the findings are important in guiding initial therapy. Signs of severe left ventricular or right ventricular dysfunction may be present (see Chapter 19, Heart Failure). The patient may have severe hypertension due to pain or, conversely, may be hypotensive. Significant tachycardia (heart rate >120 beats/min) suggests a large area of damage. On cardiac auscultation, a fourth heart sound (S_4) may be heard, denoting an ischemia-induced decrease in left ventricular compliance. New cardiac murmurs may be heard resulting from papillary muscle dysfunction. The cerebral and peripheral vasculature should be assessed. Patients with a history of cerebrovascular disease may not be eligible for thrombolytic therapy. Peripheral pulses should be examined to assess perfusion and to obtain a baseline before invasive procedures are instituted.

Diagnosis

Failure to make the appropriate diagnosis in AMI can lead to disastrous results. The list of other medical conditions that mimic the presentation of an AMI is extensive (Table 18-1). In addition to the patient's history and presentation, the diagnosis of AMI is based on the ECG and laboratory results such as cardiac enzyme changes (discussed below). Usually two of the three criteria (history, ECG changes, and cardiac enzyme findings) should be consistent with AMI before the diagnosis is made.

Table 18-1 Differential Diagnosis of Acute Myocardial Infarction

Acute cerebrovascular disease
Aortic dissection
Acute anxiety or panic attacks
Esophageal rupture or spasm
Gallbladder disease
Pancreatitis
Peptic ulcer disease
Pericarditis
Pneumothorax
Pulmonary embolism
Spinal or chest wall diseases

The ECG is an indispensable tool in the diagnosis of AMI and has become the key point in the decision pathway. The presence of ST segment elevation is used to identify patients who will benefit from thrombolytic therapy. The 12-lead ECG is helpful in determining the location of an infarct. The presence of a new Q wave, new bundle branch block, or ST segment elevation is consistent with an AMI.[2] The electrocardiographic diagnosis of an AMI is extremely difficult in the presence of a left bundle branch block. Figures 18-1 and 18-2 show the ECG in a patient presenting with AMI and after successful thrombolysis.

Patients presenting with ischemic chest pain, but without ST segment elevation and without laboratory evidence of infarction are classified as having unstable angina, a part of the acute coronary syndrome spectrum. Patients with a history consistent with ischemic chest pain, without ST segment elevation, but who develop positive enzymes within hours of presentation are also given the diagnosis of AMI (referred to as NSTEMI). Patients with NSTEMI and unstable angina continue to have some blood flow, although limited, through the affected coronary artery. Patients with NSTEMI usually have partial occlusion of the artery and/or thrombi that are made up largely of platelets and fibrinogen. Thrombolytic therapy has not been shown to be beneficial in these patients and is a major point of differentiation.

Cardiac Enzymes

When a cardiac cell is injured, enzymes are released into the circulation. The measurement of cardiac enzymes is routine in making the diagnosis of AMI. One of the standard enzymes used for the laboratory diagnosis of AMI is creatine kinase (CK). There are three isoenzymes of CK: the BB, MM, and MB bands. Of these, the CK-MB isoenzyme is the most specific for the diagnosis of AMI. It can appear in the serum within 3 to 6 hours after myocardial damage, and levels generally peak in 12 to 24 hours.[2] Serum enzymes normally are determined at admission and then repeated at least once 12 hours after the onset of chest pain. The magnitude of rise of peak CK is related to the size of the infarct, but the peak may be missed if admission is delayed. There are several conditions other than AMI in which CK-MB may be elevated (Table 18-2).[8] CK is usually reported as enzymatic activity (U/L), and CK-MB is reported as mass (ng/mL) in either plasma or serum. CK-MB is often reported as percentage of activity.

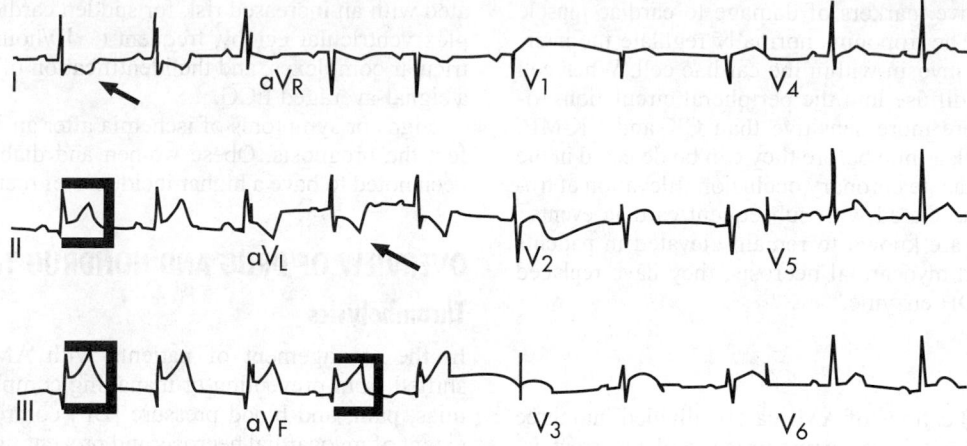

FIGURE 18-1 On this admission ECG, note the extensive ST segment elevation in leads II, III, and aV$_F$ (*brackets*), indicating an inferior wall AMI. The patient also displays reciprocal ST segment depression in I and aV$_L$ (*arrows*), which are the lateral ECG leads and are opposite the inferior leads.

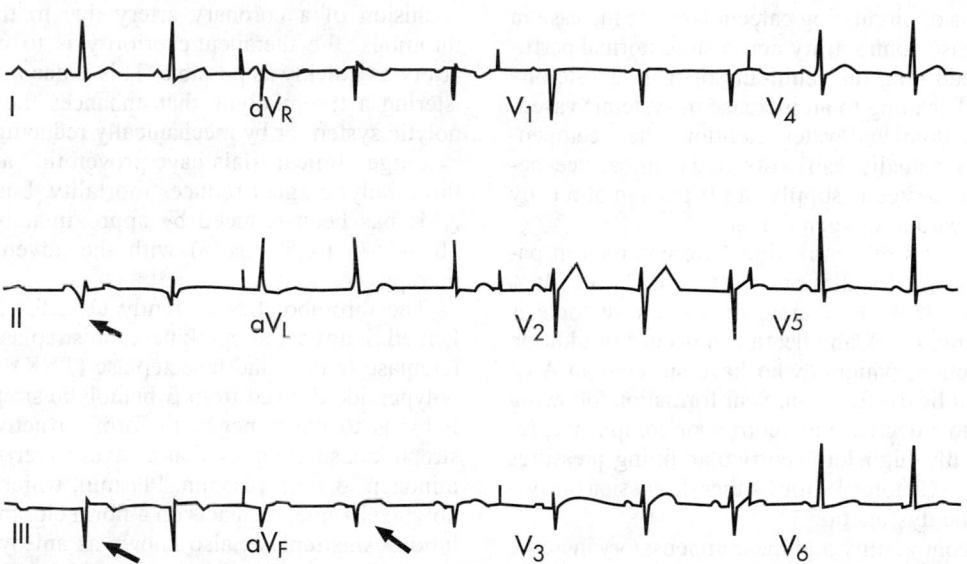

FIGURE 18-2 After successful thrombolysis, the ECG shows no ST segment changes suggestive of ischemia, but evolution of new Q waves in leads II, III, and aV$_F$ (*arrows*) is apparent.

Another laboratory change that may be seen is an increase in lactate dehydrogenase (LDH). The increase in LDH generally appears 24 to 48 hours after the onset of chest pain and peaks in 3 to 6 days. Measurement of LDH may be helpful in patients who present with a history of chest pain that began several days before admission. In these cases, the CK already may have returned to normal before the patient is evaluated. Increases in LDH also are seen in liver disease, hemolysis, leukemia, pulmonary embolism, myocarditis, and skeletal muscle disease. LDH is comprised of five isoenzymes. Since the heart muscle contains LDH$_1$, a ratio of LDH$_1$ to LDH$_2$ >1 may be helpful in distinguishing AMI from other disorders. Other nonspecific laboratory changes that occur in AMI include hyperglycemia and increases in aspartate aminotransferase (AST) and the white blood cell (WBC) count.[8]

Table 18-2	Conditions Where CK-MB Isoenzyme May Be Elevated	
Acute myocardial infarction	Alcoholism
Cardiac contusion/trauma	Carcinoma
Cardioversion (>400 J)	Acute cholecystitis
Hyper/hypothyroidism	Systemic lupus erythematosus
Myocarditis	Pericarditis
Peripartum period	Reye's syndrome
Prolonged supraventricular tachycardia	Muscular dystrophy
Skeletal muscle trauma	Polymyositis

CK, Creatine kinase.

The most sensitive markers of damage to cardiac muscle are the troponins. The troponins normally regulate the interaction of actin and myosin within the cardiac cell. When cell death occurs, they diffuse into the peripheral circulation. Although troponins are more sensitive than CK and CK-MB, they have a similar lag time before they can be detected in the blood following an acute coronary occlusion. Elevation of troponins has been associated with subsequent cardiac events.[2] Because troponins are known to remain elevated in patients who have sustained myocardial necrosis, they have replaced the less specific LDH enzyme.[9]

Complications

The primary complications of AMI can be divided into three major groups: pump failure, arrhythmias, and recurrent ischemia and reinfarction. Depression of cardiac function following an AMI is related directly to the extent of left ventricular damage. As a result of decreased cardiac output and decreased perfusion pressure associated with left ventricular dysfunction, a number of compensatory mechanisms become activated. The levels of circulating catecholamines increase in an attempt to increase contractility and restore normal perfusion pressure. In addition, the renin-angiotensin-aldosterone system is enhanced, leading to an increase in systemic vascular resistance and sodium and water retention. These compensatory mechanisms actually can worsen the imbalance between myocardial oxygen supply and consumption by increasing the myocardial oxygen demand.

Signs and symptoms of heart failure are common in patients who have abnormal wall motion affecting 20% to 25% of the left ventricle. If 40% or more of the left ventricle is damaged, cardiogenic shock and death can occur.[4] In addition to systolic dysfunction, patients who have suffered an AMI also may have diastolic dysfunction. Scar formation following an AMI may lead to a decrease in ventricular compliance, resulting in abnormally high left ventricular filling pressures during diastole. (See Chapter 19 for further discussion on systolic versus diastolic dysfunction.)

The decreased contractility and the compensatory increase in left ventricular end-diastolic volume and pressure lead to increased wall stress within the left ventricle. Left ventricular enlargement is an important determinant of mortality after AMI. Over a period of days to months following an AMI, the infarcted area may expand as a result of dilatation and thinning of the left ventricular wall. These changes are known as ventricular remodeling. In addition, hypertrophy of the noninfarcted myocardium occurs. Administration of oral angiotensin-converting enzyme (ACE) inhibitors may limit remodeling and will attenuate the progression of left ventricular dilatation.[10,11]

During the peri-infarction period, the heart is irritable and subject to ventricular arrhythmias. The continuous monitoring of patients in a coronary care unit has reduced the in-hospital mortality rate related to ventricular arrhythmias. However, patients who have had an MI have an increased risk of sudden cardiac death for 1 to 2 years following hospital discharge. The most important predictor for sudden cardiac death is an abnormal ejection fraction. The lower the ejection fraction following AMI, the worse the prognosis. Other factors associated with an increased risk for sudden cardiac death are complex ventricular ectopy, frequent (>10/hour) premature ventricular complexes, and the identification of late potentials on a signal-averaged ECG.

Signs or symptoms of ischemia after an AMI adversely affect the prognosis. Obese women and diabetic patients have been noted to have a higher incidence of recurrent infarction.[12]

OVERVIEW OF DRUG AND NONDRUG THERAPY

Thrombolytics

In the management of patients with AMI, emphasis has shifted from preventing or managing complications (arrhythmias, pain, and blood pressure [BP] control) to limiting the extent of myocardial necrosis and preventing reinfarction. The 1999 update of the ACC/AHA guidelines for the management of patients with AMI addressed the most significant advances made in the prior 2.5 years and should be used in conjunction with the 1996 guidelines.[2]

Since the majority of STEMI cases result from the sudden occlusion of a coronary artery due to the formation of a thrombus, the therapeutic priority is to open the occluded artery as quickly as possible. This is accomplished by administering a thrombolytic that enhances the body's own fibrinolytic system or by mechanically reducing the obstruction.

Large clinical trials have proven that administration of a thrombolytic agent reduces mortality. Early mortality from AMI has been reduced by approximately one third (from 10%–15% to 5%–10%) with the advent of thrombolytic therapy.[13]

The thrombolytics currently used for MI patients in the United States are streptokinase, anistreplase, alteplase (t-PA), reteplase (r-PA), and tenecteplase (TNK). Streptokinase is a polypeptide derived from β-hemolytic streptococcal cultures. It binds to plasminogen to form an active plasminogen to streptokinase complex that cleaves other molecules of plasminogen to form plasmin. Plasmin, which is an active fibrinolytic enzyme, then acts on a fibrin clot to enhance its dissolution. Anistreplase, also known as anisoylated plasminogen streptokinase activator complex (APSAC), is a combination of streptokinase and plasminogen with an anisoyl group reversibly placed within the catalytic center of the plasminogen moiety. This moiety is deacylated in the circulation at a controlled rate.[13]

Alteplase, or t-PA, is a naturally occurring enzyme produced commercially by recombinant DNA technology. t-PA cleaves the same plasminogen peptide bond that urokinase cleaves. However, t-PA has a binding site for fibrin, which allows it to bind to a thrombus and preferentially lyse it over the circulating plasminogen.

Reteplase is a genetically modified plasminogen activator that is similar to t-PA. Reteplase has a longer half-life, allowing it to be administered as two bolus injections 30 minutes apart, rather than as a bolus plus infusion.

TNK is a genetically modified form of t-PA. Compared to t-PA, TNK has a longer plasma half-life, better fibrin specificity, and higher resistance to inhibition by plasminogen-activator inhibitor.[14] The pharmacologic properties of these agents are compared in Table 18-3.

Table 18-3   Pharmacologic Comparison of Available Thrombolytic Agents[13,14]

Drug	Enzymatic Efficiency for Clot Lysis	Fibrin Specificity	Potential Antigenicity	Average Dose	Dosing Administration	Cost
Streptokinase (Streptase)	High	Minimal	Yes	1.5 MU	1 hr IV infusion	Low
Anistreplase (Eminase)	High	Minimal	Yes	30 U	2–5 min IV infusion	Moderate
Alteplase (Activase)	High	Moderate	No	100 mg	15 mg IV bolus, 50 mg over 30 min, then 35 mg over 60 min[a]	High
Reteplase (Retavase)	High	Moderate	No	10 + 10 U	10 units IV bolus, 2nd bolus 30 min later	High
Tenecteplase (TNKase)	High	High	No	30–50 mg (based on weight)[b]	Bolus over 5–10 sec	High

[a]For patients ≥65 kg; reduced doses for patients weighing <65 kg.
[b]For patients <60 kg, 30 mg; 60–69 kg, 45 mg; 70–79 kg, 40 mg; 80–89 kg, 45 mg, ≥90 kg, 50 mg.

Urokinase, although available in the United States, has not gained widespread use as a thrombolytic agent for patients with AMI. Other thrombolytic agents under investigation include staphylokinase, saruplase, and lanoteplase (n-PA).

The ideal thrombolytic would be thrombus specific, easily administered, highly efficacious, inexpensive, rapid acting, and the incidence of reocclusion and side effects would be low. Unfortunately, such an ideal thrombolytic does not exist. Three problems common to all the thrombolytics are the inability to open 100% of coronary artery occlusions, inconsistent ability to maintain good blood flow in the infarcted artery after it is opened, and bleeding complications. Good blood flow commonly is defined as TIMI (thrombolysis in myocardial infarct) grade 3 flow, which is complete reperfusion of the vessel.[13]

To minimize the risk of bleeding complications, contraindications to the use of thrombolytics must be evaluated prior to administration (Table 18-4). There are relatively few absolute contraindications to thrombolytic therapy, but each patient should be assessed carefully to ascertain whether the potential benefit outweighs the potential risk. Because of the serious nature of intracranial hemorrhage associated with thrombolytic therapy, patients should be selected carefully before receiving these agents. Generally, the diagnosis of AMI must be ensured, with a history consistent with ischemic heart disease, presence of ST segment elevation in two contiguous leads, or a new left bundle branch block on the ECG. Once the diagnosis is made, the thrombolytic should be administered immediately if there are no contraindications. The benefit derived from thrombolytic therapy is directly related to the time from the onset of chest pain to the time of administration. In the first GISSI trial (Gruppo Italiano per lo studio della streptochinasi nell'infarto miocardico), the mortality rate was lowest in the group that received the drug within 1 hour from the onset of chest pain (12.9% in the streptokinase group versus 21.2% in the control group).[15]

Antiplatelet and Anticoagulant Drugs

When thrombolysis occurs, whether due to the administration of a thrombolytic agent or through activation of the body's own fibrinolytic system, the fibrin clot begins to disintegrate. As the clot dissolves, there is a paradoxical increase in local thrombin generation and enhanced platelet aggregability, which may lead to rethrombosis. Aspirin, heparin, and low-

Table 18-4   Risk Factors Associated With Bleeding Complications Secondary to Thrombolytic Use[2,12]

Major (thrombolytics contraindicated)	Intracranial tumor or recent head trauma Known or suspected aortic dissection Previous hemorrhagic stroke at any time Nonhemorrhagic stroke or cerebrovascular events within 1 yr Active internal bleeding (excluding menses) Major surgery within 2 wks
Important (relative contraindication)	Uncontrolled hypertension (≥180 mm Hg systolic, ≥110 mm Hg diastolic) Remote thrombotic stroke Recent transient ischemic attacks Puncture of a noncompressible vessel Cardiopulmonary resuscitation for >10 min Recent trauma or major surgery (2–4 wks) Recent internal bleeding within 2–4 wks Active peptic ulcer Known bleeding diathesis or current use of anticoagulants (INR >2) Pregnancy History of chronic severe hypertension For streptokinase or anistreplase: prior exposure (especially within 2–5 days) or prior allergic reaction Diabetic retinopathy or other hemorrhagic ophthalmic conditions

molecular-weight heparin (LMWH) have been used to minimize repeat thrombosis. LMWH may offer advantages over heparin due to its ease of administration, improved bioavailability, and less need for monitoring.[16] Other agents directed toward inhibiting thrombin and reocclusion rates are being investigated. Bivalirudin, lepirudin, and argatroban are thrombin inhibitors that bind directly to thrombin and inactivate it. Results comparing direct thrombin inhibitors to heparin following thrombolytic therapy show the newer agents to be at least as effective as heparin, but in some cases they were associated with more bleeding.[17–22]

Another class of agents being used is the glycoprotein (GP) IIb/IIIa inhibitors. GP IIb/IIIa receptors are abundant on the platelet surface. Platelets become activated when patients are having an acute ischemic coronary event or are undergoing a procedure such as angioplasty. With platelet activation, the GP IIb/IIIa receptor undergoes a conformational change that increases its affinity for binding to fibrinogen. The binding of fibrinogen to receptors on platelets results in platelet aggregation, which can lead to thrombus formation. The GP IIb/IIIa receptor inhibitors prevent platelet aggregation by preventing fibrinogen from binding to GP IIb/IIIa receptor sites on activated platelets. Inhibiting fibrinogen binding to the GP IIb/IIIa receptor helps prevent the formation of a thrombus. The GP IIb/IIIa inhibitors are often used in conjunction with aspirin and heparin in patients with ischemic chest pain, usually without ST segment elevation (acute coronary syndrome patients) and in patients undergoing percutaneous coronary interventions.

β-Blockers

In addition to antiplatelet, antithrombotic, and thrombolytic agents, β-blockers are fundamental in the management of AMI. Even before the advent of thrombolytics, β-blockers were shown to be independently useful in decreasing infarct-associated morbidity and mortality. These benefits are additive to those of thrombolytics. β-Blockers decrease myocardial oxygen consumption, limit the amount of myocardial damage, and decrease some of the complications of MI, specifically myocardial rupture and ventricular fibrillation. Atenolol was compared to placebo in patients with AMI in the first ISIS (International Study of Infarct Survival) trial.[23] The mortality due to vascular causes was reduced by about 15% at the end of 7 days of treatment in this trial. Similar results have been found with metoprolol.[24] Retrospective analyses of trials using β-blockers in AMI estimate a reduction in mortality of about 13%.[25] These short-term benefits are also clearly seen with long-term use in the post-MI period.[26] Unless there are contraindications to their use, β-blocking agents should be prescribed for all patients having an AMI, and they should be continued indefinitely.[2]

Vasodilators

Other strategies for minimizing myocardial damage include the use of vasodilators in the peri-infarction period. Progressive left ventricular dilatation ("remodeling") occurs in some patients following an AMI and has become an important marker for prognosis. Vasodilators reduce oxygen demand and myocardial wall stress by reducing afterload and/or preload and can halt the remodeling process. Some vasodilators also may increase the blood supply to the myocardium by enhancing coronary vasodilatation.

ACE inhibitors have been assessed in a large number of clinical trials, and all trials using oral agents have demonstrated a benefit in mortality.[2] Only one trial has not shown a benefit.[27] Enalapril was studied in the CONSENSUS-II (Cooperative New Scandinavian Enalapril Survival Study) trial. In this study, >6,000 patients were randomized to either placebo or enalapril, which was started within 24 hours from the onset of chest pain. Enalapril was initiated by IV administration, followed by oral enalapril administration 6 hours later. In this trial, enalapril did not improve 6-month survival, but this may be because hypotension was more common in the enalapril-treated group. It would appear that early IV administration of ACE inhibitors might result in excessive hypotension, offsetting their potential benefits. The benefit of ACE inhibitors is greatest in patients with anterior infarction, signs of heart failure, tachycardia, or a history of previous infarction.[2,11] Ideally, ACE inhibitors should be started within 24 hours of diagnosis, after BP has stabilized. Initial doses should be low and then titrated as quickly as the patient will tolerate.

The effects of nitrates also have been evaluated in AMI patients. The pooled effects from several studies have shown a small but statistically significant benefit in reducing mortality in patients receiving nitrates.[2] The data suggest that nitroglycerin (NTG) is more beneficial than nitroprusside in this population.[25] IV NTG is recommended for routine use during the first 24 to 48 hours in most patients with AMI, particularly those with large anterior wall infarctions.[2,12]

Another class of vasodilators that has been investigated in the treatment of AMI is the calcium channel blockers. There are several proposed mechanisms whereby a calcium channel blocker might be beneficial. As a group, they have coronary and peripheral vasodilatory actions that could alleviate some of the coronary vasospasm present at the time of coronary thrombosis. Additionally, they are known to be effective anti-ischemic agents through their action in improving coronary blood supply and reducing myocardial oxygen demand. Since intracellular calcium overload has been observed in the ischemic myocardium, it was thought that calcium channel blockers would protect cardiac cells during the peri-infarction period. Despite these theoretical benefits, the outcomes of clinical trials have varied depending on the individual drug used and the timing of administration. The use of calcium channel blockers in the setting of AMI has declined dramatically in the past 10 years.[28]

Nifedipine is not beneficial during the immediate AMI period, and small trials evaluating its long-term effects on infarct size have been inconclusive. However, in the larger clinical trials, nifedipine had no benefit or there was a trend toward increasing mortality. Immediate-release nifedipine is thought to be particularly detrimental.[2]

There have been two large trials evaluating diltiazem in the setting of AMI. The first study evaluated the effect of oral diltiazem, started 24 to 72 hours after the onset of chest pain, on reinfarction rates in patients with non–Q-wave AMI.[29] There was a 51.2% reduction in the reinfarction rate in the diltiazem group compared to placebo after 14 days of follow-up. Diltiazem also reduced the frequency of postinfarction angina. Another trial using diltiazem for a longer period in patients with both Q-wave and non–Q-wave infarctions was published 2 years later.[30] In this trial, oral diltiazem was initiated 3 to 15 days after infarction and patients were followed for an average of 2 years. Overall, there was no difference in mortality between the two groups. However, patients assigned to diltiazem who did not have pulmonary congestion at the time of randomization had a reduced number of cardiac events compared to placebo patients. In contrast, patients who had signs of pulmonary congestion at the time of randomization had an unfavorable response to diltiazem (i.e., more deaths from cardiac causes or nonfatal reinfarctions). Diltiazem may be used to lower the heart rate or decrease angina in patients who cannot tolerate a β-blocker. However, it should be avoided in patients with signs or symptoms of pulmonary congestion, since its negative inotropic properties may worsen systolic function.

The DAVIT-II (Danish Verapamil Infarction Trial) study showed a trend toward a reduction in mortality at 18 months in patients receiving verapamil (11.1% versus 13.8% in the placebo group).[31] In patients who did not have heart failure at the time of randomization, verapamil showed a statistically significant benefit in reducing mortality (7.7% versus 11.8% in the placebo group). In contrast to the diltiazem trial, verapamil had neither a demonstrable benefit nor a detrimental effect in patients with heart failure. It has been suggested that the use of verapamil and diltiazem should be limited to patients who do not tolerate β-blocker therapy and who are not in heart failure.[2]

Analgesics

It is important to abolish the patient's pain as quickly as possible because the pain and anxiety associated with an AMI will contribute to increased myocardial oxygen demand. If the pain is not relieved by the thrombolytic and anti-ischemic medications (e.g., nitrates and β-blockers), then additional analgesia may be necessary. Morphine and meperidine are the two most commonly prescribed analgesics.

Oxygen

Many patients are modestly hypoxemic during the initial hours of an AMI. Oxygen should be administered via nasal cannula to all patients suspected of having ischemic pain. Patients with severe hypoxemia or pulmonary edema may require intubation and mechanical ventilation.[2]

Antiarrhythmics

Ventricular arrhythmias, including ventricular fibrillation, are common complications associated with myocardial ischemia and AMI. Lidocaine, procainamide, and amiodarone are the drugs of choice for the treatment of ventricular arrhythmias in the peri-infarction period.[2] The routine use of prophylactic lidocaine or other antiarrhythmic agents to prevent ventricular tachycardia and ventricular fibrillation is not recommended. Although the routine use of lidocaine may reduce the number of episodes of ventricular fibrillation, it may contribute to an increased number of episodes of asystole.[25] (See Chapter 20, Cardiac Arrhythmias.)

Suppression of ventricular ectopy following an AMI with the chronic use of oral antiarrhythmic agents is not recommended. Results of CAST-I and II (Cardiac Arrhythmia Suppression Trials) demonstrated an increase in mortality in asymptomatic patients with ventricular ectopy following an AMI who were treated with flecainide, encainide, and moricizine.[32,33]

Stool Softeners

It is common to administer agents such as docusate to prevent constipation in AMI patients, since straining causes undesirable stress on the cardiovascular system. Table 18-5 summarizes the common adjunctive therapy used in patients with AMI.

Nondrug Therapy

Direct percutaneous transluminal coronary angioplasty (PTCA) is an attractive alternative to thrombolytic therapy. PCTA consists of the insertion of a guidewire though a catheter into the occluded coronary vessel. The guidewire tip is shaped into a curve appropriate for the specific coronary anatomy. Using fluoroscopy, the wire is directed and manipulated across the stenosis. A balloon angioplasty catheter is then progressed across the guidewire to the stenosis and inflated over seconds to minutes. Balloon inflation mechanically compressed plaque in the vessel to increase lumen size.

PTCA may be used in patients with an AMI who have contraindications to thrombolytic therapy or who fail to respond to thrombolytic therapy. The disadvantages of PTCA include the longer amount of time needed to mobilize the personnel needed to prepare the catheterization laboratory, and its initial higher cost. A potential advantage of PTCA is the greater ability to achieve TIMI grade 3 flow in the affected vessel.[34] Pooled data from major trials comparing PCTA to thrombolysis have found PCTA to be associated with fewer major adverse cardiac events, irrespective of patient presentation time.[35] Therefore, many cardiologists prefer PTCA because it avoids the potential bleeding complications of thrombolytic therapy and it is more effective in opening the occluded vessel. Unfortunately, many hospitals do not have the facilities or personnel to do this procedure within 1 hour of presentation or within 12 hours of the onset of chest pain.

SIGNS AND SYMPTOMS OF ACUTE MYOCARDIAL INFARCTION

1. P.H., a 63-year-old, 80-kg man, is being admitted to the emergency department (ED) after experiencing an episode of sustained chest pain while mowing his yard (it is July and the heat index is 38.3°C). After waiting 4 hours, he called 911 and was transported to the ED. Physical examination reveals a diaphoretic man who appears ashen. Heart rate and rhythm are regular and no S_3 or S_4 sounds are present. Vital signs include BP 180/110 mm Hg, heart rate 100 beats/min, and respiratory rate 32 breaths/min. P.H.'s chest pain radiates to his left arm and jaw, and he describes the pain as "crushing" and "like an elephant sitting on my chest." He rates it as a "10/10" in intensity. Thus far, his pain has not responded to five sublingual (SL) NTG tablets at home and three more in the ambulance. His ECG reveals a 3-mm ST segment elevation and Q waves in leads I and V_2 to V_4. Based on this, P.H. is diagnosed with an anterior infarction. Laboratory values include sodium (Na), 141 mEq/L (normal, 135 to 145); potassium (K), 3.9 mEq/L (normal, 3.5 to 5.0); chloride (Cl), 100 mEq/L (normal, 100 to 108); CO_2, 20 mEq/L (normal, 24 to 30); blood urea nitrogen (BUN), 19 mg/dL

Table 18-5   Adjunctive Therapy for Acute Myocardial Infarction

Drug	Indication	Dose and Duration	Therapeutic End points	Precautions	Comments
ACE inhibitors[a]	AMI with EF <40%	Usual captopril dose 12.5–50 mg TID. Then start longer-acting ACE inhibitor. Duration indefinite	Titrate to usual doses and maintain systolic BP >90–110 mm Hg	Avoid IV therapy within 48 hr of infarct	Oral therapy in patients with EF <40%
Aspirin[a]	AMI and ischemic heart disease	160–325 mg during AMI; then 75–325 mg/day for an indefinite period	No firm end point	Active bleeding, thrombocytopenia	Unless clear contraindication exists, aspirin should be given to all AMI patients.
β-blockers[a]	General use in all AMI patients to reduce reinfarction and improve survival	Variable; titrate to HR and BP. Immediate IV therapy preferable. Duration indefinite. See Table 18-7 for specific dosing recommendations.	Titrate to resting HR approx. 60 beats/min, maintain systolic BP >100 mm Hg	Usual β-blocker contraindications. Observe HR and BP closely when given IV.	Unless clear contraindication exists, β1-selective agents such as metoprolol and atenolol should be given to all AMI patients.
Calcium channel blockers	Postinfarction angina, non–Q-wave AMI	Usual doses of calcium channel blockers are used. Duration dictated by clinical scenario. (See Chapter 17, Ischemic Heart Disease: Anginal Syndromes)	Titrate to usual doses and maintain systolic BP >90 mm Hg	Usual calcium channel blocker contraindications. Avoid in patients with pulmonary congestion or EF <40%.	a) In patients with good EF, most calcium channel blockers will exert beneficial effects. b) Some data support use of verapamil or diltiazem for non–Q-wave AMI, but not dihydropyridine types.
Clopidogrel[a]	For AMI and ischemic heart disease patients	75 mg/day	No firm end point	Active bleeding, thrombotic thrombocytopenia purpura (rare)	Reserved for patients who cannot tolerate or receive aspirin
Clopidogrel + Aspirin[a]	For NSTEMI and unstable angina patients	Clopidogrel 300 mg load, followed by 75 mg daily for 1–9 months; aspirin 75–325 mg PO daily	No firm end point	Active bleeding, thrombotic thrombocytopenia purpura (rare)	Combination may also be used prior to PCI and continued for 1–9 months
Heparin[a]	Acute anticoagulation, patients undergoing reperfusion with t-PA	Variable; 60 U/kg loading at initiation of t-PA, then 12 U/kg/hr. Usual duration 24–48 hr.	aPTT ratio 1.5–2.5 × patient's control value	Active bleeding, thrombocytopenia	Unless clear contraindication exists, heparin should be given to all AMI patients who do not receive thrombolytic therapy.
Lidocaine	Treatment of VT, VF	Variable, 1.5 mg/kg loading dose, then 1–4 mg/min. Use for <48 hr	Cessation of arrhythmia	Bradycardia. Observe for CNS toxicity.	Some data indicate increased mortality with generalized use.

Table 18-5   Adjunctive Therapy for Acute Myocardial Infarction (continued)

Drug	Indication	Dose and Duration	Therapeutic End points	Precautions	Comments
LMWH[a]	To replace heparin in STEMI and ACS	STEMI Enoxaparin: 30 mg IV bolus (optional), then 1 mg/kg SQ Q 12 hr for 7–8 days Daltaparin: 100 U/kg SQ prior to thrombolytic, then 120 U/kg SQ 12 hours later ACS: Enoxaparin: 1 mg SQ Q 12 hr for 2–8 days Daltaparin: 120 U/kg SQ Q 12 hr for 6 days	No firm end point	Active bleeding	In ACS, enoxaparin was superior to heparin for reducing mortality and ischemic events. In STEMI, compared to heparin, LMWHs may lower coronary reocclusion with variable effects on mortality.
Morphine	Treatment of severe chest pain; venodilator	2–5 mg IV Q 3–5 min PRN	Decreased chest pain and HR	Bradycardia, right ventricular infarct	Good choice for acute pain relief along with NTG
Nitrates[a]	General use in most AMI patients	Variable; titrate to pain relief or systolic BP. 5–10 mcg/min to 200 mcg/min typical regimen. Usually maintain IV therapy for 24–48 hr after infarct	Titrate to pain relief or systolic BP >90 mm Hg	Use cautiously in right ventricular infarct or large inferior infarct because of effects on preload.	Use acetaminophen, NSAIDs, narcotics for headache. NTG should be tapered gradually in ischemic heart disease patients.
Warfarin	Left ventricular thrombus	Variable; titrate to INR. Duration usually for several months.	INR 2–3 × patient's control value	Usual warfarin problems such as noncompliance, bleeding diatheses	May be useful in the presence of a left ventricular thrombus to prevent embolism

ACE, angiotensin-converting enzyme; ACS, acute coronary syndrome, AMI, acute myocardial infarction; aPTT, activated partial thromboplastin; BP, blood pressure; EF, ejection fraction; HR, heart rate; INR, International Normalized Ratio; IV, intravenous; LMWH, low-molecular-weight heparin, NSAIDs, nonsteroidal anti-inflammatory drugs; NSTEMI, non-ST segment elevation myocardial infarction; NTG, nitroglycerin; PCI, percutaneous coronary intervention; SQ, subcutaneously; t-PA, tissue plasminogen activator, VF, ventricular fibrillation; VT, ventricular tachycardia.
[a]Indicates specific drug therapies that are known to reduce morbidity and/or mortality.

(normal, 8 to 25); serum creatinine (SrCr), 1.2 mg/dL (normal, 0.6 to 1.5); glucose, 149 mg/dL (normal, 70 to 110); magnesium (Mg), 1.3 mEq/L (normal, 1.5 to 2.0); CK, 1,200 U/L (normal, 60 to 370), with a 12% CK-MB fraction (normal 0% to 5%); troponin-I, 60 ng/mL (normal <2); cholesterol, 259 mg/dL (normal, <200); triglycerides, 300 mg/dL (normal, 40 to 150). P.H. has a prior history of coronary artery disease. A previous cardiac catheterization 2 years ago revealed a lesion in his middle left anterior descending coronary artery (75% stenosis) and in the proximal left circumflex artery (30% stenosis). His ventriculogram at the time showed an ejection fraction of 58%. These lesions were deemed suitable for medical management. He also has a history of recurrent bouts of bronchitis with bronchospastic disease for 10 years; diabetes mellitus treated with insulin for 18 years with fair control; and mild hypertension with fair control for 20 years. His father died of an MI at age 70. His mother and siblings are all alive and well. P.H. has smoked one pack of cigarettes a day for 30 years and he drinks approximately one six-pack of beer a week. He has no history of IV drug use. On admission, P.H.'s medications include NPH insulin, 15 U Q AM and 10 U Q PM; albuterol inhaler, PRN; hydrochlorothiazide, 25 mg QD; NTG patch, 0.2 mg/hr; and NTG SL, 0.4 mg PRN chest pain. What signs and symptoms does P.H. have that are consistent with the diagnosis of AMI?

[SI units: Na, 141 mmol/L (normal, 135 to 145); K, 3.9 mmol/L (normal, 3.5 to 5.0); Cl, 100 mmol/L (normal, 100 to 108); CO₂, 20 mmol/L (normal, 24 to 30); BUN, 6.8 mmol/L (normal, 2.9 to 8.9); SrCr, 72 mmol/L (normal, 36 to 90); glucose, 8.3 mmol/L (normal, 3.9 to 6.1); Mg, 0.65 mmol/L (normal, 0.75 to 1.0); CK, 20 and 33.34 μkat/L, respectively (normal, 1.0 to 6.7); cholesterol, 6.7 mmol/L (normal, <5.2); triglycerides, 3.9 mmol/L (normal, 0.45 to 1.7)]

P.H. described his pain as a pressure sensation, which is common with ischemic heart disease. The chest discomfort associated with AMI is described more often as pressure or as a tight band around the chest rather than pain. Although P.H. was involved in physical exertion when his chest pain began, this is not always the case. It can begin at rest and, frequently, in the early morning hours. At least 20% of patients with AMI have no pain or discomfort; these are described as having "silent" MIs. Presentations range from asymptomatic to shortness of breath, hypotension, heart failure, syncope, or ventricular arrhythmias. Silent or atypical infarctions occur more commonly in people with diabetes or hypertension and in the elderly.[12] P.H. is diaphoretic, a common finding, but other common symptoms such as nausea and anxiety are not present. He also describes his pain as "10/10" in intensity, or perhaps "the worst pain I've ever experienced," which is typical of an AMI. The typical patient with an uncomplicated AMI has few useful physical findings. The diagnosis primarily lies in the symptoms, the ECG, and the laboratory findings.

The history of diabetes, hypertension, smoking, and a positive family history in P.H. are all risk factors for coronary disease. His admission BP is high, which could indicate poor underlying control or anxiety and stress related to his AMI. The blood sugar of 140 mg/dL is high, again indicating either poor control or a stress response. Measurement of glycosylated hemoglobin is indicated during his hospitalization to better assess his diabetes control.

Laboratory Abnormalities

2. What laboratory abnormalities can you expect to see in P.H.?

P.H. demonstrates several laboratory abnormalities commonly seen in AMI. His CK was high upon admission and the CK-MB of 12% (normally <5%) is indicative of myocardial necrosis. CK-MB rises acutely over the first 12 to 24 hours and returns to normal in 2 to 3 days. The troponin level is also increased, which is consistent with myocardial necrosis. Several other nonspecific laboratory findings should be monitored in P.H. Hyperglycemia may develop because P.H. is a diabetic, but this also can occur in nondiabetic patients. It also has been noted that total cholesterol and HDL cholesterol concentrations may fall dramatically within a few days following an AMI. Therefore, it is best to check serum lipid profiles within 24 to 48 hours.[12] Leukocytosis and an increase in the erythrocyte sedimentation rate also may be observed with AMI.[12]

STEMI Versus NSTEMI

3. P.H. was noted to have "ST segment elevation and Q waves" on the ECG. What are the implications of a ST segment elevation versus non-ST segment elevation MI?

Perhaps the most important diagnostic test in someone who is suspected to have an AMI is the ECG. The ECG is an important tool because it is noninvasive, can be performed rapidly, is readily available in most clinical settings, and adds valuable clues as to where the AMI is located (i.e., anterior, inferior, lateral) (Fig. 18-3). It also is valuable in determining

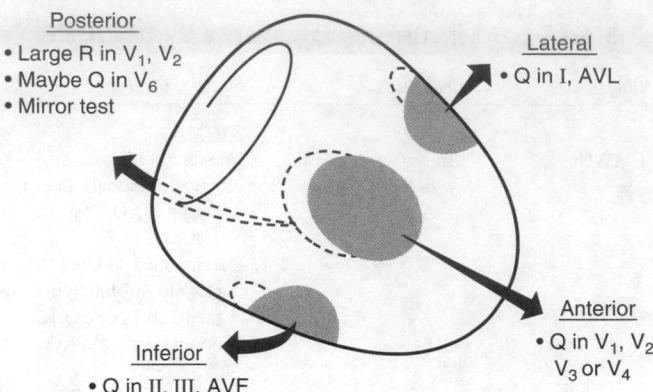

FIGURE 18-3 Location of an anterior, lateral, inferior, or posterior infarction based on the presence of Q waves in leads V_{1-6}. (With permission from Dubin D. Infarction. In Dubin D, ed. Rapid Interpretation of EKGs. 6th Ed. Tampa: COVER Publishing Co., 2000:290.)

whether a thrombolytic should be administered. While enzyme profiles are valuable, the results often are not available for hours, or the patient may present to the hospital before the cardiac enzymes are present in the serum. Therefore, enzymes allow one to confirm "retrospectively" the presence of an AMI, but do not necessarily influence the immediate therapeutic course for the patient. A thorough discussion of the ECG is beyond the scope of this chapter, but P.H. has classic ECG changes such as ST segment elevation and Q waves. Their presence in the anterior ECG leads (V_2 to V_4) indicates which part of the heart is affected and also points to the coronary arteries that are likely to be blocked.[36] P.H.'s previous left anterior descending lesion may have had a plaque rupture leading to thrombosis of the vessel.

The presence of ST segment elevation in two contiguous leads indicates severe ischemia and occlusion of the coronary artery. Every effort should be made to open the infarct-related artery as soon as possible. If the ECG showed ST segment depression instead of elevation, P.H. would not be eligible for thrombolytic therapy.

Anterior Versus Inferior Infarction

4. What are the prognostic implications of an anterior versus an inferior MI?

Damage to the anterior section of the heart is more likely to be associated with increased morbidity (e.g., left ventricular dysfunction) and mortality.[37] The patients at highest risk of death are those with an anterior AMI, left ventricular dysfunction, and complex ventricular ectopy. P.H. is at an increased risk since he has sustained an anterior AMI.

TREATMENT

Therapeutic Objectives

5. What are the immediate and long-term therapeutic objectives in treating P.H.?

The immediate therapeutic objectives in treating P.H. are to minimize the amount of myocardial necrosis that develops, to alleviate his symptoms, and to prevent his death. These objectives are achieved primarily by restoring coronary blood flow (administering a thrombolytic and/or performing an angioplasty) and lowering myocardial oxygen demand. Any life-threatening ventricular arrhythmias that develop must be treated. The long-term therapeutic objectives are to prevent or minimize recurrent ischemic symptoms, reinfarction, heart failure, and sudden cardiac death. The specific therapeutic regimens are discussed in detail in the questions that follow.

Thrombolytic Therapy

6. Is P.H. a candidate for thrombolytic therapy? Is any one agent preferred?

AMI is a medical emergency. The results of several major trials have shown unequivocally that if used appropriately, thrombolytics can reduce the mortality associated with an AMI.[38–40] Unless contraindications are present, most patients presenting with ischemic chest pain and ST segment elevation on their ECG should receive a thrombolytic. There is still controversy over which thrombolytic should be used, the period of time from the onset of chest pain during which the benefit will still outweigh the risk, the best dosing regimen, the most appropriate adjunctive therapy, and whether the risk outweighs the benefit in some subpopulations of patients (e.g., those with an inferior AMI). Each of these issues will be discussed in subsequent cases.

P.H. has a history of hypertension and at presentation his BP is 180/110 mm Hg. A BP this high is a relative contraindication to thrombolytic therapy because of an increased risk of cerebral hemorrhage; however, P.H. has an anterior MI and is very likely to benefit from thrombolytic therapy. In this case, he should receive IV NTG immediately, since the onset of pressure control with this agent usually occurs within minutes. Once his systolic BP is <180 mm Hg and the diastolic is <110 mm Hg, a thrombolytic can be administered. The NTG also will reduce the workload on his heart and may provide pain relief.

Because P.H. has very severe pain and ECG changes consistent with an anterior AMI, he is at great risk for substantial morbidity and/or mortality. t-PA or alteplase are more rapid acting and effective in restoring TIMI grade 3 blood flow than streptokinase; however, the slightly increased risk of stroke and the substantial increase in cost with t-PA may outweigh its advantages. The argument for or against a specific thrombolytic is probably less important than the decision to use an agent and to administer the medication as soon as possible after the onset of symptoms. P.H. is fortunate since he has presented within 5 to 6 hours of the onset of chest pain.

Dosage Regimens

7. "Alteplase 100 mg infused over 90 minutes" is ordered for P.H. Is this an appropriate dosage? If streptokinase, anistreplase, reteplase, or tenecteplase had been ordered, what would be an appropriate regimen?

To enhance reperfusion while minimizing bleeding complications, accelerated dosage regimens of t-PA are recommended. The recommended regimen is a 15-mg bolus followed by a 50-mg infusion over 30 minutes and then the remaining 35 mg over 60 minutes. The GUSTO (Global Utilization of Streptokinase and t-PA for Occluded Arteries) trial used this accelerated or front-loaded regimen for administration of tPA.[38] In this trial, t-PA was compared to streptokinase and a combination of streptokinase and t-PA. The results showed that t-PA alone was the most effective in reducing mortality. The 30-day mortality rate for the accelerated t-PA group was 6.3% compared to 7.3% in the streptokinase group. In GUSTO, the t-PA regimen also was weight adjusted, such that after the 15-mg bolus dose, the infusion was 0.75 mg/kg over 30 minutes followed by 0.5 mg/kg over 60 minutes. The maximum dose received was 100 mg.

Most of the large trials with streptokinase have used an IV infusion of 1.5 MU administered over 60 minutes.[15,39,40] There have been some trials in which the infusion was shortened to 30 minutes; however, there have been no large studies that have compared a 30-minute infusion to a 60-minute infusion.

Anistreplase usually is given intravenously as 30 U over 2 to 5 minutes. This convenient dosing schedule is the major advantage of this agent. It has been suggested that prehospital administration of anistreplase by emergency services personnel would reduce the amount of time from the onset of chest pain to the administration of this life-saving drug. Unfortunately, highly trained paramedics do not transport many patients with AMI to the hospital.

Reteplase was compared to t-PA in the GUSTO-III trial.[41] Reteplase has a slower clearance from the body, allowing the drug to be given as a bolus without the need for a constant infusion. In the GUSTO-III trial, reteplase was administered in two bolus doses of 10 MU, given 30 minutes apart. The mortality rate and incidence of stroke were the same in the two groups of patients.

Tenecteplase was compared to t-PA in the ASSENT-2 (Assessment of Safety and Efficacy of a New Thrombolytic) Trial. TNK was administered as a bolus of 30 to 50 mg over 5 to 10 seconds, based upon body weight (see Table 18-3). No difference existed between TNK and t-PA in 30-day mortality and stroke.[42]

Once P.H.'s BP is controlled, he should receive a thrombolytic as quickly as possible. Since he appears to be having a large anterior infarction, the added cost of t-PA, r-PA, or tenecteplase versus streptokinase may be justified. Table 18-6 summarizes the major thrombolytic trials.

Adjunct Therapy

8. Orders are written for heparin 5,000 U IV bolus, followed by 1,000 U/hr by continuous infusion. Also prescribed is aspirin 325 mg STAT. Are both these agents necessary?

The ISIS-2 trial showed that aspirin 160 mg/day alone and in combination with streptokinase reduced mortality in patients with AMI by 23% and 42%, respectively, when compared to a control group of patients who received neither aspirin nor streptokinase.[39] In doses of 160 mg or more, aspirin generates a prompt clinical antithrombotic effect as a result of its immediate and near-total inhibition of thromboxane A_2 production.[2] Thus, immediate administration of 160 to 325 mg of aspirin in patients diagnosed with AMI, whether or not they receive thrombolytics, is indicated. In the acute setting

Table 18-6   Summary of Major Thrombolytic Trials

Trial	Thrombolytics	Heparin, Aspirin, LMWH	Number of Patients	Duration of Symptoms	Results
ISIS-2 1988[39]	Streptokinase 1.5 MU over 1 hr vs. placebo	Also randomized to aspirin 160 mg/day or no aspirin. Heparin not specified.	17,187	<24 hr	Streptokinase, aspirin, streptokinase + aspirin all reduced mortality compared to placebo. Most benefit from streptokinase + aspirin. Aspirin alone and in combination with streptokinase reduces mortality. Some benefit from aspirin and/or streptokinase even administered late.
ISG 1990[44]	t-PA 100 mg over 3 hr vs. streptokinase 1.5 MU over 1 hr	Also randomized to heparin SC or no heparin. All patients received aspirin and atenolol unless contraindicated.	20,891	<6 hr	No significant difference in hospital mortality between streptokinase and t-PA. More episodes of major bleeding with streptokinase and more strokes with t-PA. Results questioned due to the use of SC heparin.
ISIS-3 1992[40]	t-PA (duteplase) 0.6 MU over 4 hr vs. streptokinase 1.5 MU over 1 hr vs. APSAC 30 U over 3 min	Also randomized to SC heparin or no heparin. All patients received aspirin 162 mg/day.	41,299	<24 hr	No significant difference in mortality between thrombolytics. More episodes of major bleeding with heparin and more strokes with t-PA. Results questioned due to the use of SC heparin.
GUSTO 1993[38]	t-PA 1.25 mg/kg (≤100 mg) over 90 min vs. streptokinase 1.5 MU over 1 hr vs. t-PA 1 mg/kg + streptokinase 1 MU over 1 hr	Aspirin 160–325 mg/day to all patients. Heparin IV with t-PA groups. Heparin IV or SC in streptokinase groups.	41,021	<6 hr	Statistically significant decrease in 30-day mortality in the t-PA group (6.3%) versus streptokinase (7.3%). More strokes in t-PA groups.
GUSTO-III 1997[41]	t-PA 100 mg over 90 min vs. r-PA 10 + 10 U	Aspirin 160 mg immediately then daily. Heparin 5,000 U bolus, 1,000 U/hr.	15,059 No upper age limit	<6 hr	Mortality rate at 30 days was 7.47% in r-PA versus 7.24% in t-PA (P = NS). Stroke occurred in 1.64% of r-PA patients versus 1.79% of t-PA patients (P = NS).
ASSENT-2 1999[42]	TNK 30–50 mg over 5-10 sec vs. t-PA 1.25 mg/kg over 90 min	Aspirin 150–325 mg and heparin 4,000 U bolus, 800 U/hr for patients ≤67 kg or 5,000 U bolus, 1,000 U/hr >67 kg	16,949	<6 hr	No significant difference in 30-day mortality, death or nonfatal stroke, or intracranial bleeding between thrombolytics. TNK had significantly fewer bleeding complications.
GUSTO-V 2001, 2002[51,52]	r-PA two 10-U boluses vs. r-PA two 5-U boluses + abciximab 0.25 mg/kg bolus, 0.125 mcg/kg/min for 12 hr	Aspirin 150–325 mg orally or 250–500 mg IV immediately, then 75–325 mg daily. For r-PA alone: heparin 5,000 U bolus, 1,000 U/hr (≥80 kg) or 800 U bolus, 800 U/hr (<80 kg). For combination therapy, heparin 60 U/kg bolus, 7 U/kg/hr.	16,588	<6 hr	No significant difference between groups in all-cause mortality at 30 days and 1 year, confirmed cerebrovascular events, or nonfatal disabling strokes. Combination therapy had a statistically significant higher rate of bleeding complications (P < 0.0001).

Table 18-6   Summary of Major Thrombolytic Trials *(continued)*

Trial	Thrombolytics	Heparin, Aspirin, LMWH	Number of Patients	Duration of Symptoms	Results
ASSENT-3 2001[53]	TNK 30–50 mg over 5 sec vs. TNK 15–25 mg over 5 sec + abciximab 0.25 mg/kg bolus, 0.125 μg/kg/min for 12 hr	Aspirin 150–325 mg orally. For full-dose TNK, patients were randomized to either enoxaparin 30 mg bolus, 1 mg/kg Q12 hr × 7 days or IV heparin 60 U bolus, 12 U/kg/hr × 48 hr. For combination therapy, 40 U bolus, 7 U/kg/hr.	6,095	<6 hr	For the composite end point of 30-day mortality, reinfarction, or refractory ischemia, event rates were 6.1% for full-dose TNK + enoxaparin, 5.2% for half-dose TNK + abciximab, 8.8% for full-dose TNK + heparin ($P < 0.0001$). No significant difference in 30-day mortality between groups. More major bleeding ($P = 0.0002$) and transfusions ($P = 0.001$) in the abciximab group compared to heparin.

APSAC, anisoylated plasminogen streptokinase activator complex; LMWH, low-molecular-weight heparin; SC, subcutaneous; t-PA, tissue plasminogen activator; TNK, tenecteplase; r-PA, reteplase.

aspirin should be chewed, since it is absorbed more quickly.[2] All patients should receive 75 to 325 mg of daily aspirin indefinitely following AMI.[43] If patients have a contraindication to aspirin, clopidogrel can be substituted.

The use of heparin as adjunct therapy to prevent reocclusion also has been evaluated. The International Study Group evaluated 20,891 patients who were randomized to either streptokinase or t-PA. Each group was further randomized to receive subcutaneous (SC) heparin or no heparin.[44] No significant differences in hospital mortality rates were found between the two thrombolytics or between the heparin or no heparin groups. The heparin group did have more major bleeding complications (1% versus 0.5%) when compared to the no heparin group, but there was no difference in the incidence of stroke or reinfarction.

The ISIS-3 trial compared three thrombolytics (streptokinase, anistreplase, and duteplase) and aspirin 162 mg/day plus heparin versus aspirin alone.[40] In this trial, heparin 12,500 U was administered SC beginning 4 hours after randomization for 7 days or until discharge. There were no statistically significant differences in mortality among the six groups of patients. Although heparin plus aspirin compared to aspirin alone had no effect on mortality measured on day 35, there was an increase in transfusions, noncerebral bleeding episodes, and definite or probable cerebral hemorrhage in the heparin + aspirin group.

The results of the International Study and ISIS-3 showed no particular benefit of adding heparin to a thrombolytic regimen; however, the route of heparin administration (IV versus SC) may have played a role. HART (Heparin-Aspirin Reperfusion Trial) evaluated 205 AMI patients with angiography 7 to 24 hours after beginning t-PA and again 7 days later.[45] Patients received t-PA (100 mg over 6 hours) in addition to either aspirin 80 mg/day or IV heparin (5,000 U bolus plus 1,000 U/hour) adjusted to achieve a partial thromboplastin time of 1.5 to 2.0 × control for 7 days. The patency rates at the first angiogram were significantly higher in the heparin group (82%)

versus the aspirin group (52%); however, there were no significant differences between the two groups at 7 days. Bleich and colleagues also found that heparin (5,000 U bolus plus 1,000 U/hour adjusted to achieve a partial thromboplastin time of 1.5 to 2.0 × control) increased the patency of infarct-related arteries when compared to no heparin 48 to 72 hours after a t-PA infusion in a small number of patients with AMI.[46]

The hypothesis that the efficacy of t-PA is influenced by the administration regimen of heparin was tested by the GUSTO trial.[38] Over 41,000 patients suspected of having an AMI were randomized within 6 hours from the onset of chest pain. Four treatments were compared: streptokinase with SC heparin, streptokinase with IV heparin, t-PA infusion (given over 90 minutes) with IV heparin, and a combination of streptokinase and t-PA with IV heparin. The patients receiving the t-PA infusion and IV heparin had the lowest mortality rate at 30 days (6.3% versus 7.2% for streptokinase with SC heparin, 7.4% for streptokinase with IV heparin, and 7.0% for the thrombolytic combination with IV heparin). The t-PA + IV heparin group and the combination thrombolytic group also had a significant increase in hemorrhagic stroke (0.72% and 0.94%, respectively) compared to the streptokinase with SC heparin (0.49%) and streptokinase with IV heparin (0.54%) groups; however, the net benefit still favored the t-PA + IV heparin group.

Overall, it appears that heparin administration offers no benefit to patients receiving streptokinase or anistreplase. However, since P.H. will receive t-PA, an IV heparin bolus followed by a continuous infusion should be started before the end of the t-PA infusion. The 1999 ACC/AHA guidelines recommend a 60-unit/kg bolus of heparin at the initiation of t-PA, followed by a maintenance infusion of 12 units/kg per hour or a maximum of a 4,000-unit bolus, followed by 1,000 units/hr.[2] The target activated partial thromboplastin time should be 1.5 to 2.0 × control (generally 50 to 75 sec). Heparin should always be considered in patients at high risk for systemic or venous embolism.

9. Would P.H. benefit from a LMWH or a GP IIb/IIIa inhibitor added to his thrombolytic regimen?

The replacement of heparin with a LMWH or the addition of an antiplatelet agent such as a GP IIb/IIIa inhibitor to thrombolytic therapy have been evaluated in patients with STEMI. In the HART II trial, which compared enoxaparin plus t-PA to IV heparin plus t-PA, coronary patency rates were similar between groups at 90-minute angiography (80.1% versus 75.1%, P = NS), but the coronary reocclusion rate was lower at 7 days in the enoxaparin group (3.1%) compared to the heparin group (9.1%) (P = 0.01). Thirty-day mortality and adverse events did not differ between groups.[47] Similar results have been demonstrated with dalteparin combined with streptokinase, but with higher bleeding risks.[48]

The TIMI-14 trial demonstrated enhanced reperfusion (TIMI 3 flow) using reduced-dose t-PA combined with abciximab (bolus 0.25 mg/kg, then 12-hour infusion of 0.125 mcg/kg per minute) compared to full-dose t-PA alone. This improvement occurred without an increase in the risk of major bleeding.[49] Similar rates of enhanced reperfusion have also been observed with the combination of double-bolus-dose eptifibatide (180/90 mcg/kg, 10 minutes apart) with a 48-hour infusion (1.33 mcg/kg per minute) plus half-dose t-PA (50 mg).[50]

In the GUSTO-V trial, 16,588 patients with STEMI were randomized to standard-dose reteplase or half-dose reteplase plus full-dose abciximab. There was no difference in death rates between the groups at 30 days or 1 year. The combination group had less reinfarction and recurrent ischemia, but this benefit was offset by more episodes of moderate and severe bleeding, especially in the elderly.[51,52]

The ASSENT-3 trial randomized 6,095 AMI patients to full-dose tenecteplase + enoxaparin, half-dose tenecteplase + heparin and a 12-hour infusion of abciximab, or full-dose tenecteplase + heparin. The addition of either abciximab or enoxaparin to tenecteplase reduced the composite endpoint of 30-day mortality, in-hospital re-infarction, or ischemia compared to heparin. More major bleeding complications were seen with abciximab compared to heparin.[53]

The ENTIRE-TIMI 23 (Enoxaparin as Adjunctive Antithrombin Therapy for ST-Elevation Myocardial Infarction) trial evaluated the use of a thrombolytic in combination with a GP IIb/IIIa inhibitor and either heparin or LMWH. In this trial, 483 AMI patients were randomized to full-dose tenecteplase or half-dose tenecteplase + abciximab. Each group was then randomized to receive either heparin or enoxaparin. Patients receiving full-dose tenecteplase plus enoxaparin exhibited lower 30-day mortality/recurrent MI rates compared to those receiving tenecteplase + heparin. Rates of major bleeding were highest with the tenecteplase, abciximab, and enoxaparin combination.[54]

In the case of P.H., there is evidence to support the use of LMWH instead of unfractionated heparin. For the LMWH, more data exist with enoxaparin. There are also data to suggest that the addition of a GP IIb/IIIa inhibitor would reduce complications of his MI; however, P.H. would be at a higher risk for bleeding complications with combination therapy. GP IIb/IIIa inhibitors are used primarily in NSTEMI and percutaneous coronary interventions. If GP IIb/IIIa inhibitors are used in conjunction with a thrombolytic agent for patients with STEMI, the dose of the thrombolytic agent is reduced by one half.

Determination of Reperfusion

10. How can you monitor for successful reperfusion in P.H. after he has received thrombolytic therapy?

Performing coronary angiography following thrombolytic therapy will reveal if the infarcted artery is open, how vigorous the blood flow is, and the extent of residual stenosis. There are several clinical indicators that correspond with reperfusion, one of which is the resolution of chest pain.[5,56] Some investigators have found the development of "reperfusion arrhythmias" to be associated with infarct-related artery patency, but neither of these clinical markers is very reliable.

Two other methods used to estimate reperfusion are the ECG and laboratory changes.[57] Since the extent of the reduction of ST segment elevation may be related to the extent of patency, 12-lead ECGs should be obtained frequently. ECGs have the advantage of being readily available, noninvasive, and inexpensive.

Early peaking of total CK and the CK-MB isoenzyme levels also may differentiate patients who have achieved reperfusion from those in whom thrombolytic therapy has failed. Lewis and colleagues found that there was an absolute rise in CK activity of 480 U/L or a relative rise of 34% within the first hour following successful thrombolysis.[58] CK-MB activity was found have a relative rise of 27% during the first hour. In the absence of reperfusion, CK activity was only increased by 15 U/L or had a relative rise of 3% over the first 2.5-hour period.

Some hospitals routinely evaluate regional wall motion using echocardiography. Unfortunately, it may take several days before improvement in wall motion is seen; therefore, it is difficult to use this test to assess the initial success of thrombolysis.

It is important to determine whether thrombolysis has been successful, since the prognosis of the patient appears to be related to the presence or absence of an open infarct-related artery.[38] If thrombolytic therapy fails to open the infarct-related artery, then the patient may benefit from mechanical revascularization such as PTCA or an emergency coronary artery bypass graft (CABG) procedure.

Time From Onset of Chest Pain

11. If P.H.'s arrival at the hospital had been delayed >6 hours from the onset of his chest pain, should he still have received a thrombolytic?

Although efforts should be directed toward administering a thrombolytic as early as possible, many patients present hours after the onset of chest pain. There are several theoretical reasons why the late administration of a thrombolytic may be helpful. Some patients present with a "stuttering" MI, which is chest pain that waxes and wanes over a period of hours or days, presumably from recurrent or ongoing ischemia. These patients should be considered candidates for thrombolytic therapy or angiographic evaluation. The magnitude of left ventricular dilatation may be diminished by reperfusion of the infarct-related artery, even if it is late. Another potential advantage of opening an infarct-related artery, even hours after an MI, is that the opened artery could become a source of collateral blood flow in the future.[59] The GISSI-1 trial enrolled patients within 12 hours from the onset of chest pain.[15] After 12 months of follow-up, the cumulative survival rate showed a statistically significant benefit from the administration of streptokinase compared to placebo. However, a subgroup analysis showed no benefit for the patients who received streptokinase after 6 hours from the onset of chest pain.

The ISIS-2 trial expanded patient enrollment to include patients admitted within 24 hours from the onset of chest pain.[39] In that trial, there was a 17% reduction in vascular death at 5 weeks in the streptokinase group treated 5 to 24 hours from the onset of chest pain, compared to a 35% reduction in the group who received streptokinase within 4 hours from the onset of pain. Although the benefit was reduced, a statistically and clinically significant benefit still was present.

Overall, there appears to be a statistically significant benefit associated with administering a thrombolytic up to 12 hours from the onset of chest pain and a trend toward benefit when given between 13 and 24 hours. Late administration may be most beneficial in patients at the highest risk for mortality. This would include the elderly, patients with large infarctions, and those with continuing pain or hypotension.[59] P.H. still may benefit from thrombolytic therapy even if he presents beyond the 6-hour time frame. If he still is having symptoms, he probably has viable myocardium at risk that may be salvaged. Streptokinase is the most cost-effective drug and the thrombolytic that has been shown to be effective in this situation.

Readministration of Thrombolytic Agents

12. This is P.H.'s first infarction. If he had a history of a previous MI that was treated with a thrombolytic agent, would he still be eligible for thrombolysis?

The need to administer a thrombolytic for a second infarction is becoming common. Many patients who are admitted to a hospital with AMI have a history of a previous infarction. Both streptokinase and anistreplase are associated with the formation of neutralizing antibodies within several days following administration. In a small study of 145 patients who had received streptokinase in conventional doses (1.5 MU), neutralizing antibodies were found in approximately 50% of patients 4 years later.[60] It is not known to what extent these antibodies could affect the efficacy of a repeat dose of streptokinase.

Another concern about repeated doses of streptokinase is the possible increased risk for allergic reactions. Major allergic reactions are rare with first-time administration of streptokinase. Based on observations made in ISIS-2, there were no reports of anaphylactic shock, and most of the allergic reactions (4.4% of individuals) consisted of shivering, pyrexia, or rashes.[39] Furthermore, the use of prophylactic corticosteroids did not seem to affect the incidence of allergic reactions.

If P.H. was presenting with a second infarction within a year and had received streptokinase for his first infarction, the thrombolytic of choice would be alteplase, tenecteplase, or reteplase. It is unclear if these agents would be the drugs of choice if the second infarction were several years later.

13. P.H. was stable initially following thrombolysis, but 48 hours later he experienced recurrent chest pain and ECG changes consistent with extension of his infarct. The attending cardiologist would like to readminister t-PA at this time. Is this a reasonable course of therapy?

Reocclusion of the infarct-related artery following initial successful thrombolysis is a major setback for this therapeutic strategy. If reocclusion occurs, mechanical intervention (e.g., angioplasty) often is attempted. There also have been attempts at reopening the infarct-related artery with repeat infusions of t-PA. In an evaluation of 52 patients who underwent repeat thrombolysis with t-PA, many patients received a second thrombolytic infusion within 1 hour of the end of the first infusion, and 44 of the 52 patients responded favorably, with resolution of pain.[61] Minor bleeding complications occurred in 19% of patients. Others have described experiences with repeat thrombolysis using t-PA within a median of 5 days. One patient developed a fatal intracranial hemorrhage within 6 hours of the second thrombolytic infusion.[62]

In the case of P.H., a repeat infusion with t-PA would probably be safe, but it may not be effective. As discussed in Question 12, repeat doses of streptokinase should be avoided. If facilities for either PTCA or surgery exist at the institution, many cardiologists would chose an invasive strategy at this time for P.H.

Use in the Elderly

14. B.T., an 85-year-old woman, presents to the ED with a history and examination that are nearly identical to P.H.'s. Should an elderly person (>70 years old) be treated any differently with regard to thrombolytic therapy?

Some of the early trials with thrombolytic therapy excluded the elderly. Although the elderly may have a higher prevalence of relative contraindications such as severe hypertension or history of stroke at presentation, they also have a higher incidence of mortality following an AMI. The 1-year cardiac mortality rate following an AMI is 17.6% in those older than 75 years compared to 12% for those ages 65 to 75.[63] In a trial using streptokinase, a higher incidence of bleeding in patients over age 70 was reported.[64] However, in the ISIS-2 trial, the greatest reduction in mortality occurred in the elderly subgroup.[39] There are no controlled trials in which thrombolytic therapy has increased mortality in the elderly.

If B.T. has no contraindications to thrombolytic therapy, she should receive it. A subgroup analysis from the GUSTO trial suggested that patients over age 70 should receive streptokinase, since there was a higher incidence of intracranial hemorrhage in elderly patients who received t-PA.[38]

Strokes Associated With Thrombolysis

15. G.M., a 45-year-old man, presents with signs and symptoms consistent with an anterolateral AMI. Upon admission, he received t-PA (100 mg over 90 minutes). He developed nystagmus, blurred vision, dysarthria, and paresthesias in his right hand 18 hours after the infusion. How often are stroke symptoms observed in patients with AMI? Is there a difference in the risk of stroke among the various thrombolytic agents?

Stroke is a very serious but infrequent complication of AMI. Before thrombolytic agents were used widely, stroke reportedly occurred in 1.7% to 3.2% of AMI patients.[65] The risk factors identified for stroke are large infarct size, anterior location, severe pump failure, atrial arrhythmias, and previous history of stroke. Large anterior wall infarcts are associated with a higher risk for mural thrombi formation. An estimated one third of patients with anterior wall infarction who do not receive a thrombolytic will develop a mural thrombus, usually within the first week of the event.[65] Many cardiologists routinely perform echocardiograms before discharge in patients who have had an anterior wall infarction to rule out a mural thrombus.

Interestingly, the overall incidence of stroke following an AMI has decreased since the use of thrombolytic agents has become widespread. This finding has occurred in both placebo- and thrombolytic-treated groups, but the reason for this decrease is unclear. In a review of six placebo-controlled trials evaluating the use of thrombolytic agents, the incidence of stroke averaged 0.86% in the patients treated with placebo and 1.06% in those receiving a thrombolytic.[65] However, these rates are only estimates, since many of the strokes in these trials were unclassified and the diagnosis may have been imprecise. Mortality rates for patients who have had a stroke also are on the decline. Better measures are needed to identify patients at risk for stroke.

The risk of stroke was analyzed from the GISSI-2 and International Study trials, where streptokinase was compared to t-PA with and without SC heparin.[66] Of the 20,768 patients who had complete records, 236 had a stroke while in the hospital. Thirty-one percent of the cases were intracerebral hemorrhage, 42% were ischemic stroke, and 26% were not classified. More hemorrhagic and ischemic strokes occurred in patients receiving t-PA (1.33% versus 0.94% for streptokinase). Elderly patients (>70 years old) had a stroke rate of 2.6% with t-PA and 1.6% with streptokinase. Patients older than age 75 had a higher incidence of death and stroke compared to patients younger than 75 in the GUSTO trial.[38] Patients older than 75 who were randomized to the t-PA group had a higher incidence of hemorrhagic stroke (2.08%) versus those randomized to either streptokinase group (1.23%). This has prompted some to suggest that patients older than age 75 should receive streptokinase rather than t-PA.[67]

Cardiopulmonary Resuscitation and Thrombolysis

16. If P.H. (the patient in Questions 1 through 13) had suffered cardiac arrest before hospitalization and had undergone cardiopulmonary resuscitation (CPR), would thrombolysis be contraindicated?

The need for CPR in the acute phase of an MI is fairly common, with a reported incidence of cardiac arrest between 10% and 16% in some trials. Patients who have a cardiac arrest during an AMI are at a high risk for death and could potentially benefit from thrombolytic therapy. A retrospective analysis of 708 patients was conducted to answer this question.[68] Fifty-nine patients who needed <10 minutes of CPR before receiving thrombolytic therapy or needed CPR within 6 hours of receiving thrombolytic therapy were assessed. The authors found that patients who required CPR were more likely to have factors present that worsened their prognosis (anterior infarctions, lower ejection fraction). The mortality rate was twice as high (12% versus 6%) in the CPR patient group. The deaths, however, were attributed to pump failure, and there were no complications as a result of the CPR. Prolonged or traumatic CPR is listed as a contraindication to thrombolytic therapy.[2] However, there are no firm data to suggest that thrombolytic therapy should be withheld from patients who require only defibrillation or a brief duration of

CPR. Therefore, P.H. would still be a reasonable candidate for thrombolytic therapy if the CPR had been brief.

Lidocaine

Risk of Ventricular Fibrillation

17. After thrombolysis, P.H. is in normal sinus rhythm with rare premature ventricular contractions (PVCs). Should he receive prophylactic lidocaine? Would G.M. (the patient with stroke symptoms in Question 15) be treated differently?

Ventricular fibrillation is a major cause of death in patients who are having an AMI. Over half of the episodes of ventricular fibrillation that occur with an AMI are within 1 hour of the onset of symptoms. Since ventricular fibrillation is estimated to occur in 4% to 18% of patients with AMI, prophylactic lidocaine has been used in an attempt to reduce this complication.[69] It was assumed initially that ventricular ectopy such as frequent PVCs or short runs of ventricular tachycardia would precede any episodes of ventricular fibrillation. Therefore, patients with these types of "warning arrhythmias" were given lidocaine prophylactically. Subsequently, it was noted that not all patients who developed ventricular fibrillation had warning arrhythmias, so it became routine to give all patients with AMI prophylactic infusions of lidocaine.[70] Although the prophylactic use of lidocaine may decrease the incidence of ventricular fibrillation, a meta-analysis of clinical trials concluded that it adversely affects the mortality rate.[71] In a summary of 14 trials, lidocaine was associated with a 35% reduction of ventricular fibrillation, but it did not reduce the overall mortality. In fact, early mortality was greater in the lidocaine-treated patients. In 7 of the 14 trials, there was an excess of asystole in the lidocaine-treated patients, although this difference was not statistically significant. Since ventricular fibrillation is treated readily with defibrillation in an intensive care unit, the risk of prophylactic lidocaine in all patients may exceed the benefit. It is desirable to avoid cardioversion because it is an unpleasant experience; therefore, it is reasonable to use prophylactic lidocaine in patients at highest risk for ventricular fibrillation. (See Chapter 20, Cardiac Arrhythmias.)

The risk of lidocaine administration would probably outweigh the benefit in G.M., since he already is demonstrating many of the symptoms often associated with lidocaine toxicity as a result of his stroke. These findings make the monitoring of lidocaine very difficult. If G.M. received lidocaine, it would complicate monitoring the symptoms of his stroke.

Risks of Using Lidocaine

18. How should lidocaine be given, and for how long? How should lidocaine be monitored?

Lidocaine should be given as a loading dose followed by a continuous infusion. Loading doses of 1 mg/kg (maximum 100 mg) are used commonly, followed by a constant infusion of 20 to 50 µg/kg per minute.[2] Patients should be monitored for the side effects of lidocaine; the most common are those associated with central nervous system toxicity. Symptoms may include drowsiness, dizziness, tremor, paresthesias, slurred speech, seizures, and coma. Massive overdoses may cause respiratory depression. Lidocaine may suppress ventricular escape mechanisms, leading to atrioventricular block or asystole. The overall incidence of side effects in studies has been approximately 15%.[69,70]

Plasma Concentrations

19. What factors following an AMI may complicate the measurement of lidocaine plasma concentrations?

The likelihood of developing adverse effects from lidocaine is dose related; however, side effects frequently are reported when plasma concentrations are within the therapeutic range. The elderly and patients with heart failure and hepatic dysfunction have reduced clearance of lidocaine and may be predisposed to lidocaine toxicity. Lidocaine is bound to α_1-acid glycoprotein (AAG) and albumin in the serum. AAG plasma concentrations have been shown to increase within 36 hours of the time of infarction.[72] Patients with AMI have an increased binding of lidocaine to AAG and a rise in total lidocaine plasma concentrations, but a reduced percentage of free lidocaine. This could result in a patient with a plasma lidocaine concentration that is above the "therapeutic range" without signs of toxicity. Therefore, plasma lidocaine concentrations may be difficult to interpret in the setting of AMI. (See Chapter 20, Cardiac Arrhythmias, for a complete discussion of lidocaine dosing and toxicity.)

Magnesium

20. Will the administration of IV magnesium be beneficial for P.H.? How is magnesium administered?

There has been considerable debate regarding the use of magnesium in the setting of AMI. The potential mechanisms by which magnesium may benefit a patient include an antiarrhythmic effect, an antiplatelet effect, reversal of vasoconstriction, reduction of catecholamine secretion, and enhancement of adenosine triphosphate production.[73,74]

In LIMIT-2, a randomized, placebo-controlled, double-blind trial of 2,316 patients with suspected AMI, IV magnesium was found to decrease mortality at 28 days by 24%.[75] However, in the MAGIC (Magnesium in Coronaries) trial, 6,213 patients with AMI were randomized to 2 g of IV magnesium sulfate given as a bolus followed by a 17-g infusion over 24 hours or matching placebo. Early administration of magnesium did not reduce 30-day mortality.[76] Similar results were also seen in the ISIS-4 study.[77]

At this time, most clinicians do not routinely administer IV magnesium to AMI patients because of the conflicting results of ISIS-4, MAGIC, and LIMIT-2. However, since P.H. has a low serum magnesium concentration (1.3 mEq/L), he could benefit from the drug. Based upon trials using magnesium in AMI, P.H. should receive 8 mmol over 5 to 15 minutes followed by 65 to 72 mmol, or 8 to 9 g, given as an IV infusion over 24 hours.[75,77]

β-Blockers

21. The physician has written orders for IV metoprolol 5 mg every 5 minutes for three doses. What are some of the benefits of administering β-blockers to P.H.? Should they be given early in his therapeutic course as IV therapy, or simply started as oral therapy a few days after the infarct?

As with thrombolytics, β-blockers offer significant benefits to the MI patient in both the acute infarct period and/or

several days later as initial oral therapy. Several large trials were designed to give early IV β-blockers (up to 24 hours after symptom onset), followed by oral therapy; other studies used oral therapy alone beginning days after the infarct.[23–26,78] Early IV administration appears to be most beneficial, with a reduction of mortality of around 25% in the first 2 days when the results of these trials are pooled.[25] However, late oral therapy alone, up to 21 days post-MI in the β-Blocker in Heart Attack Trial, also was associated with a substantial reduction in mortality (around 10%).[26]

Agents that have been studied extensively include propranolol, metoprolol, timolol, and atenolol. All have been given by early IV administration. Agents with intrinsic sympathomimetic activity such as pindolol and oxprenolol lack good efficacy data or have not been well studied. Typically, metoprolol and atenolol are used in the acute setting due to their β-1 selectivity, ease of dosing and administration, and weight of evidence. Oral carvedilol, a nonselective β- and α-blocker, has been used in the peri-infarction period specifically in patients with left ventricular dysfunction. In the CAPRICORN (Carvedilol Post-Infarction Survival Control in Left Ventricular Dysfunction) trial, carvedilol reduced all-cause and cardiovascular mortality as well as recurrent non-fatal MI.[79]

In general, if a patient has transient cardiac decompensation (e.g., hypotension, bradycardia, or worsening symptoms of heart failure) during the acute infarct period, early IV β-blockers are withheld. The patient's condition is then observed for a few days; if it stabilizes, oral therapy is initiated.[2,25] Since P.H. has experienced an uncomplicated MI and is stable, he is a candidate for early IV therapy. Acute and chronic dosing regimens for β-blockers are listed in Table 18-7.[23,24,80,81]

Use in Diabetes

22. What are some reasons for concern about the use of a β-blocker in P.H. (refer back to the data presented in Question 1)? How should this therapy be monitored?

Recall that P.H. has a longstanding history of hypertension and diabetes and that his admission BP was 180/110 mm Hg and heart rate was 100 beats/min. Some clinicians would consider the presence of diabetes a relative contraindication for β-blockade due to the adverse effects on insulin release and blunting of the hypoglycemia-associated tachycardia. However, diabetics make up a large portion of AMI patients, and many β-blocker trials contained diabetic AMI patients. Kjekshus and colleagues studied a subgroup of diabetic AMI patients and found β-blocker treatment to be beneficial.[82] Gottlieb and colleagues found that post-MI diabetic patients treated with β-blockers had a 36% reduction in mortality.[83] Due to these positive data, β-blockers would have to possess major negative effects on the diabetic condition to be considered contraindicated. Diabetic patients who are given β-blockers should receive non-intrinsic sympathomimetic activity, cardioselective agents (e.g., metoprolol, atenolol) and should be advised to monitor their blood glucose levels carefully for both hypo- and hyperglycemia after the β-blocker is initiated. Adjustments to insulin or oral hypoglycemic therapy may be required.

Table 18-7   Dosing Summary of β-Blockers in Acute Myocardial Infarction

β-Blocker	IV Dose	Chronic Dose
Atenolol[23] (Tenormin)	Administer 5 mg IV over 5 min, followed by 5 mg IV 10 min later; after 2nd IV dose, immediately begin 50 mg PO, followed by 50 mg PO 12 hr later.[a]	50–100 mg PO daily[a]
Carvedilol[79] (Coreg)	None	6.25–25 mg PO twice daily[a]
Metoprolol[24] (Toprol)	Administer 5 mg IV over 2 min for 3 doses; 15 min after the last IV dose, begin 50 mg PO Q 6 hr for 8 doses.[a]	50–100 mg PO twice daily[a]
Propranolol[80] (Inderal)	Administer 5–8 mg IV over 5 min, followed by 40 mg PO 2 hr apart, then Q 4 hr for 7 doses.[a]	180–240 mg PO daily in 2–4 divided doses[a]
Timolol[81] (Blocadren)	Administer 1 mg IV, followed by 1 mg IV 10 min later; 10 min after the 2nd IV dose, begin constant infusion of 0.6 mg/hr for 24 hr; upon completion of infusion, begin 10 mg PO twice daily.	10 mg PO twice daily[a]

IV, intravenous; PO, orally.
[a]FDA-approved dose

In a patient like P.H., a low dose of a β1-selective agent (e.g., metoprolol 25 mg BID) can be given and titrated to either adequate β-blockade or loss of diabetic control. At these doses the relative β_1 selectivity will be more likely to remain intact and is less likely than some of the nonspecific β-blockers to affect his diabetes.

Use in Hyperlipidemia
P.H. has elevated serum cholesterol (259 mg/dL) and triglyceride (300 mg/dL) levels. His low-density lipoprotein (LDL) and high-density lipoprotein (HDL) cholesterol levels are unknown. Although β-blockers have undesirable effects upon plasma lipids (they decrease HDL and increase total cholesterol and triglycerides), the evidence in support of their use in MI patients is compelling. (See Chapter 13, Dyslipidemias.) β-Blockers have reduced post-MI morbidity and mortality in hyperlipidemic patients. An appropriate lipid-lowering treatment plan should be developed and initiated as soon as possible.

Use in Heart Failure
Years ago, heart failure was considered a contraindication to β-blockade, but that is no longer the case. There are several factors to consider before withholding β-blockers. In general, patients who receive early IV β-blockade will benefit from this therapy. If the patient has a relative contraindication to β-blockade, one could consider using esmolol (500 mcg/kg IV bolus over 1 minute followed by a maintenance infusion of 50 to 300 mcg/kg per minute), which has a short duration of action. IV β-blockade should be withheld only if the patient has signs and symptoms of moderate to severe left ventricular dysfunction. However, chronic, oral therapy should be considered before discharge. As discussed previously, carvedilol has been shown to be safe and effective when initiated in the peri-infarction period and is indicated in patients post-MI with left ventricular dysfunction.[79] Both carvedilol and metoprolol are approved for use in patients with heart failure (see Chapter 19, Heart Failure). β-Blockade should be given to P.H., since he has no heart failure symptoms and his previous ejection fraction was >50%.

Use in Pulmonary Disease
P.H.'s acute situation is complicated by his history of intermittent pulmonary problems. In deciding whether to attempt use of β-blockers in patients with pulmonary disease, one must determine the nature of the pulmonary problem (i.e., reactive airways or restrictive lung disease). It also would be helpful to determine P.H.'s need for routine use of β-agonists to help quantify the severity of his disease. By history, P.H. does not use β-agonist bronchodilators routinely. No history is given regarding his pulmonary function tests or the degree of reversibility of his airway disease with bronchodilators. β_1-Selective antagonists are the drugs of choice in these patients, but at higher doses (e.g., metoprolol doses >100 mg/day), the relative β_1-selectivity may be lost. Similar to the argument regarding diabetes, a patient would need to experience significant worsening of the pulmonary disease to justify avoiding β-blockers. A better history of P.H.'s pulmonary problems should be obtained; if they are minor, low doses of metoprolol or atenolol (started in the hospital so he may be monitored closely) should be considered.

Weighing the risk versus benefit of β-blockers, one could make a case for cautiously administering IV agents to him at this time. His dose of IV metoprolol (5 mg Q 5 min for three doses) is a typical treatment plan.[25] He must have frequent monitoring of heart rate, BP, and respiratory status. Therapy should be discontinued if P.H.'s heart rate drops below 60 beats/min, systolic BP falls below 100 mm Hg, or any respiratory distress is noted. Oral metoprolol therapy could begin at 25 to 50 mg a few hours after his last IV dose. Substituting the ultra-short-acting agent esmolol for metoprolol is an option for P.H., since any adverse effects would be relatively short-lived. Unfortunately, there are no data to support the use of esmolol for an AMI.

Objective evidence of adequate β-blockade consists of a resting heart rate of 50 to 60 beats/min, an exercise heart rate of <120 beats/min, and/or a resting systolic BP of 100 to 120 mm Hg.[84] Therefore, P.H. needs a significant reduction in heart rate and BP from his admission values (100 beats/min and 180/110 mm Hg, respectively) to be considered as having achieved adequate β-blockade.

23. Several days later, a routine echocardiogram is performed on P.H. that shows hypokinesis of the anterior and lateral left ventricular walls, a slightly enlarged left ventricle, no valvular abnormalities, ejection fraction 35% to 40%, and the appearance of a thrombus in the left ventricle. Clinically, he has no signs or symptoms of heart failure. What are the therapeutic and prognostic implications of this echocardiogram?

Hypokinesis of the infarcted areas of the heart is not unusual. P.H. may have an area of "stunned" or "hibernating" myocardium; it could take several weeks to recover some of the wall motion if the area is still viable.[85] Therefore, P.H. may recover some of the wall motion and ejection fraction over time.

The presence of a thrombus in the left ventricle is a risk factor for embolization. Several studies have shown that this may increase P.H.'s risk of experiencing a later embolic event. If P.H. is thought to be compliant with his medications, he would be a candidate for warfarin therapy (titrated to an international normalized ratio [INR] of 2 to 3) for 1 to 3 months because of this thrombus. This should be enough time for the thrombus to organize and become less of an embolic threat. P.H. is a likely candidate for treatment with an ACE inhibitor and β-blocker.

Nitroglycerin

24. A.J., a 75-year-old man, presents to the ED with complaints of dizziness and chest discomfort. He is a poor historian, but it appears that his symptoms have been ongoing for >12 hours. His physician is concerned that the symptoms represent an AMI. He had a gastrointestinal bleed 6 weeks ago and has chronic obstructive pulmonary disease with a bronchospastic component. The ECG is consistent with a new anterolateral AMI. His vital signs are BP, 150/94 mm Hg; heart rate, 55 beats/min; and respiratory rate, 20/min. Physical examination reveals wheezing. What is the best treatment strategy for A.J.?

Because of the time delay since symptoms first appeared and his history of recent GI bleeding, A.J. is not a good candidate for thrombolysis. β-Blockers also should be avoided in A.J. because of his serious pulmonary disease and current physical examination. Thus, symptomatic management with IV NTG is indicated, and PTCA should be considered. NTG lowers the left ventricular filling pressure and systemic vascular resistance, thereby reducing myocardial oxygen consumption and myocardial ischemia. At lower doses (<50 μg/min), IV NTG preferentially dilates the venous capacitance vessels, which leads to a decrease in left ventricular filling pressure.[86] For patients who have signs of pulmonary congestion, IV NTG is of particular value. (See Chapter 17, Ischemic Heart Disease: Anginal Syndromes, for further discussion of NTG pharmacology.)

25. How should IV NTG be administered to A.J.? How should it be monitored?

IV NTG should be initiated with a small bolus dose of 15 mcg. A constant infusion is then delivered by a controlled infusion device, starting with 5 to 10 mcg/min, which is then increased by an additional 5 to 10 mcg/min every 5 to 10 minutes.[2] Many cardiologists routinely give patients an infusion of NTG for the first 24 to 48 hours following an AMI. Increasing doses may be required over this period to maintain the desired hemodynamic effect due to tolerance that occurs from prolonged nitrate exposure. However, if >200 mcg/min is needed to achieve the desired response, another vasodilator such as nitroprusside or an ACE inhibitor may be considered. NTG is typically administered in combination with thrombolytics and GP IIb/IIIa inhibitors in patients who require relief of myocardial ischemia. Two studies have reported that concurrent administration of NTG may impair the thrombolytic effects of t-PA, but these data have been questioned.[87,88]

Some patients may have a problem with increased sensitivity to NTG, described as development of mean BP <80 mm Hg. Of the patients who become hypotensive, many have an inferior AMI. Ferguson and colleagues noted that hypotension following NTG infusion was a common complication in patients with right ventricular infarction.[89]

NTG readily migrates into many plastics; therefore, manufactured solutions are available only in glass containers. Some filters may absorb NTG, so they should be avoided. Polyvinyl chloride (PVC) tubing may absorb NTG, especially during the early phases of infusion. Some institutions use non-PVC tubing for NTG infusions to minimize this problem.

A.J.'s BP should be monitored closely during this infusion. On admission his BP was elevated at 150/94 mm Hg and his pulse rate was low at 55 beats/min. After starting NTG, we would expect to see his BP decline; the pulse rate may or may not increase. The NTG dose should be titrated to relieve pain while avoiding hypotension. In patients with evidence of heart failure, NTG can reduce left ventricular filling pressure (preload) and improve orthopnea and venous congestion. However, excessive doses of IV NTG can reduce left ventricular filling pressure and potentially decrease cardiac output, especially in patients who do not have signs of heart failure like A.J. The end points for dose titration include relief of pain or other symptoms. The systolic BP should always be kept at ≥90 mm Hg.[2] Nitrate tolerance can be minimized by providing a nitrate-free interval to the patient. If A.J. later receives chronic nitrate therapy with either an oral agent or a transdermal delivery system, a nitrate-free interval (e.g., withholding the nighttime dose) should be used. (See Chapter 17, Ischemic Heart Disease: Anginal Syndromes.)

26. Since A.J. has an elevated BP (154/94 mm Hg), should he receive nitroprusside instead of NTG?

NTG is preferred over nitroprusside in the setting of an AMI. Although the drugs have similar hemodynamic effects, nitroprusside has been shown to increase ST segment elevation, whereas NTG decreases ST segment elevation.[90] Others have shown similar results and have proposed that nitroprusside may redistribute coronary blood flow away from the ischemic area, causing a worsening of the injury.[91]

Analgesic Use

27. A.J.'s chest pain becomes increasingly severe despite NTG, and the physician is considering use of a potent analgesic. Which analgesic would be best for A.J.?

The pain associated with AMI is due to continuing tissue ischemia surrounding the area of infarcted tissue. The relief of pain should involve efforts to optimize the myocardial blood supply and minimize myocardial oxygen demand. Pain usually is relieved with successful thrombolysis. Other interventions can include oxygen, nitroglycerin, and β-blockers. As noted previously, A.J. is not a candidate for either thrombolysis or β-blockade. If his pain continues despite administration of IV NTG, he will need an analgesic. A.J. may also need to undergo emergency revascularization with either PCTA or bypass surgery.

Morphine sulfate usually is the analgesic of choice in patients with AMI. In addition to diminishing pain and anxiety, morphine also has beneficial hemodynamic effects. By reducing pain and anxiety, the release of circulating catecholamines is diminished, possibly reducing the associated arrhythmias. Morphine also causes peripheral venous and arterial vasodilatation, which reduces preload and afterload and consequently the myocardial oxygen demand. Morphine is administered in small (2- to 4-mg) IV doses as often as every 5 minutes if needed. Cumulative doses of 25 to 30 mg may be required. The risks associated with morphine use include hypotension, bradycardia, and respiratory depression. Since A.J. already has bradycardia, meperidine may be preferred because it has vagolytic properties.

POSTINFARCTION ARRHYTHMIAS

28. **D.T., a 45-year-old man who is recovering from an AMI (onset 12 hours ago), is noted to have sustained ventricular tachycardia on the telemetry monitor in the coronary care unit. During the episode he was hemodynamically unstable (BP 80/40 mm Hg, heart rate >200 beats/min). The arrhythmia was terminated with a 100-J countershock. He now is in sinus rhythm and clinically stable. Would D.T. be a candidate for further workup of the arrhythmia? If so, what tests are appropriate?**

In the past, there was an assumption that ventricular ectopy in the immediate post-MI period would have a negative prognostic significance, especially for sudden cardiac death. Overall, ventricular arrhythmias detected with telemetry during hospitalization have not been helpful in identifying patients at high risk for sudden cardiac death on long-term follow-up.[92] Since D.T.'s arrhythmia occurred within the first 48 hours after the infarct (i.e., the peri-infarct period, when some residual ischemia may be occurring), he is not a candidate for any further specific arrhythmia workup, such as electrophysiologic testing. D.T. should receive a β-blocker and aspirin during hospitalization and after discharge to prevent reinfarction and reduce mortality.

29. **Two weeks after D.T.'s AMI, he returns to the clinic for routine follow-up. A Holter monitor (continuous ambulatory ECG monitoring) is ordered for him because he states that he has had several "skipped beats" since the MI. This is a new finding. The results of the Holter indicate that he is having >30 PVCs per hour, which are asymptomatic to mildly symptomatic. What is the appropriate antiarrhythmic therapy at this time?**

It has been known for some time that frequent PVCs in patients with organic heart disease (e.g., post-MI) were indicators for an increased risk of sudden cardiac death.[93] However, CAST showed that when PVCs were suppressed with flecainide, encainide, or moricizine, survival was significantly worse than in patients treated with placebo.[32,33] This may be related to the proarrhythmic effects of these drugs. (See Chapter 20, Cardiac Arrhythmias.) Therefore, treatment of asymptomatic or mildly symptomatic PVCs with antiarrhythmics (other than β-blockers) in this type of post-MI patient is not recommended. A pooled-data analysis of class I antiarrhyth-

mic trials in these patients also supports these conclusions.[94] Therapies should be aimed at correcting the patient's underlying ischemia and/or coexisting heart failure rather than administering antiarrhythmics. D.T. should not be given any of the class I antiarrhythmics.

There is increasing interest in using amiodarone in the post-MI patient. Several studies indicate that amiodarone prevents ventricular arrhythmias or death due to arrhythmias in some post-MI patients.[94] BASIS (Basel Antiarrhythmic Study of Infarct Survival) randomized AMI survivors with complex ventricular ectopy into three groups: physician-directed individualized treatment, amiodarone (1 g for 5 days followed by 200 mg daily thereafter), or control. At 12 months of follow-up, there was a statistically significant increase in survival among the amiodarone group compared to the control group. Importantly, no irreversible pulmonary toxicity was observed in this low-dose amiodarone group.[95] Long-term follow-up (mean 72 months) showed a sustained effect of amiodarone on survival, with continued separation in the survival curves between the amiodarone and control groups.[96] Other trials have shown either a trend toward reduced mortality in amiodarone-treated patients or no difference from placebo or control groups.[97–100] The dropout rates in the amiodarone-treated groups were high, ranging from 30% to 38%.

Ejection fraction is an important factor in predicting survival. There was a much higher (58% versus 28%) mortality rate in patients with an ejection fraction <40%, regardless of treatment group, in BASIS. At this time, D.T. should not receive empiric amiodarone because his symptoms are mild and the data do not support that treatment would prolong his life.

30. **What are some predictors of arrhythmic mortality in the post-MI patient?**

Noninvasive diagnostic tests are available to estimate a patient's mortality risk after AMI. The use of signal-averaged ECG, radionuclide ventriculography, Holter monitoring, and clinical variables to determine patient risk has been described.[101] Approximately two thirds of patients in this trial had received thrombolytic therapy. When a multivariate analysis was performed to rank the variables in order of predictability, digoxin therapy at discharge (probably representing patients with severe heart failure), abnormal signal-averaged ECG (presence of late potentials), and prior history of angina were the most powerful predictors of arrhythmic events. The presence of a poor ejection fraction (<40%) is a consistent independent predictor of mortality throughout the literature. Thus, therapy should be directed toward improving the overall function of the heart and decreasing the myocardial oxygen demand in asymptomatic patients. For patients who experienced an episode of sudden cardiac death or who have hemodynamically unstable arrhythmias beyond the peri-infarction period, antiarrhythmic therapy may be chosen based on the results of electrophysiologic studies or repeated Holter monitoring. An implantable cardiodefibrillator (ICD) is an option for some patients. (See Chapter 20 for further discussion.)

ACUTE CORONARY SYNDROMES

31. **J.W. is a 55-year-old white man who presented to the ED with chest tightness and shortness of breath. He gives a history of similar symptoms the prior day that lasted 15 minutes. He was**

given an aspirin 325 mg and started on an IV NTG infusion, which was increased to 80 mcg/min; at that time his BP was 100/60 mm Hg and his heart rate was 88. His ECG continued to show ST segment depression in the anterior leads. His shortness of breath was relieved, but he still complained of chest tightness. His past medical history is unremarkable and he was on no medications prior to admission. He has smoked a pack of cigarettes per day for the last 30 years. Blood is drawn for troponin and CK as well as routine chemistries. Based on his symptoms and ECG, the diagnosis is presumed unstable angina. Should J.W. receive an additional oral antiplatelet agent?

J.W. is presenting with signs and symptoms consistent with acute coronary syndrome (ACS). If his cardiac enzymes come back positive, his diagnosis will be NSTEMI. Clopidogrel should be added to aspirin as soon as possible on admission. It should be administered for ≥1 month and may be given for up to 9 months in patients who are not at a high risk for bleeding.

In hospitalized patients with unstable angina and NSTEMI who do not require early interventional therapy, clopidogrel may be used in combination with aspirin. In the CURE (Clopidogrel in Unstable Angina to Prevent Recurrent Ischemic Events) trial, 12,562 patients with NSTEMI presenting within 24 hours were randomized to receive placebo + aspirin (75 to 325 mg) or clopidogrel (300 mg, immediately followed by 75 mg daily) + aspirin. They were followed for approximately 9 months. Cardiovascular death, MI, or stroke occurred in 11.5% of patients in the placebo group and 9.3% in those receiving clopidogrel ($P < 0.001$). Clopidogrel was associated with reductions in severe ischemia and revascularization. Compared to placebo, an increase in major and minor bleeding was seen with clopidogrel. Based on these data, clopidogrel + aspirin should be administered immediately upon admission and continued for at least 1 month.[102]

In the PCI-CURE study, 2,658 patients from the CURE trial undergoing percutaneous coronary intervention (PCI) were randomized to receive clopidogrel or placebo in addition to aspirin. Patients were treated prior to the PCI with aspirin and study medication for a median of 10 days. After the PCI, patients received open-label clopidogrel or ticlopidine for about 2 to 4 weeks, after which the study drug was restarted for a mean of 8 months. In the clopidogrel group, there was a statistically significantly lower number of cardiovascular deaths, MIs, or urgent target-vessel revascularizations within 30 days of the PCI compared to placebo (4.5% versus 6.4%, $P = 0.03$). Overall, patients receiving clopidogrel exhibited a 31% reduction in cardiovascular death or MI compared to those receiving placebo ($P = 0.002$).[102]

In the CREDO (Clopidogrel for the Reduction of Events During Observation) trial, 2,116 patients who were to undergo elective PCI were randomized to a loading dose of 300 mg of clopidogrel 3 to 24 hours prior to the PCI or placebo. After PCI, patients in both groups then received clopidogrel 75 mg daily for 28 days. The patients receiving the loading dose continued to receive clopidogrel through 12 months. All patients received 325 mg of aspirin throughout the study. At 1 year, the patients receiving clopidogrel demonstrated a statistically significant reduction in combined risk of death, MI, or stroke compared to placebo ($P = 0.02$). However, in a subgroup analysis, only the patients who received a loading dose >6 hours before PCI demonstrated a reduction in death, MI, or urgent vessel revascularization at 28 days compared to placebo ($P = 0.051$). At 1 year, a trend toward increased major bleeding was seen in the clopidogrel group compared to placebo (8.8% versus 6.7%, $P = 0.07$).[103]

Based on these data, in patients with unstable angina and NSTEMI receiving aspirin and undergoing PCI, clopidogrel may be administered prior to the procedure, followed by ≥1 month and possibly up to 12 months of additional treatment. In patients undergoing elective CABG, clopidogrel should be discontinued for 5 to 7 days prior to the procedure.[102,103]

32. **What other antithrombotic medications should be considered for J.W.?**

The ACC/AHA guidelines recommend the use of either LMWH or unfractionated heparin for the treatment of unstable angina/NSTEMI. Enoxaparin is preferred over unfractionated heparin unless CABG is anticipated within 24 hours.[102] In the ESSENCE (Efficacy and Safety of Subcutaneous Enoxaparin) study, enoxaparin (1 mg/kg SC twice daily) was compared to unfractionated heparin (5,000 unit IV bolus followed by continued infusion titrated to an activated partial thromboplastin time of 55 to 86 sec) administered for 48 hours to 8 days. The composite outcome of death, MI, or recurrent angina at 14 days was 19.8% in the heparin group versus 16.6% in the enoxaparin group, a 20% relative risk reduction. This benefit was maintained over 1 year.[104,105]

In the TIMI-11B trial, enoxaparin (30 mg IV bolus followed by 1 mg/kg SC twice daily for 8 days) compared to unfractionated heparin (70 U/kg bolus followed by 15 U/kg per hour for 3 to 8 days) reduced the composite end point of death, MI, or need for urgent revascularization at 8 days ($P = 0.048$) and 43 days ($P = 0.048$).[106] It is not clear whether other LMWHs offer the same benefit, since no "head-to-head" trials have been done.

The addition of a LMWH with a GP IIb/IIIa inhibitor for the initial management of unstable angina/NSTEMI has been evaluated in six trials. The major finding of these trials was that major hemorrhage occurred rarely in the combination arms (0.3% to 1.8%). While not powered to detect a difference, the rates of ischemic events were noted to be similar between the LMWH and unfractionated heparin groups.[107]

33. **What is the role of a GP IIb/IIIa inhibitor in patients with ACS?**

The ACC/AHA guidelines recommend that a platelet GP IIb/IIIa inhibitor be administered, in addition to aspirin and/or clopidogrel and heparin or LMWH, to patients in whom PCI is planned. A GP IIb/IIIa inhibitor may also be administered just prior to PCI. Eptifibatide or tirofiban, when used in combination with aspirin and heparin or LMWH, is also approved for the medical management of patients with ACS. When used to treat patients medically, the GP IIb/IIIa inhibitors (in combination with the other drugs previously mentioned) are generally given for 2 to 3 days.

The GUSTO-IV-ACS trial enrolled 7,800 patients with unstable angina/NSTEMI in whom early (<48 hours) revascularization was not intended.[108] All patients received aspirin and either UFH or LMWH. They were randomized to placebo, an abciximab bolus and 24-hour infusion, or an abciximab bolus and 48-hour infusion. At 30 days, death or MI occurred in 8.0% of patients taking placebo, 8.2% of patients receiving 24-hour abciximab, and 9.1% of patients receiving

48-hour abciximab (P = NS). At 48 hours, death occurred in 0.3%, 0.7%, and 0.9% of patients in these groups, respectively (placebo versus abciximab at 48 hours, P = 0.008). Abciximab should be used only if a patient is planning to undergo PCI; it should be avoided if only medical management is intended. Major trials have been done with GP IIb/IIIa inhibitors in patients with ACS.[108–116]

LONG-TERM THERAPY

Angiotensin-Converting Enzyme Inhibitors

34. A patient with an uncomplicated MI has no signs or symptoms of heart failure. An order is written for captopril 12.5 mg TID. Is this appropriate? If so, how should the therapy be monitored?

After an AMI, the heart undergoes processes that initially compensate for the loss of contractile function, but may increase the long-term risk for development of heart failure. This is referred to as "remodeling" of the ventricle (see Chapter 19, Heart Failure, for further description of ventricular remodeling). The increase in the number of survivors of AMI has increased the number of heart failure patients.

Ventricular remodeling consists of several steps.[117] In the first few days after the AMI, the infarct is completed and early infarct expansion occurs. Factors that may increase the likelihood of infarct expansion include a large anterior infarct, absence of pre-existing ventricular wall hypertrophy, and increased intraventricular systolic pressure (i.e., increased afterload).[117,118] From days 1 to 7 post-infarct, the ventricular wall thins and the ventricle dilates; therefore, ventricular volume increases. This compensatory process can eventually lead to heart failure in some patients.

In the SAVE (Survival and Ventricular Enlargement) trial, captopril (up to 50 mg TID) had a statistically significant beneficial effect on mortality when given to asymptomatic patients with an ejection fraction <40% who were 3 to 16 days post-MI. This 4-year follow-up study also showed significant decreases in morbidity from heart failure and recurrent AMI in the captopril group. The largest risk reduction in cardiovascular death was seen in men and in patients older than 55 years.[10]

Another large trial using ramipril, the AIRE (Acute Infarction Ramipril Efficacy) study, enrolled post-MI patients with clinical evidence of heart failure (excluding New York Heart Association class IV).[119] Patients were randomized to ramipril (initially 2.5 mg BID) or placebo beginning between days 3 and 10 after their infarct. During a mean follow-up of 15 months, ramipril significantly decreased all causes of mortality. Data from the ISIS-4, GISSI-3, TRACE, and SMILE trials also have shown a benefit with the use of ACE inhibitors post-MI.[77,120,121]

Based on these studies, oral ACE inhibitor therapy should be started within the first 24 hours of an AMI, preferably after completion of thrombolytic therapy and BP stabilization (systolic BP >100 mm Hg). ACE inhibitor therapy is particularly beneficial in patients with an anterior infarction and an ejection fraction <40% (even if asymptomatic) or clinical evidence of heart failure.[2] ACE inhibitors may be used either prophylactically to prevent the occurrence of heart failure symptoms or for treatment of heart failure in the AMI patient.

However, unlike β-blockers, the use of IV ACE inhibition therapy is not recommended by the ACC/AHA guidelines.[2,27] Captopril could be given on post-infarct day 2 or 3, beginning with a test dose of 6.25 mg and then an initial maintenance dosage of 12.5 to 25 mg three times daily. BP should be monitored closely, with the systolic BP maintained at ≥90 mm Hg. Renal function and serum potassium levels should be followed closely during the first few months of therapy. In diabetics, an ACE inhibitor also may benefit long-term renal function.[122] Once it is established that the patient can tolerate an ACE inhibitor, he or she can be switched to a longer-acting agent such as lisinopril or enalapril to simplify the regimen (see Chapter 19, Heart Failure, for ACE inhibitor dosing recommendations). If the patient cannot tolerate an ACE inhibitor due to cough, an angiotensin receptor blocker may be an alternative. In the OPTIMAAL trial, losartan 50 mg daily demonstrated similar reductions in all-cause mortality compared to captopril 50 mg three times daily, with a nonsignificant trend in favor of captopril.[123]

β-Blockers

35. Should the previous patients receive a β-blocker upon discharge?

The 1999 ACC/AHA guidelines recommend β-blocker therapy indefinitely for all patients following an AMI.[2] The benefits of β-blockers in reducing reinfarctions and mortality are thought to outweigh the risk, even in patients with asthma, insulin-dependent diabetes, severe peripheral vascular disease, first-degree heart block, and moderate left ventricular dysfunction. Due to his bronchospastic disease, P.H. should be carefully titrated on a β-blocker to see if he can tolerate it. Propranolol, metoprolol, and atenolol are available as generics, making any of them a cost-effective alternative. Metoprolol or carvedilol are considered first-line choices in patients with heart failure, while atenolol or metoprolol should be considered in patients with stable asthma or bronchospastic pulmonary disorder.

Calcium Channel Blockers

36. Is there any reason to add a calcium channel blocker to any of the three patients' therapeutic regimen at this time?

As reported by Yusuf and colleagues, verapamil, diltiazem, and nifedipine all have been evaluated for use in the post-MI population.[124] Much less information is available regarding the second-generation dihydropyridine agents (amlodipine, felodipine, and isradipine). When calcium channel blockers are categorized according to agents that slow the heart rate (e.g., diltiazem, verapamil) versus agents that have no effect or that increase the heart rate (e.g., nifedipine), the data are more favorable for the former.

DAVIT-II studied 1,600 patients in a controlled, randomized manner using verapamil 360 mg/day or placebo.[31] Patients were enrolled during the second week after infarction; importantly, severe heart failure and β-blocker use were exclusion criteria. When data for the entire study were analyzed by the primary end point of mortality, no statistically significant difference was found between verapamil and placebo at 18 months of follow-up. However, the reinfarction rate was significantly lower in the verapamil group. A subgroup analysis of patients without heart failure showed a significant decrease in mortality and reinfarction.

Diltiazem was widely touted for use in non–Q-wave AMI patients. However, a frequently quoted trial showed a reduction in reinfarction only during the first 2 weeks after non–Q-wave AMI.[29] Mortality was the same in the treatment and control groups. A separate trial that studied 2,466 patients with both Q-wave and non–Q-wave infarcts showed no overall reduction in mortality or cardiac events.[30] However, this trial did show a trend for more frequent adverse cardiac events in patients with pulmonary congestion who received diltiazem. Positive data from either of these trials on long-term survival are limited since they were derived retrospectively using subgroup analyses. These trials demonstrate that the routine use of diltiazem or verapamil is not appropriate for all patients with AMI. Their use should be limited to patients without signs of pulmonary congestion or systolic dysfunction. The use of a calcium channel blocker is better justified in the patient who still has postinfarction angina. While the studies with diltiazem and verapamil suggest a lower rate of reinfarction, the benefit from β-blockers on mortality is more impressive. Verapamil and diltiazem may be considered as alternatives for patients who cannot tolerate β-blockers due to bronchospastic disease. If a patient has left ventricular dysfunction secondary to an AMI and develops angina, the newer second-generation dihydropyridine calcium channel blockers, like amlodipine, are preferable (see Chapter 19, Heart Failure).[125]

None of the patients in the cases presented needs a calcium channel blocker at this time. Consideration should be given to adding a calcium channel blocker if they develop signs or symptoms of postinfarction angina or if they are intolerant of β-blocker therapy.

Lipid-Lowering Agents

37. **Should AMI patients be started on a lipid-lowering agent?**

Although the results of a complete fasting lipid panel were not made available, P.H. had elevated total cholesterol and triglycerides as part of his routine screening laboratory tests. A complete fasting lipid profile would be helpful and should be completed within 24 hours of presenting with an AMI.[126] This is often overlooked or not done because the patient is not fasting. Most patients will require a low-cholesterol, low–saturated fat diet in addition to lipid-lowering therapy. The goal for P.H. will be to reduce his LDL to <100 mg/dL. This is most easily accomplished by using a statin as the lipid-lowering agent. When triglycerides are >200 mg/dL, drug therapy with niacin or gemfibrozil is beneficial.[2] Hormone replacement therapy is not beneficial for secondary prevention in postmenopausal women. If a patient is receiving hormone replacement therapy, it should be discontinued during the acute event (see Chapter 13, Dyslipidemias).[127]

Antithrombotic Agents

38. **Three days before P.H.'s anticipated discharge, the medical team is discussing the need to administer long-term anticoagulant therapy with warfarin in addition to antiplatelet therapy with aspirin. Is either of these therapies indicated for P.H. at this time?**

In addition to its use in the setting of AMI, aspirin is routinely prescribed for post-MI patients.[2,25,128] The prophylactic role of aspirin in asymptomatic patients has also been established by such trials as the Physicians' Health Study as well as in patients with chronic stable angina.[129,130]

Antiplatelet therapy should be life-long because of its effects on secondary prevention of reinfarction. There appears to be no difference in efficacy over a wide range of aspirin doses (75 to 1,500 mg/day), although higher doses may increase the incidence of side effects.[128] A great deal of interest exists in using lower doses of aspirin for cardiovascular disease. Most clinicians use dosages of 81 to 325 mg daily or every other day.

Long-term warfarin may be beneficial in some patients, but clinical judgment is needed to decide if the benefit is likely to exceed the risk. Kaplan reviewed data for the development of left ventricular thrombi in AMI and found an incidence of approximately 35% in patients who suffered an anterior infarct.[131] While anticoagulation will decrease the incidence of stroke, <3% of patients will develop a cerebrovascular accident following an AMI if not anticoagulated. The ACC/AHA guidelines recommend warfarin for post-MI patients unable to take aspirin, patients with a left ventricular thrombus, and those with persistent atrial fibrillation.[2] There is also consensus that post-MI patients with extensive wall motion abnormalities and those with paroxysmal atrial fibrillation will benefit from anticoagulation. Recently, data have suggested that the use of high-intensity warfarin (INR 3 to 4) or moderate-intensity warfarin (INR 2.0 to 2.5) with low-dose aspirin (75 to 100 mg) may significantly reduce subsequent cardiovascular events and death post-MI compared to aspirin (100 to 160 mg).[132,133]

P.H. probably is a good candidate for 1 to 3 months of warfarin therapy titrated to an INR of 2 to 3 because of his left ventricular thrombus. The use of low-dose aspirin in conjunction with warfarin probably will not increase his risk of bleeding.[134]

39. **Is clopidogrel more effective than aspirin in reducing the risk for further cardiovascular events?**

In patients with STEMI and NSTEMI, clopidogrel (Plavix) may be used when aspirin is contraindicated or not tolerated; however, it is significantly more expensive than aspirin. In the CAPRIE (Clopidogrel Versus Aspirin in Patients at Risk of Ischemic Events) trial, 19,185 patients with atherosclerotic vascular disease such as ischemic stroke, MI, or peripheral arterial disease were randomized to clopidogrel 75 mg once daily or aspirin 325 mg once daily and followed for 1 to 3 years. On completion of the study, an intention-to-treat analysis demonstrated a lower risk for the combined end points of ischemic stroke, MI, or vascular death in the clopidogrel group compared to aspirin (5.32% versus 5.83%, $P = 0.043$).[135] A post hoc analysis of these data found a lower rate of AMI in patients receiving clopidogrel compared to aspirin (4.2% versus 5.04%, $P = 0.008$).[136] (See Chapter 16, Thrombosis, and Chapter 55, Cerebrovascular Disorders, for further discussions of anticoagulants and antiplatelet drugs.)

40. **How would you summarize the long-term therapy needed by P.H. upon discharge?**

Appropriate discharge medications for P.H. include a β-blocker (e.g., metoprolol), aspirin 81 mg/day, an ACE inhibitor (e.g., lisinopril), and warfarin to achieve an INR of 2 to 3. He also should receive a prescription for sublingual NTG to carry with him for use as needed. Some clinicians also might choose to continue his low-dose chronic nitrate therapy. All of these agents would be continued long term except for the warfarin, which would be discontinued after a few months. His previous hydrochlorothiazide may be discontinued since his hypertension will be controlled with the β-blocker and ACE inhibitor. His insulin should be continued and his blood glucose monitored closely. The goal is to achieve a state of β-blockade that will allow P.H. to maintain a systolic BP of >100 mm Hg; therefore, the clinician must balance the hypotensive effects of the ACE inhibitor and the β-blocker. Should P.H. experience postinfarction angina, then the addition of a calcium channel blocker such as diltiazem and/or chronic nitrate therapy would be indicated. P.H. can be started on a statin drug (e.g., atorvastatin, fluvastatin, pravastatin, simvastatin) to reach his LDL goal of <100 mg/dL. Routine liver function tests should be obtained prior to initiation of therapy and periodically thereafter.

LIFESTYLE MODIFICATIONS

41. **What types of lifestyle modifications should P.H. be encouraged to pursue to reduce his risk factors?**

P.H. must be encouraged to stop smoking; this may be the most important intervention. Rosenburg and colleagues showed that the risk of AMI in men who quit smoking was reduced to that of nonsmokers within a few years after quitting.[137] (See Chapter 85, Treatment of Tobacco Use and Dependence.) Weight management, diabetic treatment, and serum lipid control also are important risk factors to address (See Chapter 13, Dyslipidemias, and Chapter 50, Diabetes Mellitus, for further information on lipid-lowering drugs and diet therapy.)

SUMMARY

The use of thrombolytics and PCI has significantly improved the survival of patients with AMI. Despite the overwhelming results favoring thrombolytic therapy in all subgroups, it is believed that these agents remain underused in patients with AMI. The major risk associated with thrombolysis is bleeding, especially within the central nervous system. Another problem associated with thrombolytic therapy is reocclusion of an artery that was initially opened. Coronary angioplasty is more effective than thrombolytic therapy; however, it is available only in hospitals with experienced invasive cardiologists, thereby limiting its availability to many patients.

Aspirin should be given to all patients with AMI; unless there is a contraindication, β-blockers should be administered as well. Clopidogrel is often used in conjunction with aspirin, especially in patients receiving stents. ACE inhibitors have been shown to be beneficial in patients who have left ventricular dysfunction (ejection fraction <40%) and are also recommended for secondary prevention. Nitrates also are useful, but care must be taken to maintain an adequate perfusion pressure. Secondary prevention emphasizing a healthy lifestyle and aggressive lipid-lowering are important components to the overall treatment plan.

REFERENCES

1. DeWood MA et al. Prevalence of total coronary occlusion during the early hours of transmural myocardial infarction. N Engl J Med 1980;303:897.
2. Ryan TJ et al. ACC/AHA Guidelines for the management of patients with acute myocardial infarction. A report of the American College of Cardiology/American Heart Association Task Force on Practice Guidelines (Committee on Management of Acute Myocardial Infarction). J Am Coll Cardiol 1996;28:1328 and J Am Coll Cardiol 1999;34:890.
3. American Heart Association. Heart Disease and Stroke Statistics, 2003 Update. Available at http: www.americanheart.org. Accessed March 1, 2003.
4. Topol EJ, Van de Werf FJ. Acute myocardial infarction: Early diagnosis and treatment. In: Topol EJ, ed. Textbook of Cardiovascular Medicine. Philadelphia: Lippincott-Raven, 1998:395.
5. Rouleau JL et al. Myocardial infarction patients in the 1990s: their risk factors, stratification and survival in Canada: The Canadian Assessment of Myocardial Infarction (CAMI) Study. J Am Coll Cardiol 1996;27:1119.
6. Haase KK et al. In-hospital mortality of elderly patients with acute myocardial infarction: data from the MITRA (Maximal Individual Therapy in Acute Myocardial Infarction) registry. Clin Cardiol 2000;23:831.
7. Phibbs B et al. Q-wave versus non-Q wave myocardial infarction: a meaningless distinction. J Am Coll Cardiol 1999;33:576.
8. Wallach J. Cardiovascular diseases. In: Wallach J, ed. Interpretation of Diagnostic Tests. Boston: Little, Brown and Company, 1996:119.
9. Jaffe AS. In search of specificity: the troponins. ACC Current Journal Review 1995;Jan/Feb:29.

10. Pfeffer MA et al. Effect of captopril on mortality and morbidity in patients with left ventricular dysfunction after myocardial infarction. Results of the Survival and Ventricular Enlargement Trial. N Engl J Med 1992;327:669.
11. ACE Inhibitor Myocardial Infarction Collaborative Group. Indications for ACE inhibitors in the early treatment of acute myocardial infarction. Systematic overview of individual data from 100,000 patients in randomized trials. Circulation 1998; 97:2202.
12. Antman EM, Braunwald E. Acute myocardial infarction. In: Braunwald E, ed. Heart Disease: A Textbook of Cardiovascular Medicine. Philadelphia: WB Saunders, 1997:1184.
13. Bizjak ED, Mauro VF. Thrombolytic therapy: a review of its use in acute myocardial infarction. Ann Pharmacother 1998;32:769.
14. Turcasso NM, Nappi JM. Tenecteplase for treatment of acute myocardial infarction. An Pharmacother 2001;35:1233.
15. Gruppo Italiano per lo studio della streptochinasi nell'infarto miocardico (GISSI). Long-term effects of intravenous thrombolysis in acute myocardial infarction: Final report of the GISSI study. Lancet 1987;2:871.
16. Kaul S, Shah PK. Low-molecular-weight heparin in acute coronary syndrome: evidence for superior or equivalent efficacy compared with unfractionated heparin? J Am Coll Cardiol 2000; 35:1699.
17. The Hirulog and Early Reperfusion or Occlusion (HERO)-2 Trial Investigators. Thrombin-specific anticoagulation with bivalirudin versus heparin in patients receiving fibrinolytic therapy for acute myocardial infarction: the HERO-2 randomized trial. Lancet 2001;358:1855.

18. Jang IK et al. A multicenter, randomized study of argatroban versus heparin as adjunct to tissue plasminogen activator (TPA) in acute myocardial infarction: Myocardial Infarction with Novastan and TPA (MINT) study. J Am Coll Cardiol 1999; 33:1879.
19. Vermeer F et al. Argatroban and alteplase in patients with acute myocardial infarction. The ARGAMI study. J Thromb Thrombolysis 2000; 10:233.
20. Neuhaus KL et al. Recombinant hirudin (lepirudin) for the improvement of thrombolysis with streptokinase in patients with acute myocardial infarction: Results of the HIT-4 trial. J Am Coll Cardiol 1999;34:966.
21. TIMI 6 Investigators. Initial experience with hirudin and streptokinase in acute myocardial infarction: results of the Thrombolysis in Myocardial Infarction (TIMI) 6 Trial. Am J Cardiol 1995;75:7.
22. Metz BK et al. Randomized comparison of direct thrombin inhibition versus heparin in conjunction with fibrinolytic therapy for acute myocardial infarction: Results from the GUSTO-IIb Trial. J Am Coll Cardiol 1998;31:1493.
23. ISIS-1 (First International Study of Infarct Survival) Collaborative Group. Randomized trial of intravenous atenolol among 16,027 cases of suspected acute myocardial infarction: ISIS-1. Lancet 1986;2:57.
24. The MIAMI Trial Research Group. Metoprolol in acute myocardial infarction (MIAMI). A randomized placebo-controlled international trial. Eur Heart J 1985;6:199.
25. Yusuf S et al. Routine medical management of acute myocardial infarction. Lessons from

overviews of recent randomized controlled trials. Circulation 1990;82(Suppl. II):II-117.

26. β-Blocker Heart Attack Trial Group. A randomized trial of propranolol in patients with acute myocardial infarction. I. Mortality results. JAMA 1982; 247:1707.

27. Swedberg K et al. Effects of the early administration of enalapril on mortality in patients with acute myocardial infarction. N Engl J Med 1992;327:678.

28. Pashos CL et al. Trends in the use of drug therapies in patients with acute myocardial infarction 1988–1992. J Am Coll Cardiol 1994;23:1023.

29. Gibson RS et al. Diltiazem and reinfarction in patients with non-Q wave myocardial infarction. N Engl J Med 1986;315:423.

30. The Multicenter Diltiazem Postinfarction Trial Research Group. The effect of diltiazem on mortality and reinfarction after myocardial infarction. N Engl J Med 1988;319:385.

31. The Danish Study Group on Verapamil in Myocardial Infarction. Effect of verapamil on mortality and major events after myocardial infarction (The Danish Verapamil Infarction Trial II-DAVIT-II). Am J Cardiol 1990;66:779.

32. Echt DS et al. Mortality and morbidity in patients receiving encainide, flecainide or placebo. The Cardiac Arrhythmia Suppression Trial. N Engl J Med 1991;324:781.

33. The Cardiac Arrhythmia Suppression Trial-II Investigators. Effect of the antiarrhythmic agent moricizine on survival after myocardial infarction. N Engl J Med 1992;327:227.

34. Ribeiro EE et al. Randomized trial of direct coronary angioplasty versus intravenous streptokinase in acute myocardial infarction. J Am Coll Cardiol 1993;32:376.

35. Zijlstra F et al. Clinical characteristics and outcome of patients with early (<2 h), intermediate (2 to 4 h) and late (>4 h) presentation treated by primary coronary angioplasty or thrombolytic therapy for acute myocardial infarction. Eur Heart J 2002;23:550.

36. Dubin D. Infarction. In: Dubin D, ed. Rapid Interpretation of EKGs. 6th Ed. Tampa: COVER Publishing Company, 2000:290.

37. Muller DWM, Topol EJ. Selection of patients with acute myocardial infarction for thrombolytic therapy. Ann Intern Med 1990;113:949.

38. GUSTO Investigators. An international randomized trial comparing four thrombolytic strategies for acute myocardial infarction. N Engl J Med 1993; 329:673.

39. ISIS-2 (Second International Study of Infarct Survival) Collaborative Group. Randomized trial of intravenous streptokinase, oral aspirin, both or neither among 17,187 cases of suspected acute myocardial infarction: ISIS-2. Lancet 1988;2:349.

40. ISIS-3 (Third International Study of Infarct Survival) Collaborative Group. ISIS-3: a randomized comparison of streptokinase vs tissue plasminogen activator vs anistreplase and of aspirin plus heparin vs aspirin alone among 41,299 cases of suspected acute myocardial infarction. Lancet 1992;339:753.

41. The Global Use of Strategies to Open Occluded Coronary Arteries (GUSTO-III) Investigators. A comparison of reteplase with alteplase for acute myocardial infarction. N Engl J Med 1997; 337:1118.

42. Assessment of Safety and Efficacy of a New Thrombolytic (ASSENT-2) Investigators. Single-bolus tenecteplase compared with front-loaded alteplase in acute myocardial infarction: the ASSENT-2 double-blind randomized trial. Lancet 1999;354:716.

43. Smith SC et al. AHA/ACC guidelines for preventing heart attack and death in patients with atherosclerotic cardiovascular disease: 2001 Update. Circulation 2001;104:1577.

44. The International Study Group. In-hospital mortality and clinical outcome course of 20,891 patients with suspected acute myocardial infarction randomised between alteplase and streptokinase with or without heparin. Lancet 1990;336:71.

45. Hsia J et al. A comparison between heparin and low dose aspirin as adjunctive therapy with tissue plasminogen activator for acute myocardial infarction. N Engl J Med 1990;323:1433.

46. Bleich SD et al. Effect of heparin on coronary arterial patency after thrombolysis with tissue plasminogen activator in acute myocardial infarction. Am J Cardiol 1990;66:1214.

47. Ross AM et al. Randomized comparison of enoxaparin, a low-molecular-weight heparin, with unfractionated heparin adjunctive to recombinant tissue plasminogen activator thrombolysis and aspirin: Second Trial of Heparin and Aspirin Reperfusion Therapy (HART II). Circulation 2001;104:648.

48. Frostfeldt G et al. Low-molecular-weight heparin (dalteparin) as adjuvant treatment to thrombolysis in acute myocardial infarction: a pilot study: Biochemical Markers in Acute Coronary Syndromes (BIOMACS II). J Am Coll Cardiol 1999;33:627.

49. Antman EM et al. Abciximab facilitates the rate and extent of thrombolysis: results of the Thrombolysis In Myocardial Infarction (TIMI) 14 Trial. Circulation 1999;99:2720.

50. Brener SJ et al. Eptifibatide and low-dose tissue plasminogen activator in acute myocardial infarction: The integrilin and low-dose thrombolysis in acute myocardial infarction (INTRO AMI) trial. J Am Coll Cardiol 2002;39:377.

51. Topol EJ et al. Reperfusion therapy for acute myocardial infarction with fibrinolytic therapy or combination reduced fibrinolytic therapy and platelet glycoprotein IIb/IIIa inhibition: the GUSTO V randomised trial. Lancet. 2001;357:1905.

52. Lincoff A et al. Mortality at 1 year with combination platelet glycoprotein IIb/IIIa inhibition and reduced-dose fibrinolytic therapy versus conventional fibrinolytic therapy for acute myocardial infarction: GUSTO V Randomized Trial. JAMA 2002; 288:2130.

53. The Assessment of the Safety and Efficacy of a New Thrombolytic Regimen (ASSENT)-3 Investigators. Efficacy and safety of tenecteplase in combination with enoxaparin, abciximab, or unfractionated heparin: the ASSENT-3 randomised trial in acute myocardial infarction. Lancet 2001;358:605.

54. Antman EM et al. Enoxaparin as Adjunctive Antithrombin Therapy for ST-Elevation Myocardial Infarction: Results of the ENTIRE-Thrombolysis in Myocardial Infarction (TIMI) 23 Trial. Circulation 2002;105:1642.

55. Califf RM et al. Failure of simple clinical measurements to predict perfusion status after intravenous thrombolysis. Ann Intern Med 1988;108:658.

56. Christian TF et al. Severity and response of chest pain during thrombolytic therapy for acute myocardial infarction: a useful indicator of myocardial salvage and infarct size. J Am Coll Cardiol 1993; 22:1311.

57. Arnold AZ, Topol EJ. Assessment of reperfusion after thrombolytic therapy for myocardial infarction. Am Heart J 1992;124:441.

58. Lewis BS et al. Usefulness of a rapid rise of initial increase in plasma creatine kinase activity as a marker of reperfusion during thrombolytic therapy for acute myocardial infarction. Am J Cardiol 1988;62:20.

59. White HD. Thrombolytic therapy for patients with myocardial infarction presenting after six hours. Lancet 1992;340:221.

60. Elliott JM et al. Neutralizing antibodies to streptokinase four years after intravenous thrombolytic therapy. Am J Cardiol 1993;71:640.

61. Barbash GI et al. Repeat infusions of recombinant tissue-type plasminogen activator in patients with acute myocardial infarction and early recurrent myocardial ischemia. J Am Coll Cardiol 1990;16:779.

62. White HD et al. Safety and efficacy of repeat thrombolytic treatment after acute myocardial infarction. Br Heart J 1990;64:177.

63. Smith SC et al. Outlook after acute myocardial infarction in the very elderly compared with that in patients aged 65 to 75 years. J Am Coll Cardiol 1990;16:784.

64. Lew AS et al. Mortality and morbidity rate of patients older and younger than 75 years with acute myocardial infarction treated with intravenous streptokinase. Am J Cardiol 1987;59:1.48.

65. Sloan MA, Gore JM. Ischemic stroke and intracranial hemorrhage following thrombolytic therapy for acute myocardial infarction: a risk-benefit ratio. Am J Cardiol 1992;69(Suppl.):21A.

66. Maggioni AP et al. The risk of stroke in patients with acute myocardial infarction after thrombolytic and antithrombotic treatment. N Engl J Med 1992;327:1.

67. Fuster V. Coronary thrombolysis—a perspective for the practicing physician. N Engl J Med 1993; 329:723.

68. Tenaglia AN et al. Thrombolytic therapy in patients requiring cardiopulmonary resuscitation. Am J Cardiol 1991;68:1015.

69. Nattel S, Arenal A. Antiarrhythmic prophylaxis after acute myocardial infarction. Drugs 1993;45:9.

70. Jaffe AS. Prophylactic lidocaine for suspected acute myocardial infarction? Heart Disease and Stroke 1992;1:179.

71. MacMahon S et al. Effects of prophylactic lidocaine in suspected acute myocardial infarction: an overview of results from the randomized, controlled trials. JAMA 1988;260:1914.

72. Routledge PA et al. Increased α-1-acid glycoprotein and lidocaine disposition in myocardial infarction. Ann Intern Med 1980;93:701

73. Shaheen BE, Cornish LA. Magnesium in the treatment of acute myocardial infarction. Clin Pharm 1993;12:588.

74. Schechter M et al. The rationale of magnesium supplementation in acute myocardial infarction. Arch Intern Med 1992;152:2189.

75. Woods KL et al. Intravenous magnesium sulfate in suspected acute myocardial infarction: results of the second Leicester Intravenous Magnesium Intervention Trial (LIMIT-2). Lancet 1992;339:1553.

76. Antman EM et al. Early administration of intravenous magnesium to high-risk patients with acute myocardial infarction in the Magnesium in Coronaries (MAGIC) Trial: a randomised controlled trial. Lancet 2002;360:1189.

77. ISIS-4: a randomised factorial trial assessing early oral captopril, oral mononitrate, and intravenous magnesium sulphate in 58,050 patients with suspected myocardial infarction. Lancet 1995; 345:669.

78. The International Collaborative Study Group. Reduction of infarct size with the early use of timolol in acute myocardial infarction. N Engl J Med 1984;310:9.

79. The CAPRICORN Investigators. Effect of carvedilol on outcome after myocardial infarction in patients with left-ventricular dysfunction: the CAPRICORN randomised trial. Lancet 2001; 357:1385.

80. Norris D et al. Prevention of ventricular fibrillation during acute myocardial infarction by intravenous propranolol. Lancet 1984;8408:883.

81. The International Collaborative Study Group. Reduction of infarct size with the early use of timolol in acute myocardial infarction. N Engl J Med 1984;310:9.

82. Kjekshus J et al. Diabetic patients and β-blockers after acute myocardial infarction. Eur Heart J 1990;11:43.

83. Gottlieb SS et al. Effect of β-blockade on mortality among high-risk and low-risk patients after myocardial infarction. N Engl J Med 1998;339:489.

84. Shub C. Stable angina pectoris: Part 3. Medical treatment. Mayo Clin Proc 1990;65:256.

85. Conti CR. The stunned and hibernating myocardium: a brief review. Clin Cardiol 1991;14:708.

86. Flaherty JT. Role of nitrates in acute myocardial infarction. Am J Cardiol 1992;70(Suppl. 8):73B.

87. Nicolini F et al. Concurrent nitroglycerin therapy impairs tissue-type plasminogen activator-induced thrombolysis in patients with acute myocardial infarction. Am J Cardiol 1994;74:662.

88. Romeo F et al. Concurrent nitroglycerin administration reduces the efficacy of recombinant tissue-type plasminogen activator in patients with acute anterior wall myocardial infarction. Am Heart J 1995; 130:692.

89. Ferguson JJ et al. Significance of nitroglycerin-induced hypotension with inferior wall acute myocardial infarction. Am J Cardiol 1989;64:311.

90. Chiariello M et al. Comparison between the effects of nitroprusside and nitroglycerin on ischemic injury during acute myocardial infarction. Circulation 1976;54:766.

91. Mann T et al. Effect of nitroprusside on regional myocardial blood flow in coronary artery disease. Circulation 1978;57:732.

92. Rosenthal ME et al. Sudden cardiac death following acute myocardial infarction. Am Heart J 1985;109:865.

93. Bigger JT et al. The relationships among ventricular arrhythmias, left ventricular dysfunction, and mortality in the 2 years after myocardial infarction. Circulation 1984;69:250.

94. Teo KK et al. Effects of prophylactic antiarrhythmic drug therapy in acute myocardial infarction. An overview of results from randomized controlled trials. JAMA 1993;270:1589.

95. Burkart F et al. Effect of antiarrhythmic therapy on mortality in survivors of myocardial infarction with asymptomatic complex ventricular arrhythmias: Basel antiarrhythmic study of infarct survival (BASIS). J Am Coll Cardiol 1990;16:1711.

96. Pfisterer ME et al. Long-term benefit of 1-year amiodarone treatment for persistent complex ventricular arrhythmias after myocardial infarction. Circulation 1993;87:309.

97. Ceremuzynski L et al. Effect of amiodarone on mortality after myocardial infarction: a double-blind, placebo-controlled, pilot study. J Am Coll Cardiol 1992;20:1056.

98. Cairns JA et al. Randomised trial of outcome after myocardial infarction in patients with frequent repetitive ventricular premature depolarisations: CAMIAT. Lancet 1997;439:675.

99. Julian DG et al. Randomised trial of effect of amiodarone on mortality in patients with left-ventricular dysfunction after recent myocardial infarction: EMIAT. Lancet 1997;439:667.

100. Elizari MV et al. Morbidity and mortality following early administration of amiodarone in acute myocardial infarction. Eur Heart J 2000;21:198.

101. McClements BM, Adgey AAJ. Value of signal-averaged electrocardiography, radionuclide ventriculography, Holter monitoring and clinical variables for prediction of arrhythmic events in survivors of acute myocardial infarction in the thrombolytic era. J Am Coll Cardiol 1993;21:1419.

102. ACC/AHA Practice Guidelines. ACC/AHA 2002 Update for the Management of Patients with Unstable Angina and Non-ST-Segment Elevation Myocardial Infarction. Found at: http: acc.org/clinical/guidelines.unstable.pdf. Accessed March 1, 2003.

103. Steinhubl S et al. Early and sustained dual oral antiplatelet therapy following percutaneous coronary intervention. JAMA 2002;288:2411.

104. Turpie AGG, Antman EM. Low-molecular-weight heparins in the treatment of acute coronary syndromes. Arch Intern Med 2001;161:1484.

105. Cohen M et al. A comparison of low-molecular-weight heparin with unfractionated heparin for unstable coronary artery disease. N Engl J Med 1997;337:447.

106. Antman EM et al. Enoxaparin prevents death and cardiac ischemic events in unstable angina/non to Q-wave myocardial infarction: Results of the Thrombolysis In Myocardial Infarction (TIMI) 11B Trial. Circulation 1999;100:1593.

107. Wong GC et al. Use of low-molecular-weight heparins in the management of acute coronary artery syndromes and percutaneous coronary intervention. JAMA 2003;289:31.

108. The GUSTO-IV-ACS Investigators. Effect of glycoprotein IIb/IIIa receptor blocker abciximab on outcome in patients with acute coronary syndromes without early coronary revascularization: the GUSTO-IV-ACS trial. Lancet 2001;357:1915.

109. The EPIC Investigators. Use of monoclonal antibody directed against the platelet glycoprotein IIb/IIIa receptor in high-risk coronary angioplasty. N Engl J Med 1994;330:956.

110. Topol E et al. Long-term protection from myocardial ischemic events in a randomized trial of brief integrin β3 blockade with percutaneous coronary intervention. JAMA 1997;278:479.

111. The EPILOG Investigators. Platelet glycoprotein IIb/IIIa receptor blockade and low dose heparin during percutaneous coronary revascularization. N Engl J Med 1997;336:1689.

112. The PRISM Investigators. A comparison of aspirin plus tirofiban with aspirin plus heparin for unstable angina. N Engl J Med 1998;378:1498.

113. The PRISM PLUS Investigators. Inhibition of the platelet glycoprotein IIb/IIIa receptor with tirofiban in unstable angina and non-Q-wave myocardial infarction. N Engl J Med 1998;378:1488.

114. The PURSUIT Trial Investigators. Inhibition of platelet glycoprotein IIb/IIIa with eptifibatide in patients with acute coronary syndromes. N Engl J Med 1998;339:436.

115. The ESPRIT Investigators. Novel dosing regimen of eptifibatide in planned coronary stent implantation (ESPRIT): a randomized, placebo-controlled trial. Lancet 2000;356:2037.

116. O'Shea JC et al. Platelet glycoprotein IIb/IIIa integrin blockade with eptifibatide in coronary stent intervention. The ESPRIT trial; a randomized controlled trial. JAMA 2001;285:2468.

117. Pfeffer JM. Progressive ventricular dilatation in experimental myocardial infarction and its attenuation by angiotensin-converting enzyme inhibition. Am J Cardiol 1991;68(Suppl.):17D.

118. Braunwald E, Pfeffer MA. Ventricular enlargement and remodeling following acute myocardial infarction: mechanisms and management. Am J Cardiol 1991;68(Suppl.):1D.

119. The Acute Infarction Ramipril Efficacy (AIRE) Study Investigators. The effect of ramipril on mortality and morbidity of survivors of acute myocardial infarction with clinical evidence of heart failure. Lancet 1993; 342:821.

120. Gruppo Italiano per lo Studio della Sopravvivenza nell'Infarto Miocardico. GISSI-3: effects of lisinopril and transdermal glyceryl trinitrate singly and together on 6-week mortality and ventricular function after acute myocardial infarction. Lancet 1994;343:1115.

121. Brown NJ, Vaughan DE. Angiotensin-converting enzyme inhibitors. Circulation 1998;97;1411.

122. Lewis EJ et al. The effect of angiotensin-converting-enzyme inhibition on diabetic nephropathy. N Engl J Med 1993;329:1456.

123. OPTIMAAL Steering Committee. Effects of losartan and captopril on mortality and morbidity in high-risk patients after acute myocardial infarction: the OPTIMAAL randomised trial. Lancet 2002;360:752.

124. Yusuf S et al. Update on effects of calcium antagonists in myocardial infarction or angina in light of the second Danish Verapamil Infarction Trial (DAVIT-II) and other recent studies. Am J Cardiol 1991;67:1295.

125. Packer M et al. Effect of amlodipine on morbidity and mortality in severe chronic heart failure (PRAISE). N Engl J Med 1996;335:1107.

126. Rosenson RS. Myocardial injury: the acute phase response and lipoprotein metabolism. J Am Coll Cardiol 1993;22:993.

127. Mosca L et al. Hormone replacement therapy and cardiovascular disease: a statement for healthcare professionals from the American Heart Association. Circulation 2001;104:499.

128. Cairns JA et al. Antithrombotic agents in coronary artery disease. Fifth ACCP Consensus Conference on Antithrombotic Therapy. Chest 1998;114 (Suppl.):611S.

129. Final report on the aspirin component of the ongoing Physicians' Health Study. N Engl J Med 1989;321:129.

130. Ridker PM et al. Low-dose aspirin therapy for chronic stable angina. Ann Intern Med 1991; 114:835.

131. Kaplan K. Prophylactic anticoagulation following acute myocardial infarction. Arch Intern Med 1986;146:593.

132. Hurlen M et al. Warfarin, aspirin, or both after myocardial infarction. N Engl J Med 2002; 347:696.

133. Es RFV et al. Aspirin and coumadin after acute coronary syndromes (the ASPECT-2 study): a randomised controlled trial. Lancet 2002;360:109.

134. Fuster V et al. Aspirin as a therapeutic agent in cardiovascular disease. Circulation 1993;87:659.

135. CAPRIE Steering Committee. A randomised, blinded, trial of clopidogrel versus aspirin in patients at risk of ischaemia events (CAPRIE). Lancet 1996;348:1329.

136. Cannon P. Effectives of clopidogrel versus aspirin in preventing acute myocardial infarction in patients with symptomatic atherothrombosis (CAPRIE trial). Am J Cardiol 2002;90:760.

137. Rosenburg L et al. The risk of myocardial infarction after quitting smoking in men under 55 years of age. N Engl J Med 1985;313:1511.

Heart Failure

Wayne A. Kradjan

Continues

INTRODUCTION

The descriptive terminology, diagnostic techniques, and treatment of heart failure (HF) have undergone significant change in the past 15 to 20 years. Since 1994, a series of consensus and evidence-based practice guidelines have been published in an effort to standardize HF management. The first was from an expert panel appointed by the Agency for Health Care Policy and Research (AHCPR) and the RAND Corporation.[1] At about the same time, the American College of Cardiology (ACC)/ American Heart Association (AHA) Task Force on Practice Guidelines published their initial recommendations.[2] The recommendations from both groups were remarkably similar and included three key principles: differentiation of HF into systolic and diastolic dysfunction, recommendation of ejection fraction measurement to determine type of HF, and establishing angiotensin-converting enzyme (ACE) inhibitors as the gold standard for the treatment of HF. The Heart Failure Society of America (HFSA) Guidelines and Consensus Recommendations by the Advisory Council to Improve Outcomes Nationwide in Heart Failure (ACTION HF) were released in 1999.[3,4] Important additions from these later guidelines include recommendation of β-adrenergic blockers for all patients with New York Heart Association (NYHA) class II and III HF and use of low-dose spironolactone (Aldactone) in class IV HF. The ACC/AHA guidelines were updated in 2001 affirming the HFSA and ACTION HF recommendations, adding new severity staging definitions, and broadening the role of β-adrenergic blockers.[5] It is highly recommended that the reader continue to monitor the release of newer guidelines and retain a copy of the latest recommendations. Two other excellent reviews have also been published.[6,7]

Epidemiology of Heart Failure

Heart failure "is a complex clinical syndrome that can result from any structural or functional cardiac disorder that impairs the ability of the ventricle to fill with or eject blood."[5] As a consequence the heart fails to pump sufficient blood to meet the body's metabolic needs. "The cardinal manifestations of HF are dyspnea (breathlessness) and fatigue which may limit exercise tolerance, and fluid retention which may lead to pulmonary congestion and peripheral edema."[5] Congestive heart failure (CHF) is a specific subset of HF characterized by left ventricular systolic dysfunction and volume excess presenting as an enlarged, blood-congested heart. Because of wide variability in the causes and clinical presentation of HF, it is recommended that the term congestive heart failure be abandoned.

It is estimated that 4.8 to 5 million people in the United States (1.5% to 2% of the population) have HF.[1-11] HF is the number one discharge diagnosis in the Medicare population, with more Medicare dollars spent for the diagnosis and treatment of HF than for any other diagnosis.[8,10] During the past 10 years the annual number of hospitalizations for HF as a primary diagnosis has increased from approximately 550,000 to nearly 900,000 and from 1.7 to 2.6 million for HF as a primary or secondary diagnosis.[12]

The incidence of HF correlates both with gender and age; the incidence is nearly twice as high in men as in women. After the age of 50, the prevalence doubles during each decade of life, with 0.8% of those age 50 to 59 and 6% to 10% of those between age 65 and 80 being afflicted.[13] Although there has been a slight decline in the incidence of HF in women during the past decade, the incidence in men has remained stable over the past 50 years.[14] More aggressive treatment of hypertension may have contributed to the lower incidence of HF in some populations, while improved survival after myocardial infarction (MI) may leave others at greater risk of developing post-infarction HF. As the size of the geriatric population increases, HF likely will become a more frequently encountered clinical entity.

Quality of life is adversely affected by progressive functional disability. Of greater consequence is the high mortality rate. Mortality rates increase with symptom severity; 30% to 50% will die within 1 year, reaching as high as 80% in 5 years.[9-11,15,16] In the most recent Framingham study reporting on patients with a new diagnosis of HF in 1990–1999, 5-year survival rates were lower in men (41%) than in women (55%).[14] Despite earlier diagnosis and aggressive medical management, the prognosis is poor. Only with the advent of ACE inhibitor and β-blocker therapy have mortality rates been reduced, although not universal to all patients. Even in survivors, quality of life continues to deteriorate.[17]

Etiology

Low Output Versus High-Output Failure

Traditionally, HF has been described as being either *low-output* or *high-output failure,* with a predominance (>90%) of cases being low-output failure (Table 19-1). In both types, the heart cannot provide adequate blood flow (tissue perfusion) to meet the body's metabolic demands, especially during exercise. The hallmark of classic low-output HF is a diminished volume of blood being pumped by a weakened heart in patients who have otherwise normal metabolic needs.

In high-output failure, the heart itself is healthy and pumps a normal or even higher than normal volume of blood. However, because of high metabolic demands caused by other underlying medical disorders (e.g., hyperthyroidism, anemia), the heart becomes exhausted from the increased workload and

Table 19-1 **Classification and Etiology of Left Ventricular Dysfunction**

Type of Failure	Characteristics	Contributing Factors	Etiology
Low output, systolic dysfunction (dilated cardiomyopathy)[a] (60% to 70% of cases)	Hypofunctioning left ventricle; enlarged heart (dilated left ventricle); ↑ left ventricular end-diastolic volume; EF <40%; ↓ stroke volume; ↓ CO; S_3 heart sound present	1. ↓ contractility (cardiomyopathy) 2. ↑ afterload (elevated SVR)	1. Coronary ischemia,[b] MI, mitral valve stenosis or regurgitation, alcoholism, viral syndromes, nutritional deficiency, calcium and potassium depletion, drug induced, idiopathic 2. Hypertension, aortic stenosis, volume overload
Low output, diastolic dysfunction (30% to 40% of cases)	Normal left ventricular contractility; normal size heart; stiff left ventricle; impaired left ventricular relaxation; impaired left ventricular filling; ↓ left ventricular end-diastolic volume; normal EF; ↓ SV; ↓ CO; exaggerated S_4 heart sound	1. Thickened left ventricle (hypertrophic cardiomyopathy) 2. Stiff left ventricle (restrictive cardiomyopathy) 3. ↑ preload	1. Coronary ischemia,[b] MI hypertension, aortic stenosis and regurgitation, pericarditis, enlarged left ventricular septum (hypertrophic cardiomyopathy) 2. Amyloidosis, sarcoidosis 3. Sodium and water retention
High-output failure (uncommon)	Normal or ↑ contractility; normal size heart; normal left ventricular end-diastolic volume; normal or ↑ EF; normal or increased stroke volume; ↑ CO	↑ metabolic and oxygen demands	Anemia and hyperthyroidism

[a]Same as congestive heart failure if symptoms also present.
[b]Heart failure caused by coronary artery ischemia or myocardial infarction classified as "ischemic" etiology. All other types combined as "nonischemic."
CO, cardiac output; EF, ejection fraction; K, potassium; MI, myocardial infarction; SV, stroke volume; SVR, systemic vascular resistance.

eventually cannot keep up with demand. The primary treatment of high-output HF is amelioration of the underlying disease. The remainder of this chapter focuses on the treatment of low-output HF.

Left Versus Right Ventricular Dysfunction

Simple classification of HF as being low-output failure does not adequately describe the complex nature of this disorder. Consequently, low-output HF is further divided into left and right ventricular dysfunction, or a combination of the two (biventricular failure). Because the left ventricle is the major pumping chamber of the heart, it is not surprising that *left ventricular dysfunction* is the most common form of low-output HF and the major target for pharmacologic intervention. Right ventricular dysfunction may coexist with left ventricular HF if damage is sustained by both sides of the heart (e.g., after MI) or as a delayed complication of progressive left-sided HF (see Question 1).

Isolated right-sided ventricular dysfunction is relatively uncommon and is usually caused by either primary or secondary *pulmonary arterial hypertension* (PAH). In these conditions, elevated pulmonary artery pressure impedes emptying of the right ventricle, thus increasing the workload on the right side of the heart.[18,19] Primary PAH is idiopathic, caused by stenosis or spasm of the pulmonary artery of unknown etiology. Secondary causes include collagen vascular disorders, sarcoidosis, fibrosis, exposure to high altitude, drug and chemical exposure, and cor pulmonale. Drug-induced sources include opioid overdoses (especially heroin), pulmonary fibrosis caused by intravenous (IV) injection of poorly soluble forms of methylphenidate (e.g., IV drug users injecting partially dissolved Ritalin tablets), and as a complication of dexfenfluramine (Redux) or the combination of phentermine and fenfluramine (Phen-Fen) used for weight loss. Cor pulmonale is defined as pulmonary hypertension, and secondary right-sided failure as a complication of chronic obstructive pulmonary disease (COPD).

Systolic Versus Diastolic Dysfunction; Ischemic Versus Nonischemic Heart Failure

Left ventricular dysfunction is further subdivided into systolic and diastolic dysfunction, with mixed disorders also being encountered (Table 19-1). In both forms, the *stroke volume* (SV) (i.e., the volume of blood ejected by the heart with each systolic contraction; normal, 60 to 130 mL) and the subsequent 1-minute *cardiac output* (CO) (i.e., SV × heart rate; normal, 4 to 7 L/min) are reduced. In diagnosing HF, a critical marker differentiating systolic from diastolic dysfunction is the *left ventricular ejection fraction* (LVEF), defined as the percentage of left ventricular end-diastolic volume expelled during each systolic contraction (normal, 60% to 70%).

In *systolic dysfunction,* the LVEF is <40%, dropping to <20% in advanced HF. Thus, systolic dysfunction is synonymous with low ejection fraction (EF) heart failure and is almost always caused by factors causing the heart to fail as a pump (decreased myocardial muscle contractility). The heart dilates as it becomes congested with retained blood, leading to an enlarged hypokinetic left ventricle.

HF caused by damage to heart muscle or valves because of chronic coronary ischemia or after MI is classified as *ischemic,* with all other types grouped as *nonischemic.* Coronary artery disease is the cause of HF in approximately two thirds of patients with left ventricular systolic dysfunction. Other causes of left ventricular pump failure include persistent arrhythmias, post-Streptococcal rheumatic heart disease, chronic alcoholism (alcoholic cardiomyopathy), viral infections, or unidentified etiology (idiopathic dilated cardiomyopathy.) Chronic hypertension, and certain cardiac valvular disorders (aortic or mitral stenosis), also precipitate systolic HF by increasing resistance to CO (i.e., a high afterload state).

In contrast, *left ventricular diastolic dysfunction* is synonymous with *normal ejection fraction HF*.[20-25] In this form of HF, cardiac muscle function (contractility) is *not* impaired and, most importantly, the EF remains >40% to 45%. However, the SV and CO are still reduced because the end-diastolic ventricular volume is less than normal. In simple terms, a high fraction of a low volume is ejected. Possible causes for diastolic failure include coronary ischemia, long standing uncontrolled hypertension, left ventricular wall scarring after an MI, ventricular wall hypertrophy, hypertrophic cardiomyopathy (formerly known as idiopathic hypertrophic subaortic stenosis), constrictive pericarditis, restrictive cardiomyopathy (e.g., amyloidosis and sarcoidosis), and valvular heart disease (mitral stenosis, acute aortic regurgitation, mitral regurgitation). These factors lead to left ventricular stiffness (reduced wall compliance) and/or an inability of the ventricle to relax during diastole, both of which result in an elevated resting pressure within the ventricle despite a relatively low volume of blood in the chamber. In turn, the elevated pressure impedes left ventricular filling during diastole that would normally occur by passive inflow against a low resistance pressure gradient. Heart size is usually (but not always) normal. To summarize, in diastolic dysfunction the EF is normal, but the SV and CO are deficient because of impaired ventricular filling and a relatively small left ventricular volume. It is estimated that 14% to 40% of patients with HF may have this form of disease.[1,5,20-25] Because coronary ischemia, MI, and hypertension are contributors to both systolic and diastolic failure, many patients have symptoms of a combined disorder.

The pathology of systolic dysfunction most closely resembles what has historically has been referred to as congestive heart failure; nevertheless, in the strictest sense, CHF only exists if the patient has both systolic dysfunction and the classic symptoms of HF. However, there is tremendous variability in the clinical presentation of both systolic and diastolic dysfunction, and both disorders can have essentially identical symptoms.[5,20] For example, some patients with either systolic or diastolic exhibit exercise intolerance, but have little evidence of fluid retention. Others may have significant edema with few complaints of exercise intolerance or shortness of breath. It is also possible to have no symptoms in the early stages of both forms of HF. For all these reasons, it is best to avoid the abbreviation *CHF,* especially since CHF has also been used to denote *chronic heart failure.* In the meantime, clinicians are strongly encouraged to obtain an EF measurement in all patients with suspected HF to help define the clinical state more fully.[1-5]

Some drugs used to treat systolic dysfunction, such as digoxin, can worsen symptoms in diastolic dysfunction. Conversely, negative inotropes (β-adrenergic blockers and calcium channel blockers) may be beneficial in diastolic dysfunction by slowing the heart and allowing the ventricles to fill more fully at low pressures.

Cardiac Workload

A common factor to all forms of HF is increased cardiac workload. Four major determinants contribute to left ventricular workload: preload, afterload, contractility, and heart rate (HR).

PRELOAD

Preload describes forces acting on the *venous* side of the circulation to affect myocardial wall tension. The relationship is as follows: as venous return (i.e., blood flowing into the heart) increases, the volume of blood in the left ventricle increases. The volume is maximal when filling finishes at the end of diastole (left ventricular end-diastolic volume [LVEDV]). This increased volume raises the pressure within the ventricle (left ventricular end-diastolic pressure [LVEDP]), which in turn increases the "stretch," or wall tension, of the ventricle. Peripheral venous dilation and decreased peripheral venous volume diminish preload, whereas peripheral venous constriction and increased peripheral venous volume increase preload.

Elevated preload can aggravate HF. For example, rapid administration of blood plasma expanders and osmotic diuretics or administration of large amounts of sodium (Na) or sodium-retaining agents can increase preload. A malfunctioning aortic valve (aortic stenosis, aortic insufficiency), resulting in regurgitation of blood back into the left ventricle, also can increase the volume of blood that must be pumped. A malfunctioning mitral valve (mitral regurgitation) may cause retrograde ejection of blood from the left ventricle back into the left atrium, with a resultant decrease in EF. In patients with systolic failure, ventricular blood is ejected less efficiently because of a hypofunctioning left ventricle; the volume of blood retained in the ventricle is thus increased, and preload becomes elevated. In diastolic failure with a stiffened left ventricle, relatively small increases in end-diastolic volume from sodium and water overload may lead to exaggerated increases in end-diastolic pressure despite normal or even reduced end-diastolic volumes.

AFTERLOAD

Afterload is the tension developed in the ventricular wall as contraction (systole) occurs. The tension developed during contraction is affected by intraventricular pressure, ventricular diameter, and wall thickness. More simply, afterload is regulated by the systemic vascular resistance (SVR) or impedance against which the ventricle must pump during its ejection and is chiefly determined by arterial blood pressure (BP). Hypertension, atherosclerotic disease, or a narrowed aortic valve opening increase arterial impedance (afterload), thereby increasing the workload on the heart. Hypertension is a major etiologic factor in the development of both systolic and diastolic HF. The Framingham group found that 75% of patients who developed HF had a history of hypertension.[11,13] The risk of developing HF was six times greater for hypertensive than for normotensive patients.

CARDIAC CONTRACTILITY

The terms *contractility* and *inotropic state* are used synonymously to describe the myocardium's (cardiac muscle's) inherent ability to develop force and/or shorten its fibers independent of preload or afterload. Myocardial contractility is decreased when myocardial fibers are diminished or poorly functioning as may occur in patients with primary cardiomyopathy, valvular heart disease, coronary artery disease, or following an MI. Defects in contractility play a major role in systolic HF, but are not a component of pure diastolic dysfunction. Occasionally, drugs such as nonselective β-adrenergic blockers or doxorubicin (Adriamycin) induce HF by decreasing myocardial contractility. (See Questions 4 and 5 for a more complete discussion of drug-induced HF.) As summarized in Table 19-1, the major contributors to systolic failure are decreased contractility and increased afterload, whereas structural abnormalities and increased preload play a greater role in diastolic failure.

HEART RATE

An increased heart rate is a reflex mechanism to improve CO as EF declines. As discussed below, the sympathetic nervous system is the major mediator of this response. Unfortunately, the workload and energy demands of a rapid heart rate ultimately place undo strain on the heart and can eventually worsen HF.

Pathogenesis

When the heart begins to fail, the body activates several complex compensatory mechanisms in an attempt to maintain CO and oxygenation of vital organs. These include increased sympathetic tone, activation of the renin-angiotensin-aldosterone system, sodium and water retention, other neurohormonal adaptations, and cardiac "remodeling" (ventricular dilation, cardiac hypertrophy, and changes in left ventricular lumen shape). Unfortunately, the long-term consequences of

these adaptive mechanisms can create more harm than good (Fig. 19-1). The relative balance of each of these adaptive processes may vary depending on the type of HF (systolic versus diastolic dysfunction) and even from patient to patient with the same type of disorder. An understanding of the potential benefits and adverse consequences of these compensatory mechanisms is essential to understanding the signs, symptoms, and treatment of HF.[26]

Sympathetic (Adrenergic) Nervous System

SV and/or CO are low in both systolic and diastolic left ventricular dysfunction, resulting in decreased tissue perfusion. The body's normal physiologic response to a decreased CO is generalized activation of the adrenergic (sympathetic) nervous system as evidenced by increased circulating levels of norepinephrine (NE) and other catecholamines. The inotropic (increased contractility) and chronotropic (increased HR) effects of NE initially maintain near-normal CO and preserve perfusion of vital organs such as the central nervous system (CNS) and myocardium. However, catecholamine-mediated vasoconstriction in the skin, gastrointestinal (GI) tract, and renal circulation decreases perfusion of these organs and ultimately increases the workload on the heart by increasing SVR. Other adverse consequences of NE activation include impaired sodium excretion by the kidneys, restricted ability of coronary arteries to supply blood to the ventricular wall (myocardial ischemia), increased automaticity of cardiac tissue to provoke arrhythmias, hypokalemia, and oxidative stress to trigger programmed cell death (apoptosis).[5]

In the long term, high levels of NE or its metabolites are potentially harmful to heart muscle because they decrease

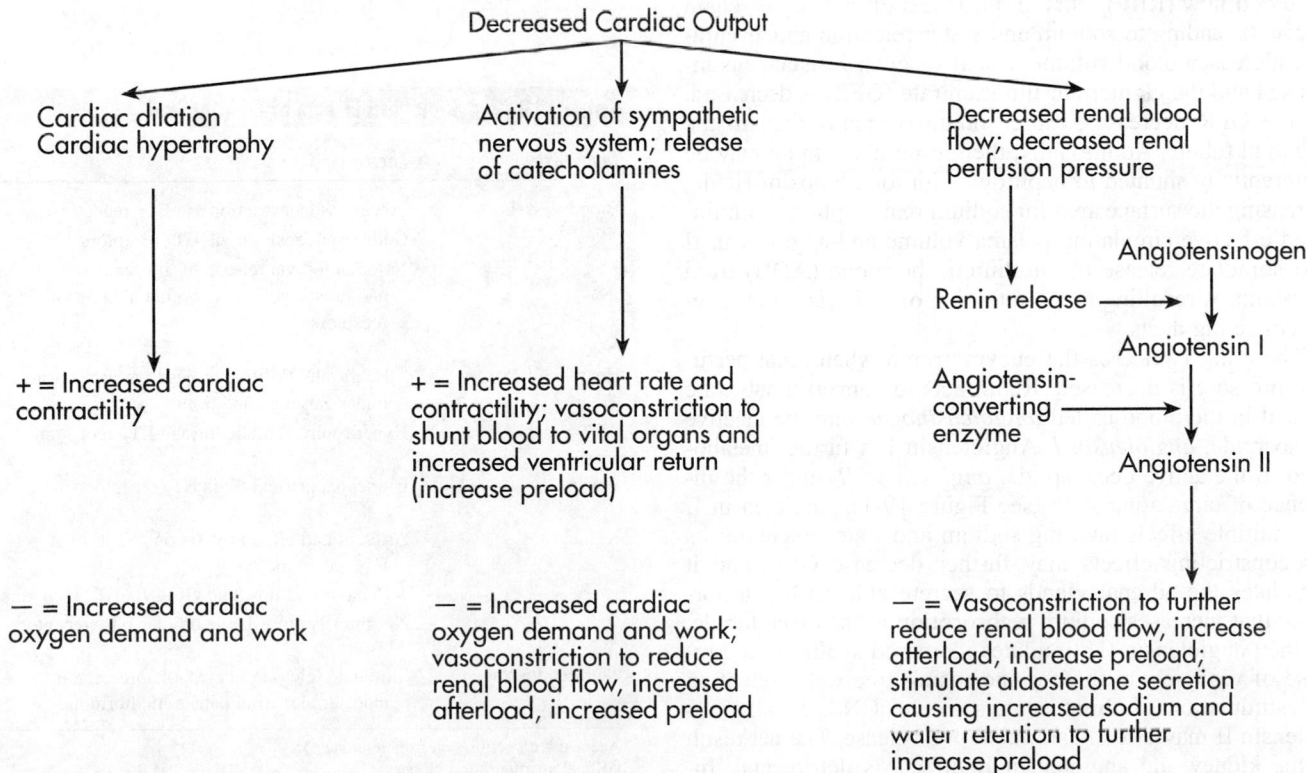

FIGURE 19-1 Adaptive mechanisms in systolic HF. +, beneficial results; −, negative (detrimental) effects.

β_1-receptor sensitivity and reduce β_1-receptor density on the surface of myocardial cells by as much as 60% to 70% in severe HF.[27–32] The normal ratio of β_1:β_2 receptors in the heart is 75–80:20–25. As a negative feedback response to overstimulation, this balance is shifted to a ratio of 60–70:30–40 in the failing myocardium by downregulation of β_1 subtype receptors. This selective downregulation of β_1-receptors is accompanied by a complex phenomenon of "uncoupling of the β_1- and β_2-receptor activity" whereby the number of β_2-receptors are unchanged and the responsiveness of these receptors in eliciting a response can be reduced by 30%.[27] Over time this leaves the myocyte less responsive to adrenergic stimuli and further decreases contractile function. At the same time, the post-synaptic α_1 subtype is upregulated in the failing heart resulting in cell growth (hypertrophy) and a positive inotropic effect. α_2 Receptors on the presynaptic side of the sympathetic nerve act to suppress NE release, providing a partial protective mechanism from adrenergic overstimulation.

Alterations in sympathetic adrenergic receptors in the heart during HF are complex and partially determined by genetic phenotype. Interestingly, among black patients with HF, there is a disproportionately high incidence of polymorphisms for variants of the β_1 receptor that are associated with increased function. Additionally, there is a variant of the α_2-receptor with defective response to adrenergic overstimulation. These combined defects are found less often in whites, perhaps partially explaining a higher incidence of HF in blacks. A better understanding of α- and β-receptor phenotyping may someday lead to improved prevention and treatment strategies for HF.[33]

Renal Function and the Renin-Angiotensin System
The combined actions of the decreased CO and vasoconstriction secondary to sympathetic tone in HF causes decreased renal blood flow (RBF). This, in turn, sets off a complex chain of events leading to sodium and water retention and, eventually, increased blood volume. Renal vascular resistance is increased and the glomerular filtration rate (GFR) is decreased. As the GFR decreases, more sodium is reabsorbed in the proximal tubule. Additionally, the glomerular filtrate may be preferentially shunted to nephrons with long loops of Henle, increasing the surface area for sodium reabsorption. A diminished effective circulating plasma volume and angiotensin II also stimulate release of antidiuretic hormone (ADH) from the pituitary, resulting in the retention of free water in the renal collecting ducts.

The kidney releases the enzyme renin when renal perfusion pressure is decreased. Renin acts to convert a substrate present in the blood called *angiotensinogen* into the inactive decapeptide, *angiotensin I*. Angiotensin I is further metabolized to the active decapeptide, *angiotensin II,* under the influence of circulating *ACE* (see Figure 19-1). Angiotensin II has multiple effects favoring sodium and water retention: its vasoconstricting effects may further decrease GFR, and it stimulates the adrenal glands to secrete aldosterone, a hormone that increases sodium reabsorption in the distal tubule. Further, angiotensin II stimulates increased synthesis and release of vasopressin, thereby increasing free water retention and stimulation of thirst centers in the CNS. Finally, angiotensin II may directly stimulate NE release. The net result of the kidney and angiotensin II effects is detrimental. Increased sodium and water retention increase preload, while

angiotensin II-induced vasoconstriction increases SVR and afterload.

Of further concern is recent evidence that angiotensin II and aldosterone can have other adverse effects that contribute to the pathophysiology of HF independent of their renal and electrolyte mechanisms.[34] These effects include coronary and vascular remodeling, endothelial cell and baroreceptor dysfunction, and inhibition of myocardial NE uptake. Morphologic studies indicate that a chronic excess of aldosterone (plus salt loading), as occurs in HF, can cause fibrosis in the atria and ventricles, kidneys, and other organs in animals and humans.[34] Thus, aldosterone may promote the remodeling of organs and fibrosis, independent of angiotensin II.

Other Hormonal Mediators
ENDOTHELINS
Several other regulatory hormones and cytokines have been identified as playing a role in the pathogenesis and/or adaptation to HF. The first of these are the endothelins, a family of 21 amino acid peptides.[35,36] Within this family, endothelin-1 (ET-1) is the most active. ET-1 was first isolated from vascular endothelial cells, but is also synthesized by vascular and airway smooth muscle, cardiomyocytes, leukocytes, and macrophages. Serum concentrations of ET-1 are elevated in HF, pulmonary hypertension, MI, ischemia, and shock and are implicated in causing vasoconstriction, potentiation of cardiac remodeling, and decreased renal blood flow and glomerular filtration. While these effects of ET-1 are detrimental in HF, its pharmacology is complex and dependent on the relative balance of two distinct G protein-coupled receptor subtypes referred to as ET_A and ET_B. As illustrated in Table 19-2, ET-1 can elicit opposing effects from each receptor, with the net effect being dependent on the relative density of the two receptors.

Table 19-2   Biological Effects of Endothelin-1

Organ System	Effect
Blood vessels	Potent vasoconstriction via ET_A receptors
	Collagen deposition via ET_A receptors
	Vasodilation via release of nitrous oxide and prostacyclin in endothelial cells via ET_B receptors
Heart	↑ Heart rate. Positive or negative inotropism under varying conditions
	Hypertrophy, remodeling via ET_A receptors
Lungs	Bronchoconstriction via ET_A receptors
Kidney	Afferent and efferent vasoconstriction via ET_A receptors
	↓ Renal blood flow and GFR via ET_A receptors
	Natriuresis, diuresis via tubular ET_B receptors
Neuroendocrine	Stimulate release of catecholamines, renin, aldosterone, atrial natriuretic hormone

Adapted with permission from reference 35.
GRF, glomerular filtration rate.

Synthesis of ET-I begins with a precursor protein called pre-proendothelin (PPET-1) and involves several enzymatic steps and intermediates. Key enzymes in its synthesis are dibasic specific endopeptidase, carboxypeptidase, and endothelin converting enzyme. Possible therapeutic implications of understanding this synthetic pathway are development of specific inhibitors of one or more of the enzymes to prevent activation of ET-1. Alternatively, selective inhibitors of ET_A receptors could shift responses toward the favorable aspects of ET_B receptor activation. Currently no such drugs exist, but bosentan (Tracleer) and tezosentan are investigational nonselective dual AT_A/ET_B antagonists. Bosentan has FDA approval for the treatment of pulmonary hypertension and is being investigated for use in HF.[18,19]

NATRIURETIC PEPTIDES

Natriuretic peptides are a family of peptides containing a common 17 amino acid ring. A-type natriuretic peptide (ANP), previously referred to as either atrial natriuretic peptide or atrial natriuretic factor, is secreted by the atrial myocardium in response to dilation and stretch. Similarly, B-type natriuretic peptide (BNP), formerly referred to as brain natriuretic peptide, is produced by the ventricular myocardium in response to elevations of end-diastolic pressure and volume. Type-C (CNP) is secreted by lung, kidney, and vascular endothelium in response to shear stress. Collectively, the natriuretic peptides have been referred to as "cardiac neurohormones" and are generally considered to be a favorable form of neurohormonal activation.[37] Among their positive attributes are antagonism of the renin-angiotensin system, inhibition of sympathetic outflow, and endothelin-1 antagonism. The net effect is peripheral and coronary vasodilation to decrease preload and afterload on the heart. As their name implies, they also have diuretic/natriuretic properties with improved renal blood flow and glomerular filtration resulting from afferent arteriolar dilation and possibly efferent arteriolar constriction. Sodium reabsorption is blocked in the collecting duct by virtue of an indirect aldosterone inhibition. Natriuretic peptides also inhibit vasopressin secretion from the pituitary gland and block "salt appetite" and thirst centers in the CNS. Each of these CNS effects contributes further to diuresis. Of note, Type-C has minimal diuretic properties.[37]

Earlier research on natriuretic peptides centered on ANP, but BNP is now receiving greater attention both for diagnostic and treatment purposes. Specifically, plasma level measurement of BNP is identified as a biologic marker for both the presence and severity of HF. BNP serum levels of greater than 200 pg/mL help to differentiate HF from other causes of dyspnea (e.g., chronic bronchitis) and edema. Moreover, the degree of elevation correlates with the severity of HF, with a mean plasma level of 241 pcg/mL in mild disease (NYHA class I patients) compared with 817 pcg/mL in severe disease (class IV patients).[38–40]

Possible therapeutic implications are synthesis of natriuretic hormone analogs or inhibitors of their metabolism as possible drug therapies. Nesiritide (Natrecor) is a recombinant produced human B-type natriuretic peptide approved by the FDA for IV management of acute HF exacerbations in hospitalized patients.[41, 42] Unfortunately, downregulation of natriuretic peptide receptors occurs during chronic HF, reducing the protective benefit of their actions and possibly limiting their usefulness as therapeutic entities.

Metabolism by neutral endopeptidase (NEP) and receptor sequestration are the primary modes of clearance of natriuretic peptides. NEP is a plasma membrane bound zinc-metalloprotease enzyme found primarily in renal tubular cells, but also in the lung, GI tract, adrenal gland, heart, brain, and peripheral vasculature. This enzyme also assists in the degradation/metabolism of bradykinin and possibly of angiotensin II. It is speculated that drugs formulated to inhibit NEP (and thus maintain protective natriuretic peptide levels) might have additive effects to ACE inhibitors in the treatment of HF and hypertension. On the other hand, administering a NEP inhibitor in the absence of a concurrent ACE inhibitor could theoretically be counterproductive by leaving unopposed angiotensin II activity.[37] As discussed in the next section, omapatrilat is a combined NEP/ACE inhibitor undergoing clinical trials. No selective NEP inhibitors are being actively investigated.

VASOPEPTIDASE INHIBITORS

Another class of drugs called vasopeptidase inhibitors have a dual action to block both ACE and NEP.[37,43,44] Drugs with this property can reduce the vasoconstrictor effects of angiotensin II and preserve the vasodilating action of endogenous natriuretic peptides and bradykinin. Omapatrilat is an investigational vasopeptidase inhibitor being evaluated for clinical use in hypertension and HF. The IMPRESS Investigators compared the effects of omapatrilat to lisinopril in 573 patients with NYHA class II–IV HF, an EF <40%, and previously stabilization with an ACE inhibitor.[43] Target doses were 40 mg and 20 mg daily for omapatrilat and lisinopril, respectively. At the end of 24 weeks, there was no difference in the primary endpoint of maximum exercise treadmill test time between the two drugs. However, there was a trend in favor of omapatrilat for the combined endpoint of death or hospitalization for worsening HF (5% versus 9%; $P = 0.052$). Diarrhea, nausea, and vomiting were more common with omapatrilat, but serious adverse events involving the cardiovascular system were less common in patients receiving omapatrilat (7%) compared to lisinopril 12%; ($P = 0.04$). Increases in serum creatinine also occurred less with omapatrilat (1.8%) than with lisinopril (6.1%; $P = 0.009$). The similarly designed OVERTURE trial compared enalapril 10 mg BID (N = 2,884) to omapatrilat 40 mg QD (N = 2,886). The primary endpoint of the combined risk of death or HF-related hospitalization was not different between the two drugs, although there was a trend for fewer deaths in the omapatrilat-treated patients. The overall incidence of side effects was similar in both groups, but more omapatrilat-treated patients developed angioedema. This was especially evident in black patients with an incidence of 5.5% for omapatrilat compared with 1.6% with enalapril.[44]

INFLAMMATORY CYTOKINES, INTERLEUKINS, TISSUE NECROSIS FACTOR, PROSTACYCLIN, AND NITROUS OXIDE

Vascular endothelial cells release various other proinflammatory cytokines, vasodilator, and vasoconstrictor substances, including interleukin cytokines (IL-1β, IL-2, IL-6), tissue necrosis factor (TNF-α), prostacyclin, and nitrous oxide (NO) (also known as endothelium-derived relaxing factor).[45–47] The exact role of these mediators in the pathogenesis of HF is unclear. Recent studies have shown that patients with HF have elevated levels of the proinflammatory cytokines

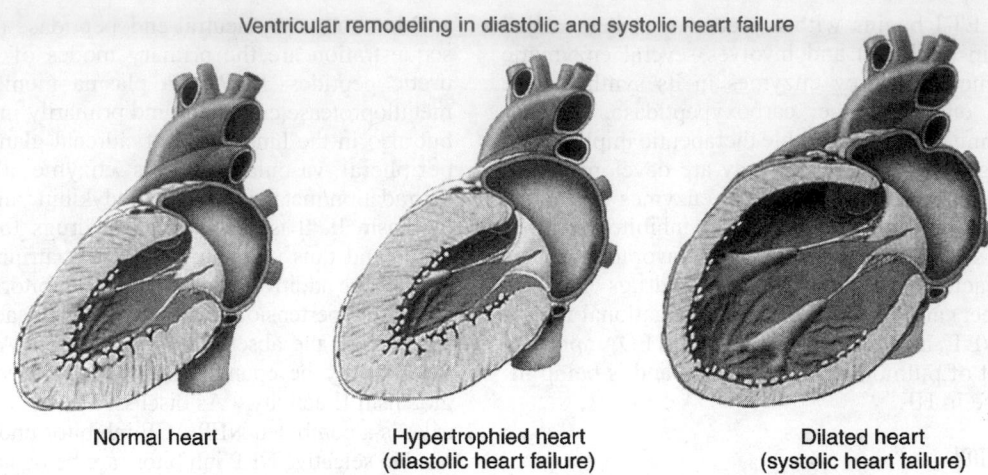

Ventricular remodeling in diastolic and systolic heart failure

Normal heart

Hypertrophied heart
(diastolic heart failure)

Dilated heart
(systolic heart failure)

FIGURE 19-2 Cardiac remodeling. (Reprinted with permission from Jessup M, Brozena S. Medical progress: heart failure. N Engl J Med 2003;348:2007. Copyright 2003 Massachusetts Medical Society. All rights reserved.)

IL-1β, IL-6, and TNF-α that correlate with the severity of disease.[47–49] Initial enthusiasm for use of the TNF-α receptor antagonist etanercept (Enbrel) as a treatment of HF has been abandoned after disappointing results in larger phase 2 and 3 clinical trials.[50] Of even greater concern is at least 47 spontaneous adverse event reports to the FDA describing new onset HF or exacerbation of existing HF with etanercept and infliximab in patients being treated for either Crohns disease or rheumatoid arthritis.[51]

Other investigators have tried using either NO or prostacyclin (epoprostenol) as therapeutic vasodilators with mixed success.[52–54] A particular concern with prostacyclin was a trend toward increased death rates despite an improved hemodynamic status in treated patients during the Flolan International Randomized Survival Trial (FIRST).[54]

Cardiac Remodeling

Progression of HF results in a process referred to as *cardiac remodeling,* characterized by changes in the shape and mass of the ventricles in response to tissue injury.[6–8] The three primary manifestations of cardiac remodeling are chamber dilation, left ventricular cardiac muscle hypertrophy, and a resulting spherical shape of the left ventricular chamber (Fig. 19-2) Cardiac remodeling starts months to years before the appearance of clinical symptoms and contributes to the progression of the disease despite treatment.

CARDIAC DILATION

Cardiac dilation results when the ventricles fail to pump an adequate volume of blood with each contraction. This is most evident in systolic dysfunction. If the rate at which blood is delivered to the heart (preload) remains the same, but the rate at which it is pumped to other tissues diminishes, residual blood will begin to accumulate in the ventricles. Thus, end-diastolic volume increases, myocardial fibers are stretched, and the ventricle(s) become dilated. In the normal heart, the end-diastolic volume is about 180 to 200 mL. With an EF of 60%, the SV is approximately 100 mL, leaving an end-systolic residual volume in the ventricle of 80 to 100 mL. Early in HF, a near normal SV of 100 mL is maintained, although

the EF may be low (e.g., 33%). Unfortunately, this leaves a 200- to 300-mL end-systolic residual volume in the ventricle. Over time, an enlarged heart will become evident on a chest radiograph, and the body cannot completely compensate. Cardiac dilation is less evident in diastolic dysfunction because normal contractility is maintained and the stiffened left ventricle is resistant to filling and not likely to enlarge (see Fig. 19-2).

FRANK–STARLING CURVE

The Frank-Starling ventricular function curve (Fig. 19-3) implies a curvilinear relationship between left ventricular myocardial muscle fiber "stretch" (wall tension) and myocardial work. As stretch increases, the volume of blood ejected with each systolic contraction (stroke volume) increases. In systolic HF, the work capacity for any degree of stretch is diminished. A simple analogy is drawn using a balloon. The greater amount of air blown into a balloon, the more it stretches and, if released, the farther it flies around a room. As the balloon gets old, it loses its elasticity and thus has less recoil when stretched. Similarly, dilation of the ventricles initially may serve as an effective compensating mechanism in systolic failure, but it becomes inadequate as the elastic limits of the myocardial muscle fibers are reached. HR may also increase to maintain CO if SV is low. The downside of cardiac

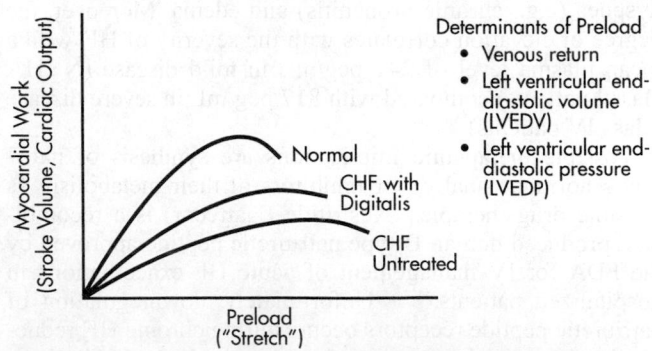

Determinants of Preload
• Venous return
• Left ventricular end-diastolic volume (LVEDV)
• Left ventricular end-diastolic pressure (LVEDP)

Myocardial Work (Stroke Volume, Cardiac Output)

Normal

CHF with Digitalis

CHF Untreated

Preload ("Stretch")

FIGURE 19-3 Representation of Frank-Starling ventricular function curve.

dilation is increased myocardial oxygen demand. Theoretically, as cardiac dilation progresses beyond a certain point, CO could decrease (as visualized on the descending limb of the Starling Curve), but this rarely is observed clinically.

CARDIAC HYPERTROPHY

Cardiac hypertrophy is a long-term adaptation to increased diastolic volume in systolic failure and represents an absolute increase in myocardial muscle mass and muscle wall thickness (Fig. 19-2) This is somewhat analogous to increased muscle mass in skeletal muscle in response to weight lifting or other forms of exercise. Cardiac hypertrophy should not be confused with cardiac dilation. Of the two, hypertrophy provides more desirable effects, but its absolute benefit is inadequate in severe disease.

Functional Limitation Classification and Stages of Heart Failure (Table 19-3)

NEW YORK HEART ASSOCIATION CLASSIFICATION

The New York Heart Association (NYHA) classification scheme identifies four categories of functional disability associated with HF.[55] Class I patients are well compensated with no physical limitations and lack symptoms with ordinary physical activity. In class II, ordinary physical activity results in mild enhancement of symptoms and imparts slight limitations on exercise tolerance. Class III patients are comfortable only at rest; even less than ordinary physical activity leads to symptoms. In class IV, symptoms of HF are present at rest and no physical activity can be undertaken without symptoms. Determination of class placement for a specific patient is highly subjective and will vary between observers. In some cases, subdivisions such as class III_A or III_B may be used to further individualize grading of severity.

A shortcoming of the NYHA classification scheme is that it does not include asymptomatic individuals who are at high risk for developing HF and who may benefit from preemptive lifestyle changes and drug therapy. The 2001 ACC/AHA Practice Guidelines introduced a new staging algorithm that can be used in conjunction with the NYHA classifications.[5] Stage A patients have hypertension, coronary artery disease, diabetes mellitus, or other conditions that, if left untreated, can result in the development of overt HF. HF symptoms or identifiable abnormalities of the myocardium or heart valves are absent in Stage A. Stage B patients remain asymptomatic but have structural defects within the heart (e.g., left ventricular hypertrophy, dilation, or valve disease) that indicate the existence of impending HF. Stage C patients exhibit varying degrees of HF symptoms corresponding to NYHA classes I–III along with structural changes in the heart consistent with systolic or diastolic HF. Stage D in the ACA/AHA scheme roughly correlates to NYHA class IV. Patients in this latter category are frequently hospitalized, dependent on IV therapy, and could be considered to have end stage disease. Table 19-3 summarizes these two classification schemes and how they overlap.

Treatment Principles

The 2001 American College of Cardiology (ACC)/American Heart Association (AHA) Task Force Practice Guidelines along with those of the Advisory Council to Improve Outcomes Nationwide in Heart Failure (ACTION HF) serve as the primary basis for recommendations within this chapter.[4,5] A clinical algorithm adapted from the 1994 AHCPR guidelines and updated with the 2001 recommendations is found in Figure 19-4.[1,5] The ACC/AHH Task Force recommends that most patients with HF should be routinely managed with a combination of four types of drugs: a diuretic, an ACE inhibitor, a β-adrenergic blocker, and (usually) digitalis.[5] An aldosterone antagonist (e.g., spironolactone) is a fifth class of drug recommended for patients with advanced HF.

The objectives of therapy for all forms of HF are to abolish disabling symptoms, avoid complications such as arrhythmias, and improve the quality of the patient's life. Increased walking distance during a 6-minute treadmill test or

---

Table 19-3   American College of Cardiology-American Heart Association (ACC/AHA) Staging and New York Heart Association (NYHA) Classification of Heart Failure.

ACA-AHA Stage	NYHA Functional Class
A. At high risk for heart failure, but without structural heart disease (normal heart exam) or symptoms of heart failure (e.g., patients with hypertension, coronary heart disease, diabetes, alcoholism, or strong family history)	No corresponding category
B. Structural heart disease present (e.g., LV hypertrophy, dilation, fibrosis, old MI), but without symptoms of heart failure	I. Asymptomatic or no limitations on normal physical activity, but symptoms with strenuous exercise.
C. Structural heart disease with prior or current symptoms of heart failure	II. Symptoms of heart failure with normal activity or with moderate exertion
	III. Symptomatic with minimal exertion; marked limitations in physical activity including activities of daily life (e.g., bathing, dressing)
	IV (or IIIB). Symptoms of heart failure at rest.
D. Refractory heart failure requiring specialized interventions	IV (or IVB). Symptoms of heart failure at rest and requiring hospitalization or intravenous inotropic support

Adapted with permission from reference 29.

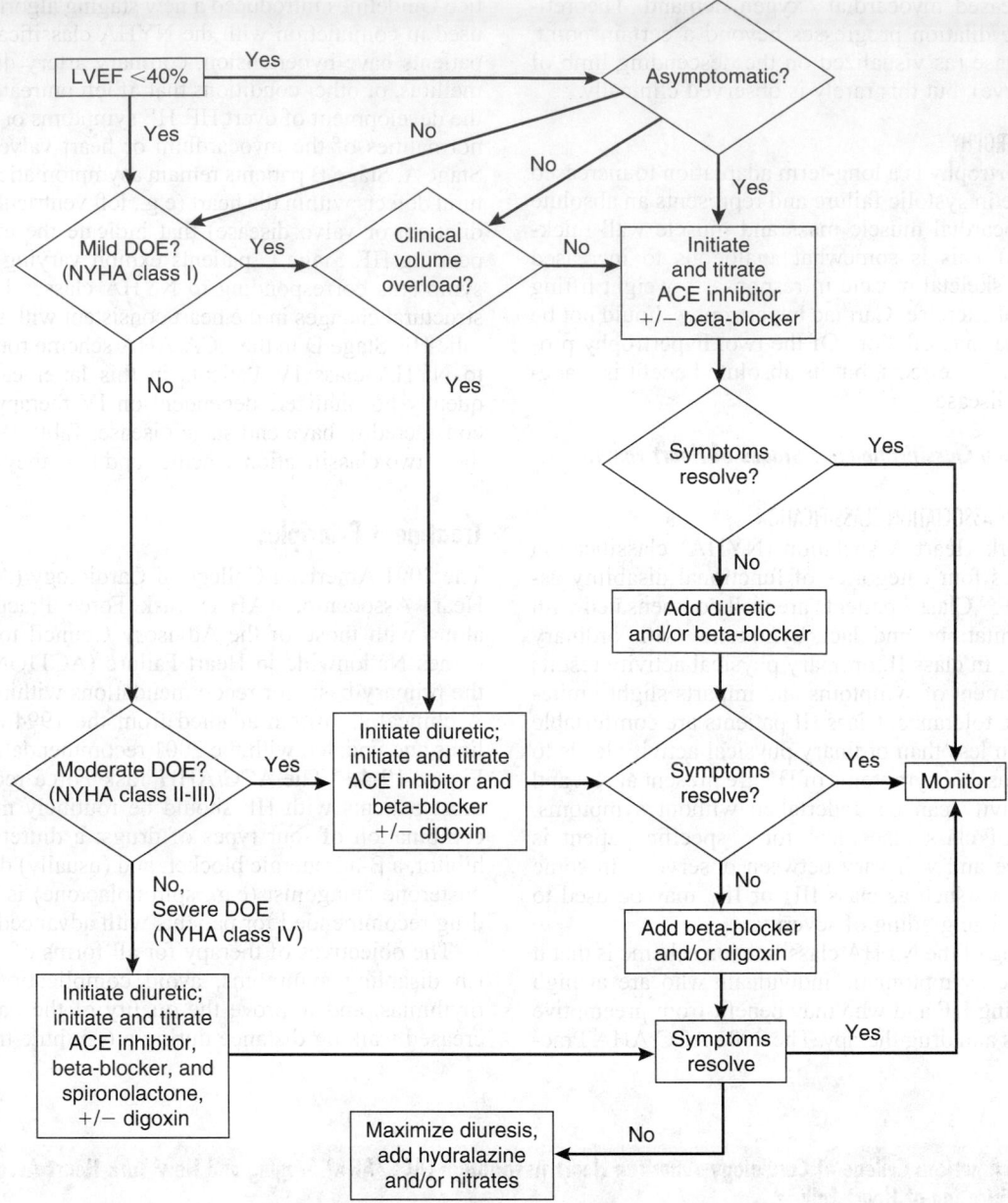

FIGURE 19-4 Heart failure treatment algorithm. DOE, dyspnea on exertion; ±, with or without.

movement to a lower NYHA symptom class are used as rough measures of success for these objectives. Specific quality of life questionnaires are also available. The ultimate goal is to prolong survival in individuals and reduce mortality rates within the population of patients with HF. Short of a heart transplant, none of the treatment measures are curative.

Nonspecific medical management of systolic HF includes addressing cardiovascular risk factors, correction of underlying disease states (e.g., hypertension, ischemic heart disease, arrhythmias, lipid disorders, anemia, or hyperthyroidism), moderate physical activity as tolerated, immunization with influenza and pneumococcal vaccines to reduce the risk of respiratory infections, and discontinuation of possible drug-induced causes. A sodium-restricted diet and diuretics are required if fluid retention is evident. Pharmacotherapeutic interventions include ACE inhibitors, certain β-blocking drugs

(e.g., carvedilol and metoprolol), digoxin, and other vasodilators (nitrates, hydralazine, or angiotensin-receptor blockers). Amiodarone is indicated in the treatment of symptomatic ventricular tachycardia and atrial fibrillation associated with HF. The role of natriuretic peptides, endothelin inhibitors, and vasopeptidase inhibitors continue to be investigated. Nondigitalis inotropic agents and TNF-α inhibitors, although theoretically valuable, have provided disappointing results and significant complications, including arrhythmias and increased mortality rates.

Treatment of diastolic failure is less well defined.[20–25] A sodium-restricted diet and diuretics are indicated for symptomatic relief of shortness breath or edema. ACE inhibitors are frequently used, although controlled trials of effectiveness are lacking. Negative inotropes such as nonselective β-blockers (e.g., propranolol) and calcium blockers (especially verapamil) are often advocated to slow HR and allow more efficient ventricular filling during diastole. Digitalis is relatively contraindicated, especially in patients with ventricular septal hypertrophy.

Physical Activity
Patients should be encouraged to maximize their activities of daily life and exercise to maintain physical conditioning. Edema can be minimized by use of elastic hosiery, which increases interstitial pressure and helps mobilize fluid into vascular spaces. During acute exacerbations, bed rest and restricted physical activity decrease the metabolic demands of the failing heart and minimize gravitational forces contributing to the formation of edema. Renal perfusion is increased in the prone position, resulting in diuresis and eventual mobilization of edema fluid.

Sodium-Restricted Diet
Reduction of dietary salt is prudent in patients with hypertension or evidence of fluid retention, but is not required in all patients. There is no evidence that salt restriction in normotensive or asymptomatic patients will prevent the onset of HF. It is convenient to remember that 1 g of sodium (Na) is equivalent to 2.5 g of salt (NaCl), and that one level teaspoon of salt weighs approximately 6 g. Similarly, 1 g Na = 43 mEq Na and 1 g NaCl = 17 mEq Na. In patients with clinically evident HF, moderate sodium restriction (<3 g Na per day) may allow patients to use lower doses of diuretics by decreasing blood volume and offsetting abnormal retention of sodium by the kidneys. If the kidney's ability to excrete sodium is not severely compromised, it is possible to approach normal balance by restricting sodium intake to match excretion. Even though <1 g of sodium chloride (NaCl) is required to meet physiologic needs, the average U.S. diet contains 10 g. Dietary sodium can be reduced to 2 to 4 g of NaCl by eliminating cooking salt. This diet is more palatable and leads to better adherence than a severely salt-restricted diet.

Diuretics: Clinical Use and Renal Pharmacology
The reader is referred to Chapter 12, Fluid and Electrolyte Disorders, for a thorough review of kidney physiology and the classification, mechanism of action, and side effects of diuretics. Only those points salient to the treatment of HF are included in this chapter. Diuretic use also is discussed in Chapter 14, Essential Hypertension.

Diuretics are indicated in both systolic and diastolic HF for patients with circulatory congestion (pulmonary and peripheral edema) and/or cardiac distension (enlarged heart on chest radiograph). They produce symptomatic relief more rapidly than other drugs for HF. However, monotherapy with diuretics is discouraged, even in patients with mild symptoms that respond well to diuretics. Because activation of the renin-angiotensin-aldosterone and sympathetics nervous systems contribute to the progression of HF, diuretics should be combined with an ACE inhibitor and a β-blocker unless contraindications exist. Conversely, continuous treatment with diuretics is not always necessary in patients with little or no evidence of fluid overload, and diuretics are relatively contraindicated in persons who are volume depleted or have compromised renal blood flow.[5]

By enhancing renal excretion of sodium and water, diuretics diminish vascular volume, thus relieving ventricular and pulmonary congestion and decreasing peripheral edema. Initially, the goal of diuretic therapy is symptomatic relief of HF by decreasing excess volume without causing intravascular volume depletion. Once excess volume is removed, therapy is aimed at maintaining sodium balance and preventing reaccumulation of new fluid, while at the same time avoiding dehydration. The rate at which edema fluid can be removed is limited by its rate of mobilization from the interstitial to the intravascular fluid compartment. If diuresis is too vigorous, intravascular volume depletion, hypotension, and a paradoxical decrease in CO (caused by compromised venous return and inadequate ventricular filling) may result. Weight loss exceeding 1 kg/day is to be avoided except in patients with acute pulmonary edema.

The effectiveness of diuretics depends on the amount of sodium delivered to their site of action in the kidney and the patient's renal function.[57,58] Proximal tubular reabsorption of sodium is increased in patients with severe HF when renal blood flow (RBF) is compromised, rendering thiazide and potassium sparing diuretics (which act primarily on the distal tubule) minimally effective. Thiazides increase the fractional excretion of sodium no more than 5% and lose their effectiveness when creatinine clearance (Cl_{Cr}) decreases to <30 to 50 mL/min. The loop diuretics (furosemide, bumetanide, and torsemide) are more potent and retain their effectiveness until the creatinine clearance is <5 mL/min. Metolazone has diuretic effects intermediate to that of the thiazide and loop diuretics and may maintain activity in patients with compromised renal function. In most HF patients, loop diuretics are preferred. In addition to having activity in the ascending limb of the loop of Henle, furosemide has vasodilating properties that decrease renal vascular resistance. It also enhances sodium excretion by shifting RBF from the long juxtamedullary nephrons to shorter superficial nephrons. In pulmonary edema, the initial beneficial effects of furosemide may be due more to dilation of venous capacitance vessels (decreasing preload) than to diuresis.[57,58]

The onset of response after an IV injection of loop diuretics is 10 minutes or less, peaking within the first 30 minutes, and usually abating within 2 hours. Natriuresis usually begins 30 to 90 minutes after the oral administration of loop diuretics; it peaks within the first or second hour and lasts for 6 to 8 hours. The usual recommended doses for the loop diuretics are found in Table 19-4.[57]

The concept of ceiling doses for loop diuretics should be understood.[57,58] This relates to the observation that the effectiveness of diuretics depends on proximal tubular delivery. Slow absorption (even if bioavailability is high) or protein binding impair tubular delivery and compromise diuretic response. However, once the drug is in the tubule, further drug delivery produces no greater diuresis. Increasing single doses beyond the ceiling dose produces no additional diuretic response. As an alternative, improved diuresis may be obtained by giving the drug more frequently.

As discussed later in this chapter, combinations of diuretics with different mechanisms (e.g., a loop diuretic and metolazone) are used in patients whose conditions are refractory to high-dose loop diuretics.[57,58] Because diuresis may lead to compensatory activation of the renin-angiotensin-aldosterone system, combining a diuretic with an ACE inhibitor and/or using spironolactone has a theoretic basis (see Question 13).

Table 19-4 Loop Diuretic Dosing

	Furosemide	Bumetanide	Torsemide
Usual daily oral dose (mg)	20–160	0.5–4	10–80
Ceiling dose (mg)			
Normal renal function	80–160 (PO/IV)	1–2 (PO/IV)	20–40 (PO/IV)
Cl_{cr}: 20–50 mL/min	160 mg (PO/IV)	2 (PO/IV)	40 mg (PO/IV)
Cl_{Cr}: <20 mL/min	200 IV, 400 (PO)	8-10 (PO/IV)	100 (PO/IV)
Bioavailability	10–100%	80–90%	80–100%
	Average 50%	Lower with food	No food effect
	Lower with food		

IV, intravenous; PO, oral.
Adapted with permission from reference 57.

Diuretics are indicated in diastolic HF, but pose a difficult challenge. This form of HF is highly volume dependent, becoming significantly worse in states of fluid overload, but responding with a rapid reduction in filling pressures and resolution of dyspnea following diuresis. Conversely, chronic diuretic use therapy runs the risk of restricting the end-diastolic volume, resulting in a significant reduction of CO. Thus, elevated filling pressure may be controlled at the expense of a greatly reduced SV such that the symptoms of dyspnea may be traded for those of fatigue and loss of exercise tolerance.[15]

Aldosterone Antagonists

Despite their profound effects on reducing HF symptoms, there are no data to substantiate that loop diuretics counteract the underlying cause of HF or modify mortality rates. The aldosterone antagonists (e.g., eplerenone and spironolactone) exert a mild diuretic effect by competitive binding of the aldosterone receptor site in the distal convoluted renal tubules. They are also referred to as potassium retaining or potassium sparing diuretics since sodium excretion at this level of the kidney is accompanied by an equimolar exchange for potassium. The Randomized Aldactone Evaluation Study Investigators found that spironolactone substantially reduced both morbidity and mortality in a select group of patients with severe HF (NYHA class III and IV).[56] However, the authors speculated that the protective effect of spironolactone was related more to a reduction in aldosterone-induced vascular damage and myocardial or vascular fibrosis than to its diuretic effect. Similarly, reduced mortality was observed in patients with left ventricular dysfunction following a recent MI treated with 25 to 50 mg of eplerenone (Inspra)[59] (See question 14). There is no evidence that the direct acting potassium sparing diuretics amiloride or triamterene exert a similar protective effect.

Angiotensin-Converting Enzyme Inhibitors and Angiotensin Receptor Inhibitors[60–63]

Drugs with vasodilating properties have become a primary treatment modality of HF. Arterial dilation provides symptomatic relief of HF by decreasing arterial impedance (afterload) to left ventricular outflow. Venous dilation decreases left ventricular congestion (preload). The combination of these two properties provides additive benefits to alleviate the symptoms of HF and increase exercise tolerance. The first vasodilator drugs to be studied were hydralazine (essentially a pure arterial dilator) and nitrates (predominately venous dilators.) By combining these two drugs, significant reductions in HF symptoms can be achieved along with a modest reduction in mortality rates. With the advent of ACE inhibitors, the use of hydralazine and nitrates has been relegated to a secondary role.

ACE inhibitors (e.g., benazepril [Lotensin], captopril [Capoten], enalapril [Vasotec], fosinopril [Monopril], lisinopril [Prinivil, Zestril], moexipril [Univasc], perindopril [Aceon], quinapril [Accupril], ramipril [Altace]), and trandolapril [Mavik]) possess both afterload and preload reducing properties (by blocking angiotensin II-mediated vasoconstriction) and volume-reducing potential (by inhibiting activation of aldosterone). They not only produce similar hemodynamic effects to the hydralazine-nitrate combination as a single agent, but they also favorably modify cardiac remodeling independent of vasodilation and have a more tolerable side effect profile. These advantages, coupled with evidence that ACE inhibitors slow the rate of mortality in HF more than the hydralazine-nitrate combination, led the authors of all the current guidelines to unequivocally recommend ACE inhibitors as the drugs of choice for initial therapy, even in patients with relatively mild left ventricular systolic dysfunction.[1–5]

The 2001 ACC/AHA guidelines state: "ACE inhibitors should be prescribed to all patients with HF due to left ventricular systolic dysfunction unless they have a contradiction to their use or have been shown to be unable to tolerate treatment with these drugs. Because of their favorable effects on survival, treatment with an ACE inhibitor should not be delayed until the patient is found to be resistant to treatment with other drugs... ACE inhibitors should not be prescribed without a diuretic in patients with current or recent history of fluid retention. Because fluid retention can blunt the therapeutic effects and fluid depletion can potentiate the adverse effects of ACE, prescribers should ensure that the appropriate doses of diuretics before and during treatment with these drugs."[5]

The pharmacologic actions of all the ACE inhibitors are essentially identical, but some of them have not been extensively studied or received FDA approval for use in HF. Their value in diastolic failure still is being investigated. Expanded discussion of ACE inhibitor use and side effects is found later in this chapter starting with question 16.

A related class of drugs are the angiotensin receptor inhibitors (candesartan [Atacand], eprosartan [Teveten], irbesartan [Avapro], losartan [Cozaar], olmesartan [Benicar], telmisartan [Micardis], and valsartan (Diovan).[60,63] The receptor inhibitors offer theoretic advantages over ACE inhibitors by being more specific for angiotensin II blockade and having a lower risk of drug-induced cough. On the other hand, indirect block of bradykinin, NE, and/or prostaglandins by some or all of the ACE inhibitors may offer an advantage over receptor inhibitors. More importantly, there is evidence that ACE inhibitors have a more favorable effect on prevention of cardiac remodeling by unclear mechanisms. Preliminary results of clinical trials with several of the angiotensin-receptor blockers (ARBs) have been encouraging, but more data are needed relative to their effects on restricting cardiac remodeling and reducing mortality.[61,63] There have been more clinical trials with losartan, but only valsartan has FDA approved labeling for treatment of HF. Currently, ARBs are reserved for use in those who fail to tolerate ACE inhibitors (e.g., angioedema or intractable cough) or during pregnancy.

β-Adrenergic Blocking Agents[27–32]

Until the mid-1990s, some variation of the following statement could be found in any standard text on the treatment of HF: "β-blockers and other negative inotropes are contraindicated." This is a logical extension of previously held belief that sympathomimetic agonists and other positive inotropes are the logical choice to counteract the hemodynamic defects of systolic failure and that negative inotropes will exacerbate HF. A better understanding of the pathophysiology of HF failure led to a rethinking of this logic.[27–32] As discussed earlier, cardiac adrenergic drive initially supports the performance of the failing heart, but long-term activation of the sympathetic nervous system exerts deleterious effects that can be antagonized by the use of β-blockers. Nonetheless, initial trials with propranolol, pindolol, and labetalol in systolic failure patients were disappointing. Much more favorable results have been achieved with metoprolol (Lopressor, Toprol XL) and bisoprolol, both of which are partially selective β_1-blockers, and carvedilol (Coreg), a mixed α1- and nonselective β-blocking agent. Extended release metoprolol (Toprol XL) and carvedilol are FDA approved for use in HF. While some patients can initially have a temporary worsening of symptoms, continued use results in improved quality of life, fewer hospitalizations, and most importantly, longer survival. The AHA/ACC guidelines state that β-blockers should be prescribed to all patients with stable HF due to left systolic dysfunction and with mild to moderate symptoms unless they have a contraindication to their use or have been shown to be unable to tolerate treatment with these drugs. Use of β-blockers should not be delayed until the patient is resistant to or intolerant of other therapies. Generally they are used in combination with diuretics and an ACE inhibitor (with or without digoxin).[5]

β-Blockers are also an important part of the treatment of patients with HF symptoms due to diastolic failure, although the specific drugs used are different. For these patients a nonselective β-blocker like propranolol can be a therapy of choice in selected patients by slowing the HR and allowing improved ventricular filling. The role of metoprolol and carvedilol is less well studied in diastolic failure. β-Blockers are discussed in greater detail in the case study portion of this chapter (see Questions 27–30 and 55).

Digitalis Glycosides (Digoxin)

Digitalis glycosides have several pharmacologic actions on the heart. Digoxin is the only drug from this family still marketed following the withdrawal of digitoxin in the late 1990s. It binds to and inhibits sodium-potassium (Na^+-K^+) adenosine triphosphatase (ATPase) in cardiac cells, decreasing outward transport of sodium and increasing intracellular concentrations of calcium within the cells. Calcium binding to the sarcoplasmic reticulum causes an increase in the contractile state of the heart.

Until recently, the primary benefit of digoxin in systolic HF was assumed to be an increase in the force of contraction (positive inotropic effect) of the failing heart to increase EF and CO. Recent evidence suggests that even at serum concentrations below those associated with positive inotropism, digoxin has beneficial neurohumoral and autonomic effects by reducing sympathetic tone and stimulating parasympathetic (vagal) responses.[5, 64–67] Inhibition of (Na^+-K^+) ATPase in vagal afferent fibers sensitizes cardiac baroreceptors to reduce sympathetic outflow from the CNS. Similarly, inhibition of (Na^+-K^+) ATPase in renal cells reduces renal tubular reabsorption of sodium and indirectly suppresses renin secretion. This has led to the suggestion that the positive benefits of digoxin can be obtained with a lower risk of side effects by using smaller than traditional doses.[5]

In addition to effects on contractility, digoxin decreases the conduction velocity and prolongs the refractory period of the atrioventricular (AV) node. This AV node–blocking effect prolongs the PR interval and is the basis for use of digoxin in slowing the ventricular response rate in patients with atrial fibrillation and other supraventricular arrhythmias (see Chapter 19, Cardiac Arrhythmias). Unfortunately, at higher serum concentrations digoxin increases cardiac automaticity and irritability and decreases the refractory period of the atrial and ventricular myocardium, all of which predispose the patient to a multitude of unwanted heart rhythm disturbances.

Before the advent of ACE inhibitors, the emphasis of HF management was to stimulate the failing heart with inotropes. Digoxin was considered the obvious drug of choice, particularly for patients with coexistent HF and supraventricular arrhythmias. This was followed by a period when the role of digoxin was challenged, especially in patients with normal sinus rhythm, with critics proclaiming it as being minimally effective and having a high risk for toxicity. As evidence mounted that vasodilators could improve survival rates, no such data existed for digoxin. In the past few years, several studies have confirmed a clinical benefit for digoxin in improving HF symptoms, independent of rhythm status, but survival data are still not convincing (see Question 15). As a result, the latest clinical guidelines state that digoxin should be considered to improve the symptoms and clinical status of patients with HF, in combination with diuretics, an ACE inhibitor, and a β-blocker.[1–5] Digoxin can be used early to reduce symptoms in patients who have started, but not yet responded to, treatment with an ACE inhibitor and a β-blocker. Alternatively, treatment with digoxin can be delayed until the patient's response to an ACE inhibitor and β-blocker has been defined and used only for those patients who remain symptomatic despite the other drugs.[5] Monotherapy with digoxin or in combination with only a diuretic is no longer recommended. Digoxin can also be considered in patients with HF who also have chronic atrial fibrillation, although β-blockers may be more effective than digoxin in controlling the ventricular response, especially during exercise. It is also important to document the patient's EF before considering the use of digoxin because the digitalis glycosides are not useful in diastolic HF and, in fact, may worsen this form of left ventricular dysfunction. Further discussion of the controversies surrounding digoxin use and detailed dosing guidelines are found in the case studies.

DIGOXIN PHARMACOKINETICS (TABLE 19-5)

Digoxin is a polar glycoside that is adequately but incompletely absorbed. Studies from the 1970s indicated that absorption of oral tablets varied between manufacturers and from lot to lot of the same product.[68–72] (The reader should consult the sixth edition of *Applied Theraputics: The Clinical Use of Drugs* for the citations and abstracts of older articles.)

In some instances, the differences were only in the *rate* of absorption but not necessarily in the *extent* of absorption (i.e., bioavailability). At least part of the variability correlated to differences in vitro dissolution. For this reason, most clinicians prefer to use the brand name product (Lanoxin), but published data regarding the lack of equivalence of current generic products are lacking. Two manufacturers (Bertek and Qualitest) now market generic versions of digoxin that have been given an AB rating (one under the brand name of Digitek).

Bioavailability of digoxin also depends on the dosage form given. Again, most published information is from the 1970s and is subject to such limitations as differences in methodology between studies (single-dose versus multiple-dose studies) and use of nonspecific assays. The original studies appear to underestimate digoxin bioavailability.[68–72] As summarized by Reuning and others and based on studies using improved

Table 19-5 Digoxin Pharmacokinetics

Parameter	Value
Bioavailability (F)	
Tablets	0.75 (0.5–0.9)[a]
Elixir	0.80 (0.65–0.9)
Liquid-filled capsules	0.95 (0.8–1.0)
Half-Life (t½)	
Normal	1.6–2 days
Renal failure	≥4.4 days
Children	0.7–1.5 days
Volume of Distribution (Vd)[b]	
Normal	6.7 (4–9) L/kg
Renal failure	Smaller: 4.7 (1.5–8.5) L/kg
Clearance (Cl)	
Normal	$1.02\ Cl_{Cr} + 57$ mL/min *or* 2.7 L/min/kg
Severe HF	$0.88\ Cl_{Cr} + 23$ mL/min
% Renally Cleared Unchanged	PO: 50–60%
	IV: 70–75%
% Nonrenal Elimination	40% (20–55%)
% Eliminated/Day	$14\% + Cl_{Cr}/5$
% Enterohepatic Recycling	6.8%
Protein Binding	20–30%
Therapeutic Serum Concentration[c]	0.5–1.2 ng/mL
Digitalizing (loading) dose[d]	0.5–1 mg or 0.01–0.02 mg/kg
Usual Maintenance Dose[e]	0.125–0.25 mg/day
Pediatric Dosing	
Neonate loading	0.01–0.03 mg/kg IV
Infant loading	0.01–0.05 mg/kg PO
>2-year-old load	0.05 mg/kg PO
Premature maintenance	0.001–0.009 mg/kg/day
Neonate maintenance	0.01 mg/kg/day
Infant maintenance	0.015–0.025 mg/kg/day
>2-year-old maintenance	0.01–0.015 mg/kg/day

[a]Mean value with range in parentheses.
[b]Volume of distribution decreases in renal failure, possibly because of change in protein binding.
[c]Digoxin serum concentration and effect are poorly correlated. Levels drawn <6 hr after a dose may be falsely elevated. Spironolactone and endogenous digoxin-like substances in the blood of neonates and renal failure patients can result in falsely elevated levels. Resting concentrations may be higher than those taken after exercise.
[d]Loading doses not recommended except for patients in acute distress, but it takes several days (5 half-lives) to reach steady state with maintenance dose. A more specific loading dose can be calculated by multiplying the desired steady-state concentration by the volume of distribution.
[e]The dosage should be adjusted lower in the elderly or those with renal insufficiency by first estimating Cl_{Cr} to calculate an estimated digoxin clearance. The dosage is estimated by multiplying the target serum concentration times the estimated clearance.
Cl_{Cr}, creatine clearance; HF, heart failure; IV, intravenous; PO, by mouth.

assay methods, the bioavailability of conventional tablets ranges from 70% to 80% (mean, 75%), while that of the commercially available elixir is slightly greater, ranging from 75% to 85%.[71] Nonetheless, considerable interpatient and intrapatient variability exists. Higher bioavailability of solutions reported in some studies might be of little clinical relevance because the solutions used were prepared extemporaneously from solutions for injection.

Lanoxicaps are a liquid-filled soft gelatin capsule form of digoxin with improved bioavailability averaging 90% to 100%. However, the digoxin content of these capsules is 80% of the corresponding tablet. Thus, a 0.2-mg Lanoxicaps is approximately equal to a 0.25-mg digoxin tablet. Because of high cost relative to conventional tablets, use of the capsules usually is reserved for those cases when the response achieved with the tablets has been erratic.

Digoxin's rapid onset of action (30 to 60 minutes) corresponds with peak plasma levels. Maximum effects from a single dose are observed 5 to 6 hours after drug administration, a time at which drug distribution in the body is complete. Digoxin has a steady-state volume of distribution averaging 6.7 L/kg of lean body weight (range, 4 to 9 L/kg).[68,71,72] Only 23% is protein bound, but the volume of distribution may be decreased significantly in renal failure (see Questions 46 and 47). A serum level of 0.8 to 2 ng/mL was recommended in older guidelines as being the therapeutic target, but new evidence indicates therapeutic benefit and greater safety by targeting serum concentrations in the range of 0.5 to 1.2 ng/mL (see Questions 34 and 36).

Digoxin has a half-life ($t\frac{1}{2}$) of 1.6 to 2 days (36 to 40 hours) and is characterized by first-order pharmacokinetics.[68,70–72] With renal impairment, the half-life of digoxin is prolonged, reaching 4.4 days or more in total anuria.[71–73] The renal clearance of digoxin (1.86 mL/min per kg) is slightly greater than creatinine clearance, indicating a component of tubular secretion. Many have the erroneous impression that nonrenal excretion of digoxin is unimportant. In fact, anywhere from 20% to 40% of a given digoxin dose is excreted nonrenally, either as metabolites or in the feces,[68,70–72] corresponding to a nonrenal clearance of 40 to 60 mL/min (0.82 mL/min per kg). In a few individuals, up to 55% of a dose is eliminated as metabolites, primarily as inactive dihydrodigoxin.[71–73] Little digoxin (6.8%) enters the enterohepatic circulation, and its metabolism is unaltered in patients with cirrhosis.

Digoxin absorption, bioavailability, and elimination are partially mediated by P-glycoprotein (PGP), a multidrug transporter that acts as a drug efflux pump across cell membranes in epithelial and endothelial cells of the intestine, kidney, and liver.[72,74] For drugs and toxins affected by PGP, the net effect is to reduce bioavailability (by transporting drugs from the blood back into the gut lumen) and promote clearance (e.g., by enhancing renal tubular secretion.) For digoxin, this system comes into play when certain drugs that block the action of PGP are taken along with digoxin.[74,75] For example quinidine blocks intestinal and renal PGP, thus increasing digoxin bioavailability and reducing renal clearance. As a result, digoxin serum levels rise. This and other digoxin drug interactions are considered in greater detail in Questions 38–40.

In approximately 10% of patients given digoxin, a substantial portion of the drug can be metabolized by bacteria in the GI tract to cardioinactive reduced metabolites.[72,73,76] In isolated cases, significantly increased requirements for digoxin dosage may be seen in patients who excrete large amounts of digoxin by this route. The resulting reduced bioavailability of digoxin is more of a problem when slowly absorbed generic tablets are used as opposed to rapidly absorbed solutions or Lanoxin brand tablets. In addition, concurrent use of certain oral antibiotics (e.g., erythromycin or clarithromycin) can lead to increased digoxin toxicity. This was initially ascribed to altered intestinal metabolism by the antibiotics, but with better understanding of the role of PGP in digoxin absorption and excretion, a probable explanation is that these antibiotics inhibit renal PGP, thus reducing enhanced digoxin renal clearance (See Question 40).

Jelliffe and colleagues present digoxin elimination in a slightly different context by describing the percent elimination in 24 hours.[77] By plotting creatinine clearance versus percent of drug eliminated per day (Fig. 19-5), they found a linear relationship between 24-hour drug excretion and renal function. As can be seen from the figure, the best-fit equation of the line ($y = b + mx$) is:

$$\% \text{ Digoxin eliminated/day} = 14 + \frac{Cl_{Cr}}{5} \quad \textbf{(19-1)}$$

where the y intercept (b), representing nonrenal elimination, is 14%, and the slope of the line (m), representing that portion of daily elimination dependent on renal elimination, is one-fifth. At a creatinine clearance of 100 mL/min, the percent eliminated per day is 35%, whereas at a creatinine clearance of 0 (i.e., anuria), the percent eliminated per day is 14%, all via nonrenal clearance mechanisms.

Other Vasodilating Drugs: Hydralazine and Nitrates

Although ACE inhibitors have become the vasodilator drug of choice, the first vasodilators to be used in patients with HF were hydralazine and nitrates. Hydralazine (Apresoline) is a potent arterial dilating agent that provides symptomatic relief of HF by decreasing arterial impedance (afterload) to left ventricular outflow. Nitrates (e.g., nitroglycerin [NTG], isosorbide dinitrate, and isosorbide mononitrate) have venous dilating properties that decrease left ventricular congestion (preload). Used in combination, these two agents have additive benefits in alleviating the symptoms of HF and increasing exercise tolerance. Importantly, the hydralazine-isosorbide dinitrate combination was the first treatment regimen to show

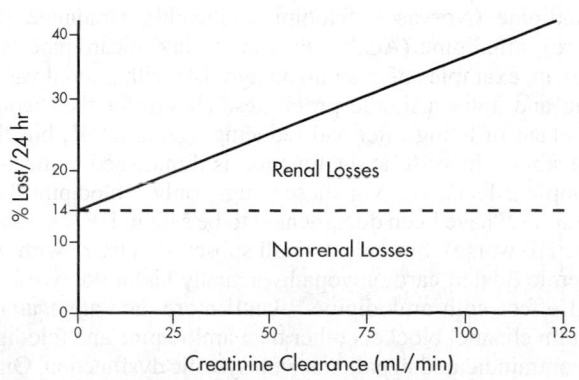

FIGURE 19-5 Relationship of digoxin elimination to renal function.

improved survival in severe HF compared with placebo (while patients continued their previous diuretic and/or digitalis therapy). Current recommendations identify hydralazine and nitrates as secondary agents, reserved for use in patients who do not tolerate ACE inhibitors or angiotensin receptor inhibitors. In refractory cases, hydralazine and/or a nitrate may be added to an ACE inhibitor. The role of these vasodilators in diastolic failure is not well studied. IV NTG and nitroprusside (a mixed arterial and venous dilator) are also used in hospitalized patients with acute HF exacerbations (see Questions 49 and 50).

Other Inotropic Agents

Previous doubt about the clinical effectiveness of digitalis derivatives and concern over their potential for toxicity prompted a search for alternative positive inotropic drugs. Dopamine and dobutamine, both of which are sympathomimetics, are commonly used in acute cardiac emergencies, but their use is limited by the need for IV administration. (See Chapter 22, Shock, for a more detailed discussion of these drugs.) Amrinone and milrinone, nonsympathomimetic inotropes (phosphodiesterase inhibitors), are associated with an unacceptably high incidence of side effects (thrombocytopenia and increased death rates) when given orally, but are available in parenteral form for short-term use (see Question 53).

Enoximone, flosequinan, ibopamine, imozodan, pimobendan, vesnarinone, and xamoterol are all orally active positive inotropic drugs with varying degrees of vasodilating properties investigated for use in HF, but never marketed.[78,79] Despite differing mechanisms of action to produce their cardiac stimulatory effect (primarily sympathomimetics or phosphodiesterase inhibitors), and whether or not the drug also has vasodilating properties (e.g., flosequinan), a disturbing trend emerged: initial positive hemodynamic effects during the first few weeks to months of therapy with all of these drugs was followed by a trend toward increased mortality compared with placebo with continued therapy. The explanation for these unexpected findings are related to an overall undesirability of further enhancing sympathetic tone, overstimulation of an already fatigued heart, and/or proarrhythmic effects of some of the drugs. Whatever the mechanism, the enthusiasm for using inotropic therapy has waned. It is important, however, not to extrapolate these results to digoxin in light of the newer findings that digoxin also has neurohumoral modulating effects. All inotropes are relatively contraindicated in diastolic HF.

Calcium Channel Blockers

Amlodipine (Norvasc), felodipine (Plendil), isradipine (DynaCirc), nifedipine (Adalat, Procardia), and nicardipine (Cardene) are examples of calcium antagonists with arterial vasodilating and antispasmodic properties. They offer the theoretic advantage of being afterload-reducing agents in HF, but their applicability in systolic dysfunction is diminished by negative inotropic effects. Among these drugs, only amlodipine[80] and felodipine[81] have been documented to be safe in HF (i.e., do not make HF worse), but only a small subset of patients with nonischemic dilated cardiomyopathy actually had a positive beneficial effect with amlodipine.[80] Until more data are available, calcium channel blockers other than amlodipine and felodipine are contraindicated in patients with systolic dysfunction. On the

other hand, the negative inotropic effects of some calcium antagonists, especially that of verapamil (Calan, Isoptin, Verelan), is an indication for use in diastolic HF.

PATIENT EVALUATION

Signs and Symptoms

1. A.J., a 58-year-old man, is admitted with a chief complaint of increasing shortness of breath (SOB) and an 8 kg weight gain. Two years before admission, he noted the onset of dyspnea on exertion (DOE) after 1 flight of stairs, orthopnea, and ankle edema. Since that time, his symptoms have progressed despite intermittent hydrochlorothiazide (HCTZ) therapy. Three weeks before admission, he noted the onset of episodic bouts of paroxysmal nocturnal dyspnea (PND). Since then he only has been able to sleep in a sitting position. A.J. notes a productive cough, nocturia (2 to 3 times/night), and mild, dependent edema.

A.J.'s other medical problems include a long history of heartburn; a 10-year history of osteoarthritis, managed with various nonsteroidal anti-inflammatory drugs (NSAIDs); chronic headaches; and hypertension, which has been poorly controlled with HCTZ and propranolol (Inderal). A strong family history of diabetes mellitus is also present.

Physical examination reveals dyspenia, cyanosis, and tachycardia. A.J. has the following vital signs: BP, 160/100 mm Hg; pulse, 100 beats/min; and respiratory rate, 28 breaths/min. He is 5'11" tall and weighs 78 kg. His neck veins are distended. On cardiac examination an S3 gallop is heard; point of maximal impulse (PMI) is at the sixth intercostal space (ICS), 12 cm from the midsternal line (MSL). His liver is enlarged and tender to palpation, and a positive hepatojugular reflux (HJR) is observed. He is noted to have 3+ pitting edema of the extremities and sacral edema. Chest examination reveals inspiratory rales and rhonchi bilaterally.

The medication history reveals the following current medications: HCTZ (Hydrodiuril) 25 mg QD; propranolol (Inderal) 80 mg TID; ibuprofen (Motrin) 600 mg QID; ranitidine (Zantac) 150 mg HS; and Mylanta Double Strength 15 mL as needed up to QID. He has no allergies and no dietary restrictions.

Admitting laboratory values include the following: hematocrit (Hct), 41.1% (normal, 40% to 45%); white blood cell (WBC) count, 5,300/mm³ (normal, 5,000 to 10,000/mm³); Na, 132 mEq/L (normal, 136 to 144 mEq/L); potassium (K), 3.2 mEq/L (normal, 3.5 to 5.3 mEq/L); chloride (Cl), 90 mEq/L (normal, 96 to 106 mEq/L); bicarbonate, 30 mEq/L (normal, 22 to 28 mEq/L); magnesium (Mg), 1.5 mEq/L (normal, 1.7 to 2.7 mEq/L); fasting blood sugar (FBS), 120 mg/dL (normal, 65 to 110 mg/dL); uric acid, 8 mg/dL (normal, 3.5 to 7 mg/dL); blood urea nitrogen (BUN), 40 mg/dL (normal, 10 to 20 mg/dL); serum creatinine (SrCr), 0.8 mg/dL (normal, 0.5 to 1.2 mg/dL); alkaline phosphatase, 120 U (normal, 40 to 80 U); and aspartate aminotransferase (AST), 100 U (normal, 0 to 35 U). The chest radiograph shows bilateral pleural effusions and cardiomegaly.

What signs, symptoms, and laboratory abnormalities of HF does A.J. exhibit? Relate these clinical findings to the pathogenesis of the disease and to left-sided or right-sided HF.

[SI units: Hct, 0.411 (normal, 0.4 to 0.45); WBC count, 5.3 10⁹/L (normal, 5.0 to 10.0); Na, 132 mmol/L (normal, 136 to 144); K, 3.2 mmol/L (normal, 3.5 to 5.3); Cl, 90 mmol/L (normal, 96 to 106); bicarbonate, 30 mmol/L (normal, 22 to 28); Mg, 0.1 mmol/L (normal, 0.85 to 1.35); FBS, 6.661 mmol/L (normal, 3.608 to 6.106); uric acid, 475.84 mmol/L (normal, 208.18 to 416.36); BUN, 14.28 mmol/L (normal, 3.57 to 7.14); SrCr, 70.72 mmol/L (normal, 44.2 to 106.08); alkaline phosphatase, 120 U (normal, 40 to 80); and AST, 100 U (normal, 0 to 0.58 mkat/L)]

The signs and symptoms of HF observed in A.J. are easily visualized if one recalls that the work of the left ventricle is the major determinant of CO and that blood flows from the left ventricle into the arterial system, through capillaries into the venous system, and back into the right heart. From the right heart, the blood circulates through the pulmonary tree and back into the left ventricle. Thus, left-sided ventricular dysfunction primarily causes pulmonary symptoms because of back-up of blood into the lungs, whereas right-sided ventricular dysfunction causes mostly signs of systemic venous congestion. Although left ventricular failure usually develops first, most patients, including A.J., present with signs of combined left- and right-sided failure. The signs and symptoms of both left-sided and right-sided ventricular dysfunction are summarized in Table 19-6.

Left-Sided Heart Failure (Left Ventricular Dysfunction)

Weakness, fatigue, and cyanosis result from decreased CO and compromised tissue perfusion. If the left ventricle is not emptied completely, blood backs up into the pulmonary circulation. SOB, dyspnea (labored or uncomfortable breathing) on exertion (DOE), a productive cough, rales (crackles in the lung during auscultation), pleural effusions on chest radiograph, and cyanosis all result from pulmonary congestion. Pulmonary symptoms are aggravated in the reclining position, which minimizes the gravitational effects on excess fluids in the extremities and improves venous return to the heart and lungs. SOB in the prone position (orthopnea) is quantified by the number of pillows the patient must lie on to sleep comfortably. A.J., for example, could only sleep sitting upright. Paroxysmal nocturnal dyspnea (PND; also called cardiac asthma) is characterized by severe SOB that awakens the patient from sleep and is alleviated by an upright position. PND results from pulmonary vascular congestion that has advanced to pulmonary edema and bronchospasm while the patient sleeps.

Left ventricular hypertrophy (LVH) and cardiac dilation are caused by an increased end-diastolic volume (see Pathogenesis). These effects are observed on chest radiography as an enlarged heart silhouette. The PMI corresponds to the apex of the left ventricle and is visualized as an external pulsation on the left side of the chest. It is displaced laterally and downward from its normal location at the fifth intercostal space, <10 cm from the midsternal line. An S_3 gallop rhythm denotes a third heart sound often heard in close time proximity to the second heart sound (closing of the aortic and pulmonary valves) in HF. Rapid filling of the ventricles causes the S_3 sound and, in an adult, usually indicates decreased ventricular compliance. In patients with mitral valve regurgitation, an S_3 heart sound is common and denotes systolic dysfunction and elevated filling pressure. *Tachycardia* is due to compensatory increases in sympathetic tone.

Weight gain and *edema* reflect sodium and water retention resulting from decreased renal perfusion (see Pathogenesis). As RBF and GFR decrease, a disproportionate amount of BUN may be retained. This phenomenon is termed *prerenal azotemia* and may be detected by an elevated BUN-to-serum creatinine ratio of >20:1. A.J. has a ratio of >40:1. Prerenal azotemia also can be caused by dehydration and overuse of diuretics. Frequency of urination at night (*nocturia*) is due to improved perfusion of the kidney when the patient is lying down.

Right-Sided Heart Failure (Right Ventricular Dysfunction)

The signs and symptoms of right ventricular dysfunction are related to either hypervolemia or the backup of blood from the right ventricle into the peripheral venous circulation. The overall effect is development of *systemic venous hypertension.*

Dependent pitting edema results from increased venous and capillary hydrostatic pressure, causing a redistribution of fluid from the intravascular to interstitial spaces. Ankle and pretibial edema are common findings after prolonged standing or sitting because fluid tends to localize in the dependent portions of the body secondary to gravitational forces. Sacral edema can be present in patients at bed rest. Edema is subjectively quantified on a 1+ (minimal) to 4+ (severe) scale. A.J. has 3+ pitting edema.

Hepatomegaly, hepatic tenderness, and ascites (fluid in the abdomen) arise from hepatic venous congestion and increased portal vein pressure. Metabolism of drugs highly dependent on the liver for body elimination may be notably impaired by both the backward venous congestion of the liver from right-sided failure and the decreased arterial perfusion of the liver from left-sided failure. Congestion of the GI tract makes the patient *anorectic.*

Neck vein distention, primarily seen as internal jugular venous distention (JVD), denotes an elevated jugular venous pressure (JVP). How high the neck veins are distended while the patient is lying down and how much his head has to be raised before the JVD disappears give the clinician a rough

Table 19-6	Signs and Symptoms of HF	
	Left Ventricular Failure	*Right Ventricular Failure[a]*
Subjective	DOE	Peripheral edema
	SOB	Weakness, fatigue
	Orthopnea (2-3 pillows)	
	PND, cough	
	Weakness, fatigue, confusion	
Objective	LVH	Weight gain (fluid retention)
	↓ BP	
	EF <40%[b]	Neck vein distention
	Rales, S_3 gallop rhythm	
	Reflex tachycardia	Hepatomegaly
	↑ BUN (poor renal perfusion)	Hepatojugular reflux

[a]Isolated right-sided failure occurs with long-standing pulmonary disease (cor pulmonale) or after pulmonary hypertension.
[b]Ejection fraction normal in patients with diastolic dysfunction.
BP, Blood pressure, BUN, blood urea nitrogen; DOE, dyspnea on exertion; EF, ejection fraction; HF, heart failure; LVH, left ventricular hypertrophy; PND, paroxysmal nocturnal dyspnea; SOB, shortness of breath.

estimate of the patient's central venous pressure (CVP). Jugular distension in centimeters is measured as the vertical distance from the top of the venous pulsation down to the sternal angle. Neck vein distension of less than 4 cm when the patient is lying with the head elevated at a 45° angle is considered normal for an average, healthy adult. Applying pressure to the liver can cause further distention of the neck veins if hepatic venous congestion is present. This phenomenon is termed *hepatojugular reflux.*

Ejection Fraction Measurement

2. **Does A.J. have systolic or diastolic HF?**

SOB, crackles on auscultation, neck vein distention, edema, and nearly all of A.J.'s other signs and symptoms are common between either form of left ventricular HF. An enlarged heart on a chest radiograph increases the suspicion of systolic failure, but this finding can be absent in some patients with systolic failure and present in others with diastolic failure.

The only way to correctly differentiate systolic from diastolic failure is by measuring the LVEF. Thus it is imperative that A.J., like all patients with suspected HF, have an EF measured before beginning therapy because the treatment strategies between the two disorders are different. Two-dimensional echocardiography coupled with Doppler flow studies (Doppler echocardiogram) is the diagnostic test of choice for measuring EF. This procedure uses sound waves, similar to sonar technology, to visualize and measure ventricular wall thickness, chamber size, valvular functioning, and pericardial thickness. EF is visually estimated based on changes in ventricular chamber size between diastole and systole. This method of EF measurement is not as technically accurate as that provided by ventriculography, but the procedure is more comfortable for the patient, and the correlation of the measured EF to that of the other methods is acceptable. The EF results from echocardiography are graded as normal, mildly, moderately, or severely depressed.

Radionuclide left ventriculography (also called a multiple gated acquisition [MUGA] scan) uses radiolabeled technetium as a tracer to measure left ventricular hemodynamics. Although this method is the most accurate measurement of EF, it is moderately invasive because it requires venipuncture and radiation exposure. In addition, radionuclide scanning does not provide information on the architecture of the left ventricle. Magnetic resonance imaging and computed tomography are useful in evaluating ventricular mass but do not provide EF data.

Subsequently, A.J. underwent an echocardiogram. The results were reported as LVH with mild to moderate depression of EF, correlating approximately to an EF of 30% to 40%. This indicates mild systolic dysfunction. Because he has the combination of systolic dysfunction and classic congestive signs, he fits the criteria for having true CHF.

Stages of Heart Failure and New York Heart Association Classification

3. **What stage of HF does A.J. exhibit according the ACA/AHA criteria? How severe is A.J.'s disability according to the New York Heart Association (NYHA) functional classification of HF?**

The ACA/AHA staging scheme and the NYHA functional classification are described in the Pathogenesis section of this chapter and are summarized in Table 19-3.[5,55]

Because AJ has active symptoms of HF and structural changes in cardiac architecture, he is in ACA/AHA stage C. On admission, A.J. is in NYHA functional class III$_B$ or IV$_A$ as evidenced by a need to sleep upright and inability to undertake even minimal physical activity. Two years ago he would have been considered NYHA class II, and 3 weeks ago he progressed to class III$_A$. Since he will not require inotropic support, he is not in ACA/AHA stage D.

Predisposing Factors

4. **What factors contributed to the cause of A.J.'s HF?**

Age and Hypertension
A.J.'s age of 58 puts him in a high-risk category for development of cardiovascular disease. He is especially vulnerable to HF because of his poorly controlled hypertension, which places an increased afterload on his left ventricle.

β-Adrenergic Blockers
Many drugs have the potential to precipitate or aggravate systolic failure (also see Question 5). A.J. was receiving several agents that might have contributed to his HF, the most significant of which was propranolol. As previously discussed, nonselective β-adrenergic blockers like propranolol decrease myocardial contractility and slow the HR. Both of these factors can compromise the heart's ability to empty effectively. Even topically applied β-blockers (e.g., timolol eye drops for glaucoma) can cause systemic toxicity in sensitive patients.[82] On the other hand, other β-blockers including metoprolol and carvedilol are first-line treatment options for HF when used in combination with ACE inhibitors or other vasodilator drugs. This poses a dilemma for the clinician in trying to sort out the potential risk and benefit from this class of drugs. Moreover, the problem is commonly encountered because many patients with HF also are being treated for hypertension or angina.

In the case of A.J., high sympathetic tone with tachycardia and hypertension are evident. Propranolol is the least desirable β-blocker to use because of its generalized β$_1$- and β$_2$-blocking properties and its documented failure as an effective treatment for systolic failure. Metoprolol or carvedilol are better options because they potentially could control both his BP and HF symptoms. At this stage of assessment and treatment, it is appropriate to discontinue propranolol and follow a more traditional treatment plan as discussed in subsequent questions.

Nonsteroidal Anti-Inflammatory Drugs and Sodium Content
Ibuprofen used for A.J.'s arthritis could contribute to sodium overload. All NSAIDs (including the COX-2 inhibitors) have well-documented, renally mediated sodium-retaining properties, increasing the blood volume by up to 50% in some individuals (See Chapter 43, Rheumatoid Disorders).[83] NSAIDs can also counteract the beneficial response of ACE inhibitors

and diuretics by causing peripheral and renal vasoconstriction. Unless there is a compelling reason for their use, NSAIDs are contraindicated in patients with HF.

Sodium chloride for injection (e.g., normal saline) used as a diluent for IV administration of drugs is an obvious source of sodium. In addition, selected parenteral cephalosporin (e.g., cefazolin and cefotaxime) and penicillin derivatives (e.g., ampicillin, carbenicillin, methicillin, nafcillin, piperacillin, and sodium penicillin G), as well as phenytoin injection, can be an overlooked source of sodium when given in high doses. Product formulation and sodium content may vary between manufacturers, but product-specific information is usually available in the package insert.

Many older formulations of antacids were high in sodium, but most popular brands (including Mylanta taken by A.J.) have been reformulated. Likewise, most cough syrups and other oral liquids have been reformulated to contain less sodium. Unless large daily quantities of these oral liquids are consumed, they are of little concern to the HF patient. If it is determined the patient is getting more than 50 to 100 mg of sodium per day from their medications, alternatives should be sought. For example, A.J. could be instructed to use a nonprescription histamine$_2$ blocker for his heartburn. More troublesome are effervescent antacids and headache powders that contain sodium bicarbonate (e.g., Alka Seltzer products, Bromo Seltzer, Goody's Headache Powder), making them exceptionally high sources of sodium. Tables of sodium content of drugs become quickly outdated, but fortunately the information for a specific patient's medications can be determined because prescription and nonprescription drug labels now carry a disclosure of sodium content.

On admission to the hospital, both A.J.'s hypertension and HF were poorly controlled and he had gained 8 kg. He needs increased diuresis, replacing HCTZ with a loop diuretic, although careful attention must be paid to his low serum potassium. An ACE inhibitor should be added to reduce the workload on his heart and simultaneously help control his BP. Propranolol should be discontinued and replaced with either metoprolol or carvedilol for additional HF and BP control. However, some clinicians delay starting a β-blocker for 2 to 4 weeks while stabilizing the dose of the diuretic and ACE inhibitor. The ibuprofen dose is high. Lowering the dose or preferably discontinuing all NSAIDs might reduce sodium retention and edema and allow ACE inhibitor therapy to be more effective. Acetaminophen is an alternative for treating his osteoarthritis, although it lacks anti-inflammatory properties.

Diet

It is possible that A.J.'s diet contains a considerable excess of sodium from foods such as canned soups and vegetables, potato chips, or overuse of salt at mealtime. Dietary supplements (e.g., Ensure and Sustacal) and sports drinks (e.g., Gatorade) can also be rich sources of sodium. He should follow a controlled-sodium (e.g., 2 to 3 g/day) diet. If salt substitutes are used, he should be warned that they are high in potassium and could cause hyperkalemia if used concurrently with potassium supplements, an aldosterone inhibitor

(spironolactone), or other potassium-sparing diuretics (amiloride, triamterene).

Drug-Induced Heart Failure

5. β-Blockers, NSAIDs, and drugs high in sodium were noted as a possible cause of A.J.'s HF. What are the basic mechanisms by which drugs can induce HF, and how can an understanding of these mechanisms be predictive of drugs to avoid in A.J.?

Drug-induced HF is mediated by three basic mechanisms: inhibition of myocardial contractility (negative inotropic agents), proarrhythmic effects, or expansion of plasma volume (Table 19-7). The latter category includes drugs that act primarily on the kidney (to either alter RBF or increase sodium retention) or those that increase total body sodium and water because of their high sodium content.

The most recognized negative inotropic agents are the β-blockers (see also Question 4). Other well-documented negative inotropes include the calcium channel blockers, most notably verapamil (Calan, Isoptin); various antiarrhythmic agents, especially disopyramide (Norpace), quinidine, and other class IA drugs; and the anthracycline cancer chemotherapeutic agents (daunomycin and doxorubicin [Adriamycin]). The anthracyclines have a direct, dose-related cardiotoxicity that can be minimized by limiting total cumulative doses to 500 to 600 mg/m^2.[84,85] For a more detailed description of anthracycline toxicity, see Chapter 89, Adverse Effects of Chemotherapy. The final group of drugs gaining increased notoriety as cardiotoxins are the amphetamine-like drugs and cocaine when used chronically in large quantities or after an overdose.

Drugs that increase the QT interval induce proarrhythmic effects in some patients. Worsening of HF occurs if the disturbed rhythm compromises cardiac functioning. Of particular concern is drug-induced torsade de pointes. Paradoxically, class IA (quinidine, disopyramide, and procainamide), class IC (encainide, flecainide, and propafenone), and class III (amiodarone, dofetilide, ibutilide, and sotalol) antiarrhythmics are among the best-documented proarrhythmic drugs. However, a multitude of noncardiac drugs also are associated with QT interval prolongation and torsade de pointe (also see Chapter 20, Cardiac Arrhythmias).[86]

Examples of drugs that induce sodium and water retention are NSAIDs (via prostaglandin inhibition), certain antihypertensive drugs, glucocorticoids, androgens, estrogens, and licorice. Weight gain accompanied by peripheral and pulmonary edema has been observed in stable HF patients given the thiazolidinedione antidiabetic drugs pioglitazone and rosiglitazone.[87] Worsening of HF appears to be dose dependent and is presumed to be at least in part due to fluid retention. As a consequence, the FDA requires that the package insert for these two drugs recommend they not be administered to patients with NYHA class III or IV HF and that they be used cautiously in earlier stages of HF. Antihypertensive drugs either decrease RBF via direct vasodilation (e.g., hydralazine, minoxidil, diazoxide) or via inhibition of the autonomic nervous system (e.g., guanethidine, methyldopa). Glucocorticoids and licorice (glycyrrhizic acid, carbenoxolone) have an aldosterone-like action.

Table 19-7 Drugs That May Induce HF

Negative Inotropic Agents	
β-Blockers[a]	Most evident with propranolol or other non-selective agents
	Less with agents with intrinsic sympathomimetic activity (acebutolol, carteolol, pindolol); may also be caused by use of timolol eye drops
Calcium channel blockers[a]	Verapamil has most negative inotropic and AV-blocking effects; amlodipine has least
Antiarrhythmics	Most with disopyramide (Norpace); also quinidine
	Least with amiodarone
Direct Cardiotoxins	
Cocaine, amphetamines	Overdoses and long-term myopathy
Anthracycline cancer chemotherapeutic drugs	Daunomycin and doxorubicin (Adriamycin); dose related; keep total cumulative dose <600 mg/m^2
Proarrhythmic Effects	
Class IA, IB, Class III antiarrhythmic drugs	QT interval widening
	Probable torsade de pointe
	HF develops if disturbed rhythm compromises cardiac functioning
Non-antiarrhythmic drugs	Same mechanism as above
(See reference 86 for a complete list)	Often associated with drug interactions that inhibit metabolism of the offending drug leading to higher than desired plasma levels
Expansion of Plasma Volume	
Antidiabetics	Na retention with metformin, pioglitazone (Actos), and rosiglitazone (Avandia)[87]
NSAIDs	Prostaglandin inhibition; Na retention
Glucocorticoids, androgens, estrogens	Mineralocorticoid effect; Na retention
Licorice	Aldosterone-like effect; Na retention
Antihypertensive vasodilators (hydralazine, methyldopa, prazosin, minoxidil)	↓ Renal blood flow, activation of renin-angiotensin system
Drugs high in Na$^+$	Selected IV cephalosporins and penicillins
	Effervescent or bicarbonate containing antacids or analgesics
	Also liquid nutrition supplements
Unknown Mechanism	
Tumor necrosis factor antagonists	Multiple case reports of new-onset HF or exacerbation of prior HF with etanercept and infliximab in patients with Crohns disease or rheumatoid arthritis[51]

[a]β-Blockers and verapamil may be beneficial in diastolic HF. Carvedilol and metoprolol counteract autonomic hyperactivity in systolic dysfunction.
AV, atrioventricular; HF, heart failure; IV, intravenous; Na, sodium; NSAIDs, nonsteroidal anti-inflammatory drugs.

TREATMENT

Therapeutic Objectives

6. **What are the therapeutic objectives in treating A.J.?**

Cure is not a feasible therapeutic objective in patients with any form of HF. Exceptions include patients who are candidates for cardiac transplantation or in certain forms of idiopathic dilated cardiomyopathy (e.g., viral origin). The immediate objective for A.J. is to provide symptomatic relief as assessed by a reduction in his complaints of SOB and PND, an improved quality of sleep, and increased exercise tolerance. Over the next several days or weeks the goal will be to get him back to his baseline status of NYHA class II or III HF. Parameters used to measure success in meeting this objective include reduced peripheral and sacral edema, weight loss, slowing of the HR to <90 beats/min, normalization of BP, reduction of the BUN back to baseline, a smaller heart size on chest radiograph, decreased neck vein distention, loss of the S$_3$ heart sound, and an improved EF.

Long-range goals are to improve A.J.'s quality of life, including better tolerance of daily life activities, fewer future hospitalizations, avoidance of side effects of his therapy, and ultimately, an increased survival time. The achievement of these goals depends on the severity of A.J.'s disease, his understanding of his disease, and his adherence to prescribed interventions.

Diuretics

7. **Bed rest and a 3-g sodium diet were ordered. Why should A.J. continue his diuretic therapy?**

Excessive volume increases the workload of a compromised heart, and diuretics are an integral part of therapy. This is especially true if volume overload is symptomatic (e.g., pulmonary congestion) as in A.J. Diuretics produce symptomatic improvement more rapidly than any other drug for HF. They can relieve pulmonary and peripheral edema within hours or days, while the clinical effects of ACE inhibitors, β-blockers, and digoxin take weeks to months to be fully realized. However, diuretics should not be used alone in HF. Even when they are initially successful in controlling symptoms and reducing edema, they are ineffective in maintaining clinical stability for long periods without the addition of other drugs. More importantly, activation of the renin-angiotensin-aldosterone and sympathetic nervous systems in response to diuresis could possibly lead to HF progression.

Current guidelines all recommend diuretic therapy both acutely and chronically if clinical volume overload is evident, but further state that patients without peripheral or pulmonary edema can be treated either intermittently or without diuretics.[1-5] Diuretics used on an intermittent (as-needed) basis are titrated based on changes in weight gain, neck vein distention, peripheral edema, or SOB. Patients with a good understanding of their disease can be instructed to weigh themselves daily and start taking their medicine if they gain more than 1 to 2 pounds in 1 day or 5 pounds over 1 week or have leg swelling. Doses can be withheld as long as they are at their target weight. In other cases, diuretic-free intervals or weekends can be arranged. Even with these options, if the patient has experienced volume overload at some time during the course of his or her disease, either past or present, a diuretic should always be part of the regimen.[5]

Despite their remarkable initial benefits, vigorous diuretic therapy carries the risk of volume depletion and diminished CO. Abrupt worsening of renal function (increased BUN or serum creatinine) or hypotension indicates the need to consider temporarily discontinuing diuretics.

Essentially all patients with clinically evident HF require loop diuretics. A.J. has been taking large doses of hydrochlorothiazide, but still has obvious signs of volume overload, indicating a need for more vigorous diuresis with a loop diuretic. His elevated BUN is worrisome and could worsen if he becomes dehydrated, but his renal function will likely improve if his HF gets better, allowing enhanced blood flow to the kidneys.

Furosemide and Other Loop Diuretics

8. It is decided to begin a combination regimen of furosemide and an ACE inhibitor in A.J. What route, dose, and dosing schedule of furosemide should be used?

ROUTE OF ADMINISTRATION

The pharmacology and dose comparison of loop diuretics is discussed in the Treatment Principles section of this chapter and in Table 19-4. Furosemide is the most commonly used loop diuretic for HF because of greater clinical experience and low cost. Bumetanide and torsemide are preferred in some settings because of more predictable absorption.[57,58,88,89]

According to one group of investigators, HF patients treated with torsemide fare better than those receiving furosemide.[89] During their 1-year open-label trial of 234 subjects, patients receiving torsemide were less likely to be admitted to the hospital for HF (17% with torsemide versus 32% for furosemide; $P < 0.01$). Admissions for all cardiovascular causes were also lower among patients taking torsemide (44%) than patients taking furosemide (59%). However, there were no differences in all cause hospital admission between the two groups (71% torsemide, 76% furosemide). Fatigue

scores improved better in torsemide-treated patients, but there was no difference between groups in the rate of dyspnea score improvement. Because generic furosemide is much less costly to prescribe, routine switching to torsemide cannot be advocated until these results are verified by a double-blind, placebo controlled trial.

Erratic responses to furosemide are more prevalent in persons with severe HF or diminished renal function. Some patients respond promptly and vigorously to small oral doses of furosemide, while others require large IV doses to achieve only minimal diuresis. Part of these differences can be explained by the drug's pharmacokinetics.[57,90] Oral absorption of furosemide is incomplete, averaging 50% to 60% in healthy subjects and 43% to 46% in those with renal failure. When taken with a meal, absorption is delayed because of slowed gastric emptying, but the total amount absorbed does not differ significantly from that in fasting states. It has been claimed that the absorption and, therefore, effectiveness of furosemide is further diminished in patients with HF attributable to edema of the bowel and decreased splanchnic blood flow. This has been partially refuted by one investigator, who noted an average furosemide bioavailability of 61% in HF patients, the same as in normal patients.[91] However, total absorption in patients with HF varies widely (34% to 80%) and both the rate of absorption and time to peak urinary excretion are delayed for furosemide and bumetanide.[57,58,91]

When interpreting these bioavailability data, another important factor must be considered. The rate and extent of absorption are not only different among individuals (as illustrated by the examples already given), but intraindividual variability also exists. Ingestion of the same brand of furosemide by the same individual on multiple occasions can show up to a threefold difference in bioavailability. These differences are evident whether considering the innovator's brand (Lasix) or one of several generic brands.[57,58,92,93] As with digoxin, these data on bioavailability differences are old and have not been verified or refuted by newer studies.

One might infer that IV therapy is the preferred route, giving a better response for any given dose. Surprisingly, this is not always the case. In both healthy volunteers and patients with HF, total daily fluid and electrolyte loss after oral therapy and parenteral therapy are comparable. The major difference is in the time course of response. During the first 2 hours, diuresis from the IV dose far exceeds that from the oral therapy, but by 4 to 6 hours, the total urinary output is equivalent.[91,94,95] Therefore, considering the significant cost differential between oral and parenteral furosemide, the clinical advantage in using IV therapy is small. Exceptions to the rule are those patients with severe pulmonary edema who need acute symptomatic relief and those patients who have failed to respond to an adequate oral challenge.

DOSING (TABLE 19-4)

Typically, a patient's treatment is initiated with 20 to 40 mg of oral or IV furosemide given as a single dose and monitored for responsiveness. If the desired diuresis is not obtained, the dose can be increased in 40- to 80-mg increments over the next several days to a total daily dose of 160 mg/day, usually divided into two doses. For torsemide, a usual starting dose is 10 to 20 mg/day, but a ceiling effect is noted in patients with HF at a dosage of 100 to 200 mg/day.[57,96] Equivalent doses of bumetanide are 0.5 to 1.0 mg once or twice daily, titrated to a maximum of 10 mg daily. Because A.J. is not in acute distress, it could be argued that oral therapy would suffice. However, it is decided to give a single 40 mg IV dose of furosemide for immediate symptom control, followed by 40 mg each morning.

There are differing opinions as to whether furosemide should be given once daily or in multiple doses. The drug's short half-life of 2 to 4 hours implies the need for multiple dosing. Nonetheless, equivalent daily diuresis has been observed following the same dose given in single or divided doses.[97] Another investigator found better effects from divided doses.[98] Because evening and nighttime doses of diuretics often disturb patients' sleep patterns (because of nocturnal diuresis), the total daily dose usually should be given as a single morning dose. For patients with symptomatic nocturnal dyspnea, two-thirds of the dose is given in the morning and one-third in the late afternoon or, if necessary, at night. Torsemide (Demadex) has a slightly longer half-life and generally can be given once daily.

Adverse Effects

9. Examine A.J.'s laboratory values (see Question 1). Can any of the abnormal values be attributed to the HCTZ A.J. was taking? What is the significance of these abnormalities?

More thorough discussions of diuretic-induced side effects are found in Chapter 12, Fluid and Electrolyte Disorders and Chapter 14, Essential Hypertension. Those findings pertinent to A.J.'s case are discussed below.

AZOTEMIA

A.J. has an elevated BUN (40 mg/dL) but a normal serum creatinine (0.8 mg/dL). Normally, a BUN-to-creatinine ratio of 10 to 20:1 is seen. Progressive renal failure is characterized by an elevation of both BUN and creatinine. A disproportionately elevated BUN relative to creatinine is indicative of prerenal azotemia, the major causes of which are dehydration (e.g., overdiuresis) or poor renal perfusion (e.g., HF). Serum creatinine will also rise in some patients with prerenal azotemia but will quickly return to normal with rehydration.

A.J.'s laboratory values reflect prerenal azotemia, but his edematous state and elevated BP point to a cause other than dehydration. The most probable cause of his azotemia is decreased RBF secondary to uncompensated HF. Diuretics should not be withheld, and in fact, judicious diuresis should improve his HF and help lower his BUN. Caution must be exercised because prolonged overdiuresis and dehydration can cause renal ischemia, leading to true renal damage. If this happens, the serum creatinine also will begin to rise (see also Question 23).

HYPONATREMIA

A marginally low serum sodium of 132 mEq/L is noted. However, low serum sodium is *not* necessarily a sign of overdiuresis. Serum sodium reported by the laboratory is the *concentration* of sodium in the serum. A person may be significantly overdiuresed (dehydrated) with a large body deficit of sodium, but if that sodium is lost isotonically, the serum sodium concentration will be normal. Conversely, a person such as A.J. can be volume overloaded (edema and hypertension), indicating excessive body sodium, but the serum

sodium concentration may be normal or even low as explained below.

Hyponatremia (low serum sodium concentration) reflects the dilutional effect of extra free water in the plasma on sodium concentration. The most common causes of dilutional hyponatremia are excess antidiuretic hormone (ADH) production or excessive water drinking (i.e., electrolyte-free fluids). Persons following a severely sodium-restricted diets can develop hyponatremia. Likewise, patients given too much diuretic and who are then given salt-free fluids and/or who have compensatory ADH release by the body can become hyponatremic. Dilutional hyponatremia, resembling the syndrome of inappropriate antidiuretic hormone (SIADH) secretion, has been described following treatment with thiazide and loop diuretics. Patients with HF or hepatic cirrhosis are more likely to develop diuretic-induced dilutional hyponatremia because of preexisting defects in free water clearance. The exact cause of hyponatremia in A.J. is unknown, but his marginally low serum sodium does not contraindicate continued diuretic therapy.

HYPOKALEMIA

A.J. has a serum potassium of 3.2 mEq/L. Hypokalemia reflecting total body potassium depletion is a well-described, but often over emphasized, side effect of thiazide and loop diuretics. Using a definition of hypokalemia as a serum potassium <3.5 mEq/L, the incidence is 15% to 40% in patients receiving 50 to 100 mg/day of HCTZ.[99,100] If lower dosages of diuretic are given or if one accepts serum levels >3.0 mEq/L as normal, the incidence is even lower. Several groups of investigators found little clinical or electrocardiographic (ECG) evidence to suggest that a serum potassium level between 3.0 and 3.5 mEq/L is harmful.[101–103] However, other studies showed increased ectopic activity in persons with serum levels between 3.0 and 3.5 mEq/L.[104–106] These latter studies have been criticized for including patients at high risk for complications.[107] Perhaps more important than serum levels is the measurement of actual tissue and body stores of potassium. Two reports indicate only a 3% to 7% deficit of total body potassium in a group of diuretic-treated patients.[108, 109] This deficit did not differ significantly from that found in a control group of subjects not taking diuretics.

One also must take into account the serum potassium concentration in patients before therapy, as well as the actual degree of fall in serum potassium. The incidence of hypokalemia usually is less in patients with HF than in patients with hypertension, because patients with HF have a higher serum potassium concentration before treatment.[110] A subgroup of HF patients with poor RBF and secondary hyperaldosteronism may have more hypokalemia. The opposite is true in renal failure, which can be associated with hyperkalemia in the absence of diuretic therapy.

Somewhat unexpectedly, furosemide has been observed to produce a lesser degree of hypokalemia than thiazides.[110,111] This seems paradoxical when one considers that furosemide blocks tubular reabsorption of sodium to a greater degree than thiazides, allowing more sodium to be presented to the distal tubule for exchange with potassium and hydrogen ions. The reason for this anomaly is not well explained. It is speculated that furosemide's shorter duration of activity, relative to the thiazides, allows greater potassium recovery between doses.

A.J.'s serum potassium of 3.2 mEq/L falls in the gray area between 3.0 and 3.5 mEq/L. Although the risk may be low, he will be receiving increased doses of diuretics over the next several days and has started receiving an ACE inhibitor. In addition, he could start digoxin in the future. Because low serum potassium levels predispose a patient to digitalis toxicity (see Questions 41–43), potassium replacement is warranted for A.J. (see Question 10).

HYPOCHLOREMIC ALKALOSIS

A.J.'s low serum chloride of 90 mEq/L concurrent with an elevated serum bicarbonate (total CO_2) of 30 mEq/L signifies hypochloremia with a metabolic alkalosis. When sodium is lost in the urine, electroneutrality must be maintained by the concomitant loss of an anion (chloride) or the reabsorption of a cation (hydrogen). Because diuretic therapy increases sodium excretion, concomitant chloruresis is unavoidable. Moreover, diuretic programs often include salt restriction, which further decreases chloride intake (see also Chapter 11, Acid-Base Disorders). The therapy for both hypochloremia and metabolic alkalosis is potassium chloride replacement.

HYPOMAGNESEMIA

A.J.'s serum magnesium level is 1.5 mEq/L. This could either be a result of magnesium diuresis induced by his diuretic therapy or malabsorption secondary to binding of magnesium ions in the intestines by his antacids. Severe hypomagnesemia can lead to somnolence, muscle spasms, a decreased seizure threshold, and cardiac arrhythmias, effects similar to those seen with hypocalcemia and hyperkalemia. Some investigators have claimed that many of the arrhythmias previously ascribed to diuretic-induced hypokalemia were actually caused by diuretic-induced hypomagnesemia.[112] Concurrent hypokalemia and hypomagnesemia can be especially dangerous. A.J. should be given 1 g of $MgSO_4$ IV and observed for changes in his magnesium level. If needed, he could be given oral supplements of magnesium.

HYPERGLYCEMIA

A.J. has a fasting blood sugar of 120 mg/dL, which is only slightly elevated and, in fact, may be normal if the sample was not taken in the fasting state. It also could represent a stress-related diabetic reaction. However, hyperglycemia and glucose intolerance have been reported to occur during treatment with thiazide diuretics (see Chapter 50, Diabetes Mellitus). Because A.J. has a family history of diabetes, he could be at increased risk. At this time A.J.'s blood sugar needs further monitoring, but no specific therapy is required.

HYPERURICEMIA

Increases of 1 to 2 mg/dL in uric acid levels are common during thiazide administration. Rarely, 4- to 5-mg/dL elevations have been reported. A.J. shows an increase of 1 mg/dL.

Most patients who develop elevated uric acid levels during treatment with diuretic agents remain asymptomatic and need not be treated. Only those with uric acid levels persistently >10 mg/dL, as well as those with a history of gout or a familial predisposition, should be considered for treatment with urate-lowering agents (See also Chapter 42, Gout and Hyperuricemia).

LIVER FUNCTION

A.J.'s elevated alkaline phosphatase and AST probably are not indicative of any drug-related toxicity. Although cholestatic jaundice has been reported with thiazide diuretics, the elevated liver function tests most likely are the result of hepatic congestion from right-sided HF.

Potassium Supplementation

10. The physician gave A.J. one 1-g dose of magnesium sulfate and three 20-mEq doses of potassium chloride IV. This raised his serum magnesium to 2.0 and his potassium to 3.9 mEq/L. Should he receive prophylactic magnesium or potassium supplementation? What is the best drug and appropriate dose?

At this time A.J. does not need further magnesium replacement, but his serum magnesium level should be remeasured after he has been receiving furosemide for a few days. If the level drops again, maintenance therapy with oral magnesium oxide tablets can be started.

Potassium supplementation is not required in all patients receiving diuretics. They should be monitored frequently in the first few months of diuretic therapy to determine their potassium requirements. Prophylactic or therapeutic potassium replacement should be given only when the therapeutic gains of treatment are balanced against its risks. A fall in serum potassium concentration can be seen within hours of the first dose of a diuretic, and the maximum fall usually is reached by the end of the first week of treatment. When diuretics are stopped, it can take several weeks for serum potassium to return to normal. Therefore, it is possible that A.J.'s admitting potassium level of 3.2 mEq/L reflects the nadir of his response to HCTZ. His initial response to potassium supplementation shows that his hypokalemia will be easily controlled. It might be argued that he should be observed for a few days and not given further supplements, but because his diuresis is to be increased and digitalis therapy may later be considered, potassium supplementation is warranted.

DIETARY SUPPLEMENTS AND DOSAGE FORMS

Potassium replacement can be accomplished by one or more of the following: dietary supplementation with potassium-containing foods, pharmacologic replacement with various oral potassium salts, or use of potassium-sparing diuretics. Table 19-8 lists the potassium content of selected foods. Inclusion of these foods in the patient's diet may be all that is required to maintain potassium balance, especially in the 60% to 90% of people who are not prone to hypokalemia in the first place. Unfortunately, the food products listed are expensive and many are high in sodium, which makes them difficult to use for people following low-salt diets. Salt substitutes are another exogenous source of potassium. Patients using these products liberally may get adequate potassium replacement; in fact, they can contribute to hyperkalemia. Some patients object to the taste of salt substitutes.

If potassium replacement is prescribed, only *potassium chloride* (KCl) should be used because all potassium-wasting diuretics can cause hypochloremic alkalosis (see Question 9); if the chloride ion is not replaced, alkalosis and hypokalemia will persist, even if large quantities of potassium are given.

Slow K and Kaon-Cl are slow-release solid dosage forms of KCl crystals imbedded in a wax matrix. They are equal to

Table 19-8   Potassium Content of Selected Foods (400 mg Potassium is Approximately Equal to 10 mEq K+)^a

Food	Quantity	Potassium Content (mg) (Approximate)
Meats		
Beef chuck	3 oz	200–400
Beef round	3 oz	200–400
Hamburger	3 oz	200–400
Rib roast	3 oz	200–400
Chicken fryer	4 oz	>400
Turkey	4 oz	200–400
Vegetables		
Artichoke	1 medium	200–400
Avocado	½ uncooked	200–400
Baked potato	1 medium	>400
Sweet corn	½ cup	200–400
Dried beans	8 oz (1 cup) cooked	>400
Lima beans	½ cup	200–400
Tomato	1 medium raw or 4 oz (½ cup) cooked	200–400
Brussels sprouts	½ cup	200–400
Broccoli	4 oz (½ cup cooked)	200–400
Collard greens	4 oz (½ cup cooked)	200–400
Spinach	4 oz (½ cup cooked)	200–400
Winter squash	4 oz (½ cup cooked)	>400
Fruits		
Banana	1 medium	>400
Orange	1 medium	200–400
Grapefruit	1 cup	200–400
Apricot	3 medium	>400
Peach	1 medium	200–400
Nectarine	1 large	>400
Cantaloupe	8 oz (1 cup)	>400
Honeydew melon	8 oz (1 cup)	>400
Watermelon	8 oz (1 cup)	200–400
Raisins	½ cup	>400
Prunes	4 medium	200–400
Dates	4 oz (½ cup)	>400
Juices and milk		
Orange	8 oz (1 cup)	>400
Grapefruit	8 oz	200–400
Pineapple	8 oz	200–400
Prune	8 oz	>400
Tomato	8 oz	>400
Milk	8 oz (1 cup)	200–400

^{a}39 mg K+ = 1 mEq.

KCl solution in bioavailability and are associated with less GI bleeding, ulceration, and stricture formation than enteric-coated potassium tablets. The major drawback to their use is high cost and the large number of tablets needed per day. Slow K has only 600 mg (8 mEq) per tablet. Other products (Kaon-CL, Klotrix, K-Tab, and K-Dur) contain 750 mg (10 mEq) per tablet. Slow-release potassium tablets should be avoided in patients with impaired GI motility, and enteric-coated potassium tablets should be avoided at all times.

A slow-release, microencapsulated form of KCl (Micro K, multiple generics) was originally postulated to produce fewer GI mucosal ulcerations than wax matrix slow-release tablets.[113] However, other investigators could not detect any difference between the two formulations,[114,115] and the Boston Collaborative Drug Surveillance Program could not find a positive association between wax matrix potassium use and significant upper GI bleeding.[116]

Another sustained-release potassium product, K-Dur, available as either 750 mg (10 mEq) or 1500 mg (20 mEq) tablets, can either be swallowed whole or dissolved in water. It offers the advantage of being tasteless even when prepared as a solution. The only patient complaint is that the capsules dissolve in the mouth if not swallowed quickly.

DOSE REQUIREMENTS

It is difficult to predict the dose of KCl that will be required to maintain proper potassium balance. Many patients do well with 20 mEq/day, but it is questionable how many of these need any supplement at all. People with well-documented hypokalemia can require anywhere from 20 to 120 mEq of KCl/day.[99,100,117] Those patients with disease states associated with high circulating aldosterone levels require doses of potassium in excess of 60 mEq/day.

POTASSIUM-SPARING DIURETICS

11. **Would use of a potassium-sparing diuretic such as triamterene offer any advantage over a potassium supplement to prevent or treat hypokalemia? What dose should be used?**

The potassium-sparing diuretics (amiloride and triamterene) may be more effective in preventing or correcting the fall in serum potassium than potassium supplements.[118,119] These agents reduce urinary potassium losses, minimize alkalosis, and mobilize edema. Approximate equivalent doses are amiloride 20 mg and and triamterene 200 mg. At these doses, potassium replenishing capacity is similar to that observed with a 10- to 20-mEq KCl supplement.[118]

Dyazide (or generic equivalent) and Maxzide are popular products that contain a combination of triamterene plus HCTZ. Although these products are effective in most cases, their cost is warranted only in a patient with documented hypokalemia with thiazide use alone. In one study, one full-strength Maxzide tablet (50 mg thiazide; 75 mg triamterene) was equivalent to 20 to 40 mEq of KCl.[119] Moduretic (a combination of amiloride plus a thiazide) could also be used.

Hyperkalemia is the major toxicity from all the potassium-sparing diuretics and could occur even when they are used in combination with potassium-wasting diuretics. As a general rule, potassium-sparing diuretics should not be used together with either KCl, ACE inhibitors, or ARBs. However, their combined use is warranted in those patients requiring more than 50 mEq/day of KCl. Judicious monitoring is necessary to avoid hyperkalemia. (Also see Question 14 for additional considerations for using spironolactone in patients with severe HF.)

Monitoring

12. After a single 40 mg IV dose of furosemide, A.J. is begun on 40 mg of furosemide each morning and KCl tablets 20 mEq BID. How should his therapy be monitored?

A.J. needs to be monitored for both an improvement in his HF and for side effects (see Tables 19-6 and 19-9). Subjectively, the clinician should monitor for decreased pulmonary distress and an increased exercise tolerance, demonstrating control of HF. Objective monitoring parameters for disease control include weight loss (ideal, 0.5 to 1 kg/day until ideal dry weight is achieved), a decrease in edema, flattening of neck veins, and disappearance of the S_3 gallop and rales. Because A.J. has hypertension, his BP also requires monitoring with a goal to reduce to <120/80 mm Hg.

Patients are sometimes instructed to record their weight each day and are allowed to adjust their diuretic dose based on changes observed. If they are at their ideal "dry weight," they may reduce their dose of diuretic by 50% or even hold one or more doses. If weight increases more than 1 or 2 pounds in a day or 5 pounds per week, edema increases, or SOB returns, the dose of diuretic is temporarily increased.

Dizziness and weakness are subjective indices of volume depletion, hypotension, or potassium loss. Muscle cramps and abdominal pain could indicate rapid changes in electrolyte balance. Objectively, a lowering of BP, especially on standing, and a rising BUN (prerenal azotemia) signify overdiuresis. As discussed in Questions 9 and 10, serum sodium, potassium, chloride, bicarbonate, glucose, and uric acid should be monitored routinely. Questioning the patient with regard to the onset of diuresis (relative to drug ingestion) and the duration of the diuretic effect helps develop the most convenient schedule for the patient.

Refractory Patients: Combination Therapy

13. You are consulted on another patient whose initial history was similar to A.J.'s. After nearly 2 years of relatively good HF control on a regimen of 40 mg furosemide, 20 mg QD lisinopril, 200 mg QD metoprolol extended release, and 0.125 mg QD digoxin, urinary output diminished about 1 week ago and edema increased significantly. Nonadherence to drug therapy and salt restriction was ruled out. The dose of furosemide was increased to 80 mg 2 days ago without much effect. Should the dose of furosemide be increased further? Could another diuretic be added to the therapy?

As described in the pharmacology of diuretics section earlier in the chapter, all loop and thiazide diuretics must reach the tubular lumen to be effective. Because these drugs are highly bound to serum proteins and endogenous organic acids, they cannot enter the tubular lumen by glomerular filtration. For diuresis to begin, they must be transported into the proximal tubule by active secretion from the blood into the tubule. If this active transport is blocked, diuretics will not reach their site of action. This can lead to a diminished diuretic response in patients with either renal insufficiency or decreased RBF associated with uncompensated HF. In particular, patients with renal insufficiency or poor RBF often require large doses of diuretics to achieve a desired response. Endogenous organic acids also can accumulate during renal insufficiency, avidly binding the drug and preventing its access to the site of action.[57,58]

Both the total amount of drug delivered to the tubule and the rate of delivery of the drug to the tubule determine the magnitude of diuretic response elicited.[57,58] This explains why 80 mg of furosemide yields more diuresis than a 40-mg dose and why an IV injection provides a more rapid and vigorous diuresis than an oral dose. However, once a threshold concentration (ceiling dose) is achieved within the tubule, higher concentrations produce no greater intensity of effect, but the duration of action may be prolonged. (See Question 8 for an expanded discussion about loop diuretic bioavailability and the concept of "gut wall edema.")

In addition to these explainable causes, many patients develop a blunted diuretic response with continued therapy for unknown reasons. Generally, alternative treatment plans are pursued when the dose given approaches the ceiling doses for each drug listed in Table 19-4. Continuous infusions of furosemide (2.5 to 3.3 mg/hour), bumetanide (1 mg/hour), or torsemide (3 mg/hour) can be more efficacious than intermittent bolus doses in patients with severe HF or renal insufficiency.[57,58,120–124] Even higher doses are recommended by one clinician: 0.25 to 1 mg/kg per hour for furosemide, 0.1 mg/kg per hour for bumetanide, and 5 to 20 mg/hr for torsemide.[125] Another institution uses an aggressive protocol of a 100 mg IV bolus of furosemide followed by a continuous IV infusion at a rate of 20 to 40 mg/hr, which is doubled every 12 to 24 hours in nonresponding patients to a maximum infusion rate of 160 mg/hr to attain a diuresis rate of 100 mL/hr or higher.[126]

In some instances, switching from one loop diuretic to another can overcome the problem.[58,59,125] For example, torsemide might work when furosemide fails because of more reliable absorption with torsemide.[88,89] If this maneuver fails, a combination of diuretics can be tried. The most effective regimens combine drugs that work at two different parts of the tubule.[58,59] For example, a loop diuretic that works on the ascending limb of the loop of Henle is added to metolazone that

---

Table 19-9   Monitoring Parameters with Diuretics

↓ CHF symptoms (see Table 19-6)

Weight loss or gain; goal is 1-2 pound weight loss/day until "ideal weight" achieved[a]

Signs of volume depletion
  Weakness
  Hypotension, dizziness
  Orthostatic changes in BP[b]
  ↓ Urine output
  ↑ BUN[c]

Serum potassium and magnesium (avoid hypokalemia and hypomagnesemia)

↑ uric acid, glucose

[a]Weight loss may be greater during first few days when significant edema is present.
[b]A ↓ in systolic BP of 10–15 mm Hg or a ↓ in diastolic BP of 5–10 mm Hg.
[c]A rising BUN can be caused by either volume depletion from diuretics or poor renal flow from poorly controlled HF. Small boluses of 0.9% saline can be given cautiously to differentiate a rising BUN from volume depletion versus poor cardiac output. If volume depletion is present, saline will cause an ↑ in urine output and a ↓ in BUN. However, if the patient has severe HF, the saline could cause pulmonary edema.
BP, blood pressure; BUN, blood urea nitrogen; HF, heart failure; K, potassium; Mg, magnesium.

blocks sodium reabsorption in the distal tubule. Various thiazide diuretics, including chlorthalidone (Hygroton), chlorothiazide (Diuril), and HCTZ, have been reported to effectively enhance diuresis when combined with a loop diuretic, but it is unclear if the responses are simply additive or truly synergistic. Rarely, triple therapy regimens of metolazone, loop, and potassium-sparing diuretics are used to optimize diuresis and electrolyte control.

Most clinicians choose a combination of metolazone plus furosemide or bumetanide based on demonstrated value in the literature and clinical experience. A small dose of metolazone (5 mg) is first added to the furosemide therapy, doubling the dose of metolazone every 24 hours until the desired diuretic response is achieved. If the synergism desired is seen with the first dose, the dose of the loop diuretic should be decreased. Metolazone's longer duration of action can cause a greater than predicted diuresis and electrolyte loss when combined with a loop diuretic. Thus, careful monitoring of weight, urine output, BP, and BUN is required. Since there is no parenteral form of metolazone, chlorothiazide, at a dose of 500 to 1,000 mg once or twice daily, is the only option for a non–loop diuretic that can be given intravenously.

Nondiuretic Effect of Spironolactone: Effect on Mortality

14. We return now to A.J. who was treated in Questions 1 to 12. It has been 2 days since he started furosemide, potassium supplements, and an ACE inhibitor. He complains of gastric cramping after each dose of potassium, even when taken with food. It is decided to discontinue the potassium supplement and start spironolactone at a dosage of 50 mg/day. Does this therapy offer any advantages other than diuresis and a source of potassium repletion?

Aldosterone contributes to HF through the increased retention of sodium and the depletion of sodium. Likewise, the diuretic and potassium-sparing actions of spironolactone are attributed to inhibition of aldosterone.[118] Until recently, it was believed that optimal doses of ACE inhibitors fully suppressed the production of aldosterone since angiotensin II is a potent stimulus for aldosterone production. However, it is now recognized that aldosterone levels can remain elevated through a combination of nonadrenal production and reduced hepatic clearance. In addition, it has become clear that both angiotensin II and aldosterone have other negative effects on the cardiovascular system including myocardial and vascular fibrosis, direct vascular damage, endothelial dysfunction, oxidative stress, and prevention of norepinephrine uptake by the myocardium.[34,127] This led the Randomized Aldactone Evaluation Study (RALES) investigators to test the hypothesis that low doses of spironolactone might impart a cardioprotective effect in patients with severe HF independent of diuresis or potassium retention.[56] In this trial, 1,663 patients with a history of NYHA class IV HF within the previous 6 months (but in class III or IV on study entry), an EF of 35% or less, and continued treatment (unless contraindicated or not tolerated) with a loop diuretic (100%), an ACE inhibitor (94%), and digoxin (74%) were randomized to receive either spironolactone 25 mg (N = 822) or placebo (N = 841). The dose of spironolactone could be increased to 50 mg if HF worsened without evidence of hyperkalemia.

The study was discontinued prematurely after a mean follow-up of 24 months when a statistically significant reduction in mortality was observed. There were 386 deaths in the placebo group (46%) compared with 284 (35%) with spironolactone. These differences were first evident at 2 to 3 months after starting treatment. The greatest risk reduction was in cardiovascular deaths. In addition, more subjects had symptomatic improvement (as evidenced by moving to a lower NYHA class) and fewer had symptomatic worsening with the active drug. Hospitalization rates were lower in the patients treated with spironolactone. Serum creatinine and potassium concentrations were somewhat higher with active drug, but the changes were not considered clinically significant. Hyperkalemia developed in 2% of spironolactone patients and 1% of placebo subjects. Gynecomastia was reported in 10% of men treated with spironolactone compared with only 1% of those receiving placebo.

It is important to emphasize that nearly all subjects had continuing HF symptoms despite maximal drug therapy with multiple drugs, including an ACE inhibitor. Although ACE inhibitors indirectly suppress aldosterone at therapeutic doses, the inhibition is not as complete as with spironolactone. Thus, this study provided the first clinical evidence that spironolactone protects against myocardial and vascular fibrosis and/or alters hemodynamic or hormonal mediators of HF.

Subsequently, the aldosterone receptor inhibitor eplerenone (Inspra) was studied in 6,632 patients with left ventricular dysfunction following MI. In the EPHESUS study, subjects were randomized to receive either eplerenone 25 mg QD initially, titrated to 50 mg QD, or placebo.[59] Concurrent therapy included diuretics (60%), ACE inhibitors (87%), β-blockers (75%), and aspirin (88%). During a mean follow-up of 16 months, there were 478 deaths (14.4%) in the active treatment group compared with 554 deaths (16.7%) with placebo (relative risk, 0.85; P = 0.008). The majority of deaths were due to cardiovascular causes. Similar to spironolactone, more subjects experienced hyperkalemia with eplerenone than with placebo. However, because eplerenone does not block progesterone and androgen receptors, gynecomastia and sexual dysfunction may be less.[59,127] Eplerenone was initially approved by the FDA for hypertension, and gained labeling for post MI patients in late 2003.

Because A.J. had NYHA class III symptoms when first seen, he fits the profile of the subjects in the RALES study, although he had not been taking his ACE inhibitor long enough to obtain the full therapeutic benefit. Starting A.J. on spironolactone is appropriate because of his intolerance of potassium supplements and it might provide cardiovascular protection. In the RALES study, the starting dose of spironolactone was 25 mg QD. The dose of 50 mg was chosen for A.J. because he has a history of hypokalemia that required potassium supplementation. This dose may or may not be enough to normalize his serum potassium. He will need to be followed to determine whether larger doses of spironolactone will be necessary or if a small dose of a potassium supplement might need to be restarted. If gynecomastia develops, triamterene or amiloride could replace spironolactone for potassium retention, but there is no evidence that these drugs protect against HF complications. Eplerenone is another possible alternative.

Drug of First Choice After Diuretics

Vasodilators and ACE Inhibitors: Comparison With Digoxin

15. After 3 days of furosemide and an ACE inhibitor, A.J.'s doctor wants to start digoxin. A.J.'s PND has resolved, but he still has difficulty walking without SOB and fatigue. His lower extremity edema is only slightly reduced. His current BP is 145/90 mm Hg and his weight has dropped to 73 kg after diuresis. Repeat laboratory measurements include the following: Na, 139 mEq/L; K, 4.3 mEq/L; Cl, 98 mEq/L; CO_2, 27 mEq/L; BUN, 27 mg/dL; and SrCr, 0.6 mg/dL. Is digoxin an appropriate choice of therapy?

Debates raged for years about whether digitalis glycosides or vasodilators should be the drug(s) of first choice for treating HF. By the time the AHCPR and first ACC/AHA guidelines were published in 1994 to 1995, a clear consensus was evident.[1-2] Vasodilators are first-line therapy, with digoxin being added in patients with either supraventricular arrhythmias, failure to achieve symptomatic relief with vasodilators alone, or intolerable side effects from vasodilators. ACE inhibitors are preferred over other vasodilators because of proven efficacy, convenience of dosing, and fewer side effects. By 1999 experts also recommended starting β-blocker therapy earlier in the treatment plan.[3,4] This latter point is discussed later.

To understand the reason for the increased emphasis on ACE inhibitors and secondary role of digoxin requires an historical overview. A partial review is given here, but the reader should consult the sixth edition of *Applied Therapeutics: The Clinical Use of Drugs* for the citations and abstract of older articles.

CONTROVERSY OVER EFFICACY OF DIGOXIN

Correction of the underlying defect is a rational approach to the treatment of any disease. If one considers HF solely as "pump failure" with a weakened myocardial muscle, then digitalis is the logical choice by improving cardiac contractility, CO, and renal perfusion. By focusing on symptom relief and increased exercise tolerance as markers of benefit, digoxin is effective. However, critics raised concerns that symptom relief was less in patients with normal sinus rhythm than in those with supraventricular arrhythmias. The most vocal critics claimed that the risk of digitalis toxicity did not warrant using this class of drugs in patients with normal sinus rhythm.

Using multivariate analysis, one group of investigators concluded that a third heart sound (S_3 gallop rhythm), an enlarged heart, and a low EF best predict those patients with normal sinus rhythm who will derive a beneficial response from digoxin.[128] Several other meta-analyses and critical reviews of the literature later concurred that many of the original trials were designed improperly or lacked proper controls and that digoxin therapy provides a beneficial effect, especially in patients with severe symptomatic ventricular systolic dysfunction.[129,130]

VASODILATORS IMPROVE SURVIVAL (TABLE 19-10)

While these debates were ongoing, recognition of the contributions of the renin-angiotensin-aldosterone system and the sympathetic nervous system in perpetuating the defects of HF brought initial interest in vasodilators. Again, the focus was on symptom relief. First hydralazine and nitrates, then their combination, and finally ACE inhibitors were all shown to be effective in improving the symptoms of HF. Nonetheless, digitalis was usually used first, especially in those patients with either supraventricular arrhythmias and/or an S_3 gallop rhythm. Vasodilators were added to those patients failing a combined regimen of a diuretic and digoxin.

Finally, investigators began focusing on the more important issue of improving survival in patients with HF. The first evidence for decreased mortality came from the First Veteran's Administration Cooperative Study (V-HeFT I) that showed combined hydralazine/isosorbide dinitrate (hydral-iso) treatment reduced mortality to a greater extent than placebo in patients with NYHA class III or IV HF.[131] All subjects continued their previously prescribed diuretic and digitalis regimens. Active intervention consisted of combination hydralazine (300 mg/day) plus isosorbide dinitrate (160 mg/day). Cumulative mortality rates over an average of 2.3 years were significantly lower in the combination therapy group (38.7%) than with placebo (44%). Exercise tolerance and LVEF were improved with combination therapy at both the 8-week and 1-year follow-up, but not in the placebo group.

The Cooperative North Scandinavian Enalapril Survival (CONSENSUS) study was the first to show improved survival in patients with HF treated with an ACE inhibitor.[132,133] Two hundred and fifty-three men and women with severe HF (NYHA class IV) were treated with either enalapril or placebo. Digitalis, diuretics, and other vasodilators were continued. At the end of 6 months, 42% of patients in the enalapril group showed symptomatic improvement compared with 22% of placebo patients. The mortality rate was 26% in patients treated with enalapril compared with 44% in the placebo group, a 40% reduction. Follow-up at 2 years showed a sustained effect with mortality being 47% with enalapril and 74% with placebo, a 37% reduction. Almost all deaths were cardiac in origin.

Although the results from both studies were encouraging, the high rate of mortality in the vasodilator groups (even when combined with diuretics and digoxin) is evidence of the poor outcome in patients with advanced HF. This is a sobering reminder of the poor prognosis associated with the later stages of HF despite aggressive therapy. In addition, both V-HeFT I and Consensus I left several questions unanswered: Does vasodilator therapy work without digitalis? Would patients with less advanced HF (NYHA class I or II) show similar benefit? Which is the better treatment regimen, hydral-iso or an ACE inhibitor?

The SOLVD study addressed the issue of treating patients with less severe disease.[134] Subjects with NYHA class II or III HF and an EF <35% were treated with either enalapril at a dosage of 2.5 to 20 mg/day (N = 1,284) or placebo (N = 1,285) in addition to conventional therapy over an average of 41.4 months. Mortality rate was 35.2% in the enalapril group compared with 39.7% in the placebo group, with the greatest benefit being from deaths attributed to progressive HF. Two lessons can be gained from this trial: patients with less severe disease also experience symptom improvement from vasodilator therapy, as well as experiencing lower mortality rates.

Next, the second Veteran's Administration Cooperative Study (V-HeFT II)[17,135] sought to answer the question of

Table 19-10 Clinical Trials of ACE Inhibitors in Left Ventricular Dysfunction[61]

Study	Patient Population	ACE Inhibitor	Time Started After MI	Treatment Duration	Outcome	Reference
Studies in LV dysfunction						
CONSENSUS	NYHA IV (N = 253)	Enalapril vs placebo		1 day–20 mo	Decreased mortality & HF	130, 131
SOLVD-Treatment	NYHA II/III (N = 2,569)	Enalapril vs placebo		22–55 mo	Decreased mortality & HF	132
V-HeFT II	NYHA II/III (N = 804)	Enalapril vs hydralazine, isosorbide		0.5–5.7 yr	Decreased mortality & sudden death	17, 133
SOLVD-Prevention	Asymptomatic LV dysfunction (N = 4,228)	Enalapril vs placebo		14.6–62 mo	Decreased mortality & HF hospitalizations	181
Studies in LV dysfunction after MI						
SAVE	MI, decreased LV function (N = 2,331)	Captopril vs placebo	3–16 days	24–60 mo	Decreased mortality	183
CONSENSUS II	MI (N = 6,090)	Enalaprilat/enalapril vs placebo	24 hr	41–180 days	No change in survival; hypotension with enalaprilat	182
AIRE	MI and HF (N = 2,006)	Ramipril vs placebo	3–10 days	>6 mo	Decreased mortality	144, 184
ISIS-4	MI (N = >50,000)	Captopril vs placebo	24 hr	28 days	Decreased mortality	
GISSI-3	MI (N = 19,394)	Lisinopril vs placebo	24 hr	6 wk	Decreased mortality	
TRACE	MI, decreased LV function (N = 1,749)	Trandolapril vs placebo	3–7 days	24–50 mo	Decreased mortality	145
SMILE	MI (N = 1,556)	Zofenopril vs placebo	24 hr	6 wk	Decreased mortality	146

Adapted with permission from reference 61.

relative benefit of hydral-iso versus enalapril. Patients receiving diuretics and digoxin for HF of varying degrees of severity (primarily functional class II or III) were randomized to either enalapril at a fixed dose of 20 mg/day or the hydral-iso combination at a dosage of 300 mg hydralazine plus 160 mg of isosorbide. Mortality rates were lower in the enalapril group (18%) than with combination therapy (28%), with the greatest benefit in both groups being in patients with less severe disease (functional class I or II). Although a placebo group was not included in this trial, the survival rate with hydral-iso was the same as seen in V-HeFT I,[131] inferring a beneficial effect with hydral-iso in V-HeFT II as well. In addition, treatment with hydral-iso was more effective than enalapril in improving patients' exercise tolerance and body oxygen consumption during peak exercise. EF also increased faster (but not necessarily to a greater extent) with hydral-iso than with enalapril. In both V-HeFT I[131] and V-HeFT II,[135] enalapril was better tolerated than hydral-iso. In summary, a trend toward better symptom control occurred with hydral-iso, but improved survival and fewer side effects were seen with enalapril. Although not specifically studied in this trial,

these trends suggest a possible benefit to using all three drugs in combination together.

In all these trials, the investigators were careful to include only patients with systolic failure as evidenced by an EF <40%. Thus taken as a whole, they provide convincing evidence for the value of vasodilators in systolic failure.

DIGOXIN WITHDRAWAL TRIALS

In 1993, two digoxin withdrawal trials, PROVED[136] and RADIANCE,[137] were published. Both attempted to determine whether patients with HF who are already treated with digoxin will show deterioration of control or remain stable after discontinuation of digoxin. In both studies, patients had documented systolic failure (LVEF <35% by radionuclide ventriculography), mild to moderate symptoms (NYHA class II or III), were in normal sinus rhythm, and were stable for at least 3 months with a treatment regimen of a diuretic and digoxin (baseline digoxin level 0.9 to 2.9 ng/mL). A significant difference was that patients in the RADIANCE trial were also stabilized on an ACE inhibitor in addition to the diuretic and digoxin.[136] A 12-week, double-blind, placebo-controlled treatment period followed initial stabilization in both studies. Patients in the active treatment groups continued digoxin at their previous dose. Those in the placebo groups were withdrawn from digoxin and given an identical looking placebo.

In PROVED,[136] 42 subjects continued digoxin and 46 were given placebo. There were 29% treatment failures in the withdrawal group compared with only 19% in those still taking digoxin. Treatment failure was defined as worsening HF symptoms requiring a therapeutic intervention (e.g., increased diuretic dosage or addition of a new drug), an emergency department (ED) visit or hospitalization for HF, and/or death. Exercise tolerance worsened in more patients taking placebo. Those taking digoxin tended to maintain lower body weight and HRs as well as higher EFs. In the RADIANCE study, 85 subjects continued digoxin therapy and 93 were switched to placebo.[137] Over the 12-week follow-up period, only 4 of the subjects taking digoxin (4.7%) developed worsening symptoms compared with 23 (24%) of the placebo-treated patients. More of the placebo-treated patients had worsening of the EF and lower quality of life scores. The finding that deterioration in symptoms after discontinuing digoxin often was delayed for several weeks offers a possible explanation as to why earlier clinical trials using shorter observation periods failed to establish a benefit from digoxin. When comparing the two trials directly, fewer patients deteriorated in both arms in the RADIANCE study. Whether this is attributed to a greater benefit from combining an ACE inhibitor with a diuretic compared with using a diuretic alone cannot be established.

These studies establish a beneficial effect of digoxin, even in those patients receiving concurrent ACE inhibitors in RADIANCE. However, there are at least two factors that limit extrapolation to all patients with HF. First, the investigators only assessed the value of therapy indirectly by using a withdrawal design instead of initiating therapy in patients previously untreated with digoxin. Second, the patients had advanced disease as evidenced by NYHA class II or III symptoms despite triple drug therapy. Thus, the benefit of digoxin as initial monotherapy in early disease is still open to debate.

EFFECT OF DIGOXIN ON MORTALITY

An obvious missing link was whether treatment with digoxin improves survival rates. The seminal study to answer this question is the Digitalis Intervention Group (DIG) study.[138] In this study 6,800 patients with HF from 302 centers in the United States and Canada were randomized to receive either digoxin (N = 3,397) or placebo (N = 3,403). Eligibility requirements included an EF of 45% or less (mean, 28% in both treatment groups), normal sinus rhythm, and clinical evidence of HF. Most subjects were in NYHA class II or III HF, although a small number of both class I and class IV subjects were included. Concurrent therapies were diuretics (82%), ACE inhibitors (94%), and nitrates (42%). Of subjects in both groups, 44% were taking digoxin before randomization. The starting digoxin dose (or matching placebo) was based on age, weight, and renal function, with subsequent adjustments made according to plasma level measurements. Approximately 70% of subjects in both groups ended up taking 0.25 mg/day, compared with 17.5% taking 0.125 mg/day and 11% receiving dosages of 0.375 mg/day or higher. By 1 month, 88.3% of subjects on active drug had serum levels between 0.5 and 2.0 ng/mL, with a mean of 0.88 ng/mL. Patients

were followed for an average of 37 months (range, 28 to 58 months).

For the primary outcome of total mortality from any cause, 34.8% of digoxin patients and 35.1% of placebo patients died; corresponding cardiovascular deaths were 29.9% and 29.5%, respectively. While neither of these differences is statistically different, there was a trend toward fewer HF-associated deaths and statistically fewer hospitalizations (risk ratio, 0.72) with active treatment. As would be expected, cases of suspected digoxin toxicity were greater in the active treatment group (11.9% versus 7.9%), but the incidence of true toxicity was low. These results can be interpreted either as disappointing in that overall mortality is not reduced, or as positive in that hospitalizations were fewer in the digoxin group and there is no increase in mortality as reported with nondigitalis inotropes.

This study improves on the PROVED and RADIANCE trials because it added digoxin to other therapy as opposed to being a withdrawal study and also because of the larger study population. However, because nearly all patients were receiving concurrent vasodilator therapy, the value of digoxin as monotherapy on mortality rates remains unanswered.

DIRECT COMPARISON OF DIGOXIN TO VASODILATORS

Surprisingly, little data are available to directly compare digoxin to an ACE inhibitor.[139–141] Two widely quoted studies are the Captopril-Digoxin Multicenter Research Group Study[140] and the Canadian Enalapril versus Digoxin Study Group trial.[141] Similarities between these two trials are inclusion of NYHA class II or III patients, all of whom had a reduced EF and were in normal sinus rhythm. All subjects continued to take diuretics, but other vasodilator therapy was discontinued. About half of the patients had an S_3 gallop rhythm, and about 60% were taking digoxin before entry into the studies. After an appropriate run-in period during which time diuretic doses were stabilized and previous digoxin therapy was discontinued, patients were randomized to receive either digoxin or an ACE inhibitor.

In the Captopril-Digoxin study, both drugs were superior to placebo as measured by symptom scores and treadmill exercise time.[140] The trend toward a more favorable functional improvement with captopril (41% improving with captopril, 31% with digoxin, 22% with placebo) was nonsignificant. The increase in the EF in the digoxin group was greater. Six-month mortality was unchanged with either drug compared with placebo. More minor side effects were associated with captopril (44% versus 30%), but more patients had to discontinue digoxin because of side effects (4.2% versus 2.9%).

In the Enalapril-Digoxin study, more patients in the enalapril group showed functional improvement at 4 weeks (18% versus 10%) and fewer showed functional deterioration (12.5% versus 23%).[141] However, by the end of 14 weeks, an equal number of patients had improved with both drugs (19%), but more patients continued to show deterioration with digoxin (30% versus 12.5%). No differences in the more objective measurements of exercise time, left ventricular function, BP, pulse, and ECG changes were noted between the two groups. More patients withdrew from the digoxin arm because of side effects.

Taken in the aggregate, these studies show no clear benefit of one class of drug versus the other; ACE inhibitors may be slightly more rapid in onset of effect and associated with better tolerance of side effects, but digoxin may improve EF to a greater extent. Mortality differences were undetectable in the Captopril-Digoxin study because of the relatively mild disease in the patients at the outset resulting in mortality rates of only 6% to 8% in either study group. A larger sample size and longer duration of observation would be required to detect a significant difference in mortality.

To summarize, based on clinical outcomes (resolution of symptoms and improved cardiac function), both vasodilators and digitalis glycosides are effective in patients with documented systolic dysfunction. The documented improvement in survival rates with both hydral-iso and ACE inhibitors, coupled with the neutral findings of the DIG study, tip the balance in favor of ACE inhibitors as initial therapy in all stages of HF. The use of both classes of drugs, plus diuretics, is indicated for severe HF.

The latest clinical guidelines state that digoxin should be considered to improve the symptoms and clinical status of patients with HF, in combination with diuretics, an ACE inhibitor, and a β-blocker.[5] Digoxin may be used early to reduce symptoms in patients who have started, but not yet responded to, treatment with an ACE inhibitor and a β-blocker. Alternatively, treatment with digoxin may be delayed until the patient's response to an ACE inhibitor and β-blocker has been defined and used only for those patients who remain symptomatic despite the other drugs. Monotherapy with digoxin or in combination with only a diuretic is no longer recommended.[5]

In the case of A.J., his physician should be discouraged from starting digoxin at this time. Instead, he should be counseled to continue with the already prescribed ACE inhibitor in addition to continuing the furosemide. A strong argument can be made for starting a β-blocker such as metoprolol or carvedilol now or within the next few days. Based on your advice, A.J.'s doctor has decided to withhold digoxin and assess the response to just one drug (i.e., the ACE inhibitor) for now.

Angiotensin-Converting Enzyme Inhibitors

Agents of Choice

16. The formulary for A.J.'s insurance company only covers four ACE inhibitors: benazepril, captopril, enalapril, and lisinopril. Benazepril is being promoted because the current contract makes it the least expensive of the four drugs. Is there a preference for any specific agent to order for A.J.?

As a general rule, formulary decisions are first based on comparative pharmacologic activity, efficacy, and safety of the drugs. Other factors to consider are labeled (FDA approved) indications, convenience of dosing schedule, and—all else being equal—the cost to the pharmacy (or institution) and the patient (or insurance carrier). A confounding factor is that hypertension is the primary labeled indication for all of the ACE inhibitors and was the initial basis for placing these drugs on formularies. The indication for HF was added after initial marketing and does not appear in the FDA-approved labeling for all of the drugs. Each of these factors are considered below.

The basic mechanism of action of all ACE inhibitors is the same and is described in the pathogenesis section of this chapter.[60–62,142] They inhibit ACE (also called kinase II), thereby reducing the activation of angiotensin II, a major contributor to the undesired hemodynamic responses to HF. Decreased circulating levels of norepinephrine, vasopressin, neurokinins, luteinizing hormone, prostacyclin, and NO also have been noted after administration of ACE inhibitors.

In addition, ACE is responsible for degradation of bradykinin, substance P, and possibly other vasodilatory substances unrelated to angiotensin II. Thus, part of the beneficial effects of ACE inhibitors is caused by the accumulation bradykinin (Fig. 19-6). After attaching to bradykinin-2 (B_2) receptors, vasodilation is produced by stimulating the production of arachidonic acid metabolites, peroxidases, nitric oxide, and endothelium-derived hyperpolarizing factor in vascular endothelium. In the kidney, bradykinin causes natriuresis through direct tubular effects.

The net effect is that ACE inhibitors regulate the balance between the vasoconstrictive and salt-retentive properties of angiotensin II and the vasodilatory and natriuretic properties of bradykinin. The physiologic consequences of the pharmacologic effects of ACE inhibitors are reduced pulmonary capillary wedge pressure (preload) and lowered systemic vascular resistance and systolic wall stress (afterload). CO increases without an increase in heart rate. ACE inhibitors promote salt excretion by augmenting renal blood flow and reducing the production of aldosterone and antidiuretic hormone. The beneficial effects on RBF coupled with the drug's indirect inhibition of aldosterone lead to a mild diuretic response, a distinct benefit over other vasodilator compounds such as hydralazine.

Vasodilation and diuresis are not the only value of ACE inhibitors in HF. Angiotensin II enhances vascular remodeling (referred to as trophic effects on cardiac myocytes), while bradykinin impedes this process.[60,143] In experimental models, ACE inhibitors impede ventricular remodeling by blocking the trophic effects or angiotensin II on cardiac myocytes. Evidence as to whether preserving bradykinin levels effects remodeling is inconclusive, although it might attenuate the progressive deposition of collagen during the chronic phase of post-MI cardiac remodeling.

As of this writing, *captopril (Capoten), enalapril (Vasotec), fosinopril (Monopril), lisinopril (Prinivil, Zestril), quinapril (Accupril), and ramipril (Altace)* have FDA-labeled approval for symptomatic relief of HF symptoms (Table 19-11). However, evidence exists that other agents such as *benazepril (Lotensin)* also increase exercise capacity and quality of life in patients with chronic HF.[145] There does not seem to be a significant difference in side effects between agents either. Based on these factors, no one drug is preferred over another.

Numerous placebo-controlled trials have documented the favorable effects of ACE inhibitor therapy on hemodynamic variables, clinical status, and symptoms of HF.[142,144] Multiple studies demonstrate a consistent 20% to 30% relative reduction in HF mortality that is superior to other vasodilator regimens including the hydralazine-nitrate combination or angiotensin receptor inhibitors (see Question 15). The benefits of ACE inhibitors are independent of the etiology of HF (ischemic versus nonischemic) or the severity of symptoms (NYHA class I through class IV).

Table 19-10 provides a brief summary of the results of the key ACE inhibitor HF trials.[60–62,131–135,144] Many of these were reviewed previously in Question 15. Of the six approved

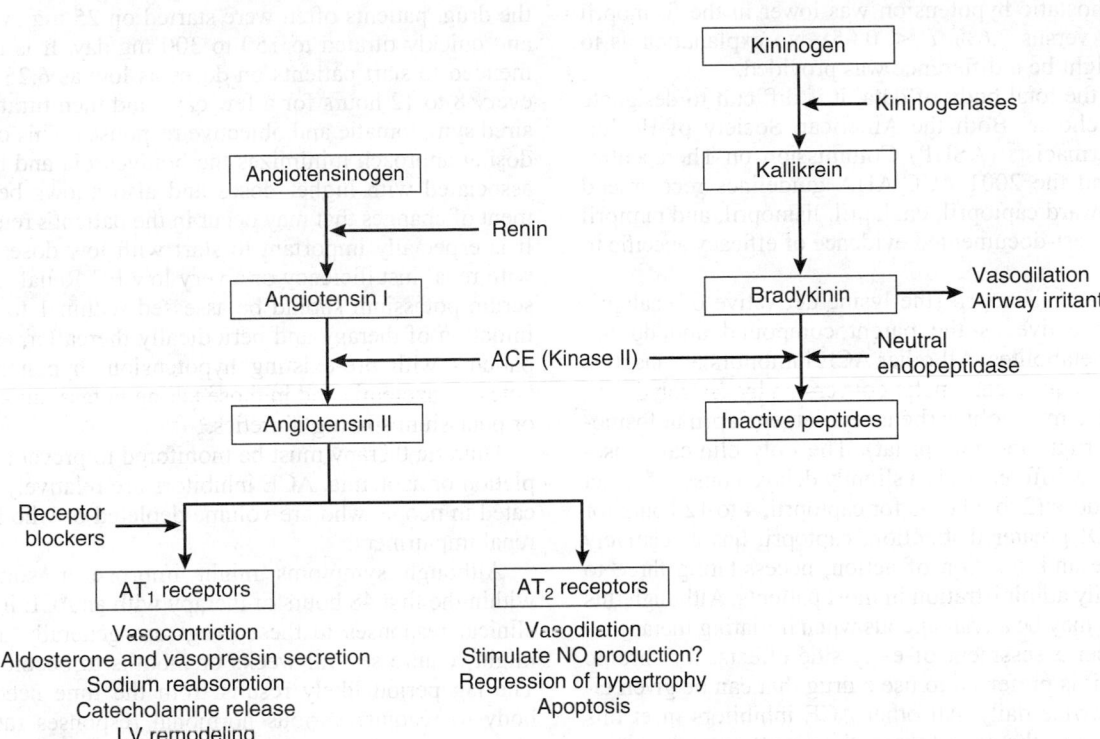

FIGURE 19-6 Angiotensin receptor blocker mechanism. ACE, angiotensin-converting enzyme; LV, left ventricular; NO, nitrous oxide

agents, the most evidence for improved survival is available for enalapril in both chronically symptomatic patients (NYHA classes II–IV) and asymptomatic patients (NYHA class I) with evidence of an impaired EF after an MI.[131–135] A 3-year follow-up to the Acute Infarction Ramipril Efficacy (AIRE) Study reported mortality rates of 27.5% in ramipril-treated subjects (target dose, 5 mg twice daily) compared with 38.9% with placebo, a 36% risk reduction.[146] Published data are also available for a positive effect on reducing short-term mortality with captopril, lisinopril, trandolapril, and zofenopril, primarily in relatively small populations of patients with chronic symptoms or in patients with new onset HF symptoms following an MI.[61,147,148]

Direct comparison of different ACE inhibitors is limited to three trials. The first two comparing lisinopril (5 to 20 mg QD) to either captopril (12.5 to 50 mg daily in two divided doses)[149] or enalapril (5 to 20 mg daily)[150] were only 12 weeks in duration. Exercise duration improved significantly with all three drugs at weeks 6 and 12. There were no statistically significant differences between drugs for NYHA class changes, HF symptoms, or side effects, although there was a trend toward greater exercise duration at week 12 with lisinopril compared with enalapril. In the third study, fosinopril 5 to 20 mg was compared to enalapril 5 to 20 mg daily for 1 year.[151] The fosinopril group had significantly fewer patients who were hospitalized for HF or who died (19.7%) than did the

Table 19-11 ACE Inhibitor Dosing in Systolic Dysfunction[a]

Drug	Dosage Form	Starting Dose[b]	Target Dose[c]	Maximum Dose
Captopril[d] (Capoten, generic)	12.5, 25, 50, 100 mg tablets	6.25–12.5 mg TID	50 mg TID	100 mg TID
Enalapril (Vasotec)	2.5, 5, 10, 20 mg tablets	2.5–5 mg QD	10 mg BID	20 mg BID
Fosinopril (Monopril)	10, 20, 40 mg tablets	5–10 mg QD	20 mg QD	40 mg QD
Lisinopril (Prinivil, Zestril)	2.5, 5, 10, 20, 40 mg tablets	2.5–5 mg QD	10–20 mg QD	40 mg QD
Quinapril (Accupril)	5, 10, 20, 40 mg tablets	5–10 mg QD	20 mg BID	20 mg BID
Ramipril (Altace)	1.25, 2.5, 5, 10 mg capsules	1.25–2.5 mg QD	5 mg BID	10 mg BID

[a]Benazepril, cilazapril, moexipril, trandolapril not labeled for use in HF.
[b]Start with lowest dose to avoid bradycardia, hypotension, or renal dysfunction. All but captopril given QD in AM at starting doses. Increase dose slowly at 2- to 4-week intervals to assess full effect and tolerance.
[c]Enalapril, quinapril, ramipril could possibly be given QD instead of BID based on half-life.
[d]Captopril is short acting. Start with a 6.25- or 12.5-mg test dose, then 6.25 to 12.5 mg TID.
Adapted from reference 6 and 62.

enalapril group (25%; $P = 0.028$). Nearly 60% of patients in the fosinopril group improved their NYHA class. The incidence of orthostatic hypotension was lower in the fosinopril group (1.6% versus 7.6%, $P < 0.05$). No explanation as to why there might be a difference was provided.

Based on the total body of data, it is difficult to designate an agent of choice. Both the American Society of Health-Systems Pharmacists (ASHP) Commission on Therapeutics guidelines and the 2001 ACC/AHA guidelines recommend preference toward captopril, enalapril, lisinopril, and ramipril based on the best-documented evidence of efficacy specific to HF.[5,62]

Captopril and lisinopril (the lysine derivative of enalaprilat) are both active as the parent compound and do not have active metabolites. All other ACE inhibitors are inactive prodrugs that require enzymatic conversion by esterolytic enzymes to active metabolites (benazeprilat, enalaprilat, fosinoprilat, quinaprilat, and ramiprilat). The only clinical consequence of these differences is a slightly delayed onset of effect with the first dose (2 to 6 hours for captopril, 4 to 12 hours for the others). Of greater distinction, captopril has a relatively short half-life and duration of action, necessitating three to four times daily administration in most patients. Although this characteristic may be advantageous when initiating therapy by allowing closer assessment of early side effects, for chronic maintenance it is preferred to use a drug that can be given either once or twice daily. All other ACE inhibitors meet this criterion, either as the parent drug (lisinopril) or as the active metabolite (all others). Based solely on half-life data there would be no expected difference between any of the longer-acting agents. Theoretically, they could all be administered once daily. However, package insert labeling and common standards of practice have led to twice daily dosing, especially at higher doses, for enalapril and ramipril.

We can conclude that A.J. should start captopril for 1 to 2 days for initial dosage titration, but then quickly transfer to a longer-acting drug if he has a good response to the captopril. Because of the lack of demonstrated superiority of one agent over the other, cost does become a factor in choosing a long-acting ACE inhibitor. Because costs are often site- or agency-specific, reflecting interplay between institutional or managed care purchasing contracts and insurance company or drug benefit manager policies, it is not possible to identify the single cheapest agent. A.J.'s doctor decides not to use benazepril, even though it is the least expensive drug, because it does not have FDA approval for HF. Instead, he chooses to start enalapril based on evidence for clinical efficacy, improved survival, and availability of a reduced-cost generic.

Dosage

17. A captopril dosage of 25 mg TID was ordered for A.J. How will this dosage be titrated in preparation for conversion to enalapril? How should he be monitored?

CAPTOPRIL DOSING

Continued experience with captopril has led to a better understanding of dose-response relationships and more rational therapy. Complete inhibition of ACE is achieved with 10 to 20 mg, but larger doses prolong the duration of action. Early single-dose studies suggested that large doses (25 to 150 mg)

were needed for maximal improvement of HF symptoms. Thus, until a better understanding was gained on how to use the drug, patients often were started on 25 mg every 8 hours and quickly titrated to 150 to 300 mg/day. It is now recommended to start patients on doses as low as 6.25 to 12.5 mg every 8 to 12 hours for a few days and then titrate to the desired symptomatic and objective responses. This conservative dosing approach minimizes the bradycardia and hypotension associated with higher doses and also allows better assessment of changes that may occur in the patient's renal function. It is especially important to start with low doses in persons with renal insufficiency or a very low EF. Renal function and serum potassium should be assessed within 1 to 2 weeks of initiation of therapy and periodically thereafter, especially in patients with pre-existing hypotension, hyponatremia, diabetes, or azotemia and in those taking potassium supplements or potassium sparing diuretics.[5]

Diuretic therapy must be monitored to prevent volume depletion or azotemia. ACE inhibitors are relatively contraindicated in people who are volume depleted or who have severe renal impairment.

Although symptoms might improve in some patients within the first 48 hours of therapy with an ACE inhibitor, the clinical responses to these drugs are generally delayed and might require several weeks or months to become apparent. The lag period likely results from the time needed for the body to readjust various hormonal responses rather than a pharmacokinetic or pharmacologic phenomenon. Even if symptoms do not improve, long-term treatment with an ACE inhibitor should be maintained because these drugs can reduce the risk of hospitalization or death independent of their effect on symptoms. Abrupt withdrawal can lead to clinical deterioration and should be avoided unless life-threatening side effects such as angioedema or renal failure are evident.[152]

Reviewing A.J.'s history (Question 1) and repeat vital signs and laboratory values (Question 15), we recall that he was hypertensive and had an elevated BUN at the time of his hospitalization. Both of these problems improved after starting furosemide, but his BUN is now still slightly above normal, although he is not hypotensive. We are, therefore, less concerned about the risk of hypotension, but we are unsure of how the ACE inhibitor will affect his renal function. If CO increases as desired, his renal function should improve; but if he becomes hypotensive, renal function may get worse. The 25-mg dose as currently ordered is probably safe in a stable patient like A.J. However, it is prudent to recommend lowering A.J.'s dosage of captopril to 12.5 mg as a single dose on the first morning. For less stable patients, a starting dose of 6.25 mg should be used. If A.J.'s BP and renal function remain stable after the test dose, he can get a total of three doses, approximately 8 hours apart, of 12.5 mg on the first day. On day 2, the dose can be raised to 25 mg TID. If he again remains stable on day 3, his regimen can be converted to enalapril, using a single daily dose.

CAPTOPRIL COMPARED WITH ENALAPRIL

18. After 2 days of taking captopril, A.J.'s exercise capacity and lower extremity edema are further improved, but his HF is not optimally controlled. He is assessed to have between NYHA class II and III symptoms. BP values throughout the day have fluctuated in the range of 127–145/80–95 mm Hg and his weight is down to 70 kg. Repeat laboratory measurements include the following: Na, 139 mEq/L; K, 4.7 mEq/L; Cl, 98 mEq/L; CO_2, 27 mEq/L; BUN, 24 mg/dL; and SrCr, 0.6 mg/dL. An order is written to begin 2.5 mg/day of enalapril. Is this an appropriate choice of therapy? What is the target dose for him?

DOSE-RESPONSE RELATIONSHIPS

Cumulative evidence from all the clinical trials indicates a relationship between the degree of improvement in HF symptoms and the dose of drug given. Larger doses are more likely to improve the patient's quality of life and reduce the incidence of hospital stays. This relationship is less clear relative to mortality data. At the same time, higher doses are associated with a greater risk of side effects. Based on these principles, proposed recommended starting, target, and maximal doses for the ACE inhibitors are listed in Table 19-11.[5,62] Bioavailability and renal clearance of ACE inhibitors may be reduced in HF necessitating caution in establishing an appropriate dose.

In general, the guidelines can be summarized as "start low and titrate to the maximum tolerated dose." Supporting this principle are the results of the ATLAS Trial.[153,154] Lisinopril was given to 3,164 patients hospitalized during the previous 6 months and with NYHA class II–IV HF and an LVEF <30%. Open label lisinopril 2.5 to 5 mg was given for first 2 weeks, then 12.5 to 15 mg for an additional 2 weeks. If the initial doses were tolerated, subjects were randomized to daily therapy with lisinopril 2.5 to 5 mg (low dosage) or 32.5 to 35 mg (high dosage). All-cause mortality was not different between the two groups (8% lower in the highest dose group compared to the lowest dose; $P = 0.128$). In the high dosage group, hospitalizations and the combined endpoint of death and hospitalization were reduced by 24% ($P = 0.003$) and 12% ($P = 0.002$), respectively. The higher dosage was tolerated by 90% of patients assigned this dose.

Despite these recommendations for using the highest tolerated doses, there is also evidence that lower doses are beneficial. For example, the UK Heart Failure Network Study found that 10 mg twice daily enalapril was no more effective than 2.5 mg twice per day.[155] In this study enalapril was given in low (2.5 mg BID), moderate (5 mg BID), and higher (10 mg BID) dosages to patients with NYHA class II–III HF. The primary combined endpoint (death, hospitalization from HF, and worsening HF incidence) occurred in 12.3%, 12.9%, and 14.7%, respectively, of patients receiving low, moderate, and higher enalapril dosages. None of the between group differences were statistically different. Mortality, evaluated separately, was 4.2%, 3.3%, and 2.9%, respectively. Again, none of the between group comparisons was statistically significant. Further dosing, pharmacologic, and pharmacokinetic information regarding the ACE inhibitors is found in Chapter 14, Essential Hypertension.

For enalapril, the recommended starting dosage is 2.5 to 5 mg/day. For older patients or those with other risk factors (i.e., systolic BP <100 mm Hg, those taking large doses of either loop diuretics or potassium-sparing diuretics, or those with pre-existing hyponatremia, hyperkalemia, or renal impairment), the starting dosage of 2.5 mg/day would be more appropriate. This dosage, or an equivalent with one of the other drugs, should also be considered if the patient is being started

directly on a long-acting drug without prior titration on captopril. However, for a patient like A.J. who has already been treated with captopril for 2 days with no evidence of intolerance, a 5-mg dose is recommended. His current order for 2.5 mg/day can either be changed immediately or within the next few days.

The long-term target dosage of enalapril for A.J. is 10 to 20 mg BID. No clear formula exists for deciding how quickly to titrate to this dose. It depends on several factors, including the degree of improvement in his HF symptoms, side effects, and his motivation to take the medicine. Whenever dosage adjustments are made, it may take as little as 24 hours for the patient to perceive symptom improvement, but generally full hemodynamic steady state is not reached for 1 to 2 months. On the other hand, hypotension and other side effects are more immediate. A.J. could have his dose changed today to 5 mg and then be reassessed in 1 to 2 weeks to determine whether he can tolerate a dosage increase to 5 mg BID. Thereafter, an extra 5 mg/day could be added every 2 to 4 weeks. Thus, it could take 6 months or more to titrate upward to 20 mg BID. If his symptoms are not responding well and he has no side effects, the rate of titration could be made faster, either by shortening the assessment periods (e.g., every week) or by using larger dosage increments (e.g., 10 mg increase).

One study comparing long-term treatment with 50 mg TID of captopril versus 20 BID of enalapril showed more hypotensive episodes and compromised cerebral and renal function in the patients treated with enalapril.[156] From this, it was postulated that the more sustained hypotensive effect of enalapril may actually be a disadvantage. However, a potential confounding variable is that the 40-mg daily dose of enalapril may have been disproportionately high compared with the 150 mg/day dose of captopril.

ACE Inhibitor—Induced Cough

19. After 6 weeks of enalapril therapy, A.J. has been titrated up to a dose of 10 mg BID. He continues to take 40 mg Q am of furosemide and 50 mg of spironolactone. His symptoms are much improved. However, about 2 weeks ago, he developed an annoying nonproductive cough that persisted throughout the day and also made it difficult for him to fall asleep at night. After about 1 week, he went to see his primary care physician who told him that he had bronchitis and recommended that he use a guaifenesin and dextromethorphan containing cough syrup. During a routine clinic visit today, he still is bothered by his "bronchitis." A chest examination reveals no evidence of wheezing, the S_3 heart sound has disappeared, and he still has a few crackles, but much less than when he was first admitted. His neck veins are only minimally elevated over normal, his ankle edema is 1+, and his weight is still 70 kg. BP today is 140/90 mm Hg. All laboratory values are normal, except that his potassium is borderline high at 4.9 mEq/L. BUN and creatinine are 19 mg/dL and 0.6 mEq/dL, respectively. Could the cough and "bronchitis" be a symptom of his HF? What do you recommend?

Cough can be a sign of HF in patients with pulmonary congestion. In extreme cases, patients demonstrate "cardiac asthma" with severe air hunger, wheezing, and dyspnea. However, A.J.'s HF is much improved as evidenced by the objective data. The absence of wheezing and no prior history of asthma or smoking make an obstructive airways disease (asthma or COPD) unlikely. It is possible that he does have bronchitis, but he does not recall having a cold or other respiratory illness preceding the cough. Without other causes, one must be suspicious of an enalapril-induced cough.

This side effect occurs with all ACE inhibitors.[157] Case reports indicate a possible lower incidence with fosinopril (Monopril), but this has not been confirmed under controlled conditions.[158] Specific to A.J., cough is a well-established complication of enalapril. ACE inhibitor–induced cough presents as a dry, nonproductive cough sometimes described as a "tickle in the back of the throat." This complication can arise within the first few weeks to months of starting an ACE inhibitor and persists until the drug is stopped. Symptoms disappear within 1 to 2 weeks of discontinuing treatment and recur within days of rechallenge with either the original or a different ACE inhibitor.

Various reports have found an incidence of cough in 3% to 15% of all patients, even those taking relatively low doses.[157,159] One investigator found a 5% to 10% incidence in white patients of European descent that rose to nearly 50% in Chinese patients.[159] There may also be a higher incidence in women and African American populations.[157]

Accumulation of bradykinin within the upper airway and/or decreased metabolism of proinflammatory mediators such as substance P or prostaglandins are proposed mechanisms of ACE inhibitor–induced cough. These chemicals then act as irritant substances in the airways to increase bronchial reactivity and induce coughing. Bradykinin stimulates unmyelinated afferent sensory C fibers by type J receptors involved in the cough reflex. Bradykinin is also a potent bronchoconstrictor, but pulmonary function remains unchanged, and persons with asthma are no more prone to the reaction than those who do not have asthma. Substance P, also degraded by ACE, has been implicated since it is a neurotransmitter for afferent sensory fibers, specifically C fibers. Because this is a pharmacologic effect rather than an allergic reaction, dosage reduction or switching from one ACE inhibitor to another is generally not helpful. Likewise, dosage reduction is often not helpful. The only way to definitively diagnose the drug-induced cough is to discontinue therapy. Even then, false-positive results may occur if the patient had a mild case of bronchitis that spontaneously resolved at about the same time that the ACE inhibitor was discontinued. If the cough persists after drug discontinuation, other causes should be investigated.

A.J. can continue taking enalapril and followed for another month to determine whether the cough will resolve on its own. Arguing in favor of this action is the symptom improvement in HF he has obtained from the drug, the potential long-term survival benefits of ACE inhibitors, and because the cough is no more than an annoyance. He is not at risk for developing asthma or other airway problems. On the other hand, it would be desirable to find a therapy that is not only effective, but causes fewer side effects for him. Possibilities include an alternative form of vasodilator such as an ARB or hydralazine-isosorbide.

Angiotensin Receptor Antagonists

20. A.J. is disturbed enough by his cough that he has requested discontinuing enalapril. Because he has had such good success with the ACE inhibitor, his physician wants to replace enalapril with valsartan 40 mg BID. What evidence indicates that valsartan or other angiotensin-receptor blocking drugs are effective in treating HF? Are these drugs still associated with causing a cough?

Angiotensin II that is normally activated by the renin-angiotensin cascade interacts with several different membrane-bound receptors, two of which include angiotensin type 1 (AT_1) and type 2 (AT_2) receptors (Fig. 19-6).[60,63,160] Attachment to AT_1 is responsible for most of the unwanted cardiovascular actions of angiotensin II, including vasoconstriction, activation of aldosterone, and stimulation of norepinephrine release. Angiotensin-receptor antagonists all preferentially bind to AT_1 to competitively inhibit attachment by endogenous angiotensin II, thus blocking angiotensin II activity.

As described previously, ACE inhibition affects not only angiotensin II production, but also impairs the metabolism of bradykinin, substance P, and other vasoactive substances.[60,63,160] These substances do not interact with either of the angiotensin receptors, but may independently be associated with production of the cough and first-dose hypotension seen with ACE inhibitors. By giving an AT_1 receptor antagonist, the positive benefits of blocking the cardiovascular effects of angiotensin II are achieved while sparing alteration of the kinin metabolism. Indeed, nearly all trials using various ARBs to treat hypertension or HF have shown a reduced incidence of cough relative to the ACE inhibitors, with prevalence no greater than that of placebo. Of further interest is preliminary information that angiotensin II attachment to the AT_2 receptor might actually lead to beneficial effects, including vasodilation and protection of the vascular wall from proliferative atherosclerotic effects. These responses should remain intact with AT_1 receptor antagonists, but are at least partially blunted by ACE inhibitors.

Evidence for a therapeutic benefit of the receptor antagonists in modifying HF symptoms is mounting[60,160–169] A recent meta-analysis combined data on all-cause mortality and HF related hospitalizations from 17 clinical trials that compared an ARB with either placebo or an ACE inhibitor in patients with HF.[161] Most of the trials also assessed short-term clinical endpoints such as exercise tolerance and EF. In total, 12,469 patients participated and 5 ARBs (candesartan, eprosartan, irbesartan, losartan, and valsartan) were tested, assuming a class effect for all ARBs. ARBs favorably improved exercise tolerance and EF compared to placebo. However, they were not superior to ACE inhibitors in reducing all-cause mortality or hospitalizations for HF. The combination of an ARB and an ACE inhibitor was superior to ACE inhibitor monotherapy in reducing hospitalizations for HF but not in improving survival. In patients not receiving an ACE inhibitor (but receiving other HF drugs), there was a nonsignificant trend favoring ARBs over placebo for both reductions in all-cause mortality and hospitalizations for HF.

The first major clinical trial comparing an ARB to an ACE inhibitor in patients with HF was the Evaluation of Losartan in the Elderly (ELITE) study.[165] Among the strengths of this trial are (1) a relatively large population (722 subjects) who were all ACE inhibitor–naive, (2) comparison of the receptor antagonist to an ACE inhibitor (captopril), and (3) an adequate duration (48 weeks) to allow a preliminary outcome evaluation of frequency of hospitalizations and incidence of death. All subjects were 65 years of age or older with NYHA class II–IV HF, had an EF of 40% or less (mean, 31%), and were not previously treated with either an ACE inhibitor or an ARB. Diuretics were used by 75% of the subjects, with 55% taking digoxin and 40% taking a non–ACE inhibitor vasodilator. Losartan was started at 12.5 mg/day in 352 patients and titrated to a dose as high as 50 mg/day in 300 of them. The 370 subjects randomized to captopril began therapy at 6.25 mg three times daily and were titrated to a maximum dose of 50 mg three times daily (N = 310). For the primary study endpoint, a sustained increase in renal function decline, the two drugs performed identically with 10.5% of subjects in each group having a >0.3 mg/dL rise in serum creatinine. Similarly, functional ability increases were equal in both groups, and only 5.7% of both groups were hospitalized for worsening HF. In an unexpected finding, there was a non-significant trend toward more deaths due to all-causes in the captopril group (N = 32, 8.7%) compared with losartan (N = 17; 4.8%). Also, more subjects discontinued captopril than losartan because of adverse effects (20.8% versus 12.2%). In particular, 3.8% of captopril patients stopped the drug because of cough compared with none of the losartan patients.

Several limitations of this study should be noted: (1) by design, the patients were all elderly; (2) 40% of the subjects were taking other vasodilators as a confounding variable; and (3) the primary endpoint was renal function changes, not hospitalization or death. Nonetheless, the study provided evidence that losartan is at least as effective as the reference ACE inhibitor (captopril) and that patients with HF have equal or fewer side effects with losartan, especially less cough.

The follow-up ELITE II Trial was specifically designed to test the hypothesis that losartan is superior to captopril in terms of reduction in mortality and morbidity in patients 60 years or older.[166] Inclusion criteria and the dosages of losartan and captopril were identical to the first ELITE Trial. By enrolling a larger number of subjects (N = 3,162), it was powered to assess the primary end point of all-cause mortality. The intent was to continue the study until a combined total of 510 deaths occurred between the two treatment groups. After a mean follow-up of 1.5 years, there was no significance difference in all-cause mortality (17.7% losartan versus 15.9% captopril), sudden death (9% versus 7.3%), or all-cause mortality plus hospitalization (47.7% versus 44.9%) between the two treatment groups. Although ARB treatment was not clinically superior to ACE-inhibitor therapy, it was better tolerated with a withdrawal rate of 9.4%, as compared with 14.5% with ACE-inhibitor therapy (P < 0.001). Specifically, significantly fewer patients experienced cough with the ARB.

Candesartan has also been compared to an ACE inhibitor in HF management. In the Randomized Evaluation of Strategies for Left Ventricular Dysfunction (RESOLVD) study, 768 subjects were randomized to receive enalapril (up to 20 mg/day), candesartan (up to 16 mg/day), or the combination of both drugs added to diuretics and/or digoxin for an average of 43 weeks.[1,167] Inclusion criteria included NYHA class II–IV HF, LVEF <40%, and a 6-minute walking distance <500 meters. As in the ELITE trials, all the subjects were ACE inhibitor–naïve. The combination of candesartan and enalapril was more beneficial for preventing left ventricular dilation and suppressing neurohormonal activation than either

candesartan or enalapril alone. No differences were found among any of the three treatment groups in either hospitalization or mortality rates. Though not powered as a mortality trial, mortality rates were higher in the subjects receiving candesartan alone (6.1%) or candesartan combined with enalapril (8.7%) than in the group that received enalapril alone (3.7%).

A second study of candesartan produced similar disappointing findings.[168] The SPICE Trial was a multicenter, double blind, parallel group study of 270 ACE inhibitor–intolerant patients with NYHA class II–IV disease and LVEF <35%. The reasons for ACE inhibitor intolerance were cough (67%), hypotension (15%), and renal dysfunction (11%). Subjects were randomized to treatment with candesartan 4 mg/day (N = 179) or placebo (N = 91) for only 12 weeks. During that time, candesartan was titrated up to the target dose 16 mg/day in 69% of subjects. Concurrent medications included diuretics (74%), digoxin (61%), and a β-blocker (20%). No difference in morbidity (worsening HF, MI, or hospitalization for HF) or mortality was observed between groups. Relevant to AJ, candesartan was well tolerated despite prior intolerance (predominately cough) to ACE inhibitor in the study subjects. Further insight as to the role of candesartan will be provided by the CHARM trial, in progress at the time this chapter was written.[169]

The Val-HeFT Trial was a double-blind, placebo-controlled study to measure the morbidity and mortality in NYHA class II–IV HF patients given valsartan.[170] In contrast to the ELITE and RESOLVD studies, 93% of subjects were already taking an ACE inhibitor at the time of randomization, 35% were taking a β-blocker, and 30% were taking both drugs. Patients were randomized to receive valsartan (N = 2,511) or placebo (N = 2,499) twice daily. The starting dose of valsartan was 40 mg BID that was then titrated up to 160 mg BID by doubling the dose every 2 weeks. The target dose was achieved in 84% of patients taking the active drug. After a mean follow-up of 23 months (range, 0 to 38 months), no significant difference was observed in all-cause mortality between the valsartan group (19.7%) and the control group (19.4%). The combined endpoint of mortality and morbidity (including hospitalization from HF, cardiac arrest with resuscitation and need for IV support) was significantly reduced among patients receiving with valsartan (723 events, 28.8%) as compared to those receiving placebo (801 events, 32.1%), a 13% reduction (P = 0.009). Adverse events were low leading to discontinuation of valsartan in 9.9% of subjects compared to 7.2% with placebo. Dizziness, hypotension, and renal impairment all occurred more frequently in the valsartan treated subjects.

Subgroup analysis of the VAL-HeFT study data raises interesting questions. For example, the observed reduction in the combined endpoint of morbidity and mortality was most pronounced in the small subgroup of only 226 patients (7% of the total study population) not receiving an ACE inhibitor compared to patients on the combination of an ACE inhibitor and valsartan. Further post hoc analysis found that within the 35% of subjects (N = 1,610) taking the combination of an ACE inhibitor and a β-blocker at baseline, the addition of valsartan as a third drug was associated with a trend toward increased morbidity and a statistically significant increase in the combined endpoint of mortality and morbidity. The clinical significance of these findings is unknown.

The overall study results suggest that a combination of valsartan and an ACE inhibitor reduces morbidity, but not mortality. Despite the intriguing results of the subgroup analysis, it is difficult to determine the independent effect of valsartan (i.e., when not combined with an ACE or β- blocker) on morbidity or mortality. More worrisome is the implication that the three-drug combination of valsartan, an ACE inhibitor, and a β-blocker adversely affects morbidity and mortality. Further study is required to determine if the three-drug combination should be avoided in all patients. Some of the answers may be provided by the VALIANT trial currently in progress.[171] In the meantime, the FDA approved valsartan as the first ARB with the labeled indication for management of HF.

Based on this information, it is considered that the angiotensin-receptor antagonists offer little therapeutic advantage over ACE inhibitors, but cough and other side effects may be less. The limited data available indicate that losartan or valsartan may be preferred over candesartan. Only valsartan is FDA approved for HF, but it should not be combined as part of a three-drug regimen with an ACE inhibitor and β-blocker until the findings of the VAL-HeFT trial are refuted. Because A.J. is not tolerating his current regimen, discontinuation of his enalapril and initiation of valsartan is justified. The starting dose of 40 mg BID is consistent with the VAL-HeFT trial protocol. Because of his prior use of large doses of enalapril with no evidence of hypotension, A.J. should tolerate this dose of valsartan. He should be evaluated in 2 weeks for resolution of his cough. The reader is referred to Chapter 14, Essential Hypertension, for further information on the mechanisms of action, metabolism, and dosing of ARBs.

Other ACE Inhibitor and Angiotensin Receptor Blocker Side Effects
HYPERKALEMIA

21. Based on the data in Question 19, what other ACE inhibitor–induced side effects are occurring in A.J.? Will changing from enalapril to valsartan reduce the risk of these side effects?

ACE inhibitors are indirect-acting aldosterone inhibitors because angiotensin II stimulates aldosterone production by the adrenals. In turn, attenuated aldosterone activity can contribute to development of hyperkalemia. For most patients, the magnitude of the increase in serum potassium concentration is small, but the risk for developing hyperkalemia is greater if the patient has compromised renal function or is taking potassium supplements or potassium-sparing diuretics along with the ACE inhibitor. Concurrent use of a potassium-losing diuretic (e.g., a thiazide or loop diuretic) may counteract the potassium retention leading to either normokalemia or hypokalemia. Thus, each patient must be assessed individually regarding their personal response to various drug combinations and whether they need potassium supplements or a reduction in their ACE inhibitor dose.

Such a drug interaction may be occurring in A.J. He was hypokalemic on admission to the hospital in Question 1, possibly because of his prior thiazide therapy. He required potassium supplementation that was continued after he was switched from the thiazide to furosemide. He is now on 50 mg of spironolactone, having discontinued potassium supplements because of GI intolerance. Since starting on enalapril, his serum potassium concentration has slowly risen to 4.9 mEq/L (see Question 19). If A.J. had continued on enalapril, his dose of spironolactone should have been reduced to 25 mg. With the substitution of valsartan for enalapril, the spironolactone dose will still most likely have to be lowered because ARBs block the effects of aldosterone in the kidney identical to ACE inhibitors. On the other hand, if he were switched to a hydralazine-nitrate combination in place of the enalapril, his spironolactone should be continued both for its potassium sparing and disease modifying effects.

ANGIOEDEMA

22. R.S. is a 65-year-old African American man who recently experienced new onset HF with presenting symptoms or shortness of breath while playing golf and edema. Until then, he was healthy and taking no medications. He does not smoke, has no history of asthma or COPD, and no known allergies to food or drugs. R.S. has been taking furosemide 40 mg QD and lisinopril 10 mg QD for 3 weeks. He woke up this morning complaining of difficult breathing, neck swelling, and a "thick tongue." Could this be an abnormal presentation of HF? What drug side effect may be occurring?

Angioedema (angioneurotic edema) is a severe, potentially life-threatening complication of ACE inhibitor treatment.[172–174] Characterized by facial and neck swelling with obstruction to air flow by laryngeal and bronchial edema, this reaction resembles an anaphylactic attack. These symptoms are compatible with those being experienced by R.S. The mechanism of ACE inhibitor induction of angioedema is unknown, but is thought to be related to hypersensitivity to accumulated vasodilating kinins, similar to the cough reaction.

Some, but not all persons with drug-induced angioedema have a history of familial angioedema associated with a genetic defect in their complement system. ACE inhibitors are contraindicated in this population. In one series of case reports, 22% of the reported angioedema reactions occurred within 1 month of starting therapy, with the remaining 77% arising from several months to years later.[173] African Americans and females may have a higher prevalence. The timing of when R.S. started lisinopril and his being African American are consistent with the diagnosis of drug-induced angioedema.

Of concern is the observation that ACE inhibitor–induced angioedema is often misdiagnosed.[174] Several of the patients described in one series had been re-treated with the same or a different ACE inhibitor followed by a repeat episode of angioedema. It is prudent to avoid all ACE inhibitors in any patient with a prior history of angioedema from any cause.

Since the mechanism of ACE-induced angioedema is speculated to be caused by kinin accumulation, changing R.S. to an ARB might be an option.[175] However, several case reports have implicated candesartan, losartan, and valsartan as possible causative agents of angioedema.[172,176–179] In some cases, the subjects had previously experienced angioedema with an ACE inhibitor (indicating possible cross reactivity), while others were ACE inhibitor–naïve. One author claims that ARB-induced angioedema usually manifests after long-term administration (late onset) and with milder symptoms compared to relatively earlier onset with ACE inhibitors. This and other conclusions regarding risk will require further observation. For now, it is prudent not to start an ARB in R.S. Options including starting a β-blocker or hydralazine-isosorbide. As discussed in Case 52, hydralazine-isosorbide might be a better choice for an African American man.

EFFECTS OF ACE INHIBITORS AND ARBS ON KIDNEY FUNCTION

23. B.N., a 62-year-old man, was admitted to the cardiac care unit (CCU) with a 2-day history of breathlessness causing him to sleep upright in a chair and preventing him from walking to the bathroom. Physical examination showed 4+ pitting edema of the legs, scrotal and sacral edema, and significantly distended neck veins. He had a central venous pressure (CVP) of 26 mm Hg (normal, 12). Laboratory values were urine output, <20 mL/hr; BUN, 48 mg/dL; SrCr, 2.0 mg/dL; and serum potassium, 3.2 mEq/L. Home medications, faithfully administered by his wife, included furosemide 240 mg/day, KCl 40 mEq/day, hydralazine 75 mg Q 6 hr, isosorbide dinitrate 20 mg Q 6 hr, metoprolol XL 200 mg QD, and digoxin 0.125mg/day. He was not taking either an ACE inhibitor or and ARB because of a history of fluctuating serum creatinine while taking both of these drugs.

A 100-mg IV bolus of furosemide in the ED resulted in a urine output of 600 mL over 2 hours, but with a subsequent rise of his BUN to 65 mg/dL. Finally, B.N. began captopril 12.5 TID. Within 2 days, B.N.'s breathing improved, his CVP was down to 16 mm Hg, and he was diuresing briskly. He was discharged 1 week later with mild SOB on exertion, 2+ ankle edema, and a reduction of his BUN to 28 mg/dL. Discharge medications included furosemide 120 mg/day, lisinopril 10 mg QD, isosorbide dinitrate 20 mg Q 6 hr, metoprolol XL 200 mg QD, and digoxin 0.125 QD.

B.N. had a BUN of 48 mg/dL and an SrCr of 2.0 mg/dL when he started captopril. The BUN first went up while he was in the hospital and later declined. Explain why these changes occurred. Is the use of ACE inhibitors contraindicated in patients with renal insufficiency? Can they be used safely with diuretics in patients with renal insufficiency?

[SI units: BUN, 17.14, 23.21 and 9.99 mmol/L, respectively; SrCr, 176.9 mmol/L; K, 3.2 mmol/L]

Note: The CVP measurement in this question refers to central venous pressure, an indicator of the right ventricular filling pressure or preload. Refer to Chapter 22, Shock, and Question 48 in this chapter for a more thorough review of this and other cardiac hemodynamic monitoring parameters. His initial CVP of 26 mm Hg was significantly elevated and the repeat value of 16 mm Hg was returning toward the normal value of 12 mm Hg.

The effects of ACE inhibitors and ARBs on RBF and renal function are complex. As seen in Figure 19-7, glomerular filtration is optimal when intraglomerular pressure is maintained at normal pressures. The balance between afferent flow into the glomerulus and efferent flow exiting the glomerulus determines the intraglomerular pressure. A drop in afferent flow or pressure occurring as a result of hypotension, volume loss (e.g., blood loss or overdiuresis), hypoalbuminemia, decreased CO (e.g., HF), or obstructive lesions such as renal artery stenosis all may significantly lower intraglomerular pressure and lead to a loss of renal function. Similarly, longstanding hypertension can damage glomerular basement membrane capillaries and cause renal insufficiency.

In the case of low-pressure or low-flow states, the renin-angiotensin-aldosterone system is activated to maintain intraglomerular pressure. A key factor in preserving glomerular

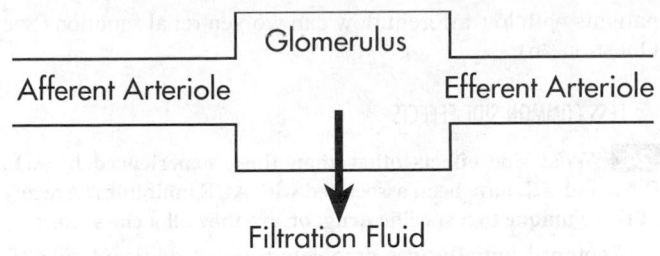

| Glomerulus | | |

Afferent Arteriole | Efferent Arteriole

Filtration Fluid

↓ Afferent flow to glomerulus caused by:

↓ Cardiac output
Systemic hypotension
Blood loss
Overdiuresis, dehydration
Renal artery stenosis (obstruction)
Inhibition of PGE from NSAIDs

↑ Afferent flow to glomerulus caused by:

Systemic hypertension

↑ Efferent pressure to maintain glomerular pressure if:

↑ Production of angiotensin II via activation of renin-angiotensin system

↓ Efferent pressure to protect glomerular pressure if:

ACE inhibitors block angiotensin II production

FIGURE 19-7 Factors affecting renal blood flow. Glomerular filtration is optimal when adequate hydrostatic pressure is maintained in the glomerulus. Governing factors include the blood flow rate to the glomerulus and the balance of afferent and efferent arteriole dilation/constriction. ACE, angiotensin-converting enzyme; NSAIDs, nonsteroidal anti-inflammatory drugs; PGE, prostaglandin E.

pressure is *efferent vasoconstriction* mediated by angiotensin II. Increased efferent pressure helps to maintain intraglomerular pressure by impeding blood flow out of the glomerulus. When patients with low-pressure states are given ACE inhibitors or ARBs, the protective mechanism of efferent vasoconstriction is inhibited and renal function can significantly and rapidly worsen. Conversely, in patients with hypertensive renal disease, glomerular function actually can improve because the ACE inhibitors lower afferent pressure and help protect the kidney. ACE inhibitors slow the progression of diabetic nephropathy and reduce proteinuria independent of their effect on BP (See Chapter 50, Diabetes Mellitus).

Patients with HF present with a complex picture. By decreasing afterload and preload, CO hopefully will improve after ACE inhibitor or ARB therapy, thus preserving or even enhancing RBF. This is obviously the desired effect. If, however, starting ACE inhibitors or ARBs leads to a rapid decrease in systemic BP that is not followed by an increase in cardiac output, worsening renal function may ensue. Because it is impossible to predict which event will occur, ACE inhibitor or ARB therapy needs to be started with low doses and careful monitoring of the BP and renal function as dosage is increased. Diuretics are not contraindicated, but the dosage may need to be reduced to avoid volume depletion and hypotension.

These events are illustrated in B.N. When he was first diuresed, the BUN increased. Addition of an ACE inhibitor and isosorbide in combination with a furosemide led to significant clinical benefit, including improved renal function. For now B.N. is tolerating captopril and is obtaining the desired effect. However, because he has a history of fluctuating renal function with both ACE inhibitors and ARBs, he will require frequent observation. NSAIDs also must be used with caution because inhibition of vasodilating renal prostaglandins in patients with low afferent flow can worsen renal function (See Question 26).

LESS COMMON SIDE EFFECTS

24. What side effects other than those experienced by A.J., B.N., and R.J. have been associated with ACE inhibitors? Are any of these unique to a specific drug, or are they all a class effect?

Captopril initially was associated with significant side effects. Ten to fifteen percent of subjects in early studies developed skin eruptions or fever. These effects were associated primarily with higher dosage (average, 683 mg/ day) and are less frequent when the drug is used in lower doses (<225 mg/day). Skin reactions may be edematous, urticarial, erythematous, maculopapular, or morbilliform in nature. The fact that the rashes disappear with continued therapy in some patients suggests that they may be caused by potentiation of kinin-mediated skin reactions. Transient loss of taste (ageusia), reflex tachycardia, and hypotension also are common at high doses. None of these have occurred in any of the patients in our cases.

Proteinuria, a transient rise in serum creatinine (independent of the mechanisms described in the previous question), agranulocytosis, neutropenia, and fatal pancytopenia[180] also have been attributed to captopril therapy. The marrow toxicity is minimized by keeping total daily doses below 75 mg and avoiding the use of captopril in patients with advanced renal failure.

A theoretic advantage of the newer ACE inhibitors over captopril is the lack of a sulfhydryl group as part of their clinical structures. The sulfhydryl group (also found in penicillamine) is associated with a high incidence of rashes, ageusia, proteinuria, and neutropenia. The clinical significance of this difference remains to be determined, especially because captopril side effects have declined since clinicians have begun to use lower doses.

All ACE inhibitors are contraindicated in pregnancy.[181] Teratogenic effects, including kidney failure and skull and facial deformities, have been reported when taken during the second or third trimester of pregnancy. Risk of use during the first trimester is less clear.

One report described captopril-induced inhibition of digoxin renal clearance, resulting in increased serum digoxin levels.[182] As with many of the other digoxin interactions described elsewhere in this chapter, the clinical significance of this interaction remains to be defined.

ACE Inhibitors in Asymptomatic Patients

25. W.N. is a 44-year-old white man diagnosed with an acute MI by ECG changes and enzyme changes 3 days ago following an episode of acute chest pain while driving his car. He was immediately treated with IV NTG and morphine and underwent thrombolytic therapy with streptokinase within 2 hours of the pain. He has no prior history of angina or hypertension, but was told that he had a high cholesterol level during a screening program 2 years ago. He was taking no medication before this event. Of note, W.N. has a strong family history of coronary artery disease and hyperlipidemia.

His hospital course has been unremarkable with only one episode of mild chest pain responding to sublingual NTG. BP is 130/83 mm Hg, pulse is 80 beats/min with a regular rhythm. He has no ectopy, no complaints of SOB, and no evidence of edema.

Lung sounds are normal as is his chest radiograph. All laboratory values have been normal except for an elevated CK and LDH on the day of admission, a total cholesterol of 245 mg/dL, and an LDL of 180 mg/dL. In preparation for discharge, he underwent repeat angiography and EF was measured by radionuclide ventriculography. His coronary arteries remain patent, but the EF is 35%. Discharge medications include aspirin 82 mg QD and simvastatin 5 mg pm. Propranolol is being withheld because of the low EF.

W.N. has evidence of left ventricular dysfunction based on his EF but is asymptomatic. How would his HF be staged in the ACC/AHA scheme and in the NYHA classification? Should he be started on a diuretic and/or an ACE inhibitor?

This case exemplifies a patient with asymptomatic (NYHA symptom class I) left ventricular dysfunction. An EF <40% indicates systolic dysfunction following heart muscle damage from the MI. These abnormalities would place him in stage B by the ACC/AHA guidelines (Table 19-3). An absence of edema, SOB, or other clinical symptoms argues against the need for diuretics. However, the ACC/AHA guidelines recommend starting patients like W.N. on both an ACE inhibitor and a β-blocker.[5]

Evidence supports use of ACE inhibitors in asymptomatic patients with early left ventricular dysfunction to slow the progression of the disease, possibly by retarding the remodeling effects on the cardiac muscle that may otherwise occur. This is best exemplified by the results of the SOLVD prevention trial.[182] Subjects enrolled in this study were actually a subset of the original SOLVD study[134] with one important difference; although they had an EF of <35%, they were asymptomatic at the time of entry into the trial. Patients received either placebo (2,117 subjects) or enalapril titrated to a dose of 2.5 to 20 mg/day (2,111 subjects). Diuretics and all other active drugs were withheld unless the patient developed overt HF. Over the 37.4-month study period, 20% of the enalapril-treated patients developed symptoms of HF compared with 30% in the placebo group, a 37% reduction. The treatment group also had fewer hospitalizations for anginal symptoms and MI. As would be expected in this relatively low-risk population, mortality rates were low (14.9% to 15.8%) and not statistically significant between the two groups. However, the death rates became more divergent in favor of enalapril late in the study as more patients developed overt HF. Because W.N. has no contraindications to using an ACE inhibitor, he should be started on 5 mg/day of enalapril and titrated to a target dose of 20 to 40 mg/day.

The reader also is referred to Chapter 18, Myocardial Infarction, for a related discussion on the early use of ACE inhibitors in symptomatic patients following infarction (CONSENSUS II, SAVE, and AIRE trials).[184–186] Chapter 18 also thoroughly reviews the rationale for prescribing β-blockers in all post-MI patients unless contraindications exist. W.N.'s physician chose not to use propranolol because of his low LVEF. This is an acceptable choice, but metoprolol should be substituted for propranolol. Metoprolol reduces morbidity and mortality following MI and also slows the onset and progression of HF.

DRUG INTERACTION OF ACE INHIBITORS WITH ASPIRIN

26. Enalapril was started in B.N. for the reasons stated in question 25. Aspirin, 82 mg QD, has also been prescribed. What are the potential benefits and risks of this combination of drugs?

Aspirin is recommended for all patients following MI (See Chapter 18, Myocardial Infarction). Several studies suggest that aspirin may attenuate the beneficial affects of ACE inhibitors when given together in patients with HF and other cardiovascular disorders. The proposed mechanism is inhibition of prostaglandin formation by aspirin, thus counteracting the clinical effects of ACE inhibitors that rely in part on prostaglandins to elicit their positive hemodynamic effects. The significance of this interaction is still being debated. The reader is referred to two comprehensive reviews of this interaction.[187,188] Both conclude that there is insufficient data to firmly establish or refute an adverse clinical outcome associated with the combination of aspirin and an ACE inhibitor in patients with HF.

The most widely quoted supporting evidence for a possible adverse effect comes from subgroup analysis of the SOLVD trial that compared enalapril to placebo in patients with HF.[134] Overall, patients taking aspirin and other antiplatelet drugs at the beginning of the trial had lower mortality rates. However, antiplatelet drugs were of benefit primarily only in patients taking placebo as opposed to those taking enalapril. The combination of enalapril with an antiplatelet agent was not associated with a mortality benefit, whereas combining placebo with aspirin was associated with reduced mortality (0.68 hazard ratio; 95% confidence interval [CI], 0.58 to 0.80). Similarly, the mortality benefit of enalapril was primarily in patients not taking antiplatelet agents (0.77 hazard ratio; 95% CI, 0.657–0.87) as opposed to those who were taking them (1.10 hazard ratio; 95% CI, 0.93–1.30). These observations are limited because it was a post hoc, retrospective analysis of the study data, and continuing use of antiplatelet drugs at the end of the trial was not assessed. Four other small published trials and two abstracts indicate a possible interaction with aspirin, all of which are limited by small sample sizes, short duration of assessment (single dose to several weeks), and reliance on hemodynamic measures such as peripheral vascular resistance and pulmonary responses instead of HF clinical outcomes.[187,188] In these trials, the interaction appeared to be limited to aspirin and various ACE inhibitors, but was not observed between aspirin and losartan or between ticlopidine (which does not affect prostaglandins) and ACE inhibitors. Conversely, one published trial and two abstracts cited in the review articles suggest no interaction between aspirin or ifetroban (a thromboxane A$_2$ receptor antagonist) and an ACE inhibitor.[187,188] In the largest of these trials (317 patients with ischemic cardiomyopathy and LVEF <35%) and with the longest follow-up (mean, 5.7 years), use of aspirin was associated with lowered risk of mortality and hospital readmission, regardless of whether an ACE inhibitor was prescribed. One of the reviewers arrived at two generalizations.[187] Dosages of aspirin of 100 mg per day or less interact little with ACE inhibitors, whereas higher dosages may carry a higher risk. Some patients, for unknown reasons, are more susceptible to the interaction.

The ACC/AHA practice guidelines claim that many physicians believe that the data supporting the existence of an adverse interaction between aspirin and ACE inhibitors are not sufficiently compelling to justify altering the current practice of prescribing the two agents together.[5] In contrast, other physicians would consider the withdrawal of aspirin (because there are no data indicating it can reduce the risk of ischemic events in patients with HF) or use of an alternative antiplatelet agent such as clopidogrel, which does not interact with ACE inhibitors and which may have superior effects in preventing ischemic events.[5]

Use of β-Blockers in Systolic Heart Failure

27. Returning to the case of A.J., we are now 6 weeks into his treatment, and as indicated in question 20, his regimen was changed to valsartan 40 mg BID in place of enalapril. After starting valsartan, his cough disappeared over the next 7 to 10 days. During that same time, he noted more fatigue and increased nighttime dyspnea. These symptoms improved after his dose of valsartan was increased incrementally to 80 mg BID. At the same time, his physician wants to reconsider the need to start a β-blocker. Is this a good time to start a β-blocker?

The physiologic basis for the use of β-blockers in HF and the changes observed in receptor sensitivity is described in greater detail in the pathophysiology section of this chapter.[27–32]

β-Blockers have been evaluated during randomized clinical trials in more than 10,000 patients with varying degrees of systolic HF.[27–32] Five meta-analyses have arrived at the same conclusions: the use of β-blockers is associated with a consistent 30% reduction in mortality and a 40% reduction in hospitalizations in patients with HF.[189–193]

The 2001 ACC/AHA guidelines state that because metoprolol and carvedilol have been shown to reduce HF symptoms and reduce mortality, they should be prescribed to all patients with stable HF due to left ventricular systolic dysfunction, unless there is a contraindication to their use.[5] They should be part of the primary treatment plan, usually in combination with a diuretic, and ACE inhibitor and often with digoxin. Contrary to the practice of some clinicians, the use of β-blocker drugs should not be delayed until the patient is found to be resistant to treatment with other drugs. Another common misperception is that patients who have mild symptoms or who appear clinically stable on diuretics and ACE inhibitors (with or without digoxin) do not require additional treatment. However, even these patients should receive a β-blocker to slow the rate of disease progression and reduce the risk of sudden death. Similarly, patients need not be taking high doses of ACE inhibitors before being considered for treatment with a β-blocker. To the contrary, in patients taking a low dose of an ACE inhibitor, the addition of a β-blocker produces a greater improvement in symptoms and reduction in the risk of death than an increase in dose of dose of an ACE inhibitor. Only those clinically unstable patients who are hospitalized in an intensive care unit, are requiring IV positive inotropic support, have severe fluid overload or depletion, have symptomatic bradycardia or advanced heart block (unless treated with a pacemaker), or a history of poorly controlled reactive airways disease should not be given a β-blocker.[5]

Based on all these factors, there is no question that A.J. should start a β-blocker. In fact, one could strongly argue that he should have started a β-blocker 6 weeks ago when he began treatment with an ACE inhibitor, or within the first 1 to 2 weeks after the ACE inhibitor was started.

Treatment with a β-blocker should be initiated at low doses, followed by gradual increments in dose every 1 to 2 weeks as tolerated by the patient. Transient bradycardia, hypotension, and fatigue are not uncommon during the first 24 to 48 hours when β-blockers are first started or during subsequent incremental increases in dosage. Thus, patients should be monitored daily for changes in vital signs (pulse and blood pressure) and symptoms during this up-titration period. Bradycardia, heart block and hypotension can be asymptomatic and require no intervention other than instructing the patient not to arise too quickly from a lying position to avoid postural changes. If either of these complications is accompanied by dizziness, lightheadedness, or blurred vision, dose reduction of the β-blocker and/or ACE inhibitor or slower up titration may be necessary. The sense of lassitude generally resolves within several weeks without other intervention, but may be a reason to slow up-titration of the dose and rarely to reduce the dose or discontinue therapy. In patients where benefits are especially apparent, but bradycardia or heart block is a concern, insertion of a pacemaker should be considered.

Because initiation of β-blocker therapy can also cause fluid retention, patients should be instructed to weigh themselves daily and to adjust concomitantly administered diuretics as appropriate. Conversely, diuretic doses should be decreased temporarily if the patient becomes hypotensive or their BUN begins to rise. Planned increments in the dose of a β-blocker should be delayed until any side effects observed with lower doses have been disappeared. In clinical trials up to 85% of patients are able to tolerate short and long term treatment with these drugs and achieve the maximum planned dose.

Metoprolol and Bisoprolol

28. Extended release metoprolol 12.5 mg is prescribed for A.J. Is this a good choice of agent and starting dose? What other similar drugs have been used to treat HF?

Several clinical trials substantiate the clinical benefits of metoprolol, a relatively selective β₁-receptor blocker, in HF.[194-197] By blocking β₁ receptors in the myocardium, heart rate, contractility, and CO are reduced at rest and during exercise, without a compensatory increase in peripheral vascular resistance. The relative sparing of β₂-receptors in the peripheral vasculature and lungs reduces vasoconstrictive and bronchospastic complications. In contrast to bucindolol and carvedilol, metoprolol has been shown to upregulate myocardial β₂-receptors.[27]

In the Metoprolol in Dilated Cardiomyopathy (MDC) study, 383 patients with nonischemic dilated cardiomyopathy and class II or III HF were randomized to immediate-release metoprolol (initiated at 5 mg BID and titrated to 100 to 150 mg/day in divided doses) or placebo.[197] All were continued on standard therapy with diuretics, vasodilators, and digoxin as tolerated. In this trial a nonstatistically significant trend toward both decreased mortality and listing for heart transplantation in the active treatment group was noted.

Of greater interest is the Metoprolol CR/XL Randomized Intervention Trial in Heart Failure (MERIT HF) in which a 35% reduction in all-causes of mortality was observed with sustained-release metoprolol.[197] In this trial, 3991 patients, most of whom had either NYHA class II or III HF, were randomized to metoprolol controlled-release/extended-release (CR/XL) or placebo. The starting dose of metoprolol was 12.5

to 25 mg/day and gradually increased every two weeks to the target dose of 200 mg per day. Conventional therapy with diuretics, ACE inhibitors and digoxin was continued. At the end of the trial, 64% of subjects assigned to active drug had reached the target dose. Planned follow-up was for 2 years, but the study was halted prematurely because of a statistically significant decrease in all-cause mortality in the metoprolol arm. Specifically, there was a 34% reduction in total mortality with a 38% decrease in cardiovascular mortality, a 41% reduction in sudden death, and a 49% reduction from death due to worsening HF. All-cause hospitalization was also reduced by 18% and hospitalization for worsening HF was decreased by 35%. Although the number of subjects was too small to detect a statistical difference, patients with severe (class IV) HF seemed to benefit as well. Up to 15% of subjects had clinical worsening of HF, even at these low doses.

Encouraging results have also been seen with another relative β₁-selective drug, bisoprolol fumarate (Zebeta).[198,199] In the first Cardiac Insufficiency Bisoprolol Study (CIBIS I), 641 subjects with moderate to severe HF were randomized to placebo or bisoprolol (starting dose, 1.25 mg/day; maximum dose, 5 mg/day) added to conventional therapy for an average of 23 months.[198] A statistically significant reduction in HF-associated hospitalization with the active drug and a non-significant trend toward reduced mortality were noted. In the larger Second Cardiac Insufficiency Bisoprolol Study (CIBIS II), reduction in both hospitalization and mortality in the bisoprolol-treated patients was significant.[199] A total of 2,647 patients were admitted to the second trial and doses were increased to as high as 10 mg/day. The study was stopped prematurely (average follow-up, 1.3 years) due to 34% reduction in total mortality with bisoprolol. Post hoc analysis showed a 44% reduction in sudden death and a 26% reduction in death due to worsening HF. As in the MERIT HF study, the number of patients with severe (class IV) HF was inadequate to determine the value of β-blocker therapy in this population.

Two dosage forms of metoprolol are marketed: metoprolol succinate extended release (Toprol XL) and metoprolol tartrate immediate release (Lopressor and generic). Only the extended release form is approved for HF in the United States, indicated for patients with mild to moderate (NYHA class II or III) HF of ischemic, hypertensive, or cardiomyopathic origin. The starting dose of 12.5 mg of extended release metoprolol prescribed for A.J. is consistent with the clinical trials and manufacturer's package insert labeling. If the initial dose is tolerated, the dose can be doubled to 25 mg twice daily for an additional 2 to 4 weeks. The final target dose is 150 to 200 mg daily either as 100 mg BID or 200 mg QD.

An alternative is to use immediate release metoprolol (Lopressor) even though it is not approved for this indication in the United States. Following a 6.25-mg test dose, the starting dose is 6.25 mg four times daily for 1 or 2 weeks. Because the smallest immediate release tablet size available is 50 mg and because of the need for three to four times daily therapy, the extended release product is used almost exclusively for treating HF. However, maintenance with a generic form of the immediate release product is less expensive (but still more complicated) than brand name extended release.

When choosing among the various formulations of metoprolol, pharmacokinetic and bioavailability differences should be considered.[194,195] Metoprolol succinate extended release is available as 25, 50, 100, and 200 mg tablets. Each tablet contains many tiny metoprolol succinate pellets, each individually coated with an ethylcellulose polymeric membrane. GI fluid penetrates the membrane of each pellet and slowly dissolves the drug. The saturated metoprolol solution is then released at a constant rate over 20 hours, consistent with zero-order kinetics, and provides β-blockade for 24 hours. The extended release formulation retains its release characteristics even if the scored tablet is divided in half, but it should not be crushed or chewed.

Absorption of metoprolol tartrate is approximately 95%, but bioavailability of the IR product is only 50% because of extensive first pass metabolism.[194,195] Systemic bioavailability of the extended release product is even lower, averaging 70% of the immediate release preparation. This is likely due to greater opportunity for first pass metabolism during slow absorption and less opportunity to saturate the metabolizing enzyme system. Because extended release metoprolol has consistently reduced bioavailability compared to immediate release metoprolol tartrate, there is concern that if a patient is receiving IR metoprolol and is switched to the same dosage of the ER formulation, the patient will in effect receive approximately 25% less drug. However, clinical studies indicate that the β-blocking effects are similar, perhaps due to the prolonged action of the ER product. The higher peak concentrations obtained with the immediate release formulation is accompanied by a greater potential for hypotension compared with extended release metoprolol. Since the dosage has to be titrated to each individual patient anyway, these differences may not be relevant unless the patient is being switched from one product to the other.

Metoprolol has several metabolic routes of elimination that can affect dosing and drug interactions. The major routes of elimination are via α-hydroxylation, O-demethylation, and N-dealkylation.[194,195] A smaller portion is metabolized by cytochrome P450 2D6, and drugs that inhibit metabolism of that isoenzyme may affect the drug's plasma levels. Approximately 10% of patients are poor metabolizers, resulting in higher drug plasma concentrations in these patients.

A.J. should be advised that clinical response to metoprolol is usually delayed and may require 2 to 3 months to become apparent. Even if symptoms do not improve, long-term treatment should be maintained to reduce the risk of major clinical events. Abrupt withdrawal of treatment with a β-blocker can lead to clinical deterioration and should be avoided.[200]

Bisoprolol is FDA approved for treatment of HF. However, dosage size limitations restrict its clinical use of this drug. For example, the starting dose of bisoprolol is 1.25 mg/day while the smallest commercially available dose is a 5 mg scored tablet. Attempting to break the tablet into quarters is not practical.

Carvedilol

29. **Might carvedilol be a better alternative than metoprolol for A.J.? What would be an appropriate dose and dosing schedule?**

Carvedilol (Coreg), a mixed α- and β-blocker, was the first drug of this class to obtain FDA approval for management of HF.[201] It might also have antioxidant effects to protect against loss of cardiac myocytes and to act as a scavenger of oxygen

free radicals that could potentiate myocardial necrosis. The correlation of these findings to clinical outcome is unknown.

Two pivotal studies support the use of carvedilol. The first was the U.S. Carvedilol Heart Failure Study.[202-206] Subjects were almost equally divided between class II and III HF and all had an EF of 35% or less (mean, 22%) despite diuretics (95%), digoxin (90%), and an ACE inhibitor (95%). Subjects with a major myocardial event in the previous 3 months were excluded. After an initial open-label period when all patients received 6.25 mg twice daily of carvedilol, subjects were stratified based on severity of their HF and then randomized to either placebo (N = 398) or carvedilol (N = 690). The maximum dose given was 50 mg twice daily. Using an intention-to-treat analysis, 7.8% of deaths occurred in the placebo group over an average of 6.5 months compared with only 3.2% in the active treatment group, a statistically significant 65% risk reduction ($P < 0.001$). Most notably, death due to progressive HF or sudden cardiac death was reduced. The patients treated with carvedilol also had fewer HF-related hospitalizations (19.6% versus 14.1%). The most common side effect with carvedilol was dizziness, usually during the first few days of therapy, but more patients discontinued placebo for worsening HF or side effects than with carvedilol.

In the Australia/New Zealand Carvedilol Study, 415 patients with chronic stable HF (NYHA class II or III, 85% taking concurrent ACE inhibitors, and average EF of 28%) were randomized to placebo (N = 208) or carvedilol (N = 207).[207] As in the U.S. study, those with severe symptoms were excluded, although 88% had a history of MI. Maintenance doses in subjects randomized to carvedilol ranged from 6.25 to 25 mg twice daily with an average follow-up of 19 months.

After 12 months, EF had increased by 5.3% and heart size was reduced in the carvedilol group compared with essentially no change in the placebo group. However, no differences between groups were found in treadmill exercise time, change in NYHA classification, or HF symptom scores. Only 26% of carvedilol patients and 28% of those receiving placebo had improved NYHA symptom scores, with the majority (58% in both groups) having neither improvement nor worsening of symptoms.

At 19 months, the frequency of episodes of worsening HF was similar in the two groups. Total deaths in the carvedilol group (N = 20) were less than the placebo group (N = 26), but most of the difference in mortality was attributed to noncardiovascular deaths. No difference was found in death from HF, MI, or total cardiac-related deaths. On a more positive note, there were 68% fewer hospital admissions for HF in the carvedilol group (N = 23) than for the placebo group (N = 33). Overall, these findings could be interpreted as being evidence for safety with either no overall benefit or a modest improvement with carvedilol.

The original FDA-approved indication for carvedilol was to reduce the progression of HF in patients with mild to moderate (NYHA class II or III) HF of ischemic or cardiomyopathic origin and whose conditions are stabilized with other drugs (digitalis, diuretics, and ACE inhibitors). In keeping with the exclusion of unstable patients from the study protocols, carvedilol was not approved for use in NYHA class IV decompensated cardiac failure. As discussed in the next case, later studies confirmed the value of carvedilol in NYHA class IV HF. As with any β-blocker, carvedilol is not recommended for use in patients with asthma, COPD, or poorly controlled diabetes.

The starting dose of carvedilol is 3.125 mg twice daily, with a doubling of the dose every 2 weeks as needed or tolerated up to a maximum of 25 mg twice daily in patients weighing <85 kg and 50 mg twice daily in larger patients. Hypotension, bradycardia, fluid retention, and worsening HF symptoms may occur in the first few weeks of therapy necessitating additional diuretics and/or a reduction of dose or discontinuation of carvedilol. Taking carvedilol with food slows the rate of absorption and reduces the incidence of orthostatic hypotension, which occurs in up to 10% of patients taking the drug.

Because carvedilol is metabolized by the cytochrome P450 2D6 (CYP2D6) enzyme system, several potential drug interactions should be considered.[201,208] The best documented are inhibition of metabolism by cimetidine and decreased carvedilol serum concentrations when taken with rifampin. Known inhibitors of CYP2D6 such as quinidine, fluoxetine, paroxetine, and propafenone may increase the risk of toxicity (especially hypotension), but substantiating data are lacking. Carvedilol has also been reported to increase serum digoxin levels by 15% by an unknown mechanism. Other sources of intrasubject variability in carvedilol response may be caused by differences in the extent or rate or absorption, stereospecific metabolism of the two isomers of the drug (carvedilol is a racemic mixture of S[-] and R[+] isomers), and impaired metabolism in the 10% of the population who lack CYP2D6 activity.[208]

Choice of β-Agonist: Metoprolol Versus Carvedilol

There is no consensus as to the relative superiority of one β-blocker compared to another. While the additional properties of carvedilol (e.g., α_1 blockade and antioxidant properties) provide a theoretical basis for selecting carvedilol over metoprolol or bisoprolol, the data from clinical trials provides conflicting conclusions. In one small head-to-head trial, carvedilol showed greater improvement in hemodynamic response during peak exercise and EF but no difference in symptom scores or exercise tolerance.[209] Another reported 30 HF patients with persistent symptoms despite at least 1 year of combined metoprolol and an ACE inhibitor.[210] They were enrolled in an open-label, parallel trial and randomized either to continue with metoprolol (mean dose, 142 ± 44 mg/day) or to cross over to maximum tolerated doses of carvedilol (mean dose, 74 ± 23 mg/day.) At the end of 12 months, patients randomized to carvedilol showed a greater decrease in end-diastolic volume, more improvement in LVEF, and fewer ectopic beats on electrocardiogram. However, there was no significant difference in symptoms or quality of life measures and a negative effect of carvedilol on peak oxygen consumption.

One meta-analysis attempted a comparison of carvedilol to metoprolol using the surrogate endpoint of LVEF as a comparator.[211] Nineteen randomized, placebo or concurrent-controlled trials involving a total of 2,184 patients with impaired LVEF were reviewed. Patients received a mean dose of 58 mg of carvedilol or the equivalent of 162 mg of extended release metoprolol. Combined results from the placebo controlled trials showed that both drugs significantly improved LVEF, with carvedilol found to be significantly better than metoprolol. Carvedilol increased LVEF 0.065% more than placebo compared to a 0.038% increase with metoprolol. These differences persisted when patients with ischemic HF

were compared to those with nonischemic cardiomyopathy. In head to head comparative trials, carvedilol once again raised LVEF greater than metoprolol. However, there was no apparent difference between the two drugs based on improvements in symptom scores or exercise tolerance. The authors caution that EF is only one of several endpoints one can measure, and the question of superiority in clinical outcomes such as mortality rates remains unanswered.

Since publication of the meta-analysis, the results of the COMET trial became available.[212] In this multicenter, double-blind trial, 3,029 patients with NYHA class II–IV HF and EF <35% were randomized to either carvedilol (target dose, 25 mg BID) or metoprolol tartrate (target dose, 50 mg BID). Diuretics and ACE inhibitors were continued in all subjects if tolerated. All-cause mortality was 34% for carvedilol compared to 40% with metoprolol ($P = 0.0017$). The composite endpoint of mortality or all cause hospital admissions was not statistically significant between groups (74% carvedilol and 76% metoprolol). One criticism of this study was use of immediate release metoprolol instead of the FDA approved extended release form.

Side effects and patient tolerance is similar between β-blockers in most trials. One investigator observed that carvedilol caused more hypotension and dizziness than metoprolol or bisoprolol, possibly due to α_1 blockade or more rapid absorption.[213] Thus, metoprolol or bisoprolol may be preferred in patients with hypotension or with complaints of dizziness. Conversely, carvedilol may be preferred in patients with inadequately controlled hypertension.

Whether carvedilol is a better choice for A.J. cannot be definitely answered. A starting dosage of 3.125 mg twice daily of carvedilol could be used in place of metoprolol. Because of lower cost, it is decided to continue metoprolol and reserve use of carvedilol only if A.J. has difficulty tolerating metoprolol.

β-Blockers in Severe Heart Failure

30. The original clinical trials of β-blockers excluded patients with severe (NYHA class IV) HF at the time of randomization. For this reason the FDA limited the original approval of carvedilol for use in class II–III HF. Likewise, the ACC/AHA guidelines strongly support the use of β-blockers in class II–III HF but are less definitive about severe HF. What evidence supports or refutes the use of β-blockers in class IV HF?

The COPERNICUS Study demonstrated clear benefit of carvedilol without undue side effects in patients with severe HF.[214] Conversely, the BEST Trial reported unimpressive results with another drug, bucindolol.[215] Details of these two trials are provided below.

The COPERNICUS study was a double-blind, placebo-controlled trial designed to test carvedilol in the of 2,289 patients with advanced HF (NYHA class IIIB/IV).[214] Subjects had symptoms of HF at rest or with minimal exertion and an EF of 25% or less despite diuretics (99%), ACE inhibitors (97%), and digoxin (67%). Subjects who required intensive care, had significant fluid retention, were hypotensive, had evidence of renal insufficiency, or were receiving IV vasodilators or positive inotrope drugs were excluded. The starting dose of carvedilol was 3.125 mg twice daily, which was increased every 2 weeks to a target dose of 25 mg twice daily.

Sixty-five percent of those in the carvedilol group achieved the target dose, with the mean dose being 37 mg at the end of the first 4 months of the trial. The trial was discontinued prematurely after an average patient follow-up of 10.4 months because of a significant survival benefit from carvedilol. There were 130 deaths in the carvedilol group and 190 deaths in the placebo group, a 35% decrease in the risk of death with carvedilol (95% CI, 19% to 48%; $P = 0.0014$). For the secondary endpoint of all deaths and hospitalizations combined, there were 425 events with carvedilol compared with 507 in the placebo group, a 24% decrease (95% CI, 13% to 33%, $P < 0.001$.). Fewer patients in the carvedilol group (14.8%) than in the placebo group (18.5%) withdrew because of adverse effects at 1 year ($P = 0.02$).

A concern over using β-blockers in class IV HF patients is that they may be predisposed to more side effects during the initiation phase of therapy. One study retrospectively analyzed the outcomes of 63 patients who were NYHA class IV compared with 167 subjects ranging from class I through III.[216] Adverse events occurred more frequently in the class IV patients (43%) than in the other subjects (24%; $P < 0.0001$) and more often resulted in permanent withdrawal of the drug (25% versus 13%). Conversely, more carvedilol treated class IV patients improved by more than one NYHA functional class than in the less symptomatic group (59% versus 37%.) A reanalysis of the COPERNICUS study data did not confirm a higher rate of intolerance over the first 8 to 12 weeks of carvedilol compared to placebo.[217] There was no difference between carvedilol and placebo in terms of death, hospitalizations, or withdrawal due to adverse events during the first 8 weeks of therapy.

The BEST Investigators failed to demonstrate that bucindolol, a nonselective β-blocker with vasodilator properties, improved overall survival in patients with NYHA class III–IV HF.[215] They randomized 2,708 patients to receive either bucindolol or placebo. Although the active drug yielded a significant decrease in norepinephrine levels and improvement in left ventricular function, the study was stopped prematurely because of the low probability of showing any significant cardiovascular mortality benefit over placebo. A possible explanation is that bucindolol has intrinsic sympathomimetic activity that may counteract some of the benefits of β-blockade. Moreover, subgroup analysis suggested that black patients might have fared worse with bucindolol, raising concerns that β-blockers may not be effective therapy for black patients with advanced HF (see Question 52 for further discussion of possible racial differences in drug response).

It can be concluded that β-blockers are safe and effective in class IV HF. The best data exist for carvedilol. Bucindolol should be avoided.

Digitalis Glycosides

Preparation for Treatment

31. Over the next 2 months, A.J.'s dose of extended release metoprolol was gradually increased to 200 mg per day. Other than some episodes of fatigue and lassitude during each dosage increment, he tolerated metoprolol well and, over time, he was more functional than he had been for several years. Unfortunately, over the ensuing 9 months, he again had several episodes

of HF symptoms that necessitated a gradual increase of his furosemide dose to 120 mg in the morning and 40 mg in the mid-afternoon. A potassium supplement was reinstituted because his potassium levels were beginning to fluctuate as his furosemide was increased.

Today, his wife brought him to the ED because she could no longer care for him. His chief complaints are weakness, dizziness, extreme SOB, and inability to get out of bed. His weight has increased to 80 kg. His BP is considerably lower at 128/83 mm Hg with a postural drop to 112/75 mm Hg. Abnormal laboratory values on admission are BUN, 31 mg/dL and serum creatinine, 1.4 mg/dL. His K is 4.3 mEq/dL. An ECG shows a HR of 98 beats/min, NSR, and LVH, but no T wave changes or ectopy. His valsartan is held for 24 hours while he is diuresed with several 40- and 80-mg boluses of IV furosemide and maintained on an NTG drip titrated to lower his PCWP below 15 and to keep his systolic BP >100 mm Hg. The plan is to reinstitute valsartan and to begin a digitalis glycoside. Is digitalis indicated for A.J.? What digitalis preparation should be prescribed?

Digoxin is the only digitalis glycoside marketed in the United States. The arguments for and against its use are presented in Question 15. Most of the recommendations stem from the Digoxin Intervention Group (DIG) trial that found in patients who had primarily class II or III symptoms, treatment with digoxin for 2 to 5 years had little effect on mortality but modestly reduced the combined risk of death and hospitalization.[138]

As presented earlier in this chapter, the ACC/AHA guidelines indicate that digoxin can be used early to reduce symptoms in patients who have been started on, but not yet responded symptomatically to an ACE inhibitor or β-blocker.[5] Alternatively, digoxin can be delayed until the patient's response to ACE inhibitors and β-blockers has been defined and used only in patients who remain symptomatic despite neurohormonal antagonists. A.J. fits the latter situation and thus is a logical candidate for adding digoxin as a fourth therapeutic intervention. It could be argued that both a β-blocker and digoxin should have been started at the onset of his treatment a year ago, but A.J.'s physician was reluctant to make multiple interventions simultaneously.

Digoxin is also prescribed routinely in patients with HF and concurrent chronic atrial fibrillation, but β-blockers may be more effective in controlling the ventricular response, especially during exercise. Digoxin should be avoided if the patient has significant sinus or atrioventricular block, unless the block is treated with a permanent pacemaker. It should be used cautiously in patients taking other drugs that can depress sinus or AV nodal function (e.g., amiodarone or β-blockers), although patients usually will tolerate this combination.

When A.J. entered the hospital today, he initially required IV furosemide and a NTG drip, but quickly stabilized. Digoxin is not indicated as primary therapy for stabilization of patients with acutely decompensated HF. Such patients should first receive appropriate treatment including IV medications as A.J. did. Thereafter, digoxin can be started as part of a long-term treatment strategy.

Gender Differences in Response to Digoxin

32. If AJ had been a woman, would it have made in any difference in the determination to prescribe digoxin?

Until recently, there was no indication that gender-based differences existed relative to prognosis of HF or in response to drugs such as digoxin. Two interesting reports published in 2002 sparked interest in this topic. The first was an extension of the Framingham Heart Study and was previously referenced in the epidemiology section of this chapter.[14] It was observed that over the past 5 decades the incidence of HF has been constant in men, but has declined by 31% to 40% in women during the last decade. During the last decade, survival rates for HF patients have improved in both men and women, although the mortality rate is higher in men than in women. The more aggressive use of drugs such as ACE inhibitors and β-blockers are likely contributors to the improved outcomes. The authors speculate that the differences observed between men and women may reflect different etiologies of HF. For example, hypertension is a predominate cause of HF in women, whereas more men have prior MI as a contributor to HF.

The second report (a review article) more directly addresses the question of use of digoxin in men compared with women.[218] As previously discussed, the Digitalis Investigation Group (DIG) Trial reported approximately equal mortality rates (35%) in subjects with HF randomized to either placebo or digoxin, while continuing usual doses of diuretics and ACE inhibitors.[138] There was a 12% reduction in the rate of death due to HF in the digoxin group, but there was a corresponding increase in death presumed to be due to arrhythmias. Upon retrospective post hoc analysis of the DIG study data, it was discovered that women overall had a lower death rate from any cause than men (31.0% versus 36.1%, $P < 0.001$), an absolute difference of 5.8%.[218] The rate of death was also lower among women in the placebo group than among men taking placebo (28.9% versus 36.9%; $P = <0.001$). Likewise, women taking digoxin had a lower death rate than men taking active drug (33.1% versus 35.2%), but this difference was not statistically different (P = 0.034). A surprising finding was that women taking digoxin had a higher death rate than women taking placebo (33.1% versus 28.9%), whereas death rates in men where essentially equal in both groups. The authors speculate that a possible mechanism for the increased risk of death among women taking digoxin is an interaction between hormone-replacement therapy and digoxin. Progesterone might increase serum digoxin levels by inhibiting PGP, thus reducing digoxin renal tubular excretion. Consistent with this hypothesis, digoxin serum concentrations after 1 month of digoxin intervention were higher in women than in men. Unfortunately, the study investigators did not routinely gather data on estrogen and hormone replacement therapy or consistently measure serum digoxin levels later in the trial. Because these observances are a retrospective, it is difficult to establish the clinical significance of the data and it is premature to argue against the use of digoxin in women. Nonetheless, it is prudent to recommend keeping serum digoxin concentrations less than 1.0 to 1.2 ng/mL in all patients and avoid hormone replacement therapy in women with HF when taking digoxin.

Loading Dose

33. **Can A.J. he be started with a properly chosen digoxin maintenance dose, or is a loading (digitalizing) dose necessary?**

Loading doses of digoxin are rarely necessary. Slow initiation of therapy with maintenance doses of digoxin in lieu of a loading dose is the method of choice for ambulatory or non-acutely ill patients with normal renal function. Even in the acute care setting, there is no indication for loading doses of digoxin for HF alone. The exception might be if the patient has atrial fibrillation and it is desired to control ventricular response as quickly as possible. Even then, alternative drugs are likely to be used (See Chapter 20, Cardiac Arrhythmias).

The main disadvantage to foregoing a loading dose is the delay in accumulating maximum body glycoside stores and achieving therapeutic effects. The length of time required to achieve 92% of plateau concentrations of a drug administered on a routine basis at maintenance doses is 4 half-lives. Thus, a patient with normal renal function ($t\frac{1}{2} = 1.8$ days) given a daily dose of 0.125 mg of digoxin will reach peak serum concentration in approximately 7 days. If the same patient was anephric ($t\frac{1}{2} = 4.4$ days), it would take 17 days to reach plateau, and the maximum concentration would be approximately 2.5 times that of a normal patient receiving the same dose. Slow digitalization can delay the onset of toxic signs, which could go unrecognized if the patient is at home.

A further argument against using a loading dose is that there is no evidence that achieving a steady state serum concentration quicker has any demonstrable effect on the time to reduction of HF symptoms. In any case, the full benefit of digoxin may be delayed for several days or weeks. Thus, clinicians should avoid rapidly increasing doses. For example, it would be improper to increase a patient's maintenance dose after 3 days if no clinical improvement were observed.

A.J. is in moderate to severe HF and in the hospital. It could be argued that a loading dose of digoxin would be safe in this environment and possibly could speed his therapeutic response. Nonetheless, the logical decision is to forgo a loading dose.

Serum Level Interpretation

34. **What is the target serum digoxin concentration for A.J.?**

The target therapeutic serum digoxin concentration is 0.5 to 1.2 ng/mL (mean, 0.75 ng/mL). Many older textbooks, review articles, and clinical trials contain the prior standard of targeting serum digoxin concentrations in the range of 0.8 to 2 ng/mL, or a mean of 1.0 ng/mL. These older recommendations should be abandoned. Factors driving this change are information suggesting that the positive hemodynamic and neurohormonal effects of digoxin can be achieved at lower serum concentrations than those needed to induce a positive inotropic effect (see digoxin pharmacology discussion in the introduction to this chapter),[64–67] use of digoxin as an adjunct to vasodilator therapy instead of as the primary intervention, and allowance for possible overestimation of the patient's renal function because of fluctuating control of HF. The correlation between serum digoxin concentrations and both therapeutic and toxic responses is considered in greater detail in Questions 36 and 41.

Maintenance Dose

35. **As predicted, A.J.'s renal function improved with diuresis and IV NTG. The latest values are BUN 24 mg/dL and SrCr 0.8 mg/dL. Determine the appropriate maintenance dose of digoxin for A.J.**

The usual maintenance doses of digoxin have traditionally ranged from 0.125 to 0.25 mg/day. With the increased emphasis on targeting lower serum concentrations, more patients are now empirically started at 0.125 mg/day. For example, because A.J. is of average body size, is relatively young, and has essentially normal kidney function, he empirically would have been started on a 0.25 mg/day maintenance dose in the past. However, a 0.125 mg dose is recommended for him now. It is safest to start with a conservative dose and assess his needs after 1 to 2 weeks.

In all cases, smaller doses of digoxin are given to patients with impaired excretion rates (e.g., those with renal failure, older patients) or small-framed individuals. For example, a totally anuric patient may receive only 0.0625 mg/day. Because of the long half-life of digoxin, all patients are given a single daily dose. A more detailed discussion of digoxin dosing in renal failure is found in questions 46 and 47.

Monitoring Parameters

36. Even after hearing the dosing principles from the prior question, A.J.'s physician decided to use a dose of 0.25 mg/day of digoxin because of his experience in using this size dose previously. How should his digitalis therapy be monitored? How useful are digoxin serum levels in monitoring therapy?

No clear therapeutic endpoint exists for digitalis therapy. Nonspecific ECG changes (ST depression, T-wave abnormalities, and shortening of the QT interval) correlate poorly with both toxic and therapeutic effects of the drug.[71,72] Although digoxin serum levels are readily available from most clinical laboratories, no "therapeutic level" and corresponding "toxic level" are clearly defined.

SERUM LEVEL INTERPRETATION

As stated in Question 34, a serum digoxin concentration of 0.5 to 1.2 ng/mL is now considered therapeutic because the beneficial parasympathomimetic and antiadrenergic effects of digoxin occur at lower concentrations than the inotropic effects. Interestingly, a recent post hoc analysis of the Digitalis Intervention Group (DIG) trial, found that patients with serum digoxin concentrations in the range of 0.5 to 0.8 ng/mL had lower all cause mortality rates than patients with serum concentrations in either the 0.9 to 1.1 ng/mL range or >1.2 ng/mL.[138,219] A small number of patients, especially if they are hypokalemic or hypomagnesemic, will manifest apparent signs of toxicity when serum digoxin concentrations are <1 ng/mL. At the other extreme, some patients tolerate concentrations exceeding 2 ng/mL with no signs of overt toxicity. Such overlap between therapeutic concentrations and toxic levels limits the absolute value of serum level monitoring. Serum levels may be used as a guide in confirming suspected toxicity or in explaining a poor therapeutic response, but clinical evaluation ultimately remains the best therapeutic guide. The correlation between serum digoxin concentrations and toxicity is considered in greater detail in Questions 40 and 41.

When interpreting serum digoxin concentrations, several procedural problems and patient characteristics must be taken into account. These include proper timing of sample collection, the effects of exercise, assay technique, and possible interfering substances in the patient's blood. A discussion of each of these factors follows.

Following an IV bolus dose or a single oral dose, equilibration of digoxin between the blood and tissues is slow. Because of this slow distribution phase, digoxin levels obtained <6 to 8 hours after the last dose may be falsely elevated and can lead to a misdiagnosis of toxicity. At steady state, serum digoxin concentrations obtained after 24 hours (just before the next dose) are considered most reliable. If a sample is obtained randomly, the time of the last dose should be carefully noted.

Physical activity increases binding of digoxin to skeletal muscle; by redistributing the drug from the blood to the tissue, a lower serum digoxin concentration is observed clinically.[220,221] The more strenuous the exertion, the greater the magnitude of effect, but even daily physical activity such as walking may decrease serum digoxin concentration by 20%.[221] About 2 hours of supine rest is required for digoxin levels to reach a new steady state. Clinical consequences of this effect might be to inappropriately increase the digoxin dose or failure to identify a possible toxic level in a patient who has a serum digoxin concentration drawn soon after walking briskly.

Similarly, a patient's serum digoxin concentration while hospitalized might be higher than serum digoxin concentrations drawn as an outpatient even with no dose change. Conversely, other investigators concluded that the changes in concentration are not clinically relevant during everyday activity and may only be of consequence for patients with large differences in activity level in the time surrounding the blood draws.[221] Obviously, a standardized approach to obtaining blood samples is key to the appropriate interpretation of results.

INTERFERING SUBSTANCES

In addition to the poor correlation between serum digoxin concentration and clinical effect, both endogenous and exogenous substances can interfere with the digoxin assay.[222–225] This is complicated further by the existence of a multitude of different assay methodologies, some of which are more susceptible to interference than others. All the tests are based on immunoassay methods, including several different radioimmune assays and numerous enzymatic immunoassays (e.g., ELISA, EMIT, TDx, Stratus, Advance). Among potential interfering substances are drugs and chemicals that are structurally similar to digoxin, most notably spironolactone (Aldactone) and possibly corticosteroids. Some assays also measure accumulated digoxin metabolites.

Other patient groups may have "endogenous digoxin-like substances" in their blood, imparting falsely elevated measurements. This has been noted in liver and renal failure patients, pregnant women, and 2- to 6-day-old neonates. One theory is that excess bile acids in neonates or patients with liver or renal disease may be a source of endogenous digoxin-like immunoreactive factors (DLIFs).[223] In some of these patient groups "digoxin levels" as high as 1.4 ng/mL may be measured without any drug in the body. It is essential that anyone monitoring serum digoxin levels be aware of which assay method is used in their laboratory and which substances may cause false-positive reactions. Most authors have found that radioimmune assay techniques are more susceptible to interference by DLIFs than enzymatic immunoassays.[222,224–225]

CLINICAL EVALUATION

As with diuretic and vasodilator therapy, clinical monitoring is the key to evaluating adequacy of digitalis therapy. As A.J. begins to improve, he should become less dyspneic and complain less of orthopnea; venous distention and signs of pulmonary congestion will diminish or disappear; diuresis (monitored through urinary output and weight loss) may increase; and a lower HR may be observed.

The response of HR to digitalis may vary depending on the patient's underlying disease. Because bradycardia and other rhythm disturbances may herald digitalis toxicity, daily monitoring of A.J.'s pulse will be needed until his condition and serum levels have reached a steady state. Ankle edema does not mobilize immediately and is a poor therapeutic endpoint.

Factors That Alter Response

37. Two days after starting digoxin, A.J. was discharged from the hospital. After 10 days of taking a maintenance dose of 0.25 mg, a serum digoxin level drawn during a clinic visit was reported as 0.7 ng/mL. Examination in the outpatient clinic 2 weeks later revealed that he had become progressively dyspneic and edematous since his hospital discharge. A STAT serum digoxin level at 3:00 PM was 0.3 ng/mL. A.J. had taken his dose of digoxin at 8:00 AM. What are some possible explanations for these events?

As stated in Question 36, serum levels are not an absolute guide to monitoring digitalis therapy. A partial explanation could be that A.J. was not at rest when the level was drawn. However, in this case, the low serum levels are accompanied by deterioration in his symptoms of HF. We can be reasonably sure of the accuracy of the serum concentration measured because it was drawn at the appropriate time (i.e., at steady state and at least 6 to 8 hours after the last dose); further, A.J.'s responses were compatible with the reported level. However, when doubt exists regarding the reliability of a reported serum level, the laboratory should be asked to repeat the measurement.

PATIENT ADHERENCE

Patient adherence must definitely be taken into consideration whenever unusually low serum concentrations or lack of response to any drug are observed. It is possible that A.J. is a poor complier because his BP was high on his first admission. He should be carefully counseled on the proper use of his medications.

DIGOXIN MALABSORPTION

Alteration of the absorption of digoxin following oral administration in patients with malabsorption syndromes has been studied.[69,226] It was found that poor and erratic absorption occurred in patients with malabsorption states such as sprue, short-bowel syndrome, and rapid intestinal transit. Other investigators studied digoxin bioavailability in malabsorptive states, but could not demonstrate large differences in serum digoxin concentrations. However, they found that use of more soluble forms, such as liquid-filled capsules, gave a better absorption than conventional tablets.[69]

ALTERED DIGOXIN METABOLISM

Altered digoxin metabolism is rare, but should be considered. One patient has been described who required 1 to 2 mg digoxin daily to control atrial fibrillation.[227] Although her half-life for digoxin was the same as control subjects, she metabolized a greater percentage of digoxin to cardioinactive

products. Also, as previously stated, approximately 10% of persons given digoxin demonstrate bacterially mediated metabolism of the drug in the GI tract leading to a relative decrease in total amount of drug absorbed.[76]

Concurrent metabolic abnormalities may decrease the responsiveness of digoxin. Hypocalcemia has been reported to cause a digitalis resistance, as has hyperthyroidism[71,72] (See Chapter 49, Thyroid Disorders).

Drug Interactions
QUINIDINE

38. As suspected, A.J. was found to have been taking his digoxin only sporadically. After being counseled on the importance of good adherence, he was restarted on 0.25 mg/day. He did well for the next 6 months until he noted the onset of palpitations, which were diagnosed by ECG as atrial fibrillation. A digoxin level drawn at that time was 1.2 ng/mL, but all other laboratory tests were normal. He began quinidine sulfate at a dosage of 200 mg QID with rapid resolution of the atrial fibrillation. Four days later, during a follow-up clinic visit, he was noted to have bradycardia with a pulse rate of 50 beats/ min. He also complained of nausea, dizziness, and weakness. His digoxin level was 2.0 ng/mL. What factors could be contributing to the apparent digitalis toxicity in A.J.?

In the past, quinidine and digoxin were frequently used adjunctively in the treatment of atrial fibrillation (AF): digoxin to control ventricular response by decreasing AV node conduction, and quinidine to decrease atrial irritability. With the advent of newer drugs, this combination has largely fallen out of favor. Reports show that more than 90% of patients previously stabilized by digoxin who subsequently begin quinidine experience a 2- to 2.5-fold increase in serum digoxin levels.[228–230] The actual magnitude of effect is highly variable and may depend on the dose of quinidine administered. Little change is seen with quinidine doses of <500 mg/day. Serum digoxin concentrations usually begin to rise within 24 hours of starting quinidine and reach a new steady state in about 5 days. Conversely, when quinidine is discontinued, digoxin concentrations return to pre-quinidine levels in about 5 days.

Several conflicting effects of quinidine on digoxin pharmacokinetics have been observed.[72,75] The most consistent finding is a 40% to 50% decrease in total body clearance of digoxin; much of this change is accounted for by decreased renal clearance.

The nonrenal clearance of digoxin also is affected by quinidine as evidenced by up to a doubling of digoxin plasma levels after addition of quinidine in patients with chronic renal failure.[231,232] A reduced volume of distribution has been observed in some individuals, but this is not a consistent finding. Digoxin's half-life does not change, probably because the changes in distribution and clearance tend to counterbalance each other. A unifying mechanism to explain all of these observations is the ability of quinidine to inhibit PGP mediated drug transport in the kidney, intestine, and possibly the liver.[72,74,75] Under usual conditions, digoxin enters the renal tubule via both glomerular filtration and renal tubular secretion, the latter mechanism being under the influence of PGP-mediated transport. Inhibition of PGP by quinidine in the kidney partially blocks the tubular secretion step, thus decreasing renal clearance of the digoxin. In the intestines, PGP facilitates active transport of absorbed digoxin back into the intestinal tract. The net effect of inhibition of gut PGP by quinidine is increased bioavailability of digoxin.

Digoxin is found in only small concentrations in the plasma, with most of the drug being distributed to lean body tissues (e.g., skeletal and cardiac muscle). Despite clear evidence that serum digoxin levels are increased with quinidine, much less is known about the importance of this interaction on the heart and the clinical effects that ensue. Since both of these drugs can individually cause GI intolerance (e.g., nausea, vomiting, diarrhea), AV block, and bradycardia, it is difficult to differentiate simple additive effects from a true drug interaction without measuring serum level changes. One 9-month study of hospital admissions for suspected digitalis toxicity observed that 50% of patients treated with the quinidine–digoxin combination had ECG evidence of digoxin toxicity compared with 5% of patients taking digoxin alone or in combination with verapamil or amiodarone.[233] Conversely, many patients tolerate the increased serum levels of digoxin with no apparent adverse consequences.

Faced with the complexity of this interaction, it is difficult for the clinician to plan a course of action when using these two drugs together. It has been suggested that the dose of digoxin be reduced by 50% when adding quinidine. Although this might minimize bradycardia, ventricular tachyarrhythmias, and GI effects, it also can lead to a loss of desired neurohormonal or positive inotropic effects. A more rational approach is to use smaller doses of digoxin in all patients, whether or not they are taking quinidine. Then when adding quinidine, patients can maintain their previous digoxin dose with careful clinical monitoring for undesirable side effects. If necessary, a serum digoxin level can be obtained after 5 to 7 days of concurrent therapy. If it exceeds 1.2 ng/mL, the dose can be decreased. Concentrations in excess of 2.0 ng/mL are a definite cause for concern. A.J. should have his digoxin dose reduced to 0.125 mg QD.

Treatment of Supraventricular Arrhythmias in Heart Failure
DIGOXIN DRUG INTERACTION WITH AMIODARONE AND PROPAFENONE

39. Quinidine was started in A.J. because of atrial fibrillation. What alternatives to quinidine and digoxin could be recommended for A.J.? What other potential drug interactions does this present?

Supraventricular arrhythmias are frequently encountered in HF because volume or pressure overload can cause atrial distention and irritability. Specifically, atrial fibrillation is present in 25% to 50% of patients with advanced HF, contributing to reduced exercise capacity, increased risk of pulmonary or systemic emboli, and worse long-term prognosis.[5,234] As in any patient with these arrhythmias, drug therapy should be aimed at controlling ventricular rate and prevention of thromboembolic events. Cardioversion to normal sinus rhythm is unlikely to be successful. Fortunately, left ventricular function and clinical status frequently improve after controlling atrial fibrillation, whether or not normal sinus rhythm is restored.

Digoxin slows the ventricular response associated with atrial fibrillation and thus is a logical choice in patients with concurrent HF. A potential limiting factor is that digoxin's AV blocking properties are most evident at rest, but are less reli-

able during exercise. Hence, digoxin may be ineffective at controlling exercise-induced tachycardia that limits the patient's functional capacity. β-Blockers are more effective than digoxin during exercise.[235–237] Propranolol is the β-blocker of choice in non-HF patients, but metoprolol is a better choice in those with HF because of its proven role in HF management. If digoxin and/or β-blockers are ineffective, amiodarone is another useful alternative. Verapamil and diltiazem are not appropriative choices for rate control in HF patients because of their negative inotropic effects.

The benefits of restoring sinus rhythm remain unclear (See Chapter 20, Cardiac Arrhythmias.) The majority of patients who are electrically cardioverted revert to atrial fibrillation in a short time. The use of most other antiarrhythmic agents (e.g., quinidine, procainamide, propafenone, and other class II antiarrhythmics) except amiodarone is associated with worse prognosis due to proarrhythmic effects and should be avoided. Warfarin is required for patients with atrial fibrillation, but not for other patients with HF. Finally, atrioventricular nodal ablation may be needed if tachycardia or bothersome symptoms persist despite aggressive pharmacologic intervention.

A.J. developed atrial fibrillation while already taking a relatively high dose of digoxin (0.25 mg/day) and metoprolol. As discussed above, quinidine is not the best choice because of its drug interaction potential and side effects, most notably the potential to cause other life-threatening arrhythmias. One alternative is to discontinue quinidine, keep the digoxin dose at 0.25 mg QD, and continue metoprolol. If his atrial fibrillation–associated palpitations persist, amiodarone should be started. (See Chapter 20, Cardiac Arrhythmias, for dosing of amiodarone in supraventricular tachyarrhythmias.) Because amiodarone is also a PGP inhibitor with a documented ability to reduce digoxin clearance in a manner similar to that described with quinidine, A.J.'s digoxin dose will need to be lowered to 0.125 mg.[72,74] The onset of the interaction may not be apparent for a prolonged time because of the long half-life of amiodarone. As serum concentrations of amiodarone slowly increase, digoxin clearance and bioavailability will be changing simultaneously. The net effect may be easily overlooked, but can result in increased serum concentrations of 30% to 60%. Similarly, propafenone increases digoxin steady state concentrations by 30% to 60% in a dose dependent fashion over the range of 450 to 900 mg per day of propafenone.[72,238]

Other Digoxin Drug Interactions

40. What other potential drug interactions with digoxin might affect A.J.'s therapy?

Two comprehensive reviews of cardiac glycoside drug interactions have been compiled.[228,239] Since publication of these earlier reviews, a greater understanding of PGP-mediated drug interactions has evolved.[74,75] A brief summary of all digoxin interactions is found in Table 19-12. Two of the better-documented interactions (quinidine and amiodarone) were discussed in the previous cases. Others drugs recently recognized as raising digoxin serum concentrations through PGP inhibition include atorvastatin (increased intestinal absorption),[240] calcium channel blockers (especially verapamil and diltiazem),[241] erythromycin and clarithromycin (reduced renal digoxin clearance),[242,243] and cyclosporine. Conversely, rifampin[244] and St.

Table 19-12   Digoxin Drug Interactions[a]

Drug	Effect
Drugs Lowering Serum Digoxin Concentration	
Antacids	↓ Bioavailability via adsorption in gut
Cancer chemotherapy	Possible ↓ bioavailability (especially combinations of cyclophosphamide and vincristine)
Cholestyramine (Questran)	↓ Bioavailability via adsorption in gut
Colestipol (Colestid)	↓ Bioavailability via adsorption in gut
Kaolin-pectin	↓ Bioavailability via adsorption in gut
Laxatives	↓ Bioavailability via gut hypermotility
Metoclopramide (Reglan)	↓ Bioavailability via enhanced gastric emptying (slow-release digoxin only)
Neomycin	Malabsorption of digoxin
Psyllium hydrophilic mucilloid (Metamucil) and dietary bran fiber	Possible ↓ bioavailability via adsorption in gut
Rifampin[244]	Probable induction of intestinal P-glycoprotein causing ↓ bioavailability. ↓ Serum concentration after oral, but not IV digoxin. No change in digoxin renal clearance or half-life.
St. John's Wort[245]	Possible induction of P-glycoprotein
Sulfasalazine (Azulfidine)	Malabsorption of digoxin
Drugs Raising Serum Digoxin Concentration	
Alprazolam[248]	↑ Serum digoxin levels by unknown mechanism
Amiodarone (Cordarone)[72, 74]	↑ Serum digoxin levels by unknown mechanism
Atorvastatin[240]	20% increase in serum digoxin concentration with 80 mg dose, minimal effect with 20 mg dose. Speculated to inhibit intestinal P-glycoprotein, but not proven
Calcium channel blockers[72, 74, 241] (See Question 56)	Inhibition of P-glycoprotein. Best documented with verapamil.
Captopril[182]	Inhibition of digoxin renal clearance by unknown mechanism
Clarithromycin[242, 243]	Inhibition of P-glycoprotein, decreased digoxin renal clearance
Cyclosporine[72, 74]	Inhibition of P-glycoprotein, decreased digoxin renal clearance
Erythromycin	↑ Bioavailability in persons who normally metabolize digoxin in intestinal tract. May also inhibit P-glycoprotein in gut.
Itraconazole[249]	↑ Serum digoxin levels by unknown mechanism
Omeprazole[246, 247]	↑ Bioavailability (slight) due to altered gut metabolism
Propafenone[72, 238]	Inhibition of P-glycoprotein
Quinidine (see Question 38)[72, 74, 75, 228-233]	Inhibition of P-glycoprotein; decreased digoxin renal clearance and increased bioavailability.
Propantheline (Pro-Banthine)	↑ Bioavailability via slowed gastric emptying (slow-release digoxin only)
Telmisartan[250]	Unknown mechanism. Increased peak serum concentration 3-4 hr after dose, but only slight increase in 24 hr AUC or trough serum concentration

AUC, area under curve.
[a]References 72, 228, and 239 include a discussion of many of these interactions that do not include a specific reference citation.

John's Wort[245] reduce oral digoxin bioavailability and serum concentrations via induction of intestinal PGP. Mylanta is the only drug listed in Table 19-12 that A.J. was taking. He should be counseled to avoid antacids within 1 or 2 hours before or 1 hour after a dose of digoxin or to use a nonprescription histamine$_2$ receptor blocker.

Digitalis Toxicity
SIGNS AND SYMPTOMS

41.   Digoxin was prescribed for Z.T., a 70-year-old man with mild HF. The label on his prescription bottle instructed him to take 1 tablet (0.25 mg) BID for 3 days, then 1 tablet daily there-after. Ten days later Z.T. returned to the clinic complaining of extreme fatigue, anorexia, nausea, and a "funny" heart beat. Close questioning and a "tablet count" disclosed that Z.T. failed to decrease his digoxin to 0.25 mg/day. An ECG revealed multiple premature ventricular contractions (PVCs) and second degree AV block. A STAT serum digoxin level was 2.8 ng/mL. What signs and symptoms in Z.T. are consistent with digitalis toxicity? What are some other adverse effects of digitalis?

This case illustrates a risk of using digoxin loading doses and one of several ways that digitalis toxicity might present. The clinical presentation of digitalis toxicity is unpredictable. In some cases, a high serum digoxin level without any appreciable adverse effects is the only clue to possible digitalis toxicity. In other patients, such as Z.T., a multitude of symptoms can be present, including both non-cardiac signs (e.g., GI complaints) and rhythm disturbances (e.g., palpitation, heart block, arrhythmias).

The most important adverse effects are those relating to the heart. A common misperception is that GI or other non-cardiac signs will precede cardiac toxicity. To the contrary, cardiac symptoms precede non-cardiac symptoms of digitalis toxicity in up to 47% of cases. Frequently (26% to 66%), non-specific arrhythmias are the only manifestation of toxicity with estimates that rhythm disturbances occur in 80% to 90% of all patients with digitalis toxicity.[251] On the other hand, rhythm disturbances in patients taking digitalis are not always related to toxicity. In one study of 100 consecutive patients with suspected digitalis-induced arrhythmias, only 24 were confirmed as being toxic as defined by resolution of cardiac irritability following drug withdrawal. In the other 76 patients, the dysrhythmia persisted long after drug removal.[252]

Most known arrhythmias can occur as a result of digoxin toxicity. Decreased conduction velocity through the AV node presents as a prolonged P-R interval (first-degree AV block) and is seen in many patients with therapeutic levels of digitalis. However, as exemplified in Question 38, higher concentrations of digitalis can impair conduction and result in brady-cardia or a variable block (second-degree AV block). With severe toxicity, complete (third-degree) AV block results in dissociation of the atrial and ventricular rates with a slow idioventricular rate predominating. AV block also may predispose patients to accelerated junctional rhythms. Increased automaticity of the atria can cause multifocal atrial tachycardia (MAT) with block, paroxysmal atrial tachycardia (PAT) with block, or atrial fibrillation.

Ventricular arrhythmias (as seen in Z.T.) are among the most common rhythm disturbances caused by digitalis toxicity and include unifocal and multifocal PVCs, bigeminy (every other beat is a PVC), trigeminy, ventricular tachycardia, and ventricular fibrillation. Comprehensive reviews are available on the topic of digitalis-induced arrhythmias.[251,252]

Hyperkalemia can develop as a consequence of massive digitalis poisoning.[253] Toxic doses of digitalis severely poison the Na^+-K^+-ATPase system, causing inhibition of the uptake of potassium by the myocardium, skeletal muscle, and liver cells. The shift of potassium from inside to outside the cell can result in significant hyperkalemia, especially in patients with underlying renal insufficiency. These same patients also are likely to accumulate digoxin in the body because of decreased clearance of the drug. Cardiac ectopy can be potentiated by the increase in serum potassium, especially when the potassium concentration exceeds 5 mEq/L. Paradoxically, in patients with good renal function, hyperkalemia can enhance renal excretion of potassium, resulting in a deficit in total body potassium despite the continued high serum concentration of potassium.

Vague GI symptoms characteristic of digitalis toxicity are difficult to evaluate because anorexia and nausea are also part of HF's clinical picture. During one prospective clinical study, an equal frequency of anorexia and nausea occurred in both toxic and nontoxic patients taking digoxin.[255] Anorexia may be the earliest symptom, followed in 2 to 3 days by nausea. More than 25% of patients have GI symptoms for >3 weeks before diagnosis. Nonspecific abdominal pain and bloating caused by nonocclusive mesenteric ischemia secondary to digitalis-induced vasoconstriction also has occurred.

CNS symptoms of digitalis are common, possibly associated with potassium depletion in neural tissue. Chronic digitalis intoxication resulting from misformulation was observed in 179 patients.[255] Acute extreme fatigue and/or visual disturbances were a complaint in 95% of these patients. Approximately 80% experienced weakness of the arms and legs, and 65% had psychic disturbances in the form of nightmares, agitation, listlessness, and hallucinations. Hazy vision and difficulties in both reading and red-green color perception frequently were present. Other complaints included glitterings, dark or moving spots, photophobia, and yellow-green vision. Disturbances in color vision returned to normal 2 or 3 weeks after discontinuation of digitalis.

Interestingly, six elderly patients had apparent digitalis-induced visual disturbances at serum concentrations below those considered to be toxic (all <1.5 ng/mL; range, 0.2 to 1.5 ng/mL).[256] Five of the reactions were described as photopsia (seeing lights not present in the environment) and one person had decreased visual acuity. Color vision disturbances or seeing color lights, both well-described with digitalis toxicity, were absent. The symptoms went away in all but one subject when digoxin was discontinued.

Some prospective studies showed a good correlation between serum digoxin levels and toxicity,[254,255,257] whereas other investigators found a poor correlation.[258,259] In one study, 87% of digitalis-toxic patients had levels >2 ng/mL and 90% of nontoxic patients had levels <2 ng/mL. Conversely, other investigators found that nearly 50% of subjects with a serum digoxin level exceeding 3 ng/mL were clinically stable without signs of digitalis toxicity.[258] In the largest series studied to date, the average serum digoxin concentration in documented toxic patients (i.e., those with a suspected digitalis-induced arrhythmia that disappeared after drug withdrawal) was 2.9 ng/mL compared with 1.0 ng/mL in patients with suspected digitalis toxicity, but in whom the arrhythmia persisted after drug withdrawal.[252] Approximately 38% of documented toxic patients, however, had serum digoxin concentrations <2 ng/mL (false-negative tests). Once levels exceed 6 ng/mL, there is a greatly increased risk of mortality.[260]

Because a significant overlap between toxic and therapeutic levels exists, serum level determinations are currently most useful as an aid in confirming suspected digitalis toxicity and in individualizing dosing regimens so that toxicity might be avoided. In particular, subjects with low serum potassium concentrations can demonstrate digitalis toxicity at lower serum digoxin concentrations.[261]

Allergic reactions to digitalis are rare. Unilateral or bilateral gynecomastia is observed during chronic digoxin administration and is reversible upon withdrawal of the drug. This latter effect may occur in addition to the gynecomastia seen with spironolactone.

PREDISPOSING FACTORS

42. B.V., a 64-year-old alcoholic man, is admitted to the hospital with a 3-day history of epigastric pain radiating to the back and associated with nausea and vomiting. B.V. also has cirrhosis of the liver and mild HF that is well controlled with furosemide 80 mg/day, ramipril 2.5 mg BID, and digoxin 0.25 mg/day. He has a 3-year history of severe rheumatoid arthritis, which is moderately relieved with NSAIDs and prednisone 15 mg/day.

Because the initial impression was acute pancreatitis, B.V. was placed on a nasogastric suction and 3 L of D51/4 NS daily. The next evening the laboratory report disclosed the following: Na, 136 mEq/L (normal, 136 to 144 mEq/L); K, 2.3 mEq/L (normal, 3.5 to 5.3 mEq/L); Cl, 90 mEq/L (normal, 96 to 106 mEq/L); bicarbonate, 32 mEq/L (normal, 23 to 28 mEq/L); Mg, 1.3 mEq/L (normal, 1.7 to 2.7 mEq/L); creatinine, 0.8 mg/dL (normal, 0.5 to 1.2 mg/dL); AST, 80 U (normal, 40 U); alkaline phosphatase, 130 U (normal, 80 U); amylase, 1,200 U (normal, 4 to 25 U); digoxin, 1.8 ng/mL; and Cl_{Cr}, 100 mL/min (normal, 100 to 125 mL/min). An ECG showed a HR of 70 beats/min with occasional PVCs and runs of bigeminy. What factors predispose B.V. to digitalis toxicity?

[SI units: Na, 136 mmol/L (normal, 134 to 144); K, 2.3 mmol/L (normal, 3.5 to 5.3); Cl, 90 mmol/L (normal, 96 to 106); bicarbonate, 32 mmol/L (normal, 23 to 28); Mg, 0.65 mmol/L (normal, 0.85 to 1.35); creatinine, 70.72 mmol/L (normal, 44.2 to 106.08); AST, 80 U/L (normal, 40); alkaline phosphatase, 130 U/L (normal, 80); amylase, 1,200 U/L (normal, 4 to 25); and Cl_{Cr}, 1.67 mL/sec (normal, 1.67 to 2.08)]

This is an example of a subtle presentation of digitalis toxicity. The serum level is in the high end of the therapeutic range. Nevertheless, B.V. shows clinical signs of digitalis toxicity (e.g., PVCs and bigeminy). His renal function is normal, so digoxin excretion should not be significantly altered. The major contribution to toxicity in B.V. is hypokalemia.

The association between digitalis toxicity and hypokalemia is well recognized. It has been observed that twice as much digitalis is required to produce toxicity in patients with serum potassium of 5 mEq/L than in those with a serum potassium of 3 mEq/L.[261] A small number of patients will develop signs of toxicity with serum digitalis concentrations as low as 1.5 ng/mL if hypokalemia is present. Therefore, drugs, diseases, and medical maneuvers that induce hypokalemia or reduce the serum potassium from elevated to normal levels may unmask digitalis toxicity. A low serum potassium has been observed to increase the uptake of digitalis by the myocardial tissue.[262]

B.V. is taking furosemide. All diuretics, with the exception of potassium-sparing diuretics, can cause hypokalemia through kaliuresis. In addition, prednisone in high doses promotes potassium excretion in the distal portion of the renal tubule. B.V.'s prednisone dose should be tapered and eventually discontinued while one of the newer disease modifying drugs is started (See Chapter 43, Rheumatic Disorders). Similarly, diseases in which mineralocorticoid activity is high (e.g., Cushing's disease, hyperaldosteronism) are associated with low serum potassium levels. B.V.'s history of cirrhosis could lead to development of portal hypertension and ascites, both of which are associated with hyperaldosteronism.

Other causes of hypokalemia in B.V. include vomiting and nasogastric suction. Similarly, hypokalemia can result from diarrheal losses, including drug-induced diarrhea (e.g., amoxicillin, quinidine).

Although the relationship of hypokalemia to digitalis toxicity is stressed, hyperkalemia is also a risk factor.[253] A bimodal effect of potassium on the AV node has been observed, whereby both hypokalemia and hyperkalemia may delay AV nodal conduction resulting in bradycardia and compensatory ventricular ectopy.

B.V. has metabolic alkalosis (HCO_3^-, 32 mEq/L) from the combined effects of diuretic therapy, vomiting, and nasogas-tric suctioning of hydrogen ion. Alkalosis results in the redistribution of potassium intracellularly and an increased renal excretion of potassium, thereby potentiating effects of hypokalemia (See Chapter 11, Acid–Base Disorders). In addition, alkalosis in and of itself has been associated with an increased incidence of digitalis toxicity. This is attributed to an intracellular depletion of potassium caused by increased urinary excretion and a relative increase in the ratio of extracellular to intracellular potassium.[262] This has the same effect on the membrane potential as digoxin.

Another metabolic problem that could contribute to digitalis toxicity in B.V. is hypomagnesemia. The causes are the same as for hypokalemia, including diuretic therapy, nasogastric suction losses, and chronic alcoholism. The prevalence of hypomagnesemia is higher in digitalis-toxic patients; magnesium sulfate has been used successfully in the treatment of digitalis toxicity.[263]

Although not illustrated by B.V., hypercalcemia theoretically can predispose patients to digitalis toxicity. The electrical and contractile effects of calcium on the myocardium are similar to those of digitalis. For this reason, rapid IV infusions of calcium can facilitate the development of digitalis toxicity, and normal or low doses of digitalis can induce toxicity in patients with hypercalcemia (e.g., hyperparathyroidism or metastatic cancer). The clinical significance of calcium-induced digitalis toxicity is questionable; there have been no reports of digitalis toxicity secondary to oral administration of calcium-containing products.

Age may be an important predisposing factor in the production of digitalis toxicity in B.V. The same IV dose of digoxin administered to elderly and young patients produces higher serum concentrations of digoxin in the elderly. The higher levels and prolonged half-life observed in these patients are likely caused by diminished renal clearance of the drug and this population's smaller body size. It is important to emphasize that although the serum creatinine of elderly patients may be within normal limits, the mean creatinine clearance is reduced.

The response to digitalis also may be altered in the very young (see Question 45). Lower doses are recommended in premature infants and neonates (younger than 1 month) because of the decreased renal function normally observed in newborns.[264] Although absorption, tissue distribution, and excretion of digoxin in infants are similar to those observed in adults, infants excrete a smaller percentage of digoxin metabolites than adults.

TREATMENT OF DIGITALIS TOXICITY

43. How should B.V.'s digitalis toxicity be treated?

Withholding Digitalis and Electrolyte Replacement

For many patients without life-threatening arrhythmias or major electrolyte imbalances, simple withdrawal of digitalis is the only treatment required. Although it may take five half-lives for the drug to be totally eliminated from the body, the serum concentration will drop to a safe level after one to two half-lives (2 to 3 days for digoxin) in most individuals.

B.V. does not have significantly elevated digoxin levels, so his ectopy should disappear rapidly with drug withdrawal. His major problem is related to hypokalemia that must be corrected. As a general rule, potassium replacement should be considered in any patient with digitalis-induced ectopic beats who has low or normal serum potassium levels. Oral administration is acceptable unless the patient cannot take medication orally or has life-threatening ectopy. If digitalis-induced arrhythmias are severe enough to warrant intravenously administered potassium, the maximum recommended rate of administration is 40 mEq/hr (preferably 10 mEq/hr) at a concentration not exceeding 80 to 100 mEq/L. A total of several hundred mEq of potassium might be required to replete body stores. Potassium should be administered with caution in patients who have conduction disturbances characterized by second-degree or complete AV block because high doses can further depresses conduction velocity in the AV node.

B.V. has a significant potassium deficit with potentially dangerous arrhythmias but no contraindications to potassium therapy. He should receive 80 to 120 mEq of IV potassium over the next 24 hours and then be switched to an appropriate oral dose. He should be monitored for signs and symptoms of potassium toxicity with frequent ECG tracings (look for tall, peaked T waves; prolonged PR interval) and serum potassium determinations.

It is important to obtain a serum magnesium concentration when measuring potassium levels. Patients with a low serum magnesium level (<1.5 mEq/L) or whose condition fails to respond after potassium repletion should receive a 20 mg/kg (2 g in an adult) loading dose of magnesium sulfate administered as a 10% solution over 20 minutes, followed by a continuous infusion at a rate of 0.5 to 2 g/hr to maintain a serum magnesium level of at least 4 to 5 mEq/L. Magnesium is relatively contraindicated in patients with renal failure, hypermagnesemia, or a high-level AV block. The infusion should be discontinued if deep tendon reflexes are diminished or serum concentrations of magnesium exceed 7 mEq/L.

Antiarrhythmic Agents

Patients with bradycardia because of second- or third-degree AV block should be given IV atropine. The usual atropine dose is 0.5 to 1 mg over 1 to 2 minutes with a repeat in 15 to 30 minutes if the patient does not respond. Doses <0.5 mg can paradoxically worsen the AV block. Atropine should be used with caution in patients with prostatic hypertrophy because significant urinary retention and postrenal azotemia may occur. Alternatively, a temporary pacemaker can be placed. Because B.V.'s HR is 70 beats/min, atropine is not indicated.

Virtually all of the antiarrhythmic agents have been used to treat digitalis-induced arrhythmias. Lidocaine and phenytoin have a theoretic advantage over quinidine-like agents because they do not further depress AV conduction. Phenytoin is particularly efficacious in the suppression of digitalis-induced tachyarrhythmias with or without first- or second-degree AV block. For B.V., potassium replacement will probably be all that is required. However, because of his bigeminy, lidocaine could be administered for a few hours until he has been given sufficient potassium supplementation. (See Chapter 20, Cardiac Arrhythmias, for dosing guidelines for lidocaine and phenytoin.)

Peritoneal and hemodialysis are ineffective in removing digoxin from the body, but charcoal hemoperfusion is used for life-threatening overdoses in patients with renal failure.[265]

Digoxin Immune Fab

44. All the treatments above are symptomatic. When is a specific antidote such as digoxin immune Fab indicated?

Most treatment regimens for digitalis toxicity are supportive only, either by counteracting the pharmacologic effects of digitalis or by interfering with further absorption of ingested tablets. A more definitive treatment consists of administration of digoxin specific antibodies that bind digoxin molecules, rendering them unavailable for binding at receptors in the heart and other areas of the body.[266–271] The antibodies bind intravascular digoxin and also diffuse into interstitial spaces to bind free digoxin. As the extracellular unbound (free) digoxin concentration decreases, intracellular digoxin diffuses into extracellular fluid and becomes available to be bound to the antidigoxin antibodies. A concentration gradient is thus created that promotes release of digoxin from binding sites. Ultimately, the digitalis-antibody complex is excreted in the urine. The official name of this product is digoxin immune Fab, ovine sold under the brand names of Digibind and DigiFab.

The use of digoxin Fab products is restricted to potentially life-threatening intoxications (severe arrhythmias or hyperkalemia) that are either refractory to more conservative therapy or associated with extremely high serum concentrations. The major reason for this approach is the high cost of digoxin Fab.

Digoxin immune Fab is supplied as a lyophilized powder (38 mg/vial of Digibind, 40 mg/vial of DigiFab) that, after reconstitution with 4 mL of sterile water for injection, yields a 10 mg/mL solution that should be used within 4 hours. One mg of digoxin immune Fab binds 12.5 µg of digoxin. Thus, the contents of one vial will bind approximately 0.5 mg of digoxin. The actual dose administered varies according to the estimated amount of digitalis glycoside in the body. For digoxin, the amount of drug in the body can be estimated by the formula:

$$\text{Body load in mg} = \frac{5.0(\text{SDC})(\text{Weight in kg})}{1,000} \quad \text{(19-2)}$$

where 5.0 is the volume of distribution of digoxin in L/kg. An oral absorption of approximately 80% for digoxin is assumed. From this estimate, the total number of vials required for neutralization is calculated by dividing the total body load by 0.5 mg/vial. Patients with renal failure have a smaller volume of distribution of digoxin and thus have higher serum concentrations for any given dose.

In cases of extremely large single-dose ingestions for which the results of digoxin serum concentrations are not available, an empiric dose of 380 to 400 mg (10 vials) is given to an adult. An additional 380 to 400 mg can be given if needed. For patients with toxicity during chronic therapy, 228 to 240 mg (6 vials) is adequate to treat most adults, whereas 38 to 40 mg (1 vial) is appropriate for children weighing <20 kg. The antibody usually is administered IV over 30 to 45 minutes, but it can be given more rapidly if the patient is in acute distress. It is recommended that the drug be infused through a 0.22-micron filter. Efficacy and safety is the same in children as in adults.[267]

Clinical improvement in the signs and symptoms of digitalis intoxication should occur within 30 minutes of antibody administration, with complete reversal of symptoms in 4 hours. If, after several hours, toxicity has not been adequately reversed or symptoms reappear, an additional dose can be given. In patients with renal insufficiency, the digitalis-antibody complex can be retained in the body for prolonged time. If retained long enough, Fab fragments could be degraded by the reticuloendothelial system, releasing active digitalis glycosides back into the circulation and necessitating retreatment. For this reason, it has been proposed to give 50% of the calculated dose immediately over 15 minutes, then the remaining 50% as a continuous infusion over 7 hours.[268]

Immediately after treatment with digoxin-specific Fab, the active (free or unbound) digitalis concentration decreases to nearly undetectable levels, but the total (free plus antibody-bound) digoxin concentration increases. In <1 hour, the total concentration increases by 10- to 20-fold; peaking in about 10 hours at concentrations often exceeding several hundred ng/mL. The monitoring of serum digoxin levels following treatment with Digibind is of no value because most clinical laboratories only measure "total" serum concentrations of digitalis glycosides, a composite of both "free" and bound (to protein or Fab) drug.[269,270]

The Fab fragment-digoxin complex is excreted via the kidneys. It takes several days before the entire complex is removed, allowing routine digoxin assays to once again become reliable. In one study of patients with varying degrees of renal function, the half-life of the initial phase of total digoxin decline was 11.6 hours and the half-life of the second, or terminal, elimination phase was 118 ± 57 hours.[270] Unbound digoxin serum levels rebound to a mean maximum free digoxin concentration of 1.7 ± 1.3 mmol/L in 77 ± 46 hours, but are delayed to a greater extent in anephric patients.[269] Paradoxical return of toxicity may either be caused by release of digoxin from the Fab-digoxin complex or late redistribution of digoxin from tissue stores into the plasma.[268, 270] As long as antibodies remain in the system, further therapy with digitalis preparations is compromised because of binding of any new doses. Thus, monitoring of unbound concentrations is necessary.

Side effects to digoxin-specific Fab antibodies are uncommon, but several cautions must be heeded.[271] HF or atrial fibrillation can be precipitated by the removal of the pharmacologic effects of the digitalis glycoside. Similarly, as Na^+-K^+-ATPase enzyme activity is restored, hypokalemia can develop. Serum potassium concentrations must be monitored frequently for the first several hours after Fab administration because potassium levels can drop precipitously as potassium shifts back into cells. This may require immediate potassium supplementation.

The incidence of hypersensitivity or other allergic reactions after Fab administration is rare, but the risk after repeated ingestions is unknown.[271] Skin testing according to the directions in the digoxin immune Fab package insert should be followed in high-risk individuals, especially in patients with known allergies to sheep serum or in whom digoxin-specific Fab has been administered previously. If an accelerated allergic reaction occurs, the drug infusion should be discontinued and appropriate therapy initiated, including antihistamines, corticosteroids, and airway management. Epinephrine should be used cautiously in patients with arrhythmias.

Pediatric Dosing

45. H.H., a 3-year-old girl with a congenital heart defect, is displaying increased symptoms of HF. She is awaiting surgery for repair of a ventricular septal defect and a damaged aortic valve. In the meantime, she is to receive digoxin therapy. All laboratory values, including renal function and electrolytes, are within normal limits. She weighs 28 lb (12.7 kg). Should digoxin dosing for H.H. be formulated using the same guidelines as for an adult? What loading dose and maintenance dose should H.H. be given?

Although many of the general principles that apply to use of digoxin in adults also apply to children, certain practical considerations and changes in pharmacokinetic parameters must be considered.[264] Dosing in children is complicated by rapid changes in body size and tissue distribution, GI motility, and maturation of the liver and kidney.

Most children cannot swallow conventional tablets or capsules and must be given the liquid (elixir) dosage form. Although the pediatric population does not differ significantly from adults in their ability to absorb digoxin, large individual variability is noted and the elixir is generally more bioavailable than the tablets.

An important difference is noted between children and adults in regard to tissue uptake and volume of distribution of digoxin. As noted previously, the average adult has a steady-state digoxin Vd of 6.7 L/kg. Greater variability is seen in very young to older children with Vd reported to be 7.5, 16.3, and 16.1 L/kg in neonates, 11-month-old infants, and children, respectively.[264] Children have slightly higher digoxin protein-binding than adults, but neither group has a high enough percentage bound (i.e., <50%) to significantly affect tissue concentrations of the drug.

As in adults, clearance and half-life of digoxin in children are highly dependent on renal function and to a lesser degree on metabolism and biliary excretion. Elimination data in children are limited by the small number of available reports and the absence of studies in healthy pediatric subjects; nonetheless, a few generalizations can be made. Total body clearance is significantly impaired in premature and term neonates (with $t_{1/2}$ ranging from 61 to 170 hours). Older children and adolescents clear the drug at approximately the same rate as adults. These findings are consistent with poorly developed renal function in premature or young newborns, but the kidney becomes highly functional by 1 month of life and function approaches that of an adult by 1 year of age.

From these data, one can surmise that after the first year of life and through early childhood, children will need a *larger* dose on a per-kilogram basis than adults. This is based on a larger apparent volume of distribution, not altered drug clearance. Although no clear consensus is available on dosing of digoxin in children, the following guidelines have been published[264]: premature and term neonates should be digitalized with 0.01 to 0.03 mg/kg IV; infants should be given 0.04 to 0.05 mg/kg orally. For maintenance, the premature neonate can be given 0.001 to 0.009 mg/kg per day, neonates 0.010 mg/kg per day, and infants (1 month to 2 years) 0.015 to 0.025 mg/kg per day. For children older than 2 years of age, the loading dose is 0.05 mg/kg orally followed by a daily maintenance dose of 0.01 to 0.015 mg/kg. As in adults, doses are adjusted based on clinical signs, renal function, and serum levels (Table 19-5).

For H.H., an argument can be made for starting a maintenance dose without a loading dose because she is not in acute distress. If a loading dose is required, an oral elixir could be used at 0.05 mg/kg (0.6 to 0.65 mg), split into two doses. Maintenance would be started at 0.01 mg/kg or approximately 0.125 mg/day. These doses are surprisingly large and reflect the large volume of distribution in children.

Dosing Digoxin in Renal Failure
LOADING DOSE

46. R.D. is an 84-year-old woman admitted to the hospital in acute distress with breathlessness, significantly distended neck veins, and in atrial fibrillation. She has been an insulin-dependent diabetic for 35 years and has progressively deteriorating renal function that has never required hemodialysis. Home medications include torsemide 6 mg QD, enalapril 20 mg BID, metoprolol XL 200 mg QD, and NPH insulin 30 units/day. Pertinent admitting laboratory values and physical examination reveal the following: Na, 140 mEq/L; K, 5.1 mEq/L; Cl, 101 mEq/L; bicarbonate, 24 mEq/L; glucose (fasting), 180 mg/dL; BUN, 48 mg/dL; creatinine (SrCr), 3.8 mg/dL; weight, 82 kg; height, 5'6"; pulse, 118 beats/min and irregular.

She is given furosemide 80 mg IV and 20 mEq of KCl with each dose of furosemide. Because of her distress and the presence of new onset atrial fibrillation, it is decided to give her an IV loading dose of digoxin. Calculate the loading dose for R.D. Do any alterations have to be made in the loading dose because of her decreased renal function?

[SI units: Na, 140 mmol/L; Cl, 101 mmol/L; bicarbonate, 24 mmol/L; glucose, 9.99 mmol/L; BUN, 17.5 mmol; creatinine, 335.92 mmol/L]

Theoretically, loading doses for renally excreted drugs do not have to be altered in renal failure because a loading dose only fills up the body tissue stores and is independent of elimination. However, the volume of distribution for digoxin may vary substantially in patients with a creatinine clearance <25 mL/min. One group of investigators observed volumes of distribution ranging from 195 to 489 L/1.73 m² in seven patients with renal failure.[272] Others calculated volumes of distribution for renal failure patients reported in the literature and found a range of 230 to 380 L/1.78 m², 30% to 50% *less* than that observed in subjects with normal renal function.[70] An average value for Vd of 330 L/70 kg or 4.7 L/kg in patients with renal failure can be used (Table 19-5).

As the volume of distribution decreases, the theoretic loading dose also decreases. Unfortunately, it is usually not possible to know what a given patient's volume of distribution is until the drug has already been administered and serum levels are measured. A report of 22 patients with renal failure showed no toxicity using an IV digoxin loading dose of 0.01 mg/kg.[273] Using the adjusted value for Vd, we can use the following standard equation for calculating a loading dose for R.D. is used:

$$\text{IV loading dose} = (Vd)(Cp) \qquad \textbf{(19-3)}$$

A desired *Cp* of 0.75 ng/mL is assumed. In calculating *Vd*, we must correct R.D.'s weight to ideal body weight (IBW) because she is obese (82 kg).

$$\text{IBW (males)} = 50 \text{ kg} + 2.3 \text{ kg/inch over 5 feet} \qquad \textbf{(19-4)}$$
$$\text{IBW(females)} = 45.5 \text{ kg} + 2.3 \text{ kg/inch over 5 feet} \qquad \textbf{(19-5)}$$

For R.D., who is female,:

$$\text{IBW} = 45.5 \text{ kg} + 2.3 \text{ kg(6 feet)} = 59.3 \text{ kg} \qquad \textbf{(19-A)}$$

Therefore, her loading dose will be:

$$
\begin{aligned}
\text{IV LD} &= (Vd)(Cp) \\
&= [(4.7 \text{ L/kg})(59.3 \text{ kg})]\,(0.75 \text{ ng/mL}) \\
&= 209{,}033 \text{ ng or } 209 \text{ μg} \\
&= {\sim}\,0.2 \text{ mg}
\end{aligned} \qquad \textbf{(19-B)}
$$

This IV loading dose is considerably smaller than one would use in a person with normal renal function because we assumed a smaller volume of distribution. A corresponding oral loading dose would be approximately 0.3 mg after correcting for an average bioavailability of 75%. When using larger loading doses, the total dose is often divided into two portions, giving two thirds of the dose to start and the remaining one third 6 to 8 hour later. However, since the dose for R.D. is small, the entire 0.2 mg can be given at once. If after 8 to 12 hours she is still in atrial fibrillation, an extra 0.1 mg could be given safely since we only targeted a serum concentration of 0.75 ng/mL.

MAINTENANCE DOSE

47. Calculate a maintenance dose for R.D.

Patients like R.D. who are older and/or have impaired renal function require reduced maintenance doses of digoxin. Advanced HF can also influence digoxin dosing requirements by reducing both renal and hepatic blood flow, thus reducing digoxin clearance. While empiric dosage reductions can be made, pharmacokinetic principles should be applied to obtain more rational dosing.

The first step is to make an estimate of the patient's creatinine clearance. While several methods are available, we will use the method of Cockcroft and Gault[274]:

$$Cl_{Cr}(\text{males}) = \frac{\text{IBW}(140 - \text{Age})}{72\text{SrCr}}$$

$$Cl_{Cr}(\text{females}) = 0.85\, Cl_{Cr}(\text{males}) \qquad \textbf{(19-6)}$$

For R.D., who is female:

$$
\begin{aligned}
Cl_{Cr} &= 0.85(59.3 \text{ kg})(140-84)/72(3.8 \text{ mg/dL}) \\
&= 10.32 \text{ mL/min}
\end{aligned} \qquad \textbf{(19-C)}
$$

The second step is to estimate the patient's digoxin clearance. A good method of estimating digoxin clearance is to use equations derived by Scheiner and associates[275] from pooled data of several hundred patients:

$$Cl_{digoxin} = 1.02(Cl_{Cr}) + 57 \text{ mL/min} \qquad \textbf{(19-7)}$$

where 1.02 (Cl_{Cr}) represents the renal clearance of digoxin and 57 mL/minute represents the nonrenal (hepatic and biliary) clearance of digoxin for a 70-kg man. The equation must be adjusted in patients with severe HF to account for decreased renal and hepatic perfusion. The adjusted equation is:

$$Cl_{digoxin} = 0.88(Cl_{Cr}) + 23 \text{ mL/min} \qquad \textbf{(19-8)}$$

R.D.'s creatinine clearance is significantly depressed and her HF is poorly controlled. Thus, the equation for digoxin clearance in severe HF is used:

$$
\begin{aligned}
Cl_{digoxin} &= 0.88(Cl_{Cr}) + 23 \text{ mL/min} \\
&= 0.88(10.3 \text{ mL/min}) + 23 \text{ mL/min} \\
&= 33 \text{ mL/min} \quad \text{(19-D)} \\
&= 47.5 \text{ L/day}
\end{aligned}
$$

Once clearance is determined, the maintenance dose is calculated using the general pharmacokinetic equation:

$$
MD = \frac{(Cl)(Cpss\ ave)(\tau)}{F} \quad \text{(19-9)}
$$

where *Cpss ave* is the average desired plasma level at steady state. Using the clearance value obtained from Scheiner's method (Equation 19-8) and a targeted serum concentration of 0.75 ng/mL:

$$
\begin{aligned}
MD &= \frac{(47.5 \text{ L/day})(0.75 \text{ ng/mL})(1 \text{ Day})}{0.75} \\
&= 47{,}250 \text{ ng/day or } 47.2\ \mu g/day \\
&= 0.047 \text{ mg/day}
\end{aligned}
$$

Only a limited number of digoxin tablet sizes are available (0.125, 0.25, and 0.5 mg). This makes administering a 0.047 mg dose difficult. There are several options: give 0.125 mg every second or third day, dividing a 0.125-mg tablet in half every day, or administering 0.05 mg/day using a pediatric elixir or digoxin capsules. Capsules and elixir may be absorbed better than the tablets.

As presented in the introduction, Jelliffe applies pharmacokinetic principles in a different way.[77] He first calculates the amount of drug lost from the body in a 24-hour period and then replaces this same amount as the daily dose. He estimates the percent of total body stores (drug in the body, *Ab*), which is lost per day by the equation:

$$
\% \text{ Eliminated} = \frac{14 + Cl_{Cr}}{5} \quad \text{(19-E)}
$$

The *amount* of drug lost per day (i.e., the desired dose) is then calculated by multiplying the maximum amount of drug you wish to achieve in the body after each dose (i.e., *Ab*) by the percent *lost* per day. The desired *Ab* can be estimated by multiplying the desired plasma (serum) level (e.g., 0.75 ng/mL) by the volume of distribution. Therefore, the equation defining an oral maintenance dose is:

$$
MD = \frac{(Vd)(Cp)(\% \text{ Eliminated daily})}{F} \quad \text{(19-10)}
$$

The reader is encouraged to refer to the 7th edition of *Applied Therapeutics: The Clinical Use of Drugs* or basic texts on clinical pharmacokinetics for further description of the Jelliffe dosing method.[70–72] The principles used by Scheiner and colleagues[275] to calculate clearance appear to be the most valid because they eliminate the need to estimate the volume of distribution, which can vary widely among patients.[71,72]

Critical Care Management of Heart Failure
Non-ACE Inhibitor Vasodilator Therapy

48. L.M., a 50-year-old African American man, was admitted several days ago with severe, progressive, and debilitating symptoms of HF. His history is significant in that his father and two brothers died of heart attacks shortly after the age of 40. L.M. has a 12-year history of HF that is symptomatic despite treatment with full therapeutic doses of furosemide, enalapril, carvedilol, and digoxin. He has no history of hypertension, but previous studies suggested a diagnosis of cardiomyopathy with an EF of 18%. Over the previous 8 months, L.M.'s DOE became progressively worse, and for the month before admission he was confined to bed because of extreme fatigue. He awoke once or twice nightly with PND.

Physical examination on this admission revealed a dyspneic, cyanotic man in obvious distress but with no complaints of chest pain. His BP was 100/66 mm Hg and his pulse was 105 beats/min. Significant JVD, bilateral rales, hepatomegaly, and 3+ peripheral edema also were observed. Chest radiograph revealed cardiomegaly and pulmonary congestion. L.M. was admitted to the CCU where a Swan-Ganz catheter was passed from an antecubital vein to the pulmonary artery.

Before therapy, L.M.'s PCWP was 27 mm Hg (normal, 5 to 12 mm Hg) and his cardiac index (CI) was 1.9 L/min/m² (normal, 2.7 to 4.3 L/min/m²). Several doses of IV furosemide were given, and IV nitroprusside was initiated at a dosage of 16 μg/min and eventually increased to 200 μg/min. At this dose, L.M.'s PCWP decreased to 15 mm Hg and his CI increased to 2.5 L/min/m². He was eventually discharged home with furosemide 80 mg BID, spironolactone 50 mg QD, enalapril 20 mg BID, carvedilol 25 mg BID, digoxin 0.125 mg/day, hydralazine 75 mg QID, and isosorbide dinitrate 40 mg Q 6 hr. Categorize L.M.'s HF by NYHA class and ACC/AHH staging.

On admission L.M. was in NYHA class IV HF despite maximal doses of the recommend four-drug therapy with a loop diuretic, ACE inhibitor, β-blocker, and digoxin. He was approaching ACC/AHA stage D as well. His PCWP was high and his CI was low, reflecting pulmonary vascular congestion (elevated preload) and poor CO, respectively (See Chapter 22, Shock for a more thorough review of principles of Swan-Ganz catheterization and hemodynamic monitoring. Also see the introduction to this chapter to review the concepts of afterload, preload, and the relative contributions of arterial and venous dilation to these hemodynamic changes.) The immediate objective of therapy is to provide symptomatic relief by decreasing the PCWP and increasing the CO.

Most patients with acute HF can be classified into one of four hemodynamic profiles using relatively simple assessment techniques[276–279] (Fig. 19-8). When using this scheme, patients are assessed for the presence or absence of elevated venous filling pressures (wet versus dry patients) and adequacy of vital organ perfusion (warm versus cold patients.) Elevated filling pressure can be assessed at the patient's bedside by observing orthopnea, jugular venous distension, the presence of a third heart sound (S_3), peripheral edema, and ascites. Presence or absence of rales on auscultation is not considered a reliable indicator.[279] Hypotension, weak peripheral pulse, a narrow pulse pressure (<25%), cool forearms and legs, decreased mental alertness, and rising BUN and serum creatinine are indicators of decreased organ perfusion. In one se-

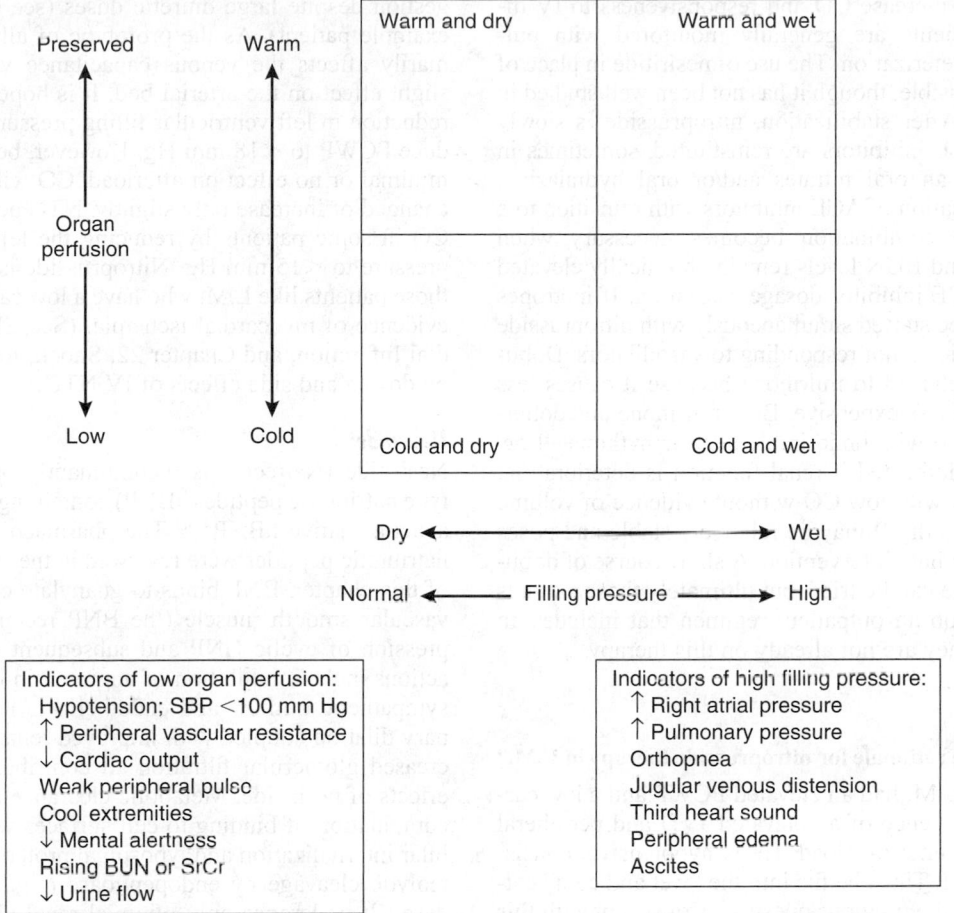

Indicators of low organ perfusion:
Hypotension; SBP <100 mm Hg
↑ Peripheral vascular resistance
↓ Cardiac output
Weak peripheral pulse
Cool extremities
↓ Mental alertness
Rising BUN or SrCr
↓ Urine flow

Indicators of high filling pressure:
↑ Right atrial pressure
↑ Pulmonary pressure
Orthopnea
Jugular venous distension
Third heart sound
Peripheral edema
Ascites

FIGURE 19-8 Hemodynamic profiles of acute heart failure. (Adapted with permission from Nohria A et al. Medical management of advanced heart failure. JAMA 2002;287:628.)

ries, 67% of patients admitted to the hospital with a low LVEF and class IV HF symptoms were classified as "wet and warm," with 28% assessed as "cold and wet," and only 5% as "cold and dry."[276] Few if any patients were in the "warm and dry category" since this is the status one is trying to achieve in well-compensated patients. Continuous blood pressure, ECG, urine flow, and pulse oximetry measurements are standard noninvasive monitoring for all patients. Invasive hemodynamic monitoring is used in critically ill patients when more precise measurements of filling pressure (e.g., right atrial or pulmonary artery pressure), systemic vascular resistance, and CO/cardiac index are desired. The goals are to achieve a right atrial pressure of less than 5 to 8 mm Hg, pulmonary artery pressure of less than 25/10 mm Hg, pulmonary artery wedge pressure of 12 to 16 mm Hg or less, a systemic vascular resistance of 900 to 1,400 dyn.s.m^{-5}, and a cardiac index of 2.8 to 4.2 L/min/m^2 (See Chapter 22, Shock, for more detailed discussion of hemodynamic monitoring).

For most patients presenting in the "wet and warm" category, the primary intervention is aggressive diuresis to rapidly reduce fluid overload. This is followed by optimization of the standard three-drug regimen of ACE inhibitors, β-blockers, and digoxin. In more severe cases (e.g., when pulmonary artery wedge pressure is >18 mm Hg), initial use of an IV vasodilator such as nitroglycerin or nesiritide to reduce preload may be indicated. Nesiritide offers an advantage of having

both natriuretic and vasodilatory properties and can add to the diuretic effect of furosemide in refractory patients.[42] Careful monitoring of pulmonary wedge pressure and cardiac index is necessary to avoid excessive reduction of pulmonary pressure than will then lead to deterioration of CO. In some cases, pulmonary artery pressure must be maintained somewhat above the normal range for optimal balance. Milrinone and other inotropes are not necessary for these patients, and may even cause deterioration of symptoms[280,281] (See also question 53 for further discussion of dobutamine and milrinone).

The "wet and cold" patients (like L.M.) who present with signs of both volume overload and hypoperfusion are more clinically challenging. Pulmonary artery wedge pressure is elevated and cardiac index is less than 2.2 L/min/m^2. Immediate attention must be directed toward correcting hypoperfusion followed by aggressive diuretic therapy as in the "wet and warm" patients. β-Blockers and ACE inhibitors should be temporarily withdrawn if symptomatic hypotension is present. Since these patients often have both a low CO and high systemic vascular resistance, both vasodilators (e.g., nitroglycerin and nitroprusside) and an inotropic-vasodilator (e.g., dobutamine, low dose dopamine, or milrinone) might be considered. There is not unanimous agreement as to the agent of choice. The desired effect is reduced right sided filling pressure (reduced preload via venous dilation) and reduced resistance to left ventricular outflow (reduced afterload via arterial dilation), both of which can increase CO and responsiveness to IV diuretics. These patients are generally monitored with pulmonary artery catheterization. The use of nesiritide in place of nitroprusside is possible, though it has not been well studied in this patient type. After stabilization, nitroprusside is slowly withdrawn and ACE inhibitors are reinstituted, sometimes in combination with an oral nitrates and/or oral hydralazine. Chronic discontinuation of ACE inhibitors with transition to a hydralazine-nitrate combination becomes necessary when serum creatinine and BUN levels remain chronically elevated or worsen after ACE inhibitor dosage escalation. If inotropes are used, they can be started simultaneously with nitroprusside or reserved for patients not responding to vasodilators. Dobutamine may be preferred to milrinone because it causes less hypotension and is less expensive. Both milrinone and dobutamine are associated with undesirable tachyarrhythmias. Low dose dopamine is indicated if renal function is deteriorating.

The rare patient with low CO without evidence of volume overload ("cold and dry") may be relatively stable and poses less need for immediate intervention. A short course of dobutamine or milrinone can be tried, but ultimately these patients should be placed on an outpatient regimen that includes an oral β-blocker if they are not already on this therapy.

Nitroprusside

49. **What was the rationale for nitroprusside therapy in L.M.?**

On admission, L.M. had an elevated PCWP and a low cardiac index. The presence of an elevated JVD and peripheral edema indicate volume overload. He is hypotensive, consistent with his low CI. Thus, he fits into the "wet and cold" category described in the previous question. Consistent with this diagnosis he was given vigorous diuresis and nitroprusside.

Nitroprusside dilates both arterial and venous vessels; therefore, it has the theoretic advantage of decreasing both afterload and preload. Its major disadvantages are it must be given by continuous IV infusion necessitating arterial line placement in most situations, it is unstable if exposed to heat and light after reconstitution, and it occasionally causes a profound hypotension that will decrease CO.

Patients should be initiated on small doses of nitroprusside (6 to 20 μg/min) that are increased slowly to a maximum of 300 to 800 μg/min until a decrease in the PCWP or arterial pressure is observed. When stopping nitroprusside therapy, a slow taper is recommended because a rebound increase in HF has been observed 10 to 30 minutes after drug withdrawal. (For a more thorough discussion of nitroprusside use, see Chapters 21, Hypertensive Emergencies and 22, Shock.)

50. **What other parenteral vasodilators can be used to treat HF refractory to nitroprusside?**

L.M. responded well to nitroprusside and needed no other therapy. However, IV nitroglycerin and IV nesiritide are alternatives to nitroprusside in patients with either "wet and warm" or "wet and cold" acute HF. Nitroglycerin or nesiritide can either be a substitute for nitroprusside or combined with nitroprusside.

Intravenous Nitroglycerin
Intravenous nitroglycerin (NTG) is indicated for patients with significant respiratory distress from pulmonary venous con-

gestion despite large diuretic doses (see Question 31 for an example patient). As the prototype of all nitrates, NTG primarily affects the venous capacitance vessels with only a slight effect on the arterial bed. It is hoped that the resulting reduction in left ventricular filling pressure (preload) will reduce PCWP to <18 mm Hg. However, because nitrates have minimal or no effect on afterload, CO will likely remain unchanged or increase only slightly. NTG actually can decrease CO in some patients by reducing the left ventricular filling pressure to <15 mm Hg. Nitroprusside is a better choice for those patients like L.M. who have a low cardiac index without evidence of myocardial ischemia. (See Chapter 18, Myocardial Infarction, and Chapter 22, Shock, for more information on dosing and side effects of IV NTG.)

Nesiritide
Nesiritide (Natrecor) is recombinantly produced human B-type natriuretic peptide (hBNP) containing the same 32 amino acids as native hBNP.[41,42] The pharmacologic activity of the natriuretic peptides were reviewed in the pathogenesis section of this chapter. BNP binds to guanylate cyclase receptors on vascular smooth muscle (the BNP receptor) leading to expression of cyclic GNP and subsequent vasodilation. Other actions include inhibition of angiotensin-converting enzyme, sympathetic outflow and endothelin-1. Peripheral and coronary dilation coupled with improved renal blood flow and increased glomerular filtration all contribute to the beneficial effects of nesiritide. Metabolic clearance of nesiritide is by a combination of binding to cell surfaces with subsequent cellular internalization and lyposomal proteolysis as well as proteolytic cleavage by endopeptidase (e.g., neutral endopeptidase.) It undergoes only minimal renal clearance. The mean elimination half-life is 8 to 22 minutes (mean, 18 minutes), necessitating IV infusion therapy.

In clinical trials of hospitalized patients with severe HF, nesiritide produced comparable hemodynamic effects and reduction in dyspnea scores as NTG when used in combination with IV diuretics and either dopamine or dobutamine.[41,42] Dose-dependent hypotension is the most common side effect with nesiritide, reported in 11% to 32% of patients. In some trials, nesiritide caused a higher incidence and/or longer duration of hypotension than NTG, whereas in other trials the incidence of hypotension was similar. The incidence of PVCs and nonsustained ventricular tachycardia are less with nesiritide than with dopamine, dobutamine, or milrinone. Other side effects include headache, abdominal pain, nausea, anxiety, bradycardia, and leg cramps.

Because of high cost, the use of nesiritide is generally restricted to those patients with acute HF exacerbations who are fluid overloaded and have a pulmonary capillary wedge pressure >18 to 20 mm hg despite high doses of diuretics and IV NTG. In contrast to NTG, nesiritide has natriuretic properties that are additive to those of the loop diuretics. It should avoided in patients with a systolic blood pressure <90 to 100 mg Hg or in cardiogenic shock. Dobutamine or milrinone should be added or substituted in hypotensive patients or those with a cardiac index <2.2 L/min/m².

The IV infusion of nesiritide is prepared by diluting the contents of a 1.5 mg vial to 6 μg/mL in 250 mL of 5% dextrose or 0.9% NaCl. An initial loading dose of 2 μg/kg is given intravenously over 60 seconds, followed by a continuous IV infusion at a rate of 0.01 μg/kg/min. The desired response is a reduction of PCWP of 5 to 10 mm Hg at 15 minutes. The dose can be increased in 0.005 μg/kg/min increments at 3-hour intervals to a maximum of 0.03 μg/kg/min. Dosage should be titrated to a PCWP <18 mm Hg and a systolic BP >90 mm Hg.

Hydralazine

51. **After L.M.'s condition was controlled with nitroprusside therapy, he was given his original medications plus spironolactone, hydralazine, and isosorbide dinitrate. Why were hydralazine and isosorbide used? What other forms of nitrates can be used in place of the isosorbide? Is combination therapy rational?**

L.M. had already been treated with a loop diuretic, an ACE inhibitor (enalapril), a β-blocker, and digoxin. Despite this therapy, he was still doing poorly. Spironolactone was added for reasons discussed in Question 14. A possible next step in treating a patient with this advanced stage of HF is the addition of a non-ACE inhibitor vasodilator.

Hydralazine is a direct-acting smooth muscle relaxant with significant arteriolar dilating effects in the kidneys and limbs. It has essentially no effect on the venous system or hepatic blood flow. Because its predominate action is as an arteriolar dilator, hydralazine is the prototype afterload-reducing agent. Decreasing aortic impedance (afterload) is of little benefit in a normal or minimally diseased heart, but it may greatly improve severely compromised left ventricular function. SVR is decreased predictably and this, in turn, increases cardiac output (cardiac index).[17,135,282]

Fortunately, the reflex tachycardia and hypotension that frequently accompany hydralazine therapy when used in treating hypertension are minimal or absent when it is used to treat HF. Increased CO overrides vasodilatory effects in the latter instance. However, in patients with end-stage cardiomyopathy, significant hypotension still can occur if the heart cannot respond appropriately. Another beneficial response to hydralazine is reduction of pulmonary vascular resistance in patients with severe pulmonary hypertension. This pulmonary arteriolar dilating effect of hydralazine is generally less beneficial than the venodilating effects of drugs such as nitrates and nitroprusside. Because hydralazine is devoid of venous dilating properties, CVP and pulmonary wedge capillary pressure are unchanged.[135,282]

The effect of a single dose occurs in about 30 minutes and lasts up to 6 hours. Larger doses than typically used for the treatment of hypertension may be required for HF management. The average maintenance dose is 200 to 400 mg/day (50 to 100 mg every 6 hours). L.M. required 75 mg four times a day. Unfortunately, hydralazine used as monotherapy is not associated with long-term improvement in functional status.[282] However, combination therapy of hydralazine with either nitrates or ACE inhibitors is highly effective.

Although tachyphylaxis generally is not a significant problem with prolonged courses of hydralazine, some patients require increased diuretic doses to counteract hydralazine-induced fluid retention. This latter response reflects activation of the renin-angiotensin system following vasodilation of the renal vasculature. Other side effects accompanying hydralazine include transient nausea during the first few days of therapy; headache, flushing, or tachycardia; and a lupus syndrome associated with prolonged, high doses (See Chapter 14, Essential Hypertension, for further discussion of hydralazine side effects and dosing).

Oral and Topical Nitrates

Nitrates have complementary effects to those of hydralazine.[17,135] They primarily dilate venous capacitance vessels, with minimal effects on selected arterial beds (coronary and pulmonary arteries). Venous dilation reduces preload resulting in significant reductions in PCWP and right atrial pressure. They are especially effective in reducing the symptoms of pulmonary edema. The lack of significant arterial dilation accounts for the observations that SVR is minimally reduced and CO remains unchanged. Nitrate monotherapy is indicated for HF patients with valvular defects such as mitral or aortic regurgitation. In these patients, reduction of the ventricular filling pressure reduces left ventricular congestion.

ISOSORBIDE DINITRATE

Because sublingual NTG has a short duration of response, more attention has been focused on sublingual and oral isosorbide dinitrate. Sublingual isosorbide is well absorbed and does not undergo first-pass metabolism. Its onset is rapid (approximately 5 minutes), but its effects are relatively short (1 to 3 hours). The usual starting dosage is 5 mg every 4 to 6 hours, but dosages may be titrated to 20 mg or more every 4 to 6 hours. These larger doses are associated with longer beneficial effects (approximately 3 hours), but also a high frequency of intolerable headaches and hypotension.

Previous claims of a poor response to orally administered isosorbide because of a large first-pass metabolic effect have been refuted. Large oral doses overwhelm the metabolic capacity of the liver and produce beneficial effects. Oral isosorbide has a slow onset (15 to 30 minutes), but the duration of activity is slightly longer than that associated with sublingual administration (4 to 6 hours). Oral doses of 5 mg are probably ineffective; 10 mg is the smallest effective starting dose with further titration to dosages as high as 20 to 80 mg every 4 to 6 hours. The best dose for both sublingual and oral nitrates is that which provides the desired beneficial effect with the least side effects.

TRANSDERMAL NITROGLYCERIN

An innovative approach to NTG administration is transdermal patch systems (Nitrodisc, Nitro-Dur, Transderm-Nitro, Minitran). Topical application of these systems is said to provide 24 hours of continuous cutaneous absorption with more convenience and less mess than NTG ointment. Although most published data on these dose forms are in patients with angina, several reports are on their use in HF.

The initial enthusiasm for transdermal NTG has been tempered by the suggestion that tolerance develops quickly, resulting in a benefit for much less than 24 hours following patch application. Considerable debate has arisen over this topic.[283–285] Some reviewers suggest abandoning this form of therapy, while others argue that the studies showing negative benefit were flawed. Removal of the patch during the night might lead to restoration of response the following day. It has been suggested that while the antianginal effects of NTG are attenuated with chronic therapy, the beneficial preload-reducing properties for HF are more sustained. However, large doses (20 to 40 mg/24 hr) may be required, necessitating the use of several patches per day and resulting in significant expense to the patient. (See Chapter 17, Ischemic Heart Disease: Anginal Syndromes, for a more detailed discussion on the application and controversy surrounding NTG transdermal patches.)

Hydralazine/Nitrate Combination

Combined afterload and preload reduction is clearly of benefit both in improving symptoms and in enhancing long-term survival. Compared with ACE inhibitors, the hydralazine-isosorbide combination provides more significant improvement in exercise tolerance, but the side effect profile and survival statistics are better with ACE inhibitors.[131] With combination therapy, CO is greater for any given level of ventricular filling pressure. Generally, the use of the two drugs together is not accompanied by reflex tachycardia or hypotension, but one must be careful not to compromise coronary blood flow in patients with coexistent angina.

Perhaps the most compelling argument for the use of combination hydralazine and nitrate vasodilator therapy comes from the results of the two Veterans Administration Cooperative Studies (V-HeFT I and V-HeFT II).[17,131,135] As discussed in more detail in Question 15, these two studies not only confirmed symptomatic relief and improved exercise tolerance with combination therapy, but they also showed improved survival.

In summary, nitrates alone are indicated for those patients with signs and symptoms of isolated pulmonary and venous congestion (i.e., dyspnea, increased pulmonary pressure, neck vein distention, edema). Conversely, use of an arterial dilator is more appropriate in a patient with high SVR, low CO, and normal PCWP. Most patients, like L.M., exhibit symptoms of decreased CO and elevated venous pressure, making combination therapy the most attractive option. Although the hydralazine-isosorbide combination actually improves symptoms slightly better than ACE inhibitors, the data on survival are more impressive with the ACE inhibitors. As illustrated by L.M.'s treatment regimen, a combination of an ACE inhibitor plus hydralazine and/or a nitrate is common in patients with far advanced disease.

Role of Race in the Pharmacotherapy of Heart Failure

52. L. M. is African American. Would he be expected to respond any differently to ACE inhibitors and/or hydralazine-isosorbide dinitrate than a patient who is not African American?

In general black patients develop HF at an earlier age and are more likely to have hypertension as a cause for HF. Conversely, the etiology of HF in non-black patients is more often due to ischemic heart disease. The rate of death due to HF is higher for black patients than for non-black patients.

Racial differences in response to drug therapy have been proposed, although this issue is far from resolved.[286–289] For example, a post hoc analysis of the V-HeFT trial data cited previously showed no difference in annual mortality between black (N = 180) and non-black patients (N = 450) in the placebo group (17.3% versus 18.8%).[131,267] However, black patients in the hydralazine-nitrate group had a significantly lower annual mortality rate (9.7%) than black subjects in the

placebo group (17.3%), while non-black subjects had no survival benefit from the drug combination (16.9% versus 18.8%). This implies that black patients, but not non-blacks, derive benefit from the treatment with hydralazine-isosorbide. These same investigators then reanalyzed the V-HeFT II trial results for possible racial differences between response to enalapril and the hydralazine-nitrate combination.[135,287] The outcome is difficult to interpret because of the absence of a placebo group. The all-cause annual mortality rate for blacks (N = 215) was identical in the two drug groups (12.8% with enalapril and 12.9% with hydral-iso.) In non-blacks (N = 574), the corresponding mortality rates were 11% with enalapril and 14.9% with hydral-iso. These data could be interpreted as either superior response to hydral-iso in black subjects or inferior activity of ACE inhibitors in black patients. The latter interpretation is consistent with the hypothesis that ACE inhibitors might have a lesser blood pressure lowering effect in black patients with hypertension compared to non-blacks. A similar reanalysis of the SOLVD Prevention[183] and Treatment[134] trials, both of which compared enalapril to placebo in patients with recent MI, concluded that enalapril therapy is associated with a significant reduction in the risk for hospitalization for HF among white patients (44% reduction) with left ventricular dysfunction, but not among similar black patients. Confounding variables contributing to all of the analyses presented include disproportionately low numbers of blacks in the trials, and possibly more underlying risk factors (e.g., hypertension) in the black subjects.

To address these factors, a meta-analysis of the seven major ACE inhibitor studies, representing a total of 14,752 patients was conducted.[288] The conclusion was that that relative risk for mortality when taking an ACE inhibitor compared to placebo was identical (0.89) for both black and white patients. The authors of the meta-analysis urged that ACE inhibitors not be withheld from black patients. One other consideration with ACE inhibitors is an observed higher rate, though still rare, of angioedema in blacks than in whites. While the debate continues over the preferred drug in blacks, it is interesting to note that an NDA for combination drug product containing hydralazine and isosorbide (BiDil) is undergoing FDA review with a proposed labeled indication specifically for black patients with HF. Until more data are available, ACE inhibitors should not be withheld from black patients, but careful monitoring is required to assess response.

A possible racial difference in response to β-blocker drugs has also been hypothesized based on differential effects observed in patients with hypertension.[286,288,289] However, a post hoc analysis of the various US Carvedilol Heart Failure trials[202–206] concluded that the benefit of carvedilol was apparently of similar magnitude in both black (N = 217) and non-black (N = 877) patients.[289] Using the combined endpoint of the risk of death from any cause or hospitalization, the risk reduction compared to placebo was 48% in black patients and 30% in non-black subjects. Because there were fewer black patients studied, these differences did not reach statistical significance. There was also a significant improvement in NYHA functional class, EF, and patient global symptom assessment with carvedilol in both black and non-black patients. Contradictory evidence comes from the Beta-Blocker Evaluation of Survival Trial (BEST).[215] In this trial (discussed in question 30), 2708 patients with NYHA class III (92%) or IV HF were randomly assigned to either bucindolol or placebo. Bucindolol is a nonselective β-blocker with partial agonist activity that imparts weak vasodilation. A unique characteristic of this study was that a subgroup analysis for racial differences was planned from the start. While there was a trend toward reductions in cardiovascular mortality and hospitalization with the active drug, the trial was terminated after 2 years when it was determined that there was no mortality benefit of active drug compared to placebo (33% mortality in placebo group versus 30% with bucindolol.) A subgroup analysis showed a mortality benefit in non-black subjects, but none in black subjects. Subsequently, a meta-analysis of the five major β-blocker in HF studies was conducted, representing a total of 12,727 patients.[288] When the BEST Trial was included in the meta-analysis, the relative risk for mortality when taking an ACE inhibitor compared to placebo was 0.69 in white subjects, but only 0.97 for black patients. When the BEST trial was excluded, the relative risks were reduced in both groups to 0.63 and 0.67 in whites and blacks, respectively. The difference between the two groups was not statistically significant, although the 95% confidence interval for black patients was broader and included 1.0 (0.38 to 1.16). Based on all of these factors, it is likely that black patients will derive similar benefit to β-blockers as whites when given carvedilol, metoprolol, or bisoprolol. Bucindolol should be avoided, most likely due to its partial agonist activity.

Use of Inotropic Drugs

53. B.J., a 60-year-old man, is admitted to the hospital with severe, crushing substernal chest pain after a domestic quarrel at home. He has a history of occasional chest pain for the past 3 years treated with SL NTG PRN. The admitting impression is an acute myocardial infarction (AMI). Over the next 3 hours he becomes less alert, hypotensive, diaphoretic, and has a thready pulse. PCWP is elevated to 27 mm Hg, and a chest radiograph shows pulmonary edema. He is diagnosed as having cardiogenic shock. He does not have atrial fibrillation. Should B.J. be given digitalis? What other positive inotropic agents can be used in place of digitalis? Is milrinone safer than amrinone? (See also Chapter 22, Shock.)

Controversy Regarding Use of Digitalis After Myocardial Infarction
Digitalis has a well-documented inotropic effect in patients who have had an MI, but its use in the immediate peri-infarction period may be deleterious. Enhanced contractility may increase bulging of ischemic or infarcted segments, thereby dissipating the inotropic effect digoxin exerts on undamaged myocardium.[290] Secondly, digitalis has a direct arteriolar vasoconstrictive effect after rapid (<10 min) IV injection. This increases afterload, aggravates left ventricular failure, and increases myocardial oxygen consumption.[290]

Digitalis should not be given to patients with MI who are not in cardiac failure because it may increase infarct size. In fact, the findings of two large trials suggest that cumulative survival following an MI may be lower in patients treated with digoxin than in those who are not treated.[291,292] However, patients in the digoxin-treated groups were generally much sicker initially and when the data were adjusted for factors such as atrial fibrillation and severe left ventricular failure, the differences between groups did not reach statistical significance. In patients with mild to moderate HF persisting for several days after an MI, digitalis may exert a minimal but significant increase in EF without increasing the infarct size. In patients with severe HF or cardiogenic shock, digitalis is not the initial drug of choice because of the delay in its time to peak action and its possible deleterious effect on the peri-infarction area. Nevertheless, it may have a role in the subsequent chronic treatment of HF.

Dopamine and Dobutamine
E.J. is in cardiogenic shock and, for this reason, digitalis should be avoided. Other agents are more effective and are less likely to extend the infarct. β-Adrenergic agonists such as isoproterenol have been used in cardiogenic shock, but are of limited value because they produce a high incidence of arrhythmias. IV inotropic agents (dobutamine, dopamine, milrinone, amrinone) are recommended for patients with cardiogenic shock or refractory symptoms causing acute destabilization. They may also be used in patients requiring perioperative support following cardiac and non-cardiac surgery or for those awaiting transplantation. Dopamine is more effective as an arterial dilator, especially in the kidney, whereas dobutamine has more potent inotropic properties (See Chapter 22, Shock, for further information on dopamine and dobutamine dosing).

Phosphodiesterase Inhibitors: Amrinone and Milrinone
The phosphodiesterase inhibitors, represented by the two bipyridine derivatives, amrinone (Inocor) and milrinone (Primacor), are alternatives to digoxin and the catecholamines for the short-term parenteral treatment of severe congestive failure. These agents selectively inhibit phosphodiesterase F-III, the cyclic-AMP-specific cardiac phosphodiesterase. They have direct cardiac stimulating effects, but they are not sympathomimetics or inhibitors of Na^+-K^+-dependent ATP. Enzyme inhibition results in increased cyclic AMP levels in myocardial cells and thus enhances contractility. Their activity is not blocked by propranolol. Because they are phosphodiesterase inhibitors, they also act as vasodilators. It has been suggested that at low doses they act more as unloading agents rather than inotropes; others refute this viewpoint. Their overall hemodynamic effect probably results from a combination of positive inotropic action plus preload and afterload reduction.

Amrinone initially was investigated for oral use, but it failed to gain FDA approval because of dose-dependent, reversible thrombocytopenia (up to 20% of patients), drug fever, liver function abnormalities, and possibly drug-induced ventricular arrhythmias. Amrinone remains available in an IV form for short-term use in severe HF. Therapy is initiated with a 0.75 mg/kg bolus over 2 to 3 minutes followed by a maintenance infusion of 5 to 10 μg/kg per minute. Higher doses occasionally have been given, but doses exceeding 18 μg/kg per day should be avoided. It has a half-life of approximately 2.5 to 3.5 hours in normal individuals; this is prolonged to 6 to 12 hours in patients with HF. Lower doses may need to be given in patients with renal insufficiency because amrinone is 50% excreted unchanged in the kidney. All dilutions should be made in saline (0.45% to 0.9%) because amrinone is incompatible with dextrose-containing solutions.

With IV use, the major side effects to monitor are hypotension and precipitation of arrhythmias. The prevalence of thrombocytopenia is reduced to 2.4% with parenteral use. In summary, amrinone is effective in reducing SVR and PCWP and in increasing cardiac output, but it appears to be less effective than dobutamine.

Milrinone is structurally and pharmacologically similar to amrinone.[293–295] Besides inhibiting phosphodiesterase, it also may increase calcium availability to myocardial muscle. It has both inotropic and vasodilating properties. Heart rate increases and myocardial consumption may be less with milrinone than with dobutamine.[280,281] The half-life of milrinone is short (1.5 to 2.5 hours) with renal clearance accounting for approximately 80% to 90% of total body elimination. Milrinone is about 15 to 20 times more potent than amrinone on a weight basis. A typical loading dose is 50 μg/kg administered over 10 minutes followed by a maintenance infusion of 0.5 μg/kg per minute. The infusion is adjusted according to hemodynamic and clinical responses and should be lowered in patients with renal insufficiency. The primary concern with the use of milrinone is induction of ventricular arrhythmias, reported in up to 12% of patients. Supraventricular arrhythmias, hypotension, headache, and chest pain also have been reported. Thrombocytopenia is rare, a distinct advantage over amrinone. Overall, milrinone has become the drug of choice among the phosphodiesterase inhibitors.

The OPTIME-CHF trial assessed the in-hospital management of 951 patients with acute HF exacerbation (NYHA class III or IV, mean LVEF 23%), but not in cardiogenic shock.[280,281] In addition to standard diuretic and ACE inhibitor therapy, subjects were randomized to receive either milrinone or placebo. The initial milrinone infusion rate was 0.5 μg/kg/min with no loading dose. For the primary endpoint of total numbers of days hospitalized for cardiovascular causes from the time of the start of study drug infusion to day 60, there was no difference between active drug and placebo (mean 12.3 days with milrinone and 12.5 days with placebo.) There was also no difference in the mean number of days of hospitalization during the primary event. Death rates within 60 days were 10.3% with milrinone and 8.9% with placebo (NS, $P = 0.41$).[280] Follow-up analysis categorized subjects by etiology of HF (ischemic versus nonischemic).[281] Not unexpectedly, those with an ischemic cause did less well with hospital rates of 13.0 days for ischemic patients compared to 11.7 days for those without ischemia ($P = 0.2$). Corresponding death rates over 60 days were 11.6% and 7.5% ($P = 0.03$). Importantly, within the cohort of patients with ischemia (N = 485), milrinone-treated patients tended to have worse outcomes than those treated with placebo: 13.6 hospital days with milrinone versus 12.4 days with placebo. Death occurred in 13.3% of milrinone patients compared to 10.0% of placebo patients. For the composite of patients dying or being rehospitalized, 42% of milrinone subjects had events compared to 36% with placebo ($P = 0.01$). In contrast, non-ischemic patients (N = 464) had a trend toward better outcomes with milrinone than with placebo: 10.9 hospital days for milrinone versus 12.6 days with placebo, 7.3% deaths with milrinone compared to 7.7% with placebo, and the composite of death or hospitalization occurring in 28% of subjects with milrinone versus 35% with placebo. From these data the following conclusions can be drawn. The benefits of milrinone in patients with acute exacerbations of HF are minimal and more likely to be seen in patients with a non-ischemic etiology of

HF. Worse outcomes may be seen in patients with ischemic HF. Milrinone was not associated with excess mortality.

OUTPATIENT INOTROPIC INFUSIONS

54. Are there any indications of using repeated intermittent infusions of inotropes for as part of a home care regimen?

It has been proposed to use regularly scheduled (e.g., weekly) intermittent infusions of dobutamine or milrinone in outpatient care centers or at home. However, the long-term safety and efficacy of inotropic therapy in general is regarded with skepticism. Nearly all the data on this therapeutic approach are from open-label and uncontrolled trials or studies that compare two inotropic agents without a placebo group.[296–300] It is unclear if the benefit observed was the result of more intensive patient monitoring or an actual pharmacologic benefit. It also is speculated that long-term therapy actually may be cardiotoxic, as evidenced by an acute worsening of HF upon withdrawal of the drug. The only placebo-controlled trial of intermittent infusion dobutamine was terminated because of excess mortality in the treatment group.[300] Death occurred in 32% of 31 dobutamine-treated patients and only 14% of 29 placebo-treated patients. Whether this phenomenon is due to progression of the underlying heart disease, continued drug therapy, or is a true cardiotoxic effect remains unknown. There is no corresponding data for milrinone, though as cited previously, a placebo-controlled trial with milrinone failed to support the routine use of IV milrinone as an adjunct to standard therapy in the treatment of patients hospitalized for an acute exacerbation of chronic HF.[280–281] For this reason, the ACA/AHA guidelines explicitly indicate that intermittent infusions of dobutamine and milrinone in the long-term treatment of HF, even if advanced stages should be avoided.[5] However, dobutamine is sometimes administered as long-term infusions (5 to 7.5 μg/kg per minute continuously for 48 to 72 hours) in patients with refractory HF while awaiting transplant. The infusion is repeated as often as weekly.

Left Ventricular Diastolic Dysfunction

55. D.F., a 54-year-old white man, has a 5-year history of HF symptoms, including decreased exercise capacity, SOB, and distended neck veins. He has minimal peripheral edema. History is suggestive of rheumatic fever as a child, but he does not recall having any cardiac symptoms when he was younger, other than being told he had a murmur. He has no history of angina, MI, hypertension, or rhythm disturbances. He has no other medical problems and all laboratory tests are normal. Cardiac examination reveals a prominent S_4 heart sound and murmurs consistent with both significant mitral regurgitation and mild aortic regurgitation. Noninvasive echocardiography reveals a normal EF of 50%. Prior treatment includes furosemide, most recently at 120 mg/day. Because of increasing symptoms, D.F.'s physician is considering adding either propranolol or verapamil to his therapy. Why might this consideration be appropriate?

This case exemplifies a patient with left ventricular diastolic dysfunction. Although he shows many of the classic signs of left-sided HF and some symptoms of right-sided failure, he has a near normal EF. The ideal treatment strategy for managing diastolic dysfunction has not been devised. In particular, no drug selectively enhances myocardial relaxation without having associated effects on left ventricular contractility or on the peripheral vasculature.[20-25] However, β-blockers and calcium channel blockers with negative inotropic properties (e.g., verapamil) may be efficacious by (1) slowing the HR to allow more time for complete ventricular filling (via more complete left atrial emptying), particularly during exercise; (2) reducing myocardial oxygen demand; and (3) controlling BP.

Left ventricular diastolic dysfunction initially is treated by slow diuresis, similar to other forms of HF. Diuresis decreases preload and lessens passive congestion of the ventricles. Excessive lowering of venous and ventricular filling pressures, however, can worsen cardiac output and hypotension. The role of ACE inhibitors in diastolic dysfunction has not been rigorously studied, though these drugs have been used with success in some patients.

An important principle in treating this form of HF is that inotropic agents such as digitalis are contraindicated. Paradoxically, β-blockers or verapamil can provide beneficial effects by slowing the heart and allowing greater diastolic filling. In addition, negative inotropic agents decrease myocardial contractility and can assist in overcoming the mechanical obstruction of the aortic and mitral valves during systole in patients with hypertrophic cardiomyopathy. Both agents also are beneficial in decreasing ischemia in patients with coronary artery disease. The relative benefits between a β-blocker and verapamil are not clear. Experience with β-blocking drugs is more extensive, but calcium blockers are preferred in patients with underlying pulmonary or peripheral vascular diseases.

B.N. fulfills the criteria for having diastolic dysfunction, probably on the basis of mitral and aortic regurgitation, resulting from childhood rheumatic fever. Because he has no pulmonary or peripheral vascular disease and already has been on diuretics, a trial of low-dose propranolol (40 to 80 mg/day) is warranted. His BP should be monitored closely to avoid hypotension.

Calcium Channel Blockers

56. A.F., a 48-year-old man, has a 5-year history of atrial fibrillation and mild HF stabilized with furosemide 40 mg/day and digoxin 0.25 mg/day. His previously well-controlled BP is now rising; the last pressure was 160/100 mm Hg despite good adherence with his diuretic therapy. All laboratory findings are normal. The digoxin level is 1.2 mg/mL. Is there evidence that calcium channel blockers may be helpful in controlling both hypertension and HF? If a calcium channel blocker is prescribed, will any interactions occur with his other drugs?

The arterial vasodilator properties of calcium channel blockers form the basis for their use in hypertension. A logical extension would suggest a role in HF symptom management via afterload reduction. Unfortunately, use of these drugs is limited by their negative inotropic effect, resulting from inhibition of calcium influx into heart muscle cells. This can result in a paradoxical worsening of HF.[301-303] Clinically, verapamil elicits the most negative inotropic effect and the dihydropyridine derivatives the least; diltiazem has intermediate effects. However, one should not develop a false sense of security that nifedipine or other dihydropyridines are clinically devoid of negative inotropic effects as demonstrated by the following randomized crossover trial comparing IV hydralazine (5 to 30 mg) to oral nifedipine (20 to 50 mg) in 15 patients.[302] Both drugs were equally effective in reducing BP and SVR (a sign of afterload reduction), but hydralazine was more effective in increasing SV and cardiac index. Four of the patients taking nifedipine experienced deterioration of their HF symptoms. The authors concluded that the vasodilatory properties of nifedipine are partially offset by its negative inotropic effect and that hydralazine is clinically superior.

A follow-up study using a randomized crossover design challenged 28 patients with class II or III HF with nifedipine, isosorbide, and a combination of the two.[303] Twenty-four percent of patients on nifedipine and 26% on combined therapy had deterioration of symptoms and required hospitalization compared with none in the isosorbide treatment arm.

The search for a more vascular selective calcium channel blocker has focused on the newer agents amlodipine and felodipine. In the Prospective Randomized Amlodipine Survival Evaluation (PRAISE) trial, patients with dyspnea or fatigue at rest or minimal exertion (NYHA class III or IV) and an EF of 30% or less (mean 21%), were randomized to either placebo (N = 582) or amlodipine (N = 571) and followed for a median of 13.8 months (range, 6 to 33 months.)[80] The starting dose of amlodipine was 5 mg daily and was titrated to 10 mg daily if tolerated; the average dose at the end of the trial was 8.8 mg daily. Essentially all the patients were taking a combination of a diuretic, an ACE inhibitor, and digoxin. Nitrates were allowed for chest pain management, but hydralazine was excluded. For the combined primary endpoint of death from any cause and/or a cardiovascular-related hospitalization, there was a nonstatistically different 9% risk reduction in events with amlodipine compared with placebo (39% versus 42%). For death rates alone, 33% of amlodipine patients died compared with 38% in the placebo group. Again, these differences were not statistically significant ($P = 0.07$). Changes in EF, specific symptom scores, and quality of life measures were not reported, but the frequency of hospitalization for worsening HF was similar in both groups (36% amlodipine, 39% placebo.) Peripheral edema and pulmonary edema were more frequent in the amlodipine group, but hypertension and angina were more evident in the placebo group.

Stratification of the subjects into those with evidence of ischemic heart disease versus those with nonischemic dilated cardiomyopathy showed a trend toward improved survival with amlodipine in the patients without ischemia. Overall, the results of this trial show a neutral effect of amlodipine, indicating that it could be used safely for concurrent hypertension or angina without making HF worse, but it does not appear to offer a significant advantage in actually treating the HF.

Similar findings have been reported with felodipine in the third report from the Vasodilator-Heart Failure Trial Study Group (V-HeFT III).[81] The primary objectives of this study were to evaluate the effects of extended-release (ER) felodipine (N = 224) compared with placebo (N = 226) on exercise tolerance, clinical symptoms, and clinical signs of HF for up to 39 months. Subjects were all men, with class II–III HF and an EF of <45% (mean, 30%). Before starting the study drug, subjects were optimized with an ACE inhibitor (97% with enalapril), diuretics (87% to 90%), and digoxin (75%). The starting dose for felodipine was 2.5 mg twice daily, with a goal dose of 5 mg twice daily (mean dose, 8.6 mg/day after titration). At the 3-month evaluation point, EF increased slightly (2.1 ± 7.0%) with amlodipine, compared with −0.1% ± 6% with placebo. At 12 months, there was no difference between the two groups (0.6 ± 8.6% with felodipine versus −0.6 ± 8.6% with placebo).

During the first 12 weeks of evaluation, neither felodipine nor placebo had either a positive or negative effect on time to dyspnea or fatigue on exercise testing; but thereafter, a trend toward deterioration in exercise capacity was found with placebo, but not with felodipine. In the first 3 months, slightly more patients on felodipine were hospitalized than with placebo (14.7% versus 10.6%), but overall the rate of hospitalization was identical in the two groups (42% to 43%). The study was not powered to evaluate the effect of felodipine on mortality, but the observed mortality rates were 13.8% in the felodipine arm and 12.9% with placebo.

In contrast to the PRAISE trial, treatment with felodipine had a more favorable effect in the subgroup of patients with a history of ischemia and coronary artery disease. The only adverse effect more common in the felodipine patients was edema, which was reported at least once in 21% of felodipine subjects and 12.8% of those on placebo. The conclusions are almost identical to those with amlodipine: there does not seem to be any negative consequences to using felodipine, but it has little role in the management of HF. Both the amlodipine and felodipine trials leave unanswered the question of efficacy of calcium channel blockers in patients not already taking an ACE inhibitor and/or digoxin.

Based on the previous discussion, nifedipine is not a good choice for A.F. In fact, nifedipine is contraindicated in any patient with systolic dysfunction. Likewise, verapamil is contraindicated even though it would otherwise lower his BP and control his atrial fibrillation by virtue of its AV nodal-blocking effect. Amlodipine and felodipine are safer alternatives for A.F.'s hypertension, but still not preferred. The more logical solution to A.F.'s problem is to add an ACE inhibitor and possibly a β-blocker to get a dual effect of controlling his BP and treating his HF. Digoxin can be continued for rate control of his atrial fibrillation, although as discussed in question 40, adding a β-blocker can also help in rate control.

Interaction With Digoxin

In the absence of HF, a case could be made for the use of verapamil or diltiazem together with digoxin for additive benefit in the treatment of supraventricular arrhythmias; but, as with the use of digoxin and quinidine, there is a risk of increased digoxin serum levels. The most reproducible interaction is with verapamil.[72,74,241] Steady-state concentrations of digoxin are consistently increased by 44% to 70% after the addition of verapamil. In some instances, the changes are only transient with digoxin levels returning toward baseline concentrations (but not completely) after several weeks of continued combination therapy. The interaction is more pronounced in patients taking larger doses of verapamil (240 to 360 mg/day) and in patients taking quinidine as well. Verapamil's primary action is the reduction of nonrenal digoxin clearance, at least partially mediated by increased digoxin bioavailability via inhibition of intestinal PGP by verapamil.

Several investigators also have confirmed an interaction with diltiazem, but the magnitude of the rise in serum digoxin concentrations (20% to 35%) is less than that seen with verapamil. One study reported a 45% increase in digoxin concentrations after nifedipine, while several other investigators could not detect a change in digoxin clearance. Although not confirmed, the mechanism may involve inhibition of PGP by diltiazem, thus enhancing digoxin bioavailability. In summary, an interaction between calcium channel blockers and digoxin definitely should be considered when using verapamil; it may be of some concern with diltiazem, and is probably insignificant with nifedipine.

Ventricular Arrhythmias Complicating Heart Failure

Amiodarone

57. B.J. (from Question 53) was stabilized over the next several days and discharged home with furosemide 40 mg QD, enalapril 5 mg QD, metoprolol XL 100 mg QD, aspirin 81 mg QD, and NTG 0.4 mg SL to be used as needed for chest pain. His EF after the infarction was 23%. Laboratory values were all normal. ECG monitoring during B.J.'s hospital stay showed normal sinus rhythm, but he was having 15 to 20 asymptomatic PVCs per hour. At that time, it was decided not to treat his arrhythmia other than with metoprolol because he was asymptomatic. Over the next several months, he continued to have frequent PVCs during follow-up examinations in the cardiology clinic.

It has now been 5 months since B.J.'s infarction and he is still having up to 12 to 15 PVCs/min. His exercise capacity is limited by SOB after walking about a block despite having his enalapril increased to 20 mg/day, metoprolol 200 mg/day, and adding digoxin 0.25 mg QD. The furosemide is still at 40 mg/day because he has little edema. Is an antiarrhythmic agent indicated for B.J. at this time? What is the agent of choice and what dose should be given?

PVCs and other arrhythmias are a common complication of left ventricular dysfunction and may be present regardless of whether the patient has had an MI. Approximately 50% to 70% of patients with HF have episodes of nonsustained ventricular tachycardia on ambulatory monitoring.[5] This myocardial irritability may be a result of autonomic hyperactivity and/or ventricular remodeling that accompany HF. However, it is not clear if these rhythm disturbances contribute to sudden death or simply reflect the underlying disease process. Recent studies suggest that sudden death in patients with HF is more likely due to an acute ischemic event in patients with underlying coronary artery disease or to a bradyarrhythmia or electromechanical dissociation in patients with nonischemic cardiomyopathy. More importantly, suppression of ventricular ectopy in patients with HF has not been shown to lead to a reduction of sudden death in clinical trials. B.J.'s PVCs were first noted after his MI. As discussed in detail in Chapters 18 (Myocardial Infarction) and 20 (Cardiac Arrhythmias), neither prophylactic antiarrhythmic therapy nor treatment of asymptomatic PVCs following an MI has been proven to improve outcome or survival. In fact, because of concerns over proarrhythmic effects of most class IA (e.g., quinidine) and class IC (e.g., encainide, flecainide) drugs as well as sotalol, treatment is considered contraindicated.

It has now been several months since B.J.'s infarct and he continues to have frequent PVCs along with HF symptoms that place him in the NYHA class II–III category. It is suggested that amiodarone has value in HF patients with arrhythmias because it has both antiarrhythmic properties as well as coronary vasodilating effects and α- and β-blocking properties. Thus, it may offer a dual benefit to reduce myocardial irritability and improve the hemodynamics of HF.

One meta-analysis reviewed 13 randomized controlled trial of prophylactic amiodarone in patients with either recent MI (N = 8) or HF (N = 5).[304] None of the individual trials was powered to detect a mortality reduction of 20%. After loading doses of 400 mg to 800 mg per day for two weeks, maintenance doses ranged from 200 to 400 mg per day. Taken as a whole, the authors concluded that prophylactic amiodarone reduces the rate of arrhythmic or sudden death in high-risk patients and this effect results in an overall 13% reduction in total mortality. Since this analysis combined trials of both MI and HF patients, it is helpful to look at two of the key HF trials.

In the Grupo de Estudio de la Sobrevida en la Insuficiecia Cardiaca en Argentina (GESICA) study,[305] 516 patients with class II to IV HF symptoms (79% class III or IV), an average EF of 20%, and frequent PVCs on cardiac monitoring were randomized to receive either standard treatment (diuretics, vasodilators, digoxin) or a fixed dose of amiodarone plus standard treatment. The dose of amiodarone was 600 mg daily for the first 2 weeks, then 300 mg/day for at least 1 year. Eighty-seven of 260 (33.5%) amiodarone patients died during follow-up compared with 106 of 256 (41.4%) receiving standard treatment, a statistically significant difference in favor of amiodarone (P = .02). Similarly, the number of HF-related hospitalizations was reduced with amiodarone. No data were presented on changes in EF, but a trend toward more patients in the amiodarone group being judged to have a decrease of at least one stage in NYHA class was noted.

Somewhat different outcomes were noted by the investigators in the Veteran's Administration Cooperative Survival Trial of Antiarrhythmic Therapy in Congestive Heart Failure (CHF-STAT) study.[306,307] Entry criteria to this trial were similar to the GESICA study, with a primary indicator being >10 asymptomatic PVCs per minute on 24-hour monitoring, but without sustained ventricular tachycardia. A higher dose of amiodarone was used, starting with 800 mg for the first 2 weeks, then 400 mg/day for 1 year. The dose was reduced to 300 mg/day after the first year, with the average follow-up being 45 months (4.5 years maximum). Disappointingly, no difference between groups for either all-cause mortality (39% amiodarone versus 42% placebo) or sudden cardiac death (15% amiodarone versus 17% placebo) was found. Similarly, 2-year survival was 69.4% with amiodarone and 70.8% with placebo. Higher survival in the amiodarone group after the first 2 years was a noted trend, but the number of subjects followed for longer periods was not large enough to establish significance. An encouraging finding in this study was that EF improved more in the patients treated with amiodarone, rising from a baseline average of 24.9% to posttreatment values of 33.7%. Corresponding change in the standard treatment group was from a baseline of 25.8% to 29.2% at follow-up. Despite the increase in EF, symptom scores did not differ between the two groups.

Taken as a whole, these two studies still leave unclear the role of amiodarone in patients with HF with asymptomatic arrhythmias. The encouraging finding is that amiodarone does not seem to have a negative effect on mortality as seen with other antiarrhythmic agents or with inotropic stimulants. On the other hand, the two studies cited have conflicting findings regarding value in improving survival and functional capacity of patients. In comparing the two studies, it has been noted that the patients in the GESICA study had more advanced disease (79% class III or IV; average EF 20%; 55% 2-year placebo mortality) than those in the VA study (43% class III or IV; average EF 25%; 29% 2-year placebo mortality); more patients had nonischemic cardiomyopathy in GESICA (60%) compared with 29% in the VA study; 99% of the VA subjects were men, whereas 19% of GESICA subjects were women; and the dose of amiodarone was lower in GESICA.[307] Further subgroup analysis suggests that those with more advanced disease, nonischemic cardiomyopathy, and female sex have better outcomes. Contradicting this speculation was a trend toward better outcomes in the small number of patients with class II symptoms in GESICA.[305] Other factors to consider are the potential for significant side effects with amiodarone (see Chapter 20, Cardiac Arrhythmias) and the risk that digoxin levels might increase after the addition of amiodarone (see Question 39).

The ACC/AHA guidelines do not recommend routine ambulatory electrocardiographic monitoring in HF patients to detect asymptomatic ventricular arrhythmias, and also recommend against treatment if such arrhythmias are inadvertently detected.[5] However, if symptomatic ventricular arrhythmias should arise or there is determined to be a high risk for sudden death, one of the following should be considered: a β-blocking drug, amiodarone, and/or an implantable cardioverter-defibrillator. As discussed extensively throughout this chapter, nearly all patients with HF should have a β-blocker as part of their regimen since these drugs reduce all cause mortality, not just sudden death. B.J. was started on metoprolol after his MI, but continued to have ectopy despite continued use of a β-blocker. Nonetheless, it is decided not to use amiodarone because he has ischemic cardiomyopathy and is not bothered by his arrhythmia.

Implantation of a cardioverter-defibrillator has been shown to reduce mortality in cardiac arrest survivors, but it is not well studied in the primary prevention of sudden death. At this time there is no evidence to justify the routine placement of an implantable cardioverter-defibrillator in patients with HF.

Herbal Products and Nutritional Supplements

58. W.L., a 60-year-old man with HF recently diagnosed by his naturopath, is concerned by his decreasing exercise capacity and increasing SOB during his morning walks in the local mall. His blood pressure is 170/85 mm Hg and he has 1–2+ ankle edema. He distrusts medical doctors and wants to treat his HF naturally. One time in the past he was given hydrochlorothiazide for blood pressure reduction, but stopped taking it after a few days because he did not tolerate the urinary urgency it caused. The naturopath has prescribed 200 mg per day of Hawthorn leaf and 50 mg per day of coenzyme Q. How effective is this treatment plan likely to be?

Hawthorn

Hawthorn extracts from the leaves and flowers of *Crataegus monogyna* and *C. oxyacantha* have been reported to have beneficial effects in mild HF.[308,309] Oligomeric procyanids and flavanoids are considered the key active ingredients. Hawthorn extracts have shown positive inotropic action, weak ACE inhibition, vasodilating properties, and increased coronary blood flow in vitro and in animal models. In short-term (8 weeks or less), placebo-controlled trials in patients with the equivalent of NYHA class II HF, there were modest improvements in exercise tolerance and subjective symptoms as well as decreases in heart rate and blood pressure. Patients with more advanced HF were excluded. One randomized trial compared twice-daily 450 or 900 mg of standardized hawthorn extract (18.75% oligomeric procyanidins) to placebo in NYHA class III patients taking hydrochlorothiazide and triamterene.[310] Both doses reduced subjective symptoms reported by the patients greater that placebo and the higher dose improved the maximal workload tolerated after 16 weeks of therapy. The Commission E monograph lists no side effects or contraindications. In clinical trials, side effects of hawthorn include nausea, vomiting, diarrhea, palpitations, chest pain, and vertigo. These side effects are more common when doses exceed 900 mg per day, but in some trials have not occurred more often that placebo. The risks and benefits of using hawthorn and digoxin together, both of which have positive inotropic effects, is not known.

Potential longer-term benefits of hawthorn, additive effects to conventional therapy, and effect on mortality await the results of the SPICE trial currently underway in Europe.[311] In this study, patients with NYHA class II to III HF and taking conventional therapy (diuretics, vasodilators, digoxin) are being randomized to receive either 450 mg doses BID of crataegus extract or placebo.

Coenzyme Q

Coenzyme Q, also known as ubiquinone and ubidecarenone, is an endogenously synthesized provitamin that is structurally similar to vitamin E and serves as a lipid soluble electron transport carrier in mitochondria and aids in the synthesis of adenosine triphosphate.[312,313] It might also have membrane-stabilizing properties, enhance the antioxidant effects of vitamin E, and stabilize calcium dependent slow channels. In animal models, it has positive inotropic effects, though weaker than from digoxin. As reviewed by Tran, there are over 18 open-label and double-blind, randomized clinical trials of coenzyme Q in patients with HF ranging from NYHA classes II to IV.[312] Doses varied from 50 to 200 mg per day. In contrast to Hawthorn, the patients in many of these trials were also taking diuretics, ACE inhibitors and/or digoxin. Different trials used different endpoint measurements. Positive effects on subjective symptoms, NYHA class improvement, EF, quality of life and hospitalization rates have all been observed. However, two trials failed to demonstrate significant changes in EF, vascular resistance, or exercise tolerance. None of the trials have large enough samples sizes or adequate duration of assessment to detect reduction in mortality. Side effects are consistently minimal, but include nausea, epigastric pain, diarrhea, heartburn and appetite suppression. Mild increases in lactate dehydrogenase and hepatic enzymes have been rarely reported with coenzyme Q doses in excess of 300 mg per day.

It can be concluded that hawthorn and coenzyme Q are both safe in the treatment of HF and might provide symptomatic improvement, especially in patients with mild HF (NYHA class II). Only coenzyme Q has been shown to be of benefit as an adjunct to conventional therapies. It is unknown if using hawthorn and coenzyme Q together as prescribed for WL will have an additive effect. No conclusion can be drawn about their effects on mortality rates.

W.L. has poorly controlled systolic hypertension and HF that is beginning to interfere with his activities of daily life. While there is evidence that patients with NHYA class II HF obtain symptomatic improvement with hawthorn and coenzyme Q, this does not address W.L.'s hypertension. (As reviewed by Tran and colleagues,[312] there is conflicting data on the value of coenzyme Q in lowering blood pressure.) Since he is being started on both drugs simultaneously, if he does improve it will be difficult to assess whether it is due to just one of the agents or the combination. With this in mind, it might be more logical to start hawthorn alone at a dose of 450 mg BID. If no benefit is derived after one month, hawthorn should be stopped and coenzyme Q started at 100 mg per day. If W.L. feels better with hawthorn monotherapy, but still has residual symptoms, coenzyme Q could be added as dual therapy with assessment in another month.

Even if W.L. and his naturopath both are satisfied with his responses to hawthorn and coenzyme Q, there is still significant concern of what will happen when and if his disease progresses. Even now he has edema. A diuretic should be strongly recommended and he should be counseled that the urinary frequency he experienced previously should diminish after a few days. Starting with a 20 mg dose of furosemide and titrating slowly may be one approach. For all of the reasons cited throughout this chapter, one must also argue strongly for starting an ACE inhibitor. Although not ideal, an ACE inhibitor could be used as monotherapy for his hypertension if he continues to refuse a diuretic. If the ACE inhibitor also improves his HF, the edema might be reduced, though slower than if a diuretic was used. Perhaps a compromise could be reached to use conventional therapy plus coenzyme Q since several studies have shown this to be a safe and effective regimen.

Acknowledgment
The author thanks Dr. Mark Munger, Pharm.D., for his thoughtful and thorough review of this manuscript.

REFERENCES

1. Agency for Health Care Policy and Research. Heart failure: evaluation and care of patients with left-ventricular systolic dysfunction. Clinical practice guidelines, no. 11. Public Health Service, US Department of Health and Human Services, 1994. (AHCPR Publication no. 94-0612).
2. American College of Cardiology/American Heart Association Task Force on Practice Guidelines. Guidelines for the evaluation and management of heart failure. J Am Coll Cardiol 1995;26:1376 and Circulation 1995;92:2764.
3. Adams K et al. for the Heart Failure Society of America (HFSA) Practice Guidelines Committee. HFSA guidelines for the management of patients with heart failure caused by left ventricular systolic dysfunction-pharmacologic approaches. Pharmacotherapy 2000:20:495. Also available at www.hfsa.org.
4. Packer M, Cohn J on behalf of the Steering Committee and Membership of the Advisory Council to Improve Outcomes Nationwide in Heart Failure. Consensus recommendations for the management of chronic heart failure. Am J Cardiol 1999; 83(Suppl.2A):1.
5. Hunt SA et al. ACC/AHA guidelines in the evaluation and management of chronic heart failure in the adult: a report of the American College of Cardiol-

ogy/American Heart Association Task Force on Practice Guidelines (Committee to Revise the 1995 Guidelines for the Evaluation and Management of Heart Failure). 2001. American College of Cardiology Web Site. Available at http://www.acc.org/clinical/guidelines/failure/hf_index.htm. Circulation 2001:104:2996 (executive summary).

6. Jessup M, Brozena S. Medical progress: heart failure. N Engl J Med 2003;348:2007.

7. Skrabal M et al. Advances in the treatment of congestive heart failure: new approaches for an old disease. Pharmacotherapy 2000;20:787.

8. O'Connell JB, Bristow M. The economic burden of heart failure. Clin Cardiol 2000;23(Suppl III):6.

9. American Heart Association. 2002 Heart and Stroke 2000 Statistical Update. Dallas: AHA, 2001. Available from http://americanheart.org

10. Massie BM, Shah NB. Evolving trends in the epidemiologic factors of heart failure: rationale for preventive strategies and comprehensive disease management. Am Heart J 1997;133:703.

11. Ho KK et al. The epidemiology of heart failure: the Framingham Study. J Am Coll Cardiol 1993;22(Suppl 6):6A.

12. Haldeman GA et al. Hospitalization of patients with heart failure: National Hospital Discharge Survey, 1985 to 1995. Am Heart J 1999;137:352.

13. Kannel WB, Belanger AJ. Epidemiology of heart failure. Am Heart J 1991;121:951.

14. Levy D et al. Long term trends in the incidence of and survival with heart failure. N Engl J Med 2002;347:1397.

15. Sharpe N, Doughty R. Epidemiology of heart failure and ventricular dysfunction. Lancet 1998;352 (Suppl 1):S13.

16. Schocken DD et al. Prevalence and mortality rate of congestive heart failure in the United States. J Am Coll Cardiol 1992;20:301.

17. Rector TS et al. Evaluation by patients with heart failure of the effects of enalapril compared with hydralazine plus isosorbide dinitrate on quality of life. V-HeFT II. Circulation 1993;87(Suppl VI).V171.

18. Pass S, Dusing M. Current and emerging therapy for primary pulmonary hypertension. Ann Pharmacother 2002;36:1414.

19. Chatterjee K et al. Pulmonary hypertension: hemodynamic diagnosis and management. Arch Intern Med 2002;162:1925.

20. Zile M. Heart failure with preserved ejection fraction: is this diastolic heart failure? J Am Coll Cardiol 2003;41:1519.

21. Yamamota K et al. Left ventricular diastolic dysfunction in patients with hypertension and preserved systolic dysfunction. Mayo Clin Proc 2000;75:148.

22. Gaasch WH. Diagnosis and treatment of heart failure based on left ventricular systolic or diastolic dysfunction. JAMA 1994;271:1276.

23. Ramachandran SV et al. Congestive heart failure with normal left ventricular systolic function: clinical approach to the diagnosis and treatment of diastolic heart failure. Arch Intern Med 1996;156:146.

24. Garcia M. Diastolic dysfunction and heart failure: causes and treatment options. Cleve Clin J Med 2000;67:727.

25. Kitzman D et al. Pathophysiological characterization of isolated diastolic heart failure in comparison to systolic heart failure. JAMA 2002;2144.

26. Schreier R, Abraham W. Hormones and hemodynamics in heart failure. N Engl J Med 1999;341:577.

27. Hash TW, Prisant M. β-Blocker use in systolic heart failure and dilated cardiomyopathy. J Clin Pharmacol 1997;37:7.

28. Patterson JH, Rogers JE. Expanding role of β-blockade in the management of chronic heart failure. Pharmacotherapy 2003;23:451.

29. Foody J et al. β-Blocker therapy in heart failure. Part I: Scientific review. Part II: Clinical applications. JAMA 2002;287:883 (part I) and 890 (part II).

30. Munger M, Cheang KI. β-Blocker therapy: a standard of care for heart failure. Pharmacotherapy 2000;20(Suppl):359S.

31. Goldstein S. Benefits of β-blocker therapy for heart failure. Arch Intern Med 2002;162:641.

32. Bristow MR. Mechanistic and clinical rationale for using beta-blockers in heart failure. J Card Fail 2000;6:8.

33. Small K et al. Synergistic polymorphisms of β₁ and α₂c adrenergic receptors and the risk of congestive heart failure. N Engl J Med 2002;347:1135.

34. Weiber K. Aldosterone in congestive heart failure. N Engl J Med 2001;345:1689.

35. Ergul A. Endothelin-1 and endothelin receptor antagonists as potential cardiovascular therapeutic agents. Pharmacotherapy 2002;22:54.

36. Nguyen B, Johnson, J. The role of endothelin in heart failure and hypertension. Pharmacotherapy 1998;18:706.

37. Nathisuwan S, Talbert R. A review of vasopeptidase inhibitors: a new modality in the treatment of hypertension and chronic heart failure. Pharmacotherapy 2002;22:27.

38. Maisel A et al. Rapid measurement of the B-type natriuretic peptide in the emergency diagnosis of heart failure. N Engl J Med 2002;347:161.

39. Lee C et al. Surrogate endpoints in heart failure. Ann Pharmacother 2002;36:479.

40. Troughton RW et al. Treatment of heart failure guided by plasma aminoterminal brain natriuretic peptide (N-BNP) concentrations. Lancet 2000;355:1126.

41. Vichiendilokkul A et al. Nesiritide: a novel approach for acute heart failure. Ann Pharmacother 2003;37:247.

42. Colucci W et al. Intravenous nesiritide, a natriuretic peptide, in the treatment of decompensated heart failure. N Engl J Med 2000;343:246.

43. Rouleau JL et al for the IMPRESS Investigators. Comparison of vasopeptidase inhibitor, omapatrilat, and lisinopril on exercise tolerance and morbidity in patients with heart failure. Lancet 2000;356:615.

44. Packer M et al. Comparison of omapatrilat and enalapril in patients with chronic heart failure: the omapatrilat versus enalapril randomized trial of utility in reducing events (OVERTURE). Circulation 2002;106:920.

45. Shan K et al. The role of cytokines in disease progression in heart failure. Curr Concept Cardiol 1997;12:218.

46. Kapadia S et al. The role of cytokines in the failing human heart. Cardiol Clin 1998;16:645.

47. Mabuchi N et al. Relationship between interleukin-6 production in the lungs and pulmonary vascular resistance in patients with congestive heart failure. Chest 2002;121:1195.

48. Bolger A, Anker S. Tumour necrosis factor in chronic heart failure. Drugs 2000;60:1245.

49. Herrera-Garza E et al. Tumor necrosis factor: a mediator of disease progression in the failing human heart. Chest 1999;115:1170.

50. Bozkurt B et al. Results of targeted anti-tumor necrosis factor therapy with etanercept (Enbrel) in patients with advanced heart failure. Circulation 2001;103:1044.

51. Kwon H et al. Case reports of heart failure after therapy with tumor necrosis factor antagonist. Ann Intern Med 2003;138:807.

52. Vanhoutte PM et al. Endothelium-derived relaxing factors and converting enzyme inhibition. Am J Cardiol 1995;76:3E.

53. Sueta CA et al. Safety and efficacy of epoprostenol in patients with severe congestive heart failure. Am J Cardiol 1995;75:34A.

54. Califf R et al. A randomized controlled trial of epoprostenol therapy for severe congestive heart failure: the Flolan international randomized survival trial (FIRST). Am Heart J 1997;134:44.

55. The Criteria Committee of the New York Heart Association, Inc. Diseases of the Heart and Blood Vessels: Nomenclature and Criteria for Diagnosis. 6th Ed. Boston: Little, Brown, 1964.

56. Pitt B et al. The effect of spironolactone on morbidity and mortality in patients with severe heart failure. N Engl J Med 1999;341:709.

57. Brater DC. Pharmacology of diuretics. Am J Med Sci 2000;319:38.

58. Kramer BK et al. Diuretic treatment and diuretic resistance in heart failure. Am J Med 1999;106:90.

59. Pitt B et al. Eplerenone, a selective aldosterone blocker, in patients with left ventricular dysfunction after myocardial infarction. N Engl J Med 2003; 348:1309.

60. Rodgers J, Patterson JH. The role of the renin-angiotensin-aldosterone system in the management of heart failure. Pharmacotherapy 2002;20(Suppl): 368S.

61. Brown N, Vaughan D. Angiotensin-converting enzyme inhibitors. Circulation 1998;97:1411.

62. American Society of Health-System Pharmacists. ASHP therapeutic guidelines on angiotensin-converting-enzyme inhibitors in patients with left ventricular dysfunction. Am J Health-Syst Pharm 1997;54:2999.

63. Patterson JH. Angiotensin II receptor blockers in heart failure. Pharmacotherapy 2003;23:173.

64. VanVeldhuisen D et al. Value of digoxin in heart failure and sinus rhythm: new features of an old drug. J Am Coll Cardiol 1996;28:813.

65. VanVeldhuisen D et al. Progression of mild untreated heart failure during 6 months follow-up and clinical and neurohumoral effects of ibopamine and digoxin as monotherapy. Am J Cardiol 1995;75:796.

66. Krum H et al. Effect of long-term digoxin therapy on autonomic function in patients with chronic heart failure. J Am Coll Cardiol 1995;25:289.

67. Gheorghiade M et al. Effects of increasing maintenance doses of digoxin on left ventricular function and neurohormones in patients with chronic heart failure treated with diuretics and angiotensin-converting enzyme inhibitors. Circulation 1995;92:1801.

68. Aronson JK. Clinical pharmacokinetics of digoxin therapy 1980. Clin Pharmacokinet 1980;5:137.

69. Heizer W et al. Absorption of digoxin from tablets and capsules in subjects with malabsorption syndromes. DICP, Ann Pharmacother 1989;23:764.

70. Moordian A. Digitalis: an update of clinical pharmacokinetics, therapeutic monitoring techniques and treatment recommendations. Clin Pharmacokinet 1988;15:165.

71. Reuning R et al. Digoxin. In: Evans W et al., eds. Applied Pharmacokinetics. 3rd Ed. Vancouver: Applied Therapeutics, 1992:20.

72. Bauer L. Digoxin. In: Applied Clinical Pharmacokinetics. New York: McGraw Hill, 2001:265.

73. Aronson JK. Clinical pharmacokinetics of cardiac glycosides in patients with renal dysfunction. Clin Pharmacokinet 1983;8:155.

74. Yu D. The contribution of P-glycoprotein to pharmacokinetic drug interactions. J Clin Pharmacol 1999;39:1203.

75. Fromm MF et al. Inhibition of P-glycoprotein-mediated drug transport: a unifying mechanism to explain the interaction between digoxin and quinidine. Circulation 1999;99:552.

76. Lindebaum J et al. Inactivation of digoxin by the gut flora: reversibility by antibiotic therapy. N Engl J Med 1981;305:789.

77. Jelliffe RW et al. A nomogram for digoxin therapy. Am J Med 1974;57:63.

78. Forker A. A cardiologist's perspective on evolving concepts in the management of congestive heart failure. J Clin Pharmacol 1996;36:973.

79. Carbonin P, Zuccala G. Inotropic agents in older patients with chronic heart failure: current perspectives. Aging Clin Exp Res 1996;8:90.

80. Packer M et al for the Prospective Randomized Amlodipine Survival Evaluation Study Group. The effect of amlodipine on morbidity and mortality in severe heart failure. N Engl J Med 1996;335:1107.

81. Cohn J et al for the Vasodilator-Heart Failure Trial Study Group. Effect of the calcium antagonist felodipine as supplemental vasodilator therapy in patients with chronic heart failure treated with enalapril. V-HeFT III. Circulation 1997;96:856.

82. Vander Zanden J et al. Systemic adverse effects of ophthalmic β-blockers. Ann Pharmacother 2001; 35:1633.

83. Johnson D et al. Effect of cyclooxygenase-2 inhibitors on blood pressure. Ann Pharmacother 2003;37:442.

84. Shan K et al. Anthracycline-induced cardiotoxicity. Ann Intern Med 1996;125:47.
85. Singal P, Iliskovic N. Doxorubicin-induced cardiomyopathy. N Engl J Med 1998;339:900.
86. Crouch M et al. Clinical relevance and management of drug-related QT interval prolongation. Pharmacotherapy 2003;23:881.
87. Page RL II et al. Possible heart failure exacerbation associated with rosiglitazone: case report and literature review. Pharmacotherapy 2003;23:945.
88. Risler T et al. Comparative pharmacokinetics and pharmacodynamics of loop diuretics in renal failure. Cardiology 1994;84(Suppl 2):155.
89. Murray MD et al. Torsemide more effective that furosemide for treatment of heart failure. Am J Med 2001;111:513.
90. Cutler R, Blair A. Clinical pharmacokinetics of furosemide. Clin Pharmacokinet 1979;4:279.
91. Greither A et al. Pharmacokinetics of furosemide in patients with congestive heart failure. Pharmacology 1979;19:121.
92. Straughn A et al. Bioavailability of seven furosemide tablets in man. Biopharm Drug Dispos 1986;7:113.
93. McNamara P et al. Influence of tablet dissolution on furosemide bioavailability: a bioequivalence study. Pharm Res 1987;4:150.
94. Kelly M et al. Pharmacokinetics of orally administered furosemide. Clin Pharmacol Ther 1979;15:1778.
95. Kelly M et al. A comparison of the diuretic response to oral and intravenous furosemide in diuretic resistant patients. Curr Ther Res 1977;21:1.
96. Vargo D et al. The pharmacodynamics of torsemide in patients with congestive heart failure. Clin Pharmacol Ther 1995;57:601.
97. Stallings S et al. Comparison of natriuretic and diuretic effects of single and divided doses of furosemide. Am J Hosp Pharm 1979;36:68.
98. Wilson T et al. Effect of dosage regimen and natriuretic response to furosemide. Clin Pharmacol Ther 1976;18:165.
99. Kosman ME. Management of potassium problems during long-term diuretic therapy. JAMA 1974;230:743.
100. Davidson C et al. Effect of long-term diuretic treatment on body potassium in heart disease. Lancet 1976;2:1044.
101. Papademetriou JV. Diuretics, hypokalemia and cardiac arrhythmias: a critical analysis. Am Heart J 1986;111:1219.
102. Leif P et al. Diuretic-induced hypokalemia does not cause ventricular ectopy in uncomplicated essential hypertension. Kidney Int 1984;25:203.
103. Madias J et al. Non-arrhythmogenicity of diuretic hypokalemia. Arch Intern Med 1984;144:2171.
104. Steiness E et al. Cardiac arrhythmias induced by hypokalemia and potassium loss during maintenance digoxin therapy. Br Heart J 1976;38:167.
105. Holland OB et al. Diuretic-induced ventricular ectopic activity. Am J Med 1981;770:762.
106. Hollifield JW et al. Thiazide diuretics, hypokalemia and cardiac arrhythmias. Acta Med Scand 1981;647:67.
107. Freis E. Critique of the clinical importance of diuretic-induced hypokalemia and elevated cholesterol level. Arch Intern Med 1989;149:2640.
108. Davidson S, Surawicz B. Ectopic beats and atrioventricular conduction disturbances. Arch Intern Med 1976;120:280.
109. Kassier JP et al. Diuretics and potassium metabolism: a reassessment of the need, effectiveness, and safety of potassium therapy. Kidney Int 1977;11:505.
110. Morgan DB, Davidson C. Hypokalemia and diuretics: analysis of publications. Br Med J (Clin Res) 1980;1:905.
111. Finnerty FA et al. Long-term effects of furosemide and hydrochlorothiazide in patients with essential hypertension. Angiology 1977;28:125.
112. Hollifield J. Potassium and magnesium abnormalities: diuretics and arrhythmias in hypertension. Am J Med 1987;77(5A):28.

113. McMahon FG et al. Effect of potassium chloride supplements on upper gastrointestinal mucosa. Clin Pharmacol Ther 1984;38:852.
114. Patterson DJ et al. Endoscopic comparison of solid and liquid potassium chloride supplements. Lancet 1983;2:1077.
115. Aselton PJ, Jick H. Short-term follow-up study of wax matrix potassium chloride in relation to gastrointestinal bleeding. Lancet 1983;1:184.
116. Jick H et al. A comparison of wax matrix and microencapsulated potassium chloride in relation to upper gastrointestinal illness requiring hospitalization. Pharmacother 1989;9:204.
117. Schwartz A et al. Dosage of potassium chloride elixir to correct thiazide-induced hypokalemia. JAMA 1974;230:702.
118. Sklath H, Gums J. Spironolactone: a re-examination. DICP, Ann Pharmacother 1990;24:52.
119. Schnaper H et al. Potassium restoration in hypertensive patients made hypokalemic by hydrochlorothiazide. Arch Intern Med 1989;149:2677.
120. Lahav M et al. Continuous infusion furosemide in patients with severe CHF. Chest 1992;102:725.
121. Rudy D et al. Loop diuretics for chronic renal insufficiency: a continuous infusion is more efficacious than bolus therapy. Ann Intern Med 1991;115:360.
122. Van Meyel J et al. Continuous infusion of furosemide in the treatment of patients with congestive heart failure and diuretic resistance. J Intern Med 1994;235:329.
123. Dormans T et al. Diuretic efficacy of high-dose furosemide in severe heart failure: bolus injections versus continuous infusion. J Am Coll Cardiol 1996;28:376.
124. Kramer W et al. Pharmacodynamics of torsemide as an intravenous injection and as a continuous infusion to patients with congestive heart failure. J Clin Pharmacol 1996;36:265.
125. Sica D, Gehr TW. Diuretic combinations in refractory edema states. Clin Pharmacokinet 1996;30:229.
126. Howard P, Dunn M. Aggressive diuresis is safe and cost effective for severe heart failure in the elderly. Chest 2001;119:807.
127. Jessup M. Aldosterone blockade and heart failure. N Engl J Med 2003;348:1380.
128. Lee DCS et al. Heart failure in outpatients. N Engl J Med 1982;306:699.
129. Jaeschke R et al. To what extent do congestive heart failure patients in normal sinus rhythm benefit from digoxin therapy? A systematic overview and meta-analysis. Am J Med 1990;88:279.
130. Kulick D, Rahimtoola S. Current role of digitalis therapy in patients with congestive heart failure. JAMA 1991;265:2995.
131. Cohn J et al. Effect of vasodilator therapy on mortality in chronic congestive heart failure. N Engl J Med 1986;314:1547.
132. The Consensus Trial Study Group. Effects of enalapril on mortality in severe congestive heart failure: results of The Cooperative North Scandinavian Enalapril Survival Group. N Engl J Med 1987;316:1429.
133. Kjekshus J et al. Effects of enalapril on long-term mortality in severe congestive heart failure. Am J Cardiol 1992;69:103.
134. The SOLVD Investigators. Effect of enalapril on survival in patients with reduced left ventricular ejection fractions and congestive heart failure. N Engl J Med 1991;325:295.
135. Cohn J et al. A comparison of enalapril with hydralazine-isosorbide dinitrate in the treatment of chronic congestive heart failure. N Engl J Med 1991;325:303.
136. Uretsky B et al. For the PROVED Investigative Group. Randomized study assessing the effect of digoxin withdrawal in patients with mild to moderate chronic congestive heart failure. J Am Coll Cardiol 1993;26:93.
137. Packer M et al. Withdrawal of digoxin from patients with chronic heart failure treated with angiotensin-converting-enzyme inhibitors. N Engl J Med 1993;329:1.

138. Garg R et al. on behalf of The Digitalis Intervention Group. The effect of digoxin on mortality and morbidity in patients with heart failure. N Engl J Med 1997;336:525.
139. Crozier I, Ikram H. Angiotensin converting enzyme inhibitors versus digoxin for the treatment of congestive heart failure. Drugs 1992;43:637.
140. The Captopril-Digoxin Multicenter Research Group. Comparative effects of therapy with captopril and digoxin in patients with mild to moderate heart failure. JAMA 1988;259:539.
141. Davies R et al. Enalapril versus digoxin in patients with congestive heart failure: a multicenter study. J Am Coll Cardiol 1991;18:1602.
142. White CM. Angiotensin-converting-enzyme inhibition in heart failure or after myocardial infarction. Am J Health-Syst Pharm 2000;57 (Suppl 1):S18.
143. Wollert KC, Drexler H. The kallikrein-kinin system in post myocardial infarction cardiac remodeling. Am J Cardiol 1997;80(Suppl):158A.
144. Garg R et al. Overview of randomized trials on angiotensin-converting enzyme inhibition on mortality and morbidity in patients with heart failure. JAMA 1995;273:1450.
145. Colfer H et al. Effects of once daily benazepril on exercise tolerance and manifestations of chronic congestive heart failure. Am J Cardiol 1992;70:354.
146. Hall A et al. on behalf of the AIREX Study Investigators. Follow-up study of patients randomly allocated to ramipril or placebo for heart failure after acute myocardial infarction: AIRE Extension (AIREX) Study. Lancet 1997;349:1493.
147. Kober L et al. for the Trandolapril Cardiac Evaluation (TRACE) Study. A clinical trial of the angiotensin-converting-enzyme inhibitor trandolapril in patients with left ventricular dysfunction after myocardial infraction. N Engl J Med 1995;333:1670.
148. Amrosioni E et al. The effect of angiotensin-converting-enzyme inhibitor zofenopril on mortality and morbidity after anterior myocardial infarction. N Engl J Med 1995;332:80.
149. Bach R, Zardini P. Long acting angiotensin-converting-enzyme inhibition: once daily lisinopril versus twice-daily captopril in mild to moderate heart failure. Am J Cardiol 1992;70:70C.
150. Zannad F et al. Comparison of treatment with lisinopril versus enalapril for congestive heart failure. Am J Cardiol 1992;70:78C.
151. Zannad F et al. for the Fosinopril in Heart Failure Study Investigators. Differential effects of fosinopril and enalapril in patients with mild to moderate chronic heart failure. Am Heart J 1998;136:672.
152. Pflugfelder PW et al. Clinical consequences of angiotensin-converting enzyme inhibitor withdrawal in chronic heart failure: a double-blind, placebo-controlled study of quinapril. The Quinapril Heart Failure Trial Investigators. J Am Coll Cardiol 1993;22:1557.
153. Hobbs RE. Results of the ATLAS study. High or low doses of ACE inhibitors for heart failure? Cleve Clin J Med 1999;65:539.
154. Packer M et al. Comparative effects of low and high doses of the angiotensin-converting enzyme inhibitor, lisinopril, on morbidity and mortality in chronic heart failure. Circulation 1999;100:2312.
155. The Network Investigators. Clinical outcome with enalapril in symptomatic chronic heart failure; a dosage comparison. Eur Heart J 1998;19:481.
156. Packer M et al. Comparison of captopril and enalapril in patients with severe chronic heart failure. N Engl J Med 1986;315:847.
157. Luque C, Ortiz M. Treatment of ACE inhibitor induced cough. Pharmacotherapy. 1999;19:804
158. Sharif MN et al. Cough induced by quinapril with resolution after changing to fosinopril. Ann Pharmacol Ther 1994;28:720.
159. Woo KS, Nicholls MG. High prevalence of persistent cough with angiotensin-converting enzyme inhibitors in Chinese. Br J Clin Pharmacol 1995;40:141.

160. Martineau P, Goulet J. New competition in the realm of renin-angiotensin axis inhibition: the angiotensin II receptor antagonists in congestive heart failure. Ann Pharmacother 2001;35:71.

161. Jong P et al. Angiotensin receptor blockers in heart failure: a meta- analysis of randomized controlled trials. J Am Coll Cardiol 2002;39:463.

162. Riegger GAJ et al. Improvement in exercise tolerance and symptoms of congestive heart during treatment with candesartan cilexetil. Circulation 1999;100:2224.

163. Havranek EP et al. Dose-related beneficial long-term hemodynamic and clinical efficacy of irbesartan in heart failure. J Am Coll Cardiol 1999;33:1174.

164. Dickstein K et al. Comparison of the effects of losartan and enalapril on clinical status and exercise performance in patients with moderate to severe heart failure. J Am Coll Cardiol 1995;26:438.

165. Pitt B et al. Randomized trial of losartan versus captopril in patients over 65 with heart failure. Lancet 1997;349:747.

166. Pitt B et al. for the ELITE II Investigators. Effect of losartan compared with lisinopril on mortality in patients with symptomatic heart failure: randomized trial—the losartan heart failure survival study ELITE II. Lancet 2000;355:1582.

167. McKelvie RS et al for the RESOLVD Pilot Study Investigators. Comparison of candesartan, enalapril, and their combination in congestive heart failure: randomized evaluation of strategies for left ventricular dysfunction (RESOLVD) pilot study. Circulation 1999;100:1056.

168. Granger C et al. Randomized trial of candesartan cilexetil in the treatment of patients with congestive heart failure and a history of intolerance to angiotensin-converting enzyme inhibitors. Am Heart J 2000;139:609.

169. Swedberg K, for the CHARM Progamme Investigators. Candesartan in heart failure-assessment and reduction in mortality and morbidity (CHARM): rationale and design. J Card Fail 1999;5:276.

170. Cohn J, Tognoni G for the Valsartan Heart Failure Trial Investigators. A randomized trial of the angiotensin-receptor blocker valsartan in chronic hear failure. N Engl J Med 2001;345:1667.

171. Pfeffler MA et al. for the VALIANT Investigators. Valsartan in acute myocardial infarction trial (VALIANT): rationale and design. Am Heart J 2000;140:727.

172. Vleeming W et al. ACE inhibitor-induced angioedema. Incidence, prevention, and management. Drug Safety 1998;18:171.

173. Brown NJ et al. Black Americans have an increased risk of angiotensin converting enzyme inhibitor associated angioedema. Clin Pharmacol Ther 1996;60:8.

174. Brown NJ et al. Recurrent angiotensin converting enzyme inhibitor associated angioedema. JAMA 1997;278:832.

175. Gavras I, Gavras H. Are patients who develop angioedema with ACE inhibition at risk for the same problem with AT-1 receptor blockade? Arch Intern Med 2003;163:240.

176. Abdi R et al. Angiotensin II receptor blocker-associated angioedema. On the heels of ACE inhibitor angioedema. Pharmacotherapy 2002; 22:1173.

177. Lo KS. Angioedema associated with candesartan. Pharmacotherapy 2002;22:1176.

178. Van Rijnsoever EW et al. Angioneurotic edema attributed to the use of losartan. Arch Intern Med 1998;158:2063.

179. Frye C, Pettigrew T. Angioedema and photosensitive rash induced by valsartan. Pharmacotherapy 1998;18:866.

180. Gavras I et al. Fatal pancytopenia associated with the use of captopril. Ann Intern Med 1981;94:58.

181. Hanssens M et al. Fetal and neonatal effects of treatment with angiotensin-converting enzyme inhibitors in pregnancy. Obstet Gynecol 1991;78:128.

182. Cleland J et al. The effects of captopril on serum digoxin and urinary urea and digoxin clearances in patients with congestive heart failure. Am Heart J 1986;112:130.

183. The SOLVD II Investigators. Effect of enalapril on mortality and the development of heart failure in asymptomatic patients with reduced left ventricular ejection fractions. N Engl J Med 1992; 327:685.

184. Swedberg K et al. Effects of the early administration of enalapril in mortality in patients with acute myocardial infarction (CONSENSUS II). N Engl J Med 1992;327:628.

185. Pfeffer M et al. Effect of captopril on mortality and morbidity in patients with left ventricular dysfunction after myocardial infarction: the Survival and Ventricular Enlargement Trial (SAVE). N Engl J Med 1992;327:669.

186. The Acute Infarction Ramipril Efficacy (AIRE) study Investigators. Effect of ramipril on mortality and morbidity of survivors of acute myocardial infarction with clinical evidence of heart failure. Lancet 1993;342:821.

187. Nawarskas J, Spinler S. Update on the interaction between aspirin and angiotensin-converting enzyme inhibitors. Pharmacotherapy 2000;20:698.

188. Olson K. Combined aspirin/ACE inhibitor treatment for HF. Ann Pharmacother 2001;35:1653.

189. Avezum A et al. Beta-blocker therapy for congestive heart failure. Can J Cardiol 1998;14:1045.

190. Lechat P et al. Clinical effects of beta-adrenergic blockade in chronic heart failure. Circulation 1998;98:1184.

191. Doughty R et al. Effects of beta-blocker therapy on mortality in patients with heart failure. Eur Heart J 1997;18:560.

192. Heidenreich PA et al. Effects of beta-blockade on mortality in patients with heart failure. J Am Coll Cardiol 1997;30:27.

193. Brophy J et al. Beta-blockers in congestive heart failure: a Bayesian meta-analysis. Ann Intern Med 2001;134:550.

194. Gattis W. Metoprolol CR/XL in the treatment of chronic heart failure. Pharmacotherapy 2001; 21:604.

195. Tangeman H, Patterson JH. Extended-release metoprolol succinate in chronic heart failure. Ann Pharmacother 2003;37:701.

196. Waagstein F et al. for the Metoprolol in Dilated Cardiomyopathy (MDC) Trial Study Group. Beneficial effects of metoprolol in idiopathic dilated cardiomyopathy. Lancet 1993;342:1441.

197. Merit HF Study Group. Effect of metoprolol CR/XL in chronic heart failure: metoprolol CR/XL randomized intervention trial in congestive heart failure (MERIT HF). Lancet 1999;353:2001.

198. CIBIS Investigators and Committees. A randomized study of β-blockade in heart failure: the cardiac insufficiency bisoprolol study. Circulation 1994;90:1765.

199. CIBIS II Investigators and Committees. The cardiac insufficiency bisoprolol study II: a randomized trial. Lancet 1999;353:9.

200. Waagstein F et al. Long term beta-blockade in dilated cardiomyopathy: effects of short- and long-term metoprolol treatment followed by withdrawal and readministration of metoprolol. Circulation 1989;80:551.

201. Bleske B et al. Carvedilol: therapeutic application and practice guidelines. Pharmacotherapy 1998; 18:729.

202. Packer M et al for the US Carvedilol Heart Failure Study Group. The effect of carvedilol on morbidity and mortality in patients with chronic heart failure. N Engl J Med 1996;334:1349.

203. Bristow MR et al. for the MOCHA Investigators. Carvedilol produces dose related improvements in left ventricular function and survival in subjects with chronic heart failure. Circulation 1996;94: 2807.

204. Packer M et al. for the PRECISE Group. Double-blind, placebo-controlled study of the effects of carvedilol in patients with moderate to severe heart failure. Circulation 1996;94:2793.

205. Colucci WS et al for the US Carvedilol Heart Failure Study Group. Carvedilol inhibits clinical progression in patients with mild symptoms of heart failure. Circulation 1996;94:2800.

206. Conn J et al. for the US Carvedilol Heart Failure Study Group. Safety and efficacy of carvedilol in heart failure. J Card Fail 1997;3:173.

207. Australia/New Zealand Heart Failure Research Collaborative Group. Randomised, placebo controlled trial of carvedilol in patients with congestive heart failure due to ischemic heart disease. Lancet 1997;349:375.

208. Meadowcroft A et al. Pharmacogenetics and heart failure: a convergence with carvedilol. Pharmacotherapy 1997;17:637.

209. Kukin ML et al. Prospective randomized comparison of effect of long-term treatment with metoprolol or carvedilol on symptoms, exercise, ejection fraction, and oxidative stress in heart failure. Circulation 1999;99:2645.

210. Di Lenarda A et al. Long-term effects of carvedilol in idiopathic dilated cardiomyopathy with persistent left ventricular dysfunction despite chronic metoprolol. J Am Coll Cardiol 1999; 33:1926.

211. Packer M et al. Comparative effects of carvedilol and metoprolol on left ventricular ejection fraction: results of a meta-analysis. Am Heart J 2001;141:899.

212. Poole-Wilson PA et al. Comparison of carvedilol and metoprolol in clinical outcomes in patients with chronic heart failure in the Carvedilol or Metoprolol European Trial (COMET). Lancet 2003;362:7.

213. Metra R et al. A prospective, randomized, double blind comparison of the long-term effects of metoprolol versus carvedilol. Circulation 2000;102:546.

214. Packer M et al for the Carvedilol Prospective Randomized Cumulative Survival Study Group (COPERNICUS). Effect of carvedilol on survival in chronic severe heart failure. N Engl J Med 2001;344:1651.

215. BEST Investigators. A trial of the beta-blocker bucindolol in patients with advanced chronic heart failure. N Engl J Med 2001;344:1659.

216. Macdonald P et al. Tolerability and efficacy of carvedilol in patients with New York Heart Association class IV heart failure. J Am Coll Cardiol 1999;33:924.

217. Krum H et al. Effects of initiating carvedilol in patients with severe chronic heart failure: results from the COPERNICUS Study. JAMA 2003;289:712.

218. Rathorne S et al. Sex-based differences in the effect of digoxin for the treatment of heart failure. N Engl J Med 2002;347:1403.

219. Rathore S et al. Association of serum digoxin concentration and outcomes in patients with heart failure. JAMA 2003;289:871.

220. Hall P et al. The effect of everyday exercise on steady state digoxin concentrations. J Clin Pharmacol 1989;29:1083.

221. Teague AC et al. The effect of age and everyday exercise on steady-state plasma digoxin concentrations. Pharmacotherapy 1995;15:502.

222. Karbosk J et al. Marked digoxin-like immunoreactive factor interference with an enzyme immunoassay. Drug Intell Clin Pharm 1988;22:703.

223. Toseland P et al. Tentative identification of the digoxin-like immunoreactive substance. Ther Drug Monit 1988;10:168.

224. Schrader B et al. Digoxin like immunoreactive substances in renal transplant patients. J Clin Pharmacol 1991;313:1126.

225. Morris R et al. Interference from digoxin like immunoreactive substances in commercial digoxin kit assay methods. Eur J Clin Pharmacol 1990;39:359.

226. Hall WH et al. Titrated digoxin XXII. Absorption and excretion in malabsorption syndrome. Am J Med 1974;56:437.

227. Luchi RJ et al. Unusually large digitalis requirements: a study of altered digoxin metabolism. Am J Med 1968;37:263.

228. Hooymans P, Merkus F. Current status of cardiac glycoside drug interactions. Clin Pharm 1985; 4:404.

229. Fitchtl B, Doering W. The quinidine-digoxin interaction in perspective. Clin Pharmacokinet 1983;8:137.
230. Bigger JT, Leahy E. Quinidine and digoxin: an important interaction. Drugs 1982; 24:229.
231. Fenster P et al. Digoxin-quinidine interaction in patients with chronic renal failure. Circulation 1982;66:1277.
232. Doering W et al. Quinidine-digoxin interaction: evidence for involvement of an extra-renal mechanism. Eur J Clin Pharmacol 1982;21:281.
233. Mardel A et al. Quinidine enhances digitalis toxicity at therapeutic serum digoxin levels. Clin Pharmacol Ther 1993;53:457.
234. Stevenson WG et al. Improving survival for patients with advanced heart failure. J Am Coll Cardiol 1995;26:1417.
235. Matsuda M et al. Effects of digoxin, propranolol and verapamil on exercise in patients with chronic isolated atrial fibrillation. Cardiovasc Res 1991; 25:453.
236. David D et al. Inefficacy of digitalis in the control of heart rate in patients with chronic atrial fibrillation: beneficial effects of an added beta-adrenergic blocking agent. Am J Cardiol 1979;44:1378.
237. Farshi R et al. Ventricular rate control in chronic atrial fibrillation during daily activity and programmed exercise: a crossover open-label study of five drug regimens. J Am Coll Cardiol 1999;33:304.
238. Nolan P et al. Effects of co-administration of propafenone on the pharmacokinetics of digoxin in healthy volunteer subjects. J Clin Pharmacol 1989;29:46.
239. Rodin S, Johnson B. Pharmacokinetic interactions with digoxin. Clin Pharmacokinet 1988;11:227.
240. Boyd RA et al. Atorvastatin coadministration may increase digoxin concentrations by inhibition of intestinal P-glycoprotein-mediated secretion. J Clin Pharmacol 2000;40:91.
241. Verschraagen M et al. P-glycoprotein system as a determinant of drug interactions. The case of digoxin-verapamil. J Pharmacol Res 2001;40:301.
242. Tanaka H et al. Effect of clarithromycin on steady-state digoxin concentrations. Ann Pharmacother 2003;37:178.
243. Wakasugi H et al. Effect of clarithromycin on renal excretion of digoxin: interaction with P-glycoprotein. Clin Pharmacol Ther 1998;64:123.
244. Greiner B et al. The role of intestinal P-glycoprotein in the interaction of digoxin and rifampin. J Clin Invest 1999;104:147.
245. Johne A et al. Pharmacokinetic interaction of digoxin with an herbal extract from St. John's wort (Hypericum perforatum). Clin Pharmacol Ther 1999;66:338.
246. Cohen AF et al. Effect of omeprazole on digoxin bioavailability [Abstract]. Br J Clin Pharmacol 1991;31:656P.
247. Oosterhuis B et al. Minor effect of multiple dose omeprazole in the pharmacokinetics of digoxin after a single oral dose. Br J Clin Pharmacol 1991;32:569.
248. Guven H et al. Age related digoxin alprazolam interaction. Clin Pharmacol Ther 1993;54:42.
249. Sachs M et al. Interaction of itraconazole and digoxin. Clin Infect Dis 1993;16:400.
250. Stangier J et al. The effects of telmisartan on the steady-state pharmacokinetics of digoxin in 12 healthy male volunteers. J Clin Pharmacol 2000;40:1373.
251. Kelly R, Smith T. Recognition and management of digitalis toxicity. Am J Cardiol 1992;69:108G.
252. Bernabei R et al. Digoxin serum concentration measurements in patients with suspected digitalis arrhythmias. J Cardiovasc Pharmacol 1980;2:319.
253. Relsdorff E et al. Acute digitalis poisoning: the role of intravenous magnesium sulfate. J Emerg Med 1986;4:463.
254. Beller GA et al. Digitalis intoxication: a prospective clinical study with serum level correlations. N Engl J Med 1971;284:989.
255. Lely AH et al. Non-cardiac symptoms of digitalis intoxication. Am Heart J 1972;83:149.
256. Butler V et al. Digitalis induced visual disturbances with therapeutic digitalis concentrations. Ann Intern Med 1995;123:675.
257. Lee T, Smith T. Serum digoxin concentration and diagnosis of digitalis toxicity. Clin Pharmacokinet 1983;8:279.
258. Park G et al. Digoxin toxicity in patients with high serum digoxin concentrations. Am J Med Sci 1987;30:423.
259. Shapiro W. Correlative studies of serum digitalis levels and the arrhythmias of digitalis intoxication. Am J Cardiol 1978;41:852.
260. Ordog G et al. Serum digoxin levels and mortality in 5100 patients. Ann Emerg Med 1987;16:32.
261. Jelliffe RW. Factors to consider in planning digoxin therapy. J Chronic Dis 1971;24:407.
262. Brater C et al. Digoxin toxicity in patients with normokalemic potassium depletion. Clin Pharmacol Ther 1977;22:21.
263. Young IS. Magnesium status and digoxin toxicity. Br J Clin Pharmacol 1991;32:717.
264. Bendayan R, McKenzie M. Digoxin pharmacokinetics and dosage requirements in pediatric patients. Clin Pharm 1983;2:224.
265. Marbury T et al. Advanced digoxin toxicity in renal failure; treatment with charcoal hemoperfusion. South Med J 1979;72:279.
266. Antman E. Treatment of 150 cases of life threatening digitalis toxicity. Circulation 1990;81:1744.
267. Woolf A et al. The use of digoxin-specific Fab fragments for severe digitalis intoxication in children. N Engl J Med 1992;326:1739.
268. Borron S et al. Advances in the management of digoxin toxicity in the older patient. Drugs Aging 1997;10:18.
269. Ujhelyi MR, Robert S. Pharmacokinetic aspects of digoxin-specific FAB therapy in the management of digitalis toxicity. Clin Pharmacokinet 1995;28:483.
270. Ujhelyi MR et al. Influence of digoxin immune Fab therapy and renal dysfunction on the disposition of total and free digoxin. Ann Intern Med 1993; 119:273.
271. Hickey AR et al. Digoxin immune Fab in the management of digitalis intoxication: safety and efficacy results of an observational surveillance study. J Am Coll Cardiol 1991;17:590.
272. Koup JR et al. Digoxin pharmacokinetics: role of renal failure in dosage regimen design. Clin Pharmacol Ther 1975;18:9.
273. Gault M et al. Loading doses of digoxin in renal failure. Br J Clin Pharmacol 1980;9:593.
274. Cockcroft DW, Gault MH. Prediction of creatinine clearance from serum creatinine. Nephron 1976;16:31.
275. Scheiner LB et al. Estimation of population characteristics of pharmacokinetic parameters from routine clinical data. J Pharmacokinet Biopharm 1977;5:455.
276. Nohria A et al. Medical management of advanced heart failure. JAMA 2002;287:628.
277. Grady KL et al. Team management of patients with heart failure: a statement for healthcare professionals from the Cardiovascular Nursing Council of the American Heart Association. Circulation 2000;102:2443.
278. Stevenson LW et al. Optimizing therapy for complex or refractory heart failure: a management algorithm. Am Heart J 1998;135(Suppl):S293.
279. Stevenson LW et al. The limited reliability of physical signs for estimating hemodynamics in chronic heart. JAMA 1989;261:884.
280. Cuffe M et al. Short term intravenous milrinone for acute exacerbations of chronic heart failure: a randomized controlled trial. JAMA 2002;287:1541.
281. Felker G et al. Heart failure etiology and response to milrinone in decompensated heart failure. Results from the OPTIME-CHF study. J Am Coll Cardiol 2003;41:997.
282. Mulrowe J, Crawford M. Clinical pharmacokinetics and therapeutic use of hydralazine in congestive heart failure. Clin Pharmacokinet 1989;16:86.
283. Earle G et al. Intravenous nitroglycerin tolerance in patients with ischemic cardiomyopathy and congestive heart failure. Pharmacotherapy 1998; 18:203.
284. Roth A et al. Early tolerance to hemodynamic effects of high dose transdermal nitroglycerin in responders with severe chronic heart failure. J A Coll Cardiol 1987;9:858.
285. Jordan RA et al. Rapidly developing tolerance to transdermal nitroglycerin in congestive heart failure. Ann Intern Med 1986;104:295.
286. Kalus J, Nappi J. Role of race in the pharmacotherapy of heart failure. Ann Pharmacother 2002;36:471.
287. Carson P et al. Racial differences in response to therapy for heart failure: analysis of the Vasodilator-Heart Failure Trials. J Card Fail 1999;5:178.
288. Shekelle P et al. Efficacy of angiotensin-converting enzyme inhibitors and beta-blockers in the management of left ventricular systolic dysfunction according to race, gender and diabetic status: a meta-analysis of major clinical trials. J Am Coll Cardiol 2003;41:1529.
289. Yancy C et al. Race and the response to adrenergic blockade with carvedilol in patients with chronic heart failure. N Engl J Med 2001;344: 1358.
290. Marcus F. Use of digitalis in acute myocardial infarction [Editorial]. Circulation 1980;62:17.
291. Bigger JT et al. Effect of digitalis treatment on survival after acute myocardial infarction. Am J Cardiol 1985;55:263.
292. Muller E et al. Digoxin therapy and mortality after myocardial infarction: experience in the MILIS study. N Engl J Med 1986;314:265.
293. Hillerman D, Forbes W. Role of milrinone in the management of congestive heart failure. DICP, Ann Pharmacother 1989;23:357.
294. DiBianco R et al. A comparison of oral milrinone, digoxin and their combination in the treatment of patients with chronic heart failure. N Engl J Med 1989;320:677.
295. Packer M et al. (PROMISE study research group). Effect of milrinone on mortality in severe chronic heart failure. N Engl J Med 1991;325:1468.
296. Cesario D et al. Beneficial effects of intermittent home administration of the inotrope/vasodilator milrinone in patients with end-stage congestive heart failure: a preliminary study. Am Heart J 1998;135:121.
297. Leier CV et al. Parenteral inotropic support for advanced congestive heart failure. Prog Cardiovasc Dis 1998;41:207.
298. Marius-Nunez AL et al. Intermittent inotropic therapy in an outpatient setting: a cost-effective therapeutic modality in patients with refractory heart failure. Am Heart J 1996;132:805.
299. Applefeld NM et al. Outpatient dobutamine and dopamine infusions in the management of chronic heart failure: clinical experience in 21 patients. Am Heart J 1987;114:589.
300. Elis A et al. Intermittent dobutamine treatment in patients with chronic refractory heart failure: a randomized, double-blind, placebo-controlled study. Clin Pharmacol Ther 1998;63:682.
301. Reicher-Reiss H, Barasch E. Calcium antagonists in patients with heart failure, a review. Drugs 1991;42:343.
302. Elkayam U et al. Differences in hemodynamic response to vasodilators due to calcium channel antagonism with nifedipine and direct acting antagonism with hydralazine in chronic refractory congestive heart failure. Am J Cardiol 1984; 54:126.
303. Elkayam U et al. A prospective randomized, double blind crossover study to compare the efficacy and safety of chronic nifedipine therapy with that of isosorbide dinitrate and their combination in the treatment of chronic congestive heart failure. Circulation 1990;82:1954.
304. Amiodarone Trials Meta-Analysis Investigators. Effect of prophylactic amiodarone on mortality after acute myocardial infarction and in congestive heart failure: a meta-analysis of individual data from 6500 patients in randomized trials. Lancet 1997;350:1417.

305. Doval CH et al. Randomized trial of low-dose amiodarone in severe congestive heart failure. Eurupo de Estudio de la Sobreivida en la Insuficiencia Cardiaca en Argentina (GESICA) Lancet 1994;344:493.

306. Singh S et al. Amiodarone in patients with congestive heart failure and asymptomatic ventricular arrhythmia. Survival Trial of Antiarrhythmic Therapy in Congestive Heart Failure. N Engl J Med 1995;333:77.

307. Massie B et al. for the CHF-STAT investigators. Effect of amiodarone on clinical status and left ventricular function in patients with congestive heart failure. Circulation 1996;93:2128.

308. De Smet P. Herbal remedies. N Engl J Med 2002;347:2046.

309. American Botanical Council. Hawthorn leaf with flower. Excerpted from Herbal Medicine: Expanded Commission E Monographs. 2000. http://www.herbalgram.org/)

310. Tauchert M. Efficacy and safety of crataegus extract WS 1442 in comparison with placebo in patients with chronic stable New York Heart Association class III heart failure. Am Heart J 2002;143:910.

311. Holubarsch CJ et al. Survival and prognosis: investigation of crataegus extract 1442 in congestive heart failure (SPICE)- rationale, study design and study protocol. Eur J Heart Fail 2000;2:431.

312. Tran MT et al. Role of coenzyme Q_{10} in chronic heart failure, angina, and hypertension. Pharmacotherapy 2001;21:797.

313. Pepping J. Alternative therapies: coenzyme Q. Am J Health-Syst Pharm 1999;56:519.

CHAPTER 20

Cardiac Arrhythmias

C. Michael White, Jessica C. Song, Moses S.S. Chow

Adequate blood pumping depends on a continuous, well-coordinated electrical activity within the heart. An arrhythmia results when disturbances of the rate and/or rhythm occur, leading to abnormal contraction or, in the worst case, cardiac standstill. This chapter reviews and discusses cardiac electrophysiology, arrhythmogenesis, common arrhythmias, and antiarrhythmic treatment.

Electrophysiology

Cellular Electrophysiology
An electrical potential exists across the cell membrane, and the electrical potential changes in a cyclic manner that is related to the flux of ions across the cell membrane, principally K^+, Na^+, Ca^{2+}, and Cl^-. If the change in the membrane potential is plotted against time in a given cycle of His-Purkinje fiber, a typical action potential results (Fig. 20-1).

The action potential can be described in five phases. Phase 0 is related to ventricular depolarization resulting from sodium entry into the cell through rapid sodium channels. On a surface electrocardiogram (ECG), phase 0 is represented by the QRS complex. Phase 1 is the overshoot phase where calcium enters the cell and contraction occurs. During phase 2, the plateau phase, inward depolarizing currents through slow sodium and calcium channels are counterbalanced by outward repolarizing potassium currents. Phase 3 constitutes repolarization, which on the ECG is represented by the T wave. During phase 4, sodium moves out of the cell and potassium

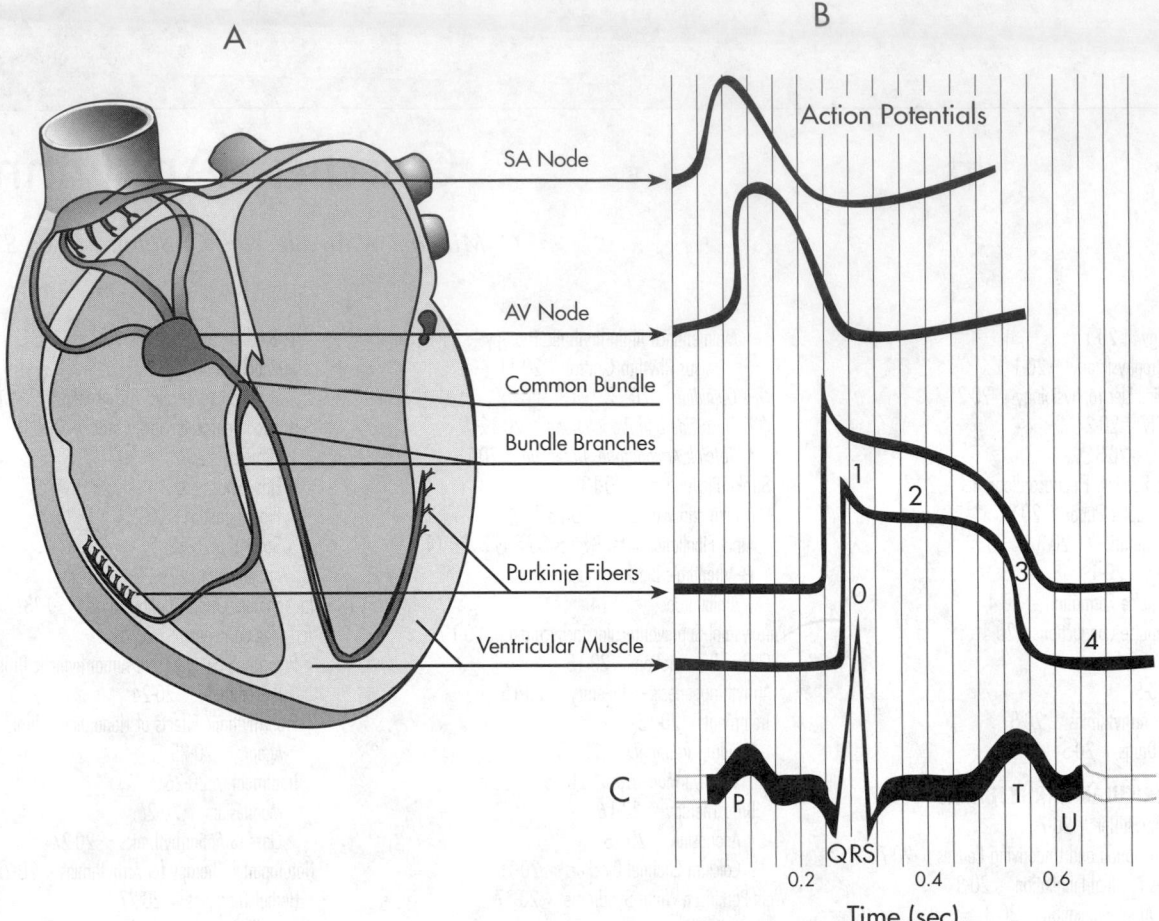

FIGURE 20-1 The cardiac conduction system. A. Cardiac conduction system anatomy. **B.** Action potentials of specific cardiac cells. **C.** Relationship of surface electrocardiogram to the action potential.

moves into the cell via an active pumping mechanism. During this phase, the action potential remains flat in some cells (e.g., ventricular muscle) and does not change until it receives an impulse from above. In other cells (e.g., sinoatrial [SA] node), the cell slowly depolarizes until it reaches the threshold potential and again spontaneously depolarizes (phase 0). The shape of the action potential depends on the location of the cell (see Fig. 20-1). In both the SA and atrioventricular (AV) nodes, the cells are more dependent on calcium influx than sodium influx, resulting in a less negative resting membrane potential, a slow rise of phase 0, and the capability of spontaneous (automatic) phase 4 depolarization (see Fig. 20-1).

The upward slope of phase 0, referred to as V_{max}, is related to the conduction velocity. The steeper the slope, the more rapid the rate of depolarization. Another influence on V_{max} is the point at which depolarization occurs. The less negative the threshold potential, the slower V_{max} will be, and hence conduction velocity is slowed. Drugs can affect V_{max} and conduction velocity by blocking the fast sodium channels or by making the resting membrane potential less negative (e.g., class I agents).

The action potential duration (APD) is the length of time from phase 0 to the end of phase 3. The effective refractory period is the length of time that the cell is refractory and will not propagate another impulse. Both of these measurements

can be obtained from intracardiac recordings of the action potential. Class Ia and III agents prolong the refractoriness of the heart.

Normal Cardiac Electrophysiology

Normal cardiac electrical activity begins with automatic impulse generation (automaticity) at the SA node and then normal impulse conduction through the heart.

AUTOMATICITY

Automaticity is the ability of cells (often referred to as pacemaker cells) to depolarize spontaneously. These cells are located in the SA and AV nodes and the His-Purkinje system. The SA node is normally the dominant pacemaker because it reaches the threshold faster than other nodes in a normal heart, resulting in 60 to 100 depolarizations per minute. The innate AV node and Purkinje rate of depolarization is 40 to 60 and 40 depolarizations per minute, respectively. In the healthy heart, the AV node and Purkinje fibers are prevented from spontaneous depolarization (overridden) by the more frequent impulses from the SA node. If the normal conduction system is disrupted (e.g., after a myocardial infarction [MI]), the AV node or Purkinje fibers may temporarily become the dominant pacemaker.

CONDUCTION

An impulse normally originates in the SA node and travels down the specialized intranodal pathways to activate the atrial muscle and the AV node. The AV node holds the impulse briefly before releasing it to the bundle of His. It then travels to the right and left bundle branches and out to the ventricular myocardium via the Purkinje fibers. The ECG tracing consists of a series of complexes that correspond to electrical activity in a specific location or anatomic site. By convention, these electrical deflections have been labeled the P wave, QRS complex, and T wave. The P wave represents depolarization of the atria, whereas the QRS complex reflects ventricular depolarization. The T wave reflects repolarization of the ventricles. To evaluate the intact conduction system, conduction intervals at different sites can be obtained. The normal intervals as measured by ECG or intracardiac electrodes are shown in Table 20-1. Drugs and ischemia can alter the conduction and hence the ECG intervals. The effects of antiarrhythmic agents on the ECG are described in Table 20-2.

An Approach to Reading Electrocardiograms

Electrocardiographic Paper

Calculation of the various intervals and widths is facilitated by recording the ECG waveforms on graph paper consisting of large squares defined by heavier lines, which in turn are composed of smaller squares. Each small square is 1 mm long

and represents 0.04 seconds. The larger squares are composed of five small squares (5 mm in length) and represent 0.20 seconds (Fig. 20-2).

Rhythm Interpretation

ECG tracings are evaluated through a systematic review as described below:

1. Is the rate fast or slow? A simple method to determine the rate is to count the number of complexes occurring within 6 seconds and multiply by 10. Most ECG recording paper places vertical lines at the top of the grid, 3 seconds apart. Therefore, if eight complexes appear within a 6-second length of strip, the rate is 80 beats/min.

2. Are there P waves before each QRS complex, and is their configuration normal? Are the P wave–to–P wave and R wave–to–R wave intervals regular or irregular? If the rhythm is irregular, is the pattern of irregularity consistent (regularly irregular) or totally random (irregularly irregular)? P waves appearing before the QRS complex usually indicate that the impulse originated in the SA node and subsequently was conducted to the ventricle. Abnormal-appearing P waves indicate that an atrial site other than the SA node is initiating the beat. Irregular rhythms may be due to an impulse originating from a site other than the SA node before the normal pacemaker can fire (premature beat); they also may result from failure to conduct impulses from the atria.

Table 20-1 Normal Electrophysiologic Intervals

Interval	Normal Indices (msec)	Electrical Activity	Measured By
P-R	120–200	Atrial depolarization	Surface ECG
QRS	<140	Ventricular depolarization	Surface ECG
QTc[a]	≤400	Ventricular repolarization	Surface ECG
J-T[b]	—	Ventricular repolarization	Surface ECG
A-H[c]	<140	—	Intracardiac lead
H-V[d]	<55	—	Intracardiac lead

[a]QTc interval is the Q-T interval corrected for heart rate. A common method for calculating QTc is the Q-T interval/(R-R interval)$^{1/2}$ (Bazett's formula).
[b]J-T interval is obtained by subtracting the QRS interval from the Q-T interval.
[c]A-H interval is the time it takes for an impulse to travel from the SA node to the bundle of His.
[d]H-V interval is the time it takes for an impulse to travel from the bundle of His to the Purkinje fibers.
ECG, electrocardiogram.

Table 20-2 Pharmacologic Properties of Antiarrhythmics

Type	Surface ECG P-R Interval	QRS Interval	Q-T Interval	Conduction Velocity	Refractory Period
IA	0/↑	↑	↑↑	↑↓[a]	↑
IB	0	0	0	0/↓	↓
IC	↑	↑↑	↑	↓	0
II	↑↑	0	0	↓[b]	↑[b]
III	0[c]	0	↑↑	0	↑
IV	↑↑	0	0	↓[b]	↑[b]

[a]Conduction increases at low dosages and decreases at higher dosages.
[b]On atrial and atrioventricular nodal tissue
[c]May cause P-R prolongation independent of class III antiarrhythmic activity
ECG, electrocardiogram.

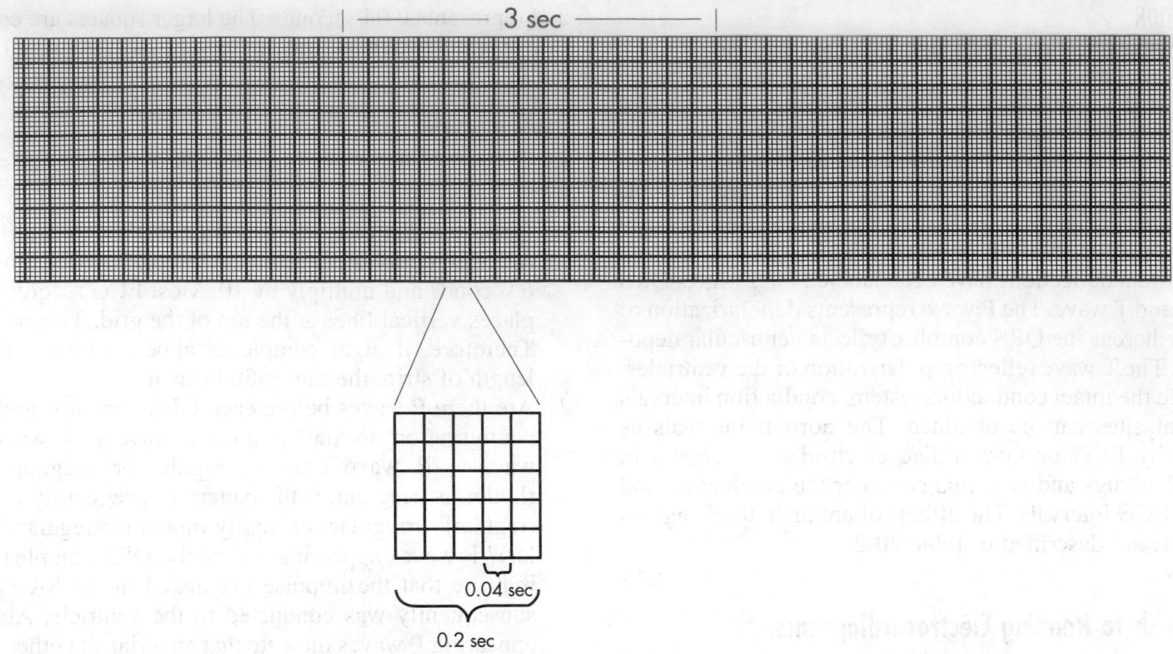

FIGURE 20-2 Electrocardigram recording paper.

3. Are the P-R and QRS complexes within normal limits? Is the QRS complex normal in its configuration? Impulses originating above the ventricles with normal conduction through the bundle branches and myocardium produce a normal-appearing, narrow QRS complex. Impulses originating in the ventricle give rise to wide, bizarre-appearing QRS complexes.

Pathophysiology

Abnormal Impulse Formation

Abnormal impulse formation can arise from abnormal automaticity or triggered activity originating from the SA node (e.g., sinus bradycardia) or other sites (e.g., junctional or idioventricular tachycardia). Causes of abnormal automaticity include hypoxia, ischemia, or excess catecholamine activity.

Triggered activity occurs when there is an attempted depolarization before or after the cell is fully repolarized, but not by a pacemaker cell (Fig. 20-3). These after-depolarizations may occur in phase 2 or 3 (early) or phase 4 (delayed) of the action potential. Early after-depolarizations (EAD) arise from a reduced level of membrane potential and may require a bradycardic state. Torsades de pointes (TdP), a form of polymorphic ventricular tachycardia (VT), is thought to be initiated by EAD. Delayed after-depolarizations (DAD), often seen with digoxin toxicity, are thought to be secondary to an overload of intracellular free calcium.

Abnormal Impulse Conduction

RE-ENTRY

The most common abnormal conduction leading to arrhythmogenesis is re-entry. A re-entrant circuit is formed as normal conduction occurs down a pathway that bifurcates into two pathways (e.g., AV node or left and right bundle branches). The impulse travels along one pathway (Fig. 20-4,

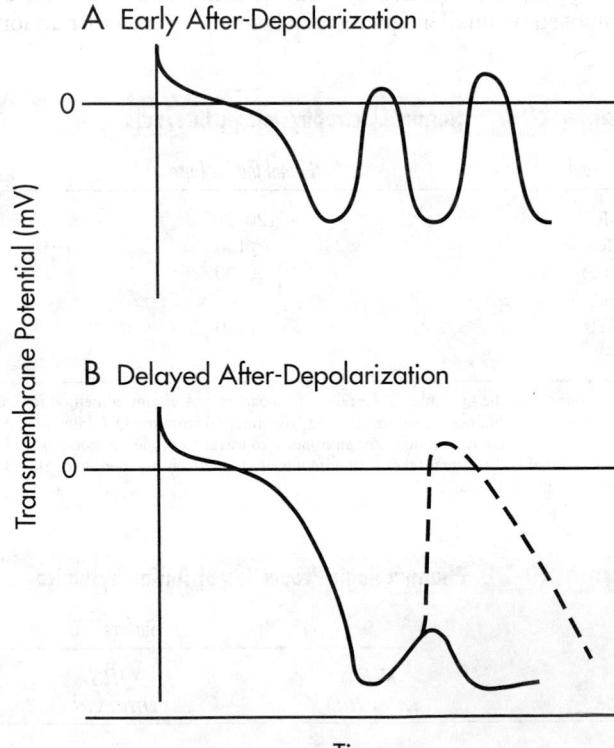

FIGURE 20-3 Triggered activity. A. Early after-depolarizations; repolarization is interrupted by secondary depolarization. Such responses may excite neighboring fibers and be propagated. **B.** Delayed after-depolarizations; after full repolarization is achieved, the cell transiently depolarizes. If the delayed after-depolarization reaches threshold, a propagating response can be seen (– – –). (Reproduced with permission from reference 135.)

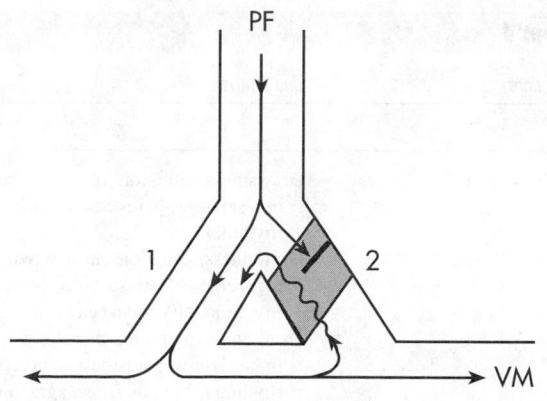

FIGURE 20-4 Re-entrant circuit of the ventricle. A branched Purkinje fiber (PF) terminates on a strip of ventricular muscle (VM). The shaded area in branch 2 represents a depolarized area that is the site of a one-way block; thus, the sinus impulses are blocked in this area, but retrograde impulses are propagated. Retrograde conduction in branch 2 is slow enough for the cells in branch 1 to recover and respond to the re-entry impulse. (Reproduced with permission from reference 135.)

pathway 1), but encounters unidirectional antegrade block in the other pathway (see Fig. 20-4, pathway 2). The impulse that passed through the unblocked pathway propagates in a retrograde manner (i.e., moves backwards) through the previously blocked pathway. This abnormal impulse can travel down the first pathway again when it is not refractory. Supraventricular and monomorphic VT are both examples of re-entrant arrhythmias (see Question 20).

BLOCK

Another form of abnormal impulse conduction occurs when the normal conducting pathway is blocked and the impulse is forced to travel through non-pathway tissues to cause depolarization. Common examples are left and right bundle branch blocks in the ventricles. A block in one path necessitates retrograde conduction through the opposite bundle to stimulate both ventricles. Typically, the non-pathway tissue conducts the electrical impulse more slowly than conduction tissues.

Classification of Arrhythmias

All arrhythmias originating above the bundle of His are referred to as supraventricular arrhythmias. These may include sinus bradycardia, sinus tachycardia, paroxysmal supraventricular tachycardia, atrial flutter, atrial fibrillation (AF), Wolff-Parkinson-White (WPW) syndrome, and premature atrial contractions (PACs). All of these arrhythmias are characterized by normal QRS complexes (i.e., normal ventricular depolarization) unless there is a bundle branch block. Not all of these rhythm changes are necessarily a sign of pathology. For example, athletes with a well-conditioned heart and large stroke volume commonly have slow heart rates (sinus bradycardia). Vigorous exercise commonly is accompanied by transient sinus tachycardia.

Arrhythmias originating below the bundle of His are referred to as ventricular arrhythmias. These include premature ventricular contractions (PVCs), ventricular tachycardia (VT), and ventricular fibrillation (VF). Conduction blocks often are categorized separately based on their level or location, which can be a supraventricular site (e.g., first-, second-, or third-degree AV block, see Question 27) or in the ventricle (e.g., right or left bundle branch block). An alternative method of classifying arrhythmias is based on the rate: bradyarrhythmia (<60 beats/min) or tachyarrhythmia (>100 beats/min).

Antiarrhythmic Drugs

Based on their electrophysiologic and pharmacologic effects, there are four Vaughn-Williams antiarrhythmic drug classes. Class I drugs, sodium channel blockers, are subdivided further depending on the duration of channel blockade (class IA is intermediate, IB is quick, and IC is long). Class II drugs are β-adrenergic blockers, class III drugs are potassium channel blockers, and class IV drugs are calcium channel blockers. The classification, pharmacokinetics, and adverse effects of these agents are summarized in Table 20-3.

Table 20-3 Vaughn-Williams Classification of Antiarrhythmic Agents

Drug and Classification	Pharmacokinetics	Indications	Side Effects
Class IA			
Quinidine sulfate (83% quinidine; SR: Quinidex) Quinidine gluconate (62% quinidine; SR: Quinaglute)	t1/2 = 6.2 ± 1.8 hr (affected by age, cirrhosis); Vd = 2.7 L/kg (↑ in HF); liver metabolism, 80%; renal clearance, 20%; Cp = 2–6 µg/mL, CYP3A4 substrate, CYP2D6 inhibitor, digoxin interaction	AF (conversion or prophylaxis), WPW, PVCs, VT	Diarrhea, hypotension, N/V, cinchonism, fever, thrombocytopenia, proarrhythmia
Procainamide (Pronestyl; Pronestyl SR, Procan SR)	t1/2 = 3 ± 0.6 hr; Vd = 1.9 ± 0.3 L/kg; liver metabolism, 40%; renal clearance, 40–60%; active metabolite (NAPA)[a] Cp = 4–10 µg/mL	AF (conversion or prophylaxis), WPW, PVCs, VT	Hypotension, fever, agranulocytosis, SLE (joint/muscle pain, rash, pericarditits), headache, proarrhythmia
Disopyramide (Norpace; SR: Norpace CR)	t1/2 = 6 ± 1 hr; Vd = 0.59 ± 0.15 L/kg; liver metabolism, 30%; renal clearance, 70%; Cp = 3–µg/mL	AF, WPW, PSVT, PVCs, VT	Anticholinergic (dry mouth, blurred vision, urinary retention), HF, proarrhythmia

Continued

Table 20-3   **Vaughn-Williams Classification of Antiarrhythmic Agents—cont'd**

Drug and Classification	Pharmacokinetics	Indications	Side Effects
Class IB[b]			
Lidocaine (Xylocaine)	t1/2 = 1.8 ± 0.4 hr; Vd = 1.1 ± 0.4 L/kg; liver metabolism, 100%; Cp = 1.5–6 µg/mL	PVCs, VT, VF	Drowsiness, agitation, muscle twitching, seizures, paresthesias, proarrhythmia
Mexiletine (Mexitil)	t1/2 = 10.4 ±2.8 hr; Vd = 9.5 ±3.4 L/kg; liver metabolism, 35–80%; Cp = 0.5–2 µg/mL	PVCs, VT, VF	Drowsiness, agitation, muscle twitching, seizures, paresthesias, proarrhythmia, N/V, diarrhea
Tocainide (Tonocard)	t1/2 = 13.5 ±2.3 hr; Vd = 3 ±0.2 L/kg; liver metabolism, 60–65%; Cp = 6–15 µg/mL	PVCs, VT, VF	Drowsiness, agitation, muscle twitching, seizures, paresthesias, proarrhythmia, N/V, diarrhea, agranulocytosis
Class IC			
Flecainide (Tambocor)	t1/2 = 12–27 hr; liver metabolism, 75%; renal clearance, 25%; Cp = 0.4–1 µg/mL	AF, PSVT, severe ventricular arrhythmias	Dizziness, tremor, lightheadedness, flushing, blurred vision, metallic taste, proarrhythmia
Propafenone (Rythmol)	t1/2 = 2 hr (extensive metabolizer); 10 hr (poor metabolizer); Vd = 2.5–4 L/kg, CYP2D6 substrate/inhibitor, digoxin interaction	PAF, WPW, severe ventricular arrhythmias	Dizziness, blurred vision, taste disturbances, nausea, worsening of asthma, proarrhythmia
Moricizine (Ethmozine)	t1/2 = 1.3–3.5 hr; Vd > 300 L	Severe ventricular arrhythmias	Nausea, dizziness, perioral numbness, euphoria
Class II			
β-Blockers Acebutolol (Sectral) Esmolol (Brevibloc) Propranolol (Inderal)	See chapters on Essential Hypertension and Hypertensive Emergencies	AF, A flutter, PSVT, PVCs	See chapters on Essential Hypertension and Hypertensive Emergencies
Class III			
Amiodarone (Cordarone)	t1/2 = 40–60 days; Vd = 60–100 L/kg; erratic absorption; liver metabolism, 100%; oral F = 50%, Cp = 0.5–2.5 µg/mL, CYP1A2, 2D6, 2C9 inhibitor, digoxin interaction	AF, PAF, PSVT, severe ventricular arrhythmias, VF	Blurred vision, corneal microdeposits, photophobia, skin discoloration, constipation, pulmonary fibrosis, ataxia, hypo/hyperthyroid, hypotension, N/V
Sotalol[c] (Betapace)	t1/2 = 10–20 hr; Vd = 1.2–2.4 L/kg; renal clearance, 100%	AF (prophylaxis), PSVT, severe ventricular arrhythmias	Fatigue, dizziness, dyspnea, Bradycardia, proarrhythmia
Dofetilide (Tikosyn)	t1/2 = 7.5–10 hr; Vd = 3 L/kg; renal elimination, 60% (GFR and active tubular secretion), CYP3A4 substrate	AF or atrial flutter conversion and prophylaxis	Chest pain, dizziness, headache, proarrhythmia
Bretylium (Bretylol)	t1/2 = 8.9±1.8 hr; Vd = 5.9±0.3 L/kg; renal clearance, 80–90%	VT, VF	Hypotension, N/V, light-headedness, dizziness, transitory hypertension, tachycardia
Ibutilide (Corvert)	t1/2 = 6 (2–12) hr; Vd = 11 L/kg, Cp = undefined	AF or atrial flutter conversion	Headache, nausea, proarrhythmia
Class IV			
Calcium channel blockers Verapamil (Isoptin) Diltiazem (Cardizem)	See chapters on Ischemic Heart Disease, Essential Hypertension, and Hypertensive Emergencies	AF, A flutter, PSVT	See chapters on Ischemic Heart Disease, Essential Hypertension, and Hypertensive Emergencies

[a]N-acetylprocainamide (NAPA) is 100% renally eliminated and possesses class III antiarrhythmic activity.
[b]Phenytoin is classified as a class IB antiarrhythmic.
[c]Possesses both class II and III antiarrhythmic activity.
AF, atrial fibrillation; A flutter, atrial flutter; Cp, steady-state plasma concentration; CR, controlled release; HF, heart failure; N/V, nausea and vomiting; PAF, paroxysmal atrial fibrillation; PSVT, paroxysmal supraventricular tachycardia; PVCs, premature ventricular contractions; SLE, systemic lupus erythematosus; SR, sustained release; t1/2, half-life; Vd, volume of distribution; VF, ventricular fibrillation; VT, ventricular tachycardia; WPW, Wolff-Parkinson-White syndrome.

Class Ia and class III antiarrhythmics increase repolarization time, the QTc interval, and the risk of TdP. Class II and IV antiarrhythmics can decrease the heart rate (may cause bradycardia), decrease the force of ventricular contractility (may decrease stroke volume), and prolong the PR interval (may cause second- or third-degree AV block). Class Ib antiarrhythmics work only in ventricular tissue, so they cannot be used in AF or atrial flutter. Class Ic antiarrhythmic agents are useful, but should never be used after an MI or with heart failure (HF) or severe left ventricular hypertrophy (classified as structural heart diseases) because increased mortality can result. These drugs are discussed in greater detail later.

SUPRAVENTRICULAR ARRHYTHMIAS

Supraventricular arrhythmias include all arrhythmias that originate from above the bifurcation of the bundle of His. The specific arrhythmias include (1) those primarily atrial in origin, such as AF, atrial flutter, paroxysmal sinus tachycardia, ectopic atrial tachycardia, and multifocal atrial tachycardia; and (2) AV nodal re-entrant tachycardia (AVNRT) and AV re-entrant tachycardia (AVRT) involving accessory pathways within the atria and/or ventricle. AVNRT and AVRT often self-terminate and are paroxysmal (episodic) in nature; thus, they are commonly referred to as paroxysmal supraventricular tachycardias (PSVT). The most common supraventricular arrhythmias are AF, atrial flutter, and PSVT.

Atrial Fibrillation/Flutter

AF is characterized by rapid, ineffective writhing of the atrial muscle with a classic "irregularly irregular" ventricular rate.

The source of the arrhythmia is one or more ectopic areas (foci) that act as independent pacemakers and fire at such a rate as to suppress normal impulse generation from the SA node. On the ECG, no identifiable P waves are present (Fig. 20-5). In contrast, atrial flutter (Fig. 20-6) is characterized by typical sawtooth atrial waves, at a rate of 280 to 320 beats/min and a variable ventricular rate, depending on the nature of the AV block present (e.g., 2:1, 3:1, or 4:1 block). In most cases, the ventricular rate is approximately 150 beats/min. Patients with atrial flutter often progress to AF. The underlying diseases and treatments of atrial flutter and AF are similar. The arrhythmogenic mechanism of AF may be due to multiple re-entrant wavelets, occurring in a paroxysmal, chronic, or acute pattern. The most common presentation is paroxysmal atrial fibrillation (PAF), which can progress to chronic AF; thus, the two overlap. An example of PAF is presented in the following section.

Clinical Manifestation and Underlying Causes

1. J.K., a 66-year-old man, presents with complaints of dyspnea on exertion (DOE) and palpitations for the last 2 weeks. He experienced palpitations of shorter duration three times in the last year, but these were not associated with DOE. His medical history includes non–insulin-dependent diabetes mellitus (NIDDM) for the past 5 years, and gout. There is no history of rheumatic heart disease, MI, HF, pulmonary embolism, or thyroid disease. Medications include glyburide (Diabeta) 5 mg BID, ibuprofen (Motrin) 600 mg QID, and allopurinol (Zyloprim) 300 mg/day. J.K. does not smoke or drink alcohol. Physical examination reveals a blood pressure (BP) of 136/84 mm Hg, pulse of

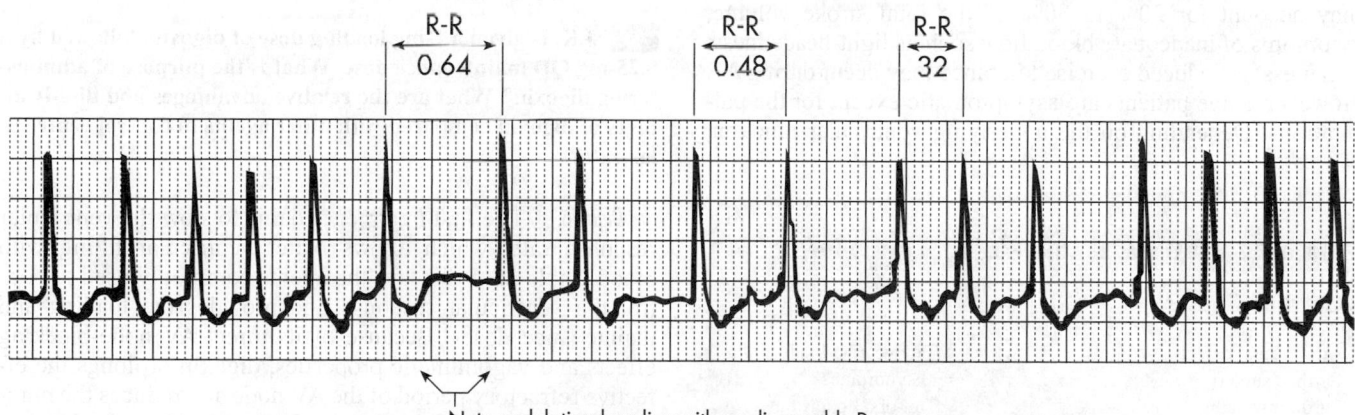

Note undulating baseline with no discernable P waves.

FIGURE 20-5 Atrial fibrillation. Note the irregularly irregular R-R intervals, undulating baseline without definitive P waves, normal width of the QRS complexes, and the ventricular rate of 140 beats/min.

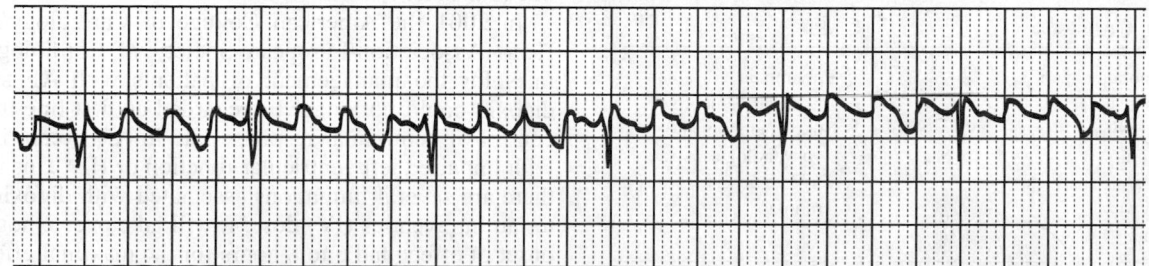

FIGURE 20-6 Atrial flutter. Note the sawtooth appearance of the rhythm strip. (Reproduced with permission from reference 204.)

154 beats/min with an irregularly irregular pattern, respiratory rate of 16 breaths/min, and temperature of 98.2°F. His chest has rales at both bases. Cardiac examination reveals an irregularly irregular rhythm without murmurs, gallops, or rubs. His jugular vein is distended 4 cm, but no organomegaly is found. His extremities have 1+ pitting edema. The ECG shows AF (see Fig. 20-5) and the chest radiograph is compatible with mild HF. A cardiac echocardiogram reveals the atrial size to be <5 cm (normal). In view of his history and previous episodes, J.K. is diagnosed with paroxysmal atrial fibrillation (PAF). Which of J.K.'s other medical problems may predispose him to AF development? What other conditions commonly are associated with AF?

AF is commonly associated with or a manifestation of other diseases or disorders (Table 20-4.[1]) When treatable underlying causes are present, they should be corrected because this may resolve the AF. In a small percentage of patients like J.K. who do not have underlying heart disease, their AF is called "lone" AF, which usually has a more benign course.

Consequences of Atrial Fibrillation

2. What clinical findings demonstrated by J.K. typically are associated with AF? What are the likely consequences of his AF?

The most common complaint in AF, as with J.K., is chest palpitations (the sensation of the heart beating rapidly or unusually in the chest). This is a result of the rapid ventricular contraction rate, which typically ranges from 100 to 160 beats/min. The H-R and R-R interval (time from the R wave in one QRS complex to the R wave in the next complex) is irregularly irregular (random irregularity). During AF, the atrial kick, or the atria's contribution to stroke volume (via the Frank-Starling mechanism), is lost. Because the atrial kick may account for 20% to 30% of the total stroke volume, symptoms of inadequate blood flow such as light-headedness, dizziness, or reduced exercise tolerance may occur during AF. However, some patients are asymptomatic except for the palpitations. Depending on the underlying ventricular function,

Table 20-4 Causes of Atrial Fibrillation and Flutter

Cardiac Causes

Atrial septal defect	Tachycardia-bradycardia
Cardiac surgery	syndrome
Cardiomyopathy	Tumors, lipomatous
Ischemic heart disease	hypertrophy
Mitral valve disease	Wolff-Parkinson-White
Nonrheumatic heart disease	syndrome
	Pericarditis

Systemic Causes

Alcohol ("holiday heart")	Pneumonia
Cerebrovascular accident	Pulmonary embolism
Chronic pulmonary disease	Sudden emotional or
Defibrillation	psychological stress
Electrolyte abnormalities	Thyrotoxicosis
Fever	Trauma
Hypothermia	

Reproduced with permission from reference 23.

signs of HF, such as DOE and peripheral edema, may develop, as experienced by J.K. Conversely, underlying HF may precipitate AF.

Patients with AF are at risk for thrombotic stroke.[2,3] With the chaotic movement of the atria, normal blood flow is disrupted and atrial mural thrombi may form. The risk of stroke increases following restoration of normal sinus rhythm, which allows more efficient cardiac contractility and expulsion of the thrombus. Patients with nonvalvular AF have a fivefold increase in the risk of stroke; this risk increases as patients have an increased number of associated risk factors. Other concurrent diseases that may increase the risk of stroke are HF, cardiomyopathy, thyrotoxicosis, congenital heart disease, and valvular heart disease.

Treatment of Atrial Fibrillation
GOALS OF THERAPY

3. What are the therapeutic goals and general approaches used to treat AF in patients like J.K.?

The two primary goals of treatment are to relieve symptoms and reduce the risk of stroke. Slowing the ventricular rate during AF, restoring normal sinus rhythm, and preventing AF recurrences can help accomplish the first goal; anticoagulation can help achieve the second goal if it is indicated. Patients who remain in normal sinus rhythm following cardioversion may not require long-term treatment with anticoagulants. Since prolonged maintenance of normal sinus rhythm cannot be guaranteed, treatment with anticoagulation may be necessary.

VENTRICULAR RATE CONTROL

4. J.K. is given a 1-mg loading dose of digoxin, followed by a 0.25-mg QD maintenance dose. What is the purpose of administering digoxin? What are the relative advantages and disadvantages of digoxin compared with other agents to control ventricular rate?

Digoxin. The first treatment goal is to slow the ventricular response rate, which allows better ventricular filling with blood. Table 20-5 displays the agents commonly used to control the ventricular response and provides the loading and maintenance doses. Because of its direct AV node-blocking effects and vagomimetic properties, digoxin prolongs the effective refractory period of the AV node and reduces the number of impulses conducted through the AV node (negative dromotropy).[4,5] Cardioversion to normal sinus rhythm can be delayed unless the patient is hemodynamically compromised due to the AF.

In 2001 the American College of Cardiology/American Heart Association/European Society of Cardiology Guidelines for the management of patients with AF stated that digoxin could no longer be regarded as first-line therapy for control of ventricular response rate in AF, except in patients with impaired left ventricular function or HF.[6] This is because there are several limitations associated with digoxin use. After an intravenous (IV) dose, it will take over 2 hours for the onset of effect and 6 to 8 hours for the maximal effect, which is markedly slower than other negative dromotropes.[7] Secondly, digoxin therapy may prolong AF episodes.[5] In one

Table 20-5 Agents Used for Controlling Ventricular Rate in Supraventricular Tachycardias

Drug	Loading Dose	Usual Maintenance Dose	Comments
Digoxin (Lanoxin)	10–15 μg/kg LBW up to 1–1.5 mg IV or PO over 24 hr (e.g., 0.5 mg initially, then 0.25 mg Q 6 hr)	PO: 0.125–0.5 mg/day; adjust for renal failure (see Chapter 19, Heart Failure)	Maximum response may take several hours; use with caution in patients with renal impairment
Esmolol (Brevibloc)	0.5 mg/kg IV over 1 min	50–300 μg/kg/min continuous infusion with bolus between increases	Hypotension common; effects additive with digoxin and calcium channel blockers
Propranolol (Inderal)	0.5–1.0 mg IV repeated Q 2 min (up to 0.1–0.15 mg/kg)	IV: 0.04 mg/kg/min PO: 10–120 mg TID	Use with caution in patients with HF or asthma; additive effects seen with digoxin and calcium channel blockers
Metoprolol (Lopressor)	5 mg IV at 1 mg/min	PO: 25–100 mg BID	Use with caution in patients with HF or asthma; additive effects seen with digoxin and calcium channel blockers
Verapamil (Isoptin, Calan)	5–10 mg (0.075–0.15 mg/kg) IV over 2 min; if response inadequate after 15–30 min, repeat 10 mg (up to 0.15 mg/kg)	IV: 5–10 mg/hr PO: 40–120 mg TID or 120–480 mg in sustained-release form daily	Hypotension with IV route; effects are additive with digoxin and β-blockers; may increase digoxin levels
Diltiazem (Cardizem)	0.25 mg/kg IV over 2 min; if response inadequate after 15 min, repeat 0.35 mg/kg over 2 min	IV: 5–15 mg/hr PO: 60–90 mg TID or QID or 180–360 mg in extended-release form daily	Response to IV therapy occurs in 4–5 min; hypotension; effects additive with digoxin and β-blockers

HF, heart failure; IV, intravenously; LBW, lean body weight; PO, orally.

study of 72 patients with PAF, the relative risk of longer AF episodes associated with digoxin was 4.3 compared with other negative dromotropic agents ($P < 0.01$). This may be because digoxin shortens the refractory period of atrial muscle, which increases AF susceptibility.[5] Thirdly, digoxin is less effective than β-blockers and nondihydropyridine calcium channel blockers during states of heightened sympathetic tone (e.g., exercise or emotional stress), a common precipitant of PAF.[4,5,8,9] Finally, digoxin serum concentrations may be increased when combined with P-glycoprotein inhibitors such as verapamil, quinidine, propafenone, flecainide, and amiodarone.[10–13] Normally, P-glycoprotein in the brush border membrane of intestinal enterocytes pumps digoxin into the lumen of the gut and reduce its bioavailability. When digoxin is given with inhibitors, more complete absorption occurs (see Chapter 19, Heart Failure, for further discussion of digoxin and digoxin drug interactions).

5. J.K. has diabetes, which increases the risk for diabetic nephropathy. Would the dosing be changed if J.K. had renal dysfunction?

J.K.'s renal function is normal. If he had renal dysfunction, only the maintenance dose would need to be altered. Remember that a loading dose is used to achieve a therapeutic level and, therefore, needs to overcome the volume of distribution, not clearance. The digoxin maintenance dose, however, is highly dependent on renal clearance, because digoxin is 50% to 75% eliminated unchanged in the urine. (See Chapter 19, Heart Failure, for further discussion of digoxin dosing in patients with normal and impaired renal function.)

6. What other drugs can be used for ventricular rate control, and what are their relative advantages and disadvantages compared with digoxin?

β-Adrenergic Blocking Agents. β-Adrenergic blocking agents are another class of negative dromotropes used in AF. Propranolol, metoprolol, and esmolol are available for IV administration. Each agent rapidly controls the ventricular rate both at rest and during exercise. β-Blockers are the first choice in high catecholamine states such as thyrotoxicosis and postcardiac surgery. However, given their negative inotropic effects, β-blockers should not be used to acutely control the ventricular response in patients with HF. Even though β-blockers are used to treat HF (e.g., bisoprolol, carvedilol, and metoprolol), they need to be started at low doses and titrated prudently over several weeks to therapeutic doses.[14–16] (See Chapter 19, Heart Failure.) When trying to achieve rate control, more aggressive dosing may be needed. β-Blockers should also be avoided in patients with asthma because of their β₂-blocking properties, and blood sugar levels should be monitored more closely in patients with diabetes mellitus because the signs and symptoms of hypoglycemia (except sweating) can be masked.

Calcium Channel Blockers. Calcium channel blockers are also effective in slowing ventricular rate at rest and during exercise. Both verapamil and diltiazem can be administered IV for a rapid (4 to 5 minutes) reduction in heart rate.[17,18] They work through their effect on slow calcium channels within the AV node. Although the duration of action produced by bolus dosing is short, both agents can be administered either as a continuous drip or orally. Given the ability of calcium channel blockers to cause arteriolar dilation, a transient decrease in blood pressure can be expected. IV calcium pretreatment can be used to attenuate the blood pressure decrease among patients with hypotension, near hypotensive blood pressure, or left ventricular dysfunction. Calcium pretreatment does not appear to diminish the negative dromotropic effects of nondihydropyridine calcium channel blockers.[19–22] Verapamil and diltiazem should be used with caution in HF, and verapamil can increase the concentrations of other cardiovascular drugs such as digoxin, dofetilide, simvastatin, and lovastatin.[23] Verapamil and diltiazem are good alternatives to β-blockers in asthmatics.[6]

For chronic therapy, oral negative dromotropes (usually a β-blocker or nondihydropyridine calcium channel blocker) are recommended. If higher-dose monotherapy with one of these drugs is needed to control symptoms, but is associated with intolerable side effects, combining lower-dose digoxin with a β-blocker or calcium channel blocker might work.[9,24–26]

J.K. has signs of HF, so digoxin is a reasonable choice. IV verapamil and β-blockers may worsen the signs and symptoms of HF and the β-blockers may mask signs of hypoglycemia in J.K. The goal of rate control should be a resting and an exercising heart rate below 90 and 140 beats/min, respectively.[26]

CONVERSION TO NORMAL SINUS RHYTHM

7. J.K. is scheduled for elective cardioversion in 3 weeks. Warfarin treatment is begun and J.K.'s prothrombin time is to be maintained at an international normalized ratio (INR) of 2 to 3. Why is warfarin therapy being used?

J.K. is to be maintained on warfarin for 3 weeks before cardioversion to prevent the embolization of any atrial clots. These atrial clots form most often in small side pouches on the atria called appendages.[6,27] Since the frequency of right atrial appendage thrombosis is half that of left atrial appendage thrombosis in AF patients, the risk of stroke is enhanced much more than the risk of pulmonary embolism.[27] Studies in patients with AF showed that those who were anticoagulated before cardioversion had a lower incidence (0.8%) of emboli than those who were not anticoagulated (5.3%).[28] Warfarin is recommended during the 3-week period before cardioversion for patients who have been in AF for >2 days.[29] The dose should be titrated to produce an INR of 2 to 3. If cardioversion is successful, patients should remain on warfarin for 4 weeks because normal atrial activity/function may not return for up to 3 weeks, and patients may be at risk of late embolization.[30] J.K. has had AF for a minimum of 2 weeks; thus, he should be maintained on warfarin for 3 weeks before he is scheduled for cardioversion.

Chemical Conversion—Ibutilide, Propafenone, Flecainide

8. After anticoagulation, the patient will be brought into the hospital for chemical cardioversion with ibutilide. If therapy fails, the patient will be electrically cardioverted later in the day. How does ibutilide therapy compare with the other therapeutic choices for chemical cardioversion?

After achieving ventricular rate control, more definitive treatment can be given in an attempt to convert the patient to normal sinus rhythm. This step is more likely to be taken in a patient like J.K. with an acute onset of symptoms.

Many class I and III antiarrhythmic agents have been evaluated for efficacy in placebo-controlled trials for conversion of AF or atrial flutter to normal sinus rhythm. The best-studied agents include IV ibutilide, oral propafenone, IV or oral flecainide, oral quinidine, oral sotalol, oral and IV amiodarone, and oral dofetilide. This section will focus on ibutilide, propafenone, and flecainide.

IV ibutilide, a class III antiarrhythmic agent with potassium channel–blocking and slow sodium channel–enhancing effects, was the first agent that the U.S. Food and Drug Administration (FDA) approved for the termination of recent-onset AF/atrial flutter.[31] Ibutilide is administered as a 1-mg infusion over 10 minutes, followed by another 1-mg infusion over 10 minutes if conversion has not occurred by 10 minutes after the infusion. The conversion rate for recent-onset AF is 35% to 50%; the conversion rate is 65% to 80% in atrial flutter. In a recent retrospective study of hospital inpatients with either AF or atrial flutter, 50% of patients converted initially (41% conversion AF, 65% atrial flutter), but only 33% of patients left the hospital in sinus rhythm. If the duration of AF/atrial flutter before cardioversion was <15 days, significantly more patients remained in sinus rhythm at discharge compared with patients who had AF/atrial flutter for >15 days before cardioversion.[32] As is the case with most class III antiarrhythmic agents, the main adverse effect is TdP, which occurred in approximately 4% of patients. Aside from the risk of TdP, therapy is well tolerated.[33–36]

There is preliminary evidence that magnesium may enhance the efficacy of ibutilide. In a multicenter cohort study called the Treatment with Ibutilide and Magnesium Evaluation (TIME), adjunctive magnesium (2.2 ±1g) plus ibutilide was compared to ibutilide alone. In this study of 323 patients, the successful chemical conversion rate went from 60.3% with ibutilide alone to 71.6% ($P = 0.04$) in the adjunctive magnesium group. The risk of TdP was also reduced 33% with adjunctive magnesium therapy, but the study was not powered to determine this endpoint ($P = 0.388$). Whether adjunctive magnesium would be of benefit with other class Ia or III antiarrhythmics is not known.[37]

Propafenone is a class IC agent with β-blocking properties. When given in doses of 450 to 750 mg orally (600 mg was the most-used dose), the initial conversion rate in patients with AF ranged from 41% to 57%. In contrast to ibutilide, no patients experienced ventricular arrhythmias (including TdP), but a risk of hypotension, bradycardia, and QRS prolongation was noted.[38–40]

Oral flecainide is another class IC antiarrhythmic agent. In one study, 300 mg oral flecainide converted 68% of patients to sinus rhythm within 3 hours and 91% of patients by 8 hours. Another study using 2 mg/kg IV flecainide over 10 minutes followed by 200 to 300 mg orally demonstrated a 71% conversion rate. The efficacy in atrial flutter has yet to be established. Sinus node dysfunction, prolongation of intraventricular rhythm, dizziness, weakness, and gastrointestinal (GI) disturbances have been reported.[41,42]

Dofetilide

9. Why is dofetilide unique among the antiarrhythmic drugs used in AF and atrial flutter? What drug interactions limit its use?

Oral dofetilide is a class III antiarrhythmic agent that inhibits the delayed rectifier potassium current (IKr).[43,44] It is the only class III agent indicated for both acute cardioversion of AF/atrial flutter and maintenance of normal sinus rhythm. However, the risk of TdP has prompted its manufacturer to mandate a minimum of 3 days of ECG monitoring in a properly equipped facility during therapy initiation. Dofetilide has been shown to be an effective pharmacologic agent for conversion to and maintenance of normal sinus rhythm. Two clinical trials, EMERALD (European and Australian Multicenter Evaluative Research on Atrial Fibrillation Dofetilide)[45] and SAFIRE-D (Symptomatic Atrial Fibrillation Investigation and Randomized Evaluation of Dofetilide)[46] have shown AF/atrial flutter patients to have conversion rates of 30% on higher doses of dofetilide. Patients failing chemical conversion received electrical conversion. If this conversion succeeded, they were continued on dofetilide for 1 year. At 1 year 60% of those converted were still in sinus rhythm with the 500-µg dose. Also, dofetilide appears to exert neutral effects on mortality rates in HF and post-MI patients.[47,48]

The dofetilide dose is based on the patient's creatinine clearance (Cl_{cr}); the doses are 500, 250, and 125 µg twice daily with Cl_{cr} above 60 mL/min, 40 to 60 mL/min, and 20 to 39 mL/min, respectively. The QTc interval must be measured (using a 12-lead ECG) 2 to 3 hours after the first dose. If the QTc interval does not increase by >15% or if it does not surpass 500 msec (550 msec in patients with ventricular conduction abnormalities), the QTc interval still needs to be measured 2 to 3 hours after each subsequent dose, but not with a 12-lead ECG. If the QTc interval exceeds the above parameters, the subsequent dose should be reduced by 50%. If the QTc interval measured 2 to 3 hours after the first adjusted dose (using a 12-lead ECG) is still above the acceptable range, dofetilide should be discontinued. If the QTc interval is within an acceptable range following the first adjusted dose, all subsequent postdose QTc intervals do not need to be measured with a 12-lead ECG. All patients must be ECG monitored by at least a single lead for 3 days.[49]

Drug interactions pose a significant problem with dofetilide. Cimetidine, ketoconazole, prochlorperazine, megestrol, and trimethoprim (including in combination with sulfamethoxazole) inhibit active tubular secretion of dofetilide and can elevate dofetilide plasma concentrations.[44,49] Since the incidence of TdP is directly related to dofetilide plasma concentrations, concomitant use with these agents is contraindicated.[49] Concomitant administration of dofetilide with verapamil or hydrochlorothiazide increases the incidence of TdP by an unknown mechanism and is contraindicated as well.[44] Concurrent use of agents that can prolong the QTc interval is not recommended with dofetilide.[49] Dofetilide also undergoes metabolism by the CYP3A4 isoenzyme to a minor extent. Therefore, inhibitors of this isoenzyme (e.g., azole antifungal agents, protease inhibitors, serotonin reuptake inhibitors, amiodarone, diltiazem, nefazodone, quinine, zafirlukast) should be coadministered with caution with dofetilide. Other agents that can potentially increase dofetilide levels (through inhibition of tubular secretion) include metformin, triamterene, and amiloride. Hence, these agents should be cautiously coadministered with dofetilide.[49]

Quinidine

10. **J.K. is brought into the hospital after 3 weeks of warfarin therapy, and 1 mg of ibutilide is used followed by another milligram 10 minutes later. He does not convert to normal sinus rhythm after ibutilide. If an agent like quinidine is used to convert the patient to normal sinus rhythm, why would it be especially important to attempt ventricular rate control first?**

The effects of quinidine and other type IA antiarrhythmic agents on the AV node are bimodal. At low concentrations, AV node conduction may be enhanced by the drug's antivagal properties. If this occurs before normal sinus rhythm is achieved by quinidine, the ventricular rate actually may increase. At higher concentrations, the type IA agents slow AV node conduction. Because it is difficult to predict which effect on the AV node will predominate in a given patient, it is prudent to initiate a rate-controlling agent first.

Electrical Conversion

11. **J.K. is scheduled for electrical cardioversion in 6 hours. What is electrical cardioversion? How efficacious and safe is it? Is it safe to cardiovert patients who are digitalized?**

Direct current (DC) cardioversion quickly and effectively restores 85% to 90% of patients with AF to normal sinus rhythm.[30] If DC conversion alone is ineffective, it can be repeated in combination with antiarrhythmic drugs.[50] In one study, the success rate of electrical cardioversion was significantly higher in AF patients (duration of AF averaged 119 days) with ibutilide pretreatment (1 mg) compared to those without pretreatment (100% versus 72%, $P < 0.001$).[51] This is because ibutilide pretreatment lowered the energy requirement for atrial defibrillation by 27% ($P < 0.001$). TdP occurred in 3% of patients, all of whom had an ejection fraction below 20%. Other studies have found class Ia antiarrhythmic agents to be promising; flecainide data were contradictory; and amiodarone was effective, but the several days needed to load the amiodarone was inconvenient.[56]

Chemical conversion generally is preferred for initially attempting cardioversion because DC conversion requires general anesthesia (short-acting benzodiazepine, barbiturate, or propofol), but DC cardioversion is indicated for patients who are hemodynamically unstable. From a managed care perspective, attempting chemical conversion first with ibutilide, with all failures subsequently receiving electrical cardioversion, is more cost-effective (saving $138/patient) than just electrically cardioverting all patients.[32]

It was once thought that digoxin should be held for 2 to 3 days before DC cardioversion because it placed patients at an increased risk of arrhythmia. This may be true for patients who have toxic digoxin concentrations, but has not been noted in patients on usual maintenance therapy.[52] If a patient shows signs of digoxin toxicity, cardioversion should be started at a low energy (10 J) and increased as needed. At the time of cardioversion, J.K. had no clinical signs of digoxin toxicity.

Maintenance Antiarrhythmic Therapy—Rate Control Versus Rhythm Control

12. **After 3 weeks of anticoagulation, J.K. is converted to normal sinus rhythm using a single 200-J electric shock. He is discharged from the hospital on digoxin and warfarin and advised to follow up with a cardiologist 4 weeks later. Within 2 weeks,**

J.K. experiences several episodes of brief, symptomatic, and self-terminating palpitations. His physician prescribes oral dofetilide and informs J.K. that he will be admitted to the hospital for the first 3 days of treatment to determine a safe and effective dose. What type of patient is likely to remain free of AF recurrence following cardioversion and while on maintenance therapy? Should rate control without rhythm control be considered for J.K.?

Conversion to and maintenance of normal sinus rhythm is determined by the duration of the arrhythmia, underlying disease processes, and left atrial size.[53] Duration of AF for >1 year significantly reduces the chances of maintaining a normal sinus rhythm.[54] When the atrial size exceeds 5 cm, there is a <10% chance of maintaining normal sinus rhythm at 6 months.

J.K.'s chance of being maintained in normal sinus rhythm is good because the duration of his AF is short and the echocardiogram revealed only slight enlargement of his left atrium.

Recently, two trials comparing rate control to rhythm control were published.[54,55] The North American AFFIRM study (Atrial Fibrillation Follow-up Investigation of Rhythm Management), a randomized, multicenter comparison of rate control and rhythm control, enrolled 4,060 patients with AF and a high risk of stroke.[55] The primary endpoint was all-cause mortality. Antiarrhythmic drugs were chosen at the discretion of the treating physician, but >60% of the patients received amiodarone or sotalol as the initial antiarrhythmic agent. Rate control agents included digoxin, β-blockers, and nondihydropyridine calcium channel blockers. After a mean follow-up of 3.5 years, there was a trend toward lower overall mortality ($P = 0.08$) with significant reductions in hospitalizations (10% lower, $P < 0.001$) and TdP (300% lower, $P < 0.007$) in the rate control group. A smaller European study enrolled 522 patients with persistent AF and a history of at least one previous cardioversion.[56] The primary endpoint was the composite of severe adverse effects of antiarrhythmic drugs, the need for implantation of a pacemaker, bleeding, thromboembolic complications, death from cardiovascular causes, and HF. The initial antiarrhythmic agent was sotalol; other antiarrhythmic agents included flecainide, propafenone, and amiodarone. After a mean follow-up of 2.3 years, no significant difference was noted between the rhythm control and rate control treatment groups with regard to the primary endpoint.

In conclusion, using rhythm control in patients with AF rather than rate control does not improve outcomes and increases the risk of hospitalizations and TdP. This suggests that a majority of patients can simply be managed with rate control and, if indicated, anticoagulation.

13. Evaluate the use of an antiarrhythmic agent to maintain J.K. in normal sinus rhythm. What are the risks and benefits of the different antiarrhythmic agents used for this purpose?

Whether J.K. should be placed on an antiarrhythmic is a judgment of benefit versus risk. There is no doubt that various antiarrhythmics can prevent episodes of AF. However, J.K.'s need for antiarrhythmic therapy should be weighed against the potential for adverse effects. Overall, both strategies lead to similar rates of overall mortality, but the risk of hospitalization and TdP is higher with rhythm control. Hence, if adequate rate control can control J.K.'s symptoms, that is the preferred strategy. If symptoms are limiting his quality of life or adequate rate control cannot be achieved, rhythm control is a valuable option. In this case the physician has chosen rhythm control, and there are no compelling reasons to try to persuade him otherwise given the symptomatic nature of the AF episodes. The question now becomes how to choose the best antiarrhythmic agent for J.K. To do this, the efficacy and adverse effect profiles for each agent should be reviewed.

Class IA, IC, and III antiarrhythmics (see Table 20-2 for electrophysiologic and ECG effects and Table 20-3 for pharmacokinetics and side effects) prevent the recurrence of AF. Quinidine, flecainide, sotalol (Betapace AF), and dofetilide are approved by the FDA for maintenance of sinus rhythm; propafenone and amiodarone are commonly used as well.

Quinidine.   If quinidine is used, sustained-release (SR) formulations such as quinidine sulfate (Quinidex) or quinidine gluconate (Quinaglute) are preferred because they produce smaller peak-to-trough fluctuations than rapid-release products and can be administered twice daily to enhance compliance.[57] Nausea, vomiting, and diarrhea occurring early in therapy are reported in up to 30% of patients receiving quinidine, requiring 10% to discontinue therapy. A unique symptom complex referred to as cinchonism occurs when quinidine blood levels exceed 5 μg/mL. This disorder is characterized by disturbed hearing (tinnitus, decreased auditory acuity), visual abnormalities (blurred vision, altered color perception, diplopia), and central nervous system (CNS) alterations (headache, confusion, delirium). Quinidine raises digoxin serum concentrations, which is important in J.K., but it is also a potent inhibitor of the CYP2D6 isoenzyme, which affects the metabolism of propafenone, carvedilol, codeine, and desipramine. HF and older age also raise quinidine concentrations, which would be a confounder for J.K. Use of quinidine is limited to third-line therapy for this indication based on a meta-analysis showing improved maintenance of sinus rhythm but nonsignificant increases in mortality (3.2% mortality versus 0.8%).[58]

Flecainide and Propafenone.   The class IC agents flecainide and propafenone are effective in suppressing AF.[59–63] The efficacy rate may be as high as 61% to 92% for flecainide.[64] Flecainide and possibly other class IC agents may cause arrhythmias, especially in patients with structural heart disease, and they should be avoided in such patients. Propafenone, a class IC agent with β-blocking properties, is as efficacious as flecainide and is relatively safe in patients without ischemic heart disease and an ejection fraction above 35%; it may be preferred in patients who require additional AV blockade. In a direct comparison with flecainide (200 to 300 mg/day), propafenone (450 to 900 mg/day) was equally safe and effective. Over 12 months, a similar percentage of patients (approximately 12% in each group) did not have adequate control of their arrhythmia. Adverse events were comparable with those associated with propafenone and occurred in 10.3% of patients on flecainide and 7.7% of patients on propafenone. Of all the adverse events noted, only one patient who was receiving propafenone developed a ventricular arrhythmia. Another 1-year comparative study of propafenone versus flecainide demonstrated similar efficacy, but this study showed a trend toward better tolerability in the flecainide group.[65,66] In comparison with quinidine (average dose 1,067 mg), propafenone (average dose 615 mg) was significantly better at reducing the occurrence of AF and at reducing the ventricular rate when AF occurred. A 75% reduction in symptomatic arrhythmic attacks occurred in 75% of the propafenone group versus 46% of the quinidine group. Both therapies were well tolerated, with 4% of patients in both groups withdrawing. Dizziness was the most common reason for discontinuation in the propafenone group, whereas GI disturbances were most common in the quinidine group.[67]

Sotalol, Amiodarone and Dofetilide. Class III agents (sotalol, dofetilide, and amiodarone) prolong refractoriness in the atria, ventricle, AV node, and accessory pathway tissue and can prevent recurrence of AF. The efficacy of sotalol in delaying the recurrence of AF was evaluated in a double-blind, placebo-controlled, multicenter, randomized trial that enrolled 253 patients with AF or atrial flutter.[68] The median times to recurrence were 27, 106, 229, and 175 days with placebo, sotalol 160 mg/day (divided in two doses), sotalol 240 mg/day (divided in two doses), and sotalol 320 mg/day (divided in two doses), respectively. In one comparative study, sotalol was as effective as quinidine in maintaining sinus rhythm after cardioversion.[69] Because of its β-blocking property, sotalol can reduce the ventricular rate and may be better tolerated than quinidine. However, because sotalol may be arrhythmogenic in high doses, the risk of inducing TdP has prompted its manufacturer to mandate a minimum of 3 days of ECG monitoring in a properly equipped facility during therapy initiation.[70] Further, during initiation and titration, QTc intervals should be monitored 2 to 4 hours after each dose, and sotalol is contraindicated in patients with a Cl_{cr} below 40 mL/min. In a comparative study versus propafenone, sotalol had similar efficacy (79% of patients on propafenone versus 76% on sotalol) and tolerability (4.8% of patients on propafenone had intolerable side effects versus 10.5% on sotalol). Bradycardia, dizziness, and GI disturbances were the most common intolerable side effects.[71]

Amiodarone is more effective than quinidine,[72] sotalol,[73] and propafenone.[74] The Canadian Trial of Atrial Fibrillation (CTAF) compared the ability of low-dose amiodarone (200 mg/day) versus propafenone (450 to 600 mg/day) and sotalol (160 to 320 mg/day) to prevent recurrence of atrial fibrillation in 403 patients with a recent episode of AF (within the preceding 6 months).[73] After a mean follow-up of 16 months, 35% of the amiodarone-treated patients had a recurrence of AF versus 63% in the combined group with sotalol and propafenone ($P < 0.001$). Low doses of amiodarone (200 to 400 mg/day) have a high rate of efficacy and a reduced incidence of the serious adverse effects often associated with high doses of this drug.[74] In view of its unusual pharmacokinetics and potential serious adverse effects, however (see Table 20-3 and Question 29), amiodarone is usually reserved for patients with HF, where it has specific safety data, or when other agents such as sotalol, propafenone, or dofetilide have failed.[6,75]

Dofetilide is another class III agent that has been shown to be effective for the maintenance of sinus rhythm after conversion and safe in heart failure patients (see Question 8 for dosing in renal impairment, critical drug interactions, and monitoring).

In view of J.K.'s new onset of HF and frequent uncomfortable episodes of AF, dofetilide and amiodarone are logical first choices with proven efficacy and studies in HF patients showing relative safety.

Stroke Prevention
ASPIRIN AND WARFARIN

14. J.K. is discharged from the hospital on dofetilide 500 μg BID, which is appropriate given his Cl_{cr} of 92 mL/min. He has been doing fine for 2 weeks after discharge. Should J.K. remain on warfarin therapy? Should aspirin be added or substituted?

Patients with nonvalvular and valvular AF have a 5- and 17-fold increased risk for stroke compared with patients without AF, respectively.[2,3] Stroke can lead to death or significant neurologic disability in up to 71% of patients, with an annual recurrence rate as high as 10%.[76] In three large, randomized trials, patients with nonvalvular atrial fibrillation benefited from antithrombotic therapy.[77–79] In the Stroke Prevention in Atrial Fibrillation (SPAF) study, both aspirin 325 mg/day and warfarin (titrated to an INR 2.0 to 4.5) reduced the risk of stroke significantly with an acceptable level of hemorrhagic complications.[79] The results of SPAF II, a direct comparison of warfarin and aspirin, indicated that warfarin was more effective than aspirin in preventing stroke.[80] These results were verified by the Copenhagen AFASAK study, which found warfarin to be significantly better than aspirin and placebo at preventing cerebral emboli and overall vascular deaths (cerebral and cardiovascular).[81]

Although greater efficacy was derived from warfarin therapy in the SPAF II study, a higher incidence of bleeding complications was noted with warfarin in patients older than 75 years of age, especially those with risk factors for bleeding (previous thromboembolism, GI or genitourinary bleeding).[80] Subsequent analysis of the first SPAF trial determined that patients below 60 years of age without hypertension, recent heart failure, or prior thromboembolism had a low risk of thromboembolism and did not benefit from warfarin therapy.[82] In view of the beneficial effect of aspirin and the bleeding risk of warfarin, a subsequent study was carried out comparing warfarin therapy, maintained at an INR of 2.0 to 3.0, with a low-dose therapy (INR 1.2 to 1.5) plus aspirin 325 mg. This study was stopped early owing to the significantly increased incidence of primary events (ischemic stroke and systemic embolism) in the combination therapy group. The rates of major bleeding were not significantly reduced by combination therapy.

This suggests that patients younger than 60 who have "lone" AF should be maintained on aspirin alone. This is because the bleeding risk with warfarin is maintained, but the benefits are reduced. These patients have a better risk/benefit profile with aspirin therapy. Older patients and those with thromboembolic risk factors should receive warfarin since the benefits of therapy far outweigh the risks, and the patient should maintain an INR of 2.0 to 3.0.[78–83]

Because J.K. has a low bleeding risk (no history of thromboembolism, GI or genitourinary bleeding, no diastolic hypertension) and an increased risk of stroke due to his age (66 years), he should continue to receive warfarin therapy without concomitant aspirin. Even though J.K. is in normal sinus rhythm on dofetilide at this time, in the AFFIRM trial, only

73% and 63% of patients remained in sinus rhythm at 3 and 5 years, respectively.[54] These patients did not necessarily know when they went back into AF.

An oral direct thrombin inhibitor called ximalagatran is being investigated for AF versus warfarin, but results from these studies were unavailable when this chapter was written. The reader may want to review the literature to determine if this option would offer advantages or disadvantages for patients such as J.K. once more is known.

15. M.P. is a 38-year-old woman who has had chronic atrial flutter for the past 2 years. She has no other medical history and is taking metoprolol 50 mg BID. She does not want to take the drug any more because it reduces her exercise tolerance. Is there a nonpharmacologic therapy for atrial flutter? Does the treatment of atrial flutter differ from the treatment of AF? Is radiofrequency catheter ablation an acceptable nonpharmacologic option for M.P.?

As mentioned previously, atrial flutter is an unstable rhythm that often reverts to sinus rhythm or progresses to AF. If atrial flutter is episodic, its underlying cause should be identified and treated if possible. If a patient remains in atrial flutter, the treatment goals (control of ventricular rate, return to normal sinus rhythm) are the same as those for AF. Similar agents and doses can be used to control the ventricular response. Chemical conversion, low-energy (<50 J) DC cardioversion, or rapid atrial pacing may acutely convert atrial flutter back to sinus rhythm, but the recurrence of atrial flutter is high. Anticoagulation is not usually needed in chronic atrial flutter because the atria are still able to contract.

Radiofrequency catheter ablation therapy is a nonpharmacologic treatment of atrial flutter. Electrophysiologic studies are performed initially to determine the optimal site for ablation. Various sections of the atria and pulmonary veins (where they intersect with the atria) are probed with a catheter that delivers cardiac pacing. Once an area is stimulated with pacing and an atrial ectopic/re-entrant focus is recognized, the area is ablated. Ablation destroys atrial or pulmonary vein tissue integral to the initiation or maintenance of the atrial flutter by delivering electrical energy over electrodes on the catheter. This procedure is successful in 75% to 90% of cases and can be recommended for patients with atrial flutter who are drug-resistant or drug-intolerant, or do not desire long-term therapy.

Radiofrequency ablation therapy may be suitable for M.P. However, if exercise intolerance is her primary complaint, this can be relieved by switching M.P. to another drug such as verapamil.[84,94]

Atrial Fibrillation After Bypass Surgery
β-BLOCKERS AND AMIODARONE

16. H.L., a 55-year-old woman with triple vessel disease, is scheduled for coronary artery bypass surgery (CABG) in 3 days. Her medical history includes exercise-induced angina treated with nitrates, metoprolol, and diltiazem. What is the incidence of AF after CABG surgery? Should H.L. be treated with a drug to prevent the postoperative occurrence of AF?

Over 750,000 CABG or heart valve surgeries (cardiothoracic surgery) are performed annually in the United States.[85] Without prophylaxis, AF develops in up to 65% of patients,

and two thirds of the cases occur on postoperative day 2 or 3.[86] The underlying mechanism is unknown, but may be related to sympathetic activation, pericarditis, or atrial dilation from volume overload.[87] The arrhythmia usually converts spontaneously, but can result in temporary symptomatology (lightheadedness), a higher risk of cerebrovascular accident, and a longer hospital stay.

β-Blockers were the first proven prophylactic strategy against post-cardiothoracic surgery AF. In a meta-analysis of clinical trials, β-blockers reduced postoperative AF, but the incidence remained at about 30%.[88]

The Atrial Fibrillation Suppression Trial (AFIST) evaluated the use of amiodarone in addition to standard of care (e.g., use of a β-blocker) versus standard of care alone.[88] Patients with ≥5 days before surgery received a total of 7 g amiodarone over 5 preoperative days (200 mg three times daily) and 5 postoperative days (400 mg twice daily) or matching placebo. Those with <5 days before surgery received a total of 6 g amiodarone, given as 400 mg QID 1 day prior to surgery, 600 mg BID on the day of surgery, and 400 mg BID for 4 postoperative days, or matching placebo. The 30-day risk of AF was 41% less, symptomatic AF was reduced by 77%, and cerebrovascular accidents were decreased by 76% with amiodarone plus standard therapy versus standard therapy alone.[88] When each amiodarone-loading regimen was evaluated separately versus placebo, the 5-day preoperative loading group had better qualitative results than the 1-day preoperative loading group.[89]

In the recently presented AFIST II trial, a hybrid IV and oral amiodarone regimen was evaluated versus placebo. In this study IV amiodarone (1,050 mg) given over 24 hours after surgery and then oral drug (400 mg three times daily) was given for 4 postoperative days (equal to 7 g oral drug given over 5 days). Amiodarone or placebo was in addition to standard-of-care treatment with β-blockers. In this study, amiodarone reduced the 30-day risk of AF by 42.7% and symptomatic AF by 68.3%.[90]

17. H.L.'s metoprolol therapy is discontinued and she is not treated prophylactically. She undergoes the surgery without complications. On postoperative day 2, she develops AF with a ventricular response rate of 142 beats/min and a BP of 126/75 mm Hg. How should H.L. be managed?

The decision to treat H.L.'s AF depends on her heart rate and how well she tolerates the arrhythmia; antiarrhythmics are often not needed in the short-term management of this disorder. For many years, digoxin has been used to control the ventricular response. However, following surgery, patients have a high sympathetic tone, and digoxin often is ineffective. β-Blockers are effective and preferred if there are no other contraindications.[91] They are especially preferred in patients like H.L. who have been taking β-blockers preoperatively, because withdrawal of β-blockers can increase the occurrence of postoperative AF.[91,92]

H.L.'s rapid ventricular rate should be controlled. Propranolol 1 mg IV every 5 minutes (up to 0.1 mg/kg), metoprolol 5 mg IV repeated at 2-minute intervals (up to a total dose of 15 mg), esmolol 0.5 mg/kg bolus followed by a continuous infusion at a rate of 50 to 300 μg/kg per minute, or verapamil 5 to 10 mg IV every 1 to 4 hours are all options for H.L., who appears to be hemodynamically stable. If one of these therapy choices is ineffective, a loading dose of digoxin can be administered IV as adjunctive therapy with the β-blocker or verapamil.

18. Metoprolol is started and ventricular rate control is achieved 4 minutes after administering the second 5-mg dose. The patient receives 50 mg oral metoprolol therapy an hour later, converts to normal sinus rhythm spontaneously the next day, and is preparing for discharge. The metoprolol therapy is discontinued. Should an antiarrhythmic agent be initiated for H.L. to prevent recurrence of AF?

Using prophylactic antiarrhythmic agents after discharge in patients with AF within a few days of CABG surgery does not seem to protect against recurrent AF. In one trial, all patients with AF after CABG surgery were given verapamil, quinidine, amiodarone, or placebo at discharge and were then followed with Holter monitoring for 90 days. There was no difference in the occurrence of AF between the placebo group (3.3% incidence) and the other groups (6.7% incidence for each treatment group).[93] Since H.L. was treated with metoprolol for angina pectoris before the surgery, therapy can be reinitiated if the anginal pain resumes with exercise.

Paroxysmal Supraventricular Tachycardia

Clinical Presentation

19. B.J., a 32-year-old woman, presents to the emergency department (ED) complaining of fatigue and palpitations. She has had similar episodes approximately twice a year for the past 2 years, but has not sought medical attention for them. She is in no apparent distress and has a temperature of 98.0°F, HR of 205 beats/min, BP of 95/60 mm Hg, and respiratory rate (RR) of 12 breaths/min. Her ECG (Fig. 20-7) shows regular rhythm with HR of 185. The P waves cannot be found and the QRS complex is 110 msec (normal, <120). The diagnosis is PSVT. What is the clinical presentation of PSVT, and what are the consequences of this arrhythmia?

PSVT often has a sudden onset and termination. At the time of PSVT, the heart rate is usually 180 to 200 beats/min. As illustrated by B.J., patients experience palpitations as well as nervousness and anxiety. In patients with a rapid ventricular rate, dizziness and syncope (near-fainting) can occur, and the rhythm may degenerate to other serious arrhythmias. Depending on the underlying heart function, angina, HF, or shock may be precipitated. It has not been demonstrated that patients with episodes of PSVT are at an increased risk of stroke.

Arrhythmogenesis—Re-entry

20. What is the arrhythmogenic mechanism of PSVT?

AV nodal re-entry is the most common mechanism of paroxysmal supraventricular arrhythmias (see Fig. 20-4). Under certain conditions, such as following an acute MI, atrial impulses will be blocked in one of the two AV nodal pathways in a unidirectional manner (antegrade block). After the impulse reaches the distal end of one pathway, it will conduct in a retrograde fashion through the other pathway, setting up a circular movement causing tachycardia.

Reciprocating tachycardias occur when there is an accessory pathway. Orthodromic AV reciprocating tachycardia is a re-entry tachycardia involving antegrade conduction through the AV node and retrograde conduction through a bypass tract. Antidromic AV reciprocating tachycardia is a re-entry tachycardia involving antegrade conduction through an accessory pathway and retrograde conduction via the AV node or another accessory pathway (e.g., WPW syndrome) (Fig. 20-8). Antidromic reciprocating tachycardias manifest as wide QRS complexes resembling ventricular arrhythmias.

Treatment

21. B.J. tries the Valsalva maneuver and her ventricular rate is reduced to 198 beats/min; the other parameters are unchanged. She is given adenosine 6 mg as an IV bolus, administered over 1 minute, with no effect on the PSVT rate. Another dose of adenosine 12 mg has no effect. No side effects are noted from therapy. What treatment options can be used if B.J. is hemodynamically unstable? What is the Valsalva maneuver? What is a probable reason for B.J.'s unresponsiveness to adenosine? Are there any drug interactions that might diminish adenosine's effect?

NONDRUG TREATMENT
Valsalva Maneuver. Although her BP is low at 95/60 mm Hg, B.J. is maintaining an adequate perfusion pressure, so nondrug treatment or vagal maneuvers should be attempted first. Two common vagal techniques are pressure over the bifurcation of the internal and external carotid arteries and the Valsalva maneuver (forcible exhalation against a closed glottis; similar to bearing down to have a bowel movement). The increase in pressure induced by these maneuvers is sensed by the baroreceptors, causing a reflex decrease in sympathetic tone and an increase in vagal tone. The increase in vagal tone will increase refractoriness and slow conduction in the AV node, thereby slowing the heart rate; the arrhythmia will ter-

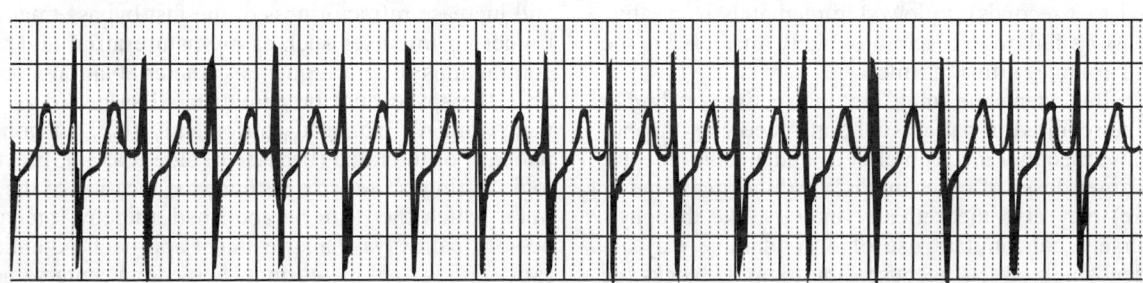

FIGURE 20-7 Supraventricular tachycardia. (Reproduced with permission from reference 204.)

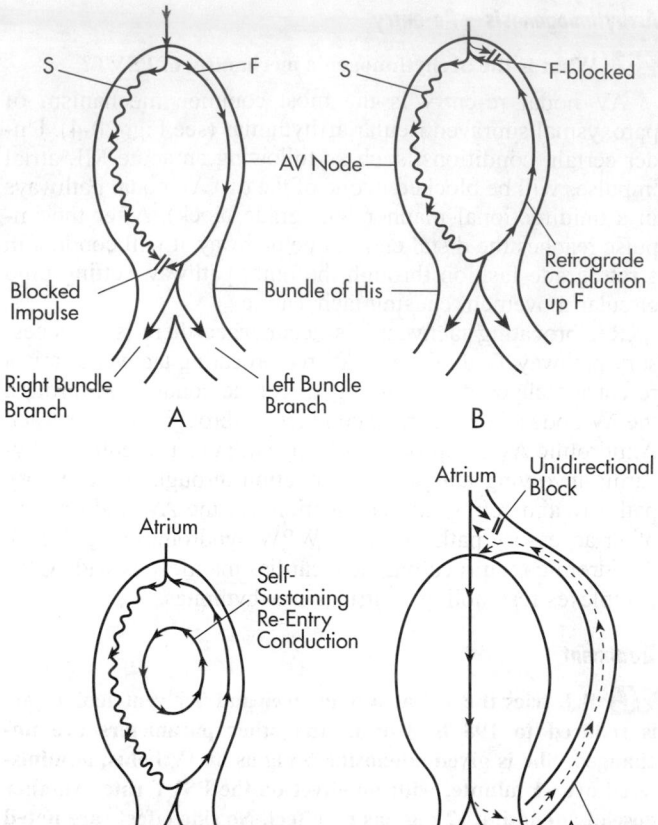

FIGURE 20-8 The AV node in PSVT and WPW syndrome.

minate in 10% to 30% of cases.[94] If B.J. is hemodynamically unstable or becomes hemodynamically unstable, she should receive synchronous DC cardioversion.

DRUG THERAPY

Adenosine. Drug therapy involves blocking the AV node, because most PSVT rhythms involve a re-entry circuit within this area. Adenosine, a purine nucleoside that exerts a transient negative chronotropic and dromotropic effect on cardiac pacemaker tissue,[95] is considered the drug of choice for the acute treatment of PSVT because of its rapid and brief effect. An initial 6-mg IV bolus is given; if this is unsuccessful within 2 minutes, it can be followed by one or two 12-mg IV boluses, up to a maximum of 30 mg. Because of its short half-life (9 seconds), adenosine should be administered as a rapid bolus (over 1 to 3 seconds), followed immediately by a saline flush. Thus, B.J.'s failure to respond is likely attributed to the prolonged (1-minute) infusion time.

Theoretically, adenosine may be ineffective or higher doses may be required in patients who are receiving theophylline, because theophylline is an effective adenosine receptor blocker.[96] Larger doses of other methylxanthines (caffeine or theobromine) may also theoretically interact like theophylline. Conversely, concomitant use of dipyridamole may accentuate adenosine's effects because dipyridamole blocks the adenosine uptake (and subsequent clearance).[96]

22. B.J. is given 12 mg adenosine IV over 2 seconds, followed by a 20-mL normal saline flush. Thirty seconds later, she complains of chest tightness and pressure. Is B.J. experiencing a heart attack? Is this response a result of a drug interaction between adenosine and another medication?

B.J. is experiencing a common side effect of adenosine.[96] Patients receiving adenosine should be warned that they may feel transient chest heaviness, flushing, or a feeling of anxiety. SOB and wheezing may be observed in patients with asthma. Lower doses are usually required in heart transplant patients, and caution should be observed when administering adenosine to these patients.

Calcium Channel Blockers.

23. B.J. is still in PSVT. What other acute therapeutic options should be considered at this time?

Nondihydropyridine calcium channel blockers, verapamil and diltiazem, can be used in patients with PSVT. Verapamil (2.5 to 5 mg IV given over 2 minutes) achieves peak therapeutic effects in 3 to 5 minutes after dosing and can be repeated at 10- to 15-minute intervals to a maximum dose of 20 mg if needed. The elderly should receive the verapamil infusion over 3 minutes. Patients aged 8 to 15 should receive 0.1 to 0.3 mg/kg as an IV bolus over 1 minute. A repeat dose of 0.1 to 0.2 mg/kg can be administered 15 to 30 minutes later if the effect was inadequate.[96] Diltiazem is given as a 0.25-mg/kg IV bolus over 2 minutes, and a second bolus of 0.35 mg/kg can be given 15 minutes later if the effect is inadequate. Both of these calcium channel blockers have an 85% conversion rate.[97] However, verapamil should not be used in patients with wide complex tachycardia of unknown origin, because it may lead to hemodynamic compromise and, potentially, VF.

β-Blockers and digoxin can be used if calcium channel blockers or adenosine fail.

24. B.J. is given 5 mg IV verapamil over 1 minute, followed by an additional 5 mg 10 minutes later. She converts to normal sinus rhythm 3 minutes after the second dose. Because she has experienced symptoms that could be attributed to PSVT in the past, she may be a candidate for chronic therapy to slow conduction and increase refractoriness at the AV node. Which agents have been evaluated for this indication? Is there a role for radiofrequency catheter ablation therapy for PSVT like there was for atrial flutter?

On a long-term basis, PSVT is managed with agents that slow conduction and increase refractoriness in the AV node, thereby preventing a rapid ventricular response. These include oral verapamil, diltiazem, β-blockers, or digoxin. Class IA, IC, and III agents are used occasionally to slow conduction and increase refractoriness of the fast bypass tract to prevent triggering impulses such as premature atrial and ventricular contractions. Radiofrequency catheter ablation is indicated if drug therapy cannot be administered safely (e.g., in a pregnant woman), managed conveniently (e.g., in noncompliant patient), or tolerated (because of side effects). Electrophysiologic testing is used to determine the location of the re-entrant tract, which then can be abolished, thereby interrupting accessory pathways. This treatment approach potentially is curative and is used increasingly in medical centers under the direction of a specially trained electrophysiologist.

B.J. has had a few episodes of PSVT in the past, but has not been on any suppressive therapy. This history suggests that chronic suppressive therapy should be tried first. Because she responded to IV verapamil, oral SR verapamil (Isoptin SR) was prescribed at a dosage of 240 mg/day.

Wolff-Parkinson-White Syndrome

25. **M.B., a 35-year-old man, presents to the ED with a chief complaint of chest palpitations for 4 hours. He relates a history of many similar self-terminating episodes since he was a teenager. He took an unknown medication 5 years ago that decreased the occurrence of the palpitations, but he stopped taking it due to side effects. M.B.'s vital signs are BP, 96/68 mm Hg; pulse, 226 beats/min, irregular; RR, 15 breaths/min; and temperature, 98.7°F. A rhythm strip confirms AF, with a QRS width varying from 0.08 to 0.14 sec. To control the ventricular rate, 10 mg IV verapamil is administered over 2 minutes. Within 2 minutes, VF is noted on the monitor. M.B. is defibrillated to normal sinus rhythm. A subsequent ECG demonstrates a P-R interval of 100 msec (normal, 120 to 200) and delta waves, compatible with WPW. What is WPW syndrome?**

WPW is a pre-excitation syndrome in which there is an accessory bypass tract (known as a Kent bundle) connecting the atria to the ventricle (see Fig. 20-8). An impulse can travel down this pathway and excite the ventricle before the expected regular impulse through the AV node arrives (hence the term pre-excitation). If there is antegrade conduction over the bypass tract while the patient is in normal sinus rhythm, the ECG will demonstrate a short P-R interval (<100 msec), a delta wave that represents a fused complex from pre-excitation, and the regular QRS complex following AV conduction. WPW can occur in children and adults without overt cardiac disease. Paroxysmal AV reciprocating tachycardias and AF occurs in these patients at a higher incidence than in the general population of the same age.[98] Similar to M.B., the rapid heart rate experienced during the tachycardia may cause palpitations, light-headedness, and fatigue. When patients with WPW develop AF, there is a danger that impulses will be conducted directly to the ventricle, causing a rapid ventricular rate that may evolve into VF.

26. **Why did verapamil cause VF in M.B.? What drug or drugs would be appropriate for M.B., and what drugs should be avoided?**

Verapamil can block AV conduction by increasing the effective refractory period, allowing all impulses from the atrial area to conduct down the bypass (Kent) tract. Because M.B. had AF, the rapid atrial impulses were conducted directly down the bypass tract to the ventricle, causing VF. In addition, verapamil may enhance conduction over the accessory pathway by shortening its effective refractory period. Also, peripheral vasodilation can induce a reflex sympathetic discharge that can, in turn, decrease the effective refractory period of the accessory pathway.[99,100]

The most common presentation of WPW syndrome involves normal antegrade conduction down the AV node and retrograde conduction back up through the accessory pathway. This will manifest as orthodromic reciprocating re-entrant tachycardia. Thus, drugs that inhibit antegrade impulse conduction through the AV node (e.g., verapamil, digoxin) will terminate the re-entrant tachycardia and can be suitable in the absence of AF. The less common variety of WPW is antegrade conduction through the accessory pathway with retrograde transmission up through the AV node, resulting in an antidromic re-entrant tachycardia. Similarly, AV nodal blocking agents will terminate this type of re-entrant tachycardia. In some situations, such as experienced by M.B., rapid AF with an accessory pathway occurs, which can lead to VF and cardiac arrest.

The antiarrhythmic drugs used to treat patients with AF who have an accessory pathway, such as M.B., include those that depress conduction and increase the effective refractory period of the fast sodium channel–dependent tissue of the accessory pathway. This includes most class I antiarrhythmics, with the class IB agents being least effective. Procainamide, an FDA-approved drug for this indication, is a reasonable first choice.[101] Propafenone and flecainide are also effective and may be preferred over procainamide.[102–105] Amiodarone and sotalol may also be effective, but clinical experience is limited.[106–108] Radiofrequency ablation of the bypass tract is used more frequently for these patients to prevent VF.

Further therapy for M.B. may not be useful at this time. However, if he has recurrent AF or other symptomatology associated with WPW, radiofrequency catheter ablation or drug therapy as outlined previously could be indicated.

CONDUCTION BLOCKS

Various arrhythmias can result from blockage of impulse conduction. These can occur above the ventricle, such as first-, second-, and third-degree (complete) AV block. Others, such as right or left bundle branch block (RBBB or LBBB) and trifascicular block, originate below the bifurcation of the His bundle. Although conduction blocks can be classified as either supraventricular or ventricular arrhythmias, they are discussed as a separate group because their mechanism of arrhythmogenesis is similar and their treatment is different from other arrhythmias.

27. **H.T., a 63-year-old man, was admitted to the coronary care unit (CCU) 12 hours ago with an acute inferior wall MI. He has remained stable. On admission, he had the rhythm strip shown in Figure 20-9 (left bundle branch block). Twelve hours later, it has changed to the rhythm strip shown in Figure 20-10 (Wenckebach or type I, second-degree AV block). Are these rhythms potentially hazardous to H.T.? How is second-degree AV block different from first- or third-degree AV block?**

H.T.'s rhythm strip revealed a diagnosis of LBBB. Bundle branch block occurs when the electrical impulse cannot be conducted along the left or right fascicle of the His-Purkinje

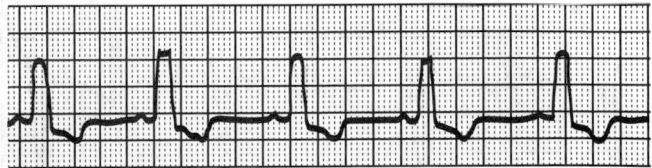

FIGURE 20-9 Bundle branch block. Note that the QRS interval is prolonged. A 12-lead ECG is required to make the diagnosis of left bundle branch block. (Reproduced with permission from reference 204.)

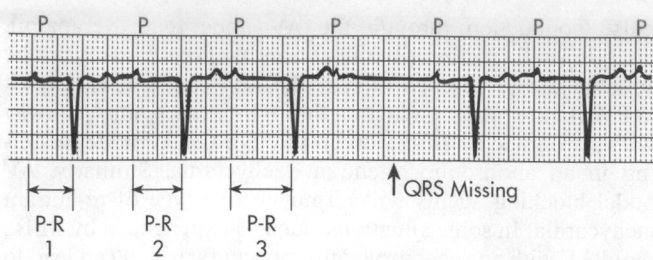

FIGURE 20-10 *Second-degree AV block type I (Wenckebach).* The P-R interval progressively prolongs until, after the third complex, a QRS complex is not conducted. (Reproduced with permission from reference 204.)

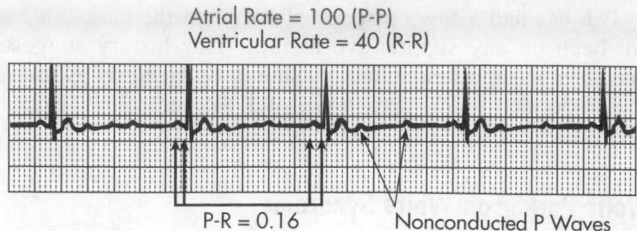

FIGURE 20-11 *Second-degree AV block type II (3:1 fixed block).*

system (see Fig. 20-1). In H.T., the impulse travels down the right bundle normally, and the right ventricle contracts at the normal time. The left bundle is blocked and, therefore, the left side is depolarized from an impulse conducted from the right ventricle. This impulse must travel through atypical conduction tissues (with slower conduction), and hence the left side depolarizes later. This is revealed on the ECG by a widened QRS complex. Bundle branch blocks, particularly in the left fascicle, are associated with coronary artery disease, systemic hypertension, aortic valve stenosis, and cardiomyopathy.[109] Typically, they do not lead to clinical cardiac dysfunction on their own. Because H.T. has LBBB, he can develop complete heart block (third-degree block) if for any reason his right fascicle is damaged.

First-degree AV block usually is asymptomatic. The ECG will show P waves with a prolonged P-R interval (normal, >200 msec), but each wave is followed by a normal QRS complex. First-degree AV block is a common finding in patients taking digoxin, verapamil, or other drugs that slow AV conduction.

Second-degree heart block consists of two types. Mobitz type I (Wenckebach) is characterized by progressive lengthening of the P-R interval with each beat and a corresponding shortening of the R-R interval until finally an impulse is not conducted; the cycle then starts over again. Mobitz type II (Fig. 20-11) impulse conduction is blocked in a fixed, regular pattern (e.g., 3:1 block, where for every three P waves, only one is conducted).

Third-degree heart block (complete heart block) occurs when none of the impulses from the SA node are conducted to the ventricles. During third-degree block, the ventricle must develop its own pacemaker (escape rhythm), which may be too slow to provide adequate cardiac output, causing the patient to become symptomatic. A mechanical pacemaker is needed for

treatment of third-degree AV block. AV blocks can be caused by drugs, acute MI, amyloidosis, and congenital abnormalities.[110]

Atropine

28. **How should H.T.'s heart block be treated?**

H.T. is experiencing a Wenckebach rhythm, which often is transient following an inferior wall MI. As long as he is hemodynamically stable, he should be monitored closely. If his heart rate and BP drop, atropine 0.5 mg IV bolus (maximum 2 mg) can increase the heart rate. This is only a short-term therapy; if the hemodynamic compromise persists, a pacemaker must be inserted to initiate the impulse to control the heart rate.

VENTRICULAR ARRHYTHMIAS

Recognition and Definition

Ventricular arrhythmias arise from irritable ectopic foci within the ventricular myocardium. Impulses from these ectopic foci generate wide, bizarre-looking QRS complexes leading to PVCs (Fig. 20-12). PVCs can arise from the same ectopic site (unifocal) or can be multifocal in origin. They can be simple (e.g., isolated or infrequent) or complex (e.g., R on T, in which the R wave of a PVC falls on top of a normal T wave). Other presentations include runs of two or more beats, bigeminy (every other beat is a PVC), or trigeminy (every third beat is a PVC). Three consecutive PVCs usually are defined as ventricular tachycardia (VT), which can be nonsustained or sustained. Ventricular flutter, VF, and TdP are other serious forms of ventricular arrhythmias (Figs. 20-13 to 20-16). The presentation, etiology, treatment, and ion channels associated with TdP are discussed separately.

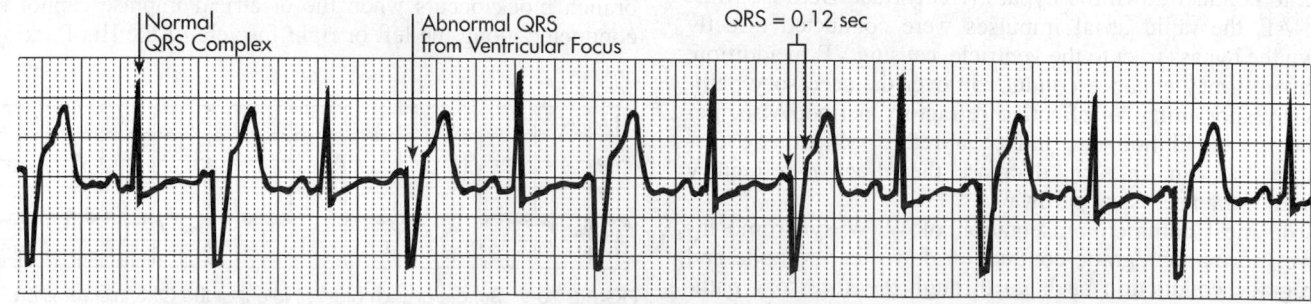

FIGURE 20-12 *Premature ventricular contraction (PVC).* Every other beat is a premature ventricular (ectopic) contraction.

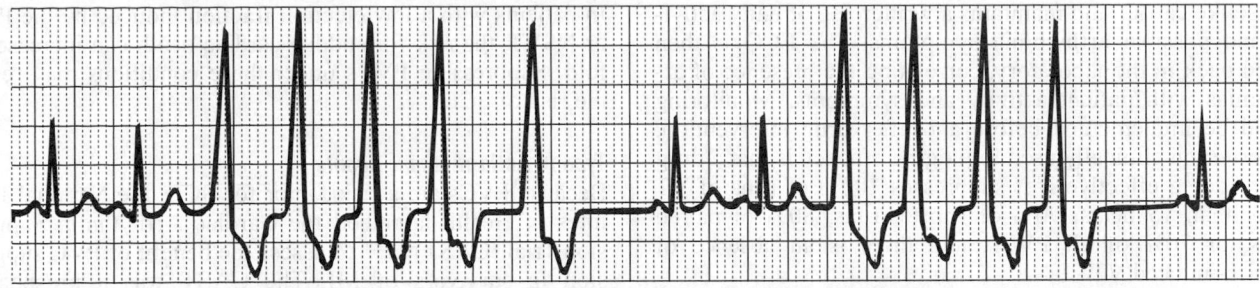

FIGURE 20-13 Nonsustained ventricular tachycardia. (Reproduced with permission from reference 205.)

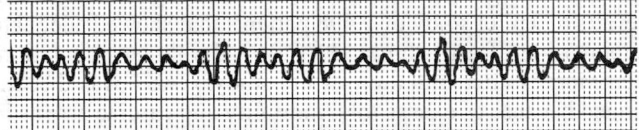

FIGURE 20-14 Ventricular fibrillation.

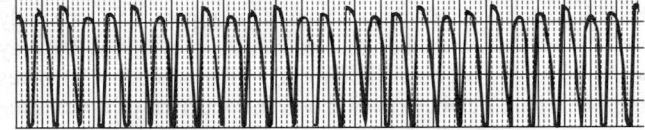

FIGURE 20-15 Sustained ventricular tachycardia.

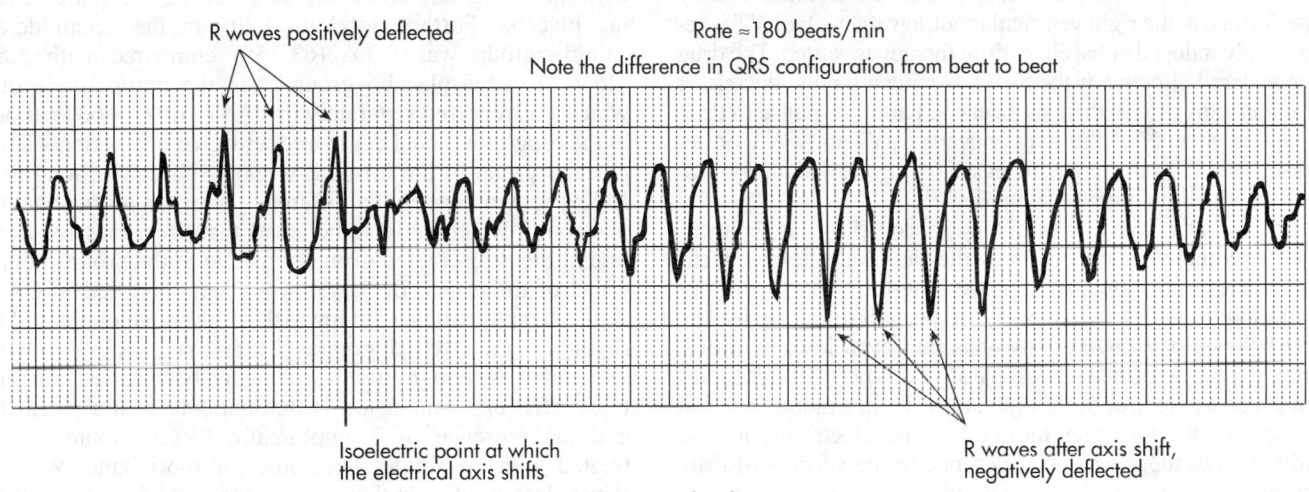

R waves positively deflected

Rate ≈180 beats/min
Note the difference in QRS configuration from beat to beat

Isoelectric point at which
the electrical axis shifts

R waves after axis shift,
negatively deflected

FIGURE 20-16 Torsades de pointes.

Nonsustained ventricular tachycardia (NSVT) (see Fig. 20-13) commonly is defined as three or more consecutive PVCs lasting <30 seconds and terminating spontaneously. Sustained VT (SuVT) is defined as consecutive PVCs lasting >30 seconds, with a rate usually in the range of 150 to 200 beats/min. P waves are lost in the QRS complex and are indiscernible. SuVT (see Fig. 20-15) is a serious development because it can degenerate into VF. Ventricular flutter is characterized by sustained, rapid, regular ventricular beats (normal, >250/min) and usually degenerates into VF. VF (see Fig. 20-14) is characterized by irregular, disorganized, rapid beats with no identifiable P waves or QRS complexes. It is thought to be triggered by multiple re-entrant wavelets in the ventricle. There is no effective cardiac output in patients with VF.[109,110]

Etiology

Common factors that cause ventricular arrhythmias are ischemia, the presence of organic heart disease, exercise, metabolic or electrolyte imbalance (e.g., acidosis, hypokalemia or hyperkalemia, hypomagnesemia), or drugs (digitalis, sympathomimetic amines, antiarrhythmics). It is essential to identify and remove any treatable cause (e.g., metabolic or electrolyte imbalance and proarrhythmic drugs) before initiating antiarrhythmic drug therapy.

Evaluation of Life-Threatening Ventricular Arrhythmias

An episode of life-threatening ventricular arrhythmia (i.e., SuVT, TdP, VF) carries a significant risk of morbidity and mortality. Adequate documentation of the arrhythmia and its suppression by either drugs or a mechanical device are essential. Patients suspected of having or documented to have symptoms of a life-threatening arrhythmia (e.g., syncope, out-of-hospital cardiac arrest) should be admitted to the hospital and evaluated. At present, two approaches are used to evaluate the arrhythmia and the effectiveness of therapy: ambulatory (Holter) monitoring and electrophysiologic studies.[109,110]

Holter Monitoring

Holter monitoring is continuous ECG monitoring, usually for 24 to 48 hours, with or without exercise (e.g., treadmill exercise). The patient wears a portable ECG monitoring device in a purselike carrier and maintains a written log of daily activities and possible arrhythmia symptoms. The ECG is then played back in the laboratory, correlating the presence of arrhythmias with patient activity and symptoms. Monitoring should be implemented before and after drug intervention. One criterion clinically used in judging efficacy is that a drug is considered effective if it suppresses 100% of runs of VT longer than 15 beats, 90% of shorter runs, 80% of paired PVCs, or 70% of all PVCs, and there is an absence of exercise-induced VT.[111]

Electrophysiologic Studies

Electrophysiologic studies are the second approach in evaluating the efficacy of antiarrhythmic drugs. This approach is especially useful in patients with sporadic ventricular arrhythmias that may be missed by short-term monitoring. This procedure involves right ventricular catheterization and introduction of up to three electrical stimuli at the right ventricular apex of the heart to induce baseline VT.[112] If the arrhythmia is not reproducibly induced, repeated stimulation with up to three extra stimuli usually is performed at the right ventricular outflow tract. Once VT is reproducibly induced at baseline, drug therapy is started. The drug is considered effective if the SuVT is rendered noninducible or occurs in runs of less than six beats. A partial response to drug therapy is obtained if the drug converts SuVT to NSVT or decreases the VT rate (e.g., increases VT cycle length by 100 msec), with elimination of symptoms.[113]

Drugs that achieve satisfactory response by Holter technique or complete suppression by the electrophysiologic technique have been shown to improve long-term survival in uncontrolled trials.[114–116] Similarly, a partial response by the electrophysiologic method also has improved long-term outcome.[117] In a randomized, comparative study of Holter monitoring versus electrophysiologic study, Holter monitoring led to a prediction of efficacy more often than electrophysiologic study, though there was no difference in the success of drug therapy as selected by either method.[116]

Premature Ventricular Contractions

29. A.S., a 56-year-old woman, is admitted to the CCU with a diagnosis of acute anterior wall MI. Her vital signs are BP, 115/75 mm Hg; pulse, 85 beats/min; and RR, 15 breaths/min. Auscultation of the heart reveals an S_3 gallop. Her electrolytes include potassium (K) 3.8 mEq/L (normal, 3.5 to 5.0), and magnesium (Mg) 1.4 mEq/L (normal, 1.6 to 2.4). Otherwise, her examination is within normal limits. Two days later, an echocardiogram estimates her ejection fraction to be 35% (normal, ≥50%). During her stay in the CCU as well as the step-down unit, multiple PVCs (15/min) were noted on the bedside monitor. No antiarrhythmic agent was ordered. Should A.S.'s multiple PVCs be treated with a class I antiarrhythmic drug?

[SI units: K, 3.8 mmol/L (normal, 3.5 to 5.0); Mg, 0.72 mmol/L (normal, 0.8 to 1.2)]

Occasional PVCs are a benign, natural occurrence, even in a healthy heart, and are not an indication for drug therapy. Similarly, asymptomatic simple forms of PVCs, even in patients with other cardiac disease, usually are not an indication for treatment. However, the presence of frequent PVCs is a well-described risk factor for sudden cardiac death (SCD).[118]

In patients with a low ejection fraction induced by the PVCs or NSVT, the risk for sudden cardiac death can increase 13-fold. Suppressing PVCs under these conditions may reduce the risk of SCD.

Type IC Antiarrhythmic Agents

Because PVCs are a risk factor for SCD, the National Institutes of Health launched the Cardiac Arrhythmia Suppression Trial (CAST)[119,120] to assess the benefit of PVC suppression in survivors of MI. The CAST was a prospective, randomized, placebo-controlled trial that evaluated three antiarrhythmic agents: flecainide, encainide, and moricizine (all class IC agents). The choice of these drugs was based on results of a pilot study of 1,498 patients that showed adequate suppression of arrhythmia (PVCs) in the target population. Ten months after initiation of the study, CAST was discontinued because of excess total mortality and cardiac arrests in patients receiving flecainide and encainide. Forty-three of 755 patients in the flecainide/encainide group died of arrhythmia or cardiac arrest versus 16 of the 743 patients taking placebo. Further, total mortality in the flecainide/encainide group was 8.3% (63/755) compared with 3.5% (26/743) in the placebo group.[119] In the moricizine group, which was reported separately in CAST II, 16 of 660 patients in the drug group died compared with 3 of 668 patients in the placebo group in the initial 2 weeks. Subsequent long-term follow-up did not show a difference between moricizine and placebo.[120] It generally is believed that the excessive death rate in the drug-treated groups was due to the proarrhythmic effect of the drugs. Because the patients enrolled in CAST were asymptomatic and at low risk for the development of arrhythmias, they were at greater risk for drug toxicity (relative to benefit). Although many issues have been raised concerning CAST, one conclusion is that patients with a recent MI and the presence of asymptomatic PVCs should not be treated with encainide, flecainide, or moricizine. Whether other class I antiarrhythmics will produce similar results is unknown. Thus, the decision not to treat A.S.'s PVCs with class I antiarrhythmic medications was a sound one. The proarrhythmic effects of the drug may outweigh the potential danger of PVCs at this time.

30. What alternatives to class I antiarrhythmics should be considered for A.S.?

β-Blocking Agents

A β-blocker should be considered in this patient and in all patients with an acute MI unless specific contraindications exist. β-Blocking drugs have been shown to reduce the risk of reinfarction and cardiac arrest when started early in the course of an MI and continued for ≥7 to 14 days. In pooled analyses from 28 clinical trials on β-blockers, the mortality rate was decreased by 28% at 1 week, with most of the benefit obtained within the first 48 hours. An 18% reduction in reinfarction and a 15% reduction in cardiac arrest were also documented.[121–123] A recent substudy looking specifically at patients with new signs of mild to moderate HF and acute MI determined that IV metoprolol (5-mg bolus every 5 minutes repeated three times to deliver 15 mg over 15 minutes) followed by 200 mg/day of oral metoprolol reduced overall mortality significantly at 3 months and 1 year.[124] This suggests that a reduced ejection fraction after MI (as in A.S.) or a large MI is not a contraindication to β-blocker therapy.

The importance of the β-blocking effect after MI is further illustrated by the results of two MI sotalol trials. The first trial of sotalol, a class III antiarrhythmic agent with β-blocking properties, showed an 18% reduction in overall mortality, which was similar to that seen in other β-blocking trials.[125] The second trial, the Survival With Oral D-Sotalol (SWORD) trial, evaluated the d-isomer of sotalol only. This isomer does not have β-blocking properties, and this trial was stopped early because the mortality rate was significantly increased.[126] The American Heart Association and the American College of Cardiology recommend the routine use of IV β-blockers (followed by oral therapy) to prevent the early occurrence of VF.[127] (See Chapter 18, Myocardial Infarction.)

Amiodarone

In high-risk patients with MI who are not candidates for β-blockade, alternative antiarrhythmic therapy with amiodarone can be considered. Amiodarone is a class III antiarrhythmic agent, but also has antiadrenergic, class I, and class IV activity. The first trial evaluating the use of amiodarone in patients who had specific contraindications for β-blockade was conducted in Poland. Treatment with amiodarone (800 mg/day for 7 days followed by 400 mg/day for 6 days of the week for a year) was associated with a significant reduction in cardiac mortality and significant ventricular arrhythmias. Overall mortality showed a trend toward benefit, but statistical significance was not achieved.[128] An evaluation of amiodarone in post-MI patients with frequent PVCs (≥10 per hour) or at least one run of VT was conducted in the Canadian Amiodarone Myocardial Infarction Arrhythmia Trial (CAMIAT).[129] In this trial amiodarone (10 mg/kg per day for 14 days, then 300 to 400 mg/day for 16 months) significantly reduced the incidence of VF or arrhythmic death by 48.5% compared with placebo. Arrhythmic death alone was reduced by 32.6% and all-cause mortality was reduced by 21.2%, but statistical significance was not achieved for these endpoints. Patients with heart failure or a previous MI had a majority of the benefit from amiodarone therapy.

A complementary study, the European Myocardial Infarct Amiodarone Trial (EMIAT), evaluated MI survivors with a reduced ejection fraction (<40%).[130] Based on the results of this study, amiodarone (800 mg for 14 days, then 400 mg for 14 weeks, and then 200 mg for the rest of the study) significantly reduced arrhythmic deaths by 35% compared with placebo. However, this study did not demonstrate any trend toward reduced mortality (mortality was 13.86% with amiodarone versus 13.72% with placebo). This suggests that amiodarone should not be used in all patients with a reduced ejection fraction after an MI, but that it could benefit patients in whom antiarrhythmic therapy is indicated. Hence, if A.S. reports problematic symptoms associated with the PVCs or develops additional risk factors for arrhythmia while on β-blockade, antiarrhythmic therapy with amiodarone can be given without an increased risk of overall mortality.[128–130] (See Chapter 18, Myocardial Infarction.)

Nonsustained Ventricular Tachycardia

31. D.S., a 62-year-old man, was admitted recently for an inferior wall MI. Following the infarction he has been free of further pain and does not exhibit signs of HF. An echocardiogram shows an ejection fraction of 48%, but D.S. does experience runs of VT (see Fig. 20-13) lasting from three beats to 20 seconds in length. D.S. states that he feels his heart racing during the longer episodes. Should D.S.'s VT be treated? If so, what are the treatment options?

D.S. is experiencing NSVT, which can occur in patients with underlying heart disease, both ischemic and nonischemic (idiopathic dilated cardiomyopathy, hypertrophic cardiomyopathy). It is not clear which of these patients is at high risk for SCD. The Multicenter Unsustained Tachycardia Trial (MUSTT) used electrophysiologic testing to see if laboratory inducibility of sustained monomorphic ventricular tachycardia could predict the duration or frequency of NSVT in patients with NSVT, coronary artery disease, and a reduced ejection fraction. No significant difference in the frequency or duration of spontaneous NSVT was noted and no clinically important differences were noted between the groups with or without laboratory inducibility.[131]

The present treatment guidelines are based on the underlying left ventricular function.[132] If a patient has an ejection fraction above 40% and no symptoms, therapy is not indicated. If symptoms are present (e.g., palpitations, light-headedness), a β-blocker is preferred unless it is contraindicated by the presence of uncompensated HF or asthma/chronic obstructive airways disease (COAD). In addition to controlling symptoms, β-blockers reduce the incidence of cardiac death in post-MI patients with and without PVCs.[133] If the patient has a reduced ejection fraction (<40%), it is uncertain what the best treatment should be. However, oral β-blocker therapy, with careful titration of dosage, may be considered because β-blockade is now an approved therapeutic approach in HF patients.

Because D.S. is symptomatic, but has preserved ventricular function, he should certainly be started on a β-blocker. Pindolol or any β-blocker with intrinsic sympathomimetic activity should be avoided because they have not been shown to be "cardioprotective" following an MI. The results from the CAMIAT study suggest a role for amiodarone in this patient if β-blockers are contraindicated or inadequate.[129]

Sustained Ventricular Tachycardia

Treatment

32. S.L., a 64-year-old woman, presents to the ED with a chief complaint of palpitations. Her medical history includes hypertension controlled with a diuretic and an inferior wall MI 6 months ago. She is pale and diaphoretic but able to respond to commands. Her vital signs are BP, 95/70 mm Hg; pulse, 145 beats/min; and RR, 10 breaths/min. When telemetry monitoring is established, S.L. is found to be in SuVT (see Fig. 20-15). S.L. states she has a history of allergy to Novocain. How should she be treated?

The acute treatment of patients with SuVT depends on their hemodynamic stability. If unstable, patients should receive synchronous cardioversion, which will decrease the chance of triggering VF. If the patient is conscious, a short-acting benzodiazepine (e.g., midazolam) should be administered before the procedure.

LIDOCAINE

In patients with stable BP, IV agents such as lidocaine or procainamide are used to abolish the tachycardia. Lidocaine can be administered as a 1-mg/kg bolus, no faster than 50 mg/min. More rapid rates can cause hypotension and asystole. If the initial bolus does not "break" the tachycardia, additional boluses of 0.5 mg/kg are administered 8 to 10 minutes apart until a total dose of 3 mg/kg is given. The need for a supplemental bolus dose at 8 to 10 minutes is based on the rapid distribution half-life (8 minutes) of lidocaine. At one distribution half-life, the plasma concentration is reduced by 50% and the concentration at the effective site (the central compartment) is also reduced by 50%.[134]

PROCAINAMIDE

Procainamide is an alternative agent if lidocaine is ineffective or is not tolerated. A loading dose of 12 mg/kg is administered at a rate of 50 mg/min. Hypotension often is the rate-limiting factor and can be minimized by administering the drug at a slower rate (20 to 35 mg/min). Once the patient has converted to normal sinus rhythm, a continuous infusion (dosage, 1 to 4 mg/min) can be started. The infusion should be reduced in renal failure because the parent drug and the active metabolite, N-acetyl procainamide (NAPA), can accumulate. NAPA itself has class III antiarrhythmic activity and is eliminated entirely by the kidneys.[135]

S.L. is hemodynamically stable at this time, so lidocaine should be given in an attempt to abolish the tachycardia. Lidocaine can be used even though S.L. reports an allergy to procaine (Novocain). Procaine is an ester-type local anesthetic, whereas lidocaine and procainamide are amide-type local anesthetics; thus, there is no cross-reactivity between the two types.

33. A 1-mg/kg lidocaine bolus is given at 50 mg/min and two additional boluses of 0.5 mg/kg are given at 10-minute intervals before normal sinus rhythm is restored. A continuous infusion of lidocaine is started at 4 mg/min and continued for 48 hours. How should lidocaine concentrations be monitored over the next 12 to 24 hours?

Once converted to normal sinus rhythm, S.L. can be maintained on a continuous lidocaine infusion at a rate based on the estimated clearance of the drug (1 to 4 mg/min). Lidocaine clearance can be reduced by HF, acute MI, advanced age, significant liver disease, and drugs such as propranolol or cimetidine.[134,136,137] Under these conditions, a lower infusion rate should be used and the plasma lidocaine concentration determined in 12 to 24 hours (see average therapeutic concentration in Table 20-3). The lidocaine concentration also should be obtained after 24 hours if a prolonged infusion is anticipated, because lidocaine clearance decreases in this situation. Phenobarbital and phenytoin may increase lidocaine clearance, thereby lowering the plasma concentration.[138]

34. After 17 hours of the lidocaine infusion, S.L. is having difficulty manipulating a spoon to eat her Jello. She is becoming increasingly agitated and is inaccurately saying that people keep coming into her room and taking her things. Could these side effects be a result of lidocaine toxicity?

S.L. is probably exhibiting CNS side effects from lidocaine. If longer-term antiarrhythmic therapy is needed, it should be with another agent that is administered orally.

Lidocaine toxicity typically presents as alterations in the CNS such as dizziness, drowsiness, paresthesias, visual disturbances, tinnitus, slurred speech, trembling, loss of coordination, confusion, somnolence, hallucinations, unresponsiveness, seizures, or agitation. Cardiovascular toxicity (conduction disturbances, bradyarrhythmias, and hypotension) is rare and usually occurs when serum concentrations exceed 9 μg/mL. Lidocaine also possesses weak negative inotropic activity, which clinically is most evident during prolonged infusions or in patients with a pre-existing depressed myocardium (e.g., acute MI).[139] In those at-risk individuals, negative inotropy could reduce cardiac output and cause or worsen HF symptoms. It is likely that S.L. is experiencing lidocaine toxicity, and her infusion should be reduced to 2 mg/min or lidocaine therapy discontinued.

SOTALOL

35. S.L.'s attending physician believes that she should undergo further testing, and an electrophysiologist is consulted. It is determined that electrophysiologic testing is necessary because S.L. has a history of SuVT. On baseline testing, SuVT at a rate of 220 beats/min was induced twice with the catheter placed at the right ventricular apex. Sotalol 80 mg BID is prescribed. Describe sotalol's properties and adverse effects. How effective is sotalol in this situation? Is it the right choice for S.L.?

Sotalol is a unique agent that possesses nonselective β-blocking activity (class II) and prolongs repolarization (class III activity).[140] The immediate effect of sotalol in suppression of inducible VT or fibrillation is modest, generally averaging response rates of 30% to 35% using Holter monitoring, but as high as 56% in one report.[116] On the other hand, a randomized, comparative trial called the Electrophysiologic Study Versus Electrocardiographic Monitoring (ESVEM) study, using both Holter monitoring and electrophysiologic testing, demonstrated that sotalol treatment produced a significantly lower probability of recurrence of arrhythmia, death from any cause, death from a cardiac cause, and death from arrhythmia compared with other drugs.[116] Thus, the initial or acute efficacy of sotalol, though not impressive, can lead to better long-term results than many other drugs. The adverse effects associated with sotalol (e.g., fatigue, bradycardia, hypotension, TdP) are covered in the AF and TdP sections, respectively.

Because S.L. has no contraindications and had an MI 6 months ago, sotalol is a suitable initial choice. Sotalol can be initiated at 80 mg twice daily and advanced to a maximum recommended dose of 640 mg/day. The half-life of sotalol is 8 to 18 hours. Because it is cleared by the kidneys, its clearance is reduced and its half-life prolonged in patients with renal dysfunction. S.L.'s BP, heart rate, and ECG should be monitored. If her rate-related ("corrected") Q-T (QTc) interval becomes prolonged (see section on TdP), the dose should be reduced or the drug discontinued.

AMIODARONE

36. Sotalol is discontinued because S.L. developed a QTc interval above 500 ms. What is the role of amiodarone for S.L.'s arrhythmia based on its efficacy and safety? If S.L. is to be treated with amiodarone, how should it be initiated and monitored?

Amiodarone exhibits properties of classes I, II, III, and IV antiarrhythmic agents. Although it has class II effects on the heart, amiodarone is virtually devoid of antiadrenergic effects outside the heart and is not contraindicated in patients with asthma. The antiadrenergic effects arise from inhibition of adenylate cyclase, the enzyme that catalyzes production of the second messenger product cyclic adenosine monophosphate [cAMP]. Amiodarone can also cause a reduction in β-1 receptor density.[141-143]

This drug has unique pharmacokinetic properties. Its apparent volume of distribution is 5,000 L. Because it is extensively bound to tissue and is lipophilic, its half-life after long-term administration is 14 to 53 days. The main metabolite of amiodarone is desethylamiodarone. Although this metabolite is active, its contribution to the overall antiarrhythmic activity is not clearly delineated.

Because of the extremely long half-life of amiodarone, loading doses are used to accelerate the onset of drug effect. One to 2 g/day (200 to 500 mg four times daily) is given over a 1-week period; after that time, a maintenance dose can be established. Typically, for treating ventricular arrhythmias, 300 to 400 mg/day is used for maintenance, but doses may range from 100 to 800 mg/day. Although a concentration–effect relationship is hard to determine for amiodarone, levels above 2.5 mg/L are associated with an increased incidence of adverse effects.[141-143]

Amiodarone has many serious adverse effects involving a variety of organ systems, the most serious and life-threatening of which is pulmonary fibrosis. This historically occurred in 5% to 10% of the population given chronic doses of 600 to 1,200 mg QD for amiodarone, with a 5% to 10% mortality rate for those who developed it.[144] Large-scale, multicenter, double-blind, placebo-controlled clinical trials in HF and after MI have provided much information on the safety of amiodarone using new and lower dosages (e.g., maintenance doses of 300 to 400 mg QD). From these trials, comprising 2,250 patients who received amiodarone for 1 or 2 years, there were three deaths from pulmonary fibrosis in the EMIAT study (0.4% incidence in this study), and no deaths were reported in the other studies. Severe pulmonary fibrosis was reported in 0.3% of patients in a Polish study and in 1.2% of patients in the CHF STAT trial (compared with 0.9% in the placebo group).[75] Unspecified pulmonary disorders were reported in 5.2% of patients in the EMIAT study (compared with 4% in the placebo group) and in 3.8% of patients in the CAMIAT study (compared with 1.2% in the placebo group). The dosage regimens and beneficial effects of therapy from the Polish, EMIAT, and CAMIAT studies were reported in the section on the treatment of PVCs. Briefly, the dosage for all studies ranged from 600 to 800 mg/day for 7 to 14 days as a loading dose followed by maintenance regimens of 300 to 400 mg/day.

Despite the lower incidence of adverse pulmonary events observed in these studies, it is still necessary to monitor for the development of pulmonary fibrosis. A baseline chest radiograph and pulmonary function tests (diffusion capacity in particular) are recommended. The chest radiograph should be repeated at 6- to 12-month intervals, but pulmonary function tests need be repeated only if symptoms (dyspnea, nonproductive cough, weight loss) occur. Patients should be specifically questioned about these symptoms because early detection can decrease the extent of lung damage.[75,128-130,145,146] (See Chapter 26, Drug-Induced Pulmonary Disorders.)

Liver toxicity can range from an asymptomatic elevation of transaminases (two to four times normal) to fulminant hepatitis. Thus, liver enzymes should be monitored at baseline and every 6 months. (See Chapter 30, Adverse Effects of Drugs on the Liver.) The most common GI complaints are nausea, anorexia, and constipation.

Both hypothyroidism and hyperthyroidism have been reported, although hypothyroidism is more common. The thyroid complications are a consequence of amiodarone's large iodine content and its ability to block the peripheral conversion of thyroxine (T_4) to triiodothyronine (T_3).

Other bothersome side effects are corneal deposits (usually asymptomatic); blue-gray skin discoloration in sun-exposed areas; photosensitivity; exacerbation of HF; and CNS effects that include ataxia, tremor, dizziness, and peripheral neuropathy. Other than an eye examination and pulmonary function tests, which should be repeated when the patient is symptomatic, all other blood tests should be repeated every 6 months for routine monitoring.[144]

37. S.L. is placed on amiodarone 400 mg BID for 7 days. On day 2 of amiodarone therapy, her INR is 2.5. On day 8 she is switched to 400 mg/day of amiodarone for maintenance therapy. Her INR on day 16 of amiodarone therapy is 4.2, and warfarin is held. Why is her INR above normal?

Amiodarone is a potent enzyme inhibitor of the cytochrome P450 enzyme system. Two of the most significant interactions associated with amiodarone are with warfarin and digoxin. Warfarin is composed of two isomers, R and S.[147] The R-isomer is eliminated through the cytochrome P450 1A2 system, whereas the S-isomer is eliminated through the cytochrome P450 2C9 system. The S-isomer is five times more potent than the R-isomer. Amiodarone inhibits the elimination of warfarin's isomers through both enzyme sites. However, the time course of the interaction is somewhat different than other enzyme inhibitors due to amiodarone's long half-life.[147] When amiodarone is added to stable warfarin therapy, close monitoring (at least weekly) is needed for up to 4 weeks.[148] Usually, dosages of warfarin are reduced by 30% to 50% after amiodarone is instituted.[148]

Amiodarone inhibits the elimination of digoxin as well. Digoxin levels increase approximately 50% by day 5 and 100% by day 14.[149] (See Chapter 19, Heart Failure.) Close monitoring is required for ≥2 weeks after digoxin initiation.[149] Even if amiodarone is discontinued, it can continue to interact with other drugs for more than a month (depending on the dose delivered) due to its long half-life.[12] Amiodarone may substantially increase the levels of quinidine, whereas ritonavir (Norvir) may potently inhibit the elimination of amiodarone.[148]

Implantable Cardiac Defibrillators

38. After 2 weeks on amiodarone, S.L. develops a run of VT lasting about 2 minutes. She is admitted for placement of an implantable cardioverter-defibrillator (ICD). What is an ICD, and how does it work?

ICDs are machines implanted under the skin with wires or patches that are advanced or attached so they are in direct contact with the ventricular myocardium. The ICD has sensing, pacing, and defibrillation capabilities. When an arrhythmia is sensed, the ICD will first try to pace the heart out of the arrhythmia. This is most effective (80% successful) when the ventricular tachycardia rate before pacing is below 180 beats/min. If pacing fails to terminate the arrhythmia, a generator will turn on and create a certain number of joules (J) of energy. Unlike external paddle defibrillators, which deliver 100 to 360 J of energy, the energy delivered by an ICD to defibrillate the heart is usually 5 to 30 J. This is adequate for two main reasons. The ICD delivers energy directly to the heart rather than having to pass the energy through skin, bone, and other organs. The use of a biphasic waveform in an ICD rather than a monophasic waveform also reduces the energy needed to defibrillate.

As the energy needed to defibrillate the heart with an ICD is increased, the amount of time the generator needs to create the energy is also increased. This is problematic, since long charge times leave the patient in the arrhythmia for a longer period of time and may cause syncope. As such, the lowest energy needed to defibrillate the patient (the defibrillation threshold) is determined experimentally. To do this, the patient has an arrhythmia started by the electrophysiologist and the machine is set to shock at different energies to determine the lowest successful defibrillation energy. The electrophysiologist then sets the energy output at 10 J above that level (a safety margin).[150] Using the "DFT + 10 J" rule prolongs battery life and reduces syncopal episodes associated with arrhythmia recurrence versus always using the ICD's maximal energy output.

However, the impact of drugs, herbals, and endogenous substances on the DFT are not well described. If a drug significantly increases the DFT, then it may reduce the effectiveness of a 10-J safety margin.

The first major results from a randomized trial came in 1996 with the publication of the MADIT (Multicenter Automatic Defibrillator Implantation Trial) study.[151] This study enrolled 196 patients with prior MI; left ventricular ejection fraction 35% or below; documented asymptomatic nonsustained ventricular tachycardia; and inducible, nonsuppressible, ventricular tachyarrhythmia on electrophysiologic testing. The effect of ICDs versus conventional medical therapy (the majority of patients received amiodarone) on the primary endpoint, all-cause mortality, was followed for an average of 27 months. There were 39 deaths in the conventional medical therapy group and 15 deaths in the ICD group (hazard ratio for the ICD was 0.46; 95% confidence interval, 0.26 to 0.82; $P = 0.009$).

A few years later, the results from the Multicenter Unsustained Tachycardia Trial (MUSTT) extended the evidence that ICD therapy may have beneficial effects on mortality in patients at high risk for sudden death.[152] This larger study (n = 704) had similar inclusion criteria to the MADIT trial with the exception of a slightly higher ejection fraction cut-off (≤40%). The primary endpoint was cardiac arrest or death due to arrhythmia. Patients were randomized to electrophysiologically guided therapy or to no antiarrhythmic therapy. Of the patients who received electrophysiologically guided therapy, nearly half received antiarrhythmic drugs (mostly class I agents) and the remainder were given ICDs. The primary endpoint was achieved in 25% of patients receiving electrophysiologically guided therapy and in 32% of patients who did not receive antiarrhythmic therapy (relative risk, 0.73; 95% confidence interval, 0.53 to 0.99).

The Antiarrhythmics Versus Implantable Defibrillators (AVID) study compared ICDs to therapy with amiodarone or sotalol. This study investigated a population at high risk (they had already experienced VF and been cardioverted previously, or they had documented VT with syncope or another serious complication and an ejection fraction <40%). Overall, 1,016 patients were randomly assigned to either antiarrhythmics or ICDs. This study was stopped early (after 18 months) because the incidence of overall mortality was significantly lower in the ICD group (15.8%) than in the antiarrhythmic group (24.0%).[153]

Patients with ICDs who have frequent bouts of ventricular arrhythmogenesis are at high risk of developing ICD anxiety (known as ICD psychosis). They live in fear of their ICD going off again because it causes pain and they are forced to think of their own mortality. Use of antiarrhythmic agents to reduce the number of times the ICD goes off per month usually helps alleviate this anxiety.

Whether ICDs could be used in patients at high risk of arrhythmia (post-MI with a left ventricular ejection fraction <30%), but without past ventricular arrhythmic events was investigated in the Multicenter Automatic Defibrillator Implantation Trial II (MADIT II). ICD implantation plus conventional therapy was compared with conventional therapy alone. Conventional therapy consisted of β-blockers, angiotensin-converting enzyme (ACE) inhibitors, lipid-lowering drugs, diuretics, and digoxin in approximately 60% to 80% of patients in both groups. The ICD group had a 31% lower overall mortality rate than the conventional therapy group. If this therapy becomes standard of care for this population, approximately 3 to 4 million patients will be eligible, and 400,000 new patients will be eligible each year.[154]

Clearly, S.L. should have the device placed: it is the best chance for prolonging long-term survival at this point. Depending on the number of times the machine discharges per month and the patient's response, adjunctive antiarrhythmics may be needed.

Torsades de Pointes

Proarrhythmic Effects of Antiarrhythmic Drugs and Clinical Presentation

39. G.G. is a 71-year-old woman who is taking sotalol 80 mg BID for a previous episode of SuVT. At baseline, her QTc interval was 445 ms and her Cl_{cr} was 52mL/min. Four weeks after therapy was initiated, she complained of bouts of dizziness. She came to her cardiologist's office earlier today, and an ECG was performed by the ECG technician. She was released and told that the cardiologist would call her later in the day after she read the ECG. While driving home 10 minutes ago, she passed out and hit a parked car. When the paramedics arrived, the ECG strip showed TdP with a ventricular rate of 110 beats/min. She is now awake and alert. The ECG taken in the physician's office shows a QTc interval prolonged at 540 ms. What is QTc interval prolongation? Why does QTc interval prolongation indicate an increased risk of TdP? Could an antiarrhythmic agent such as sotalol cause this arrhythmia? How does Cl_{cr} factor into this?

The QT interval denotes ventricular depolarization (the QRS complex in the cardiac cycle) and repolarization (from the end of the QRS complex to the end of the T wave). Certain ion channels in phases 2 and 3 of the action potential are vital in determining the QT interval (see Fig. 20-1). An abnormal increase in ventricular repolarization increases the risk of TdP. TdP is defined as a rapid polymorphic VT preceded by QTc interval prolongation. TdP can degenerate into VF and as such can be life-threatening (see Fig. 20-16).[155]

Since there is tremendous variability in the QT interval resulting from changes in heart rate, the QT is frequently corrected for heart rate (QTc interval). Several correction formulas for the QT interval exist and give similar results at most heart rates. The most common correction formula uses QT and RR intervals measured in seconds as follows: [$QTc = QT/(RR^{0.5})$].

The Committee for Proprietary Medicinal Products suggests that a QTc interval over 500 ms or a level that has increased as a result of medications by over 60 ms from baseline is a cause for concern of enhanced risk of TdP. Increases of 30 to 60 ms from baseline are a potential concern.[155] The American College of Cardiology, American Heart Association, and European Society of Cardiology produced combined AF guidelines that address this issue as well. They suggest that agents prolonging the QTc interval through potassium channel blockade, with the possible exception of amiodarone, should be dosed to keep the QTc in sinus rhythm below 520 ms.[6] As an aside, amiodarone is unique among class III antiarrhythmic agents in that it blocks both IKr and the slow IK channel (IKs). This provides less heterogeneity in ventricular repolarization and reduces the risk of TdP over agents that prolong the QTc interval solely by IKr blockade.

G.G. was in excess of the acceptable QTc interval of 500 ms shortly before the time when TdP occurred. This QTc interval is much higher than would be expected in a subject without drug therapy or other risks of TdP. In a 150-subject trial, the average QTc interval of patients without comorbid diseases or concurrent medications was 403 ±28 ms. The QTc interval was 13 ms lower in men than women (397 ±27 and 410 ±28 ms, respectively). This is backed up by epidemiologic studies where 70% of TdP was found to occur in women. The QTc interval also increases with aging. Within the age categories of 20 to 40 years, 41 to 69 years, and >69 years, the QTc intervals were 397 ±27, 401 ±28, and 412 ±28 ms, respectively.[156] Hence, G.G.'s increased age and female gender probably contributed to her higher baseline QTc interval of 445 ms, but this is still below the baseline 450 ms cut-off for using sotalol.

Sotalol is known to cause QTc interval prolongation in a dose-dependent manner. Total daily doses of 160, 320, 480, and >640 mg gave patients a steady-state QTc interval of 463, 467, 483, and 512 ms, and the incidence of TdP was 0.5%, 1.6%, 4.4%, and 5.8%, respectively.[70]

It is likely that G.G.'s reduced renal function put her at high risk for sotalol accumulation and accentuated QTc interval prolongation. In patients with a Cl_{cr} above 60 mL/min, the sotalol dose of 80 mg BID is appropriate, but in patients like G.G. with a Cl_{cr} <40 to 60 mL/min, the starting dose should be 80 mg daily owing to sotalol's predominant renal clearance.

40. **What transient conditions or other disorders can increase the risk of TdP in patients on class Ia or III antiarrhythmics?**

Hypokalemia, hypomagnesemia, and hypocalcemia are important transient causes of QTc interval prolongation. Follow-up ECG monitoring is advised if a patient on a class Ia or III antiarrhythmic has a disorder that radically alters

electrolytes, such as severe diarrhea, metabolic acidosis, or ketoacidosis. Also, patients with renal failure have dramatic electrolyte shifts occurring during dialysis that may cause QTc changes. As such, avoidance of these antiarrhythmics or close ECG monitoring is warranted.

All class III and class Ia antiarrhythmic agents except amiodarone and ibutilide exhibit IKr potassium channel reverse use dependence: this means that they block IKr potassium channels when the channels are in their inactive state. As such, the QTc interval will tend to shorten at faster heart rates and lengthen at slower heart rates. Hence, patients with an acceptable QTc interval while in AF may have an elevated QTc interval after they convert back to sinus rhythm if the ventricular rate markedly slows. A second ECG should be taken once sinus rhythm is restored to avoid this complication. Proper ventricular rate control with class II or IV antiarrhythmics before using chemical cardioversion can reduce the chances of dramatic heart rate reductions after conversion to sinus rhythm. In addition, patients who develop a bradycardic disorder should be monitored very closely. Finally, patients with vasovagal syncope usually experience transient vagally mediated bradycardia during a syncopal episode. This can increase the QTc interval and may make therapy more dangerous.

Investigators have discovered gene mutations responsible for hereditary long QTc interval syndrome,[157,158] an inherited cardiac disorder that predisposes patients to syncope, seizures, and sudden death. Sudden death in long QTc interval syndrome is usually secondary to TdP, which degenerates into VF.[157,158] Drug therapy with QTc-prolonging agents would be risky in this population.

Because G.G. did not have a family history of hereditary long QT syndrome, but was being treated with sotalol (an agent known to be associated with TdP) in renal dysfunction, it can be assumed that sotalol therapy was responsible for her arrhythmia.

Proarrhythmic Effects of Nonantiarrhythmic Agents

41. **Which nonantiarrhythmic agents cause TdP? What is the mechanism of TdP initiation in this situation?**

Nonantiarrhythmic agents can also exhibit potassium channel inhibition and can prolong the QTc interval. For example, erythromycin, fluoroquinolones, and antipsychotics cause QTc interval prolongation by inhibiting the IKr ion channel.[155,159–161] Unfortunately, the ionic basis for QTc prolongation of other nonantiarrhythmic agents have not been adequately studied.

In general, nonantiarrhythmic agents increase the QTc interval in relation to the dosage administered and the blood concentration attained.[160,161] However, the antipsychotic ziprasidone seems to have a plateau effect for QTc prolongation. The placebo group had a 2.6 ±21.2 ms reduction in the QTc interval, compared to increases of 0.6 ±21.4 to 9.7 ±19.3 ms over the range of approved doses of ziprasidone (<80 to 160 mg/day). When doses above 200 mg/day were given, the QTc interval increases were 6.4 ±20.8 ms on average, suggesting a plateau effect. This is underscored by the experience with the drug to date, where 10 cases of overdose (>300 mg single dose) were reported, with no QTc interval exceeding 500 ms.[162]

In most subjects, the QTc interval prolongation for nonantiarrhythmic agents is less than the 30-ms increase from baseline that consensus groups have defined as being a potential concern for TdP. The lack of concern for a general population receiving normal doses of antiarrhythmics is underscored by data on terfenadine. Terfenadine has been shown to increase random ECG QTc intervals by 4 to 18 ms in most studies. In addition, when its metabolism is blocked via CYP3A4 enzyme inhibitors such as itraconazole and ketoconazole, QTc interval increases of 41 and 82 ms resulted, respectively.[155] Terfenadine underwent the largest evaluation of the risk of life-threatening ventricular arrhythmias to date, the COMPASS study. This cohort trial compared the incidence of life-threatening arrhythmic events in 597,189 patients from four Medicaid databases. Terfenadine was compared to over-the-counter (OTC) antihistamines, typified by diphenhydramine, ibuprofen, and clemastine (the active ingredient in Tavist). In this trial terfenadine was shown to have significantly fewer life-threatening arrhythmic events (0.037%) than the OTC antihistamines (0.085%, $P < 0.05$) and ibuprofen (0.057%, $P < 0.05$), and similar events to clemastine (0.021%). However, when the subgroup of patients receiving ketoconazole with terfenadine were evaluated, the adjusted relative risk was 23.55 times that of terfenadine alone ($P < 0.001$), a substantial risk.[163] Hence, the risk of arrhythmogenesis was not realized without the pharmacokinetic drug interaction, which in previous studies had been shown to increase the QTc interval into the zone for concern or of potential concern. This does not mean that a patient with renal failure, dialysis therapy, severe electrolyte disturbances, or hereditary long QTc interval syndrome can also be excluded from risk based on these evaluations, because these patients were not rigorously studied and would theoretically be at greater baseline risk.

Drug interactions accentuating the blood concentrations and subsequently the risk of TdP led to the withdrawal of terfenadine, astemizole, and cisapride from the U.S. market.[164,165]

Interestingly, erythromycin is not only metabolized through the cytochrome P450 3A4 system, but its active metabolite can also inhibit the cytochrome P450 3A4 system. Because the metabolite of erythromycin must be enzymatically activated and accumulate in the plasma before inhibiting the 3A4 system, it does not usually affect its own elimination (autoinhibition), but it can affect other drugs eliminated through this metabolic route.[164,165]

The antipsychotics are unique in that inhibitors of their metabolism do not result in appreciable increase in the QTc interval. The most comprehensive evaluation of antipsychotics and their impact on the QTc interval was Study 054. In this trial, several atypical antipsychotics (ziprasidone, risperidone, olanzapine, and quetiapine) and two typical antipsychotics (thioridazine and haloperidol) were evaluated. Therapy was given for over 21 days to allow steady state to occur, and maximal doses in the package inserts were used for all drugs except thioridazine, for which half the maximum dose was given. The ECGs used to compare the QTc interval changes from baseline between agents were obtained at the time corresponding to each drug's T_{max}. This was to ensure that the maximum effect of these agents on the QTc interval was assessed. In the second phase of the study, a CYP metabolic inhibitor was added to assess the impact of drug interactions on the QTc interval. Again, the T_{max} ECG was the one used for intergroup comparisons. In phase I of the trial, only thioridazine had QTc interval increases above 30 ms (average 35.6 ms, 95% confidence interval, 30.5 to 40.7 ms). None of the other agents had an average or an upper limit of the 95%

confidence interval for the QTc interval change exceeding 30 ms. In phase II, the use of a specific CYP enzyme inhibitor did not cause a significant increase in the QTc interval for any agent compared to phase I, and again only thioridazine had 95% confidence intervals exceeding 30 ms (average 28.0 ms, 95% confidence interval 21.6 to 34.5 ms).[166]

A list of nonantiarrhythmic agents implicated in causing QTc interval prolongation or TdP at the time this chapter was written is given in Table 20-6, but an up-to-date list can be found at any time on www.torsades.org or www.Qtdrugs.com.[161,167]

Because G.G. was not taking nonantiarrhythmic agents that are associated with TdP, sotalol is still the most likely culprit.

Treatment

42. How should TdP be treated? What treatments should be considered for L.S.?

If the patient is significantly hemodynamically compromised (frequently associated with a ventricular rate >150 beats/min and unconsciousness) while in TdP, electrical cardioversion is the therapy of choice and should be given immediately. Stepwise increasing shocks of 100 to 200 J, 300 J, and 360 J (monophasic energy) can be tried if earlier shocks are unsuccessful.

MAGNESIUM

In the hemodynamically stable patient, magnesium is frequently considered the drug of choice to restore normal sinus rhythm.[96,158,168] It benefits patients whether they have hypomagnesemia or normal serum magnesium levels. However, magnesium is not effective for patients with polymorphic VT without TdP and with normal QT intervals.[96,168] A common magnesium regimen is 1 to 2 g given over 5 to 10 minutes (in 50 mL D5W) as a loading dose and then 1 g/hour for up to 24 hours. However, loading doses of 1 to 6 g given over several minutes followed by an IV infusion for 5 to 48 hours at a rate of 3 to 20 mg/min have also been used. The exact mechanism of action for magnesium in TdP is not known, but it reduces the occurrence of triggered activity such as early afterdepolarizations and has L-type calcium channel and IK1 blockade during phase 3 of the action potential.

Table 20-6 Nonantiarrhythmic Agents Implicated in QTc Interval Prolongation or Torsades de Pointes

Drug Class	Agent
Dopaminergic agents	Amantadine
Antidepressants	Maprotiline, tricyclic antidepressants
Antibiotics	Erythromycin (lactobionate and base)
	Fluoroquinolones
	Trimethoprim-sulfamethoxazole
	Pentamidine isethionate
Antipsychotics	Typical and atypical
Antimalarial	Quinine
Other	Arsenic
	Organophosphates

CLASS IB ANTIARRHYTHMICS

The second class of drugs commonly used to abolish TdP is the class IB antiarrhythmic agents (e.g., mexiletine, lidocaine, tocainide). Unlike quinidine and the class III antiarrhythmic agents, the class IB agents do not inhibit potassium outflow during phases 2 and 3.[160,167] In addition, the blockade of inward sodium channels causes a shortening of the QT interval in some patients. Preliminary data suggest that class IB antiarrhythmic agents have considerable benefit in patients with sodium channel–activated QT prolongation, but virtually no effect on patients with potassium channel blockade–induced QT prolongation.[169,170] In a landmark trial, mexiletine was given to patients who had hereditary long QT syndrome,[169] and the patients were analyzed by their genetic etiology of long QT. The group with a deficient gene for the potassium channel had no QT shortening, whereas those with a defective sodium gene had significant shortening of the QT interval. These divergent responses were confirmed in an in vitro study using mexiletine with either clofilium, a potassium channel blocker, or amkolant, a pure sodium channel activator.[170]

Cardioacceleration with isoproterenol (1 to 4 μg/min) or cardiac pacing has also been shown to be beneficial.[160,168,171] As previously described, sotalol, quinidine, and N-acetyl procainamide's ability to prolong the action potential duration is diminished at faster heart rates (reverse use dependence).[172] The more the IKr potassium channels are activated, the less susceptible the channels are to inhibition by potassium channel–blocking drugs.

Since G.G. has regained consciousness and is hemodynamically stable, a bolus injection of 2 g magnesium should be administered over 10 minutes. If it is successful, a continuous infusion of magnesium (1 g/hour for up to 24 hours) should be given and the serum potassium level should be determined. If hypokalemia is present, it should be corrected. If the arrhythmia recurs, cardiac pacing should be used. If the patient becomes hemodynamically unstable again, electrical cardioversion with 200 J is warranted. Future drug therapy with appropriately dosed sotalol, amiodarone, or ICD therapy will need to be determined subsequently.

Naturopathic Therapy for Arrhythmias

43. D.B. is interested in natural products to replace his antiarrhythmic therapy, which he says is too expensive. Are there any herbal or natural agents that can prevent or treat arrhythmias?

Herbal Therapies

Many herbal remedies have been touted as beneficial in "normalizing heart rhythm," but actual in vitro or in vivo data are lacking for most agents. Herbal substances with preliminary data suggesting an antiarrhythmic effect include hawthorn extract, changrolin (an isolate from *Radix dichroa*), berberine (an alkaloid isolate of huang lian), and ba li ma (dried ripe Chinese azalea). Unfortunately, outcome data are lacking, and their use cannot be recommended.[173–179]

Food Supplements and Minerals

Food supplements and minerals have also been investigated for antiarrhythmic effects. Omega-3 fatty acids and magnesium are the best-studied alternative and complementary therapies for arrhythmias and are described below. In addition, dietary deficiencies of taurine and selenium may predispose to arrhythmias. If deficiencies are found, supplementation seems promising.[180–183]

The largest prospective randomized controlled trial to test the efficacy of omega-3 fatty acids for secondary prevention of coronary heart disease was the Grupo Italiano per lo Studio della Spravvivenza nell'Infarcto Miocardico (GISSI) prevention study.[184] In this trial, 11,324 patients with coronary heart disease were randomized to 300 mg vitamin E, 850 mg omega-3 fatty acids (given as eicosapentaenoic acid [EPA] and docosahexanoic acid [DHA] ethyl esters), both, or neither. After 3.5 years, the group given omega-3 fatty acids had a 20% reduction in overall mortality and a 45% reduction in sudden death. Vitamin E was ineffective. Limitations to this study were that it was not placebo-controlled, and the dropout rate was 25%. However, a prospective cohort study, a case-control study, and four prospective dietary intervention trials also demonstrated a reduction in sudden cardiac death from increases in sources high in omega-3 fatty acids (such as fatty fish). A nested case-control study showed that patients with MI and subsequent sudden death had lower levels of both EPA and DHA in their blood than MI patients without sudden death.[185]

Animal experiments show that pretreatment with omega-3 fatty acids before inducing MI reduces the extent of cardiac damage. Less damage may mean less myocardial scar tissue, which is important for establishing re-entry arrhythmias. Omega-3 fatty acids in vitro prevented calcium overload by maintaining the activity of L-type calcium channels after periods of stress. In addition, omega-3 fatty acids are potent inhibitors of voltage-gated sodium channels in cultured neonatal cardiac myocytes, which may provide antiarrhythmic effects.[186]

Magnesium has been evaluated as a rate controller in AF. In a small study, IV magnesium (MgSO$_4$, 2 g over 1 minute then 1 g/hour for 4 hours) reduced the heart rate by 16% within 5 minutes and then maintained the heart rate. No heart rate change occurred in the placebo group. All patients receiving magnesium reported some flushing, warmth, and tingling initially.[187] In a direct comparative trial versus verapamil (5 mg plus 5 mg IV followed by an infusion of 0.1 mg/min), verapamil was significantly better as a rate controller (28% of patients had a heart rate <100 beats/min with magnesium versus 48% for verapamil). However, the magnesium group had significantly better conversion to normal sinus rhythm (58% in the magnesium group versus 23% in the verapamil group).[188] Combination therapy with digoxin and magnesium versus digoxin alone was investigated in a small study. Digoxin use alone resulted in 50% of patients achieving a ventricular rate of below 90 beats/min at 24 hours. However, combination therapy with MgSO$_4$ (2 g over 15 minutes, then 8 g MgSO$_4$ over 6 hours) and digoxin resulted in 100% of patients achieving the ventricular rate goal.[189] There is some indication that magnesium can also benefit patients on digoxin chronically for AF who have frequent PVCs. Magnesium glycerophosphate 570 mg daily (23.4 mmol elemental magnesium) or placebo was given over the course of 4 weeks. The use of magnesium reduced the incidence of PVCs by 56%. No difference was noted for the patients randomized to placebo over the 4 weeks.[190] Future studies should be conducted to further evaluate this potentially cost-effective therapy.

In summary, omega-3 fatty acids may provide protection against ventricular arrhythmias in patients with ischemic heart disease. How it interacts with other antiarrhythmic agents is not well studied. In AF magnesium can improve the rate-controlling effects of digoxin, but it should be used only when digoxin alone cannot adequately control the ventricular response. Magnesium does not seem to inhibit spontaneous cardioversion and may have some efficacy in chemical cardioversion.

CARDIOPULMONARY ARREST

Cardiopulmonary Resuscitation

Cardiac arrest from VF, pulseless VT, pulseless electrical activity, and asystole are life-threatening emergencies. Table 20-7 reviews commonly used drugs used for these indications and their dosing. This section will review important aspects of therapy and will give clinical pearls, but the reader should also review the national consensus source document for these disorders, which includes more detail than can be given here.[96]

Treatment

44. M.N., a 52-year-old man, is visiting his wife, who is hospitalized for pneumonia. He goes into the bathroom and 2 minutes later his wife hears a dull thud. She calls out for her husband, but he does not respond. After an additional 2 minutes, health care workers open the bathroom door and find M.N. unresponsive and pulseless. Cardiopulmonary resuscitation (CPR) is initiated and a Code Blue is called. The ECG shows VF (see Fig. 20-14), and there is no BP. In addition to CPR, what initial therapy is available?

Determining the underlying rhythm disturbance is important because it directs health care workers to follow the Advanced Cardiac Life Support algorithm for pulseless VT or VF. This algorithm calls for electrical defibrillation first, but other clinicians should work to establish IV access in case defibrillation fails.[96]

External Defibrillation

Immediate external defibrillation at the 200-J energy setting is used initially because it has a chance at being successful in terminating VF, but produces less myocardial damage than higher energy settings.[96] Further, it is associated with a lower incidence of bradyarrhythmia and heart block when the rhythm is reversed.[191] If this shock fails to cause a return of spontaneous circulation, a second shock of 300 J is used; if that is unsuccessful, a 360-J shock is warranted. A significant percentage of patients can be converted to an organized

Table 20-7 Commonly Used Cardiopulmonary Resuscitation Drugs

Drug	Dosage	Rationale/Indications	Comments
Amiodarone	300-mg IV bolus; if fails, can repeat with 150 mg	First-line antiarrhythmic drug for VF (used after arteriole vasoconstrictor therapy fails in VF)	Dilute in NS or D5W before administering to reduce phlebitis
Atropine	1.0 mg IV push over 20–30 sec repeated at 3- to 5-min intervals up to 0.04 mg/kg	Blocks parasympathetic activity due to excessive vagal activity; useful in asystole, PEA	Must be given rapidly to avoid paradoxical vagal activity
Bretylium	*Initial bolus:* 5–10 mg IV push; may repeat in 10 min up to total of 30 mg/kg *Continuous infusion:* 1–2 mg/min	Second- or third-line antiarrhythmic therapy for VF behind amiodarone	Questionable use in digitalis toxicity; catecholamine release initially, followed by hypotension
Calcium Chloride	8–16 mg/kg	Reverses the direct effects of potassium on myocardial tissue, used in PEA due to calcium channel blocker overdose or hyperkalemia	Avoid in digitalis toxicity; flush lines before and after administration; do not mix with sodium bicarbonate
Epinephrine	1 mg IV push; may be repeated in 3–5 min	Cardiac stimulant; arteriole constrictor useful in asystole, PEA, VF	See text regarding high-dose administration and endotracheal use
Lidocaine	1-mg/kg IV bolus over 30–60 sec; repeat 0.5 mg/kg if needed; *Infusion:* 1–4 mg/min	Second-line antiarrhythmic therapy for VF behind amiodarone	Decrease loading dose by 50% in heart and/or liver failure; no infusion indicated during CPR
Procainamide	100 mg IV push over 5 min up to 1 g; *Infusion:* 1–4 mg/min	Second- or third-line antiarrhythmic therapy for VF behind amiodarone	Limit loading dose to 0.5 g in heart failure, decrease infusion by 50% in renal failure; may cause hypotension
Vasopressin	40 U IV bolus	Arteriole vasoconstrictor, useful in VF	Used in place of epinephrine if cardiac arrest duration is long

CPR, cardiopulmonary resuscitation; HR, heart rate; PEA, pulseless electrical activity; PRN, as needed; VF, ventricular fibrillation.

rhythm with repeated shocks in rapid succession (called stacked shocks), but the chance of success drops off rapidly after the third shock. Finer VF (seen on an ECG as only slight wavering fibrillatory waves) is harder to electrically defibrillate than coarse VF (larger fibrillatory waves).[96]

The 200-, 300-, and 360-J shocks are specifically for monophasic waveform defibrillators. Several less commonly used defibrillators apply other waveforms and have a specific shock intensity that is equal to a monophasic waveform. Choose the equivalent shock intensity when using these machines.[96]

45. Stacked shocks fail to cause a return of spontaneous circulation in M.N. An IV line is established in a peripheral arm vein. The algorithm now calls for epinephrine or vasopressin, but which one should be used?

Epinephrine/Vasopressin

Although epinephrine stimulates β-1, β-2, and α-1 adrenoreceptors, it is the α-1 adrenoceptor effects that are most closely associated with efficacy in VF or pulseless VT.[96,192] Applying α-1 adrenoceptor stimulation increases systemic vascular resistance (via vasoconstriction), during chest compression, which elevates aortic diastolic pressure and coronary perfusion pressure. This increase in coronary perfusion pressure is most likely the key to enhancing the return of spontaneous circulation after subsequent electrical defibrillation. Epinephrine may convert fine VF to a coarse variety that may be more amenable to defibrillation.

The recommended dose of epinephrine is 1 mg (10 mL of 1:10,000 dilution) given by IV push. The dosage can be repeated at 3- to 5-minute intervals during resuscitation. If the drug is given IV via a peripheral line, which in this case includes a "peripherally inserted central catheter" (PICC), then a 20-mL flush with normal saline is recommended to ensure delivery into the central compartment. Only chest compressions cause blood circulation in VF or pulseless VT, so movement of drugs from the periphery to the heart (where the benefit will occur) is severely impaired. An electrical countershock should be given within 30 to 60 seconds of drug administration.

The optimal dose for epinephrine has been questioned by clinicians and researchers.[193] Results of animal experiments demonstrate that higher doses of epinephrine are required to improve hemodynamics and achieve resuscitation.[194] Clinical case series and retrospective studies support this finding; however, randomized clinical trials in humans do not confirm a statistically significant improvement in overall rate of return of spontaneous circulation, survival to hospital discharge, or neurologic outcome between patients treated with a standard dose of epinephrine (0.02 mg/kg or 1 mg) and those treated with high doses (0.2 mg/kg or 7 mg).[195–198] Because of this, if the first dose of epinephrine with subsequent defibrillation fails, then the clinician can choose to continue 1-mg epinephrine doses every 3 to 5 minutes or give higher doses before subsequent shocks (up to 0.2 mg/kg).

ENDOTRACHEAL ADMINISTRATION

If IV access is not available, endotracheal administration of epinephrine is acceptable. Many agents (lidocaine, epinephrine, atropine, or naloxone ["LEAN"]) can be delivered via this route.[96,199,200] The patient should be horizontal rather than in the Trendelenburg position. A catheter should be passed beyond the tip of the endotracheal tube, at which point chest compressions should be stopped. The drug solution should be sprayed quickly down the endotracheal tube, followed by 5 to 10 rapid ventilations with a respirator bag. Medications should be diluted in 10 mL of normal saline or distilled water. Endotracheal absorption is greater with distilled water than with normal saline, but distilled water has a more negative effect on PaO_2. In general, the total bioavailability by the endotracheal route is reduced compared with the direct IV route; therefore, 2 to 2.5 times the usual dose should be given.

If IV or endotracheal routes are not available, then intracardiac injection could be used. Potential problems with the intracardiac route include pneumothorax, inability to perform chest compressions while the intracardiac drugs are being given, and coronary artery laceration. Intramuscular or subcutaneous administration is not appropriate because poor peripheral perfusion leads to unpredictable absorption.

Vasopressin is exogenously administered antidiuretic hormone. In supraphysiologic doses, vasopressin stimulates V1 receptors and causes peripheral vasoconstriction. Vasopressin use during CPR causes intense vasoconstriction to the skin, skeletal muscle, intestine, and fat, with much less constriction of coronary vascular beds. Cerebral vasodilation occurs as well.[96]

In a small clinical trial of 40 patients with out-of-hospital cardiac arrest, vasopressin 40 U IV produced better return of spontaneous circulation and 24-hour survival versus epinephrine 1 mg, although no survival advantage to hospital discharge occurred. A larger (n = 200) evaluation showed no difference in 1-hour or hospital discharge survival for vasopressin 40 U versus epinephrine 1 mg. These dichotomous findings are explained by the development of acidosis in longer-duration cardiac arrest. Animal trials and in vitro studies found that acidosis blunts the adrenergic vasopressor response seen with epinephrine, but vasopressin's vasoconstrictor effect, which does not occur via sympathetic adrenoceptor stimulation, remains intact.[96]

Vasopressin 40 U IV is the recommended dose in VF and pulseless VT. Vasopressin has not been studied via endotracheal delivery, and with its large molecular size it may not be readily absorbable by this route. The duration of action of vasopressin is longer than that of epinephrine, and it should only be redosed every 20 minutes in VF and pulseless VT.[96]

46. Since M.N. has an IV site and the time from cardiac arrest to ACLS was brief, epinephrine was chosen and a 1-mg bolus was given, followed with a 20-mL normal saline flush. The arm was elevated for 20 seconds to ensure adequate delivery. Thirty seconds after administration a 360-J shock is given, but it fails to convert VF. What can be done now?

Epinephrine at 1 mg or larger doses (up to 0.2 mg/kg) can be given every 3 to 5 minutes, with shocks 30 to 60 seconds after delivery, but in addition to this M.N. should receive intravenous amiodarone.

IV Amiodarone

Amiodarone's effect in VF or pulseless VT was studied in the ARREST (Amiodarone for Resuscitation of Refractory Sustained Ventricular Tachyarrhythmias) trial. This study was conducted in patients who experienced cardiac arrest in an out-of-hospital situation with therapy given by paramedics in the field. Patients who failed three stacked shocks and one dose of epinephrine with an electrical countershock were randomized to amiodarone 300 mg IV bolus or placebo. This was followed by other antiarrhythmics used in ACLS (lidocaine, procainamide, or bretylium) if the clinicians desired. Amiodarone significantly increased the chances of arriving alive to the hospital by 29%, but survival to hospital discharge was not changed. Of note, 66% of patients received antiarrhythmic drug treatment for pulseless VT or VF after amiodarone administration.[201]

The ALIVE (Amiodarone Versus Lidocaine in Ventricular Ectopy) trial directly compared IV amiodarone 300 mg to lidocaine 1- to 1.5-mg/kg bolus.[184] In this trial patients needed to fail three stacked shocks and epinephrine plus an additional shock to be eligible for randomization to either amiodarone or lidocaine. Amiodarone was given as an initial dose of 5 mg/kg followed by a shock. If unsuccessful, a dose of 2.5 mg/kg was given followed by a subsequent shock. Lidocaine was given as a 1.5-mg/kg bolus followed by a shock. If therapy failed, then a second bolus of 1.5 mg/kg was used with a subsequent shock. If the first antiarrhythmic drug failed, other routine antiarrhythmic drugs for cardiac arrest (e.g., procainamide, bretylium) could be tried. Patients given amiodarone were 90% more likely to be admitted alive than those given lidocaine. Unfortunately, no significant advantage to hospital discharge occurred (5% versus 3%).

Based on these trials, amiodarone is the only antiarrhythmic agent with proven ability to improve return of spontaneous circulation and short-term survival versus other antiarrhythmic therapy. However, it has not yet been shown to improve survival to hospital discharge and may only postpone the inevitable.[201,202]

Amiodarone 300 mg IV should be drawn into a syringe and diluted from 6 mL to 20 mL using normal saline or 5% dextrose in water. This will reduce the risk of injection site phlebitis upon bolus administration. Dilution does not preclude flushing the line with 20 mL of normal saline or D5W after administration to ensure that the drug reaches the central compartment. In addition, IV amiodarone has several drug incompatibilities and can precipitate when it comes in contact with agents such as aminophylline, cefamandole naftate, cefazolin, heparin, sodium bicarbonate, or floxacillin. This underscores the need to flush the line after administration. Finally, if it takes 3 to 5 minutes from the last defibrillation attempt to draw up the amiodarone dose, another shock should be given first, followed by amiodarone and a follow-up shock 30 to 60 seconds later. Drug administration should not delay electrical defibrillation attempts.[96]

47. Amiodarone 300 mg followed by electrical defibrillation fails to cause a return of spontaneous circulation in M.N. A subsequent 150-mg dose is also unsuccessful. However, M.N. did convert for a very short period to normal sinus rhythm (9 seconds), but then went back into VF. Should resuscitation be discontinued, or should additional therapies be given?

M.N. is at serious risk of death due to VF. ACLS recommendations suggest that as long as the patient remains in VF, a clinician can continue to try active therapy. If the patient has prolonged VF and the rhythm degenerates into asystole (lack of any heart rhythm, seen as a flat line on the ECG), then the code should be called. A patient who has had only brief cardiac arrest that degenerates into asystole should follow the asystole pathway, and active treatment should be continued (see Question 51). However, the guidelines also say that if a patient is temporarily converting to sinus rhythm before returning to VF, that is a good sign, that future antiarrhythmic strategies could be successful.[96]

Lidocaine

48. Since the patient is still in VF and had a brief time in sinus rhythm, a 1.5-mg/kg bolus of lidocaine is given. Is it necessary to give additional supplemental bolus doses or start a lidocaine infusion at this time?

Recommendations for lidocaine in non-cardiac arrest VT have stressed the need for multiple boluses of lidocaine coupled with an IV infusion to establish and maintain a therapeutic concentration. The recommendation for multiple boluses is based on the assumption that rapid distribution of the drug into the peripheral compartment results in low central compartment or intravascular concentrations. Although this is true under normal conditions, it may not be so during CPR. During external chest compression, the cardiac output is only 15% to 20% of normal, decreasing perfusion to the peripheral compartment. Administration of pressor agents, which constrict the peripheral vasculature, further decreases peripheral perfusion. Under these conditions, the serum concentration of lidocaine achieved with bolus administration may not decline as rapidly.[203] This suggests that multiple boluses are not required during the period of chest compression. An IV infusion is also unnecessary during the period of chest compression because liver perfusion, and thus liver clearance, is severely impaired.[96]

M.N. converts to sinus rhythm, and it is maintained after the electrical defibrillation attempt. He is still unconscious and has three broken ribs, and his subsequent mental functioning or long-term survival is unknown at this time. The health care team initiates an infusion of lidocaine at 2 mg/min and searches for the underlying trigger for the arrhythmia (e.g., myocardial ischemia, hypokalemia).

Pulseless Electrical Activity and Calcium

49. J.D. is an 80-year-old woman who experiences cardiac arrest in the hospital. A rhythm is noted on the monitor, but no femoral pulse is felt. M.N. is in pulseless electrical activity. How should she be treated?

The clinical situation in which there is organized electrical activity on the monitor without a palpable pulse is called pulseless electrical activity (PEA). Although electrical activity is present, it fails to stimulate the contractile process. Virtually all patients in true PEA die. However, not all patients who present with a rhythm and no pulse are in true PEA. Therefore, it is important to rule out treatable causes in patients who appear to be in PEA. The major treatable causes are hypovolemia, acidosis, hyperkalemia, hypokalemia, hypothermia, cardiac tamponade, pulmonary embolism, acute coronary syndrome, and drug overdose. Temporary pacing, epinephrine, isoproterenol, or glucagon can be used to treat β-blocker overdose. A nondihydropyridine calcium channel blocker overdose can be reversed by IV calcium (to raise systemic vascular resistance) and pacing, epinephrine, isoproterenol, or glucagon (to reverse myocardial effects).[96] In the absence of an identifiable treatable cause, epinephrine 1 mg every 3 to 5 minutes or atropine 1 mg every 3 to 5 minutes to a total dose of 0.04 mg/kg can be used empirically.

In establishing the diagnosis of PEA, two points should be made. First, the carotid artery is the preferred site to check for a pulse. A systolic pressure of 80 mm Hg is required to generate a radial pulse, 70 mm Hg for a femoral pulse, and 60 mm Hg for a carotid pulse. A Doppler ultrasound can be used to more accurately determine if blood flow is present. Second, it may be useful to interrupt CPR and listen for heart sounds. The presence of sounds indicates that the heart valves are opening and closing and that contraction is occurring. Thus, one should intensify the search for a treatable cause. The absence of heart sounds does not confirm a lack of contraction.

If M.N. has PEA, epinephrine and atropine as described above should be administered to increase the coronary perfusion pressure during CPR.

Asystole

50. K.K. is a 73-year-old man who experiences cardiac arrest. The ECG shows a flat line and the patient is determined to be in asystole (Fig. 20-17). Is this rhythm treatable?

Lack of electrical activity or asystole, like PEA, carries a grave prognosis. Its development usually indicates a prolonged arrest, which may explain its poor response to treatment. However, a few patients will go directly from a sinus rhythm into asystole and may be resuscitated. Enhanced parasympathetic tone, possibly due to a vagal reaction, ma-

nipulation of the airway from intubation, suctioning or insertion of an oral airway, or chest compression, may play a role in inhibiting supraventricular and ventricular pacemakers. Therefore, anticholinergic or parasympatholytic drugs that block vagal activity may be beneficial.

Epinephrine is the initial agent of choice to improve coronary blood flow and generate a rhythm. If conventional dosing does not produce results, alternative dosing methods can be used (intermediate dose, 2 to 5 mg IV every 3 to 5 minutes; escalating dose, 1 to 3 to 5 mg IV every 3 to 5 minutes; or high dose, 0.1 mg/kg IV every 3 to 5 minutes). Atropine 1 mg may be repeated every 3 to 5 minutes (shorter intervals may be needed in asystolic arrest) until a total of 0.04 mg/kg has been administered.[96]

When all else fails, ventricular pacing may be tried, although this has not been shown to improve outcome. The patient should be evaluated for adequate oxygenation and ventilation or the presence of severe metabolic imbalances. Electrical defibrillation to rule out fine VF may be tried, but defibrillation of asystole is of no benefit. When VF and asystole are terminated, it is common for the patient to become hypotensive. Fluids and inotropic and vasopressor support then are required.

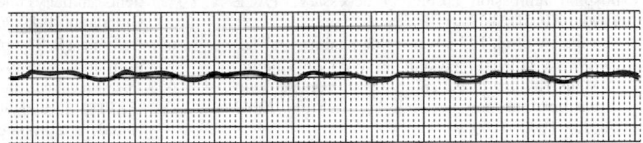

FIGURE 20-17 Asystole.

REFERENCES

1. Gereats PR, Kienzie MG. Atrial fibrillation and atrial flutter. Clin Pharm 1993;12:121.
2. Wolf PA et al. Epidemiologic assessment of chronic atrial fibrillation and the risk of stroke. The Framingham Study. Neurology 1978;28:973.
3. Albers GW et al. Stroke prevention in nonvalvular atrial fibrillation. Ann Intern Med 1991;115:727.
4. Falk RH et al. Digoxin for converting recent onset atrial fibrillation—a randomized double-blind trial. Ann Intern Med 1987;106:503.
5. Rawles JM et al. Time of occurrence, duration, and ventricular rate of paroxysmal atrial fibrillation: the effect of digoxin. Br Heart J 1990;63:225.
6. Fuster V et al. ACC/AHA/ESC guidelines for the management of patients with atrial fibrillation: a report of the American College of Cardiology/American Heart Association Task Force on Practice Guidelines and the European Society of Cardiology Committee for Practice Guidelines and Policy Conferences (Committee to Develop Guidelines for the Management of Patients With Atrial Fibrillation). J Am Coll Cardiol 2001;38:1266I.
7. Roberts SA et al. Effectiveness and costs of digoxin treatment for atrial fibrillation and flutter. Am J Cardiol 1993;72:567.
8. Beasley R et al. Exercise heart rates at different serum digoxin concentrations in patients with atrial fibrillation. Br Med J 1985;290:9.
9. Farshi R et al. Ventricular rate control in chronic atrial fibrillation during daily activity and programmed exercise: a crossover open-label study of five drug regimens. J Am Coll Cardiol 1999;33:304.
10. Woodland C et al. The digoxin–propafenone interaction: characteristics of a mechanism using renal

tubular cell monolayers. J Pharmacol Exp Ther 1997;283:39.
11. Fenster PE et al. Pharmacokinetic evaluation of the digoxin–amiodarone interaction. J Am Coll Cardiol 1985;5:108.
12. Freitag D et al. Digoxin–quinidine and digoxin–amiodarone interactions: frequency of occurrence and monitoring in Australian repatriation hospitals. J Clin Pharm Ther 1995;20:179.
13. Weiner P et al. Clinical course of acute atrial fibrillation treated with rapid digitalization. Am Heart J 1983;105:223.
14. White CM. Catecholamines and their blockade in congestive heart failure. Am J Health-Syst Pharm 1998;55:676.
15. Ikram H et al. Therapeutic controversies with use of β-adrenoceptor blockade in heart failure. Am J Cardiol 1993;71(Suppl C):54c.
16. Currie PJ et al. Oral β-adrenergic with metoprolol in chronic severe dilated cardiomyopathy. J Am Coll Cardiol 1984;3:203.
17. Salerno DM et al. Efficacy and safety of intravenous diltiazem for treatment of atrial fibrillation and atrial flutter. The Diltiazem-Atrial Fibrillation/Flutter Study Group. Am J Cardiol 1989;63:1046.
18. Waxman HL et al. Verapamil for control of ventricular rate in paroxysmal supraventricular tachycardia and atrial fibrillation or flutter: a double-blind randomized cross-over study. Ann Intern Med 1981;94:1.
19. Smallwood RA. Some effects of the intravenous administration of calcium in man. Aust Ann Med 1967;16:126.

20. Hariman RJ et al. Reversal of the cardiovascular effects of verapamil by calcium and sodium: differences between electrophysiologic and hemodynamic response. Circulation 1979;59:797.
21. Lang J et al. Effect of gradual rise in plasma calcium concentration on the impairment of atrioventricular nodal conduction due to verapamil. J Cardiovasc Pharmacol 1986;8:6.
22. Salerno DM et al. Intravenous verapamil for treatment of multifocal atrial tachycardia with and without calcium pretreatment. Ann Intern Med 1987;107:623.
23. Pauli-Magnus C et al. Characterization of the major metabolites of verapamil as substrates and inhibitors of p-glycoprotein. J Pharmacol Exp Ther 2000;293:376.
24. Falk RH, Leavitt JF. Digoxin for atrial fibrillation: a drug whose time has gone? Ann Intern Med 1991;114:573.
25. Zarowitz BJ, Gheorghiade M. Optimal heart rate control for patients with chronic atrial fibrillation: are pharmacologic choices truly changing? Am Heart J 1992;123:1401.
26. Rawes JM. What is meant by a "controlled" ventricular rate in atrial fibrillation? Br Heart J 1990;63:157.
27. de Divitiis et al. Right atrial appendage thrombosis in atrial fibrillation: its frequency and its clinical predictors. J Am Coll Cardiol 1999;34:1867.
28. Bjerkelund CJ, Oining OM. The efficacy of anticoagulant therapy in preventing embolism related to DC electrical conversion of atrial fibrillation. Am J Cardiol 1969;23:208.
29. Laupacis A et al. Antithrombotic therapy in atrial fibrillation. Chest 1992;102(Suppl.):426S.

30. Falk RH, Podrid PJ. Electrical cardioversion of atrial fibrillation. In: Falk RH, Podrid PJ, eds. Atrial Fibrillation: Mechanisms and Management. New York: Raven Press Ltd., 1992:181.

31. Kowey PR. Acute treatment of atrial fibrillation. Am J Cardiol 1998;81(5A):16c.

32. Dunn A et al. Efficacy and cost-analysis of ibutilide. Ann Pharmacother 2000;34:1233.

33. Stambler BS et al. Efficacy and safety of repeated doses of ibutilide for rapid conversion of atrial flutter or fibrillation. Circulation 1996;94:1613.

34. Ellenberg KA et al. Efficacy of ibutilide for termination of atrial fibrillation and flutter. Am J Cardiol 1996;78(Suppl 8A):42.

35. Naccarelli GV et al. Electrophysiology and pharmacology of ibutilide. Am J Cardiol 1996;78(Suppl 8A):12.

36. Kowey PR, VanderLugt JR. Safety and risk/ benefit analysis of ibutilide for acute conversion of atrial fibrillation/flutter. Am J Cardiol 1996(Suppl 8A):46.

37. Kalus JS et al. Does magnesium prophylaxis alter ibutilide's therapeutic efficacy in atrial fibrillation patients? Circulation 2002;106:II-634.

38. Boriani G et al. Oral propafenone to convert recent-onset atrial fibrillation in patients with and without underlying heart disease: a randomized, controlled trial. Ann Intern Med 1997;126:621.

39. Azpitarte J et al. Value of single oral loading dose of propafenone in converting recent-onset atrial fibrillation: results of a randomized, double-blind, controlled study. Eur Heart J 1997;18:1649.

40. Botto GL et al. Conversion of recent onset atrial fibrillation with single loading dose of propafenone: is hospital admission absolutely necessary? PACE 1996;19(Pt II):1939.

41. Capucci A et al. Effectiveness of loading oral flecainide for converting recent onset atrial fibrillation to sinus rhythm in patients without organic heart disease or with only systemic hypertension. Am J Cardiol 1992;70:69.

42. Goy JJ et al. Restoration of sinus rhythm with flecainide in patients with atrial fibrillation. Am J Cardiol 1988;62:38D.

43. Singh BN. Current antiarrhythmic drugs: an overview of mechanisms of action and potential clinical utility. J Cardiovasc Electrophys 1999; 10:283.

44. Kalus JS, Mauro VF. Dofetilide: a class III-specific antiarrhythmic agent. Ann Pharmacother 2000; 34:44.

45. Greenbaum RA et al. Conversion of atrial fibrillation and maintenance of sinus rhythm by dofetilide. The EMERALD (European and Australian Multi-center Evaluative Research on Atrial Fibrillation Dofetilide) Study [abstract]. Circulation 1998;98 (Suppl):I-633.

46. Singh S et al. Efficacy and safety of oral dofetilide in converting to and maintaining sinus rhythm in patients with chronic atrial fibrillation or atrial flutter. The Symptomatic Atrial Fibrillation Investigative Research on Dofetilide (SAFIRE-D) Study. Circulation 2000;102:2385.

47. Torp-Pedersen C et al. Dofetilide in patients with congestive heart failure and left ventricular dysfunction. N Engl J Med 1999;341:857.

48. Kober L et al. Effect of dofetilide in patients with recent myocardial infarction and left ventricular dysfunction: a randomised trial. Lancet 2000;356:2052.

49. Song JC, White CM. Dofetilide (Tikosyn). Conn Med 2000;64:601.

50. Marcus GM, Sung RJ. Antiarrhythmic agents in facilitating electrical cardioversion of atrial fibrillation and promoting maintenance of sinus rhythm. Cardiology 2001;95:1.

51. Oral H et al. Facilitating transthoracic cardioversion of atrial fibrillation with ibutilide pretreatment. N Engl J Med 1999;340:1849.

52. Mann DL et al. Absence of cardioversion induced ventricular arrhythmias in patients with therapeutic digoxin levels. J Am Coll Cardiol 1988;5:882.

53. Keefe DL et al. Supraventricular tachyarrhythmias: their evaluation and therapy. Am Heart J 1986; 111:1150.

54. Morris JJ et al. Electrical conversion of atrial fibrillation: immediate and long-term results. Ann Intern Med 1966;65:216.

55. The Atrial Fibrillation Follow-up Investigation of Rhythm Management (AFFIRM) Investigators. A comparison of rate control and rhythm control in patients with atrial fibrillation. N Engl J Med 2002;347:1825.

56. Wyse DG for the AFFIRM Investigators. A comparison of rate control and rhythm control in patients with recurrent persistent atrial fibrillation. N Engl J Med 2002;347:1834.

57. Chow MSS. Sustained-release quinidine preparations: pharmacokinetic considerations. Hosp Formul 1992;27(Suppl. 1):26.

58. Coplen SE et al. Efficacy and safety of quinidine therapy for maintenance of sinus rhythm after cardioversion: a meta-analysis of randomized control trials. Circulation 1990;82:1106.

59. Hammill SC et al. Propafenone for atrial fibrillation. Am J Cardiol 1988;61:473.

60. Porterfield JG, Porterfield JM. Therapeutic efficacy and safety of oral propafenone for atrial fibrillation. Am J Cardiol 1989;63:114.

61. Pritchett EL et al. Propafenone treatment of symptomatic paroxysmal supraventricular arrhythmias: a randomized placebo-controlled, crossover trial in patients tolerating oral therapy. Ann Intern Med 1990;114:539.

62. Pietersen A et al. Usefulness of flecainide for prevention of paroxysmal atrial fibrillation and flutter. Am J Cardiol 1991;67:713.

63. Anderson JL et al. Prevention of symptomatic recurrences of paroxysmal atrial fibrillation in patients initially tolerating antiarrhythmic therapy. Circulation 1989;80:1557.

64. Bolognesi R. The pharmacologic treatment of atrial fibrillation. Cardiovasc Drug Ther 1991;5:617.

65. The Flecainide and Propafenone Italian Study (FAPIS) Investigators. Safety of long-term flecainide and propafenone in the management of patients with symptomatic paroxysmal atrial fibrillation: report from the Flecainide and Propafenone Italian Study investigators. Am J Cardiol 1996;77:60A.

66. Aliot E et al. Comparison of the safety and efficacy of flecainide versus propafenone in hospital outpatients with symptomatic paroxysmal atrial fibrillation/flutter. Am J Cardiol 1996;77:66A.

67. Lee SH et al. Comparisons of oral propafenone and quinidine as an initial treatment option in patients with symptomatic paroxysmal atrial fibrillation: a double-blind, randomized trial. J Intern Med 1996;239:253.

68. Benditt DG et al. Maintenance of sinus rhythm with oral d,l-sotalol therapy in patients with symptomatic atrial fibrillation and/or atrial flutter. Am J Cardiol 1999;84:270.

69. Juul-Moller S et al. Sotalol vs. quinidine for the maintenance of sinus rhythm after direct current conversion of atrial fibrillation. Circulation 1990;82:1932.

70. Product information. Betapace AF. Wayne, NJ: Berlex Laboratories, 2001.

71. Lee SH et al. Comparison of oral propafenone and sotalol as an initial treatment in patients with paroxysmal atrial fibrillation. Am J Cardiol 1997;79:905.

72. Vitolo E et al. Amiodarone vs quinidine in the prophylaxis of atrial fibrillation. Acta Cardiol 1981;26:431.

73. Roy et al. Amiodarone to prevent recurrence of atrial fibrillation. N Engl J Med 2000;342:913.

74. Gosselink ATM et al. Low-dose amiodarone for maintenance of sinus rhythm after cardioversion of atrial fibrillation or flutter. JAMA 1992;267:3289.

75. Singh SN et al. Amiodarone in patients with congestive heart failure and symptomatic ventricular arrhythmia: Survival Trial of Antiarrhythmic Therapy in Congestive Heart Failure. N Engl J Med 1995;333:77.

76. Brass LM et al. Warfarin use among patients with atrial fibrillation. Stroke 1997;28:2382.

77. Peterson P et al. Placebo-controlled, randomized trial of warfarin and aspirin for prevention of thromboembolic complications in chronic atrial fibrillation. The Copenhagen AFASAK Study. Lancet 1989;1:175.

78. Boston Area Anti-Coagulation Trial for Atrial Fibrillation Investigators. The effect of low-dose warfarin on the risk of stroke in patients with non-rheumatic atrial fibrillation. N Engl J Med 1990;323:1505.

79. Stroke Prevention in Atrial Fibrillation Investigators. SPAF study: final results. Circulation 1991;84:527.

80. Warfarin vs. aspirin for prevention of thromboembolism in atrial fibrillation: Stroke Prevention in Atrial Fibrillation II Study. Lancet 1994;343:687.

81. Petersen P et al. Placebo-controlled, randomized trial of warfarin and aspirin for prevention of thromboembolic complications in chronic atrial fibrillation. Lancet 1989;1:175.

82. The STROKE Prevention in Atrial Fibrillation Investigators. Predictors of thromboembolism in atrial fibrillation. Clinical features of patients at risk. Ann Intern Med 1992;116:1.

83. Stroke Prevention in Atrial Fibrillation Investigators. Adjusted-dose warfarin versus low-intensity, fixed-dose warfarin plus aspirin for high-risk patients with atrial fibrillation: Stroke Prevention in Atrial Fibrillation III randomized clinical trial. Lancet 1996;348:633.

84. Zipes DP. Specific arrhythmias: diagnosis and treatment. In: Braunwald E, ed. Braunwald's Heart Disease: A Textbook of Cardiovascular Medicine, vol I, 5th ed. Philadelphia: WB Saunders, 1997:640.

85. American Heart Association. 2002 Heart and Stroke Statistical Update. Dallas: American Heart Assoication, accessed 12/2/2002.

86. Maisel WH et al. Atrial fibrillation after cardiac surgery. Ann Intern Med 2001;135:1061.

87. Lauer MS et al. Atrial fibrillation following coronary artery bypass surgery. Prog Cardiovasc Dis 1989;31:367.

88. Giri S et al. Oral amiodarone for the prevention of atrial fibrillation after open heart surgery, the Atrial Fibrillation Suppression Trial (AFIST): a randomized placebo-controlled trial. Lancet 2001;357:830.

89. White CM et al. A comparison of two individual amiodarone regimens to placebo in open-heart surgery patients. Ann Thorac Surg 2002;74:69.

90. White CM et al. Impact of an intravenous and oral amiodarone regimen in the post-open heart surgery Atrial Fibrillation Suppression trial II (AFIST II) [abstract]. Pharmacotherapy 2002;22:1328.

91. Rubin DA et al. Predictors, prevention and long-term prognosis of atrial fibrillation after CABG operation. J Thorac Cardiovasc Surg 1987;94:331.

92. Salazar C et al. Beta-blockade therapy for supraventricular tachyarrhythmias after coronary surgery: a propranolol withdrawal syndrome? Angiology 1979;30:816.

93. Yilmaz AT et al. Long-term prevention of atrial fibrillation after coronary artery bypass surgery: comparison of quinidine, verapamil, and amiodarone in maintaining sinus rhythm. J Cardiac Surg 1996;11:61.

94. Sager PT. Narrow complex tachycardias: differential diagnosis and management. Cardiol Clin 1991;9:619.

95. Faulds D. Adenosine. An evaluation of its use in cardiac diagnostic procedures, and in the treatment of PSVT. Drugs 1991;41:596.

96. Advanced Cardiac Life Support Writing Group. Guidelines 2000 for cardiopulmonary resuscitation and emergency cardiovascular care. Circulation 2000;102:I1-291 [Supplement].

97. Garrat C et al. Comparison of adenosine and verapamil for termination of paroxysmal junctional tachycardia. Am J Cardiol 1989;64:1310.

98. Sung RJ et al. Mechanism of spontaneous alternation between reciprocating tachycardia and atrial flutter/fibrillation in the Wolff-Parkinson-White syndrome. Circulation 1977;56:409.

99. Gulamhusein S et al. Acceleration of the ventricular response during atrial fibrillation in the WPW syndrome after verapamil. Circulation 1982; 65:348.

100. Falk RH. Proarrhythmia in patients treated for atrial fibrillation or flutter. Ann Intern Med 1992;117:141.
101. Gaita F et al. Wolff-Parkinson-White syndrome: identification and management. Drugs 1992; 43:185.
102. Camm AJ et al. Effects of flecainide on atrial electrophysiology in the Wolff-Parkinson-White syndrome. Am J Cardiol 1992;70:33A.
103. O'Nunain S et al. A comparison of intravenous propafenone and flecainide in the treatment of tachycardias associated with the Wolff-Parkinson-White syndrome. PACE 1991;14(Part II):2028.
104. Chen X et al. Efficacy of ajmaline and propafenone in patients with accessory pathways: a prospective randomized study. J Cardiovasc Pharmacol 1994;24:664.
105. Auricchio A. Reversible protective effect of propafenone or flecainide during atrial fibrillation in patients with an accessory atrioventricular connection. Am Heart J 1992;124:932.
106. Mitchell LB et al. Electropharmacology of sotalol in patients with Wolff-Parkinson-White syndrome. Circulation 1987;76:810.
107. Feld GK et al. Clinical and electrophysiologic effects of amiodarone in patients with atrial fibrillation complicating the Wolff-Parkinson-White syndrome. Am Heart J 1988;115:102.
108. Kunze KP et al. Sotalol in patients with Wolff-Parkinson-White syndrome. Circulation 1987;75:1050.
109. Goldschlager N, Goldman MJ. Principles of Clinical Electrocardiography. Norwalk, CT: Appleton and Lange, 1989:74.
110. Zipes DP. Specific arrhythmias: diagnosis and treatment. In: Braunwald E, ed. Heart Disease. Philadelphia: WB Saunders, 1992;714.
111. The ESVEM Investigators. Determinants of predicted efficacy of antiarrhythmic drugs in the electrophysiologic study vs. electrocardiographic monitoring trial. Circulation 1993;87:323.
112. Tisdale JE et al. Efficacy of class 1C antiarrhythmic agents in patients with inducible ventricular tachycardia refractory to therapy with class 1A antiarrhythmic drugs. J Clin Pharmacol 1993; 33:623.
113. Bleske BE et al. Acute effects of combination of 1B and 1C antiarrhythmics for the treatment of ventricular tachycardia. J Clin Pharmacol 1989;29:998.
114. Graboys TB et al. Long-term survival of patients with malignant ventricular arrhythmia treated with antiarrhythmic drugs. Am J Cardiol 1982;50:477.
115. Wilber DJ et al. Out-of-hospital cardiac arrest: use of electrophysiologic testing in the prediction of long-term outcome. N Engl J Med 1988; 318:19.
116. Mason JW et al. A comparison of electrophysiologic testing with Holter monitoring to predict antiarrhythmic-drug efficacy for ventricular tachyarrhythmias. N Engl J Med 1993;329:445.
117. Waller TJ. Reduction in sudden death and total mortality by antiarrhythmic therapy evaluated by electrophysiologic drug testing: criteria of efficacy in patients with sustained ventricular tachyarrhythmia. J Am Coll Cardiol 1987;10:83.
118. Bigger JT et al. The relationships among ventricular arrhythmias, left ventricular dysfunction, and mortality in the 2 years after myocardial infarction. Circulation 1984;69:250.
119. Echt DS et al. Mortality and morbidity in patients receiving encainide, flecainide, or placebo. N Engl J Med 1991;324:781.
120. The Cardiac Arrhythmia Suppression Trial II Investigators. Effect of the antiarrhythmic agent moricizine on survival after myocardial infarction. N Engl J Med 1992;327:227.
121. Beta-Blocker Heart Attack Research Group. A randomized trial of propranolol in patients with acute myocardial infarction. JAMA 1982; 247:1707.
122. Lau J et al. Cumulative meta-analysis of therapeutic trials for myocardial infarction. N Engl J Med 1992;327:248.

123. Rogers WJ. Contemporary management of acute myocardial infarction. Am J Med 1995;99:195.
124. Herlitz J et al. Effect of metoprolol on the prognosis for patients with suspected acute myocardial infarction and indirect signs of congestive heart failure (a subgroup analysis of the Goteberg Metoprolol Trial). Am J Cardiol 1997;80:40J.
125. Julian DG et al. Controlled trial of sotalol for 1 year after myocardial infarction. Lancet 1982;82:1142.
126. Waldo AL et al. Preliminary mortality results from the Survival with Oral d-Sotalol (SWORD) trial [abstract]. J Am Coll Cardiol 1995;20:15A.
127. Ryan TJ et al. ACC/AHA guidelines for the management of patients with acute myocardial infarction. J Am Coll Cardiol 1996;28:1328.
128. Ceremuzynski L et al. Effect of amiodarone on mortality after myocardial infarction: a double-blind, placebo-controlled, pilot study. J Am Coll Cardiol 1992;20:1056.
129. Cairns JA, for the Canadian Amiodarone Myocardial Infarction Arrhythmia Trial. Randomised trial of outcome after myocardial infarction in patients with frequent or repetitive ventricular premature depolarisations: CAMIAT. Lancet 1997;349:675.
130. Julian DG, for the European Myocardial Infarction Amiodarone Trial. Randomised trial of effect of amiodarone on mortality in patients with left-ventricular dysfunction after recent myocardial infarction: EMIAT. Lancet 1997;349:667.
131. Buxton AE, for the MUSTT Investigators. Nonsustained ventricular tachycardia in coronary artery disease: relation to inducible sustained ventricular tachycardia. Ann Intern Med 1996;125:35.
132. Pires LA, Huang SKS. Nonsustained ventricular tachycardia: identification and management of high risk patients. Am Heart J 1993;126:189.
133. Friedman CM et al. Effect of propranolol in patients with myocardial infarction and ventricular arrhythmias. J Am Coll Cardiol 1986;7:1.
134. Winter ME. Lidocaine. In: Koda-Kimble MA, ed. Basic Clinical Pharmacokinetics, 3rd ed. Vancouver, WA: Applied Therapeutics, Inc., 1994:242.
135. Bigger JT, Hoffman BF. Antiarrhythmic drugs. In: Gilman AG et al, eds. Goodman and Gilman's The Pharmacological Basis of Therapeutics. New York: Pergamon Press, 1990:853.
136. Lalka D et al. Lidocaine pharmacokinetics and metabolism in acute myocardial infarction patients. Clin Res 1980;28:329A.
137. Abernathy DR et al. Impairment of lidocaine clearance in elderly male subjects. J Cardiovasc Pharmacol 1983;5:1093.
138. Conrad KA et al. Lidocaine elimination: effects of metoprolol and of propranolol. Clin Pharmacol Ther 1983;33:133.
139. Pharand C et al. Prophylactic lidocaine for lethal ventricular arrhythmias following acute myocardial infarction: 8- vs 48-hour infusion [abstract]. J Am Coll Cardiol 1993;21:451A.
140. Singh B. Electrophysiologic basis for the antiarrhythmic actions of sotalol and comparison with other agents. Am J Cardiol 1993;72:8A.
141. Nokin P et al. Cardiac-adrenoceptor modulation by amiodarone. Biochem Pharmacol 1983;32:2473.
142. Gagnol JP et al. Amiodarone. Biochemical aspects and haemodynamic effects. Drugs 1985;(suppl 3):1.
143. Sharma AD, Corr PB. Modulation by amiodarone of cardiac adrenergic receptors and their electrophysiologic responsivity to catecholamines [abstract]. Circulation 1983;68(suppl 3):99.
144. Wilson JS, Podrid PJ. Side effects from amiodarone. Am Heart J 1991;121:158.
145. Burkart F et al. Effect of antiarrhythmic therapy on mortality in survivors of myocardial infarction with asymptomatic complex ventricular arrhythmias: Basel Antiarrhythmic Study of Infarct Survival (BASIS). J Am Coll Cardiol 1990;16:1711.
146. Doval HC, for the Grupo de Estudio de la Sobrevida en la Insuficiencia en Argentina (GESICA). Randomised trial of low-dose amiodarone in severe congestive heart failure. Lancet 1994; 344:493.

147. Hirsh J. Oral anticoagulant drugs. N Engl J Med 1991;324:1865.
148. Tatro DS, ed. Drug Interaction Facts. St. Louis, MO: Facts and Comparisons, Inc., 2003.
149. Nademanee K et al. Amiodarone–digoxin interaction: clinical significance, time course of development, potential pharmacokinetic mechanisms and therapeutic implications. J Am Coll Cardiol 1984;4:111.
150. Saksena S, Madan N. Management of the patient with an implantable cardioverter-defibrillator in the third millennium. Circulation 2002;106:2642.
151. Moss AJ et al. Improved survival with an implanted defibrillator in patients with coronary disease at high risk for ventricular arrhythmia. N Engl J Med 1996;335:1933.
152. Buxton AE et al. A randomized study of the prevention of sudden death in patients with coronary artery disease. N Engl J Med 1999;341:1882.
153. The Antiarrhythmics Versus Implantable Defibrillators (AVID) Investigators. A comparison of antiarrhythmic drug therapy with implantable defibrillators in patients resuscitated from near-fatal ventricular arrhythmias. N Engl J Med 1997; 337:1576.
154. Moss AJ et al. Prophylactic implantation of a defibrillator in patients with myocardial infarction and reduced ejection fraction. N Engl J Med 2002;346:877.
155. Bednar MM et al. The QT interval. Prog Cardio Dis 2001;43:1.
156. Tran H et al. An evaluation of the impact of gender and age on QT and QTc dispersion among normal individuals. Ann Noninvasive Electrocardiol 2001;6:129.
157. Curran ME et al. A molecular basis for cardiac arrhythmia: HERG mutations cause long QT syndrome. Cell 1995;80:795.
158. Wang Q et al. SCN5A mutations associated with an inherited cardiac arrhythmia, long QT syndrome. Cell 1995;80:805.
159. Daleau P et al. Erythromycin inhibition of potassium channels. Circulation 1992;86:1276.
160. Goodman JS, Peter CT. Proarrhythmia: primum non nocere. In: Mandel WJ, ed. Cardiac Arrhythmias: Their Mechanisms, Diagnosis, and Management, 3rd ed. Philadelphia: JB Lippincott, 1995:173.
161. Tran HT. Torsades de pointes induced by non-antiarrhythmic drugs. Conn Med 1994;58:291.
162. Weiden PJ et al. Best clinical practice with ziprasidone: update after one year of clinical experience. J Psych Pract 2002;8:81.
163. Pratt CM et al. Risk of developing life-threatening ventricular arrhythmias associated with terfenadine in comparison with over-the-counter antihistamines, ibuprofen and clemastine. Am J Cardiol 1994;73:346.
164. Landrum-Michalets E. Update: clinically significant cytochrome P-450 drug interactions. Pharmacotherapy 1998;18:84.
165. Cupp MJ, Tracy TS. Role of the cytochrome P450 3A subfamily in drug interactions. US Pharmacist 1997;22:HS9.
166. Glassman AH, Bigger JT. Antipsychotic drugs: prolonged QTc interval, torsades de pointes, and sudden death. Am J Psychiatry 2001;158:1774.
167. Symanski JD, Gettes LS. Drug effects on the electrocardiogram: a review of their clinical importance. Drugs 1993;46:219.
168. Schwartz PJ et al. Long QT syndrome patients with mutations of the SCN5A and HERG genes have differential responses to Na+ channel blockade and to increases in heart rate: implications for gene specific therapy. Circulation 1995;92:3381.
169. Priori SG et al. Differential response to Na+ channel blockade, beta-adrenergic stimulation, and rapid pacing in a cellular model mimicking the SCN5A and HERG defects in the long QT syndrome. Circ Res 1996;78:1009.
170. Napolitano C et al. Torsades de pointes: mechanisms and management. Drugs 1994;47:51.
171. Miwa S et al. Monophasic action potentials in patients with torsades de pointes. Jpn Circ J 1994;58:248.

172. Whalley DW et al. Basic concepts in cellular cardiac electrophysiology: Part II: Block of ion channels by antiarrhythmic drugs. PACE 1995;18:1686.

173. Poppings S et al. Effect of a hawthorn extract on contraction and energy turnover of isolated rat cardiomyocytes. Arzeimittel Forschung 1995; 45:1157.

174. Lu LL et al. Electrophysiological effects of changrolin, an antiarrhythmic agent derived from *Dichroa febrifuge*, on guinea pig and rabbit heart cells. Clin Exp Pharmacol Physiol 1995;22:337.

175. Huang KC. Antiarrhythmic herb. In: Huang KC, ed. The Pharmacology of Chinese Herbs. Boca Raton, FL: CRC Press, 1993:63.

176. Sheng WD et al. Treatment of chloroquine-resistant malaria using pyrimethamine in combination with berberine, tetracycline or cotrimoxazole. East Afr Med J 1997;74:283.

177. Chi JF. Effects of 8-oxoberberine on sodium current in rat ventricular and human atrial myocytes. Can J Cardiol 1997;13:1103.

178. Wang YX. Ionic mechanism responsible for prolongation of cardiac action-potential duration by berberine. J Cardiovasc Pharmacol 1997;30:214.

179. Wang YX. Inhibitory effects of berberine on ATP-sensitive K+ channels in cardiac myocytes. Eur J Pharmacol 1996;316:307.

180. Huxtable RJ, Sebring LA. Cardiovascular actions of taurine. Prog Clin Biolog Res 1983;125:5.

181. Lake N. Effects of taurine deficiency on arrhythmogenesis and excitation-contraction coupling in cardiac tissue. Adv Exp Med Biol 1992;315:173.

182. Wang GX et al. Antiarrhythmic action of taurine. Adv Exp Med Biol 1992;315:187.

183. Lehr D. A possible beneficial effect of selenium administration in antiarrhythmic therapy. J Am Coll Nutr 1994;13:496.

184. Grupo Italiano per lo Studio della Spravvivenza nell'Infarcto Miocardico Investigators. Dietary supplementation with omega-3 polyunsaturated fatty acids and vitamin E after myocardial infarction. Lancet 1999;354:447.

185. Albert CM et al. Blood levels of long-chain omega-3 fatty acids and the risk of sudden death. N Engl J Med 2002;346:1113.

186. Kris-Etherton PM et al. Fish consumption, fish oil, omega-3 fatty acids, and cardiovascular disease. Circulation 2002;106:2747.

187. Hays JV et al. Effect of magnesium sulfate on ventricular rate control in atrial fibrillation. Ann Emerg Med 1994;24:61.

188. Gullestad L et al. The effect of magnesium versus verapamil on supraventricular arrhythmias. Clin Cardiol 1993;16:429.

189. Brodsky MA et al. Magnesium therapy in new-onset atrial fibrillation. Am J Cardiol 1994;73:1227.

190. Lewis RV et al. Oral magnesium reduces ventricular ectopy in digitalised patients with chronic atrial fibrillation. Eur J Clin Pharmacol 1990;38:107.

191. Weaver WD et al. Ventricular defibrillation: a comparative trial using 175-J and 320-J shocks. N Engl J Med 1982;207:1101.

192. Otto CW et al. Mechanism of action of epinephrine in resuscitation from asphyxial arrest. Crit Care Med 1981;9:321.

193. Otto C, Yakaitis R. The role of epinephrine in CPR, a reappraisal. Ann Emerg Med 1987;16:743.

194. Kosnik JW et al. Dose-related response of centrally administered epinephrine on the change in aortic diastolic pressure during closed chest massage in dogs. Ann Emerg Med 1985;14:204.

195. Paradis NA, Koscove EM. Epinephrine in cardiac arrest: a critical review. Ann Emerg Med 1990;19:1288.

196. Gonzalez ER, Ornato JP. The dose of epinephrine during cardiopulmonary resuscitation in humans: what should it be? DICP 1991;25:773.

197. Brown CG et al. A comparison of standard-dose and high-dose epinephrine in cardiac arrest outside the hospital. The Multicenter High-Dose Epinephrine Study Group. N Engl J Med 1992; 327:1051.

198. Stiell IG et al. High-dose epinephrine in adult cardiac arrest. N Engl J Med 1992;327:1045.

199. Raehl CL. Endotracheal drug therapy in cardiopulmonary resuscitation. Clin Pharm 1986;5:572.

200. Hasegawa EA. The endotracheal administration of drugs. Heart Lung 1986;15:60.

201. Kudenchuk PJ et al. Amiodarone for resuscitation in out-of-hospital cardiac arrest due to ventricular fibrillation. N Engl J Med 1999;341:871.

202. Dorian P et al. Amiodarone as compared with lidocaine for shock-resistant ventricular fibrillation. N Engl J Med 2002;346:884.

203. Chow MSS et al. The effect of external cardiopulmonary resuscitation on lidocaine pharmacokinetics in dogs. J Pharmacol Exp Ther 1983;224:531.

CHAPTER 21

Hypertensive Emergencies

Robert Michocki, Omar Badawi

The term *hypertensive crisis* is arbitrarily defined as a severe elevation in blood pressure (BP), generally considered to be a diastolic pressure >120 mm Hg.[1] If these disorders are not treated promptly, a high rate of morbidity and mortality will ensue.[2] These disorders are divided into two general categories: *hypertensive emergencies* and *hypertensive urgencies* (Table 21-1).[3,4] Signs and symptoms of these disorders are nonspecific and may overlap. The distinction usually depends on the clinical assessment of the life-threatening nature of each episode. The term *hypertensive emergency* describes a clinical situation in which the elevated BP is immediately life-threatening and needs to be lowered to a safe level within a matter of minutes to hours.[1,3] The level to which the BP is elevated does not in itself represent a true emergency. A *hypertensive urgency* is less acute and can be accelerated or even malignant. It is not immediately life-threatening, and a reduction of BP to a safe level can occur more slowly over 24 to 48 hours.[1,5]

Hypertensive crises usually are characterized by an acute and marked elevation of arterial pressure, arteriolar spasm, necrotizing arteriolitis (necrosis in the media of the arterioles), and secondary organ damage. Hypertensive emergencies generally occur in patients with pheochromocytoma, renal vascular disease, or accelerated essential hypertension. Acute life-threatening elevations of BP also can occur in previously normotensive individuals with acute glomerulonephritis, head injury, severe burns, or eclampsia, as well as from abrupt drug withdrawal, drug–drug interactions (including herbal medications), erythropoietin administration, or drug–food interactions (i.e., patients receiving monoamine oxidase inhibitors who ingest foods rich in tyramine).[6–8]

Rapid, severe BP elevation is not always the hallmark of a hypertensive emergency. Indeed, even moderate elevations of arterial pressure in the context of multiple disease states demand prompt treatment. Examples include acute left ventricular failure, intracranial hemorrhage, eclampsia, dissecting aortic aneurysm, and postoperative bleeding at suture sites.

Hypertensive emergencies rarely develop in previously normotensive patients.[9] Most commonly, they complicate the accelerated phase of poorly controlled, chronic hypertension.[1] In several studies of patients with hypertensive emergency, a history of hypertension was previously diagnosed in >90% of the patients, suggesting that hypertensive emergencies are almost entirely preventable.[9,10] Effective management of chronic hypertension has lowered the number of patients who present with hypertensive emergencies to <1%.[11] A recent study reported that cerebral infarction and acute pulmonary edema were the most common types of end-organ damage in patients with hypertensive emergencies.[9]

However, even with effective therapy, the mortality for patients with a history of hypertensive crisis continues to be significant. Hypertensive emergencies occur more often in Blacks than in Whites, among patients who have no primary care physician, and among those who do not adhere to their treatment regimens.[12]

Table 21-1 Hypertensive Emergencies Versus Urgencies

Emergencies	Urgencies
Severely elevated blood pressure (diastolic >120 mm Hg)[a]	Severely elevated blood pressure (diastolic >120 mm Hg)[a]
Potentially life-threatening	Not life-threatening
End organ damage present or high risk:	Minimal end-organ damage with no pending complications
CNS (dizziness, N/V, encephalopathy, confusion, weakness,	Accelerated malignant hypertension
intracranial or subarachnoid hemorrhage, stroke)	Optic disc edema
Eyes (ocular hemorrhage or funduscopic changes,	Coronary artery disease
blurred vision, loss of sight)	Post- or perioperative hypertension
Heart (left ventricular failure, pulmonary edema, MI,	Pre- or post-kidney transplant
angina, aortic dissection)	
Renal failure/insufficiency	
Pheochromocytoma crisis	
Drug-induced hypertensive crisis	
MAOI–tyramine interactions	
Overdose with PCP, cocaine, or LSD	
Drug interaction–induced hypertension	
Clonidine withdrawal	
Eclampsia (complicated pregnancy)	
Requires immediate pressure reduction	Treated over several hours to days
Requires IV therapy (see Table 21.2)	Oral therapy or slower-acting parenteral drugs preferred. (see Table 21.3)

[a]Degree of blood pressure elevation less diagnostic than rate of pressure rise and presence of concurrent diseases or end organ damage. See Chapter 14, Essential Hypertension, for staging of hypertension.
LSD, lysergic acid diethylamide; MAOI, monoamine oxidase inhibitor; N/V, nausea and vomiting; PCP, phencyclidine.

Accelerated and Malignant Hypertension

The terms *accelerated* and *malignant hypertension* have been used to describe severe hypertension accompanied by specific funduscopic changes.[4] Accelerated hypertension is characterized by the presence of retinal hemorrhages, exudates, and arteriolar narrowing and spasm (grade III Keith-Wagener-Barker classification). The incidence of accelerated hypertension among ambulatory patients is diminishing, and mortality from it is declining.[13] Malignant hypertension, an extension of the accelerated form, is remarkable for the presence of papilledema.[11] It occurs more commonly in middle-aged hypertensive patients, with a peak prevalence in the 40- to 60-year age range. If malignant hypertension occurs with no previous history of hypertension or in a patient who is younger than 30 or older than 60, a secondary cause should be suspected. Despite the funduscopic changes, the terms *accelerated* and *malignant* often are used synonymously. It is now also known that the clinical outcomes do not differ on the basis of funduscopic findings, suggesting that they are part of the same process.[13] Although hypertensive emergencies are much less common than hypertensive urgencies, it is sometimes difficult to know whether end-organ dysfunction is new or has progressed without a thorough patient history.

Signs and Symptoms

Symptoms associated with hypertensive crisis are highly variable and reflect the degree of damage to specific organ systems. The primary sites of damage are the central nervous system (CNS), heart, kidneys, and eyes.

Central Nervous System

CNS damage can present solely as a severe headache or may be accompanied by dizziness, nausea, vomiting, and anorexia.

Mental confusion with apprehension indicates more severe disease, as does nystagmus, localized weakness, or a positive Babinski sign (i.e., upward extension of the great toe and spreading of the smaller toes when moderate pressure is applied along a curve from the sole to the ball of the foot). CNS damage may be rapidly progressive, resulting in coma or death. If a cerebrovascular accident has occurred, slurred speech or motor paralysis may be present.

Other Complications

Cardiac complications of hypertensive crisis include heart failure (HF) and angina pectoris. Myocardial infarction (MI) also can be precipitated. Ocular symptoms of hypertensive crisis usually are related to changes in visual acuity. Complaints of blurred vision or loss of eyesight often are associated with funduscopic findings of hemorrhages, exudates, and occasionally papilledema. Renal complications include hematuria, proteinuria, pyelonephritis, and elevated serum blood urea nitrogen (BUN) and creatinine levels.

Principles of Treatment

Oral Versus Parenteral Therapy

Accelerated hypertension, malignant hypertension, or elevated BP in the absence of life-threatening signs or symptoms is not an indication for parenteral treatment. Oral antihypertensive loading regimens are more appropriate for the management of these urgent cases. In contrast, hypertensive emergencies require immediate hospitalization, generally in an intensive care unit, and the administration of parenteral antihypertensive medications to reduce arterial pressure. Effective therapy greatly improves the prognosis, reverses symptoms, and arrests the progression of end-organ damage. Treatment reverses the vascular changes in the eyes and slows or arrests the progressive deterioration in renal function. Treatment of malignant hypertension can transiently worsen renal function. However, after 2 to 3 months of adequate medical therapy, renal function may gradually improve to the pre-malignant level of renal insufficiency or to a new, slightly deteriorated level. The time required for recovery of renal function ranges from 2 weeks to 2 years. A low serum creatinine level, in the absence of marked cardiomegaly or renal shrinkage, has been associated with a good chance for recovery of renal function.[14] In patients with mild encephalopathy, neurologic symptoms resolve within 24 hours after treatment.[15] Resolution of papilledema occurs in 2 to 3 weeks, whereas funduscopic exudates can require up to 12 weeks for complete resolution.[16] Whether treatment can completely reverse end-organ damage is related to two factors: how soon treatment is begun, and the extent of damage at the initiation of therapy.

There are two approaches to managing the patient with hypertensive emergencies. The first and more traditional approach (which this chapter will focus on) is centered on two fundamental concepts. First, immediate and intensive therapy is required and takes precedence over time-consuming diagnostic procedures. Second, the choice of drugs will depend on how their time course of action and hemodynamic and metabolic effects meet the needs of the crisis situation. Alternatively, a mechanistic approach to managing hypertensive emergencies based on patient-specific pathophysiology has been proposed. In this approach, patients are diagnosed with having either R-type (renin-angiotensin–dependent) or V-type (volume-dependent) predominant hypertension. Once the mechanism is determined, treatment is focused on medications that are effective against either R- or V-type hypertension.[17,18] This chapter will focus on the traditional methods of treating hypertensive emergencies, although it is extremely important to recognize the pathophysiology behind a patient's hypertensive crisis as well as to recall the antihypertensive mechanism behind each class of drug so as not to waste critical time with similar drugs during refractory cases. Drug classes effective against R-type hypertension include β-blockers (through decreased renin secretion), angiotensin-converting enzyme (ACE) inhibitors, and angiotensin receptor blockers. Drug classes effective against V-type hypertension include diuretics, calcium channel blockers, and α-blockers.

If encephalopathy, acute left ventricular failure, dissecting aortic aneurysm, eclampsia, or other serious conditions are present, the BP should be lowered promptly with rapid-acting, parenteral antihypertensive medications such as diazoxide (Hyperstat), esmolol (Brevibloc), enalaprilat (Vasotec IV), fenoldopam (Corlopam), hydralazine (Apresoline), labetalol (Normodyne, Trandate), nicardipine (Cardene IV), nitroglycerin (Tridil, Nitrostat IV, Nitro-Bid IV), nitroprusside (Nipride), or trimethaphan (Arfonad)[1,3,4,11,19–21] (Table 21-2). If a slower BP reduction over several hours or days is acceptable, rapid-acting oral therapy using captopril (Capoten), clonidine (Catapres), prazosin (Minipress), labetalol, or minoxidil (Loniten) may be used[4,11,21,22,23] (Table 21-3).

Goals of Therapy

The rate of BP lowering must be individualized because ischemic damage to the heart and brain can be provoked by a precipitous fall in BP.[24–28] Antihypertensive drugs should be used cautiously in patient groups at high risk for developing hypotensive complications, such as the elderly and patients with severely defective autoregulatory mechanisms. The latter group includes those with autonomic dysfunction or fixed sclerotic stenosis of cerebral or neck arteries.[29] In addition, patients who have chronically elevated BP are less likely to tolerate abrupt reductions in their BP, and the amount of reduction appropriate for those patients is somewhat less than for those whose BP is acutely elevated. In patients with hypertensive encephalopathy, cerebral hypoperfusion may occur if the mean BP is reduced by >40%.[30] Thus, it has been suggested that the mean pressure be lowered by no more than 20% to 30%.[30,31] For hypertensive emergencies, it is recommended that the mean arterial pressure be reduced initially by no more than 25% (within minutes to 2 hours), then toward 160/100 mm Hg within 2 to 6 hours.[3] A diastolic pressure of 100 to 110 mm Hg is an appropriate therapeutic goal.[1] Lower pressures may be indicated for patients with aortic dissection.

HYPERTENSIVE URGENCIES

Patient Assessment

1. M.M. is a 60-year-old Black man with a long history of mild heart failure, poorly controlled hypertension thought to be the result of nonadherence, and a history of MI. He was referred from a community health center this morning for a thorough evaluation of his elevated BP. He has not taken his captopril (Capoten), amlodipine (Norvasc), or hydrochlorothiazide for the past 7 days. M.M. is completely asymptomatic. Physical examination reveals a BP of 180/120 mm Hg and a pulse of 92 beats/min. The funduscopic examination is pertinent for mild arteriolar narrowing, without hemorrhages or exudates. The discs are flat. The lungs are clear, and the cardiac examination is unremarkable. The electrocardiogram (ECG) indicates normal sinus rhythm (NSR) at a rate of 90 beats/min with first-degree AV block. The chest radiograph is interpreted as mild cardiomegaly. Serum electrolytes, BUN, and serum creatinine (SrCr) are within normal limits. A urinalysis (UA) is significant for 2+ proteinuria. What is the therapeutic objective in treating M.M.? How quickly should his BP be lowered, and what therapeutic options are available?

M.M. has severe hypertension with a BP of 180/120 mm Hg.[3] However, the absolute magnitude of BP elevation does not in itself constitute a medical emergency requiring an acute reduction in BP. There is no evidence of encephalopathy, cardiac decompensation, chest pain, or rapid change in renal function. Therefore, no evidence exists to indicate a rapid deterioration in the function of target organs.

As is often the case, M.M.'s lack of BP control is related to medication nonadherence. The magnitude of his blood pressure elevation requires that his BP be lowered over the next several hours, while being careful not to induce hypotension. Rapid-acting oral agents can be used for this purpose; parenteral therapy is not warranted. A number of different oral regimens using clonidine, captopril, labetalol, prazosin, and minoxidil are available. In M.M., restarting his medications in a controlled manner so as not to drop his BP too rapidly may also be a reasonable option for treatment. Later, he can be converted to a regimen designed to enhance outpatient compliance by selecting medications with once-daily dosing. For

Table 21-2 Parenteral Drugs Commonly Used in the Treatment of Hypertensive Emergencies

Drug (Brand Name)	Dose/Route	Onset of Action	Duration of Action	Major Side Effects (All Can Cause Hypotension)	Mechanism of Action	Avoid or Use Cautiously in Patients with These Conditions
Nitroprusside[a] (Nitropress) 50 mg/2 mL (Most commonly used)	IV infusion[a]: Start: 0.5 µg/kg/min Usual: 2–5 µg/kg/min Max: 8 µg/kg/min	Seconds	3–5 min after D/C infusion	Nausea, vomiting, diaphoresis, weakness, thiocyanate toxicity,[b] cyanide toxicity (rare)[c]	Arterial and venous vasodilator	Renal failure (thiocyanate accumulation), pregnancy, increased intracranial pressure
Diazoxide (Hyperstat IV) 300 mg/20 mL	50–150 mg IV Q 5 min or as infusion of 7.5–30 mg/min[d]	1–5 min	4–12 hr	Hyperglycemia, Na retention,[d] tachycardia, painful extravasation	Arterial vasodilator	Angina pectoris, MI, aortic dissection, pulmonary edema, intracranial hemorrhage
Enalaprilat[e] (Vasotec IV) 1.25 mg/mL 2.5 mg/2 mL	0.625–1.25 mg IV Q 6 hr	15 min (max, 1–4 hr)	6–12 hr	Hyperkalemia	ACE inhibitor	Hyperkalemia. Renal failure in patients with dehydration or bilateral renal artery stenosis. Pregnancy (teratogenic)
Esmolol[f] (Brevibloc) 100 mg/10 mL 2,500 mg/10 mL concentrate	250–500 µg/kg × 1 min 50–100 µg/kg/min × 4 min, may repeat	1–2 min	10–20 min	Nausea; thrombophlebitis; painful extravasation	β-Adrenergic blocker	Asthma, bradycardia, decompensated HF; advanced heart block
Fenoldopam (Corlopam) 10 mg/mL 20 mg/2 mL 50 mg/5 mL	0.1–0.3 µg/kg/min	<5 min	30 min	Tachycardia, headache, nausea, flushing	Dopamine-1 agonist	Glaucoma
Hydralazine[g] (generic) 20 mg/mL	10–20 mg IV 10–50 mg IM	10–30 min (IV) 20–40 min (IM)	2–6 hr	Tachycardia, headache, angina	Arterial vasodilator	Angina pectoris, MI, aortic dissection
Labetalol[h] (Normodyne) 20 mg/4 mL 40 mg/8 mL 100 mg/20 mL 200 mg/20 mL	2 mg/min IV or 20–80 mg Q 10 min up to 300 mg total dose	≤5 min	3–6 hr	Abdominal pain, nausea, vomiting, diarrhea	α- and β-Adrenergic blocker	Asthma, bradycardia, decompensated HF
Nicardipine[i] (Cardene IV) 25 mg/10 mL	IV loading dose 5 mg/hr increased by 2.5 mg/hr Q 5 min to desired BP or a max of 15 mg/hr × 15 minutes, followed by maintenance infusion of 3 mg/hr	2–10 min maximum 8–12 hr	40–60 min after D/C infusion	Headache, flushing, nausea, vomiting, dizziness, tachycardia; local thrombophlebitis—change infusion site after 12 hr	Arterial vasodilator (Ca channel blocker)	Angina, decompensated HF, increased intracranial pressure

Drug	Administration	Onset	Duration	Adverse Effects	Mechanism	Precautions/Contraindications
Nitroglycerin/[j] (Tridil, Nitro-Bid IV, Nitro-Stat IV) 5 mg/mL 5 mg/10 mL 25 mg/5 mL 50 mg/10 mL 100 mg/20 mL	IV infusion pump 5-100 µg/min	2-5 min	5-10 min after D/C infusion	Methemoglobinemia, headache, tachycardia, nausea, vomiting, flushing, tolerance with prolonged use	Arterial and venous vasodilator	Pericardial tamponade, constrictive pericarditis, or increased intracranial pressure
Trimethaphan (Arfonad) 500 mg/10 mL	IV infusion pump 0.5-5 mg/min	1-5 min	10 min after D/C infusion	Tachyphylaxis, ileus, constipation, urinary retention, pupillary dilation	Ganglionic blocker	Postoperative glaucoma
Phentolamine (Regitine)	1-5 mg IV initially, repeat as needed	Immediate	10-15 min	Chest pain, nausea, vomiting, dizziness, headache, nasal congestion, arrhythmia	Alpha-adrenergic blocker	Angina, coronary insufficiency, MI or history of MI, hypersensitivity to mannitol

[a]Nitroprusside is drug of choice for acute hypertensive emergencies. Supplied as 50 mg of lyophilized powder that is reconstituted with 2-3 mL of D_5W, yielding a red-brown solution. The contents of the vial are added to 250, 500, or 1,000 mL of D_5W to produce a solution for IV administration at a concentration of 200, 100, or 50 µg/mL, respectively. The container should be wrapped with metal foil to prevent light-induced decomposition. Under these conditions, the solution is stable for 4-24 hours. A rising blood pressure may indicate loss of potency. A change in color to yellow does not ↓ effectiveness. The appearance of a dark brown, green, or blue color indicates loss in activity. The drug is more effective if the head of the bed is slightly raised. When changing to a new bag, the administration rate may require adjustment.

[b]Thiocyanate levels rise gradually in proportion to the dose and duration of administration. The $t^{1/2}$ of thiocyanate is 2.7 days with normal renal function and 9 days in patients with renal failure. Toxicity occurs after 7-14 days in patients with normal renal function and 3-6 days in renal failure patients. Thiocyanate serum levels should be measured after 3-4 days of therapy, and the drug should be discontinued if levels exceed 10-12 mg/dL. Thiocyanate toxicity causes a neurotoxic syndrome of toxic psychosis, hyperreflexia, confusion, weakness, tinnitus, seizures, and coma.

[c]Signs of cyanide toxicity include lactic acidosis, hypoxemia, tachycardia, altered consciousness, seizures, and the smell of almonds on the breath. Concurrent administration of sodium thiosulfate or hydroxycobalamin may reduce the risk of cyanide toxicity in high-risk patients.

[d]Diazoxide is administered as a bolus dose (13 mg/kg Q 5 minutes to a max of 150 mg/injection) or as a slow infusion (15-20 mg/min) until a diastolic pressure of 100 mm Hg is reached. Significant fluid retention following diazoxide can cause HF and pulmonary edema. Concurrent loop diuretics are recommended (e.g., furosemide 40 mg IV) if diazoxide is given by rapid IV bolus. Reflex ↑ in heart rate and stroke volume are potentially dangerous in patients with angina or MI. Concurrent β-blockers may be protective.

[e]Not approved by the Food and Drug Administration for treatment of acute hypertension.

[f]Approved for intraoperative and postoperative treatment of hypertension.

[g]Parenteral hydralazine is an intermediate treatment between oral agents and more aggressive therapies such as nitroprusside or diazoxide. It can be given IV or IM, but there is no appreciable difference in onset of action (20-40 min) between the two routes. This slow onset minimizes hypotension.

[h]Labetalol is contraindicated in HF due to its β-blocking properties. A solution for continuous infusion is prepared by adding two 100-mg ampules to 160 mL of IV fluid to give a final concentration of 1 mg/mL. Infusions start at 2 mg/min and are titrated until a satisfactory response is achieved or a cumulative dose of 300 mg.

[i]Indicated for short-term treatment of hypertension when the oral route is not feasible or desirable.

[j]Requires special delivery system due to drug binding to PVC tubing. Also see Chapter 17, Ischemic Heart Disease, and Chapter 18, Myocardial Infarction, for further information regarding nitroglycerin.

ACE, angiotensin-converting enzyme; Ca, calcium; D_5W, 5% dextrose in water; D/C, discontinued; HF, heart failure; MI, myocardial infarction; Na, sodium.

Table 21-3   Oral Drugs Commonly Used in the Treatment of Hypertensive Urgencies

Drug (Brand Name)	Dose/Route	Onset of Action	Duration of Action	Major Side Effects[a]	Mechanism of Action	Avoid or Use Cautiously in Patients With These Conditions
Captopril[b] (Capoten) 12.5-, 25-, 50-, 100-mg tablets	6.5–50 mg PO	15 min	4–6 hr	Hyperkalemia, angioedema, ↑ BUN if dehydrated, rash, pruritus, proteinuria, loss of taste	ACE inhibitor	Renal artery stenosis, hyperkalemia, dehydration, renal failure, pregnancy
Clonidine (Catapres) 0.1-, 0.2-, 0.3-mg tablets	0.1–0.2 mg PO initially, then 0.1 mg/hr up to 0.8 mg total	0.5–2 hr	6–8 hr	Sedation, dry mouth, constipation	Central α-2 agonist	Altered mental status, severe carotid artery stenosis
Labetalol (Normodyne, Trandate) 100-, 200-, 300-mg tablets	200–400 mg PO repeated Q 2–3 hr	30 min–2 hr	4 hr	Orthostatic hypotension, nausea, vomiting	α- and β-adrenergic blocker	Heart failure, asthma, bradycardia
Minoxidil (Loniten) 2.5-, 10-mg tablets	5–20 mg PO	30–60 min. Max response in 2–4 hr	12–16 hr	Tachycardia, fluid retention	Arterial and venous vasodilator	Angina, Heart failure
Nifedipine[c] 10-, 20-mg capsules	10–20 mg PO May repeat in 20–60 min. Avoid bite and chew.	60 min PO 15–30 min bite and chew	3–5 hr	Burning paresthesias, flushing, headaches, palpitations, edema	Calcium entry blocker	Severe aortic stenosis, coronary artery disease, cerebrovascular disease

[a]All may cause hypotension, dizziness, and flushing.
[b]Other oral ACE inhibitors too slow in onset to be useful, but can be used for maintenance.
[c]Nifedipine not recommended for acute treatment because of serious side effects (angina, MI, stroke) associated with rapid-onset calcium blockers. Biting and chewing a perforated capsule and then swallowing the liquid contents may hasten the hypertensive effect (also risk of serious side effects) by ↓ the dissolution time of the gelatin outer coating. Nifedipine is not well absorbed buccally or sublingually.
ACE, angiotensin-converting enzyme; BUN, blood urea nitrogen; PO, orally.

example, lisinopril or another long-acting ACE inhibitor would be preferred for outpatient maintenance instead of the captopril previously prescribed. Good patient counseling will be required to help M.M. better understand the severity of his disease and the need to take his medications.

Oral Drug Therapy

Rapidly Acting Calcium Channel Blockers

2. M.M.'s physician has ordered nifedipine to be given 10 mg sublingually. Is this appropriate therapy to acutely lower his BP?

Clonidine, labetalol, prazosin, minoxidil, and captopril have all been used to lower BP acutely. These oral agents take several hours to adequately lower pressure and are, therefore, useful in treating hypertensive urgencies, but not emergencies. Oral ACE inhibitors, other than captopril, are not useful for acutely lowering BP because their onset of action is too slow. The immediate-release calcium channel blockers, including diltiazem, verapamil, and nicardipine, can rapidly lower BP; however, the most extensive experience is with nifedipine. Nifedipine, when given orally or by the "bite and swallow" method, was previously recommended as a rapid-acting alternative to parenteral therapy in the acute management of hypertension. However, its use has been associated with life-threatening adverse events of ischemia, MI, and stroke.[24–28] The prompt absorption of rapidly acting calcium channel blockers is followed by a sudden and precipitous decrease in BP as a result of peripheral vasodilation. This reduces coronary perfusion, induces a reflex tachycardia, and increases myocardial oxygen consumption.[26,32] Elderly patients with underlying coronary or cerebrovascular disease, history of MI, volume depletion, or concurrent use of other antihypertensive drugs are at increased risk for significant adverse events. Currently, no outcome data are available to critically assess the safety or efficacy of this therapeutic intervention. In addition, the risks associated with high pressures without acute or progressive end-organ damage are unclear.[32] Therefore, until more data become available, neither sublingual, bite and chew, nor swallowing of the intact immediate-release nifedipine capsules or other rapidly acting calcium channel blockers is recommended.

Other adverse effects associated with nifedipine are minor and include a burning sensation in the face and legs (6%), facial flushing (5%), palpitations (4.6%), sporadic premature ventricular contractions (3.7%), ankle edema (2%), dryness of the mouth (1%), postural hypotension (0.3%), and urticaria (0.3%).

The cavalier use of rapid-release nifedipine to acutely lower BP is potentially dangerous and should be discouraged. M.M. should not be given immediate-release nifedipine by any administration method to acutely lower his BP. His age, history of MI, absence of symptoms, and lack of new or progressive target organ damage do not warrant the acute and potentially dangerous drop in BP. M.M.'s BP can be managed safely using other oral medications. Captopril, labetalol, or clonidine can be used to lower his BP, and he can be restarted on his oral maintenance regimen with appropriate follow-up care.

Clonidine

3. A decision is made not to use nifedipine or any other rapidly acting calcium channel blocker, but rather to give M.M. oral clonidine. What is an appropriate starting dose? What is the correlation between the loading dose and the maintenance dose?

Clonidine is considered a safe, effective first-line therapy for a hypertensive urgency. It is a centrally acting, α_2-adrenergic agonist that inhibits sympathetic outflow from the CNS. After acute administration, clonidine reduces mean arterial pressure, cardiac output, stroke volume, and cardiac rate. There is little change in the total peripheral resistance or renal plasma flow. The initial reduction in cardiac output is caused by decreased venous return to the right side of the heart secondary to venodilation and bradycardia, not secondary to decreased contractility. Guanabenz (Wytensin) has a similar mechanism of action, but documented efficacy in the acute treatment of hypertension is lacking.

The BP can be lowered gradually over several hours using oral clonidine. Usually, an initial oral loading dose (0.1 to 0.2 mg) is followed by repeated doses of 0.1 mg each hour until the desired response is achieved or until a cumulative dose of 0.5 to 0.8 mg is reached.[33–35] A significant reduction in BP is first seen within 1 hour, and the mean arterial pressure decreases by 25% in most patients after several hours. Clinical trials of clonidine in hypertensive urgencies resulted in response rates of >80% within 2 hours after oral administration.[34–37] Anderson and colleagues reported a 94% response rate to an oral loading dose.[34] Patients required a mean total dose of 0.45 mg, and the maximum response occurred 5 to 6 hours after the start of therapy. Doses should be reduced in patients with volume depletion, those who have recently used other antihypertensive drugs, and the elderly.[1,20]

The acute response to oral clonidine loading is not predictive of the daily dose required to maintain acceptable BP control. Maintenance oral therapy with clonidine is somewhat empiric. Some authors have recommended giving 80% to 100% of the cumulative loading dose per day in split doses morning and evening.[34,38] The major portion is given at bedtime to minimize daytime sedation.

ADVERSE EFFECTS AND PRECAUTIONS

4. What precautions should be exercised when using the oral clonidine loading regimen?

Oral clonidine is generally well tolerated. Adverse effects include orthostatic hypotension, bradycardia, sedation, dry mouth, and dizziness. Sedation is a particularly troublesome side effect, and because of this, clonidine should not be used in patients in whom mental status is an important monitoring parameter. Because clonidine can decrease cerebral blood flow by up to 28%, it should not be used in patients with severe cerebrovascular disease.[19,39] Clonidine also should be avoided in patients with HF, bradycardia, sick sinus syndrome, or cardiac conduction defects,[20] as well as patients at risk for medication nonadherence due to the rapid rise in BP that can occur with sudden drug withdrawal.[40,41]

Other Oral Drugs
CAPTOPRIL

5. M.M. has a history of mild heart failure and normal renal function on admission. Based on these findings, would captopril be a reasonable choice for initial treatment? How should it be given? What if his BUN or SrCr were elevated?

Captopril, an orally active ACE inhibitor, has been used both orally and sublingually to acutely lower BP.[42-44] Captopril decreases both afterload and preload, increases regional blood flow, and lowers total peripheral vascular resistance.[20] For this reason, captopril and other ACE inhibitors are often considered the drugs of choice in patients with heart failure (see Chapter 19, Heart Failure, for a discussion of the use of ACE inhibitors in heart failure). Captopril also may be useful in the treatment of severe hypertension associated with scleroderma.[20,23] Given that M.M. appeared to be well controlled on his ACE inhibitor prior to arbitrarily stopping his medications, it is reasonable to restart an ACE inhibitor and reinforce medication adherence issues.

After oral administration, the onset of action of captopril occurs within minutes and peaks 30 to 90 minutes after ingestion. When captopril (25 mg) is given sublingually, dissolution of the tablet occurs within 2 to 4 minutes, BP reduction starts within 10 to 15 minutes, and the effect persists for 2 to 6 hours. Sublingual captopril is as effective as nifedipine in acutely reducing mean arterial pressure in both urgent and emergent conditions.[23,43,45]

Despite these beneficial effects, captopril, as well as all ACE inhibitors, must be used with caution in patients with renal insufficiency or volume depletion. In most cases, an elevated BUN or SrCr will provide a clue to the existence of these conditions; however, captopril also can induce severe renal failure in patients with bilateral renal artery stenosis or renal artery stenosis in a solitary kidney. Such conditions may not be easy to detect in the context of an acute hypertensive emergency. Therefore, in patients in whom these conditions can be excluded, captopril can be considered for therapy. First-dose hypotension is a common limiting factor with the use of oral or sublingual captopril. This complication is most likely to occur in patients with high renin levels, such as those who are volume depleted or those receiving diuretics. Under these circumstances, initial doses should not exceed 12.5 mg, with repeat doses an hour or more later if necessary. These same patients may also be more predisposed to captopril-induced renal function changes. Although he was not taking his diuretic, M.M. is still likely to be have high renin levels due to his history of HF. Therefore, captopril would be a reasonable choice as initial therapy in M.M., which can later be replaced by a longer-acting ACE inhibitor. In addition, fewer side effects are associated with captopril than with nifedipine.

MINOXIDIL, PRAZOSIN, AND LABETALOL

6. What other oral agents are used to acutely lower BP?

Minoxidil, a potent oral vasodilator, has been used successfully in the treatment of severe hypertension.[46-48] An oral loading dose of 10 to 20 mg produces a maximal BP response in 2 to 4 hours and can be followed by a dose of 5 to 20 mg every 4 hours if necessary. Unfortunately, its onset of action is slower than that of clonidine or captopril. Another complicating factor is that β-blockers and loop diuretics generally must be used concomitantly to counteract minoxidil-induced reflex tachycardia and fluid retention.[48] Therefore, minoxidil should be used only in patients who are refractory to other forms of therapy or who have previously been taking this agent.[38]

Prazosin has been used to a limited degree to treat hypertensive urgencies. An oral loading dose of 5 mg maximally reduced BP within 60 to 120 minutes.[49] However, hypotension can be a significant limiting factor. More controlled studies are required before this drug can be recommended.

Several investigators have suggested that oral labetalol can be used acutely to treat severe hypertension.[50-53] Initial doses of 100 to 300 mg may provide a sustained response for up to 4 hours.[51] Labetalol (200 mg given at hourly intervals to a maximum dose of 1,200 mg) was comparable to oral clonidine in reducing mean arterial pressure.[53] An alternative regimen using 300 mg initially followed by 100 mg at 2-hour intervals to a maximum of 500 mg was also successful in acutely lowering BP.[52] However, Wright and colleagues[54] were unable to achieve an adequate BP response in a small series of patients using a single loading dose of 200 to 400 mg.

Oral labetalol is an alternative to oral clonidine or captopril for the acute treatment of hypertension, but the most appropriate dosing regimen remains to be determined. Because it can cause profound orthostatic hypotension, patients should remain in the supine position and should be checked for orthostasis before ambulation. In addition, because it lacks β[2] specificity, labetalol should be avoided in patients with asthma, bradycardia, or advanced heart block. Caution should also be used in patients with end-stage renal disease because case reports have documented hyperkalemia after labetalol administration in these patients.[55]

Following initial treatment with oral captopril, M.M.'s BP was reduced to 150/100 mm Hg. His oral medications were then restarted; captopril was switched to lisinopril; and he was scheduled for follow-up in 1 week.

HYPERTENSIVE EMERGENCIES

Patient Assessment

7. M.R., a 55-year-old Black man, presents to the emergency department (ED) with a 3-day history of progressively increasing shortness of breath (SOB). Over the past 2 days, he developed a severe headache unrelieved by ibuprofen (Advil), as well as substernal chest pain, anorexia, and nausea. His medical history includes asthma and a 5-year history of angina, which, 2 months before admission, resulted in hospitalization for an acute inferior MI. He has been taking albuterol via metered-dose inhaler (MDI) (Proventil, Ventolin), furosemide (Lasix), isosorbide dinitrate (Isordil Titradose, Sorbitrate), felodipine (Plendil), and lisinopril (Prinivil, Zestril), but discontinued these medications on his own 3 weeks ago.

Physical examination reveals an anxious-appearing man who is alert, oriented, and in moderate respiratory distress. His vital signs include pulse, 125 beats/min; respiratory rate, 36 breaths/min; BP, 220/145 mm Hg without orthostasis; and a normal body temperature. Funduscopic examination shows arteriolar narrowing and AV nicking without hemorrhages, exudates, or papilledema. There is no jugular venous distention, but bilateral carotid bruits are present. Chest examination reveals decreased breath sounds with bilateral rales extending to the tip of the scapula. M.R.'s heart is displaced 2 cm left of the midclavicular line with no thrills or heaves. The rhythm is regular with an S[3] and an S[4] gallop; no murmurs are noted. The remainder of M.R.'s examination is within normal limits.

Significant laboratory values include sodium (Na), 142 mEq/L (normal, 136 to 144); potassium (K), 4.9 mEq/L (normal,

3.5 to 5.5); chloride (Cl), 101 mEq/L (normal, 96 to 106); bicarbonate, 23 mEq/L (normal, 23 to 28); BUN, 30 mg/dL (normal, 10 to 20); creatinine, 1.2 mg/dL (normal, 0.5 to 1.2); hematocrit (Hct), 38% (normal, 40 to 45%); hemoglobin (Hgb), 13.0 g/dL (normal, 14 to 18); white blood cell (WBC) count and differential, within normal limits. UA shows 1+ hemoglobin and 1+ protein. Microscopic examination of the urine reveals 5 to 10 red blood cells (RBCs) per high-power field (HPF) and no casts. Pulse oximetry reveals an oxygen saturation of 88%. An ECG demonstrates sinus tachycardia and left ventricular hypertrophy. The chest radiograph shows moderate cardiomegaly and bilateral fluffy infiltrates.

What aspects of M.R.'s history and physical examination are characteristic of an emergent need to immediately lower his BP?

[SI units: Na, 142 mmol/L (normal, 136 to 144); K, 4.9 mmol/L (normal, 3.5 to 5.5); Cl, 101 mmol/L (normal, 96 to 106); bicarbonate, 23 mmol/L (normal, 23 to 28); BUN, 10.71 mmol/L urea (normal, 3.57 to 7.14); creatinine, 106 mmol/L (normal, 44.2 to 106.08); Hct, 0.38 (normal, 0.40 to 0.45); Hgb, 130 g/L (normal, 140 to 180)]

As discussed earlier, hypertensive crisis occurs most often in Black men and individuals between the ages of 40 and 60. M.R. meets all of the characteristics of this population. Further, many patients who present with hypertensive emergencies have a recent history of discontinuing the use of their antihypertensives,[12] as is the case with M.R.

Recent-onset severe headache, nausea, and vomiting are consistent with CNS signs of severe hypertension, as are the acute onset of angina (substernal pain) and HF (SOB, increased pulse and respiratory rate, cardiomegaly, S₃, and chest x-ray findings of pulmonary edema). The absence of signs of right-sided HF such as jugular venous distention or hepatomegaly suggests an acute onset of HF caused by hypertension as opposed to a gradual worsening of chronic HF. M.R.'s urinary sediment is relatively unimpressive at this time, especially in light of his history, and his ocular complications are minimal.

Parenteral Drug Therapy

Nitroprusside

8. M.R. is to be started on nitroprusside. Is this an appropriate choice of drug? What alternatives to nitroprusside are available?

M.R.'s arterial pressure should be lowered with parenteral medications, which have a rapid onset of action. Nitroprusside, fenoldopam, intravenous (IV) nitroglycerin, and trimethaphan all decrease total peripheral resistance rapidly with minimal effect on myocardial oxygen consumption and heart rate. Of these agents, either nitroprusside or fenoldopam would be preferred in patients with hypertension accompanied by acute left ventricular failure in the absence of MI. Parenteral nitroglycerin can be used to lower BP in patients with ischemic heart disease (see Question 24). IV nitroglycerin is similar to nitroprusside except that it has relatively greater effect on venous circulation and less effect on arterioles. It is most useful in patients with coronary insufficiency, MI, or hypertension following coronary bypass surgery (see Question 24). Trimethaphan is not an acceptable choice because rapid tolerance develops to its hypotensive action and its use is

associated with many side effects (see Question 31). Fenoldopam and nitroprusside are equally efficacious in acutely lowering BP.[56–58] Both drugs have an immediate onset, are easily titratable, have a short duration of action, and are relatively well tolerated. Fenoldopam also may increase renal blood flow, thereby reducing the risk for worsening renal function.[59–62] Unlike nitroprusside, fenoldopam does not cause cyanide or thiocyanate toxicity, but it is considerably more expensive than nitroprusside.

Therefore, in the absence of any significant renal or liver disease, nitroprusside is the preferred treatment for M.R.

HEMODYNAMIC EFFECTS

Nitroprusside has many pharmacologic effects that should improve M.R.'s condition. It dilates both venous and arterial vessels, thereby increasing venous capacitance and decreasing the venous return or preload on the heart (see Chapters 19, Heart Failure, and 22, Shock). A decrease in the pulmonary capillary wedge pressure and ventricular filling pressure will ultimately improve M.R.'s pulmonary edema. Afterload also is decreased as a result of arterial dilation. This action increases cardiac output, reduces arterial pressure, and increases tissue perfusion.

CONCURRENT USE OF DIURETICS

9. Should M.R. be given a diuretic before nitroprusside therapy is begun?

Administration of potent IV diuretics is relatively ineffective in the acute treatment of hypertension except in patients with concomitant volume overload or heart failure.[63] Many patients with hypertensive emergencies are vasoconstricted and have normal or reduced plasma volumes; therefore, diuretics have little effect and may actually aggravate renal failure or cause other adverse effects.[14,63,64] Further, when diuretics are given acutely in combination with other antihypertensive agents, profound hypotension can occur.

The value of diuretics in acute HF is related more to their hemodynamic effects (venodilation) than to diuresis. Venodilation following IV diuretic administration decreases right-sided cardiac filling pressures, decreases pulmonary artery and wedge pressures, and increases cardiac output before diuresis occurs.[65] Therefore, the presence of HF and severely elevated BP in M.R. warrants the IV administration of either furosemide 20 to 40 mg or bumetanide (Bumex) 1 mg.

DOSING AND ADMINISTRATION

10. How should nitroprusside be prepared and administered? What dose should be used initially?

Because of its extreme potency, sodium nitroprusside must be prepared in exact concentrations, administered at precisely calculated rates using a controlled infusion device, and closely monitored with intra-arterial BP recording. Sodium nitroprusside is supplied in units of 50 mg of lyophilized powder. The powder is reconstituted with 2 to 3 mL of 5% dextrose in water (D5W), shaking gently to dissolve.[66] The contents of the vial are then added to 250, 500, or 1,000 mL of D5W to produce a solution for IV administration with a drug concentration containing 200, 100, or 50 μg/mL. This solution should have a slight brownish tint.

Nitroprusside decomposes on exposure to light, so the solution should be shielded with an opaque sleeve. It is not necessary to protect the tubing from light as well. Although it was previously recommended that solutions of sodium nitroprusside be discarded 4 hours after reconstitution, when adequately protected from light, reconstituted solutions are stable for 24 hours. A change in the solution's color from light brown to dark brown, green, orange, or blue indicates a loss in activity, and the solution should be discarded.

Effective infusion rates range from 0.25 to 10 μg/kg per minute. Cyanide toxicity may occur with prolonged administration or with infusion rates greater than 2 to 3 μg/kg per minute.[67,68] For M.R., an infusion of nitroprusside should be initiated at a rate of 0.25 μg/kg per minute, using a microdrip regulator or an infusion pump. The dose should be increased slowly by 0.25 μg/kg per minute every 5 minutes until the desired pressure is achieved. A maximum infusion rate of 10 μg/kg per minute has been recommended. If adequate BP reduction is not achieved within 10 minutes following maximum dose infusion, nitroprusside should be discontinued.[3] The dosage must be individualized according to patient response using continuous intra-arterial BP recording and signs or symptoms of toxicity.

THERAPEUTIC ENDPOINT

11. **A nitroprusside infusion of 0.25 μg/kg per minute is started. What is the goal of therapy?**

M.R.'s arterial pressure should be reduced to near-normal levels; however, because he has cerebral occlusive disease (carotid bruits), excessive reduction of his BP should be avoided. Overly aggressive reduction of BP in the presence of major cerebral vessel stenosis may decrease cerebral blood flow and produce strokes or other neurologic complications.

Normal cerebral blood flow remains relatively constant over a wide range of systemic BP measurements through autoregulatory mechanisms.[39,63,69] The autoregulatory effects can prevent gross alterations in cerebral blood flow from either slow or rapid changes in systemic arterial pressures. In addition, the BP required to maintain cerebral perfusion is higher in hypertensive patients than in normotensive individuals. If M.R.'s BP is reduced excessively, cerebral blood flow may decrease sharply. Therefore, a diastolic BP of 100 to 105 mm Hg would be a reasonable initial therapeutic goal for him. If hypotension does occur, nitroprusside should be discontinued and M.R.'s feet should be elevated.

CYANIDE TOXICITY

12. **M.R. is being treated with nitroprusside. However, over the last 36 hours, dose titration to 7 μg/kg per minute has been necessary to control his BP. Is he at risk for developing cyanide toxicity? What indices of toxicity should be monitored? Should thiosulfate or hydroxocobalamin be given to prevent toxicity?**

A major concern when using sodium nitroprusside is toxicity secondary to the accumulation of its metabolic byproducts, cyanide and thiocyanate. Sodium nitroprusside decomposes within a few minutes after IV infusion. Free cyanide, which represents 44% of nitroprusside by weight, is released into the bloodstream, producing prussic acid (hydrogen cyanide), which is responsible for the acute toxicity.[70] The amount of hydrogen cyanide released is directly proportional to the size of the dose.[71] Endogenous detoxification of cyanide occurs through a mitochondrial rhodanese system, which, in the presence of a sulfur donor such as thiosulfate, converts cyanide to thiocyanate.[70] This enzymatic detoxification of cyanide exhibits zero-order pharmacokinetics and is dependent on the enzyme rhodanese and an adequate supply of thiosulfate. A healthy person can eliminate cyanide hepatically at a rate equivalent to the cyanide production during a nitroprusside infusion of up to approximately 2 μg/kg per minute.[72] Theoretically, cyanide can be expected to accumulate in the body when the rate of the sodium nitroprusside infusion exceeds 2 μg/kg per minute for a prolonged period. This rise can be prevented by administering sodium thiosulfate simultaneously.[73,74] A mixture of 0.1% sodium nitroprusside plus 1% sodium thiosulfate is as effective as sodium nitroprusside alone and is substantially less toxic.[73] For this reason, some clinicians have recommended that all patients receiving nitroprusside receive concomitant thiosulfate infusions.[75,76] IV boluses of thiosulfate may be effective, but they require frequent dosing. Rindone and Sloane[71] noted that 10 mg of sodium thiosulfate for every 1 mg of nitroprusside should be considered in high-risk patients (e.g., those with malnutrition) or when large doses of nitroprusside are administered (>3 μg/kg per minute). The presence of hepatic or renal failure also may predispose the patient to cyanide toxicity.[72,77] However, no studies have assessed the chemical compatibility of nitroprusside and sodium thiosulfate.

It is generally stated that symptomatic cyanide toxicity occurs infrequently, although several deaths have been reported after the use of sodium nitroprusside.[76] Cyanide toxicity occurs most commonly when large doses (total dose 1.5 mg/kg) of nitroprusside are administered rapidly to patients undergoing a surgical procedure that requires induction of hypotension. However, cyanide toxicity and mortality associated with nitroprusside exceed 3,000 and 1,000 cases per year, respectively, according to two sources.[76,78] The increasing concern about cyanide toxicity has resulted in a revision of the product label, which warns that sodium nitroprusside administration increases the body's concentration of cyanide ion to toxic and potentially fatal levels, even when given within the range of recommended doses. The revised labeling further states that infusions at the maximum recommended dose can overwhelm the body's ability to buffer the cyanide within 1 hour.

Although concurrent sodium thiosulfate administration has been recommended in high-risk patients, no clinical data are available to indicate that it reduces overall mortality. Further, this intervention may result in the accumulation of thiocyanate, particularly if sodium thiosulfate is given at high infusion rates or to patients with renal insufficiency. A 1-year retrospective review at a tertiary care teaching hospital with a level 1 trauma center found that none of the patients receiving nitroprusside at infusion rates >2 μg/kg per minute were concurrently treated with sodium thiosulfate.[79]

Hydroxocobalamin also has been used to reduce cyanide toxicity secondary to nitroprusside infusions.[77] The concurrent administration of a continuous infusion of hydroxocobalamin (25 mg/hour) lowers RBC and plasma cyanide concentrations.[80] Hydroxocobalamin combines with cyanide to form cyanocobalamin, which is nontoxic and excreted in the urine. Approximately 2.4 g of hydroxocobalamin is required to neutralize the cyanide released from 100 mg of nitroprusside. Therefore, its use is limited because of poor availability and cost considerations. Importantly, unlike hydroxocobalamin, cyanocobalamin is not effective in reducing or preventing cyanide toxicity.

To summarize, the use of hydroxocobalamin or sodium thiosulfate is likely to be of greatest value in patients receiving large doses of sodium nitroprusside acutely or in patients receiving high infusion rates or over an extended period. However, with the availability of safer alternatives (e.g., fenoldopam, IV labetalol, IV nicardipine) for use in high-risk patients, the use of hydroxocobalamin or thiosulfate is rarely required.

Cyanide toxicity can be detected early by monitoring M.R.'s metabolic status. Lactic acidosis is an early indicator of toxicity because the progressive inactivation of cytochrome oxidase by cyanide results in increased anaerobic glycolysis.[81] A low plasma bicarbonate concentration and low pH, accompanied by an increase in the blood lactate or lactate-to-pyruvate ratio, and an increase in the mixed venous blood oxygen tension could indicate cyanide toxicity.[81] Additional signs of cyanide intoxication include tachycardia, altered consciousness, coma, convulsions, and the occasional smell of almonds on the breath.[71,81] Hypoxemia resulting from pulmonary arterial shunting also has been reported during nitroprusside therapy. Measuring serum thiocyanate levels is of no value in detecting the onset of cyanide toxicity. If toxicity develops, the infusion should be stopped and appropriate therapy for cyanide intoxication should be instituted. The need for such a high-dose infusion of nitroprusside to maintain M.R.'s pressure may increase his risk for cyanide toxicity, warranting close monitoring of his acid–base balance.

THIOCYANATE TOXICITY

13. Explain the difference between cyanide toxicity and thiocyanate toxicity. What is M.R.'s risk for thiocyanate toxicity? Is monitoring of serum thiocyanate concentrations necessary?

Sodium nitroprusside is more likely to produce thiocyanate toxicity. Although this complication also is rare, patients with renal failure who receive prolonged infusions are particularly susceptible. The cyanide released from nitroprusside is normally metabolized to thiocyanate via sulfation by thiosulfate in the liver. This conversion of cyanide to thiocyanate proceeds relatively slowly, and thiocyanate levels rise gradually in proportion to the dose and duration of sodium nitroprusside administration. The half-life of thiocyanate is 2.7 days with normal renal function and 9 days in patients with renal failure.[75] When sodium nitroprusside is infused for several days at moderate dosages (2 to 5 μg/kg per minute), toxic levels of thiocyanate can occur within 7 to 14 days in patients with normal renal function and 3 to 6 days in patients with severe renal disease.[70] A total daily dose of up to 125 mg is nontoxic in patients with normal renal function, whereas 1,000 mg/day may produce toxicity within 24 to 48 hours. Unfortunately, infusion of sodium thiosulfate, which helps reduce cyanide toxicity, can result in accumulation of thiocyanate, resulting in clinical toxicity, especially in patients with renal failure.[77]

Thiocyanate causes a neurotoxic syndrome manifested by psychosis, hyperreflexia, confusion, weakness, tinnitus,

seizures, and coma.[72,75] Prolonged exposure to thiocyanate can suppress thyroid function through inhibition of iodine uptake and binding by the thyroid.[75] Routine measurement of blood levels of thiocyanate is unnecessary and is recommended only in patients with renal disease or when the duration of the nitroprusside infusion exceeds 3 or 4 days. Nitroprusside should be discontinued if serum thiocyanate levels exceed 10 to 12 mg/dL.[82,83] Life-threatening toxicity is of concern when blood thiocyanate levels exceed 20 mg/dL.[75] In emergency cases, thiocyanate can be readily removed by hemodialysis.[75]

For M.R., the potential for thiocyanate toxicity is low because his renal function is normal and the infusion time is relatively short. Therefore, measurement of thiocyanate levels is not indicated at this time. Other side effects associated with nitroprusside therapy include nausea, vomiting, diaphoresis, nasal stuffiness, muscular twitching, dizziness, and weakness. These effects usually are acute and occur when nitroprusside is administered too rapidly. They can be reversed by decreasing the infusion rate.

14. M.R.'s serum chemistries and arterial blood gas values indicate a metabolic acidosis. Should the nitroprusside infusion be continued at 7 μg/kg per minute? What alternative is available?

Although the duration of M.R.'s nitroprusside therapy has been short, tolerance to the antihypertensive effect requires the use of a high-dose infusion to maintain BP control. Thus, acidosis may represent toxicity as a result of cyanide accumulation. The nitroprusside infusion should be discontinued at this time, and another rapidly acting, easily titratable parenteral antihypertensive such as fenoldopam or IV nicardipine should be initiated.

Fenoldopam

15. What are the advantages and disadvantages of fenoldopam compared with sodium nitroprusside?

HEMODYNAMIC EFFECTS

Fenoldopam is a parenteral, rapidly acting, peripheral dopamine-1 agonist used to manage severe hypertension when a rapid reduction of BP is required.[84–87] Stimulation of the dopamine-1 receptors vasodilates coronary, renal, mesenteric, and peripheral arteries.[88] Vasodilation of the renal vasculature increases renal blood flow in hypertensive patients,[59,60,62] a property that may be particularly advantageous in patients with impaired renal function.[61,89] However, no outcome data are available to document that this effect reduces morbidity and mortality in patients with severe hypertension. Fenoldopam also has been used to control perioperative hypertension in patients undergoing cardiac bypass surgery because, relative to nitroprusside, it either maintains or increases urinary output.[90,91] Fenoldopam is as effective as sodium nitroprusside for the acute treatment of hypertension and does not cause either cyanide or thiocyanate toxicity.[56–58] However, its cost is a major limiting factor. In summary, fenoldopam is as efficacious as, less toxic than, but considerably more expensive than sodium nitroprusside. Outcome studies will be required to assess the impact of fenoldopam on increasing renal blood flow and urine output in the management of patients with hypertensive emergencies. Until such time, it should be used only as an alternative to nitroprusside in patients like M.R., who are at high risk for cyanide or thiocyanate toxicity.

DOSING AND ADMINISTRATION

16. **How should fenoldopam be administered?**

Fenoldopam is administered as a continuous infusion (without a bolus dose) beginning at a rate of 0.1 μg/kg per minute. It is then titrated upward, according to BP control, in increments of 0.05 to 0.1 μg/kg per minute at 15-minute intervals. The maximum dose is 1.6 μg/kg per minute. Clearance of fenoldopam is not altered by renal or liver disease. Like nitroprusside, fenoldopam also has a short duration of action, with an elimination half-life of approximately 5 minutes, thus allowing for easy titration.

ADVERSE EFFECTS

17. **M.R. is converted to a continuous infusion of fenoldopam, and his BP is well controlled on 0.3 μg/kg per minute. What monitoring parameters should be followed?**

Fenoldopam is well tolerated and relatively free of side effects. BP and heart rate should be followed closely to avoid hypotension and dose-related tachycardia. The vasodilating effect may also cause flushing, dizziness, and headache. Serum electrolytes should be monitored, and in some cases potassium supplementation is required. Fenoldopam should be used cautiously in patients with glaucoma or intraocular hypertension due to a dose-dependent increase in intraocular pressure.[92,93]

18. **Which antihypertensive agents should be avoided in M.R.? Why?**

Labetalol, a potent, rapidly acting antihypertensive with both α- and β-blocking activity, is very effective in the treatment of various hypertensive emergencies,[94–100] but it should not be used in M.R. (see Question 19). Hemodynamically, labetalol reduces peripheral vascular resistance (afterload), BP, and heart rate, with almost no change in the resting cardiac output or stroke volume.[101] It does not cause the reflex tachycardia and redistribution of coronary blood flow that is experienced with nitroprusside. These qualities make labetalol ideally suited for BP reduction in patients with underlying coronary artery disease, angina, or acute infarction, as well as after vascular surgical procedures.[5] In addition, labetalol may be better tolerated than nitroprusside by patients with hepatic or renal insufficiency because toxic nitroprusside metabolites accumulate in these situations.

M.R. is experiencing chest pain, and he is tachycardic; these signs and symptoms are most likely caused by his severely uncontrolled hypertension and the presence of acute left ventricular failure. Even though labetalol might improve M.R.'s angina, the negative inotropic action could acutely compromise his left ventricular dysfunction, an effect that outweighs the potential benefit of afterload reduction. In addition, even though labetalol is one of the safest β-blocking drugs when used in patients with asthma,[102] no β-blocker should be used as initial treatment in patients with asthma. Labetalol should be used only if alternative methods of reducing M.R.'s pressure fail.

Diazoxide, a potent, rapidly acting hypotensive agent closely related to the thiazide group of drugs, also should be avoided in M.R. for several reasons (see Questions 25 through 27). The hypotensive action is caused by a reduction in peripheral vascular resistance through direct relaxation of arterioles. As arterial pressure is lowered, baroreceptor reflexes are activated, leading to cardiac stimulation with increased heart rate, stroke volume, and cardiac output. The cardiostimulating effect of diazoxide could be potentially dangerous in patients such as M.R., who have ischemic heart disease and a recent history of MI. An early report indicated that 50% of the patients receiving diazoxide for hypertensive emergencies had significant ST- and T-wave changes.[103] Neurologic and cardiovascular symptoms may occur with rapid administration of diazoxide. The combination of slow infusion diazoxide preceded by a β-blocker has been recommended to prevent reflex tachycardia.[104] However, with M.R.'s history of HF and asthma, β-blockers should be avoided.

There are other reasons why diazoxide should be avoided or used cautiously in M.R. Although diazoxide has a thiazide-like structure, it causes significant sodium and water retention, which could be deleterious in a patient such as M.R. with severe HF and pulmonary edema.[105,106] The exact mechanism for this effect is unknown, but it may be through an activation of the renin system or a direct antinatriuretic effect on the renal tubules. Generally, it is recommended that a potent diuretic such as furosemide be administered before diazoxide. However, this is not necessary if diazoxide is administered by the mini-bolus or slow infusion method (see Question 26) and HF is absent.

Diazoxide decreases urate excretion and increases uric acid levels. In patients like M.R. with normal renal function, this effect can be reversed with the use of uricosurics.

Labetalol

19. **C.M., a 52-year-old White man, is admitted to the hospital with a 3-day history of increasing exertional substernal chest pain (without SOB), diaphoresis, nausea, and vomiting. His history is significant for poorly controlled hypertension, glaucoma, and angina pectoris. Prior medications include dorzolamide ophthalmic drops (Trusopt), atenolol (Tenormin), hydrochlorothiazide, and oral nitrates. Physical examination reveals an anxious White man who is alert and oriented. He has a BP of 210/146 mm Hg without orthostasis and a regular pulse of 115 beats/min. Bilateral hemorrhages and exudates are present on funduscopic examination. The lungs are clear and the heart is enlarged, but there are no murmurs or gallops. Examination of the abdomen is unremarkable, and there is no peripheral edema. The neurologic examination is normal.**

Significant laboratory values include the following: Na, 140 mEq/L (normal, 136 to 144); Cl, 109 mEq/L (normal, 96 to 106); bicarbonate, 18 mEq/L (normal, 23 to 28); BUN, 49 mg/dL (normal, 10 to 20); and creatinine, 2.8 mg/dL (renal function previously noted to be within normal limits). UA shows proteinuria and hematuria. The ECG demonstrates sinus tachycardia with left axis deviation, left ventricular hypertrophy, and nonspecific ST-T–wave changes. The chest radiograph reveals mild cardiomegaly.

C.M. is given nitroglycerin sublingually (Nitrostat), and 1 inch of nitroglycerin ointment (Nitrol Paste) is applied topically.

He is started on IV labetalol. Is this choice of treatment reasonable, considering C.M.'s angina and acute renal failure?

[SI units: Na, 140 mmol/L (normal, 136 to 144); Cl, 109 mmol/L (normal, 96 to 106); bicarbonate, 18 mmol/L (normal, 23 to 28); BUN, 17.493 mmol/L urea (normal, 3.57 to 7.14); creatinine, 247.52 mmol/L (normal, 44.2 to 106.08)]

The presence of chest pain, grade III retinopathy, new-onset renal disease, and the magnitude of the BP elevation in C.M. warrant a prompt reduction in BP. The combination of sublingual and topical nitroglycerin may help in acutely lowering his BP and relieving his chest pain while waiting for more definitive treatment to be implemented.

IV labetalol is a potent antihypertensive drug that has been used successfully in various hypertensive emergencies.[94–100] Labetalol blocks both α- and β-adrenergic receptors and also may exert a direct vasodilator effect. The β-blockade is nonselective with a β-to-α potency of 3:1 for oral and 7:1 for IV labetalol. Labetalol is particularly advantageous in C.M. because the immediate onset of action will reduce peripheral vascular resistance without causing reflex tachycardia. Myocardial oxygen demand will be reduced and coronary hemodynamics will be improved, making this agent an excellent choice for patients like C.M. who have coronary artery disease or MI. In addition, IV labetalol does not significantly reduce cerebral blood flow; therefore, it may be useful in patients with cerebrovascular disease.[1,20,63]

Fenoldopam or nitroprusside also could be used to treat C.M. Fenoldopam could potentially benefit renal function by increasing renal blood flow, but C.M.'s history of glaucoma would preclude its use. In addition, equally effective, but less costly alternatives are available. Treatment with nitroprusside would expose C.M. to the potential risk of cyanide and thiocyanate toxicity with his new-onset renal failure. Labetalol, on the other hand, has been used successfully in patients with renal disease without deleterious side effects.[107,108] Labetalol is eliminated by glucuronidation in the liver, with <5% of the dose being excreted unchanged in the urine. The presence of renal disease in C.M. will not necessitate an alteration in the dose of labetalol.

CONTRAINDICATIONS

20. What cautions should be exercised when using labetalol in C.M.?

Labetalol's disadvantages are primarily related to its β-blocking effects, which predominate over its α-blocking effects. Therefore, it should not be used in patients with asthma, heart block greater than first degree, or sinus bradycardia, and it should be used with caution in patients with severe uncontrolled HF[95,101,109] (see Question 18). None of these is present in C.M. Like other β-blockers, labetalol may mask the symptoms of hypoglycemia in insulin-dependent diabetic patients; it also should be used with caution in patients with intermittent claudication or Raynaud's syndrome.[109] Labetalol has been effective in the treatment of hypertension associated with pheochromocytoma and excess catecholamine states.[110] However, because labetalol is primarily a β-blocker, paradoxical hypertension may occur in patients with pheochromocytoma because they excrete high amounts of norepinephrine due to relatively unopposed α-receptor stimulation.[111] More clinical experience is required before labetalol can be recommended in patients with pheochromocytoma.[5,94] Labetalol also may be particularly useful for the treatment of antihypertensive withdrawal syndromes.[11,63]

21. Will C.M.'s age or prior use of antihypertensives affect his response to labetalol?

There appears to be a positive correlation between age and response to labetalol. Older patients achieve a greater reduction in BP and, therefore, require smaller doses.[112,113] Failure to lower BP also has been observed.[114–116] This phenomenon was thought to be related to single-bolus administration or prior treatment with β- and α-blocking drugs.[109] However, subsequent studies have confirmed labetalol's effectiveness in patients pretreated with antihypertensives, including β-blockers.[117]

22. How should parenteral labetalol be given to C.M.?

For acute BP reduction, C.M. should be placed in the supine position. IV labetalol can be given by pulse administration or continuous infusion.[94–99] Small incremental bolus injections are administered, beginning with 20 mg given over 2 minutes, followed by 40 to 80 mg every 10 to 15 minutes until the desired response is achieved or a cumulative dose of 300 mg is reached. The desired response usually is achieved with a mean dose of 200 mg in 90% of patients.[95] Following IV injection, the maximal effect occurs within 5 to 10 minutes,[97] and the antihypertensive response may persist for ≥6 hours.[117] Because the rate of BP reduction is accelerated with an increase in infusion rate,[97] a controlled continuous infusion may provide a more gradual reduction in arterial pressure with less frequent adverse effects.[63,99,118] A solution for continuous infusion (0.5 to 2.0 mg/minute) is prepared by adding two ampules (200 mg total) to 160 mL of IV fluid to give a final concentration of 1 mg/mL. The infusion can then be started at a rate of 2 mg/min and titrated until a satisfactory response is achieved or until a cumulative dose of 300 mg is reached.

PARENTERAL/ORAL CONVERSION

23. C.M. was treated with a labetalol infusion and required a cumulative dose of 180 mg to achieve a diastolic pressure of 100 mm Hg. His anginal symptoms resolved almost immediately, but 3 hours after the infusion, C.M. became faint and dizzy while ambulating. Should oral labetalol be withheld? When oral labetalol is given, what adverse effects can be expected?

Postural hypotension and dizziness are dose-related and are more commonly associated with the IV route of administration.[101,109] C.M. should remain in a supine position following the IV administration of labetalol, and his ability to tolerate an upright position should be established before permitting ambulation. Oral labetalol can be given to C.M. when his supine diastolic BP increases by 10 mm Hg. There is no correlation between the oral maintenance dose and the total initial IV dose. C.M. should be started on an empirical dose of 100 to 200 mg oral labetalol twice daily, and this should be titrated as necessary. Other side effects commonly associated with labetalol include nausea, vomiting, abdominal pain, and diarrhea in up to 15% of the patients.[109] Scalp tingling is an unusual side effect that has been reported in a few patients after IV administration; it tends to disappear with continued treatment. Other side effects include tiredness, weakness, muscle cramps, headache, ejaculation failure, and various skin rashes.

Nitroglycerin

24. **Would parenteral nitroglycerin be an acceptable alternative to labetalol for C.M.?**

Severe, uncontrolled hypertension in the setting of unstable angina or MI requires an immediate reduction in BP. Nitroprusside has been used successfully, but IV nitroglycerin can have more favorable effects on collateral coronary flow in patients with ischemic heart disease.[119] By diminishing preload, nitroglycerin decreases left ventricular diastolic volume, diastolic pressure, and myocardial wall tension, thus reducing myocardial oxygen consumption.[120] These changes favor redistribution of coronary blood flow to the subendocardium, which is more vulnerable to ischemia. At high dosages, nitroglycerin dilates arteriolar smooth muscles, and this reduction in afterload also decreases myocardial wall tension and oxygen consumption.[121]

IV nitroglycerin has a rapid onset of action, has a short duration, and is easily titratable. It is generally appropriate to begin IV nitroglycerin at dosages in the range of 5 to 10 μg/min, increased as needed to control pressure and symptoms. The usual dose is in the range of 40 to 100 μg/min. The major limiting side effects are headache and the development of tolerance. In general, IV nitroglycerin is well suited for use in patients like C.M. who have unstable angina or in patients who have hypertension associated with MI or coronary bypass surgery.

Diazoxide

25. **R.N., a 32-year-old Black woman, is admitted to the hospital with a 2-day history of nausea, blurred vision, confusion, and an intractable generalized headache. Her medical history is remarkable for asthma and diet-controlled diabetes mellitus. Physical examination reveals an alert but disoriented Black woman with a BP of 220/160 mm Hg (without orthostasis) and a pulse of 110 beats/min. There is no evidence of heart failure, but the neurologic examination reveals an altered mental status. Serum electrolytes, BUN, creatinine, UA, chest x-ray, and ECG are within normal limits. R.N.'s plasma glucose level is 275 mg/dL. The assessment at this time is hypertensive encephalopathy. Diazoxide is ordered. Are any special precautions required in the use of diazoxide in R.N.?**

PRECAUTIONS

Diazoxide induces a significant rise in the blood glucose level. Several mechanisms have been postulated, including a direct increase in catecholamine levels, decreased peripheral glucose utilization, and direct inhibition of insulin release. However, the predominant and most important effect of diazoxide is its inhibition of insulin secretion from pancreatic β cells. Although hyperglycemia occurs frequently, it is usually mild and does not preclude the use of the drug. In one study of 700 patients treated with diazoxide, a mild transitory elevation of serum glucose occurred in 40% of the nondiabetic subjects and in 75% of diabetic subjects 1 to 4 hours after treatment was initiated.[122] In another study of 41 patients who received diazoxide, the mean glucose values increased by only 6 mg/dL during the first 48 hours.[123]

Because R.N. has a history of diabetes, her blood glucose levels should be monitored. If necessary, treatment with insulin or oral hypoglycemics may be required. Failure to recognize and treat significant hyperglycemia could result in ketoacidosis or hyperglycemic hyperosmolar coma. This occurs most often in patients with renal failure, adult-onset diabetes mellitus, or liver disease and patients recovering from general anesthesia.

DOSING AND ADMINISTRATION

26. **How should diazoxide be administered to R.N. to achieve an optimal hypotensive response? Under what circumstances is diazoxide preferred over other agents?**

Originally, it was recommended that diazoxide be administered as an IV bolus (5 mg/kg or 300 mg in <30 seconds). Theoretically, this method of administration produced a higher concentration of unbound, or free, diazoxide, which activated vasodilator receptors on the arterioles. However, it has since been found that this method results in abrupt declines in BP, resulting in cerebral and cardiovascular hypoperfusion. Because R.N. already has evidence of encephalopathy, cerebral flow should not be further compromised.

It is now recommended that diazoxide be administered as a smaller bolus or by slow infusion. Studies confirm that diazoxide can be administered safely and effectively as a minibolus[124] (1 to 3 mg/kg every 5 to 15 minutes to a maximum of a 150 mg in a single injection) or by slow infusion (15 to 30 mg/min)[104,125] until a diastolic BP of 100 mm Hg is achieved. Single-dose injections of >150 mg should not be used. Evidence indicates that minibolus or slow infusion diazoxide quickly lowers BP with little risk of hypoperfusion. Diazoxide also can be given by repetitive infusions according to the following schedule: loading dose of 7.5 mg/kg IV over 1.5 hours (which usually decreases mean arterial pressure by 25%), followed by 10% of the loading dose every 6 hours for maintenance.[126] In general, diazoxide should be used only in patients who (1) cannot tolerate labetalol (e.g., asthma or advanced heart block), (2) require a more gradual lowering of BP than that produced by nitroprusside, and (3) require a more rapid and certain drop in BP than that which can be produced by oral antihypertensive agents.[125]

ONSET AND DURATION OF ACTION

27. **R.N. is given 150 mg of diazoxide by IV injection over 30 seconds. When will the maximum hypotensive effect occur, and how long will this persist? What should be done if there is no substantial decrease in pressure?**

The hypotensive effects of diazoxide begin within 1 minute, and maximum effects occur within 2 to 5 minutes. Over the next 20 minutes, the BP gradually increases as a result of a reflex increase in heart rate and cardiac output. The patient should remain recumbent for 15 to 30 minutes after the injection of each dose of diazoxide, and the BP should be monitored every 5 minutes for the first 30 minutes. The duration of action is variable in that the BP gradually increases to the pretreatment level in 3 to 15 hours. In a small series of patients given 100 to 150 mg of diazoxide every 5 minutes,

20% of the patients required a single dose and 75% needed two or three injections.[124] Only one patient required more than three injections. Diazoxide, when given by slow infusion, produces a maximum reduction in mean arterial pressure of 25% in 25 to 30 minutes, which lasts up to 8 hours.[124,125] If R.N. fails to respond to the first dose, repeated doses should be given at 10-minute intervals until a cumulative dose of 600 mg is reached.

A major disadvantage of diazoxide is the occurrence of reflex tachycardia, which can precipitate or worsen angina in patients with coronary artery disease. Small IV doses of propranolol (0.2 mg/kg) can be used in situations in which tachycardia is dangerous.[125]

Hydralazine

28. T.M., a 30-year-old man with a history of chronic glomerulonephritis and poorly controlled hypertension, came to the ED complaining of early morning occipital headaches during the past week. He has no other complaints. He has not taken any BP medication in a month. Physical examination revealed an afebrile male in no acute distress with a BP of 160/120 mm Hg without orthostasis and a regular pulse of 90 beats/min. Funduscopic examination revealed bilateral exudates without hemorrhages or papilledema. The lungs were clear. Cardiac examination was pertinent for cardiomegaly and an S_4 gallop. The remainder of the physical workup was normal.

Laboratory results include Hct, 32%; BUN, 40 mg/dL; creatinine, 2.5 mg/dL; and bicarbonate, 18 mEq/L. UA reveals 2+ protein, 2+ hemoglobin with 4 to 10 RBCs/HPF. The ECG demonstrates NSR with left ventricular hypertrophy. The chest radiograph is unremarkable.

T.M. was given 20 mg hydralazine intramuscularly (IM), and a repeat BP after 1 hour was 150/100 mm Hg. What are the advantages and disadvantages of parenteral hydralazine, and when should it be used to acutely lower BP?

[SI units: Hct, 0.32; BUN, 14.28 mmol/L urea; creatinine, 221 mmol/L; bicarbonate, 18 mmol/L]

Hydralazine is a direct vasodilator that reduces total peripheral resistance through relaxation of arterial smooth muscle. It rarely is used to treat hypertensive emergencies, excluding eclampsia, because its antihypertensive response is less predictable than that of other parenteral agents. It is not consistently effective in controlling crises associated with essential hypertension.

Contraindications

Hydralazine should not be used in patients with coronary heart disease because the reflex tachycardia causes an increase in myocardial oxygen demand, which may result in the development or worsening of ischemic symptoms. In addition, hydralazine should be avoided in patients with aortic dissection because of its reflex cardiostimulating effect. On the other hand, hydralazine can be useful in patients like T.M. who have chronic renal failure because the reflex increase in cardiac output is accompanied by an increase in organ perfusion. In addition, there is considerable experience with the use of hydralazine in patients with eclampsia who are less likely to have underlying coronary artery disease (see Chapter 46, Obstetrics).

DOSING AND ADMINISTRA[...]

Parenteral hydralazi[...] ate treatment between [...] apy with such agents as [...] side. It can be given IV [...] slowly over 20 to 40 m[...] acute hypotension. Paren[...] than oral doses because of inc[...]

Other Parenteral Drugs

29. Are there alternatives to hydralazine [...] ment of hypertensive urgencies?

INTRAVENOUS ENALAPRILAT

Enalaprilat, the active metabolite of the oral prodrug enalapril (Vasotec), is approved by the U.S. Food and Drug Administration for the treatment of hypertension when oral therapy is not feasible. Although not approved for the treatment of hypertensive crisis, enalaprilat has been used to treat severe hypertension.[127–132] The initial dose is 0.625 to 1.25 mg IV; this is repeated every 6 hours if necessary. The initial dose should not exceed 0.625 mg in patients receiving diuretics or in patients with clinical evidence of hypovolemia. The onset of action is within 15 minutes, but the maximum effect may take several hours. Because only 60% of the patients respond to BP reduction within 30 minutes, it cannot be used reliably to acutely lower pressure in emergent cases.[133] Although higher doses have been used to achieve BP control, recent evidence indicates that doses >0.625 mg do not alter the magnitude of enalaprilat's antihypertensive effect.[132] However, the concomitant use of diuretic therapy may enhance the response. Because ACE inhibitors do not impair cerebral blood flow, enalaprilat may be useful for the hypertensive patient at risk for cerebral hypoperfusion. Enalaprilat also is beneficial in patients with HF, but it is no better than sublingual nitroglycerin in the treatment of hypertensive patients with pulmonary edema.[131] Precautions for the use of enalaprilat are similar to those of captopril (see Question 5). Because of the prolonged time required to achieve an adequate response, limited clinical experience, and variable response rates (especially in Blacks), enalaprilat cannot be recommended for the routine treatment of patients with hypertensive emergencies.[130,133]

INTRAVENOUS ESMOLOL

Esmolol is a parenteral cardioselective β-blocker with a rapid onset and short duration of action. It has been used primarily in perioperative settings to control tachycardia induced by various surgical stimuli, including endotracheal intubation.[134] Esmolol also has been used to manage supraventricular tachyarrhythmias.[135,136] It has been particularly useful in treating postoperative hypertension, especially if it is associated with tachycardia. In a small series of patients undergoing cardiac bypass surgery, the antihypertensive effect of esmolol was comparable to that of nitroprusside.[137]

Hypotension is the most commonly reported adverse event and is directly related to the duration of esmolol administration.[138] However, because of the short half-life, resolution of hypotension occurs within 30 minutes of discontinuing the infusion. Like other β-blockers, esmolol is contraindicated in patients with asthma, advanced heart block, or severe HF.

of hypertension, esmolol should be ... e of 500 μg/kg per minute for 1 minute, ...nute maintenance infusion of 50 to 100 ...ute. This can be repeated if necessary. Irrita... ...ation, and induration at the infusion site occur in ...% of patients.

INTRAVENOUS CALCIUM CHANNEL BLOCKERS

Parenteral verapamil (Isoptin), diltiazem (Cardizem), and nicardipine (Cardene IV) are effective in the treatment of hypertensive emergencies and urgencies.

Intravenous Verapamil.   IV verapamil (5 to 10 mg) produces a significant reduction in BP, which occurs within 15 minutes and persists for 6 to 8 hours. However, the use of this drug in hypertensive emergencies has not been studied extensively.

Intravenous Diltiazem.   IV diltiazem is approved for temporary control of the ventricular rate in atrial fibrillation or atrial flutter and for rapid conversion of paroxysmal supraventricular tachycardia.[139–141] Parenteral diltiazem also has been used to control hypertension that occurs intraoperatively and postoperatively[142,143] and in patients with acute coronary artery disease.[144,145] However, published experience with the use of IV diltiazem for the treatment of severe hypertension is limited. Onoyama and collegues[146] administered a continuous infusion of diltiazem at a dosage of 5 to 40 μg/kg per minute to a small group of patients with hypertensive crisis. A normotensive level was achieved within 6 hours without any signs of organ ischemia. In a follow-up study,[147] a continuous infusion of diltiazem averaging 11 μg/kg per minute resulted in a 25% reduction in both systolic and diastolic BP measurements within 30 minutes. The magnitude of the decrease was directly correlated with the pretreatment BP level. Atrioventricular nodal conduction abnormalities were noted in both studies and resolved when the infusion was discontinued. Patients receiving IV diltiazem require continuous monitoring by ECG and frequent BP checks. This form of therapy should be avoided in patients with sick sinus syndrome or advanced degrees of heart block. Until additional information is available, caution should be exercised in using parenteral diltiazem to lower BP acutely.

Intravenous Nicardipine.   IV nicardipine, a dihydropyridine calcium channel antagonist, is a potent cerebral and systemic vasodilator and a useful therapeutic option in the management of severe hypertension. Unlike other dihydropyridines, nicardipine is photoresistant, is water soluble, and can be administered IV. Its onset of action is within 1 to 2 minutes, and its elimination half-life is 40 minutes.[148] Hemodynamic evaluations demonstrated that IV nicardipine significantly decreased mean arterial pressure and systemic vascular resistance and significantly increased cardiac index with little or no change in heart rate.[149] Titratable IV nicardipine has been studied extensively for use in controlling postoperative hypertension,[149–153] as well as severe hypertension.[154–156]

In the treatment of postoperative hypertension,[149,151] IV nicardipine was administered as an infusion titrated in the following manner: 10 mg/hour for 5 minutes; 12.5 mg/hour for 5 minutes; 15 mg/hour for 15 minutes, followed by a maintenance infusion of 3 mg/hour thereafter. The mean response time and infusion rate were 11.5 minutes and 12.8 mg/hour,

respectively. Ninety-four percent of the patients responded, and adverse effects included hypotension (4.5%), tachycardia (2.7%), and nausea and vomiting (4.5%).

The efficacy and safety of IV nicardipine for the treatment of severe hypertension have been documented in a double-blind, placebo-controlled multicenter trial.[154] The patients achieved a diastolic pressure ≤95 mm Hg. Serious adverse effects were uncommon; the most common, headache, occurred in 24% of the patients. Local thrombophlebitis can be avoided by changing the infusion site after 12 hours. Initial therapy of IV nicardipine was begun with dosages of 1 to 15 mg/hour, and adjustments were made as indicated until the therapeutic endpoint was achieved. Maintenance therapy was continued for 8 to 24 hours.[156,157] The mean dosage of IV nicardipine at the end of maintenance therapy was 7.85 mg/hour. In individual patients, the dosage of nicardipine necessary for BP control ranged from 3 to 15 mg/hour. Investigators noted that nicardipine blood levels in severe hypertension appeared to reach steady state at 8 to 12 hours after the onset of the infusion, although significant therapeutic effects were seen within 1 hour. Compared with sodium nitroprusside, IV nicardipine was as effective with fewer adverse effects.[157]

In summary, IV nicardipine is an alternative to sodium nitroprusside for the immediate treatment of severe and postoperative hypertension.[11] It has a rapid onset of action, with sustained BP control over the infusion period. It is easily titratable, with a predictable response, and is relatively free of severe adverse effects. It may be useful in patients with cerebral insufficiency or peripheral vascular disease. Because of the potential for reflex tachycardia, it should be used with caution in patients with coronary ischemia.

INTRAVENOUS PHENTOLAMINE (REGITINE)

IV phentolamine is primarily used in the management of hypertensive emergencies induced by catecholamine excess, as seen in pheochromocytoma. The mechanism of action is through nonselective competitive antagonist at α-adrenergic receptors.[158] Phentolamine is dosed in 1- to 5-mg boluses and should be given cautiously due to the risk of causing hypotension. The onset of action is almost immediate and the duration of action is short (<15 minutes). IV infusions are not recommended due to unpredictable drops in BP. As BP control is achieved, an oral α-adrenergic blocking agent such as phenoxybenzamine (Dibenzyline) can be given if needed.[159]

Aortic Dissection

Treatment

30. **B.S., a 68-year-old White man with a long history of hypertension, asthma, and noncompliance, presents to the local ED complaining of the sudden onset of severe, sharp, diffuse chest pain that radiates to his back between his shoulder blades. Significant findings on physical examination include a pulse of 100 beats/min, BP of 200/120 mm Hg, grade II K-W changes, clear lungs, and an S_4 without murmurs. The laboratory data are unremarkable. The ECG results are interpreted as sinus tachycardia with left ventricular hypertrophy, but no acute changes are noted. The chest radiograph is significant for widening of the mediastinum. An emergency aortogram reveals a dissection at the arch of the aorta. What antihypertensive medication would be most appropriate for B.S., and why?**

Dissection of the aorta occurs when the innermost layer of the aorta (the intima) is interrupted so that blood enters and separates its layers. The ultimate treatment for dissection of the aorta depends on its location and severity; however, the first principle of therapy is to control any existing hypertension with agents that do not increase the force of cardiac contraction.[11] This lessens the force that the cardiac impulse transmits to the dissecting aneurysm.

THERAPEUTIC CONSIDERATIONS

The aim of antihypertensive therapy is to lessen the pulsatile load or aortic stress by lowering the BP. Reducing the force of left ventricular contractions, and consequently the rate of rise of aortic pressure, retards the propagation of the dissection and aortic rupture.[160] The treatment of choice for aortic dissection has classically been trimethaphan or sodium nitroprusside in combination with a β-blocker.[160–162] Labetalol monotherapy has been used as an alternative. These drugs decrease BP, venous return, and cardiac contractility.

One common regimen is a combination of IV sodium nitroprusside (25 to 50 µg/minute) and IV propranolol (0.05 to 0.15 mg/kg every 4 to 6 hours).[162] An equivalent dose of esmolol may be used in place of propranol.[163] The concurrent administration of a β-blocking agent with nitroprusside is desirable because the latter may induce reflex tachycardia in response to vasodilation.

Trimethaphan's advantage over sodium nitroprusside is that it reduces both arterial pressure and its rate of increase; therefore, it does not require concurrent administration of β-blockers. However, the major disadvantages are tachyphylaxis, urinary retention, and ileus. Direct vasodilators such as diazoxide and hydralazine should be avoided because they increase stroke volume and left ventricular ejection rate. These effects augment the pulsatile flow and accentuate the sharpness of the pulse wave. This increases mechanical stress on the aortic wall and may lead to further dissection.

Depending on the location of the dissection, surgical intervention may be required.[162] However, until a definitive diagnosis is made, the primary goal is to lower the BP and depress myocardial contractility. The ultimate objective of acute medical therapy for aortic dissection is to reduce the BP to the lowest level compatible with the maintenance of adequate renal, cerebral, and cardiac perfusion.[159] In aortic dissection, the systolic BP should be lowered to 100 to 120 mm Hg or a mean arterial pressure <80 mm Hg.[164]

The drug of first choice for B.S. is trimethaphan. Although labetalol[164] or a combination of nitroprusside with either propranolol or esmolol[165] has been used successfully in the antihypertensive treatment of dissecting aortic aneurysms, B.S.'s medical history of asthma precludes the use of β-blockers.

TRIMETHAPHAN

31. How should trimethaphan be administered, and what indices of toxicity should be monitored?

Trimethaphan is a ganglionic blocking drug that inhibits sympathetic nervous effects on the arterioles, veins, and heart. The hypotensive effect is immediate. Because minor changes in the infusion rate can produce dramatic changes in BP, the rate must be carefully regulated (preferably by a constant infusion pump) and the BP must be monitored continuously.

The drug usually is prepared in a concentration of 500 mg/L of D5W. The infusion is initiated at 0.5 to 1 mg/min and the rate is increased every 3 to 5 minutes until the desired response is obtained. The hypotensive effect is most pronounced when the patient is upright, and it is often necessary to elevate the head of the bed to achieve an optimal effect. Therapy with oral antihypertensive agents should begin simultaneously, and an attempt should be made to discontinue the ganglionic blocker within 48 hours before significant tolerance renders the patient resistant to its action.

The prolonged use of trimethaphan is limited by its important sympathoplegic side effects as well as the rapid development of tachyphylaxis. Urinary retention often occurs with prolonged therapy, necessitating insertion of an indwelling catheter. Constipation and paralytic ileus may occur, as well as paralysis of visual accommodation. Severe hypotension after administration of trimethaphan may last for 10 to 15 minutes. To correct the hypotension, the infusion should be discontinued and the patient should be placed in the Trendelenburg position, where the head is kept lower than the trunk.

REFERENCES

1. Calhoun DA, Oparil S. Treatment of hypertensive crisis. N Engl J Med 1990;323:1177.
2. Ault MJ, Ellrodt AG. Pathophysiologic events leading to the end organ effects of acute hypertension. J Emerg Med 1985;3(Suppl 2):10.
3. Joint National Committee on Detection, Evaluation, and Treatment of High Blood Pressure. The Seventh Report of the Joint National Committee on Detection, Evaluation and Treatment of High Blood Pressure. Publication 03-5233. Bethesda, MD: National Institutes of Health, 2003.
4. Bales A. Hypertensive crisis: how to tell if it's an emergency or an urgency. Postgrad Med 1999;105:119.
5. Vidt DG. Current concepts in treatment of hypertensive emergencies. Am Heart J 1986;111:220.
6. Abo-Zena RA et al. Hypertensive urgency induced by an interaction of mirtazapine and clonidine. Pharmacotherapy 2000;20:476.
7. Patel S et al. Hypertensive crisis associated with St. John's wort. Am J Med 2002;507.
8. Novac BL et al. Erythropoietin-induced hypertensive urgency in a patient with chronic renal insufficiency: case report and review of the literature. Pharmacotherapy 2003;23:265.
9. Zampaglione B et al. Hypertensive urgencies and emergencies: prevalence and clinical presentation. Hypertension 1996;27:144.
10. Bennett NM, Shea S. Hypertensive emergency: case scenarios, sociodemographic profile, and previous care of 100 cases. Am J Public Health 1988;78:636.
11. Ram CV. Immediate management of severe hypertension. Cardiol Clin 1995;13:579.
12. Shea S et al. Predisposing factors for severe uncontrolled hypertension in an inner-city minority population. N Engl J Med 1992;327:776.
13. Webster J et al. Accelerated hypertension: patterns of mortality and clinical factors affecting outcomes in treated patients. Q J Med 1993;86:485.
14. Bakir A, Dunea G. Accelerated and malignant hypertension: experience from a large American inner city hospital. Int J Artif Organs 1989;12:675.
15. McNair A et al. Reversibility of cerebral symptoms in severe hypertension in relation to acute antihypertensive therapy. Acta Med Scand 1984;6935:107.
16. Winer N. Hypertensive crisis. Crit Care Nurs Q 1990;13:23.
17. Laragh JH, Blumenfield JD. The management of hypertensive crises: the scientific basis for treatment decisions. AJH 2001;14:1154.
18. Laragh JH. Laragh's lessons in pathophysiology and clinical pearls for treating hypertension; lesson XXV: how to mechanistically diagnose and correctly treat a hypertensive crisis. AJH 2001;14:837.
19. Hirschl MM. Guidelines for the drug treatment of hypertensive crisis. Drugs 1995;50:991.
20. Murphy C. Hypertensive emergencies. Emerg Med Clin North Am 1995;13:973.
21. McKindley DS, Boucher BA. Advances in pharmacotherapy: treatment of hypertensive crisis. J Clin Pharm Ther 1994;19:163.
22. Gales MA. Oral antihypertensives for hypertensive urgencies. Ann Pharmacother 1994;28:352.

23. Komsuoglu B et al. Treatment of hypertensive urgencies with oral nifedipine, nicardipine, and captopril. Angiology 1991;42:447.
24. Psaty BM et al. The risk of myocardial infarction associated with antihypertensive drug therapies. JAMA 1995;274:620.
25. Leavitt AD, Zweifler AJ. Nifedipine, hypotension, and myocardial injury. Ann Intern Med 1988;108:305.
26. O'Mailia JJ et al. Nifedipine-associated myocardial ischemia or infarction in the treatment of hypertensive urgencies. Ann Intern Med 1987;107:185.
27. Schwartz M et al. Oral nifedipine in the treatment of hypertensive urgency: cerebrovascular accident following a single dose. Arch Intern Med 1990;150:686.
28. Fami MJ et al. Another report of adverse reactions to immediate-release nifedipine. Pharmacotherapy 1998;18:1133.
29. Bertel O et al. Effects of antihypertensive treatment on cerebral perfusion. Am J Med 1987;82(Suppl 3B):29.
30. Dinsdale HB. Hypertensive encephalopathy. Neurol Clin 1983;1:3.
31. Waldman R et al. Treatment of hypertensive encephalopathy. Neurology (NY) 1983;33:118.
32. Grossman E et al. Should a moratorium be placed on sublingual nifedipine capsules given for hypertensive emergencies and pseudoemergencies? JAMA 1996;276:1328.
33. Cohen IM et al. Oral clonidine loading for rapid control of hypertension. Clin Pharmacol Ther 1978;24:11.
34. Anderson RJ et al. Oral clonidine loading in hypertensive urgencies. JAMA 1981;246:848.
35. Spitalewitz S et al. Use of oral clonidine for rapid titration of blood pressure in severe hypertension. Chest 1983;83(Suppl 2):404.
36. Marks AD et al. Oral clonidine for rapid control of accelerated hypertension. J Clin Pharmacol 1987;27:193.
37. Zeller KR et al. Rapid reduction of severe asymptomatic hypertension. A prospective, controlled trial. Arch Intern Med 1989;149:2186.
38. Vidt DG et al. Roundtable discussion. Am Heart J 1986;111:229.
39. Reed WG et al. Effects of rapid blood pressure reduction on cerebral blood flow. Am Heart J 1986;111:226.
40. Stewart M, Burris JF. Rebound hypertension during initiation of transdermal clonidine. Drug Intell Clin Pharm 1988;22:573.
41. Vernon C, Sakula A. Fatal rebound hypertension after abrupt withdrawal of clonidine and propanolol. Br J Clin Pract 1979;33:1112.
42. Damasceno A et al. Efficacy of captopril and nifedipine in black and white patients with hypertensive crisis. J Hum Hypertens 1997;11:471.
43. Misra A et al. Sublingual captopril in hypertensive urgencies. Postgrad Med J 1993;69:498.
44. Pujadas R et al. Comparison of sublingual captopril and nifedipine in hypertensive crisis. Arch Intern Med 1987;147:175.
45. Angeli P et al. Comparison of sublingual captopril and nifedipine in immediate treatment of hypertensive emergencies. Arch Intern Med 1991;151:678.
46. Wood BC et al. Oral minoxidil in the treatment of hypertensive crisis. JAMA 1979;241:163.
47. Bauer JH et al. Rapid reduction of severe hypertension with minoxidil. J Cardiovasc Pharmacol 1980;2(Suppl 2):S189.
48. Alpert MA, Bauer JH. Rapid control of severe hypertension with minoxidil. Arch Intern Med 1982;142:2099.
49. Hayes JM. Prazosin in severe hypertension. Med J Aust 1977;2(Suppl 2):30.
50. McDonald AJ, Yealy DM. Oral labetalol versus oral nifedipine in hypertensive urgencies. Ann Emerg Med 1989;18:461.
51. Gonzalez ER et al. Dose response evaluation of oral labetalol in patients presenting to the emergency department with accelerated hypertension. Ann Emerg Med 1991;20:333.
52. Zell-Kanter M, Leikin JB. Oral labetalol in hypertensive urgencies. Am J Emerg Med 1991;9:136.
53. Atkin S et al. Oral labetalol versus oral clonidine in the emergency treatment of severe hypertension. Am J Med Sci 1992;303:9.
54. Wright SW et al. Ineffectiveness of oral labetalol for hypertensive urgency. Am J Emerg Med 1990;8:472.
55. Hamad A et al. Life-threatening hyperkalemia after intravenous labetalol injection for hypertensive emergency in a hemodialysis patient. Am J Nephrol 2001;21:241.
56. Panacek E et al. Randomized, prospective trial of fenoldopam vs. sodium nitroprusside in the treatment of acute severe hypertension. Acad Emerg Med 1995;2:959.
57. Pilmer B et al. Fenoldopam mesylate versus sodium nitroprusside in the acute management of severe systemic hypertension. J Clin Pharmacol 1993;33:549.
58. Reisin E et al. Intravenous fenoldopam versus sodium nitroprusside in patients with severe hypertension. Hypertension 1990;15(Suppl 1):I59.
59. Garwood S, Hines R. Perioperative renal preservation: dopexamine, and fenoldopam: new agents to augment renal performance. Semin Anesth Periop Med Pain 1998;17:308.
60. Murphy M et al. Augmentation of renal blood flow and sodium excretion in hypertensive patients during blood pressure reduction by intravenous administration of the dopamine-1 agonist, fenoldopam. Circulation 1987;6:1312.
61. Shusterman N et al. Fenoldopam but not nitroprusside improves renal function in severely hypertensive patients with impaired renal function. Am J Med 1993;95:161.
62. Elliott W et al. Renal and hemodynamic effects of intravenous fenoldopam versus nitroprusside in severe hypertension. Circulation 1990;81:970.
63. Houston MC. Pathophysiology, clinical aspects, and treatment of hypertensive crisis. Prog Cardiovasc Dis 1989;32:99.
64. McKinney TD. Management of hypertensive crisis. Hosp Pract 1992;27:133.
65. Brater DC et al. Prolonged hemodynamic effect of furosemide in congestive heart failure. Am Heart J 1984;4:1031.
66. USPDI. Nipride. Micromedex: 2003.
67. Hirschl M. Guidelines for the drug treatment of hypertensive crises. Drugs 1995;50:991.
68. Nightingale S. New labeling for sodium nitroprusside emphasizes risk of cyanide toxicity. JAMA 1991;265:847.
69. Lavin P. Management of hypertension in patients with acute stroke. Arch Intern Med 1986;146:66.
70. Schultz V. Clinical pharmacokinetics of nitroprusside, cyanide, thiosulphate and thiocyanate. Clin Pharmacokinet 1984;9:239.
71. Rindone JP, Sloane EP. Cyanide toxicity from sodium nitroprusside: risks and management. Ann Pharmacother 1992;26:515.
72. Friederich J, Butterworth J. Sodium nitroprusside: twenty years and counting. Anesth Analg 1995;81:152.
73. Schultz V et al. Hypotensive efficacy of a mixed solution of 0.1% sodium nitroprusside and 1% sodium thiosulphate. J Hypertens 1985;3:485.
74. Baskin S et al. The antidotal action of sodium nitrite and sodium thiosulfate against cyanide poisoning. J Clin Pharmacol 1992;32:368.
75. Curry SC, Capell-Arnold P. Toxic effects of drugs used in the ICU: nitroprusside, nitroglycerin, and angiotensin converting enzyme inhibitors. Crit Care Clin 1991;7:555.
76. Robin E, McCauley R. Nitroprusside-related cyanide poisoning: time (long past due) for urgent, effective interventions. Chest 1992;102:1842.
77. Zerbe NF, Wagner BK. Use of vitamin B_{12} in the treatment and prevention of nitroprusside-induced cyanide toxicity. Crit Care Med 1993;21:465.
78. Sarvotham S. Nitroprusside therapy in post-open heart hypertensives: a ritual tryst with cyanide death. Chest 1987;91:796.
79. Johanning R et al. A retrospective study of sodium nitroprusside use and assessment of the potential risk of cyanide poisoning. Pharmacotherapy 1995;15:773.
80. Cottrell JE et al. Prevention of nitroprusside-induced cyanide toxicity with hydroxocobalamin. N Engl J Med 1978;298:809.
81. Kayser SR et al. Hydroxocobalamin in nitroprusside-induced cyanide toxicity. Drug Intell Clin Pharm 1986;20:365.
82. Stumpf JL. Drug therapy in hypertensive crises. Clin Pharm 1988;7:582.
83. Dwyer M, Morris C. Toxicity of sodium nitroprusside. Conn Med 1993;57:489.
84. Fenoldopam. Med Lett Drug Ther 1998;40:57.
85. Ellis D et al. Treatment of hypertensive emergencies with fenoldopam, a peripherally acting dopamine (DA_1) receptor agonist. Crit Care Med 1998;26(1 Suppl):A23.
86. Brogden R, Markham A. Fenoldopam: a review of its pharmacodynamic and pharmacokinetic properties and intravenous clinical potential in the management of hypertensive urgencies and emergencies. Drugs 1997;54:634.
87. Post J, Frishman W. Fenoldopam: a new dopamine agonist for the treatment of hypertensive urgencies and emergencies. J Clin Pharmacol 1998;38:2.
88. Nichols A et al. The pharmacology of fenoldopam. Am J Hypertens 1990;3:116S.
89. White W, Halley S. Comparative renal effects of intravenous administration of fenoldopam mesylate and sodium nitroprusside in patients with severe hypertension. Arch Intern Med 1989;149:870.
90. Oparil S et al. A new parenteral antihypertensive: consensus roundtable on the management of perioperative hypertension and hypertensive crises. Am J Hypertens 1999;12:653.
91. Goldberg M, Larijani G. Perioperative hypertension. Pharmacotherapy 1998;18:911.
92. Everitt D et al. Effect of intravenous fenoldopam on intraocular pressure in ocular hypertension. J Clin Pharmacol 1997;37:312.
93. Piltz J et al. Fenoldopam, a selective dopamine-1 receptor agonist, raises intraocular pressure in males with normal intraocular pressure. J Ocul Pharmacol Ther 1998;14:203.
94. Cressman MD et al. Intravenous labetalol in the management of severe hypertension and hypertensive emergencies. Am Heart J 1984;107:980.
95. Wilson DJ et al. Intravenous labetalol in the treatment of severe hypertension and hypertensive emergencies. Am J Med 1983;75(Suppl):95.
96. Smith WB et al. Antihypertensive effectiveness of intravenous labetalol in accelerated hypertension. Hypertension 1983;5:579.
97. Dal Palu C et al. Intravenous labetalol in severe hypertension. Br J Clin Pharmacol 1982;13(Suppl 1):97S.
98. Lebel M et al. Labetalol infusion in hypertensive emergencies. Clin Pharmacol Ther 1985;37:615.
99. Vidt DG. Intravenous labetalol in the emergency treatment of hypertension. J Clin Hypertens 1985;2:179.
100. Patel RV et al. Labetalol: response and safety in critically ill hemorrhagic stroke patients. Ann Pharmacother 1993;27:180.
101. Kanto JH. Current status of labetalol, the first alpha- and beta-blocking agent. Int J Clin Pharmacol Ther Toxicol 1985;23:617.
102. George RB et al. Comparison of the effects of labetalol and hydrochlorothiazide on the ventilatory function of hypertensive patients with asthma and propranolol sensitivity. Chest 1985;88:815.
103. Kanada S et al. Angina-like syndrome with diazoxide therapy for hypertensive crisis. Ann Intern Med 1976;84:696.
104. Huysmans FT et al. Combined intravenous administration of diazoxide and beta-blocking agent in acute treatment of severe hypertension or hypertensive crisis. Am Heart J 1982;103:395.

105. Vidt DG et al. Safety of diazoxide administration in antihypertensive therapy: an analysis of 1,268 injections in 423 patients [abstract]. Clin Pharmacol Ther 1977;21:120.

106. Moser M. Diazoxide: an effective vasodilator in accelerated hypertension. Am Heart J 1974; 87:791.

107. Walstad RA et al. Labetalol in the treatment of hypertension in patients with normal and impaired renal function. Acta Med Scand 1982;212 (Suppl 665):135.

108. Wood AJ et al. Elimination kinetics of labetalol in severe renal failure. Br J Clin Pharmacol 1982; 13(Suppl):81.

109. MacCarthy EP et al. Labetalol: a review of its pharmacology pharmacokinetics, clinical uses and adverse effects. Pharmacotherapy 1983;3:193.

110. Abrams JH et al. Successful treatment of a monoamine oxidase inhibitor-tyramine hypertensive emergency with intravenous labetalol. N Engl J Med 1985;313:52.

111. Navaratnarajah M et al. Labetalol and phaeochromocytoma. Br J Anaesth 1984;56:1179.

112. Kelly JG et al. Bioavailability of labetalol increases with age. Br J Clin Pharmacol 1982; 14:304.

113. Eisalo A et al. Treatment of hypertension in the elderly with labetalol. Acta Med Scand 1982;665(Suppl):129.

114. McGrath BP et al. Emergency treatment of severe hypertension with intravenous labetalol. Med J Aust 1978;2:410.

115. Anderson CC et al. Poor hypotensive response and tachyphylaxis following intravenous labetalol. Curr Med Res Opin 1978;5:424.

116. Yeung CK et al. Comparison of labetalol, clonidine and diazoxide intravenously administered in severe hypertension. Med J Aust 1979;2:499.

117. Pearson RM et al. Intravenous labetalol in hypertensive patients treated with β-adrenoceptor blocking drugs. Br J Clin Pharmacol 1976; 3(Suppl 3):795.

118. Cumming AM et al. Intravenous labetalol in the treatment of severe hypertension. Br J Clin Pharmacol 1982;13(Suppl 1):93S.

119. Flaherty JT et al. Comparison of intravenous nitroglycerin and sodium nitroprusside for treatment of acute hypertension developing after coronary artery bypass surgery. Circulation 1982;65:1072.

120. Chun G, Frishman WH. Rapid-acting parenteral antihypertensive agents. J Clin Pharmacol 1990;30:195.

121. Francis GS. Vasodilators in the intensive care unit. Am Heart J 1991;121:1875.

122. Finnerty F. Hyperglycemia after diazoxide administration. N Engl J Med 1971;285:1487.

123. McDonald WJ et al. Intravenous diazoxide therapy in hypertensive crisis. Am J Cardiol 1977;40:409.

124. Ram CV et al. Individual titration of diazoxide dosage in the treatment of severe hypertension. Am J Cardiol 1979;43:627.

125. Garrett BN et al. Efficacy of slow infusion of diazoxide in the treatment of severe hypertension without organ hypoperfusion. Am Heart J 1982;103:390.

126. Ogilvie RI et al. Diazoxide concentration-response relation in hypertension. Hypertension 1982;4:167.

127. Strauss R et al. Enalaprilat in hypertensive emergencies. Clin Pharmacol Ther 1986;26:39.

128. Evans RR et al. The effect of intravenous enalaprilat (MK-422) administration in patients with mild to moderate essential hypertension. J Clin Pharmacol 1987;27:415.

129. Rutledge J et al. Effect of intravenous enalaprilat in moderate and severe hypertension. Am J Cardiol 1988;62:1062.

130. DiPette DJ et al. Enalaprilat, an intravenous angiotensin-converting enzyme inhibitor, in hypertensive crises. Clin Pharmacol Ther 1985;38:199.

131. Hirschl M et al. Sublinguales nitroglyzerin oder intraveoses enalaprilat in der praklinischen behandlung von hypertensiven patienten mit lungenodem. Z Kardiol 1999;88:208.

132. Hirschl M et al. Clinical evaluation of different doses of intravenous enalaprilat in patients with hypertensive crises. Arch Intern Med 1995; 155:2217.

133. White C. Pharmacologic, pharmacokinetic, and therapeutic differences among ACE inhibitors. Pharmacotherapy 1998;18:588.

134. Menkhaus P et al. Cardiovascular effects of esmolol in anesthetised humans. Anesth Anal 1985;64:327.

135. Allin D et al. Intravenous esmolol for the treatment of supraventricular tachyarrhythmia: results of a multicenter, baseline-controlled safety and efficacy study in 160 patients. Am Heart J 1986;112:498.

136. Anderson S et al. Comparison of the efficacy and safety of esmolol, a short-acting beta-blocker, with placebo in the treatment of supraventricular tachyarrhythmias. Am Heart J 1986;111:42.

137. Gray R et al. Use of esmolol in hypertension after cardiac surgery. Am J Cardiol 1985;56:49F.

138. Benfield P, Sorkin E. Esmolol: a preliminary review of its pharmacodynamic and pharmacokinetic properties, and therapeutic efficacy. Drugs 1987;33:392.

139. Salerno DM et al. Efficacy and safety of intravenous diltiazem for treatment of atrial fibrillation and atrial flutter. Am J Cardiol 1989;63:1046.

140. Ellenbogen KA et al. A placebo-controlled trial of continuous intravenous diltiazem infusion for 24-hour heart rate control during atrial fibrillation and atrial flutter: a multicenter study. J Am Coll Cardiol 1991;18:891.

141. Dougherty AH et al. Acute conversion of paroxysmal supraventricular tachycardia with intravenous diltiazem. Am J Cardiol 1992;79:587.

142. Koh H et al. Clinical study of total intravenous anesthesia with droperidol, fentanyl and ketamine: control of intraoperative hypertension with diltiazem. Jpn J Anesth 1991;40:1376.

143. Boylan JF et al. A comparison of diltiazem, esmolol, nifedipine, and nitroprusside therapy of post-CABG hypertension. Can J Anaesth 1990;37:S156.

144. Jaffe AS. Use of intravenous diltiazem in patients with acute coronary artery disease. Am J Cardiol 1992;69:25B.

145. Fang ZY et al. Intravenous diltiazem versus nitroglycerin for silent and symptomatic myocardial ischemia in unstable angina pectoris. Am J Cardiol 1991;68:42C.

146. Onoyama K et al. Effect of drug infusion or a bolus injection of intravenous diltiazem on hypertensive crisis. Curr Ther Res 1987;42:1223.

147. Onoyama K et al. Effect of a drip infusion of diltiazem on severe systemic hypertension. Curr Ther Res 1988;43:361.

148. Cheung D et al. Acute pharmacokinetic and hemodynamic effects of intravenous bolus dosing of nicardipine. Am Heart J 1990;119:438.

149. IV Nicardipine Study Group. Efficacy and safety of intravenous nicardipine in the control of postoperative hypertension. Chest 1991;99:393.

150. Bernard JM et al. Deliberate hypotension with nicardipine or nitroprusside during total hip arthroplasty. Anesth Analg 1991;73:341.

151. Halpern NA et al. Postoperative hypertension: a prospective, placebo controlled, randomized, double-blind trial with intravenous nicardipine hydrochloride. Angiology 1990;41:992.

152. Halpern NA et al. Nicardipine infusion for postoperative hypertension after surgery of the head and neck. Crit Care Med 1990;18:950.

153. Kaplan JA. Clinical considerations for the use of intravenous nicardipine in the treatment of postoperative hypertension. Am Heart J 1990; 119:443.

154. Wallin JD et al. Intravenous nicardipine for treatment of severe hypertension. Arch Intern Med 1989;149:2662.

155. Clifton GG, Wallin JD. Intravenous nicardipine: an effective new agent for the treatment of severe hypertension. Angiology 1990;41:1005.

156. Wallin JD. Intravenous nicardipine hydrochloride: treatment of patients with severe hypertension. Am Heart J 1990;119:434.

157. Neutel J et al. A comparison of intravenous nicardipine and sodium nitroprusside in the immediate treatment of severe hypertension. Am J Hypertens 1994;7:623.

158. Hoffman B. Catecholamines, sympathomimetic drugs, and adrenergic receptor antagonists. In: Goodman and Gilman's The Pharmacological Basis of Therapeutics, 10th ed. New York: McGraw Hill, 2001:10.

159. Varon J, Marik PE. The diagnosis and management of hypertensive crises. Chest 2000;118:214.

160. Chen K. et al. Acute thoracic aortic dissection: the basics. J Emerg Med 1997;15:859.

161. Neerukonda S et al. Aortic dissection: diagnosis and management. Hosp Pract (Off Ed) 1991; 28:66.

162. DeSanctis RW et al. Aortic dissection. N Engl J Med 1987;317:1060.

163. Lindsay J. Aortic dissection. Heart Dis Stroke 1992;2:69.

164. Laden N et al. Labetalol and MRI as initial medical and diagnostic modalities in a marfanoid patient with expanding ascending aortic aneurysm. Chest 1990;98:1290.

165. Mohindra SK, Udeani GO. Intravenous esmolol in an acute aortic dissection. DICP Ann Pharmacother 1991;25:735.

Shock

Andrew D. Barnes, Susan H. Lee

INTRODUCTION

Shock is defined in simple terms as a syndrome of impaired tissue perfusion usually, but not always, accompanied by hypotension. This impairment of tissue perfusion eventually leads to cellular dysfunction, followed by organ damage and death if untreated. The most common causes of shock are situations that result in a reduction of intravascular volume (hypovolemic shock), myocardial pump failure (cardiogenic shock), or in-creased vascular capacitance (distributive shock, sepsis). The type of treatment required depends on the etiology.

In recent years, medical support of the patient with shock has improved because of better technologies for hemodynamic monitoring, recognition of the value of vigorous volume replacement, appropriate use of inotropic and vasoconstrictive agents, and the development of better ways to treat the underlying cause of the shock syndrome. Understanding the principles of shock should further enhance prompt recognition of patients at risk, rapid initiation of corrective measures, and development of innovative treatment regimens.

CAUSES

Table 22-1 outlines the classification of shock and precipitating events.[1] It is important to understand the etiologic classification of shock because recognition of the underlying pathology is essential for managing this condition. One must realize, however, that the distinctions among subtypes of shock only apply in the relatively early stages. As the syndrome evolves and compensatory mechanisms are overwhelmed, it becomes increasingly difficult to determine the subtypes because the clinical and pathophysiologic features of advanced shock are the same for all. Also, different types of shock can occur at the same time (e.g., a patient with septic shock who is also hypovolemic).

PATHOPHYSIOLOGY

Tissue perfusion is a complex process of oxygen and nutrient delivery as well as waste removal. When perfusion is impaired, it sets up a cascade of events that can eventually end in death. Although the etiology of shock is varied, the eventual progression (if untreated) to cell death and subsequent organ dysfunction results from a common pathway of ischemia, endogenous inflammatory cytokine release, and the generation of oxygen radicals. When cells are subjected to a prolonged period of ischemia, anaerobic metabolism begins. This inefficient process results in a decrease of ATP stores and causes the buildup of lactic acid and other toxic substances which can alter the cellular machinery and can eventually result in cell death. In the advanced stages of shock, irreversible cellular damage leads to multiple organ system failure (MOSF), also known as multiple organ dysfunction syndrome (MODS).

Inflammatory cytokines are produced by the body in response to ischemia, injury, or infection. The phrase *systemic inflammatory response syndrome* (SIRS) is the recommended umbrella term to describe any acute, overwhelming inflammatory response, independent of the cause.[2] This syndrome can occur after a wide variety of insults, including hemorrhagic shock, infection (septic shock), pancreatitis, ischemia, multitrauma and tissue injury, and immune-mediated organ injury. SIRS is usually a late manifestation of hypovolemic forms of shock. It is uncommon in cardiogenic shock but is the hallmark of septic shock. SIRS is clinically characterized by profound vasodilation, which impairs perfusion, and increased capillary permeability, which can lead to reduced intravascular volume.

The following mediators have been identified as possible causes of the proinflammatory reaction underlying sepsis and multiple organ failure[3]:

- Macrophages and their products
- Cytokines: tumor necrosis factor (TNF), interleukin-1(IL-1), interleukin-6 (IL-6), and interleukin-8 (IL-8)
- Neutrophils and products of degranulation
- Platelets and the coagulation factors formed on their surfaces
- Derivatives of arachidonic acid
- T and B lymphocytes and their products

CLINICAL PRESENTATION

Independent of the pathophysiologic cause, the clinical syndrome of shock progresses through several stages. During each step, the body uses and exhausts various compensatory mechanisms to balance oxygen delivery (Do_2) and oxygen consumption (Vo_2) in an effort to maintain perfusion of vital organs. A major determinant of tissue perfusion is the systemic, or mean arterial pressure. Mean arterial pressure (MAP) is a function of the product of blood flow [cardiac output (CO)] and systemic vascular resistance (SVR). Cardiac output is the product of heart rate (HR) and stroke volume (SV) (Fig. 22-1). Vascular resistance is determined primarily by vascular smooth muscle tone, modulated by the sympathoadrenal system and by circulating humoral and local metabolic factors. These interacting factors are what contribute to the clinical syndrome seen in patients with shock.

The classic findings observed with shock include the following:

- Systolic blood pressure (SBP) <90 mm Hg (or >60 mm Hg decrease from baseline in a hypertensive patient)
- Tachycardia (HR >90 beats/min)

Table 22-1	Classification of Shock and Precipitating Events

Hypovolemic Shock
  Hemorrhagic
    Gastrointestinal bleeding
    Trauma
    Internal bleeding: ruptured aortic aneurysm,
      retroperitoneal bleeding
  Nonhemorrhagic
    Dehydration: vomiting, diarrhea, diabetes mellitus,
      diabetes insipidus, overuse of diuretics
    Sequestration: ascites, third-space accumulation
    Cutaneous: burns, nonreplaced perspiration and in-
      sensible water losses

Cardiogenic Shock
  Nonmechanical Causes
    Acute myocardial infarction
    Low cardiac output syndrome
    Right ventricular infarction
    End-stage cardiomyopathy
  Mechanical Causes
    Rupture of septum or free wall
    Mitral or aortic insufficiency
    Papillary muscle rupture or dysfunction
    Critical aortic stenosis
    Pericardial tamponade

Distributive Shock
  Septic Shock
  Anaphylaxis
  Neurogenic
    Spinal injury, cerebral damage, severe dysautonomia
  Drug-Induced
    Anesthesia, ganglionic and adrenergic blockers, and
      over-doses of barbiturates, narcotics
  Acute Adrenal Insufficiency

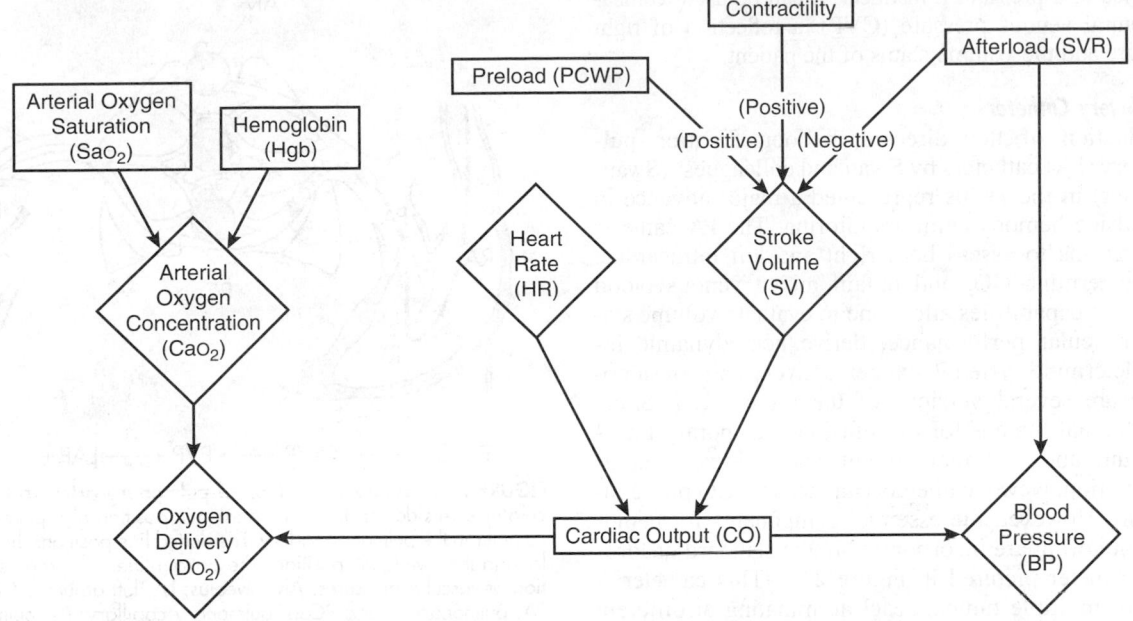

FIGURE 22-1 Determinants of blood pressure, cardiac output, and oxygen delivery.

- Tachypnea (RR >20 breaths/min)
- Cutaneous vasoconstriction: cold, clammy, mottled skin, (not typical of distributive shock)
- Mental confusion (agitation, stupor, or coma)
- Oliguria: urine output <20 mL/hour
- Metabolic acidosis (lactic acidosis secondary to anaerobic glycolysis)

Not all these described findings are encountered in every patient with shock, and considerable variability exists in both the rapidity and sequence of onset. This depends on the severity of the initiating event, the underlying mechanism, and the baseline condition of the patient, including medications that may alter the clinical presentation. Therefore, it is important to consider the patient's medical and pharmacologic history while closely monitoring for subtle clinical changes that may signal impending deterioration and necessitate immediate intervention.

HEMODYNAMIC MONITORING

Hemodynamic monitoring in the critically ill patient is mandatory to properly assess and manage various shock states. Both noninvasive and invasive monitoring techniques can be used to measure cardiovascular performance in patients and to differentiate the causes of various conditions causing hypoperfusion and organ dysfunction. The values obtained with hemodynamic monitoring should always be used in conjunction with clinical judgment.

Noninvasive Monitoring

An important part of hemodynamic monitoring in the critically ill patient involves noninvasive measures. Clinical examination and vital signs (temperature, HR, BP, RR) provide invaluable information regarding the cardiovascular system and organ perfusion. Other well-established noninvasive techniques for monitoring the hemodynamic status of patients include pulse oximetry (for measuring arterial oxygen saturation [SaO_2]) and transthoracic echocardiography, which can estimate the functional status of the heart and heart valves.

New noninvasive technologies are being developed. End tidal carbon dioxide ($EtCO_2$) monitors are used to determine oxygen consumption and help guide therapies designed to improve oxygen delivery and consumption. New devices that can measure cardiac output and tissue perfusion noninvasively (or minimally invasively), such as gastric tonometry, esophageal Doppler monitoring, thoracic bioimpedance, and others have been developed,[4,5] but are not used routinely in most ICUs. Although important, noninvasive measures have limitations, and certain hemodynamic values must be measured invasively at the present time.

Invasive Monitoring

The evaluation of critically ill patients is a complicated matter, and data that can be important in the diagnosis and assessment of illness as well as the patient's response to therapy must occasionally be obtained by invasive techniques.

Arterial Pressure Line

The arterial line is a common tool in the intensive care unit. It consists of a small catheter placed into an artery (usually the radial or femoral artery) and attached to a pressure transducer. This allows for continuous measurement of blood pressure (BP) and also provides for easy access for arterial blood gas samples to be drawn and analyzed. Arterial lines should never be used for medication administration.

Central Venous Catheter

Common in the ICU, the central venous catheter consists of a large-bore catheter usually inserted into either a subclavian or jugular vein. It can be used for infusion of fluid and medications;

when attached to a pressure transducer, it can be used to measure the central venous pressure (CVP), a reflection of right atrial pressure and the volume status of the patient.

Pulmonary Artery Catheter

The introduction of flow-directed, balloon flotation pulmonary artery (PA) catheters by Swan and colleagues[6] (Swan-Ganz catheter) in the 1970s represented a major advance in invasive bedside hemodynamic monitoring. The PA catheter enables clinicians to assess both right and left intracardiac pressures, determine CO, and obtain mixed venous blood samples. These capabilities allow one to evaluate volume status and ventricular performance, derive hemodynamic indices, and determine systemic oxygen delivery and consumption. There are several versions of the PA catheter. Some include additional lumens for IV infusions, temporary transvenous pacing, and continuous monitoring of mixed venous oxygen saturation. Newer catheters can measure CO on a continuous basis. However, the essential components for hemodynamic monitoring are incorporated in the standard quadruple lumen catheter pictured in Figure 22-2. This catheter is comprised of multiple lumens, each terminating at different points along the catheter. When properly positioned, the proximal port (C) terminates in the right atrium and is used to measure right atrial pressure, to inject fluid for cardiac output determination, and to administer IV fluids. The distal port (B), which terminates at the tip of the catheter (E), is positioned in the pulmonary artery beyond the pulmonary valve and is used to measure pulmonary artery and pulmonary capillary wedge pressure (PCWP; described below) and to obtain mixed venous blood samples. Intermittent inflation of the balloon is accomplished by inserting 1.5 mL of air into the balloon inflation valve (D). The thermistor (A) contains a temperature probe and electrical leads that connect to a computer, which calculates cardiac output by the thermodilution technique.

Although the pulmonary artery catheter is confined to the pulmonary vasculature, LV pressures can be ascertained from the PCWP. When the balloon is inflated, the PA catheter advances to a pulmonary artery branch of equal diameter and becomes lodged or "wedged" in this position. Because forward flow from the right ventricle ceases beyond the wedged PA segment, a static fluid column exists between the left ventricle and PA catheter tip during diastole when the mitral valve is open. If no pressure gradients are in the pulmonary vasculature beyond the balloon and if mitral valve function is normal, the PCWP then equilibrates with all distal pressures

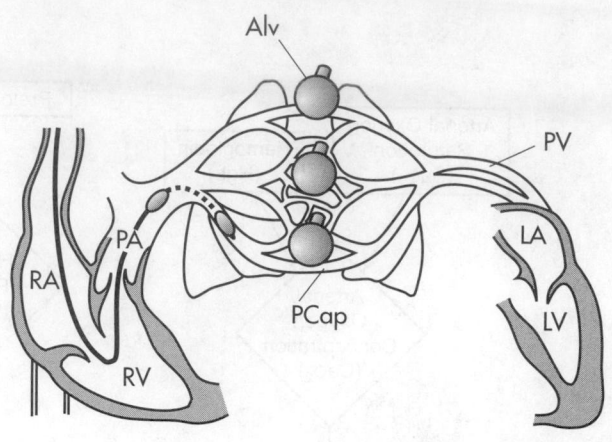

$$PAEDP \longleftrightarrow PCWP \longleftrightarrow PVP \longleftrightarrow LAP \longleftrightarrow LVEDP$$

FIGURE 22-3 Anatomic position of pulmonary artery catheter in vasculature. This demonstrates the anatomic position of a pulmonary artery catheter in the pulmonary artery. The dotted line positions the inflated balloon in the "wedged" position. The bottom line is a progressive correlation of vascular pressures. Alv, alveolus; LA, left atrium; LV, left ventricle; PA, pulmonary artery; PCap, pulmonary capillary; PV, pulmonary vein; RA, right atrium; RV, right ventricle. (From reference #115. Adapted with permission from Vender JS. Invasive cardiac monitoring. Crit Care Clin 1988;4:455.)

and thus indirectly reflects left ventricular end-diastolic pressure (LVEDP). Based on the relationship between pressure and volume, the LVEDP is equivalent to the left ventricular end-diastolic volume (LVEDV) which is also known as *preload*. Figure 22-3 illustrates the anatomic position of the pulmonary artery catheter in the pulmonary artery and the progressive correlation of distal vascular pressures (i.e., the PA end-diastolic pressure, PCWP, pulmonary vein pressure, left atrial pressure, and LVEDP).

Controversy has surrounded the use of PA catheters. Trials have failed to show a benefit in terms of mortality, and a recent study found increased mortality and complications among patients receiving PA catheterization compared with a control group matched for disease state and severity.[7] A criticism of this study is the potential for selection bias, in that only the most critically ill of patients received PA catheterization compared with controls. A large trial was recently published that randomized 1994 elderly high-risk major (noncardiac) surgery patients to treatment guided by the placement of a PA catheter or standard treatment without the use of the catheter.[8] There were no significant differences in mortality during hospitalization or at 6 and 12 months. There was a statistically greater incidence in pulmonary embolism (PE) in the catheter group (0.9% incidence in the catheter group versus in the standard treatment group). This trial raises serious concerns about the routine placement of PA catheters in this population. Whether the results can be extrapolated to other populations is unknown.

DETERMINANTS OF CARDIAC FUNCTION AND HEMODYNAMIC INDICES

The effective interpretation and management of hemodynamic parameters requires a thorough understanding of the physiologic determinants of CO and arterial pressure. Assum-

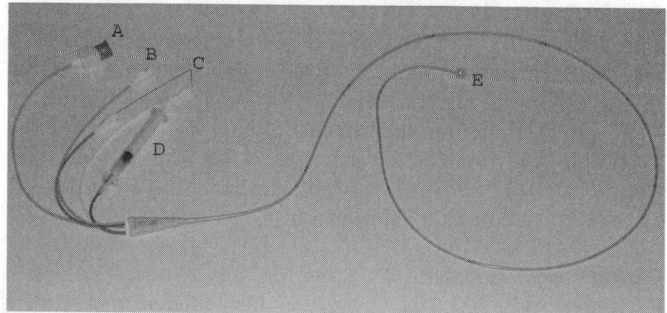

FIGURE 22-2 Pulmonary artery catheter. (See text for definitions of A, B, C, D, and E.)

ing oxygen content of blood is adequate, cardiac output and SVR are the ultimate determinants of oxygen delivery and adequate arterial pressure, and thus overall tissue perfusion. As outlined in Figure 22-1, cardiac output may be quantified as the product of SV and HR. SV is determined by preload, afterload, and contractility. The effects of these factors on hemodynamic parameters are interrelated and complex and must be assessed carefully when selecting therapeutic interventions that will produce the desired response. A good review of the determinants of cardiac performance is found in Chapter 19, Heart Failure. Table 22-2 and the glossary provide definitions of terms and normal hemodynamic indices, which are discussed in the following section.

Measured Hemodynamic Indices

Right Atrial Pressure and Central Venous Pressure

The right atrial pressure (RAP), as measured by a PA catheter, reflects the filling pressure or end-diastolic pressure of the right ventricle and is used as an index of RV preload. Central venous pressure (CVP), as determined by a catheter advanced to the superior vena cava or right atrium, is another means of measuring right ventricle filling pressure and is considered equivalent to the RAP. Vascular capacitance, circulating blood volume, and myocardial contractility maintain RAP. A low RAP usually reflects hypovolemia or vasodilation. An elevated RAP can signify increased intravascular volume, right ventricular heart failure, tricuspid regurgitation, pulmonary

Table 22-2 Normal Hemodynamic Values and Derived Indices

	Equation	Normal Value	Units
Directly Measured			
Blood pressure (BP) (systolic/diastolic)		120–140/80–90	mm Hg
Cardiac output (CO)	$CO = SV \times HR$	4–7	L/min
Central venous pressure (CVP)[a]		2–6	mm Hg[b]
Heart rate (HR) (pulse)		60–80	beats/min
Mean pulmonary artery pressure (MPAP)		12–15	mm Hg
Pulmonary artery pressure (PAP) (systolic/diastolic)		20–30/8–12	mm Hg
Pulmonary capillary wedge pressure (PCWP)		5–12[c]	mm Hg
Derived Indices			
Cardiac index (CI)	$CI = \dfrac{CO}{BSA^d}$	2.5–4.2	L/min/m²
Left ventricular stroke work index (LVSWI)	$LVSWI = (MAP - PCWP)(SVI)(0.0136)$	35–85	g/m²/beat
Mean arterial pressure (MAP)	$MAP = \dfrac{2(\text{Diastolic BP}) + \text{Systolic BP}}{3}$	80–100	mm Hg
Perfusion pressure (PP)	$PP = MAP - PCWP$	50	mm Hg
Pulmonary vascular resistance (PVR)	$PVR = \dfrac{(MPAP - PCWP)}{CO}(80)$	20–120	dynes · sec · cm⁻⁵
Stroke volume (SV)	$SV = \dfrac{CO}{HR}$	60–130	mL/beat
Stroke volume index (SVI)	$SVI = \dfrac{SV}{BSA}$	30–75	mL/beat/m²
Systemic vascular resistance (SVR)[e]	$SVR = \dfrac{(MAP - CVP)}{CO}(80)$	800–1,440	dyne · sec · cm⁻⁵
Systemic vascular resistance index (SVRI)	$SVRI = SVR \times BSA$	1,680–2,580	dyne · sec · cm⁻⁵ · m²
Oxygen delivery (Do_2)	$Do_2 = CO \times Cao_2 \; [Cao_2 = (Hgb \times Sao_2 \times 13.9)]$	700–1,200	mL/min
Oxygen consumption (Vo_2)	$Vo_2 = CO \times Hgb \times 13.9 \times (Sao_2 \times Svo_2)$	200–400	mL/min

[a]CVP is essentially synonymous with RAP.
[b]2–6 mm Hg = 3–6 cm H_2O (conversion. 1 mm = 1.34 cm H_2O).
[c]May optimally ↑ PCWP to 16–18 mm Hg in critically ill patients.
[d]BSA, body surface area = 1.7 m² (average male).
[e]SVR is synonymous with total peripheral resistance (TPR).

embolus, pulmonary hypertension, obstructive airway disease with cor pulmonale, or pericardial tamponade. In tamponade, the left ventricle filling pressure also is elevated to the same degree as the RAP.

Right-sided heart pressures are unreliable indicators of concurrent LV function.[9] In patients with cardiac or pulmonary disease or on mechanical ventilation, RAP or CVP measurements actually may vary inversely with the PCWP. Therefore, reliance on right-sided heart pressures from CVP catheters alone is adequate only in select patients.

Pulmonary Artery Systolic Pressure

Pulmonary artery systolic (PAS) pressure is obtained during systole after the opening of the pulmonic valve when blood is ejected from the right ventricle into the pulmonary artery. It measures the pressure generated by the right ventricle during contraction. Elevations in PAS pressure occur when pulmonary vascular resistance is increased. This occurs in patients with acute or chronic parenchymal pulmonary disease, pulmonary embolus, hypoxemia, or acidosis, as well as in those receiving vasoactive drugs. A low PAS pressure usually results from a reduced circulating blood volume.

Pulmonary Artery Diastolic Pressure

Pulmonary artery diastolic (PAD) pressure is measured during diastole after the closure of the pulmonic valve when the blood moves from the pulmonary artery into the pulmonary capillaries. As previously described with respect to the PCWP, the PAD pressure also may reflect LVEDP. Under normal circumstances, the PAD pressure is approximately equal (within 1 to 3 mm Hg) to the PCWP and can be used in place of the latter as an indication of LVEDP. However, because the catheter is more proximally located and is not in a "wedged" position, the PAD pressure may not correlate as well as the PCWP with the LVEDP. In conditions that increase pulmonary vascular resistance, such as those mentioned for pulmonary artery systolic pressure, the PAD may be substantially greater than the PCWP. Also, when heart rates are >120 beats/min, PAD pressure exceeds PCWP. This is because diastole is shortened and reduces the time necessary for equilibrium of blood flow.

Pulmonary Capillary Wedge Pressure

PCWP is the most reliable reflection of LVEDP measured with the pulmonary artery catheter. LVEDP, in turn, provides the closest approximation of preload, the initial end-diastolic fiber length, which is determined clinically by LVEDV. Because neither LVEDV nor LVEDP are readily measurable, PCWP is used as an indicator of preload.

Preload is an important determinant of stroke volume. The relationship between preload and stroke volume is illustrated in Figure 22-4, the Frank-Starling curve. According to this mechanism, the degree of myocardial fiber shortening, and hence SV, is proportional to the initial myocardial fiber length, or ventricular volume, at the onset of contraction. As shown in Figure 22-1, if HR remains the same, SV is proportional to cardiac output. Initially, for any given state of contractility, an increase in preload generates a contraction that results in a corresponding increase in SV. Once an optimal preload is attained, as indicated by the flat portion of the curve, further elevations in ventricular filling pressure will not enhance SV

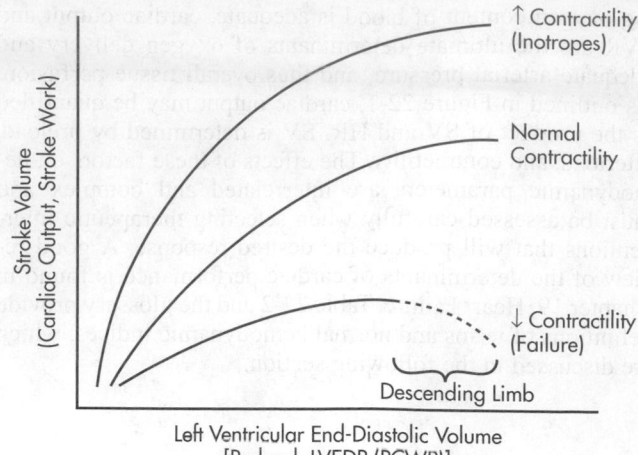

FIGURE 22-4 Ventricular function curve (general). In the normal heart, as preload (LVEDP), measured clinically by PCWP, increases, stroke volume (cardiac output, stroke work) increases, until the contractile fibers reach their capacity, at which point the curve flattens. A change in contractility causes the heart to perform on a different curve. If the contractile fibers exceed their capacity, as with severe heart failure, the heart will operate on the descending limb of the curve.

and can, in fact, result in a decline in contractility and a decrease in SV. Significant increases or decreases in the level of ventricular contractility (inotropy), independent of alterations in preload or afterload, result in shifts in the ventricular function curve, with corresponding changes in SV. As shown in Figure 22-4, enhanced myocardial contractility caused by such factors as increased sympathetic nerve activity, endogenous catecholamines, or exogenous inotropic agents, shifts the ventricular function curve upward and to the left, thus augmenting SV for a given preload. Conditions that reduce contractility, such as loss of contractile mass, use of pharmacologic depressants, systemic hypoxia, local ischemia, or acidosis, shift the curve downward and to the right, thereby diminishing SV.

Although LVEDP or PCWP can generally be substituted for LVEDV when evaluating cardiac function, the use of PCWP as a reflection of LVEDV has its limitations. In patients with mitral stenosis, pulmonary veno-occlusive disease, or high levels of positive end-expiratory pressure (PEEP) with mechanical ventilation, PCWP will exceed LVEDV and inaccurately reflect LVEDV.

The relationship between LVEDP and LVEDV is curvilinear and is determined by compliance. In conditions in which ventricular compliance is abnormal, the correlation between LVEDP to LVEDV is altered, and PCWP cannot be assumed to accurately reflect preload. Therefore, one must be aware that certain conditions or interventions can result in potential alterations in ventricular compliance and/or PCWP and interpret measurements accordingly.

The PCWP also is a useful measure of pulmonary capillary hydrostatic pressure, the major driving force for the development of pulmonary congestion. Thus, the PCWP helps the clinician determine whether pulmonary edema is cardiogenic or noncardiogenic in origin. PCWP is higher than pulmonary hydrostatic pressure with adult respiratory distress syndrome (ARDS) or elevated pulmonary vascular resistance.

Cardiac Output

CO determination involves injecting a 10-mL bolus of cold crystalloid solution through the catheter and measuring the temperature at the tip of the PA catheter via the thermistor. The relationship between the temperature change over time and blood flow allows calculation of the CO.[10] PA catheters are available that use a small heat generator and a heat sink in the catheter itself, which allows the continuous determination of CO with the same concept of thermodilution. Some conditions may make measurement of CO less reliable. Tricuspid valve regurgitation and intracardiac shunts, such as ventricular septal defects, affect the way blood flows past the tip of the thermistor and thus may give erroneous values.

Mixed Venous Oxygen Saturation

Mixed venous oxygen saturation (SVO_2) can be measured with fiberoptic sensors in newer versions of the PA catheter, or it can be measured directly from blood drawn from the catheter before oxygenation in the lungs. It can be used as an indicator of the global adequacy of perfusion and can be used to calculate the body's consumption of oxygen (VO_2, see later section). The SVO_2 may be of particular usefulness in situations in which cardiac output measurements are unreliable (such as tricuspid valve regurgitation) or in clinical situations in which oxygen consumption is increased despite normal oxygen delivery (such as septic shock).

Derived Hemodynamic Indices

Parameters that reflect cardiovascular function can be derived from the hemodynamic measurements obtained from the Swan-Ganz catheter (see Table 22-2 and Glossary).

Stroke Volume

Stroke volume (SV) is the amount of blood ejected by the ventricle with each systolic contraction, and it is directly proportional to the contractile state of the myocardium. When CO is increased by therapeutic maneuvers, it is important to know whether the increase is caused by an inotropic (SV) or a chronotropic response (HR).

Cardiac Index

Cardiac index is the CO adjusted for body surface area (BSA). Because CO is a relative measure based on size, it provides a more meaningful assessment of a person's output.

Pulmonary Vascular Resistance and Systemic Vascular Resistance

Pulmonary vascular resistance (PVR) and systemic vascular resistance (SVR, afterload) are determined by dividing the change in pressure by the flow (pressure change/cardiac output = resistance). Therapeutic maneuvers that alter SVR do not indicate a change in any specific vascular bed, such as the renal or splanchnic vascular beds; changes in SVR reflect the overall change. The systemic vascular resistance index (SVRI) is a normalized SVR for body surface area.

Left Ventricular Stroke Work Index

Left ventricular stroke work index (LVSWI) is an indication of LV contractility that takes into account preload, afterload, and CO. The constant 0.0136 is the conversion factor that changes mm Hg/mL into gram-meters. Elevation in LVSWI can be achieved by changing preload, afterload, or contractility.

Oxygen Transport Variables

Hypoperfusion associated with shock is not as readily detectable as hypotension. An imbalance between oxygen supply and demand may not be recognized until irreversible organ dysfunction has begun. Thus, it can be valuable in some patients to monitor oxygen transport variables and use these values to guide therapy.

Oxygen Delivery

Oxygen delivery (DO_2) can be calculated as the product of CO and the arterial concentration of oxygen (CaO_2). Hemoglobin concentration (Hgb) and arterial oxygen saturation (SaO_2) are the primary determinants of CaO_2. A smaller contribution to the equation is the amount of oxygen dissolved in the blood, determined by the arterial pressure of oxygen (PaO_2), which can be left out to simplify calculations:

$$Do_2 = (CO)(Cao_2)$$

where

$$Cao_2 = (Hgb)(Sao_2)(13.9)$$

Oxygen Consumption

Oxygen consumption (VO_2) estimates the oxygen demand of the body and can be calculated as the product of CO and the difference between the arterial and venous concentrations of oxygen ($CaO_2 - CvO_2$). Rearranged and simplified, the equation can be represented as follows:

$$Vo_2 = (CO)(Hgb)(13.9)(Sao_2 - Svo_2)$$

Normally consumption is independent of supply, except at low rates of Do_2. However, in some critically ill patients, consumption can depend on supply even in what would be considered "normal" Do_2 ranges. In these patients, it may be appropriate to increase the delivery of oxygen until the increase in consumption has reached a plateau.[11] This may help to "repay" some of the oxygen debt induced by hypoperfusion. Further increases in Do_2 to supranormal ranges with inotropic drugs such as dobutamine have not been conclusively shown to benefit patients and may have a detrimental effect.[12,13] A factor to consider in evaluating these values and the studies that use them is the potential for mathematic coupling of data. CO, hemoglobin, and arterial oxygen saturation are common components of both equations. Errors in the measurement of these parameters lead to errors in the calculation of both delivery and consumption of oxygen.

ETIOLOGIC CLASSIFICATION OF SHOCK AND COMMON MECHANISMS

The most common clinical conditions associated with the major forms of shock are reviewed in the following sections and detailed in Table 22-1. The pathogenesis, epidemiology, clinical, and hemodynamic manifestations for each classification are briefly discussed and further illustrated in case studies throughout the chapter. Table 22-3 describes the common hemodynamic findings for the various forms of shock.

Table 22-3   Hemodynamic Findings in Various Shock States

	Hypovolemic	Cardiogenic	Distributive (Septic)
HR	↑	↑	↑
BP[a]	↓	↑/↓	↓
CO	↓	↓	↑[b]
Preload (PCWP)	↓	↑	↑/↓
Afterload (SVR)	↑	↑	↓

[a]Patients may be in a state of compensated shock in which BP is normal but clinical signs of hypoperfusion are evident.
[b]Cardiac output is increased early in sepsis but can be decreased in late, severe sepsis.

Hypovolemic Shock

Shock secondary to a reduction in intravascular volume is referred to as hypovolemic shock. Whether the primary insult is the external loss of fluid volume (e.g., blood, plasma, or free water) or the internal sequestration of these fluids into body cavities (third spacing), the overall result is reduced venous return (decreases in CVP and PCWP) and decreased CO (see Table 22-3). The severity of hypovolemic shock depends on the amount and rate of intravascular volume loss and each person's capacity for compensation. Although responses vary, a healthy person may tolerate an acute loss of as much as 30% of his or her intravascular volume with minimal clinical signs and symptoms.[14] Compensatory mechanisms such as increases in HR, myocardial contractility, and SVR are effective enough for this loss in volume such that measurable falls in systolic BP are not detected. Losses in excess of 80% generally overwhelm compensatory mechanisms and the patient progresses to overt shock with hypotension and signs of hypoperfusion. If restorative measures are not taken immediately, irreversible shock and death may result. The most common and dramatic cause of hypovolemic shock is hemorrhagic shock in which intravascular volume depletion occurs as a result of bleeding. Trauma is responsible for most cases of acute hemorrhagic shock; other significant causes are rupture of vascular aneurysms, acute gastrointestinal bleeding, ruptured ectopic pregnancy, and postoperative bleeding. Other mechanisms for hypovolemic shock are conditions associated with either excess fluid losses from gastrointestinal or renal sources and plasma loss caused by burns or sequestration (also known as *third-space accumulation*).

Cardiogenic Shock

A shock state arising primarily from an abnormality of cardiac function constitutes cardiogenic shock. The causes of cardiogenic shock can be separated largely into mechanical and nonmechanical (see Table 22-1), although occasionally, patients may have a combination of causes. Regardless of the source, the underlying problem in cardiogenic shock is a decrease in CO that is not caused by a reduction in circulating blood volume. This decrease in CO results in the syndrome of shock: hypotension with a decrease in arterial BP, and hypoperfusion as the delivery of oxygenated blood to the tissues is reduced. Eventually organ dysfunction and death result if measures to restore perfusion are not successful.

The most common cause of cardiogenic shock is left ventricular (LV) dysfunction and necrosis as a result of acute myocardial infarction (AMI) (see Chapter 18, Myocardial Infarction). Necrosis of the left ventricle can be the result of a single massive myocardial infarction (MI), or it may follow numerous smaller events. Increases in sympathetic tone—seen clinically as increased HR and peripheral vasoconstriction—initially serve to increase CO and maintain central arterial pressure. However, when LV necrosis exceeds approximately 40% of the contractile mass of the heart, normal compensatory responses can no longer maintain CO, and hypotension and hypoperfusion result. In addition to decreased perfusion to vital tissues and organs, the decrease in CO leads to a reduction in the flow of blood through the coronary arteries, which can lead to infarct extension and a further worsening of cardiac performance.

The incidence of cardiogenic shock after AMI has remained relatively stable over the past 20 years. A recent study found an average incidence of 7.1% from 1975 to 1997.[15] The in-hospital mortality for those patients developing shock has decreased somewhat over this time frame, most likely because of coronary reperfusion strategies. The overall mortality rate, however, has remained high, with most series reporting an average of 60% to 80%.[15,16]

Cardiogenic shock caused by mechanical problems occurs relatively infrequently. In this setting the systolic function (contractile ability) of the heart may be normal, but other defects render the heart unable to eject a normal volume of blood. Pericardial tamponade and tension pneumothorax can cause cardiogenic shock by compressing the heart and decreasing the diastolic filling. Acute valvular insufficiency or stenosis prevents the normal ejection of blood. Ventricular septal or free wall rupture can occur, often in the setting of AMI, with the reduction in CO related to the inability of the left ventricle to eject a normal volume of blood during systole.

Nonmechanical origins of cardiogenic shock involve a decrease in the function of the heart muscle itself. Myocardial infarction involving the right ventricle can cause cardiogenic shock, even with normal LV systolic function. In this situation, the volume of blood reaching the left ventricle (preload) is reduced because of the right ventricle's inability to move blood to the left side of the heart. In most patients with cardiogenic shock and right ventricular (RV) infarction, significant LV dysfunction is present as well.

Patients with chronic heart failure (HF) (see Chapter 19, Heart Failure) usually can compensate for their poor cardiac function, but acute exacerbations can cause cardiogenic shock with hypotension, hypoperfusion, and organ dysfunction. Cardiac dysfunction occasionally can be seen with severe sepsis because of increases in the production of inflammatory cytokines that have a depressant effect on the myocardium. A similar picture also can be seen following cardiopulmonary bypass during heart surgery, which activates the inflammatory cascade.

The symptoms of cardiogenic shock are largely the same as for other types of shock. Hypotension and signs of inadequate tissue perfusion, such as confusion, oliguria, tachycardia, and cutaneous vasoconstriction, are present in many patients. Differentiating cardiogenic shock from distributive or hypovolemic shock requires further examination. A history of coronary artery disease or symptoms of MI are important findings. Hypovolemia occurs in up to 20% of patients in cardiogenic shock, but patients frequently have signs of volume overload because the heart cannot move blood through the circulation. Peripheral edema can be seen in the extremities; lung sounds are diminished and rales may be present as pulmonary edema develops. These findings are particularly evident in patients with severe HF, a frequent manifestation of cardiogenic shock.

Because the distinction between cardiogenic and other forms of shock can be difficult to make based on physical examination alone, further testing with invasive hemodynamic monitoring is usually required to establish the diagnosis and guide therapy. Table 22-4 lists the common laboratory, electrocardiogram (ECG), chest radiograph findings, and Table 22-3 lists the common hemodynamic findings in cardiogenic shock.

Distributive Shock

Distributive shock is characterized by an overt loss of vascular tone, causing acute tissue hypoperfusion. Although numerous events can initiate distributive shock, most cases are readily reversed by supportive measures and treatment or elimination of the underlying cause.

Table 22-4 Typical Findings of Early Cardiogenic Shock

- Arterial blood gas (ABG)
  - Hypoxemia secondary to pulmonary congestion with ventilation-perfusion abnormalities
  - Metabolic acidosis with a compensatory respiratory alkalosis

- Elevated blood lactate levels (which contributes to the acidosis)

- Complete blood count (CBC)
  - Leukocytosis
  - Thrombocytopenia (if disseminated intravascular coagulation is present)

- Elevated cardiac enzymes if myocardial infarction is present

- ECG—One or more of the following
  - T-wave changes indicating infarction
  - Left bundle-branch block
  - Sinus tachycardia
  - Arrhythmia

- Chest radiograph
  - Pulmonary edema or evidence of adult respiratory distress syndrome (ARDS)

- Echocardiography
  - Valvular or mechanical problems if present
  - Normal or decreased ejection fraction

- Hemodynamic monitoring— one or more of the following
  - Reduced cardiac output
  - Arterial hypotension
  - Elevated pulmonary capillary wedge pressure (PCWP) and pulmonary artery pressure (PAP)
  - Elevated systemic vascular resistance (SVR)

Septic Shock

Distributive shock secondary to sepsis, or septic shock, is associated with a high mortality rate, reflecting the limited therapeutic options available at this time. There are approximately 500,000 cases of sepsis syndrome annually, with mortality rates ranging from about 30% at 1 month to 50% at 5 months. Epidemiology studies show that approximately 25% of patients with sepsis syndrome progress to septic shock. Septic shock is the number one cause of death in the noncoronary ICU and the 13th most common cause of death in the United States. It has been projected that the incidence of sepsis will increase 1.5% per year mainly because of the disproportionate growth of the elderly in the U.S. population.[17–20]

The consensus conference of the American College of Chest Physicians (ACCP) and the Society of Critical Care Medicine (SCCM) defines sepsis syndrome as a systemic inflammatory response resulting from infection.[2] When there is associated organ dysfunction, hypoperfusion, or hypotension, it is termed *severe sepsis;* when hypotension persists despite adequate fluid resuscitation and requires inotropic and/or vasopressor support, it is termed *septic shock* (see Table 22-5 for definitions). More than half the cases of septic syndrome occur in the ICU, one-third occur in other currently hospitalized patients, and 10% to 15% of cases are present upon admission to the emergency department (ED).[19] Progression to septic shock occurs in about half of patients who have septic syndrome within 1 month of onset, as defined by hypotension. Persons most at risk for septic shock are immunocompromised or have underlying conditions that render them susceptible to bloodstream invasion. Groups at risk include neonates, the elderly, patients with AIDS, alcoholics, childbearing women, and those undergoing surgery or who have experienced trauma. Other predisposing factors include coexisting diseases such as diabetes mellitus, malignancies, chronic hepatic or renal failure, and hyposplenism; exposure to immunosuppressant drugs and cancer chemotherapy; and procedures such as insertion of urinary catheters, endotracheal tubes, and intravenous (IV) lines.

Septic shock is characterized initially by a normal or high cardiac output and a low systemic vascular resistance (see Table 22-3). Hypotension is caused by the low SVR as well as alterations in macrovascular and microvascular tone which result in maldistribution of blood flow and volume. Changes in the microvasculature can lead to loss of normal microvascular autoregulatory mechanisms resulting in constriction of capillaries, changes in cellular rheology, fibrin deposition, and neutrophil adherence. This causes vascular "sludging" and in some cases arteriovenous shunts that bypass capillary beds. Loss of intravascular fluid caused by increased vascular permeability and third spacing of fluid further adds to hypovolemia. In an effort to compensate for the changes in volume and SVR, the body goes into a hyperdynamic state and increases CO. Most patients develop myocardial dysfunction as manifested by decreased myocardial compliance, reduced contractility, and ventricular dilation, but maintain a normal CO due to tachycardia and cardiac dilatation. Although the cause of and mechanism for this abnormality are not fully understood, it is not believed to be caused by myocardial ischemia. Rather, it is thought to be caused by one or more circulating inflammatory mediators, such as cytokines, tumor necrosis factor-α (TNF-α), PAF, arachidonic acid, NO, and

Table 22-5 ACCP/SCCM Consensus Conference Definitions

Infection	Microbial phenomenon characterized by an inflammatory response to the presence of microorganisms or the invasion of normally sterile host tissue by those organisms.
Bacteremia	The presence of viable bacteria in the blood.
Systemic inflammatory response syndrome (SIRS)	The systemic inflammatory response to a variety of severe clinical insults. The response is manifested by two or more of the following conditions: Temperature >38°C or <36°C Heart rate >90 beats/min Respiratory rate >20 breaths/min or $Paco_2$ <32 mm Hg (<4.3 kPa) WBC >12,000 cells/mm^3, <4,000 cell/mm^3, or >10% immature (bands) forms
Sepsis	The systemic response to infection. The systemic response is manifested by two or more of the following conditions as a result of infection: Temperature >38°C or <36°C Heart rate >90 beats/min Respiratory rate >20 breaths/min or $Paco_2$ <32 mm Hg (<4.3 kPa) WBC >12,000 cells/mm^3, <4,000 cell/mm^3, or >10% immature (band) forms
Severe sepsis	Sepsis associated with organ dysfunction, hypoperfusion, or hypotension. Hypoperfusion and perfusion abnormalities may include, but are not limited to, lactic acidosis, oliguria, or an acute alteration in mental status.
Septic shock	Sepsis with hypotension, despite adequate fluid resuscitation, along with perfusion abnormalities that may include, but are not limited to, lactic acidosis, oliguria, or an acute alteration in mental status. Patients who are on inotropic or vasopressor agents may not be hypotensive at the time that perfusion abnormalities are measured.
Hypotension	A systolic BP of <90 mm Hg or a reduction of >40 mm Hg from baseline in the absence of other causes for hypotension.
Multiple organ dysfunction syndrome	Presence of altered organ function in an acutely ill patient such that homeostasis cannot be maintained without intervention.

Reprinted with permission from American College of Chest Physicians/Society of Critical Care Medicine Consensus Conference. Definitions for sepsis and organ failure and guidelines for the use of innovative therapies in sepsis. Crit Care Med 1992;20:864.

reactive oxygen species. In late septic shock, the body is no longer able to compensate because of the cardiac effects of the inflammatory mediators and myocardial edema, therefore resulting in a decreased CO. The end product of this complicated pathway is cellular ischemia, dysfunction, and eventually cellular death unless the chain of events is interrupted.

The pathogenesis of sepsis is more fully understood now, but the exact mechanisms are still not completely clear. It is known that the changes which take place during sepsis are due to the immunologic host response to infection which involves inflammatory and immunodepressive (anti-inflammatory) phases. It is unknown, however, whether these phases are sequential (inflammatory then immunodepressive) or whether immunosuppression is a primary response to sepsis rather than a compensatory response.

The inflammatory stage of sepsis is initiated by an infection with a microorganism, most commonly bacterial. Organisms can either enter the bloodstream directly (producing positive blood cultures) or may indirectly elicit a systemic inflammatory response by locally releasing their toxins or structural components at the site of infection. The lipopolysaccharide endotoxin of Gram-negative bacteria is the most potent soluble product of bacteria that can initiate a response and is the most studied, but other bacterial products can initiate the response, including exotoxins, enterotoxins, peptidoglycans, and lipoteichoic acid from Gram-positive organisms. The binding of these toxins to cell receptors promotes proinflammatory cy-

tokine production, primarily TNF-α and IL-1. These toxins stimulate the production and release of numerous endogenous mediators that are responsible for the inflammatory consequences of sepsis. The cytokines act synergistically to directly affect organ function and stimulate the release of other proinflammatory cytokines, such as IL-6, IL-8, platelet activating factor (PAF), complement, thromboxanes, leukotrienes, prostaglandins, nitric oxide (NO), and others.

The presence of these cytokines promotes inflammation and vascular endothelial injury, but also causes an overwhelming activation in coagulation. Thrombin has potent proinflammatory and pro-coagulant activities and its production is increased in sepsis. The human body normally counteracts these effects by increasing fibrinolysis, but the homeostatic mechanisms in the septic patient are dysfunctional. There are decreases in the levels of protein C, plasminogen, and antithrombin III as well as increased activity of plasminogen activator inhibitor-1 (PAI-1) and thrombin activatable fibrinolysis inhibitor (TAFI), endogenous agents that inhibit fibrinolysis.[21] The patient is in a coagulopathic state, which promotes formation of microvascular thrombi leading to hypoperfusion, ischemia, and ultimately, organ failure. Multiple organ failure is responsible for about half the deaths due to septic shock.[22]

The clinical features of septic shock are fever, chills, nausea, vomiting, and diarrhea. Characteristic laboratory findings include leukocytosis or leukopenia; thrombocytopenia with or without coagulation abnormalities; and often, hyperbilirubinemia. These features are usually readily detectable and occur within 24 hours after bacteremia develops, particularly if the bacteremia is caused by Gram-negative organisms. However, in the extremes of age or in debilitated patients, hypothermia can be present, and positive findings may be limited to unexplained hypotension, mental confusion, and hyperventilation.

In contrast to the classic progression of shock, most non-survivors of septic shock die despite a normal or elevated CO. Death within the first week after the onset of sepsis occurs as a result of intractable arterial hypotension that is secondary to a significantly depressed SVR. This causes extensive maldistribution of blood flow in the microvasculature, with subsequent tissue hypoxia and the development of lactic acidosis. Death occurring beyond the first week usually is caused by multiple organ failure that began during the acute circulatory failure. Severe, unresponsive hypotension as a result of a decreased CO does occur in a subpopulation of septic shock patients. In other words, cardiogenic shock becomes superimposed on the distributive shock of sepsis, but this is not the most common cause of death.[23]

HYPOVOLEMIC SHOCK

Acute Hemorrhagic Shock

1. B.A. is a 30-year-old man brought to the emergency department (ED) after being stabbed in the abdomen; he had significant blood loss at the scene. On arrival, he is confused and oriented only to person. His skin is pale and cool, with vital signs showing a HR of 125 beats/min, SBP of 85 mm Hg, and a RR of 30 breaths/min. Describe the physiologic changes in B.A. in response to his injury. What are the goals of resuscitation in patients with hemorrhagic shock?

B.A. has lost a significant amount of intravascular fluid directly from his stab wound and also from traumatic tissue edema. He is hypotensive with a compensatory increase in both HR and RR. His pale, cool skin indicates shunting of blood from the periphery to maintain perfusion of vital organs. Based on his clinical presentation, B.A. is in decompensated shock.

The major hemodynamic abnormality in hypovolemic shock is decreased venous return (preload) to the heart, resulting in a decrease in CO. Oxygen delivery to the tissues is reduced from this and from the loss of oxygen-carrying hemoglobin. The physiologic response of the body to a sudden decrease in volume (preload) is a release of catecholamines (epinephrine, norepinephrine). The subsequent increase in

HR and contractility help maintain CO. The peripheral vasoconstriction caused by the sympathomimetic response serves to maintain arterial pressure. In addition, fluid shifts from the interstitial spaces into the vasculature to increase preload. These responses are effective at maintaining BP in patients with a loss of up to approximately 30% of the total blood volume. B.A.'s increased HR and signs of peripheral vasoconstriction are consistent with these compensatory changes. Unfortunately, his SBP is still low and he has signs of decreased perfusion to his brain, manifested by confusion and disorientation. Given the severity of his condition, if intravascular losses are not rapidly replaced, myocardial dysfunction may ensue and lead to irreversible shock.

The goal of resuscitation of hypovolemic shock is the correction of inadequate tissue perfusion and oxygenation. HR, BP, and urine output have been traditional markers for the adequacy of resuscitation, but reliance on these end points alone is acceptable only in the initial management of hemorrhagic shock. New evidence suggests that patients may persist in a state of compensated shock even after these parameters are normalized.[24,25] Ongoing deficiencies in oxygen delivery to vital organs may progress and, if left untreated, organ dysfunction and death may result. Measurement of base (bicarbonate) deficit and lactate levels can be used to assess the global adequacy of perfusion. Metabolic acidosis can signal that resuscitation is incomplete despite normal vital signs.

Treatment
CHOICE OF FLUID IN HYPOVOLEMIC SHOCK

2. Is an intravenous saline solution adequate to compensate for BA's blood loss? What other type of fluid might be better to resuscitate this patient?

Once an adequate airway is established and initial vital signs are obtained, the most important therapeutic intervention in hypovolemic shock is the rapid infusion of IV fluids. Initially, crystalloids or colloids are used to restore blood volume as blood products may not be immediately available and are frequently unnecessary to manage mild shock (10% to 20% blood loss).[14]

CRYSTALLOIDS VERSUS COLLOIDS

Crystalloids are isotonic solutions that contain either saline (0.9% sodium chloride; "normal saline") or a saline equivalent [lactated Ringer's solution (LR)]. *Colloidal solutions* contain large oncotically active molecules that are derived from natural products such as proteins (albumin), carbohydrates (dextrans, starches), and animal collagen (gelatin) (Table 22-6).

Table 22-6 Composition and Properties of Crystalloids

Solution	Sodium (mEq/L)	Chloride (mEq/L)	Potassium (mEq/L)	Calcium (mEq/L)	Magnesium (mEq/L)	Lactate (mEq/L)	Tonicity Relative to Plasma	Osmolarity (mosm/l)
5% Dextrose	0	0	0	0	0	0	Isotonic	253
0.9% Sodium Chloride	154	154	0	0	0	0	Isotonic	308
Plasma-Lyte (Baxter)	140	103	10	5	3	8	Isotonic	312
Lactated Ringer's	130	109	4	3	0	28	Isotonic	273
7.5% Sodium Chloride	1283	1283	0	0	0	0	Hypertonic	2567

The choice of a crystalloid versus a colloid solution for the restoration of blood volume in hemorrhagic shock is controversial. The controversy primarily involves the ultimate distribution of these fluids in the extracellular compartment, which, in turn, depends on their composition. Isotonic solutions (normal saline or Ringer's solution) freely distribute within the extracellular fluid compartment, which is divided between the interstitial and intravascular spaces at a ratio of 3:1. This distribution is determined by the net forces of colloid oncotic pressure (COP) and hydrostatic pressure both inside and outside the capillary vascular space. Consequently, large volumes of crystalloid fluid are required to expand the intravascular space during resuscitation. In contrast, intact capillary membranes are relatively impermeable to colloids and, therefore, colloids effectively expand the intravascular space with little loss into the interstitium. Comparatively smaller volumes of colloids than crystalloids are thus required for resuscitation, and because these large molecules persist intravascularly, their duration of action is longer. Many of the colloidal agents, however, can cause allergic/hypersensitivity reactions as well as coagulopathic effects and colloids are much more expensive compared to crystalloids.

The proponents of crystalloids argue that in hypovolemic shock both intravascular and interstitial fluids are depleted because of the rapid shifts between the extracellular compartment. Replacement of both fluid spaces is best accomplished by using crystalloids. In addition, loss of capillary integrity in shock can cause the leak of larger molecules such as the colloidal proteins into the interstitium. The increase in the oncotic pressure in the interstitium favors fluid retention, with resultant edema.

Proponents of colloids contend that resuscitation with these solutions more rapidly and effectively restores intravascular volume following acute hemorrhage. For a given infusion volume, colloidal solutions such as albumin will expand the intravascular space two to four times more than crystalloids. Because a larger volume of crystalloid would have to be infused to restore the vascular space, the risk of developing pulmonary edema may be higher. It is also argued that large volumes of crystalloids will further dilute the plasma proteins, resulting in a decrease in the COP, which can also promote the development of pulmonary edema. This concept is based on Starling's law of capillary forces governing fluid movement, which in the pulmonary vessel wall is determined by the COP-PCWP gradient (i.e., the net force generated by the colloid oncotic pressure minus the pulmonary hydrostatic pressure [PCWP]). The normal colloid oncotic pressure is 25 mm Hg and an average PCWP is 12 mm Hg; thus, a net intravascular force of 13 mm Hg favors fluid retention in the vascular space. In critically ill patients, a COP-PCWP gradient <6 mm Hg is thought to be associated with a higher incidence of pulmonary edema.

Despite these theoretic differences, clinical studies comparing colloids with crystalloids have failed to show any differences in the development of pulmonary edema. Research suggests that certain subgroups may be at greater risk for the development of pulmonary edema, but considerable variance remains because of differences in physiologic end points, criteria for assessing pulmonary edema, and the existence or degree of shock. In an effort to find a consensus among these divergent clinical trials, a meta-analysis was performed comparing mortality rates after resuscitation with either crystalloid or colloid solutions.[26] For patients resuscitated from trauma, the mortality rate was 12.3% lower in those receiving crystalloids. In contrast, patients receiving colloids for nontraumatic shock had a 7.8% survival advantage. This finding was supported by a second meta-analysis which showed a trend toward better survival in trauma patients resuscitated with crystalloid.[27] It was concluded that the administration of crystalloids may be more efficacious than colloids in the resuscitation of shock resulting from trauma. The explanation offered for the ineffectiveness of colloids in trauma patients was that trauma causes an increase in pulmonary capillary permeability resulting in extravasation of these fluids into the lung interstitium.

In a similar analysis of randomized controlled trials involving patients with varying degrees of hypovolemia, no correlation was found between overall mortality and the type of fluid used.[28] To control for underlying pathologic conditions, patients were subdivided into three groups for further analysis: (1) surgical stress, (2) hypovolemia, and (3) severe pulmonary edema. To address the influence of increased capillary permeability on outcome, group 2 (hypovolemia) was subcategorized into those patients without sepsis or pulmonary failure (group 2.1) and those with serious hypovolemic shock with complications such as sepsis or pulmonary failure (group 2.2). When mortality rates were again compared within subgroups, differences between those patients receiving crystalloids versus those given colloids were not significant, although the sample sizes within these groups were relatively small. Patients administered colloids had a trend toward higher mortality rates as compared with those given crystalloids in all groups, with the exception of the surgical stress group in which mortality was 50% lower with colloids. A secondary cost-effectiveness analysis revealed that the cost of using crystalloid was $43.13 per life saved, as opposed to $1,493.60 per life saved with colloid. These estimates were based on an average per-patient intake of 6.57 L of fluid for the crystalloid group, at a cost of $5.95/L, and an average of 230 g of albumin in the colloid group, at a cost of $5.00/g.

Most recently, a meta-analysis of trials comparing crystalloids and colloids in critically ill patients found that the use of colloids for resuscitation was associated with a 24% mortality rate, compared with 20% in the patients receiving crystalloids.[29] This difference was not statistically significant. In contrast to the analysis by Velanovich,[26] they found no difference between trauma and nontrauma resuscitation. A meta-analysis of 30 studies with 1,419 patients showed that administration of albumin was associated with an increased risk of death and from this review, it is recommended that the use of albumin be strictly reviewed and curtailed.[30] In response to this the meta-analysis, Wilkes and colleagues conducted another review and found that use of albumin was associated with a relative risk for death of 1.1 (95% confidence interval [CI], 0.95 to 1.28).[31] They also found that the trials with higher methodologic quality were associated with relative risks less than 1.0 and, therefore, deemed albumin as being safe and effective. It is important to state that there are several limitations to these meta-analyses due to the differences in study inclusion criteria (heterogeneity), differences in fluid management, and dosages of albumin used.

Given the lack of evidence for a significant clinical difference between crystalloids and colloids and the greater expense of using albumin, guidelines for the use of resuscitation fluids were developed by the University Hospital Consortium (UHC), a nonprofit alliance of U.S. academic medical centers.[32] For the resuscitation of hemorrhagic shock, crystalloids should be the initial fluid of choice. The American College of Surgeons Advanced Trauma Life Support course[14] also recommends the rapid infusion of isotonic crystalloids for the initial fluid resuscitation of trauma patients. Thus, use of either normal saline or LR solution would be appropriate for B.A. Albumin and blood are not needed.

TIMING OF FLUID RESUSCITATION

3. When should crystalloid infusion be started in B.A.?

Current management of hypotensive trauma patients with hypovolemia follows the guidelines outlined in the American College of Surgeons Advanced Trauma Life Support course.[14] Based on these guidelines, fluid replacement should begin immediately. Recently, however, the convention of initiating fluid resuscitation before surgical correction of the hemorrhage has been challenged on the basis that aggressive administration of fluids may increase bleeding and reduce survival.[33] Postulated mechanisms for accentuated or secondary hemorrhage when fluids are given before surgical control of bleeding are hydraulic disruption of an effective thrombus, dilution of coagulation factors, and decreased blood viscosity with subsequent reduced resistance to flow around an incomplete thrombus.

One prospective, controlled trial in an urban trauma care setting compared immediate versus delayed fluid resuscitation in 598 hypotensive adults with penetrating torso injuries caused by gunshot or stab wounds.[33] The rate of survival was significantly higher in patients who did not receive fluid resuscitation until the time of operation compared with those who received traditional resuscitation before surgery (70% versus 62%). A trend toward increased intraoperative blood loss and postoperative complications in the immediate-resuscitation group was also evident. Clinical findings of increased BP, prolonged clotting times, and relative hemodilution in the immediate-resuscitation group were consistent with the proposed mechanisms for increased blood loss in this population. Although the results of this trial challenge the volume, timing, and extent of fluid resuscitation for patients with penetrating torso injuries, further controlled trials examining additional patient variables are required before this practice is adopted.[33,34] In addition, these results cannot be extrapolated to other trauma injuries or to a rural trauma care setting, in which the amount of time elapsed from the trauma scene to the operating room would be too extensive to warrant delayed resuscitation. Therefore, B.A. should be treated immediately.

CRYSTALLOIDS

4. A large-bore IV catheter is inserted into B.A.'s arm and STAT blood samples are sent for type and crossmatch, complete blood count (CBC), PT, partial thromboplastin time (PTT), and serum chemistry (BUN, creatinine, Na, K, Cl, and bicarbonate). Two liters of warmed LR solution are infused rapidly, and the operating room is notified. B.A.'s systolic BP has increased to 90 mm Hg, but the bleeding has not stopped. A Foley catheter is inserted to measure urine output. LR is continued, with 250- to 500-mL boluses ordered to be given every 10 minutes to maintain hemodynamic stability while waiting for fully crossmatched blood. How are crystalloids used in the setting of hemorrhagic shock? What clinical and objective parameters should be monitored to determine the success of fluid replacement?

Volume Requirements

Isotonic crystalloids equilibrate rapidly between the interstitial and intravascular spaces at a ratio of 3:1. For every liter of fluid infused, approximately 750 mL will pass into the interstitium, while 250 mL will remain in the plasma. Based on estimated blood loss, the "three-to-one rule" may be applied as a general guideline: for each 1 mL of blood loss, 3 mL of crystalloid is infused. Because this determination of blood loss is based solely on clinical assessment and not on quantitative measurements, treatment is best directed by the response to initial therapy rather than the initial classification. Close observation of hemodynamic status with consideration of the patient's age, particular injury, and prehospital fluid therapy is essential to avoid inadequate or excessive fluid administration and the development of pulmonary edema.

A safe and effective approach for using crystalloids in the resuscitation of patients in hemorrhagic shock is to give 1 to 2 liters of fluid as an initial bolus as rapidly as possible for an adult or 20 mL/kg for a pediatric patient.[14] Additional fluid boluses of 250 to 500 mL every 10 to 15 minutes may be necessary depending on the patient's response. Between boluses, fluids are slowed to maintenance rates (150 to 200 mL/hr), with ongoing evaluation of the patient's physiologic response for signs of continued blood loss or inadequate perfusion that would indicate the need for additional volume replacement.

Indications that circulation is improving include normalization of BP, pulse pressure, and HR. Signs that actual organ perfusion is normalizing and that fluid resuscitation is adequate include improvements in mental status, warmth and color of skin, improved acid-base balance, and increased urinary output. A urine output of approximately 50 mL/hr in an adult is a fairly reliable indicator of adequate volume replacement. Persistent metabolic acidosis in a normothermic shock patient usually indicates the need for additional fluid resuscitation; sodium bicarbonate is not recommended unless the pH is <7.2.[14]

LACTATED RINGER'S VERSUS NORMAL SALINE

5. Is there an advantage to using LR solution over normal saline?

The American College of Surgeons Committee on Trauma recommends lactated Ringer's solution as the fluid of choice for the initial resuscitation of trauma patients and normal saline as the second choice.[14] Because normal saline has a high chloride content (45 mEq more than LR), it can cause hyperchloremic acidosis, thereby worsening the tissue acidosis that occurs in the setting of hypovolemic shock. This likelihood is increased with impaired renal function. LR, in contrast, is a buffered solution designed to simulate the intravascular plasma electrolyte concentration. It contains

28 mEq/L of lactate, which is metabolized to bicarbonate in patients with normal circulation and intact liver function.[35] In situations in which hepatic perfusion is reduced (20% of normal) or hepatocellular damage is present, lactate clearance may be significantly decreased, particularly in combination with hypoxia (O_2 saturation 50% of normal).[36] In patients with shock and those undergoing cardiopulmonary bypass during surgery, the half-life of lactate, normally 20 minutes, increases to 4 to 6 hours and 8 hours, respectively.[37] Because unmetabolized lactate can be converted to lactic acid, prolonged infusion of Ringer's lactate could cause tissue acidosis in predisposed patients. In actuality, however, no differences in serum pH, electrolytes, lactate, or survival have been found in patients with hemorrhagic trauma who have received either LR or normal saline. In practice, normal saline and Ringer's lactate typically are used interchangeably because neither solution appears to be superior to the other.

HYPERTONIC SALINE

6. What is the role of hypertonic saline (HS) in the setting of hemorrhagic shock?

The use of HS (with and without dextran) for resuscitation in hemorrhagic shock has been studied extensively in animal models,[38–40] and more recently has been the focus of clinical research.[41–43] The advantage of HS as a resuscitative fluid is the smaller volume of fluid required to expand the intravascular compartment as compared with isotonic solutions. This could be a particular advantage in the prehospital setting (e.g., field rescue by emergency medical technicians) given the large volumes of fluids necessary to keep up with ongoing blood loss.

With a high concentration of sodium, HS exerts an osmotic effect, translocating fluid from the interstitial and cellular compartments to the intravascular space. Consequently, plasma volume is rapidly expanded to a greater extent than similar volumes of crystalloid solutions, and systemic BP, CO, and oxygen transport are readily increased. HS also improves myocardial contractility, causes peripheral vasodilation, and redistributes blood flow preferentially to the splanchnic and renal circulation. In addition, intracranial pressure is reduced, which may be a potential advantage in trauma patients with concomitant head injury.[38–43]

Hypertonic saline-dextran (7.5% sodium chloride in 6% dextran 70 [HSD]) was compared to isotonic crystalloid solution for prehospital resuscitation in a multicenter trial of hypotensive trauma patients.[42] Patients were randomly assigned to receive 250 mL of either HSD or a standard isotonic solution, after which fluids were given as necessary to achieve stabilization. No differences in overall survival were noted; however, there was a significant survival advantage in the HSD group requiring surgery. Fewer complications occurred in the HSD group, including a lower incidence of ARDS, renal failure, and coagulopathy. Although serum sodium levels were significantly higher in the HSD group, there were no adverse clinical symptoms of hypernatremia.

In a similar trial, the effects of resuscitation with 250-mL volumes of HS (7.5%), HSD, or normal saline were compared in trauma patients admitted to the ED in hypovolemic shock.[43] Following the initial 250-mL bolus, normal saline and blood were given as needed until the systolic pressure was >100 mm Hg. Differences in overall mortality or complication rates in the three groups were not significant. In comparison to isotonic saline, however, the hypertonic solutions significantly improved MAP and significantly decreased the volume of fluid required to restore systolic pressure.

Recent studies with HS have suggested that it may help to reduce multiple organ system failure and infections following traumatic injury. The mechanism has yet to be fully elucidated, but in animal models, HS reduces neutrophil margination,[44] which may play a role in the development of lung injury and ARDS. In another study the use of HS resulted in a decreased susceptibility to sepsis and improved survival in a murine model of hemorrhagic shock.[45]

These clinical trials suggest that HS may be safe and effective for the initial resuscitation of hemorrhagic shock and may help prevent the development of posttraumatic multiple organ system failure and sepsis. Further study is needed, however, to establish a substantial benefit before these fluids are considered for widespread clinical use.

BLOOD REPLACEMENT

7. B.A. has received 3 L of LR solution to maintain hemodynamic stability. His current vital signs are BP, 92/60 mm Hg; HR, 115 breaths/min; and RR, 28 breaths/min. He is still confused and is becoming more agitated and combative. Urine output has been 10 mL in the past 30 minutes. Laboratory results include the following: hematocrit, 23% (normal, 40 to 54%); hemoglobin, 7.6 g/dL (normal, 14 to 18 g/dL); arterial blood gas (ABG) pH, 7.18 (normal, 7.35 to 7.45); Pco_2, 35 mm Hg (normal, 35 to 45 mm Hg); Po_2, 110 mm Hg (normal, 75 to 100 mm Hg); and HCO_3^-, 17 mEq/L (normal, 23 to 29 mEq/L). Two units of packed red blood cells (PRBCs) are now available, and B.A. is being prepared for the operating room. Describe the current status of B.A.'s resuscitation and the need for blood products. What adverse effects should be anticipated with transfusion?

[SI units: Hct, 0.23 (normal, 0.40 to 0.54); hemoglobin, 1.18 mmol/L (normal, 2.17 to 2.79 mmol/L); HCO_3^-, 17 mmol/L (normal, 23 to 29 mmol/L)]

B.A. is still exhibiting signs of inadequate tissue perfusion. Although his BP has improved and his HR has decreased, his mental status has declined, urine output has been negligible, and his blood gas indicates a metabolic acidosis. B.A. has not been adequately resuscitated from his hemorrhage and should receive the available blood at this point.

The conventional approach to the transfusion of critically ill patients has been to maintain the hemoglobin above 10 g/dL or the hematocrit above 30%. Not only is this commonly used "transfusion trigger" misleading (because in acute hemorrhage the actual degree of blood loss is not accurately reflected by these values), but it also does not take into account the body's ability to compensate for the loss of oxygen-carrying capacity. Because it takes at least 24 hours for all fluid compartments to come to equilibrium, a normal hematocrit (or Hgb concentration) in the setting of hemorrhagic shock does not rule out significant blood loss or indicate adequacy of transfusion. Only when equilibrium has been reached can these measures be used reliably to gauge blood loss. On the other hand, if cardiopulmonary function is normal and if volume status is maintained, an increase in CO can compensate for a reduction in hemoglobin (O_2 content) to a certain degree (see Fig. 22-1).

Because inadequacy of tissue perfusion, and hence oxygen delivery, is the primary abnormality in shock, the need for transfusion therapy is more accurately determined by the patient's oxygen demand, rather than an arbitrary hematocrit or hemoglobin value. Calculation of Do_2 and Vo_2 can be used to determine the adequacy of perfusion. Although these values can be determined by use of a pulmonary artery catheter and arterial and venous blood samples, for practical purposes, the patient's response to initial fluid resuscitation and clinical signs of inadequate tissue perfusion are the primary determinants for blood transfusion. Patients who do not respond to initial volume resuscitation or who transiently respond but remain tachycardic, tachypneic, and oliguric, clearly are underperfused and will likely require blood transfusion.

ADVERSE EFFECTS OF TRANSFUSION

8. **After the transfusion, B.A. has a serum potassium concentration of 4.8 mEq/L (normal, 3.7 to 5.2 mEq/L) compared with 4.5 mEq/L before the transfusion. Could this be a result of the blood product? Is B.A. also at risk for contracting HIV or viral hepatitis from his transfusion of PRBCs? Would whole blood be a better choice than packed cells?**

Possible risks of blood transfusions include electrolyte abnormalities, hemolytic reactions, transmission of infectious disease, coagulopathies, and immunosuppression. Banked blood is stored with citrate anticoagulant additive. With multiple transfusions, the large amount of citrate can cause hypocalcemia and acid-base abnormalities. Hyperkalemia also can occur because transfusion of stored blood causes the release of potassium from red blood cells (RBCs). Hemolytic transfusion reactions are the most common cause of acute fatalities from blood transfusions. Astute recognition of the signs and symptoms of a transfusion reaction such as anxiety, pain at infusion site, fever, hypotension, tachycardia, hemolysis, and hemoglobinuria can prevent unnecessary morbidity and mortality. Transfusions may also cause acute lung injury due to recipient neutrophil priming by reactive lipid products from the red blood cell membrane which causes capillary endothelial damage in the lungs. The increase in serum potassium observed in B.A. may be from the blood product or it may simply reflect hemolysis of blood cells in the test tube after the blood draw. In either case, the measured serum concentration of 4.8 mEq/L in not high enough to be of concern. It is unlikely that a true hemolytic reaction is occurring.

Blood products and donors are screened for disease, thus transmission of viral illness is a small risk. It is estimated that the transmission of hepatitis B is one case for every 63,000 units transfused, hepatitis C is 1:103,000, and HIV is 1:676,000.[46]

Hemostatic abnormalities, specifically coagulopathies and thrombocytopenia, may be transiently related to dilution from administration of large volumes of crystalloids, colloids, or banked blood, but are more likely caused by the extent of injury and the development of disseminated intravascular coagulopathy. Banked whole blood contains sufficient coagulation factors (including labile factors V and VIII) to maintain hemostasis during the life span of the unit; however, it does not contain platelets because they do not survive the temperatures required for RBC storage.

Immunosuppression has also been associated with blood transfusions as evidenced by enhanced graft survival in renal transplant recipients, tumor recurrence in colorectal carcinoma patients, and in postoperative infections. The immunosuppression from transfusion is multifactorial, but it is most likely due to the infusion of donor white cells which create a competition between the donor and recipient leukocytes. This mechanism is not, however, the only cause because immunosuppression is associated with autologous blood transfusions as well as the infusion of plasma alone.

Whole blood offers no significant advantage over packed red cells as long as other less expensive fluids (crystalloids) are used for volume expansion. After extracting the red cells to provide oxygen carrying capacity, other blood elements (e.g., fresh frozen plasma and platelets, clotting factors) can be used for other patients with specialty needs. Thus, packed RBCs are an appropriate blood replacement product for B.A. His PT, PTT, platelets, electrolytes, and mixed venous blood gases, if available should be monitored frequently. These tests enable correction of any coagulopathy or electrolyte abnormality and assist in the assessment of the adequacy of tissue oxygenation. This information, in addition to the aforementioned factors, can be used to gauge his response to therapy and his need for supplemental blood products such as platelets and frozen fresh plasma.

Due to the limited supply and potential adverse effects associated with blood, research is under way to develop blood substitutes. The ideal agent would have a longer shelf life, a reduced risk of disease transmission, and less risks of transfusion reactions. The agents in various stages of clinical research include the modified hemoglobins and the perfluorocarbons. The exact role the blood substitutes would play in transfusions is unclear, and there have been problems such as short half-life and vasoconstriction associated with some of the products thus far. There are no agents approved as of yet, but research is continuing.

Postoperative Hypovolemia

Hypovolemia Versus Pump Failure

9. **J.S., a 62-year-old man, has been admitted to the ICU following surgical repair of an abdominal aortic aneurysm. He is intubated and receiving 60% oxygen. He weighs 78 kg and has a BSA of 1.8 m². He has a history of hypertension (BP, 140/100 mm Hg) for which he takes nadolol (Corgard) and hydrochlorothiazide. His ABGs are adequate and he is receiving 150 mL/hr of LR solution intravenously. His 2-hour postoperative and initial (in parentheses) hemodynamic profiles are as follows: BP (S/D/M), 90/50/63 mm Hg (130/78/95); pulse, 88 beats/min (80); CO, 3 L/min (5); RAP, 3 mm Hg (6); PCWP, 8 mm Hg (12); SVR, 1,200 dyne · sec · cm⁻⁵ (1,392); urine output, 25 mL/hr (70); temperature, 37°C (34); Hct, 32% (30). Based on the hemodynamic profile, determine whether J.S. is hypovolemic or experiencing pump failure following his surgery.**

[SI unit: Hct, 0.32 (normal, 0.40 to 0.54)]

Most of J.S.'s hemodynamic changes are consistent with hypovolemia. These include a drop in BP, CO, PCWP, and urine output. The decrease in PCWP suggests that preload is reduced, resulting in a lower CO. Urine output has declined and probably reflects a compensatory drop in renal perfusion to preserve intravascular volume. The pulse pressure is narrowed suggesting blood flow has decreased. (Changes in pulse pressure correlate with changes in SV in individual patients; that is, as pulse pressure narrows, SV decreases.) The lack of a significant increase in HR as well as a decrease in SVR is not consistent with hypovolemia. However, nadolol, a long-acting β-blocker, may have prevented a reflex increase in HR, and an increase in body temperature may account for the decrease in SVR. As the body temperature rises postoperatively, vasodilation decreases SVR and increases the intravascular space. If intravascular volume is inadequate and increased sympathetic tone cannot generate a sufficient CO, mean BP falls. The most likely explanation for the hemodynamic change in J.S. is hypovolemia, although he also should be evaluated for the occurrence of a perioperative cardiac event. Arterial blood gases should be checked to assess oxygen requirements.

Causes

10. **What are the most likely causes of hypovolemia in J.S.?**

Common causes of hypovolemia in surgical patients are postoperative bleeding, third spacing, and temperature-related vasodilation. Postoperative bleeding can produce hypovolemia; however, J.S.'s initial and 2-hour postoperative hematocrit of 30% and 32%, respectively, do not support bleeding as a cause.

Following major vascular or bowel surgery, it is not unusual for patients to "third space" significant amounts of intravascular volume. The bowel walls and interstitial space can sequester large amounts of fluids, and this can produce a state of relative hypovolemia as is occurring with J.S. This is especially apparent for the first 12 to 24 hours after the surgical procedure. J.S. is receiving 150 mL/hr of LR solution, but this is apparently not enough to maintain his intravascular volume.

Mild hypothermia is common during operative procedures. As patients warm up postoperatively, vasodilation occurs, expanding the intravascular space. If the amounts of IV fluids administered are insufficient to compensate for the increased venous capacitance, BP and CO will decline during the rewarming phase, which can range from 1 to 6 hours. J.S. has rewarmed from 34 to 37°C in 2 hours, which is not unusual after a major operative procedure. His temperature could conceivably rise as high as 38 to 38.5°C during the first 12 to 24 hours after surgery.

Other considerations include inadequate fluid administration during the operative procedure and the effects of drugs given in the operating room or in the immediate postoperative period (e.g., morphine sulfate and other narcotics) that have systemic vasodilatory properties.

Volume Replacement and Ventricular Function

11. **How will volume replacement improve J.S.'s CO and perfusion pressure?**

Starling's mechanism indicates that the volume of blood returned to the heart is the main determinant of volume pumped by the heart. Therefore, as venous return is increased, the CO also will increase within physiologic limits (see Fig. 22-1). The PCWP, which approximates left ventricular end-diastolic volume, can be used to assess venous return or preload to the left ventricle.

A ventricular function curve can be constructed by plotting a measure of cardiac pumping action (CO, SV, or LVWSI)

against a measure of preload (PCWP). A change in preload moves the ventricular output upward or downward along a given curve (see Fig. 22-4). Two hours after surgery, J.S.'s PCWP has fallen from 17 to 8 mm Hg and his CO has fallen from 5 to 3 L/min. Therefore, additional volume replacement is warranted.

12. **J.S. is given a 500-mL bolus of NS over 10 minutes and this results in the following hemodynamic profile: BP (S/D/M), 96/60/71 mm Hg; pulse, 84 beats/min; CO, 3.5 L/min; RAP, 4 mm Hg; PCWP, 10 mm Hg; SVR, 1,276 dyne · sec · cm⁻⁵. Assess J.S.'s response to the fluid challenge (see Table 22-2 for normal values).**

According to the Starling curve, a small change in PCWP in response to a volume challenge with a minimal change in CO, represents a ventricle on the flat portion of the ventricular function curve (see Fig. 22-4). Additional fluid therapy given to these patients may increase their risk for pulmonary edema without improving CO. In contrast, a large change in PCWP in response to a fluid challenge with a significant increase in CO represents a ventricle on the steep portion of the curve. In J.S., the change in PCWP from 8 to 10 mm Hg and the increase in CO show that he is still responsive to fluid; thus, it is reasonable to administer more fluid to enhance CO and renal perfusion.

Fluid Challenge

13. **One hour after the 500-mL NS bolus, J.S.'s hemodynamic profile returns to his postoperative state. ABGs are acceptable and LR solution is infusing at 200 mL/hr. J.S. is continuing to "third-space" intravascular volume. Based on this information, develop guidelines for additional fluid challenges in J.S.**

Acceptable guidelines for administering additional fluid challenges to hypovolemic patients are based on the direction and degree of changes in the various hemodynamic parameters in response to a fluid load rather than their absolute values. These include the right atrial pressure, PCWP, CO, and BP. Using the PCWP as a guide, an increase in the PCWP of 5 mm Hg after a 250- to 500-mL fluid challenge over 10 minutes implies the left ventricle is still functioning on the steep portion of the volume-pressure curve. If the PCWP rises abruptly as fluid is given, with a small change in CO, the flat portion of the ventricular function curve has been reached and the IV infusion rate should be slowed. If signs and symptoms of inadequate tissue perfusion fail to improve or worsen and if the PCWP remains >18 to 20 mm Hg, fluid challenges should be stopped and inotropic therapy initiated. J.S. is on the lower end of the curve and needs additional normal saline fluid boluses over 10 minutes every 10 to 15 minutes until the CO and PCWP are sufficient to maintain an acceptable BP and urine output (0.5 mL/kg per hour).

Generally, most critically ill patients require a CI >2.5 L/min per square meter and a PCWP of 8 to 18 mm Hg to maintain acceptable MAPs of 65 to 75 mm Hg. Ordinarily, it would be reasonable to maintain a MAP higher than 75 mm Hg. However, this is not advisable in J.S.'s case because he has a history of high BP; it is important to avoid increased arterial pressures that may jeopardize aneurysm repair.

14. **J.S. has received a total of 3.5 L normal saline in boluses over the past 6 hours and remains hemodynamically unchanged.**

His urine output has averaged 25 mL/hr for the past 4 hours, indicating volume replacement is inadequate. Given his age and the lack of response to initial crystalloid administration, the decision is made to infuse 500 mL of 6% hetastarch over the next 30 minutes. How does hetastarch compare to human serum albumin as a volume expander for J.S.?

Albumin and Hetastarch

Albumin is the predominant protein in the plasma and accounts for approximately 80% of the colloid oncotic pressure,[47] the force that maintains fluid in the intravascular space. Human serum albumin is the colloidal agent against which all others are compared for volume-expanding properties. It is prepared commercially from pooled donor plasma that is heat-treated to eliminate the potential for disease transmission. On infusion, 5% albumin increases plasma volume by approximately half the volume infused, or 18 mL/g, with an initial duration of action of 16 hours.[47] Substantial side effects primarily involve transient clotting abnormalities and anaphylactic reactions (0.5%), both of which are rare.[39] The anaphylactoid reaction is due to the pasteurization process which causes albumin to polymerize which produces an antigenic macromolecule. Albumin solutions also contain citrate, which can lower serum calcium concentrations, and which in turn could theoretically lead to decreased left ventricular function.[35] It is now generally believed that the effects on coagulation and serum calcium are related to the volume of fluid infused rather than albumin administration.[47] Albumin is available as a 5% solution that is isotonic with the plasma and a 25% solution that is hypertonic. The 5% solution is generally preferred for routine volume expansion, whereas the 25% solution is most useful in correcting hypoproteinemia or intravascular hypovolemia in patients with excess interstitial water.

Hetastarch or hydroxyethyl starch (HES) is a synthetic colloid made from amylopectin, which closely resembles human serum albumin, but is considerably less expensive. Available as a 6% solution in normal saline, HES expands the plasma volume by an amount greater than the volume infused because the high oncotic pressure draws water from the interstitial spaces. HES solutions are composed of a wide range of molecular weights which explains its complex pharmacokinetics. It has an average molecular weight of 69,000 units with a range of 10,000 units to greater than 1 million units. Smaller molecular weights are excreted more quickly in the urine, whereas larger particles remain in the circulation longer and are slowly taken up by tissues or the reticuloendothelial system. The clinical effects of HES last up to 24 hours. Hetastarch generally is well tolerated with a low incidence of side effects and allergic reactions. Dose-related reductions in platelet count and transient increases in PT and PTT have been reported with moderate infusions of HES (<1,500 mL per day) and are significant with larger volumes.[48] HES causes factor VIII levels to be lowered beyond that which can be attributed to hemodilution and also increases fibrinolysis. This places patients with von Willebrand's disease at greater risk of bleeding. There have not been any direct accounts of HES causing bleeding, but it is recommended that a maximum of 20 mL/kg/day (or 1,500 mL) be used to prevent alterations in coagulation parameters. Most patients respond to 500 to 1,000 mL so this limit does not usually impede treatment. HES can also cause elevation in serum amylase levels up to 3 times the normal level. This is because hetastarch binds to amylase and thus delays its excretion. HES does not actually interfere with pancreatic function.

Numerous clinical studies have compared albumin and hetastarch for fluid resuscitation in patients with and without shock. One study reported that HES was as effective as albumin in restoring hemodynamic stability and improving oxygen delivery in patients who were given comparable amounts of either fluid over 24 hours.[49] Other studies in hypovolemic patients have reported no difference in hemodynamic parameters when similar volumes of either HES or albumin were given as serial boluses to maintain CO and ventricular filling pressures.[50,51] In postoperative cardiac surgery patients, HES and albumin were found to be equally efficacious in restoring volume status and maintaining hemodynamic stability.[52,53]

In summary, resuscitation with moderate volumes of hetastarch is safe and hemodynamically equivalent to albumin. Either 5% albumin or 6% HES would be acceptable for intravascular volume expansion in J.S.

CARDIOGENIC SHOCK

Postoperative Cardiac Failure

Assessment by Hemodynamic Profile

15. R.G., a 62-year-old man, has undergone four-vessel coronary artery bypass graft surgery and is now in the ICU. Vital signs are stable with a MAP of 90 mm Hg. His body weight is 74 kg and his BSA is 1.7 m². R.G. has a medical history of two MIs, 6 months and 5 years before admission; unstable angina; and hypertension. His medications include NTG, metoprolol (Lopressor), and hydrochlorothiazide. Past surgical history includes a three-vessel coronary artery bypass graft (CABG) 4 years before admission. One hour after admission to the ICU, R.G.'s BP has fallen. He has the following hemodynamic profile: BP (S/D/M), 90/50/63 mm Hg; pulse, 110 beats/min; CO, 2.8 L/min (normal, 4 to 7); CI, 1.65 L/min per square meter (normal, 2.5 to 4.2); RAP, 12 mm Hg (normal, 2 to 6); PA pressure, 35/20 (S/D); PCWP, 22 mm Hg (normal, 5 to 12); SVR, 1,457 dyne · sec · cm⁻⁵ (normal, 800 to 1,440); PaO₂, 110 mm Hg (normal, 80 to 104) (on 60% inspired oxygen); PaCO₂, 28 mm Hg (normal, 35 to 45); pH, 7.32 (normal, 7.35 to 7.45); HCO₃⁻, 20 mEq/L (normal, 23 to 29); RR 26 breaths/min; urine output, 25 mL/hr; temperature, 36°C; and Hct, 35% (normal, 40 to 54%) (stable). Chest tube output is stable at 40 to 50 mL/hr. IV fluid infusion is 50 mL/hr 0.9% NS. What is your assessment of R.G.'s hemodynamic profile and clinical situation?

[SI units: HCO₃⁻, 20 mmol/L (normal, 23 to 29 mmol/L); Hct, 0.35 (normal, 0.40 to 0.54)]

The likely causes of shock in cardiac surgery patients include hypovolemia from operative and postoperative bleeding; excessive vasodilation from medications during surgery or the effects of cardiopulmonary bypass on the inflammatory cascade; tamponade; MI; or more commonly, a "stunning" of the myocardium, which can take from hours to days to resolve. A careful analysis of R.G.'s hemodynamics can help differentiate these causes and guide further therapy.

When evaluating hemodynamics, the first step should be to determine if hypovolemia is present. R.G.'s rapid pulse, low urine output, and low MAP could indicate volume depletion.

However, the data obtained from R.G.'s PA catheter show an elevated PCWP, decreased CI, and a slightly elevated SVR. These suggest that his preload is adequate, and thus hypovolemia is unlikely to be the primary problem. The elevated SVR rules out a vasodilatory form of shock. Tamponade is unlikely in R.G. because his chest tube output has remained consistent and his RAP and PA pressures are not dramatically elevated. It appears that R.G. is experiencing shock due to acute heart failure. This could be caused by a MI or stunned myocardium. An ECG and serial blood samples for analysis of cardiac enzymes should be obtained to rule out a perioperative MI.

R.G. has a PaO_2 of 110 mm Hg, a $PaCO_2$ of 28 mm Hg, and a pH of 7.32 while breathing at 26 breaths/min. This indicates that R.G. has a metabolic acidosis with respiratory compensation. The metabolic acidosis is most likely caused by his poor systemic perfusion indicated by a low CI, hypotension, and decreased urine output. A PCWP >18 mm Hg is associated with pulmonary edema and a CI of <2.2 L/min per square meter is indicative of hypoperfusion. The chest radiograph and breath sounds should be evaluated for signs of pulmonary edema.

Therapeutic Interventions

16. **The chest radiograph confirms mild pulmonary edema, and fine rales were heard throughout the lower half of lung fields on auscultation. Tamponade is not evident on the radiograph. The ECG shows ST-T–wave changes, but there is no indication of an acute MI. Cardiac enzymes are pending. BP and CO need to be improved to increase perfusion to vital organs. Three therapeutic interventions are available: fluid challenge, vasodilators, and inotropic agents. How would these choices affect R.G.'s ventricular function?**

FLUID CHALLENGE (PRELOAD INCREASE)

Augmentation of preload with a fluid challenge to improve CO is the first option. However, R.G.'s PCWP is already 22 mm Hg and increasing this value above 18 to 20 mm Hg usually does not result in further benefit.[54] Furthermore, R.G. has signs of pulmonary edema on chest radiograph and his PaO_2 is 110 mm Hg on 60% inspired oxygen (FiO_2). Therefore, elevation of intravascular volume might increase the pulmonary vascular hydrostatic pressure and worsen his pulmonary edema. If a fluid challenge is attempted to enhance preload, no more than 100 mL of normal saline should be given without repeating the hemodynamic measurements. If the PCWP rises, but the CO does not improve, fluid challenges should be discontinued. Elevating the preload without appreciably improving CO also can increase LV wall tension, which is a major determinant of myocardial oxygen consumption; consequently, myocardial ischemia could develop. Although R.G. has signs of pulmonary edema, diuretics to reduce his volume overload can be detrimental to his cardiac output and should not be used until R.G.'s hemodynamics and signs of hypoperfusion have improved.

VASODILATORS (AFTERLOAD REDUCTION)

A peripheral vasodilator also could be used. This will decrease pulmonary venous congestion by reducing preload (PCWP), and thus pulmonary vascular hydrostatic pressure. It will improve CO by decreasing the resistance to ventricular ejection (afterload) as well. With myocardial ischemia, a reduction of the LV filling pressure may improve subendocardial blood flow, reduce the myocardial wall tension, and reduce the LV radius. The resultant decrease in myocardial oxygen consumption will help prevent further depression of cardiac function. In patients with LV failure, arterial resistance is elevated because of a reflex increase in sympathetic tone in response to a fall in systemic arterial pressure. In LV failure, CO becomes increasingly dependent on resistance to outflow from the left ventricle. Lowering the SVR will shift the ventricular function curve up and to the left, depending on whether an arterial, venous, or mixed vasodilator is used, thereby improving cardiac performance at a lower filling pressure (Fig. 22-5).

R.G. appears to have LV failure with elevations in PCWP and SVR. Vasodilator therapy in this setting will probably help increase R.G.'s CO and, therefore, increase the delivery of oxygen to the tissues and prevent organ dysfunction. However, the major risk of vasodilator therapy in R.G. is further reduction of an already low MAP. Although the reduction in BP may be offset by an increase in CO, a significant drop in arterial BP could occur, which could reduce coronary pressure and thereby exacerbate or produce myocardial ischemia in addition to decreasing perfusion to other vital organ systems. Vasodilator therapy should be reserved for situations in which hemodynamic monitoring shows the patient to have LV failure with elevations in PCWP, SVR, and a systolic BP >90 mm Hg.

INOTROPIC SUPPORT

A rapid-acting inotropic agent (e.g., dopamine, dobutamine) also can be used to increase myocardial contractility and CO. This intervention shifts the ventricular function curve upward and slightly to the left (see Fig. 22-5). The disadvantage of this intervention is that improved CO is accompanied by an increased myocardial oxygen demand. Depending on the agent selected, three of the determinants of myocardial oxygen consumption could be elevated: HR, contractility, and ventricular wall tension. Therefore, inotropic support is directed at establishing or maintaining a reasonable arterial

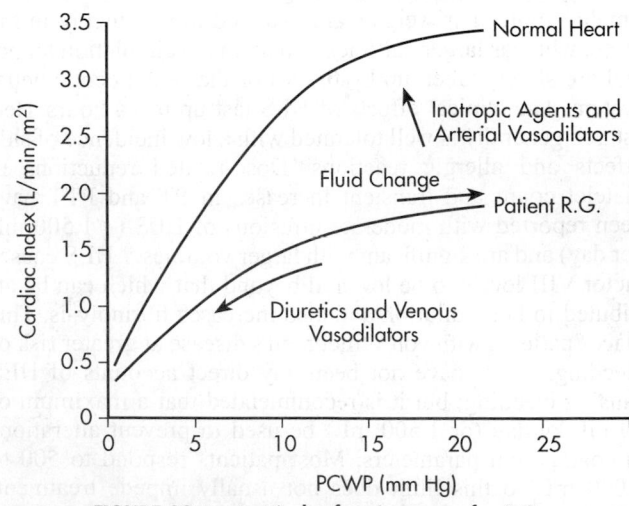

FIGURE 22-5 Ventricular function curve for R.G.

pressure and ensuring adequate tissue perfusion by improving the CO.

In summary, the most appropriate therapeutic intervention for R.G. at this time would be inotropic support. The PCWP is elevated suggesting that the preload has been maximized; therefore, fluid boluses may worsen R.G.'s pulmonary edema. Although R.G.'s SVR is slightly elevated (1,457 dyne · sec · cm^{-5}), his BP is low; therefore, initial use of a peripheral vasodilator may jeopardize perfusion. Thus, an acceptable initial therapeutic intervention to improve CO and tissue perfusion is inotropic support. After a reasonable BP has been established, addition of a peripheral vasodilator could be considered to further enhance CO if needed, and diuretics added to reduce his pulmonary edema.

Dopamine

17. Dopamine hydrochloride is prescribed for R.G. What hemodynamic changes would you anticipate?

Dopamine, a precursor of norepinephrine, has inotropic, chronotropic, and vasoactive properties, all of which are dose dependent (Table 22-7). At 0.5 to 2 μg/kg/min, dopamine stimulates dopaminergic receptors primarily in the splanchnic, renal, and coronary vascular beds, which may produce vasodilation, improved renal blood flow (controversial), and maintain natriuresis. The effect on dopaminergic receptors is not blocked by β-blockers, but is antagonized by dopaminergic-blocking agents such as the butyrophenones and phenothiazines. Depending on the clinical state of the patient, low

dosages of dopamine may slightly increase myocardial contractility, but usually will not alter HR or SVR significantly.

At 2 to 5 μg/kg/min, the improved cardiac performance produced by dopamine is through direct stimulation of β$_1$-adrenergic receptors and indirectly through release of norepinephrine from nerve terminals. Increased β$_1$-adrenergic receptor stimulation increases stroke volume (inotropic effect), HR (chronotropic effect), and consequently CO. These cardiac effects can be blocked by β-blockers.

At infusion rates of 5 to 10 μg/kg/min, the α-adrenergic receptors are activated. At this dosage, the vasoactive effects on peripheral blood vessels are unpredictable and depend on the net effect of β$_1$-adrenergic stimulation, α-adrenergic stimulation, and reflex mechanisms. MAP and PCWP usually will rise.

At doses >15 to 20 μg/kg/min, dopamine primarily stimulates peripheral α-adrenergic receptors. SVR increases, splanchnic and renal blood flow decreases, and LV filling pressure is raised. Cardiac irritability is not unusual and the overall myocardial oxygen consumption is increased. The increase in SVR limits CO; thus, infusion rates should be limited to <10 to 15 μg/kg/min in patients with cardiac failure.

18. Based on the hemodynamic dose effects described in the previous question, at what dose would you initiate a dopamine infusion in R.G.? What therapeutic outcomes are anticipated at this dose and over what time? What adverse effects may be encountered with this dose of dopamine?

R.G. has a MAP of 63 mm Hg, a CI of 1.65 L/min per square meter, a PCWP of 22 mm Hg, and an HR of 110

Table 22-7 Inotropic Agents and Vasopressors

Drug	Usual Dose	Receptor Sensitivity			Pharmacologic Effect			
		α	β$_1$	β$_2$	VD	VC	INT	CHT
Amrinone	0.75 mg/kg bolus, then 2.5–1.5 μg/kg/min	−−	−−	−−	+++	−−	++^{a}	−−
Dobutamine	2.5–15 μg/kg/min	+	+++	++	++	−−	+++^{a}	+
Dopamine	0.5–2 μg/kg/min^b (renal)	−−	−−	−−	−−^{b}	+	+	+
	2–5 μg/kg/min	−−	+	−−	−−^{b}	+	+	+
	5–10 μg/kg/min	+	++	−−	++	++	++	++
	15–20 μg/kg/min	+++	++	−−	−−^{b}	+++	++	++
Epinephrine^c	0.01–0.1 μg/kg/min	+	+++	++	+	−	+++	++
	0.1 μg/kg/min	+++	++	++	−−	+++	++	++
Isoproterenol	0.01–0.1 μg/kg/min	−−	++++	+++	+++	−−	+++	+++
Milrinone	50 μg/kg bolus, then 0.375–0.75 μg/kg/min	−−	−−	−−	+++	−−	++	−−
Norepinephrine	0.05–0.5 μg/kg/min Highly variable, titrate to desired MAP	++++	++	−−	−−	+++	+^{d}	+
Phenylephrine	0.5–5 μg/kg/min Highly variable, titrate to desired MAP	+++	−−	−−	−−	+++	−−	−−
Vasopressin^e	0.04 units/min^f	−−	−−	−−	−−	+++	−−	−−

^{a}Dobutamine, amrinone, and milrinone have more inotropic effect than dopamine.
^{b}Dopamine at 0.5–2 μg/kg/min stimulates dopaminergic receptors, causing vasodilation in the splanchnic and renal vasculature.
^{c}Epinephrine has predominant inotropic effects; norepinephrine has predominant vasoconstrictive effect. Epinephrine may vasodilate at low dosages, vasoconstrict at high dosages.
^{d}Cardiac output unchanged or may decline because of vagal reflex responses that slow the heart.
^{e}Vasopressin stimulates V$_1$ receptors to cause vasoconstriction in the periphery.
^{f}Dosing for sepsis; in other vasodilatory conditions, may be titrated from 0.01 to 0.1 units/min.
CHT, chronotropic; INT, inotropic; MAP, mean arterial pressure; SBP, systolic blood pressure; VC, peripheral vascular vasoconstriction; VD, peripheral vascular vasodilation.

beats/min. The goal of therapy is to increase the CI to at least 2.5 L/min per square meter, maintain a MAP of at least 70 mm Hg (preferably closer to 80 mm Hg, depending on clinical signs of hypoperfusion), reduce the PCWP, and maintain a HR <125 beats/min. A urine output of at least 0.5 mL/kg per hour (37 mL/hour in R.G.) is desirable. A reasonable initial infusion rate would be 3 μg/kg/min. This dose should increase cardiac contraction and CO resulting in an increase in renal blood flow. Because the onset of action is within minutes, the patient can be re-evaluated and the infusion rate can be titrated upwards by 1 to 2 μg/kg/min every 10 minutes depending on the hemodynamic data obtained. The hemodynamic response to dopamine is highly variable among patients; thus, careful titration to lowest effective infusion rate is advised.

Adverse effects encountered with dopamine infusion include increased HR, anginal pain, arrhythmias, headache, hypertension, vasoconstriction, nausea, and vomiting. Extravasation of large amounts of dopamine during infusion can cause ischemic necrosis and sloughing. At higher dosages, α_1-adrenergic effects are more prominent, causing peripheral arterial vasoconstriction and an increase in venous pressures that lead to increases in afterload, preload, and myocardial oxygen demand as well as ischemia.

EFFECT ON HEMODYNAMICS

19. **Dopamine is initiated at 3 μg/kg/min in R.G. and titrated to 8 μg/kg/min over the next 2 hours. A repeat chest radiograph shows slight worsening of pulmonary edema. The following hemodynamic profile is obtained (previous values are in parentheses): BP (S/D/M), 115/62/80 mm Hg (90/50/63); pulse, 140 beats/min (110); CO, 3.8 L/min (2.8); CI, 2.2 L/min per square meter (1.65); RAP, 10 mm Hg (12); PCWP, 20 mm Hg (22); SVR, 1,473 dyne · sec · cm^{-5} (1,457); urine output, 30 mL/hr (25); temperature, 37°C (36); and Hct, 36% (35). Do these data indicate a favorable or adverse hemodynamic effect from dopamine in R.G.?**

Dopamine at 8 μg/kg/min has established a trend in the desired direction for CI; however, the HR has increased significantly. The SVR and PCWP have not changed appreciably, and the urine flow has increased. Further analysis reveals that the stroke volume (CO/HR) has only increased from 25 mL/beat to 27 mL/beat; thus, the major increase in CO has resulted from the chronotropic rather than the inotropic effect of dopamine. As a net response, the dopamine has most likely affected the myocardial oxygen supply-demand ratio adversely; however, this cannot be established definitively. R.G. should be monitored closely for signs of myocardial ischemia.

Dobutamine

20. **The clinician decides that a HR of 140 beats/min is unacceptable in R.G., who has a history of MI. Subsequent attempts to taper the dopamine to lessen the induced tachycardia without dropping the CI and perfusion pressure are unsuccessful. Dobutamine is suggested as an alternative to dopamine. What hemodynamic changes would you expect with dobutamine in R.G.? Does dobutamine offer any advantages over dopamine?**

Dobutamine, a synthetic catecholamine, is a potent positive inotropic agent with predominant direct β_1-agonist effects and weak β_2- and α_1-effects. With greater β_2-vasodilatory than α_1-vasoconstrictive actions, dobutamine produces substantial reductions in systemic and pulmonary vascular resistances. The reduction in SVR also may be caused by a reflex decrease in vasoconstriction secondary to enhanced CO. Phenoxybenzamine blocks the α-adrenergic response and propranolol blocks the β_2-response. Unlike dopamine, dobutamine does not release endogenous norepinephrine or stimulate renal dopaminergic receptors.[55–58]

Results of studies assessing dobutamine in cardiac failure demonstrate consistent increases in CO and stroke volume, with reductions in PCWP and SVR. The reduction in filling pressures, as indicated by a lowered PCWP, results in a decrease in LV wall tension and oxygen consumption. Consequently, coronary perfusion pressure, a major determinant of coronary blood flow, improves and thus, the oxygen supply to the heart is improved (see Glossary for the definition of perfusion pressure). In comparison to dopamine, dobutamine tends to induce less tachycardia. This feature, combined with the reductions in PCWP and systemic vascular pressure, in addition to the increased perfusion pressure, tends to reduce overall myocardial oxygen consumption.

Compared with dopamine, dobutamine has equal or greater inotropic action. Dobutamine lowers PCWP and SVR with increasing doses, whereas dopamine may increase PCWP and SVR with increasing doses. The effect on HR is variable; however, evidence suggests that dobutamine is less chronotropic than dopamine at lower infusion rates. In the clinical setting, dobutamine may be preferred in patients with depressed CO, elevated PCWP, and increased SVR with mild hypotension. The increase in CO may not be sufficient to raise the BP in a patient who initially is moderately to severely hypotensive. Thus, dopamine may be preferred in the patient with depressed CO, normal or moderately elevated PCWP, and moderate or severe hypotension.

Dobutamine is a better choice than dopamine for R.G. because his initial baseline hemodynamic measurements showed a depressed CI, elevated PCWP, and increased SVR. Dobutamine also may be less chronotropic, but the response is unpredictable. Although dobutamine's positive inotropic and chronotropic effects can increase myocardial oxygen consumption, the increase will not be to the same degree as with dopamine and the decrease in PCWP and SVR ultimately produce a more favorable effect.

21. **How would you initiate therapy with dobutamine?**

Dobutamine should be started at a low dosage (i.e., 2.5 μg/kg/min). The onset of effect is rapid and the half-life short (approximately 2 minutes), with steady-state conditions generally achieved within 10 minutes of initiation of therapy. This allows dose titration every 10 minutes based on patient tolerance. The rate of infusion required to increase CO typically is between 2.5 to 10 μg/kg/min, although higher infusion rates are sometimes required (up to 20 μg/kg/min).

22. **What are the adverse effects associated with dobutamine?**

Adverse effects that can occur during dobutamine administration are arrhythmias, nausea, anxiety, and tremors. The increases in contractility and HR caused by dobutamine can cause an increase in myocardial oxygen consumption and can lead to ischemia in patients with coronary artery disease. Another limiting factor to dobutamine is tolerance to its hemodynamic effects with long-term continuous use. A decline in CO and HR has been seen after prolonged infusion and is most likely caused by downregulation of β_1-receptors.

EFFECTS ON HEMODYNAMICS

23. **Dobutamine is initiated and titrated up to 7.5 µg/kg/min. Concurrently, the dopamine is tapered down to 2.0 µg/kg/min resulting in the following hemodynamic profile (previous values in parentheses): BP (S/D/M), 122/60/80 mm Hg (115/62/80); pulse, 115 beats/min (140); CO, 4.2 L/min (3.8); CI, 2.5 L/min (2.2); RAP, 10 mm Hg (10); PCWP, 16 mm Hg (20); SVR, 1,333 dyne · sec · cm^{-5} (1,473); Pao$_2$, 115 (110) mm Hg; Paco$_2$, 38 (28) mm Hg; pH, 7.41 (7.32); HCO$_3^-$, 24 mEq/L (20); and urine output, 60 mL/hr (30). Assess the improvement in hemodynamic change and urine output with the addition of dobutamine and decreased infusion rate of dopamine.**

The CI has continued to increase and the PCWP and SVR have fallen. The increase in perfusion pressure in conjunction with the fall in afterload, preload, and HR will favorably affect the myocardial oxygen supply:demand ratio. The fall in HR with the increase in CO indicates that the stroke volume has increased significantly from 27 to 36 mL/beat. Other signs of improved systemic perfusion include the reversal of the acidosis observed initially and improved urine output.

The improved urine output can be attributed to the combined effects of dobutamine on the CO and subsequent improvement in the perfusion to the kidney and perhaps to the renal effects of dopamine, although the latter effects are controversial and have been debated vigorously. Traditionally, it was thought that the effects of low-dose dopamine on the dopaminergic receptors in the renal vasculature improves kidney blood flow and, consequently, renal function. Randomized, controlled trials have demonstrated increases in urine output with low-dose dopamine,[59] but have not been able to show a reduction in incidence or degree of renal dysfunction.[60,61] Despite the lack of convincing evidence for benefit, low-dose dopamine is widely used in critical care units. The use of low-dose dopamine often does not produce any hemodynamic changes, and adverse effects are rare.[62] Thus, its use can be considered in patients with oliguria, with the understanding that it may only have a diuretic action.

Tapering Inotropic Support

24. **R.G. has remained stable with dobutamine 7.5 µg/kg/min and dopamine 2.0 µg/kg/min for the past 4 hours. Urine output continues to be adequate. How would you taper the inotropic agents and what parameters would you monitor?**

An acceptable method is to taper dobutamine by 2 µg/kg/min every 30 to 60 minutes and maintain the dopamine at 1 to 2 µg/kg/min for its beneficial effect on urine output. Dobutamine has an elimination half-life of 2.4 ± 0.7 minutes; thus, steady-state plasma levels will occur in a short period. However, when tapering vasoactive agents, it is prudent to let the patient stabilize hemodynamically at new infusion rates for a period that exceeds the time to achieve a new steady-state plasma concentration. After each reduction in the infusion rate, hemodynamic data can be assessed. Reasonable guidelines would be to keep the mean arterial pressure at 75

to 80 mm Hg, HR at <110 beats/min, PCWP at 12 to 18 mm Hg, and CI at >2.5 L/min per square meter. After the dobutamine is discontinued, the dopamine can be discontinued as well. R.G. should be evaluated for reinstitution of the medications he was receiving before surgery.

Severe Heart Failure

Assessment by Hemodynamic Profile

25. **A.R. is a 65-year-old woman admitted to the ICU in acute respiratory distress. She has a medical history of coronary artery disease, an MI 4 years ago, hypertension, HF, and renal insufficiency. A.R. has a history of poor compliance with her medications and admits to discontinuing her usual medications (furosemide, enalapril, metoprolol, and digoxin) 5 days ago.**

A.R. is confused, in obvious distress, and cannot catch her breath. Her extremities are pale and slightly cool. Her vital signs are as follows: temperature, 36.8°C; HR, 124 beats/min; RR, 35 breaths/min; BP, 104/65; and SaO$_2$, 85% on 6 L/min of O$_2$ via a face mask. Her admission weight is 95 kg (stated home weight, 87 kg). A Foley catheter and peripheral IV are placed, and samples are sent to the laboratory for analysis. ABG values include the following: pH, 7.33 (normal, 7.35 to 7.45); Paco$_2$, 28 mm Hg (normal, 35 to 45 mm Hg); Pao$_2$, 57 mm Hg (normal, 75 to 100 mm Hg); and HCO$_3^-$, 20 mEq/L (normal, 23 to 29 mEq/L). Other laboratory results are sodium, 130 mEq/L (normal, 136 to 145 mEq/L); potassium, 5.2 mEq/L (normal, 3.5 to 5.0 mEq/L); and creatinine, 1.9 mg/dL (normal, 0.2 to 0.8 mg/dL). A pulmonary artery catheter is placed and initial hemodynamic values are RAP, 15 mm Hg (normal, 2 to 6 mm Hg); PCWP, 30 mm Hg (normal, 5 to 12 mm Hg); pulmonary artery pressure (PAP), 45/28 mm Hg (S/D); CO, 3.5 L/min (normal, 4 to 7 L/min); CI, 1.6 L/min (2.5 to 4.2 L/min) (BSA, 2.2 m^2); and SVR, 1,440 dyne · sec · m^{-5} (normal, 800 to 1,440 dyne · sec · m^{-5}). Chest radiograph shows pulmonary edema with no signs of pneumonia. ECG shows sinus tachycardia with nonspecific T-wave changes and LV hypertrophy.

Describe A.R.'s clinical situation and assess her hemodynamic variables. What initial therapies should be instituted? (also see Chapter 19, Heart Failure)

[SI units: sodium, 130 mmol/L (normal, 136 to 145); potassium, 5.2 mmol/L (normal, 3.5 to 5); creatinine, 142.5 µmol/L (normal, 15 to 61 µmol/L)]

A.R. is in respiratory distress because of pulmonary edema and acute heart failure. Her vital signs show a decreased BP and poor oxygenation. Her CO is low with high preload (PCWP, 30 mm Hg) and she has increased SVR. She has some signs of inadequate perfusion manifested by her confusion and cool skin. As described in Chapter 19, patients can be classified into four different hemodynamic categories based on volume status (wet versus dry) and organ perfusion status (cold versus warm) with subsequent treatment strategies based on which category the patients fits.[63,64] A.R would best be described as wet and warm, although she does have some early evidence of inadequate perfusion as well.

A.R.'s laboratory values (potassium, 5.2 mEq/L; creatinine, 1.9 mg/dL) show renal insufficiency, and the low serum sodium (130 mEq/L) most likely represents volume overload and hemodilution because total body sodium load in patients with HF is usually high. A.R.'s high RAP and PCWP are consistent with volume overload as well and probable cardiogenic pulmonary edema. In many patients, the onset of pulmonary congestion occurs when the PCWP is 18 to 20 mm Hg, and overt pulmonary edema can occur when the PCWP exceeds 30 mm Hg. Filling pressures are elevated secondary to activation of the renin-angiotensin system with subsequent sodium and water retention by the kidney in response to the low CO. Patients with chronic HF often can tolerate higher filling pressures (PCWP) than patients who acutely develop heart failure because the change is gradual. It is, therefore, important to follow the clinical signs, rather than treat a specific number for patients in pulmonary edema.

Improvement of A.R.'s respiratory status is the initial priority, and she should be intubated if attempts to provide supplemental oxygen via face mask are not successful in elevating her PO_2. An MI should be ruled out, although the probable precipitating event is the noncompliance with her medication regimen. In the "wet and warm" patient, diuretics should be given to reduce volume overload and pulmonary edema.

Therapeutic Interventions
FUROSEMIDE
Hemodynamic Effect of Diuretic Therapy

26. Furosemide (Lasix) is prescribed to treat A.R.'s acute pulmonary edema. What initial dose of furosemide would you recommend and how would furosemide affect A.R.'s hemodynamic status?

A.R. has not received her maintenance medications for the past week. As a consequence, she has become fluid overloaded, which has precipitated pulmonary edema and acute cardiac failure in addition to chronic HF. A loop diuretic is the drug of choice for this situation. Furosemide is used most commonly, although some clinicians prefer bumetanide or torsemide (see Chapter 19, Heart Failure, for dosing comparisons). The initial dose of furosemide used to treat acute pulmonary edema is highly variable. Patients who have been taking maintenance diuretics require larger initial doses than patients who have not. In A.R., an initial dose of 40 mg furosemide administered intravenously is reasonable. If no response is seen 1 hour after the first dose, a second IV dose of 80 mg can be administered. If still no response is elicited, dose titration of furosemide may continue at 1-hour intervals until a response is seen. In severe heart failure some patients exhibit diuretic resistance with an inadequate diuretic response. Combination therapy with a diuretic that exerts its action in another part of the nephron could be used when resistance to loop diuretics is seen.[65] An example of this would be a combination of a thiazide or metolazone and one of the loop diuretics. Significant side effects may be seen with the high dosages required if resistance to loop diuretics is present (e.g., ototoxicity with furosemide) or when a combination of different diuretic classes is used (e.g., electrolyte abnormalities). Another alternative for patients resistant to intermittent bolus administration of loop diuretics (i.e., furosemide, bumetanide, torsemide) is continuous infusion of the same agent. It has been demonstrated in patients with severe HF that continuous IV administration of a loop diuretic leads to increased diuretic and natriuretic effects compared with intermittent bolus administration.[66] See Chapter 19, Heart Failure, for further discussion of loop diuretic dosing in diuretic refractory patients.

Furosemide is a rapid-acting diuretic that also acts as a venous vasodilator. By increasing venous capacitance, venous return (preload) decreases. This combined diuresis and redistribution of intravascular fluid away from the lungs will lower the PCWP. The effect of furosemide on venous capacitance often precedes the diuresis. Reduction of LV filling pressure usually occurs within 5 minutes and peaks 15 minutes after IV furosemide administration. The reduction in PCWP usually is unaccompanied by a change in CO. The reduction in PCWP improves the myocardial oxygen supply–demand ratio but does not significantly improve systemic perfusion. The major risk of using a diuretic is excessive reduction of preload and hence, CO. In A.R., diuresis with a potent loop diuretic can be safely initiated because she has a PCWP >30 mm Hg and is fluid overloaded. A potential concern with furosemide would be a further reduction in her BP, however the benefit outweighs the risks in this patient.

VASODILATORS

27. Sixty minutes after a 40-mg IV furosemide dose, A.R. is now more confused, and her urine output has declined after an initial good response to the furosemide. A.R.'s vital signs are: HR, 110 beats/min; BP, 110/50 mm Hg; RR 20 breaths/min; and SaO_2 93% on 100% face mask O_2. The PA catheter shows a RAP of 16 mm Hg; PAP, 38/24 mm Hg; PCWP, 24 mm Hg; CO, 4.2 L/min; CI, 1.9 L/min per square meter; and SVR, 1,028 dyne · sec · m^{-5}. Laboratory results show the following: PO_2, 79; Hct, 34%; Hgb, 11.2; and SvO_2, 54%. What other therapeutic options are available for treatment of A.R.'s acute HF and pulmonary edema given the current hemodynamic values and clinical situation?

A.R.'s condition has deteriorated clinically; her calculated oxygen delivery is low (DO_2 608 mL/min) and her mixed venous oxygen saturation (SvO_2) is decreased, suggesting hypoperfusion. Improvement in A.R.'s CO is needed to increase perfusion and prevent organ dysfunction. A.R. is now best classified as "wet and cold." Vasodilators have become an accepted part of treatment for HF based on the following underlying pathophysiology (also see Chapter 19, Heart Failure). Both preload and afterload are elevated in response to a fall in CO. As CO falls, the sympathetic nervous system and renin-angiotensin system are activated to maintain circulatory stability. Arterial pressure is maintained by the excessive increase in SVR, which increases the resistance to ejection of blood from the left ventricle. Venoconstriction shifts some of the blood volume from the peripheral veins to the central circulation, which contributes to an elevation of right and left atrial pressures. A normal heart responds to the increase in preload and afterload by increasing contractility, but in HF, the heart's intrinsic capacity to increase contractility has been lost. As a result, the neurohormonal compensatory mechanism activated to maintain arterial pressure increases the work load on the heart and this leads to a further decrease in CO. Patients tend to spiral down this vicious cycle until the CO is lower and the SVR is higher than optimal to maintain perfusion pressure. Vasodilators disrupt the compensatory mechanisms that elevate preload and afterload and shift the ventricular function curve upward, which allows a greater CO at a lower LV filling pressure.

Three categories of vasodilators are available. Arterial vasodilators (e.g., hydralazine) decrease afterload thus reducing impedance to LV outflow. Venous vasodilators (e.g., NTG) primarily decrease venous return (preload), thus improving ventricular compliance, subendocardial coronary perfusion, and pulmonary hydrostatic pressure. Finally, mixed arterial and venous vasodilators have balanced effects on both preload and afterload reduction (e.g., nitroprusside, nesiritide, angiotensin-converting enzyme inhibitors). The fall in SVR from arterial vasodilation potentially may cause hypotension and a reflex increase in HR; however, this is infrequently seen in patients with HF because the decrease in SVR is counterbalanced by an increase in CO, which tends to maintain arterial pressure. Excessive preload reduction can cause deficient ventricular filling, thereby reducing the CO. The overall response in any given patient depends on their baseline hemodynamic and volume status. At this time, A.R.'s BP has improved, and she should be able to tolerate a trial of a vasodilator for afterload and preload reduction.

Initial Therapy: Nitroprusside

28. The clinician decides to begin an infusion of nitroprusside for afterload and preload reduction in A.R. How should therapy be initiated? What are the end points of therapy? What adverse effects are associated with nitroprusside infusion?

The initial infusion rate of nitroprusside should be no greater than 0.5 μg/kg/min. The infusion rate can be titrated upward by 0.25 μg/kg/min every 5 minutes until the mean arterial pressure falls 5 to 10 mm Hg. Nitroprusside will lower SVR through arterial vasodilation and will decrease PCWP through venodilation. Cardiac output will increase as the afterload is reduced. Reasonable goals of therapy in A.R. are a cardiac index of >2.5 L/min. A mean arterial pressure above 70 mm Hg will ensure adequate organ perfusion, but BP should be kept as low as A.R. tolerates clinically, because this will reflect maximal afterload reduction. A reduction in PCWP to a level that maintains CO without causing pulmonary edema is also desirable. In A.R., a goal PCWP of 16 to 18 mm Hg is reasonable.

Adverse effects associated with nitroprusside administration include excessive hypotension, reflex tachycardia, potential worsening of myocardial ischemia, thiocyanate toxicity (especially with renal dysfunction, prolonged infusions, and high infusion rates), accumulation of cyanide with subsequent cyanide toxicity, worsening arterial hypoxemia from increases in ventilation/perfusion mismatch, and, rarely, methemoglobinemia and hypothyroidism. (Also see Chapter 21, Hypertensive Emergencies, for a discussion of nitroprusside.)

HEMODYNAMIC EFFECT

29. Over the next 2 hours, A.R. received 2 doses of IV furosemide 40 mg. Nitroprusside was titrated to 1.2 μg/kg/min resulting in the following hemodynamic profile (previous values in parentheses): BP (S/D/M), 100/50/66 mm Hg (110/50/70); pulse, 94 beats/min (110); CI, 2.8 L/min per square meter (1.9); PCWP, 22 mm Hg (24); SVR, 906 dyne · sec · cm⁻⁵ (1,028); urine output, 50 mL/hr (10); Pao_2, 80 mm Hg (70); $Paco_2$, 46 mm Hg (46); pH, 7.32 (7.26); and HCO_3^-, 24 mEq/L (21). Cardiopulmonary examination reveals an S_3 gallop and bibasilar rales are present, but diminished from previous examination. The ECG shows a sinus rhythm. Evaluate the effect that nitroprusside and furosemide have had on A.R.'s hemodynamic profile and clinical status.

The CI has improved significantly (1.9 to 2.8 L/min per square meter) and the stroke volume has increased from 27 to 48 mL/beat. The improved stroke volume has decreased endogenous catecholamine levels, which, in turn, has decreased the HR (110 to 94 beats/minute) and SVR. A.R. has improved clinically and her ABGs indicate improvement of the metabolic acidosis. The increased urine output can be attributed to the combined effects of the diuretic and increased CO. Overall, A.R. has improved substantially. Supplemental oxygen still is required, but the oxygen concentration needed to maintain an adequate arterial oxygen content has been lowered.

At this point, a further reduction in preload may benefit A.R.'s respiratory function because the PCWP still is elevated at 22 mm Hg. However, the mean arterial pressure is slightly lower than acceptable and a further increase in the nitroprusside dose to reduce preload further may lower the MAP to a level that would compromise coronary and cerebral perfusion, as well as perfusion to other vital organs.

Choice of Additional Therapy

30. What therapeutic interventions are available to further reduce A.R.'s preload and improve her respiratory function?

Three options are available. The first is to continue current therapy (nitroprusside and furosemide) and wait for the diuresis to continue to reduce preload. However, because her MAP is slightly lower than desirable, signs of inadequate systemic perfusion must be monitored closely as a guide to additional or reduced diuretic therapy. The goal is to find the filling pressure (PCWP) that maximizes SV without causing pulmonary edema.

The second option to reduce preload would be the addition of intravenous nitroglycerin. An initial dose of 0.25 μg/kg/min is reasonable. Initial titration should be in 0.25 μg/kg/min increments at intervals of 3 to 5 minutes guided by patient's clinical response. If no response is seen at 1 μg/kg/min, titration increments of 0.5 to 1 μg/min may be used. See Chapter 18, Myocardial Infarction, and Chapter 19, Heart Failure, for additional discussion of intravenous nitroglycerin.

The third option is to continue the nitroprusside and add dobutamine to improve CO through inotropic support. A dobutamine infusion of 3 μg/kg/min is a reasonable initial dose. Either choice is acceptable as long as A.R. is monitored closely.

Transition to Oral Vasodilators

31. After 48 hours of nitroprusside, intermittent furosemide, and low-dose dobutamine, A.R. has remained hemodynamically stable. The decision is made to reinstitute A.R.'s previous medications (furosemide, enalapril, metoprolol, and digoxin). No evidence supports a new MI. How would you reinstitute the enalapril (10 mg BID) and taper the nitroprusside in A.R.?

Guidelines for tapering short-acting vasodilators when substituting long-acting oral agents are not strict. In this case, a reasonable approach would be to give the enalapril (Vasotec) at a lower dosage than A.R. was taking previously (e.g., 5 mg twice daily) and reduce the nitroprusside infusion rate by 25%. Then, obtain a CO and PCWP every 2 to 4 hours to assess the contribution of the enalapril to the afterload and preload reduction. If the mean arterial pressure declines excessively after the addition of enalapril, the nitroprusside dose will have to be reduced further. A smooth transition from IV therapy to oral therapy often depends on the skill of the nursing staff and their familiarity with the hemodynamic effects of the drugs. In addition, A.R. will have to be monitored for signs of renal insufficiency, a potential adverse effect of ACE inhibitors. If she develops worsening renal function, an alternative vasodilator strategy such as hydralazine and nitrate therapy may be necessary (see Chapter 19, Heart Failure).

Phosphodiesterase Inhibitors

32. **Amrinone and milrinone are noncatecholamine inotropic agents with vasodilator activity. If A.R.'s condition had failed to respond to nitroprusside and furosemide, these drugs would have been a potential therapeutic option for treatment of her acute cardiac failure. What are the considerations in choosing which agent to use? How would you dose milrinone and what adverse effects would you expect with its administration? Does milrinone offer any advantage over catecholamine inotropic agents (e.g., dobutamine, dopamine) or a pure vasodilator such as nitroprusside?**

The phosphodiesterase inhibitors (also referred to as inodilators) are a class of drugs that have the combination of inotropic and vasodilator effects. All agents in this class have basically the same mechanism of action. They inhibit intracellular phosphodiesterase, leading to an increase in the concentration of cyclic adenosine monophosphate (cAMP). This increase in cAMP causes intracellular changes that could lead to increased inotropic effects. Increased cAMP also causes relaxation of vascular smooth muscle and, therefore, decreases SVR.

The hemodynamic effects seen with phosphodiesterase inhibitors include increased inotropy, reduced SVR, and improved LV diastolic compliance. These changes result in an increase in CI and a decrease in LV afterload and filling pressures. Almost all the phosphodiesterase inhibitors have been shown to elevate CI and stroke volume index. Myocardial oxygen demand is increased by the increase in myocardial contractility and HR. On the other hand, LV filling pressures and SVR are decreased, leading to a decrease in myocardial oxygen demand. The net effect depends on the balance of the opposing forces.

Clinically, amrinone and milrinone have similar effects on hemodynamics. Adverse effects are the major clinical difference between amrinone and milrinone. Thrombocytopenia (platelet count <100,000/mm³) has been associated with amrinone,[67] but less often with milrinone.[68] However, this effect may not be clinically significant with short-term use. A study comparing amrinone with milrinone in cardiac surgery patients found no difference on hemodynamics between the agents, and concluded that the selection between the two agents could be made on considerations such as cost.[69]

MILRINONE

Milrinone is the phosphodiesterase inhibitor most often used in clinical practice. It is primarily cleared by the kidneys, and has an elimination half-life from 1 to 3 hours in patients with normal renal function. In patients with severe heart failure, or in patients with renal failure, an increase in the elimination half-life can be seen. The onset of action occurs within minutes following a loading dose.

The long half-life of milrinone compared to the catecholamine agents makes a loading dose necessary before an infusion can be started. IV milrinone usually is initiated with a 50 μg/kg loading dose administered over 10 minutes, followed by a maintenance infusion of 0.25 to 0.75 μg/kg/min. Patients with HF or renal insufficiency will have a reduced elimination rate and require dose adjustment.

IV administration of milrinone in patients with severe heart failure results in a significant increase in CO, while decreasing PVR and SVR through vasodilation. HR usually remains unaltered, although hypotension can occur when vasodilation exceeds the increase in CO and in hypovolemic patients. Theoretically, the effect of milrinone on myocardial oxygen consumption should be favorable because it does not substantially alter HR while lowering LV filling pressure. A recent placebo-controlled study of the short-term use (48-hour infusion) of milrinone in patients with acute exacerbations of heart failure found no significant differences in mortality, length of stay, or readmission, and found significant increases in arrhythmias and hypotension in the milrinone group.[70] Although patients were excluded from this trial if their treating physician felt that inotropic therapy was essential, it is important to recognize that the improvement of hemodynamic variables does not necessarily imply improved outcome.

Milrinone therapy has few serious side effects, the most significant being hypotension and arrhythmias. Because milrinone may increase arrhythmia frequency and cause sudden death, it should be used cautiously in patients with severe ventricular arrhythmias. Thrombocytopenia has also been reported with milrinone.

Compared to pure vasodilators such as nitroprusside, milrinone offers the advantage of positive inotropic action which may increase CO to a larger degree. The increased inotropy comes at a cost of increased myocardial work, or oxygen consumption, which is a potential disadvantage of PDE inhibitors.

Comparisons of the hemodynamic effects of milrinone, dobutamine, and dopamine show that milrinone is more similar to dobutamine than to dopamine. Therefore, the advantage of milrinone over dopamine would be the same as that of dobutamine over dopamine (see Question 20). In contrast to dobutamine, milrinone is a less potent inotropic agent and a more potent vasodilator. In a comparison of these agents, patients receiving dobutamine had a higher BP and PCWP compared to milrinone, reflecting the increased vasodilation with milrinone.[71] The longer duration of action poses a problem if an undesirable effect occurs, although the lack of a chronotropic effect with a resultant increase in myocardial oxygen consumption may be beneficial in A.R., who has a history of MI. Trials evaluating milrinone-based versus dobutamine-based therapy have found similar outcomes in patients with decompensated heart failure and in patients awaiting heart transplantation, with increased cost associated with milrinone.[72,73] The current cost of milrinone has decreased with the arrival of a generic product.

Because the inotropic mechanism of milrinone is independent of the β-receptor, it may be of value in patients who do not respond to catecholamine inotropic agents because of β-receptor blockade or down-regulation of β-receptors.[74] This may be an important consideration, as β-blocker therapy is becoming standard in the treatment of heart failure as evidenced by the use of metoprolol in A.R. In addition, milrinone has a different mechanism of action and therefore it may have synergistic inotropic effects with catecholamines.

Nesiritide

33. **Nesiritide is a new agent approved for the treatment of decompensated congestive heart failure. What are the hemodynamic effects of nesiritide and how does it compare to other agents used in the treatment of advanced heart failure?**

Human brain, or B-type, natriuretic peptide (BNP) is produced by the ventricle in response to increased filling pressures, and the endogenous protein has several important actions on hemodynamics. Nesiritide is a recombinant form that is identical to the endogenously produced BNP. The actions of nesiritide include mixed arterial and venous dilation, increased sodium excretion, and suppression of the deleterious effects of the renin-angiotensin-aldosterone and sympathetic nervous system.[75-77] Compared to placebo, the effect on hemodynamics are a decrease in PCWP, PA pressures, and SVR, and an increase in CO.[77] Nesiritide does not possess direct inotropic activity; the increase in CO is a result of the decrease in afterload.

The Vasodilation in the Management of Acute CHF (VMAC) study evaluated nesiritide compared with nitroglycerin in the treatment of heart failure.[78] The investigators found that nesiritide improved PCWP better than nitroglycerin, and was more effective at reducing the symptoms of dyspnea with fewer adverse effects. Compared to dobutamine in a randomized, open-label trial, nesiritide caused less tachyarrhythmias and more hypotension, with similar effects on the signs and symptoms of CHF.[78] Nesiritide is dosed as a 2 μg/kg load, followed by an infusion of 0.01 μg/kg/min. The infusion may be titrated up to a maximum of 0.03 μg/kg/min. Few data are available concerning infusions of nesiritide for longer than 48 hours. The balanced vasodilation and increased sodium excretion with nesiritide makes it an attractive option in the treatment of advanced heart failure, particularly in diuretic resistant patients with elevated filling pressures and dyspnea. Hypotension is the most common adverse effect, occurring in up to 35% of patients.[78] See Chapter 19, Heart Failure, for additional information about the clinical use of nesiritide.

Acute Myocardial Infarction

Immediate Goals of Therapy and General Considerations

34. **M.J., a 57-year-old man, is brought to the ED complaining of severe chest pain and difficulty breathing. On physical examination, M.J. has a BP of 80/40 mm Hg (normal, 120/80 mm Hg) (by cuff) with a weak pulse of 115 beats/min (normal, 60 to 80 beats/min). His RR is 24 breaths/min (normal, 18 breaths/min) and his breathing is shallow. Heart sounds include S_3/S_4 gallops, but no murmurs are heard. The jugular venous pulse is normal.**

He has diffuse rales over the lower lung fields with moderate wheezing. M.J. is cold and clammy to touch; however, his temperature is normal. He is restless, anxious, and confused about time and date. ABGs on 2 L/min oxygen via nasal prongs are PaO_2, 65 mm Hg (normal, 75 to 100 mm Hg); $PaCO_2$, 44 mm Hg (normal, 35 to 45 mm Hg); pH, 7.22 (normal, 7.35 to 7.45); and HCO_3^-, 18 mEq/L (normal, 23 to 29 mEq/L). The ECG shows ST segment elevation in the anterior lateral leads and 6 to 10 premature ventricular contractions (PVCs) per minute. Serum potassium is normal. A Foley catheter is inserted to monitor urine output. Cardiac enzymes are pending. M.J. has no known history of cardiac disease and takes no medication. What immediate goals of therapy are necessary to stabilize and treat M.J.?

[SI unit: HCO_3^-, 18 mmol/L (normal, 23 to 29)]

M.J. has signs of cardiogenic shock with decreased systemic perfusion. His BP is low, his HR is elevated, and his respiratory status is compromised. M.J. is restless, anxious, and confused, indicating poor cerebral perfusion. His ABG results indicate a component of metabolic acidosis secondary to poor systemic perfusion. The ST elevation on the ECG is consistent with an acute anterior MI.

As discussed in Chapter 18, Myocardial Infarction, most patients presenting with MI are routinely treated with aspirin, β-blockers, and thrombolytics (unless contraindicated) or immediate percutaneous coronary intervention (PCI). However, the presence of cardiogenic shock may alter the interventional strategy. Patients presenting in cardiogenic shock after MI may progress rapidly to irreversible organ system dysfunction as the compensatory mechanisms fail to maintain tissue perfusion. Treatment of these critically ill patients involves two components: (1) stabilization and (2) definitive treatment. Initial stabilization of the patient must be attained before further evaluation and treatment of the cause of cardiogenic shock can proceed. The goals are to maintain adequate oxygen delivery to the tissues and to prevent further hemodynamic compromise. Stabilization includes (1) establishing ventilation and oxygenation (arterial PO_2 should be >70 mm Hg); (2) restoring central arterial BP and CO with vasopressors and inotropic agents, if needed; (3) infusing fluids, if hypovolemic; and (4) treating pain, arrhythmias, and acid-base abnormalities, if present.

Administration of oxygen by mechanical ventilation enhances the myocardial oxygen supply and may contribute to improved ventricular performance. Mechanical ventilation is indicated when arterial oxygen saturation cannot be maintained above 85% to 90% despite 100% oxygen per face mask. Once intubated, maximal sedation should be provided to alleviate anxiety and discomfort.

The arterial pressure must be increased to provide adequate coronary and systemic perfusion to meet oxygen requirements. Some areas of ischemia in the infarct zone may be depressed but viable, provided myocardial oxygen supply exceeds demand. However, if the myocardial oxygen demands are not met, myocardial tissue necrosis will expand into the area of ischemia. This results in further hemodynamic impairment and initiates a vicious feedback cycle that can lead to intractable pump failure and irreversible shock. To be effective, treatment of cardiogenic shock should favorably influence the balance between oxygen supply and demand in the ischemic zone.

Optimizing preload to improve CO and systemic perfusion is crucial, especially in patients with RV infarction. Unfortunately, in patients with severe LV impairment caused by cardiogenic shock, increasing intravascular volume can worsen pulmonary congestion. M.J. currently has signs of pulmonary congestion and RV infarction is not immediately evident; thus, a fluid challenge must be administered cautiously or withheld until hemodynamic monitoring can be established.

Inotropic agents or vasopressors should be used to increase systemic BP and re-establish coronary perfusion in patients with cardiogenic shock and hypotension. The use of vasoactive agents, however, is not without risk because they may exacerbate ventricular arrhythmias and increase oxygen consumption in ischemic myocardium. Therefore, the minimal dose that will provide adequate perfusion pressure should be used. Achieving a MAP of 65 to 70 mm Hg is the immediate goal of therapy. Elevation of the mean arterial pressure above 80 mm Hg is unnecessary because at this level, coronary blood flow is not significantly changed, but energy expenditure is.

Correction of metabolic acidosis is best accomplished by treating the underlying cause. Improving tissue perfusion by optimizing oxygen content and increasing CO can eventually restore aerobic metabolism and eliminate lactic acid production. The use of sodium bicarbonate to correct lactic acidosis in cardiogenic shock and other critically ill patients is controversial. Sodium bicarbonate can have numerous adverse effects, such as hypernatremia, paradoxical intracellular acidosis, and hypercapnia, and conclusive data on its efficacy are lacking. Bicarbonate therapy, therefore, warrants caution and is recommended only, if at all, when severe acidemia (pH <7.2 or HCO_3^- <10 to 12 mEq/L) is present.

Because inotropic agents and vasoconstrictors can increase myocardial oxygen consumption and potentially extend the area of necrosis in patients with infarct-induced cardiogenic shock, the careful selection and titration of agents that will best preserve myocardium while sustaining systemic arterial pressure and tissue perfusion is essential. Although correction of volume deficits and early pharmacologic support may prevent the extension of myocardial damage, it must be emphasized that exclusive use of these measures does not improve survival. Therefore, drug therapy must be considered only an interim maneuver to preserve myocardial and systemic integrity while further therapeutic interventions and definitive therapy are being considered.

As mentioned before, cardiogenic shock following AMI occurs in only a small percentage of patients, but carries a high mortality rate. Reperfusion of the occluded artery is of paramount importance in these patients. Two options are available for restoring patency of the artery. Thrombolytic therapy and percutaneous transluminal coronary angioplasty, with or without stenting (See Chapter 19, Heart Failure).

Thrombolytic therapy in acute MI may reduce the incidence of subsequent cardiogenic shock, but its value may be limited in patients who have already developed shock.[79] The effectiveness of thrombolytics is reduced in this setting, possibly because of reduced delivery of the agent to the coronary artery thrombus as a result of hypotension.[80] The use of an intraaortic balloon counterpulsation pump (IABP) to augment coronary artery blood flow may improve the efficacy of thrombolytics.[81] In settings when interventional cardiac procedures such as percutaneous transluminal coronary angioplasty (PTCA) are not readily available, insertion of an IABP and thrombolytics should not be delayed if indicated.

Early percutaneous transluminal coronary angioplasty (PTCA) may be of more benefit than thrombolytics in patients with cardiogenic shock complicating acute MI. In a subset of patients with cardiogenic shock in the GUSTO-1 trial, angioplasty resulted in a reduction in 30-day mortality rate from 61% to 43%.[82] Numerous other trials have demonstrated improved outcomes with PTCA in patients with shock compared with historical controls. However, problems with subgroup analysis and nonrandomized trials include the potential for selection bias. Operator skill also is a consideration in this setting, and larger centers with greater experience may have better outcomes than smaller centers.

An early revascularization strategy with angioplasty or bypass surgery was recently compared to medical management of these patients including thrombolytics and intraaortic balloon counterpulsation.[83] There was no significant difference in mortality rate at 30 days; however, at 6 months, the mortality rate in the revascularization group was 50.3% versus 63.1% for the medical therapy group. Follow-up at 1 year also demonstrated a significant increase in survival.[84]

Assessment by Hemodynamic Profile

35. M.J. has a history of cerebrovascular disease and is thus ineligible for thrombolytic therapy. Therefore, he will require revascularization in the form of balloon angioplasty or coronary artery bypass surgery to improve his chances of survival. Meanwhile, he is given dopamine at 5 µg/kg/min to stabilize him hemodynamically before revascularization procedures are initiated. Lidocaine (100-mg IV bolus plus a 2-mg/min infusion) also is instituted to correct the PVCs. Oxygen administration is changed to 100% via face mask. Morphine sulfate, 2 mg IV, is given for chest pain. IV NTG was initiated at 0.25 µg/kg/min for myocardial ischemia, but had to be discontinued because intolerable hypotension developed. M.J. is admitted to the ICU where an arterial line and pulmonary artery line are placed, revealing the following hemodynamic profile (previous values in parentheses): BP (S/D/M), 92/46/61 mm Hg (80/40 by cuff); pulse, 122 beats/min (115); CO, 2.8 L/min; CI, 1.5 L/min per square meter; RAP, 16 mm Hg; PCWP, 26 mm Hg; SVR, 1,314 dyne · sec · cm^{-5}; PaO_2, 70 mm Hg (65); $PaCO_2$, 48 mm Hg (44); pH, 7.24 (7.22); HCO_3^-, 21 mEq/L (18); and urine output, 10 mL/hr. (M.J. weighs 82 kg and has a BSA of 1.9 m^2.) The chest radiograph shows evidence of pulmonary edema. Assess M.J.'s hemodynamic profile and response to dopamine therapy.

M.J.'s clinical and hemodynamic parameters confirm the diagnosis of cardiogenic shock. He is clearly not hypovolemic, as manifested by an elevated RAP and PCWP. Although his SBP is slightly improved, his CI (<1.8 L/min per square meter), PCWP (>18 mm Hg), and low urine output (<25 mL/hour) are all characteristic findings with this form of shock. Patients with cardiogenic shock from an acute event (such as an MI) are usually in a much more critical clinical situation than patients who have an acute exacerbation of chronic heart failure. Patients with HF have compensated over time for the increases in preload and reduced cardiac output, but patients like M.J. have not had time to develop compensatory mechanisms.

Dopamine, at an infusion rate of 5 to 10 µg/kg/min, has made M.J. more tachycardic, has not substantially enhanced CO, and the mean arterial pressure is less than optimal for coronary perfusion. M.J. has signs of pulmonary edema that are consistent with the elevated pulmonary wedge pressure. The PaO_2 of 70 mm Hg is marginally acceptable considering he is on 100% oxygen per face mask.

Therapeutic Interventions
FLUID THERAPY VERSUS INOTROPIC SUPPORT

36. The decision is made to intubate M.J. Would a fluid challenge or additional doses of dopamine improve M.J.'s status?

In M.J. a fluid challenge could exacerbate the pulmonary edema because after an AMI, ventricular compliance is decreased and a small change in LVEDV could result in a disproportionately large increase in PCWP. Thus, in patients with an AMI, the benefits of a fluid challenge must be balanced against the risk of aggravating pulmonary edema. M.J. has an elevated RAP and PCWP, indicating that he has at least adequate, if not excessive, preload. If a fluid challenge is going to be administered, no more than 100 mL of normal saline should be infused without further evaluation of hemodynamic and clinical data.

Increasing the dopamine infusion rate might improve CO and perfusion pressure, but at the expense of increasing the HR even further. The increased HR, along with the elevated PCWP, could adversely affect the myocardial oxygen supply to demand ratio. However, the increase in coronary blood flow (caused by the rise in arterial pressure) and the decrease in LV chamber size (associated with the increase in contractility) hopefully would tend to offset the increase in myocardial oxygen requirements.

It is not entirely clear which patients in cardiogenic shock will respond to dopamine. One trial of 24 patients in cardiogenic shock and found that a mean infusion rate of 9.1 µg/kg/min was required to produce beneficial effects on CO, urine output, HR, and PCWP in survivors.[85] Nonsurvivors had no change in MAP, PCWP, or HR at an average infusion rate of 17.1 µg/kg/min.

COMBINATION INOTROPIC THERAPY

37. Occasionally, a patient's hemodynamic status improves with the combined use of inotropic agents. Would the addition of dobutamine or a phosphodiesterase inhibitor to treat M.J.'s cardiogenic shock be beneficial?

The combination of dobutamine and dopamine was studied in eight cardiogenic shock patients requiring mechanical ventilation.[86] The cause of heart failure was CHF in four patients and idiopathic cardiomyopathy in the other four. None of the patients had experienced an MI within the preceding 7 days. Each patient received three infusions in a randomly assigned order: dopamine at 15 µg/kg/min; dobutamine at 15 µg/kg/min; and a combination of dopamine and dobutamine each at 7.5 µg/kg/min. All three regimens increased CI, stroke index, LVSWI, and HR similarly. MAP increased with the dopamine and dobutamine–dopamine combination but did not change with the dobutamine alone. SVR was significantly lower with dobutamine alone compared with the other two regimens. PCWP was elevated most with the dopamine infu-

sion alone as was myocardial oxygen consumption. The combination regimen offered hemodynamic superiority over either agent alone in this group of patients.

Given M.J.'s significantly low arterial BP, the addition of a phosphodiesterase inhibitor such as milrinone could be problematic. These agents tend to have more vasodilating properties than dobutamine, and their long-half lives can present difficulties in management if hypotension does develop. Until M.J.'s BP is improved, phosphodiesterase inhibitors should be avoided.

In summary, further inotropic support with dopamine or the addition of dobutamine would be indicated in M.J. at this time. The dopamine could be increased to 12.5 µg/kg/min or dobutamine could be initiated at 5 µg/kg/min. Neither maneuver is without risk. Dobutamine could lower the MAP, adversely affecting coronary perfusion pressure. Dopamine might elevate the PCWP. The addition of dobutamine or an increase in dopamine dose could increase HR even more. Any of these would adversely affect the myocardial oxygen supply to demand ratio and could further extend the area of ischemia or necrosis.

38. Despite the addition of dobutamine at a rate of 5 to 7.5 µg/kg/min and initiation of ventilatory support via tracheal intubation, M.J. continues to show signs of deterioration, with progressive obtundation and loss of bowel sounds. His systemic arterial pressure has continued to decline, and his dopamine is now up to 18 µg/kg/min. Preload reduction was attempted previously with NTG; however, the drop in BP was intolerable. A repeat hemodynamic profile shows the following (previous values in parentheses): BP (S/D/M), 86/40/55 (92/46/61); pulse, 132 beats/min (122); CO, 3.0 L/min (2.8); CI, 1.6 L/min per square meter (1.5); RAP, 18 mm Hg (16); PCWP, 24 mm Hg (26); SVR, 986 dyne · sec · cm^{-5} (1,314); urine output, 8 mL/hr (10); Pao$_2$, 75 mm Hg (70); Paco$_2$, 42 mm Hg (48); pH, 7.26 (7.24); and HCO$_3^-$, 19 mEq/L (21). The ECG shows atrial tachycardia with occasional PVCs. What therapeutic alternatives can be considered at this time?

M.J. is still in severe cardiogenic shock and his tissue perfusion continues to deteriorate as evidenced by a further reduction in urine output, a loss in bowel sounds, continuing acidosis, and central nervous system (CNS) obtundation. Because his systemic arterial pressure and tissue perfusion have declined despite the addition of dobutamine and maximal doses of dopamine, additional support with a potent vasopressor and the insertion of an intra-aortic balloon pump are indicated.

NOREPINEPHRINE
Norepinephrine is a potent α-adrenergic agonist that vasoconstricts arterioles at all infusion rates, thereby increasing SVR. Thus, systemic arterial and coronary perfusion pressures both rise. Norepinephrine also stimulates β_1-adrenergic receptors to a lesser extent, resulting in increased contractility and stroke volume. However, HR and CO usually remain constant, or may even decrease secondary to the increased afterload and reflex baroreceptor activation. Although coronary perfusion pressure is enhanced as a result of the elevation in diastolic pressure, myocardial oxygen consumption also is increased. Consequently, myocardial ischemia and arrhythmias may be exacerbated and LV function further compromised.

Infusions of norepinephrine are begun at 0.01 to 0.05 μg/kg/min and titrated upward to achieve a SBP of 90 to 100 mm Hg. Administration should be through a central IV line because local subcutaneous necrosis may result from peripheral IV extravasation. Prolonged infusion of larger doses will transiently exert a beneficial effect by diverting blood flow from the peripheral and splanchnic vasculature to the heart and brain; however, this ultimately may compromise capillary perfusion to the extent that end-organ failure, particularly renal failure, ensues.

To reduce the potential risk of end-organ damage, a reasonable approach is to add norepinephrine to the infusion of dobutamine, and reduce the dopamine infusion rate to 0.5 to 2 μg/kg/min. This will theoretically support renal and splanchnic perfusion. In addition, any deficits in plasma volume should be corrected when identified by hemodynamic monitoring.

Adverse effects of norepinephrine are related mostly to excessive vasoconstriction and compromise of organ perfusion. Worsening of ventricular function can occur because of increased afterload and tissue necrosis and sloughing may develop if extravasation occurs. Cardiac arrhythmias can emerge and HR can increase; however, in some cases the HR may slow secondary to baroreceptor-mediated reflex increases in vagal tone.

Again, it must be emphasized that in M.J. pharmacologic support, particularly the use of norepinephrine, is only an interim maneuver to temporarily maintain hemodynamic function while revascularization procedures are being considered. Patients who cannot be stabilized with pharmacologic intervention, and in whom systemic or myocardial perfusion is becoming compromised, may require further support through insertion of a mechanical circulatory assist device (e.g., intraaortic balloon pump).

INTRA-AORTIC BALLOON PUMP

When drug therapy is ineffective at stabilizing patients in cardiogenic shock, mechanical intervention should be considered. Mechanical interventions such as intra-aortic balloon counterpulsation can rapidly stabilize patients with cardiogenic shock, especially those with global myocardial ischemia or infarction complicated by mechanical defects, such as papillary muscle rupture or ventricular septal rupture. Intra-aortic balloon counterpulsation augments coronary arterial perfusion pressure during diastole and reduces LV impedance during systole. Sometimes combined inotropic support and intra-aortic balloon counterpulsation are required to maintain an acceptable BP (SBP >90 mm Hg) and CI (>2.2 L/min per square meter).

The intra-aortic balloon pump (IABP) or intra-aortic counter pulsation has been in use for over 15 years and remains the most commonly used mechanical assist device. It is designed to improve coronary perfusion and reduce afterload, thus providing short-term reperfusion of the ischemic myocardium. A 30- to 40-mL balloon catheter is inserted into an artery (usually femoral) and advanced to just below the arch of the aorta. Balloon inflation and deflation are synchronized with the ECG to inflate during diastole (after the aortic valve closes) and deflate at the onset of systole. The inflated balloon in diastole increases coronary perfusion by elevating the mean aortic pressure. The rapid deflation of the balloon at the onset of systole decreases SBP, thus reducing afterload and improving cardiac ejection. The enhanced myocardial perfusion provided by IABP may reduce vasopressor requirements, thereby further decreasing myocardial oxygen consumption. Occasionally, IABP augmentation is sufficient to allow the institution of vasodilators such as nitroprusside, or inodilators, such as amrinone and milrinone. Complications of IABP include thrombocytopenia from the mechanical destruction of platelets and the potential for limb ischemia because of reduced blood flow in the artery into which the IABP catheter is inserted. Heparin anticoagulation is usually used with IABP because the device has a large surface area that can be thrombogenic.

Recently, more advanced circulatory-assist devices (HeartMate, Novacor, Abiomed) have been developed. Mechanical assistance with these devices is used for patients with cardiogenic shock who need support while awaiting definitive, corrective therapy or as a bridging mechanism before cardiac transplantation.[87] Long-term use of some of these devices has been investigated in patients with severe cardiac failure who are not transplant candidates.[88] Implantation of a left ventricular assist device (LVAD) was compared with medical management in severe heart failure patients. Survival at one year was 52% in the LVAD group, compared to 25% in the medical management group. The high cost of these devices will undoubtedly limit the use to only the most severely ill patients.

In summary, M.J.'s condition has continued to deteriorate since his admission to the ICU. Attempts at stabilizing his hemodynamic parameters with dopamine, dobutamine, and norepinephrine have failed. This is evidenced by inadequate tissue perfusion that is reflected clinically by his continued lactic acidosis, decreased urine output, reduced bowel sounds, and CNS obtundation. M.J.'s best chance of survival is to undergo early revascularization of his ischemic myocardium with either coronary bypass surgery or PTCA.

Meanwhile, the addition of norepinephrine and intra-aortic counterpulsation can provide temporary support for M.J. before his procedure.

SEPTIC SHOCK

Clinical and Hemodynamic Features

39. **M.K., a 56-year-old man, was admitted 5 days ago with a chief complaint of acute abdominal pain of 3 days' duration associated with bloody diarrhea, fever, tachypnea, and hypotension. A diagnosis of superior mesenteric artery occlusion with necrotic bowel was made, leading to surgery for removal of necrotic bowel tissue. During postoperative days 1 through 4, there was a slight increase in serum creatinine (SCr), and he could not be completely weaned from ventilatory support. Vital signs were stable. Antibiotic therapy includes clindamycin and gentamicin in appropriate doses.**

M.K. has a history of coronary artery disease with stable angina pectoris that has been treated with lisinopril, simvastatin and NTG. He had no other medical problems before admission.

On the morning of postoperative day 5, M.K. complains of chills and has a spiking fever to 39.4°C (normal, 37°C). Physical findings include a BP of 98/60 mm Hg (normal, 120/80 mm Hg), pulse 128 beats/min (normal, 80 beats/min), and a RR of 28 breaths/min (normal, 18 breaths/min). His urine output has

dropped to 25 mL/hr and bowel sounds are absent. The chest radiograph shows an enlarged heart with bilateral pulmonary infiltrates and right lower lobe atelectasis. M.K. has become confused and disoriented. ABGs on an inspiratory oxygen concentration (FiO_2) of 40% are as follows: PaO_2, 76 mm Hg (normal, 75 to 100 mm Hg); $PaCO_2$, 34 mm Hg (normal, 35 to 45 mm Hg); HCO_3^-, 15 mEq/L (normal, 23 to 29 mEq/L); and pH, 7.31 (normal, 7.35 to 7.45). M.K. has had increased bronchial secretions over the past 2 days. Pertinent laboratory values are SCr, 1.8 mg/dL (normal, 0.2 to 0.8 mg/dL); BUN, 32 mg/dL (normal, 10 to 20 mg/dL); and WBC count, 18,000 cells/mm³ (normal, 4,500 to 11,000 cells/mm³).

Urine, sputum, and blood samples are sent for culture and sensitivity. A fluid bolus of 500 mL normal saline is given. Arterial and pulmonary artery catheters are inserted revealing the following hemodynamic profile (M.K. weighs 70 kg and has a BSA of 1.7 m²): BP (S/D/M), 90/50/63 mm Hg; pulse, 122 beats/min; CO, 6 L/min (normal, 4 to 7 L/min); CI, 3.5 L/min per square meter (normal, 2.5 to 4.2 L/min per square meter); RAP, 8 mm Hg (normal, 2 to 6 mm Hg); PCWP, 12 mm Hg (normal, 5 to 12 mm Hg); SVR, 733 dyne · sec · cm⁻⁵ (normal, 800 to 1,440 dyne · sec · cm⁻⁵); DO_2, 438 mL/min per square meter (normal, 700 to 1,200 mL/min per square meter); and VO_2, 114 mL/min per square meter (normal, 200 to 400 mL/min per square meter). What hemodynamic and clinical features of M.K. are consistent with septic shock?

[SI units: SCr, 135 μmol/L (normal, 15 to 61); BUN, 22.72 mmol/L (normal, 7.1 to 14.3); WBC count, 18 10⁹/L (normal, 4.5 to 11); HCO_3^-, 15 mmol/L (normal, 23 to 29)]

Hemodynamic signs consistent with septic shock include hypotension, tachycardia, elevated CO, low SVR, and a low PCWP. Even though the absolute value for CO is high or at the upper limits of the normal range in septic shock, it is inadequate to maintain a BP that will perfuse the essential organs in the face of a decreased SVR, evidenced by the low oxygen delivery and consumption. M.K. has a metabolic acidosis (pH 7.31 with a $PaCO_2$ 30 mm Hg, HCO_3^- 15 mEq/L), indicating anaerobic metabolism most likely due to decreased perfusion causing lactic acidosis, and a CO that is inadequate to meet the oxygen requirements of the tissues.

Other features consistent with septic shock in M.K. include worsening pulmonary function as indicated by his ABGs; declining urine output and altered sensorium, indicating decreased renal and cerebral perfusion; a rising WBC count; and a spiking fever.

Therapeutic Approach

The management of septic shock is directed toward three primary areas: (1) eradication of the source of infection, (2) hemodynamic support and control of tissue hypoxia, and (3) inhibition or attenuation of the initiators and mediators of sepsis.

Eradicating the Source of Infection

40. What factors should be considered in determining antimicrobial therapy in septic shock? What are the potential sources of infection in M.K.?

Systemic infection caused by either aerobic or anaerobic bacteria is the leading cause of septic shock. Fungal, mycobacterial, rickettsial, protozoal, or viral infections may also be encountered. Among sepsis syndromes caused by aerobic bacteria, Gram-negative organisms (e.g., *Enterobacteriaceae, Pseudomonas,* and *Haemophilus,* in decreasing order of frequency) are implicated slightly more often than Gram-positive bacteria (e.g., *Staphylococcus aureus, Staphylococcus* coagulase negative, *Streptococcus,* and *Enterococcus,* from highest to lowest frequency). However, even these trends vary, depending on the site of infection. For example, when an organism can actually be cultured in the blood, slightly more Gram-positive infections (35% to 40%) than Gram-negative infections (30% to 35%) are found. In non-bloodstream infections (e.g., respiratory tract, genitourinary system, and the abdomen, in descending order of frequency) 40% to 45% can be attributed to Gram-negative organisms and 20% to 25% are caused by Gram-positive organisms.[19] Polymicrobial infections make up the next largest group, followed by fungi, anaerobes, and others. In 10% to 30% of sepsis syndrome cases, no organisms can be isolated. Careful consideration of the patient's history and clinical presentation often reveals the most likely cause.

Eradicating the source of infection involves the early administration of antimicrobial therapy, and if indicated, surgical drainage. The use of an appropriate antibiotic regimen is associated with a significant increase in survival. In one large retrospective study, shock and mortality rates were reduced by 50%.[89] The selection of antibiotics should take into account the presumed site of infection; whether the infection is community- or hospital-acquired; recent invasive procedures, manipulations, or surgery; any predisposing conditions; and the likelihood of drug resistance. Ideally, the primary source of the infection can be determined and therapy specifically tailored to the most likely organisms. However, if the source of infection is unclear, early institution of broad-spectrum antibiotics is generally recommended while awaiting culture results. Empirical therapy is indicated, given a >50% mortality rate caused by Gram-negative sepsis within the first 2 days of illness and the increasing frequency of polymicrobial infections.[89] A combination of two antibiotics is suggested to provide for possible synergy and to reduce the emergence of resistant organisms. Recommended empiric regimens typically include an aminoglycoside plus a third-generation cephalosporin or a similar broad-spectrum agent to cover for Gram-positive cocci, aerobic Gram-negative bacilli, and anaerobes (Also see Chapter 56, Principles of Infectious Diseases).

M.K. has several potential sources of sepsis. The first is hospital-acquired pneumonia. M.K. has been intubated for 5 days, infiltrates appear on chest radiograph, and sputum production has increased over the past 2 days. Abdominal abscess or recurrent bowel ischemia also should be considered because bowel sounds are absent. Although no complaints of abdominal tenderness have been elicited, surgical exploration may be necessary. Other potential sources for infection include the urinary tract because M.K. has had an indwelling Foley catheter in place since admission. All IV catheters should be changed if possible.

Clindamycin is discontinued and imipenem and vancomycin are added to broaden M.K.'s antibiotic coverage. Imipenem should adequately cover nosocomial Gram negative pathogens such as *Pseudomonas aeruginosa* and *Acinetobacter baumannii* as well as abdominal anaerobic organisms, and vancomycin will cover *S. aureus* from possible IV contamination as well as potential Staphylococcal pneumonia. Antimicrobial therapy is adjusted once cultures are finalized.

Initial Stabilization

41. **What are the immediate goals of therapy in M.K.? How can they be achieved and assessed?**

The goals in treating septic shock, in addition to eradicating the precipitating infection, are to optimize the delivery of oxygen to the tissues and to control abnormal use of oxygen and anaerobic metabolism by reducing the tissue oxygen demand. Tissue injury is widespread during sepsis, most likely because of vascular endothelial injury with fluid extravasation and microthromboses which decrease oxygen and substrate utilization by the affected tissues. The mainstay of therapy is volume expansion to increase intravascular volume, enhance CO, and ultimately delay associated development of refractory tissue hypoxia. The therapeutic goals used for hemodynamic resuscitation are controversial. The issue is whether therapy should be directed to physiologic end points of tissue perfusion or clinical end points, such as BP, CO, and urine output. The physiologic end points include clearance of blood lactate concentrations, normalization of splanchnic perfusion, elevation to supranormal Do_2 and Vo_2, and increased CI. In most studies, interventions that have looked at the use of supranormal Do_2, Vo_2, and CI as end points in treatment have yielded inconsistent results and controversy. Although definitive evidence is lacking, a combination of these physiologic and clinical end points should be used to guide therapy.[90,91] Fluids are the mainstay of treatment because increasing CO will improve capillary circulation and tissue oxygenation by maintaining sufficient intravascular volume. If fluids do not correct the hypoxia or if filling pressures are increased, the sequential addition of inotropes and vasopressors is indicated.

Blood transfusions should be used if the hematocrit is below 21% unless there is an active source of bleeding or if there is a history of cardiac disease. Crystalloids (with electrolytes to correct imbalances) should be initiated to maintain the CI goal as well as a MAP of 65 mm Hg or a SBP of 90 mm Hg. The MAP is a better reflection of systemic arterial pressure because it considers the diastolic pressure, which is an essential component of blood flow. Although MAP and BP are not absolute measures of blood flow to all vital organs, these pressures are considered the therapeutic end points that will sustain myocardial and cerebral perfusion. After optimization with fluid therapy to a PCWP of 18 mm Hg, inotropic and vasopressor agents are indicated if the patient remains hypotensive with a low CI and if signs of inadequate tissue perfusion persist.

Continued fluid challenges to increase preload in M.K. must be approached cautiously, however, for several reasons. M.K. has a history of ischemic heart disease, and ongoing evidence suggestive of pneumonia, all of which could be made worse by overly aggressive fluid boluses. In addition, patients in septic shock are prone to developing noncardiogenic pulmonary edema or ARDS, which can cause severe deterioration in pulmonary function. Therefore, fluid boluses of no more than 500 mL normal saline over 10 to 15 minutes should be given with ongoing monitoring to determine the PCWP at which CO is maximal. This approach will avoid excessive PCWPs beyond which CO is no longer increased, thereby reducing the potential for pulmonary edema formation.

In summary, the immediate goal of therapy is to maximize oxygen delivery to the tissues. Fluid resuscitation is the mainstay of therapy and improves oxygen delivery by increasing CO; however, inotropic and vasopressor agents are often required for additional cardiovascular support. A favorable response to immediate resuscitative efforts will be reflected by a reversal or halt in the progression of the metabolic acidosis, improved sensorium, and increased urine output. In M.K., surgical evaluation for an ongoing or new abdominal process and selection of appropriate antibiotics while maintaining hemodynamic support are the clinical goals of therapy.

Oxygen Delivery
Do_2 AND Vo_2

42. **Would increasing M.K.'s oxygen delivery and consumption help improve outcome?**

The theory that improving the Do_2 and Vo_2 levels can improve survival in critically ill and septic patients has led to several clinical studies and much controversy. Critically ill patients with normal or supranormal Do_2 are more likely to survive and less likely to progress to MODS than those patients with less-than-normal Do_2. Furthermore, impaired oxygen extraction or reduced Vo_2 is associated with increased mortality. These observations have led to many randomized controlled trials aimed at improving Do_2. The analysis shows a decreased mortality in a subset of patients who achieved and maintained supranormal Do_2. Nevertheless, the relationship between treatments that improve Do_2 and outcomes has not been clearly demonstrated. Instead, it is likely that patients who survive are intrinsically or physiologically better able to respond to the manipulations rather than the result of the manipulations that account for the improvement.[92]

Hayes and colleagues[93] studied the relationship between oxygen transport patterns and outcomes in patients with sepsis syndrome or septic shock. They showed that survivors of septic shock responded with greater increases in CI, LVSWI, and Do_2, and had lower lactate concentrations. In nonsurvivors, the CI and Do_2 also increased, but they had a decrease in oxygen extraction and failed to increase Vo_2. In contrast, the survivors showed increases in Do_2 accompanied by significant increases in Vo_2. These observations suggest that patients who die from septic shock cannot increase Vo_2 and reverse tissue hypoxia. This is related to an impairment in oxygen extraction or an inability to increase aerobic metabolism, even when the oxygen supply is increased.[93] The study also suggested that survival is associated with the patient's ability to increase myocardial performance and Do_2. The nonsurvivors failed to augment cardiac function to survival levels even with high dosages of inotropic support, suggesting that these patients had a significant degree of myocardial depression. The Third European Consensus Conference in Intensive Care Medicine concluded, however, that timely resuscitation and achievement of normal hemodynamics is essential, but aggressive attempts to increase Do_2 to supranormal values in all critically ill patients are unwarranted.[92]

Hemodynamic Management
FLUID THERAPY VERSUS INOTROPIC SUPPORT

43. M.K. is given 2 500-mL fluid boluses, and norepinephrine is begun at a rate of 0.02 μg/kg per minute. Over the next 2 hours, he receives 3 L of fluid in boluses and the dopamine is increased to 0.1 μg/kg per minute to maintain his BP. Signs of pulmonary edema have become more prominent. M.K. has the following hemodynamic profile (previous values in parentheses): BP (S/D/M), 94/46/62 mm Hg (90/50/63); pulse, 124 beats/min (122); CO, 7.0 L/min (6); CI, 3.2 L/min per square meter (3.5); RAP, 13 mm Hg (8); PCWP, 18 mm Hg (12); SVR, 560 dyne · sec · cm^{-5} (733); urine output, 15 mL/hr; Pao_2, 62 mm Hg (76); $Paco_2$, 38 mm Hg (34); HCO_3^-, 19 mEq/L (15); pH, 7.30 (7.31); DO_2, 445 mL/min (438); VO_2, 118 mL/min (114); and PEEP, 5 cm H_2O. Which of the following therapeutic considerations would be reasonable for M.K. at this time: additional fluid boluses, an increase in the norepinephrine infusion rate, or initiation of a different vasopressor?

M.K. continues to be hypotensive despite a PCWP of 18 mm Hg and a norepinephrine infusion rate of 0.1 μg/kg/min. The goals of therapy remain the same (i.e., maximize arterial oxygen content and oxygen delivery to reverse cellular anaerobic metabolism).

M.K.'s Pao_2 of 62 mm Hg correlates with an oxygen-hemoglobin saturation of approximately 90%, which should provide an adequate arterial oxygen content. However, oxygen delivery still may be inadequate because the CI is <3.5 L/min per square meter, and DO_2 and VO_2 have not reached normal levels. In addition, decreased oxygen use can contribute to the continued acidosis. Thus, further attempts to enhance the CI and hence, oxygen delivery, are appropriate. However, M.K. has worsening signs of pulmonary edema and a history of cardiovascular disease that will influence the choice of therapeutic options.

Although fluid administration is the mainstay of therapy in septic shock, the elevation of M.K.'s PCWP to 18 mm Hg without a significant increase in CO suggests that an optimal PCWP has been reached. Therefore, additional fluid therapy to maintain his BP may worsen his pulmonary edema and further compromise his pulmonary gas exchange. A plot of CO versus the PCWP (ventricular function curve) would provide a more accurate assessment of the PCWP at which CO is maximal. Additional fluid boluses at this time should be used only to maintain the current level of intravascular volume status.

Vasopressors
NOREPINEPHRINE

When fluid therapy fails to maintain a satisfactory MAP despite an elevated CO, the use of a vasopressor should be considered. Norepinephrine is predominantly an α-adrenergic agonist (see Table 22-7) and is frequently used as an adjunct to therapy when inotropic agents alone are unsuccessful. Because there has been concern that excessive vasoconstriction might cause reflex decreases in CO and hypoperfusion of vital organs, the use of norepinephrine has often been limited to end-stage shock. However, studies indicate that norepinephrine alone, or in combination with inotropic agents can be beneficial in the management of septic shock.[94]

Martin and colleagues compared the ability of dopamine and norepinephrine to reverse hemodynamic and metabolic abnormalities of hyperdynamic shock.[95] They prospectively randomized 32 volume-resuscitated patients with hyperdynamic sepsis to receive either dopamine (2.5 to 20 μg/kg/min) or norepinephrine (0.5 to 5 μg/kg/min) to achieve and maintain normal hemodynamic and oxygen transport parameters for at least 6 hours. If goals were not achieved with one agent, the other agent was added. With the use of dopamine, 31% of patients met the following therapeutic goals: SVRI >1,100 dynes · sec · cm^{-5}/m^2 or mean SBP 80 mm Hg; CI 4 L/min per square meter; oxygen delivery >550 mL/min per square meter; and oxygen uptake >150 mL/min per square meter. In contrast 93% of patients treated with norepinephrine met these goals. Of the patients who did not respond to dopamine, 91% achieved the goals with the addition of norepinephrine. In this study, norepinephrine was found to be superior to dopamine, with improvement in arterial BP, urine flow, oxygen delivery and consumption, and lactate levels.

In a similar study of patients in whom previous therapy with plasma volume expansion and dopamine or dobutamine had failed, norepinephrine reversed hypotension and significantly increased MAP, SVR, and urine output.[94] The CI was increased, albeit insignificantly, in 7 of 10 patients, presumably because of stimulation of cardiac β-receptors. By limiting the SVRI to 700 dyne · sec · cm^{-5}/m^2, the investigators were able to prevent excessive vasoconstriction and promote an increased perfusion pressure to vital organs as reflected by an improved urine flow. Oxygen delivery and consumption were measured in 6 of 10 patients with variable results. Although no patient died of refractory hypotension, 4 of 10 patients died of progressive hypoxia, leading the authors to conclude that regardless of the catecholamines used, the ultimate goal of therapy should be to maximize oxygen delivery and consumption.

PHENYLEPHRINE

Occasionally, patients may respond to epinephrine or phenylephrine when other catecholamines have failed, although neither of these agents is considered to be first-line therapy. Epinephrine stimulates α-, β$_1$-, and β$_2$-adrenergic receptors (see Table 22-7). CO is augmented via increased contractility and HR, with the contribution of each being highly variable. Blood vessels in the kidney, skin, and mucosa constrict in response to α-adrenergic stimulation, while vessels in the skeletal muscle vasodilate because of β$_2$-effects. A biphasic response in SVR is observed with increasing doses as β$_2$-receptors are activated at the lower range, while β$_1$-receptors are stimulated at higher levels. The improvement in CO, therefore, may be negated by an increase in afterload at higher dosages.

Phenylephrine is a pure α-adrenergic agonist (see Table 22-7) and thus increases systolic, diastolic, and mean arterial pressures through vasoconstriction. Reflex bradycardia may occur secondarily because of the absence of β-adrenergic effects. The increase in afterload, while increasing myocardial oxygen consumption, correspondingly increases coronary blood flow because of increased perfusion pressure and autoregulation. Therefore, in patients with myocardial hypoxia, or in those experiencing atrial or ventricular arrhythmias, phenylephrine can be beneficial because it has minimal direct cardiac effects. In situations in which the CO is decreased, however, phenylephrine may be detrimental. This occurs because preload is reduced from interstitial fluid losses as a result of increased capillary hydrostatic pressure effects. This response, in addition to the reflex bradycardia may significantly impair CO (see Table 22-7).

VASOPRESSIN

Catecholamines have been the mainstay of treatment to support BP in septic patients once adequate fluid resuscitation has been achieved. Sepsis, however, can cause a decrease in responsiveness to catecholamines resulting in refractory hypotension, possibly due to downregulation of adrenergic receptors. Thus, other avenues of supportive treatment have been researched. It has been recently discovered that septic patients exhibit an increased sensitivity to vasopressin. Vasopressin is an endogenous hormone that has very little effect on BP under normal conditions, but becomes very important in maintaining BP when the baroreflex is impaired, such as in shock states. Vasopressin's direct vasoconstricting actions are mediated by the vascular V_1-receptors coupled to phospholipase C.[96,97] When these receptors are activated, calcium is released from the sarcoplasmic reticulum in smooth muscle cells leading to vasoconstriction. One study found that vasopressin levels were very low (3.1 pg/mL) in septic patients, while patients in cardiogenic shock displayed an appropriate increase in vasopressin release (22.7 pg/mL) for the degree of hypotension ($P < 0.001$).[98] The same investigators showed that a low-dose continuous IV infusion of vasopressin at 0.04U/min in 19 patients with septic shock made a statistically significant increase in vasopressin levels, systolic arterial pressure, and systemic vascular resistance when added to pre-existing catecholamine treatment. Six of ten patients were able to maintain BP on vasopressin alone. Stopping the vasopressin infusion resulted in decreases of BP to pretreatment levels, and re-institution of the infusion increased BP within minutes. It is presumed that vasopressin secretion is impaired versus enhanced vasopressin metabolism, but it is not entirely clear why this occurs. Most likely it is a combination of a deficient baroreflex-mediated secretion of vasopressin, impaired sympathetic function, and potentially depletion of the secretory stores of vasopressin.

Other studies support the vasopressor effects of vasopressin in septic patients already on catecholamines with persistent hypotension and also show a vasopressor sparing effect on catecholamines. The most recent double-blind, randomized trial showed that norepinephrine infusion could be decreased by the addition of vasopressin administration.[99] Vasopressin was compared to norepinephrine since it has already been determined that vasopressin is efficacious as a vasopressor compared to placebo. In this study, patients already receiving norepinephrine were randomized to either continue norepinephrine (titrated up to a maximum of 16 µg/min) or be started on vasopressin (titrated to a maximum dose of 0.08 units/min). The prestudy norepinephrine was then titrated down to maintain a MAP determined by the attending intensive care physician over a four hour period. The norepinephrine treatment group after titration went from a median prestudy norepinephrine infusion of 20.0 µg/min to 17.0 µg/min, and the vasopressin treatment group went from a median prestudy norepinephrine infusion of 25.0 µg/min to 5.3 µg/min ($P < 0.001$). Another statistically significant finding from this study was that the urine output increased in the vasopressin group (median, 32.5 to 65 mL/hr) compared to the norepinephrine group (median, 25 to 15 mL/hr) ($P < 0.05$), and the creatinine clearance improved as well in the vasopressin group ($P < 0.05$). It seems reasonable at this point to use vasopressin in patients with septic shock who are on high doses of catecholamines or those who need further vasopressor support. Further studies are needed to determine if treatment with vasopressin confers a mortality benefit.

M.K. has decreased MAP's despite the addition and increased titration of norepinephrine. Since it has been found that patients in septic shock have decreased endogenous levels of vasopressin, it would be reasonable to add vasopressin at 0.04 U/min to the prior dopamine infusion to increase the MAP and renal perfusion.

Inotropic Agents

Although the use of inotropic agents is well established, controlled comparative studies have not clearly determined which agent, or combination of agents, are most useful in the management of septic shock. However, because differences among the inotropic agents are significant, selection of the most appropriate drug should be guided by careful consideration of the patient's hemodynamic status.

DOPAMINE

Dopamine has frequently been the initial pharmacologic agent chosen for the treatment of septic shock. If the mean arterial pressure is low with a depressed CO and a low SVR, dopamine is an appropriate choice because its combined α-adrenergic vasoconstrictive actions and β-adrenergic inotropic effects will increase SVR and CO, thereby effectively raising the mean arterial pressure. In situations in which the PCWP is elevated or in patients with decreased ventricular compliance, the use of dopamine may be limited because it significantly increases venous return and ventricular filling pressure. In addition, dopamine increases shunting of pulmonary blood flow, leading to a decline in PaO_2. This effect may worsen hypoxemia in patients with pneumonia or ARDS.

DOBUTAMINE

Dobutamine is often advocated as the secondary inotropic agent in the management of septic shock, particularly in patients with low CO and high filling pressures. Dobutamine produces a larger increase in CO than dopamine, but also lowers SVR. In contrast to dopamine, dobutamine lowers PCWP, decreases myocardial oxygen consumption, and causes less pulmonary shunting. Because dobutamine may lower ventricular filling pressure, volume status must be monitored closely to avoid the development of hypotension and reduced MAP. Fluids should be administered as needed to maintain the PCWP at maximum tolerated levels of 16 to 18 mm Hg. With the administration of greater amounts of fluid, CO, oxygen delivery, and systemic oxygen consumption are significantly increased. Dobutamine does increase Do_2 and CI when given concurrently with or after volume resuscitation. Decreases in PaO_2 and increases in venous PO_2, as well as adverse effects on myocardium, may be evident at higher dosages (>6 µg/kg per min).[100]

Combinations of vasopressors and inotropes can also be used to achieve desired hemodynamic parameters. Since gastrointestinal perfusion can be compromised due to the vasoconstricting effects of catecholamines and may play a role in the pathogenesis of multiple organ dysfunction, the combination of norepinephrine and dobutamine has been studied to determine if there is an advantage over using norepinephrine alone and/or epinephrine alone.[101–103] One prospective study randomized thirty patients with a MAP ≤60 mm Hg despite adequate fluid resuscitation and treatment with dopamine at 20 µg/kg/min.[101] Subjects received either a constant infusion of dobutamine (5 µg/kg/min) plus norepinephrine or epinephrine monotherapy titrated to a MAP >80 mm Hg. The variables to be studied were the MAP, metabolic effects as evidenced by lactate and pyruvate concentrations, and splanchnic perfusion measured by gastric pH (pH_i) and partial pressure of carbon dioxide (PCO_2) gap. All patients achieved a MAP >80 mm Hg, but the norepinephrine-dobutamine group had decreased lactate levels at 6 hours, while the lactate levels increased in the epinephrine group. Lactic acidosis in the epinephrine group, however, returned to normal after 24 hours. The pH_i decreased and PCO_2 gap increased in the epinephrine group, but returned to normal in the norepinephrine-dobutamine group. The changes associated with epinephrine also eventually returned to normal within 24 hours. These effects were hypothesized to result from the β_2-adrenergic agonist effects which might counteract the detrimental splanchnic effects of norepinephrine. This study showed that both therapies, norepinephrine plus dobutamine and epinephrine monotherapy, were equally effective at achieving hemodynamic goals, but that treatment with epinephrine alone could worsen splanchnic oxygen utilization and potentially lead to ischemic injury.

Other investigators found that epinephrine alone and norepinephrine plus dobutamine significantly increased gastric mucosal perfusion compared to norepinephrine alone.[102] Treatment with norepinephrine-dobutamine was associated with a trend toward higher gastric perfusion compared to epinephrine, but was not statistically significant.

Most recently, the study by Seguin and colleagues[103] compared the same regimen of norepinephrine-dobutamine to epinephrine in patients with septic shock. This study produced results contradictory to the results in the previous two studies. Epinephrine produced statistically significant increases in gastric mucosal blood flow, and tended to increase cardiac index and oxygen transport more than dobutamine-norepinephrine. These results were attributed to the predominant β_1 effect that increased CI, and the attenuation of the α effects via stimulation of the β_2 receptors by epinephrine at the dosage range used. The first two studies used higher dosages of epinephrine which would cause more stimulation of the α receptors and thus would not increase CI to the same extent. Currently, it is unknown whether a specific catecholamine regimen provides a significant benefit over others. There is conflicting data about which vasopressor can increase gastric perfusion and whether this increase can alter progression to organ dysfunction.

44. **Given M.K.'s history of cardiovascular disease, what considerations must be accounted for before initiating a vasopressor agent? Outline an overall approach to maintaining adequate hemodynamic status.**

M.K. has a history of coronary artery disease and is prone to myocardial ischemia. Therefore, a careful balance must be achieved between myocardial oxygen consumption and coronary perfusion pressure. Further attempts to optimize MAP and CI with norepinephrine alone could increase myocardial oxygen consumption and precipitate ischemia. The use of a vasopressor will increase afterload and hence myocardial oxygen consumption. However, if elevations in SVR are limited to produce an adequate MAP without excessive vasoconstriction, the increase in perfusion pressure might offset the increase in myocardial oxygen consumption.

Evidence suggests that the goal of therapy in managing patients with septic shock, or any form of shock for that matter, is not to simply normalize BP, but to optimize oxygen delivery and consumption. Once anemia and hypoxia have been corrected, CO becomes the remaining parameter that can be adjusted to increase oxygen supply. Raising arterial BP and CO with inotropic agents or vasopressors before restoring adequate blood volume actually can worsen tissue perfusion. Therefore, the selection of an inotropic agent must take into consideration the patient's current hemodynamic status and the individual properties of those agents that will most effectively maintain or increase the mean arterial pressure and CO. In many instances, because of individual variability and response, more than one inotropic agent or addition of a vasopressor is required to achieve these end points.

It is important to realize that the response to exogenous catecholamines in patients with septic shock is highly variable and a successful regimen in one patient may be unsuccessful in another. In addition, septic patients often require infusion rates in the moderate-to-high range. Therefore, the goal is to use one or more agents at the dosages necessary to achieve the desired end points without unduly compromising the patient's status. The use of catecholamines, however, is only a stabilizing measure. Strict attention to all other physiologic parameters—as well as nutritional support, antibiotic modification, and ongoing surgical intervention—cannot be overemphasized.

Other Therapies

Therapies directed against the initiators and mediators of sepsis are currently the focus of intense investigation. As previously discussed, numerous exogenous and endogenous substances are involved in the pathogenesis of sepsis. Strategies under development include antioxidants and free radical scavengers, antiendotoxin therapy, inhibition of leukocytes, secondary mediators (i.e., TNF-α, IL-1, cytokine pathway), coagulation and arachidonic acid metabolites, complement and NO. Although several experimental therapies hold considerable promise for the future, controlled human data are still lacking.

CORTICOSTEROIDS

45. **What is the rationale for the use of steroids in the treatment of septic shock, and is there evidence to support its use?**

The use of steroids in sepsis and septic shock has been a controversial topic for many years. It was originally proposed as a treatment option due to its antiinflammatory properties with the hopes of attenuating the body's response to infection. More recently it has been shown that critically ill patients exhibit impaired cortisol secretion due to a relative adrenocortical insufficiency and it is suspected that these patients display a glucocorticoid peripheral resistance syndrome. Almost 50% of patients with septic shock exhibit relative adrenal insufficiency defined as a maximal change in cortisol level of less than 9 μg/dL after a 250 μg intravenous dose of corticotropin.[104]

Several clinical trials have been performed over the past few decades with varying results and meta-analyses have recommended discontinuation of high-dose corticosteroid therapy due to detrimental outcomes.[105,106] Endpoints that have been studied include time to reversal of septic shock (defined by cessation of vasopressor support) and mortality. However, older trials used different definitions of septic shock and the timing and dosing of steroids were highly variable. Most recently, the randomized, double-blind, placebo-controlled trial by Annane and colleagues[107] showed a mortality benefit after 28 days associated with the use of low doses of hydrocortisone and fludrocortisone in patients with relative adrenocortical insufficiency (nonresponders to corticotropin) and septic shock. Patients had to be randomized within 3 hours of the onset of shock and were included in the study if they met SIRS criteria and were on more than 5 μg/kg of body weight of dopamine or being treated with epinephrine or norepinephrine. The treatment group received hydrocortisone 50 mg IV Q 6 hr and fludrocortisone 50 μg per nasogastric tube daily for 7 days. All patients received a 250 μg intravenous corticotropin test before treatment with levels drawn 30 minutes and 60 minutes after the test. Relative adrenocortical insufficiency was defined as a response of 9 μg/dL or less (nonresponders). It was found that in nonresponders, 63% of the placebo group died, whereas 53% of the corticosteroid group died ($P = 0.02$). Time to cessation of vasopressor support was also shortened by the use of steroids in the treatment group compared to placebo in the nonresponders. Responders did not show any benefit or detriment due to the use of corticosteroids. Therefore, this study suggests the use of corticosteroids in vasopressor-dependent septic shock directly after the corticotropin stimulation test. Once the results of the test are available, therapy can be altered appropriately.

A corticotropin stimulation test should be administered to MK and hydrocortisone 100 mg IV TID plus fludrocortisone 50 μg PFT QD should be started after the stimulation test. Treatment can be discontinued if the results of the stimulation test show that MK is not adrenally insufficient.

DROTECOGIN α

46. **Is M.K. a candidate for recombinant activated protein C? Is there any evidence to support its use in septic shock, and what are the major risks associated with its use?**

Activated protein C (APC) is an endogenous protein that acts as one of the regulators of the coagulation cascade and also interrupts the amplification cycle of inflammation.[21] Protein C is the inactive precursor to APC, and conversion to the active form requires thrombin to complex with thrombomodulin. APC enhances fibrinolysis and has potent inhibitory effects on thrombin, which possesses thrombotic as well as inflammatory effects. Other antiinflammatory effects of APC stem from suppression of TNF-α, IL-6, and IL-1β production.

Patients in septic shock develop microvascular thrombosis which leads to organ hypoperfusion, cell dysfunction, multiple organ dysfunction, and death. The systemic response to infection activates the coagulation pathway leading to the generation of thrombin and deposition of fibrin as well as initiating an inflammatory reaction via activation of cytokines. Adult and pediatric septic patients have low levels of protein C and that there is a poor outcome for those patients with the lowest levels.[108] The deficiency in protein C is probably due to enhanced degradation as well as impaired synthesis of protein C. It is also apparent that patients in septic shock exhibit lower levels of thrombomodulin, the protein necessary for the conversion of protein C to activated protein C. Thus, the use of APC would counter the anticoagulant deficiency as well as suppress the inflammatory reaction that would normally take place due to the infection.

The Protein C Worldwide Evaluation in Severe Sepsis (PROWESS)[109] trial is the only phase 3 clinical trial that was performed to test the safety and efficacy of drotecogin α (recombinant APC). It was a randomized, double-blind, placebo-controlled, multicenter trial that was stopped early since there was a statistically significant difference in the primary endpoint, 28-day all-cause mortality, before enrollment was complete. Patients were included in the study if there was a known or suspected infection plus three or more signs of systemic inflammation and at least one organ/system dysfunction due to sepsis. Patients also had to begin treatment of drotecogin α at 24 μg/kg/hr for 96 hours within 24 hours of meeting inclusion criteria. The list of exclusion criteria was rather extensive to ensure that patients who were at higher risk for bleeding did not participate in the trial. Exclusion criteria included conditions that increased the risk of bleeding (gastrointestinal bleeding within 6 weeks, severe head trauma, evidence of active bleeding postoperatively), a known deep venous thrombosis or hypercoagulable condition, acute pancreatitis without an established source of infection, chronic liver disease or chronic renal failure, platelet count <30,000/mm³, and immunosuppressive disorders. There was no standardized protocol for the critical care provided to the patient (e.g. antibiotics, vasopressors, inotropes). D-dimer, IL-6, and protein C levels were measured and it was determined that approximately 80% of all patients had protein C deficiency (protein C <81%; normal, 81% to 173%). Treatment with APC reduced D-dimer and IL-6 levels, which indicates the attenuation of the procoagulant and inflammatory effects of sepsis, respectively. Treatment with drotecogin α was associated with a 6.1% absolute reduction in mortality at 28 days after the start of infusion ($P = 0.005$) and a decrease in the relative risk of death by 19.4%. The incidence of serious bleeding was higher in the APC group (3.5% versus 2.0%), almost reaching statistical significance ($P = 0.06$). Serious bleeding was defined as any intracranial hemorrhage, any life-threatening bleeding, any bleeding event classified as serious by the investigator, or any bleeding that required the administration of 3 units of packed red cells on two consecutive days. In both placebo and treatment groups, bleeding tended to be in patients who had an identifiable predisposition to bleeding.

M.K. meets the criteria for severe sepsis since he meets 3 of the requirements for SIRS (WBC = 18,000 cells/mm³; use of mechanical ventilation; HR > 90 beats/min) and has at least one dysfunctional organ/system since he requires vasopressor support. He also has several potential sources of infection with pulmonary infiltrates and increased secretions, and the formation of an abdominal abscess is always a possibility. His surgery was 5 days before he decompensated, so his bleeding risk should be minimal; however, the patient should be closely monitored. The cost of APC is also quite substantial: approximately $7,000 for a 70-kg person for 96 hours. M.K. is a candidate for APC use; however, the risks need to be carefully assessed since its use could lead to devastating adverse events. Because of this, the formation of institutional guidelines to determine the patient population in which this drug can be more safely administered is highly recommended.

47. What other treatment options are under research for septic shock?

ANTIENDOTOXIN THERAPIES

Because endotoxin is the initiator of the inflammatory cascade of Gram-negative sepsis, extensive research has been devoted to development and study of antibodies against the core lipid-A portion of endotoxin, which possesses most of the biologic activity.

Monoclonal antibodies to TNF-α (anti-TNF-Mab) confer significant protection in various animal models of septic shock induced by endotoxin, Gram-negative, or Gram-positive bacteremia. Investigations into anti-TNF antibodies prompted a large controlled clinical trial, by the INTERSEPT study group.[110] The results showed no difference in 28-day mortality rates between groups, and patients in the nonshock group derived no benefit. Research is still currently under way to determine whether a particular patient population will benefit with this therapy.

Another approach to blocking the effects of TNF involves the use of soluble TNF receptors, which bind to and inactivate TNF before it interacts with its cellular receptor. Although effective in primate models of sepsis, a clinical trial examining escalating doses of soluble TNF receptor in patients with sepsis syndrome revealed an increase in mortality in patients receiving higher dosages of the receptor as compared with lower-dose therapy and placebo.[111]

Continuous hemofiltration is a technique that removes proinflammatory mediators, and has potential for treatment of septic patients. The use of adsorbents in hemoperfusion columns aids in the removal of toxic compounds from the circulatory system. Experimental data show that TNF-α, IL-1, IL-6, IL-8, and endotoxin can be removed from the circulation of septic patients by continuous hemofiltration.[112,113] Many animal studies show that hemofiltration improves hemodynamic indices and human data are promising. However, no controlled, randomized clinical trials have evaluated continuous hemofiltration.

Antithrombin III (AT III) is a potent inhibitor of thrombin activity. Apart from its better known function as a regulator of the coagulation cascade, this agent also may have a direct cytokine modulation function, arresting many of the secondary sequelae of septic shock. One study showed no significant mortality benefit at 28 days and AT III was associated with a statistically significant increase in bleeding complications, particularly in those patients receiving any form of heparin.[114]

Pyridoxylated hemoglobin polyoxyethylene (PHP) is a nitric oxide synthase inhibitor that is being evaluated for the treatment of acute hypotension in patients with septic shock. Preliminary studies show an increase in SVR, decreased use of vasopressors, and maintenance of MAP.[21]

GLOSSARY

Afterload: Ventricular wall tension developed during contraction. Determined by the resistance or impedance the ventricle must overcome to eject end-diastolic volume. Left ventricular afterload is determined primarily by systemic vascular resistance; right ventricular afterload is determined primarily by pulmonary vascular resistance.

Arterial pressure (AP): Pressure in the central arterial bed; determined by cardiac output and systemic vascular resistance.

Body surface area (BSA): Average = 1.7 m².

Cardiac index (CI): Cardiac output per square meter of body surface area (BSA).

Cardiac output (CO): Amount of blood ejected from the left ventricle per minute; determined by stroke volume and heart rate. $CO = SV \times HR$.

Central venous pressure (CVP)—also called right atrial pressure (RAP): Measures mean pressure in right atrium and reflects right ventricular filling pressure. Primarily determined by venous return to the heart.

Compliance: Distensibility of the relaxed ventricle or stiffness of the myocardial wall.

Contractility: The inotropic state of the myocardium; affects stroke volume and cardiac output independently of preload and afterload.

Heart rate (HR): Number of myocardial contractions per minute; regulated by autonomic nervous system. An increase or decrease alters cardiac output in same direction.

Left ventricular stroke work index (LVSWI): Amount of work the left ventricle exerts during systole; adjusted for body surface area (BSA).

Oxygen consumption (VO₂): The amount of oxygen consumed by the body per unit time. The product of cardiac output and the difference between the arterial and venous concentrations of oxygen.

Oxygen delivery (DO₂): The amount of oxygen delivered by the body per unit time, the product of cardiac output and arterial oxygen concentration.

Perfusion pressure: The pressure gradient between the coronary arteries and the pressure in either the right atrium or left ventricle during diastole. A major determinant of coronary blood flow and oxygen supply to the heart.

Preload: End-diastolic fiber length before contraction; represented by ventricular volume (LVEDV); approximated by ventricular pressure (LVEDP) and pulmonary capillary wedge pressure (PCWP). Right ventricular preload is reflected by central venous pressure (CVP) or right arterial pressure (RAP).

Positive end-expiratory pressure (PEEP): The application of positive pressure at the end of the expiratory phase of respiration to improve oxygenation.

Pulmonary artery pressure (PAP): *Systolic (PAS):* Measures pulmonary artery pressure during systole; reflects pressure generated by the contraction of the right ventricle. *Diastolic (PAD):* Measures pulmonary artery pressure during diastole; reflects diastolic filling pressure in the left ventricle. May approximate pulmonary capillary wedge pressure (PCWP); normal gradient <5 mm Hg between PAD and PCWP.

Pulmonary capillary wedge pressure (PCWP): Measures pressure distal to the pulmonary artery; reflects left ventricular filling pressures. May optimally increase to 16 to

18 mm Hg in critically ill patients. Usually lower than or within 5 mm Hg of PAD.

Pulmonary vascular resistance (PVR): Measure of impedance or resistance within pulmonary vasculature that right ventricle must overcome during contraction; determines right ventricular afterload.

Stroke volume (SV): Amount of blood ejected from the ventricle with each systolic contraction. SV = CO/HR.

Stroke volume index (SVI): Stroke volume per square meter of body surface area (BSA).

Systemic vascular resistance (SVR): Measure of impedance applied by systemic vascular system to systolic effort of left ventricle; determined by autonomic nervous system and condition of vessels. Determinant of left ventricular afterload.

Systemic vascular resistance index (SVRI): Systemic vascular resistance adjusted for body surface area (BSA).

REFERENCES

1. Parillo JE. Approach to the patient with shock. In: Goldman L, Bennett JC, eds. Cecil Textbook of Medicine. Philadelphia: WB Saunders, 2000:496.
2. ACCP-SCCM Consensus Conference: definitions for sepsis and organ failure and guidelines for the use of innovative therapies in sepsis. Chest 1992;101:1644.
3. Bone RC. The pathogenesis of sepsis. Ann Intern Med 1991;115:457.
4. Barie PS. Advances in critical care monitoring. Arch Surg 1997;132:724.
5. Chaney JC, Derdak S. Minimally invasive hemodynamic monitoring for the intensivist: current and emerging technology. Crit Care Med 2002;30:2338.
6. Swan HJC et al. Catheterization of the heart in man with the use of a flow-directed balloon-tipped catheter. N Engl J Med 1970;283:447.
7. Connors AF Jr et al. The effectiveness of right heart catheterization in the initial care of critically ill patients. JAMA 1996;276:889.
8. Sandham JD et al. A randomized, controlled trial of the use of pulmonary-artery catheters in high-risk surgical patients. N Engl J Med 2003;348:66.
9. Boldt J. Clinical review: hemodynamic monitoring in the intensive care unit. Crit Care 2002;6:52.
10. Ganz W et al. A new technique for measurement of cardiac output by thermodilution in man. Am J Cardiol 1971;27:392.
11. Shoemaker WC. Oxygen transport and oxygen metabolism in shock and critical illness. Crit Care Clin 1996;12:939.
12. Hayes MA et al. Elevation of systemic oxygen delivery in the treatment of critically ill patients. N Engl J Med 1994;330:1717.
13. Gattinoni L et al. A trial of goal-oriented hemodynamic therapy in critically ill patients. N Engl J Med 1995;333:1025.
14. Shock. In: Advanced Trauma Life Support Program for Physicians, Instructor's Manual. Chicago: American College of Surgeons, 1997:101.
15. Goldberg RJ et al. Temporal trends in cardiogenic shock complicating acute myocardial infarction. N Engl J Med 1999;340:1162.
16. Barry WL, Sarembock IJ. Cardiogenic shock: therapy and prevention. Clin Cardiol 1998;21:72.
17. Rangel-Frausto MS et al. The natural history of the systemic inflammatory response syndrome (SIRS): a prospective study. JAMA 1995;273:117.
18. Centers for Disease Control and Prevention, National Center for Health Statistics. Mortality patterns—United States, 1990. Monthly Vital Stat Rep 1993;41:5.
19. Sands KE et al. Epidemiology of sepsis syndrome in 8 academic medical centers. JAMA 1997;278:234.
20. Angus D et al. Epidemiology of severe sepsis in the United States: analysis of incidence, outcome and associated costs of care. Crit Care Med 2001;29:1303.
21. Healy D. New and emerging therapies for sepsis. Ann Pharmacother 2002;36:648.
22. Hollenberg A et al. Practice parameters for hemodynamic support of sepsis in adult patients in sepsis. Crit Care Med 1999;27(3):639.
23. Cunnion RE, Parrillo JE. Myocardial dysfunction in sepsis. Crit Care Clin 1989;5:99.
24. Scalea TM et al. Resuscitation of multiple trauma and head injury: role of crystalloid fluids and inotropes. Crit Care Med 1994;20:1610.

25. Abou-Khalil B et al. Hemodynamic responses to shock in young trauma patients: need for invasive monitoring. Crit Care Med 1994;22:633.
26. Velanovich V. Crystalloids versus colloid fluid resuscitation: a meta-analysis of mortality. Surgery 1989;105:65.
27. Choi PT et al. Crystalloids vs colloids in fluid resuscitation: a systematic review. Crit Care Med 1999;27(1):200.
28. Bisonni RS et al. Colloids versus crystalloid in fluid resuscitation: an analysis of randomized controlled trials. J Fam Pract 1991;32:387.
29. Schierhout G, Roberts I. Fluid resuscitation with colloid or crystalloid solutions in critically ill patients: a systematic review of randomised trials. Br Med J 1998;316:961.
30. Alderson P et al. Human albumin solution for resuscitation and volume expansion in critically ill patients. The Cochrane Database of Systematic Reviews, Issue 1. 2001.
31. Wilkes M, Navickis R. Patient survival after human albumin administration. Ann Intern Med 2001;135:149.
32. Vermeulen LC et al. A paradigm for consensus. The University Hospital Consortium guidelines for the use of albumin, nonprotein colloid, and crystalloid solutions. Arch Intern Med 1995;155:373.
33. Bickell WH et al. Immediate versus delayed fluid resuscitation for hypotensive patients with penetrating torso injuries. N Engl J Med 1994;331:1105.
34. Jacobs LM. Timing of fluid resuscitation in trauma [Editorial]. N Engl J Med 1994;331:1153.
35. Wagner BK et al. Pharmacologic and clinical considerations in selecting crystalloid, colloidal, and oxygen-carrying resuscitation fluids, part 1. Clin Pharm 1993;12:335.
36. Almenoff PL et al. Prolongation of the half-life of lactate after maximal exercise in patients with hepatic dysfunction. Crit Care Med 1989;17:870.
37. McKnight CK et al. The effects of four different crystalloid bypass pump-priming fluids upon the metabolic response to cardiac operation. J Thoracic Cardiovasc Surg 1985;90:97.
38. Falk JL et al. Fluid resuscitation in traumatic hemorrhagic shock. Crit Care Clin 1992;8:323.
39. Imm A et al. Fluid resuscitation in circulatory shock. Crit Care Clin 1993;9:313.
40. Gould SA et al. Hypovolemic shock. Crit Care Clin 1993;2:239.
41. Holcroft JW et al. 3 per cent NaCl and 7.5 per cent NaCl/dextran 70 in the resuscitation of severely injured patients. Ann Surg 1987;206:279.
42. Mattox KL et al. Pre-hospital hypertonic saline-dextran infusion for post-traumatic hypotension: the USA multicenter trial. Ann Surg 1991;213:482.
43. Younes RN et al. Hypertonic solutions in the treatment of hypovolemic shock: a prospective, randomized study in patients admitted to the emergency room. Surgery 1992;111:380.
44. Angle N et al. Hypertonic saline resuscitation diminishes lung injury by suppressing neutrophil activation after hemorrhagic shock. Shock 1998;9:164.
45. Coimbra R et al. Hypertonic saline resuscitation decreases susceptibility to sepsis after hemorrhagic shock. J Trauma 1997;42:602.
46. Goodnough LT, et al. Transfusion medicine. First of two parts—blood transfusion. N Engl J Med 1999;340:438.

47. Griffel MI, Kaufman BS. Pharmacology of colloids and crystalloids. Crit Care Clin 1992;8:235.
48. Strauss RG. Review of the effects of hydroxyethyl starch on the blood coagulation system. Transfusion 1981;21:299.
49. Puri VK et al. Resuscitation in hypovolemia and shock: a prospective study of hydroxyethyl starch and albumin. Crit Care Med 1983;11:518.
50. Haupt MT et al. Colloid osmotic pressure and fluid resuscitation with hetastarch, albumin, and saline solutions. Crit Care Med 1982;10:159.
51. Lazrove S et al. Hemodynamic, blood volume and oxygen transport responses to albumin and hydroxyethyl starch infusions in critically ill postoperative patients. Crit Care Med 1980;8:302.
52. Thompson WL. Hydroxyethyl starch. Dev Biol Stand 1980;48:259.
53. Yacobi A et al. Pharmacokinetics of hydroxyethyl starch in normal subjects. J Clin Pharmacol 1982;22:206.
54. Forrester JS et al. Medical therapy of acute, myocardial infarction by application of hemodynamic subsets. N Engl J Med 1976;295(Pt 1,2):1356.
55. McGhie AI, Goldstein RA. Pathogenesis and management of acute heart failure and cardiogenic shock: role of inotropic therapy. Chest 1992;102(5 Suppl 2):626S.
56. Lollgen H, Drexler H. Use of inotropes in the critical care setting. Crit Care Med 1990;18:S56.
57. Anil OM, Hess ML. Inotropic therapy for the failing myocardium. Clin Cardiol 1992;16:5.
58. Lindeborg DM, Pearl RG. Inotropic therapy in the critically ill patient. Int Anesthesiol Clin 1993;31:49.
59. Flancbaum L et al. Quantitative effects of low dose dopamine on urine output in oliguric surgical intensive care unit patients. Crit Care Med 1994;22:61.
60. Cotte DB, Saul WP. Is renal dose dopamine protective or therapeutic? No. Crit Care Clin 1996;12:687.
61. Myles PS et al. Effect of "renal-dose" dopamine on renal function following cardiac surgery. Anaesth Intens Care 1993;21:56.
62. Carcoana OV, Hines RL. Is renal dose dopamine protective or therapeutic? Yes. Crit Care Clin 1996;12:677.
63. Grady K et al. Team management of patients with heart failure: a statement for healthcare professionals from the Cardiovascular Nursing Council of the American Heart Association. Circulation 2000;102:2443.
64. Nohria A et al. Medical management of advanced heart failure. JAMA 2002;287:628.
65. Vanky F et al. Addition of a thiazide: an effective remedy for furosemide resistance after cardiac operations. Ann Thorac Surg 1997;63:993.
66. Pivac N et al. Diuretic effects of furosemide infusion versus bolus injection in congestive heart failure. Int J Clin Pharmacol Res 1998;18:121.
67. Ansell J et al. Amrinone-induced thrombocytopenia. Arch Intern Med 1984;144:949.
68. Kikura M et al. The effects of milrinone of platelets in patients undergoing cardiac surgery. Anesth Analg 1995;81:44.
69. Rathmell JP et al. A multicenter, randomized, blind comparison of amrinone with milrinone after elective cardiac surgery. Anesth Analg 1998;86:683.
70. Cuffe MS et al. Short term intravenous milrinone for acute exacerbations of chronic heart failure: a randomized controlled trial. JAMA 2002;287:1541.

71. Feneck RO et al. Comparison of the hemodynamic effects of milrinone with dobutamine in patients after cardiac surgery. J Cardiothorac Vasc Anesth 2001;15:306.

72. Yamani MH et al. Comparison of dobutamine-based and milrinone-based therapy for advanced decompensated congestive heart failure: Hemodynamic efficacy, clinical outcome, and economic impact. Am Heart J 2001;142:998.

73. Aranda JM et al. Comparison of dobutamine versus milrinone therapy in hospitalized patients awaiting cardiac transplantation: a prospective randomized trial. Am Heart J 2003;145:324.

74. Lowes BD et al. Milrinone versus dobutamine in heart failure subjects treated chronically with carvedilol. Int J Cardiol 2001;81:141.

75. Marcus LS et al. Hemodynamic and renal excretory effects of human brain natriuretic peptide infusion in patients with congestive heart failure: a double-blind, placebo-controlled, randomized cross-over trial. Circulation 1996;76:91.

76. Abraham WT et al. Systemic hemodynamic, neurohormonal, and renal effects of a steady-state infusion of human brain natriuretic peptide in patients with hemodynamically decompensated heart failure. J Card Fail 1998;4:37.

77. Colucci WS et al. Intravenous nesiritide, a natriuretic peptide, in the treatment of decompensated congestive heart failure. N Engl J Med 2000;343:246.

78. Publication Committee for the VMAC Investigators. Intravenous nesiritide vs. nitroglycerin for treatment of decompensated congestive heart failure: a randomized controlled trial. JAMA 2002;287:1531.

79. Webb JG. Interventional management of cardiogenic shock. Can J Cardiol 1998;14:233.

80. Becker RC. Hemodynamic, mechanical, and metabolic determinants of thrombolytic efficacy; a theoretical framework for assessing the limitations of thrombolysis in patients with cardiogenic shock. Am Heart J 1993;125:919.

81. Prewitt RM et al. Intraaortic balloon counterpulsation enhances coronary thrombolysis induced by intravenous administration of a thrombolytic agent. J Am Coll Cardiol 1994;23:794.

82. Holmes D et al. Contemporary reperfusion therapy for cardiogenic shock: the GUSTO-I trial experience. J Am Coll Cardiol 1995;26:288.

83. Hochman JS et al. Early revascularization in acute myocardial infarction complicated by cardiogenic shock. N Engl J Med 1999;341:625.

84. Hochman JS et al. One year survival following early revascularization for cardiogenic shock. JAMA 2001;285:190.

85. Holzer J et al. Effectiveness of dopamine in patients with cardiogenic shock. Am J Cardiol 1973;32:79.

86. Richard C et al. Combined hemodynamic effects of dopamine and dobutamine in cardiogenic shock. Circulation 1983;67:620.

87. Frazier OH et al. Multicenter clinical evaluation of the HeartMate vented electric left ventricular assist system in patients awaiting heart transplantation. J Thorac Cardiovasc Surg 2001;122:1186.

88. Rose EA et al. Long-term mechanical left ventricular assistance for end-stage heart failure. N Engl J Med 2001;345:1435.

89. Kreger BE et al. Gram-negative bacteremia IV: re-evaluation of clinical features and treatment in 612 patients. Am J Med 1980;68:344.

90. Aztiz ME. Septic shock. Lancet 1998;351:1501.

91. Heyland DK et al. Maximizing oxygen delivery in critically ill patients: a methodologic appraisal of the evidence. Crit Care Med 1996;24:517.

92. Third European Consensus Conference in Intensive Care Medicine. Tissue hypoxia: how to detect, how to correct, how to prevent? J Crit Care 1997;12:39.

93. Hayes MA et al. Oxygen transport patterns in patients with sepsis syndrome or septic shock: influence of treatment and relationship to outcome. Crit Care Med 1997;25:926.

94. Meadows D et al. Reversal of intractable septic shock with norepinephrine therapy. Crit Care Med 1988;16:663.

95. Martin C et al. Norepinephrine or dopamine for the treatment of hyperdynamic septic shock? Chest 1993;103:1826.

96. Holmes C et al. Physiology of vasopressin relevant to management of septic shock. Chest 2001;120:989.

97. Rozenfeld V, Cheng J. The role of vasopressin in the treatment of vasodilation in shock states. Ann Pharmacother 2000;34:250.

98. Landry D et al. Vasopressin deficiency contributes to the vasodilation of septic shock. Circulation 1997;95:1122.

99. Patel B et al. Beneficial effects of short-term vasopressin infusion during severe septic shock. Anesthesiology 2002;96:576.

100. Rudis MI et al. Is it time to reposition vasopressors and inotropes in sepsis? Crit Care Med 1996;24:525.

101. Levy B et al. Comparison of norepinephrine and dobutamine to epinephrine for hemodynamics, lactate metabolism, and gastric tonometric variables in septic shock: a prospective, randomized study. Intens Care Med 1997;23:282.

102. Duranteau J et al. Effects of epinephrine, norepinephrine, or the combination of norepinephrine and dobutamine on gastric mucosa in septic shock. Crit Care Med 1999;27:893.

103. Seguin P et al. Effects of epinephrine compared with the combination of dobutamine and norepinephrine on gastric perfusion in septic shock. Clin Pharmacol Ther 2002;71:381.

104. Annane D. Resurrection of steroids for sepsis resuscitation. Minerva Anesthesiol 2002;68:127.

105. Lefering R, Neugebauer EA. Steroid controversy in sepsis and septic shock: a meta-analysis. Crit Care Med 1995;23:1294.

106. Cronin I et al. Corticosteroid treatment for sepsis: a critical appraisal and meta-analysis of the literature. Crit Care Med 1995;23:1430.

107. Annane D et al. Effect of treatment with low doses of hydrocortisone and fludrocortisone on mortality in patients with septic shock. JAMA 2002;288(7):862.

108. Dhainaut JF et al. Soluble thrombomodulin, plasma-derived unactivated protein C, and recombinant human activated protein C in sepsis. Crit Care Med 2002;30(S5):S318.

109. Bernard G et al. Efficacy and safety of recombinant human activated protein C for severe sepsis. N Engl J Med 2001;344(10):699.

110. Cohen J et al. An international, multicenter, placebo-controlled trial of monoclonal antibody to human tumor necrosis factor-α in patients with sepsis. Crit Care Med 1996;24:1431.

111. Fisher CJ et al. Treatment of septic shock with the tumor necrosis factor receptor:Fc fusion protein. N Engl J Med 1996;334:1697.

112. Bellomo R et al. Continuous hemofiltration as blood purification in sepsis. New Horizons 1995;3:732.

113. Jaber BL et al. Extracorporeal adsorbent-based strategies in sepsis. Am J Kidney Dis 1997;30(Suppl 4):S44.

114. Warren B et al. High-dose antithrombin III in severe sepsis: a randomized controlled trial. JAMA 2001;286:1869.

115. Vender JS. Invasive cardiac monitoring. Crit Care Clin 1988;4:455.

PULMONARY DISORDERS

Robin L. Corelli
SECTION EDITOR

CHAPTER 23

Asthma

Timothy H. Self

ASTHMA

According to the National Institutes of Health (NIH) Expert Panel Report[1]: Guidelines for the Diagnosis and Management of Asthma, *asthma* is now defined as a chronic inflammatory disorder of the airways in which many cells and cellular elements play a role, in particular, mast cells, eosinophils, T lymphocytes, neutrophils, and epithelial cells. In susceptible persons, this inflammation causes recurrent episodes of wheezing, breathlessness, chest tightness, and cough, particu-

larly at night and in the early morning. These episodes are usually associated with widespread, but variable, airflow obstruction that is often reversible either spontaneously or with treatment. The inflammation also causes increase in the existing bronchial hyperresponsiveness to a variety of stimuli.[2] This definition of asthma continues to evolve from earlier NIH Guidelines,[2] including the International Consensus Report[3] and the Global Initiative for Asthma[4] in the 1990s. In 2002, an Update on Selected Topics was published by the NIH Expert Panel Report.[5]

At least 15 million Americans have asthma.[1,6] It is an underdiagnosed and undertreated condition that is estimated to have overall costs exceeding $12 billion annually in the United States.[6] Asthma is the leading cause of lost school days in children and is a common cause of lost workdays among adults.

Mortality from asthma is rising for unknown reasons, and death rates are higher in inner-city minority populations. In response to the increased mortality from asthma noted in the 1980s and the enormous human and economic toll of this disease, the NIH published "Guidelines for the Diagnosis and Management of Asthma" in 1991.[2] This chapter emphasizes the 1997 NIH Guidelines and the 2002 Update on Selected Topics.[1,5] Application of the principles of these landmark reports by clinicians and patients is vital to reducing asthma morbidity and mortality.

Etiology

Childhood-onset asthma is usually associated with atopy, the genetic predisposition for the development of immunoglobulin E (IgE)–mediated response to common aeroallergens. Atopy is the strongest predisposing factor in the development of asthma.[1] A very common presentation of asthma is a child with a positive family history of asthma and allergy to tree and grass pollen, house dust mites, household pets, and molds.

Adult-onset asthma may also be associated with atopy, but many adults with asthma have a negative family history and negative skin tests to common aeroallergens. Some of these patients may have nasal polyps, aspirin sensitivity, and sinusitis. Exposure to factors (e.g., wood dusts, chemicals) at the workplace that may cause airway inflammation is also important in many adults. Inflammatory mechanisms are similar, but not the same, as in atopic asthma. Some clinicians may still refer to *intrinsic asthma* when referring to these patients and *extrinsic asthma* when discussing atopic asthma.

In addition to atopy and exposure to occupational chemical sensitizers as being major risk factors for the development of asthma, several contributing factors may increase the susceptibility to the development of the disease in predisposed individuals.[4] These factors include viral infections, small size at birth, diet, exposure to tobacco smoke, and environmental pollutants.[4]

Recent literature has focused on the "hygiene hypothesis," an imbalance of TH2- and TH1-type T lymphocytes, to explain the marked increase in asthma in westernized countries.[5,7,8] Infants who have older siblings, early exposure to day care, and typical childhood infections are more likely to activate TH1 responses (protective immunity), resulting in an appropriate balance of TH1/TH2 cells and the cytokines that they produce. On the other hand, if the immune response is predominately from TH2 cells (which produce cytokines that mediate allergic inflammation), development of diseases such as asthma is more likely. Examples of factors favoring this imbalance include common use of antimicrobial agents, urban environment, and Western lifestyle. Further insights into the pathogenesis of asthma continue to be discovered via genetic studies.[7,9]

Pathophysiology

Asthma is caused by a very complex interaction between inflammatory cells and mediators. As noted in the definition of asthma, mast cells, eosinophils, T lymphocytes, neutrophils, and epithelial cells are of central importance. Table 23-1 summarizes some of the actions of these cells and mediators (e.g., leukotrienes[10]) of airway inflammation and bronchoconstriction. Figure 23-1 depicts airway changes in asthma.

After exposure to an asthma-precipitating factor (e.g., aeroallergen), inflammatory mediators are released from bronchial mast cells, macrophages, T lymphocytes, and epithelial cells. These mediators direct the migration and activation of other inflammatory cells, most notably eosinophils, to the airways.[1,7,11] Eosinophils release biochemicals (e.g., major basic protein and eosinophil cationic protein) that cause airway injury, including epithelial damage, mucus hypersecretion, and increased reactivity of smooth muscle.[1,7,11]

An area of intense research continues to be the role of a subpopulation of T lymphocytes (TH2) in asthmatic airway inflammation.[1,4] TH2 lymphocytes release cytokines (e.g., interleukin [IL]-4 and IL-5) that at least partially control the ac-

Table 23-1 Examples of Inflammatory Cells and Mediators in Asthma

Cells	Examples of Actions
Eosinophils	Cause airway inflammation and epithelial damage by release of major basic protein, eosinophil cationic protein, and other biochemicals
TH2 lymphocytes	Release cytokines (e.g., IL-4, IL-5) that modulate eosinophil adherence, locomotion, activation
Mast cells	IgE-mediated release of inflammatory mediators (e.g., leukotrienes, histamine)
Macrophages	Release of inflammatory mediators (e.g., leukotrienes)
Neutrophils	Found in high numbers in airways of patients with sudden-onset fatal asthma
Mediators	
Leukotrienes[a]	Increase vascular permeability and mucus secretions, attract and activate inflammatory cells in the airways, contract airway smooth muscle
Histamine	Mucus secretion, increase vascular permeability, airway smooth muscle contraction
Prostaglandins[b]	Mucus secretion, increase vascular permeability, airway smooth muscle contraction

[a]For example, LTD_4 and LTE_4.
[b]For example, PGE_2 and PGD_2.
IL, interleukin.

NORMAL   ASTHMATIC

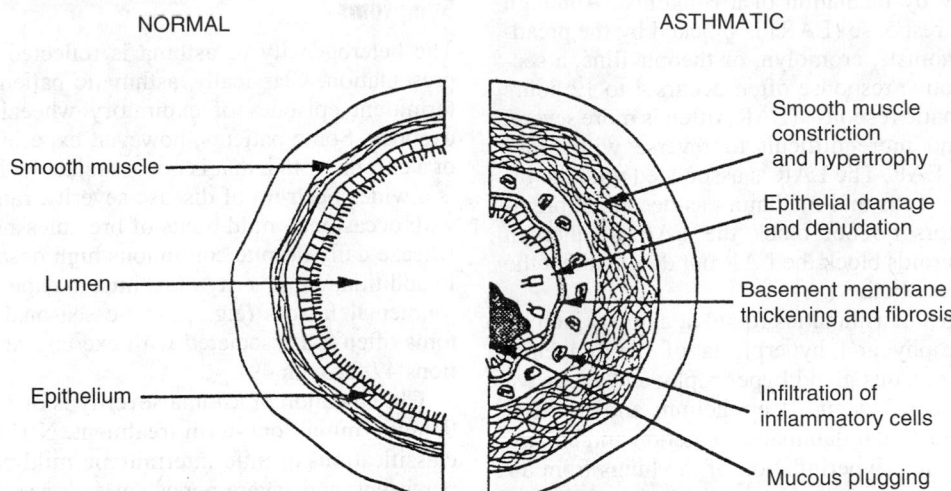

FIGURE 23-1 Diagram illustrating the histologic changes present in the airways of an asthmatic patient compared with normal. (Reproduced with permission from Herfindal ET, Gourley DR. Textbook of Therapeutics Drug and Disease Management. 7th Ed. Baltimore: Williams & Wilkins, 1996.)

tivation and enhanced survival of eosinophils.[1,4,7–11] The complexity of airway inflammation is indicated by the fact that 27 cytokines may have a role in the pathophysiology of asthma.[7] In addition, 18 chemokines (e.g., eotaxins) have been identified that are important in delivery of eosinophils to the airways.[7,12]

Other areas of research in asthma pathophysiology include adhesion molecules (which enable eosinophils to cross the venule wall and migrate to the mucosa), neural control of the airways, and the role of nitric oxide (an endogenous vasodilator and bronchodilator).[4]

Failure to adequately minimize severe and long-term airway inflammation in asthma may result in airway remodeling in some patients. Airway remodeling refers to structural changes, including an alteration in the amount and composition of the extracellular matrix in the airway wall.[1,5,13] Thus, airflow eventually may become only partially reversible.

Hyperreactivity (defined as an exaggerated response of bronchial smooth muscles to trigger stimuli) of the airways to physical, chemical, immunologic, and pharmacologic stimuli is pathognomonic of asthma.[1] Examples of these stimuli include inhaled allergens, respiratory viral infection, cold air, dry air, smoke, other pollutants, and methacholine. Endogenous stimuli that can worsen asthma include poorly controlled rhinitis, sinusitis, and gastroesophageal reflux disease.[1] In addition, premenstrual asthma has been reported, but the exact hormonal mechanism is not known.[14]

Although patients with allergic rhinitis, chronic bronchitis, and cystic fibrosis also experience bronchial hyperreactivity, these patients do not experience bronchiolar constriction as severely as patients with asthma. The degree of bronchial hyperreactivity of asthmatics correlates with the clinical course of their disease, which is characterized by periods of remissions and exacerbations. During times of remission, a more intense stimulus is required to produce bronchospasm than during times of increased symptoms. Numerous theories have been proposed to explain the bronchial hyperreactivity found in asthma, yet none fully explains the phenomenon. Inflam-

mation appears to be the primary process in the pathogenesis of bronchial hyperreactivity; however, neurogenic imbalances in the airways also may play a significant role.[4]

Inflamed airways are hyperreactive (i.e., irritable). Hyperreactivity can be measured in the physician's office by having the patient inhale small concentrations of nebulized methacholine or histamine or by exercise (e.g., treadmill). The concentration of aerosolized methacholine or histamine that decreases the forced expiratory volume in 1 second (FEV_1) by 20% is referred to as the PD_{20} or the PC_{20} (provocative dose or concentration that decreases the FEV_1 by 20%).[2] An indicator of optimal anti-inflammatory therapy is an increase in the PD_{20} over time as the airways become less inflamed and therefore less hyperreactive.

Another concept related to inflammation is "late-phase" versus "early-phase" asthma (Fig. 23-2). The inhalation of specific allergens in atopic asthmatics produces immediate bronchoconstriction (measured by a drop in peak expiratory flow [PEF] or FEV) that spontaneously improves over an hour

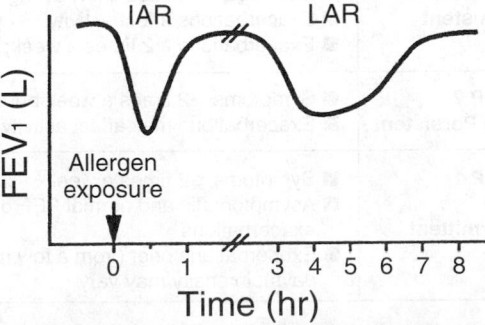

FIGURE 23-2 Typical immediate and late asthmatic responses seen after exposure to relevant allergen. Immediate asthmatic response (IAR) occurs within minutes, whereas late asthmatic response (LAR) occurs several hours after exposure. Patients may demonstrate isolated IAR, isolated LAR, or dual responses. (Reproduced with permission from Herfindal ET, Gourley DR. Textbook of Therapeutics Drug and Disease Management. 7th Ed. Baltimore: Williams & Wilkins, 1996.)

or is reversed easily by inhalation of a β-agonist. Although this early asthmatic response (EAR) is blocked by the preadministration of β-agonists, cromolyn, or theophylline, a second bronchoconstrictive response often occurs 4 to 12 hours later. This late asthmatic response (LAR) often is more severe, more prolonged, and more difficult to reverse with bronchodilators than the EAR. The LAR is associated with the influx of inflammatory cells and mediators as described previously. Bronchodilators do not block the LAR to allergen challenge; corticosteroids block the LAR but do not affect the EAR; cromolyn blocks both.[2]

Pathologic changes in asthmatics found at autopsy include (1) marked hypertrophy and hyperplasia of the bronchial smooth muscle, (2) mucous gland hypertrophy and excessive mucus secretion, and (3) denuded epithelium and mucosal edema due to an exudative inflammatory reaction and inflammatory cell infiltration.[1] Hyperinflation of the lungs from air trapping with extensive mucous plugging is found at autopsy in patients who died from acute asthma attacks, but these changes also are seen at autopsy in asthmatics dying from other causes. The bronchial smooth muscle hypertrophy and mucus hypersecretion are secondary to the chronic inflammatory response.

Symptoms

The heterogeneity of asthma is reflected best in its clinical presentation. Classically, asthmatic patients present with intermittent episodes of expiratory wheezing, coughing, and dyspnea. Some patients, however, experience chest tightness or a chronic cough that is not associated with wheezing. There is a wide spectrum of disease severity, ranging from patients with occasional, mild bouts of breathlessness to patients who wheeze daily despite continuous high dosages of medication. In addition, the severity of asthma may be influenced by environmental factors (e.g., specific seasonal allergens). Symptoms often are associated with exercise and sleep (see Questions 47 through 49).

Classification of asthma severity is of major importance in defining initial long-term treatment. NIH Guidelines use the classifications of mild intermittent, mild persistent, moderate persistent, and severe persistent asthma (Fig. 23-3). The frequency of symptoms is a key component of asthma classification.[1] For example, mild persistent asthma is defined as symptoms more than two times per week or nocturnal symptoms (including early morning chest tightness) more than two times per month. Many clinicians are unaware that this level of

Goals of Asthma Treatment
- Prevent chronic and troublesome symptoms (e.g., coughing or breathlessness in the night, in the early morning, or after exertion)
- Maintain (near) "normal" pulmonary function
- Maintain normal activity levels (including exercise and other physical activity)
- Prevent recurrent exacerbations of asthma and minimize the need for emergency department visits or hospitalizations
- Provide optimal pharmacotherapy with minimal or no adverse effects
- Meet patients' and families' expectations of and satisfaction with asthma care

Classify Severity of Asthma			
Clinical Features Before Treatment*			
	Symptoms**	**Nighttime Symptoms**	**Lung Function**
STEP 4 **Severe** **Persistent**	■ Continual symptoms ■ Limited physical activity ■ Frequent exacerbations	Frequent	■ FEV_1 or PEF ≤60% predicted ■ PEF variability >30%
STEP 3 **Moderate** **Persistent**	■ Daily symptoms ■ Daily use of inhaled short-acting beta$_2$-agonist ■ Exacerbations affect activity ■ Exacerbations ≥2 times a week; may last days	>1 time a week	■ FEV_1 or PEF >60%–<80% predicted ■ PEF variability >30%
STEP 2 **Mild Persistent**	■ Symptoms >2 times a week but <1 time a day ■ Exacerbations may affect activity	>2 times a month	■ FEV_1 or PEF ≥80% predicted ■ PEF variability 20–30%
STEP 1 **Mild** **Intermittent**	■ Symptoms ≤2 times a week ■ Asymptomatic and normal PEF between exacerbations ■ Exacerbations brief (from a few hours to a few days); intensity may vary	≤2 times a month	■ FEV_1 or PEF ≥80% predicted ■ PEF variability <20%

* The presence of one of the features of severity is sufficient to place a patient in that category. An individual should be assigned to the most severe grade in which any feature occurs. The characteristics noted in this figure are general and may overlap because asthma is highly variable. Furthermore, an individual's classification may change over time.

**Patients at any level of severity can have mild, moderate, or severe exacerbations. Some patients with intermittent asthma experience severe and life-threatening exacerbations separated by long periods of normal lung function and no symptoms.

FIGURE 23-3 **Classify Severity of Asthma.** (Reprinted from reference 1.)

symptoms is defined as persistent asthma. This classification is of major significance when selecting long-term drug therapy in that daily use of anti-inflammatory agents is an essential part of management for persistent asthma.[1]

Diagnosis and Monitoring

History

The diagnosis of asthma is based primarily on a detailed history of intermittent symptoms of wheezing, chest tightness, shortness of breath, and coughing. These episodes may be worse seasonally (e.g., springtime or late summer and early fall) or in association with exercise. History of nocturnal symptoms with awakening in the early morning is a critical component to assess. In addition, history of symptoms after exposure to other common triggers (e.g., cats, perfume, second-hand tobacco smoke) is typical. A positive family history and the presence of rhinitis or atopic dermatitis also are significant. After a careful history is obtained, skin testing may be useful in identifying triggering allergens, but it is only of supportive value in the diagnosis of asthma.

Pulmonary Function Tests

The diagnosis of asthma is based in part on demonstration of reversible airway obstruction. A brief discussion of tests to detect reversibility of airway obstruction is important. Furthermore, a short summary of arterial blood gases is pertinent here in assessing severity of asthma exacerbations.

SPIROMETRY

Lung volumes often are measured to obtain information about the size of the patient's lungs because pulmonary diseases can affect the volume of air that can be inhaled and exhaled. The classic volume displacement spirometer pictured in Figure 23-4 is used to measure lung volumes. As the patient breathes, the bell of the spirometer is displaced, and the pen deflection reflects the volume of air entering or exiting the lung. The tidal volume is the volume of air inspired or expired during normal breathing. The volume of air blown off after maximal inspiration to full expiration is defined as the vital capacity (VC). The residual volume (RV) is the volume of air left in the lung after maximal expiration. The volume of air left after a normal expiration is the functional residual capacity (FRC). Total lung capacity (TLC) is the vital capacity plus the RV. Patients with obstructive lung disease have difficulty with expiration; therefore, they tend to have a decreased VC, an increased RV, and a normal TLC. Classic restrictive lung diseases (e.g., sarcoidosis, idiopathic pulmonary fibrosis) present with decrements in all lung volumes.[15] Patients also may have mixed lesion diseases, in which case the classic findings are not apparent until the disease has advanced considerably.

The spirometer also can be used to evaluate the performance of the patient's lungs, thorax, and respiratory muscles in moving air into and out of the lungs. Forced expiratory maneuvers amplify the ventilation abnormalities produced. The single most useful test for ventilatory dysfunction is the FEV. The FEV is measured by having the patient exhale into the spirometer as forcefully and completely as possible after maximal inspiration. The resulting volume curve is plotted against time (Fig. 23-5) so that expiratory flow can be estimated.

As a result of technologic advances, standard spirometers contain pneumotachographs in the mouthpieces that can measure airflow rates directly. A number of important measures of lung function are made from the resulting flow-volume curves (Fig. 23-6). The advantages of this technique include a display of simultaneous flows at any lung volume; visual estimation of patient effort and cooperation; high reproducibility within, as well as across, individuals; and an analysis of the distribution of flow limitation.[15,16]

The FEV_1 of the forced vital capacity (FVC, the maximum volume of air exhaled with maximally forced effort from a position of maximal inspiration) commonly is measured to determine the dynamic performance of the lung in moving air. The FEV_1 usually is expressed as a percentage of the total volume of air exhaled and is reported as the FEV_1:FVC ratio. Healthy persons generally can exhale at least 75% to 80% of

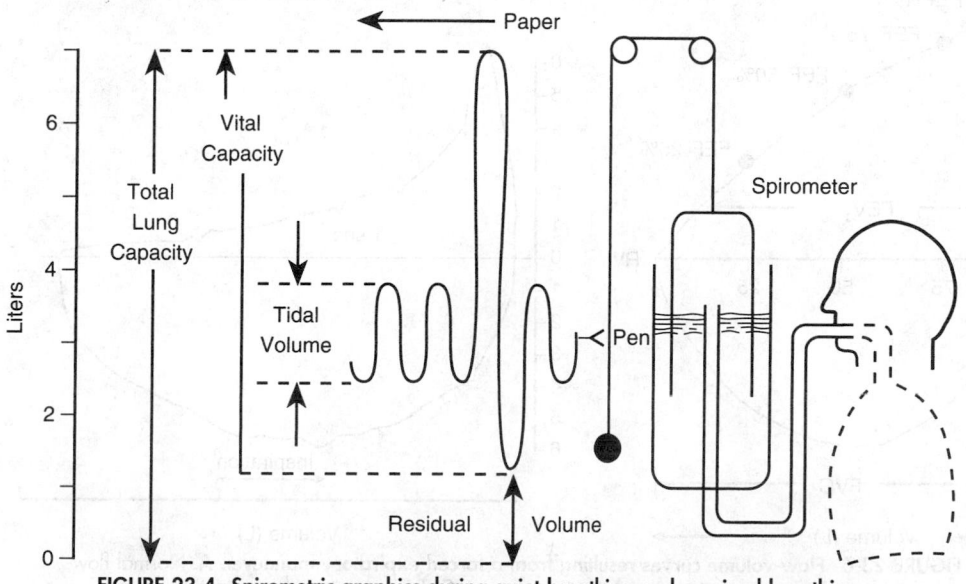

FIGURE 23-4 Spirometric graphics during quiet breathing and maximal breathing.

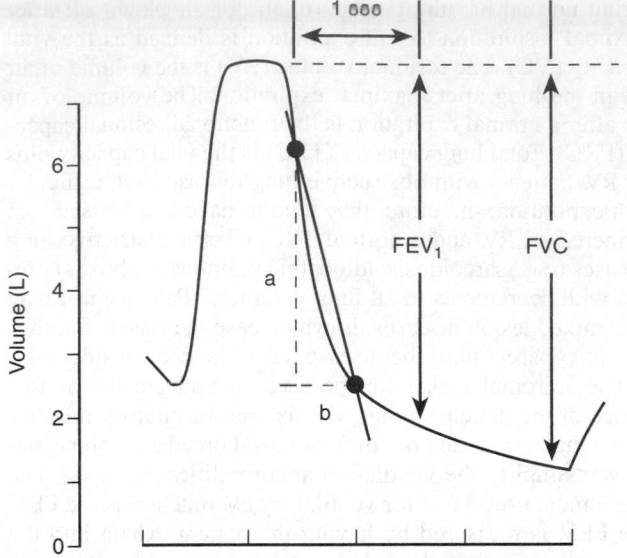

FIGURE 23-5 Volume-time curve from a forced expiratory maneuver.

their VC in 1 second and almost all of it in 3 seconds. Thus, the FEV_1 normally is 80% of the FVC. The patient's breathing ability is compared against "predicted normal" values for patients with similar physiologic characteristics because lung volumes depend on age, race, gender, height, and weight. For example, an average-sized young adult male may have an FVC of 4 to 5 L and a corresponding FEV_1 of 3.2 to 4 L. The FEV_1 and the FVC are the most reproducible of the pulmonary function tests.

The forced expiratory flow ($FEF_{25\%-75\%}$) is the mean forced expiratory flow during the middle half of the FVC and is measured as the slope of the line between 25% and 75% of FVC on the flow-volume curve. This value formerly was called the

maximal midexpiratory flow rate (MMEF) and is expressed in L/second[16] (see Fig. 23-5). Flows at less than 75% of FVC are limited by airway compressibility and therefore determined by the elastic recoil force of the lung and the resistance to flow upstream of the collapse (see Fig. 23-6A). Flows at this portion of the curve (i.e., at the middle part of expiration) are said to be independent of patient expiratory effort.[15,16] The $FEF_{25\%-75\%}$ is a more sensitive measure of airflow resistance in the small airways (e.g., those <2 mm wide).[15,16]

PEAK EXPIRATORY FLOW

The PEF is the maximal rate of flow that can be produced during the forced expiration. The PEF can be measured easily with various handheld peak flow meters (Fig. 23-7) and commonly is used in emergency departments (EDs) and clinics to quickly and objectively assess the effectiveness of bronchodilators in the treatment of acute asthma attacks. Peak flow meters also can be used at home by patients with asthma to assess chronic therapy. The changes in PEF generally parallel those of the FEV_1; however, the PEF is a less reproducible measure than the FEV_1.[4] A healthy, average-sized young adult male typically has a PEF of 550 to 700 L/minute. Commercial peak flow meters come with a chart (Table 23-2) for patients to look up their predicted normal PEFs based on their gender, age, and height. (See also Major Components of Long-Term Management.)

Obstructive versus Restrictive Airway Disease

Generally, pulmonary disorders fall into two categories: those that restrict the lungs and thorax and those that obstruct them. In simplest terms, restrictive disease limits airflow during inspiration, and obstructive disease limits airflow during expiration. Restrictive disease results from a loss of elasticity (e.g., fibrosis, pneumonia) or physical deformities of the chest (e.g., kyphoscoliosis), with a consequent inability to expand the

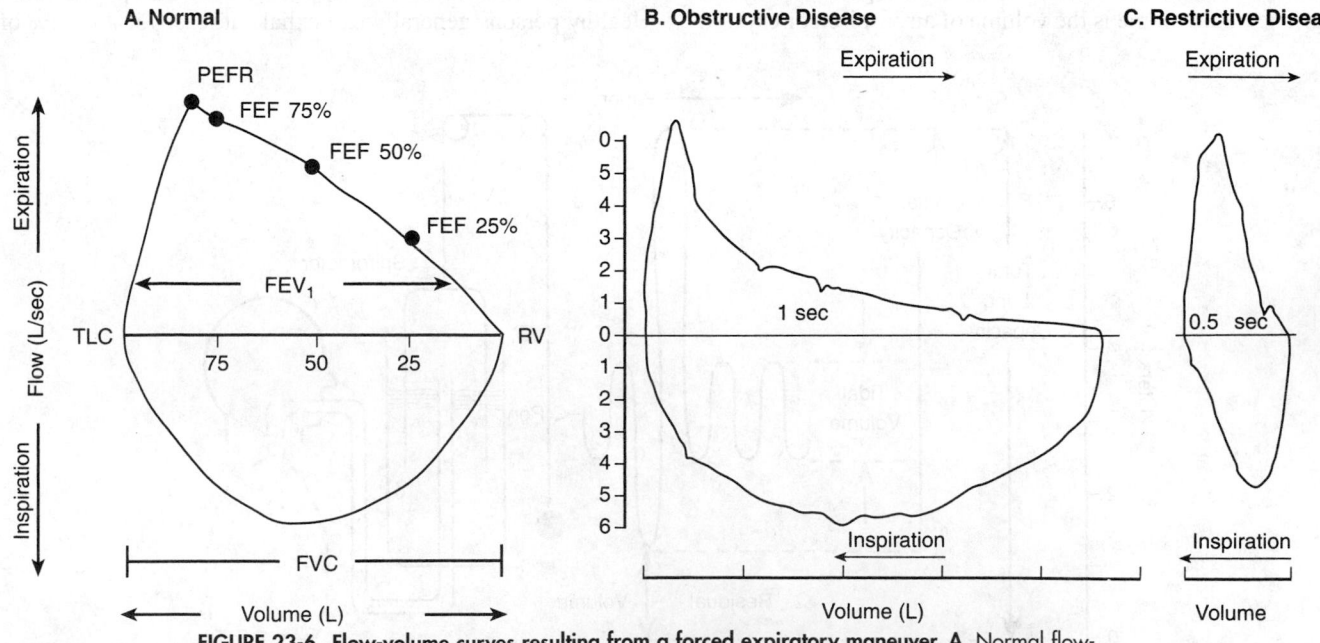

FIGURE 23-6 Flow-volume curves resulting from a forced expiratory maneuver. **A.** Normal flow-volume curve. **B.** Typical pattern for obstructive disease. **C.** Typical pattern for restrictive disease.

Table 23-2   Predicted Peak Expiratory Flow Rate (L/min)

Child and Adolescent Female: Age 6 to 20 Years

Height (in.)	42	46	50	54	57	60	64	68	72
Age 6	134	164	193	223	245	268	297	327	357
8	153	182	212	242	264	287	316	346	376
10	171	201	231	261	283	305	335	365	395
12	190	220	250	280	302	324	354	384	414
14	209	239	269	298	321	343	373	403	432
16	228	258	288	317	340	362	392	421	451
18	247	277	306	336	358	381	411	440	470
20	266	295	325	355	377	400	429	459	489

Child and Adolescent Male: Age 6 to 25 Years

Height (in.)	44	48	52	56	60	64	68	72	76
Age 6	99	146	194	241	289	336	384	431	479
8	119	166	214	261	309	356	404	451	499
10	139	186	234	281	329	376	424	471	519
12	159	206	254	301	349	396	444	491	539
14	178	226	274	321	369	416	464	511	559
16	198	246	293	341	389	436	484	531	579
18	218	266	313	361	408	456	503	551	599
20	238	286	333	381	428	476	523	571	618
22	258	306	353	401	448	496	543	591	638
24	278	326	373	421	468	516	563	611	658
25	288	336	383	431	478	526	573	621	668

Adult Female: Age 20 to 80 years

Height (in.)	58	60	62	64	66	68	70
Age 20	357	372	387	402	417	432	446
25	350	365	379	394	409	424	439
30	342	357	372	387	402	417	431
35	335	350	364	379	394	409	424
40	327	342	357	372	387	402	416
45	320	335	349	364	379	394	409
50	312	327	342	357	372	387	401
55	305	320	334	349	364	379	394
60	297	312	327	342	357	372	386
65	290	305	319	334	349	364	379
70	282	297	312	327	342	357	371
75	275	290	304	319	334	349	364
80	267	282	297	312	327	342	356

Adult Male: Age 25 to 80 years

Height (in.)	63	65	67	69	71	73	75	77
Age 25	492	520	549	578	606	635	664	692
30	481	510	538	567	596	624	653	682
35	471	499	528	557	585	614	643	671
40	460	489	517	546	575	603	632	661
45	450	478	507	536	564	593	622	650
50	439	468	496	525	554	582	611	640
55	429	457	486	515	543	572	601	629
60	418	447	475	504	533	561	590	619
65	408	436	465	494	522	551	580	608
70	397	426	454	483	512	540	569	598
75	387	415	444	473	501	530	559	587
80	376	405	433	462	491	519	548	577

From reference 181.

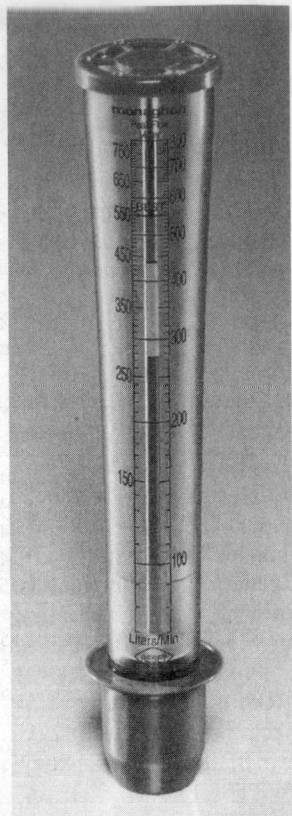

FIGURE 23-7 Peak flow meter.

lung and a reduced TLC. Therefore, a typical flow-volume curve (see Fig. 23-6C) for a patient with restrictive disease shows markedly depressed volumes with increased flow rates (when corrected for the volume).

Whereas restrictive airway diseases limit lung expansion, obstructive airway diseases (e.g., bronchitis, asthma) narrow air passages, create air turbulence, and increase resistance to airflow. In obstructive diseases, maximal expiration may begin at higher-than-normal lung volumes, and the expiratory flow is depressed (see Fig. 23-6B). Resistance to flow is increased at lower lung volumes, giving the characteristic scooped-out appearance of the obstructive flow-volume curve (see Fig. 23-6B). The $FEF_{25\%-75\%}$ or FEF_{50} can also detect early obstructive changes in the small airways before significant symptoms and hopefully while these objective changes are potentially reversible.

Reversible Airway Obstruction

Spirometry often is used to determine the reversibility of airways disease. Although many generally associate reversibility with bronchospasm, therapy can improve airflow by reversing any of the causative pathologic processes of asthma described earlier. Significant clinical reversibility produced from bronchodilators is determined by the tests outlined in Figure 23-8. Because of a high potential for variability, greater airway changes are required before the tests of small airway diseases ($FEF_{25\%-75\%}$, $FEF_{50\%}$) become significant. The FEV_1 has low variability and, during acute bronchospasm, shows the best correlation with clinical symptoms. Therefore, the FEV_1 is considered the gold standard test for determining reversibility of airway disease and bronchodilator efficacy. Significant clinical reversibility is defined as a 12% improvement in

Parameter	Restrictive	Obstructive
FVC	↓	Normal or ↓
FEV_1	Normal or ↓	↓
FEV_1/FVC	Normal or ↑	↓
$FEF_{25\%-75\%}$	Normal, ↓, ↑	↓

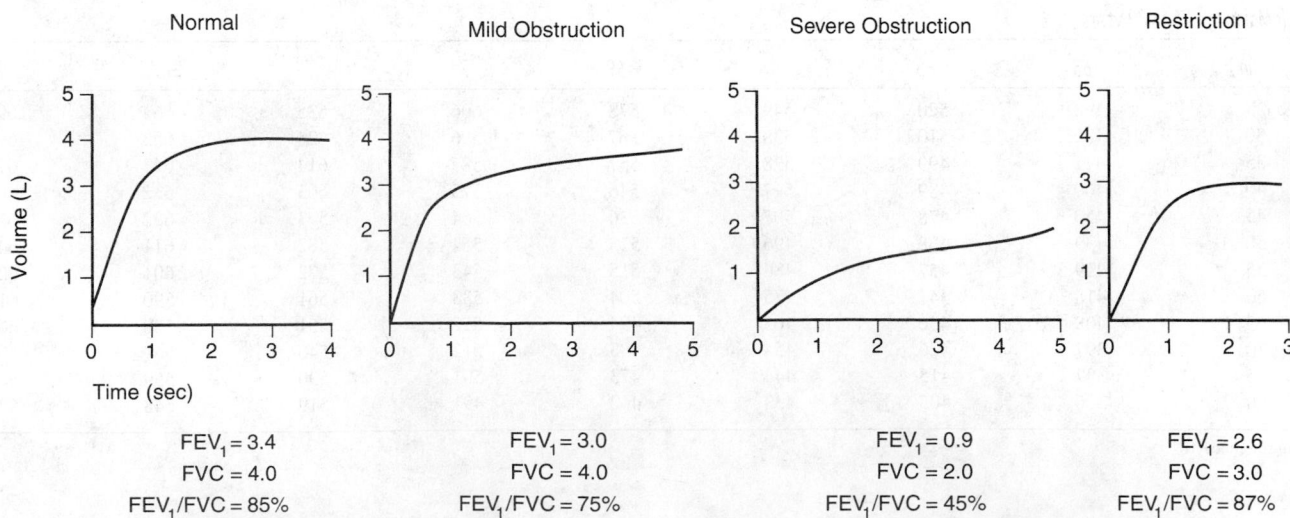

FIGURE 23-8 Interpretation of results of spirometry. The graphs depicted are for illustration only. The interpretation of flow rates may vary with the age of the patient. (Reprinted with permission from reference 2.)

FEV_1 following administration of a short-acting bronchodilator.[1] An improvement of 20% in FEV_1 provides noticeable subjective relief of respiratory symptoms in most patients. For patients with a very low baseline FEV_1 (e.g., <1 L), an absolute improvement of 250 mL sometimes is considered a better indicator of therapeutic benefit than assessing percentage of change. In either case, the patient's subjective clinical impression also should be considered when using pulmonary function testing and drug challenges as predictors for future therapy.

LIMITATIONS OF SPIROMETRY

Because the FEV_1 and the PEF are both highly effort dependent, complete patient cooperation is required for reliable results. Therefore, spirometric tests often are unobtainable in patients who are severely ill, as well as in patients who are very old or very young. The FEV_1 and PEF also are relatively insensitive to small airway changes and are therefore unable to detect early mucous plugging and inflammation in small bronchioles. Although the $FEF_{25\%-75\%}$ is a more sensitive test of small airway obstruction, it is also much more variable, requiring larger changes (30% to 40%) to be clinically significant.

Spirometric pulmonary function tests before and after administration of an inhaled bronchodilator can be useful in assessing the reversibility of airway obstruction. If significantly depressed pulmonary function tests are not reversed by the administration of a bronchodilator acutely, a 2- to 3-week trial of oral corticosteroid treatment followed by retesting might detect reversibility.[1]

If pulmonary function is normal or near normal at the time of spirometric assessment, the patient can be challenged by exercise or drugs that are known to produce bronchospasm in asthmatics (e.g., aerosolized histamine, methacholine).

Blood Gas Measurements

The best indicators of overall lung function (ventilation and diffusion) are the arterial blood gases (i.e., PaO_2, $PaCO_2$, and pH). Although arterial blood gas (ABG) measurements also are dependent on the patient's cardiovascular status, they are indispensable in assessing both acute and chronic changes in pulmonary patients. (See Chapter 11, Acid–Base Disorders, for a review of ABGs.) Another means of assessing the patient's ability to oxygenate tissues adequately is to measure oxygen saturation, which is described by the following equation:

$$O_2 \text{ saturation} = \frac{\text{Quantity of } O_2 \text{ actually bound to hemoglobin}}{\text{Quantity of } O_2 \text{ that can be bound to hemoglobin}} \times 100\%$$

According to this equation, oxygen saturation is the ratio between the actual amount of oxygen bound to hemoglobin and the potential amount of oxygen that could be bound to hemoglobin at a given pressure. The denominator in the preceding equation is the oxygen capacity. The normal oxygen saturation of arterial blood at a PaO_2 of 100 mm Hg is 97.5%; that of mixed venous blood at a PO_2 of 40 mm Hg is about 75%.[15] Oxygen saturations can be measured continuously with transcutaneous monitors. This type of monitoring is extremely helpful in determining whether supplemental oxygen therapy is indicated in patients with various chronic respiratory diseases. At a PaO_2 of <60 mm Hg, O_2 saturation begins to drop precipitously (Fig. 23-9).

Goals of Therapy

The NIH Guidelines[1] established the following goals of therapy for asthma: (1) Prevent chronic and troublesome symptoms (e.g., coughing or breathlessness in the night, in the early morning, or after exertion), (2) maintain (near) "normal" pulmonary function, (3) maintain normal activity levels (including exercise and other physical activities), (4) prevent recurrent exacerbations of asthma and minimize the need for ED visits or hospitalizations, (5) provide optimal pharmacotherapy with minimal or no adverse effects, and (6) meet patients' and families' expectations of and satisfaction with asthma care.

Major Components of Long-Term Management

To achieve these goals of therapy, the NIH Guidelines[1] also outline some general treatment principles. Asthma management has four major components, including (1) initial and periodic assessment and monitoring, (2) control of factors contributing to asthma severity, (3) pharmacologic therapy, and (4) education for a partnership in asthma care. Optimal long-term management requires a continuous care approach to prevent exacerbations and decrease airway inflammation. Early therapeutic interventions in managing acute exacerbations are very important in decreasing the chance of severe narrowing of the airways. Achieving the goals of asthma therapy also involves individualizing each patient's therapy. In addition, optimal care involves establishing a "partnership" between the patient, the patient's family, and the clinician.

Objective monitoring of lung function at home is one aspect of monitoring that can help attain the goals of asthma therapy. Monitoring PEF, initially in the morning and evening,

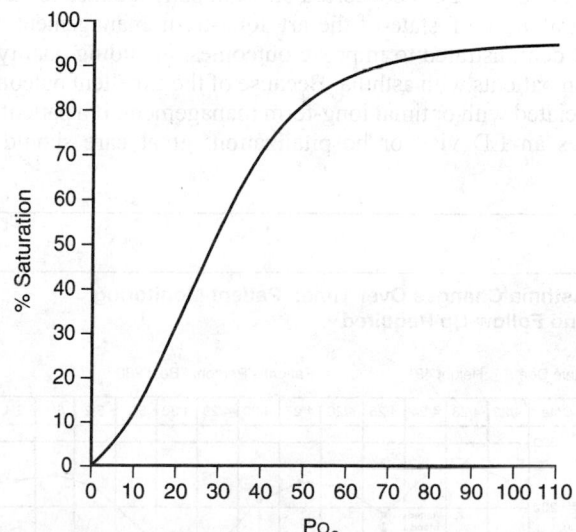

FIGURE 23-9 The oxygen dissociation curve reveals that the percent saturation of hemoglobin increases almost linearly with increases in the arterial O_2 tension until a PaO_2 of 55 to 65 mm Hg is reached. At PaO_2 values above this, the increase in hemoglobin saturation becomes proportionately less and relatively little additional oxygen is added to the hemoglobin despite large increases in PaO_2. (Reproduced with permission from reference 182.)

should be considered in patients with persistent asthma.[1] After establishing that optimal therapy has maintained the PEF in the "green zone" in the early morning, most patients can simply verify their values once daily in the early morning. Analogous to a traffic light, green, yellow, and red zones have been established to guide the patient and clinician. The *green zone* refers to a PEF that is 80% to 100% of "personal best" and generally indicates that therapy is providing good control. Before a course of optimal therapy to attain a personal best, the zones are set based on predicted values found in each peak flow meter package insert (see Table 23-2) The *yellow zone* indicates a PEF that is 50% to 79% of personal best. Patients should be instructed to call their physician or other health care provider for adjustment in preventive medication if PEF stays in yellow zone after using two puffs of a β-agonist. The *red zone* indicates a PEF that is <50% of personal best. The patient should know to call his or her health care provider immediately if use of an inhaled β-agonist does not bring return the PEF to the yellow zone or green zone.

Patients may also begin a crisis management plan if one was given to them by their health care provider or go to an ED. Use of green, yellow, and red stickers or tapes directly on the peak flow meter helps patients readily identify their zones. PEF zone values also should be written down for patients in their PEF diaries, along with a written asthma action plan.[5] A full discussion of home monitoring of PEF is beyond the scope of this chapter, and the reader is referred to more detailed sources.[1] (Also see Nocturnal Asthma and Question 49.) Figure 23-10 gives an example of PEF monitoring.

Because asthma consists of both bronchospasm and inflammation, therapy should be directed at both of these physiologic problems. Furthermore, the treatment of asthma must not be approached with timidity because the most common cause of death from asthma is undertreatment.[17] For most asthmatics, the condition can be extremely well controlled using the step-care approach recommended by the NIH Guidelines[5] (Figs. 23-11 and 23-12). A concerted effort in patient education as an integral part of state-of-the-art long-term management has been demonstrated to improve outcomes, including quality of life in patients with asthma. Because of the excellent outcomes associated with optimal long-term management, if a patient requires an ED visit or hospitalization, great care should be given to determining how the acute-care visit could have been prevented. Such events can usually be avoided.

ACUTE ASTHMA

Assessment

Signs and Symptoms

1. Q.C., a 5-year-old, 18-kg girl, presents to the ED with complaints of dyspnea and coughing that have progressively worsened over the past 2 days. These symptoms were preceded by 3 days of symptoms of a viral upper respiratory tract infection (sore throat, rhinorrhea, and coughing). She has experienced several bouts of bronchitis in the last 2 years and was hospitalized for pneumonia 3 months ago. Q.C. is not being treated with any medications at present. Physical examination reveals an anxious-appearing young girl in moderate respiratory distress with audible expiratory wheezes; occasional coughing; a prolonged expiratory phase; a hyperinflated chest; and suprasternal, supraclavicular, and intercostal retractions. Bilateral inspiratory and expiratory wheezes with decreased breath sounds on the left side are heard on auscultation. Q.C.'s vital signs are as follows: respiratory rate (RR), 30 breaths/min; blood pressure (BP), 110/83 mm Hg; heart rate, 130 beats/min; temperature, 37.8°C; and pulsus paradoxus, 18 mm Hg. Q.C. is given 2.5 mg of albuterol (Ventolin) as 0.5 mL of a 0.5% solution in 2.5 mL of normal saline by a compressed air nebulizer over 10 minutes. After the treatment, Q.C. claims some subjective improvement and appears to be more comfortable; however, wheezing on auscultation becomes louder. What signs and symptoms in Q.C. are consistent with acute bronchial obstruction? Does increased wheezing after albuterol indicate failure of the medication?

Asthma is an obstructive lung disease; therefore, the primary limitation to airflow occurs during expiration. This outflow obstruction leads to the classic findings of dyspnea, expiratory wheezes, and a prolonged expiratory phase during the ventilatory cycle.[1] Wheezing is a whistling sound produced by turbulent airflow through a constricted opening and usually is more prominent on expiration. Thus, the audible expiratory wheezing in Q.C. is compatible with bronchial obstruction. In fact, Q.C.'s obstruction is so severe that even inspiratory wheezes and decreased air movement were detected on auscultation. It is important to realize that the classic symptom of wheezing requires turbulent airflow; therefore, effective therapy of acute asthma actually may result in increased wheezing initially as airflow increases throughout the lung. As a result, Q.C.'s increased wheezing on auscultation is compatible with her clinical improvement following the albuterol nebulizer treatments.

The coughing experienced by Q.C. is another common finding associated with acute asthma attacks. The coughing may be due to stimulation of "irritant receptors" in the bronchi by the chemical mediators of inflammation (e.g., histamine) that are released from mast cells, or to the mechanics of smooth muscle contraction.

In the progression of an asthma attack, the small airways become completely occluded during expiration and air can be trapped behind the occlusion; therefore, the patient has to breathe at higher-than-normal lung volumes.[1] Consequently, the thoracic cavity becomes hyperexpanded and the di-

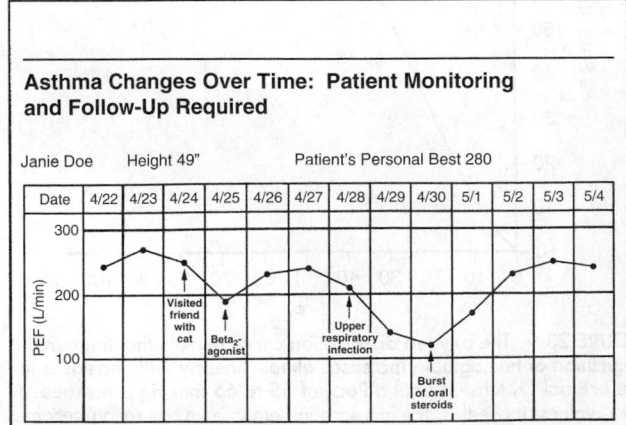

FIGURE 23-10 Asthma changes over time: patient monitoring and follow-up required. (Reproduced with permission from reference 183.)

Stepwise Approach for Managing Infants and Young Children (5 Years of Age and Younger) With Acute or Chronic Asthma

Classify Severity: Clinical Features Before Treatment or Adequate Control	Symptoms/Day Symptoms/Night	Medications Required To Maintain Long-Term Control Daily Medications
Step 4 Severe Persistent	Continual Frequent	■ **Preferred treatment:** – **High-dose inhaled corticosteroids** **AND** – **Long-acting inhaled beta₂-agonists** AND, if needed, – Corticosteroid tablets or syrup long term (2 mg/kg/day, generally do not exceed 60 mg per day). (Make repeat attempts to reduce systemic corticosteroids and maintain control with high-dose inhaled corticosteroids.)
Step 3 Moderate Persistent	Daily > 1 night/week	■ **Preferred treatments:** – **Low-dose inhaled corticosteroids and long-acting inhaled beta₂-agonists** **OR** – **Medium-dose inhaled corticosteroids.** ■ Alternative treatment: – Low-dose inhaled corticosteroids and either leukotriene receptor antagonist or theophylline. ···································· If needed (particularly in patients with recurring severe exacerbations): ■ **Preferred treatment:** – **Medium-dose inhaled corticosteroids and long-acting beta₂-agonists.** ■ Alternative treatment: – Medium-dose inhaled corticosteroids and either leukotriene receptor antagonist or theophylline.
Step 2 Mild Persistent	> 2/week but < 1x/day > 2 nights/month	■ **Preferred treatment:** – **Low-dose inhaled corticosteroid (with nebulizer or MDI with holding chamber with or without face mask or DPI).** ■ Alternative treatment (listed alphabetically): – Cromolyn (nebulizer is preferred or MDI with holding chamber) OR leukotriene receptor antagonist.
Step 1 Mild Intermittent	≤ 2 days/week ≤ 2 nights/month	■ No daily medication needed.

Quick Relief **All Patients**	■ Bronchodilator as needed for symptoms. Intensity of treatment will depend upon severity of exacerbation. – Preferred treatment: **Short-acting inhaled beta₂-agonists** by nebulizer or face mask and space/holding chamber – Alternative treatment: Oral beta₂-agonist ■ With viral respiratory infection – Bronchodilator q 4–6 hours up to 24 hours (longer with physician consult); in general, repeat no more than once every 6 weeks – Consider systemic corticosteroid if exacerbation is severe or patient has history of previous severe exacerbations ■ Use of short-acting beta₂-agonists >2 times a week in intermittent asthma (daily, or increasing use in persistent asthma) may indicate the need to initiate (increase) long-term control therapy.

Step down
Review treatment every 1 to 6 months; a gradual stepwise reduction in treatment may be possible.

Step up
If control is not maintained, consider step up. First, review patient medication technique, adherence, and environmental control.

Note
- The stepwise approach is intended to assist, not replace, the clinical decisionmaking required to meet individual patient needs.
- Classify severity: assign patient to most severe step in which any feature occurs.
- There are very few studies on asthma therapy for infants.
- Gain control as quickly as possible (a course of short systemic corticosteroids may be required), then step down to the least medication necessary to maintain control.
- Provide parent education on asthma management and controlling environmental factors that make asthma worse (e.g., allergies and irritants).
- Consultation with an asthma specialist is recommended for patients with moderate or severe persistent asthma. Consider consultation for patients with mild persistent asthma.

Goals of Therapy: Asthma Control
- Minimal or no chronic symptoms day or night
- Minimal or no exacerbations
- No limitations on activities; no school/parent's work missed
- Minimal use of short-acting inhaled beta₂-agonist (< 1x per day, < 1 canister/month)
- Minimal or no adverse effects from medications

FIGURE 23-11 Stepwise approach for managing infants and young children (5 years of age and younger) with acute or chronic asthma symptoms. (Reproduced with permission from reference 5.)

Stepwise Approach for Managing Asthma in Adults and Children Older Than 5 Years of Age: Treatment

Classify Severity: Clinical Features Before Treatment or Adequate Control			Medications Required To Maintain Long-Term Control
	Symptoms/Day Symptoms/Night	PEF or FEV$_1$ PEF Variability	Daily Medications

Step 4
Severe Persistent
	Continual
	Frequent
		≤ 60%
		> 30%
			■ **Preferred treatment:**
			– **High-dose inhaled corticosteroids**
			  AND
			– **Long-acting inhaled beta$_2$-agonists**
			  AND, if needed,
			– Corticosteroid tablets or syrup long term (2 mg/kg/day, generally do not exceed 60 mg per day). (Make repeat attempts to reduce systemic corticosteroids and maintain control with high-dose inhaled corticosteroids.)

Step 3 **Moderate Persistent**	Daily > 1 night/week	> 60% – < 80% > 30%	■ **Preferred treatment:** – **Low-to-medium dose inhaled corticosteroids and long-acting inhaled beta$_2$-agonists.** ■ Alternative treatment (listed alphabetically): – Increase inhaled corticosteroids within medium-dose range OR – Low-to-medium dose inhaled corticosteroids and either leukotriene modifier or theophylline. If needed (particularly in patients with recurring severe exacerbations): ■ **Preferred treatment:** – **Increase inhaled corticosteroids within medium-dose range and add long-acting inhaled beta$_2$-agonists.** ■ Alternative treatment: – Increase inhaled corticosteroids within medium-dose range and add either leukotriene modifier or theophylline.
Step 2 **Mild Persistent**	> 2/week but < 1x/day > 2 nights/month	≥ 80% 20–30%	■ **Preferred treatment:** – **Low-dose inhaled corticosteroids.** ■ Alternative treatment (listed alphabetically): cromolyn, leukotriene modifier, nedocromil, OR sustained release theophylline to serum concentration of 5–15 mcg/mL.
Step 1 **Mild Intermittent**	≤ 2 days/week ≤ 2 nights/month	≥ 80% < 20%	■ No daily medication needed. ■ Severe exacerbations may occur, separated by long periods of normal lung function and no symptoms. A course of systemic corticosteroids is recommended.

Quick Relief

All Patients

■ Short-acting bronchodilator: 2–4 puffs **short-acting inhaled beta$_2$-agonists** as needed for symptoms.
■ Intensity of treatment will depend on severity of exacerbation; up to 3 treatments at 20-minute intervals or a single nebulizer treatment as needed. Course of systemic corticosteroids may be needed.
■ Use of short-acting beta$_2$-agonists >2 times a week in intermittent asthma (daily, or increasing use in persistent asthma) may indicate the need to initiate (increase) long-term control therapy.

 Step down
Review treatment every 1 to 6 months; a gradual stepwise reduction in treatment may be possible.

 Step up
If control is not maintained, consider step up. First, review patient medication technique, adherence, and environmental control.

Goals of Therapy: Asthma Control

■ Minimal or no chronic symptoms day or night
■ Minimal or no exacerbations
■ No limitations on activities; no school/work missed
■ Maintain (near) normal pulmonary function
■ Minimal use of short-acting inhaled beta$_2$-agonist (< 1x per day, < 1 canister/month)
■ Minimal or no adverse effects from medications

Note

■ The stepwise approach is meant to assist, not replace, the clinical decisionmaking required to meet individual patient needs.
■ Classify severity: assign patient to most severe step in which any feature occurs (PEF is % of personal best; FEV$_1$ is % predicted).
■ Gain control as quickly as possible (consider a short course of systemic corticosteroids); then step down to the least medication necessary to maintain control.
■ Provide education on self-management and controlling environmental factors that make asthma worse (e.g., allergens and irritants).
■ Refer to an asthma specialist if there are difficulties controlling asthma or if step 4 care is required. Referral may be considered if step 3 care is required.

FIGURE 23-12 Stepwise approach for managing asthma in adults and children older than 5 years of age. (Reproduced with permission from reference 5.)

aphragm is lowered. As a result, the patient must use the accessory muscles of respiration to expand the chest wall. Q.C.'s hyperinflated chest and her use of suprasternal, supraclavicular, and intercostal muscles to assist in breathing also are compatible with obstructive airway diseases.

Occlusion of the small airways, air trapping, and resorption of air distal to the obstruction can lead to atelectasis (incomplete expansion or collapse of pulmonary alveoli or of a segment of lobe of the lung). Localized areas of atelectasis often are difficult to distinguish from infiltrates on a chest radiograph and atelectasis can be mistaken for pneumonia.

Q.C.'s history of multiple bouts of "bronchitis" is significant and typical of many young asthmatics. In any patient with recurring episodes of bronchial symptoms (i.e., bronchitis, pneumonia), the possible diagnosis of asthma should be investigated.

The increased pulse, RR, and anxiety experienced by Q.C. can be attributed both to hypoxemia and the feeling of suffocation. The hypoxemia in acute asthma is due principally to ventilation-perfusion ($\dot{V}/\dot{Q}$) mismatching.[18] Each alveolus of the lung is supplied with capillaries from the pulmonary artery for gas exchange. When ventilation is decreased to an area of the lung, the alveoli in that area become hypoxic and the pulmonary artery to that region constricts as a normal physiologic response. As a result, blood flow is shunted to the well-ventilated portions of the lung because of the need to preserve adequate oxygenation of the blood. The pulmonary arteries, however, are not constricted completely, and when a small amount of blood flows to the poorly ventilated alveoli, $\dot{V}/\dot{Q}$ mismatching is the result. Conditions of diffuse bronchial obstruction (i.e., acute asthma) increase the amount of $\dot{V}/\dot{Q}$ mismatching. In addition, some mediators of acute bronchospasm (e.g., histamine) further worsen $\dot{V}/\dot{Q}$ mismatching by constricting bronchial smooth muscle while concurrently relaxing vascular smooth muscle.

Q.C. also demonstrated a significant pulsus paradoxus. *Pulsus paradoxus* is defined as a drop in systolic blood pressure of >10 mm Hg with inspiration. In general, pulsus paradoxus correlates with the severity of bronchial obstruction; however, it is not always present.[18]

Extent of Obstruction

2. What additional tests would be helpful in assessing the extent of pulmonary obstruction in Q.C.?

Chest radiographs are not recommended routinely, but should be obtained in patients who are suspected of a complication (e.g., pneumonia).[1] Hyperinflated lungs and areas of atelectasis can be seen on a chest x-ray film; however, chest x-ray studies usually are negative and of little value in evaluating acute asthma attacks. The finding of a local decrease in breath sounds in Q.C.'s left lung may justify the need for a chest x-ray study, particularly if a significant differential in air movement persists after initial therapy. A local decrease in breath sounds may indicate pneumonia, aspiration into the lung of a foreign object, a pneumothorax, or merely thickened mucous plugging of a large bronchus.

Pulmonary function testing, particularly PEF, provides objective measurement of the degree of airway obstruction. Peak flow meters are indispensable in the ED for assessing both the severity of airway obstruction and the response to bron-

chodilator therapy. Unfortunately, infants and many young children do not have the cognitive or motor skills necessary to perform pulmonary function tests. At 5 years of age, however, Q.C. is old enough to perform the peak expiratory flow maneuver. Because of Q.C.'s initial anxiety, the PEF should be measured after bronchodilator therapy has been initiated when she may be calmer. One disadvantage of pulmonary function tests in acute asthma is that the forced expiratory maneuver can produce or worsen bronchospasm.

ABG measurements are the gold standard for assessing the severity of airway obstruction.[19] However, ABG measurements are unnecessary if other objective measures of airway obstruction (e.g., pulmonary function tests) have been monitored.[1] In acute asthma, ABG determinations usually indicate hypoxemia because of $\dot{V}/\dot{Q}$ mismatching and hypocapnia with respiratory alkalosis because of hyperventilation.[19] The degree of hypoxemia correlates with the severity of obstruction. Severe hypoxemia (PaO_2 <50 mm Hg) that is associated with an FEV_1 <15% of predicted represents severe airway obstruction.[18,19] Likewise, when the FEV_1 is <15% of the predicted value, carbon dioxide increasingly is retained and the $PaCO_2$ begins to rise into the usual normal range.[19] Because of $\dot{V}/\dot{Q}$ mismatching and the ease of correction of hypoxemia with O_2 therapy, the $PaCO_2$ is the more sensitive indicator of ventilation abnormalities in acute asthma with prolonged or chronic airway obstruction; CO_2 retention (hypercapnia) and respiratory acidosis are prominent. ABG measurements are indicated in patients who fail to respond adequately to initial therapy or in patients requiring hospitalization; they are not indicated at this time for Q.C.

Need for Hospitalization

3. Q.C. may require hospitalization. Which clinical test is predictive of the need for admission or whether Q.C. will relapse if sent home from the ED? Are Q.C.'s signs and symptoms predictive of whether she will relapse and return to the ED if not hospitalized?

The most useful predictive tool is the FEV_1 or PEF response to initial treatment. Patients who present with an FEV_1 of <30% of predicted and who do not improve to at least 40% of predicted after initial intensive therapy are more likely to have life-threatening deterioration.[1] Although Q.C. is not able to perform spirometry, she is able to do the peak flow maneuver, and the plan is to check her PEF after 1 hour of therapy. Signs and symptoms are not adequate to predict outcome of ED treatment of asthma.

Short-Acting Inhaled β-Adrenergic Agonist Therapy
Short-Acting Inhaled β-Agonists Compared with Other Bronchodilators

4. Why was a short-acting inhaled $β_2$-agonist selected as the bronchodilator of first choice in preference to other bronchodilators such as aminophylline or ipratropium for Q.C.? Could she have been given two drugs with different mechanisms of action to get an additive effect?

Because of their potency and rapidity of action, inhaled $β_2$-agonists are considered the first choice for the treatment of acute asthma.[1–4,20,21] The bronchodilatory properties of short-acting inhaled β_2-agonists are particularly effective in reversing early-phase asthma responses. In a study of 157 ED visits for acute asthma, a group of Harvard investigators found that parenteral and inhaled adrenergics were superior to aminophylline for relief of acute bronchospasm.[21] Therefore, theophylline would not be preferred over albuterol for the initial management of Q.C. in the ED. In addition, theophylline has more risks for serious side effects.

Similarly, the bronchodilation from the anticholinergic drug ipratropium is of smaller magnitude than with short-acting inhaled β_2-agonists. However, double-blind, randomized, placebo-controlled trials in the ED using changes of PEF or FEV_1 as end points have shown that ipratropium given as a nebulizer solution adds clinically significant benefit to initial doses of short-acting inhaled β_2-agonists.[22,23] For example, one study found that adult asthmatics in an ED albuterol-only group had a mean increase in PEF of 31% in 1 hour, whereas a group with ipratropium added to albuterol had a mean rise in PEF of 77%. The most severe asthmatics had a 93% increase in PEF when ipratropium was added to albuterol.[22] It is important to note that the dose of albuterol was aggressive (10 mg). Consistent with this finding, two double-blind pediatric trials found that the sickest children had a reduced rate of hospitalization if given ipratropium with albuterol in the ED.[24,25] In one trial,[24] children with baseline FEV_1 <30% of predicted value had a reduced rate of admission with ipratropium, and in the other trial,[25] children with baseline PEF <50% had a reduced rate of hospital admission. If anticholinergic agents are used, quaternary ammonium compounds such as ipratropium are preferred because of their excellent safety records. Atropine sulfate is a tertiary ammonium compound and can cause systemic side effects in large aerosol doses.[26]

Consequently, although early addition of inhaled ipratropium in adequate doses to short-acting inhaled β_2-agonists may improve pulmonary function tests, Q.C.'s physician chose to use only inhaled short-acting β_2-agonists initially because Q.C. was not severely ill and likely would not have had an improved outcome with the addition of ipratropium.

Preferred Routes of Administration

5. Why was the short-acting inhaled β_2-agonist, albuterol, administered to Q.C. by nebulizer instead of by the oral or parenteral routes of administration?

Numerous trials in stable asthmatics have shown that short-acting inhaled β_2-agonists administered by the inhaled route provide as great (Fig. 23-13) or greater bronchodilation with fewer systemic side effects than either the parenteral or oral routes.[22,27] In situations of acute bronchospasm, concerns over adequate penetration of aerosols into the bronchial tree led many clinicians to believe that the parenteral route of administration would be more effective than the inhaled route of administration. In clinical trials, however, short-acting inhaled β_2-agonists were as effective as the standard treatment of subcutaneous epinephrine for ED treatment of acute asthma in adults and children.[21,28] Therefore, short-acting aerosolized β_2-agonists now are considered the agents of choice for ED or hospital management of asthma.[1-4] β_2-Agonists should not be administered orally to treat acute episodes of severe asthma because of the slow onset of action, lower efficacy, and erratic absorption.[1,27]

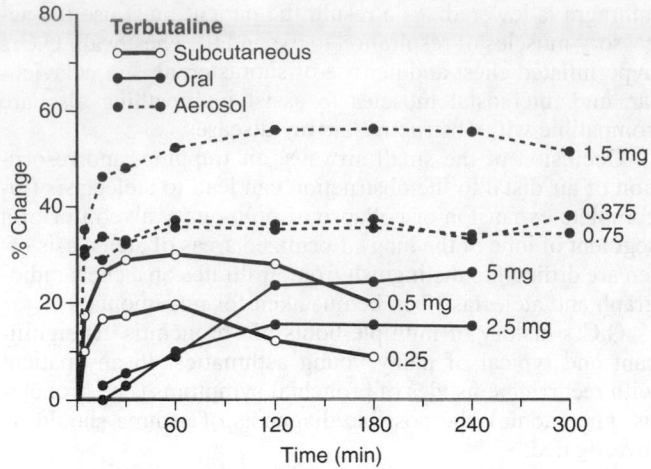

FIGURE 23-13 Time course of change in FEV_1 with different modes of administration of the β_2-selective agonist terbutaline. (Reprinted with permission from reference 27.)

6. Q.C. received albuterol by nebulization. Would intermittent positive-pressure breathing (IPPB) or metered-dose aerosol administration of the short-acting inhaled β_2-agonist have been preferred? Is the dose given by nebulization the same as that given by a metered-dose inhaler (MDI)?

Aerosols are mixtures of particles (e.g., a drug-lipid mixture) suspended in a gas. An MDI consists of an aerosol canister and an actuation device (valve). The drug in the canister is a suspension or solution mixed with propellant (e.g., chlorofluorocarbons). The valve controls the delivery of drug and allows the precise release of a premeasured amount of the product (Fig. 23-14). A second aerosol device, the air jet nebulizer, mechanically produces a mist of drug. The drug is placed in a small volume of solute (typically 3 mL of saline) and placed in a small reservoir (nebulizer) connected to an air source such as a small compressor pump, an oxygen tank, or a wall air hose. Air travels from the relatively large diameter tubing of the air source into a pinhole-sized opening in the nebulizer. This creates a negative pressure at the site of the air entry and causes the drug solution in the bottom of the nebulizer reservoir to be drawn up through a small capillary tube where it then encounters the rapid airflow. The drug solution is forced against a small baffle that causes mechanical formation of a mist (Fig. 23-15). IPPB devices aerosolize drugs in a similar manner as air jet nebulizers except that the airflow that exits the nebulizer in an IPPB device is enhanced to exceed atmospheric pressure. An ultrasonic nebulizer is a type of nebulizer that uses sound waves to generate the aerosol.

Studies comparing responses to short-acting inhaled β_2-agonists administered by nebulization versus IPPB have shown no significant advantages for the IPPB method of administration.[29] Furthermore, dose-response studies that compared nebulization with IPPB and pressurized metered-dose aerosols in stable chronic asthma patients have shown no advantage among these methods of administration when equivalent doses are administered.[4,30,31] Each method delivers approximately 10% of the beginning dose to the patient's airways.[32] Trials comparing metered-dose aerosols of short-acting inhaled β_2-agonists with the nebulization of those same drugs in acute asthma also have shown no significant advan-

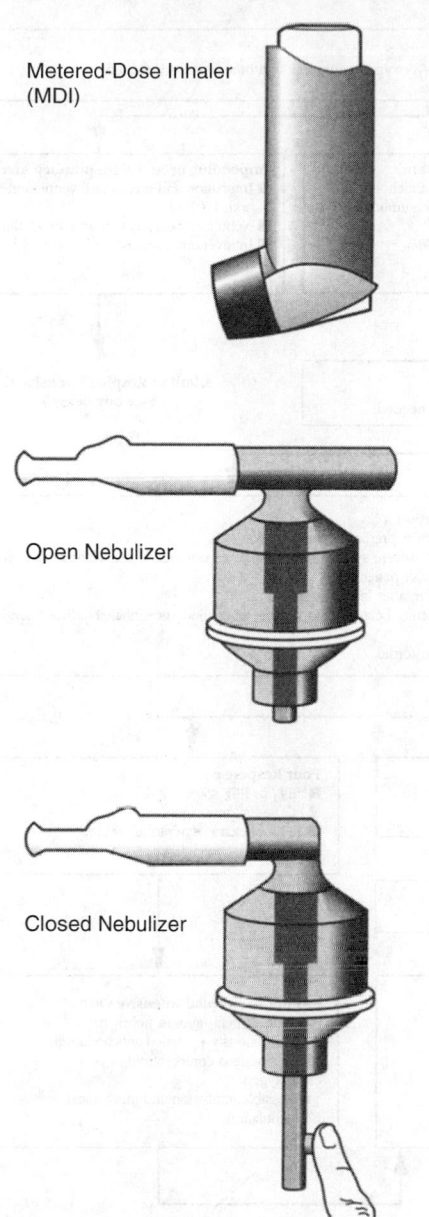

Metered-Dose Inhaler (MDI)

Open Nebulizer

Closed Nebulizer

FIGURE 23-14 Metered-dose inhaler and nebulizer.

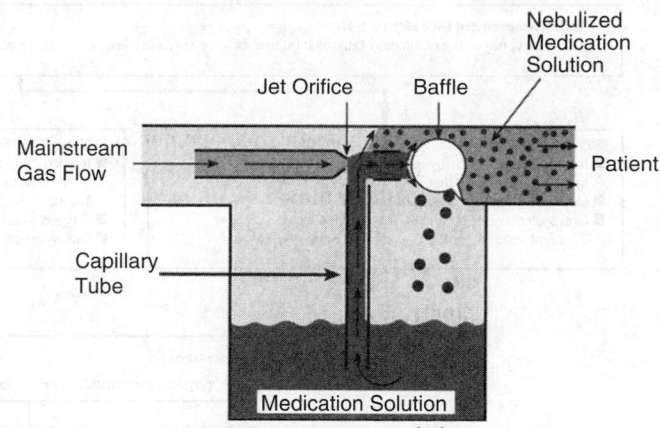

Nebulized Medication Solution

Jet Orifice   Baffle

Mainstream Gas Flow

Patient

Capillary Tube

Medication Solution

FIGURE 23-15 Air jet nebulizer.

erature. For children with mild acute asthma, 2 puffs of albuterol MDI attached to a spacer was not different from 6 to 10 puffs of albuterol or via nebulizer 0.15 mg/kg.[40] In one double-blind trial in children with a severe exacerbation, investigators used a dose ratio of 1:5 (i.e., albuterol MDI-spacer 1 mg [10 puffs]: nebulized albuterol 5 mg).[35] Nebulization of albuterol with compressed air or, preferably, oxygen was the preferred method of administration for Q.C. initially.

DOSING

7. **Because Q.C.'s symptoms were not relieved completely after the first dose of aerosolized albuterol, ABGs (on room air) were obtained with the following results: pH, 7.45; Pao$_2$, 60 mm Hg; and Paco$_2$, 28 mm Hg. Q.C.'s RR was 27 breaths/min. Starting 20 minutes after the first albuterol dose, repeated doses of 2.5 mg of albuterol were administered by nebulizer Q 20 min over the next 2 hours. After three treatments, Q.C.'s breath sounds became increasingly clear. Also, her PEF was now 65% of predicted, and discharge to home was planned.**

Were the dose and dosing interval of albuterol appropriate for Q.C.?

There are options regarding the dose or dosing interval for aerosol sympathomimetics in acute asthma. The duration of action of aerosolized short-acting inhaled β$_2$-agonists depends on the dose, physiologic state of the patient, and pharmacokinetic profile of the individual drug.[23] Patients with increased bronchiolar smooth muscle constriction will have a decreased intensity and duration of response to any given dose of a β-agonist.[20] One study indicated that a higher-dose albuterol regimen (0.15 mg/kg versus 0.05 mg/kg every 20 minutes) produced significantly greater improvement with no greater incidence of adverse effects.[41] Another study performed by Schuh and colleagues[42] demonstrated the greater efficacy of albuterol in a dose of 0.3 mg/kg (up to 10 mg) hourly over a dose of 0.15 mg/kg (up to 5 mg) hourly in children. The larger dose was tolerated as well as the 0.15 mg/kg dose. Kelly and colleagues[43] demonstrated the safety of high-dose terbutaline by continuous nebulization in children with acute severe asthma. Therefore, Q.C.'s albuterol regimen of 2.5 mg (0.14 mg/kg) nebulized every 20 minutes for 2 hours subsequent to her first dose of aerosolized albuterol was appropriate. Figure 23-16 describes the management plan for ED and hospital management of asthma from the NIH

tage for the nebulization method of administration when the metered-dose aerosolized administration was carefully supervised by experienced personnel and a spacer device was used.[33–37] However, in some younger acutely ill children, it is difficult (even with supervision) to administer an effective short-acting inhaled β$_2$-agonist with a metered-dose canister. Although some studies have found in children and adults that the first dose of short-acting inhaled β$_2$-agonists delivered by MDI with a spacer device is equivalent to nebulizer delivery, one study found that the first dose via the nebulizer was superior[38] Because many patients perceive that nebulizers provide more intensive therapy, it often is important psychologically to give at least the first dose of a short-acting inhaled β$_2$-agonist via a nebulizer. Thereafter, it is more cost-effective to use the therapeutically equivalent MDI plus spacer.[39]

The dose ratio for short-acting inhaled β$_2$-agonists delivered by MDI plus spacer versus nebulizer has varied in the lit-

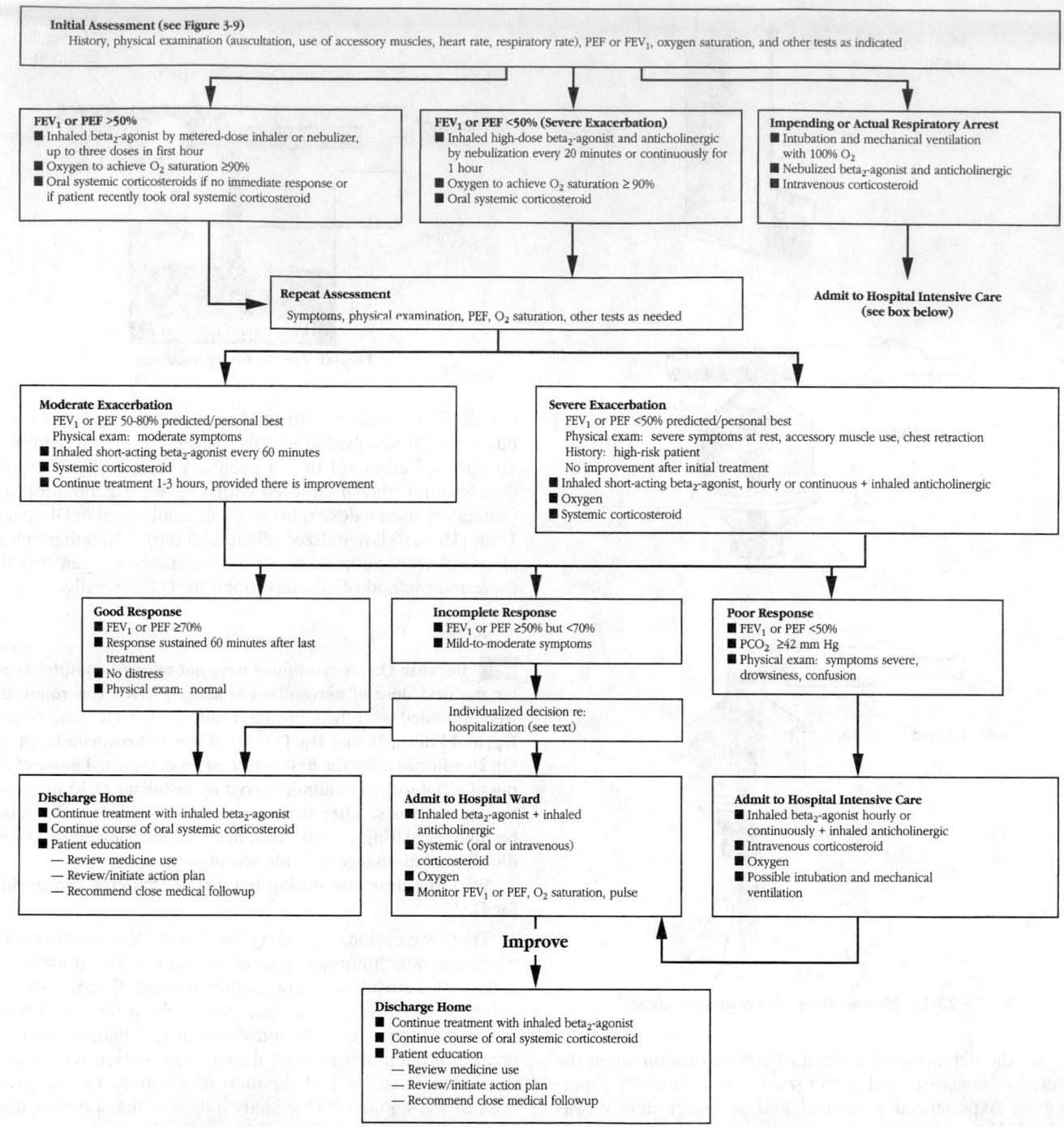

Initial Assessment (see Figure 3-9)
History, physical examination (auscultation, use of accessory muscles, heart rate, respiratory rate), PEF or FEV$_1$, oxygen saturation, and other tests as indicated

FEV$_1$ or PEF >50%
- Inhaled beta$_2$-agonist by metered-dose inhaler or nebulizer, up to three doses in first hour
- Oxygen to achieve O$_2$ saturation ≥90%
- Oral systemic corticosteroids if no immediate response or if patient recently took oral systemic corticosteroid

FEV$_1$ or PEF <50% (Severe Exacerbation)
- Inhaled high-dose beta$_2$-agonist and anticholinergic by nebulization every 20 minutes or continuously for 1 hour
- Oxygen to achieve O$_2$ saturation ≥ 90%
- Oral systemic corticosteroid

Impending or Actual Respiratory Arrest
- Intubation and mechanical ventilation with 100% O$_2$
- Nebulized beta$_2$-agonist and anticholinergic
- Intravenous corticosteroid

Repeat Assessment
Symptoms, physical examination, PEF, O$_2$ saturation, other tests as needed

Admit to Hospital Intensive Care (see box below)

Moderate Exacerbation
FEV$_1$ or PEF 50-80% predicted/personal best
Physical exam: moderate symptoms
- Inhaled short-acting beta$_2$-agonist every 60 minutes
- Systemic corticosteroid
- Continue treatment 1-3 hours, provided there is improvement

Severe Exacerbation
FEV$_1$ or PEF <50% predicted/personal best
Physical exam: severe symptoms at rest, accessory muscle use, chest retraction
History: high-risk patient
No improvement after initial treatment
- Inhaled short-acting beta$_2$-agonist, hourly or continuous + inhaled anticholinergic
- Oxygen
- Systemic corticosteroid

Good Response
- FEV$_1$ or PEF ≥70%
- Response sustained 60 minutes after last treatment
- No distress
- Physical exam: normal

Incomplete Response
- FEV$_1$ or PEF ≥50% but <70%
- Mild-to-moderate symptoms

Poor Response
- FEV$_1$ or PEF <50%
- PCO$_2$ ≥42 mm Hg
- Physical exam: symptoms severe, drowsiness, confusion

Individualized decision re: hospitalization (see text)

Discharge Home
- Continue treatment with inhaled beta$_2$-agonist
- Continue course of oral systemic corticosteroid
- Patient education
  — Review medicine use
  — Review/initiate action plan
  — Recommend close medical followup

Admit to Hospital Ward
- Inhaled beta$_2$-agonist + inhaled anticholinergic
- Systemic (oral or intravenous) corticosteroid
- Oxygen
- Monitor FEV$_1$ or PEF, O$_2$ saturation, pulse

Admit to Hospital Intensive Care
- Inhaled beta$_2$-agonist hourly or continuously + inhaled anticholinergic
- Intravenous corticosteroid
- Oxygen
- Possible intubation and mechanical ventilation

Improve

Discharge Home
- Continue treatment with inhaled beta$_2$-agonist
- Continue course of oral systemic corticosteroid
- Patient education
  — Review medicine use
  — Review/initiate action plan
  — Recommend close medical followup

FIGURE 23-16 Management of asthma exacerbations: emergency department and hospital-based care. (Reprinted with permission from reference 1.)

Guidelines[1], and Table 23-3 lists the doses for inhaled β-agonists for acute asthma as well as doses of other medications.[5]

COMPARISON OF SHORT-ACTING INHALED β$_2$-AGONISTS

8. **Would another short-acting inhaled β$_2$-agonist have been more effective in the initial therapy of Q.C.?**

Differences in the chemical structure of the various short-acting inhaled β$_2$-agonists produce differences in oral bioavailability, β$_2$-receptor selectivity, duration of action, and

molar potency.[20] If administered in equimolar potent doses, each β$_2$-agonist will produce the same degree of smooth muscle relaxation.[20] Therefore, in terms of intensity of bronchodilation, there is generally no major advantage of one short-acting β$_2$-agonist over another; however, when high dosages are required, the degree of β$_2$-selectivity becomes increasingly important. Short-acting, relatively β$_2$-specific agonists (e.g., albuterol) are preferred over nonspecific agonists (e.g., isoproterenol). Long-acting β$_2$-agonists (e.g., salmeterol) are not indicated for acute asthma. Levalbuterol (R-albuterol) be-

Table 23-3   Dosages of Drugs for Asthma Exacerbations in Emergency Medical Care or Hospital

Medications	Adult Dose	Child Dose	Comments
Inhaled Short-Acting β₂-Agonists			
Albuterol			
Nebulizer solution (5 mg/mL)	2.5–5 mg Q 20 min for 3 doses, then 2.5–10 mg Q 1–4 hr as needed, or 10–15 mg/hr continuously	0.15 mg/kg (minimum dose, 2.5 mg) Q 20 min for 3 doses, then 0.15–0.3 mg/kg up to 10 mg Q 1–4 hr as needed, or 0.5 mg/kg/hr by continuous nebulization	Only selective β₂-agonists are recommended. For optimal delivery, dilute aerosols to minimum of 4 mL at gas flow of 6–8 L/min.
Metered-dose inhaler (MDI) (90 μg/puff)	4–8 puffs Q 20 min up to 4 hr, then every 1–4 as needed	4–8 puffs Q 20 min for 3 doses, then every 1–4 hr as needed	As effective as nebulized therapy if patient is able to coordinate inhalation maneuver. Use spacer/holding chamber.
Pirbuterol			
MDI (200 μg/puff)	See albuterol dose	See albuterol dose; thought to be half as potent as albuterol on a mg basis	Has not been studied in severe asthma exacerbations.
Systemic (Injected) β₂-Agonists			
Epinephrine			
1:1,000 (1 mg/mL)	0.3–0.5 mg Q 20 min for 3 doses SC	0.01 mg/kg up to 0.3–0.5 mg Q 20 min for 3 doses SC	No proven advantage of systemic therapy over aerosol.
Terbutaline (1 mg/mL)	0.25 mg Q 20 min for 3 doses SC	0.01 mg/kg Q 20 min for 3 doses then every 2–6 hr as needed SC	No proven advantage of systemic therapy over aerosol.
Anticholinergics			
Ipratropium bromide nebulizer solution (0.25 mg/mL)	0.5 mg Q 30 min for 3 doses then Q 2–4 hr as needed	0.25 mg Q 20 min for 3 doses, then every 2–4 hr	May mix in same nebulizer with albuterol. Should not be used as first-line therapy; should be added to β₂-agonist therapy.
MDI (18 μg/puff)	4–8 puffs as needed	4–8 puffs as needed	Dose delivered from MDI is low and has not been studied in asthma exacerbations.
Corticosteroids			
Prednisone Methylprednisolone Prednisolone	120–180 mg/day in 3 or 4 divided doses for 48 hr, then 60–80 mg/day until PEF reaches 70% of predicted or personal best	1 mg/kg Q 6 hr for 48 hr, then 1–2 mg/kg/day (maximum, 60 mg/day) in 2 divided doses until PEF 70% of predicted or personal best	For outpatient "burst" use 40–60 mg in single or 2 divided doses for adults (children, 1–2 mg/kg/day; maximum, 60 mg/day) for 3–10 days

NOTE: No advantage has been found for higher-dose corticosteroids in severe asthma exacerbations, nor is there any advantage for intravenous administration over oral therapy provided gastrointestinal transit time or absorption is not impaired. The usual regimen is to continue the frequent multiple daily dosing until the patient achieves an FEV₁ or PEF of 50% of predicted or personal best and then lower the dosage to twice daily. This usually occurs within 48 hours. Therapy following a hospitalization or emergency department visit may last from 3 to 10 days. If patients are then started on inhaled corticosteroids, studies indicate there is no need to taper the systemic corticosteroids dosage. If the follow-up systemic corticosteroids therapy is to be given once daily, one study indicates that it may be more clinically effective to give the dose in the afternoon at 3:00 PM with no increase in adrenal suppression.
Modified from reference 1.

came available in the late 1990s, but further study is needed to determine whether this single isomer, higher potency drug offers any clinically significant advantages (i.e., improved outcomes) over racemic albuterol to justify its higher cost.[44]

SYSTEMIC CORTICOSTEROIDS IN THE ED FOR CHILDREN

9. Q.C. was not given any form of corticosteroid therapy as part of her ED management. Is this contrary to what is considered optimum treatment?

Yes. Because asthma is primarily an inflammatory airway disease, one should consider the degree of inflammation associated with Q.C.'s current exacerbation. Per the NIH Guidelines[1] (see Fig. 23-16), if there is not an immediate response to inhaled β_2-agonist therapy, oral systemic corticosteroids should be administered (see further discussion of this subject in Questions 14 and 15). Furthermore, if Q.C. had a peak flow meter at home, earlier objective detection of the development of this exacerbation might have prevented an ED visit. When the PEF is in the red zone (<50% of personal best) and poorly responsive to short-acting inhaled β_2-agonists, early intervention with oral corticosteroids is associated with a reduction in

ED visits[1] (Fig. 23-17; see Outcomes section at end of chapter. Q.C. and her parents should also understand that if respiratory distress is severe and nonresponsive to treatment, they should proceed to an ED or call 911. Finally, before going home from the ED, Q.C. and her parents should receive some basic education regarding asthma and its acute and long-term management. It is important to follow up with more detailed education during future clinic visits. Because Q.C. did not respond completely to the first dose of a short-acting inhaled β_2-agonist, a strong argument could be made that a short course of systemic corticosteroids as part of her discharge plan would reduce the risk of re-exacerbation.

ADVERSE EFFECTS

10. H.T., a 45-year-old, 91-kg man with a long history of severe persistent asthma, presents to the ED with severe dyspnea and wheezing. He is able to say only two or three words without taking a breath. He has been taking 4 inhalations of beclomethasone HFA (80 μg/puff) BID, and albuterol MDI, 2 inhalations QID PRN on a chronic basis. H.T. ran out of beclomethasone a week ago; since then he has been using his albuterol MDI with increas-

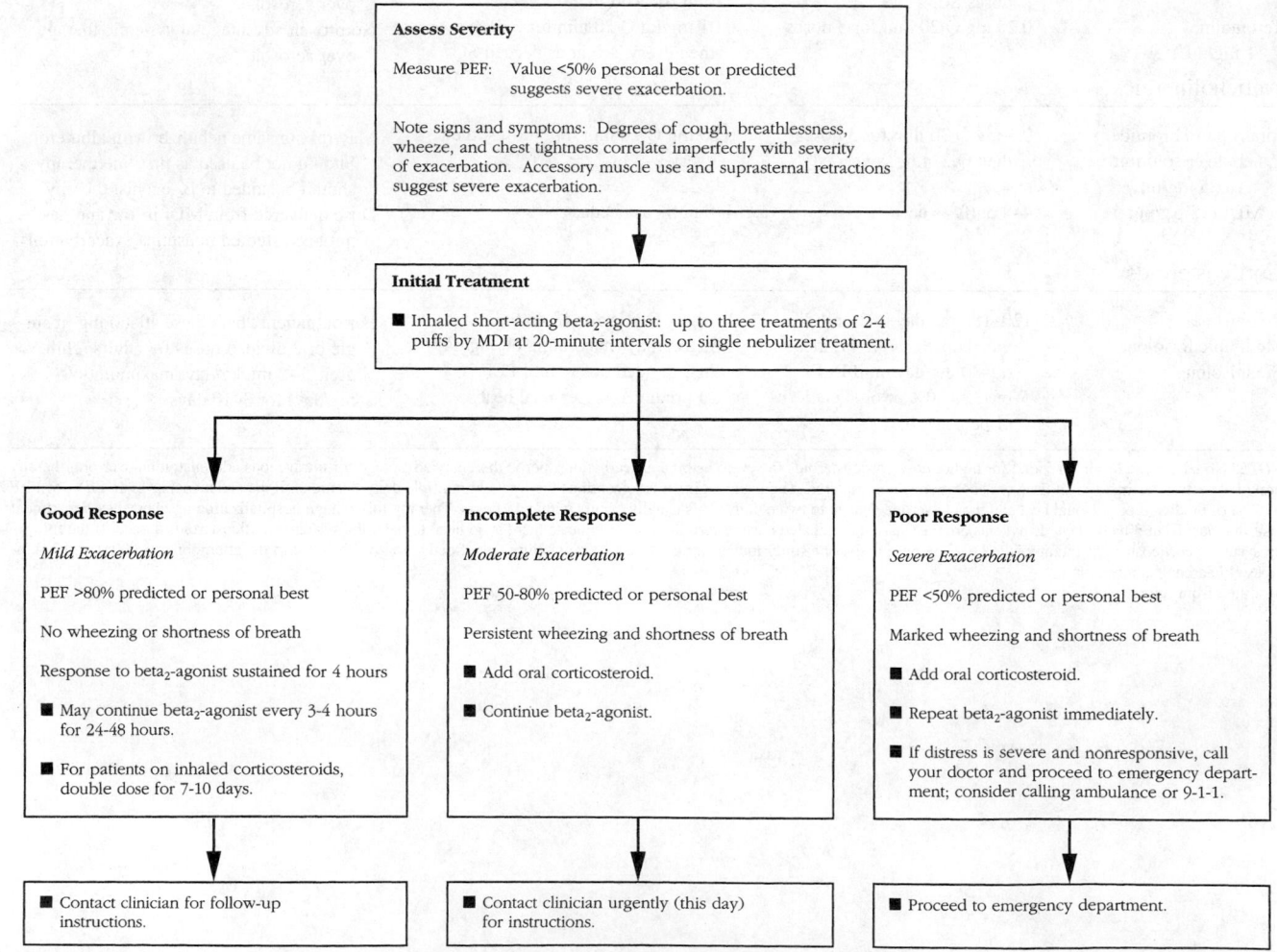

* *Patients at high risk of asthma-related death should receive immediate clinical attention after initial treatment. Additional therapy may be required.*

FIGURE 23-17 Management of asthma exacerbations: home treatment. (Reprinted with permission from reference 1.)

ing frequency up to Q 3 hr on the day before admission. His FEV_1 was 25% of the predicted value for his age and height. Vital signs are as follows: heart rate, 130 beats/min; RR, 30/min; pulsus paradoxus, 18 mm Hg; and BP, 130/90 mm Hg. ABGs on room air were as follows: pH, 7.40; Pao_2, 55 mm Hg; and $Paco_2$, 40 mm Hg. Serum electrolyte concentrations were sodium (Na), 140 mEq/L; potassium (K), 4.1 mEq/L; and chloride (Cl), 105 mEq/L. Because of the severity of the obstruction, H.T. was monitored with an electrocardiogram (ECG) that showed sinus tachycardia with occasional premature ventricular contractions (PVCs). Terbutaline 0.5 mg SC was administered with minimal improvement. H.T. then was started on O_2 at 4 L/min by nasal cannula, followed by another injection of 0.5 mg terbutaline SC. Subsequently, H.T.'s heart rate increased to 145 beats/min, more PVCs appeared on the ECG, and he complained of palpitations and shakiness. His PEF was now 25% of personal best. Laboratory values were pH, 7.39; Pao_2, 60 mm Hg; $Paco_2$, 42 mm Hg; Na, 138 mEq/L; and K, 3.5 mEq/L. What adverse effects experienced by H.T. are consistent with systemic β_2-agonist administration?

[SI units: Na, 140 mmol/L; K, 4.1 mmol/L; Cl, 105 mmol/L]

H.T. experienced palpitations, which may have been due to the widening of his pulse pressure from vasodilation or the PVCs.[2,20] Albuterol, terbutaline, and all other β-agonists are cardiac stimulants that may cause tachycardia and, very rarely, arrhythmias. Because they are relatively β_2-specific, the cardiac effects are more prominent with systemic administration (as opposed to inhalation) and at higher dosages. However, other causes of cardiac effects must also be considered, such as hypoxemia, which is also a potent stimulus for cardiac arrhythmias Therefore, H.T.'s tachycardia and PVCs may have been caused by the β_2-agonist, by the worsening of his airway obstruction (as reflected in the increase in $Paco_2$), or by both of these variables.

The decrease in the serum potassium concentration from 4.1 mEq/L to 3.5 mEq/L could be attributed to β_2-adrenergic activation of the Na^+-K^+ pump and subsequent transport of potassium intracellularly.[45,46] However, at usual doses, aerosolized albuterol and terbutaline cause relatively little effect on serum potassium. The effects may be more noticeable with systemic (oral or injectable) administration. A β_2-adrenergic-mediated increase in glucose and insulin secretion also can contribute to the intracellular shift of potassium.[45] What role, if any, the decrease in serum potassium has on the cardiac abnormalities associated with β-adrenergics is unknown.[46] H.T.'s potassium dropped from 4.1 to 3.5 mEq/L. Part of this drop may have been due to the terbutaline injections.

The shakiness (tremors) experienced by H.T. probably can be attributed to β_2-receptor stimulation of skeletal muscle. Again, this effect is most prominent with oral or parenteral administration, but some patients are very sensitive to even small doses of short-acting inhaled β_2-agonists. To minimize adverse effects, H.T. should have been given frequent high doses of inhaled albuterol rather than SC terbutaline on admission to the ED. He should have also been given nebulized ipratropium in addition to albuterol because his FEV_1 was <30% predicted.

β-Adrenergic Agonist Subsensitivity

11. Why did H.T. fail to respond to the initial therapy? Could tolerance to the β_2-agonists have contributed?

Although tolerance to systemic effects of β_2-agonists (e.g., tremor, sleep disturbances) is documented, tolerance to the airway response does not occur to a clinically significant extent.[47] Even with long-term use, the intensity of response to β_2-agonists is retained (i.e., the maximal percent increase in pulmonary function), but the duration of response with each dose may shorten. Such an effect is unlikely with intermittent use but may occur in patients who routinely use large, multiple doses daily. Possible explanations for this variability include downregulation of receptors, disease progression, or true drug tolerance. The exact contribution of each is not known. Therefore, H.T.'s failure to respond to the initial therapy most likely is due to the severity of his airway obstruction. H.T.'s history of severe chronic asthma, the slow progression of this attack, and the lack of response to his inhaled β_2-agonist also are largely due to a significant inflammatory component to this attack. Thus, bronchodilators would not be expected to immediately reverse the airway obstruction in H.T. It would be difficult to attribute his lack of initial response to therapy to β_2-adrenergic subsensitivity. In addition, it is not likely that β_2-adrenergic receptor polymorphisms could account for H.T.'s initial lack of response.[48]

Although polymorphic variations are documented to be relevant in some stable patients, further study is needed to document clinical relevance in severely ill patients.

Short-Acting Inhaled β-Agonists In Combination With Theophylline

12. When would the addition of theophylline to H.T.'s therapy be indicated?

Studies on the treatment of acute asthma in the ED have failed to demonstrate any benefit of adding theophylline to optimal, inhaled β-agonist therapy[21,49] and the NIH Guidelines do not recommended this practice.[1-4] Therefore, most clinicians would not use theophylline in H.T. Further evidence of the lack of value of theophylline in the acute-care setting emerged in the 1990s. Several double-blind, randomized, placebo-controlled studies have demonstrated that theophylline does not add benefit to intensive therapy with inhaled β_2-agonists and systemic corticosteroids in hospitalized adults[50] or children[51-54] who fail to respond to aggressive ED therapy with short-acting inhaled β_2-agonists. Note in Figure 23-16 from the NIH Guidelines[1] that theophylline is not recommended for routine management of hospitalized patients with asthma. Although one study[55] has shown a slight benefit of theophylline in hospitalized adult asthmatics, one of the authors of that study has since noted that if adequate doses of short-acting inhaled β_2-agonists and systemic corticosteroids are used, theophylline is probably not routinely indicated.[56] Although further research is needed to establish whether theophylline may add benefit to hospitalized patients who have impending respiratory failure, routine use of theophylline in hospitalized asthmatics no longer is justified.

13. Repeat measurements of PEF and ABGs indicate continued significant bronchial obstruction. What should be the next step in H.T.'s therapy?

H.T. should have had therapy initiated with short-acting inhaled β-agonists and certainly now should be changed from systemic to an aerosolized β-agonist. Because of the concern for cardiac toxicity, a β_2-selective agent such as albuterol should be selected. Three or four doses of albuterol, 5 mg by nebulizer administered every 20 minutes, should be started immediately with continuous monitoring of H.T.'s cardiac status. H.T.'s PEF also should be monitored after each nebulizer treatment. (Also see Questions 5 and 6.)

Short-Acting Inhaled β-Agonists in Combination With Corticosteroids

14. Corticosteroids are being considered for H.T. Is it rational to add them to β-agonists? When can a response be expected? By what route should they be administered? Why would corticosteroids be useful in H.T.'s initial treatment?

Corticosteroids have potent anti-inflammatory activity and are definitely indicated in H.T.[1-5] In patients like H.T. with acute asthma, corticosteroids decrease airway obstruction,[57-60] and increase the response to β_2-selective agonists.[57]

Corticosteroids are not smooth muscle relaxants (i.e., not direct bronchodilators); however, they can relieve bronchial obstruction by improving the responsiveness of β_2-receptors and by inhibiting numerous phases of the inflammatory response (e.g., arachidonic acid metabolism, cytokine production, neutrophil and eosinophil chemotaxis and migration).[1-4]

The anti-inflammatory activity of corticosteroids is delayed for about 4 to 6 hours after the dose has been administered.[4] Corticosteroid-induced restoration of responsiveness to endogenous catecholamines and exogenous β_2-agonists, however, occurs within 1 hour of administration of the corticosteroid in severe, chronic, stable asthmatics.[57] Significant improvement in objective measures (e.g., pulmonary function tests) generally occurs 12 hours after administration.[59] Consequently, the NIH Guidelines[1] advocate early initiation of corticosteroids in cases of acute severe asthma. Corticosteroids also hasten the recovery of acute exacerbations of asthma[61-65] and decrease the need for hospitalization if given early in the initial management of acute asthma in the ED.[60]

Based on his initial presentation, H.T. should have been started on systemic corticosteroid therapy immediately in the ED. Preferably, oral corticosteroids should have been started at home before H.T.'s exacerbation escalated to this degree of severity. Systemic corticosteroids should be continued throughout the hospital course and at discharge to complete a 7- to 10-day treatment course.

14. What would be an appropriate dosing regimen of corticosteroids for H.T. in the ED? Would the dose and route be the same if he were hospitalized?

Doses of corticosteroids used to treat acute asthma are largely empiric. Studies comparing very high dosages (e.g., methylprednisolone 125 mg every 6 hours intravenously in an adult) versus moderate dosages (40 mg every 6 hours) have shown no advantage with very high dosages.[1,66,67] In addition, oral therapy is as efficacious as the IV route.[1,66,67] Dosing recommendations for systemic corticosteroids in asthma patients in the ED or hospital are shown in Table 23-3. Higher corticosteroid dosages may be considered in patients with impending respiratory failure. When patients cannot take oral medication, IV methylprednisolone is preferred over hydrocortisone in patients with heart disease or fluid retention or when high dosages of corticosteroids are used; this is because it has less mineralocorticoid activity.

For patients who require hospitalization for parenteral steroid therapy, the dosage can usually be tapered rapidly to 60 to 80 mg/day for adults (1 to 2 mg/kg per day for children) as the condition improves (usually after 48 to 72 hours). Upon discharge from the hospital, prednisone 40 mg/day for <2 weeks is a common regimen in adults and the dose is then stopped abruptly. If the patient was steroid dependent before hospitalization, tapering the dose to the preadmission dosage is prudent. For patients who are discharged from the ED, 7 days or less of prednisone therapy usually is sufficient.

16. H.T. was given one dose of 125 mg methylprednisolone (Solu-Medrol) IV and three doses of albuterol 5 mg by nebulizer Q 20 min in the ED. H.T. claimed slight subjective improvement after this therapy; yet, expiratory wheezes still were audible and he still was using his accessory muscles for ventilatory efforts. His PEF improved only to 35% of predicted, and a repeat ABG measurement showed a $PaCO_2$ of 40 mm Hg. What should be done at this time?

H.T. still is significantly obstructed despite intensive therapy in the ED. As a result, he should be admitted to the intensive care unit where he can be monitored closely.

Respiratory Failure

Signs and Symptoms

17. What would be the best method of assessing the adequacy of therapy in H.T.? What are the signs of impending respiratory failure?

When patients continually must expand their chest wall with high lung volumes over a prolonged period, respiratory muscle fatigue may ensue, resulting in a decreased ventilatory effort. Clinical signs of impending respiratory failure include increased heart rate, decreased breath sounds, agitation from worsening hypoxia, or lethargy from increased CO_2 retention. These clinical signs and symptoms are relatively nonspecific and are affected by many variables. Thus, they should not be used to detect impending respiratory failure.

The best way to assess therapy is to monitor ABGs. The PaO_2 component of an ABG determination is not very helpful because of $\dot{V}/\dot{Q}$ mismatching and the administration of oxygen. The $PaCO_2$ is the best indicator of hypoventilation in acute asthma[1]; however, there is no single value for $PaCO_2$ that indicates impending respiratory failure because different $PaCO_2$ values are acceptable under different clinical circumstances. A $PaCO_2$ of 55 mm Hg 1 to 2 hours after intensive bronchodilator therapy, or an increase in $PaCO_2$ of 5 to 10 mm Hg/hour during aggressive therapy, is an ominous sign. The fact that H.T.'s $PaCO_2$ is not rising with therapy is a good sign.

β₂-Agonists and Other Potential Therapies

18. H.T. received two doses of terbutaline 0.5 mg SC and three doses of albuterol 5 mg by nebulizer Q 20 min in ED. Would the IV administration of a β-agonist be indicated in H.T. at this time? What are other potential therapies in H.T.?

Although the use of IV β-agonists for asthmatics in the intensive care unit used to be advocated, current standards of care discourage use of these agents.[1] IV albuterol is not superior to inhaled albuterol in severe asthma[68,69] and is associated with a greater risk of hypokalemia.[69] Based on current evidence, IV β-agonists are not recommended. H.T.'s history of

PVCs and response to inhaled albuterol also suggest that IV β-agonists are inappropriate at this time. As previously mentioned, H.T. should have received nebulized ipratropium initially along with inhaled albuterol and systemic corticosteroids. If these standard therapies were not sufficient, IV magnesium sulfate may benefit severely ill patients like H.T.[70] Recent research suggests that nebulized isotonic magnesium sulfate is a valuable adjunctive therapy to inhaled albuterol in the treatment of severe asthma exacerbations.[71] Further, heliox (a mixture of helium and oxygen) may also add benefit.[72]

Theophylline

19. **IV theophylline is being considered for H.T. Is theophylline likely to be of benefit in impending respiratory failure?**

It was previously stated that there is no role for theophylline in ED treatment, and its use is not justified for routine hospital admissions for asthma. However, there is a potential benefit of theophylline in the setting of impending respiratory failure. In a double-blind trial of patients requiring hospitalization for acute severe asthma, Edmunds and Godfrey[68] compared IV aminophylline with both inhaled and IV albuterol. Patients receiving either the inhaled or IV form of albuterol had a greater improvement in PEF than those receiving aminophylline over the first hour; however, the combination of aminophylline and the β2-agonist produced a greater response. Also, the addition of IV aminophylline to either route of β2-agonist administration in the second hour of therapy produced a further increase in peak flows. Based on a lack of evidence in several trials in hospitalized asthmatics,[50,54] more trials are needed to evaluate the benefit of this combination for impending respiratory failure. Two recent studies suggest a potential benefit of theophylline for some patients in the ICU with impending respiratory failure.[73–75]

Because some clinicians will choose to use theophylline in this situation and because it is a relatively high-risk drug, time is well spent examining several key aspects of theophylline use in the intensive care unit setting.

MONITORING THERAPY

20. **Because H.T. is not responding adequately to aggressive conventional therapy and is now in the intensive care unit, it is decided to initiate theophylline in H.T. How should his theophylline therapy be monitored?**

Although the therapeutic range for theophylline was formerly 10 to 20 μg/mL, close examination of the literature reveals that a more appropriate range is 5 to 15 μg/mL.[1,2,76] In 1991, the NIH Expert Panel Report recommended aiming for 5 to 15 μg/mL, which enhances safety while sacrificing little, if any, efficacy.[2] The incidence of theophylline side effects increases significantly when serum theophylline concentrations exceed 20 μg/mL.[56]

Because theophylline has a low therapeutic index, knowledge of its basic pharmacokinetics and of drugs or disease states that can alter its clearance is extremely important. A careful drug history should be taken to determine whether theophylline has been administered within the previous 24 hours. However, many patients are poor historians, and trying to estimate theophylline serum concentrations based on the history of intake during the preceding day is unreliable. In addition, there is significant interpatient variability in theophylline pharmacokinetics. Therefore, when assessing theophylline therapy, it is essential to monitor theophylline serum concentrations.[1] Clinical signs and symptoms of theophylline toxicity (e.g., tachycardia, headache, vomiting) also should be monitored carefully. However, life-threatening toxicity, including seizures and arrhythmias, may occur without warning with these minor side effects.[2]

LOADING DOSE

21. **What would be an appropriate loading dose of aminophylline for H.T.?**

A loading dose of theophylline is needed to rapidly achieve a serum concentration in the range of 5 to 15 μg/mL. The loading dose can be given intravenously or orally.[21] A rapid-release theophylline preparation (tablet or liquid) should be used if the theophylline loading dose is to be administered orally. It is imperative to administer IV loading doses slowly over 20 to 30 minutes to prevent severe cardiac arrhythmias (including cardiac arrest).[77]

The loading dose for theophylline is determined by its volume of distribution (Vd), which averages approximately 0.5 L/kg.[56] This Vd value remains relatively constant even in the presence of other diseases.

The loading dose can be calculated as follows:

$$LD = (Cp–Cp_o)(Vd) \times (Weight)$$

where LD is the calculated loading dose in milligrams, Cp is the desired serum theophylline concentration in micrograms per milliliter, Cp_0 is the existing serum concentration if previously taking theophylline, Vd is the volume of distribution in liters per kilogram, and $Weight$ is the patient's weight in kilograms.

Theophylline does not distribute into adipose tissue; therefore, either the ideal body weight (IBW) or the real body weight if it is within 20% of the ideal weight, whichever is less, should be used to calculate the loading and maintenance doses.[78] IBW in kilograms can be calculated using the following equations:

IBW males = 50 + (2.3)(Number of inches over 5 ft)
IBW females = 45.5 + (2.3)(Number of inches over 5 ft)

For children, this weight can be obtained by using standard height and weight charts. In this 5-foot, 8-inch patient, the IBW is calculated to be 68 kg [50 kg + (2.3 kg)(8)], and his real weight is 91 kg. H.T.'s IBW is less than his actual body weight; therefore, IBW should be used in the calculation of his aminophylline loading dose.

Because of the slight interpatient variability in distribution volume, it is considered prudent to target the desired serum theophylline concentration between 10 and 15 μg/mL (or mg/L) in acutely ill patients. Most clinicians would probably initially target 10 μg/mL. While the widely accepted conservative approach of targeting 10 μg/mL is appropriate for most patients, the clinicians caring for H.T. choose to target 15 μg/mL because he is extremely ill. In support of this decision, recent studies assessing the potential value of theophylline in patients with impending respiratory failure had target theophylline serum concentrations in the high therapeutic range.[73,74]

Thus, the loading dose calculation for H.T. is as follows:

$$LD = (Cp-Cp_o)(Vd)(Weight)$$
$$= (15 \text{ mg/L} - 0 \text{ mg/L})(0.5 \text{ L/kg})(68 \text{ kg})$$
$$= 510 \text{ mg theophylline}$$

If intravenous aminophylline is used, this loading dose is divided by 0.8 because aminophylline contains 80% anhydrous theophylline.

$$LD = \frac{510 \text{ mg}}{0.8}$$

$$= 637 \text{ mg or } 640 \text{ mg aminophylline}$$

As can be seen from the following equation, by assuming a distribution volume of 0.5 L/kg, every 1-mg/kg dose of theophylline will produce an approximate 2-µg/mL increase in theophylline serum concentration.

$$Cp(2 \text{ µg/mL}) = \frac{Dose(1 \text{ mg/kg})}{Vd(0.5)(L/kg)}$$

This relationship can be used to rapidly approximate loading doses for theophylline in various situations. The reader is cautioned, however, that this relationship applies only to single bolus doses for a rapid increase in serum concentration. The relationship does not apply to adjustments in maintenance doses.

MAINTENANCE DOSE (CONTINUOUS IV INFUSION)

22. **The IV loading dose of theophylline was given over 30 minutes. How is the maintenance dose determined?**

The maintenance dose is determined by the clearance of a drug according to the following relationship:

$$\text{Maintenance dose} = (Cpss)(Cl)$$

where *Cpss* represents the steady-state plasma concentration and *Cl* is the clearance.

Note that this equation is used to calculate the hourly continuous IV infusion dose of theophylline. It must be increased by a factor of 20% when using aminophylline. It also can be used to estimate intermittent oral doses by multiplying the hourly dose by the desired dosing interval.

Theophylline is cleared primarily by hepatic metabolism mediated by the cytochrome P450 mixed-function-oxidase enzyme system (CYP 1A2, 3A3, and 2E1).[56] Only about 10% of a dose is excreted unchanged in the urine, except in neonates. The metabolic clearance of theophylline is affected by age, concurrent disease states, other drugs, diet, and cigarette smoking.[1,56,79,80] The mean elimination half-life ($t_{1/2}$) in term neonates is about 24 hours.[56] The half-life of theophylline decreases gradually during infancy (as clearance increases) to a mean half-life of about 4 hours for children between 1 and 9 years old.[56] The half-life then increases in adults as clearance once again decreases to an average half-life of elimination of 7 to 8 hours in nonsmokers.[56] Smokers have a half-life ranging between 4 and 5 hours (faster clearance due to enzyme induction), and this half-life increases gradually after cessation of cigarette smoking.[80] Although there is a long-term change in theophylline half-life after smoking cessation, there also is a prompt increase in half-life 1 week after tobacco abstinence.

Lee and colleagues[80] found a 35.8% increase in theophylline half-life after smoking cessation in 14 healthy men. This initial, rapid decrease in theophylline elimination could be important clinically, especially in patients whose serum concentrations are in the higher end of the therapeutic range before smoking cessation.

A number of pathophysiologic conditions can alter the metabolism or clearance of theophylline. Disease states associated with a decreased theophylline clearance include hepatic cirrhosis, cor pulmonale, congestive heart failure, pulmonary edema, and prolonged fever associated with viral illnesses.[1,56,79]

Several pharmacokinetic dosing formulas and recommendations for the dosing of theophylline are available. Theophylline infusion doses that are calculated based on mean clearance values and dosages for corresponding ages should be used only for the uncomplicated asthma patient (Table 23-4).

In asthma patients with other complications, the method of Chiou and colleagues[81] is one approach of calculating doses that appears to be more accurate than using more empirical approaches. The Chiou method is very effective for dosing theophylline using few blood samples if (1) a constant infusion by pump is used, (2) dose (infusion rate) is constant, (3) physiologic parameters that determine theophylline clearance are not changing, (4) volume of distribution is not changing, (5) laboratory precision to measure theophylline in the serum is excellent, and (6) the patient's elimination half-life is shorter than the time interval between blood samples.[82] Equations to use with the Chiou method are as follows:

$$Cl = \frac{2 \text{ Ri}}{C_1 + C_2} + \frac{2 \text{ Vd} (C_1 - C_2)}{(C_1 + C_2)(T_2 - T_1)}$$

where *Cl* is clearance (L/kg per hour), *Ri* is infusion rate (mg/kg per hour), *Vd* is the volume of distribution (0.5 L/kg), C_1 is postloading dose serum concentration (mg/L), and C_2 is the second serum measurement. T_1 and T_2 are the times the samples were obtained. The blood samples should be obtained 4 to 6 hours apart for children and smokers or 8 hours apart in nonsmokers. The calculated clearance is then used to calculate the new infusion rate (mg/hr) needed to achieve the desired serum theophylline concentration (Cp) according to the following equation:

$$Ri = (Cp)(Cl)(Weight)$$

In conclusion, the general guidelines (see Table 23-4) are adequate for dosing theophylline in the uncomplicated asthma patient. If more precise determinations are desired, a more involved method such as that of Chiou should be used.

Because H.T. had no underlying complication known to alter theophylline clearance, a constant infusion was started using 0.6 mg/kg per hour of theophylline or 50 mg/hour of aminophylline (80% theophylline). This is greater than the recommended starting dose of 0.4 mg/kg per hour from Table 23-4 because a steady-state level >10 µg/mL is desired by H.T.'s clinician because H.T. is in the intensive care unit.[73,74] H.T. must be monitored closely for indications of theophylline toxicity at this higher dosage. Higher-than-usual doses of theophylline should not be used if serum theophylline concentrations cannot be analyzed rapidly and interpreted by practitioners well versed in theophylline kinetics. Many clinicians probably would not choose this relatively aggressive dose ini-

Table 23-4   Initial IV Maintenance Theophylline Infusion Rates

Patient Population	Average $t_{1/2}$ (hr)	Theophylline Infusion Rate (mg/kg/hr)[a]
Neonates (up to 24 days)[b,c]	20–30	0.08
Neonates (>24 days)[b,c]		0.12
Infants (6–52 wk)		0.008 (age in wk) + 0.21 mg/kg/hr
Young children (1–9 yr)[c]	3–4	0.8
Older children (9–12 yr)[c]		0.7
Adolescents (12–16 yr)		0.5
Adolescent (smoker)		0.7
Adult (>16 yr, nonsmoker)	7–8 (range, 3–16)	0.4
Adult (smoker)	3–4	0.7[d]
Elderly (nonsmoker)[c]	10	0.3
CHF, liver dysfunction, cor pulmonale, pneumonia, viral illness, high fever[e]		0.2 mg/kg/hr or ↓ above dose by 50%[e]
Cimetidine, ciprofloxacin, erythromycin, other enzyme inhibitors[f]		↓ above dose by 50%[f]
Carbamazepine, phenytoin, phenobarbital, rifampin, smoker[g]		↑ above dose by 50%[g]

[a]Doses to achieve 10 mg/L. Divide by 0.8 for aminophylline dose. Use lean body weight for obese patients.
[b]To achieve a target concentration of 7.5 mg/L for neonatal apnea.
[c]Clearance is slow in neonates due to immature hepatic function. During early childhood, clearance is most rapid. Clearance is slower in adults than in children. Clearance is further reduced with aging (>65 yr).
[d]Do not exceed 900 mg/day starting dose unless indicated by serum levels.
[e]The influence of these variables is difficult to predict. Theophylline clearance may change several times in the same patient during fluctuations in various disease processes. Do not exceed 400 mg/day starting dose unless serum levels indicate the need for larger doses.
[f]As a general rule, enzyme inhibition effects are rapid (24–48 hr), except with erythromycin. However, the magnitude of change may be both time and dose dependent. Patients with theophylline serum concentrations >13 mg/L are at greatest risk of developing side effects with combination therapy; prefer to circumvent with other agents.
[g]As a general rule, enzyme induction effects are slow (5 days–2 wk). Conversely, after stopping the drug inducer or smoking, it may take several days for the inducing effect to significantly abate.
CHF, congestive heart failure.

tially even in a very ill patient but would rather aim for 10 μg/mL and increase the dose of inhaled albuterol, systemic corticosteroid, add nebulized ipratropium, and consider other therapies previously discussed.

TIMING OF BLOOD SAMPLES

23. To use theophylline safely and optimally, serum theophylline concentrations should be monitored. When should blood samples be obtained to monitor serum concentrations?

When using the Chiou method for determining a theophylline maintenance dose, the blood samples should be obtained according to the recommendations in Question 22. When using the general guidelines in Table 23-4 for theophylline maintenance doses, an initial blood sample should be obtained 15 to 30 minutes after completion of the IV aminophylline loading dose. Another blood sample should be obtained 4 to 8 hours after starting the aminophylline constant infusion to determine the serum concentration of theophylline. It should be noted, however, that obtaining a serum level at 4 to 8 hours after starting the infusion is of little value unless there is a postloading dose concentration to use for comparison. If the aminophylline infusion dose is modified, the serum concentration of theophylline should be evaluated 12 to 24 hours after the dose change. Once the desired steady-state theophylline serum concentration has been reached (after approximately five estimated $t_{1/2}$'s), a blood sample should be analyzed for theophylline content whenever side effects are suspected, some factor that changes theophylline clearance is introduced, or there is a change in clinical response.

DOSING ADJUSTMENTS

24. H.T.'s serum theophylline concentration 30 minutes after the theophylline loading dose was 21 μg/mL. Eight hours later, while on the constant infusion, it was 15 μg/mL. H.T.'s overall clinical condition seems to have improved; however, he is still wheezing and short of breath, and his most recent $Paco_2$ is 35 mm Hg. How should H.T.'s dose of theophylline be adjusted to provide additional relief of symptoms?

The initial theophylline concentration may have been high because the loading dose was excessive (possibly because H.T.'s volume of distribution is less than estimated). Also, as with most drugs metabolized by hepatic enzymes, theophylline has the potential to saturate its metabolic enzyme system.[56] When the pathway for the hepatic metabolism of theophylline is saturated, changes in the serum concentrations of theophylline are disproportionate relative to the dose, and fine tuning of the serum concentrations of this drug can be difficult. Because of the log-linear nature of the theophylline concentration response curve, an increase above 15 μg/mL would not be expected to produce further clinically significant bronchodilation. In addition, the last $Paco_2$ measurement indicates that H.T. is improving; therefore, no dosage adjustment is necessary.

RESPONSE TO THERAPY

25. H.T. has continued to improve slowly over the last 72 hours. The nebulizer treatments with albuterol are now administered Q 4 hr and he is taking oral prednisone 80 mg/day in two divided doses. PEF measurements taken before and after the last albuterol treatment were 65% of predicted and 90% of predicted, respectively. Is H.T.'s long duration of recovery unusual?

No. In a patient such as H.T. whose condition progressively deteriorated over a long period, one should expect a slow reversal. The prolonged deterioration reflects an increasing inflammatory response in the lung. These patients require prolonged, intensive bronchodilator and anti-inflammatory therapy before maximal improvement is noted in pulmonary function tests. Thus, H.T. should continue to receive systemic corticosteroids for at least 2 weeks after such a severe acute exacerbation of asthma.

Adverse Effects of Short-Term Corticosteroid Therapy

26. H.T. has been taking corticosteroids for a total of 6 days. Long-term corticosteroid use is associated with many adverse effects (e.g., adrenal suppression, osteoporosis, cataracts). What adverse effects are related to short-term corticosteroid use?

Short courses of daily corticosteroids are usually associated with minor side effects.[61–65] Facial flushing, appetite stimulation, GI irritation, headache, and mood changes ranging from a mere sense of well-being to overt toxic psychosis are the most commonly encountered adverse effects of short-term corticosteroid therapy. Acne can be exacerbated in patients susceptible to this skin problem, and weight gain also can occur because of sodium and fluid retention. In addition, hyperglycemia, leukocytosis, and hypokalemia are possible. All these problems are transient and will disappear over time after the corticosteroids are discontinued. These short-term adverse effects are less common when small corticosteroid doses are used; however, corticosteroid doses must be adequate to prevent disease exacerbation. The minor risks of short-term use are far outweighed by the marked benefits.

Overuse of Short-Acting Inhaled β-Agonists

27. H.T.'s history of increased use of his short-acting inhaled β$_2$-agonist inhaler during the early stages of this asthma attack and the cardiac irregularities noted during admission suggest improper use of this medication. What are the risks from overuse of β$_2$-agonist?

The overuse of short-acting inhaled β-agonists as a possible risk factor for asthma death has been debated for decades, and this debate was revived in the early 1990s.[83] Because most deaths from asthma occur outside the hospital setting before the patient can reach medical assistance, the primary cause of death in asthma most probably is due to underestimation of the severity of the asthma attack by the patient and delay in seeking medical help.[17] Overuse of quick reliever medication suggests inadequate asthma control and can lead to fatal asthma.[1,83]

The association of fatal or near fatal asthma and overuse of short-acting inhaled β-agonists was greatest in patients who were using more than two canisters per month of fenoterol, a β-agonist not used in the United States. It is likely that deaths in this case-control analysis[83] were due to undertreatment of the inflammatory condition rather than to toxicity caused by the chronic use of inhaled β-agonists. In other words, patients with more severe disease were more likely to use larger doses.

Although there is no proof that use of a short-acting inhaled β$_2$-agonist four times daily is harmful, most asthma experts prefer to use as-needed rather than regularly scheduled short-acting β$_2$-agonists.[1–5] By determining the frequency of as-needed doses, the clinician has a good marker of the adequacy of inhaled anti-inflammatory therapy. For example, if the patient needs the short acting inhaled β$_2$-agonist more than two or three times a day, the clinician should increase the dose of inhaled anti-inflammatory therapy or add other controller agents per the NIH Guidelines.[1,5]

The best way to prevent asthma deaths is state-of-the-art treatment and education. Patients should be instructed on the proper use of all their medications. Frequent use of bronchodilator inhalers should be a clue to instability of the airways and increasing inflammation. Appropriate measures should be taken before the need for hospitalization occurs. Setting arbitrary absolute limits to inhaler use is not useful and may only lead to mutual dissatisfaction between the clinician and patient. Patients should be instructed verbally and in writing regarding the proper use of their inhalers during acute attacks and in recognizing when it is necessary to seek medical assistance. Patients can continue using their short-acting β-agonist inhalers on an as-needed basis until they reach medical care. H.T. should be considered at high risk because of the severity of his latest attack and should be given oral corticosteroids to self-administer at the first sign of significant deterioration.[1–5] In addition, H.T. should have a home peak flow meter so that he can objectively determine the severity of his attacks. Finally, the β-agonist controversy does not extend to use of high dosages in the acute-care setting. High dosages are essential in the ED and hospital and, as previously discussed, usually are tolerated very well.

CHRONIC ASTHMA

Classification of Severity

28. B.C., a 3-year-old, 16-kg boy with a 1.5-year history of daily recurrent wheezing, was referred to the pulmonary clinic for difficult-to-control asthma. The following medications had been prescribed for B.C.: theophylline syrup (80 mg/15 mL), 1.5 tablespoonfuls TID PRN wheezing; albuterol metered-dose aerosol inhalation QID; and prednisolone (Pediapred) oral liquid 1 teaspoonful BID for severe wheezing. B.C.'s mother had been administering the prednisolone whenever the child experienced respiratory difficulties; however, B.C. has been taking the prednisolone almost continuously over the past few months. The mother also relates that she seldom uses the theophylline because B.C. becomes "very hyper" when taking it. B.C. demonstrates the use of the inhaler with his mother's assistance. The mother holds the inhaler in B.C.'s mouth and actuates it at the end of a deep inhalation. What is the first step in deciding how to improve B.C.'s long-term drug therapy?

While keeping in mind the goals of therapy defined by the NIH Guidelines,[1] the first step here is to classify B.C.'s asthma severity (see Fig. 23-1). Because B.C. has symptoms every day, he should be classified at a minimum as "moderate persistent." Note that the presence of even one of the features of severity places the patient in that category. If we knew that B.C.'s PEF variability was >30% or if his nocturnal symptoms occurred more than once weekly, this would be further supportive evidence; but simply knowing that he has daily symptoms is sufficient to classify his asthma as moderate persistent.

Selection of Appropriate Initial Long-Term Therapy

29. **What would be a reasonable initial regimen for B.C.?**

Because B.C.'s asthma is classified as moderate persistent, the clinician is now in a position to select rational long-term therapy. The goal of the therapy is to provide maximum control of symptoms with the most convenient regimen that provides the fewest adverse effects. Using the NIH Guidelines[5] for young children (see Fig. 23-11), medium-dose inhaled corticosteroids (ICS) or low-dose ICS with a long-acting inhaled β_2-agonist with as-needed short-acting inhaled β_2-agonist would be the choice for B.C.[5] Because B.C.'s mom was not giving him regular doses of theophylline and when she did it was not well tolerated, it should be stopped at this point. If she had been giving him regular doses with a good response, it would probably be continued for a few days until the inhaled corticosteroid had time to reduce B.C.'s airway inflammation and symptoms.

The long-term use of oral corticosteroids is associated with numerous adverse effects; therefore, if possible, B.C.'s long-term prednisolone use must be tapered and ultimately discontinued. The chronic use of systemic corticosteroids can lead to hypothalamic-pituitary-adrenal (HPA) axis suppression, growth retardation in children, cushingoid appearance, diabetes, hypertension, myopathy, hirsutism, osteoporosis resulting in fractures, and postsubcapsular cataracts.[1] The degree of HPA axis suppression is both dose and duration dependent. Although B.C. has been prescribed prednisolone 5 mg twice daily, which is within the usual recommended dose (i.e., 0.5 to 2 mg/kg per day) for children, systemic steroids should be prescribed only for patients who are not responding adequately to other therapy and then as a single daily dose in the morning or every other day. To avoid growth retardation and the numerous other problems associated with long-term daily use of oral corticosteroids, every effort should be made to optimize other therapies. Subsequently, the prednisolone can be discontinued gradually as drug therapy with other medications is optimized. B.C.'s mother must be educated about the disease, its treatment, and the appropriate use of medications (e.g., proper use of inhaler devices; see Questions 50 and 51).

30. **Develop a plan to discontinue B.C.'s prednisolone.**

A structured long-term management plan, including environmental control and daily inhalation of an inhaled corticosteroid, must be established for B.C. to properly evaluate his real need for prednisolone. The initial medication program also should be aggressive in order to gain quick control of asthma and to establish confidence in the patient-clinician relationship or "partnership." Once B.C. is stabilized on an effective inhaled drug regimen, the oral corticosteroid can be discontinued by gradually decreasing the dose. To gain quick control, B.C. should receive three days of a higher dosage of prednisolone (e.g., 30 mg) concurrently with the start of ICS. Oral prednisolone should then be tapered slowly because he had already received oral therapy more than 2 weeks previously.

There are no rigid guidelines on exactly how to taper except that dosage reduction should be slow; individual patients vary in the rate that tapering is tolerated. Obviously, the higher the long-term oral dose, the longer it will take to completely stop such therapy (e.g., >3 months to completely taper off, starting with conversion to alternate-day therapy and then slowly decreasing the dose every other day).[84] B.C. was receiving 5 mg twice daily for several months. One approach to tapering in B.C. would be to convert to alternate-day therapy (20 mg [some clinicians may choose 30 mg] every other day) at 8 AM. Then, B.C.'s dose should be decreased by 5 mg per dose every 2 weeks (some clinicians prefer 2.5 mg weekly). Once 5 mg every other day is reached, tapering by smaller milligram increments (e.g., 10% weekly if tolerated) should continue over the next few weeks before cessation of therapy. Remember, B.C.'s asthma is being controlled by ICS therapy, and the slow tapering of prednisone is to allow the adrenal cortex, which was suppressed, to secrete normal amounts of cortisol. B.C.'s physician will monitor him (clinically and laboratory) during prednisolone tapering to ensure that tapering is sufficiently slow. Examples of symptoms that may occur during withdrawal include fatigue, anorexia, dizziness, or fainting. During tapering and for 1 year after, if B.C. encounters acute illness, trauma, or surgery, high dosages of systemic corticosteroids should be administered for a few days.[84]

31. **It is anticipated that because of his young age, B.C. will find it difficult to use an MDI. What alternatives can you suggest?**

Children younger than 5 five years of age have a difficult time coordinating the use of standard MDIs; therefore, the inhaled corticosteroid and short-acting β_2-agonist should be administered by another mode of delivery. For example, the as-needed β_2-agonist and scheduled inhaled corticosteroid could be administered with an inhalational aid such as InspirEase or AeroChamber, which is connected to an MDI (Table 23-5). A nebulized corticosteroid preparation (budesonide) is available for very young children.[85] Inhalation aids (also called *extender devices* or *spacers*) significantly improve the efficacy of medications that are administered by MDI, particularly in very young children who are unable to coordinate the plain inhalers correctly.[86] Studies have shown that many children as young as 2 and 3 years of age can use MDIs with spacer devices by modeling after a parent.[87,88] Spacer devices with face masks are required for some young children. Extender device-assisted delivery of aerosolized medications is as effective as nebulization in the home management of chronic severe asthma[89] and even in the ED treatment of asthma in children.[35,39,40] The InspirEase and AeroChamber are examples of devices that contain a flow indicator whistle that sounds if the patient inhales rapidly. This whistle is particularly effective in teaching the patient the appropriate slow inhalation technique. As a 3-year-old, B.C. may not need a spacer with a face mask, but the clinician should verify correct use of the device by observation of the patient and/or caregiver's administration technique.

Alternatively, the ICS could be administered to selected children using a breath-activated dry powder inhaler (e.g., budesonide [Pulmicort Turbuhaler] or fluticasone [combined with salmeterol in Advair Diskus]) (see Table 23-5). In young children, Diskus has the advantage of requiring lower peak

Table 23-5 Examples of Spacer Devices and Dry Powder Inhalers

Spacer Devices	Comments
ACE (Aerosol Cloud Enhancer) (DHD)	150-mL conical holding chamber with one-way valve at mouth-piece; flow indicator whistle
AeroChamber (Monaghan Medical)	Holding chamber; cylinder with one-way valve that releases aerosol when subject inhales; flow indicator whistle
InspirEase (Schering)	Holding chamber consisting of a collapsible bag with a flow indicator whistle
Optichamber (Health Scan)	Holding chamber; cylinder with one-way valve that releases aerosol when subject inhales; flow indicator whistle

Breath-Activated Dry Powder Inhalers

Aerolizer	Each dose of formoterol must be loaded; lactose included as carrier
Diskus	Holds 60 doses of salmeterol/fluticasone *or* salmeterol; has dose counter; lactose for taste
Rotadisk	Disk with 4 doses of flutacasone inserted into dishaler; lactose for taste
Turbuhaler	Holds 200 doses of budesonide; red indicator when 20 doses are left; no taste

inspiratory flow than Turbuhaler, and it has been used successfully in children as young as 4 years.[90] (See Question 50.)

Many pediatricians may choose a nebulizer to administer short-acting β_2-agonists to a 3-year-old child. This method is certainly acceptable and very common, but it takes longer to administer the medication (about 15 minutes), and the device must be properly cleaned. Because B.C. only recently turned 3 years old, the pediatrician chooses to initiate therapy with nebulized budesonide (Pulmicort Respules) in a moderate dose of 0.5 mg BID. The plan is to switch B.C. to a dry powder inhaler or MDI-spacer in 6 to 12 months, as soon as he and his caregiver can demonstrate correct use.

Although a selective β_2-agonist could be administered orally to B.C. as an alternative to extender device-assisted aerosolization, the advantage of ease of administration is offset by an increase in adverse effects and diminished efficacy.[27] Combining an as-needed short-acting inhaled β_2-agonist (e.g., albuterol) with an anti-inflammatory agent is basic therapy for virtually all patients with persistent asthma.[1,5]

Seasonal Asthma

32. **C.V., a 33-year-old woman, presents to the clinic with a history of asthma and seasonal allergic rhinitis (hayfever) each spring, but not the rest of the year. She describes her asthma as "mild" and intermittent. Except during springtime, her daytime symptoms occur less than once per week and she does not have nocturnal symptoms. Each spring, however, these symptoms worsen, and she requires her albuterol inhaler (her only asthma medication) TID or QID. During hayfever season, she takes a nonprescription antihistamine, which offers some relief. How can C.V.'s management be improved?**

C.V. appears to have mild, intermittent asthma during most of the year, but converts to moderate persistent asthma combined with worsening rhinitis symptoms in the springtime. This syndrome is consistent with a diagnosis of seasonal asthma and allergic rhinitis. Although as-needed albuterol is appropriate for most of the year for C.V., she needs anti-inflammatory therapy during the spring.[1] Therapy to reduce airway inflammation should begin before the onset of tree and grass pollen season and continue throughout the spring (e.g., 3 months). Per the NIH Guidelines, the preferred treatment for C.V. is low-dose inhaled corticosteroid combined with a long-acting inhaled β_2-agonist.[5] Not only are the causes and pathophysiology of allergic rhinitis and allergic asthma similar, persistent postnasal drip from poorly controlled rhinitis serves as a major asthma trigger. In addition, C.V. should also ideally receive an intranasal corticosteroid (or other intranasal agent such as cromolyn, azelastine, or ipratropium) if antihistamines (sedating or nonsedating) do not provide optimal relief of her allergic rhinitis. Intranasal corticosteroid therapy not only offer excellent relief of nasal symptoms, but also improve asthma control.[5] Good control of rhinitis is helpful in maintaining optimal asthma control.[1,2] (Also see Chapter 25, Acute and Chronic Rhinitis.) Despite precautions listed in manufacturer's literature that older (sedating) antihistamines should be avoided in asthma, these agents are safe in patients with asthma.[1,2]

Corticosteroids

33. **S.T., a 12-year-old girl with severe persistent asthma, has not been well controlled on Q 12 hr SR theophylline, flunisolide (Aerobid) one puff BID (she admits to using it only when she feels as if she needs it), and as-needed inhaled albuterol. She has been hospitalized four times in the last 2 years and has required "bursts" of prednisone with increasing frequency. S.T. has missed many days of school in the past year and has withdrawn from physical education classes and her extracurricular sports activity after school. Her parents are concerned about her increased use of prednisone now that she is approaching puberty. S.T. is just finishing a 2-week course of prednisone 20 mg/day and has a round facies appearance typical of chronic oral steroid use. On physical examination, S.T. has diffuse expiratory wheezes, and pulmonary function testing reveals significant reversibility. S.T. has been very compliant with her theophylline, and her steady-state peak theophylline serum concentrations have consistently been in the range of 10 to 12 μg/mL. What are the therapeutic alternatives for S.T.?**

Because S.T. is suffering needlessly and requiring frequent systemic corticosteroids, all efforts must be made to optimize other therapies and to minimize systemic corticosteroid toxicities. Although S.T. is receiving an inhaled corticosteroid, she has been prescribed a low dose of a low-potency agent, and she admits to poor adherence. Therefore, with her severe persistent asthma, she initially needs higher-dose ICS therapy, preferably with a more potent agent. Per the NIH Guidelines, she should also receive a long-acting inhaled β_2-agonist. Although short "bursts" of prednisone (e.g., 40 mg/day for 3 days) are very helpful occasionally, frequent short courses often indicate the need to optimize other therapies. Some patients require courses of 1 to 2 weeks. S.T. is requiring longer frequent "bursts" and is showing signs of adverse effects. Obviously, S.T. and her parents also need a concerted and persistent effort in patient education as a partnership. (See Question 48.)

ICS are chemically modified to maximize topical effectiveness while minimizing systemic toxicities. Table 23-6 is taken from the NIH Guidelines[5] and compares the dosages of ICS products. These differences in dosages (low, medium, and high) reflect differences among inhaled corticosteroids in receptor-binding affinity and topical potency. There are also differences among these agents in oral bioavailability (i.e., absorption of drug that is swallowed after inhalation) and systemic availability via absorption from the lungs. Of these two variables, absorption from the lungs is the most likely contributor to possible HPA suppression or other systemic effects. Fortunately, the total absorption has not been shown to be clinically important except at the higher recommended dosages in Table 23-6. Although the various ICS are not equipotent on a microgram-per-microgram basis, major differences in efficacy or adverse effects are not firmly established.[1,91,92] For patients with severe persistent asthma, a logical choice would be a high-potency agent that would allow for fewer puffs per day, potentially improving treatment adherence. Furthermore, the delivery system used affects pulmonary deposition. For example, the Turbuhaler delivers about twice the dose of budesonide versus an MDI and is associated with excellent efficacy if used correctly.[1,93] Clinical trials evaluating fluticasone efficacy administered via the Diskus have likewise shown excellent efficacy.[5,94] The differences between the various dry-powder inhalers is discussed later in this chapter. Addition of a spacer device to an MDI also enhances pulmonary deposition. In very high dosages

Table 23-6 Estimated Comparative Daily Dosages for Inhaled Corticosteroids

Drug	Low Daily Dose Adult	Low Daily Dose Child[a]	Medium Daily Dose Adult	Medium Daily Dose Child[a]	High Daily Dose Adult	High Daily Dose Child[a]
Beclomethasone HFA 40 or 80 μg/puff	80–240 μg	80–160 μg	240–480 μg	160–320 μg	>480 μg	>320 μg
Budesonide DPI 200 μg/inhalation	200–600 μg	200–400 μg	600–1,200 μg	400–800 μg	>1,200 μg	>800 μg
Inhalation suspension for nebulization (pediatric dose)		0.5 mg		1.0 mg		2.0 mg
Flunisolide 250 μg/puff	500–1,000 μg	500–750 μg	1,000–2,000 μg	1,000–1,250 μg	>2,000 μg	>1,250 μg
Fluticasone MDI: 44, 110, or 220 μg/puff	88–264 μg	88–176 μg	264–660 μg	176–440 μg	>660 μg	>440 μg
DPI: 50, 100, or 250 μg/inhalation	100–300 μg	100–200 μg	300–600 μg	200–400 μg	>600 μg	>400 μg
Triamcinolone acetonide 100 μg/puff	400–1,000 μg	400–800 μg	1,000–2,000 μg	800–1,200 μg	>2,000 μg	>1,200 μg

[a]Children ≤12 years of age

(the equivalent of 1,600 μg/day of beclomethasone dipropionate), all ICS produce some degree of HPA axis suppression.[91] The clinical significance of this suppression has yet to be firmly established.

Although low dosages of ICS are accepted as being quite safe, very high dosages continue to be scrutinized regarding the potential adverse effects. Clearly, for patients who require high dosages for optimal control of asthma, the benefits of therapy with these agents far outweigh the risks.[1,5,91] Systemic adverse effects of ICS have been recently reviewed.[95] A possible association between prolonged, very high dosages of inhaled corticosteroids and cataracts[96] and glaucoma[97] has been reported. The NIH Guidelines[5] have summarized recent research that has allayed concerns regarding use of ICS therapy and growth suppression in children (i.e., the decrease in growth velocity is small, not progressive, and appears to be reversible).[98,99]

34. **How would you begin S.T. on inhaled corticosteroids and what would be the optimal dosage regimen?**

In S.T., most clinicians would begin with a short course (e.g., 1 week) of high-dose systemic corticosteroids to maximally improve her pulmonary function. This approach is consistent with the NIH Guidelines[1] that emphasizes gaining quick control. Using short-course systemic therapy is logical because it is inexpensive, efficacious, and associated with low risk. One concern with gaining quick control with high-dose inhaled corticosteroids in mild persistent or moderate persistent asthma is that some clinicians may forget to "step down" the dose subsequent to an optimal response. While gaining quick control with a short course of oral corticosteroids, it is logical to start inhaled corticosteroids in many patients at a low[100] to moderate dosage (as defined in Table 23-6). Inhaled corticosteroid therapy should be initiated concomitantly with a short course of systemic corticosteroid therapy. Patient education at this time may have greater effectiveness because some patients are more attentive after having just experienced an exacerbation, and they know that change is needed to improve their health. In some patients, the psychology of emphasizing the cornerstone of therapy during the initial encounter may be significant.

Because S.T. has really struggled with her asthma and is classified as *severe* persistent, it is reasonable to start her on a moderate to high pediatric dosage of an inhaled corticosteroid (see Table 23-6 and Fig. 23-12). More aggressive therapy initially is especially important in S.T. because of her four hospitalizations in the last 2 years. In partnership with S.T. and her parents, her preference should be determined as to the delivery method (i.e., discuss options with her regarding breath-activated devices or MDI and spacer, including which spacer). Ideally, the clinician should recognize her emerging independence as a 12-year-old and talk with her alone and then with her parents. After S.T. is stabilized for 3 months, attempts should be made to slowly decrease the ICS dosage every 1 to 2 months until the lowest effective dosage is achieved. The dosages of S.T.'s other medications should not be reduced initially during corticosteroid therapy until an optimal response is seen.

Administration of the total daily-ICS dose is preferred twice daily as opposed to four times daily[1] because simplified regimens tend to improve patient adherence. All inhaled cor-

ticosteroid products in the United States are approved by the U.S. Food and Drug Administration (FDA) for twice-daily dosing. Numerous studies[101–103] have shown once-daily dosing of inhaled corticosteroids is efficacious and safe; a once-daily schedule is most likely to be successful in mild persistent and in some moderate persistent asthmatics after excellent control is established with twice-daily dosing. Similarly, using more than three to four puffs per dose should be avoided if possible. This is accomplished by using products such as double-strength (80 μg/puff) beclomethasone HFA or higher potency agents such as budesonide and fluticasone. Some patients may require three or four times daily dosing for a few days during mild exacerbations, but most do well on twice-daily doses of ICS. Adherence is a major determinant of success or failure with aerosol corticosteroids and continued patient education and contact are essential.[1–5]

Combination of Inhaled Corticosteroids and Long-Acting Inhaled β₂-Agonists

35. **Because S.T. is 12 years old, what options are appropriate to minimize the inhaled corticosteroid dosage, realizing aggressive therapy is needed? Clinicians should monitor for what local side effects in S.T. with inhaled corticosteroid therapy?**

Salmeterol has been very successful in prevention of "stepping up" the dose of inhaled corticosteroids while enhancing overall asthma control,[94,104,105] and this fact is reflected in the NIH Guidelines.[1,5] S.T.'s clinician chooses to initiate therapy with the combination of fluticasone 500 μg and salmeterol 50 μg via Diskus (Advair 500) 1 inhalation BID. The plan is to "step down" the dose of fluticasone after excellent asthma control is achieved. Another option here would be concomitant therapy with budesonide and formoterol.[93]

The most common local side effect with inhaled corticosteroid therapy is oropharyngeal candidiasis (thrush), but this problem is rare with any delivery system. With MDIs, it can be further minimized by use of a spacer device. Rinsing the mouth with water after use of any ICS is also recommended. Another possible local side effect is hoarseness (dysphonia), and spacers may not effectively reduce this problem.[106] Dry powder devices (e.g., Turbuhaler) may have less dysphonia associated with their use, but further study is required to verify this possibility.[106]

STEP-DOWN TREATMENT

36. **After being on her new therapy for 1 month, S.T. was markedly improved. She required no ED visits or hospitalizations, was sleeping through the night, and began to exercise again. She rarely required PRN albuterol. At that point, her clinician started a trial off of her SR theophylline in an effort to simplify her drug regimen. After one more month, S.T. continues to do well. Although S.T. clearly needs long-term inhaled corticosteroid therapy, after 2 months of excellent response, her clinician is now ready to step down from high-dose fluticasone. What is a prudent approach to dosage reduction? If during step down symptoms recur, what management could possibly facilitate dosage reduction of the inhaled corticosteroid?**

Initially, a dosage decrease without additional medication is appropriate. Since fluticasone 500 μg daily is considered a high ICS dose in children, Advair 250 BID is prescribed for

S.T. If a single ICS product had been started in S.T. initially, (e.g., Pulmicort, QVAR, Flovent MDI), the dosage reduction would normally proceed at a slower pace. However, fluticasone 500 μg daily, especially in combination with salmeterol, is still a large dose in a 12-year-old.

If S.T. has symptoms during dosage reduction of the inhaled corticosteroid, an approach to facilitating ICS stepdown is to add a leukotriene receptor antagonist. Montelukast (Singulair), for example, has been shown in a large, double-blind trial to result in a slight reduction in inhaled corticosteroid dose.[107] However, a review of the data from 13 trials concluded that there is insufficient evidence to promote the add-on use of leukotriene modifiers to ICS.[108] These agents combined with ICS do not provide the level of asthma control seen with long-acting inhaled β_2-agonists combined with ICS.[5] Studies are needed to assess any potential benefit of leukotriene modifiers in patients with well-documented severe persistent asthma receiving high-dose ICS in combination with a long-acting inhaled β_2-agonist.

If S.T.'s clinician had not already started salmeterol therapy, it is interesting to note that this agent may also be used to facilitate stepping-down doses of inhaled corticosteroids. One study showed a slight reduction of corticosteroid dose (17% dosage reduction) associated with salmeterol therapy.[109]

After S.T.'s dose of fluticasone was stepped down to 500 μg/day, she started requiring only slightly more PRN albuterol (but still was symptom-free most days). When she was maintained at fluticasone 1,000 μg/day, her personal best PEF was 320 L/minute, and she was staying in her green zone (260 to 320 L/minute). After step down to Advair 250 BID, her personal best PEF was 300 L/min. S.T. was continuing to be adherent to her medication schedule and had excellent inhalation technique with both Diskus and MDI.

At this point, S.T.'s clinician took the very important step of reassessment of her environmental control at home and school. It was discovered that she still did not have zippered mattress and pillow covers and that her father was smoking in the house. The father promised to ALWAYS step outside to smoke and to get purchase occlusive covers for the bedding. S.T.'s physician also added an intranasal ICS for her allergic rhinitis.

One month later, S.T. returned to the clinic and reported further improved control of her asthma, including virtually no symptoms and a new personal best PEF of 350 L/minute.

Leukotriene Modifiers

37. P.W. is a 52-year-old man with mild persistent asthma. His asthma symptoms began when he was 2 years of age, and he has never smoked. P.W. has had numerous drug regimens for his asthma over the years, but he tells his physician that he wants the simplest regimen possible and that he prefers oral medication if at all possible. What is a good choice for controller therapy in P.W.?

In patients of any age with mild persistent asthma, and certainly in children or adolescents, an oral agent such as montelukast with once-daily dosing at bedtime (or zafirlukast with twice-daily dosing) has obvious advantages. An ICS is the preferred treatment for mild persistent asthma, but in patients (adults or children) who much prefer oral therapy to inhaling

medication every day, leukotriene modifiers are a reasonable option. The simplest and safest possible oral controller regimen for P.W. is montelukast 10 mg HS (with PRN inhaled albuterol). Bedtime dosing with montelukast is recommended because it will have peak activity late at night and in the early morning hours, when asthma symptoms tend to be more frequent. It is likely that this regimen will result in very good asthma control. If on return to clinic in a few weeks, P.W. does not have good control of his asthma, switching to a low-dose ICS in the evening only would keep the regimen simple, while enhancing efficacy.

Although theoretically zileuton, a "leukotriene modifier" via 5-lipoxygenase inhibition, could also be helpful here, it is rapidly eliminated and requires four-times-daily dosing, which is undesirable in most patients. Other concerns with zileuton relate to inhibition of metabolism of some high-risk drugs (e.g., warfarin, theophylline) as well as some risk of hepatotoxicity.[1] In light of these concerns the drug was withdrawn from the U.S. market by the manufacturer in 2003.

Although some clinicians may view leukotriene receptor antagonists as appropriate for mild persistent asthma only, the NIH Guidelines also recommend these agents as *alternatives* for moderate persistent asthma in combination with ICS.

Cromolyn and Nedocromil

38. E.G. is a 7-year-old boy with mild persistent asthma. His family has just moved from the northeastern United States to the midwest. E.G.'s new pediatrician notes that he has been previously managed only by "as-needed" inhaled albuterol. E.G.'s pediatrician is aware of the NIH Guidelines[1,5] recommendation for inhaled corticosteroids in mild persistent asthma, even in small children. However, despite recent evidence in the literature regarding the safety of inhaled corticosteroids, she is concerned about the risks of these agents in children and is considering a trial of cromolyn or nedocromil therapy combined with strict environmental control. If the trial fails, she plans to switch to the lowest possible dosage of ICS. Should cromolyn (Intal) or nedocromil (Tilade) be added to E.G.'s β_2-agonist therapy? Is either agent preferred over theophylline or a leukotriene modifier in E.G.?

In studies of childhood asthma, cromolyn has been found to reduce symptoms and the need for acute-care visits, and this drug has an excellent safety profile.[5,110] Although theophylline is a relatively weak bronchodilator, it also may have very modest anti-inflammatory effects.[56] Note in Figure 23-7 from the NIH Guidelines[5] that theophylline, cromolyn, and nedocromil are *alternatives* as controller medications in mild persistent asthma (children older than 5 years and adults). Cromolyn is also an alternative to ICS in children 5 years and younger. Nedocromil is an effective anti-inflammatory agent, especially for mild persistent asthma,[5,98] and is similar to cromolyn in efficacy and tolerability.[1,5] Cromolyn and nedocromil have similar mechanisms of action as anti-inflammatory agents, and their mechanisms are compared with other agents in Table 23-7.

Based on efficacy and safety concerns and the need to monitor serum theophylline concentrations, either cromolyn or nedocromil is a better option for E.G.'s controller therapy. E.G. can learn to use an MDI plus spacer device with proper teaching, but the concern is adherence to therapy with the required QID or TID dosing schedule.

Table 23-7   Long-Term-Control Medications

Name/Products	Indications/Mechanisms	Potential Adverse Effects	Therapeutic Issues
Corticosteroids (Glucocorticoids) ***Inhaled:*** Beclomethasone dipropionate Budesonide Flunisolide Fluticasone propionate Triamcinolone acetonide	*Indications* • Long-term prevention of symptoms; suppression, control, and reversal of inflammation. • Reduce need for oral corticosteroids. *Mechanisms* • **Anti-inflammatory.** Block late reaction to allergen and reduce airway hyperresponsiveness. Inhibit cytokine production, adhesion protein activation, and inflammatory cell migration and activation. • Reverse β_2-receptor down-regulation. Inhibit microvascular leakage.	• Cough, dysphonia, oral thrush (candidiasis). • In high doses systemic effects may occur, although studies are not conclusive, and clinical significance of these effects has not been established (e.g., adrenal suppression, osteoporosis, growth suppression, and skin thinning and easy bruising)	• Space/holding chamber devices and mouth washing after inhalation decrease local side effects and systemic absorption. • Preparations are not absolutely interchangeable on a μg or per puff basis. • The risks of uncontrolled asthma should be weighed against the limited risks of inhaled corticosteroids. The potential but small risk of adverse events is well balanced by their efficacy.
Systemic: Methylprednisolone Prednisolone Prednisone	*Indications* • For short-term (3–10 days) "burst": to gain prompt control of inadequately controlled persistent asthma. • For long-term prevention of symptoms in severe persistent asthma: suppression, control, and reversal of inflammation. *Mechanisms* • Same as inhaled.	• Short-term use; reversible abnormalities in glucose metabolism, increased appetite, fluid retention, weight gain, mood alteration, hypertension, peptic ulcer, and rarely, aseptic necrosis of femur. • Long-term use: adrenal axis suppression, growth suppression, dermal thinning, hypertension, diabetes, Cushing's syndrome, cataracts, muscle weakness, and—in rare instances—impaired immune function. • Consideration should be given to co-existing conditions that could be worsened by systemic corticosteroids, such as herpes virus infections, *Varicella*, tuberculosis, hypertension, peptic ulcer, and *Strongyloides*.	Use at lowest effective dose. For long-term use, alternate-day AM dosing produces least toxicity.
Cromolyn Sodium and Nedocromil Cromolyn Nedocromil	*Indications* • Long-term prevention of symptoms; may modify inflammation. • Preventive treatment prior to exposure to exercise or known allergen. *Mechanisms* • **Anti-inflammatory.** Block early and late reaction to allergen. Interfere with chloride channel function. Stabilize mast cell membranes and inhibit activation and release of mediators from eosinophils and epithelial cells. • Inhibit acute response to exercise, cold dry air, and SO_2.	15–20% of patients complain of an unpleasant taste from nedocromil.	• Therapeutic response to cromolyn and nedocromil often occurs within 2 weeks, but a 4- to 6-week trial may be needed to determine maximum benefit. • Dose of cromolyn MDI (1 mg/puff) may be inadequate to affect airway hyperresponsiveness. Nebulizer delivery (20 mg/ampule) may be preferred for some patients. • Safety is the primary advantage of these agents.
Long-Acting β_2-Agonists ***Inhaled:*** Formoterol Salmeterol	*Indications* • Long-term prevention of symptoms, especially nocturnal symptoms, *added to anti-inflammatory therapy.* • Prevention of exercise-induced bronchospasm. • *Not to be used to treat acute symptoms or exacerbations.* *Mechanisms* • **Bronchodilation.** Smooth muscle relaxation following adenylate cyclase activation and increase in cyclic AMP producing functional antagonism of bronchoconstriction.	• Tachycardia, skeletal muscle tremor, hypokalemia, prolongation of QT_c interval in overdose. • A diminished bronchoprotective effect may occur within 1 week of chronic therapy. Clinical significance has not been established.	• *Not to be used to treat acute symptoms or exacerbations.* • Clinical significance of potentially developing tolerance is uncertain because studies show symptom control and bronchodilation are maintained. • Should not be used in place of anti-inflammatory therapy. • May provide more effective symptom control when added to standard doses of inhaled corticosteroids compared to increasing the corticosteroid dosage.

Table 23-7   Long-Term-Control Medications—cont'd

Name/Products	Indications/Mechanisms	Potential Adverse Effects	Therapeutic Issues
Long-Acting β₂-Agonists	• In vitro, inhibit mast cell mediator release, decrease vascular permeability, and increase mucociliary clearance. • Compared to short-acting inhaled β₂-agonist, salmeterol (but not formoterol) has slower onset of action (15 to 30 minutes) but longer duration (>12 hours).		
Oral: Albuerol, sustained-release			• Inhaled long-acting β₂-agonists are preferred because they are longer acting and have fewer side effects than oral sustained-release agents.
Methylxanthines Theophylline, sustained-release tablets and capsules	*Indications* • Long-term control and prevention of symptoms, especially nocturnal symptoms. *Mechanisms* • Bronchodilation. Smooth muscle relaxation from phosphodiesterase inhibition and possibly adenosine antagonism. • May affect eosinophilic infiltration into bronchial mucosal as well as decrease T-lymphocyte numbers in epithelium. • Increases diaphragm contractility and mucociliary clearance.	• Dose-related actue toxicities include tachycardia, nausea and vomiting, tachyarrhythmias (SVT), central nervous system stimulation, headache, seizures, hematemesis, hyperglycemia, and hypokalemia. • Adverse effects at usual therapeutic doses include insomnia, gastric upset, aggravation of ulcer or reflux, increase in hyperactivity in some children, difficulty in urination in elderly males with prostatism.	• Maintain steady-state serum concentrations between 5 and 15 mcg/mL. Routine serum concentration monitoring is essential due to significant toxicities, narrow therapeutic range, and individual differences in metabolic clearance. Absorption and metabolism may be affected by numerous factors (see Figure 3-5a), which can produce significant changes in steady-state serum theophylline concentrations. • Not generally recommended for exacerbations. There is minimal evidence for added benefit to optimal doses of inhaled β₂ agonists. Serum concentration monitoring is mandatory.
Leukotriene Modifiers Montelukast tablets, chewable tablets and oral granules Zafirlukast tablets	*Indications* Long-term control and preventions of symptoms in mild-persistent asthma for patients ≥12 months of age (montelukast) and ≥5 years of age (zafirlukast). *Mechanisms* **Leukotriene receptor antagonist:** selective competitive inhibitor or LTD₄ and LTE₄ receptors.	Adverse effects comparable to placebo in clinical trials and include headache, nausea, abdominal pain, influenza, diarrhea.	*Montelukast* • Administer in the evening to achieve peak plasma levels of the drug that coincide with the maximal narrowing of the airways (e.g., early AM hours). *Zafirlukast* • Administration with meals decreases bioavailability; take at least 1 hour before or 2 horus after meals. • Inhibits the metabolism of warfarin and increases the prothrombin time; competitive inhibitor of CYP2C9 hepatic microsomal isozymes.
Zileuton tablets*	*Indications* • Long-term control and prevention of symptoms in mild persistent asthma for patients ≥12 years of age. *Mechanisms* • **5-Lipoxygenase inhibitor.**	• Elevation of liver enzymes has been reported. Limited case reports of reversible hepatitis and hyperbilirubinemia.	• Zileuton is microsomal CYP1A2 and CYP3A4 enzyme inhibitor. • Monitor hepatic enzymes (ALT).

*Zileuton was voluntarily withdrawn from the U.S. market in 2003.
Modified from reference 1.

Table 23-8   Theophylline Dosing Guide for Chronic Use[a,b,c]

Starting dose for children 1–15 years <45 kg: 12–14 mg/kg/day to maximum of 300 mg/day

Starting dose for adults and children 1–15 years >45 kg: 300 mg/day

Titrate dose upward after 3 days if necessary and if tolerated to:
- 16 mg/kg/day to maximum of 400 mg /day in children 1–15 years <45 kg
- 400 mg/day in adults and in children >45 kg

Titrate dose upward after 3 more days if necessary and if tolerated to:
- 20 mg/kg/day to a maximum of 600 mg/day in children 1–15 years <45 kg
- 600 mg/day in adults and in children >45 kg

---

[a]Dose using ideal body weight or actual body weight, whichever is less. These dosages do not apply if liver disease, heart failure, or other factors documented to affect theophylline clearance are present. Doses must be guided by monitoring serum concentrations to ensure optimal safety and efficacy.

[b]Adapted from reference 114.

[c]Dosing schedule dependent on product selected; sustained-release products are much preferred if at all possible.

A much easier approach to managing mild persistent asthma in a young child (or teenager/adult) whose physician does not choose the preferred low-dose inhaled corticosteroid therapy is once-daily montelukast (note leukotriene modifiers as options for young children and older children/adults in the NIH Guidelines).[5,111,112] Taking a 5-mg cherry chewable montelukast tablet at bedtime is preferred as an option in E.G. over cromolyn, nedocromil, or theophylline.

Theophylline

Dosing

39. K.J., a 14-year-old, 40-kg girl, has a history of recurring cough and wheezing. These symptoms worsen upon vigorous running or when she has an upper respiratory infection. She has not required hospitalization for these symptoms, but has missed a few school days. She has symptoms daily and she uses her pir-

buterol inhaler more than two times daily. K.J. has a family history of asthma. A diagnosis of moderate persistent asthma is made. How should K.J. be managed?

Because K.J. has moderate persistent asthma, treatment with an anti-inflammatory agent is indicated. Low-dose ICS in combination with an inhaled long-acting β_2-agonist is the preferred treatment in children, with moderate persistent asthma. However, K.J.'s clinician opts to prescribe theophylline in combination with a low dose of budesonide via Turbuhaler. Unfortunately, K.J.'s clinician is not well versed in the NIH Guidelines and was in his residency in the early 1980s when theophylline was a widely used drug. The Guidelines do list theophylline as an *option* for moderate persistent asthma, in combination with an ICS. K.J.'s clinician is aware of a clinical trial showing that low-dose budesonide combined with theophylline provided effective therapy in patients with asthma.[113]

40.   What dosage of theophylline is appropriate for K.J.?

Low doses of budesonide combined with twice-daily theophylline that resulted in a median serum theophylline concentration of 8.7 μg/mL was superior in efficacy to high-dose budesonide as single controller therapy.[113] Thus, it is wise to give a therapeutic trial with low-dose theophylline initially, aiming for serum concentrations of 5 to 10 μg/mL. In the nonacute asthma patient in whom the theophylline dose requirement is unknown, dosages suggested for ages >1 year are listed in Table 23-8 (see Table 23-10 for infant doses). Accordingly, the initial dosage in K.J. would be 300 mg/day in divided doses (i.e., 150 mg Q 12 hr). If tolerated, the dosage is increased at 3-day intervals by about 25% to the mean dose that usually is needed to produce a peak theophylline serum concentration between 5 and 10 μg/mL. In K.J., the maximum dosage would be 600 mg/day in divided doses (i.e., 300 mg Q 12 hr). The final dose should be based on response and the absence of theophylline side effects, and it should be adjusted based on measured serum theophylline concentration. Obviously, the lowest effective dosage should be used to minimize

Table 23-9   Adjusting Doses of Theophylline Based On Serum Concentrations

Peak Theophylline Concentration (μg/mL)[a]	Approximate Adjustment in Daily Dose	Comment
<5.0	↑ by 25%	Recheck serum theophylline concentration
5–10	↑ by 25% if clinically indicated	Recheck serum concentration; ↑ dose only if poor response to therapy
10–12	Cautious 10% ↑ if clinically indicated	If asymptomatic, no ↑ needed. Recheck serum theophylline concentration before further dose changes
12–15	Occasional intolerance requires a 10% ↓	If asymptomatic, no dose change needed unless side effects present
16–20	↓ by 10–25%	Even if asymptomatic and side effects absent, a dose ↓ is prudent
20–24.9	↓ by 50%	Omit one dose even if asymptomatic and side effects absent, a dose ↓ is indicated
25–29.9	↓ by >50%	Omit next doses even if asymptomatic and side effects absent; a dose ↓ indicated; repeat serum theophylline concentration after dose adjustment
>30	Omit next doses; ↓ by 60–75%	Seek medical attention and consult regional poison center even if not symptomatic; if >60 years of age, anticipate need for treatment of seizures

[a]It is important that levels are obtained at steady state. If laboratory results appear questionable, suggest repeat measurements.

risk. If in 4 weeks K.J. does not have excellent asthma control despite peak steady state serum theophylline concentrations of 10 μg/mL (preferably 5 to 10 μg/mL) and strict adherence to budesonide (with good inhalation technique), options other than increasing the theophylline dosage should be taken. For example, switching to a long-acting inhaled β₂-agonist (versus theophylline) or a slight increase in the budesonide dose, per the NIH Guidelines, and re-examine K.J.'s environmental control measures at home and at school.

Monitoring Therapy

41. When should serum theophylline concentrations be measured for patients who are receiving chronic oral theophylline therapy?

Peak, rather than trough, theophylline serum concentrations should be measured, especially in the pediatric population or in adults who rapidly metabolize theophylline. Both the efficacy and toxicity of theophylline correlate better with theophylline peak, rather than trough, serum concentrations.

For twice-daily SR products, peak theophylline serum concentrations should be measured 4 to 6 hours after a morning dose, depending on the release characteristics of the product.[114] Monitoring of once-a-day theophylline products given in the evening (e.g., Uniphyl) typically involves obtaining a serum sample 8 hours after a dose. The final dosage can be adjusted using the guidelines listed in Table 23-9. Serum theophylline concentrations should be obtained at steady state (i.e., when there have been no missed doses and no extra doses have been taken for at least 48 hours).

Toxicity

42. M.M., a 14-year-old boy who has been treated with theophylline SR 300 mg BID, now complains of headache and difficulty in getting to sleep. Why should a theophylline serum concentration be evaluated?

Theophylline side effects can be related to excessive serum concentrations, or adverse effects can be transient and unrelated to the amount in serum. Unfortunately, it is not always possible to determine which it might be. Side effects can include headache, nausea, vomiting, irritability, or hyperactivity, insomnia, and diarrhea. With higher serum theophylline levels, cardiac arrhythmias, seizures, and death can occur.[77] Less severe symptoms may not be present before the onset of cardiac arrhythmias or seizures and cannot be relied on as a forewarning of these more serious adverse theophylline effects. It is important not to ignore any symptom consistent with theophylline toxicity. The insomnia and headaches experienced by M.M. may not be associated with excessive (i.e., out of the usual therapeutic range) serum theophylline concentrations, but a reduction in dosage should be contemplated because some patients experience toxicity when serum theophylline concentrations are within the therapeutic range. A better alternative in M.M. is a long-acting inhaled β₂-agonist (i.e., formoterol, salmeterol), assuming adequate anti-inflammatory therapy is already being given.

Guidelines for managing toxicity have been revised.[114] Major toxicity associated with theophylline is more likely with peak serum concentrations of 100 μg/mL with acute intoxication and in patients older than 60 years of age after chronic

Table 23-10 FDA Guidelines for Theophylline Dosing in Infants[a]

Premature Neonates

<24 days postnatal age: 1.0 mg/kg Q 12 hr
≥24 days postnatal age: 1.5 mg/kg Q 12 hr

Term Infants and Infants Up to 52 Weeks of Age

Total daily dose (mg) = [(0.2 × age in weeks) + 5.0] × (kg body wt)
- Up to age 26 weeks; divide dose into 3 equal amounts administered at 8-hour intervals
- >26 weeks of age; divide dose into 4 equal amounts administered at 6-hour intervals

[a]Final doses adjusted to a peak steady-state serum theophylline concentration of 5–10 μg/mL in neonates and 10–15 μg/mL in older infants. Adapted from reference 114.

overmedication, regardless of the peak toxic concentrations (e.g., concentrations >30 μg/mL).[58,114,115]

Drug Interactions
INHIBITION OF METABOLISM

43. T.R., 55-year-old woman with asthma, is well controlled on theophylline SR 300 mg BID, albuterol two puffs QID PRN, and triamcinolone (Azmacort) three puffs BID. A peak theophylline serum concentration obtained 3 months ago was 14 μg/mL. Six months ago, on the same dose of theophylline, her serum concentration was 15 μg/mL. M.M. presents with an upper respiratory tract infection, and erythromycin ethyl succinate 500 mg QID is prescribed. How should this potential drug interaction be followed?

A large number of medications inhibit cytochrome P450 isoenzymes and are capable of inhibiting the metabolism of theophylline. Because theophylline is metabolized by CYP 1A2, 3A3, and 2E1, inhibitors of these isoenzymes can cause clinically significant interactions.[56,114] Cimetidine, erythromycin, and some (but not all) of the quinolone antibiotics (e.g., enoxacin, ciprofloxacin) are well documented to inhibit theophylline metabolism.[1,56,114] Because numerous other drugs inhibit the metabolism of theophylline, all patients receiving this agent should be screened carefully for potential interactions. As with any drug interaction, mechanism, time course, management, and clinical significance should be assessed before any interventions. For example, cimetidine decreases theophylline clearance within 24 hours, and this interaction should be circumvented by using another H₂-blocker or a proton pump inhibitor (Table 23-11). Classic inducers of cytochrome P450 also affect theophylline clearance (see Table 23-11).

Erythromycin
In T.R., erythromycin has the potential to substantially reduce theophylline clearance.[1,56,114] Although some reports suggest that short-term therapy (<5 days) does not significantly decrease theophylline clearance, studies using multiple dosing over several days provide clear evidence to support such an interaction.[1,56,114,116] If erythromycin is given at a time when the patient's steady-state serum theophylline concentration is 10 μg/mL, the theophylline dosage should be decreased. The

Table 23-11   Factors Affecting Serum Theophylline Concentrations[a]

Factor	Decreases Theophylline Concentrations	Increases Theophylline Concentrations	Recommended Action
Food	↓ or delays absorption of some sustained-release theophylline (SR) products	↑ rate of absorption (fatty foods) products	Select theophylline preparation that is not affected by food.
Diet	↑ metabolism (high protein)	↓ metabolism (high carbohydrate)	Inform patients that major changes in diet are not recommended while taking theophylline.
Systemic, febrile viral illness (e.g., influenza)		↓ metabolism	Decrease theophylline dose according to serum concentration level. Decrease dose by 50 percent if serum concentration measurement is not available.
Hypoxia, cor pulmonale, and decompensated congestive heart failure, cirrhosis		↓ metabolism	Decrease dose according to serum concentration level.
Age	↑ metabolism (1 to 9 years)	↓ metabolism (<6 months, elderly)	Adjust dose according to serum concentration level.
Phenobarbital, phenytoin, carbamazepine	↑ metabolism		Increase dose according to serum concentration level.
Cimetidine		↓ metabolism	Use alternative H₂-antagonist (e.g., famotidine or ranitidine).
Macrolides: TAO, erythromycin, clarithromycin		↓ metabolism	Use alternative antibiotic or adjust theophylline dose.
Quinolones: ciprofloxacin, enoxacin, pefloxacin		↓ metabolism	Use alternative antibiotic or adjust theophylline dose.
Rifampin	↑ metabolism		Increase dose according to serum concentration level.
Ticlopidine		↓ metabolism	Decrease dose according to serum concentration level.
Smoking	↑ metabolism		Advise patient to stop smoking; increase dose according to serum concentration level.

[a]This list is not all-inclusive; for discussion of other factors, see package inserts. Modified from reference 1.

patient's serum theophylline concentration should be monitored at baseline and past 5 days of erythromycin therapy, regardless of whether toxic symptoms become apparent, because serum theophylline concentrations usually do not increase until after several days of concurrent treatment. In T.R., it would be far preferable to give an antibiotic that does not affect theophylline metabolism. For example, azithromycin should not affect theophylline metabolism.[114] Clarithromycin has a similar, but somewhat less, effect than erythromycin.[114] If a β-lactam agent or tetracycline is appropriate, theophylline metabolism would not be affected.[114] Among the quinolones, examples of agents that do not appear to affect theophylline metabolism include ofloxacin and levofloxacin.

Anticholinergics

44. R.K. is a 24-year-old graduate student with moderate persistent asthma, which has been well controlled for 10 years with Q 12 hr ICS therapy and albuterol PRN. Recently, he has noticed that his asthma symptoms tend to worsen when he has anxiety over major examinations. What drug therapy might be helpful to R.K.?

One of the myths related to asthma is that it is an emotional illness. It is true, however, that among many typical triggers (e.g., aeroallergens, exercise), emotional upset can be a precipitating factor in some asthmatics.[2] Several investigators have shown that inhaled anticholinergic bronchodilators can block this response.[120] A therapeutic trial of ipratropium given by an MDI is warranted in R.K. He probably only needs to use ipratropium a day or so before major examinations and on the day of the examination (i.e., he is well controlled all other times).

Anticholinergic bronchodilators also are useful in patients with chronic asthma who are intolerant of the side effects of other bronchodilators and in patients who are not responding adequately to standard therapies. For example, a patient who experiences nervousness or tremor with short-acting β₂-agonists could use an ipratropium MDI as an alternative. Ipratropium is slower in onset (up to 30 minutes) but may be slightly longer acting than albuterol. As a general rule, anticholinergics are inferior to β-agonists in patients with asthma and should not be used as a rescue drug. These agents also benefit some patients who have asthma and then, very unfortunately, smoke for several years and develop chronic obstructive pulmonary disease.

EXERCISE-INDUCED ASTHMA

45. T.W., a 33-year-old woman, presents to the clinic with a history of severe coughing and chest tightness after exercise. She recently joined an exercise club to lose weight, but is unable to keep up with others her own age and relative condition when jogging outside. She recalls having mild respiratory problems as a young child, but has never taken any asthma medications. She has a positive treadmill test for exercise-induced asthma (EIA). How should T.W. be treated?

During sustained exercise, at least 90% of patients with asthma experience an initial improvement in pulmonary functions quickly followed by a significant decline (Fig. 23-18). This phenomenon may be the only symptom of subclinical asthma.[1,121] Patients can be diagnosed by measuring the FEV_1 or PEF before and after exercise (6- to 8-minute treadmill or bicycle exercise test). A reduction of FEV_1 by >15% of the baseline value is a positive test.

Hyperventilation of cold, dry air increases the sensitivity to EIA and induces bronchospasm.[121] The main stimulus for EIA is respiratory heat loss, water loss, or both,[121] while breathing heated, humidified air completely blocks EIA in many patients.[121] Masks are indicated for patients with EIA in the wintertime, and patients with severe asthma with EIA also should be encouraged to swim or engage in other indoor exercise that does not promote EIA. A warm-up period before strenuous exercise is helpful in some patients. With appropriate premedication, most exercise-induced asthma can be prevented, so virtually all patients with stable asthma should be encouraged to exercise. The mechanism of bronchoconstriction after airway heat and water loss is still incompletely understood.[121]

Although several drugs inhibit EIA, inhaled short-acting β_2-agonists are generally the agents of choice for prophylaxis.[1–4,121,122] Inhaled β_2-agonists are superior to cromolyn.[122] For typical periods of exercise (e.g., <3 hours), pretreatment with agents such as albuterol 5 to 15 minutes before exercise usually provides excellent protection from EIA.

For prolonged periods of exercise, long-acting inhaled β_2-agonists (formoterol, salmeterol) provide several hours of protection.[123] Two differences in formoterol and salmeterol include the delivery systems for inhalation and the onset of action. If either of these agents is to be used to prevent EIA, it is important for the patient to inhale the medication at the proper time before exercise. Formoterol should be inhaled at least 15 minutes before exercise, and salmeterol administration should occur at least 30 minutes before vigorous activity. Obviously, for patients who are receiving Q 12 hr therapy with either drug for long-term control of asthma due to triggers other than exercise, they will already be protected. Formoterol is inhaled via the Aerolizer (single dose is loaded each time), and salmeterol is inhaled through the Diskus (multiple-dose inhaler (see Table 23-5).

Leukotriene receptor antagonists (e.g., montelukast once-daily chronic therapy) have also been demonstrated to prevent EIA.[124] Finally, it is important to point out that in persistent asthma, long-term anti-inflammatory therapy is helpful in reducing the response to most asthma triggers, including exercise.[1] For most patients who have EIA only, use of a short-acting inhaled β_2-agonist 15 minutes before exercise is the only therapy needed.

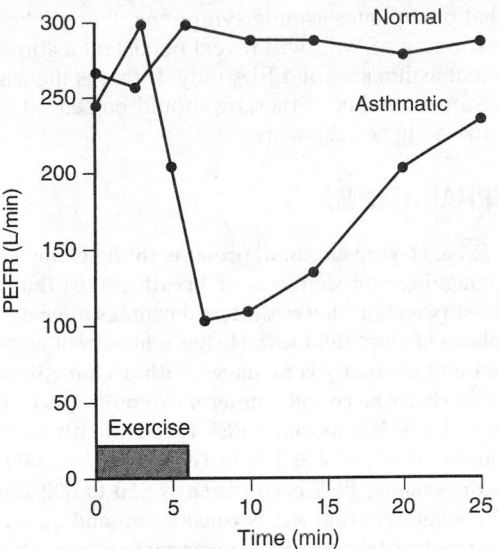

FIGURE 23-18 Changes in peak expiratory flow rate with exercise in an asthmatic and normal subject. PEFR, peak expiratory flow rate.

Because of the hyperventilation of relatively cool, dry air, jogging is a potent stimulus for EIA. A number of possible therapeutic interventions exist for T.W. She could be encouraged to swim because the inhalation of humidified warm air is less likely to produce EIA. However, if she wishes to continue jogging, two inhalations of a short-acting β_2-agonist (e.g., albuterol) from a metered-dose aerosol 15 minutes before exercise should provide adequate protection for 2 to 3 hours. If outdoor temperatures are quite cool or cold, T.W. should jog indoors. T.W. also should be counseled to take two additional inhalations if she "breaks through" the initial protection and experiences tightness.

46. W.L., a 17-year-old boy, presents to the clinic with a complaint of dyspnea and coughing that has limited his ability to keep up with his basketball teammates. He states that it is worse when playing outdoors unless the gym is cold and that it seems to be worse (occurring sooner during exercise) than a month ago. W.L. experienced several bouts of bronchitis as a young child, but has not had any problems for the past 6 years. His symptoms are consistent with EIA. How should his EIA be treated?

W.L. presents a special problem in that he is a teenager. Both for adolescents and children, peer pressure usually is extremely significant. Optimal prophylaxis is important to allow W.L. to compete at his best level. Embarrassment over not keeping up with teammates can be very hurtful now, and it has implications for setting habits of exercise into adulthood. Many adults with asthma do not exercise because they think they cannot do so based on childhood experiences. Lack of exercise can have a negative impact on physiologic and psychological well-being. W.L. should receive preventive treatment with an inhaled β_2-agonist. The question is whether he should receive a short-acting or a long-acting agent. The clinician should probe as to the duration of exercise. If W.L. exercises for >3 to 4 hours, formoterol or salmeterol administered 30 minutes before exercise would be a logical choice. Finally, the clinician should verify that exercise is the only factor that precipitates asthma symptoms. It could be that further questioning of W.L. will reveal persistent asthma or mild intermittent asthma beyond EIA only. If that is the case, long-term ICS or montelukast therapy should be started to reduce overall airway hyperresponsiveness.

NOCTURNAL ASTHMA

47. R.R., a 41-year-old man, presents to the clinic with a history of coughing and shortness of breath (SOB) that awakens him at least two nights a week. Most mornings upon awakening, he complains of chest tightness. He has a history of asthma since childhood and currently is managed with beclomethasone HFA 160 μg BID via a spacer and albuterol two puffs Q 6 hr PRN and before exercise. R.R.'s morning PEF is consistently in the yellow zone, usually at about 400 L/min (personal best, 600 L/min); whereas the evening PEF is consistently 550 to 600 L/min. The clinic physician says that she is considering adding an SR theophylline product to control the nocturnal asthma. What treatment should be recommended?

Many patients with asthma complain of symptoms that awaken them in the night or occur upon awakening in the morning. Morning cough with or without bronchospasm may be a clue to nocturnal asthma. Although nocturnal asthma may be appropriately viewed as simply another manifestation of airway inflammation, it is so common and troublesome among asthmatics that it deserves special note. Circadian rhythm in PEF is exaggerated in patients with asthma. The difference in PEF in nonasthmatics averages about 8% between 4 PM (maximal airflow) and 4 AM (minimal airflow), but in patients with asthma, the average variation can be as high as about 50%.[125,126] Several mechanisms account for this diurnal variation in PEF. The following are examples of factors that contribute to nocturnal asthma:

- Increased release of inflammatory mediators[125,126]
- Increased activity of the parasympathetic nervous system
- Lower circulating levels of epinephrine
- Lower levels of serum cortisol (lowest at about midnight)

In addition, for patients whose asthma is triggered by gastroesophageal reflux, this problem is worse at night and is another factor to consider.

The initial approach to managing nocturnal symptoms is the same as that for overall long-term therapy of persistent asthma, including adequate anti-inflammatory agents.[1,126] Inhaled corticosteroids often are effective in eliminating or reducing nocturnal asthma, including symptoms and the drop in PEF.[126] If low to moderate dosages (i.e., correctly inhaled every day) do not eliminate symptoms, a long-acting inhaled β2-agonist (salmeterol, formoterol) is indicated. Also, the basic asthma treatment principle of good control of concomitant rhinitis and environmental control, especially in the bedroom (e.g., house dust mites, household pets) should be considered in the patient with nocturnal asthma symptoms.

Bedtime doses of short-acting inhaled β2-agonists do not have sufficient duration of action to prevent early morning symptoms. Salmeterol or formoterol both of which have a 12-hour duration of action are preferred. Before the advent of long-acting inhaled β2-agonists, long-acting oral agents such as SR theophylline often were indicated.[126] Although SR theophylline is helpful, it has the potential to cause more adverse effects than inhaled agents, may interfere with sleep, and is less efficacious.[126] Before a long-acting oral agent is prescribed, adequate inhaled anti-inflammatory therapy should be ensured and then long-acting inhaled β2-agonists should be used.

Because asthma is primarily an inflammatory disease and nocturnal symptoms are due largely to airway inflammation, the first drug therapy concern in R.R. is to ensure that he is strictly adhering to his beclomethasone therapy, including not missing any doses and demonstrating excellent inhalation technique. If his use of the medication is optimal, a reasonable approach would be to add long-acting inhaled β2-agonist therapy because he is already at a moderate ICS dosage.

As part of optimal management of nocturnal asthma, R.R. also should be asked about avoiding or minimizing exposure to his asthma triggers (e.g., if he is allergic to cats, is there a cat in the bedroom?). Follow-up visits for R.R. should verify that early morning as well as the evening PEF are staying in the green zone and symptoms, both in the night and upon awakening in the morning, have been eliminated.

PATIENT EDUCATION

48. A.B., a 26-year-old woman, presents to the community pharmacy for a refill of her albuterol MDI. She has a prescription for a budesonide dry powder inhaler, but it is past due for a refill. A.B. has had asthma all of her life. She complains of symptoms most days but has not required visits to the ED or hospitalizations. The pharmacist determines that A.B. is bothered most about daily shortness of breath and worries that her condition may get worse. What should the pharmacist do in this situation?

If optimal long-term drug therapy of asthma is prescribed, treatment may still fail or be suboptimal if the patient does not receive adequate education. Patients with asthma require special educational efforts because of the use of inhalation devices and peak flow meters. In addition, it often is a major challenge to have patients and parents understand the critical importance of long-term daily controller therapy and environmental control. Of course, an important first step in educating asthmatics is to be caring and a good listener. Rather than sharing your knowledge initially, it is important to help establish a "partnership" with the patient by first asking the following question: "What is bothering you the most about your asthma?" Really listening to the patient and then addressing patient concerns is extremely important to successful education and long-term management.

Clinicians can be of invaluable assistance to the patient by repeatedly reinforcing education on the necessity to use anti-inflammatory (and long-acting inhaled β2-agonist) therapies on a regular schedule. Many patients underuse long-term preventive therapy because no health professional took the time to adequately instruct them that asthma is preventable. While underusing the most important medicines for long-term control, many patients overuse "quick relievers" (i.e., short-acting inhaled β2-agonists). Health care providers must be able to detect these problems and intervene to enhance patient care.

Because a large percentage of patients have difficulty using MDIs, teaching patients the correct use of MDIs, MDIs plus spacers, and dry powder inhalers is absolutely essential.[1,127] In one study, 89% of patients could not perform all steps for MDI use correctly.[128] Competent teaching requires *observation* of the patient using the devices initially and again on repeat visits to the clinic, hospital, or community pharmacy. Telling the patient about correct use clearly is not adequate. Health professionals must demonstrate use of the devices (live or with videotapes) for patients who cannot use the devices correctly. Although there is more than one correct way to use an MDI, Table 23-12 summarizes two commonly accepted approaches.[1,127] Many asthma experts prefer to use spacers to help ensure optimal efficacy. Spacers should be used in virtually all patients receiving ICS via a MDI, even those with perfect MDI technique, because spacers enhance efficacy and greatly reduce the risk of oropharyngeal candidiasis.[1,129,130] On the other hand, spacers do not add efficacy to correct use of a β_2-agonist MDI.[131] Although any spacer can be helpful, marketed devices that have a flow indicator whistle when inhalation is fast may be preferred (e.g., AeroChamber, InspirEase).

Studies have shown that health professionals generally are not competent in using MDIs either.[132–134] Obviously, the clinician should practice with a placebo inhaler and gain competence before teaching a patient. Among clinicians who educate asthmatics, pharmacists have been shown to be very helpful in teaching correct use of MDIs.[135] Unfortunately, one study showed that community pharmacists commonly are not providing such teaching.[136]

In addition to teaching the correct use of MDIs and spacers, clinicians should help patients via education regarding correct use of breath-activated dry powder inhalers (e.g., Turbuhaler, Diskus, Aerolizer), breath-activated MDIs (e.g., Autohaler), and nebulizing machines.[1] When using the Turbuhaler, for example, patients must clearly understand the need for a rapid (preferably 60 L/min), deep inhalation (not slow as with an MDI).[137] Such rapid peak inspiratory flow (PIF) is achievable by some young children, but many children <8 years of age have difficulty reaching PIF >60 L/min.[137] With the Diskus, PIF does not have to be as rapid as with Turbuhaler, but it should be >30 L/min.[138] In addition, patients need to breath-hold 10 seconds if possible, as with an MDI.

Objective monitoring of lung function at home by use of peak flow meters can be very helpful to patients and health care professionals. Instructing patients on the correct use of the devices, including use of the green, yellow, and red zones is essential.[1] Correct use of the peak flow meter includes standing, inhaling completely, forming a tight seal with your lips around the mouthpiece, exhaling as hard and fast as possible (blast!), and repeating this maneuver twice. The best of three attempts should be recorded. Beyond giving maximal effort when using peak flow meters, patients should be instructed to place the instrument well into the mouth on top of the tongue to avoid acceleration of air in the mouth with the tongue and buccal musculature. In essence, "spitting" into the peak flow meter, causes a dramatic "false" elevation in PEF.[139]

A.B. needs education regarding the benefits of long-term inhaled anti-inflammatory therapy. The pharmacist should explain with enthusiasm that A.B.'s budesonide is an extremely effective medicine and that it is the cornerstone of her asthma management. The slow onset and safety of inhaled corticosteroids must be stressed, as well as the requirement of regular use every day. Clearly teaching A.B. the differences between "preventers" and "quick relievers" is essential. Showing her

Table 23-12 Steps to Correct Use of Metered-Dose Inhalers[a]
1. Shake the inhaler well and remove the dust cap.
2. Exhale *slowly* through pursed lips.[b]
3. If using the "closed-mouth" technique, hold the inhaler upright and place the mouthpiece between your lips. Be careful not to block the opening with your tongue or teeth.
4. If using the "open-mouth" technique, open your mouth wide and hold the inhaler upright 1–2 inches from your mouth, making sure the inhaler is properly aimed.
5. Press down on the inhaler *once* as you start a *slow*, deep inhalation.
6. Continue to inhale slowly and deeply through your mouth. Try to inhale over at least 5 seconds.
7. Hold your breath for 10 seconds (use your fingers to count to 10 slowly). If 10 seconds makes you feel uncomfortable, try to hold your breath for at least 4 seconds.
8. Exhale *slowly*.[c]
9. Wait at least 30–60 seconds before inhaling the next puff of medicine.

[a]If using a spacer, see manufacturer's instructions. Same basic principles of slow, deep inhalation with adequate breath hold apply. With spacers, put mouthpiece on top of your tongue to ensure that tongue does not block aerosol.
[b]As long as exhalation is slow, you can exhale over several seconds. Some experts insist on exhaling only a tidal volume, but the key is to exhale *slowly*.
[c]If patient has concomitant rhinitis, exhaling through the *nose* may be of benefit when using corticosteroids, cromolyn, or ipratropium (i.e., some medication may deposit in nose).

colored pictures, models, or a video of inflamed airways can be very helpful—these teaching aids are available from several pharmaceutical manufacturers. Likewise, a peak flow meter should be given to A.B., and correct use ensured by observing her use it along with establishment of green, yellow, and red zones, coupled with a written action plan.[1,5] A.B. needs to hear from the clinicians treating her that "asthma is preventable," and in the words of a title of an NIH booklet for patients, "Your asthma can be controlled: Expect nothing less." As part of comprehensive education, such a positive message from all of her caregivers, as well as carefully listening to A.B.'s concerns, can have a major impact on A.B. who has not been managing her asthma correctly.

49. A.B. tells the pharmacist that her physician insisted that she place the albuterol MDI in front of her open mouth and spray rather than put the MDI in her mouth. She says she is confused because the package insert shows placement of the inhaler in the mouth. Also, it bothers A.B. that she cannot tell that she is receiving her budesonide dose because there is no taste. What should the pharmacist tell A.B.?

A.B. is correct that this is a confusing issue to many patients and health professionals. A small number of studies show that the "open-mouth" technique is better, but several other studies show that the "closed-mouth" technique is as good as or better than putting the MDI in front of the open mouth.[1,127] In addition, the correctly performed closed-mouth technique is as efficacious with a β_2-agonist as with a spacer[131] or nebulizer.[140] Thus, the closed-mouth technique is perfectly acceptable as is the open-mouth technique. One caution with the open-mouth technique is that misaiming the MDI may result in aerosol being sprayed onto the face or into the eyes. The pharmacist should reassure A.B. that numerous studies have shown rapid, deep inhalation with the budesonide dry powder inhaler (Turbuhaler) results in excellent efficacy even though there is no taste.

50. **For patients who are using both a bronchodilator and an anti-inflammatory inhaler, what is the proper sequencing of inhalers?**

For patients who have several inhalers, questions regarding sequencing of the inhalers are frequently asked. First, there is no well-documented evidence that outcomes are better using, for instance, a bronchodilator or an anti-inflammatory agent first. A common sense approach is that using a rapid-onset bronchodilator such as a β_2-agonist first and then an anti-inflammatory second has some appeal (i.e., quick relief and theoretically enhanced penetration of the anti-inflammatory). However, as previously discussed, short-acting β_2-agonists are preferred for *as-needed use* (and before exercise) and are not generally used on a scheduled basis. Thus, if a patient is not symptomatic at the time the anti-inflammatory is scheduled, current literature suggests the patient inhale only the anti-inflammatory agent. Therefore, it is usually NOT necessary to counsel patients regarding sequencing of inhaled medications. Because time is limited in counseling patients, teaching patients correct inhalation technique, the purpose of each medication (controllers versus quick relievers), and the need for strict adherence with controller therapies is far more important than spending precious time on the sequencing of inhalers.

DRUG-INDUCED ASTHMA

51. **M.B., 32-year-old woman with asthma, asks her community pharmacist for a refill of her ICS. As the pharmacist is reviewing the purpose of the ICS and checking her inhalation technique, he sees that M.B. has placed an over-the-counter (OTC) ibuprofen product on the counter for purchase. What should the pharmacist do?**

First, the pharmacist already should have checked the pharmacy profile to see if M.B. is aspirin sensitive. If there is no indication that she is, a double-check by asking her is important. M.B. reports that she is very sensitive to aspirin (severe wheezing). The pharmacist should counsel the patient regarding the fact that patients with asthma who are aspirin sensitive often react to other nonsteroidal anti-inflammatory drugs (NSAIDs) such as ibuprofen by developing asthma symptoms with the first dose. The pharmacist should suggest acetaminophen. If M.B. says that acetaminophen does not give adequate relief of her pain, other options are salsalate[1] or consultation with a board-certified allergist with experience in aspirin and NSAID desensitization. The pharmacist should also suggest consultation with an allergist regarding a recent study that gives strong evidence that the COX-2 inhibitor, rofecoxib, is safe in aspirin-sensitive asthma.[141] This case also points out the need for health professionals to pay attention to patient use of nonprescription medications. If the pharmacist in this situation had been "too busy" to notice the OTC purchase, the consequences could have been disastrous to M.B.

Although drug-induced asthma may present as relatively mild symptoms in some patients, fatal asthma caused by medicinal agents has been reported numerous times. Thus, it is imperative that clinicians strive to prevent this problem through education of patients and other health professionals. The most extensive literature on drug-induced asthma involves NSAIDs and β-blockers. Other drugs and drug preservatives also can induce symptoms of asthma, but because the topic is beyond the scope of this chapter, the reader is referred to other sources [142,143] and Chapter 26, Drug-Induced Pulmonary Disorders, for further discussion.

The percentage of asthmatics reported to be aspirin sensitive ranges from 4% to 28%. Clinical manifestations of aspirin sensitivity include rhinorrhea, mild wheezing, or severe, life-threatening shortness of breath. Once the reaction has occurred, there is a refractory period of 2 to 5 days.[144] If an asthmatic is aspirin sensitive, it is likely that the patient also will react to most other NSAIDs. Aspirin and other NSAIDs share common mechanisms involving the arachidonic acid pathways, including inhibition of cyclo-oxygenase, which results in more rapid synthesis and overproduction of leukotrienes.[144] Not surprisingly, because leukotrienes are an important part of the mechanism of NSAID-induced asthma, inhibitors of 5-lipoxygenase such as zileuton are generally effective in blocking this response.[145] Similarly, leukotriene receptor antagonists such as zafirlukast and montelukast are generally effective in blocking aspirin-induced asthma.[146] Because most patients with asthma do not react to aspirin and other NSAIDs, the updated NIH Guidelines recommend avoiding these agents only in patients with known sensitivity.[1] In addition, patients with severe persistent asthma or nasal polyps should be counseled regarding the risks associated with these drugs. In patients with known sensitivity, acetaminophen or salsalate are recommended for headaches and relatively minor pain.[1] For patients who are sensitive but who need to take aspirin (e.g., postmyocardial infarction [MI]) or an NSAID (e.g., arthritis), it is possible to desensitize the patient, and daily use then prevents further reaction.

When discussing drug-induced asthma, the other major consideration is β-blockers. These agents should be used with great caution in patients with asthma. Because even β_1-adrenergic blockers lose selectivity as dosages are increased, they, as well as nonselective β-blockers, should be avoided in most patients. Furthermore, ophthalmic timolol has been reported several times to cause fatal asthma and should absolutely be avoided in patients with a history of asthma.[147] Other β-blocker eye drops (e.g., betaxolol) have been reported to have less propensity to induce asthma, but all have some risk.[142,148]

Two notable exceptions to using β-blockers in patients with asthma are patients who are post-MI and patients with heart failure.[149] Because β-blockers prolong life post-MI and improve the care of patients with heart failure, benefits versus risks should be weighed. Risks outweigh benefits if a patient has severe persistent asthma.[149,150] If a post-MI patient has mild intermittent asthma or well-controlled mild persistent (and possibly moderate persistent[149]) asthma with optimal management, a low dosage of atenolol 50 mg/day is a reasonable consideration where benefits may outweigh risks.[150] Asthma patients have been shown to respond to inhaled β_2-agonists when receiving this dosage of atenolol.[150] Unfortunately, low dosages of β-blockers are not proven to prolong life after an MI, but some studies suggest efficacy of lower dosages. Chafin and colleagues[150] have recently reviewed the literature regarding β-blocker–induced asthma and potential use of these agents in post-MI patients. Although further study in post-MI and heart failure patients with moderate persistent asthma is needed, Salpeter and colleagues[149] suggest not withholding cardioselective β-blockers in patients with mild to moderate "reactive airway disease." For patients with heart failure, metoprolol CR/XL is the cardioselective β-blocker approved in the United States.

If a patient with asthma is given a β-blocker and initially reports no symptoms, subsequent exacerbations may not respond well to administration of usual doses of a β-agonist. The drug of choice for β-blocker–induced bronchospasm is ipratropium.[184] A more subtle risk with β-blockers involves the adult with allergic rhinitis and a family history of asthma. If this individual is given a β-blocker for hypertension, symptoms of asthma could be induced, especially if another trigger is introduced such as running in cold, dry air.

OUTCOMES

52. C.C. is a 36-year-old woman admitted to the hospital for asthma. This is her second hospitalization in the past 2 years, and she has had three ED visits during the same period. She also complains of frequent nocturnal awakenings and is bothered that she is gaining weight, since she cannot exercise. Lack of exercise is also troubling her because her 5-year-old daughter wants her to go outside and play with her. C.C. has been taking SR theophylline BID and flunisolide one puff BID with an AeroChamber for years along with frequent PRN albuterol. C.C. carefully controls her home environment. What could her clinicians do to improve her outcomes, including quality of life?

C.C. needs a reassessment of her long-term management considering her very poor outcomes over the past 2 years. First, her clinicians need to establish a partnership with her in education regarding asthma and its management. Clearly, she needs dosage adjustment with her anti-inflammatory therapy. Her dosage is too low, plus she is receiving a low-potency corticosteroid. Based on her recent history, she should be treated initially with high-dose ICS and a long-acting inhaled β2-agonist, preferably with a more potent ICS product that would require fewer inhalations per day (e.g., budesonide, plus formoterol or combination fluticasone-salmeterol). C.C. should have the absolute importance of daily controller therapy stressed, including the need for strict adherence and excellent inhalation technique. C.C. needs an emergency supply of prednisone (i.e., to use when her PEF is in the red zone and unresponsive to albuterol). C.C. should be told to expect a reduced need for albuterol.

Numerous studies have documented that applying the principles of the NIH Guidelines[1] results in improved clinical outcomes.[151–164] In the 1990s, several studies have documented that pharmacists who are very knowledgeable of the NIH Guidelines and who work closely with patients and physicians, improve outcomes.[153–158] Dramatic reductions in ED visits and hospitalizations have resulted from these pharmacist-initiated interventions, stressing application of NIH guidelines.[153–158] These successful studies involved highly motivated pharmacists, who were asthma experts based in university-affiliated clinics or in large private HMOs.

A recent randomized controlled trial based in community pharmacies with specially trained pharmacists has also shown very positive outcomes for patients with asthma.[165] Patients followed up for 1 year in the intervention group had significant improvements in PEF, symptom scores, quality of life, and reduced physician visits compared with the usual care group. Another randomized controlled trial based in chain drug stores with staff pharmacists did not show a benefit related to attempts at asthma care.[166] Unfortunately, the level of training and incentives did not appear optimal, and the authors pointed out that the staff pharmacists were "not universally enthusiastic" about the program. The authors also described their intervention as "cumbersome" for the pharmacists. Further study is needed to assess asthma care in this setting when pharmacists are optimally trained, given appropriate incentives, and enthusiastic about the program.

When assessing the effect of comprehensive management on clinical outcomes, quality of life measures should be assessed as well as reduction in ED visits and hospitalizations.[167] To achieve optimal outcomes, attention to each of the four major components of management is required (objective assessment, environmental control, pharmacologic therapy, and patient education as a partnership). Examples of areas that pose special challenges for inner city patients include psychosocial factors, underuse of controller medications, and passive cigarette smoke.[168–170] A recent study has emphasized again the importance of good inhalation technique with ICS.[171]

53. C.C. returns to the clinic in 2 months and is elated because she is sleeping through the night and not waking up short of breath. In addition, she is beginning to exercise again, which makes her and her child very happy. C.C. has had no further ED visits. What should the clinician do at this point?

Optimal asthma management that improves outcomes is a continuous process of education and reassessment of the overall therapy. Observation of C.C. using her peak flow meter and inhalation devices on each clinic visit is important and should be routine. Having C.C. verbalize her understanding of the role of the inhaled corticosteroid plus long-acting inhaled β2-agonist versus albuterol and the action plan with "crisis" prednisone is important. Despite her current optimism, asking C.C. what her concerns are about her asthma right now is important. Over the next month or two, a trial of slowly stepping down the inhaled corticosteroid dosage to a medium dose should be attempted. Finally, C.C. needs continued partnership with her clinician.

54. C.C. is in the clinic 2 years later, reflecting with her clinician over her total elimination of ED visits and hospitalizations as well as her improved quality of life. Her management initiated 24 months ago has continued, including environmental control, controller therapy tailored for her, PRN albuterol and, early morning PEF monitoring, and partnership with her clinician. Unfortunately, C.C. forgot to get an influenza vaccine last October and became ill with influenza in early March. Although this episode only slightly worsened her asthma symptoms, when she was almost recovered from the flu, she went to the grocery store and breathed second-hand smoke unexpectedly. In addition, early spring tree and grass pollen was affecting her allergic rhinitis. By the time she got back to her house, she was wheezing and her PEF was in the yellow zone, but it responded to three puffs of albuterol. C.C. asks what she should do if this series of events had resulted in her PEF decreasing to the red zone.

Table 23-13 Examples of Potential Future Asthma Therapies[a]

- Interleukin-4 inhibitors
- DNA vaccines
- Immunotherapy with T-cell peptide epitopes

[a]See references 7, 172–174.

C.C. needs to be re-educated regarding the action plan based on symptoms and PEF values. Referring back to the written plan for doses of albuterol and, if needed, oral corticosteroid therapy is important. Pointing out the need to put "get a flu shot" on the October calendar is obviously important here. Reinforcement of the importance of continued preventive therapy that has given such remarkable success is appropriate for C.C. and reassuring her that despite this minor setback, she is in control of her asthma. The clinician should continue to work with her to further tailor the therapy, including control of rhinitis, to maintain optimal outcomes at the lowest dosages and the simplest possible regimen.

ANTI-IMMUNOGLOBULIN E THERAPY

55. **C.C. tells her clinician that she read about a new asthma treatment called anti-IgE therapy (omalizumab, Xolair), and she asks if it would be a good treatment for her.**

Continued partnership with C.C. includes sharing with her the latest clinical research shown to improve asthma outcomes. Many patients now hear of new research in the news media and ask their clinicians what it may mean to their care; putting new research findings in the proper perspective is important, because news reports sometimes inadvertently mislead patients (i.e., patients stop current drug therapy and ask for new drug). Clinicians should anticipate continued research aimed at new targets in an effort to reduce airway inflammation (Table 23-13).[7,172–175]

Omalizumab is a humanized monoclonal anti-IgE antibody that binds to free IgE in serum. Thus, binding of IgE to high-affinity receptors on mast cells is subsequently inhibited, and the initiation of the allergic inflammatory cascade is blocked.[172–175] Omalizumab is effective in reducing oral and inhaled corticosteroid dose requirements in patients with severe asthma, and in reducing exacerbations.[172,176,177] This novel therapy is administered as a 150 to 375 mg subcutaneous injection every 2 or 4 weeks. The dose and frequency of administration are based on the serum total IgE level (IU/mL) and the patient's body weight. Common side effects associated with omalizumab include injection site reactions, upper respiratory tract infections, sinusitis, and headache. Less common, but potentially serious adverse effects, include anaphylaxis ($<0.1\%$) and the development of malignant neoplasms (0.5% of omalizumab-treated patients compared with 0.2% in controls).

Because omalizumab is expensive and must be administered as a subcutaneous injection, it should be reserved for patients with severe asthma not adequately controlled with standard therapies. Despite the high cost, anti-IgE therapy might be cost effective in selected patients with severe disease (e.g., those with frequent ED visits and hospitalizations) because an estimated $<5\%$ of asthma patients (severe disease) account for $>50\%$ of the dollars spent for asthma care.[178] Because C.C. has responded well to her current regimen, she is not a candidate for omalizumab.

COMPLEMENTARY ALTERNATIVE THERAPIES

56. **C.C. is in the community pharmacy a few months later for refills of her medications. She is continuing to have excellent control of her asthma and allergic rhinitis. C.C. asks the pharmacist her opinion of herbal remedies for asthma as well as other non-traditional approaches to treatment.**

Complementary and alternative approaches that have been used in the treatment of asthma include black tea, coffee, ephedra, marijuana, dried ivy leaf extract, acupuncture, meditation, and yoga.[1, 179,180] Despite the widespread use of alternative medications for chronic conditions, the clinician should discuss with C.C. that there is no established scientific basis for their use in the management of asthma.[1] Complementary alternative medicine cannot be recommended as a substitute for the drug therapy recommended by the NIH Guidelines and other medical literature based on randomized controlled studies.

REFERENCES

1. National Institutes of Health. Expert Panel Report 2. Guidelines for the Diagnosis and Management of Asthma, 1997; NIH publication No. 97-4051.
2. National Institutes of Health. Guidelines for the Diagnosis and Management of Asthma. National Asthma Education Program Expert Panel Report, 1991; NIH publication No. 91-3042.
3. National Institutes of Health. International Consensus Report on diagnosis and treatment of asthma, 1992; NIH publication no. 92-3091.
4. National Institutes of Health. Global Initiative for Asthma, 1995; NIH publication no. 95-3659.
5. National Institutes of Health, Guidelines for the Diagnosis and Management of Asthma—Update on Selected Topics 2002, NIH Publication No. 02-5075. J Allergy Clin Immunol 2002;110:S1-S219.
6. Weiss KB, Sullivan SD. The health economics of asthma and rhinitis. I. Assessing the economic impact. J Allergy Clin Immunol 2001;107:3.

7. Busse WW, Lemanske RF. Asthma. N Engl J Med 2001;344:350.
8. Mattes J, Karmaus W. The use of antibiotics in the first year of life and development of asthma: which comes first? Clin Exp Allergy 1999;29:729.
9. Morahan G et al. Association of IL12B promoter polymorphism with severity of atopic and nonatopic asthma in children. Lancet 2002;360:455.
10. Henderson WR Jr. The role of leukotrienes in inflammation. Ann Intern Med 1994;121:684.
11. Davis WB. Eosinophils. In: Barnes P et al, eds. Asthma and COPD: Basic Mechanisms and Clinical Management. Amsterdam: Academic Press, 2002:111.
12. Zimmerman N et al. Chemokines in asthma: cooperative interaction between chemokines and IL-13. J Allergy Clin Immunol 2003;111:227.
13. Davies DE et al. Airway remodeling in asthma: new insights. J Allergy Clin Immunol 2003;111:215.

14. Skobeloff EM et al. The effect of the menstrual cycle on asthma presentations in the emergency department. Arch Intern Med 1996;156:1837.
15. West JB. Respiratory Physiology: The Essentials. 6th Ed. Baltimore: Williams & Wilkins, 1999.
16. American Thoracic Society. Standardization of spirometry. Am J Respir Crit Care Med 1995;152:1107.
17. Benatar SR. Fatal asthma. N Engl J Med 1986;314:423.
18. McFadden ER. Clinical physiologic correlates in asthma. J Allergy Clin Immunol 1986;77:1.
19. McFadden ER, Lyons HA. Arterial blood gas tension in asthma. N Engl J Med 1968;278:1027.
20. Kelly HW, Murphy S. Beta-adrenergic agonists for acute, severe asthma. Ann Pharmacotherapy 1992;26:81.

21. Fanta CH et al. Treatment of acute asthma: is combination therapy with sympathomimetics and methylxanthines indicated? Am J Med 1986;80:5.

22. O'Driscoll BR et al. Nebulized salbutamol with and without ipratropium bromide in acute airflow obstruction. Lancet 1989;1:1418.

23. Reisman J et al. Frequent administration by inhalation of salbutamol and ipratropium bromide in the initial management of severe acute asthma in children. J Allergy Clin Immunol 1988;81:16.

24. Schuh S et al. Efficacy of frequent nebulized ipratropium bromide added to frequent high-dose albuterol therapy in severe childhood asthma. J Pediatr 1995;126:639.

25. Qureshi F et al. Effect of nebulized ipratropium on the hospitalization rates of children with asthma. N Engl J Med 1998;339:1030.

26. Kradjan WA et al. Atropine serum concentrations after multiple inhaled doses of atropine sulfate. Clin Pharmacol Ther 1985;38:12.

27. Dulfano MJ, Glass P. The bronchodilator effects of terbutaline: route of administration and patterns of response. Ann Allergy 1976;37:357.

28. Becker AB et al. Inhaled salbutamol (albuterol) vs. injected epinephrine in the treatment of acute asthma in children. J Pediatr 1983;102:465.

29. Fergusson RJ et al. Nebulized salbutamol in life-threatening asthma: is IPPB necessary? Br J Dis Chest 1983;77:255.

30. Shim CS, Williams MH. Effect of bronchodilator therapy administered by canister versus jet nebulizer. J Allergy Clin Immunol 1984;73:387.

31. Newman SP. Aerosol deposition considerations in inhalation therapy. Chest 1985;88(Suppl):152.

32. Lewis RA, Fleming JS. Fractional deposition from a jet nebulizer: how it differs from a metered dose inhaler. Br J Dis Chest 1985;79:361.

33. Turner JR et al. Equivalence of continuous flow nebulizer and metered dose inhaler with reservoir bag for treatment of acute airflow obstruction. Chest 1988;93:476.

34. Idris AH et al. Emergency department treatment of severe asthma: metered dose inhaler plus holding chamber is equivalent in effectiveness to nebulizer. Chest 1993;103:665.

35. Kerem E et al. Efficacy of albuterol administered by nebulizer versus spacer device in children with acute asthma. J Pediatr 1993;123:313.

36. Delgado A et al. Nebulizers vs metered-dose inhalers with spacers for bronchodilator therapy to treat wheezing in children aged 2 to 24 months in a pediatric emergency department. Arch Pediatr Adolesc Med 2003;157:76.

37. Cates CJ et al. Holding chamber versus nebulizer for beta-agonist treatment of acute asthma. Cochrane Database Sys Rev 2002;(2):DC00052.

38. Morley TF et al. Comparison of beta adrenergic agents delivered by nebulizer vs metered dose inhaler with InspirEase in hospitalized asthmatic patients. Chest 1988;94:1205.

39. Leversha AM et al. Costs and effectiveness of spacer versus nebulizer in young children with moderate and severe acute asthma. J Pediatr 2000;136:497.

40. Schuh S et al. Comparison of albuterol delivered by a metered dose inhaler with spacer versus a nebulizer in children with mild acute asthma. J Pediatr 1999;135:22.

41. Schuh S et al. High-versus low-dose frequently administered nebulized albuterol in children with severe acute asthma. Pediatrics 1989;83:513.

42. Schuh S et al. Nebulized albuterol in acute childhood asthma: comparison of two doses. Pediatrics 1990;86:509.

43. Kelly HW et al. Safety of frequent high dose nebulized terbutaline in children with acute severe asthma. Ann Allergy 1990;64:229.

44. Nelson HS. Clinical experience with levalbuterol. J Allergy Clin Immunol 1999;104:S77.

45. Rohr AS et al. Efficacy of parenteral albuterol in the treatment of asthma: comparison of its metabolic side effects with subcutaneous epinephrine. Chest 1986;89:348.

46. Brown MJ et al. Hypokalemia from beta$_2$-receptor stimulation by circulating epinephrine. N Engl J Med 1983;309:1414.

47. Lipworth BJ et al. Tachyphylaxis to systemic but not to airway responses during prolonged therapy with high dose inhaled salbutamol in asthmatics. Am Rev Respir Dis 1989;140:586.

48. Hall IP. Beta$_2$-Adrenoceptor Agonists. In Barnes P et al, eds. Asthma and COPD. Basic Mechanisms and Clinical Management. Amsterdam: Academic Press, 2002:521

49. Siegel D et al. Aminophylline increases the toxicity but not the efficacy of an inhaled beta-adrenergic agonist in the treatment of acute exacerbation of asthma. Am Rev Respir Dis 1985;132:283.

50. Self TH et al. Inhaled albuterol and oral prednisone therapy in hospitalized adult asthmatics: does aminophylline add any benefit? Chest 1990;98:1317.

51. Strauss RE et al. Aminophylline therapy does not improve outcome and increases adverse effects in children hospitalized with acute asthmatic exacerbations. Pediatrics 1994;93:205.

52. DiGuiulio GA et al. Hospital treatment of asthma: lack of benefit from theophylline given in addition to nebulized albuterol and intravenously administered corticosteroid. J Pediatr 1993;122:464.

53. Carter E et al. Efficacy of intravenously administered theophylline in children hospitalized with severe asthma. J Pediatr 1993;122:470.

54. Nuhoglu Y et al. Efficacy of aminophylline in the treatment of acute asthma exacerbation in children. Ann Allergy Asthma Immunol 1998;80:395.

55. Huang D et al. Does aminophylline benefit adults admitted to the hospital for an acute exacerbation of asthma? Ann Intern Med 1993;119:1155.

56. Weinberger M, Hendeles L. Theophylline in asthma. N Engl J Med 1996;334:1380.

57. Ellul-Micallef R, Fenech FF. Effect of intravenous prednisolone in asthmatics with diminished adrenergic responsiveness. Lancet 1975;2:1269.

58. Shapiro G et al. Double-blind evaluation of methylprednisolone versus placebo for acute asthma episodes. Pediatrics 1983;71:510.

59. Fanta CH et al. Glucocorticoids in acute asthma. Am J Med 1983;74:845.

60. Littenberg B, Gluck E. A controlled trial of methylprednisolone in the emergency treatment of acute asthma. N Engl J Med 1986;314:150.

61. Fiel SB et al. Efficacy of short-term corticosteroid therapy in outpatient treatment of acute bronchial asthma. Am J Med 1983;75:259.

62. Harris JB et al. Early intervention with short courses of prednisone to prevent progression of asthma in ambulatory patients incompletely responsive to bronchodilators. J Pediatr 1987;110:627.

63. Chapman KR et al. Effect of a short course of prednisone in the prevention of early relapse after the emergency room treatment of acute asthma. N Engl J Med 1991;324:788.

64. Qureshi F et al. Comparative efficacy of oral dexamethasone versus oral prednisone in acute pediatric asthma. 2001;139:20.

65. Brunette MG et al. Childhood asthma: prevention of attacks with short-term corticosteroid treatment of upper respiratory tract infection. Pediatrics 1988;81:624.

66. Connett GJ et al. Prednisolone and salbutamol in the hospital treatment of acute asthma. Arch Dis Child 1994;70:170.

67. Harrison BDW et al. Need for intravenous hydrocortisone in addition to oral prednisolone in patients admitted to hospital with severe asthma without ventilatory failure. Lancet 1986;1:181.

68. Edmunds AT, Godfrey S. Cardiovascular response during severe acute asthma and its treatment in children. Thorax 1981;36:534.

69. Salmeron S et al. Nebulized versus intravenous albuterol in hypercapnic acute asthma. Am J Respir Crit Care Med 1994;149:1466.

70. Rowe BH et al. Intravenous magnesium sulfate treatment for acute asthma in the emergency department: a systematic review of the literature. Ann Emerg Med 2000;36:181.

71. Hughes R et al. Use of isotonic nebulised magnesium sulphate as an adjuvant to salbutamol in treatment of severe asthma in adults: randomised placebo-controlled trial. Lancet 2003;361:2114.

72. Kress JP et al. The utility of albuterol nebulized with heliox during acute asthma exacerbations. Am J Respir Crit Care Med 2002;165:1317.

73. Yung M, South M. Randomized controlled trial of aminophylline for severe acute asthma. Arch Dis Child 1998;79:405-10.

74. Ream RS et al. Efficacy of IV theophylline in children with severe status asthmaticus. Chest 2001;119;1480.

75. Self TH et al. Reassessment of theophylline use for severe asthma exacerbation: Is it justified in critically ill hospitalized patients? J Asthma 2002;39:677.

76. Self TH et al. Reassessing therapeutic range for theophylline for laboratory report forms: the importance of 5-15 mcg/mL. Pharmacotherapy 1993;13:590.

77. Kelly HW. Theophylline Toxicity. In: Jenne JW, Murphy S, eds. Asthma Drugs: Theory and Practice. New York: Marcel Dekker, 1987:925.

78. Gal P et al. Theophylline disposition in obesity. Clin Pharmacol Ther 1987;23:438.

79. Self TH et al. Effect of disease states on theophylline serum concentrations: Are we still vigilant? Am J Med Sci 2000;219:177.

80. Lee BL et al. Cigarette abstinence, nicotine gum, and theophylline disposition. Ann Intern Med 1987;106:553.

81. Chiou W et al. Method for the rapid estimation of the total body clearance and adjustment of dosage regimens in patients during constant rate intravenous infusion. J Pharmacokinet Biopharm 1978;6:135.

82. Johnson M, Burkle W. Evaluation of the Chiou method for determining theophylline dosages. Clin Pharm 1983;3:174.

83. Spitzer WO et al. The use of beta agonists and the risk of death and near death from asthma. N Engl J Med 1992;326:501.

84. Helfer EL, Rose LI. Corticosteroids and adrenal suppression: characterizing and avoiding the problem. Drugs 1989;38:838.

85. Mellon M et al. Comparable efficacy of administration with face mask or mouthpiece of nebulized budesonide inhalation suspension for infants and young children with persistent asthma. Am J Crit Care Med 2000;162(2 Pt 1):593.

86. Pedersen S. Aerosol treatment of bronchoconstriction in children with or without a tube spacer. N Engl J Med 1983;308:1328.

87. Croft RD. 2 Year old asthmatics can learn to operate a tube spacer by copying their mothers. Arch Dis Child 1989;64:742.

88. Sly MR et al. Delivery of albuterol aerosol by AeroChamber to young children. Ann Allergy 1988;60:403.

89. Prior JG et al. High-dose inhaled terbutaline in the management of chronic severe asthma: comparison of wet nebulization and tube-spacer delivery. Thorax 1982;37:300.

90. Van den Berg NJ et al. Salmeterol/fluticasone propionate (50/100 μg) in combination in a Diskus Inhaler (Seretide) is effective and safe in children with asthma. Pediatr Pulmonol 2000;30:97.

91. Barnes PJ. Current issues for establishing inhaled corticosteroids as the antiinflammatory agents of choice for asthma. J Allergy Clin Immunol 1998;101:S427.

92. Kelly HW. Comparison of inhaled corticosteroids. Ann Pharmacother 1998;32:220.

93. Pauwels R et al. Effect of inhaled formoterol and budesonide on exacerbations of asthma. N Engl J Med 1997;337:1405.

94. Shapiro G et al. Combined salmeterol 50 mcg and fluticasone propionate 250 mcg in the Diskus device for the treatment of asthma. Am J Respir Crit Care Med 2000;161:527.

95. Lipworth BJ. Systemic adverse effects of inhaled corticosteroid therapy. Arch Intern Med 1999; 159:941.

96. Cumming RG et al. Use of inhaled corticosteroids and the risk of cataracts. N Engl J Med 1997;337:8.

97. Garbe E et al. Inhaled and nasal glucocorticoids and the risks of ocular hypertension or open-angle glaucoma. JAMA 1997;277:722.

98. The Childhood Asthma Management Program Research Group. Long term effects of budesonide or nedocromil in children with asthma. N Engl J Med 2000;343:1054.

99. Agertoft L, Pedersen S. Effect of long-term treatment with inhaled budesonide on adult height in children with asthma. N Engl J Med 2000;343:1064.

100. Molen TVD et al. Starting with a higher dose of inhaled corticosteroids in primary care asthma treatment. Am J Respir Crit Care Med 1998;158;121.

101. Pincus DJ et al Further studies on the chronotherapy of asthma with inhaled steroids: the effect of dosage timing on drug efficacy. J Allergy Clin Immunol 1997;100:771.

102. ZuWallack R et al. Long term efficacy and safety of fluticasone propionate powder administered once or twice daily via inhaler to patients with moderate asthma. Chest 2000;118:303.

103. Self TH, Sameri RM. Safety and efficacy of once daily inhaled corticosteroids. Am J Manag Care 2003;9:91.

104. Greening AP et al. Added salmeterol versus higher dose corticosteroid in asthma patients with symptoms on existing inhaled corticosteroid. Lancet 1994;344:219.

105. Woolcock A et al. Comparison of addition of salmeterol to inhaled steroids with doubling of the dose of inhaled steroids. Am J Respir Crit Care Med 1996;153:1481.

106. Crompton GK et al. Comparison of Pulmicort pMDI plus Nebuhaler and Pulmicort Turbuhaler in asthmatic patients with dysphonia. Respir Med 2000;94:448.

107. Lofdahl CG et al. Randomised, placebo controlled trial of effect of a leukotriene receptor antagonist, montelukast, on tapering inhaled corticosteroids in asthmatic patients. BMJ 1999;319:87.

108. Ducharme F et al. Addition of anti-leukotriene agents to inhaled corticosteroids for chronic asthma. Cochrane Database Syst Rev 2002;(1):CD003133.

109. Wilding P et al. Effect of long term treatment with salmeterol on asthma control. BMJ 1997;314:1441.

110. Adams RJ et al. Impact of inhaled anti-inflammatory therapy on hospitalizations and emergency department visits for children with asthma. Pediatrics 2001;107:706.

111. Knorr B et al. Montelukast, a leukotriene receptor antagonist, for the treatment of persistent asthma in children aged 2 to 5 years. Pediatrics 2001; 108:E48.

112. Knorr B et al. Montelukast for chronic asthma in 6 to 14 year old children. JAMA 1998;279:1181.

113. Evans DJ et al. A comparison of low-dose inhaled budesonide plus theophylline and high-dose inhaled budesonide for moderate asthma. N Engl J Med 1997;337:1412.

114. Hendeles L et al. Revised FDA labeling guidelines for theophylline oral dosage forms. Pharmacotherapy 1995;15:409.

115. Shannon M. Life threatening events after theophylline overdose: a 10-year prospective analysis. Arch Intern Med 1999;159:989.

116. Edwards DJ et al. Theophylline. In: Evans WE et al, eds. Applied Pharmacokinetics: Principles of Therapeutic Drug Monitoring. 3rd Ed. Vancouver: Applied Therapeutics, 1992.

117. Covelli HD et al. Predisposing factors to apparent theophylline-induced seizures. Ann Allergy 1985;54:411.

118. Bahls FH et al. Theophylline-associated seizures with "therapeutic" or low toxic serum concentrations: risk factors for serious outcome in adults. Neurology 1991;41:1309.

119. Dunn DW, Parekh HU. Theophylline and status epilepticus in children. Neuropediatrics 1991;22:24.

120. Neild JE, Cameron IR. Bronchoconstriction in response to suggestion: its prevention by an inhaled anticholinergic agent. BMJ 1985;290:674.

121. Tan RA, Spector SL. Exercise-induced asthma: diagnosis and management. Ann Allergy Asthma Immunol 2002;89:226.

122. Godfrey S, Konig P. Suppression of exercise-induced asthma by salbutamol, theophylline, atropine, cromolyn, and placebo in a group of asthmatic children. Pediatrics 1975;56:930.

123. Nelson JA et al. Effect of long term salmeterol treatment on exercise induced asthma. N Engl J Med 1998;339:141.

124. Leff JA et al. Montelukast, a leukotriene-receptor antagonist for the treatment of mild and exercise-induced bronchoconstriction. N Engl J Med 1998;339:147.

125. Silkoff PE, Martin RJ. Pathophysiology of nocturnal asthma. Ann Allergy Asthma Immunol 1998;81:378.

126. Holimon TD et al. Nocturnal asthma uncontrolled by inhaled corticosteroids: theophylline or long acting inhaled beta2 agonists. Drugs 2001;61:391.

127. Newman SP et al. How should a pressurized beta-adrenergic bronchodilator be inhaled? Eur J Respir Dis 1981;62:3.

128. Epstein SW et al. Survey of the clinical use of pressurized aerosol inhalers. Can Med Assoc J 1979;120:813.

129. Toogood JH et al. Use of spacers to facilitate inhaled corticosteroid treatment of asthma. Am Rev Respir Dis 1984;129:723.

130. Salzman GA, Pyszczynski DR. Oropharyngeal candidiasis in patients treated with beclomethasone dipropionate delivered by metered dose inhaler alone and with AeroChamber. J Allergy Clin Immunol 1988;81:424.

131. Rachelefsky GS et al. Use of a tube spacer to improve the efficacy of a metered dose inhaler in asthmatic children. Am J Dis Child 1986;140:1191.

132. Self TH et al. Nurses' performance of inhalation technique with metered-dose inhaler plus spacer device. Ann Pharmacother 1993;27:185.

133. Interiano B, Guntupalli KK. Metered-dose inhalers: do health care providers know what to teach? Arch Intern Med 1993;153:81.

134. Chafin CC et al. Effect of a brief educational intervention on medical students' use of asthma devices. J Asthma 2000;37:585.

135. Self TH et al. The value of demonstration and role of the pharmacist in teaching the correct use of pressurized bronchodilators. Can Med Assoc J 1983;128:129.

136. Mickle TR et al. Evaluation of pharmacists' practice in patient education when dispensing a metered dose inhaler. Drug Intell Clin Pharm 1990;24:927.

137. Toogood JH et al. Comparison of the antiasthmatic, oropharyngeal, and systemic glucocorticoid effects of budesonide administered through a pressurized aerosol plus spacer or the Turbuhaler dry powder inhaler. J Allergy Clin Immunol 1997;99:186.

138. Nielsen KG et al. Clinical effect of Diskus dry powder inhaler at low and high inspiratory flow-rates in asthmatic children. Eur Respir J 1998;11:350.

139. Strayhorn et al. Elevation of peak expiratory flow by a "spitting" maneuver: measured with five peak flow meters. Chest 1998;113:1134.

140. Mestitz H et al. Comparison of outpatient nebulized vs. metered dose inhaler terbutaline in chronic airflow obstruction. Chest 1989;96:1237.

141. Stevenson DD, Simon RA. Lack of cross-reactivity between rofecoxib and aspirin in aspirin-sensitive patients with asthma. J Allergy Clin Immunol 2001;108:47.

142. Hunt LW, Rosenow EC. Drug-induced asthma. In: Weiss EB, Stein M. eds. Bronchial Asthma: Mechanisms and Therapeutics. Boston: Little, Brown, 1993:621.

143. Meeker DP et al. Drug-induced bronchospasm. Clin Chest Med 1990;11:163.

144. Szczeklik A, Stevenson DD. Aspirin-induced asthma: advances in pathogenesis, diagnosis, and management. J Allergy Clin Immunol 2003;111:913.

145. Israel E et al. The pivotal role of 5-lipoxygenase products in the reaction of aspirin-sensitive asthmatics to aspirin. Am Rev Respir Dis 1993;148:1447.

146. Holgate ST et al. Leukotriene antagonists and synthesis inhibitors: new directions in asthma therapy. J Allergy Clin Immunol 1996;98:1.

147. Odeh M. Timolol eyedrop-induced fatal bronchospasm in an asthmatic patient. J Fam Pract 1991;32:97.

148. Dunn TL et al. The effect of topical ophthalmic instillation of timolol and betaxolol on lung function in asthmatic subjects. Am Rev Respir Dis 1986;133:264.

149. Salpeter SR et al. Cardioselective beta blockers in patients with reactive airway disease: a meta-analysis. Ann Intern Med 2002;137:715.

150. Chafin CC et al. Beta blockers after myocardial infarction: Do benefits ever outweigh risks in asthma? Cardiology 1999;92:99.

151. Mayo PH et al. Result of a program to reduce admissions for adult asthma. Ann Intern Med 1990;112:864.

152. Zeiger RS. Facilitated referral to asthma specialist reduces relapses in asthma emergency room visits. J Allergy Clin Immunol 1991;87:1160.

153. Im J. Evaluation of the effectiveness of an asthma clinic managed by an ambulatory care pharmacist. Calif J Hosp Pharm 1993;5:5.

154. Cheng B et al. Evaluation of the long term outcome of adult patients managed by the pharmacist-run asthma program in a health maintenance organization. J Allergy Clin Immunol 1999;103:51.

155. Pauley T et al. Results of a pharmacy managed, physician directed program to reduce ED visits in a group of inner city adult asthmatic patients. Ann Pharmacother 1995;29:5.

156. Kelso T et al. Educational and long term therapeutic intervention in the ED in adult indigent minority patients: Effect on clinical outcomes. Am J Emerg Med 1995;13:632.

157. Kelso T et al. Comprehensive long term management program for asthma: effect on outcomes in adult African Americans. Am J Med Sci 1996;311:272.

158. McGill KA et al. Improved asthma outcomes in Head Start children using pharmacist asthma counselors. Am J Respir Crit Care Med 1997;155:A202.

159. George MR et al. A comprehensive education program improves clinical outcome measures in inner-city patients with asthma. Arch Intern Med 1999;159:1710.

160. Greineder DK et al. A randomized controlled trial of a pediatric asthma outreach program. J Allergy Clin Immunol 1999;103:436-40.

161. Kelly CS et al. Outcomes evaluation of a comprehensive intervention program for asthmatic children enrolled in Medicaid. Pediatrics 2000;105:1029.

162. Self TH, Finch CK. Studies demonstrating improved outcomes in patients with asthma: a 10 year review. Am J Manag Care 2001;7:187.

163. Najada A et al. Outcome of asthma in children and adolescents at a specialty-based care program. Ann Allergy Asthma Immunol 2001;87:335.

164. Adams RJ et al. Impact of inhaled antiinflammatory therapy on hospitalization and emergency department visits for children with asthma. Pediatrics 2001;107:706.

165. McLean W et al. The BC community pharmacy asthma study: A study of clinical, economic and holistic outcomes influenced by an asthma care protocol provided by specially trained community pharmacists in British Columbia. Can Respir J 2003;10:195.

166. Weinberger M et al. Effectiveness of pharmacist care for patients with reactive airway disease. JAMA 2002;288:1594.

167. Becker AB. Outcomes in pediatric asthma: introduction. J Allergy Clin Immunol 2001;107:S443-44 (entire suppl).

168. Weil CM et al. The relationship between psychosocial factors and asthma morbidity in inner-city children with asthma. Pediatrics 1999;104:1274.

169. Finkelstein JA et al. Underuse of controller medications among Medicaid-insured children with asthma. Arch Pediatr Adolesc Med 2002;156:562.

170. Evans D et al. The impact of passive smoking on emergency room visits of urban children with asthma. Am Rev Respir Dis 1987;135:567.

171. Giraud V, Roche N. Misuse of corticosteroid metered-dose inhaler is associated with decreased asthma stability. Eur Respir J 2002;19:246.

172. Milgrom H et al. Treatment of allergic asthma with monoclonal anti-IgE antibody. N Engl J Med 1999;341:1666.

173. Lemanske RF et al. Omalizumab improves asthma-related quality of life in children with allergic asthma. Pediatrics 2002;110:E55-5

174. Kay AB. Allergic diseases and their treatment. N Engl J Med 2001;344:109.

175. Barnes PJ. Therapeutic strategies for allergic diseases. Nature 1999;402 (6760 Suppl):B31.

176. Busse W et al. Omalizumab, anti-IgE recombinant humanized monoclonal antibody, for the treatment of severe allergic asthma. J Allergy Clin Immunol 2001;108:184.

177. Soler M et al. The anti-IgE antibody omalizumab reduces exacerbations and steroid requirement in allergic asthmatics. Eur Respir J 2001;18:254.

178. Barnes PJ. Anti-IgE antibody therapy for asthma. N Engl J Med 1999;341:2006.

179. Blanc PD et al. Use of herbal products, coffee or black tea, and over the counter medications as self-treatments among adults with asthma. J Allergy Clin Immunol 1997;100:789.

180. Huntley A, Ernst E. Herbal medicines for asthma: a systematic review. Thorax 2000;55:925.

181. Knudsen RJ et al. Changes in the normal maximal expiratory flow-volume curve with growth and aging. Am Rev Respir Dis 1983;127(6):725.

182. Guenther CA, Welch MH. Pulmonary medicine. 2nd Ed. Philadelphia: JB Lippincott, 1982.

183. National Institutes of Health. Practical guide for the diagnosis and management of asthma. 1997;NIH publication No. 97-4053.

CHAPTER 24

Chronic Obstructive Pulmonary Disease

Dennis M. Williams, Wayne A. Kradjan

DEFINITION

Chronic obstructive pulmonary disease (COPD) is a condition characterized by limitation of airflow that is not fully reversible and does not change significantly over time. Airflow limitation is often progressive and is associated with an abnormal inflammatory response of the lungs to noxious substances.[1] It is clear that the abnormalities in the airways of COPD patients are associated with inflammation.

COPD is an umbrella term for various heterogeneous conditions, rather than a specific disease entity.[2] It most commonly refers to chronic bronchitis and emphysema. The common characteristic among conditions classified as *chronic obstructive pulmonary disease*s is longstanding airflow limitation with impairment of expiratory outflow. Asthma is not included in the definition of COPD. Older terms used synonymously for the same disorder, including *chronic obstructive airways disease* (COAD) and *chronic obstructive lung disease* (COLD), should not be used.

Epidemiology

The prevalence and mortality rate from COPD have steadily increased over the past 3 decades. An estimated 16 million people in the United States have COPD.[3] Fourteen million have chronic bronchitis and 2 million have emphysema. Many others with minimal alteration in functional ability do not seek medical care and are not included in these totals. Because of this, the true prevalence of COPD may be grossly underestimated. Indeed, the results of National Health and Nutrition Examination Survey (NHANES III) suggest the prevalence of COPD is approximately 24 million people in the United States.[4] COPD appears to be more prevalent among females compared to males and in white Americans compared to black Americans.[4] A lower rate of COPD is reported among adults ages 25 to 54 years, possibly reflecting a reduction in smoking prevalence since the 1960s.[4]

The nature, frequency, and severity of symptoms among COPD patients range from a chronic productive cough to severe, disabling dyspnea. In 1997, COPD accounted for more than 600,000 hospitalizations and nearly 14 million physician visits.[3] It is not uncommon to encounter COPD with other chronic illnesses, including cardiac, endocrine, or renal disease, presenting unique problems in the clinical management of these patients.

COPD is the fourth leading cause of death in the United States.[5] Over a 20-year period ending in 2000, mortality rates from COPD increased 67%.[4] In 1998, more than 107,000 deaths were reported from COPD. A similar number of deaths are attributed annually to pneumonia and influenza infections, both of which are complications of the disease. The increase in death rate from COPD was greater for blacks compared with whites, although the overall death rate remained higher in whites. Death rates among women tripled during this period and, in 2000, more women died of COPD than men. These latter data likely reflect the increase in smoking by women over the past 50 years compared with men.[6] COPD is predicted to become the third leading cause of death and fifth leading cause of disability worldwide within 20 years.[7]

The economic impact of COPD is also significant with estimated annual treatment costs exceeding $30 billion dollars. This includes healthcare expenditures of $14.7 billion and even greater indirect costs of $15.7 billion (e.g., lost earnings due to illness or early death).[8,9] Disability estimates are an average of 12 days annually for patients with chronic bronchitis and 68 days for patients with emphysema.

Several countries have developed treatment guidelines for COPD including the American Thoracic Society (ATS), the European Respiratory Society (ERS), and the British Thoracic Society (BTS).[2,10,11] These guidelines are remarkably similar, providing international standardization for the diagnosis and treatment of COPD. However, many of the recommendations in these guidelines are opinions and not based on evidence.[12] A critical appraisal of 15 national and international guidelines concluded that the majority of recommendations were not evidence based and were difficult to interpret.[12] In 2001, the National Institutes of Health (NIH) and the World Health Organization (WHO) collaborated to develop the Global Initiative for Chronic Obstructive Lung Disease (GOLD) guidelines.[1] These guidelines represent an international effort and the recommendations are rated based on the strength of the evidence supporting them.

Risk Factors

Risk factors for the development of COPD can be classified as environmental, behavioral, and genetic. Nearly 85% of cases of COPD are attributed to a current or past history of cigarette smoking, although only 20% of smokers develop clinically significant COPD.[1] Other risk factors for COPD include asthma, environmental and occupational exposures (e.g., grain, coal, asbestos), indoor and outdoor air pollution, and respiratory infections.[13-15] Less than 1% of patients with emphysema have an inherited deficiency of α_1-antitrypsin, a protective protein in the lung. In patients who are deficient in this enzyme, emphysema can develop at an earlier age than is common with disease associated with cigarette smoking.

The risk of COPD from cigarette smoking is related to an accelerated loss of lung function. After age 35, nonsmokers experience a decline in FEV_1 of about 20 to 30 mL/yr. In smokers, the decline may be 50 to 120 mL/yr.[16] A model of the annual decline in lung function in nonsmokers, smokers, and susceptible smokers is illustrated in Figure 24-1. Some smokers appear more susceptible to this decline based on genetic or environmental factors.

The factors that predispose some smokers to develop COPD while leaving others protected are unknown. Chronic irritation by cigarette smoke and other pollutants can increase both the number and activity level of secretory cells in the airways. Also, smoking attracts neutrophils and macrophages into the lung, promoting the release of elastases and inactivating endogenous protease inhibitors. Some evidence suggests that different patterns of smoke inhalation (e.g., depth of inhalation) may contribute to risk, but smoking in general should be considered the major risk factor.[17,18]

Components of cigarette smoke cause inflammation and increased presence and activity of proteases; however, since only 20% of smokers develop clinically apparent COPD in their lifetime, this suggests that genetic variation may be associated with an increased risk of developing COPD. Although currently unproven, in susceptible smokers, a polymorphism in the gene encoding for antiproteases can be associated with producing less protein or a protein with lower activity. Similarly, genetic variation may result in increased sensitivity to pulmonary irritants leading to an accelerated loss of lung function. These possibilities likely will represent the focus of research for the next several years.

Pathophysiology

The chronic airflow limitation of COPD is attributable to disease of small airways and parenchymal destruction. The relative involvement of these structures varies from patient to patient and, in part, explains the differing presentations of

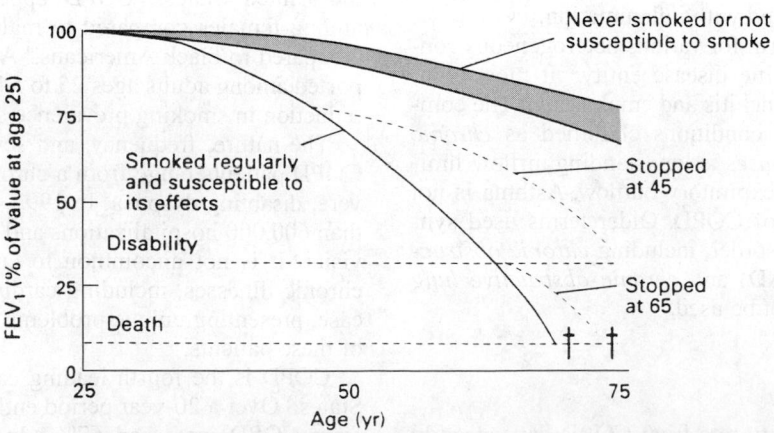

FIGURE 24-1 Model of annual decline in FEV₁ with accelerated decline in susceptible smokers. On stopping smoking subsequent loss is similar to that in healthy nonsmokers. (Modified from Fletcher C, Peto R. The natural history of chronic airflow obstruction. BMJ 1977;1:1645.)

chronic bronchitis and emphysema. These are referred to as the patient's phenotype where an individual patient's clinical presentation fits on a spectrum with symptoms of mucus hypersecretion (chronic bronchitis) at one extreme, and loss of elastic recoil and surface area for gas exchange (emphysema) at the other end. Chronic airflow limitation results from both of these processes as illustrated in Figure 24-2. Although the GOLD guidelines do not distinguish between these two entities, the classic definitions and pathophysiologic features are included here to understand the disease process.

In the simplest view, *bronchitis* is inflammation of the bronchioles. The clinical definition from the American Thoracic Society for *chronic bronchitis* is "the presence of chronic productive cough for 3 months in each of 2 consecutive years in a patient in whom other causes of chronic cough (e.g., asthma, congestive heart failure, gastroesophageal reflux) have been excluded."[2] *Emphysema* is an anatomic pathology with "abnormal permanent enlargement of the airspaces distal to the terminal bronchioles, accompanied by destruction of their walls and without obvious fibrosis."[2] As noted above, the degree of involvement of the small airways (bronchioles) or the lung parenchyma influences the clinical presentation of the patient.

Large (Central) Versus Small (Peripheral) Airways

The large airways of the lung (trachea and first generations or branches of the bronchi) are termed the central airways. This is the site of much of the airway wall inflammation and hypersecretion of mucus seen in chronic bronchitis. In response to inflammation, there is both an increase in numbers (hyperplasia) and enlargement (hypertrophy) of the submucosal glands and mucus-producing goblet cells in the surface epithelium.[10,19] Although the mucus produced in the large airways plays a major role in the symptomatic presentation of chronic bronchitis, it contributes little to the obstructive component of the disease.

Smaller bronchi down to the terminal bronchioles (the smallest branches in the lung that are not involved in gas exchange) make up the peripheral airways and are the predominate site of the increased airway resistance seen in both asthma and chronic bronchitis. Inflammation, fibrosis, and narrowing of small airways contribute to increased airway resistance and obstruction. Unique to chronic bronchitis, goblet cells proliferate in the small bronchioles of <2 mm in diameter, a site where these cells are typically absent in both asthmatics and those without pulmonary disease. This latter process, known as goblet cell metaplasia, adds significantly to the burden of secretions seen in these patients.

As described, bronchitis and mucus production alone do not cause airflow impairment. This is the case early in the process of patients with "smoker's cough." Because glandular changes are unrelated to hyperresponsiveness and bronchoconstriction, there is little effect on pulmonary function testing [e.g., forced expiratory volume in 1 second (FEV_1)] early in the disease.[2] However, prolonged periods of inflammation, edema of bronchial walls, and copious production of thick, tenacious secretions in the small and medium airways contribute to airway narrowing and eventual airflow obstruction in the later stages of COPD.

Increased mucus is an excellent medium for recurrent bronchial infections, resulting in further airway damage. The character of the mucus also changes. The mucus produced by chronic smokers is found in continuous sheets or "blankets" compared with the normal gel-like substance in distinct flakes. Finally, altered flow and adhesive properties of mucus, coupled with impaired ciliary functioning, cause reduced mucociliary clearance, pooling of secretions and possible trapping, and increased adherence of bacteria.[20] Recurrent infections result because of the inability to clear the mucus and mucous plugs.

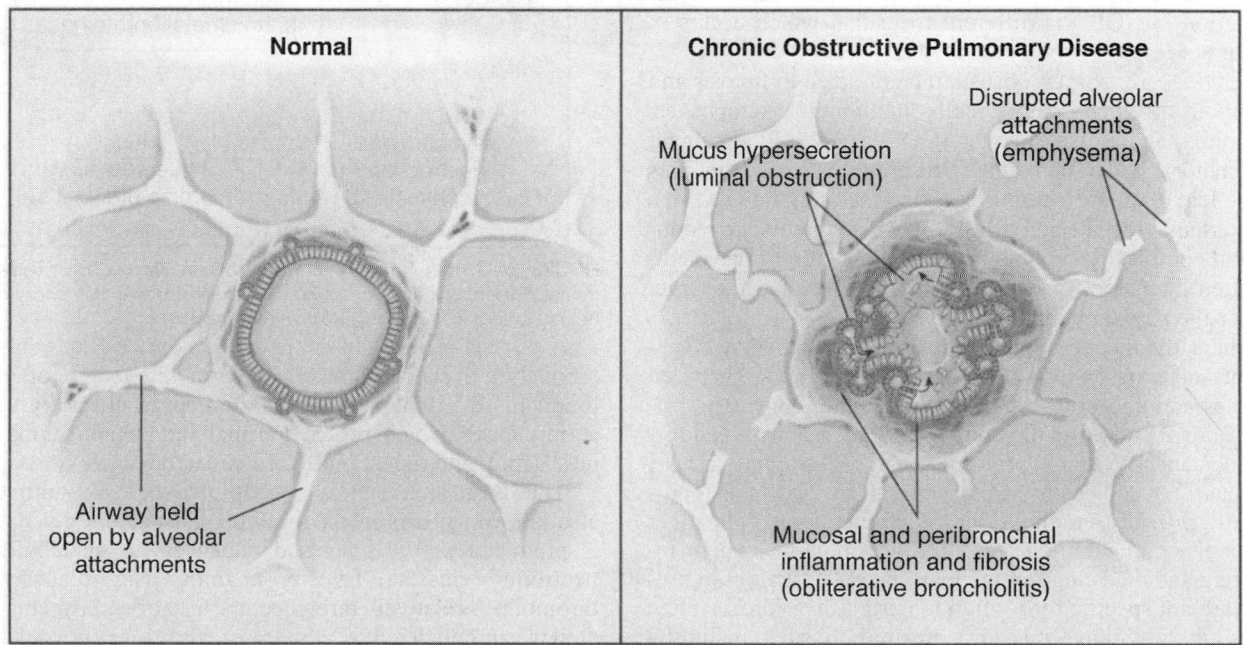

FIGURE 24-2 Mechanisms of airflow limitation in chronic obstructive pulmonary disease. (Modified from Barnes PJ. Chronic obstructive pulmonary disease N Engl J Med 2000;343(4):269 with permission.)

Parenchymal Destruction

The lung parenchyma is made up of thousands of gas-exchanging units (acini), each resembling tiny bunches of grapes. Each acinus branches from terminal bronchioles and contains respiratory bronchioles, alveolar ducts, and the alveolar sacs (the major site of gas exchange). Emphysema is characterized by destruction of the alveolar walls and enlargement of the terminal airspaces.[1,20] As the septal walls between individual alveoli are destroyed, the normal grapelike appearance becomes more rounded and the surface area for gas exchange is significantly reduced. In advanced cases, large, balloon-shaped bullae (bullous emphysema) may appear in localized areas. Rupture of these bullae leads to collapse of lung segments (pneumothorax). In panlobular (panacinar) emphysema, enlargement of the airspaces is relatively uniform throughout the entire acinus, involving the area from the respiratory bronchioles to the alveoli. The lower half of the lung is more likely to be involved. This is the type of emphysema associated with α_1-antitrypsin deficiency.[1,20] In centrilobular (centriacinar) emphysema, the primary damage is to the respiratory bronchioles, alveolar ducts, and central alveoli, with relative sparing of the terminal (distal) alveolar sacs. This is the predominant form of emphysema seen in smokers and coal workers and involves mostly the upper lobes of the lung. In either form, destruction of alveolar tissue results in loss of elastic recoil and structural support; thus, obstruction and airway collapse occur during expiration. Loss of alveolar attachments (tethering) to the terminal bronchioles as a result of the destructive changes of emphysema also contributes to small airway obstruction.[1]

Inflammation in COPD is important in the chronic progression and is driven by the interaction between several chemokines and enzymes. Numerous inflammatory mediators and cellular components exert actions that cause the resultant mucus hypersecretion, loss of alveolar structure and airway remodeling that is evident in COPD. This process is illustrated in Figure 24-3. An important point is that the nature of inflammation in COPD is different from that which occurs in asthma.

In COPD, bronchiolar obstruction is related to fibrosis and infiltration of inflammatory cells including macrophages, neutrophils, and T lymphocytes (CD8+ cells). Predominant inflammatory mediators that are present in increased amounts include leukotriene B_4, tumor necrosis factor alpha (TNF-α), and interleukin-8. The activities of these mediators are redundant and complex.[21,22] In other words, the action of one mediator often intensifies or complements another, and the target sites for the mediators may overlap.

Perhaps the most complete theory that explains the development and progression of COPD is an imbalance between proteases and antiproteases in the lung. The lungs are a primary route of entry into the body for microorganisms and foreign substances. Various proteases (e.g., neutrophil elastase, proteinase 3, cathepsins, and various matrix metalloproteinases) provide an important function, along with other components of the immune system function in the lung, by inactivating and digesting foreign material.[23] The actions of proteases are not specific for foreign material; therefore, as often occurs in immune function, normal tissue, including parenchymal tissue and alveolar attachments, can be damaged as an "innocent bystander." Proteases can also stimulate the

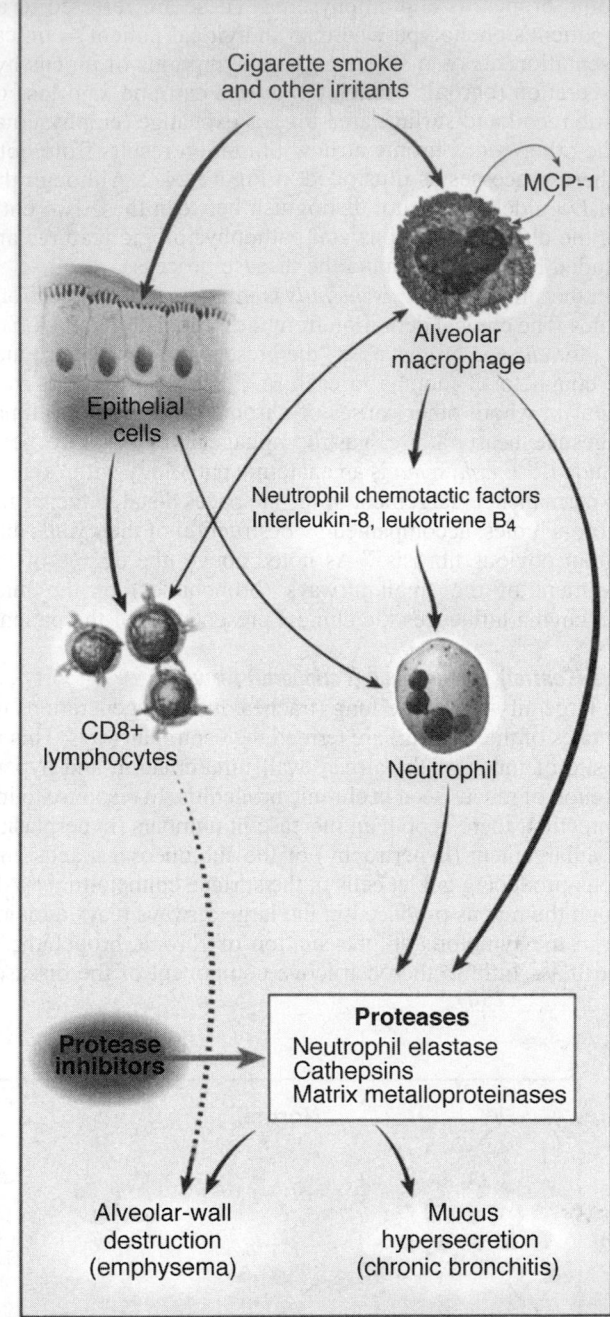

FIGURE 24-3 Inflammatory mechanisms in chronic obstructive pulmonary disease. (From Barnes PJ. Chronic obstructive pulmonary disease N Engl J Med 2000;343(4):269 with permission.)

production of mucus, which is the principle feature of chronic bronchitis. Normally, proteases are kept in check by various antiproteases which protect normal lung parenchyma from destruction and digestion by proteases.

The best characterized antiprotease is α_1-antitrypsin, also known as α_1-protease inhibitor. This serum glycoprotein is produced in the liver and enhances the metabolism of neutrophil elastase, trypsin, chymotrypsin, plasmin, and thrombin. A relatively rare genetic cause of emphysema is α_1-antitrypsin deficiency.

In COPD attributed to cigarette smoking, components of cigarette smoke attract neutrophils and macrophages into the lung, promoting release of elastases and inactivating endogenous protease inhibitors including α_1-antitrypsin, secretory leukoprotease inhibitor, elafin, and tissue inhibitors of matrix metalloproteinases.[23] This disruption of the normal balance increases the risk of tissue damage in predisposed individuals to cause the characteristic changes seen in COPD.[23,24]

In addition to the factors discussed above, environmental oxidative stress may play a role in the development of COPD.[23,25] Oxygen free radicals from cigarette smoke exert a number of effects, including increasing the concentration of inflammatory mediators and inhibiting antiprotease activity. This, in turn, sustains chronic inflammation and susceptibility to injury by protease enzymes.

In summary, COPD is primarily a disease of the small airways and adjacent alveolar structures. The obstruction and airflow limitation is generally described as being "fixed" (irreversible) because of either increased airway resistance from inflammatory and structural changes in small airways (chronic bronchitis) and/or loss of lung elastic recoil as a result of inflammation and alveolar wall destruction (emphysema). Bronchospasm and reversible airflow obstruction contribute little to the pathogenesis of COPD.

The clinical consequences of the morphologic changes are worsened obstruction, hyperinflation of the lungs, increased sputum production, reduced elastic recoil, recurrent respiratory infections, and altered gas exchange. The end results include respiratory muscle fatigue, ventilatory disorders, cardiovascular compromise, and poor quality of life.

Comparison With Asthma

Although COPD patients can have asthma concomitantly, these conditions should be considered as separate and distinct conditions. Inflammation is a key component of both conditions; however, the nature of inflammation is different. Asthma primarily involves eosinophilic inflammation. Small airway inflammation and infiltration of the bronchial mucosa with activated eosinophils are defining features of asthma. More specifically, interleukin (IL)-5—secreted by type 2 helper (CD4) T lymphocytes, mast cells, and eosinophils—plays a central role in further eosinophil recruitment that is responsible for many of the clinical manifestations of asthma.[20,26] In chronic bronchitis, inflammation is predominately neutrophilic, slower to develop, and is nonspecific, with a predominance of macrophages, IL-8, TNF-α, and type 1 helper (CD8) T cells, and a relative absence of IL-5 and eosinophils.[26]

Another example of the differences is that hypersecretion of mucus and cough are the major defining elements of chronic bronchitis but are absent in emphysema. Both can be present in asthma but only transiently during acute exacerbations. The chronicity and extent of mucus production, with eventual plugging of small airways, contributes to the airway obstruction in chronic bronchitis. Finally, hyperreactivity resulting in bronchospasm that is reversible either spontaneously or with β_2-adrenergic agonists is nearly a universal consequence of airway inflammation in asthma. In contrast, bronchospasm is an inconsistent finding in chronic bronchitis, with either no or only partial reversibility, and bronchospasm is almost always absent in emphysema. Complicating this distinction is the realization that some patients with longstanding asthma can also develop a fixed obstructive component because of chronic inflammation. A comparison of features of obstructive airways diseases (chronic bronchitis, emphysema, and asthma) is listed in Table 24-1.

Table 24-1 Clinical Features of Obstructive Airways Disease

	Asthma[a]	Bronchitis[b]	Emphysema[c]
Primary symptom	Wheezing, cough or dyspnea	Cough and sputum production	Dyspnea
Reversible with β_2-agonists	Yes	No	No
Allergic component	Frequent but not always	None	None
Inflammation	Yes (eosinophilic)	Yes (neutrophilic)	Alveoli only
Sputum production	During acute attack only	Copious, continuous	Scanty
Cough	Yes (nonproductive); morning cough may be a sign of nocturnal asthma	Yes (productive)	No
Age of onset	Often in childhood with allergies; older onset usually nonallergic	46–65 yr	55–75 yr
Chronicity	Episodic (e.g., pollen season) or continuous	Continuous	Continuous
Cigarette use	Uncommon	High incidence	High incidence
Body build	Varied	Obese	Thin, barrel chest
Hypoxia, CO_2 retention	During acute attack only	Yes (blue bloater)	No (pink puffer)
Other	Wheeze, cough, chest tightness, shortness of breath, mucous plugging, airway edema, difficulty exhaling. Often worse at night, or following exercise		

[a]Asthma is a chronic condition characterized by recurrent (intermittent) reversible bronchospasm. Reversibility may be spontaneous or after drugs. Airway inflammation and hyperresponsiveness to a variety of stimuli are important components of asthma.
[b]Chronic bronchitis is an inflammation of the bronchial tree. Chronic cough on most days for at least 3 mo/yr for 2 years. Thickened sputum and edematous bronchial walls obstruct airflow.
[c]Emphysema is a destruction of alveolar walls and capillaries by ↑ lung enzymatic activity.

α_1-Antitrypsin Deficiency

A rare cause of emphysema, implicated in less than 1% of cases, is an inherited deficiency of α_1-antitrypsin protein. In 1963, Laurell and Eriksson observed the development of diffuse panlobular emphysema in patients at a younger age than typical COPD. They attributed this problem to a hereditary deficiency of α_1-antitrypsin, a protective antiprotease found in the airways of normal individuals. α_1-Antitrypsin inhibits the activity of proteolytic enzymes, including neutrophil elastase. In the airway and lung parenchyma, it prevents tissue destruction during inflammatory reactions.

As part of this single gene inherited disease, there is a deficiency in production of α_1-antitrypsin; thus, neutrophil elastase activity in the lung is unchecked resulting in alveolar wall destruction. In normal individuals, circulating serum levels of α_1-antitrypsin are 150 to 350 mg/dL. Genes for this antiprotease can be separated by electrophoresis into phenotypes (Pi types), and individual phenotyping is based on the two-paired parental genes (alleles) inherited by the individual at birth. For example, the PiM gene confers production of normal amounts of fully functional enzyme. Accordingly, the PiMM allele is associated with normal enzyme activity. Other gene types include PiS (dysfunctional; normal serum levels of a poorly functioning enzyme), PiZ (deficient; an autosomal-recessive gene that codes for an active form of the enzyme but at a low rate of secretion), and Pi null (undetectable serum levels of enzyme). Many allele pair combinations exist. PiMZ and PiSZ are heterozygous disorders, and PiSS is a homozygous phenotype, all with >35% of normal enzyme activity and a relatively low risk of developing emphysema. PiZZ is a rare homozygous disorder characterized by accelerated lung destruction if plasma levels are <80 mg/dL (11 μM), or approximately 15% to 33% of normal. In these rare patients, the disease develops as early as age 20, but more typically in the fourth to fifth decade of life in nonsmokers, and approximately 10 years earlier in cigarette smokers. Diagnosis of α_1-antitrypsin deficiency is made by measuring circulating serum α_1-antitrypsin levels, followed by phenotyping only if necessary.

Diagnosis and Patient Assessment

COPD historically has been diagnosed based on a significant history of exposure to risk factors and patient-reported symptoms.[2,10,11] The GOLD guidelines recommend spirometry for accurate diagnosis and assessment of disease severity.[1] The diagnosis is based on a combination of subjective and objective data. A history of tobacco use should raise strong suspicion. A careful medical history should be taken, and symptoms of cough, sputum production, dyspnea, and wheezing should be confirmed with spirometry testing.

Early detection and intervention is important in slowing progression of the disease. When patients delay seeking care until symptoms are significant, benefits of therapy are limited because changes are largely irreversible. Thus, early detection of disease is essential. Cough and sputum production may be present for many years before airflow limitation develops, but not everyone with those symptoms will go on to have COPD. Dyspnea on exertion may not be present until the sixth or seventh decade.[1]

On physical examination, patients with early COPD may not exhibit any changes. Later, objective findings include the presence of a barrel chest, rales, rhonchi, prolonged expiratory phase, and cyanosis.[1,2] Symptomatic patients may present with decreased breath sounds, wheezes, and crackles on auscultation. In advanced disease, cyanosis, edema, intercostals retractions, and pursed lip breathing may be present.

Spirometry Testing

Spirometry is the gold standard measurement in assessing and monitoring obstructive lung disease.[1] It can be helpful to determine the severity, prognosis, and reversibility of the obstruction. In the evaluation of COPD, spirometry testing should be performed when the patient's condition is stable and at baseline. Spirometry testing should be performed according to the technical standards of the American Thoracic Society.[27] The two primary indicators of obstructive lung disease are a decrease in forced expiratory capacity (FEV_1) and a reduction in the ratio of FEV_1 to the forced vital capacity (FVC) to <75% (see Chapter 23, Asthma, for detailed descriptions of spirometric testing). Baseline spirometric measurements are helpful and provide information about changes in lung function over time. Early detection of changes in lung function will permit initiation of efforts to retard the progression of the disease. Peak expiratory flow (PEF), measured by a handheld peak flow meter, roughly correlate to FEV_1 testing, but should not be relied on for day-to-day monitoring. In advanced emphysema, FEV_1 can be significantly impaired, while peak flow might be only moderately reduced.

Using either FEV_1 or the FEV_1:FVC ratio, plus clinical signs, various staging guidelines have been proposed.[1,2,11,12] There has been a lack of consistency between various organizations' staging schemes, but all the methods give a rough index of disease severity (see Tables 24-2 and 24-3). The FEV_1 is the best prognostic indicator; the 5-year mortality rate is 50% when the FEV_1 is ≤1.0 L, and the mean survival is <2 years when FEV_1 is ≤0.5 L.[28,29] In contrast to asthma, reversibility of the changes in FEV_1 with bronchodilators is generally absent in COPD.

Chest radiographs are frequently obtained during the initial assessment, but are usually unremarkable except in advanced disease.[1] Nonspecific destructive changes may support the diagnosis; however, chest radiographs are most useful to rule out other causes of the patient's symptoms. Increased lung markings and peribronchial thickening are characteristic of chronic bronchitis, whereas hyperinflation, small heart size, and bullae (with loss of alveoli and wall structure) are seen with emphysema. With advanced COPD, the radiograph may show flattened diaphragms, enlarged anterior to posterior (AP) diameter, reduced vascular markings in the peripheral lung zones, and bullae. Electrocardiographic abnormalities, including premature beats and evidence of pulmonary hypertension, may be present. Arterial blood gas determinations are performed less frequently, but are helpful in certain clinical situations.

Further objective diagnosis and assessment are obtained from arterial blood gas (ABG) determinations. In stable (compensated) conditions, the pH will be normal, hypoxemia will be present in varying degrees, and mild to moderate hypercapnia (carbon dioxide retention) will be seen in many patients. Carbon dioxide retention usually develops when the FEV_1 falls to <0.8 L.[30,31] During acute exacerbations, hypercapnia worsens and respiratory acidosis is often present. The

Table 24-2   GOLD Report COPD Staging System[1]

Stage	Severity	Characteristics
0	At risk	• Normal spirometry • Chronic symptoms (cough, sputum production)
I	Mild COPD	• FEV_1/FVC <70% • FEV_1 ≥80% predicted • With or without chronic symptoms (cough, sputum production)
II	Moderate COPD	• FEV_1/FVC <70% • 50% ≤FEV_1 <80% predicted • With or without chronic symptoms (cough, sputum production)
III	Severe COPD	• FEV_1/FVC <70% • 30% ≤FEV_1 <50% predicted • With or without chronic symptoms (cough, sputum production)
IV	Very severe COPD	• FEV_1/FVC <70% • FEV_1 <30% predicted or FEV_1 <50% predicted plus chronic respiratory failure

Table 24-3   ATS COPD Staging System[2]

Stage	FEV_1	Description
I	>50% of predicted	COPD has minimal impact of health-related quality of life and results in only modest per capita health care expenditure
II	35% to 49% of predicted	COPD has significant impact on health-related quality of life and results in large per capita healthcare expenditure
III	<35% of predicted	COPD has a profound impact on health-related quality of life and results in large per capita healthcare expenditure

hemoglobin (Hgb) and hematocrit (Hct) may be elevated secondary to chronic hypoxemia. An α_1-antitrypsin concentration determination is indicated for patients developing COPD before age 50; for patients who have emphysema, but do not have a significant cigarette history; and for patients who have a family history of the genetic deficiency.

Clinical Presentation
CHRONIC BRONCHITIS

The representative patient with chronic bronchitis is a 45- to 65-year-old smoker with a chronic productive cough, moderate dyspnea, and recurrent respiratory infections. Other common features are obesity, the presence of significant hypoxemia, and cyanosis from carbon dioxide retention. These last three findings contribute to the description of a chronic bronchitis patient as a "blue-bloater." End-stage chronic bronchitis is complicated by polycythemia (increased red blood cell production) and cor pulmonale (right-sided congestive heart failure secondary to lung disease and pulmonary hypertension). Differing characteristics of chronic bronchitis and emphysema are summarized in Table 24-1.

EMPHYSEMA

Pathologically, emphysema involves destruction of alveolar walls and reduced elastic recoil. Patients commonly complain of dyspnea and exhibit fixed airflow obstruction on spirometry. Unlike chronic bronchitis, the prevalence of emphysema is higher among men compared with women.

Typical patients with emphysema are 55- to 75-year-old smokers with severe dyspnea as the primary complaint. Symptoms appear earlier in the rare patient with α_1-antitrypsin deficiency. Cough may be absent or, if present, produces only scanty sputum. Patients often are thin, barrel-chested, and breathe through pursed lips. Carbon dioxide retention usually is not a problem, and dyspnea is the most common complaint. The loss of elastic recoil that normally is responsible for exhalation increases the patient's work of breathing. With chronic symptoms, patients adapt and use accessory muscles of respiration and have a prolonged expiratory phase. Classically, emphysema patients are termed "pink-puffers" because they maintain adequate oxygenation through an increased work of breathing. Because emphysema is an anatomic disease, diagnosis often is made only during postmortem examination, especially in individuals who exhibited no significant evidence of airflow obstruction while alive.

Classification of Severity

There are two primary systems for classifying COPD in the United States.[1,2] Criteria are summarized in Tables 24-2 and 24-3. They are similar in that each is based on results of spirometry and the frequency and extent of symptoms. The American Thoracic Society (ATS) classification system represents the standard used for many years. According to the American Thoracic Society (ATS) criteria, COPD severity is staged on the basis of the degree of airflow obstruction as follows: stage I is FEV_1 ≥50% predicted; stage II is FEV_1 35% to 49% predicted; and stage III is FEV_1 <35% predicted.[2] Symptoms initially are present only on exertion, but as disease progresses will worsen to symptoms of dyspnea at rest. Patients with severe COPD have difficulty in performing daily activities without significant dyspnea. The GOLD expert panel classifies disease severity into five stages based on spirometric measurements, symptoms, and complications.[1] This staging is intended to serve as an educational tool and to guide management strategies as indicated in Table 24-4. The system recommended in the GOLD guidelines is used increasingly in clinical practice and research. The GOLD classification includes a category for asymptomatic patients with normal lung function who are at risk for developing COPD. This allows management strategies that may slow or prevent the onset for several years.

Natural Course

The natural course of COPD is highly variable, generally spanning 20 to 40 years and influenced by numerous factors, including genetic predisposition, exposure to inhaled irritants (tobacco smoke, workplace, or environmental pollutants), and repeated infections. The typical smoker who develops COPD remains asymptomatic for the first two decades of smoking, except for more frequent viral or bacterial upper respiratory tract infections. Clinical symptoms appear after significant irreversible lung damage occurs. After 25 to 30 years of smoking, mild dyspnea is noted and can be accompanied by a morning cough; however, physical examination and chest radiograph are often unremarkable.[1,2,28] As the disease progresses, loss of lung function occurs, dyspnea on exertion (DOE) develops, and sputum production and cough worsen. Ultimately, structural changes result in alveolar hypoxia and the secondary problems of pulmonary hypertension and cor pulmonale.

With continued exposure to risks (e.g., cigarette smoking), the disease progresses and patients develop increased airflow limitation and symptoms. Exacerbations, or flares, of COPD are common and can be infectious or noninfectious. Moderate to severe exacerbations may require hospitalization. Cor pulmonale is right-side heart failure that develops secondary to

lung disease. It is a late complication of COPD, especially chronic bronchitis. Acute respiratory failure is also a complication in patients with moderate to severe chronic disease. Respiratory failure can develop secondary to an acute infection, or other factors including oversedation, or heart failure.

General Management Considerations

The goals of treatment for COPD are to slow or prevent disease progression, relieve symptoms, improve exercise tolerance, improve overall health status, prevent and treat complications, prevent and treat exacerbations, and reduce mortality (Table 24-5).[1] There is no cure for COPD among currently available therapies.

Although these goals sound similar to those of asthma, there are significant differences in the degree by which they can be accomplished. The benefits of medications in COPD are generally less than those achieved in asthma. Side effects are more frequent and the presence of comorbid conditions can complicate treatment. A therapeutic goal should be to achieve a balance between the quality of life that the patient would like to accomplish and what is realistic.

In terms of functional status, an achievable goal in many patients with asthma is essentially normal functioning, including vigorous exercise. In a patient with COPD, the goals are less ambitious. One might be satisfied with making it possible to walk through the house without experiencing severe shortness of breath (SOB). Similarly, in asthma, the goal is pulmonary function test results that are >80% of the patient's predicted normal or personal best (i.e., in the green zone). A patient with far-advanced COPD may have a baseline FEV_1 that is far below 50% of normal and with minimal reversibility after bronchodilators. For this patient, the "personal best" is what would be considered in the "red zone" of pulmonary function in asthma.

Simply put, the goal is to obtain the best possible quality of life that is attainable. The success in meeting this goal is influenced by the stage of the disease when the diagnosis and interventions begin, the patient's motivation to adhere to a treatment plan, and most importantly, his or her willingness to stop smoking. On the other hand, although this is often an irreversible, progressive disease, taking an attitude of minimal intervention is not appropriate. If nothing else, disease progression may be slowed and the number of episodes of acute exacerbations with hospitalization can be reduced.

General management principles are directed toward educating the patient about his or her condition with an emphasis on understanding of the disease process and the rationale for the various components of care. The patient and health care professionals should work together to develop realistic goals,

---

Table 24-4 COPD Management Recommendations (Severity-Based)[1]

All Stages
- Avoidance of risk factor(s), especially smoking
- Influenza vaccination

0: At Risk

I: Mild chronic obstructive pulmonary disease
- I Mild: Short-acting bronchodilator when needed

II: Moderate chronic obstructive pulmonary disease
- II Moderate: Regular treatment with one or more long-acting bronchodilators
- II Moderate: Rehabilitation

III: Severe chronic obstructive pulmonary disease
- III Severe: Inhaled corticosteroids if significant symptoms and lung function response or if repeated exacerbations

IV: Very severe chronic obstructive pulmonary disease
- IV Very severe: Regular treatment
- Inhaled and lung exacerbations
- IV Very severe: Long-term oxygen therapy if respiratory failure
- Consider surgical treatment

Table 24-5 Goals for Management of COPD[1]

Prevent disease progression
Relieve symptoms
Improve exercise tolerance
Improve health status
Prevent and treat complications
Prevent and treat exacerbations
Reduce mortality

minimize unnecessary fear or anxiety, optimize strategies to improve the patient's functional abilities, and improve compliance. The main components of management in the GOLD guidelines are (1) assessing and monitoring disease, (2) reducing risk factors, (3) managing stable COPD, and (4) managing exacerbations.[1]

Smoking cessation is the most important and most effective intervention in COPD (see Chapter 85, Tobacco Use & Dependence, for more information). Successful cessation can reduce the risk of development and progression of this disease. One benefit of smoking cessation is the eventual return to an annual FEV_1 decline similar to a nonsmoker (see Fig. 24-1). Unfortunately, successful long-term smoking cessation is difficult to achieve.[1,16]

Immunizations provide protection against serious illness and death in COPD patients. The efficacy, benefit, and cost-effectiveness of vaccination against influenza among this population are significant. Data concerning the value of vaccinating against pneumococcal pneumonia is lacking, but it is recommended in the GOLD guidelines because of a favorable risk-to-benefit ratio.

The role of pulmonary rehabilitation in the management of COPD is well established. The most successful programs are interdisciplinary and designed to improve overall functional status and quality of life.[32] Common components of rehabilitation programs are listed in Table 24-6. Exercise training usually involves walking and stair-climbing exercises. Slow diaphragmatic breathing through pursed lips relieves symptoms of dyspnea and slows the respiratory rate. Resistance devices designed to improve diaphragmatic strength and endurance can reduce respiratory failure. Adequate nutrition should be maintained because high-energy requirements may be required to support the work of breathing.[33]

Efforts to optimize functional ability should be directed at maintaining quality of life and addressing specific psychosocial needs. Exercise training programs can increase oxygen utilization and overall cardiopulmonary conditioning. Exercise training should be initiated carefully with an understanding of the patient's limitations. Specifically, upper extremity exercise training can improve function and reduce dyspnea. Results from respiratory muscle training have not shown significant benefit from this activity. The patient's nutritional status should be assessed and addressed if significant nutritional deficiencies are determined. Finally, patients might benefit from biofeedback, relaxation therapy, and individual or group therapy if psychosocial stresses or other chronic diseases are interfering with their pulmonary functional capacity.

Patients with chronic obstructive airways disease can be taught proper coughing techniques, postural drainage, and chest percussion to mobilize thickened mucous secretions.

Table 24-6 Components of Pulmonary Rehabilitation Programs[1]

Patient and family education
Patient support groups
Smoking cessation strategies
Exercise programs
Breathing training and respiratory muscle conditioning
Oxygen therapy if indicated

Although adequate fluid intake generally is considered helpful in promoting health, aggressive hydration or nebulized humidification is not indicated except in acutely decompensated patients. Similarly, expectorants such as guaifenesin and iodide, which are purported to thin airway secretions, offer little clinical value.[1,34,35] The use of postural drainage and chest percussion traditionally has been included in comprehensive care regimens, but provide minimal benefit for most patients.

Pharmacotherapy

None of the currently available medications used to treat COPD alter the natural course of this condition; therefore, the primary objectives of pharmacotherapy are the relief of symptoms and minimization of airflow obstruction.[1] Bronchodilators are central in the management of COPD. These agents improve airflow by reducing bronchial airway smooth muscle tone. As a result, patients are able to exhale more fully, at rest and with exercise, thereby reducing hyperinflation.

Because of the potential for limited benefit from pharmacotherapy, a specific set of desired goals must be defined for each individual patient before therapy is initiated. Based on the nature of the disease, the initial outcomes should be realistic and developed jointly by the caregiver and the patient. If the first goals are achieved, new targets can be set.

When therapies are initiated or changed, a minimal trial period of several weeks to a few months must be used to determine their full benefit. Single-dose challenges and frequent alterations in therapy do not allow adequate assessment and can be confusing to the patient.

Evaluating the benefit of pharmacotherapy for an individual patient or a population of patients can be problematic. There is no consensus on the most appropriate outcome measure or the degree of improvement that is clinically significant. In addition, there is controversy about the irreversible nature of COPD obstruction and the appropriate method of evaluating spirometric improvement.[36]

Although the standard for assessing benefit from treatment has been a spirometric improvement in FEV_1, many patients will not demonstrate noticeable changes following either acute dosing with a β_2-agonist or a therapeutic trial of any therapy. Increasingly, clinicians are considering other measures to determine the benefit of therapy. These include improvements in quality of life, dyspnea, and exercise tolerance.[36] Other appropriate measures are COPD exacerbation rates, utilization of health care resources, and mortality. For this disease, it appears appropriate to consider numerous outcomes.

Bronchodilators

There is no clear evidence for benefit of one bronchodilator over another in the chronic management of COPD. Inhalation therapy is generally preferred over oral agents including theophylline. A short-acting, inhaled β_2-agonist or an anticholinergic (ipratropium) are rational first line treatments. Treatment should be given as needed or on a schedule depending on the frequency of symptoms.[1] In COPD, the spirometric response is often variable. The gold standard for significant improvement in FEV_1 of 12% to 15% may or may not be achieved. However, patients often feel better subjectively without evidence of objective improvement. This can be attributed to the fact that treatment facilitates emptying of the lungs and reduces thoracic overinflation at rest and during exercise.

The choice for treatment should be individualized based on cost, convenience, and individual patient response. Primary choices for inhalation include short-acting β_2-agonists, anticholinergics, or long-acting β_2-agonists (Fig. 24-4 shows a suggested treatment algorithm).

It is not unusual to find reports in the literature that suggest superiority of one bronchodilator class over another for COPD treatment. However, as is exemplified in the cases, it is difficult to predict individual responses to treatment. For some patients, β_2-agonist bronchodilators will increase airflow, improve pulmonary function test results, and reduce symptoms of dyspnea.[37] Others may achieve greater improvement with an anticholinergic compared with a β_2-agonist.[38,39] Still others do not have a reversible component with either drug, but still may perceive symptomatic benefit.[40,41] Because single-dose trials of inhaled bronchodilators are usually inadequate in predicting long-term response to bronchodilator therapy, a 1- to 2-week course of therapy should be administered before evaluating the response.[37,38,42]

In recent years, the benefit of inhaled, long-acting inhaled β_2-agonists for chronic treatment of COPD has become evident. These agents relieve symptoms as well as improve exercise tolerance and health status. For patients who require regular treatment with short-acting agents, these medications improve convenience for the patient and are used clinically with increasing frequency.

Similarly, the benefit of theophylline has been long debated.[43–45] It was once assumed that theophylline was only a bronchodilator and that failure to document a good bronchodilator response indicated drug failure. It has been postulated that other mechanisms of theophylline (e.g., stimulation of diaphragm contractility and anti-inflammatory effects) may contribute to a favorable patient response in the absence of changes in pulmonary function. Further, although no objective benefit may be evident, patients with severe COPD may report a deterioration of symptoms when theophylline is withdrawn.[45] Nonetheless, theophylline is reserved for patients who do not tolerate or fail to respond to inhaled bronchodilator therapies.

Anti-Inflammatory Therapies
Treatment of COPD with systemic corticosteroid therapy has been controversial and disappointing.[46–49] Historically, it has been evident that only 10% to 30% of patients benefit from short- and long-term anti-inflammatory therapy, and there is no reliable method to determine patients who might benefit. The risk for side effects and toxicities is substantial, and chronic systemic corticosteroid therapy is not recommended. Currently, systemic corticosteroid therapy is only indicated for short-term use during moderate to severe exacerbations of COPD.

Using the inhaled route minimizes many of the risks of long-term systemic corticosteroid therapy. Several national and international studies have been conducted to evaluate the benefit from chronic inhaled corticosteroid therapy.[50–53] Results from these trials have been disappointing in that treatment with inhaled corticosteroids had no significant effect on the progressive decline in lung function. As a result, current guidelines recommend that inhaled corticosteroids only be considered in symptomatic patients with $FEV_1 \leq 50\%$ predicted and repeated exacerbations requiring antimicrobial therapy or oral corticosteroids.[1] There is no established role for cromolyn or the leukotriene modifying drugs in the management of COPD.

Antimicrobial Therapy
Patients with COPD are chronically infected with bacteria. Acute exacerbations of COPD are infectious in approximately 50% of cases. Infectious etiologies include viruses and Gram-positive (e.g., *Streptococcus pneumoniae*) and Gram-negative bacteria (e.g., *Haemophilus influenzae*). Although the sputum of patients with COPD is often chronically colonized with bacteria, there is no evidence that prophylactic antibiotics provide any benefit. Antibiotics should be given only when an infection is documented by a predominance of a single organism on Gram's stain or culture and/or by radiologic evidence of pneumonia.[54,55]

Correcting the secondary physiologic changes of COPD includes paying attention to hypoxemia and hypercapnia and treating and managing pulmonary hypertension and cor pulmonale. The effectiveness of long-term, continuous oxygen therapy is well documented in patients who are chronically hypoxemic, with the goal of supplemental oxygen therapy being to maintain an oxygen saturation of >90%.[56–59] Chronic carbon dioxide retention (hypercapnia) may be related to reduced central drive as a result of respiratory muscle fatigue. Management for hypercapnia is directed at reducing the work of breathing by decreasing secretions, treating bronchoconstriction, and maintaining acid-base balance. Managing secondary complications of pulmonary hypertension and right-sided heart failure is difficult. Vasodilator therapy has been ineffective in treating this problem.[60]

For patients with α_1-antitrypsin-associated emphysema, plasma derived α_1-antitrypsin products are available. Patients receive weekly intravenous infusions of α_1-antitrypsin to maintain acceptable antiprotease activity and minimize the progression of lung disease. This therapy is very expensive, not well tolerated by some patients (fever, chills, allergic reactions, flu-like symptoms), and has been hampered by supply problems. Recently, two new products received FDA approval so the supply problems may be improved with the availability of three different products (Aralast, Prolastin, and Zemaira). Because the α_1-antitrypsin products are derived from pooled human plasma, there may be an increased risk for the transmission of infectious diseases (e.g., viral infections and Creutzfeldt-Jakob disease).

Acute Exacerbations

Many COPD patients experience two to four acute exacerbations annually.[61] An exacerbation is an acute worsening in health including respiratory status. Characteristics of exacerbations include increased dyspnea, cough, and sputum production. Depending on the severity of symptoms and the baseline condition of the patient, exacerbations can be managed in the ambulatory setting or may require hospitalization. For patients requiring hospitalization, the mortality rate is significant. The primary strategies for managing acute exacerbations of COPD include supplemental oxygen if indicated, intensification of combination inhaled bronchodilator regimens, short courses of systemic corticosteroids and antimicrobial therapy.

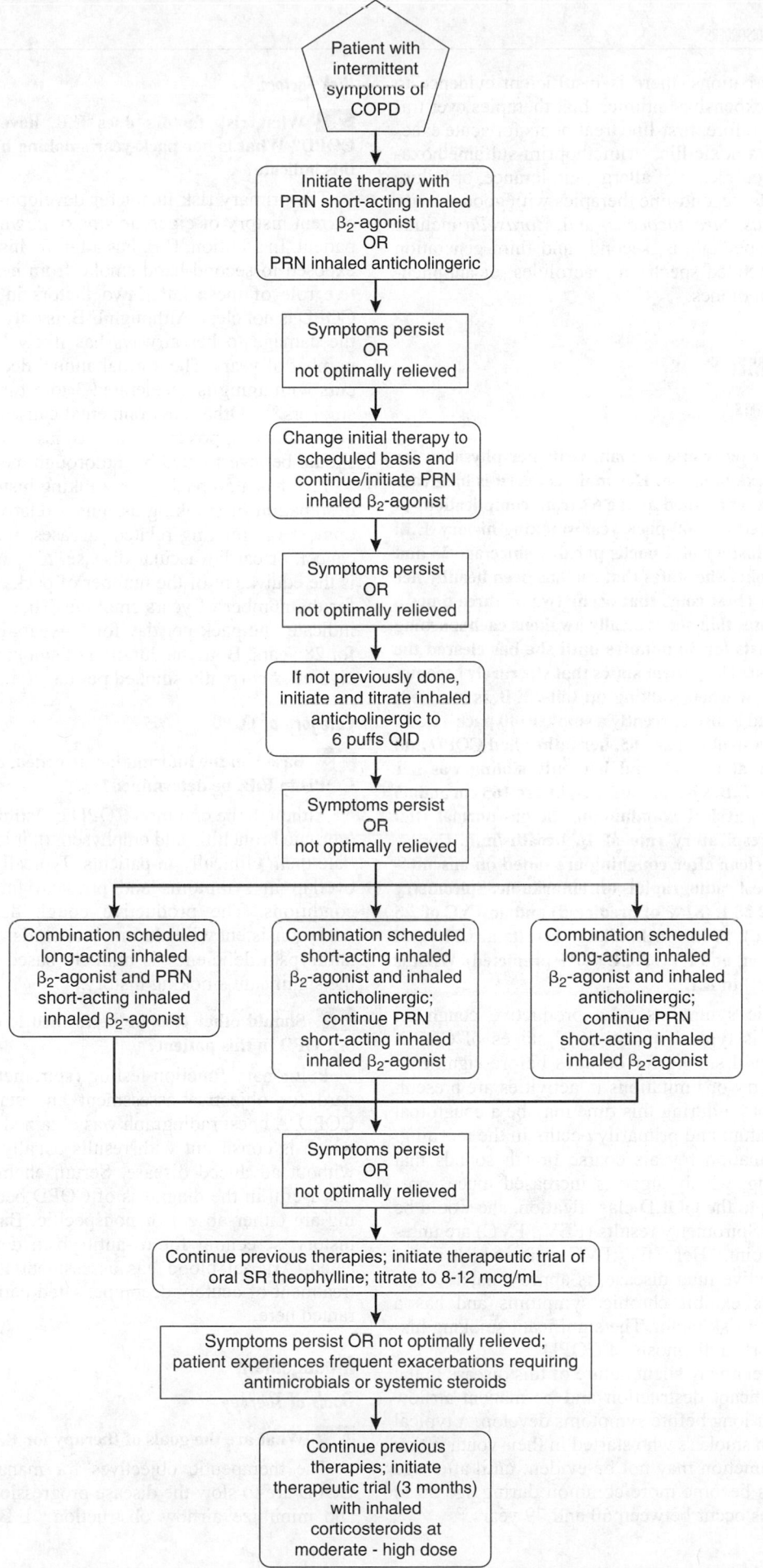

FIGURE 24-4 Approach to pharmacotherapeutic management of chronic obstructive pulmonary disease.

For acute exacerbations, there is insufficient evidence to favor newer, more expensive antimicrobial therapies over traditional agents. Therefore, first-line treatments for acute exacerbations include amoxicillin, trimethoprim-sulfamethoxazole, or doxycycline. In case of allergy, intolerance, or failure with first-line agents, second-line therapies with good activity against *Haemophilus, Streptococcus,* and *Moraxella* include β-lactamase stable penicillins, second- and third-generation cephalosporins, extended spectrum macrolides, or antipneumococcal fluoroquinolones.

CLINICAL ASSESSMENT

Signs and Symptoms

1. E.B., a 51-year-old white woman, visits her physician for an annual physical examination. Her main concern is lung cancer. E.B.'s brother recently died at age 67 from complications of lung cancer attributed to a 60-pack year smoking history. E.B. also has a smoking history of 2 packs per day since age 23 and she continues to smoke. She states that she has been healthy her entire life except for chest colds that occur two or three times a year. She also indicates that she typically awakens each morning with a cough that lasts for 30 minutes until she has cleared the mucus from her chest. The patient states that she rarely becomes short of breath except when walking up hills. E.B. is married; her husband is 59 and is also currently a smoker (40 pack-years). Her mother died of a stroke at age 65, her father had COPD and died of lung cancer at age 62, and her only sibling was her brother noted above. E.B.'s height and weight are 165 cm and 65 kg, respectively. On physical examination, she has normal vital signs, including a respiratory rate of 16 breaths/min. Coarse breath sounds that clear after coughing are noted on auscultation of her chest. Chest radiograph is unremarkable. Spirometry reveals an FEV_1 of 2.28 L (81% of predicted) and an FVC of 2.8 L (85% of predicted). Postbronchodilator results are FEV_1 of 2.44 L (87% predicted) and FVC 3.0 L (90% predicted). What is the evidence of COPD in E.H.?

E.B. has chronic symptoms of a productive cough on awakening, which is typical of the early stages of COPD. Many individuals will smoke for decades before significant changes in spirometry or limitations in activities are present. The principal symptom during this time may be a cough that is productive of sputum and primarily occurs in the morning.

Her lung examination reveals coarse breath sounds that clear after coughing, which suggests increased mucus production. According to the GOLD classification, she would be category 0: at risk. Spirometry results (FEV_1, FVC) are unremarkable at this point.[1] Her FEV_1:FVC ratio, which is the hallmark of obstructive lung disease, is approximately 81%. However, she does exhibit chronic symptoms and has a known exposure to a risk factor. The significant smoking history strongly supports a diagnosis of COPD.

Because of the relatively silent nature of this disease in the early phases, significant destruction and permanent airflow limitation can occur long before symptoms develop. A typical course for COPD in smokers who started in their youth is that a decline in lung function may not be evident until after age 40, hospitalizations become more common during age 50 to 69 years, and deaths occur between 60 and 79 years.[62]

Risk Factors

2. What risk factors does E.B. have for development of COPD? What is her pack-year smoking history, and what does this indicate?

The primary risk factor for developing COPD is a past or current history of cigarette smoking, which is present in this patient. In addition, E.B. has a family history of COPD and is exposed to second-hand smoke from her husband. The relative role of these latter two factors in the development of COPD is not clear. Although E.B. is only mildly symptomatic, the damage to her airways has likely been occurring for a number of years. The normal annual decline in FEV_1 that occurs with aging is accelerated 3 to 5 times in some cigarette smokers.[63,64] Other environmental causes of COPD, including occupational exposure to various dusts, toxins, and chemicals, should be investigated by a thorough medical history.

E.B. has a 56 pack-year smoking history. The "pack-year" designation of smoking assigns a relative risk for the development of smoking related diseases, including COPD, lung cancer, or cardiovascular disease. A "pack-year" of smoking is the equivalent of the number of packs of cigarettes per day for the number of years smoking. Thus, 56 pack years could indicate one pack per day for 56 years or two packs per day for 28 years. Both the duration of smoking and the number of cigarettes currently smoked per day are determinants of risk.

Category of COPD

3. Based on the information provided, can the precise type of COPD in E.B. be determined?

Although the common COPD constituents are well defined (chronic bronchitis and emphysema), it is difficult to differentiate them clinically in patients. Typically, there is significant overlap in symptoms and physical findings between both conditions. The productive cough described by E.B. is more consistent with chronic bronchitis. The possibility of α_1-antitrypsin deficiency is unlikely based on age of onset and the significant smoking history.

4. Should other tests be performed to confirm the diagnosis of COPD in this patient?

Pulmonary function testing (spirometry) is the gold standard for objective assessment and staging of severity of COPD. A chest radiograph was obtained but is unremarkable, which is consistent with results usually received in patients without advanced disease. Serum chemistries are generally not useful in the diagnosis of COPD because abnormal finding are either absent or nonspecific. Based on this patient's history, screening for α_1-antitrypsin deficiency is not indicated. Arterial blood gas assessment is helpful in guiding treatment of acutely decompensated patients, but is not warranted here.

Management

Goals of Therapy

5. What are the goals of therapy for E.B.?

The therapeutic objectives for managing a patient with COPD are to slow the disease progression, relieve symptoms, and minimize airflow obstruction.[1] E.B. demonstrates mild symptoms with exertion. She should be educated about COPD and its causes. Education should include information about the disease process, risk factors, and strategies to slow the progressive loss of lung function. At this point, the primary objective would be to reduce risk factors to minimize disease progression. The clinician and patient should set goals jointly.

Smoking Cessation

6. What interventions are the most important for E.B. at this time?

In addition to the education, E.B's interest and willingness in smoking cessation should be determined. Smoking cessation is the primary initial intervention in the management of COPD.[2,17] It is the only intervention with a beneficial effect on affecting the natural progression of disease and it is very cost effective.

The Agency for Health Care Policy and Research (AHCPR) has published clinical practice guidelines to assist health professionals in initiating smoking cessation programs.[65] Several resources have been published to assist health professionals in applying the guidelines and other smoking cessation techniques for their patients.[66–68]

The principles of smoking cessation are addressed in greater detail in Chapter 85, Tobacco Use and Dependence. E.B. has presented to her physician today because of concerns about smoking related diseases, so she may be receptive to smoking cessation strategies, which should include pharmacotherapy (nicotine replacement therapy and/or bupropion) for most patients in combination with behavioral counseling.[65]

Immunization

7. Should other preventive measures be considered for E.B at this time?

In addition to smoking cessation, E.B.'s immunization status should be evaluated. According to the GOLD guidelines and in the absence of contraindications, E.B. is a candidate for vaccination against influenza and pneumococcal pneumonia, even though she is in the early stages of COPD. Patients with COPD are at risk for increased morbidity and mortality if they develop either of these infectious complications.

Epidemics caused by the influenza virus result in >20,000 deaths annually. Individuals at greatest risk for significant morbidity and mortality from influenza pneumonia are those with chronic disease, including lung disease. Optimally, the influenza vaccine should be administered between October and January. This allows an adequate antibody response before the peak influenza season, which typically occurs within the first quarter of the year.

Therefore, protection against influenza virus is recommended annually. Annual vaccination against influenza is effective in reducing morbidity and mortality from influenza. E.B. also meets the age-related criterion for influenza vaccine, which was recently lowered to 50 years. Annual immunization is required to ensure adequate antibody protection against influenza virus. The influenza vaccine is administered intramuscularly; the new nasal inhalation product is not recommended for patients with COPD.

Pneumococcal polysaccharide vaccine (Pneumovax 23) is also recommended for patients with COPD.[69] This vaccine consists of antigen that provides protection against 23 common strains of *Streptococcus pneumoniae*. Candidates for this vaccine include individuals at risk for significant morbidity and mortality if they develop a pneumococcal infection, including patients with chronic lung disease. Data concerning efficacy of the vaccine in this population are lacking, but the GOLD and ATS guidelines recommend its use based on expert opinion and a favorable risk-benefit ratio. Pneumococcal polysaccharide vaccine is recommended to be administered subcutaneously or intramuscularly as a one time dose. In some cases, patients require a second dose after 5 years, commonly when the initial dose was administered before age 65.

Pneumococcal polysaccharide vaccine used for this purpose should be differentiated from the conjugated, 7-valent pneumococcal vaccine (Prevnar) that is used as a primary immunizing series for infants to provide protection against invasive pneumococcal disease. In addition, E.B.'s immunization status against tetanus should be determined. If she has not had tetanus prophylaxis in the past decade, she should be administered an adult diphtheria-tetanus booster.

Pharmacotherapy

8. What pharmacotherapy recommendations should be considered for E.B. at this point?

E.B. is experiencing early signs of COPD. Her productive cough in the morning indicates mucus hypersecretion and she is experiencing occasional shortness of breath with exertion. Among currently available medications, no therapy has been demonstrated to modify the progressive decline in lung function that is characteristic in COPD. Bronchodilators are the primary pharmacologic therapy used in the management of COPD. Although much of the airflow obstruction is fixed, many patients exhibit some reversibility. Others report subjective improvement, even if objective benefit, such as changes in pulmonary function tests, is not evident. Available bronchodilator therapies include β_2-agonists, anticholinergics, and methylxanthines (theophylline). Choices about product selection should be based on clinical experience and the specific patient situation. For initial treatment, the most common choices would be a short-acting, inhaled β_2-agonist, (e.g., albuterol) or an inhaled anticholinergic (e.g., ipratropium). Either of these therapies has a relatively short onset of action and is effective in relieving symptoms.

β_2-Agonists

β_2-Agonists produce bronchodilation by relaxing bronchial smooth muscle through activation of cyclic adenosine monophosphate (cAMP).[70] They are more effective in relieving obstruction in patients with asthma than in those with COPD, primarily because of the unpredictable reversible component of COPD. The inhalation route of delivery for bronchodilators is recommended over oral therapy based on safety and efficacy. The dose response curve among all available bronchodilators is relatively flat and similar.[1] There is no evidence that one agent is superior to another.

Albuterol is the most frequently used agent in this class. It is available as a metered dose inhaler (MDI) 90 µg/inhalation and a solution for nebulization (2.5 mg/0.5 mL). The onset of action of short-acting β_2-agonists (e.g., albuterol, pirbuterol) is rapid (within 5 minutes) and generally reaches maximal effect in 15 to 30 minutes. The duration of action is approximately 4 hours. While inhaled β_2-agonists are usually well tolerated, some patients experience adverse effects (tremors, tachycardia, or nervousness) with even low dosages. Although concern has been expressed about the safety of short-acting, inhaled β_2-agonists in patients with cardiac disease, a cohort study using the Saskatchewan Health Services database concluded that there was no increased risk for fatal or nonfatal myocardial infarction in patients using these agents.[71]

Anticholinergics

The parasympathetic (cholinergic) nervous system plays a primary role in the control of bronchomotor tone in COPD.[38,72] By inhibiting cyclic guanosine monophosphate (cGMP) in the lung, aerosolized anticholinergic drugs are effective bronchodilators. The bronchodilation produced by anticholinergics in patients with stable COPD is equal or superior to that achieved by inhaled β_2-agonists.[73–75]

Ipratropium bromide is the primary anticholinergic agent used in COPD.[1] It is marketed as both an MDI (18 μg ipratropium per puff) and as a solution for nebulization (0.5 mg ipratropium/2.5 mL). Anticholinergics have an average onset of effect within 15 minutes, with a maximum bronchodilator effect in 60 to 90 minutes, although some patients may experience more rapid symptom relief. The duration of action is 6 hours. Although some reports suggest a quicker onset of action, patients should be advised that the relief of acute symptoms will be slower compared to an inhaled β_2-agonist. A typical starting dose of ipratropium is 2 inhalations TID to QID. Based on clinical response and tolerance of side effects, the number of inhalations can be increased up to as much as 6 inhalations 4 times a day. Although well tolerated, some patients experience dry mouth, nausea, and blurred vision.

Ipratropium's anticholinergic actions are localized predominantly in the lungs, with an apparent specificity of action in the larger airways. Because it has minimal effects on sputum viscosity, there is little problem with drying of airway secretions. In addition, ipratropium's structure as a quaternary amine increases its polarity, thereby minimizing absorption from the lung and systemic side effects. These structural properties also reduce penetration across the blood-brain barrier, reducing the incidence of confusion and other CNS side effects.

Other anticholinergics that have been used clinically include atropine sulfate and glycopyrrolate. Although atropine was the first anticholinergic agent used, its benefit is limited by side effects and toxicity primarily related to its systemic absorption and, in some patients, excellent CNS penetration.[76] Atropine can produce excessive salivary drying and, at higher dosages, can cause significant CNS symptoms, including hallucinations and seizures. Glycopyrrolate, like ipratropium, is a polar anticholinergic compound, but it is not approved by the FDA for treating COPD. Its primary use is preoperatively and before diagnostic procedures to reduce secretions in the respiratory and gastrointestinal tract. The injectable form has been nebulized successfully and found to be an effective bronchodilator. However, with the availability of ipratropium in a MDI and as a solution for nebulization, there is little indication for using these other anticholinergics. With the antici-

pated FDA approval of tiotropium (Spiriva) (see Question 15) in the near future, there will be another option to patients with COPD. This long-acting anticholinergic bronchodilators has the convenience of once daily dosing.

9. Which bronchodilator therapy should be initiated in E.B.?

Trials comparing anticholinergics and β_2-agonists in patients with COPD suggest similar maximal bronchodilator efficacy in terms of relief of symptoms and improvements in lung function.[73–75,77] However, studies are often difficult to compare because some investigators exclude β_2-agonist responders before conducting their studies. Both inhaled short-acting β_2-agonists and ipratropium are well tolerated. The benefit from bronchodilator therapy may be due to improved lung emptying during expiration, which reduces hyperinflation.[78] According to the GOLD guidelines, there is no clear choice between the two bronchodilators and the decision is left to the judgment of the clinician and the clinical situation.[1]

Because of tremendous intersubject variability and even day-to-day variability within the same subject (intrasubject variability), a trial of both anticholinergics and β_2-agonists are warranted in patients with COPD. It may be helpful to obtain single-dose challenge predrug and postdrug pulmonary function tests with both drugs to aid in identifying potential drug responders, but it is more appropriate to give at least a 2-week trial of one drug or the other to look for trends in either subjective symptomatic improvement and/or morning pulmonary function. If a partial response is obtained, but the patient's goals have not been achieved, the dosage can be increased (e.g., doubled) with another assessment in 2 to 4 weeks. If no response is seen to the original two-puff regimen (or 0.5 mL nebulized), one can either try a higher dosage to see if this will elicit a benefit, or it may be decided to abandon the drug and start over with another agent such as a long-acting β_2-agonist.

Based on the frequency of E.B.'s symptoms, it is reasonable to initiate therapy with an inhaled short-acting β_2-agonist (e.g., albuterol). The most convenient form would be a metered dose inhaler. She should be instructed about the proper technique and observed using the inhaler to ensure that she benefits from this medication. The advantage of a β_2-agonist compared to the anticholinergic in this patient is a more rapid onset of action for relief of acute symptoms.

As-Needed Versus Scheduled Use

10. Should E.B. be instructed to use the β_2-agonist "as needed" or on a scheduled basis?

According to the GOLD guidelines, bronchodilator therapy can be used either as needed or on a regular schedule depending on the frequency of symptoms. There is no evidence to suggest that one strategy is superior to the other. Bronchodilator therapy does not affect the progressive decline in lung function from COPD. Albuterol has a rapid onset of action (<5 minutes), so relief of symptoms is generally prompt, even with as needed use.

There is no evidence that prolonged, regularly scheduled β_2-agonist therapy leads to exacerbations, as has been reported in asthma.[79] However, some reports suggest that regular use of β_2-agonists in patients with asthma, as well as in those with COPD, may be associated with a paradoxical increased rate of decline in lung function. One study compared regularly scheduled albuterol or ipratropium versus "on-demand" use of each.[80] The results showed that scheduled use of either bronchodilator drug was associated with a more rapid decline in FEV_1 versus on-demand use. However, changes in quality of life were not detected despite the spirometric decline. The authors concluded that effective bronchodilation might mask an ongoing decline in lung function of COPD, but that disease progression occurred because the inflammatory component of the disease was not treated. Interestingly, on follow-up over 4 years, the differences between regular and as-needed bronchodilator therapy disappeared.[81]

In another comparison, regular use of albuterol did not result in any physiologic or clinical benefit compared to as needed use in patients with COPD who were using regularly scheduled ipratropium and inhaled beclomethasone.[82] In this crossover study, subjects used almost twice as much albuterol during the regularly scheduled dosing phase compared to the as needed phase (13 puffs/day versus 7 puffs/day) without any additional benefit. Conversely, a systematic review was performed using the Cochrane Collaboration database to assess the benefit of regular use of a short-acting inhaled β_2-agonist in patients with stable COPD.[83] Small but significant improvements in lung function were noted and dyspnea was reduced. Patient preference for the active treatment was nine times higher than with placebo.

The international guidelines suggest that therapy should be prescribed as needed or on a schedule depending on the clinical situation. Another advantage to using a β_2-agonist as needed is to quantify the number of acute symptoms the patient is experiencing and/or to identify emerging patterns in disease control.

Ipratropium can also be used on an as needed basis according to the GOLD guidelines. Although the onset of effect is much slower (within 15 minutes), when compared to β_2-agonists, some patients report symptom relief faster than expected. Nonetheless, if ipratropium is prescribed as needed, patients should be advised that there might be a delay in onset of effect compared to albuterol. Several years ago, there was hope that regular use of ipratropium early in COPD would have beneficial effects on the natural course of the disease. The potential benefit of early treatment with ipratropium was evaluated in the Lung Health Study.[16] However, the addition of ipratropium used on a scheduled basis had no effect on the decline in FEV_1, thus disease progression was not altered. A slight increase in FEV_1 was observed in the first year (about 30 mL) and maintained throughout the study, but this improvement was lost when the drug was stopped after 5 years of therapy. Adherence to inhaled medication, as measured by canister weight and self-report was approximately 50%. There was no evidence of tachyphylaxis to the bronchodilating effect of ipratropium, and dry mouth was the most frequent mild side effect. Serious adverse events (cardiac symptoms, hypertension, skin rashes, and urinary retention) were reported in 1.2% of patients using ipratropium and 0.8% of patients using placebo.

Based on the frequency of her symptoms, E.B. should be instructed to use her β_2-agonist as needed for symptoms at this time. If she reports regular and frequent need for this therapy based on her symptoms, this decision can be reassessed. E.B.

also should be asked to demonstrate her inhaler technique periodically as these skills may deteriorate over time and patients with COPD may have comorbidities or physical or cognitive problems that could limit their ability to use the MDI effectively. With disease progression, she will likely needed to be converted to a scheduled regimen with this or a different drug.

Treatment of Symptomatic COPD

11. E.B. was referred to a smoking cessation program and achieved temporary success with the use of bupropion. However, after 8 months, she resumed smoking one pack per day. Her husband did not achieve a successful cessation attempt. Eight years later she returns to the physician with complaints of a chronic productive cough and increasing shortness of breath, especially with exertion. She indicates that she is not able to walk up a flight of stairs without dyspnea and that her symptoms interfere with her ability to work around the house. She continued to receive albuterol from another physician and states that she now uses this medication three or four times most days.

Her lung examination reveals scattered rhonchi throughout both lung fields and diffuse wheezing. A chest radiograph shows a slightly enlarged cardiac shadow and thickened bronchial walls. Spirometry yields an FEV_1 of 1.5 L (60% of predicted) and FVC of 2.2 L (73% of predicted). Repeat spirometry after albuterol results in an FEV_1 of 1.6 L (64%) and FVC of 2.3 L (77%). A sputum gram stain reveals numerous PMNs and mixed bacterial flora. What factors have contributed to worsening of her COPD?

COPD is characterized by a progressive decline in lung function. E.B. has continued exposure to risk factors that contributed to the development and worsening of her COPD. Relapse after quitting smoking is common. Success rates drop significantly over time, and most studies report much lower rates for successful cessation at 1 year compared with 3 months. For E.B., tobacco use has resulted in continued decline in her pulmonary function and presentation with significant disease. Continual efforts should be made toward successful smoking cessation since the advantages are still evident in patients with advanced disease.

Her complaints of cough, purulent sputum production, SOB, and decreased exercise tolerance, along with the physical examination and laboratory findings, are consistent with chronic bronchitis. The increased mucus production in the airways is an excellent medium for bacterial growth. Patients with chronic bronchitis typically are colonized with organisms such as *S. pneumoniae* and *H. influenzae*. Exacerbations are characterized by an increase in these organisms or by other bacteria. However, at this time, E.B. shows no signs of active infection. The sputum color is unchanged, and the Gram stain is consistent with normal flora.

E.B. has evidence of cardiac effects exhibited by an enlarged heart on chest radiographic examination. This can be explained by persistent hypoxemia, which results in vasoconstriction of pulmonary vessels, causing pulmonary hypertension. Subsequently, the right ventricle of the heart has to work harder to pump against this higher pressure gradient. Therefore, the chamber dilates and the heart muscle hypertrophies. The end result is cor pulmonale, defined as right-sided heart failure secondary to pulmonary hypertension and lung disease.

Interpreting Pulmonary Function Tests

12. **How do you interpret E.B.'s current pulmonary function tests? What degree of reversibility does she demonstrate after albuterol use? Is this considered a significant bronchodilator response?**

Previously this patient's spirometry showed an FEV_1 of 2.28 L (81% of predicted) and an FVC of 2.8 L (85% of predicted). The FEV_1:FVC ratio was 81%. These spirometry results were normal. Today, the baseline FEV_1 has declined to 1.5 L. This is 60% of the predicted normal (2.5 L) based on gender, age, and height and indicates moderate disease.[1] If this were a patient with asthma, an emergency department (ED) visit or hospitalization would be considered. However, obstruction of this degree is not unexpected in patients with COPD. Rather than react to the absolute value, it is helpful to consider the overall picture of no sudden change in symptoms and no evidence of infection. Thus, it can be concluded that E.B.'s disease has significantly progressed and a change in therapy is appropriate.

The FVC has also declined as well, but proportionally less than the FEV_1. This illustrates that patients with COPD may have impaired outflow during the early part of forced expiration because of mucous plugging and partial airway collapse, but over several seconds, they can achieve a near complete exhalation. The FEV_1 is typically affected to a greater degree than the FVC, which may still be reduced due to some air trapping. The FEV_1:FVC ratio today is 68%, another indicator of progression to moderate obstruction.

In traditional bronchodilator testing, reversibility of airflow obstruction is assessed by the change in FEV_1 after albuterol administration. Generally, the change in FVC is not considered. In E.B., the post-albuterol FEV_1 rose to 1.6 L or 64% of her predicted value. This is still indicative of significantly impaired airflow. It is also helpful to calculate the percent change in FEV_1 after the bronchodilator, using the following formula:

$$(FEV_1 \text{ postbronchodilator} - FEV_1 \text{ prebronchodilator}/ FEV_1 \text{ prebronchodilator}) \times 100$$

For E.B., the degree of improvement is (1.6 − 1.5 L)/1.5 L, or 6.7%. It is not accurate to calculate the change by simply subtracting the two values for percent of normal (60% to 64%). The definition of reversible airflow obstruction is usually an improvement in FEV_1 of at least 15%. The assumption here may be that E.B. has fixed, or irreversible airflow obstruction which is consistent with COPD. However, there are other factors to consider in spirometry testing for COPD.

Because patients with COPD often have low baseline FEV_1 results, a relatively large percentage improvement can be achieved with a minimal absolute increase in FEV_1. Because of this, some clinicians also utilize an absolute increase in FEV_1 of at least 200 mL to define significant reversibility in COPD.

Another consideration is the method used to assess reversibility. Traditionally, this evaluation involves baseline spirometry followed by repeat spirometry after administration of an inhaled, short-acting β_2-agonist. This is complicated in COPD because the disease is often defined by the lack of significant reversibility. Additionally, an increasing proportion of patients will demonstrate reversibility with repeated testing.[36] It is also appropriate to use both ipratropium and albuterol in combination in reversibility testing in COPD based on our knowledge of the variable response to these two agents.[84] Alternative methods of evaluating reversibility include 2-week trials of various therapies. Finally, other clinical outcome measures may be more appropriate in evaluating the benefit of therapies for COPD.[36]

For example, if the patient reported a reduction in breathlessness, it might be considered clinically relevant. Other factors to consider are day-to-day and within-day variation in baseline pulmonary function (e.g., morning versus nighttime and as symptoms wax and wane), and also in the degree of reversibility.

In summary, decisions about the appropriateness of using bronchodilators have traditionally been based on an improvement in the FEV_1 of at least 15% after an inhaled bronchodilator. Although this testing typically is performed with an inhaled β_2-agonist, reversibility following an inhaled anticholinergic agent or a combination of bronchodilators could also be assessed. Several studies have suggested that an assessment based on a single-dose challenge with either agent is not adequate. Several studies have reported a poor correlation between pulmonary function and the patient's overall quality of life, suggesting that parameters other than spirometry may be important to assess.[36]

Spirometry Goals of Treatment

13. **Based on this medical history, what goal should be set for E.B. related to spirometry?**

COPD is characterized by airflow limitation. E.B. will never be able to achieve her predicted normal FEV_1 value. She has progressive, fixed disease that will not reverse. The goal is to slow the rate of further loss and to identify her probable baseline function value to use as a target. It is also anticipated that with time she will experience acute exacerbations, during which time her FEV_1 could drop precipitously to <1.0 L. At those times, she may show more reversibility, but never to a value greater than her personal best.

Pre- and Post-Bronchodilator Testing

14. **For future evaluations, should E.B. perform pre- and post-spirometry testing?**

In COPD, pre- and post-bronchodilator testing is not performed routinely. It is useful in the initial assessment of the disease, especially to rule out asthma. However, the nature of COPD is chronic airflow limitation that does not change significantly over time.

The pre-bronchodilator pulmonary function provides an indication of the underlying airway obstruction and disease severity. The post-albuterol results identify the degree of reversibility (but the previously discussed limitations of a single test result should be considered). After an intervention is made (e.g., addition of a new drug therapy), it takes time for the underlying disease process to be modified, especially for inflammatory changes to improve. Decisions about the need for post-bronchodilator spirometry testing should be made on an individual basis depending on the clinical situation and the potential value of the information.

Additional Bronchodilator Options

15. The physician indicates that he plans to add a new agent to E.B.'s regimen and to continue the albuterol as needed. What changes should be recommended to E.B.'s drug therapy regimen?

E.B. was initially prescribed albuterol on an as needed basis. Because of her disease progression and increased frequency of symptoms, she has used this medication regularly. A change in her regimen is warranted at this point. In COPD, use of combinations of bronchodilators is a common strategy. Combining medications with different mechanisms of action offers the potential benefit of additive or synergistic improvements. In clinical practice, the use of combination bronchodilator therapy generally results in improvements in clinical symptoms and spirometry that are superior to single agents; however, these incremental improvements are usually less than additive. Further, it is not clear whether the same benefit would be achieved if the dose of the single agent were increased. Another benefit of combination therapy is the ability to use submaximal doses of each agent and avoid common side effects.[85] The combination of various bronchodilators provides additional benefit in improving lung function and health status.

E.B. was initially given albuterol. A common approach would be to add an anticholinergic (ipratropium) to the short-acting inhaled β_2-agonist regimen. There are several choices for combination therapy (see Fig. 24-4). Again, there is no clearly superior choice. Clinical trials comparing combinations report varying results. In some cases, the combinations are equivalent; in others; either one or another combination was associated with improved outcomes.[1,85,86]

Combined β_2-Agonists and Anticholinergics

The benefits of combining a β_2-agonist with an anticholinergic have not been clearly established.[85,87–91] This is most likely explained by the interpatient variability previously described. Even though a patient may respond individually to either a β_2-agonist or an anticholinergic, he or she may or may not demonstrate additive effects. For patients with proven additive benefit, it may be more convenient and less expensive to use a fixed-dose combination product (Combivent; 18 μg ipratropium bromide, 90 μg albuterol per puff) compared to using two different products together.[90] A drawback to the fixed-dose combination is that it leaves less flexibility in adjusting the dosage of the individual drugs.

Long-Acting β_2-Agonists

The role of inhaled, long-acting β_2-agonists in the chronic management of COPD has become established in recent years. Available evidence both with salmeterol and formoterol shows improved pulmonary function, reduced dyspnea, and enhanced quality of life in COPD patients. Additionally, these agents offer the convenience of a long duration of action allowing twice daily dosing. There is no benefit in exceeding the recommended dose of either agent. Therefore, salmeterol should be prescribed as 42 μg (50 μg in a dry powder device) twice daily and formoterol at 12 μg twice daily. Patients should be advised not to exceed these doses because the risk of adverse cardiac effects and electrolyte abnormalities (hypokalemia) increases with higher doses.

Inhaled, long-acting β_2-agonists improve symptoms, exercise tolerance, and health status for patients with COPD. Several studies published during the past few years have reported the value of these agents in improving spirometry and overall quality of life. Clinical evidence suggests that long-acting β_2-agonists are equally or more effective short-acting β_2-agonists or ipratropium.[92–101] Based on these results and the convenience of twice daily dosing, these agents are reasonable options for bronchodilator therapy in patients experiencing chronic persistent symptoms.

Three studies have compared the short-term responses of salmeterol with that from an anticholinergic bronchodilator.[95,100,102] In the first study, 16 COPD patients were challenged using a double-blind, placebo crossover design with albuterol (200 μg), salmeterol (50 μg), and ipratropium (40 μg).[95] All three drugs showed a greater absolute increase in FEV_1 compared with placebo. The onset was fastest with albuterol, intermediate with ipratropium, and slowest with salmeterol. The maximal increase in FEV_1 during the 4- to 12-hour periods and duration of response was greater with salmeterol than with ipratropium. The mean FEV_1 area under the curve was highest with salmeterol, intermediate with ipratropium, and lowest with albuterol. Salmeterol was also compared to ipratropium and placebo in a 12-week study.[100] Both active treatments reduced dyspnea; however, salmeterol prolonged the time to the first COPD exacerbation compared to ipratropium. In another 12-week placebo controlled comparison between salmeterol and ipratropium, each therapy produced similar maximal bronchodilation, but the effects of salmeterol persisted longer. Both treatments were well tolerated.[102]

Salmeterol has also been compared to long-acting anticholinergic agents. In a single-blind, crossover, randomized study, the responses to a single 50-μg dose of salmeterol were compared with responses to single doses of 200 and 400 μg of oxitropium bromide and placebo in 12 subjects.[96] Using the mean FEV_1 area under the curve for 12 hours as a basis for comparison, responses to salmeterol and 400 μg of oxitropium were equal, both being more effective than 200 μg of oxitropium. The onset of effect of salmeterol was slightly slower than for oxitropium, but salmeterol had a somewhat greater effect between the 10- and 12-hour observation periods.

Formoterol is another long-acting, inhaled β_2-agonist with a duration of action similar to salmeterol, but with a more rapid onset of effect (approximately 5 minutes). This agent has been compared to ipratropium in patients with COPD and found to improve quality of life, improve symptom scores, and reduce the use of albuterol.[101] In a different study, combining formoterol and ipratropium produced greater improvements in spirometry and symptoms compared to the combination of albuterol and ipratropium.[103]

In summary, it appears that inhaled long-acting β_2-agonists have a role in patients with COPD. Long-acting β_2-agonists produce similar or superior improvements in lung function, patient symptoms and quality of life measures compared to other bronchodilator therapies. A Cochrane Review of their role in treating patients with COPD concluded that small spirometric improvement were seen, but other beneficial clinical outcomes were not consistently produced.[104] They offer the convenience of twice daily dosing and are generally safe. A pooled analysis of 17 studies concluded that there was no increased risk of cardiovascular adverse events in COPD patients treated with salmeterol therapy.[105] For E.B., her pattern of use of albuterol suggests that she may benefit from a long-acting β_2-agonist. This therapy could be used in addition to, or in place of, ipratropium. The longer action of salmeterol or formoterol may smooth out the symptom pattern and allow a net decrease in the total exposure to β_2-agonists throughout the day. E.B. should be counseled that the long-acting β_2-agonist is used on a scheduled basis, every 12 hours, but not for symptomatic relief of acute symptoms. Albuterol can be continued as needed for acute exacerbations. Current recommendations are that rescue doses of albuterol should not exceed four inhalations daily with this regimen.

Long-Acting Anticholinergics

A new option on the horizon for use in COPD patients is long-acting anticholinergic agents. Tiotropium is one such agent that has been demonstrated to reduce symptoms and improve spirometry in COPD patients. Tiotropium's mechanism as a bronchodilator differs from ipratropium in than it has improved selectivity in blocking M_1 and M_3 muscarinic (acetylcholine) receptors in human airways.[106] There is less effect at the M_2 receptor where blockade increases the release of acetylcholine which might cause bronchoconstriction.[107] Tiotropium actually binds to M_1, M_2, and M_3 receptors but dissociates more rapidly from the M_2 site.[108] As a result of improved selectivity and slow dissociation from M_1 and M_3 receptors, effective bronchodilation is achieved with once a day dosing of tiotropium.[108] Studies suggest superior benefit for tiotropium compared to ipratropium.[109] Tiotropium therapy has been associated with significant improvements in symptoms, lung function, and quality of life. In addition, a reduction in the frequency of exacerbations has also been demonstrated.[110,111]

Tiotropium, 18 μg once daily, has been compared with salmeterol, 50 μg twice daily, in a 6-month trial involving 600 patients with COPD.[112] Tiotropium-treated patients achieved a statistically significant improvement in the trough (morning) FEV_1 compared with salmeterol-treated patients, although the baseline spirometry values averaged only 1.08 liters. Both treatments improved dyspnea and health related quality of life compared to placebo.

Even in the absence of an acute bronchodilator response to treatment, long-term therapy with tiotropium improves several clinical outcome parameters in patients with COPD.[111] The role of tiotropium alone or in combination with other therapies appears promising. Tiotropium has the potential to be a significant advance in the treatment of COPD as it appears to be well tolerated, may improve clinical outcomes, and offers enhanced patient convenience with once daily dosing.

Theophylline

Although inhaled bronchodilators are preferred in chronic management of COPD, another option for consideration is oral methylxanthine therapy. Theophylline has been used for more than 50 years in the treatment of pulmonary diseases, including asthma and COPD. Before the marketing of ipratropium in the mid 1980s, theophylline was commonly used in the treatment of with COPD. More recently, it is reserved for patients who do not receive adequate relief of symptoms or do not tolerate other bronchodilators. The primary concern with theophylline is the risk-benefit of use. Theophylline is a comparatively weaker bronchodilator, exhibits significant intrapatient and interpatient variability in clearance, is prone to numerous drug interactions, and can cause serious toxicities.

Although theophylline probably has no role as monotherapy for COPD management, low-dose theophylline, (targeting serum concentrations of 8 to 12 μg/mL) is indicated for patients in whom symptoms are not acceptably controlled on an inhaled bronchodilator combination. Additive bronchodilation has been demonstrated when combining theophylline to an existing dual regimen of ipratropium and a β_2-agonist.[87,113] A 2- to 4-week trial is warranted to document efficacy and tolerance. Efficacy may be judged either by improvement in pulmonary function tests or by subjective improvement in exercise capacity and dyspnea. If no improvement is noted in either of these parameters, the drug should be discontinued.

Similar to other bronchodilator therapies, theophylline therapy has variable effects on improving spirometry in patients with COPD.[45] In clinical trials, when improvements in lung function are demonstrated, the objective improvement is not always accompanied by a statistically significant change in subjective parameters such as exercise tolerance, wheezing, cough, dyspnea scores, or sense of well-being. Conversely, up to 30% to 50% of patients describe significant improvements in symptoms, but without a change in pulmonary function.[114] Similarly, when theophylline was discontinued in patients previously stabilized on the drug, up to 72% of subjects in one study had a deterioration of exercise performance, dyspnea, and quality-of-life scores in the 3 days after withdrawal, compared with only 15% of subjects who continued taking theophylline.[115] There was also a decline in pulmonary function measures in some of the patients with symptom deterioration.

The discordance between objective improvements versus subjective responses suggest that different outcome measures may be more appropriate when evaluating COPD measures. In the case of theophylline, it has also been suggested that its benefits include effects other than bronchodilation. Among the possible nonbronchodilator mechanisms are adenosine receptor antagonism, increased diaphragm muscle contractility as a result of altered calcium fluxes in muscle cells, increased central neuroinspiratory drive that augments responses to hypoxia or hypercapnia, and anti-inflammatory or immunomodulatory effects owing to alterations of various interleukin cytokines.[45,116,117] The significance of these effects and relevance to improvements in COPD patients are unclear. Currently, theophylline should be reserved for patients who continue to experience significant symptoms or have declining health despite aggressive inhaled bronchodilator therapy.

DRUG INTERACTIONS

16. C.K. is a 64-year-old woman with end-stage emphysema attributed to a 35 pack-year smoking history. She is severely limited in her physical activity because of severe dyspnea even at rest. Her home life is a "bed-to-bathroom" existence. A home health agency visits three times weekly, and Meals on Wheels brings her dinner. She requires home oxygen therapy at 1 L/min with baseline ABG measurements (on supplemental O_2) as follows: pH, 7.37; PO_2, 64 mm Hg; PCO_2, 45 mm Hg; and oxygen saturation, 91%. Her last measured FEV_1 was 0.5 L, increasing to 0.6 L after albuterol administration. Her medications include ipratropium 3 inhalations QID, salmeterol 2 inhalations BID, albuterol PRN, and sustained release theophylline 200 mg Q 12 hr. A theophylline concentration 2 months ago was 13 μg/mL. Four days ago, she began a course of ciprofloxacin 500 mg twice daily for 1 week for a urinary tract infection. Today, she visits her pulmonologist with the complaint of nausea and difficulty sleeping for the past 3 days. What is a possible cause of her complaints of nausea and difficulty sleeping?

[SI units: Po₂, 8.5 kPa; Pco₂, 6.0 kPa]

Both gastrointestinal complaints, such as nausea, and CNS symptoms, including sleep difficulty and nervousness, are consistent with theophylline toxicity. Other adverse reactions associated with methylxanthines are cardiac irritability (tachycardia or arrhythmias) and seizures. All these side effects are dose related. Gastrointestinal intolerance, nervousness, and insomnia can occur at any serum concentration, but increase in frequency when serum concentration exceeds 15 μg/mL.[117]

In C.K., the addition of the antibiotic ciprofloxacin to her regimen most likely resulted in a drug interaction causing a rise in her theophylline concentration. The potential for an interaction with theophylline varies among the available fluoroquinolone antibiotics.[118,119] Drug interactions are dependent on several factors including the dose of each agent and the baseline serum theophylline concentration. Elevations in the theophylline concentration of 25% are typical with ciprofloxacin interactions, although elevations of 50% have been observed.[118,119] In C.K., a theophylline concentration should be obtained and further doses held until results are known.

In general, theophylline metabolism is associated with significant interpatient and intrapatient variability. Patients should be monitored closely for early signs of toxicity as well as for the initiation of drugs that potentially may interact. Understanding and recognizing the potential for drug interactions can allow safe and effective therapy with theophylline.[117]

17. A theophylline serum concentration is measured for C.K. It is reported as 21 μg/ml. What action should be taken?

This serum concentration result is consistent with the interaction between theophylline and ciprofloxacin reported in the literature.[117,118] Her symptoms do not appear life-threatening at this point, so a conservative approach to management is appropriate. Theophylline should be held for one dose and then restarted at a lower dose (100 mg BID) until the ciprofloxacin therapy is completed. Alternatively, theophylline could be withheld until the antibiotic treatment is finished. C.K. should be monitored for resolution of symptoms. For a complete discussion of theophylline dosing, serum level concentration monitoring, and drug interactions, see Chapter 23, Asthma.

Oral Corticosteroids

18. Two months later, C.K. experiences a significant worsening of her pulmonary status and was hospitalized for 5 days. During that time, she received nebulized bronchodilator therapy, antibiotics, and systemic corticosteroids. She is discharged home from the hospital with her usual medications and a prednisone taper (current dose, 30 mg daily) over 2 weeks. She has recovered to her baseline level of health and function, although no significant changes were noted in her pulmonary function. Should chronic prednisone therapy be considered for C.K.?

Based on the concept of COPD as an inflammatory disease, there has been interest in the role of corticosteroids. These agents have demonstrated benefit in the management of acute exacerbations as discussed in Question 22. A short course (typically 10 days) of oral corticosteroids after an acute exacerbation is also warranted, but an attempt should be made to taper and discontinue shortly thereafter. In contrast, long-term treatment of COPD with oral corticosteroids is not recommended because of insufficient evidence of significant benefit and a substantial risk of risk of adverse effects. Only 10% to 20% of COPD patients experience a clinical response to systemic corticosteroid therapy, defined as a significant increase in FEV₁ and/or a subjective improvement in symptoms.[1]

Earlier recommendations about the role of chronic systemic corticosteroid therapy suggested that possible predictors of response were patients with a greater degree of obstruction, more bronchodilator reversibility, an elevated serum eosinophil count, and/or the presence of sputum eosinophils.[47] Caution is advised against taking these recommendations and conclusions too literally, however, since the interpretation of these measures are complex. For example, the presence of these predictors of response may indicate the presence of asthma. Additionally, a mathematical response in lung function consistent with reversibility may be achieved with relative ease in a patient with low baseline spirometry, but the clinical benefit of the improvement may be minimal.

A meta-analysis limited to studies that used an appropriate study design suggests that only 10% of patients have clinically significant improvements in pulmonary function, but failed to identify any reliable predictors.[46] Another study was designed to determine if any detrimental effects occurred with the withdrawal of chronic corticosteroid therapy in patients with COPD.[120] Patients were tapered off prednisone at a rate of 5 mg each week and followed for 6 months. Compared to a control group that continued prednisone, there were no differences in exacerbation rates, spirometry results, dyspnea, or quality of life assessments. Patients who were tapered off prednisone experienced a mean reduction in weight of almost 5 kg.

Chronic use of systemic corticosteroids is beneficial for a small minority of patients with COPD. However, all patients are susceptible to the toxicities of this therapy. Systemic corticosteroid treatment can complicate diabetes mellitus and hypertension and accelerate bone loss. Long-term treatment with systemic steroids is also associated with development of myopathy, which contributes to muscle weakness in COPD patients[48,121] (See Chapter 44, Connective Tissue Disorders: The Clinical Use of Corticosteroids).

Inhaled Corticosteroids

19. Are there other options for anti-inflammatory therapy in C.K., such as inhaled corticosteroids?

There is increasing interest in the role of inhaled corticosteroids in the management of COPD. The benefit of this therapy in asthma is well documented; however, results from several studies in COPD have yielded conflicting results.[122–129] In the middle to late 1980s several large national studies were initiated to evaluate this question.[50-53] These trials were well designed with appropriate blinding and controls, including the use of placebo treatments. Different inhaled corticosteroids were evaluated in the various studies; however, the doses employed would be classified as medium to high dose. The primary outcome in each case was the annual decline in FEV_1.

The EUROSCOP study enrolled 1,277 patients with COPD who received either placebo or budesonide 800 μg per day.[51] No significant difference was found in FEV_1 decline between the groups, although the corticosteroid-treated group experienced a modest increase in FEV_1 initially, which persisted through the study. The Copenhagen City Heart Study consisted of 290 patients with COPD randomized to either budesonide 800 to 1,200 μg daily or placebo.[50] During 3 years of follow-up, no difference was noted in the decline of FEV_1. In the Lung Health Study II, which was conducted in the United States, a total of 1,100 COPD patients received either triamcinolone 1,200 μg or placebo daily.[53] The majority of patients were followed for more than 3 years. No significant difference was detected in FEV_1 decline; however, steroid treated patients had less dyspnea, fewer new respiratory symptoms, and decreased use of health care resources.

The ISOLDE study compared fluticasone 1,000 μg daily with placebo during a 3-year evaluation involving 751 patients.[52] Of note, these patients had more severe disease, based on baseline FEV_1 than the three previous studies discussed above. Similar to other studies, there was no difference in the annual decline in FEV_1 between the groups although the steroid-treated patients did experience an initial increase in FEV_1 that persisted throughout the study. Despite the lack of a significant finding in the primary outcome, the corticosteroid group experienced 25% fewer exacerbations and the severity of exacerbations was less. Another smaller and shorter trial compared the efficacy of inhaled fluticasone (1,000 μg /day) with placebo in 281 patients.[130] All subjects were smokers or ex-smokers, met the clinical criteria for chronic bronchitis, and had experienced at least one exacerbation per year for the previous 3 years. During the 6-month follow-up, 37% of the placebo-treated patients and 32% of the fluticasone group, a nonsignificant difference, experienced at least one exacerbation in COPD. Again, the investigators noted a trend toward fewer moderate or severe exacerbations in the fluticasone group compared with the placebo-treated patients.

However, a meta-analysis conducted to evaluate the effect of inhaled corticosteroid therapy on the rate of decline in FEV_1 failed to detect any benefit even among patients with an FEV_1 ≤50%.[131] This report, which included six clinical studies involving more than 3,500 subjects, was consistent with the large scale clinical trials in concluding that inhaled corticosteroids did not modify the long-term decline in lung function in patients with COPD. Despite the lack of benefit in reducing the steady decline in FEV_1 with inhaled corticosteroids, there is evidence that suggests benefit in reducing the risk of repeat hospitalization for COPD. In a population-based study utilizing a Canadian database of more than 20,000 patients, treatment with inhaled corticosteroids at hospital discharge for a COPD exacerbation reduced repeat hospitalization within 1 year by 24%.[132] Overall mortality was also reduced by 29% in patients who received inhaled corticosteroids. The investigators in this trial suggested that these findings warrant a large scale study to validate benefit of inhaled corticosteroid in COPD.

The effect of discontinuing inhaled corticosteroid therapy following four months of treatment has also been evaluated.[134] After receiving fluticasone 1,000 μg daily for 4 months, patients were randomly assigned to continue the inhaled corticosteroid or switch to placebo for six months. Patients that discontinued the corticosteroid had a higher risk for recurrent exacerbations and experienced a decrease in health-related quality of life. These results also warrant further evaluation to determine the role for initiating and continuing inhaled corticosteroid therapy.

Based on these studies, it appears that inhaled corticosteroids do not modify the natural course of COPD as exhibited by the rate of decline in FEV_1. This is explained, in part, by the nature of inflammation that occurs in COPD. As opposed to eosinophil inflammation seen in asthma, COPD is associated with neutrophilic inflammation, which is largely unresponsive to corticosteroid treatment.[23]

Because of the cost of inhaled corticosteroids and the relative risk of toxicity with long-term treatment, the GOLD report suggests that these agents should be reserved for patients who demonstrate a significant FEV_1 response or in those with FEV_1 <50% of predicted who experience repeated exacerbations requiring treatment with antimicrobial agents or systemic corticosteroids. In evaluation of benefit from inhaled corticosteroid therapy, a therapeutic trial of 6 weeks to 3 months should be initiated.[1] Various objective and subjective assessments including spirometry and other measures of clinical improvement such as less dyspnea, reduced exacerbations, and improved quality of life and health status should be used to determine the benefit of continuing therapy.

If C.K shows spirometric improvement with corticosteroids or if she experiences repeated exacerbations requiring antibiotics or systemic corticosteroid therapy, a therapeutic trial of inhaled corticosteroids is warranted. It was previously suggested that a 2-week course of systemic corticosteroids may be useful in predicting response to inhaled corticosteroids; however, this has not been found to be a reliable strategy.[1,133]

Combinations of Bronchodilator and Inhaled Corticosteroids

20. Is there any evidence of benefit in combining bronchodilators with inhaled corticosteroids?

Combinations of bronchodilator and inhaled corticosteroid agents have been evaluated. The majority of interest has been with a combination of an inhaled, long-acting β_2-agonist (e.g., salmeterol, formoterol) and an inhaled corticosteroid. This combination has been promising in improving pulmonary function and reducing symptoms.[135]

The combination of an inhaled corticosteroid and a long acting β_2-agonist was studied in 1,465 patients in an international study entitled Trial of Inhaled Steroids and Long-acting β_2-agonists (TRISTAN).[136] Subjects with baseline FEV_1 of 25% to 70% predicted received either salmeterol monotherapy (50 μg BID), fluticasone monotherapy (500 μg BID), the combination of salmeterol and fluticasone (via the diskus device), or placebo for 12 months. Each active treatment improved lung function and reduced symptoms and exacerbations compared to placebo; however, patients in the combination group experienced greater FEV_1 improvement compared to other treatments (133 mL versus 73 and 95 mL in the monotherapy groups). The investigators concluded that the benefit from combination treatment may be attributed to enhancement of corticosteroid effects by the long-acting β_2-agonist. These results were similar to those of another trial comparing the same treatments except that the fluticasone dose was 250 μg BID.[137] The combination of agents improved the morning (trough) FEV_1 significantly compared to salmeterol and placebo, and improved the 2-hour post-dose FEV_1 compared with fluticasone and placebo.

Supplemental Oxygen Therapy

21. **A.Z., a 64-year-old woman, has a 50-pack-year smoking history and a 15-year history of chronic bronchitis. She stopped smoking 5 years ago. She also has a history of mild hypertension, which is well controlled with hydrochlorothiazide 25 mg daily. A.Z. has been hospitalized two times within the past year for acute exacerbations of her chronic bronchitis. Her medications at home are salmeterol 2 puffs BID, ipratropium inhaler 4 puffs QID, sustained-release theophylline 300 mg BID, and PRN albuterol. Her baseline pulmonary function tests show an FEV_1 of 1.3 L (51% predicted) and FVC of 2.2 L, with essentially no change after albuterol. Three days ago, A.Z. began to experience increasing symptoms of SOB on exertion, an increase in sputum production, and a change in sputum color from its normal light color to yellow. She has been using albuterol four to five times daily for the past several days. In the ED, she is very short of breath with a respiratory rate of 26 breaths/min. Her chest radiograph shows no signs of an infiltrate. A STAT ABG assessment shows the following: pH, 7.35; PaO_2, 50 mm Hg; PCO_2, 45 mm Hg; percent saturation, 80%; and bicarbonate, 26. A theophylline concentration is 9 μg/mL. She is administered 1 L of oxygen by nasal cannula. What are the indications for oxygen therapy in A.Z.? Will she require supplemental oxygen therapy at home?**

[SI units: PaO_2, 6.67 kPa; PCO_2, 6.0 kPa]

Oxygen therapy for COPD is commonly used in two situations: during an acute exacerbation of COPD associated with a drop in PaO_2 to <55 mm Hg and in patients who are chronically hypoxemic.[1,138] The goals of supplemental oxygen therapy are to correct arterial hypoxemia and prevent secondary organ damage. A PaO_2 of 55 mm Hg is equivalent to an arterial O_2 saturation of approximately 90%. Based on the slope of the oxyhemoglobin disassociation curve, a PaO_2 less than 55 to 60 mm Hg results in a dramatic drop in the saturation of hemoglobin (see Chapter 23, Asthma). Over a prolonged period, this hypoxemia results in detrimental end-organ effects, including declines in CNS, cardiac, and renal function. On the other hand, increasing the PaO_2 above 60 is associated with small changes in the saturation of hemoglobin because the curve is relatively flat in this range.

The physiologic response to hypoxemia (PaO_2 <55 mm Hg) is an increase in ventilatory drive in an attempt to raise arterial O_2 and decrease CO_2. In addition, the vascular beds supplying hypoxic tissues dilate and the heart rate increases to improve tissue oxygen delivery. Other responses include pulmonary vascular constriction to improve the match between ventilation and perfusion within the lung and release of erythropoietin to increase oxygen-carrying capacity of the blood.

Over time, many of the compensatory responses either fail to keep up with demand or cause detrimental effects. For example, a significant increase in circulating red blood cells can increase cardiac workload and worsen heart failure. Increased pulmonary vasoconstriction causes pulmonary hypertension, leading to right ventricular heart failure (cor pulmonale) with an increased risk of death.[1,56,57]

Continuous supplemental oxygen therapy at home improves pulmonary hemodynamics, reduces cardiac workload, and prolongs survival. Exercise endurance and neuropsychologic performance (judgment and short-term memory) may also improve after reversal of hypoxemia. The value of home oxygen therapy for COPD patients with chronic hypoxemia (PaO_2 <55 mm Hg) was documented in studies conducted nearly 2 decades ago.[139,140] To obtain full benefit of home oxygen therapy, it should be used 18 to 24 hours a day. In a classic study, subjects using continuous therapy (20 hr/day) had a mortality rate half as great as patients using only nocturnal oxygen (12 hr/day).[141] Symptoms of breathlessness, dyspnea, or air hunger alone are not considered accepted indications for supplemental oxygen without documented hypoxia because they often do not correlate well with the arterial blood gas. The current recommendation for patients with hypoxemia (defined as PaO_2 <55 mm Hg or and oxygen saturation <88%) is continuous, 24-hour-a-day oxygen. Patients with a PaO_2 of 56 to 59 mm Hg or an oxygen saturation of 89%, combined with either cor pulmonale or polycythemia, should also receive long-term oxygen therapy. The goal of therapy is a PaO_2 >60 mm Hg or an oxygen saturation >90%. There is less agreement as to the value of noncontinuous oxygen during exercise or exertion or during sleep in patients with nocturnal hypoxemia. Assessments should be made at 2-month intervals to determine whether oxygen therapy should be continued or whether sufficient improvement has occurred to attempt oxygen weaning. However, after discontinuation, the condition often deteriorates, necessitating reinstitution of continuous-dose oxygen.[1,138]

Administering supplemental oxygen to a patient with COPD is associated with well-defined risks. Some COPD patients with poor ventilatory capacity are categorized as "carbon dioxide retainers." In these cases, the patient no longer relies on rises in the $PaCO_2$ as the primary drive to breathe. If these patients receive too much oxygen, the rise in their PaO_2 may lead to hypoventilation. As the respiratory rate slows, they may begin to retain CO_2, which may precipitate the syndrome known as CO_2 narcosis. Clinical signs of this syndrome include somnolence, lethargy, and possibly coma. In addition, oxygen presents a significant fire hazard in the presence of heaters and furnaces. Obviously, patients and family members should refrain from smoking while oxygen is in use. Other complications are nasal irritation, drying of the airways, and cough.

In this case, A.Z. is acutely hypoxic with a PaO_2 of 50 mm Hg, but she does not appear to have a problem of chronic CO_2 retention. She has a normal pH, a slightly elevated $PaCO_2$, and normal serum bicarbonate calculated from the ABG. Supplemental oxygen therapy will be beneficial to her for this acute episode by increasing her PaO_2 and improving oxygen delivery to tissues. She should be administered oxygen therapy at 2 to 3 L/min for the next 12 to 48 hours to maintain PaO_2 >55 mm Hg. Home oxygen therapy is not warranted unless she becomes chronically hypoxemic.

Patients usually receive oxygen through a nasal cannula at a flow rate of 2 L/min, which increases the fraction of inspired oxygen (FiO_2) to 27% compared with 21% of room air. During airline travel or at higher elevations, the flow rate may be temporarily increased by an additional 1 to 2 L/min. Efficiency of delivery can be increased by using reservoir nasal cannulas, transtracheal catheters, and electronic demand devices. The review article by Tarpy and Celli includes a complete description of O_2 delivery devices and a discussion of the relative benefits of oxygen delivery as a gas, liquid, or by an oxygen concentrator.[138]

Acute COPD Exacerbations

22. **Is A.Z. experiencing an acute exacerbation of COPD? What other therapies should be considered for acute management?**

This case exemplifies the onset of an acute exacerbation of COPD following an upper respiratory infection. In some cases, the onset of symptoms is even faster (days to hours) and can also be precipitated by environmental exposure or tobacco smoke. In particular, the progressive decline of the patient's pulmonary function and PaO_2 is typical. If the exacerbation continues without treatment, she could develop progressive worsening of lung function with increasing CO_2 retention and development of respiratory acidosis.

Acute exacerbations of COPD have been defined in various ways. Common symptoms include increased shortness of breath and an increase in the amount and purulence of sputum. Hypoxemia and hypercapnia may also be present.[1] Recently, a consensus group defined exacerbation as a sustained worsening of the patient's condition from the stable state and beyond normal day-to-day variations that is acute in onset and necessitates a change in regular medication in a patient with underlying COPD.[142]

Exacerbation rates vary among patients with COPD, although many patients experience two to four exacerbations annually.[143] The impact of these episodes can be significant. For patients requiring hospitalization, the mortality rate exceeds 10% and the 1-year mortality rate approaches 45%. Further, the risk of rehospitalization within 6 months is 50%.[144]

Categorizing the severity of COPD exacerbations has been controversial as well. The most common method was proposed in 1987,[54] in which exacerbations were graded as type 1, 2, or 3 based on the presence of 1 to 3 symptoms, respectively. Symptoms are increased breathlessness, increased sputum quantity, and new or increased sputum purulence. Type 3 exacerbations present with one or more of the symptoms above combined with either sore throat or nasal discharge within the last 5 days, fever, increase in wheezing or coughing, or an increase in respiratory or heart rate of at least 20%.

The primary treatment strategies for acute exacerbations of COPD are intensification of bronchodilator therapies, systemic corticosteroids, and antimicrobial therapy. Supplemental oxygen or assisted ventilation are used in more severe exacerbations. An appraisal of recommendations in the treatment of COPD exacerbations concluded that many recommendations lacked supporting evidence and that the quality of evidence was poor in many instances.[145] Supplemental oxygen should be used if required to maintain oxygen saturations above 90% ($PaO_2 > 60$ mmHg). This must be done cautiously in patients with hypercapnia because of the risk of worsening hypoventilation.

The use of short-acting inhaled β_2-agonists and anticholinergics improve airflow obstruction during acute exacerbations of COPD. Similar improvement in FEV_1 is achieved with either drug class[145-148] with no apparent benefit in improving FEV_1 with a combination of these agents. The GOLD guidelines recommend β_2-agonists initially with the addition of anticholinergic therapy if adequate response to β_2-agonists is not achieved. Inhalation therapy can be delivered by MDI or nebulization with equal efficacy.[145,149] The benefit of bronchodilators in combination is not clearly superior but is commonly used.[61] Frequently, combinations of bronchodilators are used as submaximal doses of each agent. There is more evidence to support maximizing the dose of one agent before adding the second one if the response is not optimal or side effects are not tolerated.[61,147] Maximal doses of short-acting, inhaled β_2-agonists and ipratropium are not well defined, but in an acute situation, either of these therapies may be administered in two to three times the usual dose and given every 1 to 2 hours based on response. In this situation, the patient should be closely monitored for improvement or evidence of adverse effects.

Another bronchodilator option for management of an acute exacerbation would be intravenous theophylline. Available evidence suggests that inhaled bronchodilator regimens provide greater benefit in terms of improving spirometry. Also, the risk for toxicity with theophylline is significant.[61] A recent meta-analysis suggests there is little evidence to support the use of theophylline for acute exacerbations.[150] Despite these findings, the GOLD guidelines suggest theophylline use may be warranted in patients experiencing severe exacerbations of COPD who are not responding to other aggressive measures.

Systemic corticosteroids can improve spirometry, arterial blood gas results, and symptoms during acute exacerbations.[151,152] A commonly referenced study, The Systemic Corticosteroids in Chronic Obstructive Pulmonary disease Exacerbations (SCCOPE) trial involved 271 subjects hospitalized with an exacerbation.[151] In a randomized, double blind, placebo controlled fashion, these subject received methylprednisolone 125 mg intravenously every 6 hours for 3 days before conversion to oral prednisone and tapered. There were significantly fewer treatment failures in the steroid treatment group (23% versus 33%) and a faster spirometric response. In this study, a 2-week regimen was as effective as an 8-week regimen. The benefits of systemic corticosteroids were substantiated further in a well-controlled trial in which 147 patients discharged from the ED with a COPD exacerbation received either prednisone 40 mg orally for 10 days or placebo.[153] All subject received 10 days of antimicrobial therapy and scheduled albuterol and ipratropium. Prednisone treatment significantly reduced relapse rates at 30 days (27% versus 43%) and prolonged the time to relapse. Steroid treated patients also had greater improvements in FEV_1 and in dyspnea scores.

The optimal regimen (dose and duration) is not clear because the regimens used in clinical studies were quite variable.[145] Regimens demonstrating benefit have ranged from methylprednisolone 125 mg intravenously every 6 hours for 3 days before tapering over 2 weeks with an oral drug to prednisolone 30 mg orally daily for 2 weeks without prior intravenous corticosteroid. It is clear that regimen durations longer than 2 weeks offer no additional benefit. Unfortunately, symptoms can persist or flare for several weeks after an acute exacerbation. This can result in patients inappropriately remaining on oral corticosteroids for an excessive period. Every effort should be made to taper dosages and discontinue corticosteroids as soon as possible. The situation is compounded if symptoms worsen before the corticosteroid is withdrawn and/or the patient develops psychological dependence on the corticosteroid. Switching to inhaled corticosteroids may assist in tapering and/or removal of the oral therapy.

23. Should A.Z. start antimicrobial therapy for an acute COPD exacerbation?

The etiology of COPD exacerbations may be infectious or noninfectious. It is estimated that approximately 50% have an infectious basis and about half of these are bacterial. However, determining an infectious etiology is often hard to determine because patients are chronically colonized with bacteria. Antimicrobial therapy is most beneficial in moderate to severe exacerbations when the patient experiences a worsening in at least two of the cardinal signs. (e.g., dyspnea, quantity and purulence of sputum).

There is no clear consensus about the antibiotic of choice. The GOLD guidelines recommend that traditional antimicrobial agents with activity against the likely pathogens (*S. pneumoniae, H. influenzae* and *M. catarrhalis*) be used, including ampicillin, amoxicillin, doxycycline, and trimethoprimsulfamethoxazole. There is insufficient evidence to suggest that newer antibiotics are more effective and these therapies are relatively inexpensive. In the absence of drug allergies, treatment of COPD exacerbations with one of these traditional therapies is preferred.

Other COPD Therapies

24. What other treatments are available for the chronic management of COPD in A.Z.?

An improved understanding of the pathophysiologic basis of COPD has stimulated interest in research for new therapies. In addition to long-acting inhaled anticholinergics discussed previously, therapies directed against specific mediators of COPD inflammation have been a focus.[106] Novel anti-inflammatory agents are of interest, including protein kinase and NF-κB inhibitors, which inhibit expression of genes involved in inflammation consistent with COPD.[154] Other anti-inflammatory agents in the preliminary stages of investigation include interleukin-10, an anti-inflammatory cytokine, and blockers of adhesion molecules that recruit neutrophils and lymphocytes during inflammation. In addition, therapies that suppress the recruitment and activation of neutrophils are under investigation, including leukotriene B_4 inhibitors, interleukin-8 antibodies, and TNF-α inhibitors.

Inhibitors of phosphodiesterase 4 enzyme (PDE4 inhibitors) are the most extensively studied agents. Years ago, the mechanism of action of methylxanthines, including theophylline was attributed to inhibition of PDE4. This enzyme is responsible for the metabolism of cyclic AMP, the mediator associated with relaxation of bronchial smooth muscle through the β_2-adrenergic receptor. Other potential mechanisms for theophylline's action as a bronchodilator are more likely as discussed earlier. Phosphodiesterase enzyme, especially PDE4, is also found in neutrophils, CD8 lymphocytes, and macrophages and plays a role in modulating inflammation. Thus, inhibition of PDE is expected to reduce inflammation in COPD. Selective PDE4 inhibitors, such as cilomilast and rofumilast, have shown benefit in reducing neutrophilic inflammation in animal models.[106] PDE4 inhibitors inhibit neutrophils, CD8+ cells, and macrophages. In a short-term study, cilomilast exhibited beneficial effects in patients with COPD.[155] Compared to placebo, oral therapy with cilomilast improved lung function and symptoms. The benefits were attributed to an anti-inflammatory effect rather than a bronchodilating action. Unfortunately, the clinical utility of this class of medications is limited by gastrointestinal side effects including nausea which may be related to the drug's primary action. Cilomilast has been approved recently for treatment of COPD in the U.S.; however, its place in therapy is not well established.

Surgical Options for COPD

25. L. P. is a 66-year-old man with severe emphysema secondary to a 50-pack year history of tobacco use. He is disabled and severely limited in activities of daily living. L.P. receives chronic oxygen supplementation at 2 L/min, which maintains his oxygen saturation at 89%. His current medication regimen includes albuterol and ipratropium inhaler (Combivent) 2 puffs four times daily, theophylline sustained release 200 mg twice daily, and prednisone 5 mg daily. He complains of chronic dyspnea even at rest. Recent spirometry revealed an FEV_1 of 35% predicted and FVC of 48% predicted with no evidence of reversibility. Chest radiograph reveals thoracic hyperinflation; however, no bullae are noted. His family inquires about surgery to improve his condition. What are the options for this patient?

Surgical options include a bullectomy, lung transplantation, and lung volume reduction surgery (LVRS).[156] Bullectomy is the surgical removal of large blebs in the lung. Bullae generally don't participate in gas exchange and may increase the risk of pneumothorax (e.g., collapsed lung). Bullectomy may be beneficial if a bulla is seen on radiograph or if the patient has suffered a pneumothorax.[156] Lung transplantation in emphysema has been uncommon, although this procedure has been performed more frequently in recent years. It is typically reserved for patients younger than 60 years old and with α_1-antitrypsin associated emphysema.

A patient may be a candidate for LVRS based on the presence of thoracic overinflation. This procedure involves the removal of lung sections affected by emphysema. The objective of this surgery is to change the dynamics in the chest by improving elastic recoil and gas exchange by the remaining lung. This procedure is also favored for patients between 60 and 70 years old and with $FEV_1 > 20\%$.[156] In the National Emphysema Treatment Trial, LVRS improved exercise capacity but did not prolong survival compared to continuing medical therapy alone.[157] L.P. could be considered for LVRS if he is judged to be a good surgical candidate. A computed tomography (CT) scan should be obtained to determine the distribution of his disease.

OBSTRUCTIVE SLEEP APNEA

Signs and Symptoms

26. B.V., a 37-year-old morbidly obese (170 kg) man, is brought in by his family for evaluation. They state that he is extremely sleepy during the day with frequent spontaneous naps. Although he sleeps alone, his family states that he snores loudly, sometimes disturbing the sleep of everyone else in the house. He also often awakens with headaches in the morning. On examination, he has tachycardia (120 beats/min) with regular rhythm, an enlarged heart shadow on chest radiograph, bilateral pitting edema, and an Hct of 52% (normal, 40% to 48%). An ABG assessment shows the following: pH, 7.37; Pao_2, 50 mm Hg; $Paco_2$, 60 mm Hg; and oxygen saturation, 85%. What features of sleep apnea are present?

[SI units: Hct, 0.52; PaO_2, 6.67 kPa; $PaCO_2$, 8.0 kPa]

Sleep apnea is a breathing disorder characterized by frequent and prolonged pauses in breathing that occur during sleep.[158,159] Clinically important apnea periods generally last >15 seconds, occur repeatedly (>30 apnea episodes/night), and are associated with major reductions in arterial oxygen saturation. Three general types of apnea are described: central, obstructive, and mixed. The prevalence is estimated at 2% to 4% among middle-aged adults and is more common in obese individuals.[160] Because sleep apnea is underrecognized, the true prevalence may be significantly greater.

This syndrome is caused by disturbances of various mechanisms that maintain airway patency during sleep. Central apnea occurs because of cessation of CNS-mediated expiratory effort. Responsiveness to elevated CNS carbon dioxide concentrations (hypercapnia) is decreased, although normal responses to hypoxia are retained. During central apnea episodes, both inspiration and expiration are absent. Obstructive apnea occurs because of an occlusion in the upper airway (e.g., pharyngeal collapse), preventing airflow. There is normal inspiration (CNS-mediated) with an absence of expiration. Anatomic malformations in the upper airways and obesity are major contributing factors to obstructive apnea. Of these different forms of sleep apnea, obstructive apnea is the most prevalent, but many patients will exhibit mixed sleep apnea syndromes characterized by both obstructive and CNS components. A formal sleep study or polysomnogram is required to determine the cause.

Typical symptoms of sleep apnea syndrome include alterations in sleep pattern (sleep fragmentation) with loud snoring, gasping, or choking episodes during sleep; excessive daytime sleepiness; personality changes or cognitive difficulties related to fatigue; morning headaches; and severe shortness of breath with exertion. Sleep mates may describe episodes of no breathing followed by a heavy grunting snore as hypoxia finally stimulates breathing or the patient partially awakens. Objective signs are reduced sleep latency on electroencephalogram (EEG), pulmonary hypertension, hypoxemia, polycythemia, and hypertension.

The reported history and findings in B.V. are consistent with obstructive sleep apnea. A formal sleep study is required to confirm the diagnosis. If present, this study would reveal periods of airflow cessation of greater than 10 seconds despite ventilatory effort, at least 5 episodes each hour of sleep, and a drop in oxygen saturation of at least 4% during these episodes.[160] Several of the typical symptoms are present in this patient. His blood gases show carbon dioxide retention, and his hematocrit is elevated in an attempt to increase oxygen-carrying capacity in the blood. EEG studies have not been performed.

The risks of obstructive sleep apnea include hypertension, cardiac arrhythmias, pulmonary hypertension, heart failure, myocardial infarction, and stroke.[160,161] During periods of apnea, the arterial oxygen saturation falls and leads to local vasoconstriction in the lungs as a result of hypoxemia. Vasoconstriction leads to pulmonary hypertension, which ultimately leads to right-sided heart failure and then left-sided heart failure. This explains the enlarged heart shadow on chest radiograph and tachycardia noted in B.V.

Management

Continuous Positive Airway Pressure

27. B.V. is counseled to lose weight and has been recommended to begin continuous positive airway pressure (CPAP) therapy. Why is weight loss necessary? How is CPAP therapy administered, and what benefit does it provide?

Management approaches for the patient with sleep apnea include behavioral treatment, medical treatment, and surgery. Examples include removal of precipitating factors, CPAP breathing support, pharmacologic intervention, and surgery.[161] Simple measures should be tried first. Because many patients with sleep apnea are obese, weight loss is an essential intervention, especially if obstructive apnea is suspected. Even a 10% weight loss results in a significant decrease in the number of apneic episodes in obese patients. Patients' medications should be reviewed because respiratory depressants may worsen the problem. If possible, antihistamines, sedatives, hypnotics, or alcohol should be discontinued. Other secondary causes also should be ruled out, including hypothyroidism and heart failure. The only one of these interventions that applies to B.V. is the need for weight loss. Weight loss can significantly reduce the severity and frequency of episodes; even a small amount of weight loss provides dramatic benefit.

CPAP therapy has become the standard for treatment of obstructive sleep apnea.[159–161] This involves having the patient sleep with a nose or face mask connected to a mechanical device that delivers air or oxygen to the patient's nose throughout the night at a constant pressure that is greater than atmospheric pressure. The increased pressure is transferred to the pharynx, where it acts as a "pneumatic splint" to prevent the airway from collapsing.[159] CPAP is relatively noninvasive and often is associated with a rapid response for the patient. Symptoms of daytime sleepiness and secondary complications, such as pulmonary hypertension, dramatically improve. Adverse effects of CPAP include feelings of suffocation, excessive nasal drying, gas as a result of swallowed air, and conjunctivitis. While limiting patient tolerance of the procedure, these adverse effects are not contraindications to the use of CPAP.

CPAP machines weight about 5 pounds and can usually fit on a tabletop. Purchase costs for equipment range from $700 to $1,000, although many patients rent the machines. Usual application pressures range from 5 to 20 cm H_2O, but the optimal pressure is best tailored for individual patients in a sleep study laboratory. The goal is to establish a pressure for long-term treatment that is high enough to maintain patency of the upper airway to prevent most apneas and snoring while at the same time avoiding patient discomfort from noise, air leakage from around the mask into the eyes, and the sense of resistance to airflow during exhalation. The pressure used over time may change because of weight gain or loss, alterations in other medications, or changes in sleep patterns. A reduction in pressure may also be possible after several months of treatment. Usually, the device is used throughout the night, but some patients may use it for only a limited number of hours each night.

More recently, biphasic continuous positive airway pressure (BiPAP) has been used. This machine allows independent adjustment of pressure during inspiration and expiration, allowing lower pressures to be used in the latter instance. Because of several factors, including lower resistance to breath against during exhalation, this therapy may be tolerated better by the patient.[161] The equipment costs are two to three times that of CPAP equipment.

Other nonmedication treatments include the use of oral appliances that are worn during sleep. These devices typically manipulate tongue or mandible position to maintain airway patency. The patient's ability to tolerate these devices varies. Although the success of these therapies is widely variable, in general, fewer than 50% of patients benefit.

Drug Therapy

28. B.V. would like to avoid the cost and inconvenience of using CPAP. His doctor would like your advice regarding the value of pharmacologic agents to treat this problem. What is the role of drug therapy in obstructive sleep apnea?

Medications used to treat sleep apnea have been associated with limited benefit. Various antidepressants (e.g., protriptyline and fluoxetine) have been studied with disappointing results. The modest benefit is likely due to reductions in REM sleep in which muscle tone is decreased and obstruction is more likely.

Medroxyprogesterone and acetazolamide are both respiratory stimulants that are used in some patients with apnea. These agents are more appropriate and useful if there is a central (CNS) component of apnea. Acetazolamide stimulates ventilation by causing a metabolic acidosis, while progesterone increases ventilatory drive through stimulation of progesterone receptors in the hypothalamus.[162] Both agents have demonstrated beneficial effects on ABG parameters, although their role in obstructive sleep apnea is secondary.

Acetazolamide (Diamox), a carbonic anhydrase inhibitor, has been used to treat both central and obstructive sleep apnea

in normocapnic patients.[163–166] In addition to causing metabolic acidosis, it may exert a direct effects on brain chemoreceptor centers during long-term therapy because the body's compensatory buffering system generally corrects for drug-induced metabolic acidosis.[158] When given over a 1- to 2-week period at a dosage of 250 mg 4 times a day to six subjects with central apnea, acetazolamide produced a 69% reduction in total apnea periods.[163] At these relatively large doses, the blood pH dropped from 7.42 to 7.34. In another short-duration study, nine patients with predominantly obstructive apnea were given 250 mg of acetazolamide once daily for 1 week.[164] There was a reduction in both the number and duration of apnea episodes. A reasonable therapeutic trial of acetazolamide is 250 mg twice daily.

Medroxyprogesterone acetate (Provera) is a progestational hormone known to have respiratory stimulant properties in women during pregnancy. It may increase ventilatory response to both hypercapnia and hypoxia. It has been evaluated in a limited number of sleep apnea patients at dosages of 60 to 120 mg/day in 3 divided doses, but most patients have shown no difference in the number of nighttime apnea episodes when comparing baseline periods before therapy to active treatment with medroxyprogesterone.[161,167,168] It appears that normocapnic patients do not benefit, whereas those with hypercapnia may be more responsive secondary to an improved respiratory drive.[168] Side effects of medroxyprogesterone include sodium retention, weight gain, impotence in men, breast enlargement or tenderness, and a possible increased risk of thromboembolism.

B.V. has more of an obstructive presentation. However, central apnea cannot be ruled out from the information provided in the case. His $PaCO_2$ indicates an element of CO_2 retention. For these reasons, it is doubtful he will obtain a significant benefit from drug therapy and these options should be held in reserve in case he is intolerant or unwilling to use CPAP.

Surgical intervention may be necessary for patients with obstructive apnea who continue to have impairment despite CPAP and pharmacologic treatment. These procedures are directed toward bypassing the obstruction or preventing collapse of the tissue at the site of obstruction. Surgical options include tracheostomy and palatal or maxillofacial surgery. A tracheostomy bypasses the occlusion in the upper airway, but is not well accepted by patients because of cosmetic or psychologic reasons. Therefore, tracheostomy usually is reserved for patients whose conditions fail to respond to more conservative management. Uvulopalatopharyngoplasty involves surgical excision of excessive tissue in the oropharynx. Although this procedure has been used in some patients, it is associated with significant morbidity and has fallen out of favor in recent years. This can also be performed with lasers and is associated with fewer complications but its success if also variable.[161]

REFERENCES

1. Fabbri LM, et al. Global strategy for the diagnoses, management and prevention of chronic obstructive pulmonary disease (COPD): 2003 update. Ear Resp J 2003;22:1. Accessible at www.goldcopd.com
2. American Thoracic Society. Standards for the diagnosis and care of patients with chronic obstructive pulmonary disease. Am J Respir Crit Care Med 1995;152:s77.
3. NHLBI Data Fact Sheet. U.S. Department of Health and Human Services. Public Health Service. National Institutes of Health. May 2001. available at www.nhlbi.nih.gov/health/public/lung/other/copd_fact.htm.
4. Mannino DM. Chronic obstructive pulmonary disease surveillance: United States, 1971-2000. Sur-veillance Summaries, August 2, 2002. MMWR 2002;51(SS-6):1.
5. National Center for Health Statistics. Deaths: final data for 1999. Hyattsville, MD: U.S. Department of Health and Human Services, CDC, 2001. National Vital Statistics Report; 49: 8. Available at www.cdc.gov/nchs/releases/01facts/99mortality.htm.

6. Shopland DR. Tobacco use and its contribution to early cancer mortality with a special emphasis on cigarette smoking. Environ Health Perspect 1995; 103(Suppl 8):131.

7. Murray CJ, Lopez AD. Alternative projections of morbidity and disability by cause 1990-2020: Global burden of Disease Study. Lancet 1997; 349:1498.

8. Morbidity and Mortality: 2000 Chartbook on Cardiovascular, Lung and Blood Diseases. National Heart Lung and Blood Institute.

9. American Lung Association Fact Sheet: COPD March 2002. www.lungusa.org/diseases/copd_fact sheet.html.

10. Siafakas NM et al. A Consensus Statement of the European Respiratory Society. Optimal assessment and management of chronic obstructive pulmonary disease (COPD). Eur Respir J 1995;8:1398.

11. Standards of Care Committee of the British Thoracic Society. Summary of COPD Guidelines. Thorax 1997;52(Suppl 5):S1.

12. Lacasse Y. Critical appraisal of clinical practice guidelines targeting chronic obstructive pulmonary disease. Arch Intern Med 2001;161:69.

13. Ulrik CS, Backer V. Nonreversible airflow obstruction in lifelong nonsmokers with moderate to severe asthma. Eur Respir J 1999;14:892.

14. Becklake MR. Chronic airflow obstruction: its relationship to work in dusty occupations. Chest 1985;88:608.

15. Hogg JC. Chronic bronchitis: the role of viruses. Semin Respir Infect 2000;15:32.

16. Anthonisen MR et al. Effects of smoking intervention and the use of an inhaled anticholinergic bronchodilator on the rate of decline of FEV_1. JAMA 1994;272:1497.

17. Official Statement of the American Thoracic Society, Medical Section of the American Lung Association. Cigarette smoking and health. Am Rev Respir Dis 1985;132:1133.

18. Medici TC et al. Smoking pattern of smokers with and without tobacco-smoke related lung diseases. Am Rev Respir Dis 1985;131:385.

19. Madison J, Irwin R. Chronic obstructive pulmonary disease. Lancet 1998;352:467.

20. Jeffrey P. Structural and inflammatory changes in COPD: a comparison with asthma. Thorax 1998;53:129.

21. Keatings VM. Differences in interleukin 8 and tumor necrosis factor alpha in induced sputum from patients with chronic obstructive pulmonary disease or asthma. Am J Respir Crit Care Med 1996;153:530.

22. Hill AT et al. The interrelationship of sputum inflammatory markers in patients with chronic bronchitis. Am J Respir Crit Care Med 1999;160:893.

23. Barnes PJ. Chronic obstructive pulmonary disease. N Engl J Med 2000;343(4):269.

24. Beauchesne MF. Management of chronic obstructive pulmonary disease: a review. J Pharm Pract 2001;14(2):126.

25. Repine JE et al. Oxidative stress in chronic obstructive pulmonary disease. Am J Respir Crit Care Med 1997;156:341.

26. Humbert M. Airways inflammation in asthma and chronic bronchitis. Clin Exp Allergy 1996;26:735.

27. American Thoracic Society. Standardization of spirometry: 1994 update. Am J Respir Crit Care Med 1995;152:1107.

28. Ferguson GT, Cherniack RM. Management of chronic obstructive pulmonary disease. N Engl J Med 1993;328:1017.

29. Cooreman J et al. Mortality from chronic obstructive pulmonary disease and asthma in France, 1969-1983: comparison with the United States and Canada. Chest 1990;97(1):213.

30. Erbland ML et al. Interaction of hypoxia and hypercapnia on respiratory drive in patients with COPD. Chest 1990;97(6):1289.

31. Weinberger SE et al. Mechanisms of disease: hypercapnia. N Engl J Med 1989;321(18):1223.

32. Salman GF. Rehabilitation for patients with chronic obstructive pulmonary disease: meta-analysis of randomized controlled trials. J Gen Intern Med 2003;18:213.

33. Wilson DO et al. Nutrition and chronic lung disease. Am Rev Respir Dis 1985;132:1347.

34. Petty TL. The National Mucolytic Study: results of a double-blind, placebo-controlled study of iodinated glycerol in chronic obstructive bronchitis. Chest 1990;97:75.

35. Poole PJ, Black PN. Oral mucolytic drugs for exacerbations of chronic obstructive pulmonary disease: systematic review. BMJ 2001:322:1.

36. Gross NJ. Outcome measurements in COPD: are we schizophrenic? Chest 2003;123:1325.

37. Anthonisen NR et al. Bronchodilator response in chronic obstructive pulmonary disease. Am Rev Respir Dis 1986;133:814.

38. Gross NJ. The influence of anticholinergic agents on treatment for bronchitis and emphysema. Am J Med 1991;91(Suppl 4A):11S.

39. Lakshminarayan S. Ipratropium bromide in chronic bronchitis/emphysema: a review of the literature. Am J Med 1986;(Suppl 5A)81:76.

40. O'Donnell DE, Webb KA. Breathlessness in patients with severe chronic airflow limitation: physiologic correlations. Chest 1992;102(3):824.

41. Belman MJ et al. Variability of breathlessness measurement in patients with chronic obstructive pulmonary disease. Chest 1991;99(3): 566.

42. Nisar M et al. Acute bronchodilator trials in chronic obstructive pulmonary disease. Am Rev Respir Dis 1992;146:555.

43. Vassallo R, Lipsky J. Theophylline: recent advances in the understanding of its mode of action and uses in clinical practice. Mayo Clin Proc 1998; 73:346.

44. Ramsdell J. Use of theophylline in the treatment of COPD. Chest 1995;107:206S.

45. Barnes PJ. Theophylline: new perspectives for an old drug. Am J Respir Crit Care Med 2003; 167:813.

46. Callahan CM et al. Oral corticosteroid therapy for patients with stable chronic obstructive pulmonary disease: a meta-analysis. Ann Intern Med 1993;118:770.

47. Hudson LD, Monti CM. Rationale and use of corticosteroids in chronic obstructive pulmonary disease. Med Clin North Am 1990;74(3):661.

48. Renkema TE et al. Effects of long term treatment with corticosteroids in COPD. Chest 1996;109: 1156.

49. Eliasson O et al. Corticosteroids in COPD: a clinical trial and reassessment of the literature. Chest 1986;89:484.

50. Vestbo J et al. Long-term effect of inhaled budesonide in mild and moderate chronic obstructive pulmonary disease: a randomized controlled trial. Lancet 1999;353:1819.

51. Pauwels RA et al. Long-term treatment with inhaled budesonide in persons with mild chronic obstructive pulmonary disease who continue smoking. N Engl J Med 1999;340:1948.

52. Burge PS et al. Randomized, double-blind, placebo controlled study of fluticasone propionate in patients with moderate to severe chronic obstructive pulmonary disease: the ISOLDE trial. BMJ 2000;320:1297.

53. The Lung Health Study Research Group. Effect of inhaled triamcinolone on the decline in pulmonary function in chronic obstructive pulmonary disease. N Engl J Med 2000;343:1902.

54. Anthonisen N et al. Antibiotic therapy in exacerbations of chronic obstructive pulmonary disease. Ann Intern Med 1987;106:196.

55. Saint S et al. Antibiotics in chronic obstructive pulmonary disease exacerbations: a meta analysis. JAMA 1995;273:957.

56. Tarpy S, Celli B. Long-term oxygen therapy. N Engl J Med 1995;333:710.

57. Skwarski K et al. Predictors of survival in patients with chronic obstructive pulmonary disease treated with long-term oxygen therapy. Chest 1991; 100(6):1522.

58. Medical Research Council Working Party. Long-term domiciliary oxygen therapy in chronic hypoxic cor pulmonale complicating chronic bronchitis and emphysema. Lancet 1981;1:681.

59. Nocturnal Oxygen Therapy Trial Group. Continuous or nocturnal oxygen therapy in hypoxemic chronic obstructive lung disease. Ann Intern Med 1980;93:391.

60. Klinger JR, Hill NS. Right ventricular dysfunction in chronic obstructive pulmonary disease: evaluation and management. Chest 1991;99:715.

61. Stoller JK. Acute exacerbations of chronic obstructive pulmonary disease. N Engl J Med 2002; 346:988.

62. Rennard SI. COPD: overview of definitions, epidemiology, and factors influencing its development. Chest 1998;113(Suppl 4):s235.

63. Anthonisen NR. Prognosis in chronic obstructive pulmonary disease: results from multicenter clinical trials. Am Rev Respir Dis 1989;140:S95.

64. Owens GR. Public screening for lung disease: experience with the NIH lung health study. Am J Med 1991;91(Suppl 4A):37S.

65. Fiore MC et al. Treating Tobacco Use and Dependence, Clinical Practice Guideline. Rockville, MD: U.S. Department of Health and Human Services, Public Health Service, 2000.

66. Lancaster T et al. Training health professionals in smoking cessation. Cochrane Database Syst Rev 2000;3:CD000214.

67. Secker-Walker RH et al. The role of health professionals in a community-based program to help women quit smoking. Prev Med 2000;30:126.

68. West R et al. Smoking cessation guidelines for health professionals: an update. Thorax 2000;55: 987.

69. Williams JH, Moser KN. Pneumococcal vaccine and patients with chronic lung disease. Ann Intern Med 1986;104:106.

70. McFadden ER Jr. Clinical use of β-adrenergic agonists. J Allergy Clin Immunol 1985;76:352.

71. Suissa S et al. Inhaled short acting beta agonist use in COPD and the risk of acute myocardial infarction. Thorax 2003;58:43.

72. Gross NJ, Skorodin MS. Role of the parasympathetic system in airway obstruction due to emphysema. N Engl J Med 1984;311:421.

73. Braun S et al. A comparison of the effect of ipratropium and albuterol in the treatment of chronic obstructive airway disease. Arch Intern Med 1989; 149:544.

74. Blosser S et al. Is an anticholinergic agent superior to a β_2-agonist in improving dyspnea and exercise limitation in COPD. Chest 1995;108:730.

75. Wesseling G et al. A comparison of the effects of anticholinergic and β_2-agonist and combination therapy on respiratory impedance in COPD. Chest 1992;101(1):166.

76. Kradjan W et al. Atropine serum concentrations after multiple inhaled doses of atropine sulfate. Clin Pharmacol Ther 1985;38:12.

77. Rennard S et al. Extended therapy with ipratropium is associated with improved lung function in patients with COPD: a retrospective analysis of data from seven clinical trials. Chest 1996;110:62.

78. Bellman MJ et al. Inhaled bronchodilators reduce dynamic hyperinflation during exercise in patients with chronic obstructive pulmonary disease. Am J Respir Crit Care Med 1996;153:967.

79. Ziment I. The β-agonist controversy: impact in COPD. Chest 1995;107:198s.

80. van Schayck CP et al. Two year bronchodilator treatment in patients with mild airflow obstruction: contradictory effects on lung function and quality of life. Chest 1992;102:1384.

81. van Schayck CP et al. Continuous and on demand use of bronchodilators in patients with non-steroid dependent asthma and chronic bronchitis: 4-year follow-up randomized study. Br J Gen Pract 1995;45:239.

82. Cook D et al. Regular versus as-needed short-acting inhaled β_2-agonist therapy for chronic obstructive

pulmonary disease. Am J Respir Crit Care Med 2001;163(1):85.

83. Ram FSF, Sestini P. Regular inhaled short acting β₂-agonists for the management of stable chronic obstructive pulmonary disease: Cochrane systematic review and meta-analysis. Thorax 2003; 58:580.

84. Dorinsky PM et al. The combination of ipratropium and albuterol optimizes pulmonary function reversibility testing in patients with COPD. Chest 1999;115:966.

85. Combivent Inhalation Aerosol Study Group. In chronic obstructive pulmonary disease, a combination of ipratropium and albuterol is more effective than either agent alone: an 85-day multicenter trial. Chest 1994;105:1411.

86. van Noord JA et al. Long-term treatment of chronic obstructive pulmonary disease with salmeterol and the additive effect of ipratropium. Eur Respir J 2000;15:878.

87. Karpel J et al. A comparison of inhaled ipratropium, oral theophylline plus inhaled β-agonist, and the combination of all three in patients with COPD. Chest 1994;105:1089.

88. The Combivent Inhalation Solution Study Group. Routine nebulized ipratropium and albuterol together are better than either drug alone in COPD. Chest 1997;112:1514.

89. Campbell S. For COPD a combination of ipratropium bromide and albuterol sulfate is more effective than albuterol base alone. Arch Intern Med 1999;159:156.

90. Friedman M et al. Pharmacoeconomic evaluation of a combination of ipratropium plus albuterol compared with ipratropium alone and albuterol alone in COPD. Chest 1999;115:635.

91. Gross N et al. Inhalation by nebulization of albuterol-ipratropium combination (Dey combination) is superior to either agent alone in the treatment of chronic obstructive pulmonary disease. Respiration 1998;65:354.

92. Deltorre L et al. Effectiveness of salmeterol in patients with emphysema. Curr Ther Res 1992;52: 888.

93. Cazzola M et al. Effect of salmeterol and formoterol in patients with chronic obstructive pulmonary disease. Pulmon Pharmacol 1994;7:103.

94. Ramirez-Venegas A et al. Salmeterol reduces dyspnea and improves lung function in patients with COPD. Chest 1997;112:336.

95. Matera MG et al. A comparison of the bronchodilating effects of salmeterol, salbutamol, and ipratropium bromide in patients with chronic obstructive pulmonary disease. Pulmon Pharmacol 1995,8:267.

96. Cazzola M et al. A comparison of the bronchodilating effects of salmeterol and oxitropium bromide in stable chronic obstructive pulmonary disease. Respir Med 1998;92:354.

97. Ulrik CS. Efficacy of inhaled salmeterol in the management of smokers with chronic obstructive pulmonary disease: a single center randomised, double blind, placebo controlled, crossover study. Thorax 1995;50:750.

98. Boyd G et al. An evaluation of salmeterol in the treatment of chronic obstructive pulmonary disease (COPD). Eur Respir J 1997;10:815.

99. Jones PW, Bosh TK. Quality of life changes in COPD patients treated with salmeterol. Am J Respir Crit Care Med 1997;155:1283.

100. Mahler DA et al. Efficacy of salmeterol xinafoate in the treatment of COPD. Chest 1999;115:957.

101. Dahl R et al. Inhaled formoterol dry powder versus ipratropium bromide in chronic obstructive pulmonary disease. Am J Respir Crit Care Med 2001;164:778.

102. Rennard SI et al. Use of a long-acting inhaled β₂-adrenergic agonist, salmeterol xinafoate, in patients with chronic obstructive pulmonary disease. Am J Respir Crit Care Med 2001;163;1087.

103. D'Urzo AD et al. In patients with COPD, treatment with a combination of formoterol and ipratropium is more effective than a combination of salbutamol and ipratropium. Chest 2001;119:1347.

104. Appleton S et al. Long-acting β₂-agonists for chronic obstructive pulmonary disease patients with poorly reversible airflow limitation (Cochrane review). In: The Cochrane Library, Issue 1, 2003. Oxford: Update Software.

105. Ferguson GT et al. Cardiovascular safety of salmeterol in COPD. Chest 2003;123:1817.

106. Barnes PJ. New treatments for COPD. Nat Rev 2002;1:437.

107. Barnes PJ. The pharmacological action of tiotropium. Chest 2004;117:63s.

108. Norman P, Graul A. Tiotropium bromide. Drugs of the future 2000;25(7):693.

109. Van Noord JA et al. A randomized controlled comparison of tiotropium and ipratropium in the treatment of chronic obstructive pulmonary disease. Thorax 2000;55:289.

110. Casaburi R et al. A long-term evaluation of once daily inhaled tiotropium in chronic obstructive pulmonary disease. Eur Respir J 2002;19:217.

111. Tashkin D, Kesten S. Long-term treatment benefits with tiotropium in COPD patients with and without short-term bronchodilator responses. Chest 2003;123:1441.

112. Donohue JF et al. A 6-month placebo-controlled study comparing lung function and health status changes in COPD patients treated with tiotropium or salmeterol. Chest 2002;122:47.

113. Tsukino M et al. Effects of aminophylline and ipratropium bromide on exercise performance in patients with stable chronic obstructive pulmonary disease. Thorax 1998;53:269.

114. Murciano D et al. A randomized controlled trial of theophylline in patients with severe chronic obstructive pulmonary disease. N Engl J Med 1989;320:1521.

115. Kirsten D et al. Effects of theophylline withdrawal in severe chronic obstructive pulmonary disease. Chest 1993;104.1101.

116. Vassallo R, Lipsky J. Theophylline: recent advances in the understanding of its mode of action and uses in clinical practice. Mayo Clin Proc 1998;73:346.

117. Weinberger M, Hendeles L. Drug therapy: theophylline in asthma. N Engl J Med 1996; 334:1380.

118. Parent M, LeBel M. Meta-analysis of quinolone-theophylline interactions. DICP Ann Pharmacother 1991;25:191.

119. Hansten PD, Horn JR. Drug interactions analysis and management. Vancouver, WA: Applied Therapeutics, 1999:480.

120. Rice KL et al. Withdrawal of chronic systemic corticosteroids in patients with COPD: a randomized trial. Am J Respir Crit Care Med 2000;162(1):174.

121. Decramer M et al. Corticosteroids contribute to muscle weakness in chronic airflow obstruction. Am J Respir Crit Care Med 1994;150:11.

122. Van Schayck CP et al. Do patients with COPD benefit from treatment with inhaled corticosteroids? Eur Respir J 1996;9:1969.

123. Shim CS, Williams MH Jr. Aerosol beclomethasone in patients with steroid responsive chronic obstructive pulmonary disease. Am J Med 1985;78:655.

124. Bourbeau JR et al. A double blind randomized study of inhaled budesonide in patients with steroid responsive COPD. Am Rev Respir Dis 1993;147:A317.

125. Thompson AB et al. Aerosolized beclomethasone in chronic bronchitis: improved pulmonary function and diminished airway inflammation. Am Rev Respir Dis 1992;146:389.

126. Weiner P et al. Inhaled budesonide therapy for patients with stable COPD. Chest 1995;108:1568.

127. Bourbeau J et al. Randomized controlled trial of inhaled corticosteroids in patients with chronic obstructive pulmonary disease. Thorax 1998;53:477.

128. Overbeck S et al. Is delayed introduction of inhaled corticosteroids harmful in patients with obstructive airways disease (asthma and COPD)? Chest 1996;110:35.

129. Weir DC et al. Time course of response to oral and inhaled corticosteroids in non-asthmatic chronic airflow obstruction. Thorax 1990;45:118.

130. Paggiaro PL et al. Multicentre randomized placebo controlled trial of inhaled fluticasone propionate in patients with chronic obstructive pulmonary disease. Lancet 1998;351:773.

131. Highland KB et al. Long-term effects of inhaled corticosteroids on FEV₁ in patients with chronic obstructive pulmonary disease. A meta-analysis. Ann Intern Med 2003;138(12):969.

132. Sin DD, Tu JV. Inhaled corticosteroids and the risk of mortality and readmission in elderly patients with chronic obstructive pulmonary disease. Am J Respir Crit Care Med 2001;164:580.

133. Senderovitz T et al. Steroid reversibility testing followed by inhaled budesonide or placebo in outpatients with stable chronic obstructive pulmonary disease. The Danish Society of Respiratory Medicine. Respir Med 1999;93:715.

134. van der Valk P et al. Effect of discontinuation of inhaled corticosteroid in patients with chronic obstructive pulmonary disease. Am J Respir Crit Care Med 2002;166:1358.

135. Cazzola M et al. Additive effects of salmeterol and fluticasone or theophylline in COPD. Chest 2000;118:1576.

136. Calverley P et al. Combined salmeterol and fluticasone in the treatment of chronic obstructive pulmonary disease: a randomized controlled trial. Lancet 2003;361:449.

137. Hanania NA et al. The efficacy and safety of fluticasone propionate (250 μg)/salmeterol (50 μg) combined in the diskus inhaler for the treatment of COPD. Chest 2003;124:834.

138. Tarpy S, Celli B. Long-term oxygen therapy. N Engl J Med 1995;333:710.

139. Medical Research Council Working Party. Long-term domiciliary oxygen therapy in chronic hypoxic cor pulmonale complicating chronic bronchitis and emphysema. Lancet 1981;1:681.

140. Nocturnal Oxygen Therapy Trial Group. Continuous or nocturnal oxygen therapy in hypoxemic chronic obstructive lung disease. Ann Intern Med 1980;93:391.

141. Skwarski K et al. Predictors of survival in patients with chronic obstructive pulmonary disease treated with long-term oxygen therapy. Chest 1991;100(6):1522.

142. Rodriguez-Roisin R. Toward a consensus definition for COPD exacerbations. Chest 2000; 117(Suppl 2):398s.

143. Seemungal TAR et al. Time course and recovery of exacerbations in patients with chronic obstructive pulmonary disease. Am J Respir Crit Care Med 2000;161:1608.

144. Connors AF Jr et al. Outcomes following acute exacerbations of severe chronic obstructive lung disease. Am J Respir Crit Care Med 1996; 154:959.

145. Bach PB et al. Management of acute exacerbations of chronic obstructive pulmonary disease: a summary and appraisal of published evidence. Ann Intern Med 2001;134:600.

146. McCrory DC et al. Management of acute exacerbations of COPD: a summary and appraisal of the published evidence. Chest 2001;119:1190.

147. Snow V et al. Evidence base for management of acute exacerbations of chronic obstructive pulmonary disease. Ann Intern Med 2001;134: 595.

148. McCrory DC, Brown CD. Meta-analysis: Anticholinergic bronchodilators versus β₂-sympathomimetic agents for acute exacerbations of chronic obstructive pulmonary disease. Cochrane Database Syst Rev 2002;(4):CD003900.

149. Turner MO et al. Bronchodilator delivery in acute airflow obstruction-a meta-analysis. Arch Intern Med 1997;157:1736.

150. Barr RG et al. Methylxanthines for exacerbations of chronic obstructive pulmonary disease. Cochrane Database Syst Rev 2003;(2):CD002168.

151. Niewoehner DE et al. Effect of systemic glucocorticoids on exacerbations of chronic obstructive pulmonary disease. N Engl J Med 1999;340:1941.

152. Davies L et al. Oral corticosteroids in patients admitted to hospital with exacerbation of chronic obstructive pulmonary disease: a prospective randomized controlled trial. Lancet 1999;354:456.

153. Aaron SD et al. Outpatient oral prednisone after emergency treatment of chronic obstructive pulmonary disease. N Engl J Med 2003;348:2618.

154. Barnes PJ. New concepts in chronic obstructive pulmonary disease. Annu Rev Med 2003;54:113.

155. Compton CH et al. Cilomilast, a selective phosphodiesterase-4 inhibitor for treatment of patients with chronic obstructive pulmonary disease: a randomized dose-ranging study. Lancet 2001; 358:265.

156. Meyers BF, Patterson GA. Chronic obstructive pulmonary disease 10: bullectomy, lung volume reduction surgery, and transplantation for patients with chronic obstructive pulmonary disease. Thorax 2003;58:634.

157. National Emphysema Treatment Trial Research Group. A randomized trial comparing lung volume reduction surgery with medical therapy for severe emphysema. N Engl J Med 2003;348:2059.

158. DeBacker WA. Central sleep apnoea, pathogenesis, and treatment: an overview and perspective. Eur Respir J 1995;8:1372.

159. American Thoracic Society. Indications and standards for use of nasal continuous positive airway pressure in sleep apnea syndromes. Am J Respir Care Crit Care Med 1994;150:1738.

160. Young T et al. The occurrence of sleep-disordered breathing among middle-aged adults. N Engl J Med 1993;328:1230.

161. Strollo PJ, Roger RM. Obstructive sleep apnea. N Engl J Med 1996;334:99.

162. Wagenaar M et al. Comparison of acetazolamide and medroxyprogesterone as respiratory stimulants in hypercapnic patients with COPD. Chest 2003;123:1450.

163. White DP et al. Central sleep apnea: improvement with acetazolamide therapy. Arch Intern Med 1982;142:1816.

164. Tojima H et al. Effects of acetazolamide in patients with sleep apnea syndrome. Thorax 1988;43:113.

165. DeBacker WA et al. Central apnea index decreases after prolonged treatment with acetazolamide. Am J Respir Crit Care Med 1995;151:87.

166. Verbraecken J et al. Central sleep apnea after interrupting long term acetazolamide administration. Am Rev Respir Dis 1994;4:A929.

167. Hudgel D, Thanakitcharu S. Pharmacologic treatment of sleep-disordered breathing. Am J Respir Crit Care Med 1998;158:691.

168. Rajagopal KR et al. Effects of medroxyprogesterone acetate in obstructive sleep apnea. Chest 1986;90(6):815.

CHAPTER 25

Acute and Chronic Rhinitis

Tina Penick Brock, Dennis M. Williams

Definitions

Rhinitis is an inflammatory condition affecting the mucous membranes of the nose and upper respiratory system. The term is used broadly to encompass a syndrome of nasal symptoms characterized by periods of discharge (rhinorrhea), itching (pruritus), sneezing, congestion, and postnasal drainage. These nasal symptoms can be accompanied by ocular itching and discharge and can be exacerbated by the development/presence of sinusitis.[1,2] The most common form of rhinitis occurs in response to an allergen, although a variety of other causes have been demonstrated as well.

Practice parameters for the diagnosis and management of allergic and nonallergic rhinitis were developed and published in 1998 by a Joint Task Force representing the American Academy of Allergy, Asthma and Immunology (AAAAI), the American College of Allergy, Asthma and Immunology (ACAAI), and the Joint Council on Allergy, Asthma and Immunology.[1] In addition, the European Academy of Allergology and Clinical Immunology published a consensus state-

ment on the treatment of allergic rhinitis in 2000.[2] Most recently, evidence linking asthma and allergic rhinitis epidemiologically, pathologically and physiologically has been published.[3] These data support the tenet that upper respiratory allergic disorders and asthma may represent components of a single inflammatory airway syndrome.[4,5]

Prevalence

Relative to asthma, the literature surrounding the prevalence and cost of illness of rhinitis is rather modest and much of the data reported are associated with the allergic form of the disease.[6] Although rhinitis does not lead to the mortality associated with some common illnesses, the prevalence and negative health impact make it an important health problem in the United States.

Rhinitis is the most common allergic disorder, affecting up to 30% of adults and up to 40% of children in the United States.[7] Estimates suggest that 20 to 40 million people, excluding asthmatics with concomitant disease, experience seasonal symptoms.[8,9] Reported rates of allergic rhinitis vary, in part, because researchers' definitions and physicians' methods of diagnosing differ. In addition, rates can vary among different groups of people and even across an individual's lifetime, with symptoms being more likely to begin in childhood through young adulthood. Because rhinitis in its mildest form is largely self-managed, it is likely that health statistics underrepresent the actual scope of the problem[10] and that, in fact, the prevalence of rhinitis is increasing.[11]

In 1996, the estimated direct cost of treating allergic rhinitis in the United States was $3.4 billion, including approximately $1.6 billion for prescription medications and $1.8 billion for physician visits.[12] Considering that the prescription sales of nonsedating antihistamines alone in 2000 were $4.5 billion, the current costs are likely substantially higher.[12] These figures do not include costs spent in self-treatment, including over-the-counter medications, which are estimated to be similar to prescription expenditures.[13]

Rhinitis can lead to sleep disorders, loss of appetite, general weakness, fatigue, mood disorders, decreased concentration and difficulty learning.[1] Allergic rhinitis accounts for up to 3.5 million lost work days and 2 million missed school days.[14] The effects of indirect costs due to lost productivity or the treatment costs for complications are significant. Clearly, acute and chronic rhinitis greatly impact the physical, economic, and educational health of Americans.

Applied Anatomy and Physiology of the Nose

An understanding of the anatomy and physiology of the nose is helpful in understanding the pathophysiology and presentation of rhinitis, as well as the rationale for various pharmacotherapeutic approaches. The primary functions of the nose are smell, speech, and conditioning of inspired air. Related to the latter, the nose and upper airway warm, humidify, and filter air for delivery to the lungs.[15]

The external nose is pyramidal and consists of paired nasal bones and associated cartilage. Its base has two elliptical shaped openings called nares, or nostrils. Internally, a septum separates the nasal cavity into two halves and consists of bone and cartilage covered by a mucosal membrane.[16] The lateral walls of the internal cavity contain the conchae, or turbinates. These bony projections increase surface area substantially and contribute to turbulence of airflow, which is useful in filtering and conditioning inspired air. Sinuses and eustachian tubes open into the nasal cavity near the turbinates, as do the lacrimal drainage ducts. Figure 25-1 shows a lateral view of the head with the nasal anatomy labeled.

The membranes of the nasal cavity consist primarily of ciliated columnar epithelial cells with mucus-producing goblet cells interspersed among them. The tiny cilia beat rhythmically to transport mucus across the upper airway membrane to the nasopharynx. The cilia-lined mucous membranes of the nose provide a physical barrier of defense to microorganisms and other particles in the inspired air.[15] In addition, respiratory secretions residing on these mucous membranes contain immunoglobulin A (IgA), which serves as an immunologic defense.[16]

The autonomic nervous system controls the vascular supply and the secretion of mucus to the nasal membrane. Sympathetic activation results in vasoconstriction, which decreases nasal airway resistance. Parasympathetic stimulation results in glandular secretion and nasal congestion.[17] The mucosa is also innervated by the nonadrenergic/noncholinergic system (NANC). Neuropeptides from these nerves (e.g., substance P and neurokinins) play a role in vasodilation, mucus production and inflammation, although their significance is unclear. The trigeminal nerve also provides sensory innervation; the stimulation of which can result in sneezing and itching.[5,17]

During normal breathing, inspired air flows through the external nose before turning posteriorly almost 90 degrees into the nasopharynx. The airstream then makes another right angle turn through the pharynx and larynx toward the lower airway. The upper airway diameter is extremely narrow in places, allowing for close contact between inhaled air and mucosal surfaces. Under normal conditions, turbinates in either side of the nasal cavity swell or contract alternately, resulting in preferential airflow through the right or left nasal cavity. This process is disrupted in the presence of inflammation and congestion. Normal nasal physiology is also affected by the

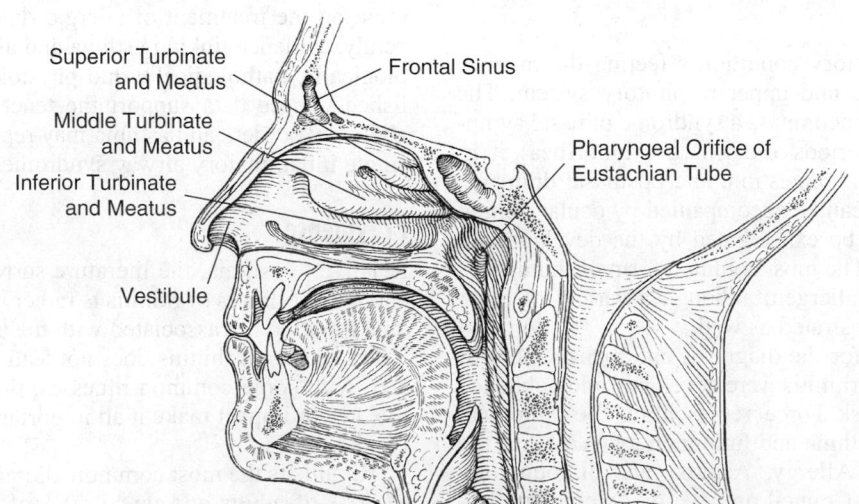

FIGURE 25-1 *Lateral view of the head with nasal anatomy.* (Reprinted with permission from the LifeArt Human Anatomy II collection.)

presence of anatomic deformities including septal deviation and/or nasal polyps.[16]

CLASSIFICATION OF RHINITIS

Rhinitis is not a single disease but rather has multiple etiologies and underlying pathophysiologic mechanisms.[7,18] Figure 25-2 depicts the common causes of acute and chronic rhinitis. Strictly speaking, some of the items in this figure are not causes of rhinitis, but rather disorders (e.g., nasal septal deviation, foreign body) that cause symptoms that mimic the inflammatory disorders of the nose.

Acute

The most common cause of acute rhinitis is viral upper respiratory infection or the common cold.[1] A bacterial infection should be suspected if the acute "cold-like" symptoms of rhinorrhea or nasal obstruction persist for more than 5 days.[1] Nasal foreign bodies, especially in young children, should be suspected when patients present with unilateral symptoms.[15] Hormonal causes of acute vasomotor rhinitis, usually associated with a clear, watery discharge without other symptoms, include hypothyroidism and pregnancy.[17] Finally, the development of rhinitis-like symptoms has been attributed to some medications. Angiotensin-converting enzyme inhibitor (ACEI)s, β-blockers, reserpine, nonsteroidal anti-inflammatory drugs (NSAIDs), oral contraceptives, and topical decongestants all have been associated with these effects.[17]

Chronic

Chronic rhinitis can be classified as allergic or nonallergic. Allergic causes are typically associated with atopy, an inherited tendency to develop a clinical hypersensitivity condition. Traditionally, allergic rhinitis has been classified as seasonal or perennial, depending on the frequency of symptoms and the allergen responsible. More recently, a system has been proposed that classifies allergic rhinitis as either intermittent or persistent based on frequency of symptoms.[5] This nomenclature more closely follows the asthma classifications as well as better describes patients who experience both seasonal and perennial symptoms. Patients with intermittent or persistent allergic rhinitis can experience symptoms ranging from mild to severe. This classification system is summarized in Figure 25-3.

Nonallergic causes of chronic rhinitis are classified as idiopathic rhinitis, nonallergic rhinitis with eosinophilia (NARES) or as anatomic abnormalities. Idiopathic rhinitis, also called vasomotor rhinitis, refers to symptoms associated with environmental stimuli including temperature changes, strong odors, tobacco smoke, stress or emotional factors. NARES occurs frequently in middle-aged patients without evidence of allergic disease except for the presence of eosinophils in the nasal smear. In these cases, increased permeability of the nasal mucosa is likely to be due to non–IgE-mediated inflammation, and neurogenic mechanisms may play a role in membrane hyperreactivity.[19]

Common anatomic causes of chronic rhinitis include nasal septum deviation, nasal polyps, tumors, choanal atresia (a congenital condition where the mouth and nose are not connected), and enlarged adenoids and tonsils. Often these anatomic abnormalities require surgical intervention.[15,17]

ETIOLOGY OF ALLERGIC RHINITIS

Both genetic factors and environmental influences are associated with the development of allergic rhinitis. Atopy is a significant predisposing factor, and the risk of a child developing allergic symptoms is 50% with one atopic parent and 66% with two atopic parents.[20] However, environmental exposures, particularly early in life are also important in the development of symptomatology.[21]

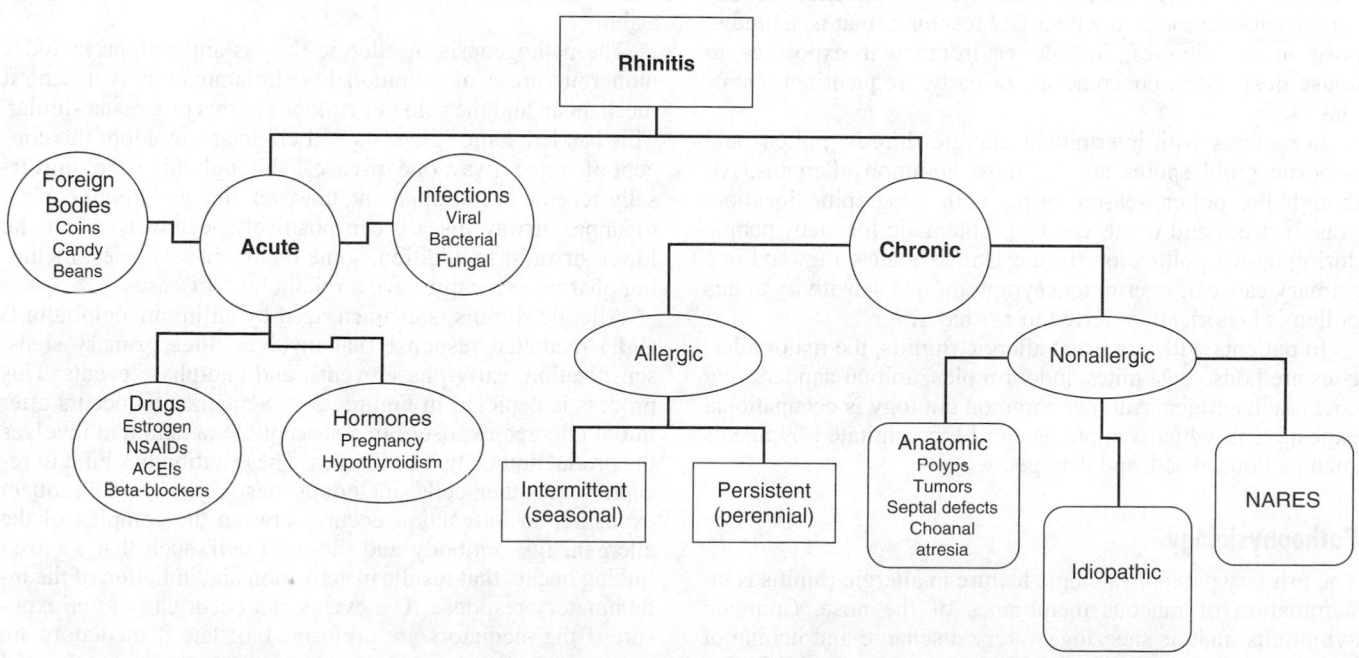

FIGURE 25-2 Possible causes of acute and chronic rhinitis. NSAIDs, nonsteroidal anti-inflammatory drugs; ACEIs, angiotensin-converting enzyme inhibitors; NARES, nonallergic rhinitis with eosinophilia syndrome.

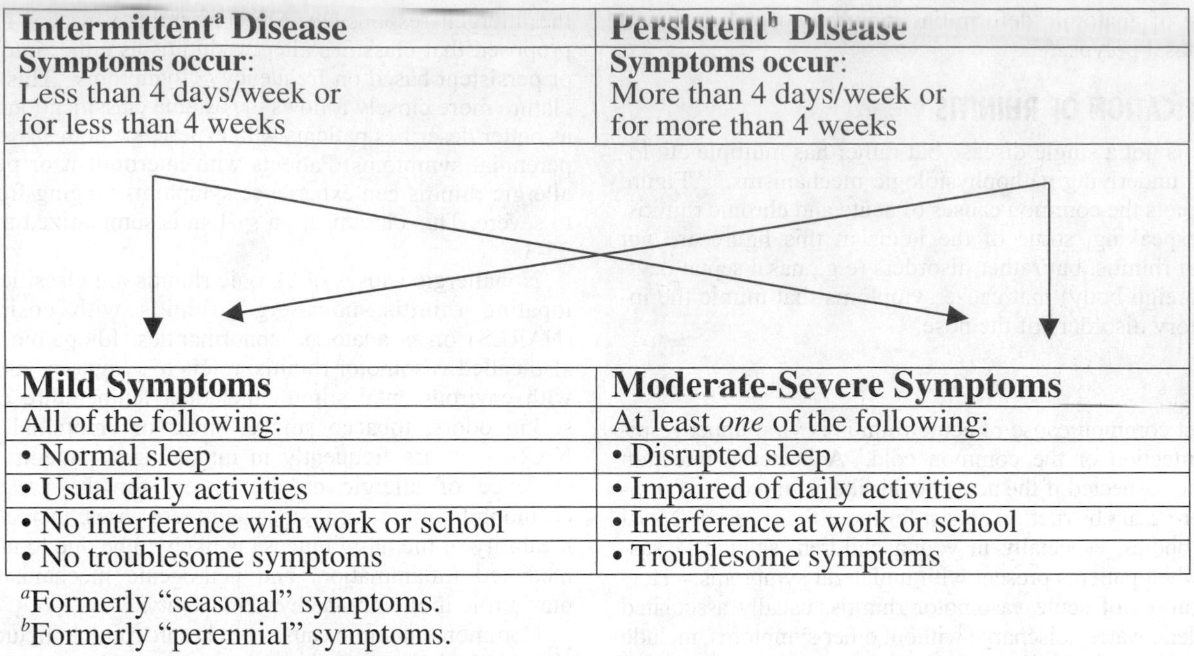

Intermittent[a] Disease	Persistent[b] Disease
Symptoms occur: Less than 4 days/week or for less than 4 weeks	Symptoms occur: More than 4 days/week or for more than 4 weeks

Mild Symptoms	Moderate-Severe Symptoms
All of the following:	At least *one* of the following:
• Normal sleep	• Disrupted sleep
• Usual daily activities	• Impaired of daily activities
• No interference with work or school	• Interference at work or school
• No troublesome symptoms	• Troublesome symptoms

[a]Formerly "seasonal" symptoms.
[b]Formerly "perennial" symptoms.

FIGURE 25-3 ARIA Classification of allergic rhinitis. ARIA, Allergic rhinitis and its impact on asthma. (Adapted from reference 5.)

One theory, referred to as the hygiene hypothesis, is that the initial differentiation of lymphocytes early in life has either positive or negative influences on the development of subsequent allergies. In the normal development of the immune system Th0 lymphocytes differentiate into either Th1 or Th2 cells based on environmental stimuli. Factors associated with a Th1 response, that is, protective against allergic conditions, include exposures to various bacteria and viruses, the presence of older siblings, and early attendance in day care. Factors associated with a Th2 response, that is, a predisposition to allergies, include environmental exposures to house dust mites, cockroaches, or early, frequent antimicrobial use.[22]

In patients with intermittent allergic rhinitis, pollens and airborne mold spores are the most common allergens. Although the pollen season varies with geographic location, grasses, trees and weeds can be problematic for many people during active pollination. In the United States, ragweed is a primary cause of intermittent symptoms and sensitivity to this pollen is historically referred to as "hay fever."

In patients with persistent allergic rhinitis, the major allergens are house dust mites, indoor molds, animal danders, and cockroach antigen. Another common etiology is occupational exposure, in which symptoms can be precipitated by agents such as flour, wood, and detergents.

Pathophysiology

The primary pathophysiologic feature in allergic rhinitis is inflammation of mucous membranes of the nose. Common symptoms include sneezing, watery discharge and itching of the nose and eyes, nasal obstruction, and postnasal dripping of secretions.[1,9]

The understanding of the pathophysiology of allergic rhinitis has improved over the last decade. There has been increasing interest in considering the relationship between the upper and lower respiratory tracts, because allergic rhinitis and asthma often coexist. Further evidence of an association includes the following: rhinitis is known to be a risk factor for asthma, some patients with rhinitis exhibit bronchial hyperresponsiveness, viral upper respiratory infections are a common cause of asthma exacerbations, and sinusitis may worsen asthma.[5]

The pathogenesis of allergic rhinitis and asthma includes numerous areas of commonality. Inflammation is a central mechanism and the role of cytokines in this process is similar. This has led some scientists and clinicians to adopt the concept of "one airway, one disease," although this is not universally accepted.[5] It is apparent, however, that good/poor control of upper airway disease can positively/negatively affect the lower airways. In addition, some treatment strategies, including pharmacotherapy, have a role in both diseases.

Allergic rhinitis is characterized by an immunoglobulin E (IgE)–mediated response that involves three primary steps: sensitization, early-phase events, and late-phase events. This process is depicted in Figure 25-4. Sensitization occurs after initial allergen exposure in a susceptible patient and involves the production of IgE antibodies. These antibodies bind to receptors on other cells, including mast cells. On subsequent exposure, an interaction occurs between the complex of the allergen, IgE antibody and the mast cell, such that a cross-linking occurs that results in activation and initiation of the inflammatory response. The events can occur early after exposure if the mediators are preformed, or late if mediators are synthesized after the process begins or are attracted to the area through chemotaxis.[23]

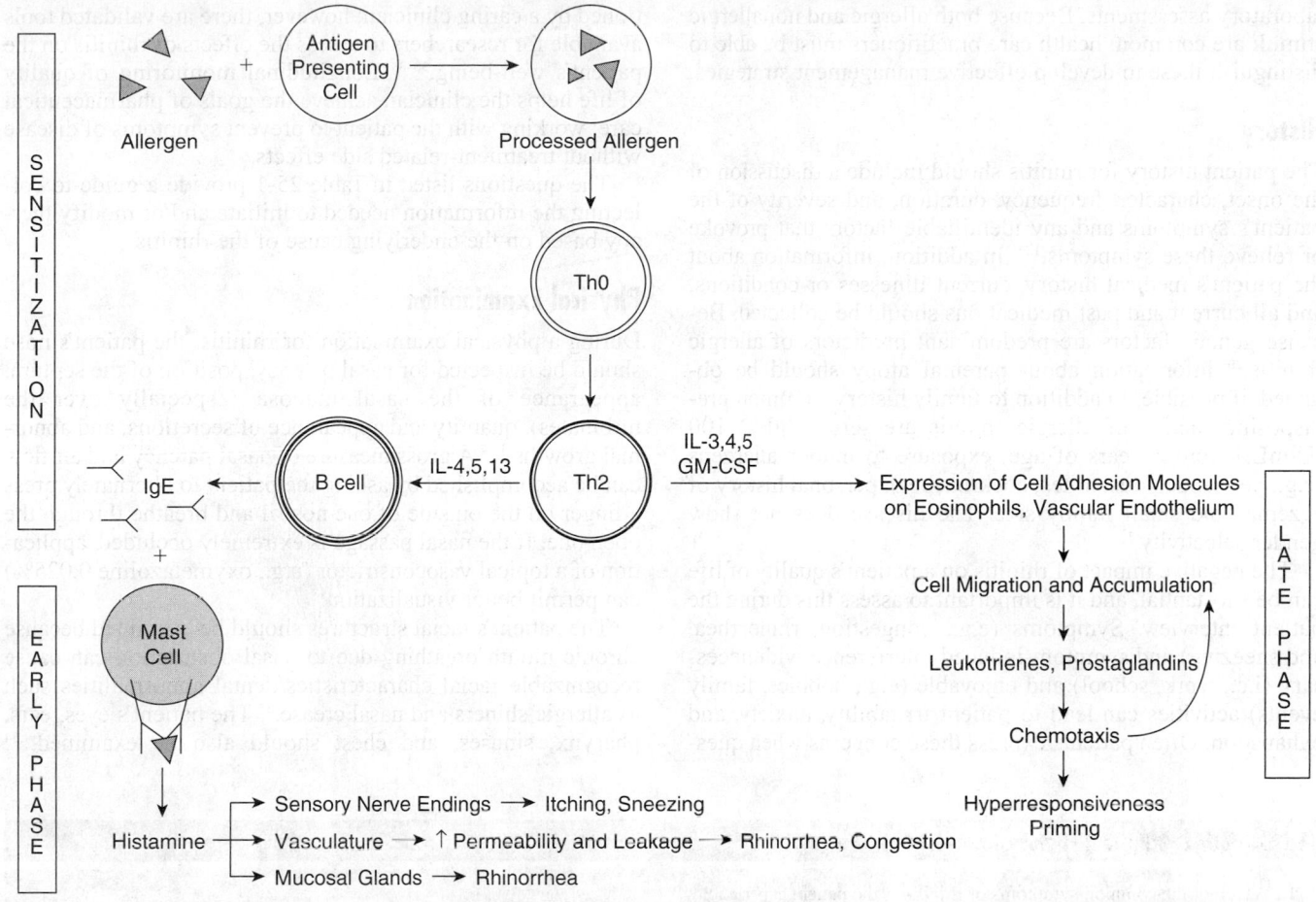

FIGURE 25-4 Pathophysiology of allergic rhinitis.

Sensitization

In an atopic patient, the result of initial exposure to allergens is production of IgE.[9,24] Following initial exposure, antigen-presenting cells of the immune system react to allergens deposited on the nasal mucosa. This results in helper T-lymphocyte differentiation into Th2 cells, which are associated with production of cytokines and other mediators of inflammation.[21] As a result, memory cells programmed for IgE production are produced.

Early Response

When a susceptible patient is exposed to an allergen to which previous sensitization has occurred, an early-phase allergic response generally occurs. This reaction is attributed largely to the interaction between the allergen, IgE and the sensitized mast cell, resulting in mast cell degranulation. Other cells, including basophils, play an important role as well. As a result, mediators of the allergic response, including histamine, are released along with various chemotactic factors, which amplify and perpetuate the allergic response. Since these mediators are already present in the mast cell, they act within minutes to cause the common symptoms of allergic rhinitis including itching, sneezing, and congestion.[24]

Histamine receptors (H_1) are present throughout the nasal mucosa and their activation results in vascular engorgement,

leading to nasal congestion, direct stimulation of mucus secretion and increased glandular secretion.[25] In addition, parasympathetic nervous system stimulation results in cholinergically mediated nasal secretions.[26] Finally, stimulation of peripheral nerve receptors results in itching and sneezing reflexes.[27]

Late Response

Up to one third of patients with allergic rhinitis also experience a late response that develops approximately 8 hours after initial exposure and may persist for up to 4 hours.[28] In this phase, the nature of inflammation is even more complex, and nasal congestion is a prominent feature. Numerous cells and mediators play important roles, including T lymphocytes, cytokines, eosinophils, neutrophils, macrophages, mast cells, and leukotrienes. These additional mediators, attracted to the area through chemotaxis, sustain the inflammatory response. Of course, this response is also perpetuated through continued exposure to the offending allergen.

DIAGNOSIS AND ASSESSMENT OF RHINITIS

The diagnosis of rhinitis is not defined by one specific laboratory test; rather it is related to the coordinated results of a thorough patient interview including medication history, pertinent physical examination, and a limited number of relevant laboratory assessments. Because both allergic and nonallergic stimuli are common; health care practitioners must be able to distinguish these to develop effective management strategies.

History

The patient history for rhinitis should include a discussion of the onset, character, frequency, duration, and severity of the patient's symptoms and any identifiable factors that provoke or relieve these symptoms.[1,29] In addition, information about the patient's medical history, current illnesses or conditions, and all current and past medications should be collected. Because genetic factors are predominant predictors of allergic rhinitis,[20] information about parental atopy should be obtained, if possible. In addition to family history, common predisposing factors of allergic rhinitis are serum IgE >100 IU/mL before 6 years of age, exposure to indoor allergens (e.g., pet dander, dust mites, cockroaches), personal history of eczema, and small family size. The disease does not show gender selectivity.[7]

The negative impact of rhinitis on a patient's quality of life can be substantial, and it is important to assess this during the patient interview. Symptoms (e.g., congestion, rhinorrhea, and sneezing) and symptom-induced interference with necessary (i.e., work, school) and enjoyable (e.g., hobbies, family events) activities can lead to patient irritability, anxiety, and exhaustion. Often patients express these concerns when questioned by a caring clinician; however, there are validated tools available for researchers to assess the effects of rhinitis on the patient's well-being.[30–33] Longitudinal monitoring of quality of life helps the clinician achieve the goals of pharmaceutical care: working with the patient to prevent symptoms of disease without treatment-related side effects.

The questions listed in Table 25-1 provide a guide to collecting the information needed to initiate and/or modify therapy based on the underlying cause of the rhinitis.

Physical Examination

During a physical examination for rhinitis, the patient's nose should be inspected for nasal patency, position of the septum, appearance of the nasal mucosa (especially over the turbinates), quantity and appearance of secretions, and abnormal growths.[1,34] A gross measure of nasal patency and air flow can be accomplished by asking the patient to alternately press a finger on the outside of one nostril and breathe through the open one. If the nasal passage is extremely occluded, application of a topical vasoconstrictor (e.g., oxymetazoline 0.025%) can permit better visualization.

The patient's facial structures should be examined because chronic mouth breathing due to nasal obstruction can cause recognizable facial characteristics/dental abnormalities such as allergic shiners and nasal crease.[35] The patient's eyes, ears, pharynx, sinuses, and chest should also be examined.[1,34]

Table 25-1 Patient History Interview

1. Which of the common symptoms of rhinitis is the patient experiencing?
   - Sneezing, nasal itching, runny nose, nasal congestion, postnasal drip, altered sense of smell, watery eyes, itching eyes, ear "popping"

2. What color are the nasal secretions?
   - Clear, white, yellow, green, blood-streaked, rusty brown

3. When did the symptoms first appear?
   - Infancy, childhood, adulthood

4. Were the symptoms associated with a change in state/environment?
   - After a viral upper respiratory infection, after a traumatic blow to the head or face, upon moving into/visiting a new dwelling, after obtaining a new pet

5. How often do the symptoms occur?
   - Daily, episodically, seasonally, constantly

6. For how long has this symptom pattern persisted?
   - Days, weeks, months, years

7. Which factors or conditions precipitate symptoms?
   - Specific allergens, inhaled irritants, climatic conditions, foods, drinks

8. Which specific activities precipitate symptoms?
   - Dusting, vacuuming, mowing grass, raking leaves

9. Are other members of the family experiencing similar symptoms?

10. Which of the following are prevalent in the household?
    - Carpeting, heavy drapes, foam or feather pillows, stuffed toys, areas of high moisture (basements, bathrooms), tobacco use (by patient or others)

11. Does the patient have other medical conditions that can cause similar symptoms?

12. Is the patient taking any medications that might cause or aggravate these symptoms?

13. What prescription and nonprescription medications have been used for these symptoms in the past?
    - Were they effective? Did they cause any unwanted effects?

14. What is the patient's occupation?

15. What are the patient's typical leisure activities?

16. To what extent have the symptoms interfered with the patient's lifestyle (i.e., are they disabling or merely annoying)?
    - Greatly, somewhat, not much

Gross examination of the expelled mucus for color and clarity may be helpful. Common characteristics of patients with allergic rhinitis are clear nasal discharge, swollen turbinates, and pale mucosa.[17]

Laboratory Tests

Microscopic examination of nasal secretions can be performed in patients with allergic rhinitis, but is primarily useful for differentiating allergic rhinitis from other causes. In allergic conditions, the clinician would expect numerous eosinophils to be present in the sample; however, this could also be true of NARES or nasal polyps.[1]

Although total serum IgE and peripheral eosinophil counts are of little value, laboratory determination of specific IgE antibodies to allergens of known sensitivity is helpful in guiding subsequent recommendations about environmental control and immunotherapy.[1]

The demonstration of specific IgE antibodies by skin testing or in vitro testing (e.g., radioallergosorbent testing [RAST]) can be important for confirmation of sensitivity to specific allergens.[1] In selected cases, other diagnostic tests such as sinus x-rays, computed tomography (CT), rhinomanometry, and spirometry may be useful.[15,17]

Clinical Signs and Symptoms

Patients with allergic rhinitis frequently experience symptoms such as sneezing, nasal and ocular itching, nasal and ocular discharge, nasal obstruction, and postnasal dripping of secretions. Sneezing may occur paroxysmally or may be preceded by itching of the nose, ears, eyes, and throat. Nasal discharge may be profuse and is characteristically thin and watery. Nasal obstruction is due to vascular engorgement and swollen turbinates. Congestion can be particularly problematic when it affects the senses of smell and taste. Chronic nasal congestion may lead to mouth breathing, which is associated with oral and dental malformations. In addition to itching and discharge, ocular symptoms can include redness and photophobia.[36] The negative impact of allergic rhinitis on quality of life may result in systemic complaints including irritability, fatigue, and malaise.[15]

GENERAL MANAGEMENT OF ALLERGIC RHINITIS

The goals of treatment for allergic rhinitis are to prevent or relieve symptoms while improving quality of life without prohibitory concerns about adverse effects or expense. These goals should be achievable through the establishment of a therapeutic partnership with a caring clinician. With appropriate treatment, the patient should be able to maintain a normal lifestyle and perform desired and usual activities of daily living. Effective management strategies include patient education, environmental control, and therapy with single or multiple medications.[1]

Considerations for patient education include instruction about the disease and its triggers, the range of symptoms, and the role of various treatments. An appropriate understanding of prevention versus treatment strategies is critical to successful outcomes. Figure 25-5 depicts an algorithm for the general management of allergic rhinitis.

Allergen Avoidance/Environmental Control

Environmental control measures can be very effective in preventing symptoms of allergic rhinitis, although they can be difficult to accomplish. Minimizing exposure to known allergens (e.g., pollens, house dust mites, molds, animal dander, and cockroaches), irritants (e.g., tobacco smoke) and predisposing medications should be a component of every management plan. Avoiding triggers that have already been identified for a specific patient may take the form of removing them from the daily environment (e.g., all warm-blooded animals including birds) or minimizing exposure to their effects (e.g., mattress covers).[5]

Pharmacotherapy

There are several classes of medications used effectively in the management of allergic rhinitis. Choices for therapy should be individualized based on the patient's specific symptoms and comfort with administration. In some instances, therapy can be administered orally, topically or systemically. Based on the frequency and severity of symptoms, medications may be used as needed or on a regular schedule.[1] Table 25-2 summarizes the effectiveness of agents for specific symptoms used in the treatment of allergic rhinitis.

Antihistamines

Antihistamines are effective in reducing sneezing and nasal/ocular itching and discharge; however, they are less effective on symptoms of nasal congestion. Antihistamines are available in oral, ocular and nasal formulations and can also be found in combination with oral decongestants. Antihistamines work best when administered on a regular basis and the second-generation agents are considered the first-line therapy for mild allergic rhinitis.[1,2]

Nasal Anti-inflammatory Agents

Intranasal anti-inflammatory agents include both steroidal and nonsteroidal compounds. Nasal corticosteroids are now recognized as the most effective medication class for the treatment of allergic rhinitis and are particularly useful for more severe or persistent symptoms.[17,37] Although these drugs are most beneficial when dosed on a regular schedule, new studies are demonstrating that as-needed use may also be appropriate.[37,38] In addition, nasal corticosteroids are also useful for some forms of nonallergic rhinitis.

Intranasal cromolyn, a nonsteroidal agent, acts as a mast cell stabilizer and although safe, is generally less efficacious than other therapies. Because it is administered four to six times daily and requires several weeks to be effective, it is best reserved for acute prophylaxis before exposure to a known allergen.[39]

Decongestants

Oral and nasal decongestants can effectively reduce nasal congestion produced by allergic and nonallergic forms of rhinitis.[1] Oral agents are often combined with antihistamines, but can lead to profound side effects (e.g., insomnia, nervousness, urinary retention) and should be used with caution in patients with arrhythmias, hypertension and hyperthyroidism. Nasal agents are not typically associated with these effects, but should be limited to short-term use to avoid rebound nasal congestion.[2]

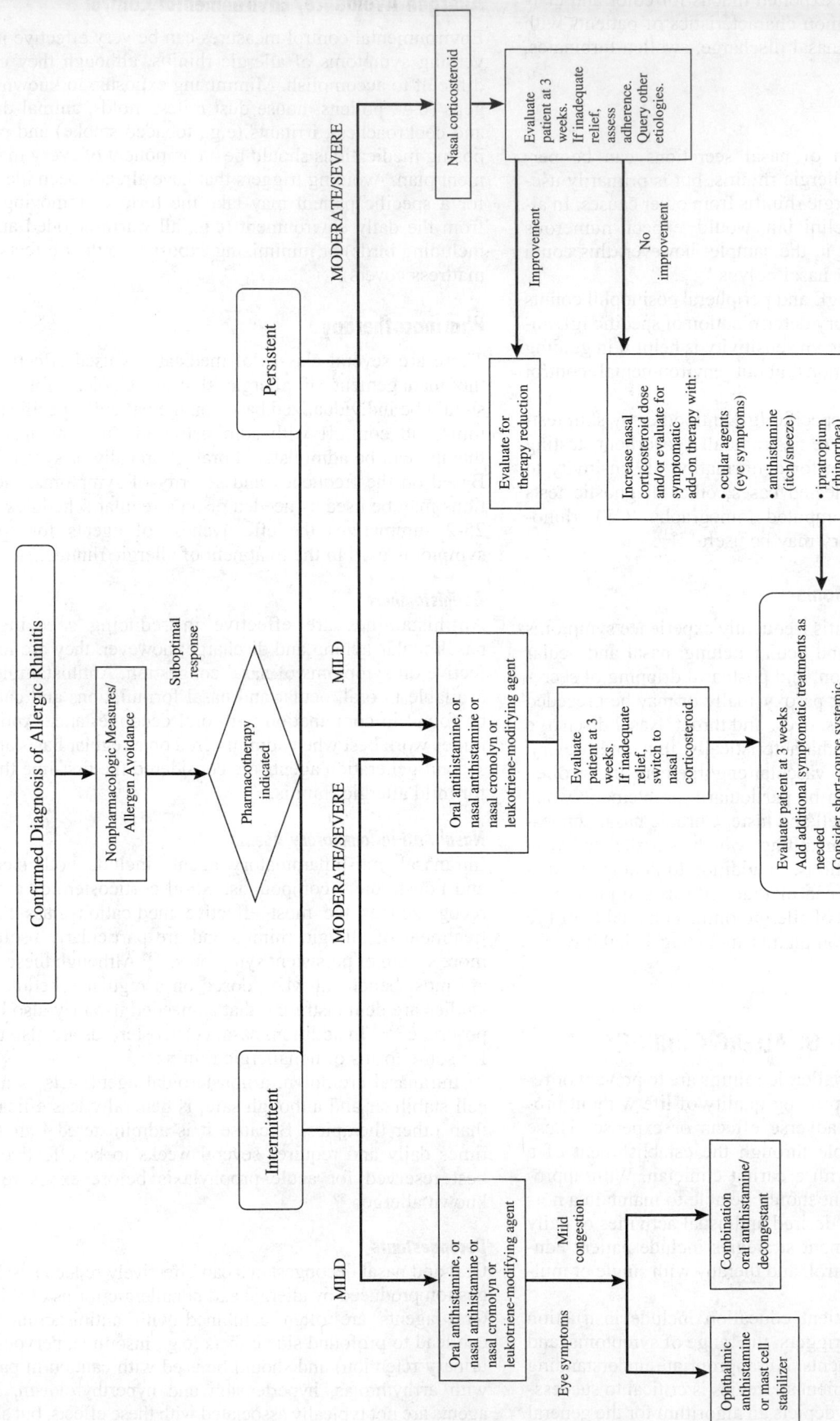

FIGURE 25-5 Treatment algorithm for allergic rhinitis. Suggested definitions for mild and moderate/severe included in Figure 25-3. Treatment should be directed at predominant symptoms (i.e., for eye symptoms in absence of other symptoms use ophthalmic preparation). Prevention strategies are more effective than treatment strategies. For intermittent symptoms, begin treatment several weeks before antigen exposure and discontinue when no longer needed. (Adapted from references 1, 5.)

Table 25-2   Effectiveness of Agents[a] Used in Management of Allergic Rhinitis

	Rhinorrhea	Nasal Pruritus	Sneezing	Nasal Congestion	Eye Symptoms	Onset
Antihistamines						
Nasal	Moderate	High	High	0/Low	0	Rapid
Ophthalmic	0	0	0	0	Moderate	
Oral	Moderate	High	High	0/Low	Moderate	
Decongestants						
Nasal	0	0	0	High	0	Rapid
Ophthalmic	0	0	0	0	Moderate	
Oral	0	0	0	High	0	
Corticosteroids						
Nasal	High	High	High	High	High	Slow (days)
Ophthalmic	0	0	0	0	High	
Mast Cell Stabilizers						
Nasal	Low	Low	Low	0/Low	Low	Slow (weeks)
Ophthalmic	Low	Low	Low	Low	Moderate	
Anticholinergics						
Nasal	High	0	0	0	0	Rapid
Leukotriene Modifiers						
Oral	Low	0/Low	Low	Moderate	Low/Moderate	Rapid

High, significant effect; moderate, moderate effect; low, low effect; 0, no efficacy.
[a]Immunotherapy may lead to significant responses in all symptom categories; however, onset of action is delayed (months).
Adapted from references 2, 133.

Anticholinergic Agents

Intranasal ipratropium bromide is an anticholinergic agent effective for reducing watery, nasal secretions in allergic rhinitis, nonallergic rhinitis, and viral upper respiratory infections.[1,5] Anticholinergic agents have no significant effect on other symptoms, however.

Leukotriene Modifiers

In recent years, the potential role of oral leukotriene modifier therapies for the management of allergic rhinitis has been explored. The basis for this interest is the relation between the upper and lower respiratory tracts, and the knowledge of common inflammatory cells and mediators in both allergic rhinitis and asthma. Leukotriene receptor antagonist monotherapy has been shown to be beneficial in reducing the frequency and severity of symptoms in allergic rhinitis and in improving quality-of-life measures.[40]

Immunotherapy

Allergen immunotherapy, or "allergy shots," should be considered an option in cases of severe or prolonged symptomatology in patients with chronic complications (e.g., asthma, otitis media, sinusitis) or when control cannot be achieved through the use of appropriate medications. It is generally unnecessary for persons with sensitivity to only one seasonal allergen when seasonal exposure is short.[2] Studies with sublingual, nasal delivery and shorter courses of subcutaneous immunotherapeutic allergens are ongoing.

Emerging Therapies

Supporting the theme of "one airway, one disease," the FDA has approved omalizumab (Xolair), an anti-IgE monoclonal antibody to treat people 12 years of age and older with moderate to severe allergy-related asthma inadequately controlled by inhaled corticosteroid treatments. Asthma caused by allergies results from the immune system's overreaction to inhaled allergens, such as dust mites or animal dander. The body forms antibodies in response to the allergen and this immune system reaction prompts inflammation and airway narrowing.

Omalizumab is a genetically engineered protein that stops an allergic reaction before it starts by blocking the release of mediators that induce inflammation. When administered as a subcutaneous injection once or twice monthly, anti-IgE has been shown to decrease the number of asthma exacerbations in patients whose allergy-related asthma has been confirmed with skin or blood tests. However, long-term studies are needed to evaluate the safety and efficacy of anti-IgE in the management of allergic rhinitis.[41,42]

SPECIFIC THERAPEUTIC OPTIONS

Antihistamine Therapy

1. L.B. is a 57-year-old man with a history of controlled hypertension for 10 years and intermittent allergic rhinitis since childhood (confirmed at one time by skin testing). L.B. presents with complaints of nasal itching, sneezing, clear rhinorrhea, and stuffiness. He usually experiences similar symptoms with added ocular itching every spring, but has noticed that the problem has become persistent since he moved into an older home in the historic district of town. In the past, L.B. has successfully self-medicated his seasonal symptoms with an over the counter antihistamine and decongestant: diphenhydramine (Benadryl) 50 mg and pseudoephedrine (Sudafed) 60 mg TID to QID as needed for symptoms, although "nothing seems to help much with the itchy eyes." L.B.'s chronic medications are hydrochlorothiazide 25 mg Q AM and extended-release diltiazem 180 mg QD. He denies any other medical problems or complaints. He has no history of adverse drug reactions or drug allergies. He does not smoke but drinks alcohol socially.

Diagnosis of Allergic Rhinitis

What elements of L.B.'s presentation indicate a probable diagnosis of allergic rhinitis?

L.B. is exhibiting the classic symptoms of persistent (perennial) allergic rhinitis with intermittent (seasonal) exacerbations: nasal itching, sneezing, watery (often profuse) rhinorrhea, and congestion.[1] His history of positive skin tests and the fact that his symptoms previously responded to antihistamine/decongestant also support the diagnosis. In the past, L.B. has experienced symptoms predictably at the onset of the tree pollination season with only minimal symptoms during the remainder of the year. Moving into an older home, however, has likely triggered latent sensitivities to dust mites and mold spores.

Environmental Control Measures

2. **What environmental control strategies could L.B. use to minimize his exposure to triggers?**

Allergen avoidance can be a very effective measure to reduce symptoms in sensitized patients. Although total allergen avoidance is often impractical to implement, simple changes that can reduce exposure to many perennial triggers, such as house dust mites, animal dander, and mold, can assist with symptom control.[1]

Dust mite avoidance (e.g., the use of impermeable covers on box springs, mattresses, and pillows) has traditionally been used as a method of reducing allergen exposure. Although this practice continues to be recommended frequently, a recent study demonstrated despite reduced exposure to antigen, this strategy alone did not improve symptoms in patients with allergic rhinitis.[43] Other methods of reducing antigen exposure include washing bedding at least weekly in hot water (greater than 130° Fahrenheit) and reducing humidity in the home to below 50%. In addition, replacing carpets with linoleum, tile, or wood floors and replacing curtains and heavy draperies with blinds that can be wiped clean have been recommended.[1]

Mold avoidance is difficult when outdoor humidity levels are high, but removing carpeting may be effective in reducing buildup. Live plants should be removed from the home to reduce mold contamination from the soil. Air conditioners should be used, and filters should be changed frequently to reduce humidity and assist with air filtration.[1]

Since L.B. has recently moved into an older home, he may not have used such strategies before. These should be the first recommendation from the clinician.

Therapeutic Objectives for Allergic Rhinitis

3. **What are the therapeutic objectives in treating L.B.?**

The therapeutic objectives for the treatment of allergic rhinitis are to control symptoms and permit all usual daily activities with no adverse side effects of therapy. In patients with seasonal exacerbations, another objective is to prevent the onset of symptoms by anticipating the patient's season of sensitivity. In L.B.'s case, he should use environmental measures to

reduce exposure and then begin chronic treatment with possible add-on therapy instituted 1 to 2 weeks before the start of pollen season.

4. **L.B. has used diphenhydramine for many years with good symptom relief and, as he recalls, only minimal daytime sedation. He asks your opinion regarding whether this is the best treatment for his allergic symptoms. He specifically requests the most cost-effective treatment available as he must pay cash for any medications.**

Choice of Therapeutic Agent

What do you recommend and how should the therapy be initiated?

Oral antihistamines are still considered the mainstay of therapy for allergic rhinitis. They reduce symptoms of nasal itching, sneezing and rhinorrhea, but have only minimal effectiveness on ocular symptoms and nasal congestion. The Allergic Rhinitis and its Impact on Asthma (ARIA) guidelines[5] indicate that oral antihistamines have a place in the treatment of mild intermittent, mild persistent, and moderate-severe intermittent disease; although if severe symptoms persist, additional or alternative treatments may be required.

For a patient like L.B. who has experienced a good response to an older "first-generation" agent such as diphenhydramine without complaints of excessive drowsiness, historically this agent would have been considered a reasonable choice because of its inexpensive cost and availability without a prescription. Nonetheless, the appropriate use of diphenhydramine and other first-generation antihistamines (FGAs), such as brompheniramine, chlorpheniramine, and clemastine, is currently the topic of much debate among clinicians and researchers. Many clinicians and patients now express a preference for newer second-generation agents, such as loratadine, desloratadine, fexofenadine, or cetirizine. Early second-generation antihistamine (SGAs) agents, astemizole (Hismanal) and terfenadine (Seldane) were withdrawn from the market because of safety concerns. These agents were associated with cardiovascular adverse events including prolongation of QTc interval and arrhythmias, usually related to higher doses and interactions with agents metabolized via the cytochrome P450 system.[4] This is not a concern with currently available SGAs. In general, SGAs include agents marketed after 1980 with one or more of the following properties: (1) improved H_1-receptor selectivity, (2) absent or reduced sedative effects, and (3) anti-allergic properties separate from antihistamine effects.[44] With the recent switch from prescription to nonprescription status, access to SGAs has increased substantially, although cost continues to be a concern.

Although traditionally the mechanism of action of antihistamines has been described as receptor blockade, recent evidence suggests that these agents may actually act as inverse agonists of the H_1-receptor, meaning that rather than physically blocking the receptor, they stabilize its inactive conformation and thus prevent histamine from causing activation.[45] Whereas all marketed antihistamines have sufficient effects on the histamine receptor to provide clinical benefits, the SGAs are more specific for the peripheral histamine receptor than are the FGAs,[46] and for this reason they present a lower risk for adverse effects, including sedation and anticholinergic effects.

The debate regarding sedation associated with the use of FGAs is long-standing. Sedation refers collectively to both drowsiness (i.e., the subjective state of sleepiness or lethargy) and impairment (i.e., an objective decrease or absence of specific physical or mental abilities).[47] A recent meta-analysis of 18 studies showed that diphenhydramine impaired performance relative to placebo and SGAs; however, the results were varied, and the methods for determining study inclusion have been scrutinized.[48]

Clinically, FGAs have been documented to be associated with increased sleepiness from single doses,[49] persistence of sleepiness after multiple doses,[50,51] and morning sleepiness following evening doses.[52] In addition to drowsiness that the patient may not perceive, an even greater percentage of individuals experience mood, cognition, and psychomotor impairment from these agents. These aspects of sedation have been identified in both self-reports and sophisticated tests of psychomotor function, including learning and driving.[50,53,54]

In light of these findings, the Joint Task Force on Practice Parameters in Allergy, Asthma and Immunology has stated ". . . many patients may not perceive performance impairment that is associated with FGAs. Consequently, SGAs that are associated with less risk or no risk for these side effects should usually be considered . . .".[1] In another expert consensus statement on the use of antihistamines in the treatment of allergic rhinitis, experts agreed that many of the FGAs produce sedation, impairment, and reduced quality of life. They acknowledge that allergic rhinitis is more appropriately treated with SGAs in all patients.[47] One exception to this is pregnant women in whom there is more long-term data on the use of FGAs and thus they are preferred by the American College of Obstetrics and Gynecology.[55] If these drugs are not tolerated, cetirizine or loratadine may be considered, ideally after the first trimester.

SGAs prevent the onset of symptoms better than they reverse symptoms that have appeared already. Also, the maximum antihistamine effects occur several hours after the drug's serum concentration peaks.[56] For maximal effect, therefore, the SGAs should be administered before allergen exposure, if possible. For the same reason, chronic dosing is preferred to intermittent dosing.

Essentially, all the antihistamines listed in Table 25-3 are equally effective.[44,57] Therefore, the choice of agent is based on duration of action, side-effect profile (especially drowsiness and anticholinergic effects), risk of drug interactions, and cost. Some patients claim that one product is more helpful in relieving their symptoms than another, and there have

Table 25-3 Oral Antihistamines

Generic Name (Product)	Available Dosage Forms/Strengths	Adult Dose	Pediatric Dose	CNS	GI	Anti
First Generation						
Azatadine (Optimine)[h]	Tablets: 1 mg 1 mg + pseudoephedrine 120 mg	1–2 mg Q 12 hr	0.5 mg–1 mg Q 12 hr *<12 yr:* Safe and effective use of combination product has not been established	++	0	++
Brompheniramine (Dimetane)	Elixir: 2 mg/5 mL Liquid gels: 4 mg Tablet: 4 mg 4 mg + pseudoephedrine 60 mg Tablet, extended release: 4 mg, 6 mg Capsule, extended release: 6 mg + pseudoephedrine 60 mg 12 mg + pseudoephedrine 120 mg Elixir: (per 5 mL) 2 mg + pseudoephedrine 30 mg 1 mg + pseudoephedrine 15 mg 4 mg + pseudoephedrine 45 mg 2 mg + phenylephrine 5 mg Caplets: 4 mg + phenylephrine 10 mg	4–8 mg Q 6–8 hr or 8–12 mg extended release Q 8–12 hr (max. 24 mg/day)	0.5 mg/ kg /day given in 3–4 divided doses Alternatively, *6–11 yr:* 2 mg Q 4–6 hr (max. 12 mg/day) *2–5 yr:* 1 mg Q 4–6 hr as (max. 6 mg/day) *Children and infants:* Do not use the extended-release dosage form.	+	0	++

Continued

Table 25-3 Oral Antihistamines—cont'd

Generic Name (Product)	Available Dosage Forms/Strengths	Adult Dose	Pediatric Dose	CNS	GI	Anti
First Generation—cont'd						
Chlorpheniramine (Chlor-Trimeton)	Capsules, extend release: 12 mg, 8 mg Syrup: 2 mg/5 mL, 1 mg/5 mL Tablet: 4 mg Tablet & capsule: 2 mg + phenylephrine 5 mg 4 mg + pseudoephedrine 60 mg 6 mg + pseudoephedrine 60 mg 8 mg + pseudoephedrine 120 mg 12 mg + pseudoephedrine 120 mg Tablet, chewable: 2 mg Tablet, extended release: 12 mg, 8 mg Tablet, sustained release: 8 mg + phenylephrine 20 mg Elixir/liquid: 2 mg + phenylephrine 5 mg per 5 mL 4 mg + phenylephrine 10 mg per 5 mL Oral Solution: 2 mg + pseudoephedrine 30 mg	4 mg Q 4–6 hr, or 8–12 mg sustained release Q 6–8hr (max. 24 mg/day)	6–12 yr: 2 mg Q 4–6 hr, or 8 mg sustained release QD (max. 12 mg/day) 2–5 yr: 1 mg Q 4–6 hr (max. 4 mg/day) <6 yr: Extended-release formulations are not recommended in this age group.	+	0	++
Clemastine (Tavist)	Syrup: 0.67 mg/5 mL Tablet: 1.34 mg, 2.68 mg	1.34–2.68 mg Q 8–12 hr (max. 8.04 mg/day)	6–12 yr: 0.67–1.34 mg Q 8–12 hr. (max. 4.02 mg/day) <6 yr: Safe dosage has not been established.	++	+	+++
Cyproheptadine (Periactin)	Syrup: 2 mg/5 mL Tablets: 4 mg	4 mg Q 8–12 hr. Increase as necessary. Usual range, 4–20 mg/day in divided doses Q 8 hr (max. 0.5 mg/kg/day or 32 mg/day)	7–14 yr 0.25 mg/kg/day in two or three divided doses or 4 mg Q 8–12 hr (max. 16 mg/day) 2–6 yr: 0.25 mg/kg/day in two or three divided doses or 2 mg Q 8–12 hr (max. 12 mg/day)	+	0	++
Dexbrompheniramine (Drixoral)[a]	Tablet, extended release: 6 mg + pseudoephedrine 120 mg	6 mg extended release Q 12 hr (max. 12 mg dexbrompheniramine + 240 mg pseudoephedrine/day)	>12 yr: 6 mg extended release Q 12 hr (max. 12 mg dexbrompheniramine 1 240 mg pseudoephedrine/day)	+	++[c]	++

Table 25-3   Oral Antihistamines—cont'd

Generic Name (Product)	Available Dosage Forms/Strengths	Adult Dose	Pediatric Dose	Side Effects		
				CNS	GI	Anti
First Generation—cont'd						
Dexchlorphenir-amine (Polar-amine)[b]	Syrup: 2 mg/5 mL Tablet: 2 mg Tablet, sustained release: 4 mg, 6 mg	2 mg Q 4–6 hr, or 4–6 mg sustained-release Q 8–10 hr or at bedtime	0.15 mg/kg given in divided doses four times a day Alternatively, *6–11 yr:* 1 mg Q 4–6 hr or 4 mg sustained release at bedtime. *2–5 yr:* 0.5 mg Q 4–6 hr	+	0	++
Diphenhydramine (Benadryl)	Capsule: 25 mg, 50 mg Elixir/Solution/Syrup 6.25 mg/5 mL, 12.5 mg/5 mL Tablet, chewable: 12.5 mg Tablets: 25 mg, 50 mg, 19 mg + pseudoephedrine 30 mg 25 mg + pseudoephedrine 60 mg Oral solution: 12.5 mg + pseudoephedrine 30 mg per 5 mL	25–50 mg Q 4–6 hr (max. 300 mg/day	*6–12 yr:* 12.5–25 mg Q 4–6 hr (max. 150 mg/day) *Up to 2–5 yr:* 6.25 to 12.5 mg Q 4–6 hr	+++	+	+++
Hydroxyzine (Atarax)[b]	Capsules (as pamoate): 25 mg, 50 mg, 100 mg Syrup: 10 mg/5 mL (as HCl) Suspension: 25 mg/5 mL (as pamoate) Tablet (as HCl): 10 mg, 25 mg, 50 mg, 100 mg	25 mg Q 6–8 hr (max. 400 mg/day)	2 mg/kg/day given in divided doses every 6–8 hr (max. 2 mg/kg/day)	++	0	+
Phenindamine (Nolahist)	Tablet: 25 mg	25 mg Q 4–6 hr (max. 150 mg/day)	*6–12 yr:* 12.5 mg Q 4–6 hr (max. 75 mg/day)	+/−	0	++
Promethazine (Phenergan)[b]	Syrup: 6.25 mg/5 mL, 25 mg/5 mL Tablet: 12.5 mg, 25 mg, 50 mg	25 mg at bedtime, or 12.5 mg Q 8 hr	*>2 yr:* 6.25–12.5 mg TID and HS	+++	0	+++
Tripelennamine (PBZ)[b]	Tablet: 25 mg, 50 mg Tablet, extended release: 100 mg	25-50 mg Q 4–6 hr or 100 mg sustained release Q 12 hr (max. 600 mg/day)	5 mg/kg/day divided into 4–6 doses. (max. 300 mg/day) Sustained-release tablets are not intended for children.	++	++ +	+/−
Second Generation						
Acrivastine (Semprex-D)[a,b]	Capsules: 8 mg + pseudoephedrine 60 mg	8 mg Q 4–6 hr (max.: 32 mg acrivastine and 240 mg pseudoephedrine/day)	*<12 yr:* Safe and effective use has not been established.	++	++[c]	++

Continued

Table 25-3   Oral Antihistamines—cont'd

Generic Name (Product)	Available Dosage Forms/Strengths	Adult Dose	Pediatric Dose	Side Effects CNS	GI	Anti
Second Generation—cont'd						
Cetirizine (Zyrtec)[b]	Syrup: 1 mg/mL, 5 mg/mL Tablets: 5 mg, 10 mg 5 mg + pseudoephedrine 120 mg (Zyrtec-D 12 Hr)	5–10 mg QD (max. 10 mg/day or 10 mg ceti-rizine and 240 mg pseudoephedrine/day)	6–11 yr: 5–10 mg QD (max. 10 mg/day) 2–5 yr: 2.5-5 mg QD or 2.5 mg Q 12 hr (max. 5 mg/day) 12–23 mo: 2.5 mg QD or 2.5 mg Q 12 hr (max. 5 mg/day) 6–11 mo: 2.5 mg QD (max. 2.5 mg/day) Infants <6 mo: Safe and effective use has not been established. <12 yr: Safe and effective use of combination product has not been established.	+/−	+/−	+/−
Desloratadine (Clarinex)[b]	Tablets: 5 mg	5 mg QD (max. 5 mg/day)	<12 yr: Safe and effective use has not been established.	+/−	+/−	+/−
Fexofenadine (Allegra)[b]	Capsule: 60 mg Tablet: 30 mg, 60 mg, 180 mg Tablet, extended release: 60 mg 1 pseudoephedrine 120 mg (Allegra D)	60 mg Q 12 hr or 180 mg QD (max. 180 mg/day) Extended release: 60 mg fexofenadine and 120 mg pseu-doephedrine Q 12 hr (max. 120 mg fexofe-nadine and 240 mg pseudoephedrine/day).	6–11 yr: 30 mg Q 12 hr (max. 60 mg/day) <6 yr: Safe and effective use has not been estab-lished. <12 yr: Safe and effective use of combination product has not been established.	+/−	0	+/−
Loratadine (Claritin, Alavert)	Syrup: 1 mg/mL Tablets: 10 mg, 10 mg rapidly disintegrating (Claritin Reditabs) 5 mg +pseudoephedrine 120 mg (Claritin-D 12 Hour) 10 mg +pseudoephedrine 240 mg (Claritin-D 24 Hour)	10 mg QD or 5 mg Q 12 hr (Claritin D-12 Hour) (max. 10 mg/day)	6–12 yr: 10 mg QD(max. 10 mg/day) 2–5 yr: 5 mg QD admin-istered as oral syrup. (max. 5 mg/day) Children <2 yr: Safe and effective use has not been established	+/−	+/−	+

[a]Available in the United States as combination product only.
[b]Currently available by prescription only.
[c]GI effects due to pseudoephedrine.
Incidence: +++, high; ++, moderate; +, low; +/−, low to none; 0, none
CNS, Central nervous system effects include sedation, and diminished mental alertness. Paradoxical CNS stimulation can occur in elderly and children. GI, Gastrointestinal ef-fects include nausea and abdominal pain. Anti, Anticholinergic effects include dry mouth, blurry vision, and urinary retention.
Adapted from reference 188.

long been reports that tolerance to specific agents can occur after consistent use. Although there is no pharmacologic explanation for these observations,[47] patients may experience benefit from switching therapies if the perception of tolerance occurs.

The major advantages of SGAs are their selectivity to the H_1-receptor and their reduced central nervous system (CNS) sedative effects. Desloratadine, fexofenadine, and loratadine at prescribed doses are reported to have an incidence of sedation no different from placebo for both somnolence and performance impairment.[58] Cetirizine and intranasal azelastine are not considered to be entirely nonsedating, although incidence of sedation is less than with FGAs.[59] Another advantage of SGAs is the fact that most products can be dosed once daily to improve patient adherence to therapy. Specific H_1-receptor antagonists are compared in Table 25-3. In the case of L.B., it would be reasonable to begin therapy with loratadine 10 mg daily, because as an SGA, it has demonstrated efficacy with minimal side effects and is also available without a prescription.

Nasal Antihistamines

5. L.B. has a friend who had side effects from antihistamines and had been given a nasal spray instead. Is it possible to give antihistamines by this route, or is L.B. confusing this with other topical therapies, such as decongestants or corticosteroids?

An aqueous intranasal solution (125 µg/spray) of azelastine (Astelin) is approved for the treatment of allergic rhinitis. This drug has an objectionable taste, making it unsuitable for oral administration, but the nasal and ophthalmic formulations have been shown beneficial in allergic rhinitis and conjunctivitis.[60-62] In studies comparing intranasal azelastine with oral antihistamines and placebo, azelastine has been found to be equal to the oral antihistamines,[63-65] although a meta-analysis comparing azelastine with nasal corticosteroids suggests that nasal corticosteroids were superior in efficacy in all but ophthalmic symptoms.[66] As with the oral agents, the intranasal formulation is less effective for nasal congestion than it is for nasal itching, sneezing, and rhinorrhea.[66] Dosing recommendations for azelastine (for adults and children >12 years) are two sprays in each nostril twice a day. Before first use and anytime when the product has not been used for 3 days or more, the dosage form must be primed. This is accomplished by pumping the spray mechanism two to four times until a consistent mist is expelled.

Surprisingly, side effects of azelastine are comparable to the FGAS in terms of somnolence (10% to 15%) and headache (15% to 30%).[60] Intranasal azelastine can also cause local side effects, including nasal irritation, dry mouth, sore throat, and mild epistaxis. Bad after taste remains a significant problem, occurring in up to 20% of patients, even those using the ophthalmic formulations. Where intranasal antihistamines fit into the treatment of allergic rhinitis has not been clearly delineated. At this time, azelastine should be considered an alternative to oral antihistamines for patients who prefer the intranasal route of administration or an alternative to cromolyn sodium for patients with milder allergic symptoms. As a prescription-only product, this alternative would be less appropriate because of its expense compared to agents available without a prescription.

Decongestant Therapy

6. What role do decongestants have in L.B.'s treatment?

Nasal congestion is often much less severe in patients who experience only intermittent symptoms, but as L.B.'s symptoms have become persistent since his move, the exact frequency and severity of his nasal congestion should be assessed before recommending drug therapy. In patients with only mild, intermittent symptoms, normal saline irrigation (administered as frequently as needed) is helpful in relieving nasal congestion by soothing and moisturizing irritated nasal mucosa. As previously noted, antihistamines do little to relieve nasal congestion; therefore, patients with moderate to severe congestion may require a combination of an antihistamine with a decongestant.[67] The combination of an antihistamine and an oral decongestant is more effective than either component alone in the treatment of allergic rhinitis.[68,69]

Both the topical (nasal) and the oral decongestants are sympathomimetics that directly stimulate α_1-adrenergic receptors, resulting in vasoconstriction. Decongestants' local effects on the nasal mucosa include decreased tissue hyperemia, decreased tissue swelling, decreased nasal congestion, and improved nasal airway patency.[67] Since phenylpropanolamine was removed from the market due to the results of the Hemorrhagic Stroke Project,[70] which found a relation between phenylpropanolamine in weight loss products and hemorrhagic stroke, pseudoephedrine is the only clinically useful oral decongestant available for allergic rhinitis. The available oral and topical decongestants, all of which are available without prescription, are compared in Table 25-4.

Pseudoephedrine can be very effective for nasal decongestion; although it is not without systemic side effects, particularly those associated with CNS stimulation (e.g., nervousness, restlessness, insomnia, tremor, dizziness, and headache). These side effects might counteract sedation when used in combination with FGAs; however, individual responses to combinations vary, ranging from sedation to "agitated sedation" to stimulation. Cardiovascular stimulation (e.g., tachycardia, palpitations, increased blood pressure) also can occur.[34,67] Reports of these effects were more commonly associated with phenylpropanolamine but results of clinical studies have been conflicting, and thus patients with hypertension should be monitored carefully while taking oral decongestants.[71] Because oral pseudoephedrine is not associated with the development of rebound congestion, in most patients, it is appropriate for chronic use. However, because of the association between pseudoephedrine and congenital defects in the abdominal wall (i.e., gastroschisis), it is not recommended for use during pregnancy.[55]

Topical administration of decongestants generally does not lead to systemic side effects; however, these agents are not appropriate for chronic use in rhinitis because of their potential for developing rebound congestion (see Question 27).

Because L.B. is complaining of nasal congestion, he will require a decongestant in addition to the loratadine. He may choose to use a fixed-dose combination product, such as Claritin-D or its generic, or to supplement the loratadine with pseudoephedrine as needed. Although L.B. has hypertension, his blood pressure is under good control, and he has used pseudoephedrine in the past without problem. Still, he should

Table 25-4   Decongestants

Generic Name (Product)	Available Dosage Forms/Strengths	Adult Dose	Pediatric Dose
Oral[a]			
Pseudoephedrine (Sudafed)	Tablet: 30 mg, 60 mg, 240 mg Tablet, extended release: 120 mg Capsule: 60 mg Liquid: 25 mg/5 mL Drops: 7.5 mg/ 0.8 mL	60 mg Q 4–6 hr, or 120 mg sustained release Q 12 hr (max. 240 mg/day)	*6–12 yr:* 30 mg Q 4–6 hr (max. 120 mg/day) *2–5 yr:* 15 mg Q 4–6 hr (max. 60 mg/day) *1–2 yr:* 0.2 mL/ kg drops Q 4–6 hr (max. 0.8 mL/kg/day) *3–12 mo:* 3 drops/kg Q 4–6 hr (max. 12 drops/day)
Topical[b]			
Naphazoline (Privine)	Solution: 0.05% Drops, 0.05% spray	1–2 drops or sprays per nostril Q 6 hr	*<12 yr:* Avoid, unless under physician direction
Phenylephrine (Neo-Synephrine)	Solution (drops): 0.125%, 0.16%, 0.25%, 0.5%, 1% Solution (spray): 0.25%, 0.5%, 1%	0.25–0.5% solution: 2–3 sprays or drops per nostril Q 3–4 hr (1% for extreme congestion)	*6–12 yr:* 0.25% solution: 2–3 sprays or drops per nostril Q 3–4 hr *6 mo–5 yr:* 0.125–0.16% solution: 1–2 drops/nostril Q 3 hr
Oxymetazoline (Afrin)	Solution (drops): 0.025%, 0.05% Solution (spray): 0.05%	0.05% solution: 2–3 sprays or drops per nostril Q 12 hr	*6–12 yr:* 0.05% solution: 2–3 sprays or drops per nostril Q 12 hr *2–5 yr:* 0.025% solution: 2–3 drops/nostril Q 12 hr
Tetrahydrozoline (Tyzine)	Solution (drops): 0.05%, 0.1% Solution (spray): 0.1%	0.1% solution: 2–4 sprays or drops Q 3–4 hr	*6–12 yr:* 0.1% solution: 2–4 sprays or drops Q 3–4 hr *2–5 yr:* 0.05% solution: 2–3 drops/nostril Q 4–6 hr
Xylometazoline (Otrivin)	Solution (drops): 0.05%, 0.1% Solution (spray): 0.1%	0.1% solution: 2–3 sprays/nostril Q 8–10 hr	*2–12 yr:* 0.05% solution: 2–3 drops/nostril Q 8–10 hr

[a]Phenylpropanolamine withdrawn from U.S. market in 2000.
[b]Limit duration of treatment to <5 days to avoid rebound congestion.
Adapted from reference 189.

be monitored closely for any cardiovascular changes caused by the therapy for his allergic rhinitis.

Ocular Therapies

7. L.B.'s new therapies are effective for his persistent nasal symptoms, however, in the spring he presents to the pharmacy with complaints that his eyes are itchy and watery and that the loratadine and pseudoephedrine do not seem to be helping. How are L.B.'s ocular symptoms related to his allergic rhinitis?

Relationship Between Ocular and Nasal Symptoms

Allergic ocular disease is a part of the full range of allergic diseases, including rhinitis, eczema, and asthma, which share a common pathophysiology and inflammatory presentation.[72,73] The most common of the allergic ocular diagnoses is seasonal (intermittent) allergic conjunctivitis, which accounts for up to 50% of all ocular allergy cases. The symptoms of both intermittent and persistent allergic conjunctivitis are identical in that they are caused by allergic response in the conjunctiva to airborne allergens. Seasonal symptoms commonly occur in response to pollens, whereas perennial symptoms are more often associated with house dust mites. The

symptoms of allergic conjunctivitis are itchy eyes with or without a burning sensation and a watery discharge or tearing. Physical examination reveals conjunctival surfaces that are mildly injected (reddened) with varying degrees of conjunctival edema. Swelling of the eyelids can also occur. The symptoms are usually bilateral, but not always symmetrical.

Because of the potential for long-term damage to vision, ocular conditions should always be assessed by a skilled specialist. Other eye problems that can be confused with allergic conjunctivitis include atopic keratoconjunctivitis, keratopathy, and giant papillary conjunctivitis (see Chapter 51, Eye Disorders).

Choice of Therapeutic Agent

8. What are the treatment options for L.B.'s allergic conjunctivitis, and how does the clinician choose between the available options?

Seasonal and perennial allergic conjunctivitis are treated similarly with only the duration of the treatment course differing (i.e., intermittent versus persistent treatment). Nonpharmacologic treatment includes avoidance of aeroallergens to the extent possible, cold compresses or the use of refrigerated eye drops, and lubrication with frequent application of normal saline or tear substitutes. Part of the effectiveness of all of the ocular preparations including lubricating eye drops is attributable to physical dilution and washout of the aeroallergens from the eye.[73]

The available therapeutic options for management of allergic conjunctivitis include topical ocular administration of antihistamines, decongestants, mast cell stabilizers, and NSAIDs (Table 25-5). These medications act by the same mechanisms to treat ocular allergies that they do for nasal symptoms. In addition, topical ophthalmic corticosteroids have a limited role in acute management; however, they are not indicated for prolonged use due to the risk of serious infectious complications in the eye.

Some patients using nasal corticosteroids or oral antihistamines may note improvement in their ophthalmic symptoms through improved ocular drainage and drying effects, particu-

larly if these symptoms are mild. Many patients, however, require add-on ophthalmic therapy to manage ocular allergies.[74] Few studies have evaluated combination therapy rigorously; however, a greater effect on ocular symptom relief was noted when using intranasal fluticasone plus topical olopatadine when compared with intranasal fluticasone plus oral fexofenadine.[75]

Several ophthalmic antihistamine-vasoconstrictor combination products are available without a prescription and at low cost. Overuse of vasoconstrictors, however, can lead to rebound conjunctivitis, similar to that occurring with nasal decongestants (see Drug-Induced Nasal Congestion). Levocabastine, emedastine and azelastine are prescription ophthalmic antihistamine formulations that do not contain a vasoconstrictor and are effective in relieving itching, hyperemia, chemosis, lid swelling, and tearing without the risk of rebound symptoms.

Table 25-5 Topical Ophthalmic Medications for Allergic Conjunctivitis

Generic Name (Product)	Available Dosage Forms/ Strength	Dose
Antihistamines		
Azelastine (Optivar)	Ophthalmic solution 0.05%	*Adults and children ≥3 yr:* 1 drop into each affected eye Q 12 hr (max 2 ophthalmic drops/day per affected eye)
Emedastine (Emadine)	Ophthalmic solution 0.05%	*Adults and children ≥3 yr:* 1 drop into affected eye(s) up to 4 times daily
Levocabastine (Livostin)	Ophthalmic suspension 0.05%	*Adults and children ≥12 yr:* 1 drop into affected eye(s) Q 4–6 hr up to 2 weeks
Antihistamine/Decongestant Combinations		
Antazoline + Naphazoline (Vasocon-A)[a]	Ophthalmic solution antazoline phosphate 0.5% naphazoline HCl 0.05%	*Adults and children ≥6 yr:* 1–2 drops into affected eye(s) Q 6 hr up to 3 days
Pheniramine + Naphazoline (Naphcon-A)[a]	Ophthalmic solution naphazoline HCl 0.025% pheniramine maleate 0.3%	*Adults and children ≥6 yr:* 1–2 drops into affected eye(s) Q 6 hr up to 3 days
Antihistamine/Mast Cell Stabilizers		
Ketotifen (Zaditor)	Ophthalmic solution 0.025%	*Adults and children ≥3 yr:* 1 drop into affected eye(s) Q 8–12 hr
Olopatadine (Patanol)	Ophthalmic solution 0.1%	*Adults and children ≥3 yr:* 1–2 drops into affected eye(s) Q 6–8 hr
Mast Cell Stabilizers		
Cromolyn sodium (Crolom)	Ophthalmic solution 4%	*Adults and children ≥4 yr:* 1–2 drops into affected eye(s) 4–6 times daily
Lodoxamide (Alomide)	Ophthalmic solution 0.1%	*Adults and children ≥2 yr:* 1–2 drops into affected eye(s) 4 times daily up to 3 months
Nedocromil (Alocril)	Ophthalmic solution 2%	*Adults and children ≥3 yr:* 1–2 drops into affected eye(s) Q 8–12 hr
Pemirolast (Alamast)	Ophthalmic solution 0.1%	*Adults and children ≥3 yr:* 1–2 drops into each affected eye(s) Q 4–6 hr (max. 2 drops/day per affected eye)
Nonsteroidal Anti-inflammatory Drugs (NSAIDs)[b]		
Ketorolac (Acular)	Ophthalmic solution 0.05%	*Adults and children ≥3 yr:* 1 drop into affected eye(s) 4 times daily
Corticosteroids		
Loteprednol (Alrex)	Ophthalmic suspension 0.2%	*Adults:* 1 drop into affected eye(s) times daily

[a]Available OTC.
[b]Other ophthalmic NSAIDs (diclofenac, flurbiprofen, suprofen) indicated for intraoperative miosis and/or postcataract surgery, but not approved for allergic conjunctivitis.
Adapted from reference 190.

Lodoxamide is an ophthalmic mast cell stabilizer found to be more effective than ophthalmic cromolyn in comparative studies.[76] Olopatadine and ketotifen are unique ophthalmic preparations in that they are antihistamines with mast cell stabilizing properties. Both agents have been shown to be effective and well tolerated, although clinical trials suggest that ketotifen may exhibit slightly better efficacy for overall symptom improvement.[77,78] However, these medications are also expensive.

Several NSAIDs have been studied for their effects in allergic conjunctivitis and one agent, ketorolac tromethamine, is approved for this use. These drugs inhibit cyclooxygenase to decrease formation of prostaglandins from arachidonic acid. The prostaglandins PGE_2 and PGI_2 appear to play a role in causing the pruritus associated with allergic conjunctivitis. Ketorolac tromethamine has been shown to significantly reduce ocular itching and irritation compared with placebo,[79] but its usefulness compared with antiallergy medications has been questioned.[80] This, along with the comparative expense of ketorolac, has limited its use in ocular allergic disease.

In the case of L.B., a trial of antihistamine-vasoconstrictor combination eye drops (e.g., Naphcon-A) for management of acute symptoms, is the best recommendation until he can follow up with his primary care provider.

Cromolyn Therapy

9. J.C. is a 10-year-old girl who recently began experiencing rhinorrhea and sneezing when visiting her father in another state a couple of times each year. Upon questioning, J.C.'s mother reveals that although J.C. has not complained of symptoms previously, her father adopted a puppy from the local animal shelter about a year ago and the symptoms correspond to the times that the child spends with the dog. J.C. will be visiting her father again next month, and she is hoping to purchase something without a prescription to prevent her from "getting sick and missing out on her summer vacation." What options are available to treat J.C.'s intermittent symptoms of allergic rhinitis?

J.C. appears to have mild allergic rhinitis triggered by exposure to animal dander. When it is possible to anticipate symptoms, as in J.C.'s case, initiating prophylactic therapy can help lessen the impact of allergen exposure.[1] J.C. appears to be a good candidate for treatment with intranasal corticosteroids or cromolyn sodium, administered regularly beginning several weeks before each trip. Because the mother indicates that she wants to select an over-the-counter product, environmental strategies plus cromolyn nasal spray would be a reasonable initial choice for therapy. The drawbacks to this are its out-of-pocket cost, its technique-dependent administration, its multiple daily dosing requirements (three to six times daily), and its reduced effectiveness compared with other treatments

10. What environmental strategies should J.C.'s father use to minimize exposure to the allergic trigger?

To minimize J.C.'s exposure to allergens, the dog should be kept out of the child's bedroom at all times and, when possible, kept outside or confined to an uncarpeted area of the home. J.C.'s father should use a high-quality air filter and should vacuum the home with a double-filter system while J.C. is out of the house. Although evidence is unclear on this topic, it may be helpful to wash the dog weekly while the child visits. The additional expense of regular, commercial cleaning of air ducts is not cost justified.[1]

Mechanism of Action

11. How does cromolyn nasal spray work in the management of allergic rhinitis?

Cromolyn sodium nasal spray (Nasalcrom) is a NSAID that stabilizes mast cells, preventing degranulation and inhibiting the release of the chemical mediators such as histamine.[1,34] Cromolyn sodium does not alter the release of mediators from basophils, nor does it block the effects of histamine already released from the mast cells or basophils. For this reason, the effect of cromolyn is critically dependent on the time it is administered prior to antigen challenge; its greatest efficacy is when it is used as a prophylactic agent.

When used correctly, intranasal cromolyn is effective for the treatment of allergic rhinitis.[39,81] Cromolyn relieves itching, sneezing, and rhinorrhea, but it may not be as effective as other treatment modalities for nasal obstruction.[82] Comparative efficacy studies indicate that cromolyn is generally less effective than intranasal corticosteroids in the treatment of allergic rhinitis, but it essentially is free of side effects.[39, 81] Because of its demonstrated efficacy and safety, the FDA has approved cromolyn for nonprescription use.

Instructions for Use

12. How should J.C. be advised to use cromolyn nasal spray to prevent her symptoms?

To be effective, cromolyn nasal spray must be dosed several times each day, which can have a detrimental effect on adherence.[39] The initial dose for the 4% cromolyn sodium nasal spray is one spray in each nostril four to six times daily. In some patients, symptom control can be maintained with dosing two to three times per day.

Cromolyn therapy should not be used intermittently and ideally should begin 2 weeks before exposure will occur and should be continued for the duration of exposure to the allergen (e.g., as long as J.C. visits her father). Patients should be informed that the full benefit from this therapy may be delayed up to 4 weeks.

Appropriate administration technique is critical to the success of intranasal cromolyn therapy, and the pharmacist should ensure that both parent and child can demonstrate this before therapy is initiated. J.C. should be instructed to gently blow her nose to remove any excess nasal secretions and then spray the cromolyn sodium solution into each nostril in a slightly upward direction, parallel to the nasal septum. On first use, the device should be primed until a consistent spray is achieved.

Topical nasal cromolyn has an excellent safety profile including minimal incidence of adverse effects. Local irritation occurs in <10% of patients, with burning, stinging, and sneezing being the most common manifestations. The risk of nasal irritation and bleeding, however, is less than that associated with using intranasal corticosteroids.[83] The safety of cromolyn has made it a popular choice as initial therapy for children with allergic rhinitis and for treating rhinitis during pregnancy.[84] Table 25-6 includes information about intranasal cromolyn dosing and availability.

Table 25-6   Additional Oral and Topical Agents for Allergic Rhinitis

Generic (Product)	Available Dosage Forms/ Strength	Adult Dose	Pediatric Dose
Oral			
Antileukotrienes[a] Montelukast[b] (Singulair)	Tablets: 10 mg Tablets, chewable: 4 mg, 5 mg Oral granules: 4 mg	10 mg QD (max. 10 mg/day)	6–14 yr: 5 mg QD (max. 5mg/day) 2–5 yr: 4 mg QD (max. 4 mg/day) <2 yr: Safe and effective use has not been established.
Topical			
Antihistamine azelastine (Astelin)	Nasal spray: 137 μg/spray	2 sprays/nostril Q 12 hr (max. 4 nasal sprays/day per nostril)	5–11 yr: 1 spray/nostril Q 12 hr (max. 2 nasal sprays/day per nostril) <5 yr: Safe and effective use has not been established.
Mast cell stabilizer cromolyn sodium[c] (Nasalcrom)	Nasal spray: 40 mg/mL (5.2 mg/spray)	1 spray/nostril Q 4–6 hr	≥2 yr: 1 spray/nostril 3–4 times daily
Anticholinergic ipratropium (Atrovent)	Nasal solution 0.03%[d]	2 sprays/nostril 2–3 times per day for up to 4 days	≥6 yr: 2 sprays/nostril 2–3 times daily up to 4 days.

[a]Other leukotriene receptor antagonists (zafirlukast) are indicated for asthma, but not approved for allergic rhinitis.
[b]Received FDA approval for the treatment of seasonal allergic rhinitis in adults and children >2 yr in 2003.
[c]Available OTC.
[d]Ipratropium nasal solution 0.06% indicated for rhinorrhea due to common cold, but not indicated for allergic rhinitis.
Adapted from reference 189.

Intranasal Corticosteroid Therapy

13. A.C. is an 8-year-old male with allergic rhinitis and asthma. He has been treated with a budesonide Turbuhaler for asthma and cromolyn nasal spray for rhinitis. His mother reports that he frequently sneezes, complains of an itchy nose and eyes, and does not sleep well at night because of nasal congestion. She also reports that she usually cannot get him to use his cromolyn more than twice a day. His asthma has been well controlled in the past; however, she is concerned that he is experiencing some shortness of breath and that this might be related to his allergies. While you are talking to him, A.C. frequently rubs his nose in an upward direction, sniffs and breathes through his mouth. When he speaks, he often snorts. You also notice slight bruising under his eyes where he has been rubbing them. What signs indicate that R.C. is experiencing allergic symptoms?

Signs and Symptoms of Allergic Rhinitis
A.C. is displaying the classic signs of allergic airways disease in children. He is sniffing and snorting in response to nasal itching and discharge. The frequent upward rubbing of the nose (generally with the palm of the hand) is known as the "allergic salute" and is caused by nasal itching. If the symptoms are long-standing, this can lead to facial abnormalities, including the formation of a transverse crease across the bridge of the nose. Infraorbital discoloration can develop with frequent rubbing of the eyes in patients with severe ocular itching and is called "allergic shiners."[35]

Role in Therapy
14. What would be the role of intranasal corticosteroids for this patient?

Intranasal corticosteroids are the most effective therapy available for the treatment of allergic rhinitis, and they are safe and well tolerated. They are highly effective in improving itching, sneezing, rhinorrhea, and congestion.[85] Nasal corticosteroids may also be beneficial in relieving cough associated with postnasal drip in patients with allergic rhinitis.[86] In addition to improving all nasal symptoms, there is also evidence that intranasal administration of corticosteroids are effective at relieving eye symptoms as well.[85] These agents also have demonstrated efficacy for nonallergic rhinitis, rhinitis medicamentosa, and nasal polyposis.[87] The currently available nasal corticosteroids are listed in Table 25-7. The benefits of intranasal corticosteroids can be attained with a minimal potential for side effects, compared with systemic corticosteroid therapy.[5]

Intranasal corticosteroids perform well compared with other therapeutic options in clinical trials. They are frequently rated as more effective than H$_1$-receptor antagonists.[88–90] In a systematic review of the medical literature performed by the Agency for Healthcare Research and Quality (AHRQ), nasal corticosteroids provided significantly greater relief of symptoms compared to antihistamines for various nasal symptoms and total nasal symptom scores.[91,18] In addition, a recent meta-analysis of nine well-controlled trials concluded that intranasal corticosteroids were more effective for nasal symptoms compared with antihistamines.[66] There were no differences in relief of ocular symptoms.

Mechanism of Action
15. How do intranasal corticosteroids work to reduce symptoms?

Table 25-7   Intranasal Corticosteroids[a,b,c]

Generic Name (Product)	Available Dosage Forms/Strengths	Adult Dose	Pediatric Dose
Beclomethasone (Beconase AQ)	Aqueous nasal spray: 42 μg/spray	1–2 sprays/nostril BID	>6 yr: 1–2 sprays/nostril BID
Budesonide (Rhinocort Aqua)	Aqueous nasal spray: 32 μg/spray, 64 μg/spray	4 sprays (32 μg/spray) or 2 sprays (64 μg/spray) per nostril QD	2 sprays (32 μg/spray) or 1 spray (64 μg/spray)/nostril QD
Fluticasone (Flonase)	Aqueous nasal spray: 50 μg/spray	2 sprays/nostril QD, or 1 spray/ nostril BID (max. 100 μg/ nostril per day)	4–17 yr: 1–2 spray/nostril QD (max. 200 μg/day)
Flunisolide (Nasalide) (Nasarel)	Propylene glycol based nasal spray: 25 μg/spray. Aqueous nasal spray: 25 μg/spray	2 sprays (25 μg/spray) in each nostril TID (max 200 μg/nostril per day)	6–14 yr: 1–2 spray/nostril TID or 2 sprays/nostril BID (max. 100 μg/nostril QD)
Mometasone (Nasonex)	Aqueous nasal spray: 50 μg/spray	2 sprays/nostril QD	2–11 yr: 1 spray/nostril QD
Triamcinolone (Nasacort AQ) (Tri-Nasal)	Aqueous nasal spray 55 μg/spray. Aqueous nasal spray 50 μg/spray	Adults and children >12 yr: 2–4 sprays/nostril QD, or 2 sprays/nostril BID	6–11 yr: 1–2 sprays/nostril QD

[a]Dosage forms containing chlorofluorocarbons removed from market in July 2003.
[b]Dosages should be reduced to lowest effective dose after symptoms controlled.
[c]May take several days for full treatment effect.
BID, twice daily; QD, once daily; TID, three times daily.
Adapted from reference 188.

Corticosteroids interact with a specific steroid receptor in the cytoplasm of a cell, and the steroid receptor complex then moves into the cell nucleus where it influences protein synthesis.[92] Among the proteins synthesized is lipocortin, which inhibits the breakdown of phospholipids to arachidonic acid; this, in turn, inhibits the formation of prostaglandins and leukotrienes. Topical corticosteroids reduce the number of eosinophils, basophils, and mast cells in the nasal mucosa and epithelium; directly inhibit the release of mediators from mast cells and basophils; reduce mucosal edema and vasodilation; stabilize the endothelium and epithelium, resulting in decreased exudation; and reduce the sensitivity of irritant receptors, resulting in decreased itching and sneezing.[34] Topical corticosteroids inhibit both the early- and late-phase reactions to antigen challenge, in contrast to systemic corticosteroids, which inhibit only the late-phase reaction in allergic rhinitis.[93]

16. Are there any specific considerations related to the use of intranasal corticosteroids in treating allergic rhinitis in a patient with concomitant asthma?

Based on the relationship between inflammation in the upper and lower airways, and the similar immunologic mechanisms involved in allergic rhinitis and asthma, it is a reasonable assumption that poor control of upper airway allergies can have a negative impact on asthma control.[94] In fact, rhinitis is a risk factor for asthma development,[95] and poorly controlled rhinitis can aggravate asthma control. In a patient with asthma, treatment of allergic rhinitis with nasal corticosteroids can reduce airway hyperresponsiveness and symptoms of asthma.[96] This patient is already receiving oral inhalation therapy with budesonide. The same agent can be added as a nasal inhaler or another intranasal corticosteroid product can be selected.

Choice of Therapeutic Agent

17. What are considerations in selecting among the various nasal corticosteroid products?

The currently available intranasal corticosteroid products have similar efficacy in relieving symptoms of allergic rhinitis. Primary differences among products include potency, dosing regimens, delivery systems, and patient preference. Each of the currently available intranasal corticosteroid products generally exhibit high topical potency with low systemic bioavailability. For allergic rhinitis, topical therapy is preferred over systemic corticosteroids for obvious advantages in the therapeutic ratio (topical to systemic ratio). Topical application is very effective in controlling nasal symptoms with minimal risks of systemic effects.[97] Generally, the current therapies are rapidly metabolized to inactive, or less active, compounds.

Currently available products differ in potency. The method to determine potency among topical corticosteroids is to measure topical vasoconstrictive activity on the skin. However, cutaneous vasoconstriction may not consistently correlate with anti-inflammatory potency in the nasal mucosa.[98] Potency may also be described as a measure of affinity for the steroid receptor or based on lipophilicity. Agents that are highly lipophilic may have faster absorption and longer residence at the receptor in the mucosa, which may contribute to potency.[98] The lowest to highest in lipophilicity among current products are flunisolide, triamcinolone, budesonide, beclomethasone, fluticasone, and mometasone.[99]

The topical to systemic potency relationship is also a consideration among the available agents. The ideal agent should exhibit high topical potency and low systemic activity. After topical administration, the corticosteroid may reach the systemic circulation by absorption across the nasal mucosa or through gastrointestinal absorption of the swallowed portion of the dose.[87,100] Among the available agents, mometasone and fluticasone have the lowest systemic bioavailability, ranging from 0.1% to less than 2%.[101] Beclomethasone may exert greater systemic effects due to its metabolism to an active metabolite (beclomethasone 17-monopropionate).[102] For this reason, newer agents are often favored over beclomethasone.

Safety

18. What criteria should be considered when choosing among the available intranasal corticosteroids? How safe are intranasal corticosteroids in this situation?

The corticosteroids currently available for intranasal administration are listed in Table 25-7. Chlorofluorocarbon (CFC)-containing intranasal corticosteroid products were removed from the U.S. market in July 2003 as part of the CFC transition plan. All these agents have the advantages of high potency (relative to hydrocortisone) and high lipophilicity. As noted previously, systemic exposure results when the medication is absorbed from the nasal mucous membrane and from the GI tract after incidental swallowing.

Among available products, intranasal corticosteroids have similar efficacy in clinical trials.[103,104] Budesonide, flunisolide, triamcinolone, and beclomethasone are indicated for ages 6 years or older. Fluticasone and mometasone are labeled for ages 4 years and older and 3 years and older, respectively.[105]

A common concern regarding the use of corticosteroids in children is the risk of growth suppression. In 1998, the FDA required new labeling on inhaled and intranasal corticosteroid preparations to alert heath care providers that use of these products in children may reduce their rate of growth. This effect was related to the dose and duration of therapy. It was specifically noted that the long-term effects of this reduction in growth velocity on final adult heights are unknown.

Two studies investigated the effects of intranasal corticosteroids on short-term (4 to 6 weeks) growth in children with rhinitis (most patients had seasonal allergic rhinitis), and both studies demonstrated significant suppression of short-term growth in children treated with intranasal corticosteroids.[106,107] However, these findings do not predict long-term effects on statural growth or ultimate adult height because short-term growth varies seasonally, and some children exhibit transient "growth spurts" and catch-up growth activity.[108] Similar effects on short term growth have been measured in children with asthma who have been treated with inhaled corticosteroids.[109] The best designed study of growth in asthmatics treated with inhaled beclomethasone dipropionate accounted for the age of the children at the time of the study and adjusted for the age of onset of puberty. This study found no significant growth suppression in the corticosteroid treated patients, and all patients achieved predicted adult height.[110] In a recent study, intranasal fluticasone at 200 μg daily did not significantly impair growth in 150 children, ages 3 to 9 years in a study of 1 year's duration.[111] In 2003, the FDA approved revised labeling for fluticasone nasal spray indicating no adverse effect on growth even with use up to 1 year's duration.

Although controversy still exists about the risk of negative effects on growth, these recent data as well as data from stud-

ies of orally inhaled corticosteroid therapy for asthma are reassuring.[111–113] Nonetheless, because growth suppression has been reported in children receiving nasal corticosteroids, it is appropriate to recommend agents with low systemic bioavailability and to use the lowest effective dose.

Prolonged topical use of intranasal corticosteroids does not impose a significant risk for mucosal atrophy.[114,115] Histologic changes in nasal mucosa have not been demonstrated, and intranasal candidiasis has never been documented.[92] Positive nasal and pharyngeal cultures for *Candida albicans* have been detected, but their relation to treatment is unknown because they also occur in placebo treated patients.[116,117]

A report from the National Registry of Drug-Induced Ocular Side Effects linked 21 cases of bilateral posterior subcapsular cataracts to the use of intranasal or inhaled corticosteroids.[118] Nine of these patients also were treated with systemic corticosteroids. The number of these patients receiving intranasal rather than inhaled corticosteroids was not reported, but many of the patients had used the beclomethasone dipropionate for >5 years, often in doses >252 mg/day. It may be important for the clinician to consider the total corticosteroid load in atopic patients who may be treated with an inhaled and/or systemic preparation for asthma, intranasal preparation for rhinitis, and dermatologic preparation for eczema, although there are no guidelines to follow in this area.

Instructions for Use

19. A.C. is given a prescription for budesonide, two actuations in each nostril BID. How should he be counseled and instructed to use this drug?

Although nasal corticosteroids have an excellent safety profile, some local adverse effects may occur. The most commonly reported side effect is epistaxis, with excessive nasal dryness and crusting possible as well.[119,120] Previously available products contained propylene glycol, which caused significant nasal stinging; however, aqueous pump products currently available are tolerated much better. A more serious concern is the risk for nasal septal perforation. Proper technique in using the nasal corticosteroid products can reduce the risks for these side effects.[1]

The delivery system for delivery of the nasal corticosteroid can influence efficacy and patient acceptance. Previously, devices contained CFC propellants that were associated with inconsistent distribution across the nasal mucosa compared with the current aqueous pumps. As noted above, propylene glycol and polyethylene glycol were used in some pump products to improve solubility of the active ingredient; however, these preparations were poorly tolerated by patients. Current pump preparations are formulated as aqueous suspensions and are well tolerated with consistent deposition on the nasal mucosa, although efficacy is generally considered to be similar to earlier CFC-containing preparations.

Patient education is important to ensure proper use of and response to the intranasal corticosteroids. A.C. should be instructed to blow his nose gently before using the nasal inhaler because copious nasal secretions cause the medication to drain back out of the nose. Severe blockage of the nasal passage may prevent deposition of the drug at the site of action. If the patient is severely congested, a short course (2 to 3 days) of topical decongestant used just before the intranasal corticosteroid may be indicated. The patient should be instructed to direct the spray away from the nasal septum. This is accomplished by pointing the applicator nozzle straight and back, parallel to the septum.

Therapeutic benefit often is perceived in 2 to 3 days, although currently available agents appear to have a faster onset of effect. Some newer agents (e.g., budesonide, mometasone, and fluticasone) may begin to relieve symptoms within hours. Fluticasone has been effective when used on as-needed basis.[38] Nonetheless, it is reasonable to advise patients that full benefit may not be realized for 2 to 3 weeks.

A.C. should be started on the maximum dose, and if his symptoms are well controlled, the dose may be tapered to the lowest effective dose. He should stay on any given dosage level for at least 1 week. If at any point his symptoms worsen after a dosage reduction, he should be instructed to increase the dose back to the last effective dose.

Systemic Corticosteroids

20. What is the role of systemic corticosteroid therapy for allergic rhinitis?

In contrast to the minimal side effects of the topical corticosteroids, systemic administration of these drugs can cause numerous, at times serious, side effects. Systemic administration, therefore, must be reserved for only short-term, adjunctive therapy in cases of severe, debilitating rhinitis. In such cases, a short course of relatively high-dose corticosteroid, so-called "burst" therapy, can be administered. Prednisone 40 mg/day for adults or 1 to 2 mg/kg per day for children (or an equivalent dose of a comparable compound) every morning for 3 to 7 days effectively relieves acute rhinitis symptoms. It should be started concurrently with the planned long-term therapy (e.g., H_1-antagonist decongestant combination, intranasal corticosteroid, intranasal cromolyn sodium).[1,23,34] Burst corticosteroid therapy rarely produces clinically important side effects.[121] An increase in appetite and mild cushingoid effects may occur toward the end of the burst with either no[122] or only transient[123] (<10 days) hypothalamic-pituitary-adrenal (HPA) axis suppression. However, four or more corticosteroid bursts a year may place some patients at greater risk for HPA axis suppression.[124]

The use of intranasal turbinate injections of corticosteroids has been reported, but the efficacy has never been studied in a controlled manner. This practice can result in serious complications, including vision loss and has been discouraged in favor of oral corticosteroid therapy for those patients requiring systemic treatment.[1,23]

If A.C. were to have a particularly severe exacerbation of his allergic rhinitis such that it interfered with sleep or ability to attend school, an oral corticosteroid burst would be indicated. This might occur if the pollen load was particularly heavy because of an unusual weather change. Incidentally, A.C. probably also will notice a remarkable improvement in nasal symptoms if he ever requires a corticosteroid burst for his asthma.

Combination Therapy

21. Would there be an advantage in combining various therapies for allergic rhinitis in this patient?

The different options used to treat allergic rhinitis have different mechanisms of action and offer the theoretical benefit of additive or synergistic actions. Combinations of antihistamines and decongestants are well studied and proven to benefit individual nasal symptoms as well as the total symptom score compared with either agent alone. Based on a systematic review of the literature, when combinations of antihistamines and nasal corticosteroids were compared with either agent alone, the combination was superior to antihistamine monotherapy but not treatment with nasal corticosteroids alone. Specific benefit has also been reported for rhinorrhea when antihistamines were combined with ipratropium; for ophthalmic symptoms of pruritus when antihistamines were combined with an ophthalmic antihistamine; and overall rhinitis symptoms when antihistamines and nedocromil were used together.[125] As noted previously, the combination of antihistamines and leukotriene modifier therapies has not consistently proved to be superior to either agent alone for allergic rhinitis. However, there may be benefit of the combination on improving asthma control in patients with concomitant diseases.[126]

Historically, the use of antihistamines was considered problematic for patients with asthma because of a theoretical concern about excessive drying of airway secretions due to anticholinergic properties of these agents. It is now clear that most patients with asthma can take any of the H_1-receptor antagonists without adverse pulmonary effects.[127]

Leukotriene-Modifying Agent Therapy

22. K.H. is a 58-year-old male with allergic rhinitis. He has experienced symptoms during ragweed pollen season for several years. He has used various antihistamines for his symptoms during this time with moderate success. At times, K.H. has self-medicated with nonprescription medications, including clemastine and diphenhydramine. This year, he initiated therapy with diphenhydramine 1 week before the pollen season, but began experiencing symptoms of urinary retention after 10 days. His physician advised him that this might be related to the anticholinergic effects of the antihistamine and his enlarged prostate and he was given a prescription for fexofenadine. After 1 week, K.H. complains that the medication is not working. After seeing an advertisement on television, he inquires about the use of a leukotriene modifier for his allergic rhinitis. What is the mechanism for the K.H.'s urinary discomfort attributed to the diphenhydramine?

K.H. is exhibiting symptoms of urinary outflow obstruction or prostatism. Common features of this are frequency, hesitancy, slow urine stream, dribbling and bladder fullness after voiding. The most common cause of obstruction is benign prostatic hyperplasia (BPH). Because the prostate is located anatomically around the urethra, enlargement of the gland can obstruct urine flow.[128]

The bladder and urethra are made up of smooth muscle tissue that is innervated by the sympathetic and parasympathetic divisions of the autonomic nervous system. The detrusor musculature is predominantly innervated by β-adrenergic and cholinergic receptors, whereas the bladder neck (or outlet) is innervated predominately by β-adrenergic receptors. Sympathetic stimulation causes relaxation of the detrusor muscle to allow bladder filling, closure of the urethra, and decreased bladder emptying. Cholinergic stimulation of the detrusor causes contraction of the detrusor to cause bladder emptying.[129] Initially, the detrusor musculature can compensate for the urethral obstruction in BPH. Eventually, however, the detrusor muscle fibers hypertrophy and decompensate, resulting in urinary retention and detrusor hyperreflexia manifesting as urinary frequency, urgency, urge incontinence, and nocturia.[128,129]

When K.H. took diphenhydramine, the anticholinergic properties of the drug blocked detrusor contraction and precipitated acute urinary retention. In this case, therapy with a second-generation antihistamine (i.e., fexofenadine) is more appropriate because these agents have little to no anticholinergic side effects.

Role in Therapy

23. **Would a leukotriene-modifying agent have a role in this case of allergic rhinitis?**

Since K.H. has experienced intolerance to first-generation antihistamines and a lack of efficacy with second-generation antihistamines, a trial with a leukotriene-modifying agent is appropriate.

In recent years, the potential role of leukotriene modifier therapies for the management of allergic rhinitis has been explored. The basis for this interest is the relationship between the upper and lower respiratory tracts, and the knowledge of common inflammatory cells and mediators in both allergic rhinitis and asthma. Leukotrienes are present in nasal secretions of patients with allergic rhinitis.

Activation of mast cells and other cells involved in the allergic response (e.g., basophils, eosinophils, and macrophages) result in the liberation of leukotrienes that are synthesized from arachidonic acid which is a component of the cell membranes. The leukotrienes that are subsequently produced are LTB4, LTC4, LTD4, and LTE4.[130] These are inflammatory mediators that result in increased vascular permeability, tissue edema, mucus secretion, and increased eosinophils. These actions lead to the symptoms of allergic rhinitis, as well as those of asthma.[40]

Efficacy

24. **What is the evidence that leukotriene modifiers are beneficial in allergic rhinitis?**

Leukotriene-modifying agents were demonstrated to be more efficacious than placebo in an initial 2-day study of 185 subjects. Zafirlukast, a leukotriene modifying agent, was effective in relieving nasal symptoms of allergic rhinitis; with a more consistent effect on symptoms of nasal congestion than rhinorrhea or sneezing.[131] Because of rare associations with eosinophilia, vasculitic rash, worsening pulmonary symptoms, cardiac complications, and/or neuropathy sometimes presenting as Churg-Strauss syndrome, this drug has not been pursued as a treatment strategy for rhinitis.

More recently, leukotriene-modifying agents have been compared with antihistamines. Two-week randomized double-blind trials in a total of more than 2,500 subjects with active seasonal allergic rhinitis found that montelukast 10 mg daily, like the active control, loratadine 10 mg daily, improved daily nasal symptom scores, night-time symptoms, daytime eye symptoms, and global evaluations by physicians and patients compared with placebo. Both active treatments improved symptoms compared with placebo, but not differently from one another.[132,133]

Using leukotriene-modifying agents in combination with nonsedating antihistamines has also been investigated. In one randomized study of 460 subjects with seasonal allergic rhinitis, taking montelukast 10 mg and loratadine 10 mg together was more effective than either drug alone, but in another study of 907 subjects, taking the two drugs in combination was not statistically significantly superior to taking either separately.[126,134] A smaller study compared monotherapy with fexofenadine to a combination of montelukast and loratadine in subjects with seasonal allergic rhinitis. Although both active treatment groups improved nasal symptoms better than placebo, there were no differences between active treatments.[135]

Collectively, these studies do not present strong evidence to support the value of combining antihistamines with leukotriene modifiers compared with therapy with either agent alone. As monotherapy, antihistamines or leukotriene-modifier therapy provide relief from numerous nasal symptoms. Clinical decisions about the value of combining treatments should be based on the specific clinical situation. For example, a patient with mild asthma and allergic rhinitis may benefit from a combination regimen with an antihistamine and a leukotriene modifier without a requirement for additional therapy.

Comparison Between Agents

25. **What is the benefit of leukotriene-modifier therapy as compared with nasal corticosteroids for allergic rhinitis?**

Leukotriene-modifier therapy has also been compared with nasal corticosteroids for patients with allergic rhinitis. Montelukast monotherapy has been compared with budesonide administered both intranasally and by oral inhalation in patients with concomitant seasonal allergic rhinitis and asthma.[136] For allergic rhinitis, both treatments improved total symptom scores and eye symptoms, but only budesonide improved nasal symptom scores.

In another 2-week study comparing once daily intranasal fluticasone 200 μg with montelukast 10 mg per day, the nasal corticosteroid was significantly more effective for individual nasal symptoms and total daytime and night-time nasal symptoms compared with montelukast treatment.[137]

In general, corticosteroid therapy demonstrates greater effects in suppressing markers of inflammation. The majority of recent studies have compared nasal corticosteroids to a combination of an antihistamine and a leukotriene modifier.[138] Intranasal fluticasone and fluticasone plus montelukast were more effective in relieving daytime symptoms compared with montelukast and placebo. Intranasal corticosteroids were more effective than all other groups, including the combination group, for night-time symptoms.

When cetirizine combined with montelukast was compared with intranasal mometasone and placebo, both active treatment groups were more effective for total nasal symptoms including nasal congestion; however, no difference was reported between the active treatments.[139]

Based on the results of these studies, nasal corticosteroids are at least as effective as, or more effective than, leukotriene-modifier therapy alone or when combined with an antihistamine.[140] Compared with other available therapies for allergic rhinitis, leukotriene modifiers offer modest benefit. Leukotrienes are known to cause nasal congestion but play a minimal role in rhinorrhea, itching, and sneezing. Therefore, the primary effect of leukotriene modifiers may be to relieve nasal congestion. This therapeutic class is an option in the overall management of patients with allergic rhinitis, although the beneficial effects are not consistently noted. This is not surprising based on the respective effects of the mediators involved.

In the case of K.H., appropriate recommendations could include a trial of another second-generation antihistamine or a nasal corticosteroid. If the patient is insistent or has concomitant asthma, a trial with a leukotriene modifier is a reasonable consideration. Table 25-6 includes information about the use and availability of montelukast.

Complementary and Alternative Therapies

26. C.L., a 25-year-old female presents to the pharmacy in mid-August complaining that her allergies are worsening daily. Symptoms are nasal discharge and obstruction, repetitive sneezing, and itching of the nose, eyes, and throat. She has fatigue and difficulty concentrating. Her symptoms have been occurring in late spring and summer since high school, and she has used a variety of medications intermittently over the years. C.L. is a competitive runner but has been unable to run as far or as often as usual owing to symptoms. A running partner mentioned that she could control her allergy symptoms with diet, exercise, and herbal remedies purchased at a local nutritional supplement shop. She asks your advice about this. What, if any, alternative treatments have been shown to be efficacious in allergic rhinitis?

Alternative treatments are common among adults with rhinitis and should be taken into account by health care providers. A survey of 300 adults indicated that herbal agents, caffeine-containing products, homeopathy, acupuncture, aromatherapy, reflexology and massage were common alternative treatments for respiratory conditions.[141] Still, because allergic rhinitis is largely a self-managed disease, it is likely that reported use of these agents is underestimated. For these reasons, patients should always be questioned specifically about the use of alternative therapies during the patient interview. Although some alternative approaches have been deemed to be safe, efficacy for many modalities has not been clearly established.[141]

Some reports have indicated that patients with allergic rhinitis may benefit from hydration and a diet low in sodium, omega-6 fatty acids, and transfatty acids, but high in omega-3 fatty acids (e.g., fish, almonds, walnuts, pumpkin, and flax seeds), and at least five servings of fruits and vegetables per day.[142] These recommendations are not without merit, because they may be beneficial for the population at large, but there is insufficient evidence to support specific value for allergic rhinitis symptoms.

There are no good clinical data on the efficacy of supplements containing vitamin C, grapeseed extract, bee pollen and honey, burdock, ginger, freeze-dried stinging nettle leaves, or quercetin (a bioflavonoid found in apples, buckwheat, grapes, red onions, red wine, and white grapefruit).[142,143] Further studies are needed to assess the efficacy of these supplements and herbs.

Menthol delivered in lozenges and rubs has been shown to have an ameliorating effect on nasal congestion; however, the effects are short-lived.[144] Other forms of aromatherapy suggested to relieve nasal congestion include massaging the essential oils of lavender and niaouli around the sinuses, or inhaling eucalyptus and peppermint oils.[145]

For the motivated patient, mind-body interventions such as yoga, hypnosis, and biofeedback-assisted relaxation and breathing exercises are beneficial for stress reduction, in general, which may improve the quality of life associated with rhinitis symptoms and treatment.[142] Acupuncture has been shown to have an attributive effect in inflammatory diseases such as rhinitis; however, there are not enough data to recommend this therapy at this time.[146] Although some studies have shown that patients with allergic rhinitis who received homeopathic dilutions of allergens had significantly better nasal air flow than those in the placebo group, overall no difference was seen in subjective measurement on a visual analog scale.[147]

Evidence regarding the use of intranasal zinc for upper respiratory symptoms has been conflicting. A randomized, double-blind, placebo-controlled trial of 160 subjects revealed that at low concentrations (0.12%), zinc sulfate nasal spray had no effect on the duration of respiratory symptoms. In another randomized, double-blind, placebo-controlled study of 80 subjects, however, results showed that zinc gluconium nasal gel 33 mmol/L shortens the duration and reduces symptom severity.

It has been suggested that herbs that support improved immune function could theoretically also help to ease symptoms of allergy.[148,149] With this in mind, echinacea has become the top-selling herbal product in the United States. Unfortunately, echinacea is closely related to sunflowers, daisies, and ragweed—all members of the Compositae/Asteraceae family.[150] The possibility that cross-sensitivity between echinacea and other environmental allergens may trigger allergic reactions is supported by an Australian review of all adverse drug reports, including cases of anaphylaxis, associated with echinacea.[151] Patients with known allergy to these plants should be cautioned regarding the use of echinacea products.

A multi-center, open-label trial on the safety and efficacy of methylsulfonylmethane (MSM) in the treatment of seasonal allergic rhinitis demonstrated that doses of 2,600 mg of MSM orally per day for 30 days were associated with improvements in respiratory symptom scores; however, the small study size (n = 55) and open-label design limit the generalizability of these findings.[152]

Although a variety of alternative remedies are widely available and used frequently in self-treatment, based on evaluation of these data, there is no firm recommendation for C.L. regarding the use of alternative therapies in allergic rhinitis.[153,154]

Immunotherapy

27. R.C. is a 25-year-old female schoolteacher who has experienced allergic symptoms since childhood, but noticed a worsening after she graduated from college and moved to a new area of the country. Although she has mild symptoms year-round, she has severe exacerbations during April–June and August–October each year. During these periods, she feels that exposure to cut grass and weeds provokes profound nasal symptoms. She also notes that when she spends more time outdoors in spring and early fall, her regular therapy, fluticasone nasal spray, is less effective. She has added loratadine, an over-the-counter nonsedating antihistamine during this time, but is frustrated by having to take so many medications while continuing to experience symptoms. R.C. asks your opinion about "allergy shots," remarking that she started them as a child with some relief, but moved after a year and never resumed treatment. Is allergen immunotherapy effective for reducing symptoms of allergic rhinitis?

Efficacy

Allergen immunotherapy (when injected, this is sometimes called "allergy shots") can be highly effective for managing allergic rhinitis symptoms in specific patients, and it represents the only approach leading to long-term symptom resolution. Traditionally, this has involved subcutaneous injection of dilute solutions of allergen extracts to increase tolerance to allergens so that the threshold for symptoms is increased (i.e., subsequent exposure elicits no or mild symptoms).

Immunotherapy administered via subcutaneous injection (SIT) has been used empirically since the early 1900s, and its efficacy has been documented in a large number of controlled trials.[155] A meta-analysis of 16 published studies involving 759 patients concluded that SIT is effective in the treatment of allergic rhinitis.[156] In addition, an extensive review of immunotherapy for allergic rhinitis in children suggested that immunotherapy may prevent the onset of asthma.[157] Taken together, these studies show that SIT should be considered a supplement to drug therapy in specific patients and possibly be used earlier in the course of allergic disease to achieve maximum benefit.[2]

Allergen Testing

28. How can the clinician determine R.C.'s specific sensitivities?

Skin testing using the modified prick test method or a prick-puncture method is used to confirm the diagnosis of allergic rhinitis and to determine specific allergen sensitivities.[34] Skin testing is a highly sensitive and relatively inexpensive objective measurement of allergen sensitivity. Small quantities of allergen are introduced into the skin by pricking or puncturing the skin in the immediate presence of the diluted allergen extract. Fifteen to 35 tests are placed on the upper portion of the back or the palmar surface of the forearms. A positive skin test produces a wheal and flare at the site within 15 to 30 minutes of application. An experienced clinician, usually an allergist, should conduct skin testing using high-quality allergen extracts and should interpret the results.

The allergens tested vary with geographic location, emphasizing the most common offending plant species that generate airborne particles. Pollen, the primary particle, is produced by trees, grasses, and weeds. Each of these plant groups generally pollinate at about the same time each year: trees in the spring, grasses from early to midsummer, and weeds from late summer into fall before the first killing frost. The onset and potency of the pollen season varies with geographic location and weather, particularly with respect to temperature and

moisture.[158] Seasonality can be misleading, however, because settled pollen particles from a previous season may be resuspended in the air following the spring snow melt or periods of heavy winds.

Mold spores also are common airborne allergens. The outdoor molds release their spores from early spring through late fall. Within this long season, spore counts increase and decrease, depending on the presence of local flora on which these molds grow, e.g., grain and other crops, forests, and orchards.[158] Some perennial allergens, such as house dust mites, insect and animal dander, and some indoor molds, occur consistently across all geographic distributions.[158] In each case, skin test results must be correlated with the patient's clinical history.[2]

R.C.'s perennial symptoms with seasonal exacerbations indicate sensitivity to the common perennial allergens with a particular sensitivity to seasonal allergens such as tree, grass, and weed pollen, but these subjective relationships should be confirmed with skin testing.

An alternative to skin testing is the radioallergosorbent test (RAST), in which the patient's serum is tested for allergen specific IgE antibodies. However, this test is less sensitive and more expensive than skin testing.[34,159] It is indicated only in selected clinical situations: when a patient consistently reacts positively to the negative control skin test (dermatographism), when antihistamine therapy cannot be discontinued, or when the patient has extensive atopic dermatitis or other skin lesions. Blood eosinophil counts and total serum IgE antibody measurements are neither sensitive nor specific enough to be useful in the diagnosis of allergic rhinitis.[160]

29. Since R.C. is currently using medications (fluticasone nasal spray and loratadine) for her symptoms, should these be discontinued before skin testing?

The H_1-receptor antagonists inhibit or blunt the wheal-and-flare reaction by blocking the effects of histamine on capillaries. Different H_1-antagonists vary in the extent to which they can blunt wheal formation and in the duration of the inhibitory effect (Table 25-8). Depending on the agent selected, antihistamines must be discontinued from 24 hours to 10 days before skin testing and even then, considerable interpatient variability exists in blocking effects.[159] For best results, R.C.'s loratadine should be discontinued 10 days before her skin testing.

Other allergy medications, including cromolyn and nasal corticosteroids, have no effect on skin tests. Likewise most asthma medications, including inhaled beta-agonists, cromolyn, theophylline, and inhaled and short-course systemic ("burst") corticosteroids have no effect on skin tests.[161] The effect of leukotriene-modifying agents has not been clearly established.[162] Oral β-agonists, long-term systemic corticosteroids, and high-potency topical corticosteroids (applied to the skin testing sites) may block cutaneous wheal-and-flare reactions, however. R.C. can continue the use of fluticasone nasal spray while she waits to be skin tested.

Other drugs also can affect allergen skin tests.[159] Tricyclic antidepressants are potent inhibitors of the wheal-and-flare reaction, and their effects can last up to 10 days. Phenothiazine-type antipsychotics and antiemetics (e.g., chlorpromazine, prochlorperazine) also can block cutaneous reactions to allergens. β-Blockers can increase skin reactivity.[159] Depending

Table 25-8 Effects of H₁-Receptor Antagonists on Allergen Skin Tests

Drug	Extent of Suppression[a]	Half-Life (hours)	Duration of Suppression (days)
Brompheniramine	+	24.9	1–4
Cetirizine	+++	7.4–11 (7)	3–10
Chlorpheniramine	+	24.4 (11)	1–4
Clemastine	++	—	1–10
Cyproheptadine	+/–	16	1–4
Desloratadine	+/++	27 (27)	3–10
Diphenhydramine	+/–	4–9	1–4
Fexofenadine	++	14 (18)	3–10
Hydroxyzine	++	20 (7.1)	1–10
Loratadine	+/++	11–24 (3.1)	3–10
Promethazine	+	12	1–4
Tripelennamine	+/–	—	1–4

[a]+++, extensive; ++ moderate; +, mild; +/–minimal to none, —unknown. Parenthetical numbers indicate half-life in children.
Adapted from references 1, 163.

on the indication for drug therapy, however, discontinuation of these drugs before skin testing is not always advisable. Additional information about skin testing is available from the American College of Allergy, Asthma and Immunology.[163]

Recommendations for discontinuing H₁-antagonists before allergen skin testing are listed in Table 25-9.

30. Is R.C. a candidate for immunotherapy injections?

SIT is indicated for patients with evidence of sustained, clinically relevant IgE-mediated disease and a limited spectrum of allergies (i.e., one or two clinically relevant allergens) and in whom pharmacotherapy and avoidance measures are insufficient.[164] Further considerations are the patient's attitude to available treatment modalities, costs of treatment, and the

Table 25-9 General Recommendations for Discontinuation of Antihistamines Before Allergen Skin Testing

1. Remind patient that allergic symptoms may return during the antihistamine-free period, but that reliable skin tests cannot be performed in a patient taking antihistamines.

2. Discontinue any short-acting antihistamine (those in Table 25-8 with a duration of suppression less than or equal to 4 days) 4 days before skin testing.

3. Discontinue longer-acting antihistamines (those in Table 25-8 with a duration of suppression greater than 4 days) at an interval appropriate to their duration of effect (e.g., hydroxyzine should be discontinued 10 days before skin testing).

4. Before applying the full battery of skin tests, apply histamine (positive) control and glycerinated diluent (negative) control tests. Application of a 1 mg/mL histamine base equivalent should yield wheal-and-flare diameters of 2–7 mm and 4.5–32.5 mm, respectively, to be considered a normal histamine reaction. A normal cutaneous reaction to histamine control suggests that accurate skin testing can be performed.

Adapted from reference 159.

quality of allergen vaccines available for treatment.[2] In the case of R.C., she has year-round symptoms with seasonal exacerbations, she has not experienced symptom relief when using appropriate therapies, and she is motivated to try immunotherapy. In addition, a previous trial in childhood was beneficial. For these reasons, skin testing and a trial of immunotherapy with specific allergens are reasonable.

Other Forms

31. Are there alternatives to injectable delivery of immunotherapy?

Traditional subcutaneous immunotherapy presents some disadvantages, such as costs, adherence, and rare systemic reactions. Because regular injections can be unacceptable to some patients, alternative methods of delivering antigens, such as sublingual immunotherapy (SLIT) and nasal immunotherapy (NIT), have been investigated.[165,166] A Cochrane Review of sublingual therapy for allergic rhinitis determined that SLIT is a safe treatment that significantly reduces symptoms and medication requirements in allergic rhinitis; however, the size of this benefit compared with that from other available therapies is not clear.[167] Currently, although sublingual and nasal methods have shown efficacy in milder disease, SIT is still optimal in severe allergic rhinitis with signs of bronchial hyperreactivity.[155]

Length of Therapy

32. If R.C. decides to proceed with immunotherapy, how long should her therapy continue?

After identification of the offending allergens via skin testing, subcutaneous immunotherapy is generally administered in two phases. During the build-up phase, increasing doses of allergen are given once or twice a week until a predetermined target or "maintenance" dose is achieved. This usually takes 3 to 4 months (e.g., 16 to 18 injections). Once this maintenance dose is reached, shots are usually administered every 2 to 3 weeks over the ensuing several years of treatment. Clinical improvement with immunotherapy usually occurs in the first year. In a small percentage of patients, there is no improvement and immunotherapy is discontinued. However, if symptoms do improve, injections are usually continued for 4 to 5 years of maintenance therapy.[168]

Although immunotherapy can lead to long-term remission of symptoms, one drawback is the lengthy treatment period. Preliminary data involving a 2-year study of 19 patients allergic to ragweed who underwent one allergy shot per week for 6 weeks before the 2001 ragweed season suggest that significant relief may be obtained from shorter-term treatment.[169]

Risks

33. **What are the risks associated with immunotherapy?**

Local adverse reactions (i.e., redness, swelling) to immunotherapy can be common, but the risk of severe reaction (i.e., anaphylaxis) is low. Still, administration should be performed by clinicians trained in resuscitation and with a clear emergency plan.[155] As pharmacists increasingly become vaccine providers, special care should be noted for those who include administering allergy shots in their scope of practice.

DRUG-INDUCED NASAL CONGESTION

34. **L. K. is a 27-year-old man who has suffered intermittent symptoms of allergic rhinitis. He reports that his symptoms are most bothersome in the spring and associated with blooming of various grasses. During these periods he typically uses chlorpheniramine, which relieves his symptoms adequately. This season, he reports that his symptoms have been more severe with sneezing, runny nose, and extreme itching in his nose. He has tried chlorpheniramine and recently switched to loratadine, with partial relief of symptoms. He also states that nasal congestion has been more of an issue with this episode and to address this he has used Afrin Nasal Spray (xylometazoline) for the past 3 weeks. Despite increasing the use of nasal spray from two to four times a day, however, he reports that the congestion is getting worse. What might be an explanation for L.K.'s increasing need for nasal decongestant?**

L.K. may be experiencing rhinitis medicamentosa or "rebound congestion." This is a common problem associated with prolonged and overuse of his topical nasal decongestant. Rhinitis medicamentosa is defined as a worsening of nasal congestion associated with overuse of topical sympathomimetic agents. For this reason, topical decongestant therapy should be limited to less than 10 days, but preferably no more than 5.[67]

Etiology

35. **Why does rhinitis medicamentosa occur?**

Sympathomimetic, or adrenergic, agents stimulate α-adrenergic receptors on blood vessels resulting in vasoconstriction. In the nasal mucosa, the therapeutic effect is relief of nasal congestion associated with edematous, congested blood vessels as a result of the allergic response. Rhinitis medicamentosa occurs as a result of a rebound phenomenon where the vessels in the nasal mucosa become more engorged and edematous as a result of overstimulation of α-adrenergic receptors. As a result, patients use the decongestant more frequently and may increase the dose for relief, creating a vi-

cious cycle. This problem is commonly reported with topical decongestants but is uncommon with oral agents.

The precise mechanism of rhinitis medicamentosa is unknown, but theories include fatigue of the constrictor muscles in the nasal vasculature; tissue hypoxemia caused by prolonged vasoconstriction, leading to a reactive vasodilation as the drug effects subside; and longer duration of the β-stimulatory effects of the drugs compared with the α-stimulatory effects, leading to secondary vasodilation.[170] It has also been suggested that benzalkonium chloride, used in topical decongestant products as a preservative, worsens rhinitis medicamentosa.[170] Whatever the subcellular mechanism, the result is a cycle of topical vasoconstrictor use followed by a profound nasal congestion necessitating repeated application of the topical agent. After only a few days of topical decongestant use, the patient can enter this cycle of use and dependence on the drug. Further, topical decongestants should never be used in infants younger than 6 months of age because they are obligate nose breathers and rebound congestion could cause obstructive apnea.

In addition to rhinitis medicamentosa, systemic medications and some drugs of abuse may cause nasal congestion or other nasal symptoms.[170,171] Table 25-10 lists drugs capable of causing nasal disease.

Strategies for Resolution

36. **What are possible strategies to recommend to L.K. to address this problem?**

There are several options to recommend to L.K. to deal with this problem. The best management for rhinitis medicamentosa is prevention.[32] Patients must be educated about the effects and potential complications of topical decongestants whenever they are prescribed or purchased without a prescription. Topical decongestant use must be limited to less than 5 days. If longer treatment is required, the patient should take a 1- to 2-day holiday during which the topical agent is not used before resuming treatment again.

In any case of drug-induced nasal congestion, the most important intervention is to discontinue the offending agent and, if necessary, substitute another therapy that will not cause nasal symptoms.[171] In the case of topical decongestants, discontinuation of the nasal spray can be difficult for the patient and presents the clinician with a therapeutic challenge. It also is important to appropriately treat the underlying cause of the nasal congestion that led to the use of the topical decongestant.

A simple strategy is to discontinue the topical decongestant spray. This can be done abruptly, but is likely to cause the patient considerable discomfort for the first 4 to 7 days after discontinuation.[170] There are also strategies to ameliorate the uncomfortable symptoms for the patient. The use of a product containing normal saline nose drops or spray can moisturize and alleviate nasal irritation. Intranasal corticosteroids often help decrease the tissue inflammation associated with rhinitis medicamentosa and can help patients in the immediate period after discontinuing the topical decongestant.[170] Oral decongestants can also be used for the recovery period. In refractory cases, a short course of systemic corticosteroids may be necessary.[170] If the patient has used the topical decongestant

Table 25-10   Drugs Capable of Causing Nasal Disease

Antihypertensives

Methyldopa
Prazosin
Reserpine
Hydralazine
β-Blockers class
ACE inhibitors class

Psychotherapeutic Drugs

Amitriptyline
Thioridazine
Perphenazine

Hormonal Products

Oral Contraceptives
Estrogen

Rebound Vasodilation After Vasoconstriction

Prolonged use of topical decongestants (rhinitis medicamentosa)

Direct Tissue Damage

Cocaine

Miscellaneous

Alprazolam
Benzalkonium chloride
Cromolyn sodium

ACE, angiotensin-converting enzyme.
Adapted from references 171, 187.

continuously for many months or years, the nasal mucosa can be damaged irreversibly.[172]

An alternative to abrupt cessation of the topical decongestant is to recommend that the patient discontinue use of the topical decongestant "one nostril at a time." In this case, the patient can continue using the topical agent in one nostril while waiting for resolution of the condition in the other nostril. When the drug is withdrawn completely from one nostril, begin decreasing the amount of drug used in the other nostril. For example, have the patient substitute normal saline nasal spray for decongestant spray in the right nostril for every other dose. Later, use saline twice for each decongestant dose. Eventually, the decongestant is discontinued totally in the right nostril and saline is substituted. Repeat the process for the left nostril. Saline can be used as often as needed throughout this process and after the topical decongestant is completely withdrawn. This method should be combined with careful patient education, support, and frequent follow-up.

IDIOPATHIC RHINITIS

37. M.S., a 29-year-old man, complains of profuse watery rhinorrhea that has been a chronic and progressively worsening problem for the past 5 years. He also experiences some nasal congestion with the rhinorrhea, but denies nasal itching or sneezing. Although the symptoms tend to remit and exacerbate, they do not occur in any definable seasonal pattern. His symptoms are worsened by exposure to tobacco smoke, strong fumes like paint or ammonia, and hot coffee and often are associated with headaches. Also, the rhinorrhea is substantially worse upon exposure to cold air. M.S. has no other medical problems and no family history for allergies. He does not smoke and drinks only occasionally. His only medication, beclomethasone dipropionate (42 μg/spray), 2 sprays in each nostril BID PRN, only partially relieves the symptoms. M.S. sniffs and blows his nose several times during the medical history. Physical examination reveals a mildly erythematous nasal mucosa and a minimally edematous inferior turbinate. Copious nasal discharge is clear and watery and air movement through the nose is relatively good. There is no sinus tenderness. The remainder of his physical examination is normal. Microscopic examination of a nasal smear demonstrates only a few neutrophils and no eosinophils. What information about M.S. supports the diagnosis of idiopathic rhinitis?

Diagnosis

Idiopathic rhinitis is a diagnosis of exclusion encompassing those patients with nasal mucous membrane inflammation with no proven immunologic, microbiologic, pharmacologic, hormonal or occupational cause.[34,173,174] Sometimes called "vasomotor rhinitis," this term implies that the origin of the disease has been identified, but that is not the case.[1,34] The prevailing theory holds that an imbalance in the autonomic nervous system exists in which the cholinergic parasympathetic activity exceeds the α-adrenergic activity in the nasal mucosa.[175] Theoretically, this is the reason that stimuli that normally increase parasympathetic activity in the nose, such as cold air and inhaled irritants, aggravate symptoms.[34,175] Still, there is substantial debate over whether idiopathic rhinitis represents a "localized" allergic response in the absence of systemic atopic markers[176,177] as well as the evidence for inflammatory pathophysiology in the disease.[178]

The symptoms of idiopathic rhinitis are variable. Most patients experience perennial nasal obstruction accompanied by profuse, watery nasal and postnasal discharge. Many patients complain of nasal obstruction as the primary symptom, while for others it is rhinorrhea. Sneezing occurs occasionally,[1,34,175] and nasal itching is uncommon. Headache may occur and usually is frontal or localized over the bridge of the nose. In patients with chronic nasal obstruction, chronic sinusitis and significant morbidity can result. In contrast to allergic rhinitis, the onset of symptoms in patients with idiopathic rhinitis usually occurs in adulthood, but before 40 years of age.

Patients report worsening of their symptoms when exposed to nonspecific irritants, including tobacco smoke, industrial pollutants, strong odors and perfumes, newsprint, chemical fumes, cold dry air, changes in humidity, and ingestion of very cold or very hot beverages or spicy foods. Most patients have no history or evidence of atopy.[175]

The appearance of the nasal mucosa also is variable. The turbinates are usually erythematous and swollen, and during an exacerbation, considerable quantities of nasal secretions usually are present. Mast cells may be present in the nasal smear, but by definition nasal eosinophilia is not present. Skin tests are usually negative.

38. M.S.'s symptoms of bothersome watery rhinorrhea, nasal congestion, and headache without itching or sneezing are typical. His complaint of worsening symptoms with exposure to noxious inhalants, cold air, and hot beverages support the diagnosis of idiopathic rhinitis. The nasal smear, which notably lacks large numbers of eosinophils, initially differentiates this disease from nonallergic rhinitis with eosinophilia syndrome (NARES). M.S. asks what causes idiopathic rhinitis and what can be done to alleviate his symptoms. What are the available nonpharmacologic and pharmacologic treatments for idiopathic rhinitis?

Choice of Therapeutic Agent

Nasal symptoms in patients with idiopathic rhinitis have been shown to be influenced by psychological factors. Some therapeutic benefit may be realized by establishing an on-going, trusting relationship between the health care provider and the patient. This should include a thorough explanation of the disease state and the realistic outcomes of therapy for most patients. Psychotherapy is helpful in some cases. In addition, patients should be instructed to avoid as many aggravating factors as possible, such as smoking, exposure to smoke or other irritants, and very cold or very hot beverages.[175] Saline irrigation is valuable as a general soothing and moisturizing treatment. Exercise may be particularly helpful for patients with idiopathic rhinitis because it increases sympathetic tone.[34]

Pharmacotherapy for idiopathic rhinitis should be directed toward the predominant symptoms of the individual patient.[175] For patients with predominant nasal congestion and minimal rhinorrhea, the intranasal corticosteroids may be helpful, although the results of clinical studies are mixed.[179,180] The addition of *oral decongestants* may improve nasal obstruction in some patients with idiopathic rhinitis, but objective measures of improvement are affected variably and side effects can be problematic.[181]

Unfortunately, M.S.'s case is typical of the often frustrating course in treating idiopathic rhinitis.[175] Commonly, multiple therapeutic plans fail, and M.S. has responded incompletely and unsatisfactorily to intranasal corticosteroids.

In patients like M.S., who suffer rhinorrhea as their predominant symptom, ipratropium bromide (Atrovent), a topically active congener of atropine, may decrease nasal secretions.[34,175] Also, systemic antihistamines may be helpful in treatment of idiopathic rhinitis because of their anticholinergic drying effects.[175] In general, though, antihistamines are less effective in the treatment of idiopathic rhinitis than for allergic rhinitis,[34] and patients may have difficulty complying with therapy. Of note, the nonsedating antihistamines have little value in idiopathic rhinitis because they lack anticholinergic properties.

39. How does ipratropium bromide work for idiopathic rhinitis and how effective is it?

Ipratropium bromide's quaternary ammonium structure makes it lipophobic; therefore, it is absorbed poorly from the nasal mucosa and GI tract and does not cross the blood-brain barrier.[182] It significantly reduces rhinorrhea (as measured by the number of nose-blowing episodes or daily number of tissues used) but has no effect on sneezing or nasal obstruction.[183] In children, it has been demonstrated to be as effective as beclomethasone in controlling rhinorrhea and diminishing the interference by rhinorrhea in school attendance, concentration on school work, and sleep, although beclomethasone was preferred for symptoms of sneezing.[179] Discontinuation of ipratropium has not been associated with rebound congestion.[184]

The recommended dose of ipratropium bromide is two sprays of the 0.03% nasal solution (42 μg) in each nostril two to three times per day.[2] If treatment with ipratropium bromide is attempted, dosage individualization is necessary because the range of doses required for symptom relief varied from 168 to 1,600 μg/ day.[185] A 0.06% nasal formulation is also available, but its use is typically reserved for short-term treatment of common cold symptoms.[186] Table 25-6 includes information about intranasal ipratropium dosing and availability.

In general, intranasal ipratropium bromide is well tolerated, though its use is associated with dose-related side effects.[1] The most common side effects are nasal dryness, nasal burning, bloody nasal discharge (epistaxis), dry or sore throat, and dry mouth.[1] Theoretically, elderly males with BPH may experience difficulty in urinating, but the risk is low because of negligible systemic absorption. No significant adverse cardiovascular or blood pressure effects have been observed.[187]

Surgical treatments have been attempted for patients in whom medical management fails. The surgical options include modification of the inferior turbinates (by turbinate displacement, electrocautery, or cryotherapy) or vidian neurectomy.

CONCLUSIONS

The initial management of acute and chronic rhinitis should be directed to prevention of symptoms, which can be achieved through a variety of pharmacologic and nonpharmacologic methods. Plans for allergic rhinitis, the most common form, should be directed toward allergen avoidance, medications, and immunotherapy, if indicated. Control of the disease process is the expected outcome—in which patients are able to live their lives comfortably without symptoms or impairment. Customizing therapy for each patient based on symptom history and response to treatments is important. Rhinitis can be controlled and effective management can greatly improve the quality of patients' lives.

Acknowledgments
The authors acknowledge the assistance of Kristan Rollins and Susan Herndon in the preparation of this chapter.

REFERENCES

1. Dykewicz MS et al. Diagnosis and management of rhinitis: complete guidelines of the Joint Task Force on Practice Parameters in Allergy, Asthma and Immunology. American Academy of Allergy, Asthma, and Immunology. Ann Allergy Asthma Immunol 1998;81(5 Pt 2):478.
2. van Cauwenberge P et al. Consensus statement on the treatment of allergic rhinitis. European Academy of Allergology and Clinical Immunology. Allergy 2000;55(2):116.
3. Vinuya RZ. Upper airway disorders and asthma: a syndrome of airway inflammation. Ann Allergy Asthma Immunol 2002;88(4 Suppl 1):8.
4. Simons FE. Allergic rhinobronchitis: the asthma-allergic rhinitis link. J Allergy Clin Immunol 1999;104(3 Pt 1):534.
5. Bousquet J et al. Allergic rhinitis and its impact on asthma. J Allergy Clin Immunol 2001;108(5 Suppl):S147.
6. Weiss KB, Sullivan SD. The health economics of asthma and rhinitis. I. Assessing the economic impact. J Allergy Clin Immunol 2001;107(1):3.
7. American Academy of Allergy, Asthma and Immunology. The Allergy Report. Milwaukee, WI: American Academy of Allergy, Asthma and Immunology, 2000.
8. National Institute of Allergy and Infectious Disease. Asthma and Allergy Statistics Fact Sheet. Bethesda, MD: National Institute of Allergy and

Infectious Disease, 2000. Available at: http://www.niaid.nih.gov.

9. Skoner DP. Allergic rhinitis: definition, epidemiology, pathophysiology, detection, and diagnosis. J Allergy Clin Immunol 2001;108(1 Suppl):S2.

10. Sly RM. Changing prevalence of allergic rhinitis and asthma. Ann Allergy Asthma Immunol. 1999;82(3):233; quiz 248.

11. Verlato G et al. Is the prevalence of adult asthma and allergic rhinitis still increasing? Results of an Italian study. J Allergy Clin Immunol 2003;111(6):1232.

12. Law AW et al. Direct costs of allergic rhinitis in the United States: estimates from the 1996 Medical Expenditure Panel Survey. J Allergy Clin Immunol 2003;111(2):296.

13. Storms W et al. The economic impact of allergic rhinitis. J Allergy Clin Immunol 1997;99S820.

14. Fireman P. Treatment of allergic rhinitis: effect on occupation productivity and work force costs. Allergy Asthma Proc 1997;18(2):63.

15. Ricketti AJ. Allergic rhinitis. In: Grammer LC, Greenberger PA, eds. Patterson's Allergic Diseases. Philadelphia: Lippincott Williams & Wilkins, 2002:159–182.

16. Lund VJ. Anatomy and physiology of the nasal cavity and paranasal sinuses. In: Raeburn D, Giembycz M, eds. Rhinitis: Immunopathology and Pharmacotherapy. Basel: Birkhauser Verlag, 1997:

17. Dykewicz MS. 7. Rhinitis and sinusitis. J Allergy Clin Immunol 2003;111(2 Suppl):S520.

18. Scadding GK. Corticosteroids in the treatment of pediatric allergic rhinitis. J Allergy Clin Immunol 2001;108(1 Suppl):S59.

19. Fokkens WJ. Thoughts on the pathophysiology of nonallergic rhinitis. Curr Allergy Asthma Rep 2002;2(3):203.

20. Bleecker ER, Meyers DA. Genetics of allergy and asthma. In: Kay AB, ed. Allergy and Allergic Disease, Vol. 2. Malden: Blackwell Science, 1997: 1196–1207.

21. Baraniuk JN. Pathogenesis of allergic rhinitis. J Allergy Clin Immunol 1997;99(2):S763.

22. Busse WW, Lemanske RF, Jr. Asthma. N Engl J Med 2001;344(5):350.

23. Naclerio RM. Pathophysiology of perennial allergic rhinitis. Allergy 1997;52(36 Suppl):7.

24. White M. Mediators of inflammation and the inflammatory process. J Allergy Clin Immunol 1999;103(3 Pt 2):S378.

25. Clark RR, Baroody FM. What drives the symptoms of allergic rhinitis? J Respir Dis 1998;19S6.

26. Hogan MB et al. Rhinitis. Ann Allergy 1994;72(4):293; quiz 301.

27. Wang D et al. An approach to the understanding of the nasal early-phase reaction induced by nasal allergen challenge. Allergy 1997;52(2):162.

28. Costa JJ et al. The cells of the allergic response: mast cells, basophils, and eosinophils. JAMA 1997;278(22):1815.

29. Urval KR. Overview of diagnosis and management of allergic rhinitis. Prim Care 1998;25(3):649.

30. Juniper EF et al. First-line treatment of seasonal (ragweed) rhinoconjunctivitis. A randomized management trial comparing a nasal steroid spray and a nonsedating antihistamine. CMAJ 1997;156(8):1123.

31. Juniper EF. Measuring health-related quality of life in rhinitis. J Allergy Clin Immunol 1997;99(2): S742.

32. Juniper EF et al. Comparison of the efficacy and side effects of aqueous steroid nasal spray (budesonide) and allergen-injection therapy (Pollinex-R) in the treatment of seasonal allergic rhinoconjunctivitis. J Allergy Clin Immunol 1990;85(3):606.

33. Juniper EF. Quality of life in adults and children with asthma and rhinitis. Allergy 1997;52(10):971.

34. International Consensus Report on the diagnosis and management of rhinitis. International Rhinitis Management Working Group. Allergy. 1994;49(19 Suppl):1-34.

35. Bresolin D et al. Facial characteristics of children who breathe through the mouth. Pediatrics. 1984;73(5):622-625.

36. Mohapatra SS, Lockey RF. Allergens. In: Kaliner MA, ed. Current Review of Allergic Diseases. Malden: Blackwell Science, 2000:

37. Dykewicz MS et al. Fluticasone propionate aqueous nasal spray improves nasal symptoms of seasonal allergic rhinitis when used as needed (prn). Ann Allergy Asthma Immunol 2003;91(1):44.

38. Jen A et al. As-needed use of fluticasone propionate nasal spray reduces symptoms of seasonal allergic rhinitis. J Allergy Clin Immunol 2000;105(4):732.

39. Meltzer EO. Efficacy and patient satisfaction with cromolyn sodium nasal solution in the treatment of seasonal allergic rhinitis: a placebo-controlled study. Clin Ther 2002;24(6):942.

40. Meltzer EO. Role for cysteinyl leukotriene receptor antagonist therapy in asthma and their potential role in allergic rhinitis based on the concept of "one linked airway disease." Ann Allergy Asthma Immunol 2000;84(2):176; quiz 185.

41. Noga O et al. Immunological and clinical changes in allergic asthmatics following treatment with omalizumab. Int Arch Allergy Immunol 2003;131(1):46.

42. D'Amato G. Therapy of allergic bronchial asthma with omalizumab—an anti-IgE monoclonal antibody. Expert Opin Biol Ther 2003;3(2):371.

43. Terreehorst I et al. Evaluation of impermeable covers for bedding in patients with allergic rhinitis. N Engl J Med 2003;349(3):237.

44. Slater JW et al. Second-generation antihistamines: a comparative review. Drugs 1999;57(1):31.

45. Leurs R et al. H_1-antihistamines: inverse agonism, anti-inflammatory actions and cardiac effects. Clin Exp Allergy 2002;32(4):489.

46. DuBuske LM. Appropriate and inappropriate use of immunotherapy. Ann Allergy Asthma Immunol 2001;87(1 Suppl 1):56.

47. Casale TB et al. First do no harm: managing antihistamine impairment in patients with allergic rhinitis. J Allergy Clin Immunol 2003;111(5):S835.

48. Bender BG et al. Sedation and performance impairment of diphenhydramine and second-generation antihistamines: a meta-analysis. J Allergy Clin Immunol 2003;111(4):770.

49. Roth T et al. Sedative effects of antihistamines. J Allergy Clin Immunol 1987;80(1):94.

50. Kay GG et al. Initial and steady-state effects of diphenhydramine and loratadine on sedation, cognition, mood, and psychomotor performance. Arch Intern Med 1997;157(20):2350.

51. Kay GG et al. Sedating effects of AM/PM antihistamine dosing with evening chlorpheniramine and morning terfenadine. Am J Man Care 1997;31843.

52. Starbuck VN et al. Functional magnetic resonance imaging reflects changes in brain functioning with sedation. Hum Psychopharmacol 2000;15(8):613.

53. Vuurman EF et al. Seasonal allergic rhinitis and antihistamine effects on children's learning. Ann Allergy 1993;71(2):121.

54. Weiler JM et al. Effects of fexofenadine, diphenhydramine, and alcohol on driving performance. A randomized, placebo-controlled trial in the Iowa driving simulator. Ann Intern Med 2000; 132(5):354.

55. The use of newer asthma and allergy medications during pregnancy. The American College of Obstetricians and Gynecologists (ACOG) and The American College of Allergy, Asthma and Immunology (ACAAI). Ann Allergy Asthma Immunol 2000; 84(5):475.

56. Simons FE, Simons KJ. The pharmacology and use of H_1-receptor-antagonist drugs. N Engl J Med 1994;330(23):1663.

57. Limon L, Kockler DR. Desloratadine: a nonsedating antihistamine. Ann Pharmacother 2003; 37(2):237; quiz 313.

58. Hindmarch I, Shamsi Z. Antihistamines: models to assess sedative properties, assessment of sedation, safety and other side-effects. Clin Exp Allergy 1999;29 Suppl 3133.

59. Howarth PH et al. Double-blind, placebo-controlled study comparing the efficacy and safety of fexofenadine hydrochloride (120 and 180 mg once daily) and cetirizine in seasonal allergic rhinitis. J Allergy Clin Immunol 1999;104(5):927.

60. Lieberman PL, Settipane RA. Azelastine nasal spray: a review of pharmacology and clinical efficacy in allergic and nonallergic rhinitis. Allergy Asthma Proc 2003;24(2):95.

61. Canonica GW et al. Topical azelastine in perennial allergic conjunctivitis. Curr Med Res Opin 2003;19(4):321.

62. James IG et al. Comparison of the efficacy and tolerability of topically administered azelastine, sodium cromoglycate and placebo in the treatment of seasonal allergic conjunctivitis and rhinoconjunctivitis. Curr Med Res Opin 2003;19(4):313.

63. Weiler JM et al. A dose-ranging study of the efficacy and safety of azelastine nasal spray in the treatment of seasonal allergic rhinitis with an acute model. J Allergy Clin Immunol 1994;94(6 Pt 1):972.

64. Gastpar H et al. Comparative efficacy of azelastine nasal spray and terfenadine in seasonal and perennial rhinitis. Allergy 1994;49(3):152.

65. Meltzer EO et al. Azelastine nasal spray in the management of seasonal allergic rhinitis. Ann Allergy 1994;72(4):354.

66. Yanez A, Rodrigo GJ. Intranasal corticosteroids versus topical H_1 receptor antagonists for the treatment of allergic rhinitis: a systematic review with meta-analysis. Ann Allergy Asthma Immunol 2002;89(5):479.

67. Naclerio R, Solomon W. Rhinitis and inhalant allergens. JAMA 1997;278(22):1842.

68. Falliers CJ, Redding MA. Controlled comparison of a new antihistamine-decongestant combination to its individual components. Ann Allergy 1980;45(2):75.

69. Meran A et al. A cross-over comparison of acrivastine, pseudoephedrine and their combination in seasonal allergic rhinitis. Rhinology 1990;28(1):33.

70. Kernan WN et al. Phenylpropanolamine and the risk of hemorrhagic stroke. N Engl J Med 2000;343(25):1826.

71. Coates ML et al. Does pseudoephedrine increase blood pressure in patients with controlled hypertension? J Fam Pract 1995;40(1):22.

72. Friedlaender MH. Management of ocular allergy. Ann Allergy Asthma Immunol 1995;75(3):212; quiz 223.

73. McGill JI et al. Allergic eye disease mechanisms. Br J Ophthalmol 1998;82(10):1203.

74. Alexander M et al. Supplementation of fexofenadine therapy with nedocromil sodium 2% ophthalmic solution to treat ocular symptoms of seasonal allergic conjunctivitis. Clin Experiment Ophthalmol 2003;31(3):206.

75. Lanier BQ et al. Comparison of the efficacy of combined fluticasone propionate and olopatadine versus combined fluticasone propionate and fexofenadine for the treatment of allergic rhinoconjunctivitis induced by conjunctival allergen challenge. Clin Ther 2002;24(7):1161.

76. Avunduk AM et al. Mechanisms and comparison of anti-allergic efficacy of topical lodoxamide and cromolyn sodium treatment in vernal keratoconjunctivitis. Ophthalmology 2000;107(7):1333.

77. Abelson MB, Spitalny L. Combined analysis of two studies using the conjunctival allergen challenge model to evaluate olopatadine hydrochloride, a new ophthalmic antiallergic agent with dual activity. Am J Ophthalmol 1998;125(6):797.

78. Ganz M et al. Ketotifen fumarate and olopatadine hydrochloride in the treatment of allergic conjunctivitis: a real-world comparison of efficacy and ocular comfort. Adv Ther 2003;20(2):79.

79. Ballas Z et al. Clinical evaluation of ketorolac tromethamine 0.5% ophthalmic solution for the treatment of seasonal allergic conjunctivitis. Surv Ophthalmol 1993;38(Suppl) 141.

80. Hingorani M, Lightman S. Therapeutic options in ocular allergic disease. Drugs 1995;50(2):208.

81. Ratner PH et al. Use of intranasal cromolyn sodium for allergic rhinitis. Mayo Clin Proc 2002; 77(4):350.

82. Bousquet J et al. Prevention of pollen rhinitis symptoms: comparison of fluticasone propionate aqueous nasal spray and disodium cromoglycate aqueous nasal spray. A multicenter, double-blind, double-dummy, parallel-group study. Allergy 1993;48(5):327.

83. Morrow-Brown H et al. A comparison of beclomethasone dipropionate aqueous nasal spray and sodium cromoglycate nasal spray in the management of seasonal allergic rhinitis. Allergol Immunopathol (Madr) 1984;12(5):355.
84. Mazzotta P et al. Treating allergic rhinitis in pregnancy. Safety considerations. Drug Saf 1999;20(4):361.
85. Bousquet J et al. Requirements for medications commonly used in the treatment of allergic rhinitis. Allergy 2003;58(3):192.
86. Gawchik S et al. Relief of cough and nasal symptoms associated with allergic rhinitis by mometasone furoate nasal spray. Ann Allergy Asthma Immunol 2003;90(4):416.
87. Szefler SJ. Pharmacokinetics of intranasal corticosteroids. J Allergy Clin Immunol 2001;108(1 Suppl):S26.
88. Ratner PH et al. A comparison of the efficacy of fluticasone propionate aqueous nasal spray and loratadine, alone and in combination, for the treatment of seasonal allergic rhinitis. J Fam Pract 1998;47(2):118.
89. Juniper EF et al. Comparison of beclomethasone dipropionate aqueous nasal spray, astemizole, and the combination in the prophylactic treatment of ragweed pollen-induced rhinoconjunctivitis. J Allergy Clin Immunol 1989;83(3):627.
90. Gehanno P, Desfougeres JL. Fluticasone propionate aqueous nasal spray compared with oral loratadine in patients with seasonal allergic rhinitis. Allergy 1997;52(4):445.
91. Management of allergic and nonallergic rhinitis. Evidence Report/Technology Assessment. Agency for Healthcare Research and Quality Publication No. 02-E023. Vol. 54, 2002:1.
92. Naclerio RM, Mygind N. Intranasal steroids. In: Mygind N, Naclerio RM, eds. Allergic and Nonallergic Rhinitis: Clinical Aspects. Philadelphia: WB Saunders, 1993:114–122.
93. Pipkorn U et al. Inhibition of mediator release in allergic rhinitis by pretreatment with topical glucocorticosteroids. N Engl J Med 1987;316(24):1506.
94. Corren J. Allergic rhinitis and asthma: how important is the link? J Allergy Clin Immunol 1997;99(2):S781.
95. Guerra S et al. Rhinitis as an independent risk factor for adult-onset asthma. J Allergy Clin Immunol 2002;109(3):419.
96. Sandrini A et al. Effect of nasal triamcinolone acetonide on lower airway inflammatory markers in patients with allergic rhinitis. J Allergy Clin Immunol 2003;111(2):313.
97. Barnes PJ et al. Efficacy and safety of inhaled corticosteroids. New developments. Am J Respir Crit Care Med 1998;157(3 Pt 2):S1.
98. Mygind N et al. Mode of action of intranasal corticosteroids. J Allergy Clin Immunol. 2001;108(1 Suppl):S16.
99. Johnson M. Development of fluticasone propionate and comparison with other inhaled corticosteroids. J Allergy Clin Immunol 1998;101(4 Pt 2):S434.
100. Corren J. Intranasal corticosteroids for allergic rhinitis: how do different agents compare? J Allergy Clin Immunol 1999;104(4 Pt 1):S144.
101. Onrust SV, Lamb HM. Mometasone furoate. A review of its intranasal use in allergic rhinitis. Drugs 1998;56(4):725.
102. Falcoz C et al. Pharmacokinetic and systemic exposure of inhaled beclomethasone dipropionate. Eur Respir J 1996;9(Suppl. 23):162s.
103. van As A et al. Once daily fluticasone propionate is as effective for perennial allergic rhinitis as twice daily beclomethasone diproprionate. J Allergy Clin Immunol 1993;91(6):1146.
104. Welsh PW et al. Efficacy of beclomethasone nasal solution, flunisolide, and cromolyn in relieving symptoms of ragweed allergy. Mayo Clin Proc 1987;62(2):125.
105. Trangsrud AJ et al. Intranasal corticosteroids for allergic rhinitis. Pharmacotherapy 2002;22(11):1458.
106. Wolthers OD, Pedersen S. Short-term growth in children with allergic rhinitis treated with oral antihistamine, depot and intranasal glucocorticosteroids. Acta Paediatr 1993;82(8):635.
107. Wolthers OD, Pedersen S. Knemometric assessment of systemic activity of once daily intranasal dry-powder budesonide in children. Allergy 1994;49(2):96.
108. Karlberg J et al. Distinctions between short- and long-term human growth studies. Acta Paediatr 1993;82(8):631.
109. Allen DB. Growth suppression by glucocorticoid therapy. Endocrinol Metab Clin North Am 1996;25(3):699.
110. Balfour-Lynn L. Growth and childhood asthma. Arch Dis Child 1986;61(11):1049.
111. Allen DB et al. No growth suppression in children treated with the maximum recommended dose of fluticasone propionate aqueous nasal spray for one year. Allergy Asthma Proc 2002;23(6):407.
112. Agertoft L, Pedersen S. Effect of long-term treatment with inhaled budesonide on adult height in children with asthma. N Engl J Med 2000;343(15):1064.
113. Long-term effects of budesonide or nedocromil in children with asthma. The Childhood Asthma Management Program Research Group. N Engl J Med 2000;343(15):1054.
114. Holm AF et al. A 1-year placebo-controlled study of intranasal fluticasone propionate aqueous nasal spray in patients with perennial allergic rhinitis: a safety and biopsy study. Clin Otolaryngol 1998;23(1):69.
115. Laliberte F et al. Clinical and pathologic methods to assess the long-term safety of nasal corticosteroids. French Triamcinolone Acetonide Study Group. Allergy 2000;55(8):718.
116. Double-blind trial comparing two dosage schedules of beclomethasone dipropionate aerosol with a placebo in the treatment of perennial rhinitis for twelve months. Brompton Hospital/medical research council collaborative trial. Clin Allergy 1980;10(3):239.
117. Sarsfield JK, Thomson GE. Flunisolide nasal spray for perennial rhinitis in children. Br Med J 1979;2(6182):95.
118. Fraunfelder FT, Meyer SM. Posterior subcapsular cataracts associated with nasal or inhalation corticosteroids. Am J Ophthalmol 1990;109(4):489.
119. Mandl M et al. Comparison of once daily mometasone furoate (Nasonex) and fluticasone propionate aqueous nasal sprays for the treatment of perennial rhinitis. 194-079 Study Group. Ann Allergy Asthma Immunol 1997;79(4):370.
120. LaForce C. Use of nasal steroids in managing allergic rhinitis. J Allergy Clin Immunol 1999;103(3 Pt 2):S388.
121. Kelly HW, Murphy S. Corticosteroids for acute, severe asthma. DICP 1991;25(1):72.
122. Shapiro GG et al. Double-blind evaluation of methylprednisolone versus placebo for acute asthma episodes. Pediatrics 1983;71(4):510.
123. Zora JA et al. Hypothalamic-pituitary-adrenal axis suppression after short-term, high-dose glucocorticoid therapy in children with asthma. J Allergy Clin Immunol 1986;77(1 Pt 1):9.
124. Dolan LM et al. Short-term, high-dose, systemic steroids in children with asthma: the effect on the hypothalamic-pituitary-adrenal axis. J Allergy Clin Immunol 1987;80(1):81.
125. Management of allergic rhinitis in the working-age population. Evidence Report/Technology Assessment. Agency for Healthcare Research and Quality Publication No. 02-E013. Vol. 67, 2003:1.
126. Nayak AS et al. Efficacy and tolerability of montelukast alone or in combination with loratadine in seasonal allergic rhinitis: a multicenter, randomized, double-blind, placebo-controlled trial performed in the fall. Ann Allergy Asthma Immunol 2002;88(6):592.
127. Meltzer EO. The use of anti-H1 drugs in mild asthma. Allergy 1995;50(24 Suppl):41.
128. Christensen MM, Bruskewitz RC. Clinical manifestations of benign prostatic hyperplasia and indications for therapeutic intervention. Urol Clin North Am 1990;17(3):509.
129. Badlani GH, Smith AD. Pharmacotherapy of voiding dysfunction in the elderly. Semin Urol 1987;5(2):120.
130. Henderson WR, Jr. The role of leukotrienes in inflammation. Ann Intern Med 1994;121(9):684.
131. Donnelly AL et al. The leukotriene D4-receptor antagonist, ICI 204,219, relieves symptoms of acute seasonal allergic rhinitis. Am J Respir Crit Care Med 1995;151(6):1734.
132. Philip G et al. Montelukast for treating seasonal allergic rhinitis: a randomized, double-blind, placebo-controlled trial performed in the spring. Clin Exp Allergy 2002;32(7):1020.
133. van Adelsberg J et al. Randomized controlled trial evaluating the clinical benefit of montelukast for treating spring seasonal allergic rhinitis. Ann Allergy Asthma Immunol 2003;90(2):214.
134. Meltzer EO et al. Concomitant montelukast and loratadine as treatment for seasonal allergic rhinitis: a randomized, placebo-controlled clinical trial. J Allergy Clin Immunol 2000;105(5):917.
135. Wilson AM et al. A comparison of once daily fexofenadine versus the combination of montelukast plus loratadine on domiciliary nasal peak flow and symptoms in seasonal allergic rhinitis. Clin Exp Allergy 2002;32(1):126.
136. Wilson AM et al. A comparison of topical budesonide and oral montelukast in seasonal allergic rhinitis and asthma. Clin Exp Allergy 2001;31(4):616.
137. Ratner PH et al. Fluticasone propionate aqueous nasal spray provided significantly greater improvement in daytime and nighttime nasal symptoms of seasonal allergic rhinitis compared with montelukast. Ann Allergy Asthma Immunol 2003;90(5):536.
138. Pullerits T et al. Comparison of a nasal glucocorticoid, antileukotriene, and a combination of antileukotriene and antihistamine in the treatment of seasonal allergic rhinitis. J Allergy Clin Immunol 2002;109(6):949.
139. Wilson AM et al. Effects of monotherapy with intra-nasal corticosteroid or combined oral histamine and leukotriene receptor antagonists in seasonal allergic rhinitis. Clin Exp Allergy 2001;31(1):61.
140. Nathan RA. Pharmacotherapy for allergic rhinitis: a critical review of leukotriene receptor antagonists compared with other treatments. Ann Allergy Asthma Immunol 2003;90(2):182; 182–190.
141. Blanc PD et al. Alternative therapies among adults with a reported diagnosis of asthma or rhinosinusitis: data from a population-based survey. Chest 2001;120(5):1461.
142. Jaber R. Respiratory and allergic diseases: from upper respiratory tract infections to asthma. Prim Care 2002;29(2):231.
143. Bernstein DI et al. Evaluation of the clinical efficacy and safety of grapeseed extract in the treatment of fall seasonal allergic rhinitis: a pilot study. Ann Allergy Asthma Immunol 2002;88(3):272.
144. Eccles R. Menthol: effects on nasal sensation of airflow and the drive to breathe. Curr Allergy Asthma Rep 2003;3(3):210.
145. Hochwald L. Natural allergy remedies. New Age 2001; March/April: 36.
146. Zijlstra FJ et al. Anti-inflammatory actions of acupuncture. Mediators Inflamm 2003;12(2):59.
147. Taylor MA et al. Randomised controlled trial of homoeopathy versus placebo in perennial allergic rhinitis with overview of four trial series. Br Med J 2000;321(7259):471.
148. Blumenthal M et al. German Commission E monographs: medicinal plants for human use. American Botanical Council. Austin, Texas, 1998
149. Wagner D. A natural approach to asthma. Natural Pharmacy 2002.
150. Gunning K. Echinacea in the treatment and prevention of upper respiratory tract infections. Western J Med 1999;171:1.

151. Mullins RJ, Heddle R. Adverse reactions associated with echinacea: the Australian experience. Ann Allergy Asthma Immunol. 2002;88(1):42.
152. Barrager E et al. A multicentered, open-label trial on the safety and efficacy of methylsulfonylmethane in the treatment of seasonal allergic rhinitis. J Altern Complement Med 2002;8(2):167.
153. Ziment I. Recent advances in alternative therapies. Curr Opin Pulm Med 2000;6(1):71.
154. Bielory L, Lupoli K. Herbal interventions in asthma and allergy. J Asthma 1999;36(1):1.
155. Malling HJ. Immunotherapy for rhinitis. Curr Allergy Asthma Rep 2003;3(3):204.
156. Ross RN et al. Effectiveness of specific immunotherapy in the treatment of asthma: a meta-analysis of prospective, randomized, double-blind, placebo-controlled studies. Clin Ther 2000;22(3):329.
157. Bousquet J, Demoly P. Specific immunotherapy for allergic rhinitis in children. Allergy Clin Immunol Int 1996;8145.
158. Wood RA. Allergens. In: Mygind N, Naclerio R, eds. Allergic and Non-allergic Rhinitis: Clinical Aspects. Philadelphia: WB Saunders, 1993: 23–31.
159. Bousquet J, Michel FB. In vivo methods for study of allergy: skin tests, techniques, and interpretation. In: Middleton E et al. eds. Allergy: Principles and Practice. St. Louis: CV Mosby, 1993: 573–594.
160. Nalebuff DJ. In vitro testing methodologies. Evolution and current status. Otolaryngol Clin North Am 1992;25(1):27.
161. Agarwal MK et al. Effect of prior medication on intradermal test response in patients with respiratory allergies. J Asthma 1988;25(5):275.
162. Sekerel BE, Akpinarli A. The effect of montelukast on allergen-induced cutaneous responses in house dust mite allergic children. Pediatr Allergy Immunol 2003;14(3):212.
163. Bernstein IL, Storms WW. Practice parameters for allergy diagnostic testing. Joint Task Force on Practice Parameters for the Diagnosis and Treatment of Asthma. The American Academy of Allergy, Asthma and Immunology and the American College of Allergy, Asthma and Immunology. Ann Allergy Asthma Immunol 1995;75(6 Pt 2):543.
164. Bousquet J et al. Allergen immunotherapy: therapeutic vaccines for allergic diseases. A WHO position paper. J Allergy Clin Immunol 1998;102(4 Pt 1):558.
165. Passalacqua G et al. Local nasal immunotherapy: experimental evidences and general considerations. Allergy 1997;52(Suppl. 32):10.
166. Andre C et al. A double-blind placebo-controlled evaluation of sublingual immunotherapy with a standardized ragweed extract in patients with seasonal rhinitis. Evidence for a dose-response relationship. Int Arch Allergy Immunol 2003;131(2):111.
167. Wilson DR et al. Sublingual immunotherapy for allergic rhinitis (Cochrane Review). Cochrane Database Syst Rev 2003(2):CD002893.
168. Weber RW. Immunotherapy with allergens. JAMA 1997;278(22):1881.
169. Rak S et al. A double-blinded, comparative study of the effects of short preseason specific immunotherapy and topical steroids in patients with allergic rhinoconjunctivitis and asthma. J Allergy Clin Immunol 2001;108(6):921.
170. Graf P. Rhinitis medicamentosa: aspects of pathophysiology and treatment. Allergy 1997;52(40 Suppl):28.
171. Mabry RL. Nasal stuffiness due to systemic medications. Otolaryngol Head Neck Surg 1983;91(1):93.
172. Fairbanks DNF, Raphael GD. Nonallergic rhinitis and infection. In: Cummings CW et al, eds. Otolaryngology-Head and Neck Surgery. St. Louis: Mosby Year Book, 1993:775–785.
173. Jones NS et al. The prevalence of allergic rhinosinusitis: a review. J Laryngol Otol 1998;112(11): 1019.
174. Carney AS, Jones NS. Idiopathic rhinitis: idiopathic or not? Clin Otolaryngol 1996;21(3):198.
175. Krasnick J, Patterson R. Vasomotor rhinitis. In: Raeburn D, Giembycz MA, eds. Rhinitis: Immunopathology and Pharmacotherapy. Basel: Burkhauser Verlag, 1997:125.
176. Carney AS et al. Atypical nasal challenges in patients with idiopathic rhinitis: more evidence for the existence of allergy in the absence of atopy? Clin Exp Allergy 2002;32(10):1436.
177. van Rijswijk JB et al. Inflammatory cells seem not to be involved in idiopathic rhinitis. Rhinology 2003;41(1):25.
178. Powe DG et al. Evidence for an inflammatory pathophysiology in idiopathic rhinitis. Clin Exp Allergy 2001;31(6):864.
179. Milgrom H et al. Comparison of ipratropium bromide 0.03% with beclomethasone dipropionate in the treatment of perennial rhinitis in children. Ann Allergy Asthma Immunol 1999;83(2):105.
180. Turkeltaub PC et al. Treatment of seasonal and perennial rhinitis with intranasal flunisolide. Allergy 1982;37(5):303.
181. Broms P, Malm L. Oral vasoconstrictors in perennial non-allergic rhinitis. Allergy 1982;37(2):67.
182. Baroody FM et al. Ipratropium bromide (Atrovent nasal spray) reduces the nasal response to methacholine. J Allergy Clin Immunol 1992;89(6):1065.
183. Kirkegaard J et al. Ordinary and high-dose ipratropium in perennial nonallergic rhinitis. J Allergy Clin Immunol 1987;79(4):585.
184. Kaiser HB et al. The anticholinergic agent, ipratropium bromide, is useful in the treatment of rhinorrhea associated with perennial allergic rhinitis. Allergy Asthma Proc 1998;19(1):23.
185. Meltzer EO et al. Ipratropium bromide aqueous nasal spray for patients with perennial allergic rhinitis: a study of its effect on their symptoms, quality of life, and nasal cytology. J Allergy Clin Immunol 1992;90(2):242.
186. Borum P et al. Ipratropium nasal spray: a new treatment for rhinorrhea in the common cold. Am Rev Respir Dis 1981;123(4 Pt 1):418.
187. Groth S et al. The absence of systemic side-effects from high doses of ipratropium in the nose. Eur J Respir Dis Suppl 1983;128 (Pt 2)490.
188. Drug Facts and Comparisons. Facts and Comparisons. St. Louis, 2001.
189. Drug Facts and Comparisons. Facts and Comparisons. St. Louis, 2002.
190. Drug Facts and Comparisons. Facts and Comparisons. St. Louis, 2000.

CHAPTER 26

Drug-Induced Pulmonary Disorders

Wendy Wilkinson Zerngast

Drug-induced pulmonary toxicity is almost always a diagnosis of exclusion. Therefore, it is imperative that the clinician be aware of the well-described clinical findings consistent with drug-induced pulmonary disorders. An understanding of the mechanism of the reaction is invaluable in selecting an alternative therapy and for avoiding or minimizing future toxicity in a given patient.

Considering the physiologic and metabolic capacity of the lung, one would expect drug-induced pulmonary disease to be encountered more commonly. The lung contains a diverse population of cells capable of various metabolic functions and is the beneficiary of the total body blood flow. Local exposure to directly acting toxins and their metabolites is the rule rather than the exception. The number of medications clearly linked to lung toxicity has more than doubled since 1972, when a comprehensive review of drug-induced pulmonary toxicity was published that identified some 20 agents.[1] In certain groups of patients, contemporary estimates of therapy-related pulmonary disease approaches 10%.[2]

Drug-induced pulmonary disorders can be subdivided into several categories based on the pathophysiologic changes that result. Table 26-1 lists the most commonly encountered pathologies and some detail on the clinical characteristics and incidence of the reaction for drugs that have been reported most often in the literature. A number of drugs that indirectly affect the lungs through other primary mechanisms (i.e., apnea through central nervous system depression or pulmonary manifestations of drug-induced lupus syndrome) are not included. For greater detail, the reader is referred to several general reviews on this topic.[2–9] The remainder of this chapter is devoted to cases representative of clinically significant drug-induced pulmonary disorders.

PULMONARY EOSINOPHILIA

1. **C.M., a 25-year-old woman, is admitted for her third episode of pneumonia this year. She complains of difficulty breathing and has a nonproductive cough. She states that she was previously treated with an oral cephalosporin with satisfactory resolution of her symptoms. Her only other significant medical problem is a history of recurrent urinary tract infections (UTIs). Physical examination shows a temperature of 39.0°C,** slight cyanosis of the extremities, and an elevated respiratory rate. Crackles are audible bilaterally on auscultation. C.M.'s blood pressure and heart rate are unremarkable. Chest radiograph reveals bilateral pulmonary infiltrates with no focal lesions. Blood and sputum are obtained and sent for culture and sensitivity testing. C.M. is given ceftriaxone 1 g Q 24 hr.

Laboratory results are as follows: Gram's stain of the sputum shows 3+ epithelial cells, 1+ Gram-positive cocci, and 1+ Gram-negative rods. A complete blood count with differential yields a white blood cell (WBC) count of 9,000 cells/mm³ and is remarkable only for a relative eosinophilia of 6%. Blood cultures are negative. Current home medications include dextromethorphan PRN for cough, a multiple vitamin, an oral contraceptive, and nitrofurantoin PRN for UTI prophylaxis. C.M. was initially diagnosed as having a possible bacterial pneumonia. What information is inconsistent with an infectious cause for her respiratory distress?

[SI unit: WBC count, 9,000 10^9 cells/L]

In an otherwise healthy individual, infectious pneumonia would be expected to cause a significant elevation of the WBC count. C.M. has a nonproductive cough, whereas a productive cough with purulent sputum would be more likely. The sputum sample obtained is nondiagnostic, reflecting only normal flora of the oropharynx (with no predominant organism) and large numbers of epithelial cells. These findings represent either a poorly obtained sample or a noninfectious cause. More importantly, the relative eosinophilia in the differential is not associated with bacterial infection, but rather points to an allergic response.

2. **A diagnosis of pulmonary eosinophilia is made. Which of C.M.'s medications is the most likely cause of respiratory illness mimicking community-acquired pneumonia?**

More than 500 cases of adverse pulmonary reactions to nitrofurantoin have been reported, most of these being acute pneumonitis, with the remainder presenting as chronic pulmonary fibrosis.

These reactions occur in <1% of those taking the medication, but the incidence is much greater in women, probably because women are more prone to UTIs. The clinical course of the acute pneumonitis reaction is characterized by onset of fever,

Table 26-1 Drug-Induced Pulmonary Disorders

Drugs, Frequency, Mechanism	Clinical Remarks
Bronchospasm Acetaminophen[31] *Frequency:* Rare *Mechanism:* Same as aspirin	Acetaminophen is a very weak cyclo-oxygenase inhibitor; therefore, <25% of patients with aspirin sensitivity will react to acetaminophen. It is considered a useful antipyretic and analgesic alternative to aspirin
Angiotensin-Converting Enzyme (ACE) Inhibitors[3,32] *Frequency:* Common *Mechanism:* Exact mechanism unknown but may involve the ability to inhibit the degradation of bradykinin, prostaglandins, and/or substance P. These products may induce airway inflammation and bronchial hyperreactivity	Cough is the predominant symptom; however, wheezing and deterioration of pulmonary function have been reported in chronic asthmatics. Reported prevalence 1% to 13%, with women affected more frequently than men. Most provocation studies demonstrate an ↑ cough reflex to capsaicin and ↑ bronchial reactivity to histamine, although standard spirometric studies remain unchanged. Cough is persistent, not episodic; dry; nonproductive; and worse at night. A tickling sensation in the throat is a frequent complaint. Cough completely disappears on discontinuation of the drug. Switching to an alternate ACE inhibitor is not helpful; however an angiotensin receptor blocker may be an acceptable alternative. Concomitant β-blockers may ↑ risk. ACE inhibitor–related cough has been treated with some success with a variety of agents including cromolyn, baclofen, NSAIDs, and local anesthetics
Aspirin[33-35] *Frequency:* Common *Mechanism:* Exact mechanism unknown, but may involve inhibition of the cyclo-oxygenase pathway of arachidonic acid metabolism resulting in increased metabolism through the lipoxygenase pathway, leading to excess production of leukotrienes which precipitate bronchospasm in susceptible individuals	Prevalence ↑ with age. Asthmatic patients >40 yr have a frequency 4× that of patients <20 yr. The classic description includes a triad of severe asthma, nasal polyps, and aspirin intolerance. Bronchospasm typically occurs minutes to hours following ingestion and is associated with rhinorrhea, flushing of head and neck, and conjunctivitis. The reaction is often life-threatening. Therapy is nonspecific; should be treated as any other acute asthma attack. Primary therapy is avoidance. Theoretically, COX-2 inhibitors may be safe alternatives. Patients can be desensitized under medical supervision if alternative therapy is unavailable. Leukotriene modifying agents (zafirlukast, montelukast, zileuton) may be protective
β-Adrenergic Receptor Blockers[8,36] *Frequency:* Common *Mechanism:* Antagonizes maintenance of normal airway tone by the sympathetic nervous system	Occurs only in patients with pre-existing bronchial hyperreactivity. Asthma attacks have been precipitated not only by nonselective β-blockers such as propranolol (Inderal), but also by cardioselective agents such as acebutolol (Sectral), atenolol (Tenormin), and metoprolol (Lopressor). Fatal status asthmaticus has occurred following topical administration of timolol maleate (Timoptic) ophthalmic solution. β-blocker–induced bronchospasm can be treated with bronchodilators including β₂-agonists, theophylline, and anticholinergics as well as discontinuation of the β-blocker
Inhalational Agents/Aerosols[37] Aerosolized acetylcysteine, aerosolized pentamidine (NebuPent), beclomethasone (QVAR), fluticasone (Flovent), flunisolide (AeroBid), cromolyn (Intal), isoetharine (Bronkosol), isoproterenol (Isuprel), racemic epinephrine	Aerosolized medications may produce cough and bronchospasm due to irritant effect of inhaled particles, propellants, and dispersants contained in MDI and/or sulfite sensitivity from sulfite-containing nebulized solutions (isoetharine, isoproterenol, and racemic epinephrine)
Nonsteroidal Anti-Inflammatory Drugs (NSAIDs)[33-35] *Frequency:* Common *Mechanism:* Same as aspirin	All NSAIDs that inhibit cyclo-oxygenase cross-react in aspirin-sensitive patients. Patients exhibit a threshold dose for cyclo-oxygenase inhibition that, if exceeded, will provoke bronchospasm. Therefore, the degree of cross reactivity is dependent on potency of cyclo-oxygenase inhibition
Sulfites[38,39] *Frequency:* Uncommon *Mechanism:* Exact mechanism unknown, but probably due to an inability to clear sulfites. As a result, H_2SO_3 is produced on the lung surface and the afferent parasympathetic receptors of the lung are stimulated	Occurs in <10% of asthmatics. Sulfites and metabisulfites are common antioxidants used to preserve wine and foods. They are in particularly high concentrations in open salad and vegetable bars in restaurants. Metabisulfites also occur in drugs as a preservative, including some bronchodilator aerosols, in concentrations high enough to produce bronchospasm. The bronchospasm is readily reversed by inhaled β₂-agonists or anticholinergics
Tartrazine (FD&C yellow #5 dye)[38] *Frequency:* Rare *Mechanism:* Unknown	Appears to occur only in aspirin-intolerant patients at a prevalence of 10% to 15%

Table 26-1   Drug-Induced Pulmonary Disorders—cont'd

Drugs, Frequency, Mechanism	Clinical Remarks
IgE-Mediated Bronchospasm and Anaphylaxis Cephalosporins, L-asparaginase (Elspar), Penicillins, Sulfonamides *Frequency:* Common Cimetidine (Tagamet) *Frequency:* Rare *Mechanism:* IgE-mediated allergic response[40,41] Neuromuscular blockers[42] Tetracyclines *Frequency:* Infrequent	Bronchospasm and anaphylaxis are the prototype disorders of the Type I hypersensitivity reaction. Although structurally unrelated, these drugs trigger the anaphylactic reaction by a common mechanism. Formation of IgE antibody B cells is induced by an allergen, in this case the specific drug, followed by release of vasoactive amines by basophils and mast cells upon a second exposure to the drug. Mast cell granules contain the primary mediators histamine, eosinophil chemotactic factor, neutrophil chemotactic factor, and neutral proteases. Result of their release is ↑ vascular permeability, vasodilation, bronchial smooth muscle contraction, and ↑ secretion of mucus. Principal organ affected is the lung, more specifically, the smooth musculature of pulmonary blood vessels and respiratory passages. Pulmonary obstruction accentuated by hypersecretion of mucus and laryngeal edema. This reaction is not dose related, although for some compounds desensitization protocols have been developed
Impairment of Respiratory Muscles Hypoventilation[43] Alcohol, narcotics, sedatives	Direct, dose-dependent centrally mediated inhibition of respiration is a well-described pharmacologic effect of these drugs
Myopathy[43] Aminocaproic acid, clofibrate, corticosteroids, diuretics, procainamide	Drug-induced necrosis (necrotizing myopathy) most commonly caused by clofibrate and aminocaproic acid. Also seen in combination therapy with statins and fibric acid derivatives for dyslipidemia. Steroid myopathy weakens respiratory muscles, as well as other striated muscles
Neuromuscular blockade[43] Aminoglycosides, calcium channel blockers, D-penicillamine, macrolides, neuro-muscular blockers, polymyxin B	Patients with myasthenia gravis and/or hepatic or renal failure at ↑ risk for drug-induced neuromuscular blockade. D-penicillamine has been reported to induce myasthenia gravis through immunologic mechanisms
Neuropathy[43] Amiodarone, captopril, gold, isoniazid, phenytoin, vincristine, vaccines	Guillain-Barré syndrome (GBS) has been reported following vaccinations. An estimated 20% to 50% of patients with GBS develop respiratory muscle paralysis. Neurotubular damage is a complication of vincristine therapy. Isoniazid neuropathy is mediated through the inhibition of pyridoxine metabolism and may be prevented by the prophylactic administration of pyridoxine (vitamin B_6)
Pseudolymphoma or Posttransplant Lymphoproliferative Disease (PTLD) Cyclosporine (Sandimmune)[44] Tacrolimus (FK506, Prograf) Muromonab (Orthoclone OKT3) *Frequency:* Rare *Mechanism:* Inhibition of T-cell function, thus preventing a cytotoxic T-cell response to Epstein-Barr virus	Incidence 5% to 35%. Lymphoproliferative disorder (or sometimes referred to as pseudolymphoma) involving the lungs occurs 2 to 6 months after transplantation. Strong correlation reported with primary or reactivation of Epstein-Barr virus and the development of this pulmonary disorder. Pulmonary findings appear as solitary or multiple nodules, seen mostly with liver, heart and heart-lung transplants. Regression of the disorder occurs after reduction of immunosuppressant dose and institution of antiviral therapy
Pulmonary Edema Contrast Media[45,46] *Frequency:* Rare *Mechanism:* Unknown	Due to injection of high concentration of this highly osmotic agent into the circulation. Previously thought to be due to acute cardiac failure as a result of intravascular volume expansion caused by hyperosmolar agents, this reaction has now been seen in with non-ionic low-osmolality agents as well
Dextran 40 (Rheomacrodex)[47] *Frequency:* Rare *Mechanism:* Unknown; probably ↑ capillary permeability; noncardiogenic	Multiple case reports despite use of dextran 1 hapten inhibition in most instances
Gemcitabine (Gemzar)[48,49] *Frequency:* Rare *Mechanism:* Capillary endothelial leak, noncardio-genic pulmonary edema	May develop after multiple doses of gemcitabine or after initial dose. Dyspnea, cough, and peripheral edema are presenting features. Treatment consists of corticosteroids and supplemental oxygen. The spectrum of pulmonary toxicity ranges from mild dyspnea on exertion to fatal ARDS
Heroin[50,55] *Frequency:* Common *Mechanism:* Due to an outpouring of edema fluid into the alveoli. Mechanism of the ↑ capillary permeability unknown	Syndrome associated with a mortality rate of approximately 10%. Usually occurs after IV administration, but has been reported to follow nasal administration ("snorting"). Patients usually present in coma with depressed respiration or marked respiratory distress. Dyspnea, tachypnea, hypotension, cyanosis, tachycardia, and severe hypoxemia common. Does not appear to be dose related, although it often may follow an overdose. Symptoms occur within 2 hours following administration and usually clear in 1 to 2 days. Radiographic evidence of resolution present in 2 to 5 days; however, significant ↓ in pulmonary function such as FVC, dynamic compliance, and diffusing capacity take much longer to improve. Treatment consists of naloxone (Narcan), respiratory support, and oxygen therapy. Secondary bacterial and aspiration pneumonias are frequent complications

Table 26-1   Drug-Induced Pulmonary Disorders—cont'd

Drugs, Frequency, Mechanism	Clinical Remarks
Hydrochlorothiazide[51,52] *Frequency:* Uncommon *Mechanism:* Unknown, noncardiogenic, nonimmu- nologic	Symptoms of pulmonary edema occur within 1 hour following oral administration of a single dose and rapidly subside within 24 hours. Radiographic evidence of resolution present within 2 to 6 days. Diffusing capacity may take a month to return to normal. Most patients had a previous history of thiazide exposure with mild reactions. This pulmonary adverse effect has not been reported with other thiazide diuretics
Interleukin-2 (IL-2 or Aldesleukin)[53,54] *Frequency:* Common *Mechanism:* ↑ capillary permeability	Pulmonary edema caused by a dose-related ↓ in cardiac contractility and VLS. VLS described as peripheral and pulmonary edema with concomitant intravascular depletion. >20% of patients treated with IL-2 will develop respiratory distress. Rarely, some patients may experience reversible bronchospasm. Most, if not all, patients regain full pulmonary function once IL-2 is withdrawn
Intravenous Fluids[7] *Frequency:* Common *Mechanism:* Cardiovascular fluid overload	Commonly occurs in trauma, septic shock and cardiac failure. Careful monitoring of central venous pressure will prevent this most common cause of iatrogenic pulmonary edema. Patients who develop ARDS from shock are particularly susceptible. These patients should be treated with ventilatory modalities specific to ARDS
Methadone[55,56] *Frequency:* Common with overdose *Mechanism:* Same as for heroin	Occurs after oral administration as much as 6 hours after dose. Symptoms and treatment same as for heroin. May take longer to improve due to a longer duration of action relative to heroin
Muromonab CD3 (OKT-3)[44,57] *Frequency:* Common *Mechanism:* Pulmonary edema due to the release of mediators by damaged T-cells, causing left ventricular overload and pulmonary edema	Occurs with the initial doses of OKT-3. Patients with fluid overload before starting OKT-3 therapy are at highest risk for developing OKT-3–induced pulmonary edema; this has not been reported in normovolemic patients. Recommended that weight gain be limited to <3% during the week before initiating OKT-3 treatment and that a chest radiograph show no evidence of volume overload
Tocolytics[58,59] Ritodrine (Yutopar), terbutaline (Brethine) *Frequency:* Infrequent *Mechanism:* Cardiovascular fluid overload	In tocolytic doses, β-agonists are postulated to cause peripheral vasodilation that is rapidly reversed when drug discontinued. As blood vessels regain normal tone, the large intravascular volume is forced into all tissues, including the lungs
Tricyclic Antidepressants (TCAs)[60,61] *Frequency:* Uncommon *Mechanism:* ↑ Capillary permeability due to degeneration of alveolar epithelium and capillary endothelium as a direct toxic effect of the TCA; ↑ levels of catecholamines caused by the TCA lead to pulmonary fat deposition or release of histamine from lung mast cells and production of bradykinin in the plasma, both of which ↑ vascular permeability	TCA-induced cases of ARDS have been reported, as well as patients with noncardiogenic pulmonary edema attributed to TCA overdose. Radiographic findings revealed diffuse bilateral opacities and interstitial edema. Autopsy results in three patients with fatal amitriptyline overdose revealed pathologic changes consistent with ARDS as well as pulmonary fat deposition, which may have interfered with gas exchange
Pulmonary Fibrosis Amiodarone (Cordarone)[1–4,6,7,24–30] *Frequency:* Common *Mechanism:* Exact mechanism unknown but thought to result from the amphiphilic (contains both hydrophilic and lipophilic portions) nature of the molecule. Amphiphilic compounds produce a phospholipid storage disorder with inflammation and fibrosis resulting from breakdown of phospho-lipid-laden macrophages	Occurs in 1% to 6% of patients and appears to be dose related; clinical toxicity rarely occurs with doses <400 mg/day. Onset of symptoms usually appears after 5 to 6 months; symptoms have occurred as soon as 2 weeks and as late as 9 years. No evidence for a cumulative dose effect. Clinical course variable. May be an acute onset with rapid progression into respiratory failure and death, or symptoms may begin with exertional dyspnea slowly developing over several months and improving when the drug is discontinued or when the dose is decreased to 200 to 400 mg/day. Radiographic changes nondiagnostic and consistent with a diffuse pneumonitis. BAL results vary. Routine pulmonary function tests not predictive for identifying patients at risk
BCNU (Carmustine)[5,62] *Frequency:* Uncommon *Mechanism:* Unknown but appears to be a dose-related toxicity	Pulmonary fibrosis developed after cumulative doses of 580 to 2,100 mg/m² were administered over 6 months to 3 years. Concomitant cyclophosphamide therapy may ↑ risk. Presents as a typical restrictive fibrosis with insidious cough, dyspnea, and hypoxemia with a diffusion defect. Corticosteroid therapy has not been effective in altering the course of the adverse effect that often is rapidly fatal

Table 26-1   Drug-Induced Pulmonary Disorders—cont'd

Drugs, Frequency, Mechanism	Clinical Remarks
Bleomycin (Blenoxane)[5,9–16] *Frequency:* Common; overall incidence estimated at 11% *Mechanism:* Direct cytotoxic injury to the lung epithelium probably due to free-radical generation following binding of drug to DNA	Clinical presentation characterized by nonproductive cough, dyspnea with occasional fever, dry basilar rales, and skin pigmentation. Onset 4 to 10 weeks after beginning therapy. The lung disease is restrictive with a severe diffusion defect. Older patients (60 to 70 years) appear to be more susceptible. Toxicity potentiated by radiation given either concomitantly or sequentially, high oxygen concentrations, cyclophosphamide, and possibly adriamycin. The disease usually insidiously progressive and irreversible. Routine monitoring of pulmonary function tests has been of questionable value. Corticosteroid therapy has been reported to be beneficial in some cases. Total cumulative dose of bleomycin should be restricted to <450 U. Bleomycin-induced pulmonary fibrosis associated with a 10% fatality rate when patients receive >550 U
Bromocriptine (Parlodel)[63,64] *Frequency:* Rare *Mechanism:* Potent vasoconstrictive effect, causing ischemia and resulting in pulmonary fibrosis	Pleural fibrosis affects approximately 2% to 3% of patients. Patients present with insidious onset of dyspnea and cough and sometimes with fatigue and chest pain. Symptoms usually start after 18 months to 2 years of treatment; however, in one case, symptoms occurred after only 2 to 3 weeks of therapy. Chest radiograph findings reveal bilateral or unilateral pleural effusions and pleural thickening. Eosinophilia and elevated ESR and C-reactive protein often seen. Symptoms slowly resolve with discontinuation; however, pleural thickening remains despite resolution of pleural effusions
Busulfan (Myleran)[5] *Frequency:* Common *Mechanism:* Exact mechanism unknown but probably due to chemical alveolitis with proliferation of granular pneumocytes and fibrosis of alveolar walls	Symptoms usually begin insidiously 3 to 4 years after therapy is initiated. The pulmonary fibrosis ("busulfan lung") presents as a dry hacking cough, tachypnea, cyanosis, dyspnea, and low-grade fever. Radiographs show diffuse interstitial and intra-alveolar infiltrates. Differential diagnosis includes opportunistic infection, leukemic infiltration, and radiation fibrosis. Pulmonary function tests are typical of restrictive lung disease with a diffusion defect. Clinical course one of progression with no reversibility. High-dose corticosteroids have been tried with little apparent benefit
Chlorambucil (Leukeran)[5] *Frequency:* Rare *Mechanism:* Unknown; probably the same as busulfan and cyclophosphamide, which are also alkylating agents	Typically occurs after 2 years of daily therapy. Symptoms and histology are the same as "busulfan lung"
Cyclophosphamide (Cytoxan)[5,65] *Frequency:* Rare *Mechanism:* Unknown; thought to be same as busulfan	Clinical picture and pulmonary function same as "busulfan lung." Pulmonary fibrosis generally detected after a long period of continuous low-dose therapy; it has occurred in children 4 to 6 years after drug has been discontinued. Fibrosis rapidly progressive
Ganglionic Blocking Agents (Hexamethonium, Mecamylamine, Pentolinium)[66] *Frequency:* Rare *Mechanism:* Unknown	Reaction merely of historical interest because these drugs are rarely used. Patients present with classic pulmonary fibrosis a few months to 1 year following initiation of therapy. Hexamethonium structurally similar to busulfan
Gold (Myochrysine)[67] *Frequency:* Uncommon *Mechanism:* Unknown; however, does not appear to be immunologically mediated	Clinical symptoms usually occur after 300 to 400 mg total dose has been given. Symptoms include dyspnea and a nonproductive cough. Radiographic studies usually compatible with diffuse interstitial fibrosis, and histologic examination is the same as for other drug-induced pulmonary fibroses. Pulmonary function tests show a restrictive pattern with a diffusion abnormality. Symptoms resolve with discontinuation of drug. Corticosteroids have no therapeutic benefit
Melphalan (Alkeran), Uracil Mustard[5] *Frequency:* Rare *Mechanism:* Same as for busulfan and cyclophosphamide	All the alkylating agents, except nitrogen mustard and thiotepa, have been associated with the syndrome. Except for busulfan, it appears to be a rare complication, but it may represent an inherent toxicity of this group of drugs. Caution should be used when these agents are given with other drugs associated with fibrosis
6-Mercaptopurine (Purinethol)[5] *Frequency:* Rare *Mechanism:* Unknown	
Methotrexate[5] *Frequency:* Uncommon *Mechanism:* Appears to be an allergic reaction with fibrosis; noncaseating granuloma formation with lymphocytic infiltrates	Mean onset of toxicity occurs 12 to 200 days after administration. No correlation with dose and 65% of the patients will have peripheral eosinophilia. Has been reported after PO, IV, and IT use. Symptoms include dry cough, dyspnea, and cyanosis. High-dose prednisone will induce a rapid remission with radiographic evidence of resolution. Appears to be completely reversible

Table 26-1   Drug-Induced Pulmonary Disorders—cont'd

Drugs, Frequency, Mechanism	*Clinical Remarks*
Methysergide (Sansert)[68] *Frequency:* Common *Mechanism:* Unknown	Fibrosis is pleuropulmonary rather than the more common interstitial fibrosis produced by other agents. Methysergide is the only drug that will produce a chronic pleural effusion as well. Onset is insidious as well as dose- and duration-related. Reaction usually occurs after at least 6 months of therapy and is a component of the retroperitoneal fibrosis induced by this drug. Symptoms include acute pleuritic pain or progressive dyspnea with radiographic changes showing either unilateral or bilateral pleural fibrosis. Syndrome usually completely reversible on discontinuation of the drug
Mitomycin (Mutamycin)[5] *Frequency:* Uncommon *Mechanism:* Unknown	Clinical presentation like that caused by bleomycin. Mitomycin-induced pulmonary fibrosis can occur with a cumulative dose as low as 40 mg/m². Toxicity appears 3 to 6 months following initiation of treatment and may occur following the second course. High oxygen tension appears to potentiate the toxicity. Postoperative patients should be ventilated with an FiO_2 ≤30%. Corticosteroids reportedly might be of some benefit in some patients, but others have died of respiratory insufficiency despite steroid therapy
Nitrofurantoin (Macrodantin)[6] *Frequency:* Rare *Mechanism:* Unknown	Long-term use of nitrofurantoin for 6 months to 6 years has resulted in cases of pulmonary fibrosis. This pulmonary reaction is rare in comparison to the acute reaction (i.e., pulmonary infiltrates with eosinophilia) described below. Clinical pattern consists of a dry cough, exertional dyspnea, and fever. Pulmonary function testing usually consistent with a restrictive disorder; and radiologic tests consistent with diffuse interstitial fibrosis and diffusion defect. Most cases have been reversible following discontinuation of the drug and institution of steroid therapy. It appears to occur most frequently in postmenopausal women
Oxygen[4] *Frequency:* Frequent *Mechanism:* Toxicity caused by the formation of superoxide anions (O_2^-) that are highly reactive and cytotoxic. These free radicals can oxidize sulf-hydryl enzymes, inactivate DNA, and result in lipid peroxidation of cellular membranes	Dose-dependent reaction that occurs following prolonged exposure to FiO_2 >50%. Clinical pathology extensive and generally presents in 2 stages: the acute or exudative state, and the chronic proliferative stage. Acute phase consists of perivascular, peribronchiolar, interstitial, and alveolar edema, as well as alveolar hemorrhage and necrosis of the pulmonary endothelium. The second or more chronic phase consists of exudate resorption, alveolar thickening, and collagen and elastin deposition in the interstitium of alveolar walls. Patient may have irreversible emphysematous and fibrotic changes. Clinical picture may be obstructive, restrictive, or mixture of the two
Paraquat (Crisquat, Ortho Paraquat CL, Gramoxone)[4] *Frequency:* Common, >175 exposures reported annually *Mechanism:* Attributed to O_2 toxicity by superoxide free radical production	Oral ingestion of as little as 15 to 20 mL can induce pulmonary fibrosis, and the mortality rate is 33% to 50%. Radiographic evidence of pulmonary edema may appear several days after ingestion and usually accompanied by complaints of progressive dyspnea. Paraquat readily inactivated by exposure to sunlight and destroyed by burning. Therefore, significant toxicity should not occur from smoking marijuana that had been sprayed with paraquat. All reported fatal cases have been from oral ingestion. Fatal outcomes are usually associated with plasma levels greater than 0.2 mg/mL at 24 hours after ingestion. Therapy is supportive, although superoxide dismutase has been shown to improve outcome in animals by preventing formation of (O_2^-) ions. A high FiO_2 in patients requiring ventilatory support will exacerbate the problem
Penicillamine (Cuprimine)[6] *Frequency:* Rare *Mechanism:* Unknown	Penicillamine-induced pulmonary fibrosis continues to be reported in the literature. Symptoms and pulmonary function tests are consistent with an alveolitis and bronchiolitis with fibrosis. A pulmonary-renal syndrome resembling Goodpasture's also has been reported
Tocainide (Tonocard)[69] *Frequency:* Rare *Mechanism:* Unknown	Severe dyspnea with diffuse pulmonary crackles appeared 4 to 6 months after the initiation of therapy. Diffuse infiltrates were noted on chest radiographs, and diffusion abnormalities were detected by pulmonary function tests. All patients recovered when drug was discontinued
Interstitial Pneumonitis Etoposide (Toposar)[70] *Frequency:* Rare *Mechanism:* Unknown	Interstitial infiltrates and respiratory failure have been reported to occur after treatment with etoposide. Symptoms improved with corticosteroid treatment and reappeared with rechallenge
Pulmonary Infiltrates With Eosinophilia (Loeffler's Syndrome) Carbamazepine (Tegretol)[6] *Frequency:* Rare *Mechanism:* Unknown	See phenytoin

Table 26-1   Drug-Induced Pulmonary Disorders—cont'd

Drugs, Frequency, Mechanism	Clinical Remarks
Dantrolene (Dantrium)[71] *Frequency:* Rare *Mechanism:* Allergic response	Chronic pleural effusions without associated parenchymal disease have been reported following long-term therapy with dantrolene. After 1 month to several years of therapy, patients develop signs of an abnormally high pleural fluid eosinophilia, peripheral eosinophilia, and unilateral pleural effusion often accompanied with pleuritic chest pain and cough. Symptomatic improvement occurs within several days following discontinuation of dantrolene; however, it may take months for radiographic findings to resolve
Fludarabine (Fludara)[72,73] *Frequency:* Rare *Mechanism:* Possibly allergic	Only one pathologically confirmed case. The range of toxic reactions varies from acute interstitial pneumonitis to acute hypoxemic respiratory failure requiring mechanical ventilation. The response to corticosteroids may be dramatic suggesting an immunologic mechanism
Minocycline (Minocin)[74,75] *Frequency:* Uncommon *Mechanism:* Allergic reaction	Many cases of minocycline-induced pneumonitis/pulmonary infiltrates and eosinophilia have been reported. Onset of pneumonitis rapid, occurring after a few days to few weeks of treatment. Symptoms described include acute chest symptoms (hacking cough, acute chest pain) and dyspnea, pulmonary infiltrates on chest radiograph, fever, hemoptysis, and eosinophilia in blood and/or bronchoalveolar lavage fluids. With continuation of minocycline, severe respiratory failure may occur. There was a definite temporal relationship between respiratory symptoms and the administration of minocycline in all cases. In addition, fever, dyspnea, and a rise in eosinophils returned upon rechallenge with the drug. This disorder carries a favorable prognosis as it quickly resolves with discontinuation of minocycline and/or administration of corticosteroids
Montelukast **Nitrofurantoin[6]** *Frequency:* Uncommon *Mechanism:* Unknown	See zafirlukast Fever, chills, cyanosis, and dyspnea begin 2 hours to 10 days following the initiation of nitrofurantoin therapy. Clinical presentation may mimic pulmonary edema or an acute asthma attack. Diffuse alveolar infiltrates with occasional small pleural effusions can be seen on chest radiograph. Eosinophilia present in one third of patients. Symptoms regress within 24 to 48 hours after discontinuation of drug (Also see Pulmonary Fibrosis in Chronic Reactions)
Para-Aminosalicylic Acid (PAS)[76] *Frequency:* Common *Mechanism:* Probably an allergic reaction	As with all the drugs known to induce Loeffler's syndrome, PAS can induce high fever, leukocytosis, eosinophilia, cough, and dyspnea. Although eosinophils may account for as much as 26% of the leukocytes in the blood, eosinophilia not noted in the sputum. Treatment of choice is discontinuation of the PAS; rechallenge with PAS usually provokes the reaction within 2 days
Penicillin[6] *Frequency:* Rare *Mechanism:* Allergic reaction	Symptoms similar to those described for the other drugs that induce Loeffler's syndrome
Phenytoin (Dilantin)[6] *Frequency:* Rare *Mechanism:* Unknown; most likely hypersensitivity	Usual symptoms of Loeffler's (e.g., cough, fever, dyspnea) develop 3 to 6 weeks after initiation of therapy. Maculopapular rash and lymphadenopathy usually present. Patients significantly improve within 1 to 2 weeks after discontinuation of drug
Procarbazine (Matulane)[5] *Frequency:* Rare *Mechanism:* Possibly an allergic reaction	Will improve with corticosteroid therapy. May progress to fibrosis
Sulfonamides[6] *Frequency:* Rare *Mechanism:* Allergic reaction	Has even been reported with sulfonamide vaginal cream. Other sulfa-like drugs (e.g., sulfonylureas and sulfasalazine) will cross-react and cause the syndrome
Zafirlukast[77] **Zileuton** *Frequency:* Uncommon *Mechanism:* Unmasking of underlying vasculitic syndrome	Leukotriene modifiers do not appear to directly cause Churg-Strauss Syndrome (CSS). Literature reports suggest these agents may have a corticosteroid sparing effect enabling dosage reduction of systemic corticosteroids. Following dosage reduction, some patients have been found to have features of eosinophilia, mono or polyneuropathy, pulmonary infiltrates, paranasal sinus abnormalities, and extravascular eosinophils in addition to moderate to severe asthma. This "unmasking" of CSS has been noted with all leukotriene inhibitors as well as with some corticosteroid inhalers

Table 26-1 Drug-Induced Pulmonary Disorders—cont'd

Drugs, Frequency, Mechanism	Clinical Remarks
Pulmonary Hypertension	
Fenfluramine (Pondimin, Ponderal), dexfenfluramine (Redux), aminorex (Menocil), appetite-suppressant drugs[78–84]	
Frequency: Rare	Clinical presentation usually late in the disease progression (dyspnea, peripheral edema, chest
Mechanism: Unknown; thought to be due to pulmonary vasoconstrictive effects of serotonin or through potassium-channel blockade	pain, syncope). Risk of development of PPH increases with >3 months of use of appetite-suppressants. In 1997 manufacturers of fenfluramine and dexfenfluramine voluntarily withdrew these drugs from the U.S. and worldwide market due to increasing reports of cardiac (primarily valvular) abnormalities. While these agents are not prescribed any longer, many patients continue to undergo long term follow-up for drug-induced complications of use before 1997. There are also many pending legal cases relating to past use of these medications.
Magnesium Trisilicate (Talc)[85]	
Frequency: Common only in drug abusers	Talc is a common inert ingredient of many oral dosage forms. When drugs that are formulated
Mechanism: Foreign body reaction	for oral use are injected intravenously by drug abusers, arteritis and angiothrombosis of the pulmonary vasculature can develop. Cornstarch from dissolved tablets also has been implicated in granuloma formation and pulmonary hypertension. The reaction also has been reported after the IV use of sympathomimetic nasal sprays

ARDS, adult respiratory distress syndrome; ESR, erythrocyte sedimentation rate; FVC, forced vital capacity; HCTZ, hydrochlorothiazide; IT, intrathecal; IV, intravenous; MDI, metered-dose inhaler; NSAID, nonsteroid anti-inflammatory drug; PEEP, positive end expiratory pressure; PO, oral; PPH, primary pulmonary hypertension; VLS, vascular leak syndrome.

chills, cough, and dyspnea a few hours to 7 to 10 days after initiation of therapy. With the first exposure, the onset may be delayed. Repeat exposures result in rapid recurrence of symptoms. Eosinophilia occurs in about one-third of these patients. Nearly 50% will manifest an elevation in the erythrocyte sedimentation rate (ESR). Bronchospasm is rare, as is pleuritic chest pain. Pulmonary infiltrates with eosinophilia sometimes is referred to as Loeffler's syndrome and is associated with para-aminosalicylic acid, methotrexate, sulfonamides, tetracycline, chlorpropamide, phenytoin, and imipramine, in addition to nitrofurantoin. The mechanism of the acute reaction is unknown, whereas pulmonary fibrosis associated with chronic toxicity is thought to be due to an oxidant reaction.

3. **What is the appropriate course of action to alleviate C.M.'s respiratory exacerbation and to prevent further recurrence?**

Resolution of symptoms within 18 to 48 hours is anticipated after the discontinuation of the offending agent. Nitrofurantoin should be discontinued and not restarted. No evidence exists that adding corticosteroids will accelerate resolution, but their addition is a consideration if there is no response to supportive care. Once infectious causes have been ruled out, ceftriaxone also can be discontinued. In many instances, it takes four or five such exacerbations before the patient or the clinician connects the medication with the reaction. A careful history elicited from C.M. might have revealed that her UTIs are associated with sexual activity; therefore, in the past year, she has used nitrofurantoin for prophylaxis only intermittently. Each time she was treated for presumed pneumonia, she discontinued taking nitrofurantoin, leading to resolution of her pneumonitis. C.M. should be followed to ensure that no other pulmonary process is occurring, and alternative prophylactic antimicrobial agents should be used to treat her recurrent UTIs.

4. **How do chronic reactions to nitrofurantoin differ from the acute pneumonitis described in C.M.?**

The chronic reaction mimics idiopathic pulmonary fibrosis clinically, radiologically, and histologically. Chest radiograph shows a diffuse interstitial process without pleural effusion. Pulmonary function testing shows a restrictive pattern without obstructive features. Bronchoalveolar lavage (BAL) generally shows a lymphocytic predominance of the cells obtained. The only notable difference from idiopathic fibrosis is that a much better response occurs after discontinuation of the drug, with resolution of the infiltrate and symptoms. The clinical picture consists of a dry cough, exertional dyspnea, and fever. The acute nitrofurantoin-induced pneumonitis and chronic fibrosis appear to be two distinct disorders. The acute reaction rarely is fatal, but the chronic one can progress to irreversible pulmonary fibrosis, respiratory insufficiency, and death. Corticosteroids are useful on a theoretical basis in cases that do not respond to withdrawal of nitrofurantoin alone. There are anecdotal reports in the literature supporting the use of corticosteroids for the purpose of accelerating the resolution of pulmonary symptoms in such instances.[3,7]

PULMONARY FIBROSIS

5. **A.E., a 35-year-old man with recently diagnosed Stage IIIC testicular cancer, has completed four cycles of PEB (cisplatin, etoposide, and bleomycin) therapy. A residual retroperitoneal mass is identified, and surgical resection under general anesthesia is scheduled. What is A.E.'s total lifetime dose of bleomycin, and how is this information relevant to his scheduled surgical procedure?**

PEB is administered every 3 weeks for 3 or 4 cycles in standard treatment of testicular cancer.[10] Thirty units of bleomycin is administered weekly for 9 to 12 doses, whereas cisplatin and etoposide are administered at 3-week intervals. Therefore, the usual lifetime dose for a patient with chemoresponsive testicular cancer is 270 U. A.E. received an additional cycle (3 doses of bleomycin) for a total of 360 U.

Pulmonary fibrosis is the dose-limiting toxicity of bleomycin. It is recommended that the cumulative lifetime dose be restricted to <450 U. Pulmonary toxicity is present in 10% of patients receiving bleomycin, and 10% of this group, or 1% of all patients who receive this drug, will die of pulmonary toxicity. The incidence increases appreciably if >450 U are given, approaching a 10% fatality rate when patients receive cumulative doses >550 U. Additional risk factors include age older than 40 and renal insufficiency.[11-13]

Furthermore, it is important to be cognizant of the total dose of bleomycin because it also will influence the anesthesiologist's management of A.E.'s inspired oxygen concentration (FiO_2) during his surgical procedure.[14,15] The combination of bleomycin and supplemental oxygen is thought to be synergistic for pulmonary toxicity.[15] There are a number of reports of adult respiratory distress syndrome (ARDS) developing in patients who have received bleomycin and subsequently have undergone general anesthesia. The onset of respiratory failure is usually 3 to 10 days after surgery and is rapidly fatal in most reported cases. It is unknown how long after administration of bleomycin that exposure to a higher inspired oxygen may precipitate toxicity, but oxygen should be given with great caution to anyone who has received this drug at any time in his or her lifetime. Patients at greatest risk include those who are older than 70 years of age, those who are recent bleomycin recipients, and those who have had prior radiation therapy. It has been conservatively recommended that patients requiring general anesthesia, such as A.E., be managed on minimal FiO_2 (i.e., 0.25), if possible, while still maintaining an appropriate target partial oxygen pressure in the blood (PaO_2). Recently some authors have challenged the need for perioperative oxygen restriction,[16] but reports of respiratory failure due to bleomycin and oxygen toxicity continue to accumulate.

6. What is the postulated mechanism for bleomycin toxicity?

Bleomycin toxicity is attributed to direct cytotoxic injury to the lung epithelium, likely caused by free-radical generation following binding of the drug to DNA. It is postulated that the relative lack of hydrolase (an enzyme necessary for degradation of bleomycin) in the lung may contribute to increased pulmonary levels of the drug with resultant toxicity. Studies in animals have confirmed that bleomycin is concentrated in the lungs and the skin.[12]

7. How can A.E. be monitored for pulmonary toxicity?

There are no pathognomonic signs or symptoms of bleomycin-related pulmonary damage. Patients usually present with dyspnea, tachypnea, and a nonproductive cough. Rales, initially at the bases and then throughout the lungs, may be present on physical examination. Signs and symptoms usually precede changes on the chest radiograph. The utility of pulmonary function tests as an indicator for the extent of the pulmonary damage produced by bleomycin is controversial. Spirometry usually shows a restrictive pattern in the presence of cytotoxic drug-induced pulmonary damage; however, such changes may not always be present in patients with subclinical bleomycin-induced pulmonary fibrosis. For this reason, pulmonary function tests are of questionable predictive value.[12]

PULMONARY COMPLICATIONS OF INTRAVENOUS DRUG ABUSE

8. J.D., a 38-year-old man known to be an intravenous (IV) drug user, presents with a 10-day history of progressive chest pain and shortness of breath. He reports that his symptoms began 1 day after attempting several bilateral "pocket shots" of heroin. Physical examination reveals a thin, wasted man with severe dyspnea and cyanosis. He is tachypneic to a rate of 30. His arms show evidence of scarred, sclerotic peripheral veins, and large bilateral bruises are noted in the neck region. Chest radiographs show severe bilateral pneumothoraces and pneumomediastinum. Lab tests are unobtainable despite multiple attempts peripherally. J.D. admits to no other prescription, nonprescription, or other illicit drug use. What is a "pocket shot?" What drug-induced pulmonary complications are illustrated by J.D.?

A "pocket shot" refers to the injection of narcotics into the great vessels of the neck. IV drug users resort to alternative access sites because of sclerosis of their peripheral veins following repeated injections of contaminated substances. Commonly selected venous routes are the pocket shot (internal jugular and subclavian veins) and the "groin hit" (femoral veins).

J.D.'s chest radiographs show the presence of both pneumothoraces and air in his chest (pneumomediastinum). His dyspnea and cyanosis are consistent with respiratory distress and poor gas exchange associated with a collapsed lung. Pneumothorax is one of the most common complications of the pocket shot.[17-19] The IV drug user often tries to "hit" the jugular vein by himself or herself or may hire a "street doc" or "hit man" to execute the more difficult subclavian injection. Because the lung is located in direct proximity to the pocket, pneumothorax occurs when the needle deviates from the desired course and punctures the lung. Pneumomediastinum follows as air leaks into the chest. Pneumomediastinum also may occur secondary to performing the Valsalva maneuver in an attempt to distend the neck veins. The increased intra-alveolar pressure ruptures alveoli, resulting in dissection of air, which can then travel and enter the mediastinum. This also has been reported with smoking crack cocaine.[20,21]

The IV drug user may delay seeking medical attention while waiting for the condition to resolve spontaneously; therefore, patients often present in an advanced stage with severe shortness of breath and cyanosis, as is the case with J.D.

9. What further pulmonary complications may result from abuse of IV opiates and other drugs?

Infectious complications are a common result of IV drug abuse. It is seldom the narcotic itself that causes the problem, but rather the nonsterile practice of drug preparation and injection. Heroin, similar to other narcotics, is only fractionally pure, having been cut with substances such as cornstarch, talc, sawdust, and other contaminants.[19] The needle, syringe, and skin often are not aseptically prepared. Therefore, all these factors, along with the common practice of sharing needles, predispose the IV drug user to a high incidence of infection. Septic thrombophlebitis, infectious endocarditis, and bone and soft-tissue infections are common complications of nonsterile injection techniques. Once an infectious nidus is established, it can serve as a source of septic pulmonary emboli.

Often, tricuspid valve vegetations are the source of infectious pulmonary emboli. Staphylococcal septic emboli may appear on a chest radiograph as multiple, solid nodular opacities; these emboli may stabilize during the course of the illness or may cavitate and then slowly resolve over several weeks. Aspiration (while the patient is in a drug stupor), necrotizing pneumonia, mycotic aneurysm, or traumatic pseudoaneurysm also have been reported secondary to IV drug abuse.[17,19]

Noncardiogenic *pulmonary edema* is a common complication of heroin and other opiate intoxication. Onset is usually within a few hours of narcotic use, although the development of symptoms may be delayed for as long as 24 hours. The typical patient is acutely ill on presentation, with constricted pupils, depressed respiration, decreased neurologic status (stupor or coma), fever, and leukocytosis. On chest radiographic examination, diffuse alveolar infiltrates may appear in a classic "butterfly" or "bat wing" symmetric distribution. The mechanism of pulmonary edema is thought to be increased pulmonary capillary permeability secondary to hypoxia from respiratory suppression, direct toxic effects of the drug itself, or secondary release of histamine induced by the opiate.[19]

Talcosis also may cause pulmonary complications. Talc, or magnesium trisilicate, is commonly used as a filler substance to decrease the purity of "mix" sold on the street.[18] It also is introduced into the blood after injection of methylphenidate (Ritalin) because ground-up and partially dissolved tablets are the only available dosage form. Magnesium trisilicate forms talc granulomas in pulmonary arteries (emboli), vessel walls, and the interstitium, leading to interstitial fibrosis or pulmonary arterial hypertension. On chest radiograph, extremely tiny, round opacities appear diffusely throughout the lungs. Numerous cases of "Ritalin lung" have been reported in the literature.[22,23] In addition, massive hemoptysis with diffuse alveolar hemorrhage, resulting in respiratory failure, has been reported with smoking freebase cocaine and in chronic heroin abusers.[20,21]

10. What are some pharmacologic treatment options for patients such as J.D. who have heroin-induced pulmonary complications?

Supportive therapy, symptomatic relief, and prevention of withdrawal are the main goals of treatment. J.D. should be supported with oxygen. Chest tubes should be inserted to re-expand his lungs, and in the absence of narcotic overdose, withdrawal symptoms should be prevented with methadone. Naloxone should be avoided unless absolutely necessary as it may precipitate withdrawal. In the setting of narcotic overdose, mechanical ventilation or naloxone may be necessary. However, it should be noted that naloxone has also been reported on rare occasions to cause noncardiogenic pulmonary edema, similar to heroin. Patients either respond with improving pulmonary function during the first 24 to 48 hours or rapidly proceed to death as a result of pulmonary edema and respiratory failure. Infectious processes should be considered, especially if patients present with fever and leukocytosis and if pulmonary edema persists after 5 days of therapy. Several weeks of supportive therapy may be required before complete resolution of pulmonary function with normal measurements of lung volumes, lung compliance, and diffusing capacity is achieved.

AMIODARONE-INDUCED PULMONARY TOXICITY

11. R.W., a 55-year-old man admitted with a 5-day history of fatigue, exertional dyspnea, and tachypnea, reports that his symptoms have progressively worsened to the point at which he can no longer walk his dog around the neighborhood without feeling "out of breath." He denies experiencing coughing or chest pain. His medical history includes two episodes of ventricular arrhythmia and a 10-year history of hypertension, controlled with benazepril. Physical examination reveals a tachypneic, tired-looking man with no signs of congestive heart failure evident on physical examination. Diffuse inspiratory crackles are audible on lung auscultation. His BP and temperature are unremarkable. The chest radiograph shows diffuse interstitial opacities. All laboratory tests are within normal limits, except for an elevated ESR. His medications on admission include amiodarone 400 mg QD (initiated 2 months previously) and benazepril 40mg QD. What signs and symptoms are consistent with a diagnosis of amiodarone-induced pulmonary toxicity in R.W.?

Pulmonary toxicity associated with amiodarone can manifest in varying ways at any time during the course of therapy. The most common presentation is an insidious progression of pulmonary symptoms, including dyspnea (especially with exertion), nonproductive cough, and fever. The chest radiograph in these cases generally reveals diffuse parenchymal infiltrates, typically in an interstitial pattern. Pleuritic chest pain, lethargy, weakness, and weight loss also may be seen. Approximately one-third of patients may present with an acute onset of symptoms associated with fever, often mimicking an infectious pneumonitis.[24] In the latter group, the chest radiograph often reveals localized opacities in a patchy acinar pattern. In addition to eliciting symptoms such as fever, tachypnea, and inspiratory crackles, a thorough physical examination is vital to exclude a diagnosis of congestive heart failure because this population is at high risk for this disorder.

Leukocytosis and an elevated ESR are also often noted in patients with amiodarone-induced pulmonary toxicity. Pulmonary function tests often reveal a decreased total lung capacity and diffusion capacity. A fall in the carbon monoxide diffusing capacity of the lung (DLCO) of 15% to 20% at any time after starting amiodarone is consistent with pulmonary toxicity. Histologic appearance of the lungs is characterized by foamy alveolar macrophages and type II pneumocytes containing lamellar inclusions.

A BAL is obtained and reveals the appearance of foamy alveolar macrophages and lamellated inclusion bodies. No alternate diagnosis is suggested by the BAL findings. R.W.'s pulmonary complaints, radiographic findings, elevated ESR, and BAL results are all consistent with a diagnosis of amiodarone-induced pulmonary toxicity.[25-27]

12. What are some risk factors that predispose patients to developing amiodarone-induced pulmonary toxicity?

The prevalence of amiodarone-induced pulmonary toxicity is reported most frequently in the range of 4% to 6% of exposed patients.[24,25] Most patients who develop pulmonary toxicity have been taking amiodarone for >4 weeks, with symptoms developing after 1 to 10 months of therapy.

Pulmonary toxicity appears to be dose related and is more likely to occur with doses >400 mg/day.[27] An abnormal chest radiograph and a low DLCO before initiating amiodarone therapy also are significant risk factors. There is no association between the cumulative lifetime dose or serum levels of amiodarone and the development of pulmonary toxicity.

Although R.W.'s amiodarone dose does not exceed 400 mg/day, he has been exposed to the upper dose limit (400 mg/day) for approximately 2 months; therefore, this may have increased his risk of developing pulmonary toxicity.

13. **What are the mechanisms by which amiodarone is thought to cause pulmonary toxicity? Which one is most likely in R.W.?**

There is evidence for two mechanisms: (1) direct chemotoxicity by inhibiting phospholipid degradation and (2) immunologically mediated destruction of lung tissue. Amiodarone is an amphophilic compound, containing both nonpolar and polar constituents. Its lipophilicity favors its concentration in adipose tissue and lipid-rich organs such as the lung and liver. In the lung, amiodarone diffuses into lysosomes, forming complexes with phospholipids. These complexes are resistant to enzymatic degradation by phospholipases, resulting in accumulation of abnormal phospholipids. It is thought that these accumulated phospholipids cause direct pulmonary damage. Thus, the characteristic finding of "foamy" alveolar macrophages and lamellar bodies is indicative of phospholipid accumulation. However, it should be noted that these findings also can occur in the lungs of patients receiving amiodarone who do not have any clinical evidence of toxicity.[3]

Alternatively, it is postulated that amiodarone induces a hypersensitivity response in the lung, resulting in indirect pulmonary toxicity.[30] BAL fluid results, showing lymphocytosis with a predominance of suppressor/cytotoxic T cells, suggest an immune-mediated or hypersensitivity mechanism. Supporting evidence comes from R.W.'s BAL findings, which are inconsistent with those observed in patients with hypersensitivity pneumonitis. In addition, findings of circulating immune complexes, increased numbers of inflammatory cells (polymorphonuclear leukocytes) and lymphocytes, and the observation that the damage responds to corticosteroids suggest an immune-mediated mechanism. Patients who present with an *acute* onset of pulmonary symptoms, often with fever, may represent those experiencing a "hypersensitivity" reaction to amiodarone. In contrast, patients who present with an insidious onset are more likely to be experiencing direct pulmonary chemotoxicity.

R.W.'s BAL findings of foamy alveolar macrophages and lamellar bodies, as well as his insidious presentation of symptoms, suggest that the pulmonary toxicity most likely developed secondary to a direct toxic effect of amiodarone on the lung resulting from an accumulation of abnormal phospholipids.

14. **What therapeutic interventions can be made?**

Amiodarone pulmonary toxicity is reversible after discontinuation of the drug. Clinical symptoms may be expected to resolve within 2 to 4 weeks; however, chest radiographic findings clear slowly over 3 months.[29] In some cases pulmonary toxicity may actually progress before it begins to resolve. This phenomenon is thought to be due to the long, 50 day, terminal half-life of amiodarone. Corticosteroids have been shown to benefit some patients with amiodarone-induced pulmonary

toxicity.[3] Typically, the patient is started on prednisone at a dose of 40 to 60 mg (or equivalent) and subsequently tapered (usually over 4 to 6 months), depending on the severity of toxicity and the clinical response achieved.

An alternative antiarrhythmic agent should be considered for R.W. However, if discontinuation of amiodarone is not feasible, the lowest effective maintenance dose should be used and corticosteroids prescribed for at least 2 to 4 months to minimize any inflammatory process that may be occurring. Despite these measures, development of irreversible pulmonary fibrosis may still occur.

GEMCITABINE-INDUCED PULMONARY TOXICITY

15. **C.B .is a 66-year-old man with non-small cell lung cancer. One year previously, he had a right upper lobe (RUL) wedge resection and radiation therapy. He now presents with a large local recurrence and enlarged bilateral mediastinal lymph nodes. Weekly intravenous gemcitabine treatments are begun. He receives gemcitabine 1 g/m^2 on days 1, 8, and 15, followed by a 2 week rest period. After the second cycle, he presents to the emergency department with complaints of dyspnea on exertion. Physical examination reveals that he has significant peripheral edema, and his vital signs are notable for an O$_2$ saturation of 82% on room air. C.B. has maintained good room air saturations at all times despite a 100 pack-year history of smoking and a history of RUL wedge resection. A chest radiograph shows increased interstitial markings. C.B. is admitted to the hospital for further workup of his dyspnea.**

How do patients with gemcitabine-induced pulmonary toxicity usually present?

Gemcitabine, a pyrimidine analogue similar to cytarabine, is a relatively well tolerated chemotherapy drug. Myelosuppression is the dose-limiting toxicity, manifesting significantly in approximately 25% of patients but necessitating discontinuation of treatment in only 1%. Common side effects include mild to moderate nausea and vomiting, rash, fever, elevation of transaminases, flu-like symptoms, and peripheral edema. Patients with pulmonary toxicity manifestations may complain of mild dyspnea or progress to fatal acute respiratory distress. Ten percent to 40% of patients will have peripheral edema thought to be due to capillary endothelial leakage. A common complaint is weight gain in conjunction with swelling of the distal extremities and dyspnea on exertion. Often, resting oxygen saturations on room air will be less than 90%. Patients are usually afebrile. Pulmonary toxicity may develop with the first dose of gemcitabine but more commonly develops after multiple cycles.

16. **How is gemcitabine-induced pulmonary toxicity diagnosed?**

As with other drug-induced pulmonary toxicities, this is a diagnosis of exclusion. Temporal association is important, as is ruling out other causes such as infection, metabolic causes, cardiac compromise, lymphangitic spread, and disease progression. Typical radiologic features include diffuse interstitial and alveolar changes on chest radiograph. Computed tomography (CT) shows a ground-glass appearance in conjunction with increased interstitial markings. Histologic features include interstitial changes and proliferation of atypical pneumocytes.

17. **What is the mechanism of gemcitabine-induced pulmonary toxicity?**

The mechanism of gemcitabine-induced lung toxicity is unknown. Cytarabine, another pyrimidine analog, has been known to cause a syndrome of noncardiogenic pulmonary edema in 13% to 28% of patients and develops after treatment with conventional and high-dose regimens. Histopathologic studies of these patients show interstitial and intraalveolar proteinaceous edema consistent with ARDS. It is postulated that damage to the capillary endothelial cells causes the leakage of the fluid resulting in pulmonary edema. In view of the structural and metabolic similarities between the two drugs, it is possible that they share the same mechanism of pulmonary injury.

18. **Describe risk factors that predispose patients to the development of pulmonary toxicity after receiving gemcitabine.**

In case reports of pulmonary toxicity attributed to gemcitabine, there is a subset of patients that appears to be more prone to developing pulmonary symptoms. Individuals older then 65 years of age, men, those with a significant smoking history, and exposure to previous radiation therapy are more likely to develop pulmonary toxicity.[48,49] More than half of these patients had a primary lung neoplasm. Studies done with concurrent radiation therapy and gemcitabine have also shown a higher incidence of pulmonary side effects. The number of gemcitabine doses received before the onset of pulmonary symptoms has ranged from 1 to 12, with a median of 5.4 doses.[48,49]

19. **Is gemcitabine related pulmonary toxicity reversible?**

Preventing a severe course of this syndrome depends on early recognition. If gemcitabine is not discontinued, pulmonary toxicity my be fatal, culminating in ARDS. Patients with prior resection of lung parenchyma and lung irradiation have less pulmonary functional reserve. If identified early, discontinuation of gemcitabine and administration of supplemental oxygen and corticosteroids has resulted in complete clinical and radiologic resolution in many cases. Prednisone 40 to 100 mg daily for 2 weeks followed by a taper has been advocated. Diuretics, such as furosemide, can be used as adjuncts to diminish symptomatic pulmonary edema in the short term. Pulmonary toxicity due to gemcitabine appears to have been underestimated. Case series continue to be published emphasizing the importance of a high index of suspicion for toxicity.

REFERENCES

1. Rosenow EC. The spectrum of drug-induced pulmonary disease. Ann Intern Med 1972;77:977.
2. Rosenow EC. Drug-induced pulmonary disease. Dis Mon 1994;40:253.
3. Cooper JA. Drug-induced lung disease. Adv Intern Med 1997;42:231.
4. Seaton A. Drug-induced lung disease, oxygen toxicity and related syndromes. In: Seaton A, ed. Crofton and Douglas's Respiratory Diseases. 5th Ed. Oxford: Blackwell Science, 2000;2:1458.
5. Tanoue LT. Pulmonary toxicity associated with chemotherapeutic agents. In: Fishman AP, ed. Pulmonary Diseases and Disorders. 2nd Ed. New York: McGraw-Hill, 1998;1:1003.
6. Zitnik R. Drug-induced lung disease due to nonchemotherapeutic agents. In: Fishman AP, ed. Pulmonary Diseases and Disorders. 2nd Ed. New York: McGraw-Hill, 1998;1:1017.
7. Keaney NP. Respiratory disorders. In: Davies DM, ed. Textbook of Adverse Drug Reactions. 4th Ed. New York: Oxford University Press, 1991:172.
8. Limper AH, Rosenow EC. Drug-induced pulmonary disease. In: Murray JF et al., eds. Textbook of Respiratory Medicine. 3rd Ed. Philadelphia: WB Saunders, 2000:1971.
9. Camus P et al. Adverse pulmonary effects of drugs and radiation. In: Gibson J et al., eds. Respiratory Medicine. London: Harcourt Health Sciences, 2001;1.
10. Williams SD et al. Treatment of disseminated germ-cell tumors with cisplatin, bleomycin, and either vinblastine or etoposide. N Engl J Med 1987;316(23):435.
11. Sleijfer S. Bleomycin pneumonitis. Chest 2001; 120:617.
12. O'Sullivan JM et al. Predicting the risk of bleomycin lung toxicity in patients with germ-cell tumours. Ann Oncol 2003;14:91.
13. Simpson AB et al. Fatal bleomycin pulmonary toxicity in the west of Scotland 1991-95: a review of patients with germ cell tumours. Br J Cancer 1998;78(8):1061.
14. Blum S. A clinical review of bleomycin-a new antineoplastic agent. Cancer 1972;32:903.
15. Waid-Jones MI, Coursin DB. Perioperative considerations for patients treated with bleomycin. Chest 1991;99:993.
16. Donat SM, Levy DA. Bleomycin associated pulmonary toxicity: is perioperative oxygen restriction necessary? J Urol 1998;160(4):1347.
17. McCarroll KA et al. Lung disorders due to drug abuse. J Thorac Imaging 1991;6(1):30.
18. Alcantara AL. Radiologic study of injection drug use complications. Infect Dis Clin North Am 2002;16(3):713.
19. Heffner JE et al. Pulmonary reactions from illicit substance abuse. Clin Chest Med 1990;11(1):151.
20. Haim DY et al. The pulmonary complications of crack cocaine: a comprehensive review. Chest 1995;107:233.
21. Thadani PV. NIDA Conference report on cardiopulmonary complication of "crack" cocaine use, clinical manifestations and pathophysiology. Chest 1996;110(4):1072.
22. Schmidt RA et al. Panlobular emphysema in young intravenous Ritalin abusers. Am Rev Respir Dis 1991;143:649.
23. Stern EJ et al. Panlobular emphysema caused by IV injection of methylphenidate (Ritalin): findings on chest radiographs and CT scans. Am J Roentgenol 1994;162:555.
24. Zitnik RJ. Drug-induced lung disease: antiarrhythmic agents. J Respir Dis 1996;17:254.
25. Martin WJ, Rosenow EC. Amiodarone pulmonary toxicity, recognition and pathogenesis (part 1). Chest 1988;93:1067.
26. Kanji Z et al. Amiodarone-induced pulmonary toxicity. Pharmacotherapy 1999;19:1463.
27. Jessurun GA et al. Amiodarone-induced pulmonary toxicity: predisposing factors, clinical symptoms and treatment. Drug Safety 1998;18:339.
28. Coudert B et al. Amiodarone pneumonitis: bronchoalveolar lavage findings in 15 patients and review of the literature. Chest 1992;102:1005.
29. Ohar JA et al. Bronchoalveolar lavage cell count and differential are not reliable indicators of amiodarone-induced pneumonitis. Chest 1992; 10(4):999.
30. Akoun GM et al. Amiodarone-induced hypersensitivity pneumonitis: evidence of an immunological cell-mediated mechanism. Chest 1984;85(1):133.
31. Settipane RA. Prevalence of cross-sensitivity with acetaminophen in aspirin-sensitive asthmatic subjects. J Allergy Clin Immunol 1995;96(4):480.
32. Luque CA, Vazquez Ortiz M. Treatment of ACE inhibitor-induced cough. Pharmacother 1999;19:804.
33. Szczeklik A. Aspirin-induced asthma: advances in pathogenesis and management. J Allergy Clin Immunol 1999;104(1):5.
34. Szczeklik A, Stevenson DD. Aspirin-induced asthma: advances in pathogenesis, diagnosis, and management. J Allergy Clin Immunol 2003; 111(5):913.
35. Babu KS et al. Aspirin and asthma. Chest 2000;118:1470.
36. Fraunfeder FT, Barker AF. Respiratory effects of timolol. N Engl J Med 1984;311:1441.
37. Meeker D et al. Drug-induced bronchospasm. Clin Chest Med 1990;11:163.
38. Simon RA. Adverse reactions to food and drug additives. Immunol Allergy Clin North Am 1996; 16(1):137.
39. Asmus MJ. Bronchoconstrictor additives in bronchodilator solutions. J Allergy Clin Immunol 1999;104(2 pt 2):S53.
40. Kemp SF. J Allergy Clin Immunol 2002; 110(3):341.
41. Cotran RS. Disorders of immunity. In: Cotran RS, ed. Robbins Pathologic Basis of Disease. 6th Ed. Philadelphia: WB Saunders, 1999:188.
42. Heier T, Guttormsen AB. Anaphylactic reactions during induction of anaesthesia using rocuronium for muscle relaxation: a report including 3 cases. Acta Anesthesiol Scand 2000;44(7):775.
43. Aldrich T et al. Adverse effects of drugs on the respiratory muscles. Clin Chest Med 1990;11:177.
44. Cronin DC 2nd. Modern immunosuppression. Clin Liver Dis 2000;4(3):619.
45. Goldsmith NR et al. Noncardiac pulmonary edema induced by nonionic low-osmolality radiographic contrast media. J Allergy Clin Immunol 1995;96(5 pt 1):698.
46. Marshall GD. Anaphylactoid reactions to radiocontrast agents. Immunol Allergy Clin North Am 1998;18(4):799.
47. Hein KD et al. The adult respiratory distress syndrome after dextran infusion as an antithrombotic agent in free TRAM flap breast reconstruction. Plast Reconstr Surg 1999;103(6):1706.
48. Gupta N et al. Gemcitabine-induced pulmonary toxicity. Am J Clin Oncol 2002;25:96.

49. Foerger M et al. Gemcitabine-related pulmonary toxicity. Swiss Med Wkly 2002;132:17.

50. Sporer KA et al. Heroin-related noncardiogenic pulmonary edema: a case series. Chest 2001; 120(5):1628.

51. Kavaru MS et al. Hydrochlorothiazide induced acute pulmonary edema. Cleve Clin J Med 1990;57:181.

52. Bernal C et al. Hydrochlorothiazide-induced pulmonary edema and associated immunologic changes. Ann Pharmacother 1999;33:172.

53. Siegel JB, Puri RK. IL-2 toxicity. J Clin Oncol 1991;9:694.

54. Mann H. Vascular leak syndrome associated with interleukin-2: chest radiographic manifestations. Radiology 1990;176(1):191.

55. Frand UI et al. Methadone-induced pulmonary edema. Ann Intern Med 1972;76:975.

56. Alderman EM. Opiates. Pediatr Rev 1997; 18(4):122.

57. Costanzo-Nordin MR. Cardiopulmonary effects of OKT3: determinants of hypotension, pulmonary edema, and cardiac dysfunction. Transplant Proc 1993;25(2 s1):21.

58. Pisani RJ, Rosenow EC. Pulmonary edema associated with tocolytic therapy. Ann Intern Med 1989; 110:714.

59. Rizk NW. Obstetric complications in pulmonary and critical care medicine. Chest 1996;110(3):791.

60. Varnell RM et al. Adult respiratory distress syndrome from overdose of tricyclic antidepressants. Radiology 1989;170:667.

61. Dahlin KL. Acute lung failure induced by tricyclic antidepressants. Toxicol Appl Pharmacol 1997; 146(2):309.

62. Schmitz N. Carmustine and the lungs. Lancet 1997;349(9067):1712.

63. Comet R et al. Pleuropulmonary disease as a side effect of treatment with bromocriptine. Respir Med 1998;92:1172.

64. Todman DH et al. Pleuropulmonary fibrosis due to bromocriptine treatment of Parkinson's disease. Clin Exp Neurol 1990;27:79.

65. Segura A et al. Pulmonary fibrosis induced by cyclophosphamide. Ann Pharmacother 2001;35:894.

66. Perry HM et al. Pulmonary disease following chronic chemical ganglionic blockade. Am J Med 1957;22:37.

67. Tomioka H et al. Gold-induced pulmonary disease: clinical features, outcome, and differentiation from rheumatoid lung disease. Am J Respir Crit Care Med 1997;155:1011.

68. Pfitzenmeyer P et al. Pleuropulmonary changes induced by ergoline drugs. Eur Respir J 1996;9:1013.

69. Feinberg L et al. Pulmonary fibrosis associated with tocainide: report of a case with literature review. Am Rev Respir Dis 1990;141:505.

70. Gurjal A. Etoposide-induced pulmonary toxicity. Lung Cancer 1999;26(2):109.

71. Antony VB. Drug-induced pleural disease. Clin Chest Med 1998;19(2):331.

72. Stoica GS et al. Corticosteroid responsive fludarabine pulmonary toxicity. Am J Clin Oncol 2002;25:340.

73. Garg S et al. Multiple pulmonary nodules: an unusual presentation of fludarabine pulmonary toxicity: case report and review of literature. Am J Hematol 2002;70(3):241.

74. Sitbon O et al. Minocycline pneumonitis and eosinophilia: a report on eight patients. Arch Intern Med 1994;154:1633.

75. Dykhuizen RS et al. Minocycline an pulmonary eosinophilia. BMJ 1995;310(6993):1520.

76. Miller et al. Loeffler's syndrome due to para-aminosalicylic acid. Dis Chest 1962;42:100.

77. Wechsler ME. Churg-Strauss syndrome in patients receiving montelukast as treatment for asthma. Chest 2000;117(3):708.

78. McGinnis JM et al. Actual causes of death in the United States. JAMA 1993;270:2207.

79. Daly PA et al. Risk Modification in the Obese Patient: Prevention of Myocardial Infarction. New York: Oxford University Press, 1996:203.

80. Gurtner HP. Aminorex and pulmonary hypertension. Cor Vasa 1985;27:160.

81. Douglas JG et al. Pulmonary hypertension and fenfluramine. BMJ 1981;283:881.

82. Abenhaim L et al. Appetite suppressant drugs and the risk of primary pulmonary hypertension. N Engl J Med 1996;335:609.

83. Naeiji R et al. Effects of dexfenfluramine on hypoxic pulmonary vasoconstriction and embolic pulmonary hypertension in dogs. Am J Respir Crit Care Med 1995;151:692.

84. Johannes L, Stocklai S. Dieting dilemma: withdrawal of Redux spotlights predicament FDA faces on obesity. Wall Street Journal, Sept 16, 1997.

85. Nan DN. Talc granulomatosis: a differential diagnosis of interstitial lung disease in HIV patients. Chest 2000;21(4):849.

GASTROINTESTINAL DISORDERS

Robin L. Corelli
SECTION EDITOR

CHAPTER 27

Upper Gastrointestinal Disorders

John K. Siepler, Candace Smith-Scott

Upper gastrointestinal (GI) disorders encompass a variety of conditions that can cause gastric discomfort, including dyspepsia, peptic ulcer disease (PUD), and gastroesophageal reflux disease (GERD). This chapter addresses four topics in the following order: dyspepsia, PUD (including Zollinger-Ellison [ZE] syndrome), GERD, and prophylaxis of stress-related mucosal lesions.

The term *dyspepsia* refers to symptoms thought to originate in the upper GI tract and is used commonly to refer to persis-tent or recurrent pain or discomfort centered in the upper abdomen.[1] This pain includes ulcer-like, GERD-like, and dysmotility-like discomfort. Discomfort is defined as a subjective, unpleasant feeling that the patient does not interpret as pain but that can include symptoms such as fullness, bloating, or nausea.[1,2] It is estimated that 25% to 55% of the U.S. population will experience some form of dyspepsia in their lifetime (Fig. 27-1). Dyspepsia of some kind accounts for approximately 60% of all upper GI complaints in the U.S. population.

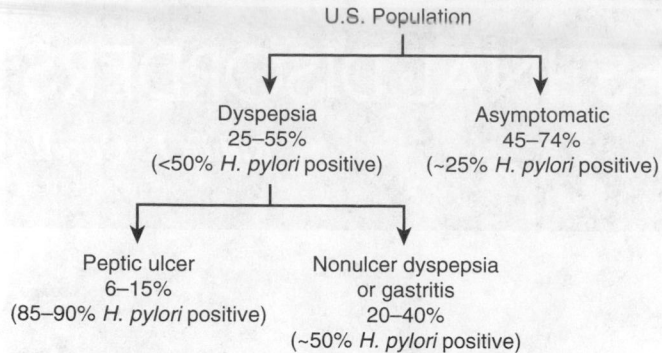

FIGURE 27-1 Prevalence of dyspepsia and peptic acid disease in the United States.

Approximately 4% to 10% of all Americans will develop a peptic ulcer during their lifetime, and the prevalence of active disease is approximately 3%.[3] The incidence of PUD varies with the type of ulcer (e.g., gastric or duodenal), geographic location, gender, age, and a variety of environmental factors. Race, socioeconomic status, and psychological stress do not correlate with the development of PUD.[4] As discussed in more detail later, three factors stand out as being the most important to the development of PUD: bacterial GI infection with *Helicobacter pylori (H. pylori),* ingestion of nonsteroidal anti-inflammatory drugs (NSAIDs), and cigarette smoking.[4] It is estimated that up to 90% of peptic ulcers, in the absence of NSAID exposure, are associated with *H. pylori* infection. However, one should avoid the false impression that the presence of *H. pylori* colonization is an indication that an ulcer will develop. As illustrated in Figure 27-2, a high proportion (approximately 40%) of the general population tests positive for *H. pylori* colonization, but only 15% to 30% of those with positive test results will develop PUD at some time in their life.

GERD is defined as the presence of heartburn two or more times weekly that is associated with a change in lifestyle.[5] It is associated with a backflow (i.e., reflux or regurgitation) of GI contents into the esophagus resulting in heartburn and regurgitation symptoms. The classic symptom of reflux is "heartburn," which is described commonly either as a pain in the center of the chest (which may mimic cardiac angina), or as a sensation of "burping up" stomach contents into in the mouth. Patients with chronic, persistent heartburn are more likely to develop esophageal adenocarcinoma.[6] Esophagitis is associated with GERD and is the presence of inflammation in the esophagus. The most common causes of GERD are inappropriate lower esophageal sphincter (LES) relaxation and reduced resting pressure in the sphincter: both facilitate the regurgitation of acid from the stomach into the esophagus. Although it is normal for the esophageal and lower esophageal sphincters to relax to allow food passage, relaxation of these sphincters at other times is abnormal. A hiatal hernia (a defect in the diaphragm that allows the stomach to slide into the chest cavity) does not cause GERD but may exacerbate the situation by decreasing the ability of gastric acid from draining back through the sphincter because of differences in the pressure gradient within the abdomen. Some drugs (e.g., vcrapamil, theophylline) also may cause the lower esophageal sphincter to relax.

Terminology can sometimes be misleading; therefore, think of *GERD* as a disease, *heartburn* as a symptom, and *esophagitis* as an endoscopic finding. These disorders are not mutually exclusive, and effective treatment of one disorder does not guarantee that the patient will be symptom free. This principle is most relevant to the treatment of PUD. With the realization that peptic ulcer often has an infectious cause, it is now possible to talk of treatment in terms of "cure" of the ulcer after antibiotic therapy, not just symptom relief or temporary healing. The presence of continued symptoms could indicate coexistence of nonulcer dyspepsia, GERD, or both.

DYSPEPSIA

Dyspepsia is usually the main complaint for patients who present with upper GI problems. As defined above, dyspepsia occurs in approximately 26% of the population in the United States and in as many as 41% in England.[1,2] As dyspepsia is a symptom complex that may apply to several patient conditions, the exact cause can be one or several different disorders. Once investigated, approximately 50% of patients have a specific problem (e.g., PUD or GERD). In the remainder, no cause is often discovered.

There have been several attempts to define dyspepsia,[1,7] and it can be classified into several subclassifications which attempt to associate the type of dyspepsia with a cause. Patients who present with dyspepsia but have not undergone any diagnostic tests are said to have "uninvestigated" dyspepsia. In addition, patients with a heartburn-like dyspepsia are said to have "GERD-like" dyspepsia, those with dyspepsia that is

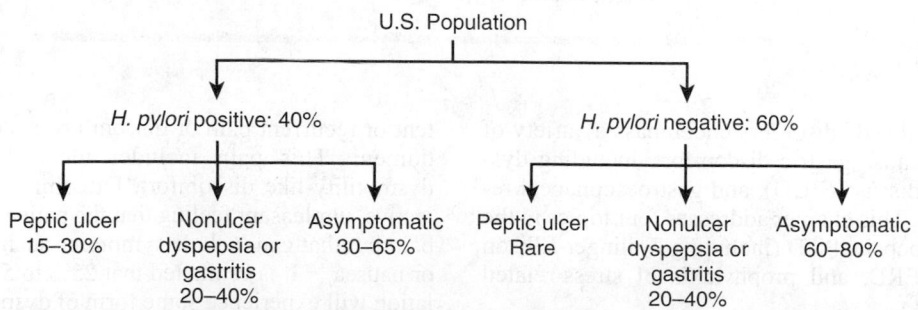

FIGURE 27-2 Relationship of *Helicobacter pylori* to peptic ulcer and nonulcer dyspepsia.

described as crampy are said to have "dysmotility-like" dyspepsia, and those with abdominal pain that is burning and relieved by meals are said to have "ulcer-like" dyspepsia. Some disagree with the inclusion of heartburn in dyspepsia classifications and would consider dyspepsia to be limited to ulcer-like or dysmotility-like. Despite these classifications, the predictive value of dyspepsia for specific pathology is poor. Understanding these classifications is essential to understanding studies that investigate this problem. When evaluating studies, close attention must be paid to the authors' definitions and inclusion criteria for study subjects when attempting to review results.

Diagnosis for a patient with a new complaint of dyspepsia is usually directed at the suspected cause. Thus, a patient who complains of "GERD-like" dyspepsia will be diagnosed and treated like a patient with GERD, and a patient who complains of "ulcer-like" dyspepsia will be diagnosed and treated like a patient with PUD. Once a patient has undergone diagnostic procedures (usually endoscopy) without finding a specific cause for their dyspepsia, it will be classified as "nonulcer" dyspepsia.

The management strategy for patients who have dyspepsia of unknown cause or are classified as having nonulcer dyspepsia varies and has been the subject of numerous studies. For treatment, most of these patients will receive H. pylori testing and eradication, antisecretory medications (either H_2-antagonists or proton pump inhibitors), or a combination of both. The remainder of this section reviews the efficacy of these strategies.

Management Strategies

Perhaps the first management option is whether empiric treatment or further diagnosis followed by a specific treatment is the most effective course of action.[8] Several trials examined whether H. pylori testing and eradication would provide better symptom control than a strategy that based treatment on results of endoscopy.[9–11] The entry criteria for the largest of the three trials included patients who presented to their primary care practitioners with dyspepsia. These patients had truly uninvestigated dyspepsia. Symptoms were controlled better in the endoscopy-directed treatment group. The remaining two trials, which enrolled patients referred for endoscopy, failed to find a difference in symptoms. It is likely that the patients in the two unsuccessful studies were selected by an initial empiric trial by their primary care practitioner.[10,11]

If the initial treatment strategy is empiric treatment, acid suppression is often the first choice. There are numerous trials that compare the various options in this area. Three trials comparing PPIs and H_2-antagonists found patients receiving PPIs to have significantly better symptom control.[12–14] In these studies, PPIs appear to offer superior control of heartburn-like dyspepsia. However, the Cochrane Database review concludes that there is insufficient evidence to make the claim that PPIs are superior to H_2-antagonists.[8]

Whereas the role of H. pylori is widely accepted in PUD, its role in other GI conditions such as dyspepsia is not clear. When patients infected with H. pylori are queried, a broad range of symptoms are reported including dyspepsia and heartburn. Until recently, studies designed to determine the role of H. pylori in nonulcer dyspepsia have not studied appropriate outcomes. Recently several studies comparing H. pylori eradication with alternate therapy have been published that used appropriate end points. Most of these trials find no significant difference in symptom resolution between the H. pylori eradication group and the control subjects. However, McColl and colleagues reported a significant improvement in symptoms in nonulcer dyspepsia patients who had H. pylori eradicated (with antisecretory and antimicrobial agents) compared to those receiving 4 weeks of PPI monotherapy.[15] This study used a continuous symptom assessment tool that patients recorded for 12 months, but they also included many patients who may have had PUD. While the overall success favored H. pylori eradication, symptom resolution was low and observed in only 27% of patients compared with 12 % for the PPI-treated group. In contrast, Blum and colleagues evaluated H. pylori eradication versus 4 weeks of a PPI and evaluated symptoms at 1 year.[16] Control of symptoms was similar in the two groups (26% to 30%). One main difference between the McColl and Blum studies is that Blum excluded patients with a history of peptic ulcer or GERD. This may explain some of the different results as PPIs would be expected to be superior in patients with GERD as their origin of their dyspepsia.

It appears that both H. pylori eradication and PPIs provide symptom control in patients with nonulcer dyspepsia. Studies arriving at different conclusions regarding empiric treatment are likely dependent on patient selection. One clear conclusion is that overall symptom control is poor, with less than one-third of patients being free of symptoms with either treatment regimen.

Treatment Recommendations

Patients with dyspepsia should receive appropriate diagnosis to determine the cause of their symptoms. If the cause is determined to be peptic ulcer, GERD, an NSAID-associated ulcer, or another condition, appropriate treatment should be initiated. If no specific cause is found, it appears that PPIs or H. pylori testing and (if positive) eradication should be tried. As studies demonstrate only modest efficacy, appropriate follow-up is important.

PEPTIC ULCER DISEASE

Peptic ulcers are lesions in the stomach or duodenum that occur as a result of the activity of acid and pepsin. Zollinger-Ellison syndrome (ZES) is a rare form of PUD resulting from hypersecretion as a result of a gastrin secreting tumor.

Epidemiology

Incidence and Prevalence

During the beginning of the 20th century, the incidence of PUD significantly increased, reaching a peak in the early 1950s.[17] Over the past two decades, both outpatient episodes of duodenal ulcers and ulcers requiring hospitalization have declined. Whether this decline reflects an actual decrease in the incidence of ulcer disease or the combined influences of more effective therapy, changes in hospital diagnostic practices or criteria, and institution coding changes is unclear. Although hospitalization for duodenal ulcers has declined, hospitalization for gastric ulcers has remained stable. The lack of decline in gastric ulcers may be attributable to aging and the use of NSAIDs.

Geographic Variation

PUD occurs worldwide with significant geographic variation. In Japan, the incidence of gastric ulcer is approximately 5 to 10 times more common than duodenal ulcer; however, in most European countries and the United States, duodenal ulcers are approximately twice as common as gastric ulcers.[18]

Gender

In the United States through the 1970s, more women than men developed PUD.[19,20] The incidence of gastric ulcers is approximately the same for men as for women; however, hospitalizations for women with gastric ulcers have increased significantly for patients older than 65.[19]

Age

Gastric ulcers rarely develop before age 40, and the peak incidence occurs from ages 55 to 65.[20] In contrast, the incidence of duodenal ulcers increases with age until the age of approximately 60 years.[2] The prevalence of *H. pylori* associated ulcers is low in children, but the incidence also increases with age.

Morbidity and Mortality

Mortality caused by PUD has declined over the past 20 years. Fewer than 2% of ulcer patients receiving therapy are expected to have a serious complication including bleeding, perforation, or obstruction. Nevertheless, PUD remains one of the most common GI diseases that results in loss of work and high-cost medical services.[20]

Physiology of the Upper Gastrointestinal Tract

The stomach consists of three anatomically and functionally distinct regions: the cardia, the body, and the antrum (Fig. 27-3). The body, which makes up approximately 80% to 90% of the stomach, contains the parietal cells, which secrete acid and intrinsic factor which is required for vitamin B_{12} absorption. The body of the stomach also contains chief cells, which secrete pepsinogen. The antrum constitutes approximately 10% to 20% of the stomach and contains the G-cells, which secrete the hormone gastrin.

Various stimuli can trigger the secretion of acid into the gastric lumen. Neurologic impulses, originating in the central nervous system (CNS) and initiated by the sight, smell, and taste of food, travel along cholinergic pathways to provoke the release of acetylcholine in both the parietal cell and antral G-cell areas (Fig. 27-4). Subsequently, gastric distention stimulates oxyntic and antral receptors, and food protein further stimulates antral receptors to further trigger the release of acetylcholine at nerve endings in parietal and G-cell areas. The acetylcholine in turn stimulates the antral G-cells to release the hormone gastrin. Other stimuli cause secretion of histamine in the vicinity of the parietal cells. All three mediators—acetylcholine, gastrin, and histamine—converge to activate potassium-hydrogen-adenosine triphosphatase (K^+-H^+-ATPase) located on the parietal cell surface. The secretion of acid occurs against a concentration gradient and therefore requires the K^+-H^+-ATPase proton pump.[21] As the hydrogen ion concentration increases, it inhibits further secretion of gastrin through a feedback pathway. Cholecystokinin, glucagon, and vasoactive intestinal peptide also inhibit gastrin secretion. Thus, gastric acid secretion is regulated through both positive and negative feedback mechanisms. Pepsinogen, released from the chief cells, is a proenzyme that will form pepsin under acidic conditions (pH <3.5). Pepsin combines with acid to form a proteolytic complex, which further aids in the digestive and ulcerogenic processes.[2]

Several mechanisms protect the gastroduodenal mucosa from the digestive effects of pepsin and acid. Prostaglandin E and somatostatin, located on the basolateral membrane of the parietal cell, inhibit gastric acid secretion, maintain mucosal blood flow, and stimulate production of mucus and bicarbonate.[22] The secretion of mucus by superficial epithelial cells and mucous cells throughout the stomach protects against the erosive effects of acid. Gastric mucus is a viscous gel that serves as a mucosal lubricant, a trap for micro-organisms, and a barrier to the back diffusion of hydrogen ions from the mucosa.[22]

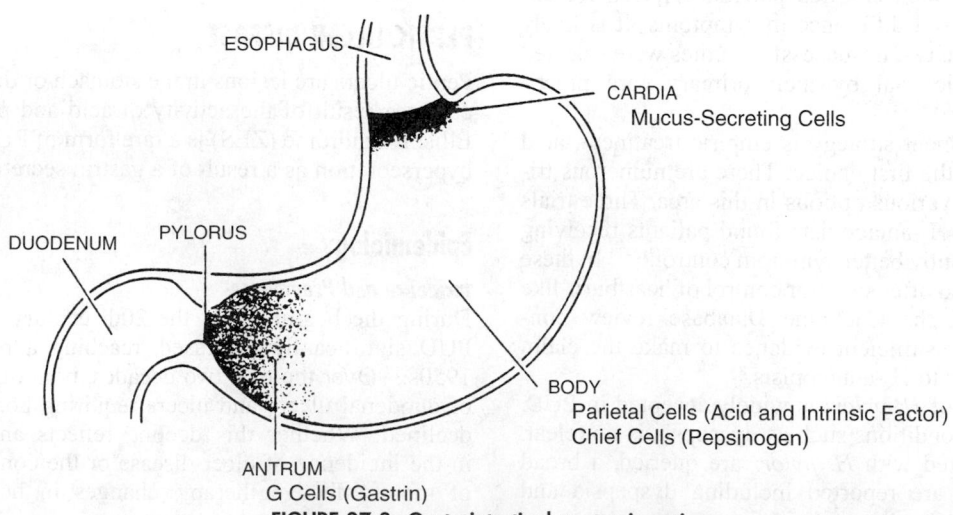

ESOPHAGUS

CARDIA
Mucus-Secreting Cells

DUODENUM PYLORUS

BODY
Parietal Cells (Acid and Intrinsic Factor)
Chief Cells (Pepsinogen)

ANTRUM
G Cells (Gastrin)

FIGURE 27-3 Gastrointestinal anatomic regions.

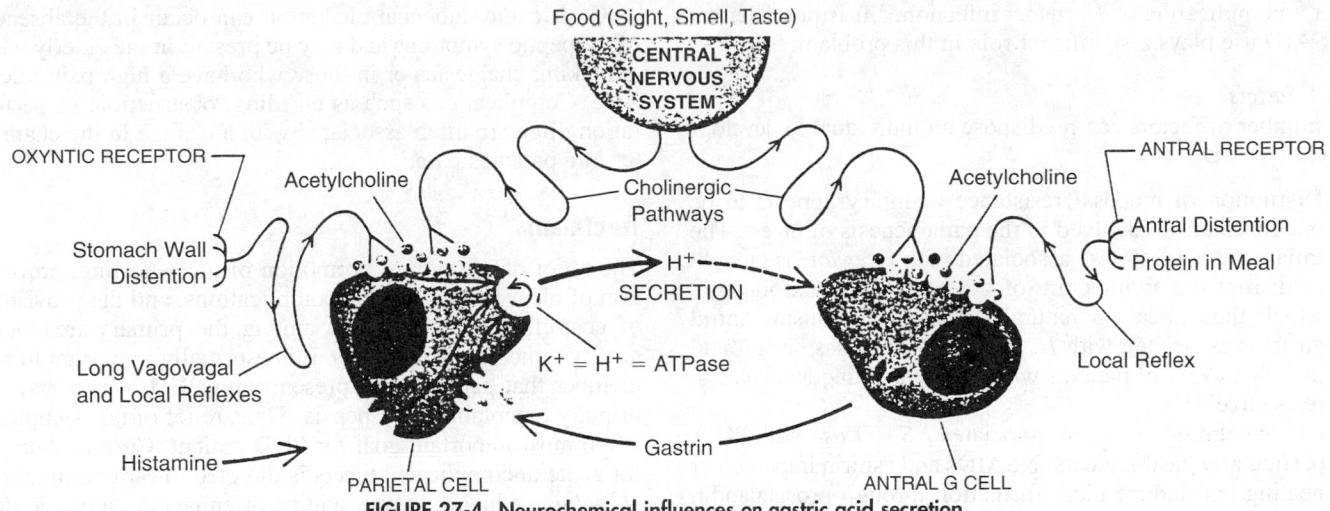

FIGURE 27-4 Neurochemical influences on gastric acid secretion.

Bicarbonate also is secreted throughout the stomach and creates a pH gradient that neutralizes the hydrogen ions.

A network of vascular capillaries beneath the surface epithelium provides yet another level of defense against gastric acid injury. Mucosal blood flow, through arterioles and capillaries, transports oxygen and substrates to the mucosa and removes acids that can be damaging to the epithelium of the stomach or duodenum.[23] The rapid and continual renewal of gastroduodenal epithelial cells also enhances resistance to injury from secreted acids. In the majority of cases, disruption of the surface epithelium can be mitigated partially by the formation of a fibrin cap over the injured area (a process known as *restitution*).[23,24] These actions of prostaglandin E, somatostatin, bicarbonate, gastric mucus, mucosal blood flow, epithelial cell regeneration, and restitution all combine to protect the gastric epithelium against injury from secreted acid.

Pathogenesis

The integrity of the upper GI mucosa depends on a balance between aggressive forces (primarily gastric acid and pepsin) and mucosal defensive factors.[24] Gastric acid is necessary for the formation of ulcers, but an alteration in the protective defenses plays a significant role as well. Patients with ZE syndrome have an increased parietal cell mass, which secretes large amounts of gastric acid. Conversely, patients with duodenal ulcers have normal acid secretion, and patients with gastric ulcers tend to have normal or low acid production.[24] These observations support the premise that other mechanisms are involved in the pathogenesis of ulcers. Studies have focused on alteration of mucosal defenses as an etiology of ulcers. For example, prostaglandin inhibitors (e.g., NSAIDs) may render the gastric mucosa susceptible to ulceration because endogenous prostaglandins protect the GI tract.[26] *H. pylori* also has a role in the pathogenesis of PUD, and eradication of this organism can alter the natural history of the PUD. As a result, many investigators have divided PUD into three etiologic groups based on pathophysiologic abnormalities: (1) ulcers associated with *H. pylori* infection, (2) those caused by NSAID use, and (3) those with acid hypersecretion (i.e., ZE syndrome).[24]

Helicobacter pylori

A Gram-negative spiral bacterium, *Campylobacter pylori*, was isolated in 1983 from patients with gastritis, and the association of this organism to the pathogenesis of PUD began to be investigated. Approximately 6 years later, the nomenclature of *Campylobacter pylori* was changed to *H. pylori* because the characteristics of this organism were more aligned with bacteria in the *Helicobacter* genus than the *Campylobacter* genus.[25,26] Approximately 40% of patients older than 60 are seropositive for *H. pylori*, whereas the prevalence in patients younger than 30 years of age is only 10%.[27]

The mode of transmission of *H. pylori* is unknown; however, person-to-person transmission is likely because of findings of familial clustering.[28] *H. pylori* can be isolated anywhere in the stomach but is found most consistently in the gastric antrum, where it is associated with inflammation. This organism is the most common cause of antral gastritis,[29] and elimination from the gastric antrum is associated with resolution of gastritis. The exact mechanism by which *H. pylori* causes gastric injury is unknown, but possibilities include production of a cytotoxin, breakdown of mucosal defenses, and adherence to epithelial cells.[30] *H. pylori* is unique in that it produces large amounts of urease. Urease catalyzes the hydrolysis of urea to form ammonia, and the accumulation of ammonia may play a role in disrupting the integrity of gastric mucosa, rendering it susceptible to ulceration.[31] In addition, *H. pylori* infected individuals have increased basal and stimulated acid secretion when compared with those not infected. Eradication of *H. pylori* can reverse this increased acid secretion to normal.[32]

H. pylori is found in approximately 90% of patients with duodenal ulcers and in 70% of those with gastric ulcers.[32] Eradication of *H. pylori* significantly decreases the recurrence rate of peptic ulcers and accelerates the ulcer healing process; therefore, *H. pylori* is implicated in the pathogenesis of PUD.[33] Nevertheless, not everyone with *H. pylori* has an ulcer, and it is often isolated from patients who do not have PUD.[33] *H. pylori* infection also is not associated with acute perforated duodenal ulcers. This latter finding suggests that perforated duodenal ulcers may have a different pathogenesis from chronic duodenal ulcer disease and that perforation is not a complication of *H. pylori* infection.[14] It is possible that NSAID use plays a significant role in this problem.

Risk Factors

A number of factors can predispose an individual to development of PUD:

- Disruption of mucosal resistance to injury appears to be one mechanism involved in the pathogenesis of ulcers. The inflammatory response associated with *H. pylori* is thought to disrupt the architecture of the gastroduodenal mucosa, which then alters its natural defense mechanism. Antral gastritis associated with *H. pylori infection* has been found in 75% to 95% of patients with gastric and duodenal ulcers, respectively.[24]
- Overwhelming evidence associates *NSAID use* with PUD, particularly gastric ulcers. NSAIDs and aspirin impair ulcer healing and induce ulcer formation through prostaglandin inhibition and directly irritate the gastric and duodenal mucosa.[36]
- *Cigarette smoking* impairs ulcer healing, promotes ulcer recurrence, and increases the likelihood of ulcer complications.[24] Cigarette smoking may cause ulcers through stimulation of gastric acid secretion and bile salt reflux,[31,32] alteration in mucosal blood flow, and reduction in prostaglandin synthesis.[4,32]
- Historically, some *foods* were believed to be factors in the development of ulcers. Although some foods and beverages (e.g., caffeine-containing foods, milk, alcohol, spicy foods) increase acid secretion and cause dyspepsia, no scientific data support the belief that diet imparts an increased risk for ulcer formation.[3] Acute *alcohol* ingestion can damage the gastric mucosal barrier, leading to acute gastric mucosal lesions and GI bleeding; however, alcohol has not been proven to cause PUD.[4]
- *Genetic predilection* appears to be a risk factor for the development of ulcers. Approximately 20% to 50% of patients with duodenal ulcers have a positive family history of PUD compared with 5% to 15% of nonulcer patients.[20]
- Although rigorous studies are lacking, *stressful life events* are thought by some to exacerbate PUD.[32]

Clinical Presentation

Patients with gastric or duodenal ulcers present with similar symptoms and cannot be differentiated on the basis of clinical findings; therefore, a definitive diagnosis requires an upper GI radiologic series or an endoscopy is needed to visualize the ulcer. The most common and often the only symptom of an ulcer is epigastric pain. Overall, the pain associated with duodenal and gastric ulcers is not well localized and usually is described as annoying, burning, gnawing, and aching.[3] Pain occurring when the stomach is empty (e.g., during the night, between meals) and when relieved by food and antacids is the most widely described characteristic of duodenal ulcer pain. Duodenal ulcer pain usually is episodic with symptomatic periods lasting for weeks followed by a period of no occurrence. The pain associated with gastric ulcers is difficult to distinguish from duodenal ulcers, but it may occur at any time of the day.

Epigastric pain does not always correlate with the presence or absence of an ulcer; asymptomatic patients have been diagnosed with ulcers, and patients with dyspeptic symptoms may not have active ulcer disease.[1,2]

Gastric and duodenal ulceration can occur in the absence of dyspeptic symptoms and may be present in the elderly who are taking analgesics or in those who have a high pain tolerance. Complications such as bleeding, obstruction, or perforation often are often associated with a change in the character of a patient's pain.[2]

Treatment

The relief of symptoms, promotion of ulcer healing, prevention of ulcer recurrence and complications, and the provision of cost-effective therapy are among the primary treatment goals of uncomplicated PUD. It is especially important to remember that patients who present with PUD usually have a primary complaint of dyspepsia. Thus, relief of this symptom is the most important goal for PUD patient. Current therapy for acute uncomplicated ulcers is directed toward eliminating *H. pylori*, reducing gastric acidity, or enhancing mucosal defenses. When patients are infected with *H. pylori*, the eradication of this organism is the primary treatment goal because of its clear association with duodenal and gastric ulcers.[35,36] Healing of and reducing recurrence of gastroduodenal lesions is associated with an effective eradication of *H. pylori*.[36] In contrast, gastric ulcers typically are associated with normal or decreased acid secretion and are less frequently associated with *H. pylori* infection. This may be due to the association of gastric ulcers to NSAID use, a potential cause that is independent of *H. pylori* infection.[35,36] Gastric ulcers can be associated with gastric carcinoma. This possibility must be addressed in the diagnosis.

Drug treatment of peptic ulcers (Tables 27-1 and 27-2) generally consists of diagnosis and eradication of *H. pylori* as well as medications that neutralize gastric acid (e.g., antacids), inhibit acid secretion (e.g., H_2-antagonists, and PPIs), and protect the gastroduodenal mucosa (e.g., sucralfate). Table 27-1 lists the antisecretory medications used, but it must be remembered that eradication of *H. pylori* is the primary treatment for PUD in infected individuals. Virtually all patients with a duodenal ulcer are infected. With the advent of antibiotic treatment for *H. pylori*, acid suppression alone is rarely indicated except for patients with bacteriologic cure and recurrent ulcers.

H_2-Antagonists
MECHANISM OF ACTION

H_2-receptor antagonists inhibit the secretion of gastric acid. Histamine, released primarily from mast cells, binds to H_2-receptors and activates adenylate cyclase, and thereby increases intracellular cyclic adenosine monophosphate (cAMP). The increased levels of cAMP activate the proton pump of the parietal cell to secrete hydrogen ions against a concentration gradient in exchange for potassium ions.[37] H_2-receptor antagonists competitively and selectively inhibit the action of histamine on the H_2-receptors of the parietal cells, thus reducing basal and stimulated gastric acid secretion.

EFFICACY

There are four H_2-receptor antagonists available in the United States. All are effective for the treatment of duodenal and gastric ulcers (see Table 27-1). Use of these medications is associated with an overall healing rate of 70% to 95% after 4 to 8 weeks of therapy. They are equally effective in the acute healing of duodenal and gastric ulcers and are equally well tolerated.[38]

Table 27-1   Antiulcer and GERD Indications

	PUD	Hypersecretory	GERD	Esophagitis	NSAID-Induced Ulcer
H₂RAs					
Cimetidine	X[a,b]	X	X	X	
Famotidine	X[a,b]	X	X	X	
Nizatidine	X[a,b]	X	X		
Ranitidine	X[b,c]	X	X	X	
Proton Pump Inhibitors					
Esomeprazole			X	X	
Omeprazole	X[a]	X	X	X	
Lansoprazole	X[b,c]	X	X	X	X[d,e]
Pantoprazole		X	X	X	
Rabeprazole	X[c]	X	X	X	
Other Agents					
Misoprostol					X[e]
Sucralfate	X[b,c]				

[a]Duodenal and gastric ulcer.
[b]Maintenance for duodenal ulcer.
[c]Duodenal ulcer.
[d]NSAID-induced ulcer healing.
[e]NSAID-induced ulcer prevention.
X, approved indication.

Table 27-2   Antiulcer and GERD Medications: Doses

	Duodenal Ulcer	Duodenal Ulcer Maintenance	Gastric Ulcer	GERD	Esophagitis	Hypersecretory	NSAID
H₂RAs							
Cimetidine	300 mg QID 400 mg BID 800 mg HS	400 mg HS	300 mg QID	800 mg BID 400 mg QID	800 mg BID 400 mg QID	300 mg QID[a]	
Famotidine	20 mg BID 40 mg HS	20 mg BID	40 mg HS	20 mg BID	20 mg BID	20 mg BID[a]	
Nizatidine	150 mg BID	150 mg BID	150 mg BID	150 mg BID	150 mg QID		
Ranitidine	150 mg BID 300 mg HS	150 mg HS	150 mg BID	150 mg BID	150 mg QID	150 mg BID[a]	
Proton Pump Inhibitors							
Esomeprazole				20 mg QD	20 mg QD	60 mg QD[a]	
Lansoprazole	30 mg QD 60 mg QD	15 mg QD	30 mg QD	30 mg QD	30 mg QD	60 mg QD[a]	30 mg QD[b]
Omeprazole	20 mg QD 40 mg QD	10 mg QD	20 mg QD 40 mg QD	20 mg QD	20 mg QD	60 mg QD[a]	
Pantoprazole				40 mg QD	40 mg QD	40 mg QD[a]	
Rabeprazole	20mg QD	20 mg QD		20 mg QD	20 mg QD	60 mg QD[a]	
Other Agents							
Sucralfate	1 mg QID 2 gm BID						
Misoprostol							200 µg QID[c]

[a]Titrate dose to acid secretory response.
[b]Prevention NSAID ulcers and NSAID ulcer healing.
[c]Prevent NSAID ulcers.
BID, twice daily; HS, at bedtime; QD, once daily; QID, four times daily.

POTENCY

Although the relative antisecretory potency on a milligram-per-milligram basis of these four agents differs (famotidine has the greatest potency, followed by nizatidine, ranitidine, and lastly, cimetidine), this issue is not clinically relevant because the formulations of these four drugs have been adjusted accordingly. The serum concentration that is necessary to inhibit 50% of pentagastrin-stimulated secretion of acid determines the dosage and frequency of administration of each H₂-receptor antagonist. Famotidine is the most potent and possess the longest duration of action.[39]

PHARMACOKINETICS

Although these agents have identical mechanisms of action and similar clinical benefits, they differ in their pharmacokinetic profiles (Table 27-3).

Oral absorption of all the H_2-receptor antagonists is rapid, and peak drug concentrations usually are achieved within 1 to 3 hours after administration.[39] The bioavailability is lower for cimetidine, famotidine, and ranitidine because they are absorbed incompletely and undergo first-pass hepatic metabolism. Ranitidine undergoes the most extensive first-pass metabolism, which accounts for the large difference between the oral and intravenous (IV) doses of this drug. Nizatidine is the only H_2-receptor antagonist that is unavailable as an IV formulation.

All four drugs are eliminated by a combination of hepatic metabolism, glomerular filtration, and renal tubular secretion.[39] Hepatic metabolism is the principal pathway for the elimination of cimetidine and ranitidine, whereas renal excretion is the major route for the elimination of famotidine and nizatidine.[39] For each of these agents, the half-life is increased, the total body clearance is decreased, and dosage reduction is recommended for patients with moderate to severe renal insufficiency. The pharmacokinetics of the H_2-receptor antagonists appear to be unaffected by hepatic dysfunction; however, in patients with hepatic failure and renal insufficiency, dosage adjustment may be necessary.

ADVERSE EFFECTS

H_2-receptor antagonists are remarkably safe and the frequency of severe adverse effects is low for all four drugs.[40] The most common adverse effects include GI discomfort (e.g., diarrhea, constipation), CNS effects (e.g., mental confusion, headaches, dizziness, drowsiness), and dermatologic effects (e.g., rashes).[40] Cimetidine has weak antiandrogenic effects, and its use in high doses has been associated with gynecomastia and impotence. Hepatotoxicity has occasionally been observed in patients taking H_2-receptor antagonists. The patients who are at greatest risk for developing adverse effects include the elderly, those taking higher doses, and those with altered renal function.

DRUG INTERACTIONS

Several drugs interact with the H_2-receptor antagonists and, in particular, cimetidine (Table 27-4). Cimetidine binds to the cytochrome (CYP) P450 mixed-function oxidase enzyme system and inhibits the biotransformation of several drugs by the liver. It primarily affects oxidative drug metabolism while conjugation generally is not affected. The magnitude of cimetidine interaction with other drugs varies from patient to patient; however, it generally will reduce the clearance of another drug by approximately 20% to 30%.[41] This interaction is most clinically significant with drugs that have narrow therapeutic ranges such as phenytoin, warfarin, and theophylline.

Although ranitidine is more potent on a molar basis, it binds less intensely to the CYP P450 system than cimetidine.[41] Therefore, when used in equipotent doses, there is less potential for ranitidine (compared with cimetidine) to interfere with the liver metabolism of other drugs.[39] In contrast, famotidine and nizatidine do not bind appreciably to the CYP P450 system and therefore have limited ability to inhibit the metabolism of other drugs.[41] Overall, ranitidine, famotidine, and nizatidine, when used in equipotent doses, are unlikely to cause clinically significant drug interactions when administered concurrently with other drugs eliminated by phase I oxidative metabolism by the liver. However, the introduction of cimetidine to a patient receiving a drug that requires the CYP P450 system for metabolism may require a downward dosage adjustment of the object drug to avoid increased serum concentrations. Patients receiving drugs known to interact with H_2-receptor antagonists should be monitored to prevent or minimize the development of an adverse drug–drug interaction.

Some of the H_2-receptor antagonists are eliminated via renal tubular secretion and therefore have the potential to compete with cationic compounds for tubular secretion.[42] Cimeti-

---

Table 27-3   **Pharmacokinetic Comparison of H_2-Receptor Antagonists**

Variable	Cimetidine	Ranitidine	Nizatidine	Famotidine
Relative potency	1	4–10	4–10	20–50
Absorption				
Bioavailability (%)[b]	30–80 (60)	30–88 (50)	75–100 (98)	37–45 (43)
Time to peak serum concentration (hr)	1–2	1–3	1–3	1–3.5
Volume of distribution (L/kg of body weight)	0.8–1.2	1.2–1.9	1.2–1.6	1.1–1.4
Elimination				
Total systemic clearance (mL/min)	450–650	568–709	667–850	417–483
Half-life in serum (hr)	1.5–2.3	1.6–2.4	1.1–1.6	2.5–4
Hepatic clearance (%)				
Oral	60	73	22	50–80
IV	25–40	30	25	25–30
Renal clearance (%)				
Oral	40	27	57–65	25–30
IV	50–80	50	75	65–80

[a]Adapted with permission from references 37–39.
[b]Average values are in parentheses.
IV, intravenous.

Table 27-4 Clinically Significant Drug Interactions With Cimetidine[a]

Drug	Effect on Serum Drug Concentration	Mechanism
Phenytoin[b]	↑	Inhibits metabolism; 140% ↑ serum levels
Nifedipine	↑	↑ AUC by 60–90%
Procainamide[b]	↑	Competition for renal tubular secretion; 44% ↑ AUC
Theophylline[b]	↑	Inhibits metabolism; 20–40% ↑ in serum levels
Warfarin	↑	Inhibits metabolism of R isomer; 20% ↑ PT
Benzodiazepines (diazepam, chlordiazepoxide)	↑	Inhibition of metabolism; 30–60%
Carbamazepine	↑	Inhibition of metabolism; variable
Propranolol	↑	Inhibition of metabolism; 1.5- to 3-fold ↑ in plasma level
Quinidine	↑	Inhibition of metabolism and may ↓ renal clearance; 14.5% ↑ AUC
TCAs (imipramine, desipramine, amitriptyline)	↑	Inhibition of metabolism; variable
Verapamil	↑	↑ clearance by up to 35%

[a]Adapted from references 40–45.
[b]There also are fewer interactions with ranitidine.
AUC, area under the curve; PT, prothrombin time; TCAs, tricyclic antidepressants.

dine and ranitidine inhibit the renal tubular secretion of procainamide and its metabolite by this mechanism.[43] Patients taking any one of these H_2-receptor antagonists have a decreased area under the concentration-time curves (AUCs) of procainamide and N-acetyl procainamide and their renal clearance is decreased. The interaction with ranitidine appears to be concentration and dose dependent; therapeutic doses of ranitidine (i.e., 300 mg/day) did not cause an interaction, whereas large doses (i.e., 750 mg/day) alter the pharmacokinetics of procainamide.[43] Although famotidine is a cationic drug that is excreted via active tubular secretion, it does not inhibit the renal elimination of procainamide or its metabolite.[44] A possible reason for this discrepancy is that the serum concentrations attained by the usual therapeutic dose (i.e., 20 mg twice a day) of famotidine may be too low to compete with other drugs at the site of renal tubular secretion.[39]

All four H_2-receptor antagonists can potentially affect the absorption and reduce the bioavailability of some drugs by altering the gastric pH.[45] By increasing the pH of the GI tract, cimetidine slows the dissolution of ketoconazole, ultimately reducing its absorption. Most H_2-receptor antagonists are weak inhibitors of gastric alcohol dehydrogenase. Thus, therapeutic doses of cimetidine, ranitidine, and nizatidine, enhance the absorption of ethanol following ingestion of moderate amounts of alcohol (approximately one or two glasses of wine or cans of beer).[45] This interaction is thought to be a result of gastric alcohol dehydrogenase inhibition. According to these findings, systemic effects of alcohol may be exacerbated and the safety of patients compromised. Famotidine has little effect on this enzyme, but in a more recent study, H_2-receptor antagonists did not alter serum ethanol levels following moderate to large alcohol consumption.[46] Until more data are available confirming the results of the latter study, possible adverse effects associated with ethanol use should be considered when selecting an H_2-receptor antagonist for patients who routinely consume alcohol.

DOSING

When cimetidine was first introduced, it was administered four times a day. However, based on clinical studies, recommendations now range anywhere from once daily to four times a day (see Table 27-2). The hypothesis that control of nighttime acid secretion is more effective in healing duodenal ulcers led to studies that compared night-time dosing with multiple-daily-dosing regimens finding similar healing rates.[47]

Proton Pump Inhibitors

MECHANISM OF ACTION

The proton pump inhibitors (PPIs) are highly specific inhibitors of gastric acid secretion. They act by irreversibly binding to K^+-H^+-ATPase (an enzyme that transports acid across the parietal cell), these drugs inhibit basal and stimulated gastric acid secretion in a dose-dependent and sustained fashion.[48–50] PPIs cause almost total elimination of acid release because they inhibit the terminal step in the acid production cycle.

EFFICACY

The PPIs (i.e., omeprazole [Prilosec], lansoprazole [Prevacid], rabeprazole [Aciphex], pantoprazole [Protonix], and esomeprazole [Nexium]) relieve symptoms and heal duodenal and gastric ulcers more quickly than the H_2-receptor antagonists (in 2 to 4 weeks compared with 4 to 8 weeks). However, the absolute healing rates for drugs in both groups are comparable (i.e., >90%) after completion of the requisite course of therapy.[51] All the PPIs inhibit >90% of gastric acid secreted in 24 hours.[52] While PPIs are indicated for the short-term treatment of active duodenal ulcers, eradication of H. pylori is the first-line treatment. PPIs are also effective in healing benign gastric ulcers, erosive reflux esophagitis, and controlling the hypersecretion associated with ZE syndrome.

PHARMACOKINETICS

The PPIs are formulated as enteric-coated granules within capsules or enteric-coated tablets because they are unstable in acid media.[53–55] Both omeprazole and pantoprazole are available in an IV formulation. Only IV pantoprazole is available in the United States. An IV formulation of lansoprazole is currently being investigated. All PPIs are rapidly absorbed after oral administration, with peak concentrations occurring 2 to 4 hours after administration of enteric-coated preparations.[55] The bioavailability of these agents ranges from 50% to 80%. Currently available PPIs serve as prodrugs for the formation of active metabolites. The parent drugs are absorbed in the small intestine and brought to parietal cells via the systemic circulation. The active metabolite of omeprazole (omeprazole sulfonamide) and the active metabolites of lansoprazole (lansoprazole sulfone and hydroxy lansoprazole) are protonated in the acidic region of the gastric parietal cell secretory canaliculi. These active metabolites then bind covalently to sulfhydryl groups on the H^+-K^+-ATPase (proton pump) to noncompetitively and irreversibly inhibit this enzyme and block release of acid. The PPIs are eliminated almost entirely by hepatic metabolism, and the elimination plasma half-lives are approximately 1 to 2 hours.[51–57] Despite the short plasma half-lives, antisecretory effect still is present 36 to 72 hours after a dose because the drugs bind covalently to the H^+K^+-ATPase in the parietal cell.[55] Dosages need not be adjusted for patients with renal impairment, but adjustment may be prudent in those with severe liver disease.[51–57] Esomeprazole, the S-enantiomer of omeprazole, has a similar pharmacokinetic profile to omeprazole.

ADVERSE EFFECTS

The adverse effects of these agents are relatively infrequent and comparable to those of H_2-receptor antagonists. Some adverse effects include GI discomfort (e.g., nausea, diarrhea, abdominal pain), CNS effects (e.g., dizziness, headache), and isolated reactions (e.g., skin rash, gynecomastia, increase in liver transaminases).[52] Theoretically, the PPIs can cause hypergastrinemia through their profound ability to inhibit gastric secretion because antral G-cells release gastrin when gastric pH increases.[53] Chronic hypergastrinemia in humans is thought to lead to hyperplasia of enterochromaffin-like cells and carcinoid tumors of the stomach; however, there is no evidence of tumors actually occurring even after several years of continued treatment with high doses in patients with esophagitis.[56]

DRUG INTERACTIONS

All PPIs bind to P450 oxidative enzymes and therefore potentially interfere with hepatic drug metabolism. Data indicate that omeprazole has a differential affinity for specific CYP P450 isoenzymes, especially CYP2C19, and can affect drugs primarily metabolized by that enzyme.[58] Omeprazole decreases the metabolism of diazepam, phenytoin, warfarin, and tolbutamide and may increase the serum concentrations of these drugs. Patients taking these drugs with omeprazole should be monitored for any potential toxic effects. Although lansoprazole has not been shown to interact with drugs that are metabolized by the CYP P450 system, there are reports of slight decreases in the AUC for theophylline; this interaction may not be clinically insignificant.[58] The bioavailability of omeprazole, lansoprazole, and probably the other PPIs may be reduced by sucralfate. Because pantoprazole also is metabolized by a cytosolic sulfotransferase, it appears to interact less with drugs that compete with the P450 enzyme system. This may explain why pantoprazole may have a lower potential for drug interactions.[58] Rabeprazole can modestly increase digoxin serum concentrations; however, no interactions have been observed with phenytoin, warfarin, or theophylline.[5] Esomeprazole may inhibit the P450 enzyme system less than omeprazole.[59]

Sucralfate
MECHANISM OF ACTION

Sucralfate (Carafate) protects ulcerated tissue from aggressive factors such as pepsin, acid, and bile salts.[60] At a pH of 2.0 to 2.5, sucralfate binds to damaged and ulcerated tissue, forming a physical barrier to injury from aggressive forces. The drug is not absorbed systemically and does not possess an antisecretory activity. However, sucralfate may have other protective actions on the mucosa that are possibly mediated by prostaglandin and gastric bicarbonate secretion.

EFFICACY

In doses of 1 g four times a day, sucralfate is more effective than placebo in healing duodenal ulcers[61]; it also appears to be as safe and effective as H_2-receptor antagonists in the treatment of acute duodenal and gastric ulcers.[62] The four-times-a-day dosing regimen for sucralfate is problematic for most patients, but studies indicate that a 2-g twice-daily regimen is as effective as 1 g four times daily in the short-term treatment of active duodenal ulcers.[63] Sucralfate is effective, but not approved by the U.S. Food and Drug Administration (FDA), for acute or maintenance therapy of gastric ulcers. Although sucralfate is generally not used in *H. pylori* eradication regimens, one recent study demonstrated an eradication rate of 75% when used with amoxicillin and clarithromycin.[64]

ADVERSE EFFECTS

Sucralfate is not appreciably absorbed systemically and therefore adverse effects are uncommon. The most common adverse side effect of sucralfate is constipation, possibly due to the aluminum content of the compound. Other side effects include dry mouth, nausea, and rashes. Sucralfate tablets are large, and some patients, particularly the elderly, may have difficulty swallowing them. Because sucralfate is available as both a tablet and a suspension, the liquid formulation can be used when patients encounter swallowing difficulties.

DRUG INTERACTIONS

The bioavailability of digoxin, fluoroquinolone antimicrobials, ketoconazole, levothyroxine, phenytoin, quinidine, tetracycline, theophylline, and warfarin may be reduced when concomitantly administered with sucralfate. The mechanism of the interaction is thought to be caused by binding of the agent with sucralfate in the GI tract. Because sucralfate may reduce the absorption of other drugs, it should be administered separately (e.g., 2 hours after other agents).

Antacids
MECHANISM OF ACTION

Antacid products contain either sodium bicarbonate, aluminum hydroxide, magnesium hydroxide, calcium carbonate, aluminum phosphate, or a combination of these agents.

Antacids relieve epigastric pain and promote healing of peptic ulcers by providing a cytoprotective effect, neutralizing gastric acid, and stimulating restitution of the gastric mucosa.[65] The cytoprotective effect of antacids may be related to the stimulation of prostaglandins involved in gastric mucosal defense.

EFFICACY

In clinical studies, antacids in various dosing regimens promoted the healing of duodenal ulcers in 46% to 88% of patients after 4 weeks of therapy compared with 24% to 45% of patients treated with placebo.[65]

Antacids need to be taken multiple times a day to neutralize gastric acid, and patient adherence to multiple-times-a-day regimens (e.g., 1 and 3 hours after meals and at bedtime) is difficult. As a result, antacids primarily are used to provide relief of ulcer pain and dyspepsia and are taken on an "as-needed" basis as often as the patient requires them. Antacids are thought to work within 5 to 15 minutes; however, the duration of relief is estimated to be only approximately 2 hours.[65] Although antacids are available in both liquid and tablet formulations, the liquid formulation has a more rapid acid-neutralizing action than the tablets. Tablet formulations should be chewed well to maximize their action.[65] Because of the inconvenient dosage regimen, the high incidence of adverse reactions (primarily diarrhea), and lack of coverage by most prescription plans, antacids are best used as a supplement to other PUD treatments for occasional dyspepsia.

ADVERSE EFFECTS

Sodium bicarbonate is a potent, rapidly acting antacid with a short duration of dyspeptic relief.[65] It should not be used for prolonged periods because systemic alkalosis can result from the accumulation of bicarbonate. *Aluminum hydroxide* commonly is combined with magnesium hydroxide or another magnesium salt because, by itself, it has low acid-neutralizing capacity compared with magnesium hydroxide or calcium carbonate. *Magnesium hydroxide* usually produces diarrhea, but when combined with aluminum, it offsets aluminum's constipating effects. Diarrhea usually predominates when large doses of aluminum- or magnesium-containing antacids are used. Small amounts of aluminum and magnesium are absorbed after antacid administration, and aluminum or magnesium levels can accumulate in patients with renal insufficiency. This is not a problem in patients with normal renal function because both are excreted effectively. Magnesium should be avoided in patients with significant renal impairment (creatinine clearance [Cl_{Cr}] <20 mL/min) because accumulation can lead to CNS effects (e.g., sedation, nausea, vomiting). *Calcium carbonate* is a rapidly acting, very effective neutralizer of gastric acidity; however, high dosages of 4 to 8 g/day also have the potential to stimulate gastric acid production and to induce the milk-alkali syndrome (i.e., hypercalcemic nephropathy with alkalosis).[62]

DRUG INTERACTIONS

Antacids, by alteration of gastric pH, can interfere with the absorption of drugs (e.g., digoxin, phenytoin, isoniazid) that require an acidic environment for dissolution and absorption.[65] Ketoconazole, a dibasic compound, requires sufficient gastric acid for dissolution and absorption, and concurrent administration of ketoconazole with antacids can decrease the plasma concentration of this antifungal drug. When antacids increase gastric pH, they also have the potential to dissolve the enteric coating of concurrently administered medications, which are designed to dissolve in an environment more alkaline than the stomach, resulting in premature dissolution of enteric-coated drugs.

By binding to concomitantly administered drugs, the calcium, aluminum, or magnesium component in antacids can interfere with the absorption of drugs that are susceptible to complexation with these salts. The bioavailability of ciprofloxacin is decreased by >50% by antacids because aluminum and magnesium ions chelate with the quinolone antibiotic to form and insoluble, inactive complex potentially leading to treatment failure. The administration of ciprofloxacin 2 hours before the antacid increases ciprofloxacin bioavailability more than when administered 2 hours after the antacid.[66] Tetracycline is another antibiotic well known to interact with antacids. Antacids containing multivalent cations (Mg^{2+}, Ca^{2+}, Al^{3+}) have a strong affinity for tetracycline, and absorption of the antibiotic can vary according to the extent of complexation.[66] Patients taking any form of tetracycline should be counseled not to take antacids for at least 2 to 3 hours after tetracycline administration. Overall, separating the administration times of each drug by 2 hours generally can minimize drug–drug interactions with antacids.

Eradication of H. pylori

We now know that most patients with a duodenal ulcer and many with gastric ulcers are colonized with *H. pylori*.[36,67] Bismuth with acid suppression was initially used in the treatment of *H. pylori*–infected patients with peptic ulcers because it is active against *H. pylori* at a minimum inhibitory concentration of 16 mg/mL,[67–69] and its use was associated with a reduction in ulcer recurrence.[67,68] Patients who remain positive for *H. pylori* have a higher recurrence rate within the first year after healing compared with patients in whom eradication of *H. pylori* is achieved. A variety of regimens have been used to eradicate H. pylori, and most currently accepted regimens use several antibiotics plus acid suppression.

MONOTHERAPY

Although FDA-approved (omeprazole or lansoprazole plus clarithromycin) regimens are available, their eradication rates are in the 70% range. This is currently considered less than acceptable by experts.[67]

COMBINATION THERAPY

Because monotherapy with antibiotics and monotherapy with acid suppressants has not been optimal, combination therapy consisting of antibiotics in conjunction with acid suppressants (PPIs or H_2-receptor antagonists) have become the primary mainstays in the management of *H. pylori*–positive ulcer patients.[71] In two prospective studies, H_2-receptor antagonists were compared with combination antimicrobial therapy to evaluate the differential contributions of decreased acid secretion to *H. pylori* eradication and on the recurrence rate of ulcers.[70,72,73] In these studies, recurrence rates for both gastric and duodenal ulcers after 1 year were significantly lower (approximately 10%) with combination therapy than with ranitidine therapy alone (approximately 85%).[71,74]

A variety of regimens have been used to eradicate *H. pylori,* each with different dosing schedules, durations of therapy, adverse effects, and costs. Several studies have evaluated antibiotic regimens for *H. pylori* eradication. Three were noted to be cost-effective and associated with good outcomes: (1) triple therapy of bismuth, metronidazole, and tetracycline for 14 days; (2) clarithromycin, PPI, and metronidazole or amoxicillin for 7 to 14 days; and (3) triple therapy of bismuth, metronidazole, and tetracycline, plus a PPI for 7 days.[70–75] For patients who cannot receive metronidazole or when resistance to metronidazole is either established or suspected, the regimen of choice is 7 to 14 days of clarithromycin, amoxicillin, and a PPI. Another therapeutic regimen (i.e., bismuth 2 tablets four times a day with meals and at bedtime, metronidazole 500 mg four times a day, and amoxicillin or tetracycline 500 mg four times a day for 14 days) results in an eradication rate of 80% to 85%.[74]

RECOMMENDED COMBINATION REGIMENS

Regardless of the regimen chosen, effective eradication of *H. pylori* requires combination therapy, and the ideal regimen contains two antibiotics combined with either a PPI or bismuth.[67,75] Recommended *H. pylori* eradication regimens can be found in Table 27-5 and are discussed in further detail below.

1. *PPIAC:* The combination of a PPI, *a*moxicillin, and *c*larithromycin is approximately 90% to 95% effective and of moderate to high expense. Patient adherence to this regimen may be good because the regimen uses twice-daily dosing and can be for a 7- to 14-day duration. This regimen (using lansoprazole) is available commercially as Prevpac in a 14-day "bingo card." When using this regimen, the PPI should be taken twice daily *before meals* for 14 days; the amoxicillin 1,000 mg twice daily should be taken *with meals* for 14 days; and the clarithromycin (Bi-

axin) 500 mg twice daily should be taken *with meals* for 14 days. More recently, 10-day PPI regimens with *a*moxicillin and *c*larithromycin have been approved by the FDA. Seven-day regimens are currently not FDA approved and are generally less effective than the 10- to 14-day regimens. All PPIs are equally effective and the choice can be determined based on cost and third-party prescription coverage. H_2-antagonists should *not* be added to regimens that contain a PPI.

2. *PPIMC:* Metronidazole at a dose of 500 mg BID can be substituted for amoxicillin with similar rates of eradication.[71,72]

3. *BMT-H_2:* The combination of *b*ismuth, *m*etronidazole, and *t*etracycline plus an H_2-antagonist may be given generically as separate medications or in a carton with 14 daily blister cards and instructions (Helidac kit). This regimen is relatively inexpensive but is complicated, requiring four drugs administered four times daily for 2 weeks followed by an additional 16 days of H_2-antagonist therapy. The bismuth is given as bismuth subsalicylate 262 mg (Pepto-Bismol) and the tablets (two) are to be chewed four times a day for 14 days with meals and at bedtime. Bismuth given on a four-times-a-day dosing schedule before meals appears to be more effective than twice-daily dosing.[74] The metronidazole is taken as 250 mg four times a day for 14 days with meals and at bedtime. The tetracycline in this regimen is given as 500 mg four times a day for 14 days with meals and at bedtime. The effect of meals in decreasing the absorption of the tetracycline is not of concern because a local, rather than systemic, action is the objective. An H_2-antagonist is needed for 30 days to enhance symptom relief and possibly enhance healing rate. A PPI taken twice daily can be substituted for the H_2-antagonist.

4. *RBC-C:* The combination of *r*anitidine, *b*ismuth *c*itrate, and *c*larithromycin is available commercially as Tritec

Table 27-5 *Helicobacter pylori* Eradication Regimens

Regimen	Agents/Dose/Frequency	Duration (days)	Efficacy (%)	Comment
PPIAC	PPI[a] BID Clarithromycin 500 mg BID Amoxicillin 1,000 mg BID	7, 10, 14	88–95	FDA approved (most PPIs); efficacy improves with increased duration of therapy; relatively simple regimen; available as "bingo card" (Prevpac)
PPIMC	PPI[a] BID Clarithromycin 500 mg BID Metronidazole 500 mg BID	7, 10, 14	88–95	Relatively simple regimen; efficacy improves with increased duration of therapy; caution with alcohol use
BMT-H_2	H_2RA[b] Bismuth two tablets QID Tetracycline Metronidazole	14–28	75–85	Complicated regimen; FDA approved ("bingo card"); efficacy less than PPIAC or PPIMC
RBC-C	Ranitidine Bismuth subcitrate[c] Clarithromycin 500 mg BID Ranitidine 150 mg BID	14	75–80	FDA approved

[a]PPI doses: omeprazole 20 mg BID; lansoprazole 30 mg BID; rabeprazole 20 mg BID; pantoprazole 40 mg BID; esomeprazole 20 mg BID.
[b]H_2RA doses: cimetidine 400 mg BID; ranitidine 150 mg BID; famotidine 20 mg BID; nizatidine 150 mg BID.
[c]Ranitidine administered for 2 weeks after completing bismuth and antibiotics.

(ranitidine 150 mg plus bismuth citrate 240 mg twice a day for 4 weeks combined with clarithromycin 500 mg three times a day for the first 2 weeks). This regimen is less effective (80% to 85% cure rates) and more costly. Moreover, the dosing schedule is complicated, the duration of therapy is longer (i.e., 4 weeks), and the regimen includes only one antibiotic. RBC may be an option in a penicillin allergic patient in whom it is desirable to avoid metronidazole due to ethanol use.

1. **M.B., a 27-year-old female executive, presents with a 1-week history of midepigastric upper abdominal pain, partially relieved both by eating and by calcium carbonate tablets (Tums), which she takes in the morning for calcium supplementation. She describes the pain as being moderately severe and different from gas pains which are associated with a bowel movement. She has not noticed darkening of the stool or the presence of blood in her stools. She has no other medical problems. In particular, she does not recall any chronic abdominal complaints such as gas, bloating, or heartburn and she has not been diagnosed previously with ulcer disease. She takes no other medications and is a nonsmoker. Her use of NSAIDs is limited to 200 to 400 mg of nonprescription ibuprofen tablets (Advil), but she does not take ibuprofen more than three times per week. What is the likelihood this patient has a peptic ulcer?**

Most patients with PUD initially present with nonlocalized epigastric pain as the only symptom, much like this patient. The relief of pain in this patient by both food and calcium carbonate makes one suspicious of a duodenal ulcer, but this in itself is not diagnostic. NSAIDs can increase the risk for the development of ulcer disease and she has been taking ibuprofen. However, her dose of ibuprofen is low, and she has used these drugs in the past without difficulty. Although a diagnosis of ulcer disease in this patient is uncertain based on her current history, she should discontinue the use of ibuprofen for now.

2. **M.B. is counseled to use acetaminophen in place of ibuprofen and is given a prescription for famotidine (Pepcid) 40 mg HS to be taken for 6 weeks. What are reasonable courses of action for the management of this patient, and is famotidine treatment appropriate before a diagnosis of PUD has been established?**

If PUD is suspected, M.B. should be tested (serology or breath test) for *H. pylori* and if positive, receive an *H. pylori* eradication regimen. Endoscopic diagnosis before starting treatment is usually not indicated in cases of PUD for patients who are not suspected of having a complication.

Endoscopy may be indicated if the patient is older than 55, if complications such as bleeding are present or suspected, if weight loss is present, or if epigastric symptoms have recurred after previous conservative treatment. It must be remembered that H. *pylori* testing alone does not diagnose the presence of an ulcer with certainty, because almost 50% of the population is colonized with this organism. A definitive workup (e.g., endoscopy, upper GI series) may be necessary if M.B. does not respond to the initial therapy, or if symptoms recur after initial therapy.

Detection of Helicobacter

3. **What available tests for the detection of *H. pylori* are appropriate for M.B.?**

H. pylori can be identified by direct testing of bacterial colonies from a culture medium or indirectly by biochemical assays and serologic tests. Because the organism is distributed unevenly throughout the gastric mucosa, at least two specimens from the antrum should be obtained.[67,74,75] Histologic identification of *H. pylori* correlates well with culture results, with a sensitivity and specificity of 85% to 100% and 50% to 100%, respectively.[67,74,75] Factors implicated in the failure to culture the organism include ingestion of simethicone, contamination of biopsy forceps with an antibacterial agent, recent treatment with antibiotics or PPIs, and biopsy in areas with low organism counts.[67] The *rapid urease test* can detect the large amounts of urease produced by *H. pylori* within 2 to 3 hours with an endoscopically obtained biopsy specimen.[67] In clinical practice, direct biopsy and culture are reserved for patients in whom other tests are nondiagnostic.

Noninvasive tests for *H. pylori* are preferred when screening for this organism.[67] The noninvasive *breath test* detects urease in the stomach subsequent to the oral administration of ^{13}C- or ^{14}C-labeled urea. If urease is present in the stomach (presumably from *H. pylori*), the carbon dioxide exhaled in the breath will contain the ^{13}C isotope (detected by mass spectrometer) and the ^{14}C isotope (detected by a scintillation counter).[67] The Meretek UBT (urea breath test) appears to be highly specific, but is costly and associated with 5% to 10% false-negative results.[67] Another noninvasive test, the *enzyme-linked immunosorbent assay* (ELISA) detects IgG and IgA antibodies to *H. pylori* in the serum. Sensitivity and specificity of these antibody tests are approximately 95%; however, a positive test can represent either past or present exposure to *H. pylori*. Serologic antibody tests may be helpful for the initial diagnosis of *H. pylori* but are more problematic for documenting eradication of this organism.[67] However, long-term serologic surveillance investigations indicate that IgG and IgA anti–*H. pylori* antibody concentrations decrease rapidly and progressively after the eradication of the infection and increase with recurrence of *H. pylori* infection. As a result, these noninvasive serologic tests are used commonly to determine the presence of *H. pylori* because of their simplicity and relative low costs.[68]

Serology testing is now commonly used because of its simplicity and relative low cost. Breath testing is more sensitive, but cost prohibitive in many situations. Direct biopsy, culture, and the rapid urease tests require endoscopy and are reserved for situations in which endoscopy is warranted. In patients with recurrent or refractory ulcers, further testing should be considered because false-negative results are sometimes encountered.[77,78] In this latter situation, other etiologies of PUD also should be evaluated. Although any of the aforementioned tests are acceptable for M.B., the most rational approach is testing with serology and eradication of *H. pylori* using one of the methods listed above. Treatment without testing for *H. pylori* has been advocated in some patients with a duodenal ulcer due to the high prevalence of *H. pylori* in patients with duodenal ulcers. However, since most duodenal ulcers are diagnosed by endoscopy, it is simple to biopsy the gastric mucosa and test for *H. pylori*.

4. **Should M.B. discontinue using Tums tablets?**

Although there is no logic for taking full-dose scheduled antacids in conjunction with PUD treatment, patients generally are instructed to continue to take antacids on an as-needed basis for breakthrough symptoms, especially for the first few days after starting treatment. In this particular situation, M.B. has been taking the Tums as a calcium supplement for osteoporosis prevention. Although she is still at low risk for osteoporosis because of her young age, there is no need to discontinue the Tums. She should be instructed to take extra doses as needed and to contact her physician or pharmacist if symptoms have not resolved within 2 weeks.

5. **PPIs are superior acid suppressants compared with H_2-antagonists. Would it be better to initiate therapy in this patient with a PPI?**

The PPIs are superior to the H_2-antagonists in acid suppression and provide more rapid symptom relief. Despite this, acute treatment of patients with PUD by either H_2-antagonists or PPIs without *H. pylori* eradication is not indicated. There is probably little, if any, role for PPIs or H_2-antagonists for acute treatment of peptic ulcers except as part of an *H. pylori* regimen. This is due to the rapid recurrence of the ulcer after completing an acute regimen.

6. **J.L., a 37-year-old woman, is in the clinic today for a routine follow-up after treatment for a second episode of suspected peptic ulcer. She relates a 14-year history of multiple GI complaints including postprandial bloating, "fullness," belching, occasional nausea, reflux, and heartburn. There is no predictable pattern to these complaints; they may be present daily for weeks at a time, while at other times they may occur just a few times per week. The heartburn and reflux may occur in the absence of the bloating, belching, fullness, and nausea and vice versa. She has taken a variety of antacids over the years including Maalox, Mylanta, generic equivalents of both, Gaviscon, and Tums, all of which give partial or complete, but temporary, relief.**

Four years ago, J.L. had one episode of increased mid-upper epigastric pain that lasted for several days. The discomfort was relieved by food and was present during the night. Bowel movements had no discernible effect on the pain. Her physician informed her that she probably had an ulcer and prescribed a 10-week regimen of cimetidine 400 mg twice a day. The abdominal pain abated, but since then she has continued to take either cimetidine or nonprescription H_2-antagonists as needed almost daily for her chronic symptoms.

Six weeks ago, a similar abdominal pain developed and she was treated empirically with clarithromycin 500 mg three times daily for 2 weeks and omeprazole 20 mg twice a day for the first 2 weeks and then 20 mg of omeprazole daily for an additional 2 weeks. Once again, the acute pain subsided, but her underlying complaints remain. She states that she was compliant most of the time, but sometimes had difficulty remembering all three doses of the clarithromycin each day. However, she continued to take them until they were all gone. She lost track of how long it took for all of the medicine to be gone.

The only other medication she has taken in the past year is an oral contraceptive, Triphasil (ethinylestradiol/levonorgestrel), which she has been taking for many years. She takes acetaminophen for headaches and avoids NSAIDs. She also relates multiple episodes of bladder/urethral and vaginal infections over the past 16 years, treated variously with trimethoprim-sulfamethoxazole, clotrimazole, and metronidazole. The last time she had any of these infections was 5 years ago.

She has no other medical problems despite a 15-year history of cigarette smoking. She has never undergone endoscopy. *H. py-* *lori* **testing was never performed before any of her treatments, but an *H. pylori* serology taken 5 days ago is positive. No other laboratory test results are available.**

Based on the data provided, is this patient's history consistent with PUD? If endoscopy were to be performed today, is it likely that an active ulcer would be found?

In the absence of endoscopy, it is impossible to know if this patient has ever had an ulcer. However, the following scenario could be hypothesized. For 14 years, she either experienced nonulcer dyspepsia, GERD, and/or PUD. The postprandial bloating, fullness, and nausea are all consistent with nonulcer dyspepsia. The reflux and heartburn could be either true GERD or a variant of nonulcer dyspepsia. In addition, PUD can also present with these symptoms. Thus, the acute change of symptoms 4 years ago, with the resolution after a course of H_2-antagonists, is consistent with an acute ulcer followed by healing. However, her symptoms continued. Six weeks ago, it appeared as though she once again developed a peptic ulcer. This is not surprising considering her failure to receive *H. pylori* eradication treatments. During this second presumed ulcer episode, her primary care provider decided to try *H. pylori* eradication with a combination of a single antibiotic and a PPI. Once again the acute symptoms resolved. Thus, one might conclude that this patient does indeed have a history of PUD, but endoscopy is needed for further diagnosis.

7. **Does the presence of a positive *H. pylori* serology 5 days ago indicate treatment failure of the antibiotic–PPI regimen?**

One should not conclude that the positive *H. pylori* serology in this patient indicates treatment failure. It should be recalled that *H. pylori* serology is the simplest and least expensive way to test for *H. pylori* infection. However, this test is limited because it only indicates the presence of antibodies to *H. pylori,* not the actual organism itself. Thus, it remains positive both in persons with an active infection and in those after successful eradication of the organism. Serology testing is most useful as a screening tool in an individual who has never received antibiotics that are active against H. pylori. In that situation, a positive test presumably is a marker of an active infection, although false-positive results may still occur. Although some data indicate that antibody titer levels decline after successful eradication, this is a less sensitive measurement tool than an enzymatic breath test that indirectly indicates the presence of living organisms, or results from a rapid urease test of endoscopically derived tissue. Furthermore, none of the confirmatory test procedures should be done within 4 to 6 weeks of the last dose of a PPI because these drugs suppress *H. pylori* growth without actually killing the organisms. In this patient, we have no prior antibody titers for comparison. The only conclusion that can be drawn from her positive serology is that she has been infected with *H. pylori* at some time in her life. She may or may not be infected now. If she had tested negative for *H. pylori* antibodies, the clinician would have suspected either a false-negative result from her recent omeprazole treatment, an ulcer not associated with *H. pylori* (which is relatively uncommon), or the absence of PUD entirely.

8. **Because of the lack of specificity of the *H. pylori* serology test, a carbon isotope urea breath test is ordered. This test indicates a continued infection. What factors may have contributed to the lack of eradication of *H. pylori* in this patient?**

Although the failure of medications to eradicate the *H. pylori* in this patient can be attributed to several variables, the issue of J.L.'s adherence to her prescribed regimen should be considered. However, she has stated that she did complete the regimen despite having missed some doses. One other explanation could perhaps be focused on a poor choice of antibiotic regimen (i.e., only one antibiotic with a PPI).

9. **Should patient J.L. be re-treated at this time? If so, what antibiotic regimen would presumably be the most appropriate?**

Although J.L. no longer has acute epigastric pain right now, she is at high risk for a recurrence of peptic ulcers if she still is infected with *H. pylori*. The most successful regimens for eradication of *H. pylori* contain either a PPI or a bismuth-containing compound (generally bismuth subsalicylate in the United States) plus two of the following antibiotics as described above. It is known that this patient had difficulty complying with her previous regimen, which was relatively simple. Thus, she may not do well with the BMT regimen of bismuth (Pepto-Bismol), metronidazole, and tetracycline, which requires a total of 16 tablets and capsules four times daily for 14 days plus an H_2-antagonist or PPI for 2 to 4 weeks. In reality, the risk of resistance may be remote because it has been several years since she took the metronidazole. Using the Helidac kit, in which the medications are supplied in a carton with 14 daily blister cards and instructions for use, could enhance compliance. A better regimen might be a PPI plus amoxicillin (or metronidazole) and clarithromycin for 10–14 days. The shorter course may enhance compliance. The most important principle is to develop a regimen with a high likelihood of success. Although cost of the medications is often foremost in the minds of third-party payers, this should not be a primary consideration because successful treatment will save much more in future costs than re-treatment, physician's visits, and hospitalization for complications. The most expensive regimen is the one that the patient does not take or that does not work.

10. **What is the likelihood that the urea breath test could have been reported back as a false-negative result? How would a negative test result alter the treatment plan for this patient?**

The single antibiotic regimen, which was chosen for this patient, is not optimal. The combination of A PPI plus amoxicillin will result in bacteriologic cure in 40% to 50% of cases. If the *H. pylori* in this patient has been eradicated, no further antibiotic treatment is necessary. A false-negative urea breath test is also possible, especially if the patient is tested too soon after the initial treatment. Nevertheless, further workup (e.g., retesting or endoscopy) is not required unless symptoms recur. As many as 40% of patients who have had successful *H. pylori* eradication will continue to require acid suppression medications to control persistent dyspeptic symptoms. Thus, clinicians should remember that bacteriologic cure might not provide complete relief of epigastric symptoms because patients also may have concurrent nonulcer dyspepsia or GERD. In this particular case, it should be recalled that this patient still has symptoms and that these may be suggestive of nonulcer dyspepsia or GERD. Dietary adjustments, simethicone, and/or H_2-antagonists may or may not help provide symptom relief for J.L.'s nonulcer dyspepsia. If GERD is suspected, endoscopy may be necessary to rule out esophagitis. If endoscopy is undertaken and if the endoscopic sample is positive for *H. pylori,* treatment is indicated because of the association between *H. pylori* infection and gastric cancer. The treatment options for GERD are presented in later cases.

Drug-Induced Peptic Ulcer Disease

Etiology and Clinical Presentation

11. **A.C., a 65-year-old woman, experienced orthostasis and diarrhea after attending a lecture. She has been in good health without any previous complaints. She has not been taking any medications other than ibuprofen 400 mg Q 4 to 6 hr PRN for headaches and arthritic knees for the past 4 weeks. Laboratory tests are unremarkable except for a hemoglobin (Hgb) of 8 g/dL, a hematocrit (Hct) of 26%, and a guaiac-positive stool. A.C. was admitted to the hospital for an endoscopy to rule out bleeding from the GI tract. Endoscopy revealed two antral ulcers (0.2 cm and 0.4 cm). What is the cause of A.C.'s GI bleeding?**

[SI units: Hgb, 4.96 mmol/L; Hct, 0.26]

A.C.'s GI bleeding probably is most likely secondary to chronic ingestion of ibuprofen, which is an NSAID. The prevalence of endoscopically confirmed GI ulcers in NSAID users is 15% to 30%.[80] Although most NSAID-induced ulcers are gastric ulcers (12% to 30%), duodenal ulcers (2% to 19%) are observed as well.[81,82] Some investigators hypothesize that duodenal ulcers associated with NSAID use may represent an exacerbation, reactivation, or complication of PUD, because there is a higher incidence of duodenal ulcers unrelated to NSAID use.[80]

12. **Why did A.C. not experience epigastric pain symptoms associated with NSAID-induced ulcers?**

Symptomatic ulcers (ulcers associated with pain, bleeding, or perforation) occur in only approximately 1% of patients after 3 to 6 months of NSAID use and in 2% to 4% of patients after 1 year of therapy.[69] NSAID-associated ulcers do not correlate well with pain possibly because the analgesic action of NSAIDs may mask the ulcer pain.[80] As illustrated by A.C., patients often take NSAIDs for chronic pain conditions such as arthritis; therefore, their perception of pain may be changed and they may tend to ignore modest epigastric pain. The reason is not clear, but NSAID ulcers in many patients are asymptomatic. Thus, complications (e.g., GI bleeding, syncope) may develop in the absence of typical symptoms. It is not unusual to find perforations, bleeding, or gastroduodenal ulcerations in asymptomatic individuals.[69] The orthostasis experienced by A.C. probably is merely reflective of volume loss secondary to GI bleeding, and epigastric pain simply was not present or was masked.

Mechanism of Action

13. **How do NSAIDs cause ulcers?**

The most common site for NSAID-associated ulcers is the antral portion of the stomach, although some occur in the gastric body and fundus.[69] NSAIDs appear to produce gastric damage by two mechanisms: a direct irritant effect and a systemic effect mediated by cyclo-oxygenase (COX) inhibition leading to a reduction in prostaglandin synthesis.[76,81,82] Therefore, both rectal and IV administration of NSAIDs can cause

GI damage despite the apparent absence of direct mucosal contact.[81] Agents that are more water soluble (e.g., aspirin) cause more topical injury.[82] Aspirin, in a dose-related fashion, disrupts the gastric mucosal barrier. When the consumption of aspirin exceeds 22 tablets a week, the occurrence of ulcers is increased.[76] Although enteric-coated tablets are designed to minimize gastric irritation, the potential for ulceration still exists but to a lesser degree.[80] Inhibition of mucosal prostaglandin synthesis is thought to be an important factor in the pathogenesis of aspirin- and NSAID-induced ulcers.[80,83] COX-1 is responsible for producing prostaglandins that protect the GI mucosa by maintaining blood flow and stimulating bicarbonate and mucus production.[76] Therefore, low levels of prostaglandin would be expected to impair the ability of the gastric mucosa to defend itself against aggressive factors. An isoform of COX-1, COX-2, is involved in the inflammatory response. Both isoforms have the same affinity to convert arachidonic acid to prostaglandin; however, the prostaglandins produced by COX-2 are associated with pain and inflammation. COX-2 inhibition is believed to be responsible for the anti-inflammatory and analgesic effects of NSAIDs, whereas inhibition of COX-1 may be associated with NSAID adverse effects including GI and renal effects.[80,83] Therefore, NSAIDs such as celecoxib (Celebrex), rofecoxib (Vioxx), and valdecoxib, which have the greatest inhibitory effects on COX-2 while maintaining minimal or no inhibition on COX-1, will have the maximum effect on inflammation and minimal (but not totally eliminated) mucosal-damaging adverse effects.[69]

Treatment

14. What therapeutic steps should be taken in the treatment of A.C.'s gastric ulcer?

When peptic ulcers develop in patients taking NSAIDs, the preferred approach is to stop the NSAID when possible. Ulcers heal slowly during treatment with H_2-antagonists when NSAIDs are continued and more quickly when they are stopped.[69]

Therefore, A.C. should discontinue or decrease the dose of the ibuprofen and she should be evaluated for *H. pylori* infection. For mild to moderate pain, acetaminophen or another analgesic option can be used. If an anti-inflammatory action is required for her arthritic knee, a COX-2 NSAID can be used.[69]

Variables that may influence the healing of NSAID-associated ulcers include continued NSAID therapy, ulcer site, ulcer size, history of PUD, and the presence of *H. pylori* gastritis.[69,84-88] Discontinuation of the NSAID may allow for mucosal restitution and more rapid ulcer healing. The continued use of NSAIDs does not appear to prevent healing of small ulcers; however, the healing process may be delayed. H_2-antagonists are generally not effective in preventing or healing NSAID-associated gastric ulcers when the NSAID is continued. An exception is famotidine given at a dose of 40 mg twice daily.[69,87] Double doses of other H_2-antagonists have not been studied.

Another option is to test for and treat for *H. pylori* (if positive). If *H. pylori* testing is negative, a PPI may provide a more rapid resolution of symptoms and quicker healing of the ulcer. If the COX-2 is not an effective alternative for A.C. and if she must continue with her NSAID for management of her arthritis, a PPI would be preferred over an H_2-antagonist. The H_2-antagonists are not very effective for healing or preventing NSAID-associated gastric ulcers during continued therapy with NSAIDs.[69]

15. A.C.'s ulcer has healed after 8 weeks of omeprazole 20 mg/day and the discontinuation of her NSAID. However, her arthritic knees continue to be a problem, and NSAID therapy needs to be reinstated. What concurrent medications should A.C. receive to minimize future ulcer formation?

Prophylactic therapy or a COX-2 NSAID should be considered for patients who are unable to discontinue NSAID therapy and who have risk factors for NSAID-associated ulcers. Patients particularly at risk include those who are taking concurrent anticoagulants or corticosteroids; those with a history of ulcer complications or ulcer disease; those who are elderly; and high-surgical risk, debilitated patients who cannot tolerate complications.[69] If a COX-2 NSAID is chosen, the clinician must remember that these agents do not provide complete freedom from ulceration and other GI-associated complications of NSAIDs.

H_2-RECEPTOR ANTAGONISTS

A few studies have examined prophylactic regimens for NSAID-associated ulcers. The H_2-receptor antagonist, ranitidine, has been associated with a decrease in the incidence of NSAID/aspirin-associated duodenal ulceration, but this association was not apparent in patients with gastric ulcers.[69,81,86] Double dose famotidine (40 mg twice daily) in another study was noted to have reduced the incidence of both gastric and duodenal ulcers compared with placebo in patients receiving long-term NSAID therapy.[87] In this study, famotidine at either 20 mg or 40 mg twice a day was more effective in preventing duodenal than gastric ulcers. Some investigators postulate that NSAID-associated duodenal ulcers represent an exacerbation of pre-existing duodenal ulcer disease.[69,87] The H_2-antagonists seem to be more effective in the prevention of NSAID-induced duodenal ulcer disease than in the prevention of NSAID-induced gastric ulcers.

Misoprostol (Cytotec), a synthetic prostaglandin E_1 analog, has both antisecretory and cytoprotective properties and can prevent both duodenal and gastric ulcers in the NSAID/aspirin user.[88-90] Despite the effectiveness of misoprostol in the prevention of duodenal and gastric NSAID-associated ulcers, it paradoxically causes GI symptoms such as diarrhea and abdominal pain.[69] Diarrhea is dose dependent and is due to stimulation of intestinal smooth muscle and fluid and electrolyte secretion. Lowering the dose to 100 μg four times a day or giving the dose less frequently (i.e., 200 μg twice daily) decreases the incidence of diarrhea, but this dose also is less effective in preventing ulcers.[69,89] Misoprostol is contraindicated in women of child-bearing age unless adequate contraceptive measures are taken, because prostaglandins are uterotonic and capable of increasing the frequency of uterine contractions, bleeding, and abortions.[90]

PROTON PUMP INHIBITORS

In one study, the efficacy of omeprazole was compared with misoprostol in 935 patients who required continuous NSAID therapy and who had gastric and/or duodenal ulcers.

At 8 weeks, treatment was successful in 76% of the patients given omeprazole 20 mg daily, in 75% of those given omeprazole 40 mg daily, and in 71% of those given misoprostol 200 μg four times a day.[91] The rates of gastric ulcer healing were significantly higher with omeprazole 20 mg daily (87%) than with misoprostol (73%). Healing rates among patients with duodenal ulcers were higher (85%) with omeprazole 20 mg daily than with misoprostol (74%), whereas healing rates among patients with erosions alone were higher with misoprostol (84% versus 77%). More patients remained in remission during maintenance treatment with omeprazole (61%) than with misoprostol (48%) and with either drug than with placebo. More adverse events were noted during the healing phase in the misoprostol group than in the groups given omeprazole.[91] The success of ranitidine, misoprostol, and omeprazole in preventing NSAID-associated duodenal ulcers suggests that acid suppression is important in the prevention of duodenal ulcers. A.C. is a candidate for prophylactic therapy because she is elderly, requires continued NSAID therapy, and has an ulcer history. The PPIs appear to be more effective in the healing of gastric ulcers than misoprostol and more effective than the H2-antagonists in healing and preventing ulcers.[69] Therefore, it would be reasonable for A.C. to receive omeprazole 20 mg daily to minimize the risk of ulcer recurrence that is associated with NSAIDs. A COX-2 NSAID may also be an option.

ZOLLINGER-ELLISON SYNDROME

Pathogenesis

ZE syndrome is a rare (occurring in fewer than 1 in 10,000 patients with DU) condition characterized by a triad of clinical findings, which include severe recurrent PUD, significant hypersecretion of gastric acid, and non–β-islet tumors (gastrinomas) of the pancreas.[92] Normally, G-cells in the antral mucosa secrete gastrin, which stimulates the parietal cells to secrete gastric acid. In ZE syndrome, an ectopic source (gastrinoma) also secretes gastrin with a subsequent hyperstimulation of gastric acid secretion.[92] Although gastrinomas are located primarily in the pancreas, they also have been found in other regions, particularly the duodenum.

Clinical Presentation

16. M.J., a 62-year-old man, was referred from his private physician for evaluation of his continuing ulcers. He has been treated for 2 to 3 years for PUD and has not experienced relief despite *H. pylori* suppression and escalating doses of various H2-receptor antagonists. M.J. was evaluated twice to rule out a possible myocardial infarction because of severe chest pain. He also complains of frequent diarrhea and abdominal pain. All routine laboratory tests were found to be within normal limits except a serum gastrin level, which was 5,243 pg/mL (normal, 0 to 100 pg/mL). Radiographic and endoscopic studies demonstrate a distal esophageal ulceration, dilation of the duodenum and jejunum with thickened folds, and a 0.1-cm ulceration in the distal duodenum. After a secretin test, his serum gastrin level was 400 pg/mL greater than the basal level. M.J. was diagnosed with ZE syndrome. Why is M.J.'s presentation consistent with ZE syndrome?

[SI unit: gastrin, 5,243 ng/L]

Diagnosis

The diagnosis of ZE syndrome is based on gastric acid hypersecretion (basal acid output >15 mmol/hr in a patient without prior gastric surgery or >5 mmol/hr in a patient with prior acid-reducing surgery) in conjunction with a fasting serum gastrin level >1,000 pg/mL.[93,94] Some healthy individuals and patients with duodenal ulcers may have marginally increased serum concentrations of gastrin.[93] Therefore, a provocative test is often used to identify patients with ZE syndrome. The secretin provocative test is the most sensitive, reliable, and simplest test for diagnosing and predicting the probability of a patient to remain disease free.[93] If a patient has ZE syndrome, IV secretin will cause a significant increase in serum gastrin.[93] A positive test, consistent with the diagnosis of gastrinoma, is defined as an absolute increase in serum gastrin of >200 pg/mL from the basal concentration.[94] M.J.'s baseline and stimulated serum gastric levels are well above normal.

Symptoms of ZE syndrome are similar to severe PUD but may be more persistent and less responsive to standard antiulcer therapy.[93–95] This is consistent with M.J.'s 2- to 3-year history of unrelenting pain despite *H. pylori* eradication and high doses of H2-receptor antagonists. Many patients have no endoscopically or radiographically detectable GI ulcers at the time of diagnosis (18% to 25%), whereas others present with solitary or multiple ulcers (as in M.J.'s case).[95] Most patients with ZE syndrome have an ulcer, usually in the duodenum or jejunum. Because the disease often presents as a routine peptic ulcer, the diagnosis of ZE syndrome may be delayed for a prolonged time.[95] M.J.'s history is consistent with this description because he was evaluated in the past for complaints resembling a severe peptic ulcer, but ZE syndrome was not considered until radiographic evidence was present.

Abdominal pain and diarrhea (both present in M.J.) are the most common symptoms at presentation and may occur in the absence of a mucosal ulcer.[95] Diarrhea occurs in approximately 30% to 50% of patients and is caused by increased amounts of gastric acid. High gastric acid levels inhibit sodium and water absorption in the jejunum and damage the GI mucosa. Abdominal pain remains the most common symptom of ZE syndrome and is localized or diffuse in nature. The pain is similar to that found in a duodenal ulcer in that food and antacids often relieve it.

Treatment

17. A PPI has been prescribed for M.J. Why would PPIs be more likely to be successful in the management of ZE compared with H2-antagonists?

Because of the excessive amounts of gastric acid produced by patients with ZE syndrome, patients have an increased chance of severe GI discomfort, bleeding, and gastroduodenal perforation. Before the routine use of acid secretory suppressant medications (H2RAs and PPIs), total gastrectomy was the treatment of choice. Now, most patients can be effectively treated using PPIs. Despite this, some patients will require a surgical excision of the gastrinoma to control symptoms associated with excessive gastric acid production that persist despite large doses of PPIs.[95] Most patients will be adequately managed with medical treatment which usually provides symptomatic pain relief and control of gastric acid secretion.

An acceptable criterion for long-term control of gastric secretion is a postdrug gastric acid secretion of <10 mEq/hr for the last hour before the next dose of medication.[95] Successful medical management requires individualized titration of the drug dose with periodic reassessment.

Histamine$_2$-antagonists were the first drugs successfully used to control gastric hypersecretion, but they are not totally effective in the medical management of ZE syndrome. Large doses and more frequent dosing than typically used to treat PUD are generally required (see Table 27-2).[95] This is due to the very high doses needed are usually inadequate to control the high gastric acid secretion.[79] It is likely that total acid suppression can never be achieved by H$_2$-antagonists alone because these drugs do not directly suppress either gastrin or acetylcholine. As a result, PPIs have become the treatment of choice for ZE.

PPIs have an advantage over H$_2$-antagonists because by selectively and irreversibly binding to H$^+$-K$^+$-ATPase, they can inhibit nearly all gastric acid production irrespective of the cause. In addition, PPIs have a long duration of action and thus require less frequent dosing than the H$_2$-antagonists. All PPIs are effective for ZE syndrome, large doses generally are necessary, and doses should be adjusted as needed.[77]

Although surgical correction of the gastrinoma is likely, M.J. should begin at least 60 mg/day of omeprazole and titrated to response. Patients frequently are seriously ill when the initial diagnosis of ZE syndrome is confirmed, and it is important that the high gastric acid secretion be controlled.[95] The total daily dose should be given in two to three divided doses initially.[78,95] Octreotide, is a potent inhibitor of gastrin and an option in the management of ZE; however, because it is only available as a parenteral product, its use is limited.[78]

Proton Pump Inhibitor Administration

18. M.J. is scheduled for surgery, and omeprazole is to be administered through an nasogastric (NG) tube. What difficulties are likely to be encountered by this order, and what are reasonable solutions?

In patients with NG tubes who are unable to take medications by mouth, drugs are often placed either directly into the NG tube or crushed and mixed with water to make a slurry/suspension. Omeprazole, lansoprazole, and esomeprazole are formulated as enteric-coated granules within gelatin capsules because they are unstable in acid media and must be absorbed to become converted to their active metabolites. Analogous to sustained-release products, the enteric-coated beads should not be chewed or crushed because they are designed to dissolve in the GI tract when the pH of the medium is >6.[95] However, when the capsules are opened, added to a bicarbonate solution, and the enteric-coated beads are not crushed, the AUC and the effectiveness of gastric acid suppression of enteric-coated omeprazole granules delivered via an NG tube can be comparable to that of encapsulated enteric-coated granules taken orally.[98] Esomeprazole has been studied by opening the capsule and suspending in water.[99] Suspensions of omeprazole and lansoprazole compounded from capsules and sodium bicarbonate solution are stable for up to 14 days at 24°C.[100,101]

When the lansoprazole gelatin capsule is opened, the intact granules can be mixed in 40 mL of apple juice and administered in a suspension of granules via the NG tube according to the manufacturer's instructions. While FDA approved, this method is difficult to administer properly, as the granules sink to the bottom of the syringe used to inject into the NG tube. This apple juice and lansoprazole granule suspension must be agitated in the syringe as it is injected into the NG tube. Failure to do this, will administer a "bolus" of granules into the NG tube and will likely clog the tube. Crushing pantoprazole tablets and preparing a suspension in sodium bicarbonate has also been studied and found to produce blood levels similar to intact tablet administration.[102]

Continuous IV H$_2$-receptor antagonists can be used to control gastric acid hypersecretion adequately in patients with ZE syndrome during surgery.[103] Frequent dosage adjustments are required may be required in the perioperative period to control gastric acid output. IV omeprazole has been available in Europe for many years. As PPIs also are more effective in controlling gastric hypersecretion, IV pantoprazole may be the most effective option for M.J. Other IV formulations of PPIs are being developed

GASTROESOPHAGEAL REFLUX DISEASE

Gastroesophageal reflux is a disorder in which reflux of gastric or intestinal contents occurs into the esophagus and results in patient complaints of heartburn and/or other symptoms (e.g., as a sensation of "burping up" stomach contents or as the taste of bitter contents in the mouth). The classic symptom of reflux is "heartburn," which commonly is described as a pain in the center of the chest that, at times, might mimic cardiac angina. An estimated 44% of adults in the United States experience heartburn at least once per month and 7% of people have daily GERD symptoms. Acid reflux is also associated with asthma and when this occurs, is called "atypical GERD." These symptoms, when accompanied by dysphagia (swallowing difficulty or a sensation of food sticking in the throat), odynophagia (severe pain on swallowing), or persistent nocturnal symptoms, usually are sufficient to make the patient aware of the need for medical attention. GERD symptoms are not necessarily associated with inflammation and tissue damage to the esophagus (esophagitis). An endoscopic examination is necessary to diagnose esophagitis. Esophagitis commonly is graded using the Savary-Miller system. This system grades esophagitis from grade 1 (mild) to grade 4 (severe, erosive changes). Although it is possible for esophagitis to be present in the absence of symptoms (and vice versa), it is important to understand that symptoms are poorly correlated with the grade of esophagitis.[104–107] Complications associated with the reflux of gastric material into the esophagus include strictures, hemorrhage, perforation, aspiration, and the development of Barrett's esophagus (see following discussion).

Infants (up to 18 months of age) can experience a form of GERD that is characterized by postmeal regurgitation or small volume vomiting, which can occur several times per day due to a poorly functioning sphincter. Esophagitis is usually absent in these children, but a small percentage may develop chronic GERD. This form of GERD may respond very well to liquid formulations of gastric motility–stimulating agents. True motility dysfunction resulting in slowed or absent esophageal food transit times are uncommon in adults with GERD.

Pathogenesis

The esophagus functions to transport food from the mouth to the stomach and to prevent the retrograde flow (i.e., "back-flow") of GI contents. As food enters the esophagus, the LES opens and remains open until the peristaltic contractions of esophageal muscles have swept the food into the stomach. Contraction of the lower esophageal sphincter after the passage of food into the stomach serves to prevent the reflux of gastric contents back into the esophagus.

The development of GERD is associated with a disruption of the balance between defensive mechanisms (e.g., LES closure, esophageal peristalsis) and aggressive factors (e.g., acid, pepsin, bile salts).[108] Three pathophysiologic mechanisms predispose a patient to reflux: (1) a spontaneous transient or sustained relaxation of the lower esophageal sphincter, (2) a low resting LES pressure, and (3) increased gastric pressure (e.g., bending over, pregnancy, obesity).[109] All these pathophysiologic mechanisms can occur in normal healthy individuals, but additional variables may contribute to the development of esophageal damage. For example, the amount of acid and pepsin that refluxes within a 24-hour period, the length of time that acid and pepsin remain in the esophagus, and the natural sensitivity of the esophageal mucosa to damage by aggressive forces all determine the susceptibility of an individual to GERD.[104]

Clinical Presentation

19. R.L., a 37-year-old, 100-kg, 68-inch tall man, has been experiencing heartburn for approximately 4 to 6 weeks. The pain usually occurs after dinner while he is lying on the couch watching television and often is accompanied by regurgitation of a warm, foul-tasting fluid into his mouth. He also has experienced these symptoms, after his night-time snack of chocolate ice cream, soon after he goes to bed. He smokes 1 to 2 packs/day of cigarettes and drinks 2 beers every evening while watching television. His symptoms are relieved by Mylanta, which he drinks directly from the bottle. What symptoms does R.L. have that are consistent with GERD?

Retrosternal burning, commonly referred to as *heartburn,* is the characteristic symptom of GERD and is caused by the contact of refluxed GI material with an inflamed esophageal mucosa.[104] The epigastric pain can be angina-like and is described as a burning, substernal pain that travels up the esophagus toward the throat.[104] In some patients, especially the elderly, no heartburn or chest pain is experienced and coughing or wheezing may be the only symptoms noted. However, the absence of symptoms does not necessarily imply the absence of esophageal damage. Symptoms of GERD often are episodic because GI contents are not refluxed continuously.[104] The frequency of heartburn symptoms and the presence of esophagitis are correlated with the duration and intensity of acid exposure (often defined in terms of percentage of time per 24 hours that the pH is <4.0).

Symptoms of GERD may be aggravated by certain foods, specific body positioning, or drugs. Foods with high-fat content (e.g., ice cream) can lead to GERD symptoms because these foods decrease the LES pressure. Other food products such as spices, onions, citric juices, and coffee can contribute to the development of GERD by direct mucosal irritation.[109]

Although symptoms of esophageal reflux can occur in any body position at any time, many patients experience symptoms primarily when they are supine or when bending over. The swallowing of saliva, water, or antacids (e.g., the Mylanta ingested by R.L.) frequently relieves the pain. R.L.'s symptoms of heartburn, the regurgitation of gastric contents soon after eating, and the association of these symptoms when he lies on the couch after dinner and when he goes to bed at night are all consistent with GERD. R.L.'s ingestion of two beers after dinner and of chocolate ice cream before bedtime and the apparent temporal relationship of these activities to the appearance of epigastric pain also are consistent with GERD. Concurrent drug therapy (e.g., alcohol, α-adrenergic agonists, β-adrenergic agonists, verapamil, diazepam, dopamine, meperidine, progesterone, prostaglandins, theophylline) also can exacerbate GERD.[110]

Treatment

Goals

20. What are the therapeutic goals for the treatment of R.L.'s GERD?

The therapeutic goals for GERD are: alleviate pain and symptoms, diminish the frequency and duration of esophageal reflux, promote healing of esophagitis (if present), avoid complications, prevent recurrence, and provide cost-effective therapy.[110,111] One concern of uninvestigated GERD is *Barrett's esophagus* (histologic change whereby the lower esophageal tissue begins to resemble the columnar epithelium similar to the lining of the stomach). Barrett's esophagus predisposes the patient to the development of esophageal cancer: the more frequent, more severe, and longer-lasting the symptoms of reflux, the greater the risk. Persons with long-standing (>20 years' duration) and severe symptoms of reflux (reflux-symptom score of >4.5) were 43.5 times more likely (95% confidence interval) for development of esophageal adenocarcinoma.[110]

Lifestyle Changes

21. What nondrug measures can improve R.L.'s symptoms?

Initially, all patients should change their lifestyle to eliminate factors that can exacerbate reflux.[110,112] Weight loss and loose-fitting clothes are recommended because obesity and tight clothes may exacerbate reflux by continuously increasing the gastroesophageal pressure gradient.[112] Cigarette smoking directly provokes acid reflux and decreases lower esophageal sphincter pressure; efforts should be initiated to discontinue cigarette smoking.[113] Foods that lower esophageal sphincter pressure (e.g., chocolate, alcohol, peppermint, fatty meals), irritate the gastric mucosa (e.g., spicy food, citric juices), or stimulate acid secretion (e.g., cola, beer) should be avoided. Most experts believe lifestyle modifications provide improved symptoms control in only approximately 20% of patients.[104,110] These measures are widely promoted in the lay press and on web sites that discuss GERD. It is likely that many patients have already tried lifestyle modification before seeking medical help, thus many clinicians fail to find significant improvements in symptoms when they ask patients to use these measures. Despite these doubts about effectiveness, all recommended lifestyle measures should be used by patients with GERD. Lifestyle modification as a sole treatment has never been demonstrated to heal esophagitis and should not be used as the sole treatment in these patients.[104]

R.L. should be instructed to lose weight, cease smoking, avoid lying on the couch in a position that increases gastric pressure, and avoid foods (chocolate ice cream, beer) that precipitate symptoms or decrease the LES pressure. He also should avoid meals 2 hours before lying down. R.L.'s symptoms appear to be the most troublesome while lying on the couch when he is watching television and at night. For patients like R.L., elevating the head of the bed with 6- to 8-inch blocks or sitting in an upright position might be helpful in enhancing the gravitational flow of gastric contents away from the esophagus.[112,113]

Drug Therapy

Because patients with GERD have frequent reflux episodes of acid, effective inhibition of gastric acid secretion is necessary to facilitate healing and relieve symptoms.[102,110,116] Antisecretory drugs, such as H_2-receptor antagonists and PPIs, are generally used and the choice of drug is based on the severity of the disease.[104,110]

ANTACIDS

Antacids can provide relief of mild symptoms associated with GERD. Antacids have short durations of action and do not promote healing of esophagitis.[104,110] Consequently, antacids are used primarily as adjunctive agents to provide daytime symptomatic relief of GERD.

H_2-ANTAGONISTS

H_2-antagonists can be effective for management of mild GERD when used in full-sized doses. Healing rates with H_2-antagonists for patients with mild esophagitis are significantly better than placebo.[111,117] The severity of the disease, the dose of the drug, and the duration of therapy affect the response to H_2-antagonists. For example, endoscopic healing was observed in 65% of patients with moderate esophagitis (grade II), in contrast to only 15% of patients with severe esophagitis (grade III) after 8 weeks of ranitidine therapy.[96,110]

Gastric acid suppression throughout the day is important in the treatment of reflux disease. As a result, H_2-antagonists administered in daily divided doses provide superior symptom relief and healing than does once-daily dosing.[110] Duration of H_2-antagonist treatment is another major determinant of esophagitis healing rates.[116] In one multicenter trial, 57% of patients with esophagitis were healed after 6 weeks of therapy, and 70% healed after 12 weeks of therapy. In another study, 45% of patients taking nizatidine experienced esophagitis healing after 6 weeks of therapy and 80% were healed after 12 weeks.[118] In both studies, symptom relief occurred earlier than esophagitis healing, confirming the poor correlation between symptom relief and presence of esophagitis. In addition, it is clear that esophagitis in some patients does not heal in response to H_2-antagonists. Some investigators attribute this lack of response to H_2-antagonist drug tolerance.[110]

PROTON PUMP INHIBITORS

PPIs such as omeprazole (Prilosec), lansoprazole (Prevacid), rabeprazole (Aciphex), pantoprazole (Protonix), or es-

omeprazole (Nexium), which can inhibit gastric acid secretion for a sustained period, are highly effective in the treatment of GERD. Normal, once-daily doses of PPIs for 4 weeks will heal approximately 85% to 90% of patients with the mild esophagitis and approximately 60% to 80% of patients with severe esophagitis (grade IV).[104,110,111] Higher doses (usually twice the "normal" dose sometimes given in divided doses twice daily) are sometimes required to heal esophagitis in patients with more severe erosive disease.

In clinical trials, PPIs heal esophagitis quicker and more effectively than H_2-antagonists. In one randomized, blinded, controlled study, healing occurred in 67% of patients after 4 weeks of omeprazole (20 mg daily) compared with 31% of patients with ranitidine (150 mg twice a day).[119] After 8 weeks, the healing rates increased further to 85% and 50% with omeprazole and ranitidine therapy, respectively. The higher healing rate for omeprazole also was accompanied by a more rapid improvement of symptoms. Omeprazole was notably more effective than ranitidine in patients with severe esophagitis.[119]

PPIs are also effective in healing esophagitis refractory to H_2-antagonists. After 12 weeks of therapy, 80% of patients with severe esophagitis experienced healing with 20 to 40 mg/day of omeprazole despite previous failures to prolonged therapy with H_2-receptor antagonists.[119,120] In another multicenter, randomized, blinded study, lansoprazole (30 mg/day) was more effective in healing erosive esophagitis in patients who were resistant to standard doses of H_2-receptor antagonists than continuation of ranitidine (150 mg twice a day).[121] The healing rate for lansoprazole was 89% at 8 weeks compared with 38% for ranitidine ($P < 0.001$). In comparative trials, PPIs have been shown to heal all grades of esophagitis in at least 65% to 90% of patients in 4 to 8 weeks.

When one compares esophagitis healing, PPIs are generally equally effective in healing mild to moderate reflux esophagitis. In one multicenter trial that evaluated healing of erosive esophagitis, lansoprazole 30mg daily and omeprazole 20 mg had similar healing rates at 8 weeks. Patients taking lansoprazole (30 mg/day) had significantly better pain relief (by 11%) than the omeprazole group in the first week.[122] Similar results have been seen with rabeprazole and esomeprazole (40mg/day) when compared with omeprazole (20 mg/day).

SUCRALFATE

Sucralfate (Carafate) appears to be effective in resolving mild cases of esophagitis but is less effective in management of severe disease.[117,123] As a result, sucralfate is not as widely used as the acid suppressants to manage GERD.

METOCLOPRAMIDE

Metoclopramide (Reglan) stimulates the motility of the upper GI tract without affecting gastric acid secretion. When administered as 10 mg, four times a day, 30 to 60 minutes before meals and at bedtime, it increases gastric peristalsis, which leads to accelerated gastric emptying.[5] Duodenal peristalsis is increased and intestinal transit time is decreased in patients with GERD.[124] Metoclopramide also increases the LES resting tone within 1 to 3 minutes following IV administration and in 30 to 60 minutes after oral administration.[116] Metoclopramide's adverse effect profile (e.g., drowsiness, diarrhea, abdominal cramps, extrapyramidal reactions) and the general lack of GI motility dysfunction in adult patients with GERD significantly limit the usefulness of this medication for the treatment of GERD. Cisapride (Propulsid) is no longer commercially available. The manufacturer (Janssen) has a special investigational limited access program for cisapride distribution which is primarily intended for patients with diabetic gastroparesis. Tegaserod, a 5-HT$_4$ receptor agonist, improves LES tone and will reduce the esophageal exposure to gastric acid when compared to placebo, but its effective use in GERD has not yet been demonstrated.[125]

22. R.L. has lost approximately 5 kg of body weight over the past 6 weeks and has discontinued drinking two beers each night and eating all spicy foods. However, he continues to smoke cigarettes despite efforts at cessation. His symptoms of reflux have continued despite his regular use of nonprescription cimetidine tablets, which were purchased at his local pharmacy. What drug therapy is appropriate for the treatment of his GERD at this time?

The traditional treatment of GERD has been based on the premise of incremental increases in the intensity of treatment options (i.e., begin first with lifestyle management and nonprescription doses of an H$_2$-antagonist, which can be replaced, if needed, by nonprescription omeprazole or prescription strength H$_2$-antagonists, and ultimately by increasing doses of a PPI in lieu of the H$_2$-antagonist). Even though R.L. has modified his lifestyle, with the exception of cigarette cessation, his condition has not responded to nonprescription cimetidine. In addition he lost weight. He should be referred for endoscopy to determine if he has an esophageal stricture or esophageal adenocarcinoma which can obstruct his esophagus resulting in dysphagia and weight loss.

If esophagitis is seen on endoscopy, he will likely be placed on a PPI. This is because PPIs are more effective than standard and high (double)-dose H$_2$-antagonists in symptom relief, healing, and maintenance of remission of esophagitis. The superiority of PPIs presumably are related to the inability of even high-dose H$_2$-antagonists to control acid secretion and possibly also due to the development of tolerance to H$_2$-antagonists. The PPIs provide quicker relief of symptoms than H$_2$-antagonists and, as a result, are possibly more of an incentive for patients to adhere to therapy.[126]

Maintenance Therapy

23. Esophagitis was noted in R.L.'s endoscopy, and he was prescribed omeprazole 20 mg twice daily. Eight weeks later, a repeat endoscopy revealed the esophagitis had healed, and the omeprazole was stopped. Since that time, he has begun to re-experience some mild symptoms occasionally. Is maintenance therapy recommended for R.L.'s occasional symptoms?

Unfortunately, even after complete healing, a large percentage of patients experience a recurrence of symptoms within 6 to 12 months after therapy is discontinued.[5,110,116,122,123,127] Therefore, maintenance therapy is often required. One recent study demonstrated that continuous maintenance treatment with a daily PPI is the most effective treatment strategy. This study compared the recurrence rates of reflux esophagitis over a 12-month period with either omeprazole 20 mg/day, omeprazole 20 mg three times a week, or ranitidine 150 mg twice daily. At 12 months, endoscopy showed sustained remission of disease in 89% of patients receiving omeprazole

daily, in 32% receiving omeprazole three times a week, and in 25% receiving ranitidine.[128] Trials using other PPIs have found similar results. Maintenance therapy with a PPI should be initiated in R.L. after further medical workup because the risk of morbidity can be high and GERD often is a chronic condition.[126]

STRESS-RELATED MUCOSAL BLEEDING

Acute stress-related mucosal lesions (SRML) are distinctly different from chronic PUD.[129] They occur in critically ill patients, are usually unrelated to a previous history of ulcer disease, and are seen within 24 to 48 hours of admission to hospital.[130] Multiple superficial ulcerative lesions can develop in the proximal stomach along the boundaries of the acid-secreting mucosa and the duodenum.[129,130] Approximately 50% of these lesions bleed, but because they are superficial, significant bleeding will occur in only 5% to 20% of untreated patients in intensive care units.[114] Patients in whom GI bleeding develops have a higher mortality rate than those critically ill patients who do not have GI bleeding.[130] During the early 1970s, stress ulcers and their complications had reached near epidemic proportions.[114] However, the occurrence of stress ulcer bleeding has decreased to <2% of the intensive care patient population due to widespread use of agents that prophylactically neutralize gastric acids and advanced medical care.[131]

Pathogenesis

Stress ulcers primarily occur because impaired protective mechanisms cause an imbalance between aggressive and defensive forces resulting in mucosal damage. Although hydrogen ions are necessary for the development of stress ulcers, large quantities of acid secretion are not necessary.[114] In fact, critically ill patients usually secrete normal amounts of gastric acid.[130] For example, trauma patients secrete normal or decreased amounts, whereas hypersecretion is found in patients with sepsis, CNS injuries, or small bowel resections.[131,132] Despite the critical role of gastric acid and other aggressive factors in the pathogenesis of stress ulceration, mucosal defenses also are important and these are often compromised in the critically ill patient. Gastric mucosal blood flow is diminished in patients with hemorrhagic, cardiogenic, and septic shock,[114] resulting in a number of unfavorable events: (1) decreased nutrient and oxygen delivery, (2) inability of the mucosa to remove or neutralize gastric acids, and (3) a decrease in bicarbonate efflux into the gastric epithelium.[130] During stressful situations, there also is a decreased rate of proliferation and cellular turnover of the gastric mucosa.[114] Furthermore, in many critically ill patients, diffusion of bile salts backward from the duodenum into the stomach and high concentrations of urea in the blood (e.g., renal failure) can disrupt the gastric barrier and contribute to stress injury. The lack of prostaglandin and mucous formation in the critically ill also may contribute to the development of stress-related damage.

Risk Factors

24. M.L., a 64-year-old woman who was admitted with diverticular disease, is transferred to the intensive care unit (ICU) because of her deteriorating respiratory condition and septic shock. She has no significant past medical history and was a healthy individual. She is in respiratory distress with a respiratory rate of 36 breaths/min, temperature of 104°F, heart rate of 120 beats/min, and a blood pressure (BP) of 60/40 mm Hg. Relevant laboratory tests include the following: sodium (Na), 147 mEq/L; potassium (K), 5.6 mEq/L; chloride (Cl), 119 mEq/L; bicarbonate, 12 mEq/L; blood urea nitrogen (BUN), 57 mg/dL; serum creatinine (SrCr), 2.7 mg/dL; and white blood cell (WBC) count, 36,000 cells/mm³. Her respiratory status deteriorates to a point that endotracheal intubation is necessary. In addition to empiric antibiotics and fluids, treatment for stress ulcers is being contemplated. M.L has no history of PUD. What are the risk factors for stress ulcers that are present in M.L?

[SI units: Na, 147 mmol/L; K, 5.6 mmol/L; Cl, 119 mmol/L; bicarbonate, 12 mmol/L; BUN, 20.3 mmol/L; WBC count, 36,000 ×10⁶ cells/L]

Numerous risk factors have been identified for stress ulcers and these include shock, burns (>30% of the body), multiple organ failure, trauma (intra-abdominal or thoracoabdominal injuries), sepsis (intraperitoneal or pulmonary infections), coagulopathy, and CNS injury. However, in a prospective multicenter study that evaluated potential risk factors for stress ulceration in 2,252 critically ill medical ICU patients, the only independent risk factors for GI bleeding were respiratory failure and coagulopathy. They concluded that prophylaxis against stress ulcers may be required only in critically ill patients who have a coagulopathy or require mechanical ventilation for >48 hours.[114] In another study, respiratory failure (mechanical ventilatory support >24 hours) and high-dose corticosteroid administration (>250 mg/day of hydrocortisone) was associated with an increased risk of stress ulcer bleeding.[131]

M.L. currently is in septic shock and will require mechanical ventilation; therefore, she should receive stress ulcer prophylaxis.

Treatment

25. What can be done to prevent the complications associated with SRML in patients like M.L.?

Despite the low occurrence of serious bleeding in critically ill patients, when it occurs, the accompanying mortality is very high. Aggressive prophylactic therapy may prevent significant complications and reduce both morbidity and mortality rates. Because alteration in defense mechanisms predisposes a patient to stress ulceration and bleeding, the most important approach is to treat the underlying disease state and physiologic conditions. The keystones are early fluid resuscitation, immediate oxygenation, early hemodynamic stabilization, prevention of infections, and effective analgesia and sedation.[114] For example, improving blood flow by correcting shock should be a priority in the management of M.L.[114,131] Other important measures are maintaining adequate nutrition and respiratory support. Some studies suggest that enteral nutrition may aid in the prevention of GI bleeding.[132] Acid-base imbalances and uremia should be corrected because of their propensity for injury to the gastric mucosa. M.L. has evidence of both a metabolic acidosis (HCO₃, 12 mEq/L) and renal insufficiency (SrCr, 2.7 mg/dL).

Adequate neutralization of gastric acid is of paramount importance because stress-associated ulceration does not occur

in the absence of acid, and if the intragastric pH is maintained between 3.5 and 4, the frequency of bleeding is lowered in stressed patients. At a pH of 4.5, pepsin is inactivated, whereas 99.9% of acid is neutralized at a pH of 5. In vitro observations demonstrate that when the gastric pH is <5 to 7, coagulation function and platelet aggregation are impaired.[130] Therefore, therapy should be directed at maintaining the gastric pH between 3.5 and 4 to prevent SRML.

26. What pharmacologic therapy can be used to prevent SRML in M.L.?

Aggressive *antacid* therapy (e.g., Mylanta 30 to 60 mL every hour) very effectively maintains the gastric pH above 3.5.[131] Numerous studies have compared H₂-antagonists with antacids for prevention of stress-related bleeding. Most have found pH control to be superior with antacids (when antacids are given hourly), but the rate of significant bleeding was not found to be different between these two treatment regimens.[133] Although antacids are effective in preventing stress ulcers, they are inconvenient to administer and are associated with accumulation of magnesium, aluminum, or calcium. Diarrhea can also occur.

H₂-Antagonists
H₂-antagonists effectively prevent stress ulcers. In an analysis of data from 16 prospective, randomized trials, cimetidine was as effective as antacids in preventing significant stress ulcer bleeding.[133] Another prospective, randomized trial compared the efficacy of several H₂-receptor antagonists (cimetidine, famotidine, and ranitidine) and antacids in the prevention of stress ulceration.[133] In a double blinded trial comparing cimetidine constant infusion (50 to 100 mg/hr) with placebo designed to prevent GI bleeding from SRML in critically ill patients, the cimetidine group had significantly fewer bleeding episodes.[134]

Proton Pump Inhibitors (PPIs)
PPIs are potent acid suppressant drugs, and in contrast to H₂-receptor antagonists, PPIs inhibit both histamine and vagally induced gastric acid secretion. Because of this, these agents should be expected to be useful in the management of stress ulcer patients. Data regarding use of PPIs to prevent bleeding associated with SRML is summarized below.

27. M.L. is to be started on ranitidine. How should it be administered?

Because the goal is to maintain the gastric pH >4.0 for the prevention of SRML and >7.0 for the treatment of bleeding ulcers, the proper administration of these agents is critical (see Table 27-6 for recommended dosing). Intermittent bolus injection has been used; however, this method of administration is labor intensive, and a continuous IV infusion of the H₂-receptor antagonists is more effective in maintaining the gastric pH above 4.[135–137] Dosages should be adjusted according to the severity of the patient's illness, renal function, and the intragastric pH. The intragastric pH can be determined with an indwelling probe or by measuring the pH of an NG aspirate. Signs of bleeding (e.g., significant bleeding out the nasogastric tube, low blood pressure, dropping Hct and Hgb) also should be assessed constantly.

Table 27-6   Stress-Related Mucosal Bleeding Prevention: Regimens and Doses

Agent	Dose and Frequency of Administration	FDA Approved
Antacid	30 mL PO/NG Q 1–2 hr	No
Cimetidine	300 mg IV Q 6–8 hr	No
	300 mg IV loading dose then 50 mg/hr continuous IV infusion	Yes
Famotidine	20 mg IV Q 12 hr	No
	1.7 mg/hr continuous IV infusion	No
Ranitidine	50 mg IV Q 6–8 hr	No
	6.25 mg/hr continuos IV infusion	No
Sucralfate	1 g PO/NG Q 4–6 hr	No
Omeprazole	20–40 mg PO/NG[b] Q 24 hr	No
Lansoprazole	30–60 mg PO/NG[b] Q 24 hr	No
Pantoprazole	40 mg IV Q 12–24 hr	No

[a]For prevention of SRMB.
[b]By suspension in bicarbonate.
IV, intravenous; NG, by nasogastric tube; PO, by mouth.

Sucralfate

28. Is there any role for sucralfate in treating M.L.?

In the critically ill patient receiving stress ulcer prophylaxis with acid-suppressing medications or neutralizing agents, growth of Gram-negative bacteria is common.[115] Because an elevated gastric pH promotes proliferation of bacteria in the stomach, aspiration of these organisms may be important in the pathogenesis of nosocomial pneumonia. Sucralfate does not alter gastric pH significantly but has generally been found to be effective in preventing SRML associated bleeding.[138,139] Several investigators have evaluated the association between SRML prophylaxis nosocomial pneumonia in the critically ill patient.[115,138,139] Most studies have failed to demonstrate a significant difference in development of nosocomial pneumonia between sucralfate and H₂-antagonists.[115,138,139] A more recent study found that in critically ill patients requiring mechanical ventilation there was no significant difference in the occurrence of pneumonia, and ranitidine was more effective than sucralfate in reducing the rate of GI bleeding.[140]

Sucralfate is available as a suspension and administration through M.L.'s NG tube would be simple; however, M.L. has decreased renal function and sucralfate can cause aluminum toxicity in renally impaired patients. Therefore, sucralfate may not be a good therapeutic option for M.L. A continuous IV infusion of an H₂-antagonist may be appropriate in this situation. The dose of the H₂-receptor should be adjusted according to M.L.'s calculated creatinine clearance (i.e., Cl_{Cr} <10 mL/ min, use 0.8 mg/hr famotidine).

29. Is there a role for PPIs in the prevention of SRML for M.L.?

PPIs administered by NG tube have been shown to provide sufficient acid suppression to prevent SRML.[98–102] In one study comparing an omeprazole suspension (in bicarbonate) administered in the NG tube with ranitidine, the NG omeprazole group had fewer GI significant bleeding episodes.[135] These authors had a very broad definition of GI bleeding (Hgb drop of 2), and the GI bleeding episodes noted may have been from non-GI sources; thus, many believe the difference noted may not be reproducible in actual practice. It is likely that NG PPIs are effective, but superiority over other regimens needs to be confirmed in further studies.

Intravenous PPIs have been used in numerous studies, but blinded, randomized trials in SRML prophylaxis have not yet been published. Thus, comparative efficacy with other options is not yet possible. Intravenous omeprazole and pantoprazole are available in Canada and most of Europe, but only pantoprazole is available for intravenous use in the US. Several trials are currently ongoing comparing IV PPIs with H₂-antagonists, but results are not available yet. It is likely they are effective at preventing SRML associated GI bleeding, but further work is necessary to determine comparative efficacy of any PPIs with the other available options.

REFERENCES

1. Corazziari E. New Rome criteria for functional gastrointestinal disorders. Dig Liver Dis 2000; 32(Suppl 3):S233.
2. Hsu P et al. Eradication of Helicobacter pylori prevents ulcer development in patients with ulcer-like functional dyspepsia. Aliment Pharmacol Ther 2001;15:195.
3. Johnsen R et al. Prevalence of endoscopic and histologic findings in subjects with and without depression. Br Med J 1991;302:749.
4. Rosenstock S et al. Risk factors for peptic ulcer disease: a population based cohort study comparing 2416 Danish adults. Gut 2003;52:186.
5. Dent J on Behalf of the Genval Workshop group. An evidenced based appraisal of reflux diagnosis and management. The Genval Workshop Report. Gut 1999;44(Suppl 2):S1.
6. Lagergren J et al. Symptomatic gastroesophageal reflux as a risk factor for esophageal adenocarcinoma. N Engl J Med 1999;340:825.
7. Barbara L et al. Definition and investigation of dyspepsia: consensus of an international ad hoc working party. Dig Dis Sci 1989;34:1272.

8. Delaney BC et al. Initial management strategies for dyspepsia. Cochrane Database Syst Rev 2003: DC001961.
9. Duggan AE et al. Does initial management of patients with dyspepsia alter symptom response and satisfaction? Gastroenterology 1999;(S4): G0654.
10. Heaney A et al. A prospective randomised trial of a "test and treat" policy versus endoscopy-based management in young H. pylori positive patients with ulcer-like dyspepsia. Gut 1999;45:186.
11. Lassen AT et al. H. pylori "test and treat" or prompt endoscopy for dyspeptic patients in primary care. A randomized controlled trial of two management strategies. Gastroenterology 1998;114:G0853.
12. Mason I et al. The management of acid-related dyspepsia in general practice: a comparison of omeprazole versus an antacid alginate/ranitidine management strategy. Aliment Pharmacol Ther 1998;12:263.
13. Meinche-Schmidt V, Krag E. Antisecretory therapy in 1017 patients with ulcer-like dyspepsia in general practice. Eur J Gen Pract 1997;3:125.
14. Jones RH, Baxter G. Lansoprazole 30 mg daily versus ranitidine 150 mg b.d. in the treatment of acid-related dyspepsia in general practice. Aliment Pharmacol Ther 1997;11:541.
15. McColl K et al. Symptomatic benefit from eradicating H. pylori infection in patients with nonulcer dyspepsia. N Engl J Med 1998;339:1869.
16. Blum AL et al. Lack of effect of treating Helicobacter pylori infection in patients with nonulcer dyspepsia. N Engl J Med 1998;339:1875.
17. Watanabe Y et al. Epidemiological study of PUD among Japanese and Koreans in Japan. J Clin Gastroenterol 1992;15:68.
18. Sonnenberg A. Temporal trends and geographical variation of peptic ulcer. Aliment Pharmacol Ther 1995;9(Suppl 2):3.
19. Katz J. The course of peptic ulcer disease. Med Clin North Am 1991;75(4):831.
20. Rosenstock S et al. Risk factors for peptic ulcer disease: a population based prospective cohort study comprising 2416 Danish adults. Gut 2003;52:186.
21. Katz J. Acid secretion and suppression. Med Clin North Am 1991;75(4):877.
22. Wallace JL. Mucosal defense—new avenues for treatment of ulcer disease? Gastroenterol Clin North Am 1990;19(1):87.
23. Schiessel R et al. Mechanisms of stress ulceration and implications for treatment. Gastroenterol Clin North Am 1990;19(1):101.
24. Shiotani A, Graham DY. Pathogenesis of gastric and duodenal ulcer. Med Clin North Am 2002;86:1447.
25. Graham DY. Treatment of peptic ulcers caused by Helicobacter pylori. N Engl J Med 1993;328:349.
26. Marshall B. Unidentified curved bacillum in gastric epithelium in active chronic gastritis. Lancet 1983;1:1237.
27. Marwick C. Helicobacter: new name, new hypothesis involving type of gastric cancer. JAMA 1990; 254:2724.
28. Drumm B et al. Intrafamilial clustering of Helicobacter pylori infection. N Engl J Med 1990; 322:359.
29. Ateshkadi A et al. Helicobacter pylori and peptic ulcer disease. Clin Pharm 1993;12:34.
30. Valle J et al. Disappearance of gastritis after eradication of Helicobacter pylori: a morphometric study. Scand J Gastroenterol 1991;26:1057.
31. Dunn BE. Pathogenic mechanisms of Helicobacter pylori. Gastroenterol Clin North Am 1993; 22(1):43.
32. Mc Gowan CC et al. Helicobacter pylori and gastric acid: biological and therapeutic implications. Gastroenterol 1996;110:926.
33. Kuipers EJ et al. The prevalence of H. pylori in peptic ulcer disease. Aliment Pharmacol Ther 1995;9(Suppl 2):59.
34. Reinbach DH et al. Acute perforated duodenal ulcer is not associated with Helicobacter pylori infection. Gut 1993;34:1344.
35. Graham DY. NSAIDs, Helicobacter pylori, and Pandora's Box. N Engl J Med 2002;347:2162.
36. National Institutes of Health (NIH) Consensus Development Panel on Helicobacter pylori in peptic ulcer disease. JAMA 1994;272:65.
37. Feldman M, Burton ME. Histamine-receptor antagonists standard therapy for acid-peptic disease. N Engl J Med 1990;323(24):1672.
38. Hurwitz A, Carter CA. The pharmacology of antiulcer drugs. Ann Pharmacother 1989;23:S10.
39. Lin JH. Pharmacokinetic and pharmacodynamic properties of histamine H2-receptor antagonist. Clin Pharmacokinet 1991;20(3):218.
40. Sax MJ. Clinically important adverse effects and drug interactions with H2-receptor antagonists: an update. Pharmacotherapy 1987;7(6 Pt. 2):110S.
41. Humphries TJ, Merritt GJ. Drug interactions with agents used to treat acid related disorders [Review]. Aliment Pharmacol Ther 1999;13(Suppl 3):18.
42. Nazario M. The hepatic and renal mechanisms of drug interactions with cimetidine. Drug Intell Clin Pharm 1986;20:342.
43. Kosoglou T, Vlasses PH. Drug interactions involving renal transport mechanisms: an overview. Ann Pharmacother 1989;23:116.
44. Christian C et al. Cimetidine inhibits renal procainamide clearance. Clin Pharm Ther 1984; 36:221.
45. Caballeria J et al. Effects of cimetidine on gastric alcohol dehydrogenase activity and blood ethanol levels. Gastroenterology 1989;96:388.
46. Raufman JP et al. Histamine2-receptor antagonists do not alter serum ethanol levels in fed, nonalcoholic men. Ann Intern Med 1993;118:488.
47. Howden CW, Hunt RH. The relationship between suppression of acidity and gastric ulcer healing rates. Aliment Pharmacol Ther 1990;4:25.
48. Jones R, Bytzer P. Acid suppression in the management of gastro oesophageal reflux disease: an appraisal of treatment options in primary care [Review]. Aliment Pharmacol Ther 2001;15:765.
49. Massoomi F et al. Omeprazole: a comprehensive review. Pharmacother 1993;13(1):46.
50. Langtry HD, Wilde MI. Lansoprazole: an update of its pharmacological properties and clinical efficacy in the management of acid-related disorders. Drugs 1997;3:473.
51. Lanza F et al. Double-blind comparison of lansoprazole, ranitidine and placebo in the treatment of acute duodenal ulcer. Am J Gastroenterol 1994;89:1191.
52. Ramakrishnan A, Katz PO. Overview of therapy for gastroesophageal reflux disease. Gastrointest Clin North Am 2003;13:57.
53. Richardson P et al. Proton pump inhibitors: pharmacology and rationale for use in gastrointestinal disorders. Drugs 1998;56(3):307.
54. Pactoflickovic D et al. Acid inhibition in the first day of dosing: a comparison of four PPIs. Aliment Pharmacol Ther 2003;17:1507.
55. Hatelbakk JG. Review article: gastric acidity—comparison of esomeprazole with other proton pump inhibitors. Aliment Pharmacol Ther 2003;17(Suppl1):10.
56. Maton PN. Omeprazole. N Engl J Med 1991; 324:965.
57. Naesdal J et al. Pharmacokinetics of 14C omeprazole in patients with impaired renal function. Clin Pharmacol Ther 1986;40:344.
58. Geeson LB, Triadafilopoulos F. Proton pump inhibitors and therapeutic drug interactions: an evidenced based approach. Eur J Gastro Hepatol 2001;13:611.
59. Johnson TJ, Hedge DD. Esomeprazole, a clinical review. Am J Health Syst Pharm 2002;59:1333.
60. Shorrock CJ, Rees WDW. Effect of sucralfate on human gastric bicarbonate secretion and local prostaglandin E2 metabolism. Am J Med 1989;86(Suppl 6A):2.
61. Martin F. Sucralfate suspension 1 g four times per day in the short-term treatment of active duodenal ulcer. Am J Med 1989;86(Suppl 6A):104.
62. Van Ness MM. Antacids. In: Van Ness MM, ed. Handbook of Gastrointestinal Drug Therapy. Boston: Little, Brown Co., 1989:7.
63. Schubert T. Twice-daily sucralfate dosing to heal acute duodenal ulcer. Am J Med 1989;86(Suppl 6A):108.
64. Vecu A et al. Amoxicillin, clarithromycin, and either sucralfate or pantoprazole for eradication of H pylori in duodenal ulcer. Wein Clin Wachlen 2001;113:935.
65. Walt RP, Langman MJS. Antacids and ulcer healing—a review of the evidence. Drugs 1991; 42(2):205.
66. Nix DE et al. Effects of aluminum and magnesium antacids and ranitidine on the absorption of ciprofloxacin. Clin Pharmacol Ther 1989;46:700.
67. Howden CW, Hunt RH. Guidelines for the management of Helicobacter pylori infection: Ad Hoc Committee on Practice Parameters of the American College of Gastroenterology. Am J Gastroenterol 1998;93:2330.
68. Barthel JS, Everett ED. Diagnosis of Campylobacter pylori infections: the "gold standard" and the alternatives. Rev Infect Dis 1990;12(Suppl 1):S107.
69. Rostom A et al. Prevention of NSAID induced gastroduodenal ulceration (Cochrane Review). Cochrane Database Syst Rev 2002;(4):C0002296.
70. Labenz J et al. Amoxicillin plus omeprazole versus triple therapy for eradication of Helicobacter pylori in duodenal ulcer disease: a prospective, randomized, and controlled study. Gut 1993;34:1167.
71. Taylor JL. Pharmacoeconomic comparison of treatments for the eradication of Helicobacter pylori. Arch Intern Med 1997;157:87.
72. Graham DY et al. Effect of treatment of Helicobacter pylori infection on the long-term recurrence of gastric or duodenal ulcer: a randomized, controlled study. Ann Intern Med 1992;116:705.
73. Hentschel E et al. Effect of ranitidine and amoxicillin plus metronidazole on the eradication of Helicobacter pylori and the recurrence of duodenal ulcer. N Engl J Med 1993;328:308.
74. Marshall BJ. Treatment strategies for Helicobacter pylori infection. Gastroenterol Clin North Am 1993;22:183
75. NIH Consensus Development Panel on Helicobacter pylori in Peptic Ulcer Disease. Helicobacter pylori in peptic ulcer disease. JAMA 1994;272:65.
76. Okam A et al. Relationship between anti-inflammatory drug use and Helicobacter pylori infection in bleeding or uncomplicated ulcers. J Gastroenterol Hepatol 2003;18:18.
77. Maton PN et al. Long-term efficacy and safety of omeprazole in patients with Zollinger-Ellison syndrome: a prospective study. Gastroenterology 1989;97:827.
78. Jensen RT, Fraker DL. Zollinger-Ellison syndrome. JAMA 1994;271:1429.
79. Jensen RT. Basis for failure of cimetidine in patients with Zollinger-Ellison syndrome. Dig Dis Sci 1998;29:363.
80. Mellem H et al. Symptoms in patients with peptic ulcer and hematemesis and/or melena related to the use of non-steroid anti-inflammatory drugs. Scand J Gastroenterol 1985;20:1246.
81. Graham DY et al. Prevention of NSAID-induced gastric ulcer with misoprostol multicentre, double-blind, placebo-controlled trial. Lancet 1988;2: 1277.
82. McCarthy DM. Nonsteroidal anti-inflammatory drug-induced ulcers: management by traditional therapies. Gastroenterology 1989;196:662.
83. Kolts B, Achem S. Gastrointestinal side effects of nonsteroidal anti-inflammatory drug use. Hosp Formul 1992;27:36.
84. Neville D et al. A comparison of omeprazole with ranitidine for ulcers associated with nonsteroidal antiinflammatory agents. N Engl J Med 1998; 338:719.
85. Ehsanullah RSB et al. Prevention of gastroduodenal damage induced by non-steroidal anti-inflammatory drugs: controlled trial of ranitidine. Br Med J 1988;297:1017.
86. Robinson MG et al. Effect of ranitidine gastroduodenal mucosal damage induced by nonsteroidal anti-inflammatory drugs. Dig Dis Sci 1989;14:424.

87. Taha AS et al. Famotidine for the prevention of gastric and duodenal ulcers caused by nonsteroidal anti-inflammatory drugs. N Engl J Med 1996;334: 1435.

88. Agrawal M et al. Misoprostol compared with sucralfate in the prevention of nonsteroidal anti-inflammatory drug-induced gastric ulcer. Ann Intern Med 1991;115:195.

89. Graham DY et al. Duodenal and gastric ulcer prevention with misoprostol in arthritis patients taking NSAIDs. Ann Intern Med 1993;119:257.

90. Raskin JB et al. Efficacy and safety of misoprostol in the prevention of NSAID-induced gastric ulcers—preliminary findings. Gastroenterology 1993;104:A177.

91. Hawkey CJ et al. Omeprazole compared with misoprostol for ulcers associated with nonsteroidal anti-inflammatory drugs. N Engl J Med. 1998;338:727.

92. Hirschowitz BI. Zollinger-Ellison syndrome: pathogenesis, diagnosis, and management. Am J Gastroenterol 1997;92(Suppl 4):44S.

93. Jensen RT. Zollinger-Ellison syndrome: current concepts and management. Ann Intern Med 1983;98:59.

94. Wolfe MM, Jensen RT. Zollinger-Ellison syndrome. N Engl J Med 1987;317:1200.

95. Roy PK et al. Gastric Secretion in Zollinger-Ellison Syndrome: correlation with clinical expression, tumor extent and role in diagnosis. A prospective NIH study of 235 patients and a review of 984 cases in the literature. Medicine 2001;80:189.

96. Johnson NJ et al. Acute treatment of reflux oesophagitis: a multicenter trial to compare 150 mg ranitidine BD with 300 mg ranitidine QDS. Ailment Pharmacol Ther 1989;3:259.

97. Bonfils S et al. Prolonged treatment of Zollinger-Ellison syndrome by long-acting somatostatin. Lancet 1986;1:554.

98. Larson C et al. Bioavailability and efficacy of omeprazole given orally and by nasogastric tube. Digest Dis Sci 1996;41:475.

99. Sostek MB et al. Esomeprazole: nasogastric tube administration of the contents of an opened capsule suspended in water compared with oral administration in healthy volunteers [Abstract]. Pharmacotherapy 2002;22:1339.

100. Quercia RA et al. Stability of omeprazole in an extemporaneously prepared oral liquid. Am J Health-Syst Pharm 1997;54:1833.

101. McAndrews KL, Eastham JH. Omeprazole and lansoprazole suspensions for nasogastric administration. Am J Health-Syst Pharm 1999;56:81.

102. Ley LM et al. Bioavailability of crushed pantoprazole tablet after buffering with sodium hydrogen carbonate or magaldrate relative to the intact enteric coated pantoprazole tablet. Meth Find Exp Clin Pharmacol 2001;23:41.

103. Saeed ZA et al. Parenteral antisecretory drug therapy in patients with Zollinger-Ellison syndrome. Gastroenterology 1989;96:1393.

104. DeVault K, Castell D, for the Practice Parameters Committee of the American College of Gastroenterology. Guidelines for the diagnosis and treatment of GERD. Am J Gastroenterol 1999;94:1434.

105. Fennerty M et al. The diagnosis and treatment of gastroesophageal reflux disease in a managed care environment. Arch Intern Med 1996;156:477.

106. Lambert R. Current practice and future perspectives in the management of gastro-oesophageal reflux disease [Review]. Aliment Pharmacol Ther 1997;11:651.

107. Faubion W, Zein N. Gastroesophageal reflux in infants and children. Mayo Clin Proc 1998;73:166.

108. Richter JE, Casterll DO. Gastroesophageal reflux. Ann Intern Med 1982;97:93.

109. Gelfand MD. Gastroesophageal reflux disease. Med Clin North Am 1991;75:923.

110. Deut J, on Behalf of the Genval Workshop Group. An evidenced based appraisal of reflux disease management: the Genval Workshop Report. Gut 1999;44(Suppl 2):S1.

111. Kozarek RA. Complications of reflux esophagitis and their medical management. Gastroenterol Clin North Am 1990;19:713.

112. Meining A, Classen M. The role of diet and lifestyle measures in the pathogenesis of gastroesophageal reflux disease. Am J Gastroenterol 2000;95:2692.

113. Kahrilas PJ, Gupta RR. Mechanisms of acid reflux associated with cigarette smoking. Gut 1990;31:4.

114. Cook DJ et al. Risk factors for gastrointestinals bleeding in critically-ill patients. N Engl J Med 1994;330:377.

115. Driks MR et al. Nosocomial pneumonia in intubated patients given sucralfate as compared with antacids or histamine type 2 blockers. N Engl J Med 1987;317:1367.

116. Sontag S. The medical management of reflux esophagitis. Gastroenterol Clin North Am 1990;19:683.

117. Hatlebakk IG, Berstad A. Pharmacokinetic optimisation in the treatment of gastro-oesophageal reflux disease. Clin Pharmacokinet 1996;31:386.

118. Quik RF et al. A comparison of two doses of nizatidine versus placebo in the treatment of reflux oe sophagitis. Aliment Pharmacol Ther 1990;4:201.

119. Klinkenberg-Knol EC et al. Double-blind multicentre comparison of omeprazole and ranitidine in the treatment of reflux oesophagitis. Lancet 1987;1:349.

120. Sontag S et al. Omeprazole for esophagitis and ulcer refractory to H₂-blockers. Gastroenterology 1989;94:A436.

121. Feldman M et al. Treatment of reflux esophagitis resistant to H₂-receptor antagonists with lansoprazole, a new H/K-ATPase inhibitor: a controlled, double-blind study. Am J Gastroenterol 1993:88;1212.

122. Klok RM et al. Meta-analysis: comparing the efficacy of proton pump inhibitors in short term use. Aliment Pharmacol Ther 2003;17:1237.

123. Ros J et al. Healing of erosive esophagitis with sucralfate and cimetidine: influence of pretreatment lower esophageal sphincter pressure and serum pepsinogen I levels. Am J Med 1991;91(Suppl 2A):107S.

124. McEvoy GK. Miscellaneous GI drugs. In: American Society of Hospital Pharmacists. AHFS Drug Information 2001. Bethesda, MD: American Society of Hospital Pharmacists, 2001.

125. Kahrilis PJ et al. Effects of tegaserod on esophageal acid exposure in gastro-oesophageal reflux disease. Aliment Pharmcol Ther 2000;14:1503.

126. Howden CW et al. Management of heartburn in a large randomized community-based study: comparison of four therapeutic strategies. Am J Gastroenterol. 2001;96:1679.

127. Blum R. Lansoprazole and omeprazole in the treatment of peptic disorders. Am J Health-Syst Pharm 1996;53:1401.

128. Howden CW et al. The rationale for continuous maintenance treatment of reflux esophagitis. Arch Intern Med 1995;155:1465.

129. Levine BA. Pathophysiology and mechanisms of stress ulcer injury. Pharmacotherapy 1987;7(6 Pt. 2):90S.

130. Tryba M, Cook D. Current guidelines on stress ulcer prophylaxis. Drugs 1997;54(4):581.

131. Tamir BM et al. Prophylaxis for stress-related gastric hemorrhage in the medical intensive care unit. Ann Intern Med 1994;121;568.

132. Ephgrave KS et al. Enteral nutrients prevent stress ulceration and increase intragastric volume. Crit Care Med 1990;18:621.

133. Lamothe HP et al. Comparative efficacy of cimetidine, famotidine, ranitidine, and Mylanta in postoperative stress ulcers. Gastroenterology 1991;100:1515.

134. Martin LF et al. Continuous intravenous cimetidine decreases frequency of upper GI hemorrhage without promoting pneumonia. Crit Care Med 1993;21:19.

135. Levy MJ et al. Comparison of omeprazole and ranitidine for stress ulcer prophylaxis. Dig Dis Sci 1997;42:1255.

136. Frank W et al. Comparison between continuous and intermittent infusion regimens of cimetidine in ulcer patients. Clin Pharmacol Ther 1989;46:234.

137. Siepler JK et al. Use of continuous infusion of histamine₂-receptor antagonists in critically ill patients. DICP 1989;23:S40.

138. Tryba M. Risk of acute stress bleeding and nosocomial pneumonia in ventilated intensive care unit patients: sucralfate versus antacids. Am J Med 1987;83(Suppl 3B):117.

139. Bresalier RS et al. Sucralfate suspension versus titrated antacid for the prevention of acute stress-related gastrointestinal hemorrhage in critically ill patients. Am J Med 1987;83(Suppl 3B):110.

140. Cook D et al. A comparison of sucralfate and ranitidine for the prevention of upper gastrointestinal bleeding in patients requiring mechanical ventilation. N Engl J Med 1998;338:791.

CHAPTER 28

Lower Gastrointestinal Disorders

Geoffrey C. Wall

OVERVIEW OF INFLAMMATORY BOWEL DISEASE
Definition and Epidemiology

Inflammatory bowel disease (IBD) is a generic classification for a group of chronic, idiopathic, relapsing inflammatory disorders of the gastrointestinal (GI) tract. IBD is common in developed countries.[1] It is estimated that more than 600,000 persons in the United States have IBD, and the prevalence of these disorders ranges from 20 to 200 per 100,000 people; however, the prevalence of IBD may actually be greater because many affected patients may be asymptomatic or have mild symptoms for which they do not seek medical attention.[2,3] By convention, IBD is divided into two major disorders: ulcerative colitis (UC) and Crohn's disease (CD).[2,4] However, approximately 10% to 15% of patients with IBD have symptoms that defy this schema.[5] Both UC and CD frequently affect a similar group of patients (Table 28-1). Whites appear to have the higher incidence of IBD compared with Asians or African Americans.[6] In particular, Jews of European descent may have up to a four-fold increase in the incidence of IBD. In addition, studies have found trends toward an increased incidence of IBD in urban compared with rural communities. Hypotheses for this trend include overcrowding, exposure to infectious agents, and lifestyle differences. Although both UC and CD are generally considered diseases of the young, with peak incidences from ages 20 to 40, about 15% of IBD cases are diagnosed in patients older than 60 years of age.[7] There seems to be no significant gender preference for IBD.

Etiology

The true cause of IBD is unclear; however, hypotheses for these disorders include a combination of genetic abnormalities, chronic infection, environmental factors (bacterial, viral, and dietary antigens), autoimmunity, and other abnormalities of immunoregulatory mechanisms.[1] Whatever the mechanism, it is now generally agreed that the symptoms of IBD result from dysregulation of the mucosal immune system. The role of genetics has been strongly supported by epidemiologic studies, showing familial aggregation, consistent ethnic differences, and an increased concordance rate in monozygotic twins. Patients with a first-degree relative with IBD are at an increased risk of developing the disorder, with a frequency of up to 40%.[8] Proponents of an environmental cause for IBD believe that similar living conditions in families may be

Table 28-1 Population Characteristics of Patients at High Risk for Inflammatory Bowel Disease Development

No sexual predilection
Peaks between ages of 15 and 30 years
European ancestry
Urban greater than rural dwellers
Whites greater than non-whites
Jews living in Europe and North America greater than non-Jews
Occurs in familial clusters

From Andres PG, Friedman S. Epidemiology and the natural course of inflammatory bowel disease. Gastro Clin North Am 1999;28:255.

responsible for this association. Recently, detailed mapping of chromosome 16 in the Human Genome Project found a strong association with the Nod2 gene and increased susceptibility to CD.[9] The fact that monozygotic twin studies showed a high, but not complete, concordance for IBD demonstrates that environmental factors also play a role. Smoking has been the most consistent and most studied environmental factor associated with IBD. Interestingly, the effects of smoking are different between UC and CD, with smokers having a decreased risk of developing UC but an increased risk for CD.[3] Use of nonsteroidal anti-inflammatory agents (NSAIDs) has been associated with exacerbation of IBD.[10]

Breast-fed infants may have a decreased risk for IBD, and appendectomy may be protective against the development of UC.[3] Although emotional stress has long been thought to play a role in IBD flares, objective evidence to support this notion remains scant. Debated for decades, the theory of an infectious etiology for IBD remains appealing.[8] Murine models of colitis have shown a decreased development of IBD in a microbe-free environment. Repeated exposure of the GI tract to a particular microorganism may trigger the immune dysregulation evident in this disease. However, some investigators believe that normal intestinal flora may be a catalyst for IBD. At various times, common intestinal organisms such as *Escherichia coli* and unusual bacteria such as *Mycobacterium paratuberculosis* have been investigated as causes of IBD, although no definitive conclusions regarding their etiologic role have been reached.[11] It appears that a complex interplay between environmental exposures and an underlying genetic predisposition are responsible for the development of IBD.

Pathogenesis

Under normal conditions, the mucosal immune system interacts with luminal antigens and mucosal bacteria on a continuous basis to maintain a state of controlled inflammation. As might be expected, the GI tract is exposed to an extremely high number of antigenic substances daily, and a delicate balance must exist for the system to operate properly. Several immune-specific genes partially determine the type of antigens that will trigger the immune response. In IBD, this immune response is perpetuated and an autoimmune cascade occurs. Thus, proinflammatory cytokines in the gut trigger an "attack" on the colonic mucosa by leukocytes and other factors leading to edema, ulceration, and destruction of the tissue. Normal immune regulators fail to halt this process and

the disease progresses. This can be due to lack of regulatory or suppressor cells, enhanced numbers of T cells, or both. The T-cell immune response is Th1 dominated, which is manifested by an increased production of interferon and tumor necrosis factor (promotes macrophage activation and development of delayed-type hypersensitivity response). In UC, Th2 response dominates with an increased production of interleukin (supports humoral mediated immunity).[12–15] Studies have demonstrated that this increase of proinflammatory cytokines, chemokines, prostaglandin, and reactive oxygen species leads to increased inflammation and tissue destruction.[5]

Clinical Presentation

UC usually presents as shallow, continuous inflammation of the colon ranging from limited forms of proctitis (rectal involvement only) to disease involving the entire colon. Crypt abscesses consisting of accumulations of polymorphonuclear neutrophil (PMN) cells adjacent to crypts, necrosis of the epithelium, edema, hemorrhage, and surrounding accumulations of chronic inflammatory cells are typical.[12,16] Fistulas, fissures, abscesses, and small bowel involvement are not present. The inflammation is limited to the mucosa, which presents as friable, granular, and erythematous, with or without ulceration. Most patients with UC experience a chronic, intermittent course of disease. Chronic, loose bloody stools are the most common symptom of UC.[2,4] Other common complaints include tenesmus (urge to defecate) and abdominal pain. Patients with pancolitis usually have more severe symptoms than those with disease limited to the rectum. Mild UC is defined as fewer than four stools a day, no systemic signs of toxicity, and a normal erythrocyte sedimentation rate (ESR). Moderate disease is characterized by more than four stools a day but minimal evidence of systemic toxicity. Severe disease is defined as more than six bloody stools a day, fever, tachycardia, anemia, and/or an ESR >30.[17,18] Proctitis is usually considered a separate type of UC for treatment purposes. Relapses and remissions are common in UC with up to 70% of patients with active disease relapsing within 1 year after induction treatment.[19,20]

CD is a chronic, transmural, patchy, granulomatous, inflammatory disease that can involve the entire GI tract, from mouth to anus, with discontinuous ulceration (so-called "skip lesions"), fistula formation, and perianal involvement. The degree of colonic involvement is variable; however, the terminal ileum is most commonly affected. Intestinal involvement is characteristically segmented and can be interrupted by areas of normal tissue. Unlike UC, the severity of the disease does not correlate directly with the extent of bowel involvement. Patients usually present with one of three patterns of disease: predominantly inflammatory, stricturing, or fistulizing. These patterns are the primary determinants of the disease course and the nature of complications.[3] The inflammatory infiltrate is made up of T and B lymphocytes, macrophages, and plasma cells.

The disease course of CD is variable. Years of frequent relapses may be followed by complete remission. Patients with IBD often require surgery to control symptoms. For patients with UC, surgery is often curative. In contrast, in patients with CD, the frequency of recurrent disease after surgery is high and anatomically correlates with the original pattern of the disease.[21]

Table 28-2 Pathophysiologic Differences Between Ulcerative Colitis and Crohn's Disease

Characteristic	Ulcerative Colitis	Crohn's Disease
Incidence (per year)	6–12/100,000	5–7/100,000
Anatomic location	Colon and rectum	Mouth to anus
Distribution	Continuous, diffuse, mucosal	Segmental, focal, transmural, rigid, thick, edematous, and fibrotic
Bowel wall	Shortened, loss of haustral markings, Generally not thickened	—
Gross rectal bleeding	Common	Infrequent
Crypt abscesses	Common	Infrequent
Fissuring with sinus formation	Absent	Common
Noncaseating granulomas	Absent	Common
Strictures	Absent	Common
Abdominal mass	Absent	Common
Abdominal pain	Infrequent	Common
Toxic megacolon	Occasional	Rare
Bowel carcinoma	Greatly increased	Slightly increased

From references 1–4, 20, and 21.

Patients usually present with abdominal pain and chronic, often nocturnal, diarrhea.[2,4,21] Weight loss, low-grade fever, and fatigue are also common. Features such as abdominal masses or abscesses as well as fistula (an abnormal communication between two organs) can make management of CD difficult and often require surgical intervention. Fistulizing disease is particularly difficult to treat and is the source of significant morbidity in CD patients. Enterocutaneous and enterorectal fistula are common, but other types, such as enterovaginal, can occur. Fistula can be excruciatingly painful, can be a source of infection, and can also exert significant psychosocial distress. Other similarities and differences in the pathophysiology of these disease states are outlined in Table 28-2.[2,3,20,21] Extraintestinal manifestations of IBD that can cause significant morbidity include reactive arthritis, uveitis, ankylosing spondylitis, pyoderma gangrenosum, and primary biliary cirrhosis. Although their incidence varies, many of the manifestations of UC and CD are similar as summarized in Table 28-3.[5,20,21]

Table 28-3 Extraintestinal Complications of Ulcerative Colitis and Crohn's Disease

Manifestation	Ulcerative Colitis (%)	Crohn's Disease (%)
Acute arthropathy	10–15	15–20
Erythema nodosum	10–15	15
Pyoderma gangrenosum	1–2	1–2
Iritis/uveitis	5–15	5–15
Ankylosing spondylitis	1–3	3–5
Sacroiliitis	9–11	9–11
Primary sclerosing cholangitis	2–7	1
Choledocholithiasis	<1	15–30
Nephrolithiasis	<1	5–10
Amyloidosis	<1	Rare

From Andres PG, Friedman S. Epidemiology and the natural course of inflammatory bowel disease. Gastro Clin North Am 1999;28:255.

A careful patient history, physical examination, and endoscopic and radiologic studies are necessary to determine the severity of IBD. Laboratory studies such as an increased ESR can also aid in the diagnosis, but no single marker (e.g., perinuclear staining antineutrophil cytoplasmic antibodies [p ANCA]) is pathognomic. Defining the severity of CD is a difficult, yet important, step in successful treatment.[22] Current guidelines from the American College of Gastroenterology define mild-moderate CD as ambulatory patients who are able to tolerate oral feeding without signs of systemic toxicity. Moderate-severe disease is defined as patients with symptoms of fever, weight loss, abdominal pain, nausea and vomiting, and/or significant anemia. Severe-fulminant disease refers to patients with persistent symptoms despite standard induction regimens or those with signs of severe systemic toxicity.[22]

Treatment

When considering IBD therapy, one must appreciate that the cause of the disease is unknown and, therefore, precludes definitive therapy. In addition, specific therapy depends on the anatomic location of the disease. Other factors to take into consideration are coexisting medical conditions, patient perception of quality of life, medication adherence behavior, lifestyle (such as smoking), dietary factors, and patient's knowledge of the disease.[4]

Medical therapy for the treatment of IBD has five primary goals: (1) providing relief of symptoms (induction of remission), (2) improving quality of life, (3) maintaining adequate nutritional status, (4) relieving intestinal inflammation, and (5) reducing the incidence of recurrent flares (remission maintenance). The ideal medications should be effective, easy to administer with few side effects, and cost-effective.[17,18,22]

Most drug therapies for IBD have been tested for both UC and CD. It is important to differentiate therapy used for acute exacerbations from those used to maintain remission.[17]

Aminosalicylates

Aminosalicylates were the first class of drugs to show benefits in IBD. The prototype agent is sulfasalazine (Azulfidine), which is composed of sulfapyridine (a sulfonamide antibiotic) linked by an azo bond to 5-aminosalicylic acid (5-ASA). It was serendipitous that attachment of 5-ASA to sulfapyridine acted as a carrier to transport 5-ASA past its primary absorption site in the upper intestine. Later, cleavage of the azo bond by lower intestinal bacteria releases 5-ASA (the active moiety) for localized action in the colon. Systemic absorption of the sulfapyridine is responsible for most of the drug's adverse effects, but contributes nothing to the therapeutic benefit.

Following oral administration, 20% to 30% of the parent compound is absorbed in the proximal small intestine.[20] The absorbed sulfasalazine is not metabolized in vivo; most of the absorbed drug is excreted unchanged in the bile and the remainder is eliminated by the kidneys. Ultimately, 75% to 85% of the oral dose reaches the distal small intestine and colon where the diazo bond is cleaved. The liberated sulfapyridine is readily absorbed and is hepatically metabolized by acetylation, hydroxylation, and glucuronidation before it is excreted in the urine as the metabolite or free drug. Because the acetylation rate of sulfapyridine is determined genetically, the half-life of elimination of the absorbed drug depends on the patient's acetylation phenotype and varies from 5 to 13 hours.[23,24] The 5-ASA liberated in the colon is poorly absorbed, although a small portion can be recovered in the urine in the acetylated form.[25] Factors that alter the normal absorption and metabolism of sulfasalazine can increase the amount of unaltered sulfasalazine excreted in the feces and decrease the amount of liberated sulfapyridine and 5-ASA. These include a rapid intestinal transit time, a sterile colon,[26] and surgical removal of the colon.[25]

About 15% of patients discontinue this medication because of dose-dependent adverse effects including nausea, vomiting, headache, alopecia, anorexia, and folate malabsorption. Other idiosyncratic adverse effects include hypersensitivity rash, hemolytic anemia, hepatitis, agranulocytosis, pancreatitis, male infertility, and colitis (Table 28-4).[27]

The dose-limiting adverse effects associated with sulfasalazine have led to the development of safer sulfa-free compounds that contain only 5-ASA. Techniques to decrease systemic absorption and maximize local delivery of 5-ASA to the lower bowel include creating pH-dependent materials to delay drug dissolution and developing hybrid or dimer molecules of 5-ASA that are activated by gut bacteria. Various synonyms and generic names have been assigned to these 5-ASA derivatives, including aminosalicylate, mesalamine, and mesalazine (in Europe). Up to 90% of sulfasalazine-intolerant patients are able to tolerate these newer agents. Mesalamine is available in three formulations: 1) Asacol, a pH-sensitive, resin-coated tablet that releases drug in the distal ileum and colon; 2) Pentasa, a capsule containing ethylcellulose-coated acid-resistant microgranules of mesalamine that releases 5-ASA in the duodenum, jejunum, ileum, and colon; and 3) Rowasa, a topical enema or suppository preparation of mesalamine that directly releases 5-ASA into the rectum and distal colon.[17] The effectiveness of these latter dosage forms is limited to digital proctosigmoiditis.[2,17,18] Administration of mesalamine by retention enemas or suppositories is significantly more effective in the treatment of active distal colitis than placebo and at least as effective as sulfasalazine given rectally or orally.[28] Olsalazine consists of two 5-ASA molecules connected by a diazo bond which is cleaved in the gut to

Table 28-4   Sulfasalazine Adverse Effects

Dose-Related Reactions
General
  Nausea, vomiting, anorexia, headache, fever, arthralgias, gastric distress
Hematologic
  G6PD-deficiency hemolytic anemia
  Leukopenia
  Thrombocytopenia
  Megaloblastic anemia
  Aplastic anemia
Other
  Cyanosis
  Male infertility (reversible)
  Neonatal kernicterus
  Tachycardia
Idiosyncratic Reactions
Hematologic
  Agranulocytosis
  Autoimmune hemolytic anemia
Dermatologic
  Skin rash
  Photosensitization
  Toxic epidermal necrolysis
  Erythema multiforme (Stevens-Johnson syndrome)
Pulmonary
  Bronchospasm, infiltrates, eosinophilia, fibrosing alveolitis, pleuritis
  Pneumonitis
Gastrointestinal
  Hepatotoxicity
  Pancreatitis
Other
  Lupus-like syndrome
  Nephrotic syndrome

From Hanauer SB. Drug therapy: inflammatory bowel disease. N Engl J Med 1996;334:841 and from Holdsworth CD. Sulfasalazine desensitization. Br Med J 1981;282:110.

release both active moieties. The newest 5-ASA agent to be approved for UC is balsalazide.[29] Similar to olsalazine, balsalazide is a 5-ASA dimer that is cleaved by gut bacteria to its active form. Despite one study that found balsalazide was superior to standard 5-ASA in achieving remission in UC patients, significant efficacy advantages of any 5-ASA drug have not been demonstrated.[29,30] Combination oral and rectal therapy for ulcerative proctitis may be superior to either modality alone.[31] 5-ASA suppositories are indicated for proctitis, while enema formulations can be useful in IBD confined to the distal colon. With the exception of abdominal pain, cramps, and discomfort (8.1%), rectally administered mesalamine is well tolerated[27,28] Enemas or suppositories should be administered in the evening and retained overnight. Mesalamine enemas are significantly more expensive than oral forms of 5-ASA. The oral 5-ASA agents are effective in inducing remission in mild CD and mild to moderate UC and for maintaining remission in UC and perhaps for mild CD confined to the colon. Adverse effects of the 5-ASA compounds include diarrhea (especially with olsalazine), headache, arthralgias, abdominal pain, and nausea. Intersitial nephritis has been rarely reported with chronic use of mesalamine but the association remains controversial. Cross-reactive allergic reactions to mesalamine in patients with a previous reaction to sulfasalazine have also been documented. An important drug interaction is the possibility of increasing 6-mercaptopurine levels in patients receiving balsalazide.[32]

Corticosteroids

Corticosteroids are the most commonly used agents in the treatment of acute flares in patients with moderate to severe IBD.[5,18,22] The anti-inflammatory actions of corticosteroids are well known, but how these translate into their full mechanism of controlling IBD is not completely understood. First-line treatment for moderate to severe active UC includes doses of corticosteroid equivalent to 40 to 60 mg of prednisone. Data are insufficient to demonstrate any difference between single versus divided oral doses or continuous versus intermittent bolus intravenous administration. Intravenous doses should be equivalent to hydrocortisone 300 mg/day or methylprednisolone 40 to 60 mg/day.[18] Although corticosteroids are effective for inducing remission in most cases of IBD, up to 30% of patients may not respond. Corticosteroids are not effective and should be avoided for maintenance therapy for both CD and UC.[2,22]

Topical steroids (enemas, foams, and suppositories) are beneficial for distal colitis and can serve as an adjunct in patients with rectal disease that also have more proximal disease and have failed topical 5-ASA therapy.[18,33] Steroids are absorbed to a significant extent from the rectum, and with long-term use, can cause adrenal suppression.[34] A new corticosteroid, budesonide, has recently been approved for the treatment of CD. Budesonide possesses a high degree of topical anti-inflammatory activity with low systemic bioavailability.[35] Commercially, budesonide is available as an enteric coated formulation that delivers drug primarily to the ileum and ascending colon. It was thought that these factors would make budesonide more effective than traditional corticosteroids while decreasing systemic side effects. Current data suggest that budesonide may be as effective or slightly less effective than traditional corticosteroids in active CD. Short-term corticosteroid-associated adverse effects may be less than with traditional agents, but adrenal suppression has been detected in study patients receiving budesonide, and its long-term safety profile remains to be determined.[36,37]

Immunomodulators

Azathioprine and 6-mercaptopurine (6-MP) are commonly used for the management of steroid-dependent and quiescent IBD. Azathioprine is converted to 6-MP, which is then metabolized to thioinosinic acid, the active agent that inhibits purine ribonucleotide synthesis and cell proliferation. It also alters the immune response by inhibiting natural killer cell activity and suppressing cytotoxic T-cell function.[34] Azathioprine (2 to 2.5 mg/kg/day) and 6-MP (1 to 1.5 mg/kg/day) are used in the treatment of active UC and CD in patients whose conditions have not responded to systemic steroids.[5,18,38] These agents are also used as maintenance therapy for both UC and CD and may be used as "steroid-sparing" agents in patients unable to be weaned from corticosteroids.[39] Because of the long onset of action of 6-MP and azathioprine, many clinicians prefer to

induce remission with either corticosteroids or infliximab and use these agents for maintaining remission. Adverse effects of 6-MP/azathioprine include rash, nausea, and diarrhea. Myelosuppression, especially neutropenia, may have a delayed onset and clinicians should monitor the complete blood count monthly for the first 3 months of treatment, then every 3 months thereafter.[22] Neutropenia necessitating discontinuation of therapy occurs in approximately 10% of patients. Despite previous concerns, it appears these agents do not increase the risk of developing lymphoma.

Methotrexate (MTX), a folate antagonist, impairs DNA synthesis. It may also reduce interleukin-1 (IL-1) production or induce apoptosis of selected T-cell populations.[27,34] These T cells can produce cytokines such as IL-2 and interferon-γ, which mediate the inflammatory response in CD.[5] MTX appears to be ineffective for induction or maintenance of UC.[40] However, recent data suggest that MTX (15 to 25 mg intramuscularly weekly) may have a role for both initial and chronic treatment of CD.[41,42] The onset of effect often takes weeks to months with MTX. Most experts reserve MTX use for patients with CD intolerant of, or refractory to, 6-MP/azathioprine treatment. Adverse effects with MTX include stomatitis, neutropenia, nausea, hypersensitivity pneumonitis, alopecia, and hepatotoxicity. MTX induced nausea and stomatitis may be prevented by the addition of folic acid 1 mg orally daily.

Cyclosporine (CSA), which selectively inhibits T-cell mediated responses, has advantages over azathioprine, 6-MP, and MTX because of its more rapid onset of action.[39] Both the oral and intravenous forms have been used to manage severe UC.[43] Due to serious adverse effects including the possible emergence of *Pneumocystis carinii* pneumonia, CSA is usually reserved for patients with severe UC refractory to corticosteroids. CSA 4 mg/kg intravenously daily has been used in severe steroid-refractory UC.[18] The role of CSA therapeutic drug monitoring for this indication has not been firmly established, but may be beneficial for toxicity monitoring. Approximately 60% of patients with corticosteroid-resistant or fistulizing CD disease respond to CSA therapy. The use of CSA for maintenance therapy or nonfistulizing disease is uncertain.

Infliximab

Early research indicating an increase in the amount of tumor necrosis factor-alpha (TNF-α) in the stool of patients with active CD, as well as an increase in the amount of lamina propria cells in the gut, led investigators to target this cytokine for treatment of CD.[44] Infliximab is a recombinant chimeric monoclonal antibody that binds to human TNF-α and neutralizes its biologic activity by binding with high affinity to both soluble cell membranes and in the blood (Fig. 28-1). Infliximab is indicated for inducing and maintaining remission in patients with moderate to severe active CD who have had an inadequate response to conventional treatment.[45,46] It is also effective for healing CD fistula, with recent data showing that chronic treatment can maintain fistula closure.[47,48] For all types of CD, infliximab is given as a 5 mg/kg intravenous infusion over 2 hours. An induction regimen, administered at 0, 2, and 6 weeks, followed by a maintenance infusion every 8 weeks is used. The response to infliximab is usually rapid, often occurring within several days, and can be dramatic in up to 60% of patents. Immediate infusion-related reactions such

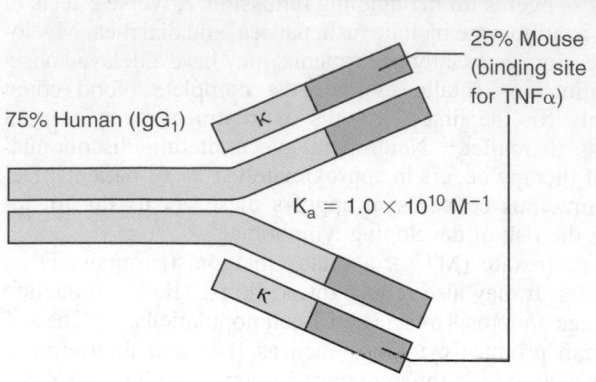

REMICADE™ (infliximab)

75% Human (IgG$_1$)

25% Mouse (binding site for TNFα)

K

K

$K_a = 1.0 \times 10^{10}\ M^{-1}$

Knight DM et al. *Mol Immunol.* 1993; 16:1443-14!

FIGURE 28-1 Structure of infliximab. Reprinted by permission from Centocor, Inc. Malvern, PA.

as fever, chills, pruritus, urticaria, and (rarely) severe cardiopulmonary symptoms can occur in about 1% of patients. Delayed hypersensitivity reactions resembling serum sickness and severe pulmonary symptoms are rarely reported and are more common in patients receiving episodic (rather than scheduled maintenance) treatment.[49] Infectious complications, including pneumonia, cellulitis, sepsis, cholecystitis, endophthalmitis, furunculosis, and reactivation of tuberculosis and histoplasmosis have also been reported.[50,51] Lupus-like symptoms, such as arthralgias, have been seen rarely and usually resolve after discontinuation of the drug. Patients with serious active infections, a history of chronic infections, a history of a neural demyelinating disorder, or severe heart failure should avoid infliximab treatment.[50] The latter two cautions are due to previous reports of exacerbations of multiple sclerosis and heart failure when patients with those diseases received anti–TNF-α therapy.

Antibiotics

Because an infectious etiology has been proposed for IBD, it stands to reason that antibiotics may have some utility.[5,11,17] All studies showing benefit of antibiotics have been in patients with CD; no consistent benefit has been demonstrated for patients with UC.[18,22,52] Metronidazole, which also has immunosuppressive properties, is the best studied antibiotic. It is especially effective in patients with perianal and post-operative CD, with benefits improving as the dosage is increased up to a maximum of 2 g/day.[53] Adverse effects with chronic, high dose metronidazole include metallic taste and peripheral neuropathy. Ciprofloxacin is also an alternative to metronidazole, with similar efficacy to mesalamine. It is beneficial in treating perianal and fistulous CD, either alone or in combination with metronidazole.[54]

Nutritional Therapies

Nutritional therapies for IBD have been used because dietary intraluminal antigens may stimulate a mucosal immune response.[8] Patients with active CD respond to bowel rest, total parenteral nutrition (TPN), or total enteral nutrition. Bowel rest and TPN are as effective as corticosteroids for inducing remission in patients with active CD in the short term.[55] En-

teral nutrition, with elemental or peptide-based preparation, appears to be as efficacious as TPN without its associated complications. Unfortunately, poor compliance often limits this modality. Neither enteral nor parenteral nutrition is effective treatment for the maintenance of remission.[21] UC is not effectively treated with either TPN or enteral nutrition. Fish oils containing omega-3 fatty acids, which inhibit the production of inflammatory cytokines, have shown modest efficacy in the treatment of both UC and CD.[56] Another approach, which is not yet generally accepted, is the topical application of short-chain fatty acids, which are important nutrients for the colonic epithelium.[57]

Supportive Therapy

Symptomatic management of IBD is important to the patient's quality of life. This includes pain relief and diarrhea control. Loperamide or diphenoxylate-atropine may be used to treat mild symptoms provided obstruction or toxicity is not evident.[27] Severe worsening of symptoms and abdominal distention may indicate toxic megacolon caused by the inability to empty rapidly produced secretory products of the bowel. Patients should be monitored for iron and vitamin B$_{12}$ deficiencies, especially if ileal involvement is extensive or resection has been performed.

Surgery

Surgery is indicated in the treatment of UC when the patient (1) fails to respond to medical management acutely or chronically, (2) develops uncontrollable drug-related complications, (3) experiences impaired quality of life from the disease or its drug therapy, (4) develops complications of a severe attack (perforation, acute dilation), (5) fails to grow and develop at a normal rate, or (6) develops carcinoma of the rectum or colon.[20] In addition, patients who have had UC for longer than 10 years or who demonstrate premalignant changes on rectal biopsy may be managed surgically as a prophylactic measure against colonic carcinoma.[58]

Generally accepted indications for surgical intervention in patients with CD include failure of medical management, incapacitation because of the disease or its drug therapy, retarded growth and development in children, intestinal obstruction, fistula formation, abscess formation, toxic megacolon, perforation and hemorrhage, and carcinoma.[20–22]

ULCERATIVE COLITIS
Pathophysiology and Clinical Presentation

1. **C.M., a 25-year-old female college student, has had episodic, watery diarrhea and colicky abdominal pain relieved by defecation for the past 9 months. Eight weeks before admission, the diarrhea increased to 3 to 5 semiformed stools daily. The frequency of the stools gradually increased to 5 to 10 times a day 1 week ago. At that time, C.M. noted bright red blood in the stools. Stool frequency has now increased to 10 to 15 per day, although the volume of each stool is estimated to be only "one-half cupful." She feels a great urgency to defecate even though the volume is small. She has not traveled outside the United States, has not been camping, and has not taken any antibiotics within the past 6 months.**

C.M. complains of anorexia and a 10-pound weight loss over the past 2 months. For the past 4 months, she has had intermit-

tent swelling, warmth, and tenderness of the left knee, which is unassociated with trauma. She denies any skin rashes or any difficulties with her vision. A review of other body systems and social and family history are noncontributory.

C.M. appears to be a slightly anxious and tired young woman of normal body habitus. Her temperature is 100°F.; her pulse rate is 100 beats/min and regular. Physical examination is normal except for evidence of acute arthritis of the left knee and tenderness of the left lower abdomen to palpation.

Stool examination shows a watery effluent that contains numerous red and white cells with no trophozoites. Stool cultures and an amebiasis indirect hemagglutination test are negative. Other laboratory values include the following: hematocrit (Hct), 32% (normal 33–43%); hemoglobin (Hgb), 8.5 g/dL (normal, 12.3 to 15.3 g/dL); white blood cell (WBC) count, 15,000/mm³ (normal, 4.4 to 11.3/mm³) with 82% PMNs (normal, 50% to 70%); ESR, 70 mm/hr (normal, <20 mm/hr); serum albumin, 2.4 g/dL (normal, 3.5 to 5.0 g/dL); and alanine aminotransferase (ALT), 35 U/mL (normal, 8 to 20 U/mL);

Sigmoidoscopy showed evidence of granular, edematous, and friable mucosa with continuous ulcerations extending from the anus to 20 cm proximally.

What is the most likely cause of C.M.'s diarrheal illness, and what is the evidence for this? How should the signs and symptoms be managed and monitored?

C.M's presentation is typical of a patient with new onset UC. Drug-induced (pseudomembranous colitis) and infectious (parasitic) causes of diarrhea have been ruled out by history (no travel outside the United States, no recent camping, no antibiotic use) and stool examination. As discussed earlier, UC is an inflammation of the mucosal layer of the colon and rectum.[20] Characteristically, the inflammation does not extend beyond the submucosa, and transmural ulcers are rare. On examination, the mucosa appears erythematous and is friable. Differentiation from CD is made by sigmoidoscopic and radiologic evidence of continuous distribution of pathology (as opposed to segmental), as well as the anatomic location (confined to colon and rectum).

C.M. presents with the classic triad of UC clinical symptoms: chronic diarrhea, rectal bleeding, and abdominal pain. The diarrhea is secondary to the decreased colonic absorption of water and electrolytes and diminished colonic segmental contractions that normally serve to decrease the flow of bowel content. A good indication of the severity of the patient's disease is the volume of stool passed per day.[18,20] C.M's disease would be classified as severe. As the severity of the disease increases, incontinence and nocturnal diarrhea commonly occur. Diarrhea can vary in severity from three to four bowel movements daily to one to two bowel movements per hour. The stools are usually soft, mushy, formed, and often contain small amounts of mucus mixed with blood, although in patients with mild, early involvement disease, blood and mucus may be totally absent. In addition to the diarrhea, the malabsorption of water and electrolytes causes dehydration, weight loss (as observed in C.M.), and electrolyte disturbances.

C.M.'s rectal bleeding is secondary to colonic mucosal erosions and occurs in most patients with UC.[20] Generally, bright red blood mixed in the stools indicates a colonic origin, whereas blood-streaked stools indicate an anal or rectal origin. The anemia associated with UC generally is secondary to

this rectal bleeding. It presents as a hemorrhagic or iron deficiency anemia, depending on the acuteness of the bleeding. Hemoglobin and hematocrit laboratory values often are decreased as in C.M.'s case. Chronic inflammatory disease induced hypoalbuminemia is often exacerbated by malnutrition.

C.M.'s abdominal pain and cramping are caused by spasm of the irritated and inflamed colon. This abdominal pain is commonly associated with urgency to defecate. As illustrated by C.M., the pain usually is relieved with defecation even though the stool volume may be small.

C.M.'s arthritis and elevated liver enzymes (alkaline phosphatase and ALT) are indicative of the extra-intestinal manifestations that occur in IBD (Table 28-3). Her nonspecific symptoms (i.e., anorexia, fatigue, weight loss, anxiety, and tachycardia) could become profound during an exacerbation of UC.[29] Fever, leukocytosis, and increased ESR are also systemic manifestations of an inflammatory disease. Rehydration is important to assure fluid balance and maintain good renal function.

2. Would it be safe to administer loperamide to C.M.?

Treatment of the diarrhea associated with UC is often difficult. In patients with mild to moderate disease, antidiarrheals, such as loperamide or diphenoxylate with atropine may help to minimize chronic diarrhea. Extreme caution must be used, however, especially in patients with severe disease, because of the chance of inducing toxic megacolon (see Question 14). For this reason, antidiarrheals are best avoided in patients with severe active disease and, if used, should be titrated according to the volume of stool produced. Bulk-forming agents, such as psyllium, may be helpful for patients suffering from constipation caused by ulcerative proctitis.[59]

Remission Induction
Corticosteroids

3. What agents can be used to induce disease remission in C.M.?

Corticosteroids are the most effective agents to induce remission of acute, severe exacerbations of UC.[18] Clinical improvement or remission occurs in 45% to 90% of patients taking 15 to 60 mg/day of prednisone, with an increased response at 40 to 60 mg/day. However, corticosteroids are not beneficial for maintaining remission. Strategies to minimize adverse effects of therapy with corticosteroids include rapid, well-defined tapering regimens. Once improvement has occurred, prednisone is tapered by 5 to 10 mg per week until the dose is 15 to 20 mg/day. The dosage is then tapered by 2.5 to 5 mg/week until the drug is discontinued. Unfortunately, a subset of patients will experience a disease flare if the steroid dosage is decreased or is tapered too quickly. Intravenous corticosteroids are an important option, especially in patients who have poor oral intake. Patients with active distal disease can be treated with hydrocortisone enemas, however 5-ASA topical therapy is as or more effective.[60]

4. Methylprednisolone at a dosage of 40 mg IV Q 6 hr is ordered. What are the treatment goals for C.M.?

The goal of parenteral corticosteroid therapy for C.M. should be to achieve a rapid therapeutic response as measured by decreased frequency of stools, decreased pain, and decreased fever and heart rate. This goal may be attained with a high initial dose followed by a gradual dosage reduction to minimize the development of corticosteroid adverse reactions. The initial dose, as well as the rate of a subsequent dosage reduction, should be individualized based on the severity of the patient's signs, symptoms, and disease course.

Poorly nourished patients in whom oral intake is expected to be absent for greater than 7 days should receive parenteral nutrition, and treatment should be continued until oral feeding is tolerated.[61] An adequate response is defined as resolution of fever, improved patient well-being, no tachycardia, and less abdominal tenderness on palpation. Diarrhea is usually considered resolved with four or fewer bowel movements daily. Stools are rarely formed at this stage, but macroscopic bleeding has stopped. Patients can then receive oral prednisone, a 5-ASA drug, and a light diet. If the patient does not respond within 72 hours of starting high-dose corticosteroids, surgery may be indicated (see Question 15). Once C.M.'s symptoms are controlled, the goal should be to switch to oral corticosteroids and discharge her from the hospital.

ORAL ADMINISTRATION

5. CM is responding well to methylprednisolone. She is afebrile, her abdominal pain is reduced (to a score of 5 on a 1 to 10 scale), and her diarrhea is decreasing. When is the oral route of corticosteroid administration indicated in UC? What are the most appropriate dosages?

Oral corticosteroids are effective for the initial treatment of mild to moderate acute UC.[27] In addition, they should be substituted for parenteral corticosteroids once a satisfactory initial response of more severe exacerbations has been achieved. In one controlled trial, 40 mg/day of prednisone was significantly more efficacious than 20 mg/ day in controlling ambulatory patients with moderately severe acute UC.[34] Prednisone doses of 60 mg/day had no additional therapeutic value, but caused more adverse effects. In addition, a single 40-mg morning dose of prednisone was as effective as and more convenient than an equivalent divided dose (10 mg four times daily). Therefore, the initial dose of corticosteroid for a patient with moderately severe acute UC is 40 mg of prednisone or its equivalent administered once daily in the morning.

TOPICAL ADMINISTRATION

6. What if CM's UC was limited to the distal colon or rectum? Would topical corticosteroids be indicated? When should other topical agents be used (e.g., 5-ASA)?

Topically administered 5-ASA and corticosteroids, in the form of suppositories, foams, and retention enemas, are effective in the management of acute, mild to moderate UC that is limited to the distal colon and rectum.[28,62,63] To justify the use of such a difficult and socially unacceptable route of administration, a clear-cut advantage of either increased efficacy or decreased side effects over other administration routes for these agents must be demonstrated.

Theoretically, 5-ASA and corticosteroids administered via this topical route provide a higher concentration of drug to the diseased mucosal area, exerting a local anti-inflammatory effect while minimizing systemic side effects. Unfortunately, variable, but significant systemic absorption (up to 90%) and

adrenal suppression occur from the topical administration of corticosteroid to the rectum and distal colon.[64] Therefore, the beneficial effects produced by topical use of these agents may accrue from systemic as well as local effects. The apparent and relatively low incidence of corticosteroid side effects associated with topical administration may be related to the low doses used and to the infrequent administration (daily to twice daily) needed to control mild acute UC. When prednisolone is given in equivalent doses orally and rectally, the incidence of side effects and therapeutic effects are similar.[64]

5-ASA suppositories and enemas are preferred over topical corticosteroids for the treatment of distal UC and proctitis because they produce higher remission rates in proctitis and effectively maintain remission of distal UC.[60,63,65] For distal UC, therapy is initiated with a nightly enema (4 g mesalamine), and the response should be evaluated in 3 to 4 weeks. If remission is attained, therapy can be tapered to one enema every third night. Simultaneous therapy with oral plus topical therapy with mesalamine showed greater efficacy than either alone in achieving remission of distal UC.[18,29] A dose of one suppository twice daily for 3 to 6 weeks of 5-ASA generally is sufficient to induce disease remission in patients with mild acute proctitis. Improvement should be seen in 2 to 3 weeks and therapy should be maintained until complete remission is achieved. Therapy can then be progressively tapered to one suppository or enema, 2 to 3 times weekly. If topical corticosteroids are to be used to manage mild, acute UC, the corticosteroid of choice would be the one with the lowest absorptive characteristics. Unfortunately, no trials have compared the absorption characteristics of all corticosteroids available for administration by this route. The available evidence indicates that, of the hydrocortisone salts, the acetate is the least absorbed.[66]

ADVERSE EFFECTS

7. What particular corticosteroid adverse effects are of importance in patients with IBD?

Corticosteroid side effects and precautions for use often limit the therapeutic effectiveness of these agents and should never be overlooked[67] (See Chapter 44, Connective Tissue Disorders: The Clinical Use of Corticosteroids, for a detailed discussion of these effects.) Certain glucocorticoid adverse effects are of particular importance in patients with IBD in that they may mimic, mask, or intensify symptoms and complications of this disease. For example, corticosteroids cause cutaneous atrophy.[35] Patients with UC are predisposed to intestinal wall perforation and drug-induced cutaneous atrophy only intensifies this predisposition. In addition, the symptoms of one of the major complications of intestinal perforation, peritonitis, may be masked by corticosteroids. Other deleterious effects of corticosteroids include hyperglycemia, avascular necrosis, cataract formation, and central nervous system effects including mood disorders, insomnia, psychoses, and euphoria.

Corticosteroids have been noted to mask the clinical signs of abdominal and pelvic abscess in CD patients resulting in septic complications. Other corticosteroid adverse effects that may be secondary to either the drug and/or IBD include retardation of growth and development in prepubescent patients, osteoporosis with secondary pathologic fractures and spinal column decompression, and hypokalemic alkalosis.[67]

Patients with IBD may have decreased bone mineral density, especially with prolonged use of corticosteroids. This is an often overlooked side effect of these drugs. A recent study suggested that even budesonide causes this adverse effect.[68] Thus, calcium, vitamin D supplements, and possibly bisphosphonates (e.g., alendronate 5 mg daily) are recommended in all IBD patients taking corticosteroids for longer than 3 months to minimize metabolic demineralization.[69]

8. CM is still responding well to oral prednisone; however, her blood glucose concentrations have ranged from 250 to 450 mg/dL (normal, 70 to 110 mg/dL). Her physician would like to try another modality for active treatment. What other drugs could be used for remission induction?

Sulfasalazine and 5-ASA

Previously, sulfasalazine was considered the drug of choice in UC exacerbation because of its demonstrated efficacy and reduced toxicity when compared to corticosteroids.[34] However, controlled trials have shown that corticosteroids may act more promptly than sulfasalazine alone, or in combination with a corticosteroid, for severe acute UC.[5,34] Sulfasalazine use has declined since the availability of better tolerated 5-ASA formulations. Clinical improvement or remission of mild to moderate UC can be attained in 40% to 74% of patients treated with oral 5-ASA in doses ranging from 1.5 to 4.8 g/day with further improved response at dosages >2 g/day.[29,70] For mild to moderate proctitis or proctosigmoiditis, topical 5-ASA has been effective in 60% to 89% of patients. Both suppositories (0.5 to 2 g/day) and enemas (1 to 4 g/day) have been used.[60] In summary, oral 5-ASA compounds are usually considered first line therapy for mild-to-moderate exacerbations of UC, with systemic corticosteroids reserved for more severe active UC or milder disease that has failed 5-ASA treatment. Even though sulfasalazine is less expensive than mesalamine compounds, the latter drugs are usually chosen because of their superior tolerability. Figure 28-2 describes a treatment approach to UC.

Remission Maintenance
Sulfasalazine

9. C.M. feels much better and claims to be "back to normal." Her abdominal pain is gone and she currently has two formed, non-bloody stools daily. Most of her laboratory parameters have returned to normal (ESR, 25 mm/hr; blood glucose, 80 mg/dL; WBC, 8,000/mm³.) She is currently taking sulfasalazine 500 mg PO TID. What drug regimen should be used to maintain disease remission in C.M.?

Oral sulfasalazine significantly reduces the incidence of relapse in UC patients who are in remission.[18,29] At 6 to 12 months, 71% to 88% of patients maintained remission taking daily doses of 1 to 4 g. In addition, the recurrence rate increases significantly if long-term sulfasalazine is stopped. Two to four grams is the recommended daily maintenance dose, although this should be individualized if adverse effects appear or if beneficial effects are not achieved. In contrast, oral and topical corticosteroids do not prevent relapse of UC once remission has occurred.

On the basis of this information, C.M.'s sulfasalazine should be increased to 500 mg PO QID and then slowly increased to 3 to 4 grams daily. If she experiences a relapse, a course of oral corticosteroids may be needed to re-achieve remission. Prophylactic therapy should be continued indefinitely unless intolerable adverse effects develop.[27]

ADVERSE EFFECTS

10. C.M.'s sulfasalazine has been increased to 1 g QID for UC maintenance therapy. Three days after starting this higher dose of sulfasalazine, C.M. developed anorexia, nausea, and occasional vomiting. What is the possible cause of C.M.'s symptoms? How can they be minimized?

C.M. appears to be experiencing adverse effects of sulfasalazine. Unwanted adverse effects occur in up to 21% of patients and can cause significant morbidity, often limiting the drug's clinical usefulness. These adverse effects appear to be of two types: dose related and idiosyncratic (Table 28-4).[34]

Most sulfasalazine adverse reactions are dose related, tend to occur early in the course of therapy, and are more frequent when the dose is 4 g/day, corresponding to serum concentrations of sulfapyridine that exceed 50 mg/mL.[71,72] Because sulfapyridine is acetylated, genetically determined slow acetylators (60% of the population) experience a higher incidence of the "dose-related" adverse effects than fast acetylators.[23,71]

Generally, sulfasalazine dose-related adverse effects occur early in the course of therapy. The concomitant use of corticosteroids may mask certain adverse effects of sulfasalazine (e.g., malaise, arthralgia, rash, fever), but these may become apparent once the corticosteroids are withdrawn.

Dose-related sulfasalazine adverse effects can be minimized by initiating the patient on a low dosage (1 to 2 g/day) and gradually increasing the amount to tolerated therapeutic levels of 3 to 4 g/day.[72] If dose-related reactions do occur, the drug should be discontinued until the symptoms subside; then, sulfasalazine may be reinstituted at a lower dosage. Although enteric-coated sulfasalazine tablets are available, they are useful only for the occasional patient who develops dyspepsia. Because they are also more expensive, their general use is unjustified.

Idiosyncratic reactions to sulfasalazine are rare but cause significantly higher morbidity and mortality. Because many of these reactions are similar to the sensitivity reactions associated with the sulfonamide derivatives, they are thought to be secondary to the sulfapyridine component of the parent compound.[20] The severe sequelae associated with these reactions may be minimized through vigilance for their occurrence, avoidance of the use of sulfasalazine in patients with documented sensitivity reactions to sulfonamides, prompt withdrawal of sulfasalazine at the first indication that such a reaction is occurring, and avoidance of sulfasalazine in the future.[71,73]

C.M.'s symptoms are probably dose-related adverse reactions to the sulfasalazine. The dosage should be decreased or the drug temporarily withheld. If tolerated, the dosage can be increased slowly as necessary or she can be switched to mesalamine.

TERATOGENICITY

11. C.M. would like to have a baby. What are the fertility and pregnancy concerns in a patient with IBD? Should she receive sulfasalazine maintenance therapy if she becomes pregnant and plans to breast-feed her baby?

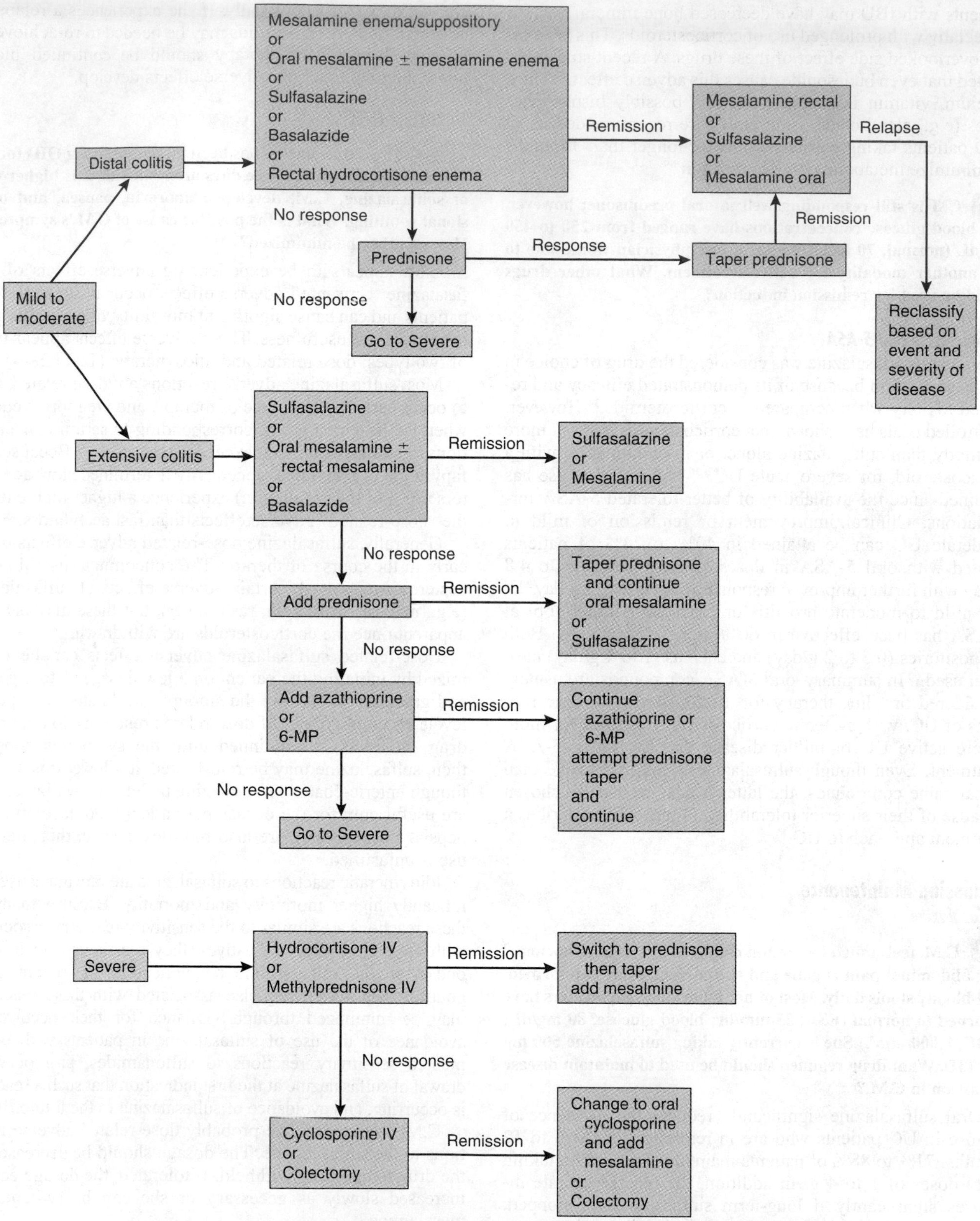

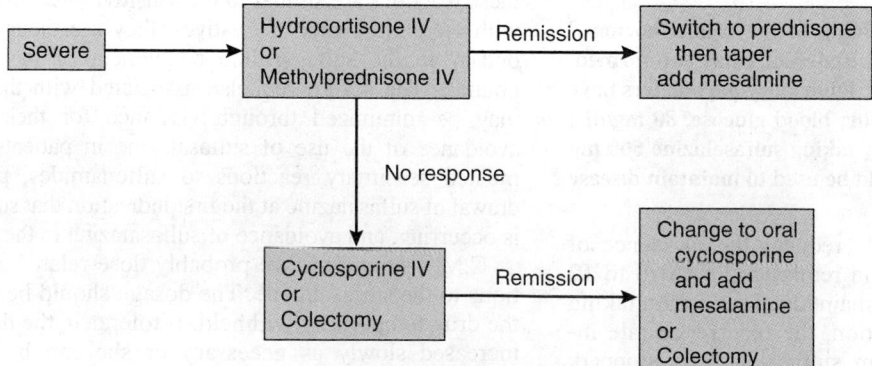

FIGURE 28-2 Treatment algorithm for ulcerative colitis. (Reprinted by permission from the American College of Clinical Pharmacy. Garnett WR, Yunker NS. The treatment of inflammatory bowel disease. In: Mueller BA et al., eds. Pharmacotherapy Self-Assessment Program. 4th Ed. Gastroenterology Model. Kansas City, MO: ACCP 2002:53.)

Fertility is generally normal in patients with IBD with the exception of active CD.[74] In males, fertility may be reduced due to azoospermia; a common adverse effect of sulfasalazine therapy. Pregnant women with UC tend to have normal outcomes, but some evidence suggests patients with CD have an increased risk for preterm delivery and babies with lower birth weights. Pregnancy itself does not seem to activate quiescent disease. Because active disease increases the chances of a complicated pregnancy, efforts to control IBD are critical. Increases in congenital defects or newborn toxicity have not been attributed to sulfasalazine or standard dose mesalamine use during pregnancy.[75] Thus UC patients being maintained on sulfasalazine can be continued on the drug during pregnancy.[76] The drug does not appear to alter the rate of prematurity or contribute to low fetal birthweight but it may interfere with folate absorption. Therefore, supplemental folate may need to be increased whenever sulfasalazine therapy is prescribed.[77] One issue to be aware of is that sulfasalazine may contribute to the nausea and vomiting that pregnant women experience, especially during the first trimester.[76]

Although listed as pregnancy category B by the Food and Drug Administration (as is sulfasalazine), high-dose mesalamine has been reported to cause interstitial nephritis in a newborn case and should be avoided if possible. Little data on olsalazine or balsalazide use in pregnancy exist.

Sulfapyridine concentrations in breast milk may reach 40% to 60% of maternal serum concentrations. Although sulfasalazine and sulfapyridine do appear in breast milk, the actual concentrations are estimated to be low.[77] In addition, the ability of sulfapyridine and sulfasalazine to displace bilirubin is minimal, which probably explains why the literature has no reports of jaundice in breast-fed babies whose mothers take sulfasalazine. Conservatively, it is appropriate to monitor bilirubin concentrations in infants nursing from mothers taking this drug. One report noted no adverse effects were observed in 16 nursing infants exposed to the drug. However, one infant experienced bloody diarrhea attributable to the mother's sulfasalazine therapy (3 g/day). The diarrhea stopped within 48 to 72 hours after the drug was discontinued[76] The American Academy of Pediatrics classifies mesalamine and sulfasalazine as agents that have produced adverse effects in a nursing infant and advises cautious use during breast-feeding because of possible allergic reactions. Thus, C.M. may continue her sulfasalazine therapy during conception and pregnancy, but she and her providers will have to weigh the risks of potential toxicity versus the benefits of breast-feeding. If C.M. decides to breast feed, she should carefully monitor the infant for signs of hypersensitivity reactions, diarrhea, and abdominal discomfort which may be related to sulfasalazine.

Other agents may be used in pregnant patients with IBD. Human studies suggest that prednisone and prednisolone are well tolerated and appear to pose a small risk to the fetus in utero. In fact, IBD is more detrimental to the fetus than corticosteroids, thus warranting continued use when necessary during pregnancy.[74] The American Academy of Pediatrics considers prednisone to be compatible with breast-feeding. The studies of metronidazole have arrived at conflicting conclusions. Several studies, case reports, and reviews have described the use of metronidazole as safe for use during pregnancy,[78] while others have shown possible associations with malformations.[79] These malformations include, but are not limited to, hydrocele (two cases), congenital dislocated hip (one case), metatarsus varus (one case), mental retardation (one case), and midline facial defects (two cases). The long-term risks from metronidazole exposure have not been fully elucidated. The Centers for Disease Control recommends that metronidazole be considered as contraindicated during the first trimester. Use in the second and third trimester for trichomoniasis may be acceptable if other therapies have failed. For other indications, the risk-benefit ratio must be considered.

Immunosuppressants are alternatives for patients with refractory IBD. These agents can cause low fetal birthweight and congenital abnormalities, but they have been used safely in pregnant transplant patients.[74] Due to a paucity of objective information concerning 6-MP/azathioprine use in pregnancy, these agents should only be utilized if absolutely necessary to maintain quiescent disease activity. Due to possible maternal toxicity the role of CSA is limited. Methotrexate is contraindicated during pregnancy[78] (see Chapter 47, Teratogenicity and Drugs in Breast Milk).

Other Agents

12. Despite lowering C.M.'s dose of sulfasalazine to 500 mg QID, she still complains of nausea and anorexia. What would be the next therapeutic alternative that would give the same beneficial effect as sulfasalazine without the accompanying adverse effects?

As mentioned above, most patients who do not tolerate sulfasalazine are likely to better tolerate other 5-ASA compounds. Because no evidence suggests that any 5-ASA is more efficacious than other members of the class, safety, cost, and disease location dictate choice of drug. If UC is confined to the distal colon or rectum, 5-ASA enemas or suppositories, respectively, are appropriate choices. Oral mesalamine is needed for more extensive disease.

A comparison of the various aminosalicylate preparations is listed in Table 28-5. Asacol is coated with a methacrylic acid copolymer B (Eudragit S), which disintegrates at a pH greater than 7. After disintegration, it releases a bolus of drug into the terminal ileum or proximal colon.[80] In controlled trials, this formulation was more effective than placebo and was at least as effective as sulfasalazine in the treatment of mild to moderate UC and in maintaining disease remission.[38,81] Pentasa contains microspheres of mesalamine encapsulated in a diffusion-dependent, semipermeable ethylcellulose membrane designed to release drug slowly and continuously throughout the small and large intestine.[82] The relatively high doses of Pentasa (4 g/day) that are necessary to treat UC are probably secondary to the release and subsequent absorption of mesalamine in the small intestine. This decreases the amount of drug that eventually is available for action in the large intestine.

13. C.M. was given Pentasa 4 g/day. After 2 weeks, C.M. continued to have nausea, diarrhea, and headache severe enough to cause her to miss classes and call in sick from her part-time job. What types of therapy should be considered at this point?

The most common adverse effects of mesalamine include abdominal cramps, headache, diarrhea, eructation, nausea, and vomiting. Although Pentasa may have a better adverse

Table 28-5 Comparison of Aminosalicylate Compounds

Generic (Trade)	Delivery System	Intestinal Site of Release	Usual Dose and Frequency
Sulfasalazine (Azulfidine)	None (cleaved in colon)	Colon	Initially 500 mg PO BID; increase to 3 to 4 g/day in divided doses
Mesalamine (Asacol)	(Eudragit S) disintegrates at a pH >7	Ileum, colon	800 mg PO TID
Mesalamine (Pentasa)	Encapsulated microspheres	Ileum, jejunum, colon	4 g daily in divided doses
Mesalamine (Rowasa)	(Eudragit L) Given rectally	Colon	4 g/60 mL enema PR QHS
Olsalazine (Dipentum)	None (cleaved in colon)	Colon	500 mg PO BID
Balsalazide (Colazal)	None (prodrug of mesalamine cleaved in colon)	Colon	750 mg PO TID

From Sandborn WJ, Hanauer SB. The pharmacokinetic profiles of oral mesalazine formulations and mesalazine pro-drugs used in the management of ulcerative colitis. Aliment Pharmacol Ther 2003;17:29 and Greeen JEB et al Balsalazide is more effective and better tolerated than mesalamine in ulcerative colitis. Gastroenterology 1998:114:15. BID, twice daily; PO, orally; PR, rectally; QHS, at bedtime; TID, three times daily.

effect profile than Asacol, some patients are unable to tolerate mesalamine and other therapies should be investigated.

IMMUNOSUPPRESSIVE AGENTS

The results of several trials suggest azathioprine and 6-MP are appropriate alternatives for patients with active UC that has not responded to systemic steroids.[18,39] These drugs are also used to maintain remission, although they are probably used more in CD than UC for this purpose (see Question 21).

CSA has also been used to treat active UC. In one clinical trial, an 82% response rate was achieved using intravenous CSA 4 mg/kg per day for severe steroid-refractory UC.[83] CSA blood levels should be obtained although correlation of clinical response and toxicity to blood levels has not been consistent. Many drug interactions and adverse effects are associated with CSA (see Chapter 35, Solid Organ Transplantation). Hypertension, gingival hyperplasia, hypertrichosis, paresthesias, tremors, headaches, electrolyte disturbances, and nephrotoxicity are common.[27] Studies using oral CSA for maintenance of remission in UC have been disappointing.[43] In C.M. a reasonable choice would be azathioprine 2.5 mg/kg/day. Monthly monitoring of white blood cell counts and periodic assessment for any signs and symptoms of pancreatitis would be appropriate.

Toxic Megacolon
SIGNS AND SYMPTOMS

14. One year has passed since C.M. last had an acute attack of UC. She has been taking azathioprine 2.5 mg/kg per day. Now she presents with a fever of 104°F, a heart rate of 110 beats/min, abdominal pain, weakness, and a sudden decrease in frequency of bowel movements. Physical examination discloses abdominal distention with nonlocalized rebound tenderness, tympany, and no bowel sounds. Abnormal laboratory values include a leukocytosis of 15,000 WBC/mm³ and serum potassium of 3.0 mEq/L (normal, 3.5 to 5.0 mEq/L). Other laboratory parameters, including serum amylase and lipase, are within normal limits. Radiographic examination of the abdomen shows the transverse colon dilated to 9 cm. What is the most probable cause of C.M.'s symptoms? What are potential sequelae of this complication of IBD?

C.M.'s signs and symptoms are consistent with an acute dilation of the colon associated with systemic toxemia. This complication of UC, commonly referred to as toxic megacolon, occurs in about 5% of patients at some time during their disease course.[20] Toxic megacolon is also a complication of Crohn's colitis and ileocolitis.

Toxic megacolon represents the most life-threatening complication of IBD and has an overall mortality rate of up to 16% with perforation. It is defined as a severe attack of colitis with total or segmental colonic dilation.[20] A patient is considered toxic if colonic dilation is present with two or more of the following symptoms: temperature >101.5°F, tachycardia with a pulse rate >100 beats/min, leukocytosis with a WBC count >10,000 cells/mm³, or hypoalbuminemia with an albumin <3.0 g/dL. Other symptoms include abdominal distention and tenderness, anemia, hypotension, and electrolyte imbalance. Signs and symptoms present in C.M. that are consistent with toxic megacolon include prostration, fever, tachycardia, electrolyte imbalance, abdominal pain and tenderness, leukocytosis, dilation of the colon to a diameter >6 cm, signs of diminished colonic peristalsis as evidenced by decreased stool frequency, and absence of bowel sounds. Other signs consistent with this diagnosis include dehydration, anemia, and hypoalbuminemia.[18]

Colonic perforation followed by peritonitis and hemorrhage is the major complication of toxic megacolon. C.M.'s condition should be considered a medical emergency.

PREDISPOSING FACTORS

15. What factors does C.M. have that predispose her to toxic megacolon? What drugs should be avoided in C.M.?

A contributing factor that predisposes C.M. to the development of toxic megacolon is hypokalemia, which decreases bowel wall muscular tone.[20,84] Other predisposing factors include the use of antispasmodics such as the opiates or anticholinergic agents; irritant cathartics such as castor oil; barium enemas; and hypoproteinemia, which produces bowel wall edema.[20,84] Although corticosteroids may be necessary for the treatment of the IBD, they may mask signs of peritonitis, a precursor to toxic megacolon.

MEDICAL MANAGEMENT

16. What medical therapeutic modalities should be considered for the treatment of C.M.'s toxic megacolon?

General supportive measures are used to arrest the necrotic process taking place in the colon. C.M.'s bowel should be allowed to rest. Nothing should be taken by mouth, and nasogastric suction should be initiated to prevent passage of swallowed air and fluid into the colon. Fluid and electrolyte imbalances must be addressed, and C.M.'s hypokalemia should be corrected as quickly as safely possible. She should also be given adequate nutritional support, including TPN, if a prolonged recovery is anticipated. High doses of intravenous corticosteroids should be initiated. C.M. is not currently taking steroids, but if she were, the dose would need to be increased to prevent adrenal insufficiency. A blood sample should be sent for culture and sensitivity, and C.M. should begin empiric antibiotic therapy because she exhibits signs and symptoms of systemic bacteremia (e.g., leukocytosis, fever, prostration). The antibiotic regimen chosen should include an agent effective against anaerobes and *Enterobacteriaceae* because both types of organisms occur in large numbers in the colon.

Other measures that may be appropriate in patients with toxic megacolon would include discontinuance of any drugs (e.g., opiates, anticholinergic agents) that decrease intestinal peristalsis and might predispose the patient to this condition. C.M. must be monitored carefully for signs of improvement or persistent dilation, perforation, peritonitis, and hemorrhage.

SURGICAL INTERVENTION

17. C.M. has been treated as previously described for 3 days. Nevertheless, her abdominal radiologic examination indicates no diminution in the caliber of the distended bowel, her temperature continues to spike to 103°F with negative blood cultures, and the abdomen remains distended and silent. Fluid and electrolyte imbalances have been restored. How should C.M. be managed at this point?

Within the first 72 hours of therapy and observation, the need for corrective surgery will be determined.[18,84] The three general patterns of response are improvement, no change, and deterioration. Those who improve with medical therapy demonstrate decreased colonic distention, a return of bowel sounds, and a decreased pulse and temperature. Medical management should be continued in these patients as long as they continue to show progress. Unfortunately, only 50% of toxic megacolon patients respond satisfactorily to medical therapy.[20]

C.M.'s course is illustrative of most patients with toxic megacolon who show fluctuating degrees of response to medical management. These patients may appear to respond initially with decreased tachycardia and fever but become toxic again in 2 to 3 days. Despite signs of improvement, change in bowel sounds or a decrease in colonic size may be variable. If these objective parameters do not improve perforation of the colon may occur unless they are managed surgically (subtotal colectomy and ileostomy). Early surgery reduces the overall mortality rate in patients such as C.M.

18. C.K. is a 49-year-old man who has had UC for 22 years. His disease is fairly well controlled with mesalamine tablets 800 mg orally three times daily. He has not had any UC flares for more than 5 years. He underwent a colonoscopy 1 week ago for routine cancer screening. Pathology results from this procedure indicate pre-metaplastic lesions in several areas of his colon. What are C.K.'s medical and surgical options for treatment of these lesions?

Of the various therapeutic modalities available for the management of UC, surgery is the most definitive form of therapy in that it is curative in most instances.[85] Because the lesions in UC are generally localized and continuous, colectomy will remove the primary focus of the disease. It will also eliminate both the extraintestinal and local complications of UC in most patients. In addition, patients may require further surgery for anastomotic leaks, intraperitoneal abscesses, adhesions, obstruction, stomal ileitis, and mechanical problems associated with the ileostomy. Patient acceptability of ileostomies is poor, and major psychologic adjustments are required of the patients and their families.[86] Patients must be given support and educated with regard to the care of their ileostomies; this includes the prevention and management of common skin problems as well as control of odor and leakage of the effluent. Therefore, even though UC can be cured by surgery, it is indicated only after all reasonable nonsurgical forms of therapy have been exhausted. Considering the degree of inflammatory damage that occurs in colonic tissue, it is probably not surprising that the risk for colon cancer is elevated in patients with UC. Therefore, surveillance colonoscopies are recommended on a regular basis (usually every 1 to 2 years after the patient has had the disease 10 years) to screen for precancerous lesions.[58] If dysplastic lesions are detected, as they have been in C.K., surgical resection is usually considered the treatment of choice. Thus, even in patients with well controlled UC, surgery may be required for cancer prevention.

CROHN'S DISEASE
Pathophysiology and Clinical Presentation

19. J.P., a 30-year-old man, was entirely well until 18 days ago when he developed crampy right lower quadrant abdominal pain associated with an increased frequency of semiformed stools (four to five per day). The pain was episodic at first, exacerbated by meals, and somewhat relieved by defecation. During this time, J.P. experienced anorexia and a 15-pound weight loss. He denied any change in vision, joint pain, or the appearance of skin rashes. He has not traveled outside the United States or taken antibiotics recently.

Physical examination is essentially normal except for soft, loose, watery stools that are streaked with fat and positive for occult blood. The abdomen is tender on palpation of the right lower quadrant. Pertinent laboratory values include: Hct, 28% (normal, 39 to 49%); Hgb, 9 g/dL (normal, 14.0 to 17.5 g/dL); WBC count, 14.0×10^9/L (normal, 4.4 to 11.3×10^9/L); and ESR, 60 mm/hr (normal, <20 mm/hr).

Results of sigmoidoscopy and rectal biopsy are negative. Stool cultures are negative, as is the examination for signs of trophozoites. A barium enema shows an edematous ileocecal valve and a terminal ileum that has a nodular irregularity of the mucosa. Follow-up endoscopy reveals a cobblestone-appearing terminal ileum with areas of normal tissue separated by diseased mucosa.

Which of J.P.'s signs, symptoms, and laboratory data are consistent with CD? Describe the pathophysiologic basis for J.P.'s clinical presentation.

J.P., like most patients with CD, presents with the classic symptom triad of abdominal pain, diarrhea, and weight loss.[21] His most frequent symptom is right lower quadrant abdominal pain, which is secondary to an indolent inflammatory process in the ileocecal area. Diarrhea is also a characteristic symptom; however, in contrast to UC, the stools usually are partly formed and gross blood is generally not visible. If the disease is limited to the colon, the diarrhea may be of the same quality and quantity as that associated with UC. If the disease is limited to the ileum, as it appears to be with J.P., the diarrhea generally is moderate, with four to six stools daily. If ileal involvement is significant, bile salt malabsorption may occur resulting in steatorrhea. Weight loss may be pronounced in patients with long-standing CD[2,21] because of anorexia and malabsorption secondary to the blind loop syndrome, bile salt malabsorption, or fistula formation, which can result in large sections of small bowel being bypassed.

Rectal bleeding often occurs in patients with CD, particularly those with colonic involvement, although it is not as common as that associated with UC. Slow blood loss may occur in patients with disease limited to the small intestine, which may cause occult blood–positive feces and, eventually, iron-deficiency anemia, as illustrated by J.P. Massive hemorrhage is usually a late complication of CD and is generally due to transmural ulceration and subsequent erosion into a major blood vessel.

J.P.'s leukocytosis and increased ESR demonstrate that, like UC, CD is a systemic disease. Extraintestinal manifestations such as arthritis, liver disease, and skin rash occur in CD with the same frequency as UC (see Table 28-2).[3] However, some types of extraintestinal disease appear to be more common in UC (e.g., primary biliary cirrhosis) than CD (e.g., pyoderma gangrenosum).[87]

Most patients with CD have recurrent, symptomatic episodes of pain and diarrhea with gradual progression of their disease to shorter and shorter asymptomatic periods. Although the clinical course is generally progressive, 10% of patients will remain essentially asymptomatic after a few acute episodes.[5] Other patients may only manifest a slight fever for years until a late complication of the disease, such as fistula formation, develops. Alternatively, CD may be rapidly progressive.

Remission Induction

20. What agents can be used to induce a remission of J.P.'s CD?

Because the clinical course of CD varies among patients, the management of this disease must be individualized. The anatomic location of the disease is also an important determinant of therapy. Most investigations evaluating the treatment of acute symptomatic CD have ignored this factor and are therefore difficult to assess or compare.[27]

Corticosteroids
Corticosteroids are the most widely used therapeutic agents for the treatment of active, symptomatic CD.[22,88] A recent systematic review of the literature confirms that steroids have a valuable role in remission induction.[35] Landmark studies have demonstrated that approximately 60% to 80% of patients with active CD will respond to a course of steroids. These agents seem to be particularly effective in ileal and ileal-colonic disease and can induce remission in even moderate-to-severe CD.

Sulfasalazine
Sulfasalazine is also widely used for treating patients with mild to moderately symptomatic CD.[22,89] Improvement generally occurs within the first 4 to 6 weeks of therapy. Sulfasalazine's beneficial effect is limited to patients with disease involving the colon or the colon and ileum; it is ineffective in patients who have small bowel disease exclusively. The effective dosage is 3 to 6 g/day and the response ranges from 38% to 62%.

Other observations concerning the use of sulfasalazine and corticosteroids in inducing remission of CD are relevant. Previously untreated patients with colonic involvement appear to respond better to sulfasalazine than to placebo or prednisone, although when anatomic distribution of disease is not considered, sulfasalazine is less effective than prednisone.[22,27] The combination of prednisone and sulfasalazine is no more effective than prednisone therapy alone and the total dose of prednisone necessary for symptomatic control is not decreased with the addition of sulfasalazine. In general, patients with mild active disease are usually started on a 5-ASA agent, while more severe disease is often treated with corticosteroids. A treatment algorithm based on guidelines[22] for the treatment of CD is depicted in Figure 28-3.

Remission Maintenance

21. After 4 weeks of prednisone 40 mg/day, J.P. experienced fewer symptoms of CD; he has one to two well-formed stools a day, increased appetite and weight, decreased abdominal pain and tenderness, and normal body temperatures. Should prednisone be discontinued? What agents are effective in maintaining remission of symptoms in patients with CD?

Corticosteroids
Once prednisone has induced remission of active symptomatic CD, attempts should be made to taper the drug.[22] The tapering schedule is usually fairly slow (typically a dose reduction of 5% to 10% per week), taking several weeks to months to complete. Several studies have demonstrated that corticosteroids are ineffective in maintaining remission in CD and many patients continue to have active disease while receiving therapy. However, a significant subset of patients (25%) with CD requires chronic administration of corticosteroids to prevent recurrence of symptoms.[90] Given the poor long-term adverse effect profile of steroids, many clinicians attempt treatment with other modalities to maintain remission.

Sulfasalazine
Large long-term studies have shown that the continued use of sulfasalazine or mesalamine in patients with symptomatic CD is not significantly more effective in preventing recurrence of symptoms than placebo, irrespective of original disease location.[89] An exception to this may be the maintenance of post-surgical CD, as a recent review concluded.[91]

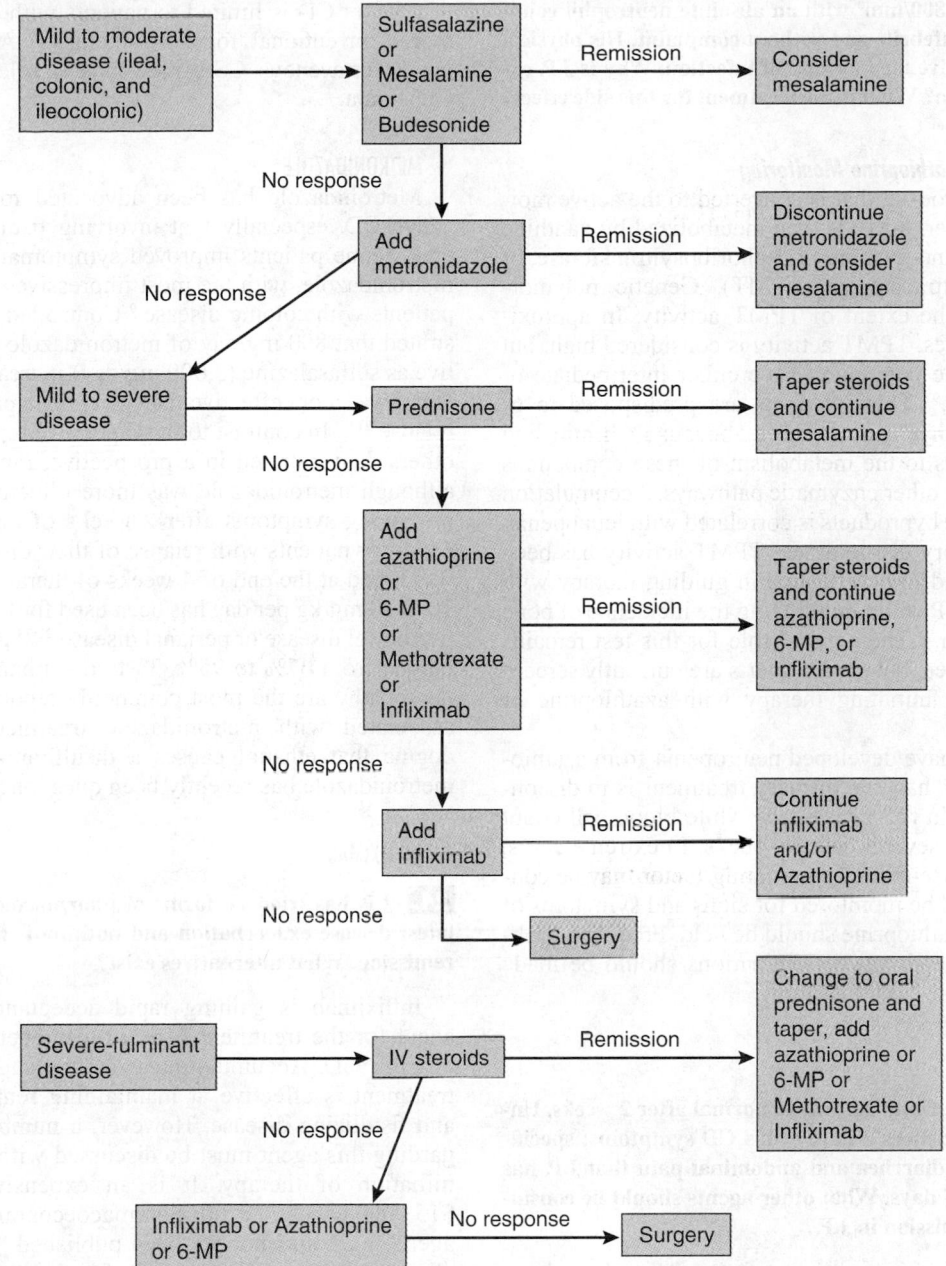

FIGURE 28-3 Treatment algorithm for Crohn's disease. (Reprinted by permission from the American College of Clinical Pharmacy. Garnett WR, Yunker NS. The treatment of inflammatory bowel disease. In: Mueller BA et al., eds. Pharmacotherapy Self-Assessment Program. 4th Ed. Gastroenterology Model. Kansas City, MO: ACCP 2002:54.)

6-Mercaptopurine/Azathioprine

Accumulating evidence suggests that both 6-MP and azathioprine have a role in maintenance treatment of CD.[92] In addition, these agents are often used as a "steroid-sparing" strategy. Most experts feel that the benefit of these drugs in decreasing recurrence of CD far outweighs possible long-term adverse effects, provided patients are appropriately monitored. Other agents with evidence to support their use in maintaining remission are MTX and infliximab.[22]

In summary, J.P.'s prednisone should be tapered as suggested above and then discontinued if possible. As the tapering regimen is started, J.P. should start 6-MP 1.5 mg/kg/day or

azathioprine 2.5 mg/kg/day. This is due to the long onset of effect for the latter drugs (usually 3 to 6 months). J. P.'s white blood cell counts should be monitored regularly and he should be counseled regarding the signs and symptoms of severe infection (e.g., fever, sore throat, or chills) and pancreatitis (e.g., severe epigastric pain and nausea).

ADVERSE EFFECTS

22. Six weeks after starting to taper J.P.'s prednisone dosage (currently 10 mg/day) and the initiation of azathioprine, he returns to the clinic for routine laboratory monitoring. His white blood cell count is 1,800/mm³ with an absolute neutrophil count of 1,100/mm³. He is afebrile and without complaint. His physical examination is negative for any sign of infection. Why is J.P. experiencing leukopenia? What is the treatment for this side effect?

6-Mercaptopurine/Azathioprine Monitoring

Azathioprine is a prodrug that is converted to the active moiety, 6-MP, in the liver. 6-MP is then metabolized by xanthine oxidase, hypoxanthine-guanine-phosphoribosyltransferase, or thiopurine-S-methyltransferase (TPMT). Genetic polymorphism determines the extent of TPMT activity. In approximately 90% of whites, TPMT activity is considered high, but the remainder of the population have either intermediate or low TPMT activity.[92] These patients are predisposed to 6-MP/azathioprine myelosuppression because diminished TPMT activity leads to the metabolism of these compounds being shunted to the other enzymatic pathways. Accumulation of the 6-thioguanine byproducts is correlated with leukopenia. Recently, a laboratory test to assess TPMT activity has been developed and found to be effective in guiding therapy with azathioprine or 6-MP while minimizing the incidence of bone marrow suppression.[93] The optimal role for this test remains to be fully determined, but some experts are currently screening patients before initiating therapy with azathioprine or 6-MP.

In patients who have developed neutropenia from azathioprine therapy, as J.P. has, the primary treatment is to discontinue azathioprine. In most cases, the white blood cell count will normalize over several days to weeks. In extreme cases, the use of granulocyte-colony stimulating factor may be considered.[94] J.P. should be monitored for signs and symptoms of infection and the azathioprine should be held. Frequent, probably daily, white blood cell determinations should be made until the count is above 3,000/mm³.

Other Agents

23. J.P.'s leukocyte count returns to normal after 2 weeks. Unfortunately, he experiences a flare of his CD symptoms; specifically, an increase in diarrhea and abdominal pain that J.P. has noted over the past 5 days. What other agents should be considered to maintain remission in J.P.?

A number of other immunosuppressive drugs have been examined in CD. Methotrexate produces and maintains remission in patients with refractory disease. Clinical improvement or reduction in corticosteroid dosages have been observed with 15 mg/week oral methotrexate or 25 mg/week of intramuscular or subcutaneous methotrexate in 39% to 54% of patients who had active bowel disease or fistulas.[95] In clinical studies, GI toxicity was the most common reason for discontinuing treatment, but neutropenia and liver enzyme elevations were also reported.[96] Many clinicians reserve methotrexate for patients who have failed or are intolerant of 6-MP/azathioprine. Some experts consider MTX to be inferior to 6-MP/azathioprine in CD, but no comparison studies have been published to date.

CSA has been studied for remission induction treatment in patients with severe, refractory CD. In general, low-dose CSA has not been shown to be effective at maintaining remission and higher dose CSA is not well tolerated. At present, the use of CSA in CD is limited to patients with disease resistant to more conventional forms of therapy.[97] As described previously, intravenous CSA may have a role in treating active CD fistula.

METRONIDAZOLE

Metronidazole has been advocated for the treatment of active CD, especially that involving fistulas or the perineal area. Some patients improved symptomatically while taking metronidazole, with the most impressive effects occurring in patients with colonic disease.[98] Controlled trials have demonstrated that 800 mg/day of metronidazole is at least as effective as sulfasalazine (3,000 mg/day) in treating active CD and that it was more effective than placebo in patients with disease relapse.[21,99] In contrast to these positive reports, Ambrose and others demonstrated in a prospective, randomized trial, that although metronidazole was more effective than placebo in improving symptoms after 2 weeks of therapy (67% versus 35%) for patients with relapse of their disease, no difference was noted at the end of 4 weeks of therapy.[100] Metronidazole 10 to 20 mg/kg per day has been used for CD patients with active bowel disease or perianal disease.[21,98] Response rates have ranged from 67% to 95%. Taste disturbances and peripheral neuropathy are the most commonly reported adverse effects associated with metronidazole treatment. The long-held dogma that ethanol causes a disulfiram-like reaction with metronidazole has recently been questioned.[101]

INFLIXIMAB

24. J.P. has tried all forms of pharmacologic therapy for his latest disease exacerbation and nothing is helping him achieve remission. What alternatives exist?

Infliximab is gaining rapid acceptance as an effective agent for the treatment of mild-to-moderate active and fistulizing CD. Accumulating evidence suggests that chronic treatment is effective at maintaining remission in standard and fistulizing disease. However, a number of concerns regarding this agent must be discussed with the patient before initiation of therapy. It is an expensive therapy (about $15,000/year) and a full pharmacoeconomic analysis of this agent in CD has not yet been published.[102] Although generally well tolerated, a number of serious adverse effects can occur. Acute and delayed hypersensitivity reactions can occur and are occasionally life threatening. Many clinicians premedicate patients with diphenhydramine, acetaminophen, or corticosteroids before an infusion; however, the most effective strategy to avoid a serious reaction is to regularly monitor vital signs during infliximab infusion and slowing the rate or stopping the infusion if any symptoms develop. The majority of reactions consist of headache, flushing, itching, and dizziness, but anaphylactoid reactions rarely occur. It is hypothesized that patients who receive regular infliximab therapy or are taking concomitant immunosuppressive drugs are at a decreased risk for these reactions.[103] Also of concern is the development of human anti-chimeric antibodies (HACA) in some patients receiving infliximab. To date no firm evidence exists that a HACA-positive patient will experience either a decreased effect or an increase in adverse reactions when treated with infliximab.

Infliximab should be avoided in patients who have a serious active infection. Due to reports that infliximab treatment may reactivate tuberculosis, all patients considered for treatment must receive a tuberculin skin test to rule out the disease (see Chapter 61, Tuberculosis). If this test is negative and, because J.P. does not appear to have any other contraindications, he would seem to be an appropriate candidate for infliximab. If latent tuberculosis is found, antitubercular treatment must be initiated before infliximab can be considered.[50] Concern that use of infliximab may increase the risk of malignancies is currently under investigation. Studies examining this issue may be difficult to interpret because CD itself may cause an increase in lymphoproliferative cancers.[44] Also, other immunosuppressant agents commonly used for CD (e.g., MTX, CSA) may increase the risk of developing cancer.[39] Current data concerning a link between infliximab use and malignancy are conflicting.[104] A recent review looking at infliximab and a similar anti–TNF-α drug, (etanercept) concluded that a possible association with anti-TNF therapy and lymphoma may exist although more data are needed to answer this question definitively.[105]

25. J.P. consents to the use of infliximab, and it is successful at keeping him symptom free. However, after 2 years of remission, J.P. is hospitalized for an acute exacerbation of right lower quadrant pain associated with abdominal distention, lack of bowel movements, and vomiting over the past 24 hours. Radiographic studies indicate partial small bowel obstruction at the terminal ileum. Is surgery indicated at this time?

SURGERY IN CROHN'S DISEASE

Because medical therapy of CD often is inadequate, 78% of patients with this disease will require surgery within 20 years of symptom onset.[6] In contrast to UC, surgical removal of the involved bowel in CD is not a definitive form of therapy. CD can recur even after extensive resections.[21] Various investigations have determined that cumulative recurrence rates after surgery for this disease are as high as 80%, depending on the surgical procedure and disease location. Therefore, multiple operations, and all their attendant risks, are often necessary over the life span of the CD patient. Depending on the amount and site of the bowel removed during surgery, specific malabsorption syndromes can occur (e.g., vitamin B_{12} malabsorption with removal of the terminal ileum). If an ileostomy is part of the surgical procedure, the patient will have to undergo significant psychologic adjustments. Therefore, surgery is indicated only for specific complications that are unresponsive to medical therapy and should be avoided if possible.[85]

Surgery is indicated at this time because of intestinal obstruction and J.P. has a well-known history of the disease that has also failed medical management using available agents. Surgery reveals that the mucosa of the terminal 40 cm of the ileum is inflamed and thickened. In all, 50 cm of the terminal ileum are removed along with the ascending colon to the hepatic flexure. The remaining small bowel is anastomosed directly to the transverse colon.

OVERVIEW OF IRRITABLE BOWEL SYNDROME

Irritable bowel syndrome (IBS) is one of the most common chronic disorders causing patients to seek medical treatment. It exerts a significant economic burden and is responsible for considerable morbidity in Western countries. Until recently, little was understood about the pathophysiology or etiology of this disorder. Indeed, some controversy exists today whether IBS is a distinct syndrome or a grouping of several chronic GI disorders. Still, investigators have made strides in understanding IBS, particularly the role of the enteric nervous system in the etiology of this disorder. As a result, new pharmacotherapeutic options are emerging for patients suffering from this often bewildering condition.

IBS can be defined as "a functional bowel disorder in which abdominal pain is associated with defecation or a change in bowel habit with features of disordered defecation and distension."[106,107] The incidence of IBS has been reported to be 15% to 20% in Western countries.[108] It is the most common disorder seen by gastroenterologists and is commonly seen by primary care clinicians as well.[109,110] Prevalence rates are dependent on IBS diagnostic criteria, which have varied over the years. A female gender predominance of about 3:1 is evident in most epidemiologic studies of IBS.[111] Some studies have demonstrated a white predominance in IBS, whereas other studies have found no such association.[112] Many patients with IBS never seek medical attention, and those who do, tend to see their physician frequently.[113] Many of these patients also suffer from other functional disorders such as fibromyalgia and interstitial cystitis and psychiatric disorders such as major depression and generalized anxiety disorder.[114] As mentioned above, the economic costs associated with IBS are considerable: it is estimated that IBS accounts for $33 billion in direct and indirect costs in the United States annually.[115]

Pathophysiology

Although knowledge of the cause of IBS remains incomplete, several theories have emerged to explain the underlying pathophysiology of this disorder. Previously, the primary cause of IBS was believed to be psychiatric or psychosomatic. This picture was at least partially validated by the finding that many IBS patients had psychiatric comorbidities. More recently, it is believed that factors such as psychological stress may exacerbate the disease, but they are not the sole cause of IBS.[116] It has long been known that IBS patients tend to exhibit visceral hypersensitivity to colonic stimulation or manipulation. Although concomitant anxiety and hypervigilance undoubtedly played a role in such observations, it is now thought that the reaction to visceral stimuli in these patients results in the perception of abdominal pain, whereas patients without IBS would have no symptoms. The etiology of this hypersensitivity is the focus of intense research efforts. Theories have emerged suggesting that the activation of silent gut nociceptors due to ischemia or infection may lead to increased abdominal pain in IBS.[116] Other experts propose that an increase in the excitability of neurons in the dorsal horn of the spinal cord lead to gut hyperalgesia. An abnormality in the processing of ascending signals from the dorsal horn may be responsible for a lower pain threshold in IBS patients. Similarly, recent findings suggest neurotransmitter abnormalities may cause the symptoms of IBS. Of particular interest is the role of serotonin (5-HT) in the etiology of this disorder. Greater than 95% of the body's 5-HT is located in the GI tract and is stored in many cells, such as enterochromaffin cells, neurons, and smooth muscle cells. When released, this 5-HT can trigger both GI smooth muscle contraction and relaxation as well as mediate GI sensory function.[117] Different 5-HT receptor subtypes may be responsible for these differing actions. Additionally, upregulation or downregulation of these receptor subtypes may produce fluctuating symptoms in some IBS patients.[107] The primary 5-HT subtypes in the GI tract are 5-HT$_3$ and 5-HT$_4$. Some data suggest that IBS patients may have higher levels of 5-HT in the colon compared with control subjects.[118] Thus, these receptors have become the target of pharmacotherapeutic manipulation for IBS.

Another proposed pathologic mechanism of IBS is altered colonic motility. Diarrhea, constipation, and abdominal bloating are common features of IBS. Patients with IBS are often categorized as having either diarrhea-predominant or constipation-predominant disease.[119] About one-half of patients with IBS report increased symptoms postprandially, and patients with diarrhea-predominant IBS (DP-IBS) have been shown to have an exaggerated response to cholecystokinin after eating, leading to increased colonic propulsions.[120] On the other hand, constipation-predominant IBS (CP-IBS) patients tend to have fewer colonic propulsions postprandially. Patients in whom bloating is the primary symptom of IBS may have gas production from poor fermentation of carbohydrates.[121] This has led investigators to search for a link between food intolerance and IBS.

Etiology

The pathogenesis of IBS is poorly understood, although consensus theories are emerging. Some investigators believe that inflammation of the GI mucosa associated with infection may be the triggering factor that results in IBS, although this notion is controversial.[122,123] Also controversial is the possible association of a history of physical or sexual abuse and the development of IBS.[116] It has been proposed that such traumatic experiences may affect the central nervous system and predispose patients to visceral hypersensitivity. Most IBS patients under emotional or psychologic stress will report an exacerbation of their symptoms, but this is not surprising considering that such stressors affect non-IBS patients' GI function as well.[123] Familial clustering of IBS patients suggests that both genetics and formative environments may play a role in the pathogenesis of this disorder.[124] Finally, food intolerances (e.g., lactose intolerance) may be involved in the etiology of IBS or may be misdiagnosed as IBS.

Diagnosis

One of the more challenging and frustrating aspects of IBS is its lack of biochemical or physical markers that are pathognomic for the disorder. Thus, the diagnosis of IBS is usually symptom based.[125] Unfortunately, this lack of "objective" criteria for diagnosis can propagate the notion that IBS is a psychological or psychosomatic disorder. Many patients express frustration with the traditional medical establishment and individual providers.[126] In addition, the lack of a definitive marker for diagnosis may lead clinicians to order excessive testing and procedures in patients with suspected IBS. To address these issues, guidelines for the diagnosis and management of IBS have been published in the United States and Canada.[125,127] Both guidelines suggest that extensive testing in IBS patients is usually unnecessary provided that patients are younger than 50 years old and do not present with any so-called "alarm symptoms" (Table 28-6). Several symptom-driven criteria have been published including the Manning criteria, the Rome I, and the Rome II criteria (Table 28-7). These diagnostic criteria have been examined for their predictive value in IBS. The U.S. guidelines recommended the Rome II criteria as the primary diagnostic schema, while the Canadian panel utilizes the Manning criteria. Both consensus panels agree that once IBS is diagnosed it should be further

Table 28-6 Alarm Symptoms Requiring Gastroenterology Consultation

Weight loss
Gastrointestinal bleeding
Anemia
Fever
Frequent nocturnal symptoms

From Fass R, et al. Evidence-and consensus-based practice guidelines for the diagnosis of irritable bowel syndrome. Arch Intern Med 2001;161:2081.

Table 28-7 Comparison of Diagnostic Criteria for Irritable Bowel Syndrome

Manning Criteria	Rome I Criteria	Rome II Criteria
Abdominal distension	>3 months of symptoms	>3 months of symptoms
Pain relief with bowel movement	Abdominal pain relieved with defecation *and/or* associated with a change of stool consistency	Abdominal pain or discomfort
More frequent stools with pain	PLUS:	PLUS:
Looser stools with pain	≥2 of the following at least 25% of the time:	≥2 of the following
Passage of mucus in stool	• Altered stool frequency	• Pain relieved with defecation *and/or*
Sensation of incomplete evacuation	• Altered stool passage	• Pain associated with a change in frequency of stool *and/or*
	• Passage of mucus in stool	• Pain associated with a change in appearance of stool
	• Bloating or feeling of abdominal distension	

From Olden KW. Diagnosis of Irritable bowel syndrome. Gastroenterology 2002;122:1701 and
Fass R, et al. Evidence-and consensus-based practice guidelines for the diagnosis of irritable bowel syndrome. Arch Intern Med 2001;161:2081.

differentiated by symptom pattern into DP-IBS, CP-IBS, or pain-predominant IBS (PP-IBS). Since there is no known cure for IBS it is logical to use these subgroups to help direct symptomatic therapy. In fact, another author suggests that a therapeutic trial of a medication may serve to diagnose and treat patients.[123] In most cases the primary clinician can successfully manage the IBS patient using the treatment algorithm depicted in Figure 28-4. However the presence of alarm symptoms or an unusual finding on routine examination (e.g., thyroid abnormality) may prompt further referrals and testing.

There are limited data concerning the natural history of IBS.[116] IBS is generally considered a benign disease with a good prognosis.[128] Patients' symptoms often wax and wane and, in some cases, the syndrome resolves spontaneously.[129]

Management

26. V.H. is a 33-year-old woman who presents with complaints of severe abdominal pain (rated 6 on a scale of 1 to 10), bloating, and the passage of hard pellet like stools about every 3 days. This has gone on for about 6 months and V.H. notices that an "attack" occurs usually after a large meal. Her past medical history is significant for a generalized anxiety disorder. Her current medications include buspirone and the Norplant birth control system.

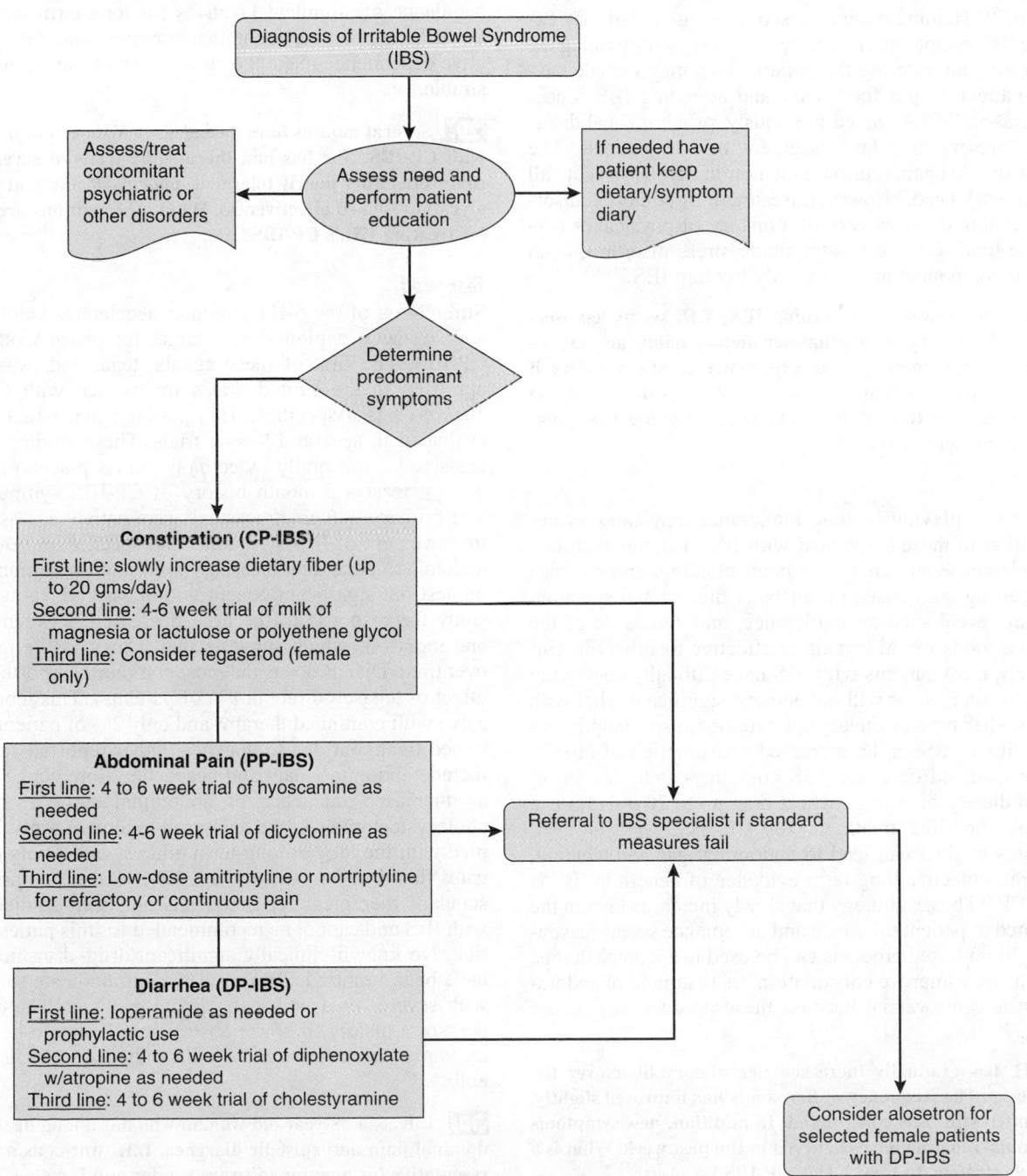

FIGURE 28-4 Treatment algorithm for irritable bowel syndrome.[123,125,127]

Her immediate family is alive and well except for a brother with depression. She drinks socially and does not smoke or use illicit drugs. V.H. is concerned that her symptoms are indicative of cancer. How should the clinician respond to V.H.'s concerns?

Patient Education

Clinicians must reassure patients with IBS that their symptoms are real. Furthermore, patients should be thoroughly counseled concerning the prognosis of IBS. Many patients are fearful that their symptoms are indicative of severe pathology such as cancer. Reassurance and education are vital to assuage fears and to reinforce the generally benign nature of this disorder. Involving patients at the earliest stages in their treatment plan is vital for patient acceptance and to avoid "doctor shopping."[113] Helping patients discover triggers that may exacerbate IBS symptoms is an effective strategy for treating the disorder and empowering the patient. This may include having the patient keep a food diary and attending IBS educational classes.[113,130] As noted previously, psychological disorders are present in a large segment of IBS patients. The clinician should again reinforce the notion that IBS is not "all in the patient's head." However, treatment of comorbid disorders, including the discovery of a history of physical or sexual abuse (and possible posttraumatic stress disorder), is an important component in successfully treating IBS.[114,131]

27. After a discussion concerning IBS, V.H. seems less worried. She relates her concern that her dietary habits are responsible for the symptoms she is experiencing. She wonders if changing her diet will "cure" her of IBS. What is the role of diet in the treatment of IBS? Will V.H. be relieved of her IBS symptoms if she changes her diet?

Diet

As mentioned previously, food intolerance may cause symptoms similar to those associated with IBS. Patients with lactose intolerance can experience pain, bloating, and diarrhea after ingesting milk-based products. A dietary and symptom diary may reveal such an intolerance, and avoidance of the implicated foods would constitute effective treatment.[113] Unfortunately, most patients with IBS have difficulty complying with exclusion diets or will not achieve significant relief with them. Another type of dietary intervention, especially in patients with CP-IBS, is the increased consumption of fiber.[132] Both the U.S. and Canadian IBS guidelines state that an increase in dietary fiber (e.g., wheat bran up to 20 g daily) is a reasonable first-line treatment for CP-IBS.[125,127] However, large doses of fiber can lead to abdominal gas and bloating, and overall objective long-term evidence of benefit in IBS is lacking.[133,134] Thus, a strategy that slowly increases fiber in the diet titrated to patient tolerance and acceptance seems reasonable. Psyllium-based products can be used to accomplish this. While this may improve constipation, its treatment of abdominal pain is controversial because these products may cause bloating.[123]

28. V.H. has gradually increased her dietary fiber over the past 6 weeks. The frequency of her stools has improved slightly, but she often still feels constipated. In addition, new symptoms of abdominal bloating have occurred in the past week. What is a reasonable strategy to treat V.H.'s CP-IBS?

Pharmacotherapy for Constipation-Predominant IBS

In patients with CP-IBS in whom fiber therapy fails, other standard laxatives may be tried for symptomatic relief.[127] Few well-designed trials looking at any laxative for IBS have been published. The Canadian IBS guidelines recommend occasional use of osmotic laxatives such as citrate of magnesia or lactulose. These agents are usually well tolerated but can occasionally cause abdominal bloating. Other adverse effects of the osmotic laxatives include diarrhea, taste disturbances, and hypermagnesemia (especially in patients with renal impairment). Some experts feel that newer laxatives containing propylene glycol may be better tolerated, but no data in IBS patients exist to support this.[116] Most authors recommend the avoidance of stimulant laxatives for long-term treatment of CP-IBS. In practice, abdominal cramping and the risk of laxative dependence make the chronic use of these agents undesirable.

29. Several months have passed since V.H. was first diagnosed with CP-IBS. She has had therapeutic trials of several agents that were either poorly tolerated (poor palatability of propylene glycol) or lacked effectiveness. What other options are available for treating V.H.'s CP-IBS?

Tegaserod

Stimulation of the 5-HT$_4$ receptor accelerates colonic transit and has been exploited as a target for pharmacotherapy of CP-IBS. The first of these agents, tegaserod, was recently approved in the United States for women with CP-IBS.[135] Tegaserod is a specific 5-HT$_4$ partial agonist that has been evaluated in several 12-week trials. These studies evaluated tegaserod 6 mg orally twice daily versus placebo in women with at least a 3-month history of CP-IBS symptoms.[136,137] The primary outcome measures were patient assessed global improvement of IBS symptoms and specific improvement in abdominal pain and bloating. The studies demonstrated a modest but significant benefit with tegaserod. In at least one study the response to the drug decreased between month 1 and month 3, which suggests that it may lose effectiveness over time. Diarrhea was the most commonly reported adverse effect of tegaserod (about 9% of patients). This tended to resolve with continued therapy, and only 2% of patients discontinued treatment due to diarrhea. Other reported side effects include abdominal pain and headache. More concerning was an increased incidence of abdominal surgeries including cholecystectomies in the tegaserod treatment arms. This coupled with the lack of long-term efficacy and safety data relegates this drug to patients with CP-IBS that has failed other standard therapies. Tegaserod has not been studied in men with IBS and cannot be recommended for this patient population. No known clinically significant drug–drug interactions have been reported. Tegaserod is contraindicated in patients with severe renal or hepatic impairment, gallbladder disorders, or a history of bowel obstruction. It should be taken on an empty stomach, as food significantly decreases its bioavailability.[138]

30. L.K. is a 38-year old woman who has a long history of abdominal pain and episodic diarrhea. L.K. works as a sales representative for a major software vendor and is called on periodically to make formal presentations. She finds that just before these presentations she develops "attacks" of abdominal pain and diarrhea. Her past medical history is significant for fibromyalgia, which manifests as chronic tiredness and fatigue. She has no other medical problems and takes no medications. She does not drink, smoke, or use illicit drugs. She has undergone an extensive workup, including colonoscopy, upper GI endoscopy with small bowel follow-through, computed tomography abdominal scans, serum electrolytes, thyroid function tests, and stool studies. All the above procedures and tests were negative, and L.K.'s gastroenterologist has diagnosed her with IBS. L.K. currently has one to two loose stools daily. They are not greasy appearing or foul smelling. She has bouts of abdominal pain (severity of 7 on a 1 to 10 scale) several times daily. She describes the pain as "stabbing" and "cramping." She has not noted any temporal relationship to meals or that certain foods exacerbate her condition. What pharmacologic options are available for L.K.'s abdominal pain? What adverse effects are associated with these medications?

Pain-Predominant IBS
Antispasmodics
Drugs that possess smooth muscle relaxation properties, usually by anticholinergic pathways, have long been used to treat IBS. In the United States, the two most commonly prescribed antispasmodics are hyoscyamine and dicyclomine, both of which possess significant anticholinergic properties.[113] Clinical trials that have examined the use of these agents in IBS have been plagued by small numbers and methodologic problems, and recently several meta-analyses have been conducted to provide insight in this area. The first analysis found that smooth muscle relaxants were superior to placebo in improving abdominal pain, although they were less effective at treating other IBS symptoms.[134] Only one of the studies examined included a drug available in the United States (dicyclomine). The second article, a systematic review, also found that antispasmodics such as cimetropium were effective in PP-IBS, but as with the first analysis, none of the agents with the highest level evidence are available in the United States.[139] A third meta-analysis reported similar results.[140] Despite this lack of objective efficacy, both the U.S. and Canadian guidelines list antispasmodics as options for PP-IBS. If prescribed, an "as needed" strategy of use is preferred to continuous dosing due to anticholinergic adverse effects.[123]

Antidepressants
Two of the meta-analyses above and the guidelines recommend the use of tricyclic antidepressants for patients with severe or continuous abdominal pain. The analgesic effects of these agents are well known, and it is thought that these agents may work by a similar mechanism in PP-IBS.[141] A separate meta-analysis that examined the use of antidepressants in IBS, found them to be effective at reducing both abdominal pain and diarrhea as well as improving global well-being.[142] A recent study examined the use of amitriptyline (in doses up to 75 mg daily) for patients with IBS.[143] It found that active treatment did improve feelings of well-being and abdominal pain, but had a large dropout rate due to adverse effects. Low doses of tricyclic antidepressants (e.g., amitriptyline 10 to 25 mg at

bedtime) are often effective in relieving abdominal pain and diarrhea. A 3-month trial at a target dose of drug (e.g., amitriptyline 50 mg) should be attempted before therapeutic failure is confirmed.[123] Anticholinergic adverse effects can be problematic, especially in patients who are experiencing constipation. Other adverse effects (sedation, dry mouth and eyes, urinary retention, and weight gain) are common and often limit the usefulness of these agents. The evidence supporting the use of other antidepressants such as fluoxetine in IBS is limited.[116]

31. Two weeks after L.K. starts nortriptyline 25 mg Q HS, she reports significant relief from both her abdominal pain and fatigue. She reports that she is sleeping better and she now rates her pain as a 2 on a 1 to 10 scale. Her diarrhea has improved somewhat; however, she still suffers from a "diarrhea attack" before each presentation she gives. What other treatments are available for DP-IBS? Are there any new agents to treat this disorder, and what are the risks and benefits of these treatments?

Diarrhea-Predominant IBS
Standard Antidiarrheals
Small bowel and colonic transit is accelerated in patients with DP-IBS; thus, drugs that slow this process should be effective in relieving diarrhea.[123] Loperamide, an opioid agonist that penetrates poorly into the central nervous system is the preferred agent for DP-IBS.[113] Meta-analyses have found loperamide to be an effective agent for improving diarrhea and in some cases improving patients' global well-being.[134,139] As with the antispasmodics, "as-needed" treatment is preferred to scheduled dosing (e.g., 2 to 4 mg orally up to four times daily as needed). Prophylactic dosing before a stressful situation or an event during which bathroom access is limited is particularly effective. Diphenoxylate with atropine is generally considered a second-line agent due to its increased risk of anticholinergic adverse effects. Finally, cholestyramine is occasionally used in refractory cases of DP-IBS, especially when bile acid malabsorption is suspected.[144] This agent is often poorly tolerated due to palatability problems. Cholestyramine also has a significant number of drug interactions of which the clinician must be aware (see Chapter 13, Dyslipidemias).

Alosetron
In February 2000, alosetron became the first drug approved by the Food and Drug Administration for the specific treatment of IBS. This was based on several clinical trials that demonstrated a mild but significant improvement in the symptoms of diarrhea, fecal urgency, and abdominal pain in female patients with IBS.[145–147] Alosetron is a highly potent 5-HT$_3$ receptor antagonist that slows colonic transit time, increases intraluminal sodium absorption, and decreases small intestinal secretions.[148] The bioavailability of the drug is about 60% and is not affected by food. It is metabolized extensively by several pathways including the cytochrome-p450 system (including the CYP 2C9 [30%] and CYP 3A4 [18%] isoenzymes), but no clinically significant interactions have been reported to date. Constipation was the most frequently reported adverse effect in these studies (approximately 30% of alosetron patients) with approximately 10% of patients withdrawing from studies

for this reason.[148] Postmarketing reports of severe constipation with cases of bowel obstructions and ischemic colitis were reported.[149] Bowel perforation and, rarely, death were also reported with alosetron use, and the drug was voluntarily withdrawn from the market in November 2000. Following extensive lobbying by several patient groups, alosetron was reintroduced to the U.S. market in June 2002 with restricted conditions for use. Prescribers must be registered with the drug manufacturer and patients must sign a patient-physician agreement and be provided with a written medication guide. The new starting dose and regimen for alosetron is 1 mg orally daily for 1 month. If, after 4 weeks, this is well tolerated but does not adequately control IBS symptoms, then the

dosage can be increased to 1 mg twice daily.[150] It is imperative that patients not start alosetron if they have a history of problems with constipation, have any history of bowel obstruction or ischemic colitis, have IBD, or a thromboembolic disorder. Patients must immediately discontinue alosetron if they become constipated or have symptoms of ischemic colitis, such as new or worsening abdominal pain, bloody diarrhea, or blood in the stool. If, after 1 month at the 1 mg BID dose patients do not have improvement of their IBS symptoms, they should discontinue treatment. Because of the serious risks involved, only patients who have had DP-IBS for longer than 6 months that has failed standard treatment should be considered for alosetron.

REFERENCES

1. Papadakis KA, Targan SR. Current theories on the causes of inflammatory bowel disease. Gastro Clin North Am 1999;28:283.
2. Botoman VA et al. Management of inflammatory bowel disease. Am Fam Physician 1998;57:57.
3. Andres PG, Friedman S. Epidemiology and the natural course of inflammatory bowel disease. Gastro Clin North Am 1999;28:255.
4. Bickston SJ, Cominelli F. Inflammatory bowel disease: short and long-term treatments. In: Schrier RW et al., eds. Advances in Internal Medicine. St. Louis: Mosby, 1998:143.
5. Podolsky DK. Inflammatory bowel disease. N Engl J Med 2002;347:417.
6. Loftus EV et al. The epidemiology and natural history of Crohn's disease in population-based patient cohorts from North America: a systematic review. Aliment Pharmacol Ther 2002;16:51.
7. Pardi DS et al. Treatment of inflammatory bowel disease in the elderly: an update. Drugs Aging 2002;19:355.
8. Fiocchi C. Inflammatory bowel disease: etiology and pathogenesis. Gastroenterology 1998;115:182.
9. Cho JH. The Nod2 gene in Crohn's disease: implications for future research into the genetics and immunology of Crohn's disease. Inflamm Bowel Dis 2001:7:271.
10. Evans JM et al. Non-steroidal anti-inflammatories are associated with emergence admission to hospital for colitis due to inflammatory bowel disease. Gut 1997;40:619.
11. Swidsinski A et al. Mucosal flora in inflammatory bowel disease. Gastroenterology 2002;122:44.
12. Elson CO, McCabe RP. Immunology of inflammatory bowel disease. In: Kirsner JB, Shorter RP, eds. Inflammatory Bowel Disease. Baltimore: Williams & Wilkins, 1995:203.
13. Targan SR. The lamina propria: a dynamic, complex mucosal compartment: an overview. Ann NY Acad Sci 1992;664:61.
14. Targan S et al. Definition of a lamina propria T cell responsive state: enhanced cytokine responsiveness of T cells stimulated through the CD2 pathway. J Immunol 1995;154:664.
15. Targan SR et al. Immunologic mechanisms intestinal diseases. Ann Intern Med 1987;106:853.
16. Konstantinos A et al. Current theories on the causes of inflammatory bowel disease. Gastro Clin North Am 1999;28:283.
17. Stotland BR et al. Medical therapies for inflammatory bowel disease. Hosp Pract 1998;33:141.
18. Kornbluth A, Sachar DB. Ulcerative colitis practice guidelines in adults. Am J Gastroenterol 1997; 92:204.
19. Langholtz E et al. Incidence and prevalence of ulcerative colitis in Copenhagen county from 1962–1987. Scand J Gastroenterol 1991;26:1247.
20. Jewell DP. Ulcerative colitis. In: Feldman M et al., eds. Gastrointestinal and Liver Disease. 6th Ed. Philadelphia: WB Saunders, 1998:1735.

21. Kornblum A et al. Crohn's disease. In: Feldman M et al, eds. Gastrointestinal and Liver Disease. 6th Ed. Philadelphia: WB Saunders; 1998:1708.
22. Hanauer SB, Sandborn W. Management of Crohn's disease in adults. Am J Gastroenterol 2001;96:635.
23. Das KM et al. Clinical pharmacokinetics of sulfasalazine. Clin Pharmacokinet 1976;1:406.
24. Klotz U et al. Therapeutic efficacy of sulfasalazine and its metabolites in patients with ulcerative colitis and Crohn's disease. N Engl J Med 1980;303:1499.
25. Sandborn WJ, Hanauer SB. The pharmacokinetic profiles of oral mesalazine formulations and mesalazine pro-drugs used in the management of ulcerative colitis. Aliment Pharmacol Ther 2003; 17:29.
26. Azad Khan AK et al. Tissue and bacterial splitting of sulfasalazine. Clin Sci 1983;64:349.
27. Stein RB, Hanauer SB. Medical therapy for inflammatory bowel disease. Gastro Clin North Am 1999; 2:297.
28. Bitton A. Medical management of ulcerative proctitis, proctosigmoiditis, and left-sided colitis. Semin Gastrointest Dis 2001;12: 263.
29. Katz S. Update in medical therapy of ulcerative colitis. J Clin Gatroenterol 2002;34:397.
30. Greeen JEB et al Balsalazide is more effective and better tolerated than mesalamine in ulcerative colitis. Gastroenterology 1998;114:15.
31. Safdi Met al. A double-blind comparison of oral versus rectal mesalamine versus combination therapy in the treatment of distal ulcerative colitis. Am J Gastroenterol 1997;92:1867.
32. Lowry PW et al. Balsalazide and azathioprine or 6-mercaptopurine: evidence for a potentially serious drug interaction. Gastroenterology 1999;116:1505.
33. Marshall JK, Irvine EJ. Rectal corticosteroids versus alternative treatments in ulcerative colitis: a meta-analysis. Gut 1997;40:775.
34. Hanauer SB et al. The pharmacology of anti-inflammatory drugs in inflammatory bowel disease. In: Kirsner JB, Shorter RP, eds. Inflammatory Bowel Disease. Baltimore: Williams & Wilkins, 1995:643.
35. Sang YX, Lichtenstein GR. Corticosteroids in Crohn's disease. Am J Gastroenterol 2002;97:803.
36. Papi C et al. Budesonide in the treatment of Crohn's disease: a meta-analysis. Aliment Pharmacol Ther 2000;14;1419.
37. Cortot A et al. Switch from systemic steroids to budesonide in steroid dependent patients with inactive Crohn's disease. Gut 2001:48:186.
38. Hanauer SB. Drug therapy: inflammatory bowel disease. N Engl J Med 1996;334:841.
39. Sandborn WJ. A review of immune modifier therapy for inflammatory bowel disease; azathioprine, 6-mercaptopurine, cyclosporin and methotrexate. Am J Gastroenterol 1996;91:423.
40. Oren R et al. Methotrexate in ulcerative colitis: a double blind, randomized Israeli multicenter trial. Gastroenterology 1996;110:1416.

41. Feagen BG et al. Methotrexate for the treatment of Crohn's disease. N Engl J Med 1995;332:292.
42. Feagan BG et al. A comparison of methotrexate with placebo for the maintenance of remission in Crohn's disease. N Engl J Med 2000;342:1627.
43. Farrell RJ, Peppercorn MA. Ulcerative colitis. Lancet 2002;359:331.
44. Blam ME et al. Integrating anti-tumor necrosis factor therapy in inflammatory bowel disease: current and future perspectives. Am J Gastroenterol 2001;96:1977.
45. Targan SR et al. A short-term study of chimeric monoclonal antibody cA2 to tumor necrosis factor alpha for Crohn's disease. N Engl J Med 1997; 337:1145.
46. Hanauer SB et al. Maintenance infliximab for Crohn's disease: the ACCENT I randomised trial. Lancet 2002;359:1541.
47. Present DH et al. Infliximab for the treatment of fistula in patients with Crohn's disease. N Engl J Med 1999;340:1398.
48. Sands B et al. Long-term treatment of fistulizing Crohn's disease: response to infliximab in ACCENT II trial through 54 weeks. [Abstract 671] Gastroenterology 2002;122:A-81.
49. Riegart-Johnson DL et al. Delayed hypersensitivity reaction and acute respiratory distress syndrome following infliximab infusion. Inflamm Bowel Dis 2002;8:186.
50. Remecade Package Insert, Centocor, Inc., Malvern, PA 2002.
51. Keane Jet al. Tuberculosis associated with infliximab a tumor necrosis factor alpha-neutralizing agent. N Engl J Med 2001;345:1098.
52. Turunen U et al. A double-blind, placebo controlled six-month trial of ciprofloxacin treatment improved prognosis in UC. Gastroenterology 1994; 106: A786.
53. Achkar JP, Hanauer SB. Medical therapy to reduce postoperative Crohn's disease recurrence. Am J Gastroenterol 2000;95:1139.
54. Greenbloom SL et al. Combination ciprofloxacin and metronidazole for active Crohn's disease. Can J Gastroenterol 1998;12:53.
55. O'Keefe SJ, Rooser BG. Nutrition and inflammatory bowel disease. In: Targan SR, Shanahan F, eds. Inflammatory Bowel Disease: From Bench to Bedside. Baltimore: Williams & Wilkins, 1994:461.
56. Stenson WF et al. Dietary supplementation with fish oil in ulcerative colitis. Ann Intern Med 1992; 116:609.
57. Patz J et al. Treatment of distal ulcerative colitis with short-chain fatty acid enemas. Am J Gastroenterol 1996;91:73.
58. Eaden JA, Mayberry JF. Colorectal cancer complicating ulcerative colitis: a review. Am J Gastroenterol 2000; 95:2710.
59. Myers S. Medical management and prognosis. In: Haubrich W, Schaffner F, eds. Gastroenterology. Philadelphia: WB Saunders, 1995:1498.

60. Marshall JK, Irvine EJ. Putting rectal 5-aminosalicylic acid in its place: the role in distal ulcerative colitis. Am J Gastroenterol 2000;95:1628.

61. Aspen Board of Directors and The Clinical Guidelines Task Force. Guidelines for the use of parenteral and enteral nutrition in adult and pediatric patients. JPEN 2002;26(1 Suppl):1SA .

62. Marshall JK, Irvine EJ. Topical aminosalicylate (ASA) therapy for distal ulcerative colitis: a meta-analysis. Gastroenterology 1994;106:A1037.

63. Marshall JK, Irvine EJ. Rectal corticosteroids versus alternative treatments in UC: a meta-analysis. Gut 1997;40:1751.

64. Peppercorn MA. Advances in drug therapy for inflammatory bowel disease. Ann Intern Med 1990; 112:50.

65. Hanauer SB. Dose-ranging study of mesalamine (Pentasa) enemas in the treatment of acute ulcerative proctosigmoiditis: results of a multi-centered placebo-controlled trial. The US Pentasa Enema Study Group. Inflamm Bowel Dis 1998;4:79.

66. Lima JJ et al. Bioavailability of hydrocortisone retention enemas in normal subjects. Am J Gastroenterol 1980;73:232.

67. Ardizzone S, Porro GB. Comparative tolerability of therapies for ulcerative colitis. Drug Saf 2002; 25:561.

68. Cino M, Greenberg GR. Bone mineral density in Crohn's disease: a longitudinal study of budesonide, prednisone and non-steroid therapy. Am J Gastroenterol 2002;97:915.

69. Anonymous. Recommendations for the Prevention and Treatment of Glucocorticoid-Induced Osteoporosis: 2001 Update. Arthritis Rheum 2001;44: 1496.

70. Hanauer S et al. Mesalamine capsules for treatment of active ulcerative colitis. Am J Gastroenterol 1993;88:1188.

71. Holdsworth CD. Sulfasalazine desensitization. Br Med J (Clin Res) 1981;282:110.

72. Kastrup EK, ed. Sulfasalazine. In: Drug Facts and Comparisons. St. Louis: Facts and Comparisons, 2000:1162.

73. Korelitz BI et al. Desensitization to sulfasalazine in allergic patients with IBD: an important therapeutic modality. Gastroenterology 1982;82:1104.

74. Alstead EM. Inflammatory bowel disease in pregnancy. Postgrad Med J 2002;78:23.

75. Diav-Citrin O. The safety of mesalazine in human pregnancy: a prospective controlled cohort study. Gastroenterology 1998;114:23.

76. Hanan IM. Inflammatory bowel disease in the pregnant woman. Comp Ther 1998;24(9):409.

77. Briggs GG et al., eds. Sulfasalazine. In: Drugs in Pregnancy and Lactation. 5th Ed. Baltimore: Williams & Wilkins, 1998:984.

78. Korelitz BI. Inflammatory bowel disease and pregnancy. Gastroenterol Clin North Am 1998;27:213.

79. Briggs GG et al., eds. Metronidazole. In: Drugs in Pregnancy and Lactation. 5th Ed. Baltimore: Williams & Wilkins, 1998:723.

80. Schroeder KW et al. Coated oral 5-aminosalicylic acid therapy for mild to moderate active ulcerative colitis: a randomized study. N Engl J Med 1987;317:1625.

81. Yu DK et al. Pharmacokinetics of Pentasa capsules in man. Pharm Res 1991;8(Suppl 10):S315.

82. Miner P et al. Maintenance of remission in ulcerative colitis patients with controlled-release mesalamine capsules (Pentasa). Gastroenterology 1992;102(4 Pt 2):A666.

83. Lichtiger S et al. Cyclosporin in severe ulcerative colitis refractory to steroid therapy. N Engl J Med 1994;330:1841.

84. Berg DF et al. Acute surgical emergencies in inflammatory bowel disease. Am J Surg 2002;184:45.

85. Becker JM. Surgical therapy for ulcerative colitis and Crohn's disease. Gastroenterol Clin North Am 1999;28(2):371.

86. Robb B, Pritts T. Quality of life in patients undergoing ileal pouch-anal anastomosis at the University of Cincinnati. Am J Surg 2002;183(4):353.

87. Gasche C. Complications of inflammatory bowel disease. Hepatogastroenterology 2000;47:49.

88. Saloman P et al. How effective are current drugs for Crohn's disease? A meta-analysis. J Clin Gastroenterol 1992;14:211.

89. Gisbert JP et al. Role of 5-aminosalicylic acid (5-ASA) in treatment of inflammatory bowel disease: a systematic review. Dig Dis Sci 2002;47:471.

90. Faubion WA et al. The natural history of corticosteroid therapy for inflammatory bowel disease: a population-based study. Gastroenterology 2001; 121:255.

91. Achkar JP, Hanauer SB. Medical therapy to reduce postoperative Crohn's disease recurrence. Am J Gastroenterol 2000;95:1139.

92. Nielsen OH et al. Review article: the treatment of inflammatory bowel disease with 6-mercaptopurine or azathioprine. Aliment Pharmacol Ther 2001;15:1699.

93. Cuffari et al. Use of erythrocyte 6-thioguanine metabolite levels to optimize azathioprine therapy in patients with inflammatory bowel disease. Gut 2001;48:642.

94. Turgeon N et al. Safety and efficacy of granulocyte colony-stimulating factor in kidney and liver transplant recipients. Transpl Infect Dis 2000; 2:15.

95. Arora S et al. A double-blind, randomized, placebo-controlled trial of methotrexate in CD. Gastroenterology 1993;102:A591.

96. Fraser AG et al. The efficacy of methotrexate for maintaining remission in inflammatory bowel disease. Aliment Pharmacol Ther 2002;16:693.

97. Sands BE. Medical therapy of steroid-resistant Crohn's disease. Can J Gastroenterol 2000; 14(Suppl C):33C.

98. Van Kruiningen HJ. On the use of antibiotics in Crohn's disease. J Clin Gastroenterol 1995;20: 310.

99. Ursling B et al. A comparative study of metronidazole and sulfasalazine for active Crohn's disease: the cooperative Crohn's disease study in Sweden. II. Results. Gastroenterology 1982;83: 550.

100. Ambrose NS et al. Antibiotic therapy for treatment in relapse of intestinal Crohn's disease. Dis Colon Rectum 1985;28:81.

101. Visapaa JP et al. Lack of disulfiram-like reaction with metronidazole and ethanol. Ann Pharmacother 2002;36:971.

102. Lombardi DA et al. Medical management of inflammatory bowel disease in the new millennium. Compr Ther 2002;28:39.

103. Panaccione R. Infliximab for the treatment of Crohn's disease: review and indications for clinical use in Canada. Can J Gastroenterol 2001; 15:371.

104. Bickston SJ et al. The relationship between infliximab treatment and lymphoma in Crohn's disease. Gastroenterology 1999;117:1433.

105. Brown SL, Greene MH. Tumor necrosis factor antagonist therapy and lymphoma: twenty-six cases reported to the Food and Drug Administration. Arthritis Rheum 2002;46:3151.

106. Drossmen DA et al. Rome II: a multinational consensus document on functional gastrointestinal disorders. Gut 1999;45(Suppl 2):1.

107. Talley NJ. Serotoninergic neuroenteric modulators. Lancet 2001;358:2061.

108. Drossman DA et al. Irritable bowel syndrome: a technical review for practice guideline development. Gastroenterology 1997;112:2120.

109. Everheart JE et al. Irritable bowel syndrome in office-based practice in the United States. Gastroenterology 1991;100:998.

110. Mirchell CM et al. Survey of the AGA membership relating to patients with functional gastrointestinal disorders. Gastroenterology 1987;92:121.

111. Sandler R. Epidemiology of irritable bowel syndrome in the United States. Gastroenterology 1990;99:409.

112. Olden KW. Diagnosis of irritable bowel syndrome. Gastroenterology 2002;122:1701.

113. Horwitz BJ et al. The irritable bowel syndrome. N Engl J Med 2001;344:1846.

114. Ballenger JC et al. Consensus statement on depression, anxiety, and functional gastrointestinal disorders. J Clin Psychiatry 2001;62(Suppl 8):48.

115. Talley NJ. Medical costs in community subjects with irritable bowel syndrome. Gastroenterology 1995;109:1736.

116. Talley NJ. Irritable bowel syndrome: a little understood organic bowel disease? Lancet 2002;360:555.

117. Kim DY et al. Serotonin: a mediator of the brain-gut connection. Gastroenterology 2000;95:2698.

118. Bearcroft CP et al. Postprandial plams 5-hydroxytryptamine in diarrhoea predominant irritable bowel syndrome: a pilot study. Gut 1998;42:42.

119. Ragnarsson G et al. Division of the irritable bowel syndrome into subgroups on the basis of recorded symptoms in two outpatients samples. Scand J Gastroenterol 1999;34:993.

120. Chey WY et al. Colonic motility abnormality in patients with irritable bowel syndrome exhibiting abdominal pain and diarrhea. Am J Gastroenterol 2001;96:1499.

121. King TS et al. Abnormal colonic fermentation in irritable bowel syndrome lancet 1998;352:1187.

122. Gwee KA et al. The role of psychological and biological factors in postinfective gut dysfunction. Gut 1999;44:400.

123. Camilleri M. Management of the irritable bowel syndrome. Gastroenterology 2001;120:652.

124. Morris-Yates AD et al. Evidence of a genetic contribution to functional bowel disorder. Am J Gastroenterol 1998;93:1311.

125. Fass R et al. Evidence-and consensus-based practice guidelines for the diagnosis of irritable bowel syndrome. Arch Intern Med 2001;161:2081.

126. Bertram S et al. The patient's perspective of irritable bowel syndrome. J Fam Pract 2001;50:521.

127. Paterson WG et al. Recommendations for the management of irritable bowel syndrome in family practice. Can Med Assoc J 1999;161:154.

128. Owens DM et al. The irritable bowel syndrome: long-term prognosis and the physician-patient interaction. Ann Intern Med 1995;122:107.

129. Janssen HA et al. The clinical course and prognostic determinants of the irritable bowel syndrome: a literature review. Scand J Gastroenterol 1998,33:561.

130. Colwell LJ et al. Effects of an irritable bowel syndrome educational class on health-promoting behaviors and symptoms. Am J Gastroenterol 1998;93:901.

131. Drossman DA. Diagnosing and treating patients with refractory functional gastrointestinal disorders. Ann Intern Med 1995;122:107.

132. Cann PA et al. What is the benefit of coarse wheat bran in patients with irritable bowel syndrome? Gut 1984;25:168.

133. WA Voderholzer et al. Clinical response to dietary fiber treatment of chronic constipation. Am J Gatroenterol 1997;92:95.

134. Jailwala J et al. Pharmacologic treatment of the irritable bowel syndrome: a systemic review of randomized, controlled trials. Ann Intern Med 2000;133:136.

135. Zelnorm product information, Novartis Pharmaceuticals, http://www.zelnorm.com/pi_hcp.jsp. Accessed November 30, 2002.

136. Muller-Lissner SA et al. Tegaserod, a 5-HT4 receptor partial agonist, relieves symptoms in irritable bowel syndrome patients, with abdominal pain, bloating, and constipation. Aliment Pharmacol Ther 2001;15:1655.

137. Novick J et al. A randomized, double-blind, placebo-controlled trial of tegaserod in female patients suffering from irritable bowel syndrome with constipation. Aliment Pharmacol Ther 2002;16:1877.

138. Appel-Dingemanse S. Clinical pharmacokinetics of Tegaserod, a serotonin 5-HT(4) receptor partial agonist with promotile activity. Clin Pharmacokinet 2002;41:1021.

139. Akehurst R et al. Treatment of irritable bowel syndrome: a review of randomized controlled trials. Gut 2001;48:272.

140. Poynard T et al. Meta-analysis of smooth muscle relaxants in the treatment of irritable bowel syndrome. Aliment Pharmacol Ther 2001;15:355.
141. Clouse RE. Antidepressants for functional intestinal syndromes. Dig Dis Sci 1994;39:2352.
142. Jackson JL et al. Treatment of functional gastrointestinal disorders with antidepressant medications: a meta-analysis. Am J Med 2000;108:65.
143. Rajagopalan M et al. Symptom relief with amitriptyline in the irritable bowel syndrome. J Gastroenterol Hepatol 1998;13:738.
144. Wilkliams AJK et al. Idiopathic bile acid malabsorption- a review of clinical presentation, diag-

nosis, and response to treatment. Gut 1991; 32:1004.
145. Camilleri M. Improvement in pain and bowel function in female irritable bowel patients with alosetron, a 5-HT receptor antagonist. Aliment Pharmacol Ther 1999;13:1149.
146. Camilleri M. Efficacy and safety of alosetron in women with irritable bowel syndrome: a randomised, placebo-controlled trial. Lancet 2000; 355:1035.
147. Camilleri M et al. A randomized controlled trial of the serotonin type 3 receptor antagonist alosetron in women with diarrhea-predominant irritable

bowel syndrome. Arch Intern Med 2001;161: 1733.
148. Talley N. Serotinergic neuroenteric modulators. Lancet 2001;358:2061.
149. Moynihan R. Alosetron: a case study in regulatory capture, or a victory for patients' rights. BMJ 2002;325:592.
150. Lotronex prescribing information. GlaxoSmithKine, Inc. September 2002.

Alcoholic Cirrhosis

Ali J. Olyaei

OVERVIEW

Cirrhosis, or end-stage liver disease, can be defined as a chronic disease of the liver with widespread hepatic parenchymal cell injury and hepatocyte destruction. Hyperplasia of fibrous connective tissue, nodular regeneration, and nonspecific inflammation around injured hepatocytes consequently develop.[1] This nonspecific pathologic process may ultimately cause anatomic and functional abnormalities of blood vessels and bile ducts, which serve as the basis for jaundice and the development of portal hypertension and the associated complications of ascites and esophageal varices. Recent advances in virology, microbiology, immunology, and hepatology have allowed more precise classification of end-stage liver diseases. Alcohol, viral illness, biliary dysfunction, metabolic disorders, inherited disorders, and drugs have all been implicated as causes of end-stage liver disease.[2,3] The most common causes of cirrhosis worldwide are viral hepatitis and alcoholism. Approximately 80% of chronic alcoholics develop fatty infiltration of the liver, up to 30% develop alcoholic hepatitis, and less than 10% develop end-stage liver disease.[4] Malnutrition and genetic factors may also contribute to the high incidence of alcohol-induced cirrhosis in the U.S. population.[5]

The objective of this chapter is to present a comprehensive and up-to date account of the pathophysiology and complications of alcoholic liver disease to health care providers. In addition, this chapter reviews the complications of cirrhosis and presents a clear and concise pharmacologic approach to their management which is consistent with practice guidelines published by the American College of Gastroenterology.[6–10] While these guidelines provide evidence-based recommendations for care, providers should use clinical judgment and experience to individualize drug therapy for patients with end-stage liver disease.

Pathogenesis

Alcohol-related liver disease includes steatosis, hepatitis, and cirrhosis. The pathogenesis of alcoholic cirrhosis is not completely understood.[11–13] Fatty infiltration of the liver is usually considered a benign and reversible condition, while progression to alcoholic hepatitis and cirrhosis is often irreversible and life threatening. Although alcohol by itself does not induce hepatocyte necrosis or acute hepatic failure, it can cause fatty infiltration and ultrastructural changes in the liver of animals and humans.[11] Approximately 80 g per day of alcohol (6 to 8 drinks) for several years is necessary to develop alcoholic liver disease. Women are at greater risk of alcoholic liver disease compared with men for any given amount of alcohol consumption. The major goals for treatment of alcoholic liver disease include alcohol abstinence, supportive care, prevention and treatment of complications of infection and portal hypertension, and aggressive nutritional support to maintain a positive nitrogen balance.

In alcoholic liver disease, the oxidation of alcohol increases the NADH:NAD [RC1]ratio, which leads to steatosis or fatty liver by increasing fatty acid and triglyceride synthesis and accumulation within the hepatocytes. These initial lesions may become necrotic with inflammatory infiltrates and fibrosis, which lead to hepatocellular injury. The continued abuse of alcohol can induce a nonspecific inflammation, which is most often reversible. This stage of alcoholic liver disease is called *alcoholic hepatitis*. In some patients, alcoholic liver disease can progress to cirrhosis, which is characterized by irreversible hepatocyte injury and the formation of scar tissue.[11–13]

Recent data suggest that the development of alcoholic liver disease is a consequence of immunologic/inflammatory host responses to alcohol injury. Cytokines, specifically tumor necrosis factor-alpha (TNF-α), play a pivotal role in hepatocyte necrosis and apoptosis. Under normal conditions, TNF-α is produced by macrophages in the liver (Kupffer cells) in response to inflammatory insults. However, following excessive exposure to hepatotoxins (e.g., alcohol), cytokines, and chemokines (produced and released from Kupffer cells) enhance infiltration of leukocytes and antibodies into the hepatocytes. This further increases the release of degradative proteins. These cytokines (TGF-β$_1$, platelet-derived growth factor, and endothelin) may also induce production of myofibroblasts and other inflammatory cytokines to increase the formation of collagen matrix in the liver (hepatic fibrosis). In addition, elevations of antibodies against lipocytes are hepatotoxic (direct antibody production against self-antigens).[14–16]

As stated earlier, up to 30% of alcoholics develop alcoholic hepatitis, but not all progress to hepatic fibrosis or alcoholic cirrhosis. It is difficult to predict in which patients end-stage liver disease will develop. Genetic predisposition, exposure to other hepatotoxins, and viral hepatitis are risk factors for the development of cirrhosis in individuals. Women develop alcoholic hepatitis in a shorter period than men. Patients who are infected with hepatitis C virus and who drink alcohol chronically are at a greater risk for cirrhosis development.[17]

At one time, the development of alcoholic liver disease was considered to be influenced by nutritional deficits. Although a high-fat, low-carbohydrate diet may promote the hepatotoxic effect of alcohol, improved nutrition and vitamin supplements do not prevent or improve alcohol-induced lesions in humans. In fact, both excessive weight and anorexia nervosa are associated with increased risk of end-stage liver disease in alcoholic individuals.[18]

Clinical Features
Common Symptoms
There is no pathognomonic pattern of physical signs and symptoms for alcoholic liver disease. Alcoholic fatty liver is predominantly an asymptomatic condition that develops in response to a short duration (a few days) of alcohol abuse. The spectrum of early stage alcoholic liver disease encompasses a wide variety of symptoms including anorexia, nausea, abdominal discomfort, weakness, weight loss, and malaise. Severe alcoholic hepatitis is characterized by advanced symptoms secondary to portal hypertension including gastrointestinal (GI) bleeding, ascites, and hepatic encephalopathy.

The clinical presentation for end-stage alcoholic liver disease is similar to other causes of liver damage. Some patients with chronic alcohol abuse and advanced liver disease present with extrahepatic manifestations including peripheral neuropathy, dementia, cardiomyopathy, and poor nutritional status.[18]

On physical examination, enlargement of the liver and spleen and evidence of portal hypertension (e.g., ascites, peripheral edema, jaundice) may be noted. Spider angiomas (branched, fiery red dilated capillaries in the skin consisting of a central point from which superficial arterioles radiate, giving the appearance of a spider's legs) are often observed in patients with advanced liver disease.[2,3] Palmar erythema, another nonspecific finding in patients with advanced liver disease, occurs more commonly with cirrhosis caused by alcohol than by other causes. It manifests as an intense diffuse flushing of the skin over the "meaty" part of the palm opposite from the thumb.[2,3]

Portal Hypertension
The portal vein collects venous blood from the splanchnic circulation (GI tract, pancreas, and spleen) and transports blood to the liver (Fig. 29-1). Portal blood contains high concentrations of oxygen, nutrients, and bacterial waste, which must cross a high-resistance capillary system within intrahepatic sinusoids. In a healthy liver, approximately 1,500 mL of blood pass through the portal vein every minute providing a detoxifying mechanism for ingested toxins and contributing to the presystemic ("first pass") metabolism of certain drugs. Normal portal pressure is between 5 to 10 mm Hg.[2,3] When portal blood flow is impeded and portal pressure exceeds 12 mm Hg, the term *portal hypertension* can be applied. Therefore, portal

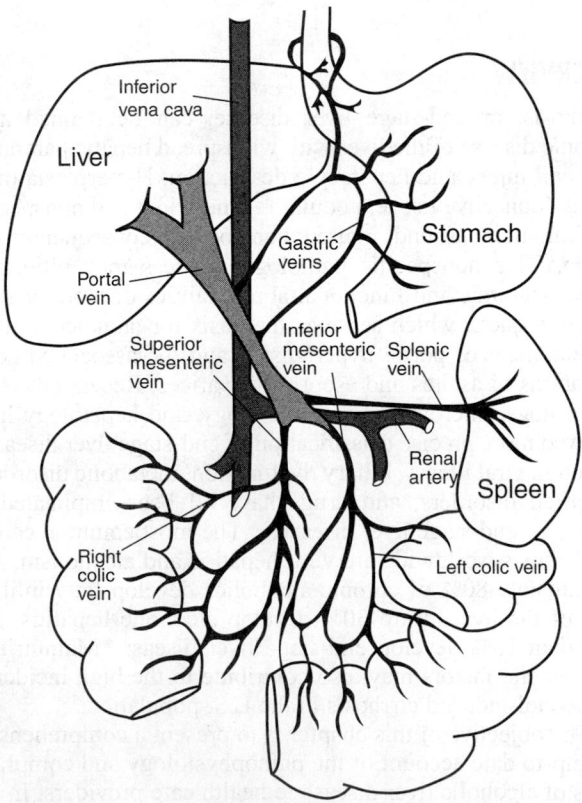

FIGURE 29-1 Schematic diagram of portal venous system.

hypertension is a hemodynamic complication of liver disease. Some studies suggest that alcohol directly increases portal pressure through an increase in vascular resistance, even in the absence of cirrhosis.[13] Fatal complications of advanced liver disease generally are related directly to portal hypertension.

Portal hypertension can be further classified as prehepatic portal hypertension, intrahepatic portal hypertension, or posthepatic portal hypertension. Splenic vein thrombosis and portal vein thrombosis are examples of prehepatic portal hypertension. In patients with cirrhotic liver disease, fibrosis and nodular regeneration of the liver with distortion of the hepatic veins is the main cause of intrahepatic portal hypertension. Hepatic venous obstruction (Budd-Chiari syndrome), as well as inferior vena caval obstruction and right-sided heart failure, are the most common causes of posthepatic portal hypertension. Persistent portal hypertension may change both blood flow and lymphatic circulation and lead to hyperfiltration and ascites formation. Persistently elevated portal pressures lead to the development of increased collateral circulation and increase the risk of *esophageal and gastric bleeding*. These forms of bleeding are medical emergencies, require prompt intervention, and are the most common life-threatening complication of portal hypertension. Hepatic encephalopathy and hepatorenal syndrome are other major complications associated with portal hypertension in patients with advanced cirrhosis.[19–21]

Laboratory Findings

Laboratory evaluations may not reflect the extent of the parenchymal necrosis, cellular regeneration, and fibrotic nodular scarring in cirrhotic liver disease. Conventional liver "function" tests are actually better characterized as liver "injury" tests and are modestly helpful to the clinician in recognizing chronic liver disease when clinical manifestations of chronic liver disease are not readily apparent. Although not specific for alcoholic cirrhosis, tests such as the serum aminotransferases (aspartate aminotransferases [AST, formerly known as *SGOT*], alanine aminotransferases [ALT, formerly known as *SGPT*]), and alkaline phosphatase are tools that aid in the early diagnosis, prognosis, and response to treatment when inflammation or injury is ongoing. However, these tests do not quantitatively measure the functional capacity of the liver. The aminotransferases are released during the normal turnover of liver cells (see Chapter 2, Interpretation of Clinical Laboratory Tests). Persistently high serum concentrations of aminotransferases suggest leakage of these enzymes from injured, rather than dead, hepatocytes. Thus, the serum concentrations of AST and ALT may not be extraordinarily high when liver dysfunction is the result of hepatocellular necrosis.

Because alkaline phosphatase is present in high concentrations in biliary canaliculi (as well as bone, intestines, kidneys, and WBCs), an increase in the serum concentration of alkaline phosphatase to greater than three times the normal value usually suggests a biliary (rather than a parenchymal) component to the hepatotoxic process. Alkaline phosphatase serum concentrations usually increase with age, and an increase of 30% to 50% above the upper limits of normal is not unusual in geriatric patients. When fractionation demonstrates high concentrations of the hepatic isoenzyme of alkaline phos-

phatase or when AST and ALT serum concentrations are elevated, hepatic toxicity is suggested. High serum concentrations of gamma glutamyl transpeptidase or of unconjugated bilirubin are also suggestive of hepatocellular dysfunction (versus obstruction).[6,7]

Serum concentrations of nonspecific proteins, such as albumin, or more specific proteins, such as factor V and VIII, can provide insight into the functional capacity of the liver. Although the hepatic parenchymal cells synthesize albumin, changes in albumin concentration are nonspecific and can be influenced by other factors including poor nutrition, renal wasting (proteinuria), and GI losses. Regardless of the cause, a low serum albumin concentration (<3 g/dL) that is unchanged after improved nutrition and treatment of other medical problems indicates an unfavorable prognosis. Prolongation of the prothrombin time (PT) due to chronic obstructive jaundice, celiac disease, or hypovitaminosis K usually improves within 24 hours after a 10 mg subcutaneous or oral dose of vitamin K, except in patients with diffuse hepatocellular disease. A prolonged PT that is unresponsive to parenteral vitamin K is a poor prognostic sign.[22]

A blood urea nitrogen (BUN) <5 mg/dL may be observed in patients with alcoholic cirrhosis but it is uncommon in other forms of cirrhosis. The low BUN is attributed to inadequate protein intake accompanied by a depressed hepatic capacity to synthesize urea. The interpretation of BUN test results in the alcoholic cirrhotic patient is difficult when other possible causes such as renal insufficiency, hemorrhage, hypervolemia, or hypovolemia are present.

A number of the factors described above have been incorporated into the *Child-Pugh Classification* of liver disease severity (Table 29-1).[19-21,23] This classification yields a scoring system to help clinicians grade disease severity and predict the long-term risk of mortality. This scoring system applies to a variety of chronic liver diseases. A score of "Grade A" is considered relatively low risk, whereas "Grade C" carries a poor prognosis. The overall 1-year survival rate is approximately 30% for Grade C and 80% for Grades A and B. Abstinence from alcohol may improve the clinical outcome and halts progression of alcoholic liver disease.

Treatment

Abstinence from alcohol and nutritional repletion are the mainstays of treatment for alcoholism.[16,17,24,25] Although a small amount of alcohol (e.g., cooking wine) does not have any direct harmful (hepatotoxicity) effect in patients with mild liver disease, most treatment protocols require a complete abstinence from alcohol due to the psychodynamics of alcohol abuse. Patients who recover from alcoholic hepatitis and remain abstinent may continue to show improvement in the clinical manifestations of alcoholic liver disease. However, continued alcohol use results in a 7-year mortality rate of 50% compared with less than 20% in those who discontinue alcohol consumption. In addition, survival is adversely effected by the presence of cirrhosis and its common complications including bleeding esophageal varices, refractory ascites, hepatic encephalopathy, and hepatorenal syndrome.[16,17,24,25] Treatment of alcoholic liver disease and addiction may be improved through a multidisciplinary approach, including an addiction specialist, primary care physician, psychiatrist, and

Table 29-1 Child-Pugh Classification of Severity of Liver Disease

Score	1 Point	2 Points	3 Points
Bilirubin (mg/dL)	<2	2–3	>3
Albumin (mg/dL)	>3.5	3–3.5	<3
Ascites	None	Easily controlled (mild)	Poorly controlled (moderate)
Encephalopathy (grade)	None	Mild (1 and 2)	Advanced (3 and 4)
Nutritional status	Excellent	Good	Poor

Grade A, <7 points; Grade B, 7–9 points; Grade C, 10–15 points.

pharmacist. Nutritional deficiency is common among alcoholics with liver disease. Lack of folic acid in the diet can result in megaloblastic anemia, which can be corrected by the administration of oral folic acid (1 mg) daily. Because most vitamins are stored intracellularly, plasma levels do not correlate with nutritional deficiencies. A single multivitamin with folic acid usually is sufficient to replenish deficiencies of thiamine (B_1), cyanocobalamin (B_{12}), riboflavin, nicotinic acid, and pyridoxine (B_6) in patients with cirrhosis.[18]

Pharmacologic treatment of alcoholic cirrhosis with currently available drugs is ineffective. There is no specific drug therapy for cirrhosis, but drugs commonly are used to treat the secondary complications of cirrhosis. Penicillamine, propylthiouracil, azathioprine, and colchicine are proposed disease-modifying drugs, but none have been shown to significantly reduce morbidity or mortality. A recent meta-analysis indicated no significant improvement in mortality rate with colchicine and a higher incidence of adverse drug reactions was noted in the colchicine-treated patients.[26] A separate meta-analysis reached a similar conclusion for treatment with propylthiouracil.[27] The reminder of this chapter addresses management of the secondary complications associated with alcoholic cirrhosis.

1. R.W. is a 54-year-old man with a 2-week history of nausea, vomiting, and lower abdominal cramps without diarrhea. Despite chronic anorexia, he has managed to eat about two meals a day and drink a fifth of vodka (750 mL) a day for the past 2 years. During this time, he experienced a 30-lb weight loss. He began drinking 9 years ago when his wife became disabled following diagnosis of a brain tumor. Two years ago, his alcohol consumption increased from one pint to a fifth daily. Recently, he has noted bilateral swelling of his legs, an increased tenseness and girth of his abdomen, and yellowing of his skin and the sclera of his eyes. His medical history is otherwise noncontributory.

Physical examination reveals an afebrile, jaundiced, and cachectic male in moderate distress. Spider angiomas were found on his face and upper chest, and palmar erythema was noted. Abdominal examination reveals prominent veins on a very tense abdomen. The liver edge is percussed below the right costal margin and ascites is noted by shifting dullness and a fluid wave. The spleen is not palpable. On neurologic examination, R.W. is awake and oriented to time, date, and place. Cranial nerves II to XII are grossly intact, but a decrease in vibratory sensation of the lower extremities is noted bilaterally. Admission laboratory data are as follows: sodium, 135 mEq/L; chloride, 95 mEq/L; potassium, 3.8 mEq/L; bicarbonate, 25 mEq/L; BUN, 15 mg/dL; serum creatinine, 1.4 mg/dL; glucose, 136 mg/dL; hemo-

globin, 11.2 g/dL; hematocrit, 33.4%; AST, 212 IU (normal, 29 IU); alkaline phosphatase, 954 IU (normal, 110 IU); PT, 13.5 seconds with a control of 12 seconds; total/direct bilirubin, 18.8/10.7 mg/dL (normal, 1.0/<0.5 mg/dL); albumin, 2.3 g/dL (normal, 3.5 to 4.0); and stool guaiac, positive. On admission to the hospital, the impression is alcoholic cirrhosis, ascites, and heme-positive stools.

Why did R.W. present with cachexia and a history of weight loss despite eating two meals daily?

[SI units: Na, 135 mmol/L; Cl, 95 mmol/L; K, 3.8 mmol/L; bicarbonate, 25 mmol/L; BUN, 5.36 mmol/L urea; SrCr, 123.76 mol/L; glucose, 7.55 mmol/L; Hgb, 112 g/L; Hct, 0.334; AST, 3.53 μkat/L; alkaline phosphatase, 159 μkat/L; bilirubin, 321.48:182.97 mol/L; albumin, 23 g/L].

Muscle wasting and dietary protein deficiency are the most common causes of weight loss in patients with alcoholic cirrhosis. Long-term alcohol abuse may impair hepatic gluconeogenesis and contribute to the depletion of liver glycogen stores (see Chapter 84, Alcohol Abuse).

In the cirrhotic patient, the demand for glucose as a source of energy leads to mobilization of amino acids from muscles and subsequent muscle wasting. A high-protein diet is unnecessary to maintain a positive nitrogen balance in the cirrhotic patient and increases the risk for development of encephalopathy symptoms. A normal protein intake of 35 to 50 g/day is sufficient to keep cirrhotic patients in protein equilibrium or positive nitrogen balance.[28]

Clinical Presentation

2. What subjective and objective evidence are compatible with alcoholic cirrhosis in R.W.?

R.W.'s liver "function" tests and physical findings (an enlarged, palpable liver edge; jaundice; spider angiomas on his face and upper chest; palmar erythema; and cachexia) are all consistent with advanced alcoholic cirrhosis in a patient with a history of chronic alcohol abuse. The prolonged PT and hypoalbuminemia suggest impaired hepatic synthesis of both albumin and vitamin K–dependent clotting factors. No evidence is available to indicate if the PT will improve with vitamin K administration. The presence of ascites (an enlarged fluid-filled abdomen) and prominent abdominal veins are suggestive of portal hypertension. A biopsy of the liver may confirm/establish the presence and severity of cirrhosis. R.W.'s prolonged PT, however, may increase the risk of bleeding from a liver biopsy. The presence of a normal BUN and an elevated direct or conjugated serum bilirubin suggest some hepatic parenchymal function remains. The increase in the serum concentrations of alkaline phosphatase and conjugated bilirubin, coupled with a history of declining nutritional intake, are also consistent with alcoholic liver disease. At this time there is no evidence of bleeding esophageal varices or hepatic encephalopathy.

Pathogenesis

3. What physiologic mechanism predisposes R.W. to fluid accumulation in the peritoneal cavity?

Ascites, or accumulation of fluid in the peritoneal cavity, is the most commonly encountered clinical symptom of cirrhosis.[29] This complication can be detected during the physical examination when greater than 1 to 3 liters of fluid has accumulated. In addition to an obviously enlarged abdomen, R.W. was found to have a positive fluid wave and shifting dullness indicating that the abdominal enlargement is not simply obesity. The fluid wave can be observed by having the patient lie on his or her back. While supporting one side of the abdomen with one hand, use the second hand to tap the opposite side of the abdomen. A wave of fluid moving across the abdomen should be visible. Once ascites develops, the 1-year survival rate decreases to 50%.[29]

Four theories explain the pathophysiology of accumulation of ascitic fluid in patients with end-stage liver diseases.[29] According to the classic (underfill) theory, formation of ascites results from a combination of increased hydrostatic pressure in the portal venous system and decreased plasma oncotic pressure (e.g., R.W.'s low serum albumin concentration). In cirrhosis, the hepatic venous outflow is blocked, resulting in an increase in the portal vein backpressure and an increase in the splanchnic blood volume (e.g., R.W.'s prominent abdominal veins). Exudation of fluid from the splanchnic capillary bed and the liver surface when the drainage capacity of the lymphatic system is exceeded also contributes to ascites. R.W.'s hypoalbuminemia (2.3 g/dL), due to impaired hepatic albumin synthesis, favors the formation of ascites by decreasing the ability to contain fluid within the vascular space.

An important consequence of portal hypertension and low plasma oncotic pressure is a reduced arterial blood supply to vital organs. Vasoconstriction and reduced circulation to the kidneys may activate the renin-angiotensin-aldosterone system.[30] Increased aldosterone enhances the distal tubular reabsorption of sodium and water, thus expanding total blood volume. This compensatory increase in circulating blood volume can also aggravate portal hypertension, increase splanchnic blood volume, and establish a vicious cycle.

In some patients, the underfill theory is sometimes conflicting, because these patients have normal aldosterone levels. Therefore, the overfill theory has been proposed for the formation of ascites. In this theory, sodium retention and plasma volume expansion precedes ascites formation. In the overfill theory, excess fluid overflows into the peritoneal cavity across the vasculature from the congested portal system.

The third explanation for the development of ascites is the lymph imbalance theory. Visceral edema from an imbalance in lymphatic flow is suggested as the primary stimulus to retention of salt and water by the kidney. Subsequent expansion of the extracellular fluid volume leads to increases in visceral lymph production that eventually exceeds lymph return, resulting in ascites.

A fourth theory describing the pathogenesis of ascites incorporates features from both the underfill and overfill theories. This hypothesis suggests that peripheral arterial vasodilation is the initiating event that causes a decrease in effective blood volume and a compensatory increase in sodium and water retention by the kidney.[31,32]

Goals of Therapy

4. What are the therapeutic goals in the management of R.W.'s ascites?

The goals of treatment for R.W.'s ascites are to mobilize ascitic fluid; to diminish abdominal discomfort, back pain, and difficulty in ambulation; and to prevent major complications (e.g., bacterial peritonitis, hernias, pleural effusions, hepatorenal syndrome, and respiratory distress). Treatment of ascites in R.W. should be undertaken cautiously and gradually because acid-base imbalances, hypokalemia, or intravascular volume depletion caused by overly aggressive therapy may lead to compromised renal function, hepatic encephalopathy, and death.[31,33] The initial medical management of ascites involves restriction of sodium and water intake and the use of diuretics to promote salt and water excretion.[31,33]

Fluid and Electrolyte Balance

5. The 24-hour urinary electrolytes for R.W. were Na, 10 mEq/L and K, 28 mEq/L. Why would sodium or water restriction be appropriate (or inappropriate) for R.W.?

Urinary Na:K Ratio

Normally, the urine concentration of electrolytes mirrors the serum concentration of electrolytes (i.e., sodium concentration is greater than that of potassium). A reversal of this pattern (i.e., potassium excretion exceeding sodium excretion) may indicate a relative hyperaldosteronism secondary to diminished renal blood flow and low oncotic pressure. If urine electrolyte monitoring is to be meaningful, the first sample must be obtained before initiating diuretic therapy.[34,35]

Sodium Restriction

Severe sodium restriction (20 mEq/day) can result in diuresis in some patients with cirrhosis and ascites; the degree of success depends on the duration of sodium restriction and the extent of hepatic injury. Cirrhotic patients with a high urine sodium concentration (i.e., >10 mEq/L) are most likely to respond to bed rest and restriction in sodium intake. R.W. should benefit from sodium restriction because his urine sodium concentration of 20 mEq/L suggests a borderline renal capacity to excrete free water. Excessive sodium intake may worsen the condition and decrease the efficacy of diuretic therapy.

Water Restriction

Water restriction is effective in cirrhotic patients who have dilutional hyponatremia (serum Na <130 mEq/L). Sodium restriction is desirable for R.W.; however, water restriction should be avoided as part of the initial treatment because his serum sodium concentration is within normal limits (135 mEq/L). Most patients with a low urine sodium concentration (<10 mEq/L) and normal renal function appear to benefit from diuretic therapy. Patients with reduced 24-hour urinary excretion of sodium, glomerular filtration rate, and free water clearance are commonly resistant to medical treatment and have a poor prognosis.[21,32,36]

Role of Aldosterone

Spironolactone, an aldosterone-antagonist, can normalize urinary electrolytes after several days of treatment at pharmacologically effective doses (100 to 300 mg daily). Diuretic agents with natriuretic properties may affect the value of monitoring urinary electrolytes. Even a single dose of hydrochlorothiazide or furosemide may cause excessive urinary sodium loss even in the presence of continued hyperaldosteronism.[37]

Diuretic Therapy
Choice of Agent

6. **R.W. was prescribed sodium and free water restriction after initial evaluation. Spironolactone 100 mg/day and furosemide 20 mg/day were ordered to induce diuresis. Why is spironolactone preferred over other potassium-sparing diuretics in the treatment of ascites?**

Many patients with advanced liver disease have high circulating levels of aldosterone. High serum concentrations of aldosterone may be attributable to both increased production and decreased excretion of the hormone. Increased portal pressure, ascites, depletion of intravascular volume, and decreased renal perfusion may lead to activation of the renin-angiotensin-aldosterone system.[38] In addition, hepatic shunting also increases aldosterone production by decreasing renal blood flow. The liver also metabolizes aldosterone, and hepatic impairment prolongs the physiologic half-life of aldosterone. Most cirrhotic patients have a low serum concentration of albumin, and because aldosterone is highly bound to albumin, these patients have higher free, active concentrations of aldosterone available to receptors.

Spironolactone is a rational diuretic choice for R.W. because it is an agent with anti-aldosterone and potassium-sparing effects. Although the usual dose of spironolactone for the treatment of hypertension is only 25 mg once or twice daily, much larger doses (100 to 200 mg/day) are generally necessary to antagonize the high circulating levels of aldosterone present in patients with ascites. If the diuretic response is unsatisfactory, the dosage can be increased slowly (every 2 to 4 days because of the long half-life of active spironolactone metabolites). Spironolactone dosages of up to 400 mg/day are sometimes needed. The diuretic effect is enhanced when spironolactone is combined with sodium restriction (0.5 to 2 g per day), but even then, only 20% to 50% of patients have an adequate response. As discussed below, combinations of spironolactone with other diuretics are often necessary. Furosemide (20 mg) can be also started to minimize the risk of hyperkalemia and enhance the onset of diuresis. Triamterene and amiloride, both potassium-sparing diuretics without antialdosterone activity, can be used as less-efficacious alternatives to spironolactone if intolerable side effects (e.g., gynecomastia) occur.[8,39,40]

Monitoring
CLINICAL RESPONSES

7. **What clinical responses should be monitored to ensure the therapeutic effectiveness of spironolactone therapy for R.W.?**

Monitoring body weight, urine output, and abdominal girth are important. The goal is a weight loss of 0.5 to 2 kg/day, which corresponds to a net fluid volume loss of about 0.5 to 2 L. Because ascitic fluid is slow to re-equilibrate with vascular volume, any diuresis exceeding this rate of fluid loss is associated with a risk of volume depletion, hypotension, and compromised renal function.

Diuresis may be approached more aggressively if peripheral edema is present. Weight loss of 2 kg/day is considered safe in edematous patients because the excess fluid in the peripheral tissues buffers against volume depletion by replacing vascular fluid losses. Once edema has resolved, the goal of weight loss should be reduced to 0.75 kg/day to minimize the risk of renal insufficiency induced by plasma volume contraction and other diuretic-induced complications. Ideally, urine output should exceed fluid intake by about 300 to 1,000 mL/day, but these measurements are often inaccurate and do not account for nonrenal fluid losses. Abdominal girth measurements with a tape measure reflect the actual change in ascitic volume, but are again subject to errors in measurement, especially if the tape measure is not placed over the same part of the abdomen with each subsequent measurement. If feasible, the same person should measure abdominal girth each day to minimize errors in measurement, and the same reference point (e.g., umbilicus) should be used consistently.[8]

LABORATORY PARAMETERS

8. **What laboratory parameters could be monitored to assess the therapeutic efficacy of R.W.'s spironolactone treatment?**

Serum concentrations of creatinine and urinary chemistries (sodium and potassium) should be monitored to define and guide the need for increasing doses of spironolactone. In addition, urinary concentrations of electrolytes reflect renal function. A low baseline urinary Na:K ratio (<1.0) indicates high intrinsic mineralocorticoid (e.g., aldosterone) activity and suggests that large dosages of 200 to 400 mg/day of spironolactone may be needed. Because R.W.'s urinary Na:K ratio is <1.0, the initial spironolactone dose of 100 mg/day could have been initiated with a higher dosage (e.g., 150 to 200 mg/day). Generally, if there is still no response following reversal of the urinary Na:K ratio or if diuresis remains insufficient after 4 or more days of increasingly larger doses of spironolactone, a thiazide (e.g., hydrochlorothiazide 25 mg/day), metolazone (5 mg/day), or furosemide (20 mg/day) can be added on a continuous or intermittent basis. If necessary, doses of the adjunctive diuretic may be doubled after approximately 2 days.[38]

Complications

9. **The spironolactone dosage was increased to 200 mg/day. Three days later, R.W.'s urinary sodium and potassium concentrations were 48 and 30 mEq/L, respectively. Fluid intake was 1,400 mL and urinary output was 750 mL. Because of insufficient diuresis, supplemental treatment with furosemide is being considered. What potential complications from the diuretic therapy might arise in R.W.? Suggest guidelines to minimize these complications.**

HYPOKALEMIC-HYPOCHLOREMIC METABOLIC ALKALOSIS AND HYPONATREMIA

Hypokalemic-hypochloremic metabolic alkalosis and hyponatremia occur frequently in untreated cirrhosis.[38,41] Many cirrhotic patients initially have a deficit in total body potassium secondary to vomiting, diarrhea, and hyperaldosteronism. Hypokalemic alkalosis generally can be corrected with potassium chloride supplementation. Because R.W. has some degree of renal impairment (SrCr, 1.4 mg/dL) and is being given spironolactone, his serum potassium level should be monitored closely. Hyponatremia, if present, usually can be corrected by temporary withdrawal of diuretics and free water restriction.

PRERENAL AZOTEMIA

Acute renal failure (prerenal azotemia) usually results from overdiuresis with subsequent compromise of intravascular volume and decreased renal perfusion. A gradual rise in serum creatinine and BUN are a warning to slow the rate of diuresis. Salt restriction alone can mobilize only 300 mL of ascitic fluid every day. Patients with both edema and ascites can mobilize up to 1,440 mL of ascitic fluid per 24-hour period, but at the expense of plasma volume contraction and renal insufficiency. Although diuretic agents enhance fluid mobilization, only about 930 mL/day of ascitic fluid is lost at the most as compared to about 4,700 mL/day of non-ascitic fluid. Thus, the fluid loss during diuresis is chiefly at the expense of non-ascitic (primarily intravascular) fluid. The maximal daily fluid loss should be limited to <750 mL/day for patients with ascites alone and to <2 L/day for those with both ascites and edema to prevent plasma volume depletion and decreased renal perfusion. If faster removal of ascites is required due to respiratory distress, large-volume paracentesis is more effective than rapid diuresis (see Question 10).[35,36,42]

Because R.W. presented with both edema and ascites, an initial fluid loss of up to 2 L/day would be reasonable. The rate of weight loss should be reduced to 0.5 to 0.75 kg/day when the edema become less pronounced. Gradual diuresis avoids diuretic-induced depletion of extracellular fluid volume by permitting ascitic fluid to equilibrate with plasma volume. Using these guidelines, untoward effects from diuretic therapy, which may occur in as many as 75% of diuretic-treated cirrhotic patients with ascites, can be minimized. Therefore, the spironolactone dosage should be increased to 300 to 400 mg/day before furosemide is started. If the desired diuresis is still not achieved after 3 to 5 days, a low dosage (40 mg) of furosemide could be started. Furosemide can be started earlier if hyperkalemia develops or if R.W.'s condition is such that he cannot wait for the slow onset of spironolactone. The response to thiazide diuretics is unpredictable and they are generally not recommended.

Paracentesis

10. Over the next several days, R.W.'s spironolactone dosage was increased to 400 mg/day. Subsequently, furosemide 40 mg orally per day was started and gradually increased to 80 mg BID without major improvement in his diuresis. Laboratory data revealed that R.W.'s SrCr had increased to 3.2 mg/dL and his BUN had increased to 45 mg/dL. Serum electrolytes were as follows: K, 3.1 mEq/L; Na, 130 mEq/L; Cl, 88 mEq/L; and bicarbonate, 32 mEq/L. R.W. became progressively short of breath because of restricted diaphragmatic movement secondary to his significantly enlarged abdomen. What therapeutic measures are appropriate for diuretic-resistant ascites?

[SI units: SrCr, 282 mol/L; BUN, 16.07 mmol/L urea; Na, 3.1 mmol/L; Cl, 88 mmol/L; bicarbonate, 32 mmol/L]

Patients with cirrhosis experiencing respiratory or cardiac symptoms despite diuretic and fluid restriction warrant more aggressive second-line treatment including large volume paracentesis and shunting procedures. Paracentesis involves the removal of ascitic fluid from the abdominal cavity with a needle or a catheter. Although paracentesis can remove large amounts of ascitic fluid (e.g., 10 L), removal of as little as 1 L of fluid may provide considerable relief from the painful stretching of skin and the respiratory distress that occurs with massive ascites. The ascitic fluid often re-accumulates rapidly after paracentesis due to transudation of fluid from the interstitial and plasma compartments into the peritoneal cavity; therefore, paracentesis is not considered a definitive treatment for ascites. The major complications of overaggressive, large-volume paracentesis include hypotension, shock, oliguria, encephalopathy, and hepatorenal syndrome. Other potential complications of paracentesis are hemorrhage, perforation of the abdominal viscera, infection, and protein depletion. The risk of bacterial peritonitis also may be increased by large volume paracentesis.[8]

Albumin

11. R.W. continues to re-accumulate ascitic fluid and is exhibiting signs of declining renal function. A 5 L paracentesis coupled with a 50 g albumin infusion is ordered. Why are albumin infusions used in conjunction with paracentesis?

Large volume paracentesis (greater than 4 liters) should be performed for patients with tense ascites or spontaneous bacterial peritonitis. However, paracentesis alone is associated with a significantly high incidence of paracentesis-induced circulatory dysfunction (PICD).[43] PICD is characterized by a reduction in systemic vascular resistance and significant increase in plasma renin activity and plasma norepinephrine.[43] Following paracentesis, there is a period of impaired circulatory function which manifests as a reduction in the cardiac output and worsening renal function 24 to 48 hours after the procedure.[44] Intravenous albumin infusions are commonly administered to prevent PICD following large volume paracentesis. The usual dose is 50 mL of a 25% albumin solution per liter of ascites removed. Contrary to common belief, circulatory dysfunction following paracentesis is not spontaneously reversible and is associated with a shorter survival rate. In addition, administration of albumin allows for expansion of plasma volume and improves the natriuretic response of diuretics. Finally, patients with advanced cirrhosis complicated by spontaneous bacterial peritonitis, when treated with plasma volume expanders (IV albumin), have a lower incidence of renal failure and mortality compared with the standard antibiotic alone.[45] Although albumin is costly and often in short supply, it is an appropriate treatment in conjunction with paracentesis.[46] When patients treated with paracentesis (4 to 6 L/day) and intravenous (IV) albumin (40 g after each tap) were compared with patients treated with paracentesis and saline solution, the incidence of PICD was significantly higher in the saline-treated group versus the albumin-treated group (33.3% versus 11.4%, respectively). The prevalence of PICD after this procedure also depends on the amount of ascites removed. Saline solution can be used in combination with small volume paracentesis (less than 2 to 3 L) in hemodynamically stable patients.[46] Use of albumin in combination with large volume paracentesis in hemodynamically unstable patients produces a sustained expansion of circulating blood volume, increases cardiac output, and significantly suppresses release of rennin and norepinephrine. Thus, albumin remains the preferred plasma expander following large volume paracentesis.[44] In another study, patients with spontaneous bacterial peritonitis were randomized to receive IV antibiotic alone or IV antibiotic and albumin. At 3 months, the overall mortality rates were 41% and 22% in the control and albumin groups, respectively. The rate of hospital mortality rate was 29% in the control group as compared with 10% in the albumin-treated group.[45]

Dextran 70 and Other Plasma Expanders

Due to the high cost and often limited supply of albumin, the use of synthetic plasma expanders in combination with large volume paracentesis has been explored as a therapeutic option for patients with ascites refractory to diuretics and fluid restriction. In one small study (N = 10), dextran 70 was combined with paracentesis in patients with ascites.[47] Dextran 70 was found to be effective in mobilizing ascites and was found to be more cost effective. However, two patients developed hyponatremia and one patient died from GI bleeding. Although dextran 70 can partially prevent hemodynamic abnormalities, albumin appears to be more effective in the prevention of PICD.[48,49] In a second study, patients with refractory ascites to pharmacologic interventions were randomized to paracentesis plus albumin, dextran 70, or polygeline.[50] More patients treated with dextran 70 (34.4%) or polygeline (37.8%) versus those receiving albumin (18.5%) experienced PICD. In contrast to albumin-treated patients, PICD was more persistent and shorter survival rate was observed in the non–albumin-treated patients.[50]

Hydroxyethyl starch, an effective colloid agent for intravascular volume expansion, should not be used in patients with chronic liver disease as repeated administration of this agent to patients with cirrhosis can cause severe portal hypertension, acute liver failure, and sepsis.[51]

Alternative Therapy

12. What alternative treatments are available for management of refractory ascites? How would these alternatives be applied in R.W.'s case?

Transjugular Intrahepatic Portosystemic Shunt

In consideration of R.W.'s increasing serum creatinine concentration, rising BUN, and the grave prognosis of hepatorenal syndrome, transjugular intrahepatic portosystemic shunt (TIPS) is a reasonable therapeutic alternative at this time. TIPS is another option for patients refractory (unresponsive) to the pharmacologic interventions described above. TIPS surgery involves opening a drainage channel between the hepatic vein and intrahepatic segment of the portal vein with an expandable metal stent placed during an angiographic procedure. This low-resistance channel allows blood to return to the systemic circulation and corrects portal (sinusoidal) hypertension. In addition, TIPS may improve urinary sodium excretion. The major complications of TIPS include severe encephalopathy renal failure and shunt occlusion. Encephalopathy occurs in approximately 30% of patients following TIPS, is similar to that reported after surgical inter-

vention. Hepatic encephalopathy is a metabolic disorder of the central nervous system (CNS) and occurs in patients with end-stage liver disease. Encephalopathy is a consequence of shunting blood from the portal to the systemic circulation (see question 20). Because of poor prognosis, liver transplantation should be considered in all patients refractory to pharmacologic treatment and or stent placement.[52] This procedure is preferred to surgical intervention in this patient.

Peritoneovenous Shunt

A peritoneovenous shunt consists of a surgically implanted valve in the abdominal wall, an intra-abdominal cannula, and an outflow tube tunneled subcutaneously from the valve to a vein that empties directly into the superior vena cava. In this manner, ascitic fluid can be withdrawn from the abdominal cavity and be re-instilled back into the vascular space. This procedure is contraindicated in the presence of peritonitis, recurrent coma, severe coagulopathy, significant cardiac failure, and acute alcoholic hepatitis. Peritoneovenous shunts are rarely used because of a number of surgical complications. Peritoneovenous shunt should not be considered in transplant candidates, since scarring of peritoneal area increases the surgical complication during and following orthotropic hepatic transplantation.[53]

Because R.W.'s PT is prolonged, vitamin K and fresh frozen plasma should be administered before surgery. Resistant ascites has been treated successfully, and the usually fatal hepatorenal syndrome has been reversed with the use of a peritoneovenous shunt. However, the basic hepatic abnormalities remain unchanged, and whether the overall survival rate is improved remains to be established. Pulmonary edema can occur after peritoneovenous shunt placement from the increased volume of fluid returning to the heart. IV furosemide is usually administered during the first 2 to 3 days after surgery to augment diuresis. Other possible complications of peritoneovenous shunt placement include consumption coagulopathy, fever, wound infection, septicemia, and GI bleeding. A mortality rate as high as 25% has been noted in the first months, and early shunt failure occurs in approximately 10% of patients. Long-term shunt patency has also been found to be problematic.[54] Currently, a peritoneovenous shunt should be considered in patients with refractory ascites that fails to respond to TIPS or diuretics and large volume paracenteses.

Peritoneovenous shunting has been compared with standard medical treatment in patients with persistent or recurrent severe ascites. Patients who received shunts had a shorter hospital stay and a longer time interval between ascites reoccurrence. However, no survival benefit was observed. When peritoneovenous shunting was compared with paracentesis plus albumin infusions, the former appeared to be more effective in the long-term management of ascites as reflected by a longer period before readmission, a lower number of readmissions for ascites, and lower diuretic requirements. However, peritoneovenous shunting did not improve survival over paracentesis, and the probability of shunt occlusion was 52% after 2 years.[55] In summary, the lack of survival benefit and high risk of shunt occlusion suggest peritoneovenous shunting should be reserved for patients with ascites and fairly well-preserved renal and hepatic function in whom more standard therapies fail.

ESOPHAGEAL VARICES
Treatment

13. C.V., a 55-year-old, pale-looking woman with known primary alcoholic cirrhosis, was admitted for a chief complaint of hematemesis. C.V. has a history of recurrent upper GI bleeding and documented esophageal varices. She has no other significant medical history. On examination, her blood pressure (BP) was 78/40 mm Hg, pulse rate was 110 beats/min, and respiratory rate was 22 breaths/ min. Her skin was cold, chest and cardiac examinations were within normal limits, and abdominal examination revealed ascites and a palpable spleen. Bowel sounds were normal. Laboratory values included the following: Hgb, 7 g/dL (normal, 11.5 to 15.5); Hct, 22% (normal, 33 to 43); albumin, 3.0 g/dL (normal, 4 to 6); AST, 160 IU (normal, 0 to 35); ALT, 250 IU (normal, 0 to 35); alkaline phosphatase, 40 IU (normal, 30 to 120); and creatinine, 2.0 mg/dL (normal, 0.6 to 1.2). The PT was 18 seconds with a control of 12 seconds. Serum electrolytes were all within normal limits. An electrocardiogram (ECG) revealed sinus tachycardia. What are the immediate goals of therapy and treatment measures of the highest priority in managing C.V.'s hematemesis?

[SI units: Hgb, 70 g/L; Hct, 0.22; albumin, 30 g/L; AST, 2.67 μkat/L; ALT, 4.17 at/L; alkaline phosphatase, 0.67 μkat/L; creatinine, 176.8 /L]

Goals of Therapy

Most patients with cirrhosis develop portal hypertension, which in turn can progress to bleeding varices (dilated veins in the upper GI tract). Thirty percent of patients with compensated cirrhosis (no evidence of ascites, encephalopathy, or severe jaundice) develop esophageal varices, as compared with 60% of patients with decompensated cirrhosis. Unless varices bleed, they do not cause significant complications or symptoms in cirrhotic patients.

The progression and severity of varices is a direct consequence of portal hypertension. The two major sites of concern in portal hypertension are the left gastric vein, supplying the esophagus and upper GI tract, and the portal vein, supplying the spleen and lower GI tract. The scarring and fibrosis associated with cirrhosis initially lead to an increase in portal vein pressure (PVP). The PVP may eventually rise above a threshold pressure (greater than 12 mm Hg), causing backflow of blood supply and subsequent pressure in the left gastric vein. Hyperkinetic circulation in the gastric vein raises the esophageal transmural pressure and increases the risk of upper GI bleed in the intraepithelial zone. Since the gastric vein is adopted for low-pressure circulation (5 to 8 mm Hg) and generally cannot tolerate a sustained hyperdynamic circulation, gastric and esophageal varices are hemodynamic compensatory mechanisms for a shunted, high pressure blood supply that—in the absence of portal hypertension—is readily drained through the portal vein.[56]

The consequence of bleeding varices is usually seen in cirrhotic patients with advanced disease (severe liver dysfunction and large varix or "red signs"). Varices can only be visualized during a diagnostic endoscopy. Once detected, varices are classified based on size (grade 1, 2, and 3) and location (type 1 and type 2). Grade 3 varices present in patients with a larger varix and are associated with a higher risk of bleeding. Type 1 varices appear contained within the esophagus and represent up to 75% of reported cases, whereas type 2 varices extend from the esophagus into the fundus and represent 25% of the cases.[56]

Prevention of variceal bleeding is critical because of the high mortality rate with each episode of variceal hemorrhage. New varices develop at a rate of 5% to 10% per year in cirrhotic patients. Once varices develop, they enlarge by 4% to 10% each year.[57]

Despite improvement in the management of portal hypertension, massive bleeding from esophageal and/or gastric varices is the leading cause of death in patients with cirrhosis.[58,59] Each episode of variceal hemorrhage carries a 20% to 30% risk of death, and if untreated up to a 70% risk of mortality.[58,59] Acute variceal bleeding is considered a medical emergency and should be managed immediately. Treatment goals include volume resuscitation, acute treatment of bleeding, and prevention of recurrence of variceal bleeding. Approximately 10% of patients are refractory to any endoscopic and medical intervention and may require life-saving portal decompressive shunt surgery or TIPS.[60]

General Management

Resuscitation is the first priority in patients with acute bleeding episodes. An indwelling nasogastric tube should be placed and saline or tap water lavage of the stomach with suctioning of the gastric contents should be initiated promptly to prevent airway complications such as aspiration pneumonia.[61,62] Obtunded or unconscious patients should be intubated to maintain and protect the airway. Pharmacologic treatment should be initiated immediately to reduce bleeding and the risk of hypotension-induced renal failure. If the PT is >15 seconds, as in this case, vitamin K (10 mg IV/PO/SC) administration is recommended. Rapid infusion or IV push of vitamin K can cause severe hypersensitivity reactions or anaphylaxis. When this route is necessary (intubated patients or patients with low muscle mass), the dose of vitamin K should be diluted in 50 to 100 mL 0.9% sodium chloride or D5W and the rate of administration should *not* exceed 0.5 mg/min. However, dilution and slow administration does not prevent the risk of hypersensitivity reactions completely. The patient should be also monitored for any abnormal electrolyte and metabolic chemistries (e.g., potassium, sodium, bicarbonate), hypoxia (e.g., PO_2, pH), and decreased urinary output.[62]

Following the initial episode, bleeding stops spontaneously in approximately 50% of patients. Rebleeding is most likely to occur within the first 48 hours in patients with large varices and in patients with advanced liver disease (i.e., Child-Pugh class C; see Table 29-1). Factors associated with early rebleeding include age older than 60 years, acute renal failure, and severe initial bleeding defined by hemoglobin <8 g/dL at presentation.[63] Risk factors for late rebleeding are severe liver failure, continued alcohol abuse, large variceal size, renal failure, and hepatocellular carcinoma.[63]

Hypovolemia

Hypovolemia should be immediately managed to keep the hematocrit >30% without increasing the degree of portal hypertension. C.V.'s pallor, cold and clammy skin, rapid pulse, and a systolic blood pressure <80 mm Hg suggest significant hypotension and hypovolemia needing correction with whole blood or packed red cell transfusion. Fresh blood is preferable because of its homeostatic properties and should constitute one-third or one-fourth of the total number of units administered, if possible.[63,64]

14. Three units of whole blood and one unit of fresh frozen plasma were transfused initially. C.V.'s stomach was lavaged with saline, and the gastric aspirate from the nasogastric (NG) tube continued to be strongly positive for blood. Vitamin K (Aqua-Mephyton) 10 mg in 100 mL normal saline was administered over 1 hour. Four hours later, her bleeding still persisted. What other pharmacologic interventions can be used to control C.V.'s bleeding esophageal varices?

Several vasoconstricting drugs have been used in the past to control variceal bleeding. The first, and at one time the gold standard, was vasopressin (Pitressin).[65,66] This naturally occurring hormone (also known as 8-arginine vasopressin, antidiuretic hormone, and ADH) is produced by the posterior pituitary and was originally derived for the treatment of diabetes insipidus in persons with pituitary insufficiency. Its use to control variceal bleeding or to treat refractory septic shock is a non–FDA-labeled use that takes advantage of its intense smooth muscle and vasoconstrictive properties. Because efficacy of vasopressin for treatment of esophageal bleeding is limited and side effects are common, it has largely been replaced by octreotide and somatostatin in most practice sites. Nonetheless, some clinicians still prescribe vasopressin.

Vasopressin

Vasopressin (Pitressin) is a powerful but nonspecific vasoconstrictor that reduces blood flow in all splanchnic beds. It is effective in reducing or terminating bleeding in approximately 60% of patients with variceal hemorrhage.[65,66] Common side effects of vasoconstrictor therapy include abdominal cramping, skin blanching, phlebitis, and hematoma at the site of the infusion. Of greater concern are worsening of hypertension and reports of patients developing angina, arrhythmias, and even experiencing myocardial infarction while receiving vasopressin.

Because of its short half-life, vasopressin must be given as a continuous IV infusion. To minimize dose-related adverse effects, the lowest effective dosage should be used when possible. The most common regimen is an IV bolus dose of 20 U, followed by a continuous infusion of 0.2 to 0.4 U/min, increasing to 0.9 U/min if necessary. Higher doses should be avoided because doses up to 1.2 to 1.5 U/min fail to control hemorrhage in patients who are unresponsive to lower dosages. When the bleeding is controlled, it is customary to taper the vasopressin dose over 24 to 48 hours, but tapering the dose does not appear to decrease the incidence of rebleeding or side effects.[65] Rarely, intra-arterial infusions directly into the bleeding site have been used at doses of 0.1 to 0.5 U/min.

Because nonspecific vasoconstriction complicates the use of vasopressin, nitroglycerin has been advocated as an adjunct to counteract the systemic side effects of vasopressin. Nitroglycerin administration (sublingually, intravenously, or transdermally) also may enhance the reduction in portal pressure and reduce the adverse vascular and cardiac effects.[65,67] Transdermal nitroglycerin (10 mg/day) is the most convenient method of administration; however, absorption may vary. When given by IV infusion, the nitroglycerin dose is 40 to 200 μg/min. The efficacy of vasopressin plus nitroglycerin in controlling variceal bleeding is about 70%.

Vasopressin should be avoided in patients with serious cardiovascular complications and only used for a short time only as necessary.

Terlipressin

Terlipressin (Glypressin), a synthetic analog of vasopressin (which is not available in the United States), effectively reduces bleeding in 80% of patients. It is slowly metabolized in vivo to lysine vasopressin. Terlipressin has a longer half-life than vasopressin, eliminating the need for continuous IV infusions. The standard dose is 2 mg as an IV bolus every 6 hours. Fewer cardiovascular side effects have been associated with terlipressin than with vasopressin.[68] However, studies with equipotent doses of terlipressin and vasopressin have not consistently reported a difference in heart rate, blood pressure, and cardiac output.

Somatostatin and Octreotide

15. C.V.'s physician is concerned about the technical difficulties of administering vasopressin and the potential for side effects. He would like to learn more about somatostatin and octreotide. How should they be dosed? Are they safer than vasopressin?

Somatostatin is a complex hormone produced by the hypothalamus, other CNS sites, pancreas, and the intestinal tract. In simple terms, it can be considered as a hormone that suppresses a variety of other hormones. For example, it is a potent inhibitor of pituitary derived growth hormone and was initially developed for the treatment of acromegaly. Insulin, glucagon, and digestive enzyme secretion are all inhibited within the pancreas. Effects on the GI tract include suppression of gastric acid, pepsin, and vasoactive intestinal protein (VIP) secretion; slowing of gastric emptying time; reduction of smooth muscle contractions; and impaired intestinal blood flow. Diarrheal syndromes related to carcinoid tumors and VIP secreting tumors are responsive to somatostatin. Shunting of intestinal blood flow served as the basis for its early investigational use in the treatment of esophageal varices, administered as a continuous IV infusion of 250 to 500 μg/hr after a bolus of 50 to 250 μg. Somatostatin is available in Europe but is substituted with octreotide in the United States. Octreotide is a synthetic analog of the somatostatin with essentially identical pharmacologic properties but a slightly longer half-life. The elimination half-life of octreotide is 1.7 hours compared with 2 to 3 minutes for somatostatin.

Octreotide (Sandostatin) is a selective and potent vasoconstrictor that reduces portal and collateral blood flow by constricting splanchnic vessels.[65,67,69] Octreotide is shown to be effective for controlling acute variceal bleeding and appears comparable in efficacy to vasopressin and balloon tamponade, with fewer side effects. Octreotide is administered as a 50 μg bolus followed by an infusion of 25 μg/hr for 18 hours to 5 days. In one study patients with portal hypertensive and upper GI bleed were randomized to receive octreotide or vasopressin. Complete bleeding control was achieved in all patients receiving octreotide after 48 hours of therapy compared with 64% of vasopressin-treated patients. Patients receiving vasopressin also experienced more side effects (abdominal cramps, nausea, tremor decreased cardiac output, myocardial ischemia, and bronchial constriction) than those receiving octreotide.[70] In the patients with bleeding not controlled within 48 hours by vasopressin, complete bleeding control was subsequently achieved by octreotide.

In a meta-analysis of octreotide versus vasopressin in the management of acute esophageal variceal bleeds, octreotide appeared to be more effective in controlling acute bleeding with a significantly more rapid onset of action, reduced transfusion requirements, and more favorable side effect profile.[71]

In general both somatostatin and octreotide are considered very safe agents. Diarrhea, hyperglycemia, and injection site pain are the most common side effects. Hypoglycemia has also been observed. Other side effects may include constipation, rectal spasms, abnormal stools, and QT prolongation (in patients with acromegaly). The choice between using vasopressin and octreotide is influenced by local practice. In most centers, octreotide has become the agent of choice.[71]

Sclerotherapy

16. **Vasopressin and octreotide are nonspecific vasoconstrictors that require continuous IV infusion and carry a risk of systemic side effects. What is sclerotherapy, and why is this procedure replacing vasoconstrictors in many hospitals?**

After successful resuscitation, endoscopy should be performed to establish the cause of bleeding. At least 30% of patients with suspected variceal bleeding do not have varices and require different treatment approaches. Fiberoptic esophagoscopy allows direct visualization of the esophagus and location of the bleeding sites. Those with actively bleeding varices can be treated with sclerotherapy, balloon tamponade, or endoscopic band ligation.[72]

Sclerotherapy involves insertion of a flexible fiberoptic esophagoscope to directly visualize the esophageal varices and injection of 0.5 to 5 mL of a sclerosing agent (e.g., concentrated saline—11.5% NaCl or ethanolamine oleate [Ethamolin]) into each varix at points about 2 cm apart to induce immediate hemostasis.[73] Sodium tetradecyl sulfate was used commonly in the past but is no longer marketed. Injection of the sclerosing agent into the bleeding varix leads to an intense irritant and inflammatory response within the intimal endothelium of the vein. This results in fibrosis, thrombus formation, and ultimately occlusion of the vein leading to cessation of bleeding within 2 to 5 minutes. Permanent destruction of the vessel will occur over several days. This procedure may need to be repeated several times over the next few weeks to several months until all the bleeding sites have been identified.

Sclerosing agents can be injected intravariceally or paravariceally. The aim of intravariceal sclerotherapy is to induce variceal thrombosis, whereas the goal of paravariceal injection is to thicken the overlying mucosa. The most common complications associated with sclerotherapy include esophageal ulceration, stricture formation, esophageal perforation, retrosternal chest pain, and temporary dysphagia. Sclerotherapy is considerably more effective than either pharmacologic interventions (vasopressin or octreotide) or balloon tamponade and is now considered the treatment of choice for esophageal variceal bleeding because it controls acute variceal bleeding in up to 95% of patients.[74]

Alternative Treatment Modalities

17. **Immediate intravariceal and paravariceal sclerotherapy procedures were undertaken for C.V. Although these procedures were transiently successful, variceal bleeding has developed again. What alternative treatment modalities could be used in lieu of a second course of sclerotherapy?**

Patients who do not respond to two courses of sclerotherapy generally continue to deteriorate and die, with a mortality rate approaching 90%. When sclerotherapy fails, there are several alternatives to further repeated sclerotherapy. These include balloon tamponade, endoscopic band ligation, and surgery.[64,75,76] Poor responders often require surgical correction of the underlying portal hypertension after temporary balloon tamponade to temporarily control the bleeding.[75,76]

Balloon Tamponade

In balloon tamponade, bleeding is controlled by direct compression of the varices at the gastroesophageal junction or at the bleeding site.[72,77] In this approach, a tube known as a Sengstaken tube or Lintern tube (gastric varices only) is passed through the mouth and into the stomach. The tube contains two balloons: an esophageal balloon and a gastric balloon. The gastric balloon is inflated and applies compression to the varices. The esophageal balloon is inflated only if bleeding is not controlled by the gastric balloon. It is important to remember that balloon tamponade is only a temporary measure and may cause pressure necrosis after 48 to 72 hours. Thus, the balloon should be deflated after 12 to 24 hours. Balloon tamponade will achieve temporary control of the bleeding and allow time for onset of other measures to work. This technique is effective in 90% of patients. An additional procedure generally is required within the first 24 hours to prevent rebleeding. Complication rates are poorly documented. However, aspiration (>10% incidence), pneumonitis, esophageal ulceration and rupture, and chest pain, as well as asphyxia, have been reported. Aspiration may be minimized by endotracheal intubation and continued aspiration of oropharyngeal secretions. Also, deflation and removal of the tube may result in removal of the fibrin scab at the bleeding site, resulting in rebleeding.

Endoscopic Band Ligation

Endoscopic band ligation is a procedure in which an elastic band is placed around the mucosa and submucosa of the esophageal area containing the varix. This leads to strangulation and fibrosis of the varix and, ideally, its obliteration. Ligation appears to be as effective as sclerotherapy in controlling acute bleeding and is associated with fewer complications. Rebleeding may occur less often in patients treated by ligation compared to sclerotherapy. Further experience may establish this as the procedure of choice in preventing variceal bleeding.

Surgery

Surgical creation of a portacaval shunt has been effective in reducing portal pressure and in preventing recurrent bleeding. However, these shunts are associated with a high incidence of hepatic encephalopathy and may exacerbate hepatic parenchymal dysfunction by shunting blood away from the liver. Mesocaval shunts and distal splenorenal shunts also are effective in preventing variceal rebleeding and may be associated with a lower incidence of hepatic encephalopathy. Generally, these procedures are reserved for patients in whom endoscopic therapy fails.[78]

Transjugular Intrahepatic Portal Systemic Shunting

Transjugular intrahepatic portal systemic shunting (TIPS) is a newer interventional (nonsurgical) technique for establishing a shunt in patients with portal hypertension. During this procedure, a needle is advanced through a catheter via a transjugular approach into a hepatic vein. Coursing through the hepatic parenchyma of the perforating wall of the hepatic vein, an intrahepatic branch of the portal vein is then punctured to create a tunnel between the two veins. Finally, after balloon dilation of this intraparenchymal tract connecting the hepatic (systemic) vein to the portal vein branch, an expandable metal stent is placed in the tract to maintain the patency of the tract and decompress the portal system. TIPS has the advantage of being less invasive, faster, safer, and less expensive than surgically created portal systemic shunts. Long-term patency of TIPS, however, remains problematic, and their use is generally confined to patients not eligible for surgical shunt procedures.[79,80]

18. **C.V. subsequently recovered from her acute episode of variceal bleeding. Her physician wants to start secondary treatment to prevent further variceal hemorrhage. What are the long-term objectives for the management of C.V.? What agents can be used?**

Secondary prevention, also called *secondary prophylaxis,* is the terminology used to describe therapy to prevent rebleeding once the primary event has been terminated. At 1 year 25% of Child's grade A, 50% of Child's grade B, and 75% of Child grade C will experience a rebleeding episode from the same site.[81] Prevention of bleeding is difficult in most patients. Clinical studies on the prevention of recurrence of the disease have produced conflicting results. Furthermore, interpretation of the clinical outcomes from various studies is often difficult because of the heterogeneous patient population studied: differing etiologies of esophageal varices (e.g., cholestatic versus alcoholic cirrhosis), location of the flow obstruction (e.g., presinusoidal versus sinusoidal), and severity of liver disease.[82] β-Blockers are the best studied drugs for this indication.

β-Blockers

Propranolol and other β-blockers have been used after the initial bleeding has stopped to help reduce hepatic blood flow and portal pressure.[83] β-Blockers are most beneficial in the patients whose cirrhosis is secondary to alcoholism, but who have less advanced disease and who stop drinking after the first bleeding episode. In one study, 94 patients were randomized to propranolol (32 patients), atenolol (32 patients), or placebo (30 patients). Propranolol was given orally at 10 mg four times a day in increasing doses until the resting pulse rate was reduced by approximately 25%. Atenolol was given at a fixed dose of 100 mg/day. The incidence of rebleeding was significantly lower in patients receiving propranolol compared with those in placebo group. Atenolol was less effective than propranolol.[76]

Although β-blockers in most studies significantly reduce rebleeding from esophageal varices, they do not decrease mortality in most of the studies.[82] Abrupt discontinuation of β-blockers may lead to rebleeding. Although some data suggest treatment with β-blockers is effective, not all studies have observed positive results.[81]

19. **All interventions up to this point were aimed at either terminating the acute bleeding episode or preventing a recurrence (secondary prevention). Could a β-blocker or other drug therapy have helped prevent the first episode of bleeding from C.V.'s esophageal varices?**

Mortality rates associated with bleeding esophageal varices ranges from 15% to 40%. Therefore, a better strategy in patients with known cirrhosis and portal hypertension would be to prevent the initial episode of variceal bleeding. Such a treatment intervention is termed *primary prevention or primary prophylaxis.* Theoretically, minimizing the complications of portal hypertension should improve both quality of life and survival rates, although there is little data to substantiate this theory.[84]

The most frequently studied drug class for primary prevention of bleeding is again the β-blockers, including both propranolol and nadolol. Only nonselective β-blockers have an adrenergic dilatory effect in mesenteric arterioles which results in a decrease in portal blood circulation and pressure.[84] Therefore, only propranolol and nadolol are recommended for primary prophylaxis against a first bleeding episode. Isosorbide mononitrate, either as monotherapy or combined with a β-blocker, has also been studied for this indication.

Nonselective β-blockers, titrated to achieve a 25% reduction in heart rate or hepatic venous pressure gradient, can reduce the risk of initial variceal bleeding to about 22% compared with approximately 45% with no intervention or placebo.[84] The usual starting dosages are propranolol 10 mg three times a day or nadolol 20 mg every day. The greatest success with propranolol has been in alcoholic patients with small varices and grade B or C Child-Pugh scores.[84] Selective β-blockers such as atenolol and metoprolol have not been demonstrated to be effective in primary prophylaxis, and the effect on mesenteric arterioles is not dramatic.[85]

Despite strong evidence that propranolol and other nonselective β-blockers prevent first-episode variceal bleeding in selected patients, there is not a consensus on their ability to increase short-term (1 month) or long-term (1 year or longer) survival. Meta-analysis indicates that patients with alcoholic cirrhosis, small varices, good compliance, and no medical contraindications may derive the most benefit from prophylactic β-blockers.[84,86] Because only 25% to 40% of cirrhotic patients will bleed from esophageal varices and the survival benefit of β-blocker therapy is not definitively established in all patients with varices, these drugs may not be warranted in all patients with cirrhosis and portal hypertension.

Isosorbide-5-Mononitrate

Isosorbide-5-mononitrate has been shown to reduce portal pressure in patients with cirrhosis.[87] When combined with propranolol, isosorbide-5-mononitrate causes a greater reduction in the hepatic venous pressure gradient than propranolol alone.[88] One study comparing isosorbide-5-mononitrate and propranolol for the prevention of first variceal bleeding showed similar efficacy with regard to bleeding and survival.[89] Patients were randomized to receive isosorbide-5-mononitrate, 20 mg twice a day and slowly titrated to 20 mg three times a day. Other patients were randomized to receive propranolol, titrated to the maximum tolerated dose (120 mg daily) given three times daily or until heart rate was less 55 beats/min. The 1- and 2-year rates of patients free of bleeding were 90.8% and 82.2% in the isosorbide-5-mononitrate-treated subjects and 93.9% and 85.8% in the propranolol-treated group, respectively. However, the mean propranolol dose used in this study was lower than that used in most other clinical trials. Thus, the role of isosorbide-5-mononitrate monotherapy requires further clarification.[90]

Other investigators have examined the value of combining a β-blocker (nadolol) and a nitrate (isosorbide mononitrate) for primary prevention of variceal bleeding.[91] Patients in the nadolol monotherapy group received between 40 and 160 mg/day titrated to achieve a 20% to 25% decrease in resting heart rate. Patients receiving both drugs received nadolol and isosorbide mononitrate 10 to 20 mg orally twice daily. The overall risk of variceal bleeding was 18% in the nadolol group compared with 7.5% in the combined treatment group. This study indicated that nadolol plus isosorbide mononitrate is significantly more effective than nadolol alone in the primary prophylaxis of variceal bleeding.

Sclerotherapy

Sclerotherapy has been evaluated for primary prophylaxis of variceal bleeding. Although the data are conflicting, one study showed a higher mortality in sclerotherapy-treated patients with alcoholic cirrhosis. Therefore, prophylactic sclerotherapy is not recommended for routine use at this time.[92]

HEPATIC ENCEPHALOPATHY

20. R.C., a 57-year-old man, was admitted to the hospital because of nausea, vomiting, and abdominal pain. He had a long history of alcohol abuse, with multiple hospital admissions for alcoholic gastritis and alcohol withdrawal. Physical examination revealed a cachectic male with clouded mentation who was not responsive to questions about name and place. Tense ascites and edema were noted, and the liver was percussed at 9 cm below the right costal margin. The spleen was not palpated, and no active bowel sounds were heard. Laboratory results on admission included the following: Na, 132 mEq/L; K, 3.7 mEq/L; Cl, 98 mEq/L; bicarbonate, 27 mEq/L; BUN, 24 mg/dL; SrCr, 1.4 mg/dL; Hgb, 9.2 g/dL; Hct, 24.1%; AST, 520 IU (normal, 5 to 29); alkaline phosphatase, 218 IU (normal, 22 to 110); lactate dehydrogenase (LDH), 305 IU (normal, 82 to 226); and total bilirubin, 3.5 mg/dL. PT was 22 seconds with a control of 12 seconds.

A 60-g protein, 2,000-kcal diet was ordered. Furosemide 40 mg IV BID was ordered in an attempt to reduce the edema and ascites. Morphine sulfate and prochlorperazine (Compazine) were ordered for his abdominal pain and nausea, respectively. Two days after admission, R.C. had an episode of hematemesis.

He became mentally confused and at times nonresponsive to verbal command. An NG tube was inserted and produced coffee ground material upon continuous suctioning. Saline lavage was continued until the aspirate became clear. The next morning, R.C. was still in a confused mental state. He demonstrated prominent asterixis, and fetor hepaticus was noted in his breath. On the second day of his hospitalization, laboratory data were as follows: Hgb, 7.4 g/dL; Hct, 21.2%; K, 3.1 mEq/L; SrCr, 1.4 mg/dL; BUN, 36 mg/dL; PT, 22 seconds; and stool guaiac, 4% positive. Impending hepatic encephalopathy and upper GI bleeding were added to the problem list.

What aspects of R.C.'s history are compatible with a diagnosis of hepatic encephalopathy?

Hepatic coma or encephalopathy is a metabolic disorder of the CNS and occurs in patients with either advanced cirrhosis or fulminate hepatic failure. It is commonly accompanied by portal systemic shunting of blood. The clinical features (as seen in R.C.) include altered mental state, asterixis, and fetor hepaticus.

During the early phase of encephalopathy, the altered mental state may present as a slight derangement of judgment, personality, or change of mood. Drowsiness and confusion become more prominent as the encephalopathy progresses. Finally, unresponsiveness to arousal and deep coma ensue.

Asterixis, or flapping tremor, is the most characteristic neurologic abnormality in hepatic encephalopathy. This tremor can be demonstrated by having the patient hyperextend his or her wrist with the forearms outstretched and fingers separated. It is characterized by bilateral, but synchronous, repetitive arrhythmic motions occurring in bursts of one flap (twitch) every 1 to 2 seconds. Asterixis is not specific for hepatic encephalopathy and may also be present in uremia, hypokalemia, heart failure, ketoacidosis, respiratory failure, and sedative overdose.

Fetor hepaticus, a peculiar sweetish, musty, pungent odor to the breath, is believed to be due to circulating unmetabolized mercaptans. A staging scheme for grading the severity of hepatic encephalopathy is found in Table 29-2.[93,94] As discussed in the questions that follow, the pharmacologic management of encephalopathy is guided both by an understanding of the pathogenesis of this disorder and the stage of severity demonstrated by each individual patient. In most cases, hepatic encephalopathy is fully reversible; therefore, it

Table 29-2   Stages of Encephalopathy

Physical Sign	Stage I Prodrome	Stage II Impending Coma	Stage III Stupor	Stage IV Coma	Stage V Coma
Mental status	Alert; slow mentation; euphoria, occasional depression, confusion; sleep pattern reversal	Stage I signs amplified; lethargic, sleepy	Arousable but generally asleep; significant confusion	Unarousable or responds only to pain	Unarousable
Behavior	Restless, irritable, disordered speech	Combative, sullen, loss of sphincter control	Sleeping, confusion, incoherent speech	None	None
Spontaneous motor activity	Uncoordinated with tremor	Yawning, grimacing, blinking	Decreased, severe tremor	Absent	None
Asterixis	Absent	Present	Present	Absent	Absent
Reflexes	Normal	Hyperactive	Hyperactive + Babinski	Hyperactive + Babinski	Absent

is probably a metabolic/neurophysiologic rather than an organic disorder.[93]

Pathogenesis

21. What is the pathogenesis of hepatic encephalopathy?

There are several theories about the pathogenesis of hepatic encephalopathy. The predominant ones involve abnormal ammonia metabolism and an altered ratio of branched chain to aromatic amino acids. Other neurotransmitters such as γ-amino butyric acid (GABA) and serotonin may be associated with hepatic encephalopathy.[95]

Ammonia

Ammonia is a byproduct of protein metabolism, and a large portion is derived from dietary ingestion of proteins or presentation of protein-rich blood into the GI tract (e.g., from bleeding esophageal varices). Bacteria present in the GI tract digest protein into polypeptides, amino acids, and ammonia. These substances are then absorbed across the intestinal mucosa, where they are either further metabolized, stored for later use, or used for production of new proteins. Ammonia is readily metabolized in the liver to urea (BUN), which is then renally eliminated. When blood flow and hepatic metabolism are impaired by cirrhosis, serum and CNS concentrations of ammonia are increased. The ammonia that enters the CNS combines with α-ketoglutarate to form glutamine, an aromatic amino acid. Although high serum ammonia and cerebrospinal glutamine concentrations are characteristic of encephalopathy, they may not be the actual cause of this syndrome.[96]

Amino Acid Balance

Body stores of branched chain and aromatic amino acids are affected by their rate of synthesis from protein metabolism (both in the GI tract and in the liver), their utilization in the resynthesis of new proteins within the liver, and their utilization by various tissues for energy. The normal ratio of branched chain amino acids (e.g., valine, leucine, isoleucine) to methionine and aromatic amino acids (e.g., phenylalanine, tyrosine, tryptophan) in plasma is 4.6:1. In both acute and chronic liver failure, the serum concentration of aromatic amino acids significantly increases, the serum concentration of branched chain amino acids either remains the same or decreases, and the ratio of the branched chain to aromatic amino acids is altered as a result.

The utilization of branched chain amino acids for skeletal muscle metabolism during liver failure partially explains the decrease in branched chain amino acids. At the same time, the blood–brain barrier appears to be more permeable to aromatic amino acid uptake into the cerebrospinal fluid (CSF). Once in the CSF, some aromatic compounds are metabolized into chemicals that disrupt normal CSF neurotransmitter balance. For example, phenylalanine is converted to octopamine, and tryptophan is converted to serotonin. Both octopamine and serotonin can compete with norepinephrine for normal CNS function.[95,96]

γ-Aminobutyric Acid

The GABA receptor forms a supramolecular complex with both the benzodiazepine (BZ) receptor and chloride ionophore. Activation of the GABA receptor results in increased chloride permeability, hyperpolarization of the neuronal membrane, and inhibition of neurotransmission. In 1982, Schafer and Jones proposed that in liver disease, gut-derived GABA escapes hepatic metabolism, crosses the blood–brain barrier, binds to its postsynaptic receptor sites, and causes the neurologic abnormalities associated with hepatic encephalopathy.[97] Others hypothesize that endogenous benzodiazepine-like substances, via their agonist properties, contribute to the pathogenesis of hepatic encephalopathy by enhancing GABA-ergic neurotransmission. The role of GABA and the endogenous benzodiazepines still is not clearly defined and requires further clarification.[98,99]

An altered ratio of branched chain to aromatic amino acids and increased concentrations of ammonia, GABA, mercaptans, and weak neurotransmitters have all been implicated in the pathogenesis of hepatic encephalopathy. Other postulated factors include increased susceptibility to various "toxins" because of the altered permeability of the blood–brain barrier, as well as the absence of some protective substances normally produced by the healthy liver. Nevertheless, none of these has been incriminated as the single cause and the pathogenesis of hepatic encephalopathy is likely to be multifactorial.

Of all the toxins suspected to cause hepatic coma, ammonia and certain aromatic amino acids are the most commonly studied and are generally held responsible. Other precipitating factors (Table 29-3) increase the serum ammonia or produce excessive somnolence in patients with impending hepatic coma. Excess nitrogen load and metabolic or electrolyte abnormalities may increase ammonia levels.[100,101]

22. What are the probable precipitating causes of hepatic encephalopathy in R.C.?

The most apparent precipitating cause of the encephalopathy in R.C. was the sudden onset of upper GI bleeding. The bacterial degradation of blood protein in the gut results in absorption of large amounts of ammonia and possibly other toxins into the portal system. Other important contributory factors in this case are diuretic-induced hypovolemia (BUN:serum creatinine, >20), hypokalemia (potassium, 3.1 mEq/L), and metabolic alkalosis (e.g., hypokalemia, continuous nasogastric suction). Overzealous diuretic therapy enhances hepatic encephalopathy by inducing prerenal azotemia and, more importantly, by promoting hypokalemia and metabolic alkalosis. Hypokalemia increases the concentration of ammonia in renal venous blood. Alkalosis, often associated with hypokalemia, promotes diffusion of nonionic ammonia and other amines into the CNS. The associated intracellular acidosis "traps" the ammonia by converting it back to ammonium ion (NH_4^+).[102,103]

Sedating drugs also may be hazardous in patients with cirrhosis. Drugs that have been associated with hepatic encephalopathy are opioids (e.g., morphine, methadone, meperidine, codeine), sedatives (e.g., benzodiazepines, barbiturates, chloral hydrate), and tranquilizers (e.g., phenothiazines). Encephalopathy precipitated by most drugs can be explained by increased CNS sensitivity and decreased hepatic clearance with subsequent drug accumulation. In addition, the effects of morphine, chlorpromazine, and diazepam may be increased in liver disease because of decreased plasma protein binding. Thus, the morphine and prochlorperazine that were prescribed for R.C. also may have contributed to the development of his hepatic encephalopathy.

Table 29-3   Factors That May Precipitate Hepatic Encephalopathy

Causes	Therapeutic Considerations
Excess Nitrogen Load	
Bleeding from GI and esophageal varices	Avoid gastric irritants; correct hypoprothrombinemia with vitamin K; give stool softener to
Hemorrhoidal bleeding	prevent variceal bleeding from straining; evacuate blood in bowel with lactulose or magne-
Peptic ulcer	sium citrate
Excess dietary protein	Limit protein intake to 1 g/kg: avoid protein with high ammoniagenic potential
Azotemia	Avoid overdiuresis; use neomycin or lactulose prophylactically to decrease gut ammonia
Diuretic-induced hypovolemia	genesis from urea
Uremia or renal failure	
Excessive enterohepatic circulation of BUN	
Infection: tissue catabolism	Treat infection with appropriate antibiotics
Constipation: ↑ ammonia generation	Use stool softener and laxatives prophylactically
due to ↓ gut transit time	
Metabolic and Electrolyte Abnormalities	
Hypokalemia	Avoid overdiuresis; KCl replacement; control diarrhea; spironolactone therapy for ascites
Diuretic-induced	
Dietary deficiency	
Excessive diarrhea	
Hyperaldosteronism	
Alkalosis	Correct hypokalemia and alkalosis; antiemetic therapy
Hypokalemia-induced	
Excessive nausea and vomiting	
Drug-Induced CNS Depression	
Sedatives	Avoid long-acting sedatives
Tranquilizers	Avoid phenothiazines because of association with hepatotoxicity
Narcotic analgesics	Avoid hypoxia from respiratory depression

BUN, blood urea nitrogen.

Although not applicable to this case, excessive dietary protein, tissue catabolism from severe infections, and constipation also can contribute to excess nitrogen load and the genesis of hepatic coma (see Table 29-3).

Treatment and General Management

23. **What steps should be taken to manage R.C.'s hepatic encephalopathy?**

After identifying and removing precipitating causes of hepatic coma, therapeutic management is aimed primarily at reducing the amount of ammonia or nitrogenous products in the circulatory system. Protein intake should be stopped completely or significantly limited at the onset of encephalopathy. Dietary protein can then be gradually increased at 10 to 20 g/day every 2 to 5 days depending on the clinical response. Vegetable protein may be better tolerated than animal protein because vegetable protein contains fewer methionine and aromatic amino acids that are less ammoniagenic.[10,104]

24. **How are lactulose and neomycin used in hepatic encephalopathy? Which agent would be more appropriate for R.C.?**

Lactulose

Lactulose is highly efficacious in the treatment of hepatic encephalopathy. This disaccharide is broken down by GI bacteria to form lactic, acetic, and formic acids. It is believed that acidification of colonic contents converts ammonia into the less readily absorbed ammonium ion. There also may be back diffusion of ammonia from the plasma into the GI tract. The net result is a lower plasma ammonia concentration. The absorption of other protein breakdown products (e.g., aromatic amino acids) also may be reduced. Lactulose-induced osmotic diarrhea also decreases the intestinal transit time available for ammonia production and absorption.

DOSING

Lactulose syrup (10 g/15 mL) has been used successfully in both acute and chronic hepatic encephalopathy. In the acute situation, initial doses of 30 to 45 mL are given three times daily and titrated to either the resolution of symptoms or the production of three soft stools per day. When the oral route of administration is not possible, as in the treatment of comatose patients, it may be necessary to administer the drug through a NG tube. Alternatively, a rectal retention enema (300 mL in 1 L water) retained for 1 hour can be administered. The beneficial clinical effect of lactulose occurs within 12 to 48 hours. Although most patients are weaned off lactulose after a few days or weeks, long-term administration is sometimes necessary for patients with recurring encephalopathy. The chronic administration of lactulose permits better dietary protein tolerance and is well tolerated if doses are kept low enough to avoid diarrhea.

Care should be taken not to induce excessive diarrhea that could lead to dehydration and hypokalemia, both of which have been associated with exacerbation of hepatic encephalopathy. Although lactulose is generally well tolerated, 20% of patients may complain of gaseous distention, flatulence, or belching. Diluting it with fruit juice, carbonated beverages, or water can reduce the excessive sweetness of the syrup.[94]

Neomycin

Neomycin, at dosages of 1 to 2 g orally four times daily, or as a 1% solution given as a retention enema for 20 to 60 minutes four times daily, is effective in reducing plasma ammonia levels (presumably by decreasing protein-metabolizing bacteria in the GI tract). Approximately 1% to 3% of a dose of neomycin is absorbed, and chronic use in patients with renal failure may rarely cause ototoxicity or nephrotoxicity. Routine monitoring of the serum creatinine, the presence of protein in the urine, and estimation of creatinine clearance are advisable for patients receiving high dosages for long periods. Neomycin therapy may also produce a reversible malabsorption syndrome that not only suppresses the absorption of fat, nitrogen, carotene, iron, vitamin B_{12}, xylose, and glucose, but also decreases the absorption of various drugs such as digoxin, penicillin, and vitamin K.[94] As with lactulose, most patients are only given neomycin for a few days until the acute episode of hepatic encephalopathy clears following treatment of the underlying cause. Because of concerns over side effects cited above, lactulose is much preferred for long-term use.

Comparison With Lactulose

Lactulose and neomycin are essentially interchangeable with equal effectiveness in the treatment of hepatic encephalopathy. In the treatment of an acute exacerbation, neomycin may produce a faster response than lactulose, but for the most part, lactulose has become the drug of choice. Occasionally, a patient who does not respond to one will respond to the other.

The interference of vitamin K absorption by neomycin may further impair R.C.'s already compromised coagulation status (PT, 22 seconds). In addition, while use of neomycin during this acute exacerbation should be safe, long-term use of neomycin is not recommended for R.C. because the combination of his decreased renal function (SrCr, 1.4 mg/dL) and the 1 to 3% absorption of neomycin could result in accumulation and a risk of toxicity over time. Therefore, lactulose is preferred for R.C. To hasten the onset of response, the first doses of lactulose can be large (i.e., 30 to 40 mL every hour) until catharsis occurs. If R.C. does not have a gag reflex, lactulose should be administered by rectal enema because the oral syrup can provoke nausea.

Neomycin in Combination With Lactulose

25. Would the combined use of neomycin and lactulose have any additive beneficial effect for R.C.?

The American College of Gastroenterology guidelines state combination therapy of lactulose and neomycin is reasonable for patients who do not respond to monotherapy.[10] In some cases, the combination may be more effective than either drug alone. Why the two drugs have additive effects is unclear, but it is probable that either degradation of lactulose may not be essential for reduction of ammonia level or there are other unknown mechanisms for the activity of lactulose. Lactulose should be tried first, and if satisfactory results do not occur, neomycin alone should be given a trial. If both agents fail when used singly, the two agents can then be tried together. Although combined use of lactulose and neomycin is beneficial, lactulose alone may be more desirable for long-term use because it is potentially less toxic.

26. Why would the benzodiazepine antagonist flumazenil be used to treat chronic encephalopathy?

Flumazenil

Based on the theory of increased GABA-ergic neurotransmission in hepatic encephalopathy, flumazenil (Romazicon), a benzodiazepine antagonist, has been evaluated for its role in treatment. Several trials have demonstrated both clinical and electrophysiologic improvement in patients with acute and chronic liver disease. In one study, 60% of patients had transient neurologic improvement after the administration of flumazenil 0.5 mg intravenously administered over 1 minute.[105] Another study suggested a response to flumazenil might be a favorable prognostic marker, as it suggests the encephalopathy is potentially reversible.[106] Chronic hepatic encephalopathy has also been successfully treated with orally administered flumazenil (25 mg orally twice daily). There is concern in some trials, however, that exogenous benzodiazepines and their metabolites may not have been detected in patients before treatment with flumazenil.[107] Therefore, a positive response to flumazenil may be attributed to reversal of the benzodiazepine effect and not a true improvement in encephalopathy. Conversely, lack of improvement with flumazenil may be associated with other metabolic abnormalities or CNS complications, such as cerebral edema or increased intracranial pressure. Despite the potential benefit of flumazenil, additional randomized, controlled trials are needed to determine its clinical role in the treatment of hepatic encephalopathy.[107]

27. When should liver transplantation be considered for the treatment of hepatic encephalopathy?

Liver transplantation has been advocated in patients with end-stage liver disease and severe hepatic encephalopathy. The current shortage of organ donors for transplantation increases the need to apply strict selection criteria. Many criteria should be evaluated in deciding whether a patient should be placed on a waiting list for transplantation. Most transplant centers accept alcoholic disease as an indication for liver transplantation after complete psychological and socioeconomic evaluations and require a 6- to 12-month period of abstinence before transplantation. Although the early result of liver transplantation for alcoholic liver disease are similar to those for other indications, well-designed controlled trails must be performed to predict the long-term risk of posttransplant recidivism in this patient population.[108] (See Chapter 35, Solid Organ Transplantation, for further information on the indications for liver transplantation.)[109]

REFERENCES

1. Anand BS. Cirrhosis of liver. West J Med 1999;171:110.
2. Williams EJ, Iredale JP. Liver cirrhosis. Postgrad Med J 1998;74:193.
3. Lieber CS. Hepatic and other medical disorders of alcoholism: from pathogenesis to treatment. J Stud Alcohol 1998;59:9.
4. Nanji AA. Role of Kupffer cells in alcoholic hepatitis. Alcohol 2002;27:13.
5. Purohit V, Russo D. Cellular and molecular mechanisms of alcoholic hepatitis: introduction and summary of the symposium. Alcohol 2002;27:3.
6. Dufour DR et al. Diagnosis and monitoring of hepatic injury. II. Recommendations for use of laboratory tests in screening, diagnosis, and monitoring. Clin Chem 2000;46:2050.
7. Dufour DR et al. Diagnosis and monitoring of hepatic injury. I. Performance characteristics of laboratory tests. Clin Chem 2000;46:2027.
8. Runyon BA. Management of adult patients with ascites caused by cirrhosis. Hepatology 1998;27:264.
9. Carithers RL Jr. Liver transplantation. American Association for the Study of Liver Diseases. Liver Transplant 2000;6:122.
10. Blei AT, Cordoba J, The Practice Parameters Committee of the American College of Gastroenterology. Hepatic encephalopathy. Am J Gastroenterol 2001;96:1968.
11. Menon KV et al. Pathogenesis, diagnosis, and treatment of alcoholic liver disease. Mayo Clin Proc 2001;76:1021.
12. de la M Hall et al. Models of alcoholic liver disease in rodents: a critical evaluation. Alcohol Clin Exp Res 2001;25:254S.
13. Neuman MG et al. Mechanisms of alcoholic liver disease: cytokines. Alcohol Clin Exp Res 2001; 25:251S.
14. Tsukamoto H et al. How is the liver primed or sensitized for alcoholic liver disease?. Alcohol Clin Exp Res 2001,25.171S.
15. Casey CA et al. Alcoholic liver disease and apoptosis. Alcohol Clin Exp Res 2001;25:49S.
16. Szabo G. New insights into the molecular mechanisms of alcoholic hepatitis: a potential role for NF-κ activation? J Lab Clin Med 2000;135:367.
17. McClain CJ et al. Cytokines in alcoholic liver disease. Semin Liver Dis 1999;19:205.
18. Schenker S, Hoyumpa AM. New concepts of dietary intervention in alcoholic liver disease. J Lab Clin Med 1999;134:433.
19. Lata J et al. Management of acute variceal bleeding. Dig Dis 2003;21:6.
20. Yeung E, Wong FS. The management of cirrhotic ascites. Medscape Gen Med 2002;4:8.
21. Sherman DS et al. Assessing renal function in cirrhotic patients: problems and pitfalls. Am J Kidney Dis 2003;41:269.
22. Henderson JM et al. Portal hypertension. Curr Prob Surg 1998;35:379.
23. Friedman SL. Efficacy of abstinence and specific therapy in alcoholic liver disease. In: UpToDate, Rose BD (Ed), UpToDate: Wellesley, MA, 2003.
24. Bosch J. Medical treatment of portal hypertension. Digestion 1998;59:547.
25. Palmer BF. Pathogenesis of ascites and renal salt retention in cirrhosis. J Invest Med 1999;47:183.
26. Rambaldi A. Colchicine for alcoholic and nonalcoholic liver fibrosis or cirrhosis. Liver 2001;21:129.
27. Rambaldi A, Gluud C. Meta-analysis of propylthiouracil for alcoholic liver disease: a Cochrane Hepato-Biliary Group Review. Liver 2001;21:398.
28. Santolaria F et al. Nutritional assessment in alcoholic patients. Its relationship with alcoholic intake, feeding habits, organic complications and social problems. Drug Alcohol Depend 2000;59:295.
29. Krige JE, Beckingham IJ. ABC of diseases of liver, pancreas, and biliary system: portal hypertension-2. Ascites, encephalopathy, and other conditions. BMJ 2001;322:416.
30. Jalan R, Hayes PC. Hepatic encephalopathy and ascites. Lancet 1997;350:1309.

31. Suzuki H, Stanley AJ. Current management and novel therapeutic strategies for refractory ascites and hepatorenal syndrome. QJM 2001;94:293.
32. Gentilini P et al. Ascites and hepatorenal syndrome. Eur J Gastroenterol Hepatol 2001;13:313.
33. Moore KP et al. The management of ascites in cirrhosis: report on the consensus conference of the International Ascites Club. Hepatology 2003; 38:258.
34. Biswas KD, Jain AK. Hepatorenal syndrome. Trop Gastroenterol 2002;23:113.
35. Gentilini P et al. Update on ascites and hepatorenal syndrome. Dig Liver Dis 2002;34:592.
36. Wong F. Liver and kidney diseases. Clin Liver Dis 2002;6:981.
37. Zervos EE, Rosemurgy AS. Management of medically refractory ascites. Am J Surg 2001;181:256.
38. Runyon BA. Albumin infusion for spontaneous bacterial peritonitis. Lancet 1999;354:1838.
39. Yamamoto S. Disappearance of spironolactone-induced gynecomastia with triamterene. Intern Med 2001;40:550.
40. Runyon BA. Treatment of patients with cirrhosis and ascites. Semin Liver Dis 1997;17:249.
41. Runyon BA. Historical aspects of treatment of patients with cirrhosis and ascites. Semin Liver Dis 1997;17:163.
42. Wong F, Blendis L. New challenge of hepatorenal syndrome: prevention and treatment. Hepatology 2001;34:1242.
43. Ruiz-del-Arbol L et al. Paracentesis-induced circulatory dysfunction: mechanism and effect on hepatic hemodynamics in cirrhosis. Gastroenterology 1997;113:579.
44. Arroyo V, Colmenero J. Ascite and hepatorenal syndrome in cirrhosis: pathophysiology basis of therapy and current management. J Hepatol 2003; 38(SI):69.
45. Sort P et al. Effect of intravenous albumin on renal impairment and mortality in patients with cirrhosis and spontaneous bacterial peritonitis [Comment]. N Engl J Med 1999;341:403.
46. Sola-Vera J et al. Randomized trial comparing albumin and saline in the prevention of paracentesis-induced circulatory dysfunction in cirrhotic patients with ascites. Hepatology 2003;37:1147.
47. Terg R et al. Dextran administration avoids hemodynamic changes following paracentesis in cirrhotic patients. Dig Dis Sci 1992;37:79.
48. Terg R et al. Pharmacokinetics of Dextran-70 in patients with cirrhosis and ascites undergoing therapeutic paracentesis. J Hepatol 1996;25:329.
49. Zeerleder S et al. Effect of low-molecular weight dextran sulfate on coagulation and platelet function tests. Thromb Res 2002;105:441.
50. Gines A et al. Randomized trial comparing albumin, dextran 70, and polygeline in cirrhotic patients with ascites treated by paracentesis. Gastroenterology 1996;111:1002.
51. Christidis C et al. Worsening of hepatic dysfunction as a consequence of repeated hydroxyethyl starch infusions. J Hepatol 2001;35:726.
52. Sanyal AJ. The management of the cirrhotic patient after transjugular intrahepatic portosystemic shunt. Semin Gastrointest Dis 1997;8:188.
53. Tueche SG, Pector JC. Peritoneovenous shunt in malignant ascites. The Bordet Institute experience from 1975-1998. Hepato-Gastroenterology 2000;47:1322.
54. Zervos EE et al. Peritoneovenous shunts in patients with intractable ascites: palliation at what price? Am Surg 1997;63:157.
55. Guardiola J et al. Prognosis assessment of cirrhotic patients with refractory ascites treated with a peritoneovenous shunt. Am J Gastroenterol 1995;90:2097.
56. Sarin SK, Agarwal SR. Gastric varices and portal hypertensive gastropathy. Clin Liver Dis 2001;5:727.
57. de Franchis R, Primignani M. Natural history of portal hypertension in patients with cirrhosis. Clin Liver Dis 2001;5:645.
58. Arguedas MR. The critically ill liver patient: the variceal bleeder. Semin Gastrointest Dis 2003; 14:34.

59. Seewald S et al. Variceal bleeding and portal hypertension: has there been any progress in the last 12 months? Endoscopy 2003;35:136.
60. Wu JC, Sung JJ. Update on treatment of variceal hemorrhage. Dig Dis 2002;20:134.
61. Therapondos G, Hayes PC. Management of gastro-oesophageal varices. Clin Med 2002;2:297.
62. Chung S. Management of bleeding in the cirrhotic patient. J Gastroenterol Hepatol 2002;17:355.
63. Bhasin DK, Malhi NJ. Variceal bleeding and portal hypertension: much to learn, much to explore. Endoscopy 2002;34:119.
64. McKiernan PJ. Treatment of variceal bleeding. Gastrointest Endosc Clin North Am 2001;11:789.
65. Goulis J, Burroughs AK. Role of vasoactive drugs in the treatment of bleeding oesophageal varices. Digestion 1999;60(Suppl 3):25.
66. Iwao T et al. Effect of vasopressin on esophageal varices blood flow in patients with cirrhosis: comparisons with the effects on portal vein and superior mesenteric artery blood flow. J Hepatol 1996;25:491.
67. Law AW, Gales MA. Octreotide or vasopressin for bleeding esophageal varices. Ann Pharmacother 1997;31:237.
68. Bruha R et al. Double-blind randomized, comparative multicenter study of the effect of terlipressin in the treatment of acute esophageal variceal and/ or hypertensive gastropathy bleeding. Hepato-Gastroenterology 2002;49:1161.
69. de Franchis R. Longer treatment with vasoactive drugs to prevent early variceal rebleeding in cirrhosis. European J Gastroenterol Hepatol 1998;10:1041.
70. Imperiale TF et al. A meta-analysis of somatostatin versus vasopressin in the management of acute esophageal variceal hemorrhage. Gastroenterology 1995;109:1289.
71. Zhou Y et al. Comparison of the efficacy of octreotide, vasopressin, and omeprazole in the control of acute bleeding in patients with portal hypertensive gastropathy: a controlled study. J Gastroenterol Hepatol 2002;17:973.
72. Helmy A, Hayes PC. Review article: current endoscopic therapeutic options in the management of variceal bleeding. Aliment Pharmacol Ther 2001; 15:575.
73. Tatemichi M et al. Differences in hemostasis among sclerosing agents in endoscopic injection sclerotherapy. Dig Dis Sci 1996;41:562.
74. Dagher L, Burroughs A. Variceal bleeding and portal hypertensive gastropathy. Eur J Gastroenterol Hepatol 2001;13:81.
75. Nevens F, Rutgeerts P. Variceal band ligation in the management of bleeding oesophageal varices: an overview. Dig Liver Dis 2001;33:284.
76. Luketic VA. Management of portal hypertension after variceal hemorrhage. Clin Liver Dis 2001;5:677.
77. Gow PJ, Chapman RW. Modern management of oesophageal varices. Postgrad Med J 2001;77:75.
78. Jovine E et al. Splenoadrenal shunt: an original portosystemic decompressive technique. Hepato-Gastroenterology 2001;48:107.
79. Tripathi D et al. The role of the transjugular intrahepatic portosystemic stent shunt (TIPSS) in the management of bleeding gastric varices: clinical and haemodynamic correlations. Gut 2002;51:270.
80. Hidajat N et al. Transjugular intrahepatic portosystemic shunt and transjugular embolization of bleeding rectal varices in portal hypertension. AJR 2002;178:362.
81. Wu CY et al. Pharmacologic efficacy in gastric variceal rebleeding and survival: including multivariate analysis. J Clin Gastroenterol 2002;35:127.
82. Bernard B et al. Propranolol and sclerotherapy in the prevention of gastrointestinal rebleeding in patients with cirrhosis: a meta-analysis. J Hepatol 1997;26:312.
83. Rossle M. Prevention of rebleeding from oesophageal-gastric varices. Eur J Gastroenterol Hepatol 2001;13:343.
84. Brett BT et al. Primary prophylaxis of variceal bleeding in cirrhosis. Eur J Gastroenterol Hepatol 2001;13:349.

85. Uribe M et al. Portal-systemic encephalopathy and gastrointestinal bleeding after cardioselective beta-blocker (metoprolol) administration to patients with portal hypertension. Arch Med Res 1995;26:221.

86. Lowe RC, Grace ND. Primary prophylaxis of variceal hemorrhage. Clin Liver Dis 2001;5:665.

87. Lui HF et al. Primary prophylaxis of variceal hemorrhage: a randomized controlled trial comparing band ligation, propranolol, and isosorbide mononitrate. Gastroenterology 2002;123:735.

88. Vorobioff J et al. Propranolol compared with propranolol plus isosorbide dinitrate in portal-hypertensive patients: long-term hemodynamic and renal effects. Hepatology 1993;18:477.

89. Morillas RM et al. Propranolol plus isosorbide-5-mononitrate for portal hypertension in cirrhosis: long-term hemodynamic and renal effects. Hepatology 1994;20:1502.

90. Garcia-Pagan JC et al. Propranolol plus placebo versus propranolol plus isosorbide-5-mononitrate in the prevention of a first variceal bleed: a double-blind RCT. Hepatology 2003;37:1260.

91. Merkel C et al. Randomised trial of nadolol alone or with isosorbide mononitrate for primary prophylaxis of variceal bleeding in cirrhosis. Lancet 1996;348:1677.

92. D'Amico G et al. Emergency sclerotherapy versus medical interventions for bleeding oesophageal varices in cirrhotic patients. Cochrane Database of Systematic Reviews 2002;CD002233.

93. Ong JP, Mullen KD. Hepatic encephalopathy. Eur J Gastroenterol Hepatol 2001;13:325.

94. Abou-Assi S, Vlahcevic ZR. Hepatic encephalopathy. Metabolic consequence of cirrhosis often is reversible. Postgrad Med 2001;109:52.

95. Als-Nielsen B et al. Branched-chain amino acids for hepatic encephalopathy. Cochrane Database of Systematic Reviews 2003;CD001939.

96. James JH. Branched chain amino acids in hepatic encephalopathy. Am J Surg 2002;183:424.

97. Schafer DF, Jones EA. Potential neural mechanisms in the pathogenesis of hepatic encephalopathy. Prog Liver Dis 1982;7:615.

98. Jones EA, Basile AS. The involvement of ammonia with the mechanisms that enhance GABA-ergic neurotransmission in hepatic failure. Adv Exp Med Biol 1997;420:75.

99. Basile AS, Jones EA. Ammonia and GABA-ergic neurotransmission: interrelated factors in the pathogenesis of hepatic encephalopathy. Hepatology 1997;25:1303.

100. Butterworth RF. Hepatic encephalopathy: a neuropsychiatric disorder involving multiple neurotransmitter systems. Curr Opin Neurol 2000;13:721.

101. Haussinger D et al. Hepatic encephalopathy in chronic liver disease: a clinical manifestation of astrocyte swelling and low-grade cerebral edema? J Hepatol 2000;32:1035.

102. Gerber T, Schomerus H. Hepatic encephalopathy in liver cirrhosis: pathogenesis, diagnosis and management. Drugs 2000;60:1353.

103. Blei AT. Diagnosis and treatment of hepatic encephalopathy. Best Pract Res Clin Gastroenterol 2000;14:959.

104. Jones EA. Pathogenesis of hepatic encephalopathy. Clin Liver Dis 2000;4:467.

105. Laccetti M et al. Flumazenil in the treatment of acute hepatic encephalopathy in cirrhotic patients: a double blind randomized placebo controlled study. Dig Liver Dis 2000;32:335.

106. Goulenok C et al. Flumazenil vs. placebo in hepatic encephalopathy in patients with cirrhosis: a meta-analysis. Aliment Pharmacol Ther 2002; 16:361.

107. Als-Nielsen B et al. Benzodiazepine receptor antagonists for acute and chronic hepatic encephalopathy. Cochrane Database of Systematic Reviews 2001;CD002798.

108. Lucey MR. Is liver transplantation an appropriate treatment for acute alcoholic hepatitis? J Hepatol 2002;36:829.

109. Neuberger J et al. Transplantation for alcoholic liver disease. J Hepatol 2002;36:130.

CHAPTER 30

Adverse Effects of Drugs on the Liver

Curtis D. Holt, Edgar Arriola

INTRODUCTION

Hepatotoxicity may be defined as liver injury caused by drugs and chemicals, whereas adverse drug reactions (ADRs) are harmful, unwarranted effects that occur as a result of routine drug therapy. ADRs affecting the liver may be present when biochemical tests such as the serum aspartate (AST) and alanine (ALT) aminotransferases, serum alkaline phosphatase (SAP), gamma-glutamyl transferase (GGT), or bilirubin increase to more than double their normal values.[1] However, some of these tests are nonspecific; thus, abnormalities may sometimes indicate an adaptive response between a drug and hepatocytes or may reflect the effects of the drug on other parts of the body. In addition, drugs exhibit varying patterns of injury. If the injury is primarily hepatocellular, ALT and AST may be up to five times as high as normal, whereas cholestatic injury may lead to elevation in SAP, GGT, or bilirubin. Therefore, because the severity of liver injury may vary from nonspecific structural and functional changes to acute liver failure or cirrhosis, the term *drug-induced liver disease* (DILD) should be reserved until liver injury has been confirmed histologically. In the past few years, there has been a heightened awareness of DILD in the United States. This is a result of drugs being withdrawn from the market by the food and Drug Administration (FDA) and the fact that DILD is responsible for more than 50% of all cases of acute liver failure, with more than 75% of these reactions leading to liver transplantation.[2]

Before World War II, DILD was an issue of minor proportions, but with the introduction of a large number of new drugs during the following 25 years, a notable increase in the instances of DILD was observed.[3] More than 900 drugs have been implicated in cases of hepatic injury; thus, recognizing DILD is an important, but challenging, task for clinicians. Recent data suggest that ADRs cause a larger number of liver diseases than previously reported.[4]

Hepatotoxicity appears to be responsible for between 2% and 5% of cases of jaundice or acute hepatitis and for even fewer cases of chronic liver disease.[2-8] However, certain patient populations may have a greater incidence of DILD.[9] For example, reports indicate that in geriatric hospitals, drug-induced jaundice occurred in up to 20% of patients.[10] Similarly, these findings have been confirmed by a large liver disease center in France, which reported a 10% incidence of drug-induced "hepatitis" in patients younger than 50 years compared with rates of >40% in those older than 50.[11] In another population-based study conducted in France from 1997 to 2000, investigators reported that the crude incidence of hepatotoxicity was 13.9 cases per 100,000 patients per year.[12] The agents most often responsible for hepatotoxicity in this report included antimicrobials (25%), psychotropic agents (22.5%), lipid lowering agents (12.5%), and nonsteroidal anti-inflammatory drugs (10%). The authors noted that the observed frequency of hepatotoxicity was 16 times greater than that typically reported to the drug regulatory authorities as part of the post-marketing surveillance system. Based on these findings, the authors speculated that the incidence and severity of drug-induced liver dysfunction is grossly underestimated in the general population. Also, in hospitals with a large number of patients receiving psychoactive[13] or antitubercular agents,[14] the relative incidence of DILD is higher.

Previously, the Danish Committee on Adverse Drug Reactions reported that hepatic injury accounted for 6% of all ADRs and 14.7% of lethal ADRs between 1978 and 1987. This is almost double the number reported during the previous decade.[5] The drugs most commonly suspected in hepatic injury were halothane, carbamazepine, cotrimoxazole, disulfiram, and valproic acid. Furthermore, among cases of acute liver failure, drugs have been responsible for 15% to 25% of cases, with case fatality rates ranging from 10% to 50%.[7,15-18] However, fatality rates associated with cholestatic injury are much lower.[6,7]

Until recently, a paucity of data has existed with respect to the incidence and outcome of DILD or acute liver failure in the United States. This was due to the relatively rare occurrence of the condition, the unusual patient referral systems in North America, and the lack of an organized data registry. Subsequently, a consortium of liver centers was developed to prospectively define the etiologies and outcomes of patients with acute liver failure.[2,19] Over a 41-month period beginning in 1998, 308 patients ($\geq$15 years) with acute liver failure from 17 tertiary care liver centers were studied.[19] Results showed that most of these patients were women (73%) with a median age of 38 years. The primary cause of acute liver failure was acetaminophen overdose (39% of cases), followed by idiosyncratic drug reactions (13%). Short-term transplant free-survival was 68% and 25% for patients with acute liver failure secondary to acetaminophen ingestion or an idiosyncratic drug reaction, respectively.

EPIDEMIOLOGY AND RISK FACTORS

Epidemiologic reports have described the low prevalence of DILD with available agents. For example, the risk of liver injury secondary to nonsteroidal anti-inflammatory drugs (NSAIDs) and cimetidine use is 1 to 10 per 100,000 exposed individuals,[7,20-23] and the combination of amoxicillin with clavulanic acid has been associated with hepatitis in 1 to 5 per 1 million exposed individuals.[20,24,25] Isoniazid-induced liver injury may occur in as many as 100 per 100,000 exposed persons, possibly because of its ability to exert a metabolic type of hepatotoxicity,[14,23] whereas the rate of acute liver failure with lovastatin is 1/1.14 million patient-treated years.[26] Furthermore, the incidence of significant elevation in ALT or AST associated with the use of protease inhibitors (PIs) in combination with other antiretroviral agents has been reported to be up to 9.5% in the randomized controlled registration trials.[27] However, the reported rate of ADRs may be a poor indicator of risk because it depends on case recognition and definition as well as the motivation of observers to report ADRs.

Recent methodology such as prescription event monitoring, medical record linkage, and case-controlled studies have better defined the true risk of an agent's association with DILD.[23,28-30] In many circumstances, drugs are the only cause of liver injury, whereas in other cases, they may augment the relative risk for types of liver injury that could potentially occur even without drug exposure. For example, salicylates are associated with Reye's syndrome, oral contraceptives have been linked to hepatic veno-occlusive disease, and methotrexate may exacerbate hepatic fibrosis in patients with coexisting alcoholic and diabetic types of fatty liver disease.[2,7,31]

1. C.W. is a 63-year-old woman, 5'1" tall and weighing 75 kg, with a history of chronic urinary tract infections for which she had previously taken prophylactic trimethoprim-sulfamethoxazole. C.W. also has a history of generalized tonic-clonic seizures after her involvement in an auto accident 7 years ago. For the previous 18 months, her seizures have been well controlled while receiving valproic acid 1 g Q 8 hr. Of note, C.W. has recently been initiated on venlafaxine 50 mg twice daily for treatment of depression. On a routine visit to the neurology clinic, she was noted to have ALT, 66 U/L (normal, 5 to 40); AST, 88 U/L (normal, 5 to 40); alkaline phosphatase, 85 U/L (normal, 21 to 91); and total bilirubin, 0.8 mg/dL (normal, 0.1 to 1.2). What nonpharmacologic risk factors does C.W. have for DILD?

Several host factors affect the risk of DILD (Table 30-1). As previously described, most hepatic ADRs occur in adults rather than in children.[10,32] In the adult population, the relative risk of hepatotoxicity induced by isoniazid,[14,33] halothane,[34] erythromycin estolate and its analogues,[2,7,35-37] and diclofenac[38] is greater in patients older than 40 years of age. Generally, the increased frequency of ADRs observed in adults may correspond with an increased exposure, ingestion of multiple agents, or altered drug disposition. Exceptions to these findings include valproic acid- or salicylate-induced hepatotoxicity, which occurs most commonly in children younger than 3 years of age.[39,40]

Gender may also be related to risks for DILD. For example, female gender has been associated with an increased risk of hepatotoxicity, especially from agents such as halothane,[34] nitrofurantoin,[41,42] methyldopa,[7] and sulfonamides.[5,43]

In addition to age and gender, genetic factors may also have an impact on the ability to metabolize or eliminate drugs, encode pathways of bile excretion, and modulate the immune response. Although rarely encountered, a familial predisposition to hepatic ADRs from agents such as halothane[44] and phenytoin[45] has been shown.

Other factors that have an impact on DILD risk include a previous history of ADRs and ingestion of multiple drugs. The mechanism of DILD in the latter appears to be enhanced cytochrome P450-mediated metabolism of the second agent to toxic intermediates (i.e., acetaminophen, isoniazid, and valproic acid). Chronic excessive ingestion of alcohol may also enhance the risk of DILD from agents such as acetaminophen by reducing the body's stores of glutathione, which essentially lowers the dose threshold for hepatotoxicity. Other concomitant diseases or conditions such as rheumatoid arthritis, diabetes, hyperthyroidism, obesity, pregnancy, or renal dysfunction may also place patients at risk for DILD, whereas pre-existing liver disease rarely predisposes patients to adverse hepatic reactions.[46-52] Furthermore, drug dose, concentration, and duration of intake may be additional determinants in DILD.

Thus, C.W.'s age, gender, and obesity appear to be nonpharmacologic risk factors for developing DILD. However, because C.W. is asymptomatic and does not have manifestations of DILD, her baseline laboratory values are not reported, and the current hepatic enzyme elevation is less than three times normal, she should undergo close monitoring of her liver function tests within the next 2 to 4 weeks and return to clinic for follow-up.

Table 30-1   Risk Factors for Developing Drug-Induced Liver Disease[2,7,10,33–40]

Factor	Examples of Drugs Affected	Comments
Age	Isoniazid, nitrofurantoin, halothane	Increased incidence/severity with age >60 yr
	Valproic acid, salicylates	Higher incidence in children
Sex	Halothane, methyldopa, nitrofurantoin	Higher incidence in females
	Flucloxacillin, azathioprine	Higher incidence in males
Dose	Acetaminophen, aspirin	Higher blood concentrations associated with risk of hepatotoxicity
	Methotrexate, vitamin A	Total dose, frequency, and duration associated with hepatotoxic risk
Genetic factors	Halothane, phenytoin, sulfonamides, isoniazid	Numerous familial cases; defective epoxide hydrolases increase susceptibility to phenytoin and halothane associated injury; acetylator phenotype may predispose to isoniazid hepatotoxicity
	Valproic acid	Familial cases, correlation with mitochondrial enzyme abnormalities
History of other drug reactions	Halothane, enflurane; erythromycins; diclofenac, ibuprofen	Rare incidence of cross-sensitivity reported between drug classes
Other drugs	Acetaminophen	Isoniazid, zidovudine may lower toxic dose threshold for hepatotoxicity
	Busulfan, azathioprine	Increased risk of hepatic veno-occlusive disease
	Valproic acid	Other antiepileptic drugs increase risk of hepatotoxicity
Excessive alcohol use	Acetaminophen	Lowered dosage threshold
	Isoniazid, methotrexate	Increased liver injury and enhanced fibrosis
Other diseases		
Obesity	Halothane hepatitis, methotrexate	Increased liver injury and enhanced fibrosis
Fasting	Acetaminophen	Increased risk of hepatotoxicity
Renal failure	Tetracycline, methotrexate	Increased liver injury and enhanced fibrosis
Pre-existing liver disease	Niacin (nicotinamide), methotrexate	Increased risk of liver injury
Organ transplantation	Azathioprine, busulfan	Increased risk of vascular toxicity
AIDS	Dapsone, trimethoprim-sulfamethoxazole, oxacillin	Increased risk of liver injury; hypersensitivity
Diabetes	Methotrexate	Increased risk of hepatic fibrosis

PATHOPHYSIOLOGY OF HEPATIC INJURY

Having a general understanding of the pathophysiology and pathways of hepatic injury secondary to phase I–mediated cytochrome P450 (toxification) and phase II (detoxification) conjugation reactions, as well as biochemical mechanisms of cellular injury or death, are important aspects of assessing DILD and are reviewed in the following discussion.

The liver is an extremely resilient organ and is well equipped to resist toxic insults because of its unique cellular attributes (e.g., cell cooperation, acute-phase response, synthesis of hepatoprotective substances). Despite this resiliency, the liver is vulnerable to injury because it is frequently exposed to agents in their most reactive, thus toxic, forms. Since the liver is located between the absorptive lining of the gastrointestinal tract and drug targets within the body, orally administered drugs enter the portal circulation and undergo "first-pass metabolism," leading to significant exposure of the drug or its metabolites to the hepatocytes. Several factors promote the close contact between hepatocytes, blood, and drugs, including (1) the structure of the hepatic sinusoids, (2) the fenestrated hepatic endothelium, and (3) the enhanced overall surface area of the hepatocytes.[53] The liver may also be rapidly exposed to intravenously administered drugs because it receives approximately 25% of the cardiac output.

Hepatic uptake of drugs is thought to occur through passive diffusion, carrier-mediated uptake, facilitated transport, or active transport. Once drugs have entered the hepatocytes, back diffusion out of the cells may be minimized through cytosolic transfer proteins such as glutathione S-transferase, fatty acid–binding proteins, and 3α-hydroxysteroid dehydrogenase.[54] Drugs are thereby transferred to either the endoplasmic reticulum, where they are metabolized, or to the canalicular membrane, where transporters actively secrete endogenous or exogenous substances into the bile. Because most drugs are primarily lipophilic, they are not readily excreted in the urine or bile and must be converted to a more excretable hydrophilic form. The liver is responsible for this biotransformation either through phase I–mediated cytochrome P450 oxidative metabolism and formation of potentially hepatotoxic metabolites (toxification)[55] or through phase II conjugation (detoxification)[55] reactions.

In drugs undergoing oxidative metabolism, an activated oxygen molecule is integrated into lipophilic substrates resulting in the formation of reactive electrophiles, free radicals, and reduced oxygen compounds.[55] Reactive electrophiles can bind to cellular membranes, disrupt their function, and subsequently lead to hepatocellular necrosis.[56] Examples of causes of this type of liver injury include isoniazid and acetaminophen. Free radical formation from agents such as carbon tetrachloride (CCl_4) may lead to peroxidative injury of membrane lipids and necrosis,[7,57] whereas activated oxygen appears to be primarily associated with pulmonary injury rather than with DILD.[56] Several cytochrome P450 isoenzymes exist that have different substrates and can be expressed differently based on increasing age, genetic, and environmental conditions.

Because cellular function is overwhelmingly disrupted through these cytochrome P450-mediated mechanisms, cellular death is a common result. This process occurs through the following mechanisms: (1) plasma membrane alteration and disruption of the cytoskeleton (e.g., loss of ionic gradients), (2) mitochondrial dysfunction (e.g., decline in adenosine triphosphate levels and disrupting fatty acid oxidation), (3) loss of intracellular homeostasis, and (4) activation of degradative enzymes.[55] Additional mechanisms causing hepatocellular death are immunoallergenic (antibody-mediated cytotoxicity or induction of direct cytolytic T-cell responses). Another response involving cytokines (e.g., interferon, tumor necrosis factor-α), nitric oxide, complement activation, and other immune cells (e.g., Kupffer's, thymus, sinusoidal endothelial cells) has also been postulated, which results in inflammation and neutrophil-mediated hepatotoxicity.[2,55,58,59] Finally, apoptosis (programmed cellular death) may occur simultaneously with immune-mediated injury. A second means of drug metabolism is by phase II (detoxification) conjugation reactions. Phase II reactions occur through binding drug metabolites to glutathione, glucuronate, or sulfate, which leads to the formation of nontoxic, readily excretable hydrophilic products.[55,59] Inadequate detoxification due to reduced binding substance concentrations (e.g., inadequate glutathione stores) may lead to a greater concentration of a reactive metabolite. An example of phase II–induced liver injury may arise from the inability to detoxify phenytoin metabolites. In addition, the combination of phase I– and phase II–induced liver injury may occur in situations resulting in both formation of toxic metabolites and inadequate detoxification (e.g., acetaminophen).

Overall, the pathogenesis of hepatotoxic drug reactions is likely a result of a "multihit" process.[2] Several genetic P 450 isoenzyme variants that result in toxic metabolites, the involvement of suppressor and attenuator pathways modulating the hepatotoxic effects, cell-mediated and antibody-induced immune responses, cell surface neoantigens and cytokines expression (interleukin-10 and TNF (tumor necrosis factor)-α), inadequate detoxification pathways and individual genetic predisposition all may contribute to DILD. Ultimately, a series of events beginning with intracellular hepatocyte disruption, cellular necrosis, and apoptosis, followed by an immune inflammatory response have been proposed to cause DILD. The actual incidence and resolution of a DILD event may rely on the adaptive phenotypes of the host, which likely is a function of their genetic predisposition. The emerging field of pharmacogenomics could help predict and identify patients with aberrant gene polymorphisms or P450 alleles that affect drug concentrations leading to DILD.

Histopathologically, there are no absolute definitive features of DILD. However, certain patterns suggest a drug etiology. These include (1) zonal necrosis or fatty changes that are associated with mitochondrial injury and (2) mixed histologic manifestations of necrosis and cholestasis. The presence of neutrophils and/or eosinophils within destructive bile duct lesions is suggestive of DILD.[2]

Classification of Drug-Induced Injury

The nature of drug-induced hepatic injury may mimic several known liver diseases, but classification is challenging because of overlap between categories and the fact that some drugs may be associated with more than one syndrome. Often there is discordance between the clinical and laboratory features of the liver disease and hepatic histology. For these reasons, it is important to realize that identifying specific patterns or syndromes is only a clue to the diagnosis of DILD, and it is not as important as recognition of the temporal relationship between drug administration and liver injury or exclusion of other causes of liver disease. Therefore, drugs are often classified as predictable or unpredictable hepatotoxins, and as a result, the terms *intrinsic hepatotoxicity* and *idiosyncrasy* have evolved to help clinically characterize the proposed drug-induced mechanism of hepatic injury. Briefly, intrinsic hepatotoxicity generally is dose dependent and has a short and consistent latency period between drug exposure and liver injury, whereas idiosyncratic reactions are unpredictable and result from a hypersensitivity reaction (immunologic) or metabolic aberration (altered drug metabolism).

However, because the aforementioned terms may not fully elucidate all forms of DILD, the nature of the hepatic injury has been further delineated based on the time frame in which it occurs (i.e., acute versus chronic), or it may be classified based on whether the drug-induced liver insult is confined to the hepatocytes (hepatocellular injury) or involves areas such as the biliary tract, liver parenchyma, or hepatic vasculature. Finally, several types of drug-induced lesions resulting from acute or chronic administration of drugs are recognized histologically. Along with the proposed mechanism for liver injury and the time frame of occurrence, the histologic characterization of hepatic lesions is also useful in describing DILD and is reviewed next.

Intrinsic and Idiopathic Reactions to Drugs as Causes of Hepatic Injury

From a clinical perspective, the terms used for identifying and describing drug-induced hepatic injury are *intrinsic hepatotoxicity* and *idiosyncrasy* (Table 30-2). Intrinsic or true hepatotoxins (e.g., chloroform) have the inherent property of predictably injuring the liver. Idiosyncratic or unpredictable hepatotoxins (e.g., halothane) cause hepatic damage only in a small number of uniquely susceptible individuals. The major differences between these two types of drug-induced hepatic injury are listed in Table 30-3.

Intrinsic Hepatotoxicity

Intrinsic hepatotoxins can be subdivided into direct and indirect toxins. Direct intrinsic hepatotoxins (e.g., carbon tetrachloride) destroy hepatocytes by a physicochemical attack, mostly

Table 30-2 Mechanisms of Drug-Induced Hepatotoxicity[2,7,8,20]

Classification	Lesion	Incidence
Intrinsic Hepatotoxicity		
Direct hepatotoxins	Necrosis or steatosis	High
Indirect hepatotoxins		
Cytotoxic	Steatosis or necrosis	High
Cholestasis	Bile casts	High
Host Idiosyncrasy		
Hypersensitivity	Hepatocellular or cholestatic	Low
Metabolic abnormality	Hepatocellular or cholestatic	Low

Table 30-3 Characteristics of Intrinsic versus Idiosyncratic Hepatotoxins

Intrinsic	Idiosyncratic
Distinctive histologic pattern observed for any given drug	Variable histologic pattern of lesions
Dose-dependent hepatotoxicity	Dose-independent hepatotoxicity
Elicited in all individuals	Only a small fraction of exposed individuals affected
Reproducible in experimental animals	Cannot be reproduced in experimental animals
Predictable appearance of lesions and usually a brief latent period following exposure	Appearance of lesions bears no temporal relationship to the institution of drug therapy
No extrahepatic manifestations of hypersensitivity	Lesions often accompanied by extrahepatic manifestations of hypersensitivity (e.g., fever, rash, eosinophilia)

through the toxic effects of their metabolites. There are no known direct hepatotoxins that are used as therapeutic agents.[7]

In contrast, indirect hepatotoxins (e.g., antimetabolites) induce structural changes in the hepatocytes by competitive inhibition of essential metabolites or by interference with selective metabolic or secretory processes of the hepatocytes. These changes in the hepatocytes can be due to either cytotoxic or cholestatic mechanisms. Indirect intrinsic hepatotoxins that produce cytotoxic changes include tetracycline, mechlorethamine, alcohol, acetaminophen, and mercaptopurine.[6–8,20] Indirect intrinsic cholestatic hepatotoxins produce jaundice and hepatic dysfunction by interfering with mechanisms for the excretion of bile from the liver (e.g., C-17 alkylated anabolic steroids and C-17 ethinylated contraceptive steroids).[7,20,57]

2. One month after her initial visit, C.W. returns to clinic with a 1-week history of jaundice, anorexia, fever, and nausea while continuing to take her valproic acid (seizures still well controlled with no change in pattern). Upon obtaining an additional medication history, C.W. states that she briefly reinitiated her trimethoprim-sulfamethoxazole for a couple of days during the last 4 weeks for a recurrence of her urinary tract infection, and increased her venlafaxine dose 100 mg twice daily. Laboratory values are immediately obtained and are reported as follows: ALT, 164 U/L (normal, 5 to 40); AST, 177 U/L (normal, 5 to 40); alkaline phosphatase, 105 U/L (normal, 21 to 91); and total bilirubin, 2.3 mg/dL (normal, 0.1 to 1.2). Biopsy results are pending. What type of liver injury could C.W. have?

Idiosyncrasy

Like intrinsic hepatic injuries, idiosyncratic injuries may be cytotoxic, cholestatic, or mixed.[2,7,20] Most idiosyncratic drug reactions cause damage to hepatocytes throughout the hepatic lobule, with various degrees of necrosis and apoptosis. Hepatic injury due to host idiosyncrasy can be caused by hypersensitivity reactions or by other mechanisms (e.g., an aberrant metabolic pathway for the drug in the susceptible patient). The liver injury may be tentatively attributed to hypersensitivity when it develops after a "sensitization" period of 1 to 5 weeks and is accompanied by systemic characteristics of rash, fever, and eosinophilia.[2,7] These hallmarks of an immunologic reaction suggest that the hepatic injury is caused by drug allergy, especially when they reappear in response to a subsequent challenge dose of the drug. Examples of drugs causing allergic hepatic dysfunctions are methyldopa, phenytoin, *para*-aminosalicylic acid, chlorpromazine, erythromycin estolate, rarely clarithromycin, and sulfonamides.[5,7,35–37] Thus, C.W.'s recent elevation of liver function tests could be explained as an apparent "idiosyncratic" reaction to her trimethoprim-sulfamethoxazole (Table 30-4). Furthermore, the second-generation nonselective serotonin reuptake inhibitor venlafaxine has also been identified as a possible cause of hepatic injury. Two cases of venlafaxine-associated "hepatitis" have been reported in the literature.[60,61] The first case occurred in a 44-year-old woman receiving 150 mg/day within 7 months of initiating therapy, whereas the second case was reported in a 78-year-old man within 1 month of a dosage increase from 37.5 mg/day to 150 mg/day. In both cases, discontinuation of venlafaxine resulted in resolution of liver function tests within 5 weeks, and 4 months, respectively. Thus, C.W. should be advised to discontinue trimethoprim-sulfamethoxazole and venlafaxine, and the clinician should monitor her liver function tests closely for the next several weeks to months. Generally, the recovery from a

Table 30-4 Drug-Induced Hepatotoxicity

Drug		Clinical Remarks
Azathioprine		Only a few isolated instances of cholestatic jaundice have been attributed to azathioprine. Jaundice starts 3 weeks to 6 months after initiation of therapy. Generalized pruritus, widespread abdominal pain, and hypochromic greasy diarrhea may be present. Although azathioprine has been used in the treatment of chronic active hepatitis, worsening of the hepatic disease also may occur.
I:	Rare	
M:	Cholestasis; minor hepatocellular injury; veno-occlusive disease	Azathioprine is the most common drug in the United States implicated in causing VOD; ~20% of bone marrow and renal transplant patients may be affected with a mortality rate of 50%. VOD results from a nonthrombotic concentric occlusion of the lumen of small intrahepatic veins, also known as *bush tea disease.*
Mech:	Hypersensitivity[168–175]	
Benoxaprofen		See nonsteroidal anti-inflammatory drugs
Bromfenac		See nonsteroidal anti-inflammatory drugs.
Captopril		Hepatotoxicity, usually cholestatic in nature, has been reported with captopril, enalapril, and lisinopril use. Cross-sensitivity also has been reported. Jaundice was the most common finding, followed by pruritus, nausea, other GI symptoms, fever, rash, and confusion. Onset of symptoms varied from 5 days to 12 months (mean, 14 weeks; median, 1 month). Doses used were variable. Hepatotoxicity usually resolves in 2 weeks to 9 months after ACE inhibitors are stopped but may progress to liver failure and death if treatment is continued.
I:	Rare	
M:	Mostly cholestasis; mixed hepatocellular and cholestatic injury; pure hepatocellular injury—rare	
Mech:	Hypersensitivity and modulation of eicosanoid metabolism by inhibition of kininase II with increased hepatic bradykinin activity[175–178]	
Carbamazepine		Hepatotoxic syndrome resembles that observed with phenytoin. Onset of injury is usually within the first 8 weeks of taking the drug in 80% of cases. Hepatic injury is associated with modest hyperbilirubinemia, fever, rash, and eosinophilia. Morphologic features are hepatocellular, cholestatic, or mixed. Fatality rates are less than those reported with phenytoin and range from 7% to 12%.
I:	<1%	
M:	Hepatocellular, cholestatic, mixed	
Mech:	Hypersensitivity; idiosyncrasy; toxic metabolites[176–182]	
Carmustine (BCNU)		Nitrosoureas apparently act as alkylating agents and produce hepatic injury in up to 25% of patients taking therapeutic doses of BCNU. Hepatic injury produced by BCNU has ranged from reversible jaundice and abnormal levels of AST to severe hepatic necrosis.
I:	Dose related	
M:	Cytotoxic	
Mech:	Intrinsic hepatotoxin[183]	
Chlorpromazine (CPZ)		In ~80% of cases, icterus develops between 1–5 weeks of CPZ treatment. In rare instances, jaundice has developed after the first dose. Prodromal symptoms consist of fever, itching, abdominal pain, anorexia, and nausea. Skin rash is observed only in ~5% of reported cases. CPZ jaundice often resembles extrahepatic obstructive jaundice.
I:	0.1–0.2%	
M:	Cholestasis; scattered focal areas of necrosis	Severe pruritus common and may be the first evidence of hepatic injury in some patients. Serum alkaline phosphatase and cholesterol levels often markedly elevated. Serum transferase levels increased slightly to moderately in almost all patients. Eosinophilia has been noted in 25–50% of cases reported. Cholestatic jaundice associated with CPZ often resolves within 8 weeks but occasionally may continue for a year or longer. Some of the patients with prolonged cholestasis have developed a syndrome resembling that of primary biliary cirrhosis. The clinical syndrome is characterized by itching, xanthoma, hepatomegaly, and splenomegaly. Although it has been suggested that this syndrome is often benign and reversible, at least two cases of irreversible cirrhosis and fatality due to CPZ have been described.
Mech:	Hypersensitivity; idiosyncrasy[84,100,184–186]	Other phenothiazines also have been reported to cause cholestatic jaundice, but no reliable estimate of the incidence is available. Because there is a potential for cross-sensitivity between chlorpromazine and other phenothiazines, it is best to avoid using any agent in this class for patients who have had CPZ jaundice. Cholestasis also has been associated with almost all other phenothiazines, and the clinical manifestations reported are similar to those seen with chlorpromazine.

Chlorpropamide (and other sulfonylurea oral hypoglycemics)

I: 0.1–0.5%

M: Mixed cholestatic-cytotoxic injury

Mech: Hypersensitivity, hepatotoxicity[187–192]

Host factors that modify the susceptibility to hepatic injury unknown. Onset of jaundice usually between 2–6 weeks of chlorpropamide therapy. Initial symptoms are anorexia, nausea, and vomiting. Soon thereafter, dark urine, jaundice, and clay-colored stools appear. Pruritus and hepatomegaly are common. Fever, rash, and eosinophilia occur frequently but not in all cases. Complete recovery generally occurs within 1–3 months after chlorpropamide is stopped. Patients who recover from chlorpropamide jaundice apparently do not relapse when given tolbutamide. Other sulfonylureas in clinical use (i.e., acetohexamide, tolbutamide, glibenclamide, and tolazamide) also have been reported to cause jaundice, but the incidence appears to be very low. Fatal hepatotoxicity in an elderly woman has been apparently induced by glibenclamide.

Chlortetracycline See tetracyclines.

Ciprofloxacin See fluoroquinolones.

Clarithromycin See erythromycin.

Cloxacillin See oxacillin.

Contraceptive steroids (OCs)

I: Dose related 1:10,000 in Europe and North America; 1:4,000 in Chile and Scandinavia

M:
1. Cholestasis[193–196]

   1. Estrogens can selectively interfere with bilirubin excretion by the liver. The phenolic character of ring A and the addition of an alkyl group at the C-17 position of the estrogen molecule seem to be responsible for the injury. Progesterone has little or no demonstrable adverse effect on hepatic function by itself but may enhance the hepatic injury produced by the estrogens. Transient hepatic dysfunction occurs much more frequently and may be as high as 40–50% of patients taking these agents, but the overall incidence of jaundice appears to be much lower (i.e., 1 per 4,000–10,000). Postmenopausal women appear to be more susceptible to hepatic dysfunction induced by estrogen than younger women are. Certain ethnic groups (Swedes, Chileans) seem to be more prone to develop anicteric dysfunction than others. Susceptibility to estrogen-induced cholestasis probably is related to a genetic factor because of the strong link with recurrent cholestasis of pregnancy. The jaundice usually is noted during the first 6 months of therapy and often during the first cycle. Jaundice is preceded by nonspecific symptoms, including malaise, anorexia, nausea, and pruritus. Splenomegaly not seen, and hepatomegaly is uncommon. Serum concentrations of bilirubin levels increased moderately in most cases (≥10 mg/dL), but values >20 mg/dL have been described. Other biochemical features resemble the jaundice produced by the C-17 alkylated anabolic steroids. Prognosis of the cholestatic jaundice good. In most individuals, the clinical syndrome resolves completely within 1 month.

2. Adenoma, peliosis hepatis[197–203]

   2. Hepatic adenoma was a very rare tumor before the widespread use of contraceptive steroids. Since then, the increase in incidence of adenoma seems to have paralleled the increased use of OCs. Women taking contraceptive steroids for periods >5 years appear to be at higher risk of developing an adenoma than those who have taken the drug <3 years. One-third to one-half of patients found to have adenoma remain asymptomatic. Approximately one-third may present with a painful, tender mass. The remaining one-fourth to one-third of reported patients often present with a sudden life-threatening intraabdominal hemorrhage secondary to rupture of the adenoma. Prognosis is good if the adenoma can be resected before rupture. For patients with hemoperitoneum, the outlook is fair if the diagnosis is made promptly and the tumor resected. Otherwise, death may result from hemorrhagic shock, coagulation abnormalities, and related complications. Peliosis hepatis is a rare complication from contraceptive steroids and often occurs along with the adenoma.

3. Budd-Chiari syndrome[204,205]

   3. Budd-Chiari syndrome is characterized by acute or subacute development of abdominal pain, hepatomegaly, portal hypertension, ascites, edema, and moderate jaundice. This syndrome is caused by thrombosis and subsequent occlusion of the hepatic veins. Although this complication is very rare, an extremely high mortality rate is observed.

4. Carcinoma[206–209]

   4. Several types of malignant tumors have been associated with the use of OCs; >100 cases have been reported, but the incidence is low when compared with the widespread use of OCs. Hepatic carcinoma may be more likely in women who use the OCs for >8 years.

Mech: Indirect hepatotoxin; genetic predisposition

Table 30-4 Drug-Induced Hepatotoxicity—cont'd

Drug	Clinical Remarks
Cyclosporine I: Uncommon M: Cholestasis Mech: Direct toxic effect on bile secretion[2,7,212]	Increased serum transferase and gamma-glutamyl transferase concentrations and increased serum bilirubin concentration are signs of cyclosporine hepatotoxicity. Elevated LFTs have been observed in ~4% of renal transplant, 7% of heart allograft, and 4% of liver transplant recipients, usually during the first month of cyclosporine therapy. Reduction of cyclosporine dosage usually reverses its hepatotoxic effects. Several cases of cholestasis have been reported. There was a significant increased incidence of VOD among patients who received cyclosporine and methotrexate (CYC-MTX) versus those who received cyclosporine and methylprednisolone (70 versus 18%) as prophylaxis against graft-versus-host disease after allogenic bone marrow transplantation. Incidence of early deaths due to VOD was significantly higher in the CYC-MTX group (25 versus 4.5%).

Dantrolene
I: Hypertransferasemia
  1. Without jaundice (1.8%)
  2. Overt hepatic injury (0.6%)
M: Severe viral hepatitis-like; submassive and massive necrosis
Mech: Idiosyncrasy; toxic metabolites[213]
	The incidence and severity of the hepatic injury appear to be related to the duration of therapy and patient age. Clinical onset of hepatic injury has been delayed for at least 45 days after starting the drug in almost all cases. In a study of 1,044 patients, all fatalities have occurred in patients >30 years and after at least 2 months of therapy. Females have a higher fatality rate than males. Dosages >300 mg/day are more likely to produce hepatic injury than lower dosages and dosages of ≤200 mg/day rarely lead to liver damage. Injury is mainly hepatocellular with a pattern of either acute, subacute, or chronic hepatitis. The fatality rate of 28% is high.

Desipramine	See tricyclic antidepressants.
Didanosine	See zidovudine.
Diltiazem I: Rare M: Granulomatous Mech: Idiosyncrasy[214-222]	Mild to marked elevations in liver function test results have been reported in <1% of patients taking diltiazem, and drug discontinuation was not required. Six case reports of hepatocellular injury, usually early in the therapy (1–8 weeks), have been published. Eight reported cases of hepatic injury have been associated with nifedipine, each producing acute hepatocellular, cholestatic, or a mixed hepatocellular picture. Three additional chronic cases have been documented beginning 9–72 months after initiation of therapy. These cases were characterized by steatosis and the presence of Mallory-like bodies. Nicardipine, a similar agent, has also been associated with hepatocellular injury. Verapamil-induced hepatocellular injury has been reported in ~6 cases. Hypersensitivity was the proposed mechanism of the injury.
Enflurane	See halothane and methoxyflurane.
Erythromycin I: 3.6/100,000 M: Cholestasis; mixed cholestatic-cytotoxic injury Mech: Hypersensitivity[2,7,8,25-37,84]	Erythromycin-associated cholestasis may be due to the estolate salt as well as the ethylsuccinate and propionate derivatives. Nevertheless, the estolate salt has been implicated most frequently. Children may be less susceptible than adults. Onset of cholestatic jaundice is usually 1–3 weeks after exposure; however, patients previously exposed may exhibit symptoms within 2 days. Abdominal pain occurs in ~75% of the cases. Icterus may precede or accompany GI complaints, such as anorexia, nausea, and vomiting. Fever occurs in ~60% of patients, and rash is often absent. Eosinophilia often occurs (45–80%). Serum bilirubin values generally are <100 mmol/L. Response to a challenge dose of the same erythromycin derivative is usually prompt. The hepatic injury is reversible, and jaundice often subsides within 2–5 weeks after the drug is discontinued. Cholestatic jaundice has also been reported with clarithromycin and in seven cases of patients receiving roxithromycin.
Felbamate I: <1% M: Submassive necrosis? Mech: Idiosyncrasy[181,182]	Twenty-three cases of hepatic failure have been reported following the use of felbamate. Of these, 13 of these were not clearly related to felbamate therapy. Of the remaining 10 cases, 5 deaths were attributable to felbamate. The overall incidence appears to be 1 per 26,000–34,000 exposed. The drug remains available; close biochemical and hematologic monitoring has been recommended. Liver dysfunction has also been reported with *lamotrigine*.

Flucoxacillin

See oxacillin.

Fluconazole

See ketoconazole.

Fluoroquinolones

I: Rare
M: Cholestasis; centrilobular necrosis
Mech: Idiosyncrasy?[223-229]

Elevations in aminotransferase, bilirubin, and alkaline phosphatase levels were observed in 1.8–2.5% of patients who received fluroquinolones. Sporadic cases of drug-induced hepatitis had appeared in the literature for ciprofloxacin, enoxacin, ofloxacin, and norfloxacin. Fatal hepatis has also been reported with levofloxacin. Hepatic injury due to fluoroquinolones apparently is not dose related and generally is reversible when the drug is stopped. However, 1 fatal case of hepatic failure, apparently due to oral ciprofloxacin, was reported.

The broad-spectrum fluoroquinolome trovafloxacin has also been associated with >100 cases of hepatotoxicity, 14 of which involved acute liver failure, with liver transplantation required in 4 of these. An immunoallergenic mechanism has been suggested as a cause. The drug remains available in the United States for very restricted indications.

Fluoxetine

I: Very low
M: Cholestatic
Mech: Hepatocellular?[230]

Three published reports of fluoxetine-induced liver disease. Patients generally presented with elevated bilirubin, ALT, and AST. Patients generally required from several weeks to months before liver function tests normalized.

Glibenclamide

See chlorpropamide.

Glucocorticoids

I: Dose related
M: Steatosis
Mech: Cholestatic Hepatotoxicity[231-232]

Hepatic steatosis secondary to glucocorticoids usually is of little clinical consequence. However, occasionally, this may lead to fat embolism in the vascular bed of major organs (e.g., lung), resulting in tissue damage and fatality.

Haloperidol

I: Low
M: Cholestasis
Mech: Hypersensitivity[323,324]

Incidence has been estimated to be between 0.2–3% of recipients. Most reported cases of jaundice appear to be cholestatic.

Halothane

I: 1. Mild form >25%
   2. Severe 1:35,000–1:3,500
M: Centraxonial necrosis; steatosis; massive necrosis
Mech: Metabolic idiosyncrasy; hypersensitivity[234-245]

Halothane exposure may be followed by two distinct types of hepatotoxicity: asymptomatic with abnormal laboratory values only or severe acute hepatitis with massive hepatic necrosis. The reactive metabolites of halothane, trifluoroacetyl acid chloride (TFA) and free radicals, cause mild, self-limiting hepatotoxicity by binding to macromolecules, resulting in subclinical damage. The rarer form of fulminant hepatitis is believed to result from the binding of TFA to subcellular free amino groups and neoantigens, resulting in an autoimmune reaction to halothane upon repeated exposure. The incidence and severity appear to be greater in females and enhanced by obesity. Susceptibility is particularly enhanced by previous exposure to halothane, especially if the interval between the exposures is <3 months. Incidence may be increased as much as 10-fold with repeated exposure to halothane or isoflurane. Irradiation also may increase susceptibility to halothane-induced hepatitis. Jaundice is rare in children and young adults <30 years. The clinical syndrome of halothane-induced liver disease often consists of a history of unexplained delayed fever postoperatively (>3 days) after halothane anesthesia. There is usually a latent period of 5–14 days between the anesthetic episode and the appearance of hepatic injury, but it may appear as early as 1 day after the operation in patients who have had multiple prior exposures to halothane. Fever with or without chills, aching, anorexia, nausea, and abdominal distress preceded jaundice in 75% of the patients. Once jaundice appears, other manifestations of serious hepatocellular damage often develop rapidly. Coagulation abnormalities, ascites, renal insufficiency, GI bleeding, and encephalopathy may follow.

Values for serum transferases are markedly elevated (≥3,000 U/L), whereas alkaline phosphatase is increased only modestly. Eosinophilia has been observed in 20–50% of reported cases. Rash is uncommon. Mortality rate for halothane hepatitis ranges from 14–67%.

Serologic testing for antibodies specific to halothane-altered antigens is positive in ~75% of patients and can be used as a diagnostic aid along with the drug history and clinical presentation.

Table 30-4 Drug-Induced Hepatotoxicity—cont'd

Drug	Clinical Remarks
Ibuprofen	See nonsteroidal anti-inflammatory drugs.
Imipramine	See tricyclic antidepressants.
Indinavir	See zidovudine.
Isoflurane	See halothane.
Isoniazid (INH)[2,7,8,14,33]	See Chapter 59, Tuberculosis. Fast and slow acetylators may be equally susceptible to the hepatotoxic effects of INH. It appears that specific P450 isoenzymes may be involved because of the enhanced hepatotoxicity by alcohol, other drugs (rifampicin), and advancing age.
Itraconazole	See ketoconazole.
Ketoprofen	See nonsteroidal anti-inflammatory drugs.
Ketoconazole	Serum transferase concentrations without overt clinical symptoms can be increased in 8–12% of patients. Symptomatic hepatic injury is rare and often presents as a mixed or cholestatic jaundice. Fulminant hepatitis also is possible. Hepatitis more common in females, especially those >40 years, and usually occurs after 10 days to 26 weeks of therapy. Hypersensitivity manifestations usually absent.
I:	0.03–0.1%
M:	Hepatocellular necrosis; mixed cholestasis-hepatocellular
Mech:	Metabolic idiosyncrasy[246–251] Fluconazole and itraconazole have also been implicated in cases of hepatic injury, but the overall incidence is extremely low.
Lamotrigine: See Felbamate	
Levofloxacin: See Fluoroquinolones	
Lovastatin	In 613 patients who received lovastatin during controlled trials, the most common laboratory abnormalities were elevations in hepatic enzymes. Serum concentrations of ALT, AST, and CPK were increased by 7.3, 5.9, and 5.1%, respectively. Serum aminotransferase concentrations were increased by >3-fold in ~1.9% of all patients. The risk of developing increases in transferase levels has been reported in patients with the homozygous form of familial hypercholesterolemia and may be dose related. Hepatitis, fatty change in the liver, cholestatic jaundice, and chronic active hepatitis have been reported rarely. Liver function test abnormalities usually are reversible after a few weeks following discontinuation, but recovery may be delayed for up to 21 months. Rechallenge can result in elevations of aminotransferases in ~50% of patients. Lovastatin should be avoided in patients who have liver disease or a history of alcohol abuse. Pravastatin and simvastatin also have been reported to cause increases in aminotransferases that may lead to cessation of therapy. Simvastatin has also led to at least five cases of presumed hepatitis.
I:	Very rare
M:	Mild focal hepatitis; cholestasis
Mech:	Hepatocellular[2,7,252–257]
Mercaptopurine (6-MP)	Liver injury with jaundice has been reported in 6–40% of leukemic patients treated with 6-MP. Adults appear to be more susceptible to hepatic injury than children. Onset of overt hepatic injury is usually within 1–2 months of receiving the drug. Jaundice commonly appears as the first sign, followed by pruritus. Serum transferase values generally are <250 U/L. Alkaline phosphatase values are moderately to markedly elevated. Doses >2.5 mg/kg are more likely to cause hepatic injury. Prognosis depends on the degree of cytotoxic injury, but mortality may reach ≥10%.
I:	Dose related
M:	Cholestasis with fatty hepatic necrosis
Mech:	Indirect intrinsic hepatotoxin[258]
Methimazole	Onset of the syndrome is usually during the first 4 months of therapy but may be as late as 3 months. Rash, fever, lymphadenopathy, and agranulocytosis may occur in various combinations. The cholestatic jaundice associated with methimazole is reversible. Death appears to have been the result of concomitant agranulocytosis and bone marrow depression, rather than the hepatic injury. (Also see propylthiouracil.)
I:	Rare
M:	Cholestasis
Mech:	Hypersensitivity[259]
Methoxyflurane	The clinical syndrome and hepatic lesions from methoxyflurane and enflurane are very similar to those observed in halothane hepatitis, but with a lower incidence. Cross-sensitivity of halothane with methoxyflurane and enflurane is probable. Isoflurane, which is minimally metabolized, and nitrous oxide may be safer alternatives.
I:	Rare, but often fatal
M:	Similar findings as in halothane hepatitis
Mech:	Hypersensitivity; metabolic aberration[260-262]

Methotrexate (MTX)

I: Dose, frequency, and duration related

M: Macrovesicular steatosis and portal inflammation; necrosis; chronic steatosis may lead to fibrosis and cirrhosis

Mech: Indirect intrinsic hepatotoxin[2,263–267]

MTX often causes steatosis and portal inflammation in the liver when it is used in the acute treatment of leukemia, choriocarcinoma, and other neoplastic diseases. Overt clinical symptoms occasionally accompany these lesions. Prolonged use of MTX in patients with psoriasis may lead to fibrosis and cirrhosis, but apparently not in those with rheumatoid arthritis. The likelihood of hepatic injury probably is directly related to the total dose and duration of therapy; it is inversely related to the time interval between doses. Other risk factors include age, obesity, diabetes, alcoholism, and perhaps severity of psoriasis. Serum concentrations of AST and ALT usually are increased for 1–2 days after a single dose of MTX; however, cirrhosis can develop insidiously without increases in the liver enzyme concentrations. Serial liver biopsies at yearly intervals are highly recommended for patients with psoriasis to facilitate the discovery of cirrhosis and its complications, which can progress without overt clinical symptoms. Some of these patients may progress to hepatic failure and death. Early recognition of this syndrome can decrease irreversible hepatic damage and improve long-term survival. Preventive measures include giving intermittent rather than small daily doses of MTX. Single weekly dosing regimens of <15 mg have been successful in reducing the incidence of significant hepatic injury.

Methyldopa

I: Low

M: Cytotoxic injury; subacute or bridging necrosis; rare cholestasis; chronic active hepatitis

Mech: Toxic metabolites; hypersensitivity[96,268,270]

Incidence of methyldopa-induced hepatic injury is difficult to estimate. In some patients, serum enzyme levels have returned to normal despite continued therapy with methyldopa. Methyldopa-induced hepatitis usually is hepatocellular, rarely mixed or cholestatic. The incidence of severe cytotoxic injury is estimated to be <0.1–0.5% of recipients.

Methyldopa hepatitis occurs more commonly in patients >35 years and predominantly affects females. Acute hepatic injury has appeared within 4 weeks of therapy in 50% of the patients reported and within 4–12 weeks in 25% of the cases. Others may have a latent period for several years. The syndrome of methyldopa-induced hepatic injury resembles acute viral hepatitis. There usually has been a prodromal period of fever, chills, malaise, anorexia, nausea, vomiting, occasional right upper quadrant tenderness, and pruritus. Jaundice, dark urine, and hepatomegaly usually follow in severe cases. Rash, lymphadenopathy, and arthralgia have been rare. Biochemical features resemble those of cytotoxic injury. Rechallenge usually leads to recurrence of hepatitis and can result in fatalities. The fatality rate from acute hepatic injury is estimated to be 10%. For these patients who survive, withdrawal of the drug results in rapid recovery in most cases.

Chronic active hepatitis induced by methyldopa resembles "autoimmune" type CAH. Biopsy of the liver has revealed subacute hepatic necrosis with confluent areas of lobular collapse, intense inflammatory response in the portal and periportal areas, and in some cases, evidence of cirrhosis. Positive Coombs' test, LE factor, and antinuclear and anti-smooth muscle antibodies may be observed. Clinical presentation may be a mixture of acute and chronic hepatitis. In some patients, hepatosplenomegaly and spider angiomas may develop when the syndrome is first recognized.

To prevent irreversible liver injury or death, it is advisable to monitor liver enzyme tests regularly during the first 3 months of therapy, particularly in females. Periodic checks for the first 3 years also may be recognized.

To prevent irreversible liver injury or death, it is advisable to monitor liver enzyme tests regularly during the first 3 months of therapy, particularly in females. Periodic checks for the first 3 years also may be indicated.

Monoamine oxidase inhibitors (MAOIs) (iproniazid, isocarboxazid, phenelzine)

I: ≈1%

M: Hepatocellular damage

Mech: Metabolic idiosyncrasy; autoimmune[273–275]

Iproniazid, the first antidepressant to produce hepatic injury, was withdrawn from the market because of many reported cases of fulminant hepatic failure. Severe hepatitis has been encountered in patients given phenelzine for periods of 18 days to 5 months. The clinical features and the histologic findings in the liver are indistinguishable from those of severe viral hepatitis. The reported mortality rate is ~15%. Tranylcypromine, a nonhydrazine MAOI, rarely causes jaundice similar to that of hydrazine derivatives.

Naproxen

See nonsteroidal anti-inflammatory drugs.

Table 30-4   Drug-Induced Hepatotoxicity—cont'd

Drug	Clinical Remarks
Nevirapine	See zidovudine.
Niacin (Nicotinic acid) I: Occasional M: Hepatic necrosis; cholestasis Mech: Unknown; dose related? Direct toxicity? Formulation related?[276-278]	Nicotinic acid-induced hepatitis has been associated with high-dose regimens (>3 g/day) given for several months to years. SR formulation of niacin seems to induce hepatotoxicity at lower dosages within days to weeks. Symptoms included nausea, vomiting, diaphoresis, anorexia, and jaundice. Elevated hepatic enzyme levels were observed in most patients and normalized upon withdrawal. Fulminant hepatocellular failure has been attributed to the SR form more often than to the crystalline form. Rechallenge with regular formulation of niacin does not produce recurring hepatocellular damage.
Nifedipine	See diltiazem.
Nonsteroidal anti-inflammatory drugs (NSAIDs) I: 1:100,000 recipients M: Cholestasis, cytotoxic, or mixed Mech: Hypersensitivity; reactive metabolites[279-291]	Hepatocellular injury, or cholestasis, has occurred in patients taking benoxaprofen and is associated with a high fatality rate. Benoxaprofen is more hepatotoxic in elderly females and in those with renal dysfunction. Benoxaprofen was therefore withdrawn from the market. Two-thirds of the cases of sulindac-induced hepatic injury had clinical hallmarks of hypersensitivity. Ratio of females to males was 3.5:1, with 69% of patients >50 years. Most commonly reported clinical features of sulindac-induced hepatitis were jaundice (67%), nausea (67%), fever (55%), rash (48%), pruritus (40%), and eosinophilia (35%). Other features included hepatomegaly, lymphadenopathy, splenomegaly, myalgia, pharyngitis, edema, thyroid disorders, interstitial nephritis, somnolence, and ulcerative stomatitis. Onset ranged from 1 day to 3 years, but mostly <8 weeks. Rechallenge led to recurrence in a few days, thus suggesting an allergic mechanism. Complete recovery occurred in all patients 2–3 weeks after drug discontinuation. Severe cholestatic hepatitis, which can progress to subacute hepatic necrosis, has been reported with piroxicam. Patients >60 years seem to be more prone to piroxicam-induced cholestasis. Liver enzymes may take 3–4 months to return to normal levels after piroxicam is discontinued. Other NSAIDs such as naproxen, diclofenac, ketoprofen, and ibuprofen also have been implicated. Fatal fulminant hepatic failure was reported in a female patient taking bromfenac 25 mg PO QID for 3 months. This idiosyncratic response along with other cases of serious hepatotoxicity resulted in bromfenac's removal from the market. Although cases of NSAID-induced hepatitis are rare, they can be fatal. Most cases of hepatitis secondary to NSAIDs occur within the first few months of treatment.
Nitrofurantoin I: Rare M: Mixed cholestatic-cytotoxic injury; chronic active hepatitis Mech: Hypersensitivity; reactive metabolites[97,292,293]	The onset of symptoms of hepatic injury are usually abrupt, with fever (60%), rash (30%), and eosinophilia (70%). Approximately two-thirds of patients have had previous exposure to nitrofurantoin. The latent period before the development of symptoms ranges from 2 days to 5 months, but usually within the first 5 weeks. Cholestatic jaundice is the most common acute injury observed with nitrofurantoin. The prognosis of nitrofurantoin-induced jaundice is good. Biochemical abnormalities and jaundice are generally reversible when the drug is discontinued. CAH of the "lupoid" type is rare and may be accompanied by pulmonary lesions. Most patients have a low serum albumin concentration and a high gamma-globulin serum concentration. Antinuclear and/or anti-smooth muscle autoantibodies are found in most patients. Few cases of cirrhosis have been reported.
Oxacillin and its derivatives I: Low M: Cholestasis Mech: Hypersensitivity? Idiosyncrasy[294-297]	Oxacillin has been associated with rare cholestatic jaundice and numerous cases of anicteric hepatic dysfunction. Liver transferase levels can be as high as 1,000 U/L in some cases. Alkaline phosphatase levels are only modestly elevated, and serum bilirubin remains normal in most patients. Eosinophilia accompanies only ~25% of cases. Upon cessation of oxacillin, liver enzyme values generally return to normal within 2 weeks. Apparently, there is no cross-hepatotoxicity between oxacillin and other penicillins. Nafcillin or penicillin G often can be substituted without recurrence of liver injury. Cloxacillin and flucloxacillin also have been associated with severe cholestatic jaundice. Occasionally, the cholestatic injury may last for months to years even after the drug is stopped. Estimated incidence of flucloxacillin-induced liver dysfunction ranged from 1:11,000 to 1:30,000 prescriptions. Higher risk was associated with female sex, age, large daily doses, and duration of >2 weeks.

Oxytetracycline

See tetracycline.

Penicillin
I: Very rare
M: Necrosis; granuloma; "lupoid" hepatitis
Mech: Hypersensitivity[300-304]

Only a few cases of hepatic dysfunction have been associated with penicillin G. Almost all cases were associated with systemic hypersensitivity reactions such as urticaria, rash, anaphylactic shock, systemic granulomatous response, serum sickness, or exfoliative dermatitis. Carbenicillin, ampicillin, amoxicillin, mezlocillin, and oxacillin also have been associated with increased serum transferase levels.

Phenelzine

See monoamine oxidase inhibitors.

Phenindione
I: <0.5%
M: Mixed cholestatic-cytotoxic
Mech: Hypersensitivity[305,306]

Overt hepatic injury induced by phenindione always is associated with generalized allergic reactions such as rash, fever, eosinophilia, lymphocytosis, renal injury, and occasionally thrombocytopenia. Onset usually is during the third or fourth week of drug administration. Hepatic injury appears to be the mixed cytotoxic and cholestatic type. Values for serum transferases usually are <500 U/L. Alkaline phosphatase serum concentrations moderately to markedly increased. As a rule, hepatitis subsides following withdrawal of phenindione. The case fatality rate of patients with phenindione jaundice is estimated to be 10% and is probably the result of severe generalized hypersensitivity, rather than that of hepatic failure. Coumarin derivatives are preferred.

Phenylbutazone
I: 0.25%
M: 1. Granulomatous form
2. Severe necrosis with or without cholestasis
Mech: Hypersensitivity; intrinsic toxicity[307]

Onset of illness often occurs within the first weeks of therapy but occasionally can occur after 12 months of therapy. Hypersensitivity probably is responsible for the hepatic injury due to the accompanying fever and/or rash. Allergic symptoms, however, are found in only 50% of patients. Because an apparent relationship between dose and toxicity was observed more frequently with large doses of phenylbutazone, the intrinsic toxicity of the drug also may play a role. Fever, rash, arthralgia, nausea, vomiting, and abdominal pain may precede or accompany the jaundice. About two-thirds experienced cytotoxic injury with or without cholestasis and steatosis. In ~30% of patients, cholestasis with little or no parenchymal injury has been observed. Granuloma also may be found in some cases with minor liver cell necrosis. A fatality rate of 12% has been reported in patients with hepatic necrosis. Patients with cholestasis and granulomatous lesion generally recover, although the lesion may take up to 4 months to resolve.

Phenytoin
I: <1%
M: Submassive necrosis; lobular hepatitis; cholestatic hepatitis; granulomatous hepatitis
Mech: Hypersensitivity; idiosyncrasy; toxic metabolites[7,8,308-312]

Subclinical hepatic enzyme elevation is common with phenytoin, but overt hepatitis is much less common. Children seem to be less vulnerable to hepatic injury from phenytoin. Almost 80% of cases involved adults >20 years. Symptoms generally occur after 1-5 weeks of therapy. Fever, rash, lymphadenopathy, and eosinophilia appear in almost all patients. Jaundice then follows. Leukocytosis with lymphocytosis and atypical lymphocytes is common. The syndrome resembles that of serum sickness or infectious mononucleosis. Biochemical features are similar to those of severe viral hepatitis. Values for AST and ALT are very high (200-4,000 U/L), and the serum concentrations of alkaline phosphatase usually is only modestly increased. A case mortality rate of ~30% is due partly to accompanying severe hypersensitivity reactions (e.g., exfoliative dermatitis) and partly to resulting hepatic failure. A single case of phenytoin-induced chronic persistent hepatitis, which was verified by histology and rechallenge, was reported.

Piroxicam

See nonsteroidal anti-inflammatory drugs.

Plicamycin (Mithramycin)
I: Dose related
M: Necrosis
Mech: Intrinsic hepatotoxins[271,272]

Biochemical evidence of hepatic injury has been found in 25-100% of recipients on "full" oncotherapeutic doses. Values for AST and ALT may be as high as 1,000 U/L. Hepatocellular jaundice may occur. Hepatotoxicity appears to be less with the doses used to treat Paget's disease and hypercalcemia. An alternate-day regimen used to treat carcinomas also seems to have an acceptable level of hepatotoxicity.

Pravastatin

See lovastatin.

Prochlorperazine
I: Rare
M: Cholestasis
Mech: Hypersensitivity[27,313]

See chlorpromazine.

Propylthiouracil (PTU)
I: Rare
M: Hepatocellular injury; chronic active hepatitis; cholestasis; granuloma
Mech: Hypersensitivity; toxic metabolites?[299,314-319]

Asymptomatic and transient elevations of liver enzymes are common in patients receiving PTU (up to 28% in one study). However, ALT levels decrease after dosage reduction and normalize in most cases. Signs and symptoms of hepatocellular damage usually appear within 2-4 weeks after initiation of the drug and often are accompanied by rash, fever, and lymphadenopathy. CAH and cholestatic jaundice secondary to PTU have been described. Fatal cases of PTU-induced jaundice have been attributed to hepatic necrosis or accompanying granulocytosis. (Also see methimazole.)

Table 30-4   Drug-Induced Hepatotoxicity—cont'd

Drug	Clinical Remarks
Quinidine I: Rare; M: Mixed hepatocellular; granulomata; Mech: Hypersensitivity[320–322]	Mild hepatic injury induced by quinidine most commonly occurs within 6–12 days of initiation of treatment and is usually anicteric. Quinidine-induced hepatitis usually heralded by fever in association with increased AST, ALT, LDH, and alkaline phosphatase levels. Discontinuation of the drug usually results in rapid resolution of fever and laboratory abnormalities. Upon rechallenge with a single dose of quinidine, most patients have promptly developed fever and increased concentrations of serum transferases, thereby supporting hypersensitivity as a mechanism.
Rifampin	See Chapter 59, Tuberculosis.
Simvastatin	See lovastatin.
Sulfamethoxazole-trimethoprim (co-trimoxazole) I: Very low; M: Cholestasis; few hepatocellular; Mech: Idiosyncrasy[323–327]	Twelve cases of co-trimoxazole–induced liver injury have been reported. The cholestasis can be severe and might last for >12 months, even after the drug was stopped. One case of fulminant hepatic failure was fatal. Prominent features are pruritus, fever, skin rash, arthralgias, and eosinophilia.
Sulfonamides I: 0.5–1% cholestatic jaundice; M: Mixed hepatocellular injury; subacute hepatic necrosis with cirrhosis; chronic active hepatitis; granulomatous hepatitis; Mech: Hypersensitivity; idiosyncrasy[63–68]	Clinical presentation of hepatic injury often occurs within 5–14 days but occasionally presents as late as several months. Approximately 25% of the patients with hepatic dysfunction have had prior exposure to sulfonamides. The reaction is characterized by fever, rash, and signs of visceral and bone marrow injury. The clinical and morphologic features of such reactions resemble those of serum sickness. Usually, the onset of symptoms is sudden, with fever, anorexia, nausea, vomiting, and sometimes rash. Jaundice appears on the third to sixth day after the onset of fever but may be delayed for as long as 2 weeks. Dark urine and acholic stools are common, and hepatomegaly may be noted. Prognosis depends on the extent of cytotoxic injury. Case fatality rate is reportedly >10%. Patients who survive generally recover slowly over a period of several weeks to months. Fatal massive necrosis has been described with pyrimethamine-sulfadoxine (Fansidar). Slow acetylators are more susceptible to sulfonamide-induced hepatic injury because of a possible genetic defect in a protective mechanism against sulfonamides.
Sulfonylurea oral hypoglycemics	See chlorpropamide.
Sulindac	See nonsteroidal anti-inflammatory drugs.
Tetracyclines I: Low; M: Microvesicular fat droplets in hepatocytes; fatty degeneration; Mech: Intrinsic hepatotoxicity[328–330]	Chlortetracycline, oxytetracycline, and tetracycline have been reported to produce hepatic steatosis. The development of clinically significant fatty liver appears to depend on the presence of high blood levels of the drug. High dosages (>1.5 g/day) of tetracycline, especially when given IV to pregnant women or individuals with renal disease, may give rise to severe hepatic injury. Clinical manifestations usually appear 4–10 days after initiation of tetracycline therapy. Early symptoms include nausea, vomiting, abdominal pain, hematemesis, and headache. Mild jaundice then follows. Hemorrhagic complications, azotemia, hypotension, shock, and coma may develop subsequently. Tetracycline-induced massive steatosis does not differ clinically or morphologically from the spontaneous form of fatty liver of pregnancy. Mortality rate from this syndrome is ~80%. This serious untoward reaction can be avoided by using safer alternative antibiotics whenever possible or by keeping the IV dosage of tetracycline <1 g/day.
Tolbutamide	See chlorpropamide.
Tranylcypromine	See monoamine oxidase inhibitors.
Tricyclic antidepressants (TCAs) (amitriptyline, imipramine, desipramine) I: Rare to infrequent; M: Cholestasis; hepatic necrosis; Mech: Hypersensitivity plus slight toxicity[2,7,8,80,331–336]	TCAs usually cause a mixed hepatitis with either the necrotic or the cholestatic component predominating, depending on the agent. Jaundice appears within 1 week to 4 months. Hypersensitivity manifestations are seen in some patients. Severe hepatic necrosis and death are rare. Prolonged cholestasis and progressive hepatic fibrosis have been reported in a few cases. Newer anti-depressants such as nafazodone have also been associated with life-threatening hepatic failure.

Trifluoperazine

I: Rare

M: Cholestasis

Mech: Hypersensitivity[337]

See chlorpromazine.

Troglitazone

I: Very low

M: Hepatocellular, cholestasis

Mech: Idiosyncrasy?[139-146]

Several cases of troglitazone-associated liver failure have been reported. Significant increases in ALT (>20× the upper limit of normal) were reported to occur between the third week and several months (mean, 147 days; range, 17–287) following initiation of therapy. In patients who had therapy discontinued, ALT usually returned to baseline (mean, 55 days; range, 8–142). Patients generally may not have symptoms of liver dysfunction (i.e., fatigue, nausea, and abdominal pain), yet jaundice may be present in some instances. Liver transplantation may also be required in some cases.

Pioglitazone and Rosiglitazone, thiazolidenedione oral antidiabetic agents, may also be associated with idiosyncratic hepatotoxicity. Case reports describe ALT and AST elevations following initiation of therapy with rapid normalization following discontinuation.

Trovafloxacin

See fluoroquinolones.

Valproic acid

I: 0.05–0.1%

M: Microvesicular steatosis; focal or massive necrosis

Mech: Toxic metabolites; idiosyncrasy?[2,8,71-78]

Valproic acid can increase the serum transferase concentration in 6–44% of patients without overt clinical symptoms. Numerous cases of fatal and nonfatal liver disease due to valproic acid have been reported. Infants and young children (<2 years) are at much higher risk than adults. Lethargy, lassitude, anorexia, nausea, vomiting, edema, facial puffiness, and a frequent change in the pattern of convulsions may precede jaundice, ascites, and hemorrhage. Severe hepatic necrosis can result in coma and azotemia. Prothrombin time is prolonged, serum ammonia concentrations are increased, and hypoglycemia may occur. The hepatotoxicity is thought to be related to an inherited or acquired deficiency in the β-oxidation of valproate resulting in increased formation of a toxic metabolite (4-envalproate). This toxic metabolic pathway seems to be cytochrome P450 enzyme dependent and is inducible by other drugs such as phenobarbital and phenytoin.

Verapamil

See diltiazem.

Vitamin A

I: Dose related

M: Fat-storing cell hyperplasia and hypertrophy; nonspecific hepatocellular degeneration; fibrosis; cirrhosis

Mech: Intrinsic hepatotoxin[338-341]

Chronic vitamin A intoxication results from intake of large amounts (25,000–1,200,000 IU/day) of the vitamin for months to years. Systemic manifestations of the syndrome include anorexia, weight loss, fatigue, mild fever, pallor, psychiatric symptoms, polyuria, polydipsia, and night sweats. Pruritus, dry skin, hair loss, as well as pain and tenderness of bone are characteristics. Hepatomegaly is associated with symptoms of portal hypertension such as splenomegaly, ascites, or variceal hemorrhage in 80% of affected patients. Jaundice is rare. Laboratory studies may reveal anemia, leukopenia, increased sedimentation rate, and proteinuria. Hepatic injury may be evidenced by increased serum concentration of alkaline phosphatase and AST, hypoalbuminemia, and hypoprothrombinemia. The prognosis of patients with impaired hepatic function and hepatomegaly is usually good if the vitamin A intake is discontinued. However, once ascites and portal hypertension are present, the syndrome may persist even after cessation of the vitamin. Current restrictions in the vitamin A content of nonprescription preparations may limit the likelihood of overdose.

Zidovudine

I: Very low

M: Macrovesicular steatosis

Mech: Idiosyncrasy?[2,7,342-346]

Patients generally present with weakness, malaise, abdominal discomfort, prolonged coagulation time, acidosis, increase in ALT, hyperbilirubinemia, and hepatomegaly following several months of therapy. The primary injury is macrovesicular steatosis, but cholestasis has also been seen. Discontinuation of therapy may only reverse acidosis.

Didanosine and nevirapine have also caused macrovesicular steatosis and have led to several cases of fulminant hepatic failure. Of the protease inhibitors, indinavir has been reported to produce hepatic injury.

Table 30-4   Drug-Induced Hepatotoxicity—cont'd

Drug	Clinical Remarks
Zileuton[a] I: Low M: Unknown Mech: Idiosyncrasy?[347,348]	The reported incidence of liver enzyme elevation is ~2% following administration of zileuton. Hepatic injury appears to occur within the first 3 months, with LFTs returning to normal values following discontinuation of therapy. Patients who have active liver disease or elevation of LFTs equal to or exceeding three times the upper limit of normal should not receive zileuton.

[a]Zileuton was withdrawn from the U.S. Market in 2003.

ACE, angiotensin-converting enzyme; ALT, alanine aminotransferase; AST, aspartate aminotransferase; CAH, chronic active hepatitis; GI, gastrointestinal; I, incidence; IV, intravenous; LDH, lactate dehydrogenase; LFTs, liver function tests; M, morphology; Mech, mechanism; OCs, oral contraceptives; RA, rheumatoid arthritis; SLE, systemic lupus erythematosus; SR, sustained release; VOD, veno-occlusive disease.

sulfonamide-induced injury depends on the extent of the cytotoxic injury but usually occurs over a period of weeks to months.[64–68]

Idiosyncratic hepatic injury also can be caused by toxic metabolites (e.g., isoniazid, halothane, valproate, ketoconazole, methyldopa).[6,7,69,70] The idiosyncratic or unpredictable hepatic injury that results from a metabolic aberration rather than hypersensitivity usually develops after variable latent periods of 1 week to ≥12 months and usually is not accompanied by fever, rash, eosinophilia, or histologic findings of eosinophilic or granulomatous inflammation in the liver. In addition, reproduction of the hepatic injury requires administration of the drug for a period of days or weeks, rather than for only one or two doses, presumably to allow for accumulation of toxic metabolites.

Furthermore, C.W.'s clinical presentation could also be explained by her chronic ingestion of valproic acid (see Table 30-4). The hepatotoxicity associated with valproic acid is thought to be related to an inherent or acquired deficiency in the β-oxidation of valproic acid, resulting in formation of a toxic metabolite (4-envalproate).[7,20,70–78] However, infants and children younger than 2 years of age are at much higher risk than adults for valproic acid–induced liver disease. In addition, there appears to be a change in the pattern of the seizure frequency, which generally precedes clinical manifestations (jaundice, anorexia, fever, and nausea) of valproic acid–induced liver disease. Although possible, it is unlikely that C.W.'s DILD is from valproic acid because of her age (>2 years). Thus, it should be continued with close monitoring for resolution of clinical symptoms and liver function tests as described previously.

The classification of the mechanism of hepatic injury by an individual drug into either intrinsic, predictable hepatotoxicity, or unpredictable idiosyncrasy can sometimes be impossible, and in many instances, both major types of mechanisms may have a role. Thus, toxic hepatitis may occur after large overdoses of an intrinsically hepatotoxic drug or in an idiosyncratic manner after therapeutic doses. The reasons for the unique susceptibility of some patients are still poorly understood, and both genetic and acquired factors are likely to be involved.[2,6,7,20,35,36]

FORMS OF DRUG-INDUCED LIVER DISEASE

In addition to classifying DILD as a result of intrinsic hepatotoxicity or idiosyncratic reactions, the nature of the hepatic lesion can be used to categorize a specific type of liver injury. However, there are several limitations to fully differentiating the number and forms of DILD based on the nature of the hepatic lesion. These limitations may include an inability to completely analyze the histologic, clinical, and biochemical characteristics of the offending agent or the lack of recognition and confidence in implicating a potentially hepatotoxic agent due to the sporadic nature of ADR reporting. Other limitations may include the concomitant use of additional hepatotoxic agents, pre-existing hepatic diseases, and the inability to rechallenge a patient with the agent in question. Despite these concerns, drug-induced hepatic injury continues to be classified according to the morphology of the liver injury, the presumed mechanism, or the circumstances of drug-induced damages.

Drug-induced hepatic lesions can also generally be characterized as either acute (clinical or histologic evidence present <3 months) or chronic (clinical or histologic evidence present >3 months). Although acute injuries have received the most attention, chronic DILD has become increasingly prevalent. Both types of injury (acute and chronic), along with the characteristic lesion(s), are discussed in the following sections.

Acute Drug-Induced Liver Disease

Acute hepatic injury produced by drugs can be hepatocellular, cholestatic, or mixed (Table 30-5). Hepatocellular injury can be either cytotoxic or cytolytic, and it results in damage to the

Table 30-5   Features of Acute Drug-Induced Acute Hepatic Injury[2,7,8,63,102–107]

Lesion	Syndrome	Clinical Presentation	Biochemical Markers ALT/AST	ALK Phos	Examples of Offending Agents
Hepatocellular					
NECROSIS	Acute hepatitis	A, N, V	8–200×	3×	Isoniazid, diclofenac, halothane
Sinusoidal beading	Pseudomononucleosis	A, N, V, L, S	8–200×	Variable	Phenytoin, dapsone
Massive	Acute liver failure	A, N, V, L, S, C, E	25–200×	<3×	Same as above
Subacute	Prolonged hepatitis	A, N, V, J, FG	8–25×	<3×	Propylthiouracil, diclofenac
Spotty	Subclinical	None	2–5×	<3×	Isoniazid, diclofenac
STEATOSIS, MICROVESICULAR	Reye-like	N, V, E	–15×	<3×	Tetracycline
Cholestatic Injury					
HEPATOCANALICULAR					
Bile casts + spotty necrosis					
Portal inflammation	Obstructive jaundice	A, N, J, PR, FV, R, P	8×	>3×	Carbamazepine, erythromycin, estolate, sulfonylureas
CANALICULAR Bile casts	Obstructive jaundice	PR, J, P	<5×	<3×	Anabolic steroids Oral contraceptives

A, anorexia; ALK Phos, alkaline phosphatase; ALT, alanine aminotransferase; AST, aspartate aminotransaminase; C, coagulopathy; E, encephalopathy; FG, fatigue; FV, fever; J, jaundice; L, lymphadenopathy; N, nausea; P, pain; PR, pruritus; S, splenomegaly; R, rash; V, vomiting.

liver parenchyma. The lesions responsible for hepatocellular injury can be due to necrosis, steatosis, or a combination thereof. Cholestatic injury depicts arrested bile flow with jaundice and is associated with minimal or no parenchymal injury. Most cases of DILD have a "mixed" pattern, with features of both hepatocellular and cholestatic injury.[2,7,79]

Hepatocellular Injury
NECROSIS

Drug-induced hepatocellular necrosis may primarily involve cells in either a centrilobular (zonal) pattern (e.g., acetaminophen, CCl_4, enflurane, ferrous sulfate, halothane), a diffuse (nonzonal) pattern, or hepatocytes similar to that of viral hepatitis (e.g., methyldopa), or it may affect significant portions of the entire liver (e.g., valproic acid).[2,7,20] Additional agents reported to cause hepatocellular injury include trazodone, diclofenac, nefazodone, venlafaxine, and lovastatin.[2,7,20] Biochemical markers (serum aminotransferases) are the hallmark of hepatic damage. The serum AST and ALT in patients with hepatic necrosis are elevated from 8 to 500 times the upper limit of normal, whereas values for alkaline phosphatase usually are increased modestly to no more than three times normal.[2,6–8,20,79–82] Blood cholesterol concentrations are often normal or sometimes low. These biochemical patterns resemble those observed in acute viral hepatitis; thus, hepatocellular necrosis is often referred to as *drug-induced* or *toxic hepatitis*.[2,7,79,82] Clinical features include fatigue, anorexia, nausea, and jaundice. With increasing degrees of liver cell necrosis, patients may experience manifestations of acute liver failure such as deep jaundice, coagulopathy, ascites, hepatic encephalopathy, coma, and death.[7,15,18,20]

A final clinical presentation of drug-induced acute hepatitis may mimic infectious mononucleosis.[7,20,79] In addition to hepatocellular injury, lymphadenopathy, lymphocytosis, and circulating lymphocytes may be present. This presentation has been associated with the use of phenytoin, dapsone, sulfonamides, and *para*-aminosalicylic acid.[7,20,79]

STEATOSIS

A second type of acute drug-induced lesion is steatosis, which can be microvesicular or macrovesicular. In microvesicular steatosis, the hepatocytes are filled with many tiny droplets of fat that do not displace the nucleus (e.g., valproic acid, tetracycline, aspirin overdose).[40,83,84] In macrovesicular steatosis, the hepatocyte contains a large fat droplet that displaces the nucleus to the periphery (ethanol, methotrexate). Drugs such as corticosteroids resulting in lipid deposition in the liver also can cause steatosis. Generally, acute toxic steatosis is likely to be microvesicular, whereas chronic steatosis is usually macrovesicular (e.g., amiodarone, tamoxifen). Although microvesicular steatosis results in enlargement of the liver, routine liver function tests often remain normal. In contrast, fatty degeneration caused by drugs such as valproic acid may result in irreversible cell damage reflected by increased AST and ALT serum concentrations of 100 to 500 U/mL.[7,40] Elevations in aminotransferase levels in patients with drug-induced hepatic steatosis are not as high as those reported with hepatocellular necrosis. The histologic picture of drug-induced fatty degeneration is similar to that observed with fatty liver of pregnancy or Reye's syndrome.[2,7,20,83,84] Certain drugs (e.g., high dosages of estrogens)

also can induce a form of degenerative, necrotizing liver damage known as *fatty liver hepatitis,* which can eventually result in micronodular cirrhosis.[2,7,84] Fatty liver hepatitis is often asymptomatic, and the appearance of malaise, diarrhea, fever, jaundice, leukocytosis, ascites, or edema may indicate that the damage is already irreversible with a poor prognosis.

Cholestatic Injury
CANALICULAR AND HEPATOCANALICULAR

Cholestatic injury has been associated with two prominent types of lesions.[2,7,20,79,80] These are manifested by bile stasis without inflammation and with minimal parenchymal injury (i.e., bland, pure, or steroid cholestasis) or by cholestasis with inflammation and slight parenchymal injury (i.e., cholestatic hepatitis, pericholangitis, cholangiolitic cholestasis, or sensitivity cholestasis). The former can be characterized as *hepatocanalicular* (i.e., combined with hepatocyte injury), whereas the latter is referred to as *canalicular* (i.e., portal inflammation).

Canalicular cholestasis is characterized by AST and/or ALT elevations less than eightfold above normal, normal cholesterol, alkaline phosphatase elevations less than threefold above normal, in a patient who is jaundiced or has a serum bilirubin level >42 μmol/L. In contrast, hepatocanalicular cholestasis usually presents with AST and/or ALT levels less than eightfold elevated, increased cholesterol, and alkaline phosphatase 3- to 10-fold above normal. Patients with AST, ALT, and alkaline phosphatase levels in the canalicular range but with a serum bilirubin level <42 μmol/L are categorized as "indeterminate type" because these values could reflect either minor hepatocellular injury or anicteric injury of the cholestatic type. Hepatocanalicular injury is typically seen in chlorpromazine jaundice, and the canalicular type usually is observed in cases resulting from anabolic or contraceptive steroids.[2,6,7,20,79,84]

Drug-induced canalicular and hepatocanalicular cholestatic injury often resembles extrahepatic obstructive jaundice both clinically and biochemically.[2,6,7,20,79,84] Pruritus, jaundice, pale stools, and dark urine are the primary clinical manifestations. Other patient complaints may include upper abdominal pain or dull aching. The serum bilirubin level is increased in all cases of drug-induced cholestasis, but it usually is <170 μmol/L (normal, 2 to 17), although on occasion, it can be >800 μmol/L.[84] The serum aminotransferase concentrations are generally only moderately increased. The serum concentrations of alkaline phosphatase usually are increased more than threefold when cholestasis is caused by oral hypoglycemic agents, some antithyroid drugs, erythromycin estolate and its derivatives, or chlorpromazine (hepatocanalicular), but they do not increase as much when the cholestasis is not accompanied by cellular injury (e.g., anabolic and contraceptive steroids).[2,6,7,20,79,84]

The immediate prognosis in patients with either hepatocanalicular or canalicular injury is good. The mortality rate for pure cholestasis is much lower than when the cholestasis is accompanied by cytotoxic damage and is believed to be <1%.[2,6,7,20,80] However, a syndrome of chronic intrahepatic cholestasis with clinical, biochemical, and histologic features that resemble primary biliary cirrhosis (PBC) has been observed following acute drug-induced cholestasis [79,85,86] (Table 30-6). These cases of PBC-like disease are likely to resolve,

Table 30-6   Drug-Induced Chronic Cholestasis Compared With Primary Biliary Cirrhosis[7,8,20,108,109]

Characteristics	Drug-Induced Chronic Cholestasis	Primary Biliary Cirrhosis
Associated disease	Irrelevant	Sicca syndrome
Drug intake	Phenothiazines, organic arsenicals	None
Clinical symptoms	Pruritus, early severe jaundice, xanthomas, hepatomegaly, splenomegaly, cirrhosis	Pruritus, latent mild jaundice, xanthomas, hepatomegaly, splenomegaly, meloderma, cirrhosis
Laboratory Markers		
Bilirubin	1–20 mg/dL	1–5 mg/dL
ALT/AST	2–8×	2–8×
Alkaline phosphatase	3–10×	3–10×
Histologic Markers		
Ductopenia	Slight	Remarkable
Nonsuppurative cholangitis	Absent	Present
Hepatic granulomas	Absent	Present

ALT, alanine aminotransaminase; AST, aspartate aminotransaminase.

yet a permanent and fatal PBC-like syndrome (vanishing bile duct syndrome) has been identified.[2,7,85,86]

Mixed Injury

Mixed forms of drug-induced injury can be primarily hepatocellular with significant cholestatic characteristics, or they can be primarily cholestatic with significant hepatocellular features and appear to be more consistent with a drug-induced etiology rather than with viral hepatitis. Biochemical markers for mixed cholestatic injury may be defined by elevations in ALT, AST (values more than eight times the upper level of normal), and alkaline phosphatase levels (values more than three times the upper level of normal).

Several drugs appear to exhibit a distinct relationship between their therapeutic class and the type of injury they elucidate.[2,7,20,79] For example, some antiepileptic drugs (i.e., phenytoin, carbamazepine) tend to produce hepatocellular or mixed hepatocellular jaundice. Most neuroleptic agents tend to produce cholestatic (hepatocanalicular) jaundice, whereas hydrazide antidepressants cause hepatocellular jaundice, and tricyclic antidepressants primarily cause cholestatic injury.

Nevertheless, most drugs do not exhibit a distinct relationship between their therapeutic class and the type of injury they induce. Specifically, some oral hypoglycemic agents such as acetohexamide produce mixed hepatocellular injury, whereas others such as chlorpropamide, tolbutamide, and tolazamide cause cholestatic jaundice.[2,7,20,79] Second-generation hypoglycemic agents such as glyburide and glipizide have rarely been associated with causing cholestatic jaundice. Also, the antimicrobial agent nitrofurantoin and the NSAID sulindac may cause either cholestatic or hepatocellular injury.[70] Gold compounds appear to be associated with cholestatic rather than hepatocellular jaundice, but this relationship is not consistent. Other agents that lead to mixed injury include para-aminosalicylic acid, sulfonamides, amoxicillin-clavulanate, cyclosporine, methimazole, carbamazepine, troglitazone (no longer available) and herbs.[2,7,20] The mortality rate of the mixed form seems to depend on the extent of cytotoxic injury.

Chronic Drug-Induced Liver Disease

Chronic adverse effects of drugs on the liver generally can be categorized based on the type of lesion or on similarity to clinical syndromes (Table 30-7). These categories include parenchymal lesions secondary to chronic hepatitis, subacute hepatic necrosis, chronic steatosis, phospholipidosis (PL), or fibrosis and cirrhosis. Also included are two forms of cholestatic lesions either from chronic intrahepatic cholestasis or biliary sclerosis. In addition, vascular, granulomatous, and neoplastic lesions may also lead to chronic hepatic disease.[2,7,10,20]

Parenchymal Disease
CHRONIC HEPATITIS

Formerly categorized as chronic active or persistent hepatitis, all chronic necroinflammatory disease of the liver is now referred to as *chronic hepatitis* (CH).[87] In addition to viral etiologies (e.g., hepatitis B virus, hepatitis C virus), autoimmune hepatitis (AIH), Wilson's disease, and cryptogenic cirrhosis, drug-induced hepatic parenchymal lesions have been reported. Drug-induced lesions appear to mimic AIH because they predominantly affect females and are accompanied by hyperglobulinemia, antinuclear antibodies, anti–single-strand DNA, and other serologic autoimmune markers.[2,7,20] Drugs associated with this syndrome include dantrolene, diclofenac, fenofibrate, methyldopa, minocycline, nitrofurantoin, sulfonamides, and drugs of abuse such as ecstasy. Acetaminophen and isoniazid also have been incriminated in causing chronic active viral hepatitis-like disease, perhaps owing to continued toxic injury rather than an autoimmune response.[2,6,7] To date, at least 24 drugs have been associated with CH, and although the overall presentation is not homogeneous, they have been categorized into four separate types of injury.[6,88]

The first group (type 1) consists of drugs that induce liver injury that resembles autoimmune hepatitis.[79,89] Drugs associated with this from of injury are often taken for prolonged periods and are continued beyond the initial liver insult. The

Table 30-7 Features of Drug-Induced Chronic Hepatic Injury[2,7,8,20,110-127]

Lesion	Associated Syndrome	Biochemical Markers		Examples of Offending Agents
		ALT/AST	ALK Phos	
Hepatocellular				
Necroinflammatory	Chronic hepatitis	3–50×	1–3×	Nitrofurantoin, minocycline, methyldopa
Steatosis	Alcoholic steatosis	1–3×	1–3×	Methotrexate, glucocorticoids
Phospholipidosis	Alcoholic hepatitis	1–5×	Variable	Amphophilic agents
Pseudoalcoholic	Alcoholic hepatitis	1–5×	Variable	Amiodarone, perhexiline
Cholestatic Injury				
Cholangiodestructive	Primary biliary cirrhosis	1–3×	3×20×	Carbamazepine, haloperidol
Biliary sclerosis	Sclerosing cholangitis	1–5×	3–20×	Floxuridine
Granulomatous	Hepatomegaly; hepatitis	1–3×	3–20×	Allopurinol, carbamazepine, hydralazine, quinine
Vascular Lesions				
Peliosis	Hepatomegaly	1–3×	<3×	Anabolic steroids, oral contraceptives
Budd-Chiari syndrome	Congestive hepatopathy	2–20×	Variable	Oral contraceptives
Veno-occlusive	Congestive hepatopathy	2–20×	Variable	Pyrrolizidine alkaloids, azathioprine
Sinusoidal dilation	Hepatomegaly	3×	Variable	Oral contraceptives
Pericellular/sinusoidal fibrosis	Noncirrhotic portal HTN	1–3× Variable	Vitamin A	
Neoplasm				
Adenoma, carcinoma	Asymptomatic hepatic mass	Variable	Variable	Oral contraceptives, anabolic steroids

ALK Phos, alkaline phosphatase; ALT, alanine aminotransaminase; AST, aspartate aminotransaminase; HTN, hypertension.

overall incidence of this "type" appears to be <5%. Unique clinical features in this group includes a high incidence in women (>90% of cases reported), hypergammaglobulinemia, autoantibodies, and a chronic necroinflammation rich in plasma cells.

Type 2 drug-induced chronic hepatitis is characterized by antibody formation against isoforms of cytochrome P450 or other microsomal proteins, which apparently leads to "neoantigen" production during biotransformation.[2,6,79,90-92] Compared with type 1, hyperglobulinemia is not a prominent feature of this entity. Only two drugs (dihydralazine and tienlic acid) have led to this type of drug-induced CH.

Drugs such as etretinate, lisinopril, sulfonamide, and trazodone make up a third form of drug-induced CH, but the serologic markers of autoimmune disease are absent.[7,88] Patients with type 3 injury often have elevations in their aminotransferases with histologic evidence of chronic hepatitis.

Type 4 of drug-induced CH consists of agents such as acetaminophen, aspirin, and dantrolene, which produce chronic toxicity rather than the chronic necroinflammatory disease that resembles chronic hepatitis.[20,93-95]

Overall, the clinical picture of drug-induced CH has mixed characteristics, with features of both acute and chronic hepatic injury. Patients may first present with either features of acute hepatocellular injury or clinical evidence of cirrhosis. Physical examination often reveals a firm, enlarged liver; splenomegaly; and spider angiomas with or without ascites. Jaundice, anorexia, and fatigue are common. Arthralgias or "arthritis" may occur. Serum transferase levels are usually moderately increased; hypoalbuminemia and coagulopathy are common.[96,97] Recognition of drug-induced CH is extremely important because withdrawal of the responsible drug may lead to marked improvement and complete resolution of the injury within 4 weeks. However, continuation of these agents may lead to cirrhosis, fulminant hepatic failure and death.

SUBACUTE HEPATIC NECROSIS

Subacute hepatic necrosis (toxic cirrhosis) is different from acute necrosis and CH in that the clinical deterioration is slower than that seen in acute injury, yet it progresses faster than that associated with CH. Manifestations include a progressive, serious liver disease with deep jaundice and evidence of cirrhosis. Drugs that have been associated with this type of presentation include isoniazid,[20,34] methyldopa,[98] and propylthiouracil.[99]

CHRONIC STEATOSIS

Compared with the acute microvesicular type of drug-induced steatosis, chronic steatosis is usually macrovascular and has minimal clinical manifestations. Ethanol, glucocorticoids, and a number of antineoplastic agents such as methotrexate (which all primarily lead to hepatomegaly) are agents associated with this type of insult.[7,100] Glucocorticoid-induced steatosis appears to be benign, whereas methotrexate-induced steatosis can progress to cirrhosis. However, in some instances, the lesions seen in chronic steatosis may be microvesicular and lead to prominent hepatic disease (i.e., necrosis). This presentation has been reported with asparaginase and valproic acid. Valproic acid not only can induce microvesicular lipid deposits in the liver, but also causes fatty degeneration that can result in chronic liver failure with encephalopathy and a fatal outcome.[2,7,100]

PHOSPHOLIPIDOSIS

PL occurs frequently and is caused by an amphophilic drug (i.e., a drug that is both lipophilic and hydrophilic) that accumulates within the lysosomes. PL is usually clinically silent or causes only mild liver dysfunction. Hepatomegaly is the predominant feature of PL with or without other organ injury (e.g., PL of peripheral nerves, lungs, thyroid, and skin). Pseudoalcoholic liver disease (PALD) or nonalcoholic steatohepatitis (NASH) consisting of steatosis, focal necrosis, inflammatory aggregates, and Mallory bodies in association with PL have also been reported. These lesions have progressed to cirrhosis in several instances after long-term administration of amiodarone[2,107,100–102] This clinical presentation of PALD or NASH can include hepatomegaly, ascites, spider angiomas, wasting syndrome, neuropathy, and moderate increase in aminotransferases (less than five times the upper limit of normal).

FIBROSIS AND CIRRHOSIS

CH, PL-associated PALD, chronic cholestatic injury, lesions affecting hepatic outflow, and chronic injury from methotrexate and etretinate all can lead to hepatic fibrosis and cirrhosis. Portal hypertension and its associated complications are the main characteristics in advanced cases.

Cholestatic Lesions

CHRONIC INTRAHEPATIC CHOLESTASIS

One form of drug-induced chronic intrahepatic cholestasis has features that resemble PBC, but it does not have some of the defining characteristics of PBC such as late-onset jaundice or antimitochondrial antibodies.[7,85,86] Common clinical findings associated with this form of lesion are pruritus, early-onset jaundice, and elevated serum bilirubin and alkaline phosphatase levels, but only moderately increased AST and ALT levels. In advanced stages, xanthomatosis, ascites, edema, and portal hypertension may occur. Bile duct destruction and portal inflammation are less significant from chronic cholestatic-associated drug-induced injury compared with PBC, and it may lead to a unique form of the vanishing bile duct syndrome. Drugs reported to cause this syndrome include carbamazepine, haloperidol, imipramine, phenothiazines (chlorpromazine, prochlorperazine), sulfamethoxazole-trimethoprim, thiabendazole, and tolbutamide.[7,80,85,86]

BILIARY SCLEROSIS

A second form of cholestatic cholestasis is biliary sclerosis, which has been observed in cases of bile duct injury produced by intrahepatic arterial infusion of floxuridine.[103] The incidence of injury due to floxuridine appears to be high. Clinical features include upper abdominal pain, anorexia, weight loss, and jaundice. Alkaline phosphatase levels are more than three times normal, whereas the aminotransferases are less than five times the normal limit.

Vascular Lesions

Four significant drug-induced vascular lesions have been reported, including hepatic vein thrombosis, hepatic venule occlusion, peliosis hepatitis, and hepatoportal sclerosis. Vascular injury that affects efferent blood flow (e.g., portal blood flow) to the liver leads to hepatic vein thrombosis. Budd-Chiari syndrome can be manifested by symptoms such as hepatomegaly, abdominal pain, ascites, moderate elevations in serum aminotransferases, and occasionally, jaundice.[32] Rapid deterioration and death may soon follow. This type of injury can be caused by oral contraceptives (OCs), and although the incidence remains low compared with the large number of women taking OCs, case-controlled studies demonstrate that women taking these agents have greater than double the risk compared with other women of developing this lesion.[2,7,105,106]

Veno-occlusive disease as a result of injury and fibrotic occlusion of the terminal hepatic venules has clinical symptoms similar to those of Budd-Chiari syndrome and may result in death or can be followed by complete recovery. This type of hepatic injury has historically been associated with pyrrolizine alkaloids (e.g., comfrey) or alkaloid derivatives (e.g., etoposide, vincristine, vinblastine), but agents such as thioguanine, azathioprine, chemotherapeutic agents (busulfan, cyclophosphamide, dactinomycin, methotrexate and mitomycin) and radiation injury serve as common etiologies.[2,7,107] Additional etiologies of this type of injury include herbal medications or dietary supplements that are often obtained in natural food stores.[108]

Peliosis Hepatitis

Peliosis hepatis, a rarely encountered blood-filled cyst in the liver, can be caused by anabolic or contraceptive steroids, as well as related agents such as danazol.[7,29,109] Most cases with this type of injury are often associated with hepatic tumors or with cholestatic jaundice induced by the offending drug. Clinical manifestations include hepatomegaly, jaundice, or liver failure.[110] Occasionally, the cyst may rupture and result in a syndrome of hemoperitoneum.

Drug-induced portal hypertension may occur without evidence of cirrhosis.[2,7,20] An example is hepatoportal sclerosis after chemotherapeutic or immunosuppressive therapy.[2,7,111] Additional causes of this lesion include chronic exposure to inorganic arsenicals, copper sulfate, and vinyl chloride, as well as vitamin A intoxication.[2,6,7,112] Clinically, splenomegaly, leukopenia, thrombocytopenia, pancytopenia, or esophageal varices may be present.

Granulomatous Hepatitis (Drug Induced)

Granulomatous reactions are a common presentation of DILD and account for 2% to 29% of cases of granulomatous hepatitis. The clinical presentation includes fever, malaise, headache, and myalgia between 10 days and 4 months after the initiation of treatment, with splenomegaly present in up to 15% of cases. Hepatic granulomas are always noncaseating and can be surrounded by eosinophils. Hepatic granulomas can be accompanied by cytotoxic or cholestatic injury as part of a hypersensitivity reaction (e.g., allopurinol, methyldopa, penicillin, phenytoin, quinidine, sulfonamides) or without any clinical evidence of hepatic injury (e.g., gold salts).[6,7,20,113] Up to 60 drugs have been associated with hepatic granulomas.[2,7]

Neoplastic Lesions

Several associations between pharmacologic agents and liver tumors have been depicted, but causality has been difficult to prove because of the infrequent nature of these events. Hepatocellular adenoma and carcinoma, although rare, are clearly associated with the use of OCs and anabolic (C-17 alkylated) steroids.[2,7,20,114] Several cases of hepatic adenomas have involved women, virtually all of whom had a history of OC use. The results of two large, case-controlled studies suggest that the incidence is between 3 and 4 per 100,000 exposed persons annually. This represents a relative risk (compared with patients not receiving OCs) of approximately 20-fold in those patients ingesting OCs for <10 years and more than 100-fold in those exposed for >10 years.[2,115] Similarly, some cases have been associated with anabolic steroid use in men.[116] Danazol has been associated with causing hepatocellular adenoma and carcinoma in humans, whereas griseofulvin, hyacanthone, and isoniazid have been known to produce hepatocellular carcinoma in experimental animals.[2,7] OCs have also been associated with causing hepatocellular carcinomas[7,117,118] and possibly focal nodular hyperplasia.[7,119]

In general, prognosis of drug-induced hepatotoxicity is good when the offending agent is withdrawn; however, the prognosis clearly is affected by the type of liver injury, the duration of the insult, and whether the hepatic damage is irreversible.[2,6,7,100] The more cytotoxic the injury, the more likely that hepatic failure and death will ensue; the more cholestatic the injury, the better the prognosis.

HERBAL MEDICATION-INDUCED HEPATOTOXICITY

3. H.D. is a 48-year-old woman with a history of chronic back pain secondary to an auto accident 3 years ago. She previously had taken oral Vicodin (hydrocodone 5 mg/acetaminophen 500 mg), 1 to 2 tablets Q 6 hr for pain relief, but recently, she discontinued the drug because of constipation; subsequently, the pain became worse. After several months of acupuncture as primary therapy, she began seeking another analgesic agent. According to her husband, she began taking the herbal supplement Jin Bu Huan per the recommendation of her mother, who claimed, based on her own experience, that the agent was an exceptional analgesic. However, after taking the herbal remedy for 2 months, H.D. began experiencing fever, fatigue, and mild abdominal pain. Her husband noticed that H.D. had also become "jaundiced" around that time; as a result, he brought her to the emergency department for treatment. Upon obtaining a careful medication history, laboratory tests revealed that H.D.'s ALT, AST, and total bilirubin were 1,378 U/L, 1,333 U/L, and 3,9 mg/dL, respectively. A biopsy was also obtained, and the results are pending. What is the association between herbal medications and hepatotoxicity?

Previous reports indicated that 3% of the population of the United States had taken herbal medications for a variety of reasons (e.g., analgesia, sedation, nutrition, weight reduction, skin disorders).[108,124,125] Recent studies show that 42% of Americans take some form of complementary and alternative medicine, and that herbal medicine use is now estimated to be 12.5%. In addition, 20% to30% of patients attending hepatology clinics use herbal remedies.[126,127] Although herbal remedies have historically been considered benign, a plethora of information has suggested that many agents are associated with toxic effects (Table 30-8). Some include asafetida, chaparral leaf, camphor, carp capsules, comfrey, dai-saiko-to (TJ-9), gentian, germander, greater celandine, hops, impila, isabgol, kava, mistletoe, mother wart, pennyroyal oil, senna fruit extract, skullcap, and valerian.[108,128–132] These effects usually manifest when the recommended threshold for toxic doses are surpassed, although the duration of therapy may also be a factor. Currently, the range of herbal-induced liver injury includes minor transaminase elevations, acute and chronic hepatitis, steatosis, cholestasis, zonal or diffuse hepatic necrosis, hepatic fibrosis and cirrhosis, veno-occlusive disease, and acute liver failure requiring liver transplantation.[108]

In one representative report, seven adult patients ingesting Jin Bu Huan, a traditional herbal remedy used primarily as a sedative and analgesic, presented with fever, fatigue, nausea, pruritus, abdominal pain, jaundice, and hepatomegaly at a mean time of 20 weeks (range, 7 to 52 weeks) after ingestion of normal doses of this agent.[133] Serum transaminases were increased 20- to 50-fold in most cases. One patient who had taken the agent for 12 months underwent a liver biopsy, which showed lobular hepatitis with microvesicular steatosis. Resolution of liver injury occurred within 8 weeks after the cessation of therapy. Other than a female predominance, no predisposing risk factors for developing liver disease were evident

Table 30-8 Selected Herbal Medications/Remedies Associated With Hepatic Injury[154–168]

Herb	Proposed Use	Toxic Ingredient	Feature of Hepatic Injury
Comfrey	Health tonic	Pyrrolizidine alkaloids	Veno-occlusive disease
Gordolobo yerba tea			
Mate tea			
Chinese medicinal tea	Health tonic	T'u-san-chi'i (Compositae)	Veno-occlusive disease
Jin bu huan	Sedative, analgesic	*Lycopodium serratum*	Hepatocellular injury: hepatitis, fibrosis, steatosis
Chinese herbs	Eczema, psoriasis	Many	Nonspecific hepatic injury
Germander (tea, capsules)	Weight reduction, health tonic	*Teucrium chamaedrys*	Hepatitis: necrosis, fibrosis
Chaparral leaf	Herbal remedy	*Larrea tridenta*	Hepatic necrosis
Mistletoe/skullcap/valerian	Herbal tonic, cathartic	Senna, podophyllin, aloin	Elevated liver function tests
Margosa oil	Tonic	*Melia azadirachta indica*	Reye's syndrome
Pennyroyal oil (squawmint)	Abortifacient, herbal remedy	Labiatae plants (possibly diterpenes)	Elevated liver function tests
Oil of cloves	Dental pain	Unknown	Dose-dependent hepatotoxin

in this case. However, it appears that concomitant agents that induce cytochrome P450 enzymes may also increase susceptibility to developing liver disease. In summary, because herbal agents are readily available, are not subject to rigorous purity testing or regulation, and may often contain small amounts of arsenic or cadmium, it is critical for clinicians to obtain a detailed medication use history when evaluating atypical cases of liver injury. H.D. should discontinue this agent and, pending the biopsy results, be followed closely for the next few weeks for resolution of her liver injury. However, if her symptoms worsen, liver transplantation may be necessary.

PATIENT ASSESSMENT

4. K.V., a 52-year-old woman with a 12-year history of non–insulin-dependent diabetes, is admitted with a 2-week history of nausea, anorexia, fatigue, and intense generalized pruritus. She noted dark urine, light-colored stools, and yellow pigmentation of the skin about 10 days ago, which has gotten progressively worse. She had no fever, rash, vomiting, abdominal pain or fatty food intolerance. She denies use of alcohol or recreational drugs and has never had a blood transfusion. Her medical history includes diabetes controlled by diet and pioglitazone (for the past 18 months) and hypertension treated with hydrochlorothiazide (HCTZ) and lisinopril for the past 4 years. One month ago, K.V. was started on a 10-day course of amoxicillin-clavulanic acid (Augmentin) for acute otitis media.

On admission, K.V. appears weak and icteric. Other significant findings include scratch marks and a slightly tender, but normal-sized, liver. Vital signs are all within normal limits. Laboratory findings show the following: serum AST, 430 U/L; serum ALT, 294 U/L; alkaline phosphatase, 1,230 U/L; total: direct (T:D) bilirubin ratio, 7.251 mg/dL:106 mol/L (normal, up to 0.994 mg/dL for total; up to 14 mol/L for direct); and albumin, 4.1 g/dL. All other chemistry data are within normal limits. Complete blood count (CBC) and differential count are normal. Serologic tests for hepatitis A, B, and C all are negative. Ultrasound shows a normal biliary tract system, with no obstruction in the bile ducts or gallbladder or near the end of the pancreas. Liver biopsy showed preserved normal liver architecture, marked centrilobular cholestasis with bile pigment in hepatocytes and canaliculi, and a mild portal inflammatory infiltrate with an excess of eosinophils.

K.V. is placed on a 1,200-calorie daily diet, with no added salt, and regular insulin before meals titrated to a pre-meal glucose level of 100 to 150 mg/dL. All other drugs are discontinued. Cholestyramine (Questran) 4 g PO TID is started for itching. By the fifth day of hospitalization, her laboratory values are as follows: AST, 85 U/L; ALT, 214 U/L; alkaline phosphatase, 288 U/L; and bilirubin T:D, 2.456 mol/L:29mol/L. Her blood pressure increased to 190/105 mm Hg and HCTZ 25 mg QD is restarted with a plan to add a calcium channel blocker if this does not adequately control her blood pressure. What signs and symptoms are suggestive of hepatitis in K.V.? Is the evidence suggestive of a cytotoxic origin or cholestatic involvement?

[SI units: AST, 7.168 and 1.41695 μkat/L; ALT, 4.90098 and 3.56738 μkat/L; alkaline phosphatase, 20.5041 and 4.80096 μkat/L; T:D bilirubin ratio, 124 μmol/L:106 and 42 μmol/L:29 μmol/L (normal, up to 17 μmol/L for total; up to 14 μmol/L for direct); albumin, 41 g/L]

Routine screening of serum aminotransferases in patients taking potentially hepatotoxic drugs generally is not recommended because the changes in laboratory tests often are delayed or erratic in onset, making detection of abnormalities difficult. Elevations of less than three times normal may reflect normal variations or spurious laboratory results. On the other hand, minor elevations that continue to trend upward on repeat evaluations or that are more than three times normal indicate a cause for concern.

In K.V., weakness, anorexia, dark urine, light-colored stools, icterus, pruritus, hyperbilirubinemia, and a high serum alkaline phosphatase concentration suggest cholestatic jaundice. The slightly tender liver and the high serum concentrations of AST and ALT suggest hepatocellular damage. K.V.'s clinical presentation is consistent with that of a mixed cholestatic-cytotoxic hepatic injury.

Etiology

5. How can the potential etiology of drug-induced hepatitis be determined, and what was the most likely etiology in K.V.?

Drug-induced hepatic injury should be suspected in every patient with jaundice. A negative history of fever, abdominal pain, and fatty food intolerance rule out gallbladder disease in K.V. She has no history of alcoholism and her viral hepatitis serologic tests are negative. In addition, negative ultrasound studies rule out the possibility of extrahepatic obstructive jaundice.

The presence of dark urine ruled out unconjugated hyperbilirubinemia, which may be associated with hemolysis. AST elevations alone may be seen in injury to cardiac and skeletal muscles, but together with increased ALT, as in K.V., usually indicate hepatic origin. The presence of eosinophils in the liver biopsy, together with the rapid decline of serum aminotransferases, alkaline phosphatase, and bilirubin concentrations toward normal when all drugs are withdrawn, supports the assessment of drug-induced hepatitis in K.V.

There are four possible causes for K.V.'s drug-induced hepatitis including, amoxicillin-clavulanic acid, pioglitazone, hydrochlorothiazide, and lisinopril. Hydrochlorothiazide is an unlikely candidate because allergic cholestatic jaundice is very rarely associated with thiazide diuretics, and K.V. has taken the drug for 4 years. Lisinopril, like other angiotensin-converting enzyme inhibitors, can cause acute hepatocellular injury with mostly mixed hepatocellular and cholestatic injury; pure hepatocellular injury is rare. Furthermore, most cases of lisinopril-induced hepatic injury occur within the first 14 weeks of exposure.[134–138] Thus, lisinopril, which is known to cause mixed hepatocellular injury, is probably not the causative agent in K.V. based on the time frame of the presentation of hepatic injury. Pioglitazone, on the other hand, has been reported to cause a mixed cholestatic-cytotoxic injury, but not to the same degree as its predecessor, troglitazone which was previously withdrawn from the market due to over 90 cases of hepatotoxic effects (68 fatalities and 10 required liver transplantation).[139–145] There is only one report of pioglitazone associated hepatotoxicity. In this case, a 49-year-old male was taking 30 mg day for 6 months was found to have an ALT level three times the upper limit of normal, and a serum bilirubin concentration five times the upper limit of normal.[145] Therefore, it is unlikely in K.V. because she had been taking pioglitazone for 18 months and her ALT elevation is not consistent with those previously reported. Amoxicillin-clavulanic acid, a semisynthetic penicillin-β-lactamase inhibitor combination drug, has been reported to cause hepatic dysfunction and jaundice in a number of patients.[146] The latent period between the initiation of the drug and onset of jaundice or hepatic dysfunction ranged from 2 to 45 days, with a mean of 27 days. In review of K.V.'s recent history of amoxicillin-clavulanic acid intake and the physical and laboratory findings, amoxicillin-clavulanic acid seems to be the most probable cause. Nevertheless, the possibility of hydrochlorothiazide- or pioglitazone-induced hepatic injury cannot be ruled out without an inadvisable rechallenge test with one or both of these drugs.

Procedure to Determine

To determine the cause of drug-induced hepatic injury, a detailed drug history should be obtained for all patients with jaundice. OC use should not be overlooked. Special attention should be paid to the duration of exposure to a specific drug and its relationship to the onset of symptoms. A history of taking OCs, nonprescription drugs such as laxatives and vitamins, and illicit drug use should be sought. Predisposing factors to drug-induced hepatitis, if any, should be noted (see Table 30-1). The presumptive diagnosis of drug-induced hepatic injury requires a history of exposure to a drug, awareness of the characteristic syndromes produced by various agents, and a search for supportive evidence. If the liver injury is accompanied by fever, rash, and eosinophilia, the likelihood of drug-induced disease increases. In some instances, these features may be associated with lymph node enlargement, lymphocytosis, and atypical circulating lymphocytes, leading to a syndrome that mimics infectious mononucleosis and serum sickness. Additional plausible systemic manifestations are listed in Table 30-9. Lack of these features, however, does not exclude the possibility of drug-induced disease.[7,15] Differentiation of drug-induced hepatocellular injury from viral hepatitis involves evaluation of the epidemiologic circumstances; serologic studies to detect hepatitis A, B, or C antigens or antibodies; and determination of whether a history of receiving blood transfusions or injection with a contaminated syringe exists. Distinction between drug-induced cholestatic jaundice and extrahepatic obstructive jaundice often requires radiographic or ultrasonic studies. If liver biopsy reveals cholestasis with an eosinophil-rich portal inflammation, as observed in K.V., drug-induced causes are more likely.

Rechallenge With Offending Agent

6. Should K.V. be given a challenge dose of amoxicillin-clavulanic acid to confirm the cause of her drug-induced hepatitis?

Confirmation of the cause may be obtained by giving a rechallenge dose of the incriminated drug. Recurrence of hepatic dysfunction or hyperbilirubinemia after a test dose offers valuable support for the diagnosis. Failure to develop abnormalities, however, does not preclude drug-induced dysfunction because only 40% to 60% of patients show a recurrence of hepatic injury after a test dose.[80] Furthermore, some drugs will produce the hepatic injury only after an extended period (1 to 12 weeks) of readministration. Testing for the effect of a challenge dose can be potentially dangerous if the drug is known to cause hepatocellular injury, whereas rechallenge is considered safe if the drug usually leads to cholestasis alone. Therefore, risk must be weighed against benefit before giving a challenge dose of an incriminated drug to a patient.

Rechallenge of K.V. with amoxicillin-clavulanic acid is potentially dangerous because of her clinical picture of hepatocellular injury. Rapid occurrence of jaundice and liver enzyme abnormalities following rechallenge with amoxicillin-clavulanic acid suggests an immunoallergic type of idiosyncrasy.[2,7,20] Because alternative antibiotics can be used to manage K.V.'s infection, rechallenging with amoxicillin-clavulanic acid is not recommended.

Treatment

7. Was K.V. treated appropriately for her suspected drug-induced hepatic injury?

Once diagnosis has been made, the presumed offending drug should be withdrawn. In K.V.'s case, all medications taken before admission were discontinued. The management of drug-induced jaundice is similar to the treatment of other hepatic diseases. Treatment usually includes a diet high in carbohydrates, moderately high in protein, and adequate in calories (e.g., 2,000 to 3,000 calories/day). However, a lower caloric diet was prescribed for K.V. because of her diabetes. Treatment of jaundice is mainly supportive. If itching is severe, the use of cholestyramine to enhance the rate of bile acid excretion may alleviate the symptoms. If possible, the use of

Table 30-9 Extrahepatic Manifestations of Drug-Induced Liver Disease[6–8]

Manifestations	Example of Offending Agent
Allergic (rash, fever, eosinophilia)	Sulindac, dapsone, phenytoin
Pseudomononucleosis	*Para*-aminosalicylic acid, phenytoin, dapsone
Antinuclear antibodies	Methyldopa, nitrofurantoin, minocycline, oxyphenisatin
Antimicrosomal antibodies	Ticrynafen, halothane, dihydralazine
Hematologic (bone marrow injury, aplastic/hemolytic anemia, thrombocytopenia)	Phenylbutazone, phenytoin
Renal injury	Methoxyflurane, sulindac
Gastrointestinal (ulcer, pancreatitis)	Phenylbutazone, tetracycline

amoxicillin-clavulanic acid should be avoided in future therapy for K.V., and appropriate alternative drugs should be used instead.

If present, ascites, esophageal variceal bleeding, and other complications are treated accordingly. The use of large doses of glucocorticoids (e.g., 1,000 mg hydrocortisone a day) in acute hepatic failure is largely empirical and may have a role in hypersensitivity related cases but otherwise is not recommended.[6,17,18] There was no indication of these complications in K.V.

DRUGS REPORTED TO CAUSE CLINICALLY SIGNIFICANT HEPATIC DYSFUNCTION

There are many reports of drug-related hepatitis in the literature. Most of these are reports of single cases involving one drug and are difficult to evaluate (see Intrinsic and Idiopathic Reactions to Drugs as Causes of Hepatic Injury). Furthermore, hepatic drug effects that occurred early after exposure may differ in character from those that occurred later (e.g., chlorpromazine). In addition, certain drugs may cause various types of morphologic responses via different mechanisms (i.e., hepatotoxic versus idiosyncratic). In an attempt to summarize and facilitate discussion of the vast amount of information on this subject, only drugs that have been implicated in causing significant liver dysfunction are listed in Table 30-4. The hepatotoxicity of acetaminophen (see Chapter 5, Managing Acute Drug Toxicity), antituberculous agents (see Chapter 61, Tuberculosis) and certain antiretrovirals (see Chapter 69, Pharmacotherapy of Human Immunodeficiency Virus Infection) are included in other chapters. The types of morphologic findings and presumed mechanisms of hepatotoxicity for each drug are presented in Table 30-4. References are listed so that more detailed information may be obtained if desired. In the column labeled "Clinical Remarks," prominent clinical features such as clinical presentation, dose and duration of therapy associated with the adverse effect, pertinent laboratory data, and prognosis are summarized.

REFERENCES

1. Pratt DS et al. Evaluation of abnormal liver-enzyme results in symptomatic patients. N Engl J Med 2000;342:1266.
2. Lee WM. Drug-induced hepatotoxicity. N Engl J Med 2003;349:474.
3. Sameshine Y et al. Clinical statistics on drug-induced liver injuries: drug-induced liver injuries in Japan in the last 30 years. Jpn J Gastroenterol 1974;71:799.
4. Lazarou J et al. Incidence of adverse drug reactions in hospitalized patients. JAMA 1998;279:1200.
5. Friis H et al. Drug-induced hepatic injury: an analysis of 1100 cases reported to the Danish Committee on Adverse Drug Reactions between 1978 and 1987. J Intern Med 1992;232:133.
6. Zimmerman HJ. Hepatotoxicity: Adverse Effects of Drugs and Other Chemicals on the Liver. 2nd Ed. Philadelphia: Lippincott Williams & Wilkins, 1999.
7. Zimmerman HJ. Drug-induced liver disease. Clin Liver Dis 2000;473.
8. Kaplowitz N. Drug-induced liver disorders. Drug Safety 2001;24:483.
9. Clarkson A et al. Surveillance for fatal suspected adverse drug reactions in the UK. Arch Dis Child 2002;87:462.
10. Eastwood HOH. Causes of jaundice in the elderly: a survey of diagnosis and investigation. Gerontol Clin 1971;13:69.
11. Benhamou JP. Drug-Induced Hepatitis: Clinical Aspects. In: Fillastre JP, ed. Hepatotoxicity of Drugs. Rouen: University of Rouen, 1986:23.
12. Sgro C et al. Incidence of drug-induced hepatic injuries: a French population-based study. Hepatology 2002;36:451.
13. Graham GS. Chlorpromazine jaundice in a general hospital. Br Med J 1957;2:1080.
14. Durand F et al. Hepatotoxicity of antitubercular treatments. Drug Safety 1996;15:394.
15. Hoofnagle JH et al. Fulminant hepatic failure: summary of a workshop. Hepatology 1995;21:240.
16. Berstein D et al. Fulminant hepatic failure. Crit Care Clin 1998;14:181.
17. Lee WM. Acute liver failure. N Engl J Med 1993;329:1862.
18. Shakil AO et al. Fulminant hepatic failure. Surg Clin North Am 1999;79:77.
19. Ostapowicz G et al. Results of a prospective study of acute liver failure at 17 tertiary care centers in the United States. Ann Intern Med 2002;137:947.
20. Larrey D. Drug-induced liver disease. J Hepatology 2000;32 (suppl 1):77.

21. Manoukian AV et al. Nonsteroidal anti-inflammatory drug-induced hepatic disorders. Drug Safety 1996;15:64.
22. Garcia-Rodriguez LA et al. The risk of acute liver injury associated with cimetidine and other acid suppressing anti-ulcer drugs. Br J Pharmacol 1997;43:183.
23. Garcia-Rodriguez LA et al. A review of the epidemiologic research on drug-induced acute liver injury using the general practice research data base in the United Kingdom. Pharmacotherapy 1997;17:721.
24. Larey D et al. Hepatitis associated with amoxicillin-clavulanic acid combination: report of 15 cases. Gut 2002;33:368.
25. Nathani MG et al. An unusual case of amoxicillin/clavulanic acid-related hepatotoxicity. Am J Gastroenterol 1998;93:1363.
26. Tolman KG. The liver and lovastatin. Am J Cardiol 2002;89:1374.
27. Sulkowski MS. Hepatotoxicity associated with antiretriviral therapy containing HIV-1 protease inhibitors. Semin Liv Dis 2003;23:183.
28. Waller PC. Measuring the frequency of adverse drug reactions. Br J Clin Pharmacol 1992;33:249.
29. Edwards IR. International Drug Monitoring. In: Aronson JK, Van Boxtal, CJ, eds. Side Effects of Drugs. Amsterdam: Excerpta Medica, 1994:468.
30. Waller PC. Postmarketing surveillance: the viewpoint of a newcomer to pharmacoepidemiology. Drug Inform J 1991;25:181.
31. Hurwitz ES et al. Public health service study of Reye's syndrome and medications. JAMA 1987;257:1905.
32. Valla D et al. Drug-induced vascular and sinusoidal lesions of the liver. Baillere's Clin Gastroenterol 1998;2:481.
33. Black M et al. Isoniazid-associated hepatitis in 114 patients. Gastroenterology 1975;69:289.
34. Stock JGL et al. Unexplained hepatitis following halothane. Anesthesiology 1985;63:424.
35. Braun P. Hepatotoxicity of erythromycin. J Infect Dis 1973;119:300.
36. Fox JC et al. Progressive cholestatic liver disease associated with clarithromycin treatment. J Clin Pharmacol 2002;42:676.
37. Brown BA et al. Clarithromycin-induced hepatotoxicity. Clin Infect Dis 1995;20:1073.
38. Banks AT et al. Diclofenac-associated hepatotoxicity: analysis of 180 cases reported to the Food and Drug Administration as adverse reactions. Hepatology 1995;22:820.

39. Zimmerman HJ. Effects of aspirin and acetaminophen on the liver. Arch Intern Med 1981;141:333.
40. Dreifuss FE et al. Valproic acid hepatic fatalities: analysis of United States Cases. Neurology 1986;36(Suppl 1):133.
41. Stricker BC et al. Hepatic injury associated with the use of nitrofurans: a clinicopathological study of 52 reported cases. Hepatology 1988;8:599.
42. Sharp JR et al. Chronic active hepatitis and severe hepatic necrosis associated with nitrofurantoin. Ann Intern Med 1980;92:14.
43. Lindgren A et al. Liver reactions from trimethoprim. J Int Med 1994;236:281.
44. Hoft RH et al. Halothane hepatitis in three pairs of closely related women. N Engl J Med 1981;304:1023.
45. Gennis M et al. Familial occurrence of hypersensitivity to phenytoin. Am J Med 1991;91:631.
46. Lewis JH et al. Methotrexate-induced chronic liver injuries: guidelines for detection and prevention. The AGC committee on FDA-related matters. Am J Gastroenterol 1988;83:1337.
47. O'shea D et al. Effect of fasting and obesity in humans on the 6-hydroxylation of chlorzoxazone: a putative probe of CYP2E1 activity. Clin Pharmacol Ther 1994;56:35a.
48. Spracklin DK et al. Cytochrome P-4502E1 is the principal catalyst of human oxidative halothane metabolism in vitro. J Pharmacol Exp Ther 1997;281:400.
49. Benson GB. Hepatotoxicity following the therapeutic use of antipyretic analgesics. Am J Med 1983;75:85.
50. Frank AK et al. Isoniazid hepatitis among pregnant and postpartum Hispanic patients. Publ Health Rep 1989;104:151.
51. Smith AC et al. Characterization of hyperthyroidism enhancement of halothane-induced hepatotoxicity. Biochem Pharmacol 1983;32:3531.
52. McDonald GB et al. Veno-occlusive disease of the liver after bone marrow transplantation: diagnosis, incidence, and predisposing factors. Hepatology 1994;4:116.
53. Wisse E et al. The liver sieve: considerations concerning the structure and function of endothelial fenestra, the sinusoidal wall and the space of Disse. Hepatology 1985;5:683.
54. LeBlanc GA. Hepatic vectorial transport of xenobiotics. Chem Biol Interact 1994;90:101.
55. Losser MR et al. Mechanisms of liver damage. Semin Liver Dis 1996;16:357.

56. Mitchell JR et al. Acetaminophen-induced hepatic injury: protective effect of glutathione in man and rationale for therapy. Clin Pharmacol Ther 1974; 16:676.
57. Kaplowitz N et al. Drug-induced hepatotoxicity. Ann Intern Med 1986;104:826.
58. Luster MI et al. The role of tumor necrosis factor in chemical induced hepatotoxicity. Ann New York Acad Sci 2002;220.
59. Jaeschke H et al. Mechanisms of hepatotoxicity. Toxicol Sci2002;65:166.
60. Cardona X et al. Venlafaxine associated hepatitis. Ann Intern Med 2000;132:417.
61. Horsmans Y et al. Venlafaxine-associated hepatitis. Ann Intern Med 1999;130:994.
62. Spigset O et al. Hepatic injury and pancreatitis during treatment with serotonin reuptake inhibitors: data from the World Health Organization (WHO) databse of adverse drug reactions. Int Clin Psychopharmacol 2003;18:157.
63. Shear NH et al. Differences in metabolism of sulfonamides predisposing to idiosyncratic toxicity. Ann Intern Med 1986;105:179.
64. Sotolongo RP et al. Hypersensitivity reaction to sulfasalazine with severe hepatotoxicity. Gastroenterology 1978;75:95.
65. Abi-Mansur P et al. Trimethoprim-sulfamethoxazole induced cholestasis. Am J Gastroenterol 1981; 76:356.
66. Thies PW, Dull WL. Trimethoprim-sulfamethoxazole-induced cholestatic hepatitis. Inadvertent rechallenge. Arch Intern Med 1984;144:1691.
67. Tanner AR. Hepatic cholestasis induced by trimethoprim. Br Med J (Clin Res) 1986;293:1072.
68. Zitelli BN et al. Fatal hepatic necrosis due to pyrimethamine-sulfadoxine (Fansidar). Ann Intern Med 1987;106:393.
69. Mitchell JR et al. Metabolic activation. Biochemical basis for many drug-induced liver injuries. Prog Liver Dis 1976;5:259.
70. Dybing E. Activation of methyldopa, paracetamol and furosemide by human liver microsomes. Acta Pharmacol Toxicol (Copenh) 1977;41:89.
71. Eadie MJ et al. Valproate-associated hepatotoxicity and its biochemical mechanisms. Med Toxicol 1988;3:85.
72. Zimmerman HJ, Ishak KG. Valproate-induced hepatic injury. Analysis of 23 fatal cases. Hepatology 1982;2:591.
73. Donat JF et al. Valproic acid and fatal hepatitis. Neurology 1979;29:273.
74. Suchy FJ et al. Acute hepatic failure associated with the use of sodium valproate. N Engl J Med 1979; 300:962.
75. Gerber N et al. Reye-like syndrome associated with valproic therapy. J Pediatr 1979;95:142.
76. Young RSK et al. Reye-like syndrome associated with valproic acid. Ann Neurol 1980;7:389.
77. Levin TL et al. Valproic-acid-associated pancreatitis and hepatic toxicity in children with endstage renal disease. Pediatr Radiol 1997;27:192.
78. Konig SA et al. Fatal liver failure associated with valproate therapy in a patient with Freidreich's disease: review of valproate hepatotoxicity in adults. Epilepsia 1999;40:1036.
79. Zimmerman HJ. Drug-Induced Liver Disease. In: Schiff ER, Sorrell MF, Maddrey WC, eds. Schiff's Diseases of the Liver. New York: Lippincott-Raven, 1998:973.
80. Larrey D, Erlinger S. Drug-induced cholestasis. Clin Gastroenterol 1988;2:422.
81. Amacher DE. Serum transaminase elevations as indicators of hepatic injury following administration of drugs. Reg Toxicol Pharmacol 1998;27:119.
82. Nomura F et al. Effects of anticonvulsant agents on halothane induced liver injury in human subjects and experimental animals. Hepatology 1986;6:952.
83. Starko KM et al. Hepatic and cerebral findings in children with fatal salicylate intoxication: further evidence for a causal relationship between salicylate and Reye's syndrome. Lancet 1983;1:326.
84. Neuberger J. Drug-induced jaundice. Clin Gastroenterol 1989;3:447.
85. Desmet VJ. Vanishing bile duct syndrome in drug-induced liver disease. J Hepatol 1997;26(Suppl 1):31.
86. Forbes GM et al. Carbamazepine hepatotoxicity: another cause of the vanishing bile duct syndrome. Gastroenterology 1992;102:1385.
87. Ishak KG. Chronic hepatitis: morphology and nomenclature. Mod Pathol 1994;7:690.
88. Lewis JH et al. Drug-Induced Autoimmune Liver Disease. In: Krawitt EL, Weisner RH, Nishioka M, eds. Autoimmune Liver Disease. 2nd Ed. New York: Elsevier, 1998:629.
89. Lungren R et al. Pulmonary lesions and autoimmune reactions after long term nitrofurantoin treatment. Scand J Respir Dis 1975;56:208.
90. Homberg JC et al. Drug-induced hepatitis associated with anticytoplasmic organelle autoantibodies. Hepatology 1985;5:722.
91. Beaunc PH et al. Human endoplasmic reticulum autoantibodies appearing in a drug-induced hepatitis are directed against a human liver cytochrome P450 that hydroxylates the drug. Proc Natl Acad Sci USA 1987;84:551.
92. Bourdi M et al. Anti-liver endoplasmic reticulum autoantibodies are directed against human cytochrome P450 I A2. J Clin Invest 1990;85:1967.
93. Bonkonsky HL et al. Chronic hepatic inflammation and fibrosis due to low doses of paracetamol. Lancet 1978;1:1016.
94. Utili R et al. Dantrolene-associated hepatic injury. Gastroenterology 1977;72:610.
95. Seaman WE et al. Aspirin-induced hepatotoxicity in patients with systemic lupus erythematous. Ann Intern Med 1974;80:1.
96. Rodman JS et al. Methyldopa hepatitis. A report of six cases and review of the literature. Am J Med 1976;60:941.
97. Black N et al. Nitrofurantoin-induced chronic active hepatitis. Ann Intern Med 1980;92:62.
98. Schweitzer IL et al. Acute submassive hepatic necrosis due to methyldopa: a case demonstrating possible initiation of chronic liver disease. Gastroenterology 1974;66:1203.
99. Mihas AA et al. Fulminant hepatitis and lymphocyte sensitization due to propylthiouracil. Gastroenterology 1976;70:770.
100. Thaler H. Fatty change. Clin Gastroenterol 1988; 2:453.
101. Simon EB et al. Amiodarone hepatotoxicity simulating alcoholic liver disease. N Engl J Med 1984;311:167.
102. Harris L et al. Side effects of long-term amiodarone therapy. Circulation 1983;67:45.
103. Ludwig J et al. Floxuridine-induced sclerosing cholangitis: an ischemic cholangiopathy? Hepatology 1989;9:215.
104. Belghiti J et al. Caustic sclerosing cholangitis: a complication of the surgical treatment of hydatid disease of the liver. Arch Surg 1986;121:1162.
105. Valla D et al. Risk of hepatic vein thrombosis in relationship to recent use of oral contraceptives: a case control study. Gastroenterology 1986;90: 807.
106. Maddrey WC et al. Hepatic vein thrombosis (Budd-Chiari syndrome): possible association with the use of oral contraceptives. Semin Liver Dis 1987;7:32.
107. McDonald GB et al. Veno-occlusive disease following bone marrow transplantation: a cohort of 355 patients. Ann Intern Med 1993;118:255.
108. Stedman C. Herbal toxicity. Semin Liver Dis 2003;22:195.
109. Cassi E et al. Splenic peliosis after danazol therapy for idiopathic thrombocytopenia purpura [Letter]. Hematologica 1985;70:549.
110. Bagheri SA et al. Peliosis hepatis associated with androgenic-anabolic steroid therapy: a severe form of injury. Ann Intern Med 1974;81:610.
111. Shepard P et al. Idiopathic portal hypertension associated with cytotoxic drugs. J Clin Oncol 1990; 43:206.
112. Villeneuve JP et al. Idiopathic portal hypertension. Am J Med 1976;61:459.
113. Ishak KG, Zimmerman HJ. Drug-induced and toxic granulomatous hepatitis. Clin Gastroenterol 1988;2:463.
114. Lisker-Melman M et al. Conditions associated with hepatocellular carcinoma. Med Clin North Am 1989;73:999.
115. Edmondson HA et al. Liver-cell adenomas associated with the use of oral contraceptives. N Engl J Med 1976;294:470.
116. Mays ET et al. Hepatic tumors induced by sex steroids. Semin Liv Dis 1994;4:147.
117. Westaby D et al. Androgen-related primary hepatic tumors in non-Fanconi patients. Cancer 1983;51:1947.
118. Neuberger J et al. Oral contraceptive and hepatocellular carcinoma. Br Med J 1987;292:1355.
119. Kerlin P et al. Hepatic adenoma and focal nodular hyperplasia: clinical, pathologic and radiologic features. Gastroenterology 1983;84:994.
120. Falk H et al. Review of four cases of childhood angiosarcoma: elevated environmental arsenic exposure in one case. Cancer 1981;47:382.
121. Zafrani ES et al. Drug-induced vascular lesions of the liver. Arch Intern Med 1983;143:495.
122. Harrison R et al. Case studies in environmental medicine: vinyl chloride toxicity. Clin Toxicol 1990;28:267.
123. Simanto L et al. A collaborative study of cancer incidence and mortality among vinyl chloride workers. Scand J Work Environ Health 1991; 17:159.
124. Kane JA et al. Hepatitis caused by traditional Chinese herbs: possible toxic components. Gut 1995;36:146.
125. Delbanco TL. Bitter herbs: mainstream magic and menace. Ann Intern Med 1994;121:803.
126. Seef LB et al. Complementary and alternative medicine in chronic liver disease. Hepatology 2001;34:595.
127. Berk BS et al. Comparison of herbal therapy for liver disease:1996 versus 1999. Hepatology 1999; 30:478A.
128. Katz M et al. Herbal hepatitis: subacute hepatic necrosis secondary to chaparral leaf. J Clin Gastroenterol 1990;12:203.
129. Ridker PM et al. Hepatic veno-occlusive disease associated with the consumption of pyrrolizidine-containing dietary supplements. Gastroenterology 1985;88;1050.
130. Larrey D et al. Hepatitis after germander (Teucrium chamaedrys) administration: another instance of herbal medication hepatotoxicity. Ann Intern Med 1992;117:129.
131. Sullivan JB et al. Pennyroyal oil poisoning and hepatotoxicity. JAMA 1979;242:2873.
132. Beuers U et al. Hepatitis after chronic abuse of senna [Letter]. Lancet 1991;1:372.
133. Woolf GM et al. Acute hepatitis associated with the Chinese herbal product Jin Bu Huan. Ann Intern Med 1994;121:729.
134. Zimran A et al. Reversible cholestatic jaundice and hyperamylasemia associated with captopril treatment. Br Med J (Clin Res) 1983;287:1676.
135. Rahmat J et al. Captopril-associated cholestatic jaundice. Ann Intern Med 1985;102:56.
136. Hagley MT et al. Hepatotoxicity associated with angiotensin-converting enzyme inhibitors. Ann Pharmacother 1993;27:228.
137. Larrey D et al. Fulminant hepatitis after lisinopril administration. Gastroenterology 1990;99: 1832.
138. Hilburn RB et al. Angiotensin-converting enzyme inhibitor hepatotoxicity: further insights [Letter]. Ann Pharmacother 1993;27:1142.
139. Murphy EJ et al. Troglitazone-induced fulminant hepatic failure. Acute liver failure study group. Dig Dis Sci 2000;45:549.
140. Kohlroser J et al. Hepatotoxicity due to troglitazone: report of two cases and review of the literature. Am J Gastroenterol 2000;95:272.
141. Gitlin N et al. Two cases of severe clinical and histologic hepatotoxicity associated with troglitazone. Ann Intern Med 1998;129:36.

142. Forman LM et al. Hepatic failure in a patient taking rosiglitazone. Ann Intern Med 2000;132:118.
143. Al-Salman J et al. Hepatocellular injury in a patient receiving rosiglitazone. Ann Intern Med 2000;132:121.
144. Isley WL et al. Hepatotoxicity of the thiazolidinediones. Diabetes, Obesity, Metab 2001;3:389.
145. Gale EA. Lessons from the glitazones: a story of drug development. Lancet 2001;357:1870.
146. May LD et al. Mixed hepatocellular-cholestatic liver injury after pioglitazone therapy. Ann Intern Med 2002;136:449.
147. Limauro DL et al. Amoxicillin/clavulanate-associated hepatic failure with progression to Stevens-Johnson syndrome. Ann Pharmacother 1999;3:560.
148. Silvain C et al. Granulomatous hepatitis due to combination of amoxicillin and clavulanic acid. Dig Dis Sci 1992;37:150.
149. Hebbard GS et al. Augmentin-induced jaundice with a fatal outcome. Med J Aust 1992;156:285.
150. Butler RC et al. Acute massive hepatic necrosis in a patient receiving allopurinol. JAMA 1977;237:437.
151. Favre M et al. Allopurinol-induced fulminant hepatitis. Semin Hosp 1990;66:2095.
152. Simon JB et al. Amiodarone hepatotoxicity simulating alcoholic liver disease. N Engl J Med 1984;311:167.
153. Kalantzis N et al. Acute amiodarone-induced hepatitis. Hepatogastroenterology 1991;38:71.
154. Harrison RF et al. Amiodarone-associated cirrhosis with hepatic and lymph node granulomas. Histopathology 1993;22:80.
155. Snir Y et al. Fatal hepatic failure due to prolonged amiodarone treatment. J Clin Gastroenterology 1995;20:265.
156. Nadell J et al. Peliosis hepatis. Twelve cases associated with oral androgen therapy. Arch Pathol Lab Med 1977;101:405.
157. Johnson LF et al. Association of androgenic-anabolic steroid therapy with development of hepatocellular carcinoma. Lancet 1972;2:1273.
158. Bagheri SA et al. Peliosis hepatis associated with androgenic-anabolic steroid therapy. A severe form of hepatic injury. Ann Intern Med 1974;81:610.
159. Karasawa T et al. Peliosis hepatis. Report of nine cases. Acta Pathol Jpn 1979;29:457.
160. Athreya BH et al. Aspirin-induced abnormalities of liver function. Am J Dis Child 1973;126:638.
161. Rich RR et al. Salicylate hepatotoxicity in patients with juvenile rheumatoid arthritis. Arthritis Rheum 1973;16:1.
162. Seaman WE et al. Aspirin-induced hepatotoxicity in patients with systemic lupus erythematosus. Ann Intern Med 1974;80:1.
163. Wolfe JD et al. Aspirin hepatitis. Ann Intern Med 1974;80:74.
164. Miller JJ et al. Correlations between transaminase concentrations and serum salicylate concentrations in patients with juvenile rheumatoid arthritis. Arthritis Rheum 1976;19:115.
165. Seaman WE et al. The effect of aspirin on liver tests in patients with rheumatoid arthritis or systemic lupus erythematosus and in normal volunteers. Arthritis Rheum 1976;19:155.
166. O'Gorman T et al. Salicylate hepatitis. Gastroenterology 1977;72:726.
167. Lopez-Morante AJ et al. Aspirin-induced cholestatic hepatitis. J Clin Gastroenterol 1993;16:270.
168. Aguilar HI et al. Azathioprine-induced lymphoma manifesting as fulminant hepatic failure. Mayo Clin Proc 1997;72:643.
169. Lemley DE et al. Azathioprine-induced hepatic veno-occlusive disease in rheumatoid arthritis. Ann Rheum Dis 1989;48:342.
170. DePinho RA et al. Azathioprine and the liver. Evidence favoring idiosyncratic, mixed cholestatic-hepato-cellular injury in humans. Gastroenterology 1984;86:162.
171. Ware AJ et al. Spectrum of liver disease in renal transplant recipients. Gastroenterology 1975;68:755.

172. McDonald GB et al. Veno-occlusive disease of the liver after bone marrow transplantation: diagnosis, incidence, and predisposing factors. Hepatology 1984;4:116.
173. Read AE et al. Hepatic veno-occlusive disease associated with renal transplantation and azathioprine therapy. Ann Intern Med 1986;104:651.
174. Perini GP et al. Azathioprine-related cholestatic jaundice in heart transplant patients. J Heart Transplant 1990;9:577.
175. Meys E et al. Fever, hepatitis and acute interstitial nephritis in a patient with rheumatoid arthritis. Concurrent manifestations of azathioprine hypersensitivity. J Rheumatol 1992;19:807.
176. Hazdie N et al. Acute liver failure induced by carbamazepine. Arch Dis Child Mar 1990;65:315.
177. Williams SJ et al. Carbamazepine hepatitis: the clinicopathological spectrum. J Gastroenterol Hepatol 1986;1:159.
178. Luke DR et al. Acute hepatotoxicity after excessively high doses of carbamazepine on two occasions. Pharmacother 1986;6:108.
179. Zucker P et al. Fatal carbamazepine hepatitis. J Pediatr 1977;91:667.
180. Hopen G et al. Fatal carbamazepine-associated hepatitis: report of two cases. Acta Med Scand 1981;210:333.
181. Pellock JM. Felbamate: 1997 update. Epilepsia 1997;38:1261.
182. Oversteet K et al. Fatal progressive hepatic necrosis associated with lamotrigine treatment. Dig Dis Sci 2002;47:1921.
183. Lessner HE et al. Toxicity study of BCNU (NSC-409962) given orally. Cancer Chemother Rep 1974;58:407.
184. Watson RPG et al. A proposed mechanism for chlorpromazine jaundice. J Hepatol 1988;7:72.
185. Ishak KG et al. Hepatic injury associated with the phenothiazines. Clinicopathologic and follow-up study of 36 patients. Arch Pathol Lab Med 1972;93:283.
186. Derby LE et al. Liver disorders in patients receiving chlorpromazine or isoniazid. Pharmacotherapy 1993;13.353.
187. Haunz EA et al. Liver function in chlorpropamide therapy. Five-year clinical study of 181 patients. JAMA 1964;188.237.
188. Goldstein MJ et al. Jaundice in a patient receiving acetohexamide. N Engl J Med 1966;275:97.
189. Baird RW et al. Cholestatic jaundice from tolbutamide. Ann Intern Med 1960;53:194.
190. Van Thiel DH et al. Tolazamide hepatotoxicity. Gastroenterology 1974;67:506.
191. Rigberg LA et al. Chlorpropamide-induced granulomas. JAMA 1976;235:409.
192. Van Basten JP et al. Glyburide-induced cholestatic hepatitis and liver failure. Case-report and review of the literature. Neth J Med 1992;40:305.
193. Reyes H. The enigma of intrahepatic cholestasis of pregnancy. Hepatology 1982;2:87.
194. Kreek MJ. Female sex steroids and cholestasis. Semin Liver Dis 1987;7:8.
195. Kern F et al. Effect of estrogens on the liver. Gastroenterology 1978;75:512.
196. Lindberg MC. Hepatobiliary complications of oral contraceptives. J Gen Intern Med 1992;7:199.
197. Baker AL et al. Liver adenoma associated with oral contraceptive pill administration. Dig Dis Sci 1978;23:53S.
198. Berg JW et al. Hepatomas and oral contraceptives. Lancet 1974;2:349.
199. Edmondson HA et al. Liver cell adenomas associated with the use of oral contraceptives. N Engl J Med 1976;294:470.
200. Klatskin G. Hepatic tumors. Possible relationship to use of oral contraceptives. Gastroenterology 1977;73:386.
201. Kerlin P et al. Hepatic adenoma and focal nodular hyperplasia: clinical, pathologic and radiologic features. Gastroenterology 1983;84:994.
202. Marks WH et al. Failure of hepatic adenomas (HCA) to regress after discontinuance of oral contraceptives. Ann Surg 1988;208:190.

203. Van Erpecum KJ et al. Pelio hepatis and cirrhosis after long term use of oral contraceptives: case report. Am J Gastroenterol 1988;83:572.
204. Hoyumpa AM Jr et al. Budd-Chiari syndrome in women taking oral contraceptives. Am J Med 1971;50:137.
205. Capron JP et al. Portal vein thrombosis and fatal pulmonary thromboembolism associated with oral contraceptive treatment. J Clin Gastroenterol 1981;3:295.
206. Ham JM et al. Hepatocellular carcinoma possibly induced by oral contraceptives. Dig Dis Sci 1978;23:38S.
207. Henderson BE et al. Hepatocellular carcinoma and oral contraceptives. Br J Cancer 1983;48:437.
208. Goodman ZD, Ishak KG. Hepatocellular carcinoma in women: probable lack of etiologic association with oral contraceptive steroids. Hepatology 1982;2:440.
209. Forman D et al. Cancer of the liver and the use of oral contraceptives. Br Med J 1986;292:1357.
210. Klintmalm GBG et al. Cyclosporin A hepatotoxicity in 66 renal allograft recipients. Transplantation 1981;32:488.
211. Essell JH et al. Marked increase in veno-occlusive disease of the liver associated with methotrexate use for graft-versus-host disease prophylaxis in patients receiving busulfan/cyclophosphamide. Blood 1992;79:2784.
212. Kassianides C et al. Liver injury from cyclosporine A. Dig Dis Sci 1990;35:693.
213. Ogburn RM et al. Hepatitis associated with dantrolene sodium. Ann Intern Med 1976;84:53.
214. Tartalione TA et al. Diltiazem: a review of its clinical efficacy and use. Drug Intell Clin Pharm 1982;16:371.
215. Pool PE et al. Diltiazem as monotherapy for systemic hypertension: a multicenter, randomized, placebo-controlled trial. Am J Cardiol 1986;57:212.
216. Sarachek NS et al. Diltiazem and granulomatous hepatitis. Gastroenterology 1985;88:1260.
217. Shallcross H et al. Fatal renal and hepatic toxicity after treatment with diltiazem. Br Med J 1987;295:1236.
218. Richter WO et al. Serious side effect of nifedipine. Arch Int Med 1987;147:1850.
219. Babany G et al. Alcohol-like liver lesions induced by nifedipine. J Hepatol 1989;9:252.
220. Isoard B et al. Pseudoalcoholic hepatitis during treatment with nicardipine. Presse Med 1988;17:647.
221. Stern EH et al. Possible hepatitis from verapamil. N Engl J Med 1982;306:612.
222. Brodsky SJ et al. Hepatotoxicity due to treatment with verapamil. Ann Intern Med 1981;94:490.
223. Halkin H. Adverse effects of the fluoroquinolones. Rev Infect Dis 1988;10(Suppl):S258.
224. Blum A. Ofloxacin-induced acute severe hepatitis. South Med J 1991;84:1158.
225. Grassmick BK et al. Fulminant hepatic failure possibly related to ciprofloxacin. Ann Pharmacother 1992;26:636.
226. Lopez-Navidad A et al. Norfloxacin-induced hepatotoxicity. J Hepatol 1990;11:277.
227. Villeneuve JP et al. Suspected ciprofloxacin-induced hepatotoxicity. Ann Pharmacother 1995;29:257.
228. Chen JL et al. Acute eosinophilic hepatitis from trovafloxacin. N Engl J Med 2000;342:359.
229. Spahr L et al. A fatal hepatitis related to levofloxacin. J Hepatol 2001;35:308
230. Qiang C et al. Acute hepatitis due to fluoxetine therapy. Mayo Clin Proc 1999;74:692.
231. Hill RB Jr. Fatal fat embolism from steroid-induced fatty liver. N Engl J Med 1961;165:318.
232. Wald JA et al. Abnormal liver-function tests associated with long-term systemic corticosteroid use in subjects with asthma. J Allergy Clin Immunol 1991;88:277.
233. Crane GE et al. A review of clinical literature on haloperidol. Int J Neuropsychiatry 1967;3(Suppl):5111.

234. Neuberger JM. Halothane and hepatitis. Incidence, predisposing factors and exposure guidelines. Drug Saf 1990;5:28.
235. Neuber J, Williams R. Halothane anesthesia and liver damage. Br Med J 1984;289:1135.
236. Nomura F et al. Effects of anticonvulsant agents on halothane-induced liver injury in human subjects and experimental animals. Hepatology 1986;6:952.
237. Klion FM et al. Hepatitis after exposure to halothane. Ann Intern Med 1969;71:467.
238. Hughes M et al. Recurrent hepatitis in patients receiving multiple halothane anesthetics for radium treatment of carcinoma of the cervix uteri. Gastroenterology 1970;58:790.
239. Carney FMT et al. Halothane hepatitis. A critical review. Anesth Analg 1972;51:135.
240. Trowell J et al. Controlled trial of repeated halothane anesthetics in patients with carcinoma of the uterine cervix treated with radium. Lancet 1975;1:821.
241. Schlipper W et al. Recurrent hepatitis following halothane exposure. Am J Med 1978;65:25.
242. Shipton EA. Halothane hepatitis revisited. S Afr Med J 1991;80:261.
243. Hubbard AK et al. Immunological basis of anesthetic-induced hepatotoxicity. Anesthesiology 1988;69:814.
244. Gunza JT et al. Postoperative elevation of serum transaminases following isoflurane anesthesia. J Clin Anesth 1992;4:336.
245. Slayter KL et al. Halothane hepatitis in a renal transplant patient previously exposed to isoflurane. Ann Pharmacother 1993;27:101.
246. Lewis JH et al. Hepatic injury associated with ketoconazole therapy. Analysis of 33 cases. Gastroenterology 1984;86:503.
247. Stricker BH et al. Ketoconazole-associated hepatic injury. A clinicopathological study of 55 cases. J Hepatol 1986;3:399.
248. Chien RN et al. Hepatic injury during ketoconazole therapy in patients with onychomycosis: a controlled cohort study. Hepatology 1997;25:103.
249. Findor JA et al. Ketoconazole-induced liver damage. Medicine 1998;58:277.
250. Samonis G et al. Prophylaxis of oropharyngeal candidiasis with fluconazole. Rev Infect Dis 1990;12(Suppl 3):S364.
251. Mann SK et al. Itraconazole-induced acute hepatitis [Letter]. Br J Dermatol 1993;129:500.
252. Tobert JA. New developments in lipid-lowering therapy: the role of inhibitors of hydroxymethylglutaryl coenzyme A reductase. Circulation 1987;76:534.
253. Grimbert S et al. Acute hepatitis induced by HMG-CoA reductase inhibitors. Dig Dis Sci 1994;39:2032.
254. Haria M et al. Pravastatin: a reappraisal of its pharmacological properties and clinical effectiveness in the management of coronary heart disease. Drugs 1997;53:299.
255. Walker JF. HMG CoA reductase inhibitors: current clinical experience. Drugs 1988;3:83.
256. Roblin X et al. Simvastatin-induced hepatitis. Gastroenterol Clin Biol 1992;16:101.
257. Boccuzzi SJ et al. Long-term experience with simvastatin. Drug Invest 1993;5:135.
258. Shorey J et al. Hepatotoxicity of mercaptopurine. Arch Intern Med 1968;122:54.
259. Schmidt G et al. Methimazole-associated cholestatic liver injury: case report and brief literature review. Hepatogastroenterology 1986;33:244.
260. Joshi PH, Conn HO. The syndrome of methoxyflurane-associated hepatitis. Ann Intern Med 1974;80:395.
261. Judson JA et al. Possible cross-sensitivity between halothane and methoxyflurane. Anesthesiology 1971;35:527.
262. Lewis JH et al. Enflurane hepatotoxicity. A clinicopathologic study of 24 cases. Ann Intern Med 1983;98:984.
263. Shergy WJ et al. Methotrexate-associated hepatotoxicity: retrospective analysis of 210 patients with rheumatoid arthritis. Am J Med 1988;85:771.
264. Zachariae H et al. Methotrexate-induced liver cirrhosis. Dermatology 1996;192:343.
265. Dahl MGC et al. Methotrexate hepatotoxicity in psoriasis—comparison of different dose regimens. Br Med J (Clin Res) 1972;1:654.
266. Lewis JH, Schiff ER. Methotrexate-induced chronic liver injury: guidelines for detection and prevention. Am J Gastroenterol 1988;83:1337.
267. Bridges SL Jr et al. Methotrexate-induced liver abnormalities in rheumatoid arthritis. J Rheumatol 1989;16:1180.
268. Maddrey WC et al. Severe hepatitis from methyldopa. Gastroenterology 1975;68:351.
269. Rehman OU et al. Methyldopa-induced submassive hepatic necrosis. JAMA 1973;224:1390.
270. Neuberger J et al. Antibody-mediated hepatocyte injury in methyldopa-induced hepatotoxicity. Gut 1985;26:1233.
271. Kennedy BJ. Mithramycin therapy in advanced testicular neoplasms. Cancer 1970;26:755.
272. Ryan WG. Mithramycin in Paget's disease of bone. Lancet 1973;1:1319.
273. Benack RT et al. Jaundice associated with isocarboxazid therapy. N Engl J Med 1961;264:294.
274. Griffith GC et al. Jaundice and hepatitis in patients who have received hydrazine-base monamine oxidase inhibitors. Am J Med Sci 1962;244:592.
275. Bandt C et al. Liver injury associated with tranylcypromine therapy. JAMA 1964;188:752.
276. Henkin Y et al. Rechallenge with crystalline niacin after drug-induced hepatitis from sustained-release niacin. JAMA 1990;264:241.
277. Etchason JA et al. Niacin-induced hepatitis: a potential side effect with low-dose time-release niacin. Mayo Clin Proc 1991;66:23.
278. Dalton TA et al. Hepatotoxicity associated with sustained-release niacin. Am J Med 1992;93:102.
279. Daniele B et al. Sulindac-induced severe hepatitis. Am J Gastroenterol 1988;83:1429.
280. Mitchell MR, Lietman PS. Evidence for the role of reactive metabolites in hepatotoxicity of benoxaprofen and other non-steroidal anti-inflammatory drugs (NSAIDs). Hepatology. 1983;3:808.
281. Wood LJ et al. Sulindac hepatotoxicity: effects of acute and chronic exposure. Aust NZ J Med 1985;15:397.
282. Victorino RMM et al. Jaundice associated with naproxen. Postgrad Med J 1980;56:368.
283. Jick H et al. Liver disease associated with diclofenac, naproxen, and piroxicam. Pharmacotherapy 1992;12:207.
284. Hepps KS et al. Severe cholestatic jaundice associated with piroxicam. Gastroenterology 1991;101:1737.
285. Sherman KE et al. Hepatotoxicity associated with piroxicam use. Gastroenterology 1992;103:354.
286. Ouellette GS et al. Reversible hepatitis associated with diclofenac. J Clin Gastroenterol 1991;13:205.
287. Scully LJ et al. Diclofenac induced hepatitis. Dig Dis Sci 1993;38:744.
288. Nores JM et al. Acute hepatitis due to ketoprofen. Clin Rheumatol 1991;10:215.
289. Tarazi EM et al. Sulindac-associated hepatic injury: analysis of 91 cases reported to the Food and Drug Administration. Gastroenterology 1993;104:569.
290. Rabkin JM et al. Fatal fulminant hepatitis associated with bromfenac use. Ann Pharmacother 1999;33:945.
291. Fontana RJ et al. Acute liver failure associated with prolonged use of bromfenac leading to liver transplantation. Liver Transplant Surg 1999;5:480.
292. Paiva LA et al. Long-term hepatic memory for hypersensitivity to nitrofurantoin. Am J Gastroenterol 1992;87:891.
293. Schattner A et al. Nitrofurantoin-induced immune-mediated lung and liver disease. Am J Med Sci 1999;317:336.
294. Pollock AA et al. Hepatitis associated with high dose oxacillin therapy. Arch Intern Med 1978;138:915.
295. Onorato IM et al. Hepatitis from intravenous high dose oxacillin therapy. Ann Intern Med 1978;89:497.
296. Taylor C et al. Oxacillin and hepatitis. Ann Intern Med 1979;90:857.
297. Turner IB et al. Prolonged hepatic cholestasis after flucloxacillin therapy. Med J Aust 1989;151:701.
298. Olsson R et al. Liver damage from flucloxacillin, cloxacillin and dicloxacillin. J Hepatol 1992;15:154.
299. Fairley CK et al. Risk factors for development of flucloxacillin-associated jaundice. Br Med J 1993;306:233.
300. Maraqa NF et al. Higher occurrence of hepatotoxicity and rash in patients treated with oxacillin compared with those treated with nafcillin and other commonly used antimicrobials. Clin Infect Dis 2002;34:50.
301. George DK et al. Antibacterial induced hepatotoxicity. Drug Safety 1996;15:79.
302. Goldstein LI et al. Hepatic injury associated with penicillin therapy. Arch Pathol Lab Med 1974;98:114.
303. McArthur JE et al. Stevens-Johnson syndrome with hepatitis following therapy with ampicillin and cephalexin. NZ Med J 1975;81:390.
304. Hargreaves JE et al. Severe cholestatic jaundice caused by mezlocillin. Clin Infect Dis 1992;15:179.
305. Perkins J. Phenindione sensitivity. Lancet 1962;1:127.
306. Perkins J. Phenindione jaundice. Lancet 1962;1:125.
307. Benjamin SB et al. Phenylbutazone liver injury: a clinical-pathologic survey of 23 cases and review of the literature. Hepatology 1981;1:255.
308. Spielberg SP et al. Predisposition to phenytoin hepatotoxicity assessed in vitro. N Engl J Med 1981;305:722.
309. Lee TH et al. Diphenylhydantoin-induced hepatic necrosis. Gastroenterology 1976;70:422.
310. Campbell CB et al. Cholestatic liver disease associated with diphenylhydantoin therapy. Am J Dig Dis 1977;22:255.
311. Parker WA et al. Phenytoin hepatotoxicity. A case report and review. Neurology 1979;29:175.
312. Roy AK et al. Phenytoin-induced chronic hepatitis. Dig Dis Sci 1993;38:740.
313. Mechanic RC et al. Chlorpromazine-type cholangitis. Report of a case occurring after the administration of prochlorperazine. N Engl J Med 1958;259:778.
314. Ichiki Y et al. Propylthiouracil-induced severe hepatitis: a case report and review of the literature. J Gastroenterol 1998;33:747.
315. Ozenirler S et al. Propylthiouracil-induced hepatic damage. Ann Pharmacother 1996;30:960.
316. Amerbein JA et al. Granulocytopenia, lupus-like syndrome, and other complications of propylthiouracil therapy. J Pediatr 1970;74:54.
317. Eisen MJ. Fulminant hepatitis during treatment with propylthiouracil. N Engl J Med 1963;249:814.
318. Seidman D et al. Propylthiouracil-induced cholestatic jaundice. J Toxicol Clin Toxicol 1986;24:353.
319. Liaw YF et al. Hepatic injury during propylthiouracil therapy in patients with hyperthyroidism. A cohort study. Ann Intern Med 1993;118:424.
320. Chajek T et al. Quinidine-induced granulomatous hepatitis. Ann Intern Med 1974;81:774.
321. Koch MJ et al. Quinidine toxicity. A report of a case and a review of the literature. Gastroenterology 1976;70:1136.
322. Geltner D et al. Quinidine hypersensitivity and liver involvement. A survey of 32 patients. Gastroenterology 1976;70:650.
323. Burkhard S et al. Fulminant hepatic failure in a child as a potential adverse effect of trimethoprim-sulfamethoxazole. Eur J Pediatr 1995;154:530.
324. Munoz SJ et al. Intrahepatic cholestasis and phospholipidosis associated with the use of trimethoprim-sulfamethoxazole. Hepatology 1990;12:342.
325. Oliver RM et al. Intrahepatic cholestasis associated with co-trimoxazole. Br J Clin Pract 1987;41:975.

326. Alberti-Flor JJ et al. Fulminant liver failure and pancreatitis associated with the use of sulfamethoxazole-trimethoprim. Gastroenterology 1989;84:1577.

327. Kowdley KV et al. Prolonged cholestasis due to trimethoprim-sulfamethoxazole. Gastroenterology 1992;102:2148.

328. Schultz JC et al. Fatal liver disease after intravenous administration of tetracycline in high dosage. N Engl J Med 1963;269:999.

329. Whalley PJ et al. Tetracycline toxicity in pregnancy. JAMA 1964;189:357.

330. Kunelis CT et al. Fatty liver of pregnancy and its relationship to tetracycline therapy. Am J Med 1965;38:359.

331. Ilan Y et al. Hepatic failure associated with imipramine therapy. Pharmacopsychiatry 1996;29:79.

332. Horst DA et al. Prolonged cholestasis and progressive hepatic fibrosis following imipramine therapy. Gastroenterology 1980;79:550.

333. Powell WJ et al. Lethal hepatic necrosis after therapy with imipramine and desipramine. JAMA 1968;206:642.

334. Short MH et al. Cholestatic jaundice during imipramine therapy. JAMA 1968;206:1791.

335. Yon J et al. Hepatitis caused by amitriptyline therapy. JAMA 1975;232:833.

336. Warning on Serzone. JAMA 2002;287:1102.

337. Margulies AI et al. Jaundice associated with the administration of trifluoperazine. Can Med Assoc J 1968;98:1063.

338. Muenter MD et al. Chronic vitamin A intoxication in adults. Am J Med 1971;50:129.

339. Muenter MD. Hypervitaminosis A. Ann Intern Med 1974;80:105.

340. Russell RM et al. Hepatic injury from chronic hypervitaminosis A resulting in portal-hypertension and ascites. N Engl J Med 1974;291:435.

341. Geubel AP et al. Liver damage caused by therapeutic vitamin A administration: estimate of dose-related toxicity in 41 cases. Gastroenterology 1991;100:1701.

342. Acosta BS et al. Zidovudine-associated type B lactic acidosis and hepatic steatosis in an HIV-infected patient. South Med J 1999;92:421.

343. Olano JP et al. Massive hepatic steatosis and lactic acidosis in a patient with AIDS who was receiving zidovudine. Clin Infect Dis 1995;21:973.

344. Sundar K et al. Zidovudine-induced fatal lactic acidosis and hepatic failure in patients with acquired immunodeficiency syndrome: report of two patients and review of the literature. Crit Care Med 1997;25:1425.

345. Cattelan AM et al. Severe hepatic failure related to nevirapine treatment. Clin Infect Dis 1999;29:455.

346. Brau N et al. Severe hepatitis in three AIDS patients treated with indinavir. Lancet 1997;349:924.

347. Wenzel SE et al. Zileuton: the first 5-lipoxygenase inhibitor for the treatment of asthma. Ann Pharmacother 1996;30:858.

348. Lazarus SC et al. Safety and efficacy of zileuton in patients with chronic asthma. Am J Manag Care 1998;4:841.

RENAL DISORDERS

Thomas J. Comstock
SECTION EDITOR

CHAPTER **31**

Acute Renal Failure

Donald F. Brophy

DEFINITION

Acute renal failure (ARF) is characterized clinically by an abrupt decrease in renal function over a period of hours to days, resulting in the accumulation of nitrogenous waste products *(azotemia)* and the inability to maintain and regulate fluid, electrolyte, and acid–base balance.[1] Many attempts have been made to objectively quantify ARF based on laboratory data, daily urine output, or the need for renal replacement therapy (RRT), but a consensus using these parameters has not been attained. Traditionally, ARF has been defined as an increase in serum creatinine (SrCr) of >0.5 mg/dL when the baseline SrCr is <2.5 mg/dL, and an increase in SrCr of >1.0 mg/dL when the baseline SrCr is >2.5 mg/dL.[1] These criteria are often inaccurate, though, because SrCr and glomerular filtration rate (GFR) do not follow a linear relationship. Diagnosing ARF solely on creatinine concentration is problematic because many patients are in high catabolic states as a result

of their critical illness. Catabolism leads to the accumulation not only of creatinine but also of noncreatinine waste products (urea nitrogen), organic acids, water, and electrolytes. Thus, ARF should be suspected when the kidney is unable to regulate fluid, electrolyte, acid–base, or nitrogen balance, even in the presence of a normal SrCr concentration.

EPIDEMIOLOGY

ARF commonly occurs in hospitalized patients and has been reported to account for nearly two-thirds of all nephrology consultations in a major referral hospital.[2] The incidence of *community-acquired ARF* (development of ARF before hospitalization) is 1%; approximately 75% of these admissions result from decreased kidney blood flow, termed *prerenal azotemia.* Other less common causes include obstructive uropathy (17%) and intrinsic renal disease (11%).[3] Community-acquired ARF can usually be reversed by correcting the underlying problems of volume status or obstruction. Hospital-acquired ARF is much more common, and the incidence and severity vary based on intensive care unit (ICU) or non-ICU setting.[4,5] The incidence of ARF in general medicine patients is approximately 2% to 5%, with the most common causes being prerenal azotemia, postoperative complications, or nephrotoxin exposure. These patients can experience one or more of these renal insults throughout their hospitalization. Conversely, ICU-acquired ARF is more prevalent and severe. A recent prospective study in ICU patients documented an ARF incidence of approximately 25%, stemming from multiple risk factors, including older age, infection, male gender, multiorgan dysfunction, and the need for mechanical ventilation.[6] Of all ARF patients, 20% to 60% require initial dialysis therapy,[7,8] and 25% of these patients progress to end-stage renal disease requiring long-term dialysis.[9]

PROGNOSIS

Despite recent advances in dialysis delivery and the development of sophisticated continuous RRTs, ARF continues to have a grim prognosis. Indeed, several recent studies have demonstrated that ARF and its complications are independently associated with increased mortality.[5,10–12] The mortality rate of ARF has declined minimally during the last 50 years. This slow decline may be explained in part by three important factors. First, patients are older when they develop ARF. Second, patients are often afflicted with serious underlying medical illnesses beyond ARF.[1] Third, the clinical severity status of the patient is much higher now than ever before.[4] Before the widespread availability of RRTs, the most common causes of death in patients with ARF were fluid and electrolyte disorders and advanced uremia. Today, the most common causes of death are infection, bleeding, cardiopulmonary failure, and withdrawal of life support.[4,13] Established ARF without other organ dysfunction bears a 40% to 60% mortality rate. However, the mortality rate increases with the number of failed organ systems.[5] When ARF is accompanied by more than three failed organ systems, the mortality rate exceeds 80%.[4,5,9]

CLINICAL COURSE

Three distinct phases of ARF exist. The *oliguric phase* generally occurs over 1 to 2 days and is characterized by a progressive decrease in urine production. Urine production of <400 mL/day is termed *oliguria,* and urine production of <50 mL/day is termed *anuria.* The oliguric stage may last from days to several weeks. *Nonoliguric renal failure* (>400 mL of urine output per day) carries a better prognosis compared with oliguric renal failure, although the exact reason remains unknown. Similarly, the shorter the duration of oliguria, the higher the likelihood of successful recovery. This is probably because the renal insults in these cases are less severe (e.g., dehydration, nephrotoxin exposure, postrenal obstruction). Strict fluid and electrolyte monitoring and management are required during this phase until renal function normalizes.

After the oliguric phase, a period of increased urine production occurs over several days; this is called the *diuretic phase.* This phase signals the initial repair of the kidney insult. The diuretic phase may result, in part, from a return to normal GFR before tubular reabsorptive capacity has fully recovered.

The elevated osmotic load from uremic toxins and the increased fluid volume retained during the oliguric phase may also contribute to the diuretic phase. Despite the increased urine production, patients may remain markedly azotemic for several days. Daily modifications in the fluid and electrolyte requirements are necessary based on urine output.

The *recovery phase* occurs over several weeks to months, depending on the severity of the patient's ARF. This phase signals the return to the patient's baseline kidney function, normalization of urine production, and the return of the diluting and concentrating abilities of the kidneys.

PATHOGENESIS

The production and elimination of urine requires three basic physiologic events.

1. Blood flow to the glomeruli
2. The formation and processing of ultrafiltrate by the glomeruli and tubular cells
3. Urine excretion through the ureters, bladder, and urethra

Many conditions can alter the above physiologic events leading to ARF. These are classified as *prerenal azotemia, functional, intrinsic,* and *postrenal* ARF (Table 31-1). It is possible for more than one of these categories to coexist.

Normal renal function depends on adequate renal perfusion. The kidneys receive up to 25% of the cardiac output, which is >1 L of blood flow per minute. Prerenal azotemia occurs when blood flow to the kidneys is reduced. Major causes include decreased intravascular volume (e.g., hemorrhage, dehydration), decreased effective circulating volume states (e.g., cirrhosis or congestive heart failure [CHF]), hypotensive events (e.g., shock or medication-related hypotension), and renovascular occlusion or vasoconstriction. Because there is no structural damage to the kidney parenchyma per se, correcting the underlying cause rapidly restores GFR. However, sustained prerenal conditions can result in glomerular ischemia causing acute tubular necrosis (ATN).

Functional ARF results when medical conditions or drugs impair glomerular ultrafiltrate production or intraglomerular hydrostatic pressure. Blood travels through the afferent arteriole and enters the glomerulus, where it is filtered, and exits through the efferent arteriole (Fig. 31-1). The afferent and efferent arterioles work in concert to maintain adequate glomerular capillary hydrostatic pressure to form ultrafiltrate. Many medications can drastically reduce intraglomerular hydrostatic pressure and GFR by producing afferent arteriolar vasoconstriction or efferent arteriolar vasodilation (Fig. 31-2).

Intrinsic ARF can occur at the microvascular level of the nephron, glomeruli, renal tubules, or interstitium. Vasculitic diseases (e.g., Wegener's granulomatosis, cryoglobulinemic vasculitis) involve the small vessels of the kidney. Glomerulonephritis and systemic lupus erythematosus, although relatively uncommon, result in glomerular damage. ATN is by far the most common cause of intrinsic ARF.[15] In fact, the term *acute tubular necrosis* is often used interchangeably with *ARF.* ATN occurs in part because the renal tubules require high oxygen delivery to maintain their metabolic activity. Consequently, any condition that causes ischemia to the tubules (e.g., hypotension, decreased blood flow) can induce

Table 31-1   Causes of Acute Renal Failure

Classification	Common Clinical Disorders
Prerenal azotemia	*Intravascular Volume Depletion*
	Hemorrhage (surgery, trauma)
	Dehydration (gastrointestinal losses, aggressive diuretic administration)
	Severe burns
	Hypovolemic shock
	Sequestration (peritonitis, pancreatitis)
	Decreased Effective Circulating Volume
	Cirrhosis with ascites
	Congestive heart failure
	Hypotension, Shock Syndromes
	Antihypertensive vasodilating medications
	Septic shock
	Cardiomyopathy
	Increased Renal Vascular Occlusion or Constriction
	Bilateral renal artery stenosis
	Unilateral renal stenosis in solitary kidney
	Renal artery or vein thrombosis (embolism, atherosclerosis)
	Vasopressor medications (phenylephrine, norepinephrine)
Functional acute renal failure	*Afferent Arteriole Vasoconstrictors*
	Cyclosporine
	Nonsteroidal anti-inflammatory drugs
	Efferent arteriole vasodilators
	Angiotensin-converting enzyme inhibitors
	Angiotensin II–receptor antagonists
Intrinsic acute renal failure	*Glomerular Disorders*
	Glomerulonephritis
	Systemic lupus erythematosus
	Malignant hypertension
	Vasculitic disorders (Wegener's granulomatosis)
	Acute Tubular Necrosis
	Prolonged prerenal states
	Drug induced (contrast media, aminoglycosides, amphotericin B)
	Acute Interstitial Nephritis
	Drug induced (quinolones, penicillins, sulfa drugs)
Postrenal acute renal failure	*Ureter Obstruction (Bilateral or Unilateral in Solitary Kidney)*
	Malignancy (prostate or cervical cancer)
	Prostate hypertrophy
	Renal calculi

ATN. Moreover, the tubules may be exposed to exceedingly high concentrations of nephrotoxic drugs (e.g., aminoglycosides). Interstitial nephritis, inflammation within the renal parenchyma, is most often associated with drug administration (e.g., penicillins).

Postrenal ARF occurs when there is an outflow obstruction in the upper or lower urinary tract. Lower tract obstruction is most common and can be caused by prostatic hypertrophy, prostate or cervical cancer, or renal calculi. Upper tract obstruction is less common and occurs when both ureters are

LIVERPOOL
JOHN MOORES UNIVERSITY
AVRIL ROBARTS LRC
TEL. 0151 231 4022

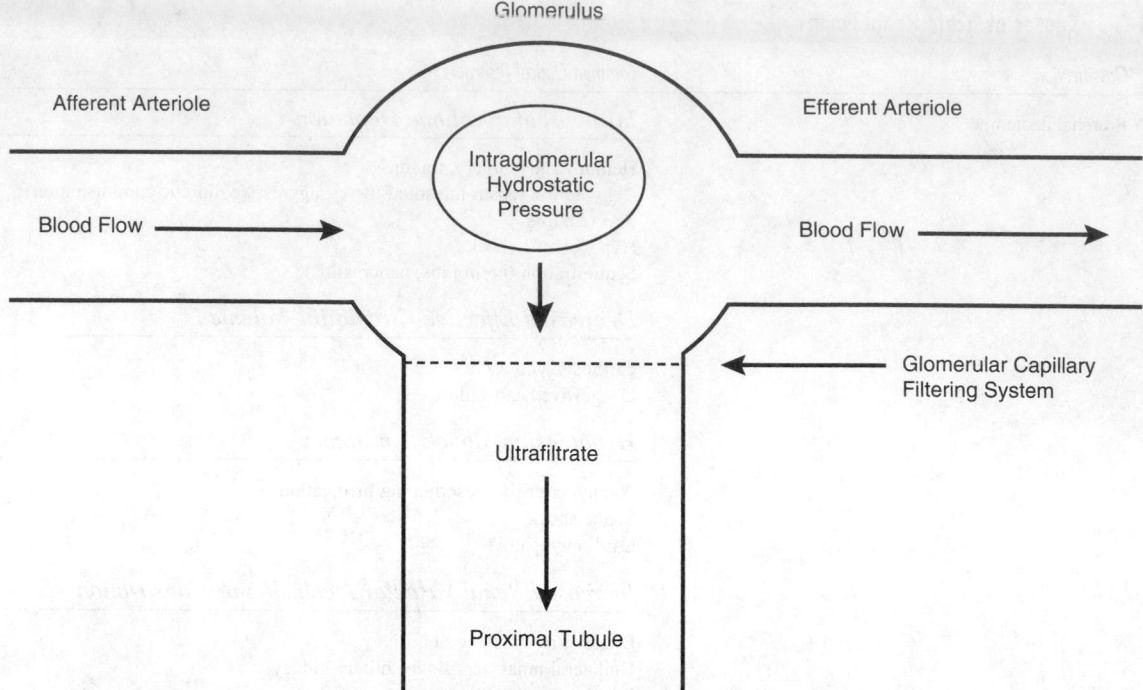

FIGURE 31-1 Schematic of renal blood flow. Blood enters the glomerulus via the afferent arteriole. The intraglomerular hydrostatic pressure leads to ultrafiltration across the glomerular into the proximal tubule. The unfiltered blood leaves the glomerulus via the efferent arteriole. In conditions of decreased renal perfusion, efferent arteriolar vasoconstriction occurs to increase intraglomerular hydrostatic pressure and maintain ultrafiltrate production. Afferent arteriolar vasodilation also occurs to improve blood flow into the glomerulus.

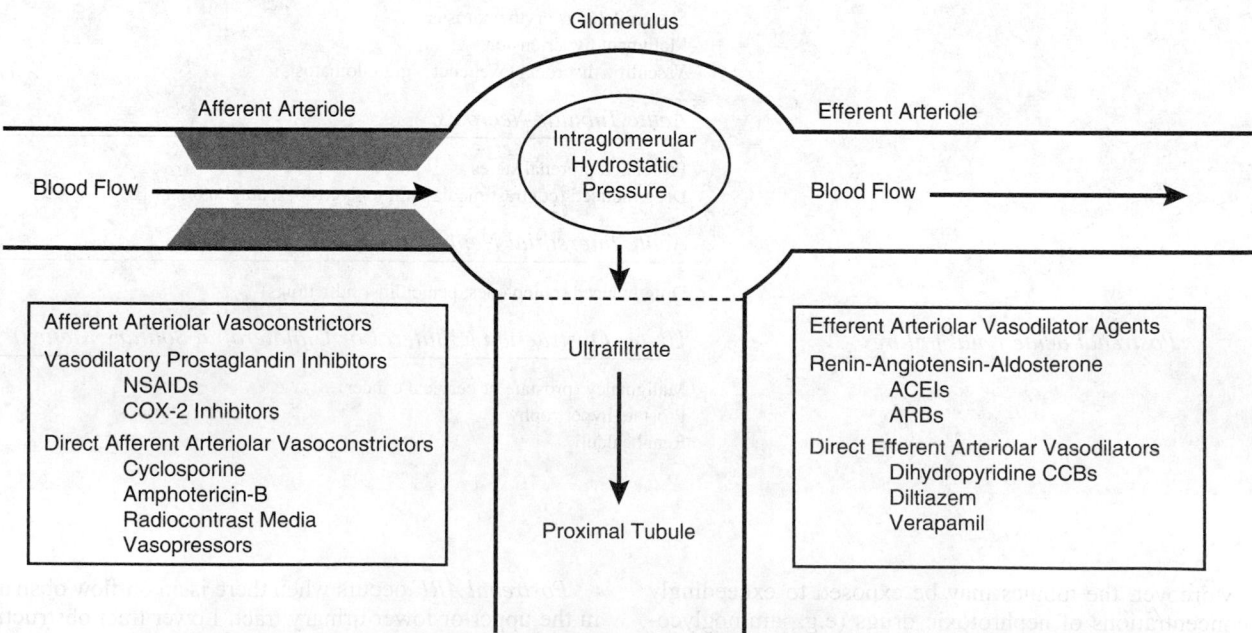

FIGURE 31-2 Drugs that alter renal hemodynamics by causing afferent arteriole vasoconstriction or efferent arteriole vasodilation. ACEIs, angiotensin-converting enzyme inhibitors; ARBs, angiotensin II–receptor blockers; CCBs, calcium channel blockers; COX-2, cyclooxygenase-2; NSAIDs, nonsteroidal anti-inflammatory drugs.

obstructed or when one is obstructed in a patient with a single functioning kidney. Postrenal ARF usually resolves rapidly after the obstruction has been removed. Postobstructive diuresis can be dramatic (e.g., 3 to 5 L/day).

CLINICAL EVALUATION
History and Physical Examination

A detailed history and physical examination often reveal the cause(s) of ARF. The clinician's responsibility is to ask specific, open-ended questions regarding the patient's chief complaint; history of present illness; medical history; family, social, and allergy history; and current prescription and nonprescription medication use. Probing for pertinent information regarding recent surgery, nephrotoxin exposure, or concurrent medical conditions can aid in rapidly determining the etiology of ARF. For example, does the patient have pre-existing conditions that point toward prerenal azotemia, such as CHF or liver disease? Did the patient receive prophylactic antibiotics before surgery? Did the patient hemorrhage or have protracted hypotension during surgery? Furthermore, assessment of the vital sign flowchart for documented weight loss, hypotensive events, fluid intake, and urine output may also prove useful.

A thorough physical examination, when used in conjunction with the history, can be invaluable in confirming the cause of ARF. The patient's volume status should be evaluated first. Evidence of dehydration (e.g., syncope, weight loss, orthostatic hypotension) or decreased effective circulating volume (e.g., ascites, pulmonary edema, peripheral edema, jugular venous distention) usually indicates prerenal azotemia. However, the presence of edema in a patient with normal cardiac function can signal the early signs of nephrotic syndrome. Concurrent rash and ARF associated with recent antibiotic exposure suggests drug-induced allergic interstitial nephritis. The clinician should suspect rhabdomyolysis in a patient with trauma or crush injuries and ARF. An enlarged prostate, painful urination, or wide deviations in urine volume can suggest obstructive ARF causes. Flank and lower abdominal pain suggest upper obstruction, whereas urinary frequency, hesitancy, dribbling, and abdominal fullness indicate lower obstruction.

Laboratory Evaluation
Quantifying Glomerular Filtration Rate

Estimating the GFR is an essential component of the assessment of patients with ARF. The total kidney GFR is equal to the sum of the filtration rates of all of the functioning nephrons and represents the total functional mass of the kidney. It is a reliable index that can be used to evaluate the severity and progression of renal disease.

Markers that are freely filtered at the glomerulus are the best indicators for the accurate measurement of GFR. The ideal GFR marker is filtered freely at the glomerulus without secretion, reabsorption, metabolism, or production by the renal tubules. Exogenous markers such as inulin and iothalamate are commonly used in clinical investigations to measure GFR.[15] Radiolabeled markers such as ^{51}Cr-EDTA, ^{131}I-iothalamate, and ^{99m}Tc-DTPA have also been used to accurately measure GFR, but unnecessary radiation exposure risks and hazardous waste disposal issues preclude their widespread use. Although these substances possess the desired properties needed to accurately measure GFR, they are cumbersome and difficult to use in the clinical setting.

One of the most widely used clinical measures for estimating GFR is determination of creatinine clearance (Cl_{Cr}). Creatinine is produced at a relatively constant rate by nonenzymatic hydrolysis of muscle stores of creatine and phosphocreatine. An individual's muscle mass, age, and sex are predictors of creatinine production. Under steady-state conditions, the urinary excretion of creatinine equals the creatinine production rate, and the SrCr concentration remains relatively stable. Creatinine is freely filtered at the glomerulus, with about 10% to 20% eliminated by active tubular secretion. Consequently, the Cl_{Cr} overestimates the true GFR by 10% to 20%. As GFR declines further, tubular creatinine secretion can account for up to 50% of creatinine elimination, which may overestimate actual GFR by as much as 100%. Commonly used drugs such as cimetidine and trimethoprim can inhibit the secretion of creatinine. Accordingly, administration of these agents can increase the SrCr and decrease Cl_{Cr} without affecting GFR.[16] Various methods for determining Cl_{Cr} have been developed, including urine and nonurine methods. All these methods have potential limitations and pitfalls when used in patients with ARF.

Clinicians commonly use nonurine methods for estimating kidney function. The Cockcroft-Gault (CG) equation is one commonly employed method for estimation of Cl_{Cr}[17]:

$$Cl_{Cr} = \frac{(140 - Age)\,(IBW)}{(72)\,(SrCr)} \qquad \textbf{(31-1)}$$

where age is in years, *IBW* is ideal body weight in kilograms [male IBW = 50 + (2.3 × height over 60 inches); female IBW = 45 + (2.3 × height over 60 inches)], and *SrCr* is the serum creatinine concentration (mg/dL). For women, equation 31-1 is multiplied by 0.85 to account for decreased muscle mass. The CG equation should not be used to estimate GFR in patients with rapidly changing SrCr concentrations because it was derived from normal, healthy subjects with stable renal function. The CG equation produces falsely high Cl_{Cr} estimates in the early stages of ARF and falsely low Cl_{Cr} estimates when ARF is resolving. An example of this is a patient who develops ATN and anuria. Within the first few days, the creatinine level may increase slightly because it takes time for the serum creatinine concentration to achieve a new steady state. In fact, the calculated Cl_{Cr} may even remain in the normal range, although the true GFR is substantially lower. The converse is true with patients recovering from ATN. As the diuretic phase of ATN begins, urine output can be dramatic, but patients may remain markedly azotemic for several days. Using the CG equation in this setting will produce a falsely low Cl_{Cr} estimate. The CG equation is also inaccurate in populations that have little muscle mass, such as elderly, obese, or cachectic patients.

Equations have been developed to determine GFR in patients with rapidly changing renal function.[18-20] These equations, such as the *average SrCr method,* which follows, are more precise estimations of GFR because they measure SrCr and urine creatinine at different points in time:

$$Cl_{Cr}(mL/min) = \frac{(U_V)\,(U_{Cr})}{0.5\,(SrCr_1 + SrCr_2)\,(Time)} \qquad \textbf{(31-2)}$$

where U_v is the urine volume (mL) produced over the collection interval time, U_{Cr} is the urine creatinine concentration (mg/dL), $SrCr_1$ and $SrCr_2$ are the serum creatinine concentrations (mg/dL) at the beginning and end of the urine collection, and *time* is the collection interval in hours.

Although this method should be very accurate in theory, it has important limitations. This calculation is only as accurate as the urine collection process. Errors in accurate urine collection (e.g., nursing collection error or patients not completely voiding before and at the completion of the designated interval) can give false Cl_{Cr} estimates. Timed collections of shorter duration (2 to 8 hours) have been shown to give more accurate results[18] and may be more user-friendly to the clinician than the standard 24-hour collection.

Blood Tests

Assessment of the blood urea nitrogen (BUN) and creatinine concentrations is crucial for guiding the diagnosis, treatment, and monitoring of ARF. The BUN:SrCr ratio can delineate prerenal causes from intrinsic and postrenal etiologies. Urea reabsorption is inversely proportional to the urine flow rate. The normal steady-state BUN:SrCr ratio is approximately 10:1. In prerenal conditions, the BUN:SrCr ratio is >20:1 because sodium and water are actively reabsorbed in the renal tubules to expand the effective circulating volume. Urea, an ineffective osmole, is reabsorbed as a result of increased water reabsorption, whereas creatinine is not reabsorbed. Whereas the SrCr may increase due to decreased glomerular filtration, BUN increases to a greater degree as a result of increased proximal reabsorption.

The presence of hypercalcemia or hyperuricemia can indicate a hematologic malignancy. *Tumor lysis syndrome* is a condition that occurs in leukemia patients after chemotherapy induction. The destruction of cancerous cells results in the release of large quantities of cellular contents (e.g., potassium, uric acid) into the bloodstream, which can overwhelm the kidney's functional ability, especially in dehydrated states.

Other elevated enzymes may also aid in the diagnosis of ARF. An increased level of creatine kinase or myoglobin in the face of ARF usually indicates rhabdomyolysis. Eosinophilia may suggest acute allergic interstitial nephritis from drug exposure. High levels of circulating immune complexes in the presence of ARF suggest glomerulopathies.[1]

Urinalysis

The urinalysis is an important diagnostic tool for differentiating ARF into prerenal azotemia, intrinsic, or obstructive ARF (Table 31-2). The presence of highly concentrated urine, as determined by elevated urine osmolality and specific gravity, suggests prerenal azotemia. During dehydrated states, *vasopressin (antidiuretic hormone [ADH])* is secreted, and the renin-angiotensin-aldosterone (RAA) system is activated. These mechanisms promote the reabsorption of water and sodium at the collecting duct of the nephron, which serves to expand the effective circulating volume in an attempt to restore renal perfusion. As a result of diminished urine volume, the urine osmolality and specific gravity increase dramatically. Patients with prerenal azotemia and oliguria often have a urine osmolality >500 mOsm/kg. The maximum urine osmolality can exceed 1,200 mOsm/kg.

The presence of proteinuria or hematuria can indicate glomerular damage. Nephrotic syndrome is characterized by urinary protein losses >3.5 g/1.73 m² per day. Proteinuria can also result from tubular damage. However, the protein loss is rarely >2 g/day. The protein content can be used to differentiate glomerular versus tubular damage. The low-molecular-weight protein, β_2-microglobulin is freely filtered at the glomerulus and reabsorbed at the proximal tubule. Therefore, the presence of excessive β_2-microglobulin in the urine suggests a tubular source of ARF, such as ATN. Conversely, albumin is not readily filtered at the glomerulus; hence, the presence of heavy albuminuria suggests a glomerular source of ARF.

Microscopic examination of the urine provides helpful clues for determining the source of ARF (Table 31-3). Pigmented granular casts are generally seen with ischemic or nephrotoxin-induced ARF. White blood cells (WBCs) and WBC casts can indicate an inflammatory process in the glomerulus, such as acute interstitial nephritis (AIN) or pyelonephritis. Red blood cells (RBCs) and RBC casts can result from strenuous exercise or can indicate glomerulonephritis. Allergic interstitial nephritis can be detected by the presence of urinary eosinophils. Obstructive ARF causes, such as nephrolithiasis, can be identified by the presence of crystals in the urine. Cystine, leucine, and tyrosine crystals are considered pathologic. The presence of calcium oxalate crystals may suggest toxic ingestion of ethylene glycol.

Urinary Chemistries

Analyzing urine electrolyte concentrations and simultaneously comparing them with serum sodium and creatinine concentrations is useful for differentiating between prerenal azotemia and ATN (see Table 31-2). The fractional excretion of sodium (FE_{Na+}) is a measurement of how actively the kidney is reabsorbing sodium, and it is calculated as the fraction of filtered sodium excreted in the urine using creatinine as a measure of GFR. In normal conditions, the proximal tubule reabsorbs 99% of filtered sodium. The FE_{Na+} formula is listed as follows:

$$FE_{Na+} (\%) = \frac{(U_{Na})(SrCr)}{(U_{Cr})(S_{Na})} \times 100 \qquad (31\text{-}3)$$

Table 31-2 Urinary Indices in Acute Renal Failure

Component	Prerenal Azotemia	Acute Tubular Necrosis	Postrenal Obstruction
Urine Na⁺ (mEq/L)	<20	>40	>40
FE_{Na+}	<1%	>2%	>1%
Urine/plasma creatinine	>40	<20	<20
Specific gravity	>1.010	<1.010	Variable
Urine osmolality (mOsm/kg)	Up to 1,200	<300	<300

Table 31-3 Clinical Significance of Urinary Sediment in Acute Renal Failure

Cellular Debris	Clinical Significance
Red blood cells	Glomerulonephritis
	IgA nephropathy
	Lupus nephritis
White blood cells	Infection (pyelonephritis)
	Glomerulonephritis
	Acute tubular necrosis
Eosinophils	Drug-induced acute interstitial nephritis
	Pyelonephritis
	Renal transplant rejection
Hyaline casts	Glomerulonephritis
	Pyelonephritis
	Congestive heart failure
Red blood cell casts	Acute tubular necrosis
	Glomerulonephritis
	Interstitial nephritis
White blood cell casts	Pyelonephritis
	Interstitial nephritis
Granular casts	Dehydration
	Interstitial nephritis
	Glomerulonephritis
	Acute tubular necrosis
Tubular cell casts	Acute tubular necrosis
Fatty casts	Nephrotic syndrome
Myoglobin	Rhabdomyolysis
Crystals	Nonspecific

where U_{Na} is the urine sodium concentration (mEq/L), $SrCr$ is the serum creatinine concentration (mg/dL), U_{Cr} is the urine creatinine concentration (mg/dL), and S_{Na} is the serum sodium concentration (mEq/L).

In prerenal azotemia, the functional ability of the proximal renal tubule remains intact. In fact, its sodium-reabsorbing abilities are markedly enhanced because of the effects of circulating vasopressin and activation of the RAA system. Both the FE_{Na+} and urinary sodium concentration become markedly low ($<1\%$ and <20 mEq/L, respectively) in prerenal conditions. In contrast, these indices are elevated in ATN because the renal tubules lose their ability to reabsorb sodium; the FE_{Na+} is $>2\%$, and the urine sodium is >40 mEq/L. FE_{Na+} values between 1% and 2% are generally inconclusive. The clinician should ensure that the patient is not receiving scheduled diuretic therapy when the FE_{Na+} is calculated. Diuretics increase natriuresis, thereby making the results difficult to interpret.

PRERENAL AND FUNCTIONAL ACUTE RENAL FAILURE
Congestive Heart Failure and Nonsteroidal Anti-Inflammatory Drug Use

1. A.W. is a 71-year-old man who had a Q-wave myocardial infarction (MI) 2 months ago. His ejection fraction is currently 15% (normal, 50% to 60%). He presents today for his 2-month follow-up clinic appointment complaining of shortness of breath, dyspnea on exertion, and inability to produce much urine. His medical history is significant for longstanding hypertension, coronary artery disease, osteoarthritis, and recent-onset CHF after his MI. His home medications include digoxin 0.25 mg PO QD, simvastatin 40 mg PO QD, and naproxen sodium 550 mg PO BID. With the exception of naproxen, A.W. often forgets to take his medications. Physical examination reveals lower leg 3% pitting edema, pulmonary crackles and wheezes, positive jugular venous distention, and an S_3 heart sound. His vital signs are significant for a blood pressure (BP) of 198/97 mm Hg and a weight gain of 4 kg since his last visit 2 months ago. Last month, his BUN and SrCr were 23 (normal, 5 to 20) and 1.2 mg/dL (normal, 0.5 to 1.2), respectively. What are A.W.'s risk factors for ARF?

[SI units: BUN, 8.2 mmol/L (normal, 1.8 to 7.1); SrCr, 106 mol/L (normal, 44.2 to 106)]

A.W.'s risk factors for ARF are CHF with poor cardiac output (ejection fraction, 15%) that resulted from his MI and his medication, naproxen sodium. CHF is a major cause of functional ARF.[21] A.W.'s diminished cardiac output has resulted in decreased effective circulating volume and activation of the RAA system, which are impairing his renal perfusion. In states of decreased renal perfusion, prostaglandins E_2 and I_2 compensate for the afferent arteriole vasoconstriction and stimulate afferent arteriole vasodilation, enhancing renal blood flow. Prostaglandin synthesis is mediated predominantly by cyclooxygenase-1 (COX-1) and perhaps cyclooxygenase-2 (COX-2). Nonsteroidal anti-inflammatory drugs (NSAIDs), such as naproxen, are often overlooked as causes of ARF.[22,23] NSAIDs exert their pharmacologic effect by inhibiting prostaglandin synthesis, thereby negating compensatory vasodilation. NSAIDs induce abrupt decreases in GFR in at-risk patient populations, specifically those with CHF, liver disease, the elderly, or dehydrated patients. Indomethacin is associated with the highest risk of NSAID-induced renal ischemia, whereas aspirin appears to have the lowest risk. Naproxen, ibuprofen, piroxicam, and diclofenac are considered intermediate in their relative capacities to acutely compromise renal perfusion.[23] Sulindac may offer a "renal-sparing" effect. Sulindac is a prodrug that is converted to its active sulfide metabolite by the liver and then becomes reversibly oxidized back to its parent compound in the kidney; renal prostaglandin synthesis is essentially unaltered by sulindac. However, note that there have been case reports of sulindac-induced renal dysfunction when administered to patients with cirrhosis and ascites.

COX-2 inhibitors are a relatively new anti-inflammatory drug class that also inhibit prostaglandin synthesis. Gertz and colleagues assessed the comparative renovascular effects of rofecoxib, a selective COX-2 inhibitor, to traditional nonselective NSAIDs in patients with osteoarthritis.[24] The results demonstrated similar renovascular effects. These data suggest that COX-2 selectivity does not offer any benefit over nonselective NSAIDs with regard to renovascular effects. Figure 31-2 illustrates common medications that alter renal hemodynamics by causing either afferent arteriole vasoconstriction or efferent arteriole vasodilation.

2. A.W.'s cardiologist obtains a stat digoxin level, electrolyte panel, urinalysis, and urine electrolyte panel. The digoxin level was reported as "not detectable" (normal, 0.5 to 2.0 ng/mL). The significantly abnormal serum laboratory values were BUN of 56 mg/dL (normal, 5 to 20) and creatinine of 1.5 mg/dL (normal, 0.5 to 1.2). The urinalysis was significant for a urinary osmolality of 622 mOsm/kg (normal, 300 to 500 mOsm/kg), and specific gravity of 1.092 (normal, 1.010 to 1.020). The urine electrolytes were significant for Na⁺ of 12 mEq/L (normal, 20 to 40) and creatinine of 87 mg/dL. What laboratory findings suggest functional ARF?

[SI units: BUN, 20 mmol/L (normal, 1.8 to 7.1); SrCr, 132.6 mol/L (normal, 44.2 to 106); urine Cr, 7,691 mol/L]

A.W. has classic laboratory findings that suggest poor renal perfusion (see Table 31-2). It is important to compare the current and previous laboratory data to assess acute changes in renal function. Compared with last month, A.W.'s renal function has deteriorated based on the BUN and SrCr concentrations. Both concentrations have increased substantially; BUN has increased nearly twofold and creatinine by 25%. The BUN:SrCr ratio is >20:1, suggesting poor renal blood flow, which is corroborated by other urinary indices such as the urinary Na⁺, 40; specific gravity (elevated), 1.090; urine osmolality, 622 mOsm/kg; and the calculated FE_{Na+}, 0.16%. These values reflect the ability of the renal tubules to respond to vasopressin and aldosterone in an attempt to expand effective circulating volume and restore renal perfusion.

3. How should A.W.'s prerenal azotemia be treated?

The presence of volume overload in the face of prerenal azotemia suggests a decreased effective circulating volume, most likely from CHF. Restoring and improving A.W.'s cardiac output and renal perfusion will rapidly correct the prerenal azotemia. This can be achieved by (1) improving cardiac contractility, (2) controlling BP to a goal of <135/85 mm Hg by decreasing both preload and afterload, and (3) modifying any drug therapy that has deleterious effects on the renal hemodynamics (e.g., NSAIDs). The specific therapies for controlling hypertension and improving cardiac output are presented in Chapter 14, Essential Hypertension, and Chapter 19, Heart Failure. Naproxen should be discontinued and substituted with acetaminophen to treat his osteoarthritis. Normal renal function should return in a few days after correction of the underlying causes.

Angiotensin-Converting Enzyme Inhibitor– and Angiotensin Receptor Blocker– Induced Acute Renal Failure

4. G.B. is a 53-year-old white woman with hypertension, coronary artery disease, peripheral vascular disease, and diabetes, for which she had been taking hydrochlorothiazide 25 mg

PO QD, atorvastatin 10 mg PO QD, aspirin 325 mg PO QD, and NPH insulin 30 U SC Q AM and 15 U SC Q PM. At last week's clinic visit, she had two consecutive BP readings of 187/96 and 193/95 mm Hg, respectively, measured 20 minutes apart. At that time, G.B.'s primary care physician discontinued her hydrochlorothiazide and started her on lisinopril 5 mg PO QD. She returns to the clinic today for her 1-week follow-up appointment complaining of dizziness, very little urine production over the past week, and swelling in her ankles. Her BP is 98/43 mm Hg. A stat serum electrolyte panel was obtained and was significant for a BUN of 62 mg/dL (normal, 5 to 20) and an SrCr of 6.1 mg/dL (normal, 0.5 to 1.2). Why is G.B. experiencing ARF?

[SI units: BUN, 22.1 mmol/L (normal, 1.8 to 7.1); SrCr, 539 mol/L (normal, 44.2 to 106)]

Inhibition of the renin-angiotensin-aldosterone (RAA) system in patients with compromised renal blood flow is a common cause of functional ARF. A basic understanding of the effects of the RAA system on renal hemodynamics is necessary in this situation (Fig. 31-3). When renal perfusion is impaired, the juxtaglomerular cells of the kidney secrete renin into the plasma and lymph. Renin cleaves circulating angiotensinogen to form angiotensin I (AT I), which is further cleaved by angiotensin-converting enzyme (ACE), to form angiotensin II (AT II). AT II induces two physiologic events to improve renal perfusion. First, it directly causes systemic vasoconstriction, which shunts blood to the major organs, and indirectly increases intravascular volume through aldosterone- and vasopressin-mediated activity. Second, it preferentially vasoconstricts the efferent arteriole to maintain adequate intraglomerular hydrostatic pressure. Under conditions of decreased arterial pressure or effective circulating volume, the RAA system is activated and plasma renin and AT II activity are increased.[25]

G.B. has extensive atherosclerotic disease indicated by the presence of coronary artery and peripheral vascular disease. Atherosclerosis not only affects major blood vessels, but also the macro- and microvasculature of the kidney; indeed, atherosclerosis is a major cause of renal artery occlusion and decreased renal perfusion. This activates the RAA system, which causes sodium and water reabsorption and AT II–mediated efferent arteriole vasoconstriction, in an attempt to restore normal renal perfusion and intraglomerular hydrostatic pressure.

The administration of ACE inhibitors directly inhibits the formation of AT II, which is necessary for efferent arteriole

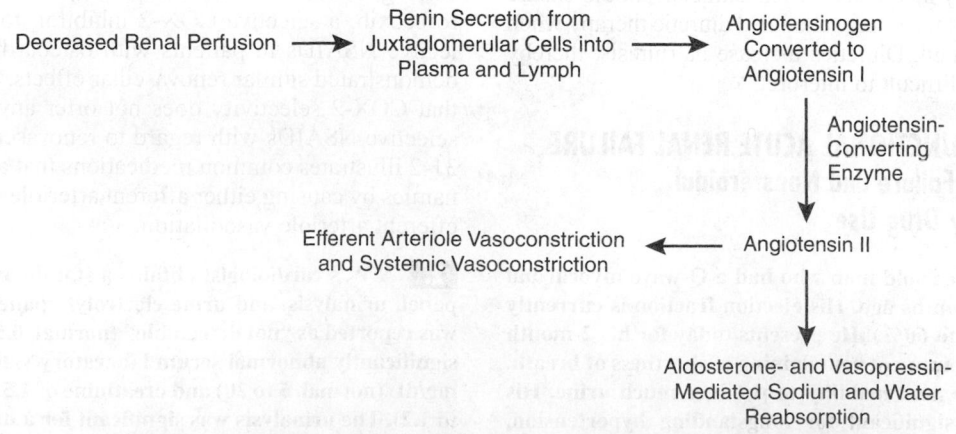

FIGURE 31-3 Compensatory hormonal mechanisms of decreased renal perfusion.

vasoconstriction. Consequently, the compensatory physiologic event that maintains G.B.'s renal blood flow is inhibited, thereby reducing her intraglomerular hydrostatic pressure and GFR. ACE inhibitors are contraindicated in patients with bilateral renal artery stenosis or unilateral stenosis in patients with a single functioning kidney.[25]

5. **Are there other factors that predispose patients to ACE inhibitor–induced ARF?**

In addition to the above situation, there are three other general scenarios that will result in the development of ARF with ACE inhibitors. First, conditions of sodium and water depletion (e.g., dehydration, overdiuresis, poor fluid intake, low-sodium diet) can increase the dependency of the efferent arteriole on AT II. When ACE inhibitors are given in these situations, GFR can fall dramatically, and SrCr rises. ARF can be averted by withholding the ACE inhibitor (and/or diuretic) for a day and repleting the intravascular fluid volume. The ACE inhibitor can be restarted at the same dose after adequate hydration. Second, ACE inhibitors can decrease the mean arterial pressure to such a degree that renal perfusion cannot be sustained. This is more likely to occur with long-acting agents or in situations in which the pharmacologic half-life of the ACE inhibitor is prolonged (e.g., pre-existing renal disease).[26] Finally, ACE inhibitors may precipitate ARF in patients who are taking concomitant drugs with renal afferent arteriole vasoconstricting effects, most notably cyclosporine and NSAIDs.[27]

6. **How is ACE inhibitor–induced ARF managed?**

Patients who are receiving ACE inhibitors should be monitored judiciously with regard to their serum creatinine and electrolyte concentrations. Fortunately, ARF related to ACE inhibitors is usually reversible,[25] principally because the ARF is caused by inadequate glomerular capillary pressure, which is restored as soon as sufficient AT II is produced. This normally takes 2 to 3 days to re-equilibrate. Anecdotally, ARF appears to develop more commonly in hypotensive patients or those with intravascular volume depletion (e.g., heart failure patients receiving high-dose diuretics). In these conditions, it is prudent to replete the intravascular fluid volume, and/or temporarily discontinue diuretic therapy.[25] In addition, ACE inhibitor therapy should be temporarily discontinued and reinstituted when the patient has a normalized intravascular volume and is hemodynamically stable.

7. **Do angiotensin II–receptor blockers (ARBs) cause less ARF compared with ACE inhibitors?**

ARBs competitively inhibit the angiotensin II receptor. There are at least two subtypes of the angiotensin II receptors: AT_1 and AT_2. The ARBs exert their pharmacologic effect at the AT_1 receptor subtype, which is responsible for most, if not all, of the cardiovascular effects of angiotensin II, such as vasoconstriction, aldosterone release, and β-adrenergic stimulation.[28]

The Evaluation of Losartan in the Elderly (ELITE) study compared losartan with captopril with the primary endpoint being development of renal dysfunction.[29] There was a 10.5% incidence of losartan-induced renal dysfunction in CHF patients without history of renal dysfunction, which was essentially identical to captopril. In summary, there are no data to suggest that ARBs are better tolerated than ACE inhibitors with respect to renal dysfunction.

INTRINSIC ACUTE RENAL FAILURE

Intrinsic ARF is a general term that connotes damage at the parenchymal level of the kidney. The term *acute tubular necrosis* is often used to describe this type of ARF, but this is a histologic diagnosis that describes only one of several intrinsic disorders. Pragmatically, intrinsic ARF can be subdivided into vascular, glomerular, or tubular disorders.

Disorders involving the large renal vessels are relatively uncommon. Acute renal artery or vein occlusion can be caused by vasculitis, atheroembolism, thromboembolism, dissection, or clamping of the ascending aorta during surgery. To affect serum BUN and creatinine, occlusion must be bilateral, or it can be unilateral in patients with concomitant renal insufficiency or one functioning kidney. Reduced blood flow to the renal microvasculature and glomeruli also can result in ARF. Common examples are rapidly progressing glomerulonephritis (RPGN) and vasculitis. If these conditions become severe enough, they can cause ischemia, resulting in superimposed ATN. Any disorder that produces tubular ischemia, such as prolonged hypotension or shock syndromes, can result in ATN.

Nephrotoxic drugs are a common cause of ATN, especially when given in septic or volume-contracted patients. There are various mechanisms by which drugs can cause ATN, which are explained in detail later in this chapter. Although relatively uncommon, drug-induced AIN is another type of intrinsic ARF. This is a hypersensitivity reaction that results from the formation of drug–antibody complexes that subsequently deposit in the glomerular membrane.

Acute Glomerulopathies
Poststreptococcal Glomerulonephritis

8. **B.M. is an 18-year-old male college freshman in otherwise good health who recently developed strep throat. He received a 10-day course of amoxicillin, which cleared the infection. He returns to the student health center after completing his 10-day course complaining of "puffy eyes," swelling in his legs, a cough productive of clear sputum, and decreased urine output that appears "tea-colored." Other than the amoxicillin, he is not on any medication. Baseline records from a routine physical examination 2 months ago revealed a serum BUN and creatinine of 10 mg/dL and 0.8 mg/dL (normal, 5 to 20 and 0.5 to 1.2), respectively, and a BP of 120/80 mm Hg. Today, the physical examination is significant for a BP of 176/95 mm Hg, 2% peripheral edema, and bilateral pulmonary rales. The urinalysis is significant for gross hematuria, nephritic-range proteinuria, RBC and WBC casts, and epithelial cells. B.M.'s SrCr has increased to 7.1 mg/dL. Based on the history, physical examination, and laboratory findings, what is the most likely cause of ARF in this patient?**

[SI units: BUN, 3.6 mmol/L (normal, 1.8 to 7.1); SrCr, 70.7 and 627.6 mol/L, respectively (normal, 44.2 to 106)]

B.M.'s recent history of a streptococcal infection with the development of ARF suggests poststreptococcal glomerulonephritis (PSGN), which results from the formation of antibodies against streptococcal antigens. The streptococcal–

antigen immune complexes are deposited in the glomerulus, resulting in complement, cytokine, and clotting cascade activation; neutrophils and monocytes attack the glomerulus causing glomerulonephritis. The onset of PSGN is usually 7 to 21 days after the start of the pharyngeal infection. PSGN is the most common acute-onset, immune-mediated, diffuse glomerulopathy. It primarily affects children, although it can affect any age group and is more prevalent in males than in females. Only certain serologic subtypes of group A β-hemolytic streptococci, known as *nephritogenic* strains, cause PSGN. Strains that follow pharyngeal infections (e.g., strep throat) include types 1, 3, 4, 6, 12, 25, and 49. Type 49 is the most prevalent strain worldwide. Positive diagnosis of PSGN requires identification of a nephritogenic group A β-hemolytic streptococcal strain; objective urinalysis findings suggestive of glomerular damage such as proteinuria, hematuria, and casts; and elevated streptococcal antibody titers.

B.M. exhibits the classic physical and laboratory findings associated with PSGN. The pertinent positive physical findings include periorbital, pulmonary and peripheral edema, tea-colored urine, hypertension, and decreased urine output. Edema is a common manifestation, with periorbital edema typically being the first to appear. Reduced GFR, proteinuria, and sodium retention by the kidney all contribute to edema formation. When protein, principally albumin, is lost in the urine, the intravascular oncotic pressure declines, causing a shift of fluid into the extravascular space. The loss of intravascular volume stimulates sodium and water reabsorption by the kidney via aldosterone and vasopressin, which often produces stage 1 to 2 hypertension.

Pertinent laboratory data in B.M. include elevated SrCr, and urinalysis positive for hematuria, proteinuria, WBC casts, and epithelial cells. Hematuria, which is found in almost all patients with PSGN, accounts for the reddish-brown tea-colored urine. Other commonly found urine sediments include cellular casts and hyaline and granular casts. Oliguria is common in PSGN, but anuria is rare.

9. **Are there other tests that can be used to confirm this diagnosis?**

Given that B.M. has received a 10-day course of amoxicillin, it is unlikely that throat cultures for the nephritogenic group A β-hemolytic streptococcal strain will be positive. However, cultures of close contacts may be positive for the streptococcal strain, even if they are asymptomatic. The presence of circulating antibodies to the nephritogenic streptococcal strains indicates recent exposure. The anti-streptolysin O (ASO), anti-hyaluronidase (AHase), anti-deoxyribonuclease B (ADNase B), and anti-nicotyladenine dinucleotidase (NADase) antibody titers can be measured clinically. ASO titers begin to rise 2 weeks after pharyngeal infection, peak at 4 weeks, and slowly decline over 1 to 6 months. There is no correlation between degree of ASO rise and nephrogenicity. In fact, ASO titers may not be elevated at all if early antibiotic treatment is initiated or in cases of streptococcal skin infections. The use of ADNase and AHase titers is more specific to detect recent infection in these situations.

The streptozyme test, which can be used clinically for rapid screening purposes, uses several antistreptococcal antibody assays. Unfortunately, false-positive and false-negative results are common because of cross-reactivity between the antibody and normal collagen.

Serial complement determinations may be of value in diagnosing PSGN. Decreased levels of C_3 protein and hemolytic complement activity (CH_{50}) are observed in nearly all patients with active PSGN. Serum C_3 levels can fall by nearly 50% of normal in the first weeks of infection and return to normal within 8 weeks after infection. However, no correlation exists between the degree of C_3 depression and severity of nephritis. Circulating antibody complexes of C_3 can be found in patients with acute infection.

Rarely is there a need for renal biopsy, but it may be prudent in patients that present with atypical symptoms such as anuria, prolonged oliguria, marked azotemia, hematuria for >3 weeks, or in those who have no streptococcal antibody titers.

10. **What are the therapeutic goals and treatment options for PSGN?**

The therapeutic goals are to minimize further kidney damage and to provide symptomatic relief for B.M. The underlying streptococcal infection should be treated with appropriate antibiotics, but as illustrated by B.M., this has no effect in preventing PSGN. Family members and close contacts of the infected patient should receive antibiotic prophylaxis as well. Restriction of protein to 0.8 g/kg per day may be beneficial in patients with marked proteinuria, and antihypertensive drugs can be used on a short-term basis to control BP. Sodium and water restriction is beneficial in reducing edema, and loop diuretics may be used as needed for symptomatic pulmonary or peripheral edema. Close monitoring of electrolytes is warranted if diuretics are used. Dialysis is rarely required.

Rapidly Progressive Glomenularnephritis (RPGN)

11. **Are there other glomerulopathies that cause ARF?**

Yes. RPGN, also called *crescentic glomerulonephritis,* is a clinical syndrome of rapid decline in renal function (from days to weeks) combined with the hallmark findings of gross hematuria, proteinuria, and the presence of extensive glomerular crescents (>50% of glomeruli) on renal biopsy. It is not uncommon for RPGN patients to have a 50% decline in GFR in only a few weeks. RPGN is a medical emergency, and treatment success depends on how early therapy is initiated. If left untreated, progression to end-stage renal disease or death is almost certain.

Idiopathic RPGN is divided into three categories based on immunofluorescence microscopy. Type I idiopathic RPGN is characterized by linear deposition of immunoglobulins, primarily IgG, along the glomerular basement membrane (GBM) indicating anti-GBM antibodies. Type II idiopathic RPGN is identified by granular immunoglobulin and complement depositions in the glomerular microvasculature and mesangium suggesting immune complex deposition. Type III idiopathic RPGN is also called *pauci-immune* because there are no hallmark immunoglobulin or complement findings on immunofluorescence microscopy. Type III idiopathic RPGN is identified by the presence of circulating antineutrophil cytoplasmic antibodies.

Multisystem vasculitic disorders that result in glomerular capillary inflammation are the most common cause of RPGN.[31] Many of these patients present with nonspecific flu-like symptoms such as fever, weight loss, myalgia, and malaise with proteinuria and hematuria. Uremic symptoms can occur with severe disease. The presence of ARF with pulmonary congestion, cough, hemoptysis, or dyspnea suggests *Wegener's granulomatosis*. The treatment for autoimmune RPGN generally involves immunosuppressive agents, such as prednisone, azathioprine, or cyclophosphamide. A more detailed discussion of glomerulonephritis is presented in Chapter 32, Chronic Kidney Disease.

NSAID-Induced Glomerulopathy

12. **What drugs cause glomerulonephropathy?**

Minimal-change disease and *membranous nephropathy* have been associated with NSAID use.[30–33] The mechanism is probably related to NSAID-induced inhibition of the cyclooxygenase pathway, which leads to increased arachidonate catabolism and increased proinflammatory leukotriene production. The hallmark feature of NSAID-induced nephropathy is nephrotic-range proteinuria. The nephropathy resolves slowly over several months once the NSAID is discontinued.

TUBULOINTERSTITIAL DISEASES
Acute Tubular Necrosis

ATN arises most often from ischemia or drug-induced causes.[34] Prolonged prerenal conditions such as hypotension, surgery, overwhelming sepsis, or major burns can lead to ischemic ATN. Unlike prerenal azotemia, tubular cell death occurs in ATN, and immediate volume resuscitation will not re-

verse the damage. The pathophysiology of ATN is complex and remains unclear.[35] It is currently thought that when tubular cells die, they slough off into the tubule lumen and contribute to cast formation. The casts completely obstruct the tubule lumen and increase intratubular pressure, which causes a backleak of ultrafiltrate across the tubular basement membrane[2] (Fig. 31-4). The aforementioned processes are mediated by a variety of substances, including calcium, phospholipases, and perhaps growth factors as well as free radical and protease activation.[34,35]

Treatment With Diuretics and Dopamine

13. **Do diuretics and dopamine have a role in treating established ATN?**

It is well documented that patients with nonoliguric renal failure have significantly better outcomes compared with those with oliguria.[4] This is probably because nonoliguric patients have less extensive renal damage and are better able to maintain fluid and electrolyte balance. Loop diuretics are commonly used in established ATN in an attempt to convert patients with oliguria to a nonoliguric state. However, many clinical trials have failed to demonstrate improved mortality or duration of azotemia in oliguric patients who receive loop diuretics, despite improved urine output.[36–40] A recent cohort study in ICU patients with ARF suggested that patients treated with aggressive diuretic therapy had an increased risk of death and nonrecovery of renal function, despite adjustment for age, severity of disease, comorbidities and urine out-

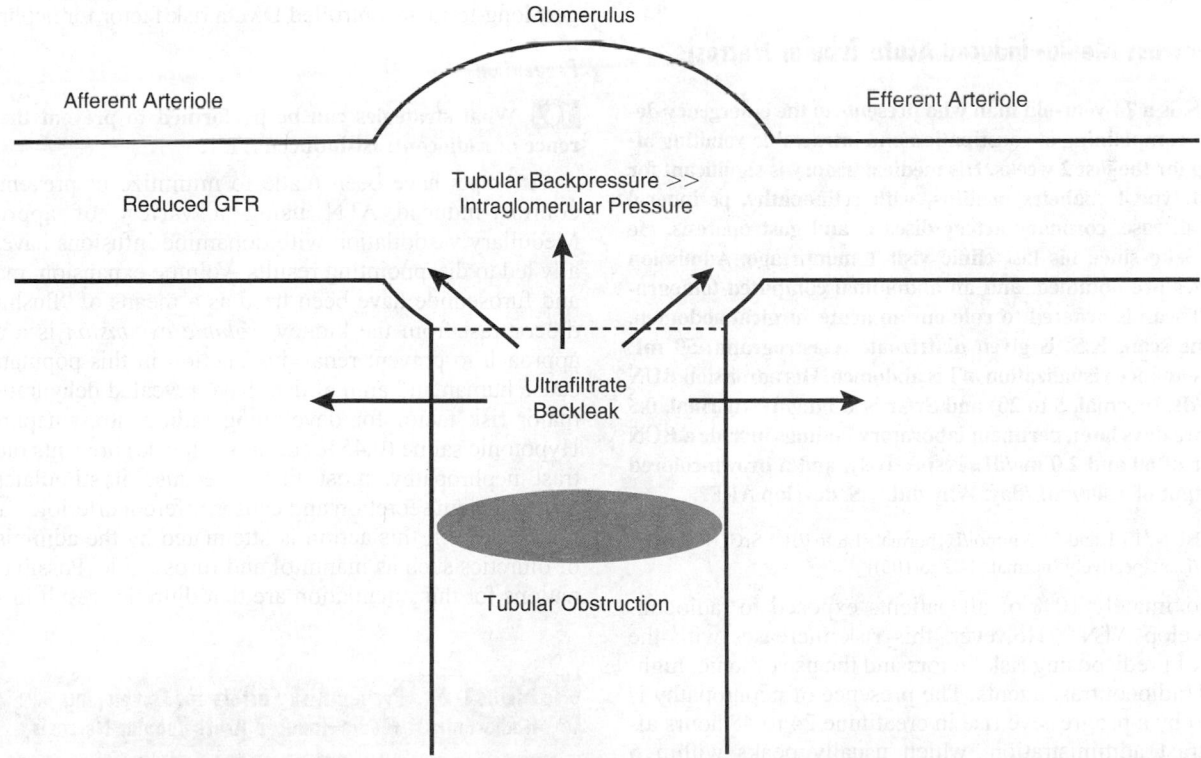

FIGURE 31-4 Schematic of acute tubular necrosis (ATN). The process is initiated by ischemia or nephrotoxin exposure that leads to tubular cell death. The cellular debris sloughs off and obstructs the proximal tubule lumen. Once the nephron is obstructed, there is a backleak of the glomerular ultrafiltrate across the tubular basement membrane and impairment of glomerular filtration. During the recovery phase of ATN, the obstructive cellular casts are released into the urine and filtration begins to normalize. GFR, glomerular filtration rate.

put.[36] These data suggest that even though nonoliguric patients generally have better outcomes, converting a patient from oliguria to nonoliguria through pharmacologic intervention does not improve patient outcomes. Currently, the only role that diuretic administration has in patients with established ATN is to increase urine output, which facilitates fluid, electrolyte, and nutritional support. Diuretic administration does not appear to alter the course or outcome of established ATN.

Another controversy that has been debated extensively in the literature is the use of dopamine in patients with established ATN. Dopamine is a catecholamine that stimulates dopaminergic receptors at low dosages (1 to 3 μg/kg per minute), and α- and β-receptors at higher dosages (5 to 20 μg/kg per minute). Animal and human studies have demonstrated that low-dose dopamine improves renal blood flow by inducing afferent arteriolar vasodilation. However, no data support the use of dopamine in the treatment of established ARF. A recent meta-analysis of 58 clinical trials conducted over the past 20 years failed to detect any significant improvement in variables such as occurrence of ARF, need for renal replacement therapy, or mortality.[41]

Another large, multicenter trial studied the clinical usefulness of low-dose dopamine in critically ill patients with systemic inflammatory response syndrome.[42] Dopamine had no clinical benefit in preventing the occurrence or reducing the severity of ARF. Furthermore, cardiac arrhythmias and myocardial ischemia have been reported in patients treated with low-dose dopamine infusions.[43] Unequivocally, dopamine has no role in preventing or treating ARF.

Radiocontrast Media–Induced Acute Tubular Necrosis

14. **K.S. is a 74-year-old man who presents to the emergency department complaining of constipation and intractable vomiting after eating for the last 2 weeks. His medical history is significant for advanced type 1 diabetes mellitus, with retinopathy, peripheral vascular disease, coronary artery disease, and gastroparesis. He has lost 5 kg since his last clinic visit 1 month ago. Admission chemistries are obtained, and an abdominal computed tomography (CT) scan is ordered to rule out an acute surgical abdomen. Before the scan, K.S. is given diatrizoate (Gastrografin) 50 mL orally to enhance visualization of his abdomen. His admission BUN is 37 mg/dL (normal, 5 to 20) and SrCr is 1.5 mg/dL (normal, 0.5 to 1.2). Two days later, pertinent laboratory findings include a BUN and SrCr of 60 and 2.0 mg/dL, respectively, and a brown-colored urine output of <400 mL/day. Why did K.S. develop ARF?**

[SI units: BUN, 13.1 and 21.3 mmol/L (normal, 1.8 to 7.1); SrCr, 132.6 and 176.8 mol/L, respectively (normal, 44.2 to 106)]

Approximately 10% of all patients exposed to radiocontrast develop ATN.[44] However, this risk increases with the number of predisposing risk factors and the use of ionic, high-osmolar radiocontrast agents. The presence of nephropathy is indicated by a progressive rise in creatinine 24 to 48 hours after contrast administration, which usually peaks within 5 days. The degree of creatinine rise and the presence of oliguria are widely variable.

The mechanisms by which radiocontrast media induce ARF are complex. Initially, the radiocontrast medium produces renal vasodilation and an osmotic diuresis. However,

this is followed by intense vasoconstriction in the medullary portion of the kidney, which has been demonstrated by significant decreases in medullary PO_2 after contrast administration. The ischemia is compounded by the increased medullary O_2 consumption because of the osmotic diuresis. Consequently, a dysequilibrium exists between O_2 supply and demand creating ischemic ATN. Various vasoactive substances are suspected of decreasing medullary blood flow, including oxygen free radicals, prostaglandins, endothelin, nitric oxide, angiotensin II, and adenosine.[44,45] Endothelin and adenosine are potent vasoconstrictors that are directly released from endothelial cells upon exposure to radiocontrast media.

15. **What are the risk factors for radiocontrast-induced ATN?**

The documented risk factors for radiocontrast-induced ATN are listed in Table 31-4. Any condition that decreases renal blood flow increases the risk of nephropathy. At-risk patient populations include individuals with underlying diabetic nephropathy or chronic renal insufficiency, CHF, volume depletion, or those receiving aggressive diuretic regimens. The use of the ionic, high-osmolar contrast products also increases the risk of nephropathy, as well as the previously discussed medications that markedly reduce renal perfusion (e.g., NSAIDs, COX-2 inhibitors, ACE inhibitors).

K.S. was at high risk for developing radiocontrast-induced ATN. He was volume depleted, as evidenced by his admission BUN:SrCr ratio, which was >20:1. Second, it is very likely that K.S. had underlying diabetic nephropathy, as evidenced by his elevated admission SrCr. The presence of retinopathy, coronary artery disease, and peripheral vascular disease suggest long-term uncontrolled DM, a risk factor for nephropathy.

Prevention

16. **What strategies can be performed to prevent the occurrence of radiocontrast-induced ATN?**

Attempts have been made to minimize or prevent radiocontrast-induced ATN using a variety of approaches. Medullary vasodilation with dopamine infusions have generally led to disappointing results. Volume expansion, mannitol, and furosemide have been tried as a means of "flushing" radiocontrast from the kidney. *Volume expansion* is a rational approach to prevent renal dysfunction in this population because human and animal data have revealed dehydration as a major risk factor for developing radiocontrast nephropathy. Hypotonic saline (0.45% sodium chloride) prevents radiocontrast nephropathy, most likely because it stimulates renal prostaglandin secretion and causes afferent arteriole vasodilation. However, this action is attenuated by the administration of diuretics such as mannitol and furosemide. Possible explanations for this attenuation are that diuretics result in volume

Table 31-4 Proven Risk Factors for Developing Radiocontrast Media–Induced Acute Tubular Necrosis

Diabetic nephropathy
Chronic renal failure
Severe congestive heart failure
Volume depletion/hypotension
Dosage and frequency of contrast administration

depletion and increase oxygen demand in the medullary portion of the kidney when diuresis occurs.

Relatively small trials using the adenosine antagonist *theophylline* have recently demonstrated a renoprotective effect in patients who have underlying chronic kidney disease.[46,47] However, large-scale clinical trials are lacking. Although the use of calcium channel blockers theoretically seems rational to prevent contrast-induced ATN, there are limited clinical data.[48,49]

There has been recent interest in the use of *N-acetylcysteine (NAC)* and fenoldopam for the prevention of radiocontrast-induced ATN. NAC is a potent antioxidant that scavenges oxygen free radicals,[44] whereas fenoldopam is a selective dopamine 1 receptor agonist.[50] The data for NAC have consistently demonstrated at least a 40% decrease in the incidence of ATN in patients with underlying chronic renal insufficiency who are undergoing radiographic studies or cardiac catheterizations.[51–55] Another positive benefit of NAC is that it is a relatively inexpensive and innocuous agent (i.e., it has a very limited side-effect profile). Therefore, it appears to be unnecessary to limit its use to specific patient populations. In patients considered at high risk for developing radiocontrast-induced nephropathy (e.g., diabetes, pre-existing chronic kidney disease), the recommended dose of NAC is 600 mg PO BID, for a total of three doses before the procedure and one dose after the procedure, along with concomitant volume expansion with IV 0.45% or 0.9% saline.[56]

The data for *fenoldopam* are less clear at this time. Three small nonrandomized trials have demonstrated modest renoprotection in patients receiving radiocontrast for radiologic procedures.[57–59] However, fenoldopam is expensive, and its use requires admission to an intensive care unit for close patient monitoring. Given the paucity of clinical efficacy data and the added expense of therapy, the routine use of fenoldopam is not advocated. Figure 31-5 summarizes recommendations for the prevention of radiocontrast-induced ATN in high-risk populations. When possible, alternative imaging studies that do not require radiocontrast should be attempted. If this is not practical, the lowest effective dose of nonionic, low-osmolar radiocontrast media should be used. Concomitant drug therapy that can impair renal perfusion such as diuretics, NSAIDs, COX-2 inhibitors, ACE inhibitors, and ARBs should be discontinued 1 day before and 1 day after radiocontrast administration. Incidentally, metformin should also be discontinued before giving radiocontrast media and held for at least 48 hours because it can cause lactic acidosis if patients develop ARF.[60] If patients are receiving calcium channel blockers for underlying cardiovascular disease, no change in therapy is warranted. All patients should be well hydrated with hypotonic saline before and after radiocontrast administration.

17. What treatment options are available for established radiocontrast-induced ATN?

Unfortunately, few data exist regarding treatment of existing radiocontrast-induced ATN. The acute management largely involves supportive care that includes strict fluid and electrolyte management to prevent undue sequelae. Approximately 25% of patients will require temporary dialysis therapy; oliguric patients generally require long-term dialysis therapy. As already noted, attempts to convert oliguria to nonoliguria with furosemide and mannitol have been largely unsuccessful.

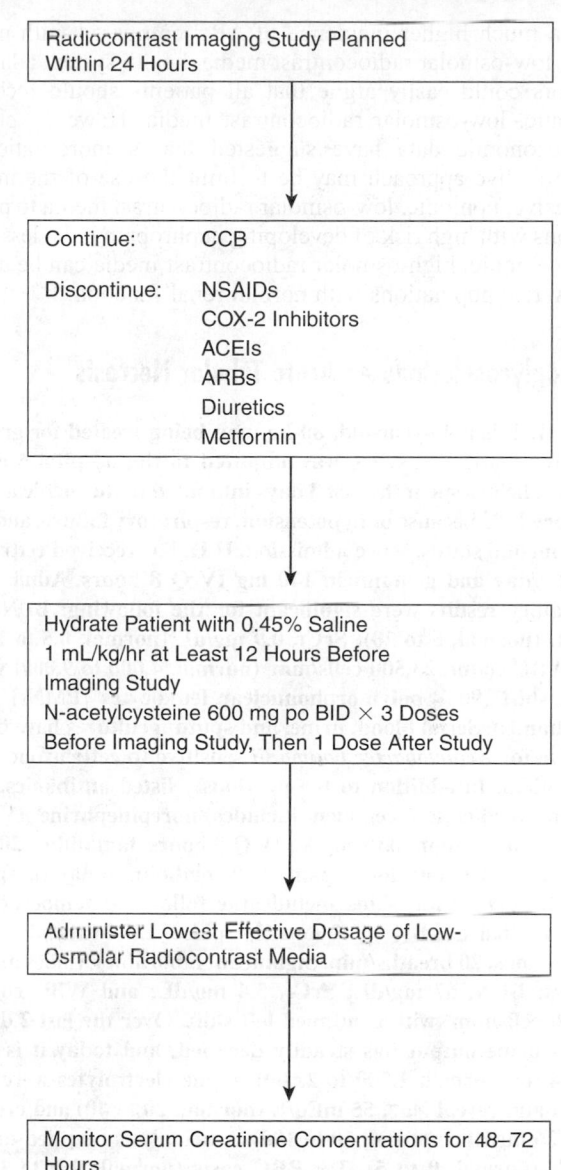

FIGURE 31-5 Prevention of radiocontrast-induced acute tubular necrosis in high-risk populations. ACEIs, angiotensin-converting enzyme inhibitors; ARBs, angiotensin II–receptor blockers; CCB, calcium channel blocker; COX-2, cyclooxygenase-2; NSAIDs, nonsteroidal anti-inflammatory drugs.

18. Given the high incidence of ARF caused by ionic, high-osmolar radiocontrast media, should nonionic, low-osmolar radiocontrast media be administered to all patients?

This is a cost-to-benefit issue because the relative costs of similar volumes of ionic, high-osmolar radiocontrast media compared with nonionic, low-osmolar radiocontrast are approximately $5 and $50 to $100, respectively. Although this is a substantial difference if one looks only at the drug acquisition cost, a more global perspective should be considered when comparing total costs of care. For example, ARF can easily extend hospitalization by at least 3 to 5 days at the cost of $1,500 per day. This does not include costs associated with dialysis, nephrology consultations, or ICU placement. Because ionic, high-osmolar radiocontrast media are associated with a much higher incidence of ARF compared with non-ionic, low-osmolar radiocontrast media, health system administrators could easily argue that all patients should receive nonionic, low-osmolar radiocontrast media. However, pharmacoeconomic data have suggested that a more rational cost-effective approach may be to limit the use of the more expensive, nonionic, low-osmolar radiocontrast media to populations with high risk of developing nephropathy; the less expensive, ionic, high-osmolar radiocontrast media can be used in low-risk populations with normal renal function.[61]

Aminoglycoside-Induced Acute Tubular Necrosis

19. H.H. is a 43-year-old, 80-kg man being treated for gram-negative septic shock. He was admitted to the hospital 6 days ago, but he has spent the last 3 days intubated in the medical respiratory ICU because of hypotension, respiratory failure, and altered mental status. Since admission, H.H. has received ceftriaxone 2 g/day and gentamicin 140 mg IV Q 8 hours. Admission laboratory results were significant for the following: BUN, 13 mg/dL (normal, 5 to 20); SrCr, 0.9 mg/dL (normal, 0.5 to 1.2); and WBC count, 23,500 cells/mm³ (normal, 4,000 to 9,000) with a left shift (90% polymorphonuclear leukocytes [PMNs] and 12% bands). Serial blood, urine, and sputum cultures have been positive for *Acinetobacter baumanii* sensitive to ceftriaxone and gentamicin. In addition to the previously listed antibiotics, his current medication regimen includes norepinephrine IV 18 g/min, pancuronium 0.02 mg/kg IV Q 3 hours, famotidine 20 mg IV Q 12 hours, and lorazepam IV 2 mg/hour. Today (hospital day 7), H.H.'s vital signs include the following: temperature, 101.5°F (38.6°C); BP, 90/40 mm Hg; pulse, 135 beats/min; and respirations, 20 breaths/min. Significant laboratory values are as follows: BUN, 67 mg/dL; SrCr, 5.4 mg/dL; and WBC count, 16,700 cells/mm³ with continued left shift. Over the last 2 days, H.H.'s urine output has steadily declined, and today it is 700 mL/24 hr (normal, 1,500 to 2,500). Urine electrolytes were obtained and reveal Na⁺, 55 mEq/L (normal, 20 to 40) and creatinine, 26 mg/dL (normal, 50 to 100). A urinalysis revealed many WBCs (normal, 0 to 5), 3% RBC casts (normal, 0% to 1%), brush-border cells (normal, negative), and granular casts (normal, negative) with an osmolality of 250 mOsm/kg (normal, 400 to 600). Serum gentamicin concentrations obtained with the last dose reveal a peak of 15 mg/dL (normal, 6 to 10) and a trough of 9.1 mg/dL (normal, <2.0). Given the history and laboratory data, what is the likely source of H.H.'s ARF?

[SI units: BUN, 4.6 and 24 mmol/L (normal, 1.8 to 7.1); SrCr, 79.6 and 477.4 mol/L (normal 44.2 to 106); WBC count, 23.5 and 16.7 × 10⁹ (normal, 4.0 to 9.0); urine creatinine, 2,298 μmol/L (normal, 4,419 to −8,838)]

The source of ARF in this situation is likely multifactorial (see Table 31-1). First, H.H. is experiencing diminished renal perfusion from profound hypotension and septic shock. As a result, he is receiving high-dose norepinephrine, a potent vasopressor. Consequently, the combination of these variables reduces renal perfusion further, resulting in prolonged renal ischemia. Second, H.H. has received 1 week of gentamicin, a well-known nephrotoxic antibiotic. The risk factors for developing aminoglycoside nephrotoxicity are listed in Table 31-5. The latest gentamicin trough concentration of 9.1 mg/L is far higher than the target value of <2 mg/L for a traditional three-times-daily dosing regimen. Given the laboratory data (see Table 31-2) and the clinical course of prolonged hy-

Table 31-5 Risk Factors for Developing Aminoglycoside Nephrotoxicity
Patient Factors
Elderly
Underlying renal disease
Dehydration
Hypotension/shock syndromes
Hepatorenal syndrome
Aminoglycoside Factors
Aminoglycoside choice: gentamicin > tobramycin > amikacin
Therapy >3 days
Multiple daily dosing
Serum trough >2 mg/L
Recent aminoglycoside therapy
Concomitant Drug Therapy
Furosemade
Amphotericin B
Vancomycin
Cisplatinum
Cyclosporine
Radiocontrast media
Forcarnet

potension, vasopressor, and aminoglycoside administration, nonoliguric ATN is the most likely diagnosis.

Presentation

20. How does aminoglycoside-induced ATN present, and what are the mechanisms of toxicity?

H.H. illustrates the typical presentation of aminoglycoside-induced nephrotoxicity. Generally, the onset occurs after 5 to 7 days of treatment and presents as a hypo-osmolar, nonoliguric renal failure with a slow rise in SrCr.[62] Because of the tubular necrosis that occurs, the urinalysis is often positive for low-molecular-weight proteins, tubular cellular casts, epithelial cells, WBCs, and brush-border cells.[63] H.H.'s plasma and urinary laboratory indices are consistent with those listed for ATN in Table 31-2.

The mechanism of aminoglycoside-induced ATN is complex. Approximately 5% of filtered aminoglycoside is actively reabsorbed by the proximal tubule cells. These agents are polycationic and bind to the negatively charged brush-border cells within the tubule lumen. Once attached, these agents undergo pinocytosis and enter the intracellular space, setting off complex biochemical events that result in the formation of myeloid bodies. With continued formation of myeloid bodies, the brush-border cells swell and burst, releasing large concentrations of aminoglycoside and lysosomal enzymes into the tubule lumen, thereby beginning a cascade of further tubular destruction.[62,64] The following rank order of nephrotoxicity has been collated from human and animal data: neomycin > gentamicin ≥tobramycin ≥amikacin ≥netilmicin > streptomycin.[63,64]

Extended-Interval Dosing

21. Is "extended-interval" aminoglycoside dosing less nephrotoxic than multiple daily dosing regimens?

Extended-interval aminoglycoside dosing entails the administration of one large daily aminoglycoside dose. This dosing scheme takes advantage of the concentration-dependent killing activity and postantibiotic effect observed with aminoglycosides while minimizing time-dependent toxicity. The net effect of this dosing scheme, purportedly, is greater efficacy with reduced toxicity. Aminoglycoside nephrotoxicity is a function of drug exposure, and it may be minimized with extended-interval dosing because of saturable uptake kinetics in the proximal tubule. That is, only a maximal amount of aminoglycoside is transported into the tubule cell, no matter how much aminoglycoside is present in the tubule. Consequently, once saturation occurs, the remaining aminoglycoside concentration passes through the proximal tubule without being absorbed, and is excreted in the urine. Accumulation is therefore averted.[65] This concept is supported by studies demonstrating that continuous-rate gentamicin infusions, which produce sustained low plasma concentrations, result in greater proximal tubule uptake and nephrotoxicity than extended-interval regimens. This is probably because the achieved drug concentrations are well below those required to saturate the uptake mechanism.[66] Extended-interval dosing results in very high peak concentrations to improve efficacy and generally undetectable trough concentrations before the next dose, thus minimizing accumulation.

At least 30 controlled clinical trials and 9 meta-analyses have compared the efficacy and toxicity of extended-interval aminoglycoside dosing with conventional multiple daily dosing regimens. Many of these meta-analyses concluded that less nephrotoxicity was associated with extended-interval aminoglycoside dosing. However, given the inherent biases of meta-analyses, these results must be interpreted cautiously. For example, meta-analyses combine results from different clinical trials, which can differ in patient population, severity of illness scores, degree of underlying renal dysfunction, and dosing regimen and duration of therapy. Most of the clinical trials did not show a clinically or statistically significant difference in efficacy or toxicity between regimens. The most current recommendations suggest that patients should receive extended-interval aminoglycoside dosing unless they have specific contraindications.[67]

In summary, extended-interval aminoglycoside dosing appears to result in similar or greater efficacy, with similar or reduced toxicity. This dosing schedule is also less costly when considering therapeutic drug monitoring, preparation, and administration costs. One study calculated that extended-interval dosing costs are approximately one-half those of multiple daily dosing.[68] The cost savings is even greater if ARF is avoided.[69]

Amphotericin B–Induced Nephrotoxicity

22. H.H. remained febrile for the next several days despite being covered by broad-spectrum antibiotics. His ceftriaxone and gentamicin were stopped 3 days ago, and imipenem 500 mg IV Q 12 hours was started. Today, he is febrile to 102.3°F (39°C). Blood fungal cultures, which were obtained 5 days ago, are positive for *Candida tropicalis,* sensitive only to amphotericin B (AmB). His current serum chemistries are significant for a BUN of 72 mg/dL (normal, 5 to 20), SrCr of 6.1 mg/dL (normal, 0.5 to 1.2), and a WBC count of 17,500 cells/mm³ (normal, 4,000 to 9,000) with a continued left shift. All other laboratories are noncontributory. His urine output has remained around 600 mL/day for the last 3 days. Are there any concerns with administering AmB to H.H. if he still remains in ATN?

[SI units: BUN, 25.7 mmol/L (normal, 1.8 to 7.1); SrCr, 539.2 mol/L (normal, 44.2 to 106); WBC count, 17.5 × 10⁹ (normal, 4.0 to 9.0)]

AmB is considered the drug of choice for the treatment of systemic fungal infections. However, its use is associated with severe nephrotoxicity, which is manifested by a marked decrease in GFR, azotemia, loss of tubular concentrating ability, renal tubular acidosis, and potassium and magnesium wasting. The incidence of AmB nephrotoxicity has been estimated to be as high as 80%.[70] The exact mechanism of AmB nephrotoxicity is not fully understood, but acute renal vasoconstriction is known to occur, and it appears that the distal tubule epithelial cells are preferentially damaged. Nephrotoxicity likely develops because AmB binds to the sterols in the renal vasculature and epithelial cells. This binding alters the cellular membrane permeability and may stimulate cytokine release and other biochemical reactions within the tubule, resulting in eventual cellular death.[71] Fortunately, preventive therapies such as sodium loading and the development of lipid-based AmB products have helped minimize AmB nephrotoxicity. Because H.H. remains in ATN, sodium loading with normal saline is contraindicated because of the potential for volume overload. Therefore, administration of a lipid-based AmB product is indicated.

23. How do lipid-based AmB products reduce nephrotoxicity?

The exact mechanism(s) by which lipid-based AmB reduces nephrotoxicity is unknown. Five potential mechanisms have been postulated.[72] One theory suggests that after systemic administration, the lipid-based AmB is taken up by macrophages, which are usually present at the fungal infection site. The macrophages liberate the AmB from the lipid encasing and release it preferentially at the site of infection, thus preventing systemic AmB exposure.[73] A second theory suggests that the AmB encapsulated liposomes have a stronger affinity for fungal ergosterol than human ergosterol, and hence are more likely to translocate at fungal cells. Studies have demonstrated that a lipid-based AmB preparation remained intact until it attached to a fungal cell membrane.[74] Third, in vitro data have suggested that lipid-based AmB products do not stimulate the release of the toxic cytokines' tumor necrosis factor-α and interleukin-1, which are associated with standard AmB preparations.[75] Other investigators have theorized that fungal cells produce extracellular phospholipases that hydrolyze the lipid encasing, thus releasing AmB at the site of fungal infection.[76] Finally, AmB that is bound to high-density lipoprotein cholesterol (HDL-C) may be less nephrotoxic compared with unbound drug or those that bound to low-density lipoprotein cholesterol (LDL-C) because there are relatively few HDL-C receptors in the kidney.[77] The mechanism for reduced nephrotoxicity is probably different for each of the different lipid-based formulations, and nephrotoxicity rates vary from 8% to 28%, depending on the product.[72]

Drug-Induced Acute Interstitial Nephritis

Drug-induced AIN accounts for approximately 1% to 3% of all ARF cases. A variety of antibiotics, such as penicillins, cephalosporins, quinolones, sulfonamides, and rifampin, as well as NSAIDs have been implicated as major causes of drug-induced AIN. The pathophysiology of this reaction is not well understood. However, it is suspected that either humoral or cell-mediated immune mechanisms or both are involved.[78] Humoral immune reactions occur within minutes to hours of drug exposure and involve the drug or its metabolite acting as a hapten that binds to host proteins, making them antigenic. The drug-protein antigens become lodged in the renal tubules, which initiate the inflammatory cascade. Cell-mediated injury can occur days to weeks after drug exposure and is identified by the presence of mononuclear inflammation and the lack of detectable immune complexes. This suggests a delayed hypersensitivity rather than a direct cytotoxic effect from a given drug. Both immune mechanisms probably contribute to the development of drug-induced AIN.

Penicillin-Induced AIN

24. **J.S. is a 50-year-old woman who developed a right-hand cellulitis 3 days after a car door was closed on her hand. She was admitted to the hospital, where blood and wound cultures were found to be positive for methicillin-sensitive *Staphylococcus aureus*. She received 2 full days of nafcillin 2 g IV Q 4 hours before being discharged to complete a 14-day course with dicloxacillin 500 mg PO QID. Ten days after discharge, J.S. returned to the emergency department complaining of malaise, fever, diffuse rash, hematuria, and reduced urine output. The following laboratory values were significant: BUN, 39 mg/dL (normal, 5 to 20); SrCr, 2.3 mg/dL (normal, 0.5 to 1.2); and WBC count, 18,500 cells/mm³ (normal, 4,000 to 9,000) with 18% eosinophils. The urinalysis was positive for elevated specific gravity, WBCs, RBCs, eosinophiluria, and a FE$_{Na+}$ of 3%. What are the objective data that suggest drug-induced AIN?**

[SI units: BUN, 13.9 mmol/L (normal, 1.8 to 7.1); SrCr, 203.3 mol/L (normal, 44.2 to 106); WBC count, 18.5 × 10⁹ (normal, 4.0 to 9.0)]

J.S.'s onset of symptoms are suggestive of drug-induced AIN. As illustrated by this case, the median onset of penicillin-induced AIN generally occurs 6 to 10 days after drug exposure. Hallmark subjective symptoms of AIN include fever, macular rash, and malaise. Fever is present in nearly all patients with AIN, whereas rash occurs in 25% to 50% of patients. J.S.'s objective laboratory data that suggest AIN include azotemia, elevated SrCr, proteinuria, cellular urinary sediment, eosinophilia, and eosinophiluria. Her FE$_{Na+}$ of 3% suggests intrinsic renal disease and her eosinophiluria and eosinophilia indicate an immune-mediated allergic reaction. Drug-induced AIN is generally nonoliguric, but oliguria can develop in severe cases of AIN.

25. **How should J.S.'s drug-induced AIN be treated?**

The dicloxacillin should be stopped immediately because most patients recover normal kidney function once the offending agent is discontinued. General supportive measures that maintain fluid and electrolyte balance are necessary. Corticosteroids have been used with variable results to shorten the duration of ARF, but no clinical guidelines have been developed to delineate when to administer them and for how long. Some administer prednisone 1 mg/kg for 7 days and then gradually taper the dose over the next several weeks. The response to corticosteroids may be delayed or absent in some patients. Dialysis may be needed in oliguric patients, but it is usually not required for nonoliguric patients. The clinician should document J.S.'s allergic reaction to penicillins because repeated exposure is likely to result in similar reactions.

POSTRENAL ACUTE RENAL FAILURE

Any condition that results in the obstruction of urine flow at any level of the urinary tract is termed postrenal ARF. Common causes of postrenal ARF are stone formation, underlying malignancies of the prostate or cervix, prostatic hypertrophy, or bilateral ureter strictures. Conditions that result in bladder outlet obstruction (e.g., prostatic hypertrophy) are the most common causes of postrenal ARF. The onset of signs and symptoms is generally gradual; it often presents as decreased force of urine stream, dribbling, or polyuria. Drugs can also result in insoluble crystal formation in the urine and should be included in the differential diagnosis.[79]

Nephrolithiasis

Kidney stones are relatively common and affect 5% to 10% of North Americans.[80] A strong genetic predisposition appears to exist in this population. Recent epidemiologic data have found that men with stones were three times more likely to have parents or siblings with a history significant for stones.[81] In addition to genetics, other underlying risk factors exist for stone development (Table 31-6). Nephrolithiasis has a male:female incidence of 3:1, and whites are twice as likely as blacks to develop stones. Kidney stones generally consist of uric acid, cystine, struvite (also called magnesium ammonium phosphate or triple phosphate nephrolithiasis), and calcium salts. Of these, calcium stones are by far the most prevalent.

Calcium Stones

Calcium nephrolithiasis constitutes approximately 70% to 80% of all kidney stones,[81] with calcium oxalate and calcium phosphate stones making up the majority of these. Genetic factors appear to play an important role in the development of calcium nephrolithiasis; the stereotypical patient is a male in his third to fifth decade of life. Other risk factors for developing calcium nephrolithiasis are low urine output, hypercalciuria, hyperoxaluria, hypocitraturia and hyperuricosuria, and distal renal tubular acidosis. Generally, more than one of these conditions is present simultaneously.

Struvite Stones

Magnesium ammonium phosphate crystallization, termed struvite stones, represent the second most common type of nephrolithiasis (approximately 2% to 20% of cases). Struvite stones can result in significantly high morbidity and mortality because they tend to recur and can result in irreversible kidney damage.[82] These stones often fill the renal collecting ducts and assume a "staghorn" appearance. Struvite stones generally result when existing stones are colonized with *Proteus,* a bacteria that produces urease, an enzyme that hydrolyzes urea

Table 31-6	Risk Factors for Nephrolithiasis
Low urine volume	
Hypercalciuria	
Hyperoxaluria	
Hyperuricosuria	
Hypercitruria	
Chronically low or high urinary pH	

and alkalinizes the urine. The alkaline environment promotes the formation of insoluble crystals of ammonium, calcium, and phosphate. In vitro, simply alkalinizing the urine results in the immediate precipitation of amorphous struvite stones.[82] Populations at risk for developing struvite stones include obese women, patients with frequent urinary tract infections or pyelonephritis, and patients with genitourinary tract abnormalities that promote bacterial colonization or make eradication of infection difficult. However, the most problematic form of stone disease develops in paralyzed patients with indwelling Foley catheters. Recurrent nephrolithiasis is one of the most common causes of death in spinal cord injury patients.[83] Treatment of struvite stones can consist of surgical intervention; prolonged courses of broad-spectrum antibiotics; administration of acetohydroxamic acid, which inhibits bacterial urease; or shock-wave lithotripsy.[82]

Uric Acid Stones

Uric acid stones commonly occur in patients whose uric acid metabolism is altered because of various medical conditions. In particular, patients with gout and those receiving chemotherapy are prone to these stones. This topic is discussed further in Chapter 42, Gout and Hyperuricemia.

Cystine Stones

Cystinuria is a rare autosomal-recessive hereditary disorder of amino acid transport in the renal tubules that results in the urinary excretion of large amounts of cystine. These stones form when the cystine excretion rate exceeds the urinary solubility limit. The calculi form staghorns in the renal tubules and can cause urinary obstruction, infection, and ARF. Therapy of cystine stones is targeted at reducing the urinary cystine excretion while increasing its urinary solubility. This can be accomplished by diet modification, increased fluid intake, urine alkalization, and drug therapy.[84] Low-sodium diets decrease cystine excretion, and restriction of methionine, a cystine precursor, may reduce cystine excretion. However, it may also result in depletion of other important amino acids. To decrease the urinary cystine concentrations, urine volume should be increased by maintaining a fluid intake of >4 L/day. The solubility of cystine in urine also can be increased by alkalinizing the urine. Pharmacologic therapy is indicated when the above nondrug measures have failed. Drug therapy is targeted at increasing the urinary solubility of cystine, which can be achieved by forming a thiol-cysteine disulfide bond. D-Penicillamine and tiopronin are the most commonly used drugs, although tiopronin appears to be better tolerated than D-penicillamine.

Presentation and Treatment

26. T.C. is a 48-year-old man who presents to the emergency department complaining of sharp flank pain radiating to the groin, gross hematuria, and dysuria. He states that these symptoms have been present for 4 hours and that they are similar to previous episodes of calcium nephrolithiasis he has had. Serum chemistries are ordered and are significant only for a BUN of 34 mg/dL (normal, 5 to 20) and a SrCr of 1.5 mg/dL (normal, 0.5 to 1.2), which are up from his baseline values of 15 and 0.9 mg/dL, respectively. A urine sample was obtained and visualized with microscopy. It was determined that T.C. passed a kidney stone, based on the large amount of calcium oxalate crystals found in the urinary sediment. On questioning, he admits that he has not been drinking much fluid over the past week owing to a busy

work schedule, and his urine volume has been markedly lower than usual. What are the common subjective and objective data that suggest nephrolithiasis, and how can this be prevented from occurring in the future?

[SI units: BUN, 12.1 and 5.3 mmol/L (normal, 1.8 to 7.1); SrCr, 132.6 and 79.5 mol/L, respectively (normal, 44.2 to 106)]

T.C. illustrates the classic presentation of nephrolithiasis: acute, severe flank pain that radiates to the groin. It is usually accompanied by gross or microscopic hematuria, dysuria, or frequency. Fortunately, 90% of symptomatic calculi pass spontaneously, as in T.C.'s case, and invasive surgical treatment is rarely necessary.[85] The risk factors that predispose T.C. to stone recurrence include a previous episode of nephrolithiasis, age within the fourth decade, and decreased fluid intake and urine output.

Preventive measures should be taken by T.C. to reduce the likelihood of stone recurrence. Many randomized trials have demonstrated that nondrug and pharmacologic mechanisms can prevent stone formation. The most cost-effective way to prevent stone formation is to increase fluid intake. A 5-year randomized study compared a "high fluid intake" group (>2 L/day) to one that had "normal" daily fluid intake (approximately 1 L/day). The results demonstrated a significantly longer time to stone recurrence (39 versus 25 months) in the "high fluid intake" group.[86] Dietary modifications remain controversial. Although it makes sense that limiting protein, calcium, and sodium intake should decrease the likelihood of recurrent nephrolithiasis, the data are conflicting.[87] Poor study designs that did not assess confounding variables such as fluid intake and oxalate restriction make the data difficult to interpret. In summary, a high calcium intake probably increases the risk of nephrolithiasis but only in patients with absorptive hypercalciuria and not in normal patients.

Pharmacologic control of calcium oxalate stones has been tried with thiazide diuretics.[88] Thiazide diuretics promote calcium reabsorption in the distal tubule, which decreases the concentration in the lumen. Thiazides also may decrease intestinal calcium absorption in patients with absorptive hypercalciuria, although this remains unclear. Patients receiving thiazide diuretics should be sodium restricted because excessive sodium intake negates their hypocalciuric effect. Allopurinol has been used successfully to prevent recurrent calcium oxalate nephrolithiasis, presumably by inhibiting purine and uric acid metabolism.[88] Alkalization of the urine with potassium citrate and potassium-magnesium citrate also prevents recurrent calcium oxalate nephrolithiasis.[89]

T.C. should be instructed to drink at least 2 liters of fluid (approximately eight 8-ounce glasses) daily. Given his busy work schedule, a thiazide diuretic probably is not the most convenient option for T.C., and noncompliance is likely. Allopurinol 200 mg orally once daily is probably the most convenient preventive strategy for T.C., and data suggest it is effective in preventing recurrent nephrolithiasis. Alternatively, urinary alkalinization with potassium citrate or potassium-magnesium citrate is likely to be beneficial for T.C., but it may be less convenient because it needs to be administered two to four times daily.

Drug-Induced Nephrolithiasis

27. Can drugs crystallize in the urine and cause ARF?

Many commonly prescribed drugs are insoluble in urine and crystallize in the distal tubule (Table 31-7). Risk factors

Table 31-7 Commonly Used Drugs That Cause Crystal-Induced Acute Renal Failure

Acyclovir
Sulfonamides
Triamterene
Methotrexate
Indinavir

that predispose patients to crystalluria include severe volume contraction, underlying renal dysfunction, or acidotic or alkalotic urinary pH.[90] In conditions of renal hypoperfusion, high concentrations of drug become stagnant in the tubule lumen. Drugs that are weak acids (e.g., methotrexate, sulfonamides) precipitate in acidic urine; drugs that are weak bases (e.g., indinavir, other protease inhibitors) precipitate in alkaline urine. Prevention of crystal-induced ARF is targeted at dosage adjustment for patients with underlying renal dysfunction, volume expansion to increase urinary output, and urine alkalization. Similarly, for established crystal-induced ARF, the above general supportive measures of urinary alkalization and volume expansion should be performed. Dialysis may be necessary in a small percentage of patients. Fortunately with appropriate pharmacotherapy, crystal-induced ARF is usually reversible without long-term sequelae.

SUPPORTIVE MANAGEMENT OF ACUTE RENAL FAILURE

28. What is the "supportive management" of ARF?

Despite years of study, there remains no pharmacologic "cure" for ARF. Therefore, supportive therapy is directed at preventing its morbidity and mortality. This is achieved by close patient monitoring; strict fluid and electrolyte management; treatment of life-threatening conditions, such as pulmonary edema, hyperkalemia, and metabolic acidosis; avoidance of nephrotoxic drugs; and the initiation of dialysis or continuous renal replacement therapies (CRRTs).

Clinicians should closely monitor patient vital signs (e.g., weight, temperature, BP, pulse, respirations, and fluid intake and output) at least once every shift. Daily weights can forewarn the clinician of edematous weight gain. The patient's medication profile should be reviewed daily to assess for appropriate dosage adjustment in renal dysfunction. Because estimation of Cl_{Cr} is difficult in patients with rapidly changing renal function, therapeutic drug monitoring should be performed when using drugs with narrow therapeutic indices. When possible, nephrotoxic drugs should be avoided, but this may be difficult in patients who are septic or hypotensive and require nephrotoxic antibiotics and vasopressors. Preventive measures to reduce the likelihood of ARF should be used, such as ensuring adequate hydration, using dosing strategies or products that are associated with less nephrotoxicity, and avoiding drug therapy combinations that enhance nephrotoxicity (e.g., NSAIDs, aminoglycosides). If ARF patients are receiving total parenteral nutrition, close monitoring of serum chemistries is needed to identify fluid and electrolyte abnormalities.

Supportive drug therapy may be used to reduce ARF symptoms. As previously discussed, diuretics currently have no role in preventing ARF progression or reducing mortality, but they can prevent complications, such as pulmonary and peripheral edema, and they may prevent tubular obstruction from ATN.

The patient's volume status should be assessed daily, and fluids should be adjusted based on laboratory chemistries, urine output, and gastrointestinal and insensible losses. Dietary sodium restriction of 2 to 2.5 g/day should be instituted to prevent edema formation.

Diuretics for Edema in ARF

If edema occurs, intravenous furosemide is preferred because of its potency and pulmonary vasodilation properties. Oral furosemide therapy should be avoided because gut edema may limit its bioavailability. *Torsemide,* a relatively new loop diuretic, has excellent oral bioavailability and is unaffected by gut edema. Unfortunately, its cost is approximately 20 times that of furosemide, making it cost-prohibitive in many medical centers. Torsemide should be reserved for patients with demonstrated bioavailability problems with furosemide. The dosage of diuretic needed is highly patient specific, especially in those with frank proteinuria, glomerulonephritis, or the nephrotic syndrome. Furosemide is highly protein bound, and thus binds to filtered protein, which negates its pharmacologic effect on the kidneys. Combinations of loop and thiazide diuretics may be needed in ARF patients if they become diuretic resistant. This combination acts synergistically to block sodium and water reabsorption in both Henle's loop and the distal convoluted tubule. Other alternatives include continuous loop diuretic infusions, such as furosemide 1 mg/kg per hour. The infusion rate should not exceed 4 mg/minute because these rates are associated with ototoxicity, especially when given in combination with aminoglycoside antibiotics.[91] Close monitoring of potassium, magnesium, and calcium is necessary when giving large doses of loop diuretics.

Hyperkalemia commonly occurs in patients with ARF because potassium homeostasis is regulated by the kidneys. Acute therapy of hyperkalemia is discussed in Chapter 12, Fluid and Electrolyte Disorders. In cases in which conventional pharmacologic treatment is not feasible, emergency hemodialysis should be performed.

Metabolic acidosis is a common manifestation of ARF because the kidneys are responsible for excreting organic acids. As GFR declines to <30 mL/minute, organic acids accumulate and clinical symptoms can occur. Severe metabolic acidosis should be corrected with dialysis, but early initiation of oral sodium bicarbonate may prolong or obviate the need for dialysis.

Extracorporeal Continuous Renal Replacement Therapy

Renal replacement therapy is not always indicated in ARF. It is reserved for patients with severe acid-base disorders, fluid overload, hyperkalemia, symptomatic uremia, or drug intoxications. RRT can be divided into intermittent hemodialysis or CRRTs such as continuous peritoneal dialysis or extracorporeal CRRT. The decision to use one over the other is most often decided by the nephrologist's experience and comfort level. Extracorporeal CRRT differs from peritoneal and hemodialysis in its mechanism of solute removal; dialysis modalities rely exclusively on solute diffusion across a semipermeable membrane, whereas CRRT relies primarily on convective ultrafiltrate production. This discussion will be limited to extracorporeal CRRT therapies. (See Chapter 33, Renal Dialysis, for a complete overview of peritoneal and hemodialysis.)

Not all *extracorporeal CRRT* is alike; many variations exist and include modalities such as continuous arteriovenous

Table 31-8   Comparison of Extracorporeal Continuous Renal Replacement Therapies

Parameter	Continuous Venovenous Hemofiltration (CVVH)	Continuous Arteriovenous Hemofiltration (CAVH)	Continuous Venovenous Hemodialysis (CVVHD)	Continuous Venovenous Hemodiafiltration (CVVHDF)
Volume control in hypotensive patients	Good	Variable	Good	Good
Solute control in highly catabolic patients	Adequate	Inadequate	Adequate	Adequate
Blood flow rates in hypotensive patients	Adequate	Poor	Adequate	Adequate
Ease of drug dosing	Published recommendations	Difficult	Difficult	Difficult
Dialytic solute clearance	None	None	Moderate	Moderate
Convective solute clearance	Good	Good	Minimal	Moderate
Corresponding GFR (mL/min)	15-17	10-15	17-21	25-26
Blood pump required	Yes	No	Yes	Yes
Replacement fluid required	Yes	Yes	Yes	Yes
Pharmacy expense	High	High	High	High

GFR, glomerular filtration rate.
Adapted with permission from reference 93.

hemofiltration (CAVH), continuous venovenous hemofiltration (CVVH), continuous venovenous hemodialysis (CVVHD), and continuous venovenous hemodiafiltration (CVVHDF).[92] Differences between these modalities are illustrated in Table 31-8.[93] Drug dosing can be difficult in patients receiving these therapies, especially in those who are undergoing both dialysis and hemofiltration modalities (i.e., CVVHDF).

CAVH and CVVH are CRRT modalities that rely solely on convective solute removal. Convection is simply the movement of water and solutes across a high-flux dialyzer or hemofilter. Because it does not depend on the molecular weight (MW) of a given solute, small solutes (MW, <500 D) and middle MW solutes (MW, 500 to 15,000 D) are removed to the same extent if they fit through the membrane pore. Drugs and solutes <15,000 D are removed very well. Most penicillin, cephalosporin, and aminoglycoside antibiotics have MWs <500 D, and vancomycin's MW is 1,450 D. Continuous convective modalities are much better than dialysis for middle molecule and low-molecular-weight protein removal. CRRT is also better able to maintain a constant total body water volume. These therapies allow for a more gradual removal of large fluid volumes (3 to 5 L/day), which is not possible with conventional dialysis therapies.

Continuous Arteriovenous Hemofiltration (CAVH)

CAVH was the first extracorporeal therapy developed in the late 1970s. In this technique, a patient's blood is accessed through an artery and systemic BP and cardiac output are used as the driving forces to pump it through a high-flux hemofilter (Fig. 31-6).[93] Heparin is infused prefilter to prevent clot formation within the hemofilter. Blood flow rates are modest at 90 to 150 mL/minute. The mean arterial pressure (MAP) generates a transmembrane pressure (TMP) that filters plasma water and dissolved solutes (urea, creatinine, and drugs) across the hemofilter membrane.[94] Most of the filtered solution, or ultrafiltrate, is replaced by a solution that contains normal electrolyte concentrations. In volume-overloaded patients, a desired volume of plasma can be maintained by adjusting the volume of replacement fluid returned to the patient. The primary disadvantage of CAVH is that arterial access is often complicated by bleeding, aneurysm, ischemia, or embolism. Second, because blood flow and ultrafiltration depend on the MAP, volume and solute control become difficult in patients who become hypotensive or hypercatabolic.[95]

These disadvantages have been averted to a degree through the introduction of venovenous access and the addition of blood roller pumps.

Continuous Venovenous Hemofiltration (CVVH)

CVVH is a major advancement in extracorporeal CRRT. Venous access is obtained by inserting a dual-lumen catheter into a central vein (e.g., internal jugular or subclavian), and a roller pump provides a constant driving force for the blood to enter the hemofilter (Fig. 31-7).[94] The pressure generated by the roller pump results in continuous ultrafiltrate production. The blood flow rate is considerably increased by the roller pump, achieving rates of 100 to 200 mL/minute, which provides adequate ultrafiltrate, even in hypotensive or hypercatabolic patients. The ultrafiltrate production rate is generally started at 1 L/hour, which corresponds to a GFR of approximately 16 mL/minute. On exiting the hemofilter, the blood is returned through the second lumen of the venous access; a replacement solution containing normal electrolyte concentrations is also infused. Like CAVH, the patient's volume status can be controlled by adjusting the volume of replacement solution. A common example is a patient with volume overload of 20 L after surgery who develops ARF. A reasonable goal in such a patient is a net fluid loss of 5 L/day. If the CVVH ultrafiltration rate is 1 L/hour, the total daily volume of fluid removal will be 24 L/day. To achieve a net loss of 5 L/day, the volume of replacement solution needs to be 19 L. Hence, the replacement solution should be infused at 792 mL/hour. At this rate, if all variables remain constant, the patient will achieve euvolemia within 4 days.

Combined Modalities (CAVHDF, CVVHDF)

CRRT modalities that combine hemofiltration with dialysis (e.g., *CAVHDF, CVVHDF*) are technically more difficult to perform and require sophisticated equipment. Although the same ultrafiltration principles described previously apply, a dialysis component that promotes additional solute diffusion across the high-flux hemofilter is added. In the case of CVVHD, the process is initiated as for CVVH with blood flow rates of 50 to 200 mL/minute, but a dialysis solution is run countercurrent along the hemofilter at 10 to 35 mL/minute, resulting in diffusion of solutes. This makes drug dosing extremely difficult because clinicians must account for both diffusive and convective drug removal.

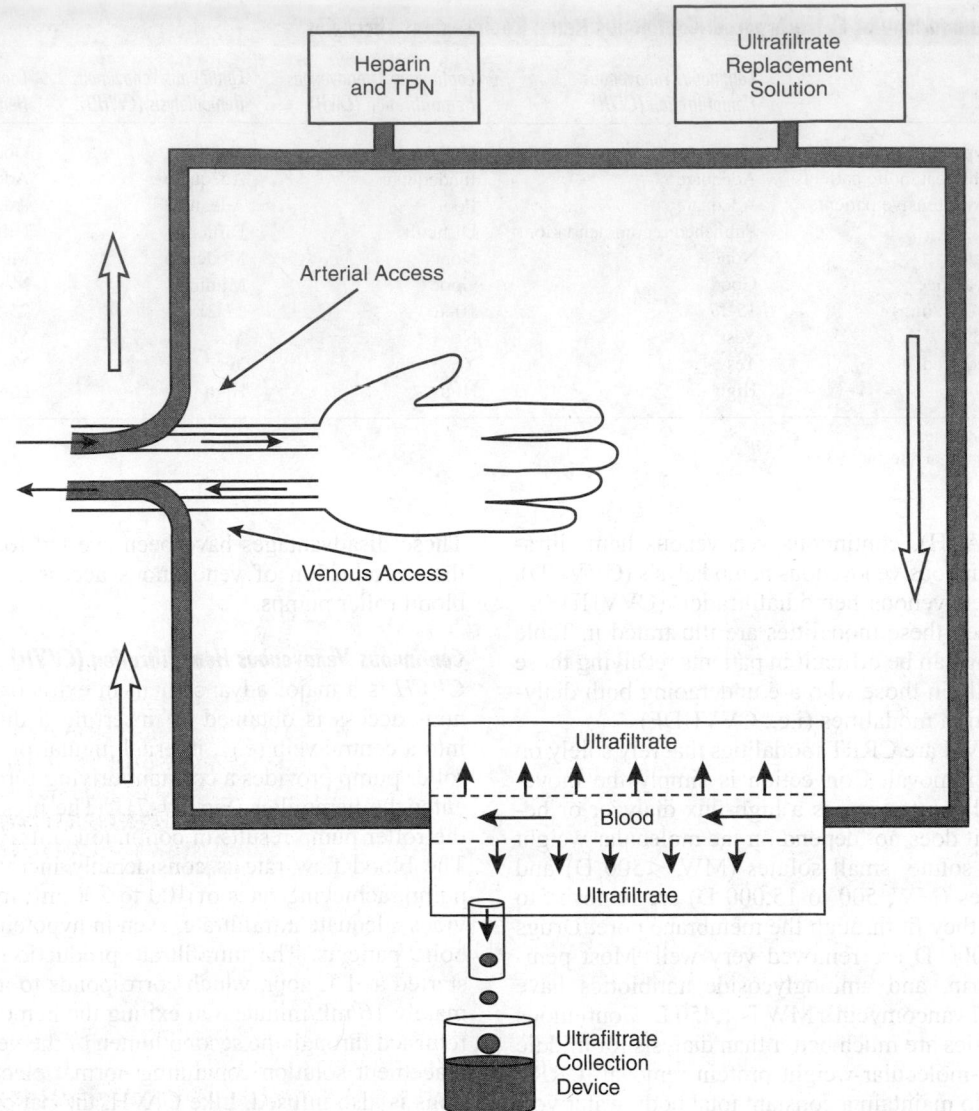

FIGURE 31-6 Schematic of continuous arteriovenous hemofiltration (CAVH). An arterial catheter is placed where blood travels through the extracorporeal hemofilter circuit and returns to the body through a separate venous catheter. The patient's mean arterial pressure provides the hydrostatic pressure required for ultrafiltrate production; hence, hypotensive episodes result in little solute removal. Patients receiving CAVH are most often in the intensive care unit and often receive concomitant total parenteral nutrition. Heparin is infused prefilter to prevent clot formation within the circuit. The ultrafiltrate replacement solution is provided back to the patient at a rate that achieves a desired total body water volume. (Reproduced with permission from reference 93.)

Estimating Drug Removal

29. **Are there ways to calculate drug removal in extracorporeal CRRT modalities?**

Several good reviews exist for drug dosing in CRRT.[96–98] The principles for drug removal in hemofiltration are basically identical with those for removal in hemodialysis. For example, drugs with a small volume of distribution and low protein binding are removed readily by these modalities. The *sieving coefficient* (SC) of a drug is the non–protein-bound fraction of the drug that is in plasma. For example, an SC of 0.8 means that 80% of the drug is unbound in plasma. Drug SCs can be obtained from the literature or by measuring concentrations simultaneously in the prefilter blood and ultrafiltrate. The ratio of the ultrafiltrate concentration to plasma concentration is the SC. Drug clearance can be calculated by multiplying the SC by the ultrafiltration rate. For example, if a patient is receiving CVVH at an ultrafiltration rate of 1 L/hour, and he or she is receiving vancomycin (which has an SC of 0.8) 1 g/day, the vancomycin clearance while receiving CVVH is 0.8 × 1,000 mL/hour = 800 mL/hour or 13 mL/minute.

Calculating drug clearance is much more difficult in hemodiafiltration modalities (CAVHDF, CVVHDF) because both convection and diffusion account for drug clearance and it is difficult to precisely predict drug clearance. The use of SCs can be useful for small-molecular-weight drugs, but the accuracy declines with larger drug molecules like vancomycin.[99] When possible, therapeutic drug monitoring should be performed to maintain therapeutic concentrations and to maximize drug therapy.

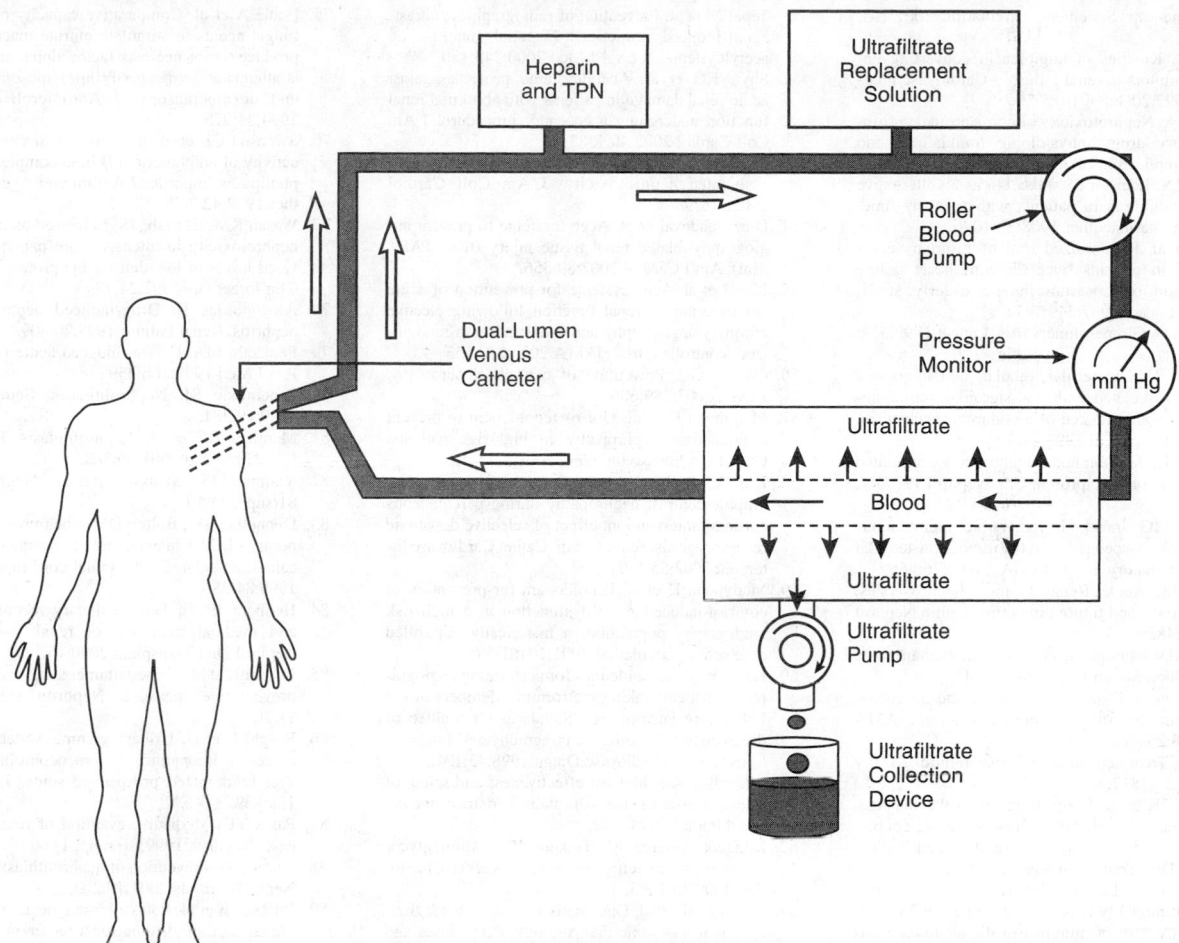

FIGURE 31-7 Schematic of continuous venovenous hemofiltration (CVVH). Blood is accessed by a dual-lumen catheter in a central vein and is pumped through the extracorporeal circuit by a roller blood pump. The blood pump maintains a constant hydrostatic pressure to create ultrafiltration, even in hypotensive conditions. Patients receiving CVVH are most often in the intensive care unit and often receive concomitant parenteral nutrition. Heparin is infused prefilter to prevent clot formation within the circuit. The ultrafiltrate replacement solution is provided back to the patient through a second venous catheter port at a rate that achieves a desired total body water volume. (Reproduced with permission from reference 93.)

REFERENCES

1. Singri N et al. Acute renal failure. JAMA 2003;289:747.
2. Vijayan A et al. Acute renal failure: prevention and nondialytic therapy. Semin Dial 1998;18:523.
3. Kaufman J et al. Community-acquired acute renal failure. Am J Kidney Dis 1991;17:191.
4. Liano F et al. Outcomes in acute renal failure. Semin Nephrol 1998;18:541.
5. Levy EM et al. The effect of acute renal failure on mortality: a cohort analysis. JAMA 1996;275:1489.
6. Guerin C et al. Initial versus delayed acute renal failure in the intensive care unit. A multicenter prospective epidemiological study. Rhone-Alpes Area Study Group on Acute Renal Failure. Am J Respir Crit Care Med 2000;161:872.
7. Turney JH. Why is mortality persistently high in acute renal failure? Lancet 1990;335:971.
8. Woodrow G et al. Cause of death in acute renal failure. Nephrol Dial Trans 1992;7:230.
9. Brivet FG et al. Acute renal failure in intensive care units: causes, outcome and prognostic factors of hospital mortality: a prospective, multicenter study. Crit Care Med 1996;24:192.
10. Liano F et al. Epidemiology of acute renal failure: a prospective, multicenter, community-based study.

Madrid Acute Renal Failure Study Group. Kidney Int 1996;50:811.
11. de Mendonca A et al. Acute renal failure in the ICU: risk factors and outcome evaluated by the SOFA score. Intensive Care Med 2000;26:915.
12. Chertow GM et al. Independent association between acute renal failure and mortality following cardiac surgery. Am J Med 1998;104:343.
13. Pruchnicki MC et al. Acute renal failure in hospitalized patients: Part I. Ann Pharmacother 2002; 36:1261.
14. Esson ML. Diagnosis and treatment of acute tubular necrosis. Ann Intern Med 2002;137:744.
15. Dowling TC et al. Comparison of iothalamate clearance methods for measuring GFR. Pharmacotherapy 1999;19:943.
16. Andreev E et al. A rise in plasma creatinine that is not a sign of renal failure: which drugs can be responsible? J Intern Med 1999;246:247.
17. Cockcroft DW, Gault MH. Prediction of creatinine clearance from serum creatinine. Nephron 1976;16:31.
18. O'Connell MB et al. Accuracy of 2- and 8-hour urine collection for measuring creatinine clearance

in the hospitalized elderly. Pharmacotherapy 1993; 13:135.
19. Jellife RW et al. A computer program for estimation of creatinine clearance from unstable serum creatinine concentration. Math Biosci 1972;14:17.
20. Chiou WL et al. A new simple rapid method to monitor renal function based on pharmacokinetic considerations of endogenous creatinine. Res Commun Chem Pathol Pharmacol 1975;10:15.
21. Behrend T et al. Acute renal failure in the cardiac care unit: etiologies, outcomes, and prognostic factors. Kidney Int 1999;56(1):238.
22. Brater DC. Antiinflammatory agents and renal function. Semin Arthritis Rheum 2002;32 (3 suppl 1):33.
23. Whelton A. Nephrotoxicity of nonsteroidal antiinflammatory drugs: physiologic foundations and clinical implications. Am J Med 1999;106(5B):13S.
24. Gertz BJ. A comparison of adverse renovascular experiences among osteoarthritis patients treated with rofecoxib and comparator non-selective nonsteroidal anti-inflammatory agents. Curr Med Res Opin 2002;18:82.
25. Schoolwerth AC et al. Renal considerations in angiotensin converting enzyme inhibitor therapy:

AHA Scientific Statement. Circulation 2001;104: 1985.

26. Sica DA. Kinetics of angiotensin converting enzyme inhibitors in renal failure. J Cardiovasc Pharmacol 1992;20(suppl 10):S13.

27. Whelton A. Nephrotoxicity of non-steroidal anti-inflammatory drugs: physiologic foundations and clinical implications. Am J Med 1999;106:13S.

28. Esmail ZN, Loewen PS. Losartan as an alternative to ACE inhibitors in patients with renal dysfunction. Ann Pharmacother 1998;32:1096.

29. Pitt B et al. Randomized trial of losartan versus captopril in patients over 65 with heart failure (Evaluation of Losartan in the Elderly study, ELITE). Lancet 1997;349:747.

30. Couser WG. Glomerulonephritis. Lancet 1999;353: 1509.

31. Ravnskov U. Glomerular, tubular, and interstitial nephritis associated with non-steroidal antiinflammatory drugs. Evidence of a common mechanism. Br J Clin Pharmacol 1999;47:203.

32. MacKay K. Membranous nephropathy associated with the use of flurbiprofen. Clin Nephrol 1997;47: 279.

33. Radford MG Jr. et al. Reversible membranous nephropathy associated with the use of nonsteroidal anti-inflammatory drugs. JAMA 1996;276:466.

34. Paller MS. Acute Renal Failure: Controversies, clinical trials, and future directions. Semin Nephrol 1998;18:482.

35. Myers BD. Pathogenic processes in human acute renal failure. Semin Dial 1996;9:444.

36. Mehta R et al. Diuretics, mortality, and nonrecovery of renal function in acute renal failure. JAMA 2002;288:2547.

37. Star RA. Treatment of acute renal failure. Kidney Int 1998;54:1817.

38. Shilliday IR et al. Loop diuretics in the management of acute renal failure: a prospective, double-blind, placebo-controlled, randomized study. Nephrol Dial Transplant 1997;12:2592.

39. Papadimitriou M et al. Acute-renal failure—which treatment modality is best? Ren Fail 1998;20:651.

40. Kellum JA. Use of diuretics in the acute care setting. Kidney Int 1998;53(suppl 66):S67.

41. Kellum JA et al. Use of dopamine in acute renal failure: a meta-analysis. Crit Care Med 2001;29:1526.

42. Bellomo R et al. Low-dose dopamine in patients with early renal dysfunction: a placebo-controlled randomized trial. Australian and New Zealand Intensive Care Society (ANZICS) Clinical Trials Group. Lancet 2000;356:2139.

43. Power DA et al. Renal-dose (low-dose) dopamine for the treatment of sepsis-related and other forms of acute renal failure: ineffective and probably dangerous. Clin Exp Pharmacol Physiol Suppl 1999;26:S23.

44. Brophy DF. Role of N-acetylcysteine in the prevention of radiocontrast-induced nephropathy. Ann Pharmacother 2002;36:1466.

45. Asif A et al. Radiocontrast-induced nephropathy. Am J Ther 2003;10:137.

46. Kapoor A et al. The role of theophylline in contrast-induced nephropathy: a case-control study. Nephrol Dial Transplant 2002;17:1936.

47. Huber W et al. Effect of theophylline on contast material-induced nephropathy in patients with chronic renal insufficiency: controlled, randomized, double-blinded study. Radiology 2002;223:772.

48. Dishart MK et al. An evaluation of pharmacological strategies for the prevention and treatment of acute renal failure. Drugs 2000;59:79.

49. Esnault VL. Radiocontrast media-induced nephrotoxicity in patients with renal failure: rationale for a new double-blind, prospective, randomized trial testing calcium channel antagonists. Nephrol Dial Transplant 2002;17:1362.

50. Chu VL et al. Fenolopam in the prevention of contrast media-induced acute renal failure. Ann Pharmacother 2001;10:1278.

51. Tepel M et al. Prevention of radiographic-contrast-agent-induced reductions in renal function by acetylcysteine. N Engl J Med 2000;343:180.

52. Shyu KG et al. Acetylcysteine protects against acute renal damage in patients with abnormal renal function undergoing a coronary procedure. J Am Coll Cardiol 2002;40:1383.

53. Briguori C et al. Acetylcysteine and contrast agent-associated nephrotoxicity. J Am Coll Cardiol 2002;40;298.

54. Diaz-Sandoval et al. Acetylcysteine to prevent angiography-related renal tissue injury (the APART trial). Am J Cardiol 2002;89:356.

55. Kay J et al. Acetycysteine for prevention of acute deterioration of renal function following elective coronary angiography and intervention: a randomized, controlled, trial. JAMA 2003;289:553.

56. Curhan GC. Prevention of contrast nephropathy. JAMA 2003;289;606.

57. Madyhoon H et al. Use of fenoldopam to prevent radiocontrast nephropathy in high-risk patients. Cathet Cardiovasc Intervent 2001;53:341.

58. Kini AS et al. A protocol for prevention of radiographic contrast nephropathy during percutaneous coronary intervention: effect of selective dopamine receptor agonist fenoldopam. Cathet Cardiovasc Intervent 2002;55:169.

59. Madyhoon H et al. Fenoldopam for prevention of contrast-induced renal dysfunction in a high risk angiography population: a historically controlled case series. Circulation 2001;104:II-585.

60. Heupler FA Jr. Guidelines for performing angiography in patients taking metformin. Members of the Laboratory Performance Standards Committee of the Society for Cardiac Angiography and Interventions. Cathet Cardiovasc Diagn 1998;43:121.

61. Michalson A et al. Cost-effectiveness and safety of selective use of low-osmolality contrast media. Acad Radiol 1994;1:59.

62. Mingeot-Leclercq M, Tulkens PM. Aminoglycosides: nephrotoxicity. Antimicrob Agents Chemother 1999;43:1003.

63. Barclay ML et al. Once daily aminoglycoside therapy: is it less toxic than multiple daily doses and how should it be monitored? Clin Pharmacokinet 1999;36:89.

64. Swan SK. Aminoglycoside nephrotoxicity. Semin Nephrol 1997;17:27.

65. Rybak MJ et al. Prospective evaluation of the effect of an aminoglycoside dosing regimen on rates of observed nephrotoxicity and ototoxicity. Antimicrob Agents Chemother 1999;43:1549.

66. Verpooten GA et al. Once daily dosing decreases renal accumulation of gentamicin and netilmicin. Clin Pharmacol Ther 1989;45:22.

67. Freeman CD. Once-daily dosing of aminoglycosides: review and recommendations for clinical practice. J Antimicrob Chemother 1997;39:677.

68. Mithani H, Brown G. The economic impact of once-daily versus conventional administration of gentamicin and tobramycin. Pharmacoeconomics 1996;10:494.

69. Eisenberg J et al. What is the cost of nephrotoxicity associated with aminoglycosides? Ann Intern Med 1987;107:900.

70. Hoeprich PD. Clinical use of amphotericin B and derivatives: lore, mystique, and fact. Clin Infect Dis 1992;14(suppl 1):S114.

71. Fanos V et al. Renal transport of antibiotics and nephrotoxicity: a review. J Chemother 2001;13:461.

72. Slain D. Lipid-based amphotericin B for the treatment of fungal infections. Pharmacotherapy 1999;19:306.

73. Mehta et al. Phagocyte transport as a mechanism of enhanced therapeutic activity of liposomal amphotericin B. Chemotherapy 1994;40:256.

74. Adler-Moore J. AmBisome targeting to fungal infections. Bone Marrow Transplant 1994;14 (suppl 5):S3.

75. Louie A et al. Comparative capacity of four antifungal agents to stimulate murine macrophages to produce tumor necrosis factor alpha: an effect that is attenuated by pentoxifylline, liposomal vesicals, and dexamethasone. J Antimicrob Chemother 1994;34:975.

76. Swenson CE et al. In vitro and in vivo antifungal activity of amphotericin B lipid complex: are phospholipases important? Antimicrob Agents Chemother 1998;42:767.

77. Wasan KM, Conklin JS. Enhanced amphotericin B nephrotoxicity in intensive care patients with elevated levels of low-density lipoprotein cholesterol. Clin Infect Dis 1997;24:78.

78. Alexopolous E. Drug-induced acute interstitial nephritis. Renal Failure 1998;20:809.

79. Perazella MA. Crystal-induced acute renal failure. Am J Med 1999;106:459.

80. Scheinman SJ. Nephrolithiasis. Semin Nephrol 1999;19:381.

81. Manthey DE et al. Nephrolithiasis. Emerg Med Clin North Am 2001;39:383.

82. Rodman JS. Struvite stones. Nephron 1999; 81(suppl 1):50.

83. Donnellan SM, Bolton DM. The impact of contemporary bladder management techniques on struvite calculi associated with spinal cord injury. BJU Int 1999;84:280.

84. Heilberg IP. Update on dietary recommendations and medical treatment of renal stone disease. Nephrol Dial Transplant 2000;15:117.

85. Borghi L et al. Urine volume: stone risk factor and preventative measure. Nephron 1999;81(suppl 1):31.

86. Borghi L et al. Urinary volume, water, and recurrences in idiopathic calcium nephrolithiasis: a 5-year randomized prospective study. J Urol 1996; 155:839.

87. Pak CYC. Medical prevention of renal stone disease. Nephron 1999;81(suppl 1):60.

88. Pearle MS. Prevention of nephrolithiasis. Curr Opin Neph Hypertens 2001;10:203.

89. Ettinger B et al. Potassium-magnesium citrate is an effective prophylaxis against recurrent calcium oxalate nephrolithiasis. J Urol 1997;158:2069.

90. Perazella MA. Crystal-induced acute renal failure. Am J Med 1999;106:459.

91. Suki WN. Use of diuretics in chronic renal failure. Kidney Int Suppl 1997;59:S33.

92. Joy MS. A primer on continuous renal replacement therapy for critically ill patients. Ann Pharmacother 1998;32:362.

93. Mueller BA. Acute renal failure. In: DiPiro JT et al, eds. Pharmacotherapy: A Pathophysiologic Approach, 5th Ed. New York, NY: McGraw-Hill, 2002:771.

94. Palevsky PM et al. The Acute Dialysis Quality Initiative—part V: operational characteristics of CRRT. Adv Ren Replace Ther 2002;9:268.

95. Bellomo R et al. The Acute Dialysis Quality Initiative—part V: operational characteristics of CRRT. Adv Ren Replace Ther 2002;9:255.

96. Golper TA et al. Drug dosing adjustments during continuous renal replacement therapies. Kidney Int 1998;53(suppl 66):S165.

97. Bohler J et al. Pharmacokinetic principles during continuous renal replacement therapy: drugs and dosage. Kidney Int 1999;56(suppl 72):S24.

98. Keller F et al. Individualized drug dosage in patients treated with continuous hemofiltration. Kidney Int 1999;56(suppl 72):S29.

99. Brunet S et al. Diffusive and convective solute clearances during continuous renal replacement therapy at various dialysate and ultrafiltration flow rates. Am J Kidney Dis 1999;34:486.

CHAPTER 32

Chronic Kidney Disease

Joanna Q. Hudson, Curtis A. Johnson

INTRODUCTION

Chronic kidney disease (CKD) describes the continuum of kidney dysfunction from early to late-stage disease. Glomerular filtration rates (GFRs) range from 90 mL/min in the early stages to 15 mL/min in the late stages of disease. The most severe stage occurs when the GFR is less than 15 mL/min and is known as end-stage renal disease (ESRD).[1] Patients with ESRD require renal replacement therapy in the form of dialysis or transplantation to sustain life. Secondary complications associated with CKD increase the complexity of the condition and include fluid and electrolyte abnormalities, anemia, cardiovascular disease, hyperparathyroidism, bone disease, and malnutrition. Optimal management of patients with CKD is best achieved using a multidisciplinary approach to address the concurrent medical problems and complex pharmacotherapeutic regimens. Alterations in drug disposition that occur with kidney impairment and the subsequent need for dosage adjustments are additional considerations when determining rational pharmacotherapy in this population.

Definitions

CKD is characterized by a progressive deterioration in kidney function ultimately leading to irreversible structural damage to existing nephrons. Based on the progressive nature of this condition, a staging system has been established to classify kidney disease according to the GFR, which is estimated clinically using creatinine clearance (Cl_{Cr}) (Table 32-1).[1] Specifically, CKD is defined as kidney damage with a normal or a mildly decreased GFR (Stages 1 and 2) or a GFR <60 mL/min/1.73 m² for at least 3 months with or without evidence of kidney damage (Stages 3 to 5). Kidney damage is indicated by pathologic abnormalities or markers of injury, including abnormalities in blood or urine tests and imaging studies.[1] The presence of protein in the urine (defined as *proteinuria, albuminuria,* or *microalbuminuria* based on protein type and amount) is an early and sensitive marker of kidney damage.

A substantial decline in kidney function also leads to *azotemia,* the condition resulting from accumulation of nitrogenous wastes such as urea (blood urea nitrogen [BUN]), and an increased risk for developing secondary complications of CKD. Uremic signs and symptoms from accumulation of nitrogenous wastes and other toxins lead to a myriad of complications affecting most major organ systems. Laboratory abnormalities include azotemia, hyperphosphatemia, hypocalcemia, hyperkalemia, metabolic acidosis, and worsening anemia. Clinical signs of CKD and its associated complications, including hypertension and uremic symptoms (e.g., nausea, anorexia), and bleeding are observed as the disease advances to stages 3 to 5. Interventions to slow the progression of kidney disease and potentially reverse the disease process are critical, because patients with a decline in GFR to <30 mL/min (Stage 4), in general, will progress to ESRD.

Epidemiology of Chronic Kidney Disease
Incidence and Prevalence

Data to characterize incidence and prevalence of Stages 1 to 4 CKD are scarce; however, the Third National Health and Nutrition Examination Survey (NHANES III), a national study of more than 18,000 persons 12 years or older conducted from 1988 through 1994, does provide information on ranges of serum creatinine (SrCr) in the U.S. population.[2] From these data it is estimated that 800,000 Americans have serum creatinine levels ≥2.0 mg/dL and 6.2 million people have creatinine levels ≥1.5 mg/dL. Although there are limitations in using serum creatinine alone to assess kidney function, these data do provide a general idea of the population at risk for CKD. When extrapolated to the larger U.S. population, approximately 20 million people are estimated to be at risk for CKD.[1]

Data describing the ESRD population are made available annually by the U.S. Renal Data System (USRDS). The reports characterize the development, treatment, morbidity, and mortality associated with ESRD in the United States and include data from patients with kidney transplants. Based on the most recent data from the USRDS, more than 370,000 patients were receiving renal replacement therapy for ESRD at the end of 2000, with approximately 96,000 new patients starting treatment during that year.[3] A continued increase in incidence rates of ESRD has been observed over the past decade, although this rate has decreased to approximately 3% to 5% per year over the past 5 years.[3] The continued increase in incidence rates of ESRD, in conjunction with a relatively stable death rate for this population, accounts for the overall increase in the prevalence of ESRD. CKD has been identified as one of the focus areas for the Healthy People 2010 national health initiative; one of the specific objectives is to reduce the number of new cases of ESRD.[4]

Populations at increased risk for developing ESRD include males and the older population, particularly patients 65 years and older. More than 51% of incident hemodialysis patients in 2000 were age 65 or older, a much larger percentage than for the peritoneal dialysis and transplant populations.[3] Racial distribution of the dialysis population shows that the prevalence is greatest in whites (60%) and blacks (32%), followed by Hispanics (11%) and Asians (4%). Blacks and Native Americans have a three to four times greater incident rate of kidney failure than white individuals.[3]

Etiology

CKD most often results from a progressive loss of functioning nephrons caused by a primary kidney disease or as a secondary complication of certain systemic diseases, but it may also result from an acute event causing irreversible damage to the kidneys. The leading causes of ESRD in patients newly diagnosed in 2000 were diabetes mellitus (43%), hypertension (26%), and chronic glomerulonephritis (8.4%).[3] Among Native Americans, diabetes is the predominant etiology, accounting for nearly two-thirds of the ESRD cases. Diabetes also accounts for higher rates of ESRD in blacks and Hispanics than in whites. Another of the Healthy People 2010 national health objectives for CKD is to focus on efforts to reduce the incidence of ESRD in blacks, Hispanics, and Native Americans.[4] Hypertension remains the most common cause

---

Table 32-1 Staging of Chronic Kidney Disease Based on GFR

Stage	Description	GFR (mL/min/1.73 m2)
—	At increased risk	≥90 (with CKD risk factors)
1	Kidney damage with normal or ↑ GFR	≥90
2	Kidney damage with mild ↓ GFR	60–89
3	Moderate ↓ GFR	30–59
4	Severe ↓ GFR	15–29
5	Kidney failure	<15 (or need for renal replacement therapy)

Adapted with permission from the National Kidney Foundation. NKF-K/DOQI Clinical Practice Guidelines for Chronic Kidney Disease: Evaluation, Classification, and Stratification. Am J Kidney Dis 2002;39:S1.

of ESRD among blacks, with approximately one-third of cases attributed to this disease. A variety of etiologies are responsible for the remaining cases of ESRD, among which are cystic kidney disease, other urologic causes, and AIDS nephropathy.

Mortality
Advances in dialysis and transplantation have improved patient care; however, mortality rates during the first year of ESRD have not improved over the past decade (first-year adjusted death rate 177 per 1,000 patient years in the year 2000 for prevalent ESRD patients).[3] Patients with cardiovascular disease on dialysis have a fivefold greater risk of all-cause mortality when compared with the general Medicare population and with patients with CKD not yet requiring renal replacement therapy. Comorbidities, low albumin, malnutrition, and anemia at initiation of dialysis are strong predictors of mortality. Life expectancy is 20% to 25% of the general population's. Cardiovascular-related events, particularly myocardial infarction, are the leading causes of death in the ESRD population. This is not surprising given the high prevalence of coexisting cardiac disorders in ESRD patients and the elevated risk for mortality associated with these conditions. The Healthy People 2010 initiative for CKD will also focus on decreasing deaths from cardiovascular disease.[4] Infection (predominantly septicemia) and cerebrovascular disease are also substantial contributors to overall mortality in patients with ESRD.[3]

Drug Induced Causes of Kidney Disease
Analgesic Nephropathy
Analgesic nephropathy is a form of tubulointerstitial kidney disease characterized by renal papillary necrosis as a primary lesion and chronic interstitial nephritis as a secondary lesion resulting from habitual ingestion of a mixture of two antipyretic analgesics and usually caffeine and/or codeine.[5] Analgesic nephropathy is part of the *analgesic syndrome,* including such nonrenal complications as anemia, peptic ulcer disease, urinary tract infection, and atherosclerosis.[5,6] Phenacetin, an acetaminophen prodrug, was the first agent to be incriminated. Currently in the United States, most cases are caused by long-term use or misuse of compound analgesics containing acetaminophen and aspirin along with caffeine or codeine.[6] Similar findings in terms of the effect on kidney function have also been observed with nonsteroidal anti-inflammatory drugs (NSAIDs), with both acute and chronic manifestations associated with long-term use.[7] The cumulative amount (at least 1 to 2 kg of acetaminophen), rather than the duration of analgesic intake, is the primary risk factor for developing chronic analgesic nephropathy.[8] Recommendations made by the National Kidney Foundation (NKF) on analgesic use have been published.[5]

Analgesic nephropathy is more prevalent in females, with a female-to-male ratio of 5–7:1. The peak incidence occurs between the fourth and the fifth decades of life.[5,8] Patients usually complain of chronic pain syndromes and, in most cases, psychiatric manifestations indicative of an addictive behavior are observed. At presentation, patients may have a reduced GFR and findings consistent with CKD. During acute necrosis, patients may suffer from flank pain, pyuria, and

hematuria. As necrosis progresses, cellular debris may cause ureteral obstruction. Kidney dysfunction is characterized as a salt-wasting nephropathy, with a substantial reduction in urine-concentrating and urine-acidifying capabilities. The exact mechanism for kidney damage is uncertain; however, it is thought that because acetaminophen accumulates in the renal medulla, its oxidative metabolite produced by the medullary cytochrome P450 enzyme system may bind to macromolecules causing cellular necrosis. Although the reduced form of glutathione in the medulla can prevent this process, agents that reduce medullary glutathione content (e.g., aspirin) may promote kidney damage. This mechanism may explain a lack of analgesic nephropathy associated with acetaminophen alone. NSAIDs, which attenuate prostaglandin-mediated vasodilation, may induce an ischemic state within the renal medulla, leading to papillary necrosis.[7]

The long-term management of analgesic nephropathy primarily involves strict abstinence from NSAIDs and combination analgesics. If possible, patients should be encouraged to maintain a high fluid intake to prevent obstruction of the tubules with necrotic debris and to reduce the risk of urinary tract infection. If such patients develop ESRD, management is similar to those with kidney disease due to other causes. For patients requiring analgesics, aspirin or propoxyphene taken alone may be reasonable alternatives. Acetaminophen as a single agent may be safe, although habitual use may contribute to progression of kidney disease.[9] Patients requiring chronic analgesic therapy should use the lowest dose to control pain, avoid combination products when possible, and maintain adequate hydration.

Lithium Nephropathy
Although lithium use has been associated with alterations in kidney function secondary to acute functional and histologic changes, its role in the development of chronic changes (i.e., chronic interstitial nephritis) is less clear. Both the concentrating ability within the kidney and the GFR may decline with long-term lithium use.[10] In addition, chronic interstitial changes may develop in patients receiving lithium, particularly those with high serum lithium concentrations. Despite these findings, however, others have failed to implicate lithium as a chronic nephrotoxic agent.[11] In patients taking lithium chronically, close monitoring of serum lithium concentrations is advised, and SrCr measurements should be obtained annually to detect changes in kidney function.

Treatment Options
Treatment of patients with Stage 1 to 4 CKD focuses on reducing risk factors for progression of CKD (e.g., uncontrolled hypertension and diabetes) and providing interventions that delay progression. Management of secondary complications, including fluid and electrolyte abnormalities, anemia, hyperphosphatemia, secondary hyperparathyroidism, metabolic acidosis, and malnutrition, is necessary once patients progress to Stage 3 CKD and beyond. Renal replacement therapies including hemodialysis (HD), peritoneal dialysis (PD), and kidney transplantation are treatment options for patients with ESRD. As recently as the 1950s, a patient diagnosed with ESRD faced unavoidable death with a life expectancy of days to weeks. Continued development of treatment options for

ESRD introduced in the 1960s dramatically reduced ESRD-related morbidity and mortality. At the end of 2000, 64% of ESRD patients were undergoing HD, 27% had a functioning transplant, and 6% were receiving PD.[3]

Medication Use

Data regarding medication use in dialysis patients, including HD and PD patients, reveal that these patients are prescribed a total of 8 to 11 medications per patient.[12,13] According to the USRDS, antihypertensive agents were prescribed for 75% of patients, with calcium channel blockers and angiotensin-converting enzyme (ACE) inhibitors as the most common agents. Approximately 80% of dialysis patients were prescribed phosphate-binding agents with a similar percentage of patients requiring erythropoietin. These patterns of medication use are reflective of the prevalence of secondary complications in the latter stages of CKD. The extent of medication use and the complexity of prescribed drug regimens contribute to nonadherence and drug-related problems in the ESRD population.[14,15] Intervention by a clinical pharmacist in some dialysis facilities has proven to be a cost-effective means to address such problems.[15,16] Although not routine in all dialysis centers, regular involvement of a clinical pharmacist is rational given the extent of medication use in this population.

Data on medication prescribing patterns in the earlier stages of CKD have not been well documented; however, the etiologies of CKD and the associated comorbidities and secondary complications indicate that medication use may be similar in these patients if such complications are identified early and treated appropriately with pharmacologic therapy.

Economics

The cost of treating patients with ESRD is substantial, with most of this cost paid by the federal government. In 2000, the cost was $12.4 billion dollars, 5.8% of the Medicare budget.[3] This amount reflects a consistent increase from prior years and an increase in the percentage of the Medicare budget dedicated to ESRD care. The increase is most likely associated with the higher prevalence of ESRD, changes in the standard of care, reimbursement structure, and types of patients being treated (e.g., diabetic patients versus nondiabetic patients). Higher costs of treatment were associated with diabetes and patients with low hemoglobin values at initiation of dialysis. Outpatient pharmacy-related costs accounted for approximately $66.3 million of the ESRD Medicare budget for 2000.[3]

PROGRESSIVE KIDNEY DISEASE
Pathophysiology

Progression of kidney disease to ESRD generally occurs over months to years and is assessed by the rate of decline in GFR. There are approximately 1 million nephrons per kidney, each maintaining its own single nephron GFR. Progressive loss of nephron function results in adaptive changes in remaining nephrons to increase single nephron GFR, a phenomenon called the *intact nephron hypothesis*.[17] Over time the compensatory increase in single nephron GFR leads to hypertrophy and an irreversible loss of nephron function from sustained increases in glomerular pressure. Glomerulosclerosis develops from prolonged elevation of glomerular capillary pressure

and increased glomerular plasma flow leading to a continuous cycle of nephron destruction. Regardless of the etiology, a predictable and continuous decrease in kidney function occurs in patients when the GFR drops below a "critical" value, to approximately <25% of normal.[18] The rate of decline remains fairly constant for an individual, but may vary substantially among patients and disease states. A more rapid rate of decline in kidney function has been associated with black race, lower baseline GFR, male gender, older age, and smoking. Compared to hypertensive kidney disease, conditions associated with a faster decline include diabetic kidney disease, glomerular diseases, and polycystic kidney disease.[1] Progressive disease is typically identified by persistent proteinuria, decreasing kidney function, and the development of glomerulosclerosis. Although early changes in kidney function can be detected through routine laboratory monitoring, most patients do not develop symptoms of uremia until they have progressed to the more severe stages (Stages 4 and 5 CKD). Appropriate medical management will often alleviate uremic symptoms until kidney function is approximately 5% to 10% of normal (Stage 5 CKD), at which time dialysis or transplantation is required to sustain life.

As the leading causes of ESRD in the United States, diabetes, hypertension, and glomerular diseases have been the focus of research to identify their associated mechanisms of kidney damage. Diabetes accounts for the majority of cases of ESRD, which are due not only to poor glycemic control, but also to hypertension.[19] Excess filtration of glucose and contact with glomerular and tubular cells results in increased cellular osmotic pressure and thickening of the capillary basement membrane. The resulting glomerulopathy may or may not result in proteinuria. Systemic hypertension is a potent stimulus for the progression of kidney disease because of its association with increased single nephron GFR.[17,20] Coexistent diabetes and hypertension increase the risk of developing ESRD by 5- to 6-fold compared to persons with hypertension alone. Proteinuria, one of the initial diagnostic signs, may also contribute to the progressive decline in kidney function with a more rapid rate of progression associated with higher protein excretion.[21] Immunologic and hemodynamic mechanisms have been identified to explain the glomerular injury and increase in renal plasma flow associated with proteinuria and high protein intake. Inflammatory cytokines may be responsible for fibrosis and renal scarring ultimately resulting in loss of nephron function.

Dyslipidemias are common in patients with CKD and are often observed concurrently with proteinuria. Increased low-density lipoprotein (LDL) cholesterol, total cholesterol, and apolipoprotein B as well as decreased high-density lipoprotein (HDL) cholesterol have been observed in patients with progressive kidney disease.[22] Hypercholesterolemia has been associated with loss of kidney function in patients with and without diabetes.[23,24] Accumulation of apolipoproteins in glomerular mesangial cells contributes to cytokine production and infiltration of macrophages and has been implicated in the progression of CKD, primarily in the presence of previous kidney disease or other risk factors such as hypertension.[25] LDL is thought to promote glomerular damage by initiating a series of cellular events in mesangial cells and through oxidation to a more cytotoxic derivative once within these cells. Although serum total cholesterol, triglycerides, and apolipoprotein B all correlate with the rate of decline in GFR, it is not clear that they directly increase the rate of progression of kidney disease, particularly when present with concomitant conditions that also cause kidney damage. There is, however, some evidence to suggest that treatment of hypercholesterolemia with statin therapy (atorvastatin) in patients with CKD may reduce proteinuria and progression of CKD.[26]

Clinical Assessment

Evaluation of Kidney Function

Estimation of GFR is the most reliable and practical means available to determine baseline kidney function and monitor progression of kidney disease over time. The best marker of GFR is a nontoxic substance that is freely filtered at the glomerulus and not secreted, reabsorbed, or metabolized by the kidney. Inulin and exogenous radioactive markers have been used to assess GFR since they meet these criteria; however, they are not readily available, require intravenous (IV) administration, and are costly. Creatinine is an endogenous substance that is derived from the breakdown of muscle creatine phosphate. Creatinine is excreted primarily by glomerular filtration; thus, creatinine clearance (Cl_{Cr}) has been used as a reasonable surrogate for GFR. There are limitations to consider when using methods to assess GFR that incorporate creatinine. Creatinine is eliminated not only through glomerular filtration but also via tubular secretion. As nephron function declines, tubular secretion of creatinine contributes more substantially to overall elimination of creatinine such that Cl_{Cr} overestimates true GFR. As a result, disease progression may be underestimated. Administration of cimetidine to patients before measurement of Cl_{Cr} may provide a more accurate assessment since cimetidine blocks tubular secretion of creatinine.[27]

Serum creatinine (SrCr) alone is used clinically as an index of kidney function; however, there are limitations to this practice. In the initial stages of kidney disease, SrCr may remain within the normal range. Consequently, SrCr may be relatively insensitive in detecting early kidney disease and is not accurate for estimating the progression of the disease. Generation of creatinine is also proportional to total muscle mass and is affected by diet, notably by the ingestion of meats. Use of creatinine to assess kidney function in patients with liver disease may also lead to overestimation of GFR.[28] This may be attributed to decreased production of creatine, the precursor to creatinine, by the liver or increased secretion of creatinine by the kidney. There is also substantial variation in the calibration of SrCr among laboratories that may result in differences in measured SrCr. Although SrCr can provide a rough estimate of kidney function, other means of assessing GFR should be used when a more accurate determination is necessary. Other markers of early kidney damage, such as proteinuria, should be evaluated in patients at risk for kidney disease also.

Several equations have been developed to estimate GFR that incorporate SrCr and other variables. The most commonly used equation is the Cockcroft-Gault equation that provides an estimate of Cl_{Cr} in patients with stable kidney function[29] (see Chapter 31, Acute Renal Failure). The Jelliffe[30] equation is also used to assess GFR in adults. More recently a prediction equation was developed using data from the Modification of Diet in Renal Disease (MDRD) study, a multicen-

ter trial that evaluated the effects of dietary protein restriction and blood pressure (BP) control on progression of kidney disease.[31] This equation, referred to as the MDRD equation, may provide a better estimate of GFR based on the fact that the equation was derived using GFR measured directly by urinary clearance of a radiolabeled marker (^{125}I-Iothalamate) as opposed to creatinine, and included a relatively large and diverse population (>500 European American and African American individuals with varying degrees of kidney disease) for derivation and validation of the equation. The MDRD equation[31] is as follows:

$$\text{Estimated GFR (mL/min/1.73m}^2 = 170 \times (\text{SrCr})^{-0.999} \times$$
$$(\text{Age})^{-0.176} \times (\text{BUN})^{-0.170} \times (\text{Alb})^{+0.318} \times \quad \textbf{(32-1)}$$
$$(0.762 \text{ if female}) \times (1.18 \text{ if African American})$$

An abbreviated version has also been developed[1]:

$$\text{Estimated GFR (mL/min/1.73m}^2) = 186 \times$$
$$(\text{SrCr})^{-1.154} \times (\text{Age})^{-0.203} \times (0.742 \text{ if female}) \times \quad \textbf{(32-2)}$$
$$(1.21 \text{ if African American})$$

The Schwartz[32] equation is used to assess GFR in children as follows:

$$\text{Creatinine clearance (mL/min)} = [k \times \text{length (in cm)}]/\text{SrCr}$$
where k is dependent on age: infant (1 to 52 weeks)
$$k = 0.45; \text{ child (1 to 13 years) } k = 0.55; \text{ adolescent male}$$
$$k = 0.7; \text{ and adolescent female } k = 0.55. \quad \textbf{(32-3)}$$

Use of the Cockcroft-Gault or MDRD equation is recommended for assessment of GFR in adults.[1]

While historically accepted as a more accurate method, calculation of Cl_{Cr} using 24-hour urine collection methods has not been proven more reliable than the equations presented to estimate GFR. Problems with urine collection methods include incomplete urine collection, diurnal variation in GFR, and variation in creatinine excretion. Despite these limitations smaller collection times or spot untimed urine samples may be useful to determine creatinine excretion. Populations in whom estimation of GFR using a 24-hour urine collection is more reasonable include patients with variation in dietary intake of creatine sources, such as vegetarians, or persons with poor muscle mass (e.g., malnourished individuals or amputees).[1]

Estimation of GFR is used not only to follow the progression of kidney disease, but to estimate the appropriate doses of drugs that are eliminated by the kidney. Frequent assessment of drug selection and dosage regimen design should be integral to the evaluation of a patient with progressive kidney disease.

Proteinuria

In patients who have or are at risk for kidney disease, additional assessment of kidney function should include evaluation of urinary protein excretion, which has been shown to be predictive of progression. Protein is not normally filtered at the glomerulus and is present only in trace amounts in the urine. With glomerular damage, proteinuria is generally observed. Proteinuria may precede elevations in SrCr and should be considered as an early marker of kidney damage. *Microalbuminuria* is defined as an albumin excretion rate of 20 to 200 μg/min or 30 to 300 mg/24 hr. Specific assays with increased sensitivity relative to standard assays are required for detecting quantities of protein in the range defined as microalbuminuria. *Proteinuria* is defined as a total protein excretion rate exceeding 200 μg/min or >300 mg/24 hr (referred to as *albuminuria* if albumin is the only protein measured). Total protein includes albumin and other proteins such as low molecular weight globulins and apoproteins. Assessment of albuminuria is a better indicator of early kidney disease since it is primarily indicative of glomerular damage as opposed to total protein, which is not as specific for glomerular damage. Other tests, including urinalysis, radiographic procedures, and biopsy, may also be valuable in further assessing kidney function.

Quantification of albumin may be done using timed urine samples. Typically, a 24-hour collection period is used, although a timed sample collected overnight may be more reliable since protein excretion may vary throughout the day and with postural changes (i.e., orthostatic proteinuria). Untimed or "spot" urine samples for measurement of protein- or albumin-to-creatinine ratios are often more convenient. As opposed to measuring protein or albumin in a timed collection, this method corrects for variations in hydration status and may be more accurate because protein excretion is normalized to glomerular filtration. The albumin and creatinine concentrations in the urine are measured from a spot urine sample, preferably from a first morning urine sample, since it correlates best with 24-hour protein excretion. If a first morning urine sample is not available, a random sample is acceptable. Factors associated with proteinuria, such as ingestion of a high-protein meal and vigorous exercise, must be considered when evaluating urinary protein. Screening for albuminuria may also be done using urine dipstick testing of a spot urine sample. Reagent strips are available from several commercial test products and differ with regard to the specified testing procedure and the sensitivity and specificity for detecting albuminuria. The Micral, Micral II, and ImmunoDip are immunochemical test strips that give a semiquantitative estimation of urinary albumin.[33,34] Patients with a positive dipstick screening test should have a subsequent quantitative assessment of the protein- or albumin-to-creatinine ratio to confirm proteinuria.

According to the NKF Kidney Disease Outcomes Quality Initiative (K/DOQI) Clinical Practice Guidelines for CKD, persistent proteinuria is diagnosed by at least two positive quantitative tests spaced by at least 1 to 2 weeks. The American Diabetes Association (ADA) defines microalbuminuria as a positive test on at least two of three quantitative measurements performed within a 3- to 6-month period.[35] ADA criteria specify albumin-to-creatinine ratios of 30 to 300 μg/mg as consistent with microalbuminuria, whereas higher values are indicative of albuminuria.[35] The K/DOQI Guidelines for CKD provide criteria for diagnosis of proteinuria and albuminuria based on testing method and gender (Table 32-2).[1]

Staging of Chronic Kidney Disease

Historically the term *chronic renal insufficiency* was used to describe patients with decreased kidney function not requiring dialysis. This included a broad range of patients from the earlier stages of the disease, with GFRs >60 mL/min, as well as those patients with more severe disease, with GFRs <30 mL/min. Failure to distinguish patients at these differing levels of kidney function also resulted in failure to recognize differences in management approaches required at these levels of GFR. Only recently has a uniform classification system been adopted to describe the various stages of kidney dysfunction, similar to the rationale for staging or classifying other chronic disease (e.g., hypertension). This staging system was developed to promote a more consistent dialogue when referring to patients with kidney dysfunction and use of terminology associated with a more objective description. Kidney disease is classified into five stages based on the GFR (Table 32-1).[1] A patient with Stage 1 or 2 CKD would have some pathologic abnormality indicative of kidney damage (See "Definitions"), since their GFR is relatively normal. Continued screening and interventions to delay progression are essential at these stages. Patients with Stages 3 to 5 CKD are diagnosed with the disease based on GFR alone (GFR <60 mL/min). It is at these stages that management of secondary complications becomes a standard of care. Stage 5 is the most severe stage when the GFR is <15 mL/min and dialysis or transplantation is necessary.

Secondary Complications

Secondary complications begin to develop as kidney disease progresses, most often when patients progress to Stage 3 CKD and the GFR is <60 mL/min. Among these complications are fluid and electrolyte abnormalities, anemia, hyper-

Table 32-2 Diagnostic Criteria for Proteinuria and Albuminuria.

	Total Protein			Albumin		
	24-Hour Collection (mg/day)	Spot Urine Dipstick (mg/dL)	Spot Urine Protein-SrCr Ratio (mg/g)	24-Hour Collection (mg/day)	Spot Urine Dipstick (mg/dL)	Spot Urine Albumin-SrCr Ratio (mg/g)
Normal	<300	<30	<200	<30	<3	<17 (men) <25 (women)
Microalbuminuria	NA	NA	NA	30–300	>3	17–250 (men) 25–355 (women)
Albuminuria or clinical proteinuria	>300	>30	>200	>300	NA	>250 (men) >355 (women)

Adapted with permission from National Kidney Foundation. NKF-K/DOQI Clinical Practice Guidelines for Chronic Kidney Disease: Evaluation, Classification, and Stratification. Am J Kidney Dis 2002;39:S1.

phosphatemia, hyperparathyroidism, metabolic acidosis, cardiovascular complications, and poor nutritional status. Often, these complications go unrecognized or are inadequately managed during the earlier stages of CKD, leading to poor outcomes by the time a patient is in need of dialysis therapy. Hypoalbuminemia and anemia were identified in more than 50% of a population of patients new to dialysis therapy, and these findings were associated with a decreased quality of life.[36] Late referral to a nephrologist to manage specific kidney disorders and associated complications has also been associated with increased mortality in the ESRD population.[37] These and similar reports underscore the need for early and aggressive therapy to manage secondary complications. These secondary complications will be presented in more detail throughout this chapter. Complications associated with dialysis therapy are discussed in Chapter 33, Renal Dialysis.

Prevention

Appropriate management of CKD includes measures to prevent or slow progression of the disease and regular evaluation of kidney function to assess changes in disease severity and to monitor therapy. This includes aggressive strategies to manage the disorders that cause kidney disease or are known to accelerate the disease process, such as diabetes, hypertension, high protein intake, and dyslipoproteinemias (see Chapter 13, Dyslipidemias; Chapter 14, Essential Hypertension; and Chapter 50, Diabetes Mellitus).

Antihypertensive Therapy

The association between BP and kidney disease is difficult to establish because hypertension is both a cause and a result of kidney failure. Hypertension, whether the primary cause of kidney disease or a coexisting disease in the presence of other etiologies, may promote kidney damage through transmission of elevated systemic pressure to glomeruli. The result is glomerular capillary hyperperfusion and hypertension leading to progressive kidney damage as continued nephron destruction occurs. Glomerular ischemia induced by damage to preglomerular arteries and arterioles may also occur. Antihypertensive therapy prevents kidney damage and slows the rate of progression of CKD in both diabetic and nondiabetic patients.[38,39] The added benefit of reduced cardiovascular mortality further supports the use of antihypertensive therapy in patients at risk for progressive CKD. Despite what is known about the beneficial effects of BP control in patients with CKD, data from NHANES III indicate that only 11% of individuals with hypertension and elevated SrCr had BPs below 130/85 mm Hg (the previous goal BP in patients with CKD) and just 27% had BPs less than 140/90 mm Hg.[1,2]

The target BP for patients with or at risk for kidney disease differs from that recommended for the general population with hypertension. Evidence now exists to support lowering BP beyond the generally advocated target of <140/90 mm Hg. According to the Seventh Report of the Joint National Committee on Prevention, Detection, Evaluation, and Treatment of High Blood Pressure (JNC-7) and recommendations from the NKF Hypertension and Diabetes Executive Committee, the goal BP for individuals with CKD and/or diabetes is: <130/80 mm Hg.[40,41] Results from the MDRD study showed that further lowering BP to <125/75 mm Hg (or a

mean arterial pressure <92 mmHg) was more beneficial than usual BP control in patients with higher rates of urinary protein excretion (>1 g proteinuria/day).[21,38] The effects of more aggressive BP lowering on progression of kidney disease were also studied in the African American Study of Kidney Disease and Hypertension (AASK) trial.[42] In this population, there was some evidence in support of a lower BP goal in patients with higher baseline proteinuria; however, the effect on GFR did not reach statistical significance. Changes in GFR over a 4-year evaluation period did not differ significantly between patients with a mean BP of 141/85 mm Hg and those with stricter control to a mean BP of 128/78 mm Hg.[42] While it is clear that control of BP is important to delay progression of kidney disease, whether more aggressive BP lowering is necessary in patients with more severe proteinuria is debatable.

BP reduction with any agent or combination of agents is reasonable in patients with CKD with the exception of dihydropyridine calcium channel blockers (e.g., amlodipine), which may contribute to worsening kidney disease when used alone.[43]Among the available classes of antihypertensive agents, ACE inhibitors (e.g., enalapril, captopril, lisinopril) and angiotensin receptor blockers (ARBs; e.g., losartan, irbesartan, candesartan) may afford additional benefits in preserving kidney function. In conditions of decreased kidney function and GFR, angiotensin II primarily causes compensatory vasoconstriction of the efferent arteriole, thereby increasing glomerular capillary pressure (P_{GC}) and GFR (Fig. 32-1). This effect is beneficial in conditions of acute renal failure; however, sustained increases in P_{GC} cause hypertrophy of individual nephrons and progressive kidney disease. ACE inhibitor and ARB therapy prevents this chronic increase in glomerular pressure mediated by angiotensin II. Benefits of ACE inhibitors have been demonstrated in patients with diabetes who had some degree of proteinuria, suggesting that use of ACE inhibitors be considered in this population regardless of BP.[39,44-46] In patients without diabetes, ACE inhibitors have been shown to reduce BP, decrease proteinuria, and slow the progression of kidney disease when compared with other agents.[42,47-49] An initial and mild decrease in GFR is expected with ACE inhibitor therapy; therefore, an increase in SrCr of approximately 30% within the first 2 months of therapy is acceptable.[50] Hypotension, acute kidney failure, and severe hyperkalemia are reasons to consider discontinuing therapy.

Angiotensin II receptor blockers offer similar benefits to ACE inhibitors based on their ability to decrease efferent arteriolar resistance by blockade of the angiotensin type 1 (AT_1) receptor. In patients with type 2 diabetes mellitus, losartan decreased the incidence of a doubling of SrCr by 25% and of ESRD by 28% when compared to placebo after a mean of 3.4 years of therapy.[51,52] Similar effects were observed in the Irbesartan Diabetic Nephropathy Trial (IDNT) with a 23% decreased risk of ESRD observed in irbesartan-treated patients.[53] In both studies, these beneficial effects were independent of reduction in BP. Reduction in the degree of proteinuria has also been demonstrated with candesartan and valsartan.[54,55] Combination therapy with an ARB and an ACE inhibitor may confer additional benefits than either therapy used alone.[56]

Calcium channel blockers have been considered for preventing progression of kidney disease because of their effects

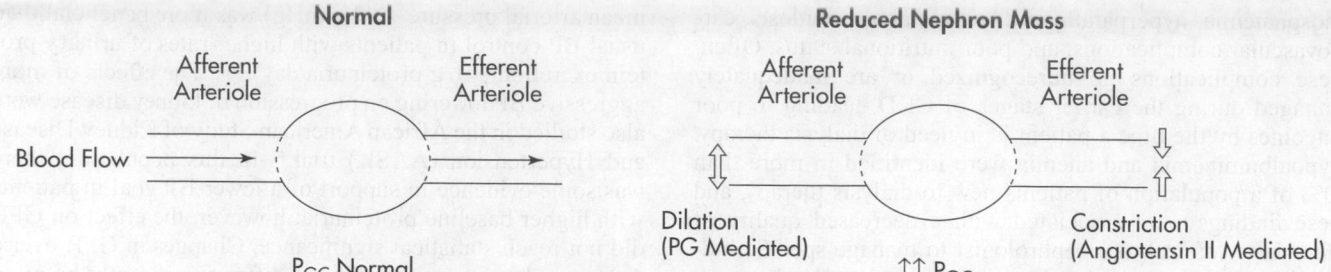

FIGURE 32-1 Renal hemodynamics: dependent on afferent and efferent arteriolar tone and glomerular capillary pressure (P_{GC}). With reduced nephron mass, afferent arteriolar vasodilation (mediated primarily by prostaglandins PGI_2 and PGE_2) and efferent arteriolar constriction (mediated primarily by angiotensin II) occur with remaining functioning nephrons to compensate. This leads to an increase in blood flow, intraglomerular capillary filtration pressure (P_{GC}), and hyperfiltration (increased single-nephron GFR). Sustained increases in plasma flow and hydrostatic pressure lead to hyperfiltration injury and glomerular sclerosis. Over time, these changes contribute to continued loss of nephron function (i.e., progression of kidney disease). ACE inhibitors and ARBs prevent vasoconstriction of the efferent arteriole and reduce the P_{GC}.

on renal hemodynamics and cytoprotective and antiproliferative properties, which prevent mesangial expansion and renal scarring. The nondihydropyridine agents (i.e., diltiazem and verapamil) have been beneficial in reducing proteinuria when compared with dihydropyridines (e.g., nifedipine), although these findings are not consistent.[57–59] Combination therapy with ACE inhibitors resulted in greater reductions in proteinuria in patients with diabetes than with either agent alone, suggesting that it may be rational to use multiple agents in this population.[60,61]

β-Blockers may offer benefits in the treatment of diabetic nephropathy as demonstrated by the United Kingdom Prospective Diabetes Study, which showed similar effects of atenolol and captopril on decreasing the incidence of albuminuria in patients with diabetes.[62]

Dietary Protein Restriction

Proteinuria was identified as the most significant predictor of ESRD in patients with type 2 diabetes and early CKD.[52] Evidence such as this has led to investigation of measures to decrease the degree of proteinuria. In addition to controlling the primary etiologies of kidney disease (e.g., diabetes, hypertension, glomerulopathies, etc) and use of ACE inhibitor and ARB therapy, dietary protein restriction has been evaluated as a strategy for reducing proteinuria and delaying progression of kidney disease. Increases in protein ingestion have been associated with a rise in GFR, potentially due to structural changes of the glomerulus and changes in renal plasma flow with increased protein load.[63]

A number of studies have investigated the effect of protein restriction on progression with varying results.[38,64,65] These conflicting conclusions may be due to differences in study design, patient populations, methods to assess kidney function, degrees of protein restriction, and dietary compliance. Evidence of the beneficial effects of protein restriction is primarily from nondiabetic patients and individuals with type 1 diabetes with protein restricted to approximately 0.6 to 0.8 grams of protein per kilogram of body weight per day.

In the MDRD study, the effects of protein and phosphorus restriction on progression of kidney disease were evaluated.[38] Nondiabetic patients with what is now considered Stage 3 to 4 CKD (GFR 25 to 55 mL/min) received either a normal pro-

tein (1.3 g/kg per day) or low-protein (0.58 g/kg per day) diet, whereas those with more severe kidney disease (GFR 13 to 24 mL/min) were randomized to a low-protein or very-low-protein diet (0.28 g/kg per day). Within each protein category, patients were either maintained at a normal or low mean arterial pressure. After a mean follow-up of 2.2 years, no significant difference was found in terms of the decline in GFR for each group. A faster initial decline (during months 0 to 4) in kidney function was observed for the low-protein and low BP groups compared with the normal protein and normal blood pressure groups, followed by a slower subsequent decline (4 months to end). A secondary analysis of this trial, which accounted for dietary compliance, revealed more encouraging results, suggesting that patients with severe kidney disease (GFR <25 mL/min) could benefit from protein restriction to 0.6 g/kg per day.[64] A meta-analysis of randomized controlled trials including just over 1,900 patients found only a small reduction in the rate of decline in GFR (0.53 mL/min/yr) suggesting that therapies with a more substantial effect on delaying progression are preferred.[65]

The potential benefits of protein restriction in patients with CKD must be weighed against the potentially adverse effect on overall nutritional status. Malnutrition is prevalent in patients with CKD starting dialysis and is a predictor of mortality in this population.[66] The decision to restrict protein should be done with referral to a dietitian and frequent monitoring of nutritional status.

Treatment of Dyslipoproteinemia

Lipoprotein metabolism is altered early in the course of kidney disease and becomes pronounced with more advanced disease, making hyperlipidemia common in patients with CKD. Elevated triglyceride, total cholesterol, LDL cholesterol, and decreased HDL cholesterol levels are generally observed. The predominance of triglyceride-rich apo-B lipoproteins may contribute to the progression of kidney disease and is also a risk factor for the development of cardiovascular morbidity and mortality.[67]

The role of antihyperlipidemic drug therapy in preventing progression of CKD is uncertain. Use of statin therapy has been associated with decreased proteinuria and preservation of GFR in a small number of patients with CKD.[26,68] A meta-analysis of trials, predominantly in patients with diabetes and CKD, showed that lipid lowering therapy slowed the rate of decline in GFR.[69] Despite uncertainty of therapy to delay progression, treatment of dyslipidemia should be considered since abnormal lipid metabolism predisposes patients to cardiovascular disease. The question of whether strategies used to prevent and treat hyperlipidemia in the general population should be extrapolated to the population with kidney disease has been addressed by the NKF Task Force on Cardiovascular Disease.[67] This group supported application of the National Cholesterol Education Program (NCEP ATP III) guidelines to the population with kidney disease and classified these patients in the highest risk group.[70] Guidelines for management of dyslipidemias in patients with CKD have recently been made available (NKF-K/DOQI guidelines).[71] These guidelines also support classifying patients with CKD in the highest risk category for cardiovascular disease, equivalent to the risk for patients with coronary heart disease. The choice of the specific antihyperlipidemic agent should be based on the individual lipid profile. In general, NCEP guidelines should be followed, with particular consideration of the effect of such interventions on patients with CKD, such as dietary restrictions and use of agents that are renally eliminated. Given that elevated triglycerides are often observed as a lipid abnormality in patients with CKD, fibric acid derivatives such as gemfibrozil may be preferred, although HMG-CoA reductase in-

hibitors are necessary to lower LDL cholesterol and may have added cardiovascular benefits. Clofibrate must be used cautiously because it accumulates in patients with kidney disease, which may lead to serious adverse effects such as myositis (see Chapter 13, Dyslipidemias).

END-STAGE RENAL DISEASE (STAGE 5 CHRONIC KIDNEY DISEASE)
Clinical Signs and Symptoms

Despite efforts to prevent or delay worsening of kidney function, many patients progress to the latter stage, or Stage 5 CKD. It is during Stages 4 and 5 that patients may develop the more severe signs and symptoms associated with advanced kidney disease, often referred to as the uremic syndrome. The manifestations and metabolic consequences of advanced kidney disease are listed in Table 32-3. These manifestations certainly may develop in the earlier stages of CKD, underscoring the importance of early intervention, but become more prominent as the disease worsens. The pathogenesis of these disorders has been attributed, in part, to the accumulation of uremic toxins. The search for these uremic toxins has led to the identification of nitrogenous compounds that are consistently observed in the serum of patients with kidney disease. Unfortunately, a cause-and-effect relationship between these compounds and the clinical manifestations of uremia has not

---

Table 32-3 Metabolic Effects of Uremia

Fluid, Electrolyte, and Acid-Base Effects	**Musculoskeletal**
Fluid retention	Renal bone disease
Hyperkalemia	Amyloidosis
Hypermagnesemia	Extraskeletal calcifications
Hyperphosphatemia	**Gastrointestinal**
Hypocalcemia	Anorexia
Metabolic acidosis	Nausea, vomiting
Hematologic	Delayed gastric emptying
Anemia	GI bleeding
Hemostatic abnormalities	Ulcers
Immune suppression	**Neurologic**
Cardiovascular	Lethargy
Hypertension	Depressed sensorium
Congestive heart failure	Tremor
Pericarditis	Asterixis
Atherosclerosis	Muscular irritability and cramps
Arrhythmias	Seizures
Endocrine	Motor weakness
Calcium-phosphorous imbalances	Peripheral neuropathy
Hyperparathyroidism	Coma
Metabolic bone disease	**Dermatologic**
Altered thyroid function	Altered pigmentation
Altered carbohydrate metabolism	Pruritus
Hypophyseal-gonadal dysfunction	**Psychologic**
Decreased insulin metabolism	Depression
Erythropoietin deficiency	Anxiety
	Psychosis
	Miscellaneous
	Reduced exercise tolerance

GI, gastrointestinal.

been clearly established. Many of these compounds originate from protein degradation; therefore, the extent of their accumulation depends on protein intake. The rate of accumulation of urea, the end product of amino acid catabolism, serves as an index of the accumulation of all nitrogenous waste products.

Treatment

Dialysis and Transplantation

As ESRD becomes inevitable, the appropriate dialysis modality must be selected based on patient preference and options for vascular access for HD or peritoneal access for PD. Early planning for dialysis therapy and timely initiation may lower patient morbidity and mortality. Indications for dialysis and considerations in selection of modality are discussed in Chapter 33, Renal Dialysis. Kidney transplantation is an option for all ESRD patients without specified contraindications if a suitable organ match is available (see Chapter 35, Solid Organ Transplantation).

Pharmacotherapy

Pharmacotherapy in the patient with ESRD involves interventions to manage comorbid conditions and secondary complications. The extent of medication use, including medications administered during dialysis therapy, contributes to the potential for drug interactions, adverse reactions, and nonadherence to therapy.[13] The effect of decreased kidney function on absorption, distribution, metabolism, and elimination of pharmacologic agents, in addition to the contribution of dialysis to drug removal, further complicates pharmacotherapy in this population (see Chapter 34, Dosing of Drugs in Renal Failure). Appropriate pharmacotherapeutic management includes choice of rational agents based on the indication, a regular comprehensive review of all medications, and frequent reevaluation to adjust regimens relative to kidney function.

DIABETIC NEPHROPATHY

1. M.R. is a 32-year-old, African American female (weight, 63kg; height, 5′8″), with a 15-year history of type 1 diabetes mellitus who presents to the diabetes clinic with a 1-week history of nausea, vomiting, and general malaise. She has been noncompliant with regular appointments and her blood glucose has generally remained >200 mg/dL on prior evaluations, with an A1C of 8% (goal, <7%) 2 months ago. M.R. has been treated for peptic ulcer disease for the past 6 months. The workup revealed the following pertinent laboratory values: serum sodium (Na), 143 mEq/L (normal, 135 to 147 mEq/L); potassium (K), 5.3 mEq/L (normal, 3.5 to 5.0 mEq/L); chloride (Cl), 106 mEq/L (normal, 95 to 105 mEq/L); CO_2 content, 18 mEq/L (normal, 22 to 28 mEq/L); SrCr, 2.9 mg/dL (normal, 0.6 to 1.2 mg/dL); BUN, 63 mg/dL (normal, 8 to 18 mg/dL); and random blood glucose, 220 mg/dL (normal, 140 mg/dL). Physical examination revealed a BP of 155/102 mm Hg, mild pulmonary congestion, and 2+ pedal edema. Additional laboratory studies showed serum phosphate, 7.6 mg/dL (normal, 2.5 to 5.0 mg/dL); calcium (Ca), 8.8 mg/dL (normal, 8.8 to 10.4 mg/dL); magnesium (Mg), 2.8 mEq/L (normal, 1.6 to 2.4 mEq/L); and uric acid, 8.8 mg/dL (normal, 2.0 to 7.0 mg/dL). Hematologic studies showed hematocrit (Hct), 26% (normal, 36% to 46%); hemoglobin (Hgb), 8.7 g/dL (normal, 12 to 16 mg/dL); and white blood cell (WBC) count, 9,600/mm³

(normal, 3,200 to 9,800/mm³). Red blood cell (RBC) indices were normal. Platelet count was 175,000/mm³ (normal, 130,000 to 400,000/mm³). M.R.'s reticulocyte count was 2.0% (normal, 0.1% to 2.4%). Her urinalysis (UA) showed 4+ proteinuria, later quantified as a urinary albumin of 700 mg/24 hr (normal, <30 mg/day). What subjective and objective data in M.R. are consistent with a diagnosis of advanced kidney disease?

[SI units: Na, 143 mmol/L (normal, 135 to 147); K, 5.3 mmol/L (normal, 3.5 to 5.0); Cl, 106 mmol/L (normal, 95 to 105); CO_2, 18 mmol/L (normal, 22 to 28); SrCr, 256 μmol/L (normal, 50 to 110); BUN, 22 mmol/L of urea (normal, 3.0 to 6.5); glucose, 12.2 mmol/L (normal, <11 mmol/L); phosphate, 2.45 mmol/L (normal, 0.8 to 1.60); Ca, 2.2 mmol/L (normal, 2.2 to 2.6); Mg, 1.4 mmol/L (normal, 0.8 to 1.20); uric acid, 524 μmol/L (normal, 120 to 420); Hct, 0.26 (normal, 0.36 to 0.46); Hgb, 87 g/L (normal, 120 to 160); WBC count, 9,600 × 10⁶/L (normal, 3,200 to 9,800); platelet count, 175 × 10⁹/L (normal, 130 to 400); reticulocyte count, 0.02 (normal, 0.001 to 0.024), urinary albumin, 0.7 g/day (normal, <0.03)]

M.R.'s abnormal values for SrCr, BUN, serum potassium, magnesium, phosphate, uric acid, CO_2 content, hemoglobin, and hematocrit are all consistent with kidney disease and its associated complications. Assuming relatively stable kidney function (i.e., no acute changes in kidney function), her estimated Cl_{Cr} is approximately 28 mL/min based on the Cockcroft-Gault equation, and she is classified with Stage 4 CKD (GFR 15 to 29 mL/min). As the GFR declines to the degree observed in M.R., normal regulation of fluids and electrolytes is impaired. Elevations in SrCr, BUN, sodium, potassium, magnesium, phosphate, and uric acid as well as signs of fluid accumulation are observed. Although potassium is mildly elevated in M.R., overall potassium balance is usually maintained within the normal range until more severe kidney disease develops (i.e., GFR <10 mL/min). The substantial degree of proteinuria observed in M.R. is consistent with more advanced glomerular damage. Volume overload from continued intake and decreased sodium and water excretion leads to weight gain (although likely not observed in M.R. due to her recent onset of nausea and vomiting), hypertension, congestive pulmonary disease, and edema. Metabolic acidosis results from impaired synthesis of ammonia by the kidney, which buffers hydrogen ions and facilitates acid excretion. Anemia associated with CKD is primarily due to decreased erythropoietin production by the kidneys, but it may also be due to increased bleeding from uremia and her peptic ulcer disease. M.R.'s recent onset of nausea, vomiting, and malaise may be a consequence of the accumulation of uremic toxins (azotemia) from the decline in kidney function, although such symptoms are generally associated with BUN values greater than that observed in M.R.

2. What is the cause of M.R.'s advanced kidney disease?

Based on M.R.'s presentation, her kidney disease is most likely due to diabetic nephropathy from her 15-year history of type 1 diabetes mellitus. Her history of noncompliance with regular appointments, elevated blood glucose concentration, and high A1C values support poor control of diabetes and diabetic nephropathy as the primary etiology. Diabetic nephropathy rarely develops within the first 10 years after onset of type 1 diabetes. The annual incidence is greatest after approximately 20 years' duration of diabetes and declines thereafter.[72] ESRD develops in 50% of type 1 diabetic patients within 10 years and in >75% of patients within 20 years.[35] M.R. fits this pattern in that she has diabetic nephropathy after a 15-year history of diabetes, although her nephropathy was likely evident several years previously. M.R. may also be at increased risk for developing ESRD because African Americans have a higher risk of ESRD relative to non-Hispanic whites.[3]

Diabetic nephropathy is a microvascular complication of diabetes resulting in albuminuria and a progressive decline in kidney function. Diabetic nephropathy develops in approximately one-third of all patients with type 1 and type 2 diabetes, with a larger percentage of patients with type 1 diabetes progressing to ESRD. However, since type 2 diabetes is more prevalent, these patients account for the majority of diabetic patients starting dialysis.[35] With the increased prevalence of diabetes and the increase in life expectancy of this population, it is likely that diabetic nephropathy will remain the leading cause of ESRD in the United States.[3,4] Whereas most research has focused on the pathophysiology, prevention, and treatment of diabetic nephropathy in type 1 diabetes, it is reasonable to extrapolate available evidence on prevention of diabetic nephropathy to the population with type 2 diabetes.

The exact mechanisms leading to the development of diabetic nephropathy are not clearly defined; however, several predictive factors for the development and progression of kidney damage have been identified. These include elevated BP, plasma glucose, glycosylated hemoglobin, and cholesterol; smoking; advanced age; male gender; and potentially, high protein intake.[73,74] Insulin deficiency and increased ketone bodies have also been proposed as contributors to the pathogenesis. Advanced glycosylation end products (AGEs) that form in conditions of hyperglycemia have also been implicated as a cause of end organ damage. The accumulation of these AGEs is associated with the severity of kidney disease in patients with diabetic nephropathy.[75] A genetic predisposition exists in that higher rates of diabetes and nephropathy, hypertension, cardiovascular events, albuminuria, and elevated BP have been observed in relatives of patients with type 2 diabetes.[73,76] Certain genes and polymorphisms have also been associated with development of diabetic nephropathy, and further exploration into this area may prove beneficial in identifying high-risk patients.[77]

3. What is the significance of M.R.'s albuminuria?

Albuminuria is the earliest sign of kidney involvement in patients with diabetes mellitus and correlates with the rate of progression of kidney disease. For most patients, GFR begins to decline once proteinuria is established. Because of this association, annual testing for the presence of microalbuminuria is indicated in patients who have had type 1 diabetes for more than 5 years and in all patients with type 2 diabetes starting at diagnosis.[35] The presence of albuminuria indicates irreversible kidney damage. M.R. has likely reached the point at which such damage is inevitable, because her urinary protein exceeds ranges normally observed at the earlier stages of kidney disease. M.R.'s current laboratory data suggest that she has substantial kidney disease and has developed associated complications of the disease. Although progression to ESRD is generally inexorable at this stage, appropriate intervention can extend the time period until M.R. will require dialysis therapy.

Management

4. How should M.R.'s kidney disease be managed?

Since reversal of M.R.'s kidney disease is unlikely, the primary goals are to delay the need for dialysis therapy as long as possible and to manage secondary complications. The three main risk factors for the progression of incipient nephropathy to clinical diabetic nephropathy are poor glycemic control, systemic hypertension, and high dietary protein intake (>1.5 g/kg body weight per day). M.R.'s current random blood glucose concentration of 220 mg/dL, history of elevated glucose on prior visits, and increased A1C indicate poorly controlled diabetes, which will accelerate progression of her diabetic nephropathy. Thus, her blood glucose concentrations need to be maintained within target concentrations while avoiding hypoglycemia. M.R.'s elevated BP is likely the result of kidney disease and changes in intravascular volume; reduction of BP may prevent further damage to functioning nephrons. Similarly, protein intake should be less liberal in an attempt to reduce the rate of further progression, although this needs to be evaluated in the context of her overall nutritional status.

Intensive Glucose Control

Strict glycemic control is clearly indicated to reduce proteinuria and to slow the rate of decline in GFR.[35,78] The Diabetes Control and Complications Trial (DCCT) was a multicenter trial in 1,441 patients, which was designed to address how rigidly blood glucose concentrations should be controlled to reduce diabetic complications.[78] The DCCT evaluated the effect of intensive insulin treatment for type 1 diabetes on the development and progression of long-term complications, including diabetic nephropathy. Patients were randomized to receive either conventional insulin treatment (one to two insulin doses a day) or intensive treatment (three or more insulin doses a day). The goal of the intensive regimen was to maintain fasting blood glucose concentrations between 70 and 120 mg/dL, with postprandial blood glucose concentrations <180 mg/dL. After a mean follow-up of 6.5 years, the intensive insulin regimen reduced the overall risk of microalbuminuria (defined as urine albumin ≥40 mg/24 hours) by 39%, and albuminuria (defined as urine albumin ≥300 mg/24 hours) by 54%. However, stricter glycemic control was associated with an increased incidence of hypoglycemic episodes.[78] The effect of intensive glycemic control has also been studied in patients with type 2 diabetes. Over a 10-year treatment period, glucose control with either insulin or an oral sulfonylurea reduced microvascular complications, including albuminuria, when compared with conventional dietary therapy.[79]

Based on this information and the need to minimize risk of hypoglycemia, the American Diabetes Association's recommended goals in the adult diabetic population are a preprandial plasma glucose of 90 to 130 mg/dL, peak postprandial plasma glucose of <180 mg/dL, and an A1C <7%.[35] M.R. will benefit from intensive insulin therapy and achievement of these goals despite her advanced kidney disease. M.R. should be counseled on appropriate techniques for insulin administration and home glucose monitoring, particularly given her history of noncompliance. Compliance with this regimen will require motivation as well as encouragement from M.R.'s family and health care providers (see Chapter 50, Diabetes Mellitus, for a more complete discussion of intensive insulin therapy and counseling).

Antihypertensive Therapy

Systemic hypertension usually occurs with the development of microalbuminuria in patients with type 1 diabetes and is present in about one-third of patients at the time of diagnosis of type 2 diabetes. The coexistence of these disorders further increases the risk of cardiovascular events. Hypertension may be a result of underlying diabetic nephropathy and increased plasma volume or increased peripheral vascular resistance. Regardless of the etiology, virtually any level of untreated hypertension (either systemic or intraglomerular) is associated with a reduction in GFR. As such, the control of systemic and/or intraglomerular BP is perhaps the single-most important factor for retarding the progression of kidney disease and has been shown to increase life expectancy in patients with type 1 diabetes.[35,39]

Patients with diabetes and hypertension develop elevated systemic vascular resistance and increased vasoconstriction from angiotensin II, which are in large part responsible for the glomerular damage characteristic of diabetic nephropathy. Although the management of hypertension with virtually any agent can attenuate the progression of kidney disease, ACE inhibitors, which inhibit the synthesis of angiotensin II, and ARBs, which block angiotensin II AT_1 receptors, are preferred due in part to the effects of these agents on renal hemodynamics (Fig. 32-1). Reductions in proteinuria and a decreased rate of decline in GFR have been observed with ACE inhibitors and ARBs in patients with type 1 and type 2 diabetes (see also the Prevention section in Progressive Kidney Disease in this chapter).[39,44–46,51–56] As a result of these and other studies, ACE inhibitors or ARBs should be considered for all patients with diabetes (particularly type 1 diabetes) and microalbuminuria, even if their BP is normal.[35] Data comparing these two classes of agent are lacking.

The primary goal in M.R. is to delay development of ESRD and to reduce the risk of cardiovascular complications and death. Treatment with an ACE inhibitor such as enalapril should be initiated since she has substantial albuminuria (700 mg/day) and an elevated BP. An ARB (e.g., losartan) is a reasonable alternative to an ACE inhibitor. The initial product selected is generally based on tolerance to therapy and cost. A goal BP for M.R. based on the fact that she has type 1 diabetes and kidney disease is a BP <130/80 mm Hg.[40,41] Since the beneficial effects of ACE inhibitor therapy occur over months to years, M.R. must be monitored on a long-term basis for changes in kidney function and albuminuria and for side effects of therapy such as hyperkalemia. An increase in SrCr of up to 30% is acceptable with initiation of therapy with ACE inhibitors or ARBs.[50] Contraindications for the use of ACE inhibitors and ARBs include bilateral renal artery stenosis and pregnancy. The risk of hyperkalemia must also be weighed against the potential beneficial effects of these agents.

Some evidence suggests that a nondihydropyridine calcium channel blocker (e.g., diltiazem, verapamil) may be beneficial alone or in combination with an ACE inhibitor.[58,59,61] Diuretics may be considered for patients with diabetic nephropathy and edema depending on their degree of kidney function. For patients with kidney disease as extensive as that observed in M.R. (Cl_{Cr} <30 mL/min), loop diuretics are generally preferred because, unlike thiazide diuretics, they may retain their effect at this reduced GFR level (see Chapter 12, Fluid and Electrolyte Disorders and Chapter 14, Essential Hypertension). Other antihypertensive agents may be considered based on response to initial therapy and changes in kidney function.

Dietary Protein Restriction

High protein consumption accelerates the progression of diabetic nephropathy, presumably due to increased glomerular hyperfiltration and intraglomerular pressure. In patients with overt albuminuria, there is some evidence that the rate of decline in GFR, as well as urinary albumin excretion, can be blunted by restricting protein intake to 0.6 to 0.8 g/kg body weight per day and maintaining an isocaloric diet.[38,64] There is, however, limited evidence indicating a beneficial role of dietary protein restriction in diabetic patients with microalbuminuria. Nonetheless, given the potential benefits to delay progression of kidney disease, M.R. should be advised to maintain an isocaloric diet with a protein intake of 0.8 g/kg body weight per day (approximately 10% of daily calories).[35] The decision to decrease this intake even further to 0.6 g/kg body weight per day must be based on the rate of decline in GFR and her nutritional status. Because the typical Western diet is high in protein, some patients may have difficulty complying with such a low-protein diet due to its perceived unpalatability. Intervention by a dietitian is recommended to design a feasible dietary regimen limited in protein yet consistent with nutritional requirements in a diabetic patient.

FLUID AND ELECTROLYTE COMPLICATIONS
Sodium and Water Retention

5. Assess M.R.'s sodium and water balance. What interventions may be used to address this problem?

As illustrated in M.R., patients in the latter stages of CKD commonly retain sodium and water. This is supported by M.R.'s elevated BP, 2+ pedal edema, and mild pulmonary congestion. Sodium and water retention also lead to weight gain, although this may not be evident in M.R. due to volume loss from her recent onset of nausea and vomiting. Early in the course of CKD, glomerular and tubular adaptive processes develop, such as an increase in the fractional excretion of sodium (FE_{Na}). These mechanisms enable patients to maintain relatively normal sodium and water homeostasis. As M.R.'s normal serum sodium concentration indicates, this value is of little use in establishing the diagnosis of total body sodium and fluid excess because retention of sodium and water usually occurs in an isotonic fashion, leaving the serum sodium concentration relatively normal. Eventually, however, patients with advanced kidney dysfunction exhibit signs of sodium and fluid retention, as sodium balance is maintained at the expense of increased extracellular volume, which results in hypertension. Expansion of blood volume, if not controlled, may cause peripheral edema, heart failure, and pulmonary edema. Thus, management of sodium and water retention is essential. To achieve control, most patients with more advanced kidney disease will be placed on sodium restriction (approximately 2 to 4 g/day) and fluid restriction (approximately 2 L/day). These restrictions will depend on the current dietary intake, extent of volume overload, and urine output and should be altered according to the special needs of the patient. The primary consideration in CKD is that the kidney cannot adjust quickly to changes in sodium intake; therefore, any dietary intervention should be initiated gradually. Because M.R. has edema and hypertension, initial restriction of salt to 4 g/day, which is essentially a no-added-salt diet, is reasonable at this stage.

Because some patients with more advanced kidney disease produce normal amounts of urine, whereas others may produce less (or no urine if the patient has ESRD), fluid restrictions must be based on urine output. Diuretic therapy, usually with loop diuretics (e.g., furosemide, bumetanide, torsemide), is often required. Combination therapy with two different types of diuretics (i.e., loop and thiazide) may be successful in patients resistant to a single agent; however, limitations in efficacy of diuretics exist under certain conditions (e.g., a reduced GFR and hypoalbuminemia), and these situations must be considered when designing a diuretic regimen. Thiazide diuretics as single agents are generally not effective when the Cl_{Cr} is less than 30 mL/min, as in M.R. The possible exception is use of the thiazide-like diuretic, metolazone, which may retain its effect at reduced GFRs.[80] As kidney failure progresses, manifestations of excess fluid accumulation develop that are resistant to more conventional interventions, and dialysis will be required to control volume status.

Hyperkalemia

6. **M.R. has a serum potassium concentration of 5.3 mEq/L. Describe the mechanisms by which potassium imbalance occurs in patients like M.R. who have progressive CKD.**

[SI unit: K, 5.3 mmol/L]

Hyperkalemia may result from a combination of factors, including diminished renal potassium excretion, redistribution of potassium into the extracellular fluid due to metabolic acidosis, and excessive potassium intake. In M.R., all these mechanisms are likely to be contributing to hyperkalemia, although in the short-term dietary intake of potassium may not be substantial due to her recent onset of nausea and vomiting.

Potassium normally is filtered at the glomerulus and undergoes nearly complete reabsorption throughout the renal tubule. Distal tubular secretion is the primary mechanism by which potassium is excreted in the urine. A variety of factors affect this distal secretion of potassium, including aldosterone, sodium load presented to the distal reabsorptive site, hydrogen ion secretion, the amount of nonresorbable anions, urinary flow rate, diuretics, mineralocorticoids, and potassium intake.[81] Serum potassium concentrations are relatively well maintained within normal limits in patients with CKD. At GFRs >10 mL/min hyperkalemia is rare without an endogenous or exogenous load of potassium. This balance is maintained despite a decreasing nephron population and an overall drop in GFR, because the remaining nephrons undergo adaptive changes to enhance the distal tubular secretion of potassium per nephron (i.e., increased fractional excretion of potassium, FE_K).[82] GI excretion of potassium is also important as increased GI excretion and fecal losses may account for up to 50% of the daily potassium loss in patients with severe kidney disease. M.R.'s estimated Cl_{Cr} of 28 mL/min is above the "threshold" value for adequate potassium homeostasis, but this must be cautiously interpreted given that Cl_{Cr} values may overestimate GFR as kidney disease becomes more severe. Manifestations of hyperkalemia in M.R. should be carefully watched for as her kidney disease progresses.

Additional factors that alter potassium homeostasis include metabolic or respiratory acidosis. Acidotic conditions may cause a redistribution of intracellular potassium to the extracellular fluid. M.R. has metabolic acidosis as indicated by a serum bicarbonate of 18 mEq/L. This condition may account for her mildly elevated potassium concentration. Correction of metabolic acidosis may lower her potassium concentration. For each 0.1-unit change in blood pH, there is an average corresponding opposite change of approximately 0.6 mEq/L in the serum potassium concentration (see Chapter 11, Acid-Base Disorders).

M.R. is not taking any drugs that could contribute to hyperkalemia, although the influence of ACE inhibitors and ARBs must be considered because they are now advocated for M.R. to delay progression of kidney disease. Potassium-sparing diuretics such as spironolactone (Aldactone), triamterene (Dyrenium), and amiloride (Midamor) should be avoided in patients with severe CKD because they decrease tubular secretion of potassium. Some diabetic patients with only mild degrees of kidney disease may develop hyperkalemia from these diuretics because they have low plasma renin activity and, as a result, lower aldosterone concentrations.

7. **Is treatment of M.R.'s potassium indicated? How should severe hyperkalemia be managed?**

Treatment of hyperkalemia depends on the serum concentration of potassium as well as the presence or absence of symptoms and electrocardiographic (ECG) changes. Manifestations of hyperkalemia include weakness, confusion, and muscular or respiratory paralysis. However, these symptoms may be absent, especially if hyperkalemia develops rapidly. Early ECG changes include peaked T waves, followed by a decreased R-wave amplitude, widened QRS complex, and a prolonged P-R interval. These changes may progress to complete heart block with absent P waves and, finally, a sine wave. Ventricular arrhythmias or cardiac arrest may ensue if no effort to lower serum potassium is initiated. Hyperkalemic ECG changes are uncommon at potassium concentrations of <7 mEq/L but occur regularly at concentrations >8 mEq/L.

M.R. has a mild elevation in potassium to 5.3 mEq/L; therefore, no specific treatment is required. Generally, treatment is unnecessary if the potassium concentration is <6.5 mEq/L and there are no ECG changes. Although this serum potassium concentration does not require immediate intervention, close monitoring for hyperkalemia and its manifestations is necessary. This would be particularly important after starting ACE inhibitor therapy, which may contribute to development of hyperkalemia by decreasing aldosterone production. If potassium concentrations rise above 6.5 mEq/L, and especially if they are accompanied by neuromuscular symptoms or changes in the ECG, treatment should be instituted.

Goals of therapy include prevention of adverse events related to excessive potassium and reduction of serum potassium concentrations to a relatively normal range (4.5 to 5.5 mEq/L). Chronic management involves prevention of hyperkalemia by limiting potassium intake and the use of agents that could elevate potassium levels. This requires regular monitoring of potassium concentrations. Acute management involves reversal of cardiac effects with calcium administration and reduction of serum potassium. The latter can be achieved by shifting potassium intracellularly with administration of glucose and insulin, β-adrenergic agonists, or alkali therapy (if metabolic acidosis is a contributing factor) and by removing potassium using exchange resins or dialysis (See Chapter 12, Fluid and Electrolyte Disorders).

Metabolic Acidosis

8. Assess M.R.'s acid-base status. How should her acid-base disorder be managed?

M.R.'s low blood CO_2 content and high chloride concentration are consistent with metabolic acidosis that occurs with CKD. Normal buffering of hydrogen ions by the bicarbonate/carbonic acid system as well as other extracellular and intracellular buffers, including proteins, phosphates, and hemoglobin, is essential for maintaining normal acid-base balance (i.e., normal pH). Normal metabolism of ingested food produces approximately 1 mEq/kg of metabolic acid daily, which must be excreted by the kidneys (primarily as ammonium ion) to maintain acid-base balance. The kidney is responsible for reabsorption of bicarbonate and excretion of hydrogen ions through buffering by ammonia (produced by the kidney) and filtered phosphates. Reduced bicarbonate reabsorption and impaired production of ammonia by the kidneys are the major factors responsible for development of metabolic acidosis in advanced kidney disease. As nephron function declines, production of ammonia is increased to compensate for a decrease in secretion of hydrogen ions; however, once the maximum capacity for ammonia production is reached, acidosis develops. Mild hyperchloremia is generally observed in the earlier stages. As kidney disease progresses, metabolic acidosis with an elevated anion gap is observed due to accumulation of organic acids (see Chapter 11, Acid-Base Disorders). Bone carbonate stores serve as a source of alkali, but over time cannot compensate for changes in acid-base balance. Metabolic acidosis may contribute to bone disease by promoting bone resorption, and it may also influence nutritional status by decreasing albumin synthesis and promoting a negative nitrogen balance.[83]

M.R.'s mild acidosis should be treated with a goal of normalizing the plasma bicarbonate concentration or at least achieving bicarbonate levels near 20 to 22 mEq/L. Treatment includes use of preparations containing sodium bicarbonate or sodium citrate. Each 325-mg tablet of sodium bicarbonate provides 4 mEq of sodium and 4 mEq of bicarbonate. Shohl's solution and Bicitra contain 1 mEq of sodium and the amount of citrate/citric acid to provide 1 mEq of bicarbonate/mL. These latter agents may be used in patients who experience excessive GI distress with sodium bicarbonate from production and elimination of carbon dioxide. If a patient such as M.R. is sodium and fluid overloaded, one must consider that sodium bicarbonate may exacerbate this problem. Polycitra, or potassium citrate, is a possible alternative; however, the potassium content limits its use in patients with more severe kidney disease. Citrate also promotes aluminum absorption and should not be used in patients taking aluminum-containing agents. The amount of sodium bicarbonate required to normalize M.R.'s serum bicarbonate can be determined by the volume of distribution of bicarbonate (0.5 L/kg) and her base deficit (relative to the normal concentration of 24 mEq/L), as shown in the following equation:

$$\text{Dose of sodium bicarbonate (mEq)} = (0.5 \text{ L/kg}) \times \text{Patient weight (kg)} \times (24 \text{ mEq/L} - \text{Serum bicarbonate}) \tag{32-4}$$

M.R. will require approximately 190 mEq of bicarbonate followed by regular administration of 0.5 mEq/kg per day in divided doses. The initial amount should be administered over several days to prevent excessive sodium intake.

Once dialysis therapy is initiated in patients with kidney disease, IV and oral supplementation with bicarbonate or citrate/citric acid preparations is generally not required. At this point, dialysis therapy is used to chronically manage metabolic acidosis through use of dialysate baths containing bicarbonate. Bicarbonate is added to the dialysate solution and is delivered through the process of diffusion from the dialysate bath into the plasma (see Chapter 33, Renal Dialysis). If dialysis therapy is initiated in M.R., the continued need for oral bicarbonate supplementation should be reassessed.

Other Electrolyte and Metabolic Disturbances of Chronic Kidney Disease

9. What other electrolyte and metabolic disturbances are exhibited by M.R.?

The mild degree of hypermagnesemia seen in M.R. is a common finding in patients with CKD due to decreased elimination of magnesium by the kidney. Magnesium is eliminated by the kidney to the extent required to achieve normal serum magnesium concentrations until Cl_{Cr} is <30 mL/min. Serum magnesium concentrations <5 mEq/L rarely cause symptoms. Higher concentrations may lead to nausea, vomiting, lethargy, confusion, and diminished tendon reflexes while severe hypermagnesemia may depress cardiac conduction. The risk of hypermagnesemia can be reduced by avoiding magnesium-containing antacids and laxatives and by use of magnesium-free dialysate in patients with Stage 5 CKD requiring dialysis.

M.R.'s hyperphosphatemia is a result of decreased phosphorus elimination by the kidneys (see Questions 17 and 18 for a more detailed discussion of hyperphosphatemia). Based on the NKF-K/DOQI guidelines for bone metabolism, patients should reduce dietary phosphorus to 800 to 1,000 mg per day while maintaining adequate nutritional needs.[84] Phosphorus-containing laxatives and enemas should also be avoided. Hyperphosphatemia is associated with low serum calcium concentrations, not a current finding in M.R.

M.R. also has mild hyperuricemia. Asymptomatic hyperuricemia frequently develops in patients with kidney disease due to diminished urinary excretion of uric acid. In the absence of a history of gout or urate nephropathy, asymptomatic hyperuricemia does not require treatment.

ANEMIA OF CHRONIC KIDNEY DISEASE

10. What findings in M.R. are consistent with the diagnosis of anemia of CKD, and what is the etiology of this disorder?

M.R.'s hemoglobin of 8.7 g/dL and hematocrit of 26% are substantially lower than the normal range for premenopausal females (hemoglobin, 12 to 16 g/dL; hematocrit, 36% to

46%) indicating that she has anemia.[85] Her normal RBC indices suggest her red cells are of normal size, but the absence of an elevated reticulocyte count suggests an impaired bone marrow response for her degree of anemia. Her recent history of peptic ulcer disease may also have contributed to the observed drop in hemoglobin/hematocrit as a result of blood loss. Her complaint of general malaise is also consistent with the symptoms of anemia.

Characteristics and Etiology

Anemia affects the majority of patients with CKD and is caused by a decreased production of erythropoietin (EPO), a glycoprotein that stimulates red blood cell production in the bone marrow and is released in response to hypoxia. Approximately 90% of the total EPO is produced in the peritubular cells of the kidney; the remainder is produced by the liver. EPO concentrations in patients with kidney failure are lower than individuals with normal kidney function who have the same degree of anemia and therefore the same stimulus for EPO production and release.[86]

Anemia appears as early as Stage 3 CKD and is characterized by normochromic (normal color) and normocytic (normal size) red blood cells unless a concomitant iron, folate, or B_{12} deficiency exists. A direct correlation between GFR and hematocrit has been demonstrated with a 3.1% decrease in hematocrit for every 10 mL/min/1.73m^2 decline in GFR;[87] a higher prevalence of anemia occurs in the population with a GFR <60 mL/min.[1] Pallor and fatigue are the earliest clinical signs, with other manifestations developing as anemia worsens progressively with declining kidney function. A significant consequence of anemia is development of left ventricular hypertrophy (LVH), further contributing to cardiovascular complications and mortality in patients with CKD. LVH has been observed in approximately 30% of patients with GFRs 50 to 75 mL/min (Stages 2 and 3 CKD) and in up to 74% of patients at the start of dialysis (Stage 5 CKD).[88,89] These findings support the need for early and aggressive treatment of anemia of CKD before the development of Stage 5 CKD.

A more complete work-up for anemia of CKD is recommended for patients with a SrCr >2 mg/dL, although use of GFR criteria of <60 mL/min has been more recently advocated due to problems with use of SrCr alone (see "Evaluation of Kidney Function").[1,85] This work-up includes monitoring of hemoglobin and hematocrit, assessment of iron indices with correction if iron deficiency is present, and evaluation for sources of blood loss such as bleeding from the GI tract. This work-up should be done regularly as CKD progresses because of the association between anemia and the progressive decline in GFR.

Iron deficiency is the leading cause of resistance to therapy with exogenous erythropoietic therapy and must be corrected before such therapy is implemented (see Treatment). Iron deficiency may develop as a result of increased requirements for RBC production with exogenous EPO administration and from chronic blood loss due to bleeding or hemodialysis. Identification and management of iron deficiency through regular follow-up testing and iron supplementation is essential for adequate RBC production (see Treatment and also Chapter 86, Anemias).[85] M.R.'s iron status should be assessed at this time to determine if iron supplementation is needed.

Other factors that contribute to anemia include a shortened RBC life span secondary to uremia, blood loss from frequent phlebotomy and hemodialysis (HD), GI bleeding, severe hyperparathyroidism, protein malnutrition, accumulation of aluminum, severe infections, and inflammatory conditions.[85] Substances present in the plasma of patients with CKD, collectively termed "uremic toxins," may inhibit the production of EPO, the bone marrow response to EPO, and the synthesis of heme. The negative effects of these substances on RBC production are supported by improvement in erythropoiesis with dialysis, which removes these uremic toxins. This uremic environment also causes a decrease in the RBC life span, from a normal life span of 120 days to approximately 60 days in patients with severe CKD. A shortened RBC life span has been observed in uremic patients transfused with RBCs from individuals with normal kidney function, whereas RBCs from uremic individuals have a normal survival time when transfused into patients without kidney failure.[90]

Blood loss also contributes to anemia of CKD, particularly in patients requiring HD. With each HD session, generally performed three times per week, blood loss occurs. In addition, these patients are usually administered heparin during dialysis or antiplatelet drugs to prevent vascular access clotting, which further increases the risk of bleeding. Although a stool guaiac test was not performed in M.R., many patients with uremia and CKD will have a positive guaiac reaction due to the risk of bleeding from uremia itself. M.R. also has a peptic ulcer, which increases her potential for blood loss.

Other deficiencies may contribute to anemia of CKD. Deficiency of folic acid, as evidenced by low serum folate concentrations and macrocytosis, is relatively uncommon in patients with early kidney disease but occurs most often in dialysis patients since folic acid is removed by dialysis. Therefore, the daily prophylactic administration of the water-soluble vitamins, including 1 mg of folic acid, is recommended. Routine use of the fat-soluble vitamin A is discouraged, because hypervitaminosis A may develop, contributing to anemia.[91] Several multivitamin preparations devoid of vitamin A (e.g., Nephrocaps) are available for patients with kidney failure. Pyridoxine (vitamin B_6) deficiency may also occur in both dialyzed and nondialyzed CKD patients. There are significant similarities between this deficiency and the symptoms of uremia, which include skin hyperpigmentation and peripheral neuropathy. Current multivitamin products for patients with Stage 5 CKD contain adequate amounts of pyridoxine to prevent deficiency.

Goals of Therapy

11. What are the goals of therapy for anemia of CKD in M.R.?

Target Hemoglobin/Hematocrit

K/DOQI guidelines recommend target ranges of 11 to 12 g/dL for hemoglobin and 33% to 36% for hematocrit in patients receiving erythropoietic therapy.[85] It is at these targets that benefits such as increased survival, exercise capacity, quality of life, cardiac output, cognitive function, and decreased risk of LVH were observed in the CKD population.[85] Although these values were initially advocated for patients with Stage 5 CKD receiving dialysis, it seems prudent to apply them to the CKD population as a whole until more specific studies in patients in the earlier stages of CKD conclude otherwise.

Hemoglobin should be used to evaluate anemia in this population for several reasons. Hematocrit is dependent on volume status, which may be problematic for patients with fluctuations in plasma water (e.g., dialysis, volume overload). In addition, a number of variables can affect the hematocrit value, including temperature, hyperglycemia, the size of the red blood cell, and the counters used for the test. These variables do not significantly affect hemoglobin, making it the preferred test for anemia.[85]

Once M.R.'s iron status is evaluated, and corrected if necessary, EPO therapy may be started (see Treatment).

Iron Status

Since iron deficiency is the primary cause of resistance to erythropoietic agents, assessment of iron status is essential before initiating erythropoietic therapy. The two tests that best evaluate iron status are the transferrin saturation percent (TSat), a measure of iron immediately available for erythropoiesis, and serum ferritin, a measure of storage iron.[85] Transferrin is a carrier protein and its concentration depends on nutritional status. The TSat indicates the saturation of the protein transferrin with iron and is determined as:

$$\frac{\% \ TSat = serum \ iron \ (\mu g/dL)}{TIBC \ (\mu g/dL)} \times 100 \qquad \text{(32-5)}$$

where TIBC is the total iron binding capacity of the transferrin protein. Serum ferritin is a marker for iron reserves, which are stored primarily in the reticuloendothelial system (e.g., liver, spleen). The goal of iron replacement therapy is to maintain the TSat between 20% and 50% and a serum ferritin of 100 to 800 ng/mL to provide sufficient iron for erythrocyte production while preventing iron overload.[85] Values below these targets are indicative of absolute iron deficiency. A functional iron deficiency may exist when these values are within the target range, yet anemia persists despite appropriate erythropoietic therapy. In these cases, iron supplementation may lead to improved erythropoiesis. Other tests, including the percentage of hypochromic red cells, reticulocyte hemoglobin content, serum transferrin receptor, red cell ferritin, and zinc protoporphyrin have been proposed as indicators of iron status.[85] Although some of these markers have demonstrated predictive value in assessing iron status, either alone or in conjunction with other laboratory data, further investigation is warranted to determine their utility and to make such testing procedures readily available.

Treatment

12. Describe the options available to treat anemia of CKD and achieve the goals of therapy in M.R.

Iron Therapy

Before initiating erythropoietic therapy, M.R.'s iron indices should be determined. If M.R. is iron deficient, as indicated by the TSat and serum ferritin and other supporting laboratory data (see Chapter 86, Anemias), supplemental iron therapy should be administered. If iron deficiency is the cause of anemia, M.R. may benefit from iron supplementation alone (i.e., without erythropoietic therapy) to increase hemoglobin/

hematocrit. Peptic ulcer disease will need to be evaluated as a source of blood loss. Given the poor bioavailability of oral iron and patient noncompliance, oral iron is usually inadequate for repletion of iron in patients receiving HD who experience chronic blood loss.[92] For the population with early CKD and for patients receiving peritoneal dialysis (PD), an initial trial of oral iron may correct the deficiency since these patients do not have the same degree of blood loss. Oral iron also is more convenient because these patients do not have regular IV access. For some patients, however, IV therapy will be required to replete iron and meet the increased demands once erythropoiesis is stimulated with epoetin or darbepoetin therapy.

The data regarding the use of IV iron in patients with early CKD are conflicting.[93,94] In a retrospective evaluation of patients with early CKD who received at least 125 mg of sodium ferric gluconate intravenously along with erythropoietic therapy, erythropoiesis improved.[93] In contrast, monthly administration of IV iron sucrose (300 mg per month) to patients with early CKD did not improve hemoglobin response or reduce epoetin dose requirements in another study.[94] To resolve this controversy, ongoing studies are evaluating the safety and efficacy of available IV iron preparations in patients with early-stage CKD. This is consistent with efforts to promote early and aggressive treatment of anemia in this population.

Despite the controversy over the best strategy for iron supplementation in patients with early CKD, current recommendations support reserving IV iron for patients in whom oral iron has failed.[85,95] Therefore, a trial of oral iron is reasonable for M.R. Oral iron supplementation with 200 mg of elemental iron per day should be started to address iron deficiency, if present, and this regimen should be continued to maintain sufficient iron status while receiving erythropoietic therapy. Many oral iron preparations are available, and their iron content varies as will the number of tablets or capsules that must be taken per day to provide the required elemental iron (Table 32-4). Some oral formulations include ascorbic acid to enhance iron absorption. A heme iron product, Proferrin-ES, has recently been approved. Heme iron is more readily absorbed; however, a large number of tablets are required to supply the 200 mg elemental iron (Table 32-4). M.R. should be advised to take oral iron on an empty stomach to maximize absorption, unless side effects prevent this strategy. She also should be counseled on potential drug interactions with oral iron (e.g., antacids, quinolones) and GI side effects (nausea, abdominal pain, diarrhea, constipation, dark stools, etc). Noncompliance with therapy is a primary cause of therapeutic failure with oral iron.

If M.R.'s condition does not respond to oral therapy, as indicated by either persistent iron deficiency based on iron indices or inadequate response to what is considered and adequate dose and duration of erythropoietic therapy, IV iron is necessary. The IV iron preparations currently available are iron dextran (InFeD, DexFerrum), sodium ferric gluconate complex in sucrose (Ferrlecit), and iron sucrose (Venofer). The dextran products have caused anaphylactic reactions and, as a result, have a black box warning that requires administration of a 25 mg test dose followed by a 1-hour observation period before the total dose of iron is infused.[96] The dextran component is believed to be the cause of such reactions. The dose of IV iron recommended to correct absolute iron deficiency is a total dose of 1 g administered in divided doses or

Table 32-4   Oral Iron Preparations

Preparation	Common Brand Names	Commonly Prescribed Unit Size[a] (Amount Elemental Iron in mg)	Number of Units/Day To Yield 200 mg Elemental Iron
Ferrous sulfate	Slow FE, Fer-In-Sol	325 (65)	3 tablets
Ferrous gluconate	Feratab	325 (36)	5 tablets
Ferrous fumarate	Femiron, Feostat	200 (66)	3 capsules
Iron polysaccharide	Niferex, Nu-Iron	150 (150)	2 capsules
Heme iron polypeptide	Proferrin-ES Proferrin-Forte	12 (12)	17 tablets

[a]Unit size reflects common tablet/capsule sizes prescribed and not necessarily that of the brand names listed.

over a prolonged period to minimize the risk of adverse effects.[85] For iron dextran the approved dose is 100 mg increments, administered over 10 dialysis sessions for HD patients to provide a total of 1 g.[96] Larger doses of 500 mg up to the total 1 g dose have been safely administered over a longer infusion period of 4 to 6 hours.[85,97]

Sodium ferric gluconate and iron sucrose have recently been approved in the United States and have been advocated as safer IV iron preparations for the CKD population. These products were used in Europe for many years before approval in the United States. Both the ferric gluconate and iron sucrose products have been used successfully in patients who have experienced allergic reactions to the dextran products and there is evidence that they are safer: 8.7 adverse events per million doses for dextran versus 3.3 adverse events for gluconate.[98] To provide the recommended total dose of 1 g, ferric gluconate is administered as 125 mg (10 mL) over 8 consecutive dialysis sessions for HD patients. The dose may be administered as a slow IV injection at a rate of up to 12.5 mg/min or diluted in 100 mL of normal saline and infused over 1 hour.[99] Administration of 125 mg over 10 minutes (without a test dose) was determined to be a safer alternative to dextran preparations in HD patients and is an approved dosing strategy.[99,100] Doses up to 250 mg over 1 hour have been administered safely.[101] The flexibility of administering larger doses of iron is an important factor in achieving care efficiencies in the outpatient setting for patients with early CKD and those receiving PD.

Iron sucrose (Venofer) is a polynuclear iron hydroxide sucrose complex. The recommended dose of iron sucrose is 100 mg (5 mL) over 10 consecutive hemodialysis sessions to provide the total dose of 1 g.[102] The dose may be administered by a slow IV injection over 5 minutes or diluted in 100 mL of normal saline and infused over at least 15 minutes. As with sodium ferric gluconate, a test dose is not required. Iron sucrose doses of 250 to 300 mg have been safely administered over 1 hour and found to be as effective as sodium ferric gluconate administration in maintaining hemoglobin in patients receiving epoetin.[103,104]

Smaller doses of IV iron, in increments of 25 to 200 mg, may be administered on a weekly, every 2 week, or a monthly basis, to patients without absolute iron deficiency. These doses will sustain adequate iron stores, maintain target hemoglobin values, and potentially reduce the required dose of the erythropoietic agent.[85,105] This regimen is most convenient for HD patients who have regular IV access and increased iron needs due to chronic blood loss. Maintenance iron therapy re-

places these losses and minimizes the need for the more aggressive 1-g total doses of IV iron required for absolute iron deficiency. If HD is started in M.R. in the future, regular dosing of IV iron during dialysis is the most reasonable way to maintain adequate iron required for sustained erythropoiesis. Iron indices should be monitored at least every 3 months to ensure that TSat and ferritin values do not exceed 50% and 800 ng/mL, respectively, and iron therapy should be discontinued if these upper limits are exceeded.[85] This is because too much iron can lead to development of hemosiderosis, which in turn may increase the potential for infection (although controversial) and organ dysfunction secondary to iron deposition in the heart, liver, and pancreas.

Erythropoietic Therapy

Recombinant human EPO is the primary treatment option for patients like M.R. with anemia of CKD. Regular dialysis may improve this anemia, but it will not restore the hemoglobin/hematocrit to normal since the primary cause of anemia is reduced EPO production by the kidneys. Although blood transfusions were once the mainstay of treatment, they are now avoided, if possible, because they are associated with a risk for viral diseases (hepatitis, HIV), iron overload, and further suppression of erythropoiesis. Transfusions may be required in certain patients with substantially low oxygen-carrying capacity, substantial blood loss, and in those patients exhibiting persistent symptoms of anemia. M.R. is currently not a candidate for transfusions based on her hemoglobin of 8.7 g/dL (hematocrit 26%) and the absence of significant symptoms on presentation. Androgens were at one time used to treat the anemia of CKD because they directly or indirectly raise EPO concentrations. However, their routine use is not recommended because the erythropoietic response is inconsistent, they cause many adverse effects, and recombinant EPO is now available.

EPOETIN ALFA

Human erythropoietin orepoetin, the exogenous form of EPO, is produced using recombinant technology. Epoetin alfa is available in the United States, whereas epoetin β is available primarily outside the United States. Since it became available in 1989, epoetin alfa (Epogen, Procrit) has provided an effective treatment option for anemia and has substantially decreased the need for RBC transfusions. Epoetin alfa stimulates the proliferation and differentiation of erythroid progenitor cells, increases hemoglobin synthesis, and accelerates the release of reticulocytes from the bone marrow.

For patients like M.R. who do not yet require dialysis and patients receiving PD, epoetin alfa is generally administered by subcutaneous (SC) injection. HD patients often receive epoetin alfa by IV administration because IV access is established. According to the K/DOQI guidelines for anemia management, SC administration is preferred because lower doses can be administered less frequently and cost is lower than IV administration.[85,106] Starting doses for SC administration are 80 to 120 units/kg/wk (approximately 6,000 units/wk), whereas IV starting doses are 120 to 180 units/kg/wk (approximately 9,000 units/wk). Based on the half-life of epoetin alfa (8.5 hours IV, 24.4 hours SC), the total weekly dose is usually divided into smaller doses, administered one to three times per week with SC administration and three times per week for IV administration in HD patients.[107] For patients being converted from IV to SC administration whose hemoglobins are within the target range, the SC dose is usually two-thirds the IV dose.[85] For patients not yet at the target hemoglobin, a SC dose equivalent to the IV dose is recommended. Patients receiving epoetin alfa SC should be instructed on the appropriate administration technique, which includes rotating the sites for injection (e.g., upper arm, thigh, abdomen).

Extended dosing intervals for SC administration of epoetin alfa have been evaluated in patients with CKD who are not undergoing dialysis.[108–110] Once weekly doses of 10,000 units improve erythropoiesis and reduce transfusion requirements in early CKD patients with initial hemoglobins <10 g/dL.[108,109] Monthly dosing intervals for epoetin alfa SC have also been effective in maintaining target hemoglobin values in this population.[110] Such dosing strategies may provide more convenient therapy for CKD patients who are not yet undergoing dialysis but must come to the clinic for erythropoietic therapy.

DARBEPOETIN ALFA

Darbepoetin alfa (Aranesp) was approved in 2001 for the treatment of anemia of CKD, whether or not the patient required dialysis. Darbepoetin is a hyperglycosylated analogue of epoetin alfa that stimulates erythropoiesis by the same mechanism. Instead of the three N-linked carbohydrate chains on epoetin alfa, darbepoetin has five, which increase the capacity for sialic acid residue binding on the protein. The increased protein binding slows total body clearance and increases the terminal half-life to 25.3 hours and 48.8 hours following IV and SC administration, respectively.[111] Darbepoetin alfa's longer half-life relative to epoetin alfa offers the potential advantage of less frequent dosing to maintain target hemoglobin values.

Studies in patients with early CKD (Stages 3 and 4) determined that starting SC doses of 0.45 μg/kg administered once per week and 0.75 μg/kg once every other week were effective in achieving target hemoglobin and hematocrit values in patients who had not previously received erythropoietic therapy.[112,113] In dialysis patients converted from epoetin alfa to darbepoetin alfa (IV and SC), darbepoetin maintained target hemoglobin values when administered less frequently (i.e., once every week in patients previously receiving epoetin alfa three times per week and once every other week in patients previously receiving epoetin once weekly).[114–116] The approved starting dose of darbepoetin alfa in patients who have not received epoetin therapy is 0.45 μg/kg given either IV or SC once weekly.[117] Patients who have been receiving epoetin therapy may be converted to darbepoetin alfa based on the weekly total epoetin dose (Table 32-5).[117] For patients prescribed epoetin alfa two to three times per week, darbepoetin alfa may be administered once weekly. Patients who were receiving epoetin alfa once weekly should receive darbepoetin alfa once every 2 weeks. To determine the darbepoetin dose in this case, the weekly epoetin alfa dose should be multiplied by 2 and that value used in Table 32-5. For example, a patient receiving epoetin 6,000 units per week should receive 40 μg of darbepoetin alfa once every 2 weeks (6,000 × 2 = 12,000, which corresponds to a darbepoetin dose of 40 μg).[117]

Epoetin alfa and darbepoetin alfa are generally well tolerated, with hypertension being the most common adverse event reported. Although elevated BP is not uniformly considered a contraindication to therapy, it should be monitored closely so that changes in antihypertensive therapy and/or the dialysis prescription are made if justified. Failure to elicit a response to erythropoietic therapy requires evaluation of factors that cause resistance such as iron deficiency, infection, inflammation, chronic blood loss, aluminum toxicity, malnutrition, and hyperparathyroidism. Resistance to erythropoietic therapy has been observed in patients receiving ACE inhibitors, although there are conflicting data.[118,119] Rare cases of antibody formation to epoetin therapy have been reported.[120,121] Neutralizing anti-EPO antibodies were identified in 13 patients with pure red-cell aplasia who required blood transfusions after a course of therapy with epoetin alfa or beta.[120] Similar cases have been reported, primarily with one epoetin alfa product manufactured outside the United States, Eprex. Some evidence supports cross reactivity of these antibodies with darbepoetin, although the information is currently limited.[122] While the clinical implications of antibody formation in patients receiving erythropoietic therapy are uncertain, clinicians should be aware of these reports when evaluating response to therapy.

Treatment of M.R.'s anemia must be initiated, given the chronic nature of her kidney disease and her current hemoglobin/hematocrit. Patients with hemoglobin values <10g/dL (hematocrit, <30%), such as M.R., are the best candidates for erythropoietic therapy. It is also important to

Table 32-5 Estimated Darbepoetin Alfa Starting Doses Based on Previous Epoetin Alfa Dose

Previous Weekly Epoetin Alfa Dose[a,b] (<2,500 U/wk)	Weekly Darbepoetin Alfa Dose (6.25 μg/wk)
2,500–4,999	12.50
5,000–10,999	25.00
11,000–17,999	40.00
18,000–33,999	60.00
34,000–89,999	100.00
≥90,000	200.00

[a]Darbepoetin alfa should be administered weekly for patients receiving epoetin alfa two or three times per week and every other week for patients receiving epoetin alfa once per week.

[b]For patients requiring darbepoetin alfa every other week, the weekly dose of epoetin alfa should be multiplied by 2 and this dose used in the conversion chart to determine the appropriate darbepoetin alfa dose.

Adapted with permission from Aranesp (darbepoetin alfa) package insert. Thousand Oaks, CA: Amgen Inc, July 19, 2002.

identify and correct any iron or folate deficiency and perform a stool guaiac test to rule out active GI bleeding. Iron supplementation is indicated not only if M.R. is iron deficient, but also to maintain iron status while receiving erythropoietic therapy (see Iron Therapy). While administration of iron alone may improve her anemia, epoetin alfa or darbepoetin alfa will likely be required based on the severity of the anemia and the progressive nature of her kidney disease. M.R. may start epoetin alfa at a dose of 6,000 units (approximately 100 units/kg) administered SC once per week or divided into two weekly doses of 3,000 units, assuming her iron status is appropriate (see Iron Status). Another option would be darbepoetin alfa administered at a dose of 25 μg (0.45 μg/kg) SC once per week. She also should be instructed on how to administer SC epoetin alfa or darbepoetin alfa. Dose adjustments should not be made more frequently than once every 4 to 6 weeks for either agent because of the time course for response (i.e., the pharmacodynamic effects on RBC homeostasis). The time it takes to reach a new steady state, when RBC production is equal to RBC destruction, is dependent on the life span of the red cell, which is approximately 60 days in patients with kidney failure. Therefore, it will take approximately 2 to 3 months to reach a plateau in measured hemoglobin/hematocrit. Dose adjustments should be made based on M.R.'s hemoglobin and hematocrit, which should be monitored every 1 to 2 weeks after initiation of therapy or following a dose change. If a rapid increase in hemoglobin/hematocrit is observed (hemoglobin >1.0 g/dL, hematocrit >3% to 4%, over a 1- to 2-week period) or the target hemoglobin/hematocrit is exceeded, then doses of either agent should be decreased by approximately 25%. If response is inadequate (hemoglobin increase <1 g/dL, hematocrit increase <2% to 3%, in 2 to 4 weeks), then the doses should be increased by approximately 50% for epoetin alfa and 25% for darbepoetin alfa.[85,117] Once stable, the hemoglobin/hematocrit should be monitored every 2 to 4 weeks. If a response is not observed despite appropriate dose titration, M.R. should be evaluated for possible reasons for nonresponse (i.e., iron deficiency, bleeding, aluminum intoxication, hyperparathyroidism, infection).

CARDIOVASCULAR COMPLICATIONS

13. H.B. is a 65-year-old white male with Stage 5 CKD, who has just started chronic HD. He comes in today for his third HD session (dialysis scheduled three times per week, 4-hour duration). He has a history of hypertension, which has been poorly controlled over the past 4 months (BP ranges 150 to 190/85 to 105 mm Hg), and has complained of shortness of breath and a significant weight gain over the past month. His pertinent medical history includes hypertension for the past 14 years. H.B.'s current medications include metoprolol 50 mg BID, furosemide 80 mg BID, calcium carbonate 500 mg TID with meals, and Nephrocaps 1 PO QD. H.B's predialysis BP was 175/98 mm Hg, and his postdialysis BP was 158/90 mm Hg. A recent ECG showed evidence of left ventricular hypertrophy (LVH).

Predialysis laboratory values were as follows: serum sodium (Na), 140 mEq/L (normal, 135 to 147 mEq/L); potassium (K), 5.1 mEq/L (normal, 3.5 to 5.0 mEq/L); chloride (Cl), 101 mEq/L (normal, 95 to 105 mEq/L); CO_2 content, 23 mEq/L (normal, 22 to 28 mEq/L); SrCr, 8.8 mg/dL (normal, 0.6 to 1.2 mg/dL); BUN,

84 mg/dL (normal, 8 to 18 mg/dL); phosphate, 5.2 mg/dL (normal, 2.5 to 5.0 mg/dL); Ca, 8.6 mg/dL (normal, 8.8 to 10.4 mg/dL); serum albumin, 3.0 g/dL (normal, 4.0 to 6.0 g/dL); cholesterol (nonfasting), 345 mg/dL (normal, <200 mg/dL); triglycerides, 285 mg/dL (normal, <200 mg/dL); Hct, 27% (normal, 39% to 49%); and Hgb, 9.0 g/dL (normal, 13 to 16 g/dL). H.B. has a urine output of 50 mL/day. What conditions evident in H.B. put him at increased risk of cardiovascular complications and mortality?

[SI units: Na, 140 mmol/L (normal, 135 to 147); K, 5.1 mmol/L (normal, 3.5 to 5.0); Cl, 101 mmol/L (normal, 95 to 105); CO_2, 23 mmol/L (normal, 22 to 28); SrCr, 778 μmol/L (normal, 50 to 110); BUN, 30 mmol/L of urea (normal, 3.0 to 6.5); phosphate, 1.68 mmol/L (normal, 0.8 to 1.60); Ca, 2.15 mmol/L (normal, 2.2 to 2.6); serum albumin, 30 g/L (normal, 40 to 60 g/L); cholesterol, 8.9 (normal, <5.2); triglycerides, 3.2 (normal, <2.3); Hct, 0.27 (normal, 0.39 to 0.49); and Hgb, 90 g/L (normal, 130 to 160 for males)]

H.B. has uncontrolled hypertension that is not being adequately managed with his current drug therapy or HD. Hypertension is associated with LVH, ischemic heart disease, and heart failure, all of which are contributing factors to overall mortality in patients with Stage 5 CKD who are undergoing dialysis.[3] H.B.'s ECG evidence of LVH should trigger additional evaluation to determine the extent of cardiac involvement and diagnosis of heart failure, which is associated with increased mortality in both diabetic and nondiabetic patients (See Chapter 19, Heart Failure). LVH develops early in the course of CKD and progresses as kidney disease progresses.[88,89] H.B. is in the most severe stage of CKD and has greatest likelihood of developing LVH. Anemia contributes substantially to the development of LVH and heart failure as well. H.B.'s hemoglobin of 9.0 g/dL (hematocrit 27%) is below the target value and requires treatment with erythropoietic therapy and iron supplementation based on evaluation of his iron indices (see Anemia).

Additional factors that increase risk of cardiovascular complications and mortality in H.B. include the elevated cholesterol and triglycerides levels as well as hypoalbuminemia (serum albumin, 3.0 g/dL). Increased levels of homocysteine are common in patients with kidney failure and have been associated with increased risk of coronary artery disease (CAD).[123] Since elevated concentrations of homocysteine have been observed in conjunction with decreased folate and vitamin B_{12} levels, more aggressive supplementation of these vitamins in this population has been suggested. Since H.B.'s total corrected calcium (corrected for hypoalbuminemia) is 9.4 mg/dL, his calcium, calcium-phosphorus product, and use of a calcium-containing phosphate binder will need to be monitored frequently. Calcifications are common in patients with kidney disease and also are associated with cardiovascular complications.

Cardiovascular disease and complications continue to be the leading cause of mortality in patients with kidney failure. According to data from a large population of dialysis patients, cardiovascular disease increases the risk of all-cause mortality five fold when compared to the general Medicare population without kidney disease.[3] All-cause death rates are almost four times greater in dialysis patients age 65 and older, such as H.B., than in the general Medicare population.[3] For these reasons, the risk of CAD should be evaluated regularly in patients with ESRD.

Hypertension

14. What options are available to treat H.B.'s hypertension considering his other cardiac complications and BP goal?

Dialysis

Hypertension is common in patients with CKD with a prevalence that varies depending on the cause of CKD and residual kidney function. Prevalence of hypertension has been estimated to be 80% in HD and 50% in PD patients.[124] Multiple factors are involved in the development of hypertension in the CKD population, including extracellular volume expansion from salt and water retention and activation of the renin-angiotensin-aldosterone system.[125] Increased sympathetic tone also has been observed with an increase in norepinephrine activity.

Since H.B. is just beginning dialysis therapy, it is difficult to assess the degree to which volume removal will ultimately affect his BP. To control BP related to volume changes, dialysis therapy should be adjusted as needed to achieve H.B.'s *dry weight*, the postdialysis weight at which symptoms of hypervolemia and hypovolemia are absent. H.B. has had recent findings consistent with worsening volume status (shortness of breath, weight gain) that should be considered when modifying his dialysis prescription; further workup is needed to determine if H.B. has systolic or diastolic heart failure. It is also important to counsel H.B. on the importance of salt and fluid intake restriction between HD sessions to minimize weight gain, volume expansion, and hypertension. Restriction of salt intake to 2 to 3 g/day and fluid to 1 L/day is appropriate and will require regular follow up by a dietitian.

Antihypertensive Therapy

Antihypertensive therapy should be used in conjunction with dialysis therapy in H.B. to achieve a BP <140/90 mm Hg.[124] For some patients, initiation of dialysis alone may achieve this goal and antihypertensive therapy may be withdrawn. The BP goal in patients with Stage 5 CKD should minimize cardiovascular complications, but it should not increase the risk for hypotension and its associated complications during dialysis. If patients experience hypotensive symptoms during HD, the goal BP can be increased, but they also should be evaluated for other cardiovascular disorders. Since the BP between dialysis sessions varies due to volume changes, the ideal time to measure BP relative to dialysis (i.e., predialysis versus postdialysis) is unclear, but predialysis BP has been favored.

Diuretics are commonly used in patients in the early stages of CKD. As previously discussed, the effectiveness of diuretics depends on the amount of sodium delivered to their site of action in the renal tubule and on the patient's kidney function. For example, a decrease in the GFR from 125 to 25 mL/min, theoretically, could result in an approximate 80% decrease in the amount of sodium filtered. Early in the course of kidney failure, thiazides or thiazide-like diuretics are effective antihypertensive agents. As GFR is further reduced (Cl_{Cr} <30 mL/min), the thiazide diuretics become essentially ineffective. Potassium-sparing diuretics are also ineffective and may increase the risk of hyperkalemia in this population. Loop diuretics (e.g., furosemide), which function more proximally are indicated in patients with Stage 4 CKD (GFR 15 to 29 mL/min).[126] These drugs can be effective for BP and volume control in patients with advanced kidney disease if residual kidney function is substantial (urine output >100 mL/day). Their effect must be frequently reevaluated based on urine output and any effect on volume control. H.B.'s urine output should be assessed to determine the rationale for continued use of furosemide and the current dose should be assessed, since doses higher than his current dose of 80 mg BID are often required in patients with this degree of kidney dysfunction. It is likely that furosemide will need to be discontinued as H.B. residual renal function declines.

Given the role of the renin-angiotensin-aldosterone system in the development of hypertension in patients with CKD, ACE inhibitors are a logical choice for antihypertensive therapy. ACE inhibitors are effective antihypertensive agents in patients with CKD and have been shown to reverse LVH.[127] They are, however, underused in this population. Response must be assessed individually to determine if renin-angiotensin-aldosterone activity is a predominant etiology of hypertension. Initiating therapy with low doses is prudent to evaluate patient response and tolerance. Use of these agents in combination with other antihypertensives is often required for adequate BP control. Most of these agents may be administered once daily; however, due to the renal elimination of the parent drug or active metabolite, dosage adjustments are necessary in patients with CKD. Fosinopril is the exception because it undergoes substantial hepatic elimination. ACE inhibitors should also be used cautiously in patients dialyzed with the polyacrylonitrile (AN69) membrane. This is because ACE inhibitors decrease the breakdown of bradykinin. Bradykinin production is increased in patients who experience systemic or immune-mediated reactions when blood comes in contact with the dialyzer, which can lead to anaphylactic reactions. Such reactions are common with AN69 due to its composition; therefore, ACE inhibitor use in combination with this dialyzer should be avoided.

Although ARBs effectively lower BP in patients without kidney disease,[128] less is known about their effectiveness in patients with kidney failure. These agents may offer an alternative to ACE inhibitors in patients experiencing kinin-mediated adverse effects; however, similar side effects have been reported with ARBs. The combined use of ARBs with other antihypertensive agents may be rational when patients are unresponsive to other regimens. One ARB, valsartan, has been approved for use in heart failure and this may offer an advantage in patients with concurrent heart failure[129]; however, this concept must be studied in a CKD population.

Calcium channel blockers are effective antihypertensives in patients with CKD. However, because the nondihydropyridine agents (i.e., diltiazem, verapamil) have negative chronotropic and inotropic effects, they should be used with care in patients with heart disease. Generally, dosage adjustment is not required in patients with kidney disease.

Other agents used to treat hypertension in the CKD population include β-blockers, centrally acting agents (e.g., clonidine, methyldopa), vasodilators (e.g., minoxidil, hydralazine), and α_1-adrenergic blockers (prazosin, terazosin, doxazosin). β-Blockers inhibit release of renin and may be useful in hypertension associated with CKD. Risk versus benefit should be evaluated when β-blockade is considered in conjunction with other comorbid conditions such as asthma, heart failure, and lipid abnormalities. Dosage adjustment is required for the less lipophilic agents (i.e., atenolol, acebutolol, nadolol).

H.B. is currently taking the β-blocker, metoprolol, and the loop diuretic, furosemide. It is likely that his diuretic will need to be discontinued as his residual kidney function decreases and response to therapy is inadequate. While an effective antihypertensive, metoprolol may not be the best single agent for H.B. and its use must be reassessed based on the recent evidence of LVH and whether systolic or diastolic dysfunction is diagnosed on further work up. If changes in H.B.'s HD prescription to improve volume control and achieve his dry weight do not reduce his BP, another antihypertensive regimen should be selected. A reasonable antihypertensive regimen would include an ACE inhibitor (e.g., enalapril) with or without β-blocker therapy or a calcium channel blocker based on cardiac findings. The selection will depend substantially on follow up results of his cardiac disease, BP control with HD, and the development of adverse effects (see Chapter 14, Essential Hypertension, and Chapter 19, Heart Failure).

Dyslipidemia

15. How should H.B.'s lipid abnormalities be treated?

H.B. has elevated serum cholesterol and triglyceride concentrations, a common finding in patients with CKD. Dyslipidemia and increased oxidative stress contribute to premature atherogenesis in these patients. Several atherogenic factors in patients with CKD have been postulated, including arterial wall injury, platelet activation and adherence, smooth muscle cell proliferation, and intra-arterial accumulation of cholesterol. Whether lowering of serum lipids will improve long-term morbidity and mortality remains to be determined, but treatment should be consistent with NCEP ATP III guidelines and the K/DOQI guidelines for treatment of dyslipidemias.[70,71] Dietary intervention successfully reduces triglyceride and cholesterol concentrations, and many drugs are available to treat lipid abnormalities in patients with Stage 5 CKD (see Chapter 13, Dyslipidemias). Statin use has been supported by recent evidence associating these agents with a decrease in cardiovascular mortality and all-cause mortality in patients on dialysis.[130] Because many β-adrenergic blocking drugs may elevate triglyceride concentrations, antihypertensive drugs with insignificant or beneficial effects on serum lipids (e.g., ACE inhibitors, calcium channel blockers, clonidine, prazosin) may be preferable.

SECONDARY HYPERPARATHYROIDISM AND RENAL OSTEODYSTROPHY

16. D.B. is a 42-year-old white female who has a 24-year history of type 1 diabetes mellitus with complications of diabetic nephropathy, retinopathy, and neuropathy. She has hypothyroidism and was diagnosed with Stage 5 CKD 4 years ago. She started continuous ambulatory peritoneal dialysis (CAPD) at that time. Her current dialysis prescription is four exchanges per day with a 1.5% dextrose dialysate solution. Her current medications include levothyroxine 0.1 mg/day, metoclopramide (Reglan) 10 mg TID before meals, regular insulin 160 U/day (given intraperitoneally), docusate 100 mg QD, calcium carbonate 1500 mg PO TID with meals, EPO 5,000 U subcutaneously twice weekly, ferrous sulfate 325 mg TID, and Nephrocaps 1 capsule QD. At a recent clinic visit, findings on physical examination included a BP of 128/84 mm Hg, diabetic retinopathic changes with laser scars bilaterally, a peritoneal catheter in the abdomen, and diminished sensation bilaterally below the knees. Her laboratory values were as follows: normal serum electrolytes; a random blood glucose of 175 mg/dL (normal, 140 mg/dL); BUN, 45 mg/dL (normal, 8 to 18 mg/dL); SrCr, 8.9 mg/dL (normal, 0.6 to 1.2 mg/dL); Hct, 30% (normal, 36% to 46%); Hgb, 10 g/dL (normal, 12 to 16 g/dL); WBC count, 6,200/mm³ (normal, 3,200 to 9,800/mm³); Ca, 9.0 mg/dL (normal, 8.8 to 10.4 mg/dL); phosphate, 6.8 mg/dL (normal, 2.5 to 5.0 mg/dL); intact PTH, 450 pg/mL (normal, 5 to 65 pg/mL); total serum protein, 5.0 g/dL (normal, 6.0 to 8.0 g/dL); serum albumin, 3.1 g/dL (normal, 4.0 to 6.0 g/dL); and uric acid, 8.9 mg/dL (normal, 2.0 to 7.0 mg/dL). Previous radiographs for D.B. revealed bone density changes consistent with early signs of renal osteodystrophy. Describe the etiology of D.B.'s abnormal bone, calcium, phosphorus, and PTH findings.

[SI units: blood glucose, 9.7 mmol/L (normal, <11 mmol/L); BUN, 16.1 mmol/L of urea (normal, 3.0 to 6.5); SrCr, 787 μmol/L (normal, 50 to 110); Hct, 0.30 (normal, 0.36 to 0.46); Hgb, 100 g/L (normal, 120 to 160); WBC count, 6,200 × 10⁶/L (normal, 3,200 to 9,800); Ca, 2.25 mmol/L (normal, 2.2 to 2.6); phosphate, 2.19 mmol/L (normal, 0.8 to 1.60); total serum protein, 50 g/L (normal, 60 to 80); serum albumin, 31 g/L (normal, 40 to 60 g/L); uric acid, 529 μmol/L (normal, 120 to 420)]

Etiology

Renal osteodystrophy (ROD) is the term used to describe the skeletal manifestations that occur as kidney function declines. Collectively, ROD refers to specific bone abnormalities that include osteitis fibrosa (most common pattern), osteomalacia, osteosclerosis, and osteopenia. Hyperphosphatemia, hypocalcemia, hyperparathyroidism, decreased production of active vitamin D, and resistance to vitamin D therapy are all frequent problems in CKD that may lead to the secondary complication of ROD.

The interrelationships between phosphorus, calcium, vitamin D, and PTH have been reviewed extensively.[131,132] Retention of phosphorus and secondary hyperparathyroidism (sHPT) play a major role in the development of osteitis fibrosa or high-turnover bone disease. The "trade-off" hypothesis best describes the events leading to changes in bone metabolism.[131] As GFR decreases, phosphorus excretion by the kidney decreases resulting in hyperphosphatemia. Hyperphosphatemic conditions lead to a corresponding decrease in ionized calcium concentration, a primary stimulus for release of PTH from the parathyroid gland. Higher concentrations of PTH decrease renal tubular reabsorption of phosphorus and promote its excretion. Both serum phosphorus and calcium concentrations are corrected depending on the degree of remaining kidney function, but this occurs at the expense of an elevated PTH concentration (the "trade off"). As kidney disease becomes more severe (GFR <30 mL/min), the phosphaturic response to PTH diminishes and sustained hyperphosphatemia and hypocalcemia develop. In response to hypocalcemia, calcium is mobilized from the bone, a mechanism largely controlled by PTH. Virtually all patients with kidney failure develop sHPT. Decreased PTH degradation by the kidney may also contribute to the hyperparathyroid state in patients with kidney disease.

The kidney is the principal organ responsible for vitamin D production and, as such, vitamin D metabolism is altered in the presence of uremia. Persistent hyperphosphatemia inhibits the normal conversion of 25-hydroxyvitamin D_3 to its biologically active metabolite, 1,25-dihydroxyvitamin D_3, by 1-α-hydroxylase. The enzyme is present in proximal tubular cells of the kidney and is necessary for conversion of vitamin D to the active form. This active form of vitamin D, also known as calcitriol, increases gut absorption of calcium and interacts with vitamin D receptors on the parathyroid gland to suppress PTH release. As a result of decreased calcitriol production, the absorption of dietary calcium in the gut is diminished, contributing to hypocalcemia. Decreased suppression of PTH release by vitamin D in conjunction with hypocalcemia promotes continued stimulus for mobilization of calcium from bone. Furthermore, uremic patients require a higher extracellular calcium concentration to suppress secretion of PTH. This is also described as an increase in the calcium "set point" or the concentration of calcium required to inhibit 50% of maximal PTH secretion.[131]

The chronic effects of hyperparathyroidism on the skeleton lead to bone pain, fractures, and myopathy. In children, these effects may be particularly severe and usually retard growth. The metabolic acidosis of kidney disease also contributes to a negative calcium balance in the bone.

D.B.'s presentation is consistent with ROD based on the observed changes in bone architecture and abnormalities in serum phosphorus, calcium, and PTH; all can be attributed to her kidney disease.

Treatment

17. What are the goals of therapy for D.B.'s calcium, phosphorus, and PTH abnormalities? What options are available to treat these disorders?

The management objectives for D.B. are to (1) maintain near-normal serum calcium and phosphorus concentrations, (2) prevent secondary hyperparathyroidism, and (3) restore normal skeletal development without inducing adynamic bone disease (or low bone turnover). The K/DOQI guidelines for bone metabolism and disease suggest target levels for serum calcium and phosphorus, the calcium and phosphorus product (Ca-P), and intact PTH for each stage of CKD.[84,133] These goals are best achieved with dietary phosphorus restriction, appropriate use of phosphate-binding agents, vitamin D therapy, and dialysis.

Dietary Restriction of Phosphorus

In general, serum phosphorus should be maintained at near normal levels in the earlier stages of CKD (approximately 2.7 to 4.6 mg/dL), with the higher range (3.5–5.5) accepted in patients with Stage 5 CKD.[84] Dietary phosphorus restriction can prevent hyperphosphatemia and maintain target phosphorus concentrations. Protein restriction will also limit phosphorus intake, because high-protein foods tend to contain high amounts of phosphorus (Table 32-6).[134] The challenge is in tailoring a diet that fulfills these criteria while providing adequate nutrition. During the early stages of kidney disease (Cl_{Cr}

Table 32-6 Phosphorus Content of Select High-Protein Foods

Food	Portion Size	Phosphorus Content (mg)
Black-eyed peas, cooked	1 cup	288
Cheese, American	4 ounces	1,200
Cheese, cheddar	4 ounces	545
Cheese creamed cottage	4 ounces	150
Cheese, Swiss	4 ounces	800
Chicken, cooked	3½ ounces	190
Chocolate candy	2 ounces	130
Egg	1 large	100
Fish, cooked	4 ounces	400
Hamburger, ground sirloin	3½ ounces	186
Ice cream	8 ounces	163
Kidney beans, cooked	1 cup	278
Lamb	3½ ounces	200
Liver, chicken	3½ ounces	312
Milk, whole or skim	8 ounces (1 cup)	278
Peanut butter	2 tablespoons	118
Peanuts	3½ ounces	466
Pork tenderloin	3½ ounces	301
Salmon, canned	3½ ounces	344
Sardines, canned in oil	3½ ounces	434
Shrimp	3½ ounces	156
Soybeans	1 cup	322
Steak, sirloin	4 ounces	282
Tofu	3½ ounces	128
Tuna fish, canned	3½ ounces	250
Turkey	3½ ounces	200
Yogurt, plain	8 ounces	270

Data from Bowes AP, Church HN. Bowes & Church's Food Values of Portions Commonly Used. Philadelphia: Lippincott-Raven, 1998.

<60 mL/min), dietary phosphorus should be reduced to 800 to 1000 mg/day (approximately 60% of normal) through restriction of meat, milk, legumes, and carbonated beverages to achieve normal phosphorus concentrations.[84,135] Patients requiring dialysis have less dietary phosphorus restriction with a recommended phosphorus intake of approximately 800 to 1,200 mg/day.[135] While phosphorus is removed to some extent by dialysis, neither HD nor PD removes adequate amounts to warrant complete liberalization of phosphorus in the diet. Regular dietary counseling by a renal dietitian is necessary to reinforce the importance of phosphorus restriction and other dietary recommendations.

Phosphate-Binding Agents

Significant reduction of serum phosphorus may be difficult to achieve with dietary intervention alone, particularly in patients with more advanced kidney disease (GFR <30 mL/min). For these patients, phosphate-binding agents used in conjunction with dietary restriction are necessary. Phosphate-binding agents limit phosphorus absorption from the GI tract by binding with the phosphorus present from dietary sources. Therefore, these agents must be administered with meals. Available binders include products that contain calcium, aluminum, or magnesium cations or the polymer-based agent, sevelamer hydrochloride (Renagel).

CALCIUM-CONTAINING PREPARATIONS

Calcium-containing preparations, especially calcium carbonate and calcium acetate, are frequently used to prevent hyperphosphatemia in patients with kidney disease. The many preparations available vary in their calcium content (Table 32-7). Correction of hypocalcemia is an added beneficial ef-

fect of the calcium-containing preparations; however, there is a risk of hypercalcemia and calcifications associated with the prolonged use of these agents.[136] Compared with calcium carbonate, calcium acetate binds about twice the amount of phosphorus for the same amount of calcium salts. This may be due to the increased solubility of calcium acetate in both acidic and alkaline environments.[137] However, despite the reduction in the dose of elemental calcium required with the acetate product, the incidence of hypercalcemia does not differ.[138] Calcium citrate is a calcium salt with a phosphate-binding capacity similar to that of calcium carbonate; however, because it also increases aluminum absorption from the GI tract, its use is not recommended in patients with kidney disease.

Although calcium-containing binders have an added benefit of correcting hypocalcemia, the potential for hypercalcemia must be frequently evaluated in patients receiving these agents chronically. Simultaneous administration of vitamin D preparations and calcium also increases the risk of hypercalcemia. Serum calcium and the Ca-P product should be determined before therapy is started and at regular intervals thereafter. Serum calcium should be maintained at near normal levels in the earlier stages of CKD. A narrower range is recommended in patients with stage 5 CKD (upper range of approximately 9.5 mg/dL) to prevent both hypocalcemia and hypercalcemia.[84] Based on the increased risk of mortality associated with an elevated Ca-P product and the potential for calcifications, the ideal Ca-P product target has been decreased to <55 mg^2/dL^2.[84] This is much lower than the former recommendation of <65 to 70 mg^2/dL^2 and more difficult to achieve. When the Ca-P exceeds the target value, the patient should be switched to a noncalcium-based phosphate binder. Other alternatives include sevelamer and other cations such as aluminum or magnesium preparations, although these metal-

Table 32-7 Phosphate-Binding Agents

Product	Select Available Agents[a]	Content of Compound	Starting Dose
Calcium carbonate (40% calcium)	Tums	200, 300, 400 mg	0.8–2 g elemental Ca with meals
	Os-Cal-500	500 mg	
	Nephro-Calci	600 mg	
	Caltrate 600	600 mg	
	Calcarb HD (powder)	2,400 mg/packet	
	$CaCO_3$ (multiple preparations)	200–600 mg	
Calcium acetate (25% calcium)	Phos-Lo 667 mg	169 mg	2–3 tablets with meals
Sevelamer hydrochloride (polymer-based)	Renagel (tablet, capsule)	403 mg (capsule) 400, 800 mg (tablet)	800–1,600 mg with meals
Aluminum hydroxide[b]	AlternaGel (suspension)	600 mg/5 mL	300–600 mg with meals
	Amphojel (tablet and suspension)	300, 600 mg (tablet) 320 mg/5 mL (suspension)	
	Alu-Cap (capsule)	400 mg	
	Alu-Tab	500 mg	
	Basaljel (tablet, capsule, and suspension)	500 mg (tablet, capsule) 400 mg/mL (suspension)	
Magnesium carbonate[b]	Mag-Carb (capsule)	70 mg	70 mg with meals
Magnesium hydroxide[b]	Milk of Magnesia (tablet and suspension)	300, 600 mg (tablet) 400, 800 mg/5 mL (suspension)	300–400 mg with meals

[a]Tablet unless noted otherwise.
[b]Not first-line choice as a phosphate binder for chronic use.

based products are associated with their own toxicities. For patients requiring dialysis, reducing the calcium concentration of the dialysate bath may decrease the risk of hypercalcemia. While avoiding hypercalcemia should reduce the risk of calcifications, they still may occur due to other contributing factors in the CKD population.

Nausea, diarrhea, and constipation are other side effects of calcium-containing products. Because calcium-containing binders may interact with other drugs, timing of their administration relative to other agents must be considered. Fluoroquinolones and oral iron, for example, should be taken at least 1 or 2 hours before calcium-containing phosphate binders. Importantly, if the calcium products are being used as supplementation to treat hypocalcemia or osteoporosis, they should be taken between meals to enhance intestinal absorption. This is in contrast to their administration with meals if they are being used as phosphate binders. Starting doses of common calcium-containing phosphate binders are listed in Table 32-7.

SEVELAMER HYDROCHLORIDE

Sevelamer hydrochloride (Renagel) is a nonabsorbed, polymer-based product that binds phosphorus in the GI tract.[139] The benefit of lowering phosphorus without significantly affecting serum calcium has led to the increased use of sevelamer in patients with CKD, and it is now considered a first-line agent in patients with Stage 5 CKD.[84] Sevelamer also lowers LDL and total serum cholesterol, a substantial benefit considering the increased risk of cardiovascular events in this population.[140] The combined use of sevelamer and calcium supplementation has been evaluated. Coadministration of calcium (900 mg elemental calcium per day) with sevelamer resulted in greater decreases in both phosphorus and PTH than either agent alone without significant increases in serum calcium.[141] This may prove to be a useful way to control phosphorus and PTH, while avoiding both hypocalcemia and hypercalcemia.

Sevelamer is available as a 403 mg capsule and as 400 mg and 800 mg tablets. The starting dose is variable and depends on the baseline serum phosphorus concentration (800 mg TID with meals if serum phosphorus is <7.5 mg/dL; 1,600 mg TID with meals if serum phosphorus is >7.5 mg/dL).[142] Gradual adjustments can be made at 2-week intervals based on serum phosphorus levels. Dosing guidelines for sevelamer are also available for patients being converted from calcium acetate. Based on studies showing similar reductions in serum phosphorus, 800 mg of sevelamer is considered equivalent to 667 mg of calcium acetate (169 mg elemental calcium).[142]

Data regarding drug interactions with sevelamer are limited; however, in recent evaluations no drug interactions with digoxin, warfarin, metoprolol, and enalapril were observed.[143,144] The current prescribing information recommends administering sevelamer 1 hour before or 3 hours after administration of other agents with narrow therapeutic indices.[142] The administration of sevelamer to hemodialysis patients has been associated with a lowering of serum bicarbonate, although additional studies are needed to confirm this effect.[145]

OTHER PHOSPHATE BINDERS

Aluminum preparations bind dietary phosphorus in the GI tract from both dietary sources and enterohepatic secretions and form an insoluble aluminum–phosphate complex that is excreted in the stool. Although these products were once used as first-line agents to decrease phosphorus, their use has lost favor due to accumulation of aluminum in CKD patients. Elevated serum aluminum concentrations and aluminum deposition in bone and other tissues of patients with kidney disease have been associated with osteomalacia, microcytic anemia, and a fatal neurologic syndrome, referred to as *dialysis encephalopathy*.[146,147] Treatment of aluminum toxicity requires chelation with deferoxamine. Aluminum-containing agents should only be considered on a short-term basis (up to 4 weeks) for patients with an elevated Ca-P product; however, sevelamer is generally preferred in these situations. Sucralfate, used primarily for the treatment of ulcers, also contains aluminum and should be used cautiously in patients with kidney disease.

Magnesium agents (magnesium hydroxide, magnesium carbonate) may be beneficial, but as with aluminum their use should be limited, because at the high doses required to control serum phosphorus concentrations, severe diarrhea and hypermagnesemia invariably result. However, its use might be considered in patients whose serum phosphorus concentrations cannot be controlled adequately by other phosphate-binding agents. In this instance, a magnesium-containing phosphate binder may be added in conjunction with a reduction in the dialysate magnesium concentration (in the dialysis population). These agents should not be considered first-line therapy for control of phosphorus and careful monitoring of magnesium is warranted if therapy is started.

Lanthanum carbonate is another agent currently being investigated as an alternative phosphate-binding agent. Initial studies have shown this agent to be effective in controlling serum phosphorus and it is well tolerated.[148] Additional data from clinical trials are needed to determine the potential role of this elemental compound in clinical practice.

D.B.'s corrected calcium is approximately 9.7 mg/dL and the Ca-P is 66 mg^2/dL^2. More aggressive control of serum phosphorus is needed to achieve a phosphorus level <5.5 mg/dL. Currently she is receiving 1,800 mg of elemental calcium (4500 mg × 40% = 1,800 mg). Although presumably much of this calcium will be bound to phosphorus in the GI tract, there is potential for calcium absorption. Since her Ca-P product is above the threshold of 55 mg/dL, she is at increased risk for calcifications and adverse outcomes. The total dose of elemental calcium provided by binders should not exceed 1500 mg/day (or 2000 mg/day from binders and diet).[84] Therefore, calcium carbonate should be discontinued and sevelamer started to minimize her calcium exposure and decrease her phosphorus levels. Sevelamer should be started at a dose of 1,600 mg TID with meals and titrated based on follow-up of calcium, phosphorus, and Ca-P values. Adjustments should also be considered in conjunction with vitamin D therapy (see Vitamin D below). D.B. should be instructed to take her phosphate binder with meals and to separate administration of her ferrous sulfate and binder by at least 2 hours. This regimen should be implemented in conjunction with a restricted-phosphorus diet. Regular reinforcement of the importance of compliance is necessary, because nonadherence with prescribed dietary phosphorus restriction and drug therapy is one of the most significant factors associated with treatment failure. It is also important to make certain D.B. is undergoing her PD exchanges regularly, since some phosphorus elimination occurs with this treatment modality. Use of a low-calcium dialysate may also help decrease her risk of hypercalcemia.

Vitamin D
CALCITRIOL

Vitamin D is available as ergocalciferol (vitamin D_2) and cholecalciferol (vitamin D_3)—both vitamin D precursors requiring activation by the kidney—and calcitriol (l,25-dihydroxycholecalciferol), the active form of vitamin D. The response to vitamins D_2 and D_3 can vary depending on the degree of kidney function and the ability of the kidney to convert these vitamins to the biologically active forms. For patients in the earlier stages of CKD, decreased levels of 25-hydroxyvitamin D (the precursor to the active form of vitamin D) have been observed.[149] Altered vitamin D metabolism that occurs in this population may warrant measurement of 25-hydroxyvitamin D and supplementation with vitamin D precursors such as ergocalciferol.[84] Oral therapy with active vitamin D (oral calcitriol) or an analog (oral doxercalciferol) is likely warranted only when PTH remains elevated despite normal 25-hydroxyvitamin D levels.[84,149] As the final, active metabolite of vitamin D, calcitriol is required in patients with more severe kidney disease (Stage 5 CKD).

Administration of active vitamin D, in conjunction with control of serum phosphorus and calcium, is necessary in many patients with CKD to control PTH and prevent ROD. Calcitriol interacts with the vitamin D receptor (VDR) located in the parathyroid gland, intestines, bone, and kidney. It is thought to decrease PTH mRNA resulting in decreased PTH secretion, and it lowers the calcium set point for PTH release in CKD patients with sHPT, most likely through a direct effect on calcium receptors within the parathyroid gland.[131] In addition, calcitriol stimulates calcium absorption from the GI tract to correct hypocalcemia and prevent sHPT. To avoid hypercalcemia, the lowest-effective dose should be used and the patient's serum calcium and the Ca-P should be closely monitored. Furthermore, control of serum phosphorus is critical before calcitriol is initiated, since this agent also increases GI phosphorus absorption.

Calcitriol is available as an oral formulation (Rocaltrol) or IV formulation (Calcijex). Administration of calcitriol by either the oral or IV route may be based on conventional dosing (usually 0.25 to 0.5 μg/day) or pulse dosing (intermittent dosing of 0.5 to 2.0 μg 2 to 3 times per week). Higher doses (e.g., 4 μg three times per week) are generally required to reduce PTH secretion in more severe sHPT (PTH >1,000 pg/mL). Daily dosing of 0.25 to 0.5 μg may be preferred in patients with hypocalcemia since this regimen primarily works to stimulate calcium absorption from the GI tract. Intermittent dosing of IV calcitriol is more routine in the HD population since administration is coordinated with dialysis. In contrast, oral dosing is more convenient in patients with CKD who are not undergoing dialysis and the PD population. Intact PTH (iPTH) and serum calcium concentrations are used to determine starting doses and dosing adjustments for calcitriol. Acceptable iPTH ranges of 3 to 4 times normal have been proposed in patients with Stage 5 CKD to prevent sHPT while avoiding adynamic bone disease.[133,150] Lower iPTH ranges of 1 to 2 times normal may be more reasonable in patients with Stage 4 CKD.[84]

Intact PTH (1-84 PTH) is the biologically active form of this hormone and is 84 amino acids in length. This hormone is metabolized into smaller, less active fragments (e.g., 7-84 PTH) with activity that is not well characterized. These fragments are cleared from the circulation by the kidney and may accumulate in patients with CKD. Assays used for iPTH measure the intact structure as well as the biologically active and inactive PTH fragments. Thus, proposed ranges for iPTH in current guidelines are based on these assays. Recently, assays that measure only the biologically active form, or 1-84 PTH have become available. When iPTH is measured using both methods, there is roughly a 2:1 ratio between the nonspecific and specific assay results. For example, the current guidelines for iPTH in patients with Stage 5 CKD state a value of 150 to 300 pg/mL (i.e., 3 to 4 times normal); this would correspond to a 1-84 PTH of approximately 75 to 150 pg/mL measured by the new methods.[151] These newer assays have not yet been adopted for the majority of the CKD population; however, they are being used in some clinical settings. Clearly, the clinician must know which assay has been used in order to appropriately interpret the results, establish the desired PTH range, and correctly adjust therapy.

Dose adjustments of calcitriol are generally made in 0.5- to 1.0-μg increments every 2 to 4 weeks in the early stages of therapy until iPTH and serum calcium are maintained at target levels. If hypercalcemia develops, the decision to withhold therapy or to switch to a vitamin D analog (see Vitamin D Analogs) must be made. Serum iPTH should be monitored every 3 to 6 months, and dose adjustments of calcitriol should be made to maintain the goal iPTH and to prevent hypercalcemia and hyperphosphatemia.

VITAMIN D ANALOGS

The unique interactions of vitamin D with the vitamin D receptor (VDR) have led to the development of vitamin D analogs, which vary in their affinity for the VDR. In the case of treatment for sHPT, some were developed to retain the suppressive effect on PTH release while decreasing the potential for hypercalcemia relative to calcitriol. Currently approved agents for managing sHPT in the United States are paricalcitol (Zemplar), also referred to as 19-nor-1,25-dihydroxyvitamin D_2, and doxercalciferol (Hectorol), or 1-α-hydroxyvitamin D_2. Doxercalciferol requires conversion to the active form (1-α-,25-dihydroxyvitamin D_2) by the liver.

In patients with sHPT, paricalcitol significantly decreases iPTH without significantly increasing calcium, phosphorus, or Ca-P.[152–154] In one such study, a significant rise in calcium concentration (within the normal range) was observed after 12 weeks of paricalcitol therapy at a maximum dose of 0.12 μg/kg. Patients experiencing transient episodes of hypercalcemia (calcium >11 mg/dL) were evaluated with regard to their corresponding iPTH levels. An iPTH level <100 pg/mL was associated with an increase in serum calcium concentration equal to or beyond the upper limits of normal, indicating that these events were caused by inappropriate dosing and over suppression of PTH.[152,153] Based on these data, the recommended initial dose of paricalcitol is 0.04 μg/kg to 0.1 μg/kg IV administered with each dialysis session or every other day.[155] Doses may be titrated by 2- to 4-μg increments every 2 to 4 weeks based on iPTH values. Some data have also suggested paricalcitol dosing based on initial PTH levels (paricalcitol dose = PTH/80), rather than weight, as a reasonable dosing strategy.[156]

The recommended conversion ratio for calcitriol to paricalcitol is 1:4 (i.e., for every 1 μg of calcitriol, 4 μg of paricalcitol should be administered). This information is based on similar efficacy observed when patients treated for secondary hyperparathyroidism with calcitriol were switched to paricalcitol using this dosing strategy.[153] A lower ratio of 1:3 also has been proposed in patients resistant to therapy with calcitriol.[157] Although data comparing paricalcitol with calcitriol are currently limited, one study reported fewer cases of hyperphosphatemia with paricalcitol at doses that had equivalent efficacy with regard to PTH suppression. There also was a trend toward more rapid suppression of PTH in paricalcitol treated patients.[158] Currently, paricalcitol is available only in an IV formulation making it most convenient for use in HD patients. An oral form of paricalcitol is currently under investigation, which may be beneficial for the population with early CKD.

Doxercalciferol is another vitamin D analog that has provided an alternative to the active form of vitamin D and has been studied in patients with Stage 5 CKD on dialysis.[159,160] Intermittent oral therapy were administered to HD patients with hyperparathyroidism (iPTH, >400 pg/mL) in a multicenter trial. In this study 10 μg of oral doxercalciferol was administered three times per week with HD.[159] Of the 99 patients completing the study, 83% achieved the target iPTH; higher doses and longer therapy was required for patients with more severe sHPT (PTH > 1,200 pg/mL). Hypercalcemia occurred in a larger percent of patients in the doxercalciferol group compared with placebo, and this was corrected by lowering the doxercalciferol dose or by reducing calcium containing phosphate binders. In another study, intermittent IV therapy was compared with intermittent oral administration.[160] The doses were 4 μg IV or 10 μg orally three times per week with HD. Oral and IV therapy were both effective in reducing iPTH levels in patients with sHPT; however, there was some evidence that intermittent IV therapy may result in less hypercalcemia and hyperphosphatemia than oral intermittent therapy. Comparisons with calcitriol have not been reported.

The recommended starting dose of doxercalciferol for dialysis patients is 4 μg IV or 10 μg orally administered three times per week with dosing titration based on changes in iPTH.[161] Availability as both oral and IV formulations provides flexibility in using this analog in patients with CKD at all stages and in the PD population as indicated.

Vitamin D analogs offer an alternative for patients in whom persistent hypercalcemia develops with calcitriol therapy. Use of these agents is increasing in clinical practice due to the concerns of hypercalcemia and its adverse consequences. As more information is gathered through formal evaluation and clinical experience, the long-term advantages and potential disadvantages of these new agents will be defined more clearly.

Calcimimetics

The discovery of extracellular calcium-sensing receptors (CaRs) has prompted research using compounds known as calcimimetics, agents that interact with CaRs to modulate their activity. CaRs have been identified in the parathyroid gland, thyroid, nephron, brain, intestine, lung, and other tissues. A calcimimetic agent that enhances the affinity of CaRs for extracellular calcium and suppresses PTH secretion may prove beneficial in the treatment of secondary hyperparathyroidism. The calcimimetic AMG 073 (or Cinacalcet) is under investigation in patients with kidney failure. This agent has demonstrated efficacy in lowering PTH concentrations and Ca-P in HD patients with sHPT.[162] Continued research may result in approval of this agent for sHPT in patients with CKD.

Parathyroidectomy

The parathyroid glands enlarge as a compensatory response to disturbances of phosphorus, calcium, and calcitriol metabolism in patients with CKD. Timely administration of vitamin D therapy to prevent parathyroid hyperplasia is crucial, because treatment with vitamin D cannot adequately reverse established hyperplasia.[135] Under circumstances in which severe sHPT cannot be controlled by dietary phosphorus restriction and drug therapy, parathyroidectomy is considered. Parathyroidectomy may be subtotal, total, or total with autotransplantation. One of the major complications of parathyroidectomy is the early development of postsurgical hypocalcemia. Clinical symptoms of hypocalcemia include muscle irritability, fatigue, depression, and memory loss. Patients should be monitored closely following parathyroidectomy, and all patients with signs or symptoms of hypocalcemia should be treated with calcium supplementation (see Chapter 12, Fluid and Electrolyte Disorders). In patients who have undergone subtotal parathyroidectomy, the remaining parathyroid tissues will start functioning adequately, so that the acute hypocalcemia is only transient, lasting only a few days. However, with total parathyroidectomy, hypocalcemia is permanent, necessitating long-term treatment with calcitriol and oral calcium supplements (1 to 1.5 g of elemental calcium/day).

Appropriate treatment of D.B. should be based on assessment of her serum calcium, phosphorus, and iPTH values. She currently has an elevated iPTH (approximately 7 times normal); therefore, therapy with vitamin D should be started in conjunction with her dietary phosphorus restriction and phosphate-binder regimen. Since her current Ca-P is well above the target of 55 mg^2/dL^2, it is reasonable to use a vitamin D analog. The question of whether to wait until her Ca-P is below the target often arises. Initiating therapy with oral doxercalciferol may be reasonable in an attempt to decrease iPTH and minimize her risk of worsening hypercalcemia and hyperphosphatemia. Oral calcitriol may be more likely to increase GI absorption of calcium and is not the best agent based on D.B.'s current laboratory data. If the calcium and/or phosphorus continue to increase with doxercalciferol, her phosphate binder regimen should be re-evaluated and vitamin D therapy may need to be discontinued until the Ca-P is better controlled. Substitution of the calcium-containing phosphate binder with sevelamer is reasonable to lower phosphorus and the Ca-P product. Short-term aluminum (as a potent phosphate binder) may be another alternative if more aggressive lowering of phosphorus is necessary. Regular monitoring of labs and patient counseling to enforce compliance are essential for successful treatment of sHPT.

OTHER COMPLICATIONS OF CKD
Endocrine Abnormalities Caused by Uremia

18. Does D.B.'s hypothyroidism have any relationship to her CKD? What other endocrine abnormalities are associated with uremia?

Disturbances in thyroid function commonly are encountered in patients with CKD because the kidney is involved in all aspects of peripheral thyroid hormone metabolism. Common laboratory abnormalities include reduced serum concentrations of total thyroxine (T_4) and 3,5,3`-triiodothyronine (T_3) and a low free thyroxine index (FTI). The thyroid-stimulating hormone (TSH) concentration is usually normal, but peripheral conversion of T_4 to T_3 is reduced in uremic patients.[163] Despite these abnormalities, clinical hypothyroidism does not occur solely as a result of kidney disease, probably because the amount of free thyroid hormone in serum remains normal. Hypothyroidism in patients with kidney failure should be confirmed by the presence of an elevated serum TSH concentration and a low serum concentration of free T_4.

Other endocrine abnormalities that have been observed in patients with CKD include gonadal dysfunction leading to impotence, diminished testicular size, menstrual abnormalities, and cessation of ovulation.[164] Decreased libido and infertility occur in both sexes. Uremic women should avoid becoming pregnant, because there is a low likelihood of successful delivery. In children with kidney disease, growth retardation occurs despite normal or elevated growth hormone. Hyperprolactinemia and altered vasoactive hormone activity are other endocrine disturbances that may occur in patients with CKD.[163]

Altered Glucose and Insulin Metabolism

19. Other than the obvious effect of D.B.'s diabetes mellitus on blood glucose, are there any effects of kidney disease itself on glucose metabolism?

Uremia often is associated with glucose intolerance early in the course of kidney disease in nondiabetic patients and this may be referred to as "pseudodiabetes." Specifically, patients with CKD often exhibit an abnormal response to an oral glucose challenge and have sustained hyperinsulinemia.[165] The fasting blood glucose is typically within normal limits. Diminished tissue sensitivity to the action of insulin is also observed. Although their exact role is unclear, several uremic toxins—including urea, creatinine, guanidinosuccinic acid, and methylguanidine—have been implicated as causes for insulin resistance. Elevated concentrations of growth hormone, PTH, and glucagon also may contribute to glucose intolerance. Most nondiabetic patients with kidney disease do not require therapy for hyperglycemia, and dialysis therapy can correct these abnormalities in glucose metabolism.[163]

Patients with diabetes mellitus and advanced kidney disease may experience improved glucose control and decreased insulin requirements. This is because the kidney is responsible for a substantial amount of daily insulin degradation, and the disease progresses, less insulin is cleared, and its metabolic half-life is increased.[163] A decreased clearance of insulin by muscle tissue also may occur in patients with uremia. Thus, in diabetic patients with progressive kidney disease, blood glucose concentrations should be monitored and insulin doses adjusted to avoid hypoglycemia. D.B. has Stage 5 CKD and is receiving her insulin in the peritoneal dialysate solution. Hyperglycemia is also a concern in D.B. because the glucose present in her CAPD fluid to promote fluid removal will be absorbed systemically. Insulin dosage adjustments should

be made on the basis of repeated home blood glucose measurements, changes in the CAPD prescription, and glycosylated hemoglobin determinations.

Gastrointestinal Complications

20. One month before her current clinic visit, D.B. complained of nausea and vomiting of partially digested food. Metoclopramide (Reglan) was begun at that time. Could D.B.'s nausea and vomiting have been caused by her kidney failure? Was the appropriate therapy selected?

GI abnormalities are extremely common in patients with CKD and include anorexia, nausea, vomiting, hiccups, abdominal pain, GI bleeding, diarrhea, and constipation.[166] Diminished gastric motility may occur from uremia; however, this problem may improve with adequate HD. Dyspeptic complaints and gastroparesis may be more prevalent in the PD population than in the HD population and in the earlier stages of CKD.[167] D.B has diabetes and diabetic neuropathy, which also contributes to the delayed gastric emptying (diabetic gastroparesis) and retention of food in the upper intestinal tract. This frequently causes distention, nausea, and vomiting. Metoclopramide is recommended to relieve these symptoms, although the risk for extrapyramidal side effects should be considered. A lower dose of 5 mg before meals may be warranted for D.B. Cisapride (Propulsid), a prokinetic agent that has restricted access, is contraindicated in patients with kidney disease because its use is associated with the development of arrhythmias in this population.

Severe uremia also causes nausea and vomiting, and these can be initial presenting symptoms of kidney failure. Although antiemetics such as prochlorperazine (Compazine) are used, dialysis is the preferred therapy. Drug-induced nausea and vomiting always should be considered, because patients with CKD often take multiple drugs and are at risk for drug toxicity due to diminished kidney function (e.g., digitalis intoxication).

Bleeding

21. During her clinic visit, D.B. reports that her bowel movements have become black and tarry in appearance. A rectal examination reveals guaiac-positive stools. Is GI bleeding related to kidney failure?

D.B. should be evaluated for peptic ulcer disease and lower GI bleeding. Uremic patients are at risk for bleeding from mucosal surfaces such as the stomach. D.B.'s hemoglobin and hematocrit are below the target values (11 to 12 g/dL for hemoglobin, 33% to 36% for hematocrit), despite therapy with epoetin, and it is likely that bleeding is contributing to poor responsiveness to therapy. Angiodysplasia of the stomach and duodenum as well as erosive esophagitis are the most common causes of bleeding in patients with CKD.[168] Treatment of upper GI bleeding in uremic patients usually consists of cautious use of antacid therapy and H_2-receptor antagonists, which should be given in reduced doses according to the degree of kidney function. Proton pump inhibitors are primarily eliminated by nonrenal routes and may be administered at standard doses (see Chapter 27, Upper Gastrointestinal Disorders). Use of H_2-receptor antagonists has generally replaced chronic antacid use for treatment of dyspepsia in patients with CKD.

Peptic Ulcer Disease

22. Is peptic ulcer disease more likely in D.B.? What treatment options for peptic ulcer disease are appropriate in patients with kidney disease?

The relationship between peptic ulcers and kidney disease remains controversial. Gastric acid production is variable and is elevated in some studies but diminished in others. The Gram-negative bacterium *Helicobacter pylori* has been implicated as a factor in the pathogenesis of peptic ulcer disease that is not due to NSAID use. No conclusive evidence supports an increased prevalence of *H. pylori* infection in the CKD population when compared with the general population. Further evaluation of peptic ulcer disease should be considered in D.B. based on criteria for *H. pylori* testing (see Chapter 27, Upper Gastrointestinal Disorders). The multiple-drug therapy used to treat *H. pylori* in patients with normal kidney function is acceptable in patients with kidney disease if appropriate dosing adjustments are made.[169] Bismuth compounds, included in some of the available treatment regimens, should be avoided because of the potential for bismuth accumulation and toxicity.

Neurologic Complications

23. S.H., a 64-year-old, 72-kg, African American male, went to his primary care physician because of weakness, nausea, lethargy, decreased exercise tolerance, and general malaise that has developed over the past few weeks. S.H. had not been seen by a physician for >10 years. His past medical history was unremarkable except he recalls being told approximately 5 years ago that he had borderline hypertension. He was taking no medications. The physician's examination revealed a BP of 168/92 mm Hg, and funduscopic examination showed grade III hypertensive changes. On neurologic examination, S.H. was slightly confused, appeared somnolent, and had diminished sensation to pinprick in both lower extremities; asterixis was present. Examination of the skin showed pallor and excoriations across the abdomen, legs, and arms. Pertinent laboratory values were as follows: Hct, 20% (normal, 39% to 49%); Hgb, 6.7 g/dL (normal, 13 to 16 g/dL); WBC count, 9,100/mm³ (normal, 3,200 to 9,800/mm³); serum Na, 135 mEq/L (normal, 135 to 147 mEq/L); K, 5.8 mEq/L (normal, 3.5 to 5.0 mEq/L); Cl, 109 mEq/L (normal, 95 to 105 mEq/L); CO_2 content, 16 mEq/L (normal, 22 to 28 mEq/L); random blood glucose, 121 mg/dL (normal <140 mg/dL); BUN, 199 mg/dL (normal, 8 to 18 mg/dL); SrCr, 19.8 mg/dL (normal, 0.6 to 1.2 mg/dL); Ca, 8.5 mg/dL (normal, 8.8 to 10.4 mg/dL); phosphate, 11.1 mg/dL (normal, 2.5 to 5.0 mg/dL); intact PTH, 830 pg/mL (normal, 5 to 65 pg/mL); uric acid, 11.9 mg/dL (normal, 2.0 to 7.0 mg/dL); and albumin, 3.0 g/dL (normal, 4.0 to 6.0 g/dL).

Renal ultrasonography revealed no obstruction and small kidneys bilaterally. Subsequent kidney biopsy showed chronic glomerular scarring. S.H. was diagnosed with Stage 5 CKD, likely due to chronic, untreated hypertension. What is the likely explanation for S.H.'s altered mental status? What treatment, if any, is indicated for his neurologic findings?

[SI units: Hct, 0.20 (normal, 0.39 to 0.49); Hgb, 67 g/L (normal, 130 to 160); WBC, 9,100 × 10⁶/L (normal, 3,200 to 9,800); Na, 135 mmol/L (normal, 135 to 147); K, 5.8 mmol/L (normal, 3.5 to 5.0); Cl, 109 mmol/L (normal, 95 to 105); CO_2, 16 mmol/L (normal, 22 to 28); blood glucose, 6.7 mmol/L (nor-

mal, <11 mmol/L); BUN, 71.0 mmol/L of urea (normal, 3.0 to 6.5); SrCr, 1,750 μmol/L (normal, 50 to 110); Ca, 2.12 mmol/L (normal, 2.2 to 2.6); phosphate, 3.58 mmol/L (normal, 0.8 to 1.60); uric acid, 708 μmol/L (normal, 120 to 420); and albumin, 30 g/L (normal, 40 to 60)]

Disorders of the central nervous system (CNS) that occur in patients with untreated kidney disease and in those receiving dialysis are referred to collectively as *uremic encephalopathy*. Symptoms generally occur when the GFR is less than 10% of normal. Although S.H.'s altered neurologic function is most likely due to uremia, a careful drug history should exclude the possibility of drug effects. Symptoms of uremic encephalopathy include alterations in consciousness, thinking, memory, speech, psychomotor behavior, and emotion. Patients or their family members may note easy fatigability, daytime drowsiness, insomnia, diminished cognitive abilities, slurred speech, vomiting, and emotional volatility. The patient also may complain of being cold, having "restless legs," or "burning feet." The encephalopathy may progress to ataxia, vertigo, nystagmus, coma, and convulsions. Electroencephalograms (EEGs) of patients with CKD usually show diffuse abnormalities.

Evidence supports PTH as a major contributing factor to the altered neurologic status of patients with ESRD; however, other uremic toxins may play a role in this disorder.[170] PTH may enhance the entry of calcium into the brain and peripheral nerves, but it also may be directly neurotoxic. In all likelihood, S.H.'s altered mental status will improve with dialysis and correction of his hyperparathyroidism, although additional factors, such as his advanced age, must be considered.

The peripheral nervous system also shows abnormal function in many patients with advanced CKD, as illustrated by S.H., who has loss of sensation in his legs by pinprick examination. Typically, the peripheral neuropathy will be slowly progressive, distal, and symmetrical, usually first involving sensory function. The abnormalities seen usually are indistinguishable from other types of neuropathy, especially diabetic neuropathy, and nerve conduction studies often reveal abnormalities preceding clinical symptoms. Treatment generally consists of measures to alleviate symptoms with agents such as tricyclic antidepressants (e.g., amitriptyline) and anticonvulsants (e.g., phenytoin, gabapentin). Increasing the intensity of dialysis does not seem to affect the neuropathy; however, successful renal transplantation may ameliorate nerve dysfunction.

Abnormalities of the autonomic nervous system also have been observed in patients with kidney failure and present as postural hypotension, impotence, impaired sweating, and alterations in gastric motility. HD may be more likely to correct autonomic dysfunction in nondiabetic patients.

Dermatologic Complications

24. Why does S.H. have excoriations on his skin? What therapy would be useful?

Several dermal abnormalities have been observed in patients with CKD including hyperpigmentation, abnormal perspiration, dryness, and persistent pruritus. Of these, *uremic pruritus* can be the most bothersome for the patient and may lead to repeated scratching and skin excoriation. Hyperparathyroidism, hypervitaminosis A, and dermal mast cell proliferation with subsequent histamine release have been suggested as causes of pruritus.[171]

Treatment of pruritus often is a frustrating experience for the patient and clinician. Although many therapies have been advocated, few have provided sustained benefit. A trial-and-error approach is recommended. Efficient dialysis therapy relieves pruritus in some patients and pharmacologic therapy may be avoided.[172] When necessary, initial pharmacologic treatment usually consists of oral antihistamines such as hydroxyzine. Topical emollients or topical steroids may provide benefit if antihistamine therapy is not completely successful. If pruritus is still present, other treatment options may be tried. These include cholestyramine, ultraviolet (UVB) phototherapy, and oral administration of activated charcoal. Ondansetron and oral naltrexone have also been studied for pruritus without success.[173,174] Control of calcium and phosphorus concentrations and prevention of secondary hyperparathyroidism are also advocated to reduce pruritus in patients with CKD.

GLOMERULAR DISEASE

Glomerular diseases lead to many secondary complications that result from disruption of normal glomerular structure and function. Several clinical syndromes of glomerular disease exist; however, glomerulonephritis, characterized as proliferation and inflammation of the glomerulus, is observed most frequently. According to the most recent USRDS report, glomerulonephritis as a broad category remains the third leading cause of ESRD in the United States, accounting for approximately 8.4% of new cases and a higher proportion of the PD population (14.6%) when compared with the HD population (8%).[3] In developing countries, glomerulonephritis is more common as a cause of kidney failure since various infectious processes responsible for glomerulonephritis are more common.[175]

Nephrotic Syndrome

Severe proteinuria can lead to nephrotic syndrome. Nephrotic syndrome is characterized by proteinuria of greater than 3 g/day, hypoalbuminemia, edema, and hyperlipidemia. In more severe conditions, hypercoagulable conditions may be present due to loss of hemostasis control proteins including antithrombin III, protein S, and protein C. This syndrome may occur with or without a change in glomerular filtration rate. Nephrotic syndrome may be due to a primary disease such as membranous glomerulopathy, which is characterized by deposition of immune complexes, or other systemic diseases including diabetic glomerulosclerosis and amyloidosis. Elevated serum cholesterol and triglycerides are observed in patients with this degree of proteinuria (>3 g/day). This hyperlipidemic condition also predisposes patients with nephrotic syndrome to accelerated atherosclerosis. Hyperlipidemia itself may also contribute to progression of kidney disease. Since nephrotic syndrome is associated with numerous causes, further evaluation of the patient for systemic causes is required to then determine the course of therapy and prognosis.

Chronic Glomerulopathies

Glomerulonephritis may occur as a primary disease that is idiopathic in origin or as a secondary manifestation of other systemic disease (lupus nephritis, Goodpasture's disease, Wegener's granulomatosis). Renal biopsy is often required for definitive diagnosis. Glomerular lesions associated with glomerulopathies may be characterized as diffuse, focal, or segmental depending on the extent of involvement of individual glomeruli. Pathologic changes are characterized as proliferative, membranous, and sclerotic based on the pattern observed. Proliferative changes usually involve an overgrowth of the epithelium or mesangium, whereas membranous changes are typically described as a thickening of the glomerular basement membrane. Signs and symptoms of glomerulonephritis include hematuria, proteinuria, and decreased kidney function. Autoimmunity is the predominant pathogenic process leading to most forms of primary and secondary glomerulonephritis. Although a number of autoantibodies are associated with glomerulonephritis, their exact role in the pathogenesis of glomerulonephritis is still unclear. Nonetheless, analysis of autoantibodies in the clinical setting can aid in early diagnosis of glomerulonephritis.[176]

Glomerular damage generally occurs in two phases: acute and chronic. During the acute phase, immune reactions occur within glomeruli that stimulate the complement cascade, ultimately resulting in glomerular damage. Nonimmune mechanisms that occur in response to loss of nephron function and hyperfiltration of remaining nephrons are characteristic of the chronic phase.

Glomerulonephritis often causes acute renal failure. Patients with damage to >50% of glomeruli in the presence of rapid loss in kidney function (over days to weeks) are classified as having *rapidly progressive glomerulonephritis* (RPGN).[175] If kidney involvement is severe, signs and symptoms of uremia may develop. RPGN may be classified based on the immunopathogenic etiology of the glomerular damage: (1) anti–glomerular basement membrane antibody formation (e.g., Goodpasture's syndrome), (2) immune complex deposition (e.g., lupus nephritis), and (3) nonimmune deposit-mediated mechanism (e.g., Wegener's granulomatosis).[176] This chapter focuses on the treatment of the most common forms of chronic glomerulonephritis (i.e., lupus nephritis, Goodpasture's syndrome, Wegener's granulomatosis).

Lupus Nephritis

Systemic lupus erythematosus (SLE) is a multisystem autoimmune disease characterized by abnormalities in cell-mediated immunity such as B-cell hyperresponsiveness and defective T-cell–mediated suppressor activity. In certain predisposed individuals, SLE may lead to the development of lupus nephritis, a secondary form of glomerulonephritis. Lupus nephritis is the prototypical immune complex-mediated kidney disease, characterized by deposition or in situ formation of autoantibody–antigen complexes along the glomerular capillary network. Lupus nephritis remains an important cause of mortality. Up to 60% of adults with SLE have some degree of kidney involvement later in the course of their disease, discernible from clinical evidence of kidney damage: heavy proteinuria, hematuria, decreased GFR, and hypertension. Early in the disease, laboratory abnormalities indicative of kidney involvement are seen in approximately 25% to 50% of patients.[177]

25. C.W., a 34-year-old African American female with a 7-year history of SLE, presents to the nephrology clinic for a follow-up of her lupus nephritis. Pertinent laboratory values are as follows: serum Na, 146 mEq/L (normal, 135 to 147 mEq/L); K, 4.2 mEq/L (normal, 3.5 to 5.0 mEq/L); Cl, 100 mEq/L (normal, 95 to 105 mEq/L); CO₂ content, 25 mEq/L (normal, 22 to 28 mEq/L); SrCr, 2.0 mg/dL (normal, 0.6 to 1.2 mg/dL); BUN, 20 mg/dL (normal, 8 to 18 mg/dL); and WBC count, 9,600/mm³ (normal, 3,200 to 9,800/mm³). RBC indices were normal. Platelet count was 175,000/mm³ (normal, 130,000 to 400,000/mm³). Her 24-hour urine contained 2.3 g of albumin (normal, <30 mg/day), and her UA showed 12 RBC/high-power field (HPF) (normal, 0 to 3). Compared with her visit of a week ago, C.W's kidney function and urinary indices (proteinuria, hematuria) showed substantial worsening of her nephritis. C.W. was hospitalized, and a kidney biopsy showed inflammation of 40% of the glomeruli. What subjective and objective data in C.W. are consistent with a diagnosis of lupus nephritis, and what is the stage of her nephritis?

[SI units: Na, 146 mmol/L (normal, 135 to 147); K, 4.2 mmol/L (normal, 3.5 to 5.0); Cl, 100 mmol/L (normal, 95 to 105); CO₂, 25 mmol/L (normal, 22 to 28); SrCr, 177 μmol/L (normal, 50 to 110); BUN, 7.14 mmol/L of urea (normal, 3.0 to 6.5); WBC, 9,600 × 10⁶/L (normal, 3,200 to 9,800); platelet count, 175 10⁹/L (normal, 130 to 400); urinary albumin, 2.3 g/day (normal, <0.03)]

C.W. has clinical evidence of kidney damage as demonstrated by her proteinuria, hematuria, and increased SrCr concentration. Glomerular damage is most evident by the presence of RBCs or red cell casts in the urine, a finding observed in C.W.

CLASSIFICATIONS

The World Health Organization has classified lupus nephritis based on the patterns of glomerular disease (Table 32-8).[177] This and other classification schemes provide a reasonable correlation among histopathology, outcome, and response to treatment. C.W. has proteinuria, hematuria, and inflammation of <50% of her glomeruli, and she is diagnosed as having class III (focal proliferative) glomerulonephritis.

TREATMENT

26. Should C.W.'s lupus nephritis be treated?

Lupus nephritis may present in various histologic forms, and patients may transform from one form to another.[178] Unlike nonrenal manifestations of SLE, serologic markers of disease correlate poorly with lupus nephritis. Therefore, eleva-

tions in SrCr, and worsening of proteinuria and hematuria, as seen in C.W., are used as primary markers of disease activity.

Treatment of lupus nephritis must address both management of the acute disease process and maintenance therapy for the more stable chronic disease process. There is a general consensus that patients, such as C.W., who present with focal or diffuse proliferative glomerulonephritis (class III or IV), should be treated aggressively, with the primary goal of preventing irreversible kidney damage. The prognosis of kidney function in patients with SLE has improved. The likelihood of developing ESRD or dying within 10 years of diagnosis has decreased from greater than 80% to less than 20%; however, the prognosis is worse in African Americans when compared with the white population treated for SLE.[178] Advances in pharmacologic therapy (i.e., safer immunosuppressive regimens, antihypertensives, etc) have contributed to this improved prognosis for the population as a whole.

The treatment of lupus nephritis is somewhat empiric but is based, to some extent, on histologic findings. Although appropriate treatment can improve patient outcomes, vigorous attempts to suppress SLE activity may lead to serious drug-related complications. Because the primary strategy in the treatment of lupus nephritis involves suppression of the immune system with corticosteroids and cytotoxic agents, such as cyclophosphamide and azathioprine, clinicians need to be aware of the potential complications associated with therapy. Therefore, careful monitoring of patients is essential in determining the indication for treatment and improving prognosis. Toxicities associated with immunosuppressive agents depend on both the dose and the duration of therapy. Abnormalities in hematopoiesis, such as neutropenia and thrombocytopenia, are the most common adverse effects associated with cytotoxic agents. Immunosuppression, in general, increases a patient's susceptibility to a vast array of infections and to lymphocytic malignancies. In addition, the alkylating agent cyclophosphamide can cause nausea and vomiting, hemorrhagic cystitis, and alopecia. The antimetabolite azathioprine can cause pancreatitis and abnormalities in liver function.

Corticosteroids

Corticosteroids represent the cornerstone of therapy, especially in patients with a mild form of lupus nephritis. Low-dose prednisone should be given to patients with stable lupus nephritis. In patients with a more severe form of lupus nephritis (diffuse proliferative), prednisone 1 to 2 mg/kg per day for 4 to 8 weeks, as a single morning dose, may be initiated. Due to the long-term complications of high-dose corticosteroid

Table 32-8 1995 World Health Organization Classification of Lupus Nephritis

Class	Histologic Characterization	Usual Clinical Presentation
I	Normal renal histology	No urine abnormalities
II	Mesangial proliferative glomerulonephritis	Mild proteinuria and urine sediment abnormalities
III	Focal and segmental proliferative glomerulonephritis	Proteinuria and hematuria
IV	Diffuse proliferative glomerulonephritis	Heavy proteinuria; active sediment; hypertension; renal failure
V	Membranous glomerulonephritis	Proteinuria; often nephrotic syndrome
VI	Advanced sclerosing glomerulonephritis	Proteinuria; renal failure; nephrotic syndrome

Data from the 1995 World Health Organization Classification of Lupus Nephritis.[177]

therapy, a lower starting dosage of prednisone (1 mg/kg per day) may be reasonable. Gradual tapering of prednisone to a low-dose regimen of 0.2 to 0.4 mg/kg per day must be attempted once glomerulonephritis has stabilized.

For the treatment of acute exacerbations of lupus nephritis, high-dose pulse therapy with methylprednisolone may be warranted. Given that C.W.'s lupus nephritis has worsened she should receive 3 days of therapy with pulse methylprednisolone (0.5 to 1 g IV, not to exceed 1 g) for 3 days in an attempt to reduce the degree of proteinuria and improve kidney function.[177] Suppression of C.W.'s active lupus nephritis should be demonstrated by a reduction in proteinuria and hematuria and an increase in her Cl_{Cr}. Although generally well tolerated, rapid methylprednisolone injections may cause transient tremor, flushing, and altered taste sensation. To reduce the risk of adverse effects associated with the rate of injection, C.W. should receive methylprednisolone over 30 minutes. After a course of pulse methylprednisolone therapy, oral prednisone at a dose 10 to 20 mg daily may be initiated.[177] Once the acute flare resolves (generally in up to 12 weeks), low-dose, maintenance steroid therapy with 5 to 15 mg/day of prednisone can be initiated in combination with cytotoxic therapy. The lowest effective dose of prednisone should be maintained to minimize the risk of side effects associated with long-term corticosteroid use.

Cytotoxic Agents

Controversy exists regarding the superiority of cytotoxic agents, such as cyclophosphamide or azathioprine, to oral corticosteroid monotherapy. Evidence in support of cytotoxic therapy during the acute phase given the potential toxicities is not compelling; however, more information in favor of the combination of cytotoxic agents with corticosteroids for treatment during the chronic phase of lupus is available.[179] In a meta-analysis assessing the efficacy of therapeutic agents used to treat lupus nephritis, improved outcomes (total mortality and ESRD) were associated with use of oral prednisone in combination with IV cyclophosphamide.[179] No differences in clinical outcome have been observed in patients treated with cyclophosphamide (oral or IV) when compared to patients treated with therapy including azothiaprine.[177] An additional benefit of combination therapy with immunosuppressive agents is their steroid-sparing effect and, potentially, lower risk of steroid toxicity. Adverse effects of cytotoxic therapy include bone marrow suppression and, with chronic therapy, lymphocytic malignancies. In addition, cyclophosphamide can cause nausea, vomiting, sterile hemorrhagic cystitis, gonadal toxicity, and alopecia. Oral doses of 1 to 3 mg/kg per day of cyclophosphamide can be used based on the degree of kidney function. The addition of cyclophosphamide or azathioprine along with corticosteroid therapy should be considered in C.W. once the acute lupus flare resolves.

Because of the low therapeutic index of oral cyclophosphamide and the associated bladder and gonadal toxicity with prolonged use, IV monthly pulse doses have been advocated. The effectiveness of pulse cyclophosphamide therapy has been demonstrated in trials comparing this regimen with pulse methylprednisolone.[180] Before, and for 24 hours after initiating IV cyclophosphamide, the patient must be well hydrated to prevent bladder toxicity. The starting dose of cyclophosphamide is 0.5 to 1 g/m² of body surface, infused over 30 to 60 minutes, with the lower doses reserved for patients with severe kidney disease. This regimen is repeated monthly for 6 months and then administered quarterly for up to 2 years. The need for a more prolonged course of therapy must be assessed on an individual basis. Combination therapy with cyclophosphamide and steroids for maintenance treatment of lupus has been successful but is associated with increased toxicity.[180] After treatment with prednisolone and cyclophosphamide for 12 weeks during the maintenance phase, patients may be switched to prednisolone in combination with azathioprine to reduce exposure to cyclophosphamide.[177] Doses of 2 to 2.5 mg per day of azathioprine have been used successfully.

In a search for alternative therapies to decrease use of cytotoxic agents, mycophenolate has been evaluated in combination with prednisolone therapy.[181] This combination was determined to be as effective as cyclophosphamide and prednisolone followed by azathioprine and prednisolone. Cyclosporine in doses of 5 mg/kg per day may also provide an alternative therapy to treat lupus in the maintenance phase.[177]

Goodpasture's Disease (Anti–Glomerular Basement Membrane Antibody–Mediated Nephritis)

Several diseases are associated with pulmonary hemorrhage and RPGN. These include autoimmune, malignant, and kidney disorders. Approximately one-third of these "pulmonary-renal syndromes" are associated with the presence of anti–glomerular basement membrane antibodies. Most other cases are associated with systemic vasculitis (e.g., Wegener's granulomatosis). The term *Goodpasture's syndrome* denotes the syndrome of pulmonary hemorrhage and RPGN with or without anti–glomerular basement membrane antibodies.[176] In this discussion Goodpasture's *syndrome* refers to the syndrome of pulmonary hemorrhage and RPGN resulting from any cause, whereas Goodpasture's *disease* denotes the syndrome in association with anti–glomerular basement membrane antibodies.

In the dialysis era, most early deaths with Goodpasture's disease are due to fulminate pulmonary hemorrhage, whereas most deaths occurring later are due to secondary infections. Once significant kidney disease develops, rapid progression to ESRD is possible. The etiology of Goodpasture's disease is due primarily to the development of anti–glomerular basement membrane (or anti–GBM) antibodies against basement membranes of the glomeruli and the pulmonary alveolar septa. The resulting damage may lead to diffuse hemorrhage of the capillaries into the acinar portion of the lungs and formation of crescentic necrotizing glomerulonephritis in the kidneys. Anti–GBM antibodies can cause glomerular damage; however, for alveolar damage to occur, other inciting factors (e.g., cigarette smoking, toxic chemical exposure, influenza A) need to be present to either increase capillary permeability or augment binding of the antibodies to the alveolar basement membrane.

Approximately half of patients have a recent history of upper respiratory infection. Alveolar hemorrhage typically precedes clinical manifestations of kidney disease. Symptoms include hemoptysis, exertional dyspnea, cough, and in severe cases, acute respiratory failure. The renal manifestations of Goodpasture's disease include RBCs, RBC casts, and protein in the urine. Azotemia may develop in 50% of cases. Hypertension is an uncommon finding.[175,176]

The diagnosis of Goodpasture's disease requires the demonstration of either circulating or tissue-fixed anti–GBM antibodies because of the many causes of pulmonary-renal syndrome and the nonspecific glomerular changes seen on biopsy. Due to the potentially rapid and fulminate progression of the disease, however, treatment should not await biopsy or serum antibody titer results.

27. J.M. is a 42-year-old white male who presents to the clinic with a 1-month history of anorexia, fatigue, cough, and dyspnea on exertion (DOE). Over the past week, he has noted bright red blood in his phlegm, which has worsened in the past 3 days. Social history includes the following: he owns a local gasoline station and smokes 1 pack of cigarettes/day. On physical examination, he appeared pale and in mild respiratory distress. Pertinent laboratory values are as follows: serum Na, 143 mEq/L (normal, 135 to 147 mEq/L); K, 5.1 mEq/L (normal, 3.5 to 5.0 mEq/L); Cl, 102 mEq/L (normal, 95 to 105 mEq/L); CO_2 content, 24 mEq/L (normal, 22 to 28 mEq/L); SrCr, 2.8 mg/dL (normal, 0.6 to 1.2 mg/dL); and BUN, 41 mg/dL (normal, 8 to 18 mg/dL). Hematologic studies revealed an Hct of 35% (normal, 39% to 49%); a Hgb of 11.7 g/dL (normal, 13 to 16 g/dL); mean corpuscular volume (MCV), 69 mm³ (normal, 76 to 100 mm³); mean corpuscular Hgb (MCH) concentration, 24% (normal, 33% to 37%); and reticulocyte count, 1.9% (normal, 0.1% to 2.4%). During last year's physical checkup visit, his SrCr and BUN were within the normal range. His 24-hour urine contained 3.8 g of albumin (normal, <30 mg) and revealed a Cl_{Cr} of 24 mL/min. His urine also contained many RBC casts and 16 RBC/HPF (normal, 0 to 3 RBC/HPF). Chest radiograph showed alveolar shadowing spreading from the hilar region. Based on his subjective and objective data, which of the chronic glomerulopathies is J.M. likely to have?

[SI units: Na, 143 mmol/L (normal, 135 to 147); K, 5.1 mmol/L (normal, 3.5 to 5.0); Cl, 102 mmol/L (normal, 95 to 105); CO_2, 24 mmol/L (normal, 22 to 28); SrCr, 247 μmol/L (normal, 50 to 110); BUN, 14.6 mmol/L of urea (normal, 3.0 to 6.5); Hct, 0.35 (normal, 0.39 to 0.49); Hgb, 117 g/L (normal, 130 to 160); MCV, 69 fL (normal, 76 to 100); MCH, 0.24 (normal, 0.33 to 0.37); reticulocyte count, 0.019 (normal, 0.001 to 0.024); Cl_{Cr}, 0.40 mL/sec]

J.M's cough, hemoptysis, respiratory distress, and chest radiograph findings are suggestive of alveolar hemorrhage. He also has clinical evidence of kidney damage, as demonstrated by proteinuria, hematuria, and increased SrCr concentration. Thus, it is likely that J.M. has a pulmonary-renal syndrome, presumably exacerbated by his daily exposure to hydrocarbons superimposed on his daily tobacco use. However, the definitive diagnosis of Goodpasture's disease requires the demonstration of either circulating or tissue-fixed anti–GBM antibodies.

TREATMENT

28. Should J.M.'s pulmonary-renal syndrome be treated?

Although J.M's pulmonary-renal syndrome has not been definitively diagnosed as Goodpasture's disease, treatment should not await biopsy or serum antibody titer results because of the potentially rapid and fulminate progression of the disease. Therefore, J.M. requires aggressive treatment to prevent rapid and irreversible kidney damage.

29. J.M. was hospitalized, and kidney biopsy results showed inflammation of 50% of the glomeruli. The results of the serum anti–GBM antibodies titer are not yet available. What are the goals of therapy and how should J.M. be treated?

The goals of treatment for Goodpasture's disease are to rapidly control alveolar hemorrhage and prevent irreversible damage to the extrapulmonary organs, especially the kidneys. These goals may be accomplished by removing the circulating anti–GBM antibodies with plasma exchange (plasmapheresis) and by preventing antibody synthesis with chemotherapy. Nonetheless, the probability of recovery of kidney function can be predicted with reasonable certainty. Progression to ESRD may be inevitable in individuals who have one or more of the following: (1) SrCr concentration >6 to 7 mg/dL, (2) total anuria, or (3) damage to >85% of the glomeruli.[182] Given the risks of immunosuppressive chemotherapy, patients with one or more of the aforementioned criteria should be treated only when pulmonary hemorrhage is present or in preparation for kidney transplantation. Dialysis-dependent patients who are not anuric and who do not have crescent formation in most of the glomeruli still may respond to aggressive treatment. Because J.M. does not meet any of the aforementioned criteria, he is likely to benefit from immunosuppressive therapy.

Plasma Exchange

30. The ELISA test for anti–GBM antibodies was positive. How will this change J.M.'s therapy?

Plasmapheresis combined with immunosuppressive therapy is the cornerstone of treatment for anti–GBM antibody–mediated nephritis. The rationale for this approach is to rapidly remove the antibodies with plasmapheresis while preventing their synthesis with the immunosuppressive agents. This combination can rapidly suppress the alveolar hemorrhage within 24 to 48 hours and retard the progression of kidney disease.[183] Therefore, J.M. should receive daily plasmapheresis for 14 days or until the circulating anti–GBMs are suppressed. To prevent fluid loss, 5% human albumin solution must be administered during plasma exchange.

Pulse Methylprednisolone

Immunosuppressive therapy is essential to prevent the synthesis of anti–GBM antibodies. High-dose pulse IV methylprednisolone therapy (30 mg/kg on alternate days for three doses) may be beneficial in treating J.M.'s alveolar hemorrhage.[175] A lower dose of 1 mg/kg daily for several months in combination with plasmapheresis and cyclophosphamide is indicated for suppression of antibody production.

Oral Cyclophosphamide Plus Corticosteroids

Conventional therapy for Goodpasture's syndrome with kidney involvement includes the combination of oral cyclophosphamide and prednisolone or prednisone. J.M. should receive oral cyclophosphamide 2.5 mg/kg per day plus prednisolone or prednisone 1 mg/kg per day (maximum daily dose, 60 mg).[184] Patients older than 55 years may be given lower cyclophosphamide doses (2 mg/kg per day). The dose should be reduced by 25% for patients with GFRs <10 mL/min. Therapy should continue until anti–GBM antibodies are no longer present (generally after several months of therapy), after which withdrawal of both agents may be safely accomplished in the absence of disease activity or circulating titers of anti–GBM antibodies.

32. How should J.M.'s therapy be monitored?

Once therapy is initiated, serial anti–GBM antibodies titer, urinalysis, and SrCr measurements must be obtained to monitor for disease relapse. Alveolar hemorrhage may be exacerbated by cigarette smoking, circulatory volume overload, and exposure to hydrocarbons and other toxic chemicals. Once the autoimmune activity subsides, as evidenced by a complete absence of circulating anti–GBM antibodies, recurrence is uncommon.[175]

Wegener's Granulomatosis

32. The result of J.M.'s cytoplasmic-staining anti–neutrophil cytoplasmic antibody (c-ANCA) is negative. The nephrologist has ruled out Wegener's granulomatosis. What is Wegener's granulomatosis, and what is the significance of this finding?

Wegener's granulomatosis is a primary systemic vasculitis characterized by granulomatous inflammation of the upper and lower respiratory tract and secondary glomerulonephritis.[175] Primary systemic vasculitic syndromes, such as Wegener's granulomatosis, often cause glomerulonephritis. Although vasculitis involves inflammation of blood vessels of any size, the small- and medium-size vessels are most commonly affected.[185] The etiology of Wegener's granulomatosis is unclear; however, autoimmunity is suspected mainly for two reasons. First, Wegener's granulomatosis is a systemic inflammatory disease without a known infectious etiology. Second, good treatment response can be obtained with immunosuppressive therapy.

The clinical features of Wegener's granulomatosis include upper airway disease, such as sinusitis, epistaxis, and nasopharyngitis, as well as otitis media due to blockage of the eustachian tube. Constitutional symptoms include fever, night sweats, arthralgia, anorexia, and malaise. After a few months, weakness may progress, severely limiting physical activity. Although the lungs are invariably affected, most patients remain asymptomatic; however, cough and hemoptysis may be present. The laboratory signs also are nonspecific and indicate the presence of a systemic inflammatory process. They include an elevated erythrocyte sedimentation rate in virtually all patients, anemia of chronic disease, and thrombocytosis.[175] Hematuria and proteinuria can be prominent features of Wegener's granulomatosis and are present on initial presentation in 80% of patients. The presence of severely diminished kidney function, seen in approximately 10% of patients, is an ominous sign, with nearly one-third of these patients progressing to ESRD. All patients with Wegener's granulomatosis are at risk for developing irreversible, rapidly progressive kidney failure. Renal histologic findings are nonspecific, with most patients exhibiting necrotizing crescentic glomerulonephritis.[185]

Wegener's granulomatosis is diagnosed primarily by the presenting signs and symptoms. According to the American College of Rheumatology 1990 classification, a person is diagnosed with Wegener's granulomatosis if any two of the following four criteria are present: (1) nasal or oral inflammation, (2) abnormal chest radiograph, (3) microhematuria (>5 RBCs/HPF) or RBC casts in the urine sediment, or (4) granulomatous inflammation on biopsy.[186]

The discovery of c-ANCA and its strong association with Wegener's granulomatosis has permitted a more certain diagnosis. Because of the substantial rise in titer that commonly precedes relapse of Wegener's granulomatosis, the c-ANCA test is best used to follow the course of disease activity and guide induction of therapy. Treatment with cyclophosphamide and corticosteroids results in improvement in kidney function in approximately 80% to 85% of patients, versus 75% with pulse steroids alone.[175] The main predictive factors for treatment success are the extent of kidney damage before therapy starts and how long therapy is delayed after symptoms develop.

TREATMENT

Cyclophosphamide

Because Wegener's granulomatosis is considered an autoimmune inflammatory disease, immunosuppressive therapy is the mainstay of treatment. Therapy is generally indicated for 6 months if remission occurs and up to 12 months in resistant cases.[187] On diagnosis of active Wegener's granulomatosis, oral cyclophosphamide 2 mg/kg per day, as a single morning dose, should be initiated to prevent irreversible glomerular scarring. With a more fulminate form of the disease, higher doses (4 to 5 mg/kg per day) may be used, although the potential for toxicities must be carefully considered. High fluid intake (>3 L/day) reduces the risk of hemorrhagic cystitis. Regular urinalysis should be performed (every 3 to 6 months) to detect hematuria caused by hemorrhagic cystitis.

Induction treatment with pulse IV boluses of cyclophosphamide is not satisfactory due to high relapse rates and increased toxicity. However, there are two conditions for which IV cyclophosphamide may be considered: (1) patients whose conditions have not responded to conventional treatment and (2) patients in whom severe kidney dysfunction developed initially, including those requiring dialysis. In the former, IV cyclophosphamide 1 g/m² in 150 mL of saline may be administered over 60 minutes. The dose must be reduced by 25% in patients with a GFR <10 mL/min. This regimen may be administered monthly for 6 months, after which a dosage reduction may be attempted.[188]

Corticosteroids

The main role of corticosteroids is to induce remission of the disease. On diagnosis of active Wegener's granulomatosis, prednisone 1 mg/kg per day must be initiated, along with oral cyclophosphamide, and continued for 2 to 4 weeks until the immunosuppressive effect of cyclophosphamide becomes evident. Over the next 2 months, the dose may be tapered to 60 mg every other day to reduce the risk of infection. Then the dose can be tapered by 5 mg/week to discontinue prednisone over 3 to 6 months. For patients with a more fulminate form of the disease, pulse methylprednisolone 1 g/m² per day for three doses is administered. The dose can be repeated in 1 to 2 weeks if progression is uncontrolled.

Azathioprine

Because of its poor efficacy, azathioprine should not be used as a first-line agent to treat active Wegener's granulomatosis. However, if remission is induced with cyclophosphamide and the patient cannot tolerate long-term treatment with that agent, azathioprine 2 mg/kg per day may be substituted.

Alternative Agents

Other agents have been studied as alternatives to cyclophosphamide. Use of trimethoprim-sulfamethoxazole over 1 year was evaluated for patients in remission or after treatment with cyclophosphamide and prednisolone.[189] A reduction in relapse rate was demonstrated compared with placebo. Methotrexate may be beneficial for patients with milder disease, although one study demonstrated high relapse rates in patients treated initially with weekly methotrexate and daily prednisone; disease was controlled in only select patients.[190]

REFERENCES

1. National Kidney Foundation. NKF-K/DOQI Clinical Practice Guidelines for Chronic Kidney Disease: Evaluation, Classification, and Stratification. Am J Kidney Dis 2002;39:S1.
2. Jones et al. Serum creatinine levels in the U.S. population: Third National Health and Nutrition Examination Survey. Am J Kidney Dis 1998;32:992 [correction in Am J Kidney Dis 2000;35:178].
3. U.S. Renal Data System, USRDS 2002 Annual Data Report: Atlas of End-Stage Renal Disease in the United States, National Institutes of Health, National Institute of Diabetes and Digestive and Kidney Diseases, Bethesda, MD, 2002.
4. U.S. Department of Health and Human Services. Healthy People 2010. 2nd Ed. With Understanding and Improving Health and Objectives for Improving Health. 2 vols. Washington, DC: U.S. Government Printing Office, November 2000.
5. Henrich WL et al. Analgesics and the kidney: summary and recommendations to the Scientific Advisory Board of the National Kidney Foundation from an Ad Hoc Committee of the National Kidney Foundation. Am J Kidney Dis 1996;27:162.
6. Gault MH, Barrett BJ. Analgesic nephropathy. Am J Kidney Dis 1998;32:351.
7. Bennett WM et al. The renal effects of nonsteroidal anti-inflammatory drugs: summary and recommendations. Am J Kidney Dis 1996;28 (Suppl 1):S56.
8. Perneger TV et al. Risk of kidney failure associated with the use of acetaminophen, aspirin, and nonsteroidal antiinflammatory drugs. N Engl J Med 1994;331:675.
9. Barrett BJ. Acetaminophen and adverse chronic renal outcomes: an appraisal of the epidemiologic evidence. Am J Kidney Dis 1996;28:S14.
10. Bendz H et al. Kidney damage in long-term lithium patients: a cross-sectional study of patients with 15 years or more on lithium. Nephrol Dial Transplant 1994;9(9):1250.
11. Kallner G, Petterson U. Renal, thyroid and parathyroid function during lithium treatment: laboratory tests in 207 people treated for 1–30 years. Acta Psychiatr Scand 1995;91:48.
12. U.S. Renal Data System, USRDS 1998 Annual Data Report. National Institutes of Health, National Institute of Diabetes and Digestive and Kidney Diseases, Bethesda, MD, 1998.
13. Manley HJ et al. Factors associated with medication-related problems in ambulatory hemodialysis patients. Am J Kidney Dis 2003;41:386.
14. Curtin RB et al. Hemodialysis patients' noncompliance with oral medications. ANNA J 1999;26:307.
15. Grabe DW et al. Evaluation of drug-related problems in an outpatient hemodialysis unit and the impact of a clinical pharmacist. Clin Nephrol 1997;47:117.
16. Manley HJ, Carroll CA. The clinical and economic impact of pharmaceutical care in end-stage renal disease patients. Semin Dial 2002;15:45.
17. Remuzzi G, Bertani T. Mechanisms of disease: pathophysiology of progressive nephropathies. N Engl J Med 1998;339:1448.
18. Mackenzie HS, Brenner BM. Current strategies for retarding progression of renal disease. Am J Kidney Dis 1998;31:161.
19. Nelson RG et al. Kidney disease in diabetes. In: Diabetes in America, National Institutes of Health Publication No. 95-1468. 2nd Ed. Bethesda, MD: National Institutes of Health, 1995;349.

20. Klag MJ et al. Blood pressure and end-stage renal disease in men. N Engl J Med 1996;334:13.
21. Peterson JC et al. Blood pressure control, proteinuria, and the progression of renal disease. The Modification of Diet in Renal Disease Study. Ann Intern Med 1995;123:754.
22. Attman PO et al. Abnormal lipid and apolipoprotein composition of major lipoprotein density classes in patients with chronic renal failure. Nephrol Dial Transplant 1996;11:63.
23. Ravid M et al. Main risk factors for nephropathy in type 2 diabetes mellitus are plasma cholesterol levels, mean blood pressure, and hyperglycemia. Arch Intern Med 1998;158:998.
24. Yang WQ et al. Serum lipid concentrations correlate with the progression of chronic renal failure. Clin Lab Sci 1999;12:104.
25. Samuelsson O et al. Complex apolipoprotein B-containing lipoprotein particles are associated with a higher rate of progression of human chronic renal insufficiency. J Am Soc Nephrol 1998;9:1482.
26. Bianchi S et al. A controlled, prospective study of the effects of atorvastatin on proteinuria and progression of kidney disease. Am J Kidney Dis 2003; 41:565.
27. Hellerstein S et al. Creatinine clearance following cimetidine for estimation of glomerular filtration rate. Pediatr Nephrol 1998;12:49.
28. Caregaro L et al. Limitations of serum creatinine level and creatinine clearance as filtration markers in cirrhosis. Arch Intern Med 1994;154:201.
29. Cockcroft DW, Gault MH. Prediction of creatinine clearance from serum creatinine. Nephron 1976; 16:31.
30. Jelliffe RW. Creatinine clearance: bedside estimate [Letter]. Ann Intern Med 1973;79:604.
31. Levey AS et al. A more accurate method to estimate glomerular filtration rate from serum creatinine: a new prediction equation. Modification of Diet in Renal Disease Study Group. Ann Intern Med 1999; 130:461.
32. Schwartz GJ et al. The use of plasma creatinine concentration for estimating glomerular filtration rate in infants, children, and adolescents. Pediatr Clin North Am 1987;34:571.
33. Fernandez I et al. Rapid screening test evaluation for microalbuminuria in diabetes mellitus. Acta Diabetol 1998;35:199.
34. Lum G. How effective are screening tests for microalbuminuria in random urine specimens. Am Clin Lab Sci 2000 ;30:406.
35. American Diabetes Association: Clinical Practice Recommendations 2003. Diabetes Care 2003;26: S94.
36. Walters BA et al. Health-related quality of life, depressive symptoms, anemia, and malnutrition at hemodialysis initiation. Am J Kidney Dis 2002;40: 1185.
37. Stack AG. Impact of timing of nephrology referral and pre-ESRD care on mortality risk among new ESRD patients in the United States. Am J Kidney Dis 2003;41:310.
38. Klahr S et al. The effects of dietary protein restriction and blood-pressure control on the progression of chronic renal disease. Modification of Diet in Renal Disease Study Group. N Engl J Med 1994;330:877.
39. Lewis JB et al. Effect of intensive blood pressure control on the course of type 1 diabetic nephropathy. Am J Kidney Dis 1999;34:809.

40. Chobanian AV el al. The Seventh Report of the Joint National Committee on prevention, detection, evaluation, and treatment of high blood pressure. JAMA 2003; 289:2560.
41. Bakris GL et al. National Kidney Foundation hypertension and diabetes executive committee working group. Preserving renal function in adults with hypertension and diabetes. Am J Kidney Dis 2000;36:646.
42. Wright JT et al. Effect of blood pressure lowering and antihypertensive drug class on progression of hypertensive kidney disease: results from the AASK trial. JAMA 2002;288:2421.
43. Ruggenenti P et al. Effects of dihydropyridine calcium channel blockers, angiotensin-converting enzyme inhibition, and blood pressure control on chronic, nondiabetic nephropathies. J Am Soc Nephrol 1998;9:2096.
44. Laffel LM et al. The beneficial effect of angiotensin-converting enzyme inhibition with captopril on diabetic nephropathy in normotensive IDDM patients with microalbuminuria. North American Microalbuminuria Study Group. Am J Med 1995;99:497.
45. Parving HH et al. Long-term beneficial effect of ACE inhibition on diabetic nephropathy in normotensive type 1 diabetic patients. Kidney Int 2001;60:228.
46. Vijan S, Hayward RA. Treatment of hypertension in type 2 diabetes mellitus: blood pressure goals, choice of agents, and setting priorities in diabetes care. Ann Intern Med 2003;138:593.
47. Maschio G et al. Effect of the angiotensin-converting-enzyme inhibitor benazepril on the progression of chronic renal insufficiency. N Engl J Med 1996;334:939.
48. Giatras I et al. Effect of angiotensin-converting enzyme inhibitors on the progression of nondiabetic renal disease: a meta-analysis of randomized trials. Ann Intern Med 1997;127:337.
49. Ruggenenti P et al. Renoprotective properties of ACE-inhibition in non-diabetic nephropathies with non-nephrotic proteinuria. Lancet 1999;354(9176): 359.
50. Bakris GL, Weir MR. Angiotensin-converting enzyme inhibitor-associated elevations in serum creatinine: is this a cause for concern? Arch Intern Med 2000;160:685.
51. Brenner BM et al. Effects of losartan on renal and cardiovascular outcomes in patients with type 2 diabetes and nephropathy. N Engl J Med 2001; 345:861.
52. Keane WF. Recent advances in management of type 2 diabetes and nephropathy: lessons from the RENAAL study. Am J Kidney Dis 2003;41(3 Suppl 2):S22.
53. Lewis EJ et al. Renoprotective effect of the angiotensin-receptor antagonist irbesartan in patients with nephropathy due to type 2 diabetes. N Engl J Med 2001;345:851.
54. Kurokawa K. Effects of candesartan on the proteinuria of chronic glomerulonephritis. J Hum Hypertens 1999;13(Suppl 1):S57.
55. Suzuki et al. Renoprotective effects of low-dose valsartan in type 2 diabetic patients with diabetic nephropathy. Diabetes Res Clin Pract 2002;57:179.
56. Mogensen CE et al. Randomised controlled trial of dual blockade of renin-angiotensin system in patients with hypertension, microalbuminuria, and

non-insulin dependent diabetes: the candesartan and lisinopril microalbuminuria (CALM) study. BMJ 2000;321:1440.

57. Bakris GL et al. Calcium channel blockers versus other antihypertensive therapies on progression of NIDDM associated nephropathy. Kidney Int 1996;50:1641.

58. Tarif N, Bakris GL. Preservation of renal function: the spectrum of effects by calcium-channel blockers. Nephrol Dial Transplant 1997;12:2244.

59. Smith AC et al. Differential effects of calcium channel blockers on size selectivity of proteinuria in diabetic glomerulopathy. Kidney Int 1998; 54:889.

60. Bakris G, White D. Effects of an ACE inhibitor combined with a calcium channel blocker on progression of diabetic nephropathy. J Hum Hypertens 1997;11:35.

61. Ritz E et al. Angiotensin converting enzyme inhibitors, calcium channel blockers, and their combination in the treatment of glomerular disease. J Hypertens Suppl 1997;15:S21.

62. UK Prospective Diabetes Study Group. Efficacy of atenolol and captopril in reducing risk of macrovascular and microvascular complications in type 2 diabetes: UKPDS 39. BMJ 1998;317:713.

63. Brandle E et al. Effect of chronic dietary protein intake on the renal function in healthy subjects. Eur J Clin Nutr 1996;50:734.

64. Levey AS et al. Effects of dietary protein restriction on the progression of advanced renal disease in the Modification of Diet in Renal Disease Study. Am J Kidney Dis 1996;27(5):652.

65. Kasiske BL et al. A meta-analysis of the effects of dietary protein restriction on the rate of decline in renal function. Am J Kidney Dis 1998;31:954.

66. Bergstrom J, Lindholm B. Malnutrition, cardiac disease and mortality: an integrated point of view. Am J Kidney Dis 1998;32:834.

67. Levey AS et al. Controlling the epidemic of cardiovascular disease in chronic renal disease: what do we know? What do we need to learn? Where do we go from here? National Kidney Foundation Task Force on Cardiovascular Disease. Am J Kidney Dis 1998;32:853.

68. Lam KS et al. Cholesterol-lowering therapy may retard the progression of diabetic nephropathy. Diabetologia 1995;38:604.

69. Fried LF et al. Effect of lipid reduction on the progression of renal disease: a meta-analysis. Kidney Int 2001;59:260.

70. Third Report of the National Cholesterol Education Program (NCEP) Expert Panel on Detection, Evaluation, and Treatment of High Blood Cholesterol in Adults (Adult Treatment Panel III) final report. Circulation 2002;106:3143.

71. K/DOQI Clinical practice guidelines on managing dyslipidemias in chronic kidney disease. Am J Kidney Dis 2003;41(4 Suppl 3):S1.

72. Breyer J. Diabetic nephropathy. In: Greenberg A, ed. Primer on Kidney Diseases. 2nd Ed. San Diego: Academic Press, 1998:215.

73. Keller CK et al. Renal findings in patients with short-term type 2 diabetes. J Am Soc Nephrol 1996;7:2627.

74. Ravid M et al. Main risk factors for nephropathy in type 2 diabetes mellitus are plasma cholesterol levels, mean blood pressure, and hyperglycemia. Arch Intern Med 1998;158(9):998.

75. Vlassara H, Palace MR. Diabetes and advanced glycation endproducts. J Intern Med 2002;251:87.

76. Strojek K et al. Nephropathy of type II diabetes: evidence for hereditary factors? Kidney Int 1997;51(5):1602.

77. Krolewski AS. Genetics of diabetic nephropathy: evidence for major and minor gene effects. Kidney Int 1999;55(4):1582.

78. The Diabetes Control and Complications Trial Research Group. The effect of intensive treatment of diabetes on the development and progression of long-term complications in insulin-dependent diabetes mellitus. N Engl J Med 1993;329:977.

79. UK Prospective Diabetes Study (UKPDS) Group. Intensive blood-glucose control with sulphonylureas or insulin compared with conventional treatment and risk of complications in patients with type 2 diabetes (UKPDS 33). Lancet 1998;352:837.

80. Sica DA, Gehr TWB. Diuretic combinations in refractory oedema states. Clin Pharmacokinet 1996;30:229.

81. Ahmed J, Weisberg LS. Hyperkalemia in dialysis patients. Semin Dial 2001;14:348.

82. Gennari FJ, Segal AS. Hyperkalemia: an adaptive response in chronic renal insufficiency. Kidney Int 2002;62:1.

83. Ballmer PE et al. Chronic metabolic acidosis decreases albumin synthesis and induces negative nitrogen balance in humans. J Clin Invest 1995;95:39.

84. Eknoyan G, Levin A, Levin NW. Bone metabolism and disease in chronic kidney disease. Am J Kidney Dis 2003; 42(4 Suppl 3):1–201.

85. National Kidney Foundation. K/DOQI Clinical Practice Guidelines for Anemia of Chronic Kidney Disease. Update 2000 Am J Kidney Dis 2001;37(Suppl 1):S182 [erratum in Am J Kidney Dis 2001;38:442].

86. Erslev AJ. Erythropoietin. N Engl J Med 1991; 324:1339.

87. Kazmi WH et al. Anemia: an early complication of chronic renal insufficiency. Am J Kidney Dis 2001;38:803.

88. Levin A et al. Left ventricular mass index increase in early renal disease: impact of decline in hemoglobin. Am J Kidney Dis 1999;34:125.

89. Foley RN et al. Clinical and echocardiographic disease in patients starting end-stage renal disease therapy. Kidney Int 1995;47:186.

90. Himmelfarb J. Hematologic manifestations of renal failure. In: Greenberg A, ed. Primer on Kidney Diseases. 2nd Ed. San Diego: Academic Press, 1998:465.

91. Fishbane S et al. Hypervitaminosis A in two hemodialysis patients. Am J Kidney Dis 1995; 25:346.

92. Markowitz GS et al. An evaluation of the effectiveness of oral iron therapy in hemodialysis patients receiving recombinant human erythropoietin. Clin Nephrol 1997;48:34.

93. Panesar A, Agarwal R. Safety and efficacy of sodium ferric gluconate complex in patients with chronic kidney disease. Am J Kidney Dis 2002;40:924.

94. Stoves J et al. A randomized study of oral vs intravenous iron supplementation in patients with progressive renal insufficiency treated with erythropoietin. Nephrol Dial Transplant 2001;16:967.

95. European best practice guidelines for the management of anaemia in patients with chronic renal failure. Working Party for European Best Practice Guidelines for the Management of Anaemia in Patients with Chronic Renal Failure. Nephrol Dial Transplant 1999;14(Suppl 5):1.

96. Schein Pharmaceutical, Inc. INFeD (iron dextran injection, USP) package insert. Sorham Park, NJ: Schein Pharmaceutical, Inc., 2001.

97. Ahsan N. Infusion of total dose iron versus oral iron supplementation in ambulatory peritoneal dialysis patients: a prospective, cross-over trial. Adv Perit Dial 2000;16:80.

98. Faich G, Strobos J. Sodium ferric gluconate complex in sucrose: safer intravenous iron therapy than iron dextrans. Am J Kidney Dis 1999;33:464.

99. Watson Pharmaceuticals, Inc. Ferrlecit (sodium ferric gluconate complex in sucrose injection) package insert. Corona, CA: Watson Pharmaceuticals, Inc., 2001.

100. Michael B. Sodium ferric gluconate complex in hemodialysis patients: adverse reactions compared to placebo and iron dextran Kidney Int 2002;61:1830.

101. Folkert VW et al. Chronic use of sodium ferric gluconate complex in hemodialysis patients: safety of higher-dose (> or = 250 mg) administration. Am J Kidney Dis 2003;41:651.

102. American Reagent Laboratories, Inc. Venofer (iron sucrose injection) package insert. Shirley, NY: American Reagent Laboratories, Inc., 2000.

103. Kosch M et al. A randomized, controlled parallel-group trial on efficacy and safety of iron sucrose (Venofer) vs iron gluconate (Ferrlecit) in haemodialysis patients treated with rHuEpo. Nephrol Dial Transplant 2001;16:1239.

104. Chandler G et al. Intravenous iron sucrose: establishing a safe dose. Am J Kidney Dis 2001;38: 988.

105. Fishbane S et al. Reduction in recombinant human erythropoietin doses by the use of chronic intravenous iron supplementation. Am J Kidney Dis 1995;26:41.

106. Besarab A et al. Meta-analysis of subcutaneous versus intravenous epoetin in maintenance treatment of anemia in hemodialysis patients. Am J Kidney Dis 2002;40:439.

107. Ateshkadi A et al. Pharmacokinetics of intraperitoneal, intravenous, and subcutaneous recombinant human erythropoietin in patients on continuous ambulatory peritoneal dialysis. Am J Kidney Dis 1993;21:635.

108. Austrian Multicenter Study Group. Effectiveness and safety of recombinant human erythropoietin in predialysis patients. Nephron 1992;61:399.

109. Provenzano R et al. Once-weekly Procrit is effective in treating the anemia of chronic kidney disease: final results from the POWER study [Abstract]. J Am Soc Nephrol 2002:13:641A.

110. Germain M et al. Retrospective review of alternate procrit dosing (RAPID) in chronic kidney disease patients: interim analysis [Abstract]. Am J Kidney Dis 2003;41:A19.

111. Macdougall IC et al. Pharmacokinetics of novel erythropoiesis stimulating protein compared with epoetin alfa in dialysis patients. J Am Soc Nephrol.1999;10:2392.

112. Locatelli F et al. Novel erythropoiesis stimulating protein for treatment of anemia in chronic renal insufficiency. Kidney Int 2001;60:741.

113. Suranyi MG et al. Treatment of anemia with darbepoetin alfa administered de novo once every other week in chronic kidney disease. Am J Nephrol 2003;23:106.

114. Vanrenterghem Y et al. Randomized trial of darbepoetin alfa for treatment of renal anemia at a reduced dose frequency compared with rHuEPO in dialysis patients. Kidney Int 2002;62:2167.

115. Nissenson AR et al. Randomized, controlled trial of darbepoetin alfa for the treatment of anemia in hemodialysis patients. Am J Kidney Dis 2002;40:110.

116. Locatelli F et al. Treatment of anaemia in dialysis patients with unit dosing of darbepoetin alfa at a reduced dose frequency relative to recombinant human erythropoietin (rHuEpo). Nephrol Dial Transplant 2003;18:362.

117. Aranesp (darbepoetin alfa) package insert. Thousand Oaks, CA: Amgen Inc, July 19, 2002.

118. Onoyama K et al. Worsening of anemia by angiotensin converting enzyme inhibitors and its prevention by antiestrogenic steroid in chronic hemodialysis patients. J Cardiovasc Pharmacol 1989;13(Suppl 3):S27.

119. Abu-Alfa AK et al. ACE inhibitors do not induce recombinant human erythropoietin resistance in hemodialysis patients. Am J Kidney Dis 2000; 35:1076.

120. Casadevall N et al. Pure red-cell aplasia and antierythropoietin antibodies in patients treated with recombinant erythropoietin. N Engl J Med 2002;346:469.

121. Prabhakar S, Muhlfelder T. Antibodies to recombinant human erythropoietin causing pure red cell aplasia. Clin Nephrol 1997;47:331.

122. Weber G et al. Allergic skin and systemic reactions in a patient with pure red cell aplasia and anti-erythropoietin antibodies challenged with different epoetins. J Am Soc Nephrol 2002;13(9): 2381.

123. Prichard S. Risk factors for coronary artery disease in patients with renal failure. Am J Med Sci 2003;325:209.

124. Mailloux LU, Levey AS. Hypertension in patients with chronic renal disease. Am J Kidney Dis 1998;32(5 Suppl 3):S120.

125. Rosenberg ME et al. The paradox of the renin-angiotensin system in chronic renal disease. Kidney Int 1994;45:403.

126. Suki WN. Use of diuretics in chronic renal failure. Kidney Int Suppl 1997;59:S33.

127. Cannella G et al. Prolonged therapy with ACE inhibitors induces a regression of left ventricular hypertrophy of dialyzed uremic patients independently from hypotensive effects. Am J Kidney Dis 1997;30:659.

128. Burnier M, Brunner HR. Comparative antihypertensive effects of angiotensin II receptor antagonists. J Am Soc Nephrol 1999;10(Suppl 12):S278.

129. Cohn. Improving outcomes in congestive heart failure: Val-HeFT. Valsartan in heart failure trial. Cardiology 1999;(Suppl 1):19.

130. Seliger SL et al. HMG-CoA reductase inhibitors are associated with reduced mortality in ESRD patients. Kidney Int 2002;61:297.

131. Llach F. Secondary hyperparathyroidism in renal failure: the trade-off hypothesis revisited. Am J Kidney Dis 1995;25:63.

132. Sakhaee K, Gonzalez GB. Update on renal osteodystrophy: pathogenesis and clinical management. Am J Med Sci 1999;317:251.

133. Block GA, Port FK. Re-evaluation of risks associated with hyperphosphatemia and hyperparathyroidism in dialysis patients: recommendations for a change in management. Am J Kidney Dis 2000;35:1226.

134. Bowes AP, Church HN. Bowes & Church's Food Values of Portions Commonly Used. Philadelphia: Lippincott-Raven, 1998.

135. Delmez JA. Renal osteodystrophy and other musculoskeletal complications of chronic renal failure. In: Greenberg A, ed. Primer on Kidney Diseases. 2nd Ed. San Diego: Academic Press, 1998:448.

136. Goodman WG et al. Coronary-artery calcification in young adults with end-stage renal disease who are undergoing dialysis. N Engl J Med 2000; 342:1478

137. Lau AH et al. Phosphate-binding capacities of calcium and aluminum formulations. Int J Artif Organs 1998;21:19.

138. Almirall J et al. Calcium acetate versus calcium carbonate for the control of serum phosphorus in hemodialysis patients. Am J Nephrol 1994;14:192.

139. Slatopolsky EA et al. Renagel, a nonabsorbed calcium- and aluminum-free phosphate binder, lowers serum phosphorus and parathyroid hormone. Kidney Int 1999;55:299.

140. Chertow GM et al. Long-term effects of sevelamer hydrochloride on the calcium phosphate product and lipid profile of haemodialysis patients. Nephrol Dial Transplant 1999;14:2907.

141. Chertow GM et al. A randomized trial of sevelamer hydrochloride (RenaGel) with and without supplemental calcium. Strategies for the control of hyperphosphatemia and hyperparathyroidism in hemodialysis patients. Clin Nephrol 1999; 51:18.

142. Renagel package insert. Geltex Pharmaceuticals. July 2000.

143. Burke S et al. Sevelamer hydrochloride (Renagel), a nonabsorbed phosphate-binding polymer, does not interfere with digoxin or warfarin pharmacokinetics. J Clin Pharmacol 2001;41:193.

144. Burke SK et al. Sevelamer hydrochloride (Renagel), a phosphate-binding polymer, does not alter the pharmacokinetics of two commonly used antihypertensives in healthy volunteers. J Clin Pharmacol 2001;41:199.

145. Marco MP et al. Treatment with sevelamer decreases bicarbonate levels in hemodialysis patients. Nephron 2002;92:499.

146. Caramelo CA et al. Mechanisms of aluminum-induced microcytosis: lessons from accidental aluminum intoxication. Kidney Int 1995;47:164.

147. Malluche HH. Aluminum and bone disease in chronic renal failure. Nephrol Dial Transplant 2002;17(Suppl 2):21.

148. D'Haese PC et al. A multicenter study on the effects of lanthanum carbonate (Fosrenol) and calcium carbonate on renal bone disease in dialysis patients. Kidney Int 2003;63(Suppl 85):73.

149. Ishiura E. Serum levels of 1,25-dihydroxyvitamin D, 24,25-dihydroxyvitamin D, and 25-hydroxyvitamin D in nondialyzed patients with chronic renal failure. Kidney Int 1999;55:1019.

150. Slatopolsky E et al. A novel mechanism for skeletal resistance in uremia. Kidney Int 2000;58:753.

151. Goodman WG et al. Parathyroid hormone (PTH), PTH-derived peptides, and new PTH assays in renal osteodystrophy. Kidney Int 2003;63:1.

152. Martin KJ et al. 19-Nor-1-alpha-25-dihydroxyvitamin D2 (Paricalcitol) safely and effectively reduces the levels of intact parathyroid hormone in patients on hemodialysis. J Am Soc Nephrol 1998;9:1427.

153. Martin KJ et al. Therapy of secondary hyperparathyroidism with 19-nor-1alpha,25-dihydroxyvitamin D2. Am J Kidney Dis 1998;32(2 Suppl 2):S61.

154. Lindberg J et al. A long-term, multicenter study of the efficacy and safety of paricalcitol in end-stage renal disease. Clin Nephrol 2001;56:315.

155. Zemplar Package Insert. Abbott Laboratories Inc, Abbott Park, IL. April 1998.

156. Martin KJ et al. Paricalcitol dosing according to body weight or severity of hyperparathyroidism: a double-blind, multicenter, randomized study. Am J Kidney Dis 2001;38(Suppl 5):S57.

157. Llach F, Yudd M. Paricalcitol in dialysis patients with calcitriol-resistant secondary hyperparathyroidism. Am J Kidney Dis 2001;38(Suppl 5):S45.

158. Sprague SM et al. Suppression of parathyroid hormone secretion in hemodialysis patients: comparison of paricalcitol with calcitriol. Am J Kidney Dis 2001;38(Suppl 5):S51.

159. Frazao JM et al. Intermittent doxercalciferol (1alpha-hydroxyvitamin D(2)) therapy for secondary hyperparathyroidism. Am J Kidney Dis 2000;36:550.

160. Maung HM et al. Efficacy and side effects of intermittent intravenous and oral doxercalciferol (1α-hydroxyvitamin D₂) in dialysis patients with secondary hyperparathyroidism: a sequential comparison. Am J Kidney Dis 2001;37:532.

161. Hectorol package insert. Madison, WI: Bone Care International, Inc. [Oral June 1999, Intravenous April 2000].

162. Quarles LD et al. The calcimimetic AMG 073 as a potential treatment for secondary hyperparathyroidism of end-stage renal disease. J Am Soc Nephrol 2003;14:575.

163. Kovalik EC. Endocrine manifestations of renal failure. In: Greenberg A, ed. Primer on Kidney Diseases. 2nd Ed. San Diego: Academic Press, 1998:472.

164. Palmer BF. Sexual dysfunction in uremia. J Am Soc Nephrol 1999;10:1381.

165. Fliser D et al. Insulin resistance and hyperinsulinemia are already present in patients with incipient renal disease. Kidney Int 1998;53:1343.

166. Etemad B. Gastrointestinal complications of renal failure. Gastroenterol Clin North Am 1998; 27:875.

167. Schoonjans R et al. Dyspepsia and gastroparesis in chronic renal failure: the role of Helicobacter pylori. Clin Nephrol 2002;57:201.

168. Tsai CJ, Hwang JC. Investigation of upper gastrointestinal hemorrhage in chronic renal failure. J Clin Gastroenterol 1996;22:2.

169. Mak SK et al. Efficacy of a 1-week course of proton-pump inhibitor-based triple therapy for eradicating Helicobacter pylori in patients with and without chronic renal failure. Am J Kidney Dis 2002;40:576.

170. Fraser CL. Neurological manifestations of renal failure. In: Greenberg A, ed. Primer on Kidney Diseases. 2nd Ed. San Diego: Academic Press, 1998:459.

171. Robertson KE, Mueller BA. Uremic pruritus. Am J Health Syst Pharm 1996;53:2159.

172. Hiroshige K et al. Optimal dialysis improves uremic pruritus. Am J Kidney Dis 1995;25:413.

173. Ashmore SD et al. Ondansetron therapy for uremic pruritus in hemodialysis patients. Am J Kidney Dis 2000;35:827.

174. Pauli-Magnus C et al. Naltrexone does not relieve uremic pruritus: results of a randomized, double-blind, placebo-controlled crossover study. J Am Soc Nephrol 2000;11:514.

175. Couser WG. Glomerulonephritis. Lancet 1999; 353(9163):1509.

176. Jennette JC, Falk RJ. Diagnosis and management of glomerular diseases. Med Clin North Am 1997;81:653.

177. Cameron JS. Lupus nephritis. J Am Soc Nephrol 1999;10:413.

178. Balow JE. Renal manifestations of systemic lupus erythematosus and other rheumatic disorders. In: Greenberg A, ed. Primer on Kidney Diseases. 2nd Ed. San Diego: Academic Press, 1998:208.

179. Bansal VK, Beto JA. Treatment of lupus nephritis: a meta-analysis of clinical trials. Am J Kidney Dis 1997;29:193.

180. Gourley MF et al. Methylprednisolone and cyclophosphamide, alone or in combination, in patients with lupus nephritis: a randomized, controlled trial. Ann Intern Med 1996;125:549.

181. Chan TM et al. Efficacy of mycophenolate mofetil in patients with diffuse proliferative lupus nephritis. Hong Kong-Guangzhou Nephrology Study Group. N Engl J Med 2000;343:1156.

182. Holdsworth S et al. The clinical spectrum of acute glomerulonephritis and lung haemorrhage (Goodpasture's syndrome). Q J Med 1985;55:75.

183. Levy JB, Pusey CD. Still a role for plasma exchange in rapidly progressive glomerulonephritis? J Nephrol 1997;10:7.

184. Salama AD. Goodpasture's disease. Lancet. 2001;358(9285):917.

185. Jennette JC, Falk RJ. Renal involvement in systemic vasculitis. In: Greenberg A, ed. Primer on Kidney Diseases. 2nd Ed. San Diego: Academic Press, 1998:200.

186. Leavitt RY et al. The American College of Rheumatology 1990 criteria for the classification of Wegener's granulomatosis. Arthritis Rheum 1990;33:11.

187. Falk RJ, Jennette JC. ANCA small-vessel vasculitis. J Am Soc Nephrol 1997;8:314.

188. Specks U, DeRemee RA. Granulomatous vasculitis: Wegener's granulomatosis and Churg-Strauss syndrome. Rheum Dis Clin North Am 1990; 16:377.

189. Stegeman CA. Trimethoprim-sulfamethoxazole (Co-Trimoxazole) for the prevention of relapses of Wegener's granulomatosis. N Engl J Med 1996; 335:16.

190. Stone JH et al. Treatment of non-life threatening Wegener's granulomatosis with methotrexate and daily prednisone as the initial therapy of choice. J Rheumatol 1999;26:1134.

Renal Dialysis

Thomas J. Comstock

Dialysis and transplantation are the two treatments available for the management of patients with end-stage renal disease (ESRD). The prevalence of ESRD in the United States at the end of 2000 was estimated to be 379,000, compared with 308,000 in 1997 and continues to rise.[1,2] There were approximately 96,000 new patients with ESRD during 2000. Although the incidence of ESRD continues to increase each year, the rate of increase has fallen from approximately 10% to 3% to 5% over the past 10 years. The reasons for this decline are unknown but may be due to reporting or a true change in the incidence rate. In 2000, 65% of patients with ESRD were treated with hemodialysis, 6.1% were receiving peritoneal dialysis, and 24.7% had a functioning transplant. The shortage of donor kidneys and the existence of ESRD patients who are unacceptable transplant recipients sustain the demand for dialysis. Kidney transplantation is further discussed in Chapter 35, Solid Organ Transplantation.

The two primary modes of dialysis therapy are *hemodialysis* (HD) and *peritoneal dialysis* (PD). Variations of PD include *continuous ambulatory peritoneal dialysis* (CAPD) and *automated peritoneal dialysis* (APD), an increasingly common modality that permits greater patient flexibility with dialysis. Without dialysis or transplantation, patients with ESRD will die of the metabolic complications of their renal failure. Among the nearly 270,000 dialysis patients in the United States, 91% undergo HD. The majority of these patients receive dialysis three times a week in a center designed primarily for stable, ambulatory patients at either a hospital-based or a free-standing dialysis facility.[1] Home HD accounts for <1% of dialysis patients. Patients undergoing PD also are managed through dialysis centers for routine care, although less often than HD patients.

Several factors are considered in the selection of the type of dialysis for each patient. Often, the overriding consideration is the suitability of the procedure for the patient's lifestyle. A patient who needs flexibility and freedom from a rigid schedule may prefer PD over HD to avoid the necessity of being at a dialysis center three times weekly for a 3- to 4-hour dialysis treatment. Other considerations include the availability of a vascular access site for HD, or a patient's ability to perform self-care for dialysate exchanges with PD. Overall morbidity and mortality are generally similar for both HD and PD; however, the first-year death rate is higher for HD than PD, and is reported to be 280 versus 249 deaths per 1,000 patient years. Second-year death rates are similar, at 268 and 286 deaths per 1,000 patient years for HD and PD, respectively. Patient characteristics and comorbid conditions influence the death rate, including age (increased with increased age), race (increased in white patients), and primary cause of ESRD (increased for diabetes and hypertension compared to glomerulonephritis).[3] The expected survival of the patient undergoing chronic dialysis compared with the average life expectancy in the United States is significantly reduced. For example, at 60 years of age the average survival is approximately 4 years for the dialysis patient compared to 21 years for the average population. Among dialysis patients, those with diabetes (the most common cause of ESRD) or hypertension have a higher mortality rate than patients without these conditions. The all-cause mortality rates are 370 and 382 deaths per 1,000 patient years, for diabetes and hypertension, respectively, compared to 311 and 215 for patients with chronic nephritis and cystic kidney disease. Other factors associated with mortality include body mass index (decreased with increased BMI) and serum albumin (decreased with increased albumin).[1] Summary reports and analysis of survival and mortality are included as part of the annual report of the USRDS.[1]

These demographic characteristics of the ESRD population are based primarily on data from the Centers for Medicare and Medicaid Services (CMS), because patients with ESRD are eligible for Medicare benefits. Coverage for ESRD began in 1973, when Congress enacted the End-Stage

Renal Disease Program as an amendment to Medicare.[4] Total Medicare expenditures in 2000 were approximately $219 billion, of which $12.7 billion, or 5.8%, were for the ESRD program. This represents an increase in the fraction expended for ESRD from 4.5% in 1991. The cost per member per month (PMPM) is approximately $5,447 for nondiabetic HD patients and $5,998 for patients with diabetes. [1] The PMPM for PD is approximately 15% less per month, and it can be diminished with improvement of certain clinical indicators such as albumin (11% decreased cost per 1 g/dL increase) and hemoglobin (3.6% decreased cost for values >11 g/dL compared to 10 to 11 g/dL). These costs for ESRD do not include other expenses such as those for most outpatient drugs and for lost productivity.[1]

The rapid growth of the number of patients undergoing dialysis calls attention to the need for practitioners who understand the processes and therapies for these patients. Both HD and PD were developed as methods for the removal of metabolic waste products across a semipermeable membrane. HD is an extracorporeal process, whereas PD uses the patient's peritoneal membrane for the clearance of water and solutes. This chapter will address the fundamental clinical aspects of both HD and PD, including principles, complications, and management. Throughout the chapter, reference will be made, when appropriate, to the clinical practice guidelines developed by the National Kidney Foundation, originally published in 1997, and updated in 2000. The initial guidelines focused on dialysis issues, the Dialysis Outcomes Quality Initiative (DOQI), and included four workgroups: Hemodialysis Adequacy,[5] Peritoneal Dialysis Adequacy,[6] Vascular Access,[7] and Anemia.[8] The updated clinical practice guidelines have been renamed the Kidney Disease Outcomes Quality Initiative (K/DOQI) to reflect the broader nature and impact of renal impairment. Additional clinical practice guidelines developed under K/DOQI include Nutrition of Chronic Renal Failure[9] and Chronic Kidney Disease: Evaluation, Classification, and Stratification.[10] The latter guideline is addressed in Chapter 32, Chronic Kidney Disease.

HEMODIALYSIS
Principles and Transport Processes

Dialysis is a process that facilitates the removal of excess water and toxins from the body, which accumulate as a result of inadequate kidney function. During HD, a patient's anticoagulated blood and an electrolyte solution (dialysate) are perfused through a dialyzer (artificial kidney) to opposite sides of a semipermeable membrane; metabolic waste products are removed from the patient's blood by diffusing down their concentration gradients into the dialysate. The blood and dialysate flow in opposite directions to maximize the concentration gradient for toxin exposure to the membrane (Fig. 33-1). The rate of removal of toxins from the blood is influenced by blood and dialysate flow, concentration gradient across the membrane, membrane characteristics, and properties of the toxin being removed.

Solutes from the blood are removed through diffusion and convection. *Diffusion* is the process whereby the molecule moves down its concentration gradient by passing through pores in the dialysis membrane.[11,12] Once equilibrium is achieved, the net movement is zero because the rate of move-

ment from the blood to dialysate compartment is equal to the rate from the dialysate to the blood compartment. For most substances, equilibrium is not achieved, either because the blood and dialysate flow rates are too rapid, or the molecule is too large to easily move through the pores. Urea (60 D) is a marker of small-molecule transport across the dialysis membrane and serves as a measure of dialysis adequacy because it distributes freely throughout body water and is cleared rapidly by HD. [13–16] The rate-limiting step for the removal of urea is blood flow. A larger-molecule, vitamin B_{12} (1,355 D), also has been used as a measure of dialysis efficiency. The clearance of vitamin B_{12} is less dependent on blood flow than urea because it is too large to easily cross the conventional dialysis membrane, much like the antibiotic vancomycin (1448 D), which is not cleared by these membranes. The overall removal of vitamin B_{12} and vancomycin depends on the type of membrane and the duration of dialysis.

Convection is the process that removes toxins during dialysis[11,12] through the ultrafiltration of plasma water from the blood compartment. A controlled pressure difference across the semipermeable membrane permits water movement through the membrane pores, which carries with it solute into the dialysate, thereby further enhancing solute removal. The removal of solutes by convection during ultrafiltration generally is small relative to their elimination through diffusion.

Patients undergoing chronic HD typically are dialyzed for 3 to 4 hours, three times a week, either Monday-Wednesday-Friday or Tuesday-Thursday-Saturday. During the interdialytic period, fluids ingested and produced through metabolic processes are retained in the patient, and the excess fluid is removed during the subsequent dialysis session. Although patients generally are on fluid-restricted diets, accumulation of 1 to 5 kg of fluid is common between sessions and must be removed during the dialysis treatment.

1. R.W., a 55-year-old man with a 25-year history of hypertension and kidney insufficiency, presents to the renal clinic for reassessment of his kidney function. He is 70 inches tall and weighs 70 kg. Since his last visit 3 months ago, his creatinine clearance (Cl_{Cr}) has decreased from 22 to 12 mL/min (normal, 75 to 125 mL/min) and the blood urea nitrogen (BUN) has increased to 89 mg/dL (normal, 8 to 18 mg/dL). The serum potassium (K) is 4.5 mEq/L (normal, 3.5 to 5.0 mEq/L) and HCO_3 is 17 mEq/L (normal, 24 to 30 mEq/L). He has selected HD as his form of therapy until a suitable donor kidney is available and is expected to begin dialysis within the next 1 to 3 months. When he begins dialysis, he will be dialyzed three times a week for 4 hours each treatment, using a Fresenius F-60A dialyzer, with blood and dialysate flows of 400 and 500 mL/min, respectively, and bicarbonate-containing dialysate. What characteristics of the Fresenius F-60A dialyzer make it a good choice for R.W.? What determines the composition of the dialysate?

[SI units: Cl_{Cr}, 0.37 and 0.2 mL/sec, respectively (normal, 1.24 to 2.08); BUN, 31.8 mmol/L (normal, 3 to 6.5); K, 4.5 mmol/L (normal, 3.5 to 5)]

The Fresenius dialyzer uses one of a class of membranes classified as high flux.[17] This polysulfone membrane is a synthetic membrane with larger pore sizes than conventional cellulose membranes. The F-60A has a KUf, the ultrafiltration coefficient (volume of water removed/mm Hg across the membrane per hour of dialysis), of 40 mL/mm Hg per hour, indicating a high ultrafiltration capability; an in vitro KoA_{urea}

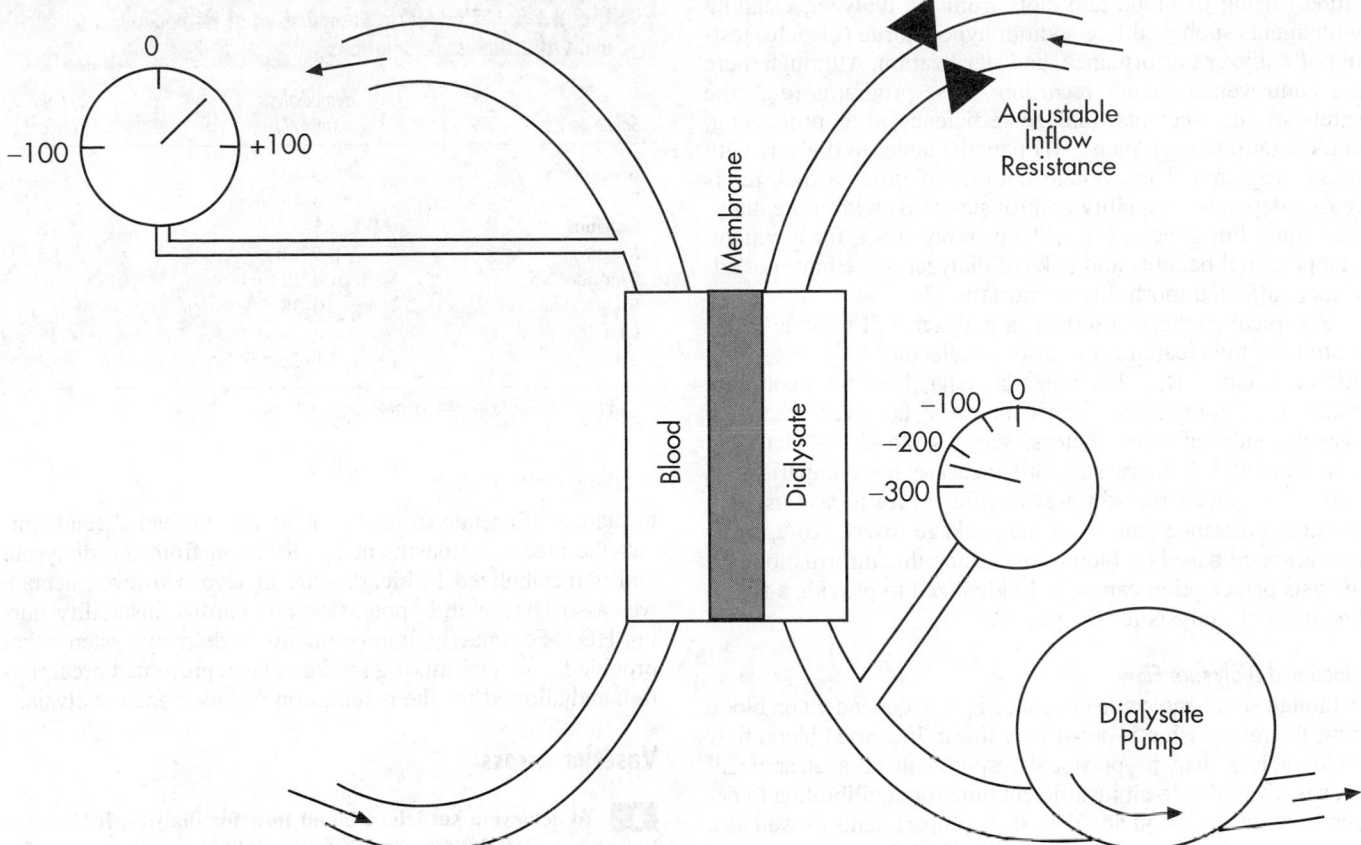

FIGURE 33-1 Representation of hemodialysis with blood flowing in one direction and dialysate in the opposite, separated by a semipermeable membrane. Note pressure monitors and dialysate pump with variable inflow resistance to create negative pressure for ultrafiltration from the blood compartment. (Reproduced with permission from Daugirdas JT, Van Stone JC. Physiologic principles and urea kinetic modeling. In: Daugirdas JT et al., eds. Handbook of Dialysis. 3rd Ed. Philadelphia: Lippincott, Williams & Wilkins, 2001:15.)

(the urea mass transfer area coefficient) of 760, a measure of dialyzer efficiency for urea removal; urea clearance of 244 mL/min and vitamin B_{12} clearance of 118 mL/minute at blood flows of 300 and 200 mL/min, respectively; and a surface area of 1.3 m^2. This information can be located in the product literature from the manufacturer or summary tables from common dialysis references.[17] These data are used to individualize the dialysis prescription for a patient.

Dialyzer Characteristics

Dialyzers are characterized by many factors, such as membrane composition, size, and ability to clear solutes. Their primary component is the dialysis membrane, made of cellulose (e.g., cuprammonium cellulose), substituted cellulose (e.g., cellulose acetate, cellulose triacetate), cellulosynthetic (e.g., Hemophan), or synthetic polymer (e.g., polysulfone, polyacrylonitrile [PAN], polymethylmethacrylate [PMMA]).[17] Membranes may differ not only by composition, but also by surface area, thickness, and configuration within the dialyzer. The most common configuration is the hollow fiber dialyzer, whereby the membrane is formed as thousands of hollow fibers that run the length of the dialyzer. Blood flows through the fibers and the dialysate flows in the space surrounding the fibers within the dialyzer cartridge. Another, less common design is the parallel-plate configuration, whereby blood and

dialysate flow between alternating sheets of the membrane. Functionally, the dialysis filters can be differentiated based on their ability to remove water and solutes. *High-efficiency* membranes generally have a large surface area and are able to clear large quantities of small molecules, such as urea, whereas *high-flux* membranes have larger pore sizes and are able to clear larger molecules (e.g., middle molecules and drugs such as vancomycin or vitamin B_{12}, with molecular weights in the range of 1,000 to 5,000.) more effectively than membranes with smaller pores. High flux membranes also have a greater permeability to water, as reflected in a KUf value >10 mL/hr/mm Hg. Membranes also differ in their degree of biocompatibility. Cellulose membranes are not biocompatible and will evoke complement response and cytokine release, which may lead to hypotension, fever, and platelet activation in patients.[18] The substituted cellulose, cellulosynthetic, and synthetic membranes are more biocompatible than the unsubstituted cellulose membranes. The use of synthetic membranes has become predominant and has also led to the reuse of dialyzers in many centers due to their increased cost. High-flux membranes are more expensive than conventional cellulose, but when reuse systems in which the filter is cleansed and sterilized are put in place, the cost per dialysis session is reduced substantially.[19] Both manual and automated systems are used to reprocess dialyzers. These systems include rinsing of blood and clots from the dialyzer, cleaning with agents such as dilute sodium hypochlorite (bleach), testing of dialyzer performance, and sterilization. Although there are controversial issues regarding reuse programs (e.g., the safety of disinfectants, dialyzer efficiency after processing, and contamination), many HD patients undergo dialysis with reuse programs. The average number of times a dialyzer is reused depends on quality control standards within the dialysis center, but generally it is 10 or more times for a patient. The potential benefits and risks of dialyzer reuse have not adversely affected morbidity or mortality.[19]

A typical package insert for a dialyzer will provide information on the clearance of various molecules (e.g., urea, creatinine, vitamin B_{12}). Urea clearance has become a common measure of comparison for membranes; however, clearance also depends on other factors, such as blood and dialysate flow rates.[11,12] A more standard measure for comparison is KoA_{urea}, the mass transfer area coefficient for urea. Based on the urea clearance data from the package insert, KoA_{urea} can be estimated based on blood flow. Using this information, the dialysis prescription can be individualized to provide a specified dose of dialysis for the patient.[13]

Blood and Dialysate Flow

Although small-molecule clearance is very dependent on blood flow, the relationship is not strictly linear. Increased blood flow yields a less than proportional response in urea clearance.[13] This is likely due to an insufficient time for equilibration to occur between the blood and dialysate compartments as well as a greater membrane resistance to diffusion from an increased stagnant layer. A typical blood flow rate for dialysis is 400 to 500 mL/min but is dependent on the vascular access site and the cardiovascular status of the patient. Some patients are not able to tolerate this rate, and a lower blood flow rate may be necessary. Dialysate flow rates generally are 500 mL/min and may be increased to 800 mL/min for high-flux dialysis, which will increase urea clearance by approximately 10%.[20]

Dialysate Composition

Dialysate composition usually is standardized within certain limits of electrolyte content, yet allows for individualization as necessary. Water is obtained through the public water system, which then undergoes treatment by reverse osmosis, followed by ion exchange with activated charcoal to remove contaminants such as aluminum, copper, and chloramines, as well as bacteria and endotoxins.[21] The dialysate solution does not require sterilization because the dialysis membrane separates the blood and dialysate compartments. Nevertheless, pyrogen reactions may occur, and there may be greater risk with high-flux membranes because of the increased pore size. The final dialysate solution is prepared in the dialysis machine by proportioning a dialysate concentrate with the purified water, resulting in a final product, which typically contains those elements listed in Table 33-1. Before delivery, the dialysate is heated to 37°C to maintain body temperature and avoid hemolysis, which can occur with excessive heating. Metabolic acidosis, which is associated with ESRD due to an inability to excrete the daily obligatory load of acid, is controlled with the addition of bicarbonate buffer to the dialysate solution.[17] Precipitation of calcium carbonate had been a problem with the addition of bicarbonate to the dialysate in the past, which led

Table 33-1 Electrolyte Composition of Hemodialysis and CAPD Dialysate Solutions

Solute	Hemodialysis (mEq/L)	CAPD (mEq/L)
Sodium	135–145	132
Potassium	0–4	0
Calcium	2.5–3.5	3.5
Magnesium	0.5–1.0	1.5
Chloride	100–124	102
Bicarbonate	30–38	
Lactate		35
pH	7.1–7.3	5.5

CAPD, continuous ambulatory peritoneal dialysis.

to the use of acetate to control acidemia instead. Acetate enters the blood compartment by diffusion from the dialysate and is metabolized to bicarbonate in vivo. However, acetate was associated with hypotension and cardiac instability during HD.[17] Fortunately, improvements in delivery systems that provide for special mixing methods have prevented precipitation and allowed for the resumption of bicarbonate dialysis.

Vascular Access

2. To achieve a sufficient blood flow for dialysis, R.W. must have a vascular site for chronic access. What are the options for chronic vascular access in R.W.?

Vascular access to achieve the blood flow rates necessary for chronic HD requires creation of an arteriovenous (AV) fistula or insertion of an AV graft, a synthetic tube made of polytetrafluoroethylene (PTFE), which connects the artery and vein. The K/DOQI guidelines for vascular access advocate placement of a fistula at the location of the wrist (radial-cephalic), then elbow (brachial-cephalic), as the preferred vascular access sites. If neither of these is feasible for the patient, insertion of an arteriovenous graft or creation of a transposed brachial basilica vein fistula is recommended. Central venous catheters are discouraged for chronic vascular access. The permanent vascular access site provides for easy access to high blood flow, which could not be achieved through routine venipuncture of superficial veins. The fistula is preferred due to its longer survival of approximately 75% at 3 years, compared with 30% for the arteriovenous graft.[22] Although preferred, the fistula may not be suitable for the patient with poor vasculature, such as elderly patients or those with diabetes, atherosclerosis, or small vessels. The fistula should preferably be created 3 to 4 months before its intended use to allow the vein to mature. The graft can be used soon after insertion, although 2 weeks will allow for healing at the anastomosis sites and may prolong patency. If R.W. has adequate vasculature, a fistula should be created for chronic access based on the higher long-term graft survival. Vascular access is critical for chronic HD and often has been labeled the "Achilles' heel" of dialysis therapy. Complications associated with vascular access are a significant problem in patients undergoing chronic HD. The most common is thrombosis, usually the result of venous stenosis.[7] If not treated, thromboses will result in loss of the access. Access-related complications are a major cause of hospitalization, and therefore attention to these problems is important clinically and economically.

Anticoagulation

3. Recommend a reasonable anticoagulation regimen to begin for R.W. with the initiation of his HD. What are alternatives for patients at high risk for bleeding?

Most patients undergoing HD will be anticoagulated with intravenous (IV) heparin during the dialysis treatment. Anticoagulation is necessary to prevent blood from clotting in the extracorporeal circuit for patients undergoing HD. Several methods have been used in an attempt to provide adequate anticoagulation without increasing the risk of bleeding. Approaches include the administration of heparin in adequate quantities to anticoagulate the patient during the dialysis procedure either by intermittent bolus injections or an initial bolus followed by a continuous infusion.[23] Modern HD delivery systems have incorporated heparin infusion devices that can be programmed to provide the desired infusion rate during dialysis.

If there is no evidence of a bleeding disorder, recent surgery, or other risk factors for heparin anticoagulation, therapy should be initiated with a 2000 U bolus of heparin intravenously 3 to 5 minutes before initiation of dialysis, followed by an infusion of 1,000 U/hour.[23] The target activated clotting time (ACT) is 40% to 80% above the average baseline for the dialysis unit (e.g., 200 to 250 seconds, for normal values of 90 to 140 seconds). Monitor for signs of bleeding and measure the ACT at 1-hour intervals during dialysis. Discontinue the heparin 1 hour before the end of dialysis to prevent excessive bleeding following dialysis. The normal elimination half-life for heparin is 50 minutes for the aforementioned dose, and heparin has a linear dose-response relationship for target ACTs within the previously stated range.[23]

Patients at increased risk of bleeding include those with recent surgery, retinopathy, gastrointestinal (GI) bleeding, and cerebrovascular bleeding. For these patients, the goal is to prevent clot formation within the dialysis circuit as well as to minimize the risk of active bleeding. This may be accomplished by the use of minimal-dose heparin (tight ACT control), no heparin, or regional anticoagulation. The minimal heparin approach individualizes therapy to achieve ACT values 40% above baseline following an initial bolus of 750 U.[23,24] The ACT is measured 3 minutes after the bolus dose of heparin to allow for distribution. Subsequent bolus doses of heparin are adjusted based on the expectation of a linear response, and additional heparin may be administered to achieve the desired effect. The initial heparin maintenance infusion rate of 600 U/hr can be modified according to results from monitoring the ACT at 30-minute intervals to ensure an adequate response. The infusion rate should be proportionate to the bolus dose needed to maintain the ACT at 40% above baseline. Samples collected for determination of ACT should be obtained from the arterial line, before the infusion of heparin, to reflect systemic anticoagulation effects.

An alternative to heparinization for patients undergoing dialysis with high blood flow rates is a no-heparin regimen.[23,25] This approach requires pretreatment of the dialyzer with heparin in normal saline, which then is rinsed before a rapid increase of blood flow to >250 mL/min. During dialysis, the dialyzer is flushed with normal saline every 15 to 30 minutes to rinse away microclots that may have formed. The incidence of clotting with this approach is approximately 5%. Regional anticoagulation of the dialysis circuit can be accomplished by the use of heparin administration into the arterial side with protamine neutralization on the venous side. This approach has fallen out of favor due to the propensity for rebound anticoagulation following dialysis as heparin dissociates from the heparin-protamine complex.

Low-molecular-weight heparins (LMWHs) have been studied as alternatives to heparin for anticoagulation. In a randomized, crossover study comparing the safety and efficacy of enoxaparin with standard heparin, a 1.0-mg dose of enoxaparin produced less minor fibrin/clot formation in the dialyzer, but more frequent minor hemorrhage between dialyses. Enoxaparin dose reduction to 0.7 mg resulted in similar efficacy and eliminated the minor hemorrhage.[26] Tinzaparin also has been shown to be effective as an anticoagulant during HD, using an IV dose of 75 IU/kg just before dialysis.[27]

Another class of agents with potential use in patients requiring anticoagulation during HD are the direct thrombin inhibitors, lepirudin (Refludan) and argatroban. Lepirudin is produced through recombinant DNA technology, based on the antithrombin product hirudin, which is isolated from the saliva of leeches. Because lepirudin is significantly cleared by the kidneys, doses should be individualized based on residual renal function.[28,29] There are no established dosage regimens, as elimination is substantially delayed; monitoring should be performed using a target aPTT of 2.0 to 2.5 times baseline. Argatroban is a synthetic derivative of L-arginine that was approved by the FDA for use in patients susceptible to thrombosis who also have heparin-induced thrombocytopenia (HIT). Because it is eliminated by nonrenal routes, the dosing in patients undergoing dialysis is similar to those with normal kidney function.[29] Reports in small numbers of patients have recommended different dosage regimens but consist of an initial bolus dose followed by a continuous infusion during dialysis. O'Shea and colleagues use a regimen of 0.1 mg/kg followed by an infusion of 0.1 to 0.2 mg/kg/hr to maintain the aPTT at 1.5 times baseline.[29] HIT is reported to occur in 0% to 12% of HD patients receiving heparin for anticoagulation. Further studies are necessary to define the role of these newer agents in patients undergoing chronic HD.

The regional administration of trisodium citrate through the arterial line is an alternative to systemic anticoagulation. It binds free calcium, which is necessary for the coagulation process. The calcium citrate complex is removed by the dialysate and, based on plasma calcium values, calcium chloride is administered on the venous side to replace the citrate-bound calcium to prevent hypocalcemia or hypercalcemia. Some of the administered citrate is returned to the patient and is metabolized to bicarbonate, leading to metabolic alkalosis in some cases. Regional citrate anticoagulation is reserved for patients who are at risk for bleeding and requires additional monitoring to adjust the dual infusions.[23]

Dialysis Prescription

Individualization of the dialysis prescription has undergone several advances during the past decade as a result of the quantification of the dose of dialysis delivered to the patient.

In 1981, the report of the National Cooperative Dialysis Study (NCDS) showed a relationship between the degree of dialysis delivered to the patient and morbidity.[14,15,30] Four groups of patients were randomized to different combinations of time-averaged serum urea concentrations (50 or 100 mg/dL) and length of dialysis (2.5 to 3.5, or 4.5 to 5.0 hours). There were no differences in mortality during the 1-year study; however, patients with higher urea exposure experienced a greater withdrawal rate from the study and more hospitalizations compared with patients with lower urea concentrations. These data suggested that urea kinetics could be used to model dialysis therapy and that urea could be used as a surrogate marker for the adequacy of dialysis. Because it is well recognized that other uremic toxins also contribute to the overall morbidity among these patients, surrogate markers of their removal by dialysis have been used in an attempt to better define the adequacy of dialysis. Creatinine (MW 113 D), which is slightly larger than urea, has been used as a marker but it otherwise distributes similarly and offers no additional benefits. As already noted, vitamin B_{12} is a marker for the class of middle molecules thought to be responsible for many of the uremic complications in ESRD. Vitamin B_{12} is eliminated in a different manner than urea by dialysis, because it is larger and not cleared easily by membranes with smaller pores than high-flux membranes. The utility of vitamin B_{12} as a surrogate for dialysis adequacy has not been established.[11]

Further analysis of the NCDS data by Gotch and Sargent[15] using a pharmacokinetic-like term, Kt/V, demonstrated a relationship between morbidity and Kt/V. The Kt/V term is based on the predialysis and postdialysis BUN values, distribution of urea, and duration of dialysis. K is the urea clearance (mL/min), t is time (minutes), and V is distribution volume for urea (mL). The term has no units and represents the quantity of dialysis delivered to the patient, or the total volume of blood cleared of urea, relative to the urea distribution volume in a given patient. Its basic relationship depends on the first-order elimination of urea, as seen in the following general equations:

$$BUN_{post} = BUN_{pre} (e^{-Kt/V})$$
$$Kt/V = - \ln(BUN_{post}/BUN_{pre})$$

The patients with a Kt/V <0.9 had a 54% failure rate, defined as death, hospitalization, or withdrawal from the study for medical reasons, whereas those with a Kt/V >0.9 had a 13% failure rate on dialysis. Based on these data, it was recommended that patients receive a dialysis "dose" of Kt/V >1.0 when undergoing dialysis three times weekly.

Several refinements of the Kt/V relationship have been made to better approximate the actual observations in HD patients. These include corrections for ultrafiltration of fluid during dialysis; access and cardiopulmonary recirculation, which result in dilution of the arterial urea concentration in vivo; and single-pool, variable volume model for urea. Timing of blood sample collection is very important, to avoid diluted samples and postdialysis rebound of the plasma urea concentration.[13] Redistribution of urea may occur for 30 to 60 minutes after dialysis treatment, and the greatest change will be evident in the first few minutes following dialysis. The effect of redistribution on Kt/V is a reduction in the apparent dose of dialysis provided to the patient.[5]

Observations after the NCDS have suggested a discrepancy between the prescribed dialysis and actual delivered dialysis, with conclusions that some patients are not receiving adequate dialysis.[31] The K/DOQI clinical practice guidelines for HD adequacy address the issue in detail and recommend formal urea kinetic modeling to determine the appropriateness of the patient's dialysis prescription. The minimum delivered dose of dialysis should be a Kt/V of at least 1.2, which corresponds to an average urea reduction ratio (URR, the percent reduction of plasma urea following an HD treatment) of 65%. To achieve this delivered dose, the guidelines further recommend that the prescribed dose be based on a Kt/V of 1.3 or a URR of 70%.[5]

4. **What are the variables that determine the Kt/V for R.W.?**

Based on a target Kt/V of 1.3 and known characteristics of the dialysis system, it is possible to develop a dialysis prescription to achieve that value.[5,13] The operative variables include the type and size of dialysis membrane with known urea removal characteristics, blood and dialysate flow rates, and duration of treatment. The membrane usually is determined based on the type of dialysis delivery equipment in the facility and economic factors. The size of the filter to be used is determined by the size of the patient, with larger patients generally being dialyzed using membranes with larger surface area. Blood flow rate is maximized based on the type of equipment and pump capability, as well as the patient and the ability of the cardiovascular system to tolerate a high blood flow. High-flux dialysis usually is carried out with a blood flow rate of 400 to 500 mL/min and rapid- and high-efficiency dialysis blood flow rates of 300 to 500 mL/min.[11,12] The last variable, time, is important to consider in providing adequate dialysis therapy to the patient. Longer dialysis sessions allow for greater Kt/V values, and it is unknown whether an upper limit exists for ideal therapy. With the introduction of high-flux membranes, dialysis treatment times were initially reduced to provide therapy to patients in a more cost-efficient manner. The total removal of urea was considered to be similar with higher urea clearance and shorter dialysis sessions, thereby allowing for reductions in personnel to manage the center and the ability to dialyze more patients.

Concern regarding increased morbidity and mortality in the United States in the early 1990s, compared with other industrialized nations, resulted in an examination of our dialysis practices. Many factors were thought to contribute to this situation, including an older dialysis population, patients with more comorbid conditions being accepted to dialysis programs, and a shorter dialysis duration. Independent of the use of high-flux membranes and higher blood flow rates, the duration of dialysis appears to be a very important factor. This may be related to the clearance of uremic toxins other than urea and the removal of fluid, which contributes to hypertension in the dialysis population. One dialysis center in Tassin, France, has reported improved patient survival with dialysis sessions of 8 hr/day, three times weekly. The mean Kt/V is 1.67, and the survival rate is 87% at 5 years, 75% at 10 years, and 55% at 15 years.[32] Although these data are promising, a major dilemma in U.S. centers is insufficient funding for prolonged dialysis and the unwillingness of many patients to commit the time required for more prolonged dialysis treatment on a chronic basis. Newer approaches for longer, slow dialysis are under investigation, including overnight HD in the home.[33]

Fluid Removal

In addition to solute removal, the artificial kidney must be used to maintain fluid balance in the patient without renal function. Most patients will become anuric once stabilized on HD, requiring control of ingested fluids between treatment sessions. Fluid removal during dialysis then is necessary to achieve the "dry weight," or weight below which the patient would become symptomatic from volume depletion. The dry weight for R.W. has been set at 69.1 kg. Below this weight, R.W. exhibited symptoms of orthostasis. Achieving the dry weight is accomplished by ultrafiltration, through adjustment of the transmembrane pressure. Negative pressure on the dialysate side of the membrane results in movement of fluid across the membrane from the blood compartment.[11,12] Dialysate membranes are characterized by their water permeability, or KUf. Most membranes have values in the range of 2.0 to 8.0 mL/mm Hg per hour, although high-flux membranes may have values as high as 60 mL/mm Hg per hour. Adjustment of the transmembrane pressure will provide the desired ultrafiltration rate, based on the amount of fluid to be removed (predialysis weight + IV saline + ingested fluids during dialysis − dry weight). For patients undergoing dialysis three times weekly, weight gains of 1 to 5 kg are common between sessions. For membranes with KUf values >10 mL/mm Hg per hour, volumetric circuitry in newer dialysis machines should be used to avoid errors in rates of fluid removal based on transmembrane pressure. Modern hemodialyzers have built-in functions to adjust the transmembrane pressure and remove fluid at a predetermined rate.

Complications
Hypotension

5. **The dry weight for R.W. is 69.1 kg. During his most recent dialysis session, he complained of nausea and light-headedness 3 hours into the procedure. His diastolic pressure had dropped from 85 to 60 mm Hg. Ultrafiltration was discontinued, and he recovered without further event. His postdialysis weight was 69.9 kg. What are possible etiologies for his hypotension?**

Many complications may occur in patients undergoing HD. The most common is intradialytic hypotension (IDH), which can produce a variety of clinical signs and symptoms, including nausea and vomiting, dizziness, muscle cramps, and headache. The reported incidence of hypotension is 10% to 30%, and even higher in patients with specific risk factors such as autonomic dysfunction with diabetes and cardiac disease. It primarily is caused by excessive fluid removal from the vascular compartment at a rate exceeding mobilization of fluid stores.[34] As a consequence, patients with an inadequate hemodynamic response to intravascular volume depletion will develop a decrease in blood pressure and other symptoms. It may be necessary to adjust the dry weight upward if the patient is volume depleted and symptomatic following dialysis. Another cause of hypotension is related to excessive heating of the dialysate, which can produce vasodilation. Cooling of the dialysate to slightly below body temperature may correct this problem, although many patients are uncomfortable and do not tolerate the cooling effect. The use of acetate as the buffer in the dialysate also has been associated with hypotension due to its direct vasodilating effects. Switching the patient to a bicarbonate dialysate will correct this problem.[17] Antihypertensive therapy before dialysis may exacerbate hypotensive episodes as well; in some patients, these drugs may need to be withheld until after the dialysis session. Immediate treatment of the hypotensive episode can be accomplished by placing the patient in the Trendelenburg position, administering a small (100 mL) bolus of normal saline into the venous blood line, and reducing the ultrafiltration rate.

Several pharmacologic agents have been proposed for the management of IDH, including ephedrine, fludrocortisone, caffeine, vasopressin, L-carnitine, sertraline, and midodrine. Perazella reviewed these agents for their potential use in the treatment of IDH and concluded that only midodrine, sertraline and L-carnitine have shown potential benefit in patients.[35] Midodrine is an oral prodrug that is converted to desglymidodrine, a selective alpha-1 agonist. Doses of 10 to 20 mg, 30 minutes before dialysis are effective for most patients, but the presence of active myocardial ischemia is a major contraindication.[35] Sertraline is a selective serotonin reuptake inhibitor that has shown promise in IDH at daily doses of 50 to 100 mg/day. The mechanism is proposed to be through attenuation of paradoxical sympathetic withdrawal. L-carnitine has also been shown to have potential benefit for treatment of IDH with intravenous doses of 20 mg/kg at dialysis. Its mechanism of action is not known but may be related to improvements in vascular smooth muscle and cardiac functioning.[35]

Because the volume status of R.W. is associated with his weight, another consideration is a change in his lean mass. R.W. has noted an improvement in his appetite lately, and as a result, added a few extra pounds. It is important to consider "real" weight changes when assessing the dry weight and volume status. Without appropriately increasing the dry weight with "real" weight gain, R.W. became volume depleted and hypotensive. His dry weight should be adjusted upward to the point at which he no longer is symptomatic (to approximately 70 kg).

6. **What other hemodialysis related complications must be watched for and how can they be treated?**

Muscle Cramps

Perhaps also related to fluid shifts, muscle cramps developing during dialysis may be induced by excessive ultrafiltration resulting in altered perfusion of the affected tissues. Several treatments have been attempted, including reduced ultrafiltration and infusion of hypertonic saline or glucose to improve circulation.[36,37] Long-term therapy may be directed at prevention with the use of vitamin E 400 IU at bedtime.[38] Exercise and stretching of the affected limbs also may be beneficial.

Hypersensitivity

Reports of anaphylactic reactions to dialyzer membranes, particularly on initial exposure, may be directly related to the membrane itself, or to ethylene oxide, which is commonly used to sterilize the dialyzer.[39,40] Membranes most commonly responsible for reactions are unsubstituted cellulose membranes (bioincompatible) or the high-flux polyacrylonitrile membrane when used in conjunction with angiotensin-converting enzyme (ACE) inhibitors.[41] This latter reaction is thought to be related to the inhibition of bradykinin metabolism by ACE inhibitors, resulting in an anaphylactoid reaction.

Dialysis Disequilibrium

Dialysis disequilibrium is a syndrome that has been recognized since the initiation of HD more than 30 years ago. Its etiology is related to cerebral edema, and patients new to HD are at a greater risk due to the accumulation of urea.[42] Rapid removal of urea from the extracellular space lowers the plasma osmolality, thereby leading to a shift of free water into the brain. Lowering of intracellular pH, as can occur during dialysis, has been suggested as an etiology as well. Clinical manifestations occur during or shortly after dialysis and include central nervous system (CNS) effects such as headache, nausea, altered vision, and in some cases, seizures and coma. Treatment is aimed at prevention by initiating dialysis gradually by using shorter treatment times at lower blood flow rates in new patients. Direct therapy can be provided in the form of IV hypertonic saline or mannitol.[42]

Some of the long-term complications associated with HD include thrombosis or infection of the access site, aluminum toxicity, and amyloidosis.

Thrombosis

Access loss is most often the result of thrombosis, which is usually a consequence of venous stenosis. Prospective monitoring of access function (e.g., intra-access flow; static or dynamic venous pressures; measurement of access recirculation; and physical findings such as swelling of the arm, clotting of the graft, prolonged bleeding after needle removal, or altered character of the pulse or thrill) is paramount to the prevention of thrombosis. Fistula patency generally is much greater than synthetic graft patency; yet, thrombosis and loss of function may occur in both.[7,43] The stenosis may be corrected by percutaneous transluminal angioplasty (PTA) or, if necessary, surgical revision of the access site. Successful correction is effective as a means to prevent thrombosis. Once it occurs, thrombosis is managed by surgical thrombectomy or with pharmacomechanical or mechanical thrombolysis. Thrombolytic therapy, administered by pulse spray technique of urokinase or streptokinase, combined with mechanical thrombectomy is as effective as surgical thrombectomy.[44] More recently, due to the potentially life-threatening adverse events associated with streptokinase and the non-availability of urokinase, clinicians have evaluated the use of alteplase as an alternative thrombolytic agent.[45] Alteplase and reteplase appear to be effective for thrombomechanical lysis of the vascular access site.[45,46] Thrombolytic therapy should be avoided in those patients with an increased risk of bleeding.

In an attempt to prevent thrombosis from occurring in patients, chronic low-intensity warfarin therapy has been suggested. Crowther and colleagues evaluated graft survival with a regimen of warfarin to achieve a target INR of 1.4 to 1.9 in a randomized, placebo-controlled trial. There was no significant difference in the likelihood of graft survival between the groups, with significantly more major bleeding episodes in the warfarin group. Patients with arteriovenous grafts should not be administered warfarin for thrombosis prevention.[47]

Infection

Usually involving grafts to a greater extent than a native fistula, access infections are predominantly caused by *Staphylococcus aureus* or *S. epidermidis,* although infection with Gram-negative organisms as well as *Enterococcus* may oc-

cur.[ ] Access infections may lead to bacteremia and sepsis with or without local signs of infection. Treatment usually is initiated with vancomycin, administered as a single, 1-g dose, repeated as necessary, depending on the type of dialysis being used, or cefazolin 20 mg/kg three times weekly, and gentamicin 2 mg/kg with appropriate serum concentration monitoring.[48] High-flux dialysis results in greater removal of vancomycin than conventional dialysis and therefore may require more than a single dose for adequate treatment.[49,50] K/DOQI clinical practice guidelines for vascular access also advocate surgical incision and resection of infected grafts. Fistula infections rare and should be treated as subacute bacterial endocarditis with 6 weeks of antibiotic therapy.[7]

Aluminum Toxicity

Aluminum accumulation in patients undergoing HD was a significant problem before water sources were adequately treated to remove aluminum.[21] Major complications of aluminum toxicity include CNS manifestations such as dementia, aluminum bone disease, and anemia. Aluminum accumulation still occurs in patients treated with aluminum-containing antacids as binding agents for phosphate in the GI tract, although not to the degree associated with water supplies.[51] Aluminum toxicity is diagnosed by clinical signs and symptoms associated with the aforementioned conditions, and a serum aluminum concentration of >200 ng/mL or a deferoxamine-stimulated serum aluminum concentration increase of >200 ng/mL.[52] Deferoxamine chelates with serum aluminum and the shift in equilibrium results in movement of aluminum from tissue storage sites. The complex can be removed by dialysis (600 D), and high-flux membranes are capable of removing the complexed aluminum in a single dialysis session, minimizing systemic exposure to deferoxamine and its potential adverse effects. The latter include mucormycosis as well as ocular, auditory, and neurologic toxicity.[53,54] Deferoxamine generally is continued until the stimulated aluminum concentration is <50 ng/mL, which may require 1 year of therapy.[55]

Amyloidosis

A relatively new complication of HD is amyloidosis, caused by the deposition of β-2-microglobulin–containing amyloid in joints and soft tissues over prolonged periods.[56] The incidence of amyloidosis is approximately 50% after 12 years of dialysis and nearly 100% after 20 years. β-2-Microglobulin (MW 11,800 D) normally is eliminated by filtration and metabolism in the intact nephron. Renal failure leads to reduced elimination and accumulation of this substance even during dialysis. High-flux membranes are more effective than conventional membranes for the removal of β_2-microglobulin but they have not been in use long enough to evaluate their role in preventing amyloidosis. Carpal tunnel syndrome, manifested as weakness and soreness in the thumb from pressure on the median nerve, is the most common symptom. Bone cysts also appear along with joint deposition of amyloid, which can impair mobility.[56] The type of membrane used for dialysis also has been implicated in increasing the rate of production of β_2-microglobulin, in that some seem to cause more rapid amyloid deposition. Biocompatible membranes are proposed to stimulate production to a lesser degree, but prospective studies demonstrating their long-term benefit have not been conducted.[57]

Malnutrition

Chronic kidney disease produces a catabolic state in patients and, along with the multifactorial complications of ESRD, leads to malnutrition. Serum albumin concentrations <3.0 g/dL are associated with an increased mortality rate compared with higher values. Inadequate dietary intake and losses of amino acids by dialysis contribute to protein malnutrition, which can in turn lead to additional complications such as impaired wound healing, susceptibility to infection, and others (see Chapter 32, Chronic Kidney Disease, for further discussion).

L-CARNITINE

L-Carnitine supplementation has been advocated in patients with ESRD to relieve intradialytic symptoms. It is a metabolic cofactor that facilitates transport of long-chain fatty acids into the mitochondria for energy production. This cofactor is found in both plasma and tissue as free carnitine, the active component, or bound to fatty acids as acylcarnitine. The primary source of carnitine is dietary intake, primarily from red meat and dairy products. Patients with renal failure may have what appear to be normal or elevated total carnitine concentrations but low levels of free carnitine. Accumulation of acylcarnitine, decreased carnitine synthesis, reduced dietary intake, and dialytic losses may account for the normal to elevated total concentrations in this population.[58,59]

The potential benefits of correcting this relative carnitine deficiency have been primarily studied in patients undergoing chronic HD. Recommended doses of carnitine are 10 to 20 mg/kg IV after each HD treatment. Although there have been suggestions that carnitine benefits muscle cramps and hypotension during dialysis, lack of energy, skeletal muscle weakness, cardiomyopathy, and anemia resistant to large does of erythropoietic therapy, there is no evidence to support its routine use in patients undergoing chronic HD.[9]

PERITONEAL DIALYSIS

PD is performed using several different modalities, including the most common, continuous ambulatory peritoneal dialysis (CAPD). Development of specialized devices to facilitate the exchange process and improve patient convenience has led to processes referred to as *automated peritoneal dialysis* (APD), including *continuous cycling peritoneal dialysis* (CCPD) and *nocturnal intermittent dialysis* (NIPD). CAPD is the most common method for chronic PD, but the APD methods are rapidly growing. The number of patients with ESRD undergoing treatment with PD in the United States increased from approximately 10,000 in 1985 to a peak of about 32,000 in 1995 and has been on the decline, with 27,000 in 2000.[1]

Principles and Transport Processes

CAPD is performed by the instillation of 2 to 3 L of sterile dialysate solution into the peritoneal cavity through a surgically placed resident catheter. The solution dwells within the cavity for 4 to 8 hours, and then is drained and replaced with a fresh solution. This process of fill, dwell, and drain is performed three to four times during the day, with an overnight dwell by the patient in his or her normal home or work environment[60-62] (Fig. 33-2). Conceptually, the process is similar to HD in that uremic toxins are removed by diffusion down a concentration gradient across a membrane into the dialysate solution. A primary difference is that because the dialysate solution is resident, the result is a very slow dialysate flow rate of approximately 7 mL/min when 10 L of fluid are drained per day. Solute loss occurs by diffusion for small molecules, and through convection for larger, middle molecules.

Blood and Dialysate Flow

HD provides constant perfusion of fresh dialysate, thereby maintaining a large concentration gradient across the dialysis membrane throughout the dialysis treatment. During a typical dwell period for CAPD, urea and other substances increase in the dialysate relative to unbound plasma concentrations. For a daytime dwell period of 4 hours, urea achieves nearly equal concentrations with plasma; therefore, the rate of elimination can become very small (Fig. 33-3). Instillation of fresh dialysate solution will re-establish the diffusion gradient leading to an increased rate of urea removal. For a patient making four exchanges of 2 L each per day, assuming the urea dialysate concentration equals the plasma concentration, and 2 L are removed by ultrafiltration, the urea clearance would be approximately 7 mL/min. This is substantially lower than urea clearances achieved with HD; therefore, CAPD must be performed continually throughout the week to achieve adequate urea removal. Clearance depends on blood flow; dialysate flow; and peritoneal membrane characteristics, such as size, permeability, and thickness. Dialysate flow is the only easily adjusted variable to alter clearance and has been used effectively in acute PD to achieve relatively high clearances with 30- to 60-minute dwell periods in a cycling system. CCPD uses this concept of shorter dwell periods during the sleeping hours with automatic fill, dwell, and drain periods, leaving a high-dextrose dialysate in the peritoneal cavity throughout the day until the next cycling session. NIPD is similar, with nightly exchanges, but the peritoneum is left unfilled, or dry, during the daytime. As a result, urea clearance is lower with NIPD, but may be suitable for many patients, and preferable to the volume load in the peritoneal cavity throughout the day with CCPD.[60] Electrolyte concentrations in the dialysate solution are near physiologic concentrations to prevent substantial shifts in serum electrolyte levels (see Table 33-1). A potential advantage of PD compared with HD is the continuous dialysis of larger, middle molecules that may exert toxic effects. These molecules are cleared through convection and follow water as it is removed through ultrafiltration. Clearance of these molecules depends less on flow and more on duration of dialysis. The continuous process of PD, albeit associated with low clearance values, provides for a more physiologic condition in patients, rather than the intermittent treatment provided with HD.

Fluid Removal

Fluid is removed by ultrafiltration through adjustment of the transmembrane pressure during HD. Because this pressure is not easily adjusted in PD, fluid is removed by altering the osmotic pressure within the dialysate. This is accomplished by the addition of dextrose monohydrate to the dialysate in varying concentrations, depending on the degree of fluid removal necessary in the patient. Concentrations of dextrose in commercially available solutions include 1.5%, 2.5%, and 4.25%,

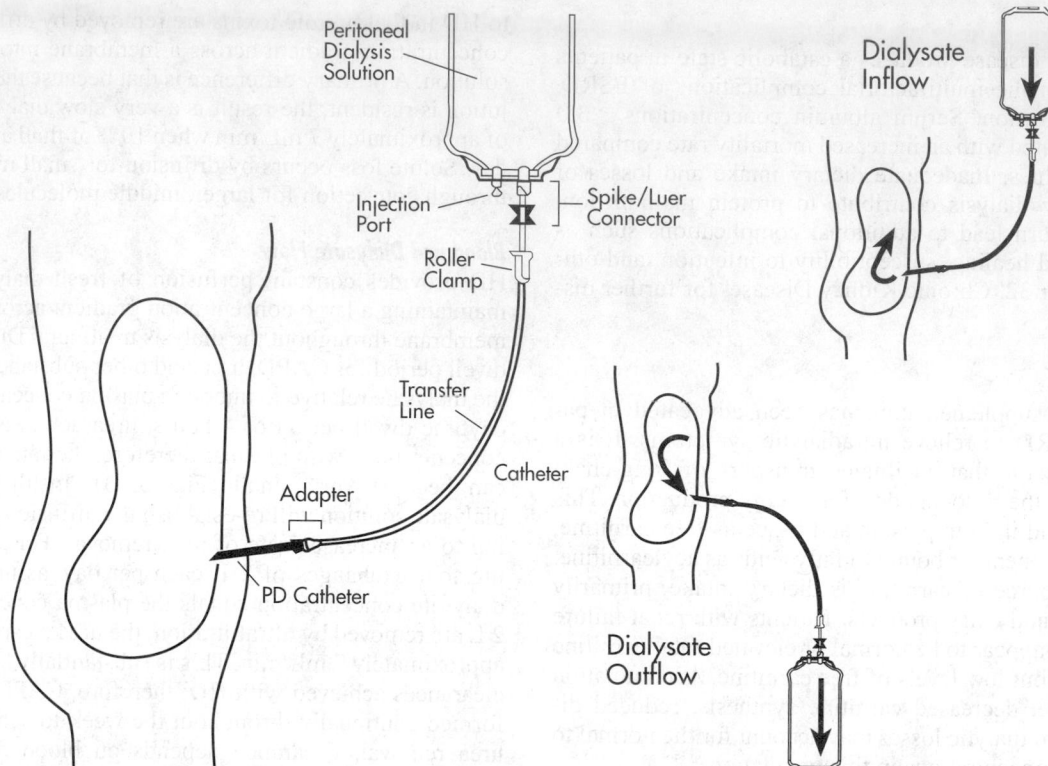

FIGURE 33-2 Schematic representation of CAPD components and techniques of inflow and outflow. (Reproduced with permission from Schoenfeld P. Care of the patient on peritoneal dialysis. In: Cogan MG, Schoenfeld P, eds. Introduction to Dialysis. 2nd Ed. New York: Churchill Livingstone, 1991:200.)

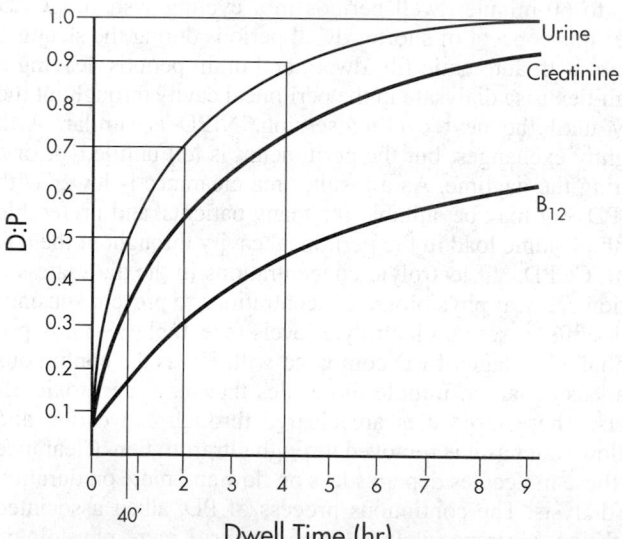

FIGURE 33-3 Rate of entry into peritoneal dialysate of urea, creatinine, and vitamin B_{12}. The y-axis indicates the ratio of dialysate to plasma concentration (D:P). (Reproduced with permission from Blake PG, Daugirdas JT. Physiology of peritoneal dialysis. In: Daugirdas JT et al., eds. Handbook of Dialysis. 3rd Ed. Philadelphia: Lippincott, Williams & Wilkins, 2001:281.)

with net fluid losses during a 4-hour dwell period of 200 and 400 mL for the 1.5% and 2.5% solutions, respectively, and approximately 700 mL for the 4.25% solution following an overnight dwell.[63] As the dwell time persists, the dextrose is absorbed and is diluted by the movement of fluid from the

vascular space, so that the majority of ultrafiltration occurs early during the dwell period.

Acid-base balance is achieved through the absorption of lactate from the dialysate, which subsequently is metabolized to bicarbonate in vivo. Bicarbonate is not compatible with the calcium and magnesium in the dialysate and would lead to precipitation.

Access

Delivery of dialysate into the peritoneal cavity is accomplished through an indwelling catheter inserted through the abdominal wall. The most common design is the Tenckhoff catheter, made of silicone rubber or polyurethane; it consists of a tube, straight or curled, with many holes in the distal end for fluid inflow and outflow.[64] The catheter also has a single or double cuff, which serves to anchor it to the internal and external attachment sites by promoting fibrous tissue growth; this also serves as a barrier to bacterial migration. Several modifications to the original catheter have appeared on the market, mostly in an attempt to overcome problems related to outflow of dialysate. Maintaining an unobstructed outlet port is essential for successful PD.

Delivery of dialysate through the catheter can be accomplished in several modes. A straight transfer set uses tubing attached to the catheter at one end, and to the bag of dialysate at the other, via a spike. The transfer set usually is changed every 1 to 2 months in the dialysis clinic. For each dialysate exchange, the patient attaches a bag of fresh dialysate, warmed to body temperature, to the transfer set and infuses the solution. The tubing is clamped and rolled up with the attached bag and placed into a pouch carried on the patient. The primary purpose for maintaining the connection is to prevent contamination and the development of peritonitis. Following the dwell period, the patient unrolls the bag and tubing, places it on the floor, unclamps the tubing and awaits drainage of the fluid, usually 5 to 15 minutes. Using aseptic technique, the patient changes the dialysate bag and infuses fresh solution to repeat the process. This process is used rarely today and has been replaced by Y sets and double bag systems. The Y transfer set employs three limbs, with fresh dialysate attached to the upper arm of the Y, an empty bag to the lower arm, and the stem connected to the catheter.[64] Clamping the inflow arm and opening the stem and outflow arm allows dialysate to drain from the peritoneum into the empty bag. Reversing the clamps then permits infusion of the fresh dialysate solution after a small rinse of the line is performed with the fresh solution. Clamping of the catheter allows removal of the Y transfer set and bags from the patient. The double bag system employs pre-attached bags to both limbs and the patient and makes only a single connection to the catheter. Use of the Y transfer set has reduced episodes of peritonitis from approximately 1 for every 9 to 12 patient-months to 1 for every 24 to 36 patient-months.[65] PD performed with the cycler involves only two disconnections of the system, compared with four for CAPD.

Dialysis Prescription

The initial CAPD prescription for most patients consists of three exchanges during the day with 1.5% dextrose and a fourth, overnight exchange with 4.25% dextrose. This would be expected to achieve fluid removal of approximately 1,300 mL, based on 200 mL from each daytime exchange and 700 mL overnight. Based on assessment of the patient's fluid status, it may be necessary to increase or decrease the dialysate prescription to achieve fluid balance. Fluid retention is solved by increasing the dextrose content of the daytime exchanges, beginning with 2.5% in place of one of the 1.5% solutions. This is expected to result in an additional removal of 200 mL, and therapy can be further adjusted as necessary. For patients with excessive fluid removal, it may be possible to decrease the number of exchanges per day as long as adequate solute removal is present. If four exchanges are needed, the fluid intake may be liberalized to maintain adequate hydration.

Patients undergoing CCPD will generally need three to five exchanges, each lasting approximately 2 hours, using a cycler while the patient sleeps. During the daytime hours, the patient maintains a reservoir of dialysate in the peritoneal cavity, then repeats the process at night. Six to eight exchanges are performed at night for patients undergoing NIPD, because they do not continue dialysis during the day. Dwell times are generally 1 to 2 hours for each exchange, resulting in a higher clearance for small molecules due to the increased dialysate flow rate.[60]

An alternative to dextrose as the osmotic agent in the dialysate solution is icodextrin (Extraneal). It was recently approved for use in the United States in patients undergoing CAPD or APD during the long dwell period.[66] It is a starch-derived, water-soluble, glucose polymer that is approximately 40% absorbed and subsequently metabolized to maltose oligosaccharides. It is superior to 1.5% and 2.5% dextrose solutions for ultrafiltration and similar to 4.25% dextrose.[67] Its use may be most beneficial in those patients characterized as low transporters.

6. **M.J., a 27-year-old woman, has a 14-year history of insulin-dependent diabetes mellitus. She is 5′2″ tall and weighs 52 kg. One result of the diabetes has been development of ESRD necessitating dialysis. She has been undergoing CAPD for 1 year and, until now, has done well without any complications. Her dialysis prescription consists of three exchanges with 1.5% dextrose during the day and a fourth, overnight exchange with 4.25% dextrose. She has a double-cuff Tenckhoff catheter and uses a Y transfer set for her exchanges. Her blood pressure is controlled and she shows no evidence of edema. She has no residual renal function. Her most recent serum laboratory results showed a calcium (Ca) of 10.9 mg/dL (normal, 8.8 to 10.2 mg/dL) and K of 3.2 mEq/L (normal, 3.5 to 5.0 mEq/L). Calculate the prescribed amount of dialysis for M.J.**

[SI units: Ca, 2.7 mmol/L (normal, 2.2 to 2.6); K, 3.2 mmol/L (normal, 3.5 to 5)]

The K/DOQI clinical practice guidelines for PD adequacy recommend a weekly creatinine clearance normalized to 1.73 m^2 body surface area and total weekly Kt/V_{urea} for determination of the weekly delivered dose of PD.[6] Residual kidney function should also be included in the overall assessment of function. This should be based on renal Kt/V_{urea} and an estimation of the glomerular filtration rate as the mean of the urea and creatinine clearance rates. The weekly delivered dose of PD should be a total Kt/v_{urea} ≥ 2.0 and Cl_{Cr} of at least 60 L/wk/1.73 m^2 for high and high-average transporters, and 50 L/wk/1.73 m^2 for low and low-average transporters (see below). For NIPD and CCPD, the weekly delivered dose should be a total Kt/V_{urea} of ≥ 2.2 and 2.1 and a weekly Cl_{Cr} ≥ 66 and 63 L/1.73 m^2, respectively.[6] Determining the number of exchanges needed for solute removal is based on the clearance of urea as a surrogate for uremia. Based on dialysate urea achieving 90% of plasma urea at the end of the dwell period, and four exchanges per day, the fluid removal would be approximately 9,300 mL/ day, or a urea clearance of 59 L/wk. For M.J., body water content (urea distribution volume) is approximately 29 L (0.55 L/kg); therefore, the dialysis prescription would provide a weekly Kt/V of 2.03. Based on her dialysis prescription, M.J. should achieve the target dose. The evidence for a Kt/V ≥ 2.0 is based on the assumptions that the patient has no residual renal function, there is full equilibration between dialysate and plasma with respect to urea, the target urea concentration is 60 mg/dL, and the normalized protein catabolic rate (nPCR) is between 1.0 and 1.2 g/kg per day, indicating adequate nutrition. A prospective analysis of Kt/V and the relative risk of death showed that a decrease of 0.1 in weekly Kt/V was associated with a 5% increase in the relative risk of death.[68] A similar trend was observed for creatinine clearance. Larger patients may need a larger volume for each exchange (up to 3 L) or an additional exchange per day to achieve the target Kt/V. The increased volume is preferable due to the inconvenience of an additional exchange.

M.J. also is noted to have an elevated serum calcium concentration of 10.9 mg/dL, probably as a result of her calcium carbonate requirements to serve as a binder of dietary phosphate. Dialysate preparations with a low calcium concentration (2.5 mEq/L) compared with the standard concentration of

3.5 mEq/L can help control hypercalcemia associated with increased oral calcium intake. Potassium is not present in the dialysate solution but may be supplemented in patients who are not able to maintain potassium within the normal range. M.J. has a somewhat low serum potassium concentration of 3.2 mEq/L. Therefore, providing a dialysate concentration of 4 mEq/L will sustain normal concentrations and prevent hypokalemia. This is particularly important for patients receiving digitalis preparations.

Assessment of Dialysis Adequacy

7. Assess the actual dialysis provided to M.J., based on a 24-hour collection of 9,130 mL dialysate with a urea concentration of 54 mg/dL and serum urea concentration of 60 mg/dL.

Following stabilization of the patient on the new dialysis prescription, it is necessary to assess the adequacy of the delivered dialysis dose. This is accomplished by taking into account both the peritoneal and residual renal clearance of urea, and comparing these with the target Kt/V. Dialysis urea clearance is determined by collecting and measuring the dialysate, as well as urine output, for a 24-hour period.[6,69] Clearance is calculated by standard methods: rate of elimination divided by average plasma concentration. The sum of the two urea clearances then is multiplied by 7 to determine the volume cleared per week, and then divided by the urea distribution volume (estimated from total body water content). This value then is compared with the target weekly Kt/V value for assessment and adjustment of the prescription. For M.J., the urea clearance was 5.7 mL/min, or 57.5 L/wk. Based on her estimated urea distribution volume of 29 L, her weekly Kt/V is approximately 1.98, near the target of 2.0, and not accounting for any residual renal function that may be present.

Another test of peritoneal function is the Peritoneal Equilibration Test (PET).[70] It is a standardized semiquantitative test of peritoneal membrane transport function, and is useful to assess membrane function over time as well as to provide guidance for the appropriate mode of PD for a patient. Based on the ratio of dialysate to plasma concentration of a solute at 2 hours into a 4-hour dwell, the patient is characterized as a high, high-average, low-average, or low transporter. Glucose absorption also is assessed by comparing the dialysate concentration at 2 hours with the baseline. High transporters are those who equilibrate rapidly, and would benefit from NIPD therapy with rapid overnight exchanges. Low transporters could be treated with standard CAPD, as long as the Kt/V was sufficient to meet their needs.

Complications

8. M.J. now presents to the dialysis clinic with complaints of abdominal tenderness and cloudy effluent. Examination of the dialysate revealed a white blood cell (WBC) count of 330 cells/mm³ with 62% neutrophils. Gram's stain was positive for Gram-positive cocci. Her diabetes has been controlled by the addition of 10 units of regular insulin to each daytime bag and 15 units to the overnight bag. How should M.J.'s infection be treated?

[SI unit: WBC, 0.33 × 10⁹ cells/L (normal, <0.05 × 10⁹)]

Peritonitis

The most significant complication among patients undergoing PD is peritonitis, which is frequently caused by *S. epidermidis* (30%) or *S. aureus* (10%).[6,62,71] The patient usually presents with abdominal pain, nausea and vomiting, and/or fever with or without a cloudy effluent. Bacterial peritonitis generally is accompanied by an elevated dialysate WBC count, >100/mm³ with >50% neutrophils. A positive Gram's stain should be followed by culture, with therapy initiated in the interim. For lower cell counts or negative Gram's stain, a culture should be obtained followed by treatment for positive cultures and continued observation for negative results. Specific consensus recommendations of the Advisory Committee on Peritonitis Management of the International Society for Peritoneal Dialysis are located at www.ispd.org.[71]

The increasing prevalence of vancomycin-resistant organisms has resulted in a shift in empiric therapy away from vancomycin, toward first-generation cephalosporins: cefazolin or cephalothin. Without a Gram's stain, therapy should be initiated with a combination of cefazolin or cephalothin and ceftazidime, co-administered in the same dialysate solution at a dose of 1 gram/bag for both drugs, once daily, given intraperitoneally. An aminoglycoside may be used in place of ceftazidime but is not recommended initially, in an attempt to preserve residual renal function. Gentamicin, tobramycin, or netilmicin are given at doses of 0.6 mg/kg/bag, once daily, and for amikacin, 2 mg/kg/bag once daily. In addition to antibiotics, heparin 500 to 1,000 U/L may be added to each exchange to prevent the formation of fibrin clots, which may result in catheter failure.[71] Subsequent antibiotic therapy should be based on culture and sensitivity results, incorporating specific dosage regimens based on the treatment guidelines.[71]

This is M.J.'s first episode of peritonitis. The most likely pathogen, a *Staphylococcus* species, is consistent with the positive Gram's stain. Her treatment should consist of cefazolin or cephalothin alone. Vancomycin should not be used for empiric therapy. Instead, it should be reserved for MRSA infections or MRSE if M.J. does not respond to empiric therapy. Heparin 1,000 U/L should be added to the dialysate to prevent fibrin clots from forming and obstructing outflow from the peritoneal cavity. Her blood glucose should be monitored, since infection causes insulin resistance and peritonitis will increase glucose and insulin absorption. Inability to control the blood glucose concentration may require temporary discontinuation of the IP insulin and administration by another route.

For patients undergoing APD, the choice of first-line antibiotics is the same as for CAPD since the likely organisms are similar. Drug dosage regimens, however, may differ because CCPD and NIPD patients undergo PD only during the night-time hours, and NIPD patients do not have residual peritoneal fluid during the day. For aminoglycoside antibiotics, once daily dosing is preferred for the foregoing reasons, as well as their longer duration of action due to the post-antibiotic effect (see Chapter 32, Chronic Kidney Disease). Vancomycin and other glycopeptides can be administered intermittently because of their prolonged elimination half-life in patients with ESRD. Due to the lack of clinical trials with other antibiotics in patients undergoing APD, extrapolation from the CAPD literature may be necessary. A review addresses the current knowledge and issues surrounding the pharmacokinetics of antibiotics in patients with peritonitis undergoing APD.[72]

Exit-Site Infection

Separate from peritonitis are catheter exit-site infections, most often caused by *S. aureus* and *Pseudomonas* species.[69] Local erythema alone can be treated with topical agents (e.g., chlorhexidine, mupirocin, hydrogen peroxide), whereas purulent drainage indicates more significant infection and the need for systemic antibiotics.[71] Gram-positive organisms are treated with first-generation oral cephalosporins, penicillinase-resistant penicillin, or sulfamethoxazole trimethoprim. Rifampin may be added at 300 mg twice daily for nonresponding infections with positive cultures after 1 week of appropriate therapy. Further lack of response requires evaluation for catheter removal. Gram-negative organisms may be treated with ciprofloxacin 500 mg orally twice daily.[71] Scheduling of the quinolone dose is important so that co-administration with foods or other drug therapies that may chelate the quinolone in the gut is avoided. Potentially chelating agents include calcium products, iron, multivitamins, antacids, zinc, sucralfate, and dairy products.

Weight Gain

Dextrose is present in dialysate solutions primarily to serve as an osmotic agent for the removal of fluid during each exchange. Higher concentrations are expected to result in greater fluid removal. Approximately 500 to 1,000 kcal/day are absorbed as glucose from PD solutions, which can lead to weight gain in patients. Some patients may require modification of oral caloric intake to avoid excessive weight gain. Insulin requirements generally are increased in patients with diabetes as a result of the additional calories, and when administered intraperitoneally, usually are two to three times the normal subcutaneous dose due to their reduced bioavailability of 20 to 50% by this route.

REFERENCES

1. U.S. Renal Data System, USRDS 2002 Annual Data Report. National Institutes of Health, National Institute of Diabetes and Digestive and Kidney Diseases, Bethesda, MD, 2002.
2. U.S. Renal Data System, USRDS 1999 Annual Data Report. National Institutes of Health, National Institute of Diabetes and Digestive and Kidney Diseases, Bethesda, MD, 1999.
3. U.S. Renal Data System, USRDS 2001 Annual Data Report. National Institutes of Health, National Institute of Diabetes and Digestive and Kidney Diseases, Bethesda, MD, 2001.
4. Pastan S, Bailey J. Dialysis therapy. N Engl J Med 1998;338:1428.
5. I. NKF K/DOQI Clinical Practice Guidelines for Hemodialysis Adequacy: Update 2000. Am J Kidney Dis 2001;37(Suppl 1):7.
6. II. NKF-K/DOQI Clinical Practice Guidelines for Peritoneal Dialysis Adequacy: Update 2000. Am J Kidney Dis 2001;37(Suppl 1):65.
7. III. NKF-K/DOQI Clinical Practice Guidelines for Vascular Access: Update 2000. Am J Kidney Dis 2001;37(Suppl 1):137.
8. IV. NKF-K/DOQI Clinical Practice Guidelines for Anemia of Chronic Kidney Disease: Update 2000. Am J Kidney Dis 2001;37(Suppl 1):182.
9. NKF-K/DOQI Clinical Practice Guidelines for Nutrition of Chronic Renal Failure. I. Adult Guidelines. Am J Kidney Dis 2000;35(Suppl 2):S17.
10. NKF-K/DOQI Clinical Practice Guidelines for Chronic Kidney Disease: Evaluation, Classification, and Stratification. Am J Kidney Dis 2002;39:S1-S266.S1.
11. Denker BM et al. Hemodialysis. In: Brenner BM, Rector FC, eds. Brenner and Rector's The Kidney. 6th Ed. Philadelphia: WB Saunders, 2000.
12. Daugirdas JT, Van Stone JC. Physiologic principles and urea kinetic modeling. In: Daugirdas JT et al., eds. Handbook of Dialysis. 3rd Ed. Philadelphia: Lippincott, Williams & Wilkins, 2001:15.
13. Daugirdas JT, Depner TA. A nomogram approach to hemodialysis urea modeling. Am J Kidney Dis 1994;23:33.
14. Laird NM et al. Modeling success or failure of dialysis therapy. The National Cooperative Dialysis Study. Kidney Int 1983;13(Suppl):S101.
15. Gotch FA, Sargent JA. A mechanistic analysis of the National Cooperative Dialysis Study (NCDS). Kidney Int 1985;28:526.
16. Shinaberger JH. Quantitation of dialysis: historical perspective. Semin Dial 2001;14:238.
17. Daugirdas JT et al. Hemodialysis apparatus. In: Daugirdas JT, Blake PG, Ing TS, eds. Handbook of Dialysis. 3rd Ed. Philadelphia: Lippincott, Williams & Wilkins, 2001:46.
18. van Ypersele de Strihou C. Are biocompatible membranes superior for hemodialysis therapy? Kidney Int 1997;52(Suppl 62):S101.
19. National Kidney Foundation Report on Dialyzer Reuse. Task Force on Reuse of Dialyzers, Council on Dialysis, National Kidney Foundation. Am J Kidney Dis 1997;30:859.
20. Hauck M et al. In vivo effects of dialysate flow rate on Kt/V in maintenance hemodialysis patients. Am J Kidney Dis 2000;35:105.
21. Wathen RL et al. Water treatment for hemodialysis. In: Cogan MG, Schoenfeld P, eds. Introduction to Dialysis. 2nd Ed. New York: Churchill Livingstone, 1991:45.
22. Churchill DN et al. Canadian hemodialysis morbidity study. Am J Kidney Dis 1992;18:214.
23. Hertel J et al. Anticoagulation. In: Daugirdas JT et al., eds. Handbook of Dialysis. 3rd Ed. Philadelphia: Lippincott, Williams & Wilkins, 2001:182.
24. Lohr JW, Schwab SJ. Minimizing hemorrhagic complications in dialysis patients. J Am Soc Nephrol 1991;2:961.
25. Schwab SJ et al. Hemodialysis without anticoagulation. One-year prospective trial in hospitalized patients at risk for bleeding. Am J Med 1987; 83:405.
26. Saltissi D et al. Comparison of low-molecular-weight heparin (enoxaparin sodium) and standard unfractionated heparin for hemodialysis anticoagulation. Nephrol Dial Transplant 1999;14:2698.
27. Hainer JW et al. Intravenous and subcutaneous weight-based dosing of the low molecular weight heparin tinzaparin (Innohep) in end-stage renal disease patients undergoing chronic hemodialysis. Am J Kidney Dis 2002;40:531.
28. Bucha E et al. R-hirudin as anticoagulant in regular hemodialysis therapy: finding of therapeutic R-hirudin blood/plasm concentrations and respective dosages. Clin Appl Thromb Hemost 1999;5:164.
29. O'Shea SI et al. Alternative methods of anticoagulation for dialysis-dependent patients with heparin-induced thrombocytopenia. Semin Dial 2003; 16:61.
30. Lowrie EG et al. Effect of the hemodialysis prescription on patient morbidity: report from the National Cooperative Dialysis Study. N Engl J Med 1981;305:1176.
31. Delmez JA et al. Hemodialysis prescription and delivery in a metropolitan area. The St. Louis Nephrology Study Group. Kidney Int 1992;41:1023.
32. Charra B et al. Survival as an index of adequacy of dialysis. Kidney Int 1992;41:1286.
33. Pierratos A. Nocturnal home hemodialysis: an update on a 5-year experience. Nephrol Dial Transplant 1999;14:2835.
34. Daugirdas JT. Dialysis hypotension: a hemodynamic analysis. Kidney Int 1991;39:233.
35. Perazella MA. Pharmacologic options available to treat symptomatic intradialytic hypotension. Am J Kidney Dis 2001;38(Suppl 4):S26.
36. Canzanello VJ, Burkart JM. Hemodialysis-associated muscle cramps. Semin Dial 1992;5:299.
37. Sherman RA. Acute therapy of hemodialysis-related muscle cramps. Am J Kidney Dis 1982;2:287.
38. Roca AO et al. Dialysis leg cramps : efficacy of quinine vs vitamin E. ASAIO J 1992;38:M481.
39. Tielemans C. Immediate hypersensitivity reactions and hemodialysis. Adv Nephrol 1993;22:401.
40. Lemke H-D et al. Hypersensitivity reactions during hemodialysis: role of complement fragments and ethylene oxide antibodies. Nephrol Dial Transplant 1990;5:264.
41. Pegues DA. Anaphylactoid reactions associated with reuse of hollow-fiber hemodialyzers and ACE inhibitors. Kidney Int 1992;42:1232.
42. Arieff AI. Dialysis disequilibrium syndrome: current concepts on pathogenesis and prevention. Kidney Int 1994;45:629.
43. Hakim R, Himmelfarb J. Hemodialysis access failure: a call to action. Kidney Int 1998;54:1029.
44. Valji K et al. Pulse-spray pharmacomechanical thrombolysis of thrombosed hemodialysis access grafts: long-term experience and comparison of original and current techniques. Am J Roentgenol 1995;164:1495.
45. Cooper SG. Pulse-spray thrombolysis of thrombosed hemodialysis grafts with tissue plasminogen activator. Am J Roentgenol 2003;180:1063.
46. Falk A et al. Reteplase in the treatment of thrombosed hemodialysis grafts. J Vasc Interv Radiol 2001;12:1257.
47. Crowther MA et al. Low-intensity warfarin is ineffective for the prevention of PTFE graft failure in patients on hemodialysis: a randomized controlled trial. J Am Soc Nephrol 2002;13:2331.
48. Lentino JR, Leehy DJ. Infections. In: Daugirdas JT et al., eds. Handbook of Dialysis. 3rd Ed. Philadelphia: Lippincott, Williams & Wilkins, 2001:495.

49. DeSoi CA et al. Vancomycin elimination during high-flux hemodialysis: kinetic model and comparison of four membranes. Am J Kidney Dis 1992;20:354.

50. Pollard TA et al. Vancomycin redistribution: dosing recommendations following high-flux hemodialysis. Kidney Int 1994;45:232.

51. DeBroe ME et al. New insights and strategies in the diagnosis and treatment of aluminum overload in dialysis patients. Nephrol Dial Transplant 1993; 8(Suppl 1):47.

52. Chazan JA et al. Plasma aluminum levels (unstimulated and stimulated): clinical and biochemical findings in 185 patients undergoing chronic hemodialysis for 4 to 95 months. Am J Kidney Dis 1989;13:284.

53. Boelaert JR et al. Mucormycosis during deferoxamine therapy is a siderophore-mediated infection: in-vitro and in-vivo studies. J Clin Invest 1993; 91:1979.

54. Olivieri NF et al. Visual and auditory neurotoxicity in patients receiving subcutaneous deferoxamine infusion. N Engl J Med 1986;314:869.

55. Felsenfeld AJ et al. Deferoxamine therapy in hemodialysis patients with aluminum-associated bone disease. Kidney Int 1989;35:1371.

56. Koch KM. Dialysis-related amyloidosis. Kidney Int 1992;41:1416.

57. Diaz RJ et al. The effect of dialyzer reprocessing on performance and β2 microglobulin removal using polysulfone membranes. Am J Kidney Dis 1993; 21:405.

58. Hurot J et al. Effects of L-carnitine supplementation in maintenance hemodialysis patients. J Am Soc Nephrol 2002;13:708.

59. Bellinghieri G et al. Carnitine and hemodialysis. Am J Kidney Dis 2003;41(Suppl 1):S116.

60. Brophy DF, Mueller BA. Automated peritoneal dialysis: new implications for pharmacists. Ann Pharmacother 1997;31:756.

61. Gokal R, Mallick NP. Peritoneal dialysis. Lancet 1999;353:823.

62. Burkart JM, Nolph KD. Peritoneal dialysis. In: Brenner BM, Rector FC, eds. The Kidney. 5th Ed. Philadelphia: WB Saunders, 1996:2507.

63. Blake PG, Diaz-Buxo JA. Adequacy of peritoneal dialysis and chronic peritoneal dialysis prescription. In: Daugirdas JT et al., eds. Handbook of Dialysis. 3rd Ed. Philadelphia: Lippincott, Williams & Wilkins, 2001:343.

64. Gokal R et al. Peritoneal catheters and exit-site practices toward optimal peritoneal access: 1998 update. Perit Dial Int 1998;18:11.

65. Port FK et al. Risk of peritonitis and technique failure by CAPD connection technique: a national study. Kidney Int 1992;42:967.

66. Baxter Healthcare Corporation. Extraneal package insert. Deerfield, IL: November 2002.

67. Wolfson M et al. Review of clinical trial experience with icodextrin. Kidney Int 2002;62(Suppl 81):S46.

68. Canada-USA (CANUSA) Peritoneal Dialysis Study Group. Adequacy of dialysis and nutrition in continuous peritoneal dialysis: association with clinical outcomes. J Am Soc Nephrol 1996;7:198.

69. Chatoth DK et al. Morbidity and mortality in redefining adequacy of peritoneal dialysis: a step beyond the National Kidney Foundation–Dialysis Outcomes Quality Initiative. Am J Kidney Dis 1999;33:617.

70. Twardowski ZJ. Peritoneal equilibration test. Perit Dial Bull 1987;7:138.

71. Keane WF et al. Adult peritoneal dialysis-related peritonitis treatment recommendations: 2000 update. Perit Dial Int 2000;20:396.

72. Manley HJ, Bailie GR. Treatment of peritonitis in APD: pharmacokinetic principles. Semin Dial 2002;15:418.

73. Abraham G et al. Natural history of exit-site infection (ESI) in patients on continuous ambulatory peritoneal dialysis (CAPD). Perit Dial Int 1988; 8:211.

74. Amair P et al. Continuous ambulatory peritoneal dialysis in diabetics with end-stage renal disease. N Engl J Med 1982;303:625.

75. Chan E, Montgomery PA. Administration of insulin by continuous ambulatory peritoneal dialysis. Pharmacotherapy 1993;13:455.

CHAPTER 34

Dosing of Drugs in Renal Failure

David J. Quan, Francesca T. Aweeka

BASIC PRINCIPLES

An increasing amount of information is available on the disposition of drugs in renal disease. It is important to design specific therapeutic regimens for patients with renal impairment. Many of these patients are treated with multiple medications that may require dose adjustment. Without careful dosing and therapeutic drug monitoring in these patients, accumulation of drugs and/or toxic metabolites may occur, causing serious adverse effects.

In addition to altered drug elimination, a number of factors associated with kidney disease predispose patients to the potential for drug toxicity. Renal disease can affect the pharmacokinetic disposition as well as the pharmacodynamic effect of drugs. For example, the physiologic changes associated with uremia can alter drug absorption, protein binding, distribution, or elimination. These physiologic changes can alter drug concentrations in the plasma or blood, and at the targeted tissue site of activity, thereby affecting drug efficacy and toxicity.

Little is known about the effect of renal disease on drug pharmacodynamics. Pharmacodynamics (or "what the drug does to the body") quantitatively describes the pharmacologic or toxicologic effects of drugs relative to the drug concentration. Patients with renal disease may have a different response to a given drug concentration than a patient with normal renal function.

Data in the area of pharmacodynamics and renal disease are limited. Patients with renal disease can be more sensitive to some drugs, and can experience an increased frequency of adverse drug reactions with or without dosing modifications.

Figure 34-1 illustrates the relationship between pharmacokinetics and pharmacodynamics. The dose of drug produces a drug concentration, which results in a pharmacologic or toxic effect. Figure 34-2 illustrates how different components of drug disposition influence the ability of a drug to exert its pharmacologic effect at the site of action.

Effect of Renal Failure on Drug Disposition
Bioavailability
Although several factors can affect drug absorption in patients with kidney disease, only limited data are available that definitively document altered bioavailability. The absorption of drugs in patients with renal disorders could be inhibited by gastrointestinal (GI) disturbances present with uremia (e.g., nausea, vomiting, diarrhea), uremic gastritis, and pancreatitis. Edema of the GI tract, which can occur in patients with

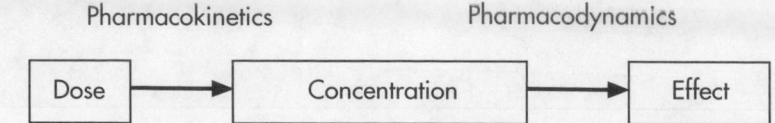

FIGURE 34-1 Relationship between pharmacokinetics and pharmacodynamics and the relationship of these two scientific principles to drug dose and concentration, and drug concentration and effect.

nephrotic syndrome, can cause impaired absorption. Gastric and intestinal motility as well as gastric emptying time can be altered by the neuropathy that is commonly associated with uremia. Uremia also can increase gastric ammonia, leading to an increased gastric pH. Drugs that require an acidic environment for absorption, such as ferrous sulfate, may be less bioavailable.[1] Calcium-containing antacids that often are used by renal failure patients for GI symptoms and hyperphosphatemia will neutralize the hydrochloric acid in the stomach and increase the gastric pH. These antacids also can complex with drugs, thereby decreasing their absorption.

The bioavailability of orally administered drugs also depends on the extent to which the drug is eliminated by first-pass (presystemic) metabolism. For example, the first-pass hepatic metabolism of oral propranolol is reduced in patients with renal disease, leading to increased bioavailability.[2] However, subsequent studies have attributed these observed increased concentrations of propranolol in renal failure to a significant increase in the blood/plasma ratio.[3] Not only can decreased first-pass metabolism contribute to increased bioavailability, but decreased intestinal P-glycoprotein activity as well.[4] Additional drugs exhibiting increased bioavailability in renal disease include cloxacillin, propoxyphene, dihydrocodeine, encainide, and zidovudine (AZT). For example, the area under the curve (AUC) of dihydrocodeine is increased 70% in those patients with impaired renal function.[5]

Protein Binding and Volume of Distribution

The extent to which a drug exerts its pharmacologic effects is related to the amount of free or unbound drug available for distribution to the target tissues. Patients with renal failure often have alterations in plasma protein binding, which can increase the amount of unbound drug.[6] Although this generally is true for acidic drugs, the binding of basic drugs is usually unchanged or possibly decreased in renal disease. Clinically, this is most important for highly protein-bound drugs (>80%). Decreased protein binding of these drugs results in increases in the free fraction of drug. This leads to an increase in the apparent volume of distribution (Vd), and plasma clearance for drugs with a low-extraction ratio. An increase in both the Vd and clearance would result in little or no change in the elimination half-life ($t_{1/2}$) of these drugs. Alternatively, the Vd of high-extraction ratio drugs can increase without a concomitant change in clearance. In this situation, the elimination half-life would increase, based on the relationships:

$$Kd = Cl/Vd$$
$$t_{1/2} = 0.693 \times Vd/Cl$$

In patients with renal failure, uremic toxins may alter protein binding. When the free fraction of drugs that are highly protein bound changes, the interpretation of the total drug concentration must also be considered. That is, with increasing free fraction, the total drug concentration necessary to exert the desired pharmacological effect is lower than that needed under normal conditions.

Hypoalbuminemia is a common complication of renal failure. Because acidic rather than basic drugs are bound to albumin, their protein binding tends to be altered in patients with renal failure (Table 34-1).[7] Patients with uremia accumulate acidic byproducts that may inhibit binding, or displace acidic drugs from albumin binding sites. This is supported by the observed improvement in protein binding following removal of

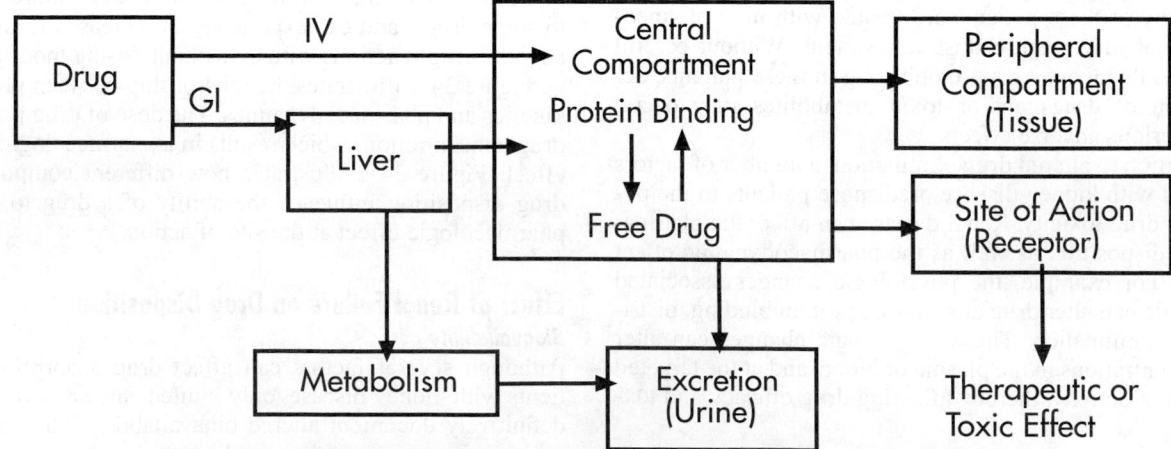

FIGURE 34-2 Factors influencing drug disposition and therapeutic/toxic effects. Following drug administration, a number of factors can influence pharmacokinetic parameters such as bioavailability, volume of distribution, clearance, and target tissue binding. These factors may include first-pass metabolism, protein binding, and renal and/or liver function.

Table 34-1   Plasma Protein Binding (%) of Acidic Drugs in Renal Failure

Drug	Normal	Renal Failure
Cefazolin	85	69
Cefoxitin	73	25
Clofibrate	97	91
Diazoxide	94	84
Furosemide	96	94
Pentobarbital	66	59
Phenytoin	88–93	74–84
Salicylate	87–97	74–84
Sulfamethoxazole	66	42
Valproic acid	92	77
Warfarin	99	98

these uremic byproducts by hemodialysis. Finally, the conformation or structural arrangement of albumin is altered in renal disease, which may reduce the number and/or affinity of binding sites for drugs. Studies have demonstrated differences in the amino acid composition of albumin between healthy people and patients with uremia.[8]

The anticonvulsant, phenytoin, is an important example of a drug whose protein binding is altered in renal disease.[9] This is discussed in more detail later in this chapter.

Renal disease may change the Vd of various drugs. The Vd or "apparent volume of distribution" is the "volume" or size of a compartment necessary to account for the total amount of drug in the body if it were present throughout the body at the same concentration as that found in plasma. A decrease in the plasma protein binding of highly protein-bound drugs, such as phenytoin, leads to an increase in the apparent Vd.

Drugs that are not highly protein bound (e.g., gentamicin, isoniazid) have little change in their Vd in renal disease. Digoxin is a unique exception in that its Vd is decreased in renal disease. This is attributed to a decrease in myocardial tissue uptake of digoxin, leading to a decrease in the myocardial or tissue to serum concentration ratio.[10]

Elimination

Drugs are eliminated primarily through renal excretion or hepatic metabolism. The extent to which renal disease affects the elimination of a drug depends on the amount of drug normally excreted unchanged in the urine and the degree of renal impairment. As kidney disease progresses, the kidney's ability to excrete uremic toxins diminishes. Consequently, the ability to eliminate certain drugs that are renally excreted also decreases. If the dose of these drugs are not modified for patients with renal dysfunction, these drugs will accumulate leading to an increase in the pharmacologic effect and the potential for toxicity.

The kidney eliminates drugs primarily by filtration or active secretion. Characteristics of a drug that determine its ability to be filtered include its affinity for protein binding and its molecular weight. Drugs with low protein binding or those that are displaced from proteins in the setting of renal disease (e.g., phenytoin) are filtered more readily. Molecules with a high molecular weight (>20,000 daltons) are not readily filtered due to their large size. The reasons for how renal disease selectively alters the process of glomerular filtration or tubular secretion of specific drugs are not well understood. The renal elimination of drugs in patients with renal disease usually is estimated by measuring the ability of the kidney to eliminate substances such as creatinine (i.e., creatinine clearance [Cl_{Cr}]) (See Chapter 31, Acute Renal Failure).

Renal disease can also have an important impact on the elimination of drugs that are primarily metabolized by the liver.[11] Metabolic processes, such as hydroxylation and glucuronidation, often produce inactive, more polar compounds that can be eliminated by the kidney. The metabolites of some drugs (e.g., meperidine, morphine, procainamide) are pharmacologically active or toxic. In patients with renal disease, these metabolites may accumulate, leading to an increase in pharmacologic activity and/or adverse effects.[12,13] For example, the central nervous system (CNS) toxicity observed in renal disease has been attributed to accumulation of the morphine metabolite, morphine-6-glucuronide. Therefore, careful dosing modifications or avoidance of these drugs are warranted in patients with renal impairment. Metabolic enzymes have been found within renal tissue, and may play a role in the metabolism of some of these drugs.[14,15] For example, the nonrenal clearance of drugs such as acyclovir decreases in patients with renal impairment, and is believed to be due to a decrease in "renal" metabolism.[16]

While renal and hepatic dysfunction may alter the metabolism and excretion of many drugs, the disposition of excipients used to formulate medications should also be considered. The pharmacokinetics of itraconazole and voriconazole are not significantly altered in the setting of renal dysfunction. The parenteral formulations of itraconazole and voriconazole contain the solubilizing agent, β-cyclodextrin. Cyclodextrin is rapidly eliminated by glomerular filtration, but can accumulate in patients with renal impairment, causing GI disturbances.[17]

Drug Removal by Dialysis

The effect of dialysis on the removal of a specific drug must be considered when using medications in patients undergoing dialysis. Patients may need supplemental doses of a medication after a dialysis procedure or alteration in their dosage to maintain therapeutic drug concentrations. Dialysis also can be initiated to hasten drug removal from the body in some cases of drug overdose.

When using dialysis to manage a drug overdose, patients may respond clinically to factors unrelated to dialysis of the drug. For example, declining plasma concentrations may be due to concurrent drug elimination by hepatic metabolism or renal excretion, which are independent of the dialysis procedure itself. Furthermore, clinical improvement may be due to removal of active metabolites by dialysis rather than the parent compound.

The primary literature should be used to determine if any information is available about the ability of dialysis to remove drug. Unfortunately, the application of data from the literature to a specific clinical situation often is difficult, and information pertaining to the dialysis of a specific drug may be limited. Anecdotal case reports in the primary literature seldom provide quantitative information. The effectiveness of dialysis is often based on a positive clinical outcome rather than on objective measurements of drug concentrations in the plasma and dialysate.

When applying information from the primary literature to a specific patient, the specifics of the dialyzer (e.g., type of machine, membrane surface area, pore size, and blood and dialysis flow rates) must be considered. Furthermore, patient-specific information (e.g., time of drug ingestion, liver and renal function) from case reports in the literature also should be evaluated appropriately. The method used to calculate dialysis clearance also should be considered. In addition, clinical investigators often use predialysis and postdialysis serum drug concentrations for estimating drug dialyzability without considering the contributing effects of drug metabolism and excretion on drug elimination.

Drug-Specific Properties

The physical and chemical characteristics of drugs can be used to predict the effectiveness of dialysis on drug removal.[18–20] Low-molecular-weight (MW) compounds are more readily dialyzed by conventional hemodialysis procedures because they can pass with greater ease across the dialysis membrane. Using cuprophane dialysis membranes, compounds with a MW ≤500 are more likely to be significantly dialyzed than compounds with a high molecular weight (e.g., vancomycin, MW ≈ 1,400). Newer high-flux dialyzers using polysulfone membranes more effectively remove large chemical compounds (see High-Flux Hemodialysis and Chapter 33, Renal Dialysis). In addition, the water solubility of a compound can also help predict drug dialyzability because water-soluble drugs are removed more readily than lipid-soluble compounds.

Pharmacokinetic characteristics (e.g., Vd, protein binding) also can affect drug dialyzability. A drug with a large Vd that distributes widely into the peripheral tissues resides minimally in the plasma and therefore is not substantially removed by dialysis. This is particularly true for highly lipid-soluble drugs such as digoxin (Vd = 300 to 500 L), and amiodarone (Vd = 60 L/kg). In addition, drugs that are highly protein bound, such as warfarin (99%) and ceftriaxone (83% to 96%), are not significantly removed by dialysis because the large protein–drug complex is unable to pass through the dialysis membrane.

The plasma clearance of a drug should also be compared to the dialysis clearance. Clearance values are additive. Dialysis clearance must contribute substantially to the patient's own clearance in order to enhance drug elimination. For example, zidovudine has a large plasma clearance in patients with severe renal disease (≈1,200 mL/min). Therefore, despite a hemodialysis clearance of 63 mL/min, the contribution of dialysis to zidovudine removal is negligible.

High-Flux Hemodialysis

High-flux hemodialysis utilizes a higher blood and dialysate flow rates compared with conventional methods. The enhanced efficiency of high-flux dialysis and the larger pore size of the polysulfone membranes allows for small- and mid-molecular-weight compounds such as vancomycin to be partially removed. Drugs such as gentamicin and foscarnet, which are removed by conventional dialysis are also efficiently removed by high-flux hemodialysis.[21,22] In many cases, the net amount of drug removed during a high-flux dialysis session is greater than the amount removed during conventional dialysis due to the use of higher blood flow rates. The principal difference is the greater efficiency and the ability to clear drugs of larger molecular weight compared to conventional dialysis.

Continuous Ambulatory Peritoneal Dialysis

Continuous ambulatory peritoneal dialysis (CAPD) uses the patient's peritoneum as the dialysis membrane. Patients maintained with CAPD undergo infusion of a dialysate solution via a catheter inserted into the peritoneal cavity; the solution is allowed to dwell in the cavity for several hours. The accumulated fluid and uremic byproducts diffuse from the blood into the dialysate solution, which is exchanged every 4 to 8 hours (see Chapter 33, Renal Dialysis).

Some drugs, such as antibiotics, may be administered intraperitoneally in CAPD patients. This is particularly useful for patients with peritonitis who require high intraperitoneal concentrations of antimicrobial agents to treat this infection. Following intraperitoneal administration of drugs, such as the aminoglycosides, plasma and intraperitoneal drug concentrations will eventually reach equilibrium. Despite systemic absorption of these drugs from the peritoneal fluid, peritoneal dialysis usually is inefficient at removing drugs from the plasma.[23] Because CAPD contributes little to the overall elimination of most drugs, dosage modifications are not always necessary in patients undergoing this procedure.

Continuous Renal Replacement Therapies

Continuous arteriovenous hemofiltration (CAVH) and continuous venovenous hemofiltration (CVVH) are forms of continuous renal replacement therapy (CRRT) used in the critically ill patient with acute renal failure. These therapies are typically reserved for patients who are unable to tolerate hemodialysis due to hemodynamic instability. Like hemodialysis, this procedure removes fluid, electrolytes, and low- and mid-molecular-weight molecules from the blood. Using a hollow-fiber that is made of a semipermeable membrane, water and solutes are filtered by hydrostatic pressure. A countercurrent dialysate can be added to the circuit to improve solute removal (CAVHD or CVVHD).

Limited data are available on the effect of CAVH or CVVH on the removal of drugs. Drugs that have a high sieving coefficient (permeability of a drug through a semipermeable membrane), such as the aminoglycosides, ceftazidime, vancomycin, and procainamide, are readily removed by CAVH or CVVH.[24,25] Data concerning the removal of drugs by hemodialysis cannot be extrapolated to CAVH or CVVH because of differences in the membranes used, blood flow rates, ultrafiltration rate, dialysate flow rate, and the continuous nature of the procedure compared with intermittent hemodialysis.

Hemoperfusion

Hemoperfusion is another method of drug removal that may be used to facilitate the elimination of a drug in the setting of an overdose.[26,27] During the hemoperfusion procedure, blood is passed through a column of adsorbent material (e.g., activated charcoal or resin) to bind drug. Hemoperfusion can be particularly useful for removing large-molecular-weight compounds or highly protein-bound drugs that are not removed efficiently by hemodialysis. Large compounds and drug-protein complexes are adsorbed onto the high-surface-area resin as blood passes through the adsorbent column. Hemoperfusion can also be used to remove lipid-soluble drugs not easily removed by hemodialysis. Lipid-soluble drugs often have a large Vd. Removal of drugs by hemoperfusion is of limited value because a significant amount of these lipophilic compounds reside in peripheral tissues.

Pharmacodynamics and Renal Disease

Few studies have investigated the pharmacodynamics of drugs in patients with renal disease. There are clinical observations that patients with renal disease are more sensitive to various drugs. For example, morphine has been associated with increased neurologic depression in patients with renal failure.[28,29] The ability of morphine to potentiate the CNS depressant effects of uremia may be due to an alteration in the permeability of the blood–brain barrier that results in higher CNS levels of morphine and morphine-6-glucuronide.

Another example of altered drug response in uremia is that of nifedipine, which, at similar unbound plasma concentrations, has an increased antihypertensive effect in patients with renal disease.[30] The mean E_{max} (maximal effect change in diastolic blood pressure) values in the control group and in severe renal failure patients were 12% and 29%, respectively. Therefore, the dose of nifedipine needs to be adjusted in patients with renal disease because of changes in drug effects rather than pharmacokinetic alterations.

PHARMACOKINETICS AND PHARMACODYNAMICS OF SPECIFIC DRUGS IN RENAL FAILURE
Ceftazidime
Dosage Modification: Factors to Consider

1. G.G., a 31-year-old, 70-kg woman with a 3-year history of systemic lupus erythematosus (SLE), presents to the emergency department (ED) with a 5-day history of fatigue, weakness, and nausea as well as worsening of her facial rash and a fever of 40°C. Her SLE had been moderately controlled until this acute flare. Her admission laboratory workup now reveals the following pertinent values: potassium (K), 6.0 mEq/L (normal, 3.6 to 4.8 mEq/L); sodium (Na), 142 mEq/L (normal, 135 to 144 mEq/L); serum creatinine (SrCr), 3.4 mg/dL (normal, 0.6 to 1.3 mg/dL); and blood urea nitrogen (BUN), 38 mg/dL (normal, 7 to 20 mg/dL). Complete blood count (CBC) reveals a hematocrit (Hct) of 32% (normal, 35% to 45% [females]) and a hemoglobin (Hgb) of 9.2 g/dL (normal, 11.8 to 15.4 g/dL [females]). The platelet count was 50,000/mm³ (normal, 140,000 to 300,000) and her erythrocyte sedimentation rate (ESR) was 35 mm/hr (normal, 0 to 20). Physical examination was significant for a blood pressure (BP) of 136/92 mm Hg and 2+ pedal edema. Prednisone is started at a dose of 1.5 mg/kg per day.

Two weeks into her hospital course, G.G.'s condition worsens and signs of sepsis develop. *Pseudomonas aeruginosa* is cultured from her urine. Therapy with ceftazidime is initiated at a dose of 1 g Q 8 hr, a dose commonly used for patients with good renal function. Considering that G.G.'s renal function has remained stable and that she has an estimated Cl_{Cr} of 27 mL/min, what factors should be considered before modifying her dose? What would be an appropriate dose of ceftazidime for G.G?

[SI units: K, 6.0 mmol/L (normal, 3.6 to 4.8); Na, 142 mmol/L (normal, 135 to 144); SrCr, 300.56 μmol/L (normal, 53.04 to 114.92); BUN, 13.57

mmol/L urea (normal, 2.5 to 7.14); Hct, 0.32 (normal, 0.35 to 0.45); Hgb, 92 g/L (normal, 118 to 154); platelet count, 50 × 10⁹/L (normal, 140 to 300); ESR, 35 mm/hr (normal, 0 to 20)]

Before modifying the dose of any drug, its route of elimination should be established. The elimination of most drugs that primarily are cleared by the kidneys will be decreased in the setting of renal impairment. The degree to which renal impairment affects elimination depends on the percentage of unchanged drug that is excreted by the kidney. For many drugs that are cleared by the kidneys, relationships between some measurement of renal function (e.g., Cl_{Cr}) and some parameter of drug elimination (e.g., plasma clearance or half-life) have been established to help the clinician determine the appropriate dosing modifications in patients with renal disease.

In contrast, the clearance of drugs that are eliminated primarily by nonrenal mechanisms (e.g., hepatic metabolism) is not altered significantly in patients with renal disease. However, limited data indicate that the kidney may play a role in drug metabolism. Enzymes with metabolic capacity have been found within renal tissue (see question 12). The clinical importance of this elimination pathway is unclear.

Of clinical significance is the role of the kidney in eliminating pharmacologically active or toxic metabolic products. Despite the metabolism of the parent drug and the lack of renal elimination of unchanged drug, the formation of active, more water-soluble metabolites that may accumulate with renal dysfunction warrants dosage adjustment or avoidance of the drug entirely (e.g., meperidine; see question 22).

Another factor important to consider is the "therapeutic window" for a given drug. The therapeutic window is the range of drug concentrations thought to be most effective. Drug concentrations below this range are usually subtherapeutic, whereas concentrations above this range can lead to a greater incidence of adverse effects. For drugs with a wide therapeutic window, the difference between toxic and therapeutic concentrations is large. Drugs that are cleared primarily by the kidney may require dosing modifications in patients with renal dysfunction. However, aggressive dose reduction may not be necessary for drugs with a large therapeutic window, particularly if the adverse effects are relatively mild (e.g., fluconazole). This is in contrast to drugs, such as the aminoglycosides, vancomycin or foscarnet, that are eliminated primarily by the kidney and have narrow therapeutic windows. For these drugs, the toxic plasma concentrations are very close to the therapeutic drug concentrations, with little room for dosing error. Table 34-2 summarizes the pharmacokinetics and dosing guidelines for drugs commonly used in patients with renal failure.

Ceftazidime is a cephalosporin that has excellent activity against most strains of *Pseudomonas* sp. Like most cephalosporins, ceftazidime primarily is cleared by the kidneys, with little nonrenal or hepatic elimination. The correlation between the clearance of ceftazidime and Cl_{Cr} in mL/min is represented by the following equation[31]:

$$Cl_{ceftaz} \text{ (mL/min)} = (0.95)(Cl_{Cr}) + 6.59 \qquad \text{(34-1)}$$

Using Equation 34-1, the clearance of ceftazidime in G.G. is estimated to be 32 mL/min compared with an average normal clearance of approximately 100 mL/min. Because her

Table 34-2 Pharmacokinetics and Dosing Guidelines for Drugs Commonly Used in Renal Failure[139]

Drug	Oral Availability (%)	Protein Binding (%)	Vd (L/kg)	Metabolism and Excretion	$t_{1/2}$ (hr)	Normal Dose $Cl_{Cr} > 50$ mL/min	Dose Change With Renal Failure Cl_{Cr} (mL/min)	Effect of Dialysis
Acyclovir	15–30	15	0.7	76–82% excreted renally; 14% hepatic	Normal: 2.1–3.2 Anephric: 20	5 mg/kg Q 8 hr	10–50: 5 mg/kg Q 12–24 hr <10: 2.5 mg/kg Q 24 hr	Dialyzed; 80 mL/min
Allopurinol	90	0	0.6	Metabolized to active oxypurinol metabolite, which is excreted renally; 6–12% excreted unchanged renally	Normal: 1.1–1.6 Anephric: no change; 7 days oxypurinol	300 mg QD	10–50: 200 mg QD <10: 100 mg QD	Oxypurinol; moderately dialyzed
Amikacin	Parenteral	<5	0.2–0.3	94–99% excreted renally	Normal: 2–3 Anephric: 36–82	See section on aminoglycoside pharmacokinetics	See section on aminoglycoside pharmacokinetics	Dialyzed; 22–38 mL/min
Amphotericin B	Parenteral	90–95	4	95–97% hepatic metabolism or inactivation in body tissue; 3.5–5.5% excreted unchanged renally	Normal: Initial: 24–48; Terminal: 15 days Anephric: No change	0.3–1 mg/kg Q 24 hr	10–50: 100% Q 24 hr <10: 100% Q 24–48 hr (to minimize azotemia)	Not dialyzed: large Vd
Ampicillin	32–76	29	0.3	73–92% excreted renally; 12–24% hepatic metabolism or biliary elimination	Normal: 0.8–1.5 Anephric: 20	1–2 g Q 4–6 hr	10–50: 1–1.5 g Q 6 hr <10: 50% 1 g Q 8–12 hr	Moderately dialyzed
Atenolol	50	<5	1.2	75% excreted renally; 10% hepatic; 10% feces	Normal: 5–6 Anephric: 42–73	50–100 mg QD	10–50: ↓ 50% and titrate <10: ↓ 50% and titrate	Moderately dialyzed
Aztreonam	Parenteral	50–60	0.15–0.38	60–70% excreted renally; 12% hepatic	Normal: 1.3–2.2 Anephric: 6–9	1–2 g Q 6–8 hr	10–50: 1–2 g Q 8–12 hr <10: 1 g Q 12–24 hr	Moderately dialyzed
Captopril	65	30 (↓R)	0.7	36–42% excreted renally; 50% hepatic	Normal: 1.7–1.9 Anephric: 21–32	6.25–12.5 mg Q 8–12 hr	10–50: No change <10: ↓ 25% and titrate	Moderately dialyzed; 80–120 mL/min
Cefazolin	Parenteral	84–92	0.2	>95% excreted renally; 3–5% hepatic	Normal: 1.8–2.6 Anephric: 12–40	1–2 g Q 8 hr	10–50: 0.5–1.5 g Q 12 hr <10: 0.5–1 g Q 24 hr	Moderately dialyzed

Drug	Route / % absorbed	% Protein binding	V_d	Elimination	Half-life (hr)	Dose	Dosage adjustment (mL/min)	Dialysis
Cefepime	Parenteral	20	0.23	>80% renally excreted	Normal = 2 hr; Anephric = 13–18 hr	1–2 g Q 8–12 hr	30–60 mL/min = 1–2 g Q 12–24 hr; 10–29 mL/min = 0.5–2 g Q 24 hr; <10 mL/min = 0.25–1 g Q 24 hr	Moderately dialyzed
Cefixime	50	69	0.1–1.0	20–40% excreted renally; 50% excreted by nonrenal mechanisms	Normal: 3.5; Anephric: 12–15	200–400 mg Q 12–24 hr	10–50: No change; <10: 50% Q 12–24 hr	Not dialyzed
Cefoperazone	Parenteral	87–93	0.16	70–85% excreted unchanged in bile; 15–30% excreted renally	Normal: 1.6–2.6; Anephric: 2.5	1–2 g Q 8–12 hr	10–50: No change; <10: ↓ with concurrent hepatic disease	Slightly dialyzed
Cefotaxime	Parenteral	38	0.22–0.36	40–60% hepatic (desacetyl active metabolite; 25% activity of parent compound); 40–65% excreted renally	Normal: 0.9–1.1; Anephric: 2.3–3.5, 12–20 (metabolite)	1–2 g Q –12 hr	10–50: 1–2 g Q 12 hr	Moderately dialyzed
Cefotetan	Parenteral	75–91	0.13	50–88% excreted renally; 12% excreted in bile	Normal: 3–4.2; Anephric: 13	1–2 g Q 12 hr	10–50: 1–2 g Q 24 hr; <10: 0.5–1 g Q 24 hr	Slightly/moderately dialyzed
Cefoxitin	Parenteral	65–79	0.27	85% excreted renally; up to 15% biliary and/or hepatic	Normal: 0.7–0.8; Anephric: 12–24	1–2 g Q 6–8 hr	10–50: 1–2 g Q 12–24 hr; <10: 0.5–1 g Q 24 hr	Moderately dialyzed
Ceftazidime	Parenteral	20–30	0.2–0.3	73–84% excreted renally	Normal: 1.6–2; Anephric: 13–25	1–2 g Q 8 hr	10–50: 1–2 g Q 12–24 hr; <10: 0.5 g Q 24 hr	Dialyzed
Ceftizoxime	Parenteral	17–25	0.2–0.4	78–92% excreted renally	Normal: 1.4–1.7; Anephric: 19–30	1–2 g Q 8–12 hr	10–50: 1–2 g Q 12–24 hr; <10: 0.5 g Q 24 hr	Moderately dialyzed
Ceftriaxone	Parenteral	83–96 (concentration dependent)	0.1	40–67% excreted renally; 40% excreted in bile	Normal: 6.5–8.9; Anephric: 12	1–2 g Q 12–24 hr	10–50: 1–2 g Q 24 hr; <10: 1–2 g Q 24 hr	Not dialyzed
Cefuroxime	Parenteral and 40–50 (as axetil salt)	33	0.19	90–95% excreted renally	Normal: 1.1–1.7; Anephric: 15–17	0.75–1.5 g Q 6–8 hr	10–50: 50–75% Q 8–12 hr; <10: 25–50% Q 24 hr	Moderately dialyzed
Cephradine	90–100	6–20	0.25–0.33	80–95% excreted renally; 5–20% hepatic metabolism or biliary/fecal elimination.	Normal: 0.7–0.9; Anephric: 8–15	250–500 mg Q 6 hr	10–50: 250–500 mg Q 12 hr; <10: 250–500 mg Q 24 hr	Moderately dialyzed

Table 34-2 Pharmacokinetics and Dosing Guidelines for Drugs Commonly Used in Renal Failure[139]—cont'd

Drug	Oral Availability (%)	Protein Binding (%)	Vd (L/kg)	Metabolism and Excretion	$t_{1/2}$ (hr)	Normal Dose $Cl_G > 50$ mL/min	Dose Change With Renal Failure Cl_G (mL/min)	Effect of Dialysis
Cimetidine	62	20	0.9–1.1	40–80% excreted renally; some metabolism	Normal: 1.5 Anephric: 3.3–4.6	PO: 400 mg Q 12 hr IV: 300 mg Q 8 hr	10–50: ↓ 25% <10: ↓ 50%	Slightly dialyzed
Ciprofloxacin	50–85	22	2.2	62% excreted renally; the rest cleared hepatically, in the bile and via intestinal mucosa	Normal: 4 Anephric: 8.5	250–750 mg Q 12 hr (PO)	10–50: 250–500 mg Q 12 hr <10: 250–750 mg Q 24 hr	Slightly dialyzed
Clindamycin	50	94	0.6	85% hepatic to active and inactive metabolites; 10% excreted renally; 5% feces	Normal: 2–4 Anephric: 1.6–3.4	600–900 mg Q 6–8 hr	10–50: No change <10: No change	Not dialyzed
Codeine	40–70	7	3–4	Hepatic with some active metabolites; little renal elimination (5–17%)	Normal: 2.9–4 Anephric: 19	No change		?
Cyclosporine	<5–89	>96	3.5	Extensively metabolized to active and inactive metabolites; <1% excreted renally	Normal: 6–13 Anephric: 16	No change	10–50: ↓ 25% and titrate <10: ↓50% and titrate	Not dialyzed
Digoxin	70	25 (↓R)	5–8 (↓R)	70% excreted renally	Normal: 36–44 Anephric: 80–120	No change	10–50: No change <10: No change	Not dialyzed
Enalapril[a]	36–44	<50	1	61% excreted renally; 33% excreted in feces	Normal: 5–11 Anephric: 36	No change	10–50: ↓ 50% <10: ↓ 75%	Slightly/moderately dialyzed
Erythromycin	30–65 (varies with salt)	84–90	0.9	85–95% hepatic to inactive metabolites; 5–15% excreted renally	Normal: 1.4–2 Anephric: 4	0.25–1 g Q 6 hr	10–50: ↓ 50% and titrate <10: ↓ 50% and titrate	Slightly dialyzed
Ethambutol	75–80	<5	1.6	65–80% excreted renally and 20% in feces; 8–15% hepatic	Normal: 3.1 Anephric: 18–20	15 mg/kg Q 24 hr	10–50: No change <10: No change	Slightly dialyzed
Fluconazole	>85	11–12	0.8	70% excreted renally; some hepatic metabolism	Normal: 20–50 Anephric: 98	100–200 mg Q 24 hr	10–50: 7.5–10 mg/kg Q 24 hr <10: 5 mg/kg Q 24 hr	Slightly dialyzed
							10–50: 50–200 mg Q 24 hr <10: 50–100 mg Q 24 hr	Moderately dialyzed

Drug					Half-life (hr)	Dose	Adjustment for GFR	Dialysis
Foscarnet	Parenteral	14–17	0.4–0.7	>80% excreted renally	Normal: 2–3 Anephric: >100	>80 mL/min: 60 mg/kg Q 8 hr 50–80 mL/min: 50 mg/kg Q 12 hr	10–50 mL/min: 60 mg/kg Q 24–48 hr <10 mL/min: 60 mg/kg Q 48 hr	Moderately dialyzed
Ganciclovir	5–9	1–2	0.5	>90% excreted renally	Normal: 2.5–3.6 Anephric: 11.5–28	>80 mL/min: 5 mg/kg Q 12 hr 50–80 mL/min: 2.5 mg/kg Q 12 hr	10–50: 1.25–2.5 mg/kg Q 24 hr <10: 1.25 mg/kg Q 24 hr	Dialyzed
Gentamicin	Parenteral	5–10	0.31	90–97% excreted renally	Normal: 1.5–3 Anephric: 20–54	See section on aminoglycoside pharmacokinetics	See section on aminoglycoside pharmacokinetics	Dialyzed; 24–50 mL/min
Ibuprofen	>80	99	0.15	Primarily metabolized; 45–60% excreted unchanged and as metabolites	Normal: 2 Anephric: No change	200–600 mg Q 4–6 hr	10–50: No change <10: No change	Not dialyzed
Imipenem	Parenteral	10–20	0.23–0.42	60–75% excreted renally; 22% hepatic to inactive metabolites	Normal: 0.8–1.3 Anephric: 2.9–3.7	5–10 mg/kg Q 6–8 hr	10–50: 5–10 mg/kg Q 8–12 hr <10: 5–10 mg/kg Q 12 hr	Moderately dialyzed
Indomethacin	98	90	0.26	Hepatic metabolism to inactive metabolites; <15% excreted unchanged	Normal: 2.6 Anephric: No change	25–50 mg Q 8–12 hr	10–50: No change <10: No change	?
Ketoconazole	50–76	99	0.36	51% hepatic; 45% excreted unchanged in feces; 3% renally	Normal: 3–8 Anephric: No change	200–400 mg Q 24 hr (depends on severity of infection)	10–50: No change <10: No change	Not dialyzed
Labetalol	20–38	50	8–10	5% excreted renally, 95% hepatic	Normal: 5 Anephric: ? prolonged	No change	10–50: No change <10: No change	Not dialyzed
Levofloxacin	99	24–38	0.92–1.36	60–87% renally excreted	Normal: 6–8 hr Anephric: 76 hr	250–750 mg QD	20–49 mL/min: 500–750 mg × 1, then 250–750 mg Q 24–48 hr <20 mL/min: 500 to 750 mg × 1, then 250–500 mg Q 48 hr	Not dialyzed

Table 34-2 Pharmacokinetics and Dosing Guidelines for Drugs Commonly Used in Renal Failure[139] —cont'd

Drug	Oral Availability (%)	Protein Binding (%)	Vd (L/kg)	Metabolism and Excretion	t₁/₂ (hr)	Normal Dose Cl_Cr >50 mL/min	Dose Change With Renal Failure Cl_Cr (mL/min)	Effect of Dialysis
Lidocaine	Parenteral	50–70	1.7 (↑H)	Hepatic metabolism to inactive and active metabolites (glycyl xylidide)	Normal: 1.5–1.8 Anephric: No change	Maintenance dose: 2–4 mg/min	10–50: No change <10: No change	Not dialyzed
Linezolid	100	31%	0.64–0.96	30% renally excreted	Normal: 5 hr Anephric: No change	600 mg BID	No change	30% removed by hemodialysis, give dose after dialysis
Lithium	100	0	0.5–0.8	95% excreted renally	Normal: 22–29 Anephric: Prolonged	Variable (titrate with Cl_Cr to therapeutic levels of 0.4–0.8)	10–50: ↓ 25–50% <10: 50–75%	Moderately dialyzed/ dialyzed
Meperidine	48–53	58	4.4	Hepatic hydrolysis and conjugation, active normeperidine metabolites; 10% excreted renally	Normal: 3–7 Anephric: ?	50–100 mg Q 3–4 hr (IV, IM)	10–50: 75–100% Q 6 hr <10: 50% Q 6–8 hr (use cautiously)	?
Meropenem	Parenteral	2	0.26	70% renally excreted	Normal: 1 hr Anephric: 15.7 hr	1g Q 8 hr	26–50 mL/min: 1 g Q 12 hr 10–25 mL/min: 1 g Q 24 hr <10 mL/min: 500 mg Q 24 hr	Moderately dialyzed
Methotrexate	16–95 (dose dependent)	50	0.4–0.8	>90% cleared renally; 10% metabolized to 7-OH-MTX	Normal: α 1.5–3.5; β 8–15 Anephric: Prolonged	No change	10–50: Adjust according to serum concentration <10: Avoid	Not/slightly dialyzed
Metoprolol	38	13	4	90% hepatic; 10% excreted renally	Normal: 3–4 Anephric: No change	50–200 mg QD	10–50: No change <10: No change	Metabolites dialyzed
Mezlocillin	Parenteral	26–42	0.2	45–65% excreted renally; 35–55% excreted hepatobiliary	Normal: 0.8–1.2 Anephric: 3–6	50 mg/kg Q 4–6 hr	10–50: 100% Q 6–8 hr <10: 50% Q 8 hr	Slightly/moderately dialyzed; 29 mL/min
Moxifloxacin	90	50	1.7–2.7	20% renally excreted	Normal: 12 hr Anephric: 14.5 hr	400 mg QD	No change	Unknown

Drug								
Nadolol	34	20	2	75% excreted renally; 25% hepatic	Normal: 15–20 Anephric: 45	40–80 mg QD	10–50: ↓ 50% and titrate <10: ↓ 50% and titrate	Moderately dialyzed
Nafcillin	50	85–90	0.35	Up to 70% hepatic; 25–30% excreted renally	Normal: 1–1.5 Anephric: 1.9	1–2 g Q 4–6 hr	10–50: No change <10: No change	Not dialyzed
Nifedipine	45	98	0.8–1.1	100% hepatic	Normal: 2–4 Anephric: 3.8	No change	10–50: No change <10: No change (? ↑ response in renal failure patients)	?
Penicillin G	15–30	60	0.9–2.1	50% excreted renally; 19% hepatic	Normal: 0.4–0.9 Anephric: 4–10	2–3 MU Q 4 hr	10–50: Dose (MU/D) = $3.2 + Cl_{cr}/7$ <10: Dose (MU/D) = $3.2\ \%\ Cl_{cr}/7$	Moderately dialyzed; 46 mL/min
Pentamidine	Parenteral	69	12	<5% eliminated renally over 24 hr	Normal: 6 (5–9 days, urine data); Anephric: ?	4 mg/kg/day (IV)	10–50: No change <10: 100% QD–QOD	Probably not dialyzed
Phenobarbital	100	48–59	0.6	Hepatic metabolism; renal excretion: 10–40% unchanged and active metabolites	Normal: 100 Anephric: ?	No change	10–50: No change <10: Slight ↓	Moderately dialyzed/ dialyzed
Phenytoin	>90	85–95 (↓R, H)	0.5–0.7 (↑R)	Hepatic metabolism; <5% excreted unchanged; 75% as inactive p-HPPH metabolites; concentration-dependent kinetics	Normal: 10–30 Anephric: 6–10	300–400 mg QD (titrate)	10–50: No change <10: No change (lower therapeutic level)	Not dialyzed
Piperacillin	Parenteral	16–22	0.2–0.47	50–60% excreted renally; up to 30–40% excreted in bile	Normal: 0.8–1.4 Anephric: 4–6	50 mg/kg Q 4–6 hr	10–50: 100% Q 6 hr <10: 50–75% Q 8 hr	Moderately dialyzed
Procainamide	75–95	15	1.7–2.3	Hepatic metabolism to active NAPA; 50–60% excreted renally	Normal: 2.5–4.7 (NAPA: 6) Anephric: 11–16 (NAPA: 42)	0.5–1.5 g Q 4–6 hr	10–50: 100% Q 6–12 hr <10: 100% Q 12–24 hr	Moderately dialyzed
Propranolol	36–40	88–94	2.9	Primarily hepatic; <1% excreted renally	Normal: 3–5 Anephric: No change	10–40 mg Q 6 hr (PO) and titrate	10–50: No change <10: No change	Not dialyzed
Ranitidine	52	15	0.8–1.1	70% excreted renally; some hepatic	Normal: 1.4–2.4 Anephric: 5–10	300 mg Q HS	10–50: ↓ 25% <10: ↓ 50%	Slightly dialyzed

Table 34-2 Pharmacokinetics and Dosing Guidelines for Drugs Commonly Used in Renal Failure[139]—cont'd

Drug	Oral Availability (%)	Protein Binding (%)	Vd (L/kg)	Metabolism and Excretion	$t_{1/2}$ (hr)	Normal Dose Cl$_G$ >50 mL/min	Dose Change With Renal Failure Cl$_G$ (mL/min)	Effect of Dialysis
Sulfamethoxazole	90–100	50–70 (↓R)	0.14–0.36 (↑R)	65–80% hepatic to inactive compounds; 20–30% excreted renally	Normal: 7–12 Anephric: 10–50	Q 6–12 hr	10–50: Q 12–24 hr <10: Q 24 hr	Slightly/moderately dialyzed
Tobramycin	Parenteral	<10	0.33	90–97% excreted renally	Normal: 2.5 Anephric: 33–70	See section on aminoglycoside pharmacokinetics	See section on aminoglycoside pharmacokinetics	Dialyzed; 50–60 mL/min
Trimethoprim	85–90	40–70	1–2	53–80% excreted renally; 20–35% hepatic	Normal: 8–16 Anephric: 24–62	Q 6–12 hr	10–50: Q 12–24 hr	Slightly/moderately dialyzed
Vancomycin	<10	10–55	0.5–0.7	80–90% excreted renally; 10–20% hepatic metabolism	Normal: 4–9 Anephric: 129–190	See section on vancomycin pharmacokinetics	See section on vancomycin pharmacokinetics	Conventional: not dialyzed; high flux: moderately dialyzed
Zidovudine	64	34–38	1.4	Primarily hepatic to inactive GAZT metabolite; 18% excreted renally	Normal: 0.8–2.9 Anephric: No change	100–200 mg Q 8 hr	10–50: No change <10: Possible ↓	Not dialyzed

*Pharmacokinetic values are for the active enalaprilat metabolite.

drug clearance is approximately one-third of normal, she would require about one-third of the normal daily dose (i.e., 1 g every 24 hours). Failure to reduce the dose from a normal dose of 1 g every 8 hours might lead to accumulation of ceftazidime, predisposing G.G. to seizures and other adverse effects associated with toxic beta-lactam antibiotic plasma levels.[32,33] Like other cephalosporins, ceftazidime has a large therapeutic window.[34] This is in contrast to the aminoglycosides, which must be dosed based upon specific pharmacokinetic calculations. Therefore, more generalized or empirical dosage modifications can be made with ceftazidime.

Aminoglycosides

2. G.G.'s medical team decides that the addition of an aminoglycoside antibiotic is now necessary to treat her infection. Considering that her renal function has remained stable, how should the gentamicin be dosed in G.G.? Is it best to alter the dose or the dosing interval for this drug?

Alteration of Dose Versus Dosing Interval
The aminoglycosides (e.g., tobramycin, gentamicin, amikacin) are effective in the treatment of serious systemic infections caused by Gram-negative organisms such as *Pseudomonas* sp. However, unlike the cephalosporins and penicillins, the aminoglycosides have a relatively narrow therapeutic window. Using pharmacokinetic principles, a dose regimen can be designed to produce specific peak and trough serum concentrations. Peak serum concentrations (Cp_{peak}) (e.g., gentamicin or tobramycin 5 to 8 mg/L) correlate best with therapeutic efficacy, whereas toxicity tends to correlate with elevated trough levels (Cp_{trough}), which reflects prolonged exposure to high drug concentrations. To minimize the risk of toxicity, trough levels of <2 mg/L should be maintained. In patients with normal renal function, these target serum aminoglycoside concentrations are usually obtained following standard doses (e.g., 1.5 mg/kg) administered every 8 hours. For most patients, peak and trough levels are usually measured once steady state is achieved, which is typically within 24 hours.[35-38]

Many clinicians now utilize once-daily dosing of the aminoglycosides (e.g., 5 mg/kg every 24 hours) for patients with normal renal function in an attempt to minimize aminoglycoside accumulation and nephrotoxicity. The rationale for this regimen is based on the aminoglycosides' concentration-dependent killing and post-antibiotic effect. This approach is not recommended for patients with renal impairment, however. When once-daily dosing is used, peak concentrations are less helpful; however, trough concentrations should be monitored, and are usually below the limit of analytical detection (<1 mg/L). The discussion regarding aminoglycoside dosing in renal impairment that follows is based on the traditional every-8-hour dosing regimen.

Aminoglycosides are almost completely eliminated by the kidneys; thus, the clearance of these drugs essentially is equal to the glomerular filtration rate (GFR). The pharmacokinetic properties of gentamicin and tobramycin are similar. A close correlation exists between Cl_{Cr} and gentamicin total body clearance. As renal function deteriorates, aminoglycoside doses must be modified to maintain the desired peak and trough plasma concentrations. Failure to appropriately adjust the dosage of aminoglycosides in renal insufficiency can lead to high drug plasma levels that can result in ototoxicity and nephrotoxicity.

In many cases, the aminoglycoside dose can be modified by extending the dosing interval rather than simply reducing the dose. This permits maintenance of adequate peak plasma concentrations to ensure efficacy, while allowing for sufficient elimination between doses to produce trough levels <2 mg/L. The advantages and disadvantages of adjusting the dosing interval versus reducing the dose are summarized in Table 34-3.

Figure 34-3 illustrates the effect of increasing the dosing interval in a patient such as G.G. with renal function that is 30% of normal. Although this is the preferred method for adjusting the dose of aminoglycosides, for many other drugs requiring dose adjustments in renal disease, simple dosage reduction is sufficient (see Table 34-2).

Determination of Appropriate Dose
A number of methods have been developed to determine the appropriate aminoglycoside dose for patients.[39] One method is Bayesian forecasting, in which pharmacokinetic data obtained in the individual patient are integrated with population parameters. Initially, a dose is used that is based on population parameter values adjusted for such characteristics as increased SrCr. Drug concentrations for the individual patient are measured at specific times (e.g., peak and trough measurements) and these are compared to the expected values from the population data. Individualized pharmacokinetic parameter estimates are subsequently derived using Bayes' theorem to calculate a more patient-specific dosing regimen.[40]

Alternatively, the "Rule of Eights" method is used for dose adjustment. In this case, the usual maintenance dose (1 to 1.5 mg/kg ideal body weight [IBW]) is administered at a dosing

Table 34-3 Advantages and Disadvantages of General Approaches to Dosing Adjustments in Renal Disease

Method	Advantages	Disadvantages
Variable Frequency Use the same dose but ↑ the dosing interval	Same Cp_{ave}, Cp_{max}, Cp_{min} Normal dose	Levels may remain subtherapeutic for prolonged periods in patients requiring dosing intervals >24 hr
Variable Dose With Fixed Cp_{ave} ↓ dose to maintain a target Cp_{ave}; keep the dosing interval the same	Same Cp_{ave} Normal dosing interval	↓ peak levels, which may be subtherapeutic; ↑ trough levels, which may ↑ potential for toxicity

Cp_{ave}, average plasma concentration; Cp_{max}, maximum plasma concentration; Cp_{min}, minimum plasma concentration.

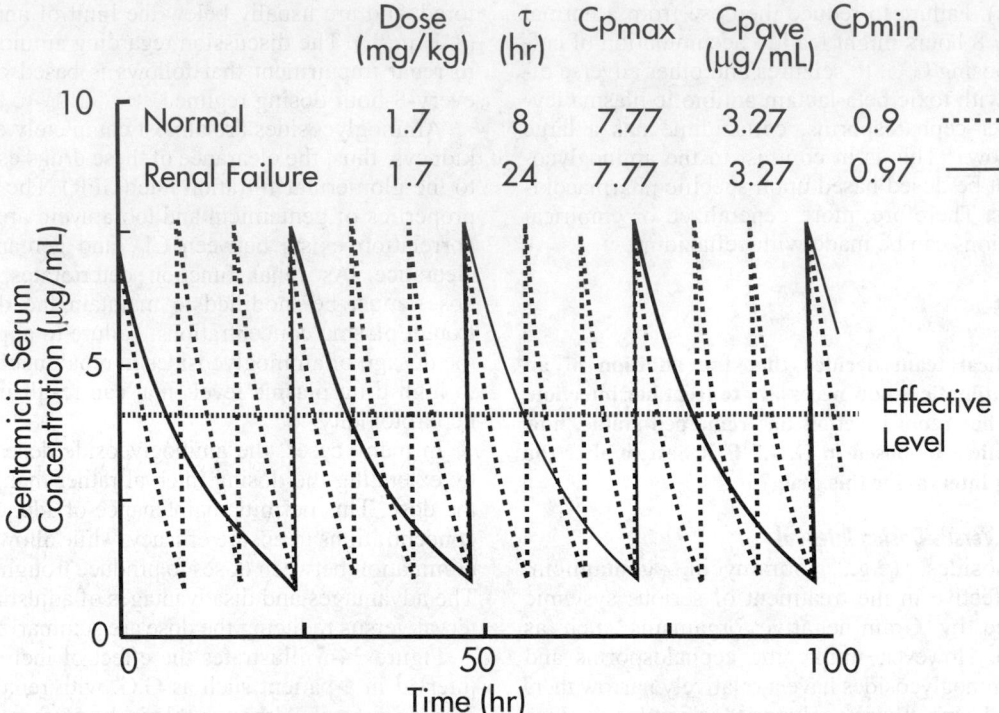

Renal Function 30%

	Dose (mg/kg)	τ (hr)	Cp$_{max}$	Cp$_{ave}$ (µg/mL)	Cp$_{min}$	
Normal	1.7	8	7.77	3.27	0.9	······
Renal Failure	1.7	24	7.77	3.27	0.97	——

FIGURE 34-3 Serum concentration versus time profile for a patient with renal function 30% of normal in whom the interval of drug administration has been extended for dose adjustment. Advantages to this method are summarized in Table 34-3. (Reproduced with permission from Brater DC. Drug Use in Renal Disease. Sydney: ADIS Health Science Press, 1983.)

interval derived by multiplying the SrCr by 8.[39] The appropriate interval is established by rounding the result to the most convenient interval (e.g., 8 hours, 12 hours, 24 hours). In G.G., a dose of 70 mg every 24 hours would be recommended if this method were used. However, this method only approximates a regimen for G.G.

Because there is wide interpatient variability in aminoglycoside pharmacokinetic parameters and the therapeutic index for these drugs is narrow, doses should be adjusted based on pharmacokinetic principles (e.g., Bayesian calculations or methods described later in this chapter) and plasma concentrations that are specific for this patient.

PATIENT-SPECIFIC METHODS

Sawchuk and Zaske developed a method to derive patient-specific estimates of Vd and clearance (Cl) based on the patient's size and estimated Cl$_{Cr}$.[37] These parameters can be used to calculate a specific dose for G.G. that will produce the desired gentamicin peak and trough concentrations. If steady-state serum concentrations of gentamicin are known, they can be used to calculate even more specific parameters. To initiate gentamicin therapy, pharmacokinetic parameters should first be estimated from population values.

The clearance of gentamicin (Cl$_{gent}$) can be calculated based on G.G.'s Cl$_{Cr}$. Using the Cockroft and Gault equation,[41] the Cl$_{Cr}$ can be estimated as follows:

$$Cl_{cr} \text{ (males)} = \frac{(140 - age)(IBW)}{(SrCr)(72)} \quad \textbf{(34-2)}$$

$$Cl_{cr} \text{ (females)} = \frac{(140 - age)(IBW)}{(SrCr)(72)}(0.85) \quad \textbf{(34-3)}$$

With a SrCr of 3.4 mg/dL, an ideal body weight of 70 kg, and an age of 31, G.G.'s estimated Cl$_{Cr}$, is 27 mL/min.

The relationship between gentamicin clearance (Cl$_{gent}$) and Cl$_{Cr}$ can be characterized by the following equation[42]:

$$Cl_{gent} \text{ in mL/min/kg} = (0.65)[Cl_{cr} \text{ in mL/min/kg}] + 3.7 \quad \textbf{(34-4)}$$

However, for practical purposes, Cl$_{gent}$ is usually considered equivalent to Cl$_{Cr}$. Therefore, Cl$_{gent}$ also is approximately 27 mL/min or 1.6 L/hour. The Vd of gentamicin (Vd$_{gent}$) is approximately 0.25 L/kg in patients with normal or impaired renal function.[37,42,43]

The Vd$_{gent}$ will be different in obese patients or those who are fluid overloaded. Although G.G. does have some fluid retention, this is minimal and should not affect her Vd$_{gent}$ significantly. Therefore, the Vd$_{gent}$ for G.G. is as follows:

$$\begin{aligned} Vd_{gent} &= (0.25 \text{ L/kg})(\text{Body Weight}) \\ &= (0.25 \text{ L/kg})(70 \text{ kg}) \quad \textbf{(34-5)} \\ &= 17.5 \text{ L} \end{aligned}$$

The loading dose of gentamicin can be determined using the following equation:

$$LD_{gent} = (Vd_{gent})(\text{desired } Cp_{peak}) \quad \textbf{(34-6)}$$

For treatment of infections due to *Pseudomonas* sp., a peak level of approximately 6 to 8 mg/L is desired:

$$LD_{gent} = (17.5\ L)(7\ mg/L)$$
$$= 122.5\ mg\ or\ round\ off\ to\ 120\ mg \quad (34\text{-}6A)$$

Using Cl_{gent} and Vd_{gent}, the elimination rate constant (Kd) and half-life for gentamicin can be estimated as follows:

$$Kd = \frac{Cl_{gent}}{Vd_{gent}}$$
$$= \frac{1.6\ L/hr}{17.5\ L}$$
$$= 0.091\ hr^{-1} \quad (34\text{-}7)$$
$$t_{1/2} = \frac{0.693}{Kd}$$
$$= \frac{0.693}{0.091\ hr^{-1}}$$
$$= 7.6\ hr$$

For the aminoglycosides, the dosing interval (τ) is determined by doubling the half-life because by the end of two half-lives, 75% of the drug will have been eliminated. This will usually lead to a desired trough level of <2 mg/L. Therefore, gentamicin should be administered at least every 16 hours. For convenience, an interval of 24 hours can be used, which also will achieve the desired trough concentration.

Gentamicin is usually infused over 30 minutes. To determine the peak gentamicin concentration, serum samples are drawn 30 minutes after the infusion has been completed. Because the estimated elimination half-life of gentamicin in G.G. (7.6 hours) is much longer than the infusion time (0.5 hours), the intravenous bolus model can be used to calculate an appropriate maintenance dose.

To achieve the peak concentration of 7 mg/L, the following equation can be used:

$$Dose = \frac{(Cp_{peak})(1 - e^{-Kd\tau})(Vd_{gent})}{(e^{-Kdt_{sample}})}$$
$$= \frac{(7\ mg/L)(1 - e^{-(0.091hr^{-1})(24hr)})(17.5L)}{(e^{-(0.091hr^{-1})(1hr)})} \quad (34\text{-}8)$$
$$= 119.2\ mg$$
$$= or\ round\ off\ to\ 120\ mg$$

where t_{sample} usually equals 1 hour (30 minutes following a 30-minute infusion).

The expected trough level in G.G. can now be estimated by the following equation:

$$Cp_{trough} = (Cp_{peak})(e^{-Kdt_{sample}})$$
$$= (7\ mg/L)(e^{-(0.091hr^{-1})(24\ hr)}) \quad (34\text{-}9)$$
$$= 0.8\ mg/L$$

Although not the case for G.G., patients with normal renal function may eliminate a significant amount of gentamicin during the 30-minute infusion. In these patients, the intermittent infusion model should be used to account for this loss of drug, where t_{in} is the duration of the infusion:

$$Dose = \frac{(Cl_{gent})(Cp_{peak})(1 - e^{-Kd\tau})(t_{in})}{(1 - e^{-Kdt_{in}})(e^{-Kd\tau})} \quad (34\text{-}10)$$

Revised Parameters

3. After 72 hours of gentamicin therapy, G.G.'s peak and trough levels are 7.6 and 2.6 mg/L, respectively. Her physician attributes this to a gradual decline in renal function. (Her most recent SrCr is 4.8 mg/dL.) How would you revise G.G.'s dosing regimen based on these levels?

A gentamicin trough level of >2 mg/L suggests that G.G.'s dosing interval is too short. Although her peak concentration is within the normal range of 5 to 8 mg/L, her trough concentration indicates that she is at a potentially toxic level. Her pharmacokinetic parameters can be revised based on these values, and a new Kd can be estimated from the equation:

$$Kd = \frac{\ln(Cp_1 - Cp_2)}{\Delta t}$$
$$= \frac{\ln(7.6\ mg/L - 2.6\ mg/L)}{23\ hr} \quad (34\text{-}11)$$
$$= 0.047\ hr^{-1}$$

Because little change in G.G.'s Vd_{gent} is expected, a new Cl_{gent} ($Cl_{revised}$) can be estimated from her revised elimination constant (if necessary, a revised Vd_{gent} could be calculated, keeping Cl_{gent} constant, although the clearance is more likely to change than the volume of distribution):

$$Cl_{revised} = (Vd_{gent})(Kd)$$
$$= (17.5\ L)(0.047\ hr^{-1}) \quad (34\text{-}12)$$
$$= 0.82\ L/hr$$

These revised values for Kd and Cl can now be used to calculate a revised maintenance dose to maintain the Cp_{trough} at <2 mg/L using Equation 34-8:

$$Dose = \frac{(7\ mg/L)(1 - e^{-(0.047\ hr^{-1})(48hr)})(17.5L)}{e^{-(0.047\ hr^{-1})(1hr)}}$$
$$= 115\ mg \quad (34\text{-}12A)$$
$$Cp_{trough} = (7\ mg/L)(e^{-(0.047\ hr^{-1})(48hr)})$$
$$= 0.73\ mg/L$$

The revised dose is now 115 mg (or approximately 110 mg) every 48 hours.

4. What are some limitations in calculating G.G.'s Cl_{Cr} based on her SrCr? Can this estimate safely be used to predict gentamicin clearance?

For patients with stable renal function, Cl_{Cr} can be estimated from SrCr using the Cockroft and Gault equation (see Equations 34-2 and 34-3). Other methods are discussed in Chapter 32, Chronic Kidney Disease. However, in a patient such as G.G. whose renal function has diminished during the hospital course, estimation of renal function based on her increasing SrCr becomes more difficult. Because her SrCr does not reflect a steady-state level, the previous equations can no longer be used to accurately estimate her renal function. Since G.G.'s SrCr has increased rapidly from 3.4 to 4.8 mg/dL over the past few days, her Cl_{Cr} is probably much lower than that estimated using the Cockroft and Gault method. A rising SrCr may represent a decline in renal function manifesting as an accumulation of creatinine.

Effect of Hemodialysis
Conventional Dialysis
GENTAMICIN

5. G.G.'s renal function continues to deteriorate to the extent that she requires hemodialysis. What additional alterations in her gentamicin dosing regimen are necessary when she is dialyzed?

Gentamicin has a molecular weight of about 500 and is significantly removed by conventional hemodialysis.[38] Gentamicin has a relatively low Vd, averaging 0.25L/kg, and is about 10% bound to proteins. The dialysis clearance of gentamicin using conventional methods depends on the actual filter used as well as the blood and dialysate flow rates. Dialysis clearance averages 45 mL/min compared with an average plasma clearance of 5 mL/min in patients with end-stage renal disease (ESRD).[44,45] Therefore, G.G.'s gentamicin dose must be adjusted to compensate for the amount of drug that will be removed by dialysis. Because drug removal represents a combination of drug elimination by the body and dialysis, the following equation can be used:

$$Cl_{total} = Cl_{dial} + Cl \qquad (34\text{-}13)$$

where Cl_{total} is the total clearance of the drug during dialysis, Cl_{dial} is the clearance by dialysis, and Cl is plasma clearance. If dialysis clearance is high relative to plasma clearance, drug removal will be enhanced by the dialysis procedure. The total clearance of gentamicin in a patient with severe renal dysfunction during dialysis is 50 mL/min (45 mL/min + 5 mL/min) or 10 times the clearance while off dialysis. Plasma clearance and dialysis clearance are related to the elimination half-life by the following equation:

$$t_{1/2} = \frac{(0.693)(Vd)}{Cl_{dial} + Cl} \qquad (34\text{-}14)$$

Thus, assuming a constant Vd of 17.5 L (i.e., 0.25 L/kg × 70 kg), the elimination half-life on dialysis is approximately 4 hours compared with 40 hours off dialysis. In addition, the extent of drug removal can be predicted from the following equation:

$$FD = 1 - e^{-(Cl+Cl_{dial})(t/Vd)} \qquad (34\text{-}15)$$

where t is the duration of dialysis. Therefore, the fraction of gentamicin removed (FD) during a 4-hour conventional dialysis procedure is approximately 50%. If specific data are not available for dialysis and plasma clearance, the following equation will predict fraction removal using the elimination half-life data alone obtained during dialysis:

$$FD = 1 - e^{-(0.693/t_{1/2on})(t)} \qquad (34\text{-}16)$$

The estimated value of 50% removal is consistent with literature values indicating that 50% to 70% of a dose of gentamicin is removed during a 4-hour dialysis procedure. However, a limitation of this equation is that it does not consider the redistribution of drug from the tissues back into the plasma following the dialysis procedure.

These data suggest that one-half the dose of gentamicin should be given to G.G. following each dialysis session.

It generally is difficult to calculate an appropriate maintenance dose for patients undergoing hemodialysis that will maintain peak and trough concentrations similar to patients with normal renal function. Sustained plasma concentrations >2 mg/L can increase the incidence of toxicity; however, dosing gentamicin to achieve trough concentrations of <2 mg/L may lead to prolonged periods of subtherapeutic concentrations. Therefore, in patients receiving hemodialysis, gentamicin doses are given to achieve a predialysis trough concentration of approximately 3 mg/L. A maintenance gentamicin dose of 1 mg/kg after each dialysis session commonly is used to achieve this desired concentration.

CEFTAZIDIME

6. Why does the dose of ceftazidime in G.G. have to be adjusted because of her hemodialysis when this drug has such a large therapeutic window?

Because only 21% of ceftazidime is protein bound and its Vd is 0.2 L/kg, it should be readily removed by hemodialysis. The mean dialysis clearance of ceftazidime is 55 mL/min, with 55% of the drug removed during 4 hours of conventional hemodialysis.[46] A supplemental dose of ceftazidime should be given to G.G following each hemodialysis session to maintain a therapeutic concentration. Half of the daily ceftazidime dose should be administered after each dialysis session.

High-Flux Hemodialysis

7. G.G.'s physician is considering changing her from a conventional dialysis system to a high-flux system that uses high efficiency polysulfone membranes. How does the dialyzability of gentamicin and ceftazidime differ with high-flux hemodialysis compared with conventional hemodialysis?

High-flux hemodialysis is more effective than conventional dialysis at removing certain pharmacologic agents (see Chapter 33, Renal Dialysis) because the membranes are more efficient and the blood flow through the dialyzer is increased. Although limited data are available, a greater fraction of drugs, such as aminoglycosides, ceftazidime, and vancomycin, are removed by high-flux versus conventional hemodialysis.[47,48] Approximately 50% to 70% of gentamicin is removed during a 2.5-hour, high-flux dialysis session.[49,50] The clearance of ceftazidime by high-flux dialysis is 75 to 240 mL/min compared with 55 mL/min for conventional hemodialysis.[47] Thus, further dosage adjustments for gentamicin and ceftazidime may be necessary when she is converted from conventional hemodialysis to high-flux hemodialysis.

Continuous Venovenous Hemofiltration

8. What changes would be necessary in her gentamicin dosing if she were to start a continuous renal replacement therapy such as CVVH?

Because of the continuous nature of CVVH and CAVH, the extent of drug eliminated by continuous renal replacement therapies will be different from intermittent modes such as hemodialysis. The clearance of a drug in a patient receiving CVVH can be described in a fashion similar to Equation 34-13, where Cl_{dial} is replaced with Cl_{cvvh}.

$$Cl_{total} = Cl + Cl_{cvvh} \qquad (34\text{-}17)$$

In G.G., the $Cl_{revised}$ from Equation 34-12 can be used for the plasma clearance (Cl). The clearance by CVVH can be described by Equation 34-18:

$$Cl_{cvvh} = Fu \times UFR \qquad (34\text{-}18)$$

where *Fu* is the fraction of drug unbound, and *UFR* is the ultrafiltration rate. Gentamicin exhibits low plasma protein binding (Fu = 0.95). Typical ultrafiltration rates for CVVH are approximately 1L/hr, but can vary.

$$
\begin{aligned}
Cl_{cvvh} &= Fu \times UFR \\
&= 0.95 \times 1 \text{ L/hr} \\
&= 0.95 \text{ L/hr}
\end{aligned} \qquad (34\text{-}18A)
$$

$$
\begin{aligned}
Cl_{total} &= Cl_{revised} + Cl_{cvvh} \\
&= 0.82 \text{ L/hr} + 0.95 \text{ L/hr} \\
&= 1.77 \text{ L/hr} \\
&= 29.5 \text{ mL/min}
\end{aligned} \qquad (34\text{-}18B)
$$

Since the clearance of gentamicin approximates that of creatinine clearance, G.G.'s total clearance is approximately one-third the normal clearance of 100 mL/min. Therefore, the gentamicin dose should be approximately one-third of the normal dose. G.G. should be given 1.5 mg/kg/day or 100 mg of gentamicin as a single daily dose (normal dose is approximately 5 mg/kg/day). Gentamicin trough concentrations should be monitored, and her dose adjusted to maintain a trough concentration of <2 mg/L.

Continuous Ambulatory Peritoneal Dialysis

9. J.J., a 24-year-old man with ESRD, is maintained with CAPD. He presents to the ED with a fever of 38.2°C and complains of severe abdominal pain. He also reports that his peritoneal dialysate has become cloudy over the past few days. All these symptoms are consistent with peritonitis, a frequent complication of CAPD. His culture results reveal *Escherichia coli*, sensitive to gentamicin. How should gentamicin be dosed in this patient?

Management of dialysis-related peritonitis may vary from one institution to another. Antibiotics often are administered intraperitoneally with or without systemic antibiotic therapy. For less severe cases, intraperitoneal (IP) administration is often considered sufficient. With IP administration, the goal is to deliver a concentration of drug similar to the desired plasma concentration for the treatment of systemic infections. Therefore, 8 mg of gentamicin into each liter of dialysate (or 16 mg into a 2 L bag of dialysate) is recommended. Once equilibrium or steady state is achieved, the dialysate concentration will be comparable to the concentration of gentamicin in the plasma. Despite a more rapid transfer of drug into the plasma due to increased permeability of the peritoneal membrane in patients with peritonitis, there will still be a substantial lag time before steady-state is reached. For more serious cases of peritonitis, concomitant systemic antibiotics should be given.

10. Is gentamicin eliminated by CAPD?

In general, most drugs are not well removed via CAPD. This is particularly true for drugs that are highly protein bound or for drugs with a large Vd. Gentamicin and other aminoglycosides, on the other hand, are removed by CAPD. Gentamicin exhibits low protein binding and has a small Vd. It is estimated that 10% to 50% of gentamicin is removed by CAPD.[51]

Acyclovir
Renal Clearance

11. D.M., a 28-year-old man with acquired immune deficiency syndrome (AIDS), presents with a severe herpetic infection requiring intravenous (IV) acyclovir. Due to other complications associated with his human immunodeficiency virus (HIV) infection, D.M. has developed renal insufficiency during his hospital course. His SrCr is 4.5 mg/dL (normal, 0.6 to 1.4 mg/dL), and his Cl_{Cr} is 20 mL/min (normal, 80 to 110 mL/min). What are important considerations for dosing acyclovir in D.M. now, and if he required dialysis?

[SI units: SrCr, 397.8 μmol/L (normal, 53.04 to 123.76); ClCr, 0.33 mL/sec (normal, 1.33 to 1.83)]

Acyclovir is used to prevent or treat a variety of viral infections, such as those caused by herpes simplex and varicella zoster viruses.[52] Acyclovir is cleared primarily by the kidneys, with approximately 70% to 80% excreted unchanged in the urine. Dosage adjustment is necessary in patients with renal disease.[16,53] Renal tubular secretion in addition to filtration contributes to the elimination of acyclovir, which explains why the renal clearance of acyclovir is about 3 times greater than the estimated Cl_{cr}.

Acyclovir also can precipitate in the renal tubules and exacerbate D.M.'s renal failure. This is more likely to occur when high doses are infused too rapidly to patients with renal dysfunction.[53] To minimize nephrotoxicity, the patient should be adequately hydrated to maintain good urine flow, and the acyclovir dose should be infused over 1 hour. Nephrotoxicity is usually reversible upon discontinuation of the drug or reduction of the dose.

In addition, acyclovir-associated neurotoxicity correlates with elevated plasma concentrations, and further underscores the need for adequate dosage adjustments in patients with renal dysfunction.[54]

The clearance of acyclovir correlates closely with the Cl_{Cr} according to the following relationship:

$$
\begin{aligned}
&Cl_{acyclovir} \text{ in mL/min/1.73m}^2 \\
&= (3.4)(Cl_{cr} \text{ in mL/min/1.73m}^2) + 28.7
\end{aligned} \qquad (34\text{-}19)
$$

In patients with normal renal function, the clearance of acyclovir ranges from 210 to 330 mL/min; in patients with ESRD, the clearance is 29 to 34 mL/min.[16,53,55] Although this change in clearance is primarily due to decreased renal clearance of the drug, nonrenal clearance of acyclovir also decreases in these patients.[16,55] As a result, the elimination half-life increases significantly from approximately 3 hours in patients with normal kidney function to 20 hours in patients with ESRD. Therefore, doses should be reduced proportionately from a normal daily dose of 15 mg/kg body weight (5 mg/kg given every 8 hours) for serious herpes simplex infections to doses as low as 2.5 mg/kg per day (given as a single daily dose) in patients with ESRD.[56] Because D.M. has a

Cl_{Cr} of 20 mL/min and an estimated $Cl_{acyclovir}$ of 97 mL/min (approximately one-third of normal), a single daily dose of 5 mg/kg (one-third of normal) would be appropriate to treat this infection (see Table 34-2).

Dialysis

Acyclovir is moderately removed by conventional hemodialysis, with plasma concentrations decreasing by 60% after 6 hours of dialysis.[57] The elimination half-life on and off dialysis is 6 and 20 hours respectively, while the dialysis clearance averages 80 mL/min. Therefore, a supplemental dose of 2.5 mg/kg following dialysis is recommended to replace the amount of drug removed by hemodialysis. No data are available on the removal of acyclovir by high-flux dialysis hemodialysis.

Effect of Renal Dysfunction on Metabolism

12. **Does D.M.'s renal dysfunction affect the metabolism of acyclovir? Are there other drugs that are affected similarly?**

Approximately 20% of acyclovir is cleared by nonrenal mechanisms.[16,55] The only significant metabolite that has been isolated is 9-carboxymethoxymethylguanine, which accounts for 9% to 14% of an administered dose. It is believed that this metabolite is a product of hepatic metabolism; however, the kidney may also play an important role.[16] Whether renal dysfunction alters hepatic metabolism or metabolic enzymes present within the kidney is unclear. Recent studies have shown that renal tissue contains many of the same metabolic enzymes found in the liver. Mixed-function oxidases have been found in segments of the proximal tubule, whereas other metabolic processes, such as glucuronidation, acetylation, and hydrolysis, also occur within the kidney.[14,15]

Several studies have examined the effect of renal failure on hepatic metabolic enzyme activity.[58,59] Most of these investigations were carried out in animals that had diminished microsomal, mitochondrial, and cytosolic enzyme activities. Renal dysfunction substantially alters the nonrenal clearance of certain cephalosporins, such as ceftizoxime and cefotaxime,[60–63] as well as the benzodiazepines, diazepam, and desmethyldiazepam.[64,65]

Zidovudine (AZT)
Dosage Adjustment

13. **D.M. also is being treated with AZT for his HIV disease. Will his AZT doses need to be adjusted?**

Zidovudine was the first drug approved for treatment of HIV infection and is still used as part of an antiretroviral regimen. However, because it has potent bone marrow–suppressive effects,[66] the dose of AZT is usually adjusted based on the patient's clinical response and the development of toxicity.

AZT is metabolized primarily by the liver to the inactive glucuronide metabolite, GAZT, which is eliminated by the kidneys. Only 18% of AZT is eliminated unchanged by the kidneys. There is little change in AZT clearance and elimination half-life in patients with renal failure. Two studies report only slight increases in the elimination half-life (from 1.0 to 1.4 hours, and from 1.4 to 1.9 hours in patients with renal failure),[67,68] while another case report measured a half-life of 2.9 hours in a single patient with renal impairment.[69] Although GAZT accumulates in renal disease, this is not clinically important.[67]

Despite little change in AZT plasma levels, patients with renal failure are predisposed to bone marrow suppression because their kidneys produce less erythropoietin. In addition, their white blood cell (WBC) counts are also decreased. Therefore, AZT should be used more cautiously in these patients, with lower starting doses, and careful titration (see Chapter 69, Pharmacotherapy of Human Immunodeficiency Virus Infection).

Hemodialysis

14. **Is AZT significantly removed by dialysis?**

A number of reports describe the removal of AZT by dialysis.[67–69] Based on the chemical characteristics, one would expect that AZT would be dialyzable: it has a low molecular weight of 267, a relatively small Vd (1 to 2.2 L/kg), and low protein binding (34% to 38%). However, the dialysis clearance of AZT is minimal when compared with its plasma clearance in patients with renal failure. Clearance by dialysis averages 63 mL/min compared with a plasma clearance (following oral administration) of approximately 1,200 mL/min. There is little change in the AZT plasma levels during dialysis; however, the elimination of GAZT may be enhanced.[67]

Penicillin
Dosage Adjustment

15. **T.H., a 57-year-old, 85-kg man with chronic renal failure secondary to poorly controlled hypertension, presents to the ED with a 24-hour history of fever (39°C), altered mental status, nausea, and vomiting. On physical examination he was found to have nuchal rigidity and a positive Brudzinski sign. Laboratory analysis revealed the following: WBC count, 22,000/mm³ with 89% neutrophils; BUN, 45 mg/dL; and SrCr, 4.4 mg/dL. A lumbar puncture revealed cerebrospinal fluid (CSF) with a WBC count of 2,000/mm³ (90% polymorphonuclear neutrophils), a glucose concentration of 36 mg/dL, and a protein concentration of 280 mg/dL. Gram-positive diplococci were seen on CSF smear. A diagnosis of meningococcal meningitis was made, and potassium penicillin G was ordered. What dose should be used?**

[SI units: WBC count, 2.2×10^9/L and 0.2×10^9/L, respectively; BUN, 16.065 mmol/L urea; SrCr, 388.96 μmol/L; glucose, 1.998 mmol/L; protein, 2.8 g/L]

Meningococcal meningitis can be treated with 20 to 24 MU (million units) of IV penicillin G in patients with normal renal function. Like many β-lactam antibiotics, penicillin is primarily excreted unchanged in the urine with little or no evidence of hepatic metabolism. Thus, the elimination half-life, which averages <1 hour in patients with normal kidney function, increases to 4 to 10 hours in ESRD patients.[70–72]

Methods to modify the dose of penicillin in renal insufficiency have been developed by numerous investigators. The clearance of penicillin correlates closely to Cl_{Cr} according to the following equation[72]:

$$Cl_{pen} \text{ in mL/min} = 35.5 + 3.35\, Cl_{Cr} \text{ in mL/min} \quad \textbf{(34-20)}$$

This correlation is based on data from patients with varying degrees of renal impairment. An equation to estimate the total daily dose for patients with renal failure to achieve serum levels similar to those produced by high-dose penicillin (20 to 24 MU/day) in patients with normal renal function has been developed for patients with an estimated Cl_{Cr} of <40 mL/min. The dose for T.H. should be given in equal divided doses at 6- or 8-hour intervals:

$$Dose_{pen} \text{ in MU/day} = 3.2 + (Cl_{Cr}/7) \qquad (34\text{-}21)$$

Using the Cockroft and Gault method, T.H.'s Cl_{Cr} is approximately 20 mL/min. Therefore, his daily dose of penicillin should be 6 MU. A dose of 2 MU every 8 hours would be appropriate for T.H.

As is true for many agents, these dosing recommendations are empiric and based on pharmacokinetic principles for patients in renal failure. These recommendations have not been subject to carefully designed clinical trials that establish therapeutic efficacy. Therefore, other factors that can influence host response also should be considered when designing an individualized therapeutic regimen. These include the host's immune status, the presence of other medical conditions, microbial sensitivity patterns, and changes in pharmacokinetic disposition (e.g., concomitant liver disease, fluid overload, dehydration).

Penicillin-Induced Neurotoxicity

16. The medical intern fails to consider T.H.'s renal dysfunction when he prescribes penicillin, and begins a dose of 4 MU Q 4 hr. Four days later, T.H. is encephalopathic (confused, disoriented, and difficult to arouse), with some twitching that is noted on the right side of his face. Are these toxic symptoms associated with high-dose penicillin? What predisposing factors may contribute to this neurotoxicity?

T.H. is experiencing signs of neurotoxicity that are consistent with elevated penicillin concentrations in the plasma and CSF. Penicillin usually produces few serious adverse effects. However, when large doses are used in patients with renal impairment, toxic symptoms such as those exhibited by T.H. can result. Signs and symptoms of penicillin-induced CNS toxicity include myoclonus, complex or generalized seizure activity, and encephalopathy progressing to coma.[32,33]

PREDISPOSING FACTORS

T.H.'s advanced age and renal dysfunction predispose him to penicillin-induced neurotoxicity. In a review of 46 cases of penicillin-associated neurotoxicity, decreased renal function was present in 35 patients.[33] There are several possible explanations for this observation. First, penicillin accumulates in patients with renal failure. Second, the binding of acidic drugs (such as penicillin) to albumin is decreased, resulting in an increased fraction of "free" or active drug that can pass into the CSF. Third, an alteration in the blood–brain barrier has been observed in uremic patients, which can further lead to increases in CSF drug levels.[32] Finally, high plasma concentrations of penicillin per se may contribute to changes in the blood–brain barrier permeability of this drug.[32] All these factors, together with the increased sensitivity of renal failure patients to centrally acting agents, make CNS toxicity more likely. Like penicillin, the carbapenem antibiotic combination, imipenem/cilastatin, is associated with a higher incidence of seizures in patients with renal dysfunction.[73,74]

Antipseudomonal Penicillins
Piperacillin

17. M.H., a 44-year-old, 70-kg woman with acute nonlymphocytic leukemia, is admitted to the oncology ward for placement of a Hickman catheter for her chemotherapy. Seven days following treatment with cytarabine (Ara-C) and daunorubicin, her temperature spiked to 39.4°C. Other physical findings consistent with sepsis included a BP of 109/70 mm Hg, pulse rate of 102 beats/min, and a respiratory rate of 27 breaths/min. M.H. is neutropenic with a WBC count of 1,400/mm³ (3% polymorphonuclear leukocytes, 70% lymphocytes, and 22% monocytes). Her platelet count is 16,000/mm³. M.H. also has renal dysfunction as reflected by a SrCr and BUN of 2.6 and 38 mg/dL, respectively. Empiric therapy for sepsis is started with tobramycin, piperacillin/tazobactam, and vancomycin. How should piperacillin/tazobactam be dosed in M.H.?

[SI units: platelet count, 16 × 10⁹/L; SrCr, 229.84 μmol/L; BUN, 13.566 mmol/L urea]

Piperacillin is an antipseudomonal penicillin that is often used in combination with the aminoglycosides to treat serious infections caused by Gram-negative organisms.[75] Piperacillin is commonly given as a combination with tazobactam, a β-lactamase inhibitor.[76] In patients with normal renal function, piperacillin is primarily excreted unchanged by the kidney with a clearance of 2.6 mL/min per kg, and a half-life of approximately 1 hour.[77,78] Doses of piperacillin/tazobactam can be as high as 4.5 g every 6 hours for the treatment of serious *Pseudomonal* sp. infections. In patients with ESRD, mean piperacillin clearance and half-life values are 0.7 mL/min per kg and 3.3 hours, respectively.[77–79] Although these parameters are significantly different, they are less than those expected for a drug primarily cleared by the kidneys, suggesting that some other compensatory mechanism for elimination must be present. Piperacillin is partially cleared by biliary excretion, a route of elimination that is increased in patients with renal failure.[79,80] Therefore, aggressive dosage reductions in M.H. are unnecessary. An appropriate dose of piperacillin/tazobactam for M.H. would be 3.375 g every 8 hours (see Table 34-2).

Vancomycin
Pharmacokinetic Dosage Calculations

18. In addition to the aforementioned regimen, vancomycin therapy is initiated at 500 mg Q 24 hr to cover the possibility of an infection resistant to antistaphylococcal penicillins such as nafcillin. Is this an appropriate dosing regimen for M.H.?

Vancomycin is a bactericidal antibiotic with excellent activity against most Gram-positive organisms such as methicillin-resistant *Staphylococcus aureus* (MRSA) and *Streptococcus* sp. including some isolates of *Enterococcus faecalis*.[81] It is used empirically in the febrile neutropenic patient, because the incidence of infection secondary to resistant organisms is much higher in this patient population. However, cases of vancomycin-resistant enterococci (VRE) have emerged at rates as high as 50%, raising concern and reducing its empiric use.[82]

Vancomycin is poorly absorbed by the oral route and must be administered intravenously when used to treat systemic infections. Like many other antibiotics, vancomycin primarily is cleared by the kidneys.[83] Significant toxicities have been associated with elevated serum concentrations, making careful dosing modification in renal failure necessary.[84]

As with the aminoglycosides, pharmacokinetic calculations are used to individualize a dosing regimen to produce the desired peak and trough plasma levels. Unlike the aminoglycosides, the therapeutic range for vancomycin is less clear. Normally, doses are designed to achieve peak levels of 25 to 40 mg/L and trough levels of 10 to 15 mg/L.[85,86] The correlation between vancomycin toxicity (such as ototoxicity) and plasma levels is not well defined. However, some clinicians have suggested that plasma levels ≥80 mg/L may correlate with auditory dysfunction.

Vancomycin has an elimination half-life of 3 to 9 hours in patients with normal renal function.[87] This increases to 129 to 189 hours in patients with ESRD.[88–90] Using pharmacokinetic principles and considering that the plasma clearance of vancomycin is approximately 60% to 70% of Cl_{Cr}[85] and the Vd averages 0.7 L/kg,[87,91,92] the estimated Vd_{vanco} and Cl_{vanco} can be calculated using the following equation:

$$Cl_{cr} = 30.5 \text{ mL/min (calculated from Eq. 34-3)}$$

$$
\begin{aligned}
Cl_{vanco} &= (0.65)(Cl_{cr}) \\
&= (0.65)(30.5 \text{ mL/min}) \\
&= 19.8 \text{ mL/min } or \text{ rounded off to 1.2 L/hr}
\end{aligned}
\tag{34-22}
$$

$$
\begin{aligned}
Vd_{vanco} &= (0.7 \text{ L/kg})(\text{Body Weight}) \\
&= (0.7 \text{ L/kg})(70 \text{ kg}) \\
&= 49 \text{ L}
\end{aligned}
\tag{34-23}
$$

Based on estimated values for Cl_{vanco} and Vd_{vanco}, the elimination rate constant can be calculated using the following equation:

$$
\begin{aligned}
Kd &= \frac{Cl_{vanco}}{Vd_{vanco}} \\
&= \frac{1.2 \text{ L/hr}}{49 \text{ L}} \\
&= 0.024 \text{ hr}^{-1}
\end{aligned}
\tag{34-24}
$$

$$
\begin{aligned}
Cp_{peak} &= \frac{\dfrac{\text{Dose}}{Vd_{vanco}}}{1 - e^{-Kd\tau}} \\
&= \frac{\dfrac{500 \text{ mg}}{49 \text{ L}}}{1 - e^{-(0.024 \text{ hr}^{-1})(24 \text{ hr})}} \\
&= 23 \text{ mg/L}
\end{aligned}
\tag{34-25}
$$

$$
\begin{aligned}
Cp_{trough} &= Cp_{peak}(e^{-Kd\tau}) \\
&= 23 \text{ mg/L}(e^{-(0.024/hr^{-1})(24hr)}) \\
&= 13 \text{ mg/L}
\end{aligned}
\tag{34-26}
$$

Because M.H.'s estimated peak concentration is <40 mg/L and her trough falls within the range of 10 to 15 mg/L, the starting dose of 500 mg every 24 hours is appropriate for M.H.

Routine monitoring of plasma vancomycin concentrations in patients with normal renal function is controversial because the likelihood that toxicity will develop in this group is relatively low. However, in patients with renal failure, such as M.H., it is advisable to measure vancomycin levels several days after initiation of therapy to ensure that they are within an acceptable range.[87,89,90,93] This is prudent if an extended course of therapy is anticipated. Vancomycin is usually infused over 60 minutes. Because there is a distribution phase, plasma samples should be drawn at least 30 minutes after the end of the infusion.

Hemodialysis

19. **Unfortunately, M.H.'s renal function begins to deteriorate so that she requires hemodialysis. How should her regimen now be altered?**

Patients with ESRD may have measurable vancomycin levels for up to 3 weeks following a single dose despite conventional hemodialysis.[90] This suggests that the ability of these patients to eliminate vancomycin is minimal and that little of the drug is removed by conventional hemodialysis. The elimination half-life for vancomycin in these individuals averaged 5 to 7 days, which is consistent with a residual vancomycin clearance in these patients of 3 to 4 mL/min.[88–90] Only about 5% of vancomycin is metabolized hepatically in patients with normal renal function.

Conventional hemodialysis removes about 7% of vancomycin during a typical 4-hour dialysis run.[94] The elimination half-life on and off dialysis, and plasma levels of the drug before and after hemodialysis are not significantly different. The poor removal of vancomycin by conventional hemodialysis is due to its large molecular weight of 1,400.

Patients receiving conventional hemodialysis are typically given a single, 1 g dose every 7 to 10 days.[87,90,93] Based on M.H.'s estimated Vd of 49 L, this dose will produce an initial peak plasma level of approximately 20 mg/L. If vancomycin is administered weekly, steady-state peak and trough levels of 40 and 16 mg/L, respectively, would be predicted.

Vancomycin is removed to a greater extent by high-flux hemodialysis than by conventional hemodialysis. As a result, more frequent dosing is necessary to maintain therapeutic vancomycin concentrations. High-flux dialysis clearance of vancomycin using the Fresenius polysulfone dialyzer is 45 to 160 mL/min and varies with membrane surface area.[48,95] Up to 50% of a dose of vancomycin is removed over 4 hours by high-flux hemodialysis compared with 6.9% using conventional dialysis. A rebound phenomenon following dialysis suggests that the total amount of drug removed may be less than initially reported.[96,97] In any case, the efficiency of high-flux procedures in removing vancomycin is greater than that of conventional dialysis. Therefore, plasma levels should be monitored carefully in these patients, and the necessity for postdialysis replacement doses of around 500 mg (approximately 10 to 15 mg/kg) should be anticipated.

Amphotericin
Dosing

20. **M.H. continues to be febrile despite her triple antimicrobial regimen. Amphotericin therapy is started empirically for a potential fungal infection. In addition, pentamidine is begun to cover *Pneumocystis carinii* pneumonia. How should amphotericin be administered in patients like M.H. with renal dysfunction?**

Amphotericin is an antifungal agent used to treat serious infections such as invasive Aspergillosis and cryptococcal meningitis. The exact mechanism of elimination for this drug is unclear but may involve hepatic metabolism or inactivation in body tissues. Small amounts of amphotericin are gradually excreted in the urine for several weeks following its discontinuation.[98] This slow elimination may be due to the extensive distribution of amphotericin into peripheral tissue and its large Vd (4 L/kg).[98,99] The drug appears to bind to cholesterol-containing cytoplasmic membranes of various tissues, resulting in a very long elimination half-life of 15 days. Pharmacokinetic studies report no significant change in the disposition of amphotericin in patients with renal or liver disease. Therefore, no dosage adjustments are required in patients with renal dysfunction.

Amphotericin is associated with acute tubular necrosis (ATN), which is believed to be dose dependent.[100–102] To prevent exacerbation of nephrotoxicity, lower doses often are administered to patients with decreased renal function. Administration of amphotericin every other day often is suggested for patients with renal failure. In addition to conventional amphotericin, a liposomal (liposomal amphotericin) or lipid-based formulation is available.[18] Lipid-based formulations have reduced distribution to the kidneys, and are associated with a lower incidence of nephrotoxicity.[103]

Hemodialysis

Amphotericin is not removed significantly by hemodialysis because it is a very large compound and distributes widely into peripheral tissues. Therefore, little drug remains in the plasma to be removed by dialysis. Studies have found that <5% of amphotericin is removed during a 4-hour conventional hemodialysis period.

Phenytoin
Protein Binding

21. R.S., a 24-year-old man with ESRD from rapidly progressive glomerulonephritis, is managed by hemodialysis three times weekly. He has a 7-year history of generalized tonic-clonic seizures and has been treated with phenytoin. He presents to the ED after having suffered a seizure lasting about 5 minutes. His mother states that he ran out of phenytoin 4 weeks ago. Because his plasma phenytoin concentration on admission was <2.5 μg/mL, R.S. is given an IV loading dose of phenytoin: 15 mg/kg over 30 minutes. Additional admission laboratory work includes the following: SrCr, 8.6 mg/dL (normal, 0.6 to 1.4); BUN, 110 mg/dL (normal, 7 to 20); potassium, 5.4 mEq/L; calcium, 9 mg/dL; and albumin, 2.9 g/dL. Eight hours after administration of phenytoin, his level is 5 μg/mL. Is this level subtherapeutic?

[SI units: phenytoin, <10 and 19.82 μmol/L, respectively; SrCr, 760.24 μmol/L (normal, 53.04 to 123.76); BUN, 39.27 mmol/L urea (normal, 2.5 to 7.14); potassium, 5.4 mmol/L; calcium, 2.24 mmol/L; albumin, 29 g/L]

R.S. has severe renal disease, which will affect how the total (bound plus free) phenytoin concentrations are measured. Decreased plasma protein binding will result in lower measured total phenytoin concentrations, and the calculated apparent volume of distribution may increase. In patients with normal renal function, approximately 90% of the measured phenytoin is bound to albumin, and 10% is free. The free fraction of phenytoin is increased to about 20% to 25% in patients with uremia.[9,104–108] Since the free fraction for phenytoin is increased in patients with uremia, lower plasma concentrations will produce therapeutic effects which will be equivalent to

those produced by higher phenytoin concentrations in patients with normal renal function.[6,109] Phenytoin is an acidic drug that is bound primarily to albumin. A number of mechanisms have been proposed that account for the decreased binding, including (1) decreased albumin concentration, (2) accumulation of uremic by-products that displace acidic drugs from their binding sites, and (3) alteration in the conformation or structure of albumin in uremic patients, resulting in a reduced number of binding sites or decreased affinity for drugs (see Chapter 54, Seizure Disorders). Other acidic drugs with altered protein binding in renal disease are listed in Table 34-1.

Figure 34-4 illustrates changes in phenytoin levels when uremic and nonuremic patients are given equivalent doses.[110]

The following equation should be used to correct for R.S.'s altered binding due to his renal dysfunction and hypoalbuminemia.[107]

$$Cp_{Normal\ Binding} = \frac{Cp'}{(0.48)(1 - \alpha)\left(\dfrac{P'}{P_{NL}}\right) + \alpha} \quad \text{(34-27)}$$

where Cp′ is the measured plasma concentration reported by the laboratory, and $Cp_{NormalBinding}$ is the corrected plasma concentration that would be seen if the patient had normal renal function and normal albumin. Alpha (α) is the normal free fraction (0.1), P' is the patient's serum albumin, and P_{NL} is normal albumin (4.4 g/dL). The factor 0.48 was derived from hemodialysis patients and represents the decreased affinity of phenytoin for albumin.

For R.S., 5 μg/mL is comparable to 12 μg/mL in a patient without renal failure. Because this falls within the phenytoin's therapeutic range of 10 to 20 μg/mL, his measured level is not subtherapeutic.

The factor 0.48 should be used only to estimate changes in protein binding for patients with ESRD receiving hemodialysis. Data for patients with moderate renal disease are limited, and it is unclear what changes exist in the binding of phenytoin to albumin.[107] For patients with normal or moderate renal

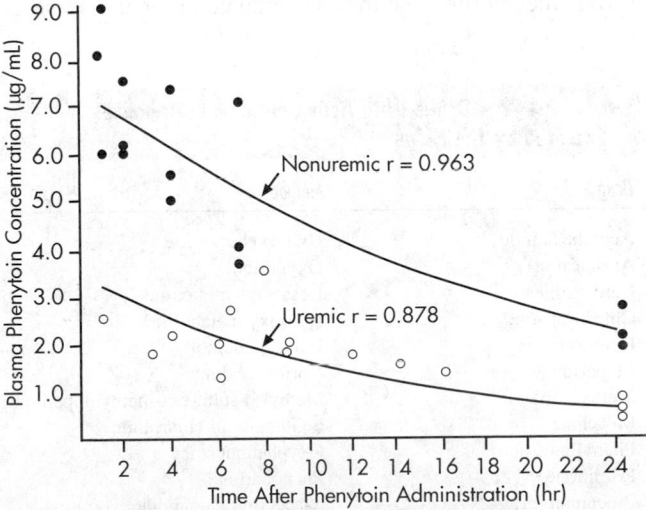

FIGURE 34-4 Plasma phenytoin concentrations in uremic (o) and nonuremic (•) patients following 250 mg of IV phenytoin. (Reproduced with permission from Letteri JM et al. Diphenylhydantoin metabolism in uremia. N Engl J Med 1971;285:648.)

impairment, the following equation should be used only if the serum albumin is low; the factor 0.48 should be omitted:

$$Cp_{\text{Normal Binding}} = \frac{Cp'}{(1 - \alpha)\left(\dfrac{P'}{P_{NL}}\right) + \alpha} \qquad (34\text{-}28)$$

EFFECT OF RENAL FAILURE ON METABOLIZED DRUGS
Meperidine

22. F.G., a 56-year-old woman, is admitted for a cervical laminectomy. She has a history of chronic renal insufficiency (Cl_{Cr} = 20 mL/min) and arrhythmias that are treated with procainamide. Her admission laboratory values are as follows: SrCr, 4.4 mg/dL (normal, 0.6 to 1.3 mg/dL); BUN, 66 mg/dL (normal, 7 to 20 mg/dL); Hct, 34%; and Hgb, 12.6 g/dL.

Following surgery, she complains of severe pain and is treated with meperidine 50 to 100 mg IM Q 3 to 4 hr. Three days postoperatively, F.G. experiences a generalized tonic-clonic seizure. She has no history of seizures. What might be responsible for this sudden event?

[SI units: SrCr, 388.96 μmol/L (normal, 53 to 114.92); BUN, 23.6 mmol/L urea (normal, 2.5 to 7.14); Hct, 0.34 1; Hgb, 126 g/L]

Meperidine is a narcotic analgesic commonly used to control acute pain. It is metabolized hepatically via *N*-demethylation to normeperidine, a metabolite known to accumulate in renal insufficiency.[12,111] Although meperidine has both CNS excitatory and depressant properties, normeperidine is a very potent CNS stimulant that can cause seizures in renal failure patients receiving multiple doses of the parent drug.[112] In a study of 67 cancer patients treated with meperidine, 48 developed neurologic adverse effects; 14 of these 48 patients had renal dysfunction defined as a BUN >20 mg/dL.[112] Because the renal clearance of normeperidine correlates significantly with Cl_{Cr}, renal dysfunction can lead to its accumulation, resulting in neurologic toxicity. In another study, the normeperidine:meperidine plasma concentration ratio was consistently higher in patients with renal failure, averaging 2.0 compared with a mean of 0.6 for patients with good renal function.[112] Table 34-4 lists examples of additional drugs that have active or toxic metabolites that may accumulate in renal disease.

Table 34-4	Drugs With Active or Toxic Metabolites Excreted by the Kidney
Drug	**Metabolite**
Acetohexamide	Hydroxyhexamide
Allopurinol	Oxypurinol
Cefotaxime	Desacetylcefotaxime
Chlorpropamide	Hydroxy metabolites
Daunorubicin	Daunorubicinol
Meperidine	Normeperidine
Methyldopa	Methyl-o-sulfate-α-methyldopamine
Morphine	6-Glucuronide morphine
Phenylbutazone	Oxyphenbutazone
Primidone	Phenobarbital
Procainamide	*N*-acetylprocainamide
Propoxyphene	Norpropoxyphene
Rifampicin	Desacetylated metabolites
Sodium nitroprusside	Thiocyanate
Sulfonamides	Acetylated metabolites

Narcotic Analgesics

23. Are the pharmacokinetics or pharmacodynamics of other narcotic analgesics altered in patients with renal insufficiency?

Morphine
The pharmacokinetic disposition of morphine does not appear to be altered in patients with renal failure;[113] however, its active metabolite, morphine-6-glucuronide as well as its principal metabolite, morphine-3-glucuronide, do accumulate in renal disease. The elimination half-life of morphine-6-glucuronide increases from 3 to 4 hours in normal subjects to 89 to 136 hours in subjects with renal failure.[114] This metabolite penetrates the blood brain barrier more readily, has a greater affinity for CNS receptors, and has analgesic activity that is 3.7 times greater than morphine.[115] Therefore, accumulation of morphine-6-glucuronide may be responsible for the morphine-induced narcosis reported in patients with severe renal disease.[28,29]

Codeine
Other analgesics that have been associated with CNS toxicity in patients with renal failure include codeine, propoxyphene, and dihydrocodeine.[116] The disposition of orally administered codeine does not appear to be altered in renal failure; however, two cases of codeine-induced narcosis have been reported.[117] Even though the dose of codeine did not exceed 120 mg/day, CNS and respiratory depression persisted for up to 4 days after discontinuation of codeine, and naloxone administration.

Guay and colleagues[118] reported a prolonged terminal elimination half-life for intravenous codeine in chronic hemodialysis patients of 18.7 ± 9 hours versus 4 ± 0.6 hours in subjects with normal renal function. Although the total body clearance was not significantly decreased, the Vd for codeine was approximately twice as large in the dialysis group. The clinical significance of these alterations is not known.

Propoxyphene
Propoxyphene and its metabolite, norpropoxyphene accumulate in renal insufficiency. Norpropoxyphene is eliminated by the kidneys, and its elimination half-life is prolonged in patients with renal failure; however, the half-life of propoxyphene remains unchanged. Accumulation of propoxyphene is thought to be due to decreased first-pass metabolism or systemic clearance. Similar pharmacokinetic changes have been observed in patients experiencing dihydrocodeine-associated narcosis.[119,120] The accumulation of these compounds may be associated with CNS and cardiac toxicities in subjects with renal failure, especially after multiple doses.[115] Therefore, these drugs also should be avoided in patients with renal failure.

Procainamide

24. F.G.'s procainamide level is 9 μg/mL (normal, 4 to 8 μg/mL) and her *N*-acetylprocainamide (NAPA) level is 34 μg/mL (normal, 10 to 20 μg/mL). How is the disposition of procainamide affected in patients with renal disease?

[SI units: procainamide level 38.24 mmol/L (normal, 17 to 34)]

The pharmacokinetics of procainamide in patients with renal insufficiency are complex. Fifty to 70% of the parent drug is excreted unchanged in the urine, and it can accumulate in patients with renal disease because plasma clearance values are reduced by as much as 70%.[121] Procainamide (PA) is also partially acetylated to NAPA, which has antiarrhythmic properties similar to procainamide and is primarily excreted by the kidneys.[122,123] Figure 34-5 summarizes the elimination of procainamide and NAPA. The half-life of NAPA is longer, especially in patients with renal impairment, increasing from 6 hours in control subjects to as long as 40 hours in patients with ESRD.[121,122] Because significant cardiac toxicity has occurred in some patients with NAPA levels >30 μg/mL, plasma level monitoring of NAPA as well as procainamide is recommended. When procainamide is used in patients with renal failure, appropriate dosage reduction of procainamide may be necessary. It also is important to realize that the time required to reach steady-state for NAPA in patients with renal failure may be as long as 5 days. Therefore, plasma levels measured early in therapy must be interpreted carefully, as these concentrations may be considerably lower than those that will be achieved under steady-state conditions.

Nonsteroidal Anti-Inflammatory Drugs

25. **F.G.'s physician would like to manage her pain with ibuprofen 400 mg Q 6 hr PRN. What factors should be considered when treating renal failure patients with nonsteroidal anti-inflammatory drugs (NSAIDs)?**

Because NSAIDs have been associated with nephrotoxicity, they should be used cautiously in patients with renal disease.[124] The clinical features of nephrotoxicity are variable, and can present acutely or chronically with or without oliguria. Pathologic changes due to these drugs also are variable and range from interstitial nephritis to acute tubular necrosis.[124,125] Mechanisms for NSAID-induced nephrotoxicity include inhibition of renal prostaglandin synthesis, leading to altered renal blood flow and ischemia.[126,127] Renal impairment may be more likely to occur in patients who have abnormally high plasma levels of vasoconstrictor hormones (e.g., angiotensin II and catecholamines).[125] Since there is a compensatory increase in the synthesis of vasodilatory renal prostaglandins to counteract the vasoconstriction, blockade of this increase by an NSAID can lead to ischemic changes and acute renal failure (See Chapter 31, Acute Renal Failure).

A second proposed mechanism involves an autoimmune response that is triggered by changes in cell-mediated immunity.[128] These changes are due to similar alterations in prostaglandin synthesis by NSAIDs. Although data are limited, sulindac is a NSAID believed to have renal-sparing effects. Unlike other NSAIDs, studies suggest that this drug does not inhibit synthesis of renal prostaglandins.[129]

NSAIDs accumulate in renal insufficiency, an interesting finding because renal elimination is negligible for these drugs.[130] These compounds primarily are metabolized to an acyl-glucuronide metabolite that accumulates in renal failure patients. This metabolite is unstable, and can deconjugate, leading to increased levels of parent drug. This phenomenon is represented in Figure 34-6. Of additional importance is the fact that many of the NSAIDs are available as racemic mixtures, with the pharmacologic activity residing primarily with the S-enantiomer. The R-enantiomer can convert selectively to the S-enantiomer particularly at elevated levels, leading to even greater pharmacologic activity in patients with renal dysfunction.[131,132] This reconversion phenomenon also has been reported for clofibric acid.[133]

Enoxaparin

26. **Since F.G. is not ambulating well after her surgery, her physician would like to initiate deep vein thrombosis prophylaxis with enoxaparin. Are there any dosing considerations for enoxaparin in this patient?**

Enoxaparin is a low-molecular weight heparin (LMWH) that is used to prevent and treat various thromboembolic

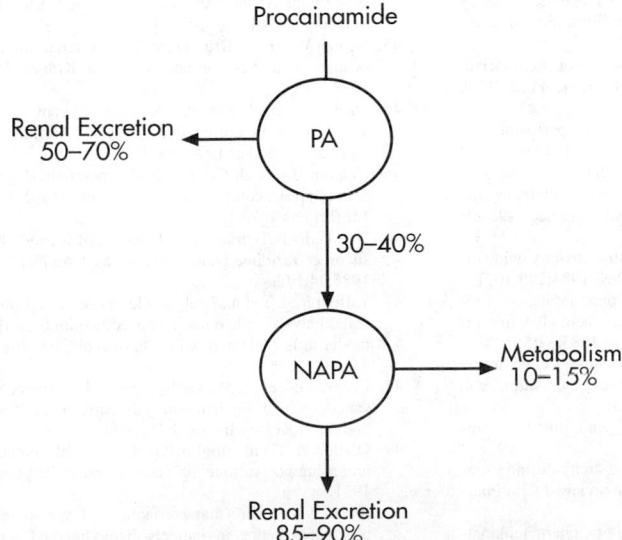

FIGURE 34-5 Elimination of procainamide (PA) and *N*-acetylprocainamide (NAPA) in subjects with normal renal and liver function.

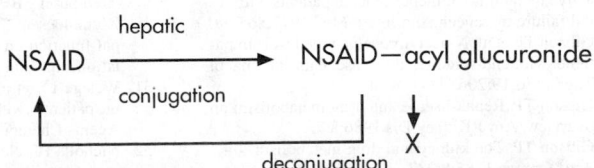

FIGURE 34-6 Schematic representation of pathways of elimination of acyl-glucuronide metabolites or arylpropionic nonsteroidal anti-inflammatory drugs. (Reproduced with permission from Brater DC. Renal disease. In: Williams R et al., eds. Rational Therapeutics. New York: Marcel Dekker, 1990. Copyright 2001 Massachusetts Medical Society. All rights reserved.)

disorders such as deep venous thrombosis, unstable angina, and non–Q-wave myocardial infarction. The kidneys play a major role in the clearance of enoxaparin,[134] and there is a higher incidence of bleeding complications associated with the use of enoxaparin in patients with renal dysfunction.[135] The elimination half-life of enoxaparin is prolonged in patients with ESRD, although the other pharmacokinetic parameters are similar to healthy subjects.[136,137] The increased incidence of bleeding complications cannot be completely attributed to pharmacokinetic changes, but may also be related to the effects of enoxaparin on anti-factor IIa and antithrombin III, as well as the effects of uremia on hemostasis.[138]

Enoxaparin should be used cautiously in patients with a $Cl_{cr} < 30$ mL/min. Although monitoring the anticoagulant effect by anti-Xa activity is not necessary in clinically stable patients, it may be warranted in patients with renal dysfunction as well as those who have other factors that may increase the risk of bleeding complications.

SUMMARY

The kidneys play a vital role in maintaining homeostasis by regulating the excretion of water, electrolytes, and metabolic byproducts. In addition, the kidneys are the primary route of elimination for many drugs. Pharmacokinetic changes such as altered bioavailability, protein binding, drug distribution, and elimination can occur with many drugs in patients with renal failure. Pharmacodynamic changes such as altered sensitivity or response to medications can also occur in this patient population. Renal replacement therapies such as hemodialysis, continuous ambulatory peritoneal dialysis, and continuous arteriovenous hemofiltration will not only aid in the removal of fluid, electrolytes, and metabolic byproducts, but drugs as well. Data from clinical trials provide valuable information about the disposition of drugs in patients with renal failure. Pharmacokinetic principles should be applied when appropriate to determine the optimal dose of drugs for patients with renal failure.

REFERENCES

1. Gambertoglio JG. Effects of renal disease: altered pharmacokinetics. In: Benet LZ et al., eds. Pharmacokinetic Basis for Drug Treatment. New York: Raven Press, 1984.
2. Bianchetti GM et al. Pharmacokinetics and effects of propranolol in terminal uremic patients and patients undergoing regular dialysis treatment. Clin Pharmacokinet 1978;1:373.
3. Wood AJ et al. Propranolol disposition in renal failure. Br J Clin Pharmacol 1980;10:562.
4. Pichette V, Leblond FA. Drug metabolism in chronic renal failure. Curr Drug Metab 2003;4:91.
5. Barnes JN et al. Dihydrocodeine in renal insufficiency: further evidence for an important role of the kidney in handling of opioid drugs. Br Med J 1985;290:740.
6. Reidenberg MM. The binding of drugs to plasma proteins and the interpretation of measurements of plasma concentrations of drugs in patients with poor renal function. Am J Med 1977;62:466.
7. Lam FYW et al. Principles of drug administration in renal insufficiency. Clin Pharmacokinet 1997;32:30.
8. Boobis SW. Alteration of plasma albumin in relation to decreased drug binding in uremia. Clin Pharmacol Ther 1977;22:147.
9. Reidenberg MM et al. Protein binding of diphenylhydantoin and desmethylimipramine in plasma from patients with poor renal function. N Engl J Med 1971;285:264.
10. Jusko WJ, Weintraub M. Myocardial distribution of digoxin and renal function. Clin Pharmacol Ther 1977;16:448.
11. Verbeeck RK et al. Drug metabolites in renal failure. Clin Pharmacokinet 1981;6:329.
12. Szeto HH et al. Accumulation of normeperidine, an active metabolite of meperidine, in patients with renal failure or cancer. Ann Intern Med 1977;86:738.
13. Gibson TP et al. N-acetylprocainamide levels in patients with end-stage renal disease. Clin Pharmacol Ther 1976;19:206.
14. Gibson TP. Renal disease and drug metabolism: an overview. Am J Kidney Dis 1986;8:7.
15. Gibson TP. The kidney and drug metabolism. Int J Artif Organs 1985;8:237.
16. Laskin OL et al. Acyclovir kinetics in end-stage renal disease. Clin Pharmacol Ther 1982;31:594.
17. Willems L et al. Itraconazole oral solution and intravenous formulations: a review of pharmacokinetics and pharmacodynamics. J Clin Pharmacol Ther 2001;26:159.

18. Boswell GW et al. AmBisome (liposomal amphotericin B): a comparative review. J Clin Pharmacol 1998;38(7):583.
19. Gibson TP, Nelson HA. Drug kinetics and artificial kidneys. Clin Pharmacokinet 1977;2:403.
20. Gwilt PR, Perrier D. Plasma protein binding and distribution characteristics of drugs as indices of their hemodialyzability. Clin Pharmacol Ther 1978;24:154.
21. Amin NB et al. Characterization of gentamicin pharmacokinetics in patients hemodialyzed with high-flux polysulfone membranes. Am J Kidney Dis 1999;34:222.
22. Aweeka FT et al. Effect of renal disease and hemodialysis on foscarnet pharmacokinetics and dosing recommendations. J AIDS Retrovirol 1999;20:350.
23. Keller E et al. Drug therapy in patients undergoing continuous ambulatory peritoneal dialysis: clinical pharmacokinetic considerations. Clin Pharmacokinet 1990;18(2):104.
24. Bickley SK. Drug dosing during continuous arteriovenous hemofiltration. Clin Pharm 1988;7:198.
25. Golper TA et al. Removal of therapeutic drugs by continuous arteriovenous hemofiltration. Arch Intern Med 1985;145:1651.
26. Pond S et al. Pharmacokinetics of hemoperfusion for drug overdose. Clin Pharmacokinet 1979;4:329.
27. Panzarino VM et al. Charcoal hemoperfusion in a child with vancomycin overdose and chronic renal failure. Pediatr Nephrol 1998;12(1):63.
28. Bigler D et al. Prolonged respiratory depression caused by slow release morphine. Lancet 1984;1:1477.
29. Shelly MP, Park GR. Morphine toxicity with dilated pupils. Br Med J (Clin Res) 1984;289:1071.
30. Kleinbloesem CH et al. Nifedipine: influence of renal function on pharmacokinetic/hemodynamic relationship. Clin Pharmacol Ther 1985;37:563.
31. Welage LS et al. Pharmacokinetics of ceftazidime in patients with renal insufficiency. Antimicrob Agents Chemother 1984;25:201.
32. Nicholls PJ. Neurotoxicity of penicillin. J Antimicrob Chemother 1980;6:161.
33. Fossieck B, Parker RH. Neurotoxicity during intravenous infusion of penicillin: a review. J Clin Pharmacol 1974;14:504.
34. Gentry LO. Antimicrobial activity, pharmacokinetics, therapeutic indications and adverse reactions of ceftazidime. Pharmacotherapy 1985;5(5):254.

35. Dahlgre JG et al. Gentamicin blood levels: a guide to nephrotoxicity. Antimicrob Agents Chemother 1975;8:58.
36. Goodman EI et al. Prospective comparative study of variable dosage and variable frequency regimens for administration of gentamicin. Antimicrob Agents Chemother 1975;8:434.
37. Sawchuk RJ et al. Kinetic model for gentamicin dosing with the use of individual patient parameters. Clin Pharmacol Ther 1977;21:362.
38. Zaske DE et al. Gentamicin pharmacokinetics in 1,640 patients: method for control of serum concentrations. Antimicrob Agents Chemother 1982;21:407.
39. McHenry MC et al. Gentamicin dosages for renal insufficiency. Ann Intern Med 1971;74:192.
40. Sheiner LB et al. Forecasting individual pharmacokinetics. Clin Pharmacol Ther 1979;26:294.
41. Cockroft DW, Gault MH. Prediction of creatinine clearance from serum creatinine. Nephron 1976;16:31.
42. Matzke GR, Keane WF. Use of antibiotics in renal failure. In: Peterson PK, Verhoef J, eds. The Antimicrobial Agents Annual. Amsterdam: Elsevier Science, 1986:472.
43. Bennet WM et al. Drug prescribing in renal failure: dosing guidelines for adults. Am J Kidney Dis 1983;3:155.
44. Danish M et al. Pharmacokinetics of gentamicin and kanamycin during hemodialysis. Antimicrob Agents Chemother 1974;6:841.
45. Halpren BA et al. Clearance of gentamicin during hemodialysis: comparison of four artificial kidneys. J Infect Dis 1976;133:627.
46. Nikolaidis P, Tourkantonis A. Effect of hemodialysis on ceftazidime pharmacokinetics. Clin Nephrol 1985;24:142.
47. Toffelmire EB et al. Dialysis clearance in high flux hemodialysis with reuse using ceftazidime as the model drug [abstract]. Clin Pharmacol Ther 1989;45:160.
48. Lanese DM et al. Markedly increased clearance of vancomycin during hemodialysis using polysulfone dialyzers. Kidney Int 1989;35:1409.
49. O'Hara K, Gambertoglio JG. Removal of gentamicin using polysulfone dialyzers. Unpublished data. 1991.
50. Amin NB et al. Characterization of gentamicin pharmacokinetics in patients hemodialyzed with high-flux polysulfone membranes. Am J Kidney Dis 1999;34:222.

51. Somani P et al. Unidirectional absorption of gentamicin from the peritoneum during continuous ambulatory peritoneal dialysis. Clin Pharmacol Ther 1982;32:113.

52. Richards DM et al. Acyclovir: a review of its pharmacodynamic properties and therapeutic efficacy. Drugs 1983;26:378.

53. Blum MR et al. Overview of acyclovir pharmacokinetic disposition in adults and children. Am J Med Acyclovir Symposium 1982;73:186.

54. Almond MK et al. Avoiding acyclovir neurotoxicity in patients with chronic renal failure undergoing hemodialysis. Nephron 1995;69:428.

55. Laskin OL et al. Effect of renal failure on the pharmacokinetics of acyclovir. Am J Med Acyclovir Symposium 1982;73:197.

56. Jayasekara D et al. Antiviral therapy for HIV patients with renal insufficiency. J AIDS Hum Retrovirol 1999;21(5):384.

57. Krasny HC et al. Influence of hemodialysis on acyclovir pharmacokinetics in patients with chronic renal failure. Am J Med Acyclovir Symposium 1982;73(1A):202.

58. Patterson SE, Cohn VH. Hepatic drug metabolism in rats with experimental chronic renal failure. Biochem Pharmacol 1984;33:711.

59. Van Peer AP, Belpaire FM. Hepatic oxidative drug metabolism in rats with experimental renal failure. Arch Intern Pharmacodyn Ther 1977; 228:180.

60. Ings RMJ et al. The pharmacokinetics of cefotaxime and its metabolites in subjects with normal and impaired renal function. Rev Infect Dis 1982; 4(Suppl):S379.

61. Fillastre JP et al. Pharmacokinetics of cefotaxime in subjects with normal and impaired renal function. J Antimicrob Chemother 1980;6(Suppl):S103.

62. Cuttler RE et al. Pharmacokinetics of ceftizoxime. J Antimicrob Chemother 1982;10(Suppl):S91.

63. Gibson TP et al. Imipenem/cilastatin: pharmacokinetics profile in renal insufficiency. Am J Med 1985;78:54.

64. Ochs HR et al. Clorazepate dipotassium and diazepam in renal insufficiency: serum concentrations and protein binding of diazepam and desmethyldiazepam. Nephron 1984;37:100.

65. Ochs HR et al. Diazepam kinetics in patients with renal insufficiency or hyperthyroidism. Br J Clin Pharmacol 1981;12:829.

66. Richman DD et al. The toxicity of azidothymidine (AZT) in the treatment of patients with AIDS and AIDS-related complex: a double-blind, placebo-controlled trial. N Engl J Med 1987;317:192.

67. Singlas E et al. Zidovudine disposition in patients with renal impairment: influence of hemodialysis. Clin Pharmacol Ther 1989;46:190.

68. Garraffo R et al. Influence of hemodialysis on zidovudine (AZT) and its glucuronide (GAZT) pharmacokinetics: two case reports. Int J Clin Pharmacol Ther Toxicol 1989;27:535.

69. Tartaglione TA et al. Zidovudine disposition during hemodialysis with acquired immunodeficiency syndrome. J AIDS Hum Retrovirol 1990;3:32.

70. Barza M, Weinstein L. Pharmacokinetics of the penicillins in man. Clin Pharmacokinet 1976;1:297.

71. Gambertoglio J et al. Use of drugs in patients with renal failure. In: Schrrew RW, Gottschalk CW, eds. Diseases of the Kidney. 5th Ed. Boston: Little, Brown, 1993:3211.

72. Bryan CS, Stone WJ. "Comparably massive" penicillin gm therapy in renal failure. Ann Intern Med 1975;82:189.

73. Calandra G et al. Factors predisposing to seizures in seriously ill infected patients receiving antibiotics: experience with imipenem/cilastatin. Am J Med 1988;84:911.

74. Norby SR. Carbapenems in serious infections: a risk-benefit assessment. Drug Saf 2000;22:191.

75. Reyes MP, Lerner AM. Current problems in the treatment of infective endocarditis due to Pseudomonas aeruginosa. Rev Infect Dis 1983;5:314.

76. Perry CM, Markham A. Piperacillin/tazobactam: an updated review of its use in the treatment of bacterial infections. Drugs 1999;57(5):805.

77. Aronoff GR et al. The effect of piperacillin dose on elimination kinetics in renal impairment. Eur J Clin Pharmacol 1983;24:453.

78. Welling PG et al. Pharmacokinetics of piperacillin in subjects with various degrees of renal function. Antimicrob Agents Chemother 1983;23:881.

79. Thompson MI et al. Piperacillin pharmacokinetics in subjects with chronic renal failure. Antimicrob Agents Chemother 1981;19:450.

80. Giron JA et al. Biliary concentrations of piperacillin in patients undergoing cholecystectomy. Antimicrob Agents Chemother 1981;19:309.

81. Fejkety R. Vancomycin. Med Clin North Am 1982;284:1508.

82. Austin DJ et al. Vancomycin-resistant enterococci in intensive-care hospital setting; transmission dynamics, persistence, and the impact of infection control programs. Proc Natl Acad Sci U S A 1999; 96(12):6908.

83. Moellering RC et al. Pharmacokinetics of vancomycin in normal subjects and in patients with reduced renal function. Rev Infect Dis 1981; 3(Suppl):S230.

84. Farber BF, Moellering RC Jr. Retrospective study of the toxicity of preparations of vancomycin from 1974 to 1981. Antimicrob Agents Chemother 1983; 23:138.

85. Rotschafer JC et al. Pharmacokinetics of vancomycin: observations in 28 patients and dosage recommendations. Antimicrob Agents Chemother 1982; 22:391.

86. MacGowan AP. Pharmacodynamics, pharmacokinetics, and therapeutic drug monitoring of glycopeptides. Ther Drug Monit 1998;20(5):473.

87. Matzke GR et al. Clinical pharmacokinetics of vancomycin. Clin Pharmacokinet 1986;11:257.

88. Tan CC et al. Pharmacokinetics of intravenous vancomycin in patients with end-stage renal failure. Ther Drug Monit 1990;12:29.

89. Golper TA et al. Vancomycin pharmacokinetics, renal handling and non-renal clearances in normal human subjects. Clin Pharmacol Ther 1988;43:565.

90. Cunha BA et al. Pharmacokinetics of vancomycin in anuria. Rev Infect Dis 1981;3(Suppl)S269.

91. Krogstad DJ et al. Single-dose kinetics of intravenous vancomycin. J Clin Pharmacol 1980; 20:197.

92. Rotschafer JC et al. Pharmacokinetics of vancomycin: observations of 28 patients and dosage recommendations. Antimicrob Agents Chemother 1982;22:391.

93. Masur H et al. Vancomycin serum levels and toxicity in chronic hemodialysis patients with staphylococcus aureus bacteremia. Clin Nephrol 1983; 20:85.

94. Lanese DM, Molitoris BA. Removal of vancomycin by hemodialysis: a significant and overlooked consideration. Semin Dialys 1989;2:73.

95. Foote EF et al. Pharmacokinetics of vancomycin when administered during high flux hemodialysis. Clin Nephrol 1998;50(1):51.

96. Torras J et al. Pharmacokinetics of vancomycin in patients undergoing hemodialysis with polyacrylonitrile. Clin Nephrol 1991;36:35.

97. Quale JM et al. Removal of vancomycin by high-flux hemodialysis membranes. Antimicrob Agents Chemother 1992;36:1424.

98. Daneshmend TK, Warnock DW. Clinical pharmacokinetics of systemic antifungal drugs. Clin Pharmacokinet 1983;8:17.

99. Starke JR et al. Pharmacokinetics of amphotericin B in infants and children. J Infect Dis 1987; 155:766.

100. Stamm AM et al. Toxicity of amphotericin B plus flucytosine in 194 patients with cryptococcal meningitis. Am J Med 1987;83:236.

101. Sacks P, Fellner SK. Recurrent reversible acute renal failure from amphotericin. Arch Intern Med 1987;147:593.

102. Antoniskis D, Larsen RA. Acute, rapidly progressive renal failure with simultaneous use of Amphotericin B and pentamidine. Antimicrob Agents Chemother 1990;34:470.

103. Brogden RN et al. Amphotericin-B colloidal dispersion. A review of its use against systemic fungal infections and visceral leishmaniasis. Drugs 1998; 56(3):365.

104. Tiula E et al. Serum protein binding of phenytoin and propranolol in chronic renal disease. Intern J Pharmacol Ther Toxic 1987;23:545.

105. Allison TB, Constock TJ. Temperature dependence of phenytoin-protein binding in serum: effects of uremia and hypoalbuminemia. Ther Drug Monit 1988;10:376.

106. Asconape JJ, Penry JK. Use of antiepileptic drugs in the presence of liver and kidney disease: a review. Epilepsia 1982;23(Suppl 1):S65.

107. Liponi DF et al. Renal function and therapeutic concentrations of phenytoin. Neurology 1984; 34:395.

108. Osar-Cederlof I et al. Kinetics of diphenylhydantoin in uremic patients: consequence of decreased protein binding. Eur J Clin Pharmacol 1974;7:31.

109. Browne TR. Pharmacokinetics of antiepileptic drugs. Neurology 1998;51(5 Suppl 4):S2.

110. Letteri JM et al. Diphenylhydantoin metabolism in uremia. N Engl J Med 1971;285:648.

111. Davies G et al. Pharmacokinetics of opioids in renal dysfunction. Clin Pharmacokinet 1996;31 (6):410.

112. Kaiko RE et al. Central nervous system excitatory effects of meperidine in cancer patients. Ann Neurol 1982;13:180.

113. Chan GLC, Matzke GR. The effects of renal insufficiency on the pharmacokinetics and pharmacodynamics of opioid analgesics. Drug Intell Clin Pharm 1987;21:773.

114. Osborne RJ et al. Morphine intoxication in renal failure: the role of morphine-6-glucuronide. Br Med J (Clin Res) 1986;292:1548.

115. Shimomura K et al. Analgesic effects of morphine glucuronides. Tohoku J Exp Med 1971;105:45.

116. Davies G et al. Pharmacokinetics of opioids in renal dysfunction. Clin Pharmacokinet 1996;31(6):410.

117. Matzke GR et al. Codeine dosage in renal failure. Clin Pharm 1986;5:15.

118. Guay DRP et al. Pharmacokinetics and pharmacodynamics of codeine in end-stage renal disease. Clin Pharmacol Ther 1987;43:63.

119. Barnes JN, Goodwin FJ. Dihydrocodeine narcosis in renal failure. Br Med J (Clin Res) 1983; 286:438.

120. Redfern N. Dihydrocodeine overdose treated with naloxone infusion. Br Med J (Clin Res) 1983; 287:751.

121. Gibson TP et al. Kinetics of procainamide and NAPA in renal failure. Kidney Int 1977;12:422.

122. Stec GP et al. N-acetylprocainamide pharmacokinetics in functionally anephric patients before and after perturbation by hemodialysis. Clin Pharmacol Ther 1979;26:618.

123. Winkle RA et al. Clinical pharmacology and antiarrhythmic efficacy of N-acetylprocainamide. Am J Cardiol 1981;47:123.

124. Pirson Y, van Ypersele de Strihou C. Renal side effects of nonsteroidal anti-inflammatory drugs: clinical relevance. Am J Kidney Dis 1986;8:338.

125. Clive DM, Stoff JS. Renal syndromes associated with nonsteroidal anti-inflammatory drugs. N Engl J Med 1984;310:563.

126. Whelton A. Nephrotoxicity of nonsteroidal anti-inflammatory drugs: physiologic foundations and clinical implications. Am J Med 1999;106(5B):13S.

127. Delmas PD. Non-steroidal anti-inflammatory drugs and renal function. Br J Rheumatol 1995;34 (Suppl 1):25.

128. Bender WL et al. Interstitial nephritis, proteinuria and renal failure caused by nonsteroidal anti-inflammatory drugs. Am J Med 1984;76:1006.

129. Davies NM, Watson MS. Clinical pharmacokinetics of sulindac; a dynamic old drug. Clin Pharmacokinet 1997;32:437.

130. Meffin PJ, Sallustio BC, Purdie YJ, Jones ME. Enantio-selective disposition of 2-arylpropionic acid non-steroidal anti-inflammatory drugs. I. 2-phenylpropionic acid disposition. J Pharmacol Exp Ther 1986;238:280.

131. Evans AM. Comparative pharmacology of S(+)-ibuprofen and RS-ibuprofen. Clin Rheumatol 2001;20(Suppl 1):S9.

132. Grubb NG et al. Stereoselective pharmacokinetics of ketoprofen and ketoprofen glucuronide in end-stage renal disease: evidence for a "futile" cycle of elimination. Br J Clin Pharmacol 1999;48:494.

133. Gugler R et al. Clofibrate disposition in renal failure and acute and chronic liver disease. Eur J Clin Pharmacol 1979;15:341.

134. Buckley MM, Sorkin EM. Enoxaparin: a review of its pharmacology and clinical applications in the prevention of treatment of thromboembolic disorders. Drugs 1992;44:465.

135. Gerlach AT et al. Enoxaparin and bleeding complications: a review in patients with and without renal insufficiency. Pharmacotherapy 2000;20:771.

136. Cadroy Y et al. Delayed elimination of enoxaparine in patients with chronic renal insufficiency. Thromb Res 1991;63:385.

137. Brophy DF et al. The pharmacokinetics of subcutaneous enoxaparin in end-stage renal disease. Pharmacotherapy 2001;21:169.

138. Norris M, Remuzzi G. Uremic bleeding: closing the circle after 30 years of controversies? Blood 1999;94:2569.

139. Schrier RW, Gambertoglio JG, eds. Handbook of Drug Therapy in Liver and Kidney Disease. Boston: Little, Brown, 1990.

140. Brater DC. Drug Use in Renal Disease. Sydney: ADIS Health Science Press, 1983.

141. Brater DC. Renal disease. In: Williams R et al., eds. Rational Therapeutics. New York: Marcel Dekker, 1990.

SOLID ORGAN TRANSPLANTATION

David J. Taber
SECTION EDITOR

CHAPTER 35

Solid Organ Transplantation

David J. Taber, Robert E. Dupuis

Continued

Solid organ transplantation is an important therapy for patients with end-stage heart, liver, lung, and kidney disease. For many of these patients, it is the only option. Solid organ transplantation has continued to prove successful. One-year patient survival for these major organs is between 80% and 90%, with some being over 90%. One-year graft survival approaches these figures as well.[1] Pancreas or combined pancreas–kidney transplantation is available as a treatment for diabetic patients with end-stage renal failure. Intestinal transplantation is also performed in a limited number of patients. Pediatric and elderly patients are transplantation candidates, increasing the pool of potential recipients. Surgical techniques involving multiorgan transplantation (e.g., heart with lung, liver, kidney), pancreatic islet cell and liver cell transplantation, intestinal transplantation, living-related and unrelated and segmental human organ transplantation (e.g., kidney, liver, lung, pancreas), domino heart and heart–lung transplantation along with improvements in mechanical assist devices (e.g., for heart transplant candidates) have made the transplantation of organs an increasingly viable treatment option. Research and progress continues in overcoming the immunologic barriers from xenotransplantation (animal to human).

Despite these approaches, many more patients are in need of transplantation than there are organs available. In 2002, 14,722 kidney (6,232 living donors), 5,327 liver, 2,153 heart, 1,042 lung, 903 kidney–pancreas, and 546 pancreas-only transplantations were performed; however, only 5,799 cadaveric and 4,274 living donors were available in the United States. There are large numbers of people waiting for organs; for example, over 50,000 people populate kidney transplant lists, and waiting times are long. Consequently, a significant number of candidates die while waiting for a transplant.[1]

During the 1960s, drugs such as azathioprine, prednisone, antilymphocyte serum, and antilymphocyte globulin (ALG) made possible the success of kidney transplantation. In the late 1970s, the introduction of cyclosporine created a new era in solid organ transplantation, and in the 1980s the first monoclonal antibody approved for human use, OKT3, was introduced.

In the mid-1990s, a number of new and unique agents were approved. These include tacrolimus, mycophenolate mofetil, sirolimus (formerly rapamycin); new monoclonal antibodies, such as daclizumab and basiliximab; and the new polyclonal antibody, thymoglobulin. Other additions include modified cyclosporine, generic modified cyclosporine and generic azathioprine. A number of new agents are undergoing investigation. These provide more individualized, specific, and selective therapies for solid organ transplant recipients.

Although transplantation has had a significant positive impact on the quality of life in most patients with end-stage disease, issues such as retransplantation due to graft failure or recurrence of disease, donation source (living—related and unrelated—neonatal organs, animal organs), and costs to individuals, insurers, and society continue to be discussed with vigor. Costs during the initial transplantation period range from $30,000 for kidney transplants up to $250,000 for heart, liver, or lung transplants. In addition, routine follow-up monitoring and drug therapy for the first year can be $5,000 to $60,000 a year. The ability of transplant patients, particularly those who are years out from their transplant, to pay for their medications is a major issue. Also the cost-effectiveness and side effects of new immunosuppressive agents are important issues.

The goal of immunosuppressive therapy is to prevent organ rejection and prolong graft and patient survival. Short-term (i.e., 1- to 2-year) survival after transplantation has improved dramatically. Long-term survival also has improved, but not to the same degree. The current immunosuppressive regimens have not produced a permanent state of tolerance (i.e., when the transplanted organ is seen as "self"). Although some encouraging data suggest that some selected patients may not require lifetime immunosuppression, these are in a minority, and more definitive studies must be done. As patients live longer after transplantation, the focus of therapy has shifted toward survival and management of long-term complications. Current immunosuppressive drug therapies are associated with significant long-term complications, including nephrotoxicity, hypertension, hyperlipidemia, osteoporosis, and diabetes, as well as graft loss secondary to infection, malignancy, and noncompliance. Although rates of acute rejection are significantly lower, there is still a problem, along with chronic rejection. The search for safer and more effective immunosuppressive regimens continues, along with a better understanding of long-term immunosuppression. This chapter addresses the immunology of transplantation and rejection, indications for solid organ transplantation, appropriate use of immunosuppressive agents, and the management of postoperative and long-term complications in the patient who receives a solid organ transplant. Many of these issues are similar for the various types of solid organ transplantations; yet there can be significant differences. This chapter addresses some of these issues as they relate to kidney, pancreas liver, heart, and lung transplantation.

TRANSPLANTATION IMMUNOLOGY

Successful organ transplantation has come from a greater understanding and application of pharmacology, microbiology, molecular and cellular biochemistry and biology, genetics, and immunology. Suppression of the host's immune system and prevention of rejection are vital for host acceptance of the transplanted organ. The ultimate goal is permanent acceptance or tolerance, a situation in which the new organ is seen as "self" by the host's immune system. In general, the currently used immunosuppressive drugs provide a nonpermanent form of tolerance. A basic understanding of the immune system and the mechanisms of rejection is key to the effective use of immunosuppressive drugs in organ transplantation.

Major Histocompatibility Complex and Human Leukocyte Antigen

The degree to which allogeneic grafting (i.e., a transplanted organ from a genetically different donor of the same species) is successful depends on the genetic similarities or differences between the organ of the donor and the immune system of the recipient. The recipient recognizes the transplanted graft as either self or foreign. This recognition is based on the host's reaction to alloantigens or antigens (i.e., substances that initiate an immune response that can lead to rejection of the transplanted organ). These substances also are known as histocompatibility antigens and play a very important role in organ transplantation. Another group of substances that also plays an important role is the ABO blood group system of red blood cells. In general, the donor and recipient must be ABO compatible; otherwise, immediate graft destruction occurs because of antibodies directed against the ABO antigens.

Histocompatibility antigens are glycoproteins that are located on the surface of cell membranes. These are encoded by the major histocompatibility complex (MHC) genes located on the short arm of chromosome 6. In humans, the MHC is called the *human leukocyte antigen* (HLA). The gene products encoded on the HLA are divided into classes I, II, and III based on their tissue distribution, antigen structure, and function. Class I antigens (HLA-A, HLA-B, and HLA-C) are present on all nucleated cell surfaces and are the primary targets for cytotoxic T-lymphocyte reactions against transplanted cells and tissues. The three class II antigens (HLA-DR, HLA-DQ, HLA-DP) have a more limited distribution and are found on macrophages, B lymphocytes, monocytes, activated T lymphocytes, dendritic cells, and some endothelial cells, all of which can act as antigen-presenting cells (APCs). Individual HLA loci are extensively polymorphic. Each individual possesses two A, B, and DR antigens, one from each parent. This is called a *haplotype*. Recognition of these polymorphic loci by host T lymphocytes appears to account for rejection events seen in vivo. Class III antigens (C4, C2, and Bf) are part of the complement system and do not play a specific role in the graft rejection process.

Rejection of a transplanted organ is the outcome of the natural response of the immune system to a foreign substance, or antigen, and is a complex process in which our understanding continues to evolve. This process, in some cases segmental and simultaneous, involves an array of interactions between foreign antigens, T lymphocytes, macrophages, cytokines (soluble mediators secreted by lymphocytes, also called *lymphokines, interleukins, cytokines*), adhesion molecules (also referred to as *costimulatory molecules*), and membrane proteins expressed on a wide variety of cells that enhance binding of T cells, and B lymphocytes. This process of organ rejection ultimately can involve all elements of the immune response (Fig. 35-1), but it is predominantly T-cell–mediated. This process can be divided into several important steps, which include antigen presentation as well as T-cell recognition, activation, proliferation, and differentiation of the various components of the immune response.

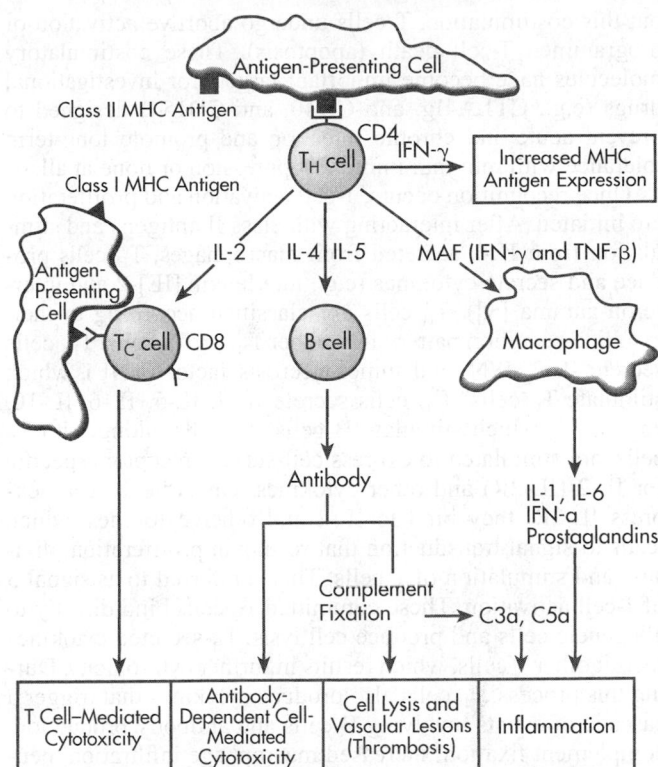

FIGURE 35-1 Activation of the acute rejection response.

For foreign antigens to interact with recipient T cells and B cells, they must be prepared for presentation by APCs. These APCs (see Fig. 35-1) usually are recipient macrophages, although donor cells—referred to as *dendritic cells* or *passenger leukocytes* and *graft endothelial cells*—also can serve as APCs. This phase takes place within the blood, lymph nodes, spleen, and the transplanted organ.

The next step involves T-cell recognition of the HLA molecules presented on the surface of the APC. The primary site for this to occur is at the CD3–T-cell receptor complex (TCR) on recipient T lymphocytes. This step involves the binding of the antigen, MHC, and TCR for T-cell activation. These T lymphocytes also express other molecules (clusters of differentiation [CD]) on their surfaces that, along with CD3, recognize and respond to different types of antigens. These T cells are known as *CD4+ cells* (T_H or helper/inducer T cells) and *CD8+ cells* (T_C or cytotoxic/ suppressor T cells). CD4+ cells interact with class II antigens. CD8+ cells interact with class I antigens.

In addition, proteins known as adhesion molecules or costimulatory molecules promote T-cell signaling and activation. For T-cell activation to occur, binding of these costimulatory molecules as well as binding of the TCR with the presented antigen and MHC is required. Examples of these molecules include intercellular adhesion molecule (ICAM)-1 on APCs, which bind with lymphocyte function–associated antigen (LFA) expressed on the surface of T cells; LFA-3 on APCs with CD2 on T cells; B7 on APCs with either CD28 or CTLA4 on T cells; CD40 on APCs with CD40 ligand (now called *CD154*) on T cells.

The binding of these molecules are critical to T-cell activation and are referred to as signal 2 for T-cell activation. Without this costimulation, T cells undergo abortive activation or programmed T-cell death (apoptosis). These costimulatory molecules have become important targets for investigational drugs (e.g., CTLA4Ig, anti-CD40, anti-CD154) designed to prevent acute and chronic rejection and promote long-term tolerance with minimal immunosuppression or none at all.

Once recognition occurs, T-cell activation and proliferation are initiated. After interacting with class II antigens and stimulation from IL-1 secreted from macrophages, T_H cells produce and secrete cytokines (e.g., interleukin [IL]-2 and interferon-gamma [γ]). T_H cells are classified according to their cytokine-secretion pattern into either T_{H1} or T_{H2} cells. T_{H1} cells secrete IL-2, IFN, and tumor necrosis factor (TNF), which stimulate T_C cells. T_{H2} cells secrete IL-4, IL-5, IL-6, IL-10, and IL-13, which stimulate B cells. T_H cells, along with T_C cells, are stimulated to express cell-surface receptors specific for IL-2 (IL-2R) and other cytokines. Once the T_C cells express IL-2R, they bind to IL-2 and other cytokines, which leads to signal transduction that results in proliferation, division and stimulation of T cells. This is referred to as signal 3 of T-cell activation. These committed T_C cells bind directly to allogeneic cells and produce cell lysis. T_H-secreted cytokines recruit other T cells, which results in further cytotoxicity. During this process, T_H cells also produce cytokines that trigger a cascade of events involving B cells and antibody production, complement fixation, increased macrophage infiltration, neutrophil involvement, fibrin deposition, platelet activation and release, prostaglandin release, and inflammatory response at the graft site. These delayed-type hypersensitivity and humoral responses occur in conjunction with one another and are not mutually exclusive. This results in cellular and tissue graft destruction (see Fig. 35-1).[2,3]

The antibodies produced by plasma cells, which are transformed B cells under the influence of cytokines, bind to the target antigenic cells. This leads to local deposition of complement and results in immune complexation and injury to the graft (complement-mediated cell lysis). The newly formed antibodies cause a series of interactions to occur with T cells, which lead to cytotoxicity (antibody-dependent, cell-mediated cytotoxicity). These cell-mediated and humoral immunologic events can impair organ function so significantly that without therapeutic intervention, complete organ graft dysfunction may occur. Under certain circumstances, which are not clear, the T_C cells can actually down-regulate the immune response to alloantigen. These cells are known as *suppressor T cells,* which express CD8+. These cells, when present in significant quantities, appear to be associated with prolonged graft survival and may play a role in the effectiveness of some immunosuppressive agents.[4]

Human Leukocyte Antigen Typing

The genetic compatibility between donor and recipient can have an impact on graft survival. For example, in kidney transplantation, the closer the HLA matching is between recipient and donor, the better the outcome, particularly over the long term.[3] To determine this compatibility, a number of laboratory tests, including serologic, flow cytometric, genetic DNA based, and cellular assessments of donor and recipient serum and lymphocytes, are needed before organ transplantation. This process is referred to as tissue typing.[4] Lympho-

cytes are typed for HLA-A, HLA-B, and HLA-DR. Typing for HLA is performed using the donor and recipient lymphocytes for serology-based techniques and any tissue or fluid containing nucleated cells.

A lymphocyte cross-match is also performed. In this case, the patient's serum is cross-matched to determine whether preformed antibodies to the donor's lymphocytes are present. A positive cross-match indicates the presence of recipient cytotoxic IgG antibodies to the donor. In solid organ transplantation, this positive cross-match would be considered a contraindication. In liver transplantation, a positive cross-match is not an absolute contraindication because the need is urgent and because the liver appears to be more resistant immunologically to this type of reaction. However, these liver transplant recipients can develop significant complications and experience early acute rejection.

The panel reactive antibodies (PRAs) test also is commonly used to assess organ compatibility because recipients may have HLA antibodies from previous exposure to antigenic stimuli (e.g., blood transfusions, previous transplantation, pregnancy). In this test, the recipient's serum is tested against a cell panel of known HLA specificities that are representative of possible donors in the general population. The percentage of cell reactions (recipient with donor) determines a recipient's PRA.[5] The potential recipient with a higher percentage of PRAs (>20% to >50%) is at higher risk for rejection.

ABO blood typing is one of the most critical of all evaluations when determining the genetic compatibility for all solid organ transplants. Transplantation of an organ with ABO incompatibility would result in a hyperacute rejection and destruction of the graft.

Because of the significant donor shortage and long wait times, investigations are underway in living-donor kidney transplantations, with the use of pre- and post-transplantation modalities, such as plasmapheresis, immunoglobulins, splenectomy, along with aggressive imunosuppression, in an attempt to overcome either the ABO incompatibility and/or positive cross-match barriers.[6]

IMMUNOSUPPRESSIVE AGENTS

Improved and increased experience with surgical techniques, better postoperative care and monitoring, and more effective immunosuppressive agents also have played significant roles in the success of organ transplantation. The use of these immunosuppressives, based on an improved understanding of their mechanisms of action and the mechanisms of rejection, has had the most significant impact on patient graft survival. The number of currently approved immunosuppressives has significantly increased since 1995 (Table 35-1), and a significant number of newly developed, more selective immunosuppressives are under investigation. Sites of action of the currently used agents, along with some of the investigational agents, are represented in Figure 35-2.

Azathioprine

Azathioprine is a prodrug of 6-mercaptopurine (6-MP). Azathioprine and 6-MP are purine antagonist antimetabolites. The introduction of cyclosporine, tacrolimus, mycophenolate, and

Table 35-1 Currently Used Immunosuppressive Agents

Drug (Brand Name)	Usual Dose (How Supplied)	Therapeutic Use(s)	Adverse Effects
Azathioprine (Imuran)	1–3 mg/kg/day (50-mg tab; 100-mg vial for injection)	As maintenance agent to prevent acute rejection	Leukopenia, thrombocytopenia, hepatotoxicity, nausea and vomiting, diarrhea, pancreatitis, infection
Antithymocyte globulin, equine (Atgam)	10–20 mg/kg/day (250 mg/5 mL ampule for injection)	Treat acute rejection (including severe or steroid-resistant forms); as induction agent in high-risk patient to prevent acute rejection	Anemia, leukopenia, thrombocytopenia, arthralgia, myalgias, nausea and vomiting, diarrhea, fevers/chills, hypotension, tachycardia, anaphylaxis, infection
Antithymocyte globulin, rabbit (Thymoglobulin)	1.5 mg/kg/day (25 mg/5 mL vial for injection)	Treat acute rejection (including severe or steroid-resistant forms); as induction agent in high-risk patient to prevent acute rejection	Fever/chills, nausea and vomiting, hypotension, neutropenia, flushing, rash/itching, joint pain/myalgias, thrombocytopenia, infection
Basiliximab (Simulect)	20 mg × 2 doses 10 mg × 2 doses for children if <35 kg (10- and 20-mg vial for injection)	As induction agent to prevent acute rejection	Abdominal pain, dizziness, insomnia, hypersensitivity reaction (rare)
Cyclosporine (Sandimmune)	Oral 5–10 mg/kg/dose BID Intravenous 1.5–2.5 mg/kg/dose (100 mg/mL oral solution; 25- and 100-mg cap; 250 mg/5 mL ampule for injection)	As maintenance agent to prevent acute rejection	Nephrotoxicity, hypertension, neurotoxicity, hair growth, gingival hyperplasia, hyperglycemia, hyperkalemia, dyslipidemia hypomagnesemia, infection, neoplasm
Cyclosporine (Neoral, Gengraf, various others)	4–8 mg/kg/day BID (100 mg oral solution; 25-, 50-, and 100-mg cap)	As maintenance agent to prevent acute rejection; conversion agent from tacrolimus in patients with intolerance or inefficacy	Same as above
Daclizumab (Zenapax)	1 mg/kg × 5 doses (25 mg/5 mL vial for injection)	As induction agent to prevent acute rejection	Headache, infection, hypo/hypertension
Methylprednisolone sodium succinate (Solu-medrol, various others)	10–1,000 mg/dose (40-, 125-, 250-, 500-, 1,000- and 2,000-mg vial for injection)	As induction and maintenance agent to prevent acute rejection; to treat acute rejection	Hyperglycemia, psychosis/euphoria, impaired wound healing, osteoporosis, acne, peptic ulcers/gastritis, fluid/electrolyte disturbances, leukocytosis, cataracts, cushingoid state, infection, insomnia, irritability
Mycophenolate mofetil (Cellcept)	1.5–3.0 g/day BID (250-mg cap; 500-mg tab; 200 mg/mL oral suspension; 500-mg vial for injection)	As maintenance agent to prevent acute rejection; conversion agent from azathioprine and sirolimus in patients with intolerance or poor response	Diarrhea, nausea and vomiting, neutropenia, dyspepsia/ulcers, infection, thrombocytopenia
OKT3 (Orthoclone)	2.5–5 mg/dose (5 mg/5 mL ampule for injection)	Treat acute rejection (including severe or steroid-resistant forms); as induction agent in high-risk patients to prevent acute rejection	Pulmonary edema, fever/chills, hypotension, weakness/fatigue, muscle/joint pain, aseptic meningitis, altered mental status, infection
Prednisone (Deltasone, others)	5–20 mg/day (1-, 2.5-, 5-, 10-, 20-, 50-, and 100-mg tab)	As maintenance agent to prevent acute rejection	See methylprednsiolone
Sirolimus (Rapamune)	2–10 mg/day (1- and 2-mg tab; 1 mg/mL oral solution)	As maintenance agent to prevent acute rejection; conversion agent from CNI or mycophenolate or azathioprine in patients with intolerance or poor response	Dyslipidemia, thrombocytopenia, neutropenia, anemia, diarrhea, impaired healing, mouth ulcers, hypokalemia, arthralgias, infection
Tacrolimus (Prograf)	Oral 0.15–0.3 mg/kg/day BID IV 0.025–0.05 mg/kg/day as continuous infusion (0.5-, 1-, and 5-mg cap; 5 mg/mL ampule for injection)	As maintenance agent to prevent acute rejection; conversion agent from cyclosporine in patients with intolerance	Nephrotoxicity, hypertension, neurotoxicity, alopecia, hyperglycemia, hyperkalemia, dyslipidemia hypomagnesemia, infection, neoplasm

CNI, calcineurin inhibitor.

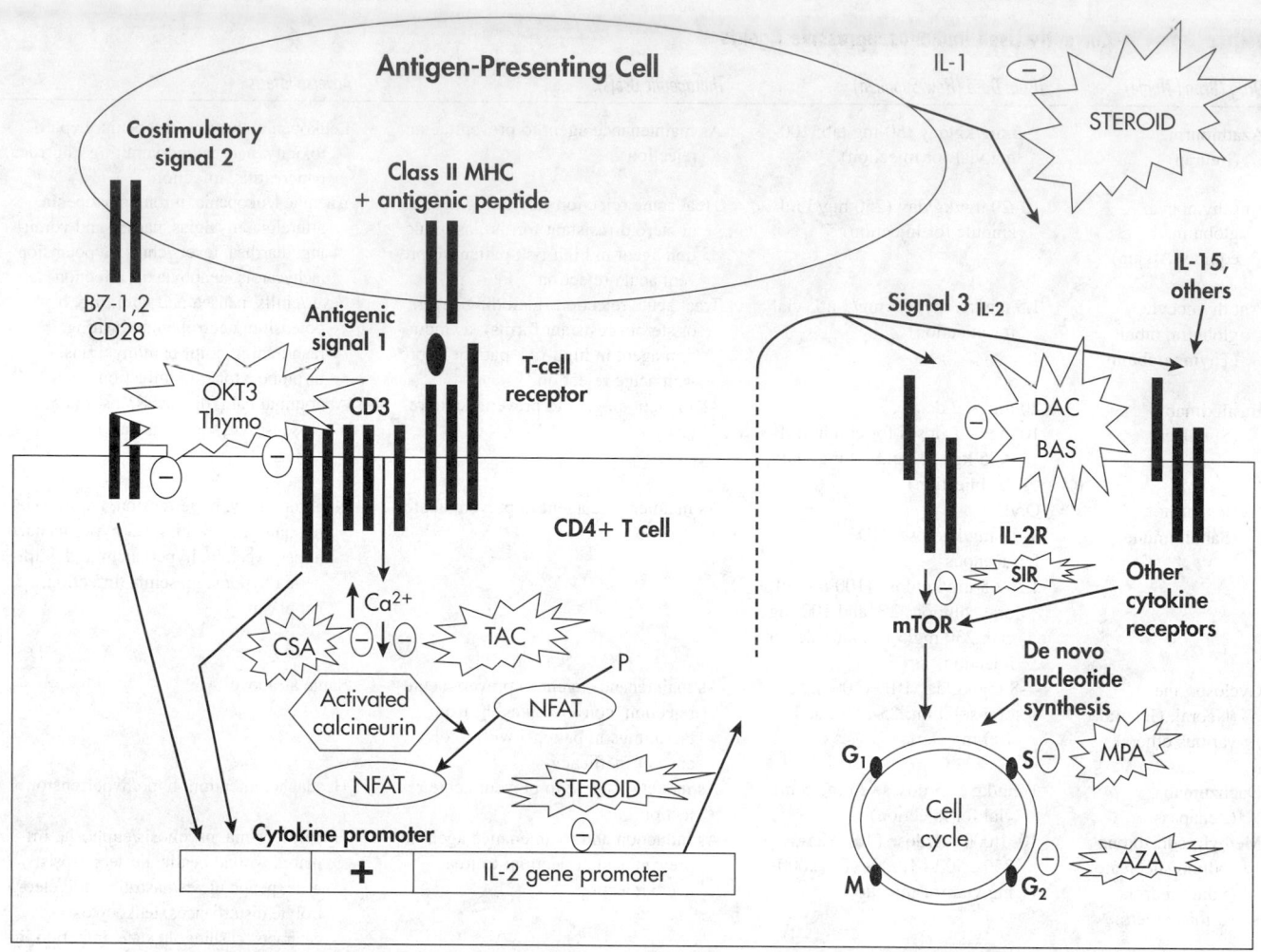

FIGURE 35-2 Schematic representation summarizing the mechanisms of action of approved and investigational immunosuppressive agents. AZA, azathioprine; BAS, basiliximab; CSA, cyclosporine; DAC, daclizumab; TAC, tacrolimus; IL, interleukin; MPA, mycophenolic acid; SIR, sirolimus; TNF. (Reprinted with permission from reference 302.)

sirolimus has led to a reduction of azathioprine use or its elimination altogether in immunosuppressive protocols.

Azathioprine, considered a nonspecific immunosuppressive agent, affects both cell-mediated (i.e., T cell) and humoral-directed (i.e., B cell) immune responses. Azathioprine inhibits the early stages of cell differentiation and proliferation. Therefore, azathioprine is useful for the prevention of rejection, but it is ineffective for the treatment of acute rejection. Active metabolites of 6-MP are incorporated into DNA and RNA, thereby interfering with the intracellular formation of thioguanine nucleotides (TGNs). 6-MP is intracellularly converted by hypoxanthine phosphoribosyl transferase (HPRT) to thioinosinic acid and then to thioguanine nucleotides. 6-MP may have two separate immunosuppressive effects: inhibition of cellular proliferation and cytotoxicity. A decrease in the levels of intracellular purine ribonucleotides decreases cellular proliferation, and incorporation of TGN into DNA mediates cytotoxicity.[7]

Azathioprine can be given intravenously (IV) or orally. Oral absorption is rapid but incomplete. The usual dose is 1 to 3 mg/kg per day. The mean bioavailability of azathioprine in renal transplant recipients is approximately 40% to 60%. Nevertheless, oral doses usually are not doubled when converting from IV to oral route. The clinical significance of not taking this into consideration has not been determined.

The half-lives for azathioprine and 6-MP are estimated to be 10 to 12 minutes and 40 to 60 minutes, respectively. Major metabolic conversion of azathioprine to 6-MP is via nucleophilic attack by glutathione. The liver and red blood cells are thought to be major tissue sites for this metabolic conversion. The 6-MP formed by this reaction can be metabolized further to thiopurine ribonucleosides and ribonucleotides. Azathioprine pharmacokinetics are not affected by renal dysfunction, but there are higher 6-TGN metabolite concentrations. In contrast, azathioprine's immunosuppressive activity is absent in patients with severe hepatic dysfunction.[8]

The most common adverse effect of azathioprine is bone marrow suppression, which presents as leukopenia or, less commonly, as thrombocytopenia and megaloblastic anemia. Myelosuppression is dose dependent and typically observed after 7 to 14 days of therapy. Bone marrow suppression may be related to a genetic deficiency of the enzyme, thiopurine methyltransferase (TPMT). Low activity of this enzyme is rare but does lead to greater availability of 6-MP, elevated 6-thioguanine levels, and susceptibility to myelosuppression. Low levels of TPMT have been associated with severe azathioprine myelotoxicity in some transplant recipients.[9] Hepatitis, cholestasis, and reversible and irreversible liver damage have been reported with azathioprine use. The irreversible liver damage appears histologically compatible with central vein phlebitis and occlusion, fibrosis, lobular necrosis, and biliary stasis.[10]

The white blood cell (WBC) count should be maintained at >5,000/mm³. If it decreases to 3,000 to 5,000/mm³, the azathioprine dosage should be reduced by 50%. If the dose reduction fails to keep the WBC count above 3,000/mm³, azathioprine should be discontinued and reinstituted at the lower dose when the leukopenia is resolved, if needed. A similar approach should be taken if thrombocytopenia occurs. If hepatotoxicity or other serious side effects occur, azathioprine is discontinued.

Pancreatitis has been associated with azathioprine. Long-term azathioprine administration also has been associated with the occurrence of non-Hodgkin's lymphoma, squamous cell skin cancer, primary hepatic tumors, fever, rigors, rash, headache, myalgia, tachycardia, hypotension, polyarthritis, and acute hypersensitivity reactions. Anorexia, nausea, and vomiting also occur.

Mycophenolate Mofetil

As a result of several comparative trials in kidney transplant patients, mycophenolate mofetil (MMF) has replaced azathioprine in many transplantation protocols. Studies in other transplantation populations have shown positive results as well. MMF is used as adjunctive therapy in combination with cyclosporine or tacrolimus, prednisone, sirolimus, and monoclonal and polyclonal antibodies to prevent acute rejection. It is also used as rescue therapy when patients have not responded to or cannot tolerate the side effects of other immunosuppressive agents.

MMF, like azathioprine, can be classified as an antiproliferative antimetabolite in that it also inhibits purine synthesis, but in a more selective manner. Unlike azathioprine, MMF interferes with the de novo pathway for purine synthesis.

MMF is the mopholinoethyl ester prodrug of mycophenolic acid (MPA), which is the active component. MPA selectively, noncompetitively, and reversibly blocks an enzyme known as inosine monophosphate dehydrogenase (IMPDH) found primarily in actively proliferating T and B lymphocytes. T and B lymphocytes rely on this enzyme and the de novo purine pathway to produce purine nucleotides for DNA and RNA synthesis. Thus, MPA interferes with T- and B-cell proliferation. MPA also may affect cytokine production. Other secondary effects include inhibition of B-lymphocyte antibody production, decreased adhesion molecule expression, decreased smooth muscle proliferation and recruitment, and infiltration of neutrophils.[11,12]

MMF is rapidly converted to MPA upon IV or oral administration. It is well absorbed. MPA is metabolized almost entirely by the liver to MPA-glucuronide, which undergoes enterohepatic recirculation and is ultimately excreted renally as MPAG.[13] Another mycophenolic acid derivative, enteric-coated mycophenolate sodium has been developed and is undergoing clinical trials.

Corticosteroids

Prednisone, methylprednisolone, and prednisolone—synthetic analogs of hydrocortisone—are the primary corticosteroids used to prevent and treat rejection of transplanted organs. Although an important part of immunosuppression, a goal of most transplantation programs is to minimize, eliminate, or avoid corticosteroid use because of their numerous and significant side effects.[14]

Corticosteroids have multiple effects on most cells and tissues of the body, but it is their anti-inflammatory and, more important, immunosuppressive properties that serve as the basis for their use in organ transplant patients. These effects are exerted through specific intracellular glucocorticoid receptors. The corticosteroids bind with these receptors and interfere with RNA and DNA synthesis as well as transcription of specific genes. Cell function is altered, resulting in suppression or activation of gene transcription. Corticosteroids also affect RNA translation, protein synthesis, production and secretion of cytokines, and protein and cytokine receptor expression.

Even after a single dose, corticosteroids cause marked lymphocytopenia by redistribution of circulating lymphocytes to other lymphoid tissues, such as the bone marrow, rather than by cell lysis; they also transiently increase the number of circulating neutrophils. Corticosteroids inhibit IL-1 and IL-6 production from APCs, a number of events associated with T-cell activation, and IL-2 production. They interfere with the action of IL-2 and IL-2R on activated T cells, resulting in the inhibition of helper and suppressor T-cell function. Moderate-to high-dose corticosteroids also inhibit cytotoxic T-cell function by inhibiting cytokine production and lysis of T cells. They can inhibit early proliferation of B cells but have a minimal effect on activated B cells and immunoglobulin-secreting plasma cells. The corticosteroids affect most cells and substances associated with acute allograft rejection and inflammatory reactions. They inhibit accumulation of leukocytes at sites of inflammation; inhibit macrophage functions, including migration and phagocytosis; inhibit expression of class II MHC antigens induced by interferon-γ; block release of IL-1, IL-6, and TNF; inhibit the upregulation and expression of adhesion molecules and neutrophil adhesion to endothelial cells; inhibit secretion of complement protein C3; inhibit phospholipase A_2 activity; and decrease production of prostaglandins.[15]

The plasma half-lives of prednisone and methylprednisolone are much shorter than their biologic half-lives. Prednisone is a prodrug that is rapidly converted to its active form, prednisolone. Bioavailability in transplant recipients is rapid and complete and similar to healthy subjects. In transplant recipients, plasma half-lives are approximately 2.5 to 4 hours for prednisolone and methylprednisolone. Prednisolone is metabolized extensively. Prednisolone and methylprednisolone are 70% to 90% protein bound. Clearance of the unbound fraction is reduced in renal and liver transplant patients. These agents usually are given in fixed doses with little regard for pharmacokinetic differences, despite the fact that significant variability exists.[16,17]

Calcineurin Inhibitors

Cyclosporine

The introduction of cyclosporine as an immunosuppressive agent has been the single most important factor in the current success of organ transplantation. Its use has increased patient and graft survival, reduced morbidity associated with rejection and infection, and extended the types and numbers of organ transplantations performed. Cyclosporine or tacrolimus are the primary agents used in almost all transplant recipients. In contrast to azathioprine and mycophenolate, cyclosporine has relatively nonmyelotoxic, immunosuppressive effects. It has been considered the prototype for agents like tacrolimus and sirolimus, as well as some investigational immunosuppressive drugs.

Cyclosporine is an 11-amino acid undecapeptide metabolite extracted from a soil fungus, *Tolypocladium inflatum gams*. The activity of cyclosporine is mediated through a reversible inhibition of T-cell function, particularly helper T cells. Its major effect is inhibiting the production of IL-2 and other cytokines, including interferon-γ. These actions result in an inhibition of the early events of T-cell activation, sensitization, and proliferation. Cyclosporine has little effect on activated mature cytotoxic T cells. Therefore, it has little usefulness in the treatment of acute rejection. Its site of action is within the cytoplasm of T cells after antigenic recognition and signaling occurs. Cyclosporine binds to an intracellular protein (immunophilin) called *cyclophilin*. Although binding to cyclophilin is required, it is not sufficient for immunosuppression. This cyclosporine-cyclophilin complex binds to a protein phosphatase, calcineurin. This is thought to prevent activation of nuclear factors involved in the gene transcription for IL-2 and other cytokines, including IFN.[18] Also, because of this inhibition, cyclosporine indirectly impairs the activity of other cells, macrophages, monocytes, and B cells in the immune response. Cyclosporine has no effect on hematopoietic cells or neutrophils. Cyclosporine is metabolized extensively in the liver to >25 metabolites. Two of these metabolites, AM1 (formerly M17) and AM9 (formerly M1), can elicit an immunosuppressive effect in vitro, but have much lower activity than cyclosporine. The role of these metabolites in the development of toxicity with cyclosporine is unclear.[18]

Tacrolimus

Tacrolimus (formerly FK506) is isolated from a soil fungus, *Streptomyces tsukubaensis*. It is a macrolide with a different molecular structure than cyclosporine. Tacrolimus is as effective as cyclosporine in liver, kidney, kidney–pancreas or pancreas, heart, and lung transplantation patients as the primary immunosuppressant in combination with corticosteroids and/or mycophenolate, azathioprine, sirolimus and/or antibodies. It also is effective as rescue treatment in liver, kidney, kidney–pancreas or pancreas, heart, and lung transplant recipients experiencing acute or chronic rejection resulting from failure of standard immunosuppressive therapy.

The activity of tacrolimus is similar to that of cyclosporine, but the concentrations of tacrolimus needed to inhibit production of IL-2, which is its major effect, are 10 to 100 times lower than those of cyclosporine. Tacrolimus also inhibits production of other cytokines, including IL-3, IL-4, and interferon-γ, TNF, and granulocyte-macrophage colony-stimulating factor

(GM-CSF). It has variable effects on B-cell response and also has anti-inflammatory effects. The action of tacrolimus on T cells is more difficult to reverse than cyclosporine. Like cyclosporine, tacrolimus binds to an intracellular, although different, protein: FK binding protein 12 (FKBP12). This protein that interacts with calcineurin, inhibits gene transcription of cytokines and interferes with T-cell activation.[19] Further pharmacologic and pharmacokinetic descriptions of tacrolimus are presented in Questions 37 to 41.

Sirolimus

Sirolimus, formerly known as *rapamycin* (Rapamune), is the newest FDA-approved agent for prevention of acute rejection in kidney transplantation. It was isolated from soil samples in Rapa Nui (Easter Island) and is a macrolide, structurally related to tacrolimus. In multicenter clinical trials, sirolimus combined with cyclosporine and prednisone significantly reduced acute rejection episodes in kidney transplant recipients when compared with a combined regimen of cyclosporine, azathioprine, and prednisone. The rejection rate was decreased from approximately 30% to 40% to <20% to 30%. Positive results for sirolimus also have been observed in other transplantation populations; in situations in which it is used in combination with other agents, including antibodies, tacrolimus and mycophenolate; and when it has been used for rescue therapy.[20]

Unlike tacrolimus and cyclosporine, which work earlier in the T-cell activation cycle and inhibit cytokine production, sirolimus is an inhibitor of late T-cell activation. It does not block cytokine production; rather, it inhibits signal transduction, which blocks the response of T cells and B cells to cytokines like IL-2.

Like tacrolimus, sirolimus binds to intracellular proteins. Specifically, sirolimus binds to the same immunophilin bound by tacrolimus, *FK binding protein* (FKBP). This complex interferes with the action of certain enzymes or proteins. Both cyclosporine and tacrolimus inhibit calcineurin, whereas sirolimus influences a protein called the *mammalian target of rapamycin* (mTOR). Sirolimus also inhibits an enzyme called *P7056 protein kinase,* which is involved in microsomal protein synthesis. These effects result in cell-cycle arrest, blockage of mRNA production, and blockage of cell proliferation.[21] Early in its development, in vitro studies indicated that tacrolimus and sirolimus were antagonistic. In vivo data indicate that this is not true. Sirolimus and cyclosporine or tacrolimus appear to work synergistically. Sirolimus also inhibits proliferation of smooth muscle cells and may, although it is too early to tell, reduce the development of chronic rejection.[20]

Antithymocyte Globulin

Before monoclonal antibody preparations were developed to prevent and treat rejection, polyclonal antilymphocyte preparations such as antilymphocyte globulin (ATG) were available. Products used today are administered intravenously and include equine (Atgam, lymphoglobulin) and rabbit (Thymoglobulin) globulin.

ATG preparations made in goats and sheep also have been synthesized for investigational study. However, the following discussion is limited to the products produced in horses (Atgam) and rabbits (Thymoglobulin). Regardless of the species from which they are produced, all ATG products have similar pharmacologic effects. However, their potency and antibody specificity vary from batch to batch and between products.[22] The production of polyclonal equine or rabbit antibody begins with the injection of homogenized human spleen or thymus preparations into the animals. This injection induces an immune response in the animals directed against human T lymphocytes; serum containing antibodies to T cells is collected from the animals and purified. Unfortunately, other antibodies to human cells are produced as well. These antibodies bind to all normal blood mononuclear cells in addition to T lymphocytes and B lymphocytes, resulting in depletion of lymphocytes, platelets, and leukocytes from the peripheral circulation. The mechanism of action of these agents is thought to be linked to lysis of peripheral lymphocytes, uptake of lymphocytes by the reticuloendothelial system, masking of lymphocyte receptors, apoptosis and immunomodulation.[23] These agents contain antibodies to a number of cell-surface markers on lymphocytes, including CD2, CD3, CD4, CD8, CD11a, CD25, CD44, CD45, HLA-DR, and HLA class I antigens. They also interfere with leukocyte adhesion and trafficking.[24] ATG preparations can produce a rapid and profound depletion of circulating T cells, often within 24 hours of the initial dose. The duration of the effect can last several weeks after a course of therapy, particularly with thymoglobulin. Antibodies can be produced to these products as well. However, the clinical significance is not known.[25] The clinical use of Atgam and thymoglobulin is described further in Question 29.

Murine Monoclonal Antibody

Muromonab-CD3 (Orthoclone OKT3), the first therapeutic murine monoclonal antibody produced for use in humans, was developed to suppress T-cell–mediated rejection. It is used for induction therapy (prophylaxis) or to treat acute graft rejection.[26] With the introduction of thymoglobulin, daclizumab, and basiliximab, the prophylactic use of OKT3 has significantly declined, although some centers still use it but in lower doses.

Murine monoclonal antibodies are formed by immunizing a mouse with a specific antigen (in this case, human T lymphocytes). After the mouse produces B lymphocytes against the injected antigen, it is sacrificed and the spleen is removed. All the lymphocytes derived from the spleen are suspended and mixed with mouse myeloma cells, a tumor cell line that can grow indefinitely in culture. The two cell types are mixed with polyethylene glycol (PEG), which allows the cells to fuse together. This mixture of mouse spleen cells, myeloma cells, and hybridomas (fused spleen and myeloma cells) is grown in a medium that allows only hybridomas to grow. Hybridoma colonies that are producing the desired antibody are cloned, and the antibodies they produce are harvested from cell supernatants. Another method used to produce large amounts of monoclonal antibody is to inject the appropriate hybridoma into the peritoneum of a mouse. After 10 to 21 days, the ascitic fluid, which contains secreted antibodies, is harvested and purified to obtain the desired monoclonal antibody.

OKT3 is an intravenously administered IgG_{2a} immunoglobulin that binds to the CD3 (cluster of differentiation 3) structure on CD3+ T lymphocytes located near the T-cell receptor complex. All mature T cells express CD3 and either the CD4 or CD8 surface antigen. Once OKT3 is bound to the CD3 region of T cells, it is thought to be opsonized and removed from the circulation by the reticuloendothelial system of the liver and the spleen. This removal occurs within minutes after IV administration. However, the first one to two doses activate T cells thereby producing significant adverse effects known as the cytokine release syndrome. OKT3 also can modulate the antigen-recognition complex of T cells, which alters normal T-cell function. The third mechanism involves blocking killer T cells attached to the allograft. This occurs when high levels of OKT3 are achieved and the killer T cells are coated and rendered inactive. Once therapy is stopped, CD3+ cells return to measurable levels quickly, often within 24 hours.

CD3+ cell counts of $<20/mm^3$ represent an appropriate response in most patients. Adequate response to OKT3 is delayed by up to 5 to 7 days after a second course, which is due to a neutralizing antibody against OKT3.[26] Patients sometimes require two to three times the initial dose. See Question 30.

Interleukin-2 Receptor Antagonists
Daclizumab and Basiliximab

Daclizumab (Zenapax) and basiliximab (Simulect) are two monoclonal antibodies approved for use in combination with other immunosuppressives to prevent acute cellular rejection in kidney transplantation. They are not considered treatment for acute rejection. Daclizumab is a humanized monoclonal antibody, which contains 90% human and 10% murine antibody sequences. Basiliximab is a chimeric antibody that contains both murine and human antibody sequences. In contrast to daclizumab, it contains higher amounts of murine antibody sequences.[27] These agents reduce episodes of acute rejection in kidney transplant patients.[28] Their use in combination with other agents is being studied in other transplant populations. Comparative studies between these agents or with other antibodies like OKT3, Atgam, and thymoglobulin are limited. Advantages over these older agents include ease of administration, minimal side effects, low immunogenicity, no greater infections or malignancy rates, and fewer required doses. However, these agents cost approximately $1,200 per dose. To date, the only perceived clinical difference between daclizumab and basiliximab is the dosing regimen. Daclizumab is given as 1 mg/kg on day 0 of the transplant and then every 2 weeks for four more doses. This regimen creates issues related to compliance, outpatient administration, and reimbursement. Basiliximab is given as a 20-mg dose on days 0 and 4 after transplantation. There are a number of reports evaluating daclizumab regimens of 1, 2, or 3 doses.[27]

Both daclizumab and basiliximab appear to have similar mechanisms. They bind to the α-subunit of the IL-2R, also known as *CD25* or the *TAC subunit,* which is expressed only on the surface of activated T cells; this subunit is critical to IL-2 activation of T cells in the acute rejection process. Daclizumab and basiliximab prevent the IL-2R from binding with IL-2 thereby blocking T-cell activation.[27]

There are differences in the elimination half-life and duration of receptor saturation with these two agents, the significance of which remains to be determined. Daclizumab has a terminal half-life of 11 to 38 days, whereas basiliximab's is shorter: 4 to 14 days. Daclizumab, using the approved five-dose regimen, saturates the IL-2R for about 120 days. Basiliximab, with the two-dose regimen, saturates the receptor for 36 days. Duration of IL-2 saturation was also found to be shorter in liver transplant patients than that reported in kidney transplant patients. The half-life and clearance of daclizumab and basiliximab have been shown to be shorter and faster, respectively, in liver transplant recipients. Total body clearance correlates positively with the volume of postoperative blood loss; basiliximab also is cleared through postoperative ascitic fluid.[29]

Investigational Agents

A number of agents are in various stages of development. These include everolimus (SDZ-RAD), mycophenolate sodium, FTY720, deoxyspergualin, brequinar, mizoribine, leflunomide, FK-778, and campath-1M. These agents have more specific activity directed at T-cell and B-cell function. Everolimus is an analogue of sirolimus. FTY-720 interferes with lymphocyte migration from the lymph nodes. Leflunomide and its analogs, FK778, HMR715, HMR279, belong to a class of agents called malanitriloamides and target pyrimidine synthesis. Mizoribine and brequinar are inhibitors of DNA synthesis. Deoxyspergualin inhibits cell activation and maturation. In addition, a number of monoclonal antibodies and peptides have been developed and are undergoing investigation. The targets of these antibodies and peptides are antigen-binding sites, adhesion molecules, and cytokines. Examples include AllotrapHLA, CTLA4IgG, anti-CD154 BMA 031, anti-T12, anti-ICAM, T10B9, and OKT4A monoclonal antibodies.[30,31]

KIDNEY TRANSPLANTATION
Indications and Evaluation

1. G.P., a 52-year-old, 72-kg African-American man, has end stage renal disease (ESRD) secondary to non–insulin-dependent diabetes mellitus and hypertension. He has been undergoing hemodialysis three times a week for 4 years. Other medical problems include anemia, hypocalcemia, and hyperphosphatemia. G.P.'s medications include amlodipine 10 mg QD, ramipril 10 mg BID, Tums 2 tablets TID with meals, HS and in between meals, NPH insulin 30 units BID, regular insulin 8 units BID, and erythropoietin 8,000 units IV TIW. He has been on the kidney transplant waiting list for 2 years. He is called by the transplant coordinator and admitted for a possible cadaveric kidney transplant. G.P. has the same blood type as the donor. His most recent PRA is 10%. Cross-match is negative, and HLA typing reveals a 3-antigen match (A1, A2, B35) between donor and recipient. On admission to the hospital, his laboratory values are as follows: Na, 141 mEq/L (normal, 135 to 145); potassium (K), 4.7 mEq/L (normal, 3.4 to 4.6); Cl, 102 mEq/L (normal, 95 to 105); bicarbonate (HCO₃), 23 mEq/L (normal, 22 to 28); blood urea nitrogen (BUN), 44 mg/dL (normal, 8 to 18); serum creatinine (SrCr), 13.9 mg/dL (normal, 0.6 to 1.2); calcium (Ca), 7.8 mEq/L (normal, 8.8 to 10.3); phosphorus, 6.2 mg/dL (normal, 2.5 to 5.0); glucose, 225 mg/dL (normal, 65 to 110); WBC count, 8.4 cells/mm³ (normal, 4,000 to 10,000); hemoglobin (Hgb), 10.8 g/dL (normal, 14 to 18); and Hct, 32% (normal, 39% to 49%). His serology is negative for HIV, hepatitis B surface antigen, hepatitis C, and cytomegalovirus (CMV) and is positive for anti-HBs. What are the indications for and potential benefits of kidney transplantation in G.P.?

[SI units: Na, 141 mmol/L (normal, 135 to 145); K, 4.7 mmol/L (normal, 3.4 to 4.6); Cl, 102 mmol/L (normal, 95 to 105); HCO₃, 23 mmol/L (normal, 22 to 28); BUN, 15.7 mmol/L (normal, 3.0 to 6.5); SrCr, 1,228.8 μmol/L (normal, 50 to 110); Ca, 1.95 mmol/L (normal, 2.20 to 2.58); P, 2.0 mmol/L (normal, 0.77 to 1.45); glucose, 12.5 mmol/L (normal, 3.9 to 6.1); WBC count, 8.4 × 10⁶ cells/L (normal, 4,000 to 10,000); Hgb, 108 g/L (normal, 115 to 155); Hct, 0.32 (0.39 to 0.49)]

All patients with ESRD are potential candidates for kidney transplantation unless contraindicated. The contraindications (absolute or relative) are determined by the individual transplant center. Absolute contraindications include current malignancy, active infection, active liver disease, HbsAg-positive, severe or symptomatic cardiac and/or pulmonary disease, specific renal diseases with an accelerated recurrence rate, substance abuse, and abnormal psychosocial and non-compliant behavior. Relative contraindications for the recipient of a kidney transplant include chronic liver disease, active infection, positive for hepatitis C, HIV-positive, morbid obesity, current positive cross-match, and age over 70 years.[32] The relative contraindication for the elderly with ESRD is controversial because approximately 40% of the ESRD population is older than 65 and an increasing number of these patients are undergoing kidney transplantation. Patients with ESRD need not wait until they are receiving dialysis before being considered for a kidney transplant because transplantation is associated with lower costs and a better quality of life than dialysis. Survival rates for both dialysis and renal transplant recipients appear similar, but comorbid factors can influence survival. For example, diabetic transplant recipients have a higher survival rate than diabetic dialysis patients awaiting transplantation. The primary diseases leading to ESRD and transplant are diabetes, glomerulonephritis, polycystic kidneys, and arterionephrosclerosis.[33]

In G.P., diabetes and/or hypertension would be the most likely causes of his ESRD. For G.P., a renal transplant should return his renal function to near normal, improve his quality of life, and correct the complications of renal dysfunction such as anemia, hypocalcemia, and hyperphosphatemia, but not diabetes or hypertension.

When evaluating a patient for any organ transplantation, the risk-to-benefit ratio must be considered. In general, kidney, kidney–pancreas and pancreas transplantations are performed to improve the quality of life. In other words, the disease itself may not be immediately life threatening in patients such as G.P., but a transplant will free him from dialysis, insulin injections, or both. In contrast, patients who are candidates for heart, lung, and liver transplantations will die if these vital organs fail. Therefore, the criteria established for organ transplantation must be evaluated carefully before it is offered to any patient.

Donor and Recipient Matching

2. What criteria are important in determining a good match between the donor and G.P.?

G.P. underwent a series of serologic tests to determine his genetic compatibility with the donor. He had a negative cross-match and low PRA of 10%, indicating that he is not already sensitized to this donor's antigens, which should result in a more favorable post-transplantation course. HLA matching also indicated a three-antigen match between G.P. and the donor. Matching of donor and recipient at the HLA-A, HLA-B and HLA-DR loci is associated with better graft survival and longer half-lives for both living-related and cadaveric kidney transplants. Half-lives are longer with living donors (13 to 15 years) compared with cadaveric donors (8 to 20 years).[31] For a group of recipients with a match similar to G.P., the 1-year and 3-year graft survival for a first cadaveric transplant is projected to be >90% and >80%, respectively. However, these positive factors may be offset by his African-American ethnicity. Patient and graft survival after kidney transplantation is reduced in this ethnic population compared with others owing to immunologic, medical, pharmacologic, pharmacokinetic, and socioeconomic reasons.[34] Along with African-American race, other risk factors associated with decreased survival include advanced donor age, recipient age <15 and >50 years, retransplantation, a high PRA (>20% to >50%), and delayed graft function. Recipients who fall into these categories are referred to as high-risk patients.[33,35]

Immunosuppressive Therapy

3. Before the transplant procedure, G.P. receives MMF 1 g PO and cefazolin 1 g IV. During surgery, he is given methylprednisolone 500 mg IV, and furosemide 100 mg IV after the kidney has been transplanted. Methylprednisolone 250 mg IV is to be given on the day after surgery. The methylprednisolone dose is to be decreased to 100 mg IV on the second postoperative day for one dose. Prednisone 65 mg (1 mg/kg per day) PO is to be given on the subsequent day for one dose and tapered by 0.3 mg/kg per day to 20 mg QD by day 7 after surgery. Cyclosporine (Neoral) NG (nasogastric)/PO 6 mg/kg per day or 175 mg Q 12 hr will be started within 12 hours after surgery. The dosage will be adjusted according to cyclosporine whole blood trough concentrations. MMF will be continued at 1g PO BID. G.P. is also to receive cefazolin 1 g IV Q 8 hr for two doses, ranitidine 50 mg IV Q 12 hr, nystatin 10 mL swish and swallow (S&S) TID, and sliding scale regular insulin. Why is G.P. being treated with this immunosuppressive regimen?

The major goal of immunosuppressive therapy is to prevent rejection and infection with minimal adverse side effects and to ensure long-term patient and graft survival. Less than 50% of kidney transplant recipients experience an acute allograft rejection episode. With newer agents, acute rejection rates are <20% during the first year after transplantation. Most of these episodes respond to acute antirejection therapy.

There is no consensus on the best immunosuppressive regimen, and the numerous dosing regimens in use primarily depend on the program and the specific organ to be transplanted. Although a number of studies have attempted to evaluate the superiority of various regimens, comparisons are hampered by variables such as differences in donor selection and condition, organ preservation and procurement, organ ischemic (cold and warm) time, recipient's pretransplant conditions, comorbid and high or low risk factors, surgical procedures and individual surgical techniques, postoperative management and monitoring, and length of follow-up. Another important consideration is that many of the newer agents show significant effects during the first year, but fail to show significant impact on long-term effects such as chronic rejection. The choice of a particular regimen may depend on the risk

factors present at the time of transplantation. During this early time period, the number of agents and doses used are higher than later on after transplantation.[36]

Most starting immunosuppressive drug regimens for the management of solid organ transplantations rely on three to four agents, although mono or dual therapy has been used, depending on organ type. These combination regimens include a calcineurin inhibitor (cyclosporine or tacrolimus) and MMF or sirolimus, or azathioprine and prednisone with or without a monoclonal antibody (OKT3, daclizumab, basiliximab) or polyclonal antibody (Atgam or Thymoglobulin). Several regimens are being studied that avoid the use of steroids and calcineurin inhibitors, use a short course in the early transplantation period, or are withdrawn sometime after transplantation in an attempt to avoid the long-term side effects of these agents.[37]

With cadaveric kidney transplants, triple therapy often is used with either cyclosporine or tacrolimus as the foundation of this type of regimen. Tacrolimus is used in >50% of new kidney transplant recipients.[38] In HLA-identical, living-related kidney transplants, conventional dual therapy such as azathioprine or mycophenolate and prednisone gives excellent results; however, acute rejection can still occur, and some programs may use dual therapy that contains either cyclosporine or tacrolimus. Triple or quadruple therapy is used to take advantage of different mechanisms of action and to reduce drug toxicity by using sequential therapy and smaller doses of multiple agents rather than larger doses of any agent used alone. However, these multidrug combinations can lead to increased drug costs, compliance issues, a higher incidence of infection and malignancy, and difficulty in assessing adverse effects.

In G.P., triple or quadruple therapy would be used. In some centers, an antibody would be added to his current triple therapy, since G.P. is considered a high-risk recipient because he is African American.

After the initial transplantation period, drug dosages are reduced over time and maintained at a stable dose for 6 months to 1 year. Cyclosporine, tacrolimus, MMF, azathioprine, or the corticosteroid may be discontinued. Although the discontinuation of a drug may reduce adverse effects, it is counterpoised against the risk of acute rejection and graft loss. This requires identification of the appropriate patient. With the newer agents such as tacrolimus, MMF and/or sirolimus, this may be less problematic. Monotherapy may be achieved in kidney, liver, and heart transplant recipients at some point after transplantation. After transplantation, most patients require lifetime immunosuppression, although studies in a small number of carefully selected patients demonstrate that some appear to be able to discontinue therapy at some time after transplant. These patients require long-term follow-up to assess the impact of this approach.

Postoperative Course and Delayed Graft Function

4. G.P. is admitted to the transplant ward for initial post-transplantation management. His urine output during the next 3 hours has decreased from 300 to 40 mL/hr. He is receiving IV fluids at a rate equivalent to his urine output. He had received 3 L of fluids in the operating room (OR). His blood pressure (BP) is 140/83 mm Hg, heart rate is 87 beats/min, and temperature 36.9°C; he has no signs of dehydration. His BUN is 56 mg/dL (normal, 8 to 18), and his SrCr is 12.8 mg/dL (normal, 0.6 to 1.2). Another dose of furosemide 100 mg IV increased his urine output to 140 mL/hr, but his urine output returned to <40 mL/hr in a few hours. Fluids and IV furosemide were given again with similar results. Renal ultrasound indicates no urine leaks, fluid collections, or ureteral obstruction. A DPTA (diethylenetriamine penta-acidic acid) renal scan indicates good perfusion, but decreased accumulation and clearance. Over the next 2 days, G.P.'s BP is 150/93 mm Hg, weight is 76 kg (4 kg higher than before the transplantation), urine output has fallen to <200 mL/day, and relevant laboratory values are as follows: BUN, 85 mg/dL; SrCr, 13.2 mg/dL; and K, 5.8 mEq/L (normal, 3.4 to 4.6). The decision is made to institute hemodialysis. What has happened to G.P.'s renal function? What is the most likely diagnosis?

[SI units: BUN, 20 mmol/L, 30.3 mmol/L (normal, 3.0 to 6.5); SrCr, 1131.5 μmol/L, 1166.9 μmol/L (normal, 50 to 110); K, 5.8 mmol/L (normal, 3.4 to 4.6)]

After kidney transplantation, recipients require management and monitoring for fluid and electrolyte imbalance, BP and blood glucose changes, surgical complications, gastrointestinal (GI) complications, infection, rejection, immunosuppressive dosing and toxicity, and, most important, kidney function. If all goes well, recipients should be discharged from the hospital within 5 days after transplantation.[39]

The initial renal function after kidney transplantation can reflect excellent, moderate, slow graft function (SGF), or delayed graft function (DGF). In recipients with excellent function, a good diuresis begins immediately and continues, and the serum creatinine rapidly declines to <2.5 mg/dL within the first few days after transplantation. Most living-related transplants and only about 30% to 50% of cadaveric transplants generally experience this excellent graft function pattern. Kidney transplant recipients with moderate graft function usually experience a slower decline in serum creatinine, which stabilizes within the first week. Recipients with DGF usually experience anuria or oliguria, require dialysis in the early period, and take days to weeks to recover. DGF is most common in cadaveric transplant recipients, occurring in approximately 20% to 60% of cases.[35]

The diagnosis of DGF is based on clinical, laboratory, and diagnostic criteria that may vary among centers. DGF has been defined at some centers simply as the need for dialysis in the early transplantation period, whereas at others, the definition may be based on both a lack of improvement in the serum creatinine (e.g., it does not fall below 2.5 to 4 mg/dL or by 25% to 30% from pretransplantation) and the presence of anuria or oliguria, after other causes of acute tubular necrosis (ATN) are ruled out, within the first 6 to 24 hours. SGF is another term that has been used to describe a lag in improvement and does not involve dialysis. DGF is influenced by conditions affecting the donor (age, condition of organ, prolonged ischemic time), intraoperative conditions (hypotension, fluid imbalance), and recipient (prior transplantation, postoperative hypovolemia or hypotension, and nephrotoxic drugs).

In G.P., poor urine output in the first hours after transplantation and subsequent oliguria, the exclusion of other causes of ATN, the results of the renal scan, the lack of improvement in BUN and serum creatinine, and the need for dialysis are indicative of DGF. DGF reduces kidney graft survival, increases the risk of acute rejection, and influences a patient's early management by requiring dialysis, increasing the length of hospital stay, and increasing the costs of therapy. It also may make the assessment of acute rejection more difficult because the patient already has impaired renal function. In DGF, a renal biopsy is obtained if no improvement in serum creatinine is seen by day 7.[40]

Induction and Sequential Therapy

5. What adjustments, if any, should be made in G.P.'s immunosuppressive drug regimen?

The adverse renal effects of calcineurin inhibitors (CNIs) can contribute to the onset of DGF as well as prolong its duration. Therefore, cyclosporine should be discontinued temporarily or its dose significantly reduced. Because of this effect, induction and sequential immunosuppressive protocols do not include CNIs or use them only in low doses for the first 1 to 2 weeks after a renal transplantation. These protocols include antibodies and provide more intense immunosuppression early after transplantation when the risk of acute rejection is highest. The use of polyclonal antibodies or OKT3 in patients with DGF is appropriate because they have shortened the duration of DGF and the need for dialysis when compared with the CNIs. Although time to first rejection appears to be increased with either polyclonal antibodies or OKT3, the preferred antibody still is a matter of debate.[41] These agents have a positive impact on DGF but have failed to show a positive effect on long-term graft survival compared with standard therapies such as calcineurin inhibitors.[42] The trend is to reserve induction therapy for those considered at high risk for rejection because the drugs included in these regimens are expensive, are associated with a significant number of adverse effects, and might increase the patient's susceptibility to CMV infections and malignancy, like post-transplantation lymphoproliferative disease (PTLD) (see Question 23). Another potential option would be to use one of the new IL-2R inhibitors, daclizumab or basiliximab, which have been shown to reduce acute rejection rates and extend the time to first rejection. However, they have been used primarily in low-risk patients. Their use in high-risk patients (African Americans, retransplantations, high PRA, prolonged ischemic time, DGF) is based primarily on single-center and retrospective studies with encouraging results, but there are no prospective studies that demonstrate effectiveness equal to other antibodies.[43,44]

In G.P., an antilymphocyte preparation—either polyclonal or monoclonal antibodies such as Thymoglobulin or OKT3—would be administered for 5 to 10 days along with his current regimen of prednisone and mycophenolate. His cyclosporine would be discontinued and reintroduced 2 to 3 days before stopping the antibody. A cyclosporine dosage of 2.5 to 3 mg/kg orally twice a day would be reasonable in G.P. with a goal of achieving trough concentrations of 150 to 300 ng/mL.

Rejection

6. G.P. was given Thymoglobulin, initially 1.5 mg/kg QD as a 6-hour IV infusion with further dosages to be adjusted to maintain CD3+ lymphocyte counts of <20 cells/mm³ for a total of 7 days along with his prednisone taper and MMF. He received 3 doses of Thymoglobulin. Cyclosporine PO 175 mg BID (3 mg/kg/dose) was initiated on the fourth day of Thymoglobulin therapy. G.P.'s urine output has increased gradually to approximately 1,600 mL/day 1 week after stopping Thymoglobulin. His weight has decreased to 73 kg, BP is 142/84 mm Hg, heart rate is 82 beats/min, temperature is 36.7°C, BUN is 23 mg/dL (normal, 8 to 18), SrCr is 2.3 mg/dL (normal, 0.6 to 1.2), and K is 4.6 mEq/L (normal, 3.4 to 4.6). He is on a regular diet and taking all oral medications. His current medications include MMF 1 g BID, prednisone 10 mg QD, cyclosporine 225 mg BID, ranitidine 150 mg QHS, dioctyl sodium sulfosuccinate 100 mg BID, nystatin S&S 10 mL TID, amlodipine 10 mg QD, NPH insulin 28 units BID, regular insulin 10 units BID, valganciclovir 450 mg QD, and trimethoprim-sulfamethoxazole (TMP-SMX) 1 tablet on Mondays, Wednesdays, and Fridays. Twenty days after stopping Thymoglobulin, G.P.'s weight increased to 74.6 kg, and his BP was 160/94 mm Hg, heart rate was 98 beats/min, temperature was 37.6°C, BUN was 30 mg/dL, SrCr was 3.4 mg/dL, K was 4.8 mEq/L, trough whole blood cyclosporine concentration (monoclonal TDx) was 110 ng/mL, and urine output decreased over the last 24 hours to 850 mL. He feels tired and has a decreased appetite, but his fluid intake has been adequate over the past day. What evidence is consistent with rejection in G.P.?

[SI units: BUN, 8.2 mmol/L, 10.7 mmol/L (normal, 3.0 to 6.5); SrCr, 212.2 μmol/L, 300.6 μmol/L (normal, 50 to 110); K, 4.6 mmol/L, 4.8 mmol/L (normal, 3.4 to 4.6)]

Although significant improvements in graft survival have occurred over the past decade, graft rejection continues to be a major reason for graft loss in kidney transplants.[33,45] Rejection episodes in all solid organ transplantations can be categorized as hyperacute, accelerated, acute, or chronic.

Hyperacute Rejection

Hyperacute rejection occurs within minutes to hours after transplantation of the allograft and is the result of preformed cytotoxic antibodies against donor-specific class I antigens. This type of rejection is associated with a poor prognosis but is rare because of ABO matching and improved HLA typing. Clinically, the patient presents with anuria, hyperkalemia, hypertension, metabolic acidosis, pulmonary edema and, in some cases, disseminated intravascular coagulopathy. Diagnostic scan of the kidney would indicate no uptake. If other causes of anuria are excluded and this diagnosis is made, then the transplanted kidney must be removed.

Accelerated Rejection

Accelerated rejection usually occurs within 2 to 6 days after organ transplantation. This is a result of prior sensitization to antigens that are similar to those of the donor and newly developed donor-specific antibodies. Accelerated rejections of transplanted kidneys occur primarily in recipients who have had prior transplantation, multiple pregnancies, or blood transfusions. These patients usually maintain good renal function for a few days before developing acute renal failure. Accelerated organ rejections generally are more resistant to pharmacologic therapy.

Acute Rejection

Acute rejection is the most common type of kidney rejection in transplant recipients and the only type of rejection that responds to therapy. Acute rejection of a transplanted kidney significantly reduces the half-life and survival of both living and cadaveric transplants. The half-life refers to the time it takes for half of the grafts that survive the first year to eventually fail. Acute rejection can occur in the first 5 to 10 days after kidney transplantation. However, the prophylactic use of antibody preparations may delay the onset for several weeks, as illustrated by G.P.'s case. If acute rejection occurs, its onset is almost always within the first year, with most episodes occurring within the first 60 days after transplantation. The clinical presentation of patients with acute rejection of a kidney ranges from an asymptomatic patient with mild renal dysfunction, as indicated by an elevated serum creatinine, to patients presenting with a flulike illness and acute oliguric renal failure.[45]

G.P. presents with subjective complaints of malaise or tiredness and lack of appetite. Such nonspecific complaints occur often in patients with rejection and can be accompanied by myalgias as well as pain and tenderness at the graft site in some cases. Objectively, G.P.'s fever, increased weight, hypertension, decreased urine output, and increase in serum creatinine are consistent with acute kidney rejection. In addition, the cyclosporine concentration and mycophenolate dose are low, suggesting inadequate immunosuppressive coverage. Acute rejection of a transplanted kidney must be distinguished from CNI nephrotoxicity, and infections (e.g., pyelonephritis, CMV) also must be ruled out. Although the clinical evidence in G.P. probably represents an acute rejection, a kidney biopsy is the gold standard for establishing the diagnosis. Biopsy results usually are available within 6 to 8 hours. If there is acute rejection, the renal biopsy will show an interstitial infiltration of mononuclear cells with tubulitis or intimal arteritis in more severe cases. The severity of rejection would be classified and graded according to standardized pathologic criteria.[46]

Humoral Rejection

Humoral rejection is an acute rejection mediated by antibodies; it differs histologically from acute cellular rejection in that there is no lymphocyte infiltration on biopsy. Presence of positive staining for the complement component C4d suggests antibody-mediated rejection. Humoral rejection usually occurs in the first week to 3 months after transplantation. Antibody-mediated rejection often is associated with hemodynamic compromise and is more resistant to drug therapy.[47]

Chronic Rejection and Chronic Allograft Nephropathy

Chronic rejection is the major cause of long-term kidney graft loss after the first year and occurs in 30% to 40% of patients.[48] An immunologic cause for chronic allograft nephropathy (CAN) is most probable, but the exact cause is unknown. Nonimmunologic causes also play a role in CAN, a term that is often used to describe this overall process of graft deterioration. Another term, chronic renal allograft dysfunction (CRAD) is the functional result of CAN.[46] It is a slow, insidious process that usually manifests as an increase in serum creatinine after about 1 year, although it can occur as early as 3 months after transplantation. The characteristic signs of chronic rejection are hypertension, proteinuria, and a progressive decline in renal function leading to renal failure. Immunologic factors that increase the likelihood of chronic rejection include history of acute rejection, inadequate immunosuppression, noncompliance with immunosuppressive therapy, previous infection such as CMV. Nonimmunologic factors are donor related (age, hypertension, diabetes), increased ischemic times, recipient hypertension, hyperlipidemia, CNI nephrotoxicity, and elevated body mass index.[48,49] CRAD is irreversible and unaffected by increased immunosuppressive therapy.

Therapy is supportive (e.g., dialysis in the case of a kidney transplantation). Ultimately, retransplantation is needed. Data suggest that some patients may benefit from some of the newer agents, such as mycophenolate and sirolimus, which are considered non-nephrotoxic, but this requires further study. The diagnosis of chronic rejection is determined by clinical signs and biopsy findings indicative of obliterative fibrosis of hollow structures and vessels within the graft. The chronic rejection of a kidney must be distinguished from chronic CNI nephrotoxicity, chronic infection, and recurrence of the original kidney disease.

Acute Rejection Treatment

7. A biopsy of G.P.'s transplanted kidney shows grade 2, moderate acute rejection. G.P. is started on methylprednisolone 500 mg QD IV for three doses. His maintenance oral prednisone is discontinued, but his other medications are maintained. He will be placed on a high-dose oral prednisone tapering regimen after his IV doses. Why is the methylprednisolone therapy of G.P.'s first acute episode of rejection appropriate?

High-dose, or "pulse," IV methylprednisolone, IV OKT3, IV Thymoglobulin, IV ATG, or oral prednisone are several of the options used to treat acute rejection in all types of solid organ transplants. A high-dose corticosteroid (usually IV methylprednisolone) is considered first-line therapy because it works very quickly in decreasing lymphocyte responsiveness, is easy to administer, and reverses at least 75% of acute rejection episodes.[50] Thymogloglobulin and OKT3 are usually reserved for steroid-resistant rejection. IVIG has also been used as an alternative for resistant rejection.[51] The ideal corticosteroid dosage, route, and regimen are unknown, and the number of corticosteroid protocols is as varied as the number of transplantation programs. IV methylprednisolone and oral prednisone are equally effective in reversing rejection, but oral corticosteroids are given for a longer period and have been associated with a higher incidence of adverse effects. Although as little as 50 mg of IV methylprednisolone has a similar lymphocyte suppressive effect as a 1-g IV dose of this drug, most programs use methylprednisolone 250 to 1,000 mg IV every day for three doses and adjust the pre-rejection oral prednisone regimen accordingly. An example of an oral prednisone regimen is 100 to 200 mg/day tapered over 1 to 3 weeks to baseline maintenance dose.[50]

For G.P., IV methylprednisolone is appropriate because corticosteroids are considered first-line therapy for acute rejection of a transplanted kidney, and first rejection episodes (such as G.P.'s) are very responsive. In addition, G.P. has received a prophylactic course of Thymoglobulin recently. Corticosteroids provide benefits similar to those from OKT3. Furthermore, Thymoglobulin, ATG, or OKT3 therapy is associated with a higher risk of CMV infection and malignancy, is more difficult to administer, requires more intensive monitoring, is more expensive, and usually is held in reserve for cases of corticosteroid-resistant rejection.

Nevertheless, high-dose corticosteroids are not without risk. They increase the risk of infection, and long-term ther-

apy can induce ocular, bone, cardiovascular, and endocrine abnormalities. Although G.P will be receiving high-dose IV methylprednisolone for only 3 days, he should be monitored for hyperglycemia and a change in his insulin requirements because corticosteroids can significantly alter glucose metabolism. Short-course methylprednisolone also can mask signs of infection (e.g., fever, changes in WBC counts, pain associated with inflammation) and delay the diagnosis. Insomnia, nervousness, euphoria, mood shifts, acute psychosis, and mania also can occur with short-term corticosteroid use. If this methylprednisolone regimen is effective in reversing the acute rejection of G.P.'s transplanted kidney, his serum creatinine concentration should decline within 2 to 5 days and his urine output should improve.

In addition, it would be appropriate to increase G.P.'s cyclosporine dosage to 250 mg twice a day because the concentration is low and there is a relationship between concentration and effect. Since small changes in cyclosporine dose can increase levels disproportionately, a trough whole blood concentration should be re-evaluated in 3 days. The mycophenolate dose could be increased to 1.5 g BID, since this dose in combination with cyclosporine has reduced acute rejection in African Americans. Another option is to change cyclosporine to tacrolimus.[52]

Calcineurin Inhibitor–Induced Nephrotoxicity

8. G.P.'s acute kidney rejection has been treated successfully, and his serum creatinine has decreased to 2.0 mg/dL within 1 week of steroid therapy. Because of this rejection episode, G.P.'s cyclosporine and MMF doses were increased to 275 mg BID and 1.5 g BID, respectively. Prednisone was reinstituted at 20 mg QD. One week later, his weight is 74.5 kg, BP is 148/94 mm Hg, heart rate is 83 beats/min, and he is afebrile. His SrCr is 2.3 mg/dL (normal, 0.6 to 1.2), K is 5.5 mEq/L (normal, 3.5 to 5.0), uric acid is 9.3 mg/dL (normal, 2.0 to 7.0), magnesium (Mg) is 1.4 mEq/L (normal, 1.6 to 2.4), and cyclosporine blood concentration is 370 ng/mL. How would you explain these findings in G.P.?

[SI units: SrCr, 88.4 μmol/L, 203.3 μmol/L (normal, 50 to 110); K, 5.5 mmol/L (normal, 3.5 to 5.0); uric acid, 553.2 μmol/L (normal, 120 to 420); Mg, 2.8 mmol/L (normal, 0.8 to 1.2)]

G.P. already has experienced an episode of acute rejection of his transplanted kidney. Some of the signs of rejection he previously demonstrated such as weight gain, increased BP, edema, decreased urine output, and an increased serum creatinine concentration are present again, but these are not specific for rejection. They also are associated with CNI-induced nephrotoxicity. In the case of acute rejection, the serum creatinine concentration usually is higher and rises more acutely and fever is generally present. With CNI nephrotoxicity, the rise in the serum creatinine concentration is more gradual and not as high as that seen with rejection. The serum concentrations of potassium and uric acid are usually increased, and the magnesium is decreased with CNI nephrotoxicity. CNI concentrations may be elevated, although some patients may experience CNI nephrotoxicity even with levels below or within the targeted therapeutic range. Acute CNI nephrotoxicity is more likely to occur in the first months after transplantation in most patients receiving therapeutic doses because CNI doses and levels are highest and are being adjusted at this time. Two forms of CNI nephrotoxicity have been identified: functional or acute renal dysfunction and chronic nephrotoxicity.[53]

Functional renal dysfunction is the most common form of renal dysfunction and is characterized by rapid reversal when the CNI dosage is held or reduced. This syndrome typically is not associated with histopathologic abnormalities, which suggests that it is related to severe vasoconstriction of the renal afferent arterioles. Repeated episodes of transient acute renal dysfunction can result in protracted acute renal dysfunction. Recovery of renal function after repeated episodes usually is not complete even when CNI is withdrawn. Protracted acute renal dysfunction can be associated with the development of thrombosis of glomerular arterioles or diffuse, interstitial fibrosis. Alternatively, cyclosporine may exacerbate intravascular thrombus formation or may serve as a stimulus to interstitial cell proliferation. Another syndrome is a chronic, usually irreversible, nephropathy, which often is associated with mild proteinuria and tubular dysfunction. Renal biopsies in allograft patients with chronic cyclosporine-related nephropathy showed tubulointerstitial abnormalities, sometimes with focal glomerular sclerosis.[53]

Nephrotoxicity is one of the most common adverse effects associated with CNIs and occurs to some degree in all patients. The pathophysiology of cyclosporine or tacrolimus-induced transient acute renal failure is not understood completely but seems to be related to its effects on renal vessels. For example, CNIs can induce glomerular hypoperfusion secondary to vasoconstriction of the afferent glomerular arteriole, thereby reducing glomerular filtration. One possible explanation for these effects is that cyclosporine alters the balance of prostacyclin and thromboxane A_2 in renal cortical tissue. Increased thromboxane A_2 results in renal vasoconstriction. Endothelin release from renal vascular cells stimulated by CNIs also may contribute to this acute effect through its potent vasoconstrictive properties. CNIs also can cause a reversible decrease in tubular function. The alterations in tubular function reduces magnesium reabsorption and decreases potassium and uric acid secretion. This may be a result of direct tubular toxicity and possibly the result of thromboxane A_2 stimulation of platelet activation and aggregation. A chronic nephropathy, usually seen after >6 months of therapy, can also occur and may become irreversible. In this situation, renal function progressively declines to a point that dialysis is required.[54]

Chronic allograft nephropathy, which can result from chronic rejection and/or chronic CNI nephrotoxicity is usually seen after 6 to 12 months. Clinically and histologically, chronic nephrotoxicity can be difficult to distinguish from chronic rejection. CAN has been reported to occur in 20% to 60% of patients with 5% to 10% developing ESRD after kidney and other types of organ transplantation.[55,56] Concern for chronic nephropathy has led to the development of cyclosporine or tacrolimus withdrawal or substitution protocols, using agents such as mycophenolate or sirolimus, or protocols using low doses of cyclosporine or tacrolimus.[57]

G.P.'s rise in serum creatinine and hypertension in conjunction with a high cyclosporine level suggests acute cyclosporine toxicity as the most likely cause of his findings. In this case, the total cyclosporine dose should be lowered by approximately 25% to 225 mg twice a day, and G.P. should be monitored closely for resolution of the symptoms or worsening if rejection results from lowering the dose. His elevated potassium, uric acid, and low magnesium should correct themselves with this dose reduction if it is acute CNI toxicity. In any case, magnesium should be replaced to maintain a level >1.5 mEq/L. If the nephrotoxicity is caused by cyclosporine, a decrease in the serum concentration of creatinine may be evident when the cyclosporine dose is reduced. If no such reduction occurs or if the serum concentration of creatinine continues to increase, then a renal biopsy is needed to rule out rejection, nephrotoxicity, or other causes.

Calcineurin Avoidance, Withdrawal, or Minimization

9. G.P.'s serum creatinine did decrease over the next several days to 2.0 mg/dL. Over the next 12 months, his serum creatinine has slowly risen to 2.6 mg/dL. Besides the increase in Scr, he has proteinuria and hypertension that have become more difficult to control. He is receiving Neoral (modified cyclosporine) 150 mg BID, Cellcept (mycophenolate) 1.5 g BID, and prednisone 10 mg QD. His last cyclosporine trough level was 85 ng/mL. He has had no further episodes of acute rejection. A kidney biopsy was consistent with chronic allograft nephropathy and cyclosporine-induced nephrotoxicity. Would it be appropriate to withdraw cyclosporine in G.P.? If attempted, how could this be accomplished?

Cyclosporine and tacrolimus are associated with a number of metabolic, cardiovascular, neurologic and cosmetic side effects. Certainly, the most concerning is nephrotoxicity, which contributes to chronic allograft nephropathy and graft loss. The potential benefit of withdrawing cyclosporine would be to reduce these toxicities, while minimizing the risk for rejection, graft loss, and toxicities of replacement agents.

IL-2R antibodies, sirolimus, and mycophenolate, which are not associated with nephrotoxicity, are being evaluated in protocols that attempt to avoid, minimize, or withdraw CNIs. Alternative regimens that have included sirolimus, mycophenolate, and steroids[58]; sirolimus and steroids[59]; and daclizumab, mycophenolate, and steroids[60] have been compared with cyclosporine-based regimens or historical data. Studies, which were usually done in low-risk populations, generally produced reduced serum creatinines and CNI-induced toxicities, but were associated with high rates of acute rejection (30% to 50%). More recent trials in small numbers of patients that compared combinations of thymoglobulin or basiliximab, sirolimus, mycophenolate and steroids with either cyclosporine- or tacrolimus-containing regimens have shown equal effectiveness with acute rejection rates of <15%.

In the case of cyclosporine withdrawal, there appears to be a 10% to 20% increased risk of acute rejection, but no change in graft survival according to a meta-analysis.[61] Several protocols are being developed that either withdraw the CNI or at least reduce the dose to a minimal level. Many are attempting to do this earlier after transplantation in the hope that the nephrotoxic effects can be reversed before significant chronic damage occurs. These approaches add mycophenolate or sirolimus as the CNI is withdrawn or reduced in dose. Most protocols have been tested in small numbers of low-risk patients. However, there has been one large multinational study using a low-risk population. All patients received cyclosporine, sirolimus, and corticosteroids as their initial immunosuppressant regimen. In one arm, at 3 months after transplantation, cyclosporine was decreased and withdrawn over 6 to 8 weeks while sirolimus and steroids were maintained. In the other arm, cyclosporine, sirolimus, and corticosteroids were continued throughout the study period. Acute rejection rates were 9.8% in the CNI withdrawal group compared with 4.2% in the nonwithdrawal group. Renal function was better and BP lower, in the withdrawal group. However in the withdrawal group, side effects associated with sirolimus, such as thromboctopenia, hypokalemia, hyperlipidemia, and elevated liver function tests, were more frequent.[62] In a mycophenolate-based study, in which cyclosporine was withdrawn, improvements were seen in patients who did not develop acute rejection. Acute rejection episodes occurred in 10% in the withdrawal group with no graft loss and lower lipid profiles.[63] Usually, when sirolimus is added to the CNI regimen, the CNI dose is reduced by 50% initially and in some cases slowly withdrawn altogether over several weeks to months. Improvement in serum creatinine may be seen initially, but this may be due primarily to diminution of the CNI vasoconstrictive effects.

This approach may not reverse CAN as seen on G.P.'s biopsy, but it may slow the rate of deterioration of his renal function. Because G.P. is currently receiving mycophenolate, one approach would be to continue to reduce his cyclosporine and maintain his mycophenolate and steroids. Another approach would be to replace the mycophenolate with sirolimus, maintain steroids, and reduce or withdraw the cyclosporine. The best regimen for someone with CAN has not been established. The long-term consequences of these changes are not known. If this approach is attempted, G.P. should be watched carefully for acute rejection, since he is black and has had a prior acute rejection episode. Side effects of these agents and infections should be closely monitored. In addition, good BP control as well as control of hyperlipidemia and hyperglycemia are also important in minimizing renal injury.[65]

Steroid Avoidance or Withdrawal

10. D.T. is a 35-year-old African-American woman who received a cadaveric kidney transplant 9 months ago. Three months after transplantation, she had an episode of steroid-responsive acute rejection. She is currently receiving Neoral 100 mg BID, mycophenolate 1 g BID and prednisone 10 mg QD. Her serum creatinine is 2.3 mg/dL. Her glucose control and BP control continue to be a problem. She also has hyperlipidemia, which is currently controlled with a 3-hydroxy-3-methylglutaryl coenzyme A (HMG-CoA) reductase inhibitor. In addition, she recently had a DEXA scan that showed osteoporosis. Would D.T. be a candidate for steroid withdrawal?

Another important issue after kidney transplantation is the role of short- and long-term steroid use. Most transplant protocols incorporate steroid therapy. The concept of either avoiding or discontinuing corticosteroids is appealing because they cause a significant adverse effects as described in Question 7: diabetes, cataracts, infection, hypertension, hyperlipidemia, osteoporosis, avascular necrosis, psychiatric, neurologic and cosmetic effects.[66,67] However, steroid withdrawal or avoidance could increase the risk of acute rejection, compromise long-term graft function, and necessitate higher doses of the other immunosuppressives.

In the case of steroid avoidance, studies are small with short-term follow-up, but results are encouraging. Preliminary studies suggest no adverse impact on short-term graft survival and no need for higher doses of other immunosuppressives when corticosteroids are not included in maintenance regimens. These protocols have included regimens such as daclizumab or basiliximab or Thymoglobulin, mycophenolate, and cyclosporine or tacrolimus.[68,69]

Steroid withdrawal in the era of cyclosporine (Sandimmune) and azathioprine based regimens was associated with a high rate of acute rejection and late graft loss.[70] With the introduction of newer agents, steroid avoidance or withdrawal has taken on a renewed interest and several studies are re-evaluating this option.

Steroid withdrawal has been successful in at least 50% of kidney,[66] heart,[71] and liver[72] transplant recipients resulting in reductions in BP and lipid levels. Some protocols have withdrawn corticosteroids within the first few days to weeks after the initial transplantation period, whereas others attempt to withdraw them 3 to 6 months or later after transplantation. The rate of success depends on not only the immunosuppressives used, but the population (high risk versus low risk) and timing of withdrawal. Regimens that appear most successful include an antibody with cyclosporine or tacrolimus, mycophenolate, or sirolimus.[66,73,74] In terms of population, African Americans, pediatric patients, retransplanted individuals, highly sensitized patients, and patients with high serum creatinine (>2.5 mg/dL) and a recent rejection episode are more difficult to withdraw from steroids, particularly early (<3 months) after transplantation; withdrawal in these cases is associated with a higher rate of rejection. Later withdrawal may be attempted, but the benefits in terms of side effect profile may not be as great. Low-risk populations are candidates for early withdrawal.[66,75] First-time transplantation, living-donor, or well-matched transplantation, older age, and stable graft function without rejection are factors associated with a positive response to steroid withdrawal.

Steroid withdrawal may be attempted; however, D.T. has two risk factors. She is African American and has had an acute rejection episode, although this occurred 6 months ago. If attempted, steroid doses should be reduced over a 3- to 6-month period with close monitoring for signs of another rejection. If the steroid cannot be discontinued completely, the lowest possible dose should be used; alternate-day regimens may be feasible in some patients. D.T. also should be monitored for signs of adrenal insufficiency (e.g., lethargy, hypotension) as corticosteroids are reduced and withdrawn.

Long-Term Complications

All transplant recipients must be followed up closely after transplantation to prevent rejection, minimize drug toxicity (e.g., nephrotoxicity), and maintain good-quality organ function. Just as important is the prevention and management of a number of other long-term complications that can occur after transplantation. These include cardiovascular disease, glucose intolerance, bone and bone marrow conditions, nutrition and obesity, cancer, infections and compliance/nonadherence. These contribute significantly to morbidity and mortality after transplantation. This applies to all types of organ transplantations.[76,77]

Post-Transplantation Cardiovascular Disease

11. H.G., a 36-year-old man who had a cadaveric renal transplantation 1 year ago, has been enrolled in an exercise and diet program to keep his weight, BP, cholesterol, and diabetes under control. His vital signs are as follows: BP, 164/95 mm Hg; heart rate, 88 beats/min; temperature, 36.9°C; and weight, 70 kg. His BP has ranged between 150/900 to 170/94 mm Hg. The results from H.G.'s laboratory tests are as follows: Na, 135 mEq/L (normal, 135 to 147); K, 4.4 mEq/L (normal, 3.4 to 4.6); Cl, 101 mEq/L (normal, 95 to 105); CO_2, 25 mEq/L (normal, 22 to 28); BUN, 15 mg/dL (normal, 8 to 18); creatinine, 1.3 mg/dL (normal, 0.6 to 1.2); uric acid, 11.3 mg/dL (normal, 2.0 to 7.0); glucose, 110 mg/dL; A1c, 6.8% (normal, 4% to 6%). His most recent fasting lipid panel is as follows: cholesterol, 360 mg/dL (normal, <150); low-density lipoproteins (LDL), 192 mg/dL (normal, <130); and triglycerides, 250 mg/dL (normal, 1 to 249). His cyclosporine blood concentration is 160 ng/mL. H.G.'s medications include cyclosporine 175 mg BID; prednisone 15 mg QD; MMF 1 g BID; NPH Insulin 30 U SC Q AM; regular insulin 10 U SC Q AM and Q PM; felodipine 10 mg QD; furosemide 20 mg QD; ranitidine 150 mg QHS; and aspirin 81 mg QD. What risk factors does H.G. have, and what impact could they have on graft survival?

[SI units: Na, 135 mmol/L (135 to 147); K, 4.4 mmol/L (normal, 3.4 to 4.6); Cl, 101 (normal, 95 to 105); CO_2, 25 mmol/L (normal, 22 to 28); BUN, 5.35 mmol/L (normal, 3.0 to 6.5); uric acid, 672.1 μmol/L (normal, 120 to 420); cholesterol, 9.30 mmol/L (normal, <5.2); high-density lipoproteins (HDL), 2.1 mmol/L (normal, 0.8 to 1.8); LDL, 5.0 mmol/L (normal, 1.3 to 4.9); triglycerides, 2.8 mmol/L (normal, <180)]

H.G. is not unlike many other transplant recipients who have significant cardiovascular disease after transplantation. Cardiovascular disease is the major cause of death among kidney transplant recipients and a significant cause of morbidity and mortality in all organ transplant recipients.[78] After kidney transplantation, cardiovascular disease has been reported as the cause of graft loss in 16% to 36% of cases and a major cause of death with graft function (DWGF) in approximately 40%.[79,80] This is especially the case in kidney or heart transplant recipients. H.G. has several risk factors that will ultimately have a negative influence on his survival and graft survival. He had ESRD requiring a transplantation. Many of these patients already have significant cardiovascular disease by the time they get to transplantation, including ischemic heart disease, peripheral vascular disease, hypertension, hyperlipidemia, and diabetes. Other factors may also contribute to cardiovascular disease after transplantation, including age, family history, obesity, smoking, left ventricular hypertrophy (LVH), and hyperhomocysteinemia. Many patients develop these conditions after transplantation, or they are exacerbated by the immunosuppressive agents used and/or organ dysfunction.[81] Approaches to prevent and manage cardiovascular disease are similar to those used in the general population, although there are certain immunosuppressive-related considerations in the transplant population.

Post-Transplantation Hypertension

12. What approaches should be taken to control H.G.'s BP?

It is not surprising that H.G. has developed arterial hypertension, which occurs in recipients of all types of solid organ transplantation regardless of age. For example, some reports suggest a prevalence of hypertension after transplantation ranging from 40% to 100%.[82] A discouraging aspect of hypertension is that prevalence of this condition increases with time after transplantation. Hypertension has a negative impact on both the patient and graft survival.[76]

Hypertension results in large part from the type of organ transplanted and the immunosuppressive regimen used. Kidney and heart transplant recipients have a higher prevalence of hypertension after transplantation compared with liver and lung transplant recipients. The higher prevalence in kidney and heart transplant recipients may be attributed to preexisting uncontrolled hypertension that led to end-organ failure (kidney failure or heart failure). Hypertension in the donor organ (kidney) may play some role in contributing to post-transplantation hypertension as well. Other risk factors include a family history of hypertension or major cardiovascular complications, such as MI, stroke, or ischemic heart disease; older age at time of transplantation; male gender; kidney disease or impairment of renal function, which may occur with the use of specific immunosuppressive regimens after transplantation; obesity; and endocrine disorders such as hyperaldosteronism, hyperparathyroidism, pheochromocytoma, thyroid disease, acromegaly, and Cushing's disease. Any of these conditions that are reversible and diagnosed after transplantation should be treated to reduce the risk for hypertension.

Cyclosporine contributes to the already high incidence of post-transplantation hypertension. It can induce hypertension in kidney, liver, heart, and bone marrow transplant recipients as well as nontransplanted patients who may use cyclosporine for immune-related disorders. A variety of mechanisms have been proposed to explain the hypertensive effect of cyclosporine. These include volume expansion, increased sympathetic tone, increased endothelin concentrations, stimulation of the renin-angiotensin system, and prostaglandin interference. Other mechanisms include renal arteriolar vasoconstriction and smooth muscle vasoconstriction, mediated by some of the aforementioned factors, as well as promotion of intracellular calcium influx. Hypomagnesemia, which results from cyclosporine's nephrotoxic effect, can increase peripheral vascular resistance and induce hypertension as well. Cyclosporine-induced hypertension usually develops within the first week to 6 months of therapy. It appears to be dose dependent, but some patients are resistant to antihypertensive medications, regardless of cyclosporine dose.[83]

Tacrolimus is another immunosuppressive agent with a mechanism of action and adverse effect profile similar to cyclosporine. For example, both cyclosporine and tacrolimus are associated with nephrotoxicity and hypertension. For these reasons, these two agents are never used together to prevent rejection. However, the prevalence of hypertension and the need for antihypertensives in patients receiving tacrolimus are lower than those in patients receiving cyclosporine for primary immunosuppression. This has also been shown in patients who are converted from cyclosporine to tacrolimus.[19,84] Corticosteroids have also been implicated as a causative factor in hypertension; sodium retention and increased plasma volume are well-known effects of these agents.

When the diastolic BP is >90 mm Hg and/or the systolic BP is >140 mm Hg, transplant recipients usually are treated with diet and behavior modification along with antihypertensive drugs. A large percentage of transplant recipients require more than one antihypertensive medication to adequately control BP. Experience indicates that many transplantation patients switch antihypertensive therapies at least three or more times the rate than their nontransplanted hypertensive counterparts. Currently, there is no single best agent or regimen. The best approach is to individualize antihypertensive therapy to the specific patient, based on response and adverse effects.[85]

Traditionally, calcium channel blockers have been considered the drugs of choice for transplantation hypertension because of their preferential effect on afferent arterioles, their ability to induce renal and peripheral vasodilatation, and their renal-protective properties that may counteract the effects of a CNI.[86] Diltiazem, verapamil, nicardipine, and possibly amlodipine appear to inhibit the metabolism of cyclosporine, which can increase its concentration. Nifedipine, isradipine, felodipine, and nitrendipine do not appear to interact pharmacokinetically to any significant degree with CNIs.[87] Diltiazem has been added intentionally to cyclosporine regimens in an effort to reduce the dosage of cyclosporine and reduce the cost of therapy.[88] A 30% to 40% reduction in CNI (both cyclosporine and tacrolimus) dose is required when diltiazem or verapamil is administered concurrently.

Angiotensin-converting enzyme (ACE) inhibitors and probably angiotensin-II blockers also are effective antihypertensive agents in transplant recipients and have particular beneficial effects in patients with heart failure, proteinuria, diabetes, or erythrocytosis.[89] Although ACE inhibitors must be used cautiously in patients with renal dysfunction, these agents are not contraindicated in transplant recipients such as H.G.[303] β-Blockers (e.g., atenolol, metoprolol, labetalol) are also useful agents, especially in patients with coronary heart disease Centrally acting α-agonists (e.g., clonidine), peripherally acting α-blockers (e.g., prazosin), and diuretics (e.g., furosemide, hydrochlorothiazide) may be used as well. In difficult-to-treat patients, vasodilators such as minoxidil or hydralazine may be required. None of these agents should be prescribed without due concern for adverse effects (e.g., hyperlipidemia, azotemia, hyperuricemia, hypo- or hyperkalemia, anemia).[85]

Because H.G. is already receiving felodopine, an increase in his dosage would be appropriate. Another possibility is to discontinue the furosemide and add an ACE inhibitor, since he is diabetic and his serum uric acid and lipid concentrations are elevated. The treatment of hypertension is presented in Chapter 14, Essential Hypertension.

Monitoring the effectiveness of antihypertensive medications in this group is challenging because transplant recipients have abnormal circadian variations in their BPs. The absence of a nocturnal fall and even an increase in mean systolic and diastolic BP during sleep have been reported. In healthy subjects, the BP falls 20% on average during sleep, but transplantation patients have a blunted response to the nocturnal decline in BP. Some authors have correlated abnormalities in nocturnal BP with a corresponding increase in LVH, which is an important and common predictor of the risk of death. For these reasons, BP measurement should be documented both during daytime and nighttime hours to establish the effectiveness of antihypertensive regimens. Ambulatory BP monitoring in some patients may be useful.[90]

In addition to treating H.G.'s hypertension, consideration should be given to altering his immunosuppressive regimen, if possible. A reduction in his cyclosporine and/or prednisone dosage may contribute to a reduction in BP. Another alternative is to convert cyclosporine to tacrolimus. This may lower BP and also allow a further reduction in steroid dosing.[91]

Hyperlipidemia

13. How should H.G.'s hyperlipidemia be managed?

Hyperlipidemia, is another common cardiovascular finding after transplantation, occurring in 30% to 80% of transplant recipients.[93] Increased concentrations of total cholesterol, LDL, and triglycerides and decreased HDL often are seen within 3 to 6 months and later after transplantation. Dyslipidemia is a significant risk factor for atherosclerosis, cardiovascular events, peripheral vascular disease, chronic allograft nephropathy, chronic allograft vasculopathy and death after transplant.[94]

The prevalence of post-transplantation hyperlipidemia (similar to post-transplantation hypertension) is often a function of the type of organ transplanted and the immunosuppressive protocols used to prevent rejection. Heart and kidney transplant recipients may have a higher prevalence of post-transplant hyperlipidemia because of pre-existing conditions, such as atherosclerosis and diabetes mellitus, which led to end organ failure. Pre-existing hyperlipidemia is a major risk factor for hyperlipidemia after transplantation, even in liver transplant recipients. Other risk factors include development of post-transplant diabetes mellitus and/or hypertension, genetic predisposition (positive family history of hyperlipidemia in both the transplant recipient and the allogeneic donor organ), renal dysfunction, dietary influences, as well as smoking, obesity, older age (possibly older than 50), male gender, underlying medical conditions such as hypothyroidism, and any medications (e.g., diuretics, β-blockers). Reversible medical conditions and pharmacologic agents that may adversely affect the lipid profile should be thoroughly explored as potential targets for control of post-transplant hyperlipidemia.[95]

Immunosuppressive agents have been identified as significant causes of post-transplantation hyperlipidemia. Cyclosporine may have an independent as well as synergistic effect with prednisone and sirolimus on elevating lipid concentrations. Cyclosporine interferes with the conversion of cholesterol to bile acids, binds to the LDL cholesterol receptor, thereby promoting increased serum concentrations of LDL cholesterol, and induces peripheral insulin resistance.[83] Cyclosporine-based immunosuppression is associated with higher serum cholesterol concentrations than regimens using tacrolimus, and conversion to tacrolimus is associated with a reduction in lipid levels.[96–98]

One of the strongest predictors of elevated lipids is the cumulative dose of prednisone. Prednisone increases the hepatic synthesis of very low-density lipoproteins (VLDLs), promotes insulin resistance and hyperinsulinemia, enhances the activity of acetyl-coenzyme A carboxylase and free fatty acid synthetase, down-regulates LDL-receptor activity, increases the activity of HMG-CoA reductase, and inhibits lipoprotein lipase. These effects increase VLDL, total cholesterol, and triglyceride concentrations and decrease HDL concentration.[88] In several studies, lipid concentrations were reduced when the dose of prednisone was lowered or therapy was discontinued. Because of the potential for multiple metabolic adverse effects (e.g., hypertension, hyperlipidemia, obesity, diabetes mellitus) from long-term use of corticosteroids, the goal is to use the lowest possible doses or to discontinue them completely.[66]

Sirolimus appears to have the most profound effect on lipid levels whether used alone or in combination with other agents. As noted previously, sirolimus is often used in combination with cyclosporine and corticosteroids to prevent acute rejection episodes in kidney transplant recipients. Its synergistic effect with cyclosporine is important because sirolimus does not seem to cause nephrotoxicity, neurotoxicity, or diabetes, which occur commonly in patients treated with cyclosporine or tacrolimus. Furthermore, sirolimus may afford some protection against chronic rejection (at least in kidney transplant recipients), although more data are needed.[99] Nevertheless, sirolimus has been associated with a significant increase in the incidence of and need for treatment of hyperlipidemia.[109] This effect is dose dependent, and with lower dosages, lipid concentrations (specifically, triglycerides) return to baseline values.[99] The mechanism of this drug-induced hyperlipidemia is unclear, but one hypothesis suggests that sirolimus inhibits insulin and insulin-like growth factor signals, thereby retarding the uptake or accelerating the secretion of fatty acids into the systemic circulation. It also decreases VLDL and LDL metabolism and increases fatty acid production.[100]

A variety of HMG-CoA inhibitors (statins) have been used successfully in many types of organ transplantations (kidney, liver, heart) to reduce cholesterol concentrations. A few studies indicate that statins combined with immunosuppressive regimens in heart transplant recipients may reduce acute rejection episodes.[101,102] This favorable effect has not been noted in kidney transplant recipients.[103,104] Because of the potential for liver toxicity associated with statins, there was concern over their routine use in liver transplant recipients with hyperlipidemia; however, no significant hepatic adverse events were reported with statins.[105] At one time, statins were not used in transplant recipients because of reports of severe rhabdomyolysis and subsequent acute renal failure in transplant recipients. This was attributed to cyclosporine-induced inhibition of lovastatin metabolism; however, these adverse effects occurred with high dosages (>40 mg/day) of lovastatin or with concurrent fibric acid derivative therapy (gemfibrozil). Low doses of lovastatin (10 to 20 mg/day) are safe and effective in transplant recipients, as are other drugs in this class. Atorvastatin, simvastatin, and pravastatin are the most commonly used agents in transplant recipients. Nevertheless, caution must be used when higher doses of these statins are used, which is not unusual in some transplant recipients. This is because some statins are metabolized by the same P450 isoenzyme as CNIs and the drug sirolimus, which may result in higher concentrations of the statins and an increased risk of myopathies.[105] Pravastatin is not metabolized by this isoenzyme and is often preferentially used, although other statins have been used safely in these patients.[106] Other available cholesterol-lowering agents are available, but some may present problems in transplant recipients as well. For example, cholestyramine and colestipol can adversely affect the absorption of cyclosporine, mycophenolate, and possibly other medications these patients require. Nicotinic acid could exacerbate existing hyperuricemia, and gemfibrozil and fenofibrate can cause myositis and further exacerbate myalgia. Ezetimibe inhibits cholesterol absorption, and when used with a statin it allows for a reduced dose of statin with an additive effect on lipid levels. Ezetimibe has a milder side effect profile and does not seem to interact with other drugs. Although it has not been evaluated in transplant recipients, it may offer an alternative to these other agents. Therefore, the lipid-lowering agents of choice for transplant recipients are the statin agents.

The treatment of H.G.'s hyperlipidemia should consist of weight control, dietary modification, and exercise, according to the National Cholesterol Education Program guidelines (see Chapter 13, Dyslipidemias). Very few transplant recipients respond to these lifestyle changes alone and require drug therapy. A statin, such as atorvastatin 10 mg QD or pravastatin 20 mg QD, should be initiated and monitored appropriately. Finally, any drugs that may increase lipid concentrations should be discontinued, if possible. An attempt could be made to reduce the dose of cyclosporine and to slowly withdraw prednisone. Another option would be to convert cyclosporine to tacrolimus.

Post-Transplantation Diabetes Mellitus

Another common problem, which appears to be on the increase in transplant recipients, is post-transplantation diabetes mellitus (PTDM). Diabetes significantly affects morbidity and mortality in transplant recipients. It is often a pre-existing condition in renal transplant recipients and a cause of ESRD. In recipients of other organs such as livers, diabetes is common as well, both as a pre-existing condition and as a post-transplantation complication. The definition of PTDM varies among studies. It has been based on symptoms and plasma glucose, oral glucose challenge results, or the need for insulin or oral antidiabetic drugs after transplantation. Reported rates range from 3% to 40%, with most cases of PTDM occurring within the first year. Risk factors, besides pre-transplantation diabetes, include advanced age, family history, CMV infection, certain HLA phenotypes, race (African American or Hispanic), and increased body weight.[107]

The most critical factor in the development of PTDM is the immunosuppressive regimen. Cyclosporine, tacrolimus, and prednisone are all diabetogenic through a multitude of mechanisms. The CNIs appear to be have a direct toxic effect on the pancreatic beta cells leading to decreased insulin synthesis and secretion; this effect seems to be dose related and generally reversible.[108] A major debate is whether tacrolimus or cyclosporine is more likely to cause PTDM. Some studies indicate that tacrolimus may cause PTDM more frequently; however, other studies have shown no difference in the diabetogenic action of these two drugs. Nevertheless, conversion from tacrolimus to cyclosporine has been useful in some patients with PTDM.[109] In evaluating these studies, other factors such as CNI drug concentrations, steroid doses, African-American race, transplant type, and time lapsed following transplantation must be considered.[110] As with diabetes in the general population, a similar intensive approach in controlling blood glucose should be undertaken. Also, other conditions such as hypertension and hyperlipidemia should be managed aggressively. Another step includes reducing or withdrawing diabetes-inducing immunosuppression as much as possible without jeopardizing graft function or using agents that are nondiabetogenic, such as mycophenolate or sirolimus if appropriate.[108,111]

Post-Transplantation Osteoporosis

Osteoporosis is another common post-transplantation disorder that must be evaluated, prevented, and treated. Osteoporosis, a silent disease, is characterized by low bone mass and microarchitectural deterioration of bone tissue, which increases bone fragility and eventually leads to fracture. Various epidemiologic and cross-sectional studies estimate that up to 7% to 11% of nondiabetic kidney transplant recipients, 45% of diabetic kidney transplant recipients, 18% to 50% of heart transplant recipients, and 24% to 65% of liver transplant recipients develop atraumatic fractures resulting from osteoporosis in the post-transplantation period.[112]

RISK FACTORS

Osteoporosis risk factors are similar to those in the general population and include menopausal status, family history, smoking, alcohol use, lack of physical activity, poor nutritional status, and ingestion of various medications such as corticosteroids, phenytoin, thyroxine, heparin, warfarin, and loop diuretics.[112] Additional factors responsible for bone loss in organ transplant recipients depend on the underlying disease state and the particular organ system transplanted. For example, patients with end-stage renal failure commonly have at least some evidence of renal osteodystrophy, which includes hyperparathyroidism, osteomalacia, osteosclerosis, and adynamic or aplastic bone disease. Hypogonadism can also be present. Many renal transplant recipients have already been exposed to medications that can affect bone and mineral metabolism, such as corticosteroids, cyclosporine for immune complex disease, loop diuretics, or aluminum-containing phosphate binders.[113] Potential heart transplant recipients with congestive heart failure (CHF) suffer from specific conditions that may contribute to low bone mineral densities. These include vitamin D deficiency, dietary calcium deficiency, therapy with loop diuretics, prerenal azotemia, hepatic congestion, and hypogonadism. Potential lung transplant recipients are at increased risk for osteoporosis because of decreased mobility, hypoxemia, malnutrition, vitamin D deficiency, tobacco use, hypogonadism, and corticosteroid therapy, as well as pancreatic insufficiency and calcium malabsorption in cystic fibrosis.[112,114]

Low bone mass and abnormal mineral metabolism are common in patients with several forms of chronic cholestatic liver disease, such as biliary cirrhosis. Therefore, liver transplant recipients are prone to this problem.[115]

Drugs used to prevent organ rejection predispose patients to osteoporosis, especially the corticosteroids.[116] Unfortunately, most transplant recipients require steroids in combination with other immunosuppressive agents to prevent rejection. Corticosteroids reduce net intestinal calcium absorption, increase urinary calcium excretion, increase parathyroid hormone, decrease production of skeletal growth factors, and decrease androgen and estrogen synthesis in the gonads and adrenal gland. They also decrease bone formation by osteoblasts and increase bone resorption.[116] The most dramatic reduction in bone loss after transplantation occurs within the first 3 to 6 months, when high doses of steroids are tapered to prednisone doses equivalent to 7.5 to 10 mg every day. Areas of the skeleton rich in trabecular or cancellous bone, such as the ribs, vertebrae, distal ends of long bones, and the cortical rim of the vertebral body, are most at risk for osteoporotic fracture because a greater degree of bone remodeling or bone turnover occurs here and because this is a target of corticosteroid activity.[112] Most studies suggest a minor effect from CNI on bone. Other currently used agents appear to be have little or no effect.[113]

TREATMENT

Because rapid bone loss and fractures can occur during the first few months postoperatively, strategies to prevent bone loss and fractures should be initiated immediately after transplantation and if possible before transplantation. Most recommendations are based on the American College of Rheumatology's (ACR's) guidelines for the prevention and treatment of corticosteroid-induced osteoporosis.[121] These recommendations focus on providing calcium (1,500 mg elemental calcium three times a day) and vitamin D (various dosing depending on kidney function and liver function) to patients who will be receiving continuous corticosteroid therapy. If patients are diagnosed with low bone mineral density (osteopenia) or even osteoporosis with bone mineral density scans using DEXA scans, calcium and vitamin D analogs are recommended in conjunction with either a bisphosphonate or calcitonin.[116]

Clinical trials are currently underway to determine whether alendronate will prevent osteoporosis that occurs after heart, liver, and kidney transplantation.[120] Because nearly all patients lose bone mass after transplantation, some clinicians advocate the use of calcitonin or bisphosphonates (alendronate, risedronate, etidronate, pamidronate) for all, regardless of bone mineral density. Alternatively, treatment with these agents could be limited to patients with lumbar spine bone mineral densities below age-matched bone mineral density values. Either calcitonin or the bisphosphonates are relatively safe in this population, and there is significant data to support their efficacy in corticosteroid-induced osteoporosis.[113,115]

A DEXA scan should be performed in H.G., and he should be given calcium and vitamin D since he is receiving steroids. Based on the results of the DEXA scan, he should receive either a bisphosphonate or intranasal calcitonin and continue calcium and vitamin D. A repeat DEXA scan should be performed in 6 months to 1 year. H.G. should be carefully counseled on how to take his medicine correctly to minimize adverse effects and he should be monitored for hypercalcemia.

HEART TRANSPLANTATION
Indications

14. R.B., a 55-year-old, 65-kg man with end-stage ischemic heart disease and functional class IV failure (according to New York Heart Association [NYHA]), is in the intensive coronary care unit, where he has been receiving continuous inotropic therapy for 1 month. He is on the heart transplant waiting list (status 1). He had an acute myocardial infarction (MI) in 1985, coronary artery bypass graft in 1986 and, in 1996, several admissions for exacerbation of CHF over the past year, and an episode of sudden death 1 month ago. His most recent multiple gated acquisition (MUGA) scan to evaluate left ventricular function reveals a left ventricular ejection fraction (LVEF) of 14%, and echocardiography shows extensive anterior, septal, lateral, and apical akinesia, and severe mitral regurgitation. Right-sided heart catheterization shows mild pulmonary hypertension with a pulmonary vascular resistance of 2.8 Woods units. VO_2 (volume of oxygen) is 8 mL/kg per minute. Medical history also includes hypertension and hypercholesterolemia. He currently is being treated with dobutamine IV infusion, enalapril 20 mg BID, warfarin 2.5 mg QD, furosemide 80 mg BID, KCl 10 mEq BID, metoprolol 50 mg BID, digoxin 0.125 mg QD, and simvastatin 20 mg QD. His vital signs are as follows: BP, 122/82 mm Hg; heart rate, 75 beats/min; respiratory rate (RR) 24 breaths/min; and temperature, 36.6°C. His laboratory values are as follows: Na, 136 mEq/L (normal, 135 to 145); K, 4.3 mEq/L (normal, 3.4 to 4.6); Cl, 94 mEq/L (normal, 95 to 105); CO_2, 32 mEq/L (normal, 24 to 30); BUN, 23 mg/dL (normal, 8 to 18); SrCr, 1.1 mg/dL (normal, 0.6 to 1.2); total bilirubin, 1.7 mg/dL (normal, 0.1 to 1.0); aspartate aminotransferase (AST), 40 U/L (normal, 0 to 35); alanine aminotransferase (ALT), 16 U/L (normal, 0 to 35); lactate dehydrogenase (LDH), 267 U/L (normal, 50 to 150); alkaline phosphatase, 100 U/L (normal, 30 to 120); 24-hour creatinine clearance (Cl_{Cr}), 60 mL/min (normal, 75 to 125); cholesterol, 225 mg/dL (normal, <200); triglycerides, 99 mg/dL (normal, 1 to 249); HDL, 71 mg/dL (normal, 28 to 71); and LDL, 134 mg/dL (normal, <130). His other laboratory tests are negative for hepatitis B, HIV, and Epstein-Barr virus (EBV), but positive for CMV. What makes R.B. an appropriate candidate for heart transplantation?

[SI units: Na, 136 mmol/L (normal, 135 to 145); K, 4.3 mmol/L (3.4 to 4.6); Cl, 94 mmol/L (normal, 95 to 105); CO_2, 32 mmol/L (normal, 24 to 30); BUN, 8.2 mmol/L (normal, 3.0 to 6.5); SrCr, 97.2 μmol/L (normal, 50 to 110), total bilirubin, 29.1 μmol/L (normal, 2 to 18); AST 0.67 μkat/L (normal, 0 to 0.58); ALT, 0.27 μkat/L (normal, 0 to 0.58); LDH, 4.45 μkat/L (normal, 0.82 to 2.66); alkaline phosphatase, 1.67 μkat/L (normal, 0.5 to 2.0); Cl_{Cr}, 1.0 mL/sec (normal, 1.24 to 2.08); cholesterol, 5.82 mmol/L (normal, <5.20); triglycerides, 1.12 mmol/L (normal, 0.01 to 2.8); HDL, 1.83 mg/dL (normal, 0.72 to 1.83); LDL, 3.47 mmol/L (normal, 0.26 to 3.34)]

The success of heart transplantation has had a significant impact on the survival of patients with end-stage heart disease (ESHD). The 1- and 5-year survival rates are 85% to 90% and approximately 70%, respectively. In contrast, the 1-year survival rate for patients with severe ESHD without transplant is 20% to 40%. Cardiomyopathy and coronary artery disease account for 45% and 45%, respectively, of those undergoing transplant. Pediatric patients (0 to 18 years of age) and patients older than 55 have been the fastest-growing segment of the population undergoing heart transplantation.[117]

The best candidates for heart transplantation are those who are least likely to survive without a transplant; that is, those with a life expectancy of 1 year and a high likelihood of a good quality of life after transplantation. The criteria for the selection of patients for heart transplantation vary from center to center, but general criteria for selection of appropriate candidates include NYHA functional class III or IV, having intolerable symptoms in spite of maximal medical and surgical management, lack of reversible factors, and a 1-year life expectancy of <50%. An ejection fraction of <20% alone is not an indication for transplantation. Secondary comorbid conditions also affect the selection of suitable patients for heart transplantation (e.g., irreversible renal, hepatic, or pulmonary disease; severe cerebrovascular or peripheral vascular disease; active infection; current malignancy; acute pulmonary embolus or pulmonary infarction; active GI disease; insulin-dependent diabetes mellitus with end-organ damage; coexisting illness with poor prognosis; morbid obesity; severe osteoporosis; substance abuse; acute psychological disorder; noncompliance). One hemodynamic exclusion criterion specific for the heart is an elevated pulmonary vascular resistance >4 Wood units or a transpulmonary gradient >15 mm Hg that does not reverse with treatment. This indicates severe irreversible pulmonary hypertension. Also, a PRA and crossmatch should be performed before transplantation. Patients with this characteristic are excluded as candidates for heart transplantation because they generally experience a poor outcome in the immediate post-transplantation period. However, these patients could be candidates for heart-lung transplants.[118]

R.B. has considerable evidence for a progressively failing heart. His increasing number of admissions for CHF, an admission for sudden death, his need for chronic IV inotropic support, and his poor LVEF and VO_2 provide clear indications for heart transplantation. The status of his organ function and his negative infectious serology should clear the way for placement on the waiting list for transplantation. The placement of R.B. into the appropriate status category for receipt of a transplanted heart would take into consideration his severity of illness, ABO blood type, time on waiting list, and length of the waiting list.

Postoperative Course

15. R.B. receives mycophenolate 1 g PO, cyclosporine 200 mg PO, and cefuroxime 1.5 g IV before surgery. During reperfusion of his new heart, methylprednisolone 500 mg IV was given, and IV infusions of dopamine, nitroglycerin, dobutamine, and isoproterenol were started. A temporary pacemaker was placed in the new heart. R.B. is placed in the cardiac thoracic ICU for post-transplantation care. The following medications were given intravenously: cefuroxime 1.5 g BID for 2 days, furosemide 20 mg QID, ranitidine 50 mg Q 8 hr, methylprednisolone 125 mg Q 8 hr, mycophenolate 1 g NG/PO BID, OKT3 5 mg QD for 7 days, Neoral 250 mg NG/PO BID, and ganciclovir 150 mg IV QD. He also is maintained on continuous IV infusions of nitroglycerin, dobutamine and milrinone. Why would R.B. require vasopressor and inotropic therapy perioperatively and postoperatively?

Most heart transplant recipients recover rapidly from the transplantation procedure, and most are extubated and are off vasopressor/inotropic support within 24 to 48 hours. However, during the early postoperative period, the cardiac, respiratory, and fluid and electrolyte status of the patient must be monitored intensively. The transplanted heart becomes denervated, and contractility and sinus node function are temporarily impaired to varying degrees based on the condition of the donor heart, quality of preservation, ischemic time, surgical technique, myocardial depletion, and elevated pulmonary artery pressure. Soon after transplantation, both left and right ventricular dysfunction often are present with elevated right and left heart filling pressures. For the first few days after transplantation, the heart depends on direct stimulation from exogenously administered catecholamines for inotropic and chronotropic support. At this time, the heart is especially sensitive to β-agonists, such as isoproterenol or dobutamine, because of upregulation of β-adrenergic receptors.[119] Therefore, inotropic and chronotropic therapy should be guided by hemodynamic monitoring results (see Chapter 22, Shock). In addition, low-dose dopamine and/or diuretics may be needed to maintain adequate fluid balance and urine output.

For recipients like R.B., inotropic and chronotropic agents usually are started in the operating room when the new heart is being reperfused and cardiopulmonary bypass is being discontinued. The choice of agent or combination of agents is based on the aforementioned hemodynamic parameters, which would be monitored continuously. The patient is eventually weaned off these agents. Isoproterenol, milrinone, and epinephrine are the primary agents used to maintain a heart rate between 110 and 130 beats/minute to maximize cardiac output. Dobutamine is used for its inotropic effect to increase cardiac output, reduce left ventricular dysfunction, and reduce systemic vascular resistance. Dopamine, at low dosages, could improve renal blood flow. Nitroglycerin or nitroprusside will reduce pulmonary arterial pressure and afterload. Temporary atrial pacing also may be used to maintain heart rate as well. In cases in which elevated pulmonary artery pressures are unresponsive to these agents, resulting in sustained right ventricular failure, IV prostaglandin E_1 and norepinephrine may be required. If these interventions fail, insertion of a mechanical assistance device may be effective.[120]

Sinus Node Dysfunction

16. **Two days later, R.B. is extubated and hemodynamically stable. Vasopressors are discontinued, and IV medications are switched to oral formulations. On day 9, his heart rate has decreased to a rate of 50 to 60 beats/min. A continuous IV infusion of milrinone was restarted because R.B.'s temporary pacemaker had been removed 2 days earlier, resulting in a heart rate of 80 to 110 beats/min. TheoDur 150 mg BID is started and the dosage adjusted. Why is this appropriate therapy of R.B.'s bradycardia?**

Sinus node dysfunction, which presents as nodal or sinus bradycardia and episodes of sinus arrest, is common in the early postoperative period. The donor sinus node serves as the heart's pacemaker, but because it is denervated, the transplanted heart cannot respond to cholinergic or vagal stimulation. Therefore, atropine, which commonly is used to treat bradycardia, is not effective in a heart transplant recipient. In most patients, the denervation is transient, and temporary use of isoproterenol or a pacemaker is needed. If resistance to vagal stimulation persists (as it does in approximately 5% to 20%), placement of a permanent pacemaker has been the traditional approach. The insertion of a permanent pacemaker may increase the risk of infection and interfere with the endomyocardial biopsy (EMB) procedure that is used to assess the status of rejection. Ultimately, up to 70% of patients with a permanent pacemaker return to normal sinus rhythm within 12 months.[121]

Theophylline use has been associated with a restoration of normal vagal response, fewer days of temporary pacing, fewer days of hospitalization and a decreased need for a permanent pacemaker. Theophylline may antagonize the negative chronotropic and dromotropic effects of adenosine and/or increase catecholamine levels. The catecholamines may stimulate the transplanted heart because of its increased sensitivity to catecholamines.[122]

Because R.B.'s temporary pacemaker was removed a few days earlier, the use of IV milrinone or isoproterenol, followed by theophylline, is appropriate as long as he is hemodynamically stable. Although there are no specific dosing guidelines in this situation, an aminophylline IV infusion of 0.5 mg/kg per hour or oral TheoDur 150 mg every 12 hours are appropriate starting regimens. These regimens should be adjusted based on heart rate and achievement of therapeutic theophylline serum concentrations (10 to 15 mg/mL). A response should be evident within 4 days; if supraventricular tachyarrhythmias occur, the dosage of theophylline should be reduced and the drug may have to be discontinued. Terbutaline is an alternative agent. Some patients ultimately may require a permanent pacemaker, particularly those with unexplained syncope or near syncope.

Cardiac Denervation

17. **What is the effect of denervation on the physiology of the heart and what are the pharmacodynamic effects of cardiac medications after heart transplantation?**

Although the transplanted heart usually functions very well, physiologic changes result in different responses to various stimuli when contrasted to the normal innervated heart. The transplanted heart has a higher resting heart rate than normal because of the loss of vagal tone. Therefore, as already noted, drugs that work via the parasympathetic pathway (e.g., atropine) will be ineffective. The transplanted heart also accelerates more slowly during exercise, usually by taking several minutes to reach a maximal heart rate, which is still less than the normal innervated heart during exercise. Acute reflex changes in heart rate do not occur in response to increases or decreases in BP in the denervated transplanted heart, and the ability to feel anginal pain is lost. Therefore, the clinical response to antianginal medications is masked. Cardiac output and BP usually are normal in the nonrejecting heart.[119] The adrenergic system remains intact in the transplanted denervated heart. Therefore, drugs such as isoproterenol, milrinone, epinephrine, norepinephrine, dopamine, phenylephrine, glucagon, and β-blockers still exert cardiac effects. The indirect chronotropic effect of digoxin on the sinus and atrioventricular nodes will not be manifested in the denervated heart, but the inotropic effect will be maintained. The usual increase in heart rate secondary to nifedipine lowered BP usually is muted as well, and responses of the denervated heart to verapamil, diltiazem, quinidine, and disopyramide also may be altered.[121] Because the effect of nonprescription sympathomimetics on the transplanted heart has not been determined, these agents should be used cautiously.[123] Reinnervation has been reported in some patients.

Immunosuppression

18. **What was the justification for using quadruple immunosuppressive therapy (i.e., OKT3, cyclosporine, methylprednisolone, and mycophenolate) in R.B.?**

After heart transplantation, as with other solid organ transplantations, immunosuppressive therapy with three or four drugs is administered aggressively during the early transplantation period when the risk of organ rejection is greatest. Regimens of azathioprine with prednisone, or azathioprine with prednisone and antithymocyte globulin, were associated with survival rates of 50% and 60%, respectively. The addition of cyclosporine led to an 80% to 90% rate of organ survival. When it was first introduced into the immunosuppressive regimen, the large IV or oral bolus doses of 15 to 18 mg/kg given preoperatively and in the initial postoperative period resulted in a significant degree of acute renal failure. Current initial regimens use cyclosporine doses of 2.5 to 10 mg/kg per day orally, or approximately 1.5 to 2.5 mg/kg per day as a continuous IV infusion. Thereafter, the dosage is adjusted based on targeted cyclosporine concentrations. However, with the introduction of Neoral, the use of IV cyclosporine has decreased. Regimens containing oral tacrolimus (initial regimen of 0.05 mg/kg BID) have shown similar efficacy to Neoral based regimens but with reduced hypertension and hyperlipidemia. [124] Because MMF (initial doses of 1 to 1.5 g BID) are associated with lower rejection rates and improved survival, it has replaced azathioprine in heart transplantation.[125,126] Furthermore, data in patients converted from mycophenolate to azathioprine later after transplant show a high rate of acute rejection.[127]

Alternatively, preoperative and early postoperative use of cyclosporine may be avoided entirely until renal function and urine output are appropriate and stable. The introduction of OKT3, antithymocyte globulins, and daclizumab has led to the development of induction regimens in which these agents, combined with other agents, either replace cyclosporine or are used with lower dosages of cyclosporine or tacrolimus to minimize renal dysfunction in the early postoperative period. Induction, in contrast to standard regimens containing only azathioprine, prednisone, and cyclosporine, is associated with a delay in the onset of the first rejection episode without differences in the frequency or severity of rejection or survival. The use of induction therapy, although not required, which is used by approximately 50% of programs, may allow for a more rapid discontinuation of maintenance corticosteroids.[128-130] Adverse effects of antibody induction include increased infection rates and potential for malignancy secondary to overimmunosuppression. IV OKT3 5 mg every day or IV ATG 10 to 15 mg/kg every day or Thymoglobulin 1.5 mg/kg is usually given for 10 days, although shorter course of 5 to 7 days is as effective. IL-2R antibodies, such as daclizumab, may also be effective in preventing acute rejection.[131]

Transplant recipients older than 65 might experience lower rejection rates and higher rates of infections, malignancy, and toxicities, although this requires further study in a larger population. Because OKT3 and antithymocyte globulin seem to be equally effective, the use of OKT3, along with mycophenolate, methylprednisolone, and cyclosporine, seems appropriate for R.B. Other alternative regimens could include tacrolimus, mycophenolate, and prednisone or cyclosporine, mycophenolate, and prednisone with or without IL-2R antibodies. Because his preoperative serum creatinine is <1.2 mg/dL, the early use of cyclosporine is not contraindicated. Over time, the maintenance doses of cyclosporine and prednisone will be reduced. The corticosteroid eventually might be discontinued within the first year depending on R.B.'s clinical course. Several reports have indicated that steroid withdrawal generally begun > 6 months after transplant is possible in many patients who are considered low risk, such as whites with fewer and less severe acute rejection episodes.[132]

However, there is always a risk of late rejection and the impact on long-term survival has not been thoroughly evaluated.[133,134]

Acute or Chronic Rejection

19. R.B. is discharged after 20 days in the hospital and returns for a routine clinic visit and scheduled endomyocardial biopsy (EMB). Current medications include cyclosporine 225 mg BID; prednisone 15 mg QD; mycophenolate 1.5 g BID; valganciclovir 900 mg QD; TMP-SMX double strength 1 tablet Mondays, Wednesdays, and Fridays; Cardizem CD 180 mg QD; ranitidine 150 mg QHS; TheoDur 200 mg BID; pravastatin 40 mg QD and aspirin 81 mg QD. R.B.'s BP readings, which he monitors at home, have been 140 to 150 mm Hg/85 to 90 mm Hg. Laboratory test results are as follows: Na, 134 mEq/L (normal, 135 to 147); K, 4.3 mEq/L (normal, 3.5 to 5.0); Cl, 103 mEq/L (normal, 95 to 105); CO_2, 26 mEq/L (normal, 22 to 28); BUN, 16 mg/dL (normal, 8 to 18); creatinine, 1.4 mg/dL (normal, 0.6 to 1.2); cyclosporine trough level, 233 ng/mL; and theophylline level, 14 mg/mL. His vital signs are as follows: heart rate, 105 beats/min; BP, 155/84 mm Hg; and temperature, 36.8°C. Biopsy results indicate mild grade 1 rejection of his transplanted heart. His cyclosporine dose is increased to 250 mg BID. A repeat EMB 1 week later now shows moderate rejection. What signs and symptoms indicate that R.B. is experiencing acute rejection of his transplanted heart?

[SI units: Na, 134 mmol/L (normal, 135 to 147); K, 4.3 mmol/L (normal, 3.5 to 5.0); Cl, 103 mmol/L (normal, 95 to 105); CO_2, 26 mmol/L (normal, 22 to 28); BUN, 5.7 mmol/L (3.0 to 6.5); creatinine, 173.3 μmol/L (normal, 50 to 110)]

As described in the answer to Question 6, organ rejection can be classified as hyperacute, accelerated, acute, vascular, and chronic. Current data indicate that acute rejection rates are <30% after heart transplantation. Approximately 50% of these occurred within the first 6 weeks and 90% within the first 6 months, although rejection can occur at any time.[120] Acute rejection of a transplanted heart accounts for approximately 15% of deaths after transplantation.[117] Risk factors for acute rejection include younger recipient age, female gender (donor and/or recipient), donor heart ischemic time, number of HLA mismatches, and retransplantation.

Most rejection episodes are asymptomatic. However, if clinical signs are present, they can include nonspecific signs of fatigue, malaise, and a low-grade temperature. In some cases, one can see dyspnea and weight gain. Unlike kidney transplant recipients who might experience pain at the graft site, heart patients do not experience cardiac pain because it is denervated. However, when patients with a heart transplant present with significant cardiovascular symptoms (e.g., hypotension, increased jugular venous distention, S_3 sounds, rales), these may indicate advanced severe rejection. Patients experiencing an acute rejection of a transplanted heart also may present with new-onset arrhythmias and CHF, although these occur late in the process.[120] Therefore, acute rejection of a transplanted heart must be determined by an internal jugular transvenous EMB, the gold standard for diagnosis. A set of histologic criteria have been developed to standardize the severity of rejection. A grading scale of 0 to 4 is used to describe the degree of damage to cardiac tissue. Grade 0 indicates no rejection, whereas grade 4 is severe acute rejection.[135]

Vascular or humoral rejection, which is an antibody-mediated process, also may occur, usually in the first 3 months after transplantation. This form of rejection is associated with a higher incidence of cardiac allograft vasculopathy and increased mortality rate and is more difficult to treat.

R.B. is asymptomatic, which is consistent with the majority of patients who have biopsy-proven evidence of acute rejection but do not present with clinical symptoms. Although patients with mild, grade 1 rejection often are asymptomatic, 20% to 30% can go on to develop moderate, grade 2 to 3, rejection.[136] When rejection of a transplanted heart is detected, the EMB should be repeated within 1 week. A number of other noninvasive electrophysiologic, echocardiographic, immunologic, radioisotopic, and biochemical methods are being investigated for their value in detecting acute rejection of a transplanted heart.

Chronic rejection of a transplanted heart is called *cardiac allograft vasculopathy* (CAV) and is sometimes referred to as *transplant coronary artery disease* (CAD), *accelerated CAD,* or *graft arteriosclerosis*. It is the leading cause of death after the first year in heart transplant recipients.[117] Despite immunosuppressive therapy, approximately 15% of patients experience chronic rejection of a heart transplant within the first year, and this increases to at least 50% within 5 years. The clinical presentation is insidious, nonspecific, and similar to the clinical presentation associated with acute rejection. Chest pain is nonexistent. However, the first presenting signs may be CHF, arrhythmias, MI, or sudden death.[137] Therefore, patients must undergo routine coronary angiography or intravascular ultrasound, which is more sensitive, shortly after the heart transplantation and every year subsequently. On angiography, chronic rejection of a transplanted heart diffusely affects both arteries and veins. The pathogenesis of this condition, which results in endothelial damage and a cascade of other related events, is unknown, but a number of immunologic (acute rejection), infectious (CMV), and nonimmunologic factors (graft ischemia, hyperlipidemia, hypertension, glucose intolerance, smoking, obesity) are associated with its development.[137]

Pharmacologic therapy has been directed toward prevention of this condition. Antiplatelet agents, such as the aspirin used by R.B., are used routinely, but have not been shown to alter progression of the condition.[138] Diltiazem, which R.B. also is receiving for hypertension, inhibits progressive coronary obstruction as well.[139] Other maneuvers include diet modification, BP control, and lipid control. Pravastatin and simvastatin initiated in the first days to weeks, have been shown to decrease coronary artery disease and improve survival after transplantation.[101,102,140] Although the preceding pharmacologic interventions hold some promise, retransplantation is the only effective therapy for chronic rejection.

Treatment of Acute Rejection

20. What approach should be taken in the treatment of R.B.'s grade 1 acute cardiac rejection?

Acute cardiac rejection is graded based on the histologic findings in the biopsy samples. It often is referred to as mild, moderate, or severe, with or without hemodynamic symptoms. This classification forms the basis for selecting pharmacologic management. Although the individual drugs usually are given as high doses over a short period, the doses, routes, and regimens vary from program to program. High-dose corticosteroids are the primary agents used to treat moderate to severe rejection, and IV methylprednisolone 1 g every day for 3 days is effective in 85% of the initial episodes of acute cardiac rejection.[141]

When R.B. was asymptomatic and had a grade 1 mild rejection, no treatment was indicated because many of these episodes resolve without intervention. An adjustment in maintenance immunosuppression is appropriate, and an increase in R.B.'s cyclosporine dose is reasonable, especially because his blood concentration of cyclosporine was lower than desired. Nevertheless, some programs treat mild rejection of a transplanted heart because of the concern for progression of the rejection in some patients. As was done with R.B., a follow-up EMB, usually within 1 week of the initial diagnosis, should be performed. In R.B.'s case, the grade 1 mild acute rejection of his transplanted heart progressed to moderate rejection or grade 2. In this situation, high-dose methylprednisolone 500 to 1,000 mg IV or 10 mg/kg every day for 3 days would be given, and his maintenance prednisone regimen would be reinstituted. Alternatively, a high-dose prednisone regimen with a gradual dosage reduction could be instituted after the 3-day course of methylprednisolone was completed.[142] Oral prednisone 50 mg twice a day for 2 to 5 days and tapered over 7 to 14 days to the previous maintenance dose is another alternative because R.B. already is on prednisone, and hemodynamic compromise is not evident.[143]

After a course of high-dose methylprednisolone, R.B. should be monitored for any hemodynamic and functional changes that might indicate further progression of rejection, and the biopsy should be repeated. If R.B.'s moderate rejection progresses to severe rejection, he may receive another regimen of IV methylprednisolone.

Alternatively, therapy could be initiated with Thymoglobulin, Atgam, or OKT3, although he has already received OKT3. Before starting on OKT3, an anti-OKT3 antibody titer should be obtained. When these antilymphocyte antibodies (i.e., Thymoglobulin, Atgam, and OKT3) are used for patients unresponsive to corticosteroids, the treatment is known as *rescue therapy*. Thymoglobulin, ATG, and OKT3 are equally advantageous in this situation. A typical regimen would be Thymoglobulin 1.5 mg/kg per day or Atgam 10 mg/kg IV every day for 7 to 10 days or IV OKT3 5 mg every day for 7 to 10 days. As many as 90% of corticosteroid-refractory episodes of acute rejection of a transplanted heart respond to OKT3.[144]

In some patients, an acute rejection episode can be refractory to high-dose corticosteroids, ATG, and OKT3. Treatment for refractory or recurrent rejection includes conversion from cyclosporine to tacrolimus or from azathioprine to mycophenolate.[145] Other therapies for this type of rejection, particularly vascular rejection, include sirolimus,[146] methotrexate,[147] and tacrolimus.[148]

LUNG TRANSPLANTATION
Postoperative Course

21. B.U., a 33-year-old, 54-kg man with a 12-year history of cystic fibrosis, is admitted for a double-lung transplantation. He had been doing reasonably well until 2 years ago. Since that time, he has been hospitalized five times for acute pulmonary exacerbations caused by *Pseudomonas aeruginosa*. In addition, he has been hospitalized twice in a 6-month period over the past year for hemoptysis secondary to pulmonary infarcts. He now requires continuous oxygen at 3 L/min via nasal cannula for daily living. Other medical problems include diabetes mellitus, gastroesophageal reflux disease, pancreatic insufficiency, and sinusitis. His current medications are DNase 2.5 mL nebulizer BID, albuterol nebulizer BID, (vitamins) ADEK 1 tablet BID, ranitidine 150 mg BID, ultralente insulin 10 units QD, and pancrease with meals and snacks. While on 3 L/min of oxygen, his oxygen saturation is 100%, forced expiratory volume in 1 second (FEV$_1$), 1.11 (22% predicted), forced vital capacity (FVC), 2.04 (34% predicted). His vital signs are as follows: temperature, 36.5°C; BP, 120/90 mm Hg; RR, 20 breaths/min; and heart rate, 96 beats/min. His laboratory results are as follows: Na, 137 mEq/L (normal, 135 to 147); K, 4.2 mEq/L (normal, 3.5 to 5.0); Cl, 100 mEq/L (normal, 95 to 105); CO$_2$, 28 mEq/L (normal, 22 to 28); BUN, 24 mg/dL (normal, 8 to 18); SrCr, 1.2 mg/dL (normal, 0.6 to 1.2); glucose, 104 mg/dL (normal, 80 to 120); Ca, 9.0 mg/dL (normal, 8.8 to 10.3); protein, 8.3 g/dL (normal, 6.0 to 8.0); albumin 3.9 g/dL (normal, 4.0 to 6.0); bilirubin, 0.3 mg/dL (normal, 0.1 to 1.0); AST, 40 U/L (normal, 0 to 35); ALT, 46 U/L (normal, 0 to 35); WBC count, 8,000 (normal, 4,000 to 10,000); Hct, 30% (normal, 39% to 49%); Hgb, 9.5 mg/dL (normal, 14.0 to 18.0); platelets, 340,000 (normal, 130,000 to 400,000); prothrombin time, 11.6 sec (normal, 9 to 12); and partial thromboplastin time, 26.4 sec (normal, 22 to 37). He is CMV antibody–negative. In the operating room, B.U. was given preoperative azathioprine 200 mg IV, tobramycin 200 mg intravenously, piperacillin 3 g IV, ranitidine 50 mg IV, and metoclopramide 10 mg IV.

B.U. underwent a 12-hour surgery for double-lung transplantation. During the procedure, he received 8 L of fluids and dopamine to correct hypotension. He was admitted to the ICU on a ventilator, where he received cyclosporine 4 mg/hr IV, azathioprine 125 mg QD IV, methylprednisolone 30 mg QD IV, furosemide 10 to 20 mg QID, D$_5$1/2 NS at a rate to keep the vein open, insulin infusion, IV infusion dopamine 3 mg/kg per minute, epidural and patient-controlled analgesia (PCA) morphine, tobramycin 200 mg QD IV, piperacillin 3 g Q 6 hr IV, ranitidine 50 mg BID IV, ganciclovir 125 mg IV QD, CMV immunoglobulin, cotrimoxazole QD, and albuterol nebulizer QID. The donor was CMV-positive. What complications can occur in B.U. during the early postoperative period?

[SI units: Na, 137 mmol/L (normal, 135 to 147); K, 4.2 mmol/L (normal, 3.4 to 4.6); Cl, 100 mmol/L (normal, 95 to 105); CO$_2$, 28 mmol/L (normal, 22 to 28); BUN, 8.6 mmol/L (normal, 3.0 to 6.5); SrCr, 106.1 (μmol/L (normal, 50 to 110); glucose, 5.8 mmol/L (normal, 3.9 to 6.1); Ca, 3.7 mmol/L (normal, 2.2 to 2.5); protein, 83 g/L (normal, 60 to 80); albumin, 39 g/L (normal, 40 to 60); bilirubin, 5.13 μmol/L (normal, 2 to 18); AST, 40 U/L (normal, 0 to 35); ALT, 46 U/L (normal, 0 to 35); WBC count, 4,000 × 10^6 cells/L (normal, 4,000 to 10,000); Hct, 0.3 (normal, 0.39 to 0.49); Hgb, 95 g/L (normal, 140 to 180); platelets, 340 × 10^9/L (normal, 130 to 400)]

Lung transplantation is a therapeutic option for end-stage pulmonary disease; >1,500 lungs worldwide are transplanted each year. The 1- and 5-year survival rates are approximately 75% and 45%, respectively. Some centers have reported a 1-year survival rate of >80%. Chronic obstructive pulmonary disease (COPD), idiopathic pulmonary fibrosis, and alpha$_1$-antitrypsin deficiency are the primary indications for a single-lung transplant. The primary indications for a double-lung transplant are cystic fibrosis and COPD. Double-lung trans-

plants also are referred to as bilateral single-lung transplants.[117]

B.U.'s cystic fibrosis–associated pancreatic and GI problems will not be corrected by a double-lung transplantation. However, his pulmonary function should improve significantly, achieving normal levels within 3 to 12 months. One would expect that after a double-lung transplantation B.U. would no longer require oxygen, would achieve normal exercise capacity, and could expect a return to a good quality of life.

Patients like B.U. usually leave the operating room under mechanical ventilation and should be extubated within 24 to 48 hours. In the early postoperative period, the transplanted lung(s) is prone to pulmonary edema, hemorrhage, dehiscence at the anastomotic sites, airway leaks, infection, and rejection. Hemorrhage, ischemic/reperfusion injury, and dehiscence have decreased as a result of improved donor preservation and surgical techniques. The most common serious complications are airway complications, reperfusion ischemic pulmonary edema, acute rejection, and infection. Significant incisional pain, which occurs in all patients, also can affect how quickly B.U. recovers. Altered GI function, such as gastroparesis, also is a typical problem in the initial period.[149]

Infection

Infection is the leading cause of death in the first 60 days after lung transplantation and contributes significantly to the number of deaths thereafter. There are several reasons for this problem. These patients usually have had several pulmonary infections before transplantation and may be colonized with organisms along the upper airways and sinuses. The donor lung may contain organisms at the time of transplantation, and the transplanted organ may have ischemic damage. After lung transplantation, patients lack a cough reflex because of denervation. Consequently, pulmonary secretions that accumulate can serve as a medium for bacterial growth. Furthermore, the transplanted lung mucociliary clearance may be impaired, alveolar macrophages may not function properly, and patients are receiving several immunosuppressives. Most infections present as bacterial sepsis or pneumonia, associated primarily with *P. aeruginosa*, *Enterobacter*, other gram-negative organisms, and staphylococci. In patients with cystic fibrosis, *Candida* and *Aspergillus* infections also are common. At least 50% of lung transplant recipients develop infection despite prophylaxis. CMV infections also occur but are more common after the initial post-transplantation period.[150]

The ideal prophylactic antibiotic regimen has not been established, but it usually is directed against gram-negative organisms and staphylococci and is based on the patient's previous antimicrobial experiences before transplantation. B.U. was given tobramycin and piperacillin based on previous culture and sensitivities obtained during his past pseudomonal infections. Antibiotics also may be selected based on the donor's previous bacterial cultures and sensitivities, if available. Ceftazidime, ciprofloxacin, or imipenem and/or tobramycin often are prescribed for gram-negative coverage, including nebulized tobramycin or colistin, and vancomycin, nafcillin, or clindamycin are given for gram-positive coverage. Antibiotics generally are administered for 4 to 10 days. B.U. was also placed on CMV prophylaxis with IV ganciclovir and CMV immunoglobulin because he is considered high risk and susceptible to CMV pneumonitis.[150,151] In some programs in which fungal infections are problematic, antifungals such as azoles and/or aerosolized amphotericin B are used prophylactically.[152]

Acute Rejection

Rejection, both acute and chronic, occurs in lung transplant recipients. Acute rejection is common in the early postoperative period, with >90% of patients having at least one episode within the first month in spite of aggressive immunosuppressive therapy. Nevertheless, acute rejection can occur at any time.[153] The diagnosis of acute rejection is made on clinical and histologic criteria. Standardized criteria have been established for histologic grading of tissue from transbronchial biopsies (TBBXs), which are scheduled routinely.[154] Clinical signs of acute rejection of a transplanted lung include fever, cough, dyspnea, rales, wheezes, infiltrates, and a decline in FEV_1. The FEV_1 and FVC are assessed daily by the patient using a hand-held spirometer. As little as a 10% decline in pulmonary function (i.e., FEV_1, FVC) can be significant in the absence of other causes of respiratory decline, particularly infection. Treatment for acute rejection may be initiated based on clinical signs only, although they are not always accurate.[153] If clinical evidence of acute rejection is present, a TBBX is needed to firmly establish the diagnosis of rejection. The diagnosis of lung transplant rejection still can be established even in the face of a negative TBBX if other causes are ruled out.[154]

The primary treatment for acute rejection is methylprednisolone 500 to 1,000 mg/day IV or 10 to 15 mg/kg per day every day for 3 days. The dose of oral prednisone also can be increased to 1 mg/kg per day and tapered down to the maintenance dose over 2 to 3 weeks. More than 90% of acute rejection episodes of transplanted lungs respond to corticosteroid therapy, with clinical response seen within 2 days in most patients.[153] OKT3, Atgam, Thymoglobulin, tacrolimus, and experimental aerosolized cyclosporine have been used for refractory cases.[155–157]

Chronic Rejection

Chronic rejection also occurs in these patients and is referred to as bronchiolitis obliterans (OB) or bronchiolitis obliterans syndrome (BOS). OB is based on histologic findings of a fibroproliferative process of the small airways, which leads to progressive airway obstruction. BOS is defined as an otherwise unexplained and sustained fall in FEV_1 of 80% or less of the peak value after transplantation. It is uncommon during the first 6 months after transplantation, but it can occur as early as 3 months after transplantation in at least 20% of patients and is a major cause (along with infection) of late deaths. The diagnosis of OB is based on clinical, physiologic, and histologic features.[158] Pulmonary function and exercise capacity progressively decline as a result of inflamed small airways and destruction of bronchioles. It is found in 40% at 2 years and 60% to 70% of patients who survive at least 5 years.[158]

There is no evidence of superiority of one drug treatment over another for OB or BOS. The primary treatment of chronic rejection relies on short courses of high-dose corticosteroids, ATG, or OKT3 to stabilize and improve the patient's condition for a short time. Therapy generally stabilizes and slows down this process, but does not reverse it. Shortly after a course with one of these agents, there is a high rate of relapse and CMV infection. Therefore, antimicrobial prophylaxis should be considered for CMV. Inhaled cyclosporine, antibodies, tacrolimus, mycophenolate, and methotrexate also have been used.[158] Sirolimus has been used in a small number of patients with little effect, but with a significant number of side effects.[159] Recently, a black box warning has been issued for sirolimus after lung transplantation.

Immunosuppression

B.U. is on the most commonly used regimen for immunosuppression of lung transplants, which consists of cyclosporine, azathioprine and steroids.[117] Immunosuppressive induction could include OKT3, ATG, Thymoglobulin, or daclizumab in combination with cyclosporine, azathioprine, and steroids.[160,161] Other regimens could include tacrolimus, mycophenolate, and prednisone. Tacrolimus and cyclosporine have similar graft survival, but tacrolimus was associated with fewer episodes of acute rejection.[162] Early, low-dose prednisone (0.5 mg/kg per day tapered to 0.15 mg/kg per day) is used. B.U.'s cyclosporine regimen would be adjusted to maintain a whole blood concentration of 250 to 350 ng/mL (by monoclonal TDx). If tacrolimus was used in place of cyclosporine, an initial starting oral or nasogastric dosage of 0.15 mg/kg per day would be used with target trough concentrations of 10 to 20 ng/mL.[163] Mycophenolate, in place of azathioprine, would be started at 1 g two times a day, although its outcomes are equivalent to azathioprine's.[164]

Pain

Pain associated with lung transplantation has not been studied formally, but all lung transplant recipients seem to require analgesia after surgery. Morphine or fentanyl is given either intravenously or via an epidural catheter in the first few days. However, the agent, route of administration, and regimen vary. B.U. was put on epidural morphine and a PCA pump. If the patient is sufficiently alert, a PCA pump may be used, but epidural administration is more likely to produce a longer duration of relief. Pain relief with narcotic analgesics should not hinder ventilatory status and should allow a more successful recovery. Over several days to weeks, B.U. will be placed on less potent oral analgesics (e.g., oxycodone with acetaminophen). Analgesics should be discontinued as soon as possible.

Gastrointestinal

Because of cystic fibrosis, diabetes mellitus, and the surgical procedure, B.U. has a predisposition for postoperative ileus and gastric outlet obstruction that may be aggravated further by narcotics. B.U. also has a history of gastroesophageal reflux that may require treatment with H_2-antagonists, proton pump inhibitors, and metoclopramide. Lactulose or polyethylene glycol–electrolyte solutions (e.g., Colyte, GoLYTELY) can be used to increase intestinal motility and maintain bowel function. Pancreatic enzymes must be reinstituted when B.U. begins to eat because cystic fibrosis patients are susceptible to meconium ileus and malabsorption. Because cystic fibrosis patients often are malnourished, parenteral or enteral nutrition usually is needed until adequate solid food intake is achieved. After the initial postoperative period, B.U. should expect to see his appetite and GI function improve.[149]

Renal Dysfunction

Acute and chronic renal dysfunction also can occur in lung transplant recipients.[165] B.U. has several risk factors that could produce an acute decline in renal function. He became hypotensive during surgery, which could lead to a decrease in renal blood flow. His renal perfusion potentially can be compromised because he is fluid restricted and receiving diuretics. He also is receiving other nephrotoxins such as cyclosporine and tobramycin. However, B.U. may benefit from the dopamine infusion because low doses of dopamine can enhance renal blood flow. In B.U., the need for diuretics, fluid restriction, and tobramycin should be evaluated continually, and these interventions should be discontinued when feasible. Aminoglycoside kinetics, immediately after transplantation differ significantly from pre-transplant in cystic fibrosis and generally require an extended dosing interval.[166] Antimicrobials less nephrotoxic than tobramycin should be considered based on culture and sensitivities. If tobramycin must be continued, evaluations of serum concentrations are probably more sensitive markers for adjustments in tobramycin dosing than the SrCr concentration.

Cyclosporine Bioavailibility

22. B.U. now is receiving all of his medications orally 3 weeks after transplantation and is ready to be discharged from the hospital. He has an excellent appetite, his lung function is very good, and he has no GI complaints. His medications include cyclosporine 500 mg BID, azathioprine 100 mg QD, prednisone 15 mg BID, ranitidine 150 mg QHS, ADEKs BID, pancrease with meals and snacks, NPH insulin 20 units BID, regular insulin 8 units BID, ganciclovir 500 mg TID, and TMP-SMX S&S QD. He experienced one rejection episode, which was treated with high-dose pulse corticosteroids. His most significant problem at this time is his low trough cyclosporine blood concentrations, which have been consistently <250 ng/mL (target range by whole blood monoclonal TDx is 300 to 400 ng/mL) despite several increases in dosage. Evaluate B.U.'s maintenance immunosuppressive regimen. What are possible explanations for B.U.'s low cyclosporine concentrations?

B.U.'s maintenance immunosuppressive regimen consists of azathioprine, prednisone, and cyclosporine. His azathioprine dose of 2 mg/kg per day (100 mg) has been adjusted to maintain a WBC count >5,000/mm^3. His prednisone dose of 15 mg twice a day should be tapered over the next 6 months to 15 mg every other day if possible; the withdrawal of corticosteroids with lung transplants is rare. His oral cyclosporine regimen was initiated at 5 mg/kg twice a day after the IV line was discontinued, although some programs overlap IV and oral cyclosporine therapy by reducing the IV dosage by 50% when oral cyclosporine is started. The target cyclosporine whole blood concentration should be the same as during the initial period and should be maintained at the same level for the first 6 months before reducing the targeted concentration to 250 to 350 ng/mL (by monoclonal TDx). These target cyclosporine concentrations should be adjusted for nephrotoxicity and other toxicities, if necessary.

The low cyclosporine levels could be a result of inappropriate drug administration, altered GI function, noncompliance, assay error, poor absorption characteristics of the drug itself, drug interactions, or concurrent disease states. The

most likely reason for B.U. is poor absorption because he has cystic fibrosis, which is associated with malabsorption of fat-soluble substances, and cyclosporine is a fat-soluble substance. The mean bioavailability of Sandimmune in heart-lung candidates with cystic fibrosis was reported to be <20%, which is lower than most other populations. With the introduction of Neoral, which is a microemulsion with improved absorption characteristics over Sandimmune, there has been an improvement in cyclosporine concentration in lung transplant recipients. In general, the T_{max} for Neoral is shorter, the C_{max} is higher, and the AUC (area under the curve) is greater.[167] In patients with cystic fibrosis, the use of Neoral has decreased dosing requirements by approximately 50%, from an average of 20 mg/kg per day with Sandimmune to 10 mg/kg per day with Neoral. In some cases, TID dosing may be required to minimize high peaks and potential toxicities and to maintain an adequate trough concentration. Despite this new formulation, patients like B.U. can still have problems with absorption in the early post-transplantation period, although altered clearance cannot be ruled out.

Secondary Malignancy

POST-TRANSPLANTATION LYMPHOPROLIFERATIVE DISORDER

Risk Factors

23. A.L., a 17-year-old, 42-kg girl with cystic fibrosis, had a double-lung transplantation 1 year ago. She now presents with low-grade fever, malaise, pain, redness and swelling at her Port-A-Cath site and a 1-week history of decreased appetite. She has experienced four episodes of rejection that were treated with 1 to 2 g of methylprednisolone each time. She also received ATG, azathioprine, prednisone, and cyclosporine after transplantation and has been on the latter three agents chronically along with ketoconazole, TMP-SMX, lactulose, and pancrease. She has just finished the last of two courses of IV ganciclovir (6 weeks) for CMV infection. The donor was CMV-positive and she is CMV-positive. Her EBV IgG-VCA titer is now elevated, although at the time of transplantation it was negative (<1:40). On physical examination, she was noted to have mediastinal adenopathy. She denies chills, sweats, nausea, vomiting, or diarrhea. Chest computed tomography (CT) scan revealed a mediastinal mass. Vital signs and all laboratory tests are within normal limits. Her cyclosporine level is 221 ng/mL. Seven days after admission, a biopsy of this mass shows a thoracic lymphoproliferative lesion identified as a thoracic immunoblastic lymphoma adherent to the right heart. Ten days later, she developed tachy/brady syndrome and a pacemaker was implanted. Given the location of her lymphoma and symptoms, surgery and radiation therapy are not viable options, and chemotherapy is started the next day. What clinical signs and risk factors in A.L. are associated with lymphoma?

A.L. has developed a post-transplantation lymphoproliferative disorder (PTLD), one of many types of malignancies that have been reported after solid organ transplantation. The exact etiology of this condition is unclear and probably multifactorial. The presentation of PTLD varies significantly. Patients can present asymptomatically, with mild mononucleosis-like symptoms or with multiorgan failure. A.L. presents with fever, lymphadenopathy, malaise, and lack of appetite. Although these symptoms are consistent with PTLD, they also are consistent with infection and episodes of rejection. Because PTLD can involve various organ systems, patients can present with organ-specific symptoms (e.g., acute abdominal pain, perforation, obstruction, bleeding if a tumor is in the GI tract). Depending on its location, a tumor can impinge on the function of other organs as seen in A.L.[168]

Besides immunosuppression, two factors that have been strongly associated with PTLD are the presence of EBV and the age of the patient. Children have a higher incidence of PTLD.[169] A.L. had an elevated positive EBV titer, which was previously negative, indicating that she had been exposed to this virus at the time of transplantation or afterward. EBV also can be transmitted from the donor lung and/or blood products. Also, patients who are EBV-positive at the time of transplantation can experience reactivation of this virus as a result of immunosuppression.

A.L. received a significant amount of immunosuppression. This could lead to an inability to suppress an active viral infection by cytotoxic T cells and result in uncontrolled B-cell proliferation and polyclonal and monoclonal expansion. In addition to this T-cell defect, an imbalance or alteration in cytokine production in response to EBV, which infects B lymphocytes, may contribute to the exaggerated B-cell expansion and transformation. The majority is classified as non-Hodgkin's lymphomas primarily of B-cell origin. However, a small percentage are of T-cell origin.[170]

The incidence and detection of PTLDs has increased. Newer, more potent agents used in different combinations, increased numbers of transplantation procedures, and closer monitoring certainly contribute to this phenomenon. When cyclosporine-based regimens were compared with azathioprine-based or cyclophosphamide-based regimens, lymphomas made up 26% and 11% of all cancers, respectively. The lymphomas occurred, on average, within 15 months in the cyclosporine group versus 48 months in the azathioprine group. One-third of these malignancies occurred in the first 4 months in the cyclosporine group compared with only 11% in the latter group.[170]

When a specific T-cell antibody (e.g., OKT3) is given as induction therapy for treatment of acute rejection or as rescue therapy, the incidence of lymphoma increases and appears to be related to a cumulative dose and multiple courses. The occurrence of PTLDs also is affected by the time of OKT3 administration in relation to the activation or reactivation of EBV. EBV shedding (which is correlated with PTLD) increases in the second month after transplantation, which usually corresponds to the time that a second course of OKT3 is given for acute rejection. ATG also has been associated with PTLD. PTLD is not caused by any single agent but probably reflects the intensity of immunosuppression with multiple agents. Chronic antigenic stimulation by foreign antigens, repeated infections, genetic predisposition, and indirect or direct damage to DNA are other variables that might affect the development of PTLD.[170] A.L. had two recent CMV infections that also could have contributed to this process.

PTLD, as a percentage of all malignancies, occurs more commonly in thoracic than in renal transplant recipients and is even more common in children.[169] Lymphomas develop in about 1% of renal transplantations, 2% of liver transplantations, 2% to 10% of heart transplantations, and 5% to 9% of lung transplantations. These tumors can often appear early and progress rapidly. The overall prevalence of malignancies in the transplantation population averages about 6%, and the risk of cancer increases with time after a transplantation. Major organ transplant recipients are 100 times more likely to have cancer than the general population.[171] Furthermore, the most common types of cancer observed in transplant recipients (e.g., lymphomas, cancer of the skin and lips) are uncommon in the general population. The development of skin and lip cancers in the transplant population has been attributed partially to exposure to sunlight and sensitization of skin to sunlight by an azathioprine metabolite, methylnitrothioimidazole.[172]

TREATMENT AND OUTCOMES

24. **What are the therapeutic maneuvers and outcomes that would be expected in A.L.?**

Treatment of a PTLD depends on timing, presentation, symptoms, extent of involvement, histologic type, and transplant type. Early experiences with PTLD indicated that reduction or discontinuation of immunosuppression led to regression of the cancer. Therefore, the first step in treating PTLD is to consider the discontinuation of all immunosuppressives. However, this course of action is not feasible for A.L. because her transplanted lungs are essential for her life. The discontinuation of immunosuppressive therapy also is not an option for heart and liver transplants, but immunosuppressive drugs can be discontinued in kidney transplant recipients because dialysis is available. A.L. will need chemotherapy for her cancer. Therefore, her azathioprine probably should be discontinued to minimize the potential for severe bone marrow toxicity. If her cyclosporine levels were high, a reduction in dose could be attempted, but her cyclosporine concentration of 221 ng/mL is in the lower range for this type of transplantation, and prednisone is reduced to the lowest dose possible. If her immunosuppressive drug therapy is diminished, she should be monitored closely for rejection of her transplanted lungs.

Antiviral therapy with IV acyclovir or ganciclovir has been used to inhibit EBV replication in an effort to treat PTLD. Response is variable and may depend on the type and extent of PTLD. A.L. already has received ganciclovir for 6 weeks during which time she presented with PTLD. Surgery, radiation therapy, and chemotherapy are used to treat PTLD depending on the situation. Interferon-α and immune globulin have been effective in a few cases that appeared unresponsive to other therapies. Monoclonal or immunoblastic, disseminated, rapidly progressive PTLD responds poorly to traditional therapy, which has a mortality rate as high as 70%.[173] Preliminary investigation with an anti–B-cell, anti-CD20 antibody, rituximab, has shown positive results in some patients with PTLD.[174] A.L.'s prognosis is poor given the type and extent of her PTLD, which is more likely to respond to therapy if diagnosed early before it has metastasized. Polyclonal PTLD responds well to reduction or discontinuation of immunosuppression and high-dose acyclovir or ganciclovir therapy for several weeks to months. The roles of prophylactic antivirals, immunoglobulins, and EBV polymerase chain reaction (PCR) monitoring in the prevention of PTLD are currently under study.[175,176]

PANCREAS TRANSPLANTATION
Indications and Evaluation

25. D.A. is a 42-year-old woman with a 24-year history of type 1 diabetes mellitus. She developed ESRD, neuropathy, retinopathy, and gastric esophageal reflux disease secondary to long-standing poorly controlled diabetes. She has been receiving hemodialysis three times a week for 2 years. Other medical problems include hypertension, anemia, hypocalcemia, and hyperphosphatemia. D.A.'s medications include diltiazem CD 360 mg PO QD, sevelamer 1,600 mg TID with meals, metoclopramide 10 mg PO before meals and at bedtime, gabapentin 300 mg PO BID, insulin glargine (Lantus) 45 U SC every night, and sliding-scale insulin lispro (Humalog) with meals, depending on fasting blood glucose concentration and the meal's carbohydrate load. She has been on the kidney–pancreas transplant waiting list for approximately 1.5 years. She is called by the transplant coordinator and admitted for a possible cadaveric simultaneous pancreas–kidney transplantation. On admission to the hospital, her laboratory values are as follows: Na, 138 mEq/L (normal, 135 to 145); K, 4.9 mEq/L (normal, 3.4 to 4.6); Cl, 99 mEq/L (normal, 95 to 105); HCO_3, 20 mEq/L (normal, 22 to 28); BUN, 48 mg/dL (normal, 8 to 18); SrCr, 7.8 mg/dL (normal, 0.6 to 1.2); Ca, 8.2 mEq/L (normal, 8.8 to 10.3); phosphorus, 5.9 mg/dL (normal, 2.5 to 5.0); glucose, 189 mg/dL (normal, 65 to 110); WBC count, 6.2 cells/mm³ (normal, 4,000 to 10,000); Hgb, 8.9 g/dL (normal, 14 to 18); and Hct, 23.4% (normal, 39% to 49%). Her serology is negative for HIV, hepatitis B and C, and CMV. What are the indications for and potential benefits of simultaneous pancreas–kidney transplantation in D.A.?

[SI units: Na, 141 mmol/L (normal, 135 to 145); K, 4.7 mmol/L (normal, 3.4 to 4.6); Cl, 102 mmol/L (normal, 95 to 105), HCO_3, 23 mmol/L (normal, 22 to 28); BUN, 15.7 mmol/L (normal, 3.0 to 6.5); SrCr, 1,228.8 (μmol/L (normal, 50 to 110); Ca, 1.95 mmol/L (normal, 2.20 to 2.58); phosphorus, 2.0 mmol/L (normal, 0.77 to 1.45); glucose, 12.5 mmol/L (normal, 3.9 to 6.1); WBC count, 8.4 × 10⁶ cells/L (normal, 4,000 to 10,000); Hgb, 93 g/L (normal, 115 to 155); Hct, 0.24 (0.39 to 0.49)]

Despite strong evidence demonstrating that type 1 diabetes and its related complications are associated with a high incidence of morbidity and mortality, pancreatic transplantation is not considered a life-saving procedure. Rather, it provides an improvement in the patient's quality of life. Selection criteria must carefully weigh the patient's risk factors for post-surgical complications with the benefits received from producing normal glucose homeostasis. An indication for simultaneous pancreas–kidney transplantation is type 1 diabetes with ESRD. Pancreas transplantation is not considered in patients with type 2 diabetes, because this disease is strongly related to insulin resistance rather than absence of insulin production within the pancreas. Other options for patients who have type 1 diabetes without associated nephropathy are pancreas transplantation alone (PTA) or pancreas after kidney transplantation (PAK), although these procedures are less commonly performed compared with simultaneous pancreas–kidney transplantation. Usually, patients awaiting pancreas–kidney transplantation also have developed other complications of longstanding diabetes, such as retinopathy and neuropathy. Contraindications to pancreas transplantation include malignancy, active infection, active substance abuse, and uncontrolled psychiatric illness. Most centers consider severe cardiovascular disease, severe obesity, age above 60, complete blindness, major amputation, active smoking, and a history of noncompliance to be strong, but not absolute, contraindications to pancreas transplantation. The procedure eliminates the need for both hemodialysis and insulin injections and reduces and even reverses diabetic neuropathy; however, it has little effect on severe retinopathy or vasculopathy. Because D.A. has demonstrated long-standing type 1 diabetes with ESRD and has no contraindications to transplantation, she is considered a good candidate for simultaneous pancreas–kidney transplantation.[177–181]

26. A.D. is considered a good match with the donor. Before the transplantation procedure, ampicillin/sulbactam (Unasyn) 3 g IV is given. Intraoperatively, IV methylprednisolone 500 mg and IV basiliximab 20 mg are administered right before reperfusing the pancreas transplant. Methylprednisolone 250 mg IV is to be given on the day after surgery and decreased to 125 mg IV on the second postoperative day for one dose. Prednisone 100 mg PO is to be given on the subsequent day for one dose and tapered daily to 20 mg QD by day 14 after surgery. She will receive one follow-up dose of IV basiliximab 20 mg on postoperative day 4. Tacrolimus (Prograf) 1 mg NG or PO BID is started postoperatively. The dosage of tacrolimus will be adjusted according to tacrolimus whole blood concentrations (goal 15 to 20 ng/L). MMF is started at 1 g IV BID immediately postoperatively, and converted to the PO dosage form. A.D. also is to receive Unasyn 3 g IV Q6 hr for 3 days, famotidine 20 mg IV Q12 hr, and fluconazole 200 mg IV QD. Is this the appropriate immunosuppressive regimen in A.D.?

Immunosuppression

Probably because of the higher immunogenicity of the pancreas, acute rejection rates in patients who receive a simultaneous pancreas–kidney transplantation, PTA, or PAK are substantially higher than in patients who receive only kidney transplants. Because of this, most transplantation centers use either triple or quadruple immunosuppressant regimens in pancreas transplant recipients. Acute rejection rates with triple therapy using cyclosporine, MMF, and steroids are approximately 30%.[182] Triple immunosuppressive regimens using tacrolimus in place of cyclosporine have reduced acute rejection rates to roughly 20%.[183] The use of antibodies as induction agents also reduces acute rejection rates and possibly improves graft survival.[184,185] This is why A.D. received a quadruple immunosuppressant regimen consisting of the antibody induction agent basiliximab, as well as the maintenance immunosuppressant regimen of tacrolimus, MMF, and corticosteroids. The overall intensity of immunosuppression will be slowly and gradually reduced over the next several months to years as the patient gets further out from her transplantation. This is accomplished by reducing the doses of all the agents and, in some cases, completely stopping one or two agents, such as MMF or corticosteroids.

Daclizumab and Basiliximab

27. A.D. received induction therapy with two 20-mg doses of IV basiliximab given immediately postoperatively and on the fourth postoperative day. What are basiliximab and daclizumab and how are they used in transplantation?

The newest agents approved for use as induction therapy in kidney transplantations are the IL-2R antibodies, daclizumab and basiliximab. Even though they are approved for use in kidney transplantations only, they are being used and studied in other organ transplant recipients as well. Most studies with these agents have been in combination with cyclosporine and steroids with or without an antimetabolite, such as azathioprine or MMF.[186] One major concern is the expense of these agents because both cost about $1,200 per dose. Thus, administration in the outpatient setting and reimbursement for this agent can be an issue.

Another important issue is the role of these agents in high-risk populations, such as patients with high PRA or long ischemic times, blacks, patients who have received another transplant, and children. One could also include kidney–pancreas transplants in this group. In these patients, induction with monoclonal or polyclonal antibodies is used in most centers. The large initial trials with these IL-2R antibodies included very few of these high-risk patients or excluded them altogether. More potent agents, such as Thymoglobulin or OKT3, may still be preferred in high-risk patients, whereas IL-2R antibodies would be conserved for low- to intermediate-risk patients.

Rejection

28. **A.D. has a routine postoperative hospital course. Her serum glucose concentrations normalized hours after the transplantation and remained stable throughout her hospitalization. Her kidney function improved such that her serum creatinine concentration was 1.4 mg/dL by the fifth postoperative day. On the sixth postoperative day, she developed good bowel sounds and was passing flatus. Her MMF, famotidine, and fluconazole were all converted to PO administration, and she continues on PO tacrolimus. A.D. is discharged on the ninth postoperative day. Several weeks later, on a routine follow-up visit, A.D. complains of tiredness, low-grade fevers of 100.1°F, and higher-than-normal blood glucose concentrations (180 to 290 mg/dL), which she monitors with her home glucometer. Her laboratory values reveal the following: Na, 136 mEq/L (normal, 135 to 145); K, 4.8 mEq/L (normal, 3.4 to 4.6); Cl, 97 mEq/L (normal, 95 to 105); HCO$_3$, 23 mEq/L (normal, 22 to 28); BUN, 23 mg/dL (normal, 8 to 18); SrCr, 1.9 mg/dL (normal, 0.6 to 1.2); Ca, 9.3 mEq/L (normal, 8.8 to 10.3); phosphorus, 3.9 mg/dL (normal, 2.5 to 5.0); glucose, 299 mg/dL (normal, 65 to 110); amylase 210 IU/L (normal 27 to 130); lipase 290 IU/L (normal 10 to 50); WBC count, 8.7 cells/mm^3 (normal, 4,000 to 10,000); Hgb, 11.4 g/dL (normal, 14 to 18); and Hct, 33% (normal, 39% to 49%). She is admitted to the hospital, where a percutaneous biopsy of her kidney reveals severe acute rejection. She will receive either IV Thymoglobulin 1.5 mg/kg per day or OKT3 5 mg per day for 7 to 14 days. What evidence is consistent with pancreas rejection in A.D., and is either of these treatments appropriate?**

Acute rejection and subsequent graft loss constitute a significant problem after pancreas transplantation. Rates of acute rejection within the first year after transplantation are approximately 20% to 40%, depending on the immunosuppressive regimen being used. Graft loss due to acute rejection at 1 year after transplantation is roughly 2% in simultaneous pancreas-kidney transplantation, 7% in PAK, and 9% in PTA patients.[180,184] Early and accurate diagnosis of pancreas rejection

is important for preventing graft loss, but it remains a challenge. Monitoring of serum amylase and lipase are the most important ways to follow post-transplant pancreatic function, but these values are not always specific for diagnosing acute rejection. Serum glucose concentrations also are important in monitoring and diagnosing acute rejection. However, they often lag behind the acute rejection episode, so that by the time the serum glucose concentrations are elevated in a pancreas transplant recipient, the patient is already days to even weeks into an acute rejection episode. If the patient has received a simultaneous pancreas–kidney transplantation, then monitoring of the serum creatinine concentrations to evaluate kidney function and possible rejection of the renal allograft is important as well, because rejection of the kidney often occurs simultaneously with the pancreas rejection. Because A.D. has received a pancreas–kidney transplantation and her serum creatinine, amylase, lipase, and glucose concentrations all have dramatically increased over the past week, the diagnosis of acute rejection is likely in this patient. In addition, symptoms such as graft tenderness and low-grade fever, both of which she is demonstrating, are consistent with acute rejection.[180,181]

Similar to treatment for other organ transplant rejections, treatment of acute rejection of the pancreas usually requires a course of intense immunosuppression, either with pulse-dose corticosteroids, or antibody preparations such as Thymoglobulin or OKT3. In mild-to-moderate acute rejections, corticosteroids are usually considered first-line therapy, but in patients with severe acute rejection, antibody preparations are often preferred. Because A.D.'s kidney tissue biopsy revealed a severe acute rejection and because rejection of the pancreas usually occurs simultaneously with the kidney, use of Thymoglobulin or OKT3 to treat her acute rejection episode is appropriate. Efficacy is demonstrated by resolution of symptoms and a return of the laboratory values to baseline.

Thymoglobulin and Antithymocyte Globulin (Atgam)$_{32}$

29. How would thymoglobulin be administered and monitored in A.D.?

DOSING AND ADMINISTRATION

Both Thymoglobulin and antithymocyte globulin are effective as induction therapy or as treatment of acute rejection. In general, Thymoglobulin appears to be more effective than antithymocyte globulin.[187,188] Thymoglobulin, when used for induction, also has been reported to result in improved survival, fewer side effects, and less infection compared with OKT3.[189] The dose of Thymoglobulin is 1.5 mg/kg per day, and the dose of antithymocyte globulin is 10 to 20 mg/kg per day. These drugs can be diluted in 0.9% sodium chloride for injection and administered over 4 to 6 hours. Both are usually infused into a high-flow central vein to reduce pain, erythema, and phlebitis at the injection site. However, peripheral administration has been used successfully with Thymoglobulin by adding heparin and hydrocortisone to the IV solution.[190] Skin testing is recommended before horse-derived antithymocyte globulin use. Patients previously sensitized to horse serum are at risk for an anaphylactoid reaction, but the prevalence of anaphylaxis has diminished with improved purification of this product. Patients with a positive pretherapy skin test could undergo desensitization, but alternatives such as Thymoglobulin and OKT3 are available. Skin testing is not required for rabbit-derived Thymoglobulin.

DURATION OF THERAPY

Duration of therapy with Thymoglobulin and antithymocyte globulin ranges from 3 to 10 days for induction therapy. Protocols used to treat rejection commonly use a 7- to 14-day course of therapy.

ADVERSE EFFECTS

A number of adverse effects have been related to the use of Thymoglobulin or antithymocyte globulin. Local phlebitis and pain usually can be avoided by administering the drug through a high-flow central vein. Anaphylaxis is rare. Chills and fever, erythema, rash, hives, pruritus, headache, leukopenia, and Thrombocytopenia are commonly encountered.[187,188] Fever, chills, nausea, and vomiting may be due to the release of cytokines, such as tumor necrosis factor and IL-6, from lysed lymphocytes.[191] These symptoms can be minimized by premedication with acetaminophen and diphenhydramine before each dose. Methylprednisolone, up to 500 mg, is given 1 hour before Thymoglobulin for the first two doses to minimize infusion reactions. Serum sickness leading to acute glomerulonephritis, hypotension, and acute respiratory distress also has been associated with these agents. It may not be evident until the seventh day of therapy or within 2 weeks of discontunuation.[192] An increase in opportunistic infections of both viral, particularly CMV, and fungal origin is the predominant delayed side effect.

MONITORING

General precautions during Thymoglobulin and antithymocyte globulin administration include daily monitoring of WBC and platelet counts and at least hourly monitoring of vital signs during infusion. If the patient's WBC count drops to <3,000 cells/mm³ or if the platelet count drops to <100,000 cells/mm³, the dose of drug is decreased by 50% or held entirely until the counts return to desired levels. The decision to decrease or hold the dose is based on the status of the patient's rejection and the degree of thrombocytopenia and leukopenia.

Dosages also can be adjusted based on absolute lymphocyte counts or lymphocyte subsets as a way of maximizing efficacy and minimizing infectious complications. For example, the dose can be adjusted by using a target absolute T-lymphocyte count (CD2 or CD3) of <25 to 50 cells/mm³.[192,193] This latter approach results in a lower dose, lower costs, and lower rate of viral infection.[194] Thymoglobulin produces a more profound and longer duration of effect on lymphocytes than antithymocyte globulin, but there is no negative effect on infection and malignancy.[195]

Muromonab (OKT3)
ADVERSE EFFECTS

30. Another treatment option for A.D.'s severe acute rejection episode is muromonab-CD3 (Orthoclone-OKT3; OKT3). OKT3 is a monoclonal antibody that binds to the CD3 receptor and effectively clears the body of T cells. It is indicated to prevent and treat rejection and is effective to treat severe rejection and steroid-resistant rejection. One hour after receiving her first 5-

mg IV dose of OKT3, she began to experience chills, nausea, and severe muscle and joint aches. Her temperature rose from 100.8°F to a maximum of 102.1°F, and her BP dropped to 100/50 mm Hg. Which of these effects is consistent with OKT3 administration?

Unfortunately OKT3 produces many adverse effects, which occur with higher frequency after the first and second doses.[196] A.D.'s adverse reaction after her first dose of OKT3 is consistent with this finding. This complex of symptoms is referred to as the *cytokine-release syndrome*. Flu-like symptoms (e.g., fever, chills, myalgia, joint pains) are the earliest signal of this syndrome, but they can be accompanied by less common, but more specific, symptoms that reflect the involvement of various organ systems.[197] For example, CNS symptoms such as seizures, headaches, photophobia, confusion, and hallucinations have been reported, as have aseptic meningitis and encephalopathy.[198,199] Acute reversible renal dysfunction, as evidenced by a rise in the serum creatinine concentration and a decrease in urine output over the first few days of therapy, also may occur. This renal dysfunction usually resolves with continued therapy.[200] Intrarenal graft thrombosis has been reported after high doses (i.e., 10 mg) of OKT3.[201] Patients with evidence of fluid overload on chest radiograph (or >3% over their base weight) should receive furosemide and some may require dialysis before initiating OKT3, because of the possible risk of rapid pulmonary edema and respiratory distress that are caused by cytokine-induced increases in capillary permeability. Anaphylaxis is rarely reported.[202]

A proposed cause is the release of cytokines, tumor necrosis factor-α, IL-2, and interferon-γ by T cells after their initial binding with OKT3. OKT3 stimulation of cytokine production is another proposed explanation for the cause of these adverse effects. This effect is independent of cell lysis. The serum concentration of cytokines becomes acutely elevated within 1 to 4 hours after the first and second doses of OKT3, and these high concentrations correlate in time with the onset of the initial symptoms, which usually resolve in 4 to 6 hours. Furthermore, these cytokines have been associated with similar adverse effects in other patient populations.[202,203]

Cardiovascular effects, including hypotension, hypertension, and tachycardia, can occur in heart transplant recipients and present as a biphasic response. The fever, hypertension, and tachycardia are followed by hypotension, hypoxemia, and decreased vascular resistance 5 to 7 hours later.[204] The cardiopulmonary effects are secondary to a series of events involving a number of mediators, including tumor necrosis factor-α, leukotrienes, prostaglandins, thromboxane A₂, and arachidonic acid metabolites produced and released by endothelial cells, neutrophils, and muscle cells.[205]

DOSING PROTOCOL

31. What special procedures should be followed in A.D. when using OKT3 therapy?

The high incidence of side effects associated with OKT3 therapy, especially after the first two doses, has prompted strict dosing protocols in most medical institutions. If A.D. had not had a chest radiograph within the last 24 hours, such would be ordered and reviewed before initiation of OKT3 therapy. If she had evidence of pulmonary edema, a dose of

IV furosemide appropriate for the patient (commonly 40 mg in an adult) or dialysis, if appropriate, would have been administered before the first OKT3 dose. A.D. should receive a dose of methylprednisolone 7 to 8 mg/kg (approximately 500 mg) IV 60 minutes before the first dose of OKT3 and 4 mg/kg before the second dose to significantly reduce the amount of cytokine released after administration.[205] Acetaminophen 650 mg orally or rectally (10 mg/kg in children) and diphenhydramine 50 mg orally or IV (1 mg/kg in children) also are administered before the first two doses of OKT3. Prophylactic IV ganciclovir (2.5 mg/kg per day and adjusted for renal dysfunction) to prevent CMV also has been advocated.

Some transplant centers monitor peripheral T-lymphocyte populations during OKT3 therapy. IL-2R levels, antimurine titers, and CMV cultures of urine, sputum, and blood are monitored for at least 3 weeks after discontinuation of OKT3 therapy. The effectiveness of OKT3 can be evaluated by monitoring for the presence of CD3+ cells among T lymphocytes in the peripheral circulation. In some transplant centers, the number of soluble CD3+ cells is kept to <10 cells/mL,[206] whereas others are willing to accept 20 to 50 CD3+ cells/mL.

ANTIBODIES TO OKT3

32. Why would doses of A.D.'s immunosuppressive drugs need to be adjusted during OKT3 administration?

When OKT3 is administered, antibodies against OKT3 can be formed. These antibodies can be anti-idiotype, anti-isotype, or both, in most cases. Anti-isotype antibodies are formed against the murine proteins of OKT3, and anti-idiotype antibodies are formed against the specific CD3 region. In one study of renal transplant patients, 60% had an anti-idiotype response and 44% had an anti-isotype response. Overall, an antibody response was detected in 75% of patients. A reduction in the dose of azathioprine, mycophenolate, and prednisone or a reduction in the dose of cyclosporine or tacrolimus while receiving OKT3 has lowered the titers of antibody against OKT3.[207,208] Anti-idiotypic OKT3 antibodies have the potential to decrease the effectiveness of repeated courses of the drug. However, multiple courses of treatment with OKT3 have been successful, particularly if antibody titers are low (<1:100).[209]

When treatment of A.D.'s acute rejection is initiated with OKT3, her tacrolimus dose should be reduced by 50%, her MMF should be held temporarily, and her prednisone dose should remain the same. On day 5 to 7 of her OKT3 treatment, her tacrolimus dose should be increased to the dose that she was taking before OKT3 therapy was initiated, and her MMF should be re-instituted. She should be tested for an anti-OKT3 antibody titer 2 to 4 weeks after the end of OKT3 treatment.

BK Polyomavirus Infection

33. A.D. is now 8 months post-transplantation. Her post-transplantation course has been complicated by two rejection episodes. The first was severe and required Thymoglobulin therapy, and the second was a mild rejection several weeks later that was adequately treated with three pulse-doses of 500 mg of IV methylprednisolone. Her current immunosuppressant regimen consists of tacrolimus 8 mg PO BID, MMF 1 g PO BID, and prednisone 10 mg PO QD. In addition, she is receiving amlodipine 10 mg PO QD, benazipril 10 mg PO QD, pravastatin 40 mg PO QIIS, and calcium with vitamin D 500 mg PO BID. Today, she is in the transplantation clinic for a routine follow-up visit. She has no complaints and says she has been feeling "great," although she has noticed some blood in her urine over the past couple of weeks. Because of this, a urinalysis is ordered in addition to the standard laboratory values. The results are: Na, 145 mEq/L (normal, 135 to 145); K, 4.2 mEq/L (normal, 3.4 to 4.6); Cl, 104 mEq/L (normal, 95 to 105); HCO₃, 26 mEq/L (normal, 22 to 28); BUN, 32 mg/dL (normal, 8 to 18); SrCr, 2.3 mg/dL (normal, 0.6 to 1.2); Ca, 10.1 mEq/L (normal, 8.8 to 10.3); phosphorus, 4.5 mg/dL (normal, 2.5 to 5.0); glucose, 110 mg/dL (normal, 65 to 110); amylase, 50 IU/L (normal, 27 to 150); lipase, 32 IU/L (normal, 10 to 50); WBC count, 7.7 cells/mm³ (normal, 4,000 to 10,000); Hgb, 10.4 g/dL (normal, 14 to 18); and Hct, 31% (normal, 39% to 49%); urinalysis, color yellow (normal, clear to yellow); specific gravity, 1.013 (normal, 1.003 to 1.030); pH, 7.0 (normal, 5.0 to 7.0); protein 100 mg/dL (normal, negative to trace); glucose, negative (normal, negative); ketones, negative (normal, negative), bilirubin, negative (normal, negative), blood, moderate (normal, negative); nitrite, negative (normal, negative) leukocyte, negative (normal, negative); squamous epithelial cells, 3 cells/HPF (normal, 0 to 5 cells/HPF); bacteria, negative (normal, negative). Because A.D.'s serum creatinine is significantly elevated, a percutaneous kidney biopsy is performed. The pathologist reviews the histology of the tissue sample and determines that it is consistent with BK virus nephritis. What is BK polyomavirus, how is it diagnosed, and what are its clinical manifestations?

BK virus is a human polyomavirus, first isolated in 1971. Polyomaviruses are small nonenveloped viruses with a closed, circular, double-stranded DNA sequence. Little is known about the transmission or about the primary infection of BK virus. It is believed that viremia during the initial exposure results in systemic seeding and subsequently into a latent infection. The kidney is the main site of BK virus latency in healthy people.[210,211] More than 50% of the general population express BK virus antibodies by age 3. Immunosuppression after transplantation probably leads to the reactivation of the virus, but other factors such as organ ischemia and co-infection with other pathogens may contribute to reactivation. Reactivation inevitably leads to viruria, or viral shedding into the urine.[210] Asymptomatic viruria occurs in approximately 10% to 45% of renal transplant recipients.[212]

Diagnosis of BK virus nephritis is made by careful review of clinical, laboratory and histological findings. Patients are often asymptomatic, although hematuria has been noted in some patients.[211] Clinically, BK virus nephritis mimics acute rejection very closely. Increases in serum creatinine often lead clinicians to perform a tissue biopsy. Tissue histology is very similar in cases of acute rejection and BK virus nephritis, with mononuclear infiltration as the predominant finding. The abundance of plasma cells, prominent tubular cell apoptosis, collecting duct destruction, and absence of endarteritis are features that may distinguish BK virus nephritis from acute cellular rejection.[213,214] Although BK virus has been implicated in up to 5% of all cases of interstitial nephritis (of which 45% go on to suffer graft failure), it is still unclear whether asymptomatic BK viruria in the kidney transplant recipient is a poor prognostic indicator.[212]

Most cases of BK nephritis occur within the first 3 months after transplantation, although a number of cases have been reported as long as 2 years after transplantation. The major risk factor for the development of BK nephritis and subsequent graft dysfunction or loss is the degree of immunosuppression, including both the type and dose of the agents used. Studies have demonstrated an increased incidence of BK nephritis in patients receiving tacrolimus and MMF, compared with those receiving cyclosporine. In addition, accelerated graft loss has been demonstrated in patients who received antilymphocyte antibodies in the presence of BK virus nephritis misdiagnosed as an acute rejection episode.[210,211] Because A.D. has received higher doses of immunosuppression recently to treat two acute rejection episodes, she is at higher risk for developing BK virus nephritis.

TREATMENT

34. **A.D. is told to stop taking MMF and to reduce her tacrolimus dose to 4 mg PO BID. In addition, serum and urine samples are taken to determine BK viral loads. The results are as follows: qualitative urine BK virus by PCR, $>1.3 \times 10^9$ copies/mL (normal, negative); qualitative blood BK virus by PCR, 8.0×10^6 copies/mL (normal, negative). Laboratory tests are to be repeated in 1 week, and viral loads are to be repeated in 2 weeks. Why was A.D.'s immunosuppressive regimen significantly reduced?**

Because BK virus reactivation and BK nephritis are strongly associated with the degree of immunosuppression, reduction in, or removal of immunosuppressant agents should be considered first-line therapy. Beneficial clinical responses have been demonstrated in some patients when the dose of tacrolimus is reduced. Unfortunately, not all patients respond to this maneuver. In addition, reduction in immunosuppression puts patients at higher risk for an acute rejection episode. Close clinical follow-up after reduction of immunosuppression is important to ensure adequate response and to make sure the patient does not develop an acute rejection episode.[215] In A.D.'s case, we expect an improvement of renal function, as seen by a reduction in serum creatinine over time. Also, monitoring viral loads both from the urine and serum have been shown to correlate with clinical disease.

Antiviral Therapy

35. **Over the next 2 weeks, A.D.'s serum creatinine remains unchanged, and her serum and urine viral loads also remain approximately the same. Are there any additional treatment options for A.D.'s BK nephritis at this time?**

Cidofovir (vistide), an antiviral agent indicated for the treatment of CMV retinitis, inhibits polyomavirus replication in vitro; however, to date, no well-conducted clinical trials have proved this agent to be effective at treating or preventing BK virus nephritis in the transplant population. In a small number of case reports and case-series, this agent was beneficial, but the appropriate dose and frequency are still undetermined. Most reports have used very small doses (0.25 to 1.0 mg/kg/dose) given intravenously either weekly or every other week; cidofovir was continued until renal dysfunction resolved and a decrease in the viral load occurred.[216,217]

Because cidofovir has a high incidence of nephrotoxicity, especially at much higher doses, patients usually receive pre- and post-dose hydration with 0.9% NaCl boluses. Close clinical monitoring of the patient is advised if this treatment option is used. Because the doses of cidofovir currently used are approximately 5% to 10% of the standard dose used to treat CMV (5 mg/kg/dose), use of probenecid as a premedication to prevent nephrotoxicity is not advocated.[217]

LIVER TRANSPLANTATION
Indications

36. **E.P., a 58-year-old, 78-kg man, with an 18-year history of chronic liver disease secondary to hepatitis C infection, arrives at the emergency room with a 2-day history of confusion, fever up to 102.2°F, and worsening jaundice, with scleral icterus. Because the patient has severe abdominal distention, a paracentesis is performed, and seven liters of fluid are drained from his peritoneal cavity. A diagnosis of spontaneous bacterial peritonitis is made.**

E.P.'s clinical status over the next several days gradually worsens, and he is moved to the intensive care unit for closer monitoring and better supportive care. E.P. continues to be severely jaundice, with worsening liver function tests. He becomes progressively more confused, and eventually comatose, requiring intubation. Within 3 days of admission into the ICU, a suitable liver donor, matched for size and ABO blood group, is found, and E.P. receives an orthotopic liver transplant with a choledochocholedochostomy (duct-to-duct anastomosis). CMV serology for E.P. is negative, and the donor liver is CMV-positive.

After the transplantation, E.P. is started on fluid maintenance with D_5W; nystatin suspension 5 mL QID; tacrolimus 2 mg NG/PO BID; and high-dose methylprednisolone with a rapid taper: 50 mg IV Q 6 hr for four doses, 40 mg IV Q 6 hr for four doses, 30 mg IV Q 6 hr for four doses, 20 mg IV Q 6 hr for four doses, 20 mg IV Q 12 hr for two doses, then 20 mg IV QD; famotidine 20 mg IV Q 12 hr; and ganciclovir 150 mg IV QD. Ampicillin/sulbactam 1.5 g IV Q 6 hr for 48 hours was begun just before transplantation. An order also is written to limit all pain medications and sedatives. E.P. returned from surgery with three abdominal Jackson-Pratt (J-P) drains, a nasogastric tube, Foley catheter, and Swan-Ganz central venous catheter. What was the indication for E.P. to receive a liver transplant?

E.P. was diagnosed with end-stage hepatic failure (cirrhosis) due to chronic hepatitis C infection. The most common indication for liver transplantation in adults is cirrhosis from various causes. Each transplantation center varies with respect to the most common disease states that indicate transplantation, but nationwide, hepatitis C and alcohol-induced disease are the number one and two reasons for patients requiring liver transplantation. Indications for liver transplantation in adults include cholestatic liver disease (e.g., primary biliary cirrhosis and primary sclerosing cholangitis), hepatocellular liver disease (e.g., chronic viral hepatitis B or C, autoimmune, drug-induced, cryptogenic cirrhosis), vascular disease (e.g., Budd-Chiari), hepatic malignancy, inherited metabolic disorders, and fulminant hepatic failure (e.g., viral hepatitis, Wilson's disease, drug or toxin induced). Controversial indications include alcohol-induced disease and some types of hepatic malignancies. The concern with these indications is either recurrence of disease as in the case of hepatic malignancies, or recidivism in the case of alcoholics.[218,219]

Contraindications to transplantation have decreased in numbers over the past few years. Current contraindications to liver transplantation include malignancy outside the liver, cholangiocarcinoma, active infection outside the biliary system, patients with alcoholic liver disease who continue to abuse alcohol, psychosocial instability and noncompliance, severe neurologic disease, and advanced cardiopulmonary disease. Patients with active infections are considered candidates after the infection has been eradicated. HIV infection is not considered an absolute contraindication to transplantation.[220]

E.P. was within the age limitations for transplantation, had severe progressive disease, and was at risk for death if he had not received a liver transplant. Because he did not have any of the listed contraindications, a liver could be transplanted emergently. His anticipated survival after transplantation at 1 year is >80%; at 5 years it is >70%.[218]

Patient Monitoring

36. How should E.P. be monitored in the initial postoperative period?

A typical course is as follows. E.P. should be awake and alert within 12 to 24 hours after the operation, transferred from the ICU to a regular bed in 2 to 3 days, and discharged home within 10 to 14 days if he has a standard postoperative course with no severe complications. Because function of the transplanted liver is essential for the survival of the patient, extensive clinical, laboratory, and radiologic monitoring are necessary. E.P. has three Jackson-Pratt abdominal drains that must be monitored for output production. The serum concentrations of BUN, creatinine, liver function tests, albumin, potassium, sodium, magnesium, calcium, phosphate, and glucose should be monitored every 6 hours on the first postoperative day.[221] The surgical transplantation of a liver has been associated with coagulopathies and bleeding. Therefore, platelets, prothrombin time, fibrinogen, and factors V and VII also must be monitored and deficiencies rapidly corrected.[222]

Initial liver function tests are highly variable. Liver function tests can either increase for the first day or two after transplantation because of ischemic damage to the allograft, or they can decrease because of initial dilution by high-volume blood replacement. If the liver is functioning well, the liver function tests, bilirubin, and prothrombin time all should begin to trend toward normal within 4 to 5 days after the operation.

Magnesium, phosphate, and calcium levels may fall in the early postoperative period and should be monitored closely. Ionized calcium serum concentrations are monitored rather than total calcium because most patients have low serum albumin concentrations. Hypocalcemia can occur because these patients may receive large amounts of citrate through blood transfusions, which can lower serum calcium concentrations. Magnesium deficiency is common in patients with end-stage liver disease and may be exacerbated in the early post-transplantation period by tacrolimus or diuretics. Why patients develop hypophosphatemia is unclear; but increased demand for phosphate for incorporation into adenosine triphosphate is a possible explanation. Hypokalemia or hyperkalemia may occur, depending on renal function and fluid status. Electrolyte serum concentrations should be followed and electrolytes replaced if needed (see Chapter 12, Fluid and Electrolyte Disorders).

Hyperglycemia, which is a good indication of a properly functioning liver in this early period, may need to be con-trolled with a continuous IV infusion of insulin initially and then subcutaneous insulin dosed on the basis of periodic glucose measurements. In contrast, persistent hypoglycemia indicates a poorly functioning liver. Hypertension, which is multifactorial, also is seen during this time and usually is treated with calcium channel blockers, nitroglycerin, nitroprusside, or β-blockers. Renal dysfunction and neurologic complications also can occur.[221,223] Neurologic complications, including those that are drug induced, include oversedation, acute psychosis, depression, tremor, headaches, peripheral neuropathy, cortical blindness, paresthesias, paresis, and seizures.[223]

Other complications that can occur within the first 3 days to 3 weeks include respiratory distress, intra-abdominal hemorrhage, biliary tract leaks and strictures, hepatic artery thrombosis, and primary graft nonfunction. Because infection is another early postoperative concern, E.P. should be monitored for bacterial, fungal, and viral infections.

Tacrolimus
Pharmacokinetics

37. Seven days after his liver transplantation, E.P.'s J-P abdominal drains, Foley catheter, and nasogastric drain have been removed. Current medications include tacrolimus (Prograf) 2 mg PO Q 12 hr; prednisone 20 mg PO QD; nystatin suspension 500,000 units to S&S QID; amlodipine 5 mg PO QD; TMP-SMX Mondays, Wednesdays, and Fridays; and valganciclovir 900 mg PO QD. E.P.'s current laboratory values include the following: BUN, 27 mg/dL (normal, 8 to 18); SrCr, 0.9 mg/dL (normal, 0.6 to 1.2); AST, 170 U/L (normal, 0 to 35); ALT, 154 U/L (normal, 0 to 35); γ-glutamyl transferase (GGT), 320 U/L (normal, 0 to 30); total bilirubin, 3.4 mg/dL (normal, 0.1 to 1.0); and tacrolimus 9.4 ng/dL (by monoclonal whole blood TDx). What important pharmacokinetic factors should be considered when using tacrolimus after transplantation?

[SI units: BUN, 9.6 mmol/L (normal, 3.0 to 6.5); SrCr, 79.6 μmol/L (normal, 50 to 110); AST, 170 U/L (normal, 0 to 35); ALT, 154 U/L (normal, 0 to 35); GGT, 320 U/L (normal, 0 to 30); total bilirubin, 58.14 μmol/L (normal, 2 to 18)]

Tacrolimus is a very lipophilic compound that is absorbed rapidly after oral administration in most patients. Peak blood concentrations are achieved in about 0.5 to 1 hour. Some patients have slower absorption or have a lag time of up to 2 hours in their absorption profiles. Oral bioavailability is usually poor, highly variable, and ranges from 4% to 89% (mean 25%). Protein binding is approximately 75% and is mainly to erythrocytes. Whole blood concentrations are significantly higher than serum concentrations for this reason. Tacrolimus has a large volume of distribution and accumulates in high concentrations in tissues, including the lungs, spleen, heart, kidney, brain, muscles, and liver. Tacrolimus is predominantly metabolized in the liver through the cytochrome P450 3A4 isoenzyme system and is primarily eliminated from the body as several inactive metabolites. Less than 1% of tacrolimus is eliminated as the parent compound in the urine, and renal dysfunction does not alter the pharmacokinetics of this agent. The elimination half-life ranges from 5.5 to 16.6 hours, with a mean of 8.7 hours, and plasma clearance averages 143 L/hr. Varying degrees of liver dysfunction, including cirrhosis and severe cholestasis, may have dramatic effects on the metabolism and excretion of tacrolimus. Pediatric patients appear to clear tacrolimus more rapidly and have a shorter half-life and larger volume of distribution compared with adults.[224] Black patients may require higher dosages.[225]

Dosing

38. **How would you initiate the dosing of tacrolimus for E.P.?**

Although tacrolimus can be administered as a continuous IV infusion through a central or peripheral infusion after transplantation (initial dose 0.025 to 0.05 mg/kg per day), it is preferable to give it via a nasogastric tube or orally because adverse effects, such as headache, nausea, vomiting, neurotoxicity, and nephrotoxicity, occur more commonly with IV administration. If tacrolimus is given intravenously, patients should be converted as soon as possible to oral therapy (initial doses of 0.1 to 0.3 mg/kg per day in adults and 0.15 to 0.3 mg/kg per day in children divided into 12-hour intervals). Pediatric patients require two to three times the adult doses of tacrolimus.

In E.P., the initial starting dose was approximately 0.15 mg/kg per day given orally or through the nasogastric tube every 12 hours. Oral tacrolimus should be administered on an empty stomach or taken consistently in relation to meals. Most institutions extemporaneously prepare an oral solution for nasogastric tube administration because it is not commercially available.

39. **How would you convert a patient from cyclosporine to tacrolimus?**

Although E.P. was initiated on tacrolimus without prior exposure to cyclosporine, many patients are converted from cyclosporine to tacrolimus either because of a poor response (as evidenced by recurrent acute rejection episodes) or intolerance (as evidenced by persistent adverse drug reactions, most commonly gingival hyperplasia or unwanted hair growth). When switching from cyclosporine to tacrolimus, the cyclosporine should be discontinued 24 hours before initiating tacrolimus therapy or longer if cyclosporine concentrations are elevated. The concomitant administration of cyclosporine and tacrolimus has been accompanied by increases in the serum concentrations of creatinine and urea nitrogen, which declined after the discontinuation of cyclosporine. Thus, combination therapy with cyclosporine and tacrolimus is not recommended because of the additive or synergistic risk of nephrotoxicity.

Therapeutic Drug Monitoring

40. **E.P.'s tacrolimus concentrations are being measured by whole blood IMx immunoassay. Why is it important to monitor E.P.'s tacrolimus concentrations and how should his tacrolimus therapy be monitored?**

Because of the large inter- and intra-patient variability, the narrow therapeutic index, and the large number of potential drug interactions associated with this agent, tacrolimus concentrations should be monitored in all patients receiving therapy. Concentrations are monitored to prevent toxicity, optimize efficacy, and assess patient compliance to the prescribed regimen. There does appear to be a relation among concentration, efficacy, and toxicity.[226] The primary monitoring parameter used clinically is the trough concentration because, unlike cyclosporine, trough concentrations correlate well with overall total body exposure (AUC).[227] Because of accuracy in measuring the tacrolimus parent compound (without measuring inactive metabolites) and a rapid turnaround time (within hours), the IMx assay method for tacrolimus that uses whole blood is the most common one used. The target range is 10 to 20 ng/mL for the first 3 months and 5 to 10 ng/mL thereafter, but this may vary with each transplantation center's protocols.[228]

As in all cases, pharmacokinetic data must be interpreted in conjunction with the patient's clinical condition. In addition, deference always must be given to trends established by multiple tacrolimus concentrations over that of a single concentration.

Adverse Drug Reactions

41. **What are the major adverse effects associated with tacrolimus and what clinical parameters should be monitored in E.P.?**

Nephrotoxicity usually is the limiting adverse effect of tacrolimus and has been reported in >50% of patients in some studies. This may have been related to the higher dosages used in earlier trials because dose reduction usually reverses the nephrotoxicity. The clinical presentation of tacrolimus-induced nephrotoxicity is similar to that of cyclosporine. Because IV administration of tacrolimus during the first week has been associated with acute renal failure in 20% of patients, very few centers use this route or rapidly convert to oral therapy. Presumably, liver recipients with poor graft function are unable to metabolize tacrolimus rapidly and are at a greater risk for acute renal failure.[229] In a multicenter study involving 529 patients, the efficacy and toxicity of tacrolimus was compared with cyclosporine in liver transplant recipients. Both agents increased serum creatinine and decreased glomerular filtration rate comparably.[230] Thus, E.P.'s renal function should be monitored closely.

Major neurologic toxicities (e.g., confusion, seizures, dysarthria, persistent coma) occur in approximately 10% of patients. Minor neurologic toxicities occur in approximately 20% to 60% of patients and include tremors, headache, and sleep disturbances.[230] Hypertension (40%) is another common finding in patients treated with tacrolimus. However, a greater number of tacrolimus-treated patients are able to discontinue or limit their use of antihypertensives as compared with cyclosporine. Other adverse effects include diarrhea, nausea, vomiting and anorexia, hypomagnesemia, hyperkalemia, hemolytic anemia, hemolytic uremic syndrome, alopecia, increased susceptibility to infection and malignancy, and hyperglycemia. Hyperglycemia is reported to occur more often with tacrolimus. This is most likely to be seen in patients with higher tacrolimus levels or higher steroid doses and in African Americans. With reduction in tacrolimus and steroid doses, hyperglycemia appears to decrease. Hirsutism and gingival hyperplasia, in contrast to that which occurs with cyclosporine, are not complications of tacrolimus.

Rejection

42. **E.P. was discharged from the hospital. He went to stay with his brother and was followed up with laboratory tests obtained three times a week. The following laboratory values were obtained 2 weeks later: AST, 36 U/L (normal, 0 to 35); ALT, 52**

U/L (normal, 0 to 35); GGT, 65 U/L (normal, 0 to 30); and bilirubin, T/D 1.0/0.3 mg/dL (normal, 0.1 to 1.0); and another week later: AST, 158 IU/L; ALT, 322 IU/L; GGT, 321 IU/L; and bilirubin, T/D 3.6/3.2 mg/dL.

E.P. was readmitted to the transplantation center because his liver function tests suggested liver dysfunction, and a percutaneous needle liver biopsy was obtained to determine the cause. On admission, he complained of tiredness, severe headaches, a mild tremor, and some pain over the area of the transplanted liver. E.P. also stated that he had not felt like eating for the last 2 to 3 days. The pathologist interpreted the liver biopsy as moderate rejection, and E.P. was given a 1-g IV bolus of methylprednisolone followed by rapidly tapered doses. This regimen used the following IV doses of methylprednisolone: 50 mg every 6 hours for four doses; 40 mg every 6 hours for four doses; 30 mg every 6 hours for four doses; 20 mg every 6 hours for four doses; 20 mg every 12 hours for two doses; then back to the pretapered oral prednisone dose. Three days into the recycle, E.P.'s liver enzyme values had not improved and Thymoglobulin therapy was initiated. Laboratory values after 10 days of Thymoglobulin IV 1.5 mg/kg per day were as follows: AST, 35 IU/L; ALT, 108 IU/L; GGT, 169 IU/L; and bilirubin, T/D 1.0/0.6 mg/dL. The 12-hour tacrolimus trough level at the end of the treatment course was 15.2 ng/mL by IMx immunoassay. E.P. was discharged and sent home with the following medications: tacrolimus 5 mg PO BID; prednisone 20 mg PO QD; clonidine 0.3 mg PO BID; felodipine 10 mg PO QD; furosemide 20 mg PO QD; co-trimoxazole 1 tablet QD Mondays, Wednesdays, and Fridays; valganciclovir 900 mg PO QD. What subjective and objective evidence of liver rejection is present in E.P.?

[SI units: AST, 36 U/L, 158 U/L, 35 U/L (normal, 0 to 35); ALT, 52 U/L, 322 U/L, 108 U/L (normal, 0 to 35); GGT, 65 U/L, 321 U/L, 169 UL (normal, 0 to 30); bilirubin, 17.1/5.13 μmol/L, 61.56/54.72 μmol/L, 17.1/6.2 μmol/L (normal, 2 to 18)]

Rejection episodes in liver transplant recipients can be categorized as acute or chronic. Hyperacute rejection rarely occurs with liver transplantation. Treatment is supportive and retransplantation is needed.[231] Unlike other organs, though, the liver may function adequately, but survival is lower when the transplanted organ is incompatible.[232]

Acute Liver Rejection

Although acute liver rejection can occur at any time after the transplantation, it is most commonly experienced within the first week to 6 weeks in approximately 30% to 50% of patients treated with either cyclosporine or tacrolimus and prednisone.[231] Early data in patients treated with tacrolimus, mycophenolate, and prednisone indicate lower rejection rates up to 6 months after transplantation.[233,234] Late acute rejections often are a result of either a reduction in dose or a discontinuation of immunosuppressive agents. These rejection episodes, although common, rarely lead to graft loss.

E.P. presents with some of the common subjective complaints of patients experiencing rejection of their transplanted liver. Commonly, patients feel poorly and complain of anorexia, abdominal discomfort, and headache. Other symptoms, such as a low-grade fever, back pain, or respiratory distress may occur. Objective evidence for rejection in E.P. includes an abrupt rise in serum concentrations of transaminases and bilirubin and a liver biopsy that was interpreted as "moderate rejection" by the pathologist. These observations,

in conjunction with the subjective signs, point to a diagnosis of rejection. Acute rejection is associated with mononuclear cell infiltration of the graft, edema, and parenchymal necrosis. Rejection should be diagnosed by biopsy using histologic criteria. Areas most commonly damaged are the bile ducts, veins, and arteries.[235]

Chronic Liver Rejection

Chronic liver rejection, also called *ductopenic rejection,* usually develops months to years after the transplant in about 5% of recipients. Characteristics of chronic liver rejection include occlusive arterial lesions, destruction of small intrahepatic bile ducts (often referred to as *vanishing bile duct syndrome*), intense cholestasis, accumulation of foamy macrophages within the portal sinusoids, and fibrosis, which may lead to the development of cirrhosis. Chronic rejection is irreversible and unaffected by increased immunosuppressive therapy. Retransplantation has been considered the only viable alternative. However, some patients with ductopenic rejection unresponsive to cyclosporine-based therapy have responded to tacrolimus.[236]

Treatment of Rejection

43. Was the treatment of E.P.'s rejection of his transplanted liver appropriate?

E.P. was receiving maintenance immunosuppression with tacrolimus and prednisone. Double or triple therapy with tacrolimus or cyclosporine and prednisone commonly is used as chronic immunosuppressive therapy in liver transplant recipients. E.P.'s tacrolimus trough whole blood concentration was in the low normal therapeutic range (*Note:* normal values for therapeutic range vary with the institution). Although E.P.'s tacrolimus concentration appeared adequate, he was treated with a bolus dose of IV methylprednisolone because of clinical evidence that supported a diagnosis of graft rejection. This treatment decision was reasonable because high-dose corticosteroids can reverse acute rejection episodes of a transplanted liver.[231] The decision to monitor E.P.'s response to the initial bolus steroid dosage and the severity of rejection by biopsy also was appropriate before proceeding with further treatment. E.P. had experienced moderate rejection of his transplanted liver, and the subsequent initiation of another cycle of corticosteroids was reasonable because the mainstay for treatment of acute liver rejection is increased immunosuppression.

Adult liver transplant recipients usually are treated with 200 mg to 1,000 mg/day of IV methylprednisolone and tapered rapidly, as described for E.P. When patients fail to respond to recycle corticosteroid therapy, two options still are available. E.P. was begun on Thymoglobulin therapy; the other option is to use OKT3. Most centers use Thymoglobulin as a second-line agent if there is no response to high-dose corticosteroids. The typical dose is 1.5 mg/kg per day given as an infusion over 4 to 6 hours. Therapy is continued for 7 to 14 days. Treatment of corticosteroid-resistant rejection with Thymoglobulin is effective in about 70% to 80% of liver transplant recipients. Other adjustments in immunosuppression could include the addition of mycophenolate or possibly sirolimus.

Mycophenolate Mofetil

44. Following the rejection episode, E.P. is started on MMF. Describe MMF's pharmacokinetic characteristics and adverse effects. How will these characteristics affect the dosing and monitoring of MMF in this patient?

MMF is an alternative to azathioprine. In most transplantation centers, MMF has replaced azathioprine as the antiproliferative agent used in combination with antibodies, calcineurin inhibitors, and prednisone. Several studies have shown significant reductions in acute rejection rates during the first year after kidney transplant as compared with azathioprine.[237,238] However, results with longer follow-up, at 3 years, indicate no difference in survival.[239]

Pharmacokinetics

MMF is a prodrug for the active form, mycophenolic acid (MPA). MMF is well absorbed (bioavailability, 94%) and is rapidly hydrolyzed to MPA after absorption. The C_{max} for MPA occurs between 1 and 3 hours, and it is hepatically metabolized via glucuronidation to inactive mycophenolic acid glucuronide (MPAG), which is eliminated by the kidney and excreted into the bile. Once MPAG is excreted into bile, it undergoes enterohepatic recycling in the GI tract, where it is deconjugated to mycophenolic acid (MPA), which is reabsorbed back into the systemic circulation. Because of this recycling, a second peak occurs 6 to 12 hours after dosing. MPA has an elimination half-life of 17 hours on average; the volume of distribution is 4 L/kg, and it is highly protein bound to albumin (98%). Protein binding correlates well with albumin and free MPA concentrations correlate with immunosuppressive effect. Studies indicate that protein binding changes over time after transplantation, with the free fraction decreasing and total MPA concentrations increasing over time. Renal impairment, liver dysfunction, and elevated MPAG concentrations in transplant recipients can reduce protein binding. This may be a function of low albumin concentrations seen in these patients.[240]

Adverse Effects

The most commonly reported side effects for MMF are GI (anorexia, nausea, vomiting and diarrhea, gastritis), hematologic (leukopenia, thrombocytopenia, anemia), and infectious in nature. GI side effects are common, and all side effects are more common with higher dosages. If a patient complains, one could try giving the dose without other medications, giving smaller doses more frequently, or lowering the dosage and titrating upward as tolerated.[241] If the WBC count is <3,000 or absolute neutrophil count (ANC) is <1.3, the MMF dose should be reduced or discontinued.

Dosing

The usual starting dose in adults is 1 to 1.5 g twice daily. In kidney transplant recipients and patients like R.F., a 1-g twice-daily regimen is appropriate because 1 g two times a day was as effective as 1.5 g two times a day and less toxic in this population. Some advocate the higher dosage in high-risk patients (e.g., patients receiving another transplant, patients with a high PRA, blacks). Excluding the early post-transplantation period, 1 g two times a day is the recommended regimen in patients with a glomerular filtration rate <25 mL/min. In heart transplant recipients, the 1.5-g twice-daily regimen is used.

In children, 300 to 600 mg/M^2 two times a day or 23 mg/kg per day two times a day has been recommended.

Therapeutic Drug Monitoring

Monitoring MPA serum concentrations is controversial and not generally recommended at this time because there is so much intra-patient and inter-patient pharmacokinetic variability. However, some studies have shown a relation between effect and concentrations.

Data in heart transplant recipients indicate that an MPA trough level of >2.5 mg/L is required for therapeutic effect. In kidney transplant recipients, area under the concentration-time curve (AUCs) have been shown to correlate with acute rejection. Another approach is to measure free concentrations, but the primary limitation to using serum concentrations is the lack of a simple, commercially available assay. The preceding studies used a high-performance liquid chromotography (HPLC) assay; but there are ongoing investigations with an enzyme-multiplied immunoassay technique (EMIT) immunoassay.[242]

Once started on MMF, E.P. should be monitored for GI and hematologic side effects, as well as for any signs and symptoms of infection and rejection.

Drug Interactions With Immunosuppressives

45. C.C. is a 42-year-old woman who underwent a liver transplantation 5 days ago. She was noted to be febrile, with an elevated WBC. Cultures were obtained, and her J-P drainage grew *Candida albicans*. C.C. was started on fluconazole 400 mg QD. Her other medications included tacrolimus 3 mg BID, prednisone 20 mg QD, mycophenolate 500 mg BID, valganciclovir 450 mg QD, TMP-SMX one-half tablet QD, and esomeprazole 20 mg QHS. The tacrolimus trough level is 11 ng/mL. What drugs interact with immunosuppressive agents? Will the initiation of fluconoazole require any adjustments in current medication doses?

Because the immunosuppressants have complex and highly variable pharmacokinetic profiles with relatively narrow therapeutic indexes, drug-drug interactions represent a significant clinical problem in transplantation. These drug interactions can be separated into two main categories: pharmacokinetic and pharmacodynamic. Pharmacokinetic drug interactions occur when one medication alters the absorption, distribution, metabolism, or elimination of the immunosuppressant agent.[86,87,246] Table 35-2 displays the most clinically relevant pharmacokinetic drug interactions that are likely to be encountered in transplant recipients and how to manage these interactions when they do occur. These include drugs that alter either the absorption or metabolism of the immunosuppressants. This table is not comprehensive.

Pharmacodynamic drug interactions with the immunosuppressant agents represent another significant problem in transplantation. These interactions occur when one medication either potentiates an adverse effect or alters the pharmacologic effects of the immunsuppressant agent.[86] An example of this would be the use of calcineurin inhibitors (cyclosporine and tacrolimus) in combination with ACE inhibitors. Because both classes of agents can cause hyperkalemia and potentially can decrease renal function, there may be a more pronounced

Table 35-2 Immunosuppressant Drug Interactions

Immunosuppressant (IS)	Interacting Drugs	Mechanism	Consequence	Clinical Management	References
Calcineurin inhibitors (cyclosporine and tacrolimus) and sirolimus	Clarithromycin[a], erythromycin[a], ketoconazole[a], itraconazole[a], fluconazole, voriconazole[a], fluoxetine, fluvoxamine, citalopram, nefazadone[a], diltiazem[a], verapamil[a], delaviridine[a], ritonavir[a], cimetidine[a], grapefruit juice[a], amiodarone, saquinavir, nelfinavir, indinavir, amprenavir, chloramphenicol[a]	Inhibit CYP450 3A4 isoenzyme in the liver and intestines.	Increase the concentration and total AUC of the IS.	Either prospectively decrease the IS dose or monitor trough concentrations more closely and adjust doses accordingly.	85, 86, 87, 246
Calcineurin inhibitors (cyclosporine and tacrolimus) and sirolimus	Carbamazepine[a], dexamethasone, phenobarbital[a], phenytoin[a], St. John's Wort[a], rifampin[a], rifabutin[a], efavirenz[a], nevirapine[a], nafcillin, clindamycin	Induce CYP450 3A4 isoenzyme in the liver and intestines.	Decrease the concentration and total AUC of the IS.	Either prospectively increase the IS dose or monitor trough concentrations more closely and adjust doses accordingly.	86, 87, 245, 246, 247
Calcineurin inhibitors (cyclosporine and tacrolimus), sirolimus, and mycophenolate mofetil	Cholestyramine, colestipol, probucol, sevelamer, antacids (magnesium and aluminum containing)[b], iron containing products[b]	Bind to IS and prevents absorption.	Decrease the concentration and total AUC of the IS.	Avoid concomitant administration with IS and monitor trough concentrations.	86, 87, 248, 249, 250
Azathioprine	Allopurinol	Inhibits metabolism by inhibiting xanthine oxidase.	Increases the concentration and total AUC of azathioprine.	Avoid use together or prospectively reduce azathioprine dose to $^1/_3$ or $^1/_4$ normal dose and monitor for increased toxicity.	86, 251

[a]Indicates potent inhibitor or inducer.
[b]Only occurs with mycophenolate mofetil.

toxicity when these classes are given in combination.[88] Pharmacodynamic drug interactions are usually more difficult to identify and require a thorough knowledge of the pharmacologic effects, in terms of both efficacy and toxicity, for the agents being used. Often, there is little or no information in the literature on these types of interactions to guide the clinician in determining whether this drug interaction will occur.

As a general rule, if an agent is known to cause a particular toxicity that is similar to a toxicity associated with the immunosuppressant agent, then there is a high likelihood of a pharmacodynamic interaction occurring. Another example of this would be an interaction between the concomitant use of metoclopramide and MMF. Both agents are known to cause diarrhea, and it is likely that if these agents are used together, there is a higher incidence or severity of diarrhea.[86] In addition, if a drug has a pharmacologic effect that may alter the efficacy of an immunosuppressant, then a pharmacodynamic drug interaction may also occur. An example of this may be when a drug is given that has immunosuppressant properties, such as the chemotherapeutic agent cyclophosphamide.[243] This may lead to overimmunosuppression of the transplant recipient, and a higher incidence or severity of opportunistic infections. Conversely, if a drug has known immunostimulant properties, such as the herbal medication echinacea,[244] it may reduce the efficacy of the immunsuppressant agent and increase the risk of rejection in the transplant recipient.[86] Although agents that have pharmacodynamic drug interactions with the immunosuppressants are not absolutely contraindicated, transplant recipients should be closely monitored for either increased risk of drug toxicity or decreased drug efficacy when these agents are used in combination with the immunosuppressants. When a transplant patient is started on any new medication, whether by prescription, over the counter, or even herbal, it should be thoroughly researched to determine whether there is a potential for it to interact with the immunosuppressant regimen.

In C.C., the addition of fluconazole will lead to a pharmacokinetic drug interaction and significantly increase (on average double) tacrolimus concentrations. This interaction is usually evident within 2 days, and a maximal effect is seen within a week of initiating fluconazole. Therefore, C.C.'s tacrolimus dose should be reduced by 50% when fluconazole is started. Tacrolimus blood levels should be monitored, as should signs and symptoms of toxicity and rejection. Fluconazole could also influence steroid metabolism, but specific recommendations are not available. In general, drug interactions can be managed, and in some cases may require only separate administration times. In other cases, one can use an alternative agent within a pharmacologic class that does not interact with these agents.

Cyclosporine

46. B.B. is a 27-year-old, 60-kg African-American man who received a cadaveric kidney transplant. Within 12 hours of the transplantation, his immunosuppression consisted of modified cyclosporine (Neoral) 300 mg PO BID, MMF 1.5 g PO BID, and prednisone. He was taking other medicines for hypertension and infection prophylaxis. Describe the pharmacokinetic characteristics of cyclosporine. Based on this information, is B.B.'s cyclosporine regimen appropriate?

Pharmacokinetics

Cyclosporine pharmacokinetic parameters (e.g., absorption, distribution, metabolism) exhibit significant intrapatient and interpatient variability, resulting in poor dose-response relationships. A number of factors are known to influence its pharmacokinetic behavior. These include age, transplant type, underlying disease, time after transplantation, GI motility and metabolism, biliary and liver function and metabolism, body weight, cholesterol, albumin, red blood cell mass, drug interactions, and formulation.[252] These factors can change cyclosporine's absorption, distribution, metabolism, and excretion and can influence therapeutic concentrations and, ultimately, outcomes.[253,254] For example, children, African Americans, and patients with cystic fibrosis tend to have reduced absorption and/or increased clearance of cyclosporine. Patients who are obese or have decreased liver function will have reduced clearance. Oral absorption of cyclosporine, which has been characterized as slow, incomplete, and highly variable, is the parameter that is most significantly affected. Absorption can depend on the type of transplant, time after transplantation, presence of food and its composition, intestinal function (e.g., diarrhea, ileus), small bowel length, and presence or absence of external bile drainage. The mean absorption of the original cyclosporine product (Sandimmune) in adults with relatively normal liver function after a liver transplantation is 27%, which is comparable to that observed in recipients of kidney (27%), heart (35%), and bone marrow (34%) transplants. Bioavailibility ranges from <5% to 90%.[255] In most transplant recipients, cyclosporine absorption increases over time.

Dosing

Because cyclosporine (Sandimmune) absorption was so poor and erratic, it was given intravenously for the first few days after transplantation, particularly after liver transplantation. Cyclosporine was often given intravenously as a continuous infusion (2 to 3 mg/kg per day) or intermittently (2.5 mg/kg per day) over 2 to 6 hours two times a day. As the trough cyclosporine levels began to rise, the IV dose was decreased gradually, while the oral dose was maintained or increased. This route may still be required in some patients with cystic fibrosis after lung transplantation.

B.B. was given modified cyclosporine (Neoral), a readily absorbed cyclosporine formulation in a solubilized microemulsified state. Neoral's bioavailability is better than that of Sandimmune (approximately 20% higher for Neoral compared with Sandimmune), and there is less intra-patient and inter-patient variability in transplant recipients. Furthermore, Neoral absorption is much less dependent on bile and thus can be used in most liver transplant recipients early after transplant without the need for IV administration, although the doses used are initially higher (10 to 15 mg/kg per day) than those used after kidney and heart transplantation (5 to 10 mg/kg per day).[255]

Neoral and Sandimmune are not bioequivalent and therefore are not interchangeable. Neoral produces a shorter T_{max}, higher C_{max}, and higher AUC than Sandimmune. It has significantly less intra-subject and inter-subject pharmacokinetic variability, and there is a better correlation between single concentrations, such as troughs, and AUC than seen with Sandimmune. The bioavailability of Neoral is approximately 20% higher than that of Sandimmune (absolute bioavailability is 10% to 89%). When converting patients on Sandimmune to Neoral, a 1:1 dosage ratio is used unless patients are taking >10 mg/kg per day of Sandimmune. Trough concentrations are initially obtained within the first 4 to 7 days, and dosage adjustments are made accordingly. Most patients tolerate conversion well, although some develop concentrated-related headaches or tremors or elevated serum creatinine levels that resolve with dose adjustment. In most patients, the Neoral dose is 10% to 20% lower than their Sandimmune dose, but there can be as much as a 50% difference in patients taking large doses (>10 mg/kg per day) of Sandimmune.[255]

The first generic cyclosporine, SangCya, is no longer available. SangCya was bioequivalent to Neoral but not Sandimmune. Three other capsule forms are now available, which are also AB-rated bioequivalent to Neoral, Gengraf from Abbott and modified cyclosporine from Eon and Sidmak. Neoral and Sandimmune are available as both capsule and liquid.

In addition, cyclosporine is extensively distributed into red blood cells, about 60%, whereas in plasma it is highly bound to lipoproteins, about 90%. It is extensively metabolized by both the gut and liver P450 3A4 and transported by P-glycoprotein. The average half-life is about 15 to 20 hours.[252]

B.B. was started on 8 mg/kg per day BID. He is African American and may require even higher doses, because the absorption of cyclosporine has been reported to be reduced in this population.[256] His blood concentration will have to be monitored closely and adjusted if necessary. He should be watched closely for signs of rejection and toxicity.

Adverse Effects

47. What are some of the adverse effects associated with cyclosporine?

Cyclosporine can cause a number of adverse effects. Nephrotoxicity is the most frequent and most worrisome. This can be either acute or chronic (see Question 8). Other major effects include hypertension (see Question 12), hyperlipidemia (see Question 13), tremors, headaches, seizures, paresthesias, hypomagnesemia, hypo- or hyperkalemia, hyperuricemia, hyperglycemia, gout, gingival hyperplasia, hirsutism, hemolytic-uremic syndrome, and hepatotoxicity. If these occur, they generally respond to a reduction in dose or discontinuation of cyclosporine.[257]

Therapeutic Drug Monitoring

48. B.B.'s cyclosporine levels are being measured by whole blood TDx assay. How should cyclosporine levels be used to optimize his therapy?

Cyclosporine concentrations are monitored to prevent toxicity, optimize efficacy, and assess patient compliance to the prescribed regimen. Most institutions monitor trough cyclosporine levels. During the early postoperative period, cy-cl7osporine levels should be measured daily, but keep in mind that these may not reflect steady-state concentrations, and that dosage changes should be made every few days. Once B.B. is home, cyclosporine monitoring can occur less frequently and eventually every 1 to 2 months. The target trough therapeutic concentration of cyclosporine during the first 2 months is 150 to 400 ng/mL with the monoclonal whole blood TDx assay. About 1 to 6 months after transplantation, the cyclosporine trough concentration target is lowered to 150 to 250 ng/mL. After 6 months, the targeted cyclosporine trough concentration is lowered even further to 50 to 150 ng/mL. These ranges may differ among institutions and also depend on the transplant type, time after transplantation, and other agents used. For example, lung and heart transplant recipients may require higher trough concentrations than kidney and liver transplant recipients. The range is reduced over time, given that less immunosuppression is required after transplantation and that the pharmacokinetics change over time.[258]

A number of assay methods are used to measure cyclosporine concentrations, and most institutions use the method that is most familiar to their transplant physicians. The type of cyclosporine assay used by a particular institution significantly influences interpretation of results because there are significant differences between methodologies. These issues have contributed to the debate on the value of monitoring cyclosporine concentrations. The pharmacologic effects of cyclosporine metabolites and whether the concentrations of these metabolites should be monitored individually, or in combination with cyclosporine, also needs to be determined.[259]

Assays currently in use include HPLC; radioimmunoassay with polyclonal or monoclonal antibodies; EMIT, and fluorescence polarization immunoassay. Cyclosporine concentrations can be measured in either whole blood or plasma, but plasma cyclosporine levels can differ by as much as 50% if the plasma temperature is 21°C or 37°C; whole blood cyclosporine concentrations are recommended. The most commonly used assay is the whole blood monoclonal TDx.[259]

No assay appears to be superior in its ability to correlate cyclosporine trough levels with clinical events. Although many studies have attempted to correlate the clinical events of acute rejection or nephrotoxicity to trough concentrations of cyclosporine in recipients of solid organ transplants, results from these studies are conflicting. It may be that the ability to correlate a single blood level during the course of a day with a clinical event that takes place over a longer time period is influenced by too many other variables (e.g., other immunosuppressives, time since transplant, dosage regimen, route, transplant type, assay method, sample matrix, donor-recipient interaction). Nevertheless, most transplant programs, if not all, use cyclosporine concentrations to guide therapy decisions.

Because of the limitations of using a single cyclosporine level and poor correlation between AUC and trough concentration, some programs use a more intensive sampling procedure (e.g., 6 to 10 samples collected over 12 to 24 hours) when cyclosporine concentrations are expected to be at steady state. The AUC and average steady-state concentrations are calculated and used to guide cyclosporine dosage adjustments. A more limited sampling strategy involving one to three samples (1 to 4 hours after a dose at steady state) collected over a dosing interval has also been advocated.[260] The more sophisticated pharmacokinetic monitoring programs have developed better correlations between the AUC and

dose, or AUC and rejection, than correlations based on cyclosporine trough levels only. A number of studies have advocated the use of what is known as C2 monitoring of cyclosporine levels. This level is obtained 2 hours after the Neoral dose. In studies conducted in kidney and liver transplant recipients, there is a much better correlation with AUC 0-4 hour, used as surrogate marker for AUC 0-12 hour, with Neoral compared with any other time point, including a C0 or trough levels. These studies indicate that C2 levels were a more sensitive predictor of acute rejection and toxicity than C0 or trough values.[261] However, the limitation to this approach requires training and re-education of staff and patients, potentially more personnel, modification of procedures, and a narrower window for timing of dose and sampling this 2-hour level (+/-15 minutes). Also, the concentrations ranges would be higher and different for kidney and liver transplant recipients with this approach.[262] Extrapolation to other populations, such as children, African Americans, and patients with cystic fibrosis or diabetes will require further study.

As in all cases, pharmacokinetic data must be interpreted in conjunction with the patient's clinical condition. In addition, deference always must be given to trends established by multiple cyclosporine levels over that of a single level. Single levels may be erroneous because of variability in dose administration, incorrect sampling techniques (e.g., not being obtained at the correct time if drawn from an IV catheter in which IV cyclosporine had been infused), or assay error.

Sirolimus

49. Unfortunately, B.B. developed GI intolerance to MMF and cannot take it anymore. A decision is made to use sirolimus instead. Describe the pharmacokinetic characteristics of sirolimus. What would be the appropriate regimen and monitoring parameters for this agent?

Pharmacokinetics

Pharmacokinetic data are derived primarily from kidney transplant recipients. Sirolimus, like cyclosporine and tacrolimus, exhibits significant pharmacokinetic variability. It is rapidly absorbed after oral administration of the liquid with a median time to maximum concentration (T_{max}) of about 1 hour. It has an apparent average bioavailability of 15%. C_{max} and AUC are linear over a wide range of doses. It is extensively distributed, with a mean apparent volume of distribution of 12 L/kg. It distributes primarily into red blood cells and is highly plasma protein bound, approximately 92%. It also binds to lipoproteins. Sirolimus is extensively metabolized in the gut and liver by CYP 3A4 isoenzymes, and it is a substrate for P-glycoprotein. Its drug interaction profile is very similar to that of cyclosporine and tacrolimus. Renal elimination accounts for only 2% of a dose. The terminal half-life generally ranges from 57 to 63 hours; the time to reach steady state occurs in 10 to 14 days. In children, it can be shorter.[263]

Dosing

Sirolimus can be used in the early transplantation period, although reports of impaired wound healing in kidney transplantations, hepatic artery thrombosis after liver transplantations and bronchial anastamotic dehiscence in lung transplants during this time period have required reconsideration of its use. In the case of liver or lung transplantations, its use is contraindicated in the early post-transplantation period. Sirolimus can be added later, as is the practice in many centers, as replacement for or minimization of cyclosporine, tacrolimus, steroids or mycophenolate doses.[264] An initial loading dose is given followed by a once-daily maintenance dose. The starting maintenance dose range is 2 to 5 mg. The typical loading dose is 6 mg followed by 2 mg every day. In high-risk patients, such as African-Americans, a 15-mg loading dose and 5-mg daily dose is recommended along with cyclosporine. Other centers have used loading doses of 10 to 15 mg, followed by 5 to 10 mg per day for the first week with target levels of 10 to 15 ng/mL for the first month, and 5 to 10 ng/mL thereafter when used with tacrolimus.[265] Sirolimus is often given 4 hours after the morning dose of cyclosporine. If administered at the same time, sirolimus concentrations were, on average, 40% higher, than cyclosporine concentrations.[247]

Adverse Effects

Like other immunosuppressives, sirolimus is associated with a number of side effects, including oral ulcerations, diarrhea, arthralgias, epistaxis, rash, acne, leukopenia, thrombocytopenia, nausea and vomiting, lymphocele, hypokalemia, anemia, hypertension, and infection. The most concerning side effects are dose-related hypertriglyceridemia and hypercholesterolemia. This occurs within the first few weeks of therapy and is significant enough to require intervention with lipid-lowering agents, although it will respond to dosage reduction to some degree.[264]

Therapeutic Drug Monitoring

Monitoring of blood concentrations plays an important role in the dosing of sirolimus. Trough concentrations are obtained and correlate well with sirolimus AUC. Because it has a longer $T_{1/2}$ than the CNIs, concentrations are obtained less frequently and only 5 to 7 days after a dose change. The target concentration range appears to be between 5 and 15 ng/mL. However, this continues to be refined with more experience. Early studies often achieved concentrations >15 ng/mL, especially if used without a CNI, and were associated with a higher degree of immunsuppression and adverse events.[59] Because sirolimus appears to work synergistically with the CNIs, their target concentrations are reduced as well when these agents are used together. Target tacrolimus trough targets are 5 to 10 ng/mL, and the cyclosporine trough targets are 75 to 100 ng/mL.[266]

B.B. could be started on sirolimus at a loading dose of 6 mg, followed by 2 mg QD. Sirolimus blood trough concentration should be obtained 5 to 7 days after initiation. B.B.'s tacrolimus may need to be reduced if concentrations exceed 10 ng/mL. Monitoring parameters should include a fasting lipid panel, CBC, chemistries, and electrolytes.

Infection Prophylaxis

50. S.C. is a 20-year-old man who underwent liver transplantation for end-stage liver disease secondary to chronic hepatitis B. Besides his immunosuppressives, he received ampicillin/sulbactam 1.5 g Q 8 hr for 24 hours perioperatively. After transplantation, he also was started on TMP-SMX 1 tablet Mondays, Wednesdays, and Fridays; nystatin 5 mL TID; lamivudine 100 mg QD; and valganciclovir 900 mg PO QD. Hepatitis B im-

munoglobulin (HBIG) 10,000 units was started intraoperatively and given every day for 8 days after transplantation. What is the rationale for all the aforementioned agents? Should other measures be considered to prevent infection?

Infection continues to be a major source of morbidity and mortality. Transplantation patients have the same risk of infection from transplant surgery as any other immunocompromised patient undergoing a surgical procedure. The percentage of transplantation patients who develop infections has decreased since the advent of cyclosporine. However, infection rates remain high—50% in transplant recipients.[267]

Prophylactic antimicrobial therapy can decrease the risk of surgical infections in patients undergoing transplantation surgery. As with other therapies in transplantation, prophylactic regimens and antibiotic therapies are highly institution dependent.[268] Kidney transplant recipients typically receive a first-generation cephalosporin, such as cefazolin, to cover uropathogens and staphylococci both perioperatively and, in some cases, for 2 to 5 days postoperatively. Pancreas transplant recipients usually receive an antibiotic that covers both the skin flora and GI flora, such as ampicillin/sulbactam (Unasyn), because both are breached during the surgical procedure. In addition, because *Candida* is often within the GI flora and because post–pancreas transplantation candidal infections occur frequently, prophylaxis with an antifungal such as fluconazole for 3 to 7 days is commonly used. Liver transplantations are associated with the highest rate of life-threatening bacterial infection. Ampicillin/sulbactam (Unasyn) commonly is used to cover staphylococci, enterococci, and *Enterobacteriaceae*. Heart transplant recipients routinely receive a first-generation cephalosporin, such as cefazolin, at anesthesia induction and for 48 hours postoperatively. Cefuroxime or vancomycin are alternatives for resistant organisms. For lung transplant candidates, common practice is to culture the patient's sputum before transplantation, individualize the prophylactic regimen to reflect the resident flora, and include an antipseudomonal drug. Duration of therapy in these patients is individualized, based on the patient's postoperative recovery, but usually lasts 7 to 14 days.

Selective bowel decontamination regimens with nonabsorbable antibacterial agents have been used in liver transplant recipients who are susceptible to a high incidence of bacterial infections, although this practice is controversial. The goal of selective bowel decontamination regimens is to eradicate the aerobic gram-negative flora from the bowel while leaving the anaerobic bowel flora intact to prevent colonization resistance. Various regimens have been used, but they typically include polymyxin E 100 mg or colistin, gentamicin 80 mg, and nystatin 2 million U/10 mL orally four times a day. Some centers incorporate quinolones into the regimen instead of gentamicin. A low-bacterial diet (excluding raw fruit, raw vegetables, cheese, and foods that are reheated or stored at room temperature for long periods) is often instituted. Nystatin or fluconazole are also used to decrease *Candida* colonization.[269]

Infections can occur at any time after transplantation, but there are predictable time patterns for certain kinds of infections.[267] The time of highest risk for infection in a transplant recipient is during the first 6 months, because they are receiving the highest doses of immunosuppressive agents during this period. Another time of high risk is during and after treatment of acute rejection with high-dose immunosuppression. Patients can acquire new infections (*Pneumocystis carinii* pneumonia [PCP], CMV), reactivate old infections (e.g., CMV, BK virus), or develop recurrence of underlying disease (hepatitis B or C). Opportunistic infections are common during this time, as shown in Table 35-3. Because the infections shown in Table 35-3 occur at such a high rate, it is routine to provide specific prophylaxis for many of them. For example, nystatin suspension 500,000 units by "swish and swallow" (S&S) three to four times a day or fluconazole 100 mg every day are used to reduce fungal colonization of the GI tract; acyclovir, ganciclovir, valganciclovir, and/or immunoglobulins are used for CMV and herpes virus infections; and TMP-SMX is used for *Pneumocystis* prophylaxis. For patients with sulfa allergies, alternatives, such as dapsone 50 to 100 mg PO QD or inhaled monthly doses of pentamidine 300 mg, are used. These generally are given for the first 3 to 6 months after transplantation and in some cases up to 1 year or even for life.[270] In S.C., there is certainly a need to receive prophylaxis with TMP-SMX, valganciclovir, HBIG, and lamivudine or adefovir.

Hepatitis B

Another major concern for S.C. would be recurrence of hepatitis B in his new liver. Hepatitis B recurs and is associated with a poorer outcome.[271] Strategies that have been effective are the use of lamivudine or adefovir preoperatively and HBIG and lamivudine or adefovir postoperatively.[272-275] S.C. was started on lamivudine and HBIG postoperatively because monotherapy with HBIG is associated with recurrence in 10% to 50% patients, whereas HBIG with lamivudine has been associated with development of resistance in 15% to 30% per year. In patients who develop a resistant form of hepatitis B to lamivudine, adefovir has been shown to be effective.[275] The combination of an antiviral with HBIG is currently preferred. After the first week of HBIG, S.C. will continue to receive 10,000 units IV as a 1- to 2-hour infusion weekly for 4 weeks, then 10,000 units monthly for the first 6 to 12 months after transplantation. During this time, anti-HBs titers are monitored and kept >500

IU/L. Because HBIG is incredibly expensive to give in this regimen (up to $50,000 per patient per year), some transplantation centers now use lower titers (>100 IU/L) and HBIG doses of 1,500 units IM every 3 to 4 weeks with lamivudine.[273]

Hepatitis C

Another virus that is major cause for concern is hepatitis C. Hepatitis C is currently the most common reason for liver transplantation, and recurrence of hepatitis C viral replication after transplantation is universal.[276] Immunosuppression, especially overimmunosuppression can have a significant detrimental effect on this disease after transplantation. Recent epidemiologic studies indicate that patient survival rates may be significantly lower at 5 years after transplant compared with patients who received liver transplants for non–hepatitis C causes.[277] Because of this, antivirals that have been shown to be effective in the pretransplant treatment of patients with chronic hepatitis C such as ribavirin, interferon, and pegylated interferon, are currently being investigated in post-transplantation patients.[278,279]

To date, no large controlled trials have been published, but some smaller noncontrolled trials have shown the effectiveness of interferon with or without ribavirin in reducing hepatitis C viral loads and preventing histologically proven liver damage. Unfortunately, there are no standards on how or when to initiate these regimens. In addition, these agents are associated with a large number of adverse drug reactions, including flu-like symptoms, leukopenia, thrombocytopenia, depression in the case of interferon, and hemolytic anemia in the case of ribaviron. The incidence and severity of these adverse effects are augmented after transplantation because of the concomitant use of immunosuppressives. Therefore, some clinicians advocate using these therapies only when the patient demonstrates evidence of liver damage caused by the reactivation of the hepatitis C virus, whereas others believe that therapy should be given to all patients with hepatitis C who receive a liver transplant. In all cases, these patients should be closely monitored for signs and symptoms of viral reactivation. If this does occur, a liver biopsy may be warranted to determine the severity of liver damage caused by the virus. In aggressive cases, the need for antiviral therapy and reduction in immunosuppression may be warranted.

Immunization

Another important element of S.C.'s care is the need for immunization. Although immunosuppression may blunt the response to some immunizations, the benefits outweigh the risks. Once he is out at least 6 months after transplantation, he should receive a yearly flu vaccine. He also should receive the pneumococcal and hepatitis A vaccines if he has not done so yet; live vaccines should be avoided.[280]

Treatment of infection in transplantation patients should be based on principles established for other immunocompromised patients (see Chapter 68, Prevention and Treatment of Infections in Neutropenic Cancer Patients). One major difference between transplant recipients and other immunocompromised hosts is the fact that the immunocompromised condition of transplant recipients is iatrogenic, secondary to their immunosuppression. Therefore, when a transplant recipient develops a life-threatening infection, the doses of immuno-

Table 35-3   Common Opportunistic Infections After Transplantation

Organisms	Time of Onset After Transplantation
CMV	1–6 mo
HSV	2 wk–2 mo
EBV	2–6 mo
VZV	2–6 mo
Fungal	1–6 mo
Mycobacterium	1–6 mo
PCP	1–6 mo
Listeria	1 mo–indefinitely
Aspergillus	1–4 mo
Nocardia	1–4 mo
Toxoplasma	1–4 mo
Cryptococcus	4 mo–indefinitely

CMV, cytomegalovirus; EBV, Epstein-Barr virus; HSV, herpes simplex virus; PCP, *Pneumocystis carinii* pneumonia; VZV, varicella-zoster virus.

suppressants are usually decreased or in some cases discontinued. After the patient has recovered from the infection, immunosuppression can be restored to preinfection levels.

Cytomegalovirus

51. A.A. is a 58-year-old, 76-kg man with end-stage liver disease due to alcoholic cirrhosis who received an orthotopic liver transplant 16 weeks ago. He presents to the transplantation clinic with a 3-day history of generalized malaise, fatigue, nausea, vomiting, diarrhea, fever, and anorexia. At the time of transplantation, the liver he received was positive for CMV, but he had negative CMV serology. His postoperative immunosuppressant regimen included oral prednisone and tacrolimus 5 mg PO BID, with adjustments made to his dose to maintain a 12-hour trough concentration between 10 and 15 ng/mL. He was also given valganciclovir 450 mg PO QD for 3 months.

His postoperative course was complicated by an acute rejection episode on postoperative day 8, which was treated successfully with a pulse and taper of steroids. At that time, MMF 1 g PO BID was added to his immunosuppressant regimen. He was discharged from the hospital on postoperative day 12, with instructions to return to the transplant clinic in 4 days. Since then, he has done fairly well with no complaints until now, 4 months later. On admission to the hospital, a physical examination was remarkable for an oral temperature of 38.8°C, a BP of 112/79 mm Hg, a heart rate of 104 beats/min, a respiratory rate of 22 breaths/min, and a mild tremor. All other findings on his examination were benign. Pertinent laboratory findings include the following: WBC count, 3,400 cells/mm³ (normal, 4,000 to 10,000); platelet count, 34,000 cells/mm³ (normal, 150,000 to 450,000); BUN, 29 mg/dL (normal, 5 to 22); SrCr, 1.4 mg/dL (normal, 0.6 to 1.1); total bilirubin, 2.2 mg/dL (normal, 0.0 to 1.2); AST, 62 U/L (normal, 14 to 38); ALT, 126 U/L (normal, 15 to 48); CMV antigen, 500/100,000 positive cells (normal, 0/100,000); and 12-hour tacrolimus concentration, 18.3 ng/dL (normal, 5 to 15). His current medications include tacrolimus 6 mg PO BID; prednisone 10 mg PO QD; TMP-SMX 80 mg PO Mondays, Wednesdays, and Fridays; calcium carbonate 1.25 g PO TID; vitamin D 800 IU PO QD; enteric-coated aspirin 325 mg PO QD; and nizatidine 150 mg PO BID. What is the most likely diagnosis for A.A.?

A major concern in A.A. at this time after transplantation is CMV infection, an infection that is commonly encountered within 1 to 6 months after both solid organ and bone marrow transplantation. It is a ubiquitous virus belonging to the herpes virus group. In healthy immunocompetent adults, infection with the virus is usually asymptomatic; whereas in immunocompromised patients, CMV can cause significant morbidity and mortality. CMV can potentiate the risk for developing both bacterial and fungal infections and induce chronic injury to the transplanted organ (arteriosclerosis in the heart, obliterative bronchiolitis in the lungs, vanishing bile duct syndrome in the liver, and chronic arteriopathy in the kidneys).[281]

Etiology
CMV infection in transplant recipients usually occurs when latent viruses from a seropositive donor organ are reactivated owing to immunosuppression. Transmission of CMV from a positive donor to a negative recipient leads to an 80% to 100% infection rate and a 40% to 50% disease rate; a positive donor

to a positive recipient leads to a 40% to 60% reactivation rate and a 20% to 30% disease rate; a negative donor to a negative recipient leads to a 0% to 5% infection rate. Transplant recipients at highest risk for developing the disease are (1) those who are or have serologically donor +/recipient – (D+/R–) at the time of transplant, (2) elderly, (3) those who received large amounts of perioperative blood transfusions, (4) those who received antilymphocyte antibodies, (5) those who received a retransplantation because of acute rejection, and (6) those who received larger amounts of immunosuppressive agents.[281] A.A. is at high risk because of his CMV serology is D+/–R–.

Diagnosis
Diagnosis of CMV is based on both clinical and laboratory findings. Serologic diagnosis is based on positive seroconversion from a previously seronegative person or a fourfold or more increase in antibody titers in a previously seropositive person. CMV may be detected by culturing body fluids, such as bronchoalveolar lavage, urine, blood buffy coat, and biopsy tissue. CMV is contained within the host's leukocytes, which appear to have large intranuclear inclusion bodies. However, documented viral shedding or positive seroconversion is not diagnostic for active disease without clinical signs and symptoms.[281,282] A.A. certainly has laboratory criteria for the diagnosis of CMV infection: viral shedding, as indicated by the CMV antigenemia of 500 cells, leukopenia, and thrombocytopenia.

Clinical Manifestations
In healthy immunocompetent adults, the CMV-infected patient is usually asymptomatic but may present with mild complaints of malaise, fever, and myalgias, as well as abnormal liver enzymes and lymphocytosis. More severe reactions are rare.[282] However, CMV may be life threatening in the immunocompromised patient and is the most common opportunistic infection associated with solid organ transplantation. There is evidence that CMV infection is associated with graft rejection and that graft rejection in the setting of immunosuppression facilitates CMV infection. It often is unclear which comes first. The actual CMV course may be limited to fever and mononucleosis, or it may extend to organs presenting as pneumonia, hepatitis, gastroenteritis, colitis, disseminated infection, encephalopathy, or leukopenia.

A.A.'s clinical presentation meets the criteria for CMV disease: positive viral shedding with clinical signs and symptoms. At this time, it is unclear whether or not A.A. has any end-organ involvement. Certainly, the fact that his liver enzyme concentrations are elevated and he is having numerous GI symptoms may be indicative of CMV hepatitis, CMV gastroenteritis, or CMV colitis, respectively. Alternatively, the increased total bilirubin and serum transaminases may be due to acute rejection, and his GI problems may be a side effect he is experiencing from his medications (e.g., MMF). To fully differentiate among CMV hepatitis, CMV gastroenteritis, CMV colitis, acute rejection, and medication side effects, tissue biopsies should be obtained.

Treatment
52. What are the treatment options for A.A.'s diagnosed CMV disease? What doses should be used, and how should the effects of these drugs be monitored?

GANCICLOVIR

Before ganciclovir was available, CMV infection was "treated" by reducing the level of immunosuppression. This may be one of the explanations for an increased prevalence of rejection associated with CMV infections. Graft loss in kidney or pancreas recipients is undesirable; yet, it is not immediately life threatening. However, reducing immunosuppression in liver, heart, or lung transplant recipients could result in patient death due to graft loss. Treatment has been attempted in the past with acyclovir, adenine-arabinoside, and immune globulin, but all these have been largely unsuccessful. At present, ganciclovir is the first-line agent used for the treatment of CMV disease in solid organ transplant recipients, bone marrow transplant recipients, and AIDS patients. Although ganciclovir is highly efficacious in this regard, there is still a 20% potential relapse rate of CMV after ganciclovir therapy in liver transplant recipients.

Ganciclovir, a virustatic agent, is a nucleoside analog that is phosphorylated in infected cells to its active form and is then incorporated into replicating viral DNA. Although ganciclovir-resistant strains of CMV have been isolated, their occurrence is far more common in HIV patients; currently, ganciclovir-resistant CMV in solid organ transplantation is not a large concern.[283] A.A. should receive ganciclovir intravenously; oral ganciclovir should not be used because its bioavailability is <10%. However, because relapses of CMV disease after IV ganciclovir are still a concern, some suggest that patients should be placed on maintenance therapy with either oral ganciclovir, valganciclovir, or oral acyclovir after the IV course is completed.[283,284]

Dosing

The usual dose of ganciclovir in patients with normal renal function is 5 mg/kg per dose every 12 hours for 14 to 21 days. Dosage adjustment is necessary for patients with renal dysfunction: 2.5 mg/kg per dose every 12 hours for creatinine clearances 50 to 79 mL/minute, 2.5 mg/kg per dose every 24 hours for creatinine clearances 25 to 49 mL/minute, 1.25 mg/kg per dose every 24 hours for creatinine clearances <25 mL/minute. Because A.A. has an estimated creatinine clearance of 60 mL/minute, he should receive 2.5 mg/kg per dose (190 mg) IV every 12 hours for 2 to 3 weeks, followed by either low-dose IV ganciclovir (2.5 mg/kg every day), valganciclovir, or oral ganciclovir for 2 to 4 weeks.

The most common adverse effect associated with ganciclovir therapy is neutropenia, which is seen in up to 27% of patients being treated with this drug.[283] Neutropenia is defined as an absolute neutrophil count of <500 to 1,000 cells/mm³. The neutropenia usually resolves with a decrease in dosage or discontinuation of the drug, but colony-stimulating factors may help correct it.[285] Because CMV disease has a propensity to cause neutropenia as well, it is often difficult to distinguish the cause. If laboratory findings and clinical signs and symptoms of CMV disease are resolving and the patient remains neutropenic, the most likely cause is ganciclovir. Thrombocytopenia occurs in approximately 20% of ganciclovir recipients. Patients with initial platelet counts <100,000/mm³ appear to be at greatest risk. Other adverse effects include CNS effects, fever, rash, and abnormal liver function tests.[283] A.A.'s WBC and platelet counts should be assessed every 3 to 4 days during therapy, and ganciclovir should be held if neutrophils fall to <500/mm³ or platelets fall to <25,000/mm³. To monitor either the regression or progression of A.A.'s CMV disease, a weekly CMV antigen test should be obtained.

IMMUNE GLOBULINS

The use of immunoglobulins to manage CMV disease in solid organ transplantation is controversial. Immunoglobulins provide passive immunization by potentiating an antibody-dependent cell-mediated cytotoxic reaction. Basically, the immunoglobulins modify the immunologic response that damages host tissue. There is some evidence that immunoglobulins may have synergistic or additive effects with current antiviral drugs in the treatment of CMV disease.[286] Both unselective immunoglobulins and CMV hyperimmune globulin have been studied in combination with ganciclovir. CMV hyperimmune globulin is prepared from high-titer pooled sera that have a fourfold to eightfold enrichment of CMV titers compared with unscreened immunoglobulin.

Most of the literature involving combination therapy for CMV disease is in bone marrow transplant recipients. Initial response rates appear to favor the combination therapy in this group. In solid organ transplantation, the data are scarce. Most of the literature is in the form of case reports or small retrospective studies. However, it appears that the combination of CMV immunoglobulin and ganciclovir may be more efficacious than ganciclovir alone in severe CMV disease (e.g., hepatitis, pneumonitis).[286] Although it is controversial, many clinicians would use combination therapy in patients with severe disease, as indicated by end-organ involvement, or in those who are refractory to monotherapy with ganciclovir.

CMV immunoglobulin may be given as 100 mg/kg per dose every other day for 14 days. This is the dose recommended for treatment of CMV when used in combination with ganciclovir. The most common adverse effects associated with the administration of immunoglobulins appear to be infusion related and include fever, chills, headache, myalgia, light-headedness, and nausea and vomiting.

FOSCARNET

Foscarnet is a virustatic pyrophosphate analog that inhibits DNA synthesis, but unlike ganciclovir, no phosphorylation is required for activation. Because this drug has a high nephrotoxicity propensity and because most transplant recipients are already receiving drugs that are nephrotoxic, experience with the use of foscarnet in solid organ transplantation is limited. In most centers, foscarnet is a second- or third-line agent to be used only if intolerance or resistance develops with ganciclovir therapy.

The usual dosage of foscarnet is 60 mg/kg per dose every 8 hours for 14 to 21 days. The dosage should be adjusted downward in patients with renal dysfunction. The most serious adverse effect with foscarnet is nephrotoxicity, which occurs in up to 50% of patients and is probably induced by acute tubular necrosis. Therefore, prehydration is suggested to help minimize or avoid nephrotoxicity. GI effects, a decrease in hemoglobin and hematocrit, an increase in liver function tests, and alteration of serum electrolyte concentrations are other side effects of foscarnet. All these appear to be reversible upon discontinuation of the drug. SrCr should be monitored daily during therapy.[282]

Prophylaxis

53. Is there any way to prevent CMV in high-risk patients, such as A.A.?

Because of its significant consequences, efforts should be made to prevent CMV disease in the transplantation population. One way to prevent primary CMV infections is to use seronegative donor and seronegative blood products, which should greatly reduce the risk. Unfortunately, this solution is difficult if not impossible to implement because the availability of donor organs is insufficient. Therefore, CMV status is not considered in the donor-matching process. A large number of studies have tried to ascertain the easiest, most cost-effective regimen to prevent CMV disease. These studies have focused on the combined use of different agents as well as IV followed by oral therapies. Trials have also targeted high-risk patients.[283,286–292]

GANCICLOVIR

The use of both the IV and oral formulations of ganciclovir to prevent CMV disease has been studied in lung, heart, liver, kidney, and pancreas transplant recipients.[281] However, there are very few relatively large trials and most of the data in the solid organ transplantation population are from small uncontrolled trials. Another difficulty lies in the fact that there are large discrepancies between the trials with regard to the terminology used to define prophylaxis and high-risk patients. However, until the recent introduction of valganciclovir, ganciclovir has been the most widely used prophylactic agent.

Both oral and IV ganciclovir have been studied in lung transplant recipients to prevent CMV disease.[281,287] Although these studies had very small numbers of subjects, it does appear that both formulations can prevent CMV disease when used in the first 90 days after transplantation. The populations targeted in these trials were patients who were considered at risk for the development of CMV disease because of their serologic status or because antilymphocyte antibodies had been used as induction therapy. Unfortunately, long-term follow-up in these patients revealed no difference in CMV disease rates when compared with placebo. This may indicate that although ganciclovir therapy is effective in delaying CMV early in the post-transplantation period, it does not prevent the disease.

Studies using prophylactic IV ganciclovir in heart transplantation have found it to be both effective and ineffective as prophylaxis. Oral ganciclovir has been compared with other drug combinations and shown to be more effective.[288,289] Studies conducted in heart transplantation focused on patients at high risk for developing CMV disease. Most patients received antilymphocyte antibody induction therapy and were in the serologic high-risk groups as well (D+/R–, D+/R+, or D–/R+).[288,289]

The prophylactic use of ganciclovir in liver transplantation patients has been evaluated as well. Trials have shown that oral ganciclovir, given for an average of 3 to 4 months after transplantation, significantly decreases the rates of CMV disease in this population. In addition, comparative trials have concluded that oral ganciclovir is more effective than oral acyclovir. Ganciclovir prophylaxis seems most effective when used in D+/R– patients.[290,291]

When ganciclovir prophylaxis, either oral or IV, is used in high-risk renal transplant recipients, it appears to reduce the incidence of CMV disease.[291,292] As in the liver transplantation population, ganciclovir is superior to oral acyclovir. In most studies, prophylaxis is continued for approximately 12 weeks after transplantation. However, as seen in A.A., CMV can occur once prophylaxis is discontinued.

VALGANCICLOVIR

Valganciclovir was developed because oral ganciclovir has a very low bioavailability (<10%). Valganciclovir is the L-valyl ester of ganciclovir, which is a prodrug that is rapidly and completely converted into ganciclovir by hepatic and intestinal esterases once absorbed across the GI tract. The absolute bioavailability of valganciclovir is approximately 60%, so that a 900-mg single dose given with food has the equivalent AUC to a 5 mg/kg IV dose of ganciclovir. This is roughly twice the AUC achieved by 1,000 mg of ganciclovir given orally TID.[293] Although valganciclovir is currently only FDA approved for the treatment of HIV-associated CMV retinitis,[294,295] it has been studied and proved to be equally effective to oral ganciclovir in preventing CMV disease in solid organ transplant recipients.[296] Currently, there are no studies examining the agent's efficacy in treating established CMV disease; however, because of its similar pharmacokinetic profile with IV ganciclovir, there will likely be studies in this area in the near future.

Similar to ganciclovir, valganciclovir is predominantly eliminated from the body through the kidney, and dosage adjustment is required in renal impairment. The incidence of adverse drug reactions is similar to IV ganciclovir and include headache, neutropenia, nausea, diarrhea, and anemia. The incidence of neutropenia is significantly higher than oral ganciclovir, and dosage reduction or temporary withdrawal of the agent is recommended in patients with an ANC less than 1,000 cells/mm^3.[293–295]

ACYCLOVIR

Acyclovir is ineffective in the treatment of established CMV disease, but it does appear to have a beneficial preventive role. Since the introduction of oral ganciclovir, several trials have compared the prophylactic efficacy of high-dose acyclovir with oral ganciclovir.[291,292] As already noted, oral ganciclovir appears to be more effective in preventing CMV disease, especially in the D+/R– subgroup. Because of this, most consider oral acyclovir to be second-line therapy to IV or oral ganciclovir or valganciclovir as a CMV prophylactic agent.

CMV HYPERIMMUNE GLOBULIN

The role of this agent in preventing CMV disease is controversial. Many studies have combined this agent with either oral acyclovir or ganciclovir, but because of its cost and IV route, its use as a prophylactic agent has decreased. In addition, in patients who are D+/R–, results have been mixed.[281,297]

VALACYCLOVIR

One recent published meta-analysis of 12 trials that included 1,574 patients evaluated valacyclovir as a prophylactic agent in transplant patients.[298] Valacyclovir was found to be more effective than acyclovir in preventing herpes viruses, including CMV. However, most transplantation centers do not use valacyclovir for routine prophylaxis of CMV.

54. Should A.A. have received prophylactic therapy and, if so, which agent should be used?

A.A. has several risk factors that predispose him to developing CMV disease. At the time of transplantation, A.A. was CMV D+/R−, which means that he has about an 80% chance of developing CMV infection and a 40% chance of developing CMV disease. In addition, A.A. had an early acute rejection episode, which means he received higher doses of immunosuppression, which also puts him at higher risk for developing CMV disease. Because of these risk factors, A.A. should have and did receive CMV prophylaxis for at least 3 months after transplantation. Immediately postoperatively, IV ganciclovir, at a dose of 5 mg/kg every day, should be used. Once A.A. is tolerating oral medications, he can be switched to valganciclovir at a dose of 900 mg PO QD with food. Because A.A. has renal insufficiency, his valganciclovir dose was adjusted to 450 mg PO QD.[295] As illustrated by A.A.'s case, the fact that a patient has received prophylactic therapy does not preclude the possibility that this person will develop CMV disease after the prophylaxis is withdrawn or, in rare instances, during prophylactic therapy. The incidence of developing CMV disease while receiving valganciclovir is significantly lower when compared with oral ganciclovir, probably because drug exposure is roughly two times higher.[294,296]

PRE-EMPTIVE THERAPY

Because of the recent advances in the laboratory tests used to identify and quantify CMV and because prophylactic therapy is not always effective and is very expensive, pre-emptive therapy has been used in an attempt to prevent CMV disease. The technique involves withholding prophylactic therapy and monitoring laboratory tests to identify presymptomatic CMV viremia. Based on one study, the CMV antigen is the best predictor of clinical CMV disease compared with PCR, serology, and shell vial assay.[299] Once a patient develops viremia, he or she usually receives treatment with IV ganciclovir or PO valganciclovir. Although several studies have acknowledged the benefit of this strategy, the lack of uniformity among them does not allow for generalizable recommendations.[300,301]

Thus, the questions of when to initiate pre-emptive therapy and who to initiate it in remain unanswered.

REFERENCES

1. United Network for Organ Sharing (UNOS) Web site. www.unos.org. January 2003.
2. Valent JF et al. Immunobiology of renal transplantation. Surg Clin North Am 1998;78:1.
3. Halloran PF et al. In vivo immunosuppressive mechanisms. J Heart Lung Transplant 1996;15:959.
4. Gudmundsdottir H et al. T cell blockade: new therapies for transplant rejection. J Am Soc Nephrol 1999;10:1356.
5. Katznelson S et al. Histocompatibility testing, crossmatching, and allocation of cadaveric kidney transplants. In: Danovitch DM, ed. Handbook of Kidney Transplantation, 3rd Ed. Lippincott Williams & Wilkins, 2001.
6. Shishido S. ABO-incompatible kidney transplantation in children. Graft 2002;8:430.
7. Lennard L. The clinical pharmacology of 6-mercaptopurine. Eur J Clin Pharmacol 1992;43:329.
8. Chan GLC et al. Azathioprine metabolism pharmacokinetics of 6-mercaptopurine, 6-thiouric acid and 6-thioguanine nucleotides in renal transplant patients. J Clin Pharmacol 1990;30:358.
9. Soria-Royer C et al. Thiopurine-methyl-transferase activity to assess azathioprine myelotoxicity in renal transplant recipients. Lancet 1993; 19.341(8860):1593.
10. Romagnuolo J et al. Cholestatic hepatocellular injury with azathioprine: a case report and review of the mechanisms of hepatotoxicity. Can J Gastroenterol 1998;12:479.
11. Sievers TM et al. Mycophenolate Mofetil. Pharmacotherapy 1997;17:1178.
12. Allison AC. Mechanism of action of MPA. Ann NY Acad Sci 1993;696:63.
13. Bullingham RES et al. Clinical pharmacokinetics of mycophenolate mofetil. Clin Pharmacokinet 1998;34:429.
14. Hricik DE et al. Trends in the use of glucocorticoids in renal transplantation. Transplantation 1994;57:979.
15. Almawi WY et al. An alternate mechanism of glucocorticoid anti-proliferative effect: promotion of a Th2 cytokine-secreting profile. Clin Transplant 1999;13:365.
16. Frey BM et al. Clinical pharmacokinetics of prednisone and prednisolone. Clin Pharmacokinet 1990;19:126.
17. Jeng S et al. Prednisone metabolism in recipients of kidney and liver transplants and in lung recipients receiving ketoconazole. Transplantation 2003;75:792.
18. Faulds D et al. Cyclosporin. A review of its pharmacodynamic and pharmacokinetic properties, and therapeutic use in immunoregulatory disorders. Drugs 1993;45(6):953.
19. Plosker GL et al. Tacrolimus. A further update of its pharmacology and therapeutic use in the management of organ transplantation. Drugs 2000;59:323.
20. Kahan BD et al. Rapamycin: clinical effects and future opportunities. Transplantation 2001;73:1181.
21. Sehgal SN. Rapamune (RAPA, rapamycin, sirolimus): mechanism of action of immunosuppressive effect results from blockade of signal transduction and inhibition of cell cycle progression. Clin Biochem 1998;31:335.
22. Bourdage JS et al. Comparative polyclonal antithymocyte globulin and antilymphocyte/antilymphoblast globulin anti-CD antigen analysis by flow cytometry. Transplantation 1995;59:1194.
23. Bonnefoy-Berard N et al. Mechanisms of immunosuppression induced by antithymocyte globulins and OKT3. J Heart Lung Transplant 1996; 15:435.
24. Michallet MC et al. Functional antibodies to leukocyte adhesion molecules in antithymocyte globulins. Transplantation 2003;75:75.
25. Ormrod D et al. Antithymocyte globulin (rabbit). A review of the use of thymoglobulin in the prevention and treatment of acute renal allograft rejection. BioDrugs 2000;14:255.
26. ten Berge UM et al. Guidelines for the optimal use of muromonab CD3 in transplantation. Biodrugs 1999;11:277.
27. Berard JL et al. A review of Interleuken-2 receptor antagonists in solid organ transplantation. Pharmacotherapy 1999;19:1127.
28. Dwomoa A et al. Interleukin-2 receptor monoclonal antibodies in renal transplantation: meta-analysis of randomized trials. Br Med J 2003;326:789.
29. Kovarik J et al. Disposition of and immunodynamics of basiliximab in liver allograft recipients. Clin Pharmacol Ther 1998;64:66.
30. Murphy B et al. HLA-derived peptides as novel immunomodulatory therapeutics. J Am Soc Nephrol 1999;10:1346.
31. Vincenti F. What's in the pipeline? New immunosuppressive drugs in transplantation. Am J Transplant 2002;2:898.
32. Kasike BL et al. The evaluation of renal transplant candidates: clinical practice guidelines. Am J Transplant 2001;1:1.
33. Hariharan S. Improved graft survival after renal transplantation in the United States. 1988 to 1996. N Engl J Med 2000;346:605.
34. Young C et al. Renal transplantation in black Americans. N Engl J Med 2000;343:1545.
35. Ojo AO et al. Delayed graft function: risk factors and implications for renal allograft survival. Transplantation 1997;63:968.
36. Denton MD et al. Immunosuppressive strategies in transplantation. Lancet 1999;353:1083.
37. Lo A et al. Strategies to reduce toxicities and improve outcomes in renal transplant recipients. Pharmacotherapy 2002;22:316.
38. Gaston RS et al. Maintenance immunosuppression in the renal transplant recipient: an overview. Am J Kidney Dis 2001;38(Suppl 6):S25.
39. Amend WJ et al. The first two posttransplantation months. In: Danovitch DM, ed. Handbook of Kidney Transplantation, 3rd Ed. Philadelphia: Lippincott Williams & Wilkins, 2001.
40. Shokes DA et al. Delayed graft function. Influence on outcome and strategies for prevention. Urol Clin North Am 2001;28.
41. Szczech LA et al. The effect of anti-lymphocyte induction therapy on renal allograft survival: a meta-analysis. J Am Soc Nephrol 1997;8:1771.
42. Szczech LA. The effect of antilymphocyte induction therapy on renal allograft survival: a meta-analysis of individual-level data. Ann Intern Med 1998;128:817.
43. Bumgardner GL et al. Daclizumab (humanized anti-IL2R mab) prophylaxis for prevention of acute rejection in renal transplant recipients with delayed graft function. Transplantation 2001;72:642.
44. Gonwa TA et al. Immunosuppression for delayed or slow graft function in primary cadaveric renal transplantation: use of low dose tacrolimus therapy with post-operative administration of anti-CD25 monoclonal antibody. Clin Transplant 2002;16:144.
45. Rao KV. Renal transplantation. Surg Clin North Am 1998;78:1.
46. Racusen LC et al. The Banff 97 working classification of renal allograft pathology. Kidney Int 1999; 55:713.
47. Mauiyyedi S et al. Humoral rejection in kidney transplantation: new concepts in diagnosis and treatment. Curr Opin Nephrol Hypertens 2002; 11:609.
48. Kreis HA et al. Causes of late renal allograft loss: chronic allograft dysfunction, death and other factors. Transplantation 2001:71:SS5.

49. Hallorhan PF et al. Call for revolution: a new approach to describing allograft deterioration. Am J Transplant 2002;2:195.

50. Hricik DE et al. Trends in the use of glucocorticoids in renal transplantation. Transplantation 1994;57:979.

51. Bock HA et al. Steroid-resistant kidney transplant rejection: diagnosis and treatment. J Am Soc Nephrol 2001;12(Suppl 17):548–552.

52. Neylan JF et al. Racial differences in renal transplantation with tacrolimus versus cyclosporine. FK506 kidney transplant study group. Transplant 1998;65:515.

53. Johnson RWG et al. The clinical impact of nephrotoxicity in renal transplantation. Transplantation 2000;69:S14.

54. Campistol JM et al. Mechanisms of nephrotoxicity. Transplantation 2000;69:S5.

55. Fisher NC et al. the clinical impact of nephrotoxicity in liver transplantation. Transplantation 2000;69:S18.

56. Parry G et al. The clinical impact of cyclosporine nephrotoxicity in heart transplantation. Transplantation 2000;69:S23.

57. Lo A et al. Strategies to reduce toxicities and improve outcomes in renal transplant recipients. Pharmacotherapy 2002;22:316.

58. Kreis H et al. Sirolimus in association with mycophenolate mofetil induction for the prevention of acute graft rejection in renal allograft recipients. Transplantation 2000;69:1252.

59. Groth CG et al. Sirolimus(rapamycin)-based therapy in human renal transplantation: similar efficacy and different toxicity compared with cyclosporine. Transplant 1999;67:1036.

60. Vincenti F et al. Multicenter trial exploring calcineurin inhibitors avoidance in renal transplantation. Transplant 2001;71:1282.

61. Tran HT et al. Avoidance of cyclosporine in renal transplantation: effects of daclizumab, mycophenolate and steroids. J Am Soc Nephrol 2000;11:1903.

62. Kasiske BL et al. Cyclosporine withdrawal in renal transplantation. A meta-analysis. J Am Soc Nephrol 2000;11:1910.

63. Johnson RWG et al. Sirolimus allows early cyclosporine withdrawal in renal transplantation resulting in improved renal function and lower blood pressure. Transplant 2001;72:777.

64. Abramowicz D et al. Cyclosporine withdrawal from a mycophenolate mofetil containing immunosuppressive regimen in stable kidney transplant recipients: a randomized, controlled study. Transplantation 2002;74:1725.

65. Danovitch GM. How should the immunosuppressive regimen be managed in patients with established chronic allograft failure. Kid Int Suppl 2002;80:68.

66. Hricik DE et al. Steroid-free imunosuppression in kidney transplantation: editorial review. Am J Transplant 2002;2:19.

67. Citterio F et al. Steroid side effects and their impact on transplant outcome. Transplant 2001;12(Suppl):S75.

68. Cole E et al. A pilot study of steroid-free immunosuppression in the prevention of acute rejection in renal allograft recipients. Transplant 2001;72:845.

69. Birkeland SA. Steroid-free immunosuppression after kidney transplantation with antithymocyte globulin induction and cyclosporine and mycophenolate maintenance therapy. Transplant 1998;66:1207.

70. Sinclair NR et al. Low dose steroid therapy in cyclosporine treated renal transplant recipients with well functioning grafts. CMAJ 1992;147:645.

71. Taylor DO et al. Improved long term survival after heart transplantation predicted by successful early withdrawal from maintenance corticosteroid therapy. J Heart Lung Transplant 1996;15:1039.

72. Raimond ML et al. Single-agent immunosuppression after liver transplantation: what is possible. Drugs 2002;62:1587.

73. Vincenti F et al. Multicenter randomized prospective trial of steroid withdrawal in renal transplant recipients receiving basiliximab, cyclosporine microemulsion and mycophenolate mofetil. Am J Transpl 2003:3:306.

74. Mahalati K et al. An open-labeled pilot study of steroid withdrawal from kidney transplant recipients on sirolimus-cyclosporine combination. Transplant 2001:1(Suppl 1):247.

75. Vanrneterghem Y et al. Double-blind comparison of two corticosteroid regimens plus mycophenolate mofetil and cyclosporine for prevention of acute renal allograft rejection. Transplantation 2000; 70:1352; Steroid Withdrawal Study Group. Prednisone withdrawal in kidney transplant recipients on cyclosporine and mycophenolate mofetil—a prospective randomized study. Transplantation 1999;68:1865.

76. Clinical practice guidelines of the American Society of Transplantation. Recommendations for the outpatient surveillance of renal transplant recipients. J Am Soc Nephrol 2000;11:S1.

77. AASLD/ITLS. Long term management of the liver transplant patients. Liver Transpl 2001;7(Suppl 1):S1.

78. Bostom AD et al. Prevention of post-transplant cardiovascular disease—report and recommendations of an ad hoc group. Am J Transplant 2002;2:491.

79. Ojo A. Long term survival in renal transplant recipients with graft function. Kidney Int 2000;57:307.

80. Wheeler DC et al. Evolution and etiology of cardiovascular diseases in renal transplant recipients. Transplant 2000;70(Suppl):SS41.

81. Kasiske BL. Epidemiology of cardiovascular disease after renal transplantation. Transplant 2001;72(Suppl):S5.

82. Midtvedt K et al. Management strategies for posttransplant hypertension. Transplant 2000;70(Suppl):S64.

83. Miller LW. Cardiovascular toxicities of immunosuppressive agents. Am J Transplant 2002;2:807.

84. Henry ML et al. Cyclosporine and tacrolimus (FK506): a comparison of efficacy and safety profiles. Clin Transplant 1999;13:209.

85. Olyaei AJ et al. A practical guide to the management of hypertension in renal transplant recipients. Drugs 1999;58:1011.

86. Neumayer HH et al. Protective effects of calcium antagonists in human renal transplantation. Kidney Int Suppl 1992;36:S87.

87. Anaizi N. Drug interactions involving immunosuppressive agents. Graft 2001;4:232.

88. Dresser GK. Pharmacokinetic-pharmacodynamic consequences and clinical relevance of cytochrome P450 3A4 inhibition. Clin Pharmacokinet 2000;38:41.

89. Stignant CE et al. ACE Inhibitors and angiotensin II antagonists in renal transplantation; an analysis of safety and efficacy. Am J Kidney Dis 2000;35:58.

90. Calzolari A et al. Hypertension in young patients after renal transplantation. Ambulatory blood pressure monitoring versus casual blood pressure. Am J Hypertens 1998;11:497.

91. Margreiter R et al. A prospective randomized multicentre study to compare the efficacy and safety of tacrolimus and cyclosporin-microemulsion in renal transplantation. Transplant 2000;69(Suppl):S112.

92. Friemann S et al. Conversion to tacrolimus in hyperlipidemic patients. Transplant Proc 1999;31(Suppl 7A):41S.

93. Massy ZA. Hyperlipidemia and cardiovascular disease after organ transplantation. Transplant 2001;72:S13.

94. Fellstrom B et al. Impact and management of hyperlipidemia posttransplantation. 2000;70(Suppl):SS51.

95. Kobashigawa JA et al. Hyperlipidemia in solid organ transplantation. Transplantation 1997;63(3):331.

96. Johnson C et al. Randomized trail of tacrolimus (Prograf) in combination with azathioprine or mycophenolate mofetil versus cyclosporine. Transplant 2000;69:834.

97. McCune TR et al. Effects of tacrolimus on hyperlipidemia after successful renal transplantation. Transplant 1998;65:87.

98. Moore R et al. Calcineurin inhibitors and posttransplant hyperlipidemias. Drug Saf 2001;24:755.

99. Brattstrom C et al. Hyperlipidemia in renal transplant recipients treated with Sirolimus (rapamycin). Transplantation 1998;65(9):1272.

100. Hoogeveen RC et al. Effect of sirolimus on the metabolism of apoB100-containing lipoproteins in renal transplant patients. Transplant 2001;72:1244.

101. Wenke K et al. Simvastatin reduces graft vessel disease and mortality after heart transplantation: a four-year randomized trial. Circulation 1997;96(5):1398.

102. Kobashigawa JA et al. Effect of pravastatin on outcomes after cardiac transplantation. N Engl J Med 1995;333:621.

103. Holdaas H et al. Effect of fluvastatin on acute renal allograft rejection: a randomized multicenter trial. Kidney Int 2001;60:1990.

104. Kasiske BL et al. Simvastatin in kidney transplant recipients. Transplant 2002;72:2232.

105. Pasternak RC et al. ACA/AHA/NHLBI Clinical Advisory on use and safety of statins. J Am Coll Cardiol 2002;40:568.

106. Magnani G et al. Role of statins in the management of dyslipidemia after cardiac transplant: randomized controlled trial comparing the efficacy and the safety of atorvastatin with pravastatin. J Heart Lung Transplant 2000;19:710.

107. Reisaeter AV et al. Risk factors and incidence of posttransplant diabetes mellitus. Transpl Proc 2001 (Suppl 5A):8S.

108. Jindal RM et al. Impact and management of posttransplant diabetes mellitus. Transplant 2000;70(Suppl):S58.

109. Aboujjoud MS et al. Neoral rescue therapy in transplant patients with intolerance to tacrolimus. Clin Transplant 2002;16:168.

110. Weir M. Impact of Immunosuppressive regimens on posttransplant diabetes mellitus. Transpl Proc 2001;33(Suppl 5A):23S.

111. Marchetti P. Strategies for risk reduction and management of posttransplant diabetes mellitus. Transplant Proc 2001;35(Suppl 5A):27S.

112. Rodino MA et al. Osteoporosis after organ transplantation. Am J Med 1998;104:459.

113. Heaf JG. Bone disease after renal transplantation. Transplant 2003;75:315.

114. Rodino MA et al. Osteoporosis after lung transplantation. Am J Med 1998;104:459.

115. Crippin JS. Bone disease after liver transplantation. Liver Transpl 2001;7(Suppl 1):S27.

116. American College of Rheumatology Task Force on Osteoporosis Guidelines. Arthritis Rheum 1996;39(11):1791.

117. Hertz MI et al. The registry of the International Society for Heart and Lung Transplantation; Nineteenth Official Report-2002. J Heart Lung Transplant 2002;21:950.

118. Cimato TR, et al. Recipient selection in cardiac transplantation: contraindications and risk factors for mortality. J Heart Lung Transplant 2002:21:1161.

119. Young JB et al. 24th Bethesda conference: Cardiac Transplantation Task Force 4: Function of the heart transplant recipient. J Am Coll Cardiol 1993;22:31.

120. Kobashigawa JA. Postoperative management following heart transplantation. Transplant Proc 1999;31:2038.

121. Cotts WG et al. Function of the transplanted heart. Am J Med Sci 1997;314:164.

122. Redmond JM et al. Use of theophylline for treatment of prolonged sinus node dysfunction in human orthotopic heart transplantation. J Heart Lung Transplant 1993;12:133.

123. Lake KD et al. Over the counter medications in cardiac transplant recipients: guidelines for use. Ann Pharmacother 1992;26(12):1566.

124. Taylor DO et al. A randomized, multicenter comparison of tacrolimus and cyclosporine immunosuppressive regimens in cardiac transplantation: decreased hyperlipidemia and hypertension with tacrolimus. J Heart Lung Transplant 1999;18:336.

125. Kobashigawa J et al. A randomized active: controlled trial of mycophenolate mofetil in heart transplant recipients. Mycophenolate mofetil investigators. Transplantation 1998;66:507.

126. Hosenpud JD et al. Mycophenolate mofetil compared to azathioprine improves survival in patients surviving the initial cardiac transplant hospitalization: an analysis of the joint ISHLT/UNOS Thoracic Registry. J Heart Lung Transplant 2000; 19:72.

127. TAYLOR DO et al. Increased incidence of allograft rejection in stable heart transplant recipients after late conversion from mycophenolate to azathioprine. Clin Transplant 1999;13:296.

128. Wilde MI et al. Muromonab CD3: a reappraisal of its pharmacology and use as prophylaxis of solid organ rejection. Drugs 1996:51:865.

129. Copeland JG et al. Rabbit antithymocyte globulin: a 10-year experience in cardiac transplantation. J Thorac Cardiovasc Surg 1990:99:852.

130. Scnetzler B et al. A prospective randomized controlled study on the efficacy and tolerance of two antilymphocytic globulins in the prevention of rejection in first heart transplant recipients. Transpl Int 2002;15:317.

131. Beniaminovitz A et al. Prevention of rejection in cardiac transplantation by blockade of the interleukin-2 receptor with a monoclonal antibody. N Engl J Med 2000;342:613.

132. Fekel TO et al. Survival and incidence of acute rejection in heart transplant recipients undergoing successful withdrawal from steroid therapy. J Heart Lung Transplant 2002;21:530.

133. Kobashigawa JA et al. Do heart transplant patients on corticoid-free immunosuppression have less rejection? Circulation 1999;100:I-525.

134. Taylor DO et al. Improved long term survival after heart transplantation predicted by early withdrawal from maintenance steroid therapy. J Heart Lung Transplant 1996;15:1039.

135. Billingham ME et al. A working formulation for the standardization of nomenclature in the diagnosis of heart and lung rejection: Heart Rejection Study Group. The International Society for Heart Transplantation. J Heart Transplant 1990;9(6):587.

136. Yeogh TJ et al. Clinical significance of mild rejection of the cardiac allograft. Circulation 1992; 86(Suppl 2):II267.

137. Weis M. Cardiac Allograft vasculopathy: prevention and treatment options. Transpl Proc 2002;34: 1847.

138. de Lorgenil M, Boissonnat P. Low-dose aspirin and accelerated coronary disease in heart transplant recipients. J Heart Transplant 1990;9:339.

139. Schroeder JS et al. A preliminary study of diltiazem in the prevention of coronary artery disease in heart-transplant recipients. N Engl J Med 1993;328(3):164.

140. Wenke K et al. Simavastatin initiated early after heart transplantation: 8-year prospective experience. Circulation 2003:07:93.

141. Miller LW. Treatment of cardiac allograft rejection with intravenous corticosteroids. J Heart Transplant 1990;9(3 Pt 2):283.

142. Kobashigawa JA, Stevenson LW. Is intravenous glucocorticoid therapy better than an oral regimen for asymptomatic cardiac rejection: a randomized trial. J Am Coll Cardiol 1993;21:1142.

143. Lonquist JL et al. Reevaluation of steroid tapering after steroid pulse therapy for heart rejection. J Heart Lung Transplant 1992;11(5):913.

144. Haverty TP et al. OKT₃ treatment of cardiac allograft rejection. J Heart Lung Transplant 1993; 12(4):591.

145. Kirklin JK et al. Treatment of recurrent heart rejection with mycophenolate mofetil: initial clinical experience. J Heart Lung Transplant 1994; 13:444.

146. Miller L et al. Treatment of acute cardiac allograft rejection with rapamycin: a multicenter dose ranging study. J Heart Lung Transplant 1997;16:44.

147. Bourge RC et al. Methotrexate pulse therapy in the treatment of recurrent acute heart rejection. J Heart Lung Transplant 1992;11(6):1116.

148. Armitage JM et al. Clinical trial of FK 506 immunosuppression in adult cardiac transplantation. Ann Thorac Surg 1992;54(2):205.

149. Duarte Ag et al. Perioperative care of the lung transplant patient. Chest Surg Clin NA 2002;12:397.

150. Chan KM et al. Infectious pulmonary complications in lung transplant recipients. Semin Respir Infect 2002;17:291.

151. Zamora MR. Controversies in lung transplantation: management of cytomegalovirus infections. J Heart Lung Transplant 2002;21:849.

152. Kubak BM. Fungal infections in lung transplantation. Transplant Infect Dis 2002;4 (Suppl 3):24.

153. Trulock EP. Management of lung transplant rejection. Chest 1993;103(5):1566.

154. Yousem SA et al. Revision of the 1990 working formulation for the standardization of nomenclature in the diagnosis of heart and lung rejection: lung rejection study group. J Heart Transplant 1996;15:1.

155. Shenib H, Massard G. Efficacy of OKT₃ therapy for acute rejection in isolated lung transplantations. J Heart Lung Transplant 1994;13:514.

156. Iacono AT et al. Dose-related reversal of acute lung rejection by aerosolized cyclosporine. Am J Resp Crit Care Med 1997;155:1690.

157. Vitulo P et al. Efficacy of tacrolimus rescue therapy in refractory acute rejection after lung transplantation. J Heart Lung Transplant 2002;21:435.

158. Estenne M et al. Bronchiolitis obliterans after human lung transplantation. Am J Respir Crit Care Med 2002;166:440.

159. Cahill BC et al. Early experience with sirolimus in lung transplant recipients with chronic allograft rejection. J Heart Lung Transplant 2003;22:169.

160. Palmer SM et al. Rabbit antithymocyte globulin decreases acute rejection after lung transplantation: results of a randomized prospective study. Chest 1999;116:127.

161. Brock MV et al. Induction therapy in lung transplantation: a prospective, controlled clinical trial comparing OKT3, anti-thymocyte globulin, and daclizumab. J Heart Lung Transplant 2001;20:1282.

162. Treede H et al. Tacrolimus versus cyclosporine after lung transplantation: a prospective, open, randomized two-center trial comparing two different immunosuppressive protocols. J Heart Lung Transplant 2001;20:511.

163. Garrity ER et al. Suggested guidelines for the use of tacrolimus in lung transplant recipients. J Heart Lung Transplant 1999;18(3):175.

164. Palmer SM et al. Results of a randomized, prospective, multicenter trial of mycophenolate versus azathioprine in the prevention of acute lung allograft rejection. Transplant 2001;71:1772.

165. Ishani A et al. Predictors of renal function following lung or heart-lung transplantation. KI 2002; 61:2228.

166. Dupuis RE et al. Tobramycin pharmacokinetics in patients with cystic fibrosis preceding and following lung transplantation. Ther Drug Monit 1999; 21:161.

167. Kesten S et al. Pharmacokinetic profile and variability of cyclosporine versus Neoral in patients with cystic fibrosis after lung transplantation. Pharmacotherapy 1998;18:847.

168. Dror Y et al. Lymphoproliferative disorders after organ transplantation in children. Transplantation 1999;67:990.

169. Penn I. De novo malignancy in pediatric organ transplantation. Pediatr Transplant 1998;2:56.

170. Penn I. Post-transplant malignancy. The role of immunosuppression. Drug Saf 2000;23:101.

171. Penn I. The problem of cancer in organ transplant recipients. Transplant Sci 1994;4:423.

172. Euvrard S et al. Skin cancer after organ transplantation. N Engl J M 2003;348:1681.

173. Swinnen LJ. Treatment of organ transplant-related lymphoma. Hematol Oncol Clin North Am 1997;11:963.

174. Verschuuren EA et al. Treatment of posttransplant lymphoproliferative disease with rituximab: the remission, the relapse, and the complication. Transplant 2002;73:100.

175. McDiarmid SV et al. Prevention and preemptive therapy of posttransplant lymphoproliferative disease in pediatric liver recipients. Transplantation 1998;66:1604.

176. Green M et al. Serial measurement of Epstein-Barr viral load in peripheral blood in pediatric liver transplant recipients during treatment for posttransplant lymphoproliferative disease. Transplantation 1998;66:1641.

177. Hakim NS. Recent developments and future prospects in pancreatic and islet transplantation. Diabetes, Obesity, and Metabolism 2001;3:9.

178. Friedman AL. Appropriateness and timing of kidney and/or pancreas transplants in type 1 and type 2 diabetes. Adv Ren Replace Ther 2001;8:70.

179. Kahl A et al. Trends and perspectives in pancreas and simultaneous pancreas and kidney transplantation. Curr Opin Urol 2001;11:165.

180. Rosenberg L. Pancreatic and islet transplantation. Curr Gastroenterol Reps 2000;2:165.

181. Pirson Y. Kidney and kidney-pancreas transplantation in diabetic recipients. Diabetes Metab 2000; 26:86.

182. Odorico JS et al. A study comparing mycophenolate mofetil to azathioprine in simultaneous pancreas-kidney transplantation. Transplantation 1998;66:1751.

183. Kaufman DB et al. Mycophenolate mofetil and tacrolimus as primary maintenance immunosuppression in simultaneous pancreas-kidney transplantation: initial experience in 50 consecutive cases. Transplantation 1999;67:586.

184. International Pancreas Transplantation Registry. Newsletter 2000;12:4.

185. Stratta RJ. Review of immunosuppressive usage in pancreas transplantation. Clin Transpl 1999; 12:1.

186. Kahan BD et al. Reduction of the occurrence of acute cellular rejection among renal allograft recipients treated with basiliximab, a chimeric anti-interleukin-2-receptor monoclonal antibody. Transplantation 1999;67(2):276.

187. Gaber AO et al. Results of the double-blind randomized multicenter phase III clinical trial of Thymoglobulin versus Atgam in the treatment of acute graft rejection episodes after renal transplantation. Transplantation 1998;66:29.

188. Brennan DC et al. A randomized double-blinded comparison of Thymoglobulin vs. Atgam for induction immunosuppression in adult renal transplant recipients. Transplantation 1999;67:1011.

189. Bock HA et al. A randomized prospective trial of prophylactic immunosuppression with ATG-Fresenius versus OKT3 after renal transplant. Transplantation 1995;59:830.

190. Willand AM et al. Peripheral administration of thymoglobulin for induction therapy in pancreas transplantation. Transplant Proc 2001;33:1910.

191. Guttman RD et al. Pharmacokinetics, foreign protein immune response, cytokine release and lymphocyte subsets in patients receiving Thymoglobulin and immunosuppression. Transplant Proc 1997;29(Suppl 7A):24S.

192. Bielory L et al. Human serum sickness: a prospective analysis of 35 patients treated with equine anti-thymocyte globulin for bone marrow failure. Medicine (Baltimore) 1988;67(1):40.

193. Peddi VR et al. Safety, efficacy, and cost analysis of Thymoglobulin induction therapy with intermittent dosing based on CD3+ lymphocyte counts in kidney and kidney-pancreas transplant recipients. Transplantation 2002;73:1514.

194. Macdonald PS et al. A prospective randomized study of prophylactic OKT₃ versus equine antithymocyte globulin after heart transplantation—increased morbidity with OKT₃. Transplantation 1993;55(1):110.

195. Brennan DG et al. Leukocyte response to Thymoglobulin vs Atgam induction. Transplant Proc 1999;31(Suppl B):19S.

196. Thistlethwaite JR Jr et al. Complications and monitoring of OKT₃ therapy. Am J Kidney Dis 1988;11(2):112

197. Norman DJ et al. Consensus statement regarding OKT$_3$-induced cytokine-release syndrome and human antimouse antibodies. Transplant Proc 1993;25(2 Suppl 1):89.

198. Martin MA et al. Nosocomial aseptic meningitis associated with administration of OKT$_3$. JAMA 1988;259(13):2002.

199. Shihab FS et al. Encephalopathy following the use of OKT$_3$ in renal allograft transplantation. Transplant Proc 1993;25(2 Suppl 1):31.

200. Batiuk TD et al. Cytokine nephropathy during antilymphocyte therapy. Transplant Proc 1993;25 (2 Suppl 1):27.

201. Abramowicz D et al. Induction of thromboses within renal grafts by high-dose prophylactic OKT$_3$ (see comments). Lancet 1992;339(8796):777.

202. Suthanthiran M et al. OKT$_3$ associated adverse reactions: mechanistic basis and therapeutic options. Am J Kidney Dis 1989;14(5 Suppl 2):39.

203. Chatenoud L et al. In vivo cell activation following OKT$_3$ administration. Systemic cytokine release and modulation by corticosteroids. Transplantation 1990;49(4):697.

204. Constanzo-Nordin MR. Cardiopulmonary effects of OKT$_3$: determinants of hypotension, pulmonary edema, and cardiac dysfunction. Transplant Proc 1993;25(2 Suppl 1):21.

205. Stein KL et al. The cardiopulmonary response to OKT$_3$ in orthotopic cardiac transplant recipients. Chest 1989;95(4):817.

206. Chatenoud L et al. Immunologic monitoring during OKT3. Clin Transplant 1993;7:422.

207. Hricik DE et al. Inhibition of anti-OKT$_3$ antibody generation by cyclosporine—results of a prospective randomized trial. Transplantation 1990;50(2):237.

208. Kimball JA et al. Mycophenolate with cyclosporin A prevents anti-OKT3 antibody response in kidney transplant recipients. J Am Soc Nephrol 1998;16:1521.

209. Shield CF III. Consequences of anti-OKT$_3$ antibody development: OKT$_3$ reuse and long-term graft survival. Transplant Proc 1993;25(2 Suppl 1):81.

210. Mylonakis E et al. BK virus in solid organ transplant recipients: an emerging syndrome. Transplantation 2001;72:1587.

211. Reploeg MD et al. BK virus: a clinical review. CID 2001;33:191.

212. Randhawa PS et al. Nephropathy due to polyomavirus type BK. N Engl J Med 2000;342:1361.

213. Nickeleit V et al. The prognostic significance of specific arterial lesions in acute renal allograft rejection. J Am Soc Nephrol 2000;342:1309.

214. Van Gorder MA et al. Cynomolgus polyoma virus infection: a new member of the polyoma virus family causes interstitial nephritis, ureteritis, and enteritis in immunosuppressed cynomolgus monkeys. Am J Pathol 1999;154:1273.

215. Binet I et al. Polyomavirus disease under new immunosuppressive drugs: a cause of renal graft dysfunction and graft loss. Transplantation 1999;67:918.

216. Gonzalez-Fraile MI et al. Cidofovir treatment of human polyomavirus associated acute haemorrhagic cystitis. Transpl Infect Dis 2001;3:44.

217. Vats A et al. Quantitative viral load monitoring and cidofovir therapy for the management of BK virus-associated nephropathy in children and adults. Transplantation 2003;75:105.

218. http://www.optn.org/organDatasource/about.asp?display=Liver; March 2003.

219. Everson GT et al. Liver transplantation: current status and unresolved controversies. Adv Intern Med 1997;42:505.

220. Gow PJ et al. Solid organ transplantation in patients with HIV infection. Transplant 2001;72:177.

221. Reich D et al. Common medical disease after liver transplantation. Semin Gastrointest Dis 1998;9:110.

222. Porte RJ. Coagulation and fibrinolysis in orthotopic liver transplantation: current views and insights. Semin Thromb Hemostat 1993;19(3):191.

223. Wijjdicks EFM. Neurotoxicity of immunosuppressive drugs. Liver Transpl 2001;7:937

224. Venkataramanan R et al. Clinical pharmacokinetics of tacrolimus. Clin Pharmacokinet 1995;29:404.

225. Mancinelli LM et al. The pharmacokinetic and metabolic disposition of tacrolimus: a comparison across ethnic groups. Clin Pharmacol Ther 2001;69:24.

226. Kershner RP et al. Relationship of FK506 whole blood concentrations and efficacy and toxicity after liver and kidney transplantation. Transplantation 1996;62:920.

227. Holt DW et al. Clinical toxicology working group on immunosuppressive drug monitoring. Ther Drug Monit 2002;24:59.

228. Pou L et al. Therapeutic drug monitoring of tacrolimus in liver transplantation, phase III FK506 multicenter Spanish Study Group: a two-year follow-up. Ther Drug Monit 1998;20:602.

229. Porryko MK, Textons SC. Nephrotropic effects of primary immunosuppression with FK506 and cyclosporine regimens after liver transplantation. Mayo Clin Proc 1994;69:105.

230. Klintmahn GB. A comparison of tacrolimus (FK506) and cyclosporine for immunosuppression in liver transplantation. The U.S. Multicenter FK506 Liver Study Group. N Engl J Med 1994;331:1110.

231. Knechtle SJ et al. Rejection of the liver transplant. Semin Gastrointest Dis 1998;9:126.

232. Gordon RD et al. The antibody crossmatch in liver transplantation. Surgery 1986;100(4):705.

233. Fisher RA et al. A prospective randomized trial of mycophenolate mofetil with Neoral or tacrolimus after orthotopic liver transplantation. Transplantation 1998;66:1616.

234. Jani A et al. A prospective randomized trial of tacrolimus and prednisone versus tacrolimus, prednisone and mycophenolate mofetil in primary adult liver transplantation: a single center report. Transplant 2001;72:1091.

235. Demetris AJ et al. Banff schema for grading liver allograft rejection: an international consensus document. Hepatology 1997;25:658.

236. Sher LS et al. Tacrolimus as rescue therapy in liver transplantation. Transplantation 1997;64:258.

237. Sollinger HW et al. Mycophenolate mofetil for the prevention of acute rejection in primary cadaveric renal allograft recipients. Transplantation 1995;69:225.

238. Tricontinental Mycophenolate Mofetil Renal Transplantation Study Group. A blinded, randomized clinical trial of mycophenolate mofetil for the prevention of acute rejection in cadaveric renal transplantation. Transplantation 1996;61:1029.

239. Mathew TH et al. A blinded, long-term randomized multicenter study of mycophenolate mofetil in cadaveric renal transplantation: results at three years. Tricontinental Mycophenolate Mofetil Renal Transplantation study. Transplantation 1998;65:1450.

240. Bullingham RE et al. Clinical pharmacokinetics of mycophenolate mofetil. Clin Pharmacokinet 1998;34:429.

241. Behrend M et al. Adverse gastrointestinal effects of mycophenolate mofetil. Aetiology, incidence and management. Drug Saf 2001;24:645.

242. Cox VC et al. Mycophenolate mofetil for organ transplantation: does the evidence support the need for clinical pharmacokinetic monitoring. Ther Drug Monit 2003;25:137.

243. Campana C et al. Clinically significant drug interactions with cyclosporine. An update. Clin Pharmacokinet 1996;30:141.

244. Ahmed AR. Cyclophosphamide (Cytoxan). J Am Acad Dermatol 1984;11:1115.

245. Pepping J. Echinacea. Am J Health-Syst Pharm 1999;56:121.

246. Barone GW. Herbal supplements: a potential for drug interactions in transplant recipients. Transplant 2001;71:239.

247. Kelly P. Review: metabolism of immunosuppressant drugs. Cur Drug Metab 2002;3:275.

248. MFinch CK. Rifampin and rifabutin drug interactions: an update. Adv Intern Med 2002;162:985.

249. Bullingham R et al. Effects of food and antacids on the pharmacokinetics of single doses of mycophenolate mofetil in rheumatoid arthritis patients. Br J Clin Pharmacol 199641:513.

250. Morli M. et al. Impairment of mycophenolate mofetil absorption by iron ion. Clin Pharm Ther 2000;68:613.

251. Gallego C. Interaction between probucol and cyclosporine in renal transplant patients. Ann Pharmacother 1994;28:940.

252. Rundles RW, Wyngaarden JB, Hitchings GH. Effects of a xanthine oxidase inhibitor on thiopurine metabolism, hyperuricemia and gout. Trans Assoc Am Physicians 1963;76:126.

253. Lindholm Aet al. Influence of cyclosporine pharmacokinetics, trough concentrations, and AUC monitoring on outcome after kidney transplantation. Clin Pharm Ther 1993;54:205.

254. Kahan BD et al. Challenges in cyclosporine therapy: the role of therapeutic monitoring by area under the curve monitoring. Ther Drug Monit 1995;17:621.

255. Dunn CJ et al. Cyclosporin: an updated review of the pharmacokinetic properties, clinical efficacy and tolerability of a microemulsion-based formulation (neural) in organ transplantation. Drugs 2001;61:1957.

256. Min DL et al. Gender-dependent racial difference in disposition of cyclosporine among healthy African American and white volunteers. Clin Pharm Ther 2000;68:478.

257. Rossi SJ et al. Prevention and management of the adverse effects associated with immunosuppressive therapy. Drug Saf 1993;9:104.

258. Oellerich M et al. Lake Loiuse consensus conference on cyclosporine monitoring in organ transplantation: report of the consensus panel. Ther Drug Monit 1995;17:642.

259. Tsunoda SM et al. The use of therapeutic drug monitoring to optimize immunosuppressive therapy. Clin Pharmacokinet 1996;30:107.

260. Mahalati K et al. Neoral monitoring by simplified sparse sampling area under the concentration time curve: its relationship to acute rejection and cyclosporine nephrotoxicity early after kidney transplantation. Transplantation 1999;68:55.

261. Levy GA. C2 monitoring strategy for optimizing cyclosporin immunosuppression from Neoral formulation. BioDrugs 2001;15:279.

262. Cole E et al. Recommendations for the implementation of Neoral C2 monitoring in clinical practice. Transplantation 2002;73:S19.

263. MacDonald A et al. Clinical pharmacokinetics and therapeutic monitoring of sirolimus. Clin Ther 2000;22(Suppl B);B101.

264. Ingle SR et al. Sirolimus: continuing the evolution of transplant immunosuppression. Ann Pharmacother 2000;34:1044.

265. El-Sabrout et al. Improved freedom from rejection after a loading dose of sirolimus. Transplant 2003;75:86.

266. MacDonald AS. Improving tolerability of immunosuppressive regimens. Transplant 2001;72:S105.

267. Fishman JA et al. Infection in organ transplant recipients. N Engl J Med 1998;338:1741.

268. ASHP therapeutic guidelines on antimicrobial prophylaxis in surgery. Am J Health-Syst Pharm 1999;56:1839.

269. Singh N. Infectious diseases in the liver transplant recipient. Semin Gastrointest Dis 1998;9:136.

270. SM et al. Should prophylaxis for *Pneumocystis carinii* pneumonia in solid organ transplant recipients ever be discontinued? Clin Infect Dis 1999;28:240.

271. Samuel D et al. Liver transplantation in European patients with the hepatitis B surface antigen. N Engl J Med 1993;329:1842.

272. McGory RW et al. Improved outcome of orthotopic liver transplantation for a chronic hepatitis B cirrhosis with aggressive passive immunization. Transplantation 1996;61:1358.

273. Markowitz JS et al. Prophylaxis against hepatitis B recurrence following liver transplantation using combination lamivudine and hepatitis B immune globulin. Hepatology 1998;28:585.

274. Bain VG et al. Efficacy of lamivudine in chronic hepatitis B patients with active viral replication and decompensated cirrhosis undergoing liver transplantation. Transplantation 1996;62:1456.

275. Benhamou Y et al. Safety and efficacy of adefovir dipivoxil in patients co-infected with HIV-1 and lamivudine-resistant hepatitis B virus: an open-label pilot study. Lancet 2001;358:718.

276. Willems M et al. Liver transplantation and hepatitis C. Transplant International 2002;15:61.

277. Forman LM et al. The association between hepatitis C infection and survival after orthotopic liver transplantation. Gastroenterology 2002;122:889.

278. Rose HR. Hepatitis C in the liver transplant recipient: current understanding and treatment. Microbes and Infection 2002;4(12):1253.

279. Gane E. Treatment of recurrent hepatitis C. Liver Transpl 1997;8(10 Suppl 1):S28.

280. Grabenstein JD et al. Immunization and organ transplantation. Hosp Pharm 1999;34:339.

281. Hebart H et al. Management of cytomegalovirus infection after solid-organ or stem-cell transplantation: current guidelines and future prospects. Drugs 1998;55(1):59.

282. Sousha SK et al. Cytomegalovirus infection following liver transplantation: review of the literature. Clin Infect Dis 1996;22:537.

283. Noble S et al. Ganciclovir: an update of its use in the prevention of cytomegalovirus infection and disease in transplant recipients. Drugs 1998; 56(1):115.

284. Nankivell BJ. Maintenance therapy with oral ganciclovir after treatment of cytomegalovirus infection. Clin Transplant 1998;12(3):270.

285. Kutsogiannis DJ et al. Granulocyte macrophage colony-stimulating factor for the therapy of cytomegalovirus and ganciclovir-induced leukopenia in a renal transplant recipient. Transplantation 1992;53(4):930.

286. Snydman DR et al. A further analysis of the use of cytomegalovirus immune globulin in orthotopic liver transplant patients at risk for primary infection. Transplant Proc 1994;2(Suppl 1):23.

287. Avery RK. Special considerations regarding CMV in lung transplantation. Transplant Infect Dis 1999;1(Suppl 1):13.

288. Rubin RH. Prevention and treatment of cytomegalovirus disease in heart transplant patients. J Heart Lung Transplant 2000;19:731.

289. Mullen GM et al. Effective oral ganciclovir prophylaxis against cytomegalovirus disease in heart transplant recipients. Transplant Proc 1998; 30(8):4110.

290. Gane E et al. Randomized trial of efficacy and safety of oral ganciclovir in the prevention of cytomegalovirus disease in liver-transplant recipients. Lancet 1997;350.1729.

291. Turgeon N et al. Effect of oral acyclovir or ganciclovir therapy after preemptive intravenous ganciclovir therapy to prevent cytomegalovirus disease in cytomegalovirus seropositive renal and liver transplant recipients receiving antilymphocyte antibody therapy. Transplantation 1998;66(12):1780.

292. Flechner SM et al. A randomized prospective controlled trial of oral acyclovir versus oral ganciclovir for cytomegalovirus prophylaxis in high-risk kidney transplant recipients. Transplantation 1998;66:1682.

293. Brown F et al. Pharmacokinetics of valganciclovir and ganciclovir following multiple oral dosages of valganciclovir in HIV- and CMV-seropositive volunteers. Clin Pharmacokinet 1999;37:167.

294. Martin D et al. A controlled trial of valganciclovir as induction therapy for cytomegalovirus retinitis. N Engl J Med 2002;346:1119.

295. Product Information: Valcyte(TM), valganciclovir. Roche Laboratories, Inc., Nutley, NJ; 4/2001.

296. Pescovitz MD et al. Valganciclovir for prevention of CMV disease: 12 month follow up of a randomized trial of 364 transplant recipients. Am J Transplant 2003;3:575.

297. Snydman DR et al. Cytomegalovirus immune globulin prophylaxis in liver transplantation. A randomized, double-blind, placebo-controlled trial. The Boston Center for Liver Transplantation. CMVIG Study Group. Ann Intern Med 1993; 119(10):984.

298. Fiddian P et al. Valacyclovir provides optimum acyclovir exposure for prevention of c tomegalovirus and related outcomes after organ transplantation. J Infect Dis 2002;186(Suppl 1):S110.

299. Tanabe K et al. Comparative study of cytomegalovirus (CMV) antigenemia assay, polymerase chain reaction, serology, and shell vial assay in the early diagnosis and monitoring of CMV infection after renal transplantation. Transplantation 1997;64(12):1721.

300. Gomez E et al. Control of cytomegalovirus disease in renal transplant patients treated with prednisone, azathioprine, and cyclosporine using intensive monitoring and decreased immunosuppression. Nephron 1999;82(3):238.

301. Yang CW et al. Clinical course of cytomegalovirus (CMV) viremia with and without ganciclovir treatment in CMV-seropositive kidney transplant recipients. Longitudinal follow-up of CMV pp65 antigenemia assay. Am J Nephrol 1998;18(5):373.

302. Salazar TA, Aweeka FT. Transplantation. In: Herfindal ET et al, eds. Clinical Pharmacy and Therapeutics, 5th Ed. Baltimore: Williams & Wilkins, 1992:1528.

303. Baroletti SA et al. Calcium channel blockers as the treatment of choice for hypertension in renal transplant recipients: fact or fiction. AJHP 2003;(6):788.

NUTRITION ISSUES

Beverly Holcombe
SECTION EDITOR

CHAPTER **36**

Adult Enteral Nutrition

Carol J. Rollins, Yvonne Huckleberry, Pauline Cawley

Enteral nutrition refers to nutrition provided via the gastrointestinal (GI) tract. However, as the term is used commonly, enteral nutrition is synonymous with delivery of nutrients into the GI tract by tube (e.g., nasogastric or jejunostomy feeding). Tube feeding allows continued use of the GI tract when one or more steps in the normal process of obtaining nutrients from oral intake is disrupted. Although steps such as chewing or swallowing may be completely disrupted, some digestive and absorptive function must remain if tube feeding is to be a viable nutrition support option.

Patient Selection

Patients generally are considered at risk of nutrient depletion and associated increased morbidity and mortality when intake is inadequate to meet nutritional requirements for ≥ 7 days or when weight loss exceeds 10% of pre-illness weight within a 6-month period of time.[1,2] Nutrition screening programs are in place in most institutional practice sites to identify patients

who may be at nutritional risk. Parameters such as weight, height, diagnosis, recent weight loss, and serum albumin are evaluated. However, availability of these parameters in patient charts sometimes is limited.[3] A nutrition assessment expands the screen by including other laboratory data (hemoglobin [Hgb], hematocrit [Hct], creatinine, cholesterol, nitrogen balance, total iron-binding capacity [TIBC], prealbumin [transthyretin]), calculation of energy requirements, dietary history, and medical history. Completion of the nutrition assessment helps identify patients that may be candidates for enteral nutrition. (See Chapter 37, Adult Parenteral Nutrition, for further information on nutrition assessment.)

Routes of nutrition intervention may include modified oral diet, enteral nutrition by tube, or parenteral nutrition. Tube feeding is considered the route of choice in patients with a functional gastrointestinal tract whose oral nutrient intake is insufficient to meet estimated needs.[1]

The normal process of preparing nutrients for absorption includes multiple steps. Table 36-1 lists the functional

Table 36-1   Functional Units of the GI Tract

Functional Unit	Major Steps	Conditions/Diseases
Mouth and oropharynx	Chew and lubricate food; swallow	Amyotrophic lateral sclerosis, muscular dystrophy, severe RA, CVA, end-stage Parkinson's disease, paralysis, coma, anorexia due to other disease: cardiac or cancer cachexia, renal failure and uremia, liver failure, neurologic disease
Esophagus	Transport food to the stomach	Esophageal disease: ulcer, cancer, obstruction, fistula, esophagectomy, CVA
Stomach	Hold food for mixing and grinding; add acid and enzymes; release chyme to small bowel; osmoregulation	Severe gastritis or ulceration, gastroparesis, gastric outlet obstruction, gastric cancer, severe gastroesophageal reflux
Duodenum	Osmoregulation; neutralize stomach acid	Severe duodenal ulcer, duodenal fistula, cancer: gastric, pancreatic
Small bowel: jejunum and ileum	Digestion; absorption	Enterocutaneous fistula, severe enteric infection, malnutrition, malabsorption, Crohn's disease, celiac sprue, ileus and dysmotility syndrome
Pancreas	Secretion of digestive enzymes	Pancreatitis, pancreatic cancer, pancreatic injury, pancreatic fistula
Colon	Absorb fluid; ferment soluble fiber and unabsorbed carbohydrate; absorb water	Ulcerative colitis, Crohn's disease, colon cancer, colocutaneous fistula, colovaginal fistula, diverticulitis, colitis of any etiology, colon surgery

CVA, cerebrovascular accident; GI, gastrointestinal; RA, rheumatoid arthritis.

anatomic units of the GI tract along with major steps that occur in each unit and provides examples of conditions and diseases that can impair each general region. Tube feeding may be appropriate for patients with the disorders listed, depending on the extent to which normal intake, transport, digestion, and absorption of nutrients is impaired. Clinical circumstances, rather than a specific diagnosis, should be the determining factor for initiating tube feeding. Enteral nutrition should be used with caution in patients with severe necrotizing or hemorrhagic pancreatitis, enterocutaneous fistulae, GI ischemia, and partial bowel obstruction.[1] Contraindications to enteral feeding generally include diffuse peritonitis, complete bowel obstruction, paralytic ileus, intractable vomiting, diarrhea severe enough to make metabolic management difficult, severe malabsorption, and early-stage short-bowel syndrome. However, frequent reassessment is recommended because patients may be candidates for enteral nutrition as the condition improves or resolves. With advances in GI access and formula composition over the past several years, many patients once considered to require parenteral nutrition are now managed successfully with tube feeding.

Route of Tube Feeding

Several options exist for the route of tube feeding. The route is determined by the anticipated duration of tube feeding, the disrupted region or process in the GI tract, and the risk of aspiration. Figure 36-1 illustrates the two basic types of tube placement—nasal versus ostomy—and the sites available for formula delivery (i.e., gastric, duodenal, or jejunal). The name of the feeding route usually includes both the type of tube placement and the site of formula delivery. For example, *nasogastric* (NG) indicates nasal placement with gastric delivery of formula, whereas *gastrostomy* indicates ostomy placement with gastric delivery of formula.

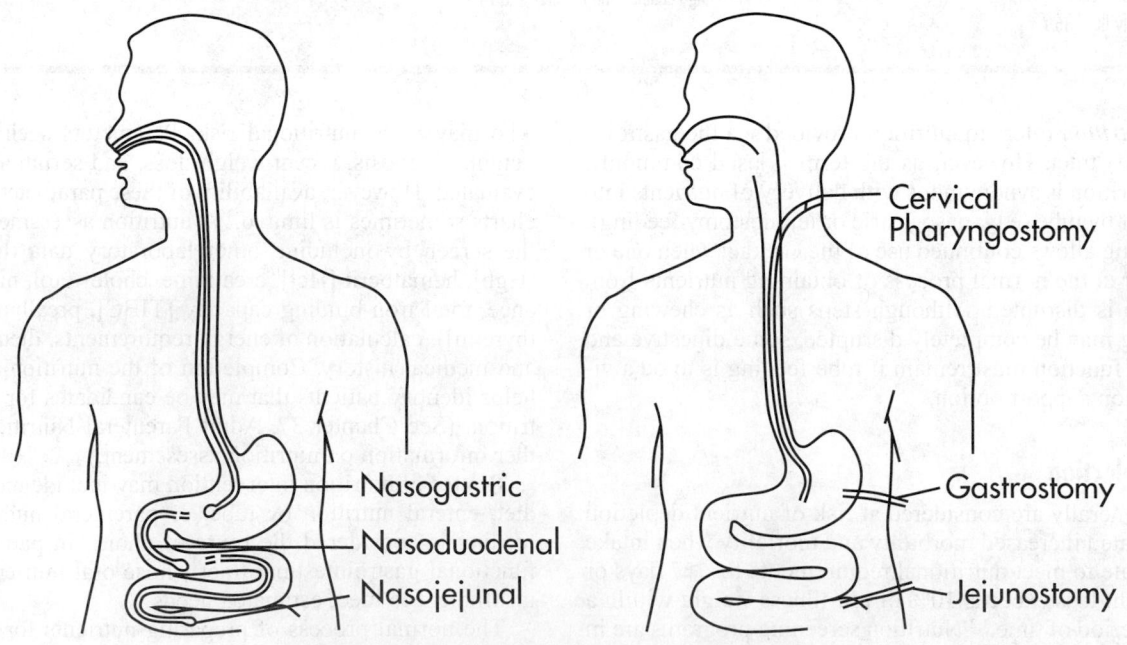

FIGURE 36-1 Nasoenteric and enterostomy feeding sites.

Tube Placement
NASAL
Nasal placement of the tube is preferred for short-term tube feeding in patients expected to resume oral feeding and without obstruction of nasal, pharyngeal, or esophageal passages. Clinically evident injury from nasal intubation appears to be very low, but up to 60% of patients may suffer ulceration or mucosal bruising of the esophagus and hypopharynx.[4] Although rare, perforation of the hypopharynx, esophagus, or stomach has been reported with tube placement. Pharyngitis, sinusitis, otitis media, and incompetence of the lower esophageal sphincter also are associated with nasoenteric tubes, especially large-bore tubes. Inadvertent pulmonary placement of small-bore feeding tubes may occur, although the actual incidence is likely 4% or less.[5,6] Radiographic confirmation of tube placement is mandatory to rule out pleural perforation and pulmonary intubation in unconscious patients, if gastric contents cannot be aspirated or if auscultation during air insufflation is uncertain in conscious and alert patients.[6,7] However, misinterpretation of radiographic images has been reported in a small percentage of patients.[5]

FEEDING OSTOMIES
Feeding ostomies (tube enterostomies) generally are reserved for long-term tube feeding. Depending on the clinical situation and the type of tube enterostomy placed, long-term feeding may be interpreted as >1 to 3 months, or up to 6 months, although nasoenteric feeding tubes occasionally are used for longer periods of time.[7] Access for enterostomies may be achieved through open surgery, laparoscopy, or percutaneously. Most surgical enterostomies require general anesthesia for placement, although some surgeons use local anesthesia for certain types of gastrostomies (Stamm gastrostomy).[7,8] Jejunostomy tubes frequently are placed while the patient is anesthetized for laparotomy or upper GI surgery, which allows early postoperative feeding.[1]

Surgical placement of an enterostomy requires that the patient be stable enough to endure the primary operation, that bacterial contamination of the primary operative site is not increased significantly, or that the patient can tolerate general anesthesia solely for enterostomy formation. Percutaneous endoscopic gastrostomy (PEG) and jejunostomy (PEJ) are performed under local anesthesia.[7,9] Most patients requiring long-term tube feeding have a PEG placed. Absolute contraindications to percutaneous endoscopic placement of a feeding tube include obstructions that prevent passage of the endoscope; relative contraindications include inability to see the endoscopic light through the abdominal wall (e.g., morbid obesity, massive ascites), peritoneal dialysis, coagulopathy, gastric varices, portal hypertension, hepatomegaly, and neoplastic or infiltrative disease of the gastric or jejunal wall.[7,9] Prior total or subtotal gastrectomy prevents PEG placement, but PEJ placement may be possible. The major advantages of percutaneous access versus surgical access appear to be the shorter time required for percutaneous tube placement and lower cost, since morbidity and mortality appear to be similar to surgical feeding tube access.[10] Major complications such as aspiration, peritonitis, hemorrhage, gastrocutaneous fistula formation, necrotizing fasciitis, gastric perforation, and migration of the tube through the gastric wall, occur in about 1% to 4% of patients.[7]

Site of Delivery
The preferred site for enteral formula delivery is the stomach because this is the most physiologically normal feeding site. Stimulation of normal digestive processes and hormonal responses associated with eating occurs with gastric feeding. The stomach serves as a reservoir that generally allows patients to tolerate bolus, intermittent, or continuous feeding. Gastric feeding, either by NG tube or gastrostomy, requires adequate gastric motility to prevent accumulation of formula in the stomach. Patients with neurologic, traumatic, or degenerative diseases that impair ingestion, chewing, or swallowing may be candidates for gastric feeding. Head and neck cancer patients often are candidates for gastric feedings, unless the cancer has invaded the stomach or lower esophagus. Patients with gastric outlet obstruction, gastroparesis, gastric distention, or gastroesophageal reflux are not candidates for gastric feeding but may be for duodenal or jejunal delivery of nutrients.

Transpyloric delivery of nutrients into the duodenum or jejunum may be appropriate when gastric dysfunction or disease is present; when the patient's risk of aspiration is high because of a need to lie flat in bed; or for early postoperative feeding when gastric emptying may be impaired. Gastroesophageal reflux and aspiration may be reduced with duodenal feeding compared with gastric feeding; however, migration of tubes from the duodenum into the stomach and equal risk of aspiration between postpyloric and intragastric tube placement has been observed.[11] Patients receiving feeding at night or those with gastric dysmotility appear to be at greatest risk for tube migration. Tube placement beyond the ligament of Treitz (i.e., jejunal placement) may be best for patients with a risk of tube migration and aspiration; however, rigorous randomized trials comparing feeding sites are lacking. Poor differentiation between aspiration of oral secretions and aspiration of feedings may result in erroneously high rates for aspiration of feedings, especially jejunal feedings.

FORMULA SELECTION
Polymeric Formulas
Enteral formula selection is based on nutrient requirements, fluid restrictions, and the extent to which nutrient digestion and absorption is impaired. More than 100 enteral formulas are available commercially; yet, practitioners can meet the needs of most patients with only a few products on the formulary. Categorizing formulas into four "generic" groups and a few subgroups, as listed in Table 36-2, simplifies the formula selection process.

Polymeric formulas are the most common type of enteral formulas. The use of whole (i.e., intact) or partially hydrolyzed proteins requires that patients have full digestive capability for proteins. The carbohydrate sources and fats used in polymeric formulas also require full digestive function. Osmolality is decreased and palatability increased by the use of relatively intact nutrient sources. Administration of approximately 1.5 to 2 L of most polymeric formulas provides 100% of Dietary Reference Intakes (DRI) for vitamins and minerals. Because 100% of DRI are provided in a typical volume consumed daily, these formulas sometimes are called "complete" formulas. Polymeric formulas tend to be the least expensive enteral formulas, although prices may vary considerably based on specific nutrient content (e.g., omega-3 fatty

Table 36-2 Generic Groups and Subgroups of Enteral Formulas

Polymeric Formulas

Nutrient Source

Blenderized
Lactose free

Fiber Content

Fiber-free
Low to moderate fiber (1–8 g/L)
Moderate to high fiber (>8 g/L)

Caloric Density

Standard density (1–1.2 kcal/mL)
Moderate density (1.5 kcal/mL)
Calorically dense (2 kcal/mL)

Protein or Nitrogen Content

Low nitrogen (6–9% of kcal)
Standard nitrogen (11–15% of kcal)
High nitrogen (16–25% of kcal)

Oligomeric Formulas

Elemental
Peptide based

Specialized Formulas

Renal Failure

Essential amino acid enriched
Low protein and electrolytes

Hepatic Failure (BCAAs)

Stress/Critically Ill

Branched-chain enriched
High nitrogen plus conditionally essential nutrients
Immune modulating

Pulmonary Disease

Glucose Control

Modular Components

Carbohydrate
Protein
Fats

BCAAs, branched-chain amino acids.

Table 36-3 Relative Cost of Enteral Formulas[a]

Type of Formula	Relative Cost (dollars)
Polymeric Formulas	
Blenderized	3.6
Lactose free, standard caloric density, standard nitrogen content plus	
Fiber free[b]	1
Low to moderate fiber (1–8 g/L)	1.2
Moderate to high fiber (>8 g/L)	1.2
Lactose free, standard nitrogen content, fiber-free plus	
Standard caloric density (1–1.2 kcal/mL)[b]	1
Moderate density (1.5 kcal/mL)	1
Calorically dense (2 kcal/mL)	0.9
Lactose free, standard caloric density, fiber-free plus	
Low nitrogen (6–10% of kcal as protein); low electrolyte	3.9
Standard nitrogen (11–15% of kcal as protein)[b]	1
High nitrogen (16–25% of kcal as protein)	1.3
Oligomeric Formulas	
Elemental (free amino acids)	13.8
Peptide-based	13.5
Specialized Formulas	
Renal failure	
Essential amino acid enriched	15
Low protein and electrolytes	3.9
Hepatic failure (branched-chain amino acids)	25
Stress/critically ill	
Branched-chain enriched	22
High nitrogen plus conditionally essential nutrients	8.9
Immune modulating	24
Pulmonary disease	2.8
Glucose control	2.9

[a]Based on average cost per 1,000 calories for equivalent formulas on contract from 1998–2003.
[b]Index product; given a relative value of 1.

acids, fiber). Table 36-3 provides a relative cost summary for enteral formulas.

Nutrient Source

Polymeric formulas can be divided into blenderized and lactose-free formulations. *Blenderized* products are formulated from table foods that are processed and packaged to provide more consistent nutrient content and lower risk of bacterial contamination compared with foods blenderized in the home. These "natural" food formulas are generally reserved for patients with GI intolerance or allergic reactions to the more common semisynthetic formulas, although other interventions are often implemented before changing to a blenderized feeding. The high viscosity of blenderized formulas may require a large-bore feeding tube and use of an enteral infusion

pump. Other disadvantages include possible lactose content, higher cost than other polymeric formulas, and reluctance of some third-party payers to cover the cost of blenderized food. *Compleat* is a typical blenderized formula.

Most enteral products are *lactose-free,* and these formulas are the standard for tube-fed patients in most hospitals and nursing facilities owing to presumed lactose intolerance in many patients with serious injury or illness.[12] Reduced disaccharidase production during fasting, malnutrition, and various diseases of the GI tract contribute to lactose intolerance in hospitalized patients.[13] In addition, most ethnic groups, except those from northern Europe, tend to have reduced lactase production in adulthood, leading to lactose intolerance. Lactose may cause bloating, flatulence, abdominal cramps, and watery diarrhea in patients with permanent or transient lactose intolerance. Several formulas, such as Boost and Isocal HN Plus, contain milk protein concentrate with lactose removed; thus, they do not cause lactose intolerance. Lactose-free formulas leave little residue in the colon and their viscosity is low unless fiber is added.

Fiber Content

Fiber content provides a second criterion for subdividing polymeric formulas. Fiber has potential physiologic benefits including increased fecal bulk, decreased transit time in patients prone to constipation, increased transit time in patients with diarrhea, reduction of serum cholesterol, and improved glycemic control in patients with diabetes. *Fiber-supplemented formulas* generally contain 5 to 15 g of fiber per liter. Recommended fiber intake is 20 to 35 g/day, although actual intake appears to be half of this for the average American.[14,15]

Fiber is added to enteral formulas primarily to reduce the intestinal transit associated with fiber-free formulas.[16] Insoluble fiber is associated with changes in fecal bulk and transit time, whereas soluble fiber tends to be responsible for effects on cholesterol and glycemic control. Enteral formulas may contain one or more sources of fiber, as indicated in Table 36-4. Use of soluble fibers, such as pectin, psyllium, and certain gums, may be limited by their tendency to form gels; therefore, they are seldom used as a single fiber source.

The most common fiber source for enteral formulas is soy polysaccharide, or soy fiber, which provides benefits associated with both soluble and insoluble fibers. Soy polysaccharide contains approximately 75% dietary fiber, 6% of which is soluble fiber and 94% insoluble fiber.[17] Despite the low level of soluble fiber, soy polysaccharide lowers serum cholesterol levels and improves glycemic control.[18] As expected from its insoluble fiber content, soy polysaccharide increases fecal weight and water content in healthy subjects and noncritically ill patients.[19] However, studies do not provide clear evidence of improved bowel function in patients receiving fiber-supplemented enteral formulas, especially in critically ill patients.[17]

Given the current data, long-term stable tube feeding patients appear to be most likely to benefit from fiber-supplemented formulas. Some patients receiving short-term tube feeding who do not have GI pathology, experience altered stool consistency and may benefit from fiber supplementation. However, the effect of fiber on patients with bowel pathology is less clear.

Addition of fiber to enteral formulas creates some potential problems. Fiber tends to increase formula viscosity and fiber-containing formulas may require a pump for administration through a feeding tube. GI symptoms from fiber may include increased gas production and abdominal discomfort.[17] Gradual introduction of fiber may help reduce these symptoms. Bezoar formation also has been reported in a patient receiving fiber-containing tube feedings and medications that suppressed GI motility.[20] Caution is thus advised for the use of fiber-containing formulas in patients with poor GI motility or underlying GI dysfunction. Inadequate fluid intake may also contribute to the risk of bezoar formation and intestinal blockage with fiber.

Decreased mineral absorption from enteral formulas supplemented with fiber is a concern. Decreased folate, zinc, copper, and iron absorption has been reported with the addition of soy fiber to fiber-free formulas.[17] The clinical significance of reduced mineral absorption is questionable, however. Formulas generally contain minerals in excess of the DRI, and the effect of fiber on mineral balance appears to be mitigated by higher mineral content in the product.[21]

Fructo-oligosaccharides (FOS) are naturally occurring sugars that are added to some enteral formulas (e.g., Optimental, Jevity Plus). Glycosidic linkages between fructose units and glucose in the FOS are not split by GI enzymes but can be fermented to short-chain fatty acids by *Bifidobacterium* in the colon.[22] Soluble fibers also are fermented to short-chain fatty acids by bacteria in the colon.[17] Short-chain fatty acids stimulate colonic blood flow, enhance fluid and

Table 36-4 Fiber Sources for Selected Enteral Formulas

| Formula Name | Total Dietary Fiber (g/L) | Primarily Insoluble Fiber | | | | Primarily Soluble Fiber | | | | |
		Soy Fiber; Soy Polysaccharide	Cellulose Gum, Gel, or Microcrystalline	Oat Fiber	Gum Arabic	Acacia	Partially Hydrolyzed Guar Gum	Pectin	Fructooligo-saccharides
Advera	8.9	x							
Boost with fiber	11	x	x			x			
Choice dm Tube Feeding	14.4	x	x			x			
Complete	4.3								Fruits and vegetables
Diabetisource AC	10	x					x		Fruits and vegetables
Ensure fiber with FOS	12	x		x			x		x
FiberSource	10		x				x		
FiberSource HN	10						x		
Glucerna	14.4						x		
Glytrol	15	x			x			x	
Impact with fiber	10	x					x		
IsoSource VHN	10	x							
Jevity 1 Cal	14.4	x	x						
Jevity 1.5 Cal	22	x	x	x	x				x
NuBasics with fiber	14	x							
Nutren 1.0 with fiber	14	x							
ProBalance	10	x			x				
Promote with fiber	14.4	x		x					
Protain XL	9.1	x							
Replete with fiber	14	x							
ReSource Diabetic	12.8		x				x		
Ultracal	14.4	x	x						

electrolyte absorption, and provide a trophic effect in the colon, which may account for the association between soluble fibers and beneficial effects on colonocytes (e.g., regulation of cell growth and adhesion, including inhibition of neoplastic cell growth). Improvement in constipation has been noted with FOS administration; however, intake of >45 g/day may cause diarrhea.[23] The role of FOS in enteral formulas is not yet well defined, but FOS appear to offer the benefits of soluble fiber without the same physiochemical limitations.

Caloric Density

Caloric density is another method of subdividing polymeric enteral formulas. The standard caloric density is 1 to 1.2 kcal/mL. Moderate density formulas contain approximately 1.5 kcal/mL, and calorically dense formulas contain 2 kcal/mL. Increased caloric density reduces gastric emptying and increases formula osmolality, either of which may result in feeding intolerance.[24] GI intolerance (e.g., nausea, flatulence, abdominal discomfort) also may occur if the capacity of intestinal enzymes is overwhelmed by infusion of a calorically dense formula. The risk of dehydration increases with increasing caloric density. However, standard caloric density formulas may result in fluid overload in patients with congestive heart failure, renal failure, or other fluid-sensitive conditions.

Protein Content

The fourth method of subdividing polymeric formulas is on the basis of protein content, either as a percentage of calories from protein or as the nonprotein calorie:nitrogen ratio (NPC:N). Protein calories are related directly to nitrogen content because protein is about 16% nitrogen by weight. However, individual amino acids vary in nitrogen content, and the overall nitrogen in enteral formulas enriched with specific amino acids may vary from 13% to 20% of protein. Grams of protein multiplied by 4 equals protein calories, and grams of protein divided by 6.25 equals grams of nitrogen, assuming protein is 16% nitrogen. Protein needs increase disproportionately to caloric needs during injury and critical illness. High-nitrogen enteral formulas, designed to supply this increased protein requirement provide approximately 16% to 25% of calories from protein. The NPC:N ratios in these formulas range from 75:1 to 130:1. Standard protein content is 11% to 15% of calories, with NPC:N approximately 140:1 to 200:1. Low-nitrogen formulas with 6% to 9% of calories from protein and a ratio >250:1 are available for patients requiring protein restriction.

Oligomeric Formulas

Oligomeric formulas, also called *monomeric* or *chemically defined formulas,* require minimal digestive function and produce little residue in the colon. Pancreatic enzyme activity is required for digestion of oligosaccharides and fats. Brush-border disaccharidase activity also is required. However, little to no digestion is required for the hydrolyzed protein and medium-chain triglyceride components. These formulas may be used for patients with pancreatic insufficiency, reduced mucosal absorption, or reduced hydrolytic ability. Patients most likely to benefit from oligomeric formulas are those with severe pancreatic insufficiency or short bowel syndrome.[1] Pancreatic enzyme supplementation with a polymeric formula may be tried before an oligomeric formula for some patients with pancreatic insufficiency (e.g., cystic fibrosis).

Two subgroups of oligomeric formulas can be differentiated based on the protein source. True "elemental" formulas contain free amino acids, whereas "peptide-based" formulas contain oligopeptides plus dipeptides and tripeptides from hydrolysis of protein. Free amino acids also may be included in peptide-based formulas. Amino acids require no digestion, but the sodium-dependent active transport mechanism responsible for absorption appears to be somewhat slow and inefficient compared with small peptide absorption. Dipeptides and tripeptides are absorbed by specific carriers located in small bowel mucosa. Sodium is not required for the noncompetitive transport process associated with small peptides.[25] However, peptides longer than three amino acid units require further hydrolysis within the lumen of the small bowel before they are absorbed. Most peptide-based formulas contain a significant portion of peptides requiring hydrolysis before absorption.

Enteral diets high in peptides have been associated with an increase in serum albumin concentrations; however, the extent of peptide absorption in critically ill patients is unclear. Studies have reported no difference in occurrence of diarrhea between patients receiving intact protein and those receiving peptide-rich formulas.[26,27] Based on current data, it is difficult to know when a peptide-based formula should be selected rather than an elemental formula. Cost and fat content may be factors that help determine which type of oligomeric formula to select. Fat content varies from 1% to 30% of calories, with elemental formulas generally having the lowest fat content. Availability of a formula in ready-to-use form versus powder requiring reconstitution may also influence the choice of formula, especially for patients on home enteral nutrition where water sources and mixing techniques are a concern.

Elemental formulas (e.g., Tolerex, Vivonex T.E.N., Vivonex Plus) are available only in a powdered form. Dehydrated formulas limit the reaction between carbohydrates and free amino acids, and extend the shelf life. Peptide-based formulas, which have a lower free amino acid concentration than elemental formulas, may be available as a ready-to-use liquid or as a powder requiring reconstitution. Alitraq, Criticare HN, Crucial, Peptamen products, Perative, Reabilan, Reabilan HN, Peptinex DT, Subdue, and Vital HN are examples of formulas containing peptides.

Oligomeric formulas tend to be hypertonic due to their partially digested nature, although peptide-containing formulas tend to be only slightly hypertonic. Osmotic diarrhea may occur because of the hyperosmolality. Taste and cost also are disadvantages of these formulas. Although flavoring packets are available and new flavors with better patient acceptance have been developed in recent years, patients commonly complain of a bitter taste when these formulas are taken by mouth. In general, it is unrealistic to expect a patient to take more than a small percentage of their daily nutritional requirements by mouth as an oligomeric formula. As shown in Table 36-3, oligomeric formulas tend to cost several times more than polymeric formulas.

Specialized Formulas

Specialized formulas are designed for specific disease states or conditions. However, the use and clinical benefit of these products are controversial. The formulas generally have a good theoretical basis for use, but lack conclusive clinical evidence of improved efficacy compared with standard formulas. Well-designed studies showing a difference in outcome between specialized and standard enteral formulas providing equal nitrogen and equal calories are difficult to find. Given the high cost of most specialized formulas, it often is difficult to justify their use without evidence of improved clinical efficacy compared with standard formulas.

Renal Failure

Specialty enteral formulas designed for patients with renal failure contain either essential amino acids plus histidine or a higher-than-normal concentration of essential amino acids in combination with nonessential amino acids. Theoretically, recycling of urea nitrogen for nonessential amino acid synthesis reduces the accumulation of blood urea nitrogen (BUN).[28,29] Unfortunately, clinically significant recycling of nitrogen and incorporation into nonessential amino acids does not appear to occur. Essential amino acid formulas may be appropriate for chronic renal failure patients with glomerular filtration rates <25 mL/minute per 1.73 m^2 who are receiving very-low-protein diets and for whom dialysis is not an option.[1,28] They are not appropriate for patients in acute renal failure or for those receiving hemodialysis or peritoneal dialysis. The NPC:N is generally >300:1 in these formulas. Vitamin and mineral supplements appropriate to the patient's condition must be provided with essential amino acid formulas because the formulas themselves are incomplete. Some formulas require reconstitution with water before use. Renalcal contains higher-than-normal essential amino acids in combination with nonessential amino acids, whereas Amin-Aid contains essential amino acids plus histidine.

Polymeric enteral formulas designed for renal failure or renal insufficiency are the standard in many facilities. These formulas are not enriched with essential amino acids and use a lower NPC:N ratio (e.g., 140:1 or 160:1) than essential amino acid–enriched formulas. Furthermore, these formulas contain lower-than-normal concentrations of potassium, phosphorus, and magnesium, as well as a higher caloric concentration (2 kcal/mL) to minimize fluid and electrolyte problems. Polymeric enteral formulas meet 100% of the DRI with <2,000 mL/day. Examples of intact protein renal formulas include Magnacal Renal, Nepro, and NovaSource Renal.

Hepatic Failure

Hepatic failure formulas contain 45% to 50% of protein as branched-chain amino acids (BCAA), compared with 15% to 20% in standard formulas. These formulas also contain lower-than-normal concentrations of aromatic amino acids (AAA), especially phenylalanine. Theoretically, an increase in BCAA and a decrease in AAA improves hepatic encephalopathy by reducing inhibitory and/or false neurotransmitter formation.[28,29] Prospective, randomized, controlled trials that compare BCAA-enriched formulas with comparable enteral formulas with standard protein sources are limited. Most studies have not shown a clear advantage for hepatic failure formulas, especially with respect to mortality, and most patients with liver disease can receive formulas with standard protein sources.[1,28] Some of these formulas, such as Hepatic-Aid II, require supplementation with vitamins and minerals. Hepatic-

Aid II is a powdered formula requiring reconstitution before use, whereas NutriHep is a ready-to-use formula containing appropriate vitamin content for end-stage liver disease patients.

Stress/Critically Ill

Specialized *stress formulas* designed for critically ill, hypercatabolic patients generally contain a NPC:N ratio of <100:1 (i.e., a high nitrogen content) and >35% of the protein content of BCAA, without reduced AAA concentrations. Thus, stress and hepatic failure formulas are not therapeutically interchangeable. These stress formulas are based on the theory that since BCAA are used preferentially for energy production in skeletal muscle of critically ill patients, exogenous provision of BCAA will reduce skeletal muscle breakdown and improve protein synthesis.[28,29] Studies evaluating the effectiveness of BCAA in stressed patients have primarily involved parenterally administered BCAA, although results for both parenteral and enteral routes of administration are conflicting and controversial, with no significant improvement in clinical outcome, including morbidity and mortality.[1,28,29] Objective criteria for defining critical illness and determining entry into the studies may have contributed to the inconclusive and controversial results when these studies are viewed as a group.[30]

Enteral formulas having a NPC:N ratio of 125:1 or less, but without BCAA supplementation, are commonly marketed as stress or critical care formulas. Several of these formulas, as listed in Table 36-5, also contain arginine, glutamine, or nucleic acid supplementation and/or a modified fat component. Such formulas are often referred to as "immune-modulating" formulas due to proposed beneficial modulation of the biologic responses to stress. The use of immunonutrition in critically ill patients is a relatively recent development and studies are not conclusive for the role of these formulas. Table 36-6 summarizes the properties of each of the main immunonutrition substrates that are discussed below.

Arginine. Enhanced wound healing and immune function response to test antigens has been demonstrated with dietary arginine supplementation in normal volunteers, including elderly subjects.[31] Enhanced T-lymphocyte response and increased CD4 (clusters of differentiation) counts also have been reported.[32] Similar results for immune response plus improved nitrogen balance were reported in postoperative patients with cancer who were tube-fed with a formula containing supplemental arginine, nucleic acids, and omega-3 fatty acids.[33] However, effects of arginine on nitrogen balance remain inconclusive.[34] The efficacy of supplemental arginine to reduce wound infections, duration of hospitalization, and mortality in burn patients has been demonstrated.[35] The potential for enhanced immune function is exciting, but much investigation is needed before the safety and efficacy of arginine supplementation can be determined conclusively. Concerns remain regarding the possible metabolic effects when large doses of a specific amino acid are administered to critically ill patients. Arginine is a precursor of nitric oxide, a potent vasodilating agent. There is concern that arginine may enhance the systemic inflammatory response and increase the incidence of hypotension in septic patients.[36] This is of particular concern when patients already require vasopressor support to maintain blood pressure. The metabolic effects of administering the hydrochloride salt in which arginine is

Table 36-5   Selected High-Protein Enteral Formulas With Altered Protein and/or Fat Sources[a]

Formula (Manufacturer)	kcal/mL (mOsm/kg)	% Free Water	Protein g/L (% kcal)	NPC:N Ratio	Protein Source	ARG g/L	GLN g/L	Approx. % Protein as BCAAs
Advera (Ross)	1.28 (680)	80	60 (18.7)	108:1	Soy protein hydrolysate; sodium caseinate	4.1	5.4	15.5
AlitraQ (Ross)	1.0 (575)	85	52.5 (21)	94:1	Soy hydrolysate; whey; lactalbumin hydrolysate; free amino acids	4.5	15.5	18.5
Crucial (Nestle)	1.5 (490)	77	94 (25)	67:1	Hydrolyzed casein; L-arginine	15	7.2	17.6
Fibersource HN (Novartis)	1.2 (490)	81	53 (18)	115:1	Soy protein isolate and concentrate	2.0	5.9	20.9
Impact (Novartis)	1.0 (375)	85	56 (22)	71:1	Sodium and calcium caseinates; nucleic acids; L-arginine	12.5	5.9	17
Impact with fiber (Novartis)	1.0 (375)	85	56 (22)	71:1	Sodium and calcium caseinates; nucleic acids; L-arginine	12.5	5.9	17
Immune-Aid (McGaw)	1.0 (460)	82	80 (32)	53:1	Hydrolyzed lactalbumin; BCAAs; nucleic acids	15	12.5	36
IntensiCal (Mead Johnson)	1.3 (550)	80	81 (25)	75:1	Casein hydrolysate; L-arginine	6.5	NA	NA
Isocal HN Plus (Mead Johnson)	1.2 (390)	81	54 (18)	114:1	Milk protein concentrate	NA	NA	NA
IsoSource HN (Novartis)	1.2 (490)	82	53 (18)	115:1	Soy protein isolate	2.3	5.8	20.6
IsoSource 1.5 (Novartis)	1.5 (650)	78	68 (18)	113:1	Sodium and calcium caseinates	NA	NA	NA
IsoSource VHN (Novartis)	1.0 (300)	85	62 (25)	75:1	Sodium and calcium caseinates	NA	NA	NA
Jevity 1 Cal (Ross)	1.06 (300)	843	44 (16.7)	125:1	Sodium and calcium caseinates; soy protein isolates	1.5	4-5.8	19
Lipisorb Liquid (Mead Johnson)	1.35 (630)	80	57 (17)	125:1	Sodium and calcium caseinates	2.3	7.3	23
Optimental (Ross)	1.0 (540)	83.5	51 (20.5)	97:1	Soy protein hydrolysate; partially hydrolyzed sodium caseinate; free amino acids	5	NA	NA
Osmolite 1 Cal (Ross)	1.06 (300)	84	44 (16.7)	125:1	Sodium and calcium caseinates; soy protein isolates	1.7	NA	19
Osmolite 1.2 Cal (Ross)	1.2 (360)	82	55.5 (18.5)	110:1	Sodium and calcium caseinate	NA	NA	NA
Oxepa (Ross)	1.5 (493)	78.5	62.5 (16.7)	125:1	Sodium and calcium caseinates	NA	NA	NA
Peptamen VHP (Nestle)	1.0 (300)	84	62.5 (25)	75:1	Hydrolyzed whey	1.9	4.6	21
Peptinex DT (Novartis)	1.0 (460)	83	50 (20)	115:1	Casein hydrolysate; free amino acids	5	4.7	30
Perative (Ross)	1.3 (385)	79	66.6 (20.5)	97:1	Partially hydrolyzed sodium caseinate; lactalbumin hydrolysate; L-arginine	6.5	5.4	18
ProBalance (Nestle)	1.2 (350)	82	45 (18)	114:1	Calcium and potassium caseinates	2	4.6-6.9	21
Protain XL (Mead Johnson/ Sherwood)	1.0 (340)	83	57 (22)	85:1	Calcium and sodium caseinates	2	5.5	21
Replete (Nestle)	1.0 (350)	84	62.5 (25)	75:1	Calcium-potassium caseinate	2.4	5.4	21
Replete with fiber (Nestle)	1.0 (390)	84	62.5 (25)	75:1	Calcium-potassium caseinate	2.4	5.4	21
Subdue (Mead Johnson)	1.0 (330)	84	50 (20)	100:1	Hydrolyzed whey	NA	NA	NA
TraumaCal (Mead Johnson)	1.5 (560)	78	82 (22)	91:1	Sodium and calcium caseinates	NA	NA	NA
Ultracal HN Plus (Mead Johnson)	1.2 (370)	81	54 (18)	114:1	Milk protein concentrate	NA	NA	NA

Table 36-5   Selected High-Protein Enteral Formulas With Altered Protein and/or Fat Sources[a]—cont'd

Fat g/L (% kcal)	Fat Sources	% Fat kcal as MCT	% Fat as n-3 Fatty Acid (ratio of n-6 to n-3)	Fiber g/L	Carnitine mg/L	Taurine mg/L
22.8 (15.8)	Canola oil; MCT oil; sardine oil	20	5.4 (2.9:1)	8.9	127	212
15.5 (13)	MCT oil; safflower oil	53	10 (4.2:1)	None	100	200
67.5 (39)	Soybean oil; MCT oil; fish oil; lecithin	50	6 (2:1)	None	150	150
39 (29)	Canola oil; MCT oil	50	4.4 (2.4:1)	10	None	None
28 (25)	Palm kernel oil (MCT); sunflower oil; menhaden oil	27	6.5 (1.4:1)	None	None	None
28 (25)	Palm kernel oil (MCT); sunflower oil; menhaden oil	27	6.5 (1.4:1)	10	None	None
22 (20)	Canola oil; MCT	50	5.5 (1.8:1)	None	200	100
42	Canola oil; MCT oil; high-oleic safflower; corn oil; menhaden oil	25	5 (3.4:1)	None	160	160
40 (29)	Canola oil; MCT oil; high-oleic sunflower oil; corn oil	NA	NA	None	150	150
39 (29)	Canola oil; MCT oil	50	4.4 (2.4:1)	None	None	None
65 (38)	Canola oil; MCT oil; soybean oil	NA	NA	8	110	110
29 (25)	Canola oil; MCT oil	50	4.4 (2.4:1)	10	80	80
35 (29)	High-oleic safflower oil; canola oil; MCT oil; lecithin	20	3.3 (4.2:1)	14	115	115
57 (35)	Soy oil; MCT oil	85	<1 (±8:1)	None	194	194
28 (25)	Structured lipid with sardine oil (EPA, DHA) and MCT; canola oil, soy oil	28	NA	6 (FOS)	110	110
35 (29)	High-oleic safflower oil; canola oil; MCT oil; lecithin	20	3.0 (5:1)	None	115	115
39 (29)	High-oleic safflower oil; canola oil; MCT oil; lecithin	19	NA (5:1)	None	115	115
94 (55)	Canola oil; MCT oil; sardine oil; borage oil	25	NA	None	181	316
39 (33)	MCT oil; soybean oil	70	NA (8:1)	None	100	100
17 (15)	MCT oil; soybean oil; lecithin	NA	NA	None	100	200
37.4 (25)	Canola oil; MCT oil; corn oil	40	4.5 (4.7:1)	None	140	140
34 (30)	Canola oil; MCT oil; corn oil; lecithin	20	5.5 (4:1)	8.3	83	83
30 (26)	Canola oil; high oleic sunflower oil; MCT oil; corn oil	20	NA (4.8:1)	9.1	150	150
34 (30)	Canola oil; MCT oil; lecithin	25	6.6 (3:1)	None	100	100
34 (30)	Canola oil; MCT oil; lecithin	25	6.6 (3:1)	14	100	100
34 (30)	MCT oil; canola oil; high-oleic sunflower oil; corn oil	50	NA	None	80	101
68 (40)	Soy oil; MCT oil	NA	NA	None	NA	NA
40 (29)	Canola oil; MCT oil; high-oleic sunflower oil; corn oil	NA	NA	10	150	150

ARG, arginine; BCAAs, branched-chain amino acids; DHA, docosahexaenoic acid; EPA, eicosapentaenoic acid; GLN, glutamine; HN, high nitrogen; MCT, medium-chain triglycerides; NA, not available; NPC:N, nonprotein calorie to nitrogen; n-3FA, omega-3 fatty acids; n-6FA, omega-6 fatty acids; VHP, very high protein; VHN, very high nitrogen.
[a]Changes periodically occur in nutrient sources and/or content; therefore, this table should be used as a general reference only and not for specific patient care issues.

Table 36-6   Role of Immunonutrients

Substrate	Role in Normal Health	Postulated Role in Critical Illness
Arginine (amino acid)	Synthesized by urea cycle during detoxification of ammonia Nonessential, since normally available in sufficient quantities for growth and tissue repair	Endogenous synthesis may become inadequate in metabolic stress Decreased arginine concentrations may result in reduced cellular growth and lymphocyte blastogenesis.
Nucleic acids (components of DNA and RNA, adenosine triphosphate [ATP], and multiple coenzymes)	Not usual component of non–immune-modulating enteral formulations	Maintenance of cellular immune function in metabolic stress
Glutamine (amino acid)	Intermediate in numerous metabolic pathways including gluconeogensis and renal ammonia-genesis Primary fuel source for epithelial cells, actively dividing lymphocytes, and enterocytes	Aids maintenance of intestinal mucosal integrity and may prevent bacterial translocation
Omega-3 fatty acids (primarily as eicosapentaenoic acid [EPA], docosahexa-enoic acid [DHA])	Present in fish oils, these are precursors to "3" series prostaglandins, prostacyclins, and thromboxanes, and to "5 series leukotrienes Less inflammatory and more vasodilatory than compounds from omega-6 fatty acids	Some evidence of decreased mortality and infection rates in selected patient populations; however, there is evidence of harm in other patients. Safety and efficacy are still to be determined.

provided also must be evaluated carefully, especially in patients at risk of acidosis from their illness.

Nucleic acids, or *nucleotides.* Animals fed nucleotide-free diets demonstrate reduced cellular immunity and increased susceptibility to bacterial challenges as compared with animals receiving a nucleotide-supplemented diet.[29] Other studies have not noted a beneficial effect of oral nucleoside-nucleotide mixtures on animal survival after intravenous (IV) bacterial challenge.[37] Studies to confirm these observations in humans are lacking.

Glutamine. Improved healing of radiation-induced small bowel lesions and prevention of pancreatic atrophy and fatty liver during enteral feeding has been shown with glutamine supplementation.[38,39] Improved nitrogen retention also has been demonstrated with parenteral glutamine supplementation following surgery and bone marrow transplantation.[40–42] However, study results are controversial and conflicting; thus, the role of glutamine in maintaining GI tract integrity and preventing bacterial translocation in humans is unclear and the benefit of enteral glutamine is uncertain, especially for critically ill patients.[43–45] As with arginine, the potential of glutamine is exciting, but further research is needed to better define potential risks (e.g., increased serum ammonia) from supplemental glutamine. Despite this, glutamine supplementation is widely used, often without adequate monitoring for potential complications.

Protein-bound glutamine is present in all enteral formulas. However, only powdered formulas contain supplemental free glutamine because of glutamine stability problems in ready-to-use formulas. Glutamine content in enteral formulas ranges from approximately 5% to 13% of protein by weight.[46] The source of protein, processing, and protein concentration influence the glutamine content of formulas. Additional research is needed to determine whether physiologic effects, especially effects on the GI tract and ammoniagenesis, are equivalent for protein-bound and free glutamine.

The potential for glutamate to substitute for glutamine with respect to maintenance of GI integrity is of interest. Like glutamine, glutamate is an amino acid that functions in transamination and nitrogen homeostasis. Dietary glutamate is well absorbed and highly catabolized by enterocytes.[47] Catabolism of glutamate produces less ammonia than catabolism of glutamine, an advantage from the waste-disposal standpoint. Glutamate has the advantage of being stable in water, a limiting factor for glutamine incorporation into ready-to-use enteral formulas. Available data are inadequate to conclude that glutamate can maintain GI integrity in humans, although it does appear to maintain GI tract integrity in some species.[48]

Alteration in the fat component of enteral formulas. Stress or critical care and immune-modulating formulas contain different sources of fat to alter the type of fatty acids provided. Medium-chain triglycerides commonly are included as a fat source, along with long-chain fatty acids. Canola oil, high oleic oils, or fish oils are used as a source of long-chain fatty acids in these formulas, whereas the usual polyunsaturated vegetable oils (i.e., corn, soy, and safflower oils) are avoided or provided in relatively small quantities. Polyunsaturated vegetable oils contain fatty acids from the omega-6 family, which are precursors to arachidonic acid and therefore to dienoic or "2" series prostaglandins, prostacyclins, and thromboxanes, and to "4" series leukotrienes. These compounds, taken as a whole, are potent inflammatory, vasoconstrictive, and platelet-aggregating agents. High concentrations of prostaglandin E_2 appear to suppress lymphocyte function thereby creating immunosuppressive effects.[49,50]

Fish oils, including menhaden oil, provide fatty acids primarily from the omega-3 family, with eicosapentaenoic acid (EPA) and docosahexanoic acid (DHA) predominating. These compounds are precursors to "3" series prostaglandins, prostacyclins, and thromboxanes, and to "5" series leukotrienes. These compounds generally are less inflammatory and more vasodilatory than compounds from omega-6 fatty acids. This may be beneficial in critically ill patients but few data are available that evaluate effects of only fat modification. Animal studies suggest that survival following endotoxin challenge is increased with a combination of omega-6 and omega-3 fatty acids (e.g., polyunsaturated vegetable oils and fish oils) than with either type of fatty acid alone.[51] Studies in humans have focused primarily on burn patients, where decreased wound infections and reduced mortality have been demonstrated with low-fat diets containing 50% of fat as fish oil.[35]

Further research is needed to determine the safety and efficacy of omega-3 fatty acids in various disease states. The effect of omega-3 fatty acids on antioxidant levels, especially vitamin E, and the need for supplementation needs to be studied. Appropriate quantities of omega-3 fatty acids and the most beneficial ratios of omega-3 and omega-6 fatty acids also must be determined before routine supplementation with omega-3 fatty acids can be recommended beyond modifying the diet to include foods rich in omega-3 fatty acids (i.e., fish such as salmon).

Canola oil and high oleic oils are other fat sources used in enteral formulas. These oils are common in standard formulas, as well as those for stress and critical illness. Canola oil contains approximately two-thirds monounsaturated fatty acids, compared with no more than one-fourth monounsaturated fatty acids in polyunsaturated vegetable oils. High-oleic safflower and sunflower oils also contain increased monounsaturated fatty acid content. Monounsaturated fatty acids have been popularized by reports of low cardiovascular disease in populations using olive oil, but further research is needed to determine the safety and efficacy of these fatty acids in patients requiring nutrition support. The combination of canola oil and high-oleic oil also increases the content of linolenic acid, an essential fatty acid.

Medium-chain triglycerides (MCTs) are included in enteral formulas to improve fat absorption. Absorption of MCTs is relatively independent of pancreatic enzymes and bile salts; thus, MCTs may be absorbed in patients experiencing malabsorption of the long-chain triglycerides found in polyunsaturated vegetable oils. Rapid, carnitine-independent metabolism occurs with MCTs, whereas long-chain triglycerides require carnitine for metabolism. Therefore, use of long-chain triglycerides is compromised when carnitine deficiency occurs, but MCT metabolism is unaffected. Many enteral formulas contain part of the fat calories as MCTs. Formulas containing a relatively large percentage of fat calories as MCTs are frequently marketed for critically ill patients with malabsorption. Examples of formulas containing 50% to 65% of fat calories as MCTs include Alitraq, Crucial, Fibersource products, Immun-Aid, IsoSource products, Nutren 1.5, Reabilan products, and Subdue. Products containing 65% to 80% of fat calories as MCTs include Nutren 2.0, NutriHep, Peptamen products, and Renalcal. Portagen and Lipisorb, liquid and powder, contain over 85% of fat calories as MCTs.

Carnitine. An important compound in normal nutrition, carnitine is required for transport of long-chain triglycerides into the mitochondria for metabolism and export of acyl-CoA compounds out of the mitochondria. The normal diet provides low but adequate amounts of carnitine. Hypermetabolism, malnutrition, and administration of carnitine-free enteral or parenteral nutrient formulations can predispose patients to developing carnitine deficiency.[52,53] Therefore, carnitine is considered a conditionally essential nutrient. The suggested safe and effective amount of carnitine supplementation in adult enteral formulas is currently 185 mg/day; however, the optimal dose of carnitine in various situations needs further study.[53] Most enteral formulas contain carnitine.

Taurine. A sulfur-containing amino acid, taurine may improve fat absorption in patients with malabsorption. Micelle formation may be reduced when taurine intake is low or synthesis may be reduced because taurine is needed to form bile salts.[54] Studies of patients with cystic fibrosis given taurine supplements have shown improved fat absorption and weight gain.[55] Taurine also is essential for normal neuronal and retinal development in infants and children.[54] Therefore, major manufacturers of pediatric formulas include taurine as an essential nutrient in their formulas. Taurine is considered conditionally essential for adults. The small amounts found in the diet are adequate under normal situations. However, with catabolic illness such as cancer, chemotherapy, radiation, burns, and operative injury, low plasma and urinary taurine levels suggest inadequate intake.[56,57] Manufacturers of adult enteral formulas generally add taurine to formulas marketed for populations who may be at risk of inadequate taurine intake (e.g., formulas for stress and critical illness).

The results of clinical trials examining the effects of immune-modulating enteral formulations on mortality, hospital and intensive care unit length of stay, incidence of nosocomial infection, duration of mechanical ventilation, and GI complications are conflicting.[43,58–64] Differences in study design, patient population, enteral formulation, time to enteral nutrition commencement, and volume of formula received, make it difficult to reliably compare study results. Meta-analyses of the major studies reveal that certain subsets of patients may benefit from immunonutrition, whereas other subgroups may exhibit increased mortality; none shows a reduction in mortality.[65–68] Risk of nosocomial pneumonia does not appear to be reduced either for the studies as a whole or for the subgroup with patients undergoing surgery for GI cancer.[65] In fact, there is some indication that patients with pneumonia who receive arginine, omega-3 fatty acids, and antioxidant-supplemented feeding may be at increased risk for death.[69] Elective surgical patients appear to be most likely to benefit from immunonutrition, with significant reductions in infectious complications and lower hospital length of stay without mortality effect.[65–67]

Further research is needed to examine this controversial area of nutrition. There is a need to define which patients will benefit from immunonutrition, and the optimal enteral formulation for different patient subgroups. Until such information is available, the immune-modulating formulas must be used with caution and should not be used without careful evaluation of each individual patient.

Pulmonary Disease

The percentage of calories from fat is relatively high (40% to 55%) in formulas marketed for patients with pulmonary disease. The higher fat content is based on the premise that fat oxidation produces less carbon dioxide (CO_2) than carbohydrate oxidation, thereby reducing the work load of the lungs. Fats, particularly long-chain triglycerides, have a lower respiratory quotient (RQ) than carbohydrates. This means less CO_2 is produced per volume of oxygen consumed during fat metabolism. Studies comparing high-fat, low-carbohydrate diets with lower fat diets have shown improved respiratory parameters in ambulatory patients with chronic obstructive pulmonary disease (COPD) as well as reduced time on the ventilator and decreased arterial CO_2 concentrations in mechanically ventilated patients.[70,71] However, these effects do not demonstrate improved clinical outcomes and are unlikely to be seen in patients without excess CO_2 production and/or retention. In addition, overfeeding is more likely to be associated with excess CO_2 production than is the caloric source.[72] Delayed gastric emptying occurs with a high-fat diet, and this must be considered when evaluating the possible benefits and adverse effects of high-fat enteral formulas. Abdominal distention, increased gastric residuals, nausea, and vomiting may result from delayed gastric emptying. Delivery of the high-fat load, especially the long-chain triglycerides, into the small bowel may overwhelm pancreatic lipase activity in some patients, leading to fat malabsorption. Formulas typically classified as pulmonary formulas include NovaSource Pulmonary, NutriVent, Oxepa, Pulmocare, and Respalor.

Glucose Control

Formulas designed for patients with hyperglycemia contain between 40% and 50% of calories from fat, which is higher than the 30% of calories from fat recommended by the American Diabetes Association.[73] Some studies have demonstrated better glucose control after feeding with low-carbohydrate, high-fat, fiber-containing formulas compared with standard formulas in ambulatory patients with diabetes mellitus.[74] However, patients with stress-induced hyperglycemia have not been adequately evaluated. In addition, more recent data do not indicate a beneficial effect of such formulas on glucose control.[75] Fiber sources associated with improved glycemic control, mainly soluble fibers but also the primarily insoluble fiber of soy polysaccharide, are included in these formulas to help minimize postprandial hyperglycemia.[16] The amount of fiber provided in the volume of formula to meet 100% of the DRI falls short of the recommended fiber intake of 20 to 35 g daily in half of the formulas.[14,15] Problems with delayed gastric emptying or fat malabsorption must be weighed against possible benefits of improved glucose control when evaluating formulas for patients with diabetes mellitus. While the data supporting improved clinical outcomes with special enteral formulas marketed for patients with diabetes mellitus are limited, intensive glycemic control in critically ill patients improves outcomes.[76] Clearly, treatment goals for tube feeding patients with diabetes mellitus should include individualization of macronutrient composition, avoidance of excess calories, and maintenance of euglycemia.[1]

Modular Components

Modular components are individual nutrient substrates designed for addition to oral diets or enteral formulas. Modules allow a single macronutrient to be increased in a diet or formula without changing other components. Vitamins and minerals are not included in modular components. When major changes in nutrient ratios are needed, a formula that better meets the patient's requirements should be selected rather than adding large quantities of modular components. Formula viscosity and texture may be altered when modules are added in large quantities.

Glucose polymers are used for carbohydrate modules. These do not increase the osmolality and do not alter the flavor of foods or formulas. Powdered carbohydrate modules contain 20 to 30 kcal/tablespoon, whereas liquids contain 2 kcal/mL. The protein modules are powders containing 3 to 4 g protein/tablespoon. Most protein modules are intact protein. A fat module containing a safflower oil emulsion is available and provides 4.5 kcal/mL. MCT oil is also available as a fat module. Vegetable oils also can be added to formulas in small quantities as a modular component, but are not marketed as such and can separate from formulas because these oils are not emulsified.

TUBE-FEEDING ADMINISTRATION REGIMEN

The route of feeding, formula selected, and anticipated duration of feeding influence the administration regimen. The location of the patient (e.g., hospital, nursing facility, home) and cost should be considered in developing an administration regimen. The administration regimen includes the schedule for formula delivery, the strength or concentration of formula for initiating and advancing the feedings, and the administration method (i.e., syringe, gravity drip, pump). Limited scientific data exist regarding tube feeding administration regimens. Thus, many different administration schedules are used in various settings, all of which appear to meet the needs of the patients and personnel.

Four basic schedules for formula delivery are available: continuous infusion, cyclic infusion, intermittent infusion, and bolus delivery of formula. *Continuous infusion* provides the daily volume of formula at a continuous rate over 24 hours per day. In contrast, *cyclic infusion* provides the daily volume of formula at a continuous rate for only several hours of the day or night. *Intermittent infusion* provides the daily volume of formula in a specified number of feedings daily. Each of three to six daily feedings is administered over 30 to 60 minutes via gravity drip or infusion pump. *Bolus delivery* is similar to intermittent infusion except that each feeding is administered via a syringe, usually over 15 to 20 minutes.

Continuous Infusion

Continuous infusion can be used for feeding by any route. Intragastric continuous infusion schedules most commonly are used for hospitalized patients, although small bowel feeding may be more common in certain settings (e.g., intensive care units).[5,9] Risks of gastric distention and aspiration appear to be lower with continuous infusion compared with intermittent formula delivery into the stomach.[77-80] In addition, continuous infusion may be better tolerated as judged by stool frequency and time to attain full nutrition support, especially in the elderly and metabolically unstable patients.[77] Feeding into the duodenum or jejunum is best initiated with a continuous infusion schedule. Rapid infusion of large volumes of formula into the small bowel may result in symptoms consistent with a dumping syndrome, including sweating, lightheadedness, abdominal distention, cramping, hyperperistalsis, and watery diarrhea. However, with time the jejunum appears to adapt to larger volumes of feeding over a shorter period of time and may tolerate a cyclic schedule or longer intermittent infusions.

Cyclic Feeding

Cyclic feeding most commonly is used for patients who need supplemental nutrition because of an inability to consume adequate oral nutrients. The infusion typically is over 10 to 15 hours at night to minimize interference with oral intake during the day. Full nutrition support is often provided by cyclic enteral nutrition at night to avoid interfering with normal activities such as work or school. However, formula volume and osmolality may limit tolerance to cyclic feedings. Full nutrition support via cyclic jejunal feedings is the most difficult to achieve, and the transition from continuous infusion to cyclic infusion should be done over several days.

Intermittent or Bolus Feedings

The reservoir capacity of the stomach allows relatively large-volume feedings to be administered using an *intermittent* or *bolus schedule.* These schedules are more physiologic than continuous feeding. They also are more convenient for patients in nursing facilities and for ambulatory patients receiving enteral feedings at home. Patients frequently start on continuous infusion feedings, then transition to intermittent infusion, and eventually to the shorter administration time of bolus feedings. However, most patients need feedings over at least 15 minutes to avoid bloating, cramping, nausea, and diarrhea.[77] A rate of <60 mL/minute is suggested to minimize symptoms of GI intolerance in patients receiving bolus feedings.[81]

Initiation of Feedings

The rate and strength, or concentration, of formula used for initiating tube feeding primarily depends on the osmolality of full-strength formula, the site of feeding, and the condition of the patient's GI tract. Diluted formula and a low infusion rate were standard for initiation of intragastric tube feedings in the past and still are used in some institutions. These "starter regimens" are based on the belief that administration of full-strength formula or a large formula volume during the first few days of feeding will result in diarrhea, cramping, bloating, and/or nausea because the GI tract has not yet adapted to the formula osmolality and volume.[77] However, controlled studies have shown that diluting polymeric formulas is not necessary in patients or subjects with normal GI function fed by continuous infusion into the stomach or duodenum.[77,81] Dilution to a very low osmolality delays delivery of adequate nutrients without significantly affecting the incidence of GI intolerance. Dilution of chemically defined and elemental formulas also appears to be unnecessary. However, rapid infusion of formula may increase the incidence of nausea, cramping, and abdominal discomfort. For intermittent feeding, a rate of 200 mL to 300 mL over 30 to 60 minutes every 4 to 6 hours is generally tolerated; bolus feedings are better tolerated when the rate is <60 mL/minute.[81] For patients with abnormal GI function, it may be preferable to start intragastric feedings with the formula at an osmolality of approximately 300 mOsm/kg and/or at a rate of no more than 50 mL/hr.

Feedings into the small bowel are initiated at 10 to 40 mL/hr, with rate increases of 10 to 25 mL/hr every 8 to 24 hours until the goal rate is reached.[81,82] Isotonic formulas can be started at 30 to 40 mL/hr; hypertonic formulas may require a slower rate.[77,81] Changing the rate by 25 mL/hr every 8 hours allows a relatively quick transition to full nutrition support. When a hypertonic formula is diluted to an isotonic strength, usually half-strength, for initiation of feedings, the strength is

increased after the goal rate of infusion is achieved. A general rule for enteral feedings is not to increase both strength and rate at the same time.

MONITORING ENTERAL FEEDING

Appropriate monitoring of patients receiving enteral feeding via tube is essential to recognize and prevent tube feeding complications. Complications can be divided into three groups: mechanical, GI, and metabolic (Table 36-7).

Mechanical Complications

Mechanical complications often can be avoided with good nursing technique and careful observation of feeding tolerance. Frequent assessment of tube placement by auscultation, location of markings on the tube, and/or withdrawal of gastric contents is important in preventing pulmonary aspiration of feeding formula. Tube placement should be evaluated at least daily in patients receiving continuous feeding, or before each intermittent feeding.[81,83] Withdrawal of gastric contents through the feeding tube using a syringe allows both confirmation of tube placement and evaluation of volume in the stomach (gastric residual volume [GRV]). High GRV has been assumed to increase the risk of esophageal reflux and pulmonary aspiration. However, one review suggests GRV does not correlate with risk of gastroesophageal reflux or aspiration. These authors conclude feedings should not be interrupted for GRV <400 to 500 mL unless volumes are persistently high or a trend of rising GRV is evident.[84] Nonetheless, many institutions hold feedings for GRV above 200 mL. Evaluation of GRV every 4 to 6 hours in patients receiving intragastric feeding allows GRV trends to be monitored. However, soft, small-bore feeding tubes may collapse when GRV is checked, preventing accurate determination of the gastric residual. Residuals are not checked through a tube placed into the small bowel because of problems with tube collapse and because the small bowel does not serve as a reservoir for residual volume. If the patient has an NG tube in addition to a feeding tube in the small bowel, GRV may be checked through the NG tube to ensure that formula is not "backing-up" into the stomach. Back-up of formula also is evaluated by adding coloring to the enteral formula. Traditionally, methylene blue, blue food coloring, or sterile coloring have been used for this purpose. Appearance of the coloring in tracheal or bronchial aspirates indicated formula regurgitation into the esophagus or airway. Tube feedings were then held until the safety of feedings could be evaluated. Unfortunately, recent reports of mortality associated with the dyes bring the routine addition of coloring to enteral formulas into question.[80,85,86] Postpyloric tube placement generally is recommended if a patient has experienced aspiration. Elevating the head of the bed 30 to 45 degrees during and after feedings also is recommended to reduce the frequency and severity of aspiration.[80,87]

Gastrointestinal Complications

GI complications frequently occur with tube feeding. Diarrhea is one of the most difficult problems for nurses, patients, and caregivers to deal with. Predisposing illnesses, including diabetes mellitus, GI infections, and malabsorption syndromes, are more likely to cause diarrhea in patients receiving

Table 36-7 Complications of Tube Feeding

Complication	Cause/Contributing Factor	Treatment/Prevention
Mechanical Complications		
Aspiration	Deflated tracheostomy cuff	Inflate trach cuff before feeding; keep inflated 1 hr after feeding; consider small-bore feeding tube placed past the ligament of Treitz (into jejunum)
	Displaced feeding tube	Reinsert tube and check placement; consider hand restraints or feeding tube bridle
	Reduced gastric emptying	Check residuals Q 4–6 hr for gastric tube; raise head of bed at least 30 degrees; change to formula with lower fat content; try a medication to stimulate gastric emptying; place feeding tube into small bowel
	Lack of gag reflex; coma	Place feeding tube into small bowel beyond pylorus and ligament of Treitz (into jejunum), keep head of bed elevated to >30 degrees if possible, provide continuous feeding
Nasal or pharyngeal irritation or necrosis; esophageal erosion; otitis media	Large-bore, polyvinyl chloride tube for long periods of time	Reposition tube daily and change tape; use smaller-bore feeding tube; position tube to avoid pressure on tissues; moisten mouth and nose several times daily
Tube obstruction	Poorly crushed medications	Crush medications thoroughly and dissolve in water; use liquid medications whenever possible; check compatibility of medication with tube and formula
	Inadequate flushing after medications or thick formula	Flush tube with 50–150 mL water after medications or thick formula and Q 8 hr with 20 mL minimum
	Poorly dissolved or mixed formula	Use a blender to mix formula (check manufacturer's guidelines for mixing); check for formula clumping as poured into container for administration
	Formula mixed with low pH substance	Avoid checking gastric residuals through small-diameter feeding tubes; use the larger-diameter nasogastric tubes for checking residuals; avoid administering acidic pharmaceutic products through small-diameter feeding tubes; consider a nonacidic therapeutic alternative; flush the tube with a minimum of 30 mL water before and after administration if the acidic product must be given
Metabolic Complications		
Hyperglycemia, glycosuria (can lead to dehydration, coma, or death)	Stress response	Monitor fingerstick glucose Q 6 hr and have sliding scale insulin ordered
	High-carbohydrate formula (e.g., elemental)	
	Drug therapy (steroids)	Monitor intake and output accurately
	Diabetes mellitus	
Excess CO_2 production (high RQ)	High percentage of carbohydrate calories or excess calories from any source	Increase fat calories and/or reduce total calories
Hyponatremia	Dilutional (fluid excess, SIADH); inadequate sodium intake; excess GI losses	Use full-strength formula or change to concentrated formula with 1.5–2 kcal/mL; add salt to the tube feeding (1 tsp = 2 g Na = 90 mEq); use diuretics if appropriate; replace GI losses
Hypernatremia	Inadequate free water intake	Use diluted formula or change to 1 kcal/mL formula; monitor intake and output accurately; temperature and weight daily
	Excess water losses (diabetes insipidus; osmotic diuresis from hyperglycemia; fever)	Correct hyperglycemia and the underlying cause of fever or diabetes insipidus
Hypokalemia	Medications (diuretics, antipseudomonal penicillins, amphotericin B)	Monitor serum potassium carefully; give PO or IV potassium replacement PRN
	Intracellular/extracellular shifts (insulin therapy, acidosis)	Correct underlying problem
	Excess GI losses (NG suction, small bowel fistula, diarrhea)	
Hyperkalemia	Potassium-sparing medications (triamterene, amiloride, spironolactone, ACE inhibitors); potassium-containing medications (penicillin G potassium)	Monitor serum potassium carefully; change to medications that do not have a potassium-sparing effect or that are not potassium salts
	Renal failure	Monitor renal function; change to formula with lower potassium content
Hypercoagulability	Warfarin antagonism due to high vitamin K content of formula	Change to formula with lower vitamin K content; monitor coagulation status

ACE, angiotensin-converting enzyme; NG, nasogastric; RQ, respiratory quotient; SIADH, syndrome of inappropriate antidiuretic hormone secretion.

tube feedings than the enteral formula.[88] GI infections related to the enteral formula are a problem in tube feeding–associated diarrhea. Formulas are commercially sterile (contain no known *pathogenic* organisms) at the time of manufacture. However, once the can/package is opened contamination with pathogens may occur from water used for reconstitution or dilution, transfer to the delivery bag, formula kept in the delivery bag for a prolonged period, or poorly cleaned feeding bags or administration sets. Concurrent drug therapy is another major contributor to diarrhea in tube-fed patients.[89]

Metabolic Complications

Metabolic complications of tube feedings include hyperglycemia, electrolyte abnormalities, and fluid imbalance. Regular biochemical determinations similar to those used for parenteral nutrition are recommended to identify developing metabolic abnormalities and to allow correction before severe abnormalities occur. Baseline values for serum glucose, creatinine, BUN, and electrolytes should be available to guide selection of the enteral formula. Fingerstick glucose measurements every 6 hours may be ordered at the start of tube feeding in patients at risk for hyperglycemia, or when hyperglycemia is noted on serum glucose in other cases. After tube feeding is initiated, serum glucose, sodium (Na), potassium (K), chloride (Cl), and bicarbonate should be determined daily for at least 4 to 5 days in hospitalized patients. The frequency of monitoring is then decreased to once or twice weekly in stable hospitalized patients, but continued daily or every other day in critically ill patients. Patients discharged to home or a nursing facility before the tube feeding goal is reached should have serum glucose and electrolytes determined two to three times during the first week of therapy, then weekly for 2 to 3 weeks in stable patients with the feeding at goal rate. Serum creatinine (SrCr) and BUN are determined daily for a few days in critically ill patients, then by the same schedule as electrolytes. These laboratory values may be needed only two to three times in the first week, then weekly in relatively stable hospitalized patients.

The monitoring schedule for SrCr, BUN, calcium, phosphorus, and magnesium for patients in a nursing facility or at home is the same as for electrolytes. For hospitalized patients, calcium, phosphorus, and magnesium are determined two to three times during the first week, then once weekly if the patient is stable on tube feeding. Nutrition monitoring also is recommended, including serum albumin and prealbumin or transferrin weekly while the patient is hospitalized. For patients receiving long-term enteral feedings, laboratory monitoring gradually is decreased from the initial monitoring schedule. Laboratory monitoring should be done at least yearly in stable patients without significant medical problems. Patients with medical problems that may affect nutrient, electrolyte, or trace element requirements or tolerances should be monitored as appropriate to the medical condition.

Weight and fluid status are important parameters to monitor throughout enteral feeding therapy. For hospitalized patients, weight is primarily a reflection of fluid status. However, for long-term patients, weight is an important parameter for adequacy of caloric intake. Consistent increases or decreases from the prescribed enteral formula volume can have significant effects on weight. For example, a weight loss of approximately 12.5 pounds over a year is expected when daily formula intake of a 1-kcal/mL formula is 120 mL less than prescribed.

Fluid status must be monitored closely in patients receiving tube feeding, especially those with unusual losses or inability to recognize thirst and/or voluntarily adjust oral fluid intake. Enteral formula contains solutes, as well as water. Only the free water portion of a formula contributes toward meeting fluid requirements. The free water content of enteral formulas ranges from approximately 80% to 85% for standard caloric density formulas, and from approximately 65% to 80% for calorically dense formulas. Manufacturers generally list free water content of formulas on packages.

Water used in irrigating, or flushing, the feeding tube may contribute a significant volume of fluid daily. Tube patency is maintained by flushing the tube with fluid every 4 to 8 hours for continuous feedings or before and after each intermittent feeding. Between 20 and 60 mL of water generally is used for each flush. The tube also should be flushed before and after administering each medication through the tube. For patients with signs of fluid overload, the flush volume should be reduced to 20 to 30 mL, and the number of flushes should be kept to a minimum. Patients requiring more daily fluid may benefit from increased flush volume or number of flushes or both.

MEDICATIONS AND ENTERAL NUTRITION BY TUBE

Patients receiving nutrition through feeding tubes often receive medications through the same tube. Feeding tube occlusion, adverse effects due to changes in pharmaceutical dosage forms, and alteration of medication pharmacokinetics and pharmacodynamics are among the problems that may arise. There are also potential interactions related to the pharmacologic or physiologic effects of medications or enteral nutrients. For this reason, oral medication administration should be considered unless a strict "nothing by mouth" status is required.

The incidence of feeding tube occlusion is 6% to 38%.[83,89] Pump malfunction, lack of periodic tube flushing, formula characteristics, and tube characteristics are non–medication-related factors that may affect the incidence of tube occlusion.[89] Important tube characteristics include the inner diameter (bore size), the arrangement of formula delivery holes (ports) at the distal end, and the number of delivery ports. The most important formula characteristic in regard to tube occlusion appears to be the protein source. In vitro studies suggest that formulas containing intact protein, particularly caseinates or soy, coagulate and clump when exposed to an acidic pH.[90,91] In contrast, hydrolyzed protein formulas are compatible with acidic pharmaceutical products.[90]

Protocols for flushing feeding tubes have not been well studied. It generally is agreed that the tube should be flushed following each intermittent administration of formula or medication. The frequency and volume for tube flushes with continuous-infusion feedings varies from facility to facility, although flushing 20 mL or more of water through the tube every 8 hours is suggested to maintain tube patency.[81,83] For administering medications, a minimum of 10 to 20 mL of water before and after each medication has been recommended.[90] A minimum of 5 mL between multiple medications may be acceptable.

Medication-related factors that may influence the incidence of feeding tube occlusion include the administration method, dosage form, pH, and viscosity. Medications admixed with formula have the greatest potential for occluding feeding tubes owing to alteration of the texture, viscosity, or physical form of the medication or formula. Therefore, medications rarely should be admixed directly with formula. Stopping the enteral formula infusion, then flushing the feeding tube with water before and after medication administration, limits the contact between medications and formula, at least within the lumen of the feeding tube, and decreases the risk of tube occlusion.

Restoring Feeding Tube Patency

When a feeding tube occludes, it must be replaced unless patency can be restored. Frequent tube replacement disrupts nutrient delivery and increases patient discomfort as well as the cost of care. Tubes requiring surgical or endoscopic placement (e.g., gastrostomies, jejunostomies) are especially costly and potentially troublesome to replace; however, tube replacement through the nares can also be difficult and disruptive for the patient.

The first step generally recommended when a feeding tube occludes is to flush the tube with warm water using a syringe. A relatively large syringe, at least 20 mL but preferably 50 mL, should be used to avoid generation of excessive pressure that could cause the tube to rupture. When a specific cause for the occlusion can be identified (e.g., a specific medication) and the physiochemical characteristics of the substance responsible are known (e.g., solubility, pH), it may be possible to select a more appropriate flush preparation than water; in most cases, however, use of an acidic or basic flush preparation could make the occlusion worse. Acidic liquids (e.g., cranberry juice, diet soda, regular soda) may perpetuate or extend the occlusion, especially when proteins are contributing to the occlusion.[90] When water fails to restore patency to an occluded feeding tube, an activated pancreatic enzyme preparation may be useful.[90–92] Dissolving 1 crushed tablet of Viokase and 1 tablet of sodium bicarbonate (324 mg) in 5 mL of warm water just before instillation into an occluded feeding tube reportedly restores patency to most tubes when formula occlusion (e.g., protein denaturation) is the most likely cause of occlusion.[92] In addition, a product that contains multiple enzymes, buffers, and antibacterial agents in a powder form (Clog Zapper, Corpak Medical Systems, Wheeling, IL) is available as a pre-assembled kit for clearing occluded feeding tubes.

Solid dosage forms are the greatest challenge to administer by feeding tube. Whenever possible, a liquid dosage form should be selected, but these are not without problems. Liquids with a high viscosity may require dilution before administration. This allows easy flow through the tube and avoids a coating inside the tube that could react with enteral formula to form an occlusion. Suspensions have a tendency to coat tubes when they are thick or when the particles are relatively large and prone to settling. Unless the coating is rinsed off the tube wall and out of the ports with an adequate flush volume, occlusion will occur with repeated doses of the suspension.

Pharmaceutical syrups with a pH of 4 or less must be used with caution because immediate clumping and tackiness of formulas mixed with the syrups have been reported.[90]

For medications that are not available in liquid form, a therapeutically equivalent medication in a liquid form can be considered. Extemporaneous preparation of a solution or suspension also may be considered but may increase cost significantly. Simple compressed tablets may be crushed, then dissolved or suspended in 10 to 30 mL of water before administration through the feeding tube. Medications in a soft gelatin capsule are best delivered by dissolving the capsule in warm water before administration through the tube. Undissolved gelatin should not be administered, because this may occlude the tube. Powders in hard gelatin capsules can be poured into water and mixed thoroughly, then administered through the feeding tube. Failure to thoroughly dissolve any of these dosage forms in water before administration through the feeding tube may result in tube occlusion. Gora and colleagues[93] have listed Dyazide, ibuprofen, magnesium oxide, Metamucil, and Micro-K as medications most likely to occlude enteral feeding tubes. In a more recent survey, nurses identified omeprazole, potassium chloride, phenytoin, multivitamins, lansoprazole, protein supplements, sucralfate, pentoxifylline, zinc salts, calcium salts, and iron salts as the drugs and supplements most frequently contributing to feeding tube occlusion.[94]

Crushing a medication and dissolving or suspending the powder in water results in an altered pharmaceutical dosage form. Depending on the design and purpose of the dosage form, changes in the form may result in adverse effects on drug efficacy or patient tolerance. Simple compressed tablets are designed to dissolve rapidly in the stomach. Crushing and dissolving these tablets in water immediately before use has little affect on efficacy or patient tolerance to the medication. However, tablets and capsules designed to release medication slowly are significantly affected by crushing. Slow-release mechanisms are destroyed by crushing, resulting in the immediate release of several hours worth of the medication all at one time. An exaggerated therapeutic response may be seen initially, followed by a loss of response part way through the dosing interval. Therefore, solid dosage forms designed to release several doses of medication from one dose (e.g., sustained-release or long-acting forms) should not be crushed.[95] Alternatives to crushing these dosage forms are to use immediate-release forms of the prescribed medication with appropriate adjustment of the dose and dosing interval, therapeutically equivalent immediate-release forms, or alternate administration routes (e.g., morphine suppositories rather than slow-release morphine tablets).

Enteric-coated tablets are designed to release medication in the small bowel, because the medication is either acid labile or irritating to the stomach. Protection for the medication or stomach is lost when enteric-coated tablets are crushed and delivered via feeding tube into the stomach. The result may be decreased efficacy of the medication or increased gastric irritation. When an irritating medication must be given by tube into the stomach, diluting the medication in at least 60 mL of water is recommended.[90,93] Administering buccal or sublingual dosage forms via feeding tube may result in altered absorption and/or destruction of the medication by stomach acid. Therefore, therapeutically equivalent medications (e.g., isosorbide dinitrate rather than sublingual nitroglycerine) or an alternate route of administration (e.g., nitroglycerine ointment or transdermal system rather than sublingual nitroglycerine) should be used.

Pharmacokinetic parameters may be altered when a medication is administered by feeding tube. The site of medication delivery may affect bioavailability, although few studies address this issue. Medications taken orally are delivered to the stomach, where dissolution occurs for most dosage forms and hydrolysis of some medications may occur. Delivery into the small bowel may alter these processes, thereby affecting bioavailability. For instance, recovery of digoxin from intrajejunal dosing is reported to be higher than with oral administration, primarily because of reduced intragastric hydrolysis.[90] Bioavailability of medications also may be affected by the presence of enteral formula in the GI tract. Medications affected by the presence of food are expected to be affected in a similar manner by the presence of enteral formula. For example, administration of tetracycline when formula is present in the GI tract is expected to reduce tetracycline bioavailability because of interactions with divalent cations.[90] A similar interaction is expected between ciprofloxacin and enteral formula, although some evidence exists that a mechanism besides binding with divalent cations may be responsible for reduced ciprofloxacin concentrations with enteral feeding.[96]

Phenytoin is a particularly troublesome medication to manage in patients receiving tube feeding. Reduced phenytoin concentrations in patients receiving enteral feeding have been reported in numerous case reports and small studies since the interaction was first noted in 1982.[90,97] Methods suggested for management include using a meat-based formula, administering phenytoin capsules rather than suspension, and stopping enteral formula delivery for 1 to 2 hours before and after the phenytoin dose.[90,97] Holding formula administration before and after the phenytoin dose is usually recommended. Unfortunately, none of these methods clearly prevents low phenytoin concentrations in patients receiving tube feedings; thus, monitoring of serum phenytoin concentrations is important whenever tube feeding is started or altered. Large-scale controlled trials are needed to determine the most appropriate method for managing the phenytoin-enteral feeding interaction.

One of the most important potential interactions related to pharmacologic effects of medications or nutrients is reversal of warfarin anticoagulation by vitamin K in enteral formulas.[90] Most enteral formulas manufactured today contain vitamin K in doses that are unlikely to interfere with anticoagulation. However, inability to adequately anticoagulate a tube-fed patient with oral warfarin should prompt an evaluation of the enteral formula's vitamin K content. In addition, binding of warfarin to a component of enteral formulas, likely protein, has been proposed as a mechanism that explains warfarin resistance with formulas containing relatively low vitamin K content.[98] Stopping formula administration for an hour before and after warfarin administration appears to prevent this type of interaction.

A potential problem related to physiologic effects of medications is diarrhea secondary to hypertonicity. Hypertonic medications (e.g., potassium chloride) should be diluted with 30 to 60 mL of water before being administered through the feeding tube.[81,90,93] Dividing the medication dose and separating each smaller dose by about 2 hours also may help reduce diarrhea secondary to hypertonic medications. For example, 60 mEq of potassium chloride can be divided into three doses of 20 mEq each, with 2 hours between doses. In addition, selection of brands and dosage forms with minimal sorbitol can reduce the risk of diarrhea. Cumulative sorbitol doses above 5 g may cause bloating and flatulence while larger doses may act as a cathartic.[99]

PATIENT ASSESSMENT
Evaluation of Nutrition Status

1. M.R., a 70-year-old man, was admitted to the hospital 5 days ago after a neighbor found him semiconscious on his backyard patio. Physical examination on admission revealed right-sided paralysis and left-sided weakness. He was confused and disoriented, and his mucous membranes were dry. M.R. was diagnosed with mild dehydration and as having suffered a cerebrovascular accident (CVA). His condition has changed little since admission. M.R. is estimated to be 5′10″ tall and weighs 136.5 lb (62 kg) on a bed scale. He is receiving a maintenance IV of 5% dextrose/0.45% sodium chloride with KCl 20 mEq/L at 100 mL/hr. Laboratory evaluation today shows a serum albumin of 3.2 g/dL, down from 3.6 on admission. Other biochemical data are within normal limits: glucose, 94 mg/dL (normal, 70 to 110); creatinine, 0.9 mg/dL (normal, 0.6 to 1.2); Na, 142 mEq/L (normal, 135 to 145); K, 4.6 mEq/L (normal, 3.5 to 5.5); and Cl, 106 mEq/L (normal, 95 to 105). Assess M.R.'s nutrition status. Identify factors placing him nutritionally-at-risk. Is nutrition support indicated at this time?

M.R. appears to have mild malnutrition based on his weight for height and serum albumin concentration. He is at risk for developing more severe malnutrition during hospitalization, and possibly mortality.[100,101] The serum albumin concentration of 3.6 g/dL at the time of admission is falsely elevated due to dehydration; therefore, today's albumin should be used to evaluate visceral protein status. The mild visceral protein depletion may have resulted from metabolic stress associated with his CVA. Weight loss to 85% of ideal body weight (IBW, 73 kg), however, most likely is due to chronic deficiency in total energy intake.

At 85% of IBW, M.R. should appear underweight. If he appears to be of normal weight, the estimated height may be wrong. A better estimate of height might be obtained by using a tape measure stretched out along M.R.'s body. Based on the information presented, it is not clear when M.R.'s weight of 62 kg was obtained. If this weight is within the first 24 hours of admission, it is expected to be falsely low (by a few kilograms at most) because of M.R.'s dehydration. Records of clinic visits and hospitalizations may provide information on chronic or recent illnesses that contributed to weight loss.

Socioeconomic factors that may contribute to nutrition risk also should be considered. Home address and type of medical insurance may provide clues to his economic status. Low income is associated with food insecurity and inadequate nutrition.[102] Social conditions also may influence nutrition. M.R. appears to live alone because a neighbor reported his condition rather than a family member. In the United States, elderly men living alone are at risk of inadequate dietary intake, perhaps due in part to skipped meals.[103]

The assumption that M.R. has been without oral intake since admission is reasonable because he is unable to feed himself and is expected to have difficulty chewing and swallowing as a result of the CVA. Dextrose provided in the maintenance fluid is considered adequate nutrition for only about a week in a previously well-nourished patient with a low degree of metabolic stress. Beyond this time period, more substantial support must be considered because the dextrose provided by maintenance fluids is considerably below the amount needed to minimize protein breakdown for gluconeogenesis. Patients with inadequate intake for 7 to 14 days or patients not expected to have adequate intake for 7 to 14 days are considered candidates for specialized nutrition support.[1] Because M.R. has mild malnutrition and is not likely to take adequate nutrients by mouth within the next few days, specialized nutrition support is indicated.

Estimation of Nutrition Requirements

2. What are M.R.'s requirements for calories, protein, and fluid? Does he have any special nutrient requirements?

Because M.R. is below IBW for his height, his actual weight should be used to estimate energy and protein requirements. Use of IBW to estimate requirements for malnourished patients may result in fluid and electrolyte imbalance. Once the patient is stabilized on nutrition support, calories can be increased, if necessary, to achieve weight gain. For patients weighing between ideal and 120% of IBW, either ideal or actual weight can be used. Because the Harris-Benedict equation and several other equations used to predict caloric requirements appear to overestimate needs, it may be preferable to use IBW and adjust calories, if necessary, based on weight changes. An adjusted weight appears to be most appropriate for patients weighing >120% of ideal. Prediction equations for resting energy expenditure generally do not correlate well with measured energy expenditure for obese subjects when actual weight is used as a variable in the equation.[104] The adjustment accounts for the portion of excess weight that is metabolically active lean tissue and avoids providing calories for the relatively inert adipose tissue.

M.R.'s level of metabolic stress is relatively low. He has no surgical wounds, no fractures or skeletal trauma, no burns, and no major infections. Therefore, caloric requirements are only slightly higher than basal needs. Although the term *calorie* is used interchangeably with kilocalorie (kcal) in nutrition literature, the large "Calorie" or kilocalorie technically is correct. Thus, energy requirements generally are listed as kcal/day or kcal/kg body weight when specific numbers are given for a patient's requirements. Requirements can be estimated using the Harris-Benedict equations or one of the many other guidelines for predicting energy expenditure. Indirect calorimetry (metabolic cart measurements) is an expensive procedure and probably is unnecessary in a mildly stressed patient. Metabolic cart measurements determine energy (or "metabolic") requirements from oxygen consumption and carbon dioxide production. They account for individual variations in energy expenditure that are not adequately accounted for by Harris-Benedict calculation of BEE or by the kcal/kg method of determining energy requirements, especially in highly complex patients. An estimation of 20 to 25 kcal/kg actual weight also can be used based on M.R.'s low level of metabolic stress. However, higher caloric intake may be needed for weight gain, which occurs primarily as fat. Protein requirements are expected to be slightly higher than the DRI of 0.8 g/kg per day.

The mild visceral protein depletion and metabolic stress experienced by M.R. are expected to increase his protein needs to approximately 1 to 1.2 g/kg actual weight per day. Renal function appears adequate for M.R. to tolerate up to 1.2 g/kg per day without developing azotemia. SrCr, however, may provide a poor estimate of renal function in a patient with below-normal muscle mass such as M.R., who is only 85% of IBW. Fluid requirements for geriatric patients can be estimated at 30 to 35 mL/kg body weight per day plus replacement of excess losses from hyperthermia, vomiting, or diarrhea.[1,29] A baseline requirement of 1,500 mL for the first 20 kg of body weight plus 20 mL per each additional kg of body weight also can be used to estimate fluid requirements, although this method was developed for use in pediatric patients. Based on caloric intake, fluid requirements can be estimated as 1 mL/kcal ingested.[1,29] M.R. does not appear to have any excess fluid losses at this time; therefore, calculation of baseline fluid requirements should provide adequate fluids.

M.R.'s estimated daily requirements are approximately 1,240 to 1,550 total calories, 62 to 74 g protein, and 1,860 to 2,168 mL of fluid. These are estimated requirements that should be adjusted based on frequent reassessment of M.R.'s response to therapy and changes in his clinical situation. Additional calories and protein may be needed for repletion of weight and protein status.

M.R.'s apparently suboptimal nutrition before hospitalization increases his risk of vitamin deficiencies. In addition, poor vitamin status may contribute to reduced cognitive ability and to risk of carotid stenosis and stroke.[105–107] Vitamins of particular concern are antioxidants (i.e., vitamin C and beta carotene) and those that influence plasma concentrations of homocysteine (i.e., vitamin B_{12}, folic acid, and pyridoxine). No medical, medication, or dietary histories are available to determine nutritional risks associated with specific conditions. Factors that predispose patients to vitamin deficiencies include weight loss of >5% of usual body weight in 1 month or >10% of usual body weight in 6 months, prolonged periods of dietary restriction, high levels of physiologic stress as occurs with trauma and large areas of burn, significant alterations in biochemical tests such as serum glucose and albumin, abnormal or protracted body fluid losses, administration of medications that alter vitamin absorption or metabolism, and diagnoses associated with alteration in vitamin absorption or requirements.[108–110] Older people tend to consume less than the DRI for several nutrients, including vitamins A, E, and pyridoxine.[103] Thus, M.R.'s age, along with his acute illness and mild mixed protein-calorie malnutrition, increases his risk of vitamin deficiencies, and it is likely that he has at least some subclinical vitamin deficiencies. In addition, M.R. should receive a minimum of 100% of the DRI for vitamins and minerals daily, and up to 200% of the DRI would not be unreasonable. A daily multivitamin preparation providing 100% of the DRI should be considered in addition to vitamins and minerals from an oral diet or tube feeding. If actual deficiencies are identified, M.R. will require higher, therapeutic doses of the specific vitamins that are deficient.

Enteral Nutrition Route

3. The health care team decides to initiate specialized nutrition support via tube feeding. What route for tube feeding is most appropriate for M.R.?

With right-sided paralysis from the CVA, it is likely that M.R. has problems with chewing and swallowing, in addition to difficulty getting food to his mouth. Otherwise, M.R.'s GI tract is expected to be functional. There is no indication that M.R. has risks associated with aspiration. Some patients have poor gag reflex after a CVA, but M.R. has no reported coughing or choking. The duration of tube feeding is uncertain because M.R. may improve with time. An NG tube is the least invasive route until M.R.'s prognosis for recovery is better predicted. Measures to prevent M.R. from pulling the feeding tube may be necessary because confused and disoriented patients often pull tubes.[77,83] Confusion was reported at least periodically in all patients experiencing tube displacement. M.R.'s right side is paralyzed, so his right hand will not be a threat for the tube. However, depending on the degree of weakness, his left hand may be able to pull and remove the tube. A soft mitten or restraint placed on the left wrist may be used to prevent M.R. from grabbing the feeding tube and displacing it.

Enteral Formula Selection

4. What type of enteral formula is most appropriate for M.R.?

M.R. has full digestive capability; therefore, a polymeric formula is most appropriate. Because no history is available regarding lactose tolerance and because M.R. has been "fasting" at least 5 days, a lactose-free formula is advised for the initial tube feeding. This minimizes bloating, cramps, and diarrhea secondary to lactose intolerance.[13] A standard caloric density of 1 to 1.2 kcal/mL should be used because M.R. has no fluid restriction and no evidence of fluid overload with his maintenance IV fluid at 100 mL/hour. Using a high-nitrogen formula to meet M.R.'s caloric needs will provide protein at the upper end of the estimated requirement (1.2 g/kg per day), whereas a standard nitrogen formula will provide between 0.8 and 1 g/kg per day. A high-nitrogen formula may replete M.R.'s visceral protein status sooner than a standard nitrogen formula, but it may not provide adequate calories for weight gain. The decision to use a high- versus standard-nitrogen formula depends on the exact nutrient composition of enteral formulas on the hospital formulary.

Fiber can be included in the enteral formula if desired. However, the benefit of fiber for short-term feeding is not clearly defined, so a fiber-free formula is an equally appropriate selection at this time.[16] If a fiber-containing formula is selected initially, the formula should contain a low to moderate fiber content (5 to 7 g/L) or be started at a low rate and advanced slowly to minimize gas and abdominal distention.

Fluid Provision

5. How much fluid is necessary to meet M.R.'s estimated daily fluid requirements?

Free water content of the selected enteral formula must be calculated to determine the volume of fluid that must be provided to M.R. in addition to the formula. Formulas with 1 to 1.2 kcal/mL generally contain 80% to 85% free water. Assuming a goal volume of 1,440 mL/day (6 cans) of a 1 kcal/mL, 0.044 g protein/mL formula, approximately 1,150 to 1,225 mL of free water is provided to M.R. per day. Using 30 mL/kg per day as M.R.'s fluid requirement, he needs 1,860 mL daily. Therefore, fluid needed in addition to the enteral formula is 635 to 710 mL/day. This fluid can be provided with medications and irrigation of the tube (flushes). The feeding tube should be irrigated with a minimum of 20 mL of fluid at least every 8 hours, as well as before and after administering each medication through the tube.[29,77,81,90] Using five flushes daily with 125 mL of water each would provide 625 mL of fluid.

Selection of a 2-kcal/mL, 0.075-g protein/mL formula for M.R. would require that he receive approximately 720 mL (3 cans) of formula daily to meet caloric and protein requirements. Formulas with 2 kcal/mL contain approximately 65% to 80% free water, meaning that M.R. would receive about 470 to 575 mL of free water from the formula. M.R. would still need 1,285 to 1,390 mL of fluid to meet his daily fluid requirement, and frequent, large flushes of water would be necessary. Dilution of formula to half-strength, which would reduce the volume of water required as flushes, is not recommended owing to increased risk of error and contamination with additional manipulation of the formula. Thus, a 1 kcal/mL formula is more appropriate for M.R. than a 2 kcal/mL product.

Enteral Nutrition Administration

6. Recommend a plan for initiating and advancing M.R.'s tube feeding.

M.R. is being fed into the stomach; therefore, continuous infusion, intermittent infusion, or bolus delivery of feedings can be used. Continuous infusion most commonly is used for hospitalized patients. However, improved tolerance with continuous intragastric infusion versus intermittent infusion has not been clearly established.[77,78]

Full-strength formula should be used to initiate tube feedings. M.R. is assumed to have full digestive capacity and is being fed into the stomach; therefore, diluting the formula is not expected to improve tolerance to either an isotonic or hypertonic formula. Dilution is likely to delay reaching M.R.'s caloric and protein goals. Starting the feedings at a very low rate also is likely to delay reaching M.R.'s nutrition goals. The standard of practice in most institutions is to start continuous infusion polymeric feedings at approximately 30 to 40 mL/hr. Feedings are then advanced by 25 to 50 mL/hr every 6 to 12 hours, as tolerated, until the goal rate is achieved.

The goal volume of enteral nutrition for M.R. is 1,440 mL/day of a 1-kcal/mL formula, or 60 mL/hr continuous infusion. The infusion can be started at 30 or 40 mL/hr for 6 to 12 hours, then increased to 60 mL/hr. If M.R. experiences diarrhea, abdominal distention, or large gastric residuals, the feeding may be held at the initial rate for 24 hours, then increased only 10 to 15 mL/hr every 12 to 24 hours as tolerance permits. If the formula is not advanced to goal rate within 24 hours of initiating feedings, extra care must be taken to ensure adequate fluid intake.

Continuous infusion enteral feeding can be administered by gravity drip or by enteral pump. With gravity drip, the infusion rate must be adjusted frequently to maintain a consistent flow rate and formula flow must be checked regularly to ensure that flow has not stopped because of kinked administration tubing or an empty delivery container. There are no alarms to alert nurses to these problems with gravity infusion. Enteral pumps provide a consistent flow rate and alarms to alert nurses to problems with the infusion, but are more expensive than gravity drip. Pumps often are used for hospitalized patients to help maintain delivery of the prescribed volume of enteral formula. Either gravity drip or an enteral pump could be used for M.R., depending on the hospital's protocol for enteral feeding. If an enteral pump is used, the connector at the distal (patient) end of the delivery set is not be compatible with IV devices, which prevents inadvertent intravenous infusion of enteral formulas.[77]

Monitoring Enteral Nutrition Support

7. Recommend a plan for monitoring M.R.'s response to enteral nutrition, including clinical and biochemical parameters.

Monitoring of enteral nutrition is necessary to prevent complications and to assess appropriateness of therapy. Clinical parameters to monitor include tube placement, gastric residual, GI symptoms, respiratory status, vital signs, and weight. Tube placement should be evaluated at least daily, but preferably every 4 to 8 hours, by auscultation, location of markings on the tube, and/or withdrawal of gastric contents.[77,81,83] A tube displaced into the esophagus or pharynx could result in pulmonary aspiration of enteral formula.

Gastric residual is evaluated by measuring the volume of fluid withdrawn from the stomach through the feeding tube using a syringe. The fluid is then infused through the tube back into the stomach to avoid electrolyte imbalances. Persistently high residuals may increase the risk of esophageal reflux and pulmonary aspiration. The residual volume considered important for holding tube feeding in patients receiving NG feeding is controversial; however, 200 mL is commonly used. Setting the residual volume too low can result in inadequate nutrition because the feedings are stopped frequently. Residuals should be checked every 4 to 8 hours as long as no residual is above the volume for holding feeding. If feeding is held because of a high residual, an hourly evaluation of gastric residual is recommended until the volume is less than 200 mL and the feeding is restarted.

Assessment of GI symptoms is important for determining tolerance to enteral feeding. Abdominal distention and bloating should be evaluated at least every 8 hours while M.R. is hospitalized. Small-bore feeding tubes may collapse during withdrawal of gastric residual, resulting in falsely low residual volume. Abdominal distention may be an indication of accumulating formula. Gas formation secondary to lactose intolerance or rapid increases in fiber intake, and poor gastric emptying secondary to a high-fat formula, medications, recent surgery, critical illness, or an underlying disease such as diabetes are among the conditions associated with distention. When considerable distention is present, the formula should be held temporarily, and the patient should be evaluated further to rule out a condition that would contraindicate continued use of the GI tract. Gastric outlet obstruction, complete or partial small bowel obstruction, or ileus precludes restarting

enteral nutrition until the condition resolves. If no contraindication to using the GI tract is found, feeding can be restarted, preferably with the feeding tube placed into the small bowel, a formula with lower fat or fiber content, and/or medications to promote gastric emptying (e.g., metoclopramide or erythromycin). Feeding should be restarted at a rate of 25 to 40 mL/hour, and M.R. should be observed closely for signs of feeding intolerance. The head of the bed should be elevated 30 to 45 degrees during feeding.[87]

Nausea, vomiting, abdominal cramping, diarrhea, and constipation are other GI symptoms that are monitored as indicators of tube feeding tolerance. Of these symptoms, vomiting creates the most immediate concern because feeding tube displacement and pulmonary aspiration may occur during vomiting. Nausea and vomiting commonly occur with high gastric residuals, severe gastric distention, poor gastric emptying when feeding into the stomach, obstruction of the GI tract, and/or lack of GI tract motility. Lactose intolerance and bolus feeding into the jejunum can lead to diarrhea and abdominal cramping, as well as nausea and vomiting. Initiation of tube feeding with a hypertonic formula, a rapid rate of infusion and/or a large volume, and use of formula at refrigerator temperature are other factors often cited as causing GI symptoms.[81,88] Although controlled studies have not supported these factors as significant contributors to GI intolerance, subjective evidence suggests they are important. Constipation is most likely to occur with long-term tube feeding in nonambulatory patients. Inadequate fluid intake and lack of fiber may be factors associated with constipation.[16,19]

Respiratory status should be evaluated every 8 hours in hospitalized patients, to help recognize pulmonary aspiration and pulmonary edema. A stethoscope should be used for assessment at least a couple of times per week, but simple observation of the patient's breathing pattern is adequate at other times unless altered respirations are noted. Coughing and/or respiratory distress may be indications of aspiration or other developing respiratory problems. Vital signs also may provide clues to aspiration or other problems, such as dehydration, fluid overload, or infection.

Weight and fluid input and output should be monitored daily in hospitalized patients. Day-to-day changes in weight reflect fluid status. Increased weight for 3 to 4 consecutive days may be an indication that fluid intake needs to be reduced, whereas decreased weight may indicate a need for increased fluid. Generally, the amount of fluid provided can be adjusted by the number of times the feeding tube is flushed daily and the volume of each flush. Caloric density of the formula can be changed when altering the number or volume of flushes is not adequate for fluid control. For patients with a stable fluid status, week-to-week weight change can be used as an indicator of appropriate caloric intake. An upward trend in weight (e.g., 3 or more consecutive weeks with an increase) may indicate a need for fewer calories unless weight gain is a goal. A downward trend may indicate a need to increase caloric intake, unless weight loss is desired.

Regular monitoring of biochemical parameters is important for identifying metabolic abnormalities before they become critical problems. Serum glucose, sodium, potassium, chloride, and bicarbonate should be determined daily in M.R. for 4 to 5 days after feeding starts. Monitoring can then be decreased to once or twice weekly if M.R. has no evidence of tube feeding intolerance or metabolic abnormalities. Finger-stick glucose measurements should be ordered every 6 hours if hospital policy requires this for all patients started on specialized nutrition support. If fingersticks are not required by policy, it would be reasonable to evaluate M.R.'s serum glucose after tube feeding starts and then decide if fingersticks are needed routinely. Because M.R. has a normal serum glucose (94 mg/dL) while receiving 5% dextrose in his IV fluid and is not highly stressed, hyperglycemia is not a major concern with tube feeding.

SrCr, BUN, calcium, phosphorus, and magnesium should be monitored a minimum of three times during the first week of tube feeding. Daily monitoring of SrCr and BUN for a few days may even be considered in M.R. because of his recent dehydration. Daily calcium, phosphorus, and magnesium also may be considered for a few days in M.R. because of his low body weight. Chronic malnutrition can lead to intracellular depletion of potassium, phosphorus, and magnesium, while serum concentrations are maintained. When specialized nutrition support begins, refeeding syndrome may develop as these electrolytes move from the extracellular space into the cells, causing a decrease in serum concentrations over the first few days of feeding. Failure to monitor the patient and replace electrolytes as necessary can result in serious electrolyte abnormalities. If SrCr, BUN, calcium, phosphorus, and magnesium are stable after the first 4 or 5 days, the frequency of monitoring could be reduced to once or twice weekly.

Biochemical parameters used to monitor response to protein provision should be monitored. For example, prealbumin (i.e., transthyretin) and transferrin are monitored as short-term indicators of visceral protein response to nutrition support and can be monitored every 3 to 4 days (transthyretin) or weekly (transferrin). Albumin is a long-term indicator that requires 2 to 3 weeks to reflect response to nutrition therapy; however, it may be included on a weekly monitoring schedule to allow adjustment of serum calcium for hypoalbuminemia. Nitrogen balance can be used as an alternative to prealbumin or transferrin, but requires an accurate 12- to 24-hour urine collection to be useful.

Electrolyte Abnormalities

8. M.R. has been receiving tube feeding for 4 days. Feeding was started at 40 mL/hr for 8 hours, then increased to 60 mL/hr (goal rate). The IV fluids were stopped when tube feeding was at goal rate. M.R.'s tube feeding was stopped for approximately 5 hours a few days ago after he removed his tube, but otherwise there have been no problems. Laboratory evaluation today shows the following: K, 3.1 mEq/L (decreased from 3.6 mEq/L yesterday, 3.9 mEq/L the previous day, and 4.6 mEq/L when tube feeding started); Cl, 95 mEq/L (normal, 95 to 105); calcium, 8.2 mg/dL (normal, 9 to 11); Mg, 2.6 mEq/L (normal, 2.5 to 3.5), decreased from 3.5 mEq/L 2 days ago; phosphorus, 3.5 mg/dL (normal, 3.5 to 4.5), decreased from 4.4 mg/dL 2 days ago; and albumin, 3.0 g/dL. Micro-K (8 mEq KCl/capsule) has been ordered as 6 capsules via feeding tube and calcium carbonate (260 mg elemental calcium/tablet) as 2 tablets BID via feeding tube. Is the electrolyte replacement appropriate as ordered for M.R.? What changes, if any, should be considered for electrolyte replacement?

Calcium carbonate is a simple compressed tablet that can be crushed, suspended in 10 to 30 mL of water, and administered through the feeding tube. However, calcium salts have been identified by nurses as one of the drugs and supplements most frequently contributing to feeding tube occlusion.[94] The risk of tube occlusion from larger pieces of tablet that are not adequately crushed may be decreased by use of calcium carbonate suspension (500 mg Ca/5 mL) if this is available in the pharmacy. Administration of either the crushed and suspended tablets or the commercial suspension requires that the feeding tube be flushed with at least 30 mL of water before and after administration of medication.[83,89,90] However, diluting the suspension 1:1 with water and using a flush volume of 75 to 100 mL may be advisable because otherwise suspensions often coat the tube. The need for calcium supplementation should be questioned because M.R.'s serum calcium concentration is within normal limits when corrected for his low serum albumin concentration. Administering any medication via the feeding tube may occlude the tube. The oral route should be used for medication administration whenever appropriate. Many patients receiving tube feedings are allowed some oral intake, and oral medications are frequently acceptable. However, M.R.'s risk for aspiration may be too high at this time to allow oral medications.

Potassium is below normal today and has been decreasing since tube feeding began. Potassium supplementation should have been considered yesterday, rather than waiting until M.R. developed hypokalemia because a definite trend downward in serum potassium was evident. The selected potassium supplement is inappropriate for administration by tube because Micro-K is a slow-release product.[95] Crushing slow-release products destroys the slow-release mechanism. Potassium chloride powder for solution (3 packets with 15 mEq KCl/packet) or liquid (10% KCl 35 mL, 15% KCl 25 mL, or 20% KCl 15-20 mL) should be ordered rather than the slow-release product. Dividing the potassium dose into two or three smaller doses and diluting each dose with 60 mL of water is recommended.[90,93] Given as a single dose, 45 to 50 mEq of potassium may cause nausea, vomiting, abdominal discomfort, and/or diarrhea. These symptoms might be mistaken as intolerance to the enteral formula, resulting in the tube feeding being stopped temporarily. The larger fluid volume for administration also may help reduce the gastric irritation associated with potassium doses.

Consideration also should be given to changes occurring in other electrolytes. M.R. appears to be developing mild refeeding syndrome. Magnesium and phosphorus are within normal range, but have decreased significantly over the past 2 days. Supplements should be considered today. By starting supplementation before electrolytes are critically low, smaller daily quantities can be used. This may decrease the risk of diarrhea and GI upset from administration of magnesium and/or phosphate. Magnesium supplementation could be accomplished with a magnesium oxide tablet (400 mg or 500 mg) administered two to four times daily. These are simple compressed tablets that can be crushed and suspended for administration via feeding tube. An alternative would be magnesium hydroxide suspension 5 mL two to four times daily.

The magnesium doses are distributed through the day to avoid the cathartic effect associated with magnesium. Phosphate supplementation could be accomplished by changing part of the potassium ordered to Neutra-Phos-K, which provides 8.1 mmol of phosphate and 14.2 mEq of potassium per 250 mg capsule. The contents of each capsule are designed to be dissolved in 75 mL of water for administration, so dissolution is not a concern. One Neutra-Phos-K twice a day plus KCl liquid to provide 20 mEq potassium provides the same potassium dose as is ordered currently. The liquid KCl should be given at least 2 hours before or after the Neutra-Phos-K to minimize GI effects. The feeding tube must be flushed adequately before and after each dose of electrolyte replacement. The flush volume should be a minimum of 30 mL, although 75 to 100 mL following the magnesium dose may be better to ensure the electrolyte preparation is out of the tube.[93] Intermittent tube flushes can be accomplished with medication administration to limit total fluid intake to the estimated requirement of 1,860 to 2,168 mL, or 635 to 710 mL in addition to that provided by a 1-kcal/mL formula.

With the current electrolyte abnormalities it is important to monitor potassium, magnesium, and phosphorus for the next several days. The extent of electrolyte depletion in the body is difficult to evaluate, but 1 day of electrolyte replacement is not expected to replete intracellular stores of these electrolytes. It is difficult to provide large quantities of potassium, phosphate, and magnesium via feeding tube secondary to GI intolerance. Therefore, IV electrolyte replacement may be necessary when intracellular depletion is extensive.

Transfer to a Nursing Facility

9. M.R. has received tube feeding for 10 days. During this time he removed his feeding tube twice despite mittens to hinder his ability to grab the tube. Feedings were off for approximately 5 hours each time the tube was removed. M.R.'s electrolyte abnormalities have been corrected with 3 days of electrolyte replacement. He has tolerated his tube feeding without metabolic abnormalities or electrolyte replacement for the past 2 days. M.R. remains confused and disoriented. The prognosis for improvement in M.R.'s right-sided paralysis, and therefore his ability to feed himself, is poor. Plans are made to discharge M.R. in 1 to 2 days to a nursing facility. What changes in the care plan would be appropriate relative to nutrition support goals?

M.R. should be evaluated for surgical gastrostomy or percutaneous endoscopic gastrostomy (PEG) placement because he is expected to need tube feeding for a prolonged period. Gastrostomy placement also should solve the problem of repeated tube displacement in M.R., although this alone is not an appropriate reason to place a gastrostomy. Placement of a PEG can be accomplished with local anesthesia, which may be advantageous given M.R.'s age and lack of another reason for general anesthesia.[7] Use of local anesthesia and no requirement for an operating room decrease the cost of PEG placement compared with surgical gastrostomies. Rates for major complications of 0% to 9% and for minor complications of 0% to 24% have been reported for PEGs, but this is not significantly different from that for surgical gastrostomies.[7]

If a fiber-free formula was selected initially, a fiber-containing formula should be considered. Fiber may prevent GI tract changes associated with prolonged use of low-residue, fiber-free formulas.[16,19] Constipation is frequently a problem in elderly and bedridden patients. Increased stool weight and frequency has been demonstrated in patients with constipation who received fiber-containing formula versus fiber-free formula.[19] Starting with a low to moderate fiber content (5 to 7 g/L) may help minimize gas and abdominal distention. However, to reach the recommended fiber intake of 20 to 35 g/day, a formula containing fiber at 13 or 14 g/L is necessary.[16] By using a combination of half of M.R.'s current fiber-free formula and half of a fiber-containing formula with 14 g/L for a few days, then changing completely to the fiber-containing formula, the fiber content can be gradually increased. The fiber-free and fiber-containing formulas probably should not be mixed directly without prior in vitro observation of compatibility, unless they are "without" and "with" fiber versions of the same product (e.g., Boost or Boost with Fiber). Although the likelihood of incompatibility is low, mixing different formulas together could result in disruption of the emulsion, with gelling or separation of formula components as a consequence.

M.R. should transition to an intermittent schedule before discharge. Many nursing facilities do not routinely use enteral pumps because of increased cost. Without a pump, delivery of the prescribed volume of formula at a consistent rate may not be reliable in a nursing facility. Transitioning M.R. from 60 mL/hr continuous infusion to intermittent delivery of formula can be accomplished by various methods. Transition over approximately 48 hours can be accomplished by changing the infusion to 120 mL (½ can) every 3 hours for three or four feedings, then increasing to 240 mL (1½ can) every 6 hours for three feedings, with each feeding infused over 60 minutes. The next step is to 360 mL (1 half cans) every 6 hours. If M.R. tolerates this feeding schedule, the time between feedings can be decreased further to allow three or four feedings during the 10 to 12 hours of the day when people normally take meals. Once M.R. is at the desired schedule for feedings, the infusion time for each feeding can be decreased from 60 to 30 minutes. A slower transition can be accomplished by extending each change in the infusion to 24 hours. Ideally, the transition will be completed before M.R. is discharged to the nursing facility. To accomplish this, a more rapid transition is needed. Reducing the number of feedings at each transition step (e.g., one to two feedings at 120 mL every 3 hours rather than three to four feedings) decreases the time to complete the transition to intermittent feedings, assuming M.R. tolerates each step.

The prescription for tube feeding on discharge to the nursing facility should state clearly the desired caloric density (e.g., standard versus moderate versus calorically dense), protein content (e.g., low versus standard versus high nitrogen), fiber content (e.g., 5 to 7 g/L versus 12 to 14 g/L), and volume of the desired formula, or the daily calories, protein, fiber, and fluid to be provided by the formula. The brand name also may be included, but the nursing facility may not have the same brands of formula on their formulary as the hospital. A generic formula prescription will help to ensure that M.R. receives the desired specialized nutrition support. Any special considerations for the feeding schedule also should be communicated to the nursing facility (e.g., if M.R. tolerates feeding better in the morning or needs to have the head of the bed at 45 degrees for at least 3 hours after the last daily feeding to avoid regurgitation).

Twice-weekly monitoring of glucose, creatinine, and electrolytes should be recommended during the first week after discharge to the nursing facility. Careful monitoring of fluid status and tolerance to the intermittent delivery schedule also is recommended after discharge. M.R. will have been on the new schedule for only a short time before discharge, so a full evaluation of tolerance to the new regimen will not have been completed.

Transfer to Home on Enteral Nutrition

10. M.R.'s overall status has improved during 3 weeks at the nursing facility, and he is now ready for discharge. However, M.R. has made no progress in his ability to take an oral diet because dysphagia and aspiration continue to be severe on "per swallow" studies. M.R. is not to take solids or liquids by mouth at this time, and swallow studies are not to be repeated for 6 months. Intermittent tube feedings with a total of 1,680 mL (7 cans) of a 1 kcal/mL, 0.044 g protein/mL, fiber-containing polymeric formula daily are to continue. His weight has increased 2 kg since hospital discharge. M.R. still needs assistance with some

activities of daily living; thus, he will be staying with his sister. She is concerned about insurance coverage for the enteral nutrition therapy. Will Medicare, M.R.'s only medical insurance, cover tube feeding?

There are strict guidelines for coverage of home enteral nutrition therapy, a Medicare Part B benefit.[111] Full nutrition support delivered by a feeding tube is covered (i.e., not oral supplements and not partial provision of estimated requirements even when given by tube) when there is a functional disability of the GI tract (e.g., dysphagia, swallowing disorder) that is expected to be "permanent." The test for full support is that calories are between 20 and 35 kcal/kg per day, whereas the test of permanence is at least 90 days. M.R. meets these guidelines. In addition, the formula M.R. receives is in a category that does not require him to meet additional eligibility criteria related to the formula itself.

Enteral formulas are divided into six categories, plus one subgroup, for purposes of reimbursement by Medicare Part B (Table 36-8).[111] Most polymeric formulas containing

Table 36-8 Medicare Categories for Enteral Formulas

Category	Description	Examples (Partial Listing)
Category I	Fibersource, Fibersource HN, protein or protein isolates	Semisynthetic intact Boost, Boost w/ fiber, Ensure fiber w/ FOS, Isocal, Isocal HN, Isocal HN Plus, Isosource, Isosource HN, Jevity 1 Cal, NuBasics, NuBasic VHP, Osmolite 1 Cal, Osmolite 1.2 Cal, Ultracal, *Disease-specific formulas:* Glytrol, Resource Diabetic
Category IB[a]	Natural or intact protein or protein isolates	Compleat Documentation that **may** provide justification for this category of formula: excessive stooling on appropriate semisynthetic formulas (e.g., isotonic, low long-chain fat content, lactose free) that resolves after changing to a Category IB formula and recurs on rechallenge with semisynthetic formula.
Category II	Intact protein or protein isolates; calorically dense	Boost Plus, Deliver 2.0, Ensure Plus, Ensure Plus HN, Isocal HCN, Isosource 1.5 Cal, Novasource 2.0, NuBasic Plus, NuBasics 2.0, Nutren 1.5, Nutren 2.0 *Disease-specific formulas:* Novasource Pulmonary, Respalor
Category III[a]	Hydrolyzed protein or amino acids	Criticare HN, Isotein HN, Impact Glutamine, Optimental, Peptamen 1.5, Peptamen w/FOS/Inulin, Peptinex DT, Reabilan, Subdue, Vivonex RTF These formulas are for critically ill patients or those with malabsorption. Documentation that **may** provide justification for this category of formula: dumping syndrome, uncontrolled diarrhea, or other evidence of absorption on appropriate semisynthetic formulas (e.g., isotonic, low long-chain fat content, lactose free) that resolves after changing to a hydrolyzed protein or amino acid formula and/or documentation of the disease process leading to malabsorption
Category IV[a]	Defined formula for special metabolic need (i.e., disease-specific formulas)	Advera, AlitraQ, Amin-Aid, Choice DM Tube Feeding Liquid, Hepatic-Aid, Immune-Aid, various Impact formulas, Isosource VHN, Lipisorb, Magnacal Renal, Modulen IBD, Novasource Renal, NutriHep, NutriRenal, NutriVent, Peptamen, Peptamen VHP, Protein XL, Pulmocare, Reabilan HN, Renalcal, Replete, Replete w/ fiber, Traumacal, Vivonex Plus, Vivonex T.E.N. Documentation that **may** provide justification for this category of formula: evidence of inability to meet nutritional goals with a Category I or II product without compromising patient safety and documentation of the specific diagnosis for which a formula is intended
Category V[a]	Modular components for protein, fat, and carbohydrate	*Protein:* Beneprotein, Casec, Propac, Promix *Carbohydrate:* Benecalorie, Moducal, Polycose *Fat:* MCT oil; Microlipid Documentation that **may** provide justification for this category of formula: inability to meet specific nutrient requirements (i.e., protein, carbohydrate, or fat) with a commercially available formula
Category VI[a]	Standardized nutrients	Tolerex Documentation that **may** provide justification for this category of formula: intolerance to intact nutrient formulas, such as excessive stooling or abdominal pain or distention

[a]Failure to provide adequate documentation of medical necessity for the specific formula will likely result in denial of claim or payment at the lower Category I rate for patients with Medicare Part B insurance coverage.
MCT, medium-chain triglyceride.

semisynthetic intact proteins or protein isolates and calories at 1 to 1.2 kcal/mL are in category I. These products have the lowest reimbursement rate and do not require documentation of medical necessity for the specific formula ordered. However, clear documentation of medical necessity for the specific category of formula ordered is required to receive reimbursement at higher rates associated with certain formula categories (e.g., category IV). A statement of medical necessity for enteral nutrition must be completed to receive reimbursement from Medicare for any enteral nutrition therapy.

Evaluation of Nutrition Status

11. D.T., a 35-year-old woman, was admitted to the hospital 65 days ago with severe hemorrhagic pancreatitis and pancreatic abscess. She has required endotracheal intubation since shortly after admission, when respiratory failure occurred. Tube feeding was attempted for the first 3 days after admission but could not be advanced beyond 15 mL/hr. Therefore, parenteral nutrition was started on day 4 after admission and has continued since. D.T.'s current parenteral nutrient formulation contains 250 g dextrose, 96 g amino acid, and 50 g fat, with a rate of 70 mL/hr to provide 1,350 nonprotein calories or 1,734 total calories daily. During her hospitalization, D.T. has undergone three exploratory laparotomies and has been treated for multiple infections, including pneumonia, sepsis, and wound infection. She also has been treated for *Clostridium difficile* diarrhea but has not had diarrhea since therapy was completed 3 weeks ago. Lysis of adhesions, closure of an enterocutaneous fistula, and placement of a feeding jejunostomy tube (J tube) were done during the last laparotomy 2 weeks ago. Postoperative ileus prevented use of the J tube until yesterday, when water was started at 25 mL/hr. Enteral feeding is to start today via the J tube. D.T. is 5'4" and weighs 62 kg today, although her weight before surgery 2 weeks ago was 58 kg and her admission weight was 55 kg. Laboratory evaluation today shows the following: Na, 132 mEq/L (normal, 135 to 145); Cl, 97 mEq/L (normal, 95 to 105); glucose, 158 mg/dL (normal, 70 to 110); BUN, 30 mg/dL (normal, 8 to 20); creatinine, 0.8 mg/dL (normal, 0.6 to 1.2); triglycerides, 125 mg/dL (normal, <160); albumin, 3.1 g/dL (normal, 4 to 6); and prealbumin, 9 mg/dL (normal, 10 to 40), which has decreased from 12 mg/dL 4 days ago and 15 mg/dL a week ago. A urine collection ending last night shows a volume of 2,500 mL/24-hr collection and a urine urea nitrogen (UUN) of 560 mg/dL. D.T. has been afebrile the past week, but remains on broad-spectrum antibiotics. Assess D.T.'s nutrition status and identify factors that place her at risk nutritionally.

D.T. is obviously at risk for severe pancreatitis and multiple complications. Currently, she appears to be malnourished; although her weight is relatively stable, the visceral proteins are decreased. Large urinary nitrogen losses indicate that she is highly catabolic. This also is evident from the low serum prealbumin concentration despite a daily intake of 1.75 g protein/kg IBW. Nutrition status should have been maintained with parenteral nutrition over the past several weeks, but it appears that visceral protein status has been declining during the past week.

D.T. has an increased risk of nutrient deficiencies because of her long-term hospitalization, antibiotic therapy, highly catabolic condition, and complications. Vitamin supplementation in parenteral nutrient formulations generally is adequate for most patients, but highly catabolic patients such as D.T. may require increased vitamin C and perhaps thiamine.[1,28] Increased GI losses of zinc occur with diarrhea and GI tract fistulas, both of which were problems for D.T. before the latest laparotomy.[110] It is assumed that excess losses of vitamins and trace elements that could be reasonably anticipated or measured have been managed appropriately in the parenteral nutrient formulation. Thus, D.T. should not have overt deficiencies. Measurement of most vitamin and trace element serum concentrations is difficult in the clinical setting in metabolically unstable patients, and interpretation of values may be equally difficult. Therefore, objective measures of marginal vitamin deficiencies rarely are available. Clinical impressions must be relied on. D.T. should receive 100% to 200% of the DRI for all vitamins and minerals.

Estimation of Nutrition Requirements

12. What are D.T.'s requirements for calories, protein, and fluid?

D.T.'s current weight is a few kilograms above her IBW of 55 kg. However, looking at the weight history it appears that this extra weight most likely is water. D.T.'s admission weight is more reliable as an indicator of nutrition status than weights obtained in the intensive care unit. Certainly, in 65 days of hospitalization some change in actual weight could have occurred, but it would be very difficult to determine what is actual weight change versus fluid change. D.T.'s IBW should be used for calculations.

Calories and protein provided by parenteral nutrition give an indication of D.T.'s requirements. Because the prealbumin has been declining despite a large protein intake, the nitrogen (N) balance should be calculated to determine whether current protein intake is less than protein losses. (N balance = daily N intake from all sources minus N output that includes daily UUN and obligatory losses.) Intake of nitrogen is calculated from grams of protein assuming that protein is 16% nitrogen (g protein/6.25 = g N). The UUN for nitrogen balance is based on total urine urea loss per 24 hours. The UUN reported by the laboratory is per 100 mL of urine; therefore, UUN loss per 24-hour urine volume must be calculated as follows:

$$560 \text{ mg N/100 mL urine} \times \\ 2,500 \text{ mL urine/24 hr} = 14,000 \text{ mg N/day} \qquad \text{36-1}$$

Obligatory losses generally are estimated as 2 to 4 g of nitrogen per day. Thus, the nitrogen balance for D.T. is calculated as follows:

$$\text{N balance} = \frac{96 \text{ g protein from PN}}{6.25} - \\ (14 \text{ g N from UUN} + 3 \text{ g}) \qquad \text{36-2}$$

where N is nitrogen, PN is parenteral nutrition, and UUN is urine urea nitrogen.

This indicates that D.T. is negative by approximately 1.6 g N or 10 g of protein (1.6 g N × 6.25). In addition, because D.T. has wounds to heal, a positive nitrogen balance of approximately 3 to 5 g of nitrogen is desirable. Therefore, D.T. needs another 4.6 to 6.6 g N/day or 29 to 41 g protein/day more than the 96 g protein currently provided by parenteral nutrition.

D.T. currently is receiving 1,734 kcal daily (31.5 kcal/kg per day) of which 1,350 are nonprotein calories (24.5 nonprotein kcal/kg per day). Calories have a protein-sparing effect up to a certain point; therefore, increased calories may have some benefit if D.T. cannot tolerate the protein increase needed to reverse her negative nitrogen balance. However, with D.T.'s highly catabolic state, maintaining the current NPC:N of approximately 90:1 or slightly less (i.e., down to 75:1) is advisable as long as D.T. can tolerate the extra protein. Indirect calorimetry measurement should be performed if possible. Estimating caloric requirements in a patient such as D.T. is subject to greater error than in a patient with low metabolic stress. If a metabolic cart is not available, the total caloric intake from the parenteral nutrient formulation plus calories from another 30 g of protein should be calculated as a guideline for D.T.'s caloric requirement:

$$\text{1,734 kcal from PN} + (30 \text{ g of protein for positive balance} \times 4 \text{ kcal/g}) = 1,854 \text{ total kcal} \qquad \textbf{36-3}$$

Fluid requirements for younger patients (i.e., those < 65 years) can be estimated at 35 to 40 mL/kg body weight per day plus replacement of excess losses from hyperthermia, vomiting, diarrhea, or wound drainage. Based on this method, D.T.'s fluid requirements are 1,925 to 2,200 mL/day. Estimated fluid needs also may be based on 1 mL/kcal ingested or on 1500 mL plus 20 mL/kg over 20 kg.[1] D.T. should receive a minimum of 1 mL/kcal due to her high protein intake but she is likely to need at least 35 mL/kg/day.

Enteral Nutrition Therapy (Tube Feeding)

13. Enteral feeding is to start today via the J tube. What type of enteral formula is most appropriate for D.T.?

D.T.'s hospitalization has been unusually long and complicated. Most patients with pancreatitis requiring specialized nutrition support can be fed into the jejunum within a few days, and polymeric formulas generally are well tolerated. A small percentage of patients with complicated pancreatitis may require an oligomeric enteral formula or parenteral nutrition. D.T. may have impaired absorptive function because of her prolonged period without GI tract stimulation. She should be assumed to have lactose intolerance at this time.[13] Reduced digestive function and fat malabsorption may persist secondary to the severe pancreatitis D.T. has experienced, although pancreatitis would usually have resolved despite other complications. If the pancreatitis has not resolved, an oligomeric formula should be considered for initiating tube feeding in D.T. Selection of an elemental versus peptide-based formula is determined by calorie, protein, and fat content because studies do not show either type of formula to be superior. If a peptide-based formula is selected, a protein profile that limits pancreatic stimulation (i.e., a high dipeptide and tripeptide percentage) is preferred. To obtain the necessary NPC:N ratio, a high or very high protein formula is needed, or a modular protein component could be added to a standard formula to meet the protein goal for D.T.

The enteral formulary includes one formula categorized as very high nitrogen and one oligomeric formula. The very high

nitrogen formula has a caloric distribution of 25% protein (NPC:N = 75:1), 45% carbohydrate, and 30% fat. The medium-chain triglyceride:long-chain triglyceride ratio is 25:75. This is a polymeric formula that provides 1,000 kcal and 62.5 g protein per liter. The oligomeric formula has a caloric distribution of 20% protein (NPC:N = 115:1), 65% carbohydrate, and 15% fat. The medium-chain triglyceride:long-chain triglyceride ratio is 50:50. This is a ready to use hydrolyzed protein formula that contains peptides and free amino acids; each liter of formula provides 1,000 kcal and 50 g protein.

The oligomeric formula is selected over the polymeric formula because of the minimal need for digestion before absorption, and the low content of long-chain triglycerides that require pancreatic lipase and bile salts for absorption. The formula has an osmolality of approximately 460 mOsm/kg and contains 83% free water per the manufacturer. The goal volume for the formula is 1,920 mL (80 mL/hr) to provide 1,920 kcal, 96 g protein, and 1,594 mL fluid. The remaining fluid requirement will be met by flushing the tube three to four times daily and by the IV antibiotics D.T. is receiving. The enteral formula provides slightly more calories than were estimated to meet D.T.'s needs (see equation 36-3), but calories are within the usual upper range at 34.9 kcal/kg per day. However, the formula does not meet D.T.'s protein requirement calculated from the nitrogen balance. At some point in the transition process, the formula should be changed to a higher protein formula or a modular protein component must be added to the current formula. If D.T. remains as catabolic as she is now, 30 g of a modular protein should be added to the current formula. This is a significant amount of protein to add to a formula; thus, it would be preferable to transition D.T. to a very high nitrogen formula if she can tolerate other components of such a formula. The primary concern in transitioning to the formulary product listed earlier will be whether D.T. can tolerate 30% of calories as fat and 75% of fat as long-chain triglycerides.

Enteral Nutrition Administration

14. Recommend a plan for initiating and advancing D.T.'s tube feeding.

Tube feeding should be initiated slowly in D.T. because she has been without enteral intake for a prolonged period and may have both impaired absorption and digestion. Formula should be administered using an enteral infusion pump to maintain a consistent flow rate. In addition to providing pressure for flow, a pump has alarms to alert nurses if the infusion stops. Small-bore feeding tubes can occlude if the flow is disrupted and surgery may be required to replace the J tube.

The protein provided by parenteral nutrition may remain at the current level, or be increased to provide adequate protein for a 3- to 5-g positive nitrogen balance because transition to tube feeding is expected to be slow. Considering the length of time D.T. has been on parenteral nutrition, transitioning to enteral feeding over several days to a week would be acceptable. The selected enteral formula is hypertonic; nonetheless, full-strength formula should be tried first and the formula diluted to half-strength (approximately 230 mOsm/kg) only if full strength formula causes abdominal distention, diarrhea, or other signs of intolerance. Studies have suggested that dilution of chemically defined and elemental formulas is not required with intragastric or duodenal feeding, but these studies did not include critically ill patients.[112,113] Also, the jejunum may not adapt as easily to concentration and/or volume changes as the duodenum.

Enteral feeding via J tube in this patient is probably best started slowly with a rate of 15 mL/hr for 6 to 12 hours, then 30 mL/hr for 6 to 12 hours if starting with full-strength formula. If starting with half-strength formula, these rates can be increased every 4 to 8 hours. After tolerance to 30 mL/hr is established, the rate can be increased to 45 mL/hr for 6 to 12 hours. The next step is 60 mL/hr for 6 to 12 hours, and finally to the goal rate of 80 mL/hr. Once the tube feeding is at goal rate for 8 to 12 hours, the formula can be increased to full-strength if feeding was initiated with half-strength formula. This transition schedule assumes tolerance to the formula with each step.

A plan also must be developed to transition from the parenteral nutrition to tube feeding. Typically, the parenteral nutrient formulation is gradually decreased, as tolerance to enteral feeding is established. The sum of enteral and parenteral calories and protein should be monitored closely to avoid complications of overfeeding while ensuring that adequate nutrition is provided. For D.T., maintaining adequate protein intake is critical; thus, cumulative protein intake (i.e., protein from parenteral plus enteral intake) should be kept at 125 g/day or higher.

Tube Feeding Intolerance

15. D.T. develops diarrhea approximately 18 hours after the tube feeding is increased to 80 mL/hr. The parenteral nutrient formulation is at 20 mL/hr. What is the likely cause of the diarrhea? Should the tube feeding be stopped and the parenteral nutrient formulation increased to goal rate again?

Diarrhea in patients receiving tube feeding is a multifactorial problem with many potential causes—both those related to tube feedings and those not related to tube feedings.[83,88] Tube feeding–related causes of diarrhea include high fat content, lactose content, and bacterial contamination. Formula temperature, caloric density, osmolality, formula strength, lack of fiber content, and method of delivery also have been associated with diarrhea, although a cause-and-effect relationship for these factors is much less clear. Factors associated with diarrhea, but not related to the tube feeding include concurrent medications, especially sorbitol-containing products and antibiotics; partial small bowel obstruction or fecal impaction; bile salt malabsorption; intestinal atrophy; hypoalbuminemia; infections such as *C. difficile;* and underlying conditions such as AIDS, Crohn's disease, ulcerative colitis, celiac sprue, or pancreatitis.[88]

D.T.'s diarrhea may be related to the change in formula volume. The jejunum does not adapt as easily to changes in volume or concentration as the duodenum, and formula volume was increased <24 hours before diarrhea started. Changing the formula back to the previous volume or slightly less should decrease stool output within 24 hours if the volume change was responsible. If D.T. does not respond to the decrease in formula volume, the formula may be held for 24 hours to assess whether diarrhea decreases or stops. Diarrhea related directly to the enteral formula usually is an osmotic diarrhea that stops within 24 hours of stopping the formula.[88] The parenteral nutrient formulation rate should be increased to 80 mL/hr (goal rate) if tube feeding is stopped for more than 2 days or so. A more objective approach than stopping the formula is to measure stool osmolality. Enteral formula–induced diarrhea is associated with a large osmotic gap, whereas secretory diarrhea (e.g., infectious diarrhea) is associated with a low or negative osmotic gap.[88]

Potential causes of D.T.'s diarrhea other than the change in formula volume should be evaluated before stopping enteral feedings. The current formula is lactose free and has a low content of long-chain triglycerides, so these factors are of minimal concern in D.T. Preparation of formula from a packaged powder, as would have been required with an amino acid–based elemental formula, could lead to bacterial contamination from equipment used in mixing, improper mixing technique, and/or water used for mixing.[83] However, the current formula is a peptide formula that comes ready to use. Cleanliness during transfer of formula to the delivery bag, the period of time formula is in the bag, and methods of cleaning the delivery bag also may contribute to bacterial contamination of formula.[83] Closed enteral systems (i.e., ready-to-hang formula-filled containers) are available and virtually eliminate transfer-related contamination when proper technique is used. Any addition (e.g., medication, carbohydrate, fat or protein module, medium-chain triglyceride oil) to the prefilled container before hanging can contaminate the system, and guidelines (e.g., hang-time, set changes) for an open enteral system should be followed.

Medications appear to be a major contributor to diarrhea in tube-fed patients. However, study results associating antibiotic therapy with diarrhea have been questioned because of failure to report stool frequency and consistency and lack of a clear definition for diarrhea in studies.[83,114] Treatment of antibiotic-associated diarrhea may include administration of *Lactobacillus acidophilus* preparations via the feeding tube to restore normal GI flora, changing antibiotics or stopping therapy when appropriate to do so, or administering antidiarrheal agents. When *C. difficile* is found in the stool, treatment with oral metronidazole or other appropriate antibiotics is indicated. Antidiarrheal agents that decrease motility should not be used when *C. difficile* is present, but adsorbents such as Kaolin-Pectin or pectin-type fibers (e.g., apple flakes or banana flakes) may be beneficial.

D.T. currently is on antibiotics and has been for some time. She has been treated for *C. difficile* once. The current diarrhea may be *C. difficile;* therefore, a stool specimen should be sent for culture and/or *C. difficile* toxin. Other medications that have been associated with diarrhea include the following: sorbitol-containing products, magnesium-containing antacids, oral magnesium electrolyte replacement, potassium chloride, phosphate supplements, quinidine, digitalis, aminophylline, propranolol, and H_2-receptor antagonists.[83,88] Liquid forms of medications used for administration by tube also may contribute to diarrhea because of their high osmolality.[90]

Malnutrition and hypoalbuminemia may contribute to diarrhea in tube-fed patients. D.T. has a low serum albumin and is expected to have atrophy of the GI tract secondary to prolonged parenteral nutrition and no GI tract stimulation; however, diarrhea would have been expected within 24 to 48 hours of starting feedings if this were the primary cause of D.T.'s diarrhea. D.T.'s diarrhea developed after several days on tube feeding. Continued use of the GI tract is encouraged when malabsorption and/or hypoalbuminemia is the primary cause of diarrhea in tube-fed patients.

Pancreatitis may result in diarrhea secondary to malabsorption. D.T. currently is receiving a peptide formula, so only minimal digestive and absorptive function is needed. However, some pancreatic function still is required for the carbohydrates, fats, and peptides larger than tripeptides. Only 15% of calories in the formula are from fat and only half of these calories come from long-chain triglycerides. Therefore, fat malabsorption is unlikely to be the cause of D.T.'s diarrhea.

D.T.'s GI tract should continue to be used to the extent possible. Enteral nutrition appears to be better than parenteral nutrition for maintaining the GI tract barrier and host immunologic function.[1,115–118] The risk of sepsis is increased in patients not receiving enteral stimulation of the GI tract; whether this occurs through bacterial translocation, an unproven process in humans in which enteric bacteria and/or endotoxin cross the GI mucosa into mesenteric lymph nodes and portal circulation, or through another mechanism, is unclear.[115–117] In addition, the GI tract serves an immune function, especially with respect to IgA secretion.[119,120] Respiratory tract infections (e.g., pneumonia) may increase without proper stimulation of the GI tract owing to less effective protection from IgA. Compared with parenteral nutrition, enteral nutrition attenuates catabolism in highly stressed patients, although initiation of feedings soon after the stressing event may be required to obtain this type of response. Before a decision is made to stop enteral feedings, the possible benefits of improved fluid and electrolyte balance with stopping enteral nutrition due to diarrhea should be weighed against the potential benefits of reduced infections from continued use of the GI tract.

Medication Administration via Feeding Tube

16. It is determined that D.T. has *C. difficile* in her stool again. The tube feeding is at 30 mL/hr and the parenteral nutrient formulation is at 55 mL/hr. Kaolin-Pectin has been ordered for administration via tube feeding. Is this an appropriate order?

It generally is better to administer medication separate from the enteral formula, since interactions are more likely to occur if the medication is admixed with the formula. Many hospitals do allow addition of Kaolin-Pectin directly into the enteral formula; however, this is not advised for administration via small inner-diameter jejunostomies. To the extent possible, medications should be given by a route other than the feeding tube because of the risk of occluding the tube lumen. Occlusion of the feeding tube would be more detrimental to the overall plan of transitioning D.T. to tube feedings than stopping the tube feeding for 2 or 3 days until treatment of *C. difficile* resolves the diarrhea. The parenteral nutrient formulation should be increased to goal rate if the tube feeding is stopped due to severe diarrhea. However, stopping the tube feeding is not expected to resolve D.T.'s infectious diarrhea and Kaolin-Pectin should not be administered through the jejunostomy tube even if tube feeding is stopped. Other methods of controlling diarrhea should be investigated.

REFERENCES

1. A.S.P.E.N. Board of Directors and the Clinical Guidelines Task Force. Guidelines for the use of parenteral and enteral nutrition in adult and pediatric patients. J Parenter Enteral Nutr 2002; 26(Suppl 1):1SA.
2. Shopbell JM et al. Nutrition screening and assessment. In: Gottschlich MM, ed. The Science and Practice of Nutrition Support. Dubuque: Kendall/Hunt, 2001:109.
3. Sayarath VG. Nutrition screening for malnutrition: potential economic impact at a community hospital. J Am Diet Assoc 1993;93(12):1440.
4. American Gastroenterological Association. American Gastroenterological Association Medical Position Statement: Guidelines for the Use of Enteral Nutrition. Gastroenterology 1995;108:1280.
5. Levy H. Nasogastric and nasoenteric feeding tubes. Gastrointest Endosc Clin N Am 1998;8(3):529.
6. Metheny N et al. Detection of inadvertent respiratory placement of small-bore feeding tubes: a report of 10 cases. Heart Lung 1990;19:631.
7. Safadi BY et al. Percutaneous endoscopic gastrostomy. Gastrointest Endosc Clin N Am 1998;8(3):551.
8. Georgeson K, Owings E. Surgical and laparoscopic techniques for feeding tube placement. Gastrointest Endosc Clin N Am 1998;8(3):581.
9. Shike M, Latkany L. Direct percutaneous endoscopic jejunostomy. Gastrointest Endosc Clin N Am 1998;8(3):569.
10. Shapiro GD, Edmundowicz SA. Complications of percutaneous endoscopic gastrostomy. Gastrointest Endosc Clin N Am 1996;6:409.
11. Heyland DK, Drover JW, Dhaliwal R, Greenwood J. Optimizing the benefits and minimizing the risks of enteral nutrition in the critically ill: role of small bowel feeding. JPEN 2002;26:S51.
12. Charney P. Enteral nutrition: indications, options and formulations. In: Gottschlich MM, ed. The Science and Practice of Nutrition Support. Dubuque: Kendall/Hunt, 2001:148.
13. Sheehy TW, Anderson PR. Disaccharidase activity in normal and diseased small bowel. Lancet 1965;2(7401):1.
14. Krause RM et al. Dietary guidelines for healthy adults. Circulation 1996;94:1795.
15. Alaimo K et al. Dietary intake of vitamins, minerals, and fiber of persons aged 2 months and over in the United States: Third National Health and Nutrition Examination Survey, Phase I, 1988-1991. Advance Data, 1994:258.
16. Slavin J. Dietary fiber. In: Matarese LE, Gottschlich MM, Eds. Contemporary Nutrition Support Practice: A Clinical Guide. Philadelphia: WB Saunders, 2003:173.
17. Slavin J. Commercially available enteral formulas with fiber and bowel function measures. Nutr Clin Pract 1990;5:247.
18. Lo GS et al. Soy fiber improves lipid and carbohydrate metabolism in primary hyperlipidemic subjects. Atherosclerosis 1986;622:239.
19. Liebl BH et al. Dietary fiber and long-term large bowel response in enterally nourished nonambulatory profoundly retarded youth. J Parenter Enteral Nutr 1990;14:371.
20. McJour AC et al. Intestinal obstruction from cecal bezoar: a complication of fiber-containing tube feedings. Nutrition 1990;6:115.
21. Hosig KG et al. Comparison of large bowel function and calcium balance during soft wheat bran and oat bran consumption. Cereal Chem 1996; 73(3):392.
22. Molis C et al. Digestion, excretion, and energy value of fructooligosaccharides in healthy humans. Am J Clin Nutr 1996;64:324.
23. Speigel JE et al. Safety and benefits of fructooligosaccharides as food ingredients. Food Technol 1994;48:85.
24. Kelly DG, Fleming CR. Physiology of the gastrointestinal tract as applied to patients receiving tube enteral nutrition. In: Rombeau JL, Rolandelli RH, eds. Clinical Nutrition: Enteral and Tube Feeding, 3rd Ed. Philadelphia: WB Saunders, 1997:12.
25. Zaloga GP. Physiologic effects of peptide-based enteral formulas. Nutr Clin Pract 1990;5:231.
26. Mowatt-Larsson CA et al. Comparison of tolerance and nutritional outcome between a peptide and a standard enteral formula in critically-ill, hypoalbuminemic patients. J Parenter Enteral Nutr 1992;16:20.
27. Heimburger DC et al. Effects of small-peptide and whole protein enteral feedings on serum proteins and diarrhea in critically ill patients: a randomized trial. J Parenter Enteral Nutr 1997;21:163.
28. Matarese LE. Rationale and efficacy of specialized enteral and parenteral formulas. In: Matarese LE, Gottschlich MM, eds. Contemporary Nutrition Support Practice: A Clinical Guide. Philadelphia: WB Saunders, 2003:263.
29. Rollins CJ. Basics of enteral and parenteral nutrition. In: Wolinsky I, Williams L, eds. Nutrition in Pharmacy Practice. Washington, DC: American Pharmaceutical Association, 2002:213.

30. Heyland DK et al. Does the formulation of enteral feeding products influence infectious morbidity and mortality rates in the critically ill patient? A critical review of the evidence. Crit Care Med 1994; 22:1192.

31. Kirk SJ et al. Arginine stimulates wound healing and immune function in elderly human beings. Surgery 1993;114(2):155.

32. Daly JM et al. Immune and metabolic effects of arginine in the surgical patient. Ann Surg 1988; 508:512.

33. Daly JM et al. Enteral nutrition with supplemental arginine, RNA and omega-3 fatty acids in patients after operation: immunologic, metabolic and clinical outcome. Surgery 1992;112:56.

34. Sigal RK et al. Parenteral arginine infusion in humans: nutrient substrate or pharmacologic agent? J Parenter Enteral Nutr 1992;16:423.

35. Mayes T, Gottschlich MM. Burns and wound healing. In: Matarese LE, Gottschlich MM, eds. Contemporary Nutrition Support Practice: A Clinical Guide. Philadelphia: WB Saunders, 2003:595.

36. Suchner U, Heyland DK, Peter K. Immune-modulatory actions of arginine in the critically ill. Brit J Nutrition 2002;87:S121.

37. Adjei AA et al. The effects of oral RNA and intraperitoneal nucleoside-nucleotide administration on methicillin-resistant Staphylococcus aureus infection in mice. J Parenter Enteral Nutr 1993; 17:148.

38. Klimberg VS et al. Oral glutamine accelerates healing of small intestine and improves outcome after whole abdominal radiation. Arch Surg 1990; 125:1040.

39. Helton WS et al. Glutamine prevents pancreatic atrophy and fatty liver during elemental feeding. J Surg Res 1990;48:297.

40. Hammarqvsit F et al. Addition of glutamine to total parenteral nutrition after elective abdominal surgery spares free glutamine in muscle, counteracts the fall in muscle protein synthesis and improves nitrogen balance. Ann Surg 1989;209:455.

41. Ziegler TR et al. Clinical and metabolic efficacy of glutamine-supplemented parenteral nutrition after bone marrow transplantation. Ann Intern Med 1992;116:821.

42. Schloerb PR, Amare M. Total parenteral nutrition with glutamine in bone marrow transplantation and other clinical applications (a randomized double-blind study). J Parenter Enteral Nutr 1993; 17:407.

43. Mendez C et al. Effects of an immune-enhancing diet in critically injured patients. J Trauma 1997;42:933.

44. Houdijk APJ et al. Randomized trial of glutamine enriched enteral nutrition on infectious morbidity in patients with multiple trauma. Lancet 1998; 352:772.

45. Novak F, Heyland DK. Glutamine supplementation in serious illness: a systematic review of the evidence. Crit Care Med 2002;30:2022.

46. Swails WS et al. Glutamine content of whole proteins: implications for enteral formulas. Nutr Clin Pract 1992;7:77.

47. Wu G. Intestinal mucosal amino acid catabolism. J Nutr 1998;128:1249.

48. Hasebe M et al. Glutamate in enteral nutrition: can glutamate replace glutamine in supplementation to enteral nutrition in burned rats? J Parenter Enteral Nutr 1999;23:S78.

49. Kelley MJ. Lipids. In: Matarese LE, Gottschlich MM, eds. Contemporary Nutrition Support Practice: A Clinical Guide. Philadelphia: WB Saunders, 2003:112.

50. Schoerb PR. Immune-enhancing diets: products, components, and their rationales. J Parenter Enteral Nutr 2001;25:S3

51. Peck MD et al. Composition of fat in enteral diets can influence outcome in experimental peritonitis. Ann Surg 1991;214:74.

52. Boehm KA et al. Carnitine: a review for the pharmacy clinician. Hosp Pharm 1993;28(9):843.

53. McAdams MP, Carnitine: a review. Support Line, Newsletter of Dietitians in Nutrition Support 1993;15(5):5.

54. Laidlawsa JD, Kopple JD. Newer concepts of the indispensable amino acids. Am J Clin Nutr 1987;46:593.

55. Belli DC et al. Taurine improves the absorption of a fat meal in patients with cystic fibrosis. Pediatrics 1987;80:517.

56. Paauw JD, Davis AT. Taurine concentrations in serum of critically injured patients and age- and sex-matched healthy control subjects. Am J Clin Nutr 1990;52:657.

57. Desai TK et al. Taurine deficiency after intensive chemotherapy and/or radiation. Am J Clin Nutr 1992;52:208.

58. Bower RH et al. Early enteral administration of a formula (IMPACT®) supplemented with arginine, nucleotides, and fish oil in intensive care unit patients: results of a multicenter, prospective, randomized, clinical trial. Crit Care Med 1995;23:436.

59. Galban C et al. An immune enhancing enteral diet reduces mortality rate and episodes of bacteremia in septic intensive care unit patients. Crit Care Med 2000;28:643.

60. Caparros T et al. Early enteral nutrition in critically ill patients with a high-protein diet enriched with arginine, fiber, and antioxidants compared with a standard high-protein diet. The effect on nososcomial infections and outcome. J Parenter Enteral Nutr 2001;25:299.

61. Tepaske R et al. Effect of preoperative oral immune-enhancing nutritio supplement on patients at high risk of infection after cardiac surgery: a randomised placebo-controlled trial. Lancet 2001; 358:696.

62. Kudsk KS et al. A randomized trial of isonitrogenous enteral diets after severe trauma: an immune-enhancing diet reduces septic complications. Ann Surg 1996;224:531.

63. Saffle J, et al. Randomized trial of immune-enhancing enteral nutrition in burn patients. J Trauma 1997;42:793.

64. Moore FA. Effects of immune-enhancing diets on infectious morbidity and multiple organ failure. J Parenter Enteral Nutr 2001;29:S36.

65. Heys SD et al. Enteral nutritional supplementation with key nutrients in patients with critical illness and cancer: a meta-analysis of randomized controlled clinical trials. Ann Surg 1999;229(4):467.

66. Heyland DK, Novak F. Immunonutrition in the critically ill patient: more harm than good? J Parenter Enteral Nutr 2001;25:S51.

67. Heyland DK et al. Should immunonutrition become routine in critically ill patients? A systemic review of the evidence. JAMA 2001;286:944.

68. Beale R, Bryg DJ, Bihari DJ. Immunonutrition in the critically ill: a systematic review of clinical outcome. Crit Care Med 1999;27:2799.

69. Dent DL et al. Immunonutrition may increase mortality in critically ill patients with pneumonia: results of a randomized trial. Crit Care Med 2003; 30:A17.

70. Kuo CD, Shiao GM, Lee JD. The effects of high-fat and high-carbohydrate diet loads on gas exchange and ventilation in COPD patients of normal subjects. Chest 1993;104(1):189.

71. Al-Saady N et al. High fat, low carbohydrate enteral feeding lowers $Paco_2$ and reduces the period of ventilation in artificially ventilated patients. Intensive Care Med 1989;15:290.

72. Talpers SS et al. Nutritionally associated increased carbon dioxide production. Excess total calories vs high portion of carbohydrate calories. Chest 1992;102:551.

73. American Diabetes Association. Translation of the diabetes nutrition recommendations for health care institutions. Diabetes Care 1999;22(Suppl 1):S46.

74. Peters AL, Davidson MB. Effects of various enteral feeding products on postprandial blood glucose response in patients with type 1 diabetes. J Parenter Enteral Nutr 1992;16:69.

75. Craig LD et al. Use of a reduced-carbohydrate, modified fat enteral formula for improving metabolic control and clinical outcomes in long term care residents with type 2 diabetes: results of a pilot study. Nutrition 1998;14(6):529.

76. van den Berghe G et al. Intensive insulin therapy in critically ill patients. N Engl J Med 2001;345(19): 1359.

77. Guenter P et al. Delivery systems and administration of enteral nutrition. In: Rombeau JL, Rolandelli R, eds. Clinical Nutrition. Enteral and Tube Feeding, 3rd Ed. Philadelphia: WB Saunders, 1997:240.

78. Kirby DF, Teran JC. Enteral feeding in critical care, gastrointestinal diseases, and cancer. Gastrointest Endosc Clin N Am 1998;8(3):623.

79. Scolapio JS. Methods for decreasing risk of aspiration pneumonia in critically patients. J Parenter Enteral Nutr 2002;26(6):S58.

80. McClave SA et al. North American summit on aspiration in the critically ill patient: consensus statement. J Parenter Enteral Nutr 2002;26(6):S83.

81. Lord L et al. Enteral nutrition implementation and management. In: Merritt RJ, ed. The A.S.P.E.N. Nutrition Support Practice Manual 1998. Silver Spring, MD: American Society for Parenteral and Enteral Nutrition, 1998:5.

82. DeWitt RC, Kudsk KA. Enteral nutrition. Gastroenterol Clin N Am 1998;27(2):371.

83. Hamaoui E, Kodsi R. Complications of enteral feeding and their prevention. In: Rombeau JL, Rolandelli R, eds. Clinical Nutrition. Enteral and Tube Feeding, 3rd Ed. Philadelphia: WB Saunders, 1997:554.

84. McClave SA, Snyder HL. Clinical use of gastric residual volumes as a monitor for patients on enteral tube feeding. J Parenter Enteral Nutr 2002;26(6):S43.

85. Maloney JP, Ryan TA. Detection of aspiration in enterally fed patients: a requiem for bedside monitors of aspiration. J Parenter Enteral Nutr 2002; 26(6):S34.

86. Maloney JP et al. Systemic absorption of food dye in patients with sepsis [Letter]. N Engl J Med 2000;343(14):1047.

87. Ibanez J et al. Gastroesophageal reflux in intubated patients receiving enteral nutrition: effect of supine and semirecumbent positions. J Parenter Enteral Nutr 1992;16:419.

88. Eisenberg PG. Causes of diarrhea in tube-fed patients: a comprehensive approach to diagnosis and management. Nutr Clin Pract 1993;8:119.

89. Hofsetter J, Allen LV Jr. Causes of non-medication-induced nasogastric tube occlusion. Am J Hosp Pharm 1992;49:603.

90. Rollins CJ. General pharmacologic issues. In: Matarese LE, Gottschlich MM, eds. Contemporary Nutrition Support Practice. A Clinical Guide. Philadelphia: WB Saunders, 1998:303.

91. Marcaurd SP et al. Clearing obstructed feeding tubes. J Parenter Enteral Nutr 1989;13:81.

92. Marcaurd SP et al. Unclogging feeding tubes with pancreatic enzyme. J Parenter Enteral Nutr 1990; 14:198.

93. Gora ML et al. Considerations of drug therapy in patients receiving enteral nutrition. Nutr Clin Pract 1989;4:105.

94. Seifert CF, Johnston BA, Rojas-Fernandez C. Drug administration through enteral feeding catheters [Letter]. Am J Health-Syst Pharm 2002;59:378.

95. Mitchell JF. Oral dosage forms that should not be crushed or chewed. Hosp Pharm 2002;37:213.

96. Healy DP et al. Ciprofloxacin absorption is impaired in patients given enteral feedings orally and via gastrostomy and jejunostomy tubes. Antimicrob Agents Chemother 1996;40:6.

97. Au Yeung SC, Ensom MHH. Phenytoin and enteral feedings: does evidence support an interaction? Ann Pharmacother 2000;34:896.

98. Penrod LE et al. Warfarin resistance and enteral feedings: 2 case reports and a supporting in vitro study. Arch Phys Med Rehabil 2001;82:1270.

99. Johnson KR et al. Gastrointestinal effects of sorbitol as an additive in liquid medications. Am J Med 1994;97:185.

100. Sullivan DH et al. Protein-energy undernutrition among elderly hospitalized patients: a prospective study. JAMA 1999;281(21):2013.

101. Volpato S et al. The value of serum albumin and high-density lipoprotein cholesterol in defining mortality risk in older persons with low serum cholesterol. J Am Geriatr Soc 2001;49(9):1142.

102. Lee JS, Frongillo EA Jr. Nutritional and health consequences are associated with food insecurity among U.S. elderly persons. J Nutr 2001;131:1503.

103. Charlton KE. Elderly men living alone: are they at high nutritional risk? J Nutr Health Aging 1999;3(1):42.

104. Heshka S et al. Resting energy expenditure in the obese: a cross-validation and comparison of prediction equations. J Am Diet Assoc 1993;93:1031.

105. Gale CR et al. Antioxidant vitamin status and carotid atherosclerosis in the elderly. Am J Clin Nutr 2001;74:402.

106. Matsui T et al. Elevated plasma homocysteine levels and risk of silent brain infarction in elderly people. Stroke 2001;32:1116.

107. Selhub J et al. B vitamins, homocysteine, and neurocognitive function in the elderly. Am J Clin Nutr 2000;7(Suppl):614S.

108. Penning-van Beest F et al. Medicine use and vitamin status in elderly Europeans. J Nutr Health Aging 1998;2(3):153.

109. Suter PM et al. Diuretic use: a risk for subclinical thiamine deficiency in elderly patients. J Nutr Health Aging 2000:4(2):69.

110. Baumgartner TG ed. Clinical Guide to Parenteral Micronutrition, 3rd Ed. Fujisawa USA, Inc. 1997.

111. Health Care Financing Administration. Durable Medical Equipment Region D Carrier Manual. Washington, DC: U.S. Department of Health and Human Services.

112. Zarling EJ et al. Effect of enteral formula infusion rate, osmolality, and chemical composition upon clinical tolerance and carbohydrate absorption in normal subjects. J Parenter Enteral Nutr 1986;10:588.

113. Rees RGP et al. Elemental diet administered nasogastrically without starter regimens to patients with inflammatory bowel disease. J Parenter Enteral Nutr 1986;10:258.

114. Haddad RY, Thomas DR. Enteral nutrition and enteral tube feeding: review of the evidence. Clin Geriatr Med. 2002;18:87.

115. Deitch EA, Goodman ER. Prevention of multiple organ failure. Surg Clin N Am 1999;79(6):471.

116. Kudsk KA et al. Enteral versus parenteral feedings: effects on septic morbidity after blunt and penetrating abdominal trauma. Ann Surg 1992;215:503.

117. Sandstrom R et al. The effect of postoperative intravenous feeding (TPN) on outcome following major surgery evaluated in a randomized study. Ann Surg 1993;217:185.

118. Braunschweig CL et al. Enteral compared with parenteral nutrition: a meta-analysis. Am J Clin Nutr 2001;74:534.

119. Jackson WD, Grand RJ. The human intestinal response to enteral nutrients: a review. J Am Coll Nutr 1991;10(5):500.

120. Langkamp-Henken B et al. Immunologic structure and function of the gastrointestinal tract. Nutr Clin Pract 1992;7:100.

CHAPTER 37

Adult Parenteral Nutrition

Beverly J. Holcombe, Jane M. Gervasio

Since the mid-1600s, many efforts have been made to provide nutrients intravenously. Peripheral veins were cannulated and various feeding solutions, including salt water, cow's milk, and glucose, were administered. However, venous access through a peripheral vein necessitated administering large volumes (up to 5 L/day) of solutions with low nutrient content to provide sufficient nutrients. This method of feeding often resulted in thrombophlebitis or fluid overload.

It was not until the 1960s that Dudrick and colleagues used the technique of placing an intravenous (IV) catheter in the superior vena cava, a vessel with rapid blood flow and hemodilution, and were able to administer small volumes of solutions with high concentrations of nutrients.[1] This technique of IV feeding was then used to feed an infant for more than 6 weeks. In turn, large series of both adults and children with abnormalities of the gastrointestinal (GI) tract were fed nutrients via a central venous catheter.[2,3]

During the past four decades, many advances in techniques for IV cannulation and formulation of IV nutrient solutions have been made. Today, the IV provision of complex mixtures of nutrients, known as parenteral nutrition, is an integral part of the medical management of patients, both hospitalized and at home, who cannot eat or ingest nutrients by the GI tract.

MALNUTRITION

Adequate nutrition is important to maintain optimal health. Malnutrition occurs when there is any disorder of nutrition status, including disorders resulting from a deficiency of nutrient intake, impaired nutrient metabolism, or overnutrition. Clinically, a more useful definition of malnutrition is the state induced by alterations in dietary intake resulting in changes in subcellular, cellular, and/or organ function that exposes the individual to increased risks of morbidity and mortality and can be reversed by adequate nutritional support.[5]

The incidence of malnutrition among hospitalized patients has been reported to be as high as 55%.[6,7] In the hospitalized patient, acute malnutrition occurs when nutrient intake is inadequate in the face of injury or stress (e.g., trauma, infection, major surgery), and nutrient stores are rapidly depleted. Acute stress or injury increases energy needs to repair tissues. When this energy is not provided exogenously, the body turns to endogenous sources of energy by breaking down skeletal muscle to release amino acids for the production of glucose. This iatrogenic malnutrition can occur rapidly even in individuals who were well nourished prior to the stress. Once the illness or injury improves and normal nutrient intake is resumed, this acute malnutrition usually resolves.

In contrast, starvation or semistarvation states, without stress or injury, allow humans to adapt slowly to inadequate nutrient intake. This adaptation results in the use of endogenous fat stores for energy and a slow loss of muscle proteins. Nevertheless, energy and protein stores are not unlimited, and with total starvation, death occurs in normal-weight individuals in about 60 to 70 days.[8,9] Clearly, the patient with a history of chronic malnutrition who is faced with stress or injury is at the greatest risk of developing malnutrition.

Protein-calorie malnutrition, the most common type of nutrition deficiency in hospitalized patients, is manifested by depletion of both tissue energy stores and body proteins. Malnourished patients have prolonged hospitalizations and are at a higher risk of developing complications during therapy. These nutrition-associated complications are the result of organ wasting and functional impairment and include weakness, decreased wound healing, altered hepatic metabolism of drugs, increased respiratory failure, decreased cardiac contractility, and infections such as pneumonia and abscesses. These complications increase the length of hospital stay and costs of care.[10–12]

SPECIALIZED NUTRITION SUPPORT

Hospitalized patients with severely inadequate intake for >7 days or those with a weight loss of 10% of their pre-illness weight are considered malnourished or at risk of developing malnutrition. Nutrition intervention should be considered for these patients.[13,14] Patients who cannot meet their nutrition needs by eating enough food by mouth should be considered for some type of specialized nutrition support. *Specialized nutrition support* is the provision of specially formulated and/or delivered parenteral or enteral nutrients to maintain or restore nutrition status.[15] For those who cannot eat by mouth but who have a functional GI tract, a method of enteral nutrition or tube feeding should be considered (see Chapter 36, Adult Enteral Nutrition).

When possible, the GI tract should be used for providing nutrients. Nutrients administered enterally may be more beneficial and less expensive than those provided by the parenteral route.[16] Stimulation of the intestine with enteral nutrients maintains the mucosal barrier structure and function and has been associated with decreased infectious morbidity in critically ill patients compared with those receiving nutrients parenterally.[17–21] For these reasons, parenteral nutrition (sometimes referred to as total parenteral nutrition [TPN]) is reserved for patients whose GI tracts are not functional or cannot be accessed and patients whose GI tracts do not absorb enough nutrients to maintain adequate nutrition status.[13]

PATIENT ASSESSMENT

Assessment of a patient's nutrition status allows analysis of body composition and evaluation of physiologic function. Such an assessment is important in determining the presence and severity of malnutrition or the risk of developing malnu-

trition, and thus determines the need for specialized nutrition support and whether the goal of therapy is to maintain current nutrition status or to replete fat and lean body mass. Assessment should include evaluation of multiple factors and should not rely on one parameter.

Nutrition History

A nutrition history is critical in assessing nutrition status. Information can be obtained by interviewing the patient or the patient's family and reviewing the medical record to identify factors that may contribute to malnutrition or increase the risk of developing malnutrition.

Multiple factors can contribute to the development of malnutrition. For example, a patient who is elderly, lives alone on a fixed income, takes multiple medications, has a history of multiple intestinal surgeries for peptic ulcer disease (PUD), and is hospitalized and receiving nothing by mouth (NPO) until return of GI function after another surgery for resection of the small intestine is nutritionally at risk.

Medications can adversely affect nutrition status by decreasing the synthesis of nutrients, decreasing food intake by altering appetite and taste, altering the absorption or metabolism of nutrients, or increasing nutrient requirements. A nutrition history also should include evaluation of body weight. The components of a nutrition history are summarized in Table 37-1.

Weight History

Weight and weight history are important in evaluating nutrition status. Weight loss is a sign of negative energy and negative protein balance and is associated with poor outcome in hospitalized patients.[6,22] An unintentional weight loss of >10% is considered significant for malnutrition.[15]

A patient's current weight often is compared with a standard such as insurance tables for ideal body weight. Percentage of ideal body weight (IBW) is determined as shown in Equation 37-1:

$$\% \text{ IBW} = \frac{\text{Current weight}}{\text{IBW}} (100) \qquad \textbf{(37-1)}$$

Table 37-1 Components of a Nutrition History
Medical history
Chronic illnesses
Surgical history
Psychosocial history
Socioeconomic status
History of gastrointestinal problems (nausea, vomiting, or diarrhea)
Diet history including weight-loss or weight-gain diets
Food preferences and intolerances
Medications
Weight history
Increase or decrease
Intentional or unintentional
Time period for weight change
Functional capacity

This method of assessing weight has its shortcomings because the patient's weight is compared with a population standard rather than using the individual patient as the reference point. For example, a patient who is significantly overweight and has lost large amounts of weight may still be >100% of IBW and therefore not considered at risk for developing malnutrition. A more patient-specific method of evaluating weight is to compare current weight with the patient's usual weight. This can be determined using Equation 37-2:

$$\% \text{ Usual body weight} = \frac{\text{Current weight}}{\text{Usual body weight}} (100) \quad (37\text{-}2)$$

Using this method, the obese patient who has lost weight may be determined to be <90% of usual weight (weight loss of >10%) and therefore nutritionally at risk. It also is important to assess over what time period the change has occurred. Involuntary weight loss is considered severe if loss exceeds 5% of usual weight within 1 month, or 10% of usual weight within 6 months. The pattern of weight loss must be evaluated to determine whether the loss is continuing or stabilized. Continuing weight loss is a more serious concern than if the weight loss has stabilized. Weight gain after a significant weight loss is a positive sign.

Physical Examination

A physical examination may reveal signs of nutrition deficiencies that require further evaluation. General evidence of muscle and fat wasting (commonly noticed in the temporal area), loss of subcutaneous fat and muscle in the shoulders, and loss of subcutaneous fat in the interosseous and palmar areas of the hands are readily identifiable. Other physical parameters that may be less obvious are hair for color and sparseness; skin for turgor, pigmentation, and dermatitis; mouth for glossitis, gingivitis, cheilosis, and color of the tongue; nails for friability and lines; and the abdomen for ascites or enlarged liver.

Anthropometrics

Physical examination may include anthropometrics that measure subcutaneous fat and skeletal muscle mass. Assessment of fat stores provides information about fat loss or gain and assumes fat is gained or lost proportionally over the entire body. Approximately 50% of body fat is in the subcutaneous compartment. Triceps skinfold and subscapular skinfold thickness measurements are examples of methods used to assess subcutaneous fat and therefore estimate total body fat.

The values obtained are compared with reference standards. Somatic protein mass or skeletal muscle mass can be estimated by measuring mid-arm circumference and then calculating arm muscle circumference. These values also are compared with standards, and the amount of muscle mass is estimated.

When used for the long-term study of large, nutritionally stable populations, anthropometric measurements accurately reflect total body fat and skeletal muscle mass. However, anthropometric measurements of hospitalized patients are of little value. During acute illness and stress, changes in subcutaneous fat may not be proportional to changes in weight, and peripheral edema can result in inflated values for skinfold thickness and mid-arm circumference.[6,22]

Biochemical Assessment

Biochemical assessment of nutrition status includes measuring concentrations of serum proteins. The visceral proteins most commonly used to assess nutrition status are albumin, prealbumin, transferrin, and retinol-binding protein. These proteins are synthesized by the liver and reflect its synthetic capability. Serum concentrations decrease with hepatic insufficiency or when intake of substrates is inadequate for synthesis of these proteins. During stress or injury, inflammatory cytokines are released and substrates are shunted away from the synthesis of these proteins to synthesize other proteins such as C-reactive protein, haptoglobin, fibrinogen and others; these are the acute phase proteins.[23] Serum concentrations of proteins are altered by acute stress or inflammatory states and chronic starvation.[22,23]

Albumin is the classic visceral protein used to evaluate nutrition status and is a prognostic indicator. Serum concentrations of <3 g/dL correlate with poor outcome and increased length of stay of hospitalized patients.[24] Albumin serves as a carrier protein for fatty acids, hormones, minerals, and drugs and is necessary for maintaining oncotic pressure. Albumin has a large body pool of 3 to 5 g/kg, and 30% to 40% is localized to the intravascular space. The normal hepatic rate of albumin synthesis is 150 to 250 mg/kg per day. Because albumin has a half-life of 18 to 21 days, a decrease in serum albumin concentrations generally is not observed until after several weeks of inadequate nitrogen intake. Serum albumin concentrations decrease rapidly in response to stress (which causes albumin to shift from the intravascular to the extravascular space), burns, nephrotic syndrome, protein-losing enteropathy, overhydration, and decreased synthesis with liver disease.[22,24]

Transferrin is responsible for the transport of iron. It has a half-life of 8 to 10 days and therefore is more sensitive than albumin to acute changes in nutrition status. Normal serum concentrations for transferrin are 250 to 300 mg/dL.

Even more sensitive to changes in energy and protein intake is prealbumin (transthyretin), which has a small body pool (10 mg/kg) and a half-life of 2 to 3 days. Prealbumin transports retinol and retinol-binding protein. Normal serum prealbumin concentrations are 15 to 40 mg/dL.

Retinol-binding protein has the shortest half-life, 12 hours; normal serum concentrations are 2.5 to 7.5 mg/dL. However, because serum concentrations of retinol-binding protein change rapidly in response to alterations in nutrient intake, monitoring it has limited use in clinical practice. The visceral proteins commonly used for nutrition assessment are summarized in Table 37-2.

Table 37-2 Visceral Proteins for Nutrition Assessment

Visceral Protein	Half-Life (Days)	Normal Serum Concentration
Albumin	18–21	3.5–5 g/dL
Transferrin	8–10	250–300 mg/dL
Transthyretin (prealbumin)	2–3	15–40 mg/dL
Retinol-binding protein	0.5	2.5–7.5 mg/dL

Other proteins, such as fibronectin and somatomedin-C (insulin-like growth factor-1 [IGF-1]), are also used as markers of nutrition status. Fibronectin is a glycoprotein found in blood, lymph, and many cell surfaces. Somatomedin-C is important in regulating growth. Both fibronectin and somatomedin-C have half-lives of <1 day and respond to fasting and refeeding. Urinary measurement of 3-methylhistidine, a byproduct of muscle metabolism that is excreted unchanged, has been used to estimate skeletal muscle mass. Although these markers have potential use in nutrition assessment, they are used primarily as research tools and are not readily available for routine clinical use.[22]

The interpretation of serum protein concentrations in hospitalized patients may be difficult because factors more important than hepatic synthesis rate alter serum concentrations. These factors may include renal, hepatic, or cardiac dysfunction; hydration status; and metabolic stress. Visceral proteins, as with any nutrition assessment parameter, must be used in conjunction with other parameters and comprehensive consideration of the patient's clinical status.

Nutrition assessment based on determinations of body composition using anthropometrics and biochemical parameters has many limitations. Newer techniques (e.g., bioelectrical impedance, isotope dilution, and neutron activation) are increasingly being used to determine body composition. Other parameters such as hand-grip and forearm dynamometry may be used to assess skeletal muscle function, which relates changes in body composition to body function.[6,22]

Another nutrition assessment method, subjective global assessment (SGA), combines objective parameters and physiologic function. This method is based on a history of weight change, dietary intake, presence of significant GI symptoms, functional capacity, and physical examination to assess the loss of subcutaneous fat and muscle and edema. Using the SGA system, patients are rated as well nourished, moderately malnourished, or severely malnourished. This subjective assessment is easy to use and useful in diagnosing malnutrition.[25]

Classification of Malnutrition

Protein-calorie malnutrition is divided classically into three categories: marasmus, kwashiorkor-like, and a mixed protein-calorie. Marasmus, which means a "dying away state," is seen in individuals who have a chronic deficiency primarily in the intake of energy (calories) over a prolonged period (i.e., partial starvation). Physical examination reveals severe cachexia through loss of both fat and muscle mass; however, visceral protein (e.g., albumin, prealbumin) production is preserved.

Kwashiorkor-like malnutrition results from a diet adequate in calories but limited in protein. Insulin is produced to metabolize the carbohydrates; it also prevents lipolysis and promotes the movement of amino acids into muscle. To meet protein needs, protein is mobilized from internal organs and circulating visceral proteins such as albumin. Thus, an individual with kwashiorkor-like malnutrition has adequate fat and muscle mass but depleted serum proteins.

Hospitalized patients commonly exhibit components of both marasmus and kwashiorkor-like malnutrition and are classified as having mixed protein-calorie malnutrition. This often occurs when an injury or stress compounds chronic starvation or semistarvation, resulting in wasting of fat and muscle mass as well as depletion of serum proteins.

Estimation of Energy Expenditure

An important aspect of patient evaluation is estimating energy expenditure. Many predictive equations for estimating expenditure have been described in the literature.[26,27] The traditional method of assessing energy expenditure is to first calculate basal energy expenditure (BEE), the amount of energy (kilocalories [kcal]) needed to support basic metabolic functions in a state of complete rest, shortly after awakening, and after a 12-hour fast. BEE is most commonly calculated using the Harris-Benedict equations. Alternatively, BEE can be estimated at 20 to 25 kcal/kg per day.

Basal metabolic rate (BMR) is the energy expended in the postabsorptive state (2 hours after a meal) and is approximately 10% greater than BEE. Determination of BEE or BMR does not include additional energy needed for stress or activity. The Harris-Benedict equations can be modified to include stress and physical activity factors, or these variables can be estimated at 20 to 35 kcal/kg per day for moderate to severe stress (Table 37-3).

Another commonly used predictive equation for estimating energy expenditure of hospitalized and critically ill patients is the Ireton-Jones Energy Equation. This equation includes variables for diagnosis, obesity, and ventilatory status.[28]

Energy expenditure can be determined more accurately by indirect calorimetry, which uses a machine ("metabolic cart") to measure the patient's breathing or respiratory gas exchange. The machine measures oxygen consumption and car-

Table 37-3 Estimation of Energy Expenditure

Basal Energy Expenditure (BEE)
Harris-Benedict Equations

BEE_{men} (kcal/day) = 66.47 + 13.75 W + 5.0 H − 6.76 A
BEE_{women} (kcal/day) = 655.10 + 9.56 W + 1.85 H − 4.68 A

or

20–25 kcal/kg/day

Total Energy Expenditure (TEE)
TEE (kcal/day) = BEE × Stress factor × Activity factor

Stress or Injury Factors (% increase above BEE)

Major surgery	10–20
Infection	20
Fracture	20–40
Trauma	40–60
Sepsis	60
Burns	60–100

Activity Factors (% increase above BEE)

Confined to bed	20
Out of bed	30

or

No stress	25 kcal/kg/day
Mild stress	28 kcal/kg/day
Moderate stress	30 kcal/kg/day
Severe stress	35 kcal/kg/day

A, age in years; H, height in cm; W, weight in kg.

Table 37-4   Estimation of Protein Requirements

U.S. RDA	0.8 g/kg/day
Hospitalized patient, minor stress	1–1.2 g/kg/day
Moderate stress	1.2–1.5 g/kg/day
Severe stress	1.5–2 g/kg/day

RDA, recommended dietary allowance.

bon dioxide production when standard testing conditions are maintained. The amount of oxygen consumed and carbon dioxide produced for carbohydrate, fat, and protein is constant and known. Through a series of equations, the energy expenditure, including stress, for that point in time is calculated and then extrapolated for 24 hours.[20,30] This is the measured energy expenditure (MEE). Because the measurement usually is conducted while the patient is at rest, activity is not included in MEE.

Indirect calorimetry is available to many clinicians and is considered the gold standard for energy expenditure determination. It is especially valuable in the energy assessment of critically ill or obese patients.

Estimation of Protein Goals

Estimation of protein needs also must be included in nutrition assessment. Protein needs are calculated based on body weight, degree of stress, and disease state. The recommended dietary allowance (RDA) for the United States is 0.8 g of protein per kg per day. Hospitalized patients with minimal stress who are well nourished need 1 to 1.2 g of protein per kg per day to maintain lean body mass. The requirement for protein intake may be as high as 2 g/kg per day for a patient in a hypermetabolic, hypercatabolic state secondary to trauma or burns. In addition, patients with renal or hepatic dysfunction may require decreased protein intake as a result of altered metabolism. Guidelines for protein needs are summarized in Table 37-4.

VENOUS ACCESS SITES

When parenteral nutrition is necessary, the type of venous access must be selected. Parenteral nutrient formulations may be administered via peripheral veins or central veins, depending on the anticipated duration of parenteral nutrition therapy, nutrient requirements, and availability of venous access.[13]

Peripheral

Peripheral administration may be considered when parenteral nutrition is expected to be necessary for <10 days and the patient has fairly low energy and protein needs because of minimal stress. Candidates for peripheral parenteral nutrition must have good peripheral venous access and must be able to tolerate large volumes of fluids.[31]

Parenteral nutrient formulations for administration via peripheral veins traditionally have contained relatively low concentrations of dextrose (5% to 10%) and amino acids (3% to 5%), providing <1 kcal/mL. Therefore, several liters may be needed daily to meet energy and protein needs. Although dilute with nutrients, the osmolarity of these formulations is 600 to 900 mOsm/L. These hypertonic formulations are irritating to peripheral veins and can cause thrombophlebitis. This necessitates frequent site rotations (at least every 48 to 72 hours), which may quickly exhaust venous access sites. Caloric density can be increased with only a modest increase in osmolarity by administering IV lipids concurrently or by adding them to the dextrose and amino acid mixtures. Lipids also may protect the vein against irritation through dilution and a buffering effect.[32,33]

Central

Administration of parenteral nutrient formulations through a central vein is preferred for patients whose GI tracts are nonfunctional or should be at rest for >7 days; for patients who have limited peripheral venous access; or for those who have energy and protein needs that cannot be met with peripheral nutrient formulations.[13,31,34]

Traditionally, the central venous catheter is percutaneously inserted in the subclavian vein and threaded through the vein so that the tip rests in the upper portion of the superior vena cava (SVC) just above the right atrium. A newer catheter technique involves the use of a peripherally inserted central catheter (PICC) that is inserted in the antecubital vein and advanced until the end of the catheter reaches the upper SVC.[34,35] The internal and external jugular veins also may be used to thread a catheter into the SVC. However, maintaining a sterile dressing on these sites is more difficult than with the subclavian approach or PICC. The SVC is an area of rapid blood flow, which quickly dilutes concentrated parenteral nutrient formulations, thereby minimizing phlebitis or thrombosis. Some patients are not candidates for placement of catheters in the SVC and require a femoral vein insertion with the tip of the catheter in the inferior vena cava. There may be a greater risk for infection with catheters placed using this technique.[34]

Central venous catheters have single or multiple lumens. Multilumen catheters permit the administration of several therapies through the same IV site. Unlike peripheral venous sites, the central venous access site does not require frequent rotation. In fact, some patients requiring parenteral nutrition for months to years may have permanently placed central venous catheters.[36] Parenteral nutrient formulations designed for administration through central veins can contain relatively high concentrations of dextrose (20% to 35%), amino acids (5% to 10%), and lipids providing a caloric density of >1 kcal/mL in a solution with an osmolarity of >2,000 mOsm/L.

COMPONENTS OF PARENTERAL NUTRIENT FORMULATIONS

Parenteral nutrient formulations are very complex mixtures containing carbohydrate, protein, lipids, water, electrolytes, vitamins, and trace minerals. These admixtures must be prepared under aseptic conditions as described by the American Society of Health-System Pharmacists and U.S. Pharmacopeia standards.[37,38] Although parenteral feeding is an important adjuvant therapy for patients with many disease states, errors have occurred in managing this complex therapy, resulting in patient harm and death. This was brought to public attention in 1994 when the U.S. Food and Drug Administration issued a Safety

Alert after two deaths occurred related to errors in compounding parenteral nutrient formulations.[39] As a result of this sentinel event and other reported errors, guidelines or safe practices have been developed for the situations in which inconsistent practices have the potential to cause harm. Pharmaceutical problem areas that are addressed in the Safe Practices for Parenteral Nutrition Formulations are compounding, formulas, labeling, stability, and filtering of parenteral nutrient formulations.[40] These practice guidelines have become standards of practice for parenteral nutrition therapy.

The three macronutrients used in parenteral nutrient formulations, carbohydrate, fat, and protein, are available from various manufacturers. Water, as sterile water for injection, is also used to dilute the macronutrients to achieve the prescribed final concentrations of dextrose, amino acids, and lipids, as well as the final volume of the parenteral nutrient formulation.

Carbohydrate

Dextrose in water is the most common carbohydrate for IV use. It is available commercially in concentrations ranging from 2.5% to 70%. These dextrose solutions are mixed with other components of the parenteral nutrient formulation and diluted to various final concentrations. From these concentrations of dextrose, all parenteral nutrient formulations can be compounded. IV dextrose is monohydrated and provides 3.4 kcal/g, in comparison with dietary carbohydrate, which has a caloric density of 4 kcal/g.

Glycerol also is available (as a 3% mixture with 3% amino acids) for administration as a peripheral parenteral nutrient formulation. Glycerol has a caloric density of 4.3 kcal/g. Other carbohydrates such as fructose, sorbitol, and invert sugar have been used investigationally in parenteral nutrient formulations but are associated with adverse effects and are not available commercially.

Lipid

Lipid for IV use is supplied as emulsions of either soybean oil or a 50:50 physical mixture of soybean and safflower oils that provide long-chain fatty acids (12 to 24 carbon length). The soybean oil emulsion is available in three concentrations: 10%, 20%, and 30%. The soybean/safflower oil emulsion is available as 10% and 20%. The 10% and 20% IV lipid emulsions may be administered concurrently (IV piggyback) with dextrose/amino acid solutions or admixed with dextrose and amino acids. The 30% IV lipid emulsion is hypotonic and should not be used for IV piggyback administration. It is used exclusively for compounding formulations that combine dextrose, amino acids, and lipid in the same container.

Although lipid has a caloric density of 9 kcal/g, the caloric density of the IV lipid emulsions is increased to approximately 10 kcal/g by the addition of glycerol, which is added to adjust the osmolarity. Egg phospholipids are also added as emulsifiers. The phospholipids are derived from egg yolks; therefore, IV lipids are contraindicated in patients with severe egg allergies, especially egg yolk allergies. Phospholipids also contribute approximately 15 mmol/L of phosphorus.

Medium-chain triglycerides (MCTs) are used investigationally. MCTs are 6 to 10 carbons in length and provide 8.3 kcal/g. Physical mixtures of soybean oil and MCTs are being evaluated for potential use in the United States and already are commercially available in other countries.[41]

Amino Acids

Protein for parenteral administration is available as synthetic amino acids and serves as the source of nitrogen. Nitrogen is the building block of cell structure and is used to produce enzymes, peptide hormones, and serum proteins. Amino acid concentrations of 3.5% to 20% are available commercially and vary slightly from one product to another in the specific amounts of each amino acid, electrolyte content, and pH. Generally, amino acid products are characterized as "standard" mixtures, which provide a balanced mix of essential, nonessential, and semiessential amino acids, or "specialty" mixtures, which are modified for specific disease states. For example, the specialty amino acid mixture for use in patients with hepatic failure contains increased amounts of the branched-chain amino acids and decreased amounts of the aromatic amino acids. Protein formulations designed for critically ill patients are supplemented with branched-chain amino acids but have normal amounts of the other amino acids. Amino acid products for patients experiencing renal failure have increased amounts of the essential amino acids or provide only essential amino acids.[42] Amino acid products designed to meet the special needs of neonates also are available (see Chapter 97, Pediatric Nutrition).

Protein or amino acids have a caloric density of 4 kcal/g. Protein calories have not always been included in the calculation of energy needs for patients receiving parenteral nutrient formulations. Ideally, protein is used to stimulate protein synthesis and tissue repair and is not oxidized for energy; however, the human body cannot compartmentalize energy metabolism this way. Today, the conventional wisdom is to include the protein calories in these calculations. Table 37-5 summarizes available nutrients and their caloric density.

Micronutrients

Micronutrients are the electrolytes, vitamins, and trace minerals needed for metabolism. These nutrients are available from various manufacturers as either single entities or in combina-

Table 37-5   Caloric Density of Intravenous Nutrients

Nutrient	kcal/g	kcal/mL
Amino acids	4	—
Amino acids 5%	—	0.2
Amino acids 10%	—	0.4
Dextrose	3.4	—
Dextrose 10%	—	0.34
Dextrose 50%	—	1.7
Dextrose 70%	—	2.38
Fat	10	—
Fat emulsion 10%	—	1.1
Fat emulsion 20%	—	2
Fat emulsion 30%	—	3
Glycerol	4.3	—
Glycerol 3%	—	0.129
Medium-chain triglycerides	8.3	—

tions. For example, the trace element zinc is available commercially as a single trace element product or as a combination product with the other trace elements: copper, chromium, manganese, and selenium. It is important to be aware of the specific products available in each institution to avoid providing inadequate or excessive amounts of various micronutrients.

PARENTERAL NUTRITION

Patient Assessment: Woman in No Acute Stress

1. S.F., a 51-year-old cachectic woman, is admitted to the hospital complaining of a 3-month history of severe abdominal pain after eating and a 30-pound weight loss. Questioning reveals that she has felt hungry, but the pain after eating is so severe she prefers not to eat. S.F. denies any nausea, vomiting, or diarrhea. Her medical history is significant for PUD. Her surgical history is significant for removal of a small section of her ileum for ischemia 4 months ago. Her current medication is nizatidine 150 mg PO BID. S.F.'s social history is significant for tobacco use, but she quit smoking 2 years ago. Review of systems is positive only for the postprandial abdominal pain. When queried about her diet and weight loss, S.F. states that, at most, she eats one meal a day and then consumes only 25% to 40% of it. Tolerance to food is no better if she eats liquids or solids. Further, her weight loss has been continuous over the past 3 months. Physical examination reveals a thin woman with wasting of subcutaneous fat in the temporal area and squared-appearing shoulders. Her height is 5 foot 4 inches and her weight is 89 lb. At the time of her ileum and colon resection, her weight was 119 lb, which is her usual weight.

Admission laboratory values are sodium (Na), 135 mEq/L (normal, 135 to 145); potassium (K), 4.0 mEq/L (normal, 3.5 to 5.0); chloride (Cl), 100 mEq/L (normal, 100 to 110); bicarbonate (HCO$_3^-$), 25 mEq/L (normal, 24 to 30); blood urea nitrogen (BUN), 4 mg/dL (normal, 8 to 20); creatinine, 0.6 mg/dL (normal, 0.8 to 1.2); glucose 87 mg/dL, (normal, 85 to 110); calcium (Ca), 8.2 mg/dL (normal, 8.5 to 10); magnesium (Mg), 2.0 mg/dL (normal, 1.6 to 2.2); phosphorus (P), 3.0 mg/dL (normal, 2.5 to 4.5); total protein, 6.0 g/dL (normal, 6.8 to 8.3); albumin, 4 g/dL (normal, 3.5 to 5.0); and prealbumin, 21 mg/dL (normal, 15 to 40). Her white blood cell (WBC) count is 6,800/mm³ (normal, 4,000 to 12,000).

Based on history and physical findings, S.F.'s working diagnosis is intestinal angina (also known as mesenteric ischemia). Assess her nutrition status.

[SI units: Na, 135 mmol/L (normal, 135 to 145); K, 4.0 mmol/L (normal, 3.5 to 5.0); Cl, 100 mmol/L (normal, 100 to 110); HCO$_3$, 25 mmol/L (normal, 24 to 30); BUN, 1.43 mmol/L (normal, 3 to 6.4); SrCr, 53 μmol/L (normal, 50 to 110); glucose, 4.83 mmol/L (normal, 4.7 to 6.1); Ca, 2.04 mmol/L (normal, 2.3 to 2.7); P 0.97 mmol/L (normal, 0.81 to 1.45); albumin, 40 g/L (normal, 35 to 50); WBC count, 6.8 × 10⁹/L (normal, 4 to 12)]

Assessment of nutrition status requires evaluation of multiple factors. S.F.'s nutrition history indicates that she is not eating because of the abdominal pain, and the recent surgery on her ileum raises the question of nutrient malabsorption. Most striking about S.F.'s history is her weight loss of 30 lb in 3 months, or about 2.5 pounds per week. S.F. is now 75% of her usual weight (see Equation 37-2). Another way of analyzing this is that she has lost 25% of her original weight, which is a severe weight loss. S.F.'s physical findings of cachectic ap-

pearance, temporal wasting, and loss of subcutaneous fat and muscle in her shoulders are significant. No anthropometric measurements are available. S.F.'s visceral proteins (albumin and prealbumin) are within normal ranges.

Consideration of all of these factors leads one to conclude that S.F. is severely malnourished. Her cachectic appearance with loss of subcutaneous fat and muscle, but normal visceral proteins, would be best classified as marasmus. If S.F. were to be faced with stress or injury (e.g., major surgery, infection) necessitating use of visceral proteins for energy production, she would likely exhibit characteristics of both marasmus and kwashiorkor-like or mixed protein-calorie malnutrition in which fat, muscle, and visceral proteins all are depleted.

2. Why is S.F. a candidate for parenteral nutrition therapy?

S.F. is admitted to the hospital for tests to evaluate her severe postprandial abdominal pain. Many of the expected diagnostic tests will require that S.F. remain NPO. Although S.F. appears to have a functioning GI tract, her postprandial pain is so severe it is doubtful she would eat much even if given the opportunity. If the diagnosis of mesenteric ischemia is accurate, surgical correction will be required. With her malnourished state, continued inadequate nutrition in the hospital will result in further deterioration of her nutrition status. Parenteral nutrition should be implemented.

Goals of Therapy

3. During the first 3 days of hospitalization, S.F. undergoes multiple diagnostic tests to evaluate her abdominal pain. An arteriogram reveals occlusion of her superior mesenteric artery, which supplies blood to her small and large intestines. This occlusion compromises blood flow to the intestines when there is increased demand for flow, such as after eating. S.F. is to remain NPO until her surgery, which is scheduled in 4 days. Parenteral nutrition is planned. What is the goal of her nutrition therapy?

S.F. has lost 30 lb, and the limited time before her surgery is not adequate to replete her fat and lean body mass. Her malnutrition occurred over several months, and repletion may take just as long. The benefits of preoperative parenteral nutrition remain unclear. Although some reports describe a trend of improved outcome with preoperative parenteral nutrition,[43] other studies have not demonstrated clear benefit.[13,43–45] Ideally, preoperative parenteral nutrition should be administered for 7 to 10 days to be of any benefit in decreasing the complications associated with surgery in severely malnourished patients. Therefore, the immediate goals for S.F.'s nutrition therapy are to maintain her current nutrition status and prevent her from becoming more malnourished. If parenteral nutrition is initiated and continued after surgery, her calorie and protein goals should be adjusted to take into account the additional stress of major surgery. Finally, once she has recovered from surgery and is convalescing, a long-term goal should be weight gain to her usual weight of 119 lb.

CALORIE AND PROTEIN GOALS

4. Calculate calorie and protein goals for S.F.

S.F.'s initial calorie goals are to meet her current energy expenditure needed for basal metabolism and activity of ambulating. The first step is to calculate BEE (see Table 37-3). For this calculation, S.F.'s actual weight of 89 lb (40.5 kg) should be used because her metabolism and current energy expenditure reflect this decrease in body mass. Using usual weight or ideal body weight in patients who have severe weight loss may result in overfeeding.

Using the Harris-Benedict equation for females, S.F.'s BEE is 1,104 kcal/day. This is then modified for light hospital activity of ambulating or increased by a factor of 30%. The total estimated energy expenditure for S.F. is $1,104 \times 1.3 = 1,435$ kcal/day (see Table 37-3). Unlike most hospitalized patients, S.F. does not require a factor for stress. If S.F. requires parenteral nutrition after surgery, her energy or calorie goals should be reassessed to include a stress factor.

A simpler method to determine energy expenditure is to estimate caloric requirements at 25 to 28 kcal/kg per day: for S.F., 1,012 to 1,134 kcal/day.

The difference in these calculations of energy expenditure demonstrates that there are many methods to estimate energy expenditure, and each method gives slightly different numbers. These methods merely provide estimates of energy expenditure.

Protein goals are estimated based on weight, degree of stress, and disease state. Because S.F. has not yet had surgery and her stress is therefore minimal, her protein goal should be based on the desire to maintain her current protein status. Using the guidelines provided in Table 37-4, S.F.'s protein dose is 1 to 1.2 g/kg per day, or 41 to 49 g/day. As with energy expenditure, calculations of protein needs are only estimates; the patient's clinical course should be monitored and the protein dose adjusted accordingly. The protein source for parenteral nutrition is synthetic amino acids. Generally, 1 g of protein is equivalent to 1 g of amino acids. S.F. will need 41 to 49 g/day of amino acids.

ACCESS

5. **S.F. has a peripheral IV, and her peripheral access appears to be adequate. Is she a candidate for using a peripheral parenteral nutrition formulation?**

With good peripheral access, S.F. meets one of the criteria for peripheral parenteral nutrition. Further, she should be able to tolerate the volume of a peripheral parenteral nutrition formulation necessary to meet her goals. Because peripheral parenteral nutrition can be irritating to the veins, the addition of IV lipid to her parenteral nutrient formulation help preserve peripheral venous access. For short-term peripheral parenteral nutrition, IV lipids can be used to provide up to 60% of nonprotein calories.

FORMULATION DESIGN
Macronutrients and Micronutrients.

6. **Design a peripheral parenteral nutrient base formulation for S.F. that provides 1,300 total calories and 45 g of amino acids. The formulation should provide 60% of the nonprotein calories as lipid and have maximum dextrose and amino acid concentrations of 6% and 3%, respectively. The macronutrient components available to prepare this formulation are dextrose 20%, amino acids 8.5%, sterile water for injection, and IV lipids 10% and 20%.**

The amino acids in S.F.'s nutrient formulation provide 180 protein calories (45×4), leaving 1,120 nonprotein calories to

be provided by fat and carbohydrate. The IV lipid provides 672 ($1,120 \times 0.6$) calories. The remaining 448 nonprotein calories are provided by dextrose. Dextrose provides 3.4 kcal/g; therefore, 132 g of dextrose is required. The volume necessary to provide 132 g of dextrose as a 6% concentration is 2,200 mL.

$$mL = \frac{132 \text{ g dextrose } (1,000 \text{ mL})}{60 \text{ g}} \qquad \textbf{(37-A)}$$

$$= 2,200 \text{ mL}$$

Similarly, the volume necessary to provide 45 g of amino acids as a 3% final concentration is calculated to be 1,500 mL. To stay within the guidelines for maximum dextrose and amino acid concentrations, the larger volume of 2,200 mL is used. Therefore, the final dextrose and amino acid concentrations are 6% and 2%, respectively. This parenteral nutrient formulation is compounded using dextrose 20% 660 mL (132 g) and amino acids 8.5% 530 mL (45 g), with sterile water for injection added to achieve a final volume of 2,200 mL.

Next, the amount of fat to provide 672 kcal must be determined. Using 10% lipid emulsion with a caloric density of 1.1 kcal/mL will require 611 mL or 336 mL of the 20% lipid emulsion (2 kcal/mL) (see Table 37-5). The IV lipid can be provided in various ways. One method is to infuse the lipids as a secondary infusion or piggybacked into the dextrose/amino acid solution. If the 10% lipid emulsion is used, S.F.'s fluid intake from her parenteral feedings will be approximately 2,800 mL/day; using the 20% lipid emulsion, 2,550 mL/day is necessary.

Alternatively, many institutions mix the entire daily requirements for lipid, dextrose, and amino acids in one large container or single daily bag. This is called total nutrient admixture (TNA), triple-mix, three-in-one, or all-in-one and is the preferred method of administering parenteral nutrient formulations via peripheral veins because the iso-osmotic lipids have a diluting as well as buffering effect.[46] Further, the addition of the lipids increases the caloric density significantly with only a slight increase in osmolarity.

S.F.'s peripheral nutrient formulation should also contain standard amounts of electrolytes, as well as a daily dose of IV multivitamins and trace elements.

Fluids.

7. **The institution uses a TNA system, and S.F.'s parenteral nutrient formulation is provided in 2,200 mL/day. Will this meet S.F.'s maintenance fluid requirements?**

Maintenance fluid needs can be estimated using several methods. The simplest method uses 30 to 35 mL/kg per day as the basis. Another method is to provide 1,500 mL for the first 20 kg body weight plus an additional 20 mL/kg for actual weight beyond the initial 20 kg. Both methods provide estimates of fluid needs for basic maintenance, and additional fluid must be provided for increased losses such as vomiting, nasogastric (NG) tube output, diarrhea, or large open wounds. S.F.'s fluid needs are estimated as follows:

$$
\begin{aligned}
mL/day &= 1,500 \text{ mL} + [(120 \text{ mL/kg})(40.5 \text{ kg} - 20 \text{ kg})] \\
&= 1,500 \text{ mL} + (20 \text{ mL/kg})(20.5 \text{ kg}) \\
&= 1,500 \text{ mL} + 410 \text{ mL} \\
&= 1,910 \text{ mL}
\end{aligned}
\qquad \textbf{(37-B)}
$$

Clearly, the peripheral parenteral nutrient formulation will more than meet S.F.'s needs, and the extra fluid intake may put her at risk for becoming fluid overloaded, manifesting as hypervolemic, hypotonic hyponatremia. Therefore, she should be monitored for signs of fluid overload, including peripheral edema, shortness of breath, daily intake exceeding daily output, hyponatremia, and rapidly increasing weight.

Monitoring and Management of Complications

8. What metabolic complication is a potential concern due to S.F.'s malnutrition?

Refeeding syndrome is the term used to define the severe hypophosphatemia and associated metabolic complications that occur when malnourished patients receive a concentrated source of calories via parenteral or enteral nutrition. This phenomenon was first reported when the Holocaust victims and prisoners of war in World War II were rescued and given normal food and liquid intake. Complications coinciding with refeeding these individuals included hypertension, cardiac insufficiency, seizures, coma, and death. These complications were reported later in the 1970s and 1980s with the introduction of parenteral nutrition in chronically ill, essentially starved hospitalized patients.

Metabolic complications from refeeding are associated primarily with severe hypophosphatemia, but hypokalemia, hypomagnesemia, vitamin deficiencies, fluid intolerance, and glucose alterations may occur. In the starved, depleted individual there is a loss of lean body mass, water, and minerals. Individuals may preserve some intracellular electrolytes, including phosphorus. When these individuals are given a concentrated source of calories, the carbohydrates are converted to glucose. Glucose, in turn, results in the secretion of insulin. The release of insulin enhances the uptake of glucose, water, phosphorus, and other intracellular electrolytes. The combination of phosphorus depletion and intracellular uptake causes severe hypophosphatemia.

To minimize the risk of refeeding syndrome in S.F., any electrolyte abnormalities must be corrected before any nutrition is initiated. Since S.F.'s electrolytes are within normal range, no adjustments are necessary. Nutrition should then be implemented slowly and vitamins administered routinely. Electrolytes, including phosphorus, potassium, magnesium, and glucose should be monitored at least daily over the first week. While electrolyte and mineral abnormalities may not be avoided, careful recognition of and close monitoring for refeeding syndrome will prevent serious complications.[47,48]

9. What additional parameters should be monitored for patients receiving peripheral parenteral nutrition?

The primary calorie source in peripheral parenteral feedings is lipids. For S.F., 60% of the nonprotein calories are provided as lipid. However, for adults, the daily lipid intake should not exceed 2.5 g/kg per day. S.F.'s formulation provides approximately 65 g of lipid daily, or 1.6 g/kg per day. It is also important to monitor serum triglyceride levels to assess tolerance to this dose of IV lipid. If the blood sample is obtained while the triglycerides are infusing, as with the TNA formulation, a serum triglyceride concentration of <400 mg/dL, although elevated, is acceptable.[49] Hypertriglyceridemia sometimes can be noted quickly by gross observation of the blood sample.

10. Forty-eight hours after peripheral parenteral nutrition is started, S.F. begins to complain that the arm where she has the IV for the feeding is swollen, red, and painful. What is the most probable cause of these complaints? What measures can be taken to prevent this complication?

A common complication (up to 70%) of peripheral parenteral nutrition is phlebitis, which occurs within 72 hours.[32,50] Phlebitis usually is attributed to the acidic pH or hyperosmolarity of the nutrient formulation. The osmolarity of typical peripheral parenteral feedings ranges from 600 to 900 mOsm/L. Osmolarity of a dextrose/amino acid formulation can be approximated quickly by multiplying the final dextrose concentration by 50 and the final amino acid concentration by 100. Alternatively, the osmolarity can be estimated by multiplying the number of grams of dextrose by 5 and the number of grams of amino acids by 10, then dividing by the final volume in liters. Approximately 150 mOsm/L should be added for contribution of electrolytes, vitamins, and trace elements.

Using the first method, a formulation of 6% dextrose and 2% amino acids has an approximate osmolarity of 650 mOsm [(6% dextrose $\times$ 50 = 300 mOsm) + (2% amino acids * 100 = 200 mOsm) + 150 mOsm for additives]. Although the concurrent administration of fat emulsions decreases osmolarity, buffers the pH, and improves peripheral vein tolerance, it does not eliminate the risk of thrombophlebitis.[51]

Other efforts to minimize phlebitis include the addition of a combination of heparin and hydrocortisone to the admixture.[32,52,53] Alternatively, a glycerol trinitrate patch may be applied near the peripheral IV site to dilate the superficial veins, which constrict when there is irritation.[54]

S.F.'s peripheral IV catheter should be removed and another one placed in the other arm if she is to continue receiving the peripheral parenteral nutrient formulation. Methods to reduce thrombophlebitis should be initiated. If S.F. exhausts her peripheral venous access and continues to need parenteral nutrition, placement of a central venous catheter should be considered.

Patient Assessment: Man in Moderate Stress

11. D.C., a 38-year-old man with a 12-year history of Crohn's disease, is admitted to the hospital after being evaluated in the clinic for a complaint of increasing abdominal pain, nausea and vomiting for 9 days, and no stool output for 5 days. Questioning reveals that over the past week he has been drinking only liquids secondary to nausea and vomiting, and his weight has decreased 10 lb during that time. D.C.'s medical history is significant for frequent exacerbations of his Crohn's disease during the past 2 years. His surgical history includes an exploratory laparotomy 6 months ago for resection of 10 cm of ileum. Family and social histories are noncontributory. His current medications include mesalamine 1,000 mg PO QID and prednisone 10 mg PO QD. Review of systems is positive for severe abdominal pain. On physical examination, D.C. appears thin, and his abdomen is distended. Vital signs are notable for a temperature of 38.3°C, heart rate of 98 beats/min, and a blood pressure (BP) of 108/71 mm Hg. He is 6 feet tall and weighs 60.5 kg. His medical record indicates that 1 month ago he weighed 64 kg, and 6 months ago his weight was 70 kg. Abdominal radiographs are consistent with a small bowel obstruction.

Admission laboratory values are Na, 131 mEq/L (normal, 135 to 145); K, 3.2 mEq/L (normal, 3.5 to 5.0); Cl, 98 mEq/L (normal, 100 to 110); HCO_3^-, 28 mEq/L (normal, 24 to 30); BUN, 19 mg/dL (normal, 8 to 20); creatinine, 0.9 mg/dL (normal, 0.8 to 1.2); glucose, 118 mg/dL (normal, 85 to 110); albumin, 3.2 g/dL (normal, 3.5 to 5.0); WBC count, 10,900/mm³ (normal, 4,000 to 12,000); hematocrit (Hct), 46% (normal, 34% to 50%); alanine aminotransferase (ALT), 29 U/L (normal, 20 to 70); aspartate aminotransferase (AST), 25 U/L (normal, 20 to 55); alkaline phosphatase, 45 U/L (normal, 40 to 125); total bilirubin, 0.5 mg/dL (normal, 0 to 1.2).

D.C. is admitted with a diagnosis of a small bowel obstruction secondary to a stricture or narrowed area in his small intestine. The plan is to manage him with IV fluids, bowel rest and decompression, and possible surgery. Why is D.C. a candidate for parenteral nutrition?

[SI units: Na, 131 mmol/L (normal, 135 to 145); K, 3.2 mmol/L (normal, 3.5 to 5.0); Cl, 96 mmol/L (normal, 100 to 110); HCO_3^-, 28 mmol/L (normal, 24 to 30); BUN, 6.78 mmol/L (normal, 3 to 6.4); creatinine, 54 μmol/L (normal, 50 to 110); glucose, 6.5 mmol/L (normal, 4.7 to 6.1); albumin, 32 g/L (normal, 35 to 50); WBC count, 10.9×10^{-9}/L (normal, 4 to 12); Hct, 0.46 (normal, 0.34 to 0.50); ALT, 0.334 mkat/L (normal, 0.03 to 0.4); AST, 0.25 mkat/L (normal, 0.1 to 0.28); alkaline phosphatase, 0.75 mkat/L (normal, 0.48 to 1.5); total bilirubin, 8.5 μmol/L (normal, 0 to 20)]

Parenteral nutrition should be considered when the patient's nutrient intake has been inadequate for 7 days or longer and the GI tract is not functioning. D.C. has eaten little in the last week, and his 5% decrease in weight is of concern. Further, his weight has decreased by >10% over the past 6 months, which is considered a severe weight loss. D.C. is not expected to resume oral intake because his small bowel obstruction is being managed conservatively with bowel rest and decompression.

Assessment of weight loss should include evaluation of hydration status, especially because D.C.'s vomiting and minimal oral intake for the past week place him at risk of dehydration. Loss of lean body mass is probably less than that reflected by the decrease in weight. Although D.C. may be dehydrated, he also may have significant loss of muscle resulting from his chronic intake of prednisone, which stimulates gluconeogenesis and muscle breakdown for amino acids. In addition, D.C.'s admission serum albumin concentration is low at 3.2 g/dL, and his hydration status should be considered when evaluating this visceral protein. D.C.'s serum albumin concentration probably will decrease further after he is rehydrated.

One factor contributing to his low serum albumin is the loss of proteins from the GI tract (protein-losing enteropathy) during exacerbations of his Crohn's disease. Continued inadequate nutrient intake increases his risk of malnutrition. Some type of specialized nutrition support should be initiated, and because D.C.'s GI tract is not functioning, parenteral nutrition is indicated.

12. What type of malnutrition does D.C. have?

At this point D.C. exhibits some loss of fat and muscle, as well as depletion of visceral proteins. He has components of both marasmus and kwashiorkor-like malnutrition; therefore, he would be considered to have mixed protein-calorie malnutrition.

Calorie and Protein Goals

13. After hydration with IV fluids, D.C.'s weight is 62.5 kg. Parenteral nutrition therapy was delayed because within 24

hours after admission, D.C. developed severe abdominal pain and distention and required surgery. An exploratory laparotomy was performed, and 25 cm of ileum was resected to remove the area of bowel with severe disease as well as a stricture causing the obstruction. A small abscess near his colon was also drained. His postoperative medications include hydrocortisone 100 mg IV Q 8 hr and piperacillin-tazobactam 4.5 g IV Q 6 hr. Bowel sounds are absent. He has a right subclavian triple-lumen central venous catheter and an NG tube output of 1,800 mL/day. His urine output is 1,400 mL/day. Parenteral nutrition is to begin on postoperative day 1. Calculate energy and protein goals for D.C.

Using the Harris-Benedict equation for men, his current weight of 62.5 kg, height of 182.9 cm, and age of 38 years, D.C.'s BEE is 1,583 kcal/day (see Table 37-3). To estimate his total energy expenditure, the BEE should be modified with an activity factor for being confined to bed of 1.2 and a stress factor of 1.2 for surgery. These modifications result in an estimated energy expenditure of 40% greater than his BEE, or 2,216 kcal/day (1,583 × 1.4). Using the simpler method for moderate stress (27 kcal/kg per day) results in an estimated energy expenditure of 1,875 kcal/day. Therefore, an energy goal of 2,000 kcal/day is reasonable. In a similar manner, his protein goal (see Table 37-4) for moderate stress is 75 to 94 g/day of protein (1.2 to 1.5 g/kg per day).

Formulation Design

14. Design a single daily bag, TNA parenteral nutrient formulation for D.C. that provides 2,000 kcal and 90 g of amino acids with a nonprotein calorie distribution of 75% carbohydrate and 25% lipid. The macronutrients available on the formulary for compounding the parenteral nutrient formulations are 70% dextrose, 30% lipid emulsion, and 10% amino acids.

1. Amino acids calculation

$$\text{Calories from amino acids (protein)} = 90 \text{ g} \times 4.0 \text{ kcal/g}$$
$$= 360 \text{ kcal}$$
$$\text{mL of 10\% amino acids} = \frac{90 \text{ g}}{0.1 \text{ g/mL}} \quad \textbf{(37-C)}$$
$$= 900 \text{ mL}$$

2. Dextrose calculation

$$\text{Calories from dextrose} = (2,200 - 360)(0.75)$$
$$= 1,380 \text{ kcal}$$
$$\text{g of dextrose} = \frac{1,380 \text{ kcal}}{3.4 \text{ kcal/g}}$$
$$= 406 \text{ g} \quad \textbf{(37-D)}$$
$$\text{mL of 70\% dextrose} = \frac{406 \text{ g}}{0.7 \text{ g/mL}}$$
$$= 580 \text{ mL}$$

3. Lipid emulsion calculation

$$\text{Calories from lipid} = (2,200 - 360)(0.25) \text{ or } (1,840 - 1,380)$$
$$= 460 \text{ kcal}$$
$$\text{mL 30\% lipid emulsion} = \frac{460 \text{ kcal}}{3.0 \text{ kcal/mL}} \quad \textbf{(37-E)}$$
$$= 153 \text{ mL}$$

4. Calculation of final volume

$$
\begin{array}{l}
900 \text{ mL amino acids } 10\% \\
580 \text{ mL dextrose } 70\% \\
\underline{153 \text{ mL lipid emulsion } 30\%} \\
1{,}633 \text{ mL total volume}
\end{array} \quad \text{(37-F)}
$$

Other additives such as electrolytes, vitamins, and trace elements are included in the parenteral nutrient formulation and slightly increase the final volume to 1,800 mL/day. The infusion rate for this formulation can be calculated as follows:

$$
\text{Hourly infusion rate (mL/hr)} = \frac{1{,}800 \text{ mL/day}}{24 \text{ hr/day}}
$$
$$
= 75 \text{ mL/hr} \quad \text{(37-G)}
$$

D.C.'s parenteral nutrient formulation of 1,800 mL/day will not meet his maintenance fluid needs of 2,350 mL/day (see Question 7). He will require extra fluid to meet the remainder of his basic fluid needs plus additional fluid to replace the fluid loss from his NG tube. These additional fluids should be provided through another IV.

Some institutions neither prepare parenteral nutrient formulations as single daily bags nor use TNA; instead, standard base formulations of dextrose and amino acids are dispensed in 1-L volumes. IV lipids are not usually included in the daily parenteral nutrient regimen. A commonly employed base formulation is dextrose 250 g/L (25%) and amino acids 42.5 g/L (4.25%), which provides 1,020 kcal/L (250 g × 3.4 kcal/g + 42.5 g × 4 kcal/g). Using this type of dextrose/amino acid formulation for D.C. would require 2.2 L/day (or an infusion rate of 92 mL/hour) to approximate his calorie and protein goals.

Monitoring and Management of Complications
METABOLIC COMPLICATIONS: ESSENTIAL FATTY ACID DEFICIENCY

15. **What consequences are associated with providing only dextrose and amino acids to meet D.C.'s nutrient needs?**

A small amount of lipid is necessary to prevent essential fatty acid deficiency (EFAD). The essential fatty acids, linoleic and alpha-linoleic, are those that cannot be synthesized by humans. Of these, linoleic acid appears to be the only one required by adults. The continuous infusion of hypertonic dextrose is associated with high circulating concentrations of insulin. Because insulin promotes lipogenesis rather than lipolysis, linoleic acid cannot be released from adipose tissue.[54]

Clinical symptoms of EFAD are dry, thickened, scaly skin, hair loss, poor wound healing, and thrombocytopenia, which may be observed after a few weeks to months of lipid-free parenteral feedings.[55] Biochemical evidence of EFAD, determined by a triene:tetraene ratio of >0.4, may be seen after 1 week of lipid-free parenteral feedings and is characterized by a decrease in the serum concentrations of linoleic and arachidonic acids and an increase in the concentration of 5,8,11-eicosatrienoic acid.[54] The requirement for essential fatty acids is 1% to 4% of total caloric intake and can usually be met by the administration of 500 mL of a 10% lipid emulsion twice weekly or 500 mL of a 20% lipid emulsion once a week to patients receiving a dextrose/amino acid parenteral nutrient formulation.[13,54] The lipid emulsions should be infused at a rate of <0.11 g/kg per hour to prevent adverse effects, which include impaired hepatic, pulmonary, immune and platelet function.[41]

METABOLIC CONSEQUENCES OF EXCESSIVE DEXTROSE ADMINISTRATION

16. **What are the benefits of using a mixed-fuel system, combining dextrose and fat to meet energy needs?**

Providing a portion of nonprotein calories as fat may reduce the metabolic consequences of excessive dextrose administration. The maximum rate of dextrose metabolism in humans is 5 to 7 mg/kg per minute, or approximately 7 g/kg per day. In doses of >7 g/kg per day, dextrose is used inefficiently and is converted to fat.[55] The conversion to fat may be associated with respiratory compromise and hepatic dysfunction.[56–58] Hyperglycemia, another complication of excessive dextrose infusion, is associated with electrolyte and acid–base disturbances, osmotic diuresis, increased risk of infections (especially *Candida albicans*), and altered phagocyte and complement function. Furthermore, using a mixed-fuel system allows the administration of a small amount of IV lipid daily and avoids the need for larger boluses of lipid twice weekly to prevent EFAD. Rapid administration of IV lipids has been associated with alterations in the reticuloendothelial system that are not observed with continuous administration of small doses.[59] Typically, a mixed-fuel system provides 15% to 30% of nonprotein calories as fat, 70% to 85% as carbohydrate.

Total Nutrient Admixtures

17. **What are the advantages to combining the dextrose, fat, and amino acids in one container?**

The system of providing one container per day offers the advantage of convenience to pharmacy staff, nursing personnel, and the patient. The pharmacy department usually prepares TNA only once per day and therefore requires fewer supplies and inventory; waste of unused feeding formulations is minimized as well. Nursing time to administer TNAs is decreased because only one bag is hung per day, minimizing venous catheter interruptions and avoiding the need to manipulate a secondary infusion of lipid emulsions as well as additional IV tubing and an infusion pump.[60]

Although there are many practical benefits to using TNA parenteral feeding formulations, this system is not without concerns. These formulations must be mixed in plastic containers constructed with ethylvinylacetate. Containers with diethylhexylphthalate (DEHP) should be avoided because this toxic material may by extracted by the lipid and may harm patients. The addition of lipid to the traditional mixture of dextrose and amino acids converts this solution to a complex emulsion formulation with physiologic differences that alter the stability of the product.[61] These differences must be considered in the compounding of TNA parenteral feeding formulations. (See Question 6 for an alternative administration method for fat emulsions.)

STABILITY

18. **How stable are the TNA parenteral feeding formulations?**

IV lipid emulsions alone gradually deteriorate over time because of increased formation of free fatty acids and a resultant decrease in pH. When lipids are mixed with dextrose and amino acids, this process is accelerated, IV lipid products commercially available in the United States use an anionic egg yolk phosphatide emulsifier, which stabilizes the lipid droplets of the dispersed phase with the aqueous external phase and maintains the integrity of the dispersion. Because the emulsifier is anionic, the addition of any substance with cationic properties can neutralize the negative charge of the emulsifier and alter the emulsion's stability. When the emulsion becomes unstable or breaks down, the fat particles begin to aggregate and the particle size increases.

Destabilization of the emulsion occurs in steps that begin with creaming and end with the coalescence of the lipid particles, or "cracking" of the emulsion. A decrease in pH and the addition of divalent cations (Mg^{2+}, Ca^{2+}) increase fat particle size. Although dextrose decreases the pH, the addition of amino acids provides an adequate buffer for this variable. The amount of divalent cations added to TNAs should be limited to minimize the risk of emulsion instability. Trivalent cations such as iron should never be added to a TNA parenteral nutrient formulation. Nutrient formulations containing lipid must be assessed visually for signs of phase separation, in which the instability of the emulsion is manifested by "oiling out," indicated by a continuous layer of oil or individual fat droplets. Fat emulsion particles have an average size of 0.5 microns. A destabilized emulsion is not visibly apparent until the lipid particles are 40 to 50 microns. Fat particles as small as 5 microns may occlude pulmonary capillaries.[60,61] Therefore, the use of a 1.2-micron filter is recommended to protect against the infusion of enlarged lipid particles.[39,40,60]

Using dual-chamber bags may extend the shelf life of TNAs because they allow the lipid to be physically separated from the dextrose, amino acids, and other additives until it is time to administer the feeding. The use of dual-chamber bags has the greatest advantage for the home care setting, where up to a week's supply of parenteral feedings are prepared at one time.[60]

After preparation, TNAs should be refrigerated (4°C) to preserve stability. Once the bag is removed from the refrigerator, it should be warmed to room temperature and the contents mixed well before administration. Mixing is best accomplished by gently inverting the container up and down to ensure top-to-bottom transfer of the fluid. Vigorous shaking should be avoided because it introduces air, which can destabilize the emulsion.[60,61]

MICROBIAL GROWTH

19. How does the microbial growth in TNAs compare with that of dextrose/amino acid formulations?

Dextrose/amino acid parenteral nutrient formulations are not conducive to growth of most organisms because of their high osmolarity (>2,000 mOsm/L) and acidic pH. Lipid emulsions alone, however, are isotonic and have a physiologic pH, providing an optimal growth medium. Combining these three substrates in a TNA provides a formulation with a microbial growth potential that is intermediate between these two.[60,61] The number of central venous catheter violations or manipulations correlates strongly with the incidence of catheter-related infections. From an infection control perspective, the use of a single daily bag TNA system limits the number of manipulations of the central venous catheter to one per day,

thereby minimizing touch contamination. The Centers for Disease Control and Prevention guidelines allow TNA or dextrose/amino acid formulations to hang for up to 24 hours. However, because of concerns about the potential of lipid emulsions to support microbial growth, the hang time for lipids when administered alone is 12 hours.[60]

MICRONUTRIENTS
Electrolytes

20. D.C.'s current laboratory values are Na, 137 mEq/L; K, 4.5 mEq/L; Cl, 102 mEq/L; HCO_3^-, 26 mEq/L; BUN, 9 mg/dL; creatinine, 0.8 mg/dL; glucose, 148 mg/dL; Ca, 8.9 mg/dL (normal, 8.5 to 10.0); Mg, 1.9 mg/dL (normal, 1.6 to 2.2); P, 2.8 mg/dL (normal, 2.4 to 4.5); and albumin, 3.0 mg/dL. Which electrolytes should be included in D.C.'s parenteral nutrient formulation?

[SI units: Na, 137 mmol/L; K, 4.5 mmol/L; Cl, 102 mmol/L; HCO_3^-, 26 mmol/L; BUN, 3.2 mmol/L; creatinine, 48 μmol/L; glucose, 8.2 mmol/L; Ca, 2.22 mmol/L; Mg, 9.5 mmol/L; P, 0.9 mmol/L; albumin, 30 g/L]

Electrolytes added are sodium, potassium, chloride, acetate (which is metabolized to bicarbonate), magnesium, calcium, and phosphate. Electrolytes should be added to the parenteral nutrient formulation based on the individual patient's needs. However, patients without significant fluid and electrolyte losses, hepatic or renal dysfunction, or acid–base disturbances do well with maintenance doses of electrolytes. Electrolytes may be added individually or as commercially available combination products of maintenance doses, but the electrolyte content of the amino acid solution should be considered. General guidelines for electrolyte requirements for parenteral feedings are included in Table 37-6.

Vitamins and Trace Elements.

21. What doses of multiple vitamins and trace elements should D.C. receive in his parenteral nutrient formulation?

Vitamins and trace elements are essential for normal metabolism and should be included in a patient's daily parenteral nutrition regimen. Guidelines for the 13 essential vitamins have been established by the Nutrition Advisory Group of the American Medical Association[62] (Table 37-7).

Guidelines for daily doses of the trace elements zinc, copper, chromium, and manganese also have been developed.[63] In addition to these trace elements, many practitioners provide selenium on a daily basis. Recommended doses of the trace elements are listed in Table 37-8. As with vitamins, trace elements are available as single entities or combination products. Molybdenum and iodine also are available commercially.

Table 37-6 Guidelines for Daily Electrolyte Requirements

Electrolyte	Amount
Sodium	80–100 mEq
Potassium	60–80 mEq
Chloride	50–100 mEq[a]
Acetate	50–100 mEq[a]
Magnesium	8–16 mEq
Calcium	5–10 mEq
Phosphorus (phosphate)	15–30 mmol

[a]As needed to maintain acid–base balance.

Table 37-7 Recommended Adult Daily Doses of Parenteral Vitamins

Vitamins	Dose
Fat-Soluble Vitamins	
A	3,300 IU (990 retinol equivalents
D	200 IU (5 mg cholecalciferol)
E	10 IU (6.7 mg/dL-α-tocopherol)
K	150 μg
Water-Soluble Vitamins	
Thiamine (B₁)	6 mg
Riboflavin (B₂)	3.6 mg
Pyridoxine (B₆)	4 mg
Cyanocobalamin (B₁₂)	5 μg
Niacin	40 mg
Folic acid	0.6 mg
Pantothenic acid	15 mg
Biotin	60 μg
Ascorbic acid (c)	200 mg

Table 37-8 Recommended Daily Adult Doses of Parenteral Trace Elements

Trace Element	Dose
Zinc	2.5–4 mg
Copper	0.5–1.5 mg
Chromium	10–15 μg
Manganese	150–800 μg
Selenium	20–60 μg

22. D.C.'s daily parenteral nutrient formulation of 1,800 mL provides 2,200 calories (70% nonprotein calories as carbohydrate, 30% as fat) and 90 g of amino acids with the following additives per daily volume: NaCl, 75 mEq; K acetate, 70 mEq; phosphate as Na, 27 mmol; MgSO₄, 16 mEq; calcium gluconate, 10 mEq; and standard doses of adult multivitamins and multiple trace elements providing copper, chromium, manganese, selenium, and zinc. The infusion is initiated at a rate of 40 mL/hr. Why is this slow infusion rate selected?

Standard practice for administering parenteral nutrient formulations containing hypertonic dextrose is to begin at a slow infusion rate of <250 g during the first 24 hours for most patients, <150 g for patients with known diabetes mellitus or hyperglycemia. The infusion is increased slowly over the next 24 to 48 hours to the goal infusion rate. This initial period allows the clinician to assess the patient's ability to tolerate the nutrient formulation components and to avoid metabolic complications, primarily hyperglycemia.[54] If D.C.'s serum glucose level remains <150 mg/dL, the parenteral nutrient formulation infusion rate can be increased to his goal rate of 75 mL/hour.

Monitoring and Management of Complications
METABOLIC COMPLICATIONS

Parenteral nutrition therapy may be associated with multiple metabolic complications. The most common abnormalities are hypokalemia, hypomagnesemia, hypophosphatemia, and hyperglycemia. The plan for parenteral nutrition therapy should include routine monitoring of these serum chemistries to identify complications early and institute methods to manage or prevent complications.

23. Over the next 24 hours, D.C.'s infusion rate is increased to the goal rate of 75 mL/hr. A comparison of his intake and output reveals an overall negative fluid balance because a high volume of gastric fluid is being removed via the NG tube. Laboratory values at this time are Na, 138 mEq/L; K, 3.1 mEq/L; chloride, 91 mEq/L; HCO₃⁻, 33 mEq/L; BUN, 28 mg/dL; creatinine, 0.9 mg/dL; glucose, 279 mg/dL; Ca, 7.8 mg/dL; Mg, 1.4 mg/dL; P, 1.8 mg/dL; and albumin, 2.8 g/dL. Arterial blood gas (ABG) results are pH, 7.46 (normal, 7.37 to 7.44); PO₂, 98 (normal, 85 to 100); PCO₂, 47 (normal, 35 to 45); HCO₃⁻, 31 (normal, 24 to 30). What factors contribute to these metabolic abnormalities?

[SI units: Na, 130 mmol/L; K, 3.1 mmol/L; Cl, 91 mmol/L; HCO₃⁻, 33 mmol/L; BUN, 8.96 mmol/L; creatinine, 75 μmol/L; glucose, 15.5 mmol/L; Ca, 1.92 mmol/L; Mg, 0.8 mmol/L; P, 0.58 mmol/L; albumin, 28 g/L]

Hypokalemia. Hypokalemia, a common metabolic abnormality associated with the initiation of parenteral nutrition, usually occurs within 24 to 48 hours. Potassium moves, along with dextrose, from the extracellular to the intracellular space. Furthermore, building lean body mass (i.e., anabolism) requires approximately 3 mEq of potassium per gram of nitrogen provided by the amino acids. Administering dextrose promotes repletion of glycogen stores, which also requires potassium.[48,54,64]

D.C.'s decreased serum potassium concentration is compounded by metabolic alkalosis secondary to his loss of gastric secretions through the NG tube and the administration of hydrocortisone. With this type of metabolic alkalosis, the renal excretion of potassium is increased. Additional potassium should be administered and can be provided in D.C.'s parenteral feeding or through another IV.

Hypomagnesemia. Magnesium, like potassium, is primarily an intracellular cation and is considered an anabolic electrolyte. It is common to observe decreases in magnesium serum concentrations during the administration of parenteral nutrient formulations. Synthesis of lean tissue requires 0.5 mEq magnesium per gram of nitrogen.[48,54,64] Additional magnesium can be added to the parenteral nutrient formulation. However, when a TNA formulation is used, the amount of magnesium must stay within the guidelines for the cation content to maintain the stability of the lipid emulsion.

Hypophosphatemia. Hypophosphatemia occurs when phosphorus moves into the cells for the synthesis of adenosine triphosphate (ATP), an important energy carrier. Phosphorus is depleted quickly with the administration of hypertonic dextrose, especially in malnourished patients (see Question 8 for discussion of refeeding syndrome). The phosphorus is used for ATP synthesis, primarily in the liver and skeletal muscle. Alkalosis also decreases phosphate stores by stimulating the phosphorylation of carbohydrates. As a component of 2,3-diphosphoglycerate (2,3-DPG), found in red blood cells (RBCs), phosphorus is necessary for the disassociation of oxygen from hemoglobin.[64]

Clinical signs and symptoms of hypophosphatemia usually occur when serum concentrations fall below 1.0 mg/dL; they include lethargy, muscle weakness, impaired WBC function, glucose intolerance, rhabdomyolysis, seizures, hemolytic anemia, reduced diaphragmatic contractility, and death. Moderate to severe, complicated hypophosphatemia can be managed by administering up to 0.5 mmol/kg of phosphate IV.[48,64–66] Although D.C.'s serum phosphorus is not <1.0 mg/dL, it is low (1.8 mg/dL), and he should receive 15 to 30 mmol phosphate in the parenteral nutrient formulation per day. Additional supplements may be necessary to replete his phosphorus stores.[65]

Metabolic Alkalosis. D.C. has evidence of a metabolic alkalosis based on his ABG results, hypochloremia, and elevated bicarbonate level. The continued loss of fluid and HCl from the NG tube is the most probable cause of his metabolic alkalosis. Management of this type of metabolic alkalosis is to replace the fluid and chloride through another IV. Because acetate is converted to bicarbonate and further contributes to the alkalosis, the acetate salts in the parenteral nutrient formulation can be changed to chloride salts.[64] Nevertheless, the parenteral nutrient formulation is not the primary vehicle for adjusting and supplementing electrolytes and fluid. Generally, the fluid and electrolyte balance should be adjusted with maintenance IV fluid and electrolyte supplements.

Hyperglycemia. Hyperglycemia is a common metabolic complication of parenteral nutrition therapy, especially in stressed patients. Stress alone increases gluconeogenesis, and the administration of hypertonic dextrose compounds the potential for hyperglycemia.[67] D.C. is at particular risk for hyperglycemia because he is recovering from surgery and is receiving steroids, which increase gluconeogenesis.

Persistent hyperglycemia leads to glucosuria and an osmotic diuresis, resulting in dehydration and concomitant electrolyte abnormalities. It also compromises the immune response by causing abnormalities in chemotaxis and phagocytosis and by impairing complement function. Hyperglycemia is associated with an increased risk of infections, especially *C. albicans.* In extreme cases, hyperglycemia progresses to hyperosmolar, nonketotic acidosis and coma, a condition associated with 40% mortality.

Hyperglycemia can be minimized by limiting the dextrose infusion rate to <4 mg/kg per minute.[68] (D.C.'s parenteral nutrient formulation provides 4 mg/kg per minute.) Other measures that will minimize the risk of hyperglycemia include gradually increasing the parenteral nutrient formulation infusion rate, frequently monitoring capillary blood glucose concentrations, and advancing therapy only when the serum glucose is consistently <150 mg/dL for stable patients and <120 mg/dL for critically ill patients. Insulin therapy should be considered if serum glucose concentrations exceed these parameters and can be administered subcutaneously according to a sliding scale, IV by continuous infusion, or by adding insulin to the parenteral nutrient formulation.[69,70] Only regular insulin can be added to a parenteral nutrient formulation. A reasonable strategy for adding insulin to the parenteral nutrient formulation is to begin with 0.1 units of regular insulin per gram of dextrose. This dosage is adjusted depending on serum glucose concentrations.[69] Clinical evidence suggests that treatment of hyperglycemia and maintenance of euglycemia may reduce morbidity and mortality, length of stay, and hospital costs.[70–74]

Formulation Design

Compatibility

24. In response to these serum chemistries, the electrolytes in D.C.'s parenteral nutrient formulation are changed to the following per liter: NaCl, 90 mEq; KCl, 80 mEq; phosphate as K, 50 mmol; MgSO$_4$, 30 mEq; calcium gluconate, 20 mEq. How do the doses of calcium and phosphate compare to maintenance doses? What calcium and phosphate incompatibilities should be anticipated? Will the calcium and magnesium content alter the lipid stability?

The dose of calcium ordered for D.C. is more than three times the usual maintenance dose (see Table 37-7). This amount of calcium is not necessary because the observed hypocalcemia merely reflects D.C.'s low serum albumin concentration; therefore, less calcium is bound to albumin. D.C. probably does not have true hypocalcemia because his free (or ionized) calcium, which is critical for physiologic function, has not changed. For every 1-g/dL decrease in serum albumin concentration, there will be about a 0.8-mg/dL reduction in the serum calcium concentration.[75] For D.C., a serum calcium of 7.8 mg/dL will correct to a serum concentration of 8.8 mg/dL [(4.0 g/dL −2.8 g/dL albumin)(0.8) + 7.8 mg/dL calcium].

The amount of phosphate prescribed for D.C. at this time exceeds the usual recommended dose of 15 to 30 mmol/day (see Table 37-7). Although D.C. has a low serum phosphorus concentration and needs additional phosphate, increasing the dosage in the parenteral nutrient formulation to 40 mmol/day (22 mmol/L) may be incompatible with the calcium content, resulting in calcium phosphate precipitation. The precipitate may be visible as small "snowflakes" in a parenteral nutrient formulation of dextrose and amino acids, but in a TNA the precipitation may not be visible because the admixture is opaque. Administering a parenteral nutrient formulation containing calcium phosphate crystals may occlude blood flow, especially in the lungs, and has been associated with adverse events such as respiratory distress and death.[39,40,76]

It is important to consider the factors that affect calcium phosphate solubility and to take measures that ensure the solubility limits are not exceeded when preparing parenteral nutrient formulations. The *in vitro* precipitation of calcium phosphate depends on multiple factors, including the calcium salt, concentrations of calcium and phosphate, amino acid concentration, temperature, pH of the formulation, and infusion time. Using calcium gluconate rather than the chloride salt can enhance calcium phosphate solubility. In solution at equimolar concentrations, calcium chloride dissociates more than calcium gluconate, thereby increasing the yield of free calcium available for binding with phosphate.

The amounts of calcium and phosphorus in the formulation are critical. Multiple investigators have varied the calcium and phosphate concentrations in parenteral nutrient formulations and have developed precipitation curves to assist practitioners in determining the amounts of calcium and phosphate that can be added safely to nutrient formulations. These guidelines help predict the points at which calcium phosphate precipitation is likely to occur. However, extrapolating these data to parenteral nutrient formulations different from those described is difficult because these mixtures are extremely complex, and numerous variables affect the interrelationship between calcium and phosphate.

The solubility of calcium and phosphate must be determined based on the volume of the formulation at the time the calcium and phosphate are mixed together, not the final volume. For example, if the electrolytes including calcium and phosphate are added to 1,000 mL of a dextrose/amino acid mixture and then 300 mL of IV fat is added, the calcium phosphate solubility is based on the 1,000 mL, not the final 1,300 mL volume. In addition, some amino acid products contain phosphate ions, and these should be considered when determining calcium phosphate solubility.[39,40]

Last, calcium and phosphate should not be added to the parenteral nutrient formulation in close sequence, and during preparation the parenteral nutrient formulation should be agitated periodically and inspected for precipitates.[77] Other guidelines for improving the solubility of calcium are a final amino acid concentration of >2.5% and a pH <6. Temperature is a critical variable, and an increase in the ambient temperature can facilitate the precipitation of calcium phosphate. Formulations should be infused within 24 hours after compounding if stored at room temperature; if refrigerated, they should be infused within 24 hours after rewarming. Furthermore, slow infusions may decrease solubility. Increasing temperature and slow infusions may result in precipitation in the IV catheter even if precipitation has not occurred in the infusion container.[39,40]

The amount of divalent cations, calcium (20 mEq) and magnesium (30 mEq), exceeds the general guidelines for maximum amounts that can be added safely to a TNA without disrupting the stability of the lipid emulsion. A limit of 20 divalent cations per liter is a general guideline. The amount prescribed for D.C.'s regimen is excessive because it provides 50 divalent cations in 1.8 L (28 divalent cations/L) and may result in a potentially unstable admixture.

Last, a 1.2-micron air-eliminating filter should be used when infusing TNA parenteral nutrient formulations, and a 0.22-micron air-eliminating filter should be used for non–lipid-containing admixtures.[39,40]

Medication Additives

25. In addition to his parenteral nutrient formulation, D.C. is receiving ranitidine 50 mg IV Q 8 hr and hydrocortisone 100 mg IV Q 8 hr, and now he needs insulin. Can these medications be mixed with his parenteral nutrient formulation to simplify his medication regimen?

Patients receiving parenteral nutrition therapy often require concomitant drug therapy. Most patients have adequate venous access or have multiple-lumen central venous catheters, so that mixing medications with the parenteral nutrient formulation is not an issue. However, for some patients with limited venous access, directly added medications or piggybacking medications via a secondary infusion must be considered.

The stability of medications when mixed with parenteral nutrient formulations is a complex issue. Some medications may be added directly to the parenteral nutrient formulation, while others should be administered via a secondary infusion set (piggybacked). Many medications have been studied for physical compatibility, but few have been evaluated for pharmacologic activity. Furthermore, the study conditions vary and different nutrient formulations have been used; therefore, interpretation and application of data from a particular scientific study to a specific nutrient formulation may be difficult. This area of knowledge is growing rapidly, and current information regarding compatibility and stability is available in standard references such as *Trissel's Handbook of Injectable Drugs.*[78]

Although insulin, antibiotics, chemotherapeutic agents, H_2-receptor antagonists, and heparin have been considered for addition to parenteral nutrient formulations in some specific circumstances, the routine addition of medications to parenteral nutrient formulations is discouraged. The addition of insulin to parenteral nutrient formulations is common and is often the preferred method for managing hyperglycemia, as described in Question 23.

MONITORING PARAMETERS

26. Design a plan to monitor the adequacy of D.C.'s specialized nutrition support and to identify and prevent adverse complications.

Routine evaluation of patients receiving nutrition support should include an assessment of nutrition and the metabolic effects of therapy. Goals for nutrition therapy are estimates of a patient's needs; therefore, the adequacy of therapy to meet these needs must be evaluated. Daily monitoring parameters must include vital signs, body weight, temperature, serum chemistries, hematologic indices, nutrition intake, and fluid intake and output.

The adequacy of nutrition therapy should be assessed weekly. This may include measuring serum concentrations of visceral proteins (see Table 37-2). Because prealbumin has a half-life of only 2 to 3 days, serum concentrations of this protein should increase with adequate nutrition and improving clinical status. Albumin, with a much longer half-life, may not change for several weeks to months despite provision of adequate nutrients. In addition, it is reasonable to perform indirect calorimetry to reassess energy expenditure.

Another method to assess the adequacy of protein intake is to evaluate nitrogen balance. This test is designed to estimate the amount of nitrogen retained by comparing the amount of nitrogen administered to the amount of nitrogen excreted (amount "in" versus amount "out"). The nitrogen "in" is provided by the amino acid component of the parenteral nutrient formulation and other sources from tube feeding or an oral diet. Each commercially available amino acid formulation has a slightly different amount of nitrogen per gram of amino acids, and the manufacturer's product information should be consulted to obtain this value. An average value is 6.2 g of nitrogen per gram of amino acids.

Most of the nitrogen is excreted as byproducts of protein breakdown for energy. This nitrogen is excreted in the urine as urea nitrogen, which increases with increasing stress. To determine this value, urine must be collected for 24 hours and the amount of urea nitrogen (UUN) measured. Some laboratories have the capability of measuring total urine nitrogen (TUN), which measures all nitrogen entities in the urine. In addition, some nitrogen lost via skin, respiration, and stool is not measurable but is estimated to be 2 to 4 g/day.

Nitrogen balance = Nitrogen in − Nitrogen out

$$= \frac{AA(g)}{6.2} - (UUN(g) + 3\ g) \quad (37\text{-}3)$$

$$= \quad g$$

Achieving a positive nitrogen balance is difficult, if not impossible, in critically ill patients; therefore, the calculation may result in a negative number or zero. For convalescing patients, a nitrogen balance of +2 to 4 g is acceptable. A negative nitrogen balance prompts a reevaluation of the amount of protein and energy a patient is receiving. For patients with a negative nitrogen balance, it may be helpful to increase intake of both calories and protein.

As with all tests, assessment should include monitoring several parameters, including the patient's clinical status. Most important is the identification of trends that may alert one to impending complications. A suggested schedule for monitoring is provided in Table 37-9.

Table 37-9 Routine Monitoring Parameters for Parenteral Nutrition

Before Initiating Therapy

Body weight
Serum electrolytes (Na, K, Cl, HCO_3^-, BUN, creatinine)
Glucose
Ca, Mg, P
Albumin, transthyretin
Triglycerides
Complete blood count
Liver-associated tests (AST, ALT, alkaline phosphatase, GGT, bilirubin)
Prothrombin time, INR

Daily

Body weight
Vital signs (pulse, respirations, temperature)
Fluid intake
Nutritional intake
Output (urine, other losses)
Serum electrolytes (Na, K, Cl, HCO_3^-, blood urea nitrogen, creatinine)
Glucose

2 or 3 Times a Week

CBC
Ca, Mg, P

Weekly

Albumin, transthyretin
Liver-associated tests (AST, ALT, alkaline phosphatase, GGT, bilirubin)
Prothrombin time, INR
Nitrogen balance

ALT, alanine aminotransferase; AST, aspartate aminotransferase; Ca, calcium; Cl, chloride; GGT, gamma-glutamyl transpeptidase; HCO_3^-, bicarbonate; K, potassium; Mg, magnesium; Na, sodium; P, phosphorus.

Home Therapy

Enterocutaneous Fistulas

27. After a 10-day hospitalization, D.C. is discharged home. He returns to the clinic 3 weeks later with a fever and green, purulent fluid draining from a small hole in his previously healed incision site. D.C. is admitted to the hospital for workup of his fever and evaluation of the discharge. He has an enterocutaneous fistula, which is a communication between his intestine and the skin. The fluid loss from D.C.'s fistula is about 500 mL/day. Management will include NPO and parenteral nutrition for 4 to 6 weeks in anticipation that the fistula will heal and further surgery can be avoided. Design a plan for home parenteral nutrition therapy.

Parenteral nutrition therapy in the home has allowed patients such as D.C. to be managed at home rather than staying in the hospital. Home therapy has become much more common due to economic pressures that encourage short hospital stays. Candidates for home therapy must be physically and medically stable, have a strong support network in the home setting to assist with care, and have an appropriate home environment; they must be educated regarding the prescribed therapy.[80]

As with a hospitalized patient, the first step in designing a parenteral nutrition regimen is to estimate energy and protein needs. Since discharge, D.C.'s weight has increased only slightly to 63 kg, so his BEE has changed little, if at all. D.C.'s calorie goal includes adequate energy for daily activities at home and can be estimated at 50% to 60% greater than his BEE of 1,583 kcal, or approximately 2,400 to 2,500 kcal/day. Protein goals must include adequate nitrogen (protein) for wound healing and replacement for losses from the enterocutaneous fistula. A goal of 1.5 to 1.8 g/kg per day (95 to 115 g) is reasonable.

To simplify his nutrition and fluid regimen, all of D.C.'s fluids, including parenteral nutrients, electrolytes, vitamins, trace minerals, and water, should be provided in one container per day. D.C.'s home parenteral nutrient formulation can be provided in 2,500 mL/day to meet maintenance requirements (30 to 35 mL/kg per day) and to replace losses from his enterocutaneous fistula (500 mL/day). Nutrients provided include 105 g amino acids (420 kcal); 441 g dextrose (1,500 kcal); 33 g lipid (660 kcal); and electrolytes, vitamins, and minerals to maintain normal serum chemistries. Initially, daily intake and output must be monitored; therapy should be adjusted based on this information and D.C.'s clinical status.

Adjustments in fluids and electrolytes may be needed. Management of D.C.'s enterocutaneous fistula will include NPO because food stimulates GI secretions and increases fistula output. The fluids secreted by the GI tract are rich in electrolytes, including sodium, potassium, chloride, and bicarbonate. Measurement of the electrolyte content of the fistula fluid will determine those that must be replaced, and in what quantities. Both fluid and electrolytes should be replaced to prevent dehydration and electrolyte and acid–base imbalances.

In addition to losses of fluids and electrolytes, the trace element zinc is lost in fluid from the small intestine. Approximately 12 mg of zinc is lost in each liter of small bowel fluid, and this should be replaced to prevent zinc deficiency. Furthermore, zinc may play a role in wound healing.[80] Management of enterocutaneous fistulas may include octreotide 50 to 100 μg given subcutaneously two or three times daily or added to the parenteral nutrient formulation to decrease fistula output.[81]

A home infusion pharmacy will be responsible for preparing D.C.'s parenteral nutrient formulations. Typically, nutrient formulations for 7 days are prepared and delivered to the patient's home. These formulations must be refrigerated until administration; however, formulations should be warmed to room temperature and visually inspected for particulate matter before being administered. Because some additives such as multivitamins are not stable for long periods, the patient or caregiver must add these to the parenteral nutrient formulation just before administration.

Patients and caregivers preparing for home parenteral nutrition therapy must be taught how to manage home therapy. This includes assessment of fluid status, care of a central venous catheter, infection, and the technical aspects of administering parenteral feeding formulations.[79]

Preparation for home parenteral nutrition will include placement of a central venous access device. Various devices are available for long-term therapy.[34,36] However, because the duration of D.C.'s therapy is expected to be 4 to 6 weeks, he may be a good candidate for a PICC.

Cyclic Therapy

28. What other measures can be used to simplify D.C.'s parenteral feeding regimen and encourage ambulation?

After all of D.C.'s daily nutrient and fluid needs are consolidated and he is stable on that regimen, his parenteral nutrient regimen can be cycled. *Cycling* means infusing the parenteral nutrient formulation over <24 hours so that there is some time free from therapy. Cycling is usually done gradually and depends on the patient's ability to tolerate the changes in fluid and dextrose intake. Initially, the infusion period is decreased by 2 to 6 hours and the infusion rate is increased to compensate for the shorter infusion period. For example, a 24-hour infusion at 100 mL/hour would be changed to a 20-hour infusion at 120 mL/hour. This gradual adjustment is more likely to ensure that all nutrients are infused and well tolerated. With each incremental decrease in time, the infusion rate should be increased.

Vital signs, fluid intake and output, and serum electrolytes and glucose concentrations should be monitored during this period. The serum glucose concentration should be evaluated 30 minutes after the infusion is completed to be sure that hypoglycemia does not occur as the result of the rapid cessation of the nutrient formulation. If hypoglycemia occurs, the infusion rate can be tapered at the end of the infusion because a gradual decrease in glucose intake should minimize the potential for hypoglycemia. Furthermore, the infusion can be gradually increased to minimize sudden hyperglycemia at the beginning of the infusion. Infusion management devices used at home can automatically make these adjustments in the infusion rate. Eventually, the nutrient formulation can be infused over 10 to 12 hours during the night, leaving D.C. free from his infusion bag during the day.

METABOLIC COMPLICATIONS: ELEVATED LIVER-ASSOCIATED ENZYMES

29. After receiving home parenteral nutrition for 3 weeks, D.C.'s liver function tests are found to be elevated Current values are bilirubin, 0.8 mg/dL (normal, 0 to 1.2); AST, 70 U/L (normal, 19 to 25); ALT, 90 U/L (normal, 19 to 72); alkaline phosphatase, 100 U/L (normal, 38 to 126); γ-glutamyl transpeptidase, 85 U/L (normal, 13 to 68). Could his parenteral nutrition be contributing to these abnormalities?

Elevations in liver function tests are common in adults receiving long-term parenteral nutrition therapy and may be noted as early as 2 to 3 weeks after beginning therapy. The abnormalities are usually mild and transient and do not progress to significant liver dysfunction in adults. The predominant type of hepatobiliary dysfunction is steatosis, while other patients develop cholestasis or cholelithiasis. Liver-associated enzyme elevations usually resolve when parenteral nutrition therapy is discontinued. Rarely does this dysfunction proceed to hepatic failure.[82,83]

Although parenteral nutrition-associated liver abnormalities were first noted >30 years ago, a cause-and-effect relationship has been difficult to establish because patients have many confounding factors that also can cause liver dysfunction, including medications, inflammatory bowel disease, and sepsis. Other contributing factors are overfeeding with parenteral nutrient formulations containing high amounts of carbohydrate, amino acid deficiencies, excess fat, EFAD, carnitine deficiency, choline deficiency, toxic effects of the amino acid degradation products, bacterial overgrowth in the small intestine, and lack of stimulation of the GI tract.[82,83] Other than avoiding overfeeding with carbohydrate and lipid, there are few options to prevent or manage parenteral nutrition-associated liver abnormalities. Potential treatments include metronidazole and supplements of ursodeoxycholic acid, choline, and carnitine. Patients with progressive liver disease may be candidates for liver and small bowel transplantation.[83]

The elevations in D.C.'s liver enzymes should be monitored weekly for continued increases. Since he may not need lifelong parenteral nutrition therapy, the mild elevations are likely to resolve.

USE OF PARENTERAL NUTRITION IN SPECIAL DISEASE STATES

Hepatic Failure

30. V.G. is a 42-year-old woman with a 15-year history of alcohol abuse, cirrhosis, ascites, and esophageal varices who was admitted to the hospital 5 days ago with an upper GI bleed after a weekend drinking binge. She was supported initially with IV fluids, packed RBCs, and fresh frozen plasma. Endoscopic examination showed bleeding esophageal varices, which were banded. V.G.'s hospital course is now complicated by primary bacterial peritonitis causing a paralytic ileus. On physical examination, V.G. is cachectic, with a large protuberant abdomen and ascites; bowel sounds are absent. She is alert, oriented, and without evidence of encephalopathy. V.G. has a central venous catheter. The plan is to begin parenteral nutrition because she has not eaten in 8 days and is not expected to eat for several more days when her peritonitis resolves. Is V.G. a candidate for a specialty amino acid product specifically designed for use in hepatic failure?

Aromatic Amino Acids and Branched-Chain Amino Acids

Patients with chronic hepatic failure, especially those with alcohol-induced disease, are malnourished and prone to complications such as GI bleeding and infection. The metabolism of glucose, fat, and protein is altered in liver disease. Amino acid metabolism is particularly affected because blood is shunted around the liver.

In patients with hepatic insufficiency, adequate protein must be provided to support regeneration of the liver and other vital functions such as the immune system. However, administration of protein may result in hepatic encephalopathy, a severe complication of hepatic failure. Encephalopathy is characterized by progressive depression and impaired neurologic function. The pathogenesis of encephalopathy is controversial, although several theories have been proposed. It is probably caused by the inability of the diseased liver to remove neurotoxins, which accumulate in the brain, resulting in abnormal neurotransmitters. Substances implicated as neurotoxins include ammonia, benzodiazepines, and aromatic amino acids.

Cirrhosis and chronic hepatic failure are associated with significant protein breakdown. The branched-chain amino acids (BCAAs) (e.g., leucine, isoleucine, valine) are used in the muscle as an energy source rather than being released into the circulation. Although the BCAAs are used for energy, the aromatic amino acids (AAAs; phenylalanine, tyrosine, and free tryptophan) are released, increasing circulating concentrations of these amino acids. This results in increased plasma concentrations of the AAAs and methionine and subnormal concentrations of the BCAAs. Both AAAs and BCAAs share a common pathway across the blood–brain barrier and compete for entry into the cerebrospinal fluid (CSF). The "false neurotransmitter" theory proposes that because the concentration of AAAs is greater, more are transported across the blood–brain barrier, where they accumulate and form "false neurotransmitters" such as octopamine and serotonin, an inhibitory neurotransmitter. These compete with normal neurotransmitters for binding sites and impair normal neurotransmission and brain activity.[84]

Based on these theories, an amino acid mixture was designed to provide adequate protein for anabolism while also treating hepatic encephalopathy. To normalize the amino acid profile in the brain, specially designed products with increased amounts of BCAAs and decreased amounts of both AAAs and methionine are available (Table 37-10). Controversy exists with regard to the ability of this special amino acid mixture to improve encephalopathy by altering the amino acid profile of the CSF.[84-86] Generally, this amino acid mixture is reserved for patients with significant hepatic encephalopathy.

Because V.G. is alert, oriented, and without signs of encephalopathy, use of this product is not warranted at this time. Furthermore, protein restriction is not necessary. She should receive 1 to 1.2 g/kg per day of a standard amino acid product, and she should be monitored for signs of encephalopathy. Should she develop hepatic encephalopathy while receiving the standard amino acids, temporary protein restriction of 0.6 to 0.8 g/kg per day is reasonable while the etiology of the encephalopathy is determined and treated. The use of the increased BCAA–decreased AAA mixture may be appropriate

Table 37-10 · Amino Acid Product Comparison Table

Description	Product Name	Supplier	Available Concentrations (%)
Standard Formulations			
Contain essential[a] and nonessential[b] amino acids, some available with electrolytes[c]	Aminosyn, Aminosyn II	Abbott	3.5,[c] 5, 7,[c] 8.5,[c] 10,[c] 15
	FreAmine III	B Braun	3, 8.5, 10
	Novamine	Baxter	15
	Prosol	Baxter	20
	Travasol	Baxter	3.5,[c] 5.5,[c] 8.5,[c] 10
Hepatic Failure Formulations			
Contain essential and nonessential amino acids with an ↑ proportion of branched-chain amino acids (leucine, isoleucine, valine)	HepatAmine	B Braun	8
	Hepatasol	Baxter	8
Renal Failure Formulations			
Contain primarily essential amino acids; RenAmin also contains a complement of nonessential amino acids	Aminess	Baxter	5.2
	Aminosyn-RF	Abbott	5.2
	Nephramine	B Braun	5.4
	RenAmin	Baxter	6.5
Stress Formulations			
Contain ↑ percentages of leucine, isoleucine, and valine as well as all essential and nonessential amino acids	Aminosyn HBC	Abbott	7
	FreAmine HBC	B Braun	6.9
Supplements			
Contain only branched-chain amino acids (isoleucine, leucine, valine); must be used with a general formulation	BranchAmin	Baxter	4

[a]Essential amino acids: isoleucine, leucine, lysine, methionine, phenylalanine, theonine, tryptophan, valine, histidine.
[b]Nonessential amino acids: cysteine, arginine, alanine, proline, glycine, glutamine, aspartate serine, tyrosine.
[c]These concentrations are available with or without electrolytes.

for patients with chronic encephalopathy who are unresponsive to pharmacotherapy.[13]

31. **What other amino acid mixtures are enriched with BCAAs?**

BCAAs have metabolic properties that are considered beneficial during physiologic stress (multiple trauma, sepsis, and major surgery). BCAAs can be used as an alternative energy source by the heart, brain, and skeletal muscle. These BCAAs can increase protein synthesis in muscle and liver, decrease excessive proteolysis in muscle, and normalize abnormal plasma amino acid profiles. These unique properties led to the design of commercially available amino acid mixtures that provide about 45% of the amino acids as BCAAs. In comparison, most standard amino acid mixtures contain 19% to 25% BCAAs.

Multiple trials have evaluated the effects of BCAA-enriched amino acid formulations in critically ill patients. Although most evidence suggests that these formulations may improve nitrogen retention, they do not appear to improve clinical outcome.[87,88] It is important to appreciate the differences between the amino acid composition of the mixtures for hepatic failure and those designed for stress. They are not therapeutically equivalent, and one should not be substituted for the other.

Renal Failure

32. **O.M. is a 75-year-old man with a long history of hypertension, coronary artery disease, and peripheral vascular disease. Four days ago, he was admitted to the hospital complaining of severe abdominal pain and was diagnosed with a ruptured abdominal aortic aneurysm, which was repaired surgically. Hypotension and hemodynamic instability requiring pressors, respiratory distress necessitating endotracheal intubation and mechanical ventilation, and renal failure with oliguria have complicated his postoperative course. Furthermore, there is concern that O.M. has ischemic bowel, which precludes using his GI tract for enteral feeding. Serum chemistries are Na, 130 mEq/L; K, 5.2 mEq/L; Cl, 99 mEq/L; HCO_3^-, 15 mEq/L; BUN, 79 mg/dL; creatinine, 4.0 mg/dL; glucose, 143 mg/dL; Ca, 7.9 mg/dL; Mg, 2.4 mg/dL; P, 5.8 mg/dL; and albumin, 2.7 g/dL. The decision is made to initiate parenteral nutrition therapy via a central venous catheter. In view of O.M.'s acute renal failure, what adjustments should be made in the amount and type of protein (amino acid) provided in the parenteral feeding formulation?**

[SI units: Na, 130 mmol/L; K, 5.2 mmol/L; Cl, 99 mmol/L; HCO_3^-, 15 mmol/L; BUN, 28 mmol/L; creatinine, 240 mmol/L; glucose, 9.6 mmol/L; Ca, 1.96 mmol/L; Mg, 12 mmol/L; P, 1.9 mmol/L; albumin, 27 g/L]

The protein dose in acute renal failure should be reduced to 0.6 to 1 g/kg per day because the kidneys have a limited ability to excrete nitrogenous byproducts of protein metabolism.[89] The use of essential amino acids (EAAs) orally has been demonstrated to improve uremic symptoms. Based on this experience, parenteral amino acid mixtures containing only EAAs were investigated. These studies compared parenteral feedings containing dextrose and EAAs to the administration of only dextrose; there was an improved rate of recovery in the group that received the EAA and dextrose. Subsequent studies comparing parenteral nutrient formulations containing a standard mix of both EAAs and nonessential amino acids to EAAs alone have not demonstrated any difference in urea appearance or nitrogen balance.[89,90] The use of EAAs alone in parenteral nutrient formulations for patients with acute renal failure offers no clinical advantage over formulations providing a balanced mixture of EAAs and nonessential amino acids.

33. **What other adjustments should be made in formulating a parenteral nutrient formulation for O.M.?**

O.M.'s nutrient needs should be provided in the least amount of fluid possible. This can be accomplished by using the most concentrated macronutrients of 70% dextrose, 20% amino acids, and 30% lipid. Using these substrates, a patient's entire needs can often be provided in <1,200 mL/day. Electrolytes also should be adjusted. Initially, patients with acute renal failure may not require potassium, magnesium, and phosphorus because they cannot excrete them. However, once parenteral feedings begin and an anabolic state occurs, these patients commonly experience decreases in the serum concentrations of these minerals and will require small daily doses to maintain normal serum concentrations.

Renal Replacement Therapies

34. **O.M.'s renal failure progresses and he requires renal replacement therapy. Because of his hemodynamic instability, continuous venovenous hemodialysis (CVVHD) is initiated. How should his nutrition therapy be altered?**

Continuous renal replacement therapies (CRRT), including CVVHD, continuous arteriovenous hemodialysis (CAVHD), continuous venovenous hemofiltration (CVVHF), continuous venovenous hemodiafiltration (CVVHDF), and slow continuous ultrafiltration (SCUF) provide a means to remove large volumes of water, nitrogenous byproducts, and electrolytes, permitting unlimited quantities of fluids, nutrients, and electrolytes. Several factors must be considered in the nutritional management of a patient requiring these therapies. First, a dialysate solution of 1.5% to 2.5% dextrose may be used. If so, some dextrose is absorbed during the process and contributes to the caloric intake. A solution with a 1.5% dextrose concentration at a rate of 1 L/hour delivers approximately 5.8 g of glucose per hour. Increasing the dextrose concentration of the dialysate solution to 2.5% increases the glucose delivery to 11.5 g per hour. The amount of glucose absorbed (550 to 700 kcal/day) must be considered when designing the amount of calories that will be provided in the parenteral nutrient formulation.[89-94]

The second nutritional consideration is the loss of amino acids across the dialysis filter, which can range from 20 to 28 g of nitrogen per day. Sufficient amino acids should be provided to compensate for this daily loss of 120 to 175 g of amino acids (approximately 6.25 g of amino acids per gram of nitrogen).[89,91,93,94]

Last, the rapid loss of electrolytes must be considered. Patients may experience dramatic decreases in potassium, magnesium, and phosphorus once CRRT is initiated. This requires frequent monitoring and replacement of these electrolytes, usually as IV supplements rather than as additions to the parenteral feeding formulation.

35. After several days of CVVHD, O.M. is changed to intermittent (three times a week) hemodialysis. What alterations in his parenteral nutrition are necessary?

Hemodialysis also allows the passage of amino acids through a semipermeable membrane. The loss is approximately 1 g of amino acids for each hour of hemodialysis with a glucose-free dialysate. This loss is reduced by 50% when a glucose-containing dialysate solution is used. These losses should be considered when determining the dosage of protein that will be provided by the parenteral nutrient formulation. The recommended protein dosage for patients requiring hemodialysis is 1 to 1.2 g/kg per day.[89,93,94] In addition, hemodialysis can increase energy expenditure by increasing oxygen consumption and gluconeogenesis; therefore, energy goals should be increased to 30 kcal/kg per day.[89] Patients requiring chronic hemodialysis may require protein doses of 1.2 to 1.4 g/kg per day to maintain a positive nitrogen balance and prevent protein malnutrition. Patients requiring peritoneal dialysis have higher losses of protein through the peritoneal cavity and may need 1.2 to 1.5 g/kg per day of protein. In contrast to patients on hemodialysis, those on peritoneal dialysis require fewer calories provided by parenteral feedings because 600 to 800 calories per day may be absorbed through the peritoneal membrane from the glucose-containing dialysate.[89,93,94]

Diabetes, Obesity, and Short Bowel Syndrome

36. F.L., a 51-year-old man with a history of diabetes mellitus, is hospitalized after receiving a gunshot wound to the abdomen. His injuries included a lacerated spleen, requiring a splenectomy, and several tears in his small and large intestine, necessitating resection of these areas. A feeding jejunostomy tube is placed at the time of surgery and enteral tube feedings are begun on postoperative day 2. Five days later, F.L. is noted to have a temperature of 39.6°C, a WBC count of 18,900/mm³, and a distended, tender abdomen. He requires surgery for a small bowel perforation at the site of the feeding jejunostomy and peritonitis. The jejunostomy tube is removed, but F.L. is not expected to have return of bowel function for 7 to 10 days. Parenteral nutrition is to be initiated. F.L. is 5 foot 8 inches and his usual weight is 215 lb. What adjustments should be made in determining F.L.'s energy goals?

First, F.L. is considered obese, and an adjusted body weight should be calculated and used in nutrition calculations. Obesity is defined as weight exceeding 120% of IBW or a body mass index (BMI) of >27 kg/m². F.L. weighs 215 lb, or 98 kg, which is 142% of his IBW of 69 kg ± 10%. BMI is determined as shown by Equation 37-4.

$$\begin{aligned} \text{BMI} &= \frac{\text{Weight (kg)}}{\text{Height (m)}^2} \\ &= \frac{98 \text{ kg}}{(1.73 \text{ m})^2} \\ &= 32.7 \text{ kg/m}^2 \end{aligned} \qquad (37\text{-}4)$$

Obese patients should have their weight adjusted because adipose tissue is not metabolically active. However, about one fourth of the adipose tissue is composed of some supporting tissue that is metabolically active. Adjusted weight for obesity is calculated using Equation 37-5.[95]

$$\begin{aligned} \text{Adjusted weight} &= (0.25)(\text{Actual Weight} - \text{IBW}) + \text{IBW} \\ &= (0.25)(98 - 69) + 69 \qquad (37\text{-}5) \\ &= 76 \text{ kg} \end{aligned}$$

Using an adjusted weight will decrease the risk of overfeeding, which can further increase adipose tissue and complicate glucose management, especially in a patient with a history of diabetes mellitus. Another approach is to use the Ireton-Jones predictive equation that includes a factor for obesity. Using indirect calorimetry to obtain a MEE may more accurately assess energy expenditure and avoid overfeeding.

37. What special considerations should be addressed in designing a parenteral nutrient regimen for F.L.?

Patients without a history of diabetes mellitus may develop hyperglycemia under conditions of stress. Even greater derangements in glucose metabolism may be observed in patients with diabetes mellitus during a critical illness. Dextrose should be limited to 150 g during the first 24 hours of therapy, and the amount of dextrose should not be increased until serum glucose concentrations are consistently <150 mg/dL. It can be anticipated that F.L. will need supplemental insulin when his parenteral nutrient regimen is infused. Insulin may be added to the parenteral nutrient formulation. Initial insulin therapy of 0.1 units of regular insulin per gram of dextrose is a good starting point and should be adjusted to achieve serum glucose levels of <150 mg/dL. Alternatively, a separate insulin infusion may be used. Frequent capillary glucose monitoring is necessary in these patients, and it may be necessary to provide additional subcutaneous insulin.[71,72,96] (See Question 23 for additional discussion on management of hyperglycemia.)

38. F.L. has a prolonged hospital course complicated by multiple intra-abdominal abscesses, poor wound healing, and necrotic bowel, requiring removal of all but 55 cm of his small intestine but leaving his colon intact. F.L. is given a diagnosis of short bowel syndrome (SBS). What issues should be addressed in the nutrition and metabolic management of this patient?

SBS is characterized by maldigestion, malabsorption, dehydration, and both macronutrient and micronutrient abnormalities. Severe malnutrition will develop without adequate nutrition support. To maintain adequate nutrition status, F.L. will require parenteral nutrition until his remaining intestine begins to adapt. This adaptive period may take several weeks to months to years. Adaptation is enhanced by stimulation of the enterocytes with nutrients, which is best provided by small, frequent oral meals or tube feeding.[13,97,98]

First, F.L. should be continued on parenteral nutrition support, including therapy at home, to meet his nutrient and fluid requirements. After extensive small bowel resection, F.L. may experience severe diarrhea. This increase in GI losses may lead to dehydration and electrolyte abnormalities, including hyponatremia, hypokalemia, hypomagnesemia, hypocalcemia, and metabolic acidosis.[98] F.L.'s fluid status must be monitored and evaluated daily for clinical signs of dehydration or fluid overload.

Medication therapy plays an important role in managing fluid and electrolyte imbalances secondary to excessive GI fluid losses. H_2-receptor antagonists are useful in decreasing gastric secretion, thereby reducing fluid and electrolyte losses and enhancing absorption. Antimotility agents should be used to decrease diarrhea. Octreotide also may have a role in decreasing diarrhea in patients with SBS. Patients with extensive small bowel resections and an intact colon, such as F.L., may develop diarrhea as a result of bile salt depletion.[13,97,98]

Patients with SBS are at risk for developing vitamin deficiencies, especially folate and B_{12}. These patients should receive supplemental B_{12} and IV parenteral or oral liquid multivitamin supplements. GI losses of trace minerals, particularly zinc and selenium, are increased in SBS, and these minerals should be supplemented.[97,98]

Pancreatitis, Respiratory Failure

39. **K.R., a 59-year-old woman, is admitted to the hospital complaining of increasing abdominal pain and vomiting. She is diagnosed with pancreatitis. This is her third admission for acute pancreatitis during the last year. Her past medical history is significant for ethanol abuse and chronic obstructive airway disease (COAD). An NG tube is inserted and she is to be NPO. IV fluids are begun for hydration.**

Over the next 5 days, K.R.'s abdominal pain subsides, her pancreatitis resolves, and she is started on an oral diet. Two days after beginning an oral diet, K.R. complains of severe abdominal pain and is vomiting. She is febrile, her WBC count increases to 21,000/mm³, and she is hypotensive, requiring large volumes of IV fluids. Furthermore, she develops respiratory distress and requires endotracheal intubation and mechanical ventilation. Her most recent ABG is notable for pH, 7.36 (normal, 7.37 to 7.44); PCO_2, 51 mm Hg (normal, 35 to 45); PO_2, 88 mm Hg (normal, 85 to 100); and HCO_3, 28 mEq/L (normal, 24 to 30). This clinical presentation is consistent with severe pancreatic necrosis. A small-bore nasojejunal feeding tube is placed and enteral nutrition therapy is begun. However, K.R. develops severe abdominal pain and distention and bowel sounds are absent, so the enteral feeding is discontinued. The decision is made to begin parenteral nutrition because K.R. is not expected to have a functional GI tract in the near future and her nutrient intake has been inadequate during her hospitalization. What special considerations should be addressed in designing a parenteral feeding formulation for K.R.?

[SI unit: WBC count, 21 × 10⁻⁹/L]

Overfeeding should be avoided in all patients, especially in patients with COAD. Overfeeding with carbohydrates is particularly detrimental because of the amount of carbon dioxide (CO_2) produced relative to the amount of oxygen (O_2) consumed. This relationship is described by the respiratory quotient (RQ), which is the ratio of the amount of CO_2 produced to the amount of O_2 consumed. The RQ differs for each substrate and is 0.8 for protein oxidation, 1 for carbohydrate oxidation, and 0.7 for fat oxidation. However, when carbohydrate is converted to fat for storage, the theoretical RQ is 8.[99] This relationship is described in the following equations:

Dextrose oxidation

$$C_6H_{12}O_6 + 6O_2 \rightarrow 6H_2O + 6CO_2 \quad (37\text{-}6)$$
$$RQ = 6CO_2/6O_2 = 1$$

Fat oxidation

$$CH_3(CH_2CH_2)_7COOH + 23O_2 \rightarrow 16CO_2 + 16H_2O \quad (37\text{-}7)$$
$$RQ = 16CO_2/23O_2 = 0.7$$

Fat synthesis

$$4C_6H_{12}O_6 + O_2 \rightarrow C_{16}H_{32}O_2 + 8CO_2 + 8H_2O$$
$$RQ = 8CO_2/O_2 = 8 \quad (37\text{-}8)$$

Based on these relationships, the oxidation of dextrose produces 9.0 mmol CO_2 per calorie and the oxidation soybean oil emulsions produce 7.1 mmol CO_2 per calorie, a 21% reduction in carbon dioxide produced.[99,100] Lipogenesis or fat synthesis occurs when the amount of carbohydrate administered exceeds the maximum oxidative capacity. Complete oxidation of carbohydrate is demonstrated at dextrose infusions of 4 to 5 mg/kg per minute.[56] Infusions exceeding this rate increase CO_2 production and may cause respiratory distress. Therefore, in designing a parenteral nutrient formulation for K.R., it is important to provide a moderate calorie dose and to limit her dextrose dose to <4 mg/kg per minute.[99,100]

40. **Although the use of fat to meet K.R.'s energy needs may be beneficial in managing her COAD, is the use of fat contraindicated in patients with pancreatitis?**

Several observations have caused concern over the use of IV lipid emulsions in patients with pancreatitis. The oral ingestion of fats may stimulate pancreatic exocrine function and should be restricted in patients with pancreatitis. Although hyperlipidemia has been well described in patients with alcohol-induced pancreatitis, it is unlikely that it is primarily responsible for initiating the pancreatitis. Hypertriglyceridemia associated with acute pancreatitis is most often seen in patients with hereditary or acquired defects in lipid metabolism. Furthermore, pancreatitis alone may be associated with hypertriglyceridemia.[101]

Several investigators have evaluated the effects of parenteral nutrient formulations containing fat emulsions in patients with acute pancreatitis and have found no stimulation of pancreatic exocrine function. Furthermore, IV lipids did not result in abdominal pain or relapse in patients with a history of pancreatitis. Available data suggest that IV lipid emulsions are a safe and efficacious form of calories for patients with pancreatitis.[101]

Monitoring serum triglyceride concentrations should be part of routine management for patients with pancreatitis and those receiving parenteral nutrient formulations containing lipids. Serum triglyceride concentrations should be maintained at <400 mg/dL with a continuous infusion of lipids and <250 mg/dL when checked 4 hours after the infusion for patients receiving intermittent lipid infusions.[13,101,102] If serum concentrations exceed these parameters, consideration must be given to decreasing or eliminating the IV lipid from the parenteral nutrient regimen.

41. **K.R. is recovering from her pancreatitis, and the small-bore nasojejunal enteral feeding tube is reinserted. Tube feeding is considered because she cannot eat by mouth secondary to the endotracheal tube and mechanical ventilation. How should she be transitioned from parenteral to enteral feedings?**

Tube feedings can begin with a full-strength isotonic enteral feeding formulation at a slow infusion rate (25 mL/hour). Concurrently, the parenteral nutrient formulation should be decreased to avoid fluid overload and to keep the calorie and protein intake constant. It can be anticipated that K.R. can transition from parenteral to enteral feedings in 24 to 48 hours. (See Chapter 36, Adult Enteral Nutrition.)

REFERENCES

1. Dudrick SJ et al. Long-term parenteral nutrition with growth, development and positive nitrogen balance. Surgery 1968;64:134.
2. Wilmore DW, Dudrick SJ. Growth and development of an infant receiving all nutrients exclusively by vein. JAMA 1968;203:860.
3. Dudrick SJ et al. Can intravenous feeding as the sole means of nutrition support growth in the child and restore weight loss in an adult? An affirmative answer. Ann Surg 1969;169:974.
4. A.S.P.E.N. Board of Directors. Definitions and terms used in A.S.P.E.N. guidelines and standards. Nutr Clin Pract 1995;10:1.
5. Grant JP. Nutritional assessment in clinical practice. Nutr Clin Pract 1986;1:3.
6. Shopbell JM et al. Nutrition screening and assessment. In: Gottschlich MM, ed. The Science and Practice of Nutrition Support. Dubuque, IA: Kendall/Hunt, 2001:107.
7. McWhirter JP, Pennington CR. Incidence and recognition of malnutrition in the hospital. Br Med J 1994;308:945.
8. Leiter LA, Marliss EB. Survival during fasting may depend on fat as well as protein stores. JAMA 1982;248:2306.
9. Keys A et al. The Biology of Human Starvation. Minneapolis: University of Minnesota Press, 1950.
10. Robinson G et al. Impact of nutritional status on DRG length of stay. JPEN J Parenter Enteral Nutr 1987;11:49.
11. Reilly JJ et al. Economic impact of malnutrition: a model system for hospitalized patients. JPEN J Parenter Enteral Nutr 1988;12:371.
12. Detsky AS et al. Is this patient malnourished? JAMA 1994;271:54.
13. A.S.P.E.N. Board of Directors and the Clinical Guidelines Task Force. Guidelines for the use of parenteral and enteral nutrition in adult and pediatric patients. JPEN J Parenter Enteral Nutr 2002;26 (Suppl):18SA.
14. A.S.P.E.N. Board of Directors and Task Force on Standards for Specialized Nutrition Support for Hospitalized Adult Patients. Standards for specialized nutrition support: adult hospitalized patients. Nutr Clin Pract 2002:17:384.
15. A.S.P.E.N. Board of Directors. Definitions of terms used in A.S.P.E.N. guidelines and standards. Nutr Clin Pract 1995:10:1.
16. Lipman TO. Grains or veins: is enteral nutrition really better than parenteral nutrition? A look at the evidence. JPEN J Parenter Enteral Nutr 1998;22:167.
17. Braunschweig CL et al. Enteral compared with parenteral nutrition: a meta-analysis. Am J Clin Nutr 2001;74:534.
18. Beier-Holgersen R. Influence of postoperative enteral nutrition on postsurgical infections. Gut 1996;39:833.
19. Hernandez G et al. Gut mucosal atrophy after a short enteral fasting period in critically ill patients. J Crit Care 1999;14:73.
20. Kudsk KA et al. Enteral versus parenteral feeding. Ann Surg 1992;215:503.
21. Moore FA et al. Early enteral feeding, compared with parenteral, reduces septic complications: the results of a meta-analysis. Ann Surg 1992;216:172.
22. Charney P. Nutrition assessment in the 1990's: Where are we now? Nutr Clin Pract 1995;10:131.
23. Gabay C, Kushner I. Acute-phase proteins and other systemic responses to inflammation. N Engl J Med 1999;340:448.

24. Vanek VW. The use of serum albumin as a prognostic or nutritional marker and the pros and cons of IV albumin therapy. Nutr Clin Pract 1998;13:110.
25. Detsky AS et al. What is subjective global assessment of nutritional status? JPEN J Parenter Enteral Nutr 1987;11:8.
26. Garrel DR et al. Should we still use the Harris and Benedict equations? Nutr Clin Pract 1996;11:99.
27. Frakenfield D. Energy and macrosubstrate requirements. In: Gottschlich MM, ed. The Science and Practice of Nutrition Support. Dubuque, IA: Kendall/Hunt, 2001:31.
28. Ireton-Jones CS et al. Equations for estimation of energy expenditures in patients with burns with special reference to ventilatory status. J Burn Care Rehab 1992;13:330.
29. Brandi LS et al. Indirect calorimetry in critically ill patients: clinical applications and practical advice. Nutrition 1997;13:349.
30. McClave SA, Snider HL. Use of indirect calorimetry in clinical nutrition. Nutr Clin Pract 1992;7:207.
31. Krzywda EA, et al. Parenteral access devices. In: Gottschlich MM, ed. The Science and Practice of Nutrition Support. Dubuque, IA: Kendall/Hunt, 2001:225.
32. Payne-James J, Kwahaja HT. First choice for total parenteral nutrition: the peripheral route. JPEN J Parenter Enteral Nutr 1993;17:468.
33. Kane KF et al. High osmolality feedings do not increase the incidence of thrombophlebitis during peripheral IV nutrition. JPEN J Parenter Enteral Nutr 1996;20:194.
34. Vanek VW. The ins and outs of venous access: Part 1. Nutr Clin Pract 2002;17:85.
35. Alhimyary A et al. Safety and efficacy of total parenteral nutrition delivered via a peripherally inserted central venous catheter. Nutr Clin Pract 1996;11:199.
36. Vanek VW. The ins and outs of venous access: Part 2. Nutr Clin Pract 2002:17:142.
37. ASHP Technical Assistance Bulletin on quality assurance for pharmacy-prepared sterile products. Am J Hosp Pharm 1993;50:2386.
38. Total parenteral nutrition/total nutrient admixture. USP DI Update. United States Pharmacopeial Convention Inc., Rockville, MD, 1996:66.
39. Food and Drug Administration. Safety alert: hazards of precipitation associated with parenteral nutrition. Am J Hosp Pharm 1994;51:427.
40. National Advisory Group on Standards and Practice Guidelines for Parenteral Nutrition. Safe practices for parenteral nutrition formulations. JPEN J Parenter Enteral Nutr 1998;22:49.
41. Driscoll EF. Intravenous lipid emulsions: 2001. Nutr Clin Pract 2001;16:215.
42. Kearns LR et al. Update on parenteral amino acids. Nutr Clin Pract 2001;16:219.
43. The Veterans Affairs Total Parenteral Nutrition Cooperative Study Group. Perioperative nutrition in surgical patients. N Engl J Med 1991;325:525.
44. Torosian MJ. Perioperative nutrition support for patients undergoing gastrointestinal surgery: critical analysis and recommendations. World J Surg 1999;23:565.
45. Klein S et al. Nutrition support in clinical practice: Review of published data and recommendations for future research. JPEN J Parenter Enteral Nutr 1997;21:133.
46. Nordenstrom J et al. Peripheral parenteral nutrition: effect on a standardized compounded admixture on infusion phlebitis. Br J Surg 1991;78:1391.

47. Solomon SM, Kirby DK. The refeeding syndrome: A review. J Parenter Enteral Nutr 1990;14:90.
48. Brooks MJ, Melnik G. The refeeding syndrome: An approach to understanding its complications and preventing its occurrence. Pharmacotherapy 1995;15:713.
49. Sacks GS. Is IV lipid emulsion safe in patients with hypertriglyceridemia? Nutr Clin Pract 1997;12:120.
50. Bayer-Berger M et al. Incidence of phlebitis in peripheral parenteral nutrition: effect of the different nutrient solutions. Clin Nutr 1989;8:81.
51. Daly JM et al. Peripheral vein infusion of dextrose/amino acid solutions ±20% fat emulsion. JPEN J Parenter Enteral Nutr 1985;9:296.
52. Makarewicz PA et al. Prevention of superficial phlebitis during peripheral parenteral nutrition. Am J Surg 1986;151:126.
53. Madan M et al. A randomized study of the effects of osmolarity and heparin with hydrocortisone on thrombophlebitis in peripheral intravenous nutrition. Clin Nutr 1991;10:309.
54. Matarese LE. Metabolic complications of parenteral nutrition therapy. In: Gottschlich MM, ed. The Science and Practice of Nutrition Support. Dubuque, IA: Kendall/Hunt, 2001:269.
55. Driscoll DF. Clinical issues regarding the use of total nutrient admixtures. DICP 1990;24:296.
56. Wolfe RR. Glucose metabolism in burn injury: a review. J Burn Care Rehab 1985;6:408.
57. Delafoss BY et al. Respiratory changes induced by parenteral nutrition in postoperative patients undergoing inspiratory pressure support ventilation. Anesthesiology 1986;66:393.
58. Quigley EMM et al. Hepatobiliary complications of total parenteral nutrition. Gastroenterology 1993;286:301.
59. Seidner DL et al. Effects of long-chain triglyceride emulsions on reticuloendothelial system function in humans. JPEN J Parenter Enteral Nutr 1989;13:614.
60. Barber JR et al. Parenteral feeding formulations. In: Gottschlich MM, ed. The Science and Practice of Nutrition Support. Dubuque, IA: Kendall/Hunt, 2001:251.
61. Driscoll DF. Total nutrient admixtures: theory and practice. Nutr Clin Pract 1995;10:114.
62. Federal Register, April 20, 2000 (Volume 65, Number 77).
63. Guidelines for essential trace element preparations for parenteral use: a statement by the Nutrition Advisory Group. JPEN J Parenter Enteral Nutr 1979;3:263.
64. Baumgartner TG. Enteral and parenteral electrolyte therapeutics. Nutr Clin Pract 2001;16:226.
65. Clark CL et al. Treatment of hypophosphatemia in patients receiving specialized nutrition support using a graduated dosing scheme: Results from a prospective clinical trial. Crit Care Med 1995;23:1504.
66. Rosen GH et al. Intravenous phosphate repletion regimen for critically ill patients with moderate hypophosphatemia. Crit Care Med 1995;23:1204.
67. Mizock BA. Alterations in carbohydrate metabolism during stress: a review of the literature. Am J Med 1995;98:75.
68. Rosemarin DK et al. Hyperglycemia associated with high, continuous infusion rates of total parenteral nutrition. Nutr Clin Pract 1996;11:151.
69. McMahon MM. Management of hyperglycemia in hospitalized patients receiving parenteral nutrition. Nutr Clin Pract 1997;12:35.

70. Van den Berghe G et al. Intensive insulin therapy in the critically ill patients. N Engl J Med 2001;345:1359.

71. Van den Berghe G et al. Outcome benefit of intensive insulin therapy in the critically ill: Insulin dose versus glycemic control. Crit Care Med 2003;31:359.

72. Montori VM et al. Hyperglycemia in acutely ill patients. JAMA 2002;288:2167.

73. Furnary AP et al. Continuous intravenous insulin infusion reduced the incidence of deep sternal would infection in diabetic patients after cardiac surgical procedures. Ann Thoracic Surg 1999;67:352.

74. Zerr KJ et al. Glucose control lowers the risk of wound infection in diabetics after open heart operations. Ann Thorac Surg 1997;63:356.

75. Rose BD. Clinical Physiology of Acid–Base and Electrolyte Disorders, 4th ed. New York: McGraw-Hill, 1994:891.

76. Knowles JB et al. Pulmonary deposition of calcium phosphate crystals as a complication of home parenteral nutrition. JPEN J Parenter Enteral Nutr 1989;13:209.

77. McKinnon BT. FDA safety alert: hazards of precipitation associated with parenteral nutrition. Nutr Clin Pract 1996;11:59.

78. Trissel LA. Handbook of Injectable Drugs, 12th ed. Bethesda, MD: American Society of Hospital Pharmacists, 2003.

79. Hammond KA, et al. Transitioning to home and other alternative sites. In: Gottschlich MM, ed. The Science and Practice of Nutrition Support. Dubuque, IA: Kendall/Hunt, 2001:701.

80. Malone AM. Supplemental zinc in wound healing: Is it beneficial? Nutr Clin Pract 2000;15:253.

81. Seidner DL et al. Can octreotide be added to parenteral nutrition solutions? Point-counterpoint. Nutr Clin Pract 1998;13:84.

82. Quigley EMM et al. Hepatobiliary complications of total parenteral nutrition. Gastroenterology 1993;104;286.

83. Buchman A. total parenteral nutrition-associated liver disease. JPEN J Parenter Enteral Nutr 2002;26:S43.

84. Teran FC, McCullough AF. Nutrition in liver diseases. In: Gottschlich MM, ed. The Science and Practice of Nutrition Support. Dubuque, IA: Kendall/Hunt, 2001:537.

85. Marchesini G et al. Nutritional treatment with branched-chain amino acids in advanced liver cirrhosis. J Gastroenterol 2000;35:S1.

86. Fabbri A et al. Overview of randomized clinical trials of oral branched-chain amino acid treatment in chronic hepatic encephalopathy. JPEN J Parenter Enteral Nutr 1996;20:159.

87. Skeie B et al. Branch-chain amino acids: their metabolism and clinical utility. Crit Care Med 1990;18:549.

88. Oki JC, Cuddy PG. Branched-chain amino acid support of stressed patients. DICP 1989;23:399.

89. Wolk R. Nutrition in renal failure. In: Gottschlich MM, ed. The Science and Practice of Nutrition Support. Dubuque, IA: Kendall/Hunt, 2001:575.

90. Oldrizzi L et al. Nutrition and the kidney: how to manage patients with renal failure. Nutr Clin Pract 1994;9:3.

91. Bellomo R et al. Continuous arteriovenous haemodiafiltration in the critically ill: Influence on major nutrient balances. Intensive Care Med 1991;17:399.

92. Frankenfield DC et al. Glucose dynamics during continuous hemodiafiltration and total parenteral nutrition. Intensive Care Med 1995;21:1016.

93. Charney P, Charney D. Nutrition support in acute renal failure. In: Shikora SA, et al, eds. Nutritional Considerations in the Intensive Care Unit. Dubuque, IA: Kendall/Hunt, 2002:209.

94. Charney P, Charney D. Nutriton support in renal failure. Nutr Clin Pract 2002;17:226.

95. Choban PS et al. Nutrition support of obese hospitalized patients. Nutr Clin Pract 1997;12:149.

96. McMahon M, Rizza RA. Nutritional support in hospitalized patients with diabetes mellitus. Mayo Clin Proc 1996;71:587.

97. Bernard DKH, Shaw MJ. Principles of nutrition therapy for short-bowel syndrome. Nutr Clin Pract 1993;8:153.

98. Kelly DG, Nehra V. Gastrointestinal disease. In: Gottschlich MM, ed. The Science and Practice of Nutrition Support. Dubuque, IA: Kendall/Hunt, 2001:517.

99. Mowatt-Larssen, Brown RO. Specialized nutritional support in respiratory disease. Clin Pharm 1993;12:276.

100. Talpers SS et al. Nutritionally associated increased carbon dioxide production. Chest 1992;102:551.

101. Seidner DL, Fuhrman MP. Nutrition support in pancreatitis. In: Gottschlich MM, ed. The Science and Practice of Nutrition Support. Dubuque, IA: Kendall/Hunt, 2001:553.

102. Sacks GS. Is IV lipid emulsion safe in patients with hypertriglyceridemia? Adult patients. Nutr Clin Pract 1997;12:120.

DERMATOLOGIC DISORDERS

Allan Ellsworth
SECTION EDITOR

CHAPTER **38**

Dermatotherapy and Drug Induced Skin Disorders

Allan Ellsworth, Robert E. Smith

ANATOMY AND PHYSIOLOGY OF THE SKIN

The skin is the largest organ in the body and constitutes, on average, 17% of a person's body weight. The skin's thickness ranges from 3 to 5 mm. Figure 38-1 shows a cross-section of the anatomy of human skin. The major function of the skin is to protect underlying structures from trauma, temperature variations, harmful penetrations, moisture, humidity, radiation, and invasion of microorganisms. There are three layers of skin: the epidermis, dermis, and subcutaneous tissue.[1-6]

Epidermis

The epidermis consists of four distinct layers: stratum corneum, stratum lucidum, stratum spinosum, and stratum germinativum. The major function of the epidermis is to serve as a barrier. This layer keeps chemicals and other substances from penetrating into the body and prevents the loss of water from the skin and underlying tissues. The maturation of keratinocytes from the stratum germinativum to the stratum corneum is critical for this barrier function. As the keratinocytes migrate to the skin

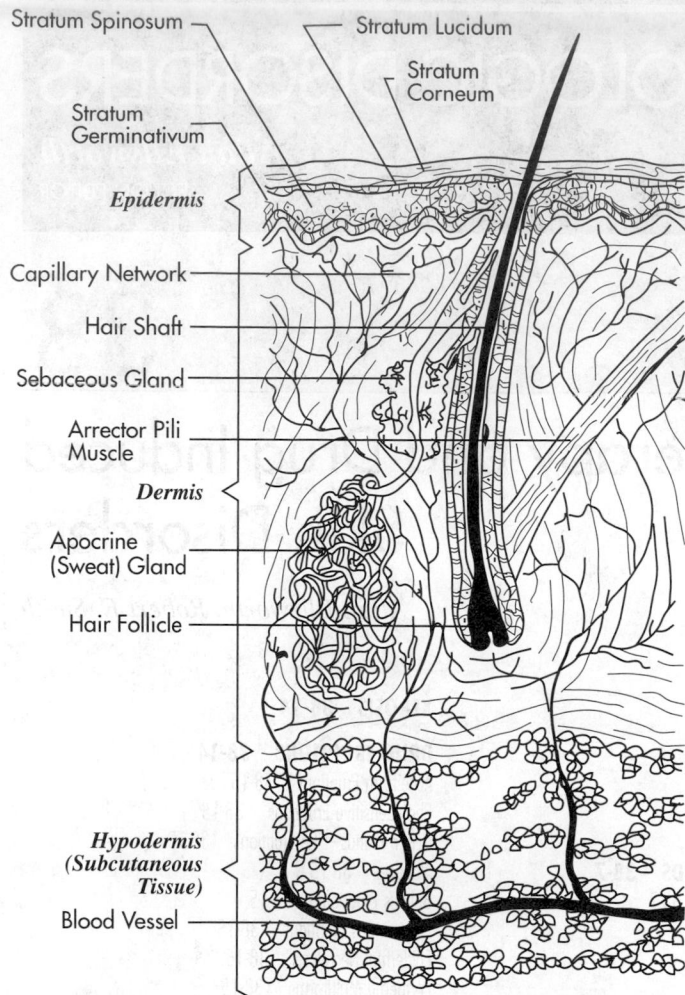

Stratum Spinosum
Stratum Lucidum
Stratum Corneum
Stratum Germinativum
Epidermis
Capillary Network
Hair Shaft
Sebaceous Gland
Arrector Pili Muscle
Dermis
Apocrine (Sweat) Gland
Hair Follicle
Hypodermis (Subcutaneous Tissue)
Blood Vessel

FIGURE 38-1 Cross-section of the anatomy of human skin.

surface, they change from living cells to dead, thick-walled, non-nucleated cells containing keratin, a hard fibrous protein. It normally takes 26 to 28 days for a keratinocyte to divide, differentiate, move up to the stratum corneum and be sloughed off.

The *stratum corneum,* which is composed of the dead cells, provides the greatest resistance to the percutaneous absorption of chemicals and drugs. It behaves as a semipermeable membrane through which drugs are absorbed by passive diffusion. Factors that can affect drug absorption are hydration of the skin and damage to the stratum corneum. In general, the greater the damage to the stratum corneum, the greater is the absorption of topically applied drugs. Skin diseases affecting only the epidermis heal without scarring.[1–6]

Dermis

The dermis, which ranges in thickness from 1 to 4 mm, is composed of collagen fibers, elastic fibers, and an extrafibrillar gel of mucopolysaccharides called *glycosaminoglycans* (formally called *ground substances*). The major function of the dermis is to protect the body from mechanical injury and to support the dermal appendages and the epidermis. It also provides a capillary, lymphatic, and nerve supply to the skin and its appendages: apocrine and eccrine sweat glands, seba-

ceous glands, and hair follicles. The capillary network plays a major role in temperature regulation and provides nutrition to the epidermis. The nerves transmit sensations of touch and pain. Finally, the dermis contains large amounts of water, thus serving as a water storage organ. All but the most superficial injuries to the dermis generally result in scarring as the wound heals.[1–6]

Drugs passing through the epidermis penetrate directly into the dermis and may be absorbed into the general circulation through the capillary network. Generally, only small amounts of topically applied drugs enter the dermis via the sweat glands or the pilosebaceous units.

Subcutaneous Layer

The subcutaneous layer supports the dermis and epidermis and serves as a fat storage area. This layer helps regulate temperature, provides nutritional support, and cushions the outer skin layers.[1–6]

INFLAMMATORY LESIONS

One of the dermatologic axioms regarding therapy is particularly useful in selecting dosage forms. "If it's wet, dry it; if it's dry, wet it." Wet dressings are most useful in drying acute, inflamed lesions, while ointment type bases are most useful for chronic, lichenified, scaling lesions. The choice of vehicle for chronic lesions is often based on what the patient has found to work best or will use. Frequently, patients with chronic dermatologic conditions use multiple types of vehicles concomitantly (e.g., cream bases [which are drying]) during the day, as they are cosmetically acceptable, and ointment bases at night (greasy, but better emollients).

Acute Lesions

Acute inflammatory lesions are characterized by vesiculation, erythema, swelling, warmth, pruritus, oozing and/or weeping. Generally, the more severe the dermatitis, the milder the initial topical therapy. For instance, cool water in the form of an aqueous vehicle, preferably a wet dressing, soak or bath, is more effective as the initial therapeutic agent than a potent topical corticosteroid applied to a warm, erythematous, weeping dermatitis. The specific approach depends on the part(s) of the body involved.

Subacute and Chronic Lesions

Subacute lesions are characterized by decreasing vesiculation and oozing and are often covered with crusts. They still require cleaning and drying with aqueous preparations, but for a shorter duration than with acute lesions. Chronic inflammatory lesions are characterized by erythema, scaling, lichenification, dryness, and pruritus. There are no absolute rules for treating chronic lesions. If the lesion is dry, an oleaginous or occlusive base should be used, perhaps with a keratolytic agent.

DERMATOLOGIC DRUG DELIVERY SYSTEMS

A range of dermatologic formulations are available: solutions, suspensions or shake lotions, powders, lotions, emulsions, gels, creams, ointments, and aerosols. Each dermatologic delivery vehicle has specific characteristics and uses based on the type, relative acuteness, and location of the lesion.

Solutions

Solutions provide evaporative cooling, vasoconstriction, and resultant mild antipruritic effects. They soothe and cool inflamed skin, dry oozing lesions, soften crusts, aid in cleaning wounds, and assist in the drainage of purulent wounds. Aqueous solutions are most useful for acutely inflamed, oozing lesions; erosions; and ulcers. In most instances, solutions should be the sole therapy until the oozing or weeping subsides. If other topical medications are applied to oozing or weeping lesions, they will be washed away and will not provide the desired effect. The most commonly used solutions are normal (0.9%) saline and aluminum acetate 5% solution (Burow's solution) diluted 1:10 to 1:40. Solutions are often applied as wet dressings. The most important component of a solution is water. Although active or inert substances may be added to solutions, the cleansing, drying and cooling effect of water provides the major therapeutic benefit. Some of the products (e.g., Burow's solution) also have *astringent* properties. These locally applied preparations alter the skin surface and interstitial spaces to cause contraction and wrinkling. Water penetration is reduced to minimize edema, inflammation, and exudation. Table 38-1 lists the most commonly used solutions. Boric acid should not be used as a topical agent because it can be absorbed through the skin, causing systemic toxicity.[7]

Depending on the affected area and its size, a patient may soak the affected area directly in the solution for 15 to 30 minutes three to six times per day. If larger areas are involved or if the affected area cannot be easily soaked (e.g., a shoulder), a clean towel or cloth soaked in the solution (lightly wrung out) is directly applied to the lesion(s) as a wet dressing. The soaked cloth should be left in place for 5 to 10 minutes, then re-soaked in the solution and reapplied. The patient may repeat this procedure for 15 to 30 minutes three times daily. Solutions applied with a cloth should have the cloth material wrapped around the lesions several times, if possible. If large areas are involved, the patient may draw a bath, add ap-

propriate amounts of medications, and soak for 15 to 30 minutes three to six times per day. It is impractical to prepare a Burow's solution bath at the 1:10 to 1:40 concentration. Again, the concentration of the Burow's solution is probably insignificant as the major effect of the solution is produced by the water. In general, no more than one-third of the body should be soaked in this manner at any time. One should be aware that evaporation can concentrate solutions, potentially making them too irritating to use. Small volumes of a 1:40 concentration of Burow's solution left standing open at room temperature after 30 to 60 minutes may yield a 1:10 solution. This problem would not be as significant with larger volumes or if the solution was stored in a closed container. For this reason, wet dressings should always be freshly prepared (i.e., within 24 hours), kept in closed containers, and never reused. Wet dressings are most comfortable if they are slightly cool or warm, depending on the patient's preference. When drying the affected area after a wet dressing has been used, care must be taken not to irritate the inflamed skin by rubbing it with a towel. The proper technique for drying the skin is to pat the area gently with a soft, clean towel.[7]

Baths

In addition to wet dressings and soaks, topical solutions can be applied to large areas of the body through bathing. In using this type of treatment, the bath should be about half full. Soothing and antipruritic colloidal bath additives may be used to treat widespread eruptions such as lichen planus, pityriasis rosea, urticaria, and other weeping or crusting dermatoses. Colloidal oatmeal (1 cup of oatmeal [Aveeno] mixed with 2 cups of cold tap water and poured into 6 inches of a lukewarm bath) produces a pleasing and soothing bath. Alternatively, a starch bath using 2 cups of hydrolyzed starch (Linit) or cornstarch mixed with 4 cups of tap water and added to a bath may be used. A mixture of equal parts baking soda and starch also may be used. Epsom salt baths, made by dissolving 3 cups of magnesium sulfate in 6 inches of lukewarm water in a tub, are useful in treating pyodermas, furuncles, and necrotic acne (especially when the back, shoulders, and buttocks are affected). Water-soluble

Table 38-1 Solutions for Wet Dressings or Drying Weeping Lesions

Agent[a]	Strength	Preparation (H₂0)	Germicidal Activity	Astringent Activity	Comments
Normal saline	0.9% NaCl	1 tsp NaCl per pint H₂0	None	None	Inexpensive; easy to prepare
Aluminum acetate (Burow's solution) (Domeboro packets/ tablets)	5%	Dilute to 1:10–1:40 (0.5–0.125%) One packet/tablet to a pint of water yields a 1:40 solution; two packets/ tablets yields a 1:20 solution	Mild Mild	+ +	– –
Potassium permanganate	65- and 330-mg tablets	Dilute to 1:4,000–1:16,000; 65-mg tablet to 250–1,000 mL; 330-mg tablet to 1,500–5,000 mL	Moderate	None	Stains skin, clothing
Silver nitrate	0.1–0.5%	1 tsp of 50% stock solution to 1,000 mL will yield a 0.25% solution	Good	+	Stains; can cause pain
Acetic acid[b]	1%	Dilute 1 pint of standard 5% household vinegar with 5 parts H₂0	Good	+	Unpleasant odor; can be irritating

[a]Although many substances are added to wet dressings, the cleansing and drying effect of the water is the major benefit.
[b]Used primarily for *Pseudomonas aeruginosa* infections.
Adapted from Reference 7.

coal tar preparations applied via a bath for the treatment of psoriasis may be the most acceptable way to apply this medication. Ointments or creams containing coal tar are malodorous and have a tendency to stain materials on contact.

A variety of bath oils are available: Alpha-Keri, Domol, Lubriderm, and Nutraderm. Adding bath oil directly to the bath is not recommended, as they make the tub slippery and potentially dangerous. The concentration of the oil in the water becomes almost insignificant anyway (5 to 10 mL in 20 to 40 gallons). Five to ten milliliters of bath oil may be applied directly to wet skin on leaving a bath and patted dry with a towel for a more significant effect. These are most useful in preventing and treating mild cases of xerosis (dry skin). With moderate to severe cases of xerosis, additional topical oleaginous products generally are required to improve the condition. Patients may make their own bath oil by adding 2 ounces of olive oil or Nivea oil to a cup of milk and applying it following a bath.[7]

Powders

Powders are drying and cooling; they absorb moisture and create more surface area for evaporation. They are used mainly in intertriginous areas (e.g., under the breasts or in skin folds) to decrease friction, which can cause mechanical irritation. They also are useful in the treatment of chafing, tinea pedis (athlete's foot), tinea cruris (jock itch), and diaper dermatitis (diaper rash). Occasionally, powders are applied on top of ointments to protect clothing from the ointment. The liberal use of powders on bedridden patients helps prevent pressure ulcers (bed sores).

Powders can be applied with a cotton puff or shaker. Care should be taken to minimize breathing the powder, because this can lead to respiratory tract irritation, particularly in infants. Powders that contain starch or cellulose should be washed off before reapplication, as continued build-up can produce mechanical irritation. Corn starch-containing powders should not be used for intertrigo because starch can serve as a substrate for *Candida albicans*. Powders should not be applied to oozing lesions because they tend to cake into hard granules, making them difficult and painful to remove and promoting maceration. Concerns regarding the association of routine cosmetic talc use and ovarian cancer and granulomatous lung changes are without convincing evidence.[8] The most commonly used powders are talc and the antifungal, nystatin.

Lotions

Lotions are suspensions or solutions of powder in a water vehicle. They are usually cooling and drying, but may provide some lubrication, depending on the formulation. Lotions are used to treat superficial dermatoses, especially if there is slight oozing. They are useful if large or intertriginous areas are affected, and they are especially advantageous in the treatment of conditions characterized by significant inflammation and tenderness. In these situations, creams or ointments may cause pain on application. Sunburn, acute contact dermatitis, or poison ivy/oak are examples of conditions in which this principle may apply. Generally, lotions are applied three or four times daily, with each fresh application placed over previous application, unless there is significant oozing present, which could promote caking of dried solid ingredients. If this

is the case, the area should be cleansed before repeat application. Because many lotions are suspensions, it is advisable to shake the lotion well before application. Generally, 6 oz of lotion covers the entire body of an average adult.[7]

Emulsions

Emulsions are solid or liquid and can be divided into two classes: *oil-in-water* and *water-in-oil*. Cream preparations are generally oil-in-water emulsions, while ointment preparations are water-in-oil emulsions. As the amount of oil increases, the viscosity of the emulsion also will increase.

The indications for liquid oil-in-water emulsions are similar to those for lotions, except that this dosage form provides greater occlusion and is more useful in conditions where dry skin predominates. Liquid water-in-oil emulsions have similar indications to ointments, except they can be applied more easily than ointments. Water-in-oil emulsions are most useful in conditions where dry skin predominates; application to hairy or intertriginous areas should be avoided. As with lotions, 6 oz of a liquid emulsion will cover all exposed skin on an average adult.[7]

Table 38-2 lists some commercially available oil-in-water and water-in-oil emulsion bases.

Gels

Gels are a form of ointment (semisolid emulsion) that contain propylene glycol and carboxypolymethylene. They are clear, nongreasy, nonstaining, nonocclusive, and quick drying. They are thixotropic, i.e., become thinner with rubbing and may sting on application. Gels are most useful when applied to hairy areas or other areas such as the face or scalp where it is considered cosmetically unacceptable to have the residue of a vehicle remain on the skin. Because of their ingredients, gels tend to be more drying.

Creams

Creams are the most commonly used vehicle in dermatology. Most are oil-in-water emulsions and are intended to be rubbed in well until they vanish (vanishing creams). Since creams do not provide much occlusiveness, they are most often recommended for subacute lesions and occasionally for chronic lesions without significant lichenification. The most common mistake made by patients when applying creams is that they use too much and/or do not rub them in fully. Generally, if the

Table 38-2	Commercially Available Emulsion Bases
Oil-in-Water	*Water-in-Oil*
Acid Mantle Cream	Aquaphor
Aquaphilic	Eucerin
Cetaphil	Lubriderm
Dermabase	Nivea Cream
Dermovan	Nutraderma
Hydrophilic Ointment USP	Polysorb
Keri Lotion	Vanicream
Lanaphilic	Velvachol
Unibase	

Adapted with permission from Reference 7.

cream can be seen on the skin after application, the patient has made one or both of these application mistakes. Ultimately, they are wasting the preparation or are not getting the full therapeutic benefits. One gram of cream should cover 100 cm² of surface area. Table 38-3 lists the approximate amount of cream required for application to various parts of the body.[7]

Ointments

Ointments are made of inert bases such as petrolatum or may consist of droplets of water suspended in a continuous phase of oleaginous material (water-in-oil emulsions). Ointments are most useful on chronic lesions, relieving dryness, brittleness, and protecting fissures due to their occlusive properties. They should not be used on acutely inflamed lesions. Ointments should not be applied to intertriginous or hairy areas because they tend to trap heat and promote maceration. Ointments are greasy and may be cosmetically unacceptable.

Aerosols

Aerosols are the most expensive and inefficient way to apply dermatologic medications. Their only advantage over other dosage forms is that they do not require direct mechanical contact with the skin and may be useful if mechanical application causes intolerable pain for the patient. If an aerosol is used, it should be shaken well before use, and the patient should be cautioned not to spray the product around the face where it could get into the eyes or nose or could be inhaled. Generally, aerosols should be sprayed from approximately 6 inches above the skin in bursts of 1 to 3 seconds. Aerosols also are useful for application to hairy areas if a special application nozzle is used. Aerosols have a drying effect and should not be used for a long period of time.

Other Delivery Systems

The addition of solvents, such as dimethyl sulfoxide (DMSO), may enhance dermal absorption, allowing the delivery of many drugs directly through the skin. Skin patch delivery systems also have been designed to deliver drugs directly through the skin. Examples include scopolamine, nitroglycerin, clonidine, nicotine, opioids, and various hormones. These dermatologic drug delivery systems, or similar ones, offer great potential for the sustained delivery of pharmaceuticals over extended periods of time.

Selection of a Delivery System

Dermatologic vehicles should be matched to the type of lesion for which they will be used. Acute lesions require aqueous vehicles until the lesions become dry. Subacute lesions also benefit from aqueous vehicles, but for shorter periods of time before switching to creams or gels. Chronic lesions usually require ointments because of their dry, lichenified characteristics. While there are exceptions, these principles are depicted on Table 38-4.

ASSESSING THE DERMATOLOGIC PATIENT

1. C.B., a 23-year-old, 66-kg woman, complains of a rash. What types of questions should C.B. be asked to help determine the appropriate diagnosis and treatment?

The diagnosis of dermatologic conditions can be simplified by considering six primary factors: morphology (what the lesions look like; pattern of the lesions); location or distribution of the lesions on the body; symptoms, both local and systemic; history of the present condition as well as related conditions; age of the patient; and patient gender. These six factors are discussed below with their significant qualifying characteristics.

Morphology

Table 38-5 provides a listing of common dermatologic lesions along with their respective definitions and some well known clinical examples. Lesions may also be classified as either primary or secondary. Primary lesions are lesions as they first appear on the skin, whereas secondary lesions develop from primary lesions. A papule (primary lesion) might progress to a pustule (secondary lesion). A pustule may also be a primary lesions if it originally developed as a pustule. The ability to recognize and describe specific lesions is critical to a successful diagnosis and communication regarding response to therapy.

In addition many lesions present in a particular distribution or pattern. Poison ivy lesions are commonly distributed linearly. Herpetic lesions are so typical that the term herpetiform is used for lesions due to other conditions that have a herpes-like distribution. The specific size of the lesion is also important in assessing a patient's condition. Dermatologic terms related to lesion distribution or pattern are shown in Table 38-6. The lesion's consistency (firm versus soft), the lesion's borders and color are also important diagnostic considerations.

Table 38-3   Amount of Topical Medication Needed for Various Dosage Regimens

Area Treated	Single Application (g)	BID for 1 week (g)	BID for 1 month(g)
Hands, head, face, anogenital area	2	28	120
On arm, anterior or posterior trunk	3	42	180
One leg	4	56	240
Entire body	30–60	420–840 (14–28 oz)	1.8–3.6 kg (60–120 oz)

Adapted from Reference 7.

Table 38-4   Appropriate Dermatologic Vehicle Selection Across the Range of Dermatologic Lesions

Range of Lesions	Range of Vehicles
Acute inflammation: Oozing, weeping, vesication, edema, pruritus ↓	Aqueous vehicles, water, then . . . . . . powders solutions, lotions, sprays, aerosols ↓
Subacute inflammation: Crusting, less oozing, pruritus ↓	Creams, gels ↓
Chronic inflammation: Lichenification, dryness, erythema, pruritus, scaling	Ointments

Table 38-5   Dermatologic Lesions, Definitions, and Clinical Examples

Name	Definition	Examples
Primary Lesions		
Macule	Nonpalpable, flat, change in color, smaller than 1 cm	Freckles, flat moles
Patch	Nonpalpable, flat, change in color, larger than 1 cm	Vitiligo, café au lait spots, chloasma
Papule	Palpable, solid mass, may have change in color, smaller than 1 cm	Verrucae, noninflammatory acne (comedone), raised nevus
Nodule	Palpable, solid mass, most often below the plane of the skin, 1–2 cm	Erythema nodosum, severe acne
Tumor	Palpable, solid mass, >2 cm, most often above and below the plane of the skin	Neoplasms
Plaque	Flat, elevated, superficial papule with surface area greater than height, larger than 1 cm	Psoriasis, seborrheic keratosis
Wheal	Superficial area of cutaneous edema, fluid not confined to cavity	Urticaria (hives), insect bite
Vesicle	Palpable, fluid-filled cavity, smaller than 1 cm, filled with serous fluid (blister)	Herpes simplex, herpes zoster, contact dermatitis
Bulla	Palpable, fluid-filled cavity, greater than 1 cm, filled with serous fluid (blister)	Pemphigus vulgaris, second-degree burn
Pustule	Similar to vesicle, but filled with purulent fluid	Acne, impetigo, folliculitis
Special Primary Lesions		
Comedone	Plugged opening of sebaceous gland	Acne, blackhead, whitehead
Cyst	Palpable lesion filled with semiliquid material or fluid	Sebaceous cyst
Abcess	Accumulation of purulent material in dermis or subcutaneous layers of skin. Purulent material not visible on surface of skin	
Furuncle	Inflammatory nodule involving a hair follicle, following an episode of folliculitis.	Small boil
Carbuncle	A coalescence of several furuncles	Large boil
Secondary Lesions		
Erosion	Loss of part or all the epidermis	Ecthyma
Ulcer	Loss of epidermis and dermis	Stasis ulcer
Fissure	Linear crack from epidermis into dermis	Tinea pedis
Excoriation	Self-induced linear, traumatized area caused by intense scratching	Atopic dermatitis, extreme pruritus
Atrophy	Thinning of skin with loss of dermal tissue	Striae
Crusts	Dried residue of pus, serum or blood from a wound, pustule or vesicle	Impetigo, scabs
Lichenification	Thickening of epidermis, accentuated skin markings, usually induced by scratching or chronic inflammation.	Atopic dermatitis

Table 38-6   Descriptive Dermatologic Terms

Term	Characteristics	Examples
Annular	Ring shaped	Tinea
Arcuate	Shaped like an arc	Syphillis
Circinate	Circular	Tinea
Confluent	Lesions run together	Psoriasis, tinea
Discrete	Lesions remain separate	Psoriasis, tinea
Eczematous	General term for vesiculation, crusting and lichenification	Contact dermatitis, atopic dermatitis
Geographic	Shaped like islands or continents; Maplike	Generalized psoriasis
Grouped	Lesions clustered together	Herpes
Herpetiform	Appears like herpes simplex	Herpes simplex
Iris	Looks like a bulls-eye, lesion within a lesion, target lesion	Erythema multiforme
Keratotic	Horny thickening	Psoriasis, corn, callus
Linear	Shaped in lines	Poison ivy
Multiform	More than one type or shape of lesion	Erythema multiforme
Papulosquamous	Papules with desquamation	Psoriasis
Serpiginous	Snakelike lesions	Cutaneuous larva migrans
Zosteriform	Appears like herpes zoster	Herpes zoster

Location

"Location, location, location" is another axiom of dermatology. Simply put, certain lesions or conditions almost always occur in certain body locations. Table 38-7 provides a list of anatomic sites with common dermatoses occurring in those locations. For example, diseases of the sebaceous glands (e.g., acne, seborrheic dermatitis and rosacea) occur only in sites with high concentrations of sebaceous glands, such as the scalp, head, neck, chest, and umbilicus. Atopic dermatitis shows a predilection for the flexor surfaces of the body (i.e., antecubital and popliteal fossae).

Symptoms

Most skin conditions have only localized symptoms with the most common symptom being pruritus. Occasionally, localized burning or pain is the predominant symptom.

History

Although a diagnosis may often be made from morphology, location, and symptoms, the patient history provides very useful diagnostic and therapeutic information. Similar to the historical information obtained for any acute medical problem, the following questions should always be asked:

1. When and how did the problem start?
2. How has it progressed or changed since its onset? Have the lesions changed in size, color, appearance or severity?
3. What is the patient's past and current medical history? Could this be a dermatologic manifestation of a systemic disease?
4. What are the patient's symptoms?
5. Does the patient have any allergies?
6. What makes the condition worse or better?
7. Are there any events or happenings associated with the onset or worsening of the condition? Has there been any increased stress, exposure to new products, recent travel or changes in climate?

8. Has the patient treated the condition and how have the treatments worked?
9. How did the patient use any previous therapy and for how long did they use it?

Age

Many conditions occur predominantly in certain age groups, such as acne in neonates and the 11- to 20-year age group, seborrheic dermatitis in neonates and those age 11 to 12 years, rosacea in those over age 30 years, and atopic dermatitis primarily in children under 6 years of age. In fact, in 95% of patients the disease begins and ends before age 6 years. It is equally important to realize that many conditions such as primary irritant and allergic contact dermatitis occur independent of age. In addition, the skin of children and patients over 65 years of age is more penetrable, thus more responsive and more susceptible to adverse effects from therapy with topical agents. Topical therapeutic agent potency and delivery systems must be carefully evaluated before usage.

Gender

While most dermatologic conditions occur in both sexes, sometimes frequency and severity are gender dependent. Rosacea occurs more frequently in females, but is often more serious in males.

TOPICAL CORTICOSTEROIDS
General Principles of Therapy

Table 38-8 lists the most common topical corticosteroid preparations by their degree of potency. The following principles are used to guide the choice of agent and application technique.

- Topical corticosteroids should be applied twice daily. Increasing the application from twice daily to four times daily does not produce superior responses and is more expensive.[9]
- Preparations should be rubbed in thoroughly and, when possible, applied while the skin is moist (e.g., after bathing).[7] Hydration of the skin increases percutaneous absorption and the resultant therapeutic effect of topical steroids.
- Appropriate-strength preparations should be used to control the condition. For maintenance, most dermatologic conditions requiring topical corticosteroids can be managed with medium- or low-strength corticosteroid preparations (i.e., 1% hydrocortisone or a low-strength fluorinated corticosteroid such as triamcinolone acetonide 0.025%).[9,10]
- Occluded areas and certain, thin-skinned areas of the body, such as the face and flexures, are more prone to the development of side effects.[9,11] If corticosteroids must be used on the face or flexures, hydrocortisone or other nonfluorinated topical steroids should be used to reduce the probability of side effects.
- Children, elderly patients, and patients with liver failure are at risk for systemic corticosteroid toxicities. In addition, patients who use the highest-potency preparations for >2 weeks are susceptible to percutaneous absorption and systemic toxicity.[9–11]

Table 38-7	Common Skin Diseases by Body Location
Location	Skin diseases
Scalp	Seborrheic dermatitis, dandruff
Face	Acne, rosacea, seborrheic dermatitis, perioral dermatitis, impetigo, herpes simplex
Ears	Seborrheic dermatitis
Chest/abdomen	Tinea versicolor, tinea corporis, pityriasis rosea, acne, herpes zoster
Back	Tinea versicolor, tinea corporis, pityriasis rosea
Genital area	Tinea cruris, scabies, pediculosis, condyloma acuminate (venereal warts)
Extremities	Atopic dermatitis
Hands	Tinea manuum, scabies, primary irritant contact dermatitis, warts
Feet	Tinea pedis, contact dermatitis, onychomycosis
Generalized or localized	Primary irritant or contact dermatitis, photodermatitis

Table 38-8   Topical Corticosteroid Preparations

Corticosteroid	Brand Name(s)	Vehicle
1 (Most Potent)		
Betamethasone dipropionate	Diprolene 0.05%	Ointment, optimized vehicle
Clobetasol propionate	Temovate 0.05%	Cream, ointment, optimized vehicle
Diflorasone diacetate	Psorcon 0.05%	Ointment
Halobetasal propionate	Ultravate 0.05%	Cream, ointment
2		
Amcinonide	Cyclocort 0.1%	Cream, lotion, ointment
Betamethasone dipropionate	Diprolene AF 0.05%	Cream
Betamethasone dipropionate	Diprosone 0.05%	Ointment
Desoximetasone	Topicort 0.25%	Cream, ointment
Desoximetasone	Topicort 0.05%	Gel
Diflorasone diacetate	Florone, Maxiflor 0.05%	Ointment
Fluocinonide	Lidex 0.05%	Cream, ointment, gel
Halcinonide	Halog 0.1%	Cream
Mometasone furoate	Elcon 0.1%	Ointment
Triamcinolone acetonide	Kenalog 0.5%	Cream, ointment
3		
Amcinonide	Cyclocort 0.1%	Cream, lotion
Betamethasone	Benisone, Uticort 0.025%	Gel
Betamethasone benzoate	Topicort LP 0.05%	Cream (emollient)
Betamethasone dipropionate	Diprosone 0.05%	Cream
Betamethasone valerate	Valisone 0.1%	Ointment
Diflorasone diacetate	Florone, Maxiflor 0.05%	Cream
Fluocinonide	Cutivate 0.005%	Ointment
Fluticasone propionate	Lidex E 0.05%	Cream
Halocinonide	Halog 0.1%	Ointment
Triamcinolone acetate	Aristocort A 0.1%	Ointment
Triamcinolone acetate	Aristocort HP 0.5%	Cream
4		
Betamethasone benzoate	Benisone, Uticort 0.025%	Ointment
Betamethasone valerate	Valisone 0.1%	Lotion
Desoximetasone	Topicort-LP 0.05%	Cream
Fluocinolone acetonide	Synalar-HP 0.2%	Cream
Fluocinolone acetonide	Synalar 0.025%	Ointment
Flurandrenolide	Cordran 0.05%	Ointment
Halcinonide	Halog 0.25%	Cream
Hydrocortisone valerate	Westcort 0.2%	Ointment
Mometasone furoate	Elocon 0.1%	Cream
Triamcinolone acetonide	Aristocort, Kenalog 0.1%	Ointment
5		
Betamethasone benzoate	Benisone, Uticort 0.025%	Cream
Betamethasone dipropionate	Diprosone 0.02%	Lotion
Betamethasone valerate	Valisone 0.1%	Cream
Clocortolone	Cloderm 0.1%	Cream
Fluocinolone acetonide	Synalar 0.025%	Cream
Flurandrenolide	Cordran 0.05%	Cream
Fluticasone propionate	Cutivate 0.05%	Cream
Hydrocortisone buryrate	Locoid 0.1%	Cream
Hydrocortisone valerate	Westcort 0.2%	Cream
Prednicarbate	Dermatop 0.1%	Cream
Triamcinolone acetonide	Aristocort 0.25%	Cream
6		
Aclometasone dipropionate	Aclovate 0.05%	Ointment
Betamethasone valerate	Valisone 0.1%	Lotion
Desonide	Tridesilon 0.05%	Cream
Fluocinolone acetonide	Synalar 0.01%	Solution
Triamcinolone acetonide	Kenalog 0.1%	Cream, lotion
7 (Least Potent)		
Hydrocortisone	Generic 0.5, 1.0, 2.5%	Cream, ointment
Dexamethasone	Decadron 0.1%	Cream

- With chronic conditions such as atopic eczema, it is best to discontinue therapy gradually. This reduces the potential for rebound flares of topical lesions.[7]

Indications

A topical corticosteroid is often the drug of choice for inflammatory and pruritic eruptions. In addition, they are useful with hyperplastic and infiltrative disorders. The following conditions generally respond well to topical corticosteroids: primary irritant and allergic contact dermatitis, alopecia areata, atopic eczema, discoid lupus erythematosus, granuloma annulare, hypertrophic scars and keloids, lichen planus, lichen simplex, lichen striatus, various nail disorders, pretibial myxedema, psoriasis, sarcoidosis, and seborrheic dermatitis.

Contraindications

The following conditions (predominantly infectious etiologies) are worsened by topical corticosteroids: acne vulgaris, ulcers, scabies, warts, molluscum contagiosum, fungal infections, and balanitis. However, during the acute phase topical corticosteroids are sometimes combined with other active ingredients (e.g., antifungal agents) for a few days if marked inflammation is present.

Side Effects

Though relatively infrequent, both localized (i.e., at the application site) and systemic side effects (from percutaneous absorption) can be caused by topical corticosteroids. The risks for adverse reactions are influenced by the potency of preparation used, frequency of application, duration of use, anatomic site of application, and individual patient factors. Any of the previously discussed factors that increase potency, such as inflammation and occlusion, increase the chances of side effects.[9]

Epidermal and dermal atrophy, telangiectasia, localized fine hair growth, bruising, hypopigmentation, and striae can result from repeated application of topical corticosteroids.[11] Epidermal changes consisting of a reduction in cell size may begin within several days of therapy and generally are reversible after therapy is stopped.[9] Exposed areas are most vulnerable to epidermal atrophy.

Dermal atrophy generally takes several weeks to occur and is rarely irreversible, depending on how long the patient has used the corticosteroid and individual host factors such as skin age. Inguinal, genital, and perianal areas are most vulnerable to dermal atrophy. Most cases of dermal atrophy are reversible within 2 months after stopping the corticosteroid.[11]

Telangiectasia, which occurs most often on the face, neck, groin, and upper chest, may not be reversible after stopping corticosteroid therapy. Striae, which occur most commonly in the groin, axillary, and inner thigh areas, are usually permanent.[11] Fine hair growth may be particularly bothersome to female patients using corticosteroid preparations on the face. This problem generally is reversible after stopping therapy. Hypopigmentation, predominantly a problem of dark-skinned patients, is generally reversible after therapy is discontinued.[11]

Prolonged (several weeks or months) of application of high-potency steroids to large areas of the body, especially if occlusion is used, can lead to systemic absorption and subsequent adrenal suppression. Rarely, typical cushingoid features are observed.

Atopic Eczema

2. **P.K., a 17-year-old young man, presents to the University Dermatology Clinic with 30% of his body covered with a pruritic, eczematous rash. There is extensive involvement of popliteal and antecubital fossae bilaterally. There is evidence of excoriation with cosmetic disfigurement in the antecubital fossae, around the neck, and on his forehead.**

Family History: P.K.'s mother and aunt have bronchial asthma; one sister (L.K.), age 15, has hay fever and atopic eczema; his father and younger brother, age 11, appear to have no atopic manifestations.

Past Medical History: A rash was first noted 1 month after birth. The scalp, face, and neck were the only areas affected, and the rash continued with varying degrees of severity until age 2½ years, when it spontaneously resolved. A similar rash reappeared at age 12, was diagnosed as atopic eczema, and has not disappeared since that time. P.K. developed hay fever at age 6 years and has had occasional attacks of asthma (last attack, age 15). He has had a difficult time trying to follow provided nondrug recommendations for eczema. He has used over-the-counter topical hydrocortisone cream to cool down flare-ups over the years. He reports a variable course; clearing in the summer and during periods of little stress, and worsening during the winter and periods of stress.

Physical Examination: P.K. is a well-nourished, well-developed, adolescent male with no physical abnormalities noted except for skin. Oozing, crusted, erythematous, hyperkeratotic, hyperpigmented, maculopapular, and fine vesicular eruptions are on his face, neck, flexor aspects of both arms and legs, hands, and chest. There is some evidence of secondary bacterial infection in both antecubital fossae and on portions of the left leg. Identify the presenting history, symptoms, and signs characteristic of eczema.

Atopic eczema can be acute or subacute, but is more commonly a chronic pruritic inflammation of the epidermis and dermis, often occurring in association with a personal or family history of allergic rhinitis or asthma. Atopic eczema is believed to be a type I (IgE-mediated) hypersensitivity reaction occurring as a result of the release of vasoactive substances from both mast cells and basophils that have been sensitized by the interaction of the antigen with IgE. An allergy workup rarely is helpful in determining the allergen. The disorder affects 0.5% to 1.0% of the general population, although its prevalence in children is 5% to 10%. In infants and young children, the dermatitis often occurs on the scalp, face, and extensor surfaces. In older children and adults, it tends to localize to the flexural areas, especially the antecubital and popliteal fossae and the neck. In addition, the rash may affect the hands and feet, sometimes in the absence of eczema elsewhere. Most patients become afflicted between infancy and age 12, with 60% being affected by the first year; another 30% are seen for the first time by age 5, with the final 10% developing atopic dermatitis between 6 and 20 years of age.

Pruritus is the hallmark of atopic eczema. The constant scratching leads to a vicious cycle of itch-scratch-rash-itch, with the rash consisting primarily of lichenification of the skin. Atopic dermatitis has been described as "the itch that rashes, rather than the rash that itches." In other words, the itching precedes the rash. Wool, detergents, soaps, a change in room temperature, and mental and/or physical stress precipitate itching. Patients tend to have dry skin (xerosis). This is due to a reduced water-binding capacity and a higher transdermal water loss. Xerosis is worsened during periods of low humidity, such as winter in northern latitudes.

P.K.'s family and medical history are classic for atopic eczema. His family history is significant for asthma, hay fever, and atopic eczema. He had his initial outbreak at 1 month and then developed hay fever and asthma. His skin examination reveals findings of both acute and chronic atopic eczema, with typical lesion location and description.

3. What are the relevant biopharmaceutic considerations for selecting a topical corticosteroid for P.K.?

Topical corticosteroids are classified into potency categories (see Table 38-8). The relative potency assigned to a topical corticosteroid is determined by the ability of the preparation to penetrate the skin after release from the vehicle, the intrinsic activity of the corticosteroid at the receptor, and the rate of clearance from the receptor. Activity of corticosteroids may be enhanced by the use of a more occlusive vehicle, the addition of penetration enhancing substances (i.e., urea, salicylic acid, propylene glycol), and modifications of the steroid molecule. Hydrocortisone was the initial local corticosteroid discovered, and since then the molecule has been modified in several ways. The addition of a fluorine atom protects the steroid ring from metabolic conversion, resulting in more potent activity. The introduction of an acetonide bond and/or lipophilic groups increases skin penetration. Many newer topical corticosteroids have incorporated one or more of these molecular changes, resulting in increased-potency agents and a growing armamentarium of agents.

It is believed that topical corticosteroids penetrate into the stratum corneum by passive diffusion, which varies considerably depending on the part of the body to which the preparation is applied. When a standard hydrocortisone preparation was applied to various parts of the body, absorption was found to be 0.14% on the plantar surface of the foot, 1% on the forearm, 4% on the scalp, 7% on the forehead, 13% on the cheeks, and 36% on the scrotum. Because penetration is high in the groin, axillae, and face, lower-potency topical preparations (hydrocortisone 0.5% to 1%) should be used on these areas.[9,10] In areas where penetration is poor, owing to thickening of the stratum corneum, such as the elbows, knees, palms, or soles, higher-strength preparations should be used.[9]

For P.K., a 1% hydrocortisone cream should be used on his face and other areas of high penetrability to reduce the possibility of complications.[9] A high-potency cream (intermediate- or higher-potency classification from Table 38-8) should be used initially on acutely inflamed areas or where high penetration is not a problem. This will "cool down" these lesions quickly.

If equal amounts of a corticosteroid are incorporated into ointments, gels, creams, and lotion bases, the gel and ointment preparations generally are more active.[9,10] The addition of certain substances enhances penetration and potency. Increasing the concentration of a corticosteroid in a preparation also increases its potency, but not in a linear fashion. Because P.K. has a fine vesicular eruption, a cream should be used initially, to facilitate drying. However, patients often express a preference (e.g., cream or gel), and this should be considered.

Occlusion

4. It has been some time since P.K.'s atopic eczema has been aggressively treated. He has many acute, inflamed lesions. Should occlusive therapy be used? What complications could develop from occlusion? How would you describe the use of occlusion to P.K.?

As discussed previously (see Dermatologic Delivery Systems), occlusion traps heat and promotes maceration. This same mechanism increases the hydration of the skin and resultant absorption of corticosteroid preparations, thus producing a heightened therapeutic effect. As a general rule, occlusion enhances the potency of corticosteroids by a factor of 10. Occlusion can be accomplished by selecting an ointment-based corticosteroid, applying a nonmedicated ointment base over another corticosteroid preparation (gel, cream, lotion, or aerosol), or by enveloping the medicated area with plastic (e.g., plastic wrap, gloves, or plastic suit [space suit]).[5,7,9,11] Several hours of occlusion are all that is necessary to increase potency; thus, relatively short periods of occlusion are clinically useful. Occlusion can be uncomfortable and can lead to sweat retention and an increased risk of bacterial and candidal infections. To reduce these problems and the chances of systemic side effects, occlusion should not be maintained for more than 12 hours in a 24-hour period. Occlusion should not be used for acute lesions, which already have increased absorptive capability and need the vasoconstrictive effects of cooling first. Occlusion is best used for chronic lesions that are thick and scaly, where drug absorption is impaired. Most patients with atopic dermatitis do not tolerate occlusion because their itch threshold is low, and heat, sweat retention, and maceration increase pruritus. The long-term benefit of occlusion in a patient with atopic dermatitis is reduced by the increased pruritus, which may lead to noncompliance. When using occlusion in patients with eczema, care should be taken not to occlude unaffected skin (because of the low itch threshold). For other chronic dermatologic conditions (e.g., psoriasis) that are not associated with severe pruritus, occlusion could be used for prolonged periods if necessary. Increasing the hydration of the skin (after a shower or bath) also increases the effects of medications immediately applied after the bath or shower. This would be an appropriate recommendation for P.K.

Product Selection
Pharmacokinetic Considerations

5. P.K. received a prescription for halcinonide (Halog) 0.1% cream, 80 g, to be applied at bedtime, with five refills. Comment on the appropriateness of this prescription based on pertinent biopharmaceutic considerations.

Corticosteroids tend to penetrate human skin very slowly, leading to a reservoir effect. With low-potency preparations, this reservoir effect persists for several days, and with the most potent preparations under occlusion, the effects may persist for up to 14 days.[9,10] The clinical implication of this reservoir effect on chronic conditions is a cumulative effect with repeated application of topical corticosteroids. As a result, the number of applications per day can be reduced, and less-potent preparations can be used after the acute inflammatory process has been brought under control. Results from P.K.'s treatment regimen might be improved by providing more frequent (twice-daily) application or a more potent preparation for twice-daily administration to control inflamed lesions. Once control is achieved, a less-potent preparation could be used for maintenance and the number of applications per day can be reduced.

Side Effects

Acne

6. After several months of continuous corticosteroid therapy in a maintenance format, P.K. presents with four pustules and two closed comedones on his forehead and multiple pustules on both cheeks. What problems could this present with the use of topical corticosteroid therapy on the face?

The face is particularly vulnerable to corticosteroid side effects because of enhanced penetration.[11] Acne, acne rosacea, and perioral dermatitis can develop after several weeks to months of application. Corticosteroid-induced conditions can generally be distinguished from naturally occurring disorders. Corticosteroid-induced acne lesions are uniformly at the same level of development and are present only in areas treated with the corticosteroid. Generally, steroid acne, acne rosacea, and perioral dermatitis resolve after discontinuing the drug. Application of corticosteroid preparations (particularly the potent preparations) to areas around the eye can lead to increased intraocular pressure, glaucoma, cataracts, increased risk of ocular mycotic infections, and exacerbation of pre-existing herpes simplex infections.[11] Hydrocortisone or nonfluorinated topical corticosteroids are often the agents of choice for facial lesions.

P.K.'s acneiform lesions may get worse secondary to the application of topical corticosteroids. He should be instructed to apply the corticosteroid preparation only to the atopic eczema and to avoid areas where acne exists. If the atopic eczema and acne lesions are in the same area and his acne gets worse after using the topical corticosteroid, P.K. must make a decision as to which of these two dermatologic conditions bothers him more, and treat the condition that is most disturbing. Some improvement in corticosteroid-exacerbated acne may be achieved by decreasing the strength of the topical product applied to the face and reducing the frequency of application. An alternative to this approach, if P.K.'s acne is severe, would be to continue topical corticosteroid therapy, but treat the acne systemically.[5,6] (See Chapter 39, Acne, for a more extensive discussion.)

Idiosyncratic/Allergic Reactions

7. P.K.'s sister, L.K., who also has atopic eczema, started using a new topical corticosteroid preparation (halcinonide) 10 days ago. She has been complaining of a burning sensation lasting for 1 hour after every application of this product. She stopped using the product 2 days ago because of this. Is it possible that she has developed an allergy to a corticosteroid-containing medication?

Cortisol is endogenously secreted by the adrenal gland and is essential to life. As a result, allergic reactions to topical corticosteroid preparations are rare. When allergic symptoms do occur, they generally are not due to the corticosteroid, but to the preservatives (e.g., paraben) or other ingredients in the formulation or the base (e.g., lanolin). Allergic sensitization can occur within 2 weeks of therapy, but may be difficult to diagnose because the corticosteroid can modify the allergic reaction.[12] One should suspect an allergic reaction if lesions change appearance after starting therapy, if healing does not occur within the expected period of time, or if the condition improves and then abruptly gets worse. Most case reports of allergic reactions (dryness, itching, burning, or irritation) to topical corticosteroids are nonspecific and have been in patients with atopic eczema.[12] Atopic individuals are more likely to react to the vehicle base than the active corticosteroid ingredient.

Because of the time course of the burning sensation in L.K. (starting the first day and lasting only 1 hour), it is doubtful that she actually is allergic to this product. However, atopic eczema patients often have "sensitive" skin that reacts idiosyncratically to a variety of topical preparations.[12] To remedy this situation, L.K. should be given another topical corticosteroid preparation with a different formulation (base and preservatives). If the reaction continues with a new product, an allergy workup may be necessary and patch testing could be considered.

Adrenal Axis Suppression/Risk of Infection

8. P.K. recently sustained a knee injury and corrective surgery is being considered. Should he receive systemic corticosteroid during the perioperative period as a precaution against adrenal insufficiency? Should he wear a Medic-Alert tag while using long-term topical corticosteroids? Is he at risk for developing an infection after surgery?

Systemic adrenal axis suppression from topically applied corticosteroids appears to be more of a theoretic risk than a clinical entity in adults, except when the highest-potency preparations are used[13] or other risk factors are present (Table 38-9). Although suppression has been reported with use of mild to moderately potent agents, these cases can be attributed to excessive use or to application of corticosteroids over large areas of the body for prolonged periods under occlusion. If suppression does occur, it reverses within 2 to 4 weeks after application is stopped. Patients using more than 45 g/week of a high-potency corticosteroid are at risk for adrenal axis suppression.[13] Therefore, the use of preparations such as clobetasol (Temovate) should be limited to no more than 45 g/week for no more than 2 weeks. In addition, these preparations should not be used under occlusion and should be reserved for dermatoses that are unresponsive to less-potent preparations.

Because young children absorb corticosteroids to a greater extent, they have a greater risk of developing adrenal axis suppression and other systemic side effects.[13] To reduce this risk, hydrocortisone topical preparations should be used in children, and their use should be limited to short periods of time. Patients whose corticosteroid clearance is impaired (e.g., liver failure) also should use hydrocortisone and be monitored closely for signs of systemic toxicity.[11]

Table 38-9   Risk Factors for Systemic Side Effects From Topical Corticosteroids

Duration of application
 Prolonged application (greater than 3–4 wk)
Potency of corticosteroid
 Weak or moderately strong, 100 g/wk without occlusion
 Very potent, greater than 45 g/wk without occlusion
Application location
 Thin stratum corneum results in easier penetration (eyelids, forehead, cheeks, armpits, groin, and genitals)
Age of patient
 Very young children and elderly people have very thin epidermis
Manner of application
 Occlusion
Presence of penetration-enhancing substances
 Propylene glycol
 Salicylic acid
 Urea
Condition of the skin
General factors
Compromised liver function

The risk of developing an addisonian crisis during surgery or at other times of stress secondary to adrenal suppression from topical steroids is extremely low. Patients who have used potent topical corticosteroids over large areas of their bodies (>30%) or those who have used occlusion are at greater risk (see previous discussion) and often are given systemic hydrocortisone prophylactically before surgery. Because P.K. is not likely to require such supplementation, a Medic-Alert tag is unnecessary.

Infection secondary to topically administered corticosteroids is also a theoretic risk, but is uncommon. Although anecdotal reports of secondary bacterial infections appear in the literature, there is scant evidence to suggest that they occur with any frequency. Topical corticosteroids do not alter normal skin flora.[14]

Topical Antibiotics With Corticosteroids

9. P.K.'s atopic eczema presentation is complicated with areas of erythematous, honey-colored, crusted lesions on his forehead, arm, and leg. Can a corticosteroid and an antibiotic preparation be used together? What are the risks associated with topical antibiotics?

It is determined that P.K. has impetigo superimposed on his chronic eczema. Combination therapy with a corticosteroid–antibiotic preparation is presumably more efficacious than either agent alone in treating impetiginized eczema. The corticosteroid suppresses the clinical signs of infection and helps re-establish the normal skin barrier function. This, in combination with an appropriate antibiotic, allows the skin's normal defense mechanisms to ward off the infection. There are commercially available topical combination products (e.g., hydrocortisone/neomycin/polymyxin B [Cortisporin]). However, many clinicians treat impetiginized eczema with oral antibiotics (penicillin, dicloxacillin, erythromycin, or cephalexin), not topical antibiotics, in combination with topical corticosteroids for the eczema.[15–17] An ongoing secondary bacterial infection will certainly delay resolution of an eczematous flare-up.

Otitis externa, certain intertriginous eruptions, and possibly seborrheic dermatitis may respond favorably to combination antibiotic-corticosteroid preparations. Table 38-10 describes the spectrum of activity of common topical antibiotics. While mupirocin may be an appropriate alternative for topical dermatologic infections, the current over-the-counter topical antibiotics (bacitracin, neomycin and polymyxin) are ineffective for most dermatologic infections and are indicated only for the prophylaxis of skin infections. Mupirocin resistance occurs with overuse.[18]

P.K. would most likely benefit from a treatment course of either topical mupirocin or an oral antibiotic.

Side Effects

There have been many reports of contact dermatitis caused by topical antimicrobials, particularly neomycin.[19] Neomycin sensitivity has been reported in 4% of the general population by patch testing and 40% in patients with a history of allergic contact dermatitis or a history of recurrent use of topical antibotics.[19,20] The corticosteroid contained in many neomycin preparations does not prevent these allergic reactions, although it may decrease the severity of the reaction.

Pruritus

10. As stated in Question 2, one of P.K.'s complaints is pruritus. What could you recommend for relief of pruritus?

Pruritus (itching) is the most common cutaneous symptom. It has many different causes and has been associated with a variety of systemic diseases, several of which are listed in Table 38-11.[5,7,21] In the absence of a cutaneous manifestation, a careful history and physical examination should be performed to rule out one of the systemic causes of pruritus. In addition, a chest radiograph, stool examination for occult

Table 38-10   Spectrum of Activity of Antibiotics Available for Topical Use

Bacitracin
Effective against all anaerobic cocci, most strains of streptococci, staphylococci, and pneumococci. Not effective against most Gram-negative organisms.

Gentamicin
Effective against most Gram-negative organisms (similar to neomycin) including *Pseudomonas* and many strains of *Staphylococcus aureus*.

Mupirocin
Very effective against *S. aureus* and does not interfere with wound healing. Currently, the only topical antibiotic that has been proved to be more effective than the vehicle based on FDA guidelines.

Gramicidin
Effective against most Gram-positive organisms. Not effective against most Gram-negative organisms.

Neomycin
Effective against most Gram-negative organisms (except *Pseudomonas*) and some Gram-positive organisms. Group A streptococci are resistant.

Polymixin B
Effective against most Gram-negative organisms (including *Pseudomonas*). Most strains of *Proteus*, *Serratia*, and Gram-positive organisms are resistant.

Table 38-11	Systemic Diseases Associated With Pruritus
Brain abscesses	Iron deficiency anemia
Carcinoid syndrome	Multiple myeloma
Carcinoma of the breast, lung, or stomach	Multiple sclerosis
Central nervous system infarct	Mycosis fungoides
Diabetes mellitus	Obstructive biliary disease
Gout	Polycythemia vera
Hodgkin's disease and other lymphomas	Pregnancy (first trimester)
	Thyroid disease (both hyper- and hypothyroidism)
Hypertension	Uremia

blood, complete blood count with differential, thyroid panel, blood urea nitrogen, creatinine, liver function panel, glucose, and urinalysis may be necessary to help screen for the aforementioned systemic diseases.[21]

Scratching, which can damage or fatigue receptor nerve endings, is the most common method of relieving pruritus. One would, therefore, expect topically applied local anesthetics or antihistamines to be effective in dulling the sensation. However, this approach is often disappointing, probably because the intact epidermis poorly absorbs the salt forms of these drugs. Also, low concentrations are used in many over-the-counter preparations. If adequate concentrations of local anesthetics are used (benzocaine 20% or lidocaine 3% to 4%), pruritus or pain may be reduced for up to 45 minutes. These agents are most useful for relieving pruritus or pain for short periods of time (e.g., when trying to go to sleep at night).[21] A drawback to the use of benzocaine, is its propensity to induce hypersensitivity.[22] Topical antihistamine preparations provide only a mild topical anesthetic effect, and they are also IgE sensitizers.[23,24]

P.K. could also try cold water or ice cubes, which effectively relieve pruritus, via vasoconstriction, as do products containing aluminum acetate (Burow's solution), tannic acid, or calamine. A cool bath may be useful for the relief of pruritus from dermatologic lesions if they are widespread.

Moisturizing mixtures such as Keri Lotion, Lubriderm, or, simply, mineral or baby oil are useful in the treatment of pruritus caused by xerosis. This problem often is encountered in the elderly and others during the winter months. Bathing should be restricted to avoid washing away normal body oils, the drying effect of water, the irritant effect of alkaline soaps, and the trauma of toweling.[7]

Topical corticosteroid applications can be very effective. They reduce inflammation and often are contained in a cream base, which helps soothe the affected area.

Systemic antihistamines are effective antipruritics, although their major beneficial effect may be due to sedation. The newer, nonsedating antihistamines are notably ineffective at relieving itch, with the exception of ceterizine.[25] There is disagreement over which antihistamine or antiserotonin agents are most effective for treatment of pruritus.[21,25,26] Many practitioners consider hydroxyzine to be the antihistamine of choice; doses of 10 to 25 mg three to four times a day are commonly used. There is little evidence that antihistamines are effective in treating non–histamine-mediated pruritus, except that their inherent sedative effect may be somewhat ben-

eficial in all pruritic conditions. Doxepin, a tricyclic antidepressant with potent H_1-blocking properties, is valuable as a second-line antihistamine topically or systemically if others fail.[27]

Nondrug Recommendations for Atopic Eczema

11. In addition to prescriptions for topical corticosteroids (triamcinolone acetonide cream 0.1%/augmented betamethasone dipropionate 0.05%) for flareups, a systemic antibiotic (erythromycin 250 mg QID ×10 days), and an oral antihistamine (hydroxyzine 25 mg, 1 to 2 tablets TID as needed), what nondrug interventions should be suggested for P.K.?

The general goals of therapy for atopic dermatitis are to decrease pruritus, suppress inflammation, lubricate the skin, and reduce anxiety. The nondrug recommendations shown in Table 38-12 are useful adjuncts and mainstays in between planes, for patients such as P.K. with eczema or any other irritant dermatitis.

P.K. should be warned to avoid people with active herpes simplex infections because severe disseminated infections can occur. Similarly, based on the anthrax bioterrorism attack in October 2001, debate has emerged on the advisability of reinitiating routine vaccination against smallpox. Vaccinia virus was the live poxvirus used throughout the world as the vaccine against smallpox. Because of the increased risk for eczema vaccinatum, vaccinia vaccine should not be administered to persons with eczema of any degree, those with a past history of eczema, household contacts who have active eczema, or household contacts who have a history of eczema.[26]

Tachyphylaxis/Specialized Corticosteroid Dosage Forms/Antihistamines

12. P.K. responded well to the treatment plan above and now requests a refill of his topical corticosteroid prescriptions. The bacterial superinfected areas have cleared. He continues to have problems with his fingers. He has applied betamethasone dipropiniate to his hands five to six time daily for the last 3 weeks without any noticeable improvement. Triamcinolone cream resolved the rash on other areas of his body. Other than occasional

Table 38-12 Nondrug Recommendations for Patients With Atopic Eczema or Other Irritant Dermatitis

- Clothing should be soft and light. Cotton or corduroy is preferred. Wools and coarse, heavy synthetics should be avoided.
- Heat should be avoided because it often makes eczema worse. The environment should be well ventilated, cool, and low in humidity (30% to 50%). Rapid changes in ambient temperature should be avoided.
- Bathing should be kept to a minimum (no longer than 5 minutes), and the patient should use a nonirritating soap (e.g., Basis soap). A colloid bath or the use of appropriate amounts of bath oil may be useful.
- The skin should be kept moist with frequent applications of emollients (e.g., Keri, Lubriderm, Nivea, Aquaphor, Eucerin, or petrolatum).
- Primary irritants such as paints, cleansers, solvents, and chemical sprays should be avoided.

sedation early on from the hydroxyzine and when he uses it intermittently, he has not had any other adverse effects. As P.K. continues to follow other nondrug recommendations, he inquires if anything else could be done for his hands. Assess P.K.'s use and response to the corticosteroids.

P.K. is overusing the potent topical corticosteroid and may have developed tachyphylaxis. Tachyphylaxis can occur within 1 week of therapy, but generally takes several weeks to a month to occur.[29] To treat this problem, P.K. should stop applying the betamethasone preparation for 4 to 7 days and then restart therapy in a more appropriate manner (i.e., twice daily). Limited courses of treatment separated by short periods of rest maybe more effective than continuous treatment. However, clinicians commonly misdiagosis tachyphylaxis. Failure of topical corticosteroids to clear difficult atopic dermatitis after an initial improvement may give the false impression of tachyphylaxis when the actual problem is a primary failure of the treatment.[30] This could be caused by either inappropriate application technique by the patient or the choice of a product with inadequate potency.

Flurandrenolide 4 mg/cm^2 tape (Cordran) may be useful after P.K. stops his other corticosteroids for 4 to 7 days. Although this product is expensive, it is effective for small areas because the tape serves as a protectant and provides occlusion. It is a good choice for use on the hands, particularly the fingers, where P.K. is having problems, because other vehicles are often quite messy when applied to the hands. When using Cordran tape, the general principles previously outlined for occlusion should be followed.

Topical tacrolimus (Protopic) is a safe and effective alternative to topical corticosteroids and is safe in children.[31,32] In addition to its inhibitory effect on cytokine production, topical tacrolimus has been shown to cause alterations in epidermal antigen-presenting dendritic cells that may result in decreased immunologic response to antigens. Transient burning, erythema, and pruritus are the most common adverse effects. Pimecrolimus cream (Elidel) 1% is an immunomodulatory agent with properties similar to those of cyclosporine and tacrolimus, but it does not appear to affect the systemic immune response and might therefore be better tolerated for long-term therapy.[33] Neither pimecrolimus nor tacrolimus causes skin atrophy, making them attractive alternatives for patients with lesions on the face and neck.

XEROSIS

13. C.R., a 64-year-old woman, requests something for dry skin on her arms and back. She has had this problem for a number of years. It is generally not a problem in the summer, with most symptoms troubling her in the winter. She has no other medical conditions and only takes an occasional aspirin for "arthritis." How would you advise C.R. to manage this condition?

C.R.'s complaints represent a common problem of the elderly, xerosis (dry skin). The seasonal cycle described is frequently called, "winter itch." Most cases of dry skin are caused by dehydration of the stratum corneum.[34] Table 38-13 gives general recommendations for the treatment of dry skin.

However, before recommending therapy, the following differential should be considered: ichthyosis vulgaris (familial history usually present), atopic eczema, psoriasis, contact dermatitis, and hypothyroidism. Usually, simple questioning can rule out these conditions.

Table 38-13 General Recommendations for the Treatment of Dry Skin
1. Use room humidifiers.
2. Keep room temperature as low as comfortable to prevent sweating and water loss from the skin.
3. Keep bathing to a minimum (every 1 to 2 days) with warm, but not hot, water. After bathing, the patient should immediately apply an emollient (see Table 38-2). When the skin is soaked for 5 to 10 minutes, the stratum corneum can absorb as much as six times its weight in water. Application of an emollient immediately after bathing will trap the water in the skin and reduce dryness.
4. Eliminate exposure to solvents, drying chemicals, harsh soaps, and cleaners. These substances remove oils from the skin and reduce its barrier function. As the barrier function is lost, water loss from the skin is increased up to 75 times above normal. Exposure to cold, dry winds also will enhance water loss.
5. Apply emollients (see Table 38-2) three to six times a day. Many patients find the use of a urea-containing product to be effective and more cosmetically acceptable because it does not leave a greasy residue on the skin after application.
6. If scaling is a problem, a keratolytic (Keralyt Gel) or a higher-strength, urea-containing preparation (20%) may be useful.
7. If inflammation is present, a mild to moderately potent topical corticosteroid may be useful (see Table 38-8). An ointment vehicle is more effective than others.

DRUG ERUPTIONS

Clinically recognizable adverse drug reactions are manifested more often on the skin than any other organ or organ system.[35,36] An estimated 1% to 5% of hospitalized patients develop a drug eruption.[36] Outpatient statistics are more difficult to obtain, but probably are within the same range. There is no correlation between age, diagnosis, or severity of illness and the likelihood of developing a drug eruption. Women appear to be twice more likely than men to develop a drug eruption.

The most common type of eruption encountered in clinical practice, and probably the one most often overlooked, is the exanthematic (bursting out) eruption. This type of reaction comprises both morbilliform (measles-like) and scarlatiniform (scarlet fever–like) eruptions. Stevens-Johnson syndrome, toxic epidermal necrolysis, hypersensitivity syndrome, vasculitis, serum sickness, coagulant-induced skin necrosis, and angioedema are the most important severe reactions and require immediate attention and management. Because drug eruptions often mimic other types of dermatitis, it is necessary to have a good understanding of the mimicked disease state to make the proper diagnosis. The diagnosis of drug eruptions is best done by identifying the type of lesions observed and associating the lesions with specific drug therapy. The most important diagnostic criteria is an accurate assessment of the skin lesions. With this critical information, the clinician can then refer to a drug information source to associate any current or past drug therapy with the specific lesions observed.

Acneiform Eruptions

Acneiform eruptions appear very much like common acne. They may be distinguished from acne by their sudden occurrence, the absence of comedones, uniform appearance (that is, all at the same stage of development), and the fact that they may occur on any part of the body. Cysts and scarring are rarely associated with drug-induced acne. Eruptions also can occur during any period of the patient's life; thus, drug-induced acne should be suspected when the lesions appear in persons outside of the typical age bracket for acne. Drugs implicated include glucocorticoids, ACTH, anabolic steroids, oral contraceptives, halogens (iodides, bromides), isoniazid, danazol, lithium, and azathoprine. For patients with acne, these drugs may worsen existing lesions (see Chapter 39, Acne).

Photosensitive Eruptions

Photosensitivity eruptions require the presence of both a drug (or chemical) and a light source of appropriate wavelength. These eruptions are divided into two subtypes: photoallergic and phototoxic. In *photoallergic* reactions, ultraviolet A (UVA) light alters the drug so that it becomes an antigen or acts as a hapten. Photoallergic eruptions require previous contact with the offending drug; are not dose related; exhibit cross-sensitivity with chemically related compounds; and may appear as a variety of lesions, including urticaria, bullae, and sunburn. These lesions usually are secondary to the use of topical agents. In *phototoxic* reactions, the light source alters the drug to a toxic form, resulting in tissue damage independent of allergic response. This eruption can occur on first exposure to a drug, is dose related, usually has no cross-sensitivity, and almost always appears as exaggerated sunburn. In some instances, a drug may produce both photoallergic and phototoxic reactions. Most phototoxic and photoallergic reactions occur fairly soon after exposure to light. Implicated drugs are numerous, including, among others, antibiotics (tetracyclines, fluoroquinolones), antidepressants (tricyclics), antihypertensives (hydrochlorothiazide, β-blockers), hypoglycemics (sulfonylureas), nonsteroidal anti-inflammatory drugs, sunscreens (PABA), oral contraceptives, and antipsychotics (phenothiazines) (see Chapter 41, Photosensitivity and Burns).

Lichen Planus—Like Eruptions

Lichen planus—like lesions appear as flat-topped papules that have a distinctive sheen. Pruritus is usually quite pronounced. Any part of the body can be affected (most commonly the arms and legs), including mucous membranes. The lesions are sometimes confused with fixed eruptions, but can easily be differentiated histologically. Implicated drugs include angiotensin-converting enzyme inhibitors, antimalarials, phenothiazine derivatives, thiazide diuretics, and sulfonylurea hypoglycemic agents among others.

Alopecia

Alopecia is not a true drug eruption, but hair may occasionally be lost when other drug reactions such as exfoliative dermatitis and erythema multiforme occur. Hair loss can be caused by a direct toxic action of a drug (e.g., a cancer chemotherapeutic agent) or from interference with the normal growth phases of hair (e.g., warfarin).

Bullous Eruptions

Bullous (blisterlike) lesions can occur in combination with other drug eruptions, such as erythema multiforme and toxic epidermal necrolysis or by themselves. The lesions may be round or irregular and contain a clear, serous fluid. The fluid-filled sacs may be tense or flaccid and can occur on both mucous membranes and skin. These lesions are very similar to those associated with pemphigus and pemphigoid reactions. Lesions usually resolve after discontinuation of the drug, but occasionally become chronic. Implicated drugs include amiodarone, barbiturates, coumarins, gold, penicillins, and sulfonamides among others.

Eczematous Eruptions

Systemic administration of a drug to a patient previously sensitized to the drug by topical application can provoke widespread eczematous dermatitis. Implicated systemically or topically administered drugs that reactivate allergic contact dermatitis include procaine/benzocaine, radiographic contrast media/iodine; and streptomycin and gentamicin/neomycin among others.

Epidermal Necrolysis

Epidermal necrolysis, a severe, life-threatening mucocutaneous and systemic reaction, may be preceded by a prodrome characterized by malaise, lethargy, fever, and occasionally throat or mucous membrane soreness. Epidermal changes follow and consist of erythema and massive bullae formations that easily rupture and peel, giving the skin a scalded appearance. Hairy parts of the body usually are not affected, but mucous membrane involvement is common. Approximately 30% of patients with toxic epidermal necrolysis succumb, often within 8 days after bullae appear. The usual cause of death is infection complicated by massive fluid and electrolyte loss. Although the skin takes on a very grave appearance, healing occurs within 2 weeks in approximately 70% of patients, usually with no scarring. In addition to drugs, certain bacterial infections and foods are believed to cause this type of eruption. Most causes of toxic epidermal necrolysis in children are due to infection (e.g., *Staphylococcus aureus)*. There appears to be a higher incidence of this type of drug eruption in HIV-positive patients. Drugs most frequently implicated include sulfa drugs, allopurinol, hydantoins, carbamazepine, phenylbutazone, piroxicam, and aminopenicillins.

Erythema Multiforme

As the name implies, erythema multiforme eruptions take on a variety of morphologic forms. The lesions characteristically are erythematous, iris-shaped papules and vesicolobullous lesions typically involving the extremities (especially the palms and soles) and the mucous membranes. Lesions take on the appearance of a circular target with a bulls-eye in the middle; thus the term, target lesion. Erythema multiforme is more common in children and young adults. Sometimes malaise, a low-grade fever, and itching or burning may accompany this type of eruption. Etiologic factors associated with erythema multi-forme include drugs, mycoplasma and herpes infections, radiation therapy, foods, and sometimes neoplasms. Sulfonamides, phenothiazines, barbiturates, and allopurinol are the drugs most often implicated in erythema multiforme eruptions.

Erythema Nodosum Eruptions

Erythema nodosum eruptions appear as red, indurated, very tender inflammatory nodules usually in the pretibial region. Occasionally, these lesions are accompanied by mild constitutional symptoms, but there is usually no mucous membrane involvement. Etiologic factors associated with the development of erythema nodosum include drugs, female gender, rheumatic fever, sarcoidosis, leprosy, certain bacterial infections (e.g., tuberculosis), and systemic fungal infections. Usually, the lesions heal slowly over several weeks after the offending agent is removed. Oral contraceptives are the most frequently implicated drug with this type of eruption. Other implicated drugs include sulfonamides and analgesics.

Exfoliative Dermatitis

Large areas of skin becoming scaly, erythematous and then sloughing off (as the name implies) characterizes exfoliative dermatitis. Hair and nails are sometimes lost. In most patients, a generalized systemic toxicity also accompanies the eruption. Secondary bacterial infections can occur, and most fatalities are due to infection. Exfoliative dermatitis also may follow other drug eruptions; thus, a less severe eruption can culminate with an exfoliative dermatitis. This type of eruption takes weeks or months to resolve, even after withdrawal of the offending agent. The most commonly implicated drugs are sulfonamides, antimalarials, phenytoin, and penicillin.

Fixed Drug Eruptions

Fixed drug eruptions, unlike the previously mentioned reactions, are caused exclusively by drugs. The lesions are erythematous and sharply bordered and have a tendency to be darker than the surrounding, unaffected skin. Eruptions can be eczematous, urticarial, vesicular, bullous, or nodular. Lesions appear 30 minutes to 8 hours after re-administration in sensitized individuals. Because these lesions have a marked propensity to recur at the same location with each drug exposure, the word *fixed* is applied. The face and genitalia are common sites for this type of drug eruption. Although the eruptions heal after withdrawal of the causative drug, there usually is a marked hyperpigmentation of the area that may take months to resolve. The mechanism by which fixed drug eruptions occur has not been elucidated, but is believed to be allergic in nature. It can be described figuratively as islands of hypersensitivity; one area of the skin having the ability to evoke an allergic response and other areas lacking this ability. Commonly implicated drugs include antimicrobial agents (tetracycline, sulfonamides, metronidazole, nystatin), anti-inflammatory drugs (salicylates, nonsteroidal anti-inflammatory drugs), barbiturates, oral contraceptives, and phenolphthalein-containing laxatives.

Maculopapular Eruptions

Maculopapular eruptions are subdivided into two groups: scarlatiniform and morbilliform. Most drug eruptions fall within one of these two groups. *Scarlatiniform* eruptions are erythematous and usually involve extensive areas of the body. They are differentiated from streptococcal-induced scarlet fever by the lack of other diagnostic signs and laboratory studies. *Morbilliform* eruptions usually begin as discrete, reddish-brown maculae that may coalesce to form a diffuse rash. These eruptions are differentiated from measles by the lack of fever and other typical clinical signs. In either type of maculopapular eruption, pruritus may or may not be present. Generally, this type of eruption appears within 1 week after the causative drug (with penicillins, 2 or more weeks) has been started and completely clears within 7 to 14 days after stopping it. Morbilliform eruptions commonly are caused by ampicillin, amoxicillin, and allopurinol.

Purpura

Purpuric lesions are characterized as hemorrhages into the skin. They are purplish and sharply bordered and have a tendency to become brownish as they get older. These lesions may or may not be associated with thrombocytopenia. Etiologic factors other than drugs that are associated with purpura are vitamin C deficiency, snake bites, and infections. The mechanism by which these lesions are produced is not known, but they have a tendency to recur with re-exposure to the causative agent. Sometimes purpura may develop concurrent with other types of eruptions, such as erythema multiforme.

Stevens-Johnson Syndrome

Stevens-Johnson syndrome is probably the most common type of severe drug eruption. The syndrome is usually a moderate mucocutaneous and systemic reaction. With more extensive involvement, clinical findings are almost indistiguishable from toxic epidermal necrolysis. The skin can become hemorrhagic, and pneumonia and joint pains may occur. Serious ocular involvement is common and can culminate in partial or complete blindness. Besides drugs, this syndrome has been associated with infections, pregnancy, foods, deep radiographic therapy, and neoplasms. Mortality is estimated to be in the range of 5% to 18%. The duration of the syndrome is usually 4 to 6 weeks. The long-acting sulfonamides are most often implicated. Allopurinol, hydantions, carbamazepine, fluoroquinolones, phenylbutazone, and piroxicam are also possible causative agents.

Urticaria

Urticarial eruptions are immediate hypersensitivity reactions and usually appear as sharply circumscribed (raised), edematous, and erythematous lesions with an abrupt onset. In most cases, the lesions disappear within a few hours, rarely last >24 hours, and are associated with an intense itching, stinging, or prickling sensation. Commonly called *hives,* urticarial eruptions frequently are associated with certain drugs, foods, psychic upsets, and serum sickness. Rarely, parasites or neoplasms can precipitate hives. Angioneurotic edema, a variation of urticaria, is a more severe form in which giant hives predominate. The most frequently implicated drugs with this type of reaction are aspirin, penicillin, and blood products.

14. D.Z., a 42-year-old man with a chronic seizure disorder and long standing anxiety was recently given a prescription for penicillin V 250 mg QID for a group A, β-hemolytic streptococcal-positive pharyngitis. Chronic medications include carbamazepine 200 mg TID, diazepam 5 mg TID PRN, and Maalox 30 mL PRN. One week later, D.Z. presents with a pruritic, sharply circumscribed, edematous, and erythematous rash on his arms and chest that appeared overnight. Is this a typical time of onset for a drug-induced dermatologic reaction? How should the drug eruption in D.Z. be managed?

Most drug eruptions occur within 1 to 2 weeks after starting therapy. Penicillins sometimes can be the exception to this rule by having a slightly more prolonged onset of up to several weeks (especially amoxicillin and ampicillin). Because D.Z. has been taking diazepam and carbamazepine chronically and has been taking penicillin for only 8 days, the temporal relationship of this drug eruption would initially lead to the conclusion that penicillin is the cause of his drug eruption.

For D.Z., a different antibiotic should be substituted for penicillin (to complete the 10 day course of therapy). The lesion should begin to clear in a day or two (if the penicillin is the cause of the drug eruption). If the rash does not begin to clear in a couple of days, another cause should be investigated.

Treatment is primarily supportive and if the reaction is severe, a 1- to 2-week course of prednisone 40 to 60 mg/day will control most symptoms within 48 hours. For less severe reactions, systemic antihistamines (if pruritus is present) can be used.

CONTACT DERMATITIS: POISON IVY/OAK/SUMAC

Poison ivy (*Rhus*) dermatitis is the major cause of allergic contact dermatitis in the United States, exceeding all other causes combined. It is estimated that 50% to 95% of the population is sensitive to the plant to some degree. The severity of the condition varies from mild discomfort to an extremely painful, debilitating condition. *Rhus* dermatitis is caused by sensitization to an allergic substance in the leaves, stems, and roots of poison ivy, poison oak, and poison sumac plants. All three plants contain the same sensitizing oleoresin, urushiol oil, which contains pentadecacatechol, the actual sensitizing agent. Therefore, the dermatitis caused by the three different plants is identical.

Direct contact with the plant is unnecessary for the rash to occur. Highly sensitive persons may develop severe dermatitis merely from exposure to *Rhus* oleoresin carried by pollen or by smoke from burning leaves. The oleoresin may remain active for months on clothing, shoes, tools, and sporting equipment. Once the toxic substance comes in contact with the skin, it can be spread by the hands to other areas of the body (e.g., genitals or eyes) or to people who may come into close contact with the exposed person. Although washing with soap and water will not prevent the dermatitis, even if it is done within 15 minutes of exposure, it will prevent spread of the oleoresin to other parts of the body.

Rhus dermatitis can be contracted throughout the year, even in winter, by contact with the roots of the plant. The virulence of the leaf sap varies little during the foliage period. The incidence of poison ivy is higher during the spring because the leaves are tender and bruise easily, and people spend more time outdoors. Sensitive individuals should be instructed to avoid contact with the offending plant. If contact is inevitable, every effort should be made to shield exposed areas of the skin with appropriate clothing, and bentoquatam (Ivy Block), a topical organoclay compound, should be considered. A 5% lotion applied to the skin 15 minutes before exposure and reapplied ever 4 hours has reduced or prevented contact dermatitis induced by experimental challenge with urushiol in sensitive individuals. Cost may limit its routine use. Exposed individuals should bathe or shower as soon as they come in from outdoors and should wash their clothes.

After an initial incubation period of 5 to 21 days, a patient would be expected to react to the oleoresin in 12 to 48 hours after re-exposure. A mild exposure to these plants in a sensitized person results in a typical erythematous, vesicular, linear, and sometimes, oozing rash after 2 to 3 days; complete clearing occurs in 1 to 3 weeks. If a large area is exposed, lesions appear within 6 to 12 hours and may appear blistered and eroded; in some cases, ulcers may appear. Healing occurs more slowly, often requiring 2 to 3 weeks for complete resolution. The following factors contribute to the development of poison ivy/oak/sumac: the concentration of the oleoresin to which the skin is exposed; area of exposure, i.e., the thickness of the stratum corneum; duration of exposure, site of exposure, genetic factors, and immune tolerance. It is important to determine the areas of the body that are affected. If the eyes, genital areas, mouth, respiratory tract, or >15% of the body is affected, the patient should receive a course of systemic corticosteroids.

Because different sites of the body differ in their sensitivity to the oleoresin and because patients spread the *Rhus* oleoresin to different parts of their bodies over a period of time, lesions often erupt over a period of several days. A common misconception many people have is that the fluid from the *Rhus*-induced vesicles will spread the disease to unaffected areas. A more likely explanation is the presence of residual resin underneath poorly washed fingernails, soiled clothes (including gloves used in yard work), and pet fur.

Treatment

15. K.P., a 27-year-old woman, has recently returned from an outing in the woods. She now has vesicular eruptions that appear in a linear pattern on one arm and hand. She believes she has poison oak and requests therapy. What should be recommended at this point? What should be recommended if the condition becomes more severe?

Weeping lesions should be treated with aqueous vehicles (e.g., Burows solution or saline) as outlined in the beginning of this chapter. Lesions that are not wet or weeping should be treated with calamine lotion applied two to four times daily. The zinc oxide in calamine lotion may act as a mild astringent, although some people find this preparation to be unacceptable because of its pink color, which can stain clothes. Alternatively, a topical corticosteroid appropriate for the body part affected could be used. If K.P.'s poison oak becomes much more severe, additional treatment with prednisone 1 mg/kg/day for at least 2 or 3 weeks will be required; such therapy should be withdrawn slowly (over 1 to 2 weeks) to prevent recurrence of the lesions.

Systemic Therapy

16. Z.T., a 19-year-old man, has just returned from a fishing trip and now has an erythematous, linear, dry eruption on his leg and arm and a generalized eruption on his hands and face. He has been in areas that have dense poison ivy and may have burned some in the campfire. Z.T. has washed himself and his clothes thoroughly. How should he be treated?

The fact that Z.T.'s facial rash is not linear (as one would expect if he had just contacted the plant) suggests that he may have contacted the smoke of a burning poison ivy plant. This can be quite serious because the oleoresin can be carried in smoke and, if inhaled, can cause severe respiratory problems. Z.T. should be observed for signs of respiratory difficulties and should be treated with a course of systemic corticosteroids.

Relapse

17. Z.T.'s physician prescribed prednisone for his rash. He was instructed to take 80 mg/day for 14 days and to decrease the dose by 5 mg/day each day thereafter. Calamine lotion (TID to affected areas) also was prescribed. After 12 days, Z.T. complains that the lesions seem to be getting worse. The lesions had cleared after 8 days of treatment, and he began rapidly tapering the prednisone at that time. Why is he experiencing a relapse?

Two weeks is the absolute minimum course of treatment when systemic corticosteroids are used for severe cases of poison ivy/oak/sumac. The oleoresin remains fixed in the skin, and if the systemic corticosteroid is withdrawn too soon, the lesions return. This is probably the most common reason for treatment failure with systemic corticosteroids.

Contact Dermatitis

18. Z.T.'s corticosteroid therapy was reinstated. After 3 weeks, most of the lesions had disappeared and the prednisone therapy was discontinued. However, Z.T. continued to complain of a rash on his hands. Further questioning revealed that he was continuing to apply an over-the-counter topical calamine lotion containing diphenhydramine. What is a potential drug-related cause of this persistent rash?

Topical application of diphenhyramine and other antihistamines may cause an allergic contact-sensitivity reaction.[24] Z.T. should stop using this product to see if his rash clears. A list of common contact sensitizers is found in Table 38-14.

The treatment for sensitivity reactions is basically the same as that outlined for poison ivy/oak/sumac.

Table 38-14   Frequent Contact Sensitizers

Substance	Found In
Ammonia	Soaps, chemicals, hair dyes
Balsam of Peru	Cosmetics
Benzyl alcohol	Medications, cosmetics
"Caine" anesthetics	Medications (e.g., OTC benzocaine products)
Carba	Rubber
Chromium	Jewelry
Epoxy resin	Glue
Ethylenediamine	Stabilizer in topical products (e.g., aminophylline)
Formaldehyde	Shoes, clothing, soaps, insulations
Mercaptobenzothiazol	Rubber
Naphthyl	Rubber
Neomycin	Topical medications (e.g., Neosporin)
Nickel sulfate	Jewelry, fasteners
Paraben	Preservative in many topicalproducts
Paraphenylenediamine	Hair dyes, leather
Potassium dichromate	Shoes, leather
Thiomersal	Preservatives, contact lens products
Thiram	Rubber products
Turpentine	Paint products
Wool alcohols	Lanolin-containing products, clothes

REFERENCES

1. Hall JC. Sauer's Manual of Skin Diseases, 8th Ed. Philadelphia: Lippincott Williams & Wilkins, 1999.
2. Hood AF et al. Primer of Dermatopathology, 3rd Ed. Philadelphia: Lippincott Williams & Wilkins, 2002.
3. Odom RB. Andrew's Diseases of the Skin, 9th Ed. Philadelphia: WB Saunders, 2000.
4. Champion RH et al. Roo/Wilkinson/Ebling's Textbook of Dermatology, 6th Ed. Oxford, England: Blackwell Scientific Publications, 1998.
5. Freedberg IM et al. Fitzpatrick's Dermatology in General Medicine, 5th Ed. New York: McGraw-Hill, 1999.
6. Habif TP et al. Clinical Dermatology: A Color Guide to Diagnosis and Therapy, 3rd Ed. St. Louis: Mosby, 19967.
7. Arndt KA et al. Manual of Dermatologic Therapies, 6th Ed. Philadelphia: Lippincott Williams & Wilkins, 2002.
8. Wehner AP. Biological effects of cosmetic talc. Food Chem Toxicol 1994;32:1173.
9. Lee NP et al. Topical corticosteroids: back to basics. West J Med 1999;171:351.
10. Giannotti B et al. Topical corticosteroids. Which drug and when? Drugs 1992;44:65.

11. Fisher D. Adverse effects of topical corticosteroid use. West J Med 1995;162:123.
12. Butani L. Corticosteroid-induced hypersensitivity reactions. Ann Allergy Asthma Immunol 2002;89:439.
13. Levin C et al. Topical corticosteroid-induced adrenocortical insufficiency: clinical implications. Am J Clin Dermatol 2002;3:141.
14. Chan HL et al. Effect of topical corticosteroid on microbial flora of human skin. J Am Acad Dermatol 1982;7:346.
15. George A et al. A systematic review and meta-analysis of treatments for impetigo.Br J Gen Pract 2003;53:480.
16. Guay DR. Treatment of bacterial skin and skin structure infections. Expert Opin Pharmacother. 2003;4:1259.
17. Brown J et al. Impetigo: an update. Int J Dermatol 2003;42:251.
18. Walker ES et al. Mupirocin-resistant, methicillin-resistant Staphylococcus aureus: does mupirocin remain effective? Infect Control Hosp Epidemiol 2003;24:342.
19. Kimura M et al. Contact sensitivity induced by neomycin with cross-sensitivity to other aminoglycoside antibiotics. Contact Dermatitis 1998;39:148.

20. Yung MW et al. Delayed hypersensitivity reaction to topical aminoglycosides in patients undergoing middle ear surgery. Clin Otolaryngol 2002; 27:365.
21. Charlesworth EN et al. Pruritic dermatoses: overview of etiology and therapy. Am J Med 2002;113(Suppl 9A):25S.
22. Prystowsky SD et al. Allergic contact hypersensitivity to nickel, neomycin, ethylenediamine, and benzocaine. Relationships between age, sex, history of exposure, and reactivity to standard patch tests and use tests in a general population. Arch Dermatol 1979;115:959.
23. Marks JG, DeLeo VA. Evaluation and treatment of patients with contact dermatitis. In: Marks JG, DeLeo VA, eds. Contact and Occupational Dermatology, 2nd Ed. St. Louis: Mosby, 1997:14.
24. Heine A. Diphenhydramine: a forgotten allergen? Contact Dermatitis 1996 Nov;35:311.
25. Dimson S, Nanayakkara C. Related articles. Do oral antihistamines stop the itch of atopic dermatitis? Arch Dis Child 2003;88:832.
26. Herman SM et al. Antihistamines in the treatment of atopic dermatitis. J Cutan Med Surg 2003; epub ahead of print.

27. Gupta MA et al. The use of antidepressant drugs in dermatology. J Eur Acad Dermatol Venereol 2001;15:512.

28. Wharton M et al. Advisory Committee on Immunization Practices: Healthcare Infection Control Practices Advisory Committee. Recommendations for using smallpox vaccine in a pre-event vaccination program. Supplemental recommendations of the Advisory Committee on Immunization Practices (ACIP) and the Healthcare Infection Control Practices Advisory Committee (HICPAC). MMWR Recomm Rep 2003;52(RR-7):1.

29. Senter TP. Topical fluocinonide and tachyphylaxis. Arch Dermatol 1983;119:363.

30. Miller JJ et al. Failure to demonstrate therapeutic tachyphylaxis to topically applied steroids in patients with psoriasis. J Am Acad Dermatol 1999; 41:546.

31. Kapp A et al. Atopic dermatitis management with tacrolimus ointment (Protopic). J Dermatol Treat 2003;14(Suppl 1):5.

32. Patel RR et al. The safety and efficacy of tacrolimus therapy in patients younger than 2 years with atopic dermatitis. Arch Dermatol 2003;139:1184.

33. Weinberg JM et al. Atopic dermatitis: a new treatment paradigm using pimecrolimus. J Drugs Dermatol 2003;2:131.

34. Norman RA. Xerosis and pruritus in the elderly: recognition and management. Dermatol Ther 2003;16:254.

35. Fiszenson-Albala F et al. A 6-month prospective survey of cutaneous drug reactions in a hospital setting. Br J Dermatol 2003;149:1018.

36. Cutaneous Drug Reaction Case Reports: From the World Literature. Am J Clin Dermatol 2003;4:727.

CHAPTER 39

Acne

Terry L. Seaton

Definition, Clinical Signs, and Symptoms

The term *acne* usually refers to acne vulgaris, a common self-limiting disease involving the pilosebaceous units of the skin (see Fig. 38-1 in Chapter 38, Dermatotherapy and Drug Induced Disorders).[1] It differs from rosacea (formerly called *acne rosacea*), which causes facial erythema, telangiectasia, and papules and occurs later in life. Severe acne variants are called *acne fulminans* and *acne conglobata*. Other terms incorporate the cause of acne vulgaris, such as occupational, cosmetica, mechanica, and so on.[2] The earliest lesions generally appear on the face, but the chest, back, or upper arms also may be affected. Acne lesions can be noninflammatory or inflammatory and vary in number. Noninflammatory lesions are called *closed comedones* ("whiteheads") or *open comedones* ("blackheads").[3] The dark pigmentation in open comedones is caused by oxidation of sebaceous material and melanin rather than dirt, a public misperception. Inflammatory lesions are typically erythematous and are usually described as pustules (lesions with a tip of pus), papules (more substantial and deeper lesions), nodules (large, very deep papules), or cysts (abscesses). Acne severity should be assessed using a consistent clinical grading scale. Available scores range from simple to more complex (e.g., 0 to 10 scale). One suggested scale rates acne with predominantly comedones as grade I, comedones plus papules as grade II, pustules as grade III, and nodulocystic acne as grade IV. Regardless of the system, acne grading is essential in determining treatment options and response.[4] Most commonly, clinicians describe acne as mild (few lesions, little or no inflammation), moderate (many lesions, significant inflammation), or severe (numerous lesions, extreme inflammation and/or cysts, presence of scarring). The newest technology used for assessing response to therapy employs polarized light photography

and videomicroscopy.[5] Lesion counts per se are not practical for clinicians, but are used by researchers.

The major long-term complication of acne is scarring that can present as "ice pick" pitting with significant disfigurement. Scarring can be exacerbated by tissue excoriation caused by picking at or squeezing the lesions.[6] This complication of acne can cause psychological distress, low self-esteem, and other psychosocial effects, especially in affected adolescents.[1] It is important to initiate effective therapy early to prevent scarring.[7,8] Excellent questionnaires have been developed to identify the psychosocial impact of acne, but fortunately, many cases of acne are mild and do not lead to scarring.[9,10]

Acne occurs in people of all ages, from neonates through the eighth or ninth decade of life. Acne vulgaris primarily afflicts teenagers and young adults.[11,12] Acne also is associated with systemic diseases such as SAPHO (synovitis, acne, pustulosis, hyperostosis, osteitis) and Apert's syndromes.[13,14] The differential diagnosis of acneiform eruptions includes acne vulgaris, rosacea, gram-negative folliculitis, mechanical folliculitis, steroid acne, and perioral dermatitis.[15] Steroid acne (acne associated with either topical or systemic corticosteroid use) has been linked to folliculitis caused by the fungus *Pityrosporum ovale* and may respond to antifungal medications.[16] Discussions of severe acne variants such as pyoderma faciale (rosacea fulminans), acne conglobata, and acne fulminans are not presented in this chapter, which focuses exclusively on acne vulgaris.[17,18]

Incidence and Prevalence

Acne vulgaris affects between 40 and 50 million people in the United States and about 90% of all adolescents.[19] It accounts for more physician visits than any other dermatologic disorder.[6] Although no gender preference exists, females typically develop acne at a younger age and have milder cases than males.[15] Acne can occur in children as young as 8 years of age; however, most cases occur in adolescents between 14 and 19 years of age.[20] Mild forms of acne may persist longer in females and may, in rare cases, remain a life-long problem.[21] Asians and blacks have a slightly lower incidence of acne.[22] Females treated with antiepileptic drugs such as phenytoin or phenobarbital experience acne more commonly than age-matched controls (80% versus 30%),[23] and cases of severe acne may be more common in some families.

Etiology

The development of acne is related to increased sebum production, abnormal keratinization within the pilosebaceous canal (also called *hypercornification*), bacterial colonization, and an immune-mediated inflammatory reaction.[24,25] Multiple exogenous and endogenous factors can affect the development of acne vulgaris. Despite rare individual exceptions, diet, psychological stress, cleanliness, and sexual activity do not contribute to severity or exacerbations of acne.[26] Premenstrual exacerbations of acne are common.[15] Sex hormone imbalance (relative androgen excess), certain cosmetics, pomades, and moisturizers also may affect the development of acne.[27,28] Hot and humid conditions that stimulate sweating often worsen acne; dry and sunny weather conditions can improve acne and its appearance.

Occupational or environmental exposure to halogenated compounds, ultraviolet light, animal fats, dioxin, or petroleum derivatives may cause "chloracne" or other acneiform lesions.[29,30] It is important to identify drug-induced acne (see Chapter 38, Dermatotherapy and Drug Induced Disorders) because treatment outcomes likely depend on drug therapy modification.[31] Mechanical skin irritation caused by headbands, hats, chin straps, backpacks, or shoulder pads also may induce acne flare-ups (known as *acne mechanica*).

Pathogenesis

The earliest stage in the development of acne lesions involves accelerated proliferation of keratinocytes and accumulation of the unusually "sticky" horny cells that line the sebaceous follicle in the pilary (hair) canal. These horny cells continue to accumulate and eventually plug the sebaceous follicle.[15] As sebum accumulates in the plugged sebaceous follicle, a clinically undetectable microcomedone is formed.[32] The microcomedone enlarges as this process continues, and a closed comedone becomes the first clinically visible lesion. With increasing keratinization and expansion, an open comedone is formed. An inflammatory reaction occurs if the follicular wall ruptures from pressure caused by accumulated sebum or from mechanical pressure. Lymphocytes, monocytes, macrophages, and cytokines such as interleukins and tumor necrosis factor in the disrupted follicular wall then mediate inflammation.[15] Both the classic and alternative complement pathways may be activated.

Androgen-enhanced sebocyte activity and bacterial colonization significantly increase comedone formation.[6] Testosterone, of testicular origin in males or ovarian and adrenal origin in females, is metabolized in the skin by 5α-reductase to dihydrotestosterone (DHT). DHT has a high affinity for sebocyte receptors. The DHT–receptor complex then is translocated within the cytoplasm to the nucleus, where sebum biosynthesis is stimulated. The microaerophilic gram-positive diphtheroid *Propionibacterium acnes* generates proteases (hyaluronidases, phosphatases, and lipases) that liberate free fatty acids from sebum.[33] These fatty acids likely stimulate local inflammation. Other skin flora, such as *Staphylococcus epidermidis* and *Malassezia furfur,* do not contribute to comedone or pustule formation, but are also harbored within the duct.[34] Finally, a genetic predisposition may exist in which patients with acne have enhanced cytochrome P450 1A1 activity, which reduces levels of protective endogenous retinoids.[35] This condition is not screened for in clinical practice.

Therapy

No known cure exists for acne, but treatment can reduce its severity. In most cases, especially in severe forms, treatment is more an "art" than a science, and therapy must be highly individualized. The goals of treatment are to relieve discomfort, improve skin appearance, prevent pitting or scarring, and alleviate psychological distress and social rejection. The cost of treating acne has dramatically increased in recent years.[36]

Treatment is largely preventive because little can be done for existing lesions. Slow improvement, often over several weeks to months, is the rule for all treatments. Resolution of 20%, 60%, and 80% of lesions can be expected within 2, 6, and 8 months, respectively, after effective therapy is begun.[15] Therefore, treatment regimens should not be modified more often than every 1 to 2 months. Patient counseling should include a basic discussion of the chronicity and natural history of acne, proper drug administration or application technique, potential adverse effects, and actions to be undertaken if adverse reactions are experienced. General treatment guidelines issued by the American Academy of Dermatology serve as the current standards of practice.[24,37] These guidelines need to be used with patient-specific data (see Table 39-1).

Nondrug Therapy

Because of its complex pathophysiology, nondrug therapy plays a minimal role in the management of acne. Twice-daily washing with warm water and mild, nonmoisturizing soap is sufficient to remove excess sebum and improve skin appear-

---

Table 39-1   Pertinent Historical Components to Be Obtained From a Patient With Acne

- Duration, including onset and peak severity
- Location and distribution
- Seasonal variation
- For *females*, relation to menstrual periods, pregnancy status, scalp hair thinning, contraceptive method if used
- Present and past treatments, topical and systemic, prescription and over the counter
- Family history, including severity
- Other skin disorders or medical problems
- Medications and drug allergies
- Occupational exposure to chemicals or oils
- Use of cosmetics, moisturizers, hairstyling products (pomades)
- Areas of skin friction or irritation

ance. Aggressive skin washing does not alter the course of acne, and antibacterial or abrasive cleansers are not recommended.[15] Manipulation (e.g., squeezing, picking) of acne lesions should be strongly discouraged. Drugs, cosmetics, or other known precipitants also should obviously be avoided. Trial and error may be necessary to find cosmetics that will not exacerbate acne. Dermatologists may use one of several physical modalities to treat acne, especially as adjuncts to medication in severe cases. These include surgical comedone extraction, dermabrasion, and cryotherapy.[6] No prospective, controlled trials comparing medical and physical measures for managing severe acne exist. Ultraviolet light and x-ray therapy are rarely, if ever, necessary. Acne scarring is treated with CO_2 laser therapy, iontophoresis, recollagenation, or dermabrasion, but systematic randomized trials are needed to fully assess safety and comparative efficacy.[38,39]

Drug Therapy

Although many drugs either alone or in combination may ultimately be used, all therapies are based on treating one or more of the primary pathogenic factors.[24,40] Effective drugs work by (1) normalizing follicular keratinization (e.g., retinoids, azelaic acid, benzoyl peroxide), (2) decreasing sebum production (e.g., isotretinoin, hormone manipulation), (3) suppressing bacterial (P. acnes) flora (e.g., antibiotics, benzoyl peroxide, azelaic acid, isotretinoin), and (4) preventing an inflammatory response (e.g., antibiotics, retinoids). Topical therapy generally is preferable for mild to moderate acne (Table 39-2).[41]

BENZOYL PEROXIDE

One of the most effective acne treatments available is topical benzoyl peroxide. It predominantly works as an antibacterial agent, but also unblocks pores by causing mild keratinolysis and increasing epithelial cell turnover.[42] Bacterial wall proteins are oxidized by oxygen free radicals that are released by the metabolism of benzoyl peroxide on the skin; bacterial resistance does not develop. Benzoyl peroxide minimally reduces sebum production, but significantly lowers free fatty acid concentrations.[24] The irritant effects of benzoyl peroxide also cause vasodilation and increase blood flow, which may hasten resolution of inflammatory lesions. Benzoyl peroxide improves both inflamed and noninflamed lesions and is similar to topically applied retinoids in improving comedonal acne.[43] Treatment is associated with a 50% to 75% reduction in inflammatory lesions in 8 to 12 weeks.[42] Its efficacy is enhanced when combined with other systemic or topical agents, especially topical erythromycin.[44-46] Benzoyl peroxide is available over-the-counter (OTC) and by prescription in a variety of dosage forms (cleansers, lotions, creams, and gels) and concentrations (2.5% to 10%). More drying gels, either water- or alcohol/acetone-based, are available by prescription.

Benzoyl peroxide has been associated with tumors in mice, but long-term use has not been associated with skin cancer.[47]

RETINOIDS

Vitamin A and its analogs have been used to treat acne for >50 years.[48,49] Tretinoin (Retin-A), also called *all-trans-retinoic acid,* is the naturally occurring form of vitamin A acid and is available for topical application as a cream (0.025%, 0.05%, 0.1%), gel (0.025%, 0.01%), and liquid (0.05%). Another topical retinoid, adapalene (Differin), is available as a gel or solution in a concentration of 0.1%.[50] It appears to bind to different receptors than tretinoin.[51] Adapalene is at least as effective as tretinoin, but may cause less skin irritation.[52-54] The newest agent in the class, tazarotene (Tazorac), is available in a 0.1% gel formulation and has a long duration of action.[55] Isotretinoin (Accutane), a synthetic 13-*cis*-isomer of tretinoin, has greater biologic activity and is administered orally as 10-, 20-, or 40-mg capsules.

Unlike benzoyl peroxide, retinoids have no in vitro antibacterial properties. Isotretinoin indirectly reduces P. acnes colonization by reducing the production of sebum, which P. acnes requires for survival.[56] Retinoids are comedolytic and normalize keratinization by decreasing horny cell cohesiveness and stimulating epidermal cell turnover. These actions combine to unplug follicles and prevent microcomedone formation.[57] In addition to decreasing sebum and P. acnes colonization, the retinoids reduce inflammation by directly inhibiting neutrophil and monocyte chemotaxis.[58,59] Because retinoids affect each of the four known pathogenic factors (previously described), they are very effective agents.

Tretinoin, adapalene, or tazarotene are often applied topically to patients with mild to moderate comedonal acne that fails to respond to benzoyl peroxide or topical antibiotics. They also may be used in combination with antibiotics to manage moderate to severe inflammatory acne or to treat fine acne scarring.[60-62]

Systemic isotretinoin (Accutane) is the only effective agent for severe cystic acne and can induce remissions for months to years after one or two courses of therapy (3 to 5 months per course).[63,64] The high cost, risk of serious adverse effects, and potential for overuse have resulted in guidelines for rational retinoid use (Table 39-3).[65,66] In fact, a specific treatment plan called S.M.A.R.T. (system to manage Accutane-related teratogenicity) must be used to prescribe and dispense the product. The process requires designated prescription stickers, standardized written information (MedGuide) for the patient, and precise documentation of avoidance of pregnancy. The use of isotretinoin for severe acne is perhaps even more cost-effective than long-term antibiotics because of superior efficacy and long-term cost savings.[67] Topical isotretinoin is not yet available in the United States.

Table 39-2	Choice of Topical Versus Oral Acne Therapy	
Clinical Characteristics	Topical Therapy	Oral Therapy
Severity	Mild to moderate	Moderate to severe
Location	Face	Back, chest, arms
Treatment resistant	In combination	Monotherapy or combined therapy
Likelihood of scarring	Not indicated	Indicated

Table 39-3 Guidelines for Isotretinoin Use in Acne

Patient Selection

Severe cystic acne
Moderate acne, but resistant to combination conventional therapies
Unusually severe acne variants (conglobata, fulminans)

Dosage

0.5–1 mg/kg/day
Use higher dosage in young patients, males, those with severe acne, patients with acne involving the trunk

Duration of Therapy

Cumulative dose of 120 mg/kg (usually 3–7 mo)

Relapse Rate

Repeat courses required in 15–20% of patients
Re-treatment usually safe and effective
Very rarely, patients may require 3–5 courses

Topical tretinoin can darken skin in dark-skinned patients. Other adverse effects associated with systemic isotretinoin are listed in Table 39-4. Although related to vitamin A, systemic effects that resemble hypervitaminosis A syndrome are uncommon.[68] Appropriate use of systemic retinoids is generally well tolerated with predictable adverse effects.[69] Retinoids *must* be avoided during pregnancy because of their well-established teratogenic effects. Contraception should be used during therapy and continued for at least 1 month after drug discontinuation.

AZELAIC ACID

A 20% concentration of azelaic acid in a cream is another alternative for acne management.[70,71] This dicarboxylic acid, originally studied for its effects on hyperpigmentation conditions such as melasma, works by at least two mechanisms: suppressing *P. acnes* and normalizing keratinization.[72,73] Azelaic acid appears to be as effective as oral antibiotics or topical tretinoin, but with potentially less skin irritation than tretinoin.[74,75] Its efficacy may be potentiated by combining it with glycolic acid, a keratolytic in cosmetic preparations that is currently under investigation.[76] A small amount of azelaic acid cream is applied to the affected area twice daily.

ANTIBIOTICS

Acne is not an "infectious" disease per se and certainly is not contagious. Rather, *P. acnes* helps transform comedones into inflammatory pustules or papules. Antibiotics do not resolve existing lesions, but they can prevent future lesions by decreasing sebaceous fatty acid metabolic byproducts that stimulate inflammation by decreasing *P. acnes* colonization. In addition, antibiotics themselves seem to suppress neutrophil chemotaxis, even at subminimal inhibitory concentrations.[77,78] No single agent is universally superior because there is significant interpatient variability in efficacy and tolerability. Antibiotics commonly used include clindamycin, the macrolides, tetracyclines, trimethoprim/sulfamethoxazole, and metronidazole. Although not yet well studied, three-times-weekly administration of the azalide azithromycin (Zithromax) has been beneficial.[79,80] Because all are equally effective, the choice of antibiotic should ultimately be based on cost, response to previous treatment, adverse effects, pregnancy status, and age.

Antibiotic Resistance

The development of antibiotic resistance by *P. acnes* is commonly recognized and correlated with treatment failure.[81] Systematic reviews reveal that rates of resistance range from 1% with minocycline to 60% with erythromycin.[82,83] Genetic mutation has been identified as the mechanism by which resistance develops to erythromycin and clindamycin.[84] Guidelines for rational antibiotic use have been suggested.[85,86] Intermittent treat-

Table 39-4 Adverse Effects of Systemic Retinoids

Body System	Adverse Effect	Management
Common, Pharmacologic		
Reproductive	Teratogenicity (birth defects, premature birth, neonatal death)	Avoid pregnancy
Skin	Dryness, peeling, pruritus, photosensitivity	Moisturizers or emollients, sunscreens, protective clothing
Hair, nails	Alopecia, nail fragility	None, discontinue drug if severe
Mucous membranes	Cheilitis (dry mouth, nose, eyes), blepharoconjunctivitis	Lip balms, sugarless gum/candy, saline nasal spray, artificial tears or ophthalmic ointment ↓ dosage if severe or bothersome
Uncommon, Toxic		
Liver	↑ Transaminases; hepatitis	Monitor if mild elevation. Avoid in patients with previous liver dysfunction. Discontinue drug if hepatitis occurs.
Bones	Pain	Monitor at each visit.
	Bone loss (osteopenia)	Routine monitoring is not recommended
Muscle, ligaments	Pain, calcifications	Monitor; discontinue if severe.
Eyes	↓ Night vision	Patients should use caution when driving.
Metabolic	↑ Triglycerides, ↑ cholesterol, ↑VLDL, ↑LDL	Reduce/eliminate alcohol; low-fat diet; consider dosage reduction or drug discontinuation.
Psychiatric	Depression, suicide	Monitor for depressed mood and suicidal thoughts

LDL, low-density lipoprotein; VLDL, very low-density lipoprotein.

ment with either topical benzoyl peroxide or oral isotretinoin also prevents clinically significant *P. acnes* resistance.[87]

Topical Antibiotics

Topically applied antibiotics are effective for mild to moderate acne.[88] Clindamycin and erythromycin are the most commonly used topical antibiotics.[89] Skin discoloration, especially with the tetracyclines, can occur in addition to tingling and stinging.[90] Combination products containing benzoyl peroxide and erythromycin are available for moderate to severe acne and are easier for patients to use. Although infrequent case reports exist, systemic adverse effects (including antibiotic-associated colitis) are rare.[91] Topical tretinoin can enhance the systemic absorption of topically applied clindamycin.[92] Oral antibiotics should be used in patients with moderate to severe acne who are intolerant or unresponsive to topical agents or those with widespread acne such as on the trunk, back, or shoulders.[24] Twice-daily dosing of all agents improves compliance and is usually as effective as more frequent dosing. The goal of chronic therapy is to use the smallest dose once daily. Long-term use of antibiotics is usually safe and effective.

COMBINATION THERAPY

Although many patients respond to monotherapy with either a topical agent or a systemic antibiotic, optimal control of moderate to severe acne often requires combination therapy.[93] Combinations may allow for lower dosages of individual drugs and are almost always more effective.[94] Rational combinations include agents with different mechanisms of action such as either topical benzoyl peroxide or a retinoid plus a topical or systemic antibiotic.[95,96] Because isotretinoin addresses virtually every pathophysiologic mechanism of acne, combining it with other medications is unnecessary.

MISCELLANEOUS TOPICAL AGENTS

Three unique topical preparations also are used to treat mild to moderate acne.[97] Salicylic acid, sulfur, and resorcinol have been used for many years, but with varying degrees of success. Topical salicylic acid, a concentration-dependent keratolytic, is more effective than placebo, but probably less effective than topical benzoyl peroxide or tretinoin.[98,99] It may augment the effectiveness of other agents when used in combination.[100] Chronic use over large body surfaces should be avoided to prevent systemic toxicity. Sulfur preparations have both antibacterial and comedolytic properties and also are clinically effective.[101,102] Disadvantages of sulfur include a displeasing odor, skin discoloration, and limited effectiveness. Sulfur also may be comedogenic.[15] Resorcinol alone is not effective and is available only in combination with sulfur preparations.[103] Although not currently available in the United States, topical nicotinamide also is effective in treating inflammatory acne.[104]

ZINC SALTS

Zinc salts are rarely used to treat acne. A reduction in granulocyte zinc concentration, which inhibits chemotaxis, appears to reduce inflammation.[105] Zinc also blocks the formation of DHT from testosterone by inhibiting 5α-reductase.[106] More supporting clinical data are necessary before zinc supplementation can be recommended routinely.

ANTIANDROGENS AND HORMONES

The critical role of androgens in the pathogenesis of acne has stimulated great interest in the use of antiandrogens.[107,108] Cyproterone (Androcur) is the only agent available in the United States and is listed as an orphan drug for treatment of severe hirsutism. Cyproterone and spironolactone (Aldactone), which also has antiandrogenic effects, are used in Europe for treatment of acne.[109,110] Safety and effectiveness data are still lacking.[111] Antiandrogens should not be used in males because gynecomastia is likely to develop. In females, these drugs usually are given with estrogens to prevent menstrual irregularities.[100]

Oral Contraceptives

Estrogen, usually administered as ethinyl estradiol in the form of a cycled combination oral contraceptive (OC) agent, may improve acne in females through its antiandrogenic effects.[113–115] Estrogen exerts this effect as a trophic hormone that stimulates protein synthesis. Specifically, estrogen increases concentrations of sex hormone–binding globulin and decreases levels of free endogenous testosterone. The accompanying progestin component of the oral contraceptive has little or no inherent antiandrogenic activity. Progestins with androgenic effects (i.e., norgestrel, levonorgestrel) may worsen acne. Acceptable progestins include norgestimate, desogestrel, and norethindrone. Ortho Tri-Cyclen is approved by the U.S. Food and Drug Administration for the treatment of moderate acne in females 15 years of age or older who have achieved menarche and are unresponsive to topical antiacne medications.[116] Indeed, the increasing prevalence of OC use may be reducing the prevalence of acne.[117]

CORTICOSTEROIDS

Although corticosteroids have been implicated as causing acne, they also can be used to treat severe acne. Intralesional injections of triamcinolone (usually diluted with normal saline to concentration of 1.25 to 5 mg/mL) markedly improve severe inflammatory acne.[118] Systemic corticosteroids have been used for both short- and long-term treatment of severe cystic acne. A 7-day course of prednisone (e.g., 20 mg/day) can be used for "prom acne," to quickly and dramatically improve acne for important events such as a prom or a wedding. Low-dose prednisone (e.g., 5 mg/day) also may have antiandrogenic effects. Topical application of corticosteroids is not effective. In treating severe acne, steroids can be used in combination with isotretinoin to decrease the inflammatory response.[15]

CLINICAL ASSESSMENT

1. L.Y., a 15-year-old freshman cheerleader, presents to her physician complaining of worsening "zits." Because several of her classmates are taking antibiotics for acne, she wants a "strong medicine" to make them go away. The first signs of acne occurred at age 13, when lesions occasionally appeared on her chin and forehead. L.Y.'s acne progressively worsened, and now she consistently has four to eight lesions, which have spread to her cheeks and nose. She has no other medical problems. Menarche occurred at age 12, with normal menstrual periods following, and her only surgery was an appendectomy at age 11. She has two older brothers with acne (one with mild and one with severe lesions). L.Y. denies alcohol, tobacco, or illicit drug use. She has a boyfriend but denies sexual intercourse. After school, she works part-time at a fast food restaurant, plays doubles on the varsity tennis team, and enjoys playing the violin. L.Y. takes no chronic prescription medications, but uses OTC Clearasil (5% benzoyl peroxide cream) as needed when her acne "gets really bad." She has used a "medicated" soap in the past, but stopped because it caused excessively dry skin. She wears a headband while playing tennis and uses a hair styling gel. Examination reveals three pustules and two closed comedones on her forehead, three excoriated lesions on her cheeks and chin (which are covered with makeup), two well-healing areas on her nose, and no open comedones. There is only one pustule on her back; her chest and arms are clear. She has no facial hair, and her voice is normal in pitch. What are the key components in the clinical assessment of L.Y.'s acne?

The clinical assessment of her acne should include evaluating each of the following factors:

• Type, number, and distribution of lesions. This patient has relatively few lesions that are mostly inflammatory (pustules) and located on the face.
• Contributing factors such as family history of acne (noted in brothers), work-related exposures (oils from fast-food restaurant), systemic or topical medications (hair gel), or mechanical pressure on the skin (headband and violin chin rest).
• Hormonal influences that indicate androgen excess or atypical menstrual cycles. This patient has no signs of virilization (normal voice and lack of facial hair), and although she has a history of early menarche, her menstrual periods are normal.
• A detailed medical history. This patient is healthy and does not have epilepsy, liver disease, alcohol abuse, or dyslipidemia.
• Effectiveness of current or past treatments. This patient's response to two therapies was suboptimal, but because she used them erratically, effectiveness is difficult to assess.
• Psychosocial impact of acne on her quality of life. This appears to be very important to her based on her plea for effective therapy.

2. What subjective and objective data support a diagnosis of acne vulgaris?

This patient's age (teenager) puts her in the highest prevalence category. The facial distribution of lesions, while sparing most other areas, further supports acne, as does a strong positive family history. The fact that her condition has waxed and waned, but progressively worsened is consistent with acne. Her condition also worsened because of mechanical irritation caused by sweatband use and violin playing. The lesion type and severity rules out more severe variants such as gram-negative folliculitis or acne fulminans.

MILD ACNE
Benzoyl Peroxide

3. Evaluate L.Y.'s current acne management.

L.Y.'s current antiacne regimen is suboptimal, which explains her progressively worsening course. Her choice of an OTC 5% benzoyl peroxide cream is excellent for mild to moderate inflammatory acne, but it was ineffective for her be-

cause she applies it infrequently to existing lesions only. Routine use over the entire susceptible areas is required for long-term acne control.

4. Why should other treatment options be avoided at this time?

Because topical antibiotics, retinoids, and azelaic acid are more expensive and may cause more skin irritation, they should be reserved for patients who fail to respond to benzoyl peroxide treatment or who cannot tolerate its effects.[119] Oral antibiotics are not yet indicated because the acne is mild and distributed in a small area. Although oral isotretinoin is likely to be very effective, it also is not warranted at this time because of high cost, significant bothersome adverse effects, need for close monitoring, and potential teratogenicity. Combination oral contraceptives would have been a reasonable choice if she was sexually active or had menstrual abnormalities.

Skin Irritation

5. How can L.Y. reduce the risk of developing skin irritation and dryness while using benzoyl peroxide (Clearasil)?

Topical application of benzoyl peroxide may cause transient warmth or stinging, significant drying, or skin irritation.[42] The benzoyl peroxide dosage form (cream) and potency currently used by L.Y. (5%) are good choices and should minimize the risk of skin irritation while still achieving the desired therapeutic effect. Mild skin redness or drying is acceptable and indicates proper dosage and optimal therapeutic response. Patients should decrease the frequency of application, perhaps to every other day, if necessary (especially when beginning therapy). The cream should be applied at bedtime and washed off in the morning (or after several hours, if excessive skin dryness or peeling occurs). Generally, they should avoid "countertreating" skin irritation with moisturizers or emollients. Factors that worsen skin irritation include increased benzoyl peroxide concentration and contact time, gels or lipophilic vehicles, thin and sensitive skin, low environmental humidity, use of irritating adjunctive therapies, and increased application frequency.[42] A lower strength (e.g., 2.5%) or less drying formulation (e.g., lotion) may also need to be used. Benzoyl peroxide lotions provide shorter contact time on the skin than creams, whereas creams are shorter acting than gels. Therefore, alcohol-based benzoyl peroxide gels cause more drying than creams. To minimize skin irritation, she should also discontinue use of medicated cleansers.

L.Y. should also be educated that contact of benzoyl peroxide with clothing, washcloths, or towels will cause bleaching or discoloration. Likewise, rugs and other areas in the bathroom may be discolored by medication that is spilled or wiped from the hands.

Allergic contact dermatitis due to benzoyl peroxide, characterized by pruritus and inflammation, occurs in up to 1% of patients.[25] Those who develop such contact dermatitis should discontinue its use.

6. How should L.Y.'s benzoyl peroxide therapy be modified if the desired effect is not achieved?

L.Y. could either increase the strength of her benzoyl peroxide to 10% or obtain a prescription product in the form of a gel, which may be more effective, but potentially more irritating. If the desired therapeutic endpoints have not been achieved after 4 additional weeks, the application frequency of benzoyl peroxide can be increased to twice daily if tolerated. The inflamed lesions usually resolve slowly, but progressively.

7. R.P., a 17-year-old boy, has been using a benzoyl peroxide 5% gel (Benzac-W) for 2 months. Since he began using this treatment, his acne has slightly improved. About 1 week ago, he began noticing significant redness and itching in the areas where he had applied the gel. He stopped using the medication until last night, when the irritation had almost resolved. During this period of resolution, R.P. spent several days at the beach and began using a new skin cleanser. Within 10 minutes after applying a small amount of gel to his forehead and nose area (also known as the T-zone because of the shape of the area), his skin became reddened and began to burn and itch. He immediately washed the area well with cool, soapy water, but the skin irritation prevented him from getting a good night's sleep. The area is better this morning, but remains red and itchy. Currently, his acne consists of some noninflammatory and many inflammatory lesions located primarily in the T-zone. Is this a typical adverse reaction to benzoyl peroxide?

No. Because sun exposure or dryness from a change in skin cleanser did not appear to provoke the skin reaction, it is unlikely due to benzoyl peroxide's direct irritating effects. The intense itching and burning following rechallenge is more consistent with an allergic-type contact dermatitis that occurs uncommonly.

Topical Antibiotics

8. This patient's treatment with benzoyl peroxide was discontinued. What alternative therapy is indicated at this time?

After the allergic reaction has resolved, this patient should begin a trial with a topical antibiotic such as clindamycin. The entire susceptible area, not just the lesions, should be treated for optimal results. Twice-daily application is most effective, and patient compliance is important. This antibiotic is selected because topical tetracyclines often cause skin discoloration. Erythromycin is associated with the development of resistance and benzoyl peroxide cannot be used concomitantly to prevent resistance. Topical metronidazole is generally reserved for managing rosacea rather than acne vulgaris. An oral antibiotic is not indicated at this time because only a small area is affected.

9. Explain why either a topical retinoid or azelaic acid is not the second-line agent of choice in R.P.

Both topical retinoids and azelaic acid are likely to be effective in this patient. Although either agent is a reasonable choice, these agents are not chosen because they are more expensive and more likely to cause skin irritation. The predominance of inflammatory lesions also makes an antibiotic a better alternative.

MODERATE ACNE

10. R.P. moved away to go to college and returns for follow-up care after 4 months. He has been applying topical clindamycin gel regularly twice daily. He plays basketball 3 nights per week, but has no other precipitating factors. Nevertheless, his lesions

have increased in number and have now appeared on his chest and back. He has one cyst on his left cheek that is painful to touch. R.P. is embarrassed by the appearance of his skin, which is exposed when he wears a basketball jersey. How would you assess his acne now? Why might his acne be worsening?

R.P.'s acne is now moderate in severity because of the extensive distribution of lesions. He also now has a more severe, cystic lesion. For unknown reasons, perhaps hormonal changes that are increasing keratinization of the pilosebaceous unit, the acne has clearly progressed. The hot and humid conditions associated with playing basketball and colonization with clindamycin-resistant *P. acnes* also may be contributing to his acne flare. It is unlikely that either the stress of college or dietary changes are factors.

Systemic Antibiotics

11. Modify R.P.'s treatment regimen to gain better control of his acne. Provide rationale for your antibiotic choice.

Because R.P.'s lesions are primarily inflammatory in nature, antibiotics remain a good choice. However, the area affected is more widespread, so oral antibiotics should now be used. Topical clindamycin should be discontinued, and oral tetracycline should be prescribed. Oral tetracycline is the first oral antibiotic of choice for moderate acne because it has been most extensively studied and is usually the least expensive. The usual dosage is 500 mg twice daily for 2 months, after which R.P. should be reassessed. At that time, if the acne is not at least 20% improved, an alternative oral antiobiotic should be substituted for the oral tetracycline. Doxycycline is less commonly used, but is also effective.

Minocycline may have some advantages over tetracycline, but is significantly more expensive and has additional toxicities.[120] Food and dairy products impair minocycline's oral absorption to a lesser extent than other tetracyclines.[121] It also can be dosed once daily, optimally with water 1 hour before a meal, because of a long duration of action. Finally, minocycline may be effective even if tetracycline has failed.[122–126] The dose should be taken with a full glass of water in an upright position to minimize the risk of the capsule lodging and dissolving in the esophagus, which can cause irritation or ulceration. This and other serious adverse effects associated with minocycline use relegate it to a second choice within the tetracycline family (Table 39-5).[127–128] When minocycline is necessary, the lowest effective dosage should be maintained to minimize the risk of adverse effects associated with long-term use.

If gram-negative folliculitis is suspected, oral trimethoprim/sulfamethoxazole (Bactrim) should be considered. R.P.'s acne is moderately severe; therefore, it is also reasonable to combine the oral antibiotic with a once-daily, bedtime application of either a topical retinoid or azelaic acid. The topical agents are generally applied only to the face because chest and back application is difficult and expensive.

12. Should any specific laboratory tests be monitored? How should R.P.'s tetracycline regimen be monitored and the dosage adjusted?

Although acne is both a chronic and a self-limiting skin disease, systemic antibiotics may be necessary for long periods. The lowest effective antibiotic dosage should be used to

Table 39-5 Potentially Serious Adverse Effects Associated With Minocycline

- Lupus-like syndrome
- Necrotizing vasculitis of uterine cervix
- Hepatotoxicity
- Eosinophilic pneumonitis
- Polyarteritis nodosa
- Arthralgia, arthritis, or other autoimmune phenomena
- Intracranial hypertension or pseudotumor cerebri
- Discoloration or hyperpigmentation of the skin or gums
- Hypersensitivity (e.g., fever, rash, neutropenia, eosinophilia)

minimize the risk of adverse effects. After R.P.'s acne is controlled, the tetracycline dosage can be reduced to 250 mg twice a day or 500 mg once a day. If his acne remains well controlled for another 2 to 3 months, the tetracycline dosage should be reduced further to a single daily dose of 250 mg. Although low-dose tetracycline therapy can be continued for several years without long-term adverse effects, discontinuation of the antibiotic should be attempted periodically. The single daily doses of tetracycline should be taken on an empty stomach without dairy products to maximize drug absorption. Potential for systemic adverse effects—mainly diarrhea, rash, photosensitivity, and vulvovaginal candidiasis—is greater with oral than with topical administration. R.P. should be counseled to contact his physician if these adverse effects occur. Routine laboratory monitoring is not necessary for most young, healthy patients receiving long-term oral tetracyclines or erythromycin because the incidence of serious adverse effects is low.[129]

Tretinoin, Adapalene, and Azelaic Acid

13. J.H., a 23-year-old red-haired, fair-skinned woman, has had acne vulgaris for the past 10 years. Over this time, she has tried several medications without much success. Benzoyl peroxide was moderately helpful, but she developed excessive skin dryness. The highest strength she was able to tolerate was only a 5% cream. J.H. also has used two different topical antibiotics, erythromycin and clindamycin, with only about a 25% improvement over 2 to 3 years. Oral erythromycin caused gastrointestinal upset, and she found taking oral tetracycline difficult because she eats lots of dairy products. Currently, she has 20 to 30 open and closed comedones on her forehead, cheeks, and chin. There are fewer than five inflammatory lesions and no cysts or nodules. Recommend a new treatment strategy for J.H.

J.H.'s story is a common one because acne is a chronic condition. It is important to obtain as many therapeutic details as possible regarding her dosages and adherence to the prescribed regimens. Because her acne is mostly of the noninflammatory, comedonal type, a topical retinoid would likely be effective. She should begin with once-daily applications at bedtime of the least irritating strength and dosage form (e.g., 0.025% tretinoin cream). Adverse effects caused by retinoids are common and occur to some extent in nearly all patients. Topical tretinoin (Retin A) causes local skin irritation characterized by dryness, redness, and peeling. Predisposing factors are similar to those for benzoyl peroxide, but true hypersensi-

tivity is rare. Sun exposure significantly intensifies skin irritation, so users should be instructed to apply sunscreen to sun-exposed areas. A new dosage form using polymers of microencapsulated tretinoin has been successful in decreasing local irritation.[130–132] Therapy should begin with single bedtime applications of the 0.01% formulation.

Some acne might appear worsened within the first 1 to 2 weeks because preclinical lesions may become visible. Mild skin redness and drying during this time are expected, and therapy should not be modified. A more concentrated formulation can be used if necessary after 4 to 8 weeks of suboptimal response.

Topical azelaic acid, a keratinolytic agent, also is an option for treating J.H.'s acne because it is equally effective as topical retinoids for comedonal acne. Cost is comparable. Anecdotally, certain individuals respond differently to these products, but unfortunately, response cannot be predicted before selection.

14. Three weeks into her 2-month trial of topical tretinoin and oral tetracycline, J.H. notices a slight improvement in the acne but complains of skin redness and irritation. This occurs when she is exposed to minimal amounts of sun, even if she applies sunscreen. Should a microencapsulated form of tretinoin be substituted?

The use of systemic tetracyclines can cause the skin to be more sensitive to ultraviolet (UV) light. J.H. should be educated to wear protective clothing when possible and to regularly apply a sunscreen with a sun protection factor (SPF) of at least 15 if she anticipates even minimal sun exposure. The sunscreen must block both UVA and UVB light. She should also be cautioned that certain sunscreens can worsen acne and that finding an optimal brand may require a trial-and-error process. If the sun continues to cause redness and irritation after preventive measures have been instituted, it is reasonable to switch to either a microencapsulated form of tretinoin or adapalene. The microencapsulated form of tretinoin minimizes irritation by delaying drug contact to the skin. Depending on the patient's insurance plan, it is possible that one of these products may not be covered on the drug formulary. Formulary status of these similar agents is often limited because of specific contract and incentive issues. Both agents are expensive, but equally effective, and do cause less skin irritation in some patients.

SEVERE ACNE
Isotretinoin
Dose

15. Four years ago, K.S., a 24-year-old female office assistant, was diagnosed with moderate noninflammatory and inflammatory acne that was primarily located on her face and back. She tried topical benzoyl peroxide and systemic erythromycin with limited success. She began taking minocycline 100 mg BID 1½ years ago and noted significant improvement about 2 months after starting this regimen. She has not been able to reduce her dosage to 100 mg daily because of predictable flare-ups. In fact, her acne has worsened over the past 3 months, and she now has at least a dozen cysts or nodules widely distributed among multiple papules and pustules on her face and back. Her medical history is significant for deep venous thrombosis 2 years ago after a long car trip across the country; this was likely secondary to combination oral contraceptives that she was taking for polycystic ovary syndrome. She stopped taking warfarin (Coumadin) about 6 months ago. K.S. is 5'6" and weighs 180 lb (81.8 kg). She has no other health problems. She does not smoke, but she occasionally drinks alcohol on weekends. She is sexually active with one partner, her husband, who uses condoms for contraception. Two months ago, blood chemistries, thyroid-stimulating hormone, complete blood count, and a lipid panel were normal. Suggest a therapeutic plan for K.S.'s acne.

K.S. has severe acne based on the large number of lesions, wide distribution on multiple body sites, and presence of multiple inflammatory lesions, including cysts and nodules. The most effective medication for K.S. will be oral isotretinoin at an initial dose of 20 mg twice daily (approximately 0.5 mg/kg). The dosage should be increased to 40 mg twice daily (1 mg/kg) as tolerated after 1 month. A single treatment course is most effective if a cumulative dose of approximately 120 mg/kg, which should take almost 5 months to complete, is attained. Higher dosages are associated with an increased risk of adverse effects. A lower dosage of 0.3 to 0.5 mg/kg per day for a longer treatment period (6 to 12 months) would be recommended if she were a child younger than 15 years of age.[133] K.S. should stop taking all other anti-acne medications. Her acne should significantly improve within the first month of therapy and gradually resolve by the third or fourth month. A second course of therapy is usually not necessary.

Adverse Effects

16. How should K.S. be counseled with regard to adverse effects of isotretinoin?

Severe sunburn can occur in any patient taking isotretinoin, and the use of protective clothing and sunscreen must be recommended. These measures are important because photosensitivity reactions to tretinoin can be debilitating. (See Chapter 41, Photosensitivity and Burns, for a more detailed discussion of sunscreens.) She also should be cautioned about limiting alcohol consumption, which can enhance isotretinoin-induced hypertriglyceridemia and hepatotoxicity. K.S. should expect significant skin and mucous membrane dryness, which is reported by virtually all patients taking isotretinoin. Another possible adverse effect is muscle or joint pain, which occurs in up to 5% of patients. Bone growth is not impaired when isotretinoin is used in recommended dosages. Refer to Table 39-4 for a complete list of potential adverse effects caused by isotretinoin.

17. The package insert for isotretinoin warns against possible drug induced depression. How significant is this risk?

In 1998, the manufacturer of Accutane revised the product labeling to include a warning that isotretinoin may cause "depression, psychosis and, rarely, suicidal ideation, suicide attempts, and suicide."[134] The caution is based on case reports and a retrospective analysis of postmarketing surveillance. It is also possible that severe acne, and not isotretinoin use, cause severe depression. Although the absolute risk of severe depression is low, all patients with severe acne, whether receiving isotretinoin or not, should be monitored for the development or worsening of depression.[135]

18. After 3 weeks of therapy, K.S. complains of dry eyes and cracks with bleeding at the corners of her mouth. How might these bothersome mucocutaneous side effects be managed?

Frequent application of a lip balm or emollient, particularly one with a sunscreen, is recommended to treat her chapped lips (cheilitis). Daytime artificial tear instillation should relieve the discomfort of her dry eyes and bedtime application of a lubricating ophthalmic ointment also may be helpful. If the symptoms become intolerable, a small reduction in the isotretinoin dose (e.g., 10 to 20 mg/day) usually decreases the intensity of skin and mucous membrane reactions. Drug discontinuation is rarely necessary.[68] Application of normal saline spray (e.g., Ocean) to the nasal mucosa also should be recommended because about 60% of isotretinoin-treated patients experience dry nasal mucosa and nose bleeds. Application of petroleum jelly to the nares should be avoided because of a small risk of developing lipoid pneumonia. About 95% of patients receiving isotretinoin also develop dry skin that should be treated with lotions, creams, or other emollients (see Chapter 38, Dermatotherapy and Drug Induced Disorders).

TERATOGENICITY

19. What should K.S. be told about getting pregnant while taking isotretinoin?

Because of isotretinoin's teratogenic effects (e.g., severe birth defects, premature birth, and neonatal death), all females of childbearing potential must have a negative pregnancy test before beginning therapy.[136] Some clinicians recommend monthly pregnancy tests in sexually active fertile females, regardless of contraceptive method used. Others have recommended a specific pregnancy prevention program.[137,138] Because K.S.'s husband is using condoms, she should be warned that condom failure can occur and that a back-up method, such as spermicides or a second barrier method, may be necessary to ensure contraception. K.S. should not become pregnant for at least 1 month after stopping isotretinoin therapy because of delayed elimination of isotretinoin from the body.[139]

Monitoring Parameters

20. What baseline and periodic monitoring parameters should be followed in this patient?

LIPIDS

A baseline, afractionated lipid panel should be ordered because of the association between isotretinoin and hypertriglyceridemia. The blood sample should be collected at least 36 hours after alcohol consumption and 10 hours after eating food. The sample measured 2 months ago will suffice for K.S. because it likely would not be different now. The panel should be repeated periodically, but there is no consensus on the frequency. Maximal lipid changes usually occur within 4 to 8 weeks after beginning isotretinoin therapy. About 30% of patients develop significant triglyceride elevations. Mild triglyceride elevations (>400 mg/dL) should be treated with diet and a reduced alcohol intake. Serum triglycerides >800 mg/dL are extremely rare but, theoretically, could cause acute pancreatitis. If severe hypertriglyceridemia occurs, isotretinoin should be discontinued or used at a reduced dosage. If pancreatitis develops, the drug must be discontinued. These lipid abnormalities usually resolve within several weeks after the dosage of isotretinoin is reduced. High-density lipoprotein (HDL) concentrations may decrease slightly, and total cholesterol concentrations may increase; however, the clinical significance is unknown.

LIVER FUNCTION

A baseline liver panel that includes serum transaminases and bilirubin should be obtained from K.S. because isotretinoin can be hepatotoxic. The tests must be repeated if clinical symptoms of hepatitis occur. Mild elevations in serum aminotransferase levels (less than twice the upper limit of normal) are harmless and occur in about 15% to 25% of patients; they rarely lead to cessation of therapy. However, isotretinoin dosage reduction or drug discontinuation should be considered in asymptomatic patients with persistent enzyme elevations greater than twice the upper limit of normal. Clinical hepatitis occurs in <1% of patients taking isotretinoin, but requires drug discontinuation if suspected.

OTHERS

Although other laboratory abnormalities may be encountered during isotretinoin therapy, no guidelines have been established requiring routine monitoring of serum concentrations of glucose and electrolytes, urinalysis, red or white blood cell counts, creatine kinase, or the erythrocyte sedimentation rate. Although osteopenia has been associated with systemic retinoid use, bone density monitoring is also not formally recommended by the manufacturer.[140] Baseline values should be obtained if clinically warranted. Measuring plasma isotretinoin and its metabolite 4-oxo- isotretinoin is feasible and may allow for dosage optimization for severe acne; however, this is not common practice.[141]

Hormonal Agents

21. **Would other treatment modalities focused on hormonal manipulation be indicated in this patient?**

The use of combination oral contraceptives is unfortunately contraindicated because of K.S.'s history of venous thromboembolism. Otherwise, it would be an excellent choice because of her relative androgen excess from the ovarian disease and the fact that she desires contraception. Progestin-only methods of contraception, such as parenteral medroxyprogesterone (Depo-Provera), are safer in women with a history of thromboembolism but may worsen her acne; in addition, they are associated with a high rate of irregular menstrual bleeding. Antiandrogens such as spironolactone and cyproterone should be reserved until after her course of isotretinoin brings her acne under better control. After isotretinoin is discontinued, the antiandrogens may be considered for maintenance therapy.

REFERENCES

1. Thiboutot DM. An overview of clinical research findings. Dermatol Clin 1997;15:97.
2. Odom RB et al, eds. Andrews' Diseases of the Skin: Clinical Dermatology, 9th Ed. Philadelphia: W.B. Saunders Company, 2000:284.
3. Cunliffe WJ. Looking back to the future—acne. Dermatology 2002;204:167.
4. Burke BM, Cunliffe WJ. The assessment of acne vulgaris—the Leeds technique. Br J Dermatol 1984;111:83.
5. Rizova E et al. Polarized light photography and videomicroscopy greatly enhance the capability of estimating the therapeutic response to a topical retinoid (adapalene) in acne vulgaris. Cutis 2001;68(Suppl 4):25.
6. Strauss JS, Thiboutot DM. Diseases of the Sebaceous Glands. In: Freedberg IM et al, eds. Fitzpatrick's Dermatology in General Medicine. New York: McGraw-Hill, 1999:769.
7. Madden WS et al. Treatment of acne vulgaris and prevention of acne scarring: Canadian consensus guidelines. J Cutaneous Med Surg 2000;4(Suppl 1):S2.
8. Layton AM. Optimal management of acne to prevent scarring and psychological sequelae. Am J Clin Dermatol 2001;2:135.
9. Niemeier V et al. Coping with acne vulgaris: evaluation of the Chronic Skin Disorder Questionnaire in patients with acne. Dermatology 1998;196:108.
10. Layton AM et al. Scarred for life? Dermatology 1997;195(Suppl 1):15.
11. Strasburger VC. Acne: what every pediatrician should know about acne treatment. Pediatr Clin North Am 1998;44:1505.
12. Cunliffe WJ. Management of adult acne and acne variants. J Cutan Med Surg 1998;2(Suppl 3):7.
13. Campanati A et al. Pronounced and early acne in Apert's syndrome: a case successfully treated with oral isotretinoin. Eur J Dermatol. 2002;12:496.
14. Koh ET. Synovitis, acne, pustulosis, hyperostosis and osteitis (SAPHO) syndrome: a brief review of a rare condition. Ann Acad Med (Singapore) 1998; 27:122.
15. Cunliffe WJ, Simpson NB. Disorders of the sebaceous glands. In: Champion RH et al, eds. Textbook of Dermatology. Boston: Blackwell Scientific, 1998:1927.
16. Yu HJ et al. Steroid acne vs. *Pityrosporum* folliculitis: the incidence of *Pityrosporum ovale* and the effect of antifungal drugs in steroid acne. Int J Dermatol 1998;37:772.
17. Jansen T, Plewig G. Acne fulminans. Int J Dermatol 1998;37:254.
18. Kligman AM. Treating severe inflammatory acne: the last word. Cutis 1996;57:26.
19. White GM. Recent findings in the epidemiologic evidence, classification, and subtypes of acne vulgaris. J Am Acad Dermatol 1998;39(Suppl 2):S34.
20. AO Lucky AW. A review of infantile and pediatric acne. Dermatology 1998;196:95.
21. DeGroot HE, Friedlander SF. Update on acne. Curr Opin Pediatr 1998;10:381.
22. Fitzpatrick TB. Disorders of sebaceous and apocrine glands. In: Fitzpatrick TB et al, eds. Color Atlas and Synopsis of Clinical Dermatology: Common and Serious Diseases. New York: McGraw-Hill, 1997:4.
23. Swart E et al, eds. Skin conditions in epileptics. Clin Exp Dermatol 1992;17:169.
24. Oberemok SS et al. Acne vulgaris, I: pathogenesis and diagnosis. Cutis 2002;70:101.
25. Burkhart CG et al. Acne: a review of immunologic and microbiologic factors. Postgrad Med J 1999;75:328.
26. Landow K. Dispelling myths about acne. Postgrad Med 1997;102:94.
27. Litt JZ. Drug Eruption Reference Manual 2001: Derm. New York: Parthenon Publishing Group, 2001:373.
28. White IR. Plant products in perfumes and cosmetics. In: Lovel CR, ed. Plants and the Skin. Oxford: Blackwell, 1993:15.
29. Marks JG et al. Contact & Occupational Dermatology, 3rd Ed. St. Louis: Mosby, 2002:306.
30. Tirado JGO et al. Chloracne in the 1990s. Int J Dermatol 1996;35:643.
31. Plewig G, Jansen T. Acneiform dermatoses. Dermatology 1998;196:102.
32. Aldana OL et al. Variation in pilosebaceous duct keratinocyte proliferation in acne patients. Dermatology 1998;196:98.
33. Webster GF. Inflammation in acne vulgaris. J Am Acad Dermatol 1995;33:247.
34. Swerlick RA, Lawley TJ. Eczema, psoriasis, cutaneous infections, acne and other common skin disorders. In: Fauci AS et al, eds. Harrison's Principles of Internal Medicine, 14th Ed. New York: McGraw-Hill, 1998:298.
35. Paraskevaidis A et al. Polymorphisms in the human cytochrome P-450 1A1 gene (CYP1A1) as a factor for developing acne. Dermatology 1998; 196:171.
36. Stern RS. Medication and medical service utilization for acne 1995-1998. J Am Acad Dermatol 2000;43:1042.
37. Drake LA et al. Guidelines of care for acne vulgaris. J Am Acad Dermatol 1990;22:676.
38. Solish N et al. Approaches to acne scarring: a review. J Cutan Med Surg 1998;2(Suppl 3):24.
39. Jordan RE et al. Laser resurfacing for facial acne scars. Cochrane Database Syst Rev 1, 2003.
40. Liao DC. Management of acne. J Fam Pract 2003;52:48.
41. Weiss JS. Current options for the topical treatment of acne vulgaris. Pediatr Dermatol 1997;14:480.
42. Ives TJ. Benzoyl peroxide. Am Pharm 1992; 33:S32.
43. Hughes BR et al. A double-blind evaluation of topical isotretinoin 0.05%, benzoyl peroxide gel 5% and placebo in patients with acne. Clin Exp Dermatol 1992;17:165.
44. Chu A et al. The comparative efficacy of benzoyl peroxide 5%/erythromycin 3% gel and ery-

thromycin 4%/zinc 1.2% solution in the treatment of acne vulgaris. Br J Dermatol 1997;136:235.

45. Eady EA et al. The effects of acne treatment with a combination of benzoyl peroxide and erythromycin on skin carriage of erythromycin-resistant propionibacteria. Br J Dermatol 1996;134:107.

46. Brown RH et al. Treatment of acne vulgaris: combination of 3% erythromycin and 5% benzoyl peroxide in a gel compared to clindamycin phosphate lotion. Int J Dermatol 1996;35:209.

47. Kraus AL et al. Benzoyl peroxide: an integrated human safety assessment for carcinogenicity. Reg Toxicol Pharmacol 1995;21:87.

48. Straumfjord JV. Vitamin A: its effects in acne vulgaris. Northwest Med 1949;42:219.

49. Shalita A. The integral role of topical and oral retinoids in the early treatment of acne. J Eur Acad Derm Venereol 2001;3:43.

50. Shroot B et al. A new concept of drug delivery. Dermatology 1998;196:165.

51. Shroot B. Pharmacodynamics and pharmacokinetics of topical adapalene. J Am Acad Dermatol 1998;39:S17.

52. Brogden RN, Goa KL. Adapalene: a review of its pharmacological properties and clinical potential in the management of mild to moderate acne. Drugs 1997;53:511.

53. Weiss JS, Shavin JS. Adapalene for the treatment of acne vulgaris. J Am Acad Dermatol 1998;39:S50.

54. Nyirady J et al. A comparative trial of two retinoids commonly used in the treatment of acne vulgaris. J Dermatol Treatment 2001;12:149.

55. Leyden J et al. Comparison of treatment of acne vulgaris with alternate-day applications of tazarotene 0.1% gel and once-daily applications of adapalene 0.1% gel: a randomized trial. Cutis 2001;67(Suppl 6):10.

56. Saurat JH. Oral isotretinoin: where now, what next? Dermatology 1997;195(Suppl 1):1.

57. Lavker RM et al. An ultrastructural study of the effects of topical tretinoin on microcomedones. Clin Ther 1992;14:773.

58. Falcon RH et al. In vitro effect of isotretinoin on monocyte chemotaxis. J Invest Dermatol 1986;86:550.

59. Pigatto PD et al. Effects of isotretinoin on the neutrophil chemotaxis in cystic acne. Dermatologica 1983;167:16.

60. Gollnick H, Schramm M. Topical drug treatment in acne. Dermatology 1998;196:119.

61. Harris DWS et al. Topical retinoic acid in the treatment of fine acne scarring [Letter]. Br J Dermatol 1991;125:81.

63. Orfanos CE, Zouboulis CC. Oral retinoids in the treatment of seborrhea and acne. Dermatology 1998;196:140.

64. Lehucher-Ceyrac D, Weber-Buisset MJ. Isotretinoin and acne in practice: a prospective analysis of 188 cases over 9 years. Dermatology 1993;186:123.

65. Ortonne JP. Oral isotretinoin treatment policy: do we all agree? Dermatology 1997;195(Suppl 1):34.

66. Kauffman RE et al. Retinoid therapy for severe dermatological disorders. Pediatrics 1992;90:119.

67. Honein MA et al. Cost-effectiveness of oral isotretinoin. Dermatology 1999;198:404.

68. Saurat JH. Side effects of systemic retinoids and their clinical management. J Am Acad Dermatol 1992;27:S23.

69. Meigel WN. How safe is oral isotretinoin? Dermatology 1997;195(Suppl 1):22.

70. Shemer A et al. Azelaic acid (20%) cream in the treatment of acne vulgaris. J Eur Acad Dermatol Venereol 2002;16:178.

71. Fitton A, Goa KL. Azelaic acid: a review of its pharmacological properties and therapeutic efficacy in acne and hyperpigmentary skin disorders. Drugs 1991;41:780.

72. Nguyen QH, Bui TP. Azelaic acid: pharmacokinetic and pharmacodynamic properties and its therapeutic role in hyperpigmentary disorders and acne. Int J Dermatol 1995;34:75.

73. Hjorth N, Graupe K. Azelaic acid for the treatment of acne: a clinical comparison with oral tetracycline. Acta Venereol (Stockh) 1989;143(Suppl):45.

74. Webster G. Combination azelaic acid therapy for acne vulgaris. J Am Acad Dermatol 2000;43(Suppl 2 Pt 3):S47.

75. Spellman MC, Pincus SH. Efficacy and safety of azelaic acid and glycolic acid combination therapy compared with tretinoin therapy for acne. Clin Ther 1998;20:711.

76. Mills O et al. Bacterial resistance and therapeutic outcome following three months of topical acne therapy with 2% erythromycin gel versus its vehicle. Acta Dermato Venereol 2002;82:260.

77. Meynadier J, Alirezai M. Systemic antibiotics for acne. Dermatology 1998;196:135.

78. Fernandez-Obregon AC. Azithromycin for the treatment of acne. Int J Dermatol 1997;36:239.

79. Gruber F et al. Azithromycin compared with minocycline in the treatment of acne comedonica and papulo-pustulosa. J Chemotherapy 1998;10:469.

80. Nishijima S et al. The antibiotic susceptibility of Propionibacterium acnes and Staphylococcus epidermidis isolated from acne. J Dermatol 1994;21:166.

81. Cooper AJ. Systematic review of Propionibacterium acnes resistance to systemic antibiotics. MJA 1998;169:259.

82. Seukeran DC et al. Benefit-risk assessment of acne therapies [Letter]. Lancet 1997;349:1251.

83. Ross JI et al. Clinical resistance to erythromycin and clindamycin in cutaneous propionibacteria isolated from acne patients is associated with mutations in 23S rRNA. Antimicrob Agents Chemother 1997;41:1162.

84. Bojar RA et al. Direct analysis of resistance in the cutaneous microflora during treatment of acne vulgaris with topical 1% nadifloxacin and 2% erythromycin. Drugs 1995;49(Suppl 2):164.

85. Eady EA et al. Antibiotic resistant propionibacteria in acne: need for policies to modify antibiotic usage. Br Med J 1993;306:555.

86. Coates P et al. Does oral isotretinoin prevent Propionibacterium acnes resistance? Dermatology 1997;195(Suppl 1):4.

87. Eady EA et al. Topical antibiotics for the treatment of acne vulgaris: a critical evaluation of the literature and their clinical benefit and comparative efficacy. J Dermatol Treat 1990;1:215.

88. Toyoda M, Morohashi M. An overview of topical antibiotics for acne treatment. Dermatology 1998;196:130.

89. Burton J. A placebo-controlled study to evaluate the efficacy of topical tetracycline and oral tetracycline in the treatment of mild to moderate acne. J Int Med Res 1990;18:94.

90. Facklam DP et al. An epidemiologic postmarketing surveillance study of prescription acne medications. Am J Public Health 1990;80:50.

91. van Hoogdalem EJ et al. Transdermal absorption of clindamycin and tretinoin from topically applied anti-acne formulations in man. Biopharm Drug Dispos 1998;19:563.

92. Berson DS et al. The treatment of acne: the role of combination therapies. J Am Acad Dermatol 1995;32(Suppl 5):S31.

93. Lookingbill DP et al. Treatment of acne with a combination clindamycin/benzoyl peroxide gel compared with clindamycin gel, benzoyl peroxide gel, and vehicle gel: combined results of two double-blind investigations. J Am Acad Dermatol 1997;37:590.

94. Leyden JJ et al. The efficacy and safety of a combination benzoyl peroxide/clindamycin topical gel compared with benzoyl peroxide alone and a benzoyl peroxide/erythromycin combination product. J Cutan Med Surg 2001;5:37.

95. Gupta AK et al. A randomized, double-blind, multicenter, parallel group study to compare relative efficacies of the topical gels 3% erythromycin/5% benzoyl peroxide and 0.025% tretinoin/erythromycin 4% in the treatment of moderate acne vulgaris of the face. J Cutan Med Surg 2003;7:31.

96. Food and Drug Administration. Topical acne products for over-the-counter human use-final monograph. Fed Regist 1991;56:41008.

97. Shalita AR. Comparison of a salicylic acid cleanser and a benzoyl peroxide wash in the treatment of acne vulgaris. Clin Ther 1989;11:264.

98. Zander E, Weisman S. Treatment of acne vulgaris with salicylic acid pads. Clin Ther 1992;14:247.

99. Billow JA. Acne products. In: Covington TR, ed. Handbook of Nonprescription Drugs. Washington, DC: American Pharmaceutical Association, 1996:569.

100. Lin AN et al. Sulfur revisited. J Am Acad Dermatol 1988;18:553.

101. Breneman DL, Ariano MC. Successful treatment of acne vulgaris in women with a new topical sodium sulfacetamide/sulfur lotion. Int J Dermatol 1993;32:365.

102. Mills OH, Kligman AM. Drugs that are ineffective in the treatment of acne vulgaris. Br J Dermatol 1983;108:371.

103. Parish LC et al. Topical nicotinamide compared with clindamycin gel in the treatment of inflammatory acne vulgaris. Int J Dermatol 1995;34:434.

104. Dreno B et al. Zinc salts effects on granulocyte zinc concentration and chemotaxis in acne patients. Acta Derm Venereol (Stockh) 1992;72:250.

105. Stamatiadis D et al. Inhibition of 5a-reductase by zinc and azelaic acid. Br J Dermatol 1988;119:627.

106. Shaw JC. Antiandrogen and hormonal treatment of acne. Dermatol Clin 1996;14:803.

107. Schmidt JB. Other antiandrogens. Dermatology 1998;196:153.

108. Shaw JC. Low-dose adjunctive spironolactone in the treatment of acne in women: a retrospective analysis of 85 consecutively treated patients. J Am Acad Dermatol 2000;43:498.

109. Gilliam M et al. Acne treatment with a low-dose oral contraceptive. Obstet Gynecol 2001;97(4):S9.

110. Farquhar C et al. Spironolactone versus placebo or in combination with steroids for hirsutism and/or acne. Cochrane Database Syst Rev 1, 2003.

111. Van Vloten WA et al. The effect of 2 combined oral contraceptives containing either drospirenone or cyproterone acetate on acne and seborrhea. Cutis 2002;69(Suppl 4):2.

112. Leyden J et al. Efficacy of a low-dose oral contraceptive containing 20 micrograms of ethinyl estradiol and 100 micrograms of levonorgestrel for the treatment of moderate acne: a randomized, placebo-controlled trial. J Am Acad Dermatol. 2002;47:399.

113. Ortho-McNeil. Ortho Tri-Cyclen package insert. Raritan, NJ: 2001 March.

114. Jemec GB et al. Have oral contraceptives reduced the prevalence of acne? A population-based study of acne vulgaris, tobacco smoking, and oral contraceptives. Dermatology 2002;204:179.

115. Brown SK, Shalita AR. Acne vulgaris. Lancet 1998;351:1871.

116. Gollnick HP et al. Topical treatment in acne: current status and future aspects. Dermatology 2003;206:29.

117. Garner SE et al. Minocycline for acne. Cochrane Database Syst Rev 1, 2003.

118. Meyer FP. Minocycline for acne. Food reduces minocycline's bioavailability [Letter]. 1996;312:1101.

119. Bodokh I et al. Minocycline induces an increase in the number of excreting pilosebaceous follicles in acne vulgaris. Acta Derm Venereol (Stockh) 1997;77:255.

120. Chosidow O et al. Comedonal diffusion of minocycline in acne. Dermatology 1998;196:162.

121. Eady EA et al. Tetracycline-resistant propionibacteria from acne patients are cross-resistant to doxycycline, but sensitive to minocycline. Br J Dermatol 1993;128:556.

122. Shubin JA. Minocycline vs. tetracycline [Letter]. J Fam Pract 1995;41:538.

123. Ferner RE, Moss C. Minocycline for acne [Letter]. BMJ 1996;312:138.

124. Goulden V et al. Safety of long-term high-dose minocycline in the treatment of acne. Br J Dermatol 1996;134:693.

125. Colvin JH et al. Minocycline hypersensitivity syndrome with hypotension mimicking septic shock. Pediatr Dermatol 2001;18:295.

126. Driscoll MS et al. Long-term oral antibiotics for acne: is laboratory monitoring necessary. J Am Acad Dermatol 1993;28:595.

127. Quigley JW, Bucks DAW. Reduced skin irritation with tretinoin containing polyolprepolymer-2, a new topical delivery system: a summary of pre-clinical and clinical investigations. J Am Acad Dermatol 1998;38:S5.

128. Ortho Pharmaceuticals. Retin-A Micro package insert. Raritan, NJ: 2002 May.

129. Webster GF. Topical tretinoin in acne therapy. J Am Acad Dermatol 1998;39:S38.

130. Ruiz-Maldonado R et al. The use of retinoids in the pediatric patient. Dermatol Clin 1998;16:553.

131. Roche Laboratories. Accutane package insert. Nutley, NJ: 2002 June.

132. Ng CH et al. Prospective study of depressive symptoms and quality of life in acne vulgaris patients treated with isotretinoin compared to antibiotic and topical therapy. Aust J Dermatol 2002;43:262.

133. Jick H. Retinoids and teratogenicity. J Am Acad Dermatol 1998;39:S118.

134. Koren G, Pastuszak A. How to ensure fetal safety when mothers use isotretinoin (Accutane). Can Fam Phys 1997;43:216.

135. Moskop JC et al. Ethical and legal aspects of teratogenic medications: the case of isotretinoin. J Clin Ethics 1997;8:264.

136. Wiegand UW, Chou RC. Pharmacokinetics of oral isotretinoin. J Am Acad Dermatol 1998;39:S8.

137. Milstone AM et al. Is retinoid-induced osteopenia reversible? Arch Dermatol. 2002;138:1516.

138. Almond-Roesler B et al. Monitoring of isotretinoin therapy by measuring the plasma levels of isotretinoin and 4-oxo-isotretinoin: a useful tool for management of severe acne. Dermatology 1998;196:176.

Psoriasis

Allan Ellsworth

Epidemiology

Psoriasis, a chronic, proliferative skin disease characterized by sharply defined, erythematous plaques covered with a distinctive silvery scale, occurs in 0.1% to 3% of the population worldwide.[1] All races are affected with the disease, but it is most common in northern Europeans and Scandinavians.[1] Seventy-five percent of patients present with symptoms of psoriasis before the age of 40 years.[2] Men and women are affected equally.[2] A family history of psoriasis is found in nearly half of patients. There does not appear to be a single major chromosomal locus for psoriasis.[3-5] Psoriasis has a strong association with the major histocompatibility complexes HLA-B and HLA-C (human leukocyte antigens).[3,5] The most significant association is with HLA Cw6, in which the likelihood of developing psoriasis can be 6 to 15 times normal. However, this antigen does not fully explain psoriasis: the disease is believed to be polygenic with a variable and irregular penetrance, and the expression is in part dependent on other external factors.[3,5]

Pathogenesis

The preponderance of evidence supports an autoimmune mechanism for psoriasis, mediated by T lymphocytes. This conclusion is based on finding T lymphocytes in early plaque infiltrates, the association with HLA antigens, the observation that anti–T-lymphocyte therapy clears the disease (as does bone marrow transplantation from a normal donor) and that purified CD4+ cells isolated from the peripheral blood of patients with psoriasis induce lesions on a nonpsoriatic skin grafts.[4,6,7] Pathogenesis involves vascular and inflammatory changes, which precede epidermal changes. The alterations in the dermal vasculature also appear to be a result of angiogenesis, similar to a number of other disease processes, including tumor growth. Many commonly used therapeutic agents for psoriasis have antiangiogenic activity.[1]

The epidermal changes of psoriasis are based on the time required for affected epidermal cells to travel to the surface and be cast off, which is markedly reduced (3 to 4 days versus normal cells, which take 26 to 28 days)[8] This sixfold to ninefold transit time decrease does not allow the normal events of cell maturation and keratinization to take place and is reflected clinically as diffuse scaling. T cells contribute to this keratinocyte hyperproliferation through the secretion of various growth factors.[9,10]

Although the precise cellular pathogenesis of psoriasis still has not been fully delineated, a model consistent with the immune-surveillance paradigm has been proposed. Memory T lymphocytes (marked with cutaneous lymphocyte antigen [CLA] to remember the anatomic site where they first encountered antigen) are recruited to skin by a number of immunologic and inflammatory triggering mechanisms released from keratinocytes after minor trauma. On entry into skin, these T cells complex with epidermal self-antigens presented by major histocompatibility complex molecules that confer the risk of psoriasis. The subsequent release of T-cell cytokines results in further inflammation, the recruitment of additional marked T cells, and ultimately the development of psoriatic lesions in susceptible persons.[6,10] The prevalence of psoriasis on the elbows, knees, and other sites of repetitive trauma is consistent with this model, as is the association of acute exacerbations of psoriasis with bacterial and fungal skin infections.

Signs and Symptoms

Most psoriatic lesions are asymptomatic, but not always. Pruritus, for example, is noted in 20% of patients. The primary psoriatic lesion is a relapsing eruption of scaling papules that rapidly coalesce or enlarge to form circumscribed, erythematous, scaly, plaques. The scale is adherent, silvery white, and reveals bleeding points when removed (called *Auspitz's sign*). Scales may become extremely dense on the scalp or macerated and dispersed in intertriginous areas.

Lesions of active psoriasis can develop at the site of epidermal trauma (*Kobner's phenomenon*). Scratch marks, sunburn, or surgical wounds may heal, leaving psoriatic lesions in their place. The elbows, knees, scalp, gluteal cleft, fingernails, and toenails are favored areas of involvement. Extensor surfaces are affected more than the flexor surfaces, and the disease usually spares the palms, soles, and face. Nail beds may show punctate pitting or profuse collections of keratotic material. A yellow-brown subungual discoloration ("oil spot") is characteristic, as are onycholysis and subungual debris. Psoriatic arthritis occurs in approximately 5% to 31% of all patients with psoriasis, with combined features of both rheumatoid arthritis and the seronegative spondyloarthropathies.[11,12]

Most patients (90%) have chronic localized disease (plaque-type or *psoriasis vulgaris*), but there are several other presentations. The most severe form of the disease is *erythrodermic psoriasis*, which describes a condition of acute inflammatory erythema and scales involving >90% of body surface area. *Pustular psoriasis* is generally localized to palms and soles, but there is also a generalized version. Both generalized *pustular psoriasis* and *erythrodermic psoriasis* can be accompanied by systemic symptoms (hyperthermia, tachycardia, edema, dehydration, shortness of breath) and can have life-threatening consequences (hypovolemia, electrolyte imbalance, septicemia) if not promptly treated appropriately.[13] *Guttate psoriasis* describes small, scaly, erythematous spots of psoriasis (classically following β-hemolytic streptococcal pharyngitis). *Flexural* or *inverse psoriasis* lacks scales and looks like intertrigo.

Prognosis

Psoriasis is lifelong and characterized by chronic recurrent exacerbations and remissions that are generally more emotionally than physically disabling ("the heartbreak of psoriasis").[14] Therefore, even when a patient has only a few asymptomatic chronic plaques, the disease can be more serious than it appears.[15] It is important to emphasize that psoriasis is a treatable disease. Optimism and encouragement are justified and make it easier for the patient to conscientiously apply sometimes awkward and messy topical treatments or take potentially toxic medications. The goal of therapy should be to achieve complete clearing of psoriatic lesions, particularly during emotionally critical times, such as the commencement of school, puberty, and the summer months. The Self-Administered Psoriasis Area and Severity Index (PASI) is a validated, structured instrument that can be used for patient assessment of the severity of psoriasis and response to therapy. It closely correlates with the standard clinician assessment instrument, Psoriasis Area and Severity Index (PASI), which includes quantification of the percentage of body involvement and severity of lesions.[16] The National Psoriasis Foundation (www.psoriasis.org) is an organization that can provide psychosocial support as well as information on treatment options to both patients and providers.[17]

TOPICAL DRUG THERAPY

Many topical and systemic therapeutic agents are available, varying from simple topical emollients to systemic, highly potent, immunosuppressant drugs for more recalcitrant conditions. Treatment modalities are chosen on the basis of disease severity, patient preference (including cost and convenience), and response. Patients with limited disease can generally be managed with topical therapy (Table 40-1). Patients with psoriasis covering >20% of the body need more specialized systemic treatment programs (Table 40-2).

Topical Corticosteroids

Topical corticosteroids are effective in the treatment of psoriasis because of their anti-inflammatory, antimitotic, immunosuppressant and antipruritic properties.[18–20] These properties are explained by a reduction in phospholipase A$_2$, DNA synthesis, and epidermal mitotic activity, as well as their vasoconstrictive actions.[18–20] They provide prompt relief, and patients find them convenient and acceptable, but expensive at times. Tachyphylaxis occurs, and long-term use after skin has returned to a normalized state leads to typical corticosteroid side effects (atrophy, telangiectasia, and striae). Thin-skinned areas (facial and intertriginous) are particularly susceptible. Psoriasis is generally a corticosteroid-resistant disease; therefore, the more potent corticosteroids are frequently necessary, with occlusion, for best results. (See Table 38-8 in Chapter 38, Dermatotherapy and Drug Induced Skin Disorders, for a listing of topical corticosteroids by potency.) Less potent agents are more appropriate in intertriginous areas, on the face, and for maintenance. Potent corticosteroids clear psoriasis in 25% of patients in 3 to 4 weeks, with 75% clearing in 50% of treated patients.[20]

Intermittent dosing or "pulse therapy" seems to yield the best long-term results and minimizes tachyphylaxis and adverse effects. An additional drawback of chronic corticosteroid therapy is an associated acute flare-up of psoriasis when corticosteroid therapy is terminated.[19] Hence, continuous application for >3 to 4 weeks should be discouraged in patients with psoriasis, and systemic corticosteroids have no place in therapy.[20,21] Topical corticosteroids occasionally can cause a reversible suppression of the hypothalamic-pituitary-adrenal (HPA) axis, as indicated by a decrease in the morning plasma cortisol level.[21] For anything more extensive than mild disease, topical corticosteroids are best used in an adjunctive role. During a flare-up, steroids help reduce inflammation, redness, and irritation and prepare the involved area for initiation of other potentially irritating, but more appropriate, maintenance topical treatments such as coal tar, anthralin, calcipotriene, or tazarotene.

Coal Tar

Crude coal tar is a complex mixture of thousands of hydrocarbon compounds.[19] It is a time honored modality for treating psoriasis. It affects psoriasis by enzyme inhibition and antimitotic action (antiproliferative and anti-inflammatory).[19] The efficacy of the combination of tar and ultraviolet B (UVB) light (i.e., Goeckerman regimen) led to tar's increased popularity beginning in the 1920s. Tar preparations of 2% to 10% are processed as creams, ointments, lotions, gels, oils,

Table 40-1   Topical Agents for the Treatment of Psoriasis (Mild to Moderate)[a]

Treatment Modality	Advantages	Disadvantages
Emollients	Basic adjunct for all treatments; safe, inexpensive, reduces scaling, itching, and related discomfort	Provides minimal relief alone
Keratolytics (salicylic acid, urea, α-hydroxy acids [i.e., glycolic and lactic acids])	Reduce hyperkeratosis; enable other topical modalities to better penetrate; inexpensive	Provide minimal relief individually; nonspecific; salicylism (tinnitus, nausea, vomiting) with salicylic acid if applied extensively
Topical corticosteroids	Rapid response; control inflammation and itching; best for intertriginous areas and face; convenient, not messy; mainstay topical treatment modality for psoriasis; cost varies widely (generics less expensive)	Temporary relief; less effective with continued use (tachyphylaxis occurs); withdrawal can produce flares; atrophy, telangiectasia, and striae with continued use after skin returns to normalized state; expensive; adrenal suppression possible
Coal tar	Particularly effective for "flaky" scalp lesions; new preparations "pleasant"; efficacy enhanced in combination with UVB (i.e., Goeckerman regimen); moderately priced	Effective only for mild psoriasis or scalp psoriasis; inconvenient—difficult to apply; stains clothing and bedding, not skin; strong smelling; folliculitis and contact allergy (bronchospasm in atopic patient with asthma after inhalation of vapor); carcinogenic in animals
Anthralin (dithranol in the United Kingdom)	Effective for widespread, refractory plaques; produces long remissions; short, concentrated programs preferred; enhanced efficacy in combination with UVB (i.e., Ingram regimen)	Purple-brown staining (skin, clothing, and bath fitments); irritating to normal skin and flexures; careful application required (inpatient?); can precipitate generalized psoriasis
Calcipotriene	As effective as topical corticosteroids, although slower onset, without long-term corticosteroid side effects; convenient, well tolerated	Slow onset; expensive; potential effects on bone metabolism (hypercalcemia); irritant dermatitis on face and intertriginous areas; contraindicated during pregnancy; more expensive than corticosteroids
Tazarotene	Extended response; convenient (QD, gel); maintenance therapy; effective on scalp and face; used in combination with topical corticosteroids	Slow onset; local irritation and pruritus; teratogenic (adequate birth control required)
UVB	Effective as maintenance therapy; eliminates problems of topical steroids	Expensive (insurance reimburses); office-based therapy; sunburn (exacerbates psoriasis); photoaging; skin cancer

[a] <20% body involvement.
UVB, ultraviolet B.

Table 40-2   Agents for the Treatment of Severe Psoriasis[a]

Treatment Modality	Advantages	Disadvantages
UVA and psoralen (PUVA)	80% efficacy; "sun tan" cosmetically desirable	Time consuming; expensive, office-based therapy (restrictive); sunburn (exacerbates psoriasis); photoaging; both nonmelanoma skin cancer and melanoma; contraindicated during pregnancy and lactation
Acitretin	Not as effective as other systemic agents; efficacy enhanced if given with PUVA or UVB (i.e., RePUVA or ReUVB); less hepatotoxic than methotrexate	Teratogenic (adequate birth control required); contraindicated with liver or renal dysfunction, drug or alcohol abuse, hypertriglyceridemia, hypervitaminosis A
Methotrexate	Gold standard for efficacy; effective for both skin lesions and arthritis as well as psoriatic nail disease	Hepatotoxicity (periodic liver biopsy?); bone marrow toxicity; folic acid protects against stomatitis (not against hepatic or pulmonary toxicity); drug interactions; contraindicated during pregnancy and lactation, drug or alcohol abuse; caution during acute infections
Cyclosporine	Toxicity reputation and short-lived remissions have relegated use to extensive disease—not responsive to other agents; however, given changing pathophysiology and increasing experience at lower dosages, role in therapy changing; increasing role in rotational therapy to induce remissions	Renal impairment; suppressive therapy (relapse occurs when discontinued); increased risk of skin cancer, lymphomas and solid tumors; phototoxic; contraindicated during pregnancy and lactation, and with hypertension, hyperuricemia, hyperkalemia, acute infections
Immunomodulatory drugs (alefacept, efalizumab, etanercept, infliximab)	Specific, targeted therapy; effective for moderate-severe both skin lesions and arthritis; maintains remission	Expensive; parenteral (often office-based) therapy; long term safety unknown; increased risk of serious infections

[a] >20% body involvement.
UVA, ultraviolet A; UVB, ultraviolet B.

shampoos, and coal tar solution (liquor carbonis detergens). Newer purified preparations, using refined coal tar, are less messy and more acceptable, but perhaps not as effective.[19] Tar may be helpful for patients with mild to moderate disease, and tar shampoos are useful for psoriasis of the scalp. Overall, the potential severity of side effects from tars is less than that from anthralin and much less than that from topical steroids. However, because tar, in every form, is messy, stains the skin, and has an odor, it has been relegated to second-line therapy for most patients, despite its moderate price.[22]

Tar preparations generally are used once or twice daily, and bedtime application (as a shampoo or cream overnight) is particularly useful in psoriasis of the scalp and overcomes some of the negative cosmetic bias. Patients should be warned about the staining properties of tar on clothing and bedding. Other side effects include photosensitivity, acneiform eruptions, folliculitis, and irritation dermatitis. Care should be taken to avoid use of tar on the face, flexures, and genitalia and with inflammatory psoriasis because of tar's irritant properties.

The polyaromatic hydrocarbons contained in coal tar may be metabolized to active carcinogens by epidermal microsomal enzymes. The incidence of hyperkeratotic lesions, including squamous-cell carcinomas, is increased after prolonged industrial exposure to tar; however, extensive reviews of patients who have used tar preparations in psoriasis have not noted an increased risk of carcinoma.[23]

Anthralin (Dithranol)

Anthralin (dithranol in the United Kingdom), a hydroxyanthrone derivative, inhibits DNA synthesis, mitotic activity, and a variety of enzymes crucial to reducing cell proliferation.[18,20] It is effective for treatment of widespread, discrete psoriatic plaques. When applied as a stiff paste (anthralin in Lassar's paste) overnight and used in conjunction with coal tar baths and UV light (i.e., Ingram regimen), anthralin is still the standard inpatient treatment regimen in the United Kingdom (although less popular in the United States). Most cases of chronic plaque psoriasis clear in 3 weeks. The primary disadvantages of anthralin are its irritant and staining properties to skin and clothing. Anthralin also can precipitate generalized psoriasis if applied to unstable psoriasis (i.e., plaque transformation to pustular form).

The standard anthralin regimen involves liberal application of gradually increasing concentrations (0.1% to 0.2% up to no more than 3% to 5%) for 8 to 12 hours (often overnight), depending on degree of irritation and clinical response. To minimize brownish to purplish staining (of hair, skin, clothing, and bedding), plastic gloves should be used as well as old sheets and bedclothes. Contact with the face, eyes, mucous membranes, and nonpsoriatic skin should be avoided because of irritant properties. Application of petrolatum ointment around the psoriatic lesion prevents perilesional irritation.[19] Removal of the anthralin application is facilitated with a bath (often containing coal tar) or mineral oil in the morning. A steroid cream may be used during the day.

Alternative, shorter contact (10 to 60 minutes twice daily) regimens (e.g., SCAT, short-contact anthralin therapy) have been developed to minimize application time and staining.

These SCAT regimens are most appropriate for the outpatient setting.[19,20,24] Higher concentrations of anthralin are used in the shorter-contact regimens and irritation is more of a problem. Both methods are used daily for clearing of psoriasis, then once or twice weekly for maintenance therapy. Short-course regimens clear 32% of lesions and produce >75% improvement in 50% of patients after 5 weeks. These regimens are comparable in effectiveness to the Ingram regimen and topical corticosteroids are associated with fewer side effects.[20,24]

Calcipotriene (Calcipotriol)

Calcipotriene (calcipotriol in Europe), a topical vitamin D_3 analog that suppresses keratinocyte proliferation and that has anti-inflammatory effects,[25–27] can be applied twice daily as a cream, ointment, or solution. Although systemic absorption is small and the vitamin D effects of calcipotriene on calcium and bone metabolism are about 100 to 200 times less that that of 1,25-dihydroxyvitamin D_3, calcium serum levels and urine calcium excretion should be monitored to prevent serious effects on calcium and bone metabolism. Other adverse effects of calcipotriene include lesional and perilesional irritation, burning, stinging, pruritus, erythema, and scaling, especially in facial and intertriginous areas.[18,25] About 30% of patients using calcipotriene develop skin irritation.[28]

Most patients see improvement, although not clearing, of psoriatic plaques when treated with calcipotriene.[18] Of treated patients, 57% experience >75% clearance of psoriatic plaques, which is comparable to that achieved with corticosteroids (albeit slower in onset and associated with more dermal irritation).[19,20,28,29] Tachyphylaxis has not been a problem.[25,30]

Tazarotene

Tazarotene is a novel, topically applied, synthetic retinoid that is rapidly converted to its biologically active metabolite, tazarotenic acid.[31] By interacting with the predominant retinoid receptors on the skin surface regulating gene transcription, the retinoic acids normalize abnormal keratinocyte differentiation, reduce hyperproliferation, and decrease inflammation associated with psoriasis.[31] Treatment success rates compare favorably with corticosteroids (52% clearing of all lesions; 70% clearing of trunk and limb lesions). The antipsoriatic effects of tazarotene are sustained for a longer period after treatment compared with corticosteroids.[20,32,33] Because local skin irritation and pruritus are common side effects of tazarotene use, combination therapy with corticosteroids not only provides additive antipsoriatic effects, but also reduces retinoid-induced irritation.[34] Oral retinoids are known teratogens, but teratogenicity has not been observed from topically applied retinoids in animal studies. Women, however, should be warned of potential risk and the need to use adequate contraception.[31,32]

PHOTOTHERAPY
Ultraviolet B

UVB light (sunburn spectrum, 290 to 320 nm) induces pyrimidine dimers, inhibits DNA synthesis, and depletes intraepidermal T cells found in psoriatic epidermis (i.e., UVB has antiproliferative and local immunologic effects).[18] UVB light, unlike ultraviolet A (UVA) light, is effective without additional sensitizers (i.e., psoralens). UVB therapy is generally considered pleasant to use and relatively nontoxic. Heat and humidity from sunlight provide additional positive effects. Aggressive UVB phototherapy may be the most rapid and effective single-agent regimen for clearing psoriasis. Typically, 60% of patients with chronic plaque psoriasis experience clearing, and an additional 34% achieve 75% clearance with treatment for 7 to 8 weeks.[20]

UVB treatments are administered three times weekly. Pretreatment removal of scales improves efficacy by decreasing the reflectance characteristics of psoriatic scale, thereby increasing light transmission into psoriatic skin. However, use of pretreatment emollients (e.g., petrolatum, mineral or "baby" oil, Eucerin) applied before UV exposure, long thought to improve results, actually inhibit the penetration of UV and should not be used.[35] After the skin clears, therapy is discontinued gradually over 2 to 4 months to prolong remissions. The risks of ultraviolet radiation and sunlight are similar: sunburn, photoaging, and skin cancer.

Regimens combining UVB with anthralin (Ingram regimen) or tar (Goeckerman regimen) have been used for years, theoretically, taking advantage of the photosensitizing properties of tar and anthralin. The Goeckerman regimen involves daily application of coal tar and exposure to UV light. The Ingram regimen combines daily application of anthralin plus tar baths with exposure to UVB light.[20] Both the Goeckerman and Ingram regimens can clear widespread psoriasis in 3 to 4 weeks, induce remissions that last for weeks to months, and may reduce the long-term adverse effects of UVB exposure.[20]

A recent development in UVB therapy involves use of a high-energy 308-nm excimer laser. Laser treatment allows exposure of only involved skin, thus higher doses of UVB can be administered during a given treatment. After only 10 twice-weekly treatments, 84% and 50% of patients achieved 75% or better and 90% or better clearing of plaques, respectively. Side effects include erythema and blistering, but are generally well tolerated.[36]

Photochemotherapy

Photochemotherapy combines psoralens with UVA light (PUVA) in the 320 to 400 nm spectrum. The psoralens (methoxsalen, 5-methoxypsoralen, and trioxsalen) are a group of photoactive compounds that upon absorption of UV light, are both antiproliferative and immunomodulatory. When photoactivated by UVA, psoralens form monofunctional adducts and crosslinks with pyrimidine bases. PUVA also inhibits cytokine release and depletes both epidermal and dermal T cells. As measured by extent of T-cell depletion and decreases in delayed hypersensitivity, PUVA has greater immunomodulatory effects in the skin than UVB.[18] Remissions are longer in duration than with UVB. Psoralens are not active without UVA.

Photochemotherapy is used to control severe, recalcitrant, disabling plaque psoriasis. After 10 to 20 treatments over 4 to 8 weeks, >80% of patients experience clearing of symptoms, which can be maintained with periodic (twice monthly) treatments.[20] UVA penetrates the skin more deeply than UVB and

may have marked effects on the dermis. The use of PUVA requires careful consideration and adherence to strict photoprotective measures. Patients unwilling to adhere to PUVA-related precautions may prefer UVB treatment because it is much less restrictive.

The peak range for UVA light's therapeutic action is between 320 and 335 nm. 8-Methoxypsoralen is the most widely used agent, taken at a dosage of 0.6 to 0.8 mg/kg of body weight, 1.25 to 1.5 hours before exposure to UVA light. The initial dose is selected based on the patient's skin type (i.e., ease of sunburn and inherent skin color).

Acute phototoxic side effects, such as erythema and blistering, are dose related and, therefore, controllable. Other acute side effects include nausea, lethargy, headaches, pruritus, and hyperpigmentation. Topical steroid therapy should be continued until the psoriasis is brought under control. If topical steroids are discontinued at the start of PUVA, an exacerbation of psoriasis usually occurs. Patients should wear protective clothing (with long sleeves and high necklines), use sunscreens that filter out both UVA and UVB, and wear sunglasses that block UVA after PUVA (see Chapter 41, Photosensitivity and Burns). Because methoxsalen has a short half-life and 80% is eliminated within 6 to 8 hours, physical barriers are most important during the 8 hours immediately following PUVA therapy.

Of greater concern are the potential long-term side effects: mutagenicity, carcinogenicity, and cataract formation. Squamous-cell carcinoma has been associated with cumulative PUVA treatments (11-fold increase in patients who receive >260 treatments compared with patients who received <160 treatments).[20] Male patients have an increased risk of developing genital squamous-cell carcinoma.[20] More controversial is the relationship of exposure to PUVA and the risk of malignant melanoma. At present, there appears to be a dose-dependent increase in the risk of melanoma associated with high-dose exposure to PUVA. The risk is first manifested ≥15 years after initial exposure to PUVA.[37–39] Long-term maintenance and high cumulative dosages should be avoided. Shielding the face and genitalia during treatment and performing annual examinations to detect skin cancer at an early stage may lessen the risk of long-term adverse effects of photochemotherapy (Table 40-3).

Table 40-3 Measures to Reduce the Toxicity of Photochemotherapy

Minimize long-term maintenance treatment and cumulative dosages of radiation (approximately 200 treatments or a total UVA dose of 1,200 j/cm² is threshold for development of skin cancer).
Shield face and male genitalia during treatment.
Perform examinations to detect skin cancer at an early age.
Instruct patient to use sunscreen, protective clothing, and sunglasses.
Use rotational therapy (i.e., alternating monotherapies, allowing extended intervals off PUVA to allow skin recuperation before repeat exposure).
Use combination therapy (i.e., RePUVA) to reduce phototherapy dosage with superior efficacy.[40]

PUVA, psoralens with UVA light; RePUVA, retinoids plus psoralens with UVA light.

Topical psoralens are extremely photosensitizing, hence difficult to administer. However, application of methoxsalen 0.1% followed by small UVA doses (i.e., ≤20% of the level of usual doses for oral PUVA) has been used to treat localized areas and to prevent gastrointestinal side effects.[20]

SYSTEMIC THERAPY
Acitretin

Second-generation systemic retinoids are effective for treatment of recalcitrant psoriatic disease. Antipsoriatic effects stem from the drug's ability to modulate epidermal differentiation and immunologic function in addition to an antiinflammatory action.[41] This latter effect may alleviate the arthritis that accompanies psoriasis.[18,41] Acitretin is the principle metabolite of etretinate. It is less lipophilic, has a considerably shorter half-life (50 hours versus 120 days),[41] and appears to have a more favorable side effect profile. (Etretinate has been removed from the U.S. market.) However, patients taking retinoids should still be monitored closely (Table 40-4).

Systemic retinoids are not as effective in psoriasis as other systemic agents. Acitretin 50 mg/day completely cleared psoriatic plaques in 11% of patients and provided >75% clearance in 40% of patients treated for 8 to 12 weeks.[20] However, when combined with PUVA (RePUVA) or UVB (ReUVB) phototherapy (about 50% of usual phototherapy dose), the oral retinoids are highly effective, resulting in superior clinical efficacy. Acitretin 30 to 35 mg/day with UVB cleared psoriatic plaques in 55% of patients and provided >75% improvement in an additional 20% of patients treated for 6 to 8 weeks.[20,40] Acitretin is indicated for patients who have received extensive radiation with PUVA, pretreatment for PUVA (1 to 3 weeks) to accelerate the response rate, for patients who fail to respond to UVB with anthralin or tar, or for patients who are not candidates for methotrexate. Liver biopsy is not a routine part of etretinate therapy.[42] Most patients require maintenance or intermittent therapy to prevent relapses.[42]

Numerous other side effects are associated with acitretin use, including hypervitaminosis A syndrome (i.e., dry skin, skin thinning and fragility, chapped lips, dry nasal mucosa, skin peeling, alopecia, and nail dystrophy), retinoid rash, extraspinal tendon and ligament calcification and bone changes in children, hyperlipidemia with elevated levels of serum triglycerides and cholesterol, and liver enzyme alteration and hepatitis.[43,44]

Many patients find the side effects to the retinoids intolerable and discontinue treatment. Topical steroids can reduce some of the cutaneous retinoid side effects. Retinoids are teratogens. With continued therapy, retinoids accumulate in adipose tissue and the liver and may be detectable in serum for >2 years after discontinuation of therapy. Appropriately, pregnancy should be avoided after treatment with acitreton for three years.[43]

Immunosuppressive Agents

Methotrexate

Methotrexate (MTX), a folic acid analog, inhibits dihydrofolate reductase needed for synthesis of several amino acids, pyrimidines, purines, and subsequently DNA, RNA, and protein synthesis. MTX therapy greatly suppresses rapidly proliferating cells, such as those in psoriatic skin. Antipsoriatic mechanisms of MTX action include inhibition of keratinocyte differentiation and immunomodulation by destruction of lymphoid cells.[18,20]

Unlike other cytotoxic drugs, MTX produces antipsoriatic effects at dosages that are much lower than those used in cancer chemotherapy. Methotrexate in 10- to 25-mg weekly doses cleared psoriatic plaques in 50% of patients treated for 3 to 4 weeks and resulted in >75% improvement in an additional 40% of patients. Prolonged remissions are expected with continued therapy.[20] MTX is relatively safe and well tolerated, but the long-term concerns for hepatotoxicity (fibrosis and cirrhosis) and the need for periodic liver biopsies discourages many patients and physicians from using it.[45] Alcohol and methotrexate are a particularly potent hepatotoxic combination. Patients

Table 40-4 Acitretin Therapy: Patient Monitoring

Type of Evaluation	Comments
Clinical evaluation (Psoriasis Area and Severity Index [PASI] score,[16] which includes the percentage of body involvement and severity of lesions)	Performed twice in first month, monthly for 6 mo, and Q 3 mo thereafter
Laboratory testing (CBC, UA, fasting glucose, renal function tests, calcium; children: calcium and phosphorus in blood and urine, vitamin D metabolism, osteocalcin, and parathyroid hormone)	Performed at each visit during first year and twice yearly thereafter *Children:* performed Q 6 mo
Liver function tests	Performed monthly for first 6 months, then Q 3 mo
Fasting lipids	Performed monthly for first 4 months, then every 2–3 months; stop acitretin if serum triglycerides >800 mg/dL to reduce risk of pancreatitis
Pregnancy test	Performed before, monthly during, and effective contraception for at least 3 yr after therapy
Radiographs	*Adults:* yearly radiograph monitoring if >40 years for vertebral abnormalities *Children:* yearly radiographic monitoring for long-term (>0.5 yr) treatment

CBC, complete blood count; UA, urinalysis.
Adapted from references 15 and 40–42.

with psoriasis receiving MTX have a 2.5- to 5-fold higher incidence of advanced liver changes than patients with rheumatoid arthritis receiving comparable regimens.[46] Methotrexate hepatotoxicity may be related to both cumulative doses and constant blood levels. Daily administration has been replaced by weekly dosage schedules for this reason. Liver surveillance chemistry tests (i.e., serum alanine aminotransferase [ALT], serum aspartate aminotransferase [AST], serum albumin, bilirubin) can be within the "normal" range even in the presence of methotrexate-induced liver disease.[45,46] Therefore, consensus guidelines (not completely evidence based) call for a liver biopsy in all patients with psoriasis after a cumulative dose of 1.0 to 1.5 g of MTX and repeat liver biopsies at intervals of approximately 1.5 g cumulative methotrexate dosing.[47] A liver biopsy is an invasive procedure and should be used conservatively. However, a high degree of vigilance is necessary in methotrexate-treated psoriatic patients (Table 40-5).

Bone marrow depletion, nausea, diarrhea, and stomatitis are other adverse effects associated with MTX. Pneumonitis may occur early in the course of treatment, particularly when MTX is given at higher dosages similar to those used in cancer chemotherapy regimens. Folic acid, 1 mg daily, may prevent some of these adverse events, but not hepatitis or pulmonary toxicities. Teratogenesis and miscarriage have occurred, and MTX may cause reversible oligospermia. A number of clinically significant drug interactions may enhance the toxicity of methotrexate (Table 40-6). Drug interactions are most likely to be clinically relevant problems in patients with decreased renal function.[47]

Relative contraindications to treatment with MTX include decreased renal function, significant abnormalities in liver function (i.e., fibrosis, cirrhosis, hepatitis), pregnancy or breast-feeding, anemia, leukopenia, thrombocytopenia, active peptic ulcer disease or infectious disease (tuberculosis, pyelonephritis), alcohol abuse, and patient unreliability.[47] Conception must be avoided during MTX therapy and for at least 3 months after cessation of MTX in men or one full ovulatory cycle in women.[47]

Hydroxyurea, thioguanine, and azothioprine are additional antineoplastic agents that have antipsoriatic activity. Their effects are not as potent as methotrexate, but they cause less hepatotoxicity with continuous use.[48,49] Dose-dependent myelo-suppression is a bigger concern with these agents compared with MTX.[20,49]

Cyclosporine

The positive dermatologic effects of cyclosporine, an immunosuppressive agent, highlight the importance of immune alterations in the pathogenesis of psoriasis. Unfortunately, the toxicity and the short duration of remissions induced by the immunosuppressant agents cyclosporine and tacrolimus limit their usefulness. Cyclosporine is generally reserved for patients with extensive psoriasis who have not responded adequately to topical agents, UVB, PUVA, and other systemic agents.

In psoriasis, cyclosporine most likely acts via its effect on lymphocytes. Cyclosporine inhibits calcineurin, which is necessary for production of interleukin (IL)-2. IL-2 amplifies helper T cells and cytotoxic lymphocytes. Decreased IL-2 production leads to a decline in activated CD4 and CD8 cells in the epidermis. Cyclosporine also inhibits tumor necrosis factor-α (TNF-α) and interferon-γ, both of which are involved in the chemotaxis of inflammatory cells; inhibits release of cytokines; and inhibits growth of keratinocytes.[50,51]

Cyclosporine is used at lower dosages for the treatment of psoriasis than for prevention of organ transplant rejection. In general, 3 to 5 mg/kg of cyclosporine is recommended for the treatment of psoriasis. Rapid improvement of plaque psoriasis is expected, with 30% of patients experiencing clearing of psoriatic plaques and 50% achieving >75% clearing of lesions within 10 weeks at 2 to 3 mg/kg per day. Increasing the dosage to 5 mg/kg per day cleared psoriatic lesions in 97% of those treated for 10 weeks.[20] Most people relapse 2 to 4 months after the discontinuation of cyclosporine therapy.[20]

Drug-induced renal impairment is common with cyclosporine use, but usually reversible. Hypertension, secondary to vasoconstrictive effects on the smooth muscle of renal blood vessels or drug-induced arteriolar hyalinosis, is dose dependent and insidious in onset. Blood pressure and serum concentrations of creatinine should be monitored closely in patients receiving cyclosporine.[52] Hypokalemia, hypomagnesemia, hyperuricemia, gingival hyperplasia, hypercholesterolemia, hypertriglyceridemia, gastrointestinal side effects, hypertrichosis, fatigue, myalgia, and arthralgia also have been attributed to cyclosporine therapy.[53] The risk of skin

---

Table 40-5 Methotrexate Therapy: Patient Monitoring

Type of Evaluation	Comments
Clinical evaluation (Psoriasis Area and Severity Index [PASI] score,[16] which includes the percent of body involvement and severity of lesions)	Performed twice in first month, monthly for 6 mo; then Q 3 mo thereafter
Laboratory testing	Weekly for first 2 wk, biweekly for next month, then Q 1–2 mo
CBC with differential and platelet count; renal function (serum creatinine, blood urea nitrogen, urinalysis), liver chemistry (AST, ALT, bilirubin, albumin)	
Hepatitis A, B, C serologies	
Liver biopsy	Baseline (first 2–4 mo of therapy) only for high-risk patients; then (or first): after 1–1.5 g cumulative dose; *repeat:* Q 1.5-g cumulative dose

ALT, serum alanine aminotransferase; AST, serum aspartate aminotransferase; CBC, complete blood count.

LIVERPOOL JOHN MOORES UNIVERSITY
LEARNING & INFORMATION SERVICES

Table 40-6   Methotrexate Drug Interactions

Mechanism	Drugs
Decreased renal elimination of methotrexate	Nephrotoxins (e.g., aminoglycosides, cyclosporine)
	Salicylates
	Sulfonamides
	Probenecid
	Cephalothin
	Penicillins
	Colchicine
	Nonsteroidal anti-inflammatory drugs
Additive or synergistic toxicity	Trimethoprim-sulfamethoxazole
Displacement of methotrexate from protein-binding sites	Salicylates
	Probenecid
	Barbiturates
	Phenytoin
	Retinoids
	Sulfonamides
	Tetracycline
Intracellular accumulation of methotrexate	Dipyridamole
Hepatotoxicity	Retinoids
	Ethanol

cancer, lymphomas, and solid tumors also can increase.[54,55] Patients should be cautioned about excessive sun exposure and should not receive concurrent UVB or PUVA treatment during cyclosporine therapy.[53] Both systemic tacrolimus and mycophenolate mofetil are also reported to be highly effective and well tolerated in the treatment of severe recalcitrant psoriasis. More clinical experience with these agents is needed.[56,57]

Immunomodulatory Drugs

Advances in biotech immunomodulatory therapy, specifically the use of anticytokines, are becoming important treatment alternatives for moderate to severe plaque type psoriasis. Promising results have been reported with two TNF-α inhibitors: infliximab (Remicade) and etanercept (Enbrel). Both produce rapid, well tolerated, beneficial responses compared with placebo.[58–60] Two other promising biologic agents, recently approved by the FDA for treatment of adult patients with chronic plaque psoriasis are the recombinant monoclonol antibodies, alefacept (Amevive) and Efalizumab (Raptiva).[61,62] These agents bind to CD2 on memory effector T lymphocytes, inhibiting their activation in plaques. Administered parenterally on a weekly regimen, lesion improvement compared with placebo is seen, and some patients have sustained clinical response after cessation of therapy.[63] All these biotech agents are expensive, estimated to cost $13,000 to $20,000 per year.

ALTERNATIVE THERAPY

Balneology (bathing in the sea) and spa therapy are not accepted as mainline dermatologic treatment modalities for psoriasis; however, these approaches are used throughout the world. The antipsoriatic properties of the Dead Sea area may be attributed to its unique climatic characteristics and natural resources. Mechanisms may involve mechanical, thermal, and chemical effects.[64,65] Favorable results of climatotherapy have been reported from specialized treatment centers along the Dead Sea, the German North Sea coast, and the Mediterranean Sea.[64,65] Climatotherapy is the combination of bathing in the sea (thalassotherapy or balneotherapy) and exposure to sunlight (heliotherapy). A major aspect of climatotherapy, in addition to daily sunbathing, is bathing in salt water (sea). Relaxation, rest, and simple topical remedies such as petrolatum are also important. When rigorously studied, there is actually little difference in therapeutic outcomes of bathing in salt water or tap water, or the application of various topical ointments (e.g., 2% salicylic acid in white petrolatum, Eucerin, or mineral oil) when used in the current UVB phototherapy protocols.[66] However, psychological factors (especially relaxation) may contribute substantially to the favorable results of natural heliobaleotheapy. If UV phototherapy is administered via artificial UV sources on an outpatient basis, the psychological effect will certainly be much less than when the patient receives this treatment far from home, when cares and social problems are left behind.[66]

Traditional Chinese medicine provides an alternative method of therapy that emphasizes the importance of using many herbs that are combined in different formulations for each individual patient. This has become quite popular among some segments of the population. Both topical and systemic use of herbs has been administered to treat psoriasis, as well as a combination of herbal medications with UVA. For example, *Radix angelicae dahuricae* combined with UVA was not significantly different from 8-methoxypsoralen and UVA.[67]

Amphiregulin is an autocrine growth factor that is overexpressed in psoriatic lesions. Keratinocytes produce protein-bound and free heparin sulfate, which function physiologically as an amphiregulin antagonist. Because glucosamine promotes keratinocyte synthesis of heparin sulfate, it may provide a therapeutic benefit in psoriasis. Clinical trials evaluating the efficacy of amphiregulin are not available.[68]

LIVERPOOL JOHN MOORES UNIVERSITY
LEARNING & INFORMATION SERVICES

MILD TO MODERATE (≤20% BODY) PSORIASIS
Classic Presentation

1. M.M., a 35-year-old man, presents with worsening psoriasis. Approximately 1 year before presentation, he was given triamcinolone 0.025% cream to apply to several thick, well-defined erythematous plaques on his elbows and knees that were covered with silvery scales. He recently returned from a trip to the Dominican Republic, where he noted gradual worsening of redness and scaling despite adherence to a twice-daily triamcinolone regimen. He is emotionally distraught because of this "flare-up," which disrupted his vacation. On examination, besides erythematous, scale-covered plaques on his elbows and knees, there are several scattered, circumscribed, erythematous, scaly plaques on the flexural surfaces of both arms and legs. A dense scale was evident on his scalp (forehead). These and other areas, demonstrating typical psoriatic involvement, including the gluteal fold and fingernails, now total approximately 20% of his body area. His medical history is noncontributory. His only medication besides the topical corticosteroid is a recently completed course of chloroquine for malaria prophylaxis during recent travel. Characterize the classic psoriatic lesions demonstrated by M.M.

The classic plaques of psoriasis appear symmetrically on the extensor surfaces of the elbows and knees as distinctive, chronic, erythematous plaques covered with silvery scales. Removal of scales reveals small, punctate areas of bleeding (Auspitz's sign). Although Auspitz's sign was not noted in M.M., he did present with several thick, well-demarcated, erythematous plaques covered with silvery scale. Patients can present a broad clinical spectrum ranging from only scalp involvement to scattered plaques on the trunk and extremities to, in the most serious cases, a generalized erythroderma accompanied by a rheumatoid factor–negative symmetric arthritis. In addition, the finding of very small pits in the nail plates of the hands and feet ("oil spots"), the presence of gluteal "pinking" (erythema and slight scaling of the intergluteal cleft), and the occurrence of lesions conforming to specific sites of skin trauma (Kobner's phenomenon) help characterize psoriatic plaques from seborrheic dermatitis and eczema. Most psoriatic lesions are asymptomatic, but pruritus is noted in 20% of patients.

2. What part does emotional support play in the total management of M.M.'s psoriasis?

Psoriasis is often more emotionally or psychologically disturbing than is recognized, and it may cause a reluctance of the patient to participate in swimming and other sports.[14] Even though exposure to sunlight helps most patients with psoriasis, there is an unwillingness to sunbathe if the lesions can be seen. Furthermore, if the psoriatic lesions become pruritic and are scratched, there is further deterioration because of the Kobner's phenomenon (i.e., the appearance of lesions of psoriasis at the site of an injury). Many patients alter their lifestyles or use nontraditional medicine (perhaps irrationally) in desperation. This is unfortunate because much can be done to control psoriasis.

Emotional support should begin with explanation of the psoriatic condition. M.M. needs to be reassured that many other people have the same affliction, that the disorder is not contagious or fatal, and that it can be controlled even though there is, as yet, no cure. The National Psoriasis Foundation website (www.psoriasis.org) contains much useful information for psoriatic afflicted patients.[17] Patients usually are com-

forted in the knowledge that a wide range of treatments are available. Clinical optimism and psychological encouragement and support are justified and make it easier for the patient to conscientiously apply sometimes awkward and messy topical treatments or to take toxic medications.

3. What are the potential causes of M.M.'s psoriatic exacerbation? List other factors that can precipitate or aggravate psoriasis.

A thorough medical history may reveal a cause for exacerbations of psoriatic lesions. Most patients report that hot weather, sunlight, and humidity help clear psoriasis, whereas cold weather has an adverse effect on its course. Anxiety or psychological stress is believed to contribute adversely. Viral or bacterial infections, especially streptococcal pharyngitis may precipitate the onset or flare-up of psoriasis. Trauma to the uninvolved skin can cause a lesion to appear at the exact site of injury (Kobner's phenomenon). Cuts, burns, abrasions, injections, and other trauma can elicit this reaction. Any drug that causes a skin eruption to develop may exacerbate psoriasis via this response.

Drug-Induced Psoriasis

A number of drugs have been reported to either exacerbate pre-existing psoriasis, induce psoriatic lesions on apparently normal skin in patients with psoriasis, or precipitate psoriasis in persons with or without a family history of psoriasis (Table 40-7).[67] Antimalarial agents such as chloroquine (taken by M.M.) may have an adverse effect on the course of psoriasis and can cause exfoliative erythroderma.[68] Hydroxychloroquine, however, has not shared this association (except for one recent case report) and usually induces a beneficial response in 75% of patients with psoriatic arthritis.[68] Therefore, hydroxychloroquine is preferred over chloroquine in psoriasis patients who need prophylactic treatment for malaria when both are effective against the particular plasmodium species in the area (see Chapter 74, Parasitic Infections).[68]

Lithium also can precipitate psoriasis and contribute to resistance to treatment through its effects on cell kinetics (increase in circulating neutrophils, accelerated neutrophil turnover, increased epidermal cell proliferation).[67] However, psoriasis is not a general contraindication to lithium therapy. More intensive psoriasis treatment can be used if these reactions occur and lithium must be continued.[67]

β-Blockers and some nonsteroidal anti-inflammatory drugs (NSAIDs) also can precipitate a psoriasiform state.[67] Because both lithium and propranolol inhibit cyclic adenosine monophosphate (cAMP), cyclic nucleosides may play a role in the onset and clinical course of psoriasis. Chemotactic substances, including 12-HETE and leukotrienes, may accumulate in the epidermis of some patients taking indomethacin, thereby precipitating psoriasis. When compared with other NSAIDs, indomethacin may selectively inhibit cyclooxygenase more than lipoxygenase pathways of arachidonic acid metabolism. As a result, indomethacin may have a more significant adverse psoriatic effect than other NSAIDs, as some have been reported to ameliorate psoriasis.[67]

Flare-ups of pustular psoriasis also can be precipitated by withdrawal from systemic steroids or withdrawal from high-potency topical steroids that are applied under occlusion to large areas.[19] Systemic steroids have virtually been abandoned as a routine treatment for psoriasis because of this problem

Table 40-7   Drugs Reported to Induce Psoriasis

Anesthetics	Procaine
Antimicrobials	Amoxicillin, ampicillin, penicillin, sulfonamides, vancomycin, terbinafine, tetracycline
Anti-inflammatory drugs	Corticosteroids (following withdrawal), nonsteroidals (oxyphenbutazone, phenylbutazone, indomethacin, salicylates)
Antimalarials	Chloroquine, hydroxychloroquine[a]
β-Blockers	Propranolol
Cardiovascular drugs	Clonidine, digoxin, amiodarone, quinidine, calcium channel blockers (dihydropyridines, verapamil, diltiazem), acetazolamide, gemfibrozil, angiotensin-converting enzyme inhibitors
H$_2$-antagonists	Cimetidine, ranitidine
Hormones	Oxandrolone, progesterone
Narcotic analgesics	Morphine
Psychotropics	Lithium carbonate, sodium valproate, fluoxetine
Miscellaneous	Potassium iodide, sulfapyridine gold, mercury, oxandrolone, progesterone, lithium

[a]Except for one case report, hydroxychloroquine (unlike chloroquine) does not adversely affect the course of psoriasis and usually induces a beneficial response in 75% of patients with psoriatic arthritis.
Adapted from reference 67.

and because fatalities have been associated with systemic corticosteroid use and withdrawal.

Chloroquine prophylaxis, a Caribbean sunburn, and triamcinolone tachyphylaxis probably all contributed to the exacerbation of M.M.'s psoriasis.[19,68]

Topical Steroids

4. Are additional potent topical steroids appropriate for treatment of M.M.'s psoriasis? Outline the place of steroids in the pharmacotherapy of psoriasis.

For isolated hyperkeratotic plaques, potent topical steroids are the most widely used initial treatment for psoriasis. They give fast relief, especially for reducing inflammation and controlling itching. Patients find them convenient and acceptable. However, their relief is temporary because they become less effective with continued use (tachyphylaxis).[19] In addition, psoriasis is a relatively steroid-resistant disease that responds only to potent or superpotent agents.[19] Long-term use of potent agents also leads to predictable side effects (atrophy, telangiectasia, and striae), and potent topical corticosteroids are quite expensive. For these reasons, topical steroids are best used in an adjunctive role unless used to treat mild disease for short periods. Continuous application of topical steroids for >3 weeks, particularly after skin normalization, should be discouraged. An interval of several weeks between successive courses of therapy is recommended. High-potency steroids produce better clinical results than low-potency steroids, but the potential for side effects is greater. Potent topical steroids can suppress the HPA axis as a result of cutaneous absorption, especially when large areas of the body are involved.[21]

A short course of potent topical steroid is appropriate for this "flare-up" of erythematous plaque psoriasis in M.M. With plastic occlusion (e.g., plastic food wrap on top of the steroid treated area), topical steroids help reduce inflammation, redness, and irritation before initiation of more appropriate chronic topical treatments such as calcipotriene, coal tar, or anthralin with UVB, all of which are potentially irritating. Topical steroids also may continue to be useful on the face and flexures, where the alternative topical agents are poorly tolerated. Potent fluorinated steroid preparations should be used cautiously and only for short periods on the face and flexures, if at all. Scalp psoriasis can be treated with steroid preparations in gels, lotions, or aerosol sprays, but a coal tar shampoo lathered into the scalp for 5 to 10 minutes then rinsed out generally is more effective for scaling and pruritus.

The response to once- or twice-daily corticosteroid application is as effective or better than that observed with more frequent regimens (steroid reservoir effect) and is much less expensive. Patients should apply steroids after a bath, at bedtime with occlusion, and possibly again during the day without occlusion. As the lesions subside, occlusion should be decreased or omitted, emollient use should increase, and steroid potency should decrease. After lesions have flattened, steroids can be continued intermittently (e.g., 1 to 2 weeks on, 1 to 2 weeks off; or on alternate days [e.g., days 1, 3, 5, 7, and so on]).

Alternative Topical Treatments

5. Assuming that a short course of potent topical steroid is effective in reducing the acute flare-up, what alternative topical therapeutic regimens are available for patients like M.M. who have localized disease (involving <20% of the body)?

There are four effective alternative topical therapies for patients with localized mild to moderate psoriasis. The two old, well-known agents are crude coal tar and anthralin. Newer topical agents are calcipotriene and tazarotene. Although anthralin has irritating properties and both coal tar and anthralin generally stain clothing and skin and are somewhat inconvenient to apply, they have stood the test of time and are still worth considering. Tachyphylaxis does not occur with chronic use of any of these alternative agents. Once corticosteroids have flattened acute psoriatic lesions and diminished erythema significantly, daily application of these alternative agents can be used until the lesions are totally clear.

Ointment vehicles are favored for patients with psoriasis because ointments help moisturize the plaques (in contrast to creams, which dry the plaques further). Moisturizers or emollients alone are often helpful for psoriasis.

Coal tar, although effective, is of low potency when compared with anthralin. Tar products such as Estar or T/Derm, which are colorless, or 1% to 5% crude coal tar ointment (messy, but more effective), are commonly applied topically at night, even during the initial corticosteroid phase. Short-contact tar therapy, unlike anthralin, generally is not effective. A number of tar shampoos and bath additives are available. The combination of tar with salicylic acid (2% to 6%) is useful in reducing scaling.

Once the inflammation and erythema have lessened with corticosteroid use or when a twice-daily, high-potency corticosteroid regimen along with bedtime application of tar is ineffective, calcipotriene ointment applied twice daily or tazarotene gel applied once daily is effective in treating flare-ups and maintaining remission.

Calcipotriene may be the topical maintenance treatment of choice in patients with generalized mild to moderate psoriasis. The drug is usually effective, relatively easy to apply, odorless, and nonstaining (cream, ointment, or scalp solution). It is generally considered about as effective as moderate- to high-potency topical steroids. There is a slower onset of action than corticosteroids, and about 10% of patients develop irritation. This irritation precludes the drug's use on the face or in intertriginous areas. Sequential or simultaneous use of topical steroids and vitamin D derivatives may provide synergy and reduce irritation. Tachyphylaxis does not occur. Calcipotriene is expensive, and patient use must be monitored to ensure that a 100 g/week limit is not exceeded; exceeding this limit results in negative effects on calcium and bone metabolism.

Similar to calcipotriene, tazarotene works slowly and can be irritating. It is formulated as a gel, which many patients find more cosmetically appealing than an ointment. It is also effective in a once-a-day regimen, which might help improve compliance. The ointment should be used in combination with a high-potency topical corticosteroid to increase efficacy and to reduce irritation. Because there is a potential for retinoids to be teratogenic, tazarotene should not be used in women who are pregnant or who are contemplating becoming pregnant.

Topical anthralin, generally reserved for resistant cases, is seldom used in the United States, but is commonly used in the United Kingdom. Anthralin clears lesions in some patients within 2 to 3 weeks. Although overnight regimens are available, short-contact therapy, which is more appealing, starts with 0.1% anthralin applied for 20 to 30 minutes and then washed off. Irritation should be checked for at least 48 hours. According to tolerance, the potency can be increased (up to 1%) and the contact time shortened, or for resistant plaques, increased. This regimen is used daily for clearing, then once or twice weekly for maintenance therapy.

In summary, the first step in treatment of mild to moderate localized disease is to start with a high-potency corticosteroid ointment twice daily along with tar ointment at night. If this is not effective, either calcipotriene ointment can be added twice daily or tazarotene gel can be used once a day for 8 weeks. Once control is achieved, patients may use calcipotriene or tazarotene without topical corticosteroids; these products do not cause steroid atrophy, and they do not have the potential for systemic side effects associated with topical corticosteroids. Topical anthralin can be used for resistant cases.

Phototherapy also is an option. UV light can be used as an outpatient modality, produces comparatively long-lasting remissions, is pleasant to use, and is relatively nontoxic. Different protocols require exposure daily or multiple times per week for varied lengths of time depending on patient variables. The optimal effect of UVB on psoriasis is a dose that produces minimal erythema at 24 hours. The usual time to induce clearing of psoriasis is approximately 4 to 6 weeks.

Both tar (Goeckerman regimen) and anthralin (Ingram's regimen) can be used in combination with UVB, with superior results. These two regimens are reported to clear plaques in 75% of patients treated for 6 weeks for chronic plaque psoriasis (versus 56% with UVB alone). The total number of treatments and the total UVB dose required for clearing are less in the combination groups.[20]

SEVERE (>20% BODY) PSORIASIS

Psoralens and Ultraviolet A Light

6. G.L., a 35-year-old man with a several-year history of psoriasis (generally fairly localized) presents with diffuse, erythematous plaque-like lesions now extending over 80% of his body surface area. The areas have become inflamed, and application of his maintenance topical medication (anthralin) causes pain and irritation. He expresses frustration with the messiness of the current topical regimen. He has reinitiated topical steroids, which helped the redness and itching but are too expensive to use long term. He is free of cardiovascular, renal, or hepatic disease and takes no systemic medications. He is self-employed as a business consultant. Which "systemic" therapy would be most appropriate for G.L. at this point?

Systemic therapies for psoriasis include PUVA; the systemic retinoid, acitretin; methotrexate; and cyclosporine. Newer biotech anticytokines, including the TNF inhibitors, infliximab and etanercept, and the recombinant human monoclonal antibodies, alefacept and efalizumab, have also been used for skin lesions. These agents prevent the activation and reduces the number of memory T-lymphocytes.

PUVA and methotrexate are used most often; however, cyclosporine and the newer immunomodulatory agents are being used increasingly as more experience is gained with them for treatment of severe psoriasis.[71] The choice of agents depends on patient and drug characteristics. Because patients with psoriasis generally have the disease for the rest of their lives, the goal of treatment is not just safe and effective resolution of disease at a specific point in time, but also safe and effective maintenance therapy for long periods. Anecdotal experience suggests that long-term maintenance of psoriasis can generally be achieved even with weaning or discontinuation of UVB, PUVA, and methotrexate. From a histologic perspective, these drugs have been shown to induce remittive cellular changes. In contrast, partial to relatively full doses of acetretin or cyclosporine are necessary to maintain the therapeutic effects of these two drugs, perhaps because they induce suppressive rather than remittive histopathologic changes. For example, most patients will relapse in a predictable manner 2 to 4 months after cyclosporine is discontinued.[72]

Rotational Therapy

No form of therapy used in psoriasis today is without toxicity. Rotational therapy involves the use of alternating monotherapies, which allows the patient to experience extended intervals off a particular treatment. When used in long-term maintenance, rotational therapy limits side effects associated with either long-term use of one specific agent or the additive or synergistic interactions when multiple therapies are used concurrently. As discussed, the relative risk of skin cancer associated with PUVA increases after 150 treatments. If a patient in remission is rotated off PUVA to another treatment after 100 exposures, the skin has time to recuperate from the light therapy, and PUVA can eventually be reinstated presumably at a smaller risk. Rotational therapy assumes that the patient can tolerate three to four alternative treatments with unrelated toxicity profiles.[71,72] By rotating each treatment after 12 to 18 months of cumulative use, the potential for long-term toxicity associated with any single treatment is minimized. With this theoretical rationale, cyclosporine could be used for a limit of possibly 3 to 6 months, thus inducing a remission. The patient could then be rotated to another treatment (e.g., methotrexate or PUVA) for maintenance.

Psoralens and UVA irradiation become noticeably effective in 80% to 90% of patients in 6 to 8 weeks.[20] The regimen is time-consuming because UV radiation treatments must be administered at least three times a week. Adverse long-term effects (premature photoaging, dyskaryotic or precancerous dermal changes, skin cancer [including melanoma], immunologic changes, and cataracts) can be minimized with appropriate patient selection and monitoring. More immediate adverse effects (e.g., itching, nausea, headache, lethargy, erythematous phototoxic reactions with overexposure, skin pain, and hyperpigmentation) are common. Male patients have increased risk of developing genital squamous-cell cancer (the groin should be shielded during therapy), wrinkling, lentigines (brown macule resembling a freckle), irregular pigmentation, and cataracts (if protective eye wear is not used). Generally, 8-methoxypsoralen is administered (0.6 to 0.8mg/kg of body weight), followed by UVA (dose selected based on skin type, ease of sunburn, and inherent skin color) about 75 to 90 minutes later when psoralen blood levels peak. PUVA-induced erythema generally appears later than with UVB therapy, reaching a peak by 48 hours. Consequently, treatment should not be administered more frequently than every second day. The time to produce clearing of psoriatic plaques with PUVA takes longer than with UVB therapy (average 10 weeks compared with ≤3 weeks for UVB).[37] PUVA treatment must be decreased slowly once clearing of plaques has been achieved (frequency of treatment is reduced over 2 to 3 months) to prevent recurrence of psoriatic plaques. In contrast, UVB therapy can be ceased abruptly. Taking time off from work three times weekly for photochemotherapy can be disruptive to some patients' work or school schedules.

PUVA should be avoided in patients with a history of skin cancer, in children, during pregnancy, in patients who are immunosuppressed, and in those who have light-colored skin that burns rather than tans. Absolute contraindications to treatment with PUVA include a history of photosensitivity diseases (i.e., lupus erythematosus, porphyria), idiosyncratic or allergic reactions to psoralens, arsenic intake, exposure to ionizing radiation, skin cancer (relative contraindication), pregnancy, and lactation. Measures that may reduce the risk of long-term adverse effects of photochemotherapy are listed in Table 40-3. Other photosensitizing drugs (e.g., fluoroquinolones, phenothiazines, sulfonamides, sulfonylureas, tetracyclines, thiazides) should be avoided in patients receiving PUVA.

In summary, PUVA is effective in 80% to 90% of patients, and G.L.'s severe, extensive, plaque psoriasis should be expected to respond accordingly. The systemic drugs (e.g., methotrexate, cyclosporine) may be preferred if G.L. had systemic symptoms (e.g., psoriatic arthritis). Although thrice-weekly PUVA treatments can be disruptive to work schedules, G.L. is self-employed and presumably has some flexibility in his working hours. Rotational therapy could be considered at a later time depending on G.L.'s response and tolerance of PUVA.

Psoriatic Arthritis

7. R.T., a 38-year-old man, is an aerospace machinist with psoriasis and increasing joint complaints. He describes a flare-up over the last month or so involving predominantly the middle finger of the right hand. He also has had arthralgias of the shoulders, knees, and the rest of his hands. Concomitantly, his skin disease has once again become active, despite nightly betamethasone dipropionate (Diprolene) administration. He has a history of chronic depression and alcoholism, although he is currently sober and not being treated with antidepressant medications. Physical examination reveals a significant amount of tenderness of the right third metacarpophalangeal joint, without a great deal of active synovitis. He also has a moderate effusion of his right knee, but the rest of the joint examination is otherwise benign. There are active psoriatic lesions on his feet, knees, elbows, and he has characteristic psoriatic nail changes. An erythrocyte sedimentation rate is mildly elevated. Which systemic therapy would be most appropriate for both R.T.'s skin and joint complaints?

Psoriatic arthritis is a distinct form of inflammatory arthritis that is usually seronegative for rheumatoid factor. In various reports, 5% to 31% of patients with psoriasis can experience arthritis, and the prevalence is increased among patients with severe cutaneous disease.[11,12] Nail involvement occurs in >80% of patients with psoriatic arthritis, as compared with 30% of patients with only cutaneous psoriasis.[73] Arthropathy is experienced in 15% of the patients before the appearance of cutaneous manifestations, in 75% after, and in 10% concurrently with the cutaneous manifestations.[74] Five clinical subsets of psoriatic arthritis have been identified: distal interphalangeal arthritis (classic, 5% to 10%, often accompanied by nail changes), arthritis mutilans (5%, starts in early age, accompanied by osteolysis with severe deformities of fingers and toes), symmetric polyarthritis (rheumatoid-like, <25% incidence, milder course), asymmetric oligoarthritis (most prevalent, 70%, proximal and distal interphalangeal joints, metacarpophalangeal joints, knee and hip), and spondylitis (5% to 40%, often asymptomatic).

Treatment of psoriatic arthritis consists of NSAIDs and local corticosteroid injections, with second-line drugs being reserved for resistant or progressively destructive clinical subsets. NSAIDs suppress symptoms, do not induce remissions, and can exacerbate cutaneous symptoms.[69] Systemic corticosteroids are avoided because they destabilize psoriasis (transformation to pustular forms), induce resistance to other effective therapies, and re-exacerbate the skin disease during withdrawal.[19,21,74,75] PUVA and acitretin have negligible antiarthritic efficacy.

Methotrexate

Methotrexate has traditionally been the drug claimed to produce benefit in both the cutaneous and the articular manifestations of psoriatic arthritis.[76] However, despite its widespread use in psoriatic arthritis, data on its effectiveness are sparse. In a meta-analysis of the published randomized trials of second-line drugs for psoriatic arthritis, only sulfasalazine (no activity against skin disease) and methotrexate were proved to be effective. Cyclosporine was not considered because no controlled study met the inclusion criteria for this particular meta-analysis.[77] Another study compared low-dose methotrexate (up to 15 mg/week) with cyclosporine. Both were found to be effective, but methotrexate was better tolerated (28% versus 41% withdrawal rate).[78] Methotrexate therapy is a reasonable second-line agent for R.L.'s arthralgias in his shoulders, knees, and hands and his active skin disease.

Therapy with methotrexate usually is initiated with a 2.5-mg test dose. If no idiosyncratic reaction occurs, doses are gradually increased to a maintenance of 10 to 25 mg/week. Methotrexate is best given in a single weekly oral dose or in three 2.5- to 7.5-mg doses at 12-hour intervals during a 24-hour period (e.g., 8 AM, 8 PM, and again at 8 AM). Folic acid 1 mg daily should be prescribed concomitantly to protect against common side effects such as stomatitis. Folate does not protect against hepatic or pulmonary toxicity, and monitoring for these complications is necessary during therapy. Regular blood counts, urinalysis, and renal and liver function tests should be evaluated. An aspiration needle biopsy of the liver should be performed at or near the initiation of treatment.[47] More practically, if there are no risk factors for hepatotoxicity, the liver biopsy can be postponed for 2 to 4 months until the drug's efficacy and lack of toxicity have been established for the patient and long-term therapy is about to be initiated. Delaying the biopsy for this period does not pose a risk because it is rare for life-threatening liver disease to develop with the first 1.0 to 1.5 g of methotrexate.[46,47]

Unfortunately, hepatotoxicity may not be apparent on routine laboratory evaluation. When liver chemistry tests are obtained, there should be at least a 1-week interval after the last methotrexate dose because liver chemistry values are often elevated 1 to 2 days after methotrexate therapy. If a significant abnormality in liver chemistry is noted, methotrexate therapy should be withheld for 1 to 2 weeks and the battery of liver chemistry tests repeated. Liver chemistry values should return to normal in 1 to 2 weeks. If significantly abnormal liver chemistry values persist for 2 to 3 months, a liver biopsy should be considered. Liver biopsy is recommended when the cumulative dosage level reaches 1.5 g and after each subsequent 1.5-g increase in the cumulative dose. Risk factors for hepatotoxicity include daily methotrexate administration, heavy alcohol intake, diabetes, obesity, intravenous drug abuse, previous exposure to hepatotoxic drugs, and pretreatment liver dysfunction. Liver function abnormalities may improve after cessation of MTX therapy for 6 months.

8. During a follow-up visit to his family doctor several months later, R.T. had several somatic complaints that lead to a diagnosis of recurrent depression. Subsequent history reveals that he also has resumed use of alcohol. He tends to drink four to five beers a night on weekends or when he is feeling low, although he does admit that his level of alcohol use is sometimes higher. His skin disease is relatively well controlled, but joint complaints have persisted. What additional options now exist for R.T.?

Methotrexate should be discontinued because the risks probably now exceed the benefits, particularly because rheumatic complaints have not been controlled and alcohol consumption has resumed. RT should be referred for physical and occupational therapy, encouraged to exercise, and (if needed) referred for orthotics. NSAIDs can be given symptomatically. Sulfasalazine and hydroxychloroquine might be beneficial for joint symptoms alone, and cutaneous manifestations may be controlled with topical agents. Alternative second-line agents include the immunomodulatory agents: cyclosporine, and the anticytokines, TNF inhibitors, infliximab, and etanercept.

Immunomodulatory Agents

Oral cyclosporine is given in divided daily doses in the range of 2.5 to 5 mg/kg, lower than for organ transplantation. Improvement is generally observed within 4 weeks. In one study, pain, number of painful and swollen joints, and duration of morning stiffness all decreased by 30% to 50%, along with 52% improvement in skin scores and serum C-reactive protien.[79] Another open-label study of 99 patients randomized to cyclosporine, sulfasalazine, or placebo reported beneficial effects from cyclosporine compared with placebo, but not sulfasalazine over 6 months, in terms of pain and tender, swollen joints counts.[80] Hypertension (5 of 36), declining renal function (10 of 36), and a variety of neurologic complaints (7 of 36) were common in the cyclosporine-treated group. Skin disease also improved more in the cyclosporine group. Close monitoring is required because these toxicities often limit the long-term use of cyclosporine.

Both methotrexate and cyclosporine reduce inflammatory joint activity in the short term, but it remains to be seen whether they actually modify the long-term disease process. Methotrexate over a period of 2 years did not afford protection from disease progression in patients with psoriatic arthritis compared with that in matched controls.[81] It is clear that better therapies for psoriatic arthritis are necessary.

TNF-α is a potent cytokine involved in inflammation and joint damage. Inhibition of this cytokine reduces direct actions as well as the action of other pro-inflammatory cytokines. Etanercept is a TNF-α receptor blocker. In a 3-month double-blind placebo-controlled study of 60 patients with psoriatic arthritis, an etanercept response was observed in 73% of patients (versus 13% with placebo) and skin improvement in 50% (versus 0% with placebo).[82] Infliximab is a human/mouse chimeric anti–TNF-α antibody. Patients given infliximab intravenously 10 mg/kg at 0, 2, and 6 weeks, reported 91% clinical response (versus 18%, placebo) at 10 weeks and 82% (versus 18%, placebo) and had at least 75% improvement in Psoriasis Area and Severity Index (PASI). The median time to response was 4 weeks. No serious adverse events occurred during this short trial.[58] In two other 1-year, open-label trials, infliximab at 5 mg/kg every 4 to 8 weeks produced significant improvement in both psoriatic skin lesions and joint symptoms, which was maintained with continued 5 mg/kg doses every 14 weeks.[83,84]

For patients like R.T., whose disease cannot be treated successfully or safely with methotrexate, proceed with an anti–TNF-α agent. If available, etanercept (25 mg subcutaneously twice a week) is preferred for convenience. Screening for tuberculosis before beginning therapy with anti-TNF agents is prudent, and those with evidence of prior tuberculous chest infection or with a positive skin test for TB should be offered prophylactic antituberculous therapy. If further study confirms the long-term effectiveness and safety of the anti-TNF treatments, these may become the preferred treatment for patients with moderate to severe disease. Increased availability and decreased cost would make the immunomodulatory therapies more attractive.

REFERENCES

1. Barker JNWN. Pathogenesis of psoriasis. J Dermatol 1998;25:778.
2. Barker J. Psoriasis. J R Coll Phys Lond 1997;31:238.
3. Nickoloff BJ. The immunologic and genetic basis of psoriasis. Arch Dermatol 1999;135:1104.
4. Griffiths CEM, Voorhees JJ. Psoriasis, T cells and autoimmunity. J R Soc Med 1996;89:315.
5. Henseler T. Genetics of psoriasis. Arch Dermatol Res 1998;290:463.
6. Robert C, Kupper TS. Inflammatory skin diseases, T cells, and immune surveillance. N Engl J Med 1999;341:1817.
7. Nickoloff BJ et al. Injection of pre-psoriatic skin with CD4+ T cells induces psoriasis. Am J Pathol 1999;155:145.
8. Leyden JJ. Therapy for acne vulgaris. N Engl J Med 1997;336:1156.
9. Bos JD, DeRie MA. The pathogenesis of psoriasis: immunological facts and speculations. Immunol Today 1999;20:40.
10. Prinz JC. Which T cells cause psoriasis? Clin Exp Dermatol 1999;24:291.
11. Ruzicka T. Psoriatic arthritis. Arch Dermatol 1996;132:215.
12. Brockbank U et al. Psoriatic arthritis is common among patients with psoriasis and family medicine clinic attendees [Abstract]. Arthritis Rheum 2001;44 (Suppl):S94.
13. Bonifati C et al. Recognition and treatment of psoriasis. Special considerations in elderly patients. Drugs Aging 1998;12:177.
14. Updike J. Personal history: at war with my skin. New Yorker 2 Sept, 1985.
15. Finlay Aye et al. Validation of sickness impact profile and psoriasis disability index in psoriasis. Br J Dermatol 1990;123:751.
16. Feldman SR et al. The self-administered psoriasis area and severity index is valid and reliable. J Invest Dermatol 1996;106:183.
17. www.psoriasis.org, The National Psoriasis Foundation, accessed, September 2003.
18. Stern RS. Psoriasis. Lancet 1997;350:349.
19. Federman DG et al. Topical psoriasis therapy. Am Fam Physician 1999;59:957.
20. Tristani-Firouzi P, Krueger GG. Efficacy and safety of treatment modalities for psoriasis. Cutis 1998;61:11.
21. Katz HI. Topical corticosteroids. Dermatol Clin 1995;13:805.
22. Thami GP, Sarkar R. Coal tar: past, present and future. Clin Exp Dermatol 2002;27:99.
23. Pion IA et al. Is dermatologic usage of coal tar carcinogenic? A review of the literature. Dermatol Surg 1995;21:227.
24. Harris DR. Old wine in new bottles: the revival of anthralin. Cutis 1998;62:201.
25. Feldman SR, Clark AR. Psoriasis. Med Clin North Am 1998;82:1135.
26. Koo J et al. Advances in psoriasis therapy. Adv Dermatol 1997;12:47.
27. Van de Kerkhof PC. An update on vitamin D3 analogues in the treatment of psoriasis. Skin Pharmacol Appl Skin Physiol 1998;11:2.
28. Kragballe K et al. Calcipotriol cream with or without concurrent topical corticosteroid in psoriasis: tolerability and efficacy. Br J Dermatol 1998;139:649.
29. Ashcroft DM et al. Systematic review of comparative efficacy and tolerability of calcipotriol in treating chronic plaque psoriasis. BMJ 2000;320:963.
30. Bleiker TO et al. Long-term outcome of severe chronic psoriasis following treatment with high dose topical calcipotriol. Br J Dermatol 1998;139:285.
31. Marks R. Pharmacokinetics and safety review of tazarotene. J Am Acad Dermatol 1998;39:S134.
32. Lebwohl M. Clinical efficacy and safety of tazarotene: optimizing clinical results. Cutis 1998;61:S27.
33. Kreuger GG et al. The safety and efficacy of tazarotene gel, a topical acetylenic retinoid, in the treatment of psoriasis. Arch Dermatol 1998;134:57.
34. Lebwohl M, Poulin Y. Tazarotene in combination with topical corticosteroids. J Am Acad Dermatol 1998;39:S139.
35. Lebwohl M et al. Effects of topical preparations on the erythemogenicity of UVB: implications for psoriasis phototherapy. J Am Acad Dermatol 1995;32:469.
36. Feldman SR et al. Efficacy of the 308-nm excimer laser for treatment of psoriasis: results of a multicenter study. J Am Acad Dermatol 2002;46:900.
37. Stern RS. Malignant melanoma in patients treated for psoriasis with PUVA. Photodermatol Photoimmunol Photomed 1999;15:37.
38. Lindelof B. Risk of melanoma with psoralen/ultraviolet: a therapy for psoriasis. Drug Saf 1999;20:289.
39. Stern RS. The risk of melanoma in association with long-term exposure to PUVA. J Am Acad Dermatol 2001;44:755.
40. Lebwohl M. Acitretin in combination with UVB or PUVA. J Am Acad Dermatol 1999;41:S22.
41. Saurat JH. Retinoids and psoriasis: novel issues in retinoid pharmacology and implications for psoriasis treatment. J Am Acad Dermatol 1999;41:S2.
42. Roenigk HH et al. Effects of acitretin on the liver. J Am Acad Dermatol 1999;41:584.
43. Ling MR. Acitretin: optimal dosing strategies. J Am Acad Dermatol 1999;41:S13.
44. Bodemer C, de Prost Y: Acitretin in children. Acta Derm Venereol 1994;186(Suppl):124.
45. Ahern MJ et al. Methotrexate hepatotoxicity: what is the evidence? Inflamm Res 1998;47:148.
46. Whiting-O'Keege QE et al. Methotrexate and histologic hepatic abnormalities: a meta-analysis. Am J Med 1991;90:711.
47. Roenigk HH et al. Methotrexate in psoriasis: consensus conference. J Am Acad Dermatol 1998;38:478.
48. Smith CH. Use of hydroxyurea in psoriasis. Clin Exp Derm 1999;24:2.
49. Jackson CG. Immunomodulating drugs in the management of psoriatic arthritis. Am J Clini Dermatol 2001;2:367.
50. Wong RL et al. The mechanisms of action of cyclosporin A in the treatment of psoriasis. Immunol Today 1993;14:69.
51. Koo J, Lee J. Cyclosporine—what clinicians need to know. Dermatol Clin 1995;13:897.
52. Powles AV et al. Renal function after 10 years' treatment with cyclosporin for psoriasis. Br J Dermatol 1998;138:443.
53. Lebwohl M et al. Cyclosporine consensus conference: with emphasis on the treatment of psoriasis. J Am Acad Dermatol 1998;39:464.
54. Paquet P, Pierard GE. Breast and lung cancers in two cyclosporin-A-treated psoriatic women. Dermatol 1998;196:450.
55. Paul C, Hornig F. Risk of malignancy associated with cyclosporin use in psoriasis. Dermatology 1999;198:320.
56. Ruzicka T et al. Tacrolimus. The drug for the turn of the millennium? Arch Dermatol 1999;135:574.
57. Nousari HC et al. Mycophenolate mofetil in autoimmune and inflammatory skin disorders. J Am Acad Dermatol 1999;40:265.
58. Chaudhari U et al. Efficacy and safety of infliximab monotherapy for plaque-type psoriasis: a randomised trial. Lancet 2001;357:1842.
59. Gottlieb AB et al. Pharmacodynamic and pharmacokinetic response to anti-tumor necrosis factor-alpha monoclonal antibody (infliximab) treatment of moderate to severe psoriasis vulgaris. J Am Acad Dermatol 2003;48:68.
60. Iyer S et al. Etanercept for severe psoriasis and psoriatic arthritis: observations on combination therapy. Br J Dermatol 2002;146:118
61. Gordon KB et al. Remitive effects of intramuscular alefacept in psoriasis. J. Drugs Dermatol 2003;2:624.
62. Lebwohl M et al. A novel targeted T-cell modulator, efalizumab, for plaque psoriasis. N Engl J Med 2003;349:1987.
63. Ellis CN et al. Treatment of chronic plaque psoriasis by selective targeting of memory effector T lymphocytes. N Engl J Med 2001;345:248.
64. Halevy S, Sukenik S. Different modalities of spa therapy for skin diseases at the Dead Sea area. Arch Dermatol 1998;134:1416.
65. Even-Paz, Z. Dermatology at the Dead Sea spas. Isr J Med Sci 1996;32(Suppl 3):11.
66. Boer J. The influence of mineral water solutions in phototherapy. Clin Dermatol 1996;14:665.
67. Koo J, Arain S. Traditional Chinese medicine for the treatment of dermatologic disorders. Arch Dermatol 1998;134:1388.
68. McCarty MF. Glucosamine for psoriasis? Med Hypotheses 1997;48:437.
69. Tsankov N et al. Drugs in exacerbation and provocation of psoriasis. Clin Dermatol 1998;16:333.
70. Vine JE et al. Pustular psoriasis induced by hydroxychloroquine: a case report and review of the literature. J Dermatol 1996;23:357.
71. Weinstein GD et al. Rational approach to therapy for moderate to severe psoriasis. J Am Acad Dermatol 1993;28:454.
72. Koo J. Systemic sequential therapy of psoriasis: a new paradigm for improved therapeutic results. J Am Acad Dermatol 1999;41:S25.
73. Gladman DD. Psoriatic arthritis. Rheum Dis Clin North Am 1998;24:829.
74. Ruzicka T. Psoriatic arthritis. Arch Dermatol 1996;132:215.
75. Salvarani C et al. Psoriatic arthritis. Curr Opin Rheum 1998;10:299.
76. Chang DJ. A survey of drug effectiveness and treatment choices in psoriatic arthritis [Abstract]. Arthritis Rheum 1999;42(Suppl):S372.

77. Jones G et al. Psoriatic arthritis: a quantitative overview of therapeutic options. Br J Rheumatol 1997;36:95.

78. Spadaro A et al. Comparison of cyclosporin A and methotrexate in the treatment of psoriatic arthritis: a one-year prospective study. Clin Exp Rheumatol 1995;13:589.

79. Mahrle G et al. Anti-inflammatory efficacy of low-dose cyclosporin A in psoriatic arthritis. A prospective multicentre study. Br J Dermatol 1996; 135:752.

80. Salvarani C et al. A comparison of cyclosporine, sulfasalazine, and symptomatic therapy in the treatment of psoriatic arthritis. J Rheumatol 2001; 28:2274.

81. Abu-Shakra et al. Long-term methotrexate therapy in psoriatic arthritis: clinical and radiologic outcome. J Rheumatol 1995;22:241.

82. Mease PJ et al. Etanercept in the treatment of psoriatic arthritis and psoriasis: a randomised trial. Lancet 2000;356:385.

83. Ogilvic AL. Treatment of psoriatic arthritis with antitumor necrosis factor-α antibody clears skin lesions of psoriasis resistant to treatment with methotrexate. Br. J Dermatol 2001;144:587.

84. Van den Bosch F et al. Effects of a loading dose regimen of three infusions of chimeric monoclonal antibody to tumour necrosis factor-α (infliximab) in spondyloarthropaty: an open pilot study. Ann Rheum Dis 2000;59:428.

CHAPTER 41

Photosensitivity and Burns

Timothy J. Ives

PHOTOSENSITIVITY
Effects of Ultraviolet Radiation

Changing lifestyles have considerably increased human exposure to sunlight: more outdoor recreational activities, more emphasis on tanning, longer life spans, and seasonal population shifts to the Sunbelt. Public attitudes toward tanning and sun exposure have not changed even though epidemiologic evidence clearly implicates sunlight as a causative factor in many skin diseases. Squamous cell carcinoma (SCC) and basal cell carcinoma (BCC), which together account for more than half of all malignancies in the United States, are linked closely to exposure to ultraviolet radiation (UVR).[1] Malignant melanoma, the incidence of which has increased >100% in the last decade, most likely is linked to UVR exposure.[2] Sun-

burn, photoaging, immunologic changes in the skin, cataracts, photodermatoses, phototoxicity, and photoallergy are other commonly encountered photosensitivity reactions. The appropriate use of sunscreens or other photoprotective behaviors can help mitigate the incidence of the adverse effects of UVR.

Ultraviolet Radiation Spectrum

UVR, the primary inducer of photosensitivity reactions in humans, is divided into ranges according to the effects of the three primary wavelengths: UVA, UVB, and UVC (Fig. 41-1). UVA, with a wavelength of 320 to 400 nm, is closest in wavelength to visible light.[3] It is considerably less likely than a comparable dose of UVB to cause a similar degree of erythema.[4-6] However, unlike UVB, UVA penetrates to the dermal layer and may cause harmful effects not caused by UVB.[3]

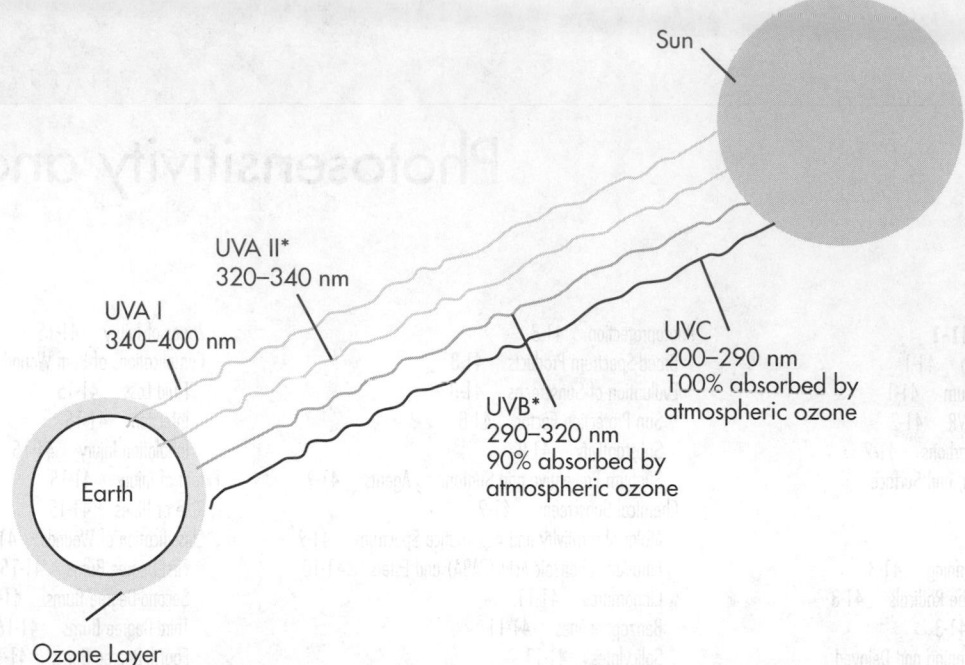

FIGURE 41-1 Ultraviolet radiation spectrum. *Erythrogenic and melanogenic bands of UVR.

About 10 to 100 times more UVA reaches the earth's surface than UVB. Consequently, UVA may contribute up to 15% of the erythemal response at midday.[3,6] UVB, in wavelengths from 290 to 320 nm, is the most erythrogenic and melanogenic of the three UVR bands.[3,7] Up to 90% of UVB is blocked by the earth's stratospheric ozone layer, and it is absorbed completely by the epidermal layer of the skin.[8,9] The only known beneficial effect of UVR in humans is exposure to small amounts of UVB, most commonly through sunlight, which converts which converts 7-dehydrocholesterol to cholecalciferol (vitamin D_3). Vitamin D enhances calcium homeostasis and has direct and indirect effects on cells involved with bone remodeling. As a result, vitamin D can decrease the risk of rickets in childhood and fractures and osteomalacia in adults.[10]

UVC wavelengths of 200 to 290 nm are absorbed completely by the earth's stratospheric ozone layer. Artificial sources of UVC have been used in the sterilization and preservation of food and in minimizing bacterial growth in laboratories and hospital operating rooms by germicidal lamps, which may cause erythema or cataracts if mishandled.[3,7]

Environmental Effects on UVR
OZONE AND CHLOROFLUOROCARBONS

The amount of UVR that reaches the earth's surface is influenced by many factors. Concern has been focused on the implications of depletion of the ozone layer.[6,9,11] In the decade after it was first detected in 1983, ozone levels above the Antarctic had fallen to 50% of normal.[11] In the early 1990s, worldwide estimates from the Environmental Protection Agency (EPA) predicted a 40% depletion of ozone by the year 2075 if controls on chlorofluorocarbons (CFCs) were not enacted. The EPA also concluded that for every 1% decrease in ozone, UVB radiation reaching the earth's surface would increase by 2% per year, possibly resulting in a 1% to 3% increase per year in nonmelanoma skin cancer.[12] In addition, UVB radiation can alter the immune system. As demonstrated by the worldwide meteorologic phenomena known as *El Nino* and *La Nina,* an impaired immune system can increase the incidence of certain cancers, including skin cancers.[9] These losses in the ozone layer are thought to be caused by man-made pollutants (e.g., nitrous oxides from jet airliners in stratospheric aviation and CFCs as propellants and refrigerants). The effect of the ban on the commercial use of CFCs by many of the industrialized nations has begun to be seen, as evidenced by a slow decline in these ozone-depleting compounds. Since ozone depletion takes place approximately a decade after CFC expression in the stratosphere, this recovery may take place later than expected.[13] Because UVA is only slightly filtered by the ozone layer, any decrease in the ozone layer would result in a disproportionate increase in UVB reaching the earth.

TIME OF DAY, CLOUD COVER, AND SURFACE REFLECTION

The time of day influences the amount of UVR reaching the earth's surface; 20% to 30% of the total daily UVR is received from 11 AM to 1 PM, with 75% between 9 AM and 3 PM. Cloud cover can decrease UV intensity by 10% to 80% and decreases infrared radiation to an even greater extent. This greater attenuation of infrared radiation by cloud cover may lead to an increased risk of UVR overexposure because less infrared radiation will be absorbed by the body and transformed into heat, resulting in less warning of overexposure to UVR. Reflection of UVR by substances (e.g., sand, water, snow) also may be important. For example, sand reflects about 25% of incident UVB radiation; therefore, sitting under an umbrella at the beach may not offer adequate protection. In general, whenever someone's shadow is shorter than his or her height, care should be taken; the shorter the shadow, the more likely a sunburn will occur. Fresh snow can reflect 50% to

95% of incident sunlight. Water reflects approximately 5% of erythemal UVR, whereas 75% of the radiation is transmitted through 2 m of water, offering swimmers little protection.[3] Seasonal changes, geographic latitude, and altitude also influence the amount of UVR reaching the earth's surface.

UV INDEX

The UV Index, offered by the EPA, the National Weather Service, and the Centers for Disease Control and Prevention, is a public health education service that is available in 58 U.S. cities.[14] This index, with a scale from 1 (minimal exposure) to 10 (very high exposure), forecasts the probable intensity of skin-damaging UVR expected to reach the surface during the noon hour when the sun is highest in the sky. Theoretically, the UV Index can range from 0 (e.g., during the night) to 15 or 16 (in the tropics at high elevations under clear skies). The higher the UV Index, the greater the dose received of skin- and eye-damaging UVR, and the less time it takes before skin damage occurs.

The amount of UVR exposure needed to damage an individual's skin is affected by the elevation of the sun in the sky, the amount of ozone in the stratosphere, and the amount of clouds present. Clear skies transmit 100% of UVR to the surface, with scattered clouds 89%, broken clouds 73%, and overcast clouds 32%. The darker an individual's skin tone, the longer (or the more UVR) it takes to cause erythema.

Erythema, Sunburn, and Tanning

ERYTHEMA AND OXYGEN-FREE RADICALS

Excessive exposure of the epidermal and dermal layers of the skin to UVR can result in an inflammatory erythematous reaction. Excess UVA and UVB causes the release of vasodilatory mediators (e.g., histamine, prostaglandins, cytokines), resulting in increased blood flow, erythema, tissue exudates, swelling, increased sensation of warmth, and a characteristic sunburn.[3,7] Severe UVR exposure, primarily UVB, may cause blister formation, desquamation, fever, chills, weakness, and shock. Erythema caused by UVB begins within 3 to 5 hours after exposure, is maximal after 12 to 24 hours, and usually resolves over the ensuing 3 days.[7] In contrast, erythema caused by UVA begins immediately, plateaus between 6 and 12 hours, and remains for 24 hours. UVA-induced changes in the dermis are characterized by greater damage to the vasculature and dense cellular infiltrates that penetrate to deeper levels of the skin.[7] The dermis also may be damaged when endogenous components of the skin absorb UVR energy and subsequently interact with oxygen to form tissue-damaging oxygen-free radicals.[9]

HISTOLOGY OF SUNBURN

The skin undergoes adaptive changes in response to UVR exposure. When keratinocytes in the epidermis are damaged and lose their typical organization, both the epidermis and the stratum corneum thicken[6] and attempt to serve as a barrier to UVR, particularly to UVB. The skin's normal protective immune response, however, is altered with exposure to UVR. Metalloproteinase proteins, proteolytic enzymes that are induced with low-dose UVR exposure, cause degradation of collagen and elastin in the dermal matrix.[15] Langerhans' cells (i.e., antigen-presenting cells in the skin) are decreased in number and function even after small doses of UVB.[15] These cells abnormally activate suppressor T lymphocytes and lose their ability to activate normal effector pathways of the immune system.

IMMEDIATE PIGMENT DARKENING AND DELAYED TANNING

Tanning is an adaptive mechanism of the skin to UVR. Tanning occurs by two different mechanisms: immediate pigment darkening (Meirsowsky phenomenon) and delayed tanning. The primary cell involved in tanning is the melanocyte, which produces the radiation-absorbing protein, melanin.[3,6] Immediate pigment darkening begins during the actual exposure to UVA and certain bands of visible light,[3,6] and the oxidation of existing melanin in the epidermis, transiently turns the skin grayish brown. The degree of immediate pigment darkening depends on the duration and intensity of exposure, the extent of previous tanning (or amount of pre-existing melanin), and the skin type of the individual.[3] Immediate pigment darkening is not protective against UVB erythema.[6]

Delayed tanning occurs 48 to 72 hours after exposure to either UVA or UVB. It is most intense 7 to 10 days after UV exposure and may last for weeks to months.[3] Delayed tanning is the result of increased production of melanin, an increase in the size and dendricity of the melanocyte, and the rate of transfer of melanosomes (particulate bodies of melanin) to keratinocytes.[3,6] The keratinocyte, now pigmented with melanosomes, migrates to the epidermis, producing the characteristic suntan. Delayed tanning caused by UVA is less protective against sunburn than delayed tanning caused by UVB, as epidermal thickening is not induced by UVA.[3]

SKIN TYPES

1. L.M., a 26-year-old female, and G.M., her 28-year-old husband, have planned a 2-week cruise to the Caribbean and are inquiring about sunscreens for the trip. L.M. has fair complexion with blonde hair and blue eyes, and G.M. has a light brown complexion with brown hair and brown eyes. On first exposure to the sun with about an hour of intense midday sunlight, L.M. almost always develops a deep red, painful sunburn, with only minimal subsequent tanning. She freckles easily when exposed to sunlight and remembers being severely sunburned on several occasions as a child. When G.M. is first exposed to the sun in the summer, he usually develops mild erythema, followed by moderate tanning. He cannot recall being severely sunburned as a child, but does recall becoming moderately tanned each summer as a child and adolescent. L.M. is employed as a receptionist for an accounting firm, and G.M. works outdoors for a construction company. Both spend considerable amounts of time participating in outdoor activities. What data in this history would influence your recommendation of a sunscreen product for G.M. and L.M.?

One of the most important pieces of information to include in the patient history is the patient's skin type.[16,17] Patients can be classified into six sun-reactive skin types based on their response to initial sun exposure, skin color, tendency to sunburn, ability to tan, and personal history of sunburn (Table 41-1). This skin typing system has been used by the U.S. Food and Drug Administration (FDA) since 1978 in its guidelines for sunscreen agents. L.M.'s fair complexion, propensity to sunburn, and minimal tanning classify her as skin type II. G.M.'s light brown complexion, minimal sunburn reaction, and moderate tanning classify him as skin type IV. Hair and

Table 41-1   Suggested SPF for Various Skin Types

Complexion	SkinType	Skin Characteristics	Suggested Product SPF
Very fair	I	Always burns easily; never tans	20–30
Fair	II	Always burns easily; tans minimally	15–20
Light	III	Burns moderately; tans gradually	10–15
Medium	IV	Burns minimally; always tans well	8–10
Dark	V	Rarely burns; tans profusely	8
Very dark	VI	Never burns; deeply pigmented	8

SPF, sun protection factor.

eye color also gives an indication as to skin reactiveness to sunlight. People who have blonde, red, or light brown hair or blue or green eyes tend to have greater skin reactivity to sunlight than people with darker-colored hair or eyes. A history of severe sunburn also may be associated with skin reactivity to sunlight, although self-reported patient histories of sunburn or tanning may not be consistently reliable, and personal interviews may be a more reliable indicator. L.M.'s propensity to freckle and her history of severe sunburns as a child may give an indication as to her skin's sun reactiveness. Other important information to consider in the patient history includes a medication history, history of sun-reactive dermatoses, history of allergies (particularly contact hypersensitivities to cosmetics or other topical agents), and the intended activities during sunscreen use.

Photocarcinogenesis
RISK FACTORS

2. What subjective and objective evidence do L.M. and G.M. exhibit that place them at risk for the long-term adverse effects of UVR? What are the risk factors for these long-term adverse effects of UVR?

The long-term effects of UVR include photocarcinogenesis and premature aging of the skin (photoaging). The associated risks for development of these long-term effects are directly related to the congenital pigmentation of an individual (which includes skin type and hair and eye color) and intensity, duration, and frequency of exposure to UVR. With a type II skin type, L.M. is at high risk for carcinogenesis and photoaging, whereas G.M., with skin type IV, may be at a lower risk. Excessive sun exposure, especially during childhood, increases the risk of nonmelanoma and melanoma skin cancers. During the first 18 years of life, the average child receives three times the dose of UVB of the average adult; consequently, most sun exposure occurs during childhood.[18,19] A history of frequent sunburn or intermittent high-intensity exposures to UVR may be associated with the occurrence of malignant melanoma, whereas large cumulative doses of UVR over a lifetime may contribute to the incidence of nonmelanoma skin cancers. L.M.'s history of several severe sunburns as a child may more than double her risk of cutaneous malignant melanoma (CMM).[18,19] Cumulative doses of UVR received unintentionally from working outdoors (as in G.M.) or from participating in outdoor recreational activities also can contribute significantly to the risk of photocarcinogenesis and photoaging.[4] A large number of moles, congenital moles >1.5 cm wide, and abnormal moles also appear to be a risk

factor for malignant melanoma.[20] Furthermore, because its use allows for a longer exposure to the sun, sunscreen use appears to be associated with the occurrence of nevi, which is a strong predictor of melanoma development.[21,22]

SQUAMOUS CELL AND BASAL CELL CARCINOMA

The association of skin cancer in humans to UVR exposure is based primarily on clinical and epidemiologic evidence. Nonmelanoma skin cancers, such as SCC and BCC, occur most commonly on areas that are maximally exposed to sunlight (e.g., the face, neck, arms, back of the forearms, and hands).[3] The prevalence of nonmelanoma skin cancers is inversely related to geographic distance from the equator and to the melanin content of the skin, with SCC more strongly linked than BCC to UVR.[3,20] Persons of skin types most sensitive to sunlight, as well as persons working outdoors, have higher incidences of nonmelanoma skin cancers.[3] Albinism, a genetic disease characterized by partial or total absence of pigment in the skin, hair, and eyes, is associated with increased and premature development of skin cancers.[3]

CUTANEOUS MALIGNANT MELANOMA

The development of CMM also may be linked to UVR exposure, specifically exposures that induce sunburn. A history of five or more severe sunburns during adolescence more than doubles the risk of CMM.[20] CMM, like nonmelanoma skin cancers, demonstrates an inverse relationship to geographic distance from the equator and melanin content of the skin.[3] Unlike nonmelanoma skin cancers, however, CMM does not demonstrate a clear relationship to the cumulative dose of UVR, and it occurs on areas of the body exposed to the sun intermittently (e.g., on the back in men and the lower legs in women). In addition, it occurs most commonly in the middle-aged and individuals who work indoors, as well as those whose sun exposure is limited to weekends and vacations.[20]

MECHANISMS OF CARCINOGENESIS

Mechanisms may include damage to DNA and alterations in immunologic status. Epidermal and dermal DNA can absorb UVR, which can contribute to abnormal formation of pyrimidine dimers. Normally, these pyrimidine dimers are excised and repaired; however, if left uncorrected, these DNA lesions can lead to interruption of transcription, with possible mutagenesis and malignancy.[22]

TANNING BOOTHS

3. B.P., a 32-year-old woman, is preparing for a business trip to Cancun. She is seeking advice about the use of a tanning bed to stimulate melanin for the prevention of sunburn while on her trip. B.P. has skin type III and light brown hair and green eyes. She recently heard, however, that a tan produced by artificial sunlight may not protect against sunburn and may even cause skin cancer. What advice will you offer her? What precautions would you recommend if she decides to visit a tanning salon?

Most tanning beds, booths, or salons use an artificial light source that emits about 95% UVA with minimal (i.e., 1% to 5%) UVB.[23,24] Although UVA is much less likely to produce photoaging and photocarcinogenic changes of the skin than UVB, high doses of UVA received during a tanning session, as well as increasing cumulative UVA doses over time, and increased exposure to sunlight in general, raise great concern over the long-term effects of UVA. UVA causes many of the same effects on the skin as UVB, including immunologic, degenerative, and neoplastic changes, as well as damage to DNA and the formation of reactive oxygen species.[25] UVA also contributes to cataract formation and the activation of herpetic lesions.[26] In addition, UVA may augment the photocarcinogenic effect of UVB.[2]

With a skin type III, B.P. may be able to gradually achieve a moderate tan with minimal burning, thus providing some protection from UVR due to increased melanization of the skin. This UVA-induced tan, however, may not be as protective as a tan achieved under normal sunlight conditions because UVA does not thicken the stratum corneum.[27] An artificially produced tan plus subsequent sun exposure has not been found to provide any net reduction in long-term damage to the skin when compared with the same amount of tan obtained by sunbathing alone.[27] For these reasons, B.P. should not use the tanning booth to obtain a protective tan, and she should use appropriate photoprotective measures during her trip.

If B.P. decides to artificially tan despite your recommendation, she should undertake some precautions. Because she has skin type III, her UVR exposure should be limited to 30 to 50 half-hour sessions a year and she should keep a record of total joules of exposure that she has received over time.[3] To minimize cataract development, B.P. always should wear protective eye wear that absorbs all UVA, UVB, and visible light up to 500 nm; simply closing her eyes or wearing regular sunglasses provides no protective effect against eye damage.

Photoaging
NORMAL AGING AND HISTOLOGY OF PHOTODAMAGED SKIN

Photoaging, or premature aging of the skin, involves skin changes that are different from those associated with normal chronologic aging.[28,29] Normal aging of the skin involves fine wrinkling of the skin, atrophy of the dermis, and a decrease in the amount of subcutaneous adipose tissue, all of which lead to a state of hypocellularity of the skin.[29] Photoaging involves a chronic inflammatory state induced by long-term exposure to sunlight, leading to a hypermetabolic state of the skin.[27] Photodamaged skin is characterized histologically by an accumulation of excessive quantities of thickened, degenerated elastic connective tissue fibers (elastosis).[29] Type I collagen predominates in normal skin, but in photodamaged skin, type III collagen increases about fourfold and the mature matrix of type I collagen slightly decreases.[25] These degenerative changes in connective tissue may be caused by hyperactive fi-

broblasts or by enzymatic degradation via cellular infiltrates in inflamed skin.[3] The elastic connective tissue then replaces the collagen in upper parts of the dermis.[27] The ground substance, composed of proteoglycans and glycosaminoglycans, also is increased considerably in photoaged skin.[3] Capillaries in the dermis become dilated and tortuous, resulting in telangiectasias, ecchymosis, and purpura.[28] The epidermis thickens, and epidermal cells become hyperplastic and possibly neoplastic. Actinic keratosis, a premalignant lesion found mostly in the older population, is a risk factor for the development of BCC, because a low percentage of these lesions transform into SCC.[28,30] Large cumulative doses of UVA, UVB, and possibly infrared radiation over the course of a lifetime are strongly implicated as the cause of these changes in photoaged skin.[3]

Photodamaged skin is characterized as being wrinkled, yellowed, and sagging. Mildly affected skin becomes irregularly pigmented, rough, and dry, with mild wrinkles. Moderately affected skin becomes deeply wrinkled, sagging, thickened, and leathery, with vascular lesions.[28] Largely irreversible, severely affected skin may become deeply furrowed, permanently (and irregularly) pigmented, and may manifest pre-malignant and malignant lesions.[28] Areas of the body most commonly affected are the face, back of the neck, back of the arms and hands, the V-line of the neck of women, and balding areas of the head of men.

TOPICAL RETINOIDS—TRETINOIN AND TAZAROTENE

4. P.B. is a 38-year-old woman who has enjoyed many outdoor activities over the years. She lives in a moderate climate, with hot, sunny summers and cold winters. She feels that she appears older than other women her age because of wrinkling and color changes of her skin. Her facial color is somewhat yellowish in appearance and the fine wrinkles at the corners of her eyes and mouth have become more obvious. She has noticed the formation of small brown spots mottling parts of her face, hands, and forearms. P.B. has skin type III; a clear complexion; and skin that is sensitive to soaps, heavy cosmetics, and perfumes. Would P.B. be an appropriate candidate for therapy with a topical retinoid product (e.g., tretinoin)?

Tretinoin (trans-retinoic acid) is available as a cream (0.025%, 0.05%, and 0.1%), gel (0.01%, 0.025%, 0.1% [in microspheres]), or liquid (0.05%). Tazarotene, another retinoic acid, is available as a 0.1% cream. These agents are effective in partially reversing some of the clinical and histologic changes of photoaging by lessening fine wrinkles, mottled pigmentation, and the tactile roughness associated with photoaged skin.[31–36] Adverse drug events include erythema, peeling, burning, and stinging, and these adverse effects, as well as the clinical and histologic improvements, are thought to be dose-dependent. Mild to moderate reactions decrease gradually after the second week of therapy. Additional benefits of retinoid therapy include the formation of new dermal collagen and vessels, reduction in the number and melanization of freckles, resorption of degenerated connective tissue fibers, and treatment of premalignant and malignant skin lesions.[37] In one of the initial trials, all subjects treated (100%) demonstrated global improvement in the signs of photoaging, with 53% showing moderate changes and the remainder having at least slight improvement. Of the clinical parameters assessed, the most impressive improvements were found with facial skin sallowness, with respondents developing a healthy, rosy glow.[34]

Patient Selection

Topical retinoid therapy is most effective for patients 50 to 70 years of age with moderate to severe photoaging and for prophylactic use in patients undergoing the initial changes of photoaging.[32] Recently, P.B. has noticed some of the skin changes consistent with early photoaging and would be a good candidate for prophylactic therapy with topical tretinoin. Treatment may improve her sallow skin color and lessen the mottling on her face, forearms, and fine wrinkles at the corners of her eyes and mouth, as well as prevent worsening of the photoaging process that she is experiencing.

Patient Counseling

5. **Recommend an appropriate therapy and provide patient counseling for P.B.**

Because both the beneficial and adverse effects of topical retinoid therapy are dose dependent, the underlying goal is to provide the maximal benefit by using the highest concentration that causes minimal skin irritation. Considering P.B.'s skin sensitivity to soaps, cosmetics, and perfumes, her skin is likely to be irritated easily by tretinoin; therefore, it would be best to initiate therapy with the lowest strength (e.g., tretinoin 0.025% cream, or tazarotene 0.1% cream). These agents are usually applied every night at bedtime, but in some instances, they are applied initially on an every-other-night basis until the skin accommodates to the irritant effects. The likelihood of irritation depends on the type of vehicle, more than on the concentration of the agent.[37] The cream formulation causes the least skin irritation and would be preferred for initiating therapy for P.B. Tretinoin is also available as an alcohol base (55%), with a tendency to be drying and irritating. It is preferred for patients with persistent acne or for those with focal actinic lesions. The vehicle in the gel formulation of tretinoin can evaporate, resulting in the potentiation of its effects. Younger patients often prefer the gel because it leaves no residue and is compatible with most cosmetics. The solution and gel may be better tolerated in older patients with oily, thick, pigmented skin.

Before applying the cream to her face at bedtime, P.B. should wash her face gently, using her fingertips and mild soap, then patting her skin dry with a towel. If gentle washing with her fingers does not remove the dry, peeling skin, a washcloth can be used gently on the face. The treated stratum corneum is fragile, and erosions could occur if P.B. is not careful when washing. After waiting about 15 minutes, she should apply a pea-sized amount of cream to her forehead and spread the cream evenly over her entire face. Care should be exercised while applying the cream to the areas adjacent to the eyes and mouth because tretinoin can cause irritation and burning of mucous membranes.

Skin irritation can be expected to start in the first 3 to 5 days of therapy and hopefully will subside in 1 to 3 months. If P.B. experiences excessive irritation, she can reinitiate the regimen on a slower timeline by applying the cream on an every-other-night or every-third-night basis for the first 2 weeks to reduce skin irritation, or she can also apply a topical corticosteroid product such as hydrocortisone 1% cream. As she begins to tolerate the therapy, her frequency of applications and strength of cream should be titrated to cause mild scaling with only occasional mild erythema. A thicker film of cream can be applied to photodamaged areas. After 9 to 12 months of therapy, she can begin maintenance therapy, which consists of application two or three nights a week indefinitely.

Because these agents can dry the skin, counseling P.B. on the use of moisturizers during the day will help decrease the dryness and irritation of the skin. Nighttime application of moisturizers should be discouraged with topical tretinoin use because the moisturizers can cause a pH incompatibility with the cream and possibly dilute the concentration of tretinoin. With a thinning of the stratum corneum, P.B.'s skin may be more susceptible to the effects of UVR. For this reason, as well as to prevent further actinic damage, P.B. should begin prophylactic daytime application of a sunscreen. Considering her skin type (III) and early photoaging changes, a sunscreen with a SPF of at least 30 would be appropriate. P.B. should be counseled not to become discouraged by any apparent lack of response; her skin damage is mild, her response to therapy will be gradual, and part of the goal of therapy is to prevent further damage. Her wrinkles may actually appear to worsen early in therapy owing to an initial buildup of the stratum corneum. P.B. should avoid facial saunas and irritating soaps and cosmetics.

Phototoxicity and Photoallergy
PATIENT HISTORY

6. **D.L., a 16-year-old, blond-haired, blue-eyed boy of skin type II, presents with a severe sunburn. He states that he started a new summer job 2 days ago with typical sun exposure. He is surprised at the severity of this sunburn, which is worse than normal for the same amount of sun exposure. What nonprescription remedies might you recommend for D.L. at this time?**

Treatment recommendations for D.L.'s sunburn are inappropriate without first obtaining additional data (e.g., a history and brief visual examination of the condition). Information that may be important in the history of the condition include the temporal relationship between sun exposure and onset of symptoms; the nature and duration of symptoms; recent ingestion or topical application of medications; possible exposure to photosensitizers, chemical irritants, or plants that may cause allergic contact dermatitis (e.g., poison ivy); and the potential for arthropod bites. Information that may be important from the physical examination includes the distribution and morphology of the reaction, as well as areas of the body spared of the reaction.

A drug-induced photosensitivity reaction most commonly appears as a sunburn of greater severity than would normally be expected or as a rash in areas exposed to the sun or tanning apparatus. With an increased emphasis on health that includes exercise and physical activity outdoors, the incidence of these reactions is common, with a greater frequency during both the summer and winter. Further, with an increase in the use of complementary/alternative medications, many people are unaware that some of these products (e.g., St. John's Wort) can also cause photosensitivity reactions. Chemicals with photosensitization potential are found in medications, cosmetics, shampoos, moisturizing lotions, hair dyes/tints, soaps, and other topically applied medications and agents.

Drug-induced photosensitivity reactions can be subdivided into phototoxic and photoallergic reactions. The same medication or agent may produce both phototoxic and photoallergic reactions, and it may at times be difficult to differentiate clinically between the two types of reactions.

PHOTOSENSITIZERS AND SYMPTOMS OF PHOTOTOXICITY

7. On further questioning, you discover that D.L. first experienced painful erythema of the extensor surface of his hands and forearms, the anterior aspect of his neck, and parts of his face within hours of starting his new job at an outdoor garden and greenhouse. Besides painful erythema, the symptoms also included an immediate prickling and burning sensation. The symptoms continued to worsen until the following morning, about 24 hours after initial exposure to the sun. D.L. does not recall orally ingesting or topically applying any medication or other preparation to his skin, nor does he recall exposure to any chemical irritants, or poison ivy or oak. The morphology of the skin lesions is that of an exaggerated sunburn. The skin lesions are patchy in distribution with greater density on his forearms and hands than on his neck and face. The posterior aspect of his neck and covered areas of his body were spared completely. What are some possible causes of his exaggerated sunburn reaction?

The most likely explanation for D.L.'s exaggerated sunburn reaction is *phototoxicity,* secondary to contact with psoralen-like chemicals from the plants at his job at the outdoor garden and greenhouse. Phototoxicity is an immediate or delayed inflammatory reaction which occurs when a compound with photosensitizing ability absorbs a sufficient concentration of UVR in or on the skin, and when the skin is exposed simultaneously to a specific wavelength of light.[38] This spectrum of offending UVR occurs from the UVB to the UVA range. These compounds include many drugs (see Table 38-8 in Chapter 38, Dermatotherapy and Drug Induced Skin Lesions) and naturally occurring psoralen-like (furocoumarin) compounds that are found in many plants (e.g., limes, parsley, celery, figs).[39] When the photosensitizing compound is deposited on the skin surface, the photosensitizer absorbs the radiologic energy and transfers the energy to surrounding molecules, which then become destructive to the surrounding tissue.[3,38]

The most common type of drug-induced photosensitivity reaction is phototoxicity, in which the offending agent is thought to act as a chromophore, absorbing UVR. When the chromophore reaches a sufficient concentration in or on the skin and when the skin is exposed to the appropriate wavelength of UVR, energy is emitted, which damages the adjacent tissue to cause a phototoxic reaction. The wavelength of radiation necessary to produce such a reaction depends on the absorption spectrum of the offending agent.

Phototoxic photosensitivity reactions are dose dependent and occur in almost any person who takes or applies an adequate amount of the offending agent. The dose necessary to produce such a reaction varies from person to person and depends on such factors as complexion, hair and eye color, usual ability to tan, and type and amount of UVR exposure. Phototoxic photosensitivity reactions are not immunologically mediated, are not allergic reactions, can occur on first exposure to the agent, and generally show no cross-sensitivity to chemically related agents.

A phototoxic reaction usually has a rapid onset, often within several hours after UVR exposure and presents as an exaggerated or intensified sunburn with erythema, pain, and prickling or burning. Blistering, desquamation, and hyperpigmentation can occur in severe cases.[38] Symptoms generally peak 24 to 48 hours after the initial exposure and are usually limited to the areas of UVR-exposed skin. Because phototoxicity reactions do not involve the immune system, prior exposure to the photosensitizer is unnecessary for this reaction to occur.

Presumably, D.L. came into contact with psoralen-containing plants and simultaneous exposure to sunlight. With an unusual distribution of lesions on his hands, forearms, neck, and face, the lack of lesions on areas not contacted by the plants or sunlight, the temporal relationship between the exposure and onset of symptoms place phototoxicity higher in the differential diagnosis.

PHOTOSENSITIZERS AND SYMPTOMS OF PHOTOALLERGY

Photoallergy is another possible cause of D.L.'s symptoms. Although much less common than phototoxicity, photoallergy requires prior or prolonged exposure to the photosensitizing compound. Photoallergy results from a similar mechanism to phototoxicity, except that the immune system is involved. Most commonly, it is caused by polycyclic photosensitizers that react with UVA to form antigenic macromolecules, evoking a delayed hypersensitivity response. Clinically, photoallergy differs from phototoxicity in that it produces an intensely pruritic, eczematous form of dermatitis.[38] The rash is preceded by pruritus and may subside within an hour. In 5% to 10% of cases, persistent hypersensitivity to light occurs, even after the offending chemical has been eliminated.[38]

In photoallergic photosensitivity reactions, the suspected medication or chemical agent is altered in the presence of UVR to become antigenic or to become a hapten (i.e., an incomplete antigen), which can combine with a tissue antigen. These antigen–antibody or immune-mediated processes differentiate photoallergic from phototoxic reactions. Photoallergic reactions do not occur on first exposure to the medication, but like other allergic reactions, they require prior or prolonged exposure (sensitization period) to the offending agent.[38] Once sensitization has occurred, subsequent exposure to even small amounts of the offending product will produce a photoallergic reaction.

Photoallergic reactions are not dose-related, and eruptions may also be caused by chemically related agents owing to a cross-sensitivity or cross-allergenicity. As a type of delayed hypersensitivity reaction, time is required to develop an immune response and the onset of a photoallergic reaction is often delayed for 1 to 3 days. These reactions may present as macular, bullous, or purpuric lesions, and acute urticaria may occur within minutes after UVR exposure. Recovery is slower than from a phototoxic reaction, and it can persist after the offending product has been removed. These reactions may present with erythema and possible edema secondary to the inflammation, but are most commonly found to be eczematous, characterized by erythema; pruritus (possible severe); papules and vesicles, with weeping, oozing, and crusting. Scaling, lichenification, and pigmentation may occur later.

In a small percentage of cases, hypersensitivity to UVR can persist after the suspected agent is discontinued. Photoallergic reactions primarily occur on the skin at sites that are exposed to UVR, but may extend to nonexposed areas. These reactions are more common in adults, usually caused by topical medications or chemicals, but also can be seen with the use of systemic medications.

D.L. is unlikely to have a photoallergic reaction because of the lack of a delayed temporal relationship between the onset of symptoms and combined exposure to plant furocoumarins and sunlight. Unlike phototoxicity reactions, photoallergic reactions can spread to areas that have not been exposed to sunlight; however, D.L.'s lesions were limited to areas of skin exposed to sunlight.

MANAGEMENT

8. **What recommendations should you give D.L. for management of his photosensitivity?**

General recommendations for the management of phototoxicity and photoallergy reactions are focused on the removal of exposure to the potential photosensitizer and reduced exposure to the sun. Patients should be counseled not to take any medications, orally or topically, without first consulting with their health care provider to minimize exposure to other photosensitizers. D.L. should try wearing long-sleeved shirts, pants, and gloves when working to limit exposure to plant photosensitizers. He also may try applying a broad-spectrum sunscreen to protect his skin from UVB and UVA radiation. If these measures do not prevent further photosensitivity reactions, D.L. should consider a different type of employment. His presenting symptoms should be managed in a manner similar to that for an exaggerated sunburn.

Photoprotection
Broad-Spectrum Products

Sunscreens are used to prevent sunburn and reduce the incidence of premature aging and carcinogenesis.[30,40,41] The original formulations were developed to protect against the effects of UVB radiation because the potential adverse effects of UVA were not yet recognized. Because UVA plays a significant role in many of the adverse effects associated with UVR exposure, broad spectrum sunscreen products with absorption spectra in the UVA range have become commercially available, in combination with UVB absorbers. These broad-spectrum products provide additional benefit for patients with photosensitivity reactions caused by wavelengths not covered by single-ingredient sunscreens.

Sunscreens should be considered as only one component of an overall program to reduce UV exposure and protect against long-term photodamage.[42] This program can be recalled with the acronym C-H-E-S-S:

C—Clothing that is sun protective (i.e., tightly woven and in dark colors)
H—Hats with wide brims all around
E—Eyeglasses that block both UVA and UVB light
S—Sunscreen with an SPF of at least 15 that is applied appropriately
S—Shade, especially between 10 AM and 4 PM

Table 41-2 lists the available sunscreen chemicals that have been judged to be both safe and effective.

Evaluation of Sunscreens
SUN PROTECTION FACTOR

The effectiveness of a sunscreen formulation is based on its sun protection factor (SPF) and its substantivity.[43] *SPF* is defined as the ratio of the minimal dose of UVR required to produce an erythemal response in sunscreen-protected skin compared with unprotected skin.[30] SPFs are based on tests of volunteers with skin types I through III, using either natural sunlight or a solar simulator that generates both UVB and UVA.[30,43] Because the SPF can be influenced by the composition, chemical properties, emollient properties, and pH of the vehicle, sunscreen formulations must be evaluated on an individual basis.[43] SPF also is influenced by the amount applied to the skin, the time of initial application before UVR exposure, the frequency of application, and environmental factors such

Table 41-2 **Sunscreens and UVR Absorbance**

Sunscreen	Absorbance
Anthranilates	
Menthyl anthranilate	260–380
Benzophenones	
Dioxybenzone	250–390
Oxybenzone	270–350
Sulisobenzone (Eusolex 4360)	260–375
Cinnamates	
Diethanolamine p-methoxycinnamate	280–310
Octocrylene	250–360
Octyl methoxycinnamate (Parsol MCX)	290–320
Dibenzoylmethanes	
Avobenzone (butyl methoxydibenzoylmethane, Parsol 1789)	320–400
Aminobenzoic Acid and Ester Derivatives	
Lisadimate (Glyceryl PABA)	264–315
Para-aminobenzoic acid (PABA)	260–313
Padimate O (octyl dimethyl PABA)	290–315
Roxadimate	280–330
Salicylates	
Homosalate	295–315
Octyl salicylate	280–320
Triethanolamine salicylate	260–320
Trolamine salicylate	260–320
Camphor Derivatives	
Benzoate-4 methylbenzylidene camphor	290–300
Mexoryl SX	290–400
Others	
Phenylbenzimidazole	290–340
Physical Sunscreens	
Red petrolatum	290–365
Titanium dioxide	290–700
Zinc oxide	290–700

UVR, ultraviolet radiation.

as photodegradation during UVR exposure; therefore, the SPF achieved during actual use can be significantly less than indicated on the label.[44-49]

In 1978, the FDA Over-the-Counter (OTC) Review Panel on sunscreens reclassified sunscreens from cosmetics to drugs intended to protect the structure and function of the human integument against actinic damage. In May 1999, the FDA finalized its regulations for OTC sunscreens. Manufacturers of cosmetic tanning preparations that do not contain a sunscreen were required to include a warning statement (see the following discussion) on their products. These regulations list the active ingredients that can be used in sunscreens, labeling and testing requirements, and also provide for uniform, streamlined labeling for all OTC products intended for use as sunscreens to assist consumers in making decisions on sun protection. The revised regulations include the following:

- Similar labeling requirements for all OTC products intended for use as sunscreens (including sunscreen–cosmetic combinations such as makeup products carrying sun protection claims) to provide good, useful information to consumers.
- Uniform, streamlined labeling for all sunscreens. Accommodations in labeling will be made for sunscreens that are labeled for use only on specific small areas of the face (e.g., lips, nose, ears, and/or around eyes).
- A list of 16 allowed sunscreen active ingredients, with zinc oxide and azobenzene being the two most recent additions.
- Both required and optional label claims, warnings, and directions.
- Required SPF testing for all agents.
- A new SPF category of "30" plus (or "30%") for SPF values above 30.
- Simplification of the previously proposed five product sun protection categories down to three: *minimum* (corresponding to the current SPF of 2 to 12), *moderate* (corresponding to an SPF of 12 to 30), or *high* (corresponding to an SPF of 30 or greater), plus optional claims to help consumers with the selection of sunscreen products.
- A "Sun Alert" statement that reflects the important role that sunscreens play in a total program to reduce the harmful effects of the sun (i.e., "Sun alert: Limiting sun exposure, wearing protective clothing, and using sunscreens may reduce the risks of skin aging, skin cancer, and other harmful effects of the sun").
- Cessation of unsupported, absolute, and/or misleading and confusing terms such as *sun block, waterproof, all-day protection, deep tanning,* and *visible and/or infrared light protection.*

In addition to the aforementioned changes, new cosmetic regulations require tanning preparations that do not contain a sunscreen ingredient to display the following warning: "Warning—this product does not contain a sunscreen and does not protect against sunburn. Repeated exposure of unprotected skin while tanning may increase the risk of skin aging, skin cancer, and other harmful effects to the skin even if you do not burn."

SUBSTANTIVITY

Substantivity is a measure of the sunscreen formulation's effectiveness. The substantivity of a sunscreen formulation is its ability to be adsorbed by, or adhere to, the skin while swimming or perspiring. In the past, labeling of a product as "waterproof" or "water-resistant" indicated that the SPF of the product was maintained after 80 minutes of moderate activity or 40 minutes while swimming, respectively. Because testing is performed indoors under close to ideal conditions (e.g., lower humidity), the effects of the actual environment where it is used and the evaporation of the vehicle may reduce considerably the overall effectiveness of the sunscreen. The substantivity of a product largely depends on the vehicle, as well as the active ingredient[50] (Table 41-3). The affinity of a sunscreen to the keratinaceous layer of the stratum corneum is directly related to the keratin/vehicle partition coefficient. The saturation of the active agent in keratin depends on the drug's lipophilicity, whereas its substantivity is independent of its lipophilicity. Sunscreen compounds with a high solubility in the product's vehicle penetrate the skin most easily. Classically, vehicles such as water-in-oil emulsions or ointments tend to have a higher degree of substantivity. Some of the newer products have improved substantivity with the addition of a polymer such as polyacrylamide to the formulation.

SUNBURN PREVENTIVE AND SUNTANNING AGENTS

Sunburn preventive agents are those active ingredients that absorb ≥95% of UVB radiation and have the potential to prevent sunburn. Suntanning agents are those with active ingredients that absorb 85% to 95% of UVB radiation, thereby allowing suntanning without significant sunburn in the average individual. Chemical sunscreens include both of the aforementioned designations. Opaque sunblocks, or physical sunscreens, are those active ingredients that reflect or scatter all UVA, UVB, and visible light, thereby preventing or minimizing sunburn and suntanning.[51]

Chemical Sunscreens

Chemical sunscreens are compounds capable of absorbing UVR, thereby protecting the skin structures from the adverse effects of the selective wavelengths absorbed.[30] After application to the skin, these aromatic compounds convert the high UVR energy into harmless longer-wave radiation, which may or may not be perceived as warmth.[30] Chemical sunscreens usually are nonopaque because they do not absorb the wavelengths of visible light.

MOLAR ABSORPTIVITY AND ABSORBANCE SPECTRUM

The molar absorptivity and absorption spectrum determine the effectiveness of an individual chemical sunscreen agent, which are determined mostly by its chemical structure. Molar absorptivity is a measure of the amount of UVR absorbed by a particular sunscreen, and it depends on the concentration of the sunscreen in the product and the amount applied to the skin. Sunscreens with an absorbance spectrum in the UVB range with a maximal absorption between 310 and 320 nm, are the most effective at preventing a sunburn.[43] Chemical sunscreens with absorption spectra in the UVB range are para-aminobenzoic acid (PABA) and its esters, cinnamates, and the salicylates. Sunscreens with absorption spectra that extend into the UVA range are the anthranilates (e.g., menthyl anthranilate), dibenzoylmethanes (e.g., azobenzene), and benzophenones (e.g., oxybenzone).

Table 41-3 Examples of Commercially Available Sunscreen Products

Name (Active Ingredients)	Formulation	SPF
Bain de Soleil All Day Waterproof Sunblock (octocrylene, octyl methoxycinnamate*, oxybenzone, titanium dioxide)	Lotion	15, 30
Bain de Soleil Oil-Free Protecteur Faces (octocrylene, oxybenzone, octisalate*, avobenzone, homosalate)	Lotion	35
Banana Boat Baby Block (octyl methoxycinnamate*, octyl salicylate*, oxybenzone, titanium dioxide)	Lotion	50
Banana Boat Maximum Sunblock (octocrylene, octinoxate*, oxybenzone, octisalate*)	Lotion	50
Banana Boat Quik Blok Kids (octyl methoxycinnamat*, homosalate, octyl salicylate*, oxybenzone, avobenzone)	Lotion	25+
Banana Boat Sport Sunblock (octyl methoxycinnamate*, octyl salicylate*, oxybenzone, octocrylene)	Lotion	50
Blistex Ultra Protection (homosalate, menthyl anthranilate*, octyl methoxycinnamate*, octyl salicylate*, oxybenzone)	Lip balm	30
Blue Lizard Australian Sunscream (octinoxate*, octocrylene, oxybenzone, zinc oxide)	Lotion	30+
Bullfrog Body Lotion (octocrylene, octyl methoxycinnamate, oxybenzone)	Lotion	45
Bullfrog For Babies (octocrylene, octyl methoxycinnamate*, oxybenzone, octyl salicylate*, titanium dioxide, menthyl anthranilate*)	Lotion	45
Bullfrog Magic Block—Disappearing Green (octyl methoxycinnamate*, octyl salicylate*, octocrylene, oxybenzone)	Lotion	30
Bullfrog Sport (octocrylene, octyl methoxycinnamate*, octyl salicylate*, oxybenzone)	Lotion	18, 30
Bullfrog Sunblock (octyl methoxycinnamate*, oxybenzone, octyl salicylate*, octocrylene)	Gel	36
ChapStick (padimate O)	Lip balm	15
ChapStick Ultra (octocrylene, octyl methoxycinnamate*, oxybenzone, octyl salicylate*)	Lip balm	30
ChapStick Sunblock (oxybenzone, padimate O)	Lip balm, or ointment	15
Coppertone BUG & SUN for Adults (with insect repellent) (homosalate, octyl methoxycinnamate*, octyl salicylate*, oxybenzone)	Lotion	15, 30
Coppertone KIDS Colorblock Disappearing Colored Sunblock (Blue or Purple Formula) (octyl methoxycinnamate*, octyl salicylate*, oxybenzone, homosalate)	Lotion/Spray	30, 40
Coppertone Moisturizing Sunblock (octyl methoxycinnamate*, octyl salicylate*, octocrylene, oxybenzone)	Lotion	45
Coppertone Shade Sunblock (homosalate, octyl methoxycinnamate*, octyl salicylate*, oxybenzone)	Lotion	45
Coppertone Spectra 3 (homosalate, octinoxate*, octocrylene, octisalate*, zinc oxide)	Lotion	30, 50
Coppertone Spectra 3 Water Babies (homosalate, octinoxate*, octocrylene, octisalate*, oxybenzone, zinc oxide)	Lotion	50
Coppertone Sport Ultra Sweatproof (octinoxate*, oxybenzone, octisalate*)	Lotion	15, 30, 48
DuraScreen (octyl methoxycinnamate*, octyl salicylate*, oxybenzone, phenylbenzimidazole, titanium Dioxide)	Lotion	15, 30
Eucerin Dry Skin Therapy Facial Moisturizing (octyl methoxycinnamate*, octyl salicylat*, titanium dioxide, zinc oxide)	Lotion	25
Fisher-Price Waterproof Sunblock (titanium dioxide)	Cream	28
Hawaiian Tropic Baby Faces Sunblock (octocrylene, octyl methoxycinnamate*, octyl salicylate*, oxybenzone, titanium dioxide)	Lotion	35, 50
Hawaiian Tropic Just For Kids (octocrylene, octyl methoxycinnamate*, octyl salicylate*, oxybenzone, titanium dioxide)	Lotion	45
Hawaiian Tropic Sunblock (octocrylene, octyl methoxycinnamate*, octyl salicylate*, oxybenzone, titanium dioxide)	Lotion	45%
Neutrogena Chemical-Free Sunblocker (titanium dioxide)	Lotion	17
Neutrogena Kids Sunblock (homosalate, octinoxate*, oxybenzone, octisalate*)	Lotion	30
Neutrogena Healthy Defense Oil-Free Sunblock (homosalate, octinoxate*, oxybenzone, octisalate*)	Lotion/Spray	30
Neutrogena Sensitive Skin Sunblock (titanium dioxide)	Lotion	17
Neutrogena Sunblock (menthyl anthranilate*, octocrylene, octinoxate*)	Cream	30
Neutrogena UVA/UVB Sunblock (octinoxate*, homosalate, octisalate*, oxybenzone, avobenzone)	Lotion	30, 45
Off! Skintastic with Sunscreen (octyl methoxycinnamate*, octocrylene, oxybenzone, benzophenone-3, plus N,N-Diethyl-m-toluamide (DEET))	Lotion	15, 30
Sundown Sport Sunblock (titanium dioxide, zinc oxide)	Lotion	15

SPF, sun protective factor.
*Interchangable terminology used by different product manufacturers.
Newer terminology—older traditional terminology: octinoxate—octyl methoxycinnamate; octisalate—octyl salicylate; meradimate—menthyl anthranilate.

PARA-AMINOBENZOIC ACID (PABA) AND ESTERS

Commonly used in the past, PABA absorbs UVR in the UVB range from 260 to 313 nm, with maximal absorbance around 290 nm;[52] its molar absorptivity is considered to be high.[43] PABA readily penetrates and binds to the stratum corneum and, after several days of application, may remain in the skin and provide protection even after swimming, perspiration, and bathing.[43] It is commonly formulated as an alcoholic mixture, which may cause stinging, dryness, or tightness, particularly when applied to the face.[52] Its major disadvantage is the causation of contact or photocontact dermatitis.[53] Responsible for more sensitivity reactions than any

other sunscreen,[48] PABA can also cause cross-sensitivity reactions with benzocaine, thiazides, sulfonamides, paraphenylenediamine (a common ingredient in hair dyes), and other PABA derivatives.[52] It may cause discoloration of clothes as well. The use of PABA in commercial sunscreens has decreased to the point where many of the newer sunscreens are promoted as being PABA-free.

PABA esters include octyl dimethyl PABA (Padimate O) and glyceryl PABA. These esters are incorporated easily into formulations, demonstrate good substantivity, and do not discolor clothing.[52] Their absorption spectra are similar to that of PABA (see Table 41-2). With a maximal absorbance of 311 nm and the lowest likelihood of the PABA/PABA esters to cause cross-sensitivity reactions or contact and photocontact dermatitis, Padimate O is used in many sunscreen agents. Glyceryl PABA can cause contact dermatitis and cross-sensitivities, both of which may be due to benzocaine impurities in the commercial products.[52,54]

CINNAMATES

Cinnamates have UVB-absorbing qualities. Ethylhexyl para-methoxycinnamate (Parsol MCX), which has high molar absorptivity and a maximal absorbance of 305 nm, is the most commonly used cinnamate.[55] Cinnamates are related chemically to balsam of Peru, balsam of Tolu, coca leaves, cinnamic acid, cinnamic aldehyde, cinnamic oil, ingredients that are used in perfumes, topical medications, cosmetics, and flavorings.[54] These agents do not bind well to the stratum corneum, leading to poor substantivity. Cinnamate-based sunscreens tend to be comedogenic because the vehicle may contain other occlusive ingredients that are added to improve the substantivity. Cinnamates, which absorb only UVB radiation, are often used in combination with benzophenones, appear to be nonstaining, and rarely cause contact dermatitis.[55]

BENZOPHENONES

Benzophenones such as oxybenzone and dioxybenzone are UVB-absorbing sunscreens that have absorbance spectra extending into the UVA range.[56] Benzophenones are also found in shampoos, soaps, hair sprays and dyes, paints, varnishes, and lacquers. The maximal absorbance for each is about 290 nm, but both are limited because of poor substantivity and sensitization.[56] Photocontact dermatitis with oxybenzone and contact dermatitis with dioxybenzone occur commonly, with the latter usually occurring as a contact urticaria.

SALICYLATES

Salicylates are weak UVB absorbers often found in PABA-free products. Topical salicylates are considered among the safest sunscreens, even though they are used in high concentrations.[57] Salicylates have low molar absorptivities, are incorporated easily into formulations, and are used to boost the SPF of combination products. Sensitization to the salicylates is rare.[57]

ANTHRANILATES

Anthranilates, such as menthyl anthranilate, are weak UVB-absorbing sunscreens with an absorbance spectrum extending into the UVA range. Like the salicylates, they have low molar absorptivity, with a maximal absorbance of approximately 336 nm.[43] Menthyl anthranilate has a low risk of sensitization and has a desirable absorbance spectrum, especially when it is used in combination with other sunscreens to give broad-spectrum protection.[57]

DIBENZOYLMETHANES

As a prototype of this class, azobenzene (butyl methoxydibenzoylmethane, Parsol 1789) has high molar absorptivity and absorption spectra exclusively in the UVA range, with maximal absorbance around 360 nm, and reported photosensitization.[58] It is commonly formulated with UVB sunscreens to broaden UVR coverage. Even though protection is provided throughout the UVA and UVB ranges in these combination products, it is unknown whether sufficient protection is available for highly UVA-sensitive patients. Avobenzone loses approximately 35% of its absorbance capacity about 15 minutes after UVR exposure, possibly because of instability of the compound.[2]

ANTIOXIDANTS

Antioxidants have received a revived interest in terms of providing a photoprotective effect, particularly because it has been determined that vitamin C levels in the skin can be severely depleted after UVR exposure.[59] Antioxidants such as vitamins C and E, either taken orally or applied topically when incorporated into a commercially available sunscreen product, may provide additive protection against both UVA- and UVB-induced photodamage.[59–61]

PHYSICAL SUNSCREENS

Physical sunscreens are opaque formulations made of particulate insoluble compounds, incorporated into a vehicle. The skin is shielded from sunlight by reflection and scattering of both UV and visible radiation; both size of the particles and thickness of the film determine the amount of protection.[62] The most effective and commonly used physical sunscreens are titanium dioxide and zinc oxide, which absorb UVR as well as reflect and scatter.[62,63] Other physical sunscreens include magnesium oxide, red veterinarian petrolatum, iron oxides, kaolin, ichthammol, and talc.

These compounds are used in conjunction with chemical sunscreens to formulate products of higher SPF and as single-ingredient sunblocks. When used alone they are usually placed in an ointment base designed specifically for vulnerable parts of the body, such as the nose, cheeks, lips, ears, and shoulders.[51] Physical sunscreens are important in individuals who are unusually sensitive to UVA and visible light, such as those with vitiligo, a skin condition with amelanotic lesions surrounded by areas of normally pigmented skin. Appropriately colored formulations can be used to camouflage and protect these vulnerable amelanotic lesions.[51] Physical sunscreen agents are preferred for persons who need absolute UVR and visible light protection (e.g., young children; persons with skin types I through IV who receive constant exposure; and persons with drug photosensitivity reactions, xeroderma pigmentosa, lupus erythematosis, and other photosensitive skin reactions).[51]

Physical sunscreens are not widely accepted because they are visible to others, messy, and occlusive when applied to the skin. They have a higher substantivity, but may melt in the heat of the sun, limiting their protection to a few hours. Physical sunscreen products tend to be so occlusive that they may cause or worsen acne or obstruction of sweat glands.[51] Neutrogena Sensitive Skin Sunblock Lotion SPF 30 (titanium dioxide 9.1%) is an example of a physical sunscreen with cosmetically appealing properties (e.g., ease of application).

Product Selection

9. **R.J. and her husband J.J. are parents of two children: P.J., a 6-month-old girl, and L.J., an 18-month-old boy. They are spending a week in August vacationing on the Outer Banks of North Carolina, with plans for time at the beach, bicycling, and sailing. R.J. is 25 years old, has type V skin, brown hair and**

brown eyes, and has no history of photosensitivity reactions or medication allergies. She has a history of contact dermatitis on her scalp and around her hairline on several occasions after dying her hair and using certain shampoos. J.J. is 27 years old and has skin type II with blonde hair and blue eyes. As a teenager, he suffered from frequent sinus infections and often was treated with trimethoprim-sulfamethoxazole (TMP-SMX [Septra/Bactrim]) because of an allergy to penicillin. He remembers developing a severe sunburn after minimal exposure to the sun while taking the sulfa-containing antibiotic. He recently has been started on hydrochlorothiazide (HCTZ), 12.5 mg PO QD, for hypertension. What considerations are important in recommending sunscreens for R.J. and J.J.? Recommend an appropriate sunscreen for each member of the family with appropriate directions for application while on vacation.

CROSS-SENSITIVITY

The first consideration for recommending an appropriate sunscreen for R.J. and J.J. is their skin type. R.J. has skin type V, suggesting that a sunscreen with an SPF of at least 8 would provide adequate protection for her (see Table 41-1). J.J. has skin type II, suggesting that a sunscreen with an SPF of 30 would be required to provide adequate protection for him. Furthermore, the history of contact dermatitis and photosensitivity reaction exhibited by R.J. and J.J., respectively, is important when providing a recommendation for use of a sunscreen. The contact dermatitis that R.J. experienced from hair dyes and shampoos may have been caused by para-phenylenediamine, an ingredient of hair dyes,[52] or a benzophenone, which sometimes is included in products such as hair dyes and shampoos.[56] Because a cross-reactivity between para-phenylenediamine and PABA or its derivatives is possible, a sunscreen for R.J. that does not contain PABA or a benzophenone should be recommended. A wide-spectrum PABA-free sunscreen that does not contain a benzophenone may be ideal for R.J. because cinnamates and anthranilates rarely cause contact dermatoses.

Because both contain sulfa moieties, the photosensitivity reaction that J.J. experienced while taking TMP-SMX may indicate that he might be susceptible to a cross-sensitivity reaction with PABA or its derivatives. This reaction to TMP-SMX also indicates that J.J. may be susceptible to a photosensitivity reaction with HCTZ. If a photosensitivity reaction is likely, it is advisable to recommend an SPF of 30. Because drug-induced photosensitivity reactions are caused by UVA, a PABA-free broad-spectrum sunscreen that absorbs UVA as well as UVB would be necessary to provide J.J. with adequate protection. Broad-spectrum chemical sunscreens commonly contain a benzophenone and a cinnamate. A broad-spectrum sunscreen containing both of these chemical classes (e.g., Shade Sunblock Lotion, with octyl methoxycinnamate, oxybenzone, homosalate, and octyl salicylate; see Table 41-3) would be an acceptable broad-spectrum product. Alternatively, because Padimate O is the least likely of the PABA ester derivatives to cause photocontact dermatitis,[52] a broad-spectrum combination product that contains Padimate O could be recommended for J.J. If the photosensitivity reaction is caused by visible light, it would also be necessary to recommend a physical sunscreen to block all sunlight or complete avoidance.[51] With all of these issues considered, it may be preferable to recommend an alternative antihypertensive medication for J.J. that would not place him at risk for a photosensitivity reaction.

APPLICATION

Because R.J. and J.J. are planning to be active on the beach, sunscreens that are water-resistant or waterproof are recommended (see Table 41-3). Before complete application of the sunscreen to the body, because of the risk of cross-sensitivity reactions, patients can perform a patch test by applying small quantity of the sunscreen to the inner aspect of the forearm and covering with a small bandage overnight. Most persons apply 20% to 60% of the required amount of sunscreen needed to achieve the SPF of their product.[49] Because of this, a method has been developed to determine an approximate volume of sunscreen product needed for adequate protection.[64] For protection in the beach environment, for example, an average-size adult should apply and rub in 2 to 2.5 ounces evenly to all exposed skin surfaces at least 30 to 45 minutes before exposure.[64] It is best to reapply the sunscreen every 1 to 2 hours or after sweating, swimming, or toweling off.

10. How long might J.J. expect to be protected with the sunscreen properly applied? Do products with an SPF >15 provide any additional benefit?

If J.J. (skin type II) normally burns after 30 minutes of exposure to the sun, a sunscreen with an SPF of 15 to 30 may provide up to 7.5 hours (0.5 hours ×15 [SPF 15]) of photoprotection from UVB. However, a high SPF product may provide only partial protection against UVA, with little or no protection from infrared radiation.[43] Because of this, sun exposure should be limited to 90 to 120 minutes for each outing after appropriate sunscreen application. Further, environmental factors such as elevated atmospheric humidity and inadequate application techniques may reduce photoprotection by as much as half.

Sunscreen formulations with SPFs as high as 50 can be made using combinations of chemical and physical sunscreen agents (e.g., Hawaiian Tropic Baby Faces Sunblock Lotion, with octyl methoxycinnamate, octocrylene, oxybenzone, octyl salicylate, and titanium dioxide; see Table 41-3).[3] Individuals who are extremely sensitive to the sun may benefit from formulations of higher SPFs, but the average fair-skinned person gains adequate protection for sunbathing or for average daily exposure from a product with an SPF of 30.[49]

Photoprotection for Children

11. What photoprotective measures should be provided for P.J. and L.J.? What nonsunscreen protection is appropriate for use with children?

AGE-RELATED RECOMMENDATIONS AND OTHER PROTECTIVE BEHAVIOR

Sun protection during childhood is very important, considering that most of a person's lifetime of sun exposure occurs in childhood and that the harmful effects of UVR are cumulative.[21] The FDA has recommended that sunscreen agents not be used for children younger than 6 months of age because of the possible chemical absorption through the skin and lowered ability of children of this age to metabolize the absorbed drug.[65] P.J. needs to be kept out of direct sunlight and, when outside, must be protected with proper clothing and shading.[66-69] The FDA has recommended that children younger than 2 years be treated with an SPF >4 because of inadequate UVR protection with lower SPF products for most individuals.[65]

L.J. should be protected with a PABA-free sunscreen with an SPF of at least 15. Regular use of a sunscreen with an SPF of at least 15 for the first 18 years of life can reduce the lifetime incidence of nonmelanoma skin cancers by about three-fourths.[67] If L.J. is in the sun during 6 hours of maximal exposure (i.e., 10 AM to 4 PM), or otherwise for an extended period, he should wear protective clothing, covering as much of his body as possible.[68] Tightly woven clothing, long sleeves, and pants protect the skin from almost all UVR, whereas loosely woven clothing or wet T-shirts can allow up to 30% of UVR to pass through to the skin. Although not complete, water is thought to reduce UVR scattering, thus decreasing its transmission. An average-weight cotton T-shirt provides only an SPF of 7 or 8.[68] The transmission of UVR through a fabric is measured using a spectrophotometer or spectroradiometer. The Ultraviolet Protection Factor (UPF), rather than SPF, has been recommended as a measure of the sun-protective properties of fabrics.[70,71] It is calculated using a formula based on UV transmission through the fabric and the erythema response for human skin. For example, if a fabric has a UPF of 20, then only 1/20 of the UVR at the surface of the fabric actually passes through it. Table 41-4 compares the UPF with the amount of effective UVR transmitted and absorbed.

No woven fabric provides complete coverage because the holes between the threads permit UVR transmission. A baseball cap shields little more than the upper central forehead. Broad-rimmed hats can protect the ears, neck, nose, and cheeks,[71,72] but may provide inadequate protection against SCC of the head or neck.[72] A newer concept that is being introduced to consumers is an ultraviolet absorbing ingredient for fabric softeners (e.g., Tinosorb-FR, Ciba). The fabric softener is added to the laundry rinse cycle, and it works by binding to laundered fibers; it accumulates to increase the UV protection through repeated wash and rinse cycles.

PRODUCT SELECTION

Two types of sunscreens are appropriate for use in children. A lotion is preferred for total body application versus an alcoholic lotion or gel because alcoholic preparations can cause stinging, burning, and irritation of the skin and eyes. Physical sunscreens (e.g., zinc oxide) are available in bright colors and are recommended for selected body areas, such as the nose, cheeks, and shoulders. PABA and its derivatives are considered potentially harmful to a child's tender skin. For adolescents with acne vulgaris, the use of an oil-free, non-comedogenic sunscreen formulation (e.g., Shade Sunblock Oil-Free Gel, or Neutrogena Healthy Defense Sunblock) and a lip balm that contains a sunscreen of at least SPF 15 (e.g.,

Table 41-4 Relative Ultraviolet Protection Factor (UPF) by Ultraviolet Ray (UVR) Transmission and Absorption

% UVR Transmitted	% UVR Absorbed	UPF	Protection Category
10	90.0	10	Moderate protection
5	95.0	20	High protection
3.3	96.7	30	Very high protection
2.5	97.5	40	Extremely high protection
<2.0	>98.0	50	Maximum protection

ChapStick or Blistex Regular (SPF 15), Blistex Ultra (SPF 30) or ChapStick Ultra (SPF 30) would be appropriate.

Photoeffects on the Eye

12. Why should R.J. and J.J. be concerned about the effect of prolonged sunlight on their eyes? Recommend appropriate protective eyewear for them while they are on vacation.

CATARACT FORMATION

Age-related opacification of the ocular lens, or senescent cataracts, has been attributed to a lifetime of exposure to sunlight. The incidence of cataracts increases steadily after age 50, reaching nearly 50% in individuals over the age of 75.[26] UVB is absorbed by the cornea and lens, which slowly results in protein oxidation and precipitation within the lens. UVA penetrates the ocular lens and can cause cumulative damage to deeper structures of the eye. Decreased transmittance and increased scattering of light by the opacified lens eventually results in blurred vision, rings or halos around lights, changes in color perception, and blindness.[73] In advanced cases, the only treatment is surgical removal of the cataract.

High exposure of the eye to UVR, which can range from a few seconds of exposure to arc welding, a few minutes of exposure to a UVC-emitting germicidal lamp, commercial tanning, or UVR reflection by snow or sand can cause photokeratitis, a painful inflammation of the cornea, or conjunctivitis. Photokeratitis usually begins 30 minutes to 24 hours after the exposure and time to onset depends upon the intensity of the exposure.[74] Conjunctivitis commonly accompanies photokeratitis and is characterized by the sensation of a foreign body or grit in the eyes. Varying degrees of photophobia, lacrimation, and blepharospasm also may accompany photokeratitis.[74] Because the corneal epithelium has a great regenerative capacity, photokeratitis tends to be transient, with regression in 24 to 48 hours. The treatment consists of cool, wet compresses and mild anti-inflammatory analgesics such as ibuprofen, aspirin, or naproxen sodium.

PROTECTIVE EYEWEAR

R.J. and J.J. should wear sunglasses when outdoors to decrease their lifelong exposure to solar radiation and while at the beach to prevent high exposure of UVR and possible photokeratitis or conjunctivitis. Many manufacturers of sunglasses label their products according to three categories: cosmetic, general purpose, and special purpose. Cosmetic sunglasses block at least 70% of UVB, at least 20% of UVA, and <60% of visible light and are appropriate for casual wear when high exposure to UVR is unlikely. General-purpose sunglasses block at least 95% of UVB, at least 60% of UVA, 60% to 92% of visible light, and are appropriate for most activities in sunny environments.[75] Special-purpose sunglasses block at least 99% of UVB, at least 60% of UVA, and at least 97% of visible light and are appropriate for very bright environments such as ski slopes or tropical beaches.[75] Special- or general-purpose sunglasses are appropriate recommendations for R.J. and J.J. to wear while on vacation.

Treatment of Sunburn

13. G.B., a 31-year-old man with skin type IV, returned a few hours ago from an afternoon of activity in the sun. His shoulders, back, neck, and arms are bright red and are beginning to feel hot, stretched, and painful. G.B. has been otherwise healthy, has no significant medical history, and has no known allergies to medications. What treatment recommendations would you give G.B. for his sunburn?

Sunburn is a self-limiting condition, and treatment is usually symptomatic. Suggested treatments that G.B. can try for his first-degree burn are oral (e.g., ibuprofen, aspirin) or topical (e.g., camphor, menthol) analgesics, topical anti-inflammatory agents (e.g., hydrocortisone cream or aloe vera gel), cooling compresses (tap water, saline, or aluminum acetate solution [Burow's]) applied to the skin, or cool protectant baths (e.g., colloidal oatmeal). Nonsteroidal anti-inflammatory drugs (NSAIDs) such as aspirin or ibuprofen may be preferred over acetaminophen because of blockade of the inflammatory prostaglandin-mediated sunburn process.[76] Topical NSAID use, commonly seen as a cream formulation of indomethacin, possesses anti-inflammatory activity, especially if applied before UVR exposure, which may prove impractical for many individuals.

Treatment beyond self-management is unnecessary unless the sunburn is extensive with constitutional symptoms (i.e., severe first- or second-degree burns), involves second-degree burns on the eyes or genitalia, or becomes infected. In such cases, referral of the patient to his/her continuity provider is indicated as a short course (i.e., up to 3 days) of an oral corticosteroid may need to be given (e.g., 1 mg/kg of prednisone or equivalent, given once daily).

Topical anesthetics, such as benzocaine or lidocaine, provide only transient analgesia for up to 15 to 45 minutes. These agents should not be used in large quantities or applied more than three or four times a day. In addition, they should not be used on raw, blistered, or abraded skin. Benzocaine has minimal systemic toxicities, but is associated with contact sensitization.[77] In contrast, lidocaine is associated with a low incidence of contact sensitization, but has the potential to cause significant systemic toxicity (e.g., cardiovascular) if adequate serum drug concentrations are reached as a result of cutaneous absorption.[78]

If G.B. desires to try one of these agents, application or administration is recommended when the pain is particularly bothersome, such as at bedtime. Topical 1% hydrocortisone, when applied to mild to moderate sunburn, may provide some additional benefit. If G.B. experiences fever, chills, nausea, vomiting, and prostration, he should be referred to his health care provider. These symptoms generally respond to oral prednisone 20 mg/day for three days. Antihistamines may help control pruritus associated with sunburn, as well as aid with sleep, if taken at bedtime.

MINOR BURNS

Burn injuries rank second only to motor vehicle accidents as the leading cause of death in children between 1 and 4 years of age and rank third after motor vehicle accidents and drowning as the leading cause of injury and death in persons between 0 and 19 years of age.[79] Of the 2 million Americans treated for burns yearly, >80,000 require hospitalization; burns cause an overall yearly mortality of approximately 6,500.[80,81] The cause of hospitalization for these cases are due to complications such as fluid and electrolyte imbalances,

metabolic derangements, respiratory failure, sepsis, scarring, and functional impairment. Most burns, however, are minor and can be managed in an ambulatory environment, provided the burned patient is evaluated carefully, the severity of the burn is assessed accurately, and proper and continuous follow-up care is ensured.

Epidemiology

Burn injuries range from relatively minor, superficial injuries to severe, extensive skin loss resulting from contact with hot solids and liquids, steam, chemical agents, electricity, or other physical agents such as UVR or infrared radiation. House fires, commonly caused by cigarettes or malfunctioning heating or electrical equipment, are responsible for 84% of fire- and burn-related deaths.[79] The peak incidence of burn injuries occurs in up to 10% of preschool-aged children, who are often scalded by or immersed into hot liquids, frequently as a result of child abuse and neglect that crosses all socioeconomic classes.[81–84] School-aged children and adolescents often are injured when experimenting with matches or gasoline or in association with cars, motorcycles, fireworks, or flammables.[79] Teenagers and adults between 17 and 30 years of age most commonly are involved in accidents with flammable liquids, but the mortality associated with clothing ignition continues to decrease as a result of the use of flame-retardant forms of fabric in clothing. Categories of individuals who have a higher reported incidence of burn injuries are very young, elderly, males, blacks, economically disadvantaged, individuals who have ingested alcohol, handicapped children, and children with previous history of burn.[80]

With the development of multidisciplinary burn centers and a better understanding of the pathophysiology of the burn wound, survival of patients with second- and third-degree burns has improved by five to six times over the last three decades.[85] An increased national focus on burn treatment and prevention, societal changes such as an overall decrease in tobacco use, decreased alcohol abuse, changes in home cooking practices, and reduced industrial employment have contributed to the lower national burn incidence.[80] The techniques of improved burn wound management that have contributed to this decline include topical antimicrobial therapy, early excision or enzymatic debridement of devitalized tissue, and skin grafting/substitutes.[85–87]

Pathophysiology
Structure and Function of the Skin

The skin constitutes approximately 15% of the average person's body weight, making it the largest organ in the body. It is composed of the epidermis, the outermost surface layer; the dermis, which contains nerves, glands, hair follicles, and blood vessels; and the hypodermis, the subcutaneous layer, which contains adipose and connective tissue (see Fig. 38-1 in Chapter 38). The skin functions as a protective barrier of the underlying organ systems from trauma, temperature variations, harmful penetrations, moisture, humidity, radiation, and invasion by microorganisms. It also is involved with carbohydrate, protein, fat, and vitamin D metabolism; produces secretions that lubricate the skin; is involved with the immune response; and provides the body with the sense of touch.

Zones of Injury

The burn wound caused by thermal injury can be described by varying zones of injury.[88] The most peripheral area of injury is the *zone of hyperemia*. The tissue in this area is characterized by inflammatory changes with minimal tissue damage. The *zone of stasis* is the next area of injury, extending inward from the zone of hyperemia. This area involves ischemic, damaged tissue, with blood vessels only partially thrombosed. The damaged endothelial linings of blood vessels within this zone of injury may trigger further thrombosis, resulting in further ischemia, cell death, and deepening of the burn wound. This process of further injury may occur 24 to 48 hours after the injury. Drying of the burn wound or infection can cause deepening of the burn wound by preventing re-establishment of circulation to injured tissue. The central-most area, or the *zone of coagulation,* is characterized by thrombosed vessels and necrosed tissue. This area absorbs the most thermal energy, resulting in the greatest tissue damage. Minor burns may involve only the most peripheral zones of injury, whereas severe burns encompass all three zones of injury.

Complications of Burn Wounds

FLUID LOSS

In severe burns, release of vasoactive mediators and capillary injury cause sequestration of large amounts of body fluid, plasma, and electrolytes in extravascular compartments, resulting in edema both locally and throughout the entire body. This redistribution of fluid is compounded by the loss of large amounts of fluid, electrolytes, and protein into the open wound. The cumulative effect is a marked decrease in blood volume, a fall in cardiac output, and decreased tissue and organ perfusion. During the first 24 to 48 hours after a severe burn injury, adequate fluid must be given to replace fluid lost from the vascular space to prevent shock and, possibly, multiple organ failure, and death.[89]

INFECTION

The most important threat to survival of the fully resuscitated patient is infection, with burn wound sepsis and pneumonia being the leading causes of death.[89] The local mechanical defenses of the skin and respiratory tract often are damaged in burn victims, making these common foci for fatal infections. Loss of circulation to the burn wound margins disallows proper functioning of cellular and humoral defense mechanisms, which increases susceptibility to infection. Devitalized tissue and tissue exudates provide an ideal environment for the proliferation of bacteria. Colonization of Gram-positive bacteria occurs if topical antimicrobial therapy is not initiated promptly, and Gram-negative bacteria may predominate by the fifth day after injury.[89] Systemic antibiotics are of limited benefit in full-thickness burns and are used only to treat infections documented by wound biopsy, which reveal $\geq 10^5$ bacteria/g of burn tissue.[89] Topical antimicrobials, local wound care, and strict infection control practices are the mainstays of controlling burn wound infections. Devitalized tissue initiates and perpetuates a sepsislike state in the absence of an identifiable focus of infection.[89] For this reason, as well as for infection control, early excision of devitalized tissue and closure of the burn wound by skin grafting/substitutes have been adopted by many burn centers.

INHALATION INJURY

Burn injuries complicated by inhalation injury are associated with greatly increased mortality rates. Injury to the tracheobronchial mucosa is caused by inhalation of smoke or flames and may result in bronchospasm, ulceration of the mucous membranes, damage to cell membranes, edema, and impairment of bacterial ciliary clearance. Even patients with minor burns can have inhalation injury and require hospital admission. The early symptoms of pulmonary injury (hoarseness, dyspnea, tachypnea, and wheezing) may not be evident for 24 to 48 hours, so patients with suspected inhalation injury (i.e., facial burns or entrapment in a closed space) must be examined carefully. Singed nasal hair, soot-coated tongue or oropharynx, and upper airway edema are indications of inhalation injury. The diagnosis is established by bronchoscopy, and management may include endotracheal intubation and mechanical ventilation. Maintenance of the patient's fluid status is essential. Corticosteroids do not influence survival rates and should not be routinely administered to inhalation patients. They can also increase morbidity and mortality associated with burns and inhalation injury by increasing the risk of infection.[89] The use of exogenous surfactant in the treatment of inhalation burns in patients with adult respiratory distress syndrome (ARDS) improves the survival of these high-risk patients.[90]

Extent of Injury

Rule of Nines

The severity of a burn is proportional to the percent of body surface area (BSA) involvement and the depth of the wound. The percent of BSA for adults can be estimated by using the "rule of nines," in which each arm constitutes 9% of the BSA, the head 9%, each leg 18%, the front and back of the torso 18% each, and the genitalia 1%. For children younger than 10 years, the determination of the percent BSA must be adjusted because their bodies have different proportions. The Lund and Browder chart has been used for this purpose.[91] At birth, the infant's head constitutes about 19% of the BSA. For each additional year of age, the head decreases by about 1% and the BSA of the legs increases by about 1% of the patient's total body surface area (TBSA), so a quick estimation of the percent BSA of a burn can be made.[82]

Classification of Wounds

Burn wounds also are classified according to the depth of tissue damage. Determining the depth of the burn wound can be difficult during the first 24 to 48 hours because of the presence of edema and continued tissue ischemia and/or infection, both of which may cause deepening of the wound. In addition, the depth of destruction may vary within the same burn, and skin surface characteristics may not match underlying tissue damage, making assessment of the burn wound difficult.[88]

FIRST-DEGREE BURNS

First-degree burns result from injury to the superficial cells of the epidermis. A common example is a mild sunburn. The burned skin does not form blisters, but it does become erythematous and mildly painful. This partial-thickness burn heals within 3 to 4 days without scarring.

SECOND-DEGREE BURNS

Second-degree burns may be superficial or deep, depending on the depth of dermal involvement. Superficial second-degree burns involve the epidermis and the upper layer of the dermis. The burn surface often is erythematous, blistered, weeping, painful, and very sensitive to stimuli. The erythema blanches with pressure, and the hair follicles, sweat, and sebaceous glands are spared. Superficial second-degree burns heal spontaneously within 3 weeks with little, if any, scarring. Deep second-degree burns involve the deeper elements of the dermis and may be difficult to distinguish from third-degree burns. The burn surface is pale, feels indurated or boggy, and does not blanch with pressure. This wound is less painful than more superficial wounds; some areas may be insensitive to stimuli. Healing occurs slowly over about 35 days with eschar formation and possible severe scarring and permanent loss of hair follicles and sweat and sebaceous glands.

THIRD-DEGREE BURNS

Third-degree burns entail complete destruction of the full thickness of the skin, including all skin elements. The wound may appear pearly white, gray, or brown and is dry and inelastic. Pain is sensed only when deep pressure is applied. If the wound is small, healing over several months can occur by epithelial migration from the margins of the injury, with scar and contracture formation. Third-degree burns are repaired most often by excision and grafting of the wound to prevent contractures of the skin.[89]

FOURTH-DEGREE BURNS

Fourth-degree burns are similar to third-degree burns except that devitalized tissue extends into the subcutaneous tissue, fascia, and bone. These burns are blackened in appearance, are dry and generally painless (because of destruction of nerve endings), and confer great risk for infection.

Triage

14. S.T., a 17-year-old, nonobese boy, has just burned the calf of his right leg on the muffler of his motorcycle. Immediately after being burned, S.T. was able to rinse his leg with cool water from a garden hose. The burn on his leg is about twice the size of the palm of his hand and appears erythematous and weeping. He sustained no other injury, but now he is in considerable pain. S.T. has no significant medical history. Should S.T. be referred to a health care provider or can he safely self-treat his burn? What patient information is necessary to consider in making this decision?

Before recommending treatment for a patient with a minor burn, it is important to accurately assess the patient to determine whether he or she can self-treat safely or whether referral or hospitalization is necessary. The location and severity of the burn, the patient's age and state of health, and the cause of the burn injury all must be considered.

American Burn Association Treatment Categories

Three treatment categories for burn injuries are recommended by the American Burn Association: major burn injuries; moderate, uncomplicated burn injuries; and minor burn injuries.[92]

- *Major burn injuries* are second-degree burns with >25% BSA involvement in adults (20% in children); all third-degree burns with ≥10% BSA involvement; all burns involving the hands, face, eyes, ears, feet, and perineum that may result in functional or cosmetic impairment; high-voltage electrical injury; and burns complicated by inhalation injury, major trauma, or poor-risk patients (elderly patients and those with debilitating disease).
- *Moderate, uncomplicated burns* are second-degree burns with 15% to 25% BSA involvement in adults (10% to 20% in children); third-degree burns with 2% to 10% BSA involvement; and burns not involving risk to areas of specialized function such as the eyes, ears, face, hands, feet, or perineum.
- *Minor burn injuries* include second-degree burns with <15% BSA involvement in adults (10% in children), third-degree burns with <2% BSA, and burns not involving functional or cosmetic risk to areas of specialized function.

Patients with minor burn injuries may be treated on an outpatient basis if no other trauma is present; if circumferential burns of the neck, trunk, arms, or legs are not present; and if the patient is able to comply with therapy. After initial evaluation by a health care provider, patients may self-treat a second- or third-degree burn only if <1% BSA is involved.

Major or moderate, uncomplicated burns necessitate hospital admission, and surgical referral is recommended for patients of all ages who have deep second- or third-degree burns covering ≥3% of the TBSA.

Both the American Burn Association and the American College of Surgeons recommend transfer to a burn center for all acutely burned patients who meet any of the following criteria[92]:

- Partial-thickness burns ≥20% TBSA in patients aged 10 to 50 years old
- Partial-thickness burns ≥10% TBSA in children aged 10 or adults aged 50 years old
- Full-thickness burns ≥5% TBSA in patients of any age
- Patients with partial- or full-thickness burns of the hands, feet, face, eyes, ears, perineum, and/or major joints
- Patients with high-voltage electrical injuries, including lightning injuries
- Patients with significant burns from caustic chemicals
- Patients with burns complicated by multiple trauma in which the burn injury poses the greatest risk of morbidity or mortality (in such cases, if the trauma poses the greater immediate risk, the patient may be treated initially in a trauma center until stable before being transferred to a burn center)
- Patients with burns who suffer an inhalation injury
- Patients with significant ongoing medical disorders that could complicate management, prolong recovery, or affect mortality
- Patients who were taken to hospitals without qualified personnel or equipment for the care of children

Burn injury in patients who will require special social/emotional and/or long-term rehabilitative support, including cases involving suspected child abuse or substance abuse

Age-Related Recommendations

Children younger than 2 years of age and elderly patients with a burn injury should be referred for evaluation because these patients may not tolerate any trauma associated with the burn.

In addition to medical issues, children with burns that result from suspected child abuse should be hospitalized for legal, psychosocial, and protective reasons. Burns in varying stages of healing, demarcated patterns of burns (e.g., stocking or glove distribution), or more than two burn sites may be clues in identifying an abused child.[84]

Disease-Related Recommendations

Burn patients with any other medical condition such as diabetes mellitus, cardiovascular disease, immunodeficiency disorders (e.g., HIV-associated disease, patients receiving cancer chemotherapy), renal disease, obesity, or alcoholism may be more susceptible to complications from the burn and may have compromised wound healing.

Etiology

The etiology of a burn should always be considered because this may provide some insight into the burn presentation and its management. Electrical burns can appear to be superficial because external injury may occur at only the entrance and exit sites of the current. These burns, however, can cause extensive damage to underlying nervous and muscle tissue that is not initially evident. Except for very minor electrical burns, these patients should be referred for further evaluation. S.T. has sustained a superficial second-degree burn over about 2% of his BSA. Even though the burn wound on his leg was caused by thermal injury and is relatively minor, S.T. should be referred for further evaluation and treatment.

Treatment

15. How should S.T.'s burn be treated? What treatment alternatives may be used for S.T.? What immunization should S.T. be questioned about?

Goals of Treatment and Immediate Care

Treatment goals for first- and second-degree burns are to relieve the pain associated with the burn, prevent desiccation and deepening of the wound, prevent infection, and provide a protective environment for healing. Immediate care of the wound should be application of cold, wet compresses or immersion in cool water. S.T. may have prevented extension of the burn to deeper layers of tissue and alleviated some of his pain from the burn by immediately irrigating the wound with cool water. Next, the area should be cleansed with a mild hypoallergenic soap (e.g., Basis, Purpose) and water. A sterile, nonadherent, fine-mesh gauze dressing that is impregnated with hydrophilic petrolatum (Xeroflo, Adaptic) should be placed over the wound. This type of dressing prevents the gauze from adhering to the wound and allows the burn exudate to flow freely through the dressing, thus preventing maceration.

A second layer of absorbent gauze should be placed over the petrolatum gauze and a supportive layer of rolled gauze can be used to keep the dressing in place. The outer layer must not be too constricting, and the dressing should be replaced every 48 hours after recleansing the area and inspecting for signs of infection. If S.T.'s wound continues to weep, it may be beneficial to soak his wound or apply a towel saturated with water, normal saline, or Burow's solution (diluted 1:20 or

1:40) for 15 to 30 minutes at least four times daily (see Chapter 38). The use of butter, grease, or similar home remedies should be avoided in the treatment of burns because these measures tend to retain the thermal energy sustained in the burn and may increase the area of thermal injury. Since burn patients are prone to secondary tetanus infections, S.T. should receive a tetanus toxoid booster if he has not been immunized within the previous 10 years.

Skin Substitutes/Synthetic Dressings

Advances in the development of skin substitutes are being used to achieve the elusive goal of finding a skin replacement to mimic completely the interaction and functions of dermis and epidermis. Although this goal has yet to be achieved, a growing number of synthetic and biologic products are available that can serve important roles in caring for burn patients.[93] Some of the current modalities are as follows.

HUMAN CADAVER SKIN

Fresh human cadaver skin (allograft) is considered the *sine qua non* for temporary closure of burn wounds. It adheres well to a healthy wound bed, resulting in reduced contamination and reduced protein, heat, and water loss. Cost, rejection, and disease transmission (e.g., hepatitis) are the most commonly perceived disadvantages of human cadaver skin, thus, appropriate cadaveric screening is essential.

EPIDERMAL SUBSTITUTE: CULTURED EPITHELIAL ALLOGRAFTS

The technique of culturing autologous human epidermal cells grown from a single full-thickness skin biopsy into confluent keratinizing sheets suitable for grafting has been available for over two decades and is especially useful for patients with large wounds.[94] A lack of mechanical stability of cultured epithelium, causing an imperfect cover, remains a major concern; therefore, the development of a dermal substitute (or a vascularized remnant of allogenic dermis) in combination with cultured epithelial allografts to increase mechanical stability and decrease wound contracture, or a laboratory-derived autologous composite continues to receive scientific investigation.

ANIMAL SUBSTITUTE: PIG SKIN

Pig skin (xenograft) has gained acceptance as a temporary dressing alternative to allograft because of its lower cost and greater availability. At 0°C, frozen pig skin has a storage life of 6 to 18 months from the date of manufacture. Like an allograft, it has the desirable properties of being able to adhere initially to a clean wound; to cover nerve endings to decrease pain; to function as an autograft test graft; and to diminish heat, protein, and electrolyte loss. A premeshed, de-epithelialized shelf-stored form is available (EZ-Derm, Brennen Medical), which is thought to be more resistant to bacterial degradation.

DERMAL SUBSTITUTES: ALLODERMAL GRAFTS

Unlike the epidermis, the dermis can be rendered acellular and still perform its basic protective and supportive functions. With removal of the dermal cells, the antigenic elements are also eliminated; therefore, an alloplastic transplantation can occur without rejection. The principle of allodermal grafting is that an ultrathin (0.01 cm) meshed autograft laid on top of the allodermis provides skin quality that is comparable to that obtained from thick partial-thickness grafts. AlloDerm (Life-Cell) is a shelf-stored, freeze-dried, acellular human cadaveric dermal matrix. Integra (Integra Life Sciences) has been approved by the FDA for use in life-threatening burns. The inner layer of this material is a 2-mm thick combination of collagen fibers isolated from bovine tissue and the glycosaminoglycan chondroitin-6-sulfate that has a 70 to 200 μm pore size to facilitate host fibrovascular ingrowth. The outer layer is a 0.009 inch polysiloxane polymer with vapor transmission characteristics that simulate normal epithelium.[86]

SEMISYNTHETIC/SYNTHETIC DRESSINGS

Biobrane (Bertek) is a bilaminar, semisynthetic, temporary skin substitute made of silicone bonded to nylon mesh. Its adherence is facilitated by collagen peptides bonded to the nylon underlayer. This substitute has been shown to be as effective as frozen human allograft for the temporary coverage of freshly excised full-thickness burn wounds before autografting.[94] Duoderm (Bristol-Myers Squibb) is a hydrocolloid dressing, whereas OpSite (Smith & Nephew) and Tegaderm (3M) are elastomeric polyurethane films. Comfeel (Coloplast) is a semipermeable polyurethane film coated with a flexible, cross-linked adhesive mass containing sodium carboxymethylcellulose (NaCMC) as the principal absorbent and gel-forming agent. This product is permeable to water vapor but impermeable to exudates and microorganisms. In the presence of an exudate, NaCMC absorbs liquid and swells to form a cohesive gel that does not disintegrate or leave residues in the wound bed.

Alternatives in treating S.T.'s second-degree burn include the use of synthetic dressings and topical antimicrobial agents. Synthetic dressings serve as skin substitutes that are applied to fresh, clean, and moist burns. They are trimmed to about the size of the burn and left in place until the burn is healed or the dressing separates from the wound spontaneously. The synthetic dressings keep the wound warm and moist, require absorbent dressings that must be changed daily, and are indicated for superficial second-degree burns. The chief advantage over gauze dressings is that synthetic dressings prevent mechanical injury from daily cleansing and dressing changes.[95]

Topical Antimicrobial Agents

SILVER SULFADIAZINE

Silver sulfadiazine (Silvadene) is the usual agent of choice because it has broad-spectrum Gram-positive and Gram-negative antibacterial activity, provides reasonable eschar penetration, and is easy and painless to apply and wash off. The cream is a 1% suspension of silver sulfadiazine in a water-miscible base. As a consequence of poor water solubility, the active agent shows only limited diffusion into the eschar. Silver sulfadiazine cream is most effective when applied to burn wounds immediately after thermal injury to prevent bacterial colonization of the burn wound surface as a prelude to intra-eschar proliferation. This agent has the advantages of being painless when applied to the wound and being free from acid-base and electrolyte disturbances. The limitations of silver sulfadiazine cream include neutropenia,[96] which usually reverses when application is discontinued; hypersensitivity, which is rare; and ineffectiveness against certain strains of

Pseudomonas organisms and virtually all strains of *Enterobacter cloacae*. This agent should not be applied around the eyes or mouth in patients with hypersensitivity to sulfonamides or in pregnant or breastfeeding women.

MAFENIDE ACETATE

Mafenide acetate (Sulfamylon) is an 11.1% cream formulation of mafenide acetate in a water-dispersible base, or a 5% powder for topical solution. As a water-soluble agent, mafenide diffuses freely to establish an effective antibacterial concentration throughout the eschar and at the interface of viable/nonviable tissue, where bacteria characteristically proliferate before invasion. Because of this characteristic, mafenide is the best agent for use if the patient to be treated has heavily contaminated burn wounds, if treatment is delayed for several days after the burn occurred, or if a dense bacterial population already exists on and within the eschar. Adverse effects include hypersensitivity reactions in 7% of patients (usually responsive to antihistamines), pain or discomfort of 20 to 30 minutes duration when applied to partial-thickness burns (seldom a cause for discontinuation), and inhibition of carbonic anhydrase. The inhibition of carbonic anhydrase may produce both an early bicarbonate diuresis and an accentuation of postburn hyperventilation. The resulting overall reduction of serum bicarbonate levels renders such patients liable to a rapid shift from an alkalotic to an acidotic state. If acidosis should develop during use of mafenide, the frequency of application should be reduced to once daily, or it should be omitted for 24 to 48 hours, with buffering used as necessary, and with efforts made to improve pulmonary function.

Either topical silver sulfadiazine or mafenide should be applied in a ⅛-inch thick layer to the entire burn wound with a sterile gloved hand immediately after initial debridement and wound care. Twelve hours later, to ensure continuous topical treatment, a ⅛-inch coat of cream should be reapplied to those areas of the burn wound from which it has been abraded by clothing. The topical cream should be cleansed gently once each day from all of the burn wound and the wound inspected. Daily debridement should be carried out to a point of bleeding or pain without the use of general anesthesia. After debridement, the wound should be covered again by the topical cream.

SILVER NITRATE

If topical antimicrobial creams are unavailable, multilayered occlusive gauze dressings, saturated with a 0.5% solution of silver nitrate, can be used. These soaks are changed two or three times each day and moistened every 2 hours. Evaporation should be avoided to prevent raising the silver nitrate concentration to cytotoxic levels within the soaks. Transeschar losses of sodium, potassium, chloride, and calcium should be anticipated and appropriately replaced. Similar to therapy with silver sulfadiazine cream, silver nitrate soak therapy is best for bacterial control in burn patients who are received immediately after injury before significant microbial proliferation has occurred. Silver nitrate is immediately precipitated on contact with proteinaceous material, does not penetrate the eschar, and consequently is ineffective in the treatment of established burn wound infection. For these reasons, it is not routinely recommended.

In S.T.'s case, *silver sulfadiazine cream* could be chosen to treat his burn on an outpatient basis if an assessment determines that he is at particular risk for infection. The cream would be applied in a thin layer over the wound and covered with absorbent gauze and wrapped with rolled gauze. The dressing must be changed twice daily to maintain an application of cream that is biologically active. Topical bacitracin and the combination of polymyxin B and bacitracin are transparent formulations that also may be used but, because of limited efficacy, may be desirable for use only on small, second-degree burns on the face.

Oral Analgesics and Topical Protectants

S.T.'s burn pain can be treated with oral OTC analgesics, aspirin, acetaminophen, or ibuprofen. If these analgesics do not provide adequate relief, oxycodone/acetaminophen (or equivalent) may be of additional benefit. Topical protectants, such as allantoin, calamine, white petrolatum, or zinc oxide are safe and effective in treating first-degree and minor second-degree burns. These agents protect the burn from mechanical irritation caused by friction and rubbing and prevent drying of the stratum corneum.

REFERENCES

1. Green A et al. Daily sunscreen application and beta carotene supplementation in prevention of basal-cell and squamous-cell carcinomas of the skin: a randomised controlled trial. Lancet 1999;354:723.
2. Howe HL et al. Annual report to the nation on the status of cancer (1973 through 1988), featuring cancers with recent increasing trends. J Natl Cancer Inst 2001;93:824.
3. Council on Scientific Affairs. Harmful effects of ultraviolet radiation. JAMA 1989;262:380.
4. Ferrini RL, Perlman M, Hill L. American College of Preventive Medicine Practice Policy Statement: Skin protection from ultraviolet light exposure. Am J Prev Med 1998;14:83.
5. Leffell DJ, Brash DE. Sunlight and skin cancer. Sci Am 1996;275:52.
6. National Institutes of Health Consensus Development Panel. National Institutes of Health summary of the consensus development conference on sunlight, ultraviolet radiation, and the skin. J Am Acad Dermatol 1991;24:608.
7. Diffey BL. What is light? Photodermatol Photoimmunol Photomed 2002;18:68.
8. McMichael AJ, Haines A. Climate change and health: implications for research, monitoring and policy. Br Med J 1997;315:870.
9. World Meteorological Organization, Scientific Assessment of Ozone Depletion: 1998, WMO Global Ozone Research and Monitoring Project—Report No. 44, Geneva, 1998.
10. Utiger RD. The need for more vitamin D. N Engl J Med 1998;338:828.
11. Thrush B. Causes of ozone depletion. Nature 1988;332:784.
12. Salawitch RJ. A greenhouse warming connection. Nature 1998;392:551.
13. Shindell DT et al. Increased polar stratospheric ozone losses and delayed eventual recovery owing to increasing greenhouse-gas concentrations. Nature 1998;392:589.
14. Coldiron BM. The UV Index: a weather report for skin. Clin Dermatol 1998;16:441.
15. Fisher GJ et al. Molecular basis of sun-induced premature skin aging and retinoid antagonism. Nature 1996;379:335.
16. Fitzpatrick TB. Ultraviolet-induced pigmentary changes: benefits and hazards. Curr Probl Dermatol 1986;15:25.
17. Fitzpatrick TB. The validity and practicality of sun-reactive skin types I through VI. Arch Dermatol 1988;124:869.
18. Gallagher RP et al. Broad-spectrum sunscreen use and the development of new nevi in white children: a randomized controlled trial. JAMA 2000; 283:2955.
19. Buller DB, Borland R. Skin cancer prevention for children: a critical review. Health Educ Behav 1999;26:317.
20. Bentham G, Aase A. Incidence of malignant melanoma of the skin in Norway, 1955-1989: associations with solar ultraviolet radiation, income and holidays abroad. Int J Epidemiol 1996;25:1132.

21. Autier P et al. Sunscreen use, wearing clothes, and the number of nevi in 6- or 7-year-old European children. J Natl Cancer Inst 1998;90:1873.
22. Wolf P et al. Phenotypic markers, sunlight-related factors and sunscreen use in patients with cutaneous melanoma: an Austrian case-control study. Melanoma Res 1998;8:370.
23. Gerber B et al. Ultraviolet emission spectra of sunbeds. Photochem Photobiol 2002;76:664.
24. Culley CA et al. Compliance with federal and state legislation by indoor tanning facilities in San Diego. J Am Acad Dermatol 2001;44:53.
25. Fisher GJ et al. Mechanisms of photoaging and chronological skin aging. Arch Dermatol 2002;138:1462.
26. West SK et al. Sunlight exposure and risk of lens opacities in a population-based study. The Salisbury Eye Evaluation Project. JAMA 1998;280:714.
27. Fisher GJ et al. Pathophysiology of premature skin aging induced by ultraviolet light. N Engl J Med 1997;337:1419.
28. Gilchrest BA. A review of skin aging and its medical therapy. Br J Dermatol 1996;135:867.
29. Uitto J. Understanding premature skin aging [Editorial]. N Engl J Med 1997;337:1463.
30. Naylor MF, Farmer KC. The case for sunscreens. A review of their use in preventing actinic damage and neoplasia. Arch Dermatol 1997;133:1146.
31. Humphreys TR et al. Treatment of photodamaged skin with trichloroacetic acid and topical tretinoin. J Am Acad Dermatol 1996;34:638.
32. Kang S, Fisher GJ, Voorhees JJ. Photoaging and topical tretinoin: therapy, pathogenesis, and prevention. Arch Dermatol 1997;133:1280.
33. Kang S, Voorhees JJ. Photoaging therapy with topical tretinoin: an evidence-based analysis. J Am Acad Dermatol 1998;39:S55.
34. Leyden JJ et al. Treatment of photoaged facial skin with topical tretinoin. J Am Acad Dermatol 1989;21:638.
35. Kang S et al. Tazarotene cream for the treatment of facial photodamage. Arch Dermatol 2001;137:1597.
36. Phillips TJ et al. Efficacy of 0.1% tazarotene cream for the treatment of photodamage. Arch Dermatol 2002;138:1486.
37. Kligman AM. Guidelines for the use of topical tretinoin (Retin A) for photoaged skin. J Am Acad Dermatol 1989;21:650.
38. Gonzalez E, Gonzalez S. Drug photosensitivity, idiopathic photodermatoses and sunscreens. J Am Acad Dermatol 1996;35:871.
39. Gonzalez E et al. Bilateral comparison of generalized lichen planus treated with psoralens and ultraviolet A. J Am Acad Dermatol 1984;10:958.
40. Darlington S et al. A randomized controlled trial to assess sunscreen application and beta carotene supplementation in the prevention of solar keratoses. Arch Dermatol 2003;139:451.
41. Hawk JLM. Cutaneous photoprotection (editorial). Arch Dermatol 2003;139:527.

42. Adam JE. Living a "shady life": sun-protective behaviour for Canadians. Can Med Assn J 1999;160:1471.
43. Gasparro FP, Mitchnick M, Nash JF. A review of sunscreen safety and efficacy. Photochemistry Photobiol 1998;68:243.
44. Bech-Thomason N, Wulf H. Sunbathers' application of sunscreens probably inadequate to obtain the sun protective factor assigned to the preparation. Photodermatol Photoimmunol Photomed 1992;9:242.
45. Robinson JK, Rademaker AW. Sun protection by families at the beach. Arch Pediatr Adolesc Med 1998;152:466.
46. Diffey BL. When should sunscreen be reapplied? J Am Acad Dermatol 2001;45:882.
47. Wright MW, Wright ST, Wagner RF. Mechanisms of sunscreen failure. J Am Acad Dermatol 2001;44:781.
48. Sayre RM, Dowdy JC. Photostability testing of avobenzone. Cosmet Toiletries 119;114:85.
49. Autier P et al. European Organization for Research and Treatment of Cancer Melanoma Co-operative Group. Quantity of sunscreen used by European students. Br J Dermatol 2001;144:288.
50. Hagedorn-Leweke U, Lippold BC. Accumulation of sunscreens and other compounds in keratinous substrates. Eur J Pharmaceu Biopharm 1998;46:215.
51. Patel NP, Highton A, Moy RL. Properties of topical sunscreen formulations. A review. J Dermatol Surg Oncol 1992;18:316.
52. Fisher AA. Sunscreen dermatitis: para-aminobenzoic acid and its derivatives. Cutis 1992;50:190.
53. Schauder S, Ippen H. Contact and photocontact sensitivity to sunscreens. Review of a 15-year experience and of the literature. Contact Dermatitis 1997;37:221.
54. Dromgoole SH, Maibach HI. Sunscreening agent intolerance: contact and photocontact sensitization and contact urticaria. J Am Acad Dermatol 1990;22:1068.
55. Fisher AA. Sunscreen dermatitis: Part II—the cinnamates. Cutis 1992;50:253.
56. Fisher AA. Sunscreen dermatitis: Part III—the benzophenones. Cutis 1992;50:331.
57. Fisher AA. Sunscreen dermatitis: Part IV—the salicylates, the anthranilates, and physical agents. Cutis 1992;50:397.
58. Gange RW et al. Efficacy of a sunscreen containing butyl methoxydibenzoylmethane against ultraviolet A radiation in photosensitized subjects. J Am Acad Dermatol 1986;15:494.
59. Humbert P. Topical vitamin C in the treatment of photoaged skin. Eur J Dermatol 2001;11:172.
60. Darr D et al. Effectiveness of antioxidants (vitamin C and E) with and without sunscreens as topical photoprotectants. Acta Derm Venereol 1996;76:264.
61. Eberlein-Konig B, Placzek M, Przybilla B. Protective effect against sunburn of combined systemic ascorbic acid (vitamin C) and d-alpha-tocopherol (vitamin E). J Am Acad Dermatol 1998;38:45.
62. Kollias N. The absorption properties of "physical" sunscreens. Arch Dermatol 1999;135:209.

63. Tan MH et al. A pilot study on the percutaneous absorption of microfine titanium for sunscreens. Australas J Dermatol 1996;37:185.
64. Schneider J. The teaspoon rule of applying sunscreen. Arch Dermatol 2002;138:838.
65. Notice of proposed rule-making on sunscreen drug products for over-the-counter use: tentative final monograph. Fed Regist 1993;58:282.
66. Emmons KM, Colditz GA. Preventing excess sun exposure: it is time for a national policy. J Natl Cancer Inst 1999;91:1269.
67. Committee on Environmental Health. American Academy of Pediatrics. Ultraviolet light: a hazard to children. Pediatrics 1999;104:328.
68. Adam JE. Sun protective clothing. J Cutan Med Surg 1998;3:1.
69. Buller DB et al. Sun protection policies and environmental features in US elementary schools. Arch Dermatol 2002;138:771.
70. Stanford DG et al. Sun protection by a summerweight garment: the effect of washing and wearing. Med J Aust 1995;162:422.
71. Gambichler T et al. Protection against ultraviolet radiation by commercial summer clothing: need for standardised testing and labelling. BMC Dermatol 2001;1:6.
72. Gambichler T et al. Role of clothes in sun protection. Recent Results Cancer Res 2002;160:15.
73. de Gruijl FR et al. Health effects from stratospheric ozone depletion and interactions with climate change. Photochem Photobiol Sci 2003;2:16
74. Longstreth J et al. Health risks. J Photochem Photobiol 1998;46:20.

75. Sliney DH. Photoprotection of the eye—UV radiation and sunglasses. J Photochem Photobiol B: Biol. 2001;64:166.
76. Hughes GS et al. Synergistic effects of oral nonsteroidal drugs and topical corticosteroids in the therapy of sunburn in humans. Dermatology 1992;184:54.
77. Sidhu SK et al. A 10-year retrospective study on benzocaine allergy in the United Kingdom. Am J Contact Derm 1999;10:57.
78. Cuesta-Herranz J et al. Allergic reaction caused by local anesthetic agents belonging to the amide group. J Allergy Clin Immunol 1997;99:427.
79. McLoughlin E, McGuire A. The causes, cost, and prevention of childhood burn injuries. Am J Dis Child 1990;144:607.
80. Brigham PA, McLaughlin E. Burn incidence and medical care use in the United States: estimate, trends, and data sources. J Burn Care Rehab 1996;17:95.
81. Ryan CM et al. Objective estimates of the probability of death from burn injuries. N Engl J Med 1998;338:362.
82. Morrow SE et al. Etiology and outcome of pediatric burns. J Pediatr Surg 1996;31:329.
83. Hultman CS et al. Return to jeopardy: the fate of pediatric burn patients who are victims of abuse and neglect. J Burn Care Rehab 1998;19:367.
84. Stratman E, Melski J. Scald abuse. Arch Dermatol 2002;138:318.
85. Demling RH. The advantage of the burn team approach. J Burn Care Rehab 1995;16:569.
86. Sheridan RL. Burns. Crit Care Med 2002;30:S500.

87. Sheridan RL, Tompkins RG. Skin substitutes in burns. Burns 1999;25:97.
88. Dziewulski P. Burn wound healing: James Ellsworth Laing memorial essay for 1991. Burns 1992;18:466.
89. Monafo WW. Initial management of burns. N Engl J Med 1996;335:1581.
90. Pallua N et al. Intrabronchial surfactant application in cases of inhalation injury: first results from patients with severe burns and ARDS burns. Burns 1998;24:197.
91. Miller SF et al. Burn size estimate reliability: a study. J Burn Care Rehab 1991;12:546.
92. American Burn Association. Hospital and prehospital resources for optimal care of patients with burn injury: guidelines for development and operation of burn centers. J Burn Care Rehab 1990;11:98.
93. Hopper RA et al. Use of skin substitutes in adult Canadian burn centres. Can J Plast Surg 1997;5:112.
94. Purdue GF et al. Biosynthetic skin substitute versus frozen human cadaver allograft for temporary coverage of excised burn wounds. J Trauma-Injury Infect Crit Care 1987;27:155.
95. Poulsen TD et al. Polyurethane film (Opsite) vs impregnated gauze (Jelonet) in the treatment of outpatient burns: a prospective, randomized study. Burns 1991;17:59.
96. Caffee F, Bingham H. Leukopenia and silver sulfadiazine. J Trauma 1982;22:586.

CHAPTER 42

Gout and Hyperuricemia

Tricia M. Russell, Lloyd Y. Young

The syndrome of gout generally is characterized by acute or chronic recurrent arthritis, deposits of monosodium urates, and association with hyperuricemia. The monosodium urate crystals may deposit into a joint and precipitate an acute, painful inflammatory response or may deposit into soft tissue and elicit no inflammatory response. Most cases of gout are manifested by the sudden appearance of severe acute monoarticular arthritis in a peripheral joint in the foot and often are associated with hyperuricemia. However, attacks of acute gouty arthritis have been documented in the presence of persistently normal serum urate levels, and many individuals who are hyperuricemic may never experience an attack of gouty arthritis (see Hyperuricemia).[1] Hence, *gout* should be considered as a clinical diagnosis and *hyperuricemia* as a bio-

chemical one. These two terms are not synonymous and are not interchangeable.

PATHOPHYSIOLOGY

Uric Acid Disposition

Uric acid serves no biologic function; it is merely the end-product of purine metabolism. Unlike other animals, humans lack the enzyme uricase, which degrades uric acid into more soluble products for excretion. As a consequence, uric acid is not metabolized in humans and must be excreted renally. Therefore, increased serum uric acid concentrations can result from an increase in the production of uric acid, a decrease in the renal excretion, or a combination of these two mechanisms.

Overproduction

Overproduction of uric acid can result from excessive de novo purine synthesis, excessive dietary purines, or excessive nucleoprotein turnover. Excessive de novo purine synthesis is associated primarily with rare enzyme mutation defects. For example, a deficiency of hypoxanthine-guanine phosphoribosyltransferase (HGPRTase) is associated not only with hyperuricemia and gout, but also with mental retardation, choreoathetosis, and self-mutilation by biting (Lesch-Nyhan syndrome).[2] Likewise, excessive purine biosynthesis leading to hyperuricemia and gout has been associated with type 1 glycogen storage disease (von Gierke's) because of the deficiency of the glucose phosphatase enzyme. Excessive dietary ingestion of yeast or liver tablets, which are high in purines, has caused hyperuricemia. However, diet generally plays only a very minor role in the development of hyperuricemia, and dietary restrictions (with the exception of alcohol) cannot be advocated in the management of hyperuricemia. Excessive nucleoprotein turnover from neoplastic diseases such as multiple myeloma, leukemias, lymphomas, and Hodgkin's disease, as well as from myeloproliferative disorders such as myeloid metaplasia or polycythemia vera, has been associated with gout and hyperuricemia.[3,4]

Underexcretion

Underexcretion of uric acid results from a defect in renal excretion. Uric acid is filtered in the renal glomerulus and is almost completely (>99%) reabsorbed in the proximal tubule by a high-capacity system. Uric acid then is secreted distal to the proximal tubular reabsorption site, and subsequently approximately 75% of the secreted urate is reabsorbed again.[5] Therefore, urinary uric acid excretion is almost entirely attributable to the tubular secretory process.

When large urate loads are filtered during hyperuricemia, urate reabsorption increases to avoid the dumping of large amounts of poorly soluble urate into the urinary tract. However, tubular urate secretion does not appear to be influenced by serum urate concentrations, and impaired tubular secretion of urate is the probable explanation for hyperuricemia.[5]

ACUTE GOUT

Clinical Features

1. W.S., a 46-year-old male professor, is seen by his physician because of a chief complaint of severe pain at the base of his left great toe and around the forward portion of his arch. This pain was first noted approximately 2 days ago, a few hours after an uneventful 4-mile run. W.S. experienced pain severe enough to awaken him from sleep that evening. The pain was more constant the next morning, and for the remainder of the day he walked with a significant limp. He was still unconcerned because he attributed the pain to a sprain from his jogging. Last night, while asleep, W.S. was awakened several times with episodes of pain around the base of his left great toe and around the instep of his left foot. The pain, which was at first moderate, became more intense. The pain was not sharp or knifelike; rather, it was a constant gnawing pain that did not abate with time. His foot felt like it was being tightened slowly in a vise, and the pain was more of a constant squeezing, pressure sensation than an acute transient phenomenon. By this morning, his foot was so exquisitely painful that he could not tolerate even the weight of the bedcovers.

Pertinent medical history includes left foot trauma during a motorcycle accident approximately 10 years ago and essential hypertension of approximately 5 years' duration. His systolic blood pressure (BP) is approximately 140 to 145 mm Hg and diastolic pressure approximately 90 to 95 mm Hg during treatment. W.S. currently is receiving hydrochlorothiazide 25 mg/day and metoprolol (Lopressor) 100 mg/day. This patient's social history is noncontributory except for a nightly bedtime glass of wine.

On physical examination, the first metatarsophalangeal joint is warm and tender to touch. The entire periarticular area is erythematous and swollen to such an extent that it is difficult to determine which joint is the focus of the inflammation.

What subjective or objective data in W.S.'s history are compatible with the clinical features of gout?

Epidemiology

The risk of gouty arthritis is approximately the same for both men and women at any given serum uric acid concentration; however, many more men are hyperuricemic. For example, men are six times more likely than women to have serum uric acid concentrations >7 mg/dL. Overall, gout occurs as often in postmenopausal elderly women as in men.[6]

The onset of gout is rare in prepubertal children and is uncommon before the age of 30. The onset is classically during middle age; in one study, the average age at the time of the first attack was 48 years.[7] The appearance of gout in a man younger than 30 years of age or in a premenopausal woman is unusual and should alert the clinician to the possibility of a renal parenchymal disease that decreases urate clearance or to an enzymatic defect that is associated with increased purine production.

A controversial epidemiologic association of gout with coronary heart disease (CHD) has gained increased credibility from the Framingham study group finding that "gout is a marker for susceptibility to coronary heart disease."[8] In a further epidemiologic evaluation, the value of hyperuricemia as a predictor of mortality and ischemic heart disease noted no correlation in men, but a significant direct relationship in women to mortality from ischemic heart disease was observed.[9] Gout may be an independent risk factor for CHD or it may serve simply as a clinical marker for increased risk of CHD without being causally related to CHD. A biologic explanation for the association of gout with CHD might be related to the activation of platelets by monosodium urate crystals and subsequent release of chemical mediators, such as serotonin and adenosine diphosphate (ADP), which have been implicated in the endothelial damage of atherosclerosis. Other epidemiologic correlations with race, intelligence, geographic locale, or genetic disposition probably contribute more confusion than clarity. However, a strong association exists between the risk of gout and lead exposure through diet (e.g., "moonshine" whiskey) or occupation (e.g., painters, plumbers, shipbuilders).[10,11] Lead exposure does not appear to be a factor in W.S.

Epidemiologically, W.S.'s age and gender are compatible with the typical profile of a gouty patient, and W.S. has a history of hypertension. The most important epidemiologic relationship of gouty arthritis for W.S., and indeed for all patients, is the association of gout and hyperuricemia (see Questions 27 and 28).

Number of Joints

Acute gout attacks usually affect a single joint, and the initial attack in 75% to 90% of patients involves a joint of the lower extremity (especially the first metatarsophalangeal joint).[4,12] Although initial gout attacks are primarily monoarticular, as many as 39% of the patients in one study experienced polyarticular involvement as their first manifestation of gout.[13] In another study, 8 of 30 (27%) patients with gout had crystal-proven polyarticular onset and 60% subsequently experienced polyarticular symptoms.[14] In a prospective investigation of 106 patients with crystal-documented gouty arthritis, 42 (40%) had articular inflammation at two or more sites.[15] In addition, radionuclide imaging has demonstrated that multiple joints can be undergoing asymptomatic, low-grade inflammatory reactions despite the presence of only one symptomatic joint.[16] Therefore, gout attacks usually are monoarticular, but polyarticular gout also is common. When the first attack of gout involves multiple joints, only two or three joints usually are affected.

Generally, recurrent attacks are of longer duration than first attacks and are more likely to be polyarticular.[12] Patients with polyarticular recurrent gout tend to experience attacks of a more smoldering onset, and these attacks are of longer duration. The polyarticular joint involvement tends to occur in an ascending and asymmetrical fashion (i.e., the joints in the upper extremities usually become involved only after several attacks involving joints in the lower extremities).[15]

W.S. seems to be experiencing polyarticular gout, because both his great toe and instep appear to be afflicted. This clinical presentation is compatible with cases of gouty arthritis that have presented as polyarticular disease.[13–16] Nevertheless, it is difficult to determine whether W.S.'s gout truly is polyarticular, because the area around the base of his left great toe is too inflamed to attribute the inflammatory process to one or multiple contiguous joints.

Podagra

An acute attack of the great toe (podagra) is the most common manifestation of acute gouty arthritis in Western societies. More than 50% of patients with gout have the initial attack in either great toe, and approximately 85% to 90% will have at least one attack of podagra sometime during the course of this disease.[1] The predilection for the big toe appears less often in non-European and non–North American populations and perhaps can be attributed to differences in traditional footwear, climate, and other variables associated with gout.[17] If the great toe is not affected, the acute attacks almost always affect other peripheral joints in the feet and ankles. The small joints in the hands usually are affected next, then the knees and elbows. Although acute gouty arthritis can occur in other joints such as the shoulders, hips, and vertebrae, occurrence in these sites is rare except in patients with established severe disease. The involvement of W.S.'s great toe is typical of the usual acute attack of gout.

An explanation for the predilection of the great toe to acute gouty arthritic attacks is based on the premise of a transient local increase in the concentration of monosodium urate in this joint.[18] Because urate diffuses more slowly across a synovial membrane than water,[19,20] resorption of synovial effusion from traumatic joints when the patient is in a recumbent position increases the urate concentration within a joint. Synovial effusions are increased in the great toe during the day because of degenerative changes in that joint: the first metatarsophalangeal joint is the most common and often the only joint affected in degenerative joint disease of the foot. According to radiographic surveys and surgical dissections, the frequency of degenerative joint disease at the base of the great toe far exceeds that in any other weight-bearing joint.[18] Although this concept explains why the great toe is most commonly affected by gout attacks, additional studies are needed to explain why all hyperuricemic individuals with presumably similar degenerative joint changes do not experience acute gouty arthritis.

It probably is not coincidental that W.S.'s left foot is afflicted, because it was this foot that was traumatized in the motorcycle accident 10 years ago. Most acute attacks have no obvious precipitating event, but trauma,[14] excessive alcohol intake (presumably due to increased serum concentrations of lactic acid),[21] or initiation of hypouricemic therapy (presumably because of mobilization of urate stores) may contribute to the development of an acute attack. In older patients, attacks often follow surgical procedures or a medical illness such as stroke, pneumonia, myocardial infarction, or urinary tract infection. The precipitation of acute gouty attacks in hyperuricemic individuals most likely involves a multitude of factors.

Physical Stress

Gouty attacks also seem to be more common during episodes of increased physical exercise. Long walks, hikes, golf games, or tight new shoes historically have been associated with the subsequent onset of podagra.[18] Thus, this painful episode of foot pain experienced by W.S. after a 4-mile run also is compatible with these clinical observations.

Nocturnal Occurrence

Acute gouty arthritis commonly begins at night. Thomas Sydenham's 18th-century classic description of an acute gouty attack begins, "The victim goes to bed and sleeps in good health. About two o'clock in the morning he is awakened by a severe pain in the great toe; more rarely in the heel, ankle, or instep."[4] According to the Simkin hypothesis,[18] small amounts of effusion fluid gravitationally enter into degenerative joints of the feet during the day, when most people are busily walking around, and are reabsorbed during the night when the lower extremities are elevated. Thus, the onset of foot pain in W.S. during the night also is typical of gout.

Pain

Sydenham continues his classical description of an acute gouty attack as follows: "This pain is like that of a dislocation. The pain, which was at first moderate, becomes more intense. After a time this comes to a height. Now it is a violent stretching and tearing of the ligaments—now it is a gnawing pain and now a pressure and tightening. So exquisite and lively meanwhile is the feeling of the part affected, that it cannot bear the weight of bedclothes nor the jar of a person walking in the room. The night is spent in torture, sleeplessness, turning of the part affected, and perpetual change of posture."[4] This description of the affected part is remarkably similar to the description presented by W.S.

Laboratory Data

2. What laboratory data should be obtained at this time if the clinical assessment is gout?

Baseline Tests

The cardiovascular and renal systems of all patients with gout should be examined because hypertension or impaired renal function is common in gouty patients. It would be especially prudent to monitor W.S.'s BP because of his history of hypertension. Preliminary laboratory investigations should include a complete blood count (CBC), urinalysis (UA), blood urea nitrogen (BUN), serum creatinine (SrCr), and serum uric acid.[1]

Infectious Component

The sudden appearance of acute swelling and tenderness of a joint without a background of arthritis, such as in W.S., can be attributed not only to gout but also to septic arthritis. If the patient is a young man, the possibility of an infectious etiology for the acute inflammation would be more seriously considered because of the lack of a history of chronicity.[3] Furthermore, the infectious organism may be presumed to be gonococcus unless another organism is suspected.[22] Although febrile reactions, leukocytosis, and elevation of the erythrocyte sedimentation rate generally can be attributed to infectious disease, such symptoms also are common to acute gouty arthritis.[14] Systemic signs are most likely to occur in patients with polyarticular attacks.[15] In view of W.S.'s age, social history, and classic clinical features, acute gouty arthritis would be the most likely cause of his pain.

Diagnosis

3. What objective data would confirm the diagnosis of gout in W.S.?

Although hyperuricemia is a precursor of gout, hyperuricemia is not a disease and by itself is not diagnostic of gout. Many hyperuricemic individuals never develop symptomatic gout, and acute gout may be present in some patients with normal serum uric acid concentrations.

Radiographic findings during the early phase of gout are nonspecific and generally characterized by asymmetric soft tissue swelling overlying the involved joint; bone mineralization and joint spaces are well preserved.[21] However, when gout has been longstanding, bony changes can be noticed, and repeated attacks can lead to calcium deposition with a resultant increase in density in the areas of soft tissue swelling.[21]

The diagnosis of acute gouty arthritis is confirmed only when large numbers of polymorphonuclear leukocytes and monosodium urate crystals are demonstrated in synovial fluid aspirated from the inflamed joint.[3,4,23] Acutely inflamed joints will have intracellular urate crystals in 85% of patients with gout, and this finding is specific for gout.[10,24]

When viewed through a microscope with normal illumination, monosodium urate crystals are long and needle-shaped.

However, a polarizing microscope with a first-order red compensator usually is needed to demonstrate these negatively birefringent urate crystals.[25] In selected cases, electron microscopic examination of synovial fluid may be needed for the initial documentation of urate crystal-induced synovitis when polarizing microscopy has failed to identify these crystals.[26]

In an occasional patient with acute gout, urate crystals cannot be found in fluid aspirated from the inflamed joint.[27–29] Therefore, a diagnosis of acute gouty arthritis cannot be ruled out with an absence of urate crystals in the initial synovial aspirate. Repeated search of other involved joints,[28] or even of the same joint a few hours later,[27,29] may demonstrate the diagnostic urate crystals. When synovial fluid was aspirated from the knees of 50 patients with asymptomatic, nontophaceous gout (synovial fluid monosodium urate crystals had been previously documented in the knees or other joints of these patients), urate crystals were found in 58% of these asymptomatic patients.[30]

W.S. should have his first metatarsophalangeal joint aspirated to confirm the clinical assessment of gout. Although his instep might be the primary focus of his acute attack, the first metatarsophalangeal joint is by far the most commonly affected. Aspiration of this joint, even if asymptomatic and never previously involved clinically, can be recommended as an aid in establishing a definitive diagnosis of gout.[31,32] The aspiration of joints, however, is difficult, and clinicians primarily have relied on patients' descriptions of the presumed gouty attacks. As a result, gout often is diagnosed by focusing on the oligoarticular nature of the attack, its finite duration, complete relief of pain after the attack, a positive response to colchicine, and the criteria described in Question 1. Nonetheless, two reports by Wolfe indicate an overdiagnosis of gout by a factor of three, and misdiagnosis by community physicians of 164 patients later seen in a rheumatology clinic.[33,34] The most common misdiagnoses were in patients with psoriatic arthritis and pseudogout. However, the American College of Rheumatology has set forth the criteria needed to establish a diagnosis of gout for epidemiologic studies. When 6 of the 11 criteria listed in Table 42-1 are present, gout can be distinguished from pseudogout with a specificity of 92.7% and an overall sensitivity of 84.8%.[10] These criteria are useful not only for epidemiologic studies, but also for clinical use when the aspiration of a joint is not viable.

Table 42-1   Criteria for Epidemiologic Diagnosis of Gout[10]

>1 acute attack of arthritis

Exquisite pain involving joint

Joint inflammation maximal within 1 day

Oligoarthritis

Erythema over involved joints

Podagra (first metatarsophalangeal joint)

Unilateral podagra

Tophi

Hyperuricemia

Asymmetric swelling within a joint on a radiologic examination

Complete termination of acute attack

Differential Diagnosis: Pseudogout

4. After a collaborative discussion with his physician, W.S. chose not to have his affected joints aspirated. Although he meets many of the criteria commonly attributed to gout, what other crystal-induced arthritides should be considered in the differential diagnosis of W.S.?

Deposition of microcrystals such as calcium pyrophosphate, calcium oxalate, and calcium hydroxyapatite into joints can cause acute or chronic arthritis in a manner similar to that caused by monosodium urate deposition.[35] The role of these microcrystals in causing acute synovitis has been greater than previously expected because new crystallographic technology (e.g., electron microscopy, x-ray diffraction) can differentiate these diagnoses from that of acute gout.

Crystal-induced diseases tend to occur in older patients because prior joint disease, especially osteoarthritis (which is generally a disease of the elderly), predisposes them to crystal deposition and acute episodes of joint inflammation. The elderly also are more prone to microcrystal-induced arthritis because these crystals generally accumulate over a long period and must attain a sufficient concentration and size before they precipitate into the synovial fluid and begin causing inflammation.[36]

CALCIUM PYROPHOSPHATE DIHYDRATE DEPOSITION DISEASE

Acute calcium pyrophosphate dihydrate deposition disease also has been referred to in the literature as *pyrophosphate gout* and *pyrophosphate arthropathy*. Although these terms connote specificity, the term *pseudogout* will no doubt remain in common use to describe the acute intermittent arthritis induced by calcium pyrophosphate dihydrate crystals. Although other crystals may mimic gouty arthritis, pseudogout is but one of a number of common syndrome names that need not be threatened by a taxonomic reclassification of the underlying deposition processes.[37] The arthropathy may be acute or chronic or may cause acute synovitis superimposed on chronically involved joints. The initial episode of pseudogout, or calcium pyrophosphate dihydrate deposition disease, usually occurs between ages 65 and 75 years and most commonly affects the knee.

CALCIUM HYDROXYAPATITE DEPOSITION DISEASE

Calcium hydroxyapatite deposition disease, or apatite gout, occurs far less often than gout or pseudogout. It usually occurs in younger persons, but people of all ages can be affected. Calcium hydroxyapatite is the primary mineral of bone and teeth.[36]

CALCIUM OXALATE DEPOSITION DISEASE

Calcium oxalate deposition disease, or oxalate gout, is a relatively new complication of end-stage renal disease. It was not until 1982 that calcium oxalate crystal deposition was noted to produce gout-like acute arthritis, usually in patients with chronic renal failure undergoing long-term hemodialysis.[35] Many of these patients have a history of taking pharmacologic doses of ascorbic acid, which is metabolized to oxalate.

The diagnosis of these nonurate microcrystal–induced arthritides can be made based on light microscopy demonstration of these crystals in synovial fluid.

Treatment of Acute Gout

Goals of Therapy

5. What is the primary goal in the treatment of this acute gout attack in W.S.?

The immediate goal in the treatment of an acute attack of gout is to relieve pain and inflammation. The immediate goal of therapy should not be aimed at decreasing the serum uric acid concentration with hypouricemic agents such as allopurinol (Zyloprim) or probenecid (Benemid). Patients most likely have been hyperuricemic for several months or years, and it is not necessary to treat the hyperuricemia immediately. Furthermore, a decrease in the serum urate concentration at this time might mobilize urate stores and precipitate yet another acute gouty attack.

Drug Therapy Overview

6. W.S.'s serum uric acid concentration is 10.5 mg/dL. His other laboratory tests (e.g., CBC, hemoglobin [Hgb], hematocrit [Hct], SrCr concentration, serum electrolytes, and UA) are within normal limits. W.S. remained unconvinced of the necessity for aspiration of his first metatarsophalangeal joint and just wanted treatment for his excruciating pain. What medications are effective in the treatment of acute gout?

[SI unit: serum uric acid, 624 μmol/L]

Acute gouty arthritis can be effectively treated in most instances by indomethacin; a nonsteroidal anti-inflammatory drug (NSAID) such as ibuprofen (Motrin), naproxen (Naprosyn), fenoprofen (Nalfon), or piroxicam (Feldene); various corticosteroids; or colchicine.

INDOMETHACIN

Indomethacin (Indocin), a first-generation NSAID, is commonly prescribed for the treatment of acute attacks of gouty arthritis, and many consider it to be the drug of choice.[38] Doses of 50 mg TID or QID should be given until there is significant relief of symptoms (usually within 2 to 3 days). This dose then should be decreased to 25 mg TID to QID until there is total resolution of the attack. Adverse effects (e.g., gastrointestinal [GI] disturbances, mental changes, headache, rash, leukopenia) are minimized when indomethacin is used in this manner. At one time, indomethacin was associated with a high incidence of adverse effects because large doses of 100 to 200 mg QID were prescribed unnecessarily. The sustained-release dosage form of indomethacin is not recommended for acute gouty arthritis.

NONSTEROIDAL ANTI-INFLAMMATORY DRUGS

NSAIDs such as ibuprofen, naproxen, and piroxicam are widely used in the management of numerous inflammatory disorders because they are highly effective and have minimal toxicities. As a result, these agents have largely replaced colchicine in the treatment of acute gout. In a multicenter study, naproxen (Naprosyn) 750 mg as a single dose followed by 250 mg three times a day was highly effective[39]; in another study, a dosing regimen consisting of an initial 750-mg dose of naproxen followed by 500 mg 8 hours later and 250 mg every 8 hours for the next 2 to 3 days had better results than a regimen that did not use large initial doses.[40] Alternatively, success also can be achieved with naproxen 500 mg for the first two doses, followed by 250 mg three times a day. Ibuprofen (Motrin) 2,400 mg/day in one patient[41] and in 10 other patients[42] resulted in rapid improvement and complete resolution of gouty arthritis within 72 hours. Fenoprofen (Nalfon) in various doses up to 3.2 g/day (800 mg three or four times daily) was effective in 27 patients with acute gouty arthritis.[43] When fenoprofen was compared in a double-blind study with phenylbutazone, both drugs were equally successful in relieving acute gouty arthritis.[44] Other NSAIDs such as piroxicam (Feldene) 40 mg/day,[45,46] flurbiprofen (Ansaid) 100 mg four times a day for 1 day followed by 50 mg four times a day,[47] ketoprofen (Orudis) 50 mg four times a day,[48] tolmetin (Tolectin) 400 mg three or four times a day,[49] meclofenamate (Meclomen) 100 mg three or four times a day,[50] and sulindac (Clinoril) 200 mg twice a day[51] have all been proven effective in the treatment of acute gouty arthritis. Adverse effects of NSAIDs have been modest. The efficacy and safety of selective cyclooxygenase-2 (COX2) inhibitors in gout has not been assessed with agents currently available in the United States. However, etoricoxib, an investigational agent, was effective in the treatment of acute gout.[52] The COX2 inhibitors are more costly and unlikely to have significantly fewer GI effects than the older NSAIDs, primarily because an acute attack of gout is seldom treated for more than a few days. (See Chapter 43, Rheumatic Disorders, for a further discussion of NSAIDs.)

CORTICOSTEROIDS

Corticosteroids probably are the most potent anti-inflammatory drugs currently available, and one would expect these drugs to be highly useful in the management of an acute gouty attack. However, their use has been dismissed by most major textbooks[4,35] and review articles[1,17] because of the alleged potential for rebound flares of arthritis when therapy was discontinued. However, at dosages of 20 to 30 mg/day of oral prednisone or its equivalent, corticosteroids are clearly effective in the treatment of acute gouty attacks. The dose of the corticosteroid should be decreased gradually over the ensuing 10 days.[53] When 100 patients with acute gouty arthritis were randomly assigned to receive a single intramuscular injection of 40 units of adrenocorticotropic hormone (ACTH) or indomethacin 50 mg four times a day, patients who received the ACTH within 24 hours of the onset of pain experienced pain relief sooner and with fewer adverse effects than those who received indomethacin.[54] Corticosteroids probably would be more widely used in the treatment of acute gout attacks if NSAIDs and indomethacin were not so effective.

COLCHICINE

At one time, colchicine was the agent of choice for the treatment of an acute attack of gout. This drug not only provided symptomatic relief to >95% of patients when administered early in the course of an attack of gout, but it also provided diagnostic confirmation because of its relative specificity for relieving only the symptoms of acute gout. For the fully developed acute attack, the traditional dose of colchicine has been one or two 0.5- to 0.6-mg tablets initially, followed by 0.5 to 0.6 mg hourly or every other hour, until joint pain was relieved or GI side effects (i.e., diarrhea, nausea, vomiting) intervened.

Choice of Agent

7. **What therapeutic intervention would be the most appropriate for W.S. at this time?**

As noted previously, many drugs can effectively manage an acute attack of gout. Indomethacin, more recent NSAIDs, corticosteroids, and colchicine are all highly effective. The pharmacodynamic differences between these agents are relatively minor when treating acute gout because these drugs are used for only a few days at a time. Therefore, the selection of the most appropriate drug for an acute attack of gout primarily depends on coexistent conditions (e.g., renal dysfunction) and physician or patient preferences.

Potent prostaglandin inhibitors such as indomethacin can inhibit diuretic-induced increases in renal sodium excretion[55-58] and decrease the hypotensive effect of diuretics and other antihypertensive drugs (e.g., β-blockers).[59,60] Although it seems doubtful that hypertensive patients will experience problems with indomethacin when it is used for only a few days, three patients reportedly have experienced hyperkalemia and renal insufficiency after taking indomethacin for treatment of gouty arthritis.[61]

The newer NSAIDs also have the potential of reversing the effects of antihypertensive drugs; however, the potential for such a drug interaction is not as great as with indomethacin and is not likely to be highly significant when the duration of therapy is <1 week.

It was decided to initiate an NSAID such as naproxen for this acute attack of gout in W.S., and it would be prudent to monitor his BP as well. Some clinicians with long-standing experience with colchicine might select it over an NSAID for W.S. if there were concern for reversal of his BP control. However, many young clinicians have not had much experience with colchicine or its potential for adverse effects when used inappropriately.[62] Although colchicine historically has been the classic drug chosen to treat patients with acute gouty arthritis, growing awareness of its potential for fatal complications has limited the selection of this drug. When the risks and benefits of colchicine for treatment of acute gout were rigorously studied, colchicine was deemed to have "the smallest benefit to toxicity ratio of drugs that are effective for acute gout."[62] The predictable diarrhea that accompanies colchicine use is especially disturbing to patients with podagra, who must hobble to the bathroom on a painful joint, and provides a further explanation for the increasing disfavor of colchicine use.

Thus, an NSAID would seem to be a reasonable choice for W.S. because it has both analgesic and anti-inflammatory effects as well as minimal adverse effects.

Delay of Hypouricemic Therapy

8. **W.S. experienced dramatic relief of pain with oral naproxen therapy. In fact, his response was much better than expected. After receiving 750 mg of naproxen, W.S. could feel that the pain at the base of his great toe was no longer worsening, and after the second dose of 500 mg, the pain began to lessen. Within 72 hours of initiating therapy, his metatarsophalangeal joint was no longer inflamed. Neither a synovial aspirate of the inflamed joint nor a 24-hour urine sample for uric acid quantification was**

obtained. Other laboratory tests were within normal limits, and W.S. was instructed to monitor his BP daily. Why should (or should not) W.S. receive hypouricemic therapy at this time?

After the initial attack of acute gout, the interval between subsequent attacks varies from a few days to several years. Some patients may never experience another acute attack of gout; however, >60% will have a second attack of gouty arthritis within 1 to 2 years of the initial presentation.[4,63] No specific therapy is required during this interval, although it often is tempting to initiate hypouricemic therapy because of the clear association of hyperuricemia with gout. However, antihyperuricemic drugs should not be prescribed indiscriminately. Once started, such therapy usually is continued indefinitely. Hypouricemic therapy should be initiated only when gouty patients have frequent acute attacks, urate tophi, or evidence of urate nephropathy (e.g., uric acid stones or renal damage). If these indications are absent, hypouricemic drug therapy should await the natural course of events because nothing is lost by waiting. The acute attack can be treated when it appears and usually resolves within days.

Long-term hypouricemic medications should not be started for W.S. at this time because these criteria for therapy are not met and, more importantly, the diagnosis of gout has not been firmly established by demonstration of urate crystals in the synovial fluid of an inflamed joint. In today's era of routine laboratory tests, there is the tendency to overdiagnose gout in hyperuricemic individuals. It is not uncommon to find a hyperuricemic patient with a musculoskeletal problem inappropriately treated with urate-lowering drugs. Therefore, W.S. should not be treated with hypouricemic drugs at this time.

Finally, antihyperuricemic drugs may not be needed in W.S. because his hyperuricemia and presumed acute gouty attack may have been the result of the hydrochlorothiazide therapy. Hyperuricemia is a common adverse effect of thiazide and other diuretics, including furosemide, ethacrynic acid, chlorthalidone, and acetazolamide.[64,65] These diuretics indirectly increase serum urate concentrations during extracellular fluid volume contraction. The volume depletion may enhance urate retention because of altered renal blood flow or changes in intrarenally generated angiotensin.[66] The volume contraction also could cause hyperuricemia by inducing a generalized reabsorption of all solutes.[67] Replacement of urinary salt and water losses prevents diuretic-induced hyperuricemia.[65] Therefore, discontinuation of hydrochlorothiazide, although it would require reformulating his antihypertensive therapy, may be all that is needed to lower W.S.'s serum urate concentration. Initiation of hypouricemic medications such as allopurinol or probenecid at this time would be premature. In any case, probenecid should not be initiated until uric acid overproduction is ruled out by urine uric acid analysis.

Nonsteroidal Anti-Inflammatory Drugs

9. After being relatively symptom-free since his first acute gouty attack 8 months ago, W.S. now complains of pain around the base of his left great toe similar to that he experienced in the past, along with some pain in several joints in his left foot, in-

cluding his left ankle. This apparent gouty attack began last night after a late evening lecture. He was awakened by acute pain and took three nonprescription Advil tablets (200 mg/tablet), which seemed to be beneficial. On physical examination, the first metatarsophalangeal joint of his left foot is markedly inflamed, tender, and brightly erythematous. His entire left foot appears inflamed and is tender to touch. Other findings are unremarkable, and his BP of 135/85 mm Hg continues to be controlled on metoprolol 100 mg/day.

Approximately 3 months before this episode he had taken three 200-mg ibuprofen tablets TID for 2 days because of some vague pain in the same region; approximately 1 month ago, similar vague discomfort responded to several 600-mg doses of ibuprofen. Why would it be reasonable (or unreasonable) to initiate therapy for acute gout with an NSAID at this time?

In W.S.'s case, presumptive evidence for a diagnosis of gout is present; however, in other cases, patients have been treated with NSAIDs for nonspecific joint pains without due consideration for gout as the primary cause of the treated disorder. In one report, the escape from detection of chronic polyarticular gout resulted in a needless dependence on NSAIDs, failure to correct the underlying problem, and in some cases progression of joint destruction. Although acute inflammation was modified in these patients, the basic pathogenic mechanisms remained unresolved and the joint disease continued.[68] By promoting misdiagnosis, the indiscriminate use of NSAIDs may prevent the effective control of gout, which is perhaps the most correctable rheumatic disorder. The spontaneous resolution of symptoms within 3 to 10 days[36] in most patients with monoarthritic or oligoarthritic disease further complicates management if the diagnosis of gout is not confirmed.

Because the diagnosis of gout has not been confirmed in W.S., aspiration of his inflamed joint would be prudent before initiating further NSAID therapy. W.S. previously responded well to naproxen and nonprescription ibuprofen tablets. Further laboratory tests (e.g., SrCr) to rule out possible underlying adverse effects from using nonprescription ibuprofen in large doses also should be considered.

Corticosteroids

10. The synovial fluid obtained from W.S.'s first metatarsophalangeal joint contains numerous polymorphonuclear leukocytes and monosodium urate crystals. A review of his laboratory tests notes a SrCr of 2.5 mg/dL and a low Hgb count that was consistent with W.S.'s complaint of considerable GI pains within the last month. Pending further evaluation of W.S.'s renal and GI system, what medication should be prescribed for this particular acute gouty attack?

[SI unit: SrCr, 221 μmol/L]

W.S.'s Hgb was normal at his last medical visit, but his history of GI distress with concurrent use of ibuprofen suggests the possibility of peptic ulcer disease. Likewise, the SrCr concentration of 2.5 mg/dL could suggest NSAID-induced renal insufficiency. Contraindications to NSAID therapy include renal insufficiency, anticoagulation, GI intolerance, or prior NSAID toxicity such as rash or wheezing; therefore, it would be prudent to treat this acute attack of gout with a medication other than an NSAID until the status of his renal and GI systems is known.

The *Textbook of Rheumatology* states, "anecdotally, rebound attacks may occur as steroids are withdrawn"; [4] however, these anecdotal reports of "rebound flare-ups" or relapses following corticosteroid discontinuance have been refuted by clinical trials.[53] In one study, 13 consecutive patients and 15 episodes of acute gout were successfully treated with systemic corticosteroids when adequate doses were administered for a sufficiently long period. When initial prednisone doses of 20 to 50 mg/day (mean, 37 mg) were decreased gradually over a mean of 11 days, 11 of 13 episodes of acute gout completely resolved within 7 days. Patients with gout involving more than five joints and patients with a prolonged duration of symptoms before the initiation of therapy required longer courses of corticosteroid therapy. All patients improved within 12 to 48 hours. One patient required treatment with a higher dosage of prednisone for 20 days because a "rebound gouty inflammation" was noted when the prednisone was tapered over a shorter period. No other patients experienced any episodes that could be construed to represent a rebound effect.[53] In another study, 8 of 144 gouty episodes (6%) needed retreatment because symptoms recurred in patients who received a single intramuscular dose of ACTH; in comparison, the incidence of relapse was higher in patients treated with 50 mg of indomethacin four times a day.[54] When 27 patients were treated with either indomethacin 50 mg three times a day or triamcinolone acetonide 60 mg given intramuscularly, efficacy was comparable and no episodes of rebound gout attacks were noted when triamcinolone acetate therapy was discontinued.[69] Therefore, the potential for relapse of gouty arthritis when corticosteroids are prescribed does not seem to be higher when compared to therapy with other anti-inflammatory drugs.

Corticosteroid adverse effects such as osteoporosis, myopathy, peptic ulcer disease, central nervous system effects, hypertension, and predisposition to infections are not expected with short courses of therapy and seldom appear unless corticosteroids are continued for a long period. Glucose intolerance, however, can occur with short-term therapy.

Because colchicine, indomethacin, and NSAIDs are associated with increased risks in patients with renal and GI disorders, this acute attack of gout in W.S. probably would be best treated with systemic corticosteroid therapy. A prednisone dose of 40 mg orally, followed by a 20-mg dose 6 to 8 hours later, would be a reasonable approach to the management of this episode of gout. Subsequently, the 20-mg/day dosage of prednisone can be decreased gradually over the next 5 to 10 days. Although intra-articular corticosteroid injections can provide quick relief when only one or two joints are involved, W.S. seems to have polyarticular involvement at this time. Injectable corticotropin or corticosteroids also could be used; however, most patients would prefer the less costly oral prednisone therapy over the more painful injections.

Colchicine

11. The repeat laboratory SrCr measurement in W.S. is normal, and the previous elevated value is attributed to laboratory error. Why might colchicine be considered as an alternative to corticosteroids in W.S.?

Colchicine, unlike general anti-inflammatory drugs, is relatively specific for relieving the symptoms of acute gout.[70] A positive therapeutic response to colchicine in a hyperuricemic patient with monoarticular arthritis is considered supportive evidence for the diagnosis of gout. Support for the diagnosis of gout is of value when synovial fluid cannot be obtained from small joints for inspection of urate crystals. For various reasons, joints are not always aspirated, and urate crystals are not found in as many of 15% of acute gouty effusions.[27–29] As a result, colchicine had been preferred by some clinicians for the first acute attack of gout because it not only provided symptomatic relief to >95% of patients when administered early in the course of an attack, but it also was a useful diagnostic tool.[70] Nevertheless, the response to colchicine must be interpreted with some caution. The arthritis that accompanies psoriasis and sarcoidosis sometimes responds to colchicine.[70] Likewise, colchicine also can prevent acute attacks of familial Mediterranean fever[71,72] and perhaps even alleviate amyloidosis.[73] As a diagnostic test, colchicine is neither so specific nor so sensitive as to be completely diagnostic. The preferred treatment of acute gout in most cases is NSAIDs.

Intravenous Use

12. Although a corticosteroid might have been preferred for W.S., his family physician has considerable experience using colchicine in this setting and has decided to treat this attack of gout with IV colchicine. What is the role for IV colchicine in the management of acute gout?

IV colchicine commonly was prescribed for the treatment of acute gout after clinical trials in the 1960s clearly established its efficacy. This route of administration was preferred over the oral route because it was considered to be associated with a lower incidence of GI adverse effects. Although IV colchicine had been used commonly for the treatment of acute gout, it is no longer frequently prescribed. According to one estimate, probably <1% of the patients with gout received parenteral colchicine in the United States in 1984, and IV colchicine is no longer licensed for clinical use in Britain.[62] A single intramuscular 7-mg dose of betamethasone can be as effective as 6 days of diclofenac,[74] and intramuscular ketorolac (Toradol) can be as effective as oral indomethacin.[75] Because IV colchicine is rarely used, the risks of toxicity with this drug outweigh its benefits when prescribed by clinicians who are inexperienced in its use. In exceptional cases when IV colchicine is the only suitable alternative, one can expect rapid relief of gouty arthritis symptoms following its administration.

Onset of Effects

13. When should the therapeutic effects of colchicine begin to become apparent?

When given parenterally, colchicine is one of the faster-acting drugs in the treatment of gout. IV colchicine provides relief from acute gout in 6 to 12 hours in most patients and in <6 hours in some patients. The onset of effectiveness of colchicine can be delayed if treatment is not initiated early. Generally, the pain, redness, and swelling resolve completely within 48 to 72 hours after the initiation of colchicine therapy. Nevertheless, there is considerable interpatient variation to this time frame for response.

Guidelines for Use

14. Because IV colchicine was prescribed for W.S., what guidelines should be followed to optimize the safe IV use of this drug?

When IV colchicine is used infrequently in hospitals, supervision of its use would be appropriate. Automatic review of IV colchicine orders by the pharmacy department can prevent the use of excessive doses. It would be advantageous to monitor the IV doses of colchicine when it is prescribed for elderly patients. As with most medications, the elderly seem to be more sensitive to therapeutic and toxic effects, even when renal or hepatic function seems to be normal. Elderly patients should not receive >2 mg of colchicine IV per attack, nor should they receive another dose until at least 3 weeks have elapsed. In young patients, no further colchicine should be administered for 1 or 2 weeks following IV colchicine.[76] Renal and hepatic dysfunction must be ruled out in all patients before IV use, and the drug should be avoided in patients in whom function is impaired.

The initial 2-mg dose of colchicine should be diluted with normal saline to 30 mL and administered slowly over a period of 5 minutes. One additional IV dose may be repeated in 6 to 8 hours if needed, but the total IV dose of colchicine should not exceed 4 mg for a given attack of gouty arthritis. The dose of IV colchicine should be restricted to no more than 1 or 2 mg (not 4 mg) if the patient has been receiving long-term oral colchicine therapy.[77] Furthermore, IV colchicine should not be substituted milligram for milligram for oral colchicine.[62]

These dosing guidelines are underscored by the death of a 70-year-old man with apparently normal renal and hepatic function who developed marrow aplasia and pancytopenia after receiving 10 mg of IV colchicine over a period of 5 days for acute gouty arthritis.[78] Other anecdotal reports of serious toxicities have been published when established dosing guidelines were significantly modified.[62,77]

IV colchicine solutions are extremely irritating, and care also must be taken to prevent extravasation during administration. The needle used to aspirate the colchicine solution into the syringe should be discarded and a new needle used for actual venipuncture to diminish the risk for phlebitis.

Concomitant Use of Opiate Analgesics

15. W.S. is in excruciating pain and requests an analgesic to supplement his antigout medication. Why might a narcotic analgesic be appropriate?

A dose or two of a narcotic analgesic may be a reasonable adjunct to blunt the pain of acute gouty arthritis while awaiting the apparent benefits of colchicine. In addition, the narcotic analgesics have the added advantage of decreasing the troublesome diarrhea that accompanies colchicine use. GI side effects such as nausea, vomiting, abdominal cramping pain, or watery diarrhea are common in patients given full therapeutic courses of colchicine.

Adverse Effects

16. What toxicities might be expected from an overdose of colchicine?

Adverse effects from colchicine usually are reversible and consist most commonly of nausea, diarrhea, abdominal pain, and vomiting. More severe toxic effects from therapeutic doses of colchicine affect the hepatic, hematopoietic, and nervous systems but occur primarily in elderly patients[79] or those with prior cardiac, hepatic, or renal disease.[80] Reports of a toxic effect of colchicine on sperm production are contradictory.[81,82]

Large overdoses or acute poisonings with colchicine can cause life-threatening multiple system disturbances. Neurologic dysfunctions have been manifested as persistent mental confusion, loss of deep tendon reflexes, ascending paralysis, and respiratory failure. GI toxicities result in abdominal pain, vomiting, severe watery diarrhea, and a hemorrhagic gastritis that has led to dehydration and shock. Hepatotoxicity and pancreatitis also may be associated with colchicine's effects on the GI system. Musculoskeletal problems such as myopathy, myoglobinuria, and large increases in muscle enzymes have been reported. Myopathy and neuropathy may be a common, unrecognized disorder in patients with renal dysfunction who take customary doses for gout.[83] The myopathy usually presents with proximal weakness and always presents with an elevated serum concentration of creatine kinase; both features remit within 3 to 4 weeks after the drug is discontinued. Hematologic abnormalities include severe leukopenia followed by recovery leukocytosis and complete bone marrow aplasia. Renal complications can be manifested as reversible azotemia or as proteinuria, myoglobinuria, or hematuria, with many hyaline casts on urinalysis. Respiratory problems may be the result of neurologic failure as well as chest wall weakening or pulmonary edema with hypoxemia.[70]

URIC ACID URINE QUANTIFICATION

17. W.S. revisited his physician approximately 6 months after his last gout attack. At this time, the clinical laboratory noted that his serum uric acid concentration was 10.4 mg/dL, and he was given instructions for a 24-hour urine collection. What is to be gained by a 24-hour urine collection for uric acid?

[SI unit: serum uric acid, 619 μmol/L]

Some believe that urine concentrations of uric acid should be measured in every hyperuricemic patient,[84] whereas most practitioners are unconvinced as to the benefit of such studies. Urinary uric acid excretion studies are of potential diagnostic benefit in defining the cause of hyperuricemia and could be useful in determining the most appropriate hypouricemic agent.

Urinary uric acid excretion usually is measured in a 24-hour collection to ascertain whether the patient overproduces or underexcretes uric acid. Patients excreting <750 mg/day of uric acid into the urine generally are considered underexcretors, and those excreting >800 mg/day are categorized as overproducers. A few overproducers of uric acid suffer from genetic defects in enzymes such as hypoxanthine-guanine phosphoribosyltransferase (HGPRTase), or from disorders such as leukemias, which are associated with increased turnover of cells. Moreover, overproducers are probably best treated with the hypouricemic drug allopurinol, which inhibits the formation of uric acid, as opposed to a hypouricemic agent such as probenecid, which increases urate excretion.

Predictions of urinary uric acid overproducers by use of uric acid:creatinine (or creatinine clearance [Cl_{Cr}]) ratios based on spot midmorning serum and urine samples[84] have been advocated because of the inherent difficulties in 24-hour urine collections.[85]

HYPERURICEMIA

Choice of Allopurinol Versus Uricosurics

18. **W.S. apparently has experienced at least two, and perhaps four, attacks of gout within the past 8 months. His thiazide diuretic was discontinued at the time of his first attack, but he is still hyperuricemic, with a serum uric acid concentration of 9.4 mg/dL. The uric acid excretion study noted that 690 mg of uric acid was excreted during the 24-hour collection. What hypouricemic medication should W.S. receive?**

[SI unit: serum uric acid, 559 μmol/L]

Two types of hypouricemic drugs have stood the test of time and are commonly used in the management of symptomatic hyperuricemia. Uricosuric drugs reduce the serum urate concentration by increasing the renal excretion of uric acid, and xanthine oxidase inhibitors decrease serum uric acid by inhibiting uric acid synthesis. The uricosuric drugs probenecid (Benemid) and sulfinpyrazone (Anturane) are the most logical hypouricemic agents for underexcretors of uric acid. The uric acid synthesis inhibitor allopurinol (Zyloprim) is the most logical agent for overproducers of uric acid. Although this strategy for managing hyperuricemia certainly seems attractive, an inhibitor of uric acid synthesis should be effective in both underexcretors and overproducers. Consequently, allopurinol is prescribed most commonly for the management of hyperuricemia because it is an effective hypouricemic in all patients, and because the relative propensities for adverse effects of uricosurics and allopurinol are comparable.

Although a 24-hour urine uric acid excretion of 690 mg would numerically label W.S. as an underexcretor, this test result actually is inconclusive. As previously stated, patients excreting <750 mg/day of uric acid generally are considered to be underexcretors; however, 24-hour urine collections are notoriously difficult,[86] and to conclude that W.S., who excretes 690 mg/day, is an underexcretor is too categorical. W.S. does not have corroborating evidence of myeloproliferative disease, tophaceous deposits, or renal insufficiency, and neither allopurinol nor the uricosuric drug probenecid is better than the other in this situation. Likewise, neither probenecid nor allopurinol is effective for the acute gouty attack, and both are effective only in the long-term management of hyperuricemia.

Allopurinol

Initiation of Therapy: Dose

19. **W.S.'s hyperuricemia is to be treated with allopurinol. What would be an appropriate dosage of this drug to initiate therapy?**

The ability of allopurinol to lower serum uric acid is a dose-related phenomenon: the higher the dose of allopurinol, the greater the decrease in uric acid serum concentration. Generally, the dosage required to normalize hyperuricemia is 200 to 300 mg/day in patients with mild disease and 400 to 600 mg/day in those with moderate or severe disease.[87] Allopurinol dosages of 300 mg/day in one study reduced the serum urate concentration to <7 mg/dL and halved the urinary uric acid excretion in approximately 70% of patients. The remaining patients needed 400 to 600 mg/day, although 200 mg/day sufficed in some.[88] Therefore, it would be reasonable to expect that 300 mg/day of allopurinol would be appropriate for W.S. In patients with normal renal function, the initial allopurinol dosage should not exceed 300 mg every 24 hours.[89] The serum urate concentration can be used as a guide for subsequent allopurinol dosages when managing hyperuricemia.[90]

Symptoms of acute gout may be slightly exacerbated during the first 6 weeks of allopurinol therapy because of uric acid mobilization from tissues. Although this claim is not well documented, allopurinol therapy should be initiated slowly simply because nothing is lost by so doing. Patients generally have been hyperuricemic for many years, and the extra week or two required to reach usual therapeutic dosages is inconsequential. Therefore, W.S. should receive 150 mg/day of allopurinol (e.g., half of a 300-mg tablet) for the first 2 weeks of therapy. Thereafter, the dosage should be increased to 300 mg/day to reduce the urate serum concentration to <6.5 mg/dL. This dosage can be increased after a period of time if needed. The gradual approach to initiating allopurinol in this situation is admittedly conservative and perhaps unnecessary.

Onset of Effects

20. **When should the hypouricemic effect from allopurinol become apparent?**

Serum uric acid levels usually begin to fall within 1 to 2 days after initiation of allopurinol therapy; maximal uric acid suppression to a given dosage usually requires 7 to 10 days.[87,88] However, serum concentrations of oxypurinol (the active metabolite of allopurinol) comparable to those achieved at steady state may be achieved within minutes after IV administration of 300 to 400 mg of allopurinol or within 1 to 3 hours of an oral dose. Therefore, therapeutic blood levels for prevention of uric acid nephropathy may be achieved quite rapidly in patients with neoplastic disease who must suddenly undergo neoplastic treatment.[90] Clinically observable improvement takes longer. After approximately 6 months, one should observe a gradual decrease in the size of established urate tophi, as well as the absence of new tophaceous deposits if these were present.

Once-Daily Dosing

21. **Why is allopurinol commonly administered once a day when its half-life is <2 hours?**

Approximately 80% of an oral dose of allopurinol is rapidly absorbed when administered by the oral route. Once absorbed (30 minutes to 2 hours), allopurinol is rapidly cleared from plasma, with a probable plasma half-life of <2 hours.[90,91] A small portion of allopurinol is excreted in the urine unchanged; the remainder is rapidly oxidized to alloxanthine (oxypurinol). Oxypurinol is eliminated slowly from the blood by renal excretion and has a serum half-life of 13 to 18 hours and perhaps as much as 30 hours in some.[90,92] Thus, oxypurinol may accumulate in patients with renal impairment.

Oxypurinol and allopurinol are not bound to plasma proteins and are filtered at the glomerulus. Therefore, factors that decrease glomerular filtration rate (GFR) would be expected to decrease the clearance of oxypurinol as well. For example, a decrease in the dietary intake of protein decreases creatinine clearance, renal blood flow, and the clearance of oxypurinol by 64%. During a low-protein diet (e.g., patients receiving prolonged IV dextrose infusions without amino acid or protein supplements), the plasma oxypurinol half-life increased almost threefold in one study from 17.3 hours to 49.9 hours.[93]

After glomerular filtration, oxypurinol, unlike allopurinol, undergoes proximal tubular reabsorption.[94] As with urate tubular reabsorption, the tubular reabsorption of oxypurinol is significantly enhanced by volume contraction.[89] For example, thiazide diuretics can inhibit the excretion of oxypurinol as they do that of uric acid.[94]

Oxypurinol also is a potent inhibitor of xanthine oxidase, and most of allopurinol's xanthine oxidase inhibitory effects are attributable to that of oxypurinol. Due to oxypurinol's long half-life, allopurinol can be administered on a once-daily basis.[92,95]

Adverse Effects

22. **What adverse effects are encountered with allopurinol therapy, and which one effect is the most clinically significant?**

Allopurinol generally is well tolerated, with few significant adverse effects. Occasionally GI intolerance, bone marrow suppression, renal or hepatic toxicities, and mild skin rash are reported. Hyperuricemic patients receiving allopurinol might be more susceptible to "ampicillin rash"[96] and to interactions with other drugs (Table 42-2). Allopurinol's interaction with azathioprine is well documented and is of major clinical significance; however, in one survey of 24 transplant patients taking both drugs, the dose of azathioprine was decreased in only 14 of 24 patients.[97] This survey exposes one weakness in our understanding of how best to adjust azathioprine dosages despite the widely acknowledged need for dosage adjustment.[17]

Whether allopurinol causes cataracts is controversial. In one study, allopurinol use for >2 years was associated with the formation of cataracts.[98] This adverse reaction has been attributed to above-average exposure to sunlight that enhances the photobinding of allopurinol in the lens, resulting in cataracts.[98] This report disputes the finding of the Boston Collaborative Drug Surveillance Program that any association between allopurinol and cataracts was coincidental.[99] However, a subsequent study found no evidence to confirm a higher risk of cataract formation in allopurinol users than in nonusers.[100]

HYPERSENSITIVITY REACTIONS

Of the adverse drug reactions sometimes encountered with allopurinol, hypersensitivity-type reactions have been the most notorious. These generally present as mildly erythematous, dusky red purpuric, or scaly maculopapular skin eruptions. When allopurinol is discontinued promptly, these hypersensitivity reactions subside without sequelae.

However, the continued administration of allopurinol to hypersensitive individuals has resulted in progression of these symptoms and several fatalities.[101–110] The cutaneous reactions often progressed to include necrosis of the skin and mucous membranes, exfoliative dermatitis, Stevens-Johnson syndrome, or toxic epidermal necrolysis. Hepatomegaly, jaundice, hepatic necrosis, and renal impairment often accompanied these reactions.[111] The hepatic and renal changes usually were reversible when the drug was discontinued, and these organ failures were not correlated with any one cutaneous reaction pattern. Patients

---

Table 42-2 Allopurinol Drug Interactions

Major Documentation

Azathioprine (Imuran). Metabolized to 6-mercaptopurine and then to inactive metabolites by xanthine oxidase. Allopurinol inhibition of xanthine oxidase ↑ the serum concentration of 6-mercaptopurine and the risk of bone marrow depression. When azathioprine (or 6-mercaptopurine) is used concurrently with allopurinol, use extreme caution, and the azathioprine dose should be ↓ to 1/4 of the recommended dose.

Mercaptopurine (Purinethol). See Azathioprine.

Moderate Documentation

ACE Inhibitors. May predispose patients to severe allopurinol hypersensitivity reactions (e.g., Stevens-Johnson syndrome). Concurrent and subclinical renal impairment may be important variables.

Anticoagulants. Occasionally, patients on oral anticoagulants and allopurinol develop enhanced anticoagulant effects; however, this interaction is unpredictable and primarily based on isolated case reports.

Cyclophosphamide. Allopurinol ↑ cyclophosphamide-induced bone marrow depression based on epidemiologic data and may inhibit cyclophosphamide clearance.

Anecdotal Documentation

Ampicillin. Dermatologic reactions occurred in 22.4% of 67 patients receiving concomitant allopurinol and ampicillin, compared with 7.5% receiving only ampicillin and 2.1% receiving only allopurinol.[96] The observations from this epidemiologic report in 1972 have not been noted subsequently.

Antacids. Aluminum hydroxide inhibited the GI absorption of allopurinol in three patients on hemodialysis; however, the interaction can be avoided by the administration of allopurinol ≥3 hr before or 6 hr after aluminum hydroxide.

Chlorpropamide. Allopurinol or its metabolites might compete with chlorpropamide for renal tubular secretion and can result in an ↑ chlorpropamide effect in an occasional patient.

Cyclosporine. Cyclosporine toxicity was reported in one patient who had a cyclosporine blood level of 325 ng/mL (baseline, 110 ng/mL) 12 days following the addition of allopurinol 100 mg to a stable immunosuppressive regimen that included cyclosporine.[147]

Phenytoin. Allopurinol inhibits the hepatic metabolism of some drugs and seemed to inhibit the metabolism of phenytoin in one patient.

Probenecid. Allopurinol can inhibit the metabolism of probenecid, and probenecid can enhance the renal elimination of the active oxypurinol.

Theophylline. Allopurinol in high doses (300 mg Q 12 hr for 14 days) can ↑ mean theophylline AUC by approximately 27% and half-life by 25%; clearance can be ↓ approximately 21%. An active metabolite (1-methylxanthine) also can accumulate.[148,149]

Vidarabine. An active metabolite of vidarabine is metabolized by xanthine oxidase, and accumulation of this metabolite can ↑ neurotoxicity.

ACE, angiotensin-converting enzyme; AUC, area under the concentration–time curve; GI, gastrointestinal.
Adapted from reference 60.

with renal insufficiency, those receiving thiazide diuretics, and those with chronic alcoholism or severe liver disease have been the most commonly afflicted with this syndrome.

The toxic syndrome generally appeared within the first 5 weeks of therapy; however, it has appeared as part of a delayed hypersensitivity reaction as late as 25 months after the initiation of therapy.[110] The mechanism by which this toxicity syndrome occurs is unknown. The cutaneous reaction and renal failure have been consistent with a diffuse systemic vasculitis, and the nonfatal cases did not improve until large steroid doses were instituted, despite the discontinuation of the allopurinol. Biopsy specimens from patients provide support for the premise that the vasculitis results from an immune hypersensitivity reaction to allopurinol.[101,104,107,111] Although no specific mechanism or causative agent producing this toxicity has been identified, the accumulation of allopurinol or a metabolite is postulated to be a primary factor, especially because 80% of patients with this syndrome had significantly impaired renal function before the initiation of allopurinol.[112] In one particular incident, allopurinol serum concentrations were 50 times normal values.[110] Therefore, maintenance dosages of allopurinol should be adjusted based on individual Cl_{cr} measurements.[89,107]

23. If a patient has recovered from an allopurinol hypersensitivity syndrome but continues to need this drug because of cytotoxic therapy for malignancy, can a smaller dose of allopurinol be prescribed?

Patients who have recovered from an allopurinol hypersensitivity syndrome should avoid the future use of this drug because most probably will experience a similar reaction on reexposure. However, a few hypersensitive individuals may tolerate low dosages (50 to 100 mg/day). If there is no reaction after a few days, the allopurinol dosage can be increased gradually. Nevertheless, severe toxic reactions have been produced by doses of allopurinol as low as 1 mg. Some hypersensitive patients have been desensitized with daily doses as small as 0.05 mg that were increased gradually over a period of 30 days. Although the cautious reintroduction of allopurinol through graded oral doses can be attempted in patients with cutaneous rash who have failed other options,[113] the risk of serious hypersensitivity is significant, and an alternative agent (e.g., rasburicase) should be considered.

Rasburicase

Uricase, an enzyme endogenous in many animal species other than humans, converts uric acid to allantoin, which is considerably more soluble in urine than uric acid. Rasburicase (Elitek) is a recombinant urate oxidase enzyme that received approval from the U.S. Food and Drug Administration in 2002 for the management of hyperuricemia in children with leukemia, lymphoma, or solid tumor malignancies who are likely to develop hyperuricemia subsequent to chemotherapy and tumor lysis. In a multicenter, randomized trial of 52 children with leukemia or lymphoma during initial chemotherapy, a 5- to 7-day course of oral allopurinol (median 300 mg/day) was compared to IV rasburicase (0.2 mg/kg once daily). Rasburicase decreased serum urate concentrations more effectively and had a more rapid onset than allopurinol.[114]

Although rasburicase is not currently approved by the Food and Drug Administration for use in adults, this drug has been shown to be safe and effective for the prophylaxis or treatment of hyperuricemia in adults with leukemia or lymphoma.[115]

Rasburicase is contraindicated in patients with glucose-6-phosphate dehydrogenase (G6PD) deficiency, a known history of anaphylaxis, hypersensitivity reactions, or hemolytic reactions. Rasburicase therapy has been associated with fever, neutropenia, respiratory distress, sepsis, and mucositis.[116] Rasburicase use also has been associated with spuriously low uric acid serum concentrations in laboratory reports because of its interference with uric acid assays. This drug should be used for a single course of treatment, given as a 0.15- or 0.20-mg/kg 30-minute infusion once daily for 5 days. Chemotherapy should be initiated 4 to 24 hours after starting rasburicase. Rasburicase should be reserved for patients who cannot undertake allopurinol therapy and who are at high risk for tumor lysis syndrome (see Chapter 90, Hematological Malignancies). Rasburicase is 3,000 times more costly than allopurinol.[117,118]

Probenecid

Initiation of Therapy

24. W.S. has not experienced any gouty attacks since the initiation of allopurinol approximately 10 months ago. During a routine yearly physical examination, his aspartate aminotransferase (AST) was noted to be slightly increased to 90 U/L. All other liver function tests are within normal limits. W.S. states that he did develop a localized rash that later subsided despite continuation of his medications. Although these findings probably do not represent allopurinol hypersensitivity, allopurinol is discontinued as a precautionary measure and probenecid is started. How should uricosuric therapy be initiated for W.S.?

[SI unit: AST, 90 U/L]

Probenecid (Benemid) is well absorbed orally, and plasma concentrations peak within 2 to 4 hours. Its biologic half-life is 6 to 12 hours and its active metabolites help prolong the uricosuria. The dosage of probenecid should be 250 mg twice daily for the first week of therapy; thereafter, 500 mg may be given twice a day. If necessary, the dosage may be increased to 2 g/day. Uricosuric therapy should begin with small doses because excretion of large amounts of uric acid increases the risk of urate stone formation in the kidney. High fluid intake to maintain urine flow of at least 2 L/day also minimizes renal stone formation. This gradual approach to the initiation of hypouricemic therapy also decreases the likelihood of precipitating an acute attack of gout.

Because the initiation of uricosuric therapy has been associated with acute attacks of gouty arthritis, prophylactic colchicine often had been prescribed concurrently (e.g., the fixed-combination product ColBenemid contains both colchicine and probenecid). Although it might seem reasonable to administer prophylactic colchicine initially, it is unreasonable to prescribe colchicine for prolonged periods of time because of its adverse effects[62,119] (see Question 16). Nonetheless, prophylactic colchicine is prescribed occasionally, with caution.[120–122]

Sulfinpyrazone (Anturane), another effective uricosuric agent, inhibits the tubular secretion of uric acid at low doses and inhibits the tubular reabsorption of uric acid at usual therapeutic doses. As with probenecid, therapy should be initiated slowly and the dosage increased gradually.

Contraindications

25. **Does W.S. have any contraindications to probenecid uricosuric therapy?**

Since uricosuric drugs do not affect the production of uric acid but merely increase its excretion, uricosurics should not be used in patients with a Cl_{cr} of <30 mL/min. Patients with a history of renal stones, patients who are gross overexcretors (>1,000 mg/day) of uric acid, and patients undergoing an acute attack of gout should not be treated with uricosurics. None of these contraindications is applicable to W.S., and probenecid can be safely prescribed for him.

Salicylate Interaction

26. **W.S. is a health-conscious individual who realizes that his hypertension and hyperuricemia increase his risk for ischemic heart disease. Therefore, to reduce the chance of a coronary event, he self-medicates with adult low-strength aspirin 81 mg/day. Would this dosage of aspirin interfere with his uricosuric therapy?**

Two 300-mg tablets of aspirin every 6 hours can completely antagonize the uricosuric effects of 2 g of probenecid. This drug interaction probably involves several mechanisms, including competition for renal tubular transport.[123] Doses of salicylate that do not produce serum salicylate levels of ≥5 mg/dL do not significantly affect probenecid uricosuria.[60] Therefore, a single daily aspirin probably will not interfere with his probenecid therapy. Interestingly, aspirin in high doses (e.g., 1.3 g four times a day) has uricosuric activity of its own. Acetaminophen (Tylenol) and NSAIDs do not interfere with probenecid and are reliable alternatives for antipyresis and mild analgesia in patients taking uricosuric agents.

Asymptomatic Hyperuricemia

Clinical Significance

27. **L.M., a 50-year-old man, is seen by his physician for a routine evaluation. His physical examination is unremarkable and his laboratory evaluations are all within normal limits except for a serum uric acid concentration of 9.5 mg/dL, which is noted on an SMA-12 panel. What is the clinical significance of this hyperuricemia?**

[SI unit: serum uric acid, 565 μmol/L]

Hyperuricemia can be drug-induced (e.g., thiazide diuretics) and can be affected by the laboratory methods of analysis for uric acid. Some common medications associated with hyperuricemia are listed in Table 42-3.

Table 42-3 Drugs Commonly Associated with Hyperuricemia

Drug	Mechanism	Comments
Certain ACE inhibitors: lisinopril, ramipril, trandolapril[150-152]	Reduced urate renal clearance	Hyperuricemia and gout have occurred at therapeutic doses. Conversely, captopril and enalapril significantly reduce serum urate levels, as does the ARB losartan; other ARBs have no effect or cause rare hyperuricemia.[153-156]
Cytotoxic chemotherapy: aldesleukin, asparaginase, busulfan, carboplatin, chlorambucil, cisplatin, cyclophosphamide, cytarabine, daunorubicin, fludarabine, hydroxyurea, mechlorethamine, melphalan, mercapto-purine, thioguanine, vinblastine, vincristine[157-173]	Rapid cell lysis	Occurs primarily with lymphomas and leukemias. Uric acid nephropathy, acute renal failure, and nephrolithiasis can result.
Cyclosporine[174,175]	Decreased urate renal clearance, either via a tubular mechanism or decrease in GFR	Cyclosporine-induced hyperuricemia may cause gout in patients with risk factors (renal dysfunction, concurrent diuretics, and male gender).
Diazoxide[176]	Decreased urate renal clearance	
Didanosine[177,178]	Catabolic effect	Uric acid blood increases of 0.5–5 mg/dL have occurred in patients receiving >9.6 mg/kg per day. Dose- and duration-dependent elevations in uric acid
Diuretics: acetazolamide, bumetanide, chlorthalidone, ethacrynic acid, furosemide, indapamide, metolazone, thiazides, torsemide, triamterene[179-183]	Secondary to volume contraction and increased uric acid reabsorption in the proximal tubules for all diuretics; thiazides may also competitively inhibit proximal tubular secretion	

Continued

Table 42-3   Drugs Commonly Associated with Hyperuricemia—cont'd

Drug	Mechanism	Comments
Ethambutol[184]	Decreased urate renal clearance	Hyperuricemia and gout have been demonstrated. A majority of patients were receiving 20 mg/kg per day orally.
Ethanol[185]	Increased uric acid production due to adenine nucleotide turnover	Associated with acute gout
Filgrastim[186]	Increased WBC production	Transient effect, seen more often with higher doses (30–60 μg/kg per day)
Fructose[187,188]	Diminished hepatic ATP synthesis and resultant acceleration of uric acid formation	Hyperuricemia seen with rapid infusion (500 mL/hr). Avoid in patients with gout and/or cirrhosis.
Glucocorticoids[189]	Tumor lysis	Seen when glucocorticoid is used as an antineoplastic agent
Isotretinoin[190]	Hypervitaminosis A	Hyperuricemia and rare gout cases have been reported.
Levodopa[191]	Inhibition of urate excretion	Patients taking therapeutic doses have experienced hyperuricemia and gout. Secondarily, interference with colorimetric assay of uric acid may contribute a false-positive increment.
Niacin[192]	?	Hyperuricemia and gout have occurred.
Pancreatic enzymes: pancreatin and pancrelipase[193]	Ingestion of pancreatic enzyme products having high purine content.	Hyperuricemia, hyperuricosuria, and uric acid crystalluria have occurred with high dosages.
Pyrazinamide[194]	Inhibition of renal tubular urate secretion	Hyperuricemia is more common with daily than with intermittent administration. Gouty attacks have occurred in those with a history of gout. Asymptomatic hyperuricemia was the only manifestation seen in one trial of pediatric patients.
Ribavirin and interferon[195]	Mechanism unclear; commonly associated with hemolysis	Nephrolithiasis developed in a patient with diabetes and hypertension. Hyperuricemia noted in 24% of those receiving with concurrent interferon.
Salicylates (low dose)[80]	Inhibition of proximal tubular secretion of urate	Dosages <2 g/day cause hyperuricemia.
Tacrolimus[196]	Reduced urate excretion	Associated with hyperuricemia. However, two case reports demonstrated resolution of polyarticular gout after switching cyclosporine to tacrolimus.
Theophylline[197,198]	Interference with uric acid assay	False-positive elevation with automated Bittner adapted method. Interference does not appear to occur with phosphotungstate assay method.

ACE, angiotensin-converting enzyme; ARB, angiotensin II receptor blocker; ATP, adenosine triphosphate; GFR, glomerular filtration rate; WBC, white blood cell.

Laboratory Tests of Uric Acid

The phosphotungstate or colorimetric method, commonly used in automated laboratory screening panels, is not as specific as the uricase method of uric acid analysis and generally provides readings that are approximately 1 mg/dL higher for the same sample.

In normal subjects, plasma becomes saturated with sodium urate at a concentration of 7 mg/dL. However, supersaturated solutions of monosodium urate form readily, and serum urate concentrations as high as 40 to 60 mg/dL are not uncommon in untreated, non-gouty patients with myeloproliferative disorders.[124] It is unclear how uric acid can remain in a supersaturated solution and then, suddenly, under certain conditions, begin to precipitate into joints and soft tissues. Nevertheless, it is known that plasma urate-binding protein deficiency, urate affinity for chondroitin sulfate, local pH changes, cold, trauma, and stress can cause seeding of urate crystals.

When maximum serum uric acid concentrations from the Framingham Heart Study[7] were analyzed, gouty arthritis occurred in 1.8% of patients with serum uric acid concentrations between 6.0 and 6.9 mg/dL and in 11.8% of those with levels between 7.0 and 7.9 mg/dL. Nevertheless, 15% of the men who actually had developed gouty arthritis did not have a serum uric acid value >6.9 mg/dL, and 81% of subjects with serum uric acid values >7 mg/dL did not develop gouty arthritis. The higher the serum concentration of uric acid, the greater the risk of developing gouty arthritis; however, a high serum uric acid concentration does not guarantee the development of gout.

Treatment

28. Should asymptomatic hyperuricemia, such as that noted in L.M., be treated?

Individuals with high serum uric acid levels are more likely to develop acute gouty arthritis than normouricemic individuals, and the magnitude of the risk increases with increasing degrees of hyperuricemia. Nevertheless, it would be excessive to treat all hyperuricemic individuals with uric acid–lowering medications for a lifetime solely to prevent acute attacks of gouty arthritis. A large percentage of hyperuricemic patients may never experience an acute attack of gout.[125] If an attack should occur, it can be treated easily within 48 to 72 hours, and after the acute episode has subsided, uric acid–lowering medications can then be considered.

The key issue in the treatment of hyperuricemia concerns the effect of uric acid on renal function. Renal disease commonly was associated with gout, and renal failure was thought to be the eventual cause of death in as many as 25% of gouty patients. Thus, treatment of asymptomatic hyperuricemia is justifiable if renal disease is prevented. However, this renal damage was noted to occur in a setting that included hypertension, diabetes, renal vascular disease, glomerulonephritis, pyelonephritis, renal calculi, or some other cause of primary nephropathy independent of gout.[126] In fact, the coexistence of gout and renal insufficiency without hypertension is so rare that its presence should raise the suspicion of chronic lead toxicity.[11,127] Therefore, the consensus now seems to be that hyperuricemia by itself has no deleterious effect on renal function.[128,129] Considering the financial costs, risks of adverse drug reactions, and practical considerations such as patient compliance, drug treatment of asymptomatic hyperuricemia is difficult to justify.[125]

The relationship of hyperuricemia to hypertension in individuals who have not had gout was studied prospectively in 124 hyperuricemic subjects. None of these patients had evidence of gout, hypertension, or cardiovascular, renal, or other diseases. After 10 years, 22.5% of these individuals with "asymptomatic hyperuricemia" had developed hypertension and 5.4% had developed atherosclerotic heart disease. The incidences of hypertension and atherosclerotic heart disease in the control group were 2.1 and 0.5%, respectively.[130] Atherosclerosis and hypertension apparently were more serious problems in this population than renal disease. Although hyperuricemia may represent an important risk factor for the development of cardiovascular disease,[8] the evidence is not sufficiently compelling to justify the treatment of asymptomatic hyperuricemia at this time.

Special Situations

Urate Nephropathy

29. Q.A., a 54-year-old man with a history of heart failure, is hospitalized with a diagnosis of acute myelogenous leukemia. On admission, his BUN was 49 mg/dL, SrCr was 2.1 mg/dL, and

serum uric acid was 16.2 mg/dL. On the following hospital day, chemotherapy is begun. His white blood cell (WBC) count decreased within a week from 90,000 cells/mm³ on admission to 7,500 cells/mm³ as a result of the cytotoxic treatment. On the seventh day, he complained of nausea, and his urine volume decreased to 35 mL/24 hr. At this time, BUN increased to 115 mg/dL, SrCr increased to 10.6 mg/dL, serum potassium (K) was 5.9 mEq/L, and serum uric acid increased to 22.6 mg/dL. IV furosemide and urine alkalinization had no effect on Q.A.'s clinical condition, and hemodialysis was started due to continued clinical deterioration.

During the ensuing 2 days, his urine output increased and then gradually returned to normal. Q.A.'s renal function continued to improve, and 16 days after hemodialysis was initiated, the SrCr was again 2.1 mg/dL. What was the probable cause for the increased serum uric acid concentration that was noted upon Q.A.'s admission?

[SI units: BUN, 17.5 and 41 mmol/L of urea, respectively; SrCr, 186 and 937 μmol/L, respectively; serum uric acid, 964 and 1,344 μmol/L, respectively; WBC, 90 × 10⁹ cells/L and 7.5 × 10⁹ cells/L, respectively; serum K, 5.9 mmol/L]

Upon superficial review, it would appear that Q.A.'s hyperuricemia is a result of both overproduction and underexcretion of uric acid. However, the major cause of hyperuricemia in this patient is most likely due to the overproduction of nucleic acids secondary to the leukemia and subsequent tumor lysis syndrome accompanying chemotherapy. Mild to moderate renal failure is not usually a cause of hyperuricemia as long as the creatinine clearance is >15 mL/min. Renal urate secretory mechanisms remain functional and do not become defective until the creatinine clearance falls to <10 mL/min. At this level of renal function, the defective secretory mechanism cannot compensate entirely for the decrease in urate reabsorption, and hyperuricemia occurs.[131,132]

Urine Alkalinization

30. Why was urine alkalinization tried in Q.A.?

Urine alkalinization was instituted because the serum uric acid was 22.6 mg/dL in the presence of oliguria. Uric acid is poorly soluble in water, but a pKa of 5.75 allows for greater solubility of the ionized form in alkaline environments. At a urine pH of 5, only 6 to 8 mg of uric acid is soluble per deciliter of urine. When urine is alkalinized to pH 7, the solubility of uric acid increases 20-fold to 120 to 160 mg/dL. Although asymptomatic hyperuricemia is not associated with renal impairment, unusually high serum uric acid concentrations in the presence of oliguria and undue acidity may result in the intrarenal and urinary precipitation of urate.[129] Thus, the desire to alkalinize the urine can be appreciated.

Urine can be alkalinized using sodium or potassium bicarbonate in an initial oral dose of 4 g followed by 1 to 2 g every 4 hours. IV sodium bicarbonate also can be used, as it was in Q.A. The urine pH should be tested (e.g., Nitrazine paper) at intervals throughout the day, and the dosage of bicarbonate should be adjusted accordingly. Potassium or sodium citrate also can be used in dosages of 1 g three to six times daily or Shohl's solution 10 to 30 mL four times daily. The citrates have the same urine-alkalinizing properties of sodium bicarbonate and neither neutralize gastric secretions nor promote a dumping syndrome. The bicarbonate and citrate doses should be divided evenly throughout the day and night. During the night, the urine becomes the most concentrated and acidic; thus, it may be necessary to add an IV dose to the IV solution during the night in hospitalized patients. Acetazolamide (Diamox) also is capable of alkalinizing urine, but it can produce a mild metabolic acidosis that is undesirable in a patient with renal decompensation.

Although an alkaline urine theoretically is desirable to increase the solubility of uric acid, it often is difficult to achieve clinically without affecting other organ systems. In Q.A., sodium intake is a problem, and the benefits from alkalinization probably are not worth the effort. In patients with hematologic malignancies, a primary goal is to prevent the hyperuricemia that developed in Q.A. Every effort should be made to identify patients at risk of tumor lysis syndrome and pretreat them with hydration, allopurinol, and urine alkalinization during the first 1 to 2 days of chemotherapy. The ability of the kidneys to excrete potassium also may be critically important. The cation content of various alkalinizing agents is listed in Table 42-4.

Hemodialysis

31. Hemodialysis was initiated in Q.A. How well is uric acid dialyzed, and would prophylaxis against an acute attack be needed?

Uric acid is readily dialyzable although it is bound to plasma proteins.[133] Apparently this urate–albumin bond is weak and influenced by many factors. In fact, hemodialysis is so efficient in removing uric acid that each 6-hour dialysis can reduce the uric acid level by 50%. In 16 patients with hyperuricemia and renal failure, each 6-hour dialysis removed 1.5 to 13.4 g of uric acid. Although 3.4 to 4.8 g of uric acid can be removed by peritoneal dialysis, hemodialysis is estimated to be 10 to 20 times more efficient in eliminating uric acid.[131] Disequilibrium does not occur even with rapid hemodialysis, and prophylaxis against an acute gouty attack is unnecessary.

Renal Transplants and Cyclosporine

32. T.M., a 42-year-old male renal transplant patient, developed an acute attack of gout localized to the great toe of the left foot while being treated with prednisone, cyclosporine, and azathioprine for maintenance immunosuppression. His cyclosporine dosage of 14 mg/kg per day during the first posttransplant week subsequently was reduced based on SrCr concentrations of <2 mg/dL and trough cyclosporine blood levels of 100 to 200 ng/mL. The prednisone dosage of 2 mg/kg per day (50 mg BID) was gradually tapered to 20 mg QD 3 months after transplant and to 10 mg/day subsequently. The azathioprine dosage of 1.5 to 2.5 mg/kg per day was adjusted to maintain a WBC count of >3,000 cells/mm³. The serum urate concentration at the time of presen-

tation was 11.8 mg/dL. Which of T.M.'s medications was most likely to cause his hyperuricemia and attack of gout?

[SI units: SrCr, <177 μmol/L ; WBC, >3 × 10⁹ cells/L; serum urate, 702 μmol/L]

The incidence of hyperuricemia in renal allograft recipients receiving azathioprine, prednisone, and antilymphocyte globulin is similar to that of the general population. However, hyperuricemia is common in cyclosporine-treated renal,[134] heart,[135] and liver transplant patients.[136]

The hyperuricemia occurs independently of cyclosporine-induced nephrotoxicity and occurs in approximately 30% to 80% of patients, depending on the definition of hyperuricemia.[137] The University of Minnesota renal transplant team noted that 105 of 131 patients (80%) treated with both cyclosporine and prednisone experienced hyperuricemia (serum uric acid, >8 mg/dL), and 13 of 131 (10%) were severely hyperuricemic (serum uric acid, >14 mg/dL).[134] Lin and colleagues at the University of Michigan reported that among the patients with stable allograft function and SrCr concentrations <3 mg/dL, hyperuricemia occurred in 84% of the cyclosporine-treated group versus 30% of the azathioprine group.[137] Despite the frequent occurrence of hyperuricemia, gout occurred in only approximately 5% to 10% of these patients.

A longitudinal study of a subgroup of the cyclosporine-treated patients revealed that hyperuricemia usually developed within 3 months after renal transplantation, and the mean length of time from transplantation to the first attack of gout was 24 months.[137] The prevalence of gout and the onset of gout may be higher in heart transplant patients because of the larger doses of cyclosporine.

MECHANISM

33. What is the mechanism of cyclosporine-induced hyperuricemia?

Whenever the serum concentration of any substance is at a greater concentration than expected, the question that must always be asked is whether the high concentration should be attributed to increased input (e.g., overproduction), decreased clearance, or a combination of decreased clearance and increased production. This principle holds true for all substances regardless of whether the problem is a high serum concentration of potassium, glucose, or uric acid. Because uric acid is produced primarily as a by-product of purine metabolism and is excreted renally, cyclosporine-induced hyperuricemia must be evaluated both as to increased production and decreased clearance.

The urate metabolism of 13 patients (6 adults with stable, functioning transplanted kidneys who were receiving cyclosporine therapy; 4 normal adults; 1 renal-transplant donor; and 2 renal-transplant recipients who were being treated with azathioprine and prednisone) was studied.[137] At least 7 days before the study, all subjects discontinued medications that were known to affect uric acid clearance and were placed on a purine-free diet. Urine samples were collected every 8 hours on the first day, every 12 hours on the second day, and then every 24 hours for the ensuing 5 days. The purine-enzyme activities of erythrocytes and the plasma concentrations of adenosine, inosine, hypoxanthine, and xanthine were measured. The rates of urate turnover were similar in all 13 pa-

Table 42-4	Cation Content of Alkalinizing Agents
Product	**mEq/g**
Na HCO₃	11.9
Na Citrate · 2H₂O	8.4
K HCO₃	9.9
K Citrate · H₂O	9.3

tients, and there was no change in purine-metabolite levels or in the activity of enzymes involved in purine metabolism. As a result, hyperuricemia was deemed to occur as a consequence of decreased urate clearance rather than overproduction of urate.[137]

Acute cyclosporine-induced prerenal nephrotoxicity is associated with intrarenal vasoconstriction and diminished GFR, and chronic renal insufficiency caused by cyclosporine is associated with renal parenchymal injury.[138] Renal tubular, glomerular, renovascular, and interstitial lesions all have been associated with cyclosporine. Because the clearance of urate in the kidney occurs by glomerular filtration, proximal tubular reabsorption, proximal tubular secretion, and postsecretory reabsorption, cyclosporine-induced renal insufficiency could modify urate clearance by affecting one or all of these processes. However, SrCr concentrations did not change significantly in the 13 patients enrolled in the University of Michigan study, and no direct correlation was noted with trough cyclosporine concentrations.[137] Nevertheless, cyclosporine-induced hyperuricemia is deemed to be the result of decreased renal urate clearance. SrCr values do not adequately reflect renal function in cyclosporine-treated patients because cyclosporine enhances Cl_{cr} relative to GFR, resulting in spuriously low SrCr concentrations despite marked reductions in GFR.[139,140]

Cyclosporine also may have an independent effect on urate transport within the tubules.[141]

TREATMENT

34. What drug-specific factors influence the selection of the most effective agent for treating acute gout in T.M.?

The drug therapy of uncomplicated acute gout with NSAIDs and corticosteroids is relatively straightforward, because all of the drugs in these categories are effective and relatively nontoxic when used for only a few days. Even colchicine, when appropriate precautions are taken, is relatively safe to use. However, the management of acute gout in transplant patients poses several special problems. Colchicine should be used with caution in patients with decreased renal function because of the increased potential for neuromuscular toxicity and bone marrow dysplasia (see Question 16). NSAIDs can reduce renal prostaglandin synthesis and can cause serious nephrotoxicity, especially in heart transplant patients who are receiving cyclosporine and perhaps diuretics as well.[135] The concurrent use of corticosteroids and cyclosporine may increase the plasma concentrations of both drugs and increase seizure activity, based on preliminary anecdotal reports.[142–145]

Because all of these drugs seem to be associated with an increased potential for toxicity, the clinical experience of others, although anecdotal, is worthy of review. Kahl and associates[135] described four patients with acute gout who experienced a prompt increase in SrCr concentrations of 0.7 to 1.7 mg/dL after only a few doses of an NSAID. Two of these cases involved the use of sulindac (Clinoril), the NSAID that was thought to have the fewest adverse effects on renal prostaglandins (see Chapter 43, Rheumatic Disorders). Although these patients experienced difficulty with NSAIDs, their gout responded to modest doses of colchicine. However, in three patients, the use of colchicine was limited by diar-

rhea, and it was withheld in two patients who were experiencing azathioprine-induced leukopenia due to the possible additive bone marrow–suppressing effects of colchicine.[135] Acute attacks of gout in six renal transplant patients were controlled with colchicine.[134] Experience with large corticosteroid doses for the treatment of acute gout in transplant patients is limited but may increase because of the newer trials in nontransplant patients.[53,54]

Treating acute gout in the transplant patient presents a serious therapeutic dilemma. All drugs carry hazards, yet patients like T.M. require relief from the pain and inflammatory discomfort of the attack. Furthermore, cyclosporine-induced gout appears to be particularly aggressive in some patients, even though clinical symptoms probably are ameliorated by the concomitant immunosuppressive and anti-inflammatory drugs being administered.[146] Because the acute attack compels treatment, the apparent option is to select an agent from among the NSAIDs, corticosteroids, or colchicine that appears the least damaging, then to dose it cautiously, closely monitor key parameters, and discontinue it as soon as possible. Pre-existing hyperuricemia before transplantation should be treated aggressively in the pretransplant waiting period. In T.M.'s case, because there is monoarticular involvement, an intra-articular injection of corticosteroid, which produces minimal systemic effects, might be a reasonable choice when supplemented with a few doses of an opiate analgesic, if needed.

RISKS

35. Is hypouricemic treatment feasible in T.M.? If so, what adverse effects must be guarded against?

The management of hyperuricemia in the transplant patient is a therapeutic dilemma because uricosuric drugs and xanthine oxidase inhibitors are relatively contraindicated.

The uricosuric drugs sulfinpyrazone (Anturane) and probenecid (Benemid) are ineffective in patients with decreased renal function (i.e., creatinine clearance <30 mL/min). Therefore, these drugs would be ineffective in many renal transplant patients and would increase the risk of intrarenal urate precipitation.

The xanthine oxidase inhibitor allopurinol is associated with a greater potential for significant adverse effects in patients with decreased renal or hepatic function.[105,107] (Also see Question 22.) Furthermore, allopurinol interacts in a clinically significant manner with azathioprine, an immunosuppressive agent commonly used in combination with cyclosporine and prednisone to prevent organ rejection in transplant recipients.

Azathioprine is first metabolized to 6-mercaptopurine and then to inactive metabolites via a metabolic pathway controlled by xanthine oxidase. Therefore, the inhibition of xanthine oxidase by allopurinol impairs the conversion of 6-mercaptopurine. Because the principal toxic effect of mercaptopurine is bone marrow depression, the increased blood concentrations of 6-mercaptopurine can exert profound toxic effects on the bone marrow and other tissues. Allopurinol and azathioprine should never be given together without meticulous attention to adjusting the dosage of the azathioprine. When allopurinol is prescribed for a patient stabilized on either azathioprine or 6-mercaptopurine, the azathioprine dose should be reduced to one-fourth the recommended dose.[60] Because pre-existing renal dysfunction predisposes patients to this drug interaction, the use of allopurinol in renal transplant recipients, who already are stabilized on azathioprine, is especially hazardous.

The dosage of allopurinol also should be adjusted in patients with renal impairment. The plasma half-life of oxypurinol, an active metabolite of allopurinol, is 18 to 30 hours in patients with normal renal function and increases in proportion to the reduction of glomerular filtration in patients with renal impairment.[79,90] The high serum concentrations of allopurinol and oxypurinol purportedly increase the intrinsic hepatotoxicity of allopurinol.[110]

REFERENCES

1. Pittman JR, Bross MH. Diagnosis and management of gout. Am Fam Physician 1999;59:1799.
2. Curto R et al. Analysis of abnormalities in purine metabolism leading to gout and to neurological dysfunctions in man. Biochem J 1998;329:477.
3. Emmerson BT. Drug therapy: the management of gout. N Engl J Med 1996;334:445.
4. Wortmann RL, Kelley WN. Gout and hyperuricemia. In: Ruddy S et al., eds. Kelley's Textbook of Rheumatology, 6th ed. Philadelphia: WB Saunders, 2001:1339.
5. Puig JG et al. Renal handling of uric acid in gout: impaired tubular transport of urate not dependent on serum urate levels. Metabolism 1986;35:1147.
6. Agudelo CA, Wise CM. Crystal-associated arthritis in the elderly. Rheum Dis Clin North Am 2000;26:527.
7. Hall AP et al. Epidemiology of gout and hyperuricemia. A long-term population study. Am J Med 1967;42:27.
8. Abbott RD et al. Gout and coronary heart disease: the Framingham study. J Clin Epidemiol 1988;41:237.
9. Freedman DS et al. Relation of serum uric acid to mortality and ischemic heart disease. The NHANES I epidemiology follow-up study. Am J Epidemiol 1995;141:637.
10. Roubenoff R. Gout and hyperuricemia. Rheum Dis Clin North Am 1990;16:539.
11. Batuman V et al. The role of lead in gout nephropathy. N Engl J Med 1981;304:520.
12. Hermann G, Bloch C. Gout. In: Taveras JM, ed. Radiology: Diagnosis, Imaging, Intervention. Philadelphia: JB Lippincott, 1994:1.
13. Hadler NM et al. Acute polyarticular gout. Am J Med 1974;56:715.
14. Baraf HSB et al. Gouty arthritis: prevalence of chronic synovitis, polyarticular attacks, and positive serological tests for rheumatoid factor. Arthritis Rheum 1978;21:544.
15. Lawry GV et al. Polyarticular versus monoarticular gout: a prospective, comparative analysis of clinical features. Medicine (Baltimore) 1988;67:335.
16. Rosenthal L, Hawkins D. Radionuclide joint imaging in the diagnosis of synovial disease. Semin Arthritis Rheum 1977;7:49.
17. Simkin, PA. Gout and hyperuricemia. Curr Opin Rheum 1997;9:268.
18. Simkin PA. The pathogenesis of podagra. Ann Intern Med 1977;86:230.
19. Simkin PA, Pizzorno JE. Trans-synovial exchange of small molecules in normal human subjects. J Appl Physiol 1974;36:581.
20. Simkin PA. Synovial permeability in rheumatoid arthritis. Arthritis Rheum 1979;22:689.
21. Cardenosa G, Deluca SA. Radiographic features of gout. Am Fam Physician 1990;4:539.
22. Fessel WJ. Distinguishing gout from other types of arthritis. Postgrad Med 1978;63:134.
23. McCarty DJ, Hollander JL. Identification of urate crystals in gouty synovial fluid. Ann Intern Med 1961;54:452.
24. Wallace SL et al. Preliminary criteria for the classification of the acute arthritis of primary gout. Arthritis Rheum 1977;20:895.
25. Becker MA. Clinical aspects of monosodium urate monohydrate crystal deposition disease (gout). Rheum Dis Clin North Am 1988;14:377.
26. Honig S et al. Crystal deposition disease. Diagnosis by electron microscopy. Am J Med 1977;63:161.

27. Schumacher HR et al. Acute gouty arthritis without urate crystals identified on initial examination of synovial fluid: report on nine patients. Arthritis Rheum 1975;18:603.
28. Abeles M, Urman JD. Acute gouty arthritis. The diagnostic importance of aspirating more than one involved joint. JAMA 1977;238:2526.
29. Romanoff NR et al. Gout without crystals on initial synovial fluid analysis. Postgrad Med J 1978;54:95.
30. Bomalaski JS et al. Monosodium urate crystals in the knee joints of patients with asymptomatic nontophaceous gout. Arthritis Rheum 1986;29:1480.
31. Agudelo CA et al. Definitive diagnosis of gout by identification of urate crystals in asymptomatic metatarsophalangeal joints. Arthritis Rheum 1979;22:559.
32. Weinberger A et al. Urate crystals in asymptomatic metatarsophalangeal joints. Ann Intern Med 1979;91:56.
33. Wolfe F. Gout and hyperuricemia. Am Fam Physician 1991;43:2141.
34. Wolfe F, Cathey MA. The misdiagnosis of gout and hyperuricemia. J Rheumatol 1991;18:1232.
35. Reginato AJ. Gout and other crystal arthropathies. In: Braunwald E et al., eds. Harrison's Principles of Internal Medicine, 15th ed. New York: McGraw-Hill, 2001:1994
36. Finch W. Acute crystal-induced arthritis. Gout and a whole lot more. Postgrad Med 1989;85:273.
37. Simkin PA. Articular oxalate crystals and the taxonomy of gout [editorial]. JAMA 1988;260:1285.
38. Rozenberg S et al. Diversity of opinions on the management of gout in France. A survey of 750 rheumatologists. Rev Rhum (Engl Ed) 1996;63:255.
39. Sturge RA et al. Multicentre trial of naproxen and phenylbutazone in acute gout. Ann Rheum Dis 1977;36:80.
40. Willkens RF et al. The treatment of acute gout with naproxen. J Clin Pharmacol 1975;15:363.
41. Franck WA, Brown MM. Ibuprofen in acute polyarticular gout. Arthritis Rheum 1976;19:269.
42. Schweitz MC et al. Ibuprofen in the treatment of acute gouty arthritis. JAMA 1978;239:34.
43. Wanasukapunt S et al. Effect of fenoprofen calcium on acute gout arthritis. Arthritis Rheum 1976;19:933.
44. Weiner GI et al. Double-blind study of fenoprofen versus phenylbutazone in acute gouty arthritis. Arthritis Rheum 1979;22:425.
45. Widmark PH. Piroxicam: its safety and efficacy in the treatment of acute gout. Am J Med 1982;72(2A):63.
46. Bluestone RH. Safety and efficacy of piroxicam in the treatment of gout. Am J Med 1982;72(2A):66.
47. Lomen PL, et al. Flurbiprofen in the treatment of acute gout. A comparison with indomethacin. Am J Med 1986; 80(Suppl. 3A):134.
48. Tamisier JN. Ketoprofen. Clin Rheum Dis 1979;5:381.
49. Petera P et al. Treatment of acute gout attacks with tolmetin. Wien Med Wochenschr 1982;132:43.
50. Eberl R, Dunky A. Meclofenamate sodium in the treatment of acute gout. Results of a double-blind study. Arzneimittelforschung 1983;33:641.
51. Karachalios GN, Donas G. Sulindac in the treatment of acute gout arthritis. Int J Tiss Reac 1982;4:297.
52. Schumacher HR et al. Randomised double blind trial of etoricoxib and indomethacin in treatment of acute gouty arthritis. Br Med J 2002;324:1488.

53. Groff GD et al. Systemic steroid therapy for acute gout: a clinical trial and review of the literature. Semin Arthritis Rheum 1990;19:329.
54. Axelrod D, Preston S. Comparison of parenteral adrenocorticotropic hormone with oral indomethacin in the treatment of acute gout. Arthritis Rheum 1988;31:803.
55. Patak RV et al. Antagonism of the effects of furosemide by indomethacin in normal and hypertensive man. Prostaglandins 1975;10:649.
56. Frolich JC et al. Suppression of plasma renin activity by indomethacin in man. Circ Res 1976;39:447.
57. Smith DE et al. Attenuation of furosemide's diuretic effect by indomethacin: pharmacokinetic evaluation. J Pharmacokinet Biopharm 1979;7:265.
58. Brater DC. Analysis of the effect of indomethacin on the response to furosemide in man: effect of dose of furosemide. J Pharmacol Exp Ther 1979;210:386.
59. Durao V et al. Modification of antihypertensive effect of beta-adrenoceptor-blocking agents by inhibition of endogenous prostaglandin synthesis. Lancet 1977;2:1005.
60. Hansten PD, Horn JR. Drug Interactions & Updates Quarterly. St Louis, MO: Facts and Comparisons, 2000.
61. Findling JW et al. Indomethacin-induced hyperkalemia in three patients with gouty arthritis. JAMA 1980;244:1127.
62. Roberts WN et al. Colchicine in acute gout. Reassessment of risks and benefits. JAMA 1987;257:1920.
63. Grahame R, Scott JT. Clinical survey of 354 patients with gout. Ann Rheum Dis 1970;29:461.
64. Demartini FE. Hyperuricemia induced by drugs. Arthritis Rheum 1965;8:823.
65. Steele TH, Oppenheimer S. Factors affecting urate excretion following diuretic administration in man. Am J Med 1969;47:564.
66. Manuel MA, Steele TH. Changes in renal urate handling after prolonged thiazide treatment. Am J Med 1974;57:741.
67. Wyngaarden JB. Diuretics and hyperuricemia [letter]. N Engl J Med 1970;283:1170.
68. Scopelitis E, McGrath H Jr. NSAID-masked gout. South Med J 1987;80:1464.
69. Alloway JA et al. Comparison of triamcinolone acetonide with indomethacin in the treatment of gouty arthritis. J Rheumatol 1993;20:111.
70. Wallace SL et al. Diagnostic value of the colchicine therapeutic trial. JAMA 1967;199:93.
71. Dinarello CA et al. Colchicine therapy for familial Mediterranean fever. N Engl J Med 1974;291:934.
72. Zemer D et al. A controlled trial of colchicine in preventing attacks of familial Mediterranean fever. N Engl J Med 1974;291:932.
73. Rubinow A, Sonnenblick M. Amyloidosis secondary to polyarticular gout. Arthritis Rheum 1981;24:1425.
74. Werlen D et al. Corticosteroid therapy for the treatment of acute attacks of crystal-induced arthritis: an effective alternative to nonsteroidal antiinflammatory drugs. Rev Rhum (Engl Ed) 1996;63:248.
75. Shrestha M et al. Randomized double-blind comparison of the analgesic efficacy of intramuscular ketorolac and oral indomethacin in the treatment of acute gouty arthritis. Ann Emerg Med 1995;26:682.
76. Putterman C et al. Colchicine intoxication: clinical pharmacology, risk factors, features and management. Semin Arthritis Rheum 1991;21:143.

77. Bonnel RA et al. Deaths associated with inappropriate intravenous colchicine administration. J Emerg Med 2002;22:385.

78. Liu YK et al. Marrow aplasia induced by colchicine: a case report. Arthritis Rheum 1978; 21:731.

79. Insel PA. Analgesics-antipyretic and anti-inflammatory agents and drugs employed in the treatment of gout. In: Gilman AG et al., eds. The Pharmacological Basis of Therapeutics, 10th ed. New York: McGraw-Hill, 2001:687.

80. Naidus RM et al. Colchicine toxicity: A multisystem disease. Arch Intern Med 1977;137:394.

81. Merlin HE. Azoospermia caused by colchicine: a case report. Fertil Steril 1972;23:180.

82. Bremner WJ, Paulsen CA. Colchicine and testicular function in man. N Engl J Med 1976;294:1384.

83. DuPont P et al. Colchicine myoneuropathy in a renal transplant patient. Transplant Intl 2002; 15:374.

84. Simkin PA et al. Uric acid excretion: quantitative assessment from spot, midmorning serum and urine samples. Ann Intern Med 1979;91:44.

85. Wortmann RL, Fox IH. Limited value of uric acid to creatinine ratios in estimating uric acid excretion. Ann Intern Med 1980;93:822.

86. Turner WJ, Merlis S. Vicissitudes in research: the twenty-four hour urine collection. Clin Pharmacol Ther 1971;12:163.

87. Rundles RW et al. Allopurinol in the treatment of gout. Ann Intern Med 1966;64:229.

88. Yu TF, Gutman AB. Effect of allopurinol [4-hydroxypyrazolo-(3,4-d)pyrimidine] on serum and urinary uric acid in primary and secondary gout. Am J Med 1964;37:885.

89. Cameron JS, Simmonds HA. Use and abuse of allopurinol. Br Med J (Clin Res) 1987;294:1504.

90. Hande K et al. Allopurinol kinetics. Clin Pharmacol Ther 1978;23:598.

91. Elion GB. Enzymatic and metabolic studies with allopurinol. Ann Rheum Dis 1966;25:608.

92. Elion GB et al. Renal clearance of oxipurinol, the chief metabolite of allopurinol. Am J Med 1968;45:69.

93. Berlinger WG et al. The effect of dietary protein on the clearance of allopurinol and oxypurinol. N Engl J Med 1985;313:771.

94. Rundles RW. The development of allopurinol. Arch Intern Med 1985;145:1492.

95. Rodnan GP et al. Allopurinol and gouty hyperuricemia. Efficacy of a single daily dose. JAMA 1975;231:1143.

96. Boston Collaborative Drug Surveillance Program. Excess of ampicillin rashes associated with allopurinol or hyperuricemia. N Engl J Med 1972;286:505.

97. Cummins D et al. Myelosuppression associated with azathioprine–allopurinol interaction after heart and lung transplantation. Transplantation 1996;61:1661.

98. Fraunfelder FT, Lerman S. Allopurinol and cataracts [letter]. Am J Ophthalmol 1985;99:215.

99. Jick H, Brandt DE. Allopurinol and cataracts. Am J Ophthalmol 1984;98:355.

100. Clair WK et al. Allopurinol use and the risk of cataract formation. Br J Ophthalmol 1989;73:173.

101. Kantor GL. Toxic epidermal necrolysis, azotemia, and death after allopurinol therapy. JAMA 1970;212:478.

102. Mills RM. Severe hypersensitivity reactions associated with allopurinol. JAMA 1971;216:799.

103. Young JL Jr et al. Severe allopurinol hypersensitivity. Association with thiazides and prior renal compromise. Arch Intern Med 1974;134:553.

104. Boyer TD et al. Allopurinol-hypersensitivity vasculitis and liver damage. West J Med 1977; 126:143.

105. Al-Kawas FH et al. Allopurinol hepatotoxicity. Report of two cases and review of the literature. Ann Intern Med 1981;95:588.

106. Lang PG Jr. Severe hypersensitivity reactions to allopurinol. South Med J 1979;72:1361.

107. Hande KR et al. Severe allopurinol toxicity. Description and guidelines for prevention in patients with renal insufficiency. Am J Med 1984;76:47.

108. Singer JZ, Wallace SL. The allopurinol hypersensitivity syndrome. Unnecessary morbidity and mortality. Arthritis Rheum 1986;29:82.

109. Rundles RW. Metabolic effects of allopurinol and alloxanthine. Ann Rheum Dis 1966;25:615.

110. Tam S, Carroll W. Allopurinol hepatotoxicity. Am J Med 1989;86:357.

111. Jarzobski J et al. Vasculitis with allopurinol therapy. Am Heart J 1970;79:116.

112. Arellano F, Sacristan JA. Allopurinol hypersensitivity syndrome: a review. DICP, Ann Pharmacother 1993;27:337.

113. Fam AG. Difficult gout and new approaches for control of hyperuricemia in the allopurinol-allergic patient. Curr Rheumatol Rep 2001;3:29.

114. Goldman SC et al. A randomized comparison between rasburicase and allopurinol in children with lymphoma or leukemia at high risk for tumor lysis. Blood 2001;97:2998.

115. Pui CH et al. Recombinant urate oxidase for the prophylaxis or treatment of hyperuricemia in patients with leukemia or lymphoma. J Clin Oncol 2001;19:697.

116. Sanofi-Synthelabo Inc. Elitek package insert. New York: July 2002.

117. Anon. Rasburicase (Elitek) for hyperuricemia. Med Lett Drugs Ther 2002;44:96.

118. Rasburicase (Elitek) for hyperuricemia (Erratum). Med Lett Drugs Ther 2002;44:106.

119. Neuss MN et al. Long-term colchicine administration leading to colchicine toxicity and death. Arthritis Rheum 1986;29:448.

120. Diamond HS. Control of crystal-induced arthropathies. Rheum Dis Clin North Am 1989; 15:557.

121. Yu TF. The efficacy of colchicine prophylaxis in articular gout: a reappraisal after 20 years. Semin Arthritis Rheum 1982;12:256.

122. Wallace SL et al. Renal function predicts colchicine toxicity: guidelines for the prophylactic use of colchicine in gout. J Rheumatol 1991; 18:264.

123. Yu TF et al. Mutual suppression of the uricosuric effects of sulfinpyrazone and salicylate: a study in interactions between drugs. J Clin Invest 1963;42:1330.

124. Smyth CJ. Disorders associated with hyperuricemia. Arthritis Rheum 1975;18(Suppl. 6):713.

125. Liang MH, Fries JF. Asymptomatic hyperuricemia: the case for conservative management. Ann Intern Med 1978;88:666.

126. Berger L, Yu TF. Renal function in gout. IV. An analysis of 524 gouty subjects including long-term follow-up studies. Am J Med 1975;59:605.

127. Reif MC et al. Chronic gouty nephropathy: a vanishing syndrome? [editorial] N Engl J Med 1981;304:535.

128. Yu TF et al. Renal function in gout. V. Factors influencing the renal hemodynamics. Am J Med 1979;67:766.

129. Yu TF, Berger L. Impaired renal function in gout: its association with hypertensive vascular disease and intrinsic renal disease. Am J Med 1982;72:95.

130. Fessel WJ et al. Correlates and consequences of asymptomatic hyperuricemia. Arch Intern Med 1973;132:44.

131. Kjellstrand CM et al. Hyperuricemic acute renal failure. Arch Intern Med 1974;133:349.

132. Steele TH. Renal excretion of uric acid. Arthritis Rheum 1975;18(Suppl. 6):793.

133. Campion DS et al. Binding of urate by serum proteins. Arthritis Rheum 1975;18(Suppl. 6):747.

134. Abdelrahman M et al. Hyperuricemia and gout in renal transplant recipients. Ren Fail 2002;24:361.

135. Kahl LE et al. Gout in the heart transplant recipient: physiologic puzzle and therapeutic challenge. Am J Med 1989;87:289.

136. Neal DAJ et al. Hyperuricemia, gout, and renal function after liver transplantation. Transplantation 2001;10:1689.

137. Lin HY et al. Cyclosporine-induced hyperuricemia and gout. N Engl J Med 1989;321:287.

138. Myers BD et al. Cyclosporine-associated chronic nephropathy. N Engl J Med 1984;311:699.

139. Tomlanovich S et al. Limitations of creatinine in quantifying the severity of cyclosporine-induced chronic nephropathy. Am J Kidney Dis 1986;8:332.

140. Ross EA et al. The plasma creatinine concentration is not an accurate reflection of the glomerular filtration rate in stable renal transplant patients receiving cyclosporine. Am J Kidney Dis 1987; 10:113.

141. Noordzij TC et al. Cyclosporine-induced hyperuricemia and gout [letter]. N Engl J Med 1990;322:334.

142. Durrant S et al. Cyclosporin A, methylprednisolone, and convulsions [letter]. Lancet 1982; 2:829.

143. Boogaerts MA et al. Cyclosporin, methylprednisolone, and convulsions [letter]. Lancet 1982; 2:1216.

144. Ost L. Effects of cyclosporin on prednisolone metabolism [letter]. Lancet 1984;1:451.

145. Klintmalm G, Sawe J. High-dose methylprednisolone increases plasma cyclosporin levels in renal transplant recipients [letter]. Lancet 1984; 1:731.

146. Burack DA et al. Hyperuricemia and gout among heart transplant recipients receiving cyclosporine. Am J Med 1992;92:141.

147. Stevens SL, Goldman MH. Cyclosporine toxicity associated with allopurinol [letter]. South Med J 1992;85:1265.

148. Manfredi RL, Vesell ES. Inhibition of theophylline metabolism by long-term allopurinol administration. Clin Pharmacol Ther 1981;29:224.

149. Grygiel JJ et al. Effects of allopurinol on theophylline metabolism and clearance. Clin Pharmacol Ther 1979;26:660.

150. Merck & Co, Inc. Prinivil package insert. West Point, PA: Jan. 2002.

151. Walter U et al. Dose-response relation of the angiotensin converting enzyme inhibitor ramipril in mild to moderate essential hypertension. Am J Cardiol 1987;59:125D.

152. Bevan EG et al. Effect of renal function on the pharmacokinetics and pharmacodynamics of trandolapril. Br J Clin Pharmacol 1993;35:128.

153. Minghelli G et al. Uricosuric effect of the angiotensin II receptor antagonist losartan in heart transplant recipients. Transplantation 1998; 66:268.

154. Wurzner G et al. Comparative effects of losartan and irbesartan on serum uric acid in hypertensive patients with hyperuricemia and gout. J Hypertens 2001;19:1855.

155. Ilson BE et al. The effects of eprosartan, an angiotensin II AT$_1$ receptor antagonist, on uric acid excretion in patients with mild to moderate essential hypertension. J Clin Pharmacol 1998;38:437.

156. AstraZeneca Pharmaceuticals LP. Atacand package insert. Wilmington, DE: Sept. 2001.

157. Chiron Corporation. Proleukin package insert. Emeryville, CA: Sept. 2000.

158. Merck & Co., Inc. Elspar package insert. West Point, PA: Aug. 2000.

159. GlaxoSmithKline. Myleran package insert. Research Triangle Park, NC: May 2002.

160. Bristol-Myers Squibb Company. Paraplatin package insert. Princeton, NJ: June 2001.

161. GlaxoSmithKline. Leukeran package insert. Research Triangle Park, NC: Aug. 2001.

162. Bristol-Myers Squibb Company. Platinol-AQ package insert. Princeton, NJ: Oct. 1999.

163. Bristol-Myers Squibb Company. Cytoxan package insert. Princeton, NJ: July 2000.

164. Bedford Laboratories. Cytarabine package insert. Bedford, OH: Aug. 2000.

165. Bedford Laboratories. Daunorubicin package insert. Bedford, OH: July 1999.

166. Berlex Laboratories. Fludara package insert. Richmond, CA: Dec. 2001.

167. Bristol-Myers Squibb Company. Hydrea package insert. Princeton, NJ: March 2001.

168. Merck & Co., Inc. Mustargen package insert. West Point, PA: March 1999.

169. GlaxoSmithKline. Alkeran package insert. Research Triangle Park, NC: Nov. 2001.

170. GlaxoSmithKline. Purinethol package insert. Research Triangle Park, NC: Nov. 2002.

171. GlaxoSmithKline. Tabloid brand thioguanine package insert. Research Triangle Park, NC: Feb. 2002.

172. Bedford Laboratories. Vinblastine package insert. Bedford, OH: Dec. 2001.

173. Faulding Pharmaceutical Company. Vincristine package insert. Paramus, NJ: Sept. 2002.

174. Laine J, Holmberg C. Mechanisms of hyperuricemia in cyclosporine-treated renal transplanted children. Nephron 1996;74:318.

175. Zurcher RM et al. Hyperuricaemia in cyclosporin-treated patients: GFR-related effect. Nephrol Dial Transplant 1996;11:153.

176. Wegienka LC et al. Clinical experience with diazoxide. Ann NY Acad Sci 1968;150:383.

177. Yarchoan R et al. Long-term toxicity/activity profile of 2′,3′-dideoxyinosine in AIDS or AIDS-related complex. Lancet 1990;336:526.

178. Cooley TP et al. Once-daily administration of 2′,3′-dideoxyinosine (ddI) in patients with acquired immunodeficiency syndrome or AIDS-related complex. Results of phase I trial. N Engl J Med 1990;322:1340.

179. Hopkinson N, Doherty M. In patients with chronic cardiac failure who have diuretic induced gout, are certain diuretics less prone at causing problems? Br J Rheum 1991;30:225.

180. Waller PC, Ramsay LE. Predicting acute gout in diuretic-treated hypertensive patients. J Human Hyperten 1989;3:457.

181. Friedel HA, Buckley MMT. Torasemide: a review of pharmacological properties and therapeutic potential. Drugs 1991;41:81.

182. Achimastos A et al. The effects of the addition of micronised fenofibrate on uric acid metabolism in patients receiving indapamide. Cur Med Res Opin 2002;18:59.

183. Curry CL et al. Clinical studies of a new, low-dose formulation of metolazone for the treatment of hypertension. Clin Ther 1986;9:47.

184. Khanna BK et al. Ethambutol-induced hyperuricaemia. Tubercle 1984;65:195.

185. Nishimura T et al. Influence of daily drinking habits on ethanol-induced hyperuricemia. Metabolism 1994;43:745.

186. Morstyn G et al. Effect of granulocyte colony stimulating factor on neutropenia induced by cytotoxic chemotherapy. Lancet 1988;1:667.

187. Mayes PA. Intermediary metabolism of fructose. Am J Clin Nutr 1993;58(Suppl. 5):754S.

188. Loguercio C et al. Intravenous load of fructose and fructose 1,6-diphosphate: effects on uricemia in patients with nonalcoholic liver disease. Am J Gastroenterol 1996;91:559.

189. Vachvanichsanong P et al. Severe hyperphosphatemia following acute tumor lysis syndrome. Med Pediatr Oncol 1995;24:63.

190. Mawson AR. Hypervitaminosis A toxicity and gout. Lancet 1984;1:1181.

191. Bierer DW, Quebbemann AJ. Effect of L-dopa on renal handling of uric acid. J Pharmacol Exp Ther 1982;223:55.

192. Knodel LC, Talbert RL. Adverse effects of hypolipidaemic drugs. Med Toxicol 1987;2:10.

193. Stapleton FB et al. Hyperuricosuria due to high-dose pancreatic extract therapy in cystic fibrosis. N Engl J Med 1976;295:246.

194. Sanchez-Albisua I et al. Tolerance of pyrazinamide in short-course chemotherapy for pulmonary tuberculosis in children. Pediatr Infect Dis J 1997;16:760.

195. Fontana RJ. Uric acid nephrolithiasis associated with interferon and ribavirin treatment of hepatitis C. Dig Dis Sci 2001;46:920.

196. Pilmore HL et al. Tacrolimus for treatment of gout in renal transplantation: two case reports and review of the literature. Transplantation 2001; 72:1703.

197. Yamamoto T et al. Theophylline-induced increase in plasma uric acid–purine catabolism increased by theophylline. Int J Clin Pharmacol Ther Toxicol 1991;29:257.

198. Shimizu T et al. Effect of theophylline on serum uric acid levels in children with asthma. J Asthma 1994;31:387.

CHAPTER 43

Rheumatic Disorders

Steven W. Chen, William C. Gong

RHEUMATOID ARTHRITIS

Epidemiology

The term *arthritis* refers to more than 100 diseases causing pain, swelling, and damage to joints and connective tissue.[1] Approximately 43 million (i.e., 1 in 6) Americans suffer from a form of arthritis, making it the most common chronic condition in persons older than 15 years of age.[2] Consequently, arthritic conditions are the single leading cause of disability in the United States.

Rheumatoid arthritis (RA) is a chronic systemic inflammatory disorder characterized by potentially deforming polyarthritis and a wide spectrum of extra-articular manifesta-

tions. Because no single chemical or laboratory finding is specific for this disease, the diagnosis of RA is primarily based on clinical criteria (Table 43-1).[3] The prevalence of RA is estimated to be 1% worldwide.[4] RA afflicts approximately 2.1 million individuals in the United States, with 1.5 million being women (RA is two to three times more common in females than in males). The onset of RA typically occurs between the third and fourth decades of life, and prevalence increases with advancing age up to the seventh decade.[1,4]

The cause of RA appears to be an interplay among multiple factors, including genetic susceptibility, environmental influences, and the effects of advancing age on somatic changes in the musculoskeletal and immune systems.[4] Support for the

Table 43-1   Criteria for Diagnosis of RA

Morning stiffness in and around joints lasting at least 1 hr before maximal involvement[a]

Soft-tissue swelling (arthritis) of three or more joint areas observed by a physician[a]

Swelling (arthritis) of the proximal interphalangeal, metacarpophalangeal, or wrist joints[a]

Symmetric arthritis[a]

Subcutaneous nodules

Positive test for RF

Radiographic erosions or periarticular osteopenia in hand or wrist joints

---

[a]Criteria 1 to 4 must be present for at least 6 weeks; 4 or more criteria must be present.
RA, rheumatoid arthritis; RF, rheumatoid factor.
Adapted from reference 3.

Table 43-2   Criteria for Complete Clinical Remission in RA

A minimum of five of the following requirements must be fulfilled for at least 2 consecutive months in a patient with RA[a]:

1. Morning stiffness not >15 minutes
2. No fatigue
3. No joint pain
4. No joint tenderness or pain on motion
5. No soft-tissue swelling in joints or tendon sheaths
6. ESR (Westergren's) <30 mm/hr (females) or 20 mm/hr (males)

---

[a]Exclusions: Manifestations of active vasculitis, pericarditis, pleuritis, myositis, or unexplained recent weight loss or fever secondary to RA prohibit designation of complete clinical remission.
ESR, erythrocyte sedimentation rate; RA, rheumatoid arthritis.
Adapted from reference 9.

concept of genetically controlled susceptibility comes from studies demonstrating an association between RA and class II gene products of the major histocompatibility complex. Although epidemiologic associations have not been clearly established, smoking may increase the production of rheumatoid factor (RF), which often precedes the clinical presentation of RA.[5] In a case–control study of 2,625 men and women (1,095 with RA, 1,530 healthy adults), a history of smoking increased risk for RA in men, but not in women.[6] A possible explanation for this gender-dependent difference is that female hormones may interfere with smoking-induced RF production and subsequent RA development.

The course of RA is variable.[7] Approximately one-third of patients initially experience mild intermittent symptoms that resolve over the course of several weeks to months. The patient may be symptom-free for several weeks to months and then experience symptoms that may be more severe than those experienced initially. Another group of patients experiences a rather sudden onset of symptoms followed by a prolonged clinical remission of disease activity, although this is relatively uncommon. The third and most common pattern of RA onset involves progressive uninterrupted disease that ultimately results in characteristic disabling joint deformities. The disease usually evolves over the course of a few months, but the rate of disease progression in this group may be rapid or slow. Patients within this group may be divided further into a subgroup that responds to "aggressive" therapy and a subgroup that does not. Patients with more aggressive disease (multiple joint involvement, positive RF) have a >70% probability of developing damage or erosions to joints within 2 years of disease onset.[8]

Before the increased use of medications capable of halting or slowing disease progression, the rate of RA disease remission was low. The development and application of standardized criteria of remission (Table 43-2)[9] in a cross-sectional evaluation of rheumatology clinic patients revealed a remission rate of about 1%.[10] Over 2.5 years in another clinic, 18% of patients were in remission at some time, including slightly >10% of patients not receiving disease-modifying (or second-line) drugs.[11] However, remissions were temporary, with <4% experiencing a remission lasting up to 2 years and only 1.2% experiencing a remission lasting up to 3 years. More recent

studies using disease-modifying drugs early in the course of RA have yielded remission rates from between 16% and 31% at 2 years with monotherapy to 37% at more than 6 years with combination drug therapy.[12–15]

In contrast to older studies, which suggested an increased mortality rate associated with RA, more recent evaluations of survival in RA patients indicate that life span is probably no different than the general population during the first 10 years of the disease.[16,17] The more aggressive use of disease-modifying drugs over the past two decades perhaps is a major contributor to this outcome. This does not, however, rule out the possibility of premature death beyond the first decade of RA.

Pathophysiology

RA-induced joint destruction begins with inflammation of the synovial lining.[18] This normally thin membrane surrounding the joint space continues to proliferate and transforms into the synovial pannus. The pannus, a highly erosive enzyme-laden inflammatory exudate, invades articular cartilage, leading to narrowing of joint spaces, erosion of bone resulting in osteoporosis, and destruction of periarticular structures (ligaments, tendons) resulting in joint deformities (Fig. 43-1).

Familiarity with basic cellular processes involved in tissue destruction and sustained inflammation in rheumatoid synovium is critical to understanding pharmacologic therapies for RA.[19] Under normal circumstances, the body can distinguish between self (proteins found within the body) and nonself (foreign substances such as bacteria and viruses). On occasion, immune cells (T or B lymphocytes) may react to a self-protein while developing in the thymus or bone marrow. These developing cells are usually killed or inactivated; however, a self-targeted immune cell can escape destruction and become activated years later, initiating an autoimmune response. Some believe the source of activation is bacteria (possibly streptococcus) or a virus containing a protein with an amino acid sequence similar to tissue protein. When this activation source reaches the joint, complex cell-to-cell interactions take place leading to RA pathology.

The initiating interaction takes place between antigen-presenting cells (APC) displaying complexes of class II major histocompatibility complex (MHC) molecules and CD4-

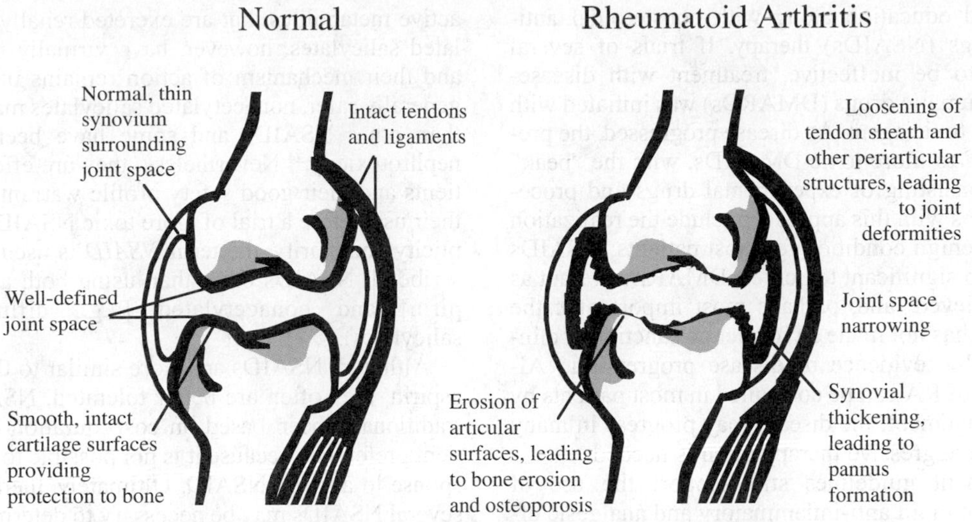

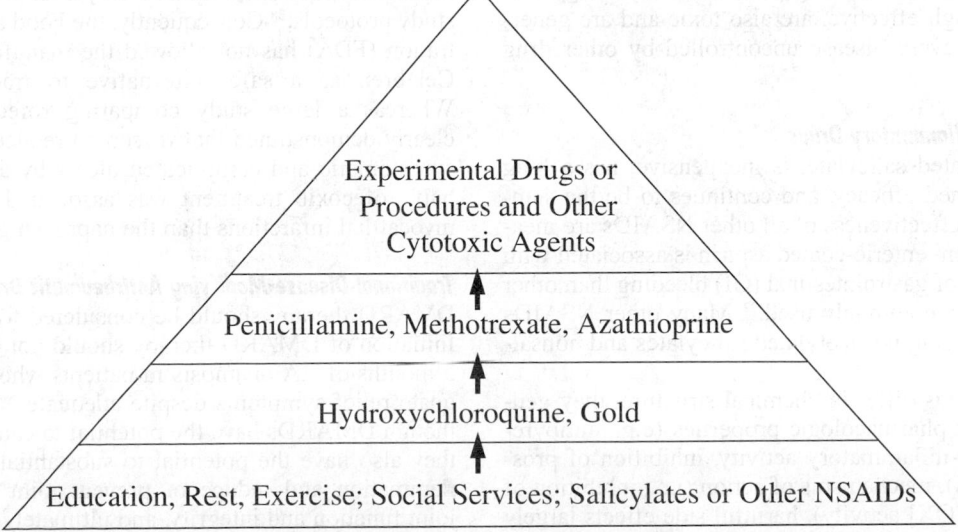

Normal   Rheumatoid Arthritis

Normal, thin synovium surrounding joint space

Intact tendons and ligaments

Loosening of tendon sheath and other periarticular structures, leading to joint deformities

Well-defined joint space

Joint space narrowing

Smooth, intact cartilage surfaces providing protection to bone

Erosion of articular surfaces, leading to bone erosion and osteoporosis

Synovial thickening, leading to pannus formation

FIGURE 43-1. Overview of joint changes in rheumatoid arthritis.

lineage T-cell lymphocytes. (Alternatively, B cells may become activated leading to antibody formation and ultimately to accumulation of polymorphonuclear leukocytes, which release cytotoxins and other substances destructive to the synovium and joint structures. T-cell activity, however, appears to be predominant in RA.) The binding together of these cells results in T-cell differentiation and the activation of macrophages with secretion of cytotoxins and cytokines. Cytotoxins can lead directly to cell and tissue destruction, while cytokines are polypeptides that serve as important mediators of inflammation. Proinflammatory cytokines such as interleukin-1 (IL-1) and tumor necrosis factor (TNF)-α stimulate synovial fibroblasts and chondrocytes in neighboring articular cartilage to secrete enzymes that lead to tissue destruction by degrading proteoglycans and collagen. In healthy individuals, the inflammatory process is regulated by balancing the ratios of proinflammatory cytokines such as IL-1 and TNF-α with anti-inflammatory cytokines such as IL-1 receptor antagonist (IL-1Ra), IL-10, IL-4, and IL-11. In the synovium of RA patients, however, this balance is heavily weighted toward the proinflammatory cytokines, leading to sustained inflammation and tissue destruction.[20]

Treatment

The treatment of RA involves a combination of interventions including rest, exercise (physical therapy), emotional support, occupational therapy, and drugs.[8] Specific treatment is individualized based on such factors as joint function, degree of disease activity, patient age, gender, occupation, family responsibilities, drug costs, and results of previous therapy. The ultimate goal of RA treatment is disease remission; however, if remission is not achieved, the goals include control of disease activity, pain relief, maintenance of activities of daily living, maximization of quality of life, and slowing of joint damage.

The old standard for treatment of RA, known as the "pyramid approach," was based on the assumption that RA is a slowly progressing, benign disease that is not life-threatening (Fig. 43-2).[21] Based on the pyramid approach, the initial treatment for any RA patient was to prescribe a basic program of

Experimental Drugs or Procedures and Other Cytotoxic Agents

↑

Penicillamine, Methotrexate, Azathioprine

↑

Hydroxychloroquine, Gold

↑

Education, Rest, Exercise; Social Services; Salicylates or Other NSAIDs

FIGURE 43-2. Traditional pyramid approach for treatment of rheumatoid arthritis. ↑ indicates worsening disease.

rest, exercise, and education along with nonsteroidal anti-inflammatory drugs (NSAIDs) therapy. If trials of several NSAIDs proved to be ineffective, treatment with disease-modifying antirheumatic drugs (DMARDs) was initiated with the relatively least toxic agent. As disease progressed, the prescriber "ascended" to more toxic DMARDs, with the "peak" of the pyramid consisting of experimental drugs and procedures. The problems with this approach include the realization that RA is not a benign condition for most patients; NSAIDs are associated with significant toxicities; DMARDs are not as toxic as once believed; and, perhaps most importantly, the pyramid approach has not made an impact on functional, clinical, or radiographic evidence of disease progression.[8] Although symptoms of RA can be controlled in most patients by conservative management, the disease may progress in many patients, and more aggressive therapy often is needed.

Current treatment guidelines still support the use of NSAIDs to provide rapid anti-inflammatory and analgesic effects.[8] However, since NSAIDs do not prevent or slow joint destruction, DMARD therapy should be initiated within the first 3 months of RA diagnosis. Traditional DMARDs (i.e., hydroxychloroquine [HCQ], sulfasalazine [SSZ], methotrexate [MTX], leflunomide [LEF], gold, azathioprine [AZA], or D-penicillamine [DPEN]) have the potential to slow disease progression. These agents, alone or in combination, should be considered as initial therapy for most RA patients. The newest class of DMARDs, biological agents (also referred to as anticytokines, biologicals, biological modifiers, or biological response modifiers), include etanercept [Enbrel], infliximab [Remicade], anakinra [Kineret], and adalimumab [Humira]. These agents target the physiologic proinflammatory and joint-damaging effects of TNF-α or IL-1. Due to high cost, biological agents should generally be reserved for RA patients who either fail to respond to, or are unable to tolerate, one or more traditional DMARDs, particularly methotrexate.[22] Glucocorticoids are potent anti-inflammatory agents that appear to slow the progression of joint damage in RA; however, they are generally reserved for brief periods of active disease (low-dose oral therapy) or for isolated joints experiencing disease flares (local intra-articular injection) because of harmful adverse effects associated with long-term use. Alkylating cytotoxic drugs, although effective, are also toxic and are generally reserved for severe disease uncontrolled by other drug therapies.

Nonsteroidal Anti-Inflammatory Drugs

Aspirin, an acetylated salicylate, is inexpensive, has a long history of established efficacy, and continues to be the standard by which the effectiveness of all other NSAIDs are measured. However, non–enteric-coated aspirin is associated with a higher incidence of gastrointestinal (GI) bleeding than other NSAIDs and is not commonly used.[23] Many other NSAIDs are available, including nonacetylated salicylates and nonsalicylate NSAIDs.

Although NSAIDs differ in chemical structure, they generally have similar pharmacologic properties (e.g., antipyresis, analgesia, anti-inflammatory activity, inhibition of prostaglandin synthesis), mechanisms of action (i.e., inhibition of cyclooxygenase [COX] activity), harmful side effects largely attributable to COX inhibition (e.g., GI intolerance, nephrotoxicity, risk of bleeding), and pharmacokinetic properties (e.g., highly protein bound and extensively metabolized to in-

active metabolites that are excreted renally).[23] The nonacetylated salicylates, however, have virtually no effect on COX and their mechanism of action remains unknown. Although generally safer, nonacetylated salicylates may be less effective than other NSAIDs and some have been associated with nephrotoxicity.[24] Nevertheless, they are effective in some patients and their good safety profile warrants consideration of their use before a trial of more toxic NSAIDs. (Note: For simplicity and clarity, the term *NSAID* is used henceforth to describe all NSAIDs other than using both acetylated [i.e., aspirin] and nonacetylated [e.g., diflunisal, salsalate] salicylates).

Although NSAIDs are more similar to than different from aspirin, they often are better tolerated. NSAID selection has traditionally been based on cost, duration of action, and patient preference because it is not possible to predict patient response to a given NSAID. Ultimately, therapeutic trials with several NSAIDs may be necessary to determine the best agent for a given patient because individual patients may respond to or tolerate one NSAID better than another. However, the identification of two COX isoforms (i.e., COX-1 and COX-2) with different physiologic effects has led to the development of COX-2–specific NSAIDs, which may be associated with fewer adverse effects than traditional NSAIDs.[25,26] These agents are commonly referred to as COX-2 inhibitors.

Whereas COX-1 is expressed in most tissues of the body, including the GI tract, kidneys, and platelets, COX-2 expression is normally low throughout the body.[27] However, inflammatory mediators such as cytokines upregulate COX-2 expression, leading to high levels of COX-2 in inflamed tissue. Selective inhibition of COX-2, therefore, is expected to produce anti-inflammatory activity with minimal adverse effect on GI mucosa as well as other structures and cells such as platelets. Examples of COX-2 inhibitors include celecoxib (Celebrex), rofecoxib (Vioxx), and valdecoxib (Bextra). Long-term safety data have been published for celecoxib and rofecoxib, and the results have not been reassuring.[28,29] Although a large study comparing celecoxib to ibuprofen and nabumetone demonstrated that celecoxib users experienced significantly less symptomatic and complicated ulcers, the published results represented only 6 of the 12- to 16-month study protocols.[28] Consequently, the Food and Drug Administration (FDA) has not allowed the manufacturer to promote Celebrex as a safer alternative to traditional NSAIDs. Whereas a large study comparing rofecoxib to naproxen clearly demonstrated that rofecoxib reduces the incidence of symptomatic and complicated ulcers by approximately one-half, rofecoxib treatment was associated with 4-fold more myocardial infarctions than the naproxen group.[29]

Traditional Disease-Modifying Antirheumatic Drugs

DMARD therapy should be considered for all RA patients.[8] Initiation of DMARD therapy should not be delayed beyond 3 months of RA diagnosis in patients who experience inadequate relief symptoms despite adequate NSAID therapy. Although DMARDs have the potential to cause serious toxicity, they also have the potential to substantially reduce joint inflammation and reduce or prevent joint damage, maintain joint function and integrity, and ultimately reduce health care costs and allow patients to remain productive.[8]

The onset of action of most traditional DMARDs is slow, ranging from 3 to 6 months; however, sulfasalazine, MTX, leflunomide, and cyclosporine produce results in as early as 1 to 2 months. Biological agents, on the other hand, can produce benefits within days to weeks.[22,30] The agent of choice is determined primarily by physician and patient preference, taking into consideration convenience of administration, monitoring requirements, medication and monitoring costs, time to therapeutic onset, and frequency and severity of adverse reactions.

Few comparative trials are available to provide objective comparisons among these agents.[31] The American College of Rheumatology (ACR) acknowledges that the best initial DMARD selection for RA treatment is not known. MTX is heavily favored by most rheumatologists for initial treatment, particularly for severe RA, because of a relatively rapid response, high response rate, and the longest sustained efficacy of all DMARDs. The probability of continuing MTX therapy at 5 years was 62% in one study.[32,33] Hydroxychloroquine and sulfasalazine are relatively safe, convenient, and inexpensive and are commonly selected as initial therapy for patients with mild RA; most studies indicate that HCQ is used more than SSZ, even though HCQ is considered to be less potent.[34-36] LEF is an attractive option for treatment of severe RA because it has an onset of effect in as soon as 4 weeks and overall efficacy (including retarding of radiographic progression) similar to MTX.[37-39]

Injectable gold is effective but can be inconvenient and causes numerous intolerable adverse side effects. Interestingly, a follow-up study of patients with early RA who discontinued injectable gold after an average of 11.3 months of treatment because of side effects found that these patients experienced sustained disease improvement (i.e., remission) for several years thereafter.[40] The rate of clinical remission among these patients was similar to that of patients who *continued* gold or MTX therapy over a 6-year period. The oral form of gold, auranofin (AUR) is rarely used because of poor GI tolerance, slow onset of action (up to 6 months), and low efficacy.

In a meta-analysis of traditional DMARD therapy, the most effective appeared to be parenteral gold, MTX, SSZ, and penicillamine.[41] HCQ was relatively less effective, and AUR was found to be least effective. Parenteral gold appeared to be most toxic while AUR and antimalarials were best tolerated. Leflunomide was not evaluated in this study. Azathioprine is effective but is usually reserved for patients with severe disease who do not respond to safer alternatives because of myelosuppression and hepatotoxicity potential. Although effective, D-penicillamine (DPEN), is probably the slowest-acting DMARD because of a slow titration schedule (i.e., dose adjustments every 3 months). As a result of this and the potential to cause rare but serious autoimmune diseases (e.g., systemic lupus erythematous, myasthenia gravis, Goodpasture's syndrome), DPEN is seldom used. Because of potential toxicity (renal insufficiency and hypertension) and cost, cyclosporine is reserved for severe, refractory RA. In organ transplant patients, cyclosporine has been associated with an increased risk of malignancy, however, this risk does not appear to be significant in RA treatment.[42]

Biological Agents

The introduction of biological agents has provided an entirely new approach to RA management. The cytokines TNF-α and IL-1 (specifically IL-1α and IL-1β) appear to be key inflammatory mediators in RA.[43] Both cytokines are abundant in rheumatoid synovial tissues and fluid. In addition, both can independently induce expression of the other, and IL-1 is capable of upregulating its own expression.[44] Excessive macrophage-produced cytokines (including TNF-α, IL-1, IL-6, and IL-8) correlates closely with RA disease activity and severity. Most importantly, RA improves when the physiologic action of TNF-α and/or IL-1 is suppressed.

TNF-α is a proinflammatory cytokine produced by activated macrophages and T cells in joints affected by RA. TNF-α also plays a role in keeping infections localized by increasing platelet activation and adhesion, resulting in local blood vessel occlusion and containment of infection. This action of TNF-α is responsible for its tumor necrosis properties, thus leading to the name.

TNF-α exerts its physiologic effects by binding to two different cell-surface receptors (i.e., receptors with portions extending from within the cell cytoplasm to the cell exterior) known as p55 and p75 (55 kD and 75 kD, respectively).[45] Both receptors are capable of binding TNF to the domains extending above the cell surface. In addition to their location on inflammatory cells, soluble forms of these receptors are found in the serum and synovial fluid and appear to play a role in regulating TNF-α.

Two approaches have been attempted to target the action of TNF-α: the use of soluble TNF receptors with high TNF binding affinity (e.g., etanercept) and antibodies against TNF-α (e.g., infliximab, adalimumab).[43] Etanercept (Enbrel) is a recombinant TNF receptor Fc fusion protein with the extracellular portion of two p75 receptors fused to the Fc portion of human immunoglubulin-G1 (IgG1).[45] Infliximab (Remicade) is a chimeric IgG antibody directed against TNF-α; adalimumab is a genetically engineered human IgG1 monoclonal antibody. All three TNF-α inhibitors (Enbrel, Remicade, Humira) render TNF biologically unavailable and are highly effective in reducing RA disease activity. It is not clear whether one agent is superior to the other. Although anti-infliximab antibodies develop with long-term use of infliximab, this appears to be effectively prevented by concomitant immunosuppression with MTX.

In healthy individuals, IL-1 overexpression is prevented by naturally occurring IL-1Ra.[44,46] Consequently, inadequate production of IL-1Ra relative to IL-1 is hypothesized to be an important contributor to active RA. In addition to proinflammatory properties, IL-1 augments cartilage damage and inhibits bone formation. While TNF-α appears to be key in RA inflammation regulation and symptomatology, IL-1 may be largely responsible for bony erosion and periarticular osteoporosis. In animal studies, the combination of IL-1-receptor antagonists (IL-1Ra) with anti-TNF-α have synergistic benefits.[47] However, the combination is not recommended due to high risk of neutropenia and severe infections.[48]

TNF-α and IL-1 serve important physiologic functions, including protection against infections.[8,44] No increase in the incidence of serious infections among patients receiving biological agents has been observed in clinical trials. However, hospitalizations and deaths among patients treated with biological agents have been reported during postmarketing surveillance, and have been associated with sepsis, tuberculosis, atypical mycobacterial infections, fungal infections, and opportunistic infections.[8,49] Although these occurred primarily among patients with significant risk factors for infection (e.g., poorly controlled diabetes, concurrent corticosteroid or

DMARD therapy), biological agents should not be given to patients with active infection, history of recurring infections, or medical conditions predisposing them to infection.

Based on clinical trials, the best candidates for biological agent monotherapy or "add-on" to traditional DMARD therapy appear to be patients who respond suboptimally to adequate doses of MTX.[43,45,48] However, no trial has determined whether this approach is superior to commonly used DMARD combinations such as MTX plus sulfasalazine and/or hydroxychloroquine.

Corticosteroids

Corticosteroids administered orally at low dosages (i.e., the equivalent of 10 mg of daily prednisone or less) or through local injections are effective in relieving symptoms of active RA.[8] Oral corticosteroids appear to slow the rate of disease progression, particularly when used for less than 1 year.[48,50,51] Long-term use, however, is associated with many serious adverse effects, including osteoporosis, weight gain, diabetes, cataract formation, adrenal suppression, hypertension, increased risk for infection, and impaired wound healing. As a result, oral corticosteroid dosing should be limited to daily doses of 10 mg prednisone or equivalent (some sources recommend 7.5 mg of prednisone or equivalent) and should be administered for as brief a time as possible. Oral corticosteroids are particularly useful when patients are waiting for the onset of DMARD action or during brief flares of active RA involving multiple joints. Local corticosteroid injections are useful when flares involve only a few joints. Frequent corticosteroid injections over an extended period have the potential to accelerate bone and cartilage deterioration; therefore, the same joint should not be injected more than once every 3 months.

Alkylating Cytotoxic Agents

Cyclophosphamide and chlorambucil are effective in the treatment of severe progressive cases of RA, but they also carry the risk of potentially serious toxicity such as malignancy and infectious complications.[21] Thus, use of these drugs is usually limited to patients with progressive RA unresponsive to more conservative management or, in some cases, potentially life-threatening complications of RA such as rheumatoid vasculitis.[48]

Other Therapies

Minocycline appears to be a useful adjunctive agent in the treatment of RA, perhaps supporting the notion that RA has an infectious origin or relationship. A double-blind, placebo-controlled trial involving 46 patients with recent onset RA evaluated the benefit of minocycline 100 mg twice daily added to conventional therapy (e.g., varying use of NSAIDs, DMARDs, corticosteroids).[52] At 4-year follow-up, eight minocycline-treated patients without DMARD or steroid therapy were in remission as defined by the American College of Rheumatology compared with one patient in the placebo group ($P = 0.02$). Perhaps even more impressive are the results of a randomized trial comparing minocycline 100 mg BID to HCQ 200 mg QD in patients with early onset RA.[53] At 2 years, significantly more minocycline-treated patients experienced relief of RA signs and symptoms, required less prednisone, and were more likely to be completely tapered off prednisone.

Apheresis with the Prosorba column is an effective therapeutic option for patients with severe RA refractory to several DMARDs.[54] The Prosorba column, a medical device, contains highly purified staphylococcal protein A bound to a silica matrix that has a high affinity for IgG and complexes of IgG and IgM, including RF and circulating immune complexes. A plasmapheresis machine is used to withdraw blood from the patient, separate blood cells from plasma, pass the plasma through the Prosorba column to remove selected immunoglobulins and immune complexes, and recombine the plasma with the blood cells for return to the patient. Removal of these immunoglobulins and immune complexes results in immunomodulation and improvement in RA symptomatology. In a randomized, double-blind, sham-controlled trial, the effect of weekly apheresis with the Prosorba column in patients with severe RA (i.e., average disease duration, 15.5 years; average number of failed DMARDs per patient, 4.2; average number of tender joints and swollen joints, 36.6 and 24.2, respectively) on improvement of symptoms was evaluated. According to American College of Rheumatology (ACR) criteria for response, 32% of the Prosorba-treated and 11.4% of the sham-treated patients improved ($P < 0.019$) at 19- or 20-week follow-up. The trial was stopped early by the data safety monitoring board because of overwhelming benefit with the Prosorba column. No differences in harmful adverse effects were found; both treatment groups experienced short-term joint pain flares and swelling after treatment, which were thought to be caused by the plasmapheresis procedure. However, because of the difficulty and expense of weekly treatments, combined with a limited duration of response, this treatment should be reserved for patients with RA refractory to multiple DMARDs.[8]

Cyclosporine is an effective treatment option, either alone or in combination with methotrexate.[8] However, cyclosporine therapy is complicated by serious side effects (particularly dose-related renal toxicity and hypertension), the inconvenience of necessary drug level monitoring, drug interactions, and high cost. As a result, consideration of cyclosporine is limited to patients with refractory RA.

Thalidomide also is a TNF-α inhibitor that is effective in treatment-resistant RA.[55] Although thalidomide is associated with serious adverse effects (e.g., teratogenesis, peripheral neuropathy), strict treatment guideline adherence and diligent monitoring make thalidomide a treatment consideration for selected cases of refractory RA.

Two new classes of NSAIDs in development may provide GI protection without COX-2 specificity.[56] Nitric oxide NSAIDs (NO-NSAIDs), also known as cyclooxygenase inhibiting nitric oxide donors, consist of standard NSAIDs linked to a nitric oxide moiety. By donating nitric oxide to the gastric mucosa, NO-NSAIDs produce the same the same gastroprotective effect as prostaglandins. A human safety study comparing nitric oxide donating naproxen to plain naproxen has verified this protective effect.[57] The second class of NSAIDs broadens the pharmacologic effects of existing NSAIDs by inhibiting both enzymatic pathways of arachidonic acid metabolism (i.e., both cyclooxygenase and 5-lipoxygenase). While cyclooxygenase inhibition is clearly associated with GI toxicity, inhibition of both enzymatic pathways of arachidonic acid metabolism has been proven to be GI-sparing in animal studies and in initial human safety studies.[58] Interestingly, both of these new NSAID classes appear to provide extended anti-inflammatory activity and, as a result, may have disease-modifying properties.[56]

Vaccine therapy has been evaluated for RA prevention. In a double-blind, placebo-controlled phase II study of a T-cell receptor peptide vaccine in 99 patients with active RA, doses of 90 or 300 µg were administered at baseline and at 4, 8, and 20 weeks. At 20-week follow-up, significantly more patients receiving the 90-µg vaccine dose demonstrated improvement in RA signs and symptoms.[59] Although both vaccine dosage groups did not improve significantly when compared with placebo, a trend toward improvement was noted and no patients withdrew because of treatment-related adverse effects.

Treatment Limitations

Numerous studies document the short-term efficacy of gold, penicillamine, antimalarials, AZA, SSZ, and MTX in attenuating clinical and laboratory manifestations of RA.[41] For example, a meta-analysis of the four published placebo-controlled trials that used strict research methodologies supports parenteral gold as an effective intervention.[60] Using a strict definition of improvement, 27% of patients treated with gold achieved 50% reduction in active joint count compared with 11% of placebo-treated patients within 6 months.[61] However, long-term, positive therapeutic outcomes have not been realized for these drugs. Sustained treatment with any of these therapies is uncommon with the exception of MTX. Fewer than 20% of individuals started with parenteral gold, penicillamine, or antimalarials continue to receive this initial therapy for up to 5 years.[62] Many discontinue therapy for loss of responsiveness and still more discontinue because of toxicity. Over a 20-year period, traditional DMARDs may improve function during the first 10 years, but considerable decline occurs during the following 10 years, resulting in severe disability.

These observations have been confirmed repeatedly. In a retrospective survey of 154 patients involving 251 second-line drug–patient exposures randomly selected from a pool of 2,320 patients with RA, 57% improved after a delay of 1 to 7 months.[63] Of those withdrawn after <2 months of therapy, 25% subsequently improved without further DMARD therapy. For those continuing DMARD therapy, the probability of uninterrupted therapy 8 months, 24 months, and 36 months after the start of treatment was 50%, 25%, and 10%, respectively. Most withdrawals were because of drug toxicity.

In another series reported over a 14-year observation period in 671 patients receiving 1,017 courses of DMARDs, the median time to discontinuation for intramuscular gold, AUR, HCQ, or penicillamine was 2 years.[64] Again, adverse reactions were the most common reason for withdrawal.

In a prospective study, long-term medication use was evaluated by survival analysis in 245 patients with recently diagnosed RA receiving 432 courses of second-line therapy: HCQ, SSZ, gold, and penicillamine.[65] When indexed for side effects, 40% of gold, 12% of HCQ, 19% of SSZ, and 13% of penicillamine regimens were discontinued at 2 years. Indexed for lack of efficacy, 61% of HCQ, 46% of SSZ, 43% of gold, and 43% of penicillamine regimens were discontinued by 2 years. These studies reveal the limited effectiveness of most traditional DMARDs in RA and provide important insight regarding the inability of relatively short-term efficacy studies

to fully characterize therapeutic outcomes achievable for chronic diseases.

Another prospective trial incorporated aggressive use of DMARDs in patients with early onset RA.[66] The strategy, known as the "sawtooth" treatment strategy, entailed early initiation of DMARD therapy and continuous use of 1 or more DMARDs for an average of 6.2 years (range, 18 to 111 months). Throughout the study, DMARD therapy was combined or substituted if a lack of efficacy was evident or adverse side effects occurred. This approach achieved a remission rate that increased with time to 32% at final follow-up. The DMARDs used in this trial included injectable gold, SSZ, HCQ, DPEN, AUR, MTX, AZA, and cyclosporine. MTX use continued to rise throughout the study period until 37% of patients were taking MTX at the end of the study. The use of all other agents either fell dramatically (particularly injectable gold) or remained constant at a low level. The authors of the study concluded that the beneficial effects of active and continual traditional DMARD therapy may persist for at least 6 years and yield better long-term outcomes than achieved in previous trials. However, this approach is far from adequate for all patients as demonstrated by the fact that RA progressed in 25% of the study patients.

Long-term experience with MTX indicate that MTX remains efficacious for a significantly longer period than other DMARDs.[67] In a study of nearly 400 patients with RA, patients were successfully treated with continuous MTX as monotherapy for an average of 42 months, with some patients continuing as long as 60 months. In another study of nearly 600 patients with RA, only half of patients taking any DMARD (except MTX) were able to continue therapy beyond 9 to 24 months.[68] On the other hand, 62% of patients receiving MTX were able to continue after 5 years of treatment. Nevertheless, MTX monotherapy rarely results in complete disease remission; only one-third of patients improve by 50% after 2 to 4 years.[69]

The long-term safety and efficacy of biological agent therapy continue to be evaluated in numerous clinical trials. Short-term study results (mostly up to 2 year follow-up) indicate that biological agents provide more rapid improvement than traditional DMARDs in signs and symptoms of RA, including radiographic evidence of slowing disease progression, both as monotherapy and in combination with methotrexate.[69] Long-term results of biological agent clinical trials, including much-needed comparisons with traditional DMARD combinations, will provide valuable information for determining when treatment with a biological agent is most appropriate.

EARLY AND PROGRESSIVE RHEUMATOID ARTHRITIS

See Questions 1 to 16 for the role of non-drug and NSAID therapy in RA treatment and Questions 17 to 46 for DMARD (traditional and biological agents) and corticosteroid therapy.

Signs and Symptoms

1. **T.W., a previously healthy 42-year-old, 60-kg woman, has been suffering from morning stiffness that persists for several hours, anorexia, fatigue, and generalized muscle and joint pain during the past 4 months. In addition, she has noted that her**

eyes seem red most of the time and are unusually dry. Her symptoms have been much worse during the past month and a half, and she has been forced to limit her physical activities. She also notes that she can no longer wear her wedding ring because of swelling of her hand.

Physical examination reveals bilaterally symmetrical swelling, tenderness, and warmth of the metacarpophalangeal and proximal interphalangeal (PIP) joints of the hands and the metatarsophalangeal joints of the feet. A subcutaneous nodule is evident on the extensor surface of the left forearm. Pertinent laboratory findings include the following: erythrocyte sedimentation rate (ESR) by the Westergren method, 52 mm/hr; hemoglobin (Hgb), 10.6 g/dL (normal, 12 to 16 g/dL); hematocrit (Hct), 33% (normal, 36% to 47%); platelets, 480,000/mm³ (normal, 140,000 to 400,000/mm³); albumin, 3.8 g/dL (normal, 4.3 to 5.6 g/dL); serum uric acid, 3.0 mg/dL (normal, 2 to 8 mg/dL); serum iron, 40 mg/dL (normal, 60 to 180 mg/dL); total iron-binding capacity (TIBC), 275 mg/dL (normal, 200 to 400 mg/dL); and positive RF performed by latex fixation method in a dilution of 1:320. Tests for antinuclear antibodies (ANA) and tuberculin sensitivity are negative. Radiographic films of the hands and feet show soft-tissue swelling, narrowing of joint spaces, and marginal erosions of the second and third metacarpophalangeal and proximal interphalangeal joints bilaterally with no evidence of tophi or calcification. Other routine laboratory data and physical findings are normal. What signs and symptoms of RA does T.W. manifest?

[SI units: Hgb, 6.6 mmol/L (normal, 7.4 to 9.9); albumin, 38 g/L (normal, 35 to 50); uric acid, 178.4 μmol/L (normal, 202 to 416); iron, 7.2 μmol/L (normal, 9 to 26.9); TIBC, 49.2 μmol/L (normal, 45 to 73)]

The presentation of RA at onset can vary, but characteristically 50% to 70% of cases have a rather insidious onset of disease over weeks to months.[7] Early nonspecific symptoms such as fatigue, malaise, diffuse musculoskeletal pain, and morning stiffness may precede more specific symptoms. Prominent features of RA in T.W. include fatigue and morning stiffness. About half of patients with RA initially experience fatigue that later in the disease serves as a useful index of disease activity. Patients usually experience prolonged morning stiffness upon awakening. This stiffness usually lasts 30 to 60 minutes but may be present all day with decreasing intensity after arising. Duration of morning stiffness also may be a useful index of disease activity.

Over time, nonspecific musculoskeletal pain localizes to the joints bilaterally. Bilaterally symmetrical joint swelling and pain, involving the metacarpophalangeal (MCP) and PIP joints of the hands and metatarsophalangeal (MTP) joints of the feet, as illustrated by T.W., are characteristic of RA. The peripheral joints of the hands, wrists, and feet usually are involved first. Although MCP and PIP joints of the hands often are affected, the distal interphalangeal (DIP) joints usually are spared. Ultimately, any or all of the diarthrodial joints may be involved, including the elbows, knees, shoulders, ankles, hips, temporomandibular joints, sternoclavicular joints, and glenohumeral joints (Fig. 43-3).

Joint involvement is characterized by soft-tissue swelling and warmth, decreased range of motion (ROM), and sometimes muscle atrophy around affected joints. Progressive disease is characterized by irreversible joint deformities such as ulnar deviation of the fingers (Fig. 43-4), boutonniere defor-

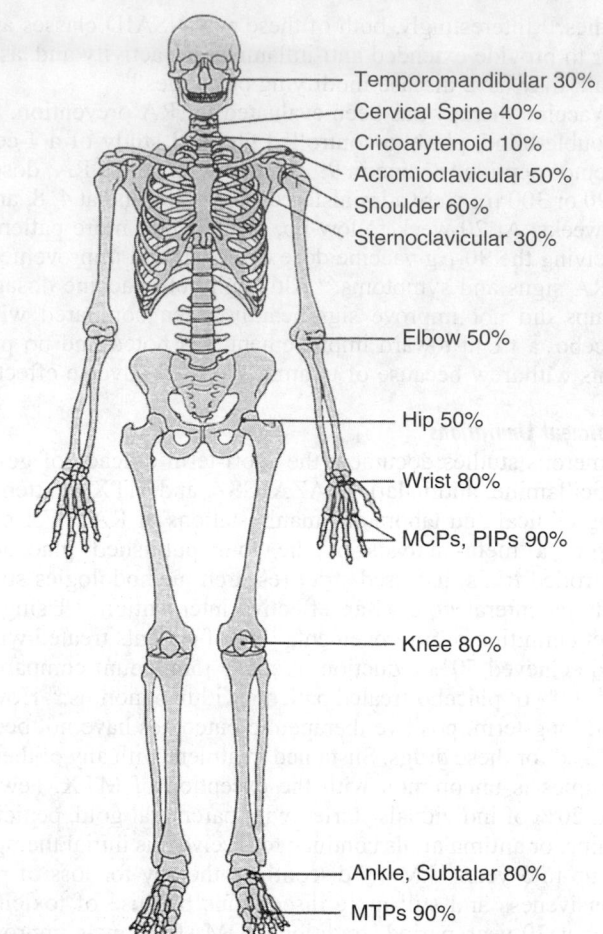

FIGURE 43-3. Frequency of involvement of different joint sites in established RA.

Temporomandibular 30%
Cervical Spine 40%
Cricoarytenoid 10%
Acromioclavicular 50%
Shoulder 60%
Sternoclavicular 30%
Elbow 50%
Hip 50%
Wrist 80%
MCPs, PIPs 90%
Knee 80%
Ankle, Subtalar 80%
MTPs 90%

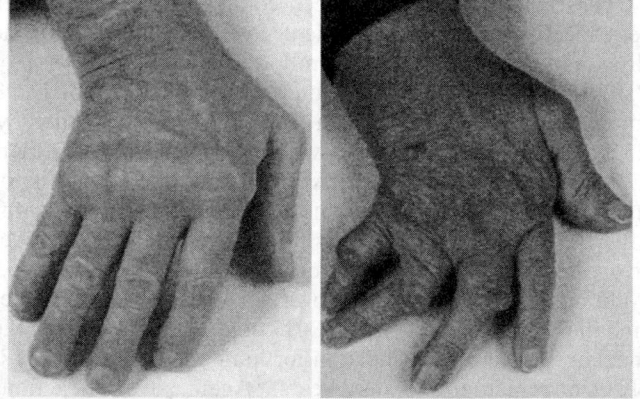

FIGURE 43-4. Ulnar deviation and MCP synovitis (left). This may progress to more marked lateral deviation with subluxation of the extensor tendons (right finger) (right).

mities (hyperextension of the DIP joint and flexion of the PIP joint), or swan neck deformities (hyperextension of the PIP joint and flexion of the DIP joint) (Fig. 43-5). Similar irreversible deformities also may involve the feet.

RA is a systemic disease, which is reflected by the extra-articular manifestations that may accompany joint involvement. *Subcutaneous nodules* are found in up to 35% of individuals with RA.[7] As in the case of T.W., these nodules usually

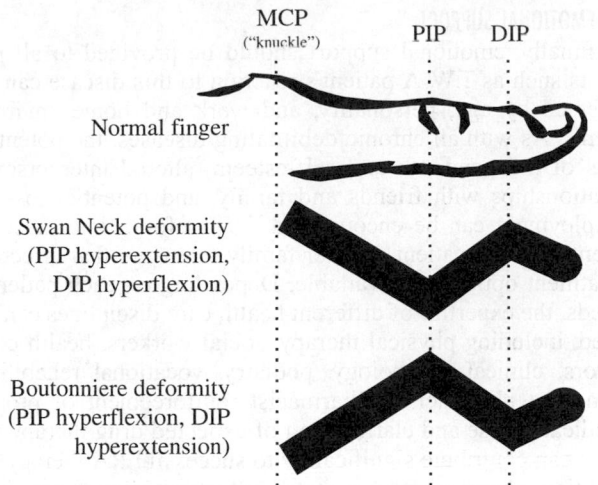

MCP
("knuckle")   PIP   DIP

Normal finger

Swan Neck deformity
(PIP hyperextension,
DIP hyperflexion)

Boutonniere deformity
(PIP hyperflexion, DIP
hyperextension)

FIGURE 43-5. Characteristic finger deformities in rheumatoid arthritis. DIP, distal interphalangeal joint; MCP, metacarpophalangeal joint; PIP, proximal interphalangeal joint.

develop along extensor surfaces (e.g., olecranon process, proximal ulna), but occasionally may be found in the hands, sacral areas, eyes, lungs, and heart. In addition, they can occur on the soles of the feet and along the Achilles tendon. Patients who develop rheumatoid nodules almost always are RF positive.

Organ system involvement may be extensive. *Pleuropulmonary manifestations* (e.g., pleuritis, development of pulmonary nodules, interstitial fibrosis, pneumonitis, and rarely arteritis of the pulmonary vasculature) also can accompany the articular involvement of RA.[7] *Cardiac involvement* can present as pericarditis or myocarditis. In addition, rheumatoid nodules can produce conduction defects or valve defects.

Some extra-articular manifestations occur as syndromes. *Sjögren's syndrome* includes dry eyes (keratoconjunctivitis sicca), dry mouth (xerostomia), and connective tissue disease.[70] T.W.'s eye complaints may be an extra-articular manifestation of her RA. *Felty's syndrome* is characterized by chronic arthritis, splenomegaly, and neutropenia; thrombocytopenia, anemia, and lymphadenopathy also may be present.[71]

Vasculitis, another extra-articular manifestation of RA, can involve any organ system and can vary in seriousness from mild to potentially life-threatening (see Chapter 44, Connective Tissue Disorders: The Clinical Use of Corticosteroids).

2. What abnormal laboratory values in T.W. could be used to monitor the efficacy of drug therapy or disease progression?

The laboratory findings in RA are characteristic of a chronic systemic inflammatory disease. No test is specific for RA. T.W.'s elevated ESR is a nonspecific indication of inflammation. Alternatively, C-reactive protein (CRP) plasma concentrations can be tested instead of ESR.[72] Levels of CRP, a plasma protein of the acute-phase response, correlate with RA disease activity better than ESR; however, CRP is also not disease specific. T.W.'s hematologic findings are consistent with a mild anemia of chronic inflammation. Although her serum iron concentration is decreased, her normal iron-binding capacity makes a diagnosis of iron-deficiency anemia unlikely. Her anemia probably results from a failure of iron release

from the reticuloendothelial tissues and would not be expected to respond to iron therapy. The mild thrombocytosis is additional evidence of a systemic inflammatory response.

The serum albumin concentration can be low in RA patients such as T.W. A low serum albumin concentration theoretically could result in decreased protein binding of salicylates and other highly protein-bound drugs and yield higher free drug serum concentrations.[73]

RF, an autoantibody (usually IgM or IgG) that reacts with the Fc portion of antigenic IgG to form an immune complex in vitro, is found in the serum of approximately 75% of patients with RA.[74] RF is not found in some patients with RA and can be present in 3% to 5% of healthy individuals as well as in patients with diseases other than RA, including almost any condition associated either with immune complex formation or with hypergammaglobulinemia (e.g., chronic infections, lymphoproliferative and hepatic diseases, systemic forms of autoimmunity). Therefore, RF does not establish the diagnosis of RA. An RF titer of at least 1:160 is considered a positive test.[75] Patients with RA typically have titers of at least 1:320. Although RF titers do not parallel disease activity, high titers (>1:512) early in the disease course are associated with more severe and progressive disease. The test for antinuclear antibodies (ANA) ruled out systemic lupus erythematosus in T.W. However, ANA can be positive in 10% to 70% patients with RA.[75]

The laboratory manifestations of inflammation should improve with effective drug therapy and, along with many of the clinical features of RA, are useful parameters for monitoring disease activity and response to therapy (Table 43-3).

Treatment
Nondrug Treatment

3. What nondrug therapy should be included in the management of T.W.'s RA?

Treatment objectives in RA are reduction of joint pain and inflammation, preservation of joint function, and prevention of deformity. This is best achieved by instructing patients on proper joint protection, energy conservation, joint range of

---

Table 43-3 Parameters Used to Assess Disease Activity and Drug Response in RA

Duration and intensity of morning stiffness
Number of painful or tender joints
Number of swollen joints; severity of joint swelling
Range of joint motion
Time to onset of fatigue
ESR or CRP
Radiographic changes: osteopenia, joint space narrowing, bony erosions
Hgb/Hct
Subcutaneous nodules, pleuritis, pneumonitis, myocarditis, vasculitis
AIMS
HAQ

AIMS, arthritis impact measure scale; CRP, C-reactive protein; ESR, erythrocyte sedimentation rate; HAQ, health assessment questionnaire; Hct, hematocrit; Hgb, hemoglobin; RA, rheumatoid arthritis.

motion and muscle strengthening exercises in combination with effective symptom-relieving and disease-modifying drug therapy.[8] Physical therapy and occupational therapy can provide valuable assistance to patients with compromised activities of daily living.

JOINT PROTECTION AND ENERGY CONSERVATION

Systemic and articular rest (achieved by splinting the affected joints) may significantly reduce inflammation.[76] Restful and adequate sleep is important for general health and particularly important in a chronic, fatigue-inducing disease such as RA. However, prolonged rest can induce negative effects such as rapid losses in strength and endurance. Therefore, RA patients experiencing acute inflammation, such as T.W., should rest often but limit daytime rest periods to 30 to 60 minutes. Splinting of joints is typically prescribed throughout the day and night during periods of active inflammation, then at night only for several weeks following cessation of inflammation.

EXERCISE AND HEAT

Passive exercise (e.g., ROM exercises) should be prescribed for T.W. until the acute inflammation subsides. Passive exercise minimizes muscle atrophy and flexion contractures and maintains joint function without increasing inflammation. The external application of heat, soaking her hands and feet in warm water, hot baths, or hot paraffin treatments, can reduce joint stiffness and allow greater benefit from passive exercise programs, although literature evidence supporting the value of these interventions is very limited.[76] Heat treatments in general should be avoided during periods of active joint inflammation, since heat can further exacerbate pain and swelling.

EMOTIONAL SUPPORT

Finally, emotional support should be provided to all patients such as T.W. A patient's reaction to this disease can be affected by age, personality, and work and home environments. As with all chronic debilitating diseases, the potential loss of independence and self-esteem, altered interpersonal relationships with friends and family, and potential loss of employment can be encountered.[77] Therefore, time must be spent with the patient and her family to ensure that effective treatment options are available. Depending on each patient's needs, the expertise of different health care disciplines can be used, including physical therapy, social workers, health educators, clinical psychology, podiatry, vocational rehabilitation, and pharmacists. Pharmacist reinforcement of proper medication use and clarification of expected drug therapy results can contribute significantly to successful RA therapy. In addition, pharmacists in capitated outpatient clinical practices may have opportunities to monitor RA drug therapy for therapeutic and adverse effects under collaborative practice agreements with prescribers.

Drug Treatment (Fig. 43-6)
NONSTEROIDAL ANTI-INFLAMMATORY DRUGS—ASPIRIN

4. T.W. will be treated with a DMARD and concurrent NSAID therapy initially to rapidly control inflammation and swelling. Why would aspirin be a reasonable (or unreasonable) consideration for T.W.?

Based on T.W.'s clinical presentation, disease-modifying antirheumatic drug therapy is indicated (see Question 17). The purpose of NSAID therapy, which has no disease-

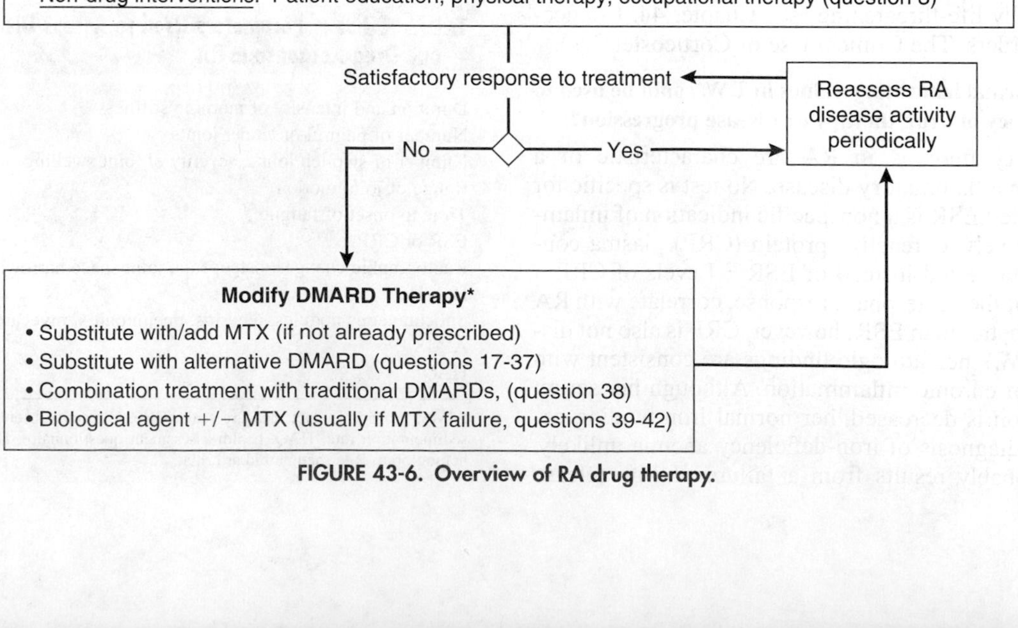

Overview: RA Drug Therapy

Initial Therapy

- Treatment of choice: DMARD (within 3 months of diagnosis)
  - *Severe RA:* Usually MTX or combination of traditional DMARDs including MTX (questions 25-31)
  - *Mild RA:* Usually hydroxychloroquine or sulfasalazine (questions 17-20)
- Treatment considerations: NSAID (questions 4-16), local corticosteroid injections (few joints, question 46), low-dose systemic steroid (multiple joints, questions 43-45)
- Non-drug interventions: Patient education, physical therapy, occupational therapy (question 3)

Satisfactory response to treatment

No — Yes →

Reassess RA disease activity periodically

Modify DMARD Therapy*

- Substitute with/add MTX (if not already prescribed)
- Substitute with alternative DMARD (questions 17-37)
- Combination treatment with traditional DMARDs, (question 38)
- Biological agent +/− MTX (usually if MTX failure, questions 39-42)

FIGURE 43-6. Overview of RA drug therapy.

modifying activity, is to provide rapid pain relief and reduction of joint inflammation.

Historically, aspirin was considered to be the first-line treatment for patients who tolerate it. Today, however, aspirin is seldom considered an NSAID of choice because of well-documented GI toxicity and the availability of safer and more convenient NSAIDs.[8,78]

Advantages of aspirin therapy include proven efficacy, low cost, and the correlation between serum salicylate levels and both efficacy and toxicity.[23] To be effective, aspirin must be prescribed at dosages sufficient to provide serum salicylate concentrations ranging from 15 to 30 mg/dL.[23] A reasonable initial daily dose is 45 mg/kg divided into 4- or 6-hour intervals. However, the dosage required to achieve optimal anti-inflammatory responses varies widely because of interindividual variation in metabolism.

After intestinal absorption, aspirin is hydrolyzed rapidly to salicylate. Salicylate (or salicylic acid) subsequently is metabolized via multiple pathways. Metabolism to salicyluric acid and salicyl phenolic glucuronide is capacity limited.[23] The serum salicylate half-life is 3.5 to 4.5 hours after a single 650-mg dose of aspirin. On the other hand, daily doses of 4.5 g/day result in a serum salicylate half-life of 15 to 20 hours. Salicylate pharmacokinetics, therefore, are complex, following both first order and Michaelis-Menten elimination processes. In anti-inflammatory doses, 5 to 7 days of therapy are needed before steady-state serum concentrations of salicylate are attained; therefore, dosage adjustments should be made no more often than every 5 to 7 days.

5. A.L., a patient with RA, had her aspirin dosage increased to 975 mg QID approximately 1 week ago. She now complains of, ". . . ringing in my ears all the time!" What is the most probable cause of this symptom?

Aspirin-induced tinnitus (i.e., a ringing or high-pitched buzzing sensation in the head) is noticeable to most patients with normal hearing at serum levels between 10 and 30 mg/dL, although one study noted that tinnitus did not occur until serum levels exceeded 25 mg/dL.[23] Therefore, when tinnitus occurs, serum salicylate concentrations usually are within the therapeutic range. Tinnitus can be used to titrate patients to therapeutic doses of aspirin; dosages are increased slowly until tinnitus is experienced, then the dosage is reduced just enough to eliminate tinnitus. However, patients with pre-existing hearing loss may not experience tinnitus despite potentially toxic concentrations.[79] Therefore, patients with known pre-existing hearing loss and older subjects who can have undetected hearing loss should be monitored by serum salicylate concentrations rather than by the occurrence of tinnitus.

Alternative Formulations

6. P.D., a man with an alleged aspirin allergy, avoids aspirin because it has upset his stomach in the past. However, he can take large doses of an enteric-coated aspirin (Ecotrin) without experiencing GI intolerance. Is this a rational alternative to regular aspirin? What are appropriate alternatives for patients who cannot tolerate therapeutic doses of aspirin?

Patients who complain of GI side effects commonly use aspirin formulations that contain buffering agents (e.g., Alka-Seltzer, Ascriptin, Bufferin). Although the antacid content in

Alka-Seltzer may be sufficient to reduce acute GI microbleeding and symptoms, Alka-Seltzer contains more than a gram of sodium for each 650 mg of aspirin, making it undesirable for chronic use. Ascriptin and Bufferin probably contain too little antacid to appreciably reduce GI microbleeding,[80] but occasionally are better tolerated than regular aspirin. All these formulations are more expensive than regular aspirin.

Enteric-coated aspirin is associated with fewer GI complaints than uncoated aspirin.[80] Although enteric coating increases the likelihood of incomplete absorption,[59] Measurin was absorbed reliably in one study involving small numbers of patients,[81] and other newer enteric-coated aspirin preparations can be absorbed reliably as well. Thus, enteric-coated aspirin can be a useful alternative to regular aspirin in some patients. Easprin enteric-coated tablets contain 975 mg of aspirin per tablet and, therefore, are available only by prescription. It provides the convenience of taking fewer tablets each day, but small adjustments in dose are not possible.

Sustained-release (SR) aspirin (e.g., ZORprin, Measurin) is intended to provide more stable salicylate concentrations with less frequent administration. Twice-daily dosing of Measurin produces average serum salicylate concentrations comparable to equal doses of aspirin administered four times daily.[82] However, the elimination half-life of regular aspirin in anti-inflammatory doses is sufficiently long that twice-daily dosing also yields relatively stable serum salicylate concentrations,[83] and some patients have been maintained on a once-daily regimen.[84] Thus, the relative advantage of SR aspirin compared with regular or enteric-coated aspirin remains unclear. Nevertheless, some patients do tolerate these expensive SR aspirin dosage forms better than regular aspirin.

In summary, various aspirin dosage forms are available. Enteric-coated preparations, despite their expense and potential for incomplete absorption, are alternatives for patients with a history of gastroduodenal ulcers or patients who develop ulcers while taking regular aspirin. Alternatively, some newer NSAIDs may offer equal efficacy with less GI toxicity (see Question 11).

Aspirin and NSAID Allergy

7. Aspirin is ordered for C.S., who was hospitalized recently for evaluation and treatment of his RA. An allergy to aspirin is noted in C.S.'s medical chart. Why is aspirin, or another NSAID, contraindicated for C.S.?

C.S. should be asked to describe his reaction to aspirin. If he describes symptoms consistent with a hypersensitivity reaction, aspirin is contraindicated. Most patients who claim to be allergic to aspirin merely experience GI distress. In these patients, aspirin may be tolerated if administered with food or if the formulation is switched to an enteric-coated preparation.

Aspirin intolerance (hypersensitivity) in association with asthma is cause for serious concern. Challenge with aspirin in these patients can precipitate an acute, life-threatening, bronchospastic reaction.[85] Approximately 10% of asthmatics have a history of aspirin-induced bronchospasm, more often women than men and rarely in children.[86] A somewhat smaller percentage of patients with recurrent rhinitis also suffer from this problem.[87] The frequency of aspirin intolerance in patients with nasal polyps is as high as 22%, and 70% of these patients have asthma.[88] All these patients experience a high degree of cross-reactivity to other chemicals, including indomethacin (Indocin), naproxen (Naprosyn), ibuprofen (Motrin), fenoprofen (Nalfon), mefenamic acid (Ponstel), sodium benzoate (a widely used preservative), and tartrazine dye (FD&C Yellow No. 5), which is used in foods and some drugs.[89–93] These substances are structurally dissimilar, but most are inhibitors of prostaglandin synthesis. Therefore, this reaction may result from an abnormal response to a common pharmacologic effect. Weak prostaglandin synthesis inhibitors, such as sodium and choline salicylate, have been administered cautiously to such aspirin-intolerant patients without untoward reactions.

Several small studies have demonstrated safe use of COX-2 inhibitors in aspirin-sensitive asthmatics.[94,95] In theory, these agents might be safer because they allow COX-1 to continue producing prostaglandin E_2. Prostaglandin E_2 is an important mediator of multiple physiologic processes, including reduction of leukotriene synthesis, suppression of the release of inflammatory mediators from mast cells, and prevention of aspirin-induced bronchoconstriction.[86]

Some patients with chronic urticaria, as well as patients with rhinitis and aspirin allergy may be at increased risk to develop urticaria or angioedema on exposure to aspirin.[88] The pathogenic mechanism for this urticarial form of aspirin intolerance is unknown.

Prolongation of Bleeding Time

8. A.C. is scheduled to have an impacted wisdom tooth removed. She states that she is taking an aspirin-like product for arthritis. Why would the specific NSAID she is taking affect this dental procedure?

Aspirin, nonacetylated salicylates, nonaspirin NSAIDs, and COX-2 inhibitors have different effects on platelet function. Aspirin alters hemostasis most significantly and, if possible, should be discontinued before any type of surgery. Several mechanisms may be responsible for altered hemostasis.[23] First and most important, low doses of aspirin irreversibly impair platelet aggregation through irreversible binding to COX and, thereby, prolong bleeding time. Because new platelets must be released into the circulation before the bleeding time will normalize, the bleeding time can be prolonged for several days following the ingestion of aspirin. Second, salicylates appear to enhance blood fibrinolytic activity. Finally, near toxic doses of salicylates can induce a hypoprothrombinemia that is reversible by vitamin K. Salicylate-induced hypoprothrombinemia usually is not clinically significant, but it can be the cause of bleeding when associated with severe liver dysfunction or malnutrition.[89] Bleeding times normalize within 3 to 6 days after discontinuation of aspirin, corresponding to the average life span of platelets. Therefore, aspirin should be discontinued about 7 days before surgery when possible.

Nonaspirin NSAIDs also can prolong bleeding times by inhibiting platelet aggregation, but they bind reversibly to COX resulting in reversible platelet inhibition.[23] The impairment of platelets is usually reversed within 2 days after nonaspirin NSAID discontinuation. A conservative approach would be to stop a nonaspirin NSAID approximately 5 half-lives before surgical procedures. Because nonacetylated salicylates have minimal effects on COX and platelet function, they are of little concern in presurgical patients.[23] Likewise, since COX-2 is not found in platelets, COX-2 inhibitors are not expected to alter platelet function; this lack of effect has been verified in clinical trials.[96]

Use in Pregnancy

9. K.H., a 28-year-old pregnant woman with RA, is concerned about the possible effects of NSAIDs on her baby. What are the risks to the fetus with uninterrupted consumption of NSAIDs? Should K.H. be concerned about maternal- and lactation-related effects of these medications?

While NSAIDs, including aspirin, are not teratogenic, they must be used cautiously in women who are pregnant and who breast-feed infants.[97] Fetal effects of NSAIDs include possible premature ductus arteriosus closure, increased cutaneous and intracranial bleeding, transient renal impairment, and a reduction in urine output. High doses of aspirin (>3 g/day) and NSAIDs can inhibit uterine contraction, resulting in prolonged labor. Other maternal effects include increased peripartum blood loss and anemia. Both aspirin and non-aspirin NSAIDs should be used only if necessary and sparingly at lowest effective doses in pregnancy; adverse fetal and maternal effects can be minimized if these medications are discontinued at least 6 to 8 weeks before delivery.

Aspirin is generally not preferred for breast-feeding women since significant serum salicylate levels have been found in breastfed neonates, raising concerns regarding the potential for metabolic acidosis, bleeding, and Reye's syndrome. A policy statement from the American Academy of Pediatrics states that the non-aspirin NSAIDs ibuprofen, indomethacin, and naproxen are usually compatible with breast-feeding.[98]

NONASPIRIN NONSTEROIDAL ANTI-INFLAMMATORY DRUGS
Choice of Agent

10. The decision is made to give T.W. (see Questions 1 through 4) NSAID therapy and initiate DMARD therapy shortly thereafter. What is the NSAID of choice for T.W.?

In general, there is no such thing as an "NSAID of choice" for treatment of RA.[8,23] There is no significant difference among the NSAIDs in efficacy, and it is impossible to predict a given patient's response to a particular NSAID. Therefore, the choice of NSAID is based primarily on safety, convenience, cost, and patient preference.[8] An adequate trial (i.e., 1 to 2 weeks) of any given NSAID at a moderate to high dose on a scheduled basis (i.e., not "as needed") is the only method of determining anti-inflammatory efficacy, as opposed to the analgesic and antipyretic effects which are relatively prompt in onset.

While aspirin is an effective and inexpensive anti-inflammatory agent, the availability of less toxic, more convenient, and relatively low-cost non-aspirin NSAIDs have limited its use[78] (Table 43-4). Included among these alternatives are salicylic acid derivatives known as nonacetylated salicylates. These products may be better tolerated than aspirin. In stud-

Table 43-4   Nonsteroidal Anti-inflammatory Drugs (NSAIDs)

NSAID Generic Name (Brand Name)	Product Availability	Usual Dosing Interval	Maximum Daily Dose (mg)	Cost/30-Day Supply ($)[a]
Salicylates (Acetylated and Nonacetylated)[b]				
Aspirin, enteric-coated (generic)[c]	Tablets: 325 mg; 325, 500, 800, 975 mg SR	QID	6,000	18.00
Salsalate (Disalcid)[c]	Tablets: 500, 750 mg	BID–TID	4,800	27.60
Diflunisal (Dolobid)[c]	Tablets: 250, 500 mg	BID	1,500	30.00
Magnesium choline salicylate (Trilisate)[c]	Tablets: 293, 362, 440, 544, 587, 725 mg	QD–TID	4,800	65.70
	Solution: 293 mg/5 mL, 362 mg/5 mL			
Sodium salicylate[c]	Tablets: 325 mg; 325, 650 mg SR	TID–QID	4,800	33.23
Propionic Acid Derivatives				
Fenoprofen (Nalfon)[c]	Capsules: 200, 300 mg	TID–QID	3,200	43.20
	Tablets: 600 mg			
Flurbiprofen (Ansaid)[c]	Tablets: 50, 100 mg	BID–QID	300	40.20
Ibuprofen (Motrin)[c]	Tablets: 200, 400, 600, 800 mg	TID–QID	3,200	13.80
	Suspension: 100 mg/5 mL			
Ketoprofen (Orudis, Orudis ER)[c]	Capsules: 25, 50, 75 mg	TID–QID	300	67.20
		ER: QD	ER: 200	ER: 67.50
Naproxen (Naprosyn)[c]	Tablets: 250, 375, 500 mg; 375, 500 mg SR	BID	1,500	22.80
	Suspension: 125 mg/5 mL			
Naproxen sodium (Anaprox)[c]	Tablets: 275, 550 mg	BID	1,375	29.40
Oxaproxin (Daypro)[c]	Tablet or capsule: 600 mg	QD	1,800	34.80
Acetic Acid Derivatives				
Diclofenac (Voltaren, Voltaren XR)[c]	Tablets: 25, 50, 75 mg; 100 mg XR	BID–TID	200	42.00
		XR: QD	XR: 100 mg	XR: 73.80
Etodolac (Lodine, Lodine XL)[c]	Capsules: 200, 300 mg	BID–TID	1,200	46.80
	Tablets: 400, 500 mg; 400, 500, 600 mg XL	XL: QD	XL: 1,000	38.70
Indomethacin (Indocin, Indocin SR)[c]	Capsules: 25, 50 mg; 75 mg SR	TID–QID	200	32.40
	Suppository: 50 mg	SR: QD–BID	SR: 150	SR: 41.70
	Suspension: 25 mg/5 mL			
Ketorolac (Toradol)[c]	Tablet: 10 mg	QID	40	100.00
Nabumetone (Relafen)	Tablet: 500, 750 mg	QD	2,000	84.00
Sulindac (Clinoril)[c]	Tablets: 150, 200 mg	BID	400	36.60
Tolmetin (Tolectin)[c]	Tablets: 200, 600 mg	TID–QID	1,800	33.30
	Capsules: 400 mg			
Anthranilic Acids				
Meclofenamate sodium (Meclomen)[c]	Capsules: 50, 100 mg	TID–QID	400	184.80
Oxicam Derivatives				
Piroxicam (Feldene)[c]	Capsule: 10, 20 mg	QD	20	39.60
Meloxicam (Mobic)	Tablets: 7.5, 15 mg	QD	15	65.40
Cyclooxygenase-2 Inhibitors				
Celecoxib (Celebrex)	Capsules: 100, 200, 400 mg	BID	400	94.20
Rofecoxib (Vioxx)	Tablets: 12.5, 25, 50 mg	QD	25	80.00
	Suspension: 12.5 mg/5 mL, 25 mg/5 mL			
Valdecoxib (Bextra)	Tablets: 10 mg, 20 mg	QD	10	85.50

[a]From reference 48. Average cost to patient based on usual dose for RA; price is for generic version if available (see footnote c below).
[b]Highly variable half-life; anti-inflammatory doses associated with salicyclate serum concentrations from 15 to 30 mg/dL.
[c]Generic version available.

ies involving small numbers of patients, the anti-inflammatory efficacy of a nonacetylated salicylate was comparable to aspirin or indomethacin.[23] Other studies, on the other hand, demonstrate that nonacetylated salicylates are slightly less potent as anti-inflammatory and analgesic agents than other NSAIDs. Aspirin irreversibly inactivates the enzyme COX via acetylation. Nonacetylated salicylates, except diflunisal (Dolobid), are weak inhibitors of COX in vitro.[99,100] Considering the favorable toxicity profile of nonacetylated salicylates, a large-scale controlled trial seems justified to clarify the relative efficacy and toxicity of these agents in the treatment of chronic inflammatory disorders. Of the nonacetylated salicylates, sodium salicylate is the least expensive. Salsalate (a salicylate prodrug) may be activated erratically, resulting in variable salicylate concentrations.[101] Nonacetylated salicylates can be useful alternatives when the antiplatelet effects of aspirin and nonselective NSAIDs are undesirable (see Question 8). In general, nonacetylated salicylates are reasonable first-line NSAIDs because of their favorable adverse effect profile but might not be as efficacious as other NSAIDs.

Other available nonsalicylate NSAIDs have important differentiating properties.[23] Indomethacin penetrates the blood–brain barrier better than any other NSAID, achieving levels in the cerebrospinal fluid of up to 50% of serum levels. As a result, the incidence of central nervous system side effects often precludes the use of optimal anti-inflammatory doses of indomethacin, particularly in the elderly.[102] Loose stools or diarrhea can be dose limiting for some patients receiving meclofenamate. Several trials report a high frequency of peptic ulcer disease (relative risk versus nonuser, 6.4; 95% confidence interval [CI], 4.8 to 8.4) and GI bleeding (relative risk, 13.7 to 18.0; 95% CI, 7.1 to 39.6) with piroxicam, a long-acting NSAID.[78] Therefore, piroxicam should seldom be prescribed. On the other hand, ibuprofen appears to be associated with one of the lowest frequencies of peptic ulcer disease (relative risk, 2.3; 95% CI, 1.8 to 3.0) and GI bleeding (relative risk, 2.9 to 2.0; 95% CI 1.4 to 5.0).

Newer NSAIDs may be associated with lower toxicity potential, but are expensive and should be considered only in patients at high risk for GI bleeding (see Question 11). Lower doses of mildly selective COX-2 inhibitors such as nabumetone and etodolac can be safer than other NSAIDs; however, lower doses are insufficient for anti-inflammatory effects.[23,25] Highly selective COX-2 inhibitors (e.g., celecoxib, rofecoxib, valdecoxib) remain selective at all doses and are widely promoted as GI-sparing; however, the largest safety trial to date evaluating celecoxib could not confirm its GI safety[28] (see discussion of NSAIDs in general treatment section).

Because T.W. is relatively young and does not have any other illnesses, a low-cost NSAID with a good safety profile such as ibuprofen is a reasonable initial selection. If convenience of administration is a more important consideration, longer-acting agents can be tried (with the exception of piroxicam). If the first agent is ineffective or not well tolerated, trials of several alternatives may be necessary to identify the optimal NSAID for T.W.

Adverse Effects

11. The decision is made for T.W. to start ibuprofen 800 mg TID with meals. Should T.W. be given misoprostol or other antiulcer therapy for prophylaxis against GI complications of NSAID therapy? Is there a correlation between dyspepsia and gastroduodenal mucosal injury? Would a COX-2–selective NSAID be preferable?

About 5% and 15% of patients with RA discontinue NSAID therapy because of dyspepsia,[25] and about 1.3% of patients taking NSAIDs for RA experience a serious GI complication.[103] As expected, the rate is somewhat lower for patients using NSAIDs for osteoarthritis (0.7%) because these patients generally use analgesics only as needed. Serious NSAID-induced GI complications account for about 103,000 hospitalizations annually in the United States and for approximately 16,500 NSAID-related deaths each year.[25] Although these figures warrant concern, most patients who experience NSAID-induced gastropathy suffer only superficial and self-limiting injury. Nevertheless, prevention of NSAID-induced GI bleeding should be an important focus, particularly in high-risk patients.

NSAID-induced gastroduodenal mucosal damage is primarily the result of COX-1 inhibition in the mucosal lining.[25] This leads to a reduction in protective mucus and bicarbonate secretion, mucosal blood flow, proliferation of the epithelium, and the ability of the mucosa to resist injury. Direct, NSAID-induced topical injury to the mucosa is thought to contribute to the damage but plays a relatively smaller role. Several methods are available to help minimize NSAID-induced GI toxicity. The management of NSAID-induced gastropathy can be divided into three categories: (1) treatment of NSAID-related dyspepsia, (2) prevention of NSAID-associated gastroduodenal ulcers, and (3) management of NSAID-related gastroduodenal ulcers.

Dyspepsia can be managed by simple measures, such as taking the NSAID with meals or a large glass of water; however, these measures are not effective in preventing GI ulcers and associated complications. In addition, dyspepsia is a poor correlate of endoscopically confirmed mucosal injury.[25] Histamine-2 (H_2)-receptor antagonists (e.g., ranitidine, famotidine) significantly reduce dyspepsia among NSAID users; however, NSAID users with RA who take a H_2-receptor antagonist may have a higher risk of developing serious GI complications compared with those who did not take these medications (odds ratio [OR], 2.14; 95% CI, 1.06 to 4.32).[104] The suppression of dyspepsia can give a false sense of security on the part of the patient and physician, leading to higher doses of NSAIDs and increased risk of major gastropathy. Therefore, H_2-receptor antagonists are not recommended for routine use in asymptomatic patients receiving NSAIDs. If NSAID-related dyspepsia is managed with a H_2-antagonists, the patient must be monitored carefully for any signs or symptoms of serious GI toxicity. Proton pump inhibitors (PPIs) such as lansoprazole (30 mg daily) and omeprazole (20 mg daily) relieve dyspepsia better than H_2-receptor antagonists and prevent the development of NSAID-induced gastroduodenal ulcers.[25,105,106] Therefore, PPIs are safe and effective for the treatment of NSAID-induced dyspepsia and can be considered if symptoms develop in T.W.

Routine concomitant antiulcer prophylactic therapy is not warranted for all patients taking NSAIDs.[8,24,25] The most effective means of preventing NSAID-related gastroduodenal ulcers is obviously to avoid their use. If NSAIDs must be used, nonacetylated salicylates should be considered (see Question 10). If nonacetylated salicylates prove to be subpotent and nonsalicylate NSAID therapy is initiated, the patient's risk for GI ulcer development must be assessed to determine the need for ulcer prevention measures.[25] Established risk factors include advancing age (particularly older than 60 years old), a history of ulcers, use of ulcer-promoting medications (corticosteroids, high-dose NSAIDs, concurrent use of more than one NSAID, anticoagulants), and serious systemic disorders such as cardiovascular disease.[4]

Risk factors for peptic ulcer disease development include concomitant *Helicobacter pylori* infection, cigarette smoking, and alcohol consumption. Although *H. pylori* eradication might reduce peptic ulcer risk in patients receiving NSAIDs, clinical trials have demonstrated only a minimal impact on preventing gastroduodenal injury.[107] If the patient is found to be at high risk, two strategies are available to help prevent gastroduodenal ulceration: use of concomitant gastroduodenal protective agents (i.e., misoprostol or PPI) or selection of NSAIDs with minimal gastropathy potential. Both misoprostol (100 to 200 mg four times daily), a prostaglandin E_1 analog, and PPIs (e.g., lansoprazole 30 mg daily, omeprazole 20 mg daily) are effective in preventing NSAID-induced gastroduodenal mucosal injury.[25,105,106] Dose-related GI upset, particularly diarrhea and abdominal pain, is a common cause of misoprostol intolerance. H_2-receptor antagonists appear to decrease the incidence of duodenal lesions but have failed to significantly prevent gastric ulcers. Sucralfate and antacids also are not beneficial.

Active NSAID-induced gastroduodenal ulcers are best treated by discontinuing the NSAID and initiating either a H_2 receptor antagonist (e.g., cimetidine 800 mg, ranitidine 150 mg, nizatidine 150 mg, famotidine 40 mg) or a PPI (same dosing as for ulcer prevention). If discontinuation of the NSAID is not feasible, ulcer healing can still be accomplished with a PPI.[25] Sucralfate, misoprostol, and antacids are ineffective treatments for NSAID-induced ulcers, and sucralfate is not effective in preventing ulcers.

The development of NSAIDs highly selective for COX-2 introduced the potential to reduce inflammation without the worrisome adverse effects of nonselective NSAIDs, particularly gastropathy (see general treatment section and Table 43-5). COX-2 selective inhibitors (e.g., celecoxib, rofecoxib, valdecoxib) do not interfere with COX-1 at therapeutic plasma concentrations in humans, but may have deleterious effects.[108–111] The concurrent use of COX-2 inhibitors may impair ulcer healing because conditions causing inflammation of the GI tract (e.g., gastric injury, healed ulcers, gastritis, inflammatory bowel disease) may induce COX-2 expression.. Although COX-2 inhibitors are associated with significantly less endoscopically confirmed gastroduodenal ulcers when compared to nonselective NSAIDs, their effect on clinically significant gastropathy is unclear.[108–110] The incidence of clinically significant gastropathy was evaluated in two large clinical trials involving celecoxib (CLASS- Celecoxib Long-Term Safety Study) and rofecoxib (VIGOR- Vioxx Gastrointestinal Outcomes Research).[28,29] Both of these trials evaluated approximately 8,000 patients and used at least double the maximum recommended dose of the COX-2 inhibitor (i.e., celecoxib 400 mg BID and rofecoxib 50 mg QD). CLASS consisted of primarily OA patients (72% OA, 28% RA) while all VIGOR patients had RA. The CLASS trial compared celecoxib to ibuprofen (800 mg TID) and diclofenac (75 mg BID), and the VIGOR trial compared rofecoxib to naproxen (500 mg BID). Up to 325 mg per day of aspirin use was allowed in CLASS (taken by 21% of patients),

but aspirin use was an exclusion criteria in VIGOR. The primary endpoint for CLASS at six months of treatment was complicated ulcers and for VIGOR at nine months of treatment was symptomatic ulcers. The secondary endpoint for CLASS included symptomatic and complicated ulcers, while VIGOR used only complicated ulcers as its secondary endpoint.

In the VIGOR study, rofecoxib was associated with significantly less symptomatic ulcers (primary endpoint) than naproxen. In the 6-month published CLASS study, only the secondary endpoint proved to significantly favor celecoxib over ibuprofen and diclofenac. These conclusions of CLASS and VIGOR are controversial. The published CLASS data consisted of no more than half of the treatment duration specified in the original study design.[112] The study design for CLASS consisted of two separate long-term comparisons with diclofenac (12 months) and ibuprofen (16 months). The reporting of only 6-months of data appears to seriously violate the study protocol. Complete results, available through the FDA's website, indicates that the two-fold reduction in combined symptomatic and complicated ulcers associated with celecoxib is only significant when compared to ibuprofen; no gastropathy advantage was identified when compared to diclofenac.[113] In fact, when an alternate definition of ulcer-related complications is applied to the CLASS trial (which was pre-planned by the FDA), a nonsignificant trend in favor of diclofenac was found.[112] Consequently, the FDA has not approved of product labeling that suggest GI-sparing advantages associated with celecoxib. The results from VIGOR, on the other hand, led to FDA approval of labeling changes reflecting the reduction in serious GI complications associated with rofecoxib. However, the FDA also required the rofecoxib labeling to reflect the higher rate of serious cardiovascular thromboembolic events (including myocardial infarction and angina) associated with rofecoxib treatment (1.8%) as opposed to naproxen treatment (0.6%).[114] This finding may be due to the lack of COX-2 expression by platelets, the platelet-inhibiting activity of naproxen (which may have provided cardioprotection), the higher risk of cardiovascular disease prevalent among RA patients, or a combination of these. The absence of increased cardiovascular events in the celecoxib group of the CLASS trial may have been related to the allowance of low-dose aspirin in study participants and the majority of patients having OA versus RA.

COX-2 inhibitors do not appear to be less renal toxic than nonselective NSAIDs (see Question 13). Because COX-2

Table 43-5 Comparison of Cyclooxygenase-1 and Cyclooxygenase-2 Isoforms[282]

Cyclooxygenase (COX) Isoform	COX-1	COX-2
Expression: continuous or induced?	Primarily continuous, although some evidence of induction	Primarily induced, but present continuously in several organs
Common organs/tissues	Nearly all organs, including stomach, kidneys, platelets, vasculature	Induced at sites of inflammation and neoplasms
		Continuously active in kidneys, small intestine, pancreas, brain, ovaries, uterus
Primary role	Housekeeping/maintenance	Inflammation, repair, neoplasia
	May be important when induced in response to inflammation	May be important in housekeeping/maintenance of organs which continuously express COX-2

appears to play a role in vascular prostacyclin production, inhibition of this enzyme may increase the incidence of vascular disease.

Without risk factors other than NSAID use, T.W. does not need an ulcer prophylaxis medication at this time.

Use in Renal Disease

12. **T.Z., a patient with congestive heart failure (CHF) previously well controlled with furosemide 40 mg/day, digoxin 0.125 mg/day, metoprolol 50 mg BID, and lisinopril 40 mg/day, returns for a prescription refill of ibuprofen 600 mg TID, which he takes for his RA. He has noted increased leg swelling over the past 2 weeks associated with a weight gain of several pounds, increasing shortness of breath (SOB), and easy fatigability. What information should be provided about potential ibuprofen side effects to T.Z.?**

Mild fluid retention occurs in approximately 5% of NSAID users, and NSAID-induced kidney disease occurs in <1% of patients.[115] NSAID therapy should be monitored carefully in patients with CHF, liver disease with associated ascites, compromised renal function, or when diuretics are administered concomitantly. In these situations, renal function highly depends on local production of prostaglandin E_2 within the kidney to offset the vasoconstrictor effects of high concentrations of angiotensin, vasopressin, and catecholamines.[116] Inhibition of COX by NSAIDs within the kidney leads to reduced prostaglandin concentrations and unopposed vasoconstriction. Consequently, urine output declines, serum blood urea nitrogen begins to rise, serum creatinine eventually increases, and fluid is retained. This phenomenon is a potential complication associated with all of the currently marketed NSAIDs.[116,117]

T.Z. should be informed that his leg swelling, weight gain, SOB, and fatigability might be caused by ibuprofen.

13. **How should this drug-related problem be managed? Why would a COX-2 inhibitor be preferred over a nonselective NSAID for T.Z.?**

Initially, ibuprofen (Motrin) should be discontinued until renal function normalizes. In several studies, sulindac (Clinoril) was associated with less adverse effects on the kidney than other NSAIDS.[118–121] The reason(s) for this are unclear, but one explanation is that the active sulfide metabolite undergoes renal metabolism and, therefore, might not achieve tissue concentrations within the kidney sufficient to reduce prostaglandin production.[122] Unfortunately, patients do not seem to benefit from sulindac as well as from other NSAIDs. Nabumetone (Relafen), an NSAID with moderate COX-2 selectivity, has less of an effect on glomerular filtration than sulindac or ibuprofen.[123] The nonacetylated salicylates have minimal prostaglandin-inhibiting activity and could be alternatives for T.Z.

COX-2 inhibitors are associated with renal complications similar to nonselective NSAIDs. Celecoxib use has resulted in a 2.1% incidence of edema, 0.8% incidence of new hypertension, and 0.6% exacerbation of preexisting hypertension postmarketing.[124] These event rates are similar to those reported with nonselective NSAIDs. Similarly, in a study comparing the incidence of edema and blood pressure elevation in elderly patients with OA receiving rofecoxib 25 mg QD or celecoxib

200 mg QD significantly more patients in the rofecoxib group experienced edema (9.5% versus 4.9% in the celecoxib group) and blood pressure elevation (17% versus 11% in the celecoxib group).[125] The relatively higher dose of rofecoxib used (12.5 mg QD is recommended for the elderly and those at risk for renal hypoperfusion) might have contributed to this difference.[109]

Regardless of the NSAID selected, close monitoring of renal function continues to be warranted.

14. **What other renal syndromes are associated with NSAID therapy?**

In addition to previously described acute renal failure, NSAIDs may produce various renally mediated complications, including nephrotic syndrome, interstitial nephritis, hyponatremia, abnormalities of water metabolism, and hyperkalemia.[126] Nephrotic syndrome, unlike NSAID-induced acute renal failure, may occur anytime (i.e., from days to years) after starting therapy; resolution after discontinuation of the NSAID also may follow a prolonged course (as short as 1 month or as long as 1 year). Hematuria, pyuria, and proteinuria without prior renal disease differentiates nephrotic syndrome from other NSAID-induced renal problems. Histologically, nephrotic syndrome is characterized by interstitial lymphocytic infiltrates, vacuolar degeneration of proximal and distal tubules, and fusion of epithelial foot processes of glomeruli.

Prostaglandin-mediated inhibition of active chloride transport, regulation of medullary blood flow within the kidney, and antagonism of antidiuretic hormone can be suppressed by NSAIDs. As a result, urine is maximally concentrated, free water clearance is limited, and water retention that is disproportionate to sodium retention can occur. The resulting hyponatremia can be severe and might be potentiated by thiazide diuretics.[127]

Local prostaglandin synthesis also can stimulate renin production within the kidney. NSAID therapy can critically attenuate this regulatory mechanism in some situations, resulting in reduced aldosterone-mediated potassium excretion and hyperkalemia.

Although the mechanism is poorly understood, some NSAIDs have been associated with sustained mean arterial pressure (MAP) increases of 5 to 6 mm Hg,[128] presumably the result of COX-2 inhibition and sodium/water retention. However, in several studies, only patients taking antihypertensive medications experienced NSAID-induced MAP elevations, while those who controlled their hypertension without medications were unaffected by NSAID therapy. It appears, therefore, that NSAIDs can interfere with the action of antihypertensive drug therapy by a mechanism that has yet to be identified.

Laboratory Test Monitoring for NSAID Therapy

15. **When should routine renal or liver function be tested during NSAID therapy?**

Patients at high risk for NSAID-induced renal disease (see Questions 12 to 14) should have their serum creatinine checked weekly for several weeks after initiation of therapy because renal insufficiency occurs early in the course of therapy.[127] NSAID-induced nephrotic syndrome and allergic interstitial nephritis occur an average of 6.6 months and 15 days after NSAID initiation, respectively.

In most cases, liver function testing is unnecessary.[127] Although NSAIDs may elevate liver enzymes, severe hepatotoxicity is rare. Abnormal liver function tests without clinical symptoms have no impact on patient outcome and have not been associated with severe hepatotoxicity. However, patients who appear to be at greater risk for hepatotoxicity are those with established or suspected intrinsic liver disease and those receiving diclofenac. These patients should have liver function tested no later than 8 weeks after initiation of therapy because liver toxicity manifests early in therapy if at all.

Patient Instructions

16. **What instructions should accompany T.W.'s (the patient from Questions 1 through 4, 10, and 11) ibuprofen prescription?**

It is important for patients to understand the purpose and proper use of NSAIDs for RA. Patients should be informed that NSAIDs are used to provide quick relief of pain and inflammation associated with RA, but do nothing to slow or stop the progression of RA. It should be explained that the latter only can be provided by a disease-modifying drug. Patients should also understand that moderate to high daily doses of NSAIDs are required for anti-inflammatory activity, as opposed to analgesic and antipyretic effects which can be achieved with single and low doses.

Patients should be instructed to keep the NSAID container tightly closed and to avoid storing NSAIDs, particularly aspirin, in moist environments (e.g., bathrooms). Aspirin is hydrolyzed to salicylic acid and acetic acid with moisture. Prescription NSAIDs and aspirin come in child-proof safety containers, but many arthritic patients have difficulty with these safety closures because of diminished grip strength and hand deformities. If an NSAID is dispensed in a conventional closure container, it is necessary to explain the hazards of accidental ingestion by children and, as required by law in most states, obtain a signed release form.

Patients should be taught to recognize the signs and symptoms of GI bleeding (e.g., nausea, vomiting, anorexia, gastric pain), GI bleeding as manifested by melena (described to the patient as "dark, tarry stool") or emesis of coagulated blood (described to the patient as, "vomiting up what appears to be 'coffee grounds'"). The patient should be instructed to contact their health care professional immediately for further instructions if any such signs or symptoms occur.

TRADITIONAL DISEASE-MODIFYING ANTIRHEUMATIC DRUGS

17. **Which traditional DMARD therapies are most appropriate for T.W.?**

Every newly diagnosed RA patient is a candidate for DMARD therapy, which should be started within 3 months of diagnosis.[8] In addition, a relatively more potent DMARD (e.g., MTX) should be chosen for initial therapy in patients with very active disease or a poor prognosis, since radiographic evidence of disease progression is most rapid in the first several years of active disease[129,130] (Fig. 43-7). Although most DMARDs are associated with potentially serious side effects, the majority of these side effects are reversible and

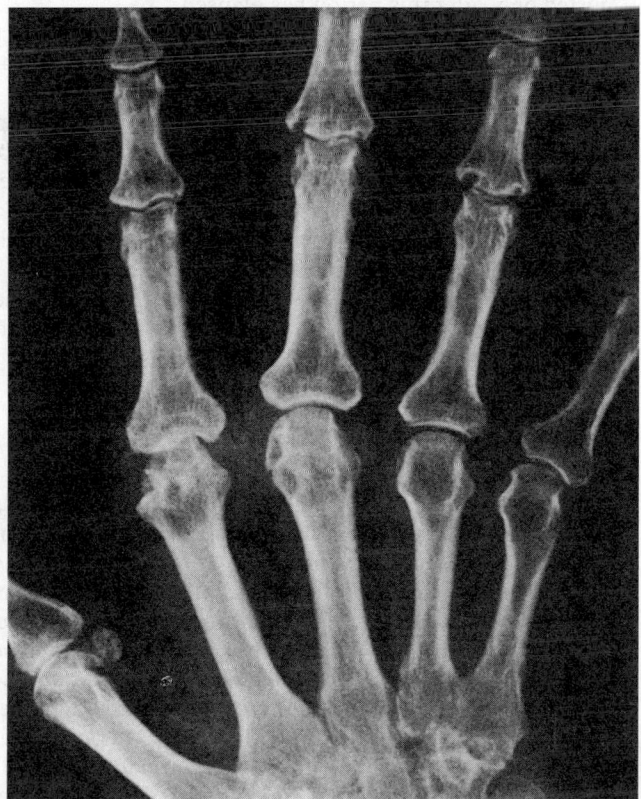
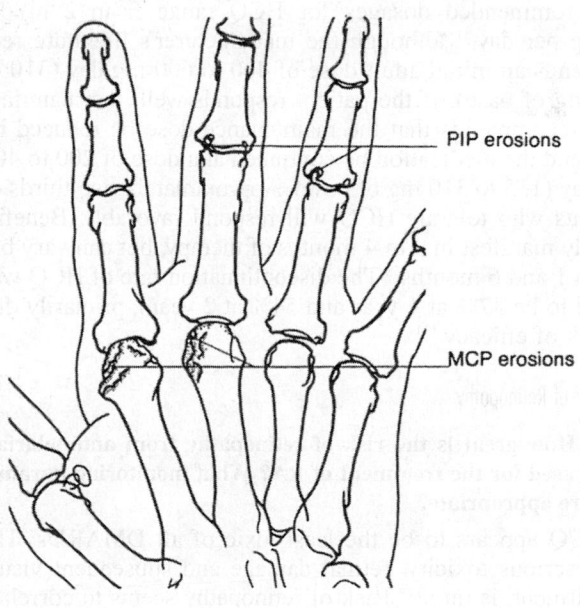

FIGURE 43-7. Radiograph of the hand in RA showing both active erosions at the metacarpophalangeal joints (MCPs) and old well-demarcated erosions at the proximal interphalangeal joints (PIPs).

seldom lead to serious complications if the patient is monitored appropriately.

Most patients with active RA receive at least one DMARD with an NSAID.[8] In addition, low-dose oral corticosteroids are often used on an "as needed" basis for brief periods of severe disease activity or while awaiting the onset of DMARD action. During periods of disease remission, NSAID therapy can be discontinued; however, attempts to discontinue DMARDs have resulted in disease reactivation or "rebound flare" and resumption of the discontinued DMARD is not always successful in re-establishing control. Therefore, successful DMARD therapy should be continued indefinitely. Although the long-term safety and efficacy of DMARDs combined with biological agents remains to be determined, use of this combination has yielded promising results and is becoming more common (see Questions 39 and 43).

DMARD selection considerations were discussed previously in the general treatment section. The selection of DMARDs and their use in combination appears to be more effective than DMARD monotherapy (see Question 38). For milder cases of RA, HCQ or sulfasalazine are reasonable first selections.[8] The response to either agent should be apparent within 1 to 4 months, at which time a change in therapy can be considered if necessary.

Antimalarials
Dosing

18. Although T.W.'s presentation may warrant a more potent DMARD, the decision is made to start HCQ. What dosages would be appropriate, and when should clinical improvement be expected?

Recommended dosages for HCQ range from 2 to 6.5 mg/kg per day,[21] although the manufacturer's literature recommends an initial adult dose of 400 to 600 mg/day (310 to 465 mg of base). If the patient responds well, the manufacturer recommends that the maintenance dose be reduced by 50% and the medication be continued at a dose of 200 to 400 mg/day (155 to 310 mg of base). Approximately two-thirds of patients who tolerate HCQ will respond favorably. Benefits usually manifest in 2 to 4 months of therapy, but can vary between 1 and 6 months.[8] The discontinuation rate of HCQ was found to be 37% at 1 year and 54% at 2 years, primarily due to lack of efficacy.[131]

Risk of Retinopathy

19. How great is the risk of retinopathy from antimalarials when used for the treatment of RA? What monitoring parameters are appropriate?

HCQ appears to be the least toxic of all DMARDs. The most serious toxicity, retinal damage and subsequent visual impairment, is rare.[127] Risk of retinopathy seems to correlate with cumulative dose (>800 g) and age (older than 70 years of age). The risk relation to age appears to be related to the increased prevalence of macular disease in the elderly. In addition, doses of HCQ exceeding 6.0 to 6.5 mg/kg can increase risk of retinal damage, particularly in patients with renal or hepatic dysfunction.

Symptoms of antimalarial retinopathy include difficulty seeing faces or entire words, glare intolerance, poor night vision, or loss of peripheral vision.[127] If any of these symptoms occur, patients should be instructed to stop therapy immediately and an ophthalmologic evaluation should be performed. The fully developed lesion of antimalarial retinopathy is seen on ophthalmoscopy as a pigmentary disturbance with a characteristic "bull's eye" appearance in the macular region. Because 4-amino-quinolines bind to melanin, they concentrate in the uveal tract and retinal pigment epithelium. They are retained for years in the retina, and retinopathy may be progressive even after stopping the drug.

Baseline eye examination is not required in patients younger than 40 years of age with no family history of eye disease. The first ophthalmologic examination is recommended after 6 months of therapy, followed by an examination with central field testing every 6 to 12 months. More frequent testing is recommended for patients with renal dysfunction or patients who have received HCQ therapy for >10 years. Benign corneal deposits of antimalarial drug may occur during therapy. Although this adverse effect may be symptomatic, it is harmless, reversible when the antimalarial drug is discontinued, and not related to the more serious and less common retinopathy.[132]

Sulfasalazine

20. If SSZ were chosen as initial therapy for T.W., when would you expect the therapeutic effects to manifest and what adverse effects would you anticipate?

The onset of SSZ effect is generally more rapid than HCQ and may be apparent within 1 month;[8] however, a clinical response may be delayed for 4 months, and doses should be adjusted only after this period has elapsed.

Compared with other DMARDs, adverse effects associated with SSZ are relatively mild, consisting of nausea, abdominal discomfort, heartburn, dizziness, headaches, skin rashes, and, rarely, hematologic effects such as leukopenia (1% to 3%) or thrombocytopenia (rare).[133] A complete blood count (CBC) is recommended every 2 to 4 weeks for the first 3 months of therapy, then every 3 months thereafter. Leukopenia more commonly manifests within the first 6 months of therapy. To minimize GI-related adverse effects, SSZ is initiated at 500 mg or 1 g daily and the dosage is increased at weekly intervals by 500 mg until 1,000 mg two or three times daily is reached.

Gold
Preparations and Adverse Reactions

21. S.S., a 41-year-old Asian woman diagnosed with RA, presents with inflammation in both hands (MCP and PIP joints), wrists, elbows, shoulders, knees, hips, ankles, and MTP joints. Objective test results include radiographic evidence of joint erosion in both hands and elbows, a positive RF (dilution of 1:1,280), and ESR of 78 mm/hr. Her symptoms were managed over the past year with ibuprofen 800 mg TID; however, pain and inflammation have progressively worsened over several months. ROM testing reveals deficits in wrist flexion and extension (20° bilaterally for both motions; normal, 90 and 70°, respectively), elbow flexion (90° bilaterally with flexion contracture; normal, 160°), shoulder abduction (70° right, 90° left; normal, 180°), and plantarflexion of both ankles (20° bilaterally;

normal, 45°). **Three firm, pea-sized, nontender moveable subcutaneous nodules are found on both elbows at the ulnar border, two on the right and one on the left. In your discussion about considering DMARD therapy, S.S. states that she does not want gold therapy ". . . because I've heard that it has terrible side effects." What gold preparations are available, and is S.S.'s concern about adverse effects warranted?**

Two parenteral gold preparations are available: gold sodium thiomalate (Myochrysine), an aqueous solution, and aurothioglucose (Solganal), an oil suspension. Although an oral gold formulation, auranofin (Ridaura), is also available, it is slow in onset (4 to 6 months) and is less efficacious.[8] The parenteral formulations, containing approximately 50% gold by weight expressed as milligrams of complex, generally are considered to be equally effective.[21] Aurothioglucose must be shaken thoroughly before withdrawal from its vial and a large bore needle is necessary to draw up this viscous suspension. Lumps at the intramuscular injection site sometimes can be troublesome to the patient.

Toxicities with both injectable gold preparations are numerous and largely responsible for their high rate of discontinuation. In a 6-year prospective trial, nearly half of patients receiving gold sodium thiomalate discontinued therapy, with 95% of those discontinuing because of toxicity.[40] The toxicity profiles of the parenteral gold preparations differ. A vasomotor reaction (also termed nitritoid reaction), which manifests as nausea, weakness, flushing, tachycardia, and/or syncope, may occur in up to 5% of patients receiving gold sodium thiomalate. These reactions generally are mild, are transient, and often can be alleviated by having the patient lie down.

Rarely, severe myocardial ischemia or infarction may result.[134] The cause of this reaction is unknown, but may be related to the vehicle or preservative in the thiomalate preparation; it has not been reported with aurothioglucose. Patients with concomitant cardiovascular disease or patients who experience a nitritoid reaction after an injection of gold sodium thiomalate, therefore, can be managed safely with aurothioglucose.

Nonvasomotor reactions, consisting of transient stiffness, arthralgias, and myalgias, developed in 15% of patients after initiation of gold sodium thiomalate therapy in one retrospective study.[135] Substituting aurothioglucose resulted in decreased severity in 40% of the patients.

Skin eruptions, stomatitis, and albuminuria are more common in patients who receive the aqueous gold sodium thiomalate preparation than in patients who received the oil suspension of aurothioglucose.[136] Aurothioglucose also is more commonly associated with renal toxicity than gold sodium thiomalate, although the overall incidence is rare.[127] Membranous nephropathy (most common), nephrotic syndrome, and interstitial nephritis have been reported. Hematuria and proteinuria may be early indicators of membranous nephropathy; however proteinuria may occur transiently in up to 50% of patients receiving aurothioglucose. Patients who develop proteinuria should have a 24-hour urinalysis performed. Gold therapy should be discontinued if protein excretion is >500 mg/24 hr.

Both parenteral gold preparations have been associated with thrombocytopenia (1% to 3%) and aplastic anemia (<1%).[137] Both reactions are believed to be idiosyncratic and may appear suddenly. Screening for urine protein and a CBC should be performed before each injection (i.e., every week) for the first 20 to 22 weeks, then before every other injection. In addition, patients should be asked about the occurrence of pruritus, skin eruptions, purpura, sore throat, and stomatitis before each dose of gold is administered.

Cutaneous reactions (e.g., pruritus, erythema, a fine morbilliform rash on the neck or extremities) may develop after the first few injections of gold. Cutaneous reactions are common, usually subside within several days, and do not seem to be affected by subsequent injections. Although a highly pruritic localized eruption resembling pityriasis rosea is common, gold dermatitis may assume many different forms, including exfoliative dermatitis.[21] Therapy should be discontinued if a pruritic dermatitis develops. Mild dermal reactions may be managed with topical corticosteroids.[137]

If discontinued, gold can be reintroduced in a reduced dosage following resolution of rashes (see Question 23). Gold treatments should be discontinued if white blood cells (WBCs) decline to <3,500 cells/mm³, if platelets fall to <100,000 cells/mm³, or if the hemoglobin concentration falls rapidly.[137] Although eosinophilia may be associated with toxic reactions, it is not a reliable predictor of gold toxicity and is not an indication to discontinue gold therapy.[138]

Thrombocytopenia may be life-threatening and sometimes is difficult to treat because of the long half-life of gold.[137] Most cases respond to cessation of gold therapy. Platelet or red cell transfusions should be judiciously administered if severe thrombocytopenia or anemia/hemorrhage occurs. Appropriate antibiotic therapy should be given for patients who develop fever and absolute neutropenia (<1,000/mm³).[137]

Other unusual but potentially serious complications of gold therapy include colitis, pneumonitis, and cholestatic hepatitis.[139–142] Corneal chrysiasis also can occur but does not lead to ocular complications.[143]

AUR capsules, containing 3 mg of gold, are 25% bioavailable.[144] The recommended AUR daily dose of 6 mg can be given either as single or divided doses. AUR is better tolerated than parenteral gold formulations, but is significantly less effective.[8] Like parenteral chrysotherapy, benefit can occur as early as 6 to 8 weeks after starting AUR, but objective benefits may not be apparent for several months. Overall, AUR has a slower onset of action when compared with gold sodium thiomalate.[145] AUR must be monitored in a manner similar to parenteral therapy. Proteinuria and bone marrow suppression occur with AUR, but the incidence is low.[146] The incidence of rashes necessitating AUR withdrawal is lower compared with parenteral gold therapy, but loose stools and diarrhea are encountered more commonly (47%).

S.S.'s concerns have merit. Although gold is an effective DMARD, none of the gold formulations are ideal. Gold sodium thiomalate is easier to administer, but is associated with more frequent side effects compared with aurothioglucose. Aurothioglucose carries a low but serious risk of nephrotoxicity. Both parenteral forms of gold are commonly discontinued because of side effects. AUR is the best tolerated gold preparation, but the least effective and is associated with significant diarrhea.

Dosing

22. **How is parenteral gold administered? Is serum drug monitoring of value in gold therapy?**

The standard treatment schedule consists of an initial intramuscular test dose of 10 mg followed by a 25 mg IM dose 1 week later. The third and subsequent weekly intramuscular injections of 25 to 50 mg should be continued until the cumulative dose reaches 1 g, toxicity occurs, or major benefit is derived.[21,137] If a satisfactory response is achieved, maintenance doses of 25 to 50 mg every other week are recommended. If the disease remains stable, doses can be administered every third and subsequently every fourth week for an indefinite period.[137]

Attempts to correlate serum gold concentrations to clinical outcomes generally have been unsuccessful.[147,148] Furthermore, toxicity has not been correlated with serum gold concentrations.[147]

23. After 10 weeks of treatment with aurothioglucose (total, 435 mg), L.T. developed pruritus and a rash on her abdomen. Gold was withheld and she was given a prescription for triamcinolone cream. Should L.T's gold therapy be discontinued?

Dermatologic reactions to gold occur in 15% to 30% of patients.[137] Because of fears of subsequent exfoliative dermatitis and the belief that dermatologic reactions recur upon rechallenge, there is a natural reluctance to continue gold treatment after the appearance of dermatitis or stomatitis. However, in one series of patients, gold treatments were reinstituted successfully in 28 of 30 patients in whom dermatologic reactions developed.[149] One of these patients who presented initially with severe exfoliative dermatitis was treated successfully with gold several years later. Gold therapy was reinstituted in these patients as follows. After waiting at least 6 weeks after the lesions had healed completely, a 1-mg test dose of gold was administered intramuscularly. Subsequent doses were increased to 2 mg, then to 5 mg, and then to 10 mg at 2- to 4-week intervals. Thereafter, 5-mg increments were added until a dose of 50 mg weekly was attained. Dermatologic reactions did not develop in any of these patients subsequently. Gold therapy, therefore, need not be abandoned in L.T.

Auranofin

24. J.M., a patient receiving gold sodium thiomalate for 1 year and responding well to a maintenance regimen of 50 mg IM Q 4 wk asks about switching to AUR. Will switching to AUR from parenteral gold maintain J.M.'s RA under good control? Can patients who have discontinued parenteral therapy because of adverse side effects be treated with AUR?

Some patients originally treated with parenteral therapy can be switched to AUR and remain well controlled.[150,151] This experience is not universal, however, and it is not possible to predict which patients can be switched successfully to oral therapy.

When parenteral gold is injected weekly, the relative cost of parenteral gold therapy (including office visits and monitoring) is more than the costs associated with daily AUR therapy. When gold injections are given every 2 to 3 weeks, the cost of parenteral and oral therapy is similar, depending on local laboratory and medical costs. When injections are given monthly, the cost of parenteral therapy usually is less than for oral therapy. Because this patient is well controlled, little is to be gained by switching from parenteral therapy to AUR, either from an economic or therapeutic standpoint.

Data are limited on the use of AUR in patients who experienced side effects from parenteral gold. Because rashes usually are mild and proteinuria is reversible if the patient is properly monitored, a trial of AUR in patients withdrawn from parenteral gold for these reasons may be justified.[152] It is inadvisable, however, to initiate AUR in patients who were withdrawn from parenteral gold because of bone marrow suppression.

Methotrexate
Dosing

25. S.S. (from Question 21) will start MTX therapy. Why is MTX a good selection for her?

MTX is currently the initial DMARD of choice among most rheumatologists, particularly for patients with severe disease.[8] S.S. has many indicators of severe disease, including a younger age of onset (because the patient has many years of life ahead, aggressive therapy is necessary to preserve joint function), positive RF with a high titer, multiple joint involvement, elevated ESR, radiographic evidence of bone erosions, and extra-articular manifestations (subcutaneous nodules). The disease prognosis for S.S. is clearly poor, and a relatively potent DMARD is indicated. MTX has a rapid onset (1 to 2 months before a "plateau" of effectiveness), a high efficacy rate, and the most predictable benefit of any DMARD.[8] To date, no DMARD has yielded longer sustained benefit in RA management; the probability of continuing MTX therapy at 5 years was 62% in one study.[33] In contrast, only half of patients taking any traditional DMARD except MTX in a different study were able to continue therapy beyond 9 to 24 months, with steady declines thereafter.[68]

Based on clinical presentation, laboratory test results, and properties of DMARDs, MTX is an appropriate selection for S.S.'s very active RA. Hydroxychloroquine, the second most commonly used DMARD, or sulfasalazine are reserved for milder cases of RA.

26. How should MTX be administered when it is used in the treatment of RA?

MTX is administered orally at an initial dose of 7.5 mg once per week. The dose may be given all at once (more common) or divided into 2.5 mg every 12 hours for a total of three doses (i.e., "pulse dosing"). The rationale for pulsing MTX doses in RA is unclear; however, it is as effective as single weekly dosing and may be associated with reduced hepatotoxicity.[153] If no objective response is obtained by 6 weeks (i.e., the time at which the plateau of therapeutic effectiveness occurs), the dosage is increased to 15 mg/week (or 5 mg every 12 hours for three doses) and therapy is continued for a minimum of an additional 12 weeks.[154] If no response is seen at this time, several options should be considered: the dosage may be increased to the maximum of 25 mg/week; the patient may be switched to the injectable (subcutaneous or intramuscular) formulation to improve bioavailability; the same dose may be continued for a longer period; or MTX may be discontinued.[8,48,155] Liquid methotrexate is a less expensive alternative to the tablet formulation and is equally efficacious.[48]

RA patients with a short disease duration (i.e., <3 years) who achieve disease remission with weekly MTX therapy appear to remain in remission when switched to every-other-week administration of the same dose (i.e., monthly dose is reduced by 50%).[156] This effect was demonstrated for up to 6 months in a clinical trial. However, it is not known whether every-other-week dosing of MTX prevents joint destruction as effectively as weekly dosing.

Adverse Effects

27. How should MTX therapy be monitored?

Frequent side effects associated with low-dose MTX therapy include nausea and other GI disturbances, malaise, dizziness, mucositis, and mild alopecia.[127] More serious but less common adverse effects include myelosuppression, pneumonitis, and hepatic fibrosis and cirrhosis.[127] Patients should have a complete blood count (CBC), liver function tests (LFTs), and serum creatinine check at baseline, monthly for the first 6 months of therapy, and every 4 to 8 weeks during therapy. Renal dysfunction can result in accumulation of MTX and higher risk of myelosuppression. Hypersensitivity pneumonitis, occurring in 1% to 2% of patients, has no known risk factors for development, although it may be more common in patients with a history of lung disease.[48] In addition, hypersensitivity pneumonitis can occur at any time during therapy and at any MTX dosage. A baseline chest radiograph is recommended within the year before MTX initiation. If the patient is found to have pre-existing lung disease, MTX treatment should be reconsidered because further pulmonary damage could be devastating to the patient. Otherwise, the patient should be monitored carefully for cough, dyspnea on exertion, and SOB at each visit.

MTX-induced liver disease is rare, but age and duration of therapy increase risk.[127] Other possible risk factors include obesity, diabetes mellitus, ethanol consumption, and a history of hepatitis B or C. MTX should be prescribed with great caution, if at all, in patients with pre-existing liver disease. Liver function test should be monitored in all patients receiving MTX as described above. LFTs should be obtained just before each scheduled round of MTX because mild increases in liver enzymes are seen commonly for 1 to 2 days after administration. MTX is withheld if liver enzymes rise to three times baseline or remain elevated for sustained periods during therapy.[157] The ability of liver function test monitoring to predict risk for serious hepatotoxicity is unclear. In psoriatic patients receiving MTX, liver enzyme elevations do not predict risk of serious hepatotoxicity.[158] It is noteworthy that in these studies liver function tests were performed only on the day of biopsy rather than at regular intervals before biopsy. Patients taking MTX should be advised to avoid alcohol and report to their health care provider if symptoms of jaundice or dark urine occur. Routine liver biopsies are not recommended (see Question 28).

28. Should a baseline liver biopsy be performed before starting MTX?

At one time, routine liver biopsies were recommended for RA patients receiving MTX. This recommendation was based on the longer experience with use of MTX in psoriasis. Cirrhosis was reported in up to 26% of psoriasis patients.[159] However, serial liver biopsies are not recommended or cost effective for monitoring hepatotoxicity in RA patients. Liver biopsy, however, is indicated in patients with suspected liver disease (a biopsy should be performed before treatment) and in patients with persistent liver function test abnormalities during, or after discontinuation of, MTX therapy (Table 43-6).[160]

29. Should either supplemental folate or folinic acid be administered along with MTX to reduce risk of drug-related toxicity?

In preliminary studies, folate supplementation was effective in preventing or treating GI disturbances, mucositis (mouth or GI ulcerations), and possibly alopecia attributable to MTX therapy.[161–166] In larger randomized controlled trials, the only adverse effect significantly reduced by either folic acid or folinic acid (leucovorin) is the incidence of alanine aminotransferase (ALT) elevation.[167,168] In a study evaluating more than 400 RA patients, folic acid (1 mg/day), folinic acid (2.5 mg/week), or placebo was added to MTX therapy (7.5 mg/week, titrated up to 25 mg/week). Hepatotoxicity leading to MTX discontinuation occurred in 26%, 4%, and 4% of patients in the placebo, folic acid, and folinic acid groups ($P < 0.001$ for treatment groups vs. placebo). Since hepatotoxicity is one of most common reasons for MTX discontinuation, the benefit of folate supplementation is clearly important.

Concerns have been raised about whether folate supplementation reduces the efficacy of MTX, which is a folate antagonist. Several trials have suggested that a slightly higher dose of MTX is needed in folate users to produce clinical benefits similar to that achieved by patients without folate supplementation.[167,168] Clinically, however, there does not appear to be a significant attenuation of MTX efficacy associated with concomitant folate supplementation and, very importantly, folate supplementation reduces the incidence of MTX discontinuation secondary to ALT elevation.

Although both folic acid or folinic acid may be used for folate supplementation, folic acid at a dosage of 1 mg/day or 7

Table 43-6   Proposed Criteria for Liver Biopsies During MTX Therapy

Baseline liver biopsy if patient has:

1. History of significant regular ethanol consumption, arbitrarily defined as 3 drinks/day
2. History of hepatitis, jaundice, or liver disease

Liver biopsy during therapy if:

1. Six of 12 monthly determinations of AST are elevated into the abnormal range
2. Baseline normal serum albumin falls to 3.3 g/dL
3. Three to 5 of 12 monthly elevations of AST are in the abnormal range for 3 consecutive years

Liver biopsy results:

Biopsy showing Roenigk class I, II, or IIIA (minimal fibrosis) would be grouped as a "benign" hepatic outcome and a repeat biopsy would be performed only if serum albumin falls to lLd3.3 g/dL. Roenigk Class IIIB (significant hepatic fibrosis) or IV (cirrhosis) would be cause to permanently discontinue MTX

AST, aspartate aminotransferase; MTX, methotrexate.
Adapted from reference 152.

mg once a week is recommended over folinic acid because of cost and ease of administration.[127]

30. S.S. starts MTX 7.5 mg along with folic acid 7 mg PO every week. Nine weeks later, she returns to the clinic with subjective and objective improvement in morning stiffness, fatigability, and joint tenderness and swelling. However, she has noted increased SOB and dyspnea over the past week. Can this be related to MTX?

As discussed in Question 27, pneumonitis is a rare but important complication of MTX therapy characterized by a nonproductive cough, malaise, and fever, progressing to severe dyspnea.[169] Recognition of this unusual reaction is important to ensure that MTX is discontinued before the pneumonitis progresses to respiratory failure. After discontinuation of MTX, pulmonary function improves. Corticosteroids can accelerate improvement in pulmonary symptoms associated with pneumonitis. S.S.'s dyspnea and SOB may be related to MTX. If appropriate tests rule out other causes for her pulmonary complaints, MTX-induced pulmonary toxicity should be considered and treatment discontinued.

31. What are considered major MTX food and drug interactions?

Concurrent NSAID therapy, which is very common for RA patients, increases MTX serum concentrations and increases risk of toxicity.[48] MTX doses should be adjusted cautiously in patients taking NSAIDs regularly. Trimethoprim may increase the risk of MTX-induced bone marrow suppression. Major liver damage, including some deaths, have been reported with the concurrent use of MTX and leflunomide; as a result, this combination is not recommended. In a small observational study of 39 RA patients treated with MTX, low caffeine consumption (<120 mg/day) was associated with 30% greater improvement in morning stiffness and joint pain when compared to high caffeine consumption (>180 mg/day).[170] Caffeine may interfere with the anti-inflammatory effects of MTX.

Leflunomide
Place in Therapy

32. B.W., a 36-year-old woman, has severe, progressive RA and is not responding sufficiently to MTX therapy. Why would LEF be a reasonable consideration for her?

Leflunomide (Arava), an oral DMARD, can slow the progression of RA; however, its long-term safety and efficacy remain to be determined, because clinical trials only were of 6 to 24 months in duration. Nevertheless, the onset of benefit (as early as 4 weeks), rate of discontinuation of therapy resulting from lack of efficacy or toxicity, overall efficacy (including slowing radiographic progression), and benefit after 24 months of treatment were similar for LEF, MTX, and SSZ.[48,171–175] However, postmarketing surveillance of LEF has resulted in the reporting of more than 130 severe liver-related adverse events, including 12 liver-related deaths likely due to this drug.[176] In one clinical evaluation, more than 75% of patients (N = 369) who received etanercept or infliximab continued with therapy after 20 months compared to only 22% of LEF-treated patients.[177] Although the incidence of hepatotoxicity was not specifically reported, adverse effects were the

primary reason for LEF discontinuation during the first 6 months of treatment.

LEF is as safe and effective as MTX or SSZ in early randomized clinical trials; however, postmarketing reports are a reminder that diligent patient monitoring is crucial. It is not known whether the addition of other DMARDs to MTX therapy is a better therapeutic option than substituting LEF for MTX (see Question 38).

Dosing

33. How would you initiate LEF in B.W.? How would you monitor B.W. for adverse effects?

The active metabolite of LEF, A771726 or M1, is responsible for virtually all the pharmacologic activity of LEF.[178] The serum half-life of the M1 metabolite is approximately 2 weeks. As a result, LEF should be initiated with a loading dose of 100 mg once daily for 3 days to reduce time to steady-state, followed by 20 mg once daily. If this dose is not tolerated, the dose should be reduced to 10 mg once daily.

Monitoring for Adverse Effects

Common adverse effects to LEF include diarrhea (20% to 30%), rash (10%), alopecia (10% to 17%), and reversible liver enzyme elevations more than three times the upper limit of normal (ULN) (2% to 4%).[172,178] Routine laboratory testing includes a baseline ALT followed by monthly ALT testing for several months. When it is evident that ALT results are stable and within normal limits, testing can be performed less often according to the clinician's judgment. Because of the risk of liver toxicity and the need for activation by the liver to the M1 active metabolite, LEF is not recommended in patients with pre-existing liver disease, including hepatitis B or C.

Potential hepatotoxicity is the greatest concern with LEF. The rate of LEF-induced liver enzyme elevation is not significantly different than MTX. Guidelines for managing potential hepatotoxicity include dosage reduction from 20 mg/day to 10 mg/day if ALT (SGPT) increases more than twofold the ULN.[178] If ALT elevations remain steady between two to three times the ULN and treatment continuation is desired, a liver biopsy is recommended. If ALT elevations are persistently more than three times the ULN despite dosage reduction and cholestyramine administration to enhance elimination (see Question 34), then the drug should be discontinued and another course of cholestyramine elimination therapy should be given.

Enhancement of Elimination With Cholestyramine

34. After 2 months of therapy, B.W. does not respond to LEF and the decision is made to discontinue treatment, especially since she is beginning to consider starting a family. What precautions must be taken when discontinuing LEF?

Leflunomide (pregnancy category X) has not been tested in pregnant women but appears to greatly increase the risk of fetal death or teratogenicity in animals receiving as little as 1% of human equivalent doses.[178] Following discontinuation of therapy, however, up to 2 years may be required to reach undetectable plasma M1 metabolite levels. As a result, an elimination procedure involving cholestyramine is recommended for all women of childbearing potential who discontinue LEF. After stopping the medication, cholestyramine 8 g three times a day is administered for 11 days (which need not be consecutive). Plasma levels of the M1 metabolite are reduced by 40% to 65% in 24 to 48 hours and should become nondetectable (i.e., <0.02 mg/L) at the end of therapy. Two blood tests should be performed at least 14 days apart to verify the absence of the metabolite. If plasma M1 levels remain >0.02 mg/L, more cholestyramine should be administered. In addition, cholestyramine can be used to enhance elimination in patients who experience hepatotoxicity or in the event of an overdose. Activated charcoal also can reduce plasma M1 levels by 50% after 48 hours, and can be an effective alternative to cholestyramine when a need arises for the management of LEF overdosages.

Azathioprine
Indications and Adverse Effects

35. In considering options for B.W., AZA is mentioned. B.W. knows someone who is using AZA for prevention of kidney transplant rejection and thinks AZA is a highly toxic drug. How can adverse effects to AZA be minimized?

Azathioprine is FDA approved for transplant rejection prophylaxis and for treatment of severe RA. The starting dose of AZA for RA is 1 mg/kg per day in single or divided doses.[8] The dose can be increased by 0.5 mg/kg/day after 6 to 8 weeks if the patient does not respond; further adjustments of the same magnitude should be made every 4 weeks if needed until a maximum dose of 2.5 mg/kg/day is reached.

The most common adverse effect of AZA is GI intolerance and about 10% of patients discontinue therapy because of this problem.[127] Myelosuppression, can occur within this dosage range, but is reversible upon discontinuation of therapy.[127] Renal insufficiency and allopurinol (decreases metabolism and elimination of AZA via inhibition of xanthine oxidase) increase risk for myelosuppression. Patients with renal insufficiency should receive a lower AZA dose, although guidelines for dosage adjustment are not provided by the manufacturer. If concomitant allopurinol therapy cannot be avoided, the dose of AZA must be reduced by 75%. Monitoring for AZA adverse effects should include a baseline CBC, renal function, and liver function tests. When AZA doses are increased, a CBC should be monitored every 1 to 2 weeks. Subsequently, a CBC should be monitored every 1 to 3 months thereafter. Although serious adverse effects have limited the use of AZA for RA; diligent laboratory and clinical monitoring can minimize risk to patients.

Penicillamine
Considerations for Use

36. Would you consider penicillamine therapy for B.W.? How is penicillamine dosed and monitored?

Penicillamine is not often used for the treatment of progressive RA because of a lengthy dose titration schedule and possible association with autoimmune diseases.[8,48]

Dosing

A "go low, go slow" approach is recommended for dosing penicillamine.[137] The usual starting dose is 250 mg/day, increased to 500 mg/day after 4 to 8 weeks. If therapeutic benefits are not observed after an additional 4 to 8 weeks, the dosage is increased to 750 mg daily, then occasionally to 1,000 mg. Up to 6 months of therapy may be necessary before therapeutic benefits become apparent.

Adverse Effects

The most common adverse effects associated with penicillamine include rash, stomatitis, and dysgeusia.[127] Myelosuppression (particularly thrombocytopenia), proteinuria, renal toxicity, and autoimmune syndromes (e.g., systemic lupus erythematosus, myasthenia gravis, polymyositis, Goodpasture's syndrome) have been reported but are rare. Gradual increases in DPEN doses of 125 to 250 mg every 3 months appear to reduce the risk of thrombocytopenia. Laboratory monitoring includes a baseline renal function test. A CBC and urine protein assay should also be obtained at baseline and every 2 weeks until dosing is stabilized, then every 1 to 3 months thereafter.

Although B.W. has failed to respond to several DMARDs, other therapeutic options with faster onset of action are preferred in light of B.W.'s RA severity.

37. A patient with RA, M.M., is allergic to penicillin. Could he receive penicillamine for RA treatment?

Metabolites of penicillin, rather than penicillin itself, are responsible for allergic reactions. The penicilloyl group is recognized as the major haptenic determinant, but other metabolites such as penicillinate, penicillate, and penicillamine groups are important. Penicillamine is an end product of metabolic processes starting with penicilloyl or penicillinic groups. The recommendation that penicillamine be given with caution, if at all, to penicillin-allergic patients is based on in vitro studies demonstrating cross-sensitivity to penicillamine in 44% to 65% of penicillin-allergic patients.[179] However, none of these patients received an oral penicillamine challenge. In a study of 40 patients giving histories of penicillin allergy, confirmed by positive skin tests in 80%, none experienced an immediate or delayed reaction after an oral dose of 250 mg of penicillamine.[180] Three patients who had positive penicillin skin test reactions also had RA. All three subsequently received penicillamine without experiencing hypersensitivity reactions during therapy. Penicillamine, therefore, need not be withheld in patients with a history of penicillin allergy. The potential for cross-reactivity, although real, appears to be small.

Traditional DMARD Combination Therapy

38. Would earlier use or combining second-line drug therapies in RA improve treatment outcomes?

Most RA patients will develop joint erosions within the first few years of disease and a goal of therapy is to slow disease progression as quickly as possible. The initiation of disease-modifying agents early in the course of therapy and using them in combination have been associated with improved patient outcomes. The rationale for combination therapy is similar to that of combination therapy for cancer, infectious diseases, hypertension, diabetes, or asthma (i.e., a combination of drugs may result in improved outcomes because of pharmacologic actions at different sites or through different mechanisms).

A combination of several drugs also may allow for use of lower doses of individual drugs, and, thereby, reduce the risk of toxicity while maintaining or increasing efficacy. On the other hand, the earlier use potent disease-modifying agents in combination also may expose the patient to increased risks of drug adverse effects. Not surprisingly, the number of published clinical trials evaluating the efficacy and safety of combination DMARD therapy are limited[31] because of the multitude of possible study designs (e.g., different DMARD combinations, variable doses, variable durations of therapy needed to fully evaluate outcomes, sufficient number of patients enrolled). Studies most applicable to clinical practice should compare the efficacy of MTX against a combination of drugs that incorporate MTX in the regimen because MTX is the single most effective traditional DMARD. Nevertheless, MTX by itself, improves only one-third of patients by 50% after 2 to 4 years.[69] In several studies of up to 2 years in duration, DMARD combinations are more effective and no more toxic than DMARD monotherapy.[181,182]

In 1997 U.S. rheumatologists used combination DMARD therapy in approximately 25% of their RA patients.[183] In another survey higher disease severity correlated with more frequent use of combination DMARDs, ranging from 3% in mild cases to 58% in severe cases.[184] The most common 2-DMARD combination used in the United States is MTX plus HCQ, followed by MTX plus SSZ.[36,43,183,184] European physicians more commonly select MTX plus SSZ as their first-choice 2-DMARD combination.[184] For 3-DMARD combinations, both European and U.S. physicians prefer MTX plus HCQ and SSZ.

The most effective DMARD combination appears to be the triple combination of methotrexate, hydroxychloroquine, and sulfasalazine.[181,182,185] In one study, this triple combination resulted in a 2-year disease remission rate of 37% versus 21% in patients treated with sulfasalazine or MTX monotherapy with no significant differences in adverse effects.[182] Another trial compared the triple drug regimen to MTX alone or the combination of HCQ and SSZ.[183] At 2-year follow-up, 77% of the triple-drug-treated patients responded significantly as compared with 33% of the patients treated with MTX monotherapy ($P < 0.001$) and 40% of the patients treated with SSZ plus HCQ ($P = 0.003$). Toxicity did not differ between the treatment groups. A follow-up abstract of the same study reported that triple drug therapy remained efficacious and safe in 36 of 58 patients (62%) after 5 years.[185]

In a randomized controlled trial of 263 MTX-treated patients with active persistent RA, the addition of leflunomide resulted in significant clinical improvement without an increase in adverse event and treatment discontinuation rates.[186] However, the publication of anecdotal reports of serious liver disease, including fatalities, have prompted some to conclude that this combination of MTX with LEF is unsafe.[48]

Aggressive DMARD therapy can be implemented through many approaches. Fries hypothesized that after an initial response to a DMARD, disease progression accelerates (even on therapy), explaining the apparent paradox of short-term improvement but failure to alter long-term outcomes in RA (Fig. 43-8).[187] DMARD treatment, therefore,

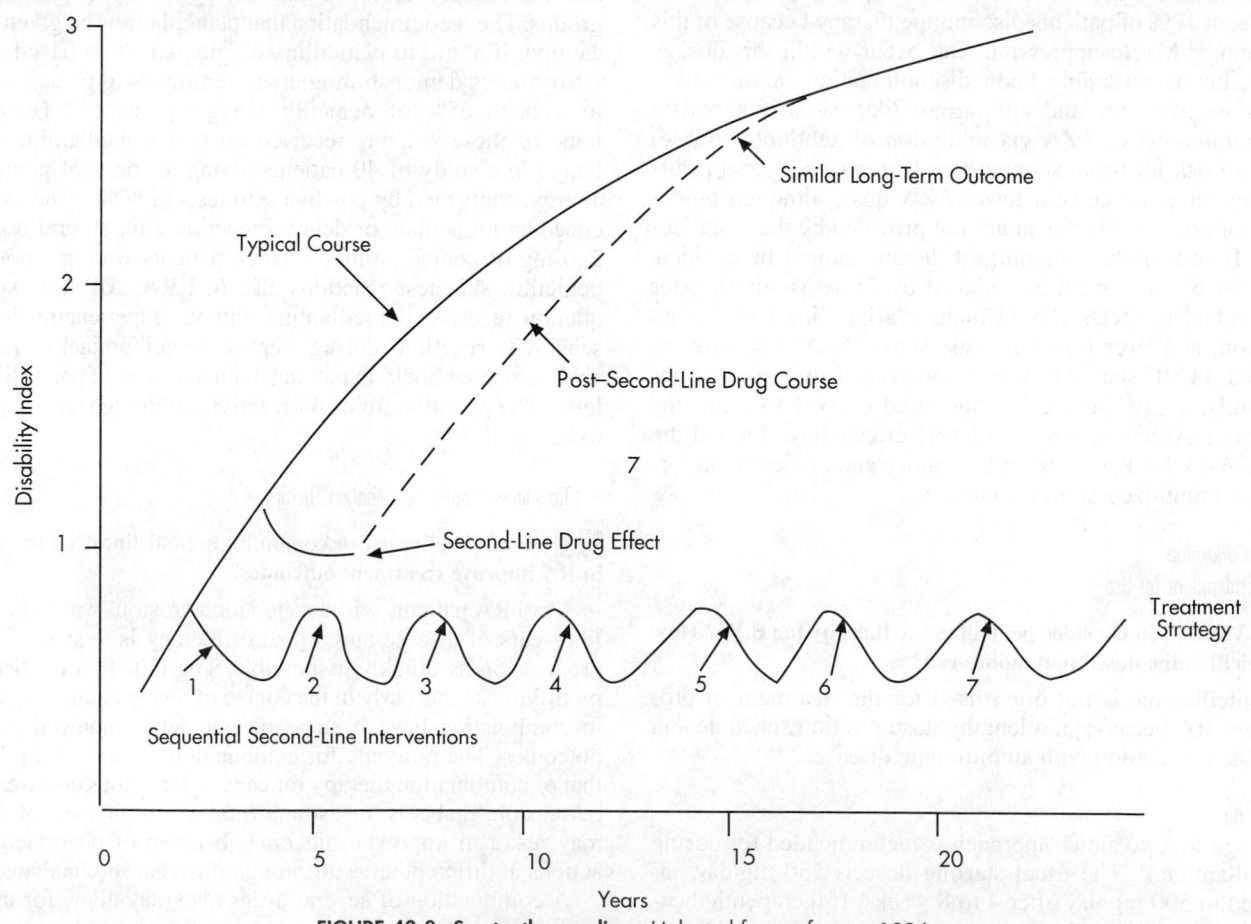

FIGURE 43-8. Sawtooth paradigm. (Adapted from reference 182.)

makes progression to disability irregular, like the tooth of a saw. To improve disease outcome and at the same time to keep overall drug toxicity near traditional levels, they proposed initiating DMARDs as soon as possible, before substantial damage to the joints occurs. One or multiple DMARDs are used continually, throughout the entire disease course, while monitoring for evidence of disease progression. A ceiling is set in terms of progression, which triggers treatment changes. DMARD therapy is changed serially, alone or in combination, at each decision point. Analgesics and NSAIDs are used only as adjunctive therapy for symptomatic relief as required.

A more aggressive approach, the "step-down bridge" paradigm, proposes initial treatment with prednisone 10 mg daily for 1 month.[188] If active RA is still evident, multiple DMARDs are added all at once to induce disease remission as quickly as possible. One DMARD at a time is then tapered and discontinued, eventually leaving a single agent as monotherapy (Fig. 43-9).

Yet another, more conservative approach is the "graduated step" paradigm. Disease severity and activity are matched to "appropriate" initial and long-term therapy (Fig. 43-10).[189] Goals of this strategy include increasing objectivity of therapeutic decision making throughout the course of disease treatment and exposing only those patients with sufficiently active disease to the risks of combination DMARD therapy. Patients are re-evaluated at 3 month intervals and disease activity is scored quantitatively (Tables 43-7 and 43-8). Patients with disease activity index values of 0 to 3 are designated as responders with inactive disease. Patients with values between 6 to 8 are considered to have active, unresponsive disease, and treatment is to be escalated. Patients with disease activity

scores of 4 to 5 are considered to have subacute RA; decisions for treatment of these patients are based on additional information beyond disease activity criteria (e.g., time of onset of afternoon fatigue, change in grip strength, change in hemoglobin concentration, onset or worsening of extra-articular disease manifestations).

Although each strategy differs in specifics, they share the concepts of starting DMARD therapy earlier and a willingness to combine DMARDs to achieve improved short-term as well as long-term outcomes. The longest prospective study of the sawtooth strategy for DMARD therapy was conducted among 135 patients over 15 years.[190] A total of 606 monotherapy or combination DMARD therapies were initiated. Five hundred twenty-eight (87.1%) of these therapies were discontinued after a median time of 10 months, with most discontinuing because of inefficacy (51.1%) rather than adverse effects (28.2%). Thus, the main factor limiting the sawtooth strategy was the loss of efficacy as opposed to harmful adverse effects. Although the sawtooth and other DMARD strategies for treatment appear to be safe over a prolonged period, more effective drug therapies are needed.

In summary, earlier intervention with DMARDs and the use of combinations of DMARDs are commonly implemented in clinical practice. Higher disease severity increases the likelihood of early DMARD use, both as monotherapy and combination DMARD therapy. Loss of efficacy and intolerable adverse effects appear to be the first and second most common reasons for DMARD discontinuation, respectively. To date, the most efficacious and sustaining traditional DMARD combination appears to be the triple combination of MTX, HCQ, and SSZ, whereas the most common 2-DMARD combination in the United States is MTX plus HCQ.

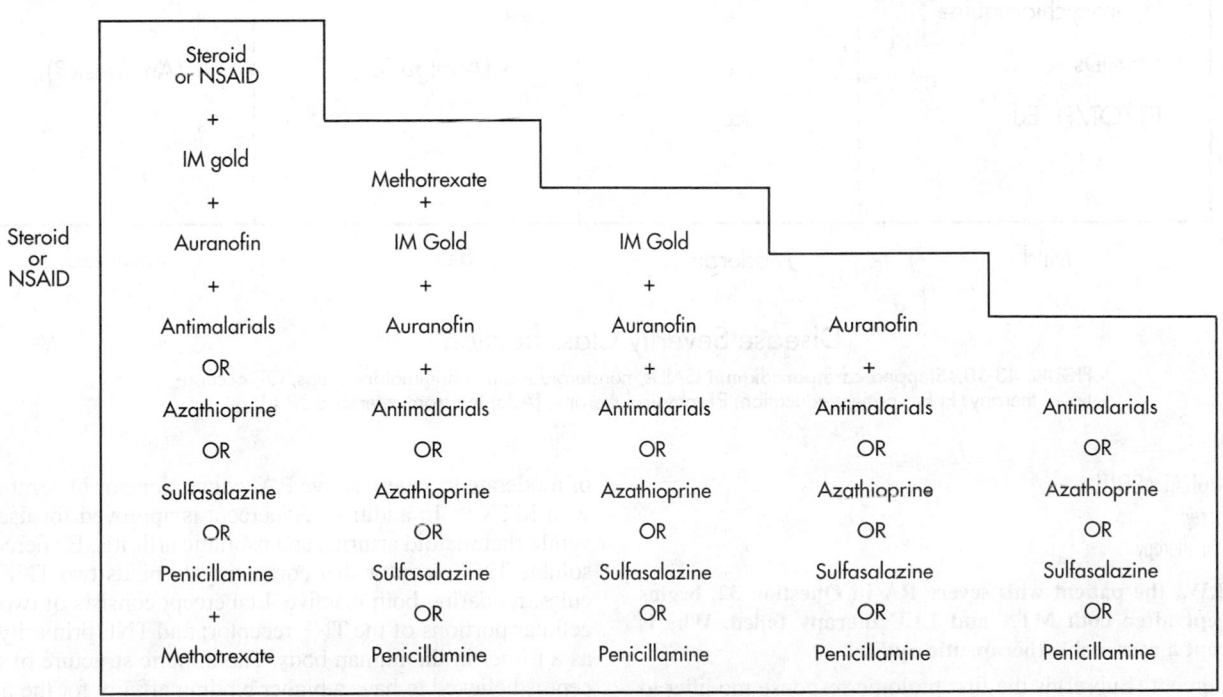

FIGURE 43-9. Step-down bridge paradigm. (Adapted from reference 183.)

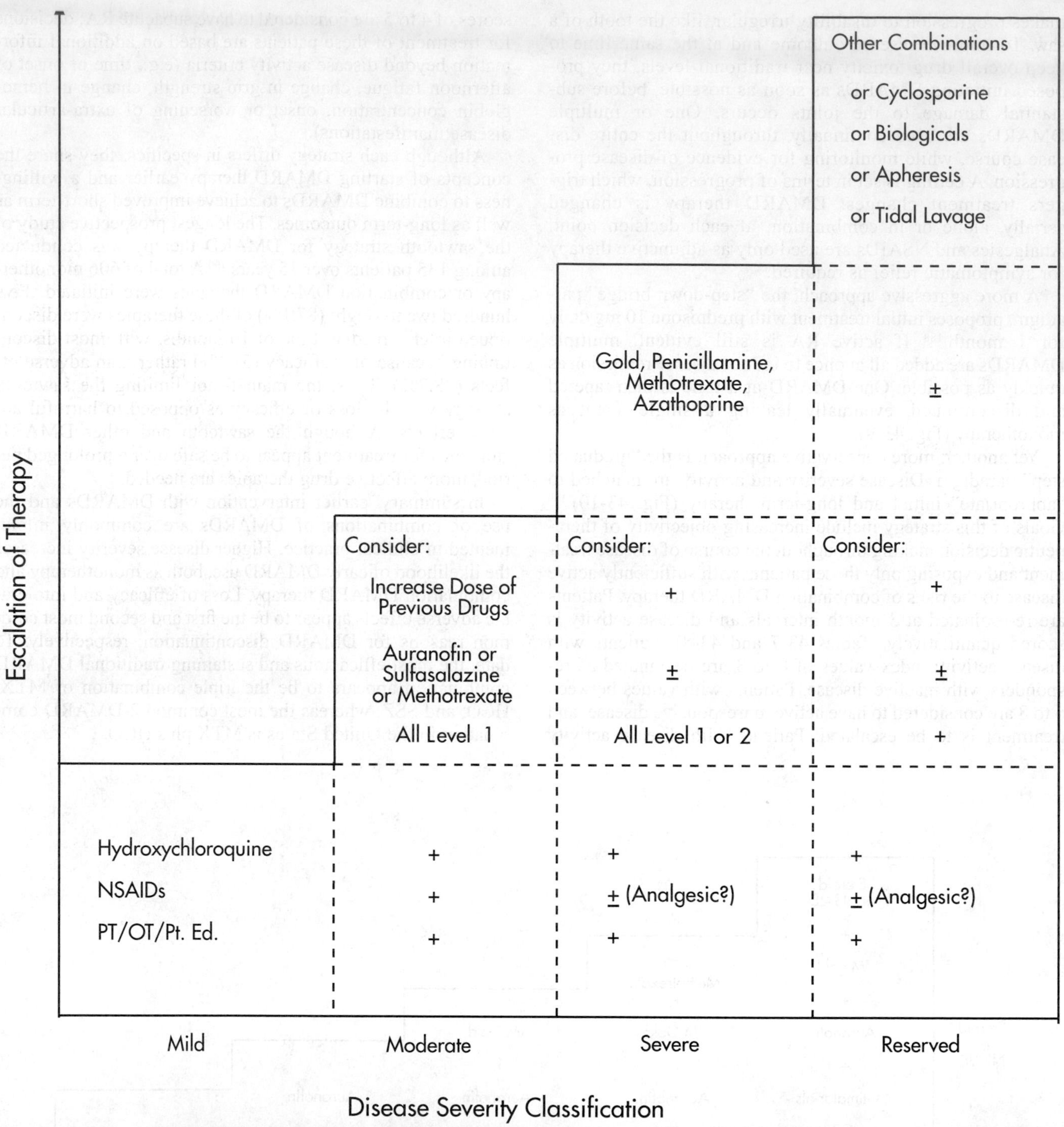

Disease Severity Classification

FIGURE 43-10. Stepped-care paradigm. NSAIDs, nonsteroidal anti-inflammatory drugs; OT, occupational therapy; Pt Ed, patient education; PT, physical therapy. (Adapted from reference 184.)

BIOLOGICAL AGENTS

Etanercept

Place in Therapy

39. **B.W., the patient with severe RA in Question 32, begins etanercept after both MTX and LEF therapy failed. Why is etanercept a reasonable therapeutic option?**

Etanercept (Enbrel) is the first biologic response modifier to be approved by the FDA for reducing the signs and symptoms

of moderate to severe active RA, either alone or in combination with MTX.[191] In addition, etanercept is approved for use in juvenile rheumatoid arthritis and psoriatic arthritis. Etanercept is a soluble TNF receptor that competitively binds two TNF molecules, rendering both inactive. Etanercept consists of two extracellular portions of the TNF receptor; and TNF primarily exists as a trimer in the human body. The dimeric structure of etanercept is believed to have a higher binding affinity for the trimeric TNF than the naturally occurring monomeric receptor.[192]

Table 43-7   Scoring Criteria for "Stepped Care" Paradigm

Disease Activity	Inactive		Subacute		Active			
	Significant Response	Score	Partial Response	Score	Poor Response	Score	Prognostic Factors	Score
Pain	None	0	Intermittent		Constant		Deteriorating function capacity	1
Morning stiffness	<15	0	15–30	1	>30	2	Sustained (6 mo) elevated ESR	1
Swollen/tender joints	0–2	0	3–5	1	>5	2	RF titer 1:640	1
ESR or	<30	0	30–45	1	>45	2	Extra-articular manifestation	1
CRP	<2.0		2.0–2.6	1	>2.6	2	Radiologic joint damage	1
Total points		0		4		8		5

CRP, C-reactive protein; ESR, erythrocyte sedimentation rate; RF, rheumatoid factor.

Table 43-8   Disease Severity Classification

Score	Classification
0–4	Mild
5–7	Moderate
8–13	Severe

In a randomized, placebo-controlled trial of 234 patients with active RA, the efficacy of etanercept 10 mg or 25 mg subcutaneously twice weekly for 26 weeks was evaluated.[193] Enrollment criteria included an inadequate response to at least one of several DMARDs. Most patients (approximately 90%) had tried MTX at one time or another, followed by HCQ (approximately 68%), injectable gold and SSZ (approximately 50% each), azathioprine (approximately 30%), and DPEN and gold (approximately 20% to 25% each). At 6-month follow-up, 20% American College of Rheumatology (ACR-20) response was compared. The definition of ACR-20 response is a 20% reduction in tender joint count and swollen joint count and 20% improvement in at least three of the following: patient's assessment of pain, patient's global assessment, physician's global assessment, patient's assessment of disability, and acute phase reactant measures (i.e., ESR or CRP). Significantly more patients receiving etanercept 10 mg (51%) and 25 mg (59%) met ACR-20 response criteria compared with placebo (11%); the differences in response rate between the two doses of etanercept was not significant. Likewise, 24% and 40% of the patients taking etanercept 10 mg and 25 mg, respectively, met ACR-50 response criteria compared with 5% of the placebo group (P < 0.001 for both doses compared with placebo, no significant difference between doses). Significant ACR-20, ACR-50, and ACR-70 responses to either etanercept dose were seen after only 2 weeks of therapy.

Another randomized, placebo-controlled trial evaluated the use of combination MTX and etanercept therapy in 89 patients with active RA refractory to at least 6 months of MTX therapy.[194] A dose of 25 mg etanercept or placebo was given subcutaneously twice weekly, and a stable dose of MTX (between 15 and 25 mg weekly) was provided to all patients. At 24-week follow-up, an ACR-20 response was found in 71% of the MTX plus etanercept group and 27% of the MTX plus placebo group (P < 0.001). Similarly, 39% of the MTX plus etanercept group met ACR-50 response criteria compared with 3% of the MTX plus placebo group (P < 0.001). Etanercept was also associated with significantly greater improvement in ESR or CRP test results. The addition of etanercept to MTX appears to provide greater clinical efficacy when compared with MTX monotherapy.

The only clinical trial to date comparing a TNF inhibitor (etanercept) with a traditional DMARD (MTX), the Early Rheumatoid Arthritis (ERA) trial, was conducted among 632 moderate to severe early RA patients.[195] Conventional dosing of etanercept (25 mg twice a week) was associated with significantly greater improvement in clinical and radiologic measures within the first 6 months of therapy, but no significant therapeutic differences were found between etanercept and MTX at 12-month follow-up. However, at the conclusion of the 24-month trial, significantly less radiographic progression of disease (as measured by the Sharp score, a composite of joint space narrowing and erosions) was found among the etanercept patients.

Etanercept appears to provide rapid and significant improvement in subjective and objective measures of RA, either alone or in combination with MTX. Etanercept prevents radiographic progression of RA better than MTX. Based on clinical trial data, etanercept appears to be an appropriate therapeutic option for many patients and may produce better long-term results than MTX. Cost is a significant consideration, but etanercept is a reasonable consideration for B.W. Clinical trials comparing biological agents with common traditional DMARD combinations are needed.

Dosing and Monitoring

40. **How would you initiate etanercept therapy and monitor B.W. for therapeutic and adverse effects?**

The FDA-approved dose of etanercept for the treatment of active RA is 25 mg subcutaneously twice weekly.[191] The medication may be self-administered after proper training by a qualified health professional. Etanercept must be reconstituted using *only* the diluent supplied; the contents should be swirled, not shaken, to avoid excessive foaming. Injection sites should be rotated and can include the thigh, abdomen, or upper arm. Clinical response usually appears within 1 to 2 weeks of treatment, and nearly all patients will respond within 3 months. Drug interaction studies have not been conducted with etanercept, but clinical trials seem to indicate that concurrent use of other arthritis medications (e.g., MTX, glucocorticoids, NSAIDs) is safe.

More commonly observed adverse effects with etanercept include injection site reactions (37% versus 10% in placebo patients), upper respiratory infections (29% versus 10% in placebo patients), and the development of autoantibodies. Injection site reactions were all described as mild to moderate and usually occurred within the first month of treatment with decreased frequency over time. Upper respiratory infections, including sinusitis, are estimated to occur at a rate of 0.82 events per patient-year in patients treated with etanercept versus 0.68 events per patient per year in the placebo group. Autoantibodies that developed during etanercept treatment included antinuclear antibodies (11% versus 5% in placebo group) and new positive anti–double-stranded DNA antibodies (15% versus 4% in placebo group). No patients developed clinical signs of autoimmune disease, and the long-term effect of etanercept on the development of autoimmune disease is unknown. Patients with severe heart failure (e.g., NYHA Class III or IV) may be at increased risk for heart failure exacerbation and mortality when taking any anti-TNF agent.[22] Although not a contraindication, caution is advised if etanercept is prescribed for patients with heart failure; the FDA is considering a class warning for all anti-TNF agents.[196] While an increased incidence of lymphoma has been observed among RA patients receiving any of the available anti-TNF agents, causation has not been established since both RA and MTX are also associated with an increased rate of lymphoma.[30] Other adverse effects, in order of decreasing frequency, include headache, rhinitis, dizziness, pharyngitis, cough, asthenia, abdominal pain, and rash.

The greatest concern with etanercept therapy is the risk of immunosuppression and subsequent serious infections, including sepsis. TNF is a key mediator of inflammation and plays a major role in regulation of the immune system. Approximately 6 months after FDA-approval of etanercept, 30 patients receiving etanercept developed serious infections.[194] Although the number of reports was not more than what was expected from clinical trials, concern was warranted because 6 of these patients died within 2 to 16 weeks of starting therapy. Postmarketing reports of other infections such as tuberculosis (a black box warning for all anti-TNF agents), mycobacterial infections, and fungal infections further reinforces the strong recommendation against the initiation of etanercept therapy in patients with sepsis or any form of active infection (i.e., chronic or localized).[8,48] *M. tuberculosis* skin testing and a baseline chest radiograph are now recommended before beginning anti-TNF therapy. Therapy should be postponed for patients identified as having latent tuberculosis until appropriate anti-tuberculosis therapy is completed. In addition, clinicians must be cautious when prescribing etanercept to other high-risk individuals such as patients with a history of

recurring infection or with underlying illnesses that predispose them to infection (e.g., diabetes).

B.W. should receive a tuberculosis skin test, undergo a chest radiograph, and be warned of the potential adverse effects of etanercept, particularly the risk of immunosuppression and subsequent infection. Any sign of infection must be reported immediately to her health care provider.

Infliximab and Adalimumab
Dosing and Place in Therapy

41. After 3 weeks of etanercept therapy, B.W. appears to respond well. However, she dislikes the subcutaneous administration of etanercept twice weekly and wants another medication that can be administered on a much more convenient basis. How do the other TNF-α inhibitors differ from etanercept, and is B.W. a candidate for one of these alternatives?

Two anti–TNF-α monoclonal antibodies are FDA-approved for the treatment of RA. The first, infliximab (Remicade), is a chimeric (mouse/human) IgG antibody directed against TNF-α that is approved for the treatment of Crohn's disease and for the treatment of RA in patients who have not responded adequately to MTX.[197] Infliximab selectively binds to and neutralizes TNF-α; etanercept, on the other hand, binds to both TNF-α and TNF-β. Whether one method of neutralizing TNF-α has an advantage over the other is not clear at this time. The usual dose of infliximab is 3 mg/kg *intravenously* at 0, 2 and 6 weeks, then every 8 weeks thereafter; thus, the convenience of infrequent dosing is tempered by the need for supervised intravenous administration. Infliximab should be given with MTX therapy to prevent the formation of antibodies to infliximab.

In a randomized, placebo-controlled trial of 101 patients with active RA who responded suboptimally to MTX therapy, the effect of different doses of infliximab with and without concomitant MTX therapy was compared.[198] Patients received one of three doses of intravenous infliximab (1, 3, or 10 mg/kg) with or without MTX 7.5 mg weekly. A control group received intravenous placebo with MTX 7.5 mg weekly. At 26-week follow-up, 60% of patients receiving 3 or 10 mg/kg of infliximab with or without MTX responded to treatment as defined by a 20% Paulus response criteria (i.e., 20% reduction in at least 4 of the following 6 criteria: number of swollen joints, number of tender joints, duration of morning stiffness, reduction in ESR, a two-grade improvement in the patient's global assessment of disease severity, and a two-grade improvement in the physician's global assessment of disease severity). Patients receiving the 1-mg/kg dose without MTX did not respond, while a significant number of patients receiving 1 mg/kg infliximab with MTX met the 20% Paulus response criteria through the 16th week of treatment; however, this response was no longer significant at week 26.

Serious adverse effects included two infections in patients treated with infliximab, which occurred 9 and 15 weeks after the last dose. The first case resulted in severe bacterial endophthalmitis, resulting in enucleation (complete removal) of the affected eye. The second case resulted in an emergency admission for staphylococcal septic shock; the patient died within 24 hours of admission. The development of antibodies to infliximab (human antichimeric antibodies [HACA]) occurred at a rate of 53%, 21%, and 7% of patients receiving the

1-, 3-, and 10-mg/kg doses of infliximab alone, respectively. These rates were lower when MTX was given concurrently (15%, 7%, and 0%, respectively). The data suggest that high doses of infliximab or concurrent use of MTX minimizes HACA formation.

An open-label trial of MTX, 10 mg/week, with intravenous infliximab at a dose of 5, 10, or 20 mg/kg every 2 months produced encouraging results at 40 weeks in 19 patients with RA.[199] These results led to the initiation of a randomized, double-blind, multicenter, placebo-controlled trial of 428 active RA patients who failed to respond adequately to at least 12.5 mg/week of MTX. The study, known as the ATTRACT trial, involved the use of infliximab 3 or 10 mg/kg or placebo every 4 or 8 weeks along with MTX therapy. The trial was unblinded after 1 year because of radiographic evidence of disease modification in patients receiving infliximab. Analysis of radiographic results after a total of 2 years of follow-up demonstrated that infliximab significantly protected against joint erosion.[200]

The newest anti–TNF-α monoclonal antibody, adalimumab (Humira), is a genetically engineered fully-humanized IgG1 monoclonal antibody, as opposed to the chimeric composition of infliximab. The usual dose of adalimumab, whether as monotherapy or in combination with traditional DMARDs including MTX, is a 40 mg self-administered subcutaneous injection every other week.[201] In a randomized controlled trial comparing both weekly and every other week adalimumab 40 mg *monotherapy* to placebo in 283 RA patients refractory to traditional DMARDs, both regimens of adalimumab resulted in significantly greater ACR-20 response rates when compared to placebo.[202] A higher response rate was observed among patients receiving 40 mg weekly versus every other week; as a result, weekly adalimumab may be more beneficial for RA patients who are not receiving concomitant MTX therapy. In a placebo-controlled trial evaluating adalimumab 40 mg every other week added to RA patients receiving stable MTX doses, significantly more adalimumab patients (67%) achieved an ACR-20 response versus placebo (15%) after 24 weeks.[203] Radiographic data reflecting 1 or 2 years of treatment indicate that adalimumab slows the progression of joint damage.[30]

Adverse Effects of Anti–TNF-α Antibodies

Infliximab and adalimumab have treatment risks and side effect profiles very similar to etanercept, including relatively minor reactions such as injection site pain, local reactions, upper respiratory tract infections, nausea, flu-like symptoms, and rash.[30] Serious adverse effects are shared as well, including serious infections and increased incidence of lymphoma. As with all anti-TNF-α agents, a tuberculosis skin test result and chest radiograph must be obtained before treatment initiation. As noted previously, the development of antibodies against infliximab occurs frequently with monotherapy due to the chimeric nature of the medication, requiring concurrent use with MTX. Interestingly, although adalimumab is a fully humanized product, approximately 5% of RA patients will develop antibodies against it at least once during therapy when used as a single agent.[201] This reaction is attenuated with weekly dosing of adalimumab or concurrent use of MTX.

B.W. appears to be a reasonable candidate for either infliximab or adalimumab therapy. Her interest in a biological agent with less frequent dosing is understandable. Although no trials have compared the biological agents to one another, key differentiating variables between infliximab and adalimumab need to be considered. While infliximab is ultimately administered every 2 months, it must be administered intravenously and in combination with MTX (or possibly at a higher dose) to minimize HACA formation. The benefits of adalimumab include ease of administration (self-injected subcutaneous injection) and infrequent dosing interval compared with etanercept (twice weekly injections) and anakinra (daily injections) but more frequent than infliximab. At FDA-approved doses, all biological agents (etanercept, infliximab, adalimumab, anakinra) are priced similarly (approximately $15,000 to $16,000 annual average wholesale price, 2003).[30] However, some clinical trial data suggest additional therapeutic benefit from weekly dosing of adalimumab. If adalimumab is administered weekly, the cost of adalimumab therapy will be considerably more than the other biological agents.

Anakinra

42. **B.W. would prefer to avoid anakinra [Kineret] since it requires daily subcutaneous injection dosing. Apart from this inconvenience, does anakinra offer any therapeutic advantages over the anti–TNF-α agents?**

Anakinra is currently the only available IL-1 receptor antagonist (IL-1RA), almost identical in composition to human IL-1RA (see biological agents in the general treatment section). The recommended dose of anakinra is 100 mg daily by self-administered subcutaneous injection.[204] Clinical trials evaluating anakinra have demonstrated significant but modest improvement in RA signs and symptoms and radiographic evidence of joint erosion.[48,205] In a study of 472 patients with serious active RA, three different doses of anakinra monotherapy (30, 75, and 150 mg daily) were compared with placebo.[206] At 24-week follow-up, 34% of patients receiving anakinra 75 mg demonstrated an ACR-20 response; however, 27% of placebo patients achieved the same response. While modest, this difference is statistically significant. Although the higher dose of 150 mg produced improvement in 43% of patients, this dose exceeds the manufacturer-recommended dose. The combination of anakinra and MTX appears to be more effective than anakinra monotherapy. A 24-week randomized controlled trial compared five different doses of anakinra (0.04, 0.1, 0.4, 1.0, and 2.0 mg/kg daily) to placebo among 419 RA patients receiving at least 3 months of fixed MTX doses.[207] Significantly more patients receiving the higher daily doses of anakinra (1.0 and 2.0 mg/kg) experienced the ACR-20 response (42% and 35%, respectively) versus placebo (23%) at 24 week follow-up. Frequent adverse effects include local injection site reactions.[48] Although neutropenia and severe infections are more commonly associated with anakinra versus placebo, there have been no reports of patients experiencing tuberculosis reactivation. Combining anakinra with an anti–TNF-α agent appears to be logical based on their different mechanisms of action; however, the combination is not recommended due to a significantly increased incidence of serious infections and leukopenia in a small open label study.[205]

Although the anti–TNF-α agents have not been compared directly, anakinra appears to be relatively less effective. In addition, the advantage of being able to self-administer anakinra is offset by the need for daily injections. Anakinra is a therapeutic alternative for RA patients in whom traditional DMARD treatment fails; however, it appears to offer no advantages and some real and potential disadvantages when compared with the anti–TNF-α agents.

Corticosteroids
Indications

43. W.M., a 57-year-old man, has progressive RA that has not been responsive to SSZ or HCQ. He is having difficulty working a full day and is seeking an alternative medication. After a discussion of therapeutic options, W.M. declines MTX therapy and asks to start penicillamine. Would it be appropriate to initiate corticosteroids concurrently?

Despite the potential for serious adverse effects with long-term therapy, the judicious use of low-dose corticosteroids represents an important component of treatment during the course of unremitting disease. In addition, low-dose corticosteroids may have disease-modifying properties, particularly in the first year or two of treatment.[8,48] Although it is hoped that W.M. will respond well to penicillamine, penicillamine is the slowest-acting DMARD and W.M.'s RA is sufficiently active that it is compromising his ability to earn an income. Thus, beginning an intermediate-acting corticosteroid such as prednisone in a daily or divided dose of 5 to 10 mg is justified.[8] The onset of action of corticosteroids is relatively rapid and their immediate benefits will allow W.M. to maintain his current employment and continue taking care of home responsibilities. The corticosteroid dose can be decreased gradually and eventually discontinued as W.M. begins to respond to penicillamine therapy. An important goal of low-dose corticosteroid treatment is to provide bridge therapy until the second-line therapy becomes effective, in hopes of then being able to taper and discontinue the corticosteroid.[21] Unfortunately, this goal is not always realized. In some cases, patients do not respond to one second-line agent and then must be started on another. In other instances, patients fail to experience sufficient benefit from any second-line agent, and discontinuation of the corticosteroid is never realized.

Dosing

44. Why are corticosteroids sometimes administered in divided daily doses rather than as single daily doses or on an every-other-day regimen when used to treat RA?

Administering intermediate- or short-acting corticosteroids as a single daily dose each morning most closely mimics the early morning physiologic secretion of cortisol, and, thereby, minimizes hypothalamic-pituitary-adrenal (HPA) axis suppression. Administering corticosteroids on alternate mornings further reduces the risk of HPA axis suppression by allowing the adrenal glands to respond to hypothalamic and pituitary mediators during the "off" day.[208] Once-a-day and alternate-day steroid therapies are most advantageous when used to prevent reactivation of diseases such as asthma, ulcerative colitis, chronic active hepatitis, and sarcoidosis.[209] In contrast, when corticosteroids are used to provide symptomatic relief in RA during periods of active, ongoing inflammation, switching patients to single daily doses or every-

other-day regimens frequently results in increased symptoms during the latter part of each day and during the "off" day. The anti-inflammatory effect of prednisone or prednisolone is attenuated after 12 hours, and is either diminished or absent after 24 hours.[15] As a result, daily prednisone doses are often divided in half and administered twice daily to ensure 24-hour anti-inflammatory activity. Although a larger single daily dose may provide comparable therapeutic benefits, dividing the daily dose of prednisone is preferable since larger doses are associated with more frequent and severe adverse effects.

Osteoporosis

45. What therapeutic interventions can prevent steroid-induced osteoporosis?

Chronic corticosteroid therapy induces osteoporosis by inhibiting bone formation and enhancing bone resorption. Steroids impair bone formation by inhibiting the production of bone-forming osteoblasts and enhance bone resorption by reducing GI calcium absorption and increasing the renal excretion of calcium.[209] In addition, corticosteroids reduce the secretion of luteinizing hormone from the pituitary, resulting in a reduction in estrogen production in women and testosterone production in men.[210] This leads to deficiencies in circulating levels of anabolic hormones (e.g., estradiol, estrone, androstenedione, progesterone), which contribute to the development of osteoporosis. Trabecular bone of the spine and ribs seems to be affected primarily by corticosteroid therapy, with most rapid skeletal wasting occurring during the first 6 months.[210]

Before starting long-term (i.e., 6 months) corticosteroid therapy at a dose of 7.5 mg of daily prednisone or equivalent, bone mineral density (BMD) should be evaluated.[210,211] Anteroposterior (AP) measurement of the lumbar spine and femoral neck by dual-energy x-ray absorptiometry (DXA) is the preferred procedure. A complete history should be obtained to identify potentially modifiable osteoporosis risk factors (e.g., smoking, alcohol consumption, other drugs that may induce osteoporosis, calcium and vitamin D intake, indicators of hormone deficiency such as menopause in women and infertility or impotence in men, lack of participation in weight-bearing exercises). Height and weight should be measured. Lifestyle changes should be encouraged to modify those risk factors that do not require drug therapy. Physical therapy referral is recommended.

Pharmacologic-related efforts to prevent corticosteroid-induced osteoporosis begins with keeping corticosteroid doses to a minimum (<7.5 mg daily if possible).[210] Alternate daily dosing does not reduce the incidence of osteoporosis. Hormone replacement therapy may be considered, but is no longer considered a first-line option for osteoporosis prevention in postmenopausal women due to major safety concerns identified in large well-designed trials.[211] Pharmacologic doses of vitamin D (800 IU daily or 50,000 IU three times per week) or calcitriol (0.5 μg/day) and calcium supplements (approximately 1,500 mg daily) can correct the decreased GI absorption of calcium in patients treated with corticosteroids and are recommended for all patients.[210] Thiazide diuretics reduce urinary calcium excretion and maintain bone mineral content.[212] A thiazide diuretic is recommended if hypercalciuria is present. Calcitonin (100 IU every day or every other day subcutaneously or 200 IU intranasally every day) or bisphosphonates also are effective in preventing corticosteroid-induced osteoporosis, although bisphosphonates are not recommended in premenopausal women and men younger than 50 years of age because of a lack of long-term safety data.

All patients with established osteoporosis must receive adequate vitamin D and calcium supplementation. For premenopausal women, estrogen-containing oral contraceptives with a minimum of 50 μg of estradiol or equivalent is recommended; if refused or contraindicated, calcitonin is an alternative. For postmenopausal women, either calcitonin or a bisphosphonate may be prescribed. Hormone replacement therapy is no longer a treatment of choice. Men with abnormally low serum testosterone should be offered testosterone replacement. If refused or contraindicated, calcitonin or bisphosphonates are alternatives. Sodium fluoride therapy may also be effective.

Intra-Articular Corticosteroids

46. **Do intra-articular corticosteroid injections provide any benefit in RA?**

Intra-articular corticosteroid injections are safe and effective for patients with RA but should only be used when flaring occurs in one or a few joints.[8] Systemic side effects are minimal when compared with oral corticosteroid therapy. Although onset of action is virtually immediate, effects are often short-lived; however, a corticosteroid injection may be all that is necessary to relieve a temporary RA flare. If the decision is made to re-inject a given joint, the injection site should be rotated and administration frequency should be no more than every 3 months.

JUVENILE RHEUMATOID ARTHRITIS

Arthritis is the most common pediatric connective tissue disease. In the United States, all chronic arthritis of childhood is known as juvenile rheumatoid arthritis (JRA). In Europe, the term used is *juvenile chronic arthritis*. JRA affects all races and afflicts approximately 250,000 children in the United States.[213,214]

By definition, JRA usually begins before the age of 16 and must present with objective signs of joint inflammation (e.g., swelling, pain, limited ROM, warmth, erythema) in at least one joint for at least 6 weeks. In addition, other conditions causing arthritis (such as infectious arthritis and malignancy) must be excluded.[214] The onset of disease is rare before 6 months of age, and the peak age of onset ranges from 1 to 3 years. However, new cases are seen throughout childhood.

Signs and Symptoms

As with adult RA, JRA begins with synovial inflammation.[214,215] Morning stiffness and joint pain probably occur in JRA as frequently as in RA; however, children should be observed carefully for symptoms because they often cannot articulate complaints. The morning stiffness and joint pain may manifest as increased irritability, guarding of involved joints, or refusal to walk. Fatigue and low-grade fever, anorexia, weight loss, and failure to grow are other manifestations. JRA may be divided into several subsets based on characteristic signs and symptoms during the first 4 to 6 months of disease.

In one classification, patients are categorized according to one of three distinct subsets of symptoms: (1) polyarticular, (2) pauciarticular or oligoarthritic, and (3) systemic disease.[214]

Patterns of Onset

JRA is classified under the subgroup "polyarticular" when the disease involves five or more joints with few or no systemic manifestations of disease. Two types of polyarticular JRA exist: seronegative (i.e., RF negative, 20% to 30% of all JRA patients) and seropositive (i.e., RF positive, 5% to 10% of all JRA patients) disease. Both affect girls more often than boys, with seronegative arthritis more common in children younger than 5 years of age and seropositive arthritis more common after the age of 8 years. Although the onset of disease in this category may be acute, it more commonly is insidious. Generally, the large, fast-growing joints such as the knees, wrists, elbows, and ankles are affected, but the small joints of the hands and feet also may be involved. Although the joints at onset usually are symmetrically involved, asymmetric patterns also may be seen. Temporomandibular joint involvement is relatively common and may lead to limitation of bite and micrognathia. Systemic manifestations of disease in children with polyarticular disease are rare and include low-grade fever, slight hepatosplenomegaly, lymphadenopathy, pericarditis, and chronic uveitis. Subcutaneous nodules are seen most typically in children with "polyarthritis onset" JRA. When present, nodules are associated with positive RF in >75% of patients. Approximately 30% to 35% of JRA presents as polyarticular.

Pauciarticular JRA or "oligoarthritis" accounts for approximately 40% to 50% of children with JRA, usually involving four or fewer joints (although cases involving up to nine joints have been reported).[214] Joint involvement in these children most commonly includes large joints in an asymmetric distribution. At least two major subgroups of pauciarticular arthritis exist: early childhood-onset (more common, usually affecting girls between the ages of 1 and 5 years of age) and late childhood-onset (less common, usually affecting boys after 8 years of age).

Approximately 20% to 30% of children with early-onset pauciarticular JRA will develop iridocyclitis (inflammation of the iris and ciliary body, also known as uveitis) within the first 10 years of the disease (see Question 53). Antinuclear antibody (ANA) testing is positive in approximately 60% of these patients. Joints commonly affected include the knees, ankles, hands (especially PIP joints), feet, and wrists; in one study, the frequency of involvement was reported to be 56%, 20%, 10%, 6%, and 4%, respectively.[216] When only one joint is involved, the knee is the most common joint affected. Hip and sacroiliac joint involvement are rare. On the other hand, children with late-onset pauciarticular JRA do not test positive for ANA, have no extra-articular manifestation of the disease, and often have hip involvement in addition to other lower-limb joints (e.g., knees, ankle, feet). Arguably, this late-onset subgroup may be grouped with the spondyloarthropathies well-known in adult patients (e.g., ankylosing spondylitis).

A smaller percentage (10% to 20%) of children experience severe systemic involvement associated with or preceding the onset of arthritis. The hallmarks of the "systemic-onset" category of JRA, which can afflict children at any age, are a high spiking fever and a rheumatoid rash. Once or twice daily, the body temperature may increase to 103° F or higher. The temperature increase may be accompanied by a rash consisting of small, discrete erythematous morbilliform macules that are seen most commonly on the trunk and proximal extremities. The lesions tend to be migratory and of short duration in any one location. Other manifestations of "systemic-onset" JRA are hepatosplenomegaly, lymphadenopathy, and pericarditis; these occur in approximately two-thirds of patients.

In contrast to adult RA, in which joint destruction is common within the first year of the disease, 70% to 90% of children with JRA experience no long-term disability. However, complete remission is uncommon, occurring in approximately one-third of all JRA patients over a 10-year period.[217] Preservation of joint function is least favorable in children with seropositive polyarticular JRA (severe arthritis in >50%). Children with pauciarticular JRA experience the least joint disease, and those with early-onset pauciarticular JRA experience the worst uveitis. Children with systemic-onset are most prone to develop life-threatening or fatal complications with approximately 25% developing severe arthritis.

Diagnosis of Systemic-Onset Juvenile Rheumatoid Arthritis

47. J.R., a 4-year-old girl, is hospitalized for high fever and arthritis. Several weeks before admission, J.R. developed a daily fever ranging from 103° to 106°F. One week before admission, her knees became painful and swollen. J.R. is listless and irritable during her physical examination. The rectal temperature is 102.4°F. She refuses to walk. The right hip is tender and the right wrist and both knees are warm, red, and swollen. Minimal generalized lymphadenopathy and splenomegaly are present. The Westergren ESR is 82 mm/hr, the WBC count 37,000 cells/mm³ with a mild left shift, and Hct 33%. Cultures of the throat, urine, stool, and blood are negative. An intermediate-strength purified protein derivative, antistreptolysin-O titer, ANA titer, and RF titer all are normal. Radiographs of the chest and involved joints all are normal. An electrocardiogram reveals only tachycardia. After hospitalization and withholding aspirin, an evanescent rash becomes apparent in conjunction with fever spikes. What signs and symptoms of JRA does J.R. manifest?

The signs and symptoms (i.e., the spiking fever episodes, evanescent rash, arthritis, lymphadenopathy, splenomegaly) that J.R. experienced are characteristic of systemic-onset JRA. These children also may have a normocytic, hypochromic anemia, elevated ESR, thrombocytosis, and leukocytosis. Leukocytosis is common and a WBC count of 30,000 to 50,000 cells/mm³ is seen occasionally. A positive RF titer is uncommon in JRA and is present in only 5% to 10% of all cases.[214] The ANA titer more often is positive and is most prevalent in young girls and children with early-onset pauciarticular arthritis and uveitis.

Treatment
Nonsteroidal Anti-Inflammatory Drugs
SELECTION AND DOSING

48. What is the initial drug therapy for treatment of JRA?

NSAID therapy is the treatment of choice for treating the joint manifestations as well as the febrile episodes in systemic-onset JRA.[214] Up to two-thirds of JRA patients achieve good disease control with NSAID therapy.[218] In most cases, at least two different NSAIDs should be tried before ruling out this group of medications; failure to respond to an NSAID in a particular chemical class does not rule out the efficacy of others in the same class. As with adults, it is not possible to predict a patient's response to any NSAID.

Some FDA-approved NSAIDs for the treatment of JRA include salicylates, tolmetin, naproxen, ibuprofen, and diclofenac. The COX-2 inhibitors (celecoxib, rofecoxib, valdecoxib) are not FDA-approved for JRA. Aspirin is initiated in divided doses totaling 60 to 80 mg/kg per day.[23] The dosage should be increased slowly to 130 mg/kg per day to achieve anti-inflammatory serum salicylate concentrations ranging from 20 to 30 mg/dL. One authority recommended initiating therapy with 1,800 to 2,500 mg/m² for children weighing over 25 kg to reduce the risk of toxicity.[23] Tolmetin 15 mg/kg per day in divided doses generally is used to initiate therapy when indicated and doses up to 30 mg/kg per day (maximum, 1,800 mg) can be used for maintenance therapy.[219] Naproxen 10 to 15 mg/kg per day (maximum, 750 mg) in two daily divided doses may be advantageous in school-age children; it is commonly used because of a convenient dosing interval and availability in liquid or tablet formulations.[23,215] Ibuprofen doses should not exceed 40 to 50 mg/kg per day. Suspensions of naproxen and ibuprofen are available for use in children. Diclofenac may be given at 2 to 3 mg/kg per day in 2 to 4 divided doses; however, the SR formulation should not be used. Although not FDA approved, oxaprozin has been used at a once daily dose of 10 to 20 mg/kg. Sulindac requires additional study in children but recommended doses are approximately 6 mg/kg per day (maximum, 400 mg).

REYE'S SYNDROME

49. Should aspirin be discontinued in a JRA patient who experiences chickenpox because of the potential for causing Reye's syndrome?

Unrelated to the mild, reversible, dose-related transaminitis, Reye's syndrome occurs in association with the use of aspirin as an antipyretic in children during the prodromal phase of viral illnesses such as influenza and chickenpox. Reye's syndrome is characterized by fatty vacuolization of the liver producing hepatic injury, vomiting, hypoglycemia, and progressive encephalopathy. The suggestion that aspirin might be a factor in the development of Reye's syndrome first was proposed in the early 1960s.[220] Subsequently, retrospective case-controlled studies revealed a statistically significant difference in the prevalence of salicylate use in patients with Reye's syndrome compared with controls.[221–223] Virtually all cases of Reye's syndrome were exposed to salicylates during an antecedent illness. In the control population, salicylate use varied from approximately 40% to 70%. Based on these findings, the Committee of Infectious Diseases of the American Academy of Pediatrics issued a statement that aspirin should not be given to febrile children who are at risk for Reye's syndrome by virtue of possible infection with either influenza virus or chickenpox.[224]

The risk of Reye's syndrome in children receiving salicylate therapy for JRA is unknown. However, in a retrospective study, 6 of 176 patients with biopsy-confirmed Reye's syndrome were treated with salicylates for connective tissue disease.[225] Three of these children experienced a preceding upper respiratory tract infection; the other three experienced no apparent prodromal illness. Therefore, patients with JRA also should avoid salicylate ingestion during febrile illnesses that represent possible infection with either influenza or chickenpox.

DMARD THERAPY

50. **When should DMARDs be used in JRA?**

The heterogeneity of JRA is an important consideration in approaching treatment. Fortunately, most children with JRA improve significantly with NSAID treatment, particularly those with pauciarticular disease. Only a small number of these patients are considered for DMARD therapy, usually because of the evolution of their condition into the polyarticular type. Patients with polyarticular, RF-positive disease and patients with early-onset polyarthritis in association with systemic-onset disease both have poor prognosis in terms of ultimate joint function and should receive early consideration for DMARD therapy. Children with polyarticular-onset, RF-negative disease generally have a better prognosis than patients with polyarticular involvement. One may wait considerably longer before introducing a DMARD for these patients.

Most DMARDs used for adult RA are not effective for JRA,[214] and D-penicillamine is no more effective than placebo. A randomized controlled trial of injectable gold has not been performed, but interest in using gold has waned because of the multitude of injections required.

MTX is clearly the DMARD of choice for JRA.[226,227] The recommended dose of MTX for JRA treatment is 5 to 15 mg/m² (0.15 to 0.5 mg/kg) orally or subcutaneously each week, although doses as large as 30 mg/m² have been used. Pediatric patients are often prescribed the injectable form of MTX for oral consumption via a suspension. Oral absorption of MTX is best when taken on an empty stomach; however, absorption is impaired with higher doses of MTX (i.e., 10 to 15 mg/m²). As a result, patients who fail to respond adequately to oral MTX should consider subcutaneous therapy, particularly if higher doses are being administered.[226] Depending on the definition of response to therapy, 33% to 100% of JRA patients respond to dosages of MTX between 7.1 and 30 mg/m² (0.15 and 1 mg/kg) per week. MTX at a dose of 10 to 15 mg/m² appears to require an average of 13 months of treatment until remission is achieved in most JRA patients. Radiologic evidence of improvement or slowing of joint damage has been demonstrated in JRA patients who responded to MTX therapy over a 2-year period.[228]

Because the prognosis of JRA-related joint damage is much better than that associated with adult RA, attempts should be made to discontinue MTX when disease remission is apparent. The optimal length of time between achievement of disease remission and MTX discontinuation, however, has not been established. Some suggest that MTX should not be discontinued sooner than 1 year after disease remission, with slower withdrawal in patients at high risk for relapse.[226,227] In one trial involving all types of JRA subgroups, MTX discontinuation was attempted approximately 6 to 8 months after disease control was achieved.[218] After 11 months, 50% of patients relapsed; patients younger than 4.5 years old at the time of diagnosis appeared to be at higher risk of relapse. However, all patients who relapsed responded to MTX re-treatment at prediscontinuation doses. In another study, patients with pauciarticular JRA who progressed to polyarticular disease were at greatest risk for relapse.[227]

Children tolerate MTX therapy well and generally experience few serious or troublesome adverse effects.[226] The most common adverse effects include transient liver enzyme elevations and nausea/vomiting. Liver biopsy studies of patients with JRA receiving cumulative MTX doses up to 5,300 mg for up to 6 years have all been normal with the exception of a single case report in 1990. Liver toxicity monitoring in JRA, therefore, is the same as the guidelines recommend for MTX therapy in adult RA, including biopsy recommendations (see Questions 27 and 28). The combination of MTX and other DMARDs has not been fully evaluated.

If MTX is not tolerated or is ineffective, SSZ is often the next DMARD selected.[215,229] SSZ is effective for pauciarticular and polyarticular JRA, but is associated with numerous adverse effects leading to discontinuation of therapy in approximately 30% of patients.[230] These adverse effects include liver enzyme elevations, leukopenia, hypoimmunoglobulinemia, hematomas, diarrhea, and anorexia. Recommended dosing of SSZ for JRA is 30 to 50 mg/kg per day in two divided doses (maximum, 2 g/day). HCQ may be considered if SSZ fails, but efficacy data from well-designed randomized controlled trials are not available.[215]

Biological Agents

51. **Are any of the biological agents effective in JRA?**

Etanercept (Enbrel), the only FDA-approved biological agent for the treatment of JRA, is indicated for patients 4 years of age and older whose conditions have failed to respond to one or more DMARDs.[191] The recommended dose is 0.4 mg/kg (maximum, 25 mg) subcutaneously twice weekly. An open-label trial of 54 patients with JRA receiving etanercept monotherapy at this dose yielded a 76% response rate according to JRA Definition of Improvement criteria (i.e., a minimum 30% improvement in at least 3 of 6 and 30% or greater worsening in no more than 1 of 6 JRA core set criteria, including physician and patient global assessment, active joint count, limitation of motion, functional assessment, and ESR). The safety of etanercept in children is comparable to adults with the exception of significantly more abdominal pain (17% of JRA patients versus 5% of adult patients with RA) and vomiting (14.5% of patients with JRA versus <3% of adult patients with RA). JRA patients should be current on immunizations before initiation of etanercept therapy because the effect of etanercept on vaccine response is unknown.

Intra-Articular Corticosteroid Therapy

52. **What is the evidence to support the use of intra-articular corticosteroid therapy in JRA?**

Intra-articular corticosteroid therapy appears to be highly efficacious in JRA. One study reported full disease remission of injected joints lasting over 6 months in 84% of patients with JRA.[231] In addition, 60% of patients receiving intra-articular corticosteroid therapy were able to discontinue all oral medications, with even greater success in patients with pauci-articular JRA (75%). No significant adverse effects were reported with the exception of two cases of self-limiting postinjection joint flare. After an average of 30 months of follow-up, long-term negative effects of corticosteroid therapy (e.g., joint stability, osteonecrosis, soft-tissue atrophy) were not encountered. As a result, intra-articular corticosteroid therapy appears to be a safe and effective option for JRA, particularly in pauciarticular disease limited to a few troublesome joints.[214]

Uveitis

53. J.R. is scheduled to be seen by an ophthalmologist every 6 months to screen for uveitis. How should her uveitis be managed?

Uveitis associated with JRA is a nongranulomatous inflammation involving the iris and ciliary body. This type of uveitis sometimes is referred to as iridocyclitis. The posterior uveal tract, or choroid, rarely is affected.[214] Chronic uveitis can progress to blindness; therefore, careful screening is necessary for early detection. Uveitis occurs most often in young girls of early-age onset with limited joint disease and who are ANA-positive serologically.

Until recently, treatment had to be supervised by an ophthalmologist and initially consisted of a topically administered corticosteroid and a short-acting mydriatic drug (e.g., tropicamide or cyclopentolate) to dilate the eye and prevent adhesion of the iris to the lens or cornea. This treatment, however, is inadequate for up to 30% to 50% of children.[214] One study demonstrated that severe JRA-associated uveitis responds well to MTX (0.5 to 1.0 mg/kg subcutaneously every week), resulting in a dosage reduction in or discontinuation of topical corticosteroid.[232]

OSTEOARTHRITIS

Osteoarthritis (OA), previously known as degenerative joint disease (DJD), is the most common form of arthritis in the United States in which approximately 21 million individuals have clinical signs and symptoms.[233] These numbers may be much higher as recent data suggest that we may have up to 69 million people affected with some type of arthritis disorders as opposed to the 43 million reported in 1997.[234]

Osteoarthritis is the single most common cause of rheumatic symptoms and results in the most loss of time from work. Patients with OA accounted for more dependence on others in climbing stairs and walking a mile than any other disease. It is second only to heart disease as the most common disability for patients to receive Social Security benefits.

OA mainly affects older individuals with the incidence going up sharply after age 45. Although men are affected more commonly in early adulthood, men and women are generally affected equally. However, at age 65 OA becomes twice as prevalent in women, and women are more likely to have proximal and DIP joint involvement presenting with Bouchard's nodes or Heberden's nodes. Although only 30% are symptomatic, more than 90% of all individuals older than age 40 have some radiographic changes in their weight-bearing joints indicative of OA.[235]

In addition to advancing age, other risk factors could lead to OA. These include obesity, quadriceps muscle weakness,[236] joint overuse/injury from vocational or sports activities, genetic susceptibility,[237] and developmental abnormalities.[235] Obesity is thought to be a problem because of the excess weight that is placed on the joints leading to the development of OA, especially in the knee. However, metabolic factors other than excess weight may also play a role in the development of OA in obese individuals. Excess adipose tissue may produce abnormal levels of certain hormones or growth factors that affect cartilage or underlying bone in such a way as to predispose one to OA.[238] A weight loss of 5 kg was found to be associated with a 50% reduction in the odds of developing symptomatic knee OA.

Quadriceps muscle weakness is strongly predictive of both radiographic and symptomatic OA of the knee. Because persons with OA tend to be obese, the quadriceps weakness is more pronounced in relation to body weight. Vocational and/or athletic activities can also contribute to OA as the result of repetitive joint use or trauma subjected to the joints. This is consistent with the old "wear and tear" concept that has persisted for years as a cause of OA. However, OA is more than just a degenerative joint disease as the chondrocytes in OA undergo active cell division and are active metabolically. Under normal conditions, chondrocytes in articular cartilage balance matrix degradation and repair. Biomechanical stress placed on the joint is believed to stimulate cytokine-mediated release of enzymes such as the matrix metalloproteinase, plasmin, and cathepsins that degrade the proteoglycan and collagen components of cartilage. Disturbances in this process can lead to OA.[235]

Signs and Symptoms

The clinical presentation of OA is variable and depends on which joints are involved. Unlike RA, which is characterized by synovial proliferation within joints and systemic disease, the symptoms of OA are limited to the involved joints in which progressive degeneration of cartilage with secondary reactive bone changes (osteophyte formation) occurs. Occasionally, secondary synovial inflammation may contribute to symptoms. The primary symptom is a deep aching pain localized to the involved joint or joints. The joints most commonly involved are the DIP (Heberden's nodes), PIP (Bouchard's nodes), first carpometacarpal, knees, hips, cervical and lumbar spine, and the first MTP joints. Other sites include shoulder, elbow and rarely, the MCP joints. Associated with joint pain are morning stiffness and stiffness after rest during the day lasting less than 20 to 30 minutes and limited to involved joints. Joint motion may be limited secondary to loss of integrity of the joint surfaces, development of osteophytes, intra-articular loose bodies, and protective muscle spasm. Crepitus, a sense of grating or crackling, may be associated with both passive and active motion in involved joints.[235]

54. G.R., a 190-lb, 60-year-old school teacher, developed painful, tender swelling in the right knee about 1 year ago. Since then, she has experienced intermittent pain in the right knee and hip. She now has moderate morning stiffness in the hip and knee and some joint stiffness after inactivity. Her pain is increased significantly by ambulation. Examination of her joints revealed Heberden's nodes in both hands, limitation of flexion of the right hip to 90°, no synovial thickening, patellar crepitus, and some tenderness at the joint margin of the right knee. Laboratory studies were all normal and an RF was negative. What signs and symptoms of OA are present in G.R.?

Symptoms of OA usually are referable to the particular joint or joints involved. Common complaints include joint pain, particularly on motion and for weight-bearing joints, stiffness after periods of rest, and aching at times of inclement weather. Crepitation on joint motion, limitation of motion, and changes in the shape of the joint may be detected on physical examination. The joint(s) may be tender to palpation, but signs of inflammation are relatively uncommon, except for effusion, which may be noted following trauma or vigorous use of the involved joint. The Heberden's nodes observed in G.R.'s hands are bony protuberances (osteophytes) at the margins on the dorsal surfaces of the DIP joints. These nodes are more common in women, tend to occur in families, and often are associated with other joint involvement. OA of the hip generally progresses and eventually ROM is lost. Knee OA is observed frequently in older women in whom obesity and weak quadriceps could be contributing factors and is associated with crepitus, loss of motion, and flexion deformities. In addition to these characteristics, most of which were observed in G.R., other manifestations often observed are vertebral column involvement and Bouchard's nodes (osteophytes on the PIP joints).

Results of laboratory studies usually are normal unless an underlying disease co-exists. In patients with generalized OA characterized by three or more joint groups with some local inflammation marked by soft-tissue swelling, redness, and warmth, the ESR may be elevated. RF is negative. The synovial fluid may show nonspecific features of mild inflammation—increased volume, decreased viscosity, mild pleocytosis, and a slight increase in synovial fluid protein.[239]

Treatment
Nonpharmacologic and First-Line Therapy

55. **How should G.R. be treated?**

Nonpharmacologic options are as important in the management of OA and need to be considered first; drugs should serve as an adjunctive role in the management of this disease. G.R. has significant pain in both the hip and knees. She should first be educated about their disease status and self-management techniques. Appropriate nonpharmacologic management activities can include non–joint stress exercises to strengthen periarticular muscles and aerobic aquatic exercises; avoidance of excessive loading of the hip or knee joints by using assistive devices such as canes, walkers, or shoes that are cushioned properly; weight reduction for obese individuals; principles in joint protection; and thermal modalities.[240]

G.R. should be made aware of physical therapists who can help in developing an exercise program appropriate for OA patients and occupational therapists who can help her in dealing with activities of daily living.

Treatment goals are normally to relieve pain, maintain or improve joint function, minimize disability, enhance quality of life and functional independence, minimize risks of therapy, and educate patients and their families. Because the cause and much of the pathophysiology pertaining to OA re-

main unexplained, drug therapy is empiric and directed toward providing symptomatic relief.

To date, no pharmacologic agent is known to prevent, delay the progression of, or reverse the pathologic changes of OA in humans. Simple analgesic is usually indicated and acetaminophen has been recognized as the first-line agent that should be initiated. The recommendation that acetaminophen should be used as a first line drug for osteoarthritis is based on the premise that it has less toxicities and is as effective as the NSAIDs for symptomatic osteoarthritis. In one 4-week study of patients with symptomatic OA of the knee,[241] acetaminophen 1 g QID was comparable to an analgesic regimen of ibuprofen (1.2 g/day) and an anti-inflammatory regimen (2.4 g/day). When naproxen 750 mg/day was compared with acetaminophen 2.6 g/day in a multicenter, randomized, double-blind, 2-year trial, no significant differences were noted between treatments except for improvement in knee flexion and walking time in the naproxen group.[242] Based on these early two studies, acetaminophen has been recommended as the initial agent prescribed at doses up to 4 g/day.[240] Acetaminophen, however, may not be as effective as originally thought. In two placebo controlled double-blinded studies diclofenac 75 mg was more effective for symptomatic treatment of osteoarthritis than was acetaminophen 1 g QID.[243,244] Another double-blinded study compared acetaminophen 4 g/day to rofecoxib 12.5 mg/day and 25 mg/day and celecoxib 200 mg/day. Rofecoxib 25 mg/day was associated with significant relief for all osteoarthritis endpoints. Rofecoxib 12.5 mg/day and celecoxib 200 mg/day also had positive numerical endpoints for improvements, but nonsignificant benefits were noted with acetaminophen.[245] In a telephone survey of 300 patients (172 had confirmed osteoarthritis), NSAIDs were preferred over acetaminophen. In comparison to ibuprofen, naproxen, and diclofenac, only 24% who took acetaminophen found it "very helpful" as compared to 31%, 30%, and 56% respectively. In addition, many patients who took acetaminophen for pain relief also took an NSAID. For patients who took these drugs for more the 24 months, 33% continued to use acetaminophen, 21% continued with ibuprofen, 17% with naproxen, and 19% with diclofenac. The higher percentage of patients who continued to use acetaminophen in comparison to these other NSAIDS was attributed to the association of fewer adverse effects with acetaminophen.[246] The discrepancies as noted in earlier studies compared to the more recent studies in the finding of beneficial effects from acetaminophen in comparison to NSAIDs may be attributed to differences in the study design, differences in the severity of the osteoarthritis in enrolled patients, and the measurement tools used to assess improvement. As a result of these studies, the preference of acetaminophen over NSAIDs for the initial treatment of osteoarthritis needs further consideration. The severity of the osteoarthritis ultimately will dictate how the disease will be treated. For patients with early or mild osteoarthritis acetaminophen still merits a trial as initial therapy at doses up to the maximum dose of 4 g/day based on its costs, efficacy, and toxicity profile.[240]

Alternatives to Simple Analgesics

56. **G.R. starts a regimen of acetaminophen 1 g QID and returns to the clinic 4 weeks later. At that time, she states that she**

is improved symptomatically and is functioning much better. Her only problem now is that her right knee really has not responded. She believes that it is more bothersome to her now than 1 month ago. What is the next best course of drug therapy for G.R.?

If joint symptoms persist despite a reasonable period of treatment with acetaminophen, topical agents such as methylsalicylate or capsaicin can be considered, especially for those who do not wish to take systemic therapy.[240] Capsaicin cream is commonly used and is derived from vanillyl alkaloids found in hot peppers and related plants. It is effective in relieving pain by depleting the local sensory nerve endings of substance P. It can reduce joint pain and tenderness when applied topically by the patients with hand or knee OA, even when used as monotherapy. Topical agents such as capsaicin could be used before or after the addition of NSAIDs.[235] For those who do not respond adequately to a topical agent such as capsaicin, the use of NSAIDs or the COX-2 inhibitors must be considered. Whatever therapy is chosen, the need for continuation of that treatment requires ongoing reassessment. If traditional NSAIDs are used, risk factors for the NSAID induced gastropathy must be considered. The use of COX-2 inhibitors would be indicated for those patients who are at risk for upper GI complications.

NSAIDs and COX-2 Inhibitors

57. What is the role of the NSAIDs and/or COX-2 inhibitors in managing G.R.'s osteoarthritis?

Because G.R. is overweight and has had her osteoarthritis for more than 1 year, her condition is most likely more than a mild form of osteoarthritis. The 2000 ACR updates on the medical management of osteoarthritis of the hip and knee recommend that patients be started first with acetaminophen. The COX-2 specific inhibitors are the next preferred agents, followed by a nonselective NSAID used in conjunction with misoprostol or a proton pump inhibitor for those who are at increased risk for upper GI events. Many patients with osteoarthritis will require a nonselective NSAID or a COX-2 inhibitor if the disease is more severe.[241,245,247] Some patients may benefit from a combination acetaminophen plus an NSAID.[248,249] This combination would allow for lower doses of NSAIDs when used with acetaminophen. In one study, acetaminophen 4 g/day in combination with naproxen 500 mg/day was as effective as naproxen alone (1,000 mg/day or 1,500 mg/day) in patients with osteoarthritis of the hip.[250] Patients with inflammatory osteoarthritis (clinically defined as having detectable effusion in their joints) may respond better to NSAIDs.[251]

The nonselective NSAIDs or the COX-2 inhibitors can be used early in the therapy of osteoarthritis, especially for patients who have not responded adequately to maximum doses of acetaminophen, patients who have moderate to severe osteoarthritis with significant pain and not likely to respond to acetaminophen, and patients with joint effusions. Although the nonselective NSAIDS are effective for controlling pain and inflammation associated with osteoarthritis, approximately 107,000 patients (44,000 patients with RA or probable RA and another 32,000 with OA or other musculoskeletal conditions) are hospitalized each year for GI complications associated with the use of NSAIDs.[252] Arthritic patients are at much greater risk of developing GI symptoms, ulceration, hemorrhage, and death as the result of NSAID use, and relative to the general population, arthritis patients are 2.5 to 5.5 times more likely to be hospitalized for these NSAID-related complications. Overall, NSAIDs are estimated to cause 16,500 deaths per year among arthritis patients. Other risks for GI complications, include NSAID dose, concurrent prednisone use, prior GI side effects, and old age.[253]

For patients with increased risks or GI complications, gastroprotective agents such as misoprostol or high doses of H_2-receptor antagonists can be taken with the traditional NSAIDs with positive outcomes in terms of reducing the rate of serious clinical GI events or the formation of endoscopic ulceration. The proton pump inhibitors are also widely used and are effective in preventing NSAID induced gastropathy even though they do not have the FDA approval for prophylaxis. When using the gastroprotective agents, there are other factors such as patient convenience, costs, adverse effects, and adherence issues that must be considered. The COX-2 inhibitors are the drugs of choice for the initial treatment of osteoarthritis for those who are at increased risks for gastropathy as they have minimal inhibition of the constitutive prostaglandins leading to fewer problems with GI complications. Although the COX-2 inhibitors have minimal impact on the protective prostaglandins in the GI tract, NSAIDs are associated with other adverse effects (e.g., fluid retention, increases in blood pressure, congestive heart failure [CHF] exacerbation). In one study NSAIDs were responsible for approximately 19% of hospital admissions with CHF. The burden of illness from NSAID-related CHF may exceed those with GI tract damage.[253]

Rofecoxib and celecoxib can cause sodium retention and decrease glomerular filtration rate similar to the nonselective NSAIDs.[254] Valdecoxib also is to be used with precaution in patients with renal impairment.[255] The COX-2 inhibitors and the nonselective NSAIDs should be with caution in patients with congestive heart failure (especially those receiving ACE-inhibitors and diuretics), renal disease, hepatic disease, or advanced age.[254,256]

The synthetic opioid, tramadol is an alternative to the nonselective NSAIDs or COX-2 inhibitors for patients who have contraindications to the cyclooxygenase inhibitors. Tramadol relieves moderate to severe pain and is comparable to ibuprofen for the treatment of osteoarthritis of the hip and knee. It is also effective as an adjunctive therapy to the NSAIDs.[240] Since tramadol is a synthetic opioid, nausea, constipation, and drowsiness are common side effects. Tramadol does not appear to be associated with any abuse potential.[257]

Influence of Treatment on Progression of OA

The 1995 ACR recommendations first introduced the concept of disease modifying OA drugs (DMOADs) which can prevent the development of further progression of structural joint damage for those who have OA. In contrast to the symptomatic treatment of the OA, the disease modifying osteoarthritis drugs (DMOADS) are aimed to inhibit the breakdown of articular cartilage by matrix metalloproteinase, or at stimulating repair activity by chondrocytes.

There has been some thought that NSAIDs could alter the course of OA. Drug therapy of OA is symptomatic, directed primarily toward relief of pain and secondary inflammation. Symptomatic improvement is not associated with suppression of the underlying pathophysiologic process that results in cartilage degeneration and bony proliferation of joint margins. In theory, a decrease in symptoms may allow the patient to increase activities that enhance the rate of joint degeneration, and in this sense, NSAIDs may enhance the progression of joint disease.

Some NSAIDs (e.g., salicylates, fenoprofen, ibuprofen), when added to culture media containing osteoarthritic cartilage, inhibit proteoglycan synthesis in a dose-dependent fashion.[258] Other NSAIDs, such as sulindac and indomethacin, do not have this effect. Thus, certain NSAIDs ultimately may prove to be preferable in the treatment of OA. However, it remains to be determined whether any of the NSAIDs have detrimental effects on cartilage metabolism *in vivo* despite, paradoxically, providing symptomatic improvement.

In summary, current NSAID regimens do not appear to deter the progression of OA. The central role of NSAIDs has been questioned because of the greater risks of toxicity from prolonged NSAID therapy in the prolonged treatment of the elderly.[252,253,258]

Corticosteroids

Systemic corticosteroids are not normally used for patients with OA because of serious side effects associated with chronic use to treat a disorder that is not life-threatening or associated with serious morbidity. Intra-articular injection of a glucocorticoid can be of value when joints with effusions are painful and swollen. The aspiration of effusion fluid followed by an injection of a corticosteroid such as triamcinolone hexacetonide (up to 40 mg) can be effective for reducing pain and increasing muscle strength. The injections can be used as monotherapy or as adjunctive therapy along with an analgesic or a nonselective NSAID or COX-2 specific inhibitor. Symptomatic improvement from intra-articular corticosteroids may last only a few days, but also may persist for a month or longer. The initial relief of pain may permit more effective use of physical therapy and appropriate balance of rest and exercise, thus attenuating the need for repeated injections.[240] The dilemma, of course, is that symptomatic improvement may lead to overuse of the joint and potentially accelerate the degenerative process. Moreover, corticosteroids may have direct effects on articular cartilage. Repeated weekly joint injections for up to 9 weeks in animals resulted in histologic evidence of cartilage degeneration and depressed collagen and proteoglycan synthesis.[259] In weight-bearing joints, these changes were associated with degenerative changes in the cartilage. After termination of corticosteroid injections, recovery and normalization of the biochemical indices occurred over a several-month period.

The intra-articular injection of crystalline steroid suspension can precipitate a flare of synovitis which usually is temporary and can be relieved with cold compresses and analgesics. Other potential, but rare, complications of intra-articular injections include tendon rupture, microcrystalline corticosteroid deposition in the synovial fluid, and joint capsule calcification.[260] Thus, frequent injections into the same joint, particularly weight-bearing joints, should be avoided. The mechanism of action of the intra-articular corticosteroid providing relief in OA is still not clear. However, patients do respond; more than 95% of rheumatologists use intra-articular corticosteroids at least "sometimes," and 53% use them "frequently."[261]

Viscosupplements

Viscosupplements, classified by the FDA as a "medical devices" are used as substitutes for the natural hyaluronic acid in the joint fluid that breaks down in patients with OA. Two viscosupplements are currently available in the United States, hyaluronan (sodium hyaluronate) and hylan. Hyaluronan, polysaccharide molecules that occur naturally in synovial fluid, help to create a viscous environment, cushion joints, and maintain normal function. The viscosupplements (derived compound from rooster combs) act as lubricants and shock absorbers in the weight-bearing joints. Hyaluronans may also have structure-modifying activity. Proposed mechanisms of actions include inhibition of inflammatory mediators such as cytokines and prostaglandins, stimulation of cartilage matrix synthesis, and inhibition of cartilage degradation. Thus, compared with currently approved products for osteoarthritis, hyaluronans may also have beneficial effects on the disease process in osteoarthritis.[240,262]

Being a "medical device," the hyaluronans are usually administered when analgesics and other measures fail for knee OA. The affected knee is first aspirated and hyaluronan is administered intra-articularly into the knee as a series of five injections on a weekly basis. In clinical trials, intraarticular hyaluronan is superior to placebo injections and comparable to that of NSAID therapy. Pain relief is evident up to 6 months after a course of treatment and comparable to that achieved with naproxen 500 mg BID for 6 months. In addition, pain relief was comparable or greater than that achieved with the glucocorticoids. Hyaluronan was well-tolerated with the major adverse event being mild to moderate pain at the injection site.[263,264] The duration of action is longer than that of the corticosteroids and the role for these products in the management of OA of the knees may given the American College of Rheumatology support for its intra-articular use. The hyaluronans are an alternative to oral analgesics for patients who cannot tolerate the nonselective NSAIDs or COX-2 specific inhibitors. The hyaluronans are also currently being studied for osteoarthritis in joints other than the knee.

Glucosamine and Chondroitin

The high level of interest in unconventional therapies to manage arthritis has been stimulated by Theodosakis's book, *The Arthritis Cure*.[265] Glucosamine has been used for years in the United States for arthritis in dogs and horses and is thought to halt and reverse OA. Endogenous glucosamine, an amino-monosaccharide synthesized from glucose, is integral to the biosynthesis of proteoglycans and the glycosaminoglycans (GAG), which are thought to be the building blocks of cartilage. Chondroitin sulfate is theorized to work by providing substrate for the formation of a healthy joint matrix and blocking the enzymes that break down old cartilage. These products are often sold as combination products for the treatment of OA, but there is no evidence that the combination produces better results than glucosamine sulfate alone.[266] Most of the earlier clinical trials of glucosamine have been unconvincing because of small sample size or other deficiencies in study design.[267]

Two meta-analyses of glucosamine and chondroitin in the treatment of OA noted substantial benefit. However, both meta-analyses provided insufficient information regarding the study design and on the methodology used in the analyses to allow definitive conclusions.[268] While some studies show moderate to large beneficial effects from glucosamine and chondroitin, these studies have been challenged. Nevertheless, there is some evidence that these agents may relieve pain and joint stiffness associated with osteoarthritis.[269] In two relatively well-controlled studies glucosamine 500 mg TID was as effective or better than ibuprofen 400 mg TID in providing pain relief.[270,271] In another study, chondroitin 400 mg TID worked as well as diclofenac 50 mg TID. Clinical symptoms reappeared after the treatment ended; however, the chondroitin group experienced relief of symptoms up to 3 months after the treatment had ended.[272]

In a randomized, double-blind placebo-controlled study of 212 patients with OA of the knee, glucosamine 1500 mg/day was capable of slowing OA disease progression At 3-year follow-up, the 106 patients in the placebo group showed an average joint space narrowing of 0.31 mm (95% confidence interval, 0.48 to 0.13), while no joint space narrowing was detectable in radiographs of patients taking glucosamine.[273] Subsequently, another randomized, double-blind placebo-controlled trial of 202 patients receiving oral glucosamine sulfate 1,500 mg once a day or placebo for knee osteoarthritis also demonstrated that glucosamine sulfate retarded the progression of knee osteoarthritis. At the end of the 3-year follow-up, there was progressive joint space narrowing of the placebo group. Conversely, there was no average joint space narrowing in the glucosamine group. There was a significant difference in the joint space narrowing for the glucosamine group compared to the placebo at the end of each year. At the end of the 3 years, there was a difference of 0.36 mm (95% confidence interval, 0.13 to 0.50 mm).[274] These two studies provide good evidence that long-term use of glucosamine reduce radiographic progression of OA of the knee. As a result, glucosamine meets the criteria to be classified as a symptom- and structure-modifying drug in osteoarthritis as established by the definition of scientific organizations[275,276] and as acknowledged by the regulatory agencies.[277,278]

A more recent study to examine the role of topical glucosamine sulfate and chondroitin was performed in 63 patients randomized to receive either a topical glucosamine and chondroitin preparation or a placebo to be used over an 8-week period. At the end of the 8-week period, the topical application of glucosamine and chondroitin sulfate was effective in relieving pain from OA of the knee and improvement was evident in 4 weeks. The patients received an average of 2.5 application of the cream per day. It was estimated that the patients received approximately glucosamine sulfate 300 mg and chondroitin sulfate 780 mg per day topically. Clinically significant improvement in pain was evident at both 4 and 8 weeks. The speed of the onset of pain relief was unexpected, and it was speculated that some of immediate pain relief may have been provided by the peppermint oil and camphor that was in formulation. However, the placebo contained peppermint oil and camphor as well.[279]

Glucosamine and chondroitin are considered natural products and appear to be well tolerated. Now we have further evidence that they may be effective in controlling and modifying osteoarthritis, something that has not been shown for the NSAIDs. There is a growing body of evidence that glucosamine and chondroitin are effective.[280] Patients still should be warned they should remain under medical supervision and be aware of the consequences of osteoarthritis. Since these products are considered natural products, they are not FDA regulated. As a result, patients who want to take these products should be cautioned that their potency, safety, purity, and efficacy (depending on the product selected) cannot be assured.

Acknowledgments

The primary author acknowledges Mircea Florea, MD, for his guidance and mentoring in the evaluation and management of arthritic disorders.

REFERENCES

1. Arthritis Foundation. Disease Center. Available at: http://www.arthritis.org/conditions/diseasecenter/default.asp, 2003.
2. Impact of arthritis and other rheumatic conditions on the health-care system—United States, 1997. MMWR 1999;42:349.
3. Arnett FC et al. The American Rheumatism Association 1987 revised criteria for the classification of rheumatoid arthritis. Arthritis Rheum 1988;31:315.
4. Felson DT. Epidemiology of the rheumatic diseases. In: Koopman WJ, ed. Arthritis and Allied Conditions [Online], Chapter 1. 14th Ed. Baltimore: Lippincott Williams & Wilkins, 2001.
5. Tuomi T et al. Smoking, lung function, and rheumatoid factors. Ann Rheum Dis 1990;49:753.
6. Krishnan E et al. Smoking-gender interaction and risk for rheumatoid arthritis. Arthritis Res Ther 2003;5:R158.
7. O'Dell JR. Rheumatoid arthritis: the clinical picture. In: Koopman WJ, ed. Arthritis and Allied Conditions [Online], Chapter 58. 14th Ed. Baltimore: Lippincott Williams & Wilkins, 2001.
8. American College of Rheumatology Subcommittee on Rheumatoid Arthritis Guidelines. Guidelines for the management of rheumatoid arthritis. Arthritis Rheum 2002;46:328.
9. Pinals RS et al. Preliminary criteria for clinical remission in rheumatoid arthritis. Arthritis Rheum 1981;24:1308.
10. Alarcon GS et al. Evaluation of the American Rheumatism Association preliminary criteria for remission in rheumatoid arthritis: a prospective study. J Rheumatol 1987;14:93.
11. Wolfe F, Hawley DJ. Remission in rheumatoid arthritis. J Rheumatol 1985;12:245.
12. Mottonen T et al. Comparison of combination therapy with single-drug therapy in early rheumatoid arthritis: a randomised trial. Lancet 1999;353:1568.
13. Mottonten T et al. Outcome in patients with early rheumatoid arthritis treated according to the "sawtooth" strategy. Arthritis Rheum 1996;39:996.
14. van Jaarsveld CFM et al. Aggressive treatment in early rheumatoid arthritis: a randomized controlled trial. Ann Rheum Dis 2000;59:468.
15. The North American Rheumatoid Arthritis Disease Management Study Group. A population-based assessment of disease activity, quality of life and cost of care in early rheumatoid arthritis. Arthritis Rheum 1998;41:S127.
16. Lindqvist E, Eberhardt K. Mortality in rheumatoid arthritis patients with disease onset in the 1980s. Ann Rheum Dis 1999;58:11.
17. Kroot EJA et al. No increased mortality in patients with rheumatoid arthritis: up to 10 years of follow up from disease onset. Ann Rheum Dis 2000;59:954.
18. Hale LP, Haynes BF. Pathology of rheumatoid arthritis and associated disorders. In: Koopman WJ, ed. Arthritis and Allied Conditions [Online], Chapter 56. 14th Ed. Baltimore: Lippincott Williams & Wilkins, 2001.
19. Arend W. The pathophysiology and treatment of rheumatoid arthritis. Arthritis Rheum 1997;40:595.
20. Feldmann M et al. Rheumatoid arthritis. Cell 1996;85:307.
21. Weinblatt ME. Treatment of rheumatoid arthritis. In: Koopman WJ, ed. Arthritis and Allied Conditions [Online], Chapter 62. 14th Ed. Baltimore: Lippincott Williams & Wilkins, 2001.
22. Furst DE et al. Updated consensus statement on biological agents for the treatment of rheumatoid arthritis and other rheumatic diseases. Ann Rheum Dis 2002;61(Suppl ii):ii2.
23. Furst DE, Hillson J. Aspirin and other nonsteroidal anti-inflammatory drugs. In: Koopman WJ, ed. Arthritis and Allied Conditions [Online], Chapter 32. 14th Ed. Baltimore: Lippincott Williams & Wilkins, 2001.
24. Greene JM, Winickff RN. Cost-conscious prescribing of nonsteroidal anti-inflammatory drugs for

adults with arthritis. Arch Intern Med 1992;152: 1995.

25. Wolfe MM et al. Medical progress: gastrointestinal toxicity of nonsteroidal anti-inflammatory drugs. N Engl J Med 1999;340:1888.

26. Cryer C, Feldman M. Cyclooxygenase-1 and cyclooxygenase-2 selectivity of widely used nonsteroidal anti-inflammatory drugs. Am J Med 1998;104:413.

27. Buttar NS, Wang KK. The aspirin of the new millennium: cyclooxygenase-2 inhibitors. Mayo Clin Proc 2000;75:1027.

28. Silverstein FE et al. Gastrointestinal toxicity with celecoxib vs nonsteroidal anti-inflammatory drugs for osteoarthritis and rheumatoid arthritis: the CLASS study: a randomized controlled trial. Celecoxib Long-term Arthritis Safety Study. JAMA 2000;284:1247.

29. Bombardier C et al. VIGOR Study Group. Comparison of upper gastrointestinal toxicity of rofecoxib and naproxen in patients with rheumatoid arthritis. VIGOR Study Group. N Engl J Med 2000;343: 1520.

30. Adalimumab (humira) for rheumatoid arthritis. In: Abramowicz M, ed. Med Lett 2003;45:25.

31. Verhoeven AC et al. Combination therapy in rheumatoid arthritis: an updated systematic review. Br J Rheum 1998;37:612.

32. Felson DT et al. Use of short-term efficacy/toxicity trade-offs to select second-line drugs in rheumatoid arthritis. Arthritis Rheum 1992;35:1117.

33. Buchbinder R et al. Methotrexate therapy in rheumatoid arthritis: a life table review of 587 patients treated in community practice. J Rheumatol 1993;20:639.

34. Nowlin NS et al. DMARDs in the nineties: the UW experience. Arthritis Rheum 1998;41:S153.

35. Suarez-Almazor ME. Practice patterns in the management of rheumatoid arthritis: increased use of combination therapy. Arthritis Rheum 1998;41: S153.

36. Wang BWE et al. Frequency of two-DMARD combinations in the treatment of rheumatoid arthritis. Arthritis Rheum 1998;41:S59.

37. Smolen JS et al. Efficacy and safety of leflunomide compared with placebo and sulphasalazine in active rheumatoid arthritis: a double-blind, randomised, multicentre trial. Lancet 1999;353:259.

38. Leflunomide (Arava) [package insert]. Bridgewater, NJ: Aventis Pharmaceuticals, April 2000.

39. Cohen S et al. Two-year, blinded, randomized, controlled trial of active rheumatoid arthritis with leflunomide compared with methotrexate. Arthritis Rheum 2001;44:1984.

40. Sander O et al. Prospective six year follow up of patients withdrawn from a randomised study comparing parenteral gold salt and methotrexate. Ann Rheum Dis 1999;58:281.

41. Felson DT et al. The comparative efficacy and toxicity of second-line drugs in rheumatoid arthritis. Arthritis Rheum 1990;33:1449.

42. Van den Borne B et al. No increased risk of malignancies and mortality in cyclosporin A-treated patients with rheumatoid arthritis. Arthritis Rheum 1998;41:1930.

43. O'Dell JR. Anticytokine therapy—a new era in the treatment of rheumatoid arthritis? N Engl J Med 1999;340:310.

44. Jenkins JK et al. Biological modifier therapy for the treatment of rheumatoid arthritis. Am J Med Sci 2002;323:197-205.

45. Moreland LW et al. Etanercept therapy in rheumatoid arthritis: a randomized, controlled trial. Ann Intern Med 1999;130:478.

46. Louie SG et al. Biological response modifiers in the management of rheumatoid arthritis. Am J Health System Pharm 2003;60:346.

47. Bendele AM et al. Combination benefit of treatment with the cytokine inhibitors interleukin-1 receptor antagonist and PEGylated soluble tumor necrosis factor receptor type I in animal models of rheumatoid arthritis. Arthritis Rheum 2000;43:2648.

48. Drugs for rheumatoid arthritis. In: Abramowicz M, ed. Treatment Guidelines from The Medical Letter 2003;1:25.

49. Ault A. Rheumatoid arthritis drug linked to infections. Lancet 1999;353:1770.

49. Conn DL. Resolved: low-dose prednisone is indicated as standard treatment in patients with rheumatoid arthritis. Arthritis Rheum 2001;45:462.

50. Saag KG. Resolved: low-dose glucocorticoids are neither safe nor effective for the long-term treatment of rheumatoid arthritis. Arthritis Rheum 2001;45:468.

51. O'Dell JR et al. Treatment of early seropositive rheumatoid arthritis with minocycline: four-year follow-up of a double-blind, placebo-controlled trial. Arthritis Rheum 1999;42:1691.

52. O'Dell JR et al. Treatment of early seropositive rheumatoid arthritis: a two-year, double-blind comparison of minocycline and hydroxychloroquine. Arthritis Rheum 2001;44:2235.

53. Felson DT et al. The Prosorba column for treatment of refractory rheumatoid arthritis. Arthritis Rheum 1999;42:2153.

54. Ossandon A et al. Thalidomide: focus on its employment in rheumatologic diseases. Clin Exp Rheumatol 2002;20:709.

55. Skelly MM, Hawkey CF. Potential alternatives to COX 2 inhibitors. BMJ 2002;324:1289.

56. Hawkey CJ et al. Gastrointestinal safety of AZD 3582: a new chemical entity with a novel multipathway mechanism of action [Abstract 446]. Gastroenterology 2002;122:a446.

57. Palmer RH et al. Licofelone (ML 3000) an inhibitor of COX-1, COX-2 and 5-LO is associated with less gastric damage than naproxen and is similar to placebo in man [Abstract 445]. Gastroenterology 2002;122:a445.

58. Moreland LW. T cell receptor peptide vaccination in rheumatoid arthritis: a placebo-controlled trial using a combination of V-beta3, V-beta14, and V-beta14 peptides. Arthritis Rheum 1998;41:1919.

59. Clark P et al. Meta-analysis of injectable gold in rheumatoid arthritis. J Rheumatol 1989;16:442.

60. Ward JR et al. Comparison of auranofin, gold sodium thiomalate, and placebo in the treatment of rheumatoid arthritis. Arthritis Rheum 1983; 26:1303.

61. Scott DL et al. Long-term outcome of treating rheumatoid arthritis: results after 20 years. Lancet 1987:1108.

62. Thompson PW et al. Practical results of treatment with disease-modifying antirheumatoid drugs. Br J Rheumatol 1985;24:167.

63. Wolfe FE et al. Termination of slow acting antirheumatic therapy in rheumatoid arthritis: a 14-year prospective evaluation of 1017 consecutive starts. J Rheumatol 1990;17:994.

64. Wijnands MJH et al. Long-term second-line treatment: a prospective drug survival study. Br J Rheumatol 1992;31:253.

65. Mottonen T et al. Outcome in patients with early rheumatoid arthritis treated according to the "saw-tooth" strategy. Arthritis Rheum 1996;39:996.

66. Ortendahl M et al. Influence of time on methotrexate in rheumatoid arthritis. Arthritis Rheum 1998;41:S156.

67. Morand EF et al. Life table analysis of 879 treatment episodes with slow acting antirheumatic drugs in community rheumatology practice. J Rheum 1992;19:704.

68. Cannella AC, O'Dell, JR. Is there still a role for traditional disease-modifying antirheumatic drugs (DMARDs) in rheumatoid arthritis? Curr Opin Rheumatol 2003;15:185.

69. Jonsson R et al. Sjogren's syndrome. In: Koopman WJ, ed. Arthritis and Allied Conditions [Online], Chapter 85. 14th Ed. Baltimore: Lippincott Williams & Wilkins, 2001.

70. Hale LP, Haynes BF. Pathology of rheumatoid arthritis and associated disorders. In: Koopman WJ, ed. Arthritis and Allied Conditions [Online], Chapter 56. 14th Ed. Baltimore: Lippincott Williams & Wilkins, 2001.

71. Blackburn WD Jr, Chatman WW. Laboratory findings in rheumatoid arthritis. In: Koopman WJ, ed. Arthritis and Allied Conditions [Online], Chapter 60. 14th Ed. Baltimore: Lippincott Williams & Wilkins, 2001.

72. Dromgoole SH et al. Rational approaches to the use of salicylates in the treatment of rheumatoid arthritis. Semin Arthritis Rheum 1981;11:257.

73. Bridges SL Jr. Rheumatoid factor. In: Koopman WJ, ed. Arthritis and Allied Conditions [Online], Chapter 61. 14th Ed. Baltimore: Lippincott Williams & Wilkins, 2001.

74. Marble DA. Rheumatic diseases. In: Traub SL, ed. Basic Skills in Interpreting Laboratory Data. 2nd Ed. Bethesda: American Society of Health-Systems Pharmacists, 1996:371.

75. Brander VA, Chang RW. Rehabilitation for persons with arthritis and rheumatic disorders. In: Koopman WJ, ed. Arthritis and Allied Conditions [Online], Chapter 46, 14th Ed. Baltimore: Lippincott Williams & Wilkins, 2001.

76. Rogers MP et al. Psychological care of adults with rheumatoid arthritis. Ann Intern Med 1982; 96:344.

77. Roth SH. NSAID gastropathy: a new understanding. Arch Intern Med 1996;156:1623.

78. Anderson RJ et al. Unrecognized adult salicylate intoxication. Ann Intern Med 1976;85:745.

79. Lanza FL et al. Endoscopic evaluation of the effects of aspirin, buffered aspirin, and enteric-coated aspirin on the gastric and duodenal mucosa. N Engl J Med 1980;303:136.

80. Orozco-Alcala JJ, Baum J. Regular and enteric coated aspirin: a reevaluation. Arthritis Rheum 1979;22:1034.

81. Karahalios WJ et al. Comparative bioavailability of sustained-release and uncoated aspirin tablets. Am J Hosp Pharm 1981;38:1754.

82. Cassell S et al. Steady-state serum salicylate levels in hospitalized patients with rheumatoid arthritis. Arthritis Rheum 1979;22:384.

83. Mann CC, Boyer JT. Once-daily treatment of rheumatoid arthritis with choline magnesium trisalicylate. Clin Ther 1984;6:170.

84. Szczeklik A. Aspirin-induced asthma. In: Vane JR, Botting RM, eds. Aspirin and Other Salicylates. London: Chapman & Hall Medical, 1993:548.

85. Szczeklik A, Stevenson DD. Aspirin-induced asthma: advances in pathogenesis and management. J Allergy Clin Immunol 1999;104:5.

86. Slepian IK et al. Aspirin-sensitive asthma. Chest 1985;87:386.

87. Settipane GA. Aspirin and allergic diseases: a review. Am J Med 1983;74(6A):102.

88. Goldsweig HG et al. Bleeding, salicylates, and prolonged prothrombin time: three case reports and a review of the literature. J Rheumatol 1976;3:37.

89. Slone D et al. Aspirin and congenital malformations. Lancet 1976;1:1373.

90. Turner G, Collins E. Fetal effects of regular aspirin ingestion in pregnancy. Lancet 1975;2:338.

91. Zierler S, Rothman KJ. Congenital heart disease in relation to maternal use of bendectin and other drugs in early pregnancy. N Engl J Med 1985; 313:347.

92. Rudolph AM. Effects of aspirin and acetaminophen in pregnancy and the newborn. Arch Intern Med 1981;141:358.

93. Woessner KM et al. The safety of celecoxib in patients with aspirin-sensitive asthma. Arthritis Rheum 2002;46:2201.

94. Martin-Garcia C et al. Safety of a cyclooxygenase-2 inhibitor in patients with aspirin-sensitive asthma. Chest 2002;121:1812.

95. May N et al. Selective COX-2 inhibitors: a review of their therapeutic potential and safety in dentistry. Oral Surg Oral Med Oral Pathol Oral Rediol Endod 2001;92:399.

96. Janssen NM, Genta MS. The effects of immunosuppressive and anti-inflammatory medications on fertility, pregnancy, and lactation. Arch Intern Med 2000;160:610.

97. Committee on Drugs. The transfer of drugs and other chemicals into human milk (American Academy of Pediatrics). Pediatrics 2001;108:776.

98. Morris HG et al. Effects of salsalate (nonacetylated salicylate) and aspirin on serum prostaglandins in humans. Ther Drug Monit 1985;7:435.

99. Cryer B et al. Comparison of salsalate and aspirin on mucosal injury and gastroduodenal mucosal prostaglandins. Gastroent 1990;6:1616.

100. Dromgoole SH et al. Availability of salicylate from salsalate and aspirin. Clin Pharmacol Ther 1983;34:539.

101. Brooks PM, Day RO. Nonsteroidal anti-inflammatory drugs—differences and similarities. N Engl J Med 1991;324:1716.

102. Sing G, Triadafilopoulus G. Epidemiology of NSAID-induced GI complications. J Rheumatol 1999;26:(Suppl 26):18.

103. Singh G et al. Gastrointestinal tract complications of nonsteroidal anti-inflammatory drug treatment in rheumatoid arthritis: a prospective observational cohort study. Arch Intern Med 1996;156:1530.

104. Ad Hoc Committee on Practice Parameters of the American College of Gastroenterology. A guideline for the treatment and prevention of NSAID-induced ulcers. Am J Gastroenterol 1998;93:2037.

105. Graham DY et al. Ulcer prevention in long-term users of nonsteroidal anti-inflammatory drugs. Arch Intern Med 2002;162:169.

106. Barkin J. The relation between *Helicobacter pylori* and nonsteroidal anti-inflammatory drugs. Am J Med 1998;105:22S.

107. Celecoxib (Celebrex) package insert. New York: Pfizer, August 2002.

108. Rofecoxib (Vioxx) package insert. Whitehouse Station, NJ: Merck, April 2003.

109. Valdecoxib (Bextra) package insert. New York, NY: Pfizer, October 2002.

110. Hawkey CJ. Cox-2 inhibitors. Lancet 1999; 353;307.

111. Juni P et al. Are selective Cox-2 inhibitors superior to traditional non steroidal anti-inflammatory drugs? BMJ 2002;321;1287.

112. Witter J. Medical Officer Review. Available at: http://www.fda.gov/ohrms/dockets/ac/01/briefing/3677b1_03_med.pdf (accessed June 2003).

113. FDA Talk Paper. FDA approves new indication and label changes for the arthritis drug, Vioxx. 2002, Available at: http://www.fda.gov/bbs/topics/ANSWERS/2002/ANS01145.htm. (accessed June 2003).

114. Dunn MJ et al. Nonsteroidal anti-inflammatory drugs and renal function. J Clin Pharmacol 1988;28:524.

115. Patrono C, Dunn MJ. The clinical significance of inhibition of renal prostaglandin synthesis. Kidney Int 1987;32:1.

116. Rossat J et al. Renal effects of selective cyclooxygenase-2 inhibition in normotensive salt-depleted subjects. Clin Pharmacol Ther 1999;66:76.

117. Ciabottoni G et al. Effects of sulindac and ibuprofen in patients with chronic glomerular disease. N Engl J Med 1984;310:279.

118. Swainson CP, Griffiths P. Acute and chronic effects of sulindac on renal function in chronic renal disease. Clin Pharmacol Ther 1985;37:298.

119. Berg KJ, Talseth T. Acute renal effects of sulindac and indomethacin in chronic renal failure. Clin Pharmacol Ther 1985;37:447.

120. Sedor JR et al. Effects of sulindac and indomethacin on renal prostaglandin synthesis. Clin Pharmacol Ther 1984;36:85.

121. Miller MJS et al. Renal metabolism of sulindac: functional hypothesis. J Clin Pharmacol Exp Ther 1984;231:449.

122. Cook ME et al. Comparative effects of nabumetone, sulindac, and ibuprofen on renal function. J Rheumatol 1997;24:1137.

123. FitzGerald GA, Patrono C. Drug therapy: the cox-ibs, selective inhibitors of cyclooxygenase-2. N Engl J Med 2001;345:433.

124. Whelton A et al. Cycloxygenase-2Ospecific inhibitors and cardiorenal function: a randomized controlled trial of celecoxib and rofecoxib in older hypertensive patients. Am J Ther 2001;8:85.

125. Clive DM, Stoff JS. Renal syndromes associated with nonsteroidal anti-inflammatory drugs. N Engl J Med 1984;310:563.

126. American College of Rheumatology Ad Hoc Committee on Clinical Guidelines. Guidelines for monitoring drug therapy in rheumatoid arthritis. Arthritis Rheum 1996;39:723.

127. Johnson AG et al. NSAIDs and increased blood pressure: what is the clinical significance? Drug Safety 1997;17:277.

128. Weinblatt ME. Rheumatoid arthritis: treat now, not later. Ann Intern Med 1996;124:773.

129. Schattner A. Treatment considerations in early rheumatoid arthritis. J Intern Med 1997;241: 445.

130. Morand EF et al. Continuation of long term treatment with hydroxychloroquine in systemic lupus erythematous and rheumatoid arthritis. Ann Rheum Dis 1992;51:1318.

131. Bernstein HN. Ophthalmologic considerations and testing in patients receiving long-term antimalarial therapy. Am J Med 1983;75(1A):25.

132. Farr M et al. Side effects profile of 200 patients with inflammatory arthritides treated with sulphasalazine. Drugs 1986;32:49.

133. Gottlieb NL, Brown HEJ. Acute myocardial infarction following gold sodium thiomalate-induced vasomotor (nitritoid) reaction. Arthritis Rheum 1977;20:1026.

134. Halla JT et al. Postinjection nonvasomotor reactions during chrysotherapy: constitutional and rheumatic symptoms following injection of gold salts. Arthritis Rheum 1977;20:1188.

135. Lawrence JS. Comparative toxicity of gold preparations in treatment of rheumatoid arthritis. Ann Rheum Dis 1976;35:171.

136. Chatham WW. Gold and d-penicillamine. In: Koopman WJ, ed. Arthritis and Allied Conditions [Online], Chapter 33. 14th Ed. Baltimore: Lippincott Williams & Wilkins, 2001.

137. Edelman J et al. Prevalence of eosinophilia during gold therapy for rheumatoid arthritis. J Rheumatol 1983;10:121.

138. Podell TE et al. Pulmonary toxicity with gold therapy. Arthritis Rheum 1980;23:347.

139. Smith W, Ball GV. Lung injury due to gold treatment. Arthritis Rheum 1980;23:351.

140. Stein HB, Urowitz MB. Gold-induced enterocolitis: case report and literature review. J Rheumatol 1976;3:21.

141. Favreau M et al. Hepatic toxicity associated with gold therapy. Ann Intern Med 1977;87:717.

142. Gottlieb NL, Major JC. Ocular chrysiasis correlated with gold concentrations in the crystalline lens during chrysotherapy. Arthritis Rheum 1978; 21:704.

143. Gottlieb NL. Comparative pharmacokinetics of parenteral and oral gold compounds. J Rheumatol 1982;9(Suppl 8):99.

144. Ward JR et al. Comparison of auranofin, gold sodium thiomalate and placebo in the treatment of active rheumatoid arthritis: response by treatment duration. In: Capell HA et al, eds. Auranofin: Proceedings of a Smith Kline & French International Symposium. Amsterdam, Excerpta Medica, 1982:115.

145. Morris RW et al. Worldwide clinical experience with auranofin. Clin Rheumatol 1984;3(Suppl 1):105.

146. Gottlieb NL. Serum gold levels. Arthritis Rheum 1975;18:626.

147. Dahl SL et al. Lack of correlation between gold concentrations and clinical response in patients with definite or classical rheumatoid arthritis receiving auranofin or gold sodium thiomalate. Arthritis Rheum 1985;28:1211.

148. Klinefelter HF. Reinstitution of gold therapy in rheumatoid arthritis after mucocutaneous reactions. J Rheumatol 1975;2:21.

149. Hull RG et al. A double-blind study comparing sodium aurothiomalate and auranofin in patients with rheumatoid arthritis previously stabilized on sodium aurothiomalate. Int J Clin Pharmacol Res 1984;4:395.

150. Wenger ME et al. Therapy of rheumatoid arthritis. Transferring treatment from injectable gold to auranofin. In: Capell HA et al, eds. Auranofin: Proceedings of a Smith Kline & French International Symposium. Amsterdam: Excerpta Medica, 1982:201.

151. Tosi S et al. Injectable gold dermatitis and proteinuria: retreatment with auranofin. Int J Clin Pharmacol Res 1985;5:265.

152. Dahl MG et al. Methotrexate hepatotoxicity in psoriasis—comparison of different dose regimens. Br Med J 1972;1:654.

153. Williams HJ et al. Comparison of low-dose oral pulse methotrexate and placebo in the treatment of rheumatoid arthritis. Arthritis Rheum 1985;28:721.

154. Kremer HM. Rational use of new and existing disease-modifying agents in rheumatoid arthritis. Ann Intern Med 2001;134:695.

155. Magdalena L et al. Comparison of two dosing schedules for administering oral low-dose methotrexate (weekly versus every-other-week) in patients with rheumatoid arthritis. Arthritis Rheum 1999;42:2160.

156. Health and Public Policy Committee AC of P. Methotrexate in rheumatoid arthritis. Ann Intern Med 1987;107:418.

157. Tobias H, Auerbach R. Hepatotoxicity of long-term methotrexate therapy for psoriasis. Arch Intern Med 1973;132:391.

158. Zachariae H et al. Methotrexate induced liver cirrhosis: studies including serial liver biopsies during continued treatment. Br J Dermatol 1980; 102:407.

159. Kremer JM. Liver biopsies in patients with rheumatoid arthritis receiving methotrexate: where are we going? J Rheumatol 1992;19:189.

160. Tishler M et al. The effects of leucovorin (folinic acid) on methotrexate therapy in rheumatoid arthritis. J Rheumatol 1988;31:906.

161. Buckley LM et al. Administration of folinic acid after low dose methotrexate in patients with RA. J Rheumatol 1990;17:1158.

162. Shiroky JB et al. Low dose methotrexate with leucovorin (folinic acid) rescue in the management of rheumatoid arthritis. Results of a multicenter randomized, double-blind, placebo-controlled trial. Arthritis Rheum 1993;36:795.

163. Weinblatt ME et al. Low dose leucovorin does not interfere with the efficacy of methotrexate in rheumatoid arthritis: an 8 week randomized placebo controlled trial. J Rheumatol 1993;20:950.

164. Morgan SL et al. The effect of folic acid supplementation on the toxicity of low-dose methotrexate in patients with rheumatoid arthritis. Arthritis Rheum 1990;33:9.

165. Stewart KA et al. Folate supplementation in methotrexate-treated rheumatoid arthritis patients. Semin Arthritis Rheum 1991;20:332.

166. van Ede AE et al. Effect of folic or folinic acid supplementation on the toxicity and efficacy of methotrexate in rheumatoid arthritis: a fort-eight-week, multicenter, randomized, double-blind, placebo-controlled study. Arthritis Rheum 2001; 44:1515.

167. Hoekstra M et al. Factors associated with toxicity, final dose, and efficacy of methotrexate in patients with rheumatoid arthritis. Ann Rheum Dis 2003; 62:423.

168. Carson CW et al. Pulmonary disease during the treatment of rheumatoid arthritis with low dose pulse methotrexate. Semin Arthritis Rheum 1987; 16:186.

169. Nesher G et al. Effect of caffeine consumption on efficacy of methotrexate in rheumatoid arthritis. Arthritis Rheum 2003;48:571.

170. Furst D et al. Onset of effect and duration of response to leflunomide treatment of active rheumatoid arthritis compared to placebo or methotrexate. Arthritis Rheum 1998;41:S155.

171. Weaver A et al. Treatment of active rheumatoid arthritis with leflunomide compared to placebo or methotrexate. Arthritis Rheum 1998;41:S131.

172. Scott DL et al. Treatment of active rheumatoid arthritis with leflunomide: two year follow-up of a double blind, placebo controlled trial versus sulfasalazine. Ann Rheum Dis 2001;60:913.

173. Sharp JT et al. Treatment with leflunomide slows radiographic progression of rheumatoid arthritis. Arthritis Rheum 2000;43:495.

174. Osiri M et al. Leflunomide for the treatment of rheumatoid arthritis: a systematic review and metaanalysis. J Rheumatol 2003;30:1182.

175. Barbehenn E et al. Petition to the FDA to ban the rheumatoid arthritis drug leflunomide (ARAVA) (HRG publication #1614) Public Citizen. March 28, 2002. http://www.citizen.org/documents/1614.pdf (Accessed June 2003).

176. Geborek P et al. Etanercept, infliximab, and leflunomide in established rheumatoid arthritis: clinical experience using a structured follow up programme in southern Sweden. Ann Rheum Dis 2002;61:793.

177. Leflunomide (Arava) package insert. Bridgewater, NJ: Aventis Pharmaceuticals, April 2000.

178. Assem ESK, Vickers MR. Immunological response to penicillamine in penicillin-allergic patients and in normal subjects. Postgrad Med J 1974;50(Suppl 2):65.

179. Bell C, Graziano F. The safety of administration of penicillamine in penicillin-sensitive individuals. Arthritis Rheum 1983;26:801.

180. O'Dell J et al. Treatment of rheumatoid arthritis with methotrexate alone, sulfasalazine and hydroxychloroquine, or a combination of all three medications. N Engl J Med 1996;1287.

181. Mottonen T et al. Comparison of combination therapy with single-drug therapy in early rheumatoid arthritis: a randomised trial. Lancet 1999; 353:1568.

182. O'Dell J. Combination DMARD therapy for rheumatoid arthritis: apparent universal acceptance. Arthritis Rheum 1997;40:S50.

183. Moreland LW et al. European (EU) and US rheumatologists (RHEUM) agree in triple but not on double or single early DMARD choice for different types of RA. Arthritis Rheum 1997;40: S218.

184. O'Dell et al. Combination DMAARD therapy with methotrexate-sulfasalazine-hydroxychloroquine in rheumatoid arthritis: continued efficacy with minimal toxicity at 5 years. Arthritis Rheum 1998;41:S132.

185. Kremer JM et al. Concomitant leflunomide therapy in patients with active rheumatoid arthritis despite stable doses of methotrexate. Ann Intern Med 2002;137:726.

186. Fries JF. Reevaluating the therapeutic approach to rheumatoid arthritis: the "sawtooth" strategy. J Rheumatol 1990;17(Suppl 22):12.

187. Wilske KR, Healey LA. Challenging the therapeutic pyramid: a new look at treatment strategies for rheumatoid arthritis. J Rheumatol 1990; 17(Suppl 25):4.

188. Wilke WS, Clough JD. Therapy for rheumatoid arthritis: combinations of disease-modifying drugs and new paradigms of treatment. Semin Arthritis Rheum 1991;21(Suppl 1):21.

189. Sooka T, Hannonen P. Utility of disease modifying antirheumatic drugs in "sawtooth" strategy. A prospective study of early rheumatoid arthritis patients up to 15 years. Ann Rheum Dis 1999;58:61.

190. Etanercept (Enbrel) package insert. Thousand Oaks, CA: Immunex, June 2003.

191. Moreland et al. Etanercept therapy in rheumatoid arthritis: a randomized, controlled trial. Ann Intern Med 1999;130:478.

192. Weinblatt M et al. A trial of etanercept, a recombinant tumor necrosis factor receptor: Fc fusion protein, in patients with rheumatoid arthritis receiving methotrexate. N Engl J Med 1999;253.

193. Ault A. Rheumatoid arthritis drug linked to infections. Lancet 1999;353:1770.

194. Bathon JM et al. A comparison of etanercept and methotrexate in patients with early rheumatoid arthritis. N Engl J Med 2000;343:1586.

195. Peterson L. FDA review of the safety of rheumatoid arthritis therapies. Trends-in-Medicine March 2003, http://www.trends-in-medicine.com/March2003/FDA-TNF033p.pdf (Accessed June 2003).

196. Infliximab (Remicade) package insert. Malvern, PA: Centocor, April 2003.

197. Ravinder MN et al. Therapeutic efficacy of multiple intravenous infusions of anti-tumor necrosis factor (alpha) monoclonal antibody combined with low-dose weekly methotrexate in rheumatoid arthritis. Arthritis Rheum 1998;41:1552.

198. Lipsky P et al. Long-term control of signs and symptoms of rheumatoid arthritis with chimeric monoclonal anti-TNF (alpha) antibody (infliximab) in patients with active disease on methotrexate. Arthritis Rheum 1998;41:S364.

199. St Clair EW. Infliximab treatment for rheumatic disease: clinical and radiological efficacy. Ann Rheum Dis 2002;61(Suppl iii):ii67.

200. Humira (adalimumab) package insert. North Chicago, IL: Abbott Laboratories, January 2003.

201. van de Putte LB et al. Efficacy and safety of adalimumab (D2E7), the first fully human anti-TNF monoclonal antibody, in patients with rheumatoid arthritis who failed previous DMARD therapy: 6-month results from a phase 3 study. Program #467. Abstract presented at: The European Congress of Rheumatology, June 12–15, 3003, Stockholm, Sweden.

202. Weinblatt ME et al. Adalimumab, a fully human anti-tumor necrosis factor-alpha monoclonal antibody, for the treatment of rheumatoid arthritis in patients taking concomitant methotrexate: the ARMADA Trial. Arthritis Rheum 2003;48:35.

203. Anakinra (Kineret) for rheumatoid arthritis. In: Abramowicz M, ed. Med Lett 2002;44:18.

204. Bresnihan B. Effects of anakinra on clinical and radiological outcomes in rheumatoid arthritis. Ann Rheum Dis 2002;61(Suppl ii):ii74.

205. Bresnihan B et al. Treatment of rheumatoid arthritis with recombinant human IL-1 receptor antagonist. Arthritis Rheum 1998;41:2196.

206. Cohen S et al. Treatment of rheumatoid arthritis with anakinra, a recombinant human interleukin-1 receptor antagonist, in combination with methotrexate: results of a twenty-four-week, multicenter, randomized, double-blind, placebo-controlled trial. Arthritis Rheum 2002;46:574.

207. Myles AB et al. Single daily dose of corticosteroid treatment. Ann Rheum Dis 1976;35:73.

208. Boumpas DT, Wilder RL. Corticosteroids. In: Koopman WJ, ed. Arthritis and Allied Conditions [Online], Chapter 40. 14th Ed. Baltimore: Lippincott Williams & Wilkins, 2001.

209. American College of Rheumatology Task Force on Osteoporosis Guidelines. Recommendations for the prevention and treatment of glucocorticoid-induced osteoporosis. Arthritis Rheum 1996;39:1791.

210. Eastell R et al. A UK consensus group on management of glucocorticoid osteoporosis: an update. J Intern Med 1998;244:271.

211. Writing Group for the Women's Health Initiative Investigators. Risks and benefits of estrogen plus progestin in healthy postmenopausal women: principal results from the Women's Health Initiative randomized controlled trial. JAMA 2002;288:321.

212. Wasnich RD et al. Thiazide effect on mineral content of bone. N Engl J Med 1983;309:344.

213. Schaller JG. Juvenile rheumatoid arthritis. Pediatr Rev 1997;18:337.

214. Warren RW et al. Juvenile idiopathic arthritis (juvenile rheumatoid arthritis). In: Koopman WJ, ed. Arthritis and Allied Conditions [Online], Chapter 64. 14th Ed. Baltimore: Lippincott Williams & Wilkins, 2001.

215. Sharma S, Sherry DD. Joint distribution at presentation in children with pauciarticular arthritis. J Pediatr 1999;134:642.

216. Fantini F et al. Remission in juvenile chronic arthritis: a cohort study of 683 consecutive cases with a mean 10 year followup. J Rheumatol 2003;30:579.

217. Gottlieb BS et al. Discontinuation of methotrexate treatment in juvenile rheumatoid arthritis. Pediatrics 1997;100:994.

218. Levinson JE. Comparison of tolmetin sodium and aspirin in the treatment of juvenile rheumatoid arthritis. J Pediatr 1977;91:799.

219. Mortimer EA et al. Varicella with hypoglycemia possibly due to salicylates. Am J Dis Child 1962; 103:583.

220. Starko KM et al. Reye's syndrome and salicylate use. Pediatrics 1980;66:859.

221. Waldman RJ et al. Aspirin as a risk factor in Reye's syndrome. JAMA 1982;247:3089.

222. Halpin TJ et al. Reye's syndrome and medication use. JAMA 1982;248:687.

223. Committee on Infectious Diseases AA of P. Aspirin and Reye syndrome. Pediatrics 1982;69:810.

224. Rennebohm RM et al. Reye syndrome in children receiving salicylate therapy for connective tissue disease. J Pediatr 1985;107:877.

225. Wallace CA. The use of methotrexate in childhood rheumatic diseases. Arthritis Rheum 1998; 41:381.

226. Cassidy JT. Outcomes research in the therapeutic use of methotrexate in children with chronic peripheral arthritis. J Pediatr 1998;133:179.

227. Ravelli A et al. Radiologic progression in patients with juvenile chronic arthritis treated with methotrexate. J Pediatr 1998;133:262.

228. Sherry DD. What's new in the diagnosis and treatment of juvenile rheumatoid arthritis. J Pediatr Orthop 2000;20:419.

229. Van Rossum MAJ et al. Salazine in the treatment of juvenile chronic arthritis: a randomized, double-blind, placebo-controlled, multicenter study. Arthritis Rheum 1998;41:808.

230. Padeh S, Passwell JH. Intra-articular corticosteroid injection in the management of children with chronic arthritis. Arthritis Rheum 1998; 41:1210.

231. Weiss AH et al. Methotrexate for resistant chronic uveitis in children with juvenile rheumatoid arthritis. J Pediatr 1998;133:266.

232. Lawrence RC et al. Estimates of the prevalence of arthritis and selected musculoskeletal disorders in the United States. Arthritis Rheum 1998;41:778.

233. Prevalence of self-reported arthritis or chronic joint symptoms among adults—United States, 2001 MMWR 2002;51:948.

234. Brandt KD. Osteoarthritis. In: Fauci AS et al, eds. Harrison's Principles of Internal Medicine. New York: McGraw-Hill, 1998:1880.

235. Slemenda C et al. Quadriceps weakness and osteoarthritis of the knee. Ann Int Med 1997; 127(2):97.

236. Holderbaum D et al. Genetics and osteoarthritis: exposing the iceberg. Arthritis Rheum 1999; 43:397.

237. Freidich MJ. Steps toward understanding, alleviating osteoarthritis will help aging population. JAMA 1999;11:1023.

238. Solomon L. Clinical features of osteoarthritis. In: Ruddy S et al., eds. Kelley's Textbook of Rheumatology. 6th Ed. Philadelphia: WB Saunders, 2001:1409.

239. Recommendations for the medical management of osteoarthritis of the hip and knee: 2000 update. American College of Rheumatology Subcommittee on Osteoarthritis Guidelines. Arthritis Rheum 2000;43:1905.

240. Case JP et al. Lack of efficacy of acetaminophen in treating symptomatic knee osteoarthritis: a randomized, double-blind, placebo-controlled comparison trial with diclofenac sodium. Arch Intern Med 2003;163:169.

241. Bradley JD et al. Comparison of an anti-inflammatory dose of ibuprofen, an analgesic dose of ibuprofen, and acetaminophen in the treatment of patients with osteoarthritis of the knee. N Engl J Med 1991;325:87.

242. Williams HJ et al. Comparison of naproxen and acetaminophen in a two-year study of treatment of osteoarthritis of the knee. Arthritis Rheum 1993;36:1196.

243. Pincus T et al. A randomized, double-blind, crossover clinical trial of diclofenac plus misoprostol versus acetaminophen in patients with osteoarthritis of the hip or knee. Arthritis Rheum 2001;44:1587.

244. Geba GP et al. Efficacy of rofecoxib, celecoxib, and acetaminophen in osteoarthritis of the knee: a randomized trial. JAMA 2002;287:64.

245. Pincus T et al. Preference for nonsteroidal anti-inflammatory drugs versus acetaminophen and concomitant use of both types of drugs in patients with osteoarthritis. J Rheumatol 2000;27:1020.

246. Pincus T. Clinical evidence for osteoarthritis as an inflammatory disease. Curr Rheumatol Rep 2001; 3:524.

247. Shamoon M, Hochberg MC. The role of acetaminophen in the management of patients with osteoarthritis. Am J Med 2001;110(Suppl 3A): 46S.

248. Schnitzer TJ. Update of ACR guidelines for osteoarthritis: role of the coxibs [discussion S31]. J Pain Sympt Manage 2002;23:S24.

249. Seideman P et al. Naproxen and paracetamol compared with naproxen only in coxarthrosis: increased effect of the combination in 18 patients. Acta Orthop Scand 1993;64:285.

250. Schumacher HR et al. Effect of a nonsteroidal anti-inflammatory drug on synovial fluid in osteoarthritis. J Rheumatol 1996;23:1774.

251. Singh G. Recent considerations in nonsteroidal anti-inflammatory drug gastropathy. Am J Med 1998;105(Suppl 1B):31S.

252. Singh G, Triadafilopoulos G. Epidemiology of NSAID induced gastrointestinal complications. J Rheumatol 1999;26(Suppl)26:18.

253. Page J, Henry D. Consumption of NSAIDs and the development of congestive heart failure in elderly patients: an underrecognized public health problem. Arch Intern Med 2000;160:777.

254. Brater DC. Renal effects of cyclooxygyenase-2-selective inhibitors [discussion S21-3]. J Pain Sympt Manage 2002;23:S15.

255. Ormrod D et al. Valdecoxib [discussion 2072-3]. Drugs. 2002;62:2059.

256. Brater DC. Anti-inflammatory agents and renal function. Semin Arthritis Rheum 2002;32:33.

257. The management of chronic pain in older persons: AGS Panel on Chronic Pain in Older Persons. American Geriatrics Society. J Am Geriatr Soc 1998;46:635.

258. Brandt KD. Should nonsteroidal anti-inflammatory drugs be used to treat osteoarthritis? Rheum Dis Clin North Am 1993;19:29.

259. Behrens F et al. Metabolic recovery of articular cartilage after intra-articular injections of glucocorticoids. J Bone Joint Surgery 1976;58:1157.

260. Gray RG et al. Local corticosteroid injection treatment in rheumatic disorders. Semin Arthritis Rheum 1981;10:231.

261. Creamer P. Intra-articular corticosteroid injections in osteoarthritis: do they work and if so, how? Ann Rheum Dis 1997;56(11):634.

262. Altman RD. Status of hyaluronan supplementation therapy in osteoarthritis. Curr Rheumatol Rep 2003;5:7.

263. Altman RD, Moskowitz R. Intraarticular sodium hyaluronate (Hyalgan) in the treatment of patients with osteoarthritis of the knee: a randomized clinical trial. Hyalgan Study Group J Rheumatol 1998;25(11):2203.

264. Altman RD. Intra-articular sodium hyaluronate in osteoarthritis of the knee. Semin Arthritis Rheum 2000;30:11.

265. Theodosakis J et al. The arthritis cure: the medical miracle that can halt, reverse, and may even cure osteoarthritis. New York: St. Martins Mass Market Paper, 1997.

266. Kelly GS. The role of glucosamine sulfate and chondroitin sulfates in the treatment of degenerative joint disease. Alt Med Rev 1998;3(1):27.

267. da Camara CC. Dowless GV. Glucosamine sulfate for osteoarthritis. Ann Pharmacother 1998; 32(5):580.

268. Deal CL, Moskowitz RW. Nutraceuticals as therapeutic agents in osteoarthritis. The role of glucosamine, chondroitin sulfate, and collagen hydrolysate. Rheum Dis Clin North Am 1999; 25(2):379.

269. McAlindon TE et al. Glucosamine and chondroitin for treatment of osteoarthritis: a systematic quality assessment and meta-analysis. JAMA 2000;283:1469.

270. Noack W et al. Glucosamine sulfate in osteoarthritis of the knee. Osteoarthritis Cartilage 1994;2:51.

271. Muller-Fabbender H et al. Glucosamine sulfate compared to ibuprofen in osteoarthritis of the knee. Osteoarthritis Cartilage 1994;2:61.

272. Morreale P et al. Comparison of the antiinflammatory efficacy of chondroitin sulfate and diclofenac sodium in patients with knee osteoarthritis. J Rheumatol 1996;23(8):1385.

273. Reginster JY et al. Long-term effects of glucosamine sulphate on osteoarthritis progression: a randomised, placebo-controlled clinical trial. Lancet 2001;357:251.

274. Pavelka K et al. Glucosamine sulfate use and delay of progression of knee osteoarthritis: a 3-year, randomized, placebo-controlled, double-blind study. Arch Intern Med 2002;162:2113.

275. Dougados M, for the Group for the Respect of Ethics and Excellence in Science. Recommendations for the registrations of drugs used in the treatment of osteoarthritis. Ann Rheum Dis 1996;55:552.

276. Altman R et al. Design and conduct of clinical trials of patients with osteoarthritis: recommendations from a task force of the Osteoarthritis Research Society. Osteoarthritis Cartilage 1996; 4:217.

277. Committee for Proprietary Medicinal Products. Points to Consider on Clinical Investigation of Medicinal Products Used in the Treatment of Osteoarthritis. London, England: The European Agency for the Evaluation of Medicinal Products, 1998.

278. Center for Drug Evaluation and Research. Clinical Development Programs for Drugs, Devices and Biological Products Intended for the Treatment of Osteoarthritis. Rockville, MD: US Food and Drug Administration, 1999.

279. Cohen M et al. A randomized, double blind, placebo controlled trial of a topical cream containing glucosamine sulfate, chondroitin sulfate, and camphor for osteoarthritis of the knee. J Rheumatol 2003;30:523.

280. Hungerford DS, Jones LC. Glucosamine and chondroitin sulfate are effective in the management of osteoarthritis. J Arthroplast 2003;18:5.

CHAPTER 44

Connective Tissue Disorders: The Clinical Use of Corticosteroids

William C. Gong

Despite new knowledge in the immunology and the pathogenesis of the different connective tissue diseases (CTDs), their etiology and classification remains elusive.[1] Different textbooks approach the connective tissues disease in varied fashions. Some textbooks group systemic lupus erythematosus (SLE), progressive systemic sclerosis, inflammatory muscle disease, Sjögren's syndrome, and the systemic vasculitides together loosely. Other textbooks put them in separate sections.[2] The diagnosis of the different CTDs is a matter of clinical judgment as patients present with constellations of symptoms, physical findings, and laboratory features that permit their recognition. Patients may present with findings consistent with more than one CTD. There is also overlap CTD representing the presence of two defined CTDs. Examples of this include SLE/RA or what is known as lupus and myositis/scleroderma resulting in sclerodermatomyositis or scleromyositis. Complicating matters, there is also the mixed connective tissue disease (MCTD), which includes examples such as myositis/scleroderma/RA/SLE first described in 1972.[1]

Sustained inflammation is the hallmark of CTDs. The inflammatory effector mechanisms can engage mast cells, platelets, neutrophils, endothelial cells, mononuclear phagocytes, and lymphocytes as well as trigger the complement, kinin, and coagulation cascades. The diversity of the potential mechanisms activated during inflammation can lead to a broad spectrum of clinical manifestations. Environmental factors can also serve as stimuli to the particular mechanism activated. For example, biologic agents such as group A β-hemolytic streptococci can lead to rheumatic fever or *Borrelia burgdorferi* leading to Lyme disease, drugs such as hy-dralazine and procainamide can lead to drug-induced lupus, and vinyl chloride can lead to progressive systemic sclerosis.[2]

GENERAL SIGNS AND SYMPTOMS

Many patients can have arthralgias and arthritis as part of the inflammatory disease associated with their CTD such as those patients with SLE. Inflammatory disease is suggested by morning stiffness of greater than 1 hour (a similar problem occurs with sitting or resting), swelling, fever, weakness, and systemic fatigue. In some patients, activities of daily living and function may be excellent despite pain and deformity; in others, because of psychologic and systemic disease, there may be poor function with minimum articular involvement. Other psychosocial aspects of their life, including sexuality, may be affected by many of the inflammatory disorders.

Dermatologic changes are often associated with a particular rheumatic disease. Examples include alopecia with SLE, onycholysis and keratoderma blenorrhagica with Reiter's syndrome, buccal or genital ulcers with SLE or Reiter's syndrome, Raynaud's phenomenon with SLE or systemic sclerosis, calcinosis and rash over the knuckles (Gottron's papule) with dermatomyositis, and sun sensitivity malar rash with SLE. The presence of nodules, tophi, telangiectasia, or vasculitic changes also may be detected, helping the clinician differentiate which inflammatory disease is present and what management is necessary.

The CTDs are commonly associated with musculoskeletal changes. Joints may display warmth, redness and effusion, synovial thickening, deformities, decreased range of motion, pain on motion, tenderness on palpation, and decreased function. Often, a patient's hand and arm function, as well as gait, may be altered. In addition to the signs and symptoms used to differentiate various rheumatic diseases, laboratory evaluation of patients with rheumatic complaints can often define the extent of disease or detect other organ systems that may be involved.

NONPHARMACOLOGIC AND PHARMACOLOGIC TREATMENT

The aim of present therapy is to provide pain relief, decrease joint inflammation, and more importantly, maintain or restore joint function and prevent bone and cartilage destruction. The current approach to treatment is to interrupt the complex inflammatory process. The general treatment program consists of patient education, balance between rest and exercise, physical and occupational therapy, adequate nutrition, local heat, use of supportive or rehabilitative devices, and orthopedic surgery. Depending on the disorder being treated, various drugs may be used, including the salicylate class of drugs, nonsteroidal anti-inflammatory drugs (NSAIDs), disease-modifying antirheumatic drugs (DMARDs), and corticosteroids. All drugs other than corticosteroids have been reviewed extensively in other chapters.

These agents and especially the corticosteroids used in the treatment of CTDs and systemic rheumatic disorders may have systemic toxicity as well. A good understanding of corticosteroids and their effects can help the clinician monitor the patient appropriately and order laboratory studies such as renal or liver function tests, complete blood counts, muscle enzyme levels, or urinalysis. More sophisticated tests may be necessary to differentiate hypothalamic-pituitary-adrenal (HPA) axis abnormalities from effects of chronic corticosteroid therapy.[3] Functional evaluation and health status outcome measurements are ultimately the most important measurement tools in evaluating treatment. Psychologic function typically is assessed in terms of affective domains such as depression and anxiety, whereas social function usually is measured in terms of social interactions and social support.

SELECTED CONNECTIVE TISSUE DISEASES

CTDs and rheumatic diseases encompass a wide range of disorders that are inflammatory in nature and related to the immune system. The following are some of the conditions that are encountered in clinical practice, which necessitates the use of corticosteroids as part of their therapy.

LUPUS ERYTHEMATOSUS: SYSTEMIC AND DISCOID

Systemic lupus erythematosus (SLE) is the most diverse of the autoimmune diseases as it is a multi-system CTD caused by several autoantibodies and immune complexes.[4] Disease manifestations depend on the tissues targeted and often have musculoskeletal involvement. It generally involves one organ system at the onset but can affect other organ systems subsequently displaying a broad range of clinical manifestations.[5] SLE is a dynamic disease in a sense that many patients have fluctuations or flare-ups that necessitate the use of steroids and other potent immunosuppressive agents. Discoid lupus erythematosus is a form of lupus erythematosus in which cutaneous lesions appear on the face and elsewhere. These are atrophic plaques with erythema, hyperkeratosis, follicular plugging, and telangiectasia. These are chronic cutaneous lesions and have few if any systemic manifestations. The lesions are usually sharply demarcated and can be round, thereby having the term discoid (or disc-like).[6]

Epidemiology

SLE generally affects women of childbearing age; this population accounts for >90% of all cases. However, SLE can affect people of all ages and gender, including children, men, and the elderly. SLE can begin at any age but occurs most frequently in women between16 and 45 years of age. It is more common in African Americans than in whites, and the mean age for diagnosis of African American females is younger than that of white females. Its prevalence ranges from 17 to 50 per 100,000 in American European white females, compared with 60 to 280 per 100,000 in African American females.[4,7] Asian and Hispanic patients are also susceptible, with the prevalence in Chinese patients being similar to that seen in whites. There are currently no published data on the incidence in Hispanic Americans.[7,8] Genetic epidemiology of SLE has generated strong evidence of hereditary predisposition to this disorder.[7]

Clinical Presentation

SLE is the prototype autoimmune disease as it can affect almost any organ system, and most patients have multi-organ involvement. Clinical signs of SLE are presented in Table 44-1.[9] The most common organ systems affected include cutaneous, musculoskeletal, and renal systems. The most com-

Table 44-1	Signs of Systemic Lupus Erythematosus
Organ System	*Sign*
Cutaneous	Malar rash, discoid rash, mouth/nasal sores, Raynaud phenomenon, cutaneous vasculitis, alopecia
Musculoskeletal	Polyarthritis, especially of the small joints of hands and wrists, myositis
Renal	Proteinuria, hematuria, red blood cell casts, nephrotic syndrome, elevated creatinine
Cardiopulmonary	Pericarditis, pleurisy, pleural effusions, pneumonitis, pulmonary emboli, pulmonary hypertension, myocardial infarction
Hematologic	Anemia, leucopenia, thrombocytopenia, elevated sedimentation rate, lupus anticoagulant, anticardiolipin
Neurologic	Seizure, psychosis, stroke, encephalopathy, transverse myelitis, mononeuritis multiplex, peripheral neuropathy
Gastrointestinal	Esophageal dysmotility, intestinal vasculitis, protein-losing enteropathy
Constitutional	Fever, weight loss, lymphadenopathy

mon sign of SLE is cutaneous involvement occurring in about 90% of the patients. Rashes are photosensitive in about 70% of the patients, and maculopapular rashes are usually indicative of disease flare-ups. The malar rash or butterfly rash is reported in 20% to 60% of the SLE patients. The rash is often precipitated by exposure to sunlight.[10] Discoid lesions occur primarily in the face but also occur in the ears and on forearms. Most patients with SLE experience fatigue and suffer from some form of arthralgias and myalgias which mimic rheumatoid arthritis with symmetrical involvements of the joints. However, unlike rheumatoid arthritis, the affected joints of lupus arthritis are rarely erosive. Renal involvement, occurring in about 50% of the whites and 75% of the African Americans with SLE, is manifested by proteinuria, hematuria, and red blood cell casts. The more severe cases of renal involvement can lead to renal failure if not controlled early. Hematologic manifestations of lupus are frequent and can be life-threatening. Anemia generally is consistent with anemia of chronic disease and iron-deficiency anemia. Leukopenia is common, but rarely severe (i.e. <2,000 cells/mm³). Mild chronic thrombocytopenia is common but can be sudden and life-threatening. Lupus patients can also present with neurologic and gastrointestinal signs as presented in Table 44-1. Vague constitutional signs of SLE (e.g., fatigue, malaise, fever, anorexia, nausea, weight loss) occur in 95% of patients during the course of their disease. Because of its multi-system organ involvement, the diagnosis of SLE may be difficult. The American College of Rheumatology has published criteria for the classification of patients having SLE. The Diagnostic and Therapeutic Criteria originally published in 1982 and updated in 1997 lists 11 characteristic signs, symptoms, and laboratory values most often associated with a positive diagnosis of SLE (Table 44-2). The presence of four or more of these criteria, either serially or simultaneously, during any period of observation, confers >97% sensitivity and 98% specificity for the diagnosis of lupus.[11-13]

Prognosis

Although disability of varying degrees is common in patients with SLE, most will live nearly normal lives. Survival rates are 90% to 95% at 2 years, 82% to 90% at 5 years, 71% to 80% at 10 years, and 63% to 75% at 20 years.[5] The prognosis is poor in patients with high serum creatinine levels (>1.4 mg/dL), hypertension, nephrotic syndrome, anemia, hypoalbuminemia, and hypocomplementemia at the time of diagnosis. Another 50% of the patients who go into remission remain in remission for decades. The leading causes of death are generally from complications of renal failure or infections.[5]

Treatment

Because there is no cure for SLE, therapy generally involves 1) controlling the acute symptoms of SLE and 2) providing maintenance therapy to prevent exacerbations and to keep clinical manifestations of SLE at acceptable levels. Approximately 25% of patients with SLE have mild symptoms without any life-threatening situations. These patients are normally treated for their symptoms of arthritis, arthralgias, myalgias, fever, and mild serositis with NSAIDs and salicylates. More potent agents and immunosuppressives are used for more active disease. Corticosteroids are used for the more severe life-threatening and severely disabling manifestations unresponsive to immunosuppressive agents.[5]

DRUG-INDUCED LUPUS

The first case of drug-induced lupus was reported in 1945 in a patient receiving sulfadiazine.[14] Since then, approximately 75 drugs have been identified that induce a lupus-like syndrome or exacerbate pre-existing SLE. Classes of drugs that have been linked to the lupus-like syndrome include antihypertensives, antimicrobials, anti-inflammatory agents, anticonvulsants, immunosuppressive agents, recombinant cytokines,

Table 44-2   1997 Revised Criteria for Classification of Systemic Lupus Erythematosus

Criteria	Explanation[a]
Malar rash	Fixed erythema, flat or raised
Discoid rash	Erythematosus raised patches with adherent keratotic scaling and follicular plugging; atrophic scarring may occur in older lesions
Photosensitivity	Skin rash resulting from an unusual reaction to sunlight by patient history or observed by physician
Oral ulcers	Painless oral or nasopharyngeal ulcers observed by physician
Arthritis	Nonerosive arthritis involving two or more peripheral joints; characterized by tenderness, swelling, or effusion
Serositis	Evidence of pleuritis or pericarditis documented by ECG or rub heard by physician or evidence of pericardial effusion
Renal disorder	As manifested by persistent proteinuria (>0.5 g/day or >3+) or cellular casts
Neurologic disorder	Seizures or psychosis occurring without any other explanation
Hematologic disorder	Leukopenia (<4,000/mm³), or hemolytic anemia, or lymphopenia (<1,500/mm³), or thrombocytopenia (<100,000/mm³)
Immunologic disorder	Anti-double stranded DNA antibody, or anti-Sm antibody, or anti-phospholipid
Antinuclear antibody	An abnormal ANA titer in the absence of drugs known to be associated with drug-induced lupus

[a]The diagnosis of systemic lupus erythematosus is made when a patient has 4 or more of the 11 criteria at any time during the course of the disease with 98% specificity and 97% sensitivity.

psychotropic agents, and antithyroid and hormonal drugs. Drug-induced LE occurs in at least two forms. One is characterized by serositis and the finding of a positive antihistone antibody. This form has been associated with procainamide, hydralazine, minocycline, and isoniazid. The second form involves positive anti-Ro (SS-A) antibody findings[15] and is most prominently linked to hydrochlorothiazide and calcium channel blockers.[16] The most common drugs causing drug-induced LE are procainamide and hydralazine followed by chlorpromazine, isoniazid, methyldopa, penicillamine, quinidine, and sulfasalazine. The most commonly reported drug associated with drug-induced lupus is procainamide, which has resulted in the syndrome in approximately one third of patients who have taken it over a 1-year period. The drug-induced lupus-like syndrome onset can occur as soon as 1 month of therapy or as late as 12 years from the initiation of procainamide. Hydralazine follows procainamide, with a prevalence of drug-induced lupus-like syndrome being reported between 2% and 21%, with the wide range reflecting differences in duration of treatment, dosage, and acetylator phenotype. Drug-induced lupus from hydralazine appears to be associated with daily dosage >200 mg or a cumulative dose of 100 g. Drug-induced cutaneous lupus erythematosus occurs in 15,000 to 20,000 people yearly in the United States and is often unrecognized.[17–19] New cases of drug-induced LE continue to occur with newer drugs such as terbinafine and celecoxib.[15,20] In particular for celecoxib, this may be another precaution to keep mind since the COX-2 inhibitors are being widely used in the treatment of rheumatic diseases. Patients who develop drug-induced lupus have symptoms (e.g., arthralgias, myalgias, fever) similar to those of patients with idiopathic SLE; however, renal disease is rare.[14,21] Fever, rash, anemia, and cardiac problems occur slightly less frequently than with spontaneous lupus. Although the lupus erythematosus (LE) cell and antinuclear antibody (ANA) titer can be positive, antibodies to native or double-stranded DNA are not found. Drug-induced lupus typically improves rapidly after discontinuation of the drug and usually does not require specific therapy. However, in some situations (e.g., symptoms present for a long time or patients are significantly symptomatic), a short course of low- to moderate-dose prednisone is beneficial.

SYSTEMIC SCLEROSIS (SCLERODERMA)

Systemic sclerosis, also called scleroderma (*skleros,* meaning hard; *derma,* meaning skin), is a multisystem disorder of connective tissues characterized by inflammation, fibrosis, and degenerative changes in the blood vessels, skin, synovium, skeletal muscle, and some internal organ systems (e.g., gastrointestinal tract, lung, heart, kidney). Systemic sclerosis is an acquired, noncontagious, rare disorder that affects all races worldwide. The incidence in the United States is 19 to 20 per million per year with a prevalence of 19 to 75 cases per 100,000.[22] Overall, females are affected three times as often as males, and the female-to-male ratio is increased during the childbearing years when the ratios of women to men may reach 7–12:1. Onset of systemic sclerosis generally begins in people between 30 and 50 years of age. It is rare in childhood and after age 80. Environmental factors including occupational silica and organic solvent exposure have been implicated in predisposing or precipitating systemic sclerosis. It is a disease of unknown etiology but most investigators believe the key players are endothelial cells, activated immune cells, and fibroblasts. It is hypothesized that the process is initiated by an immune attack on the endothelium resulting in endothelial cell activation and/or injury. This is followed by activation of the fibroblasts resulting in subendothelial connective tissue proliferation, narrowing of the vascular lumen, and Raynaud's phenomenon. T cells are then selectively activated and populate the affected areas such as the dermis and lung. These cells produce cytokines that simulate resident fibroblast to produce excessive amounts of procollagen, which is then converted extracellularly to mature collagen. Later and when the inflammatory process subsides, the fibroblasts revert back to normal.

Systemic sclerosis is divided into two major classes: diffuse cutaneous and limited cutaneous disease, which are distinguished from one another based on the degree and extent of skin involvement. The term *overlap syndrome* is used when features common in one or more of the other CTDs are also present. In most cases of limited cutaneous systemic sclerosis, the initial complaint is Raynaud's phenomenon. Patients with diffuse cutaneous systemic sclerosis most often have generalized swelling of the hands, skin thickening, or arthritis as the first manifestation. The diffuse cutaneous systemic sclerosis patients will present with fatigue or lack of energy, musculoskeletal complaints, and sclerosis of the skin and certain organs. The degree and the rate of organ involvement vary among patients. The skin is taut, firm, and edematous and is firmly bound to subcutaneous tissue; it feels tough and leathery, may itch, and later becomes hyperpigmented. The dermatologic manifestations usually precede the development of signs of visceral involvement. The combination of *C*alcinosis with *R*aynaud's phenomenon, *E*sophageal dysfunction, *S*clerodactyly, and *T*elangiectasias normally found in limited cutaneous systemic sclerosis is called the *CREST syndrome*. Patients with limited cutaneous systemic sclerosis may have Raynaud's phenomenon for years before other signs of disease become evident. They are less likely than those with diffuse cutaneous systemic sclerosis to develop severe lung, heart, or kidney disease, although all these diseases can occur. In contrast to limited cutaneous systemic sclerosis, diffuse cutaneous systemic sclerosis develops only with a short interval between the onset of Raynaud's phenomenon and significant organ involvement.

The overall course of systemic sclerosis is highly variable and unpredictable. However, once a remission occurs, relapse is uncommon. The diffuse form of the disease generally has a worse prognosis with a 10-year survival rate of 40% to 60%, compared with a greater than 70% 10-year survival rate in those with limited cutaneous systemic sclerosis. The prognosis is worse in white males and African American females. There is no specific therapy for systemic sclerosis. Supportive therapy is indicated for the organ systems affected. Because multisystem organs are involved, treatment is directed toward alleviating the affected organ systems. Because of potential toxicities, including precipitating acute renal failure, corticosteroids are not generally used and are typically restricted to patients with inflammatory myopathy or symptomatic serositis not adequately controlled with NSAIDs. D-Penicillamine significantly improves diffuse cutaneous systemic sclerosis symptoms in patients with skin thickening, reduces subsequent renal involvement, and increases survival. Vasodilators such as the calcium channel blocker, nifedipine and the angiotensin converting enzyme receptor blocking agent, losartan have proved useful in alleviating Raynaud's phenomenon. Angiotensin-converting enzyme (ACE) inhibitors are the drugs of choice to manage renal complications and hypertension associated with systemic sclerosis. Metoclopramide, erythromycin, nifedipine, proton pump inhibitors, and H_2 blockers can alleviate specific gastrointestinal symptoms.[23]

POLYMYALGIA RHEUMATICA AND TEMPORAL ARTERITIS (GIANT CELL ARTERITIS)

Polymyalgia rheumatica (PMR) and temporal arteritis or giant cell arteritis (GCA) are clinical syndromes that usually affect the elderly population, and both can occur in the same patient. The incidence of PMR and GCA increases in patients after the age of 50 and peaks in those 70 to 80 years of age.[24] The occurrence of PMR is two to five times more likely than GCA. Up to 15% of patients with PMR can have GCA, and PMR is found in 40% to 60% of patients with GCA.[25] The incidence of PMR increases with age and has been estimated to be as high as 400 cases per 100,000 in individuals older than 65 years of age.[26–28] Women are affected twice as much as men.[24] PMR generally affects whites and is uncommon in African Americans, Hispanics, Asians, and Native Americans.[25] A viral cause has been suspected but not confirmed in PMR and GCA, as the prevalence of antibodies against parainfluenza virus type 1 is increased in patients with PMR and GCA.[29]

Patients with PMR generally present with malaise, weight loss, night sweats, and occasional fever. There is intense pain and stiffness in the neck, shoulder, and buttocks, and the patient may have difficulty arising from bed in the morning. The most useful supporting evidence in support of a clinical diagnosis of PMR is the ESR. It is usually in excess of 50 mm/hr and may exceed 100 mm/hr.[25] The C-reactive protein has been found to be a more sensitive indicator of disease activity than the ESR.[24,30] Also, levels of interleukin-6 appear to be a sensitive indicator of active disease, but most clinical laboratories do not yet have the means to measure these levels.[28] As with other CTDs, the diagnosis if PMR is made based on clinical presentation despite well-recognized laboratory abnormalities. No pathognomonic laboratory test exists. Nonspecific clinical features and the frequent absence of physical signs make diagnosis difficult.

GCA is a connective tissue disorder that involves the inflammation of the medium and large arteries and almost always occurs in whites. It is more common in women and rare in African Americans. GCA rarely affects patients younger than 50 year of age, and the incidence increases with age. It is closely associated with PMR and affects many arteries throughout the body, producing symptoms and signs that mimic other medical and surgical conditions. Carotid artery involvement lends itself to the name *temporal arteritis* when the temporal arteries are distended, are tender, and pulsate early in the disease. These arteries can become occluded and lead to visual disturbances and blindness from ischemic optic neuritis. The symmetric and proximal muscle pain and stiffness of PMR are often associated with GCA.

Corticosteroids are essential for the treatment of PMR and GCA because they rapidly relieve symptoms and reduce the incidence of blindness associated with GCA. The therapeutic goal in PMR is to alleviate stiffness and constitutional features. The corticosteroids are the drugs of choice and the NSAIDs are used when PMR symptoms are mild.[25] For patients with PMR, the current recommendation is to start with prednisone 15 to 20 mg per day. Most patients respond significantly within 24 hours, but it may take up to 48 to 72 hours to achieve a good response in a few patients. The results are dramatic. If patients do not obtain relief of symptoms after a few days, another diagnosis should be considered.[24] If the patient's symptoms are not reduced by the initial dose, prednisone can be increased by an additional 10 mg/day for control. Once the symptoms are controlled, the dosage of prednisone can be decreased by 2.5 mg every 2 weeks for as long as the symptoms remain improved until 10 mg per day is reached. Afterwards, the prednisone is titrated at 1-mg decrements every 4 weeks while following the clinical response and the ESR.[25] Although patients respond quickly to the corticosteroids, treatment is often required for several years. Duration of treatment may be related to the severity of the disease as measured by the ESR. High pretreatment ESRs indicate more severe disease, and these patients require longer duration of therapy.[28] Typically, corticosteroid treatment is required for 6 to 24 months. For patients with mild PMR disease, the NSAIDs can effectively manage their symptoms.

For patients with GCA, corticosteroid treatment must be initiated immediately as soon the diagnosis is made because GCA can lead to severe visual loss and potential blindness.[24] Treatment for GCA is more aggressive than PMR and usually begins with prednisone 40 to 60 mg as a single or a divided dose. Initial pulsed intravenous does of methylprednisolone (1,000 mg every day for 3 days) may be given to patients with recent or impending visual loss. Corticosteroids may prevent but usually do not reverse visual loss.[24,25] Once the clinical symptoms and laboratory findings of inflammation have subsided for about 1 month, decreases in the prednisone dose should be initiated. Sometimes, it may take several months at doses of 15 to 25 mg per day before prednisone may be decreased. Prednisone dosages should be decreased gradually in 1- to 2-week intervals by a maximum of 10% of the total daily dose. Excessively rapid tapering of the prednisone dose may result in relapses and recurrence of symptoms.[24] The decrease in the dosage of prednisone should be based on the patient's clinical status rather than on laboratory results.[27] Treatment of GCA should be continued for 1 to 2 years to minimize the potential for relapse.[25] If the patients do not achieve clinical remission or do not respond to low doses of the corticosteroids, immunosuppressive agents such as azathioprine should be considered. Monitoring ESR or the C-reactive protein value is the most useful in determining disease activity.[24] Another study suggested that measurement of interleukin-6 levels after 4 weeks of therapy was helpful.[28] PMR and GCA are among the most rewarding diseases for a clinician to diagnose and treat because the unpleasant symptoms and serious consequences of these two disorders can be relieved rapidly and prevented by corticosteroids.[25]

REITER'S SYNDROME

Reiter's syndrome is a form of reactive arthritis defined as peripheral arthritis often accompanied by one or more extra-articular manifestations that appear shortly after certain infections of the genitourinary or gastrointestinal tracts. Reactive arthritis typically begins acutely 2 to 4 weeks after venereal infections or bouts of gastroenteritis.[31] Some evidence also suggests that respiratory infection with *Chlamydia pneumoniae* may also trigger the disease.[32] Most of the cases affect young men, with the ratio of male to female patients of 9:1. The classic triad of Reiter's syndrome is arthritis, urethritis, and conjunctivitis. Urethritis usually appears first in this syndrome, which occurs mainly in young men.[33] Mild dysuria and a mucopurulent urethral discharge are the most typical symptoms in men. Women may have dysuria, vaginal discharge, and purulent cervicitis and/or vaginitis. Reiter's syndrome has its peak onset during the third decade of life, but has been reported in children and octogenarians.[34]

There is no specific therapy for Reiter's syndrome. Interventions should include joint protection and relief of pain, suppression of inflammation, and when appropriate, eradication of infection. The arthritis is treated symptomatically with NSAIDs. Systemic corticosteroids are relatively ineffective in the routine management of patients with seronegative spondyloarthropathies such as Reiter's syndrome.[34] Aggressive and unremitting Reiter's syndrome may benefit from immunosuppressive drugs.

POLYMYOSITIS AND DERMATOMYOSITIS

Polymyositis and dermatomyositis are autoimmune diseases of unknown etiology. Polymyositis is predominately a disease of adults. Dermatomyositis affects both children and adults, and more women than men. Polymyositis includes inflammation of a number of voluntary skeletal muscles simultaneously. The onset is insidious, and patients initially complain of muscle weakness of the trunk, shoulders, hip girdles, upper arms, thighs, neck, and pharynx. These patients usually report increasing difficulties in everyday tasks requiring the use of proximal muscles such as getting up from a chair, climbing stairs, stepping onto a curb, lifting objects and combing hair. Polymyositis spares the skin; however, dermatomyositis is a progressive polymyositis condition that is associated with a skin rash. The rash accompanies or more often precedes the muscle weakness of polymyositis. The rash is erythematous, scaly, and eczematous and generally affects the eyelids, bridge of the nose, cheeks, forehead, chest, elbows, knees, and knuckles and around nail beds. One-third of these cases are associated with various connective tissue disorders such as rheumatoid arthritis, SLE, and progressive sclerosis; one-tenth are associated with a malignancy. Edema, inflammation, and degeneration of muscles characterize both polymyositis and dermatomyositis.[35]

The goal of therapy is to improve muscle weakness, thereby improving the activities of daily living. Supportive therapy such as bed rest, physiotherapy, warm baths, and moist heat applications to the affected areas can improve muscle stiffness. If mouth lesions are present, irrigation of these lesions with warm saline solution is helpful. Oral prednisone (e.g., 1 to 2 mg/kg/day) is the initial treatment of choice and should be initiated as soon as possible. Once the symptoms are brought under control in approximately 3 to 4 weeks, the dosage of the steroid is tapered slowly over a period of 10 weeks to 1 mg/kg every other day. Afterward, the dose is further decreased to the lowest possible dose to control symp-

toms and to avoid adverse effects of the corticosteroids as long-term steroid usage can cause steroid myopathy. This can further confuse the issue of whether the muscle weakness is due to increased disease activity or to adverse effects of steroid therapy. Generally, there should be objective increase in muscle strength and activities of daily living by the end of the third month of therapy. Approximately 75% of these patients may require immunosuppressive therapy if their conditions do not respond to prednisone after 3 months.[35]

CLINICAL USE OF CORTICOSTEROIDS

Corticosteroids play an important role in the treatment of a wide variety of disease states. In physiologic doses, they are used to replace deficiencies of this endogenous hormone. In pharmacologic doses, they are used to treat and, more often, provide supportive therapy for a variety of diseases. In the past 40 years, much has been learned about the corticosteroids; however, the exact mechanism by which corticosteroids exert their anti-inflammatory and immunosuppressive effects remains unclear. Corticosteroids may be used for the treatment of many rheumatologic disorders, including ankylosing spondylitis, bursitis, tenosynovitis, acute gouty arthritis, RA, osteoarthritis, dermatomyositis, PMR, acute rheumatic carditis, SLE, mixed CTD, polymyositis, and vasculitis.

Predictable Pharmacologic Effects Relative to the Corticosteroids

1. J.L., a 62-year-old man with a 1-year history of scleroderma, is being treated with prednisone 60 mg/day and azathioprine 50 mg/day. At a recent clinic visit, his vital signs and laboratory test results were as follows: weight, 292 lb; blood pressure (BP), 180/102 mm Hg; pulse, 62 beats/min and regular; and fasting plasma glucose (FPG), 196mg/dL. J.L. complains of occasional headaches, a "swollen face," a modest weight gain, and increases in urinary frequency. Based on J.L.'s presentation, are any of his symptoms related to his drug therapy?

[SI unit: FPG, 10.9 mmol/L]

His "swollen face" could represent a cushingoid feature resulting from long-term corticosteroid use. Hypercortisolism alters normal body fat distribution, resulting in moon facies, buffalo hump, truncal obesity, and other localized fatty deposits. J.L.'s complaint of headaches could be related to his increased BP (180/102 mm Hg) in part to fluid retention resulting from his corticosteroid use, even though hypertension usually is asymptomatic (see Chapter 14, Essential Hypertension). Although corticosteroids with the greatest mineralocorticoid activity are more likely to produce fluid retention and increase BP, even those without mineralocorticoid action (Table 44-3) can increase BP. Hypertension can also be induced by high-dose glucocorticoids due to the permissive effects of the glucocorticoids on the action of vasoactive substances (angiotensin II, catecholamines) on the vessel wall and myocardium that results in increased systemic vascular resistance and increased cardiac contractility.[36] A history of high BP and advanced age can predispose individuals to corticosteroid-induced increases in BP. Whether hypertension is related to the dose or duration of corticosteroid therapy is un-

Table 44-3   Comparison of Corticosteroid Preparations

Compound	Equiv. Potency (mg)	Anti-Inflammatory Potency	Na-Retaining Potency (Mineralocorticoid Activity)	Plasma $t_{1/2}$ (min)	BIOLOGIC $t_{1/2}$ (hr)
Short Acting					
Cortisone	25	0.8	2+	30	8–12
Hydrocortisone (Cortisol)	20	1	2+	80–118	8–12
Prednisone	5	4	1+	60	18–36
Prednisolone	5	4	1+	115–212	18–36
Methylprednisolone	4	5	0	78–188	18–36
Triamcinolone	4	5	0	200	12–36
Long Acting					
Dexamethasone	0.75	20–30	0	110–210	36–54
Betamethasone	0.6	20–30	0	300+	36–54

known; it rarely occurs in patients receiving alternate-day therapy. The hypertension usually resolves after discontinuation of the steroid. In J.L., however, the hypertension also can be attributed to other possible etiologies (e.g., scleroderma). J.L. also has urinary frequency and elevated fasting plasma glucose that could be attributed to using high doses of glucocorticoids. The increases in glucose are mainly mediated through decreased peripheral utilization of glucose and induction of gluconeogenesis in the liver. In patients whose glucose levels remain elevated and the continued use of the glucocorticosteroid is warranted, antihyperglycemic agents may be started.

The equivalent potency, sodium-retaining potency, plasma half-life, and biologic half-life of several synthetic analogs of cortisol are listed in Table 44-3. The corticosteroids are used primarily for their anti inflammatory, immunosuppressive, or antiallergic activity. Cortisone and hydrocortisone have the highest sodium-retaining potency and, therefore, are seldom prescribed for long-term anti-inflammatory therapy. They are useful when sodium and water retention properties are desirable (e.g., adrenal insufficiency after surgery for Cushing's syndrome). All corticosteroids are 21-carbon steroid molecules. The chemical structures of the corticosteroids have been modified, resulting in large differences in duration of action, anti-inflammatory potency, and mineralocorticoid activity.[37] The body synthesizes cortisol by converting cholesterol to pregnenolone, which in turn is converted to progesterone and ultimately to cortisol, the major corticosteroid in humans.[38]

Active Corticosteroid Compounds

2. M.H. is a 43-year-old woman with RA awaiting a liver transplant. Her total bilirubin is 3.1 mg/dL, aspartate aminotransferase (AST) is 93 U/L, and alanine aminotransferase (ALT) is 65 U/L. She has been well maintained on prednisone for her arthritis until recently, when her arthritis failed to respond despite escalating doses of prednisone. Why has prednisone seemed to have stopped being effective? What factors need to be considered when selecting an alternative corticosteroid for M.H.?

[SI units: bilirubin, 53.01 µmol/L; AST, 93 U/L; ALT, 65 U/L]

Although orally administered corticosteroids are well absorbed, exogenously administered corticosteroids, which are

11-keto compounds, are devoid of corticosteroid activity until converted in vivo into active 11 β-hydroxyl compounds.[39] Cortisone and prednisone must be converted to the active compounds, cortisol and prednisolone, respectively, in the liver.[39] M.H. has very little hepatic capacity and, theoretically, might not have been converting the prednisone to its active prednisolone metabolite. To circumvent this possibility, M.H. should be given prednisolone or perhaps a different corticosteroid (e.g., methylprednisolone). Although this explanation is logical given this patient's end stage liver disease, dosage adjustments for hepatically metabolized drugs in the setting of liver disease are difficult to predict because hepatic metabolism is complex and involves numerous oxidative and conjugative pathways that are variably affected in hepatic disease. M.H.'s ability to adhere to her medication regimen because of encephalopathic changes and other potential variables also should be considered as explanations for her decreased responsiveness to prednisone.

Approximately 95% of cortisol is bound to α-globulin transcortin or cortisol-binding globulin (CBG), and the remaining 5% is bound to albumin after this carrier is saturated.[40] However, the bond between cortisol and albumin is weak, and about 25% of the steroid disassociates from albumin and is free to circulate in the plasma. Although the dosing of corticosteroids is not a very precise science, it is important to consider adjusting dosages for patients who have decreased serum albumin concentrations. In these patients, a greater amount of free hormone will result in increased pharmacologic effects. Because albumin is synthesized by the liver, M.H. is likely to have decreased serum albumin concentrations and could be more susceptible to the pharmacologic effects of corticosteroids when given an active corticosteroid moiety.

When selecting an alternative corticosteroid to replace M.H.'s prednisone, the clinician should not base the dosing interval of the replacement corticosteroid strictly on the plasma half-lives shown in Table 44-3. Corticosteroids have biologic half-lives that are 2 to 36 times longer than their plasma half-lives. In addition, the onset of biologic effects lags behind peak plasma levels. Practitioners must always be mindful that the serum or plasma half-life of a drug might not be synonymous with the biologic half-life. For example, prednisone with a plasma half-life of only about 1 hour can be dosed on alternate days for some disorders.

Clinical Presentation of Systemic Lupus Erythematosus

3. H.R., a 33-year-old African American woman with recently diagnosed lupus erythematosus, has experienced a recent weight loss of 15 lb (down to 130 lb), joint pain, fatigue, and a worsening of her facial rash. She has a temperature of 105°F, serum creatinine (SrCr) of 2.8 mg/dL, Westergren ESR of 50 mm/hr, ANA titer of 1:320, and positive anti-dsDNA and anti-Sm tests. Urinalysis (UA) reveals 3% proteinuria and a modest amount of casts. What subjective and objective data are consistent with SLE, and would therapy be likely to reflect resolution of these signs and symptoms?

[SI unit: SrCr, 247.52 µmol/L]

According to some of the objective data (fever, increased Westergren ESR, proteinuria, weight loss, high ANA titer, increased SrCr, positive anti-dsDNA and anti-Sm tests) and subjective data (fatigue, joint pain, worsening facial rash), H.R. is experiencing a flare of her SLE (major disease activity shown on Table 44-4). Three major patterns of SLE exist. The classic pattern, one of exacerbations, or "flares" of disease activities, now is called the "relapsing remitting pattern."[18] Newly diagnosed lupus continue to evolve more than 5 years after initial diagnosis and flares of lupus occur with a median time of 12 months, even in patients with long-standing disease and treatment.[41] This disease tends to wax and wane, and the aggressiveness of therapy should be adjusted to accommodate these changes.

Role of Corticosteroids in Systemic Lupus Erythematosus

4. Why might corticosteroids be indicated for H.R.?

The general management of SLE stresses patient education through which patients need to understand their disease processes. H.R. is definitely experiencing a flare of her SLE and needs aggressive therapy to control her symptoms. Normally, she would be maintained with NSAIDs (including the COX-2 inhibitors) for her joint pains and possibly an immunosuppressive agent such as hydroxychloroquine since she was recently diagnosed.[42] H.R.'s fever, joint pain, fatigue, and worsening facial rash all reflect an inflammatory response to her SLE. These subjective symptoms along with the objective measurements of her disease activity (e.g., increased ESR, ANA, SrCr) are mediated by leukotrienes, prostaglandins, lymphocytes, and the other inflammatory responses described earlier. Therefore, corticosteroids are indicated for the treatment of H.R.

Selection of Appropriate Corticosteroid Therapy

5. What would be a reasonable corticosteroid dosage for H.R.?

Because of the great variety of clinical applications and the wide variety of corticosteroid compounds and dosages, the selection of the most appropriate dosage of a corticosteroid is as much an art as it is a science. Generally, higher dosages and shorter dosing intervals of the corticosteroid translate into an increased anti-inflammatory effect and increased side effects.[36] Therefore, the need to modify disease activity must be balanced against the need to minimize toxicities.

There are multiple dosage forms and uses of corticosteroids in SLE, including topical preparations for inflammatory rashes, intralesional injections for discoid lupus, low-dose oral therapy for mild active disease, and high-dose oral or bolus intravenous infusions for acute, severe manifestations. These indications and the corresponding dose of corticosteroid are listed in Table 44-4.[42]

A review of H.R.'s subjective and objective data suggests that her disease activity probably represents a major flare-up of her SLE. Uncontrolled disease activity can be both debilitating and life-threatening and thus demands rapid an effective intervention. Therefore, a short course of a high-dose corticosteroid regimen probably would be a reasonable treatment for this episode of SLE in H.R.

A short course of steroids or even a single treatment with a high-dose corticosteroid typically can result in prompt and complete resolution of most manifestations of lupus SLE. Pulse therapy with methylprednisolone 1,000 mg intravenously daily for 1 to 3 days has proven effective for SLE, vasculitis, and RA.[36] High-dose steroid pulses must be considered on an individualized basis because adverse effects can be more likely with this dosing regimen. Normally, the pulse methylprednisone therapy of 1,000 mg per day for 3 days is not given more frequently than at monthly intervals because high doses of glucocorticoids are invariably toxic.[36] Alternatively, the use of minipulses of oral prednisone (100 to 200 mg/day) for several days also may help in disease control. In some situations, the addition of a potent immunosuppressive agent such as cyclophosphamide in combination with the corticosteroid pulse therapy may be necessary to bring the patient under control.[43] In any case, depending on how high the dose of glucocorticoid initiated, tapering of the glucocorticoid should be initiated within one to two weeks following initiation of therapy.[36] Table 44-5 provides a summary of different steroid regimens that may be used for severe and active SLE.[44] Assuming that H.R. had been taking a higher dose of oral prednisone, the rationale for IV pulse therapy seems applicable to H.R.

6. After finishing her bolus "pulse" therapy of methylprednisolone (1 g/day IV for 3 days), H.R.'s lupus has responded well. Her joint pain is decreased, and her temperature decreased to

Table 44-4 Systemic Lupus Erythematosus Disease Activity and Use of Corticosteroids

Indication	Corticosteroid Regimen
Cutaneous manifestations	Topical or intralesional corticosteroids
Minor disease activity	Prednisone (or equivalent) at a dosage of <0.5 mg/kg in a single or divided daily dose (5–30 mg prednisone daily)
Major disease activity	Oral: Prednisone (or equivalent) at a dosage of 1–2 mg/kg in a single or divided daily dose IV bolus: Methylprednisolone (1 g or 15 mg/kg) over 30 min; dose often repeated for 3 consecutive days for life-threatening situations

Table 44-5   Usual Regimens of Systemic Corticosteroid Therapy in Severe, Active Systemic Lupus Erythematosus

Preparations	Dose	Rationale	Toxicities
Regimen 1: daily oral short-acting (prednisone, prednisolone, methylprednisolone)	1–2 mg/kg daily; begin in divided doses	Controls disease activity rapidly	High—infections, sleeplessness, mood swings, hyperglycemia, psychosis, hypertension, weight gain, hypokalemia, fragile skin, bruising, osteoporosis, osteonecrosis, irregular menses, muscle cramps, acne, hirsutism, cataracts
Regimen 2: intravenous methylprednisolone	500–1,000 mg daily for 3–5 days; Then, 1–1.5 mg/kg/day of oral corticosteroids	Controls disease activity rapidly, may achieve results more rapidly than daily oral therapy; some nonresponders to oral regimen respond to the intravenous regimen	High—same as above except more rapid taper of daily maintenance steroid dose may be possible, leading to lower cumulative doses
Regimen 3: combination of either regimen 1 or 2 with cytotoxic or immunosuppressive agent			

normal. The current laboratory test results are as follows: Westergren ESR, 22 mm/hr; SrCr, 2.5 mg/dL; ANA titer, 1:80; and positive anti-dsDNA. H.R. wishes to go home to finish her recovery. What dosage of oral corticosteroid would be reasonable to prescribe for H.R. at her discharge from the hospital?

Along with adjustments of the other medications that she may be taking (e.g., NSAIDs or other immunosuppressive agents), H.R. needs to have her IV doses of methylprednisolone converted to an oral formulation (Table 44-6) and consideration given to reducing the steroid dosage. Because the steroid dosage H.R. received is considered massive supraphysiologic, the corticosteroid effects on lymphocyte function can be expected to be prolonged. Therefore, the residual benefits from the supraphysiologic doses of methylprednisolone will be additive to the effect of the oral steroid that will be prescribed for her upon departure from the hospital. Because of this fact, H.R. does not require an oral corticosteroid dose that is equivalent to the IV dose, and a lower oral daily dose can be prescribed because she responded well to her IV doses. In some patients with presumably modest disease activity, alternate-day dosing of corticosteroids may be adequate to maintain disease suppression as there are less adverse effects associated with alternate-day dosing[36,41]. However, more study is needed to better determine the role of alternate-day dosing of corticosteroids as there is less efficacy in patients renal nephritis taking alternate-day therapy as compared to those taking daily glucocorticoids [36,41].

In the United States, prednisone is the most commonly prescribed corticosteroid for oral use in the treatment of CTDs. Prednisone is rapidly and substantially absorbed following oral administration, has an intermediate duration of action (12 to 36 hours), is available in many dosage forms and strengths, and is relatively inexpensive. The recommended dosage of prednisone for most CTDs is 1 mg/kg per day in three to four divided doses. Administration of corticosteroids in daily divided doses given two to four times per day provides a more rapid onset and a greater degree of anti-inflammatory effect. Considering the severity of H.R.'s lupus flare-up, this dosing appears appropriate. The dosing of oral corticosteroids is a balancing act to minimize toxicity while preventing flare up of disease activity.[36] For H.R., who weighs approximately 59 kg, a maintenance regimen of prednisone 20 mg three times a day (for a total of 60 mg/day) or an equivalent dose of another corticosteroid should be prescribed. H.R. also might need an immunosuppressive agent, such as azathioprine or cyclophosphamide, because of her increased SrCr and possibility of lupus nephritis. These latter drugs

Table 44-6   Routes of Administration of Various Corticosteroids

Corticosteroid	Route of Administration
Betamethasone	PO, IM, intra-articular, intrasynovial, intradermal, soft-tissue injection
Cortisone	PO, IM
Dexamethasone	PO, IM, IV, intra-articular, intradermal, soft-tissue injection
Hydrocortisone	IM, IV, PO
Methylprednisolone	PO, IM, IV
Prednisolone	PO, IM, IV, intra-articular, intradermal, soft-tissue injection
Prednisone	PO
Triamcinolone	PO, IM, intra-articular, intrasynovial, intradermal, soft-tissue injection

IM, intramuscularly; IV, intravenously; PO, oral.

would not be initiated in H.R. because she seems to be responding to her methylprednisolone without adverse sequelae thus far. The addition of immunosuppressive agents may have a "steroid-sparing" effect and could allow for steroid dosage reduction.[36]

Once-Daily Dosing

7. **H.R. was discharged from the hospital taking ibuprofen 600 mg QID with food and prednisone 20 mg TID. After 3 weeks, her flare-up has subsided and her symptoms are now back at her previous baseline. Why should a change in her medication be considered?**

Once the patient's lupus flare-up is under control and has responded to steroids, the divided daily doses of a steroid can be consolidated into a single daily dose, usually administered in the morning. Endogenous cortisol levels are normally highest at about 7 to 8 AM and decline to their lowest at midnight. Thus, a once-a-day morning corticosteroid dose coincides in time with high endogenous plasma cortisol. Because this is the time that the patient's tissues would normally be exposed to the highest levels of endogenous cortisol, suppression of the HPA axis is minimized somewhat. If the divided dose regimen has been used for <2 weeks, the dose can be combined into a single daily dose immediately; however, if the divided dose regimen has been used for >2 weeks, the dose should be converted over a 2-week period to a single daily dose because patients who have taken glucocorticoids for more than 2 weeks are candidates for more HPA suppression and their dose needs to be tapered more slowly.[45] Because H.R. received her dosage for 3 weeks, the daily dose should be converted to 60 mg each morning over a 2-week period.

Hypothalamic-Pituitary-Adrenocortical Axis Suppression

8. **R.S., a 48-year-old, 135-lb, 5'5" man, has recently been diagnosed with polyarteritis. After a recent hospitalization, R.S. was discharged home taking 15 mg prednisone QID. He has been adhering to this regimen for approximately 1 month, and his symptoms are well controlled. R.S. now is scheduled for major surgery. His laboratory test evaluation revealed the following: SrCr, 1.4 mg/dL; blood urea nitrogen (BUN), 17 mg/dL; white blood cell (WBC) count, 11,200 cells/mm³; and Westergren ESR, 29 mm/hr. Why should R.S.'s corticosteroid regimen be adjusted?**

[SI units: SrCr, 123.76 μmol/L; BUN, 6.07 mmol/L urea; WBC, 11.2 ×10³ ESR, 29 mm/hr]

The HPA axis regulates the amount of circulating cortisol.[36,45] Corticotropin-releasing factor, a hormone secreted by the hypothalamus, stimulates the release of adrenocorticotropin (ACTH) from the anterior pituitary. ACTH, in turn, stimulates the adrenal cortex to secrete cortisol.[45] As serum cortisol levels rise, a negative-feedback mechanism inhibits corticotropin-releasing factor and ACTH secretion, resulting in decreased secretion of cortisol (Fig. 44-1). Under normal conditions, about 10 to 30 mg/day of cortisol is secreted by the adrenal cortex in accordance with the circadian cycle of an individual.[39,40] Under stress and illnesses the amount of cortisol increases to up to 10-fold or 250 to 300 mg/day for patients undergoing surgery or prolonged major stress.[39,40]

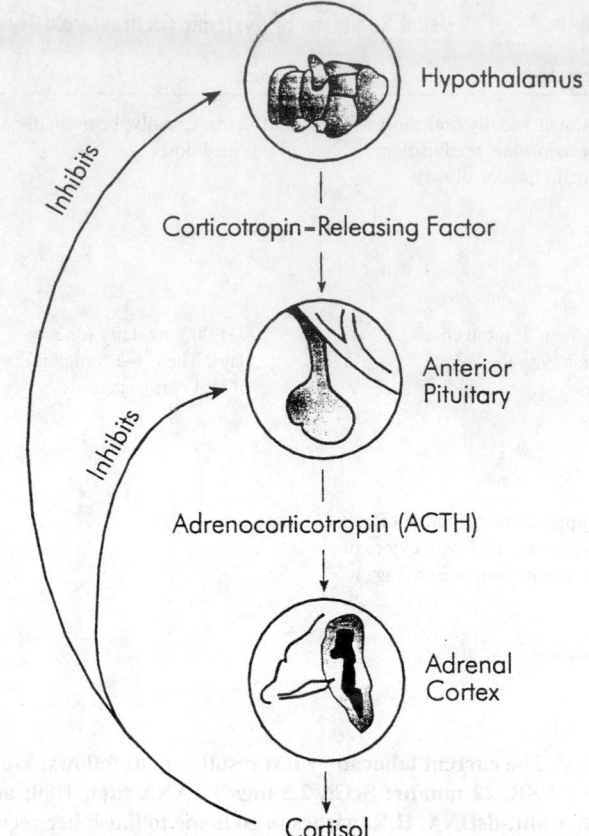

FIGURE 44-1 Hypothalamic-pituitary-adrenocortical axis regulation.

Corticosteroid doses can be classified as physiologic (i.e., replacement) or pharmacologic (i.e., supraphysiologic). A physiologic dose of a corticosteroid is equal to the amount of corticosteroid usually secreted by the adrenal cortex each day and is equal to about 5 mg/day of prednisone. A dosage of prednisone of 0.1 to 0.25 mg/kg per day is a low supraphysiologic dosage; 0.5 mg/kg per day of prednisone is a supraphysiologic dose; 1 to 3 mg/kg per day is a high supraphysiologic dose; and 15 to 30 mg/kg per day is a massive supraphysiologic dose.

Shortly after cortisone and ACTH were accepted into clinical practice, adrenocortical insufficiency and subsequent adrenal atrophy were noted in patients who received doses of exogenous corticosteroids that exceeded the normal amount needed for hormone replacement. When corticosteroids are discontinued abruptly in the patients who had been treated with supraphysiologic doses of corticosteroids for a prolonged period, the HPA axis cannot respond to situations in which there is a need for increased cortisol (e.g., illness, stress, surgery).[45] The minimum dose, dose interval, and therapy duration required to suppress the HPA axis are difficult to assess. The best predictor of HPA axis suppression is the patient's current corticosteroid dosage and duration of the corticosteroid therapy. There is a strong correlation between prednisone maintenance doses >5 mg/day and a subnormal ACTH-stimulation test result.[3] Following long-term therapy, this suppression can last up to 1 year. The duration of adrenal suppression following a short course of corticosteroid therapy is unknown. Even though there is HPA axis suppression in short-term treatment of 1 week or less, clinically evident adrenal insufficiency is probably extremely rare and the suppression lasts only for a few days.[3] Because R.S. is receiving prednisone 1 mg/kg per day, he is receiving a massive supraphysiologic dose that is capable of suppressing endogenous cortisol secretion. Surgery is a stressful event and supplemental doses of a corticosteroid with mineralocorticoid effects probably are warranted for R.S. because he most likely has some degree of HPA axis suppression. Although corticosteroids can decrease wound healing, this is a minor consideration relative to HPA axis suppression.

Adrenal Function Testing

9. How can the degree of adrenal suppression in R.S. be assessed?

The clinician has two options when HPA axis suppression is suspected. The first option is to treat the suspected patient as though adrenocortical insufficiency is present. The second is to try to quantify the adrenocortical reserves of the pituitary and hypothalamus. In today's environment of cost containment, the former approach usually is taken. There are currently five well-established stimulatory tests of HPA axis function. The most commonly used test to diagnose adrenal insufficiency is the short 250-μg ACTH (cosyntropin) stimulation test. This test directly assesses adrenal gland responsiveness to exogenous ACTH. The test measures baseline cortisol plasma concentrations both before the rapid injection of a highly supraphysiologic dose of a synthetic ACTH analog and the cortisol level 30 to 60 minutes after injection. Patients with normal adrenal gland function should be able to generate a poststimulation cortisol concentration of 20 μg/dL. Plasma cortisol concentrations of <495 nmol/L (18 μg/dL) suggest adrenal insufficiency.[40] The remaining four tests—insulin-induced hypoglycemia, overnight metyrapone, CRH stimulation, and low-dose (1 μg) ACTH stimulation—are more sensitive than the 250-μg ACTH stimulation test because they depend on a completely intact HPA axis for a normal result.[3] With the exception of the low-dose (1 μg) ACTH stimulation, these tests tend to be labor intensive and expensive. The low-dose ACTH stimulation not only measures adrenal gland responsiveness, but may be able to detect subtle degrees of adrenal atrophy caused by central adrenal insufficiency.[46,47]

Dosing During Stressful Events

10. R.S. has a cosyntropin test performed, and it demonstrates an increase of 80 mmol/L to a level of 190 mmol/L. In the consideration of this laboratory report, what dosages of corticosteroid should be ordered to prevent an addisonian crisis during R.S.'s surgery?

A normal response includes an increase in plasma cortisol of >170 mmol/L (6 μg/dL) from baseline to a level >495 nmol/L (18 μg/dL).[40] R.S. apparently has adrenal insufficiency and needs cortisol supplementation during periods of stress. Depending on the amount of stress and how prolonged the stress, recommendations for corticosteroid replacement regimen for patients with suppressed HPA axis has been somewhat arbitrary (e.g., hydrocortisone 100 mg Q 6 to 8 hours).[45] Newer recommendations propose that the amount and duration of

corticosteroid coverage should be determined by 1) the preoperative dose of corticosteroid taken by the patient, 2) the preoperative duration of the corticosteroid administration, and 3) the nature and anticipated duration of surgery.[48] Because the adrenal gland can secrete as much as 300 mg/day during acute stress, 150 mg of hydrocortisone every 6 hours is a reasonable regimen for R.S. on the day of his surgery.

Leukocytosis

11. R.S. was doing fine until 3 days after surgery when his temperature spiked to 103°F. R.S. has been back on his original prednisone dosage. Urine, blood, and sputum cultures were ordered as well as a STAT complete blood count (CBC), drawn at 4 PM. His CBC revealed an increase in WBCs, with a differential showing an increase in segmented neutrophils (granulocytes 16,000/mm³, from 11,000 at baseline) along with decreases in both total lymphocyte and monocyte count from baseline. No "left shift" was noted. What could be causing these results?

At first, it would be reasonable to assume there may be an infectious process present. The effects of prednisone on peripheral or circulating WBC counts are well documented and predictable (e.g., granulocytosis along with lymphopenia and monocytopenia). T-cell lymphocytes are decreased more than B-cell lymphocytes. The occurrence of a "left shift" (e.g., an increase in immature leukocytes, such as bands) is variable, and only slight if present. The increase in granulocytes (PMNs) and decrease in lymphocytes and monocytes is most significant 4 to 6 hours after a prednisone dose; these values return to normal in 24 hours. The decrease in monocyte accumulation at tissue sites of inflammation may persist for several days.

Prednisone increases granulocytes by an average of 4,000/mm³, with a range of 1,700 to 7,500/mm³. The increase in granulocytes results primarily from release of cells from bone marrow and secondarily from the shift of cells from the marginal or noncirculating cell pool to the circulating or peripheral pool.[49] The temporal relationship of WBC changes in patients taking multiple doses of corticosteroids is less predictable because of the constant flux in steroid effect.

The results from R.S.'s most recent CBC should be compared with his baseline CBC. The temporal relationship to his prednisone dose also should be determined. Because a STAT CBC, at the time of a temperature spike, was obtained only 7 hours after his prednisone dose was administered, the CBC changes (leukocytosis, monocytopenia, and lymphocytopenia) are difficult to interpret. Another CBC, 24 hours after his dose, was ordered to differentiate the cause of his CBC abnormalities. This CBC was normal, indicating that the abnormalities on the first CBC were probably steroid induced.

Alternate-Day Therapy

12. One month later, R.S. states he feels much better. He has recovered from his surgery, and his polyarteritis is now asymptomatic; his WBC count, BUN, SrCr, and Westergren ESR are returning toward the normal range. Why should R.S.'s prednisone dosage be adjusted at this time?

Once a stable clinical response is attained with a single daily dose of a corticosteroid, R.S.'s corticosteroid dosage should be decreased to the lowest effective dosage and, if possible, to taper the steroid to an alternate-day regimen.[3,45] If used appropriately, alternate-day corticosteroid therapy can help minimize HPA axis suppression and undesirable side effects, while allowing effective treatment of the disease process. A corticosteroid with a short or intermediate duration of action should be chosen for alternate-day therapy to minimize accumulation from subsequent doses that would negate the benefits of every-other-day dosing. If the dosing interval is substantially longer than the biologic half-life (e.g., giving prednisone every 48 hours), nearly normal hypophyseal-pituitary-adrenal function can be maintained. This can minimize the risks of daily therapy. Although alternate-day steroid dosing can be used to maintain disease suppression in chronic therapy, control of the active disease process usually necessitates more intensive dosage schedules.

Conversion to Alternate-Day Therapy

13. How would you convert R.S.'s current 60 mg/day dosage to alternate-day therapy?

Before converting a patient to alternate-day therapy, the minimum effective daily dosage must be determined. Generally, the optimum every-other-day dose is 2.5 to 3 times the minimal daily dose.[45,50] The dose on the "off" day should be tapered gradually by the equivalent of 2.5 to 5 mg of prednisone or its equivalent per week until the patient is taking the steroid every other day. Tapering of the alternate-day dosage can continue until the minimum dosage sufficient to control the underlying disorder is achieved. For R.S., one approach would be to decrease the dosage of prednisone by 5 mg/week until the minimum daily dose is reached that controls his polyarteritis. For illustrative purposes, assume this dosage is 30 mg/day. The 30-mg dose is multiplied by 2.5, so R.S. would take 75 mg on one day, alternating with 30 mg of prednisone the next. The 30-mg dose would then be tapered each week by 5 mg/week until discontinued. R.S. would then be taking 75 mg of prednisone every other day. Should R.S. be asymptomatic at this dosage, a taper of the 75 mg could then be attempted. Tapering should be 2.5 mg/week until the lowest possible dosage that will control his disease is achieved.

Discontinuation of Therapy

14. R.S. has now received prednisone 60 mg QOD for 5 months, and his polyarteritis is well controlled. What would be a reasonable dosing schedule for implementing the gradual discontinuation of R.S.'s corticosteroid?

Many methods of tapering steroid dosages have been tried.[3] Some suggest decreasing the corticosteroid dosage by the equivalent of 2.5 to 5 mg of prednisone every 3 to 7 days until the physiologic dose is reached. Another recommends the daily dose of prednisone (or its equivalent) can be decreased by 5% to 10% per week until a dose of 0.25 to 0.5 mg/kg/day is reached and more slowly thereafter, aiming for either a complete withdrawal or, if not possible, for a low dose of corticosteroid.[36] Others suggest decreasing the dosage by 2.5 mg of prednisone (or the equivalent of another corticosteroid) every 1 to 2 weeks if on daily therapy, or by 5 mg of prednisone every 1 to 2 weeks if on alternate-day therapy, until it can be discontinued. Some clinicians follow this procedure until a physiologic dose is reached and, at that time, will convert the patient to hydrocortisone 20 mg/day. After 2 to 4 weeks, this dosage can be decreased by 2.5 mg every week until 10 mg/day is achieved. At this time, the patient should have a plasma cortisol concentration measured. If this is normal, the hydrocortisone can be discontinued.[45,50] During the tapering process, disease flare-up is a definite possibility; therefore, the patient must be monitored closely. Also, if the patient is stressed during this period, exogenous corticosteroid supplementation may be necessary. Abrupt withdrawal of steroids following long-term, high-dose therapy should be avoided because this may produce a steroid withdrawal syndrome manifested by the presence of nausea, vomiting, anorexia, headache, joint pain, fever, lethargy, myalgia, hypotension, and weight loss. These symptoms are thought to occur as a consequence of rapidly falling serum corticosteroid concentrations rather than the presence of low concentrations.

R.S.'s prednisone dosage of 60 mg every other day can now be decreased by 5 mg at 1- to 2-week intervals until he is receiving 5 mg on alternate days. R.S. can then be converted to hydrocortisone 20 mg/day for 2 to 4 weeks. Weekly reductions of the hydrocortisone by 2.5 mg could be undertaken until the daily dose of 10 mg is reached. At this point, R.S.'s morning dose should be held and a cortisol level taken.

If the serum cortisol concentration is normal ($>10 \ \mu g/dL$), the hydrocortisone can be discontinued. This is but one of the many possible approaches.[45,51] All approaches to discontinuing corticosteroids must be modified based on factors such as dose, duration of therapy, disease status, patient condition, and existence of adverse effects.

Adverse Effects

In addition to suppression of the HPA axis, corticosteroid therapy produces inevitable side effects.[36,39,45] A compilation of documented complications and adverse effects associated with various organ systems is listed in Table 44-7.[52]

Osteoporosis

15. D.L., a 28-year-old, 5'4", 105-lb woman, is diagnosed with SLE. After an acute episode of lupus nephritis, D.L. has been maintained on high-dose prednisone, currently at a level of 15 mg/day. Her lupus seems well controlled, but she comes in today with complaints of back pain. A physical examination reveals no apparent joint involvement typical of a lupus flare-up. What are possible explanations for her back pain, and what additional data are needed to assist in the differential diagnosis?

A good medical history combined with a physical examination and laboratory tests should be obtained to determine whether D.L. is having arthralgias due to SLE or other etiologies. It also is important to note that osteoporosis and osteonecrosis are common adverse effects of corticosteroid therapy, and that 30% to 50% of patients treated with chronic corticosteroids develop osteoporosis. During the first 3 to 6 months of corticosteroid therapy, there is a rapid bone loss of up to 12%, which slows down to 2% to 5% annually.[36] Prednisone dosages of >10 mg/day result in a 10% to 12% annual reduction in the bone mineral content of the lumbar spine.[53,54] Dosages as low as prednisolone 7.5 mg/day appear to be the threshold dose for the development of osteoporosis.[54] Bone

Table 44-7   Adverse Effects of Corticosteroid Therapy

Organ System	Complication
Immunologic	Increased susceptibility to infections, decreased inflammatory responses, suppressed delayed hypersensitivity, neutrophilia, lymphocytopenia
Musculoskeletal	Osteoporosis, fractures, osteonecrosis, myopathy
Gastrointestinal	Peptic ulcers and gastrointestinal bleeds associated with NSAID use, pancreatitis
Cardiovascular	Hypertension, fluid retention accelerated atherosclerosis
Dermatologic	Acne, hirsutism, purple striae, skin fragility, ecchymoses
Neuropsychiatric	Altered mood, emotional lability, euphoria, insomnia, depression, psychosis, pseudotumor cerebri
Ophthalmologic	Cataracts, glaucoma
Endocrine-metabolic	Glucose intolerance, weight gain, fat redistribution (Cushing's syndrome), negative nitrogen balance, growth suppression, muscle wasting, impaired wound healing, fluid retention, hypokalemia, impotence, irregular menses, HPA suppression, acute renal insufficiency

HPA, hypothalamic-pituitary-adrenal; NSAID, nonsteroidal anti-inflammatory drug.

loss leading to fractures at sites such as the spine, hip, and ribs are well-recognized complications of corticosteroid therapy. Osteoporosis in postmenopausal women with RA is more evident at the hip than the spine, and the most important determinants of bone loss are disability and cumulative corticosteroid dose.[55]

The mechanism of corticosteroid-induced osteoporosis is uncertain, but it appears to be different from that of postmenopausal osteoporosis. Corticosteroid-induced osteoporosis is attributable, in part, to decreased osteoblast activity, decreased matrix synthesis, and decreased active life span of osteoblasts. In general, bone formation is decreased and bone resorption may be increased as well.[53] The degree of bone loss correlates to the dose of the corticosteroid and the duration of treatment; however, the absolute amount and duration of corticosteroid therapy have not been determined. When large corticosteroid doses are used, vertebral bone loss can be rapid, and compression fractures can occur within weeks to months after initiation of therapy.[53] D.L. has multiple risk factors for osteoporosis (young, female, and small stature); therefore, her bone mineral density (BMD) should be evaluated and a vertebral radiograph should be taken to look for a compression fracture. D.L.'s bone mineral density test results will determine whether she is a candidate for either primary or secondary prevention and treatment. Primary prevention with prophylactic calcium and calcitriol, with or without calcitonin, should be initiated for any patient with multiple risk factors who possibly will be maintained on the equivalent of prednisone 7.5 mg/day or more of corticosteroids.[53] Primary prevention is indicated for D.L. if her bone density is not decreased. Because D.L. has been taking prednisone 15 mg/day for an extended time, she most likely would require secondary prevention and treatment. Secondary prevention and treatment are indicated when bone density is low, regardless of whether fractures are present.[53] Primary and secondary interventions include the bisphosphonates, calcitriol (for primary prevention only), vitamin D and calcium, calcitonin, fluoride, and selective estrogen receptor modulators (e.g., raloxifene) for postmenopausal women (also see Chapter 48, Gynecological Disorders). The statins may have promise as they have been preliminarily studied to have bone anabolic activity, block osteoporosis and osteonecrosis, resulting in lower rates of fractures in human studies.[56–58] For D.L., a bisphosphonate

such as cyclical etidronate would be a good choice especially at the initiation of corticosteroid when bone loss is the worse. While there is some concern with prolonged use of these agents in young individuals, due to their long retention in bones, this should not discourage their use when they are clearly indicated in young SLE patients. The bisphosphonates should not be used in pregnancy or moderate-severe renal failure, and their discontinuation should be considered when the corticosteroids doses have been substantially tapered with stabilization of BMD.[36] If she is not able to tolerate etidronate or if safety is a concern, calcitriol may be used, although it requires regular serum calcium monitoring at 4 weeks, 3 and 6 months, and 6-month intervals afterwards.[53] The pathogenesis of osteonecrosis is not well-known. Symptoms of osteonecrosis usually take a few months to a few years to develop after exposure to corticosteroids.[59,60] The risk increases with both the dose and duration of corticosteroid therapy. Corticosteroid therapies of short-term high doses, adrenal insufficiency replacement dose, and intraarticular injections have all been implicated.[36]

Gastrointestinal

16. **C.W., a 66-year-old, 5'6", 68-kg woman, is newly diagnosed with PMR. She is an occasional drinker and smoker (1 to 2 packs/wk). She started prednisone 15 mg/day and naproxen 500 mg Q 12 hr PRN 1 week ago and has shown dramatic improvement in the muscle pain of her shoulder and pelvic girdle. She comes in today to begin a taper of her prednisone and comments she's been having some "stomach" problems. What may be the cause of her stomach problems, and how may it be addressed?**

Whether corticosteroids lead to peptic ulcer disease is controversial despite early observations of a probable correlation.[45,61,62] The prevalence of peptic ulcer disease is increased with the combined use of NSAIDs and corticosteroids.[63] Corticosteroids and NSAIDs commonly are prescribed concomitantly because many patients with connective tissue disorders have symptoms such as arthralgias, inflammation, and pain. Corticosteroids can induce tissue atrophy and probably enhance the ulcerogenic potential of other drugs. The risk also depends on the underlying disease and the dose and duration of the steroid therapy. Several risk factors can contribute to

C.W.'s stomach problems. First, she probably has been taking her prescribed naproxen, a nonspecific cyclooxygenase inhibitor (COX) for her chronic aches and pains until her diagnosis of PMR. The nonspecific COX inhibitors (see Chapter 43, Rheumatic Disorders) have been used significantly in the United States and are well documented to precipitate gastrointestinal complications. C.W. is also at increased risk for gastrointestinal complications because of her gender, advanced age, and her smoking and drinking history. At this time, she should have her naproxen switched to a COX-2 inhibitor (e.g., celecoxib, rofecoxib), which, theoretically, should be expected to decrease the potential for developing serious gastrointestinal complications, despite the paucity of substantive documentation. Because prednisone probably will be needed for an extended period by C.W., prophylactic therapy against ulceration may be reasonable.

Hyperglycemia

17. G.P., a 58-year-old man, has a medical history of dermatomyositis, type 2 diabetes mellitus (5 years), hypercholesterolemia, and obesity. G.P.'s current medications are prednisone 80 mg/day (started 2 months ago), lovastatin 20 mg Q HS, and glyburide 5 mg Q am. He came into clinic this morning with the following physical findings: weight, 285 lb; BP, 140/90 mm Hg; pulse, 50 beats/min and regular; and FPG, 189 mg/dL. G.P.'s diabetes has been controlled for 3 years. What are likely explanations for his hyperglycemia?

[SI unit: FPG, 10.5 mmol/L]

Hyperglycemia in G.P. can be attributed to corticosteroid stimulation of gluconeogenesis or impairment of peripheral glucose utilization[36]; however, other etiologies (e.g., missed glyburide dose) also should be considered. Corticosteroids can promote pancreatic glucagon secretion with resultant glycogenolysis and formation of sugar from breakdown of amino acids and lactate produced during glycogenolysis. This process is not generally ketosis producing. Corticosteroids also decrease peripheral glucose utilization by decreasing glucose cell entry and cell membrane insulin receptors. The effects of the corticosteroids on carbohydrate metabolism in susceptible patient are dose related.[36] Increases in blood glucose are usually mild and dosages of prednisone as low as 15 mg/day can cause this effect. Alternate-day therapy has been proposed to minimize, but does not prevent, this adverse effect and in fact produces alternate-day hyperglycemia. Hyperglycemia peaks 2 to 4 hours after administration of the corticosteroid and can last from 12 to 24 hours, depending on the size of the dose.

G.P.'s diabetes has been well controlled in the past; therefore, immediate medication changes are not warranted. He should self-monitor his blood glucose (SMBG) on a regular basis and report the results on the next clinic visit. Corticosteroid-induced hyperglycemia can occur in nondiabetic patients as well. Blood sugars in many nondiabetic patients will return to normal as the patient adjusts to the excess glucose concentration. G.P.'s diabetes should be managed aggressively because he is overweight and at increased risk for cardiovascular complications with hypercholesterolemia. If his fasting blood glucose remains above the American Diabetes Association (ADA) guidelines on subsequent clinic visits, his glucose control may necessitate modifications in his medication management (e.g., increasing the glyburide dosage).

Ecchymosis

18. Several weeks after discharge, R.D. began noticing large purple blotches on her arms that did not blanch upon application of local pressure. Also, these "bruises" did not seem to disappear very rapidly. Why is this dermatologic effect probably prednisone induced?

Ecchymosis, easy bruisability, is a common side effect of prolonged corticosteroid use; it occurs most often in the elderly and is associated with continued use of supraphysiological corticosteroid doses.[39] Steroids destroy the collagen support of small blood vessels, resulting in leakage of blood into surrounding tissue. The anti-inflammatory effects of steroids reduce the normal resorption of blood leakage into tissue, making the "bruise" last longer. A reduction in the dosage of prednisone or the use of an alternate-day prednisone dosing regimen should lessen the purpura.[64] Unfortunately, patients such as R.D. often are already receiving the lowest dosage of corticosteroid that is compatible with keeping the clinical condition under control.

REFERENCES

1. Alarcon GS. Unclassified or undifferentiated connective tissue disease. In: Koopman WJ et al., eds. Clinical Primer of Rheumatology. Philadelphia: Lippincott Williams & Wilkins, 2003:213.
2. Kimberly RP. Connective-tissue diseases. In: Klippel JH et al., eds. Primer of the Rheumatic Diseases. 12th Ed. Atlanta: Arthritis Foundation, 2001:325.
3. Krasner AS. Glucocorticoid-induced adrenal insufficiency. JAMA 1999;282:671.
4. Karpouzas FA et al. Systemic lupus erythematosus. In: Smolen JS et al., eds. Targeted Therapies in Rheumatology. London: Taylor & Francis Group PLC, 2003:563.
5. Hahn BH. Systemic lupus erythematosus. In: Braunwald E et al., eds. Harrison's Principles of Internal Medicine. 15th Ed. New York: McGraw-Hill, 2001:1922.
6. Callen JP. Lupus erythematosus. In: Callen JP et al., eds. Dermatological Signs of Internal Disease. 3rd Ed. Philadelphia: WB Saunders, 2003:1.
7. Rus V et al. The epidemiology of systemic lupus erythematosus. In: Wallace DJ et al., eds. Dubois's Lupus Erythematosus. 6th Ed. Philadelphia: Lippincott Williams & Wilkins, 2002:65.
8. McCarty DJ et al. Incidence of systemic lupus erythematosus. Race and gender differences. Arthritis Rheum 1995;38:1260.
9. Petri M. Systemic lupus erythematosus. In: Koopman WJ et al., eds. Clinical Primer of Rheumatology. Philadelphia: Lippincott Williams & Wilkins, 2003:164.
10. Sontheimer RD et al. Cutaneous manifestations of lupus erythematosus. In: Wallace DJ et al., eds. Dubois' Lupus Erythematosus. 6th Ed. Philadelphia: Lippincott Williams & Wilkins, 2002:575.
11. Tan EM et al. The 1982 revised criteria for the classification of systemic lupus erythematosus. Arthritis Rheum 1982;25:1271.
12. Hochberg MC. Updating the American College of Rheumatology revised criteria for the classification of systemic lupus erythematosus. Arthritis Rheum 1997;40:1725.
13. Guidelines for referral and management of systemic lupus erythematosus in adults. American College of Rheumatology Ad Hoc Committee on Systemic Lupus Erythematosus Guidelines. Arthritis Rheum 1999;42:1785.
14. Morelock SY et al. Drugs and the pleura. Chest 1999;116:212.
15. Callen JP et al. Subacute cutaneous lupus erythematosus induced or exacerbated by terbinafine: a report of 5 cases. Arch Dermatol 2001;137:1196.
16. Crowson AN et al. Subacute cutaneous lupus erythematosus arising in the setting of calcium channel blocker therapy. Hum Pathol 1997;28:67.
17. Callen JP. Drug-induced cutaneous lupus erythematosus, a distinct syndrome that is frequently unrecognized. J Am Acad Dermatol 2001;45:315.
18. Petri MA. Systemic lupus erythematosus: clinical aspects. In: Koopman WJ, ed. Arthritis and Allied Conditions: A Textbook of Rheumatology. 14th Ed. Philadelphia: Lippincott William & Wilkins, 2001:1455.
19. Rubin RL. Drug-induced lupus. In: Wallace DJ et al., eds. Dubois' Lupus Erythematosus. 6th Ed. Philadelphia: Lippincott Williams & Wilkins; 2002:885.
20. Poza-Guedes P et al. Celecoxib-induced lupus-like syndrome. Rheumatology (Oxford) 2003;42:916.

21. Yung RL et al. Drug-induced lupus. Rheum Dis Clin North Am 1994;20:61.
22. Medsger TA Jr. Systemic sclerosis and Raynaud syndrome. In: Koopman WJ et al., eds. Clinical Primer of Rheumatology. Philadelphia: Lippincott Williams & Wilkins, 2003:171.
23. Legerton CW et al. Systemic sclerosis (scleroderma). Clinical management of its major complications. Rheum Dis Clin North Am 1995;21:203.
24. Salvarani C et al. Polymyalgia rheumatica and giant-cell arteritis. N Engl J Med 2002;347:261.
25. Kumar R. Polymyalgia rheumatica and temporal arteritis. In: Koopman WJ et al., eds. Clinical Primer of Rheumatology. Philadelphia: Lippincott William & Wilkins, 2003:207.
26. Kyle V et al. Polymyalgia rheumatica/giant cell arteritis in a Cambridge general practice. Br Med J (Clin Res Ed) 1985;291:385.
27. Swannell AJ. Polymyalgia rheumatica and temporal arteritis: diagnosis and management. BMJ 1997;314:1329.
28. Weyand CM et al. Corticosteroid requirements in polymyalgia rheumatica. Arch Intern Med 1999;159:577.
29. Duhaut P et al. Giant cell arteritis, polymyalgia rheumatica, and viral hypotheses: a multicenter, prospective case-control study. Groupe de Recherche sur l'Arterite a Cellules Geantes. J Rheumatol 1999;26:361.
30. Evans JM et al. Polymyalgia rheumatica and giant cell arteritis. Rheum Dis Clin North Am 2000;26:493.
31. Amor B. Reiter's syndrome: diagnosis and clinical features. Rheum Dis Clin North Am 1998;24:677.
32. Hannu T et al. Chlamydia pneumoniae as a triggering infection in reactive arthritis. Rheumatology (Oxford) 1999;38:411.
33. Arnett FC. Seronegative spondyloarthropathies B. reactive arthritis and enteropathy arthritis. In: Kippel JH et al., eds. Primer on Rheumatic Diseases. 12th Ed. Atlanta: Arthritis Foundation, 2001:245.
34. Boulware DW et al. The scronegative spondyloarthropathies. In: Koopman WJ et al., eds. Clinical Primer of Rheumatology. Philadelphia: Lippincott Williams & Wilkins, 2003:127.
35. Dalakas MC. Polymyositis, dermatomyositis, and inclusion body myositis. In: Braunwald E et al., eds. Harrison's Principles of Internal Medicine. 15th Ed. New York: McGraw-Hill, 2001:2524.
36. Kirou KA et al. Systemic glucocorticoid therapy in systemic lupus erythematosus. In: Wallace DJ et al., eds. Dubois' Lupus Erythematosus. 6th Ed.

37. Fullerton DS. Steroids and therapeutically related compounds. In: Delgado JN et al., eds. Wilson and Gisvold's Textbook of Organic Medicinal and Pharmaceutical Chemistry. 10th Ed. Philadelphia: Lippincott-Raven, 1998:727.
38. Kehrl JH et al. The clinical use of glucocorticoids. Ann Allergy 1983;50:2.
39. Schimmer BP et al. Adrenocorticotropic hormone; adrenocortical steroids and their synthetic analogs; inhibitors of the synthesis and actions of adrenocortical hormones. In: Hardman JG et al., eds. Goodman and Gilman's The Pharmacological Basis of Therapeutics. 10th Ed. New York: McGraw-Hill, 2001:1649.
40. Williams GH et al. Disorders of the adrenal cortex. In: Braunwald E et al., eds. Harrison's Principle of Internal Medicine. 15th Ed. New York: McGraw-Hill, 2001:2084.
41. Petri M. Systemic lupus erythematosus (including pregnancy and antiphospholipid antibody syndrome). In: Weisman MH et al., eds. Treatment of Rheumatic Diseases. Philadelphia: WB Saunders, 2001:274.
42. Manzi S. Systemic lupus erythematosus: c. treatment. In: Klippel JH, ed. Primer on the Rheumatic Diseases. 12th Ed. Atlanta: Arthritis Foundation, 2001:346.
43. Illei GG et al. Combination therapy with pulse cyclophosphamide plus pulse methylprednisolone improves long-term renal outcome without adding toxicity in patients with lupus nephritis. Ann Intern Med 2001;135:248.
44. Hahn BH. Management of systemic lupus erythematosus. In: Ruddy S et al., eds. Kelley's Textbook of Rheumatology. 6th Ed. Philadelphia: WB Saunders, 2001:1125.
45. Baxter JD. Advances in glucocorticoid therapy. Adv Intern Med 2000;45:317.
46. Dickstein G et al. One microgram is the lowest ACTH dose to cause a maximal cortisol response: there is no diurnal variation of cortisol response to submaximal ACTH stimulation. Eur J Endocrinol 1997;137:172.
47. Abdu TA et al. Comparison of the low dose short synacthen test (1 microg), the conventional dose short synacthen test (250 microg), and the insulin tolerance test for assessment of the hypothalamo-pituitary-adrenal axis in patients with pituitary disease. J Clin Endocrinol Metab 1999;84:838.

48. Salem M et al. Perioperative glucocorticoid coverage: a reassessment 42 years after emergence of a problem. Ann Surg 1994;219:416.
49. Bishop CR et al. Leukokinetic studies. 13. A nonsteady-state kinetic evaluation of the mechanism of cortisone-induced granulocytosis. J Clin Invest 1968;47:249.
50. Walton J et al. Alternate-day vs shorter-interval steroid administration. Arch Intern Med 1970;126:601.
51. Kountz DS et al. Safely withdrawing patients from chronic glucocorticoid therapy. Am Fam Physician 1997;55:521.
52. Stein MC et al. Glucocorticoids. In: Ruddy S et al., eds. Kelley's Textbook of Rheumatology. 6th Ed. Philadelphia: WB Saunders, 2001:823.
53. Eastell R et al. A UK Consensus Group on management of glucocorticoid-induced osteoporosis: an update. J Intern Med 1998;244:271.
54. Eastell R. Management of corticosteroid-induced osteoporosis. UK Consensus Group Meeting on Osteoporosis. J Intern Med 1995;237:439.
55. Hall GM et al. The effect of rheumatoid arthritis and steroid therapy on bone density in postmenopausal women. Arthritis Rheum 1993;36:1510.
56. Wang PS et al. HMG-CoA reductase inhibitors and the risk of hip fractures in elderly patients. JAMA 2000;283:3211.
57. Meier CR et al. HMG-CoA reductase inhibitors and the risk of fractures. JAMA 2000;283:3205.
58. Schlienger R et al. HMG-CoA reductase inhibitors in osteoporosis: do they reduce the risk of fracture? Drugs Aging 2003;20:321.
59. Mankin HJ. Nontraumatic necrosis of bone (osteonecrosis). N Engl J Med 1992;326:1473.
60. Simkin PA et al. Osteonecrosis: pathogenesis and practicalities. Hosp Pract (Off Ed) 1994;29:73.
61. Keenan GF. Management of complications of glucocorticoid therapy. Clin Chest Med 1997;18:507.
62. Conn HO et al. Corticosteroids and peptic ulcer: meta-analysis of adverse events during steroid therapy. J Intern Med 1994;236:619.
63. Piper JM et al. Corticosteroid use and peptic ulcer disease: role of nonsteroidal anti-inflammatory drugs. Ann Intern Med 1991;114:735.
64. Yanovski JA et al. Glucocorticoid action and the clinical features of Cushing's syndrome. Endocrinol Metab Clin North Am 1994;23:487.

Contraception

Jennifer L. Hardman

The world population is about 6.3 billion. At the predicted rate of growth, the population is projected to reach 7.5 billion by 2020 and >9 billion by 2050.[1] In the United States, there are approximately 290 million people, and there is one birth every 8 seconds and 1 death every 13 seconds. This results in an increase in one person every 11 seconds.[2]

Preventing unwanted pregnancy is an important goal of contraceptive use. Is it estimated that nearly 20% of adolescents have had sex before the age of 15. About 15% of 14-year-old girls who have had sex report having been pregnant.[3]

Contraceptive policies established and implemented in this decade will help determine how quickly the population will grow in the United States and worldwide and can help reduce the number of unwanted pregnancies.

MENSTRUAL CYCLE PHYSIOLOGY

Feedback biologic mechanisms involving the hypothalamus, anterior pituitary gland, ovaries, and endometrial lining of the uterus control the average 28-day menstrual cycle.[4,5] The hypothalamus synthesizes gonadotropin-releasing hormone (GnRH) and secretes the hormone in a pulse-like manner with varying frequencies throughout the menstrual cycle. GnRH stimulates the anterior pituitary to produce and release follicle-stimulating hormone (FSH) and luteinizing hormone (LH). FSH and LH act on the ovaries to produce estrogen and progesterone. Estrogen in turn acts on the hypothalamus and anterior pituitary, in a negative feedback manner, to stop FSH and LH secretion (Fig. 45-1).

The menstrual cycle can be divided into three phases: the follicular phase, ovulation, and the luteal phase (Fig. 45-2).[4–6] The day bleeding begins is referred to as the first day (or day 1) of the menstrual cycle. Bleeding usually occurs from days 1 to 5 of the cycle. The follicular phase begins at the onset of menstruation (menstrual phase) and lasts approximately 10 to 14 days (see Fig. 45-2). At the beginning of this phase, several follicles begin to develop within the ovary. In the second half of the follicular phase, most of the developing follicles atrophy, while the dominant follicle develops further and produces estrogen in increasing amounts. Elevated estradiol levels results in a surge in LH and FSH. This LH surge is responsible for final-stage growth and maturation of the follicle, ovulation, and the formation of the corpus luteum. Ovulation usually occurs 14 days before the last day of the cycle, and is followed by the luteal phase. In 90% of women, the luteal phase is 13 to 15 days in duration and is the least variable part of the human reproductive cycle. During this progesterone-dominant phase, the corpus luteum produces progesterone and estrogen. Progesterone prepares the endometrium for implantation of a fertilized ovum. If implantation does not occur, corpus luteum regression causes a decrease in the levels of estrogen and progesterone. When these hormone levels decrease, the endometrium cannot be maintained and is sloughed off (menstrual phase). Using the average 28-day cycle as an example, day 28 is the last day of the cycle and is the day before bleeding begins again for the next menstrual cycle.

COMPARISON OF CONTRACEPTIVE METHOD EFFECTIVENESS

The effectiveness of any contraceptive method depends on its mechanism of action, availability (e.g., if a prescription is required, cost), and acceptability (e.g., side effects, ease of use, religious and social beliefs). Any or all of these reasons can account for the discrepancy between the lowest observed fail-

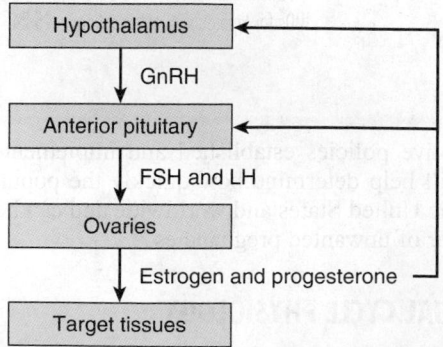

FIGURE 45-1 Menstrual cycle physiology. GnRH, gonadotropin-releasing hormone; FSH, follicle-stimulating hormone; LH, luteinizing hormone.

ure rate and the actual failure rate in typical users. Table 45-1 compares the first-year failure rates of various contraceptive methods.[5]

HORMONAL CONTRACEPTION PHARMACOLOGY

Estrogens prevent the development of the dominant follicle by suppressing FSH secretion. Estrogens also stabilize the endometrial lining to minimize breakthrough bleeding with oral contraceptives (OCs).[4,5] Progestins prevent ovulation by suppressing LH secretion. They also hamper the transport of sperm through the cervical canal by thickening cervical mucus and causing alterations in the endometrial lining (so that it is not favorable for implantation) and in the fallopians tubes (affecting ovum transport).

COMBINATION ORAL CONTRACEPTIVE PILLS

Manipulating the normal physiologic feedback mechanisms of the menstrual cycle using estrogen and progestin has proven to be an effective method of contraception. In 1960, the U.S. Food and Drug Administration (FDA) released the OC Enovid 10.[4] Enovid 10 (containing 150 μg mestranol and 9.85 mg norethynodrel) exposed the patient to much higher doses of estrogen and progestin than are in today's OCs. The resulting side effects prompted the search for better OC products. Table 45-2 lists the available brand-name and generic OCs.

The failure rate of OCs ranges from 0.1 to 5 pregnancies per 100 women-years (see Table 45-1).[5] All low-dose OCs available in the United States contain the synthetic estrogen ethinyl estradiol (EE). Mestranol is another estrogen that has been used in the United States and is used in other countries. Mestranol is inactive and must be converted in the body to EE. Mestranol 50 μg has approximately the same activity as EE 35 μg.[7] OCs contain one of the following progestins: ethynodiol diacetate, desogestrel, drosperinone, levonorgestrel, norethindrone, norethindrone acetate, norgestimate, and norgestrel (a mixture of dextronorgestrel and levonorgestrel; dextronorgestrel appears to be progestationally inert compared with levonorgestrel).[8] These progestins differ significantly in their progestational potency and also in the extent of their metabolism to estrogenic substances. Progestins have both estrogenic and antiestrogenic effects. Because the progestins have a chemical structure similar to that of testosterone, they also have varying degrees of androgenic activity (Table 45-3).[9] Minor structural changes in all of the progestins may lead to significant changes in their progestational, estrogenic, antiestrogenic, and androgenic activities, which may vary widely in effect from patient to patient (see Table 45-2).

Different terminology is used to describe the classes of pills that have been approved over the years. The OCs most commonly used today are also called low-dose OCs. They contain <50 μg of EE per day. In the literature, OCs are commonly referred to as first, second, or third generation.[4] First-generation OCs contain >50 μg EE per day. Second-generation OCs contain the progestins levonorgestrel, norgestimate, norethindrone, norethindrone acetate, or ethynodiol diacetate, along with 30 to 35 μg EE. Third-generation OCs contain desogestrel and 20 to 30 μg EE. There are also generations of progestins; first-generation progestins include norethindrone,

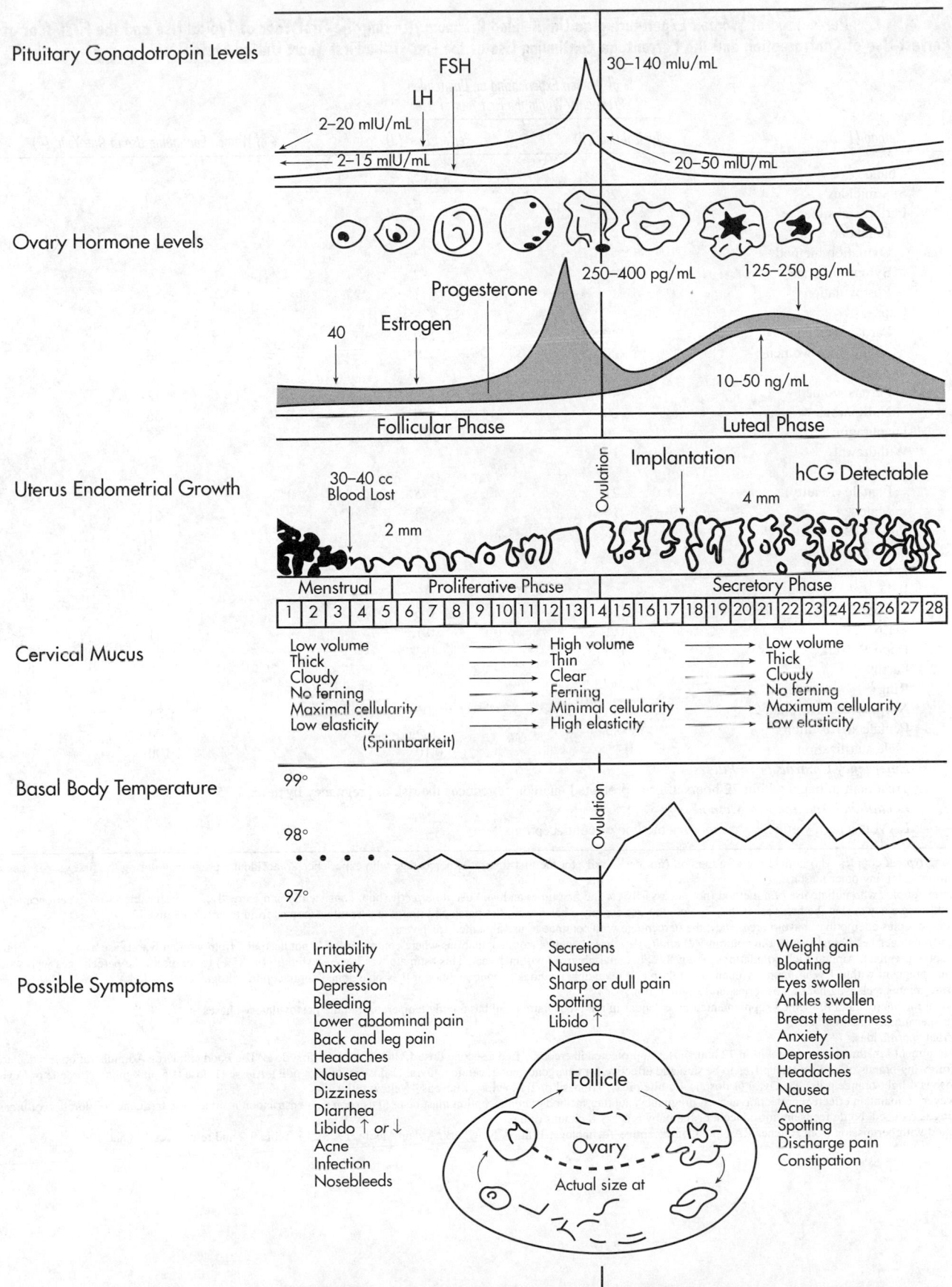

FIGURE 45-2 The menstrual cycle. FSH, follicle-stimulating hormone; hCG, human chorionic go-nadotropin; LH, luteinizing hormone. (Adapted with permission from Hatcher RA et al. Contraceptive Technology, 16th ed. New York: Irvington Publishers, 1994;41, Figure 2.2)

Table 45-1 Percentage of Women Experiencing an Unintended Pregnancy During the First Year of Typical Use and the First Year of Perfect Use of Contraception and the Percentage Continuing Use at the End of the First Year: United States

Method (1)	% of Women Experiencing an Unintended Pregnancy Within the First Year of Use		% of Women Continuing Use at One Year[c] (4)
	Typical Use[a] (2)	Perfect Use[b] (3)	
Chance[d]	85	85	
Spermicides[e]	26	6	40
Periodic abstinence	25		63
Calendar		9	
Ovulation method		3	
Symptothermal[f]		2	
Postovulation		1	
Cap[g]			
Parous women	40	26	42
Nulliparous women	20	9	56
Sponge			
Parous women	40	20	42
Nulliparous women	20	9	56
Diaphragm[g]	20	6	56
Withdrawal	19	4	
Condom[h]			
Female (Reality)	21	5	56
Male	14	3	61
Pill	5		71
Progestin only		0.5	
Combined		0.1	
IUD			
Copper T 380A	0.8	0.6	78
LNg 20	0.1	0.1	81
Depo-Provera	0.3	0.3	70
Patch		1	
Ring		1–2	
Norplant and Norplant-2	0.05	0.05	88
Female sterilization	0.5	0.5	100
Male sterilization	0.15	0.10	100

Emergency Contraceptive Pills

Treatment initiated within 72 hours after unprotected intercourse reduces the risk of pregnancy by at least 75%.[i]

Lactational Amenorrhea Method

LAM is a highly effective, *temporary* method of contraception.[j]

[a]Among *typical* couples who initiate use of a method (not necessarily for the first time), the percentage who experience an accidental pregnancy during the first year if they do not stop use for any other reason.

[b]Among couples who initiate use of a method (not necessarily for the first time) and who use it *perfectly* (both consistently and correctly), the percentage who experience an accidental pregnancy during the first year if they do not stop use for any other reason. For patch and ring, the percentage comes from the package insert.

[c]Among couples attempting to avoid pregnancy, the percentage who continue to use a method for 1 year.

[d]The percentages becoming pregnant in columns (2) and (3) are based on data from populations where contraception is not used and from women who cease using contraception to become pregnant. Among such populations, about 89% become pregnant within 1 year. This estimate was lowered slightly (to 85%) to represent the percentages who would become pregnant within 1 year among women now relying on reversible methods of contraception if they abandoned contraception altogether.

[e]Foams, creams, gels, vaginal suppositories, and vaginal film.

[f]Cervical mucus (ovulation) method supplemented by calendar in the preovulatory and basal body temperature in the postovulatory phases.

[g]With spermicidal cream or jelly.

[h]Without spermicides.

[i]The treatment schedule is one dose within 72 hours after unprotected intercourse, and a second dose 12 hours after the first dose. The Food and Drug Administration has declared the following brands of oral contraceptives to be safe and effective for emergency contraception: Ovral (1 dose is 2 white pills), Alesse (1 dose is 5 pink pills), Nordette or Levlen (1 dose is 4 light-orange pills), Lo/Ovral (1 dose is 4 white pills), Triphasil or Tri-Levlen (1 dose is 4 yellow pills).

[j]However, to maintain effective protection against pregnancy, another method of contraception must be used as soon as menstruation resumes, the frequency or duration of breast-feeding is reduced, bottle feeds are introduced, or the baby reaches 6 months of age.

Adapted with permission from Hatcher RA et al. Contraceptive Technology, 17th ed. New York: Ardent Media, 1998:216, Table 9-2 and references 133 and 134.

Table 45-2   Commercially Available Brand-Name and Generic Oral Contraceptive and Progesterone-Only Pills

Brand Name	Generic Name	Progestin Type and Dose	EE Dose (μg)	Progestin Activity	Estrogen Activity	Androgen Activity
Monophasic OCs						
Alesse	Aviane	Levonorgestrel 0.1 mg	20	L	L	L
Demulen 1/35	Zovia 1/35	Ethynodiol diacetate 1 mg	35	H	L	L
Desogen	Apri	Desogestrel 0.15 mg	30	H	I	L
Levlen	Levora, Portia	Levonorgestrel 0.15 mg	30	I	L	I
Levlite	Lessina	Levonorgestrel 0.1 mg	20	L	L	L
Lo-Ovral	Cryselle, Low-Ogestrel	Norgestrel 0.3 mg	30	I	L	I
Loestrin 1.5/30[a]	Microgestin Fe 1.5/30	Norethindrone acetate 1.5 mg	30	H	L	H
Loestrin 1/20[a]	Microgestin Fe 1/20	Norethindrone acetate 1 mg	20	H	L	I
Mircette[b]	Kariva	Desogestrel 0.15	20	H	L	L
Modicon	Brevicon, Nortel 0.5/35 Necon 0.5/35	Norethindrone 0.5 mg	35	L	H	L
Nordette	Levora, Portia	Levonorgestrel 0.15 mg	30	I	L	I
Ortho Cyclen	Sprintec, MonoNessa	Norgestimate 0.25 mg	35	L	I	L
Ortho-Cept	Apri	Desogestrel 0.15 mg	30	H	I	L
Ortho-Novum 1/35	Norinyl 1+35, Nortrel 1/35, Necon 1/35, Genora 1/35	Norethindrone 1 mg	35	I	H	I
Ovcon-35		Norethindrone 0.4 mg	35	L	H	L
Yasmin		Drosperinone 3 mg	30	No data	I	None
Biphasic OCs						
Ortho-Novum 10/11	Necon 10/11, Jenest	Norethindrone 0.5, 1 mg	35	I	H	L
Triphasic OCs						
Cyclessa		Desogestrel 0.1, 0.125 0.15 mg	25	H	L	L
Estrostep[a]		Norethindrone acetate 1 mg	20, 30, 35	H	L	I
Ortho Tri-Cyclen	Tri-Sprintec	Norgestimate 0.18, 0.215, 0.25 mg	35	L	I	L
Ortho Tri-Cyclen Lo		Norgestimate 0.18, 0.215, 0.25 mg	25	L	L	L
Ortho-Novum 7/7/7	Necon 7/7/7, Nortrel 7/7/7	Norethindrone 0.5, 0.75, 1 mg	35	I	H	L
Tri-Norinyl		Norethindrone 0.5, 1, 0.5 mg	35	L	H	L
Tri-Levlen	Enpresse, Trivora	Levonorgestrel 0.05, 0.075, 0.125 mg	30, 40, 30	L	I	L
Triphasil	Enpresse, Trivora	Levonorgestrel 0.05, 0.075, 0.125 mg	30, 40, 30	L	I	L
Progesterone Only Pills						
Micronor	Errin	Norethinedrone 0.35 mg	None			
Nor-QD	Nora-BE, Camila	Norethinedrone 0.35 mg	None			
Ovrette		Norgestrel 0.075 mg	None			

[a]Also available with iron tablets instead of placebo tablets during the usual placebo week.
[b]Has 2 days of placebo followed by 5 days of EE 10 μg during the usual placebo week.
EE, ethinyl estradiol; H, high; I, intermediate; L, low.

Table 45-3   Estrogenic, Progestogenic, and Androgenic Effects of Oral Contraceptive Pills

Estrogenic Effects	Progestogenic Effects	Androgenic Effects
• Nausea • Increased breast size (ductal and fatty tissue) • Cyclic weight gain due to fluid retention • Leukorrhea • Cervical eversion or ectopy • Hypertension • Rise in cholesterol concentration in gallbladder bile • Growth of leiomyomata • Telangiectasia • Hepatocellular adenomas or hepatocellular cancer (rare) • Cerebrovascular accidents (rare) • Thromboembolic complications including pulmonary emboli (rare) • Stimulation of breast neoplasia (exceedingly rare) (Most pills with <50 μg of ethinyl estradiol do not produce troublesome estrogen-mediated side effects or complications.)	Both the estrogenic and the progestational components of oral contraceptives may contribute to the development of the following adverse effects: • Breast tenderness • Headaches • Hypertension • Myocardial infarction (rare)	All low-dose combined pills suppress a woman's production of testosterone, which has a beneficial effect on acne, oily skin, and hirsutism. The progestin component may have androgenic as well as progestational effects: • Increased appetite and weight gain • Depression, fatigue, tiredness • Decreased libido and/or enjoyment of intercourse • Acne, oily skin • Increased breast tenderness or breast size • Increased LDL cholesterol levels • Decreased HDL cholesterol levels • Decreased carbohydrate tolerance; increased insulin resistance • Pruritus

Adapted with permission from Hatcher RA et al. Contraceptive Technology, 17th ed. NY: Ardent Media, 1998:419, Table 19-4.

second-generation progestins include levonorgestrel and norgestrel, and third-generation progestins include desogestrel and gestodene (not available in the United States).[10]

Contraindications to Oral Contraceptive Use

1.   M.F., a healthy 32-year-old woman, wants to know if she is a good candidate for OCs. She smokes a pack of cigarettes per day. What contraindications to OC therapy must be considered? Is M.F. a good candidate for OCs?

To determine if any contraindications or precautions exist, the clinician should first obtain baseline health information from M.F.[11] (Table 45-4). M.F. should be encouraged to stop smoking. She does not currently have any contraindications to OC use, but she should be informed that OCs will no longer be prescribed for her in a few years if she continues to smoke (see Question 8). Since M.F. does not have any medical problems, she is an acceptable candidate for OCs.

Choice

2.   M.F. has decided to start OCs. Which OC should be selected for her?

Confusion abounds in selecting an OC because of the multitude of OCs available, the lack of studies comparing one product with others, and managed care formulary restrictions. The information in Figure 45-3 may be used to select an initial OC for most patients and to change pills when side effects necessitate an alternative choice.[12] Any pill containing <50 μg EE can be used for M.F. because she is a healthy woman without medical complications.

However, since higher body weight (≥70.5 kg) has been associated with increased OC failure, a pill with a higher dose of EE (e.g., 35 μg) may be a better choice if M.F. is heavier.[14]

21-Day Versus 28-Day Cycle

Most 28-day OC pill packs contain 21 days of active pills (pills that contain estrogen and progestin) followed by 7 days of placebo pills. The 21-day pill packs contain only the active pills. Many clinicians prefer the use of 28-day cycle OCs to minimize confusion; the patient takes one tablet daily regardless of whether it is an active or placebo pill. After taking the last tablet of a 28-day pack of OCs, the patient should begin a new pack the next day. However, when continuous ovarian suppression is indicated to treat estrogen-dependent disorders such as endometriosis, the 21-day cycle OCs are preferred to facilitate taking active tablets continuously. Alternatively, the placebo tablets could be removed from 28-day cycle packs. M.F. will not be taking OCs continuously, so a 28-day pack is recommended.

Multiphasic Oral Contraceptives

3.   Should M.F. start a monophasic or triphasic OC? What are the advantages and disadvantages of the triphasic OCs relative to other OCs?

Because of metabolic and physiologic effects related to the progestin component of OCs, the biphasic and triphasic products were formulated to contain less progestin overall (with the exception of Mircette). These products attempt to provide adequate endometrial support while also providing adequate contraception.[14]

The multiphasic products contain varying amounts of progestin and/or estrogen during each of the active phases. Currently, Necon 10/11, Ortho-Novum 10/11, and Jenest 28 are the only biphasic OCs marketed in the United States, and they are rarely used. Mircette has been classified as a monophasic or biphasic OC. It provides a novel regimen containing 21 days of 0.15 mg desogestrel plus 20 μg EE, then only 2 days of placebo, and finally 5 days of 10 μg EE alone.

Table 45-4 Medical Eligibility Criteria for Contraceptive Use[12]

Condition	OC	CIC	POP	DMPA	Norplant	Cu-IUD	LNG-IUD
				Contraceptive Method			
			I = Initiation, C = Continuation				
Personal Characteristics and Reproductive History							
Smoking							
a) Age <35	2	2	1	1	1	1	1
b) Age >35							
(i) <15 cigarettes/day	3	2	1	1	1	1	1
(ii) >15 cigarettes/day	4	3	1	1	1	1	1
Obesity >30 kg/m² body mass index (BMI)	2	2	1	2	2	1	2
Cardiovascular Disease							
Multiple Risk Factors for Arterial Cardiovascular Disease (such as older age, smoking, diabetes and hypertension)	3/4	3/4	2	3	2	1	2
Hypertension							
a) History of hypertension where blood pressure *cannot* be evaluated (including hypertension during pregnancy)	3	3	2	2	2	1	2
b) Adequately controlled hypertension, where blood pressure *can* be evaluated	3	3	1	2	1	1	1
c) Elevated blood pressure levels (properly taken measurements)							
(i) Systolic 140–159 or diastolic 90–99	3	3	1	2	1	1	1
(ii) Systolic >160 or diastolic >100	4	4	2	3	2	1	2
d) Vascular disease	4	4	2	3	2	1	2
History of High Blood Pressure During Pregnancy (where current blood pressure is measurable and normal)	2	2	1	1	1	1	1
Deep Venous Thrombosis (DVT)/ Pulmonary Embolism (PE)							
a) History of DVT/PE	4	4	2	2	2	1	2
b) Current DVT/PE	4	4	3	3	3	1	3
c) Family history (first-degree relatives)	2	2	1	1	1	1	1
d) Major surgery							
(i) With prolonged immobilization	4	4	2	2	2	1	2
(ii) Without prolonged immobilization	2	2	1	1	1	1	1
e) Minor surgery without immobilization	1	1	1	1	1	1	1
Superficial Venous Thrombosis							
a) Varicose veins	1	1	1	1	1	1	1
b) Superficial thrombophlebitis	2	2	1	1	1	1	1
Stroke (history of cerebrovascular accident)	4	4	I 2 / C 3	3	I 2 / C 3	1	2
Known Hyperlipidemias (screening is NOT necessary for safe use of contraceptive methods)	2/3	2/3	2	2	2	1	2
Neurologic Conditions							
Headaches	I / C	I / C	I / C	I / C	I / C		I / C
a) Nonmigrainous (mild or severe)	1 / 2	1 / 2	1 / 1	1 / 1	1 / 1	1	1 / 1
b) Migraine							
(i) Without focal neurologic symptoms							
Age <35	2 / 3	2 / 3	1 / 2	2 / 2	2 / 2	1	2 / 2
Age >35	3 / 4	3 / 4	1 / 2	2 / 2	2 / 2	1	2 / 2
(ii) With focal neurologic symptoms (at any age)	4 / 4	4 / 4	2 / 3	2 / 3	2 / 3	1	2 / 3
Epilepsy	1	1	1	1	1	1	1

Continued

Table 45-4 Medical Eligibility Criteria for Contraceptive Use—cont'd

Condition	OC	CIC	POP	DMPA	Norplant	Cu-IUD I	Cu-IUD C	LNG-IUD I	LNG-IUD C
Reproductive Tract Infections and Disorders									
Unexplained Vaginal Bleeding (suspicious for serious condition)						I	C	I	C
Before evaluation	2	2	2	3	3	4	2	4	2
Endometriosis	1	1	1	1	1	2		1	
Benign Ovarian Tumors (including cysts)	1	1	1	1	1	1		1	
Cervical Intraepithelial Neoplasia (CIN)	2	2	1	2	2	1		2	
Cervical Cancer (awaiting treatment)						I	C	I	C
	2	2	1	2	2	4	2	4	2
Breast Disease									
a) Undiagnosed mass	2	2	2	2	2	1		2	
b) Benign breast disease	1	1	1	1	1	1		1	
c) Family history of cancer	1	1	1	1	1	1		1	
d) Cancer									
(i) Current	4	4	4	4	4	1		4	
(ii) Past and no evidence of current disease for 5 years	3	3	3	3	3	1		3	
Endometrial Cancer						I	C	I	C
	1	1	1	1	1	4	2	4	2
Ovarian Cancer						I	C	I	C
	1	1	1	1	1	3	2	3	2
Uterine Fibroids									
a) Without distortion of the uterine cavity	1	1	1	1	1	2		2	
b) With distortion of the uterine cavity	1	1	1	1	1	4		4	
Pelvic Inflammatory Disease (PID)									
a) Past PID (assuming no current risk factors of STDs)						I	C	I	C
(i) With subsequent pregnancy	1	1	1	1	1	1	1	1	1
(ii) Without subsequent pregnancy	1	1	1	1	1	2	2	2	2
b) PID-current or within the last 3 months	1	1	1	1	1	4	3	4	3
HIV/AIDS									
High Risk of HIV	1	1	1	1	1	3		3	
HIV-Positive	1	1	1	1	1	3		3	
AIDS	1	1	1	1	1	3		3	
Endocrine Conditions									
Diabetes									
a) History of gestational disease	1	1	1	1	1	1		1	
b) Nonvascular disease									
(i) Non-insulin dependent	2	2	2	2	2	1		2	
(ii) Insulin dependent	2	2	2	2	2	1		2	
c) Nephropathy/retinopathy/neuropathy	3/4	3/4	2	3	2	1		2	
d) Other vascular disease or diabetes of >20 years' duration	3/4	3/4	2	3	2	1		2	
Gastrointestinal Conditions									
Gallbladder Disease									
a) Symptomatic									
(i) Treated by cholecystectomy	2	2	2	2	2	1		2	
(ii) Medically treated	3	2	2	2	2	1		2	
(iii) Current	3	2	2	2	2	1		2	
b) Asymptomatic	2	2	2	2	2	1		2	
Viral Hepatitis									
a) Active	4	3/4	3	3	3	1		3	
b) Carrier	1	1	1	1	1	1		1	

Table 45-4 **Medical Eligibility Criteria for Contraceptive Use—cont'd**

Condition	OC	CIC	POP	DMPA	Norplant	Cu-IUD	LNG-IUD
				Contraceptive Method			
Gastrointestinal Conditions—cont'd							
Cirrhosis							
a) Mild (compensated)	3	2	2	2	2	1	2
b) Severe (decompensated)	4	3	3	3	3	1	3
Liver Tumors							
a) Benign (adenoma)	4	3	3	3	3	1	3
b) Malignant (hepatoma)	4	3/4	3	3	3	1	3
Anemias							
Sickle Cell Disease	2	2	1	1	1	2	1
Iron Deficiency Anemia	1	1	1	1	1	2	1

1, a condition for which there is no restriction for the use of the contraceptive method;
2, a condition where the advantages of using the method generally outweigh the theoretical or proven risks;
3, a condition where the theoretical or proven risks usually outweigh the advantages of using the method;
4, a condition which represents an unacceptable health risk if the contraceptive method is used.
CIC, combined injectable contraceptive; Cu-IUD, copper intrauterine device; DMPA, depot medroxyprogesterone acetate; LNG-IUD, levonorgestrel intrauterine device; OC, oral contraceptive; POP, progestin-only pills.
Adapted with permission from reference 12.

The patient does not need to take missed 10-μg EE doses or use a backup method when missed. The 5 days of 10 μg EE alone help minimize breakthrough bleeding with this product and may be useful for patients who have estrogen deficiency symptoms such as headaches during the hormone-free week.

The triphasic OCs (e.g., Ortho-Novum 7/7/7, Tri-Levlen, Triphasil, Ortho Tri-Cyclen) appear to support the endometrium more consistently than the biphasic OCs.[9] No studies, however, show a superiority of one triphasic over another or compared to monophasic OCs. The reduced progestin content is desirable for women complaining of side effects caused by too much progestin or women with cardiovascular disease or metabolic abnormalities.[5,9] Women with side effects related to progestin deficiency (e.g., late-cycle bleeding) or conditions necessitating progestin dominance (e.g., benign breast disease) may do better with monophasic OCs.

One drawback associated with triphasic OC use is the confusion caused by the different-colored tablets in each of the three different phases, making the missed-dose instructions more complicated. Monophasic OCs would be preferred for women who will be taking OCs continuously (i.e., skipping the placebo pills). M.F. may be started on either a monophasic or triphasic OC.

Patient Instructions

4. What instructions should be given to M.F. about her OC?

When to Start Oral Contraceptives
M.F. should start the first cycle of OCs according to the manufacturer's package instructions or according to one of the two following recommendations:[5]

1. Day 1 Start: Take the first tablet in the OC pack on the first day of menses.
2. Sunday Start: Take the first tablet in the OC pack on the first Sunday after the beginning of menstruation. If menses begins on Sunday, start that day.

A newer method for initiating OCs is the quick start method,[15] in which the patient takes her first OC tablet while still in the health care provider's office. This method can minimize the confusion that many patients have about when to start their first pack and can increase rates of method continuation. Also, the quick start method provides contraceptive protection sooner and would, therefore, likely lower the risk of unintended pregnancy. More research on and awareness about this method are needed for it to be used routinely by health care providers.

When to Use a Backup Method of Contraception
Some clinicians recommend that the woman use an alternative method of contraception for the entire first cycle. Others believe that alternative methods of contraception are unnecessary if the OC is started on or before the fifth menstrual day. Most OC package inserts state that a backup method of contraception (e.g., condoms) is not necessary if patients use the Day 1 start method.[5,7] If patients use the Sunday start method, backup contraception should be used for the first week of the OC cycle. A backup method is also recommended when doses are missed, as described in the following section. M.F. has decided to use the Sunday start method, so her partner will need to use condoms for the first week of her first cycle of pills.

Proper Pill Taking
M.F. should take the OC tablets at exactly the same time each day. If she experiences nausea with OCs, she may find that the nausea improves if she takes her pill at bedtime or with food. The best time for OCs to be taken depends on the patient. The optimal time for M.F is the time when she will have the fewest problems remembering to take her pill each day.

If a woman forgets to take one pill, she must take it as soon as she remembers and refer to the patient instructions in the package insert for further information.[5] Most manufacturers recommend that if she forgets to take one pill, she should take two pills on the day she remembers (e.g., if she forgets her pill

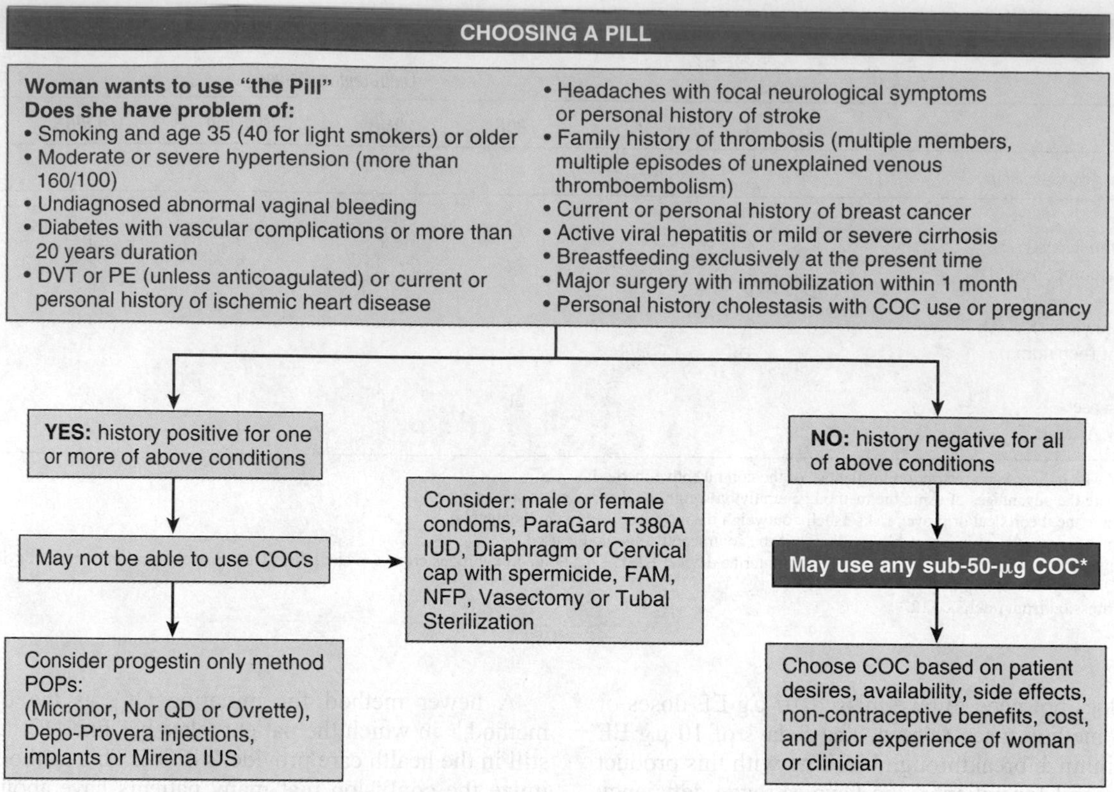

CHOOSING A PILL

Woman wants to use "the Pill"
Does she have problem of:
- Smoking and age 35 (40 for light smokers) or older
- Moderate or severe hypertension (more than 160/100)
- Undiagnosed abnormal vaginal bleeding
- Diabetes with vascular complications or more than 20 years duration
- DVT or PE (unless anticoagulated) or current or personal history of ischemic heart disease

- Headaches with focal neurological symptoms or personal history of stroke
- Family history of thrombosis (multiple members, multiple episodes of unexplained venous thromboembolism)
- Current or personal history of breast cancer
- Active viral hepatitis or mild or severe cirrhosis
- Breastfeeding exclusively at the present time
- Major surgery with immobilization within 1 month
- Personal history cholestasis with COC use or pregnancy

YES: history positive for one or more of above conditions

May not be able to use COCs

Consider progestin only method POPs:
(Micronor, Nor QD or Ovrette), Depo-Provera injections, implants or Mirena IUS

Consider: male or female condoms, ParaGard T380A IUD, Diaphragm or Cervical cap with spermicide, FAM, NFP, Vasectomy or Tubal Sterilization

NO: history negative for all of above conditions

May use any sub-50-μg COC*

Choose COC based on patient desires, availability, side effects, non-contraceptive benefits, cost, and prior experience of woman or clinician

- The World Health Organization and the Food and Drug Administration both recommend using the **lowest dose pill** that is effective. All combined pills with less than 50 μg of estrogen are effective and safe.

- There are no studies demonstrating a decreased risk for deep vein thrombosis (DVT) in women on 20-μg pills. Data on higher dose pills have demonstrated that the less the estrogen dose, the lower the risk for DVT.

- All OCs lower free testosterone. In the US, only Ortho Tri-Cyclen and Estrostep have FDA labeling indicating it as a treatment of moderate acne vulgaris, based on results of randomized, placebo controlled trials. Other formulations are under study. Class labeling in Canada for all combined pills states that use of pills may improve acne. In Canada only, Tri-Cyclen has "treatment of moderate acne vulgaris" as an indication for use.

- To minimize discontinuation due to spotting and breakthrough bleeding, warn women in advance, reassure that spotting and breakthrough bleeding become better over time.

- To attain the most favorable lipid profile, consider norgestimate, desogestrel pill or low dose norethindrone acetate, or lowest dose norethindrone (Ovcon-35) or ethnodiol diacetate (Demulen 1/35 or Zovia 35). No clinical benefits have been demonstrated to be attributable to difference in lipids caused by these pills. Estrogen has a beneficial effect on the walls of blood vessels. All currently available COCs raise triglycerides.

*The package insert for women on Yasmin states *[Berlex-2001]:* "Yasmin is different from other birth control pills because it contains the progestin drospirenone. Drospirenone may increase potassium. Therefore, you should not take Yasmin if you have kidney, liver or adrenal disease, because this could cause serious heart and health problems. Other drugs may also increase potassium. If you are currently on daily, long-term treatment for a chronic condition with any of the medications below, you should consult your health-care provider about whether Yasmin is right for you, and during the first month that you take Yasmin, you should have a blood test to check your potassium level: NSAIDs (ibuprofen [Motrin®, Advil®], naproxen [Naprosyn®, Aleve®, and others] when taken long-term and daily for treatment of arthritis or other problems); potassium-sparing diuretics (sprironolactone and others); potassium supplementation; ACE inhibitors (Capoten®, Vasotec®, Zestril® and others); Angiotensin-II receptor antagonists (Cozaar®, Diovan®, Avapro® and others); heparin."

FIGURE 45-3 Choosing a pill. Reprinted with permission from Reference 13.

on Monday, she should take two pills on Tuesday). Then she should take the remaining pills as usual. A backup method of contraception is not necessary. If she misses two tablets in a row in week 1 or 2 of her pack, she must take two pills on the day she remembers and two pills the next day. She should use an alternative method of contraception for 7 days after missing the pills.

If a woman misses two tablets in a row in the third week (for day 1 starters), she must discard the rest of the pack and start a new pack on that same day. For Sunday starters, she should keep taking one pill every day until Sunday, then start a new pack on Sunday. She must use an alternative method of contraception for 7 days after missing the pills. She may not have her menstrual period this month.

If a woman misses three or more pills in a row during the first 3 weeks (for day 1 starters), she must discard the rest of her pack and start a new pack that same day; Sunday starters should keep taking one pill every day until Sunday, start a new pack on Sunday, and use an alternative method of contraception for 7 days after missing the pills. She may not have a menstrual period this month.

Drug Interactions

Antibacterials

5. G.H. is a 26-year-old woman whose last menstrual period (LMP) was 7 weeks ago. She has a history of regular menstrual cycles both before and during the use of OCs. Six weeks ago, she developed an *Escherichia coli* urinary tract infection, which was treated with ampicillin 500 mg po QID for 7 days. This coincided with the first seven tablets of her OC cycle. She has been taking Ortho-Novum 1/35 for 3 years and tetracycline 250 mg po QD for acne. What is the clinical significance of the potential drug interactions in G.H.?

EE is conjugated in the liver, excreted in the bile, hydrolyzed by intestinal bacteria, and reabsorbed as active drug.[16] Antibiotics, by reducing the population of intestinal bacteria, interrupt the enterohepatic circulation of the estrogen, resulting in a decreased concentration of circulating estrogen. The existence of similar antibiotic interactions with contraceptive progestins is unlikely. Although this proposed mechanism for the drug interaction is not firmly established, various antibiotics have been reported to decrease OC efficacy. This interaction may cause unintended pregnancy or abnormal bleeding patterns. The antibiotics rifampin and griseofulvin are known to cause contraceptive failure, as these products also increase the metabolism of estrogen.

Theoretically, any antimicrobial with significant effects on intestinal bacterial flora could affect OC efficacy by interfering with the enterohepatic recycling of exogenous estrogen. Numerous reports of changes in bleeding patterns and contraceptive failure have been documented.[16] About 30 case reports of contraceptive failure with concomitant OC and antibiotic use have been published. The antibiotics in the case reports include rifampin, ampicillin, penicillin G, tetracycline, and minocycline. In addition, surveys conducted on patients in clinics have revealed about 20 other cases of OC failure. A major limitation of survey data is that it relies on patients' memories, which are often unreliable. The Committee on the Safety of Medicines in the United Kingdom received 63 reports of unplanned pregnancies between 1968 and 1984 in women on antibiotics and OCs. Penicillins, tetracyclines, sulfamethoxazole-trimethoprim, metronidazole, cephalosporins, and erythromycin were among the antibiotics used. Finally, >200 reports of OC failure have been documented in women seeking family planning services.

The probability of a clinically significant drug interaction between OCs and antimicrobials depends on numerous factors: the hormonal content of the OC relative to the patient's requirements, the dosage and duration of use of the interacting drug, variation in the patient's response to bacterial flora alteration, and the fertility of the couple.[17] The number and complexity of these variables make prediction of outcome in a specific patient exceedingly difficult. Even if a drug produces a several-fold increase in unwanted pregnancies in women taking OCs, the likelihood of pregnancy in a given patient still will be low. Long-term, low-dose tetracycline use for G.H.'s acne therapy (tetracycline 250 mg daily) is unlikely to interfere with her OC efficacy, but there are no data to support this supposition. Topical antibiotics often can control acne and are viable alternatives to oral tetracycline.[18]

A practical approach to managing patients taking OCs and antibiotics is to educate patients to be conservative by using a backup method of contraception until menses occurs. In addition, the clinician should discuss what little is described in the literature about these interactions (Table 45-5). Whether

Table 45-5 Oral Contraceptive Drug Interactions

Interacting Drug	Net Effect
Drugs that may reduce OC enterohepatic circulation	
Ampicillin[19–26]	
Cephalosporins[24,27]	
Chloramphenicol[28]	
Dapsone[24]	
Erythromycin[24,29]	Spotting, breakthrough bleeding, or
Isoniazid[28–31]	pregnancy
Penicillins[24,29]	
Sulfonamides[24]	
Tetracyclines[24,27,32]	
TMP-SMX[20–22,24,27,29,33]	
Drugs that may induce the metabolism of OCs	
Butabarbital[24,34,35]	
Carbamazepine[24,34,35]	
Ethosuximide[24,35,35]	
Griseofulvin[22,36]	
Nelfinavir[37]	
Phenobarbital[24,34,35]	Spotting, breakthrough bleeding, or
Phenytoin[24,34,35]	pregnancy
Primidone[24,34,35]	
Rifabutin[38]	
Rifampin[17,22,28–35,39]	
Secobarbital[40]	
St. John's wort[41,42]	
Miscellaneous drug interactions with OCs	
Amprenavir[43]	↓ concentrations of amprenavir; ↑ or ↓ concentrations of EE or progestin
Anticoagulants[44,45]	↓ anticoagulation
Atorvastatin[46]	30% ↑ norethindrone; 20% ↑ EE
Benzodiazepines[47,48]	Enhanced benzodiazepine effect
Cyclosporine[49]	Doubling of cyclosporine level
Insulin[50]	19% require ↑ insulin dose
Phenytoin[34,58]	↑ concentrations of phenytoin
Corticosteroids[51]	↓ metabolism of corticosteroids
Ritonavir[52]	40% ↓ in AUC of EE
Tacrolimus[53]	↑ tacrolimus level
Theophylline[54]	33% reduction in theophylline clearance
Tizanidine[55]	50% reduction in tizanidine clearance
Topiramate[56]	18–30% ↓ concentrations of EE

AUC, area under the time-concentration curve; EE, ethinyl estradiol; OC, oral contraceptives; TMP-SMX, trimethoprim-sulfamethoxazole.

ampicillin inhibits OC efficacy is not certain; however, all clinical data are consistent with the premise that ampicillin occasionally impairs OC efficacy. In this case, G.H. should take a pregnancy test. If she is pregnant, harm to the fetus from the OC or antibiotics is unlikely (see Question 25).

Liver Enzyme Induction

6. S.R., a 22-year-old woman, is taking phenytoin (Dilantin) 300 mg po QD and phenobarbital 60 mg po BID. Her serum concentrations of these drugs have been consistently in the therapeutic range for at least 2 years, and she has not experienced seizures for 18 months. Is S.R. a good candidate for OCs?

EE is a substrate of cytochrome P450 3A4 (CYP3A4), so drugs that induce CYP3A4 may decrease OC efficacy. In earlier years, OC efficacy was not decreased significantly by other drugs because of their high hormone content. Because the estrogen and progestin concentrations of OCs have gradually been decreasing, reports of menstrual irregularities (e.g., spotting, BTB) and unintended pregnancies attributable to drug interactions have been increasing (see Table 45-5).

Carbamazepine, phenytoin, phenobarbital, and primidone are CYP3A4 inducers and are known to cause increased metabolism of OCs. Another possible inducer of CYP3A4 is St. John's wort.[42] The newer anticonvulsants topiramate and oxcarbazepine have also been shown to lower serum levels of estrogen. Although drugs can influence the OC efficacy, OCs also can affect the activity of other drugs. OCs have been reported to increase or decrease serum levels of lamotrigine and can affect seizure control (see Table 45-5). Also, one report claims that OCs might increase serum phenytoin concentrations substantially.[57]

Unlike many drug classes that are carefully dosed to maintain a therapeutic range of monitored blood levels, contraceptive estrogen and progestin blood levels are obtained only in clinical drug studies. Therefore, patients are managed by monitoring side effects and by changes in menstrual patterns. It is no wonder, therefore, that the drug interaction literature is less than satisfactory and that patient management may be haphazard. Although some prescribers suggest using a 50-μg EE OC in patients on interacting drugs, most would recommend that S.R. use a contraceptive method other than OCs.

Oral Contraceptive Risks and Adverse Effects

Some patients may not be candidates for OCs because of the risks and adverse effects associated with their use. Other patients may experience minor side effects with OCs that may be managed by changing to an OC with different types and doses of estrogen or progestin.

Breakthrough Bleeding (BTB), Spotting, and Amenorrhea

7. V.S. comes to the family planning clinic after taking Ovcon-35 for 2 months. She had been started on Ovcon-35 to help with her acne. Her only complaint is spotting at various times during her past two menstrual cycles. What action should be taken to correct V.S.'s bleeding pattern?

Intermenstrual bleeding that requires a pad or tampon is designated BTB, while a lesser amount of intermenstrual bleeding is called spotting. Intermenstrual bleeding is the most frequent explanation for the discontinuation of OCs.[58]

Most clinicians will continue with the same OC for at least 3 months if irregular bleeding is the only complaint, since BTB usually resolves on its own.[12,59] Early-cycle intermenstrual bleeding, which usually starts before the 14th day of the menstrual cycle (or never ceases completely after menses), usually is due to insufficient estrogen. Late-cycle intermenstrual bleeding, occurring after day 14, is usually due to insufficient progestational support of the endometrium. Another cause of intermenstrual bleeding is drug interactions (see Questions 5 and 6).

The balance between estrogen and progestin components in OCs determines its endometrial activity and, therefore, the likelihood of intermenstrual bleeding problems. It is helpful to envision the estrogen component as the basic building blocks or "bricks" of the endometrium and the progestational component providing the mortar that holds the bricks together. In addition, the estrogenic activity of the progestational component increases the number of bricks, while its antiestrogenic activity decreases their numbers. If there are not enough bricks or mortar or if they are present in the wrong proportions, the wall will crumble and bleeding will ensue (see Table 45-2).

If V.S.'s intermenstrual bleeding irregularities continue late in her cycle after 3 months, another OC with the same estrogen dose and more progestin should be prescribed. Desogen/Ortho-Cept would be a good choice because progestational activity would be increased and estrogenic activity would be maintained with minimal androgenic liability (see Table 45-2). If V.S. develops intermenstrual bleeding early in the cycle after several months of use, she should be changed to a pill with a higher ratio of estrogen to progesterone or should try Mircette, which provides a low dose of estrogen during the usual placebo week.

Some patients experience amenorrhea with OCs. If this occurs, pregnancy should first be ruled out. If the patient is not pregnant and amenorrhea is acceptable to the patient, then the OC need not be changed. If the patient would prefer a monthly menstrual period, then an OC with more estrogen or less progestin or a triphasic pill should be tried.

Cardiovascular Disease

8. M.F. (from Questions 1 to 4) and her fiancé, who is with her in the health care provider's office, have been reading about the cardiovascular risks of estrogen in the lay press. What is the effect of OCs on M.F.'s risk of morbidity and mortality from cardiovascular disease?

In women who do not smoke or use OCs, the risk of death due to cardiovascular disease is 0.59 per 100,000 women <35 years old and 3.18 per 100,000 women ≥35 years.[59] This risk is increased by 0.06 and 3.03 for OC users <35 or ≥35, respectively. For OC users who smoke, the risk is increased by 1.73 and 19.4 for women <35 or ≥35, respectively.

Both the Royal College of General Practitioners and the Oxford/Family Planning Association OC studies showed that women <35 years, regardless of smoking status, taking the new low-dose OCs did not have a significantly increased mortality risk from cardiovascular disease.[60–62] The increase in mortality is concentrated in smokers >35 years of age.

Several studies have focused on the effect of OCs on serum lipoprotein concentrations because of the association between lipoproteins and atherosclerotic cardiovascular disease.[63–65]

High levels of total cholesterol (TC), triglycerides (TG), low-density lipoprotein (LDL) cholesterol, and very-low-density lipoprotein (VLDL) cholesterol serum concentrations are associated with the risk of developing atherosclerotic circulatory diseases, whereas high-density lipoprotein (HDL) cholesterol has an inverse relationship. Apolipoprotein levels also affect atherosclerotic risk (e.g., elevations in Lp(a) increase risk).

Estrogen tends to increase serum concentrations of HDL, while decreases in HDL are linked to progestin dose and potency.[63,64] Progestins can modify the composition of total HDL by changing the relative amounts of HDL_2 and HDL_3.[66,67] HDL_2 is protective against cardiovascular disease, unlike HDL_3.[68] Decreases in HDL are associated with increasing age, weight, and cigarette smoking. Increased serum triglyceride concentrations are related to the estrogen content of the OC as well as to the antiestrogenic effect of the progestin component.

Studies evaluating the effect of OCs on lipids have reported similar results.[63–65] One study found an increase in HDL from baseline with a low-androgenic progestin compared to a high-androgenic progestin.[64] Another study compared OCs with phasic EE and levonorgestrel or desogestrel.[63] After six cycles, significant increases in HDL_3 and apolipoproteins (apo A-I, apo A-II, and apo B), were seen in both groups. HDL_2 also increased significantly in the desogestrel group but decreased in the levonorgestrel group. After nine cycles, levels of TG and VLDL in both groups and HDL in the desogestrel group were significantly increased from baseline. HDL did not change significantly in the levonorgestrel group after six cycles. In another study, a reduction in the OC doses of EE and levonorgestrel by one third improved levels of LDL, TG, Lp(a), and HDL.[65]

Lipid serum concentrations also are altered in adolescent (ages 12 to 17) OC users. These adolescents had significantly higher TC levels compared to nonusers, although the type of OC used was not specified.[69]

Patients taking OCs containing levonorgestrel may be more likely to suffer a myocardial infarction (MI) than users of OCs containing desogestrel or gestodene.[70] When confounding factors for cardiovascular disease were accounted for, women taking levonorgestrel-containing OCs were 2.5 times more likely to have an MI than nonusers. Another study found the opposite effect of the two types of OCs, but the results were not significant.[71] Heavy smoking, especially in women >35 years old, increases the risk of MI.[59]

M.F. and her fiancé should understand that the risk of a cardiovascular adverse effect may be increased with OC use, but the risk is still very low no matter which OC is used. Cigarette smoking is a much more significant risk factor for MI, causing a reported 8- to 13-fold increase in risk.

Cervical Dysplasia and Cervical Cancer

9. J.M. has an older sister who had cervical dysplasia that progressed to carcinoma in situ. Her sister never took OCs. What can you tell J.M. about the risks of cervical dysplasia and cancer associated with OCs?

An estimated 12,200 new cases of cervical cancer and 4,100 deaths from cervical cancer will occur in 2003.[72] Behavior, not genetics, is the usual cause of cervical cancer. Women at highest risk for cancer are those who are positive for certain subtypes of human papilloma virus (HPV), who have certain sexual behaviors, who are immunosuppressed, or who smoke.[5] Sexual behaviors associated with cervical cancer include beginning sexual activity at a young age, having multiple male sexual partners, and having a male sexual partner who has had multiple partners. Women at low risk for cancer are those who have two or fewer partners, whose partners use condoms, and who do not smoke.

Pooled data on cervical cancer risk from eight case-control studies found that OC users positive for HPV were more likely to develop cervical cancer.[73] Women who had ever used OCs and those who had used OCs for >5 years were 1.5 and 3.4 times, respectively, more likely to develop cervical cancer. This is consistent with older studies that suggest that OC users have an increased risk of developing or dying of cervical cancer. In contrast, a large cohort study conducted in England found no significant increase in deaths due to cervical cancer in women who had ever used OCs.[74]

Epidemiologic comparisons of the prevalence of cervical cancer in OC users versus nonusers often are difficult to interpret because yearly medical examinations (e.g., Pap smears) of OC users result in early detection and treatment of precancerous lesions.[75] Health care providers may wish to perform Pap smears every 6 months in women who have used OCs for ≥5 years and who are also at a higher risk because of multiple partners or a history of sexually transmitted diseases (STDs).[4] J.M. should be counseled on the behaviors that put her at risk for cervical cancer and should be encouraged to have a Pap smear annually.

Headache

10. G.R., a 32-year-old woman, comes to the clinic complaining of headaches, which predominantly occur during the 7-day placebo phase of her 28-day cycle of Nordette. The throbbing headaches are preceded by blurred vision, nausea, and vomiting. Aspirin and acetaminophen, which normally relieve her headaches, are ineffective. Lying down in a dark room provides some relief. Her family history is pertinent because her mother and maternal grandmother have migraine headaches. Are these headaches a relative contraindication for the continued use of OCs?

Headache is a common complaint in women taking OCs. They may notice headaches while taking active pills or during the placebo week, due to the withdrawal of estrogen.[59] Women with migraines may find that their headaches either improve or worsen when OCs are initiated.

Mild headaches may improve over time or if the woman is changed to a pill with less estrogen or progestin. Headaches that occur during the placebo week can be managed by trying Mircette or taking OCs continuously (i.e., skipping placebo pills). Patients with severe headaches should discontinue OCs and should be evaluated by their health care provider.

Ischemic stoke is more likely to occur in OC users with a history of migraines, especially if they smoke.[76] Women with migraines should use OCs with caution or not at all, particularly if they smoke, are >35 years old, or have other significant medical problems. Clinical experience indicates that women who have increasing migraine attacks with OCs are not likely to improve when the OC is changed to one with a different hormone balance.

G.R.'s symptoms are typical of migraine headache and because she has a family history of migraine headaches, she may need to discontinue OCs and use another method of contraception. Subsequent to a thorough medical evaluation of her headaches, she should be monitored carefully if OCs are to be continued.

Hypertension

11. A.M., an obese 26-year-old Black woman, became hypertensive during all of her pregnancies. She restarted her Lo-Ovral after her last pregnancy and continues to smoke a half-pack of cigarettes per day. Her blood pressure (BP) prior to starting OCs was 126/76 mm Hg. Today, her BP is 146/96 mm Hg. What is the mechanism of OC-induced hypertension? How can OCs be safely used by A.M. despite her history of hypertension during pregnancy?

The underlying mechanisms for OC-induced hypertension may be sodium and water retention and increased renin activity.[77,78] Hypertension secondary to OCs may develop slowly over 3 to 36 months and may not decline for 3 to 6 months after OC discontinuation.[9]

Women taking the older and more potent oral contraceptives (e.g., OCs with ≥50 μg EE) had a two to three times higher incidence of hypertension (BP >140/90 mm Hg) than nonusers.[79–81] Small studies have found systolic BP to increase by 7 to 8 mm Hg and diastolic BP to increase by 6 mm Hg in normotensive or mildly hypertensive women.[82] Population-based, case-control studies have shown differing results on whether women with hypertension who use OCs are more likely to suffer an MI than nonusers. A small study of adolescent women showed similar systolic and diastolic BPs in users versus nonusers.[69]

In this patient it is reasonable to consider using a 20-μg EE OC such as Alesse/Apri/Levlite or an OC with less progestin and estrogen such as Ortho TriCyclen Lo. The effect of this change in medication on A.M.'s blood pressure should be monitored to determine whether continued use is warranted.

Liver Tumors

12. T.A.'s physician is concerned about the possibility of hepatic tumors. What is the risk of hepatomas in patients using OCs?

The incidence rate of benign liver tumors for women using low-dose OCs is 3.3 per 100,000 users per year compared with 0.1 per 100,000 users per year in nonusers or short-term users.[83] The incidence increases after 4 years of use. Although the tumors generally are benign, death can result from intrahepatic or extrahepatic tumor rupture and hemorrhagic shock.[84,85] Because animal studies suggest that both estrogen and progestin may accelerate abnormal liver cell proliferation, the lowest effective OC dose should be used in all patients.[83,86] A significant increase in death from liver disease or cancer was not seen in one large cohort study.[74]

Cholestatic jaundice also has been associated with OC use.[87] T.A. can monitor for signs or symptoms of cholestatic jaundice, since this disorder usually presents as malaise, nausea, anorexia, and pruritus; these usually appear 4 weeks after the initiation of OC use. Discontinuation of the OC results in complete clinical remission within a month.

Thromboembolic Events

13. B.C., a 21-year-old woman, is interested in starting OCs. After taking a complete history, the provider learns that her sister and mother have both had a deep vein thrombosis (DVT). Can OCs contribute to the development of a DVT or pulmonary embolism (PE)? If so, which patients are at the highest risk? Should B.C. start OCs?

OCs contribute to thromboembolic events by several mechanisms. Estrogens increase coagulability and thereby increase the possibility of clot formation. They may increase the serum concentrations of clotting factors VII, X, and XII and decrease the prothrombin time after one to three cycles of use.[10,63,65,82] Estrogens may also reduce antithrombin III activity and decrease the inhibitory activity of factor X. Long-term OC use is associated with an increased platelet count and increased platelet aggregation similar to that seen late in pregnancy; this is generally thought to be caused by the estrogen component. More recent data showing increased thrombosis rates in users of third-generation progestins (desogestrel and gestodene) suggest that progestin may also has a role in thromboembolism risk.[10]

The baseline risk of venous thrombosis is low, at 1 for every 10,000 person-years.[10] The best studies looking at thromboembolism in OC users found that most users have a three- to six-fold increased risk of developing superficial or deep venous thrombosis or PE. Therefore, the risk is still quite low, at approximately 3 to 4 per 10,000 person-years—less than the risk during pregnancy of 6 per 10,000 person-years. Patients requiring emergency major surgery while on OCs are more prone to thromboembolism than nonusers.[82] The risk of venous thrombosis does not seem to be associated with duration of OC use, past OC use, mild obesity, or cigarette smoking. A greater risk is associated with EE doses >35 μg.

Women with a mutation in clotting factor V (also called factor V Leiden) or a deficiency in protein C, protein S, or antithrombin are more likely to develop a venous thrombosis with OC use than women without a hereditary prothrombotic defect.[10] Women with blood types other than O may also be more susceptible to clotting due to higher levels of factor VIII.

Whether third-generation progestins are associated with a higher risk of venous thromboembolism (VTE) relative to other progestins is controversial.[10] It was believed that the risk of thrombosis with third-generation progestins would be lower than other progestins since they have more beneficial effects on HDL. However, most studies that compared the risk of thrombosis with third-generation progestins to second-generation progestins found that desogestrel and gestodene are associated with a greater VTE risk. Although the risk is increased, the overall rate of thrombosis is still low.

A prospective study from the PHARMO system database in The Netherlands compared the incidence of VTE with the second-generation OC Nordette/Levlen/Levora (2.4/10,000 person-years), the third-generation OC Apri/Desogen/Ortho-Cept, and a gestodene OC that is not available in the United States (9.0/10,000 person-years). In this study, the relative risk for third-generation OC use was 3.5 (95% confidence interval [CI], 1.4 to 8.8). The adjusted relative risk of VTE in women who had used OCs before was 1.7 (95% CI, 0.9 to 3.1).[89] The relative risk was highest in women <25 years of age who were taking OCs for the first time.

The Contraception Report gave the following advice to practitioners regarding the use of OCs containing a third-generation progestin:[90]

1. Patients already taking a desogestrel-containing OC with no VTE risk factors do not need to change OCs.
2. In new-start patients, take a personal and family history. If no VTE risk factors exist, inform the patient of a possible increased risk with a desogestrel OC.
3. Patients with a personal history of VTE should not start OCs.
4. Patients with a family history of VTE in young first- and second-degree relatives who also have other risk factors such as obesity or immobilization should consider other methods.
5. All patients using OCs should know the VTE warning signs (ACHES; Table 45-6).

The minimal risk of thrombosis associated with OCs in the general population does not justify the cost of routine screening for deficiencies in the coagulation system; however, when a patient has a family history of thrombosis, measurement of antithrombin III, protein C, activated protein C resistance ratio, protein S, anticardiolipin antibodies, prothrombin G mutation, and homocysteine levels should be considered.[10]

B.C. should be evaluated for hereditary prothrombotic defects. If any exist, she should avoid OC use. If none exist, she may still wish to consider a method without estrogen but should be educated on the signs and symptoms of thrombosis if she decides to start OCs.

Benefits of Oral Contraceptives

Acne

14. D.S., a 20-year-old woman, has had severe acne since menarche at age 13. She is currently taking no medications but wants to begin OCs. What effect, if any, would oral contraceptives have on her acne? Which OC would you recommend for D.S.?

Depending on the patient, OC use may cause acne to appear, disappear, or significantly improve.[5,9] Most patients will have improvement in acne with all available OCs, and several brands are FDA approved for this indication. Progestins with

higher androgenic activity may be more likely to increase acne since they stimulate sebaceous glands to produce more sebum. Higher doses of estrogen may decrease acne by suppressing the activity of sebaceous glands, decreasing the production of androgens, and increasing the synthesis of sex hormone binding globulin (SHBG). SHBG binds androgens and thereby diminishes their effects.[91] The triphasic OCs are modestly estrogen-dominant, and these lower-dose contraceptives can significantly reduce the overall incidence of acne. Both desogestrel- and norgestimate-containing OCs are less androgenic, thereby increasing SHBG levels and decreasing acne.[92]

D.S.'s acne should improve with OC use. Products to consider starting with are OrthoTriCyclen, Estrostep, and Ovcon 35.

Benign Breast Disease

15. A young woman has a family history of fibrocystic breast disease. What influence do OCs have on fibrocystic breast disease?

There appears to be a 50% to 75% reduction in the risk of fibroadenomas, chronic cystic breast disease, and breast biopsies in OC users.[9] Protection seems directly related to length of use. Because the progestin component may be primarily responsible for this protection, progestin-dominant OCs that contain a less estrogenic progestin such as levonorgestrel are preferred.[5,9,93] The progestin-only minipill could be of use here, except that its contraceptive effect is not as good as the OCs. In addition, it does not provide endometrial stability and other benefits of OCs such as decreased dysmenorrhea, iron deficiency anemia, acne, and hirsutism.

Dysmenorrhea and Premenstrual Syndrome

16. C.P. has a history of premenstrual syndrome (PMS) and complains of worsened menstrual cramping with an intrauterine device (IUD). What effect on PMS and dysmenorrhea might she expect from OCs?

Dysmenorrhea, or painful menstruation, may be of unknown etiology or may be due to endometriosis or uterine fibroids. Complaints of menstrual pain subsequent to OC therapy may be decreased by >60%.[9] An OC with decreased estrogenic and increased progestational activity may be the best at relieving dysmenorrhea.

Premenstrual tension has been reported to be reduced 29% in OC users, and other premenstrual symptoms seem to improve as well.[94,95] Nevertheless, the effect of OCs on PMS symptoms is inconsistent and unpredictable, probably because PMS symptoms are neither consistent nor predictable. There may be augmentation of depression and mood swings by the progestational component. Although the probability of this effect is low with a low-dose product, C.P. should be monitored for changes in her PMS symptoms. (See Chapter 48, Gynecological Disorders, for further discussion of dysmenorrhea and PMS.)

Endometrial Cancer

17. C.P. is hesitant to take OCs because her grandmother, who had been receiving estrogen replacement therapy for 5 years, died of endometrial cancer in 1970. What is the relationship between OCs and endometrial cancer?

Table 45-6 Pill Early Danger Signs (ACHES)

Signals	Possible Problem
Abdominal pain (severe)	Gallbladder disease, hepatic adenoma, blood clot, pancreatitis
Chest pain (severe), shortness of breath, or coughing up blood	Blood clot in lungs or myocardial infarction
Headaches (severe)	Stroke, hypertension, or migraine headache
Eye problems: blurred vision, flashing lights, or blindness	Stroke, hypertension, or temporary vascular problem
Severe leg pain (calf or thigh)	Blood clot in legs

Clinical data suggest that cyclic OCs contain enough progestin to prevent endometrial hyperplasia and to reduce the risk of endometrial cancer by about 50% to 70%.[76] The protection is directly related to duration of use and may persist for many years after discontinuation of the OC. A meta-analysis of 11 studies showed a 56%, 67%, and 72% reduction in endometrial cancer risk after 4, 8, and 12 years of OC use, respectively.[96]

C.P. should be reassured that OC use will not cause endometrial cancer and will likely reduce her chances of developing this disease. She may want to find out more about her grandmother's cancer, since it may have been due to treating her menopausal symptoms with estrogen alone rather than with estrogen plus a progestin.

Menorrhagia (Heavy Menstrual Bleeding)

18. **M.V. has iron deficiency anemia attributed to heavy menses secondary to her past IUD use. What will be the effect of OC use on her iron deficiency anemia?**

The total amount of menstrual flow in established OC users is decreased by $\geq$40%.[97–99] This may reflect the progressive thinning of the endometrium of OC users and the lack of irregular bleeding. Bleeding may be decreased the most by OCs that have a high ratio of progestin to estrogen, since endometrial thinning is maximized.[5] Another option would be to have the patient take OCs continuously so she has fewer menses.

Ovarian Cancer and Functional Ovarian Cysts

19. **C.P. (from Questions 16 and 17) is also concerned about ovarian cysts and cancer. Can OCs cause ovarian problems?**

The risk of developing functional ovarian cysts is decreased, pre-existing cysts are more rapidly resolved, and surgery rates for ovarian masses are reduced in women taking OCs.[97,100,101] This is likely due to reducing ovulation, suppressing androgen production, or increasing progesterone levels.

Each year of OC use decreases the relative risk of developing ovarian cancer by 7% to 9%.[100] The risk reduction continues to be seen in women using OCs for >15 years and persists after OCs are discontinued.

C.P. should be reassured that OC use will decrease, not increase, her likelihood of developing ovarian cancer.

Pelvic Inflammatory Disease and Ectopic Pregnancy

20. **M.A., a 20-year-old woman who has several sexual partners, arrives at the emergency department with a temperature of 38.2°C (normal, 37°C) and lower abdominal cramping. Examination is compatible with the diagnosis of pelvic inflammatory disease (PID), based upon her cervical motion tenderness, abdominal pain, and adnexal (ovary and fallopian tube) tenderness. She has been using a Copper-T IUD for contraception for 2 years. Why might OCs be a more suitable contraceptive for M.A.?**

Many clinicians prefer to prescribe OCs over other forms of contraception for sexually active young women with multiple sexual partners because PID has been found to be less prevalent with this form of contraception.[5,102] In one study, OC users were half as likely to develop PID as nonusers.[103] Although early studies failed to distinguish between gonococcal and nongonococcal PID, the PID protective effects of OCs may depend on the organism. A Swedish study found that OCs protect against both gonococcal and chlamydial PID.[104] In contrast, one report suggested that OCs may promote chlamydial PID; and another concluded that OC users were neither more nor less likely to develop PID.[105,106] A 1990 case-control study showed protection against symptomatic PID in women infected with chlamydia but not in those infected with gonococcus.[107]

Despite the contradictory data, it is logical that the thickening of cervical mucus caused by OCs may prevent bacteria from ascending into the uterus and fallopian tubes, thereby minimizing hospitalizations as well as deaths stemming from PID. The risk of ectopic pregnancy is greater for women who already have had PID, and OC use has been shown to prevent hospitalizations and deaths stemming from ectopic pregnancies.[108,109]

In view of these data, M.A.'s IUD should be removed and her PID treated. OCs may be initiated if no contraindications are present. Patients and clinicians should be alert for the symptoms of cervicitis or salpingitis in women who are at high risk for STDs.

Other Issues with Oral Contraceptives

Breast Cancer

21. **The medical history and physical examination of S.M. are negative for breast disease, except for a history of breast cancer in her maternal grandmother. How will OC use affect S.M.'s risk of breast cancer?**

Some studies have suggested an increased risk of breast cancer in young, nulliparous women using OCs with high progestin activity.[110,111] In addition, the Royal College of General Practitioners' Oral Contraceptive Study in 1981 reported a significant increase in risk for breast cancer in women 30 to 34 years of age who use OCs.[112] Another study found an increased risk of breast cancer in women with a first-degree family history of breast cancer who had ever used OCs.[113]

In contrast, other studies found no association between current or former OC use and breast cancer.[74,114] In addition, both the Oxford/Family Planning Association Contraceptive Study in 1977 and the Walnut Creek Contraceptive Drug Study in 1981 found no association between breast cancer and OC use in any age group.[115–117] The Centers for Disease Control Cancer and Steroid Hormone Study in 1983 reported a relative risk of 0.9 for OC users compared with never-users, despite other risk factors for breast cancer such as early menarche, later age at first birth and menopause, family history of breast cancer, or benign breast disease.[118] The ongoing Nurses' Health Study identified 3,383 cases of breast cancer from 1976 to 1992 among 1.6 million person-years of OC use and found that long-term past OC use (10 years), either overall or before a first full-term pregnancy, does not appreciably increase breast cancer risk in women >40 years of age.[119]

OC users tend to have a greater awareness of breast cancer, examine their breasts more frequently, and are examined by clinicians more often than nonusers. Thus, early detection of breast abnormalities can preclude the progression of these abnormalities into cancerous lesions.[120] OCs would not be expected to increase the risk of breast cancer in S.M. She should be instructed to perform monthly self-breast examinations and to return annually for a physical examination by her health care provider.

Depression

22. **K.G. is a 24-year-old woman with persistent mild depression. Taking into account her depression, would an OC with high or low estrogen or progestin balance be preferred for K.G.?**

Usually patients notice improved mood or premenstrual symptoms when taking an OC.[5] However, OC-related depression has been attributed to progestin or estrogen excess. Some OC users experience deterioration in mood during the pill-free period. Other causes of depression, such as hypothyroidism or vitamin B_6 deficiency, should also be considered. If depression is severe or of concern, OCs should be discontinued.

On further questioning, K.G. states that she noticed only a minor change in mood, denies suicidal or homicidal ideations, and desires to continue taking OCs. K.G.'s OC should be changed from Nordette to an OC with less estrogenic activity (e.g., Lo-Estrin 1/20), less progestational activity (e.g., Ovcon 25), or both (e.g. Alesse/Levlite/Apri) (see Table 45-2). If K.G. found that her depression was worse during the hormone-free week, then changing her to continuous-use OCs may be helpful.

Diabetes

23. **R.D., a 33-year-old woman, experienced glucose intolerance during pregnancy that resolved after delivery. She has a father and sister with diabetes. Would an OC be appropriate for R.D.?**

Generally, low-dose OCs do not alter glucose tolerance.[63,65] Results of one controlled, randomized, prospective study showed no adverse effect on carbohydrate or lipid metabolism in women with a history of gestational diabetes after 6 to 13 months of low-dose OC use.[121] Both the users and nonusers showed a significant and similar deterioration in glucose tolerance with an overall prevalence of 14% impaired glucose tolerance and 17% diabetes mellitus. The authors concluded that low-dose OCs could be prescribed safely and that serum lipids and glucose tolerance should be monitored closely, regardless of contraceptive choice.

Women with a history of gestational diabetes and those with a strong family history of diabetes in parents or siblings are at greater risk for OC-induced glucose intolerance.[5,9,82] OCs have complex effects on carbohydrate metabolism. Progestins decrease and estrogens increase the number of insulin receptors on the cell membrane. Progestins also may alter insulin receptor affinity. The different progestins in OCs have different propensities to induce glucose intolerance. Norgestrel appears to have the greatest insulin-antagonizing activity. Ethynodiol diacetate, norethindrone, norethindrone acetate, desogestrel, and norgestimate have significantly less effect. In general, carbohydrate metabolism is not affected to an important degree in most diabetic women using low-dose OCs.

For R.D., Levlen/Levora/Nordette would be poor choices because they are known to cause glucose intolerance in patients with previous gestational diabetes.[122] Interestingly, the triphasic levonorgestrel product TriLevlen/Trivora, containing

39% less progestin than the monophasic product, did not alter glucose tolerance, and Alesse/Levlite/Apri, which contains 33% less EE, also should not alter glucose tolerance. Lowering the estrogen content of an OC without changing progestin content also has improved glucose tolerance and increased insulin secretion.[123,124]

For women without diabetes, OC use may protect against developing diabetes. One large prospective, observational study found that White and Black OC users had lower fasting glucose levels and lower odds of diabetes.[125]

R.D. can be started on OCs. However, if she smokes or has other medical problems such as hypertension, nephropathy, retinopathy, or other vascular diseases, OCs should probably be avoided. It seems prudent to put R.D. on an OC with a low dose of estrogen and progesterone and to monitor for any changes in glucose control.

Gallbladder Disease

24. **L.S., a 26-year-old woman, arrives at the emergency department with acute epigastric pain accompanied by nausea, vomiting, and diarrhea. She has been taking OCs for 1 year. She is diagnosed as having gallstones. What is the association between gallbladder disease and OC therapy? What would be an appropriate OC for L.S.?**

The incidence of cholelithiasis has been reported to increase with OC use. Estrogens and progestins may contribute to bile stasis and cholelithiasis by reducing cholesterol clearance and altering bile acid composition.[9,126] The incidence of gallbladder disease has been reported to increase during the first year of use but then to decline steadily to a rate lower than that of controls.[127] In another large study, long-term OC users experienced slightly lower rates of gallbladder disease than nonusers.[128] Finally, another study found that women who had ever used OCs were not more likely to have symptomatic gallstones, but current and long-term users were. An analysis of 482 women with benign gallbladder disease from the Oxford/Family Planning Association contraception study concluded that it is unlikely that OCs cause gallbladder disease.[129]

The newer OCs with lower progestin and estrogen concentrations should have little effect, if any, on gallstone formation in normal patients. Women who are obese, young, or long-term users of OCs may be the most likely to develop gallstones.

In L.S., it is not known whether OCs were the cause of her gallstones. A history of or the current presence of gallstones is not a contraindication to OC use, so L.S. may continue to use OCs if desired.

Use During Pregnancy and Breastfeeding

25. **P.S., a 25-year-old woman, was started on Triphasil 2 months ago because of a history of abnormal menstrual periods. Unknowingly, she was pregnant at that time and continued her OC for two complete cycles. What can you tell P.S. about the possible effects of OC use on her unborn child?**

The fact that OCs are classified as pregnancy category X (contraindicated, fetal risks clearly outweigh maternal benefit) is very misleading.[130] Although an association between OC use and cardiac or limb anomalies had been reported, other studies have not noted a teratogenic effect. Simpson summarized all available data on contraceptive steroid exposure during pregnancy and concluded that OC use did not substantially increase the risk of anomalies over that expected in other uneventful pregnancies.[131]

Clearly, an OC should not be started in someone who is known to be pregnant. However, P.S. should be reassured that the risks to her fetus from the use of a low-dose OC during the first trimester should be minimal.

P.S. may use OCs after she has her baby even if she is breastfeeding, although it may be preferable for her to use a progesterone-only method.[5,130] For patients without contraindications to OCs, the American Academy of Pediatrics considers OCs to be compatible with breastfeeding.[132] However, OCs have been reported to decrease milk quantity and quality (see Question 27).[130] Therefore, many providers suggest avoiding OCs in women who are exclusively breastfeeding. If a postpartum woman would like to start OCs, she should wait to begin them until at least 3 weeks postpartum. By this time, the increased risk of thrombosis that occurs during pregnancy should be reduced to baseline.

CONTRACEPTIVE PATCH AND RING

26. K.H. is a 16-year-old who started taking OCs 3 months ago. She is very concerned about getting pregnant because she has trouble remembering to take her pill each day. She likes all the noncontraceptive benefits of OCs but is wondering if there are dosage forms other than pills. What do you tell her?

Contraceptive Patch

Contraceptive patch users experience about 1 pregnancy per 100 women-years of use (see Table 45-1). The contraceptive patch (Ortho Evra) contains 6 mg norelgestromin and 750 µg EE and delivers, transdermally, 150 µg norelgestromin and 20 µg EE daily into the bloodstream.[133] The patch is a 1.75″ square with rounded corners and is beige and thin. It is applied once weekly for 3 consecutive weeks, followed by 1 week with no patch. Then this cycle is repeated. Menses should begin during the patch-free week.

The contraceptive patch may be worn on the buttock, abdomen, upper torso, or upper outer arm.[133] K.H. should not apply the patch to the same exact spot each month, but rather rotate within or between sites. The patch should not be applied to the breasts. When applying the patch, K.H. should select the application site and be sure it is clean and dry. She should press firmly on the patch for 10 seconds and trace her finger around the edge of the patch to be sure it sticks properly. The patch should stay attached during usual activities, including exercising, swimming, and bathing. If the patch falls off for <24 hours, she should reapply it or apply a new one as soon as possible, and her patch change day will stay the same. No backup contraception is needed. If the patch is off for >24 hours, she should start a new cycle, she will have a new patch change day, and she should use backup contraception for one week.

The patch may be started using the Sunday start or Day 1 start method, and the recommendations for backup contraception are the same as described earlier with OCs.[133] If K.H. forgets to start the first patch of a cycle, she should apply it as soon as she remembers. This day will become her new patch change day, and she should use backup contraception for 1

week. If she forgets to change the patch for 1 or 2 days during week 2 or 3, she should apply a new patch as soon as she remembers. This becomes her new patch change day. No backup contraception is needed. If she forgets for >2 days, she should start a new cycle as soon as she remembers. She will need to use backup contraception for 1 week and will have a new patch change day.

Since the patch contains similar hormones to those in OCs, the risks and benefits are thought to be similar. The package insert lists the same contraindications and precautions with the use of the patch as for OCs (see Table 45-4).[133] However, since the delivery system and serum levels are different, future studies may find that there are differences in certain risks or benefits between these products. One difference with the patch is efficacy is reduced in users over 90 kg. Therefore, providers may choose to recommend another method for heavier women. The most common side effects reported with the patch are breast tenderness, headache, application site reaction, and nausea.

Contraceptive Ring

The failure rate for the contraceptive ring is one or two pregnancies per 100 woman-years. The contraceptive ring (NuvaRing) delivers 120 µg etonogestrel and 15 µg EE daily through the vaginal mucosa.[134] The ring is flexible, transparent, and has a diameter of just over 2″. The ring is inserted vaginally and kept in place for 3 weeks in a row. After 3 weeks, the ring is removed for 1 week, and then a new ring is inserted.

The ring may be placed anywhere in the vagina, so K.H. does not need to worry about its exact position.[134] To insert the ring, she should compress it so the opposite sides of the ring are touching, and gently insert it into the vagina. If she feels discomfort with the ring, it has probably not been inserted into the vagina far enough. Most women do not feel the ring once it is in place. To remove the ring, K.H. should grasp the ring between two fingers or hook one finger inside the ring and pull it out. Menses will usually begin within 3 days of removing the ring. If the ring slips out, it should be rinsed with cool water and reinserted. If the ring is out for <3 hours, backup contraception is not needed. If the ring is out for >3 hours, backup contraception should be used for 1 week. If the ring has been left in the vagina for 3 to 4 weeks, the woman should remove it, wait 1 week, then reinsert a new ring. If it has been in place for >4 weeks, the woman should remove it, confirm that she is not pregnant, reinsert a new one, and use backup contraception for 1 week.

The contraceptive ring should be inserted anytime during the first 5 days of the menstrual cycle.[134] Backup contraception should be used for the first week. When changing from OCs, the woman should insert the ring within 7 days of the last active pill. No backup contraception is needed.

As with the patch, the ring has the same contraindications and precautions as OCs (see Table 45-4).[134] The most common side effects with the ring are vaginal infections, irritation, and discharge, headache, weight gain, and nausea.

PROGESTERONE-ONLY PILL (MINIPILL)

27. P.K., a 39-year-old woman, plans to breastfeed her infant and begin some type of contraception following her discharge from the hospital. Her past experience with condoms and concurrent spermicidal foams or gels resulted in itching and burning, and an IUD caused severe cramping and bleeding. She has a strong family history of cardiac disease and smokes two packs of cigarettes a day. What are the advantages of the minipill as a contraceptive method for P.K?

Advantages

The minipill is devoid of some of the nuisance side effects (see Table 45-4) caused by estrogen (e.g., headaches, chloasma).[5] More importantly, estrogen-mediated hypertension and clotting factor changes will be avoided in this smoker, who has a strong family history of cardiovascular disease. Confusion with pill taking is minimized since there is no placebo week and all 28 tablets in each pack are the same. Therefore, the missed-dose directions are the same whenever any pill is missed. Minipills also have noncontraceptive benefits, including decreased dysmenorrhea and bleeding. They also may protect against PID and endometrial cancer.

Theoretically, progestin use in the early postpartum period may decrease milk production, since milk production is triggered by the decline in progesterone that occurs after delivery. However, no data have consistently shown this to be a problem in postpartum women.[130] Once breastfeeding has been established, progestins have not been shown to interfere with the quantity or quality of milk produced by a nursing mother. Thus, an OC containing only progestin is preferred for a patient who plans to breastfeed her infant.

Disadvantages

28. What disadvantages of the minipill should you discuss with P.K.?

The minipills, with a failure rate of 0.5% to 5%, are less effective than OCs (see Table 45-1).[5] Since minipills must be taken even more regularly than OCs, minipills are not often used in women who are not breastfeeding (see patient instructions below). Some women on minipills consistently have ovulatory cycles, and some shift back and forth between ovulatory and anovulatory cycles. Women who consistently have menses on the minipill are likely to be ovulating and should be advised to use a backup method of contraception or to change to a different method.

Irregular menses, decreased duration and amount of menstrual flow, spotting, or amenorrhea commonly occurs in women taking the minipill.[5] Because of this, patients often are concerned that they may be pregnant. Women who are exclusively breastfeeding will usually have amenorrhea. The high incidence of irregular menses associated with the minipill may mask underlying pathology. Other side effects reported with minipills include headaches, breast tenderness, mood changes, and nausea.

Minipills should be avoided if there is a personal history of breast cancer or undiagnosed vaginal bleeding. Caution should be exercised when using minipills in women with hepatic disease, certain cardiovascular conditions, a current DVT or PE, or complicated diabetes (see Table 45-4).[11]

Patient Instructions

29. What instructions should P.K. receive regarding the use of a minipill?

P.K. should begin taking the minipill on the first day of her menses.[5] Since she is breastfeeding and is less likely to have menses, she can begin taking them immediately postpartum. Alternatively, some providers recommend waiting until 3 to 6 weeks postpartum to begin minipills to minimize complaints of irregular bleeding and to confirm that milk flow is established. Backup contraception is not needed with a Day 1 start. When starting minipills on a day other than the first day of menses, a backup method of contraception should be used for 48 hours.

P.K. should be instructed to take the pill at the exact same time each day. If she is >3 hours late taking a pill, she should take the pill as soon as she remembers and should use backup contraception for 48 hours. This is quite different from the directions for OCs, so this point should be stressed with patients.

LONG-ACTING INJECTIONS: DEPO-PROVERA AND LUNELLE

Depo-Provera

30. A.K., a lactating 35-year-old woman, returns to the gynecology clinic for her second injection of depot medroxyprogesterone acetate (Depo-Provera; DMPA). She is a smoker with a history of thromboembolism. She was given her first injection 3 months ago, immediately postpartum. She is experiencing prolonged intermenstrual bleeding and a 2-lb weight gain. Is this to be expected? What are the benefits and risks of DMPA? How are the side effects managed?

DMPA is given as a 150-mg deep intramuscular injection in the deltoid or gluteus maximus every 11 to 13 weeks.[5] Since its development in the early 1960s, DMPA has been approved for use in >90 countries and has been used by >30 million women worldwide.[135] The FDA approved it in 1992. DMPA inhibits ovulation, thickens the cervical mucus, and suppresses endometrial growth, making it a very effective contraceptive.

Advantages

Depo-Provera is a good contraceptive choice for A.K. because she is at risk for estrogenic side effects. She is 35 years old, smokes, is lactating, and has a history of thromboembolism. Among its benefits are a low failure rate of 0.3% (see Table 45-1), ease of use, lack of estrogenic side effects, decreased dysmenorrhea and monthly blood loss, and a reduced risk of endometrial cancer and PID.[5,136] Other noncontraceptive benefits may include decreasing pain and frequency of sickle cell crises, reduction in seizure frequency in epileptic patients, and a possible reduction in ovarian cancer.[5,137] Furthermore, contraceptive efficacy is not reduced by the concurrent use of anticonvulsants as is seen with OCs.

Disadvantages

Patients with breast cancer should not use DMPA.[11] DMPA should be used with caution in women with undiagnosed vaginal bleeding, certain cardiovascular diseases or multiple risk factors for cerebrovascular disease, or a current DVT or PE (see Table 45-4). Some experts disagree with the Depo-Provera Contraceptive Injection U.S. package insert, which lists a history of prior thromboembolism as a contraindication, because clotting factors have not been shown to be clinically affected by DMPA.[138] Some clinicians also begin DMPA immediately postpartum rather than waiting 6 weeks postpartum, as directed by the package insert. Patients started earlier are more likely to report frequent episodes of bleeding or spotting, however.[139,140]

Estrogen production declines in women using DMPA, so A.K. should be told that DMPA may decrease bone mineral density (BMD).[141] Numerous studies have found that women receiving DMPA injection have lower BMD compared with nonusers. Other studies have found that DMPA does not affect BMD. Although there have been reports of stress fractures in DMPA users, no studies to date have documented an increased rate of hip or vertebral fractures in DMPA users.[142,143] Also, BMD has been shown to recover after discontinuation of the injections.[144]

A.K. must understand that DMPA frequently causes irregular bleeding or spotting during the first few months of use or more because estrogen is insufficient to maintain the endometrium. After 1 and 2 years of use, 55% and 68% of women experience amenorrhea, respectively. Amenorrhea leads to discontinuation of DMPA in 13% of patients.[138] All patients beginning Depo-Provera should be informed that during the first year of use, they might have menstrual changes. If unusually heavy or continuous bleeding occurs, A.K. should be evaluated. A.K. should be counseled and reassured that her intermenstrual bleeding probably will resolve in the next few months. If the bleeding is bothersome to her, a 4- to 21-day course of oral estrogen (e.g., conjugated estrogen 0.625 to 2.5 mg/day) or an OC with 20 μg EE will minimize or eliminate the bleeding.[12] However, the bleeding may recur after discontinuation of the estrogen. Low-dose estrogen may be continued if bleeding recurs. The mean weight gain after 1 year of therapy with DMPA was about 5 lb in two thirds of users. Users typically gain a total of about 8 lb over 2 years, nearly 14 lb over 4 years, and 16.5 lb over 6 years. Other side effects include mood changes, hair loss, and headaches.

Following a 150-mg DMPA injection, conception is delayed approximately 10 months after the last injection in half of users.[138] The remaining users took longer to become pregnant, with nearly all users becoming pregnant by 18 months.

Lunelle

31. A.K. is concerned about the menstrual changes with DMPA but likes the idea of an injectable method of contraception. Are there any other options for her?

Lunelle contains medroxyprogesterone 25 mg and estradiol cypionate 5 mg and is administered intramuscularly every 28 to 33 days.[145] With this injection, women may experience spotting initially but should have regular menses about 2 to 3 weeks after each injection. The first injection should be given within 5 days of menstrual bleeding, and no backup contraception is needed. Unlike DMPA, ovulation resumes within 2 to 3 months of discontinuing Lunelle. The most common side effects of Lunelle are irregular menses, weight gain (an average of 4 lb in the first year), fluid retention, breast symptoms, nausea, headache, and mood changes.

Lunelle, formerly available in vials and prefilled syringes, encountered manufacturing problems and is no longer marketed because of business reasons. Lunelle has not been available since October 2002, and it is not available as of this writing. Pfizer medical information does not know if it will ever become available again. At this time, A.K. will have to select an alternate method.

SUBDERMAL IMPLANTS

32. A.K. returns to the gynecology clinic on the first day of her flow after missing three consecutive DMPA injections because she cannot remember to come in for her shots and does not like the weight gain and prolonged intermenstrual bleeding that occurred over 6 months. A friend of hers has used Norplant in the past, and she would like to try it. What information should be given to her?

The Norplant System brand of subdermal levonorgestrel implants, approved by the FDA in 1990, consists of a set of six Silastic capsules 2.4 mm wide and 34 mm long that are implanted under the skin in the upper arm.[5] The set contains a total of 216 mg of levonorgestrel that is released at a constant rate of only 20 to 30 μg/day over 5 years, after which time they are replaced.

Unfortunately, the Norplant System is no longer available. Certain lot numbers of Norplant were recalled in 2000 due to efficacy concerns, and patients were encouraged to use backup contraception. Further research found that the recalled lots did not have reduced efficacy, so backup contraception is no longer required for the affected patients. However, Wyeth does not plan to reintroduce the system. Other implants using one or two rods (versus the six rods for Norplant) are under investigation and may be available in 2004.

INTRAUTERINE DEVICES AND INTRAUTERINE SYSTEMS
Background and Mechanism of Action

33. R.P., a 23-year-old G_0P_0 woman with hydrocephalus, is brought to the gynecology clinic by her mother, S.P., to determine the best method of contraception for her mentally impaired daughter. R.P. is in a monogamous relationship with a mentally impaired partner. According to S.P., R.P. wishes to put off pregnancy for many years, and any method of contraception that necessitates compliance is virtually impossible for the couple. DMPA has been considered but is unacceptable because of the possibility of menstrual irregularities that would upset R.P. R.P. has never heard of IUDs or intrauterine systems (IUSs) before. Counsel her on what is available and how they work.

In the 1960s and 70s, several types of IUDs were available to women in the United States (e.g., Lippes Loop, Saf-T-Coil, Copper 7, Tatum T, Progestasert).[146] The Dalkon Shield IUD was introduced in the United States in 1971. Due to increased susceptibility to PID, with subsequent tubal scarring and infertility, the Shield was removed from the market in 1974. Although the high incidence of PID was not seen with the other types of IUDs, the negative publicity hurt the use of other IUDs. By 1976, the only IUD still available was the Progestasert. The ParaGard IUD was introduced in 1988 and the Mirena IUS in 2000. Progestasert has since been discontinued and has not been available since 2001. Although the IUDs/IUSs available today are a safe and effective method of contraception, they are still not as popular in the United States (<1% of women are users) as they are worldwide (12% of married women of reproductive age are users).[147]

The ParaGard IUD, also known as the Copper-T IUD, has a polyethylene body that is wound with copper wire. Once inserted, the ParaGard may be left in place for 10 years.[5,148] The Mirena IUS also has a polyethylene body, with a levonorgestrel reservoir in the vertical stem of the T.[149] Mirena is effective for 5 years. The failure rate of ParaGard is 0.6 to 0.8 pregnancies per 100 woman-years compared with 0.1 for Mirena (see Table 45-1). IUDs/IUSs are inserted by a health care provider in their office. The procedure usually takes only a few minutes and does not require sedation. Many providers will recommend that patients take a dose of an NSAID before the insertion visit.

Possible mechanisms of action for ParaGard include prevention of fertilization and implantation and interfering with sperm transport, viability, or number.[148] Mirena is believed to work by thickening the cervical mucus, preventing sperm from entering the uterus, altering the endometrial lining, preventing ovulation, and altering sperm activity.[149]

Advantages

34. **R.P.'s mother thinks that an IUD/IUS is a good option for her daughter, but R.P. is not sure. What are the advantages of IUDs/IUSs that R.P. should be aware of?**

Both the Mirena and ParaGard are both very effective, reversible, long-term methods that are easy to comply with. The ParaGard IUD is a wonderful option for women who desire a nonhormonal method. The Mirena IUS has the advantages of reducing menstrual bleeding and cramping.

Although the initial cost of inserting an IUD/IUS is high (around $500 for the device and insertion costs), there are no monthly costs to R.P. as there are with other methods. Therefore, women who use an IUD/IUS for over 1 year have an overall lower monthly cost than women who use OCs or the contraceptive ring or patch.

Disadvantages

IUDs/IUSs are contraindicated in women with certain anatomic abnormalities of the uterus, unexplained vaginal bleeding, cervical cancer, and PID or other active genital infection and should be used with caution in women who are HIV positive or are immunosuppressed (see Table 45-4).[11] The Mirena IUS should not be used in women with active breast cancer and should be used with caution in women with a current DVT or PE or a history of breast cancer. Breast cancer is hormonally sensitive, and the disease may be worsened by the use of levonorgestrel. Although the serum levels of levonorgestrel are low with the Mirena IUS, the manufacturer currently does not recommend that women with active or past breast cancer use the device.

IUD users are more likely to develop PID than nonusers. For all patients, the greatest risk of PID occurs shortly after insertion.[150] To prevent this from occurring, all patients should be tested for gonorrhea and chlamydia prior to IUD/IUS insertion. Women who are positive for either STD should consider an alternative form of contraception. In addition,

Table 45-7	IUD/IUS Early Danger Signs (PAINS)

Period late (pregnancy) or abnormal spotting or intermenstrual bleeding
Abdominal pain or pain with intercourse
Infection exposure (e.g., gonorrhea) or abnormal vaginal discharge
Not feeling well, fever, chills
String missing, shorter, or longer

IUDs/IUSs should be reserved for women in monogamous relationships or who have strict use of condoms, since these women are least likely to acquire an STD.

If an IUD/IUS user becomes pregnant, the likelihood that the pregnancy is ectopic is higher (i.e., the ratio of ectopic to uterine pregnancies is higher in IUD/IUS users).[148,149] If a patient using an IUD/IUS becomes pregnant, her risks for spontaneous abortion, sepsis, and premature delivery are increased if the IUD/IUS is left in place.

Approximately 10% to 15% of IUDs are removed because of excessive uterine bleeding, spotting, or pain.[148,149] Another 2% to 6% of women spontaneously expel their IUD within the first year. Rarely, IUDs/IUSs may become embedded in the endometrium or partially or totally perforate the uterine wall. R.P. should be instructed to look for the warning signs of a possible complication with IUD/IUS use (Table 45-7).

DIAPHRAGM

Mechanism of Action

35. **R.C., a 16-year-old G₁P₁ girl who is breastfeeding her 6-week-old infant, will consider only a barrier method of contraception. How do diaphragms prevent pregnancy?**

The diaphragm is a soft, latex or silicone rubber cap with a metal spring reinforcing the rim.[5,12] The device is inserted vaginally and placed over the cervical os to mechanically block access of sperm to the cervix. It is held in place by the spring tension of the rim, vaginal muscle tone, and the pubic bone. Because the diaphragm does not fit tightly enough to be a complete barrier to sperm, spermicidal gel must be placed in the dome prior to use.[9]

The first-year failure rate with diaphragms is 6 to 20 pregnancies per 100 woman-years (see Table 45-1).[5] R.C. should be counseled that diaphragms are less effective than other available methods. Since breastfeeding offers some protection against pregnancy, breastfeeding women may be the best candidates for the diaphragm.

Types

36. **What types of diaphragms are available?**

Diaphragms must be properly fitted to be effective. They are made of silicone or latex and are available in different sizes (50 to 95 mm in diameter) and different styles of construction of the circular rim.[5,12] The coil spring rim diaphragm folds flat and may be used with a diaphragm introducer. These diaphragms are indicated for women with average vaginal muscle tone and for women who can tolerate the sturdy rim and firm spring strength. The rim of the arcing spring rim diaphragm arcs when folded. Most women, even those with lax vaginal muscle tone, can tolerate the firm spring strength of the arcing spring rim diaphragm. The flat spring rim diaphragm is good for women with firm vaginal muscle tone, because the rim is less firm than the other styles. The wide-seal rim diaphragm (available as an arcing spring or coil spring) has a flexible flange designed to hold spermicide in place and to create a better seal between the diaphragm and vaginal wall.

R.C. would likely be able to tolerate any of the diaphragms. Perhaps she will find that one type is more comfortable than the others when she is fitted for the diaphragm.

Fitting

37. How is a diaphragm size selected?

The goal of fitting a diaphragm is to select the largest rim size that is comfortable for the patient.[5,12] A diaphragm that is too small may become dislodged during intercourse because vaginal depth increases during sexual arousal. Conversely, a diaphragm that is too large may cause vaginal pressure, abdominal pain or cramping, vaginal ulceration, or recurrent urinary tract infections.

Patient Instructions

38. What instructions should be provided to R.C. concerning the use of a diaphragm?

The diaphragm should not remain in the vagina for >24 hours.[5,12] Toxic shock syndrome (TSS) has been associated with diaphragm use and women should be alert to its symptoms, which include fever, diarrhea, vomiting, muscle aches, and a sunburn-like rash. Allergic reactions to the latex or spermicides also have been reported.

Prior to insertion, R.C. should inspect the diaphragm for holes or puckering. R.C. should be counseled that the diaphragm should always be inserted before intercourse if contraception is to be maximized; it can be inserted as long as 6 hours before intercourse if necessary. The diaphragm should not be removed for at least 6 hours after intercourse. One teaspoon of spermicidal gel should be placed into the dome of the diaphragm prior to insertion. If intercourse is repeated, a new application of spermicide should be inserted vaginally without removal of the diaphragm.

When the diaphragm is removed, it should be washed with mild soap and water, rinsed and dried, and stored in its plastic container. Talcum or perfumed powders should not be used on the diaphragm because these may damage the diaphragm or harm the vagina or cervix. Oil-based products also may decompose the diaphragm and should not be used. Contraceptive gel, however, may be used if vaginal lubrication is needed. If R.C. gains or loses 10 to 20 lb, has a pregnancy, or has abdominal or pelvic surgery, the fit of her diaphragm should be checked.

CERVICAL CAP

39. R.C. is also interested in the cervical cap. What is it, how well does it work, and what information should be provided to cervical cap users?

The cervical cap is a small, flexible, cuplike device made of latex and designed to fit closely around the base of the cervix; it is available in 22-, 25-, 28-, and 31-mm internal rim diameter sizes.[5,12] The cervical cap is less effective in women who have delivered a child, with pregnancy rates of 26 to 40 pregnancies per 100 woman-years in nulliparous women and 9 to 20 pregnancies per 100 woman-years in parous women. Women generally prefer other methods of contraception to cervical caps. In one study, 50% of women discontinued using cervical caps after 6 months, and 50% were pregnant after 2 years of use.[151]

To use the cervical cap, R.C. should fill the cap about one-third full with spermicidal gel, insert it vaginally, and place it over the cervix.[5,12] Suction holds it in place. It should be left in place at least 8 hours after intercourse but no longer than 48 hours, according to the manufacturer. Most experts recommend removal after 24 hours because of problems with vaginal odor at 36 to 48 hours and the theoretical risk of TSS.

As with the diaphragm, patients should check the cap for holes before using. Also, R.C. should avoid using oil-based lubricants or medications when using the cervical cap.

CONDOMS

40. J.D. is a 45-year-old woman who is unmarried and has sex infrequently. For this reason, she would like a method to protect against pregnancy as well as STDs. How effective are condoms in preventing pregnancy? What types of condoms are available?

Condoms are an effective method of contraception when used properly. The failure rate with condoms is 3 to 12 pregnancies per 100 woman-years of use (see Table 45-1).[5,12] The female condom is slightly less effective, with 5 to 21 pregnancies per 100 woman-years. Many different brands of condoms are available in the United States. The brands differ in size, shape, color, material, and the presence or absence of lubricants or spermicide. Most practitioners recommend lubricated condoms with reservoir ends to collect the ejaculate and to prevent breakage.

The most commonly used male condom is made of latex.[5,12] There are also male condoms made of polyurethane and lambskin, which are recommended for men or women allergic to latex. However, polyurethane condoms are more expensive and harder to find than latex condoms, and lambskin condoms do not offer the same protection against STDs. Female condoms are made of polyurethane.

41. What are the advantages and disadvantages of condoms? How are they used?

Because the pre-ejaculatory secretions may contain sperm, the male condom should be applied before vaginal contact.[5,12] Female condoms should also be inserted before sexual contact; they may be inserted up to 8 hours before intercourse. Condoms should be used by their expiration date and should not be reused. They should be stored in a cool, dry place, not somewhere they will be exposed to prolonged periods of heat or light.

The chief noncontraceptive benefit of condoms is the prevention of STDs (including gonorrhea, chlamydia, and HIV), and they can be used for vaginal, anal, or oral sex.[5,12] Condoms are also readily available without a prescription and do not cause systemic side effects like the hormonal methods, and latex male condoms are inexpensive. However, some complain that condoms reduce sensitivity and spontaneity, and female condoms are more costly (about $3 each), can be noisy, and can be difficult to insert.[12] Condoms may also break; this is less likely with the female condom. Oil-based products can degrade latex and should be avoided when using male, latex condoms. Oil-based lubricants can be used with female condoms or male polyurethane or lambskin condoms.

When using a male condom, the man or his partner holds the tip of the condom and unrolls it down to the base of the erect penis.[5,12] The female condom consists of a smaller circular ring at one end (which secures the device around the cervix like a diaphragm) and a larger ring at the other end. The inner ring should be compressed and inserted vaginally as far as it will go, and the larger ring remains outside of the vagina, protecting the external genitalia.

VAGINAL SPERMICIDES

42. J.D. would like to use a spermicide along with condoms. What options does she have, and how effective are spermicides when used alone?

Vaginal spermicides currently are available as gels (jellies), suppositories, foams, and films.[5,12,152] Most of these products use a nonionic surfactant, nonoxynol-9, as the spermicide; the balance use octoxynol-9. The in vitro spermicidal potencies of the various preparations are highest with foam, followed by cream, jelly, and gel, respectively.[249] First-year failure rates with these dosage forms range from 6 to 21 failures per 100 woman-years of use (see Table 45-1).

43. What dosage form should J.D. use? How should she be instructed to use a vaginal spermicide? What side effects can be anticipated?

Table 45-8 compares the different spermicidal products.[5,12,152] The different characteristics of the products can help guide J.D. when selecting a dosage form. Regardless of the dosage form, a new dose of spermicide should be applied before each act of intercourse.

Spermicides may can cause genital irritation and in some patients lead to ulceration. For this reason, spermicides have been shown to increase the transmission of STDs, including HIV, gonorrhea, and chlamydia.

EMERGENCY CONTRACEPTION

Emergency Contraceptive Pills

44. B.P., a 24-year-old woman, has just returned home from a vacation in Europe. Her luggage containing her OCs was stolen 2 weeks ago, and she had unprotected midcycle intercourse 34 hours ago. What can be done to prevent an unwanted pregnancy at this time?

Emergency contraception (also known as the morning-after pill) is postcoital contraception[153] that is useful for women who did not use a contraceptive (e.g., forgot, were assaulted) or whose method failed (e.g., broken condom). Emergency contraceptive pills (ECPs) may reduce the risk of pregnancy by several mechanisms: preventing ovulation, preventing fertilization, or preventing implantation.

Although ECP use is on the rise, many women are not aware that it is available. In a 1998 survey, 686 of 1,000 women aged 18 to 44 had heard of emergency contraception.[154] Only 5% had learned about it from a health care professional, 44% identified the source as a television news program, and another 16% read about it in a magazine. Approximately 12% of obstetrician/gynecologists interviewed in the same survey feared women would use ECPs for routine contraception, and another 11% stated that they had moral or religious objections to emergency contraception.

Available Emergency Contraceptive Pills

ESTROGEN AND PROGESTIN EMERGENCY CONTRACEPTIVE PILLS

One option for patients is to use regular OCs for emergency contraception. The Yuzpe regimen of emergency contraception uses commercially available OCs to deliver 0.5 mg levonorgestrel or 1 mg norgestrel and 100 µg EE per dose.[155] Patients are instructed to take two doses 12 hours apart. Table 45-9 shows which OCs may be used and how many tablets need to be taken per dose.[152,156,157] It is very important to counsel patients about which pills to take, since the tablet color and number differ depending on the brand chosen. This makes this method less desirable than Preven and Plan B (discussed below).

The Preven Emergency Contraceptive Kit, which contains four blue tablets (each containing 0.25 mg levonorgestrel and

Table 45-8	Comparison of Vaginal Spermicides			
Formulation	Brand Name Examples	How to Use	Onset of Action	Duration of Action
Gel	Conceptrol, Gynol II	Fill applicator, insert applicator vaginally as far as it will comfortably go, press plunger of applicator to deposit spermicide near the cervix.	Immediate	1 hr
Film	VCF	Fold film in half, fold over finger, use finger to insert as far as it will comfortably go.	15 min	3 hr
Foam	Delfen, Koromex, VCF	Shake foam canister, fill applicator, insert applicator vaginally as far as it will comfortably go, press plunger of applicator to deposit spermicide near the cervix.	Immediate	1 hr
Suppository	Conceptrol, Encare	Unwrap, use finger to insert as far as it will comfortably go.	15 min	1 hr

Table 45-9 Oral Contraceptive Pills That May Be Used As Emergency Contraception

Brand	Number of Tablets per Dose	Color
Alesse	5	Pink
Aviane	5	Orange
Cryselle	4	White
Enpresse	4	Orange
Lessina	5	Pink
Levlen	4	Light-orange
Levlite	5	Pink
Levora	4	White
Lo-Ovral	4	White
Low-Ogestrel	4	White
Nordette	4	Light-orange
Ogestrel	2	White
Ovral	2	White
Ovrette	20	Yellow
Plan B	1	White
Portia	4	Pink
Preven	2	Blue
Tri-Levlen	4	Yellow
Triphasil	4	Yellow
Trivora	4	Pink

50 µg EE), a pregnancy test, and an instruction book, is a good alternative to using OCs. Patients are instructed first to read the instruction book, then to use the pregnancy test; if the pregnancy test is negative, they should take two tablets as soon as possible and two more tablets exactly 12 hours later.

Estrogen and progestin ECPs have been shown to reduce the incidence of pregnancy by about 75%.[153] The reduction in pregnancy is greatest when used within 24 hours after unprotected intercourse.

PROGESTIN EMERGENCY CONTRACEPTIVE PILLS

Plan B is a progestin-only ECP. The Plan B pack consists of two white levonorgestrel 0.75-mg tablets and patient instructions.[152,155,156] One tablet is taken as soon as possible and the second is taken 12 hours later. Progestin ECPs have been shown to be more effective than estrogen and progestin

ECPs.[157] They reduce the average risk of pregnancy by 89% after a single act of intercourse when taken within 72 hours. In the first 24 hours after intercourse, progestin ECPs can prevent 95% of expected pregnancies.

The progesterone-only pill, Ovrette, may also be used for emergency contraception.[153] However, this product is rarely used, since the patient would need to take 20 pills per dose to get the proper amount of progestin.

Patient Instructions

ECPs are most effective when taken as soon as possible after intercourse; therefore, treatment should not be delayed.[153,156,157] Although the FDA-approved indication for Preven and Plan B is for use within 72 hours after intercourse, ECPs have been shown to be effective when the first dose is taken within 5 days of unprotected sex.[158,159] The most common side effects with ECPs are nausea and vomiting. Gastrointestinal adverse effects are more likely with the estrogen and progestin ECPs than with the progestin ECPs. B.P. should be instructed that if she vomits within 1 hour of taking either dose of medication, the dose should be repeated. Providers often prescribe an antiemetic such as prochlorperazine or meclizine that patients can take 30 to 60 minutes before each dose of ECP to prevent nausea or vomiting.[153]

B.P.'s menses may come early or late, but she should take a pregnancy test if her menses does not come within 3 weeks of taking ECPs.

Patients may call the Emergency Contraception Hotline (1-888-NOT-2-Late or 1-888-668-2528) to find a provider near them who will prescribe ECPs. Patients may also find information about ECP at the Emergency Contraception website (www.not-2-late.com).

IUDs for Emergency Contraception

The copper IUD is also an effective method of emergency contraception when inserted within 5 days of unprotected sex.[13] Since some women are not good candidates for IUDs (see discussion above) and IUDs must be inserted by a health care provider, they are not used as regularly for emergency contraception. The biggest advantage of using an IUD for emergency contraception is that it provides continued contraception for the patient.

REFERENCES

1. International Programs Center, U.S. Census Bureau World POPClock. Available at *http://www.census.gov/ipc/www/worldpop.html*. Accessed May 10, 2003.
2. U.S. Bureau of the Census International Data Base. Available at *http://www.census.gov/cgi-bin/popclock*. Accessed May 9, 2003.
3. National Campaign to Reduce Teen Pregnancy. 14 and Younger: The Sexual Behavior of Young Adolescents. Washington, DC: 2003.
4. Speroff L, Glass RH, Kase NG, eds. Clinical Gynecologic Endocrinology and Infertility, 6th ed. Philadelphia: Lippincott Williams & Wilkins, 1999.
5. Drug Facts and Comparisons, 57th ed. St Louis, MO: Facts and Comparisons, 2002.
6. Hatcher RA et al. Contraceptive Technology, 17th ed. New York: Ardent Media, 1998.
7. Hatcher RA et al. Contraceptive Technology, 16th ed. New York: Irvington Publishers, 1994.
8. Goldzieher JW et al. Comparative studies of the ethinyl estrogens used in oral contraception: II: antiovulatory potency. Am J Obstet Gynecol 1975; 122:619.
9. Briggs MH. Choosing contraceptive steroids and doses. J Reprod Med 1983;28(Suppl 1):57.
10. Dickey RP. Managing Contraceptive Pill Patients, 11th ed. Dallas: Essential Medical Information Systems, 2002.
11. Vandenbroucke JP et al. Oral contraceptives and the risk of venous thrombosis. N Engl J Med 2001; 344:1527.
12. Family and Reproductive Health Programme. Improving Access to Quality Care in Family Planning. Medical Eligibility Criteria for Contraceptive Use, 2d ed. Geneva: World Health Organization, 2000.
13. Hatcher RA et al. A Pocket Guide to Managing Contraception. Tiger, GA: Bridging the Gap Foundation, 2002.
14. Holt VL et al. Body weight and risk of oral contraceptive failure. Obstet Gynecol 2002;99:820.
15. Upton GW. The phasic approach to oral contraception: the triphasic concept and its clinical application. Int J Fertil 1983;28:121.
16. Westhoff C et al. Quick start: a novel oral contraceptive initiation method. Contraception 2002; 66:141.
17. Dickinson BD et al. Drug interactions between oral contraceptives and antibiotics. Obstet Gynecol 2001;98:853.
18. Hansten PD, Horn JR. Inhibition of oral contraceptive efficacy. Drug Interactions Newsletter 1985; 5:7.
19. Hudson P. The tetracycline–oral contraceptive controversy. J Am Acad Dermatol 1982;7:269.
20. Joshi JV et al. A study of interaction of low-dose combination oral contraceptive with ampicillin and metronidazole. Contraception 1980;22:643.

21. Back DJ et al. The interaction between ampicillin and oral contraceptive steroids in women. Br J Clin Pharmacol 1982;13:280.

22. Robertson YR, Johnson ES. Interactions between oral contraceptives and other drugs: a review. Curr Med Res Opin 1976;3:647.

23. D'Arcy PF. Drug interactions with oral contraceptives. Drug Intell Clin Pharm 1986;20:353.

24. Hansten PD, Horn JR. Inhibition of oral contraceptive efficacy. Drug Interactions Newsletter 1985; 5:7.

25. Orme MLE. The clinical pharmacology of oral contraceptive steroids. Br J Clin Pharmacol 1982;14:31.

26. D'Arcy PF. Drug interactions update: nitrofurantoin. Drug Intell Clin Pharm 1985;19:540.

27. Dickey RP. Medical approaches to reproductive regulation: the Pill. ACOG Semin Fam Plan 1974;Table IX:32.

28. Friedman CI et al. The effect of ampicillin on oral contraceptive effectiveness. Obstet Gynecol 1980; 55:33.

29. Back DJ et al. Drug interactions with oral contraceptives. Int Planned Parenthood Federation Med Bull 1978;12:4.

30. Back DJ et al. Interindividual variation and drug interactions with hormonal steroid contraceptives. Drugs 1981;21:46.

31. Hempel E et al. Drug-stimulated biotransformation of hormonal steroid contraceptives: clinical implications. Drugs 1976;12:442.

32. Joshi JV et al. A study of interaction of a low-dose combination oral contraceptive with antitubercular drugs. Contraception 1980;21:617.

33. Bacon JF, Shenfield GM. Pregnancy attributable to interaction between tetracycline and oral contraceptives. Br Med J 1980;280:293.

34. Grimmer SFM et al. The effect of co-trimoxazole on oral contraceptive steroids in women. Contraception 1983;28:53.

35. McArthur J. Oral contraceptives and epilepsy. Br Med J 1967;3:162.

36. Coulam CB, Annegers JF. Do anticonvulsants reduce the efficacy of oral contraceptives? Epilepsia 1979;2:519.

37. Van Dijke CPH, Weber JCP. Interaction between oral contraceptives and griseofulvin. Br Med J 1984;288:1125.

38. Agouron Pharmaceuticals. Viracept package insert. San Diego: June 2002.

39. Pharmacia & Upjohn Company. Mycobutin package insert. Kalamazoo, MI, Feb. 2002.

40. Back DJ et al. The effect of antibiotics on enterohepatic circulation of ethynylestradiol and norethisterone in the rat. J Steroid Biochem 1978;9:527.

41. Mattson RH et al. Use of oral contraceptives by women with epilepsy. JAMA 1986;256:238.

42. Ernst E. Second thoughts about safety of St. John's wort. Lancet 1999;354:2014

43. Roby CA et al. St John's wort: effect of CYP3A4 activity. Clin Pharmacol Ther 2000;67:451.

44. GlaxoSmith Kline. Amprenavir package insert. Research Triangle Park, NC, Oct. 2002.

45. Schroggie JJ et al. Effect of oral contraceptives on vitamin K-dependent clotting activity. Clin Pharmacol Ther 1967;8:670.

46. de Teresa E et al. Interaction between anticoagulants and contraceptives: an unsuspected finding. Br Med J 1979;2:1260.

47. Pfizer Inc. Lipitor package insert. New York, Nov. 2002.

48. Abernethy DR et al. Impairment of diazepam metabolism by low-dose estrogen-containing oral contraceptive steroids. N Engl J Med 1982;306:791.

49. Stoehr GP et al. The effect of low-dose estrogen-containing oral contraceptives on the pharmacokinetics of triazolam, alprazolam, temazepam, and lorazepam [abstract]. Drug Intell Clin Pharm 1984;18:495.

50. Deray G et al. Oral contraceptive interaction with cyclosporine [letter]. 1987;1:158.

51. Steele JM, Duncan LJP. Effect of oral contraceptives on insulin requirements in diabetics. J Fam Plan Doctors 1978;3:77.

52. Boekenoogen SJ et al. Prednisone disposition and protein binding in oral contraceptive users. J Clin Endocrinol Metab 1983;56:702.

53. Abbott Laboratories. Norvir package insert. North Chicago, IL: Sept. 2001.

54. Fujisawa Healthcare. Tacrolimus package insert. Deerfield, IL: May 2002.

55. Tornatore KM et al. Effect of chronic contraceptive steroids on theophylline disposition. Eur J Clin Pharmacol 1982;23:129.

56. Athena Neurosciences. Zanaflex package insert. Dec. 1996.

57. Ortho-McNeil Pharmaceuticals. Topamax package insert. Raritan, NJ : Oct. 1999.

58. DeLeacy EA et al. Effects of subjects' sex, and intake of tobacco, alcohol, and oral contraceptives on plasma phenytoin levels. Br J. Clin Pharmacol 1979;8:33.

59. Rosenberg MJ et al. Oral contraceptive discontinuation: a prospective evaluation of frequency and reasons. Am J Obstet Gynecol 1998;179:577.

60. Schwingl PJ et al. Estimates of the risk of cardiovascular death attributable to low-dose oral contraceptives in the United States. Am J Obstet Gynecol 1999;180:241.

61. Royal College of General Practitioners' Oral Contraceptive Study. Incidence of arterial disease among oral contraceptive users. J R Coll Gen Pract 1983;33:75.

62. Vessey MP et al. Mortality in oral contraceptive users. Lancet 1981;1:549.

63. Vessey MP et al. Mortality among oral contraceptive users: 20-year follow-up of women in a cohort study. Br Med J 1989;299:1487.

64. Knopp RH et al. Comparison of the lipoprotein, carbohydrate, and hemostatic effects of phasic oral contraceptives containing desogestrel or levonorgestrel. Contraception 2001;63:1.

65. Merki-Feld GS et al. Long-term effects of combined oral contraceptives on markers of endothelial function and lipids in healthy premenopausal women. Contraception 2002;65:231.

66. Endrikat J et al. An open-label, comparative study of the effects of a dose-reduced oral contraceptive containing 20 μg ethinyl estradiol and 100 μg levonorgestrel on hemostatic, lipids, and carbohydrate metabolism variables. Contraception 2002;65:215.

67. Tikkanen MJ et al. High density lipoprotein 2 and hepatic lipase: reciprocal changes produced by estrogen and norgestrel. J Clin Endocrinol Metab 1982;54:1113.

68. Tikkanen MH et al. Reduction of plasma high-density lipoprotein-2 cholesterol and increase of post-heparin plasma hepatic lipase activity during progestin treatment. Clin Chim Acta 1981;115:63.

69. Miller NE et al. Relation of angiographically defined coronary artery disease to plasma lipoprotein subfractions and apolipoprotein. Br Med J 1981; 282:1741.

70. Paulus D et al. Oral contraception and cardiovascular risk factors during adolescence. Contraception 2000;62:113.

71. Tanis BC et al. Oral contraceptives and the risk of myocardial infarction. N Engl J Med 2001;345: 1787.

72. Dunn N et al. Oral contraceptives and myocardial infarction: results of the MICA case-control study. Br Med J 1999;318:1579.

73. American Cancer Society. Cancer Facts and Figures 2003. Atlanta: American Cancer Society, 2003.

74. Moreno V et al. Effect of oral contraceptives on risk of cervical cancer in women with human papillomavirus infection: the IARC multicentric case-control study. Lancet 2002;359:1085.

75. Beral et al. Mortality associated with oral contraceptive use: 25-year follow-up of cohort of 46 000 women from Royal College of General Practitioners' oral contraception study. Br Med J 1999; 318:96.

76. Irwin KL et al. Oral contraceptives and cervical cancer risk in Costa Rica. Detection bias or causal association? JAMA 1988;259:59.

77. Seibert C et al. Prescribing oral contraceptives for women older than 35 years of age. Ann Int Med 2003;138:54.

78. Royal College of General Practitioners' Oral Contraception Study. Oral contraceptives, venous thrombosis, and varicose veins. J R Coll Gen Pract 1978;28:393.

79. Tapla HR et al. Effect of oral contraceptive therapy on the renin angiotensin system in normotensive and hypertensive women. Obstet Gynecol 1973;41:643.

80. Fisch TR et al. Oral contraceptives and blood pressure. JAMA 1977;237:2499.

81. Fisch TR et al. Oral contraceptives, pregnancy and blood pressure. In: Ramcharan S, ed. The Walnut Creek Contraceptive Drug Study: A Prospective Study of the Side Effects of Oral Contraceptives, vol 1. Washington, DC: Government Printing Office, 1974:105. DHEW publication no. (NIH) 74-562.

82. Ramcharan S et al. The occurrence and course of hypertensive disease in users and nonusers of oral contraceptive drugs. In: Ramcharan S, ed. The Walnut Creek Contraceptive Drug Study: A Prospective Study of the Side Effects of Oral Contraceptives, vol 2. Washington, DC: Government Printing Office, 1976:1. DHEW publication no. (NIH) 74-562.

83. American College of Obstetrics and Gynecology. The use of hormonal contraception in women with coexisting medical conditions. ACOG Practice Bulletin Number 8: July 2000.

84. Rooks JB et al. Epidemiology of hepatocellular adenoma: the role of oral contraceptive use. JAMA 199;242:644.

85. Bein NN, Goldsmith HS. Recurrent massive hemorrhage from benign hepatic tumors secondary to oral contraceptives. Br J Surg 1977;64:433.

86. Klatskin G. Hepatic tumors: possible relationship to use of oral contraceptives. Gastroenterol 1977;73:386.

87. Desser-Wiest L. Promotion of liver tumors by steroid hormones. J Toxicol Environ Health 1979;5:203.

88. Ockner R et al. Hepatic effects of oral contraceptives. N Engl J Med 1967;276:331.

89. Herings RMC et al. Venous thromboembolism among new users of different oral contraceptives. Lancet 1999;354:127.

90. Venous thromboembolism and combination OCs containing desogestrel orgestodene. Where are we now? Contraception Report 1999;10(1):4.

91. Cunliffe WJ. Acne, hormones and treatment. Br Med J 1982;285:912.

92. Speroff L et al. Evaluation of a new generation of oral contraceptives. Obstet Gynecol 1993; 81:1034.

93. Brinton LA et al. Risk factors for benign breast disease. Am J Epidemiol 1981;113:203.

94. Royal College of General Practitioners. Oral Contraceptives and Health: An Interim Report From the Oral Contraception Study of the Royal College of General Practitioners. Pitman, NY: Royal College of General Practitioners, 1974.

95. Speroff L. PMS: looking for new answers to an old problem. Contemp Obstet Gynecol 1983; 21:102.

96. Schlesselman JJ. Risk of endometrial cancer in relation to use of combined oral contraceptives. A practioner's guide to meta-analysis. Hum Reprod 1997;12:1851.

97. Darney PD. Evaluating the pill's long-term effects. Contemp Obstet Gynecol 1982;20:57.

98. Barber HRK. The pill: noncontraceptive benefits. Female Patient 1982;7:12.

99. Halbert DR. Noncontraceptive uses of the pill. Clin Obstet Gynecol 1981;24:987.

100. Siskind V et al. Beyond ovulation: oral contraceptives and epithelial ovarian cancer. Epidemiology 2000;11:106.

101. Susannel G et al. Declining ovarian cancer rates in U.S. women in relation to parity and oral contraceptive use. Epidemiology 2000;11:102.

102. Sherris JD, Fox G. Infertility and sexually transmitted disease: a public health challenge. Popul Rep [L] 1983;11:113.
103. Rubin GL et al. Oral contraceptives and pelvic inflammatory disease. Am J Obstet Gynecol 1982; 140:630.
104. Wolner-Hanssen P et al. Laparoscopic findings and contraceptive use in women with signs and symptoms suggestive of acute salpingitis. Obstet Gynecol 1985;66:233.
105. Washington AE et al. Oral contraceptives, chlamydia trachomatous infection, and pelvic inflammatory disease. JAMA 1985;253:2246.
106. Cramer DW et al. Tubal infertility and the intrauterine device. N Engl J Med 1985;312:941.
107. Wolner-Hanssen P et al. Decreased risk of symptomatic chlamydial pelvic inflammatory disease associated with oral contraceptive use. JAMA 1990;263:54.
108. Ory HW. The noncontraceptive health benefits from oral contraceptive use. Fam Plan Perspect 1982;14:182.
109. Rubin GL et al. Ectopic pregnancy in the United States, 1970–1978. JAMA 1983;249:1725.
110. McPherson K et al. Oral contraception and breast cancer [letter]. Lancet 1983;2:144.
111. Pike MC et al. Breast cancer in young women and use of oral contraceptives: possible modifying effect of formulation and age of use. Lancet 1983; 2:926.
112. Royal College of General Practitioners' Oral Contraception Study. Breast cancer and oral contraceptives: findings in Royal College of General Practitioners' Study. Br Med J 1981;282:2088.
113. Grabrick DM et al. Risk of breast cancer with oral contraceptive use in women with a family history of breast cancer. JAMA 2000;284:1791.
114. Marchbanks PA et al. Oral contraceptives and the risk of breast cancer. N Engl J Med 2002;346:2025.
115. Vessey MP et al. Mortality among women participating in the Oxford/Family Planning Association Contraceptive Study. Br Med J 1977;282:731.
116. Ramcharan S et al. General summary of findings: general conclusions; implications. In: Ramcharan S et al., eds. The Walnut Creek Contraceptive Drug Study: A Prospective Study of the Side Effects of Oral Contraceptives, vol 3. An interim report: a comparison of disease occurrence leading to hospitalization or death in users and nonusers of oral contraceptives. Bethesda, MD: Center for Population Research, 1981:1.
117. Vessey MP et al. Breast cancer and oral contraceptives: findings in Oxford/Family Planning Association Contraceptive Study. Br Med J 1981; 282:2093.
118. The Centers for Disease Control Cancer and Steroid Hormone Study. Oral contraceptive use and the risk of breast cancer. JAMA 1983;249:1591.
119. Hankinson SE et al. A prospective study of oral contraceptive use and risk of breast cancer (Nurses' Health Study, United States). Cancer Causes and Control 1997;8:65.
120. Matthews PN et al. Breast cancer in women who have taken contraceptive steroids. Br Med J 1981;282:774.
121. Kjos SL et al. Effect of low-dose oral contraceptives on carbohydrate and lipid metabolism in women with recent gestational diabetes: results of a controlled, randomized, prospective study. Am J Obstet Gynecol 1990;163:1822.
122. Skouby SO. Low-dosage oral contraception in women with previous gestational diabetes. Obstet Gynecol 1982;59:325.
123. Skouby SO et al. Triphasic oral contraception: metabolic effects in normal women and those with previous gestational diabetes. Am J Obstete Gynecol 1985;153:495.
124. Briggs MH et al. Randomized prospective studies on metabolic effects of oral contraceptives. Acta Obstet Gynecol Scand 1982;105(Suppl):25.
125. Kim C et al. Oral contraceptive use and association with glucose, insulin, and diabetes in young adult women; the CARDIA Study. Diabetes Care 2002;25:1027.
126. Grodstein et al. A prospective study of symptomatic gallstones in women: relation with oral contraceptives and other risk factors. Obstet Gynecol 1994;84:207.
127. Royal College of General Practitioners' Oral Contraception Study. Oral contraceptives and gallbladder disease. Lancet 1982;2:957.
128. Ramcharan S et al. The Walnut Creek Contraceptive Drug Study: A Prospective Study of the Side Effects of Oral Contraceptives, vol 3. An interim report: a comparison of disease occurrence leading to hospitalization or death in users and nonusers of oral contraceptives. Bethesda, MD: Center for Population Research, 1981;NIH publication no. 81564:349.
129. Vessey M, Painter R. Oral contraceptive use and benign gallbladder disease; revisited. Contraception 1994;50:167.
130. Briggs GG et al., eds. A Reference Guide to Fetal and Neonatal Risk. Drugs in Pregnancy and Lactation, 6th ed. Philadelphia: Lippincott Williams & Wilkins, 2001.
131. Simpson JL. Relationship between congenital anomalies and contraception. Adv Contracept 1985;1:3.
132. Committee on Drugs, American Academy of Pediatrics. The transfer of drugs and other chemicals into human milk. Pediatrics 1994;93:137.
133. Ortho-McNeil Pharmaceuticals. Ortho Evra package insert. Raritan, NJ: Nov. 2001.
134. Organon. NuvaRing package insert. West Orange, NJ: Oct. 2001.
135. Kaunitz AM. Injectable contraception. Clin Obstet Gynecol 1989;32:356.
136. WHO Collaborative Study of Neoplasia and Steroid Contraceptives. Depot medroxyprogesterone acetate (DMPA) and risk of endometrial cancer. Int J Cancer 1991;49:186.
137. de Abood M et al. Effect of Depo-Provera or Microgynon on the painful crises of sickle cell anemia patients. Contraception 1997;56:313.
138. Pharmacia & Upjohn. Depo-Provera package insert. Kalamazoo, MI: June 2002.
139. Kaunitz AM, Rosenfield A. Injectable contraception with depot medroxyprogesterone acetate. Current status. Drugs 1993;45:857.
140. Archer B et al. Depot medroxyprogesterone. Management of side effects commonly associated with its contraceptive use. J Nurse Midwif 1997; 42:104.
141. Cundy T et al. Recovery of bone density in women who stop using medroxyprogesterone acetate. Br Med J 1994;308:247.
142. Lappe JM et al. The impact of lifestyle factors on stress fracture in female Army recruits. Osteoporosis Int 2001;12:35.
143. Harkins GJ et al. Decline in bone mineral density with stress fractures in a woman on depot medroxyprogesterone acetate. A case report. J Reprod Med 1999;44:309.
144. Cromer B. Recent clinical issues related to the use of depot medroxyprogesterone acetate (Depo-Provera). Curr Opin Obstet Gynecol 1999;11:467.
145. Pharmacia & Upjohn. Lunelle package insert. Kalamazoo, MI: July 2001.
146. Planned Parenthood Federation of America. A history of contraceptive methods. Available at http://www.plannedparenthood.org/library/birth-control/020709_bchistory.html. Accessed May 10, 2003.
147. Stanwood NL et al. Obstetrician-gynecologists and the intrauterine device: a survey of attitudes and practice. Obstet Gynecol 2002;99:275.
148. Ortho-McNeil Pharmaceuticals. ParaGard package insert. Raritan, NJ: Feb. 2002.
149. Berlex Laboratories. Mirena package insert. Montville, NJ: Dec. 2000.
150. Lee NC et al. The intrauterine device and pelvic inflammatory disease revisited: new results from the Women's Health Study. Obstet Gynecol 1988;72:1.
151. Smith GG, Lee RJ. The use of cervical caps at the University of California, Berkeley: a survey. Contraception 1984;30:115.
152. Berardi RR et al., eds. Handbook of Nonprescription Drugs, 13th ed. Washington, DC: American Pharmaceutical Association, 2002.
153. Wellbery C. Emergency contraception. Arch Fam Med 2000;9:642.
154. Demott K. ObGyns not discussing "morning-after pill." Obstet Gynecol News 1998;33(6):14.
155. Task Force on Postovulatory Methods of Fertility Regulation. Randomised controlled trial of levonorgestrel versus the Yuzpe regimne of combined oral contraceptives for emergency contraception. Lancet 1998;352:428.
156. The Emergency Contraception Website. http://ec.princeton.edu/. Accessed May 6, 2003.
157. American Pharmaceutical Association. Emergency contraception: the pharmacist's role. Washington, DC: American Pharmaceutical Association, 2000.
158. Rodrigues I et al. Effectiveness of emergency contraceptive pills between 72 and 120 hours after unprotected sexual intercourse. Am J Obstet Gynecol 2001;184:531.
159. Ellertson C et al. Extending the time limit for starting the Yuzpe regimen of emergency contracetion to 120 hours. Obstet Gynecol 2003; 101:1168.

CHAPTER 46

Obstetric Drug Therapy

Fotini K. Hatzopoulos

PREGNANCY

Good prenatal care can have a major influence on the outcome of pregnancy. In 2001, the infant mortality rate (from birth through the first year of life) for infants of mothers beginning prenatal care after the first trimester, or not at all, was 37% higher (8.5 per 1,000 live births) than the rate for infants whose mothers' prenatal care began in the first trimester (6.2 per 1,000 births).[1] Prenatal care in the United States, although much improved, is still not accessible to all women.[2] Appropriate preconception counseling and treatment of women with preexisting high risk medical conditions such as diabetes, hypertension and epilepsy (also see Chapter 54, Seizure Disorders) can greatly improve their pregnancy outcomes. Essential preconception and early prenatal care, critical for normal fetal organogenesis, may not be sought because 40% of pregnancies in an American woman's lifetime are unwanted.[2] Two-thirds of all fetal deaths in the United States were attributable to chronic hypertension, hypertensive diseases of pregnancy, diabetes, small for gestational age (SGA) births (birth weight <10th percentile for gestational age), and placental abruption (detachment of the placenta).[3] Another obstetrical complication that continues to plague pregnancies is preterm labor.

The goal of prenatal care, to promote a safe and successful pregnancy and the delivery of a healthy infant, can be achieved through education and by monitoring the health of the mother and fetus. Mothers should be educated about proper nutrition, general hygiene, and the danger signals of pregnancy. Prenatal care should begin as early as possible after pregnancy is confirmed so that women at risk for complicated pregnancies can be identified and potential problems monitored and treated. The first prenatal visit should occur no later than the second missed menstrual period, generally 8 weeks after missed menses.[2]

Placental Physiology

Conception begins with the fertilization of an ovum. The time after conception is the conceptional or developmental age. The gestational age or menstrual age, is the time from the start of the last menstrual period (LMP) and generally exceeds the developmental age by 2 weeks.[4] The fertilized ovum, or zygote, undergoes mitotic divisions that lead to the formation of the blastocyst, a hollow fluid-filled sphere.[5] The outer cell mass of the blastocyst differentiates into trophoblasts, while the internal cell mass gives rise to the embryo. About 5 to 6 days after fertilization, the blastocyst adheres to the endometrial epithelium, where it undergoes implantation between postconception day 7 to 12.[4] The outer cell mass, or trophoblasts, invades the endometrium, and the blastocyst becomes completely buried within the endometrium. Once trophoblastic invasion of the endometrium occurs, the endometrium is transformed into the decidua, the functional layer of the pregnant endometrium, and is referred to by this term throughout pregnancy.[6]

The trophoblast secretes human chorionic gonadotropin (hCG), which maintains the corpus luteum so that menstruation is prevented and pregnancy can continue.[7] (See Chapter 45, Contraception, for a detailed discussion of the menstrual cycle.) As more of the decidua is invaded, the walls of the decidual capillaries are eroded, thereby leaking maternal blood into spaces called lacunae.[5] This initial contact with the maternal blood allows hCG to enter the maternal circulation by day 11 of gestation when it can be measured to aid in the diagnosis of pregnancy.[7] The trophoblasts are the only cells of the conceptus that are in direct contact with maternal tissue or blood; embryonic cells never come in contact with maternal tissues.[5]

As the embryo within the blastocyst grows, the thickness of the decidua decreases. The part of the decidua directly below the site of implantation becomes the decidua basalis, and the part that lies over the the growing blastocyte, which separates it from the rest of the uterine cavity, is the decidua capsularis; this part of the decidua contacts the chorion leave, the extraembryonic, avascular, fetal membrane. The rest of the uterus is lined by the decidua parietalis. By 14 to 16 weeks, the gestational sac is large enough to fill the entire uterine cavity, at which time the decidua capsularis has lost its blood supply and fuses with the decidua parietalis (which is somtimes refered to as the decidua vera).[6]

The vessels (spiral arteries) supplying blood to the decidua parietalis retain their endothelium and smooth muscle wall and therefore continue to respond to vasoactive agents.[6] By contrast, the spiral arteries supplying the decidua basalis undergo trophoblastic invasion whereby they are transformed into wide-bore uteroplacental vessels that empty directly into the intervillous space in fountainlike spurts.[4,5] This process creates a low-resistance arteriolar circuit that allows maximal placental blood flow necessary for the growing fetus.[8] Unlike the rest of the maternal and fetal vasculature, the resistance within these uteroplacental vessels does not change in response to vasoactive agents. The resistance is fixed and therefore directly dependent on maternal perfusion pressure.[7] If the maternal perfusion pressure decreases, blood flow to the placenta decreases. Likewise, placental blood flow is increased when the maternal perfusion pressure is increased. Incomplete trophoblastic invasion of the spiral arteries in the myometrium results in decreased placental perfusion and ischemia. This is believed to be a factor in the pathogenesis of pre-eclampsia.[8]

The placenta has both fetal and maternal components. The placenta is made up of the amnion, chorion, chorionic villi and intervillous spaces, decidual plate, and the myometrium.[4] The fetal surface of the placenta is covered by the amnion beneath which the fetal chorionic vessels cross. Figure 46-1 describes the structure of the placenta and its maternal-fetal circulation. Maternal-fetal circulation to the intervillous space is not fully established until the second trimester.[4] Maternal uteroplacental arteries perfuse the intervillous spaces, and as the maternal blood flows around the villi, exchanges (oxygen and nutrients) occur with fetal blood contained within capillaries found inside these villi.[4] Even though the placenta serves as a strong barrier between the fetal and maternal circulations, a few cells are able to cross between the two circulations.[4] Except for pathologic conditions, fetal blood and maternal blood do not make contact. Placental blood flow reaches the fetus through a single umbilical vein. At the juncture of the placenta and umbilicus, the umbilical vein and arteries repeatedly branch and traverse the fetal surface of the placenta (between the amnion and the chorionic plate) forming capillary networks that terminate within the villi. These vessels are termed the chorionic veins and arteries. Fetal blood flow reaches the placenta through two umbilical arter-

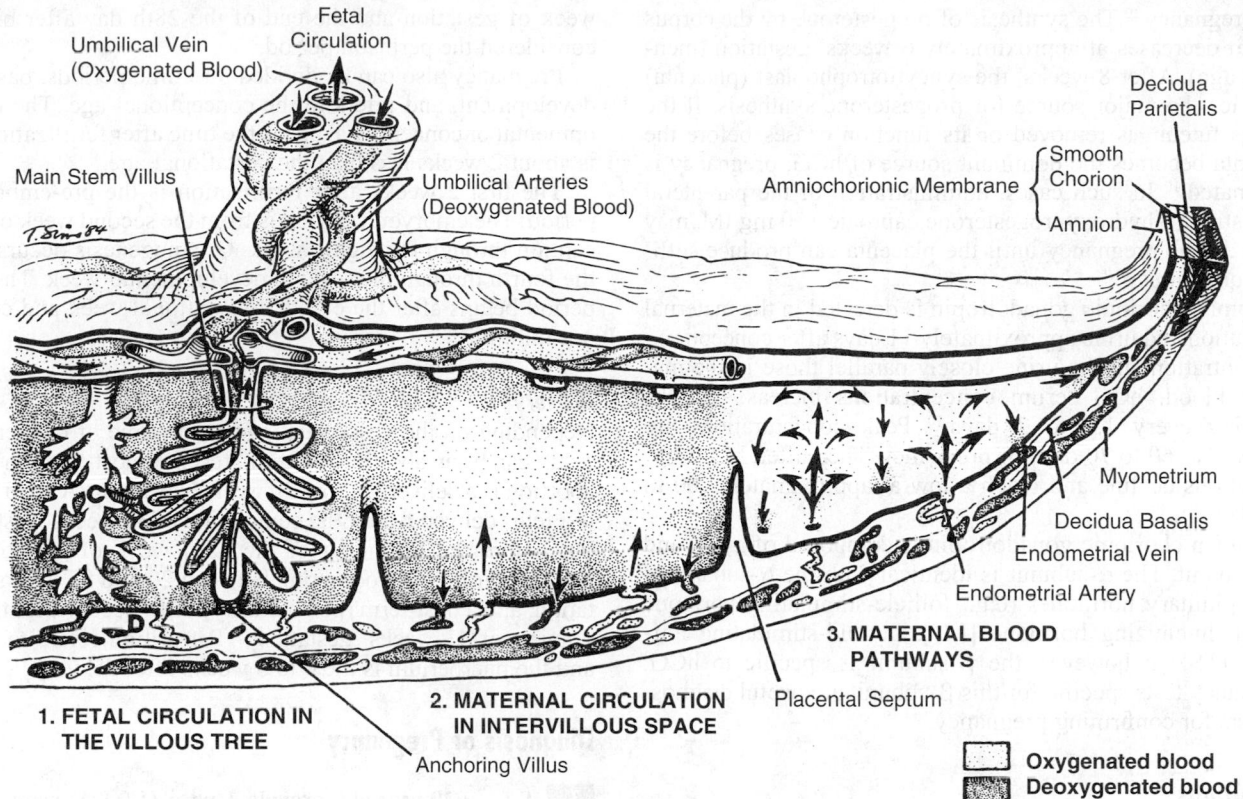

FIGURE 46-1 Term placenta. 1. The relation of the villous chorion (C) to the decidua basalis (D) and fetal placental circulation. 2. The maternal placenta circulation. Maternal blood flows into the intervillous spaces in the funnel-shaped spurts, and exchanges occur with the fetal blood as the maternal blood flows around the villi. 3. The inflowing arterial blood pushes venous blood into the endometrial veins, which are scattered over the entire surface of the decidua basalis. Note also that the umbilical arteries carry deoxygenated fetal blood to the placenta and that the umbilical vein carries oxygenated blood to the fetus. (Reprinted with permission from The placenta and fetal membranes, In: Cunningham FG et al, eds. Williams Obstetrics. New York: McGraw-Hill, 2001:102.)

ies; carbon dioxide and waste products diffuse into the intervillous spaces and are carried away by the maternal decidual veins.[4] A description of fetal circulation can be found in Chapter 94, Neonatal Therapy.

The placenta has many functions in pregnancy.[4] In addition to respiratory functions, the placenta also has excretory functions, similar to those of the postnatal kidney (e.g., maintaining water and pH balance). The placenta also has resorptive functions similar to those of the gastrointestinal (GI) tract.[4] The placenta and the fetus regulate the course of pregnancy. This fetoplacental unit functions as the endocrine portion of the fetal-maternal communication system, producing several hormones responsible for regulating and maintaining pregnancy (e.g., hCG, estrogens, progesterone, placental lactogen).[7] The placenta also produces many other hormones, enzymes, proteins, and releasing factors.[7]

Fetal Membranes

The fetal membranes are made up of an innermost membrane, the amnion, and an outer membrane, the chorion. These make up the "water bag." The amnion at term gestation is a tough but pliable membrane whose integrity is vital for the continuation and progression of pregnancy.[5] The fluid-filled space between the amnion and the embryo is the amniotic cavity. The

membranes surround the developing fetus and function to contain the amniotic fluid and assist in its formation. This fluid provides a mechanically buffered, stable environment in which the fetus develops. The amniotic fluid has both maternal and fetal sources and is the paracrine arm of the fetal-maternal coomunication unit. The maternal source is plasma filtrate and, as pregnancy advances, the fetal contribution is from urine and lung fluids. The volume of amniotic fluid increases from 50 mL at 12 weeks' gestation to a maximum of 1,000 mL at 36 weeks, and declines at term.[9] The composition of the amniotic fluid includes water, fetal cells, hormones, lecithin, sphingomyelin, electrolytes, creatinine, and urea.[9] Amniotic fluid can be obtained by amniocentesis and tested for the presence of some of these substances to aid in fetal assessment. For example, the lecithin-to-sphingomyelin ratio is used as a marker of fetal lung maturity when preterm delivery is being contemplated for obstetric reasons (e.g., severe preeclampsia).[9]

Human Chorionic Gonadotropin

Human chorionic gonadotropin (hCG), produced by the trophoblasts, is responsible for maintaining the synthesis of progesterone by the corpus luteum within the ovary until the placenta is able to synthesize the amount necessary to maintain pregnancy.[10] The synthesis of progesterone by the corpus luteum decreases at approximately 6 weeks' gestation (menstrual age). After 8 weeks, the syncytiotrophoblast (placenta) becomes the major source for progesterone synthesis. If the corpus luteum is removed or its function ceases before the placenta becomes the dominant source of hCG, pregnancy is terminated.[10] In such cases, administration of the parenteral progestin, 17-hydroxyprogesterone caproate 150 mg IM, may maintain the pregnancy until the placenta can produce sufficient quantities.[10]

Human chorionic gonadotropin is detected in the maternal circulation and urine approximately 11 days after conception.[7] Concentrations in the urine closely parallel those in the maternal blood. hCG serum concentrations increase rapidly, doubling every 1.4 to 2 days.[10] Peak concentrations are achieved at 60 to 70 days of pregnancy. Thereafter, hCG concentrations decline and reach a low at approximately 100 to 130 days.

Human chorionic gonadotropin is composed of an α- and a β-subunit. The α-subunit is identical with the α-subunit of other pituitary hormones (e.g., follicle-stimulating hormone [FSH], luteinizing hormone [LH], thyroid-stimulating hormone [TSH]); however, the β-subunit is specific to hCG. Pregnancy tests specific for this β-subunit are useful diagnostic tests for confirming pregnancy.[10]

Definitions

Parity and Gravida

Parity and *gravida* are terms used to describe a pregnant woman. Parity is the number of deliveries after 20 weeks' gestation. A delivery before the completion of 20 weeks' gestation is considered an abortion and can either be elective or spontaneous. Parity is independent of the number of fetuses delivered (live or stillborn, single fetus, or twins) or the method of delivery. The term *nullipara* describes a woman who has never delivered a fetus after 20 weeks' gestation, regardless of whether or not she aborted previously (elective or spontaneous). A *primipara* is a woman who has delivered a fetus beyond 20 weeks' gestation, and a *multipara* is a woman who has had two or more deliveries. *Gravida* refers to the number of pregnancies a woman has had regardless of the outcome. A *nulligravida* has never been pregnant, a *primigravida* has been pregnant once, and a *multigravida* has been pregnant two or more times. For example, a woman who is currently pregnant and has previously delivered one set of twins and had two spontaneous abortions is described as a gravida 4 para 1 ($G_4 P_1$). The past obstetric history can be further described by a series of digits. The first digit refers to the number of term infants delivered, the second digit refers to the number of preterm infants, the third digit refers to the number of abortions, and the fourth digit refers to the number of children currently alive. For example, a woman who has had one abortion and delivered three term infants who are still alive is described as a 3-0-1-3.[11]

Trimesters of Pregnancy

The average pregnancy is approximately 280 days or 40 weeks when calculated from the first day of the LMP. Pregnancy is typically divided into three trimesters, approximately 13 to 14 weeks each.[11] The time between the end of the 22nd week of gestation and the end of the 28th day after birth is considered the perinatal period.[2]

Pregnancy also can be divided into time periods, based on development, and refers to the conceptional age. The developmental or conceptional age is the time after fertilization and is about 2 weeks less than the gestational age.[4]

The first 2 weeks after fertilization is the pre-embryonic period. The embryonic period is from the second week of conception through the eighth week. Organogenesis occurs from the fourth through the seventh developmental week. The fetal period begins after the eighth conceptional week and continues until birth.[4]

Delivery

Depending on the gestational age at the time of delivery, the result can be an abortion, preterm, term, or post-term birth. An abortion is a delivery before 20 weeks' gestation. A term infant is a fetus delivered after the completion of 37 weeks' gestation, but before the beginning of the 43rd week of gestation. A preterm birth is one occurring between 20 and 37 weeks' gestation, and a post-term (postmaturity) birth occurs after the beginning of 43 weeks' gestation.[11] Parturition refers to labor, and the puerperium is the 6 to 8 weeks after delivery.[11]

Diagnosis of Pregnancy

1. S.C., a 29-year-old, gravida 1 para (1-0-0-1) woman, has not started her menstrual period since she had unprotected intercourse about a month ago and is worried that she may be pregnant. S.C. cannot remember the exact start date of her LMP. She asks her pharmacist for help on choosing and using an over-the-counter commercially available home pregnancy test. How do these home pregnancy tests work and how should S.C. be counseled?

Commercially available home pregnancy tests are enzyme immunoassays with monoclonal or polyclonal antibodies, which bind to hCG in the urine.[12] They are highly sensitive and provide accurate results within 1 to 2 weeks after ovulation.[10,12] There are many brand-name and generic kits available. These tests can be performed privately and quickly and are easily interpreted. The results are obtained rapidly—within 1 and 5 minutes—and are highly accurate when performed at the start of the first missed menstrual period. Although home pregnancy tests are reportedly 98% to 100% accurate when used correctly, consumer studies have documented accuracy rates as low as 50% to 75% if product directions are not precisely followed.[12] Many home pregnancy tests include a second test, which should be repeated at a specified time after the first negative test result.

S.C. should purchase a product containing two tests with features she can handle most comfortably. She should be instructed to follow the printed instructions exactly to ensure accurate results and prevent her from missing an ongoing pregnancy, thereby allowing her the opportunity to make early and appropriate decisions about lifestyle changes and prenatal care. If the first test result is negative, the pharmacist should stress the importance of repeating the test in 1 week if she does not start menstruating. False-negative results occur when testing is done before the first day of a missed period or if the urine is not at room temperature.[12] False-negative results may also occur in patients with an ectopic (outside the uterus) pregnancy or ovarian cysts and in patients receiving menotropins or chorionic gonadotropin.[12] If the test is positive, S.C. should be counseled on the possible fetal effects of any medications or herbal products she may be taking and advised to see her physician.

A positive urine or blood test result for hCG is still considered a probable diagnosis of pregnancy. The diagnosis of pregnancy is positively made with the identification of fetal heart sounds, perception of active fetal movements by examiner, or visualization of embryo or fetus by sonography or radiography.[10]

Prenatal Care

Initial Visit

During the initial prenatal visit, a medical history should be obtained and a physical examination performed to establish the health status of the mother and fetus, the gestational age, and a plan for prenatal care. The pregnancy should be confirmed. The medical history should include menstrual, obstetric, medical, social, and medication histories, and the physical examination should include a general and a pelvic examination. The pelvic examination should include a Pap smear; and, if deemed necessary, cultures for gonococci and chlamydia; and inspection for genital herpes, venereal warts, trichomoniasis, and *Candida* infection. The clinician should evaluate hematological status (e.g., a complete blood cell count [CBC], blood type, D antigen [Rh factor]); infectious history (e.g., serologic test for syphilis; rubella antibody titer; HIV testing); and urinalysis (i.e., glucosuria, proteinuria, bacteriuria).[13] Baseline maternal blood pressure (BP), body weight, and body mass index should be determined.

Maternal and fetal risks should be assessed during the initial visit. High-risk pregnancies include patients with certain pre-existing medical illnesses or conditions, a history of poor obstetric performance, or evidence of malnutrition. Women should be educated about nutrition; use of medications, tobacco, alcohol, and caffeine; general hygiene; exercise; danger signals of pregnancy (e.g., vaginal bleeding, dysuria, persisitent vomiting, marked changes in intensisty or frequency of fetal movements), signs and symptoms of preeclampsia (see Question 26); and the importance of follow-up appointments.[9,13]

Follow-Up Visits

The frequency of return visits depends on the health status of the mother and fetus. Traditionally, visits are scheduled every 4 weeks for 7 months, then every 2 weeks until the last month, then weekly until delivery.[13] On every return visit, S.C.'s weight, BP, fundal height, and urinalysis for protein and glucose should be determined and recorded. She also should be evaluated for danger signals in pregnancy. During weeks 35 to 37, S.C. may need to be screened for group B streptococci with a rectovaginal culture.[13] In the third trimester, tests for syphilis, gonorrhea, chlamydia, HIV, or hepatitis should be repeated if she is at increased risk for these infections.[9] Fetal heart rate, growth, position, and activity should be evaluated as well as the amount of amniotic fluid. In high-risk pregnancies, it may be necessary to order genetic tests and monitor the fetus for the development of complications.[13]

Date of Confinement (Due Date)

2. **What is S.C.'s "due date"?**

The assessment of gestational age is important to determine the expected date of confinement (EDC), schedule a cesarean section, or determine when it is safe to end a pregnancy prematurely. Errors in estimating the gestational age may result in delivery of a preterm neonate. Gestational age can be determined by several methods, including the date of the LMP, pelvic examination, uterine size, and measurement of fetal parameters by ultrasound. The onset date of the LMP is most commonly used to estimate the gestational age of the fetus.

The uterine fundal height should be measured and recorded at each prenatal visit. The duration of gestation is firmly established when there is consistent agreement between the EDC and fundal height.[13] Discrepancies in estimations of gestational age should alert the physician to problems such as large fetal size, multiple pregnancies, oligohydramnios (a reduction in the amount of amniotic fluid), or intrauterine growth retardation (IUGR). In such cases, an ultrasound provides valuable information.

Because the day of conception rarely is known, it is more practical to measure the duration of pregnancy from the first day of the LMP. The EDC is generally determined by adding 7 days to the first day of the LMP, counting back 3 months, and adding 1 year (Nagele's rule).[13] This method assumes that ovulation occurs on day 14 of a 28-day menstrual cycle. The problems with this method are that many pregnant women do not know the date of their LMP, and it is inaccurate in women with irregular or prolonged menstrual cycles. S.C.'s first day of her LMP was estimated to be 6 weeks ago on August 6. It is now September 17; therefore, her EDC or "due date" is May 13. Although this may not be an accurate date, a more exact date will be estimated at future visits using fundal height and sonography.

Physiologic Changes in Pregnancy

3. S.C. is now at 16 weeks' gestation. What important physiologic changes has S.C undergone that may affect drug disposition during pregnancy?

Physiologic changes occur in almost all maternal organs during pregnancy. These physiologic changes (including the placental-fetal unit) can greatly influence the pharmacokinetic parameters of drugs.[14-17] Very little is known about pharmacokinetic and pharmacodynamic changes during pregnancy before 1993 because the U.S. Food and Drug Administration (FDA) banned the participation of women of childbearing potential in phase I or phase II clinical trials. This changed with the publication of the Guidelines for Study and Evaluation of Gender Differences in the Clinical Evaluation of Drugs.[18] The placental transfer of drugs in pregnancy and potential effects of drugs on the developing fetus are presented in Chapter 47, Teratogenicity and Drugs in Breast Milk.

Pharmacokinetic changes during pregnancy primarily involve the processes of absorption, distribution, metabolism, and excretion of drugs. Important pregnancy-induced changes affecting drug absorption are (1) a decrease in intestinal motility, which is attributed to smooth muscle relaxation by progesterone and which results in a 30% to 50% increase of gastric and intestinal emptying time; (2) 40% decrease in gastric acidity, which increases gastric pH; and (3) altered bioavailability or absorption attributable to increased incidence of nausea and vomiting. Acid-labile drugs may have increased bioavailability, whereas drugs that require acid medium for stability may have decreased bioavailability. A prolonged gastric and intestinal emptying time may decrease the maximim concentration of a drug (C_{max}) and the time to reach C_{max} of a drug, whereas the decreased intestinal transit time may increase the AUC (area under the curve) and bioavailability of a drug. In contrast, pregnancy-induced vomiting may decrease amount of drug ingested; it is therefore better to schedule medications during the evening when the incidence of nausea and vomiting is lower or to use the rectal route for drug administration. In summary, the effect of pregnancy on drug absorption is variable and depends greatly on the physicochemical properties of the drug.[14] Increased blood flow to maternal skin, which helps dissipate fetal heat production, may also increase the absorption of a topically (transdermal) administered medication.[15]

Mothers generally gain approximately 11 to 14 kg (25 to 30 lb) of weight (see Question 4) by the time of a term delivery owing to increased blood volume, increased uterine and breast size, deposition of maternal fat stores, fetal and placental growth, and amniotic and interstitial fluid accumulation.[19,20] Plasma volume increases by 6 to 8 weeks' gestation and continues to expand to 40% to 50% above pregnancy volumes by 32 to 34 weeks' gestation.[14,15] Plasma volume expands even more with multiple gestations. Total body water (TBW) increases by 8 L; 40% of this increase can be attributable to the mother and 60% to the fetal-placental unit. This increase in TBW necessitates larger loading doses of water-soluble drugs (e.g., aminoglycosides) because of the increase in volume of distribution (Vd). However, increases in the Vd of drugs secondary to decreased protein binding (e.g., phenytoin) do not necessitate increasing loading doses because the unbound or free fraction (f_u) is decreased. Plasma albumin concentrations decrease during pregnancy mostly because of dilution by the increased plasma volume.[14,15]

Albumin concentrations during pregmancy may be decreased because of decreased synthesis and/or increased catabolism.[15] Total protein and α_1-acid glycoprotein concentrations remain fairly unchanged. In addition, increased concentrations of steroid and placental hormones may decrease protein-binding sites for drugs.[16] These changes in protein binding generally result in decreased protein binding, increased (f_u) fraction of drugs, and increased clearance of drugs when clearance is dependent on f_u (e.g., valproic acid, carbamazepine).[17] However, when both f_u and intrinsic clearance are increased as is the case with increased cytochrome P450 enzyme activity, both the total and free concentrations are decreased (e.g., phenytoin, phenobarbital).[17]

Renal blood flow increases by 25% to 50% early during gestation, and glomerular filtration rate (GFR) increases by 50% by the beginning of the second trimester. As a result, renal drug excretion (e.g., β-lactams) can increase.[14,20] GFR begins to increase in the first half of the first trimester.[16] The increased cardiac output and regional blood flow (e.g., renal blood flow), primarily are due to increased stroke volume and

increased heart rate, which can increase drug distribution and drug excretion.

Hepatic blood flow, as a percentage of the cardiac output, is decreased; however, the rate (L/min) remains unchanged.[15] CYP3A4 and CYP2D6 activities are increased during pregnancy.[15–17] CYP1A2, xanthine oxidase, and N-acetyltransferase activity are decreased, presumably from increased progesterone concentrations.[16,17,20] As a result, the clearance of caffeine can be decreased by 70%.[20] The activity of nonhepatic enzymes (e.g., plasma cholinesterase) is also decreased.[17]

Interpretation of pharmacokinetic data from pregnant women must be tempered by potential non-adherence to drug regimens secondary to maternal fear of fetal teratogenicity. The cardiovascular changes and the resultant pharmacokinetic changes can extend as long as 12 well weeks postpartum.[15] Altered hepatic enzyme activity may revert to normal within 24 hours or as late as a few months after delivery.

The physiologic changes that occur during pregnancy also can affect the interpretation of laboratory parameters. For example, the normal values for serum creatinine in adults is 0.6 to 1.2 mg/dL.[21] During pregnancy, the serum creatinine concentration is lower because of the increased GFR, resulting in normal serum creatinine values of 0.3 to 0.7 mg/dL in the first and second trimesters.[21] Similar changes occur with serum urea nitrogen and uric acid concentrations. These differences have important implications when assessing renal function in a pregnant patient. A serum creatinine indicative of normal renal function in a nonpregnant woman may be indicative of renal insufficiency in a woman who is pregnant in her third trimester. Generally, normal values for liver function tests are unaltered during pregnancy.[21] Clinicians should refer to an obstetric text for clinical laboratory values in pregnancy.

NUTRITION

Pregnancy increases the requirements of all nutrients, and prenatal vitamins are prescribed to help meet these needs. A low pre-pregnant weight, inadequate protein and caloric intake, and inadequate weight gain during pregnancy may result in preterm labor, IUGR, perinatal mortality, or the delivery of a low-birth-weight infant. Uneducated and low family income women are at risk for inadequate weight gain and preterm labor.[22] Poor nutrition is also more common in black, young, or unmarried women. Low-birth-weight infants have an increased risk for neurologic impairment, retarded growth, and increased perinatal mortality. Excessive maternal weight gain may result in a high-birth-weight baby (>9 pounds), increasing the risk of difficult delivery (e.g., prolonged labor, forceps or cesarean delivery) and infant morbidity (e.g., shoulder dystocia, birth trauma) and mortality (e.g., asphyxia).[23] To ensure normal fetal development and maintain maternal health, nutrition during pregnancy should stress a diet that provides an intake of protein, calories, and nutrients that allows adequate weight gain during pregnancy.

Assessing the nutritional status of a pregnant woman and providing nutritional counseling are critical early in prenatal care. The nutrition assessment should include clinical observations (physical signs of malnutrition), anthropometric data (weight, height, and possibly arm and arm muscle circumference and skinfold thickness), laboratory data (hemoglobin, hematocrit, serum albumin, and electrolytes), and history (social, medical, and obstetrical).[19] Additional tests may be needed in special populations such as other measures of protein metabolism (urinary creatinine and urine urea nitrogen), anemia (transferrin, ferritin, and total iron-binding capacity), or fat- or water-soluble vitamins.[19] A history of eclampsia, anemia, diabetes, renal or heart disease, or hyperemesis should be noted.

Some patients require special nutritional attention. Overweight women are at higher risk for pregnancy-induced hypertension, gestational diabetes mellitus, urinary tract infections, and pyelonephritis.[19] They are also more likely to have prolonged labor and are therefore more likely to need delivery by cesarean section. Requirements for calories, protein, and calcium are higher in pregnant adolescents than in pregnant adults because adolescents still are developing and growing and often have inadequate diets.[19]

Women who have multiple pregnancies over a short period of time; ingest unusual diets; or abuse alcohol, nicotine, or drugs; and women with chronic systemic diseases such as diabetes mellitus or malabsorption problems have special nutritional needs.[19]

Energy Requirements

Energy requirements increase as pregnancy progresses and resting basal metabolic rate increases.[19,24] Fetal growth needs also need consideration and are greatest during the last quarter of pregnancy. The total energy cost of pregnancy is estimated to be 85,000 kcal (i.e., about 300 more kcal/day—less during the first trimester and more during the third trimester).[19] The increase in calories to be consumed helps to ensure maternal weight gain and to provide energy required to build tissue for the developing fetus.[19] Energy can be derived from various sources. Stored maternal fat and protein and consumed fat, protein, and carbohydrates are all sources of energy. Obese women and those who continue to be physically active may require a greater energy intake.[19]

Protein Requirements

Protein is needed as a building material for new maternal and fetal cells. Although somewhat controversial, inadequate protein intake may lead to pre-eclampsia.[19] The National Research Council recommends increasing daily protein intake by about 10 g/day during pregnancy to support fetal and placental growth and to support maternal tissues (uterus and breasts), blood volume, and amniotic fluid formation.[19] The consumption of excessive protein, however, can cause premature deliveries, neonatal death, or restricted fetal growth.[19] The importance of a balanced diet must be stressed with pregnant patients.

Weight Gain

4. A nutritional assessment of S.C. reveals a 5 ft 3 in., 141 lb, healthy female. She is not taking any medications or vitamins and does not have significant medical or social history. She eats three meals a day and tries to eat fruits and vegetables when possible (about three servings per day). She is concerned that she has only gained 2 pounds during her first 6 weeks of pregnancy.

Should S.C. be eating the same types of food that she was eating before she became pregnant and is her weight gain sufficient?

On average, women gain 25 to 30 pounds during pregnancy.[19,25] The recommendations for weight gain are based on body mass index (BMI), defined as weight/height^2 (kg/m^2), rather than weight only (Table 46-1).[19,25] BMI is used as an indicator of nutritional status, assuming that thin women have low tissue reserves and obese women have excessive ones. Weight gain recommendations should be used only as a guide and are intended for singleton pregnancies. A 35- to 45-pound weight gain has been associated with a favorable pregnancy outcome in women carrying twins.[19,26]

S.C.'s BMI is 25 [64 kg/(1.6 m)^2], which is normal. During a normal singleton pregnancy, weight gain usually is minimal during the first trimester (2 to 5 pounds) and averages about 1 pound weekly during the last two trimesters.[19] Therefore, S.C. is gaining weight appropriately. Weight gains of <1 to 2 lbs or >6 lbs in the same time frame should be evaluated. S.C. should be weighed at every prenatal visit.

S.C. should be encouraged to eat four to five servings of fruits and vegetables daily, along with four or more servings of grains, bread, or cereal.[27] S.C. also may wish to speak to a nutritionist for recommendations on achieving adequate dietary protein intake.

Vitamins and Minerals

5. What vitamin and mineral supplementation would you recommend for S.C. and when should she begin taking these products?

A balanced diet that provides S.C. with multiple B vitamins, oil-soluble vitamins (A, E, D, and K), folic acid, and minerals (iron, calcium, phosphorus, magnesium, iodine, zinc) should be encouraged.

Iron Requirements

Iron requirements increase during pregnancy because of maternal blood volume expansion, fetal needs, placenta and cord needs, and blood loss at time of delivery.[19] Maternal iron deficiency can cause anemia during infancy, spontaneous abortion, premature delivery, and delivery of a low-birth-weight infant.[19]

A woman needs about 18 to 21 mg of iron/day during pregnancy, and as a result, the body compensates by increasing iron absorption from the GI tract by about 15% to 50% during pregnancy.[19] The average diet of women in the United States does not meet these requirements because only about 6 mg of iron are absorbed from 1,000 kcal of food. In addition,

Table 46-1	Recommended Weight Gain During Pregnancy

Prepregnancy Weight for Height (BMI)	Total Weight Gain Recommendations (lb)
Low: <19.8	28–40
Normal: 19.8–26	25–35
High: 26.1–29	15–25
Obese: >29	≥15

BMI, body mass index. BMI is weight/height^2 (kg/m^2).
From reference 19.

some women may already have inadequate body stores of iron before pregnancy. For these reasons, the Food and Nutrition Board of the National Research Council recommends a daily elemental iron supplementation of 30 mg during the second and third trimesters of pregnancy.[28] Prenatal vitamins usually contain 30 to 60 mg of elemental iron. Women with iron deficiency anemia should be given 60 to 120 mg of elemental iron daily. Iron deficiency anemia during pregnancy generally is associated with a hemoglobin and hematocrit <11% and 33%, respectively, during the first and third trimesters or below 10.5% and 32%, respectively, during the second trimester. The risk for iron deficiency is exacerbated by menorrhagia, multiple gestation, closely spaced pregnancies, low meat and ascorbic acid diet, chronic aspirin or nonsteroidal anti-inflammatory drug (NSAID) use, and frequent (>3 times/yr) blood donations.[30] These women may require 60 to 100 mg/day of elemental iron during the last two trimesters of pregnancy.

Iron supplementation decreases the development of iron deficiency anemia, which increases the risk for a poor pregnancy outcome. Anemic women are more likely to suffer adverse effects from blood loss during delivery, hemorrhage secondary to other causes, or infections after delivery.[30] On the other hand, iron can cause GI adverse effects (e.g., heartburn, nausea, abdominal discomfort, constipation, diarrhea, discoloration of stools). Young children may also mistake iron for candy; therefore, iron supplements should be stored carefully. Iron absorption can be enhanced by taking the supplements between meals and by avoiding the concurrent ingestion of milk, tea, coffee, or antacids. Taking iron concurrently with food can reduce adverse GI effects and should be recommended despite lower absorption (also see Chapter 86, Anemias).

S.C.'s hemoglobin and hematocrit should be assessed today and again at 26 to 28 weeks' gestation. If her hemoglobin and hematocrit are normal, she will not need more iron than what is already available in a prenatal vitamin. S.C. should be given a prescription for iron because she is not currently taking a prenatal vitamin and may need additional iron later in her pregnancy if anemia develops.

Folate Requirements

Folic acid is essential in the synthesis of DNA and RNA. Pregnant women who take 0.4 to 0.8 mg of folic acid daily during the first trimester of pregnancy are significantly less likely to have a child with neural tube defects (NTDs) such as spina bifida and anencephaly.[31,32] NTDs may lead to stillbirth, neonatal death, or serious disabilities. Approximately 4,000 pregnancies in the United States are affected by NTDs each year.[33]

NTDs can develop within the first month of pregnancy at a time when many women are unaware of their pregnancy (>50% of pregnancies in the United States are unplanned).[33,32] In 1992, the U.S. Public Health Service recommended that all women with child-bearing potential should consume 0.4 mg/day of folic acid to reduce the risk of an NTD-affected pregnancy.[32] If this practice were implemented in the United States, the incidence of NTDs could possibly be reduced by 50%.

It may be difficult to meet the RDA (recommended daily allowance) for folic acid because foods contain only a small amount of this vitamin: overcooking and high fiber diets also can reduce the amount of available folic acid from food.[19] Most prenatal vitamins contain 0.8 to 1 mg of folic acid.

Folic acid supplementation is especially important in women with a history of infants born with NTDs. Women who have had an NTD-affected pregnancy should receive genetic counseling because they have a 2% to 3% risk of having another such outcome. Women with previous NTD-affected pregnancies, who plan another pregnancy, should take 4 mg/day of folic acid at least 1 month before conception and through the first 3 months of pregnancy.[34] In one study of 1,195 women with a previous NTD pregnancy, six experienced another NTD pregnancy despite high-dose folic acid (4 mg/day) compared with 21 women who did not receive high-dose folic acid.[35]

Women, who require 4 mg/day of folic acid, should be prescribed folic acid tablets rather than combination prenatal multivitamins, which contain folic acid. When several fixed-combination multivitamin tablets are taken daily, the mother could be exposed to a potentially teratogenic dose of vitamin A. High doses of folic acid do not prevent NTDs better than 0.4 mg/day in women without a previous history of NTD-affected pregnancies and may complicate the diagnosis of a B_{12} deficiency.[32]

S.C. should be counseled about the risks for NTDs, especially because she has not been taking a folic acid–containing vitamin during the first weeks of her pregnancy. She should receive adequate folic acid during the remainder of her pregnancy from a daily prenatal vitamin.

Calcium Requirements

Calcium is needed during pregnancy for adequate mineralization of the fetal skeleton and teeth, especially during the third trimester when teeth are formed and skeletal growth is greatest.[19] The RDA for calcium during pregnancy is 1,200 mg/day.[19] Some argue that less calcium is needed because calcium absorption is enhanced and renal excretion of calcium is decreased during pregnancy.[19] Large maternal stores can provide calcium if dietary intake is inadequate; however, depleting maternal stores may put S.C. at risk for osteoporosis later in life. Foods rich in calcium (e.g., milk, cheese, yogurt, legumes, nuts, dried fruits) or calcium supplements can be used to meet the calcium RDA.[16] Calcium also has beneficial effects in reducing hypertensive disorders of pregnancy and preterm labor.[19]

Nutrition During Breast-Feeding

6. S.C. expresses the desire to breast-feed her child after delivery. What nutritional advice should be provided to her?

Breast-feeding reduces the risk of breast and ovarian cancer, saves money, and helps women to physically recover from pregnancy. Passive maternal immunity to viral and bacterial diseases can be provided to S.C.'s baby through breast-feeding, and breast-fed babies also have decreased risks of respiratory and diarrheal diseases.[36]

Breast-fed infants consume approximately 600 to 900 mL daily of breast milk.[36] Thus, the lactating woman needs a diet that supplies more nutrients compared with that of a nonlactating woman. Dietary supplements are not necessary if S.C. has a well-balanced diet. Lactation increases energy expenditures by approximately 500 kcal/day.[36] The energy costs of lactation can be met by a combination of increased caloric intake and tissue mobilization. Rapid weight loss after pregnancy may reduce ability to synthesize milk; therefore, weight loss after pregnancy should be gradual over 6 months. Once lactation has been established, modest caloric restriction does not affect milk quality or quantity. S.C. may exercise without adverse effects on her breast milk.[36]

COMMON COMPLAINTS OF PREGNANCY
Nausea and Vomiting

7. Now S.C. is 10 weeks pregnant, and the nausea and vomiting has worsened. How long is her nausea and vomiting likely to last?

Nausea and vomiting during pregnancy (NVP) are common, occur in 50% to 89% of pregnancies, usually appear by 4 to 8 weeks' gestation, and generally disappear by the 16th week of gestation.[37,38] Most women have mild nausea and vomiting, whereas about 10% experience moderate nausea and vomiting sufficiently severe to require treatment.[37] Severe intractable nausea and vomiting is referred to as hyperemesis gravidarum and occurs in 0.05% to 1% of pregnancies.[38] Hyperemesis gravidarum can lead to metabolic acidosis, ketosis, hypovolemia, electrolyte disturbances, and weight loss.[37,38]

The cause of NVP is unknown, although a combination of hormonal, psychologic, and neurologic factors have been implicated.[37,38] Elevations in hCG, which has structural similarities TSH, may be the cause of the emesis. Reductions in lower esophageal pressure, gastric peristalsis, and gastric emptying may worsen nausea and vomiting. S.C. may be evaluated for other causes of nausea and vomiting (e.g., urinary tract infection, hypercalcemia, thyrotoxicosis, diabetic ketoacidosis, hepatitis, drugs, gastritis).[38]

Nonpharmacologic Management

8. How should S.C.'s NVP be managed?

Most mild forms of NVP can be managed with psychologic support and dietary changes. A light snack upon arising can be helpful in the management of morning nausea.[37,38] Eating smaller, more frequent meals rich in carbohydrates and sipping small quantities of fluids also may help decrease nausea and vomiting. Ingestion of a high-protein drink can decrease nausea significantly better than high-carbohydrate and high-fat liquid meals during the first trimester.[39] S.C. should be instructed to avoid cooking or smelling foods that she associates with precipitating these symptoms. Foods high in fat content can delay gastric emptying; therefore, it may be helpful to avoid fatty, fried, or spicy foods until the end of the first trimester. Iron supplements can cause GI discomfort and should be discontinued if associated with S.C.'s symptoms.[37,38] Nausea and vomiting rarely continue beyond the fourth month of pregnancy.

Pharmacologic Management

9. S.C. does not respond to nonpharmacologic treatment of her nausea and vomiting. What antiemetic would be appropriate for her?

Antiemetics are indicated for the treatment of moderate nausea and vomiting that fails to respond to nonpharmacologic interventions and especially are necessary when the nausea or vomiting threatens the metabolic or nutritional status of the mother (e.g., hyperemesis gravidarum). Unfortunately, nausea and vomiting most commonly occur during the first trimester when the developing embryo is most susceptible to the teratogenic effects of drugs.[39] Most antiemetics (e.g., phenothiazines, antihistamines, promotility agents) are classified in pregnancy category B or C (Table 46-2)[40] Teratogenicity is always a concern because many drugs cross the placenta.[40,41] Antihistamines may be effective in treating S.C.'s NVP and have been used for this indication for decades. Meclizine (Antivert) 25 to 50 mg/day has not been shown to be teratogenic in humans.[40,41] Dimenhydrinate (Dramamine) 50 to 100 mg every 4 hours may be associated with cardiovascular defects or inguinal hernias in infants exposed in utero, but the overall risks of teratogenicity are low.[40,41] Congenital defects also have been reported in infants exposed to phenothiazines in utero,[40,41] but the risk of teratogenicity is small if used occasionally in low doses (see Chapter 47, Teratogenicity and Drugs in Breast Milk). Promethazine (Phenergan) 12.5 to 25 mg PO or IM BID-QID and prochlorperazine (Compazine) 5 to 10 mg PO or IM TID-QID have been used safely and effectively to manage NVP.[42]

Metoclopramide (Reglan) 5 to 10 mg PO TID, or 5 to 20 mg IV or IM TID, can control vomiting and gastric reflux associated with pregnancy.[42] No malformations have been reported in infants born to mothers given this drug and is the

Table 46-2 Pregnancy Categories for Gastrointestinal Medications

Drug	Pregnancy Category[a]
Cimetidine	B$_m$
Dimenhydrinate	B$_m$
Famotidine	B
Granisetron	B
Lansoprazole	B
Meclizine	B
Metoclopramide	B$_m$
Misoprostol	X
Nizatidine	B$_m$
Omeprazole	C$_m$
Ondansetron	B$_m$
Prochlorperazine	C
Promethazine	C
Ranitidine	B$_m$
Sucralfate	B$_m$
Trimethobenzamide	C

[a]Manufacturer's rating, when one is available, is denoted by m.
Category A: Controlled studies in women fail to demonstrate risk to the fetus.
Category B: Either animal studies have not demonstrated a risk and there are no controlled studies in women, or animal studies have shown a risk that has not been confirmed in humans.
Category C: Either studies in animals have shown an adverse effect on the fetus and there are no controlled studies in women, or no studies in women or animals are available.
Category D: There is evidence of fetal harm, but the benefit of the medication may outweigh the risk.
Category X: There is evidence of fetal harm, and no benefit of the medication outweighs the risk.
From reference 40.

antiemetic of choice in many countries.[41,42] Ondansetron (Zofran) has been used in the treatment of hyperemesis gravidarum, but has been evaluated in only small numbers of patients.[41] Trimethobenzamide (Tigan), which may be given orally or rectally, has been used in pregnancy to treat nausea and vomiting without observation of adverse effects in the fetus.[40]

Alternative therapies (e.g., vitamin B$_6$, ginger root, acupuncture, acupressure) have improved NVP in small number of patients.[38] Intravenous fluids, total parenteral nutrition, and enteral nutrition may be needed in hyperemesis gravidarum.[38] Corticosteroids may also improve nausea and vomiting symptoms.[38,41] S.C. may be started on meclizine, metoclopramide, or prochlorperazine. Drug selection for S.C. mostly depends on the tolerability of adverse effects.

Constipation and Hemorrhoids

10. During her second trimester, S.C. returns for a follow-up visit complaining of constipation and hemorrhoids. What can she do to reduce the symptoms or treat the problems?

Elevations in estrogen and progesterone, which inhibit smooth muscles in GI tract; reductions in motility, which stimulates smooth muscles in the small and large bowel; increased intestinal pressure secondary to hemorrhoids or the gravid uterus; iron supplementation; decreased activity; and dehydration are some of the multiple causes of constipation during pregnancy.[44] As a result, 10% to 30% of women experience constipation at some stage during pregnancy.[44,45]

S.C. should be instructed to drink plenty of water, exercise, and increase the bulk in her diet with vegetables, fruits, high-fiber cereals, and whole grains as nonpharmacological approaches to maintaining normal bowel function. She also should try to time her bowel movements for after a meal to take advantage of gastrocolic reflex.[44] If these nonpharmacologic interventions do not work, S.C. should try stool softeners (e.g., docusate 100 to 200 mg/day), mild laxatives (e.g., milk of magnesia 30 mL once or twice daily), or bulk-producing products (e.g., Metamucil 1 teaspoonful one to three times daily). Strong cathartics and enemas should be avoided. Use of castor oil or stimulants such as bisacodyl (Dulcolax) and senna is not recommended.[44]

Hemorrhoids produce itching, anal protrusion of a mass, pain, and occasional bleeding and occur during pregnancy because the enlarging uterus exerts pressure on the middle and inferior hemorrhoidal vessels.[37,44] In addition, a 25% to 40% increase in blood volume during pregnancy increases venous dilation and engorgement.[44] S.C. can try hemorrhoidal ointments or suppositories, which are sometimes helpful, and should use stool softeners (e.g., docusate) to minimize straining during a bowel movement, which further exacerbates her hemorrhoids. Sitz baths two to three times daily also can be used to decrease hemorrhoidal symptoms.[44]

Reflux Esophagitis

11. S.C. is now 30 weeks pregnant and no longer complains of nausea or vomiting. Her hemorrhoids have improved with the periodic use of rectal hydrocortisone and daily docusate. However, now she has heartburn that worsens when she lies down.

What causes reflux esophagitis in pregnancy and how should S.C. manage this problem?

Reflux esophagitis or heartburn occurs in >25% of pregnant women, usually in the third trimester.[46] The enlarging uterus increases intra-abdominal pressure, and estrogen and progesterone relax the esophageal sphincter. These two factors cause the reflux of stomach acid into the lower esophagus, producing symptoms of substernal burning worsened by eating, lying down, or bending over (also see Chapter 27, Upper Gastrointestinal Disorders).[46]

S.C. should avoid taking unnecessary medications because of her pregnancy and first try nondrug treatment: eating smaller, more frequent meals; avoiding meals close to bedtime; and avoiding salicylates, caffeine, alcohol, and nicotine. Elevation of the head of the bed by 4 to 6 inches is often helpful.[46] If these modifications are not successful, S.C. should try a calcium carbonate antacid. Animal studies have not shown antacids to cause teratogenic effects, and human data are limited. Sodium bicarbonate can cause metabolic alkalosis and fluid overload and should be avoided.[46] Magnesium-containing antacids may slow or stop labor and may cause convulsion if given late in pregnancy.[46] Despite evidence of fetal toxicity with aluminum, available data suggest that usual doses of aluminum-containing medications are not harmful to the fetus of a pregnant woman with normal renal function.[40]

Sucralfate (Carafate), which contains aluminum, appears to be safe in pregnancy. The American College of Gastroenterology has classified sucralfate as a medication with benefits that outweigh the risks when used in pregnant women.[40] H$_2$-receptor antagonists (see Table 46-2) can be used when necessary because most studies in animals and humans have not found fetal harm with cimetidine (Tagamet), ranitidine (Zantac), famotidine (Pepcid), or nizatidine (Axid).[40,46] Animal data with lansoprazole (Prevacid) have been positive, but little human data are available.[40] The proton pump inhibitors should be avoided during pregnancy, at least during the first trimester, but preferably during any part of gestation because birth defects have been reported in animal pregnancies in which omeprazole (Prilosec) was used.[40]

PREVENTION OF RH D ALLOIMMUNIZATION
Maternal-Fetal Rh Incompatibility

12. G.G., a 34-year-old primigravida, had her ABO blood group and Rh status determined during her initial prenatal visit. She is determined to be type O, Rh-negative. Her husband is type O, Rh-positive. What are the risks associated with Rh incompatibility that could affect G.G.'s unborn infant?

Blood group incompatibility between a pregnant female and her fetus can result in alloimmunization of the mother and hemolytic anemia in the fetus. When a female is exposed during pregnancy, labor, or delivery to a fetal erythrocyte antigen (i.e., AB, Rh-complex) that is not found on her own erythrocytes, she forms antibodies against that antigen. This is referred to as alloimmunization. Antibodies of the IgG class cross the placenta and can interact with the fetal erythrocyte antigens, resulting ultimately in their destruction and leading to hemolytic disease of the newborn (HDN).[47] Rh and ABO incompatibility are the most common causes of immune HDN in neonates.[47] ABO incompatibility occurs in 20% to 25% of all pregnancies, but HDN is clinically present in approximately 10% of fetuses. An ABO incompatibility occurs almost exclusively when a type O mother is carrying a type A (specifically A_1) or B fetus. Type O mothers produce anti-A and anti-B antibodies that are predominantly IgG, whereas antibodies produced by those who are type A or B are predominantly immunoglobulin M (IgM).[47] Only maternal IgG production results in HDN because it is the only immunoglobulin that crosses that placenta.

ABO incompatibility in the newborn is manifested clinically in the first 24 hours after birth as hemolytic anemia and hyperbilirubinemia. The problem usually is managed by following serial bilirubin serum concentrations and phototherapy. Occasionally, exchange transfusion may be required.[47] HDN secondary to ABO incompatibility rarely causes the severity of disease that is observed with Rh incompatibility. An ABO incompatibility should not be a problem for G.G.'s unborn child because both she and her husband are type O.

Rh alloimmunization is much more severe and is associated with fetal and neonatal morbidity and mortality. The Rh antigen complex is the expression of at least five antigens. Rh incompatability to the D antigen causes most of the hemolytic disease of the fetus and newborn. Therefore, Rh positivity usually is assumed to be due to the presence of the D antigen. An Rh D–negative mother becomes immunized during exposure to fetal erythrocytes that carry the D antigen.[48] The Rh D antigen is expressed on fetal red blood cells (RBCs) by 38 days after conception or 52 days from the last menstrual period. The likelihood of having an Rh D–positive offspring is determined by whether an Rh D–positive father is homozygous or heterozygous for the D antigen. If the father is homozygous for the D antigen, all of his offspring will be D positive (Rh-positive). If he is only heterozygous for the D antigen, then there is a 50% chance that his offspring will be Rh-positive.[48]

Pregnant women can produce detectable IgG antibodies to Rh antigens within 6 weeks to 6 months.[47] These antibodies can cross the placenta during subsequent pregnancies and destroy fetal Rh D–positive RBCs. Seventeen percent of Rh D–negative women become alloimmunized during pregnancy.[49] Approximately 90% of pregnancy-induced alloimmunizations result from fetomaternal hemorrhage at delivery. Ten percent of these cases are a result of spontaneous fetomaternal hemorrhage during the third trimester. As little as 0.1 mL of blood can immunize a human. A concomitant ABO incompatibility between an Rh D–positive fetus and the Rh D–negative mother can partially protect the mother against alloimmunization.[48] This is because the ABO-incompatible RBCs are rapidly hemolyzed and sequestered in the liver, where there is a lower potential for antibody production.

The severity of Rh-associated HDN or erythroblastosis fetalis depends on the concentration of antibodies the fetus is exposed to in utero. Mild disease may result only in hemolysis, but the placental transfer of significant amounts of antibody may cause substantial erythrocyte destruction. This initially results in anemia and hyperbilirubinemia with compensatory extramedullary erythropoiesis (e.g., liver, spleen). In severe hemolytic diseases, the fetus may develop hepatosplenomegaly, portal hypertension, edema, ascites, and hepatic and cardiac failure. The clinical presentation of profound anemia, anasarca, hepatosplenomegaly, cardiac failure, and circulatory collapse is termed hydrops fetalis.[48]

The fetus may be protected from high bilirubin concentrations because of maternal and placental metabolism. After birth, the neonate may become jaundiced rapidly as bilirubin concentrations exceed the newborn's capacity to metabolize bilirubin through conjugation. The resultant high concentrations of unconjugated bilirubin may exceed the albumin-binding capacity of the newborn. Unbound bilirubin can cross the blood-brain barrier and deposit in the basal ganglia of the central nervous system (CNS) leading to kernicterus.[47,48]

The severity of Rh-associated HDN also may increase with each pregnancy in the alloimmunized mother. Thus, it is important to discuss the consequences of alloimmunization with any woman who is known to be alloimmunized and wishes to have more children in the future.

$Rh_0(D)$ Immunoglobulin

13. **What interventions should be undertaken to prevent G.G. from becoming alloimmunized?**

Antepartum Prophylaxis

G.G. should have antibody screens at the beginning of each pregnancy, at 28 weeks' gestation, and postpartum. An antibody screen at 35 weeks' gestation is optional, and G.G. should be monitored closely during every pregnancy.[47]

As pregnancy progresses, both the incidence and the degree of fetomaternal hemorrhage increase. Fetomaternal hemorrhage during the third trimester accounts for nearly 2% of alloimmunization of Rh D–negative women who give birth to Rh D–positive infants.[47,49] Administrating $Rh_0(D)$ immune globulin to G.G. before or shortly after exposure to fetal Rh D–positive erythrocytes will prevent her from becoming alloimmunized. Giving $Rh_0(D)$ immune globulin at 28 to 29 weeks' gestation decreases this sensitization rate to 0.1%.

Antibody testing at 28 weeks' gestation is repeated to diagnose $Rh_0(D)$ alloimmunization because the administration of $Rh_0(D)$immune globulin is of no benefit if the patient is already alloimmunized. G.G. should be given her first dose of $Rh_0(D)$ immune globulin at 28 weeks' gestation, providing she had no major events or procedures during the first two trimesters and she tests negative for anti-$Rh_0(D)$ antibodies. G.G. can be given either one of the two parenteral formulations of human $Rh_0(D)$ immune globulin: (1) $Rh_0(D)$ IGIM (RhoGAM,HypoRho-D, Gamulin Rh) for IM use only; (or 2) $Rh_0(D)$ IGIV (WinRho SD) for both IM and IV use (Table 46-3).

The most likely mechanism by which $Rh_0(D)$ immune globulin suppresses sensitization is unknown, but it is believed to involve suppression of the primary immune response to the D antigen.[47] The anti-D immune globulin binds the D antigen, and this complex is filtered by the spleen and lymph nodes whereby it inhibits D antigen-specific B cells from proliferating.

Postpartum Prophylaxis

A second dose of $Rh_0(D)$ immune globulin should be repeated within 72 hours of delivery. A larger dose is needed if a large transplacental bleed occurs at the time of delivery (0.4% of cases). Therefore, all $Rh_0(D)$–negative women who deliver an $Rh_0(D)$–postive newborn should be tested to detect fetal RBCs in maternal blood (e.g., Kleihauer-Betke test) to calculate the correct dose of $Rh_0(D)$ immune globulin.[47,48]

Table 46-3 Recommendations for the Administration of Rho (D) Immune Globulin to an Rh₀ (D)–Negative Pregnant Woman

Clinical Event or Procedure[a]	Rh₀(D) IMIG (IM Route Only)	Rh₀(D) IVIG (IV or IM Route)
Antepartum prophylaxis at 26–28 wk	300 µg IM	1,500 U (300 µg) IV or IM
After delivery within 72 hr	300 µg IM	600 U (120 µg) IV or IM
Spontaneous or elective abortion[b], ruptured tubal pregnancy	≤12 wk : 50 µg IM	600 U (120 µg) IV or IM
	≥13 wk: 300 µg IM	
Amniocentesis, percutaneous umbilical blood sampling, chorionic villus sampling, abdominal trauma[c]	300 µg IM[d]	≤34 wk: 1,500 U IV or IM
		≥35 wk: 600 U IV or IM
Threatened abortion at any GA[c]	300 µg IM	1,500 U IV or IM
Massive fetal-maternal hemorrhage	300 µg IM per 30 ml whole blood or	IM route
	300 µg IM per 15 ml PRBC	60 U (12 µg) per 1mL whole blood or
		120 U (24 µg) per 1 mL PRBC
		IV route
		45 U (9µg) per 1 mL whole blood or
		90 U (18 µg per 1 mL PRBC
		Divide in doses of 3,000 U (600 µg) Q 8 hr

[a]Father is Rho(D)–positive or paternal status unknown.
[b]Give immediately after pregnancy termination, preferably within 3 hours but no later than 72 hours.
[c]Additional doses should be given Q 12 weeks antepartum to maintain adequate titers throughout pregnancy.
[d]If given between 13 and 18 weeks; repeat dose at 28 weeks.
IMIG, intramuscular immune globulin; IVIG, intravenous immune globulin.
From reference 50.

Adverse Effects Rh₀(D) Immune Globulin

The plasma, from which immune globulin is obtained, is tested for viral infections and the manufacturing process used to produce Rh₀(D) immune globulin inactivates viruses such as HIV, HBV, and HCV.[47–49] Adverse reactions associated with the use of anti-D immune globulin are rare. Pain and swelling at the injection site and rash are the most common adverse reactions.[48] Hypersensitivity reactions such as anaphylaxis, though rare, may occur. Patients should be monitored for such reactions immediately after administration of Rh₀(D) immune globulin IV and for at least 20 minutes after Rh₀(D) IGIM injection, and epinephrine should be readily available for the treatment of anaphylaxis.[50]

Prophylaxis for First- and Second-Trimester Events and Procedures

14. G.G. will undergo amniocentesis at 16 weeks' gestation. Will she need a dose of Rh₀(D) at that time?

Rh₀(D) immune globulin should be given after all clinical events (e.g., abortion) or procedures (e.g., amniocentesis, fetal blood sampling, or chorionic villus sampling) in which fetomaternal hemorrhage is a risk in an Rh-incompatible pregnancy. The risk of maternal alloimmunization associated with abortion during the initial trimester of pregnancy is 3% to 5.5%.[47] Although there is little evidence supporting the need for prophylaxis in early pregnancy in this type of patient, adverse effects are rare and the benefits outweigh the risks.[51] Indications and dosage regimens for Rh₀(D) immune globulin are listed in Table 46-3.

Length of Protection

15. G.G. had an amniocentesis at 16 weeks for which she received Rh₀(D) IGIM 300 µg IM. Will she need another dose at 28 weeks' gestation? How long will this dose protect G.G. against alloimmunization?

G.G. will still need a dose of 300 µg repeated at 28 weeks' gestation and within 72 hours postpartum if her infant is Rh₀(D)–positive. The half-life of Rh₀(D) immune globulin is approximately 24 to 25 days.[47,49] Without a large fetomaternal hemorrhage, a standard dose of 300 µg will protect against alloimmunization for up to 12 weeks. If >12 weeks have lapsed between receipt of anti-D immune globulin and delivery, many practitioners recommend administering another dose[48,49] (see Table 46-3).

Failure of Immunoprophylaxis

16. What are the most common reasons for Rh D alloimmunization during pregnancy?

The most common reasons for Rh D alloimmunization are (1) failure to give a dose of anti-D immune globulin at 28 to 29 weeks' gestation; (2) failure to give Rh₀(D) immune globulin in a timely manner postpartum to women who have delivered an Rh₀(D)–positive or untyped fetus; and (3) failure to recognize clinical procedures and situations that increase maternal risk for alloimmunization (i.e., amniocentesis, abortions).[49]

Thus, G.G. should be told that with proper prophylaxis with anti-D immune globulin, there is little chance for her to become alloimmunized. She need not worry about her present pregnancy or future pregnancies.

DIABETES MELLITUS

Diabetes mellitus is the most common maternal medical complication during pregnancy.[52] In the United States, 2.7% of all live births in 1999 were complicated by maternal diabetes.[53] These women are separated into two major groups: one group includes women with pre-existing diabetes, and the second group includes women diagnosed durng pregnancy. Patients with carbohydrate intolerance that develops or is recognized during pregnancy are classified as having gestational diabetes mellitus (GDM).[54,55] The diagnosis of GDM does not depend on severity of diabetes or the type of treatment necessary.[54,55]

The American College of Obstetrics and Gynecology classifies diabetes in pregnancy according to White Classification, modified to include gestational diabetes according to glycemic control.[52] The White Classification relies on age at onset, duration of diabetes, and complications for patient classification rather than the current status of diabetic control.[56] It is still used by some physicians when comparing treatment and pregnancy outcomes for women with pre-existing diabetes mellitus (Table 46-4).[52,55]

In only 10% of the pregnancies complicated by diabetes did the mother have pre-gestational diabetes.[52,53] Less than 0.5% of all pregnancies in the United States are complicated by type 1 diabetes.[57] Most affected women are insulin-dependent patients who developed diabetes during childhood, adolescence, or young adulthood. For patients who had good diabetic control before pregnancy, the first signs of pregnancy may be fluctuating glucose levels and hyperglycemia followed by hypoglycemia, thereby necessitating multiple insulin dose changes to retain carbohydrate control. A smaller number of pregnant women have type 2 diabetes. These women typically are older and obese and are treated by diet alone or diet combined with oral hypoglycemic agents. GDM is believed by some to be type 2 diabetes, which is diagnosed during pregnancy.[52]

Pre-existing Diabetes Mellitus
Fetal and Infant Risks

17. K.H., a 27-year-old, 60-kg, woman known to have type 1 diabetes since age 12, has married recently and wishes to have children. She has been conscientious in her diabetic care and self-monitors her blood glucose concentrations with a glucometer. Over the past month, her fasting blood glucose (FBG) concentrations have ranged from 90 to 140 mg/dL. Today, her FBG and HbA$_{1c}$ laboratory results are 134 mg/dL (normal, 70 to 110) and 7.8% (normal, 4.5 to 6.5), respectively. Her BP is 145/94 mm Hg, renal function is normal, serum creatinine is 0.8 mg/dL (normal, 0.6 to 1.2), and no proteinuria. K.H. is complaining of tingling and pain in her toes. Her current human insulin regimen consists of a combination of 16 units of isophane insulin (NPH) and 8 units of regular insulin 30 minutes before breakfast, and 8 units of NPH and 4 units of regular 30 minutes before supper. How will diabetes affect the health of a child she would like to conceive?

Perinatal mortality for infants of diabetic mothers has declined dramatically with strict maternal metabolic control, improved fetal surveillance, and neonatal intensive care.[58] Fetal and neonatal mortality rates are approximately 2% to 4%, and the risk of spontaneous abortion in well-controlled type 1 diabetics is equal to that of nondiabetic women.[59] The incidence of stillbirth is greatest after 36 weeks' gestation in women with poor glycemic control, fetal macrosomia (see below), maternal vascular disease, ketoacidosis, or pre-eclampsia.[52]

The incidence of major congenital anomalies is two to four times greater (about 5% to 10%) in women with type 1 diabetes compared with that in the general population.[52] The major malformations observed are NTDs and other anomalies (caudal regression and cardiac, renal, or GI defects).[52] Many of these congenital anomalies occur before the seventh week of gestation, a time when organogenesis is occurring.[60] The risk of giving birth to an infant with a major congenital anomaly correlates with the degree of glycemic control during the time just before and the 2 months after conception.[52,58] Women with higher HbA$_{1c}$ values during this time have a significantly higher incidence of infants with anomalies compared with women with HbA$_{1c}$ closer to the normal range.[59] HbA$_{1c}$ values up to 1% above normal are associated with rates of spontaneous abortions and congenital malformations similar to those of nondiabetic pregnancies.[58]

Macrosomia, defined as birth wight >4 kg, occurs in 20% to 25% of pregnancies complicated by diabetes.[52] It is thought to be caused by fetal hyperglycemia and hyperinsulinemia.[52] These infants are at greater risk for metabolic complications and trauma during delivery because of their size.[52,61] Infants of diabetic mothers (IDM) are also at increased risk for respiratory distress syndrome (RDS), hypoglycemia, hypocalcemia, hypomagnesemia, and hyperbilirubinemia during the neonatal period.[62]

K.H. should be informed that tight glucose control, especially early in the first trimester, will maximize her chance of having a healthy baby. She should be educated before pregnancy about the healthy practices she can institute now to improve a successful pregnancy outcome. Reassure K.H. that fetal ultrasounds will be performed throughout her pregnancy to evaluate fetal anatomy and to measure fetal weight and amniotic fluid volume throughout her pregnancy.

Maternal Risks

18. K.H. wants to know what health risks she might incur from becoming pregnant and what measures could minimize these risks?

Table 46-4 Modified White's Classification of Diabetes During Pregnancy

Class Gestational Diabetes Mellitus	Criteria
A$_1$	No fasting hyperglycemia Controlled by diet
A$_2$	Fasting hyperglycemia Elevated 2-hr postprandial glucose level Requires insulin
Pregestational Diabetes Mellitus	
B	Onset >20 yr Duration <10 yr Absence of vascular disease or retinopathy Insulin-dependent
C	Onset between ages 10–20 yr Duration between 10–20 yr Background retinopathy observed Insulin-dependent
D	Onset before age 10 yr Duration >20 yr Background retinopathy observed Insulin-dependent
F	Presence of diabetic nephropathy
H	Presence of cardiac disease
R	Presence of proliferative retinopathy

From references 52 and 56.

Hypoglycemia, hyperglycemia, ketoacidosis, preterm labor, maternal infections, pre-eclampsia, nephropathy, retinopathy, hydramnios, and neuropathy are common complications in pregnant women with diabetes.[57,60] A prepregnancy assessment, including a history and physical examination, is necessary to determine the risks or contraindications to pregnancy for K.H.. This patient should be evaluated for ischemic heart disease, neuropathies, or retinopathy, and her renal status must be assessed.[58] The presence of gastroparesis should be noted, because it will make controlling her glucose more difficult.[58] Potential contraindications to pregnancy for women with diabetes are ischemic heart disease, untreated proliferative retinopathy, or renal insufficiency (creatinine clearance <50 mL/minute or a serum creatinine ≥3 mg/dL).[58]

Controlling K.H's diabetes before she becomes pregnant may benefit her hypertension and neuropathies and will minimize maternal and fetal problems. Good metabolic control of her diabetes can minimize progression of her diabetes.[58]

Preconception Management

19. **What pre-pregnancy interventions relative to her general health and diabetes should K.H. undertake before she attemps to become pregnant?**

K.H. would benefit by continuing (or initiating) a healthy lifestyle (e.g., exercising, not smoking, avoiding alcohol and unnecessary medications). Her BP of 145/94 mm Hg is high and should be decreased to a diastolic BP of about 80 mm Hg to minimize risks for pre-eclampsia or exacerbation of her disorder.

She also should be started on prenatal vitamins, and re-educated about diet and glycemic control of her diabetes. Her insulin therapy should be titrated to reduce her preprandial (capillary whole blood) glucose to 70 to 100 mg/dL and her 2-hour postprandial glucose to below 140 mg/dL.[58] K.H.'s current regimen may not achieve euglycemia (see Chapter 50, Diabetes Mellitus). Although K.H. is already using a glucometer, her ability to demonstrate appropriate technique should be verified. She could also benefit from a session with a genetic counselor to discuss the maternal and fetal risks in more detail.

Treatment

20. **After lowering her BP to 125/80 mm Hg with a calcium channel blocker and HbA$_{1c}$ to 7.3% K.H. discontinues her oral contraceptive and returns to clinic 5 months later and is noted to be about 4 weeks pregnant. How should K.H.'s diabetes be managed at this time?**

GOALS OF THERAPY

The overall goals of treatment of K.H.'s diabetes are to reduce the maternal and fetal morbidity and mortality associated with diabetes. Treatment of diabetes (Chapter 50, Diabetes Mellitus), should include dietary management, appropriate maternal weight gain, insulin therapy to normalize glycemic control, and exercise.

DIETARY MANAGEMENT

The goals of dietary management for pregnant women with diabetes are directed at ensuring fetal growth and development, appropriate weight gain for the mother, and normal-izing maternal glucose concentrations. Patients often benefit from individualized diets developed by a nutritionist.[58,60] Neonatal macrosomia has been associated with high postprandial glucose levels; therefore, a reduction in postprandial hyperglycemia is an important goal.[60]

INSULIN THERAPY

Insulin is the hypoglycemic of choice during pregnancy because it does not cross the placenta and has an established safety record for both mother and fetus. Oral hypoglycemic agents are not favored because of failure to adequately control hyperglycemia and the potential to cause neonatal hypoglycemia.[40] The teratogenicity of oral hypoglycemics is uncertain because reports of congenital anomalies could be attributable to inadequate maternal glycemic control during the critical organogenesis period early in pregnancy.[40] The goal with insulin therapy is to imitate the glucose levels of a healthy pregnant woman.[60]

Insulin requirements may vary depending on the trimester. The first trimester is characterized by unstable diabetes, followed by a stable period.[52] During the first trimester, glucose and gluconeogenic substances in the blood are taken up by the fetus, which may lead to a decrease in maternal insulin requirements and an increased episodes of hypoglycemia. If K.H. experiences nausea and vomiting during this time, blood glucose control may be unstable and should be monitored closely. When K.H. reaches about 24 weeks' gestation, insulin requirements begin to increase and insulin doses may need to be adjusted every 5 to 10 days. These needs continue to increase during the third trimester to as much as twice the prepregnancy dose, in part, because of the placental hormones (i.e., lactogen, prolactin, estrogen, and progesterone), which antagonize the action of insulin.[52] An insulin regimen with three to four daily injections is most successful at maintaining adequate glucose control.

BLOOD GLUCOSE AND HBA$_{1c}$ MONITORING

K.H. should check her blood glucose daily. Although the accuracy of most glucose monitors are less depedent upon technique than in the past, her technique for testing glucose should be reviewed if her glucose measurements do not match those from the laboratory.[60] K.H. should measure her glucose before and after meals, at bedtime, if she feels symptomatic, and occasionally at 3:00 am to rule out nocturnal hypoglycemia (i.e., about five to seven times daily).

K.H. should have her HbA$_{1c}$ evaluated monthly and her blood glucose concentration at each clinic visit.[60] The laboratory glucose levels should be compared with those obtained from the patient's glucometer to validate accuracy. Two-hour postprandial glucose levels should be <140 mg/dL and fasting levels should be <95 mg/dL. Adjusting therapy based on postprandial glucose levels (as opposed to preprandial levels) can lower HbA$_{1c}$ levels and decrease the risk of macrosomia and neonatal hypoglycemia.[60]

Gestational Diabetes Mellitus
Diagnostic Criteria

21. **J.B. is a 22-year-old, Asian woman in the 26th week of her first pregnancy. She is 5 ft 2 in., 75 kg (prepregnancy weight), and her BMI is 30. At her regular prenatal visit, her obstetrician**

recommends an oral glucose-screening test for GDM. J.B. has a mother with diabetes but has had normal blood glucose concentrations and no glucosuria during pregnancy. Why is J.B. at risk for GDM?

GDM is defined as carbohydrate intolerance that develops or is recognized during pregnancy regardless of severity, needed treatment, time of onset, or persistence after pregnancy.[54,55] GDM occurs in about 7% (range of 1% to 14%), and the prevalence varies with the population and methods of detection.[54] Complications noted in the offspring of these women include macrosomia, hypocalcemia, hypoglycemia, polycythemia, and jaundice.[54] Women with GDM are more likely to develop pregnancy-induced hypertensive disorders or require a cesarean delivery. Women with GDM are at risk for type 2 diabetes later, and their children have an increased risk for obesity and diabetes later in life.[54]

Risk factors for GDM include age >25, obesity (BMI ≥ 25), family history of diabetes, previous delivery of an infant >4 kg, a history of a stillbirth, a history of glucose intolerance, or current glycosuria.[54,55] In addition, African-American, Hispanic, Asian, and Native-American women are at increased risk for GDM.[54,55] Some practitioners screen all pregnant women for GDM, whereas others do not screen women at low risk for GDM. Women considered at low risk must meet all of the following criteria: age <25 years, normal weight before pregnancy, member of a low-risk ethnic group, no history of abnormal glucose tolerance, diabetes in a first-degree relative, or poor obstetric outcome.[54] High-risk women should undergo oral glucose tolerance testing (OGTT) early in pregnancy, and the test repeated between 24 and 28 weeks' gestation in the women who do not initially meet the diagnostic criteria for GDM.[54]

A random plasma glucose concentration of >200 mg/dL or a fasting concentration >126 mg/dL is diagnostic for GDM, especially if subsequently confirmed.[54] The results from oral glucose challenge tests (see Chapter 50, Diabetes) can be used to screen for gestational diabetes mellitus. J.B. is at risk for GDM because she is Asian and obese and has a positive family history. Since she is at risk for GDM, J.B. should undergo OGTT. The diagnosis of GDM is important to the mother and the fetus because of the increased risks related to fetal hypersinsulinemia and macrosomia.[52,61] GDM does not have the same negative effect on pregnancy outcomes as pregestational diabetes.[52]

Treatment

22. J.B.'s 1-hour plasma glucose is 160 mg/dL. The results of a 3-hour test show a fasting plasma glucose of 115 mg/dL, a 1-hour of 185 mg/dL, a 2-hour of 175 mg/dL, and a 3-hour of 150 mg/dL. These results confirm that J.B. has GDM. How should she be managed?

Treatment of GDM is similar to the treatment of type-1 diabetes. The HbA$_{1c}$ levels of J.B, however, need not be monitored because she is past the first trimester.[60] Most gestational diabetics can control their glucose with dietary modifications and regular exercise; however, insulin therapy should be initiated if dietary management fails to maintain fasting plasma blood glucose concentrations ≤105 mg/dL, a 1-hour postprandial plasma concentration ≤155 mg/dL, or 2-hour postprandial plasma glucose concentrations <130 mg/dL.[54]

J.B. requires more extensive education than patients with type 1 diabetes who know about the disease before becoming pregnant. She needs to be educated about her disease, the signs and symptoms of hyperglycemia and hypoglycemia, and the use of a glucometer. If she is started on insulin, she will also need to learn about injection technique, and how to mix and store insulin.

Risk of Developing Diabetes Mellitus

23. Why is J.B. at risk for developing diabetes mellitus after delivery?

Glucose tolerance normalizes after delivery for most women. However, women with GDM have a 17% to 63% chance of developing nongestational diabetes within 5 to 16 years.[55] The highest risk is in women who are obese or were diagnosed before 24 weeks' gestation.[56] The risk of developing GDM in a future pregnancy is estimated to be 50% to 70%.

J.B. should try to minimize the potential for development of insulin resistance by exercising and maintaining a normal weight. She should also have her glucose checked 6 weeks after delivery and then at least every 3 years.[54] In addition, J.B. should be instructed about the importance of using an effective birth control method to prevent unplanned pregnancies. She also needs to schedule regular check-up appointments with her primary care physician.

HYPERTENSION AND PRE-ECLAMPSIA
Classification and Definitions

Hypertensive disease occurs in 5% to 10% of all pregnancies and is a major cause of maternal and perinatal morbidity and mortality.[62,63] About 40% of women with vascular disorders or chronic renal disease and about 20% of nulliparas develop pregnancy-related hypertensive disease.[63] As much as 25% of all perinatal deaths in developed countries have been attributed to hypertensive disorders in pregnancy. *Hypertension in pregnancy* is defined as a systolic BP ≥140 mm Hg or a diastolic BP ≥90 mm Hg on two separate occasions at least 6 hours apart.

Women with pregnancy-associated hypertension can be grouped into the following categories: chronic hypertension, pre-eclampsia–eclampsia, pre-eclampsia superimposed on chronic hypertension, and gestational hypertension.[62] *Gestational hypertension* can be further delineated as (1) transient hypertension of pregnancy if pre-eclampsia is absent during delivery and BP normalizes by 12 weeks postpartum or (2) chronic hypertension if BP remains elevated.[62] Women with transient hypertension have an increased BP "as a sign of the underlying disorder," whereas those with chronic hypertension before pregnancy have elevated BP as the "'cardinal pathophysiologic feature" of their disease.[62]

Chronic hypertension is defined as hypertension diagnosed before conception or before the 20th week of gestation, or hypertension persisting beyond 6 weeks postpartum.[62] Hypertension noted after the 20th week of gestation might be difficult to classify, particularly if a woman has had inadequate prenatal care without appropriate BP monitoring.

Pre-eclampsia is a pregnancy-specific condition usually occurring after 20 weeks' gestation and usually consisting of hypertension with edema, proteinuria, or both.[62,63] The signs and symptoms of pre-eclampsia can affect various organ systems (e.g., kidney, liver, hematologic, CNS), are often unpredictable, and can be mistaken for other disorders.[8,64] Pre-eclampsia is a consequence of progressive placental and maternal endothelial cell dysfunction, increased platelet aggregation, and loss of arterial vasoregulation.[8] A variant of pre-eclampsia is HELLP syndrome, which consists of hemolysis (H), elevated liver enzymes (EL), and low platelet count (LP). HELLP can be life-threatening despite minimal proteinuria and minimal increase in BP.[62,64]

When women with pre-eclampsia develop convulsions, the term "*eclampsia*" is applied.[62,64] Women with pre-eclampsia may unpredictably progress rapidly from mild to severe pre-eclampsia and to eclampsia within days or even hours. Eclampsia is a potentially preventable complication of pre-eclampsia (see Questions 35 and 36). About 20% of women who develop eclampsia have a diastolic BP <90 mm Hg or no proteinuria.[64]

The term "*gestational hypertension*" is used when BP is increased during pregnancy or is increased in the first 24 hours postpartum in a woman without signs or symptoms of pre-eclampsia and without pre-existing hypertension.[62] Women with gestational hypertension are at high risk of recurrence during subsequent pregnancies.

Chronic Hypertension
Clinical Presentation

24. T.D., a 37-year-old G_1P_0, obese African-American woman at 28 weeks' gestation, was diagnosed with stage 1 hypertension several months before her pregnancy (BP 135 to 145 mm Hg systolic and 90 to 95 mm Hg diastolic pressure). She had no cardiovascular risk factors (i.e., smoking, diabetes mellitus, dyslipidemias) and was prescribed a trial of lifestyle modification (i.e., weight loss and exercise). Between 16 and 20 weeks' gestation, her BP ranged from 130 to 135 mm Hg systolic pressure and 82 to 85 mm Hg diastolic pressure. Her BP today is 142/90 mm Hg. In the third trimester, her serum chemistry values were sodium (Na) 140 mEq/L (normal, 133 to 143); potassium (K) 4 mEq/L (normal, 3.2 to 4.5); chloride (Cl) 95 mEq/L (normal, 92 to 97); bicarbonate (CO_2) 22 mEq/L (normal, 18 to 25); urea nitrogen (UN) 5 mg/dL (normal, 2 to 6); creatinine (Cr) 0.6 mg/dL (normal, 0.5 to 0.6); uric acid (UA) 4 mg/dL (normal, 2.5 to 5.9). A random urinalysis did not demonstrate proteinuria. A 24-hour urine collection during the first trimester showed a protein excretion rate of 150 mg/24 hr (normal <300 mg) and creatinine clearance of 135 mL/minute (normal in first trimester 132 to 166). Ultrasound confirms an adequately growing fetus at 28 weeks' gestation. What is the likelihood T.D. has pre-eclampsia?

Women with chronic hypertension commonly have a normal BP during the first half of pregnancy because of the normal physiologic decline of BP during the second trimester.[62,64] Early in a normal pregnancy, diastolic BP decreases by an average of 7 to 10 mm Hg between 13 and 20 weeks' gestation and does not increase to prepregnancy values until the third trimester.[62,64] Systolic pressure changes minimally during pregnancy. T.D.'s diastolic pressure decreased from the prepregnancy levels of 90 to 95 mm Hg to 86 to 90 mm Hg during the second trimester. It is normal for T.D.'s BP to increase during the third trimester. These changes in BP make it difficult to differentiate chronic hypertension from pre-eclampsia during the second half of pregnancy, particularly in women with poor prenatal care and inadequate monitoring of BP. T.D. had chronic hypertension before her pregnancy. It is difficult to diagnose pre-eclampsia superimposed upon existing hypertension using BP measurements alone. A sharp increase in T.D.'s pressure of >30 mm Hg systolic or >15 mm Hg diastolic could be consistent with pre-eclampsia. However, without co-existing proteinuria (≥ 0.3 g/24-hour or $\geq 1+$ in a random urine) or evidence of renal dysfunction, a diagnosis of pre-eclampsia would be a reach.[62] T.D. has no proteinuria, and a normal serum creatinine and serum uric acid. Since an increase in BP to prepregnancy values is normal during the third trimester, it is unlikely that T.D. has pre-eclampsia at this time.

Risk Factors for Pre-eclampsia

25. What risk factors does T.D. have for developing pre-eclampsia?

A family history of pre-eclampsia is associated with a threefold increased risk of developing pre-eclampsia; and women with previous pre-eclampsia are at high risk for recurrence of pre-eclampsia in subsequent pregnancies, particularly if it developed before 30 weeks' gestation.[65] This risk increases with increased maternal age and interval between pregnancies. Chronic diseases that increase the risk for pre-eclampsia are thrombophilic disorders, which are associated with an increased risk of vascular thrombosis (e.g., antithrombin deficiency, hyperhomocystinemia), and diabetes mellitus or insulin resistance.[65] Pregnancy-associated risk factors are twin gestations, urinary tract infection, multiple congenital anomalies, certain chromosomal anomalies, and hydatiform moles.[65]

Pre-eclampsia generally occurs during first pregnancies.[65] T.D. is six to eight times more likely to develop pre-eclampsia than a multiparous woman because she is primigravida.[64] Her other risk factors are advanced age, obesity, and chronic hypertension. Chronic hypertension is T.D.'s biggest risk factor for developing pre-eclampsia in this pregnancy as well as for recurrence in subsequent pregnancies.[62] Fortunately, T.D. does not have longstanding severe hypertension or pre-existing renal or cardiovascular disease, which greatly increase the risk for developing superimposed pre-eclampsia.

MONITORING

26. What subjective and objective data should be monitored in T.D. for the development of pre-eclampsia?

T.D. is at risk for developing pre-eclampsia superimposed on her hypertension, which was diagnosed before her pregnancy. She should be monitored closely for signs, symptoms, and laboratory evidence of pre-eclampsia. T.D. should have her BP monitored frequently. Her serum concentration of creatinine should be monitored occasionally along with a urinalysis for proteinuria.[8] We know that T.D. had no evidence of renal disease at the beginning of her pregnancy because she had a normal 24-hour urinary protein excretion and creatinine clearance. If protein is detected in a random urinalysis, then a

24-hour urine collection for protein and creatinine should be repeated to determine accurately the degree of proteinuria and severity of disease.[8] Serial fetal ultrasounds should be obtained to assess fetal growth because IUGR (intrauterine growth retardation) is common in pregnant women with chronic hypertension. T.D. should be taught to recognize and immediately report all signs and symptoms of pre-eclampsia such as nondependent edema (e.g., facial and hand), which can be the result of sodium retention or hypoalbuminemia. Headaches and visual disturbances are signs of severe pre-eclampsia and may indicate impending eclampsia. Abdominal pain is also a danger sign of severe pre-eclampsia and possibly indicates pancreatitis or impending hepatic rupture.[8,66] Because T.D. has chronic hypertension, worsening of hypertension alone may not be a reliable sign of superimposed pre-eclampsia. Proteinuria is the best indicator of superimposed pre-eclampsia in a pregnant woman with chronic hypertension and no renal disease.[64]

ANTIHYPERTENSIVE DRUG THERAPY

27. Why should (or should not) T.D.'s chronic hypertension be treated with antihypertensive drugs to prevent pre-eclampsia?

The ultimate goal for T.D. is to deliver a normal, healthy, full-term infant without adverse sequelae to her own health. This goal can be achieved best by minimizing the risk of pre-eclampsia and the complications of pregnancy such as abruptio placentae (detachment of the placenta).

The goal of antihypertensive therapy for women with chronic hypertension during pregnancy is to minimize the risks of an elevated BP to the mother without compromising placental perfusion and fetal well-being.[62] A sustained diastolic BP of >100 mm Hg can cause maternal vascular damage, especially if the diastolic pressure is >105 mm Hg.[66] Morbidity is unlikely with a diastolic BP of 95 to 100 mm Hg. Therefore, many clinicians recommend treatment with antihypertensive drugs to lower diastolic pressures >100 mm Hg.[64,67] Treatment of a diastolic BP of <100 mm Hg should be reserved for women with chronic hypertension and target organ damage or underlying renal disease because antihypertensive drugs can decrease placental blood flow or cause harm to the fetus.[67] T.D. has normal renal function and her BP is <100 mm Hg; she does not need antihypertensive drug treatment at this time. If T.D. were on antihypertensive drug therapy before conception, she would have been instructed to continue with drug therapy throughout pregnancy.[62,64,67] In such cases, however, the doses of the antihypertensive agents often need to be lowered or discontinued altogether to prevent hypotension because the maternal BP naturally decreases during the second trimester. The only antihypertensive drugs contraindicated during pregnancy are angiotensin-converting enzyme (ACE) inhibitors[68] and angiotensin II–receptor blockers.[67] These drugs have been associated with fetal and newborn morbidity and mortality.[68] The use of β-blockers early in pregnancy should also be avoided because they have been associated with a high incidence of IUGR.[67,69]

Perinatal outcomes in women with untreated chronic hypertension who do not progress to pre-eclampsia are similar to those of the general obstetric population.[64] Although chronic hypertension is a major risk factor in pre-eclampsia,

treating T.D.'s uncomplicated mild chronic hypertension is unlikely to prevent the development of pre-eclampsia.

Mild Pre-eclampsia
Etiology and Pathogenesis

The cause of pre-eclampsia is unknown. Its pathogenesis begins early in pregnancy, and the disease is not clinically evident until the latter half of the pregnancy and persists until the fetus is delivered.[8,70] Incomplete physiologic placental vascular bed changes and endothelial cell dysfunction are integral to the pathogenesis of pre-eclampsia (see Placental Physiology).

PLACENTAL ISCHEMIA

Early in a normal pregnancy, the trophoblastic migration and invasion of the uterine spiral arteries result in physiologic changes within the placental vascular bed that facilitate maximal intervillous blood flow. The physiologic changes within these spiral arteries are responsible for creating a fixed low-resistance arteriolar circuit, which increases blood supply to the growing fetus. In pre-eclampsia, these physiologic changes do not occur completely, resulting in decreased perfusion and consequently, placental ischemia.[8,70,71]

ENDOTHELIAL DAMAGE

An intact vascular endothelium assists in preserving the integrity of vasculature, mediating immune and inflammatory responses, preventing intravascular coagulation, and modulating the contractility of the underlying smooth muscle cell.[71]

In normal pregnancy, prostacyclin is increased 8 to 10 times, creating an increased ratio of prostacyclin to thromboxane A_2.[70] The biologic dominance of prostacyclin along with nitric oxide play an important role in maintaining vasodilation throughout pregnancy. Prostacyclin may be responsible for vascular refractoriness to angiotensin II in normal pregnancy. In pre-eclampsia, the ratio of prostacyclin to thromboxane A_2 is reversed. Thromboxane A_2 is biologically dominant during pre-eclampsia, leading to increased vascular sensitivity to angiotensin II and norepinephrine.[70] The increased release of thromboxane A_2 is believed to be due to endothelial cell dysfunction. The end result is vasospasm, which further increases endothelial cell dysfunction, and increases BP.[8,70] Reduced activity of nitric oxide synthase and decreased nitric oxide-dependent or nitric oxide-independent endothelium-derived relaxing factor are believed to increase the vasoconstrive potential of pressors such as angiotensin II.[62]

Endothelial cell dysfunction in pregnancy is thought to be due to oxidative stress. Intermittent hypoxic and reperfusion injury that occurs as a consequence of decreased placental perfusion may increase oxidative stress.[70,71] Endothelial damage eventually leads to the disruption of the vascular lining, which causes leaking capillary membranes, allowing fluid to leak into the interstitium.[71] In severe pre-eclampsia, this results in hypovolemia, hemoconcentration, and consequently an increase in hematocrit. The loss of plasma volume, vasospasm, and microthrombi decrease perfusion of the kidney, CNS, liver, and other organs. The loss of intravascular proteins in the urine secondary to renal damage, and through damaged epithelia, decreases plasma oncotic pressure and leads to a rapid onset of nondependent edema. The imbalance of endogenous procoagulants and anticoagulants produces platelet consumption and results in thrombocytopenia and co-agulation defects.[71]

Clinical Presentation

28. T.D. returns to her obstetrician 3 weeks later at 31 weeks' gestation complaining of mild hand and leg edema. She has 1+ proteinuria by dipstick and her BP has increased to 155/102 mm Hg. A fetal ultrasound indicates a growth-restricted fetus of 31 weeks' gestation. Pertinent laboratory results are serum Na 140 mEq/L (normal, 133 to 143); serum K 4.3 mEq/L (normal, 3.2 to 4.5); serum Cl 97 mEq/L (normal, 92 to 97); serum CO_2 20 mEq/L (normal, 18 to 25); UN 8 mg/dL (normal, 2 to 6); serum Cr 0.8 mg/dL (normal, 0.5 to 0.6); UA 6.0 mg/dL (normal, 2.5 to 5.9); aspartate aminotransferase (AST) 25 U/L (normal, 0 to 35); alanine aminotransferase (ALT) 16 U/L (normal, 0 to 35); total bilirubin 0.7 mg/dL (normal, 0.1 to 1); total protein 6.0 g/dL (normal, 5.9 to 7.2); albumin 2.5 g/dL (normal, 2.3 to 4.2); platelets 230,000/mm³ (normal, 203,000 to 353,000): random urine protein 1%. What signs and laboratory evidence are consistent with pre-eclampsia in T.D.? Does she have mild or severe pre-eclampsia?

T.D.'s diastolic BP is now higher than it was before her pregnancy and has increased by 12 mm Hg in the last 3 weeks. Although an increase in BP by itself is not diagnostic for pre-eclampsia, it is ominous because T.D. now also presents with mild hand and leg edema. The most important laboratory evidence confirming the diagnosis of pre-eclampsia in T.D. is a new-onset proteinuria and an elevated serum creatinine.[62,64] Other evidence for pre-eclampsia is an elevated serum uric acid concentration, which is a sensitive marker for pre-eclampsia.[66] T.D. denies headaches, visual disturbances, and abdominal pain, which usually are experienced in severe pre-eclampsia. The liver function tests and platelet counts in T.D. are normal; therefore, HELLP syndrome can be ruled out.[62] T.D.'s clinical presentation is consistent with mild pre-eclampsia; however, a 24-hour urine collection should be obtained to measure protein excretion, quantify the urine output, and further rule out severe pre-eclampsia..

Treatment
GENERAL PRINCIPLES

29. T.D. is admitted to the hospital for observation and management. The 24-hour urine protein is 0.5 g/24 hours and creatinine clearance is 100 mL/min. Although fetal growth is mildly restricted, all other fetal testing is reassuring. How should T.D.'s mild pre-eclampsia be treated?

The delivery of the fetus is the only cure for pre-eclampsia and would be the best treatment option for T.D. if she were >37 weeks' gestation.[8] T.D. has mild disease, however, and is remote from term. Her delivery should be postponed as long as possible because premature delivery increases neonatal morbidity and mortality. T.D.'s fetus is somewhat growth restricted, which is common in women with chronic hypertension, with or without superimposed pre-eclampsia. However, if T.D.'s fetus is severely growth restricted and if subsequent fetal biophysical testing is abnormal, premature delivery would be indicated.[8,72] Since neither of these is evident in the present circumstances, T.D. should carry her fetus under close medical supervision to as long a term as possible without causing significant harm to herself.

It is appropriate for T.D. to be hospitalized for observation and assessment of the severity of pre-eclampsia. Bed rest in the lateral decubitus position may help reduce T.D.'s BP and promote diuresis by decreasing vasoconstriction and improving renal and uteroplacental perfusion.[62] Continuous bed rest is not warranted and has no increased benefit compared with periodic ambulation in decreasing the progression and severity of pre-eclampsia.[72]

T.D. should have her BP measured every 4 hours during the day.[72] Her urine should be checked for protein daily. Liver function tests, hematocrit, and platelet counts should be measured twice a week. T.D's urine output and body weight should be measured daily, and she should be monitored for worsening of her edema (i.e., facial and abdominal). She also should be assessed for symptoms of severe pre-eclampsia such as headaches, visual disturbances, epigastric or right upper quadrant pain. The well-being of the fetus should be evaluated by counting daily fetal movements, a nonstress test twice a week, and an ultrasound evaluation of fetal growth every 3 to 4 weeks.[72]

If T.D's hypertension is controlled, fetal growth is adequate, and her adherence to therapy is good, she may be managed on an outpatient basis. T.D. can be discharged from the hospital when her BP is controlled, when signs, symptoms, and laboratory evidence do not indicate worsening disease, and when reassuring evidence of continued fetal well-being exists.

ANTIHYPERTENSIVE DRUG THERAPY

30. T.D. was started on methyldopa (Aldomet) 250 mg PO Q 8 hr. After 24 hours, her BP decreased to 145/102 mm Hg. Her 24-hour urine protein excretion rate on admission was 0.5 g/24 hr and urine protein has been 1+ to 2+. Over the course of 3 to 4 days the methyldopa was increased to 750 mg PO Q 8 hr and T.D.'s BP eventually decreased to 140/94 mm Hg. T.D.'s BP remained between 138 and 142 mm Hg systolic and 90 to 95 mm Hg diastolic throughout the rest of her hospitalization. Her platelet counts remained stable at 230 × 10³/mm³ and liver function tests remained normal. Her edema was not increased, and no other signs and symptoms of pre-eclampsia were noted during the hospitalization. T.D. complained only of some dizziness and sedation. She was discharged home on the tenth hospital day. Why was this appropriate drug therapy?

A diastolic BP of >100 mm Hg during pregnancy warrants antihypertensive drug treatment.[62,67] The benefit of treating diastolic BPs between 90 and 99 mm Hg in pregnancy continues to remain controversial. Antihypertensive treatment of mild to moderate hypertension is associated with a decrease in the risk of developing severe hypertension by approximately 50%, but the overall risk of developing pre-eclampsia is unchanged.[73] Moreover, women treated with antihypertensives were more likely to develop adverse drug effects compared with those who received placebo or were untreated. Antihypertensive therapy reduces the risk of cardiovascular morbidity and stroke in pregnant women with severe hypertension (diastolic >110 mm Hg).[62,67]

Methyldopa

Methyldopa (Aldomet) is a centrally acting α-agonist that decreases sympathetic outflow to decrease BP. It is the antihypertensive most commonly used for chronic treatment of hypertension in pregnancy in the United States. The usual starting dose of 750 to 1,000 mg/day, to be administered in three to four daily divided doses, can be increased to 2 or 3 g/day if needed. Higher doses may be needed to control BP in pregnancy.[69] T.D.'s methyldopa dosage (2,250 mg/day) is within the recommended range.

Methyldopa, classified as category B for fetal risk (Chapter 47, Teratogenicity and Drugs in Breast Milk), has the longest and best safety record of all antihypertensive agents during pregnancy. Despite its common use, few adverse effects have been reported in neonates exposed to methyldopa in utero.[40] In addition, no congenital anomalies are associated with methyldopa.[40]

T.D. is experiencing dizziness and sedation, which, together with a loss of energy, are among the most common adverse effects reported by pregnant women.[69] Generally, these adverse effects occur early in therapy and tend to subside, but may recur with an increased dosage. Problems with postural hypotension do not usually occur in pregnant females.[69] T.D. should be monitored for methyldopa-induced liver damage.[64] Other drugs used to treat hypertension in pregnancy are labetalol, β-blockers, and calcium channel blockers.

Labetalol

Labetalol (Normodyne, Trandate), with combined α- and β-receptor antagonist properties, can decrease maternal BP, maintain adequate uteroplacental blood flow, decrease platelet consumption in women with pre-eclampsia, and increase fetal lung surfactant production and lung maturity.[75] Labetalol crosses the placenta, and concentrations in cord blood average 40% to 80% of peak maternal concentrations.[40] Fetal malformations are not associated with labetalol exposure, however, experience with labetalol treatment during the first trimester is limited. In a surveillance study of >200,000 completed pregnancies of Michigan Medicaid recipients during a 7-year period in which 29 neonates were exposed to labetalol during the first trimester, approximately 14% of these newborns had a major congenital defect.[40] Specific details on the malformations are not available, and other factors such as maternal disease and concomitant drug use could not be excluded as contributing factors. Most reports of labetalol exposure in utero have not documented decreased Apgar scores, decreased birth weights, decreased head circumferences, or decreased glucose control in neonates.[40] Newborns of hypertensive pregnant women treated with labetalol have significantly higher birth weights compared with newborns of women treated with atenolol.[40] One study comparing hospitalization alone with hospitalization and treatment with labetalol for the management of mild pre-eclampsia found that labetalol treatment did not improve perinatal outcome, and the incidence of IUGR was higher in the newborns exposed to labetalol.[75]

Labetalol seems to be as safe as methyldopa when used for a short time during the third trimester.[69] It appears to cause less IUGR than other β-blockers and is preferred over other β-blockers.[76] Drug-associated effects reported in infants exposed to labetalol in utero include bradycardia and hypotension.

β-Blockers

The β-adrenergic blockers (atenolol, metoprolol, nadolol, pindolol, propranolol) are effective alternatives to methyldopa for reducing BP in pregnancy; however, they are associated with an increased incidence of intrauterine fetal growth retar-

dation and are not recommended for long-term use in pregnancy.[40,67,76] Nevertheless, the incidence of respiratory distress syndrome is decreased in preterm neonates born to mothers treated with β-blockers late in the gestational period.[76]

Propranolol has been used extensively during pregnancies to treat many conditions, and fetal and neonatal adverse effects have been associated with its use during pregnancy, particularly with doses >160 mg/day.[40] In utero exposure to propranolol has been associated with IUGR (14%), hypoglycemia (10%), bradycardia (7%), hyperbilirubinemia (4%), and respiratory depression at delivery (4%).[40] Concomitant medications and maternal diseases, however, also may have contributed to these effects.

The association of IUGR with β-blockers is more common when these drugs are started early in the second trimester.[40,77] IUGR is thought to be due to β-blocker-induced increased vascular resistance in both mother and fetus.[40] The degree of growth retardation depends on the length of drug exposure. When atenolol is initiated during the third trimester, only placental weight is significantly decreased.[40] Neonates exposed to β-blockers near delivery should be observed for signs of bradycardia, hypotension, and hypoglycemia during the first 24 to 48 hours after birth.[40] As a result of the association with IUGR, the β-blockers are classified as teratogenic risk factor Category D if used in second or third trimester.[40]

Calcium Channel Blockers

Nifedipine also is classified as a teratogenic category C drug and has been used safely in all three trimesters of pregnancy. No increase in the risk of major congenital malformations was noted in a prospective, cohort study of 78 women with first trimester exposure to the calcium channel blockers (nifedipine, verapamil, diltiazem) as compared to a comparable control group.[40]

Angiotensin-Converting Enzyme Inhibitors

ACE inhibitors should not be used in pregnancy because of a high association with fetal and neonatal morbidity and mortality. Fetal renal failure is the primary event in the pathogenesis of ACE inhibitor fetopathy (fetal renal failure, oligohydramnios, limb contractures, pulmonary hypoplasia, IUGR, neonatal renal failure).[78] Angiotensin II–receptor antagonists should not be used to treat hypertension in pregnancy for similar reasons.[78]

Diuretics

Diuretics are not recommended to treat hypertension in pre-eclampsia because the maternal intravascular volume can be contracted in pre-eclampsia or eclampsia, and diuretics can further decrease uteroplacental perfusion.[62] When necessary, diuretics have been used to treat maternal pulmonary edema or heart failure. If a woman was taking a diuretic for chronic hypertension before becoming pregnant, it also would be reasonable to continue with therapy during pregnancy.[62,67]

Severe Pre-eclampsia
Clinical Presentation

31. T.D.'s BP for about 2 weeks ranged from 140 to 150 mm Hg systolic and 90 to 100 mm Hg diastolic despite bed rest and an increased methyldopa dose of 1,000 mg TID. Her proteinuria remained stable at 1+ to 2+ by dipstick. During the past 2 days

T.D.'s BP started to increase again, and today her BP is 160/112 mm Hg and her urine dipstick is 3+. She complains of headaches, dizziness, and visual disturbances and has significant edema in her face, hands, legs, and ankles. T.D. is admitted to the Labor and Delivery Unit for evaluation and treatment. Pertinent laboratory results are serum UN 20 mg/dL (normal, 2 to 6); serum Cr 1.3 mg/dL (normal, 0.5 to 0.6); serum uric acid 6.7 mg/dL (normal, 2.5 to 5.9); AST 30 U/L (normal, 0 to 35); ALT 16 U/L (normal, 0 to 35); total bilirubin 1 mg/dL (normal, 0.1 to 1); total protein 5 g/dL (normal, 5.9 to 7.2); albumin 2 g/dL (normal, 2.3 to 4.2); platelets, 95,000/mm³ (normal, 203,000 to 353,000); hematocrit 38% (normal, 32.7% to 36%); hemoglobin 13 g/dL (normal, 10.9 to 13.5); random urine protein 4+. Estimated fetal weight by ultrasound is 1,700 g, which is between the 10th and 25th percentile for a gestational age of 34 weeks. What signs, symptoms, and laboratory evidence of severe pre-eclampsia supports this diagnosis in T.D.?

T.D. has developed severe pre-eclampsia. Her systolic and diastolic BP is above 160 and 112 mm Hg, respectively. She has >3+ protein in a random urine sample and her serum creatinine is >1.2 mg/dL. She complains of headaches and visual disturbances. T.D. is also thrombocytopenic as her platelet count is 95,000/mm³. HELLP syndrome, a variant of severe pre-eclampsia associated with a high incidence of maternal and perinatal morbidity and mortality can be ruled out because her liver transaminases are normal.

Complications

32. What complications of severe pre-eclampsia would T.D. be exposed to?

T.D. is at risk for cerebral hemorrhage, cerebral edema, encephalopathy, coagulopathies, pulmonary edema, liver failure, and eclamptic seizures.[8,64] Severe pre-eclampsia is not only dangerous to T.D., but also to her fetus because uteroplacental perfusion is compromised.

T.D. requires aggressive drug treatment to lower her BP and prevent eclampsia. Deterioration in either maternal or fetal status is an indication for emergent delivery.[79] Postponing delivery for as little as 24 hours to allow for glucocorticoid (e.g., betamethasone) administration to promote fetal lung maturity decreases the development of RDS in preterm newborns <34 weeks' gestation[80] (see also Question 60 and Chapter 94, Neonatal Therapy). T.D. already is at 34 weeks' gestation is not a candidate for empiric glucocorticoid administration. If time permits, an amniocentesis may be performed to determine fetal lung maturity before the decision is made to deliver T.D.'s fetus.

Acute Treatment of Severe Hypertension
HYDRALAZINE

33. How should T.D.'s severe hypertension be treated?

The goal of antihypertensive therapy in T.D. is to prevent cerebral complications (e.g., encephalopathy, hemorrhage).[64] Although it is important to reduce the maternal BP, it must be accomplished gradually while the fetus is in utero because a large and sudden drop in maternal BP could result in an even greater reduction in uteroplacental perfusion.[64]

Hydralazine, a direct arterial smooth muscle dilator, is the drug of choice for the acute treatment of severe hypertension in pregnancy.[64,69] This drug reflexly induces a baroreceptor–mediated tachycardia and increases cardiac output, which increases uterine blood flow as the BP is lowered.[81] Hydralazine 5 mg IV over 1 to 2 minutes should be administered to T.D. and repeated in doses of 5 to 10 mg every 20 to 30 minutes to a cumulative dose of 20 mg.[8,64,81]

T.D. should have repeated measurements of her BP at 15-minute intervals. Because intervillous blood flow depends on maternal perfusion pressure, the goal is to decrease the diastolic pressure to 90 mm Hg.[8,64] Lowering the maternal BP excessively may decrease uteroplacental perfusion and compromise the fetus. The onset of antihypertensive effect for hydralazine ranges from 10 to 20 minutes and duration of action ranges from 3 to 6 hours after an intravenous dose.[79] Therefore, doses of hydralazine should not be repeated more frequently than every 20 to 30 minutes to prevent drug accumulation.[69] T.D. should also be monitored for nausea, vomiting, tachycardia, flushing, headache, and tremors. Some of these hydralazine-induced adverse effects mimic symptoms associated with severe pre-eclampsia and imminent eclampsia, making it difficult for a clinician to differentiate between drug-associated and disease-related problems and could result in inadvertent early termination of pregnancy.[69] Fetal hydralazine serum concentrations are reportedly the same as or higher than maternal serum concentrations, but drug-associated fetal abnormalities have not been reported.[40]

ALTERNATIVE ANTIHYPERTENSIVE DRUGS

34. After receiving two doses of IV hydralazine (total dose 15 mg), T.D.'s BP decreased to 150/100 mm Hg. What other antihypertensive drugs could be used to treat her severe hypertension?

Labetalol

Labetalol is the second most commonly used drug to treat severe hypertension during pregnancy and should be used only after hydralazine has failed or is not tolerated because of adverse effects.[64,81] It should be administered intravenously in increasing doses of 20, 40, and 80 mg every 10 minutes to a cumulative dose of 300 mg or until the diastolic pressure is <100 mm Hg.[81] The onset of action is within 5 minutes, and its effect peaks in 10 to 20 minutes with a duration of action ranging from 45 minutes to 6 hours.

Intravenous labetalol is as effective as intravenous hydralazine in lowering BP in patients with hypertension during pregnancy, but has fewer reported adverse effects.[69,76] In a meta-analysis of β-blocker trials for the treatment of hypertension in pregnancy, labetalol was associated with less maternal hypotension, fewer cesarean deliveries, and no increase in perinatal mortality.[76] Labetalol also does not appear to decrease uteroplacental blood flow even with a decrease in maternal BP.[69] Labetalol reduces cerebral perfusion pressure, which occurs in up to 43% of women with severe pre-eclampsia, without negatively affecting cerebral blood flow.[82] Decreased cerebral perfusion pression may prevent progression to eclampsia.[82]

Nifedipine

Nifedipine (Procardia, Adalat) often is the preferred antihypertensive agent for acute treatment of severe hypertension during pregnancy because it can be given orally.[69,81] Nifedipine is effective in decreasing BP without reducing uteroplacental blood flow or decreasing fetal heart rate.[81] Short-acting nifedipine capsules are no longer recommended for the treatment of hypertension because of the risk of stroke or myocardial infarction. However, immediate-release nifedipine continues to be used to treat hypertension in pregnancy because this unique patient population may not be at high risk for ischemic events secondary to atherosclerotic disease.[81] Calcium gluconate or calcium chloride should be available for intravenous administration in the event of sudden hypotension. Caution should be used when giving nifedipine to women concomitantly treated with magnesium sulfate because these drugs have synergistic effects, causing hypotension and neuromuscular blockade.[81,83]

Several studies comparing oral nifedipine with intravenous labetalol in hypertensive emergencies of pregnancy have found them to be equally effective in lowering BP.[84,85] Nifedipine lowers BP to <160 mm Hg systolic and <100 mm Hg diastolic earlier than labetalol,[84] but it increases cardiac index[85] (see Chapter 21, Hypertensive Emergencies).

Eclampsia
Magnesium Sulfate Prophylaxis

35. T.D. was given magnesium sulfate 4 g IV for 30 minutes and then started on a continuous IV infusion of 2 g/hr. Labor was induced approximately 12 hours later, and T.D. delivered an 1,800-g male neonate, appropriate for a gestational age of 34 weeks. Why was T.D.'s drug therapy appropriate?

Magnesium sulfate was given to T.D. to prevent eclamptic seizures during labor.[62,86,87] Although termination of the pregnancy is the definitive treatment for severe pre-eclampsia, the intrapartum and immediate postpartum periods are also the periods of greatest risk for eclampsia.[63] The incidence of eclampsia is extremely low; however, maternal morbidity and mortality are high.[86] In the United States, it is the standard of practice to treat all pre-eclamptic women with magnesium sulfate during labor and for 12 to 24 hours postpartum.[62,64] In the United Kingdom, it is common to reserve therapy with magnesium sulfate for severe pre-eclampsia.[88] The evidence for magnesium sulfate prevention of the progression of disease in mildly pre-eclamptic women had been largely anecdotal. However, in one large international study of more than 10,000 women, magnesium sulfate clearly decreased the risk of eclampsia in pre-eclamptic women by 58% compared with placebo.[88] Magnesium sulfate does not increase cesarean delivery rates, obstetric hemorrhage, nor neonatal depression.[89] In utero exposure to magnesium sulfate also may decrease the risk of cerebral palsy in preterm infants.[88]

In a prospective, randomized study, magnesium sulfate was superior to phenytoin for the prevention of eclampsia in hypertensive pregnant women.[86] In addition, magnesium sulfate was more effective than nimodipine for seizure prophylaxis in severely pre-eclamptic women.[90]

A magnesium sulfate 50% solution can be used to administer 10 g IM in two divided doses into the upper outer quadrant of each buttock followed by 5 g IM every 4 hours.[83,87] In cases of severe pre-eclampsia, an additional 4-g dose of 20% magnesium sulfate solution is administered intravenously for 5 to 15 minutes.[91] This regimen maintains serum magnesium

concentrations between 4.2 and 7.2 mg/dL.[91] A regimen of magnesium sulfate 4 to 6 g IV as a loading dose followed by a continuous infusion of 2 g/hour is the most commonly used regimen in the United States.[87] Continuous infusion of 1 g/hour has been associated with treatment failures.[92] Intravenous loading doses of 6 g followed by continuous infusions of 2 g/hour maintain therapeutically effective magnesium serum concentrations between 4 to 8 mg/dL.[92] A population pharmacokinetic-pharmacodynamic analysis of magnesium sulfate quantifying the antihypertensive effect of magnesium sulfate showed that a continuous infusion rate of 2 g/hour achieves therapeutic magnesium serum concentrations of 4.8 to 9.6 mg/dL after 10 hours.[93]

All continuous infusions of magnesium sulfate should be given through a controlled infusion pump designed to protect against free flow to prevent the accidental administration of large doses. If such an infusion pump is not available, the intramuscular route of administration should be used.

36. What is the proposed mechanism of action of magnesium sulfate in the prevention and treatment of eclamptic seizures?

The precise mechanism of anticonvulsant action of magnesium for the prevention and treatment of eclamptic seizures is unknown. The anticonvulsant activity may be partly mediated through blockade of an excitatory amino acid receptor, N-methyl-d-aspartate (NMDA).[83] Seizures are thought to be caused by decreased cerebral blood flow because of vasospasm. Magnesium sulfate is a potent cerebral vasodilator and increases the synthesis of prostacyclin, an endothelial vasodilator. It also causes a dose-dependent decrease in systemic vascular resistance, which may explain its transient hypotensive effect. Magnesium may also protect against oxidative injury to endothelial cells.[83]

Monitoring Magnesium Sulfate Therapy

37. What subjective and objective data should be monitored during treatment of T.D. with magnesium?

Deep tendon reflexes (patellar reflex), respiratory rate, and urine output should be monitored periodically during treatment with magnesium sulfate.[86] The patellar reflex should be checked before each intramuscular dose is administered and every hour during continuous intravenous administration. The loss of patellar reflexes is the first sign of magnesium toxicity and generally occurs at serum concentrations of 8 to 12 mg/dL.[86,94] The respiratory rate should be monitored hourly and should be >12 breaths per minute. Urine output should be at least 100 mL every 4 hours (or 25 mL/hr).[86] Magnesium serum concentrations are not routinely measured unless renal dysfunction is evident because magnesium is almost entirely excreted by the kidney.[83,86] Hypocalcemia and hypocalcemic tetany also can occur secondary to hypermagnesemia and can be reversed by calcium gluconate 1 g (10 mL of a10% solution) slow intravenous push over 3 minutes.[8]

Neuromuscular depression can occur in infants whose mothers received magnesium sulfate.[91] Neonatal toxicity is usually associated with maternal renal dysfunction or prolonged intravenous administration before delivery (>24 hours).[94] Parenteral magnesium sulfate is safe and rarely causes maternal or neonatal toxicity when administered properly.[86]

Treatment

38. **What is appropriate drug therapy for eclampsia?**

Diazepam, phenytoin, and magnesium sulfate have all been used to treat eclampsia. The use of magnesium sulfate to treat these seizures results in less maternal morbidity and mortality and less neonatal morbidty as well.[95] Generally, higher serum concentrations of magnesium sulfate are needed to treat than to prevent eclamptic seizures. However, the same therapeutic range guides both prophylaxis and treatment.[87] Eclampsia unresponsive to magnesium sulfate treatment should prompt an evaluation for other cerebrovascular events (e.g., cerebral hemorrhage or infarction).[87]

39. **How long should magnesium sulfate be continued in T.D.?**

Depending on the severity of pre-eclampsia, magnesium sulfate therapy usually is continued for 24 hours after delivery.[96] Attempts are being made to identify patient-specific criteria that can be used to determine the optimal duration of therapy. Women with severe pre-eclampsia or pre-eclampsia superimposed on chronic hypertension are at greater risk for disease exacerbation when magnesium sulfate is discontinued too soon.

Prevention of Pre-eclampsia

40. **What therapeutic interventions could be used to minimize the progression of pre-eclampsia in T.D.?**

Various treatments to prevent the development of pre-eclampsia have been used because pre-eclampsia continues to be an important cause of maternal and perinatal morbidity and mortality. Unfortunately, no single strategy has been successful in preventing pre-eclampsia in pregnancy. The two most studied strategies have been low-dose aspirin and calcium.

Low-Dose Aspirin

Aspirin irreversibly inhibits platelet cyclooxygenase and thromboxane A_2 production while minimally affecting vascular prostacyclin production. This "normalization" of the prostacyclin to thromboxane A_2 ratio is the basis for low-dose aspirin use in decreasing hypertension and pre-eclampsia during pregnancy.[97–99] Aspirin, selective for maternal platelet cyclooxygenase, does not affect fetal platelet function, urine output, cardiac function, nor neonatal outcome.[98]

Low-dose aspirin can reduce the prevalence of pre-eclampsia in healthy nulliparous women.[98] Aspirin (low dose), however, did not decrease perinatal morbidity and increased abruptio placentae in the mother. Therefore, low-dose aspirin should not be used routinely to prevent pre-eclampsia except in high-risk groups (e.g., those who previously had pre-eclampsia, multiple gestations, or chronic hypertension or diabetes mellitus).[98] A subsequent double-blind, placebo-controlled trial of low-dose aspirin in women at high risk for pre-eclampsia failed to reduce the incidence of pre-eclampsia or improve perinatal outcomes.[99]

Calcium

In epidemiologic studies, low calcium intake has been associated with the development of pre-eclampsia.[97] Low calcium intake purportedly stimulates the secretion of either renin or parathyroid hormone, which increase vascular tone and re-sponsiveness to vasopressors through increasing calcium uptake into the cells of vascular smooth muscle. The effect of calcium supplementation, however, on the development of hypertension and pre-eclampsia in pregnancy is unclear and doses of 2 g/day do not appear to decrease the incidence of pre-eclampsia in healthy nulliparous women.[97,100]

INDUCTION OF LABOR
Mechanisms of Term Labor

In pregnancy, many hormones and peptides, including progesterone, prostacyclin, relaxin, nitric oxide, and parathyroid hormone-related peptide inhibit uterine smooth muscle contractility. Labor at term occurs because the myometrium is released from its quiescent state.[101] For example, as progesterone concentrations decrease near-term gestation, estrogen may stimulate uterine contractility.

Uterine activity is divided into four phases: quiescence (phase 0), activation (phase 1), stimulation (phase 2), and involution (phase 3). Each of these phases is stimulated or inhibited by several factors.[101] During activation, uterotropins such as estrogen and possibly others stimulate a complex series of uterine changes (e.g., increased myometrial prostaglandin and oxytocin receptors and myometrial gap junctions), which are important for the coordination of contractions. These changes help prime the myometrium and cervix for stimulation by the uterotonins oxytocin and prostaglandins E_2 and $F_{2\alpha}$. The cervix softens, shortens, and dilates, a process referred to as cervical ripening. Uterine stimulation is responsible for the change in myometrial activity from irregular to regular contractions. During phase 3, involution of the uterus occurs after delivery and is mediated mostly by oxytocin.[101]

The exact stimulus of the biochemical scheme leading to labor in humans is unknown. The fetus may help facilitate this process by affecting placental steroid production through mechanical distention of the uterus and by activating the fetal hypothalamic-pituitary-adrenal axis. Ultimately, these lead to increased production of oxytocin and prostaglandins by the fetoplacental unit.

Labor is divided into three stages.[102] Weak, irregular, rhythmic contractions (Braxton Hicks contractions or "false labor") may happen for weeks before the onset of true labor. The first stage begins with the start of regular uterine contractions and ends with complete cervical dilation. Stage 1 is divided further into the latent phase, active phase, and deceleration phase. During the latent phase, the cervix effaces (thins) but dilates minimally. The contractions become progressively stronger and longer, better coordinated, and more frequent. The duration of the latent phase is the most varied and unpredictable of all aspects of labor and can continue intermittently for days. During the active phase, contractions are strong and regular, occurring every 2 to 3 minutes. The cervix dilates from 3 to 4 cm to full dilation, usually 10 cm. The second stage starts with complete cervical dilation and ends with the delivery of the fetus. The third stage of labor is the time between the delivery of the fetus and the delivery of the placenta.[102]

Indications, Contraindications, and Requirements

41. J.T., a 28-year-old primigravida, is admitted to the Labor and Delivery suite for labor induction. She is at 42 weeks' gestation by dates and ultrasound and has a normal obstetric examination. Cervical examination reveals an unfavorable cervix for labor induction; Bishop score is 4. What are the indications and contraindications for labor induction in J.T.?

The induction of labor involves the artificial stimulation of uterine contractions that lead to labor and delivery.[103] Induction of labor is indicated when the continuation of pregnancy jeopardizes maternal or fetal health (e.g., pre-eclampsia, chorioamnionitis [infection of the fetal membranes], fetal demise, IUGR, Rho(D) alloimmunization, maternal medical problems, post-term pregnancy).[103] Post-term pregnancy (≥42 weeks' gestation), as in J.T.'s case, is the most common indication and most commonly encountered problem leading to induction of labor.[103,104] Contraindications to labor induction are similar to those for spontaneous labor and vaginal delivery[103] and include, but are not limited to, active genital herpes infection, placenta previa (abnormally implanted placenta), prior classic uterine incision, transverse fetal lie, and prolapsed umbilical cord. If uterine activity is appropriately monitored, induced labor yields similar maternal and perinatal outcomes as those with spontaneous labor.[103]

A complete assessment of both mother and fetus should be performed before inducing labor.[103–105] Previous labor complications or cesarean deliveries in the mother should be considered. Fetal maturity must be assessed accurately before the induction of labor to avoid the inadvertent delivery of a preterm fetus.[103,105] Every attempt should be made to ensure fetal lung maturation before inducing labor when termination of pregnancy is necessary before 34 weeks' gestation; and antenatal corticosteroids should be administered.[80]

The degree of cervical ripeness and readiness for induction of labor should be assessed because the success of labor induction depends on the degree of cervical ripeness.[103,106] The state of the cervix is assessed using a pelvic scoring method. The Bishop method assigns a score based on the station of the fetal head relative to the maternal spine and the extent of cervical dilation, effacement, consistency, and position.[105,106] Bishop scores of >8 are associated with a 100% induction rate and short labor.[103,106] Bishop scores ≤4, as is documented in J.T., are associated with a high likelihood of failed inductions and cesarean deliveries.[106] Unfortunately, women with Bishop scores ≤2 who undergo cervical ripening before induction of labor still have high incidence of failure and cesarean deliveries.[106]

Cervical ripening can be accomplished by the administration of prostaglandins (E$_2$ and E$_1$) or low-dose oxytocin. Alternatively, cervical dilators or separation of the chorioamniotic membranes from the internal surface of the uterus can ripen the cervix.[103,105,106] Osmotic or hygroscopic dilators (e.g., Dilapan, Lamisil) work by absorbing cervical mucous and gradually swelling, thereby dilating the cervical canal.[105,106] The hygroscopic dilators require less monitoring of the mother when compared with the administration of prostaglandins; however, they do not appear to decrease the incidence of cesarean deliveries.[105,106] Labor induction is accomplished most commonly by amniotomy (artificial rupture of the fetal membranes) and oxytocin administration.[103,105]

Although labor induction is medically indicated in J.T. to decrease the risk of an adverse fetal outcome with continuing a post-term pregnancy, her cervix is unfavorable for induction.

Cervical Ripening
Prostaglandin E$_2$ (Dinoprostone)

42. **When should dinoprostone be used to induce labor?**

Prostaglandins (e.g., dinoprostone) induce cervical ripening and enhance myometrial sensitivity to oxytocin by promoting the breakdown of collagen and increasing the submucosal hyaluronic acid and water content.[103,105,106] A Bishop score of ≤4 is a definite indication for cervical ripening. Although not universally accepted, intermediate Bishop scores of 5 to 7 indicate a need for cervical ripening.[107] Patients with intermediate Bishop scores undergoing cervical ripening with prostaglandins are more likely to achieve labor without oxytocin.[103] Dinoprostone is the drug used most commonly for cervical ripening.[105] Up to half of the women treated with dinoprostone experience labor and deliver within 24 hours, some without oxytocin.[108–110] Dinoprostone cervical gel (Prepidil Gel) contains dinoprostone 0.5 mg/3 g (2.5 mL gel) and is to be administered endocervically. Dinoprostone vaginal insert (Cervidil) contains dinoprostone 10 mg and is to be inserted vaginally.[112] Prepidil-Gel must be refrigerated and Cervidil vaginal inserts must remain frozen until administration. Women with unfavorable cervices, such as J.T., should undergo a trial of cervical ripening with dinoprostone before labor induction. Post-term women with unfavorable cervices who receive dinoprostone have shorter duration of labor, require lower doses of oxytocin, and may have a decreased incidence of cesarean deliveries.[106,108–110]

43. **Which dinoprostone dosage form should be used in J.T.?**

Both dinoprostone products are effective for cervical ripening, leading to successful induction of labor.[106,108–110] The two dinoprostone formulations differ in dosing and application.[111,112]

DINOPROSTONE GEL (PREPIDIL)

Prepidil 0.5 mg should be administered endocervically at room temperature in or near the labor and delivery suite.[103,111] After administration, the patient should remain in a recumbent position for at least 30 minutes to minimize leakage from the cervix.[103,111] Fetal heart rate and uterine activity should be monitored before administration and continuously for at least 2 hours after administration. The cervix should be reassessed and the dose repeated every 6 hours if needed or until a maximum cumulative dose of 1.5 mg (three doses) has been administered in 24 hours.[111] Most women need more than one application, and at least 50% need three doses.[113] The average wholesale price for one dose of Prepidil Gel has been about $172 per 0.5 mg dose.[114]

Once the cervix has ripened but the patient is not in active labor, oxytocin may be started if at least 6 hours have elapsed from the time the last dinoprostone dose was administered.[112,115] Waiting at least 6 to 12 hours may decrease the incidence of uterine hyperstimulation, which is defined as uterine contractions occurring more frequently than every 2 minutes or lasting longer than 90 seconds, with or without fetal heart rate changes.[116]

DINOPROSTONE VAGINAL INSERT (CERVIDIL)

The dinoprostone 10-mg vaginal insert, Cervidil, slowly releases dinoprostone 0.3 mg per hour over a 12-hour period.[112]

The insert is contained within a knitted pouch attached to a long tape. This is a major advantage because it can be removed quickly at the beginning of active labor or in the event of uterine hyperstimulation.[112,115] The use of this vaginal insert requires continuous monitoring of fetal heart rate and uterine activity for as long as the insert is in place and for at least 15 minutes after its removal because of possible uterine hyperstimulation anytime during its administration.[109,115] The dinoprostone vaginal insert allows for a shorter dosing interval for oxytocin, which can be infused as soon as 30 minutes after the removal of the dinoprostone vaginal insert.[112] The total cost of using Cervidil may be considerably less than Prepidil.

EFFICACY OF DINOPROSTONE GEL VERSUS VAGINAL INSERT

The number of prospective, randomized trials comparing the efficacy of dinoprostone endocervical gel and the controlled-release vaginal insert for pre-induction cervical ripening are limited.[113,117] In one study, women treated with the vaginal insert experienced shorter cervical ripening and delivery times, decreased need for oxytocin, and decreased lengths of hospital stay.[113] A second prospective, randomized comparison of the two products showed no difference in the number of women delivering within 24 hours, time to delivery, or cesarean deliveries.[117] However, women treated with the vaginal insert achieved a greater change in Bishop score and active labor, negating the need for oxytocin.

ADVERSE EFFECTS

The most serious side effect associated with dinoprostone administration is uterine hyperstimulation with or without abnormal fetal heart rate tracings. The incidence of uterine hyperstimulation associated with the use of dinoprostone intravaginal insert is about 5%: the rate of occurrence for dinoprostone endocervical gel is about 1%.[104,115] Uterine hyperstimulation occurs more frequently if the Bishop score is >4 before administration of dinoprostone and can occur up to 9.5 hours after placement of the intravaginal insert.[103,104] Most episodes of uterine hyperstimulation with the use of the vaginal insert occur during active labor and resolve within a few minutes after removal of the insert.[109] Uterine contraction abnormalities may be avoided if the insert is promptly removed upon the onset of labor.[118]

Both dinoprostone formulation are associated with fever, nausea, vomiting, and diarrhea; and neither are associated with adverse neonatal outcomes.[103,111,112] Therefore, either formulation of dinoprostone is appropriate for cervical ripening in J.T. Cervidil may be more cost effective.

Misoprostol (Cytotec)

44. What advantages does misoprostol have over dinoprostone when used for cervical ripening?

Misoprostol (Cytotec) is a prostaglandin E_1 analog approved for use in the prevention of NSAID-induced peptic ulcer disease. It also has been used for cervical ripening and the induction of labor in women despite the lack of approval by the FDA for these latter indications.[118,119] In two large meta-analyses, misoprostol was more effective for cervical ripening and labor induction than either placebo or treatment with dinoprostone.[118,119] Failure to deliver within 24 hours and the need for supplemental oxytocin were both higher in women

treated with dinoprostone compared with women treated with misoprostol. Women treated with misoprostol experienced labor more often during cervical ripening and had a reduced rate of cesarean deliveries, a shorter delivery time, and a greater incidence of vaginal delivery within 24 hours, but a higher incidence of uterine contraction abnormalities.[118,119,121] In other comparisons, intravaginal misoprostol resulted in shorter times to delivery than either dinoprostone vaginal insert or dinoprostone endocervical gel.[122,123] Again, uterine hyperstimulation without fetal heart rate abnormalities was most common with misoprostol use. Maternal and neonatal outcomes were similar in both groups. The need for oxytocin is decreased significantly in women treated with misoprostol compared with women treated with dinoprostone.[124]

Misoprostol has been given both orally and intravaginally, but intravaginal doses of 25 μg every 4 hours are more effective than oral doses of 50 μg every 4 hours for cervical ripening and labor induction.[125] Misoprostol 25 μg (1/4 of a 100-μg tablet) is inserted into the posterior vaginal fornix and repeated as needed every 3 to 6 hours.[121,124] Higher doses of 50 μg are associated with increased uterine contractile abnormalities.[118,124] Continuous fetal heart rate and uterine monitoring is recommended throughout the administration of misoprostol.[123]

Misoprostol should not be used in women with previous uterine scars because of the risk for uterine rupture.[121,122] Misoprostol appears to be an effective, and much less costly method of cervical ripening, but the incidence of uterine hyperstimulation appears to be increased relative to dinoprostone, especially with higher doses. Although misoprostol is a known teratogen in the first trimester of pregnancy, there are no reports of teratogenic effects with exposure beyond the first trimester.[121] Misoprostol's low cost and ease of administration are advantages over dinoprostone; however, its lack of FDA approval for cervical ripening and induction of labor is a disadvantage.

Oxytocin (Pitocin)
Mechanism of Action

45. Twelve hours after administration of dinoprostone vaginal insert, J.T.'s cervix has responded and her Bishop score is now 9, but she has not developed a consistent pattern of uterine contractions. What drug therapy should be initiated at this point?

Synthetic oxytocin should be administered to J.T. to stimulate uterine contractions for the purpose of accomplishing delivery. Oxytocin increases the frequency, force and duration of uterine contractions.[126] The uterine response to oxytocin increases throughout pregnancy beginning at approximately 20 weeks' gestation and increases considerably at 30 weeks' gestation.[126] Oxytocin is indicated for both the induction and augmentation of labor. A prolonged latent phase or dystocia (difficult labor) caused by uterine hypocontractility in the active phase of labor is indication for augmentation with oxytocin.[127]

Dosing and Administration

46. How should oxytocin be administered to J.T.?

Oxytocin should be administered by continuous intravenous infusion using a controlled infusion device. The goal of oxytocin administration is to induce uterine contractions that dilate the cervix and aid in the descent of the fetus while avoiding uterine hyperstimulation and fetal distress.[126] There are two opposing views about oxytocin administration for the induction or augmentation of labor. One view is that oxytocin infusions should mimic physiologic doses in the range of 2 to 6 mU/minute with the goal being vaginal delivery with as little as possible uterine hyperstimulation and fetal distress.[122] The other view is that oxytocin should be used in pharmacologic doses to cause strong uterine contractions with the goals being shortened labor, timely correction of dysfunctional labor, decreased cesarean deliveries, and reduced maternal morbidity.[117,127]

Oxytocin plasma concentrations increase linearly with increasing doses and steady-state is reached within 20 to 40 minutes.[128] However, oxytocin serum concentrations correlate poorly with uterine activity.[128] Factors that may affect response to oxytocin include parity, gestational age, and cervical dilation.[127,128]

Despite many randomized controlled trials and much experience with oxytocin, the optimal starting doses, dosage increments, dosing intervals, and maximum doses are different in the various protocols (Table 46-5).[116,126,129] Starting doses range from 0.5 to 0.6 mU/minute and dose increment intervals range from 15 to 60 minutes.[103,116,129] Waiting for 30 to 40 minutes between each dosage rate increase allows time to assess the response at steady-state. Most low-dose protocols usually start oxytocin at 1 to 2 mU/minute and increase the rate of infusion by 1 to 2 mU/minute every 30 to 40 minutes.[129,130] High-dose protocols start oxytocin at 3 to 6 mU/minute with incremental increases of 3 to 6 mU/minute every 20 to 40 minutes.[129] The maximum dose of oxcytocin for augmentation of delivery and for induction of labor are 20 mU/minute and 40 mU/minute, respectively.[129] The American College of Obstetricians and Gynecologists recommends a low-dose oxytocin protocol starting at 0.5 to 2 mU per minute and increasing by 1 to 2 mU/minute every 30 to 60 minutes, using a cervical dilation rate of 1 cm/hour as a gauge of adequate progression of active labor.[103]

Oxytocin protocols using higher doses and/or shorter dose adjustment intervals (15 to 20 minutes) for augmentation of labor generally result in fewer cesarean deliveries for labor dystocia.[130–132] However, the incidence of uterine hyperstimulation during labor induction is higher with high-dose protocols (initial dose of 6 mU/minute with incremental increases of 6 mU/minute) when compared with shorter dosing adjustment intervals of 20 minutes or with longer dose adjustment intervals of 40 minutes.[130] Women undergoing labor induction with high-dose oxytocin have a higher incidence of uterine stimulation and cesarean deliveries for fetal distress, but a re-

duced incidence of failed inductions and neonatal sepsis compared with women treated with low-dose oxytocin.[131] In general, lower maximum doses are needed for augmentation of labor than for induction of labor.[129,131]

J.T. should be started on an infusion of oxytocin 10 or 20 U diluted in 1,000 mL of an isotonic solution (concentration = 10 and 20 mU/mL, respectively) at 1 mU/minute. She should have continuous uterine and fetal heart rate monitoring throughout the infusion to detect abnormal uterine contraction patterns or fetal heart rate patterns. The goal is to establish a pattern of 3 to 5 uterine contractions of 60 to 90 seconds duration per 10-minute period.[116] The oxytocin infusion should be increased by 1 to 2 mU/minute every 30 to 40 minutes as needed for inadequate progression of labor (cervical dilation rate of <1cm/ hour).[103] Fluid intake and urine output should be assessed hourly.

Adverse Effects

47. **What are the adverse effects and complications of oxytocin for which J.T. should be monitored?**

Uterine hyperstimulation with fetal heart rate deceleration is the most common adverse effect of oxytocin.[126,127] Uterine hyperstimulation, usually associated with excessive maternal dosing or increased myometrial sensitivity to oxytocin, may result in uterine rupture, vaginal and cervical lacerations, precipitous delivery, abruptio placentae, emergency cesarean delivery for fetal distress, and postpartum hemorrhage secondary to uterine atony.[116] In general, neonatal outcomes associated with oxytocin use are not different than those achieved by spontaneous labor.[116] Although oxytocin has only weak antidiuretic properties, water intoxication resulting in seizures, coma, and death have been reported.[103] Intravenous bolus administration may cause paradoxical relaxation of vascular smooth muscle leading to hypotension and tachycardia.[126]

POSTPARTUM HEMORRHAGE
Prevention

48. **What are other uses for oxytocin during delivery other than induction or augmentation of labor?**

Oxytocin is administered routinely following the delivery of the placenta to promote uterine contraction and vasoconstriction.[126,133] Uterine contraction leading to vasoconstriction is important for hemostasis.[133] Uterine atony, the condition in which the uterus fails to contract after delivery of the placenta, is the most common cause of postpartum hemorrhage.[126,133,134] Risks for uterine atony include induction with

Table 46-5	Oxytocin Regimens for Induction and Augmentation of Labor				
Regimen	Starting Dose	Incremental Increase	Dosage Interval	Maximum Dose	Reference
Low-dose	1 mU/min	1 mU/min up to 8 U/min then 2 mU/min	20 min	20 mU/min	131
High-dose	6 mU/min	6 mU/min[a]	20 or 40 min	42 mU/min	130
	4 mU/min	4 mU/min	15 min	Until adequate contractility reached	132

[a]Uterine hyperstimulation: reduce incremental increase to 3 mU/min; recurrent hyperstimulation: reduce to 1 mU/min.

oxytocin, prolonged labor, overdistended uterus and previous postpartum hemorrhage.[133–135] Oxytocin 10 to 20 U IM or diluted in 0.5 to 1 L of parenteral fluid and given as an IV infusion of 200 mU per minute until the uterus is firmly contracted reduces the risk for postpartum hemorrhage secondary to uterine atony.[126,136] Oxytocin should never be administered undiluted as a bolus dose because it can cause severe hypotension and cardiac dysrhythmias.[136]

Misoprostol

Misoprostol 400 to 600 μg PO can be administered in the third stage of labor to prevent postpartum hemorrhage.[137,138] In the presence of vaginal bleeding, the vaginal route of administration is not optimal. Misoprostol also can be administered rectally. The rectal route of administration is associated with a lower incidence of fever and shivering, which is common with orally administered misoprostol during the third stage of labor.[137] The rectal route of administration also is associated with lower maximum serum concentrations and lower time to maximal concentrations than when the drug is administered orally.

Treatment

49. Within a few hours of delivering her fetus, J.T. has visible vaginal bleeding. She has a distended uterus and the hemorrhage is attributed to uterine atony. Uterine massage and infusion of oxytocin do not control the bleeding. What other pharmacologic options are available to treat J.T.?

Ergot Alkaloids

If the postpartum hemorrhaging does not respond to oxytocin administration, ergonovine maleate (Ergotrate) and its semisynthetic derivative, methylergonovine maleate (Methergine) can be used because of their potent uterotonic effects. The intramuscular route of administration is associated with less frequent adverse effects (nausea, vomiting, hypertension, headache, chest pain, dizziness, tinnitus, diaphoresis) than the intravenous route.[134,139] Ergot alkaloids should be avoided in hypertensive and eclamptic patients because of the potential for arrhythmias, seizures, and cerebrovascular accidents.[139] The dose of both drugs is 0.2 mg administered intramuscularly every 2 hours as needed followed by 0.2 to 0.4 mg administered orally two to four times daily for 2 to 7 days to promote involution of the uterus.[139] Ergot derivatives are not frequently used in obstetric care because of their adverse cardiovascular effects.[134,135]

15-Methyl Prostaglandin F_2 (Carboprost Tromethamine)

Bleeding caused by uterine atony that is unresponsive to oxytocin can be treated with 15-methyl prostaglandin $F_{2\alpha}$-tromethamine, also known as carboprost tromethamine (Hemabate).[133,135] Carboprost tromethamine, like naturally occurring prostaglandins, stimulates uterine contraction and decreases postpartum hemorrhage; it is more potent and has a longer duration of effect than its parent compound, prostaglandin $F_{2\alpha}$.

Carboprost tromethamine is approved for intramuscular use, but also has been also administered through direct myometrial injection[133,134] and intrauterine irrigation.[133] The in-

tramyometrial route of administration has been associated with severe hypotension and pulmonary edema.[140] An initial dose of 0.25 mg IM is given followed by 0.25 mg every 15 to 90 minutes.[134,141] The dose may be increased to 0.5 mg if a patient does not respond adequately to several 0.25-mg intramuscular doses. The total cumulative dose should not exceed 2 mg.[141] Carboprost tromethamine is effective in treating 60% to 85% of women with uterine atony who have failed standard treatment.[134] Improvement in bleeding typically occurs after one to two injections.

The most common adverse effects of carboprost tromethamine (nausea, vomiting, diarrhea) can be reduced considerably by pretreatment with antiemetic and antidiarrheal agents.[141] Flushing and fever also occur frequently. Many of the adverse effects are related to the contractile effect of this drug on smooth muscle.[141] Hypertension, although rare, typically occurs in women with pre-existing hypertension or pre-eclampsia. The potent vasoconstricting and bronchoconstricting properties of carboprost can cause uterine rupture, as well as pulmonary and cardiac problems. Carboprost is contraindicated in women with active pulmonary, cardiac, renal, or hepatic disease as well as in women with acute pelvic inflammatory disease.[134,135,141]

PRETERM LABOR

Preterm labor, which begins before the end of the 37th week of gestation, occurs in approximately 7% to 10% of all births and is responsible for >85% of all perinatal morbidity and mortality.[101,142] Pregnancy ending before the 20th week of gestation generally is the result of either an elective or spontaneous abortion.[142] Despite improvements in obstetric care (see Chapter 94, Neonatal Therapy), the incidence of preterm delivery has not decreased.[142,144]

Etiology

The cause of preterm labor is multifactorial as many risk factors are associated with preterm labor and delivery.[102,142] A hostile intrauterine environment (e.g., amnionitis caused by infection) is responsible for about 30% of preterm labors.[101] Infection triggers an inflammatory response that results in the release of prostaglandins and cytokines, which stimulate uterine activity and induce preterm labor.[101] Thrombin is another strong uterotonic that has been implicated in causing preterm labor.[101] In addition, about 15% of idiopathic preterm labor has been attributed to a deficiency of the enzyme responsible for fetal membrane metabolism of prostaglandins, thus permitting prostaglandin E_2 to initiate myometrial contractions.[101]

Approximately one-third of preterm labors are the result of preterm premature rupture of the membranes (PROM).[144] Premature rupture of membranes, which consist of the amnion and chorion, is the spontaneous rupture of the fetal membranes before the onset of labor. If PROM occurs before the end of the 37th week of gestation, it is referred to as preterm PROM. The closer to term that PROM occurs, the shorter the period before delivery.[144] Labor occurs within 24 hours in 90% of women with PROM at term. In contrast, half the women with preterm PROM between 28 and 34 weeks' gestation deliver within 24 hours and 80% to 90% within 7 days.[144]

The amniotic fluid surrounding the fetus is necessary to protect the umbilical cord and the fetus from compression.[144] It is also vital to the developing fetal lungs, limb movements, and gas exchange. Amniotic fluid may be lost during PROM, leading to fetal compromise. In addition, the vagina serves as a point of entry for bacteria with PROM, increasing the risk for intra-amniotic and fetal infections, which in turn can trigger labor indirectly through the production of prostaglandins and cytokines. PROM that exceeds 24 hours is considered prolonged.[144]

Spontaneous preterm deliveries can occur without maternal or fetal illness, can follow PROM or chorioamnionitis (infection of the amnion or chorion membranes), or be the result of an incompetent cervix. Several risk factors are associated with spontaneous preterm births, including a history of a previous preterm birth.[142] When medical or obstetrical conditions place the mother or fetus at serious risk if the pregnancy is continued, preterm delivery is indicated.[142,145] The two most common conditions requiring preterm deliveries are preeclampsia and IUGR.[145]

Clinical Presentation and Evaluation

50. B.B., a 17-year-old white female, G_2P_1, 29 weeks' gestation, is admitted to the obstetrical unit with complaints of vaginal bleeding, backache, cramps, and uterine contractions. Her contractions vary in intensity, last about 30 seconds, and are approximately 8 to 10 minutes apart. B.B. has been closely followed because she had a previous preterm birth at 32 weeks' gestation. A cervical examination reveals 2 cm cervical dilation, which is increased by 1 cm from her previous prenatal visit 1 week ago, and 80% effacement without signs of PROM. Cervicovaginal secretions are positive for fibronectin. Cervical cultures for *Chlamydia trachomatis* and *Neisseria gonorrhoeae* from her previous visit are negative. Vaginal wet preparations are also negative for bacterial vaginosis and *Trichomonas vaginalis*. Vital signs, urinalysis, and CBC with differential are normal. Urine cultures show no growth. Uterine contractions and fetal heart tones are being monitored. Fetal ultrasound reveals a fetus of 30 weeks' gestation with an estimated weight of 1,200 g. What signs, symptoms and laboratory evidence suggest spontaneous preterm labor for B.B.?

B.B. has vaginal bleeding, backache, and uterine contractions, all of which are symptoms of preterm labor. Other important signs of preterm labor are a change or increase in vaginal discharge and a leaking of amniotic fluid.[143]

Preterm labor is difficult to diagnose using uterine contractions as the lone criterion because it is often confused with Braxton Hicks contractions. Contractions during preterm labor are not always painful and often are undetected by women.[143] The use of contractions alone to diagnose preterm labor result in high false-positive rates of diagnoses.[142] As a result, either the dilation or effacement of the cervix in combination with biochemical markers in the presence of persistent uterine contractions are used to diagnose preterm labor.[142,144]

Fibronectin, a protein that serves as an adhesive between the fetal membranes and decidua, is normally present in cervical secretions during the first half of pregnancy after which it disappears and then reappears again at term as labor approaches.[142] Its usefulness lies in its negative predictive value in preventing the overdiagnosis of preterm labor. A negative fibronectin test is helpful in ruling out imminent preterm delivery (i.e., within 2 weeks) when obtained from women who are at risk for preterm delivery and are 24 to 34 weeks' gestation and have intact amniotic membranes and a cervical dilation <3 cm.[146]

Persistent contractions with a dilated cervix of >2 cm, a change of ≥1 cm, are necessary to diagnose preterm labor. B.B. has the criteria necessary to establish a firm diagnosis of preterm labor.

Risk Factors

51. What risk factors does B.B. have for spontaneous preterm labor?

B.B. has several risk factors for preterm delivery. She has a twofold increased risk of preterm delivery because she has had one previous preterm delivery.[143] If this pregnancy ends in a preterm delivery, her risk for a preterm delivery during her third pregnancy will be three times higher than that in the normal population.[143] Her young age may also be a risk factor.[142,143] A maternal age younger than 18 or older than 35 years of age is also a potential risk factor for preterm labor, although it is difficult to separate age itself from the confounding factors associated with age.[142,143] Black race is an independent risk factor for both preterm labor and lower neonatal birth weight.[165] Other risk factors include low maternal weight before pregnancy, smoking, second-trimester bleeding, multiple gestation, and uterine anomalies.[101,142,143] Cervical competence is an important risk factor, and the shorter the length of the cervix, the greater the risk for preterm delivery.[142] Maternal infections such as untreated urinary tract infections and pneumonia are associated with preterm delivery.[143] In addition, genital infections such as bacterial vaginosis and those caused by group B streptococcus (GBS), *Chlamydia trachomatis*, *Neisseria gonorrhoeae*, *Ureaplasma urealyticum*, and *Trichomonas vaginalis* are also associated with preterm births.[101] Although it is important to identify women at risk for spontaneous preterm delivery, only half of the preterm deliveries occur in women with known risk factors.[142]

Tocolysis
Goals of Therapy

52. What are the goals of tocolysis?

The treatment for spontaneous preterm labor is geared toward preventing or prolonging delivery to improve neonatal outcome. Prolonging pregnancy for just 1 week may decrease neonatal morbidity and mortality up to 15%.[143] A dramatic increase in survival occurs between the gestational ages of 23 to 26 weeks.[142] Neonatal morbidity is substantially decreased once the gestational age surpasses 34 weeks.[142]

Prolongation of pregnancy can be achieved through tocolytic drugs, which interrupt or stop uterine contractions. Although tocolysis temporarily prolongs gestation, it rarely prevents preterm delivery.[150,151] Furthermore, tocolysis alone does not appear to decrease neonatal mortality or morbidity.

The goal of tocolysis is to stop contractions and prolong delivery for at least 48 to 72 hours in 75% to 80% of women.[150] Tocolysis prolongation of labor allows time for the administration of glucocorticoids to women who are between 24 and 34 weeks' gestation to improve fetal pulmonary surfactant production; allows time for antibiotic treatment of infections; or allows time for transfer of the mother to a tertiary facility equipped to care for a preterm neonate.[80,150]

Numerous factors affect the decision to arrest preterm labor with a tocolytic agent. Fetal factors precluding tocolysis include fetal distress, severe IUGR, major congenital anomalies incompatible with life, and intrauterine death.[142,143] Maternal factors include chorioamnionitis, pre-eclampsia, HELLP syndrome, and advanced labor.[142,143] Tocolysis is less likely to be effective in women with cervical dilation of >3 cm[149] and is usually unsuccessful if the patient is in advanced labor (cervical dilation >5 cm).[142,143] Because the etiology of preterm labor is multifactorial, B.B. should be evaluated thoroughly and periodically for potential causes of preterm labor and treated appropriately when diagnosed. For example, diagnosis of a urinary tract infection and treatment with antibiotics may prevent progression of preterm labor to delivery.[142] B.B. has no evidence suggestive of infection or other complications and has no contraindications to tocolysis. She does not exhibit any of the characteristics that could make her unresponsive to these agents. Prolonging gestation, even for a few days would be beneficial in B.B. because she is only 29 weeks' gestation.

Magnesium Sulfate

53. Magnesium sulfate 6 g IV loading dose for 30 minutes followed by 2 g/hr continuous IV infusion through a controlled infusion pump has been ordered for B.B.. Why was such a large dose prescribed?

Magnesium sulfate is the most frequently used parenteral tocolytic agent in the United States and also is frequently prescribed for the prevention and treatment of eclampsia.[149,151,152] Larger doses are needed to arrest preterm labor than for seizure prophylaxis in pre-eclampsia.[83]

Magnesium sulfate relaxes uterine smooth muscle and decreases myometrial contractility.[142,143,150] It is effective in stopping contractions for 48 to 72 hours in approximately 60% to 80% of preterm labor in women without PROM.[149,150] The mechanism by which it exerts this effect is not understood clearly, but it probably involves calcium antagonism at the neuromuscular junction.[142,149,150] It is interesting to note that uterine activity increases with calcium supplementation of hypocalcemic women treated with magnesium sulfate.[150]

EFFICACY

54. How effective is magnesium sulfate for tocolysis?

Despite its widespread use, the evidence for magnesium's efficacy in prolonging gestation is inadequate.[149,153] In meta-analyses of placebo-controlled trials of magnesium for tocolysis, no prolongation of pregnancy was noted.[153,154] The small sample size in this limited number of studies, however, could have precluded the ability to detect a difference in the risk of delivery between magnesium and placebo.[154] More studies have compared magnesium with β-adrenergic agonists than

to placebo.[149,154] Magnesium probably is as effective as the β-adrenergic agonists, terbutaline and ritodrine (approximately 80% to 90%), in postponing preterm delivery for 48 hours.[154,155] Because β-adrenergic agonists have proven efficacy for delaying delivery for at least 48 hours and are as effective as magnesium, magnesium is presumed to be equally effective in prolonging pregnancy. The efficacy of magnesium in delaying delivery for longer than 48 hours is unclear.[154] Maternal magnesium therapy is associated with a decreased risk of cerebral palsy and mental retardation in neonates that is not due to selective early mortality of exposed infants.[156]

Magnesium is better tolerated by women than are the β-adrenergic agonists.[154] Magnesium is contraindicated in patients with hypocalcemia, myasthenia gravis, and renal failure.[148,157]

MONITORING FOR EFFICACY AND TOXICITY

55. How should magnesium sulfate therapy in B.B. be monitored for efficacy and safety?

The hourly rate of magnesium administration for B.B. may be increased by 1 g/hour until she has ≤1 contraction per 10 minutes or a maximum of 4 g/hour is attained.[150] The deep tendon reflexes and respiratory rate of B.B. should be monitored every hour, and urine output should be measured every 2 to 4 hours because magnesium is renally eliminated. In addition, close monitoring of fluid balance is important to prevent pulmonary edema.[150] Fortunately, most women undergoing tocolysis with magnesium have normal renal function and are not at risk for renal failure as are women with pre-eclampsia (see Hypertension and Pre-eclampsia).

Magnesium serum concentrations should be evaluated every 6 to 12 hours in an effort to minimize adverse effects.[158] The patellar reflex disappears with magnesium serum concentrations between 9 and 10 mg/dL, and the presence of deep tendon reflexes can serve as a guide for determining when magnesium serum concentrations need to be monitored.[86,87,149] As long as deep tendon reflexes are present, many practitioners will not measure concentrations.[149] Myometrial contractions are inhibited in vitro with magnesium serum concentrations of 9.6 to 12 mg/dL and clinically with concentrations of 6 to 9.6 mg/dL.[150] Serum concentrations of magnesium, however, do not relate linearly to its efficacy for tocolysis.[159]

The most common side effects associated with magnesium loading doses are transient hypotension, flushing, a sense of warmth, headache, dizziness, lethargy, nystagmus, and dry mouth.[142,155,160] Other adverse effects reported with magnesium are hypothermia[149,151]; paralytic ileus[151]; and pulmonary edema, which may occur in up to 2% of patients treated with magnesium sulfate and can be a lethal complication of tocolysis.[150,171] Pulmonary edema occurs less frequently with magnesium sulfate than with β-sympathomimetics and is more commonly encountered with prolonged infusions.[150,151] Treatment consists of discontinuing magnesium sulfate and treatment with diuretics.

To prevent inadvertent overdoses, a controlled infusion device should always be used to deliver magnesium as a continuous infusion. Hypocalcemia and tetany can occur with hypermagnesemia; therefore, parenteral calcium gluconate or chloride should be available for acute treatment.[8] Neuromuscular blockade and respiratory arrest develop with magnesium serum concentrations of 15 to 17 mg/dL, and cardiac arrest develops with concentrations of 30 to 35 mg/dL.[94]

Fetal magnesium serum concentrations are similar to maternal concentrations.[150] The most common neonatal adverse effects are hypotonia and sleepiness. Hypotonia may continue for 3 or 4 days in the neonate because of decreased renal elimination of magnesium. Rarely, assisted mechanical ventilation for neuromuscular depression may be needed.[150]

β-Adrenergic Agonists
EFFICACY

56. **Could B.B. have been treated with a β-adrenergic agonist?**

β-Adrenergic agonists are second-line choices for arresting labor and prolonging pregnancy because of high costs and the maternal adverse effects described below.[149] These agents selectively bind to β_2-adrenergic receptors in uterine smooth muscle and ultimately inhibit smooth muscle cell contractility.[153,155] β-Adrenergic agents are as effective as magnesium in delaying delivery for at least 48 hours.[154] Similar to magnesium, β-agonists do not reduce the rate of preterm delivery and the effects of β-agonists on perinatal outcome are not clear.[149,153] The continued use of β-agonists can result in the development of tachyphylaxis to its effects on the myometrium and may in part explain treatment failures with these drugs.[149,163]

Terbutaline is available for IV, SC, and oral administration. One dose of terbutaline subcutaneously is often administered to women with mild contractions and cervical dilation <2 cm.[149] Intravenous β-sympathomimetics are used in cases with more severe and frequent contractions and cervical dilation >2 cm.[149]

MATERNAL AND FETAL ADVERSE EFFECTS

57. **What adverse effects are associated with terbutaline?**

β-Adrenergic agonists are not selective for myometrial β_2-adrenergic receptors, and this accounts for their high incidence of adverse effects.[149,151,155] Maternal adverse effects such as pulmonary edema, palpitations, tachycardia, myocardial ischemia, hyperglycemia, hypokalemia, and hepatoxicity result in discontinuation of therapy in up to 10% of patients.[142] Pulmonary edema is common and, if not recognized promptly, can lead to adult RDS and death.[142,151] β-Sympathomimetics should not be used in women with underlying cardiac disease or arrhythmias, hypertension, diabetes mellitus, or thyrotoxicosis.[142,156]

The most commonly reported fetal or neonatal adverse effects associated with β-agonist therapy include tachycardia, hypotension, hypoglycemia, and hypocalcemia.[155] Maternal hyperglycemia causing fetal hyperglycemia and hyperinsulinemia can lead to neonatal hypoglycemia if not properly monitored postnatally.[149] Fetal tachycardia rarely leads to fetal myocardial ischemia or hypertrophy.[149] The use of β-sympathomimetic drugs has also been associated with an increased risk of neonatal intraventricular hemorrhage.[142,145,149]

Other Tocolytic Drugs

58. **What other drugs are commonly used for tocolysis?**

INDOMETHACIN

Prostaglandins $F_{2\alpha}$ and especially E_2 are important regulators of myometrial contractility and cervical ripening.[101] Prostaglandin synthetase inhibitors (e.g., indomethacin, celecoxib) decrease prostaglandin production and thereby decrease contractions and inhibit cervical change. Indomethacin (Indocin) is as effective as magnesium sulfate and β-adrenergic agonists in delaying delivery for 48 to 72 hours.[101,164–171] In a meta-analysis of tocolytics, indomethacin was the only tocolytic agent associated with a significant decrease of preterm birth and birth weight <2,500 g.[153]

Indomethacin is often used when women have failed tocolysis with magnesium sulfate; however, this drug has been associated with neonatal necrotizing enterocolitis, intraventricular hemorrhage, renal failure, and closure of the fetal ductus arteriosus.[148,168,169] The risk for neonatal adverse effects is increased when the fetus is >34 weeks' gestation, when exposed to indomethacin for longer than 48 hours, and when delivery occurs within 24 to 48 hours of administration.[151] Since indomethacin can decrease fetal urine output leading to oligohydramnios, the amniotic fluid index (AFI) should be followed and indomethacin discontinued if it falls below 5 cm.[148] Oligohydramnios generally resolves within 48 to 72 hours of the discontinuation of indomethacin.[148] The ductus arteriosus—a fetal vessel important in maintaining fetal circulation—constricts in 25% to 50% of fetuses exposed to indomethacin in utero and generally is reversible.[149] Permanent closure of the ductus arteriosus, however, has led to intrauterine demise. An increased risk for maternal postpartum hemorrhage is also associated with indomethacin use.[153] Indomethacin should not be used in the presence of oligohydramnios or suspected fetal renal or cardiac anomaly (see Chapter 94, Neonatal Therapy).[148,157]

Dual tocolysis with magnesium and indomethacin may increase the risk for severe (grade III or IV) intraventricular hemorrhage in neonates <800 g infants.[165] It is difficult to discern whether the increased intraventricular hemorrhage was indeed associated with indomethacin or with refractory preterm labor (e.g., intra-amniotic infection).[166,169] An analysis of the risks and benefits of indomethacin justifies its continued use as second-line treatment for preterm labor in women with contraindications to other tocolytics.[169] Tocolysis with indomethacin between the gestational ages of 24 to 32 weeks resulted in a lower number of adverse neonatal outcomes compared with no tocolysis.[169] Typical dosing regimens include a loading dose of 50 to 100 mg either rectally or orally followed by maintenance doses of 25 to 50 mg orally every 4 to 8 (most commonly given every 6 hours) hours for 24 to 48 hours.[164,165,167]

COX-2 INHIBITORS

Only amniotic cyclooxygenase-2 (COX-2), and not COX-1, activity is increased during labor, and tocolysis with COX-2 specific inhibitors may result in fewer adverse effects than with indomethacin or nonspecific cyclooxygenase inhibitors.[170,171] In a randomized, double-blind, placebo-controlled trial, celecoxib was comparable to indomethacin in efficacy and did not negatively affect ductal patency when used to treat preterm labor.[170] Both drugs decreased AFI (amniotic fluid index); however, fluid reaccumulation was prolonged when indomethacin was discontinued, an effect not observed with the discontinuation of celecoxib. More studies with larger number of subjects are needed to determine the safety and efficacy of COX-2 enzyme inhibitors relative to indomethacin.

CALCIUM CHANNEL BLOCKERS

The calcium channel blockers, nifedipine and nicardipine, inhibit preterm labor by decreasing calcium influx into uterine smooth muscle and inhibiting myometrial contractions.[149] Nifedipine is equally as effective as magnesium and β-adrenergic agents in delaying pregnancy for 48 hours.[149,152,172] Maternal side effects (e.g., tachycardia, headache, flushing, dizziness, nausea, hypotension in the hypovolemic patient) are rare.[151] Nifedipine does not adversely affect uteroplacental blood flow or fetal circulation. Concurrent use with magnesium should be avoided because the combination may potentiate neuromuscular blockade.[83,151] Nifedipine appears to be an attractive alternative for short-term tocolysis. The starting dose is usually 10 mg orally with repeated doses of 10 mg every 15 to 20 minutes for persistent contractions up to a maximum of 40 mg in the first hour.[152,172] Depending on the tocolytic effect, nifedipine is then maintained at 10 to 20 mg orally every 4 to 6 hours.[152,173] The appropriate duration of treatment has not been established, but typically it is continued through the 34th week of gestation.[152,172] Maintenance therapy with oral nifedipine in women treated initially with intravenous magnesium sulfate has not significantly prolonged pregnancy.[173]

Nicardipine is a more potent inhibitor of myometrial contractions in vitro compared with nifedipine, and it achieved arrest of preterm labor more quickly than intravenous magnesium sulfate.[174] Moreover, women treated with magnesium sulfate were more likely to have recurrence of preterm labor and had a higher incidence of adverse effects such as nausea and vomiting.

Duration of Tocolysis
ACUTE THERAPY

59. **B.B. has been maintained on magnesium sulfate continuous IV infusion for approximately 48 hours. The dose was increased to 3 g/hour shortly after the start of the infusion. B.B. has had no contractions for the past 24 hours. How long does she need to be treated? Should she be "weaned" off magnesium sulfate?**

B.B.'s contractions have completely stopped for 24 hours. Some protocols maintain magnesium sulfate for 12 to 24 hours after successful tocolysis.[150] After successful acute tocolysis is achieved, the magnesium infusion often is discontinued gradually. Some protocols decrease the magnesium sulfate by 1 g/hour every 4 hours, whereas others decrease the dose by 1 g/hour every 30 minutes and therapy is discontinued when the dose has been decreased to 2 g/hour.[150,158] The weaning of magnesium sulfate, however, may not beneficial, and abrupt discontinuation of the magnesium infusion probably is safer and less costly.[158]

CHRONIC MAINTENANCE THERAPY

60. **Should B.B. be started on chronic maintenance tocolytic therapy?**

Maintenance tocolysis has been used to prevent recurrence of preterm labor and prolong gestation in women in whom preterm labor was terminated successfully with parenteral tocolytics.[175,176] The use of continuous subcutaneous low-dose terbutaline infusion through a portable pump has been used widely in outpatient tocolysis and in conjunction with home uterine activity programs.[176,177] Although continuous subcutaneous low-dose terbutaline is associated with fewer cardiopulmonary adverse effects compared with intravenous β-adrenergic therapy, the FDA issued a "Dear Colleague" letter alerting practitioners about the lack of effectiveness and danger of continuous subcutaneous terbutaline for the treatment and prevention of preterm labor.[176,181] B.B. should not be started on chronic maintenance tocolysis

Antenatal Glucocorticoid Administration

61. **While receiving the loading dose of magnesium sulfate, B.B. was given betamethasone 12 mg IM with a second dose in 24 hours. Why was betamethasone given?**

B.B. was given betamethasone to facilitate fetal lung maturation by increasing production of fetal lung surfactant, thereby reducing the incidence of RDS).[80] Antenatal corticosteroid administration (betamethasone and dexamethasone) also decreases the incidence of intraventricular hemorrhage, necrotizing enterocolitis, and neonatal death.[80] The greatest reduction in RDS occurs when delivery can be delayed 24 hours up to 7 days after starting treatment. Repeat weekly corticosteroid courses are discouraged because of the association with decreased birth weight and head circumference, hypothalamic-pituitary-adrenal axis suppression, deleterious effects on cerebral myelination and lung growth, and neonatal death (particularly in neonates born to mothers who received three or more courses).[178,179]

The National Institutes of Health (NIH) Consensus Panel and the American College of Obstetrics and Gynecology (ACOG) recommend antenatal betamethasone or dexamethasone for all women in preterm labor between 24 to 34 weeks' gestation.[80] However, betamethasone is the preferred agent because fewer IM injections are needed and because this drug is the only one associated with decreased neonatal mortality. In cases of preterm PROM, the NIH Consensus recommends that corticosteroids may be given up to 32 weeks' gestation in the absence of chorioamnionitis.[80] Women >32 weeks' gestation should have their amniotic fluid tested for presence of phosphatidylglycerol or for a lecithin-to-sphingomyelin (L/S) ratio (>2) because these are indicators of fetal lung maturation.[180] Corticosteroids are not recommended for use in pregnant women who are more than 34 weeks' gestation unless there is an indication of fetal lung immaturity (see Chapter 9, Neonatal Therapy).

Antibiotic Therapy

62. **What is the role of antibiotic therapy in the prevention and treatment of preterm births? Is B.B. a candidate for a trial of antibiotics?**

Antibiotics are given during preterm labor to treat bacterial vaginosis, occult or documented intra-amniotic infections in preterm PROM and prophylactically against neonatal group B *Streptococcus* (GBS) infection.

Bacterial Vaginosis

All pregnant women should be screened and treated for sexually transmitted diseases and bacteriuria, and women at high risk for preterm delivery should be screened and treated for bacterial vaginosis (BV) as well.[181,182] A polymicrobial overgrowth of mostly anaerobic bacteria, BV is one of the most common genital infections in pregnancy and is associated with an increased risk of preterm delivery.[145] Treatment of women with BV, who had a prior preterm delivery with oral metronidazole (Flagyl) alone or in combination with erythromycin decreases the risk of recurrent preterm delivery.[183,184] However, the treatment of asymptomatic BV in the general obstetric population does not reduce the occurrence of preterm labor, intra-amniotic or postpartum infections, neonatal sepsis, or newborn admission to the neonatal intensive care unit.[184] B.B. does not have BV; therefore, treatment with metronidazole is unnecessary (also see GBS resistance to erythromycin in Chapter 96, Pediatric Infections Disease).

Preterm Premature Rupture of Membranes

Increasing evidence associates preterm labor with intra-amniotic infections.[166,184] Twenty to 40% of preterm births may be due to an infectious-inflammatory process.[181] Intrauterine infection preceding PROM is associated with approximately 80% of early preterm deliveries.[145] Most of the bacteria found in amniotic fluid and the placenta are believed to have ascended from the vagina.[184] It has been suggested

that the microbes responsible for preterm birth are already present in the endometrium before conception, causing a chronic, subclinical infection weeks to months before eventually causing preterm PROM or labor.[142]

Antibiotic therapy during preterm labor is indicated in select cases. Untreated, preterm PROM will result in spontaneous labor and delivery within 7 days.[145] Prophylactic treatment with antibiotics helps prolong the period between preterm PROM and delivery, and in decreasing neonatal morbidity.[145] In the largest and best designed trial of antibiotic treatment of preterm PROM, women between 24 to 32 weeks' gestation treated with ampicillin and erythromycin had prolonged pregnancies and lower rates of chorioamnionitis.[185] Their newborns experienced decreased neonatal morbidity or mortality, RDS, and necrotizing enterocolitis. These effects were not due to tocolytics or corticosteroids because these were exclusionary factors. Therefore, women with preterm PROM benefit from antibiotic therapy with a broad-spectrum regimen of intravenous ampicillin plus erythromycin for 48 hours followed by 5 days of oral amoxicillin plus erythromycin for a total of 7 days treatment.[185] Clindamycin should be substituted for erythromycin if BV is present.[181,182]

The most common reason to give antibiotics to women in preterm labor with intact membranes is to prevent group B streptococcal infection in the newborn. Other broad-spectrum antibiotic therapy to prevent preterm delivery should not be

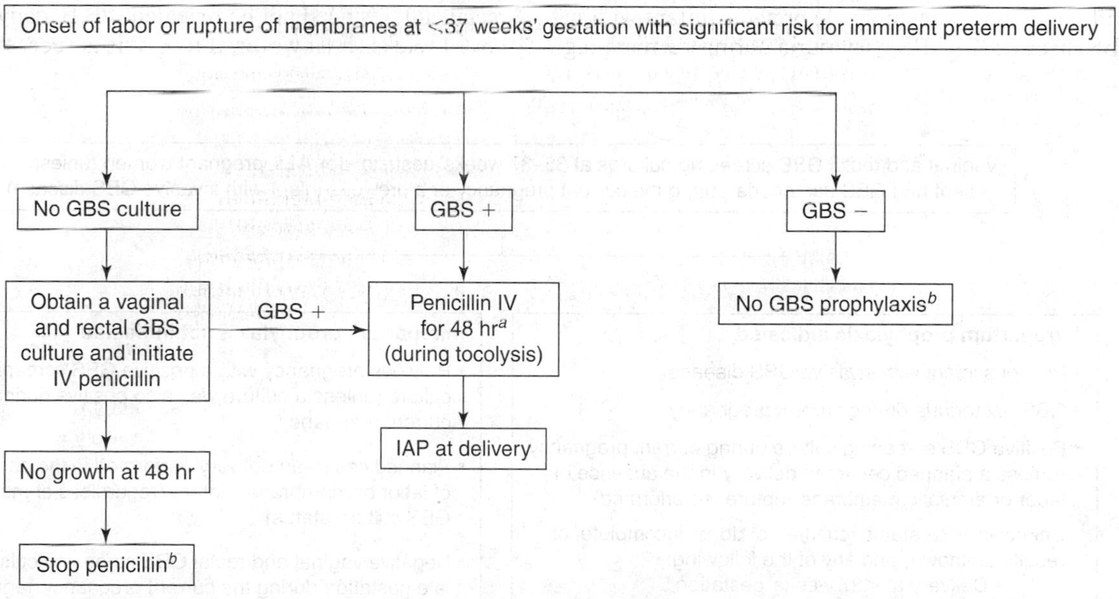

a Penicillin should be continued for a total of at least 48 hours, unless delivery occurs sooner. At the physician's discretion, antibiotic prophylaxis may be continued beyond 48 hours in a GBS culturepositive woman if delivery has not yet occurred. For women who are GBS culture positive, antibiotic prophylaxis should be reinitiated when labor likely to proceed to delivery occurs or recurs.

b If delivery has not occurred within 4 weeks, a vaginal and rectal GBS screening culture should be repeated and the patient should be managed as described, based on the result of the repeat culture.

GBS, group B streptococcus; IAP, intrapartum antibiotic prophylaxis.

Reprinted from Centers for Disease Control and Prevention. Prevention of perinatal Group B streptococcal disease. Revised guidelines. MMWR 2002;51(No. RR-11):8.)

FIGURE 46-2 Sample algorithm for group B streptococcus (GBS) prophylaxis for women with threatened preterm delivery. This algorithm is not an exclusive course of management. Variations that incorporate individual circumstances or institutional preferences may be appropriate.

given routinely to women in preterm labor with intact membranes. Antibiotics have not been proven to prevent premature births.[181,182]

Because B.B. does not have preterm PROM and/or signs of chorioamnionitis (temperature ≥100.4°F or 38°C), she should not be treated with broad-spectrum antibiotics. However, she should receive penicillin G to prevent perinatal group B streptococcus infection (Fig. 46-2).

Group B Streptococcus Intrapartum Prophylaxis

Ten to 30% of pregnant women are colonized with GBS in the vagina or rectum, and 1% to 2% of neonates born to colonized women develop early-onset invasive GBS disease. One-fourth of all cases of neonatal GBS infections occur in preterm newborns. B.B.'s fetus, therefore, is at risk for invasive GBS or *Streptococcus agalactiae* infection from vertical transmission (mother to infant) of bacteria during labor or delivery.[186,187] The mortality rate for GBS is reported to be between 5% and 20%. During pregnancy, GBS infection causes maternal urinary tract infection, amnionitis, endometriosis, and wound infection.[186]Antibiotics given to the mother during preterm labor and delivery prevent neonatal GBS disease. In the past decade, the routine administration of intrapartum antibiotic prophylaxis to certain subsets of pregnant women has led to a 70% reduction in the overall incidence of GBS disease (see Chapter 94, Neonatal Therapy). The decision to treat women with intrapartum antibiotics has been based on either a positive vaginal GBS culture or one or more of the following risk factors without culture screening: (1) previous infant with invasive GBS disease; (2) GBS bacteriuria during current preg-

nancy; (3) preterm labor of <37 weeks' gestation; (4) PROM ≥18 hours; and (5) intrapartum temperature >38°C (100.4°F).[186] This treatment algorithm prevents an estimated 85% of all early-onset GBS disease. A multistate, retrospective cohort study identified the culture-screening process as being 50% more effective than the risk-based process.[188] Consequently, the CDC and ACOG no longer recommend the risk-based approach, except in situations for which no culture results are available before delivery.[187] The new recommendations for intrapartum antibiotic prophylaxis are outlined in Figure 46-3.

Vaginal and rectal GBS cultures should be obtained from B.B., and she should be given a loading dose of penicillin G injection 5 million units, followed by 2.5 million units intravenously every 4 hours until delivery, while awaiting success of tocolysis and culture results. At least two doses before delivery are needed for maximum efficacy.[189] Penicillin G is preferred over ampicillin because it has a narrower spectrum of antimicrobial activity. Although most of the studies evaluating intrapartum antibiotics have used ampicillin, resistant *E. coli* could be problematic. If B.B. were allergic to penicillin she would be given clindamycin. Alternative antibiotic regimens for intrapartum antimicrobial prophylaxis are listed in Table 46-6.

63. B.B.'s culture results are negative for GBS growth. She is still at high risk for imminent delivery. Should penicillin G administration be discontinued?

Penicillin should be discontinued at this time. Vaginal and rectal cultures need not be repeated if B.B. delivers within the next 4 weeks.[187] However, if tocolysis is successful and deliv-

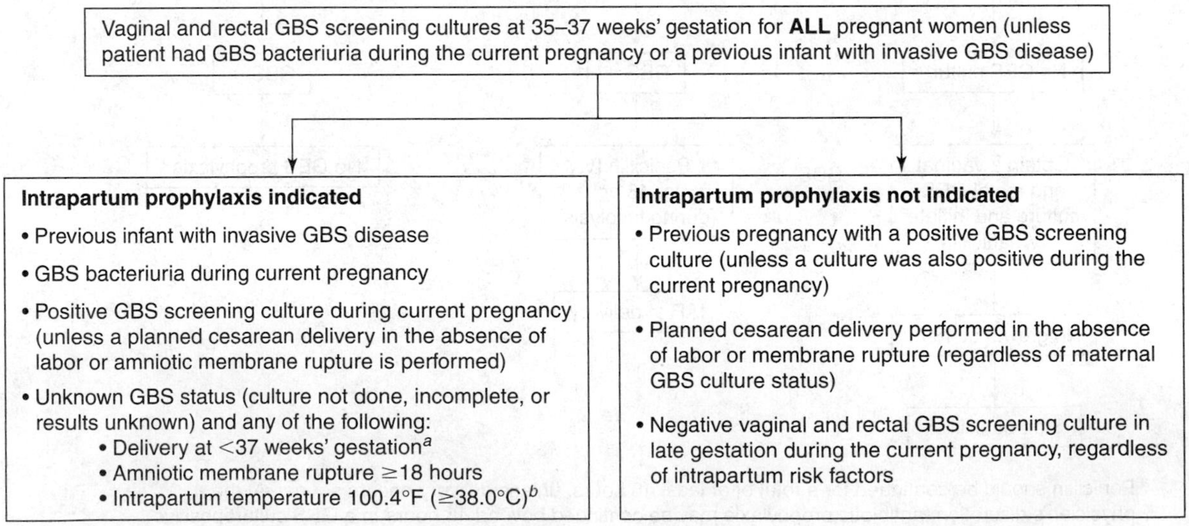

Vaginal and rectal GBS screening cultures at 35–37 weeks' gestation for **ALL** pregnant women (unless patient had GBS bacteriuria during the current pregnancy or a previous infant with invasive GBS disease)

Intrapartum prophylaxis indicated

- Previous infant with invasive GBS disease

- GBS bacteriuria during current pregnancy

- Positive GBS screening culture during current pregnancy (unless a planned cesarean delivery in the absence of labor or amniotic membrane rupture is performed)

- Unknown GBS status (culture not done, incomplete, or results unknown) and any of the following:
  - Delivery at <37 weeks' gestation[a]
  - Amniotic membrane rupture ≥18 hours
  - Intrapartum temperature 100.4°F (≥38.0°C)[b]

Intrapartum prophylaxis not indicated

- Previous pregnancy with a positive GBS screening culture (unless a culture was also positive during the current pregnancy)

- Planned cesarean delivery performed in the absence of labor or membrane rupture (regardless of maternal GBS culture status)

- Negative vaginal and rectal GBS screening culture in late gestation during the current pregnancy, regardless of intrapartum risk factors

[a] If onset of labor or rupture of amniotic membranes occurs at <37 weeks' gestation and there is a significant risk for preterm delivery (as assessed by the clinician), a suggested algorithm for GBS prophylaxis management is provided (Figure 46-2).

[b] If amnionitis is suspected, broad-spectrum antibiotic therapy that includes an agent known to be active against GBS should replace GBS prophylaxis.

Reprinted from Centers for Disease Control and Prevention. Prevention of perinatal Group B streptococcal disease. Revised guidelines. MMWR 2002;51(No.RR-11):8.

FIGURE 46-3 Indications for intrapartum antibiotic prophylaxis to prevent perinatal group B streptococcus (GBS) disease under a universal prenatal screening strategy based on combined vaginal and rectal cultures collected at 35–37 weeks' gestation from all pregnant women.

Table 46-6   Recommended Regimens for Intrapartum Antimicrobial Prophylaxis for Perinatal GBS disease Prevention[a]

Recommended: Penicillin G, 5 million units IV initial dose, then 2.5 million units IV every 4 hours until delivery
Alternative: Ampicillin, 2 g IV initial dose, then 1 g IV every 4 hours until delivery

If penicillin allergic[b]

Patients not at high risk for anaphylaxis:	Cefazolin, 2 g IV initial dose, then 1 g IV every 8 hours until delivery
Patients at high risk for anaphylaxis[c]:	
GBS-susceptible to clindamycin and erythromycin[d]:	Clindamycin, 900 mg IV every 8 hours until delivery
	or
	Erythromycin, 500 mg IV every 6 hours until delivery
GBS-resistant to clindamycin or erythromycin or susceptibility unknown:	Vancomycin,[e] 1 g IV every 12 hours until delivery

[a]Broader-spectrum agents, including an agent active against GBS, may be necessary for treatment of chorioamnionitis.
[b]History of penicillin allergy should be assessed to determine whether a high risk for anaphylaxis is present. Penicillin-allergic patients at high risk for anaphylaxis are those who have experienced immediate hypersensitivity to penicillin including a history of penicillin-related anaphylaxis; other high-risk patients are those with asthma or other diseases that would make anaphylaxis more dangerous or difficult to treat, such as persons being treated with beta-adrenergic–blocking agents.
[c]If laboratory facilities are adequate, clindamycin and erythromycin susceptibility testing should be performed on prenatal GBS isolates from penicillin-allergic women at high risk for anaphylaxis.
[d]Resistance to erythromycin is often but not always associated with clindamycin resistance. If a strain is resistant to erythromycin but appears susceptible to clindamycin, it may still have inducible resistance to clindamycin.
[e]Cefazolin is preferred over vancomycin for women with a history of penicillin allergy other than immediate hypersensitivity reactions, and pharmacologic data suggest it achieves effective intra-amniotic concentrations. Vancomycin should be reserved for penicillin-allergic women at high risk for anaphylaxis.
GBS, group B streptococcus.
(Reprinted from Centers for Disease Control and Prevention. Prevention of Perinatal Group B Streptococcal Disease. Revised guidelines. MMWR 2002;51(No. RR-11):10.)

ery is delayed for more than 4 weeks, obtaining cultures and starting penicillin G preemptively should be repeated at that time (see Fig. 46-3). Intrapartum prophylaxis is effective only if antibiotics can be given immediately before and during delivery.

LACTATION

Approximately half of the women in the United States choose to breast-feed at the time of hospital discharge. This declines to 18% by the time their infants reach the age of 6 months. Public health officials had hoped that by the year 2000, 75% of all infants born in the United States would be breast-fed, but this goal has been achieved only in the Pacific region.[190]

Lactation is controlled primarily by prolactin (PRL), but the entire process is under the intricate control of several hormones. Breast tissue maturation during pregnancy is influenced by many factors, including estrogen, progesterone, PRL, insulin, growth hormone, cortisol, thyroxine, and human placental lactogen.[191] PRL concentrations gradually increase during pregnancy, but high estrogen and progesterone concentrations inhibit milk secretion by blocking PRL's effect on the breast epithelium.[191–192] It is the dramatic decrease in progesterone that triggers lactogenesis or milk secretion for the first 3 days following delivery. Infant suckling at the breast is necessary to maintain an adequate milk supply beyond postpartum day 3 or 4. Nipple stimulation transmits sensory impulses to the hypothalamus to initiate PRL release from the anterior pituitary and oxytocin from the posterior pituitary. Prolactin stimulates the production and secretion of breast milk and oxytocin stimulates the contraction of the myoepithelial cells in the breast alveoli and ducts so that milk can be ejected from the breast (milk letdown). Oxytocin also can be secreted through other sensory pathways, which is why women can release milk upon hearing, smelling, or even thinking about their infants. Prolactin, however, is released only in response to nipple stimulation.

Prolactin synthesis and release depend on the inhibition of hypothalamic prolactin inhibitory factor (PIF) secretion. Prolactin secretion is regulated primarily by dopamine-releasing neurons. Activating the dopamine receptors on the prolactin-secreting cells of the anterior pituitary inhibits the release of prolactin. PIF is believed to be closely associated with dopamine.[191,192]

Although prolactin controls the volume of milk produced, once lactation is established, milk production is regulated by infant demand. Lactation eventually ceases if milk is not removed from the breast. Absence of suckling stops milk letdown and restores the normal production of PIF. Decreased blood flow to the breast reduces oxytocin delivery to the myoepithelium. Consequently, milk secretion stops within a few days.[191,192]

Stimulation
Nonpharmacologic Measures

64. **C.C., a 22-year-old woman, vaginally delivered her first child, a healthy term infant. C.C. plans to breast-feed and was educated about breast-feeding during obstetric visits and prenatal classes. After giving birth, C.C. tried to breast-feed in the delivery room with great difficulty. Afterward, she became extremely apprehensive and continued to have trouble breast-feeding. What can be done to encourage C.C. and help her with lactation?**

The most effective stimulus for lactation is suckling. Many women nurse in the delivery room after uncomplicated vaginal deliveries because nursing increases maternal-infant bonding and helps establish good milk production. If a mother does not nurse immediately after delivery, she should be encouraged to do so as soon as she is physically able. C.C. did try to nurse after delivery, but experienced problems that may have been related to her emotional or physical state, or to the physical state of her infant. The nursing staff should encourage and support C.C. emotionally to help her relax, be comfortable, and relieve her anxiety about breast-feeding. Health care personnel also should emphasize appropriate feeding techniques and proper positioning for breast-feeding. Allowing C.C.'s infant to sleep in her room, rather than the nursery, may help C.C. develop a breast-feeding routine.

Most new mothers who have difficulty breast-feeding initially respond to the emotional and educational support of a good obstetric nursing staff. Few require pharmaceutical intervention.

Enhancement of Milk Production

65. C.C. was successful in establishing breast-feeding. However, despite good technique and adequate nutrition, she had trouble maintaining adequate milk production after about 2 to 3 weeks and was forced to supplement her infant with formula. How can C.C.'s milk production be enhanced?

Although not an FDA-approved indication, metoclopramide is used to stimulate lactation in women with decreased or inadequate milk production.[40,193-197] Metoclopramide, a dopamine-antagonist increases prolactin secretion. This is particularly useful in women whose infants do not breast-feed effectively (e.g., preterm infants).[193] Metoclopramide 10 mg orally three times daily for 1 to 2 weeks is effective in restoring milk production.[40,193-196] Improvement in lactation occurs within 2 to 5 days of starting therapy and persists after discontinuing metoclopramide.

The estimated total daily dose of metoclopramide ingested by the nursing infant of a woman on 30 mg/day is 1 to 45 μg/kg per day.[40] This is below the maximum recommended infant daily dose of 0.5 mg/kg per day. Maternal doses of 30 mg/day do not alter PRL, thyroid-stimulating hormone, or free thyroxin serum concentrations in breast-fed infants.[197]

The only adverse effect reported in nursing infants has been intestinal gas.[40,195] The short-term use of metoclopramide for re-establishing lactation appears to be both safe and effective, even in preterm infants.[40,193,196] However, the American Academy of Pediatrics considers metoclopramide use in breast-feeding women to be of concern because of the potential for adverse CNS effects in infants.[40]

Suppression

66. After delivery, J.G., a 26-year-old G$_2$P$_2$, informs her obstetrician that she does not wish to breast-feed. What methods are available to suppress lactation?

Suppression of lactation is indicated for women who do not want to breast-feed, women who have delivered a stillborn infant, and those who have had an abortion. Both drugs and nonpharmacologic methods have been used. However, in 1988 the FDA recommended against drug-induced suppression of lactation.[198] The only drug therapy that the FDA recommends in women who are not breast-feeding are analgesics for the relief of breast pain. Bromocriptine (Parlodel) was approved for the postpartum suppression of lactation; however, the FDA rescinded its approval for that indication because of cardiovascular complications (e.g., stroke, myocardial infarction) associated with its use.[192]

If breast stimulation is avoided (with or without the use of a breast binder), breast milk production will continue, leading to engorgement and distention of breast alveoli. This leads to the termination of lactation after several days. Approximately 40% of women using this method experience breast discomfort and pain; 30% experience milk leakage from their nipples.[198,199] Ice packs may be applied to the breasts for comfort and a mild analgesic used if necessary.

REFERENCES

1. Mathews TJ et al. Infant mortality statistics from the 2001 period linked birth/infant death data set. National vital statistics reports, vol 52. Hyattsville, MD: National Center for Health Statistics, 2003:1

2. Cunningham FG et al, eds. Obstetrics in broad perspective. In: Williams Obstetrics. New York: McGraw-Hill, 2001:3.

3. Smulian JC et al. Fetal deaths in the United States: influence of high-risk conditions and implications for management. Obstet Gynecol 2002;100:1183.

4. Cunningham FG et al, eds. The placenta and fetal membranes. In: Williams Obstetrics. New York: McGraw-Hill, 2001:95.

5. Craven C, Ward K. Embryo, fetus, and placenta: normal and abnormal. In: Scott JR et al, eds. Danforth's Obstetrics and Gynecology. Philadelphia: Lippincott Williams & Wilkins, 1999:29.

6. Cunningham FG et al, eds. The endometrium and decidua: menstruation and pregnancy. In: Williams Obstetrics. New York: McGraw-Hill, 2001:69.

7. Buster JE, Carson SA. Endocrinology and diagnosis of pregnancy. In: Gabbe SG et al, eds. Obstetrics: Normal and Problem Pregnancies. New York: Churchill Livingstone, 1996:31.

8. Lockwood CJ, Paidas MJ. Preeclampsia and hypertensive disorders. In: Cohen WR, ed. Cherry and Merkatz's Complications of Pregnancy. Philadelphia: Lippincott Williams & Wilkins, 2000:207.

9. Cunningham FG et al, eds. Fetal growth and development. In: Williams Obstetrics. New York: McGraw-Hill, 2001:129

10. Cunningham FG et al, eds.. Pregnancy: overview, organization, and diagnosis In: Williams Obstetrics. New York: McGraw-Hill, 2001:15..

11. Farrington PF, Ward K. Normal labor, delivery, and puerperium. In: Scott JR et al, eds. Danforth's Obstetrics and Gynecology. Philadelphia: Lippincott Williams & Wilkins, 1999:91.

12. Rosenthal WM, Briggs GC. Home testing and monitoring devices. In: Young LL, ed. Handbook of Nonprescription Drugs. Washington: American Pharmaceutical Association, 2002:1017.

13. Cunningham FG et al, eds. Prenatal care. In: Williams Obstetrics. New York: McGraw-Hill, 2001:221.

14. Loebstein R, Koren G. Clinical relevance of therapeutic drug monitoring during pregnancy. Ther Drug Monit 2002;24:15.

15. Frederiksen MC. Physiologic changes in pregnancy and their effect on drug disposition. Semin Perinatol 2001;25:120.

16. Little BB. Pharmacokinetics during pregnancy: evidence-based maternal dose formulation. Obstet Gynecol 199;93:858.

17. McAuley JW, Anderson GD. Treatment of epilepsy in women of reproductive age. Pharmacokinetic considerations. Clin Pharmacokinet 2002;41:559.

18. Merkatz RB et al. Women in clinical trials of new drugs. A change in Food and Drug Administration policy. N Engl J Med 1993;329:292.

19. Worthington-Roberts BS. Nutrition. In: Cohen WR, ed. Cherry and Merkatz's Complications of Pregnancy, 5th Ed. Philadelphia: Lippincott Williams & Wilkins, 2000:17.

20. Harris RZ et al. Gender effects in pharmacokinetics and pharmacodynamics. Drugs 1995;50:222.

21. Bowers D, Wenk RE. Clinical laboratory referent values. In: Cohen WR, ed. Cherry and Merkatz's Complications of Pregnancy. Philadelphia: Lippincott Williams & Wilkins, 2000:873.

22. Subcommittee on Nutritional Status and Weight Gain During Pregnancy, Institute of Medicine. Summary. In: Nutrition During Pregnancy. Washington, DC: National Academy Press, 1990:10.

23. Subcommittee on Nutritional Status and Weight Gain During Pregnancy, Institute of Medicine. Effects of gestational weight gain on outcome in singleton pregnancies. In: Nutrition During Pregnancy. Washington, DC: National Academy Press, 1990:176.

24. Subcommittee on Nutritional Status and Weight Gain During Pregnancy, Institute of Medicine. Energy requirements, energy intake, and associated weight gain during pregnancy. In: Nutrition During Pregnancy. Washington, DC: National Academy Press, 1990:137.

25. Subcommittee on Nutritional Status and Weight Gain During Pregnancy, Institute of Medicine. Total amount and pattern of weight gain: physiologic and maternal determinants. In: Nutrition During Pregnancy. Washington, DC: National Academy Press, 1990:96.

26. Subcommittee on Nutritional Status and Weight Gain During Pregnancy, Institute of Medicine.

Weight gain in twin pregnancies. In: Nutrition During Pregnancy. Washington, DC: National Academy Press, 1990:212.

27. Williams SR. Nutrition assessment and guidance in prenatal care. In: Worthington-Roberts BS, Williams SR, eds. Nutrition in Pregnancy and Lactation, 6th Ed. Dubuque: Brown & Benchmark, 1997:220.

28. National Research Council. Trace elements. In: Recommended Dietary Allowances. Washington, DC: National Academy Press, 1989:195.

29. Subcommittee on Nutritional Status and Weight Gain During Pregnancy, Institute of Medicine. Iron nutrition during pregnancy. In: Nutrition During Pregnancy. Washington, DC: National Academy Press, 1990:272.

30. Cunningham FG et al, eds. Hematological disorders. Prenatal care. In: Williams Obstetrics. New York: McGraw-Hill, 2001:1307.

31. Czeizel AE, Dudas I. Prevention of the first occurrence of neural-tube defects by periconceptional vitamin supplementation. N Engl J Med 1992;327:1832.

32. Centers for Disease Control and Prevention. Recommendations for the use of folic acid to reduce the number of cases of spina bifida and other neural tube defects. MMWR Morbid Mortal Wkly Rep 1992;41:RR-14.

33. Centers for Disease Control and Prevention. Neural tube defect surveillance and folic acid intervention—Texas-Mexico border, 1993–1998. MMWR Morbid Mortal Wkly Rep 2000;49:1.

34. Centers for Disease Control and Prevention. Use of folic acid for prevention of spina bifida and other neural tube defects—1983–1991. MMWR Morbid Mortal Wkly Rep 1991;40:513.

35. MRC Vitamin Study Research Group. Prevention of neural tube defects: results of the Medical Research Council Vitamin Study. Lancet 1991;338:131.

36. Worthington-Roberts BS. Lactation: basic considerations. In: Worthington-Roberts BS, Williams SR, eds. Nutrition in Pregnancy and Lactation, 6th Ed. Dubuque: Brown & Benchmark, 1997:319.

37. Davis DC. The discomforts of pregnancy. J Obstet Gynecol Neonatal Nurs 1996;25:73.

38. Nelson-Piercy C. Treatment of nausea and vomiting in pregnancy: when should it be treated and what can be safely taken? Drug Safety 1998;19:155.

39. Koch KL. Gastrointestinal factors in nausea and vomiting of pregnancy. Am J Obstet Gynecol 2002;186:S198.

40. Briggs GG et al, eds. Drugs in Pregnancy and Lactation, 6th Ed. Philadelphia: Lippincott William & Williams 2002.

41. Boussard CN, Richter JE. Nausea and vomiting of pregnancy. Gastroenterol Clin North Am 1998;27:123.

42. Mazzotta P, Magee LA. A risk-benefit assessment of pharmacological and nonpharmacological treatments for nausea and vomiting of pregnancy. Drugs 2000;59:781.

43. Berkovitz, M. Fetal effects of metoclopramide therapy for nausea and vomiting of pregnancy. N Engl J Med 2000;343:445.

44. Bonapace ES, Fisher RS. Constipation and diarrhea in pregnancy. Gastroenterol Clin North Am 1998;27:197.

45. Marshall K et al. Incidence of urinary incontinence and constipation during pregnancy and postpartum: survey of current findings at the Rotunda Lying-in Hospital. Br J Ob Gyn 1998;105:400.

46. Katz PO, Castell DO. Gastroesophageal reflux disease during pregnancy. Gastroenterol Clin North Am 1998;27:153.

47. Scott JR, Branch DW. Immunologic disorders in pregnancy. In: Scott JR et al, eds. Danforth's Obstetrics and Gynecology. Philadelphia: Lippincott Williams & Wilkins, 1999:363.

48. Bowman JM. Hemolytic disease (erythroblastosis fetalis). In: Creasy RK, Resnik R, eds. Maternal-Fetal Medicine: Principles and Practice. Philadelphia: WB Saunders, 1999:736.

49. Anonymous. ACOG practice bulletin. Prevention of Rh D alloimmunization. Int J Gynecol Obstet 1999;66:63.

50. Rh₀(D) Immune Globulin. In: McEvoy G, ed. AHFS Drug Information. Bethesda, MD: American Society of Health-System Pharmacists, Inc., 2003:3153.

51. Jabara S. Is Rh immune globulin needed in early first-trimester abortion? A review. Am J Obstet Gynecol 2003;188:623.

52. Cunningham FG et al, eds. Diabetes In: Williams Obstetrics. New York: McGraw-Hill, 2001:1359.

53. Ventura SJ et al. Births: final data for 1999. Natl Vital Rep 2001:49:1.

54. American Diabetes Association. Gestational diabetes mellitus. Diabetes Care 2003;26:S103.

55. Kjos SL, Buchanan TA. Gestational diabetes mellitus. N Engl J Med 1999;341:1749.

56. White P. Classification of obstetric diabetes. Am J Obstet Gynecol 1978;130:228.

57. Garner P. Type I diabetes mellitus and pregnancy. Lancet 1995;346:157.

58. American Diabetes Association. Preconceptional care of women with diabetes. Diabetes Care 2003;26:S91.

59. Diabetes Control and Complications Trial Research Group. Obstetrics: pregnancy outcomes in the diabetes control and complications trial. Am J Obstet Gynecol 1996;174:1343.

60. Homko CJ, Reece EA. Ambulatory care of the pregnant woman with diabetes. Clin Obstet Gynecol 1998;41:584.

61. Brody SC et al. Screening for gestational diabetes: A summary of the evidence for the U.S. Preventive Services Task Force. Obstet Gynecol 2003;101:380.

62. National High Blood Pressure Education Program Working Group report on high blood pressure in pregnancy. Report of the national High Blood Pressure Education Program Working Group on high blood pressure in pregnancy. Am J Obstet Gynecol 2000;183(Suppl):S1.

63. Branch DW, Porter TF. Hypertensive disorders of pregnancy. In: Scott JR et al, eds. Danforth's Obstetrics and Gynecology. Philadelphia: Lippincott Williams & Wilkins, 1999:309.

64. Sibai BM. Treatment of hypertension in pregnant women. N Engl J Med 1996;335:257.

65. Dekker GA. Risk factors for preeclampsia. Clin Obstet Gynecol 1999;42:422.

66. Roberts JM. Pregnancy-related hypertension. In: Creasy RK, Resnik R, eds. Maternal-Fetal Medicine. Philadelphia: WB Saunders, 1999:833.

67. Chobian AV, et al. The Seventh Report of the Joint National Committee on Prevention, Detection, Evaluation, and Treatment of High Blood Pressure. Hypertension 2003;42:1206.

68. Shotan A et al. Risks of angiotensin-converting enzyme inhibition during pregnancy: experimental and clinical evidence, potential mechanisms, and recommendations for use. Am J Med 1994;96:451.

69. Kyle PM, Redman WG. Comparative risk-benefit assessment of drugs used in the management of hypertension in pregnancy. Drug Safety 1992;7:222.

70. Dekker GA, Sibai BM. Etiology and pathogenesis of preeclampsia: current concepts. Am J Obstet Gynecol 1998;179:1359.

71. Patrick T, Roberts JM. Current concepts in preeclampsia. MCN Am J Matern Child Nurs 1999;24:193.

72. Barton JR et al. Management of mild preeclampsia. Clin Obstet Gynecol 1999;42:455.

73. Abalos AE. Antihypertensive drug therapy for mild to moderate hypertension during pregnancy. Cochrane Database Systemic Review 2003;1:1.

74. Cockburn J et al. Final report of study on hypertension during pregnancy: the effects of specific treatment on the growth and development of the children. Lancet 1982;1:647.

75. Sibai BM et al. A comparison of labetalol plus hospitalization versus hospitalization alone in the management of preeclampsia remote from term. Obstet Gynecol 1987;70:323.

76. Magee LA et al. Risks and benefits of β-receptor blockers for pregnancy hypertension: overview of the randomized trials. Eur J Obstet Gynecol Reprod Biol 2000;8:15.

77. Butters L et al. Atenolol in essential hypertension during pregnancy. Br Med J 1990;301:587.

78. Tabacova SA, Kimmel CA. Enalapril: pharmacokinetic/dynamic inferences for comparative developmental toxicity. A review. Reprod Toxicol 2001;15:467.

79. Friedman SA et al. Expectant management of severe preeclampsia remote form term. Clin Obstet Gynecol 1999;42:470.

80. NIH Consensus Development Panel on the Effect of Corticosteroids for fetal Maturation on Perinatal Outcomes. Effect of corticosteroids for fetal maturation on perinatal outcomes. JAMA 1995;273:413.

81. Mabie WC. Management of acute severe hypertension and encephalopathy. Clin Obstet Gynecol 1999;42:519.

82. Belfort MA et al. Labetalol decreases cerebral perfusion pressure without negatively affecting cerebral blood flow in hypertensive gravidas. Hypertension Pregnancy 2002;21:185.

83. Idama TO, Lindow SW. Magnesium sulphate: a review of clinical pharmacology applied to obstetrics. Br J Obstet Gynecol 1998;105:260.

84. Vermillion ST et al. A randomized, double-blind trial of oral nifedipine and intravenous labetalol in hypertensive emergencies of pregnancy. Am J Obstet Gynecol 1999;181:858.

85. Scardo JA et al. A randomized, double-blind, hemodynamic evaluation of nifedipine and labetalol in preeclamptic hypertensive emergencies. Am J Obstet Gynecol 1999;181.862.

86. Lucas MJ et al. A comparison of magnesium sulfate with phenytoin for the prevention of eclampsia. N Engl J Med 1995;333:201.

87. Witlin AG. Prevention and treatment of eclamptic convulsions. Clin Obstet Gynecol 1999;42:507.

88. Magpie Trial Collaborative Group. Do women with pre-eclampsia, and their babies, benefit from magnesium sulphate? The Magpie Trial: a randomized placebo-controlled trial. Lancet 2002;359:1877.

89. Livingston JC et al. Magnesium sulfate in women with mild preeclampsia: a randomized controlled trial. Obstet Gynecol 2003;101:217.

90. Belfort MA et al. A comparison of magnesium sulfate and nimodipine for the prevention of eclampsia. N Engl J Med 2003;348:304.

91. Pritchard JA. The use of magnesium sulfate in preeclampsia-eclampsia. J Reprod Med 1979;3:107.

92. Sibai BM et al. Reassessment of intravenous MgSO₄ therapy in preeclampsia-eclampsia. Obstet Gynecol 1981;57:199.

93. Lu J et al. Pharmacokinetic-pharmacodynamic modelling of magnesium plasma concentration and blood pressure in preeclamptic women. Clin Pharmacokinet 2002;41:1105.

94. Sibai BM. Magnesium sulfate is the ideal anticonvulsant in preeclampsia-eclampsia. Am J Obstet Gynecol 1990;162:1141.

95. The Eclampsia Trial Collaborative Group. Which anticonvulsant for women with eclampsia? Evidence from the collaborative eclampsia trial. Lancet 1995;345(8963):1455.

96. Isler CM et al. Postpartum seizure prophylaxis: using maternal clinical paratmenters to guide therapy. Obstet Gynecol 2003;101:66.

97. Mattar F, Sibai BM. Prevention of preeclampsia. Semin Perinatol 1999;23:58.

98. Sibai BM et al. Prevention of preeclampsia with low-dose aspirin in healthy, nulliparous pregnant women. N Engl J Med 1993;329:1213.

99. Caritis S et al. Low-dose aspirin to prevent preeclampsia in women at high risk. N Engl J Med 1998;338:701.

100. Levine RJ et al. Trial of calcium to prevent preeclampsia. N Engl J Med 1997;337:69.

101. Norwitz ER et al. The control of labor. N Engl J Med 1999;341:660.

102. Farrington PF, Ward K. Normal labor, delivery, and puerperium. In: Danforth's Obstetrics and Gynecology. Philadelphia: Lippincott Williams & Wilkins, 1999:91.

103. Anonymous. ACOG technical bulletin. Induction of labor. Int J Gynecol Obstet 1996;53:65.

104. Anonymous. ACOG practice patterns. Management of postterm pregnancy. Int J Gynecol Obstet 1997;60:86.

105. Laube DW. Induction of labor. Clin Obstet Gynecol 1997;40:485.

106. Riskin-Mashiah S, Wilkins I. Cervical ripening. Obstet Gynecol Clin North Am 1999;26:243.

107. Xenakis EMJ et al. Induction of labor in the nineties: conquering the unfavorable cervix. Obstet Gynecol 1997;90:235.

108. Rayburn WF. Prostaglandin E_2 gel for cervical ripening and induction of labor: a critical analysis. Am J Obstet Gynecol 1989;160:529.

109. Witter FR et al. A randomized trial of prostaglandin E_2 in a controlled-release vaginal pessary for cervical ripening at term. Am J Obstet Gynecol 1992;166:830.

110. Rayburn WF et al. An intravaginal controlled-release prostaglandin E_2 pessary for cervical ripening and initiation of labor at term. Obstet Gynecol 1992;79:374.

111. Pharmacia & Upjohn Company. Prepidil Gel package insert. Kalamazoo, MI: 1999 April.

112. Forrest Pharmaceuticals, Inc. Cervidil package insert. St. Louis, MO: 1997 July.

113. Chyu JK, Strassner HT. Prostaglandin E_2 for cervical ripening: a randomized comparison of Cervidil versus Prepidil. Am J Obstet Gynecol 1997;177;606.

114. Cohen HE, ed. Drug Topics Red Book. Montvale, NJ: Thomson Medical Economics Company, 2002.

115. Anonymous. ACOG committee opinion. Monitoring during induction of labor with dinoprostone. Int J Gynecol Obstet 1999;64:200.

116. Shyken JM, Petrie RH. The use of oxytocin. Clin Perinatol 1995;22:907

117. Ottinger WS et al. A randomized clinical trial of prostaglandin E_2 intracervical gel and slow release vaginal pessary for preinduction cervical ripening. Am J Obstet Gynecol 1998;179:349.

118. Sanchez-Ramos L et al. Misoprostol for cervical ripening and labor induction: a meta-analysis. Obstet Gynecol 1997;89:633.

119. Hofmeyr GJ, Gulmezoglu AM. Vaginal misoprostol for cervical ripening and induction of labour. Cochrane Database Syst Rev 2003;3:1.

120. American College of Obstetricians and Gynecologists. Committee on Obstetric Practice. New U.S. Food and Drug Administration labeling on Cytotec (misoprostol) use and pregnancy. Obstet Gynecol 2003;101:1049.

121. Wing DA, A benefit-risk assessment of misoprostol for cervical ripening and labour induction. Drug Safety 2002;25:665.

122. Blanchette HA et al. Comparison of the safety and efficacy of intravaginal misoprostol (prostaglandin E_1) with those of dinoprostone (prostaglandin E_2) for cervical ripening and induction of labor in a community hospital. Am J Obstet Gynecol 1999;180:1551.

123. Sanchez-Ramos L et al. Labor induction with prostaglandin E_1 misoprostol compared with dinoprostone vaginal insert: a randomized trial. Obstet Gynecol 1998;91:401.

124. Wing DA et al. A comparison of orally administered misoprostol with vaginally administered misoprostol for cervical ripening and labor induction. Am J Obstet Gynecol 1999;180:1155.

125. Wing DA. Labor induction with misoprostol. Am J Obstet Gynecol 1999;181:339.

126. Dudley DJ. Complications of labor. In: Scott JR et al, eds. Danforth's Obstetrics and Gynecology. Philadelphia: Lippincott Williams & Wilkins, 1999:437.

127. Anonymous. ACOG technical bulletin. Dystocia and the augmentation of labor. Int J Gynecol Obstet 1996;53:73.

128. Perry RL et al. The pharmacokinetics of oxytocin as they apply to labor induction. Am J Obstet Gynecol 1996;174:1590.

129. Dudley DJ. Oxytocin: use and abuse, science and art. Clin Obstet Gynecol 1997;40:516.

130. Satin AJ et al. High-dose oxytocin: 20-versus 40-minute dosage interval. Obstet Gynecol 1994; 83:234.

131. Satin AJ et al. High- versus low-dose oxytocin for labor stimulation. Obstet Gynecol 1992;80:111.

132. Xenakis EMJ et al. Low-dose versus high-dose oxytocin augmentation of labor—a randomized trial. Am J Obstet Gynecol 1995;173:1874.

133. Ripley DL. Uterine emergencies. atony, inversion, and rupture. Obstet Gynecol Clin North Am 1999;26:419.

134. Cohen WR. Postpartum hemorrhage and hemorrhagic shock. In: Cohen WR, ed. Cherry and Merkatz's Complications of Pregnancy. Philadelphia: Lippincott Williams & Wilkins, 2000:803.

135. Alamia V, Meyer BA. Peripartum hemorrhage. Obstet Gynecol Clin North Am 1999;26:385.

136. Cunningham FG et al, eds. Conduct of normal labor and delivery. In Williams Obstetrics. New York: McGraw-Hill, 2001:309.

137. Khan RU, El-Refaey H. Pharmacokinetices and adverse-effect profile of rectally administered misoprostol in the third stage of labor. Obstet Gynecol 2003;101:968.

138. Caliskan E et al. Oral misoprostol for the third stage of labor: a randomized controlled trial. Obstet Gynecol 2003;101:921.

139. Ergonovine maleate/Methylergonovine maleate. In: McEvoy G, ed. AHFS Drug Information. Bethesda, MD: American Society of Health-System Pharmacists, Inc., 2003:3098.

140. O'Brien WF. The role of prostaglandins in labor and delivery. Clin Perinatol 1995;22:973.

141. Pharmacia & Upjohn Company. Hemabate package insert. Kalamazoo, MI: February 1999.

142. Creasy RK, Iams JD. Preterm labor and delivery. In: Creasy RK, Resnik R, eds. Maternal-Fetal Medicine. Philadelphia: WB Saunders, 1999:498.

143. Parsons MT, Spellacy WN. Preterm labor. In: Scott JR et al, eds. Danforth's Obstetrics and Gynecology. Philadelphia: Lippincott Williams & Wilkins, 1999:257.

144. Garite TJ. Premature rupture of the membranes. In: Creasy RK, Resnik R, eds. Maternal-Fetal Medicine. Philadelphia: WB Saunders, 1999:644.

145. Goldenberg RL, Rouse DJ. Medical progress: prevention of premature birth. N Engl J Med 1998;339:313.

146. Anonymous. ACOG committee opinion. Fetal fibronectin preterm labor risk test. Int J Gynecol Obstet 1997;59:164.

147. Anonymous. ACOG committee opinion. Fetal fibronectin preterm labor risk test. Obstet Gynecol 2003;101:1039.

148. Goldenberg RL. The managmentof preterm labor. Obstet Gynecol 2002;100:1020.

149. Katz VL, Farmer RM. Controversies in tocolytic therapy. Clin Obstet Gynecol 1999;42:802.

150. Gordon MC, Iams JD. Magnesium sulfate. Clin Obstet Gynecol 1995;38:706.

151. Hill WC. Risks and complications of tocolysis. Clin Obstet Gynecol 1995;38:725.

152. Glock JL, Morales WJ. Efficacy and safety of nifedipine versus magnesium in the management of preterm labor: a randomized study. Am J Obstet Gynecol 1993;169:960.

153. Gyetvai K et al. Tocolytics for preterm labor: a systematic review. Obstet Gynecol 1999;94:869.

154. Macones GA et al. Evidence for magnesium sulfate as a tocolytic agent. Obstet Gynecol Surv 1997;52:652.

155. Besinger RE, Niebyl JR. The safety and efficacy of tocolytic agents for the treatment of preterm labor. Obstet Gynecol Surv 1990;45:415.

156. Grether JK et al. Magnesium sulfate tocolysis and risk of neonatal death. Am J Obstet Gynecol 1998;178:1.

157. Anonymous. ACOG technical bulletin. Preterm labor. Int J Gynecol Obstet 1995;50:303.

158. Lewis DF et al. Successful magnesium sulfate tocolysis: is "weaning" the drug necessary? Am J Obstet Gynecol 1997;177:742.

159. Madden C et al. Magnesium tocolysis: serum levels versus success. Am J Obstet Gynecol 1990; 162:1177.

160. Cox SM et al. Randomized investigation of magnesium sulfate for prevention of preterm birth. Am J Obstet Gynecol 1990;163:767.

161. Lam F et al. Clinical issues surrounding the use of terbutaline sulfate for preterm labor. Obstet Gynecol Surv 1998;53(Suppl):85.

162. Boyle JG. Beta-adrenergic agonists. Clin Obstet Gynecol 1995;38:688.

163. The Canadian Preterm Labor Investigators Group. Treatment of preterm labor with the beta-adrenergic agonist ritodrine. N Engl J Med 1992;327:308.

164. Morales WJ, Harrish M. Efficacy and safety of indomethacin compared with magnesium sulfate in the management of preterm labor: a randomized study. Am J Obstet Gynecol 1993;169:97.

165. Iannucci TA et al. Effect of dual tocolysis on the incidence of severe intraventricular hemorrhage among extremely low-birth-weight infants. Am J Obstet Gynecol 1996;175:1043.

166. Weeks JW et al. Antenatal indomethacin exposure and neonatal intraventricular hemorrhage: a side effect or an association? [Letter]. Am J Obstet Gynecol 1997;176:1122.

167. Vermillion ST, Newman RB. Recent indomethacin tocolysis is not associated with neonatal complications in preterm infants. Am J Obstet Gynecol 1999;181:1083.

168. Norton ME et al. Neonatal complications after the administration of indomethacin for preterm labor. N Engl J Med 1995;329:1602.

169. Macones GA. The controversy surrounding indomethacin for tocolysis Am J Obstet Gynecol 2001;184:264.

170. Stika CS et al. A prospective randomized safety trial of celecoxib for treatment of preterm labor. Am J Obstet Gynecol 2002;187:653.

171. Sawdy RJ. A double-blind randomized study of fetal side effects during and after the short-term maternal administration of indomethacin, sulindac, and nimesulide for the treatment of preterm labor. Am J Obstet Gynecol 2003;188:1046.

172. Papatsonis DNM et al. Nifedipine and ritodrine in the management of preterm labor: a randomized multicenter trial. Obstet Gynecol 1997;90:230.

173. Carr DB et al. Maintenance oral nifedipine for preterm labor: a randomized clinical trial. Am J Obstet Gynecol 1999;181:822.

174. Larmon JE. Oral nicardipine versus intravenous magnesium sulfate for the treatment of preterm labor. Am J Obstet Gynecol 1999;181: 1432.

175. Sanchez-Ramos L et al. Efficacy of maintenance therapy after acute tocolysis: a meta-analysis. Am J Obstet Gynecol 1999;181:484.

176. Guinn DA et al. Terbutaline pump maintenance therapy for prevention of preterm delivery: a double-blind trial. Am J Obstet Gynecol 1998; 179:874.

177. Perry KG Jr et al. Incidence of adverse cardiopulmonary effects with low-dose continuous terbutaline infusion. Am J Obstet Gynecol 1995;173: 1273.

178. Anonymous. ACOG practice bulletin. Antenatal corticosteroid therapy for fetal lung maturation. Int J Gynecol 2002:95.

179. Crowley P. Prophylactic corticosteroids for preterm birth. The Cochrane Database of Systemic Reviews 2003;1:1.

180. Chen B, Yancey MK. Antenatal corticosteroids in preterm premature rupture of membranes. Clin Obstet Gynecol 1998;41:832.

181. Gibbs RS, Eschenbach DA. Use of antibiotics to prevent preterm birth. Am J Obstet Gynecol 1997;177:375.

182. Anonymous. ACOG committee opinion. Bacterial vaginosis screening for prevention of preterm delivery. Int Gynecol Obstet 1998;61:311.

183. Hauth JC et al. Reduced incidence of preterm delivery with metronidazole and erythromycin in women with bacterial vaginosis. N Engl Med 1995;333;1732.

184. Carey JC et al. Metronidazole to prevent preterm delivery in pregnant women with asymptomatic bacterial vaginosis. N Engl J Med 2000;342:534.

185. Mercer BM et al. Antibiotic therapy for reduction of infant morbidity after preterm premature rupture of the membranes. JAMA 1997;278:989.

186. Centers for Disease Control and Prevention. Prevention of perinatal group B streptococcal disease: a public health perspective. MMWR Morbid Mortal Wkly Rep 1996;45(No. RR-7):1.

187. Centers for Disease Control and Prevention. Prevention of perinatal group B streptococcal disease. Revised guidelines from CDC. MMWR Morbid Mortal Wkly Rep 2002;51(No. RR-11):1.

188. Schrag SJ et al. A population-based comparison of strategies to prevent early onset group B streptococcal disease in neonates. N Engl J Med 2002; 347:233.

189. Baker CJ. Group B streptococcal infections. Clin Perinatol 1997;24:59.

190. Ryan AS et al. Recent declines in breast-feeding in the United States, 1984 through 1989. Pediatrics 1991;88:719.

191. Lawrence RA. Anatomy of the human breast. In: Breastfeeding: A Guide for the Medical Profession, 4th Ed. St. Louis: Mosby-Year Book, 1994:37.

192. Neville MC, Walsh CT. Effects of drugs on milk secretion and composition. In: Bennett PN, ed. Drugs and Human Lactation, 2nd Ed. New York: Elsevier Science, 1996:15.

193. Ehrenkranz RA, Ackerman BA. Metoclopramide effect on faltering milk production by mothers of premature infants. Pediatrics 1986;78:614.

194. Gupta AP, Gupta PK. Metoclopramide as a lactagogue. Clin Pediatr 1985;24:269.

195. Kauppila A et al. A dose response relation between improved lactation and metoclopramide. Lancet 1981;1:1175.

196. Toppare MF et al. Metoclopramide for breast milk production. Nutr Res 1994;14:1019.

197. Kauppila A et al. Metoclopramide and breast feeding: efficacy and anterior pituitary responses of the mother and the child. Eur J Obstet Gynecol Reprod Biol 1985;19:19.

198. Spitz A. Treatment for lactation suppression: little progress in one hundred years. Am J Obstet Gynecol 1998;179:1485

199. Lawrence RA. Breastfeeding and medical disease. Med Clin North America 1989;73:583.

CHAPTER 47

Teratogenicity and Drugs in Breast Milk

Veronica S.L. Young

The use of drugs during pregnancy and lactation is controversial and presents great challenge to clinicians. The limited availability of scientific data from randomized trials complicates the decision to prescribe or recommend medications for pregnant or lactating women, even when they are medically necessary. The use of drugs during pregnancy is of special concern because of medical, social, and legal implications. Congenital anomalies or birth defects are the leading cause of infant mortality in the United States, accounting for 20% of all infant deaths.[1] The economic impact of anomalies from the 18 most clinically significant structural birth defects is approximately $8 billion annually.[2] This estimate does not include minor anomalies or the psychological and emotional impact to the child and family.

Drugs used in pregnancy have been implicated as causes of birth defects. Although once thought to be rare occurrences, the tragedy with thalidomide in the early 1960s highlights the detrimental effects of fetal exposure to drugs. With >7,000 cases, observed defects include various forms of limb defects, including phocomelia, as well as other major organ abnormalities.[3] The embryotoxic effects were unexpected because no teratogenicity was observed in different animal species, and only mild adverse effects were reported in human adults.

Other examples of iatrogenic major birth defects include diethylstilbestrol (DES), which causes vaginal adenocarcinoma in female offspring (detected only in later years of life), and valproic acid, which causes neural tube defects (NTDs).

Despite the significant impact of drug-induced birth defects, it is difficult and unethical to conduct randomized, controlled trials to assess the risk of fetal exposure to drugs in humans. Much of the data available are derived from epidemiologic studies, anecdotal experiences in humans, and animal studies. Because birth defects are species specific and influenced by many factors including genetic predisposition, one must carefully interpret the data and avoid overgeneralizing results.

The use of medications during lactation is another area of concern because the risk to the infant often is unknown. Despite limited definitive data, variables that can affect the excretion of drugs into breast milk have been identified and can be used to help predict the likelihood of drug passage into milk. Although these predictions do not necessarily equate with absolute risks or safety, they can be used, along with other information, to assist clinicians in weighing the risks and benefits of continuing lactation while the mother receives the necessary medication.

CONGENITAL ANOMALIES

Terminology

The term *congenital malformations* is defined as "structural abnormalities of prenatal origin that are present at birth and that seriously interfere with viability or physical well-being."[4] Although this definition is widely accepted among clinicians, some drug-induced defects relate to changes in functions or conditions that are not structural abnormalities (e.g., mental or physical growth retardation, central nervous system [CNS] depression, deafness, tumors, or biochemical changes). The broader term *congenital anomalies* (i.e., birth defects) includes both these toxicities and major and minor structural changes.[5] Except for the sections on prevalence and causes of malformations, the latter term is used throughout this chapter.

Prevalence of Congenital Malformations

The prevalence of major congenital malformations discovered at or shortly after birth in the general population is approximately 3%.[6] This number has been derived from large epidemiologic studies completed over the past several decades and depends on how terms are defined (e.g., major versus minor congenital malformations), the thoroughness with which the infant is examined, and how long the exposed person is followed after birth.[3] Although the collection of data on the occurrence of malformations would seem to be straightforward, it is in fact a complicated task subject to numerous errors and biases. Several problems cited in various studies were noted by Thelander.[7] Chief among these was the lack of consistency in reports on congenital malformations. Some studies examined only "significant anomalies," others "major malformations," while still others reported only "live births" or "single births" or "birth weights >500 g." Stillbirths and spontaneous abortions, both often associated with congenital malformations, often were excluded from epidemiologic data. Hospital records in some countries are biased because of numerous home deliveries, with only women with high-risk pregnancies being hospitalized. Also, hospitals conducting studies on congenital malformations are more likely to record these problems and hence usually report higher rates. Other inconsistencies identified involved diagnostic criteria, the lack of follow-up studies, and inadequate maternal histories.

The prevalence of defects varies widely depending on the population studied and the time period surveyed. In the early 1960s, the World Health Organization (WHO) completed a study of 421,781 pregnancies in 16 countries to determine the frequency of all malformations.[8] The prevalence ranged from 3.1 to 22.5 malformations per 1,000 births, with a mean of 12.7 per 1,000. The risk increased two-fold by 5 years of age. Other epidemiologic reports noted prevalences ranging from 0.27% to 9.41%.[7] In the United States, the reported rates of birth defects for 2000 ranged from 7.2 per 100,000 live births for microcephalus to 217 per 100,000 live births for various musculoskeletal/integumental anomalies (Table 47-1).[9]

These prevalence data generally do not include minor anomalies that may go unrecognized for years or may be discovered only at autopsy.[5] Some examples of minor malformations are umbilical and inguinal hernias, single umbilical artery, phimosis, slight malformations of the external ear, slight epispadias and hypospadias, cryptorchidism, hydrocele,

Table 47-1 Rates of Congenital Anomalies in the United States[a,b]

Congenital Anomaly	Rates[c]
Central Nervous System	
Anencephalus	10.7
Spina bifida/meningocele	20.7
Hydrocephalus	23.7
Microcephalus	7.2
Other	20.7
Circulatory/respiratory	
Heart malformations	124.9
Other	138.1
Gastrointestinal	
Rectal atresia/stenosis	8.4
Tracheo-esophageal fistula/esophageal atresia	12.1
Omphalocele/gastroschisis	29.7
Other	29.9
Musculoskeletal/integumental	
Cleft lip/palate	82.1
Polydactyly/syndactyly/adactyly	87.2
Clubfoot	57.2
Diaphragmatic hernia	10.8
Other	217.0
Genitourinary	
Malformed genitalia	84.2
Renal agenesis	13.8
Other	99.3
Chromosomal	
Down syndrome	46.9
Other	39.7

[a]Rates are calculated based on congenital anomalies reported in 2000 on birth certificates from all states (including District of Columbia) except for New Mexico.
[b]Total births reported in 2000: 4,031,591
[c]Rates are calculated per 100,000 live births.
Data from Martin JA et al. Births: final data for 2000. National Vital Statistics Reports, vol. 50, no. 5. Hyattsville, MD: National Center for Health Statistics, 2002.

abnormal dermatoglyphics, small nevus, and angioma (see Glossary at the end of this chapter). Neurodevelopmental delays and growth retardation also are potential long-term effects that will not be diagnosed in the immediate postpartum period. The prevalence of congenital anomalies is likely >3% if minor anomalies and long-term adverse effects are considered.

Drug Consumption During Pregnancy

Pregnancy is a symptom-producing condition. As a result, many drugs regularly are consumed during gestation, including some that are potential teratogens. Earlier epidemiologic studies attempting to identify patterns of drug exposure during pregnancy have estimated that women consumed on average five to nine medications. A more recent epidemiologic collaborative study, conducted under the auspices of the WHO Drug Utilization Research Group, assessed the pattern of drug use in pregnancy in 22 countries.[10] This survey of 14,778 women estimated that approximately 14% did not take any medications during pregnancy. In the group that did consume drugs, the average number of drugs taken was 2.9. Vitamin and iron supplements were the most commonly used, followed by anti-infectives and analgesics/antipyretics/anti-inflammatory agents. The proportion of women who consumed medications and the pattern of drug use varied by geographic distribution.

Placental Transfer

Placental Layers

At one time, the placenta was thought to present a barrier to the passage of drugs and noxious chemicals to the fetus. It is now known, however, that most medications cross the placenta to the fetus and, in general, what the mother consumes also is consumed by the fetus. Although the placenta acts like a biologic membrane, it initially is composed of four layers effectively separating two distinct individuals.[11] These layers are (1) the endothelial lining of fetal vessels, (2) the connective tissue in the core of the villus, (3) the cytotrophoblastic layer, and (4) the covering syncytium. During gestation, the placenta's surface area increases while its thickness decreases from approximately 25 microns during the first trimester to 2 to 6 microns at term. Both processes tend to favor the transfer of chemicals to the fetus.

Mechanisms of Substance Transfer

Drugs, nutrients, and other substances cross the placenta by five mechanisms: (1) simple diffusion (e.g., most drugs), (2) facilitated diffusion (e.g., glucose), (3) active transport (e.g., some vitamins, amino acids), (4) pinocytosis (e.g., immune antibodies), and (5) breaks between cells (e.g., erythrocytes).[11,12] The latter two mechanisms are of no practical importance in the transfer of drugs.

Factors Influencing Rate of Chemical Transfer

Several factors influence the rate of drug transfer across the placenta, including molecular weight (MW), lipid solubility, ionization, protein binding, uterine and umbilical blood flow, and maternal diseases.[12] Drugs with molecular weights <600 cross easily, while those >1,000 (e.g., heparin) cross with difficulty or not at all. Because most drugs have molecular weights <600, it is safe to assume that most drugs reaching the mother's circulatory system also will reach the fetus. Like other biologic membranes, lipid-soluble substances are transferred rapidly, with the rate of entry primarily governed by the lipid solubility of the nonionized molecule. Conversely, those molecules that are ionized at physiologic pH (e.g., the cholinergic quaternary amines) cross slowly, whereas weak acids and bases with pKa values between 4.3 and 8.5 are transferred rapidly to the fetus. The penetration of highly protein-bound drugs also is inhibited; only the free, unbound drugs cross the placenta.

Uterine blood flow, a major factor in determining the rate of drug transfer, increases throughout gestation. Several variables can affect uterine blood flow and the rate of drug transfer, including maternal blood pressure, cord compression, and drug therapy. Maternal hypotension reduces uterine blood flow and the rate at which substances are delivered to the membrane. Cord compression reduces the blood flow on the fetal side of the membrane. The use of drugs with α-adrenergic property (e.g., epinephrine) may constrict uterine vessels and thereby reduce blood flow.[13] Maternal diseases such as pregnancy-induced hypertension, erythroblastosis, and diabetes change the permeability of the placenta and may reduce or increase transfer.[12]

Fetal Development and Drug Effects

After fertilization, the development of the embryo and fetus is divided into three main stages: pre-embryonic period, embryonic period, and fetal period.[5,12] In the first 2 weeks after fertilization or the pre-embryonic period (0 to 14 days), little is known about the effects of drugs on human development. Exposure to a teratogenic agent during this period usually produces an "all or none" effect on the ovum:[14] the ovum either dies from exposure to a lethal dose of a teratogenic drug, or it regenerates completely after exposure to a sublethal dose. However, some animal studies have suggested that exposure to some drugs during the preimplantation stage can halt growth and development before implantation.[15] Although the damage can be repaired, intrauterine growth may be retarded in the offspring.

During the embryonic period (14 to 56 days after fertilization), when organogenesis occurs, the embryo is most susceptible to the effects of teratogens or other chemicals.[12] Exposure during this sensitive period may produce major morphologic changes. The stages and the time frames for the stages of human development are shown in Table 47-2. These stages of development differ significantly from other species, and knowledge of these stages is essential for the interpretation of the relationship between congenital malformations and drugs. For example, if a specific drug exposure occurs after the time of organ development, then a structural defect in that organ is less likely to be due to that specific drug.

The fetal period (57 days to term) includes most of the stages of histogenesis and functional maturation, although the latter continues for some time after birth.[5,12] Minor structural changes are still possible during histogenesis, but anomalies are more likely to involve growth and functional aspects such as mental development and reproduction.

Causes of Malformations

Classification

Causes of congenital malformations are generally classified into one of five categories: (1) monogenic origin; (2) chromosomal abnormalities; (3) multifactorial inheritance; (4) environmental factors; and (5) unknown.[5,6] Single gene and chromosomal-related defects account for approximately 25% of all congenital malformations in live-born infants (monogenetic, 7.5% to 20%; chromosomal, 5% to 6%).[4,5] *Multifactorial inheritance* refers to defects that are polygenic in origin; it has an environmental component. One surveillance program estimated that this interaction between genetic and environmental factors causes 23% of defects.[6] Congenital dislocation of the hip is an example of a defect in this category: the depth of the acetabular socket and joint laxity are genetically determined, and a frank breech malposition is one of the environmental factors.[17] In most cases, however, the environmental factors in multifactorial inheritance are unknown.

Environmental factors account for approximately 10% of malformations.[5] These include maternal conditions, mechanical effects, chemicals and drugs, and certain infectious agents. Maternal diseases associated with malformations include diabetes, phenylketonuria, virilizing tumors, and maternal hyperthermia. About 9% (range, 6.6% to 13.0%) of infants of diabetic mothers develop major congenital defects, primarily consisting of cardiovascular, neural tube, and skeletal malformations.[18] Mechanical effects such as

Table 47-2   Stages of Human Development

Blastula	4–6 days	**Excretory System**	
Implantation	6–7 days		
Primitive streak	16–18 days	Mesonephric (Wolffian) duct	4 wk
Total gestational time	267 days	Wolffian duct reaches cloaca	4.5 wk
Central Nervous System		Ureteric bud	5 wk
		Paramesonephric (Müllerian) duct	6 wk
		Müllerian duct reaches urogenital sinus	9 wk
Neural groove	3 wk	**Integumentary System**	
Neural crest	3.5 wk		
Three brain vesicles	3.5 wk	Milk hillocks	6 wk
Closure anterior neuropore	3.5 wk	Earliest hair follicles	10 wk
Closure posterior neuropore	4 wk	**Musculoskeletal System**	
Cerebral hemisphere	4.5 wk		
Cerebellum	5 wk	Anterior upper limb bud	4.33 wk
Cessation cell proliferation	6–8 mo postnatally	Myotomes	4.5 wk
Circulatory System		Epiphysis	4.5 wk
		Posterior lower limb bud	4.67 wk
Fused tubular heart	3 wk	End of somite formation	5 wk
Heart first beats	3 wk	Digits upper limb	6 wk
Aortic arches (I–VI)	3–4.5 wk	Chondrification centers	6 wk
Interatrial septum	4 wk	Digits lower limb	6.5 wk
Interventricular septum	4 wk	First indication ossification	7 wk
Spleen	5.5 wk	**Respiratory System**	
Atrioventricular valves	5.5 wk		
Aortic-pulmonary septum	6 wk	Paired lung buds	4 wk
Closure interventricular septum	6.5 wk	Closure cervical sinus	5.5 wk
Digestive System		Occlusion lower larynx	6 wk
		Completion diaphragm	7 wk
Rupture oral membrane	4 wk	**Reproductive System**	
Liver diverticulum	4 wk		
Cloacal membrane	4 wk	Gonadal fold	5 wk
Dorsal pancreas	4.5 wk	Gonadal sex differentiation	6.5 wk
Laryngotracheal groove	5 wk	Differentiation external genitalia	9 wk
Ventral pancreas	5 wk	Regression heterologous genital duct	10 wk
Tongue	5.5 wk	Vagina opens	5 mo
Fusion pancreas	6 wk	Descent testis	7 mo
Palatine shelf	6 wk	**Sense Organs**	
Beginning umbilical hernia	6 wk		
Salivary glands	6 wk	Optic vesicle	3.5 wk
Dental lamina	6.5 wk	Optic placode	3.5 wk
Upper lip	6.5 wk	Optic cup	4 wk
Hepatopancreatic duct	7 wk	Olfactory placode	4.5 wk
Rupture anal membrane	7 wk	Closure optic cup	4.5 wk
Withdrawal umbilical hernia	9 wk	Lens placode	4.5 wk
Completion of palate	10 wk	Closure lens vesicle	5.5 wk
Eruption incisor	7 mo postnatally	Pigment layer retina	5.5 wk
Endocrine System		Utriculus and sacculus	5.5 wk
		Cochlea	5.5 wk
Thyroid	4 wk	Olfactory pit	5.5 wk
Rathke's pouch	4.5 wk	Disappearance lens cavity	6.5 wk
Neurohypophysis	4.5 wk	Semicircular canals	6.5 wk
Thymus	5 wk	External auditory meatus	6.5 wk
Adrenal cortex	5 wk	Pinna	6.5 wk
Parathyroids	5.5 wk	Eyelids	6.5 wk
Adrenal medulla	5 wk	Nasolacrimal duct	7 wk
Interstitial cells in testis	17 wk	Corti's organ	7.5 wk
Primary ovarian follicles	30 wk	Closure eyelids	8 wk
		Opening external naris	24 wk
		Reopening eye lids	7–8 mo

From references 11 and 16.

intrauterine compression and abnormal cord constriction may result in fetal deformations.[5,18]

Probably the best known of the teratogenic viruses is rubella, which can cause a fetal rubella syndrome consisting of cataracts, heart disease, and deafness.[19] *In utero* exposure to rubella in the first trimester can cause defects in up to 85% of fetuses. Cytomegalovirus (CMV) infection occurs in 0.5% to 1.5% of newborns in the United States, resulting in deafness and mental retardation in 5% to 10% of these infants.[4] Characteristics of cytomegalic inclusion disease, the syndrome produced by CMV, include intrauterine growth retardation (IUGR), microcephaly, and at times chorioretinitis, seizures, blindness, and optic atrophy.[16] Herpes simplex 1 and 2 and varicella may be associated with malformations.[5] The data on varicella are controversial.[19]

The protozoan generally accepted as a teratogen is *Toxoplasma gondii*.[4] Most infants infected with *T. gondii* show no symptoms and develop normally. When toxicity does occur, the anomalies may consist of hepatosplenomegaly, icterus, maculopapular rash, chorioretinitis, cerebral calcifications, and hydrocephalus or microcephalous.[16] *Treponema pallidum* (syphilis) can cross the placenta and cause congenital syphilis as well as other defects, such as hydrocephaly, chorioretinitis, and optic atrophy.[5,19] *In utero* exposure to syphilis after the fourth month of pregnancy is associated with higher risk.

The final category, defects of unknown cause, makes up the greatest percentage of congenital malformations, accounting for about 60% to 65% of the total.[6]

Proven Human Teratogens

Numerous drugs have been associated with congenital anomalies, but only in a few cases has a consensus been reached that a specific agent is teratogenic. Table 47-3 lists those agents generally considered to be proven human teratogens. Heavy alcohol (ethanol) consumption is considered by many to produce a recognizable pattern of defects (Table 47-4, Fig. 47-1). Together, environmental chemicals and drugs may cause up to 6% of all congenital malformations.

Food and Drug Administration Risk Factors

In 1979, the U.S. Food and Drug Administration (FDA) introduced a system of rating pregnancy risks associated with pharmacologic agents. This system categorizes all drugs approved after 1983 into one of five pregnancy risk categories (Table 47-5). It establishes the level of risks to the fetus based on available animal and human data and recommends the degree of caution that should be undertaken with each drug. The risk factors assigned are sometimes difficult to interpret because they may not always reflect the latest findings.[20] Level of risks also have been described and categorized by teratology specialists, and they may or may not concur with manufacturers' ratings.[13,23] Table 47-6 lists some drugs that are considered contraindicated during pregnancy. Table 47-7 lists selected commonly used drugs and drug classes that should be used with caution. These lists are not all-inclusive, and a

---

Table 47-3   Drugs Considered Proven Human Teratogens

Aminopterin/ methotrexate	Coumarin derivatives	Phenytoin
ACE inhibitors	Diethylstilbestrol	Polychlorinated biphenyls
Antineoplastics	Ethanol (high dose)	Retinoids
Antithyroids	Iodides and radioactive iodine	Tetracycline
Barbiturates	Lithium	Thalidomide
Carbamazepine	Methyl mercury (organic)	Valproic acid
Cocaine	Misoprostol	Vitamin A (>18,000 IU/day)
	Paramethadione/trim ethadione	

ACE, angiotensin-converting enzyme.
From references 13, 16, 20, 21.

Table 47-4   Fetal Alcohol Syndrome

Craniofacial

Eyes	Short palpebral fissures, ptosis, strabismus, epicanthal folds, myopia, microphthalmia, blepharophimosis
Ears	Poorly formed conchae, posterior rotation
Nose	Short, upturned hypoplastic philtrum
Mouth	Prominent lateral palatine ridges, thinned upper vermilion border, retrognathia in infancy, micrognathia or relative prognathia in adolescence, cleft lip or palate, small teeth with faulty enamel
Maxilla	Hypoplastic

Central Nervous System

Mild to moderate retardation, microcephaly, poor coordination, hypotonia, irritability in infancy and hyperactivity in childhood (both mental and motor development are delayed)

Growth

Prenatal (affecting body length more than weight) and postnatal deficiency

Cardiac

Murmurs, atrial septal defect, ventricular septal defect, great vessel abnormalities, tetralogy of Fallot

Renogenital

Labial hypoplasia, hypospadias, renal defects

Cutaneous

Hemangiomas, hirsutism in infancy

Skeletal

Abnormal palmar creases, pectus excavatum, restriction of joint movement, nail hypoplasia, radioulnar synostosis, pectus carinatum, bifid xiphoid, Klippel-Feil anomaly, scoliosis

Muscular

Hernias of diaphragm, umbilicus or groin, diastasis recti

Other Problems Associated with Heavy Alcohol Consumption in Pregnancy

Intrauterine growth retardation, increased risk of spontaneous abortions, neonatal withdrawal

Data from reference 13.

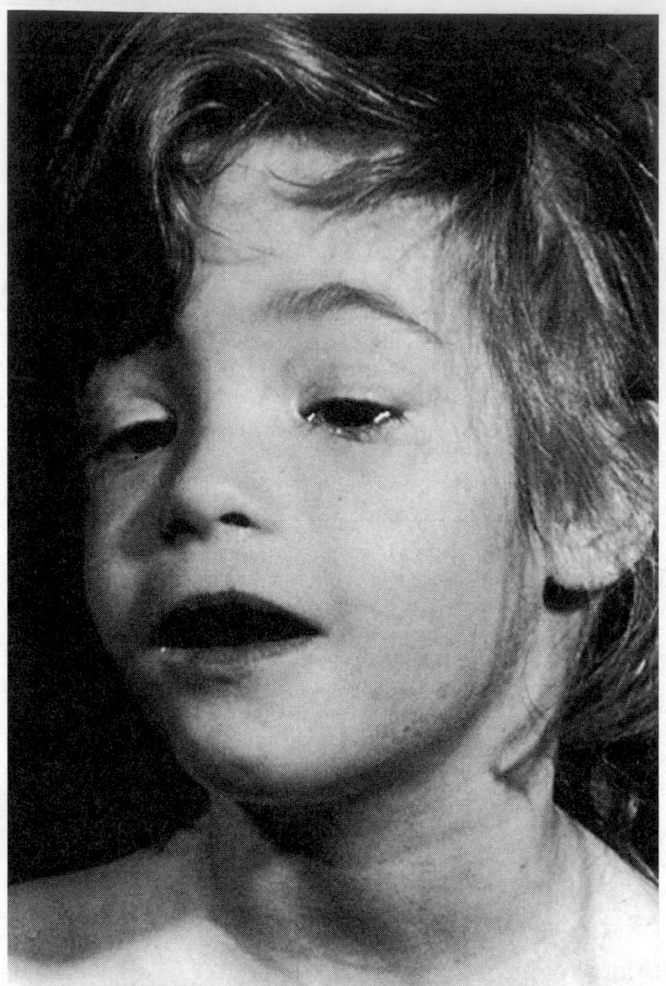

FIGURE 47-1 Fetal alcohol syndrome. Note strabismus, short palpebral fissures, long smooth philtrum, and thinned upper vermilion border. (Photo courtesy of K.L. Jones, MD, UC San Diego.)

Table 47-5 FDA Categories: Teratogenic Risks of Drugs

Category	Risk Factors
A	Controlled studies in women fail to demonstrate a risk to the fetus in the first trimester (and no evidence indicates a risk in later trimesters), and the possibility of fetal harm appears remote
B	Either animal reproduction studies have not demonstrated a fetal risk and there are no controlled studies in pregnant women, or animal reproduction studies have shown an adverse effect (other than a decrease in fertility) that was not confirmed in controlled studies in women in the first trimester (and no evidence indicates a risk in later trimesters)
C	Either studies in animals have revealed adverse effects on the fetus (teratogenic, embryocidal, or other) and no controlled studies in women are available or studies in women and animals are not available. Drugs should be given only if the potential benefit justifies the potential risk to the fetus
D	Evidence of human fetal risk is positive, but the benefits from use in pregnant women may be acceptable despite the risk (e.g., if the drug is needed in a life-threatening situation or for a serious disease for which safer drugs cannot be used or are ineffective)
X	Studies in animals or human beings have demonstrated fetal abnormalities or there is evidence of fetal risk based on human experience or both, and the risk of the drug in pregnant women clearly outweighs any possible benefit. The drug is contraindicated in women who are or may become pregnant

Adapted from reference 22.

Table 47-6 Drugs Considered Contraindicated During Pregnancy[a,b]

Drug/Drug Class	Fetal/Neonatal Effects
Acitretin	Acitretin is the active metabolite of etretinate. Use of ethanol with acitretin results in conversion of acitretin back to etretinate.[24] See etretinate.
Aminopterin	Aminopterin is a folic acid antagonist similar to MTX.[23] See MTX.
Chenodiol	Contraindicated because of potential for hepatotoxicity.[13]
Clomiphene	Used to induce ovulation. Neural tube defects and other anomalies have been reported, but most studies indicate no association with malformations. Inadvertent use in early pregnancy may have resulted in one infant with a ruptured lumbosacral meningomyelocele, and one infant with esophageal atresia with fistula, congenital heart defect, hypospadias, and absent left kidney.[13,23]
Cocaine	Maternal cocaine abuse associated with *in utero* cerebrovascular accidents, bowel atresias, and congenital defects of the GU tract, heart, limbs, and face. Other fetal and newborn consequences of maternal abuse are fetal growth retardation, and ↑ morbidity and mortality, including a possible association with SIDS. Maternal complications include shorter gestations, premature delivery, spontaneous abortions, abruptio placentae, and death.[13]

Table 47-6   Drugs Considered Contraindicated During Pregnancy^{a,b}—cont'd

Drug/Drug Class	Fetal/Neonatal Effects
Danazol	Use after the eighth week of gestation (the onset of androgen receptor sensitivity) may result in masculinization of the female fetus (i.e., pseudohermaphroditism); male fetuses usually not affected but one male had multiple anomalies after first trimester exposure.[25]
Diethylstilbestrol (DES)	An estimated 6 million pregnant women were exposed to DES from 1940–1971 to treat obstetric problems. Exposure resulted in reproductive system defects in both female and male offspring.[13] *Female:* Lower Müllerian tract: vaginal adenosis; cervical/vaginal fornix defects; cockscomb, collar, pseudopolyp, and hypoplastic cervix; vaginal defects exclusive of fornix; incomplete transverse and/or longitudinal septum. Upper Müllerian tract: uterine structural defects; fallopian tube structural defects *Male:* Altered semen ($\downarrow$ count, concentration, motility, morphology); epididymal cysts; hypotrophic testis; microphallus; varicocele; capsular induration DES exposure increases risk of developing vaginal and cervical clear cell adenocarcinoma.[26] DES exposure has not been related to defects other than those found in the reproductive system.
Estrogen and related compounds	Contraindicated in pregnancy. A study found an association between estrogen exposure and cardiovascular defects, eye and ear anomalies, and Down syndrome. Further analysis of these data failed to support the association with cardiac malformations. Other studies have also failed in finding association with congenital defects.[13]
Ethanol	Heavy consumption during pregnancy associated with IUGR and a pattern of anomalies known as the "fetal alcohol syndrome" (see Table 45-4). No known safe levels in pregnancy. Potent fetal brain toxin.[13]
Etretinate	Teratogenic effects reported include meningomyelocele, meningoncephalocele, multiple synostoses, facial dysmorphia, syndactylies, absence of terminal phalanges, malformation of hip, ankle and forearm, low-set ears, high palate, decreased cranial volume, and alterations of the skull and cervical vertebrae. Teratogenic potential can persist for years because of a long half-life of 100 days after prolonged use.[24]
HMG-CoA reductase inhibitors	One case of first trimester exposure to lovastatin with subsequent birth of an infant with constellation of malformations termed the VATER association (vertebral anomalies, anal atresia, tracheoesophageal fistula with esophageal atresia, and renal and radial dysplasias).[13] An interim evaluation of lovastatin and simvastatin exposure during pregnancy in postmarketing surveillance failed to demonstrate an increased risk of fetal anomalies.[27] A theoretic concern is that the interference of cholesterol biosynthesis by HMG-CoA reductase inhibitors may adversely impact sex steroid biosynthesis.[28]
Isotretinoin	Defects can occur with any doses and for short durations of use. Reports include defects of the skull, ear, eye, face, CNS, thymus, and cardiovasculature; cleft palate; limb reductions; low IQ scores.[23,29]
Leflunomide	It is teratogenic/embryotoxic in animals. Effects may be dose-related. Because of its long half-life of about 14–18 days, women of childbearing potential discontinued from this drug should undergo the drug elimination procedure using cholestyramine as recommended by the manufacturer.[29,30]
Leuprolide	Teratogenic in animals; no adverse fetal effects in over 100 cases of human exposure; spontaneous abortions and IUGR may occur because drug suppresses endometrial proliferation.[13]
Lysergic acid diethylamide (LSD)	Pure chemical does not cause chromosomal abnormalities, spontaneous abortions, or congenital anomalies. Reported adverse fetal effects in maternal abusers probably caused by multiple factors, including reporting bias.[13]
Menadione	Use near term or close to delivery has resulted in marked hyperbilirubinemia and kernicterus in newborn. If vitamin K needed during pregnancy, use phytonadione (K_1).[13]
Methotrexate (MTX)	MTX is a folic acid antagonist with abortifacient property. Exposure in first trimester may cause malformations that are dose-related. Anomalies reported include cranial (e.g., oxycephaly, absence of lambdoid and coronal suture), ocular (e.g., ocular hypertelorism), and skeletal defects.[13,23]
Methyl mercury	Organic mercury poisoning has occurred primarily in Japan and Iraq. Known as Minamata disease in Japan. Nonspecific neurologic symptoms after third trimester exposure were observed in about 72 known cases.[4]
Mifepristone (RU-486)	Antiprogesterone agent used to induce abortion; teratogenic potential has not been determined.[26]

Continued

Table 47-6   Drugs Considered Contraindicated During Pregnancy[a,b]—cont'd

Drug/Drug Class	Fetal/Neonatal Effects
Misoprostol	Has abortifacient properties; teratogenic potential has not been determined.[26]
Phencyclidine	Persistent irritability, jitteriness, hypertonicity, and poor feeding reported in newborns.[37]
Ribavirin	Teratogenic and/or embryotoxic in nearly all animal species tested.[26] Teratogenic risk in humans has not been determined. Pregnant health care workers or those trying to conceive should avoid or use caution when caring for these patients.
Sodium iodide(^{125}I) and (^{131}I)	Administration at 12 weeks' gestation or later will cause partial or complete destruction of fetal thyroid gland; effect is dose dependent with toxic doses 10 mCi.[13]
Thalidomide	Over 7,000 birth defects have been linked to thalidomide use during pregnancy. The most susceptible period is from days 34–50 after the first day of the last menstrual period.[3] Thalidomide embryopathy does not appear to be dose-related.[23] Limb reduction and ear defects are common. Malformations include amelia, phocomelia, bone hypoplasticity, absence of bones, anotia, micro pinna, auditory canal defects, facial palsy, anophthalmos, microphthalmos, congenital heart defects, and GI tract and genital abnormalities.[24]
Vaccines, live	Most live, attenuated virus vaccines potentially can cause fetal infection. Vaccination with smallpox in first and second trimesters has resulted in fetal death.[13]
Vitamin A (high dose)	Both deficiency and excess are thought to be teratogenic. Prolonged high dosages (>25,000 IU/day) associated with: microtia, craniofacial and CNS anomalies, facial palsy, microphthalmia/anophthalmia, facial clefts, cardiac defects, limb reductions, GI atresia, and urinary tract defects.[3,13]

[a]This list is not all-inclusive. Most drugs listed have been designated FDA risk factor X. All drugs of abuse are contraindicated in pregnancy.
[b]A glossary is provided at the end of this chapter.
CDC, Centers for Disease Control and Prevention; CNS, central nervous system; GI, gastrointestinal; GU, genitourinary; HMG CoA, hydroxymethyl-glutaryl-CoA; IUGR, intrauterine growth retardation; MTX, methotrexate; SIDS, sudden infant death syndrome.

Table 47-7   Selected Drugs That Should Be Used with Caution During Pregnancy[a,b]

Drug/Drug Class	Risk Factor[c]	Fetal/Neonatal Effects
ACE inhibitors	C/D[d]	Use in second and third trimesters has been associated with a pattern of anomalies called ACEI fetopathy with renal tubular dysplasia as the major malformation. Other reported defects include hypocalvaria, IUGR, patent ductus arteriosus, oligohydramnios, pulmonary hypoplasia, and anuria.[31–34]
Aminoglycosides	C/D[e]	Potential for VIII cranial nerve toxicity with high dosages. Prolonged therapy with kanamycin produced VIII cranial nerve damage; nine of 391 (2.3%) infants had hearing loss.[11,13] Short-term therapy with streptomycin (1 g/day for 4.5 days) combined with ethacrynic acid resulted in complete hearing loss in both mother and infant.[13]
Amiodarone	D	Complications reported include fetal hypothyroidism, low birth weight, prematurity, bradycardia, and QT prolongation.[35] Because the drug contains 75 mg iodine per 200-mg dose, newborn thyroid status should be closely monitored.[36]
Amitriptyline	D	Limb reduction defects reported, but analysis of 86 first-trimester exposures did not confirm association. Other defects observed in three infants include micrognathia, anomalous right mandible, left talipes equinovarus (1 case), swelling of hands/feet (1 case), and hypospadias (1 case). Urinary retention occurred in one newborn after nortriptyline use.[13]
Angiotensin II-receptor antagonists	C/D[d]	Acts on the renin-angiotensin system; see ACE inhibitors.
Aspirin	C/D[g]	Risk of adverse fetal effects is low if low doses are used occasionally.[23] No specific pattern of malformations has been identified. It has been used to prevent pregnancy-induced hypertension, pre-eclampsia, and eclampsia. Use of full-dose aspirin near term may prolong gestation and labor, adversely affect clotting ability of newborn by reducing collagen-induced platelet aggregation, and may increase risk in premature or low-birth-weight infants for intracranial hemorrhage.[13,23]

Table 47-7   Selected Drugs That Should Be Used with Caution During Pregnancy[a,b]—cont'd

Drug/Drug Class	Risk Factor[c]	Fetal/Neonatal Effects
Azathioprine	D	Teratogenic in animals. No specific pattern of malformation noted in humans. Examples of anomalies reported include hydrocephalus, anencephaly, cleft palate, atrial septal defect, and polydactyly.[37] Fatal neonatal anemia, thrombocytopenia, and lymphopenia reported.[23]
Benzodiazepines	D/X[e]	Congenital anomalies reported include cleft lip/palate, congenital heart disease, and defects of the CNS, lung, abdomen, GI tract, musculoskeletal system, and digits. Strength of association is controversial. Neonatal withdrawal has been reported.[38]
β-Blockers	B/C/D[e]	Reduced birth weight may result from use of some β-blockers in second and third trimesters but effect also may be due to severe maternal disease. Use of acebutolol, atenolol, or nadolol near term has caused β-blockade in newborns.[13]
Bismuth subsalicylate	C	Hydrolyzed in GI tract to bismuth salts and sodium salicylate, absorption of bismuth salts is negligible, but chronic exposure to salicylates may present fetal risk (see Aspirin). Restrict use to first half of pregnancy and do not exceed recommended doses.[13]
Busulfan	D	Used in 38 pregnancies, 22 in first trimester resulting in six infants with defects: unspecified malformations (aborted at 20 wk); anomalous deviation left lobe liver, bilobular spleen, and pulmonary atelectasis; pyloric stenosis; cleft palate, microphthalmia, cytomegaly, hypoplasia of ovaries and thyroid gland, corneal opacity, and IUGR; myeloschisis, aborted at 6 wk; IUGR, left hydronephrosis and hydroureter, absent right kidney and ureter, and hepatic subcapsular calcifications.[13]
Carbamazepine	D	May produce malformations similar to those seen with phenytoin (see Table 47-13).[13] Risk may be increased almost threefold.[39] Examples of anomalies reported include cardiac, urinary tract, and craniofacial defects, cleft palate, fingernail hypoplasia, and low birth weight. Slightly increased risk of NTD.
Chloramphenicol	C	Use with caution at term. Unconfirmed report of cardiovascular collapse (gray syndrome) in newborns exposed in final stage of pregnancy.[13,40]
Codeine	C	Major and minor anomalies have been reported, but the frequencies in affected newborns were similar to control. Examples of anomalies include congenital heart disease, respiratory malformations, GU tract defects, umbilical and inguinal hernia, hydrocephaly, and pyloric stenosis. Some retrospective studies suggested a link between codeine and cleft lip/palate.[16,23,41]
Corticosteroids	C/D[e]	Use of oral corticosteroids during the first trimester may be associated with a slightly increased risk of oral cleft.[42] Topical (drug not specified) and inhalation (beclomethasone, budesonide) use do not appear to increase risk of malformations.[43,44]
Diphenhydramine	B	Most studies did not show an increased risk of congenital anomalies with diphenhydramine versus control.[13,23] One case-control study found possible association with cleft palate after first-trimester exposure.[45]
Ephedrine	C	No evidence of teratogenicity based upon 873 exposures; ↑ in fetal heart rate and beat-to-beat variability have been observed.[13,41]
Epinephrine	C	Statistically significant association found between 189 first trimester exposures and major or minor anomalies in one study. Association also found between use anytime in pregnancy and inguinal hernia. Data may reflect serious maternal conditions requiring use of drug. After 9,719 exposures, adrenergics as a group were associated with minor anomalies, inguinal hernia, and clubfoot.[41] Adrenergics, including epinephrine, are teratogenic in some animal species.[13]
Ergotamine	X/D[f]	Small, infrequent doses may not be teratogenic; large doses or frequent use may cause teratogenicity because of disruption of fetal blood supply; oxytocic properties of drug may cause dysfunctional labor marked by prolonged contractions resulting in fetal hypoxia.[13] If possible, should be avoided in pregnancy.

Continued

Table 47-7   Selected Drugs That Should Be Used with Caution During Pregnancy[a,b]—cont'd

Drug/Drug Class	Risk Factor[c]	Fetal/Neonatal Effects
Ethosuximide	C	An association between ethosuximide and congenital anomalies has not been established. Reports of defects include patent ductus arteriosus, cleft lip/palate, and hydrocephalus. Spontaneous hemorrhage reported in 1 neonate.[13,23]
Fluconazole	C	Risk is unlikely increased when used as a single oral dose of ≤150 mg.[23] Chronic use may be teratogenic. Case reports described anomalies with structural defects of the CNS, extremities, and cleft palate; features resembled a known recessive genetic disorder.[46]
Fosphenytoin	D	This is a prodrug of phenytoin. After parenteral administration, fosphenytoin is converted to phenytoin.[29] See phenytoin.
Hydroxyurea	D	Inhibits DNA synthesis and is considered a human carcinogen and mutagen. It is teratogenic/embryotoxic in animals.[29] Human data are limited, but potential for risk is high.
Ibuprofen	B/D[g]	No evidence of teratogenicity with first trimester use, but experience limited. Use after 34–35 weeks' gestation may cause premature closure of ductus arteriosus resulting in PPHN. Naproxen use at 30 weeks' gestation associated with PPHN in three infants.[13] (see NSAIDs)
Imipramine	D	Congenital anomalies described in case reports include bilateral amelia, polydactyly, omphalocele, defective abdominal muscles, diaphragmatic hernia, exencephaly, cleft palate, adrenal hypoplasia, and renal cystic degeneration.[13,23] Early reports of limb reduction defects cannot be confirmed.
Indomethacin	B/D[g]	Used to treat premature labor; oliguric renal failure, hemorrhage, and intestinal perforation have been reported in some premature infants exposed just before delivery. Reduced fetal urine output may be therapeutic in cases of polyhydramnios. May cause constriction of the fetal ductus arteriosus, with or without tricuspid regurgitation.[13,47] (see NSAIDs)
Lithium	D	Case reports and cohort studies showed that lithium exposure in the first trimester can increase risk of Ebstein's anomaly (absolute risk of 0.05–0.1%), a rare congenital heart defect occurring in 1/20,000 live births.[48] Incidence of other CV defects range from 0.9–12%. Other anomalies reported include cyanosis, rhythm disturbances, thyroid dysfunction, hypoglycemia, lethargy, hyperbilirubinemia.[49] Use near term may cause "floppy baby syndrome" in infants with lithium toxicity.[23]
Marijuana	C	Maternal use may be associated with fetal growth retardation, but other factors such as multiple drug use, lifestyles, diseases, socioeconomic status, and nutrition may play significant role. One report has associated in utero exposure to marijuana to the development of acute non-lymphoblastic leukemia in childhood.[13,50] Contraindicated if used as drug of abuse.
Mercaptopurine (6-MP)	D	6-MP has teratogenic/mutagenic potential.[29] Adverse outcomes reported include microphthalmia, corneal opacity, hypoplasia of ovaries and thyroid, cytomegaly, cleft palate, hypospadias, polydactyly, neonatal anemia and pancytopenia.[37] Results complicated by polytherapy.
Methimazole (MMI)	D	First-trimester exposure may be associated with a small increased risk of aplasia cutis congenita (congenital scalp defect). A pattern of anomalies (MMI embryopathy) has been proposed consisting of choanal atresia, esophageal atresia with tracheo-esophageal fistula, facial and skin dysmorphology, hypoplastic nipples, psychomotor delay, and growth restriction.[51,52] Hypothyroidism and goiter have been reported in neonates exposed in utero.[23]
Methyldopa	C	No known association with congenital defects. Frequently used for treatment of pregnancy-induced hypertension. A decrease in intracranial volume after first trimester use has been reported but no relationship between small head size and retarded mental development at 4 years of age.[13]

Table 47-7   Selected Drugs That Should Be Used with Caution During Pregnancy[a,b]—cont'd

Drug/Drug Class	Risk Factor[c]	Fetal/Neonatal Effects
Methylene blue	D	Intra-amniotic injection has caused hemolytic anemia, hyperbilirubinemia, methemoglobinemia, and possibly small bowel obstructions.[53]
Metronidazole	B	Drug is mutagenic in bacteria and carcinogenic in rodents. Vaginal use does not appear to increase risk of teratogenicity.[23] Risk with systemic use is controversial. Oral cleft has been reported.[13]
Nicotine Nicotine polacrilex	C/D[e]	Smoking during pregnancy can cause fetal growth retardation, increased risk of spontaneous abortion, and perinatal mortality.[26] Use of nicotine replacement in the third trimester has been associated with decreased fetal breathing.[29] Spontaneous abortion has been reported.
Nitrofurantoin	B	Apparently safe but use with caution at term because of theoretic potential for hemolytic anemia in newborn.[13]
NSAIDs	B/D[e,g] or C/D[e,g]	Epidemiologic studies of NSAID use as a class found conflicting data. In a study of 2,557 first-trimester exposures to NSAIDs, a slightly increased risk for cardiac defects and oral cleft was noted.[54] Another study of 1,462 women exposed anytime during pregnancy did not show an increased risk for abnormalities, LBW, or preterm birth.[55] Rate of miscarriage may be increased when NSAID is used weeks before the miscarriage. Risk assessment requires further studies. (See ibuprofen, indomethacin)
Penicillamine	D	Use in pregnancy is associated with connective tissue defects (cutis laxa). Examples of other anomalies reported are pyloric stenosis, inguinal hernia, hyperflexion of hips and shoulders, and low-set ears.[13,16,23]
Phenobarbital	D	May produce malformations similar to those seen with phenytoin when used in epileptic patients (see Table 47-13). May cause early HDN. Also may cause fetal/newborn addiction.[13]
Phenylephrine	C	Anomalies were reported in studies involving >5,000 exposures, but significance of association is undetermined. Fetal hypoxia is possible. Avoid use with other pressor agents.[13] (See epinephrine)
Phenytoin	D	See Table 47-13[13]
Progesterone and related compounds	D/X[e]	In 1977 the FDA restricted use in pregnancy based on reports of cardiac malformations, CNS defects, masculinization of female fetuses, and limb defects. Re-evaluations of some of these data and new, well-designed studies have failed to show an association between these defects and progesterones. Progesterone is used frequently to prevent imminent abortion during the first trimester. Use of hydroxyprogesterone or medroxyprogesterone during early pregnancy may have been associated with esophageal atresia but the absolute risk was low (about 6/10,000 exposed lived births).[13,56]
Propylthiouracil (PTU)	D	Drug of choice for treatment of hyperthyroidism during pregnancy; anomalies reported in seven infants after *in utero* exposure, but no association between PTU and defects suggested. May produce mild hypothyroidism in fetus when used close to term, evident as a goiter and elevated levels of neonatal TSH. Goiters in two infants sufficiently massive to cause death in one infant and respiratory distress in the other.[13]
Quinolones	C	Erosions of cartilage and arthropathy have been reported in immature animals, but effects in human are unknown.[29] A cohort study of 57 women exposed to fluoroquinolones during pregnancy did not find an increased risk of congenital anomalies versus 17,259 control patients.[57] Avoid use if safer alternatives are available.[26,29]
Rifampin	C	Although not a proven teratogen, one report observed nine defects in 204 pregnancies: anencephaly (1 case), hydrocephalus (2 cases), limb malformations (4 cases), renal tract defect (1 case), and congenital hip dislocation (1 case). HDN observed in 3 infants; prophylactic vitamin K recommended.[13]

Continued

Table 47-7   Selected Drugs That Should Be Used with Caution During Pregnancy[a,b]**—cont'd**

Drug/Drug Class	Risk Factor[c]	Fetal/Neonatal Effects
SSRIs	C	Most data available are for fluoxetine. First-trimester exposure to fluoxetine does not appear to increase risk of major malformations.[58] One study suggests that minor anomalies may be increased, but this remains to be confirmed. Other SSRIs (sertaline, paroxetine, fluvoxamine, citalopram) do not appear to increase risk of major anomalies.[23,59] Withdrawal symptoms in neonates have been reported.[23,60] Safety requires further investigation.
Sulfonylureas, oral	C	Use near term may result in prolonged hypoglycemia. Not recommended in pregnancy because it will not provide better control than diet alone. Insulin is the treatment of choice during pregnancy.[13]
Tetracyclincs	D	Use after fifth month of gestation will result in permanent yellow-brown staining of teeth. Inhibition of fibula growth may occur in premature infants.[13] Based on 1,944 pregnancy exposures, possible associations with congenital anomalies found in 61 infants: hypospadias (5 cases), inguinal hernia (47 cases), limb hypoplasia (6 cases), and clubfoot (3 cases).[41]
Thiazides and related diuretics	C/D[e]	They are unlikely to be teratogenic. Other adverse outcomes reported include: neonatal thrombocytopenia in 11 newborns (with 2 deaths) following use near term of chlorothiazide, HCTZ, and methyclothiazide; hemolytic anemia in two neonates after chlorothiazide and bendroflumethiazide; fetal electrolyte disturbances when exposed during third trimester.[13,23] May decrease placental perfusion.[61]
Trimethadione	D	Phenotype exists for fetal trimethadione syndrome (see Table 47-12). Use in nine families (36 pregnancies) resulted in 25 infants with wide spectrum of defects. Not recommended in pregnancy.[13]
Trimethoprim (TMP)	C	TMP is a dihydrofolate reductase inhibitor. Exposure during first and second month of pregnancy may ↑ NTD; exposure during second and third month may ↑ cardiovascular defects and oral cleft.[51,52,62]
Valproic acid	D	Risk for NTDs is 1–2% (exposure must occur between the seventeenth and thirtieth day after fertilization). A valproic acid syndrome has been suggested to consist of anomalies involving the following: NTDs, craniofacial, digits, and urogenital. Retarded psychomotor development and low birth weight also have been observed.[13,23,63]
Warfarin	X/D[f]	Teratogenic; see Table 47-12.[13]

[a]This list is not all-inclusive. Selected drugs are listed by drug class and not by individual names.
[b]A glossary is provided at the end of this chapter.
[c]Risk factors listed for most drugs are according to the manufacturers' ratings based on FDA definitions. When this is not available, the risk factor indicated is from reference 13.
[d]Rated risk factor C in first trimester, D in second and third trimesters.
[e]Drugs within the same class may have different pregnancy category ratings.
[f]Rated risk factor X by manufacturer, rated D in reference 13.
[g]Rated risk factor D in third trimester or near delivery.
ACEI, angiotensin-converting enzyme inhibitor; CNS, central nervous system; CV, cardiovascular; ECG, electrocardiogram; FDA, Food and Drug Administration; GI, gastrointestinal; GU, genitourinary; HDN, hemolytic disease of the newborn; IUGR, intrauterine growth retardation; NSAIDs, nonsteroidal anti-inflammatory drugs; NTDs, neural tube defects; PPHN, persistent pulmonary hypertension of the newborn; SSRIs, selective serotonin reuptake inhibitors; TSH, thyroid-stimulating hormone.

review of specialty resources on drug use in pregnancy is recommended.[13,16,23] Teratogen information programs also are available in the United States and Canada to respond to questions concerning the risks of drug exposure during pregnancy. These programs are usually affiliated with medical or university settings.[20,64] Because the potential for fetal risks cannot be entirely disregarded for many drugs, the need to medicate during pregnancy should be evaluated carefully.

DRUG EXCRETION IN HUMAN MILK

Breast milk is recognized as the optimal source of nutrition for infants, with documented benefits not only to infants but also to mothers, families, and societies.[65] Evidence indicates that breast-feeding decreases the incidence or severity of many infectious processes (e.g., otitis media, respiratory infections, urinary tract infections) in infants. In children and adults who were breast-fed, the risk of developing certain medical illnesses also may decrease (e.g., obesity, inflammatory bowel disease, celiac disease, childhood leukemia).[66] Breast-feeding may also positively influence cognitive and intellectual development in children and young adults.[67] Numerous benefits to the mother also have been identified, such as decreased postpartum blood loss, more rapid uterine involution, earlier return to prepregnancy weight, and decreased risks of breast cancer, ovarian cancer, and osteoporosis.[65]

The American Academy of Pediatrics (AAP) recommends that mothers breast-feed for ≥12 months. Recognition of the importance of breast-feeding is highlighted in *Healthy People 2010,* a national health promotion and disease prevention program that helps the nation address public health issues by establishing objectives and goals. In the United States, breast-feeding during the early postpartum period increased from 54% in 1988 to 67% in 1999.[68] The percentage of women who are still breast-feeding at 6 months decreases to 31%. Although encouraging, these figures are still below the *Healthy People 2010* targets of 75% for early postpartum and 50% at 6 months.

The perception that nursing should be discontinued while the mother is medicated persists, even though only a finite number of drugs are absolutely contraindicated during lactation. This misconception is likely a result of the uncertainty surrounding the effects of exposure of many drugs in nursing infants because of the inherent difficulties in accessing risks in controlled environments (e.g., clinical trials). Unlike the use of drugs during pregnancy, when the effects of fetal exposure are difficult to predict, drug excretion in breast milk can be approximated to a certain extent. Actual measurements of drug concentrations in milk and clinical observations in breast-fed infants have been published for selected drugs. An understanding of the basic physiochemical principles of drug excretion in breast milk and the factors that affect this process allows for better prediction of the risk of drug exposure to the nursing infant.

Pharmacokinetics

Different pharmacokinetic models of drug excretion in milk have been described.[69–71] A two-compartment open model presents the maternal fluids as one compartment and breast milk as the other. After ingestion, the drug gets absorbed into the maternal compartment, with a proportion of drug passing into breast milk and the remaining portion distributed in and eliminated from the maternal system. Drugs reaching breast milk will ultimately leave this compartment either by diffusing back into maternal fluids or through milk production and nursing.[70,71] A more popular model describes drug excretion in milk using a three-compartment model that incorporates the pharmacokinetics of the mother, mammary tissues, and infant.[69,70] The overall risk to the infant depends on the amount of drug bioavailable to the mother, the amount reaching breast milk, and the actual amount of drug ingested and bioavailable to the nursing infant.

Transfer of Drugs From Plasma to Milk

Transfer of drugs from maternal plasma to milk is generally through passive diffusion.[72] Low-molecular-weight, water-soluble substances diffuse through small, water-filled pores, while lipid- soluble compounds pass through lipid membranes.[73] Many factors affect the excretion of drugs in breast milk, and they should be carefully assessed before making a recommendation (Table 47-8). The extent of drug passage into breast milk is often expressed quantitatively as the milk-to-plasma (M/P) ratio. This ratio should not be used as the sole determinant of whether a drug is safe for use during breast-feeding (see Estimating Infant Exposure).

Several parameters affect drug excretion into breast milk (see Table 47-8). The pKa of a drug partially determines how much drug can reach the milk, because only the nonionized

Table 47-8 Factors Affecting the Fate of Drugs in Milk and the Nursing Infant

Maternal parameters	• Drug dosage and duration of therapy • Route and frequency of administration • Metabolism • Renal clearance • Blood flow to the breasts • Milk pH • Milk composition
Drug parameters	• Oral bioavailability (to mother and infant) • Molecular weight • pKa • Lipid solubility • Protein binding
Infant parameters	• Age of the infant • Feeding pattern • Amount of breast milk consumed • Drug absorption, distribution, metabolism, elimination

From references 69, 72, 74, 75.

portion of free drug is transferred. Human milk, with an average pH of 7.1, is slightly more acidic than plasma. In general, drugs that are weak acids (e.g., penicillin) tend to have a higher concentration in plasma than milk (M/P <1). Conversely, the concentration of weak bases (e.g., erythromycin) in milk is more likely to be higher or to reach an equilibrium with that measured in plasma (M/P ≥1).[69,71] Once in the milk, the proportion of ionized weak base rises in the relatively acidic solution, and thus drug "trapping" occurs. Drug reabsorption has been found for some agents, and the prevention of passage back into the plasma by "trapping" may be clinically important. Lipid solubility also is determined to a large extent by the degree of ionization because drugs with relatively high lipid solubility exist in the nonionized form. Diffusion through lipid membranes is probably the most important pathway for drug transfer. Although pH, pKa, and lipid solubility are important elements, other factors may significantly modify predictions based solely on these chemical characteristics. Two of these other factors are protein binding and molecular weight.[72–74] Drugs with high molecular weights such as insulin (MW > 6,000) are less likely to transfer into breast milk, while those with molecular weights <300 transfer more readily.[75] Highly protein-bound drugs such as glyburide (99% protein bound) are less likely to be transferred into breast milk, even though infants should still be monitored for signs of hypoglycemia.

Drug transfer also is influenced by the yield of milk, which is related to blood flow and prolactin secretion.[69] Lactation is associated with a high blood flow to the breasts, but little is known about this flow during or between feedings. The milk yield (volume) differs slightly depending on the duration of lactation and the time of day. A diurnal pattern has been observed, with highest yields at 6 AM and lowest yields at 6 PM or 10 PM. The mean composition of mature human milk is approximately 87% aqueous solution, 3.5% lipids, 8%

carbohydrate (83% of which is lactose), 0.9% protein, and 0.2% nitrogen.[76] The proportions of these components may vary widely from woman to woman and even within the same woman. For example, hind milk contains four- to five-fold the fat content of foremilk, while colostrum contains little fat. Fat content also has exhibited a diurnal variation.

After a drug reaches the milk, it equilibrates between the aqueous and lipid phases. The nature of this equilibration can modify how much drug actually reaches the infant. Infant feeding patterns differ significantly from one baby to another. The time spent suckling at each breast and the volume of milk taken in also determine the amount of drug ingested, especially if the drug has partitioned into one phase more so than the other. Once the infant ingests the drug via breast milk, the pharmacologic and adverse effects on the infant will be determined by the extent of oral bioavailability, distribution, metabolism, and rate of elimination. These pharmacokinetic parameters differ depending on the infant's age and whether he or she was born prematurely or at term.

Estimating Infant Exposure

Understanding the transfer of drugs into breast milk is important because the primary objective is to minimize infant exposure to these substances. The actual amount an infant will ingest is difficult to determine due to varying maternal, drug, and infant parameters. Available data generally are from single or small numbers of case reports or pharmacokinetic studies involving few mother–infant pairs. An M/P ratio is sometimes used alone as the basis for a recommendation, but this should be avoided because its accuracy can be affected by many factors. The time of sampling after maternal ingestion (peak versus steady-state), dose, length of therapy, route of administration, and milk composition are a few of the variables that can influence the M/P ratio.[69,71,74] Sampling during maternal peak drug concentration attempts to approximate the highest amount of drug that can reach the infant. This assumption is inherently flawed because peak drug concentration in the mother does not necessarily equate with peak drug concentration in milk at that same point in time.[70,74] The amount of drug an infant actually receives also depends on the volume of milk ingested. Even if a drug has a high M/P ratio, the actual amount received by the infant could be low if only a small volume of milk was consumed. Therefore, an M/P ratio describes the likelihood of drug excretion into breast milk, but it does not indicate the level of infant exposure. In general, drugs with lower M/P ratios (<1) are preferred over those with higher M/P ratios (>1) during breast-feeding, but other parameters such as maternal condition and therapeutic efficacy should be considered.

Infant exposure to a drug via ingestion of breast milk can be estimated for some drugs. The M/P ratio is used to estimate the drug concentration in milk (Equation 47-1) and the dose the infant may ingest (Equation 47-2).[64,70,74] The variables required to calculate Equation 47-1 can be located in the published literature, but only for some drugs. The actual volume of milk ingested by the infant is difficult to estimate, but the average consumption is approximately 150 mL/kg per day.[74] The estimated infant dose can then be used to calculate a "relative infant dose" (RID) (Equation 47-3), which is expressed as a percentage of the maternal dose.[77] A RID <10% is gen-

erally interpreted as an acceptable level. However, this must be interpreted with caution, taking into account other variables such as the age and health of the infant and the safety profile of the drug. It is also important to note that these are estimated values, often based on data collected from one or only a few individuals. Unfortunately, applying these equations using measurements specific to a woman and her infant is not clinically practical. Compared to the M/P ratio, experts believe that the RID is a better estimate of infant exposure.

$$\text{Drug concentration in milk} = \text{Maternal plasma drug concentration} \times \text{M/P} \quad (47\text{-}1)$$

$$\text{Infant dose (mg/kg/day)} = \text{Drug concentration in milk} \times \text{Milk volume (mL/kg/day)} \quad (47\text{-}2)$$

$$\text{RID (\%)} = (\text{Infant dose [mg/kg/day]})/(\text{Maternal dose [mg/kg/day]}) \times 100 \quad (47\text{-}3)$$

Reducing Risk of Exposure

If pharmacologic treatment is medically necessary for a nursing mother, every attempt should be made to minimize infant exposure to the drug. Methods of reducing risks have been proposed.[70,71,78] Table 47-9 summarizes critical factors that should be considered. Except for drugs that are contraindicated during lactation, the decision to continue or discontinue nursing while receiving medication is ultimately the mother's. Therefore, patient education is an integral component in this decision-making process. The mother should be informed of

---

Table 47-9 Reducing Risk of Infant Exposure to Drugs in Breast Milk[70,71,77,78]

A drug should be used only if medically necessary and treatment cannot be delayed until the infant is ready to be weaned.

Drug Selection

Consider whether the drug can be safely given directly to the infant.
Select a drug that passes poorly into breast milk with the lowest predicted M/P ratio, and a RID <10%.
Avoid long-acting formulations (e.g., sustained-release).
Consider possible routes of administration that can reduce drug excretion into milk.
Determine length of therapy and if possible avoid long-term use.

Feeding Pattern

Avoid nursing during times of peak drug concentration.
If possible, plan breast-feeding before administration of the next dose.

Other Considerations

Always observe the infant for unusual signs (e.g., sedation, irritability, rash, decreased appetite, failure to thrive).
Discontinue breast-feeding during the course of therapy if the risks to the fetus outweigh the benefits of nursing.
Provide adequate patient education to increase understanding of risk factors.

the potential risks, or lack thereof, associated with a drug. She also should be made aware that certain risks may be minimized by altering feeding pattern and drug administration time and by carefully monitoring the infant for early signs of adverse effects.

Resources for Drugs and Lactation

Comprehensive sources reviewing drug use in lactation are available to assist clinicians in weighing the potential risks versus benefits of using medications while breast-feeding. The AAP Committee on Drugs reviews periodically the transfer of drugs and other chemicals into human milk and publishes their findings.[79] The committee identifies drugs that should be avoided during breast-feeding, drugs that should be used with caution, drugs whose effects on infants are unknown but of concern, and those considered usually compatible with breast-feeding. This rigorous review is an ongoing process, and new guidelines are published every few years; therefore, the reader should locate the latest AAP recommendations available. In addition to the AAP guidelines, several other references also offer comprehensive information and recommendations on drug use in lactation.[13,74]

Table 47-10 lists drugs that should be avoided during breast-feeding, and Table 47-11 lists some commonly used drugs and drug classes that are either considered compatible

Table 47-10 Drugs Considered Contraindicated During Lactation[a]

Drug/Drug Class	Effects on Nursing Infants
Amphetamine[b]	Accumulate in breast milk and may cause irritability and poor sleep patterns.[13,79]
Antineoplastics	Potential for immune suppression; cytotoxic effects on drugs on dividing cells in infants unknown.[79]
Cocaine[b]	Excreted in milk; contraindicated because of CNS stimulation and intoxication.[13,79,80,81]
Ergotamine	Potential for suppressing lactation; vomiting, diarrhea, and convulsions have been reported.[13] Considered contraindicated by some clinicians. AAP recommends using with caution.[79]
Heroin[b]	Possible addiction if sufficient amounts ingested.[13,79]
Immunosuppressants	Potential for immune suppression.[79]
Lithium	Milk and serum concentrations average 40% of maternal serum levels. Potential for toxicity exists.[13,82] Considered contraindicated by some clinicians. AAP recommends using with caution.[79]
Lysergic acid diethylamide (LSD)[b]	Probably excreted in milk.[13]
Marijuana[b]	Excreted in milk.[13,79]
Misoprostol	Excretion in milk has not been studied but contraindicated because of potential for severe diarrhea in infant.[29]
Phencyclidine[b]	Potent hallucinogenic properties.[13,79]
Phenindione	Massive scrotal hematoma and wound oozing after herniotomy in one infant; contraindicated.[13,79]

Requiring Temporary Cessation of Breast-Feeding

Metronidazole (after single-dose therapy)	Diarrhea and secondary lactose intolerance in one infant; mutagenic and carcinogenic in some species; AAP recommends halting breast-feeding for 12–24 hr to allow clearance of drug from the milk if single-dose therapy administered.[79,82]
Radiopharmaceuticals	Halt breast-feeding temporarily to allow clearance of radioactivity from milk. Suggested times for individual agents are[79]: Copper-64 (^{64}Cu) 50 hr; Gallium-67 (^{67}Ga) 2 wk; Indium-111 (^{111}In) 20 hr; Iodine-123 (^{123}I) 36 hr; Iodine-125 (^{125}I) 12 days; Iodine-131 (^{131}I) 2–14 days; Radioactive Sodium 96 hr; Technetium-99m (^{99m}Tc) 15 hr–3 days; (^{99m}TcO$_4$) (^{99m}Tc macroaggregates) 15 hr–3 days.

[a]This list is not all-inclusive. Selected drugs are listed by drug class and not by individual names.
[b]All drugs of abuse are contraindicated during lactation.
AAP, American Academy of Pediatrics; CNS, central nervous system.

Table 47-11 Effects of Selected Drugs Used During Breast-Feeding on Nursing Infants[a,b]

Drug/Drug Class	Effects on Nursing Infants
Acetaminophen	Maculopapular rash on upper trunk and face of a nursing infant has been reported. Usually compatible with breast-feeding.[79,83]
Acyclovir	M/P ratios from 0.6 to 4.1 have been reported. Absolute infant dose is expected to be small due to low oral bioavailability of drug.[84] Usually compatible with breast-feeding.[79,83]
Alprazolam[c]	Drug withdrawal observed in an infant exposed to drug via breast milk for 9 months.[85]
Amiodarone	Not recommended because of long elimination half-life and high proportion of iodine contained in each dose.[13] AAP recommends using with caution.[79]

Continued

Table 47-11   Effects of Selected Drugs Used During Breast-Feeding on Nursing Infants[a,b]—cont'd

Drug/Drug Class	Effects on Nursing Infants
Aminoglycosides	Potential for disrupting infant's intestinal flora.[70,78]
5-Aminosalicylic acid	AAP recommends using with caution.[79]
Aspartame	Use with caution if infant has phenylketonuria.[13,79]
Aspirin	Metabolic acidosis reported in one case. Potential for platelet dysfunction and rash exists. AAP recommends using with caution.[79]
β-Blockers	Observe exposed infants for signs of β-Blockade (e.g., hypotension, bradycardia). Acebutolol, atenolol, and nadolol are concentrated in milk; β-blockade evidenced by hypotension, bradycardia, cyanosis, hypothermia, or tachycardia observed in infants exposed to acebutolol or atenolol in breast milk.[13,86,87] Metoprolol and propranolol are usually compatible with breast-feeding.[79]
Bismuth subsalicylate	Significant amounts of bismuth in milk not expected because of poor oral absorption; salicylate portion excreted in milk (see Aspirin).[13]
Bromocriptine	Suppresses lactation in mother. Use contraindicated in the postpartum period because of severe and potentially fatal effects. AAP recommends using with caution during breast-feeding.[79]
Brompheniramine	Reports of irritability, excessive crying, and disturbed sleeping patterns.[13]
Bupropion[c]	One case report of bupropion (immediate-release) resulting in an M/P ratio of 2.51 to 8.58. Concentration in infant plasma was low.[88]
Caffeine	Accumulation may occur when mother is moderate to heavy consumer; irritability and poor sleeping habits observed. Compatible in usual amounts.[13,79]
Carbamazepine	No adverse effects reported. Usually compatible with breast-feeding.[79]
Cephalosporins	Potential for disrupting infant's intestinal flora; usually considered compatible.[70,78,79]
Chloramphenicol	Excreted in milk. Potential bone marrow depression exists; AAP recommends using with caution.[13,79]
Chlorpromazine[c]	Drowsiness and lethargy reported. May cause galactorrhea in mother.[89]
Cimetidine	Cimetidine may accumulate in milk. Potential for suppressing gastric acidity and inhibiting drug metabolism. Usually compatible with breast-feeding.[79]
Citalopram[c]	Citalopram and its metabolites are excreted in breast milk. Estimates of RID ranged from 0.2% to 6%.[82,91] No adverse effects observed in children in a small study at 1 year follow-up.[91]
Clemastine	Drowsiness, irritability, refusal to feed, neck stiffness, and high-pitched cry in one infant. AAP recommends using with caution.[13,79,90]
Clindamycin	Grossly bloody stools in an infant whose mother received clindamycin and gentamicin.[13] Usually compatible with breast-feeding.[79]
Codeine	Usually compatible with breast-feeding.[79]
Contraceptive, oral (estrogen+progestin)	Possible ↓ in milk volume and nitrogen/protein content. May shorten duration of lactation, and ↓ infant weight gain. Effects may be dose-dependent.[13,79] Consider waiting at least 6 weeks before starting.[82] Usually compatible with breast-feeding.[79]
Diazepam[c]	Lethargy and weight loss reported. Watch for accumulation in infant.[79]
Digoxin	Excreted in breast milk. Usually compatible with breast-feeding.[79]
Ethanol	Passes freely into milk. High maternal intake may cause, in nursing infants, sedation, diaphoresis, deep sleep, weakness, ↓ in linear growth, and abnormal weight gain. Chronic exposure also may be related to retarded psychomotor developments. ↓ in milk ejection reflex may occur.[13,79,82] AAP considers use compatible, but indicates large amounts is associated with adverse effects in infants.[79]
Famotidine	Potential for suppressing gastric acidity. Accumulates in milk but to lesser degree than cimetidine or ranitidine.[92] Drug has not been reviewed by the AAP.
Fluoxetine[c]	Fluoxetine and its active metabolite, norfluoxetine, are both excreted in breast milk. Symptoms of colic observed.[93]
Fluvoxamine[c]	Excreted in breast milk. RID <1.5% observed in case reports.[82,94]
Ibuprofen	Very low amounts excreted in breast milk. 90–99% protein bound. Usually compatible with breast-feeding.[26,79,95,96]
Lamotrigine	Excreted in breast milk.[13] AAP considers use as cause for concern.[79]
Metformin	Low M/P ratios reported from 0.27 to 0.71. Estimated RIDs ranging from 0.11% to 0.25%.[97] Observe infant for hypoglycemia, gastrointestinal effects, and signs of lactic acidosis.

Table 47-11   Effects of Selected Drugs Used During Breast-Feeding on Nursing Infants[a,b]—cont'd

Drug/Drug Class	Effects on Nursing Infants
Methimazole	May cause thyroid dysfunction (goiter) in nursing infant; small doses (10–15 mg/day) may be safe if thyroid function of infant monitored. Use propylthiouracil if antithyroid agent required; usually compatible with breast-feeding.[13,79]
Metoclopramide	Mild intestinal upset observed. Stimulates milk production in mother. AAP considers use as cause for concern.[13,79,89]
Morphine	Excreted in breast milk. Usually compatible with breast-feeding.[79]
Naproxen	<1% excreted in breast milk. RID <3% estimated. Usually compatible with breast-feeding.[13,79,82]
Nefazodone[c]	Drowsiness, lethargy, poor body temperature control, and poor feeding reported in one infant born prematurely at 27 weeks' gestation.[13,93] Drug has not been reviewed by the AAP.
Nicotine	Absorption via passive smoking is higher than through breast milk. Smoking in general is not recommended while breast-feeding.[78] ↓ milk production.[75]
Nitrofurantoin	Hemolytic anemia in infants with G6PD deficiency possible. Usually compatible with breast-feeding.[13,79]
Nizatidine	Potential for suppressing gastric acidity. Excreted in breast milk in low amounts.[82] Drug has not been reviewed by the AAP.
Paroxetine[c]	Average M/P ratio from 0.39 to 1.11. RID <3%.[93] No adverse effects reported.
Penicillins	Potential for allergic sensitization and disruption of infant's intestinal flora. Usually compatible with breast-feeding.[79,98]
Phenobarbital	Methemoglobinemia and sedation reported; AAP recommends using with caution.[79]
Phenytoin	Methemoglobinemia, drowsiness, and ↓ suckling activity reported. Usually compatible with breast-feeding.[13,79]
Primidone	One active metabolite of primidone is phenobarbital. AAP recommends using with caution.[79]
Propoxyphene	Usually compatible with breast-feeding.[79]
Propylthiouracil (PTU)	Excreted in breast milk. Usually compatible with breast-feeding.[79]
Pseudoephedrine	Excreted in breast milk. Usually compatible with breast-feeding.[79]
Quinolones	Use with caution because of potential for arthropathy in infants.[13] Excretion into breast milk is likely due to good oral bioavailability and low protein binding.[99] Only ciprofloxacin, ofloxacin, and nalidixic acid have been reviewed by the AAP. They are considered usually compatible with breast-feeding.[79] Nalidixic acid may cause hemolysis in infants with G6PD deficiency.
Ranitidine	Potential for suppressing gastric acidity. Concentrated in breast milk.[13] Drug has not been reviewed by the AAP.
Sertraline[c]	Excreted in breast milk.[93] No adverse effects reported.[79]
Sulfasalazine	One case of bloody diarrhea observed.[99] AAP recommends using with caution.[79] (See sulfonamides)
Sulfonamides	Use caution in infants with jaundice, G6PD deficiency, or if premature.[13]
Sulfonylureas, oral	Caution against hypoglycemia in infants.[13]
Topiramate	Excreted in breast milk.[100] Effects on neonate unknown.
Trimethoprim/ sulfamethoxazole	Excreted in breast milk. Usually compatible with breast-feeding.[79] (See sulfonamides)
Tetracyclines	Tetracyclines are not recommended for children <8 years old. Excretion in breast milk is expected to be low.[99] Only tetracycline has been reviewed by the AAP. Usually compatible with breast-feeding.[79] Some experts suggest avoiding long-term exposure.[82]
Thiazide diuretics	May suppress lactation.[13] Most are considered usually compatible with breast-feeding.[79]
Valproic acid	Usually compatible with breast-feeding.[79]
Vancomycin	Excreted in breast milk. Poor systemic absorption by infant. Drug has not been reviewed by the AAP.[79,101]
Venlafaxine[c]	Excreted in breast milk.[82] Drug has not been reviewed by the AAP.
Warfarin	Usually compatible with breast-feeding.[79]

[a]This list is not all-inclusive. Most drugs listed in this table are known to be excreted in breast milk, but effects of drug exposure to the nursing infant may not always be known. Some drugs designated as "usually compatible" may have case reports of adverse effects to infants, but these may be rare or limited only to certain types of patients. Always consider the age and medical status of the infant, and consult the latest guidelines before recommending use. Not all drugs have been reviewed by the AAP.
[b]Selected drugs are listed by drug class and not by individual names.
[c]The AAP considers use of anti-anxiety agents, antidepressants, and neuroleptics during breast-feeding as cause for concern. Long-term neurodevelopmental effects in infants exposed are unknown.
AAP, American Academy of Pediatrics; CNS, central nervous system; G6PD, glucose-6-phosphate-dehydrogenase deficiency; RID, relative infant dose.

or should be used with caution. When available, summaries of the reported adverse effects of drug exposure via breast milk are included. These lists are not all-inclusive and are meant to provide an overview for the reader. Because most drugs are excreted into breast milk to some extent, the reader is referred to specialty sources for an in-depth review of the drug in question. In addition, categories assigned to these drugs may change as new data become available for specific drugs.

THERAPEUTIC DILEMMAS IN PREGNANT AND LACTATING WOMEN

Anticoagulation

Warfarin

FETAL WARFARIN SYNDROME

1. H.P. is a 25-year-old woman with a 5-week intrauterine pregnancy. She had a mitral valve commissurotomy approximately 7 years ago, followed by a mitral valve replacement 2 years ago, both for rheumatic heart disease. Her current medications are warfarin 5 mg/day, penicillin VK 500 mg/day, and digoxin 0.25 mg/day. Do these drugs present a therapeutic problem to the fetus? If so, what changes should be made?

Neither penicillin VK (Pen-Vee K) nor digoxin (Lanoxin) presents a known fetal risk. Both drugs have been used extensively in pregnancy, including the first trimester, without causing an increase in the expected rate of fetal loss or congenital malformations (see Table 47-5). Serum digoxin concentrations should be monitored at frequent intervals because of the increased drug elimination rate that normally occurs during pregnancy.

On the other hand, warfarin (Coumadin) crosses the placenta and is generally considered contraindicated in pregnancy except under specific circumstances.[102] Use of warfarin in the first trimester has been associated with a characteristic pattern of defects collectively known as the fetal warfarin syndrome (FWS).[103] The susceptible period seems to be between weeks 6 and 12 of gestation.[103,104] Nasal hypoplasia and a depressed nasal bridge (Table 47-12, Fig. 47-2) are common to all known cases of FWS. The nares and air passages may be constricted to such a degree that respiratory distress results. As seen roentgenographically, stippling in uncalcified epiphyseal regions occurs in most newborns with FWS but may not be evident after the first year of life.[103] The axial skeleton, proximal femurs, and calcanei are the sites primarily involved in FWS, and this pattern of distribution distinguishes it from other syndromes and genetic disorders.[103] Less common features (see Table 47-12) are reduced birth weight, eye and ear defects, hypoplasia of extremities, development retardation, congenital heart disease, laryngeal calcification, and death.[23,26]

The exact incidence of warfarin-induced anomalies is unknown, but it is estimated to range from 17% to 37%.[13,105] The rate of FWS reported is approximately 3% to 10%.[13,23] Therefore, the use of warfarin in H.P. is controversial. Discontinuation of warfarin should be considered, especially during the critical period between weeks 6 and 12 of gestation. Heparin and more recently low-molecular-weight heparin (LMWH) are the preferred anticoagulants in pregnancy for most indications, including prevention and treatment of deep vein throm-

Table 47-12	Fetal Warfarin Syndrome

Exposure Sixth to Twelfth Weeks

Common Features

Nasal hypoplasia
Depressed bridge of nose
Stippling in uncalcified epiphyseal regions (axial skeleton, proximal femurs, and calcanei)

Less Common Features

Birth weight <10th percentile for gestational age
Developmental retardation
Congenital heart disease
Deafness/hearing loss
Death
Laryngeal calcification
Scoliosis
Seizures
Eye anomalies (blindness, optic atrophy, and microphthalmia)
Hypoplasia of extremities ranging from severe rhizomelic dwarfing to dystrophic nails and shortened fingers

Exposure in Second and Third Trimesters

CNS Anomalies

Dorsal midline dysplasia characterized by agenesis of corpus callosum, Dandy-Walker malformation, and midline cerebellar atrophy; encephaloceles
Ventral midline dysplasia characterized by optic atrophy

Effects of CNS Anomalies

Blindness
Deafness
Death
Growth failure
Hydrocephalus
Mental retardation
Scoliosis
Seizures
Spasticity

Adapted from references 13, 23, 26, 103

bosis.[104] The efficacy of heparin and LMWH in pregnant women with prosthetic heart valves is less clear, although they have a better safety profile for the fetus. If heparin or LMWH is used in H.P., close monitoring for thromboembolic complications is required.[106]

Heparin

2. Heparin therapy (10,000 units SC BID) is initiated, and warfarin is discontinued. What are the fetal and maternal risks of using heparin in H.P.?

Heparin is a large molecule (MW 12,000) and does not cross the placenta. According to the Sixth American College of Chest Physicians (ACCP) Consensus Conference, heparin is one of the preferred anticoagulants during pregnancy for most thromboembolic conditions because of its efficacy and more favorable safety profile compared with warfarin.[104] Although earlier cases reported that the rate of fetal complica-

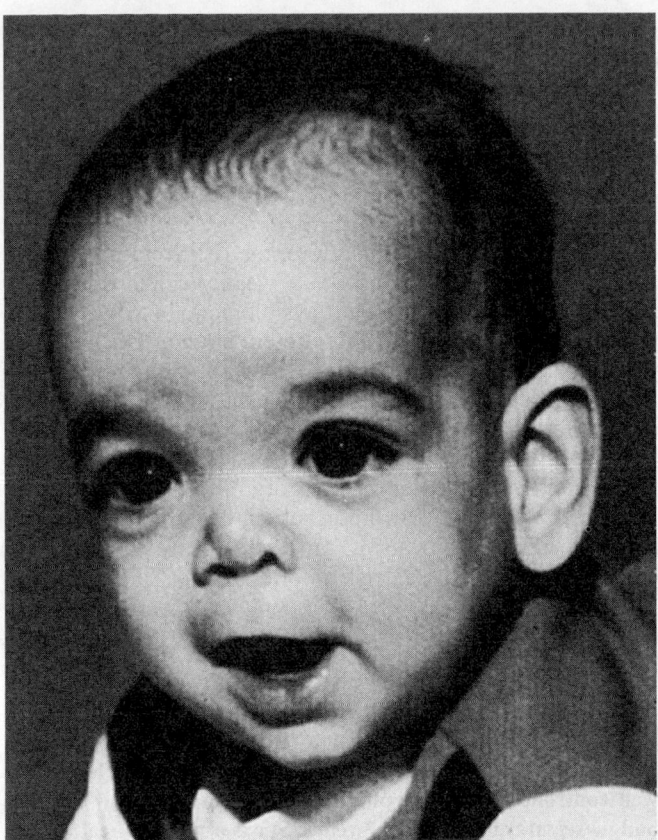

FIGURE 47-2 Fetal warfarin syndrome. Note depressed nasal bridge and nasal hypoplasia. (Photo courtesy of K.L. Jones, MD, UC San Diego.)

tions associated with heparin use may be as high as those reported with warfarin (22% versus 27%, respectively),[103] subsequent evaluations demonstrated that the rate of adverse fetal outcome with heparin therapy is comparable to that reported in the normal population.[23,105] The high incidence of fetal abnormalities reported earlier can be attributed to the use of heparin in pregnancies with comorbid conditions known to increase risks.

In a review of 186 reports that described the outcomes of 1,325 pregnancies associated with anticoagulant therapy, the rate of adverse fetal/infant outcomes for heparin was 2.5% compared with 16.8% with warfarin.[105] This lower incidence rate reflects the exclusion of cases with comorbid conditions (e.g., glomerulonephritis or eclampsia in the pregnant female), which could have accounted for the undesirable effects. The results of a retrospective cohort study of 100 pregnancies in 77 women treated with heparin were similar, with rates of fetal complications comparable to that in normal pregnancies.[107]

Nevertheless, the use of heparin during pregnancy may pose several risks to the mother. The risk of bleeding from heparin during pregnancy is approximately 2%.[104] Heparin-induced thrombocytopenia (HIT) is a well-recognized complication and may require discontinuation of therapy if it is an immune-mediated response. The frequency of HIT during pregnancy is unknown but has been estimated at 3% in non-pregnant patients.[104]

Prolonged administration of heparin (>1 month) increases the risk of developing osteoporosis. Although the occurrence of symptomatic fractures is uncommon (2% to 3%), the development of osteopenia may occur in up to one third of pregnant women on chronic heparin therapy.[108–112] This reduction in bone mineral density (BMD) may be reversible after discontinuation of heparin.[109,111] Heparin-induced osteoporosis may be associated with higher doses of heparin and longer duration of use. In a prospective, cohort study of 184 cases by Dahlman,[110] the incidence of osteoporosis was higher in women who received a mean dose of 25,000 IU/24 hours versus a mean dose of 16,500 IU/24 hours. The average duration of treatment was 25 weeks (range, 7 to 27 weeks). However, a definitive dose–response relationship cannot be confirmed because reductions in BMD have been reported with lower dosages and shorter duration of heparin use. The mechanism behind this effect is thought to be heparin inhibition of the renal activation of calcifediol (25-hydroxyvitamin D_3, a major transport form of vitamin D) to calcitriol, one of the active forms of vitamin D_3.

3. **H.P. presents again at 14 weeks' gestation complaining of mild muscle pain, tingling in the lower left extremity, and mild pleuritic pain. Laboratory workup confirmed an activated partial thromboplastin time (APTT) of 1.5 times control despite an adjusted heparin dosage of 20,000 units SC every 12 hours several weeks ago. H.P. is now in her second trimester. What subjective and objective evidence does H.P. exhibit that indicates a need to change anticoagulant therapy?**

H.P. is at increased risk for valve thrombosis and other thromboembolic complications because heparin is less effective than oral anticoagulants at preventing these complications in pregnant patients with prosthetic heart valves.[104,106,113] Factors that may contribute to this lowered efficacy include inadequate dosing, types of prosthetic heart valves, and position of valve placement.[104,106] Higher doses are generally required due to increases in plasma volume, renal clearance, heparin-binding proteins, and decreased bioavailability of heparin because of degradation by the placenta.[114] The optimal regimen for heparin during pregnancy in patients with prosthetic heart valves is not known. To minimize H.P.'s risk of developing thrombotic complications and osteoporosis, an adjusted-dose regimen with SC heparin Q 12 hours is warranted. The lowest effective heparin dose to achieve a mid-interval APTT at least two times control should be maintained.[104]

H.P.'s symptoms are consistent with thromboembolism. Her low APTT level despite a high dosage of heparin suggests an increased requirement for heparin. Because H.P. already is on high-dose heparin, prolonged administration will significantly increase her risk of osteoporosis. Of special concern is her apparent resistance to heparin therapy. An alternative anticoagulant should be considered to minimize her risk for further thrombotic complications.

Low-Molecular-Weight Heparin

4. **Is LMWH an alternative for H.P.?**

Like heparin, LMWH does not cross the placenta to the fetus. It offers more convenient dosing (once daily) and may be associated with less thrombocytopenia, bleeding, and osteoporosis.[104] Although it is an effective alternative to heparin in general, its role in preventing thromboembolic complications in pregnant women with prosthetic heart valves has not been determined. Preliminary data suggest LMWH does not increase the risk of adverse birth outcomes.[115,116] An optimal dose of LMWH has not been established. If an LMWH is considered for H.P., the Sixth ACCP recommends an adjusted-dose regimen based on weight or to maintain a 4-hour postinjection anti-Xa heparin level of 1.0 U/mL.[104] Since H.P. failed heparin therapy and has early signs of thromboembolic complications, warfarin may be a more effective alternative.[102,113]

Warfarin in the Second and Third Trimesters

5. **A decision is made to restart warfarin. What is the expected fetal risk from second- and third-trimester use of warfarin?**

Avoiding warfarin between weeks 6 and 12 of gestation decreases the risk of FWS. Warfarin exposure after this critical period may increase the risk of CNS anomalies in the fetus (see Table 47-12). These anomalies appear to be a result of abnormal growth arising from an earlier fetal hemorrhage and subsequent scarring.[103] Two distinct patterns of CNS damage may occur: (1) dorsal midline dysplasia, characterized by agenesis of the corpus callosum, Dandy-Walker malformation, midline cerebellar atrophy, and encephaloceles in some; and (2) ventral midline dysplasia, characterized by optic atrophy.[26,103] The effects of CNS defects include mental retardation (ranging from mild to severe), blindness, hydrocephalus, deafness, spasticity, seizures, scoliosis, growth failure, and death.

The incidence of adverse fetal outcome after second- and third-trimester exposure to warfarin varies among studies. A summary of cases through 1983 estimated that approximately 16% (33/208) of exposures had adverse fetal outcomes. CNS and other defects were reported in 5% of exposures, spontaneous abortions in 2%, and stillbirths or neonatal deaths in 9%.[13] The long-term effects of in utero exposure to coumarin derivatives in 274 school-aged children were assessed by Wesseling and colleagues.[117] These *in utero* exposures took place between 1982 and 1990. Compared to controls, more of the children exposed had minor neurologic dysfunction (relative risk [RR] 1.7; 95% confidence interval [CI] 1.0 to 3.0) and IQ scores <80 (RR 4.7; 95% CI 1.0 to 20.8). Fetal complications from warfarin may be dose dependent, as demonstrated in two retrospective studies.[118,119] Cotrufo and colleagues[119] observed that daily warfarin doses >5 mg were associated with more pregnancy complications, including adverse fetal outcomes.

In addition to fetal risks, the risk of bleeding to the mother is increased with warfarin therapy. If warfarin is necessary, it can be continued until the middle of the third trimester, at which time heparin should be restarted until delivery.[104] Approximately 12 hours before delivery, heparin therapy should be stopped to prevent severe maternal hemorrhage during and after delivery. H.P. should be fully informed of the risks to herself and to her fetus if the pregnancy is continued and, if she concurs, warfarin therapy restarted. Because the heparin requirement was significantly increased during H.P.'s previous trial, she should be closely monitored for signs of thromboembolic complications when heparin is restarted in the latter part of her third trimester.

Breast-Feeding

6. **After vaginal delivery, H.P. is restarted on low-dose heparin and then changed to warfarin on day 5. H.P. also is breast-feeding. Does either of these drugs present a risk to the nursing infant?**

Heparin does not cross into breast milk (see Drug Excretion in Human Milk) because of its high molecular weight (approximately 12,000). Therefore, the risk from this anticoagulant is minimal. Warfarin is a weakly acidic drug (pKa 5.05) that is highly ionized at physiologic pH (>99%) in maternal serum.[73] It also is highly protein bound (97%).[26] These pharmacokinetic parameters make warfarin unlikely to transfer into breast milk. Case reports in lactating mothers confirm that warfarin was not detected in breast milk or infant plasma, or that very low amounts were detected in breast milk.[13] The AAP lists warfarin under the category of "usually compatible with breast-feeding."[79] As a precaution, the mother should observe the infant for bruising or other signs of hemorrhage, even though the apparent risk is low.

Antiepileptic Drugs

Phenytoin

7. **L.F. is a 30-year-old woman with epilepsy who is planning to start a family. Her generalized tonic-clonic seizures have been well controlled with oral phenytoin 100 mg QID, and L.F. has had no seizures for the past 3 years. She is otherwise healthy and is not taking any medication besides phenytoin. Should L.F. become pregnant, what are the risks of phenytoin to the fetus?**

Approximately 90% of women with epilepsy who receive antiepileptic drugs (AEDs) have uneventful pregnancies. A few women have an increased risk for fetal abnormalities, with both major and minor malformations reported. There is controversy over whether maternal epilepsy increases the rate of malformations; however, newer studies suggest this increased incidence is most likely due to AED therapy.[120–122] The risk of fetal abnormalities is lowest with monotherapy and is generally considered to be two- to three-fold higher than in the general population.[123] In a prospective study by Holmes and colleagues[122] conducted between 1986 and 1993, congenital malformations occurred more frequently in infants exposed to one AED compared to controls (20.6% versus 8.5%; odds ratio [OR] 2.8; 95% CI 1.1 to 9.7). The rate was even higher for infants exposed to two or more AEDs compared to control (28% versus 8.5%; OR 4.2; 95% CI 1.1 to 5.1). Abnormalities most commonly observed with the use of AEDs are major congenital malformations (e.g., cardiac malformations, cleft lip or palate), microcephaly, hypoplasia of the midface and fingers, and growth retardation.[122,124,125] Preliminary data also proposed that children exposed to AEDs *in utero* may be more likely to have developmental delay, childhood medical problems, and behavior disorders.[126] More studies are needed to confirm these initial findings.

FETAL HYDANTOIN SYNDROME

Phenytoin (Dilantin) can cause a recognizable pattern of malformations collectively known as the fetal hydantoin syndrome (FHS). It is now recognized that this syndrome is not restricted to phenytoin use and can be linked to other AEDs.

Infants of mothers who were treated with AEDs have a 10% to 30% chance of developing some aspects of FHS, but the full-blown syndrome is less common.[127,128,164]

Common features identified with FHS are varying degrees of craniofacial malformations, including lip and palatal changes; limb anomalies such as hypoplasia of nails and distal phalanges; congenital heart disease; and mental and physical growth retardation.[13,127,128] Table 47-13 lists the characteristic defects observed in this syndrome. Figures 47-3 and 47-4 show some of these defects in a newborn.

PROPOSED MECHANISMS OF TERATOGENICITY

A study published in 1990 demonstrated a relationship between levels of activity of the enzyme epoxide hydrolase and the risk of FHS.[127] Toxic oxidative metabolites of phenytoin normally are removed by epoxide hydrolase, which appears to be regulated by a single gene with two allelic forms. The level of enzyme activity was measured using amniocytes obtained through amniocentesis. Fetuses of women with low activity of this enzyme appear to be at an increased risk from phenytoin. If further studies confirm these findings, this would be an example of an interaction between the mother's genetic predisposition and the environment (in this case, a drug). Two other AEDs, phenobarbital and carbamazepine, also are metabolized via this route.

A second proposed mechanism is altered folate concentration by AEDs. Phenytoin, carbamazepine, and barbiturates have been shown to decrease serum folate concentration. Valproic acid also decreases this by interfering with folate metabolism. Decreased folate concentration is correlated with an increased risk of developing NTDs.[121,129,130]

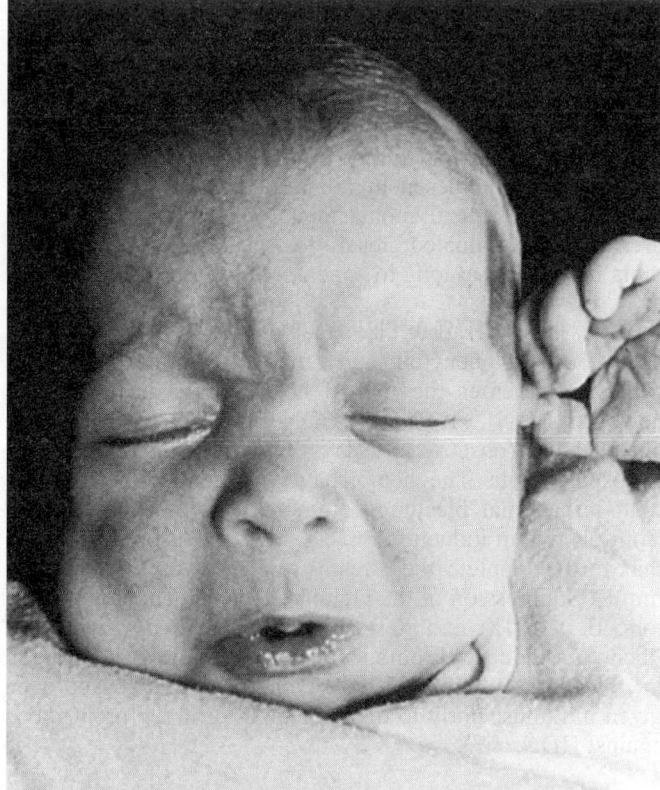

FIGURE 47-3 Fetal hydantoin syndrome. Note broad nasal bridge, short nose, and nail hypoplasia. (Photo courtesy of K.L. Jones, MD, UC San Diego.)

Table 47-13 Fetal Effects of Hydantoins

Fetal Hydantoin Syndrome

Craniofacial	Broad nasal bridge, wide fontanel, low-set hairline, ocular hypertelorism, cleft lip/palate, epicanthal folds, coloboma, broad alveolar ridge, metopic ridging, short neck, microcephaly, abnormal or low-set ears, ptosis of eyelids, coarse scalp hair
Limbs	Small or absent nails, altered palmar crease, dislocated hip, hypoplasia of distal phalanges, digital thumb
Other	Impaired growth (physical and mental), congenital heart defects

Other Birth Defects/Toxicities Associated with Phenytoin

Multiple malformations	Nearly all possible types have been reported
Tumors	Neuroblastoma, ganglioneuroblastoma, melanotic neuroectodermal, extrarenal Wilms' tumor, mesenchymoma, lymphangioma, ependymoblastoma
HDN	Involves various organ systems

HDN, Hemorrhagic disease of the newborn.
Data from reference 13.

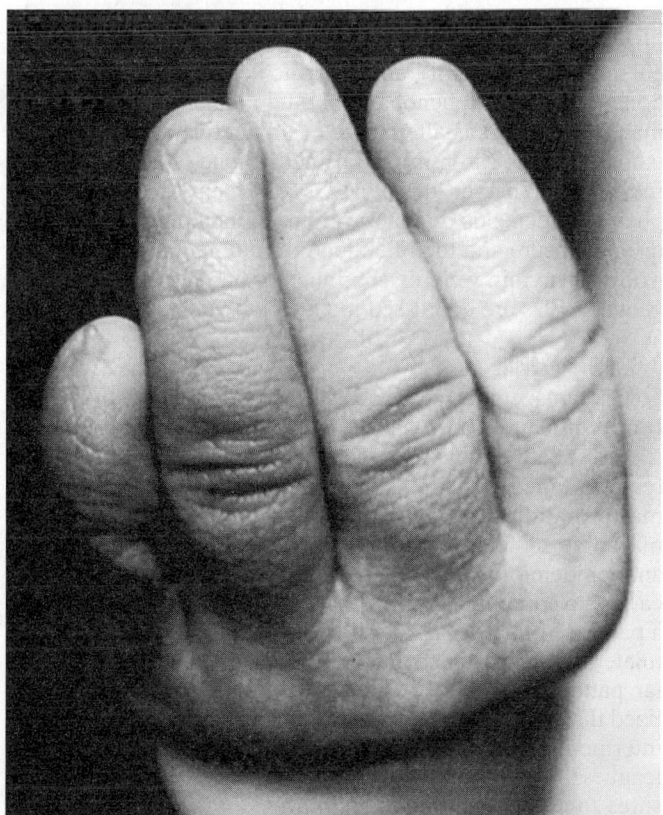

FIGURE 47-4 Fetal hydantoin syndrome. Note nail hypoplasia on far left finger. (Photo courtesy of K.L. Jones, MD, UC San Diego.)

CARCINOGENIC POTENTIAL

Phenytoin may be a human transplacental carcinogen: several tumors have been observed in children exposed to this drug during gestation.[13] The reported tumors are neuroblastoma (five cases), ganglioneuroblastoma (one case), melanotic neuroectodermal tumor (one case), extrarenal Wilms' tumor (one case), mesenchymoma (one case), lymphangioma (one case), and ependymoblastoma (one case). Exposed children must be evaluated closely for several years because tumors may take that long to appear.

HEMORRHAGIC DISEASE OF THE NEWBORN

The use of phenytoin and other AEDs during the third trimester increases the risk of hemorrhagic disease of the newborn (HDN).[13] Both early HDN (onset, 0 to 24 hours) and classic HDN (onset, 2 to 5 days) may occur in gestationally exposed infants. The hemorrhage is often life-threatening, with intracranial bleeding common. It is thought to result from phenytoin induction of fetal liver microsomal enzymes that further deplete the already low reserves of fetal vitamin K. Suppression of the vitamin K–dependent clotting factors, II, VII, IX, and X, results from the hypovitaminosis. Phenytoin-induced thrombocytopenia also may play a role in the bleeding. Vitamin K_1 (phytonadione) 1 mg should be given intramuscularly to the neonate at birth for prophylaxis against HDN.[120,128]

Teratogenicity of Nonhydantoin Antiepileptic Drugs

8. Do other AEDs offer an advantage over phenytoin in pregnancy?

For patients with generalized tonic-clonic seizures, the drugs that offer the most effective therapy are phenytoin, carbamazepine (Tegretol), and valproic acid (Depakene). Primidone (Mysoline), phenobarbital, and clonazepam (Klonopin) may be effective as alternative or adjunctive agents, whereas ethosuximide (Zarontin) and trimethadione (Tridione) are not indicated. Whether these AEDs offer any advantage over phenytoin depends on many variables, including fetal risks to drug exposure and the likelihood of maintaining seizure control if phenytoin were discontinued or another AED initiated. Newer AEDs are addressed in Question 9.

CARBAMAZEPINE

Carbamazepine, an AED structurally related to the tricyclic antidepressants, has been used frequently in pregnancy. It was once thought to be the AED of choice because earlier reviews failed to demonstrate a relationship with congenital malformations.[131,132] Evidence since has linked carbamazepine to fetal abnormalities.[13,23] Numerous case reports and epidemiologic studies have been published involving carbamazepine-induced anomalies. Earlier reports described a pattern of malformations similar to FHS.[133] It has been postulated that carbamazepine and phenytoin may cause a similar pattern of fetal abnormalities because both are metabolized through the arene oxide pathway to produce an oxidative intermediate that is embryotoxic.[133,134] Matalon and colleagues[39] conducted a meta-analysis of 1,255 in utero exposures to carbamazepine that confirmed a 2.89-fold increased risk of major congenital anomalies in exposed children compared to healthy controls. No significant difference in congenital anomalies was observed in untreated epileptic women compared to control. Anomalies reported with carbamazepine include cardiac defects, urinary tract defects, craniofacial defects, cleft palate, fingernail hypoplasia, and low birth weight.[39,133,135] In addition, exposure to carbamazepine in utero carries a 0.5% to 1% risk of developing NTDs, including spina bifida.[130,136] If possible, carbamazepine should be avoided in women with family histories of NTDs.[120]

VALPROIC ACID

In utero exposure to valproic acid is associated with a broad range of major and minor congenital anomalies often referred to as fetal valproate syndrome (FVS).[23,63] Abnormalities may involve craniofacial defects, organ malformations, and growth and developmental defects. In a review of 70 cases of valproic acid exposure, some of the more common features were small/broad nose (57%), small/abnormal ears (46%), long/flat philtrum (43%), and hypertelorism (27%).[63] Use of valproic acid during pregnancy is associated with a 1% to 2% risk of NTDs, ranging from spina bifida to meningomyelocele.[13] Other major adverse fetal effects observed with this drug include craniofacial, cardiac, digital, skeletal and limb, urogenital, skin and muscle, and miscellaneous anomalies.[13] A small observational study of nine infants from mothers who received valproic acid during pregnancy suggests that valproic acid may cause immediate and long-term (evaluated at 6 years of age) neurologic dysfunction in some children.[137] If valproic acid must be used during pregnancy, the total dose should be divided over three or four administrations per day to avoid high plasma concentrations, because NTDs may be dose dependent.[120,128,138] Dosages >1,000 mg/day may be associated with an increased risk of congenital anomalies.[63] Like carbamazepine, valproic acid should be avoided in women with a family history of NTDs.[120] High serum concentration of the free fraction of valproic acid during labor and at birth may be responsible for a fetal/newborn toxicity consisting of fetal distress and low Apgar scores.[139] Because of the high incidence of teratogenicity, valproic acid does not offer any advantage over phenytoin in L.F.

PHENOBARBITAL

Phenobarbital often is used in combination with phenytoin, although it is used much less frequently as a single agent for the treatment of the type of seizures that L.F. has. Although a recognizable pattern of malformations, such as FHS, does not occur in epileptic women treated only with phenobarbital, some of the minor anomalies composing FHS are observed.[13] In three cases, women treated during the first trimester with only primidone, a structural analog of phenobarbital, bore infants with malformations similar to those in FHS. Another pharmacologically related AED is mephobarbital (Mebaral), which is partially demethylated by the liver to phenobarbital. The teratogenic potential of mephobarbital is unknown because there is limited information about its use during pregnancy.[13]

All of these agents may induce maternal folic acid deficiency, a situation similar to that observed with phenytoin. Low folate concentration is linked to NTDs. HND has been reported after phenobarbital or primidone exposure and should be expected after mephobarbital use as well. The mechanism of this effect and its treatment are the same as that described for phenytoin.

In addition, barbiturate withdrawal has been observed in newborns exposed to phenobarbital during gestation. The average onset of symptoms was 6 days (range, 3 to 14 days) after birth, and withdrawal has been reported with daily doses as low as 64 mg.[13] Neonates should be monitored for withdrawal symptoms for 2 to 6 weeks because phenobarbital has a long elimination half-life (100 hours).[121] Recent data also suggest that infants exposed to phenobarbital in utero may experience some decline in cognitive performance.[128] Use of phenobarbital could be considered in L.F.; however, carbamazepine, valproic acid, and phenytoin are the preferred AEDs for tonic-clonic seizures.

ALTERNATIVE ANTIEPILEPTIC DRUGS

Experience with clonazepam as an AED is limited in human pregnancy. One infant exposed *in utero* and delivered prematurely at 36 weeks' gestation developed apnea, cyanosis, lethargy, and hypotonia at 6 hours of age.[140] Although congenital malformations were not evident, the toxic symptoms persisted for several days. Clonazepam usually is given in combination with other AEDs; hence, an increased rate of malformations caused by the agent would be difficult to detect. Thus, too little information is available to recommend this drug.

The fetal effects of ethosuximide are shown in Table 47-7; those of trimethadione are described in Table 47-14. As stated above, neither drug would be effective for L.F.'s seizures.

NEWER ANTIEPILEPTIC DRUGS

9. Several AEDs have been approved in the past few years. Have they been associated with teratogenicity, and do they offer any advantage over phenytoin for L.F.?

Most of the newer AEDs are approved as adjunctive therapy for partial seizures; currently, they are not first-line therapy for generalized tonic-clonic seizures. Their safety in women with epilepsy during pregnancy is yet to be determined because little information is available to assess their teratogenic potential.

Of the newer AEDs, preliminary pregnancy outcomes are available for lamotrigine (Lamictal). The manufacturer of lamotrigine, GlaxoSmithKline, initiated the International Lamotrigine Pregnancy Registry in 1992 to monitor the occurrence of major structural birth defects associated with in utero exposure to lamotrigine. As of September 30, 2001, birth outcomes for 389 pregnancies were prospectively collected and analyzed.[141] Of these, 168 infants were exposed to lamotrigine monotherapy. Three cases (1.8%) of major birth defects (esophageal malformation, cleft soft palate, right clubfoot) were observed. The occurrence of birth defects was higher in women on polytherapy, especially those who received lamotrigine and valproic acid (5/50; 10%). In comparison, the rate of major birth defects for infants exposed to lamotrigine polytherapy without valproic acid was 4.3% (5/116). Lamotrigine is rated pregnancy risk category C and has been found to cross the placenta in one case report.[142]

Other new AEDs available include felbamate (Felbatol), gabapentin (Neurontin), levetiracetam (Keppra), oxcarbazepine (Trileptal), tiagabine (Gabitril), topiramate (Topamax), and zonisamide (Zonegran). The teratogenic risk of these new agents has not been determined. They are rated pregnancy risk category C, and malformations have been reported in animals exposed to these agents.[29] The use of felbamate in any epileptic patient is limited because of the risk of aplastic anemia and acute liver failure. Until more data become available, these new AEDs do not appear to offer any advantage for L.F.

Reducing Fetal Risks

10. If L.F. chooses to become pregnant, what steps should her physician implement to lessen the risks of AED toxicity to her fetus?

Preconception planning with patient education is an extremely important component in epileptic women desiring to bear a child. Achieving good seizure control before conception is imperative. Although no clear consensus on the AED of choice during pregnancy has been reached, discontinuation of the agent should be considered in women who have been free of seizures for at least 2 to 5 years.[128] The dose should be tapered over 1 to 3 months. In patients for whom withdrawal is not an option, monotherapy is preferred, and the lowest effective dose of the appropriate AED should be used.[120,123,128] Because L.F. has had no seizure activity for the past 3 years, her phenytoin should be gradually discontinued before conception. If discontinuation is not an option, a careful reduction of her dose may be possible.

Close monitoring of phenytoin plasma concentrations is required during pregnancy to ensure maintenance of therapeutic levels and to help prevent seizures, which may increase the risk of fetal malformations. Consideration also should be given to changing L.F.'s drug therapy to another AED effec-

Table 47-14	Fetal Trimethadione Syndrome	
Cardiac	Septal defects	Patent ductus arteriosus
Limb	Simian crease, hand defects	Clubfoot
Craniofacial	Low-set, cupped/abnormal ears; high arched or cleft lip and/or palate; macrocephaly; irregular teeth	Epicanthic folds, broad nasal bridge, strabismus, low hairline, facial hemangiomata
Growth/Performance	Prenatal/postnatal deficiency, speech disorder	Mental retardation, myopia, impaired hearing
Genitourinary	Kidney/ureter defects, hypospadias, clitoral hypertrophy	Inguinal hernias, ambiguous genitalia, imperforate anus
Other	Tracheoesophageal fistula	Esophageal atresia

Data from reference 13.

tive for tonic-clonic seizures. Any change to her regimen should be initiated and seizure control achieved before conception is attempted.

SUPPLEMENTAL FOLIC ACID

Folic acid deficiency increases the risk of NTDs such as spina bifida and anencephaly. The Medical Research Council (MRC) Vitamin Study evaluated the protective effects of folic acid in 1,817 pregnant women carrying fetuses at high risk for NTDs.[143] High-dose folic acid (4 mg once daily), given from the date of randomization until 12 weeks of pregnancy, reduced the risk of NTDs by 72%. Women with epilepsy were excluded from this study because of concerns that elevated folate concentrations might interfere with AED therapy. It is now recommended that all women of childbearing age take 0.4 mg folic acid as a daily supplement. Women at high risk of having a child with NTDs should consult with their health care provider and consider supplementing with 4 mg folic acid daily from at least 1 month before conception through the first 3 months of pregnancy.[128,138] Because AEDs can significantly decrease folate concentrations, supplementation with folic acid 4 mg daily in epileptic women may be warranted to decrease the risk of NTDs.

L.F. is at risk of having a child with NTDs because of phenytoin therapy. The addition of folic acid 4 mg daily to her drug regimen should be considered, especially before conception and during the first 3 months of pregnancy.

Phenytoin in Breast Milk

11. If L.F. decides to breast-feed her newborn, would the use of phenytoin be expected to cause any problems?

Phenytoin is readily bioavailable after oral administration, but its high protein binding (95%) hinders its passage into breast milk.[26] The estimated M/P ratio of 0.13 to 0.45 is low.[74] Because an infant may receive about 5% of the maternal dose,[71] the AAP considers maternal use of phenytoin compatible with breast-feeding.[79] L.F. should be counseled on ways to reduce the risk of exposure (see Table 47-9).

Isotretinoin

12. P.J. is a 19-year-old woman with severe, recalcitrant nodular acne that has been treated with isotretinoin. After several months of therapy, P.J. suspects she is pregnant. What is the risk to P.J.'s fetus from isotretinoin exposure in early pregnancy?

Isotretinoin (Accutane), an isomer of vitamin A, was introduced in 1982 as a treatment for severe, recalcitrant nodular acne. The drug is rated pregnancy risk category X and is a known human teratogen.[29] Serious fetal abnormalities, including spontaneous abortion, can occur with any amounts, even for a short duration of use after conception. A recognized pattern of embryopathy is reported with isotretinoin[23,29] that includes defects of the skull, ear (e.g., microtia/anotia), eye (e.g., microphthalmia), face, CNS, thymus, and cardiovascular system. Other adverse outcomes reported include cleft palate, rare limb defects, and low IQ scores.

To prevent unintended pregnancies in women on isotretinoin like P.J., the manufacturer of Accutane established a more stringent prescribing program known as the System to Manage Accutane-Related Teratogenicity (SMART).[29] Both the physi-

cian and patient are required to follow the steps of this program before isotretinoin is prescribed and dispensed. In general, routine pregnancy avoidance counseling, regular pregnancy testing, and use of two forms of effective contraception are required. Pregnancy should be avoided for at least 1 month after stopping therapy. The health care provider should refer to the package insert and contact the manufacturer for details.

Isotretinoin must be discontinued immediately for P.J. She has a significant chance of spontaneously aborting her fetus. Should her pregnancy continue to term, the likelihood of delivering an infant with a major congenital malformation is high. Her health care provider must discuss these risks with P.J. and closely monitor her for adverse fetal outcomes. After this pregnancy, whether P.J. remains a candidate for isotretinoin must be carefully reassessed.

Tretinoin

13. If P.J. had been treated with topical retinoic acid (tretinoin), another vitamin A derivative used for acne vulgaris, would this have placed her fetus at risk?

Tretinoin, like other retinoids, is a potent teratogen when taken systemically. However, topical use is associated with minimal risk because, at most, only about one third of a topical dose is absorbed.[13] Assuming a 1-g/day application of a 0.1% preparation, this would amount to about one seventh of the vitamin A activity received from a typical prenatal vitamin supplement. P.J.'s fetus would not have been at risk from this degree of exposure.

Enalapril and Hydrochlorothiazide

14. A.R. is a 34-year-old woman with severe chronic (essential) hypertension that is well controlled on enalapril 20 mg/day and hydrochlorothiazide (HCTZ) 50 mg/day. She is in the first month of pregnancy. Is either of these agents likely to be harmful to her developing fetus? If so, what changes should be made?

Diuretics such as HCTZ are commonly used to manage hypertension. Although it is unlikely to be teratogenic, available data are insufficient to confirm its safety. Some clinicians are concerned with the theoretical possibility that diuretics could decrease placental perfusion, thereby preventing the normal plasma volume expansion that occurs in pregnancy.[13,61] If necessary, low dosages of HCTZ (e.g., 12.5 or 25 mg daily) should be used as add-on therapy.[61]

Exposure to enalapril or other angiotensin-converting enzyme (ACE) inhibitors in the second or third trimester of pregnancy is associated with a pattern of malformations known as ACE inhibitor fetopathy.[32] The hallmark feature is renal tubular dysplasia. Other anomalies observed include calvarial hypoplasia, oligohydramnios, pulmonary hypoplasia, IUGR, and patent ductus arteriosus (PDA).[31,32] Therefore, ACE inhibitors should be avoided during the second and third trimesters of pregnancy. No association of anomalies with ACE inhibitor use in the first trimester has been shown, but the number of cases available for review is too small to confirm their safety.

Skull Defect

The mechanism of fetal calvarial hypoplasia is thought to be related to the drug-induced oligohydramnios that allows the uterine musculature to exert direct pressure on the top of the head. This mechanical insult, combined with drug-induced fetal hypotension, inhibits peripheral perfusion and ossification of the calvaria.[144]

Renal Defect

A 1990 report described the following kidney abnormalities in a newborn who had been exposed throughout gestation to enalapril 20 mg/day, propranolol 40 mg/day, and HCTZ 50 mg/day: irregular corticomedullary junctions; glomerular maldevelopment with a decreased number of lobulations in many of the glomeruli, and some congested glomeruli; a reduced number of tubules in the upper portion of the medulla with increased mesenchymal tissue; and tubular distention in the cortex and medulla.[33] Because renal anomalies had not been reported previously, either with diuretics or β-blockers, the investigators concluded that the defects were either a result of reduced renal blood flow secondary to enalapril, or a direct teratogenic effect of the drug.

Other Toxicity

Fetal and neonatal renal failure have been reported frequently following *in utero* exposure to ACE inhibitors.[13] Fetal renal toxicity is characterized by oligohydramnios, with the resulting risk of pulmonary hypoplasia and fetal skull defects (see Skull Defects). Newborn infants may present with anuria and severe hypotension that is resistant to volume expansion and pressor agents. Dialysis may be required but may not produce a return to normal renal function. Fetal kidney failure is thought to be a result of enalapril blocking the formation of angiotensin II. During gestation, fetal renal blood flow and perfusion pressures are low.[145] High concentrations of angiotensin II may be physiologically necessary to maintain fetal renal blood flow and low perfusion pressures.

The risk associated with the continued use of enalapril and hydrochlorothiazide cannot be justified in A.R. because more appropriate alternatives are available. Other antihypertensives that could be considered include methyldopa, hydralazine, and labetalol, because more experience has been gained with these agents.

Indomethacin

Premature Labor

15. J.B. is 30 weeks pregnant when premature labor is diagnosed. Intravenous (IV) magnesium sulfate is administered to stop her uterine contractions and progressive cervical changes. Several attempts to wean her from the IV therapy onto oral terbutaline have failed. Indomethacin, 50 mg one time, then 25 mg Q 6 hr, is started as the magnesium is tapered again. No contractions or cervical changes are noted on this therapy, and the IV magnesium is discontinued. What are the risks to the fetus from indomethacin?

The use of indomethacin for tocolysis has become more common in obstetrics as experience is gained with the therapy. Its usefulness is limited by serious complications such as necrotizing enterocolitis, intracranial hemorrhage, oligohydramnios, and immature closure of the ductus arteriosus.[47,146–148] Of these, the most common fetal complication is ductal constriction, accompanied by tricuspid regurgitation in

some cases.[47,146,147] Fetal echocardiography revealed that ductal closure associated with indomethacin use occurs more frequently in fetuses at 31 weeks' gestation or later, although narrowing can occur within hours of the first dose and may not always correlate with either gestational age or maternal indomethacin serum levels.[47,146–148] Tricuspid regurgitation is likely a result of the increased pressure in the right ventricular outflow tract caused by ductal constriction; mild endocardial ischemia with papillary muscle dysfunction can result. In most cases, ductal closure is reversible within 24 to 40 hours of prompt discontinuation of indomethacin. Exposed infants also can have lower urine output and higher serum creatinine concentrations during the first 3 days of life.[148] In most cases, however, short-term therapy (24 to 48 hours) has not been associated with toxicity in the newborn if allowance is made for at least 24 hours or more between the last dose and delivery. If indomethacin is required, use should be restricted to gestational ages <32 weeks, and fetal echocardiography should be conducted to closely monitor for complications.

Polyhydramnios

16. M.M. is in 26 weeks pregnant when polyhydramnios and premature uterine contractions are diagnosed. How might the use of indomethacin in M.M. differ from that in J.B.?

One of the effects of indomethacin on the fetus is reduced renal output. In most cases, this drug effect would be considered detrimental to the fetus. In M.M., however, reduced fetal urine output is therapeutic because fetal urine is the major component of amniotic fluid. Decompression (i.e., mechanical removal of excess amniotic fluid) can be attempted, but often the condition quickly recurs. In a limited number of published and unpublished cases, long-term therapy (2 to 11 weeks) with indomethacin has resolved the condition without producing fetal or newborn toxicity.[13] Fetal echocardiography has been used in conjunction with the therapy to ensure that the ductus arteriosus remains patent.

Interaction With β-Blockers

17. T.V., a patient similar to M.M., also was being treated with atenolol for hypertension. How will β-blocker therapy change planned therapy with indomethacin?

An interaction between indomethacin and β-blockers resulted in severe maternal hypertension in two women.[149] In both cases, a marked rise in blood pressure to 240/140 mm Hg in the woman treated with propranolol and to 230/130 mm Hg in the patient treated with pindolol occurred on days 4 and 5 of combined treatment, respectively. The mechanism of the interaction is unknown, but one reference source has described several other cases of this interaction.[150] Because fetal distress occurred in both of these cases, presumably because of reduced placental blood flow, long-term therapy with indomethacin should not be attempted in patients receiving β-blockers.

The appropriateness of chronic use of atenolol in T.V. also should be re-evaluated. Data available so far do not link atenolol to congenital malformations, but information is too limited to exclude risk. Atenolol has been shown to cause IUGR and bradycardia in the neonate.[23,61] Should atenolol be continued in T.V., her fetus should be closely monitored during pregnancy and early postpartum for adverse effects.

β-Blockers and Breast-Feeding

18. **B.B., a 38-year-old woman, developed hypertension in the postpartum period and is being treated with atenolol. She is nursing her infant and has noticed that the baby has become "sluggish" over the past few days. A thorough examination of the infant revealed no significant medical problems except for mild bradycardia and lethargy, which is concerning in an otherwise healthy infant. Because the symptoms are consistent with β-blockade, is atenolol compatible with breast-feeding, and should an alternative agent be considered?**

Atenolol (Tenormin) has an estimated M/P ratio of 1.1 to 6.8 and thus has the potential to accumulate at higher concentrations in milk than in maternal plasma.[74] Based on a dosage of 100 mg/day in a 65-kg mother, calculated RIDs ranged from 6.6% to 19%.[75] This is not unexpected because atenolol is a weak base that is highly water soluble, has low protein binding (5% to 15%), and is renally excreted. Newborns are more likely to be sensitive to drugs eliminated renally because of their immature renal function.[151,152] At least one case report of atenolol use resulting in β-blockade that required discontinuation of breast-feeding has been reported.[26]

Adverse effects also have been reported with another β-blocker, acebutolol (Sectral). Acebutolol and its metabolite, N-acetylacebutolol, have high M/P ratios of 7.1 and 12.2, respectively; they can be expected to accumulate in milk to a greater extent than atenolol. Adverse reactions reported with acebutolol include hypotension, bradycardia, and transient tachypnea.[13] Both atenolol and acebutolol should be avoided in B.B. and an alternative β-blocker should be considered.

All β-blockers are distributed into breast milk to some extent. Some experts recommend avoiding the use of β-blockers that are water soluble and have low protein binding during lactation.[151,152] Metoprolol (Lopressor) and propranolol (Inderal) appear to be more compatible with breast-feeding.[71,151] The amount of metoprolol excreted in breast milk is small compared with other β-blockers. Propranolol is highly protein bound (>90%) and has a low M/P ratio of 0.5 to 0.64.[74] Accumulation in milk is low, and no adverse effects have been reported with its use. The AAP considers metoprolol and propranolol compatible with breast-feeding.[79]

Therefore, metoprolol and propranolol are safer alternatives for B.B. and may allow her to continue breast-feeding. However, because drug excretion into breast milk is possible, the infant should be monitored for signs of adverse effects such as hypotension, bradycardia, respiratory depression, and changes in blood glucose.

Methylene Blue

19. **Methylene blue has been ordered for B.D., a woman at 35 weeks' gestation. The dye is to be injected into the amniotic fluid to assist in the diagnosis of premature rupture of the membranes. Is the use of methylene blue associated with increased fetal risks?**

The dark-blue dye methylene blue has been injected intra-amniotically to help visualize the leakage of amniotic fluid into the vagina, an indication of rupture of the membranes. This use has been associated with hemolytic anemia, hyperbilirubinemia, respiratory distress, and methemoglo-

binemia in the newborn.[53] Moreover, if delivery occurs shortly after injection, the newborn will be stained a deep blue, which impairs clinical assessment of hypoxia.[153] The staining is reversible but may require several weeks to dissipate. Use of methylene blue in the second trimester by injection into one of the amniotic sacs of twin pregnancies has been associated with multiple ileal occlusions and jejunal atresia.[154–156] If a dye is necessary to help diagnose premature rupture of the membranes, a dye known as indigo carmine has been used successfully with few reported adverse effects.[53] Use of methylene blue in amniocentesis during the second trimester to distinguish the sacs of twins is not recommended. Methods that do not require the use of dye arc preferred.

Herbal Supplements

Herbs in Pregnancy

20. **T.H., a 28-year-old woman, is in general good health except for complaints of feeling chronically tired. Physical examination and complete blood work were unremarkable. Four months ago, T.H. read an advertisement promoting an herbal tea for its "tonic" properties, which help boost energy and improve overall well-being. She purchased this product and has been drinking one cup every morning before work. T.H. and her husband are planning to start a family. If T.H. continues to drink this tea during pregnancy, what are the risks to the fetus? According to the product label, this tea contains primarily echinacea, garlic, guarana, and ginseng. Other ingredients in subtherapeutic amounts include various vitamins and minerals.**

To assist T.H. in evaluating the safety of this herbal tea, she must first be informed of the status of dietary supplements in the United States. Products containing herbs, vitamins, minerals, or amino acids are referred to as *dietary supplements* in the United States. Although often used by consumers hoping to improve their health or treat minor ailments and diseases, these products are not considered drugs. Many of these products are promoted as "natural" supplements, and the public often equates "natural" with "safe." As awareness of these products increases, it has become clear that not all "natural" products are safe. Except for selected herbs, most information available is derived from in vitro and animal studies, case reports, small clinical trials, anecdotal experiences, or historical records. The lack of stringent regulations overseeing dietary supplements raises the issue of questionable product quality and purity of ingredients. (See Chapter 3, Herbs and Nutritional Supplements.)

Compared with studies on FDA-approved drugs, reports on herbs are more challenging to review. Many variables limit the interpretation of data and subsequent extrapolation to other scenarios. Examples of factors that complicate the evaluation of herbs include the following: (1) use of the common name (e.g., garlic) without listing the scientific name (*Allium sativum*); (2) no description of preparation method or the dose ingested; (3) plant misidentification; and (4) product contamination by other ingredients. When this information is missing, one is cautioned against overgeneralizing efficacy and safety data. In T.H.'s case, information can be found for the herbs in question, but because the scientific names are not available, caution should be used when evaluating the data.

ECHINACEA

Echinacea is an herb commonly promoted as an immuno-stimulant.[157] The German Commission E, an authoritative body in Germany that critically reviews the efficacy and safety of herbs, has categorized echinacea (*Echinacea pallida, Echinacea purpurea*) as an "approved" herb for use.[158] The proposed mechanisms include increases in white blood cells and enhanced phagocytic activity.[157,159] In a prospective follow-up study of 206 pregnant women exposed to echinacea for 5 to 7 days in the first trimester, the rates of malformations were similar between the echinacea and control groups.[160] The species most commonly used in this study were *E. angustifolia* and *E. purpurea*. These results are preliminary and involved women who elected to contact a teratogen information center for information on echinacea. Echinacea is generally well tolerated, although allergic reactions and gastrointestinal symptoms have been reported.[161]

GARLIC

Garlic is among the most popularly used herbs today, not only for cooking but also for its lipid-lowering effects and antimicrobial properties. Garlic (*Allium sativum*) is in the "approved" category according to the German Commission E.[158] Garlic appears to be a relatively safe herb in amounts typically used in cooking, but individuals at increased risk for bleeding should avoid garlic or use it with caution because it can inhibit platelet aggregation.[157] The clinical significance of this inhibition is unknown. Other side effects reported include gastrointestinal irritation from ingestion of raw garlic. Information on using garlic during pregnancy is limited, but it has been postulated that excess consumption may cause menstruation or uterine contractions.[161]

GUARANA

Guarana is an herb commonly found in dietary supplements for weight loss or for "boosting energy." The main constituent is caffeine (approximately 3% to 7%).[193,195] Other compounds identified include theophylline and theobromine.[159] Preliminary data suggest that it may inhibit platelets, although the mechanism is unknown. Because the amount of caffeine in guarana is twice that in coffee beans, this herb is expected to cause caffeine-like side effects. At least one source suggests that pregnant women should avoid guarana because of the high caffeine content, or should not exceed 300 mg/day of caffeine.[159] Guarana has not been addressed by the German Commission E.

GINSENG

Ginseng has been used for centuries as a tonic or adaptogen, an agent "that increases resistance to physical, chemical, and biological stress and builds up general vitality, including the physical and mental capacity for work."[163] Ginseng is currently promoted to help increase resistance to stress. Adverse effects have been reported with ginseng. Most of this information is difficult to interpret and extrapolate because in many cases, the genus and/or species of ginseng was not identified. The common name "ginseng" is used loosely to refer to Asian/Korean ginseng and Siberian ginseng, even though they belong to two different genera and possess different properties.

The safety of ginseng in pregnancy is not known. Reports of ginseng causing estrogen-like side effects have been rare, although the validity has been questioned.[164–166] The most publicized effect is ginseng abuse syndrome, consisting of diarrhea, skin eruptions, nervousness, sleeplessness, and hypertension.[167] The causal relationship of this syndrome with ginseng is questionable. There is a single published case report of ginseng use in a 30-year-old mother during her entire pregnancy.[168] She delivered a term male infant with signs of androgenization (excess hair growth over the entire forehead and in the pubic area). The ginseng reported in this case was Siberian ginseng according to the product label; however, a subsequent chemical analysis suggested that the culprit was not ginseng, but another herb misidentified for ginseng.[169] This case demonstrates the inherent difficulties in reviewing herb-induced side effects. Ginseng root (*Panax ginseng*) is recognized by the German Commission E as an approved herb.[158]

Teratogenicity associated with the use of these herbs has not been reported, but their true teratogenic potential is unknown. The absence of published case reports does not necessarily imply safety. Because of lack of information, the use of this herbal tea by T.H. during pregnancy cannot be recommended. Although the ingredients appear to be safe and their use is not absolutely contraindicated during pregnancy, T.H. should be informed of the data available to date and carefully weigh the benefits and risks of continuing this product.

Herbs and Lactation

21. **T.H. decided to stop taking this herbal tea until after her pregnancy. She gave birth to a healthy baby girl and started breast-feeding. She returned to work 2 months after delivery and her tiredness returned. She would like to restart the herbal tea because it worked well for her before. Are there any risks to the infant if T.H. decides to take this herbal tea while breast-feeding?**

In general, safety data concerning the use of most herbs during lactation are lacking. Unlike approved drugs, it is difficult to predict the excretion of herbs into breast milk because their pharmacokinetic parameters are usually unknown. Experts in the field have tried to identify those herbs that should be avoided or used with caution and only under the supervision of a qualified health care provider (Table 47-15).[158,162] This list is not comprehensive and may change as new data become available.

The use of this herbal tea cannot be recommended if T.H. continues to nurse her child. If T.H. insists on restarting this product while breast-feeding, she needs to be well informed of the risks. It has been recommended that garlic be used with caution during breast-feeding,[162] and guarana's high caffeine content makes it undesirable during lactation. There have been rare reports of toxicity and one death associated with the use of ginseng in newborns, although the validity of these reports is questionable because the source and purity of ginseng were unknown.[162] No data on echinacea use during lactation are available. If T.H. decides to use this product despite recommendations against doing so, she should watch her child for signs of caffeine excess (e.g., difficulty sleeping) and for any unusual symptoms or behavior. Because T.H.'s fatigue may be work-related, she should seek counseling and use relaxation techniques before restarting the herbal tea.

Table 47-15 Selected Herbs That Should Be Avoided or Used with Caution During Lactation[a,b]

Common Name	Scientific Name(s)[c]
Aloe	*Aloe barbadensis; A. capensis*
Black cohosh	*Cimicifuga racemosa*
Bladderwrack	*Fucus vesiculosis*
Borage	*Borago officinalis*
Bugleweed	*Lycopus americanus; L. europaeus; L. virginicus*
Buckthorn bark	*Rhamnus catharticus*
Cascara sagrada	*Rhamnus purshiana*
Coltsfoot	*Tussilago farfara*
Comfrey	*Symphytum officinale*
Ephedra	*Ephedra gerardiana; E. equisetina; E. sinica*
Garlic	*Allium sativum*
Guarana	*Paullinia cupana*
Kava Kava	*Piper methysticum*
Rhubarb	*Rheum palmatum; R. officinale; R. tanguticum*
Senna	*Senna alexandrina; S. obtusifolia*
Uva Ursi	*Arctostaphylos uva ursi*
Wormwood	*Artemisia absinthium*

[a]This list is not all-inclusive
[b]If indicated, use of these herbs should only be under the supervision of a qualified health care provider with expertise in medicinal plants.
[c]Most common names refer to numerous species within one genus.
Selected scientific names are included and may not be inclusive of all species.
Data from references 158 and 162.

GLOSSARY

Adactyly: A developmental anomaly characterized by the absence of digits on the hand or foot

Alopecia: Baldness; absence of hair from skin areas where it normally is present

Amelia: Congenital absence of a limb or limbs

Anencephaly: Congenital absence of the cranial vault, with cerebral hemispheres completely missing or reduced to small masses attached to the base of the skull

Aneuploidy: Any deviation from an exact multiple of the haploid number of chromosomes, whether few or more; individuals exhibiting aneuploidy are usually abnormal physiologically and morphologically.

Angioma: A tumor whose cells tend to form in blood or lymph vessels

Aplasia cutis: Localized failure of development of skin, most commonly of the scalp, less frequently of the trunk and limbs; the defects are usually covered by a thin translucent membrane or scar tissue, or may be raw, ulcerated, or covered by granulation tissue.

Arthrogryposis: Persistent flexure or contracture of a joint

Bifid xiphoid: Cleft of the xiphoid process into two parts

Blastula: The usually spherical structure produced by cleavage of a fertilized ovum, consisting of a single layer of cells (blastoderm) surrounding a fluid-filled cavity (blastocele)

Blepharophimosis: Abnormal narrowness of the palpebral fissure in the horizontal direction, caused by lateral displacement of the inner canthi

Brachycephaly: Disorder in which the head is short, with a cephalic index of 81.0 to 85.4

Calvaria hypoplasia: Failure of the dome-like superior portion of the cranium to form

Choanal atresia: Congenital bony or membranous occlusion of one or both choanae caused by failure of the embryonic bucconasal membrane to rupture

Coloboma: An apparent absence or defect of some ocular tissue, usually resulting from a failure of a part of the fetal fissure to close

Chorioretinitis: Inflammation of the choroid and retina

Coronal: Pertaining to the crown of the head

Corpus callosum: An arched mass of white matter found in the depths of the longitudinal fissure, composed of transverse fibers connecting the cerebral hemispheres

Cryptorchidism: A developmental defect characterized by failure of the testes to descend into the scrotum

Cutis laxa: A congenital hereditary disorder in which the skin and subcutaneous tissues hypertrophy, the skin hanging in folds as a result

Dandy-Walker malformation: Congenital hydrocephalus caused by obstruction of the foramina of Magendie and Luschka

Dermatoglyphics: Study of the patterns of ridges of the skin of the fingers, palms, toes, and soles; may be a clinical and genetic indicator, particularly of chromosomal abnormalities

Diastasis recti: Separation of the rectus muscles of the abdominal wall

Diplegia: Paralysis affecting like parts on both sides of the body; bilateral paralysis

Ebstein's anomaly: A malfunction of the tricuspid valve, the septal and posterior leaflets being attached to the wall of the right ventricle to a varying degree, and the anterior leaflet being normally attached to the annulus fibrosis

Ectromelia: Gross hypoplasia or aplasia of one or more long bones of one or more limbs; the term includes amelia, hemimelia, and phocomelia.

Encephalocele: Hernia of the brain, manifested by protrusion of brain substance through a congenital or traumatic opening of the skull

Epicanthal folds: See Epicanthus.

Epicanthus: A vertical fold of skin on either side of the nose, sometimes covering the inner canthus; it is present as a normal characteristic in persons of certain races and sometimes occurs as a congenital anomaly in others.

Epididymal cyst: A cyst of the elongated cord-like structure along the posterior border of the testis, in the ducts of which the spermatozoa are stored

Epispadias: A congenital defect in which the urethra opens on the dorsum of the penis.

Exencephaly: A developmental anomaly characterized by an imperfect cranium, the brain lying outside of the skull

Hamartoblastoma: A tumor developing from a hamartoma

Hamartoma: A benign tumor-like nodule composed of an overgrowth of mature cells and tissues that normally occur in the affected part, but often with one element predominating

Hemangioma: A benign tumor made up of newly formed blood vessels

Hydrocele: A collection of fluid in the tunica vaginalis of the testicle or along the spermatic cord

Hydrocephalus: A condition characterized by abnormal accumulation of fluid in the cranial vault, accompanied by enlargement of the head, prominence of the forehead, atrophy of the brain, mental deterioration, and convulsions

Hydronephrosis: Distention of the pelvis and calices of the kidney with urine as a result of obstruction of the ureter, with accompanying atrophy of the parenchyma of the organ

Hydrops fetalis: Abnormal accumulation of serous fluid in the entire body of the newborn

Hydroureter: Abnormal distention of the ureter with urine or with a watery fluid

Hypertrichosis lanuginosa: Excessive growth of hair on the body of the fetus

Hypognathia: Having a protruding lower jaw

Hypospadias: A developmental anomaly in the male in which the urethra opens on the underside of the penis or on the perineum

Imperforate anus: Abnormally closed anus

Klippel-Feil anomaly: A condition characterized by shortness of the neck resulting from reduction in the number of cervical vertebrae or the fusion of multiple hemivertebrae into one osseous mass; the hairline is low and motion of the neck is limited.

Macrosomia: Greatly increased body size

Meckel's diverticulum: An abnormal appendage of the ileum derived from an unobliterated yolk stalk

Megacolon: Abnormally large or dilated colon

Meningoencephalocele: Hernial protrusion of the meninges and brain substance through a defect in the skull

Meningomyelocele: Hernial protrusion of a part of the meninges and substance of the spinal cord through a defect in the vertebral column

Microcephaly: Abnormal smallness of the head, usually associated with mental retardation

Micrognathia: Unusual smallness of the jaws

Microphallus: Abnormal smallness of the penis

Microphthalmia: Abnormal smallness of the eyes

Microtia: Gross hypoplasia or aplasia of the pinna of the ear, with a blind or absent external auditory meatus

Müllerian duct: Ductus paramesonephricus; either of the paired embryonic ducts arising as a peritoneal pocket, extending caudally to join the urogenital sinus, and developing into uterine tubes and uterus

Myelomeningocele: Hernial protrusion of the spinal cord and its meninges through a defect in the vertebral canal

Myeloschisis: A developmental anomaly characterized by a cleft spinal cord, owing to failure of the neural plate to form a complete tube

Myoclonia: Any disorder characterized by myoclonus

Myoclonus: Shock-like contractions of a muscle

Myotomes: The muscle plate or portion of a somite that develops into voluntary muscle

Neuropore: The open anterior end or the posterior end of the neural tube of the early embryo; openings gradually close as the tube develops.

Nevus: A circumscribed stable malformation of the skin and occasionally of the oral mucosa that is not due to external causes; excess (or deficient) tissue may involve epidermal, connective tissue, adnexal, nervous, or vascular elements.

Ocular hypertelorism: Abnormal increase in the interorbital distance.

Oligodactyly: A developmental anomaly characterized by a smaller-than-usual number of fingers or toes

Oligohydramnios: Characterized by <300 mL of amniotic fluid at term

Omphalocele: Protrusion, at birth, of part of the intestine through a large defect in the abdominal wall at the umbilicus, the protruding bowel being covered only by a thin transparent membrane composed of amnion and peritoneum

Oxycephaly: A condition in which the top of the head is pointed

Palpebral fissures: The longitudinal opening between the eyelids

Pectus carinatum: Undue prominence of the sternum; also called chicken or pigeon breast

Pectus excavatum: Undue depression of the sternum; also called funnel breast or chest

Philtrum: The vertical groove in the median portion of the upper lip, a part of the prolabium

Phimosis: Tightness of the foreskin so that it cannot be drawn back from over the glans; also the analogous condition in the clitoris

Phocomelia: A developmental anomaly characterized by absence of the proximal portion of a limb or limbs, the hands or feet being attached to the trunk of the body by a single small, irregularly shaped bone

Pierre Robin syndrome: Micrognathia in association with cleft palate and glossoptosis, and with absent gag reflex

Placode: A plate-like structure, especially a thickened plate of ectoderm in the early embryo, from which a sense organ develops

Polydactyly: A developmental anomaly characterized by supernumerary digits (fingers or toes) on the hands or feet

Polyhydramnios: An excess of amniotic fluid; also called hydramnios

Potter facies: A facial condition resembling that seen in Potter syndrome (oligohydramnios caused by renal agenesis) and caused by a lack of amniotic fluid and resulting fetal compression

Prognathia: Having projecting jaws

Rathke's pouch: A diverticulum from the embryonic buccal cavity, from which the anterior lobe of the pituitary gland is developed

Retrognathia: Position of the jaws back of the frontal plane of the forehead

Rhizomelic dwarfing: A dwarfing pertaining to or involving the hip joint and shoulder joint

Sacculus: The smaller of the two divisions of the membranous labyrinth of the vestibule, which communicates with the cochlear duct by way of the ductus reuniens

Scoliosis: An appreciable lateral deviation in the normally straight vertical line of the spine

Simian crease: A single transverse palmar crease formed by fusion of the proximal and distal palmar creases

Somite: One of the paired, block-like masses of mesoderm, arranged segmentally alongside the neural tube of the embryo, forming the vertebral column and segmented musculature

Spina bifida: A developmental anomaly characterized by defective closure of the bony encasement of the spinal cord through which the cord and meninges may or may not protrude

Syndactyly: The most common congenital anomaly of the hand, marked by persistence of the webbing between adjacent digits, so they are more or less completely attached

Synostosis: A union between adjacent bones or parts of a single bone formed by osseous material, such as ossified connecting cartilage or fibrous tissue

Talipes: A congenital deformity of the foot, which is twisted out of shape or position; also called clubfoot

Talipes equinovarus: A deformity of the foot in which the heel is turned inward from the midline of the leg and the foot is plantar-flexed

Tetralogy of Fallot: A combination of congenital cardiac defects consisting of pulmonary stenosis, interventricular septal defect, dextroposition of the aorta so that it overrides the interventricular septum and receives venous and arterial blood, and right ventricular hypertrophy

Utriculus: The larger of the two divisions of the membranous labyrinth, located in the posterosuperior region of the vestibule; the major organ of the vestibular system

Varicocele: A varicose condition of the veins of the pampiniform plexus, forming a swelling that feels like a "bag of worms," appearing bluish through the skin of the scrotum, and accompanied by a constant pulling, dragging, or dull pain in the scrotum

Vermilion border: The exposed red portion of the upper or lower lip

Wolffian duct: Ductus mesonephricus; mesonephric duct, an embryonic duct initiated in association with rudiments of the pronephric kidney, taken over as excretory duct by the mesonephros, developed into various ducts of the reproductive system in the male and into vestigial structures in the female

Acknowledgment
The author acknowledges Gerald G. Briggs, B.Pharm., for his contributions to this chapter in earlier editions.

REFERENCES

1. Mathews TJ et al. Infant mortality statistics from the 1999 period linked birth/infant death data set. National Vital Statistics Reports, vol. 50, no. 4. Hyattsville, MD: National Center for Health Statistics, 2002.
2. Economic costs of birth defects and cerebral palsy—United States, 1992. MMWR 1995;44:694.
3. Schardein JL. Chemically Induced Birth Defects, 3rd ed. New York: Marcel Dekker, Inc., 2000.
4. Kalter H, Warkany J. Congenital malformations. Etiologic factors and their role in prevention. Part I. N Engl J Med 1983;308:424.
5. O'Rahilly R, Muller F, eds. Human Embryology & Teratology, 3rd ed. New York: Weily-Liss, 2001.
6. National Research Council. Scientific Frontiers in Developmental Toxicology and Risk Assessment. Washington, DC: National Academy Press, 2000.
7. Thelander HE. Interference with organogenesis and fetal development. Tex Rep Biol Med 1973;31:4.
8. Stevenson AC et al. Congenital malformations. A report of a study of series of consecutive births in 24 centres. WHO Bull 1966;34(Suppl):9.
9. Martin JA et al. Births: final data for 2000. National Vital Statistics Reports, vol. 50, no. 5. Hyattsville, MD: National Center for Health Statistics, 2000.
10. Collaborative Group on Drug Use in Pregnancy. Medication during pregnancy: an intercontinental cooperative study. Int J Gynecol Obstet 1992;39:185.
11. Nishimura H, Tanimura T. Clinical Aspects of the Teratogenicity of Drugs. New York: American Elsevier, 1976.
12. Polin RA, Fox WW, eds. Fetal and Neonatal Physiology, 2nd ed. Philadelphia: WB Saunders, 1998.
13. Briggs GG et al. Drugs in Pregnancy and Lactation. A Reference Guide to Fetal and Neonatal Risk, 6th ed. Philadelphia: Lippincott Williams & Wilkins, 2002.
14. Shepard TH. Teratogenicity of therapeutic agents. Curr Prob Pediatr 1979;10(2):1.
15. Fabro S et al. Chemical exposure of embryos during the preimplantation stages of pregnancy: mortality rate and intrauterine development. Am J Obstet Gynecol 1984;148:929.
16. Shepard TH. Catalog of Teratogenic Agents, 10th ed. Baltimore: Johns Hopkins University Press, 2001.
17. Carter CO. Genetics of common single malformations. Br Med Bull 1976;32:21.
18. Beckman DA, Brent RL. Mechanism of known environmental teratogens: drugs and chemicals. Clin Perinatol 1986;13:649.
19. Seaver LH, Hoyme HE. Teratology in pediatric practice. Pediatr Clin North Am 1992;39:111.
20. Koren G et al. Drugs in pregnancy. N Engl J Med 1998;338:1128.
21. Brent RL, Beckman DA. Prescribed drugs, therapeutic agents, and fetal teratogenesis. In: Reece EA, Hobbins JC, eds. Medicine of the Fetus and Mother. Philadelphia: Lippincott-Raven, 1998:289.
22. Food and Drug Administration. Federal Register 1980;44:37434.
23. Heitland G, Hurlbut KM, eds. REPRORISK System. MICROMEDEX, Greenwood Village, CO (Edition expires 6/2003).
24. Physicians' Desk Reference, 53rd ed. Montvale, NJ: Medical Economics Company, 1999.
25. Brunskill PJ. The effects of fetal exposure to danazol. Br J Obstet Gynaecol 1992;99:212.
26. McEvoy GK, ed. AHFS Drug Information 2003. Bethesda, MD: American Society of Health-System Pharmacists, 2003.
27. Ghidini A et al. Congenital abnormalities (VATER) in baby born to mother using lovastatin. Lancet 1992;229:1416.
28. Manson JM et al. Postmarketing surveillance of lovastatin and simvastatin exposure during pregnancy. Reprod Toxicol 1996;10:439.
29. Physicians' Desk Reference, 57th ed. Montvale, NJ: Thomson, 2003.
30. Brent RL. Teratogen update: reproductive risks of leflunomide (Arava), a pyrimidine synthesis inhibitor: counseling women taking leflunomide before or during pregnancy and men taking leflunomide who are contemplating fathering a child. Teratology 2001;63:106.
31. Burrows RF, Burrows EA. Assessing the teratogenic potential of angiotensin-converting enzyme inhibitors in pregnancy. Aust NZ J Obstet Gynaecol 1998;38:306.
32. Postmarketing surveillance for angiotensin-converting enzyme inhibitor use during the first trimester of pregnancy, United States, Canada, and Israel. MMWR 1997;46:240.
33. Cunniff C et al. Oligohydramnios sequence and renal tubular malformation associated with maternal enalapril use. Am J Obstet Gynecol 1990;162:187.
34. Rosa FW et al. Neonatal anuria with maternal angiotensin-converting enzyme inhibition. Obstet Gynecol 1989;74:371.
35. Joglar JA, Page RL. Treatment of cardiac arrhythmias during pregnancy. Drug Safety 1999;20:85.
36. Laurent M et al. Neonatal hypothyroidism after treatment by amiodarone during pregnancy. Am J Cardiol 1987;60:942.
37. Polifka JE, Friedman JM. Teratogen update: azathioprine and 6-mercaptopurine. Teratology 2002;65:240.
38. Iqbal MM et al. Effects of commonly used benzodiazepines on the fetus, the neonate, and the nursing infant. Psychiatr Serv 2002;53:39.
39. Matalon S et al. The teratogenic effect of carbamazepine: a meta-analysis of 1255 exposures. Reprod Toxicol 2002;16:9.
40. Oberheuser F. Praktische Erfahrungen mit Medikamenten in der Schwangerschaft. Therapiewoche 1971;31:2200. As reported in Manten A. Antibiotic drugs. In: Dukes MNG, ed. Meyler's Side Effects of Drugs, vol, VIII. New York: American Elsevier, 1975:604.
41. Heinonen OP et al. Birth Defects and Drugs in Pregnancy. Littleton: Publishing Sciences Group, 1977.
42. Park-Wyllie L et al. Birth defects after maternal exposure to corticosteroids: prospective cohort study and meta-analysis of epidemiological studies. Teratology 2000;62:385.
43. Mygind H et al. Risk of intrauterine growth retardation, malformations and other birth outcomes in children after topical use of corticosteroid in pregnancy. Acta Obstet Gynecol Scand 2002;81:234.
44. Position statement: the use of new asthma and allergy medications during pregnancy. Ann Allergy Asthma Immunol 2000;84:475.
45. Saxen I. Cleft palate and maternal diphenhydramine intake. Lancet 1974;1:407.
46. King CT et al. Antifungal therapy during pregnancy. Clin Infect Dis 1998;27:1151.
47. Moise KJ Jr et al. Indomethacin in the treatment of premature labor: effects on the fetal ductus arteriosus. N Engl J Med 1988;319:327.
48. Viguera AC et al. Managing bipolar disorder during pregnancy: weighing the risks and benefits. Can J Psychiatry 2002;47(5):426.
49. Pinelli JM et al. Case report and review of the perinatal implications of maternal lithium use. Am J Obstet Gynecol 2002;187:245.
50. Robinson LL et al. Maternal drug use and risk of childhood nonlymphoblastic leukemia among offspring: an epidemiologic investigation implicating marijuana (a report from the Children's Cancer Study Group). Cancer 1989;63:1904.

51. Shepard TH et al. Update on new developments in the study of human teratogens. Teratology 2002; 65:153.

52. Hernandez-Diaz S et al. Folic acid antagonists during pregnancy and the risk of birth defects. N Engl J Med 2000;343:1608.

53. Cragan JD. Teratogen update: methylene blue. Teratology 1999;60:42.

54. Ericson A, Kallen BAJ. Nonsteroidal anti-inflammatory drugs in early pregnancy. Reprod Toxicol 2001;15:371.

55. Nielsen GL et al. Risk of adverse birth outcome and miscarriage in pregnant users of nonsteroidal anti-inflammatory drugs: population based observational study and case-control study. Br Med J 2001; 322:266.

56. Lammer EJ, Cordero JF. Exogenous sex hormone exposure and the risk for major malformations. JAMA 1986;255:3128.

57. Larsen H et al. Birth outcome following maternal use of fluoroquinolones. Int J Antimicrob Agents 2001;18:259.

58. Addis A, Koren G. Safety of fluoxetine during the first trimester of pregnancy: a meta-analytical review of epidemiological studies. Psychol Med 2000;30:89.

59. Kulin NA et al. Pregnancy outcome following maternal use of the new selective serotonin reuptake inhibitors. JAMA 1998;279:609.

60. Dahl MI et al. Paroxetine withdrawal syndrome in a neonate [letter]. Br J Psychiatry 1997;171:391.

61. Barrilleaux PS, Martin JN. Hypertension therapy during pregnancy. Clin Obstet Gynecol 2002;45:22.

62. Hernandez-Diaz S, Mitchell AA. Folic acid antagonists during pregnancy and risk of birth defects. N Engl J Med 2001;344:934.

63. Kozma C. Valproic acid embryopathy: report of two siblings with further expansion of the phenotypic abnormalities and a review of the literature. Am J Med Gen 2001;98:168.

64. Koren G, ed. Maternal-Fetal Toxicology: A Clinician's Guide. New York: Marcel Dekker, 1990.

65. American Academy of Pediatrics. Breastfeeding and the use of human milk. Pediatrics 1997;100. 1035.

66. Zembo CT. Breastfeeding. Obstet Gynecol Clin North Am 2002;29:51.

67. Mortensen EL et al. The association between duration of breastfeeding and adult intelligence. JAMA 2002;287:2365.

68. National Center for Health Statistics. Healthy People 2000 Final Review. Hyattsville, MD: Public Health Service, 2001.

69. Wilson JT, ed. Drugs in Breast Milk. Sydney: ADIS Press, 1981.

70. Anderson PO. Drug use during breastfeeding. Clin Pharm 1991;10:594.

71. Lawrence RA, Lawrence RM. Drugs in breast milk. In: Breastfeeding: A Guide for the Medical Profession. St. Louis: Mosby, 1999;351.

72. Dillon AE et al. Drug therapy in the nursing mother. Obstet Gynecol Clin North Am 1997;24:675.

73. Breitzka RL et al. Principles of drug transfer into breast milk and drug disposition in the nursing infant. J Hum Lact 1997;12:1155.

74. Bennett PN, Jensen AA, eds. Drugs and Human Lactation, 2nd ed. New York: Elsevier, 1996.

75. Hale TW, Ilett KF. Drug therapy and breastfeeding: from theory to clinical practice. Boca Raton, FL: Parthenon Publishing Group, 2002.

76. Picciano MF. Nutrient composition of human milk. Pediatr Clin North Am 2001;48:53.

77. Begg EJ et al. Studying drugs in human milk: time to unify the approach. J Hum Lact 2002;18:323.

78. Howard CR, Lawrence RA. Drugs and breastfeeding. Clin Perinatol 1999;26:447.

79. Committee on Drugs. American Academy of Pediatrics. The transfer of drugs and other chemicals into human milk. Pediatrics 2001;108:776.

80. Shannon M et al. Cocaine exposure among children seen at a pediatric hospital. Pediatrics 1989; 83:337.

81. Chasnoff IJ et al. Cocaine intoxication in a breast-fed infant. Pediatrics 1987;80:836.

82. Hale TW. Medications and Mothers' Milk, 10th ed. Amarillo: Pharmasoft Publishing, 2002.

83. Matheson I et al. Infant rash caused by paracetamol in breast milk? Pediatrics 1985;76:651.

84. Mactal-Haaf C et al. Use of anti-infective agents during lactation, part 3: antivirals, antifungals, and urinary antiseptics. J Hum Lact 2001;17:160.

85. Anderson PO, McGuire GG. Neonatal alprazolam withdrawal: possible effects of breast feeding. Ann Pharmacother 1989;23:614.

86. Boutroy MJ et al. To nurse when receiving acebutolol: is it dangerous for the neonate? Eur J Clin Pharmacol 1986;30:737.

87. Schmimmel MS et al. Toxic effects of atenolol consumed during breast feeding. J Pediatr 1989;114:476.

88. Briggs GG et al. Excretion of bupropion in breast milk. Ann Pharmacother 1993;27:431.

89. Gabay MP. Galactogogues: medications that induce lactation. J Hum Lact 2002;18:274.

90. Kok THHG et al. Drowsiness due to clemastine transmitted in breast milk. Lancet 1982;1:914.

91. Heikkinen T et al. Citalopram in pregnancy and lactation. Clin Pharmacol Ther 2002;72:184.

92. Courtney TP et al. Excretion of famotidine in breast milk. Br J Clin Pharmacol 1988;26:639P.

93. Winans EA. Antidepressant use during lactation. J Hum Lact 2001;17:256.

94. Kristensen JH et al. The amount of fluvoxamine in milk is unlikely to be a cause of adverse effects in breastfed infants. J Hum Lact 2002;18:139.

95. Weibert RT et al. Lack of ibuprofen secretion into human milk. Clin Pharm 1982;1:457.

96. Townsend RJ et al. Excretion of ibuprofen into breast milk. Am J Obstet Gynecol 1984;149:184.

97. Gardiner SJ. Transfer of metformin to human milk. Clin Pharmacol Ther 2003;73.71.

98. Chin KG et al. Use of anti-infective agents during lactation: part 1-beta-lactam antibiotics, vancomycin, quinupristin-dalfopristin, and linezolid. J Hum Lact 2000;16:351.

99. Chin KG et al. Use of anti-infective agents during lactation: part 2: aminoglycosides, macrolides, quinolones, sulfonamides, trimethoprim, tetracyclines, chloramphenicol, clindamycin, and metronidazole. J Hum Lact 2001; 17:54.

100. Ohman I et al. Topiramate kinetics during delivery, lactation, and in the neonate: preliminary observations. Epilepsia 2002;43:1157.

101. Reyes MP et al. Vancomycin during pregnancy: does it cause hearing loss or nephrotoxicity in the infant? Am J Obstet Gynecol 1989;161:977.

102. ACOG practice bulletin: thromboembolism in pregnancy. Int J Gynecol Obstet 2001;75:203.

103. Hall JG et al. Maternal and fetal sequelae of anticoagulation during pregnancy. Am J Med 1980; 68:122.

104. Ginsberg JS et al. Use of antithrombotic agents during pregnancy. Chest 2001;119:122s.

105. Ginsberg JS et al. Risks to the fetus of anticoagulant therapy during pregnancy. Thromb Haemost 1989;61:197.

106. Stein PD et al. Antithrombotic therapy in patients with mechanical and biological prosthetic heart valves. Chest 2001;119:220s.

107. Ginsberg JS et al. Heparin therapy during pregnancy. Risks to the fetus and mother. Arch Intern Med 1989;149:2233.

108. Barbour LA et al. A prospective study of heparin-induced osteoporosis in pregnancy using bone densitometry. Am J Obstet Gynecol 1994;170: 862.

109. Dahlman TC et al. Osteopenia in pregnancy during long-term heparin treatment: a radiologic study post partum. Br J Obstet Gynaecol 1990; 97:221.

110. Dahlman TC. Osteoporotic fractures and the recurrence of thromboembolism during pregnancy and the puerperium in 184 women undergoing thromboprophylaxis with heparin. Am J Obstet Gynecol 1993;168:1265.

111. Dahlman TC et al. Bone mineral density during long-term prophylaxis with heparin in pregnancy. Am J Obstet Gynecol 1994;170:1315.

112. Douketis JD et al. The effects of long-term heparin therapy during pregnancy on bone density. Thromb Haemost 1996;75:254.

113. Chan WS et al. Anticoagulation of pregnant women with mechanical heart valves. Arch Intern Med 2000;160:191.

114. Barbour LA. Current concepts of anticoagulant therapy in pregnancy. Obstet Gynecol Clin North Am 1997;24:499.

115. Sorensen HT et al. Birth outcomes in pregnant women treated with low-molecular-weight heparin. Acta Obstet Gynecol Scand 2000;79:655.

116. Rowen JA et al. Enoxaparin treatment in women with mechanical heart valves during pregnancy. Am J Obstet Gynecol 2001;185:633.

117. Wesseling J et al. Coumarins during pregnancy: long-term effects on growth and development of school-age children. Thromb Haemost 2001;85: 609.

118. Vitale N et al. Dose-dependent fetal complications of warfarin in pregnant women with mechanical heart valves. J Am Coll Cardiol 1999;33:1637.

119. Cotrufo M et al. Risk of warfarin during pregnancy with mechanical valve prostheses. Obstet Gynecol 2002;99:35.

120. Delgado-Escueta AV, Janz D. Consensus guidelines: preconception counseling, management, and care of the pregnant woman with epilepsy. Neurology 1992;42(Suppl 5):149.

121. Nulman I et al. Treatment of epilepsy in pregnancy. Drugs 1999;57:535.

122. Holmes LB et al. The teratogenicity of anticonvulsant drugs. N Engl J Med 2001;344:1132.

123. Eller DP et al. Maternal and fetal implications of anticonvulsive therapy during pregnancy. Obstet Gynecol Clin North Am 1997;24:523.

124. Arpino C et al. Teratogenic effects of antiepileptic drugs: use of an international database on malformations and drug exposure (MADRE). Epilepsia 2000,41:1436.

125. Fonager K et al. Birth outcomes in women exposed to anticonvulsant drugs. Acta Neurol Scand 2000;101:289.

126. Dean JCS et al. Long-term health and neurodevelopment in children exposed to antiepileptic drugs before birth. J Med Genet 2002;39:251.

127. Buehler BA. Prenatal prediction of risk of the fetal hydantoin syndrome. N Engl J Med 1990; 322:1567.

128. ACOG educational bulletin: seizure disorders in pregnancy. Int J Gynecol Obstet 1997;56:279.

129. Dansky LV et al. Mechanisms of teratogenesis: folic acid and antiepileptic therapy. Neurology 1992;42(Suppl 5):32.

130. Morrell MJ. Guidelines for the care of women with epilepsy. Neurology 1998;51(Suppl 4):S21.

131. Nakane Y et al. Multi-institutional study on the teratogenicity and fetal toxicity to antiepileptic drugs: a report of a collaborative study group in Japan. Epilepsia 1980;21:633.

132. Paulson GW, Paulson RB. Teratogenic effects of anticonvulsants. Arch Neurol 1981;38:140.

133. Jones KL et al. Pattern of malformations in the children of women treated with carbamazepine during pregnancy. N Engl J Med 1989;320:1661.

134. Chang SI, McAuley JW. Pharmacotherapeutic issues for women of childbearing age with epilepsy. Ann Pharmacother 1998;32:794.

135. Diav-Citrin O et al. Is carbamazepine teratogenic? A prospective controlled study of 210 pregnancies. Neurology 2001;57:321.

136. Rosa FW. Spina bifida in infants of women treated with carbamazepine during pregnancy. N Engl J Med 1991;324:674.

137. Koch S et al. Antiepileptic drug treatment in pregnancy: drug side effects in the neonate and neurological outcome. Acta Paediatr 1996;85:739.

138. Recommendations for the use of folic acid to reduce the number of cases of spina bifida and other neural tube defects. MMWR 1992;41(RR14):1.

139. Jager-Roman E et al. Fetal growth, major malformations, and minor anomalies in infants born to women receiving valproic acid. J Pediatr 1986; 108:997.

140. Fisher JB et al. Neonatal apnea associated with maternal clonazepam therapy: a case report. Obstet Gynecol 1985;66(Suppl):34S.

141. Tennis P et al. Preliminary results on pregnancy outcomes in women using lamotrigine. Epilepsia 2002;43:1161.

142. Tomson T et al. Lamotrigine in pregnancy and lactation: a case report. Epilepsia 1997;38:1039.

143. MRC Vitamin Study Research Group. Prevention of neural tube defects: results of the Medical Research Council Vitamin Study. Lancet 1991; 338:131.

144. Brent RL, Beckman DA. Angiotensin-converting enzyme inhibitors, an embryopathic class of drugs with unique properties: information for clinical teratology counselors. Teratology 1991;43:543.

145. Guignard J-P, Gouyon J-B. Adverse effects of drugs on the immature kidney. Biol Neonate 1988;53:243.

146. Moise KJ. Effect of advancing gestational age on the frequency of fetal ductal constriction in association with maternal indomethacin use. Am J Obstet Gynecol 1993;168:1350.

147. Vermillion ST et al. The effect of indomethacin tocolysis on fetal ductus arteriosus constriction with advancing gestational age. Am J Obstet Gynecol 1997;177:256.

148. Norton ME et al. Neonatal complications after the administration of indomethacin for preterm labor. N Engl J Med 1993;329:1602.

149. Schoenfeld A et al. Antagonism of antihypertensive drug therapy in pregnancy by indomethacin? Am J Obstet Gynecol 1989;161:1204.

150. Hansten PD et al., eds. Hansten's and Horn's Drug Interactions Analysis and Management. St. Louis: Facts and Comparisons, 2000:714.

151. Anderson PO. Drugs and breast milk [letter]. Pediatrics 1995;95:957.

152. Eidelman AI, Schimmel MS. Drugs and breast milk [letter]. Pediatrics 1995;95:956.

153. Troche BI. The methylene-blue baby. N Engl J Med 1989;320:1756.

154. Nicolini U, Monni G. Intestinal obstruction in babies exposed in utero to methylene blue. Lancet 1990;336:1258.

155. Van Der Pol JG et al. Jejunal atresia related to the use of methylene blue in genetic amniocentesis in twins. Br J Obstet Gynaecol 1992;99:141.

156. McFadyen I. The dangers of intra-amniotic methylene blue. Br J Obstet Gynaecol 1992;99:89.

157. DerMarderosian A, Beutler JA, eds. The Review of Natural Products. St. Louis: Facts and Comparisons, 2003.

158. Blumenthal M et al., eds. The Complete German Commission E Monogarphs: Therapeutic Guide to Herbal Medicines [Trans. S. Klein]. Boston: American Botanical Council, 1998.

159. Gruenwald J et al. PDR for Herbal Medicines, 2nd ed. Montvale, NJ: Medical Economics Company, 2000.

160. Gallo M et al. Pregnancy outcome following gestational exposure to echinacea. Arch Intern Med 2000;160:3141.

161. Jellin JM et al. Natural Medicines Comprehensive Database, 5th ed. Stockton: Therapeutic Research Faculty, 2003.

162. McGuffin M et al., eds. American Herbal Products Association's Botanical Safety Handbook. Boca Raton, FL: CRC Press, 1997.

163. Tyler VE. Herbs of Choice. Binghamton: Pharmaceutical Products Press, 1994.

164. Punnonen R, Lukola A. Oestrogen-like effect of ginseng. Br Med J 1980;281:1110.

165. Palmer BV et al. Ginseng and mastalgia [letter]. Br Med J 1978;1:1284.

166. Hopkins MP et al. Ginseng face cream and unexplained vaginal bleeding. Am J Obstet Gynecol 1988;159:1121.

167. Siegel RK. Ginseng abuse syndrome. JAMA 1979;241:1614.

168. Koren G et al. Maternal ginseng use associated with neonatal androgenization [letter]. JAMA 1990;264:2866.

169. Awang DVC. Maternal ginseng use associated with neonatal androgenization. JAMA 1991; 266:363.

CHAPTER 48

Gynecologic and Other Disorders of Women

Louise Parent-Stevens, Rosalie Sagraves

During their reproductive years, young women commonly experience gynecologic infections (e.g., vaginitis, pelvic inflammatory disease) as well as dysmenorrhea, premenstrual syndrome, and endometriosis. In older women undergoing the transition between the reproductive and nonreproductive years, problems related to declining estrogen concentrations (e.g., hot flushes, genitourinary atrophy) are likely to be experienced, whereas postmenopausal women have an increased risk for cardiac disease, osteoporosis, and various cancers (e.g., breast cancer).

GENDER-BASED DIFFERENCES

In addition to various health problems and diseases that are unique to women, health care providers must address gender-based differences in disease states that can affect women and men, their prevention and treatment, and differences in morbidity and mortality. When examining therapies for women and men who suffer from the same disease state, differences in the response to a medication or to a specific dose may be due to gender-related pharmacokinetic and/or pharmacodynamic differences. It was only during the 1990s that gender-based differences in the metabolism of and response to medications began to be examined. We are now aware of some clinical differences between women and men in the pharmacokinetic disposition of and pharmacodynamic response to some drugs. In addition, there is a need to determine whether there are pharmacokinetic and pharmacodynamic differences that occur in women over their life spans secondary to variations in hormone status.

1. **Why have gender-based differences in drug disposition and disease states not been readily addressed?**

Before the 1993 publication of the *Guideline for Study and Evaluation of Gender Differences in the Clinical Evaluation of Drugs,* the U.S. Food and Drug Administration (FDA) banned the inclusion of women in phase I and early phase II drug trials.[1] Women were not encouraged to participate in latter-phase trials, and the FDA did not require analysis of gender effects in new drug applications submitted before 1993. The following year, the National Institutes of Health (NIH) expanded the inclusion of women as research subjects by publishing the *NIH Guidelines on Inclusion of Women and Minorities as Subjects in Clinical Research.*[2] A regulation enacted in 2000 allows the FDA to delay approval for a new drug if women, who are otherwise eligible for the study, are excluded from clinical trials because of possible reproductive risk.[3]

Because of past governmental restrictions, women have been underrepresented in clinical studies that would have helped advance knowledge about appropriate drug use. Reasons for these past restrictions included the protection of unborn fetuses in women of childbearing potential and a belief by many that metabolism and response to drugs were similar in men and women.[4] Gender-based differences in metabolism, among other factors, may affect drug pharmacokinetics and pharmacodynamics. There may also be pharmacokinetic and pharmacodynamic changes that occur over women's life cycles that are under the influence of hormones such as estrogen.

2. **What is the clinical significance of gender differences when determining drug doses for women? What are some examples of gender differences that could affect drug pharmacokinetics and pharmacodynamics?**

The clinical significance of gender-specific differences in drug metabolism needs further study. For drugs with wide therapeutic ranges, pharmacokinetic differences between women and men may not be important clinically because the magnitude of change may not be sufficient to require a dosing adjustment based on gender.[4] Conversely, gender differences could be important when calculating the doses of drugs with narrow therapeutic ranges. However, these drugs are generally titrated on a patient-by-patient basis, diminishing the need for gender-associated pharmacokinetic considerations.[4]

Information about sex differences derived during the early phases of clinical drug trials could be useful in determining dosage ranges for drugs.[4] Although documented cases of pharmacodynamic differences between women and men are few, these differences can have a significant clinical impact. Gender-based pharmacodynamic differences, along with other factors such as body size, may underlie the higher incidence of adverse drug reactions in women than men.[4] For example, women have a heightened sensitivity to developing cardiac arrhythmias when exposed to some antiarrhythmics and antihistamines.[5] This possible drug hypersusceptibility in women underscores the need for research on the mechanisms of gender-specific adverse drug events.

Drug absorption after oral dosing may be greater in women, but may be of minimal clinical consequence.[6] Some differences in drug distribution, based on tissue binding, have been reported.[4,6] The general tendency for men to have greater muscle mass and for women to have a higher percentage of body fat may account for the higher volume of distribution of fat-soluble drugs in women. A decreased renal clearance of drugs in women may be related to sex differences in glomerular filtration rates: differences in renal secretion and reabsorption have not been well characterized.[6] There may be gender differences in oxidative metabolism based on specific cytochrome P450 isozymes. In general, women appear to have greater CYP3A4 activity than men, while the opposite may be true for CYP2D6 and CYP1A2. Gender-linked differences for CYP2C19 are not apparent.[7] Conjugative metabolism may be greater in men than in women.[6]

Examples of Diseases With Possible Gender-Based Differences

3. What are some of the diseases that appear to have gender-based differences?

Although most chronic diseases affect both genders, mortality rates are typically higher for men compared with women. Women, however, experience higher rates of morbidity and short-term disability. Diseases for which gender-specific differences in clinical presentation, morbidity, and/or mortality have been observed include asthma, arthritis and other immunologic diseases, cardiovascular disease (e.g., myocardial infarction, hypertension), diabetes mellitus, depression, epilepsy, and migraine.[8–10]

VAGINITIS

Vaginal infection is one of the most common reasons women seek gynecologic care. Approximately 10 million physicians' office visits are made annually in the United States by women who believe they may have a vaginal infection.[11] The most common vaginal infections are bacterial vaginosis (30% to 35% of cases), vulvovaginal candidiasis (20% to 25% of cases), *Trichomonas* vaginitis (10% of cases), and mixed infections (15% to 20% of cases).[11] Bacterial vaginosis (BV) is a polymicrobial infection characterized by a decreased concentration of hydrogen peroxide–producing lactobacilli coupled with an increased concentration of *Gardnerella vaginalis, Mycoplasma hominis, Mobiluncus* species, and anaerobic organisms.[11–13] Species of *Prevotella, Porphyromonas, Bacteroides,* and *Peptostreptococcus* species may also be present.[12,13] *Candida albicans* is the causative organism of vulvovaginal candidiasis (VVC) in 80% to 92% of cases, with *C. (Torulopsis) glabrata* and *C. tropicalis* accounting for most of the remaining cases.[11,12] The latter organisms have been identified increasingly as the causative agents of VVC over the past two decades. *Trichomonas* vaginitis is presented in Chapter 65, Sexually Transmitted Diseases.

Vulvovaginal Candidiasis
Assessing Self-Treatment

4. L.L., a 23-year-old woman, purchases an over-the-counter (OTC) antifungal agent to relieve vaginal symptoms that she believes are caused by a vaginal yeast infection. L.L. asks the pharmacist for assistance in the selection of an antifungal agent. What information should be obtained from L.L. before a medication is recommended?

The pharmacist should ask L.L. if this is her first episode of vaginitis or whether she has experienced similar symptoms previously that have been diagnosed as a vaginal yeast infection and treated by a physician. The nonprescription antifungal agents are indicated for the treatment of VVC in women who previously were diagnosed and treated by their physicians. She should be referred to her physician if (1) this is her first episode of VVC; (2) she has had two episodes of VVC within the past 6 months; (3) she is pregnant; (4) she is younger than 16 or older than 60 years of age; (5) she currently has abnormal vaginal bleeding or lower abdominal pain; (6) she has been exposed to a sexually transmitted disease (STD); or (7) she has a malodorous vaginal discharge (Table 48-1).

Signs and Symptoms

5. L.L. has experienced two episodes of vaginal yeast infections, with the most recent case occurring approximately 1 year ago. On both occasions she was diagnosed as having VVC by her physician and responded to antifungal therapy. L.L. currently describes vaginal and vulvar itching, vaginal soreness, and vulvar burning accompanied by a thick, white vaginal discharge that has the consistency of cottage cheese. She has been unable to have sexual intercourse because of pain. These symptoms are similar to those she experienced with her previous vaginal yeast infections. L.L. has no underlying major health problems. Her current medications include oral tetracycline for acne and Ortho Tri-Cyclen for birth control. She has regular menstrual cycles and her last menstrual period ended 4 days ago. What clinical manifestations does L.L. exhibit that are consistent with VVC? What are other common manifestations?

L.L. exhibits signs and symptoms associated with VVC (i.e., vulvar and vaginal pruritus, vaginal soreness, vulvar burning, dyspareunia, a thick, white vaginal discharge that appears to be "curdlike"). Although vulvar pruritus occurs in

Table 48-1   Questions to Gain Information About Possible Candida Vulvovaginitis[a]

What symptoms are you experiencing currently? (See Question 5.)

Have you previously been diagnosed by a physician as having a vaginal yeast infection? (See Question 4.)

What symptoms did you experience with that previous yeast infection? Are the symptoms you are experiencing now the same or similar to those you had with that previous infection? (See Questions 4–6.)

If you were treated previously for a vaginal infection, what antifungal agent did you use? For how long did you use it? Was it effective?

Did you experience any adverse effects associated with use of the antifungal agent? (See Question 11.)

Are you pregnant? (See Question 8.)

Do you have any medical problems? (See Questions 8 and 14.)

Are you taking any medications? (See Question 8.)

Do you have allergies?

Do you use any vaginal preparations (e.g., feminine hygiene sprays or douches)? (See Question 7.)

If you have sexual intercourse, what contraceptive method do you use? Does your sexual partner use a condom? (See Question 7.)

You also might ask questions about tight-fitting clothes, nylon undergarments, swimming, and so on (see Question 12).

[a]A Questionnaire also might be helpful in collecting information from the patient.

Table 48-2 Characteristics of Vaginal Discharge

Characteristics	Normal	Candidiasis	Trichomoniasis	Bacterial Vaginosis
Color	White or clear	White	Yellow-green	White to gray
Odor	Nonodorous	Nonodorous	Malodorous	Fishy smell
Consistency	Floccular	Floccular	Homogeneous	Homogeneous
Viscosity	High	High	Low	Low
pH	≤4.5	4–4.5	5–6.0	>4.5
Other characteristics	—	Thick, curdlike	Frothy	Thin

From references 11, 12, and 16.

most symptomatic patients, many affected women have little or no vaginal discharge.[11] Typically, the vaginal discharge associated with VVC is a nonodorous, highly viscous, white discharge that may vary in consistency from curdlike to watery.[11] Symptoms may be worse before menses and may diminish with the onset of menses.[11]

Differential Diagnosis

6. **How can VVC be differentiated from other vaginal infections?**

VVC should be differentiated from other vaginal infections (e.g., bacterial vaginosis) because a nonprescription antifungal agent could delay the appropriate treatment of other vaginal infections. The physical appearance of the vaginal discharge may be useful in predicting VVC if it is a viscous, nonodorous, white, curdlike discharge and the patient has a normal vaginal pH (pH 4.0 to 4.5).[11–13] The quantity of the discharge may be scanty to profuse. Some women with VVC exhibit only vaginal erythema with minimal discharge or an increased amount of normal vaginal secretion. Table 48-2 characterizes the vaginal discharges associated with VVC, BV, and vaginal trichomoniasis. The vaginal discharge from a woman with signs and symptoms of VVC should be examined for the microscopic presence of *C. albicans* using a wet mount preparation with 10% potassium hydroxide (KOH) or a Gram's stain of the vaginal discharge. (The use of KOH improves the visualization of yeast or pseudohyphae that are seen in approximately 70% of women diagnosed with VVC.)[13] The patient's vaginal discharge should be cultured in an appropriate growth medium if microscopy is negative.

The mere presence of *C. albicans* in the vagina is not necessarily consistent with a yeast infection because *C. albicans* can be isolated from the vagina in 10% to 20% of asymptomatic, healthy women of childbearing age.[13] It is the proliferation of *C. albicans* or other yeasts that lead to vulvovaginitis symptoms.

BACTERIAL VAGINOSIS

BV is the most common cause of vaginosis among U.S. women of childbearing age. Women with a diagnosis of BV have decreased numbers of vaginal facultative (hydrogen peroxide–producing) lactobacilli that help maintain vaginal acidity, which is important in preventing vaginal infections.[12] They are also likely to have increased numbers of *Gardnerella vaginalis, Mycoplasma hominis, Mobiluncus* species, anaerobic Gram-negative rods (e.g., various species of *Prevotella, Porphyromonas, Bacteroides*), as well as *Peptostreptococcus*

species.[12] Many of the organisms associated with BV may be present in low numbers in the normal vagina and can be sexually transferred.[12,13]

BV can be asymptomatic or associated with mild symptoms. The vaginal discharge of BV is thin, foul-smelling (fishy odor), homogeneous, off-white to gray, and associated with an increased pH (see Table 48-2). BV is classified as vaginosis rather than vaginitis because vaginal inflammation and symptoms usually are mild. The diagnosis of BV is typically based on Amsel's criteria (Table 48-3).[12,14] The single most reliable predictor of BV appears to be the presence of clue cells.[12,14]

A vaginal culture for *G. vaginalis* is not usually recommended because 50% to 60% of asymptomatic women are colonized with *G. vaginalis*.[12,14] A Gram's stain of vaginal secretions is less subjective than most other criteria for BV but is not commonly ordered.[14] An office-based test that detects elevated pH and trimethylamine, however, is clinically useful in the diagnosis of BV.[13,14]

BV primarily occurs in women during childbearing years and is detected equally in pregnant and nonpregnant women. Maternal BV and chorioamnionitis increase the risk of premature delivery 2 and 6.9 times, respectively.[12] Races other than white and use of intrauterine devices (IUD) for birth control have been associated with a higher risk for BV.[11–13]* Although sexual intercourse with multiple partners is a risk factor, BV is not considered an STD.[13]

PHYSIOLOGIC VAGINAL DISCHARGE AND SYMPTOMATIC NORMAL PH VULVOVAGINITIS

7. **Do women such as L.L., who have an increased vaginal discharge and symptoms consistent with VVC, necessarily have a vaginal infection?**

Table 48-3 Modified Amsel's Criteria for the Diagnosis of Bacterial Vaginosis

At least three of the following signs must be present for diagnosis:
Homogeneous discharge
Fishy amine odor when 10% KOH is added (sniff test)
Clue cells (i.e., >20% on wet mount)
Vaginal pH >4.5
No lactobacilli on wet mount

KOH, potassium hydroxide.
From reference 14.

Although the possibility of vaginal infection must be addressed when a woman presents with an increased vaginal discharge with or without symptoms, other conditions are associated with an increased discharge. First, a physiologic vaginal discharge must be distinguished from a pathologic discharge. Physiologic discharges (see Table 48-2) characteristically are nonodorous, white or clear, highly viscous or floccular, and acidic (pH ~ 4.5). Physiologic discharges may become more profuse at midcycle secondary to increased cervical mucus or vaginal epithelial cells. Other conditions resulting in excessive vaginal discharge with or without VVC-like symptoms include retention of foreign bodies (e.g., tampons) and allergic reactions or contact dermatitis secondary to the use of vaginal spermicidal agents, soaps, deodorants, douches, vaginal lubricants, and condoms. Episodes of vulvovaginitis-like symptoms can be secondary to the frequent use of hot tubs, jacuzzi, or swimming pools that contain chemically treated water (e.g., high levels of chlorine).[15]

Susceptibility to Vulvovaginal Candidiasis

8. What specific groups of women are most susceptible to VVC? Would L.L. fit into any group at high risk for VVC?

Women are most susceptible to VVC during their child-bearing years. Approximately 50% of U.S. college women report having an episode of VVC between menarche and age 25.[12] An estimated 75% of U.S. women experience one episode of VVC during their lifetimes while 40 to 45% report at least two episodes.[13] Approximately 5% of women who have VVC have recurrent candidal episodes.[13]

C. albicans colonization and symptomatic VVC increase during pregnancy and when high estrogen-containing oral contraceptives are used. This increase has been attributed to estrogen enhancement of the binding affinity of vaginal epithelial cells to *C. albicans*.[16] Women with high glycogen concentrations (e.g., uncontrolled or poorly controlled diabetes mellitus); women with depressed cell-mediated immunity secondary to disease (e.g., cancer, HIV infection); and women taking broad-spectrum antibiotics or immunosuppressive drugs (e.g., cytotoxic agents, corticosteroids) may have increased susceptibility to VVC.[12,16] VVC is not described as an STD because celibate women can have VVC; however, the incidence of VVC increases when women become sexually active.[12] Individual cases of VVC, although not related to intercourse, may be related to orogenital sex.

L.L. is taking tetracycline, which may heighten her risk of developing VVC. Broad-spectrum antibiotics (e.g., tetracycline, ampicillin, cephalosporins) increase the risk for *C. albicans* overgrowth by suppression of normal vaginal flora (e.g., lactobacilli), which protect against *C. albicans*. L.L. was using a low-estrogen–containing oral contraceptive, but low-dose oral contraceptives have not been consistently associated with an increased risk of VVC.[17,18] The use of diaphragms, vaginal sponges, and IUDs also may be risk factors for VVC.[13,19]

Stress-induced VVC and an increased incidence of VVC before menstruation have been described.[16] The cause of both is currently unknown. Although various dietary factors have been postulated as a cause of vaginal yeast overgrowth, the role of diet in the development of VVC remains inconclusive.[16]

Treatment of Vulvovaginal Candidiasis
VAGINALLY ADMINISTERED AZOLES

9. What vaginally administered therapy might be effective for L.L.'s VVC?

L.L. is an appropriate candidate for OTC therapy (Table 48-4) because she had previous vaginal yeast infections with symptoms similar to those she currently is experiencing, and her VVC is uncomplicated (i.e., mild to moderate, sporadic, nonrecurring disease in a normal host).[13] When a patient's VVC appears complicated, (e.g., severe or recurrent, presence of uncontrolled diabetes, debilitation, immunosuppression, or pregnancy), she should be referred to her medical practitioner.[13] L.L. should respond to short-term topical azole (imidazole or triazole) therapy. She should ask her physician whether she should continue with oral tetracycline or be prescribed another oral antimicrobial. If L.L. had been evaluated by her physician, an azole that is available for single oral dose or 3-day vaginal therapy might have been prescribed (see Question 10).

Vaginally administered azoles are effective in treating VVC with cure rates between 80% and 90% when a full course of therapy is completed.[13,20] All the azole antifungal products listed in Table 48-4 are superior to nystatin. The azole medication to treat the VVC of L.L. should be selected based on efficacy, cost, response or failure to previous therapy, length of therapy, and L.L.'s preference for dosage form. She should select a non–oil-based product if a latex condom or a diaphragm is used for contraception (see Table 48-4).

OTHER TREATMENTS FOR VULVOVAGINAL CANDIDIASIS

Oral lactobacillus and lactobacillus-containing yogurt have long been advocated for the treatment of VVC; however, evidence in support of this treatment is inconclusive.[21] Boric acid (600-mg capsules) inserted high in the vagina at bedtime for 14 days is effective for the treatment of VVC, but vaginal burning and irritation occur in about 4% of women and boric acid is poisonous if inadvertently ingested.[21] Gentian violet preparations also have limited use in the treatment of candidiasis because they stain clothing and bed linens and cause local irritation and edema.

ORAL AZOLES

10. How effective are orally administered azoles in the treatment of an acute VVC infection such as the one L.L. is experiencing?

Fluconazole (Diflucan), administered as a single 150-mg oral dose, is the only oral antifungal agent currently approved by the FDA for the treatment of acute VVC (see Table 48-4). In two clinical studies, a single 150-mg oral dose of fluconazole was as effective as 3- to 6-day regimens of intravaginal clotrimazole.[22,23] Itraconazole (200 mg/day for 3 days or 400 mg administered as a single dose) and ketoconazole (400 mg/day for 5 days) also are effective for the treatment of VVC.[12,13] Although some women prefer an orally administered drug rather than one that is vaginally administered, their use for mild to moderate VVC is controversial because of possible systemic adverse effects, especially with ketoconazole.

Table 48-4   Products Available for the Treatment of Candida Vulvovaginitis

Drug	Availability	Trade Names	Dosing Regimens
OTC Products			
Butoconazole	2% vaginal cream[a]	Femstat 3	*Nonpregnant women:* Administer 1 applicatorful intravaginally Q HS for 3 consecutive days; may extend to 6 days of therapy if necessary *Pregnant women during second and third trimesters:* Administer 1 applicatorful intravaginally Q HS for 6 consecutive days
Clotrimazole	1% vaginal cream[a]	Gyne-Lotrimin 7; Mycelex-7; Sweet'n Fresh Clotrimazole 7; various generics	Administer 1 applicatorful intravaginally Q HS for 7 consecutive days
	100-mg vaginal tablets	Gyne-Lotrimin; Mycelex-7; Sweet'n Fresh Clotrimazole 7; various generics	Insert 1 tablet intravaginally Q HS for 7 consecutive days
	200-mg vaginal inserts	Gyne-Lotrimin 3	Insert 1 suppository intravaginally Q HS for 3 consecutive days
Miconazole	2% cream[a]	Monistat 7; Femizol-M; various generics	Administer 1 applicatorful intravaginally Q HS for 7 consecutive days
	100-mg vaginal suppositories[a]	Monistat 7	Insert 1 suppository intravaginally Q HS for 7 consecutive days
	100-mg vaginal suppositories[a] (with 2% topical cream)	Monistat 7 combination pack	Insert 1 suppository intravaginally Q HS for 7 consecutive days; apply topical cream to affected areas BID (morning and night) for 7 consecutive days
	200-mg vaginal suppositories[a]	Monistat 3	Insert 1 suppository intravaginally Q HS for 3 consecutive days
	200-mg vaginal suppositories[a] (with 2% topical cream)	Monistat Dual-Pak; M-Zole 3 Combination Pack	Insert 1 suppository intravaginally Q HS for 3 consecutive days; apply topical cream to affected areas BID (morning and night) for 7 consecutive days
Tioconazole	6.5% vaginal cream[a]	Vagistat-1, generics	Administer 1 applicatorful intravaginally at HS for 1 dose only
Prescription Products			
Fluconazole	150-mg oral tablet	Diflucan tablet	Take 1 tablet PO for 1 dose only
Nystatin	100,000 U vaginal tablet	Mycostatin; Nystatin; various generics	Insert 1 tablet intravaginally Q HS for 14 consecutive days
Terconazole	0.4% vaginal cream	Terazol 7	Administer 1 applicatorful intravaginally Q HS for 7 consecutive days
	0.8% vaginal cream	Terazol 3	Administer 1 applicatorful intravaginally Q HS for 3 consecutive days
	80-mg vaginal suppositories[a]	Terazol 3	Insert 1 suppository intravaginally Q HS for 3 consecutive days

[a]The Centers for Disease Control and Prevention states that the use of vaginally administered oil-based preparations may weaken latex products such as condoms and diaphragms.
OTC, over-the-counter.

Adverse Effects Associated With Azoles

11. **What adverse effects might L.L. experience from an azole antifungal agent administered vaginally or orally?**

When used vaginally, azoles are associated with minimal adverse reactions, many of which are similar to the symptoms women report from candidiasis infections. Thus, it can be difficult to differentiate disease symptoms from adverse drug reactions. If the vaginal symptoms seem to worsen after therapy is started, the patient should contact her health care provider. In addition, if symptoms have not improved within 3 days after initiation of therapy, the patient should contact her physician to rule out more severe disease, the treatment of the wrong disease, or drug-related adverse effects. Vulvovaginal irritation, itching, burning, and pelvic cramps are commonly associated with vaginal administration of azoles (3% to 4%).[24] Miconazole has also been associated with headaches, allergic contact dermatitis, and skin rashes; clotrimazole with vulvovaginal pruritus, dyspareunia, and bloating; butaconazole with vulvovaginal pruritus (0.9%), burning (2.3%), soreness, discharge, and swelling; terconazole with headaches (21% to 30%), dysmenorrhea (6%), genital pain (4.2%) and pruritus (2.3% to 5%); and tioconazole with burning (6%) and itching (5%).[24]

Oral fluconazole 150 mg has been associated with headache (13%), nausea (7%), abdominal pain (6%), diarrhea, dyspepsia, dizziness, taste perversion, angioedema, and rare cases of anaphylactic reactions.[24] Oral ketoconazole has been associated with nausea and vomiting (3% to 10%), diarrhea (<1%), abdominal pain (1.2%), pruritus, headache, somnolence, dizziness, photophobia, neuropsychiatric effects, anaphylaxis (rare), and reversible hepatotoxicity (1 in 10,000).[11,24] Adverse effects reported for itraconazole are similar to those noted for ketoconazole, including abnormalities in liver function tests.

Patient Counseling

12. How should L.L. be counseled about the use of a nonprescription (OTC) vaginal antifungal product?

L.L. should be instructed to read the patient information supplied with the antifungal agent and be informed of the importance of completing a full course of therapy even if her symptoms subside before that time. She should be instructed to continue the medication throughout her menstrual period. In addition, L.L. should be instructed to see her physician if her symptoms persist, if she experiences symptoms that signal a more serious problem (e.g., abdominal pain, fever, a foul-smelling or bloody vaginal discharge), or if another yeast infection recurs within 2 months.

The details of intravaginal administration should be reviewed with her, including instructions on how to clean the applicator (if one is used for drug administration) after each use. She also should be advised to use sanitary napkins to prevent staining of her clothing, and should be informed that many oil-based vaginal preparations may weaken condoms or diaphragms. L.L. also should be advised to avoid wearing tight-fitting, unventilated underwear (e.g., nylon panties or panty hose) and tight-fitting jeans because a warm, moist environment can facilitate fungal growth. However, a study addressing risk factors for VVC found no relation between type of underwear and the incidence of VVC.[19] L.L. also could be alerted to the possible relation between candidiasis and swimming in a heavily chlorinated pool or frequent use of a jacuzzi or hot tub.

Complicated Vulvovaginal Candidiasis

13. How would management of L.L.'s VVC differ if she had poorly controlled diabetes?

VVC in a woman with uncontrolled diabetes is usually considered to be complicated VVC.[13] A diagnosis of complicated VVC also is warranted when the VVC is severe, recurrent, caused by non-*albicans* species of *Candida,* or when VVC occurs in an immunosuppressed, debilitated, or pregnant woman. Approximately 10% to 20% of VVC cases can be classified as complicated. The treatment of complicated VVC varies depending on the underlying cause of complication. Severe VVC (i.e., extensive vulvar erythema, edema, excoriation, and fissures) should be treated with a 7- to 14-day course of topical azoles or two oral doses of fluconazole 150 mg given 3 days apart.[13] Infection with non-*albicans Candida* can be treated with a 7- to 14-day course of intravaginal terconazole (more effective than the imidazoles against non-*albicans Candida*) or oral itraconazole or ketoconazole (fluconazole has poor activity against non-*albicans Candida*).[20] If these traditional therapies are not effective in eradicating the infection, boric acid

vaginal capsules, 600 mg administered intravaginally once daily for 14 days, can be used.[13] See Questions 14 and 15 for treatment of recurrent VVC and VVC in pregnancy.

Recurrent Vulvovaginal Candidiasis

14. L.L. develops another case of VVC 1 month later. Does she have recurrent VVC? How should she be treated?

Most women have only occasional episodes of VVC, but approximately 5% have recurrent VVC, defined as four or more episodes per year.[13] First, to determine whether L.L. has recurrent VVC, a diagnosis of *C. albicans* needs to be confirmed by her physician. Second, underlying risk factors for VVC, such as uncontrolled diabetes mellitus, must be ruled out. Based on the timing of L.L.'s episodes and the absence of risk factors, L.L. does not meet the definition for recurrent VVC.

Even if a patient meets the criteria for recurrent VVC and is diagnosed as having *C. albicans* as the causative agent, an underlying cause of the problem may not be determined. In addition, the role of sexual transmission is not currently well understood.[12] In most patients, the pathogenesis of recurrent VVC cannot be determined.

Therapy for recurrent *C. albicans* vulvovaginitis may need to emphasize control or prophylaxis (rather than cure) after induction therapy achieves clinical remission and negative cultures. See Table 48-5 for a list of maintenance regimens.[11,25] Discontinuation of a maintenance regimen after 6 months can result in a 50% or greater relapse rate. If relapse occurs, the patient can be restarted on a maintenance azole for 12 months. Women who experience breakthrough VVC while receiving azole prophylaxis may require cultures and susceptibility testing to exclude the presence of a rare azole-resistant strain of *C. albicans* or a non-*albicans Candida* species.

Vulvovaginal Candidiasis During Pregnancy

15. Pregnant women are at increased risk for VVC. What teratogenic risks are associated with the use of azole preparations?

Vaginal colonization with *Candida* and symptomatic VVC are common during pregnancy. Asymptomatic colonization is not associated with increased maternal or fetal risks and need

Table 48-5   Maintenance Regimens for Prevention of Recurrent Vulvovaginal Candidiasis

	Dose	Frequency
Topical Agents		
Clotrimazole Vaginal Suppositories	200 mg	Twice weekly
Terconazole 0.8% Vaginal Cream	5 g	Weekly
Oral Agents		
Fluconazole tablets	100–150 mg	Weekly
Itraconazole tablets	100 mg	Daily
	400 mg	Monthly
Ketoconazole tablets	100 mg	Daily

Adapted from references 13 and 25.

not be treated.[26] However, symptomatic VVC should be treated. Although doses of oral fluconazole used to treat VVC have not been associated with increased fetal defects, higher doses may be teratogenic. Therefore, topical antifungal agents are preferred for treatment of VVC in pregnant women. Although the Centers for Disease Control and Prevention (CDC) recommends a minimum of 7 days of topical treatment of VVC during pregnancy, the standard 3-day regimen with appropriate follow-up to assess efficacy is effective for mild to moderate cases.[26] Although nystatin is classified as a category A drug during pregnancy, it is not commonly used owing to its low efficacy rate. Clotrimazole is classified as a category B drug for fetal risk, and the remaining vaginally administered azoles are designated as category C.[26] The teratogenic risks associated with these categories are described in Chapter 47, Teratogenicity and Drugs in Breast Milk

16. One year later, L.L. complains of a thin, yellow-colored vaginal discharge that has a fishy smell; she has no other symptoms. What is the most likely diagnosis and how should the problem be treated?

Bacterial Vaginosis

These symptoms described by L.L. are consistent with BV (see Table 48-2). The diagnostic criteria for BV are listed in Table 48-3. L.L. should be referred to her physician.

For treatment of BV in symptomatic, nonpregnant women, the CDC recommends metronidazole (Flagyl) 500 mg orally BID for 7 days; clindamycin (Cleocin) cream 2%, one applicatorful (5 g) intravaginally at bedtime for 7 days; or metronidazole (MetroGel Vaginal) gel 0.75%, one applicatorful (5 g) intravaginally, BID for 5 days.[13] Metronidazole 2g PO as a single dose or clindamycin 300 mg PO BID for 7 days are reasonable alternatives. Single-dose metronidazole (2 g), however, is less effective than the standard 7-day regimen. Clindamycin 100-mg vaginal ovules (Cleocin) are effective when inserted vaginally at bedtime for three consecutive nights. Vaginal administration is preferred for patients with mild to moderate disease because systemic absorption is minimal and patients may experience fewer adverse effects. The treatment of BV in an HIV-infected patient is the same as for HIV-negative women. Although BV is associated with multiple sexual partners, routine treatment of sex contacts is not recommended.[13]

Treatment of Bacterial Vaginosis in Pregnant Women

Pregnant women at high risk for preterm delivery should be screened for BV during their first prenatal visit. Asymptomatic women with BV should be treated with metronidazole 250 mg PO TID for 7 days, metronidazole 2 g PO as a single dose, or clindamycin 300 mg PO BID for 7 days.[13] All pregnant women with symptomatic BV should be treated to relieve symptoms regardless of risk for preterm delivery. The treatment regimens are the same as those used in asymptomatic pregnant women. Alternately, metronidazole gel (0.75%) 5 g administered intravaginally twice daily for 5 days can be used.[13] The CDC does not recommend the use of vaginal clindamycin by pregnant women because of an increased incidence of preterm deliveries among women who were treated with this medication.[13]

The treatment of asymptomatic BV in non–high-risk pregnant women is controversial. Some recommend treatment be-

cause BV has been associated with premature births. However, in two clinical trials, metronidazole given orally late in the second trimester did not reduce premature births in women without risk of premature delivery.[27] The lack of benefit from treatment may be attributed to inadequate doses of metronidazole or administration too late in the pregnancy. The advisability of treatment of asymptomatic BV in pregnant women not at high risk for preterm delivery is presently unclear.

Patients who receive metronidazole for BV should be counseled to avoid consuming alcohol during therapy and up to 24 hours afterward.[13] Women treated with clindamycin vaginal cream should be informed that this oil-based formulation might weaken latex condoms and diaphragms.

DYSMENORRHEA

Primary dysmenorrhea (painful menstruation) is caused by factors intrinsic to the uterus rather than by underlying pelvic pathology. Primary dysmenorrhea should be differentiated from secondary dysmenorrhea caused by pelvic inflammatory disease; endometriosis; pelvic congestion syndrome; adenomyosis; complications associated with IUD use; ovarian cysts; uterine polyps, adhesions, and fibroids; and cervical strictures or stenosis.

About 30% to 60% of women experience pain during menstruation, and 7% to 15% experience severe pain sufficient to interfere with daily activity. Primary dysmenorrhea most commonly affects women 17 to 24 years of age, and its prevalence decreases with age.[28]

Signs and Symptoms

17. J.J., a 14-year-old girl, complains of severe cramping pain associated with her menstrual cycles. The pain begins with the onset of her menstrual flow and has occurred monthly for the past year. J.J. states that she experienced her first menstrual period at age 12. The pain usually is cramplike, starting in the pelvic area radiating to her back and legs. In addition, she sometimes experiences a headache and feels extremely tired. J.J. has no nausea, vomiting, or diarrhea. She also states that her symptoms last for 1 to 2 days but are most severe during the first 12 to 24 hours, then subside somewhat with the use of aspirin. She usually takes two 325-mg tablets when her pain begins and then two tablets Q 4 to 6 hr PRN. She has taken no other medications for her symptoms and has no known allergies to medications. She has no other medical problems. Her physical examination was within normal limits. What clinical manifestations in J.J. are consistent with primary dysmenorrhea?

The diagnosis of primary dysmenorrhea is based largely on a patient's symptoms and her response to therapy rather than on a negative physical examination for pelvic diseases that could result in a diagnosis of secondary dysmenorrhea.[29] J.J.'s symptoms that are typical of primary dysmenorrhea include cramping pain in the suprapubic area, which may radiate into the back and/or thighs, headache, and fatigue. She also commonly experiences nausea, vomiting, fatigue, headache, and vertigo.[29] Irritability, nervousness, depression and insomnia may also occur.[30]

J.J. first experienced the pain 1 year after menarche. This is consistent with primary dysmenorrhea, which occurs only with ovulatory cycles. Anovulatory cycles are common for the first year after menarche. Once ovulatory cycles commence, the prevalence of dysmenorrhea increases. The time sequence of J.J.'s pain also fits the pattern of dysmenorrhea, with pain typically beginning up to 12 hours before menstrual flow, becoming most severe for 2 to 24 hours, and continuing for 24 to 72 hours.[29] The pain, often is characterized as "crampy," typically decreases with age, after the person becomes sexually active, and after childbirth.[29] J.J. had a normal gynecologic examination, which also is consistent with primary dysmenorrhea. The diagnosis of primary dysmenorrhea in J.J. can be confirmed by her response to appropriate drug therapy, such as a prostaglandin synthetase inhibitor or a combination oral contraceptive.

Pathogenesis

18. What causes the symptoms of primary dysmenorrhea that J.J. is experiencing?

Intrauterine pressure monitoring techniques indicate that uterine activity is cyclic in response to the variations in ovarian hormonal production and endometrial prostaglandin concentrations that occur during the normal menstrual cycle. During the menstrual phase (menses), women with primary dysmenorrhea have higher resting uterine tone and contraction pressures compared with women without dysmenorrhea.[29] Women with primary dysmenorrhea do not show a single abnormality in uterine activity but may have one or more of the following problems: increased resting pressure, increased active pressure, increased rate of uterine contraction, or dysrhythmic uterine activity. These alterations in uterine activity may decrease uterine blood flow, resulting in hypoxia and ischemia.[29]

Prostaglandins are strongly implicated in the etiology of dysmenorrhea. Prostaglandin $F_2\alpha$ ($PGF_2\alpha$) is a potent stimulator of smooth muscle contraction, which stimulates uterine contractions and results in ischemia and pain. The exogenous administration of $PGF_2\alpha$ produces pain and uterine contractions similar to those observed in patients with primary dysmenorrhea.[30] The administration of another prostaglandin, PGE_2, produces similar symptoms through its actions. These vasodilator and potent platelet disaggregator prostaglandins induce nausea, vomiting, and diarrhea, which are commonly encountered by women with primary dysmenorrhea. Increased concentrations of $PGF_2\alpha$, PGE_2, and the ratio of $PGF_2\alpha$ to PGE_2 occur in the endometrial and menstrual fluids of women with primary dysmenorrhea.[29,30] Endometrial $PGF_2\alpha$ concentrations are highest after exposure to luteal-phase levels of progesterone. This supports the observation that primary dysmenorrhea occurs with ovulatory cycles and explains the effectiveness of oral contraceptives in decreasing associated symptoms. In addition, nonsteroidal anti-inflammatory drugs (NSAIDs), which inhibit prostaglandin synthesis, are effective in the treatment of primary dysmenorrhea.

Women with IUDs often suffer from dysmenorrhea-like symptoms that may result from the increased production of prostaglandins by leukocytes that infiltrate areas near the IUD. These women may respond to NSAIDs, but one also must remember that a patient with an IUD in place is at risk for pelvic inflammatory disease, IUD perforation, or an unplanned pregnancy, all of which could produce similar symptoms.

Only 80% to 85% of patients believed to have primary dysmenorrhea respond to usual therapy. The remaining patients may be incorrectly diagnosed or have other factors that may be contributing to their symptoms. For example, some women with primary dysmenorrhea symptoms have normal concentrations of $PGF_2\alpha$, but increased leukotriene concentrations, which stimulate uterine contractions and symptoms of dysmenorrhea. The NSAIDs do not block the production of leukotrienes.[29]

Treatment
General Management

19. What nondrug therapies are effective for the treatment of J.J.'s manifestations of primary dysmenorrhea?

A treatment plan should include a discussion about primary dysmenorrhea, its proposed etiology, and various treatment options. Regular exercise may reduce dysmenorrhea-related symptoms; however, the studies are not well controlled. Mechanisms for this possible benefit include an increased release of β-endorphins or improved pelvic blood flow.[31] Exercise also may decrease the stress that can exacerbate dysmenorrhea. Cessation of tobacco use should be encouraged because greater risk for and severity of dysmenorrhea have been reported in smokers.[28] Because dysmenorrhea has been linked to diet, lowering dietary fat and increasing intake of omega-3 polyunsaturated fatty acids (fish oil) may decrease symptoms.[32] Local application of heat via an abdominal patch can be as effective as NSAIDs in providing pain relief of dysmenorrhea.[33] Transcutaneous electrical nerve stimulation (TENS) may provide analgesia for dysmenorrhea by decreasing the patient's ability to perceive pain or by stimulating the release of β-endorphins.[34] Although most women with primary dysmenorrhea require drug therapy, nonpharmaceutical measures, including exercise programs, relaxation techniques, and dietary modifications, are adjunctive. J.J.'s therapy should be based on her specific symptoms, response to previous therapy, and any adverse effects associated with that therapy. J.J.'s previous therapy consisted only of aspirin, which was somewhat effective.

Nonsteroidal Anti-Inflammatory Drugs
MECHANISM OF ACTION

To understand the mechanisms by which ibuprofen and other NSAIDs act to decrease prostaglandin concentrations in women with primary dysmenorrhea, it is important to have a basic knowledge of prostaglandin biosynthesis. Prostaglandins, leukotrienes, thromboxanes, and prostacyclin are synthesized via the arachidonic acid pathway (Fig. 48-1). Free, unesterified fatty acids such as arachidonic acid (derived from phospholipids, cholesterol, and triglycerides) are prostaglandin precursors. Arachidonic acid may be synthesized from phospholipids found in cell membranes of the menstruating uterus through hydrolysis by the lysosomal enzyme, phospholipase A_2. It is then metabolized by one of two enzyme systems. Lipoxygenase converts arachidonic acid to 5-hydroperoxyeicosatetranoic acid, which is converted to leukotrienes. Cyclooxygenase metabolizes arachidonic acid to unstable cyclic endoperoxides (PGG_2 and PGH_2), which are then converted to prostacyclin (PGI_2), thromboxane A_2, and the prostaglandins PGF_2 and PGE_2 by the action of prostacyclin synthetase, thromboxane synthetase, or

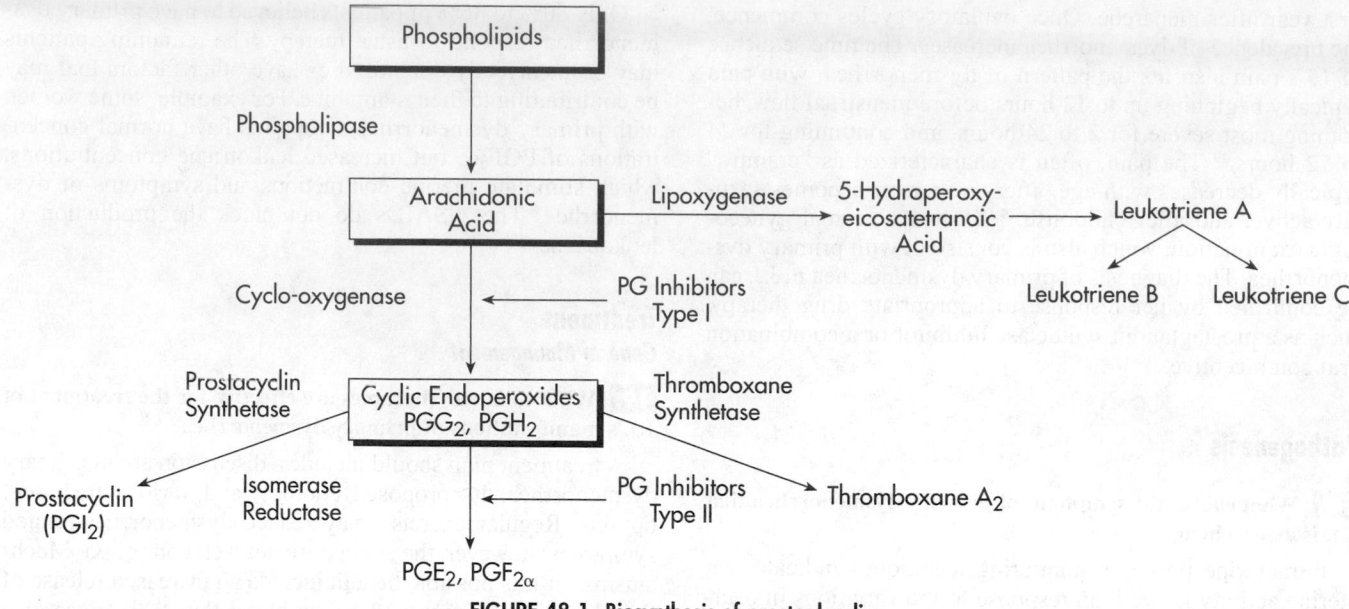

FIGURE 48-1 Biosynthesis of prostaglandins.

isomerase reductase, respectively.[35] There are two subtypes of cyclooxygenase. Cyclooxygenase I (COX-1) is responsible for the synthesis of prostaglandins involved in normal physiologic processes. Cyclooxygenase 2 (COX-2) is an inducible enzyme that produces prostaglandins involved in an inflammatory response. Although it is unclear which COX subtype stimulates the production of prostaglandins in primary dysmenorrhea, the efficacy of COX-2 selective inhibitors in the treatment of dysmenorrhea implicates COX-2–mediated prostaglandin synthesis as a factor in the condition.[36] The traditional NSAIDs inhibit the activity of both COX-1 and COX-2, whereas the COX-2 selective agents inhibit only COX-2 activity and do not affect the synthesis of prostaglandins involved in normal physiologic function.[36] In addition to the inhibition of prostaglandin synthesis, NSAIDs may relieve pain through their analgesic effects.

Choice of Agent

20. **J.J.'s gynecologist decides to start her on ibuprofen 200 mg PO at the beginning of menses, followed by 200 mg Q 4 to 6 hr thereafter for the 2 to 3 days she experiences dysmenorrhea. J.J. also is informed to telephone the clinic for an adjustment in her ibuprofen dose if she does not receive adequate relief from her symptoms. Why is the selection of ibuprofen appropriate for J.J.? What criteria should be used to select an NSAID for primary dysmenorrhea?**

IBUPROFEN

The traditional NSAIDs and the newer COX-2 selective inhibitors are effective for treatment of dysmenorrhea (Table 48-6). Initial selection of therapy should be based on effectiveness, incidence of adverse effects, cost, availability, and FDA approval for this specific indication. In multiple clinical trials, ibuprofen was significantly more effective than placebo in decreasing pain, reducing the need for additional analgesics, and reducing absenteeism and activity restriction. In these studies, ibuprofen demonstrated a low incidence of adverse effects.[37] In addition, it is available without a prescrip-

tion, and generic products are generally low cost. Therefore, the selection of ibuprofen to relieve J.J.'s primary dysmenorrhea symptoms is most appropriate.

OTHER NSAIDs

Two other NSAIDs, naproxen (as the sodium salt) and ketoprofen, are approved without a prescription for the treatment of primary dysmenorrhea. In a systematic review of clinical trials, naproxen and ibuprofen were judged to be equally efficacious in treating pain from dysmenorrhea.[37] In a separate pooled analysis, naproxen was more effective than ibuprofen.[38] However, the dose of ibuprofen used in the first analysis was 400 mg, whereas the average dose in the second review was 200 mg, which may account for the apparent difference in these results. Ketoprofen also is effective in relieving pain from dysmenorrhea.[39] Naproxen and ketoprofen offer the advantage of less frequent dosing compared with ibuprofen. Some of the studies, which demonstrated efficacy of the OTC NSAIDs for dysmenorrhea, used doses higher than the recommended dose on the labels of these OTC products.

Mefenamic acid is as effective as naproxen for control of dysmenorrhea pain. However, this product is available only by prescription.[29] Other NSAIDs approved for the treatment of dysmenorrhea are listed in Table 48-6.

Aspirin in doses of 500 to 650 mg four times a day appears minimally better than placebo in regard to pain relief and does not significantly change the need for additional analgesic therapy nor the degree of absenteeism and activity restriction.[37] Acetaminophen does not suppress prostaglandin synthesis and is of limited efficacy in the treatment of dysmenorrhea.[37]

COX-2 SELECTIVE INHIBITORS

The currently available COX-2 selective inhibitors are FDA approved for the treatment of primary dysmenorrhea. In two separate clinical trials, rofecoxib and valdecoxib were as equally efficacious as naproxen sodium in the treatment of dysmenorrhea.[40] Because of their high cost, use of the

Table 48-6 NSAIDs and Dosing Regimens for Primary Dysmenorrhea

Groups	Drugs	Dosages	Dosing Regimen/Maximum Daily Dose	Approved for Primary Dysmenorrhea
Salicylic acids	Aspirin Various[a]	325, 500, 650, 975 mg	500–600 mg PO Q 4–6 hr	No
Indole acetic acids	Diclofenac Cataflam[b]	50 mg (as potassium)	50 mg PO TID; some patients may need a first dose of 100 mg followed by 50 mg TID; (max, 150 mg/day, may give 200 mg on first day)	Yes
Propionic acids	Ibuprofen Advil[a] Motrin IB[a] Nuprin[a] Motrin[b] Other Rx and OTC products	200 mg 200 mg 200 mg 200 mg 300, 400, 600, 800 mg	400 mg PO Q 4–6 hr[c] (max, 3.2 g/day)	Yes
	Ketoprofen Orudis[b] and other Rx products	25, 50, 75 mg	25-50 mg Q 6–8 hr[d] (max, 300 mg/day)	Yes
	Orudis KT,[a] Actron[a]	12.5 mg		Yes
	Naproxen Naprosyn[b] and other Rx products	250, 375, 500 mg	500 mg PO first dose; 250 mg PO Q 6–8 hr (max, 1,250 mg/day)	
	Naproxen sodium Aleve[a]	200 mg (220 mg naproxen sodium)	550 mg (naproxen sodium) PO first dose; 275 mg (naproxen sodium) PO Q 6–8 hr (max, 1,375 mg/day [naproxen sodium])[e]	Yes
	Anaprox[b] and other Rx products	250 mg (275 mg naproxen sodium) 500 mg (550 mg naproxen sodium)		
Fenamates	Meclofenate sodium Meclomen[b]	50, 100 mg	100 mg TID for up to 6 days (max, 300 mg/day)	No Yes
	Mefenamic acid Ponstel[b]	250 mg	500 mg PO first dose; 250 mg PO Q 6 hr for 2–3 days (max, 1 g/day; may give 1.25 g on first day)	Yes
Cox-2 selective agents	Rofecoxib, Vioxx[b]	12.5, 25 mg	50 mg Q 24 hr (max, 50 mg/day)	
	Valdecoxib, Butra[b]	10, 20 mg	20 mg PO bid	Yes
	Celecoxib (Celebrex)[b]	100, 200, 400 mg	400 mg PO first dose; 200 mg BID	Yes Yes

[a]OTC product, available without prescription.
[b]Rx product available by prescription.
[c]Dosing recommended for dysmenorrhea when using the prescription product is higher than the OTC dosing of 200 mg Q 4–6 hr; may wish to start with the OTC dosing when an OTC product is used.
[d]Dosing recommended for dysmenorrhea when using the prescription product is higher than the OTC dosing of 12.5 Q 6–8 hr; may wish to start with the OTC dosing when an OTC product is used.
[e]Dosing recommended for dysmenorrhea when using the prescription product is higher than the OTC dosing of 220 mg Q 8–12 hr; may wish to start with the OTC dosing when an OTC product is used.
NSAID, nonsteroidal anti-inflammatory drug; OTC, over-the-counter.
From references 24 and 37.

COX-2 selective inhibitors should be limited to patients who have significant risk for gastric ulceration or who have failed therapy with traditional NSAIDs.

Adverse Effects

21. **What adverse effects might J.J. experience from her NSAID?**

Similar GI, central nervous system (CNS), or allergic adverse effects occur with all NSAIDs. Nausea, vomiting, indigestion, anorexia, diarrhea, constipation, abdominal pain, melena, and bloating are common GI complaints. CNS adverse effects include headache, vertigo, dizziness, visual disturbances, depression, drowsiness, irritability, excitation, insomnia, fatigue, tremors, and confusion. Patients who experience hypersensitive reactions to salicylates (e.g., bronchospasm, asthma, anaphylaxis, and acute respiratory distress) are not candidates for NSAID therapy. Rashes also have been reported with NSAID use. In addition, adverse effects also may involve cardiovascular, hepatic, renal, or hematologic systems (see Chapter 43, Rheumatic Disorders).

In a systematic review of trials of ibuprofen, mefenamic acid, aspirin, and naproxen in primary dysmenorrhea, only naproxen was associated with significantly more nausea than placebo.[37] In the studies of the COX-2 selective inhibitors, adverse effects were similar to those seen with naproxen.

Contraindications

22. **What contraindications should be considered before J.J.'s NSAID therapy is initiated?**

The primary contraindications to the use of NSAIDs include a history of hypersensitivity to salicylates or previously used NSAIDs or underlying renal disease. Persons with active or chronic ulcer disease should avoid the traditional NSAIDs, but can use a COX-2 selective agent cautiously. J.J. did not have any problems with aspirin nor does she have any medical problems that would preclude her from using an NSAID.

Initiation and Duration of Therapy

23. **When should J.J. begin taking ibuprofen and for what length of time?**

Because the absorption and onset of action of NSAIDs occurs within 30 minutes, it usually is unnecessary to start treatment before the onset of menstrual pain.[38] This practice decreases the likelihood that a sexually active woman will take the drug when she is pregnant. The NSAID should be initiated at the beginning of menses or at the onset of pain, whichever occurs first, and continued for up to 3 days because prostaglandin release is highest for the first 48 hours after the menstrual flow.[30] Loading doses are not recommended. NSAIDs prevent pain in dysmenorrhea by inhibiting prostaglandin formation; therefore, they should be taken on a scheduled basis rather than waiting until the pain recurs. A course of therapy should be tried for at least 3 months. If symptoms are not relieved or if they become worse even when NSAID doses are increased or other NSAIDs (or an oral contraceptive agent) are tried, further evaluation for causes of secondary dysmenorrhea should be considered.

Oral Contraceptives

24. **When would the use of an oral contraceptive be an appropriate therapeutic choice for J.J.?**

Oral contraceptives (OCs) suppress ovulation, decrease menstrual fluid volume, and thereby decrease prostaglandin production and uterine cramping.[41] If J.J. desires a birth control method, OCs may be especially useful. Comparisons of OCs in the treatment of dysmenorrhea do not suggest a significant difference between products.[29,41] Therefore, selection of an OC for an individual patient should be based on factors presented in Chapter 45, Contraception. OCs relieve dysmenorrhea symptoms in 50% to 80% of women within 3 to 6 months after beginning hormone therapy.[20] If J.J. has no need for contraception, she may not wish to take a drug for 3 weeks each month for a problem that occurs only 2 to 3 days monthly. Also, adverse effects associated with OCs use must be considered. Although serious complications from OC use are uncommon in young, healthy women, "nuisance" effects, (e.g., nausea, acne, breakthrough bleeding, breast soreness, depression) are frequently reported. If dysmenorrhea symptoms do not abate with OC use, a prostaglandin synthetase inhibitor alone or in combination with an OC may be effective.[29] If pain does not respond to either course of therapy, laparoscopy may be necessary to determine the cause.

Other Agents

25. **What drugs other than NSAIDs and OCs can be recommended for the treatment of J.J.'s primary dysmenorrhea?**

Currently, only NSAIDs and OCs are recommended for treating women with primary dysmenorrhea. Calcium channel blockers may decrease dysmenorrhea by reducing uterine hyperactivity.[29] Transdermal nitroglycerin ointment also can relieve dysmenorrhea for up to 4 hours.[42] β-Adrenergic agonists, vitamin B_1, magnesium, and fish oil (omega-3 fatty acids) also have some efficacy.[29,43]

ENDOMETRIOSIS

Endometriosis refers to the presence of functioning, proliferating endometrial tissue located outside the uterine cavity. The endometrial tissue most commonly is limited to the pelvic structures, but can be present anywhere in the body. The true prevalence of endometriosis is difficult to estimate because the disease can exist without significant symptoms and current diagnosis requires visual affirmation of endometrial tissue during surgery. The best estimate of the prevalence of endometriosis in the general population of women 15 to 44 years of age is 1% to 8%[44]; however, the absence of reliable noninvasive marker for the diagnosis of endometriosis makes the estimate of the true prevalence problematic. Endometriosis occurs almost exclusively in menstruating women; it rarely is observed before puberty, after menopause, or in women with amenorrhea.

Pathogenesis

The cause of endometriosis is uncertain. One proposed etiology suggests that viable endometrial tissue is delivered and implanted in the abdomen and other areas of the body by retrograde menstruation through the fallopian tubes or by hematogenous or lymphatic spread.[45] This implantation and direct transportation etiology theory account for the endometrial plaques on the organs located in the pelvic and abdominal cavities (the most common sites for endometriosis) and at distant sites such as the lungs and the extremities. It does not explain, however, why only a few women develop endometriosis when retrograde menstruation is an almost universal phenomenon, nor does it explain the more rare occurrences of endometriosis in men or nonmenstruating women. Another proposed cause of endometriosis suggests that stimulation (by an as-yet-unidentified substance) of the ovarian epithelium and the mesothelium of the pelvic peritoneum can result in their transformation into müllerian elements, which then give rise to endometrial tissue. This coelomic metaplasia and induction theory has been criticized for its failure to explain the predominance of the disease in women, the primary occurrence of the disease in the pelvis, and the age distribution of the disease.[46] Both of these theories account for some aspects of endometriosis, but each fails to explain all of its features.

A role for the immune system in the pathogenesis of endometriosis also is proposed. Autoantibodies to the endometrium, abnormal T- and B-cell activation, impaired macrophage activity, altered cytokine activity, and decreased natural killer cell activity have been noted in the immune systems of women with endometriosis.[46,47] Furthermore, characteristics of endometriosis are similar to other autoimmune diseases (e.g., changes in the immune system, multiorgan involvement, a genetic linkage, a predisposition to concomitant autoimmune diseases).[48] Alterations in the immune system also may be responsible for the increased infertility and miscarriage rates associated with endometriosis.

Once endometrial tissue becomes implanted, hormones are necessary for their continued growth. As with intrauterine endometrium, the implants of endometriosis possess estrogen, progesterone, and androgen receptors. However, the endometrial implants may respond differently to hormonal stimulation than normal endometrium. In general, estrogens stimulate the implants, whereas androgens or lack of estrogen results in implant atrophy. Because of their complex hormonal effects, progestins have variable effects on the implants.[49,50] (See Chapter 45 for the effects of estrogens and progestins on the endometrium.) Pharmacologic treatment of endometriosis is based on this hormonal response: danazol, GnRH agonist, progestins, and estrogen-progestin combination all cause endometrial tissue to atrophy.

The responsiveness of endometrial implants to ovarian hormones plays a role in the pathology of endometriosis. Withdrawal of estrogen and progesterone causes the endometrial implants to bleed, leading to an inflammatory response in the adjacent tissues. Repetitive cycles of bleeding and inflammation lead to the development of scar tissue and adhesions between adjacent peritoneal tissues. On laparoscopy, these areas of involvement appear as multiple hemorrhagic foci composed of endometrial epithelium, stroma, and glands. Ovarian endometriosis usually involves the formation of endometriomas, blood-filled cysts ("chocolate cysts") ranging in size from microscopic to 10 cm. Nodules may form on uterosacral ligaments. Fibrosis usually is present with the endometrial implants, and extensive adhesions may form between pelvic structures.[45]

Signs and Symptoms

26. J.B., a 27-year-old woman, has been married for 3 years and is currently taking low-dose oral contraceptives. She has not attempted to become pregnant. Her chief complaints are severe pelvic pain associated with menstruation and mild to moderate pelvic pain associated with some nonmenstrual days. Her menstrual history reveals menarche at age 10 with regular cycles every 26 to 27 days and heavy menses for 6 to 7 days. She experiences lower abdominal cramping and a dull backache with her menstrual periods. The occurrence of this pain has been increasing in severity and frequency over the past several months and has been poorly responsive to NSAIDs. Recently, she has begun to experience some pain during sexual intercourse. Her mother had a history of endometriosis.

A physical examination of J.B. is normal except that on pelvic examination, there is diffuse uterine and adnexal tenderness and multiple tender nodes palpated along the uterosacral ligament. J.B. is scheduled for a laparoscopy the following week. Laparoscopic examination of the pelvis and lower abdomen reveals endometriotic lesions. The involvement of the endometriosis is staged as moderate according to the Revised American Fertility Society Classification of Endometriosis. What subjective and objective evidence in J.B. is compatible with endometriosis?

J.B.'s age (27 years) and her nulliparity are consistent with the characteristics of women with endometriosis. Although endometriosis has been diagnosed in women of all ages, it most commonly occurs in women in their late 20s and early 30s who have delayed pregnancy or who have infrequent pregnancies.[51]

J.B.'s chief complaints are progressive dysmenorrhea and dyspareunia. These symptoms, though not specific for this disease, are the most common presenting complaints associated with endometriosis. Dysmenorrhea may be described as aching, cramping, or a pressure sensation located in the pelvic area or low back that seems to progress in severity with time. The pain may occur premenstrually, menstrually, or throughout the menstrual cycle. Less commonly, women may report pain during sexual intercourse (dyspareunia). These women usually have a fixed, retroverted uterus or endometriosis located in the posterior fornix of the vagina or along the uterosacral ligaments.[45]

Although it is unclear whether infertility is a problem in J.B., endometriosis occurs in 30% to 50% of women with infertility.[50] The cause of endometriosis-associated infertility is unknown. Proposed mechanisms include physical distortion of the pelvic architecture, inflammatory factors, impaired folliculogenesis, or defects in fertilization or implantation.[52] Distortion of the internal genitalia is thought to be a primary contributor to infertility in women with moderate to severe endometriosis. The cause of infertility in women with minimal to mild disease and no anatomic alterations has not been determined but may be due to defects in the immune system.

J.B.'s menstrual pattern is characteristic of women with endometriosis. Menarche at a young age and short cycle lengths (~27 days) are associated with an increased risk of endometriosis. Greater frequency of dysmenorrhea occurs in women with endometriosis but is believed to be a symptom of the disease rather than a risk factor.[51] Other symptoms associated with endometriosis depend on the organs affected. If the intestines are involved, painful defecation or rectal bleeding may be present. Hematuria, dysuria, and cyclic flank pain may occur with bladder or ureter involvement. On rare occasions, hemoptysis during menstruation may occur if endometrial lesions are located in the pleura[45] (Table 48-7).

J.B.'s physical findings of uterine and adnexal tenderness and multiple tender nodes in the area of the uterosacral ligament are common clinical findings in women with endometriosis. Other physical findings that may be present in women with endometriosis are a fixed, retroverted uterus; adnexal enlargement; fixed ovarian masses; nodules in the area of the posterior fornix of the vagina; and pelvic tenderness. Physical findings may be absent if the lesions are small and few.[45] Some symptoms and physical findings of endometriosis can be associated with other gynecologic conditions or diseases; therefore, a diagnosis of endometriosis needs to be confirmed by laparoscopy or laparotomy, which allows direct visualization of the pelvic and abdominal structures, and biopsy of the lesions.[45] Laparoscopy allows staging of the disease, which aids in selecting the appropriate method of treatment. Endometriosis currently is staged at the time of surgery according to the Revised American Fertility Society Classification of Endometriosis. The stages are minimal (stage I), mild (stage II), moderate (stage III), and severe (stage IV). Staging is determined by an accumulated point total. Points are as-

Table 48-7 Location of Endometriosis and Associated Symptoms

Sites	Symptoms
Most Common	
Pelvic	
Cervix	Abnormal uterine bleeding
Ovaries	Dysmenorrhea
Peritoneum	Dyspareunia
Rectovaginal septum	Infertility
Uterosacral ligaments	Pelvic pain
Intestinal	
Abdominal scars	Intestinal obstruction
Sigmoid colon	Midabdominal pain
Small intestines	Nausea
	Painful defecation
	Rectal bleeding
Urinary tract	
Bladder	Cyclic flank pain
Ureter	Hematuria
	Hydronephrosis
	Hydroureter
Least Common	
Miscellaneous	
Breasts	Hemoptysis
Diaphragm	Sciatica
Extremities	Subarachnoid bleeding
Gallbladder	
Pleura	
Sciatic notch	
Spleen	
Stomach	
Subarachnoid space	

From references 45, 61.

signed based on the location of the endometrial lesions, the size of the lesions, the presence of adhesions, the extent of the adhesions, and the degree of obliteration of the posterior cul-de-sac.[53] The classification system is designed to document the location and extent of endometriosis and does not predict infertility or pelvic pain, aid in treatment selection or outcomes, or predict recurrence of disease. Variability in staging may occur between evaluators as well as with different surgical procedures.[54] The diagnosis of infertility attributed to endometriosis is made after other causes of infertility such as female genital tract defects, ovarian defects, and male factors have been ruled out. Blood tests that can be used to diagnose endometriosis are not commercially available, however, antiendometrial antibodies in women with endometriosis can be highly sensitive and specific markers for endometriosis.[55] Biochemical markers (e.g., CA125, CA19-9) are not sufficiently specific to diagnose endometriosis, but have potential as markers of disease severity and of treatment efficacy.[56] Tests for these markers could greatly simplify the diagnosis and management of endometriosis.

Treatment

27. What therapeutic approaches are available for the management of J.B.'s endometriosis?

Therapy for endometriosis should be individualized for each patient after carefully considering the following factors: the patient's age, extent of the disease, severity of symptoms, presence and duration of infertility, and the patient's desire for fertility. The goals of treatment are to relieve symptoms and, if desired, to preserve or promote the woman's childbearing potential. The modalities currently available to treat endometriosis include definitive and conservative surgery, hormonal therapy with estrogen-progestin combinations or progestins alone, danazol and gestrinone (not approved for use in the United States), or the gonadotropin-releasing hormone agonists, and expectant management. With the exception of surgical removal of the uterus and ovaries, treatment should be considered temporizing only because the disease and symptoms eventually recur after surgery or once pharmacologic therapy is discontinued.

Pain Management
CONSERVATIVE SURGERY

Pharmacologic therapy and surgery are both effective in relieving most of the symptoms of endometriosis. Conservative surgery (e.g., ablation of endometriotic lesions and removal of adhesions and endometriomas) performed during a diagnostic laparoscopy can significantly decrease pain.[57] In theory, drug treatment after conservative surgery for endometriosis serves to suppress any remaining lesions, decreasing the risk of recurrence. Danazol, medoxyprogesterone acetate (MPA) and the GnRH agonists have, in some studies, prolonged the time to recurrence of endometriosis symptoms.[50,58] Although they are commonly used for this purpose, OCs have not been studied for preventing recurrence after surgery.

DEFINITIVE SURGERY

In definitive surgery, the patient undergoes a total abdominal hysterectomy and bilateral salpingo-oophorectomy, which eliminate the risk of recurrence of the disease. This radical surgery is reserved for women who have no desire for future conception or who have intractable pain unresponsive to hormonal therapy or conservative surgery.[45] Because most women with endometriosis are premenopausal, estrogen therapy (ET) has been used after surgery to relieve symptoms secondary to the hypoestrogenic state and to delay the development of osteoporosis. Short-term therapy with 0.625 mg/day of CEE (conjugated equine estrogens) usually is effective and does not appear to stimulate any residual endometriosis remaining after surgery.[49] When considering the use of ET after definitive surgery, the clinician should note that there are no studies evaluating the recurrence of endometriosis in women on postsurgical ET beyond several years.

DANAZOL

Danazol (Danocrine), a synthetic derivative of 17-ethinyl testosterone, is used to induce a pseudomenopausal state by suppressing the release of luteinizing hormone (LH) and follicle-stimulating hormone (FSH) from the anterior pituitary. It inhibits the enzymes involved in ovarian steroidogenesis and increases the metabolic clearance of estradiol; in addition, danazol may inhibit the autoimmune component of endometriosis.[59] The net effect of danazol therapy is the creation of a hypoestrogenic, hypoprogestogenic environment resulting in anovulation, amenorrhea, and atrophy of the endometrium and endometrial implants.

The goal of danazol therapy is to provide symptomatic relief. Up to 95% of women using danazol for moderate to severe endometriosis may have significant improvement in dysmenorrhea, pelvic pain, dyspareunia, and menorrhagia.[60] Regression of endometriotic lesions has also been documented.[50] Danazol 200/day is used for mild to moderate disease and 400 to 800 mg/day for more severe disease.[61] The usual duration of danazol therapy is 6 to 9 months, depending on the severity of the disease. Problems associated with danazol therapy include a high incidence of side effects, a high rate of disease recurrence once therapy is discontinued, and a high cost of therapy. In clinical trials, most women placed on danazol therapy experienced some side effects (see Question 31), and many discontinued therapy. Recurrence rates of 22% to 50% have been documented 4 to 5 years after danazol therapy, with the highest rates occurring in women with greater disease severity initially.[50]

Another testosterone derivative, gestrinone, is available in other countries for the treatment of endometriosis. Its long duration of action allows twice-weekly dosing. Side effects are similar to danazol and are related to the androgenic effects of the drug.[60]

GONADOTROPIN-RELEASING HORMONE AGONISTS

Gonadotropin-releasing hormone (GnRH) agonists prevent the pulsed release of endogenous GnRH from the hypothalamus, blocking the release of FSH and LH. Continuous use of these agents results in a decline in serum estradiol concentrations to the range found in menopausal women (<30 to 45 pg/mL). In comparison studies, the GnRH agonists were as effective as danazol in reducing endometriotic growth and relieving symptoms.[50] The dosing regimens for the GnRH agonists are listed in Table 48-8. The most common adverse effects of the GnRH agonists are secondary to the hypoestrogenic state (Table 48-9 and Question 32). Disease and symptoms recur in about 53% of patients treated with a GnRH agonist, and women with greater disease severity experience higher recurrence rates.[62]

ORAL CONTRACEPTIVES

Oral contraceptives are commonly used for the management of endometriosis-related pelvic pain because they often are better tolerated for long-term use than other agents. How-ever, studies documenting the effectiveness of low-dose OCs (<35 μg of ethinyl estradiol) compared with other treatments are limited. One study compared 3.6 mg of goserelin depot administered every 28 days to the cyclic use of a monophasic oral contraceptive containing ethinyl estradiol 20 to 30 μg and desogestrel 150 μg/tablet for 6 months in women with all stages of endometriosis. Both groups experienced significant reductions in dyspareunia, dysmenorrhea, and nonmenstrual pain. The only statistical difference between groups was greater relief of dyspareunia with goserelin.[50] In one study, the combination of an oral contraceptive with very-low-dose danazol significantly improved endometriosis over baseline and adverse effects were minimal. Nevertheless, the combination was not as effective as depot MPA at controlling dysmenorrhea.[63] The OCs are considered first-line therapy, especially in young women who have mild symptoms and do not desire immediate conception.[58]

PROGESTINS

In a systematic review of clinical studies using progestins for endometriosis, approximately 90% of women responded to treatment.[64] In trials comparing progestins with danazol or GnRH agonists, efficacy was similar between groups. However, approximately half the subjects experienced recurrence of pain within a short time after drug discontinuation.[64] Commonly used regimens include oral MPA in doses of 30 to 50 mg/day for 3 to 4 months and intramuscular administration of depot MPA (DMPA) 150 mg every 90 days. The suppression of the hypothalamic-pituitary-gonadal axis persists for 6 to 12 months after discontinuation of intramuscular MPA; therefore, women who wish to conceive soon after therapy should be treated with the oral form. Adverse effects include breakthrough or cyclic bleeding (36%); average weight gain of 1.5 kg (14% to 60%); edema or bloating (12%); breast tenderness (8%); and headache, nausea, and mood changes (7% each).[64] Although multiple studies have documented a modest decrease in bone density with DMPA use, the loss appears to be reversible.[65] Both beneficial and detrimental lipid changes have been reported with depot MPA.[24] MPA is recommended for use in women who have failed first-line therapy with NSAIDs or OCs.[58]

Clinical Application

28. J.B. wants relief from pelvic pain and wishes to delay conception at this time. What is the treatment of choice?

Table 48-8   GnRH Agonists

GnRH Agonist (Brand Name)	Strength	Dosage Form	Dosage Regimen
Nafarelin (Synarel)	2 mg/mL delivers 200 μg/spray	Intranasal	200–400 μg BID
Leuprolide (Lupron)	3.75, 7.5, 11.25 mg	IM depot	3.75 mg/month
Goserelin (Zoladex)	3.6 mg	SC implant	3.6 mg/month
Buserelin[a] (Suprefact)	300 μg/spray	Intranasal	300 μg BID to TID
Histrelin[b] (Supprelin)	120 μg/0.6 mL	SC injection	100 μg/day
	300 μg/0.6 mL		
	600 μg/0.6 mL		

[a]Not available in the United States.
[b]Not FDA approved for treatment of endometriosis.
GnRH, gonadotropin-releasing hormone; IM, intramuscular; SC, subcutaneous.

Table 48-9   Adverse Reactions With Danazol and the GnRH Agonists[24]

	Danazol (%)	Nafarelin (%)	Leuprolide (%)	Gosarelin (%)
Antiestrogenic Effects				
Hot flashes	67–69	90	84	96
Vaginal dryness/vaginitis	7–43	19	28	75
Abnormal vaginal bleeding[a]	+	+	28	+
Breast atrophy	16–42	10	6	33
Decreased libido	7–44	22	11	61
Androgenic Effects				
Weight gain	23–28	8	13	3
Voice alteration	8	NR[c]	<5	3
Hirsutism	6–7	2	<5	15
Acne	20–42	13	10	55
CNS Effects				
Sleep disturbances	4	8	<5	11
Headaches	21–63	19	32	75
Depression/emotional lability	18–60	2–15	22	54–56
Other				
Peripheral edema	34	8	7	21
Nausea	14	NR	13	8
Seborrhea	17–52	8	10	26
Nasal irritation	NR	10	NR	NR
Injection site reactions	NR	NR	<5	6
Joint pain	+	<1	8	≥

[a]Amenorrhea is expected consequence of these medications.
+, reported but percentages not given; NR, not reported.

Based on current knowledge, the treatment of choice for J.B. is unclear. Visible endometriotic lesions can be surgically ablated, and endometriomas and adhesions can be removed at the time of diagnosis; however, the relationship between these lesions and the cause of endometriosis-related pelvic pain is not established. Pain was relieved in 69% to 96% of women 1 year after surgery[60]; however, that number decreased to 23% to 69% at 5 years.[58] Conservative surgery, like medical management of endometriosis, is palliative and not curative.[60] One study reported a 40% recurrence rate of lesions at repeat laparoscopy 5 years after initial surgery.[62] Pharmacologic therapy with danazol, GnRH agonists, OCs, or progestins relieves endometriosis-related pain, and each agent appears to be equally efficacious but their side effect profiles differ. Treatment usually is continued for 6 months, but this is an arbitrary duration. A study of 3 months versus 6 months of nafarelin showed similar response and recurrence rates between the two regimens.[66] Other treatment issues that need to be addressed include the efficacy and safety of re-treatment of women whose symptoms return, the preoperative and postoperative roles of pharmacologic agents, and therapeutic direction in women who fail to respond to a particular agent. As the pathogenesis of endometriosis is better understood, well-designed studies will be needed to evaluate the efficacy of current and future treatment options.

OCs or NSAIDs are recommended for initial management of endometriosis because of their safety profile. Progestins, danazol and GnRH agonists should be reserved for women who fail or cannot use first line agents.[58] J.B. has failed both OCs and NSAIDs and is therefore a candidate for a second-line agent.

29. J.B. is 5′2″ and weighs 100 lbs. She does not smoke and drinks alcohol only occasionally. She does not have a regular exercise program, and her calcium intake is inadequate based on dietary recall. She has no risk factors for cardiovascular disease. How does this information assist in the selection of therapy for her endometriosis?

J.B. has several risk factors that increase the likelihood that she will develop osteoporosis (see Question 48). Given the increased bone loss associated with the GnRH agonists and the fact that she has no risk factors for the development of heart disease, danazol or MPA are preferable over GnRH for J.B.

Danazol

DOSING AND DURATION OF TREATMENT

30. J.B. wants relief from pelvic pain and wishes to delay conception at this time. As a result, her physician prescribes danazol therapy. How should danazol therapy be managed in J.B.?

The initial dosage recommendation for danazol therapy is 200 to 400 mg daily. Doses of 800 mg QD may be needed for women with severe disease. The optimal duration of danazol therapy has not been determined, but most clinicians usually treat patients for 6 to 9 months, depending on the severity of the disease and the patient's response. Women with severe disease may require longer treatment periods.

J.B. can be started on 200 mg BID; this dosage should be increased by 200 mg monthly until amenorrhea is achieved or a total daily dose of 800 mg is attained. Doses >800 mg/day should not be prescribed because insufficient data exist to support the use of these doses. Danazol should be initiated on the first day of the menstrual cycle (day 1 is the first day of menstrual flow). She should be advised to use a nonhormonal contraceptive agent while taking danazol because ovulation may occur in women taking lower dosages, and virilization of female fetuses occurred in women who became pregnant while taking this drug. J.B. should experience relief of symptoms within 1 to 2 months. Dysmenorrhea usually is the first symptom to disappear, followed by dyspareunia and pelvic pain. Analgesics and antiprostaglandin agents may be used to relieve dysmenorrhea in the interim if needed (see Questions 20 to 23). While J.B. is taking danazol, she should be monitored for relief of symptoms and amenorrhea as evidence of response to therapy and for the appearance of adverse effects.

ADVERSE EFFECTS

31. **J.B. returns to the clinic 6 weeks after beginning danazol therapy. She has experienced a significant decrease in pelvic pain and dysmenorrhea; however, she complains of a 10-lb weight gain, muscle soreness, facial acne flares, oily skin, hot flushes, and mild fatigue. A lipid profile shows a significant increase in low-density lipoproteins (LDLs) and a decrease in high-density lipoproteins (HDLs) from baseline values. What subjective and objective evidence in J.B. is compatible with the adverse effects of danazol therapy?**

Most women experience some adverse reactions to danazol therapy (see Table 48-9), and most usually tolerate these side effects, which may be dose related. However, adverse effects have been severe enough to cause up to 10% of women to discontinue the drug.[67]

The common side effects of danazol therapy are related to its androgenic and antiestrogenic activity. Weight gain, an androgenic effect, is the most common complaint of patients receiving danazol and may be 10 pounds or more. Other androgenic side effects include acne, oily skin and hair, hirsutism, and deepening voice.

The hot flushes J.B. reported are secondary to the antiestrogenic effects of danazol. Other side effects related to this hypoestrogenic state are similar to those reported by postmenopausal women and include irregular vaginal bleeding, decreased breast size, and vaginal dryness. Other common side effects are muscle cramps and a generalized maculopapular skin rash that may require discontinuation of the drug.

Danazol decreases HDL cholesterol by 48% and increases LDL by 19% to 41% during treatment; values return to pretreatment levels within 1 month after therapy is withdrawn. This effect on plasma lipids is undesirable, but probably is clinically insignificant, considering the short-term use of this drug. J.B.'s lipid profile should be re-evaluated after danazol is discontinued to ensure that these plasma lipid concentrations return to baseline values.[68]

The severity of the side effects J.B. is experiencing and her willingness to continue therapy should be assessed. The side effects that occur in women taking danazol must be weighed against the relief of endometriosis symptoms. If J.B. is willing to tolerate these side effects, she should be encouraged to continue therapy.

Gonadotropin-Releasing Hormone Agonists
DOSING

32. **C.B., a 30-year-old woman with significant pelvic pain secondary to moderate endometriosis, had good pain relief after surgical ablation of endometriotic lesions 3 years ago, but her symptoms have returned. She has no cardiovascular risk factors and no risk factors for the development of osteoporosis. She wishes to try a GnRH agonist. How should GnRH agonist therapy be managed in C.B.?**

Of all the GnRH agonists, only leuprolide, nafarelin, and goserelin have FDA-approved labeling for the treatment of endometriosis (see Table 48-8). Contraindications to the use of these agents are hypersensitivity to the drug, pregnancy, breastfeeding, and undiagnosed vaginal bleeding. Leuprolide and goserelin are given by injection, whereas nafarelin is available in an intranasal dosage form. Nafarelin and leuprolide are similar in efficacy; however, nafarelin is associated with a lower incidence of bone loss and vasomotor symptoms.[69] The GnRH agonists are as effective as danazol in treatment of endometriosis related-pelvic pain.[58] Patient preference can guide product selection. Leuprolide is given IM either monthly (3.75 mg) or every 3 months (11.25 mg). Goserelin is given by subcutaneous implant every 28 days, whereas nafarelin is initiated at a dose of 200 μg twice daily with one spray in one nostril in the morning and one spray in the other nostril in the evening. If menses do not stop after 2 months, then the dose of nafarelin can be increased to 800 μg/day. Strict compliance with daily inhalations is critical to the effectiveness of this product. Missed doses can result in breakthrough bleeding or ovulation and pregnancy. For sexually active women, a nonhormonal contraceptive agent should be used during GnRH agonist therapy because GnRH agents are teratogenic (FDA category X).[24] Duration of therapy is 6 months, although several studies of 3 months of treatment suggest similar benefits to 6 months.[70] Menses usually return within 1 to 2 months after a GnRH agonist has been discontinued. C.B., as all women, should be monitored for resolution of dysmenorrhea, dyspareunia, and pelvic pain.

ADVERSE EFFECTS

C.B. should be informed of the adverse effects she may experience with GnRH agonist therapy. Adverse effects of the GnRH agonists (see Table 48-9) are related to the hypoestrogenic state they induce (see Question 33). Increases in LDL and HDL cholesterol and triglycerides were observed in goserelin clinical trials.[24] No changes in hepatic function have been reported with GnRH agonist therapy. Nafarelin has been reported to increase eosinophils and decrease white blood cells but no increased susceptibility to infections has been noted.[24] Women with rhinitis who require a topical decongestant should be advised to administer it at least 2 hours after the nafarelin dose to decrease the potential for reducing drug absorption. Significant bone loss has been associated with the use of GnRH agonists (see Question 34).

Hypoestrogenic Effects

33. **What can be done for C.B. to ameliorate the hypoestrogenic effects of the GnRH agonists?**

The addition of a progestin or estrogen-progestin combination (add-back therapy) to GnRH agonist therapy can mitigate the adverse reactions related to low estrogen levels without diminishing the benefits of the GnRH agonist. Two studies evaluating the combination of norethindrone and a GnRH agonist found a significant decrease in vasomotor symptoms in women taking both medications as opposed to those taking the GnRH agonist only.[71] The addition of an estrogen-progestin combination to a GnRH agonist diminished the occurrence of hot flashes, but did not prevent the adverse lipid changes.[71]

Bone Demineralization

34. **How significant is the bone loss associated with GnRH agonists?**

Significant bone loss, primarily of trabecular bone, is associated with GnRH-agonist therapy and is evident within 3 months of administration[72] This bone loss is significant and continues for the duration of treatment. In a study of nafarelin, average loss of trabecular bone in the spine at 3 and 6 months of therapy was 4.6% and 7.2%, respectively.[73]

Dual-energy x-ray absorptiometry (DEXA) is the preferred method for assessing bone density changes secondary to GnRH agonists. Bone density should be assessed at sites with a high proportion of trabecular bone, such as the spine.[72]

At least a portion of GnRH agonist–induced bone loss is reversible, although the recovery period may be prolonged. In one study, 60% of lost bone had been recovered 12 months after completion of therapy. In a retreatment study, bone loss was reversed completely 30 months after the initial treatment. Retreatment with a GnRH agonist was associated with a recurrence of bone loss and restoration after completion of the second course.[74]

The duration of GnRH-agonist therapy should be limited to 6 months or less if the drugs are used alone because of the association of GnRH agonists with progressive bone loss and possible irreversibility of the bone loss. To increase the clinical usefulness of these drugs, combination regimens aimed at limiting bone loss have been developed. When 20 women with endometriosis were treated with leuprolide 3.75 mg IM (depot) every 28 days for 6 months and assigned randomly to receive either 5 to 10 mg/day of norethindrone or placebo, the women assigned to the norethindrone group had significantly less bone loss.[75] At the 6-month follow-up, a reversal of bone loss back to baseline occurred only in the women who received norethindrone.

In contrast, in another study no significant bone loss was noted in women who received leuprolide and norethindrone (or a combination of estrogen and norethindrone) for 1 year compared with women who received only leuprolide for the same time.[71,75] Concomitant use of the bisphosphonate etidronate also mitigates the loss of bone mass associated with GnRH agonists.[76] For women who use a GnRH agonist for more than 6 months, the addition of a progestin, estrogen/progestin, or a bisphosphonate to their regimens is recommended. These combination regimens, however, have not been evaluated beyond 1 year of treatment.[75]

Management of Endometriosis-Related Infertility

35. H.R. is a 38 year-old female with a history of endometriosis. She had conservative surgery 3 years ago with good pain re-

lief, and her current pain has been adequately controlled with NSAIDs. She has been trying without success to get pregnant for about 18 months and is getting concerned. What interventions are useful in improving infertility related to endometriosis?

Expectant Management

Current recommendations for management of women with minimal to mild endometriosis include reassurance, emotional support, antiprostaglandins for pelvic pain, and a "wait-and-see" approach for 6 to 12 months, depending on the woman's age and duration of fertility. If the woman does not conceive within this time, the next step is surgical intervention or assisted conception with ovarian stimulation.[77] Since H.R. is 38 years old and has already been attempting to conceive for more than 1 year, further intervention is appropriate.

Pharmacologic versus Surgical Intervention

Pharmacologic therapy does not appear to be effective at improving pregnancy rates in women with endometriosis-related infertility. A meta-analysis of studies comparing drug therapy versus placebo for the management of endometriosis-related infertility reported no significant difference in pregnancy rates between the two groups.[57]

Conservative surgery in women with minimal to mild endometriosis (stage I to II) modestly increases pregnancy rates, with approximately eight women requiring surgery to achieve one additional pregnancy.[57] Although no controlled clinical trials have evaluated the fertility benefits of surgery in women with moderate to severe endometriosis (stage III or IV), anecdotal data support its role in these patients.[57]

Ovulation induction, with or without intrauterine insemination, increases pregnancy rates in women with endometriosis. In vitro fertilization also increases pregnancy rates, although it is unclear at what point this intervention should be considered, especially in less severe manifestations of the disease.[57]

PREMENSTRUAL SYNDROME
Signs and Symptoms

36. J.K., a 27-year-old woman, visits her family physician complaining of significant mood changes that occur the week before her menstrual cycle. She experiences increased irritability, sadness, and sensitivity to rejection; crying episodes for no apparent reason; an intense desire to be alone and to avoid contact with friends, family, and coworkers; and increased fatigue and appetite for sweets. Sometimes these feelings lead to verbal outbursts of extreme anger that have caused problems at home and at work. During this time, her breasts swell, she feels bloated, and she gains 2 to 3 pounds. These symptoms usually subside the first or second day after her menses begin. For 2 to 3 weeks after her menstrual period, J.K. is her "normal, usual self." Her menstrual cycles are regular, occurring every 28 to 30 days with a light flow lasting 3 to 4 days.

Pelvic, cardiovascular, and neurologic examinations are normal. The following laboratory results are within normal limits: complete blood count (CBC) with differential, serum electrolytes, thyroid function tests, serum glucose, liver function tests, and urinalysis. She has a class I (normal) Pap smear, and a serum pregnancy test is negative. She has no history of an affective disorder. Her physician makes a preliminary diagnosis of premenstrual syndrome (PMS). What symptoms of PMS does J.K. have that are consistent with the diagnosis of this syndrome?

PMS is an ill-defined problem with no standard definition. The term is applied broadly to several behavioral and somatic symptoms that occur cyclically during the late luteal phase of the menstrual cycle and disappear shortly after the onset of menses. Ninety percent of menstruating women report some degree of mood and physical changes during the premenstruum and up to 30% report moderate symptoms, but most are not disabled by these symptoms.[78] However, about 3% to 5% of women report symptoms consistent with premenstrual dysphoric disorder (PMDD), the most severe form of PMS. In these women, premenstrual symptoms are severe enough to interfere with the woman's work responsibilities and/or social relationships, create legal difficulties, and cause the woman to entertain suicidal ideations or seek medical help for physical complaints.[78] Over 150 nonspecific symptoms have been reported during the premenstrual phase (Table 48-10). J.K.'s symptoms are consistent with PMS.

The true cause of PMS is unknown. Gonadotropic hormone levels are not significantly different in women with PMS compared with controls. A reduction in serotonin (5-HT) function, triggered by the normal hormonal changes of the menstrual cycle, is thought to be the primary factor in the development of PMS/PMDD. This proposed etiology is supported by the therapeutic benefit in PMS of drugs that increase serotonin levels or affect. Changes in the level or sensitivity of other neurotransmitters, including the γ-aminobutyric acid (GABA), β-endorphin and α-adrenergic systems, may also play a role in the etiology of PMS.[79,80]

For a true diagnosis of PMS, symptoms must occur during the luteal phase of the menstrual cycle. However, symptoms may develop even in the absence of a luteal phase, suggesting that the biologic triggers that lead to PMS symptoms begin in the follicular phase of the menstrual cycle. This hypothesis is supported by the elimination of PMS symptoms by the administration of GnRH agonists, which suppress ovarian hormone production throughout the menstrual cycle.[81]

Diagnosis

37. How is the diagnosis of PMS determined in patients like J.K.?

PMS is a diagnosis of exclusion; therefore, a thorough physical examination is needed to rule out dysmenorrhea, ovarian cysts, uterine fibroids, galactorrhea, thyroid dysfunction, and endometriosis (i.e., conditions that may produce symptoms similar to those observed in PMS). A medical, gynecologic, obstetric, menstrual, and psychiatric history also should be obtained. A lifetime history of affective disorders is highly associated with PMS; therefore, the possibility that the woman has an underlying affective disorder, which is exacerbated during the premenstruum, should be ruled out.[82]

The American Psychiatric Association has developed criteria for *premenstrual dysphoric disorder* (PMDD) to characterize a subset of women with PMS who experience primarily mood changes of a severity comparable to a major depressive disorder.[82] Based on these criteria (Table 48-11), a diagnosis of PMDD requires a 1-year history of symptoms associated with most menstrual cycles, and prospective documentation

Table 48-11   Diagnostic Criteria for Premenstrual Dysphoric Disorder

A. In most menstrual cycles during the past year, symptoms listed in B occurred during the last week of the luteal phase and remitted within a few days after onset of the follicular phase. In menstruating females, these phases correspond to the week before and a few days after the onset of menses. (In nonmenstruating females who have had a hysterectomy, the timing of the luteal and follicular phases may require measurement of circulating reproductive hormones.)

B. At least 5 of the following symptoms have been present for most of the time during each symptomatic late luteal phase, with at least 1 of the symptoms being either number 1, 2, 3, or 4:
1. Marked affective lability (e.g., feeling suddenly sad, tearful, irritable, or angry)
2. Persistent and marked anger or irritability
3. Marked anxiety, tension, feelings of being "keyed up" or "on edge"
4. Significantly depressed mood, feelings of hopelessness, or self-deprecating thoughts
5. Decreased interest in usual activities (e.g., work, friends, hobbies)
6. Easily fatigued or significant lack of energy
7. Subjective sense of difficulty in concentration
8. Marked change in appetite, overeating, or specific food cravings
9. Hypersomnia or insomnia
10. Other physical symptoms (e.g., breast tenderness or swelling, headaches, joint or muscle pain, a sensation of "bloating," weight gain)

C. The disturbance seriously interferes with work or with usual social activities or relationships with others.

D. The disturbance is not merely an exacerbation of the symptoms of another disorder, such as major depression, panic disorder, dysthymia, or a personality disorder (although it may be superimposed on any of these disorders).

E. Criteria A, B, C, and D are confirmed by prospective daily self-ratings during at least 2 symptomatic cycles (the diagnosis may be made provisionally before this confirmation).

Adapted from reference 82.

Table 48-10   Common PMS Symptoms

Physical Complaints	Behavioral and Psychologic Complaints
Abdominal bloating	Anger
Acne	Anxiety
Ankle edema	Crying, labile mood
Backache	↓ efficiency or work performance
Breast swelling and/or tenderness	↓ judgment
Constipation	↓ feeling of well-being
Diarrhea	Depression, sadness, or hopelessness
Fatigue, hypersomnia, insomnia	
Headache	Difficulty concentrating
↑ cravings for sweet or salty foods	Loneliness, social withdrawal
Joint and muscle pain	Irritability
Nausea and vomiting	Restlessness, agitation
Weight gain	Self-deprecating thoughts
	Tension

PMS, premenstrual syndrome.
From reference 29, 82.

of symptoms during the luteal phase for at least two cycles. Symptoms must remit during the follicular phase. At least five of the listed symptoms must be sufficiently severe to interfere seriously with the patient's work or personal relationships. These criteria exclude women with affective disorders that are exacerbated during the luteal phase and those who experience predominantly physical symptoms.

In an effort to standardize the diagnostic criteria for PMDD, the National Institute of Mental Health proposed setting the degree of symptom change between the luteal and follicular phases at 30% or greater.[83] However, this guideline is not universally used. Several validated tools are available to aid in the diagnosis of PMDD, including the Calendar of Premenstrual Experiences (COPE), the Premenstrual Assessment Form and the Prospective Record of the Impact and Severity of Menstrual Symptoms calendar.[84,85] To confirm a diagnosis of PMDD, J.K. should keep a daily diary for two consecutive menstrual cycles to demonstrate a temporal relationship between her symptoms and the luteal phase and to document the severity of these symptoms (Table 48-12). In addition, she should indicate the presence of menstrual flow, weight, and daily basal body temperature readings to help determine when ovulation occurs. The diary establishes a baseline for each patient and documents the most troublesome symptoms. Once therapy is selected for these symptoms, the diary can aid in assessing patient response.

Treatment

38. Using J.K.'s diary (see Table 48-12) and the criteria for PMDD, assess her symptoms and recommend treatment.

A review of J.K.'s diary reveals that her symptoms are related to the luteal phase because they begin after ovulation and end with menses. She has at least five symptoms required for the diagnosis of PMDD: fatigue, irritability, inability to concentrate, breast tenderness, and bloating. These symptoms are graded severe and show at least a 30% change in severity between the luteal and follicular phases.

Selecting therapy for PMS is based on patient presentation. If mild to moderate symptoms consistent with PMS are present, lifestyle modifications can be tried initially. These changes, which include salt and caffeine restriction, regular exercise, and increased intake of complex carbohydrates and tryptophan-rich foods, may provide some relief.[29,84,86] However, most of these lifestyle modifications are not well studied and, as sole intervention, are unlikely to markedly improve the severe psychological symptoms of PMDD. Because J.K. has been diagnosed with PMDD, psychotropic drug therapy targeted to her most severe symptoms should be initiated. Selective serotonin reuptake inhibitors (SSRIs), serotonergic tricyclic antidepressants, and anxiolytics have been evaluated in the treatment of affective symptoms of PMS. In controlled trials, 20% to 30% of women receiving placebo will demonstrate sustained improvement in PMS symptoms; therefore, only agents with clinically proven efficacy should be used.[87]

Selective Serotonin Reuptake Inhibitors

SSRIs are considered by some to be the drugs of choice for the treatment of PMS (Table 48-13).[85] In a meta-analysis of 15 randomized placebo-controlled trials, SSRIs overall had a 60% to 70% response rate at improving the psychological and physical symptoms of PMD. Fluoxetine and sertraline are FDA-approved for the treatment of PMS. Citalopram and paroxetine have each shown clinical efficacy in a single controlled trial. Among the SSRIs studied, only fluvoxamine did not demonstrate significant improvement compared with placebo.[88] Initial studies of SSRIs used daily dosing to good effect. Subsequently, intermittent dosing of fluoxetine, sertraline, and citalopram during the luteal phase (i.e., the 14 days before menses) was also effective, with onset of efficacy occurring within the first treatment cycle.[85,88] Fluoxetine 90 mg (enteric-coated) was significantly better than placebo when a dose was given on days 14 and 7 before onset of menses; however, a single dose given on day 7 before menses was not better than a placebo.[89] SSRIs used in the treatment of depression generally exhibit a lag time to onset of efficacy of 4 to 6 weeks. The rapid onset of efficacy with intermittent dosing in PMS suggests a different mechanism of action in this condition.[88]

Although PMS is a chronic disorder, most of the studies of SSRIs have been less than 6 months in duration. A nonblinded study evaluated use of fluoxetine in PMS patients for an average of 18 months. Although therapeutic benefit was maintained, symptoms recurred in those who discontinued treatment.[85]

ADVERSE DRUG REACTIONS

SSRIs are generally well tolerated; however, in a systematic analysis of trials, discontinuation rates in women taking SSRIs was 2.5 times higher than in those taking placebo.[88] Side effects commonly reported with SSRIs include decreased libido (45%), delayed orgasm (28%), nausea (22%), sweating (19%), weight gain (20%), headache (16%), vertigo (14%), and insomnia (12%).[85] There has not been a study directly comparing the side effects seen with daily versus luteal-phase dosing; however, some studies have noted fewer adverse reactions with intermittent dosing.[88] Withdrawal symptoms have not been reported upon discontinuation of luteal-phase dosing.[85] Lengthening or shortening of menstrual cycles has been reported in 6% to 15% of women using fluoxetine.[90]

Other Antidepressants

Non-SSRI antidepressants that affect serotonin are also beneficial in treating PMS (see Table 48-13). Clomipramine, a tricyclic antidepressant, given daily or during the luteal phase, decreases the psychological symptoms of PMS.[85] Venlafaxine, dosed daily, is significantly better than placebo at relieving psychological and physical symptoms of PMS.[85] In an open-label study, nefazodone effectively decreased symptoms compared with baseline.[91] However, a placebo-controlled trial of continuous or luteal-phase dosing with nefazodone showed no significant benefit compared with placebo for irritability, depression or tense mood. Only affect lability was significantly improved by nefazodone compared to placebo.[92] Nortriptyline 50 to 150 mg daily improved PMS symptoms over baseline, but this benefit has not been confirmed in a controlled trial.[29] In comparison trials, antidepressants that affect noradrenaline, such as desipramine and bupropion, are not as efficacious as the SSRIs in relieving symptoms of PMDD.[85]

Anxiolytics

Alprazolam, a short-acting benzodiazepine, in some trials seems to improve PMS symptoms. In one study, luteal-phase

Table 48-12 Menstrual Cycle Daily Diary Chart

Grading Severity of Symptoms:
1 = Mild; general awareness of discomfort but does not interfere with daily activities
2 = Moderate symptoms present; interferes with activities but not disabling
3 = Severe; symptoms disabling, unable to meet daily social, family, or work obligations

Each Day:
1. List the major symptoms (mood, physical, emotional, behavioral) that you experience during your menstrual cycle
2. Grade the severity of the symptom
3. Record daily weight
4. Record basal body temperature
5. Check the days of the cycle when menstrual flow occurs

Month 1

Day of month	1	2	3	4	5	6	7	8	9	10	11	12	13	14	15	16	17	18	19	20	21	22	23	24	25	26	27	28	29	30	31
Day of cycle	18	19	20	21	22	23	24	25	26	27	28	1	2	3	4	5	6	7	8	9	10	11	12	13	14	15	16	17	18	19	20
Menses												*	*	*	*																
Breast tenderness and pain				1		1	1	1	1	1	1																				
Sadness/depression				1	2	3	3	3	3	3	3	2	1																		
Fatigue				3	3	3	3	3	3	3	3	2	1																		
Irritability					2	2	3	3	3	3	3																				
Inability to concentrate							2	2	3	3	3																				
Daily weight	130	130	130	130	130	130	130	130	130	130	130	131	131	131	130	130	130	130	130	130	129	129	129	129	128	129	128	128	128	128	128
Basal body temperature	98.0	98.2	98.0	98.2	98.0	98.0	98.2	97.8	98.0	97.8	97.6					97.8	97.6	97.6	97.8	97.6	97.8	97.8	97.6	97.4	98.4	98.0	98.4	98.6	98.0	98.2	98.0

Month 2

Day of month	1	2	3	4	5	6	7	8	9	10	11	12	13	14	15	16	17	18	19	20	21	22	23	24	25	26	27	28	29	30
Day of cycle	21	22	23	24	25	26	27	28	1	2	3	4	5	6	7	8	9	10	11	12	13	14	15	16	17	18	19	20	21	22
Menses									*	*	*	*	*																	
Breast tenderness and pain				1	1	1	1	1	1																					
Sadness/depression		1	2	3	3	3	3	3	2	2	1																			
Fatigue		2	2	3	3	3	3	3	2	1	1																			
Irritability	1	2		2	2	2	3	3				1																		
Inability to concentrate										1		1																		
Daily weight	128	128	128	128	128	128	128	128	129	129	128	128	128	128	128	128	128	128	128	128	128	128	128	128	128	129	128	128	128	128
Basal body temperature	98.0	98.2	98.4	98.0	98.2	97.8	98.0	97.4					97.6	97.6	97.8	97.8	97.6	97.8	97.6	97.6	97.6	97.2	97.2	97.0	98.4	98.6	98.0	98.2	98.2	98.0

Table 48-13 Psychotropic Drugs for the Management of PMS

Drug (Brand Name)	Daily Dosing Regimen (mg)	Intermittent Dosing Regimen (mg)[a]
SSRIs		
Citalopram (Celexa)	20	10–30
Fluoxetine (Prozac)	20	20
Fluvoxamine (Luvox)	100	NS
Paroxetine (Paxil)	5–30	NS
Sertraline (Zoloft)	50–150	100
Other Serotonergic Antidepressants		
Nefazodone (Serzone)	200–600	NS
Venlafaxine (Effexor)	50	NS
Tricyclic Antidepressants		
Clomipramine (Anafranil)	25–75	25–75
Nortriptyline (Aventyl, Pamelor)	50–125	NS
Anxiolytics		
Alprazolam (Xanax)	NS	1–2[b]
Buspirone (BuSpar)	NS	25–60

[a] Day 14 until onset of menses.
[b] Dose to be tapered over 2 days after onset of menses to prevent withdrawal symptoms.
NS, not studied; SSRIs, selective serotonin reuptake inhibitors.

dosing of alprazolam 0.5 to 3.0 mg/day was effective in reducing tension, irritability, anxiety, and feelings of being out of control. However, women who had luteal-phase exacerbation of anxiety and depression that were also present during the follicular phase did not do better with alprazolam compared with placebo.[93] In another study, alprazolam 0.75 mg/day during the luteal phase, reduced physical and psychological symptoms, but overall was less effective than fluoxetine 20 mg/day.[94] A placebo-controlled trial noted a 50% or greater improvement in 37% of women taking luteal-phase alprazolam, which was significantly better than the response seen in women taking oral progesterone or placebo. In this latter study, alprozolam was most effective at improving mood, mental function and pain, but did not significantly reduce physical symptoms or food cravings.[95] A fourth study of luteal-phase administration of alprazolam, up to 2.25 mg/day, did not improve symptoms in women with PMS.[96] Daytime sedation is the most commonly reported side effect with alprazolam. Luteal-phase dosing may limit the risk of drug dependence of this benzodiazepine, but the dose should be tapered over several days to minimize mild withdrawal symptoms.

Buspirone, a partial 5HT$_{1A}$ receptor agonist, significantly reduces irritability when given daily, but does not seem to affect physical symptoms of PMS. The intermittent dosing of buspirone in one study was not significantly better than placebo. This result may have been related to the short duration of the study or the buspirone dose (20 mg/day).[92] Lightheadedness and dizziness were commonly reported with buspirone.

In summary, anxiolytics may be useful in treating women with mild symptoms, especially if related to anxiety or insomnia, or in treating women who do not respond to first-line therapy (see Table 48-13). Luteal-phase dosing of alprazolam appears more effective than daily dosing. If benzodiazepine drug dependence is a possible concern, or if intolerable side effects occur, buspirone may be tried.

39. J.K. would like to try natural products to help with her PMS symptoms. What is the evidence for the use of vitamins, minerals, or herbal products for PMS?

Calcium and Magnesium

In two small trials and one large study, calcium supplementation improved the symptoms of PMS.[97,98] Elemental calcium, 1,200 mg/day for three menstrual cycles, decreased negative affect, water retention, food cravings, and pain in 466 women with PMS.[98] Overall, the calcium-treated group had a 48% reduction in symptoms compared with a 30% reduction in the placebo group. Side effects were not significantly different between the two groups. Because calcium is well tolerated and may provide other benefits (see *Postmenopausal Osteoporosis* in this chapter), calcium supplementation should be recommended to women with symptoms of PMS.

Trials of magnesium supplementation have produced varying results. One trial found that magnesium, 360 mg/day during the luteal phase was associated with a decrease in negative affect, whereas a second trial found that magnesium 200 mg/day reduced symptoms of fluid retention but had no effect on psychological symptoms.[99] The conflicting results may be caused by differences in the dosing regimens of the magnesium and differing levels of magnesium stores in the study subjects.

Pyridoxine

A meta-analysis of nine placebo-controlled studies was unable to show any overall benefit of pyridoxine in women with PMS.[100] However, an analysis of three of the trials, which specifically examined depressive symptoms, showed that pyridoxine was more effective than placebo in improving depressive symptoms. There did not appear to be a dose-related effect from pyridoxine. Although a well-controlled trial is needed to confirm the benefits of pyridoxine, dosages of 50 to 100 mg/day can be tried in women with primarily depressive symptoms. As neuropathy has been reported with pyridoxine dosages as low as 100 mg/day, patients should be advised to monitor for neurologic symptoms and to discontinue therapy and seek medical attention if they occur.

Vitamin E

Two small, randomized, placebo-controlled studies of vitamin E 300 to 400 IU/day reported improvement in all symptom groups except fluid retention.[99] The studies were of marginal quality, but vitamin E is generally considered safe and could be recommended as part of a treatment plan.

Herbal products

Although many herbal products are promoted for the relief of PMS symptoms, good quality trials supporting their use are lacking. Four small controlled studies of evening primrose oil failed to demonstrate significant benefit over placebo.[99] Traditional uses of Chastetree or Chasteberry (agnus castus fruit, *vitex agnus castus*) include management of PMS. A randomized, double-blind, placebo-controlled trial of agnus cactus fruit extract 20 mg daily showed a treatment response rate of 52% compared with 24% for placebo. Individual symptoms of irritability, mood alteration, anger, headache, and breast fullness were improved. Bloating was not significantly altered compared with placebo. The incidence of side effects was low, but long-term safety is unknown.[101]

Combination Oral Contraceptives

40. J.K is considering starting on OCs. How might this affect her PMS? What effect do noncontraceptive hormones have on PMS?

Although OCs are commonly prescribed for PMS symptoms, some women may notice lessening of their cyclic symptoms, whereas others may experience worsening of their PMS symptoms, especially fluid retention and mood swings.[102] In one uncontrolled trial, a monophasic OC containing drospirenone, a progestin with antimineralocorticoid effects, reduced symptoms of fluid retention and negative affect.[102] For women in need of contraception, OCs may be tried cautiously, but the patient should be advised to monitor for exacerbation of PMS symptoms.

Progestins and Estrogen

Progestins and progestagens have long been advocated for the treatment of PMS based on a belief that the condition was caused by inadequate progesterone production. In the 1990s, progesterone suppositories were included in the majority of regimens for PMS.[103] For the most part, progesterone deficiency has been ruled out as the cause of PMS, but the hormone does play a role in PMS. Women who experience "medical ovariectomy" with a GnRH agonist may have a recurrence of symptoms with the additional of a progestin to their regimen.[81] A systematic review of 10 placebo-controlled trials of progestins did not support a significant benefit from either oral or vaginal administration.[103] Currently, there is little clinical support for the use of progestins for the treatment of PMS symptoms.

Exogenous estrogen, administered by patch or implant, improves premenstrual mood symptoms.[104] However, in women with an intact uterus, addition of a progestin is necessary to prevent endometrial hyperplasia, which may result in the recurrence of PMS symptoms.

41. What other therapeutic modalities are available to treat symptoms of PMS and what evidence exists to support their use?

NSAIDs

NSAIDs do not improve the mood symptoms of PMS. However, they effectively relieve physical symptoms (e.g., headache, joint pains) related to PMS.[86]

Spironolactone

In women with PMDD, spironolactone 100 mg/day given on day 14 of the menstrual cycle through the first day of menses is associated with decreased irritability, depression, breast tenderness, and food cravings compared with placebo. Intermittent use is well tolerated.[105] Other diuretics may also be effective but good clinical evidence is lacking. Intermittent, low-dose diuretic therapy may be appropriate for women who experience a documented, significant weight gain during the luteal phase.

Gonadotropin-Releasing Hormone Agonists

GnRH agonists effectively eliminate many of the physical and psychological symptoms of PMS. In 8 out of 10 double-blind, placebo-controlled trials, GnRH agonists were more effective than placebo at reducing symptoms in women with PMS. Women with premenstrual exacerbation of ongoing dysphoric symptoms did not show any significant improvement.[104]

Adverse effects of the GnRH agonists are related to their hypoestrogenic action (see Question 33). Increased rate of bone loss is the duration-limiting factor (see Question 34). In an effort to decrease the hypoestrogenic side effects and decrease or prevent bone loss, GnRH agonist therapy with a combination of estrogen and progestin (add-back therapy) has been advocated (see Question 34). Mezrow and others[106] combined placebo or leuprolide 7.5 mg IM every 4 weeks, with CEE 5 days per week and 10 days of MPA every fourth cycle of leuprolide in 10 women. PMS symptoms were significantly improved in the women receiving leuprolide compared with those receiving placebo. A nonsignificant decrease in bone mineral density occurred, but lipids were not changed in the leuprolide group; no endometrial hyperplasia was seen in the treatment group.[106] Use of a bisphosphonate (etidronate) can protect bone from the effects of a GnRH agonist.[76]

In summary, GnRH agonists can be used for the management of PMS in women who do not respond to more conservative measures. However, additional information is needed to determine the optimal regimen for these agents.

Bromocriptine and Danazol

Bromocriptine mesylate 5 to 7.5 mg/day, administered usually at mid-cycle and continued until the onset of menses, relieves the pain of cyclic mastodynia.[86] The most common side effects are nausea, vomiting, dizziness, and headaches. In a placebo-controlled study of danazol 400 mg/day, PMS symptoms were more improved in the treatment group with the exception of depression.[66] Another study compared danazol 200 mg on days 14 to 28 of the menstrual cycle with placebo in 100 women with PMS and premenstrual breast pain.[107] The intermittent danazol regimen was more effective than placebo in reducing breast pain but had no effect on other symptoms of PMS. No increase in adverse effects occurred with intermittent danazol compared with placebo. Because of the lack of efficacy data and the risk of possible side effects with danazol, its use in PMS should be limited to women who have failed other therapies.[86]

THE CLIMACTERIC AND POSTMENOPAUSE

The climacteric, or perimenopause, is the phase in the female aging process between the reproductive and nonreproductive years and is characterized by waning ovarian function and decreasing estrogen concentrations. Menopause is the last spontaneous episode of physiologic uterine bleeding and may occur several years after the beginning of the climacteric.

Although age at puberty has declined steadily and longevity has increased, the average age of women at menopause has remained approximately 51.4 years for centuries.[108] Thus, women today may spend one-third of their lives with reduced ovarian hormonal concentrations. Age at menopause may be genetically determined and does not appear to be influenced by race, physical characteristics, age at menarche, age at last pregnancy, socioeconomic status, or alcohol consumption. Cigarette smoking may decrease age of menopause by 1 to 2 years. Postulated mechanisms for this effect of cigarette smoking include an effect of nicotine on the CNS or ovaries or an increase in hormonal metabolism.[109]

Pathophysiology

The climacteric occurs in response to an age-related decline in estrogen secretion from ovarian follicles. Throughout life, the number and function of the ovarian follicles decrease secondary to ovulation and follicular atresia so that postmenopausally, ovarian weight decreases to one-third of premenopausal ovarian weight.[108] The remaining follicles require higher concentrations of FSH for follicular maturation: without maturation, estradiol-17β (E_2) production, ovulation, and progesterone secretion do not occur. Estradiol serum concentrations fall from a mean of 120 ng/L premenopausally to 18 ng/L after menopause, which leads to lengthening menstrual intervals, anovulation, oligomenorrhea, and dysfunctional uterine bleeding (all clinical manifestations of the approaching menopause).[108] The earliest pituitary-ovarian axis change during the climacteric is an increase in serum FSH concentration that continues beyond the final menstrual period, eventually exceeding serum LH concentrations, which are also elevated. Both gonadotropins reach their maximum concentrations 2 to 3 years after menopause. Although gonadotropin concentrations may be many times those observed during the reproductive years, residual ovarian follicles become refractory to gonadotropin stimulation. A declining ovarian production of estradiol-17β leads to lower circulating estradiol concentrations, an alteration in the cyclic estrogen pattern, and a decreased negative feedback to the hypothalamic-pituitary axis.[108,109]

After menopause, the primary estrogen no longer is estradiol but the less potent estrogen, estrone, which is largely derived from the peripheral conversion of the androgen, androstenedione. The aromatase enzyme responsible for this conversion is found in fat, liver, and hypothalamic nuclei and increases with age and body weight.[108]

Postmenopausally, approximately 40 μg of estrone and 6 μg of estradiol are produced daily compared with premenopausal daily production of 80 to 300 μg for estrone and 80 to 500 μg for estradiol.[109] Levels of estradiol in the postmenopausal woman result primarily from the conversion of estrone to estradiol. Estrogen concentrations do not vary in a cyclic fashion as they do in women who are in their reproductive years.

Ovarian progesterone production also is diminished during the climacteric with progesterone concentrations after menopause becoming unmeasureable.[109] These low progesterone plasma concentrations may result in unopposed estrogen effects even if estrogen levels are also low. Androgen production declines during the climacteric but to a lesser degree than the decrease in estrogen. Concentrations of androstenedione, the predominant androgen, are decreased from 1,500 pg/mL in premenopausal women to approximately 800 pg/mL after menopause.[108] Testosterone is produced by the ovary, adrenal glands, and extra-glandular conversion of androstenedione in premenopausal women. After menopause, ovarian production accounts for at least 50% of circulating testosterone.[108]

Estrogen Receptors

Two estrogen receptors (ER-α and ER-β) appear to interact with and activate the same genes. These receptors each have a DNA-binding domain and a ligand binding domain. At their DNA-binding domains, they share 97% of the same amino acids, whereas only 60% of their amino acids are the same at their ligand-binding domains.[110] Binding of a ligand to the ER can induce a change in the conformation of the receptor, triggering agonist or antagonist effects, depending on the nature of the structural change. In addition, the presence of cellular adaptor proteins, called co-activators or co-repressors, may mediate the interaction with the target gene, determining the expression of the agonist or antagonist response.[111] ER-α is expressed at a moderate to high level in the adrenal gland, kidney, ovary, pituitary, uterus and mammary glands (also in male testes), whereas ER-β exhibits activity to a higher degree in the brain, bladder, lung, ovary, and uterus (also in the male prostate). Both appear to be well expressed in bone. Finding ER-β in the brain may explain the effect of estrogen on learning and memory in postmenopausal women. As more knowledge is obtained about the interaction of estrogen and other ligands with the ER, a clearer understanding of the risks and benefits of therapy should emerge.

Target Tissues Affected by Decreased Estrogen Concentrations

Clinical symptoms in the climacteric period primarily are associated with an estrogen deficiency, which directly affects target tissues (e.g., hypothalamic-pituitary axis, ovary, endometrial lining of the uterus, vaginal epithelium, skin, bone).[108,109] Vasomotor symptoms (e.g., hot flushes), genitourinary atrophy, and osteoporosis improve with ET. Other organ systems (e.g., intestines, skin, eyes) may also be favorably affected by estrogen, but more clinical data are needed before estrogen can be recommended specifically for these targets.

Hot Flushes
Signs and Symptoms

42. **D.R., a 50-year-old woman, has been having sudden feelings of warmth over her chest accompanied by a patchy flushing of her skin and increased sweating for the past month, especially after drinking coffee or wine or if she is upset. She now visits her physician because she has been waking up shivering from a perspiration-drenched gown nightly for the past week. D.R. does not take any medications. She has not had a menstrual period for at least 6 months; her physical examination was normal for a 50-year-old woman. What is the assessment based on the data provided for D.R.?**

It appears that D.R. is experiencing hot flushes, a vasomotor symptom experienced by 50% to 85% of all women in the climacteric years.[108,109] The onset of vasomotor symptoms may precede the last menstrual period, but the prevalence is highest during the 2 years after menopause and declines over time.[109] Symptoms persist for longer than 1 year in 80% and longer than 5 years in 25% of women.[108] Of women who have had a bilateral oophorectomy before menopause, 37% to 50% also experience hot flushes.[108] Symptoms include a feeling of warmth in the chest, neck, and facial areas that may be accompanied by visible red flushing. The flushes are characteristically episodic rather than continuous.

Other vasomotor symptoms include headaches, dizziness, palpitations, nausea, vomiting, diaphoresis, and night sweats.[108] Insomnia and sleep deprivation associated with hot flushes may result in fatigue, nervousness, irritability, forgetfulness, inability to concentrate, and depression. An increased environmental temperature, the ingestion of hot liquids or alcohol, and mental stress also may provoke hot flushes. An increase in body temperature generally precedes the actual flush, triggering heat-loss mechanisms (e.g., cutaneous vasodilation, sweating) that constitute the flush and restore normal body temperature. An average hot flush is approximately 4 minutes in duration.[112]

43. **What are the underlying causes of the hot flushes associated with the climacteric?**

The exact trigger for hot flushes is unknown, but there clearly is an association between the development of hot flushes and declining estrogen concentrations that occur during the climacteric. Estrogen therapy (ET) is more effective than placebo in reducing hot flushes, and when exogenous estrogen is withdrawn, hot flushes promptly resume. Although total estrogen concentrations do not differ between women who experience hot flushes and those who do not, there may be differences in concentrations of biologically active estrogen (i.e., estrogen not bound to sex hormone-binding globulin) that cross into the CNS. Estrogen deficiency in the CNS may then affect the neurons in the hypothalamus that produce hot flushes.[108,112]

LH, adrenocorticotropic hormone, and growth hormone concentrations increase before a hot flush while an increase in cortisone levels occurs after the hot flush. These changes do not appear to cause the flush, but may be triggered by the same factors that initiate the hot flush. Alterations in the concentration and sensitivity of catecholamine or serotonin receptors can be induced by changes in gonadal hormone levels. As both these neurotransmitters are believed to be involved in temperature regulation mediated by the hypothalamus, decreasing levels of estrogen may initiate a cascade of events that culminates in a hot flush.[112]

Treatment
ORAL ESTROGEN WITH OR WITHOUT A PROGESTIN

44. **What therapeutic modalities might benefit D.R.?**

First-line treatment for hot flushes includes avoidance of known triggers (e.g., hot beverages, alcohol, warm environments), regular exercise, biofeedback, and relaxation techniques.[112] If the patient continues to experience bothersome symptoms, drug therapy should be considered. It is important to note that there is a high placebo response in clinical trials evaluating interventions for hot flushes.

Menopausal hot flushes are highly responsive to ET. The effective estrogen dose for the relief of vasomotor symptoms may vary with each individual; however, low doses seem to be as effective as higher doses.[113] Treatment for a patient such as D.R. could begin with a low dose of oral estrogen, such as 0.3 to 0.45 mg of CEE (Premarin) or an equivalent dose of another oral estrogen. The dose should then be adjusted until the lowest dose that will control symptoms is achieved. Estrogen may be administered on a continuous or a cyclic basis (e.g., 25 days per month).

Women such as D.R. with an intact uterus should receive estrogen and progestin therapy (EPT) rather than ET only. The progestin, which can be given on a continuous or cyclic basis, is added to decrease the risk of endometrial hyperplasia and the twofold or greater increase of endometrial cancer associated with unopposed estrogen use.[114] Progestin should be given for at least 10 days each month to eliminate the risk of endometrial cancer.[115] Oral progestins commonly used to antagonize the endometrial effects of estrogen are divided into three classes: natural progesterone, C-19-nortestosterone derivatives, and C-21 derivatives. MPA (Provera), a C-21 derivative, is the most commonly used progestin in the United States in HRT (hormone replacement therapy) regimens. Data suggest that 5 to 10 mg/day of oral MPA is needed for at least 12 days/month to prevent endometrial hyperplasia when used in cyclic regimens, whereas 1.5 to 5 mg/day are recommended when used in continuous regimens.[116] Oral micronized progesterone 200 mg daily for 12 days/month also decreases the risk of endometrial hyperplasia.[117] (See Table 48-14 for products used for hormone replacement and Questions 54 through 56.)

EPT administered continuously may result in variable patterns of breakthrough bleeding for the first year of therapy; however, amenorrhea should occur in 75% to 85% of women thereafter.[118] EPT administered cyclically will result in regular withdrawal bleeding. Bleeding that begins after the tenth day of progesterone in women on cyclic therapy is considered normal. Bleeding during the estrogen-only phase or during the first 10 days of progestin therapy or in a woman receiving continuous EPT requires evaluation. Continuous administration may be preferred because it should increase patient compliance in women who prefer to have as little estrogen-associated bleeding as possible.

Because hot flushes are self-limiting, discontinuation of ET/EPT should be attempted every 6 to 12 months, unless the patient needs to continue therapy for other postmenopausal problems. Before estrogen is started, a baseline histologic evaluation of the endometrium may be performed to rule out endometrial hyperplasia or adenocarcinoma. If either is revealed, estrogen should not be instituted. Obtaining a baseline histologic evaluation may not always be possible, especially in women who are extremely estrogen deficient and have little, if any, endometrial lining.

TRANSDERMAL ESTRADIOL

As an alternative to oral estrogen, D.R. can use estradiol transdermally. If a transdermal system (patch) is used, she should be started on a low dose (estradiol 0.025 or 0.05 mg/day), and only if her symptoms do not abate, should the dose be increased to 0.1 mg/day. The transdermal system should be used for at least 3 weeks each month to relieve vasomotor symptoms. The patch should be applied to a clean, dry area on the trunk such as the abdomen rather than the breasts or to skin that is oily, abraded, or irritated. In addition, the old patch should be removed before applying the new one. For a patient with an intact uterus, a progestin (either orally or transdermally in a combination patch) should be administered to prevent endometrial hyperplasia.

Table 48-14   Hormone Replacement Therapy

Drug (Brand Name)	Initial Daily Dosage
Estrogens	
Conjugated equine estrogens[a] (Premarin)	0.3 mg
Synthetic conjugated estrogens[b] (Cerestin)	0.625 mg
Estropipate[a] (piperazine estrone sulfate) (Ogen)	0.625 mg
Ethinyl estradiol[b] (Estinyl)	0.2 mg
Micronized estradiol[a] (Estrace)	0.5 mg
Estradiol transdermal system[a] (various brand name products)	0.05 mg/24-hr patch applied weekly or twice weekly
Esterified estrogen[a] (Estratab, Menest)	0.3 mg
Estradiol acetate (Femring, Estring)[b]	0.05 mg/24 hr ring inserted vaginally every 90 days
Progestins	
Medroxyprogesterone acetate[b] (various generic and brand name products)	2.5 mg for continuous regimens or 5 or 10 mg for sequential regimens
Norethindrone/norethindrone acetate[b] (various brand name products)	2.5–5 mg for continuous and sequential regimens
Progesterone[b] (Prometrium)	100–300 mg for continuous and sequential regimens
Estrogen and Progestin Combinations	
Prempro[a]	0.3 mg conjugated equine estrogens and 1.5 mg MPA
Premphase[a]	0.625 mg conjugated equine estrogens for 14 days and 0.625 mg conjugated equine estrogens and 5 mg MPA for 14 days
Combipatch[b]	0.05 mg estradiol with either 0.14 or 0.25 mg norethindrone
femhrt, Activella[a]	1 mg norethindrone acetate and 5 μg ethinyl estradiol
Prefest[a]	1 mg estradiol and 0.09 mg norgestimate
Climara Pro[a]	0.045 mg estradiol/0.015 mg levonorgestrel/24 hr patch once weekly

[a]Approved by the FDA for prevention of osteoporosis.
[b]Not approved by the FDA for prevention of osteoporosis.

PROGESTINS

Progestins given without estrogen can mitigate vasomotor symptoms. In a group of men and women with hot flushes secondary to chemotherapy, megestrol acetate 20 mg PO BID reduced hot flushes by 85% compared with a 21% reduction when placebo was used.[119] MPA 20 mg/day and depot MPA 150 mg IM every 3 months also effectively reduce hot flashes similarly.[112,120] Side effects of progestins include vaginal bleeding, bloating, weight gain, and blood clots.[112] Progestins are a reasonable alternative for women who cannot take estrogen but need highly effective therapy for hot flushes.

ANDROGENS

Although androgens do not relieve vasomotor symptoms in postmenopausal women, women with low androgen levels and symptoms of generalized fatigue, low libido and a decreased sense of well-being benefit from androgen therapy.[112,121] In women with symptoms consistent with androgen deficiency, a short-term trial of androgen therapy can be given. If the symptoms do not improve with maximal doses of the androgen, it should be discontinued.

CLONIDINE

Clonidine is modestly effective in reducing menopausal flushes but is less effective than estrogen. Clonidine 0.1 to 0.4 mg/day orally or 0.1 mg/day transdermally decreases hot flushes 20 to 46%.[112,120] This effect may be attributed to clonidine's selective stimulation of postsynaptic α_2-receptors found in the vasomotor center of the medulla oblongata and in the hypothalamus. Dry mouth, constipation, drowsiness, and orthostatic hypotension are common, especially with high clonidine doses, and limit its usefulness.

PSYCHOTROPIC AGENTS

Some serotonergic antidepressants decrease hot flushes. In placebo-controlled trials, venlafaxine, fluoxetine, and paroxetine significantly decreased frequency of hot flushes, whereas sertraline did not.[112] Gabapentin 300 mg TID significantly decreased hot flush frequency and severity compared with placebo. Side effects (e.g., dizziness, somnolence, rash, peripheral edema) were more common in the active drug group.[122]

PHYTOESTROGENS

Plant-based phytoestrogens (e.g., isoflavones in soy products) exert mild estrogenic effects. A low incidence of menopausal symptoms in populations that consume high soy diets led to the use of isoflavones for the treatment of vasomotor symptoms. Some studies noted a decrease in hot flush frequency and severity whereas others noted no clinical benefit.[123] These conflicting results may be due to differences in the source and dose of the isoflavones and study duration. Other than gastrointestinal side effects, soy protein is generally well tolerated. As they may also provide some cardiovascular protection via beneficial changes in lipid levels, dietary supplementation with soy-based foods is reasonable. At this time, data are inadequate to support a recommendation for isolated isoflavone supplements for management of menopausal symptoms.

BLACK COHOSH

Black cohosh (*cimicifuga racemosa*) is one of the most popular herbs for the management of menopausal symptoms. Three of four controlled clinical trials found it to be effective in decreasing hot flushes. The usual dose of 40 mg BID is generally well tolerated but use beyond 6 months in duration has not been evaluated.[123]

OTHER THERAPY

Data in support of the use of vitamin E, ginseng, evening primrose oil, or dong quai to manage hot flushes are lacking (see Chapter 3, Herbs and Nutritional Supplements).[123]

TRANSDERMAL ESTRADIOL VERSUS ORAL ESTROGENS

45. **What are the potential advantages associated with transdermal estradiol over oral estrogens for vasomotor symptoms?**

Orally administered estrogens are primarily metabolized to estrone because of a significant hepatic first-pass effect, which does not occur when estrogens are administered transdermally, vaginally, or parenterally. This first-pass effect produces elevations of hepatic factors such as renin substrate, sex hormone–binding globulin, cortisol-binding globulin activity, and thyroxine-binding globulin; these substances are not elevated significantly in women using transdermal estrogen.[124] The significance of these elevations is poorly understood, but increased renin substrate and an alteration in clotting factors did not appear to increase the risk of hypertension or coagulation problems in women using oral agents. Estrogen, given orally, decreases total cholesterol and LDL but increases HDL cholesterol and triglycerides. Transdermal estrogen has similar effects on lipid levels with the exception of triglyceride levels, which were decreased with transdermal estrogen.[113] Although it has been postulated that transdermal estrogen may be less likely to induce gallbladder disease because it lacks a first-pass effect, data do not support this conclusion.[125]

Genitourinary Atrophy
Signs and Symptoms

46. **R.J., a 60-year-old woman who has remarried recently, complains of debilitating pain associated with intercourse. She also complains of vaginal dryness during intercourse, pain and urgency on urination, and occasional nocturia. On physical examination, she is noted to have sparse, gray pubic hair. Her labia minora have a pale, dry appearance while the labia majora appear flattened. Her vagina is small with a pale, dry epithelium. Vaginal and urine specimens were obtained for cultures. Direct endometrial sampling also was performed for cytologic and histologic studies. How would you assess R.J.'s problem?**

R.J. appears to be experiencing symptoms associated with genitourinary atrophy, a problem that begins as estrogen levels decline. The vulva, vagina, uterus, urethra, and trigone of the bladder all are sensitive to changes in circulating estrogens and are prone to atrophic changes as estrogen stimulation diminishes with age. The vagina decreases in size and loses its rugal pattern: its mucosa becomes pale, thin, and dry. The labia minora shrink in size, whereas the labia majora are flattened because of decreased subcutaneous fat and tissue elasticity.[108] Thus, the postmenopausal vagina is traumatized more easily with intercourse. Postmenopausal women who engage in regular coital activity have less atrophic vaginal changes compared with those of similar age and estrogen levels who do not have regular intercourse.[126] Also, postmenopausal women who have breaks in their sexual intercourse patterns,

such as that experienced by R.J. between the death of her first husband and remarriage, tend to experience dyspareunia (painful coitus) with the resumption of intercourse. About 10% to 40% of postmenopausal women experience symptoms of urogenital atrophy, although many do not seek medical attention for this condition.[127]

Changes in vaginal pH from 4.5 to 5 (observed during the reproductive years) to 6 to 8 after menopause may predispose women such as R.J. to increased bacterial colonization and possible *infectious vaginitis.* Although R.J.'s problem is probably atrophic vaginitis, a vaginal culture for possible bacterial-related vaginitis may be needed.

Secondary to declining estrogen concentrations, atrophic changes also occur in the urethra and bladder trigone, which predispose postmenopausal women to the *urethral syndrome,* a recurrent, nonbacterial urethritis. Symptoms associated with the syndrome include increased dysuria (painful urination), frequency and urgency of urination, postvoid dribbling, and nocturia.[108] R.J. is experiencing many of these symptoms. However, the incidence of bacteriuria, which may cause similar symptoms, also is increased in postmenopausal women (7% to 10% versus 4% in premenopausal women).[108] A urine culture may be indicated in R.J to exclude bacteria as the cause of her symptoms.

Incontinence is another common problem in older women that can cause significant discomfort and embarrassment. Incontinence may be acute or chronic and some patients experience both forms. Chronic urinary incontinence can be divided into overflow incontinence, urge incontinence, and stress incontinence. ERs are in high concentration in the urethra and trigone of the bladder; however, conjugated equine estrogen (CEE) 0.625 mg did not ameliorate urinary symptoms, whereas CEE 2.5 mg increased maximal urethral pressures. Although vaginal administration of ET can decrease urinary symptoms, such symptoms respond slowly to ET/EPT, requiring up to 12 months of treatment for clinical benefit.[128] Combination therapy with estrogen and α-adrenergic agonists is more effective than ET alone in treating urinary symptoms.[128] Therefore, a trial of estrogen is reasonable if there are no contraindications to its use.

Treatment
VAGINALLY ADMINISTERED ESTROGENS

47. **What would be a reasonable vaginal dose of estrogen for R.J. to decrease her vaginal and urinary symptoms?**

Symptoms associated with genitourinary atrophy respond to either local or systemic ET.[108] Estrogens reverse vaginal epithelial thinning and decrease the vaginal pH. The vaginal administration of estrone, estradiol, or CEE cream may alleviate symptoms associated with atrophic vaginitis. As hormonal therapy should begin with the lowest dose that will relieve symptoms, 0.3 to 0.625 mg of CEE cream (or an equivalent dose of another vaginally administered estrogen cream) can be prescribed initially, followed by an increase to 1.25 mg daily if symptoms have not been abated with the initial dose. The cream should be applied daily intravaginally for 1 to 3 months, then intermittently for the relief of symptoms.[108] Vaginal tablets containing 25 μg of 17β estradiol used daily for 2 weeks, then twice weekly, or a vaginal ring (E-String) that releases 7.5 μg/day of estradiol over 90 days are also effective in treating genitourinary symptoms.[126] Although vaginally administered estrogen can be absorbed systemically, it is unclear whether the amount absorbed is adequate to provide protection against osteoporosis. ET should be discontinued as soon as possible unless it is needed for other menopausal problems.

The endometrium should be evaluated histologically before ET is started to rule out endometrial hyperplasia or adenocarcinoma. If either is observed, ET should not be started. Use of a progestin with vaginal ET is generally considered unnecessary.[126] Vaginal bleeding during intravaginal ET requires evaluation. (See Questions 54 to 56 for discussions of risks, benefits, contraindications, and adverse effects associated with ERT.)

ORAL AND TRANSDERMAL ESTROGENS

Oral or transdermal estrogen administration is an alternative to vaginal administration if the patient does not wish to use a vaginal cream. The urinary symptoms that R.J. has been experiencing also may respond to ERT if the urethral syndrome caused these symptoms.

OTHER TREATMENT

If a patient with genitourinary atrophy is unwilling or unable to use estrogen, a vaginal bioadhesive (Replens) is similar in efficacy to ET in providing relief from symptoms without altering vaginal cell morphology.[126] Genitourinary benefits from orally consumed herbal treatments (e.g., black cohosh, isoflavones) have not been established.

POSTMENOPAUSAL OSTEOPOROSIS

Although osteoporosis has many definitions, the World Health Organization (WHO) defines it as a disease "characterized by low bone mass and microarchitectural deterioration of bone tissue, leading to enhanced bone fragility and a consequent increase in fracture risk."[129] Other definitions have been developed to help clinicians diagnose osteoporosis. For example, a WHO Working Group defined osteoporosis as "the presence of bone mineral density (BMD) or a 'T' score that is 2.5 standard deviations (SDs) or more below the mean peak value in young, healthy adults."[130,131] Osteopenia, a lesser degree of bone loss, is defined as a T score that is between 1 and 2.5 SDs below the mean peak value in young, healthy adults. A Z score (mean value for BMD in normal subjects of the same age and sex) can help in the diagnosis of osteoporosis. For example, a z score <-1 at the lumbar spine or proximal femur indicates "a value in the lowest 25% of the reference range, a value at which the risk of fracture is approximately double. A Z score <-2 indicates a value in the lowest 2.5% of the reference range, a level associated with a considerably larger increase in the risk of fracture."[131]

Incidence and Fracture Sites

Osteoporosis is a major health problem that affects over 9.4 million people in the United States and is especially prevalent among postmenopausal white women.[132] Women in other ethnic groups may have a slightly lower risk. For example, women of Asian descent have rates of osteoporosis similar to that for White women, whereas African-Americans have a lower risk. The incidence for osteoporosis increases with age; 30% of women between the ages of 70 and 79 and 70% of women 80 years of age or older develop osteoporosis without medical intervention.[133]

Annually, 1.5 million osteoporosis-related fractures occur in elderly Americans.[134] Osteoporosis-related fracture sites predominantly include the vertebrae, distal radius (Colles' fracture), and hips. Approximately 40% of White women age 50 and older will sustain an osteoporosis-related fracture (i.e., fractures of spine, distal forearm, or hip) in their lifetime.[135] Patients who suffer hip fractures have a 12% to 20% higher mortality rate relative to persons of the same sex and similar age without fractures.[136] In addition, hip fractures result in a multitude of complications for the elderly, including prolonged hospitalization, decreased independent living, depression, fear of future falls, and lifelong disability. Vertebral fractures may be painless or result in pain that usually lasts <3 months. The initiating injury may be as minor as a cough or turning over in bed. Vertebral collapse or deformity may result in loss of height, kyphosis (dowager's hump), abdominal protuberance, decreased pulmonary function, and chronic back pain.

The annual direct cost for treating osteoporosis and osteoporosis-related fractures in the United States is estimated at $15 billion; a figure that may double in the next 30 years if prevention and early intervention measures do not reduce the incidence.[137–139] Thus, the impact of osteoporosis on the health care system as the baby-boom generation ages and lifespan increases is potentially staggering.

Physiology

Structurally, bone is either cortical or cancellous (trabecular), with the adult skeleton containing 80% cortical and 20% cancellous bone. Dense cortical bone forms the outer shell of the skeleton, whereas porous cancellous bone forms the interior structures in a honeycombed fashion. The proportions of cortical and cancellous bone vary at different sites in the skeleton, with cortical bone predominating in long bones (approximately 90%) except at their ends, which are predominantly cancellous. This type of bone is also found in the vertebrae and distal forearms. A balance between osteoblast and osteoclast activity results in a continuous remodeling process; osteoclasts resorb bone, whereas osteoblasts help reform bony surfaces and fill bony cavities.

Bone remodeling normally is a continuous process that occurs in discrete skeletal foci called *bone-remodeling units*. This process begins with bone resorption that is initiated by osteoclasts excavating lacuna found on the surface of cancellous bone, or it occurs when cavities are formed in cortical bone (Fig. 48-2). Enzymes produced in this process dissolve bone mineral and proteins. Thereafter, bone formation occurs as osteoblasts gradually refill spaces created during the resorption process. This occurs as collagen fills in bone cavities, which then are calcified.

Changes in Bone Mass

Bone mass peaks during the third decade of life. At about 35 years of age, cortical bone gradually begins to decrease 0.3% to 0.5% yearly in both women and men.[140] With menopause, the decline in 17β-estradiol concentrations further accelerates cortical bone loss by 2% to 3% per year that is superimposed

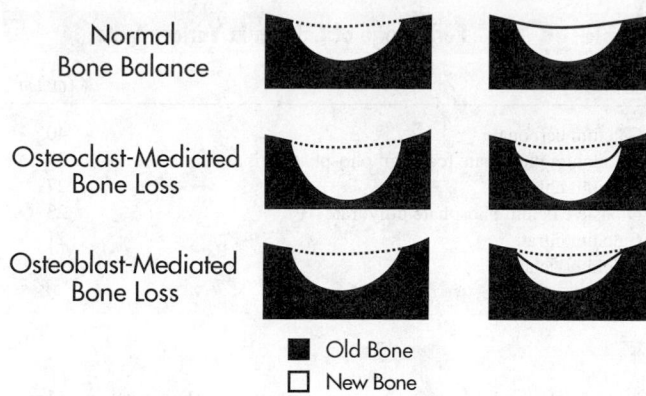

FIGURE 48-2 The bone remodeling cycle at the cellular level. In normal young adults *(top panels)*, the bone removed by the osteoclasts *(left)* is replaced completely by the osteoblasts *(right)*. In high-turnover bone loss *(middle panels)*, such as that which occurs in women soon after menopause, the osteoclasts create a deeper resorption cavity that is not refilled completely. In low-turnover bone loss *(bottom panels)*, such as that which occurs with aging, the osteoclasts create a resorption cavity of normal or decreased depth, but the osteoblasts fail to refill it. (Reproduced by permission of the New England Journal of Medicine 1992;372:621.)

on age-related bone loss. This loss gradually decreases over the next 8 to 10 years.[140] This hormone-related, accelerated bone loss can also occur after surgical oophorectomy.

Cancellous bone loss begins between the ages of 30 and 35 with yearly decreases in women of 0.6% to 0.8% (linear decrease) or 2.4% (curvilinear decrease).[140,141] Age-related cancellous losses in women appear to begin up to a decade earlier than cortical bone loss. The effect of menopause on cancellous bone loss is controversial; some studies indicate an increased rate of loss, whereas others do not.[141] Thus, early cancellous bone loss in conjunction with postmenopausal decreases in cortical (and possibly cancellous) bone may lead to increased vertebral and distal forearm fractures, which predominate early after menopause.[140] Women may lose 50% of cancellous and 30% of cortical bone over their lifetimes, whereas men may lose only 30% and 20%, respectively.[134,142] In addition, women may have an increased risk for osteoporosis because throughout life they have 30% less bone mass than men of a similar age.[143]

Classification

Osteoporosis can be defined as primary or secondary. Sometimes primary osteoporosis is further classified as type I or II. Type I, "postmenopausal osteoporosis," is associated with increased cortical and cancellous bone loss resulting from increased bone resorption. It typically occurs in women during the first 3 to 6 years after menopause. It is manifested by vertebral fractures, distal radius fractures, hip fractures, and even an increased tooth loss secondary to osteoporosis of the mandible. It may occur earlier in women who have had an oophorectomy.

Type II, senile osteoporosis, occurs in both women and men 75 years of age and older with a female:male ratio of 2:1.[141] Cortical and cancellous bone losses are proportional. These persons are at greatest risk for hip, pelvic, and vertebral fractures.

Secondary osteoporosis, occurs secondarily to the use of various medications or the presence of particular disease states (Table 48-15). This type of osteoporosis can occur at any age and is equally common in men and women.

Risk Factors

48. T.J., a 28-year-old thin White woman, is worried about developing osteoporosis. Her 75-year-old maternal grandmother has osteoporosis, and recently her postmenopausal mother (age 53) was told that she was at increased risk for osteoporosis. T.J. is 5'2", weighs 108 lb, and is in good health. She jogs and occasionally does aerobic exercise. Her diet typically consists of cereal for breakfast, a sandwich for lunch, and meat with vegetables for dinner. Her only milk consumption consists of 1 cup of skim milk on her cereal. She occasionally has a dairy product for lunch or dinner. T.J. takes no medications, vitamins, or calcium supplement routinely. She occasionally takes a medication for headache or menstrual cramps. She does not smoke cigarettes and occasionally drinks alcohol socially. Does T.J. have an increased risk for developing osteoporosis?

Table 48-15 lists risk factors associated with the development of osteoporosis. T.J. has several risk factors that could increase her risk for osteoporosis. She is a white woman of small stature and low weight, has a positive family history, and has a low calcium intake.

Gender, Race, Heredity, and Body Build

White and Asian women in the United States are generally at greater risk for osteoporosis than other ethnic or racial groups, especially those who are of small stature such as T.J. and those who are proportionally underweight for their height. The significance of heredity as a risk factor for osteoporosis is being studied. It has been proposed that approximately 75% of the genetic effect on a person's chance to develop osteoporosis is due to a particular allelic variant in the gene that is responsible for encoding the 1,25-dihydroxyvitamin D receptor.[144] This study suggests that heredity may be important in the development of osteoporosis. Women with a first-degree relative with osteoporosis typically have low bone mass.[145] In addition, women of African-American ancestry have higher BMD than do white women.

Table 48-15 Risk Factors Associated with the Development of Osteoporosis

↑ age	Predisposing medical problems (e.g.,
Female gender	chronic liver disease, chronic renal
Caucasian or Asian	failure, hyperthyroidism, primary hy-
Family history	perparathyroidism, Cushing's syn-
Small stature	drome, gastrointestinal resection, or
Low weight	malabsorption)
Early menopause or	Drugs (e.g., corticosteroids, long-term
oophorectomy	anticonvulsant therapy [e.g., phenytoin
Sedentary lifestyle	or phenobarbital], excessive use of
↓ mobility	aluminum-containing antacids, long-
Low calcium intake	term high-dose heparin, furosemide,
Excessive alcohol problems	excessive levothyroxine therapy)
Cigarette smoking	

Mobility/Physical Activity

Immobility resulting from prolonged bed rest (especially in the elderly) has been associated with decreased bone mass. Conversely, weight-bearing exercise (e.g., walking, running, step aerobics, lifting weights) helps prevent bone loss. Exercise throughout life helps maintain skeletal mass and may help reduce bone loss in postmenopausal women. Exercise appears to stimulate osteoblastic activity to help maintain bone mass.[146]

Calcium Intake

Calcium, in conjunction with vitamin D, is needed to strengthen bones, increase bone mass, and decrease fracture rates. Girls and women such as T.J. need an adequate calcium intake to achieve and help maintain optimal bone mass, but the typical American diet is low in calcium. The National Academy of Sciences published recommendations for calcium intakes based on age. For example, they recommended 1,000 mg/day of elemental calcium for women younger than 51 years of age.[147] The National Institutes of Health recommend the same amount of calcium for women in this age group.[148] Calcium is best ingested from the diet (Table 48-16 for the calcium content of various foods), but if the diet is low in calcium, supplements can be used (Table 48-17; see Questions 49, 52, and 63).

Cigarette Smoking and Alcohol Ingestion

Although T.J. does not smoke and only occasionally ingests alcohol, it is important to include questions concerning cigarette and alcohol use when obtaining a medication history from an person at risk for osteoporosis. Women who smoke, especially those who are thin, have an increased risk for fractures compared with nonsmokers.[149,150] In addition, premenopausal smokers have lower estrogen serum concentra-

Table 48-17 Percentage of Calcium in Various Salts

Salt	% Calcium
Calcium carbonate	40
Tricalcium phosphate (calcium phosphate, tribasic)	39
Calcium chloride	27
Dibasic calcium phosphate dihydrate	23
Calcium citrate	21
Calcium lactate	13
Calcium gluconate	9

tions and undergo menopause earlier than nonsmokers, whereas postmenopausal smokers using exogenous estrogen have lower estrogen serum concentrations than expected.[150]

Excessive alcohol use by both women and men may predispose them to low BMD, but it is unclear whether moderate alcohol consumption has an effect on bone mass. The mechanism may be a direct effect of alcohol on osteoblasts, or it may be secondary to nutritional compromise that could result in impaired calcium and vitamin D intakes that can result in decreased bone formation.[151] Alcoholics also may be at risk for increased falls.

Other Potential Risks
DRUGS
Various medications that may be associated with the development of secondary osteoporosis are listed in Table 48-15.

DISEASES
Patients with various diseases may be at higher risk than the general population for secondary osteoporosis (see Table 48-15 for specific diseases). In addition, women who have undergone oophorectomy before menopause have a high risk for developing osteoporosis at a younger age.

Prevention
Premenopausal Women

49. **Although T.J. is premenopausal, what recommendations could be made to decrease her future risk of developing osteoporosis?**

T.J.'s course of action should be to maximize her peak bone mass and prevent or decrease bone loss. This may be accomplished by ingesting a nutritious diet with adequate calcium and vitamin D intakes while developing a lifelong exercise program.

VITAMIN D INTAKE
Vitamin D helps regulate calcium by a complex interaction that also involves parathyroid hormone (also see Chapter 12, Fluid and Electrolyte Disorders) and having a direct effect on bone. Adult requirements for vitamin D range from 200 to 600 IU/day (200 IU/day for nonpregnant women ages 19 to 50).[147] T.J. should be able to obtain an adequate vitamin D intake from her diet and exposure to sunlight. T.J. could increase her dietary vitamin D intake by adding more milk that contains vitamin D and calcium to her diet. Other sources of vitamin D include liver and fatty fish. She could also take a multiple vitamin daily that contains vitamin D 200 IU

Table 48-16 Calcium Content of Selected Foods

Food	Serving Size	Calcium (mg)
Dairy Products		
Milk, dry nonfat	1 cup	350–450
Yogurt, low fat	1 cup	345
Milk, skim	1 cup	300
Milk, whole	1 cup	250–350
Cheese, cheddar	1 oz	211
Cheese, cottage	1 cup	211
Cheese, American	1 oz	195
Cheese, Swiss	1 oz	270
Ice cream or ice milk	½ cup	50–150
Fish		
Sardines, in oil	8 med	354
Salmon, canned (pink)	3 oz	167
Fruits and Vegetables		
Calcium fortified juices	1 cup	100–350
Spinach, fresh cooked	½ cup	245
Broccoli, cooked	1 cup	100
Collards, turnip greens	½ cup	175
Soy beans, cooked	1 cup	131
Tofu	1 oz	75
Kale	½ cup	50–150

and calcium. Current studies do not show that increased vitamin D helps prevent osteoporosis; however, higher-than-recommended doses could lead to toxicity.

EXERCISE

T.J. should be encouraged to participate regularly in weight-bearing exercises such as jogging, walking, running, biking, tennis, or weight lifting and to continue exercise appropriate for her age throughout life because weight-bearing exercise is important for the maximization and maintenance of bone. Aerobic training is important in controlling weight, increasing cardiorespiratory endurance, and decreasing the risk for cardiovascular disease.

Young women such as T.J. should be informed that excessive exercise may cause amenorrhea. Women with exercise-induced amenorrhea have been reported to have decreased bone mineralization and an increased risk for fractures.[152]

CALCIUM INTAKE

T.J.'s diet should be calcium-enriched to ensure that she receives 1,000 mg/day of elemental calcium. Optimally, calcium should be from dietary sources. Because dairy products are the major source of dietary calcium in the United States, T.J. should select low-fat dairy products to decrease her caloric intake and minimize her fat intake when possible. If T.J. were lactose intolerant, she could select dairy products containing lactase. Although nondairy sources may contain lower amounts of calcium, they may be included in a diet plan to increase calcium content, especially when a woman cannot or will not use dairy products. (See Table 48-16 for the calcium content of selected foods.) The ingestion of foods rich in phytates may decrease calcium absorption.

If T.J. cannot meet her daily calcium requirement from dietary sources, she can use a calcium supplement. Table 48-17 lists the percentage of elemental calcium available from selected calcium salts. See Question 50 for further information on calcium supplements.

MAGNESIUM

Currently, it appears that magnesium supplementation is not needed for the prevention of osteoporosis. People who might need extra magnesium beyond that found in their diets most likely are elderly women or individuals with gastrointestinal disease.[145]

ISOFLAVONES

Isoflavones are a class of phytoestrogens found in soybeans, soy products, and red clover. Although some promote their use for the prevention or treatment of osteoporosis, the current data, mostly from small studies of short duration, are insufficient to support the use of isoflavones for this purpose.[145]

SMOKING CESSATION

A woman who smokes should be encouraged to stop because cigarette smoking is associated with lowered BMD and increased fracture risk as well as other health problems.[145]

50. If T.J. needs a calcium supplement, which calcium salt should be recommended?

Calcium carbonate is usually the calcium salt recommended for women such as T.J. because it is reasonably priced and contains the highest percentage of calcium (40%); this allows for fewer tablets per day to meet a person's calcium requirement. If T.J. needs a calcium supplement, she should be advised to take it in divided doses (e.g., 500 to 600 mg/dose) to increase absorption. In addition, calcium should be taken with fluids during or after meals that are low in fiber to increase absorption. Because their absorption may be decreased, medications such as tetracyclines, iron, quinolones, and atenolol should not be taken concomitantly with calcium. T.J. should be informed that the most common adverse effects associated with calcium are constipation, GI irritation, and flatulence. Doses exceeding 2,500 mg/day of elemental calcium can result in hypercalcemia, hypercalciuria, and, possibly, urinary stones. If T.J. or any family member has a history of urinary stones, she should be under medical supervision while taking calcium.

Postmenopausal Women

51. T.J.'s mother, M.J., age 53, also is a woman of small stature and low weight. She occasionally walks in the evenings, but otherwise exercises little. She currently is taking a calcium supplement to maintain her total calcium intake (dietary plus supplementation) of about 1 g/day. She takes no medications except occasional acetaminophen for headaches. M.J. was a cigarette smoker but stopped in her late twenties; she rarely drinks alcohol. She is in good health and has had no gynecologic surgery or major diseases. Her last menstrual period was approximately 6 months ago, but she began experiencing menstrual irregularity 2 years ago. M.J. has been experiencing some menopausal symptoms such as hot flushes, but states that these are mild and occur only at night. M.J., worried about developing osteoporosis, decided to make an appointment with her gynecologist to discuss preventive measures. A dual-energy x-ray absorptiometry (DEXA) measurement of her spine was administered, which noted her T score to be a −2. In addition to the DEXA, what other information should be obtained to determine whether she is at risk for developing osteoporosis or already has osteoporosis?

A medical history (including a medication history) and physical examination are needed in addition to a risk factor analysis. Other diagnostic tests should be obtained if needed.

From her history and risk factor analysis, it is determined that M.J. shares similar risk factors for osteoporosis with her daughter, but in addition she is early in the postmenopausal phase and was a previous smoker. M.J. has no loss of height, does not complain of back pain, and does not have signs of kyphosis (abnormal curvature of the spine in the thoracic region), all of which may be signs of osteoporosis. (Women can lose 1 to 1.5 inches in height as part of the normal aging process, secondary to shrinking of intervertebral disks.[145]) Biochemical markers of bone turnover are not needed for M.J. at this time.

The North American Menopause Society (NAMS) recommends a BMD measurement in women such as M.J., who are less than 65 years of age if risk factors for osteoporosis are present (e.g., body weight of less than 127 pounds, occurrence of a nonvertebral fracture, first-degree relative with a history of a vertebral or hip fracture).[145] The National Osteoporosis Foundation recommends BMD testing for women 50 to 60 years of age when risk factors for osteoporosis are present and for women over age 60, even when risk factors are not present for osteoporosis.[153]

Although DEXA is the gold standard for determining BMD, other methods can also be used for screening but should not be used for diagnosis nor to follow a patient's response to therapy[145] (Table 48-18). For postmenopausal women who are not receiving medications for osteoporosis prevention, a DEXA may be useful no more frequently than every 3 years because it takes approximately 5 years for a 0.5 change in SD from the mean in either T or Z scores to occur.[145] In addition, it has been estimated that for every one decrease in SD from the mean, a 10% to 12% change can occur in BMD. The magnitude of this change can be translated into a 1.5-fold change in risk for fractures.[145] As a result, a BMD determination should be obtained no more frequently than every 2 years to assess the effectiveness of pharmacologic interventions for the prevention or treatment of osteoporosis in a postmenopausal woman.[145]

52. **What preventive measures would help decrease M.J.'s likelihood of developing osteoporosis?**

EXERCISE

Although M.J. goes for walks occasionally, she should begin an aerobic and weight-bearing exercise program appropriate for her age and physical condition because exercise (particularly weight-bearing exercise) in conjunction with appropriate calcium and vitamin D intake is important for maintaining healthy bones. Weight-bearing exercise improves muscular function and agility, whereas aerobic exercise helps improve cardiovascular health (also see Question 49).

VITAMIN D INTAKE

Like T.J., it is important for M.J. to have an adequate vitamin D intake from her diet and from exposure to sunlight. The RDA for vitamin D for women between 51 and 70 years of age is 400 IU/day, and those >70 years of age an intake of 600 IU/day may be needed.[147] This may be achieved from ingesting foods that contain vitamin D (e.g., vitamin D fortified milk, fatty fish) or from ingesting a daily multiple vitamin containing vitamin D. For elderly persons who have limited exposure to sunlight because of minimal outdoor activities or because they live in areas where winters are long, vitamin D supplementation may be needed. Patients with renal or hepatic disease may need supplementation with active vitamin D metabolites, which are available by prescription only. (For further information about vitamin D, see Question 49.)

CALCIUM INTAKE

Because of her postmenopausal status and other risk factors, M.J. should increase her current intake of calcium to at least 1,200 mg/day to prevent bone loss.[147] The National Institutes of Health Consensus Development Panel on Optimal Calcium Intake recommended that postmenopausal women who do not receive EPT (estrogen-progestin therapy—formerly called hormone replacement therapy or HRT) should have a daily elemental calcium intake of 1,500 mg. Although calcium has antiresorptive activity, its use alone by postmenopausal women is not an alternative to ET, EPT, bisphosphonates, or a selective estrogen receptor modulator (SERM) for osteoporosis prevention. Calcium supplementation, however, helps delay BMD loss in postmenopausal women, and its use reduces the risk of hip fractures by 25% to 70%.[154] (Also see Questions 48 and 49.)

Estrogen-Progestin Therapy

In the past, EPT would have been considered first-line prevention for osteoporosis in a postmenopausal woman such as M.J., who has a uterus and is at risk for osteoporosis (see Table 48-15) based on her risk factors and T score. Since the publication of the Heart and Estrogen/Progestin Replacement Study (HERS) I[155] and HERS II[156] and the National Institutes of Health Women's Health Initiative (WHI),[157] health care providers are less likely to prescribe EPT for only osteoporosis prevention or to continue its use after a woman no longer needs EPT for postmenopausal symptoms such as hot flushes.

HERS was not undertaken to see whether EPT would have positive effects on BMD or fracture rates but to see whether EPT use could decrease the risk of further cardiac disease in women who already had at least one cardiac event. Thus, it was really undertaken to explore hormone use as secondary prevention of cardiac disease. Likewise, the WHI was not undertaken to primarily evaluate the effects of ET or EPT on BMD or fracture risk associated with osteoporosis but to explore ET/EPT use as primary prevention of cardiac disease—to decrease the incidence of coronary heart disease (CHD), nonfatal myocardial infarction, and CHD-related deaths in women.[157] The WHI was also undertaken to help determine whether ET/EPT use could lower the incidence of colorectal cancer while also determining the extent of ET/EPT association with invasive breast cancer risk. In addition to hormone trials, other studies were undertaken to explore the effects of low-fat diets and calcium and vitamin D supplementation. Overall, 16,608 women ages 50 to 79 (average age approximately 63 years) with a uterus were enrolled in the EPT arm of the WHI (8,506 received Prempro [0.625 mg CEE and 2.5 mg MPA] with the others on placebo). Another 10,739 women who had previously had a hysterectomy were enrolled in the ET arm of the study. None of the women in either study arm was perimenopausal or less than 50 years of age.

Table 48-18 **Techniques for Measuring Bone Mineral Density**

Technique	Abbreviation	Measurement Sites
Dual-energy x-ray absorptiometry	DEXA	Hip, spine, total body bone mineral density
Peripheral dual-energy x-ray absorptiometry	PDXA	Forearm, fingers, heel
Peripheral quantitative computed tomography	PQTC	Forearm
Quantitative ultrasound	QUS	Heel, shin
Quantitative computed tomography	QCT	Spine
Single-energy x-ray absorptiometry	SXA	Heel

In May 2002, the EPT arm of the WHI was terminated prematurely after 5.2 years because overall risks for individuals enrolled in the treatment group exceeded benefits and the predetermined Global Index for risks exceeded a hazard ratio of 1 (i.e., 1.15). The ET versus placebo clinical arm of this study is to be continued until March 2005 because the level of risk noted in the EPT arm has thus far not been observed. Risks such as stroke, venous thromboembolism, and breast cancer (see individual information about these risks in the sections that follow) were at the levels anticipated for those receiving EPT, but the risk of CHD noted in WHI had not been anticipated. EPT did not appear to prevent CHD. The WHI clinical outcomes noted a CHD hazard ratio of 1.29, which translates into a relative risk of 1.29 at 5.2 years of therapy with an absolute risk of 37 cases of CHD per 10,000 women/year taking EPT versus 30 cases in the same number of women receiving placebo.[157]

A lack of cardiac protection was also noted for women in the HERS study who were in the EPT group, but these women had previous cardiac disease and the investigators were looking for secondary prevention of cardiac disease. In the WHI, the investigators were exploring the use of EPT as primary cardiac prevention. This latter point has been debated because of the older age of many of the women enrolled in WHI. In addition, some of the women were using statins (i.e., HMG-CoA reductase inhibitors) and/or aspirin at baseline. After that time, there was not a follow-up on whether medications such as these were instituted or how adherent patients were with medications. For these reasons, some of the women might have had underlying cardiac disease and thus, the prevention sought from EPT was really not just primary but also secondary cardiac prevention. In addition, younger women or those most recently postmenopausal might have responded differently to EPT than older women as to cardiac events. Currently, there is no breakdown of CHD data by age or time since menopause to address this issue. (Please see Question 57 for further information about cardiovascular disease as it relates to the WHI and HERS.)

After the findings from the EPT arm of the WHI study were published, the FDA worked with the manufacturer of the estrogen/progestin product used in the WHI EPT Study to develop new language for the product package inserts. Information inserts now have a black box warning about the use of these products for the prevention of cardiovascular disease. Approved indications for use of these products include treatment of moderate to severe vasomotor symptoms associated with menopause, treatment of symptoms associated with moderate to severe menopausal vulvar or vaginal atrophy, and/or the prevention of postmenopausal osteoporosis.[158] Information contained in these inserts states that if the product is "solely for the prevention of postmenopausal osteoporosis, therapy should be considered for women at significant risk and non-estrogen medications should be carefully considered."[158] Although there is no specific time limit for the use of estrogen-containing products for osteoporosis prevention, it is implied in the package insert that the product should be used for as short a time as possible. For example, a product should be used for the length of time a woman is experiencing menopausal symptoms. Table 48-14 lists oral and transdermal estrogens approved for the prevention of osteoporosis.

ESTROGEN EFFECTS ON BMD AND FRACTURE RATE

53. What effect does estrogen have on BMD in a postmenopausal woman such as M.J.? Can EPT or ET decrease fracture rates?

The primary effect of estrogen on BMD is related to its antiresorptive activity, which decreases bone loss and lowers fracture rates. Although not fully understood, the interplay between estrogens and their receptors may stimulate osteoblast activity and the secretion of insulin-like growth factor 1 and transforming growth factor-β. In addition, estrogens possibly inhibit interleukin-1 (IL-1), IL-6, and the release of tumor necrosis factor. Both ER-α and ER-β have been isolated from primary osteoblastic cells of neonatal rats, which if it can be translated to humans, shows that both estrogen receptors may have beneficial effects on BMD.[159] Estrogen may also affect calcium absorption and vitamin D receptors in osteoblasts.

An estimated 10% to 15% of a woman's bone mass is estrogen dependent[160]; therefore, estrogen (oral or transdermal) appears to effectively prevent osteoporosis in postmenopausal women.[145] The addition of a progestin to ET for women with a uterus does not appear to decrease estrogen efficacy as an osteoporosis preventative. Over 50 randomized, placebo-controlled clinical trials have shown that ET or EPT can increase BMD by 4% to 6% in the spine and 2% to 3% in hips.[145] These levels of BMD also have been noted to be maintained after 3 years of therapy.[145]

In the Postmenopausal Estrogen/Progestin Interventions (PEPI) Trial, a randomized, placebo-controlled, multicenter 3-year study of 875 postmenopausal women averaging 56 years of age, BMD increased in the spine 3.5% to 5% and in the hips at an average of 1.7% in all groups who received oral CEE 0.625 mg with or without a progestin (MPA or micronized progesterone [MP]).[161]

In observational studies, ET/EPT appears to reduce fracture rates in postmenopausal women. In one meta-analysis, hip fracture risk was reduced by 25% for postmenopausal women who had used ET/EPT.[162] A second meta-analysis found that the use of ET or EPT for at least 1 year significantly reduced nonvertebral fracture risk (RR 0.73). This effect on fracture rate was somewhat reduced in women who began ET or EPT after age 60 years.[163]

The Study of Osteoporotic Fractures, a large prospective cohort study, showed decreased risks for wrist and nonspinal fractures in estrogen users who were over 65 years of age and decreased risks in the incidence of hip fractures in those older than 75.[164] The relative risk for nonspinal fractures in postmenopausal women who were current estrogen users versus those not receiving ET or EPT was 0.66. Vertebral bone mass increases in women with known osteoporosis who receive ET or EPT, which can then decrease fracture rates.[165]

Although the use of EPT in the WHI resulted in risks overall exceeding benefits, women receiving EPT had significant decreases in hip and vertebral fractures compared to women in the placebo group (hazard ratio of 0.66 with a 95% adjusted CI of 0.33 to 1.33, and 0.66 with a 95% adjusted CI of 0.32 to 1.34, respectively).[157] Another way to look at this issue is in terms of absolute differences in rates of major disease end points. Over the 5.2 years of the WHI EPT study, there were 20 fewer hip fractures per every 10,000 women receiving EPT compared with a similar number of women who received placebo.

In another randomized, placebo-controlled trial that enrolled 2,763 postmenopausal women (HERS), a different outcome was noted. No reduction in fracture risk was observed, even after 4 years of EPT (CEE 0.625 mg/day and MPA 2.5 mg/day). Women enrolled in HERS had histories of cardiac disease, but many were at low risk for fractures because they did not have osteoporosis. Women were enrolled in HERS to determine whether EPT use would decrease the incidence of cardiovascular disease while fracture risk was a secondary observation.[155]

ESTROGEN PRODUCT SELECTION AND DOSING

54. Based on labeling information for ET and EPT, M.J. is most likely not a candidate for EPT for osteoporosis prevention unless a decision is made to begin EPT to decrease her menopausal symptoms such as the hot flushes. If an individual is to receive EPT for osteoporosis prevention as well as menopausal symptoms, which estrogen product should be selected and at what dose?

Although estrogen products used to control hot flushes are addressed in Questions 44 and 45, the selection of the "best" estrogen product to prevent osteoporosis is difficult because few studies have compared products directly. Oral and transdermal estrogens do not appear to have differential effects on BMD, but transdermal estrogen may have the least effect on clotting and thus could have lower incidences of thromboembolism.

Conjugated equine estrogens (CEE), or Premarin, is the most frequently prescribed estrogen in the United States for the prevention of osteoporosis. CEE 0.625 mg (or an equivalent dose of another estrogen) has proved effective for the prevention of osteoporosis and has been considered the preferred dose.[166] However, recently the FDA has approved lower doses of CEE with MPA as combination products (CEE 0.3 mg with MPA 1.5 mg and CEE 0.45 mg with MPA 1.5 mg) for the prevention of osteoporosis as well as CEE 0.3 mg and CEE 0.45 mg. (See Table 48-14 for estrogen preparations and doses.) After starting with the lowest possible dose of estrogen, the dose can be modified if needed. A progestin must also be given to protect the endometrium in a woman such as M.J. When estrogen is given with progestin in a fixed combination formulation (e.g., Prempro) in a continuous fashion, EPT induces amenorrhea in 60% to 65% of women after 6 months.[166] The newer low dose Prempro combinations (CEE 0.3 mg/MPA 1.5 mg and CEE 0.45 mg/MPA 1.5 mg) produced higher rates of amenorrhea than CEE 0.625 mg/MPA 2.5 mg. Patients experiencing no bleeding during the first 3 months of therapy were 89% in the CEE 0.3mg/MPA 1.5 mg group and were 82% in those receiving CEE 0.45 mg/MPA 1.5 mg, whereas rates from CEE 0.625 mg/MPA 2.5 mg were 66% to 72%.[167] As an alternative, estrogen can be given cyclically for 25 days each month with a progestin taken for at least 12 days of each estrogen cycle (cyclic EPT). There are several other ways to administer EPT. These include cyclic-combined EPT, continuous-cyclic EPT, continuous long-cycle EPT, and intermittent-combined EPT.[168]

The following are examples of studies in which low doses of estrogens, with or without a progestin, were used for the prevention of osteoporosis. Bone loss was prevented in postmenopausal women who received CEE 0.3 mg administered with 1,500 mg of calcium daily.[169] Low-dose CEE (0.3 mg/day), in a continuous combined formulation including MPA 2.5 mg/day, increased spinal bone density 3.5% to 5.2% in older (>65 years) postmenopausal women with low bone mass.[170] As part of the Women's HOPE Study, 822 postmenopausal women (40 to 65 years) were randomized into groups (i.e., CEE 0.625 mg with or without MPA 2.5 mg; CEE 0.45 mg with or without MPA 2.5 mg; CEE 0.45 mg with or without MPA 1.5 mg; CEE 0.3 mg with or without MPA 1.5 mg; or a placebo for 2 years).[171] All women received 600 mg/day of elemental calcium during the study period. After 2 years, all treatment patients had significant increases in spine and hip BMD from baseline levels compared to placebo. Bone mineral content was significantly increased over the placebo group in all treatment groups except for the CEE 0.3 mg group.[171]

Postmenopausal women who received esterified estrogens 0.3 mg/day without a progestin had a greater increase in BMD in their lumbar spines and hips as well as whole body BMD than did those taking a placebo.[172] These estrogen-associated changes in BMD occurred without an increase in endometrial hyperplasia. In a randomized, controlled clinical trial of unopposed transdermal 17β-estradiol, doses ranging from 0.025 to 0.1 mg/day significantly increased BMD of the spine and hip compared with placebo.[173]

CONTRAINDICATIONS TO ESTROGEN USE

55. What are contraindications to the use of ET or EPT in a postmenopausal woman?

Contraindications to ET or EPT include pregnancy; active deep vein thrombosis, pulmonary embolism or a history thereof; active or recent (e.g., within the past year) arterial thromboembolic disease (e.g., stroke, myocardial infarction); undiagnosed abnormal genital bleeding; known, suspected, or a history of breast cancer; known or suspected estrogen-dependent neoplasia; liver dysfunction or disease; or known hypersensitivity to the product or any of its ingredients.[174] In addition, women with a history of asthma, diabetes mellitus, migraine, epilepsy, systemic lupus erythematosis, porphyria, and hepatic hemangiomas may have their disease exacerbated by the use of ET/EPT. Thus, women with any of the previously mentioned diseases should be monitored closely by their physicians for potential problems.[174]

RISKS OR HARMS ASSOCIATED WITH ET OR EPT
Cancer Risks

56. M.J. was told by friends and has read in magazines that there are cancer risks associated with the use of ET/EPT, especially if it is used for 5 or more years, as might be needed for osteoporosis prevention. What are these risks or harms?

There is evidence that EPT use increases the risk for developing breast cancer, and postmenopausal women with intact uteri, such as M.J., are at an increased risk for developing endometrial cancer if estrogen is used alone. This risk increases when estrogen is used for long periods of time, such as for osteoporosis prevention. Adding a progestin to ET can prevent this latter condition. There is also a question as to whether ET/EPT will increase or decrease the risk for ovarian cancer.

Endometrial Cancer

Estrogenic receptors in the endometrium respond to exogenous estrogen stimulation by proliferation and hyperplasia of the endometrium. Approximately 12% of women with an intact uterus who use ET without concomitant progestin will experience endometrial hyperplasia. In addition, 16% to 25% of women with endometrial hyperplasia will develop endometrial adenocarcinoma.[175]

The relative risk of endometrial cancer in women with an intact uterus who are receiving estrogen replacement without a progestin is approximately 2- to 12-fold greater than for nonusers and appears dose- and duration-related.[174] Typically, there is little risk if ET is used for less than a year, whereas risks of 15- to 24-fold occur when ET is used for 5 years or longer; this risk may then persist for 8 to 15 years thereafter.[174] The use of a concomitant progestin for 12 to 14 days a month while a woman is using estrogen will decrease the risk of endometrial hyperplasia and subsequent cancer. Typically, MPA 2.5 mg is added daily to continuous estrogen, whereas doses of MPA 5 mg are typically used 12 to 14 days monthly as part of cyclical estrogen regimens. For CEE doses of 0.3 mg and 0.45 mg, the MPA dose needed is 1.5 mg (as is now commercially available), which exposes the user to lower doses of both hormones.

Breast Cancer

Because many studies have reported increases, decreases, or no change in the incidence of breast cancer in postmenopausal women who were ever users or current users of EPT/ET compared with those who were never-users, meta-analyses have been used to explore this issue.[162,176–179] Some analyses demonstrated no increased risk of breast cancer in women who were ever users,[162,176–179] whereas others revealed an increase in breast cancer for current users (RR 1.2 to 1.6).[176–179] Of these analyses, one using data from 51 studies suggested a relative risk of 1.35 (95% CI 1.21 to 1.49) for breast cancer in women who used ET or EPT for 5 years or longer compared with never-users.[178]

The EPT arm of the WHI (see Questions 52 and 53) was terminated in May 2002 because the overall risks outweighed its benefits (i.e., the predetermined Global Index exceeded a relative risk [RR] of 1 at 1.15).[157] Part of the elevated risk was an increased incidence of breast cancer (RR 1.26, 95% CI 1.00 to 1.59) in the EPT group. This can be translated into a 26% increase in breast cancer risk, which could account for 38 events annually per 10,000 women receiving EPT versus 30 events in the placebo group.[157,180] These results are similar to those that have been noted in observational studies and meta-analyses. In addition, increases in breast cancer incidence were comparable among women taking EPT over 6.8 years of follow-up in HERS (RR 1.27, 95% CI 0.84 to 1.94).[155,156]

Although in some studies, such as the WHI, no effect of EPT on breast cancer mortality was noted, some observational studies have shown a decrease in breast cancer mortality in ever- or short-term users (RR 0.5 to 1.0).[181] This difference is related to cancer type. For example, the type of breast cancer associated with EPT use was studied by following 37,105 women for 11 years in Iowa.[182] Of these women, 1,520 developed breast cancer, but investigators noted that the most common breast cancers were those with a favorable histology. Typically, <15% of breast cancers diagnosed have a favorable histologic type.

Whether estrogen combined with a progestin confers a greater breast cancer risk than estrogen alone is currently unknown. WHI investigators reported no increase in breast cancer after 5 years of therapy in women who have had a hysterectomy and were receiving estrogen alone. Possibly, EPT rather than ET increases the incidence of breast cancer, but its effects on breast cancer mortality are currently uncertain.[181]

Ovarian Cancer

In one prospective cohort study, postmenopausal use of estrogen for 10 or more years appeared to increase the risk for ovarian cancer, a risk that the authors stated lasted for up to 29 years after estrogen discontinuation.[183] Of the 211,581 postmenopausal women enrolled in the study, there were 944 ovarian cancer deaths. The relative risk for developing ovarian cancer was 2.2, 95% CI 1.53 to 3.17 for women who used an estrogen product at the study baseline and continued its use for 10 years or longer. In another cohort study, an increased relative risk of 1.8 was noted for ovarian cancer among women who had taken HRT for at least 10 years.[184] Still another study found no effect of hormones on ovarian cancer mortality.[185] Data from studies addressing ovarian cancer risk for woman using ET or EPT appear to be inconsistent according to the U.S. Preventive Services Task Force of the Center for Practice and Technology Assessment, Agency for Healthcare Research and Quality (USPSTF).[181]

Postmenopausal Cardiovascular Disease

57. M.J. asks whether information has changed about the association between cardiovascular disease and EPT use. She said that at one time she was told that EPT could help prevent cardiovascular disease, but she has heard that this was not true. She also wants to know about its effect on women who have cardiac disease. What should M.J. be told?

Cardiovascular disease (CVD) is the number one cause of death among women in the United States, resulting in nearly twice the number of deaths annually as from all causes of cancer combined.[8,186] Because the incidence of CVD increases as estrogen concentrations decline, it appeared appropriate to consider menopausal and postmenopausal women as candidates for ET or EPT because observational, primary-prevention studies had shown that ET/EPT prevented mortality from CVD[187–189] and because postmenopausal women faced other medical problems such as vasomotor symptoms and osteoporosis for which ET/EPT might be used.

In addition to observational studies, the PEPI Trial (see Question 53) evaluated 875 healthy, postmenopausal women (average age 56) over 3 years.[190] These women were divided into five groups—a placebo group and four therapy groups who received oral CEE (0.625) mg with or without a progestin (MPA or MP). Women in all therapy groups significantly raised HDL-C (high-density lipoprotein cholesterol), lowered LDL-C, and raised triglycerides compared with placebo. CEE alone and CEE plus MP were more effective at raising HDL-C than regimens with MPA. Women assigned to regimens with MPA had significantly lower levels of total cholesterol. Although the PEPI Trial looked only at markers of CVD, not disease, observational studies in postmenopausal women have found that compared with never-users, ET or EPT reduces death from cardiovascular causes, including death resulting from CHD and stroke.[187–189]

In 2002, the EPT arm of the WHI was terminated in part because of an elevated risk for CHD (see Questions 52 and 53). The increased risks for other diseases such as cancer, venous thromboembolism, and stroke were expected and were similar to what had been observed in previous studies. The increased risk for CHD was unexpected, especially when one of the major outcomes to be determined by the WHI was the benefit versus risk of ET/EPT for the prevention of CHD. Women receiving EPT in the WHI had an increased risk for CHD (nonfatal and fatal myocardial infarctions) (RR 1.29, 95% CI 1.02 to 1.63) or a 29% increased risk with an absolute risk (AR) of 0.37% versus 0.30% (37 versus 30 events annually per 10,000 women).[180] Relative risks noted in various observational studies averaged 0.61 (0.45 to 0.82); different from those for women enrolled in the WHI EPT arm.[191] It must again be noted that the ET arm of the WHI continues.

Unfortunately, observational studies for CHD appear to be less than ideal because of various factors, including the potential for selection bias. For example, one study found that women taking EPT were more likely to exercise, lose weight, have higher dietary fiber intake, better potassium and calcium intakes, and get preventive health care (cholesterol screening, rectal examination, mammogram, Pap smear) than women not using estrogen.[192] Thus, lower death and stroke rates in women receiving ET/EPT in observational studies might be attributable to healthier lifestyles. Other methodologic reasons for difference in CHD outcomes between a randomized trial such as the WHI and observational studies in addition to confounding (healthy user) bias might be compliance bias or incomplete capture of early cardiac events in observational studies.[191] Other reasons include differences in the hormone regimen used (e.g., formulation and/or dose) or characteristics of the study population.[191] As to study population, the WHI had as one of its goals the inclusion of diverse populations (e.g., participants from racial and ethnic minorities).

Thus, we need to convey to M.J. that EPT should not be considered as preventive therapy for CHD and that there are still questions to be answered. For example, why did observational studies and studies such as the PEPI Trial differ in their results compared with a randomized trial such as the WHI. It must again be noted that the ET arm of the WHI is continuing to 2005 because the risks versus benefits seen in the EPT arm have not be noted thus far.

In observational studies, EPT appears to lower the risk of recurrent cardiovascular events in patients with cardiovascular disease.[193] However, HERS found no difference in the incidence of cardiovascular deaths and nonfatal myocardial infarctions in the secondary prevention of CHD in postmenopausal women receiving EPT (CEE 0.625 mg plus MPA 2.5 mg) after an average of 4.1 years.[155] These women were of an average age of 67 years and had documented histories of CHD. Women receiving EPT were significantly more likely to have a thromboembolic or CHD event during the first year of the study, but the relative hazard declined over time. The overall outcome of HERS was as follows: nonsignificant increased risk for cardiac events, RR 1.09, CI 0.88 to 1.35.

These statistics translate into a 9% increased risk with an AR of 2.12% versus 1.95% (or 212 events versus 195 events annually per 10,000 women). Despite the lack of improved cardiovascular outcomes in HERS, EPT improved lipid profiles.

The prevention and treatment of cardiovascular disease in women are also presented in Question 61 and in Chapter 18, Myocardial Infarction.

Other Risks or Harms

An increase in the prevalence of stroke, venous thromboembolism, gallbladder disease, and dementia has been noted with ET/EPT use.[174] In addition, caution should be exercised if a postmenopausal woman with any of the following conditions wishes to use ET or EPT: hypertension (although blood pressure may not be increased, blood pressure should be monitored); hypertriglyceridemia (estrogen use can increase triglycerides, leading to pancreatitis); impaired liver function (possibly due to decreased estrogen metabolism); past history of cholestatic jaundice; or hypothyroidism.[174] Some risks associated with estrogen used for oral contraception do not apply to the use of estrogens as part of EPT in an older woman. Differences in the types and potencies of estrogens used for these two purposes may be responsible for the divergent risk rates.

Thromboemoblic Disease

Current ET/EPT users have increased risks for pulmonary emboli (twice that for nonusers)[194] and for deep venous thromboembolism.[195] In some studies there did not appear to be an increased risk in past users, only current users. In the EPT arm of the WHI, a significant risk for venous thromboembolism was noted (RR 2.11, 95% CI 1.58 to 2.82). This was about a twofold increased rate of venous thromboembolic disease, which included deep venous thrombosis and pulmonary embolism.[157,180]

On an individual basis, if it is determined that a woman who is at risk for thrombophlebitis, pulmonary embolism, or intravascular clotting needs estrogen replacement, the use of transdermal estrogen may be more beneficial than oral estrogen. The potential benefit of this route of drug delivery is related to avoidance of the hepatic first-pass effect. Skin irritation may be a problem for some women who use a transdermal estrogen product. This problem can be decreased by site rotation and possibly switching the brand of patches if there are differences in the materials from which the patches are made or the adhesives used.

Stroke

The incidence of stroke in women enrolled in the EPT arm of the WHI appears similar to incidences noted in observational studies in which similar hormone regimens were used. For example, RR of 1.45 (1.10 to 1.92) was noted for observational studies,[191] whereas in the WHI there was an increased risk (RR 1.41, 95% CI 1.07 to 1.85). This translates into a 41% increased risk.[157,180] Women in the WHI EPT arm were followed up for 4 additional months after this arm was stopped. Thereafter, 16,608 women receiving EPT or placebo were analyzed for the incidence of stroke by type. Of these women, 1.8% (151 women) in the EPT group and 1.3% (107 women) in the placebo group were diagnosed as having had a stroke with 79.8% being ischemic. The intention-to-treat hazard ratio with adjustment for adherence was 1.50 (95% CI 1.08 to 2.08) for ischemic and hemorrhagic strokes combined when comparing the EPT with the placebo group.[196]

Gallbladder Disease

RR of 2.5 for gallbladder disease has been reported for postmenopausal women receiving estrogen replacement.[175] In HERS, a significant increase in incidence of biliary tract surgery (RR 1.48, 95% CI 1.12 to 1.95) was seen. This can also be stated as an AR of 1.19% versus 1.29% or 119 versus 129 events annually per 10,000 women.[155]

Dementia

Please see comments about dementia in Question 59 below.

BENEFITS

58. **What are the benefits from ET/EPT besides relief from menopausal symptoms such as hot flushes and osteoporosis prevention?**

For information about the benefits of ET and EPT, see questions addressing vasomotor symptoms and genitourinary atrophy. In addition, some data suggest a positive association between the use of estrogen replacement and increased cognitive function as well as decreased dementia and the risk of Alzheimer's disease; however, this is controversial. For example, in one study[197] 120 elderly women with mild-to-moderate Alzheimer's disease were randomized into one of two estrogen groups or a placebo group; estrogen replacement had no beneficial effect on memory or cognitive function.

As an ancillary study to the WHI, the Women's Health Initiative Memory Study (WHIMS) was undertaken to gather information about whether EPT could protect global cognitive function in older postmenopausal women.[198] Most studies of cognitive function have been observational. The WHIMS was a randomized, double-blind, placebo-controlled trial in which 4,532 of 4,894 women (65 years and older) enrolled to receive EPT (2,229) or placebo (2,303). All appeared dementia free at baseline. At discontinuation, it was determined that EPT did not improve cognitive function. The effect of EPT on the incidence of dementia and mild cognitive impairment were determined using this same population. The probability of developing apparent dementia appeared to be two times higher in the EPT group compared with those in the placebo group at 4.2 years. In addition, the AR of probable dementia was 45 cases per 10,000 woman-years in the EPT group versus 22 per 10,000 woman-years in the placebo group.[174] There has been speculation about why the increased incidence of probable dementia occurred. One thought is that it was the result of vascular dementia, which possibly occurred because women using EPT are at increased risk of stroke even though few of the women diagnosed with dementia had a history of stroke or a clinical stroke during the study period. On the other hand, silent brain infarcts have been associated with the development of dementia.[199]

The risk of colorectal cancer in women who have received hormone therapy appears to be decreased. In a meta-analysis of 18 observational studies colon cancer was decreased (RR 0.80, 95% CI 0.74 to 0.86) among women who were ever users of ET/EPT.[200] These same investigators also noted a decreased incidence of rectal cancer (RR 0.81, 95% CI 0.72 to

0.92). Similar results were noted in the EPT arm of the WHI (RR 0.63, 95% CI 0.43 to 0.92). This is an AR of 0.10% versus 0.16%, which translates into 10 versus 16 events per 10,000 women annually.[157,180]

ADVERSE EFFECTS

59. **What are the potential adverse effects of estrogens and progestins that might be administered to a postmenopausal woman such as M.J.?**

The woman should be made aware of estrogen-related adverse effects such as nausea, vomiting, dizziness, weight gain, breast tenderness, and breast enlargement. She must also be educated about the possible return of uterine bleeding if she begins using ET or EPT. Used alone, estrogens produce dose-dependent uterine bleeding; women who received 0.625 mg/day of CEE had a 1% to 4% incidence.[175] The addition of a progestin cyclically increases the incidence of uterine bleeding, normalizes the bleeding pattern, and reduces breakthrough bleeding. The continuous administration of both hormones decreases the incidence of bleeding, but breakthrough bleeding may continue for 6 months to 1 year until the endometrium becomes atrophic.

Adverse effects associated with progestin use may depend on the type of progestin prescribed, but typically these effects include edema, increased breast size, mastalgia, rash, acne, hirsutism, alopecia, headaches, and psychological effects (e.g., irritability, fatigue, mood swings, depression).[168] Edema and mastalgia may be more commonly noted with MPA or gestodene use. Alopecia, acne and hirsutism may be more commonly noted with the use of the more androgenic agents, norethindrone and levonorgestrel.

Other Prevention Modalities
Selective Estrogen Receptor Modulators

60. **Should a selective estrogen receptor modulator (SERM) such as raloxifene be considered for the prevention of osteoporosis in M.J.?**

RALOXIFENE

Raloxifene (Evista), a SERM, may be an alternate therapeutic choice for M.J. SERMs are pharmaceutical agents that are "hormone-related" or "designer estrogens" that have estrogen agonist and/or antagonist activity in various tissues where estrogen receptors are present. These compounds are also structurally diverse. For example, benzothiophene analogs, such as raloxifene, have agonistic effects on bone and serum lipid profiles and antagonistic effects on endometrial and breast tissues. Triphenylethylene analogs, such as tamoxifen (Nolvadex), have agonistic effects on bone, serum lipid profiles, and endometrial tissue, and antagonistic effects on breast tissue.

Raloxifene at a dose of 60 mg/day is the only SERM currently approved by the FDA for the prevention of postmenopausal osteoporosis; some investigational SERMs, such as droloxifene, have estrogen receptor agonist/antagonist activity similar to that of raloxifene. SERMs are used for various health problems and disease states. For example, tamoxifen is used as an adjuvant for axillary node-negative or node-positive breast cancer in women, for metastatic breast cancer in women and men, and for the prevention of breast cancer in high-risk women. Clomiphene (Clomid) is used for ovulatory dysfunction, and toremifene (Fareston) is used to treat metastatic breast cancer in postmenopausal women.

Raloxifene's agonist activity on bone tissue is believed to occur through a reduction in bone resorption and a decreased rate of bone turnover, which then results in increased BMD. The effects appear to be mediated through action as an estrogen agonist at estrogen receptors in bone. Raloxifene activity may be mediated through transforming growth factor-β3 (TGF-β3) and suppression of cytokinase IL-6.[201]

Data supporting raloxifene's effect on BMD were collected in three clinical osteoporosis prevention trials that were conducted in North America (544 women), Europe (601 women), and internationally (619 women, all of whom had undergone hysterectomy).[202,203] The trials were all randomized, double-blind, placebo-controlled studies that lasted 2 years. Participants were postmenopausal women 45 to 60 years of age. All received calcium supplementation, and women in the treatment groups received raloxifene 60 mg/day; in the international study, there was also a CEE arm (0.625 mg/daily). The results of these studies showed loss of approximately 1% BMD in the women in the placebo groups. In contrast, those in the raloxifene groups had an increase in BMD of 1.3% to 2.4% in the hips, 1.6% to 2.5% in femoral neck, 1.3% to 2.7% in the trochanter, 1.3% to 2.4% in the intertrochanter, and 1.8% to 2.4% in the lumbar spine. The increase in BMD in the hips of women in the CEE arm of the international study was two times that noted for raloxifene.

The Multiple Outcomes of Raloxifene Evaluation (MORE) Trial enrolled 7,705 postmenopausal women ages 31 to 80 years of age. Of these women, 5,129 were randomized to either the 60 mg/day or 120 mg/day raloxifene group, whereas the remainder was in the placebo group.[204] MORE Trial outcomes after 3 years were as follows for BMD: increases in femoral neck BMD was 2.1% (60 mg/day group) and 2.4% (120 mg/day group) compared with placebo, whereas spinal BMD increased by 2.6% and 2.7% in the raloxifene groups, respectively, compared with placebo. The RR for vertebral fractures was 0.7, 95% CI 0.5 to 0.8 for those in the 60 mg/day group, whereas those in the 120 mg/day group had an RR of 0.5, 95% CI 0.4 to 0.7. This translates into a 38% and 41% reduction in vertebral fracture rate for the 60 mg/day and 120 mg/day groups, respectively.[205] No significant difference in nonvertebral fractures was noted among groups.

Another study was undertaken to ascertain whether raloxifene prescribed with alendronate would have an additive effect on biochemical markers for bone remodeling and BMD in postmenopausal women with osteoporosis.[206] Postmenopausal women ($N = 331$) who were 75 years of age or younger were divided into four groups: placebo; raloxifene 60 mg/day only; alendronate 10 mg/day only; or raloxifene plus alendronate (combination group) at 30 study sites worldwide. Markers of bone turnover (serum osteocalcin, bone-specific alkaline phosphatase, and urinary N- and C-telopeptide) were measured, as was BMD at baseline, at 6 months and then 12 months later. In the final time period, markers of bone turnover were decreased in all groups except the placebo group. These markers were reduced 1.6-fold in the alendronate-only group compared with the raloxifene-only group. No differences were noted in marker reduction at 12 months

between the alendronate-only and the combination groups, but lumbar spine BMD increased by 2.1%, 4.3%, and 5.3% from baseline for raloxifene-only, alendronate-only, and combination therapy, respectively. The increase in femoral neck BMD in the combination group was 3.7% above baseline compared with the alendronate-only (2.7%) and raloxifene-only (1.7%) groups. Total hip BMD and total body BMD were not determined. Overall, combination therapy was better than raloxifene or alendronate alone. Thus, combination therapy could be considered for individuals who do not respond to either therapy alone. In addition, markers of bone turnover and BMD appear to respond better to alendronate alone than to raloxifene alone. The study did not address fracture rates.

Differences in BMD, bone architecture, and bone turnover were determined in a 6-month study in which raloxifene 60 mg/day was compared with CEE 0.625 mg/day in 51 white women ages 55 to 85 years.[207] During this short, randomized, double-blind study, most of the markers of bone resorption/formation were decreased in both groups, but to a greater extent in those receiving CEE. Total body and lumbar spine BMD increased in both groups with a greater increase in women receiving CEE. Hip BMD was similar for both groups. Overall, CEE had a greater effect on bone, but effects were positive for raloxifene users. It should be remembered that study results were determined after only 6 months and that the number of women enrolled was small.

There is a paradox about how raloxifene can decrease vertebral fractures by up to 41% while increasing BMD by only 2% to 3%, rates that are lower than those noted for ET/EPT or alendronate. In addition, raloxifene has not been observed to have a positive effect on hip fractures. It has been postulated that the antifracture effect of raloxifene on vertebral fractures occurs secondary to its normalization of the high turnover rate of cancellous bone, which then prevents further disruption of bone microarchitecture.[208,209] This probably occurs through raloxifene binding at estrogen β-receptor sites that are predominant in cancellous bone.[208,209] In addition, a less potent antiresorptive agent such as raloxifene may help prevent vertebral fractures but not hip fractures because the threshold for preventing osteoclastic activity in cancellous bone, which is predominant in vertebrae, may be lower than in cortical bone, which predominates in hips. It should also be noted that estrogen receptors in cortical bone are predominantly alpha, whereas those in cancellous bone are typically beta. Thus, bone type and estrogen receptors are different in the hips compared with vertebrae. For these reasons, it may require a more potent antiresorptive agent to increase BMD in the hips.

Raloxifene might be considered for osteoporosis prevention in a woman such as M.J. and could be considered for osteoporosis prevention if she were at risk for breast cancer. This latter recommendation is based on results from the Multiple Outcomes of Raloxifene Evaluation (MORE) Trial. There was a 76% decrease in risk for invasive breast cancer in postmenopausal women with osteoporosis (mean age, 66.5 years) who received raloxifene for 3 years.[210] A total of 7,705 women were assigned to raloxifene groups (60 mg twice daily or 60 mg daily) or a placebo group. Of those enrolled in either raloxifene group (n = 5,129), only 13 cases of breast cancer were reported versus 27 that occurred in the 2,576 women in the placebo group.

Dosing and Pharmacokinetics

If M.J. is to use raloxifene, she should take 60 mg once daily without regard for food.[201,202] Raloxifene is approximately 60% absorbed after oral ingestion and then undergoes extensive glucuronide conjugation that results in a 2% absolute bioavailability while some circulating raloxifene glucuronide conjugates are converted back to the parent compound.[202] Raloxifene and its monoglucuronide conjugates are highly protein bound. Raloxifene is primarily excreted in feces, with <0.2% excreted unchanged and <6% eliminated in urine as glucuronide conjugates.[202] There appear to be no differences in pharmacokinetics based on age or gender. It has a mean half-life of 27.7 hours after a single dose and 32.5 hours after multiple doses.[202]

Adverse Effects

M.J. should be counseled about adverse effects of raloxifene that might pertain to her if she begins the medication. Adverse effects include an increased risk for venous thromboembolic disease and an increase in hot flushes (25% in postmenopausal raloxifene users versus 18% in those receiving placebo).[201,202] The greatest risk for thromboembolic events is during the first 4 months of therapy.[201] To decrease the risk of thrombosis associated with immobilization, raloxifene should be discontinued for at least 72 hours before immobilization such as that associated with surgery. Because M.J. is still experiencing hot flushes, raloxifene is probably not the drug of choice for her because her hot flushes could be exacerbated.

Contraindications and Potential Drug Interactions

Raloxifene is contraindicated for administration to women who are pregnant or who may become pregnant. It is also contraindicated in women with an active or past history of venous thromboembolic events.[201,202] Hypersensitivity to raloxifene or any constituent in Evista tablets is also a contraindication to its use. Patients with hepatic dysfunction may need dosage adjustments, although more information is needed to clarify doses needed.[201,202] Cholestyramine, when coadministered with raloxifene, may decrease raloxifene absorption by 60% because of its effects on enterohepatic cycling.[201,202] Women who may be receiving warfarin as well as raloxifene should be monitored closely.[201] This may also be true for some other highly protein-bound medications. It does not appear that M.J. has any contraindication to the use of raloxifene.

Other Potential Benefits of Raloxifene

61. What are other effects of raloxifene?

In addition to antagonist effects on breast tissue, raloxifene is an antagonist in the uterus. Therefore, vaginal bleeding is not likely to occur nor is endometrial hyperplasia and the risk for endometrial cancer.[201-203] A decreased incidence of breast pain, flatulence, and abdominal pain have also been reported in women with an intact uterus who were administered raloxifene versus those receiving continuous EPT.[202]

Raloxifene may be of benefit in the prevention of CVD. Most studies that have evaluated the effects of raloxifene on CVD have reported surrogate markers such as lipid serum concentrations rather than cardiovascular outcomes. For example, in the MORE study, postmenopausal women who received raloxifene had significantly fewer reports of hypercholesterolemia.[210] Total cholesterol and LDL-C concentrations in women who were using raloxifene were reduced significantly compared with those receiving placebo.[210] When compared with EPT, raloxifene showed similar reductions in LDL-C. Only EPT significantly increased HDL-C, but it also elevated triglyceride concentrations.[211] It is currently unknown whether or not these effects translate into a reduction in mortality from CVD.

In 2005, the Raloxifene Use for the Heart (RUTH) study should be completed. It is hoped that it will provide us with much-needed information about the effectiveness of raloxifene in the prevention of CVD.[212] The RUTH study is randomized and placebo-controlled. Approximately 10,000 postmenopausal women have been enrolled. The Study of Tamoxifen and Raloxifene (STAR) is also currently ongoing to compare raloxifene 60 mg daily with tamoxifen 20 mg daily in 22,000 postmenopausal women over a 7-year period. Prevention of CVD is one of the secondary end points for this study.[213]

Bisphosphonates
ALENDRONATE AND RISEDRONATE

62. Why should bisphosphonates be considered for the prevention of osteoporosis in a woman such as M.J.?

Another alternative to EPT for M.J. would be a bisphosphonate such as alendronate sodium (Fosamax) or risedronate sodium (Actonel), if osteoporosis prevention is the only reason that EPT was being considered. This is because bisphosphonates have no effects on vasomotor symptoms or genitourinary symptoms. Both drugs are FDA approved for the prevention of postmenopausal osteoporosis and the treatment of postmenopausal and glucocorticoid-induced osteoporosis. They can also be used to treat Paget's disease. Alendronate, an aminobisphosphonate, decreases bone resorption, resulting in decreased fracture rates in postmenopausal women who are at risk for osteoporosis. The amino group on alendronate appears to increase selectivity for the antiresorptive surfaces of bone. Alendronate and risedronate have high affinities for bone hydroxyapatite and can be incorporated into bone; in doing this, they can then interfere with osteoclast-mediated bone resorption. Because of their incorporation into bone, bisphosphonates have long half-lives, estimated to be 1 to 10 years. Unlike etidronate (another bisphosphonate), alendronate and risedronate do not inhibit bone mineralization, which could lead to osteomalacia.

Effects on Bone Mineral Density

For the prevention of osteoporosis, both alendronate and risedronate are approved by the FDA at doses of 5 mg/day or 35 mg once weekly.

A study of the efficacy and safety of oral alendronate (5 mg/day) for osteoporosis prevention in early postmenopausal women[214] showed BMD increases in the spine of 2.9% (range 2.3% to 3.5%) at 5 years for women receiving alendronate, whereas total body density was increased only 0.3%. In a 2-year prevention study in postmenopausal women younger than 60,[215] placebo, 2.5 mg/day alendronate, 5 mg/day alendronate, and EPT were compared. An increased BMD in the spine, total hip, and total body were observed in the alendronate groups versus the placebo group. Results from the 5-mg group were as follows: lumbar spine, 3.5% (range 3.3% to 3.7%); hip, 1.9% (range 1.8% to 2.0%); and total body, 0.7% (range 0.6% to 0.8%). These results were better than for those in the 2.5-mg group but lower than those who received estrogen; BMD for the ERT group was 1% to 2% greater than for the alendronate 5-mg group.

Another study found that women (ages 55 to 81 years) diagnosed with postmenopausal osteoporosis who were in an alendronate study group (alendronate 5 mg/day for 2 years followed by 10 mg/day for 1 year) had reduced risk for fractures at various anatomic sites compared with those in the placebo group.[216] For new vertebral fractures the RR was 0.53 (95% CI 0.41 to 0.68); hip, 0.49 (95% CI 0.23 to 0.99); and wrist, 0.52 (95% CI 0.31 to 0.87). The Fracture Intervention Trial (FIT) was a multicenter, placebo-controlled trial that enrolled 2,027 women between the ages of 55 and 81 years of age who had vertebral fractures and reduced BMD.[217] These women received placebo or alendronate 5 mg/day for 2 years and 10 mg/day during the third year. Relative to the placebo group, BMD increased by 6.2% in the spine and 4.7% in the total hip region after 3 years. Over 3 years, 18.2% of the placebo group and 13.6% of the alendronate group had fractures.

In 2000, Black and associates[218] combined the data from the previous two studies to give overall information from the FIT. The investigators believed this was appropriate because fracture reduction rates in both studies with the use of alendronate were similar. The pooled information from 3 to 4 years of alendronate versus placebo use resulted in the following fracture risk data: hip RR 0.47 (95% CI 0.26 to 0.79); radiographic vertebral RR 0.52 (95% CI 0.42 to 0.66); clinical vertebral RR 0.55 (95% CI 0.36 to 0.82); and all clinical fractures RR 0.70 (95% CI 0.59 to 0.82). The investigators concluded from these data that women with osteoporosis (T score less than –2.5), with or without previous vertebral fractures and who took alendronate, had reduced risk for fractures.

A meta-analysis was used to determine the nonvertebral fracture rate in postmenopausal women with osteoporosis who had been treated for at least 3 years with placebo or alendronate (doses used in the five trials ranged from 1 to 20 mg/day).[219] The overall results showed a 12.6% incidence of nonvertebral fracture in the placebo groups and a 9.0% incidence in the alendronate groups. This resulted in a RR of 0.71 (95% CI 0.502 to 0.997) for those receiving alendronate.

Several studies have addressed the effects of risedronate on BMD. In a study of women 40 to 60 years of age (early postmenopausal) who had normal BMD for age, those receiving risedronate 5 mg/day for 2 years had increases of 5.7% in lumbar spine and 5.4% in the hip compared with women taking a placebo.[220] In another study, postmenopausal women (mean age 69 years) who were older than those mentioned in the previous study had increases in BMD of 4.3% in the spine and 2.8% in the femoral neck when risedronate use was compared with placebo over 3 years.[221]

Many studies show the benefits of bisphosphonates in not only the prevention of osteoporosis-related fractures by increasing BMD, but also for the treatment of osteoporosis. Many of these studies have been of 3 years' duration with at least one being of 7 years' duration[222] with a 3-year extension.[223] This latter study extension noted that during years 8

through 10, 247 women receiving either alendronate 5 mg/day or 10 mg/day had similar safety and tolerance profiles as women in placebo groups. They noted that spinal BMD increased by 2.25% for those in the 10-mg/day group and 1.60% for the 5-mg/day group; hip and total body BMD was maintained at levels that were noted at 7 years; and forearm BMD was maintained in the 10-mg/day group but decreased slightly in the 5-mg/day group. Women who took alendronate for 5 years, but thereafter were in a placebo group, maintained their spinal and total body BMD over the past 5 years. Ten-year cumulative spinal BMD was 13.7% for the 10-mg/day group and 9.8% for the 5-mg/day group. Rates for nonvertebral fractures between years 8 and 10 were 8.1% for the 10-mg/day group, 11.5% for the 5-mg/day group, and 12.0% for the group who had been on alendronate for 5 years and off for the past 5 years. In addition, most bisphosphonate studies have been randomized, double-blind, placebo-controlled studies with large sample sizes. Therefore, the use of a bisphosphonate for the prevention of osteoporosis in M.J. would be a good choice.

Contraindications and Precautions

Although no dosage change is recommended for a patient with mild to moderate renal failure, alendronate use is not recommended for patients with significant renal insufficiency (e.g., creatinine clearance <35 mL/min).[24] Hypocalcemia, if it exists, should be corrected before beginning therapy. Caution should be taken in patients who have any upper GI problem such as esophageal disease, dysphasia, duodenitis, or ulcers. Sitting upright after ingesting alendronate is recommended to decrease the possibility of reflux into the esophagus and to decrease esophageal irritation as well as to ensure the absorption of alendronate, which has a low bioavailability. A patient who cannot sit upright for 30 minutes after ingesting the drug should not use alendronate. The same precautions should be considered for the use of risedronate. None of these contraindications appears to apply to M.J.

Adverse Effects

Common adverse effects associated with the use of alendronate include GI symptoms such as acid regurgitation, dysphagia, abdominal distention, gastritis, nausea, dyspepsia, flatulence, diarrhea, and constipation.[24] Although rare, esophageal adverse effects such as esophagitis, esophageal ulcers, and erosions have occurred and have been followed by esophageal stricture. This last adverse effect is one of the reasons a patient should sit upright for 30 minutes after ingesting alendronate. In addition, musculoskeletal pain, headaches, and rash have been noted.[24] Adverse effects noted for risedronate are similar to those noted for alendronate.

Dosing

If M.J. takes alendronate, she can be prescribed 5 mg daily or 35 mg once weekly. It might be more convenient to take the medication once weekly, and this might also increase her adherence to therapy. M.J. should be instructed to take her medication with 6 to 8 ounces of water early in the morning on arising and at least 30 minutes before ingesting food, beverage, or other medications. She should not lie down, but should stay fully upright for at least 30 minutes after ingesting alendronate to prevent esophageal irritation or ulceration and to ensure appropriate bioavailability. A patient using alendronate should ingest adequate calcium and vitamin D, but should not take the calcium or vitamin D at the same time as the alendronate. Dosing of risedronate is 5 mg daily or 35 mg once weekly. The aforementioned information about the administration of alendronate applies to risedronate.

Treatment

63. T.J.'s 75-year-old grandmother, M.B., was diagnosed as having osteoporosis 5 years ago when she broke her distal forearm. In addition, she has lost 2 inches in height (current height 5' and weight 100 lb) and has mild kyphosis. M.B. denies severe back pain but occasionally uses acetaminophen or a NSAID for mild back pain. A recent bone scan revealed significantly decreased vertebral and forearm bone mass. M.B. had her last menstrual period before her hysterectomy approximately 25 years ago. Her only major medical problem is mild congestive heart failure (CHF) for which she receives hydrochlorothiazide 25 mg/day PO and digoxin 0.125 mg/day PO. In addition, M.B. takes CEE 0.625 mg PO daily and calcium carbonate 1,200 mg/day in divided doses with meals. Does M.B. have any clinical signs of osteoporosis? What changes, if any, should be made in her treatment plan? What other medications might be considered for the treatment of osteoporosis?

Clinical signs of osteoporosis exhibited by M.B. include a loss of 2 inches in height and the presence of mild kyphosis. She also has mild back pain that may be associated with osteoporosis. (See Question 51 for further information about osteoporosis clinical signs and symptoms.)

A treatment plan for M.B. should be aimed at preventing further bone loss and minimizing falls, which could lead to fractures.

Calcium and Vitamin D Intake

Calcium is an antiresorptive agent that decreases bone demineralization. Calcium supplementation can slow or prevent further bone loss. M.B.'s calcium intake, which should be at least 1,200 mg/day of elemental calcium, is adequate according to National Academy of Sciences,[147] but information from the National Institutes of Health recommends 1,500 mg/day of elemental calcium for women such as M.B. who are age 65 and older.[148] Calcium absorption may be decreased in older people because of lower gastric acid secretion, decreased 1,25-dihydroxyvitamin D_3 serum concentrations, and decreased endogenous estrogen serum concentrations. To overcome this problem, M.B. should continue taking her calcium in divided doses with meals or use a more soluble calcium product such as calcium citrate. Questions 49, 50, and 52 further discuss calcium requirements, supplementation, and product selection and the use of vitamin D for postmenopausal women.

Estrogens

In light of the results from the EPT arm of the WHI and the previously published HERS, estrogen use is in question, especially if used long term, although the results of the ET arm of the WHI will not be available until 2005.[155,157] As discussed in Question 52, EPT has positive effects on BMD and fracture rates but does not appear to prevent CHD (WHI) nor prevent further cardiovascular events in individuals with a history of heart disease (HERS).[155,157] Thus, M.B. and her physician should discuss whether she should continue ET or be switched to another drug for treatment of her osteoporosis.

Exercise and Prevention of Falls

M.B. should continue an exercise routine (particularly a weight-bearing exercise) that is appropriate for her age and physical condition. Exercise helps maintain bone mass, function, and agility. The prevention of falls, which often result in fractures, also should be considered part of M.B.'s therapy.

Thiazides

M.B. currently is receiving hydrochlorothiazide for mild heart failure, but thiazides may also increase calcium retention. Whether this effect has a long-term benefit on calcium balance is debated. Data from a meta-analysis of 11 studies (none were prospective) established an RR of 0.82 (95% CI 0.73 to 0.91) for hip fractures and 0.88 (0.77 to 1.02) for all fractures related to osteoporosis in people taking thiazides.[224] In most of these studies, patients were 65 or older. It also appears that longer use of thiazides had a greater effect on the prevention of fractures. Thus, M.B.'s thiazide therapy may have a positive effect on her BMD. The North American Menopause Society (NAMS) does not believe that thiazides prevent bone loss or fracture risk, although in the elderly there may be some benefit.[145]

Because M.B. has a history of fractures, she should continue calcium supplementation (possibly increasing it to 1,500 mg/day), hydrochlorothiazide (as long as it is needed for another health problem), and an adequate vitamin D intake. A decision needs to be made about her ET. If it is decided that she should not continue ET, then a decision should be made as to whether a bisphosphonate or raloxifene might be an alternative. If ET is discontinued, it would most likely be best to taper her off estrogen and not stop it abruptly. There are no guidelines as to how to taper estrogen but NAMS recommends one of two ways to do this: either skip progressively more days between doses or lower the dose of estrogen every 4 to 6 weeks until the hormones have been successfully tapered.[180] It must be remembered that if ET is discontinued and another medication not added for the treatment of osteoporosis, M.B. could begin to lose BMD but the rate of loss should be lower than for a younger postmenopausal woman who is taken off ET or EPT without another medication added.

Selective Estrogen Receptor Modulators

Raloxifene might be considered for M.B. because of her need for osteoporosis treatment and her history of CVD (see Question 61). Raloxifene is FDA approved for the treatment of postmenopausal osteoporosis. Ettinger and coworkers[204] noted that at 3 years, women (ages 31 to 80) with postmenopausal osteoporosis who received raloxifene (60 mg or 120 mg daily) had increased BMD in the femoral neck (2.1% and 2.4%, respectively) compared with placebo. They also had increased BMD in their spines 2.6% and 2.7%, respectively, compared with placebo, but they also had an RR of 3.1 (95% CI 1.5 to 6.2) for venous thromboembolism versus those in the placebo group. In another study that compared raloxifene 60 and 120 mg/day with placebo,[225] increases in

BMD were noted in the total hip and ultradistal radius in the 60-mg/day group. Nonsignificant trends over placebo were noted for the lumbar spine, total body, and total hip in the 120-mg/day group. In addition, results showed a lower increase in BMD when compared with estrogen studies. (See Questions 61 and 62 for additional information about raloxifene.)

Bisphosphonates

ALENDRONATE AND RISEDRONATE

A bisphosphonate such as alendronate or risedronate can be an alternative to ET if another benefit of ERT (e.g., genitourinary) is not needed or can be provided by another medication.

In addition to the alendronate and risedronate clinical studies described in Question 63, the following studies address the use of alendronate and risedronate in the treatment of postmenopausal osteoporosis. In 1995, Liberman and colleagues[226] performed a multicenter, double-blind, placebo-controlled study in which 994 postmenopausal women, ages 45 to 80 years with osteoporosis were enrolled. Alendronate 5 mg or 10 mg or placebo was administered daily for 3 years followed by 20 mg for 2 years, and then 5 mg/day for 1 year. All study participants received calcium 500 mg/day. Increases in BMD of 8.8 ±0.4% were noted in lumbar spine, 5.9 ±0.5% in the femoral neck, and 7.8 ±0.6% at trochanter in those in the alendronate 10-mg group. Vertebral fractures occurred in 6.2% of those receiving placebo and in 3.2% of those receiving alendronate (48% reduction in fracture rate). In another study, increases in lumbar spine BMD of 0.65%, 3.5%, and 5.7% were noted in elderly women who received 1, 2.5, or 5 mg of alendronate over 2 years with calcium supplements versus those receiving placebo.[227] A meta-analysis that compared the results of five studies performed in postmenopausal women between the ages of 42 and 85 documented that alendronate, when given in doses of 10 mg/day for 3 years, increased BMD over placebo administration as follows: spine 8.8%, femoral neck 5.9%, and trochanter 7.8%.[228]

In two clinical trials,[221,229] the use of risedronate 5 mg daily for 3 years reduced vertebral fractures in postmenopausal women with osteoporosis by 41% and 49%, respectively. The incidence of nonvertebral fractures was reduced by 39% over the same time period.[221] McClung and associates[230] studied two groups of women (5,445 women ages 70 to 79 with confirmed osteoporosis and 3,886 women age 80 years or older who had risk factors for osteoporosis or low BMD at the femoral neck) to determine whether risedronate could decrease the risk for hip fractures. All women were randomly assigned to receive risedronate 2.5 mg/day, 5 mg/day, or placebo for 3 years. In the osteoporosis group (i.e., women 70 to 79 years of age), the overall incidence of hip fracture in the risedronate groups was 1.9% with a rate of 3.2% among those in the placebo group (RR 0.6, 9% CI 0.4 to 0.9). Among the women age 80 years and older, the incidence of hip fractures was 4.2% among risedronate users and 5.1% in those in the placebo group. Thus, risedronate significantly reduced the risk of hip fracture in women diagnosed with osteoporosis but not in the women over age 80 who had risk factors for osteoporosis and low BMD but not osteoporosis.

A study to investigate the use of alendronate 70 mg once weekly for the treatment of osteoporosis showed that its effects on BMD in the lumbar spine and total hip were similar to that produced by alendronate 10 mg daily after 1 year.[231] The study addressed convenience of therapy while making sure that efficacy was not diminished. Alendronate is approved for the treatment of postmenopausal osteoporosis in doses of 10 mg daily or 70 mg once weekly. Risedronate is approved for the treatment of osteoporosis in doses of 5 mg daily or 35 mg once weekly. Alendronate and risedronate are discussed in detail in Question 63.

A bisphosphonate would be an alternative to ET for M.B. if only osteoporosis treatment is considered and not her cardiac problems. Overall, it must be noted that bisphosphonates have a greater effect on BMD than does raloxifene.

ETIDRONATE

Etidronate (Didronel), another bisphosphonate available in the United States, inhibits bone resorption mediated by osteoclasts. It is not FDA approved for the treatment (nor for the prevention) of postmenopausal osteoporosis, but it is approved for the treatment of Paget's disease in the United States and for the treatment of osteoporosis in Canada. Studies have shown that although etidronate has positive effects on fracture prevention, there is concern about the development of osteomalacia. To overcome this potential problem, alternating regimens of etidronate 400 mg/day for 2 weeks followed by a 13-week (3 months) course of calcium and vitamin D have been used.[232] Etidronate administration to women receiving EPT, calcium, and vitamin D has resulted in an additive effect on BMD in hips and spines.[233]

A meta-analysis was used to evaluate 13 clinical trials of etidronate administration in an intermittent, cyclical fashion as therapy for postmenopausal osteoporosis (administered 2 weeks, every 3 months).[234] Results showed that, relative to controls, with 1 to 2 years of etidronate therapy at 400 mg/day, BMD was increased by 4.1% in the lumbar spine and 2.3% in the femoral neck. It was suggested that use of etidronate could reduce vertebral fractures by 37%, but not the risk for nonvertebral fractures.

Calcitonin

Calcitonin acts directly on osteoclasts to inhibit bone resorption primarily from vertebral and femoral sites. It is approved for the treatment but not the prevention of postmenopausal osteoporosis by injection or as an intranasal spray. It also is effective in reducing corticosteroid-induced osteoporosis. It typically is recommended for postmenopausal osteoporosis for those who have been diagnosed for at least 5 years.

Calcitonin may increase BMD in the lumbar spine (cancellous bone) by 1% to 3%, but its use has little effect on cortical bone. In one study, new fractures were reduced. This resulted in an RR of 0.23 (CI 0.7 to 0.77).[235] Various intermittent regimens of calcitonin are being used investigationally to see whether they can help prevent a decrease in effectiveness that occurs after 1 to 2 years. Calcitonin is used in some patients because of its analgesic effects on bone pain, especially for those who suffer from vertebral compression fractures.[145]

A large, randomized, double-blind, placebo-controlled study (Prevent Recurrence of Osteoporotic Fracture [PROOF]) explored the effectiveness of intranasal calcitonin at a dose of 200 IU/day for 5 years versus other doses.[236] It was determined that it decreased the risk of developing new vertebral fractures in women with osteoporosis by 33%. Doses of 100 and 400 IU/day administered in this same trial did not result in positive results. No significant effect on hip BMD occurred at any dose.[236]

When used intranasally, calcitonin (Miacalcin) is dosed at 200 IU daily in alternating nares; given subcutaneously or intramuscularly (Calcimar) the dose is 100 IU/day.[24] A patient using calcitonin should have adequate intake of calcium and vitamin D.

Adverse effects associated with intranasal calcitonin include nasal symptoms, such as rhinitis and epistaxis. Other adverse effects include arthralgia, headache, and back pain. When calcitonin therapy is administered by injection, adverse effects such as flushing, nausea, and vomiting as well as local irritation at the injection site (10%) may occur.[24] Flushing typically occurs on the hands and face and is noted in approximately 2–5% of patients. Nausea and/or vomiting occur in about 10%. These latter reactions most commonly occur when therapy is initiated and usually subside with time. Injectable calcitonin should be refrigerated when not in use. The intranasal preparation should be refrigerated until it is opened for use; thereafter, it is stable for 30 days at room temperature.[24]

Other Therapies

64. What other agents (both FDA approved and investigational) are possible alternative or additive therapies for the treatment of postmenopausal osteoporosis?

PARATHYROID HORMONE

Parathyroid hormone (PTH) works differently from other medications discussed thus far because it stimulates new bone formation, which then results in increased BMD, primarily in cancellous bone. This can be accomplished by administration of recombinant human PTH in women with postmenopausal osteoporosis with or without ET/EPT.[145] For example, in one study of 1,637 postmenopausal women who had previously sustained vertebral fractures, therapy (19 months of PTH 20 or 40 μg daily subcutaneously) resulted in a reduction of new vertebral fractures by 65% and 69%, respectively, and a reduction of new nonvertebral fractures by 53% and 54%, respectively.[237]

The FDA has approved the PTH derivative teriparatide (Forteo) for use by women and men with osteoporosis who do not adequately respond to other therapies. In addition, those diagnosed as having severe osteoporosis and who are at an increased risk for fracture may be considered for therapy. Teriparatide 20 μg should be given once daily subcutaneously in the thigh or abdomen.[238]

Because osteosarcomas were noted in study animals that received teriparatide, the FDA has required a black box warning for this medication even though no osteosarcomas have been observed in patients.[238] This information may also be found in a Medication Guide that should be given to all patients receiving teriparatide. Children, adolescents, and indi-

viduals with Paget's disease are not candidates for teriparatide because those with growing bones are at increased risk for developing osteosarcomas.

Adverse effects that have been noted to be associated with teriparatide use include hypercalcemia, leg cramps, nausea, and dizziness.[238]

INVESTIGATIONAL BISPHOSPHONATES AND SERMS

In the next few years, new bisphosphonates and SERMs should be approved for the prevention and treatment of diseases such as osteoporosis that affect postmenopausal women. An example of these new agents is the bisphosphonate, zoledronic acid. Because this agent has low bioavailability and significant GI intolerance, it is being studied for intravenous administration.

In a randomized, double-blind, placebo-controlled trial, zoledronic acid was administered for 1 year to 351 postmenopausal women who had low BMD.[239] The study population was divided into five treatment groups and a placebo group. Doses of zoledronic acid 0.25 mg, 0.5 mg, 1 mg, or placebo were administered at 3-month intervals, whereas 4 mg of the drug was administered as a single dose or as two doses of 2 mg at 6-month intervals. Increases in BMD were as follows: spine BMD for treatment patients ranged from 4.3% to 5.1% above placebo; femoral neck BMD was 3.1% to 3.5% greater than placebo. When looking at nonvertebral BMD, results were not as good as those noted for vertebral BMD. In the distal radius, BMD was only slightly greater for the treatment groups than for the placebo group at 1 year (range 0.8% to 1.6% compared with placebo, which decreased about 0.8%). Differences between treatment groups and the placebo group in terms of total body BMD were 0.9% to 1.3% higher for the treatment groups (significant for all except the 0.5 mg-every-3-month group). No vertebral fractures were noted during the study period. Nonvertebral fractures were noted in the group who received four doses of 1 mg (two fractures) and one fracture was noted in each of the other groups except the group who received four doses of 0.25 mg of zoledronic acid. Dropout rates were similar for treatment and placebo groups. Because the duration of the study did not extend beyond 1 year, data from longer time studies are needed.

FLUORIDE

Fluoride is an agent that can stimulate osteoblasts to increase the bone formation that can be more resistant to resorption, but which may not be as strong as normal bone. The effect of fluoride appears more likely to increase cancellous bone mass than cortical bone. Calcium supplementation in conjunction with fluoride administration can help prevent mineralization abnormalities that occur when fluoride is used without adequate calcium. Past use of high-dose sodium fluoride (75 to 100 mg) has been replaced with sustained-release products that are investigationally administered at doses of 25 mg twice daily. Pak[240] demonstrated the positive effects of sustained-release fluoride (25 mg twice daily) given orally for two 14-month cycles with a washout period (2 months) between cycles when compared with women receiving placebo. Both groups also received calcium citrate 400 mg twice daily. Those in the fluoride group had increased femoral neck density (4.1% and 2.1% during the two study periods), and fracture rates were decreased. A later article stated that the sustained-release product helped maintain fluoride in the therapeutic serum concentration range of 95 to 190 ng/mL.[241]

GI irritation and musculoskeletal pain may be less when sustained-release fluoride is used in low doses. Patients with underlying renal disease may require adjustment in fluoride doses. Those using fluoride must have a diet that has adequate dietary calcium or calcium supplementation. Timing of calcium and fluoride administration is important because fluoride absorption can be adversely affected by concomitant use of calcium, antacids, or dairy products.

TIBOLONE

This synthetic hormone has androgenic, estrogenic, and progestogenic activities that may help prevent cortical and cancellous bone loss. It has an effect on serum lipid concentrations that is lower than that noted for ET on HDLs and LDLs; however, it also decreases triglycerides, lipoprotein (a), and total cholesterol.[242]

STATINS

When it was discovered that bisphosphonates might suppress osteoclastic activity by inhibiting a step in the cholesterol synthesis pathway, speculation followed as to whether agents such as HMG CoA-reductase inhibitors (i.e., statins) might display similar effects.[145] In laboratory studies, statins inhibit osteoclastic-related bone resorption. It is unknown whether lipid-reducing doses of statins, which are used clinically, can have an effect on bone. Study results thus far have not presented consistent results and prospective clinical trials are needed.[145]

PHYTOESTROGENS

The effect of phytoestrogens for the treatment of osteoporosis is currently unknown. (See Question 44 and 49.)

Acknowledgment
We would like to thank Dr. Jennifer Hardman, Clinical Assistant Professor, University of Illinois at Chicago College of Pharmacy, and Dr. Nancy Letassy, Clinical Associate Professor, College of Pharmacy, University of Oklahoma Health Sciences Center, for their outstanding work on previous editions of this chapter.

REFERENCES

1. Merkatz RB et al. Women in clinical trials of new drugs. A change in Food and Drug Administration policy. N Engl J Med 1993;329:292.
2. NIH guidelines on inclusion of women and minorities. Available from: www.nih.gov/grants/guide/1994/94.03.18/notice-nih-guideline008.html.
3. Investigational new drug applications: amendment to clinical hold regulations for products intended for life-threatening diseases and conditions. Federal Register Vol 66 No 106 June 1, 2001 34963-71.
4. Harris RZ et al. Gender effects in pharmacokinetics and pharmacodynamics. Drugs 1995;50:222.
5. Drici MD, Clement N. Is gender a risk factor for adverse drug reactions? An example of drug-induced long QT syndrome. Drug Saf 2001;24:575.
6. Schwartz JB. The influence of sex on pharmacokinetics. Clin Pharmacokinet 2003;42:107.
7. Berg MJ et al. Pharmacologic issues. In: U.S. Department of Health and Human Services, Public Health Service, National Institutes of Health. Agenda for Research on Women's Health for the 21st Century: a report of the Task Force on the NIH Women's Health Research Agenda for the 21st Century, Volume 2. Bethesda: National Institutes of Health. NIH Publication No. 99-4386. 1999;147.
8. Mosca L et al. Cardiovascular disease in women: a statement for healthcare professionals from the American Heart Association. Circulation 1997;96:2468.
9. Ensom MHH. Gender-based differences and menstrual cycle-related changes in specific diseases: implications for pharmacotherapy. Pharmacotherapy 2000;20:5239.
10. Case AM, Reid RL. Effects of the menstrual cycle on medical disorders. Arch Intern Med 1998;158:1404.
11. Ries AJ. Treatment of vaginal infections: candidiasis, bacterial vaginosis, and trichomoniasis. JAPhA 1997;37:563.
12. Sobel JD. Vaginitis. N Engl J Med 1997;337:1896.
13. Centers for Disease Control and Prevention. Sexually Transmitted Diseases Treatment Guidelines—2002. MMWR 2002;51(RR-06):1.
14. Sobel JD. Bacterial vaginosis. Annu Rev Med 2000;51:349-56.
15. Sobel JD. Vulvovaginitis: when Candida becomes a problem. Dermatol Clin 1998;16:763.
16. Carr PL et al. Evaluation and management of vaginitis. J Gen Intern Med 1998;13:335.
17. Eckert LO et al. Vulvovaginal candidiasis: clinical manifestations, risk factors, managment algorithm. Obstet Gynecol 1998;92:757.
18. Gieger AM et al. The epidemiology of vulvovaginal candidiasis among university students. Am J Public Health 1996;85:1146.
19. Otero L et al. Vulvovaginal candidiasis in female sex workers. Int J STD AIDS 1998;9:526.
20. Tobin MJ. Vulvovaginal candidiasis: topical vs. oral therapy. Am Fam Physician 1995;51:1715.
21. Van Kessel K et al. Common complementary and alternative therapies for yeast vaginitis and bacterial vaginosis: a systematic review. Obstet Gynecol Surv 2003;58:351.
22. O-Prasertsawat P, Bourlert A. Comparative study of fluconazole and clotrimazole for the treatment of vulvovaginal candidiasis. Sex Transm Dis 1995;22:228.
23. Mikamo H et al. Comparative study on the effectiveness of antifungal agents in different regimens against vaginal candidiasis. Chemotherapy 1998;44:364.
24. Drug Facts and Comparison. St. Louis: Facts and Comparison, 2002 (updated monthly).
25. Ringdahl EN. Treatment of recurrent vulvovaginal candidiasis. Am Fam Physician 2000;61:3306.
26. Sobel JD. Use of antifungal drugs in pregnancy: a focus on safety. Drug Saf 2000;23:
27. Ugwumada AHN. Bacterial vaginosis in pregnancy. Curr Opin Obstet Gynecol 2002;14:115.
28. Harlow SD, Ephross SA. Epidemiology of menstruation and its relevance to women's health. Epidemiol Rev 1995;17:265.
29. Parent-Stevens L, Burns E. Menstrual disorders. In: Smith MA, Shimp LA, eds. 20 Common Problems in Women's Health Care. New York: McGraw-Hill 2000:381.
30. Deligeorglou E. Dysmenorrhea. Ann N Y Acad Sci 2000;900:237.
31. Golomb LM et al. Primary dysmenorrhea and physical activity. Med Sci Sports Exerc 1998;30:906.
32. Harel Z et al. Supplementation with omega-3 polyunsaturated fatty acids in the management of dysmenorrhea in adolescents. Am J Obstet Gynecol 1996;174:1335.
33. Akin MD et al. Continuous low-level topical heat in the treatment of dysmenorrhea. Am Coll Ob Gyne 1997;343.
34. Kaplan. Transcutaneous electrical nerve stimulation (TENS) as a relief for dysmenorrhea. Clin Exp Obstet Gynecol 1994;21:87.
35. Parente L, Perretti M. Advances in the path physiology of constitutive and inducible cyclooxygenases: two enzymes in the spotlight. Biochem Pharmacol 2003;65:153.
36. Morrison BW et al. Rofecoxib, a specific cyclooxygenase-2 inhibitor, in primary dysmenorrhea: a randomized controlled trial. Obstet Gynecol 1999;94:504.
37. Zhang WY, Li Wan Po A. Efficacy of minor analgesics in primary dysmenorrhea: a systematic review. Br J Obstet Gynecol 1998;105:780.
38. Milsom T et al. Comparison of the efficacy, and safety of nonprescription doses of naproxen and naproxen sodium with ibuprofen, acetaminophen, and placebo in the treatment of primary dysmenorrhea: a pooled analysis of five studies. Clin Ther 2002;24:1384.
39. Ezcurdia M et.al. Comparison of the efficacy and tolerability of dexketoprofen and ketoprofen in the treatment of primary dysmenorrhea. J Clin Pharmacol 1998;38:S65.
40. Hayes EC, Rock JA. COX-2 inhibitors and their role in gynecology. Obstet Gynecol Surv 2002;57:768.
41. Proctor ML et al. Combination oral contraceptive pill (OCP) as treatment for primary dysmenorrhea. Cochrane Database Syst Rev 2001;1.
42. Ghazizadeh S et al. Local application of glyceril trinitrate ointment in primary dysmenorrhea. Int J Gynecol Obstet 2002;79:43.
43. Proctor ML, Murphy PA. Herbal and dietary therapies for primary and secondary dysmenorrhea. Cochrane Database Syst Rev 2003;1.
44. Martin DC, Ling FW. Endometriosis and pain. Clin Obstet Gynecol 1999;42:664.
45. Schenken RS. Endometriosis. In: Scott JR et al, eds. Danforth's Obstetrics and Gynecology, 8th Ed. Philadelphia: Lippincott Williams & Wilkins, 1999;669.
46. Johnson KM. Endometriosis: the case for early, aggressive treatment. J Reprod Med 1998;43:309.
47. Giudice LC et al. Status of current research on endometriosis. J Reprod Med 1998;43:252.
48. Gleicher N, Pratt D. Abnormal (auto) immunity and endometriosis. Int J Gynecol Obstet 1993;40(Suppl):S21.
49. Barbieri RL. Endometriosis and the estrogen threshold theory: relation to surgical and medical treatment. J Reprod Med 1998;43:287.
50. Rice VM. Conventional medical therapies for endometriosis. Ann N Y Acad Sci 2002;955:343.
51. Cramer DW, Missmer S. The epidemiology of endometriosis. Ann N Y Acad Sci 2002;955:11.
52. Mahutte NG, Arici A. New advances in the understanding of endometriosis related infertility. J Reprod Immunol 2002;55:78.

53. American Fertility Society. Revised American Fertility Society for Reproductive Medicine classification of endometriosis: 1996. Fertil Steril 1997; 67:817.

54. Lin SY et al.Reproducibility of the revised American Fertility Society classification of endometriosis using laparoscopy or laparoscopy. Int J Gynecol Obstet 1998;60:265.

55. Mathur SP. Autoimmunity in endometriosis: relevance to infertility. Am J Reprod Immunol 2000;44:89.

56. Harada T et al. Usefulness of CA19-9 versus CA125 for the diagnosis of endometriosis. Fertil Steril 2002;78:733.

57. Olive DL, Pritts EA. Treatment of endometriosis. N Engl J Med 2002;345:266.

58. Gambone JC et al. Consensus statement for the management of chronic pelvic pain and endometriosis: proceedings of an expert panel consensus process. Fertil Steril 2002;78:961.

59. Vigano P et al. Immunosuppressive effect of danazol on lymphocyte-mediated cytotoxicity toward human endometrial stromal cells. Gynecol Endocrinol 1994;8:13.

60. Donnez J. Today's treatments: medical, surgical and in partnership. Int J Gynecol Obstet 1999; 64:S5.

61. Valle RF. Endometriosis: current concepts and therapy. Int J Gynecol Obstet 2002;78:107.

62. Donnez J et al. The efficacy of medical and surgical treatment of endometriosis-associated infertility and pelvic pain. Gynecol Obstet Invest 2002; 54(Suppl):2.

63. Vercellini P et al. Depot medroxyprogesterone acetate versus an oral contraceptive combined with very-low-dose danazol for long-term treatment of pelvic pain associated with endometriosis. J Obstet Gynecol 1996;175:396.

64. Vercellini P et al. Progestins for symptomatic endometriosis: a critical analysis of the evidence. Fertil Steril 1997;68:393.

65. Westhoff C. Bone mineral density and DMPA. J Reprod Med 2002;47(Suppl):795.

66. Hornstein MD et al. Prospective randomized double-blind trial of 3 versus 6 months of nafarelin therapy for endometriosis associated pelvic pain. Fertil Steril 1995;63:955.

67. Hahn PM et al. A randomized, placebo-controlled, crossover trial of danazol for the treatment of premenstrual syndrome. Psychoneuroendocrinology 1995;20:193.

68. Burry KA et al. Metabolic changes during medical treatment of endometriosis: nafarelin acetate versus danazol. Am J Obstet Gynecol 1989;160:1454.

69. Agarwal SK et al. Nafarelin vs. leuprolide acetate depot for endometriosis: changes in bone mineral density and vasomotor symptoms. J Reprod Med 1997;42:413.

70. Heinrichs WL, Henzl MR. Human issues and medical economics of endometriosis: three- vs. six-month GnRH-agonist therapy. J Reprod Med 1998;43:299.

71. Hornstein MD et al. Leuprolide acetate depot and hormonal add-back in endometriosis: a 12-month study. Obstet Gynecol 1998;91:16.

72. Agarwal SK. Comparative effects of GnRH agonist therapy: review of clinical studies and their implications. J Reprod Med 1998;43:293.

73. Cann CE. Bone densitometry as an adjunct to GnRH agonist therapy. J Reprod Med 1998; 43(Suppl):321.

74. Adamson CD et.al. Therapeutic efficacy and bone mineral density response during and following a three-month re-treatment of endometriosis with nafarelin (Synarel). Am J Obstet Gynecol 1997; 177:1413.

75. Surrey ES. Add-back therapy and gonadotropin-releasing hormone agonists in the treatment of patients with endometriosis: can a consensus be reached? Fertil Steril 1999;71:420.

76. Mukherjee T et al. A randomized, placebo-controlled study on the effect of cyclic intermittent etidronate therapy on the bone mineral density changes associated with six months of gonado-

77. Falcone T et al. Endometriosis: medical and surgical intervention. Curr Opin Obstet Gynecol 1996;8:178.

78. Korzekwa MI, Steiner M. Premenstrual syndromes. Clin Obstet Gynecol 1997;40:564.

79. Halbreich U et al. Low plasma GABA during the late luteal phase of women with premenstrual dysphoric disorder. Am J Psychiatry 1996;153:718.

80. Steiner M, Pearlstein T. Premenstrual dysphoric disorder and the serotonin system: pathophysiology and treatment. J Clin Psychiatry 2000; 61(Suppl):17.

81. Schmidt PJ et al. Differential behavioral effects of gonadal steroids in women with and in those without premenstrual syndrome. N Engl J Med 1998;338:209.

82. American Psychiatric Association. Diagnostic and Statistical Manual of Mental Disorders, 4th Ed. Washington, DC: American Psychiatric Association, 1994.

83. Endicott J. History, evolution and diagnosis of premenstrual dysphoric disorder. J Clin Psychiatry 2000;61(Suppl):5.

84. Grady-Weliky TA. Premenstrual dysphoric disorder. N Engl J Med 2003;348:433.

85. Pearlstein T. Selective serotonin reuptake inhibitors for premenstrual dysphoric disorder: the emerging gold standard? Drugs 2002;62:1869.

86. Bhatia SC, Bhatia SK. Diagnosis and treatment of premenstrual dysphoric disorder. Am Fam Physician 2002;66:1239.

87. Freeman EW, Rickels K. Characteristics of placebo responses in medical treatment of premenstrual syndrome. Am J Psychiatry 1999;156:1403.

88. Dimmock PW et al. Efficacy of selective serotonin-reuptake inhibitors in premenstrual syndrome: a systematic review. Lancet 2000;356:1131.

89. Miner C et al. Weekly luteal-phase dosing with enteric-coated fluoxetine 90mg in premenstrual dysphoric disorder: a randomized, double-blind, placebo-controlled clinical trial. Clin Ther 2002; 24:417.

90. Steiner M et al. Effect of fluoxetine on menstrual cycle length in women with premenstrual dysphoria. Obstet Gynecol 1997;90:590.

91. Freeman EW et al. Nefazodone in the treatment of premenstrual syndrome: a preliminary study. J Clin Psychopharmacol 1994;14:180.

92. Landen M et al. Compounds with affinity for serotonergic receptors in the treatment of premenstrual dysphoria: a comparison of buspirone, nefazodone and placebo. Psychopharmacology 2001; 155:292.

93. Berger CP, Presser B. Alprazolam in the treatment of two sub samples of patients with late luteal phase dysphoric disorder: a double-blind, placebo-controlled crossover study. Obstet Gynecol 1994;84:379.

94. Diegoli MSC et al. A double-blind trial of four medications to treat severe premenstrual syndrome. Int J Gynecol Obstet 1998;62:63.

95. Freeman EW et al. A double-blind trial of oral progesterone, alprazolam, and placebo in treatment of severe premenstrual syndrome. JAMA 1995;274:51.

96. Schmidt PJ et al. Alprazolam in the treatment of premenstrual syndrome. A double-blind, placebo-controlled trial. Arch Gen Psychiatry 1993;50:467.

97. Ward MW, Holimon TD. Calcium treatment for premenstrual syndrome. Ann Pharmacother 1999;33:1356.

98. Thys-Jacobs S et al. Calcium carbonate and the premenstrual syndrome: effects on premenstrual and menstrual symptoms. Am J Obstet Gynecol 1998;179:444.

99. Stevinson C, Ernst E. Complementary/alternative therapies for premenstrual syndrome: a systematic review of randomized trials. Am J Obstet Gynecol 2001;185:227.

100. Wyatt KM et al. Efficacy of vitamin B-6 in the treatment of premenstrual syndrome: systematic review. Br Med J 1999;318:1375.

101. Schellenberg R. Treatment for the premenstrual syndrome with agnus castus fruit extract: prospective, randomized, placebo controlled study. BMJ 2001;332:134.

102. Brown C, Ling F, Wan J. A new monophonic oral contraceptive containing drospirenone: effect on premenstrual symptoms. J Reprod Med 2002; 47:14.

103. Wyatt K et al. Efficacy of progesterone and progestogens in management of premenstrual syndrome: systematic review. BMJ 2001;232:776.

104. Pearlstein T, Steiner M. Non-antidepressant treatment of premenstrual syndrome. J Clin Psychiatry 2000;61(Suppl)22.

105. Wang M et al. Treatment of premenstrual syndrome by spironolactone: a double-blind, placebo-controlled study. Acta Obstet Gynecol Scand 1995;74:803.

106. Mezrow G et al. Depot leuprolide acetate with estrogen and progestin add-back for long-term treatment of premenstrual syndrome. Fertil Steril 1994;62:932.

107. O'Brien PMS, Abukhalil IEH. Randomized controlled trial of the management of premenstrual syndrome and premenstrual mastalgia using luteal phase-only danazol. Am J Obstet Gynecol 1999;180:18.

108. Hammond CB. Climacteric. In: Scott JR et al, eds. Danforth's Obstetrics and Gynecology, 8th Ed. Philadelphia: Lippincott Williams & Wilkins, 1999:677.

109. Sowers MR, La Pietra MT. Menopause: its epidemiology and potential association with chronic diseases. Epidemiol Rev 1995;17:287.

110. McDonnell DP et al. Analysis of estrogen receptor function in vitro reveals three distinct classes of antiestrogens. Mol Endocrinol 1995;9:659.

111. Diel P. Tissue-specific estrogenic response and molecular mechanisms. Toxicol Lett 2002, 127:217.

112. Stearns V et.al. Hot flushes. Lancet 2002; 360;1851.

113. Rice VM. Hormone replacement therapy: optimizing the dose and route of administration. Drugs Aging 2002;19:807.

114. Grady D et al. Hormone replacement therapy and endometrial cancer risk: a meta-analysis. Obstet Gynecol 1995;85:304.

115. Pike MC, Ross RK. Progestins and menopause: epidemiological studies of risks of endometrial and breast cancer. Steroids 2000;65:659.

116. Rosenfeld JA. Update on continuous estrogen-progestin replacement therapy. Am Fam Physician 1994;50:1519.

117. The Writing Group for the PEPI Trial. Effects of hormone replacement therapy on endometrial histology in postmenopausal women: the postmenopausal estrogen/progestin interventions (PEPI) trial. JAMA 1996;275:370.

118. Archer DF et al. Bleeding patterns in postmenopausal women taking continuous combined or sequential regimens of conjugated estrogens with medroxyprogesterone acetate. Obstet Gynecol 1994;83:686.

119. Loprinzi CL et al. Megestrol acetate for the prevention of hot flashes. N Engl J Med 1994; 331:347.

120. Lucero MA, McCloskey WW. Alternatives to estrogen for the treatment of hot flashes. Ann Pharmacother 1997;31:915.

121. Braunstein GD. Androgen insufficiency in women: summary of critical issues. Fertil Steril 2002;77(Suppl):S94.

122. Guttuso T et.al. Gabapentin's effects on hot flashes in postmenopausal women: a randomized controlled trial. Obstet Gynecol 2003;101:337.

123. Kronenberg F, Fugh-Berman A. Complementary and alternative medicine for menopausal symptoms: a review of randomized, controlled trials. Ann Intern Med 2002;127:805.

124. Chetkowski RJ et al. Biologic effects of transdermal estradiol. N Engl J Med 1986;314:1615.

125. Uhler ML et al. Comparison of the impact of transdermal versus oral estrogens on biliary

markers of gallstone formation in postmenopausal women. J Clin Endocrinol Metab 1998;83:410.

126. Willhite LA, O'Connell MB. Urogenital atrophy: prevention and treatment. Pharmacother 2001; 21:464.

127. Cardoso L, Robinson D. Special considerations in premenopausal and postmenopausal women with symptoms of overactive bladder. Urology 2002;60(Suppl):64.

128. Freedman MA. Quality of life and menopause: the role of estrogen. J Womens Health 2002;11:703.

129. World Health Organization. Assessment of Fracture Risk and Its Application to Screening for Postmenopausal Osteoporosis: report of a WHO Study Group. Geneva, Switzerland: World Health Organization, 1994:2. Technical Report Series 843.

130. Kanis JA et al. The diagnosis of osteoporosis. J Bone Miner Res 1994;9:1137.

131. Eastell R. Treatment of postmenopausal osteoporosis. N Engl J Med 1998;338;736.

132. Melton LJ III. How many women have osteoporosis now? J Bone Miner Res 1995;10:175.

133. Prestwood KM, Weksler ME. Osteoporosis: up-to-date strategies for prevention and treatment. Geriatrics 1997;52:92.

134. Riggs BL, Melton LJ III. The prevention and treatment of osteoporosis. N Engl J Med 1992; 327:620.

135. Cosman F. Skeletal effects of selective estrogen receptor modulators. Am J Managed Care 1999; 5:S169.

136. Cummings SR et al. Epidemiology of osteoporosis and osteoporotic fractures. Epidemiol Rev 1985;7:178.

137. Consensus development conference: prophylaxis and treatment of osteoporosis. Am J Med 1991;90:107.

138. Ray NF et al. Medical expenditures for the treatment of osteoporotic fractures in the United States in 1995: report from the National Osteoporosis Foundation. J Bone Miner Res 1997;12:24.

139. Gold DT, Lee LS, Tresolini CP, eds. Working with Patients to Prevent, Treat and Manage Osteoporosis: A Current Guide for the Health Professions, 3rd Ed. Durham, NC: Center for the Study of Aging and Human Development, Duke University Medical Center, 2001.

140. Mazess RB. On aging bone loss. Clin Orthop 1982;165:239.

141. Riggs BL, Melton LJ III. Involutional osteoporosis. N Engl J Med 1986;314:1676.

142. Willhite L. Osteoporosis in women: prevention and treatment. JAPhA 1998;38:614.

143. Gallagher JC. Pathophysiology of osteoporosis. Semin Nephrol 1992;12:109.

144. Morrison NA et al. Prediction of bone density from vitamin D receptor alleles. Nature 1994; 367:284.

145. The North American Menopause Society. Management of postmenopausal osteoporosis: position statement of The North American Menopause Society. Menopause 2002;9:84.

146. Gutin B, Kasper JM. Can vigorous exercise play a role in osteoporosis prevention? A review. Osteoporos Int 1992;2:55.

147. Institute of Medicine, National Research Council. Summary statement on calcium and related nutrients. 1997;S1. Available from www.nas.edu/new.

148. NIH Consensus Development Panel on Optimal Calcium Intake. Optimal calcium intake. JAMA 1994;272:1942.

149. Baron JA, Farahmand BY, Weiderpass E et al. Cigarette smoking, alcohol consumption, and risk for hip fracture in women. Arch Intern Med 2001;161:983.

150. Morley JE et al. UCLA geriatric grand round: osteoporosis. J Am Geriatr Soc 1988;36:845.

151. Moniz C. Alcohol and bone. Br Med Bull 1994;50:67.

152. Cummings DC. Exercise induced amenorrhea, low bone density and estrogen replacement therapy. Arch Intern Med 1996;156:2193.

153. Eddy DM et al. Osteoporosis: review of the evidence for prevention, diagnosis and treatment and cost-effectiveness analysis. Osteoporos Int 1998;8 (Suppl 4):S7.

154. Cummings RG, Nevitt MC. Calcium for prevention of osteoporotic fractures in postmenopausal women. J Bone Miner Res 1997;12:1321.

155. Grady D et al. Heart and estrogen/progestin replacement study (HERS): design, methods and baseline characteristics. Control Clin Trials 1998;19:314.

156. Grady D, Herrington D, Bittner V et al. Cardiovascular disease outcomes during 6.8 years of hormone therapy: heart and estrogen/progestin replacement study follow-up (HERS II). JAMA 2002;288:49.

157. Writing Group for the Women's Health Initiative Investigators. Risks and benefits of estrogen plus progestin in healthy postmenopausal women: principal results from the Women's Health Initiative Randomized Controlled Trial. JAMA 2002;288:321.

158. Kusiak V. FDA approves prescribing information for postmenopausal hormone therapies. Wyeth Pharmaceuticals: Philadelphia, January 6, 2003 (letter to health care professionals).

159. Kuiper GGJM et al. The estrogen receptor beta subtype: a novel mediator of estrogen action in neuroendocrine systems. Front Neuroendocrinol 1998;19:253.

160. Ettinger B et al. The waning effect of postmenopausal estrogen therapy on osteoporosis. N Engl J Med 1993;329:1192.

161. The Writing Group for the PEPI. Effects of hormone therapy on bone mineral density: results from the Postmenopausal Estrogen/Progestin Interventions (PEPI) Trial. JAMA 1996;276:1389.

162. Grady D et al. Hormone therapy to prevent disease and prolong life in postmenopausal women. Ann Intern Med 1992;117:1016.

163. Torgerson DJ, Bell-Syer SE. Hormone replacement therapy and prevention of nonvertebral fractures: a meta-analysis of randomized trials. JAMA 2001;285:2891.

164. Cauley JA et al. Estrogen replacement therapy and fractures in older women: Study of Osteoporotic Fracture Research Group. Ann Intern Med 1995;122:9.

165. Lufkin EG et al. Treatment of postmenopausal osteoporosis with transdermal estrogen. Ann Intern Med 1992;117:1.

166. Sagraves R et al. Therapeutic options for osteoporosis. APhA Special Report. Washington, DC: American Pharmaceutical Association, 1993.

167. Archer DF et al. Effects of lower doses of conjugated equine estrogens and medroxyprogesterone acetate on endometrial bleeding. Fertil Steril 2001;75:1080.

168. The North American Menopause Society. Role of progestogen in hormone therapy for postmenopausal women: position statement of The North American Menopause Society. Menopause 10;113:2002.

169. Ettinger B et al. Menopausal bone loss can be prevented by low-dose estrogen combined with calcium supplements. In: Update on Postmenopausal Osteoporosis. New York: Biomedical Information, 1984:63.

170. Recker RR et al. The effect of low-dose continuous estrogen and progesterone therapy with calcium and vitamin D on bone in elderly women: a randomized, controlled trial. Ann Intern Med 1999;130:897.

171. Lindsay R et al. Effect of lower doses of conjugated equine estrogens with and without medroxyprogesterone acetate on bone in early postmenopausal women. JAMA 2002;287:2668.

172. Genant HK et al. Low-dose esterified estrogen therapy: effects on bone, plasma estradiol concentrations, endometrium, and lipid levels. Arch Intern Med 1997;157:2609.

173. Weiss SR, Ellman H, Dolker M. A randomized controlled trial of four doses of transdermal estradiol for preventing postmenopausal bone loss. Transdermal Estradiol Investigator Group. Obstet Gynecol 1999;94:330.

174. PremproTM and Premphase® package insert. Wyeth Pharmaceuticals:Philadelphia, May 23, 2003.

175. Hammond CB, Maxson WS. Estrogen replacement therapy. Clin Obstet Gynecol 1986;29:407.

176. Colditz GA et al. Hormone replacement therapy and risk of breast cancer: results from epidemiologic studies. Am J Obstet Gynecol 1993;168:1473.

177. Sillero-Arenas M et al. Menopausal hormone replacement therapy and breast cancer: a meta-analysis. Obstet Gynecol 1992;79:286.

178. Collaborative Group on Hormonal Factors in Breast Cancer. Breast cancer and hormone replacement therapy: collaborative reanalysis of data from 51 epidemiological studies of 52,705 women with breast cancer and 108,411 women without breast cancer. Lancet 1997;350:1047.

179. Roy JA et al. Hormone replacement therapy in women with breast cancer: do the risks outweigh the benefits? J Clin Oncol 1996;14:997.

180. The North American Menopause Society. Amended report from the NAMS Advisory Panel on Postmenopausal Hormone Therapy. Menopause 2003;12:10.

181. U.S. Preventive Services Task Force. Postmenopausal hormone replacement therapy for the primary prevention of chronic conditions: recommendations and rationale. Center for Practice and Technology Assessement, Agency for Healthcare Research and Quality: Rockville, MD, www.preventiveservices.ahrq.gov.

182. Gapstur SM et al. Hormone replacement therapy and risk of breast cancer with a favorable histology. Results of the Iowa Women's Health Study. JAMA 1999;281:2091.

183. Rodriguez C et al. Estrogen replacement therapy and ovarian cancer mortality in a large prospective study of US women. JAMA 2001;285:1460.

184. Lacey JJ et al. Menopausal hormone replacement therapy and risk of ovarian cancer. JAMA 2002;288:334.

185. Persson I et al. Cancer incidence and mortality in women receiving estrogen and estrogen-progestin replacement therapy—long-term follow-up of a Swedish cohort. Int J Cancer 1996;67:327.

186. American Heart Association. 1999 Heart and stroke statistical update. Dallas, TX: American Heart Association, 1998.

187. Grodstein F et al. Postmenopausal hormone therapy and mortality. N Engl J Med 1997;336:1769.

188. Henderson BE et al. Decreased mortality in users of estrogen replacement therapy. Arch Intern Med 1991;151:75.

189. Sullivan JM et al. Estrogen replacement and coronary artery disease: effect on survival in postmenopausal women. Arch Intern Med 1990;150:2557.

190. The Writing Group for the PEPI Trial. Effects of estrogen or estrogen/progestin regimens on heart disease risk factors in postmenopausal women: the postmenopausal estrogen/progestin interventions (PEPI) trial. JAMA 1995;273:199.

191. Grodstein F, Clarkson TB, Manson JE. Understanding the divergent data on postmenopausal hormone therapy. N Engl J Med 2003;348:645.

192. Barrett-Connor E. Postmenopausal estrogen and prevention bias. Ann Intern Med 1991;115:455.

193. Hulley S et al. Randomized trial of estrogen plus progestin for secondary prevention of coronary heart disease in postmenopausal women. JAMA 1998;280:605.

194. Grodstein F et al. Prospective study of exogenous hormones and risk of pulmonary embolism in women. Lancet 1996;348:983.

195. Daly E et al. Risk of venous thromboembolism in users of hormone replacement therapy. Lancet 1996;348:977.

196. Wasserheil-Smoller S et al. Effect of estrogen plus progestin on stroke in postmenopausal women.

The Women's Health Initiative: a randomized trial. JAMA 2003;289:2673.

197. Mulnard RA et al. Estrogen replacement therapy for treatment of mild to moderate Alzheimer disease. JAMA 2000;283:1007.

198. Rapp SR et al. Effect of estrogen plus progestin on global cognitive function in postmenopausal women. The Women's Health Initiative Memory Study: a randomized controlled trial. JAMA 289:2663.

199. Yaffe K. Hormone therapy and the brain, déjà vu all over again? JAMA 2003;289:2717.

200. Grodstein F, Newcomb P, Stampfer M. Postmenopausal hormone therapy and the risk of colorectal cancer: a review and meta-analysis. Am J Med 1999;106:574.

201. Eli Lilly and Company. Introducing new Evista (raloxifene HCl). Indianapolis, IN, 1997.

202. Eli Lilly and Company. Evista package insert. Indianapolis, 1997.

203. Delmas PD et al. Effects of raloxifene on bone mineral density, serum cholesterol concentrations, and uterine endometrium in postmenopausal women. N Engl J Med 1997;337:1641.

204. Ettinger B et al. Reduction of vertebral fracture risk in postmenopausal women with osteoporosis treated with raloxifene: results from a 3-year randomized clinical trial. JAMA 1999;282:637.

205. Sarkar S et al. Relationships between bone mineral density and incident of vertebral fracute risk with raloxifene therapy. J Bone Miner Res 2002; 17:1.

206. Johnell O et al. Additive effects of raloxifene and alendronate on bone density and biochemical markers of bone remodeling in postmenopausal women with osteoporosis. J Clin Endocrinol Metab 2002;87:985.

207. Prestwood KM et al. A comparison of the effects of raloxifene and estrogen on bone in postmenopausal women. J Clin Endocrinol Metab. 2000;85:2197.

208. Riggs L, Hartmann LC. Selective estrogen-receptor modulators—mechanisms of action and application to clinical practice. N Engl J Med. 2003; 348:618.

209. Riggs BL, Melton J III. Bone turnover matters: the raloxifene treatment paradox of dramatic decreases in vertebral fractures without commensurate increases in bone density. J Bone Miner Res. 2002;17:11.

210. Cummings SR et al. The effect of raloxifene on risk of breast cancer in postmenopausal women: results from the MORE Randomized Trial. JAMA 1999;281:2189.

211. Walsh BW et al. Effects of raloxifene on serum lipids and coagulation factors in healthy postmenopausal women. JAMA 1998;279:1445.

212. Mosca L. Cardiovascular effects of selective estrogen receptor modulators. Am J Managed Care 1999;5(Suppl):S156.

213. Jordan VC, Morrow M. Raloxifene as a multifunctional medicine? Current trials will show whether it is effective in both osteoporosis and breast cancer. Br Med J 1999;319:331.

214. Weiss et al. Five-year efficacy and safety of oral alendronate for prevention of osteoporosis in early postmenopausal women [Abstract]. J Bone Min Res 1997;12 (Suppl 1):165.

215. Hosking MD et al. Prevention of bone loss with alendronate in postmenopausal women under 60 years of age. N Engl J Med 1998;338:485.

216. Black DM et al. Randomised trial of effect of alendronate on risk of fracture in women with existing vertebral fractures. Lancet 1996;348:1535.

217. Cummings S et al. Effect of alendronate on risk of fracture in women with low bone density but without vertebral fractures: results from the Fracture Intervention Trial. JAMA 1998;280:2077.

218. Black DM et al. Fracture risk reduction with alendronate in women with osteoporosis: the fracture intervention trial. J Clin Endocrinol Metab 2000;85:4118.

219. Karpf DB et al. Prevention of nonvertebral fractures by alendronate: a meta-analysis. JAMA 1997;277:1159.

220. Mortensen L et al. Risedronate increases bone mass in an early postmenopausal population: two years of treatment plus one year of follow-up. J Clin Endocrinol Metab 1998;83:396.

221. Harris ST et al. Effects of risedronate treatment on vertebral and nonverbetral fractures in women with postmenopausal osteoporosis: a randomized controlled trial. JAMA 1999;282(14):1344.

222. Tonino RP et al. Skeletal benefits of alendronate: 7-year treatment of postmenopausal osteoporotic women. J Clin Endocrinol Metab 2000;85:3109.

223. Emkey R et al. Ten-year efficacy and safety of alendronate in the treatment of osteoporosis in postmenopausal women. ASBMR 24th Annual Meeting, San Antonio, TX, September 22, 2002 (Abstract).

224. Jones G et al. Thiazide diuretics and fractures: can meta-analysis help? J Bone Miner Res 1995; 10:106.

225. Lufkin EG et al. Treatment of established postmenopausal osteoporosis with raloxifene: a randomized trial. J Bone Miner Res 1998;13:1747.

226. Liberman UA et al. Effect of oral alendronate on bone mineral density and the incidence of fractures in postmenopausal osteoporosis. N Engl J Med 1995;333:1437.

227. Bone HG et al. Dose-response relationships for alendronate in osteoporotic elderly women. J Clin Endocrinol Metab 1997;82:265.

228. Merck & CO., Inc. Fosamax package insert. Whitehouse Station, NJ, 1999.

229. Reginster J et al. Randomized trial of the effects of risedronate on vertebral fractures in women with established postmenopausal osteoporosis. Vertebral Efficacy with Risedronate Therapy (VERT) Study Group. Osteoporos Int 2000; 11(1):83.

230. McClung MR et al. Effect of risedronate on the risk of hip fracture in elderly women. N Engl J Med 2001;344:333.

231. Schnitzer T et al. Therapeutic equivalence of alendronate 70 mg once weekly and alendronate 10 mg daily in the treatment of osteoporosis. Aging Clin Exp Res 2000;12:1.

232. Storm T et al. Five years of clinical experience with intermittent cyclical etidronate for postmenopausal osteoporosis. J Rheumatol 1996;23: 1560.

233. Wimalawansa SJ. A four-year randomized controlled trial of hormone replacement and bisphosphonate, alone or in combination, in women with postmenopausal osteoporosis. Am J Med 1998;104:219.

234. Cranney A et al. A meta-analysis of etidronate for the treatment of postmenopausal osteoporosis. Osteoporosis Research Advisory Group. Osteoporos Int 2001;12:140.

235. Silverman SL. Calcitonin. Am J Med Sci 1997; 313:13.

236. Chesnut CH III et al. A randomized trial of nasal spray salmon calcitonin in postmenopausal women with established osteoporosis: The Prevent Recurrence of Osteoporotic Fractures Study. PROOF study group. Am J Med 2000;109:267.

237. Neer RM et al. Effect of parathyroid hormone(1-34) on fractures and bone mineral density in postmenopausal women with osteoporosis. N Engl J Med 2001;344:1434.

238. Schuna AA, Dong BJ (section advisors). Teriparatide provides useful option in severe osteoporosis. APhA Drug Info Line 2002;3(12):1.

239. Reid IR et al. Intravenous zoledronic acid in postmenopausal women with low bone mineral density. N Engl J Med 2002;346:653.

240. Pak CYC et al. Slow-release sodium fluoride in the management of postmenopausal osteoporosis. A randomized controlled trial. Ann Intern Med 1994;120:625.

241. Pak CYC et al. Sustained-release sodium fluoride in the management of established postmenopausal osteoporosis. Am J Med Sci 1997;313:23.

242. Bjarnason NH et al. Tibolone: prevention of bone loss in late postmenopausal women. J Clin Endocrinol Metab 1996;81:2419.

CHAPTER 49

Thyroid Disorders

Betty J. Dong

OVERVIEW

Thyroid disease is common, affecting approximately 5% to 15% of the general population. Females are three to four times more likely than males to develop any type of thyroid disease. The typical thyroid disorders emphasized in this chapter are hypothyroidism, hyperthyroidism, and nodular disease. Thyroid cancer is discussed briefly. The reader is referred to standard medical textbooks for more detailed medical and diagnostic information.

Triiodothyronine (T_3) and thyroxine (T_4) are the two biologically active thyroid hormones produced by the thyroid gland in response to hormones released by the pituitary and hypothalamus. The hypothalamic thyrotropin-releasing hormone (TRH) stimulates release of thyrotropin (i.e., thyroid-stimulating hormone [TSH]) from the pituitary in response to low circulating levels of thyroid hormone. TSH in turn promotes hormone synthesis and release by increasing thyroid activity. When sufficient synthesis has occurred, high circulating thyroid hormone levels block further production by inhibiting TSH release. The intrapituitary deiodination of T_4 to T_3 also plays a critical role in the inhibition of TSH secretion. As the serum concentrations of thyroid hormone decrease, the hypothalamic-pituitary centers again become responsive by releasing TRH and TSH.

T_3 is four times more potent than T_4, but its serum concentration is lower. T_4 is the major circulating hormone secreted by the thyroid. In contrast, about 80% of the total daily T_3 production results from the peripheral conversion of T_4 to T_3 through deiodination of T_4. T_4 has intrinsic biologic activity and does not function solely as a prohormone. Approximately 35% to 40% of secreted T_4 is converted peripherally to T_3; another 45% of secreted T_4 undergoes peripheral conversion to inactive reverse T_3 (rT_3). Certain drugs and diseases can modify the conversion rate of T_4 to T_3 and decrease the serum T_3 levels (Table 49-1; see Question 2).

T_3 and T_4 exist in the circulation in free (active) and protein-bound (inactive) forms. About 99.97% of circulating T_4 is bound: 70% to thyroxine-binding globulin (TBG), 15% to thyroxine-binding prealbumin (TBPA), and the rest to albumin. Only 0.03% exists as the free form. This affinity for plasma proteins accounts for T_4's slow metabolic degradation and long half-life ($t_{1/2}$) of 7 days. In contrast, T_3 is considerably less strongly bound to plasma proteins (99.7%); about 0.3% exists as free hormone. The lower protein-binding affinity of T_3 accounts for its threefold greater metabolic potency and its shorter half-life of 1.5 days.

Hypothyroidism is a clinical syndrome that results from a deficiency of thyroid hormone. The prevalence of hypothyroidism is 1.4% to 2% in females and 0.1% to 0.2% in males. The incidence increases in persons >60 years of age to 6% of women and 2.5% of men. Hypothyroidism can be caused by either primary (thyroid gland) or secondary (hypothalamic-pituitary) malfunction. Primary hypothyroidism is more common than secondary causes.

Hashimoto's thyroiditis, an autoimmune disorder, is the most common cause of primary hypothyroidism and appears to have a strong genetic predisposition. The pathogenesis of Hashimoto's thyroiditis results from an impaired immune surveillance, causing dysfunction of normal "suppressor" T lymphocytes and excessive production of thyroid antibodies by plasma cells (differentiated B lymphocytes). The destruction of thyroid cells by circulating thyroid antibodies produces

Table 49-1 Factors That Can Significantly Alter Thyroid Function Tests in Euthyroid Patients	
↑ TBG Binding Capacity	Drugs/Situations
↑ TT_4	Estrogens,[4,21,22] tamoxifen[24],
↑ TT_3	raloxifene[23]
↓ RT_3U	Oral contraceptives[4]
Normal TSH	Heroin[20]
Normal FT_4I, FT_4	Methadone maintenance[20]
Normal FT_3I, FT_3	Genetic ↑ in TBG
	Clofibrate
	Active hepatitis[1]
↓ TBG Binding Capacity/Displacement T_4 from Binding Sites	
↓ TT_4	Androgens[4]
↓ TT_3	Salicylates,[4,12,13] disalcid,[13] salsalate[13]
↑ RT_3U	High-dose furosemide
Normal TSH	↓ TBG synthesis-cirrhosis/
Normal FT_4I, FT_4	hepatic failure
Normal FT_3I, FT_3	Nephrotic syndrome[1,4]
	Danazol[1,4]
	Glucocorticoids[1,4]
↓ Peripheral T_4→T_3 Conversion	
↓ TT_3	PTU
Normal TT_4	Propranolol[142]
Normal FT_4I, FT_4	Glucocorticoids[3,4]
Normal TSH	
↓ Pituitary and Peripheral T_4→T_3	
↓ TT_3	Ipodate, iopanoic acid[127–130]
↑ TT_4	Amiodarone[25,26]
↑ TSH (transient)	Euthyroid sick syndrome[5–7]
↑ FT_4I	
↑ T_4 Clearance by Enzyme Induction/↑ Fecal Loss	
↓ TT_4	Phenytoin[14–15]
↓ FT_4I	Phenobarbital[14]
Normal or ↓ FT_4	Carbamazepine[14–19]
Normal or ↓ TT_3	Cholestyramine, colestipol[74]
Normal or ↑ TSH	Rifampin[14]
↓ TSH Secretion	
	Dopamine[1,4] dobutamine[27]
	Levodopa[13] cabergoline[28]
	Glucocorticoids[3,4]
	Bromocriptine[3,4]
	Octreotide[2]
↑ TSH	Metoclopramide[1,3,4]
	Domperidone[1,3,4]

FT_3, free triiodothyronine; FT_4, free thyroxine; FT_3I, free triiodothyronine index; FT_4I, free thyroxine index; PTU, propylthiouracil; RT_3U, resin triiodothyronine uptake; TBG, thyroxine-binding globulin; T_3, triiodothyronine; T_4, thyroxine; TSH, thyroid-stimulating hormone; TT_3, total triiodothyronine; TT_4, total thyroxine.
From references 1–4, 12–15, 20–28.

an underlying defect or block in the intrathyroidal, organobinding of iodide. As a result, inactive hormones or insufficient amounts of active hormones are synthesized, and this eventually produces hypothyroidism. However, the clinical presentation of Hashimoto's thyroiditis can be variable, depending on the time of diagnosis. Although the typical presentation is hypothyroidism and goiter (thyroid gland enlargement), patients can present with hypothyroidism and no goiter, with euthyroidism and a goiter, or rarely (<5%) with hyperthyroidism (Hashi-toxicosis).

Hashimoto's thyroiditis might be related to Graves' disease, a common cause of hyperthyroidism. Both diseases share similar clinical features: positive antibody titers, a goiter with lymphocytic infiltration of the gland, a familial tendency, and a predilection for women. Both diseases can coexist in the same gland. Thyrotoxicosis can precede the onset of Hashimoto's hypothyroidism, and the end result of Graves' hyperthyroidism often is hypothyroidism. These common clinical features suggest that Graves' disease and Hashimoto's thyroiditis might be the same disease manifesting in different ways.

Other common causes of hypothyroidism are presented in Table 49-2 and include iatrogenic destruction of the gland after radioiodine therapy or surgery and hypothyroidism secondary to nontoxic multinodular goiter. Drug-induced hypothyroidism (e.g., iodides, amiodarone, lithium, interferon-α) occurs in susceptible persons (i.e., Hashimoto's thyroiditis) with a pre-existing thyroid abnormality.

The typical symptoms of hypothyroidism include weight gain, fatigue, sluggishness, cold intolerance, constipation, heavy menstrual periods, and muscle aches. A goiter might or might not be present. Patients with end-stage hypothyroidism, or myxedema coma, also can present with hypothermia, confusion, stupor or coma, carbon dioxide retention, hypoglycemia, hyponatremia, and ileus. Symptoms of "slowing down" would be expected because thyroid hormone is essential for the function and maintenance of all body systems and metabolic processes. In general, the more severe the degree of hypothyroidism, the greater the number of clinical findings. The exception is the older patient with hypothyroidism, who often presents with minimal or atypical symptoms (e.g., weight loss, deafness, tinnitus, carpal tunnel syndrome). Patients with mild and subclinical hypothyroidism also might have few or no symptoms. Laboratory findings that are diagnostic for overt hypothyroidism include elevated TSH and low free thyroxine levels; those for subclinical or early hypothyroidism are elevated TSH and normal free thyroxine levels. The common clinical symptoms, physical findings, and laboratory abnormalities of overt hypothyroidism are summarized in Table 49-3.

Table 49-2   Causes of Hypothyroidism

Nongoitrous (No Gland Enlargement)

Primary Hypothyroidism (Dysfunction of the Gland)

Idiopathic atrophy
Iatrogenic destruction of thyroid
   Surgery
   Radioactive iodine therapy
   X-ray therapy
Postinflammatory thyroiditis
Cretinism (congenital hypothyroidism)

Secondary Hypothyroidism

Deficiency of TSH due to pituitary dysfunction
Deficiency of TRH due to hypothalamic dysfunction

Goitrous Hypothyroidism (Enlargement of Thyroid Gland)

Dyshormonogenesis: defect in hormone synthesis, transport, or
   action
Hashimoto's thyroiditis[a]
Drug-induced: iodides, lithium,[b] thiocyanates, phenylbutazone,
   sulfonylureas,[c] amiodarone,[d] interferon-α
Congenital cretinism: maternally induced
Iodide deficiency
Natural goitrogens: rutabagas, turnips, cabbage

---

[a]Most common cause, an autoimmune disease; intrathyroidal organo binding of iodine is blocked; can also present as hyperthyroidism
[b]Goiter with or without hypothyroidism can occur in a small percent of patients after 5 months–2 yr of therapy. Most affected individuals have personal or family history of thyroid disease. Inhibits release of thyroid hormone and also may affect the pituitary-thyroid axis. *Effect on thyroid tests:* low TT_4 and FT_4I; elevated TSH and RAIU. Goiter responds to discontinuation of lithium or suppression with thyroid. Discontinuation of lithium can unmask underlying hyperthyroidism.
[c]Large doses of tolbutamide or chlorpropamide (exceeding usual therapeutic range) can inhibit thyroid formation.
[d]Prevalence 6%–16%. Mechanism may be related to high iodine content (37.5 mg organic 1/100 mg) or altered metabolism of T_4 to reverse T_3. Rarely causes hyperthyroidism.

Table 49-3   Clinical and Laboratory Findings of Primary Hypothyroidism

Symptoms	Physical Findings	Laboratory
General: weakness, tiredness, lethargy, fatigue	Thin brittle nails	↓ TT_4
Cold intolerance	Thinning of skin	↓ FT_4I
Headache	Pallor	↓ FT_4
Loss of taste/smell	Puffiness of face, eyelids	↓ TT_3
Deafness	Yellowing of skin	↓ FT_3I
Hoarseness	Thinning of outer eyebrows	↑ TSH
No sweating	Thickening of tongue	Positive antibodies (in Hashimoto's)
Modest weight gain	Peripheral edema	↑ Cholesterol
Muscle cramps, aches, pains	Pleural/peritoneal/pericardial effusions	↑ CPK
Dyspnea	↓ DTRs	↓ Na
Slow speech	"Myxedema heart"	↑ LDH
Constipation	Bradycardia (↓ HR)	↑ AST
Menorrhagia	Hypertension	↓ Hct/Hgb
Galactorrhea	Goiter (primary hypothyroidism)	

AST, aspartate aminotransferase; CPK, creatinine phosphokinase; DTRs, deep tendon reflexes; FT_3I, free triiodothyronine index; FT_4I, free thyroxine index; Hct, hematocrit; Hgb, hemoglobin; HR, heart rate; LDH, lactate dehydrogenase; Na, sodium; TT_3, total triiodothyronine; TT_4, total thyroxine.

Levothyroxine is the preferred thyroid replacement preparation. Several brand-name and generic preparations are available, and they are interchangeable in most patients. The signs and symptoms of hypothyroidism can be reversed easily in most patients by the administration of levothyroxine on an empty stomach at average oral replacement dosages of 1.6 to 1.7 μg/kg per day. Exceptions include older patients, patients with severe and longstanding hypothyroidism, and patients with cardiac disease, in whom administration of full replacement doses might cause cardiac toxicity (Table 49-4). In such patients, minute thyroxine doses should be started initially and the dosage titrated upward as tolerated; complete reversal of hypothyroidism might not be indicated or possible. In myxedema coma, intravenous (IV) therapy with large initial doses of levothyroxine (e.g., 400 μg) is necessary to increase the active free hormone level by saturating the empty thyroid-binding sites, and to prevent the 60% to 70% mortality rate. In subclinical hypothyroidism, it is controversial whether thyroxine replacement therapy is beneficial. There is no justification for treating patients with hypothyroid symptoms and normal laboratory findings with thyroxine.

The goal of therapy is to reverse the signs and symptoms of hypothyroidism and normalize the TSH and free thyroxine levels. Some improvement of hypothyroid symptoms is often evident within 2 to 3 weeks of starting thyroxine therapy. Overreplacement of levothyroxine (manifested by below-normal or suppressed serum concentrations of TSH) is associated with osteoporosis and cardiac changes. The optimal thyroxine replacement dosage must be administered for ≥6 to 8 weeks before steady-state levels are reached. Evaluation of thyroid function tests before this time is misleading. Once a euthyroid state is attained, laboratory tests can be monitored every 3 to 6 months for the first year, and then yearly thereafter. Medications that interfere with thyroxine absorption (e.g., iron, aluminum-containing products, some calcium preparations, cholesterol resin binders, raloxifene) should not be coadministered with thyroxine.

Table 49-4   Treatment of Hypothyroidism

Patient Type/Complications	Dose (l-thyroxine)	Comment
Uncomplicated adult	1.6–1.7 μg/kg/day; 100–125 μg/day average replacement dose; usual increment 25 μg Q 6–8 weeks	*Onset of action:* 2–3 weeks; *max effect:* 4–6 weeks. Reversal of skin and hair changes may take several months. An FT$_4$ or FT$_4$I and TSH should be checked 6–8 weeks after initiation of therapy because T$_4$ has a half-life of 7 days and 3–4 half-lives are needed to achieve steady state. Levels obtained before steady state can be very misleading. Since 80% bioavailable, adjust IV doses downward. Small changes can be made by varying dose schedule (e.g., 150 μg QD except Sunday)
Elderly	≤1.6 μg/kg/day (50–100 μg/day)	Initiate T$_4$ cautiously. Elderly may require less than younger patients. Sensitive to small dose changes. A few patients >60 yr require ≤50 μg/day
Cardiovascular disease (Angina, CAD)	Start with 12.5–25 μg/day. ↑ by 12.5–25 μg/day Q 2-6 weeks as tolerated.	These patients very sensitive to cardiovascular effects of T$_4$. Even subtherapeutic doses can precipitate severe angina, MI, or death. Replace thyroid deficit slowly, cautiously, and sometimes even suboptimally.
Longstanding hypothyroidism (>1 year)	Dose slowly. Start with 25 μg/day. ↑ by 25 μg/day Q 4-6 weeks as tolerated.	Sensitive to cardiovascular effects of T$_4$. Steady state may be delayed because of ↓ clearance of T$_4$.[b] Correct replacement dose is a compromise between prevention of myxedema and avoidance of cardiac toxicity.
Pregnant	Most will require 45% ↑ in dose to ensure euthyroidism.	Evaluate TSH, TT$_4$, and FT$_4$I. *Goal:* normal TSH and TT$_4$/FT$_4$I in upper normal range to prevent fetal hypothyroidism
Pediatric (0–3 months)	12–17 μg/kg/day	Hypothyroid infants can exhibit skin mottling, lethargy, hoarseness, poor feeding, delayed development, constipation, large tongue, neonatal jaundice, pig-like facies, choking, respiratory difficulties, and delayed skeletal maturation (epiphyseal dysgenesis). The serum T$_4$ should be increased rapidly to minimize impaired cognitive function. In the healthy term infant, 37.5 to 50 μg/day of T$_4$ is appropriate. Dose decreases with age (Table 49-9).

CAD, coronary artery disease; FT$_4$I, free thyroxine index; TSH, thyroid-stimulating hormone; T$_4$, thyroxine; TT$_3$, total triiodothyronine; TT$_4$, total thyroxine.
[b]In severely myxedematous patients, steady state may require ≥6 months. In patients who are clinically euthyroid but have ↑ TT$_4$ and FTI, use TT$_3$ and TSH as guide to dose adjustments.

Hyperthyroidism or thyrotoxicosis is the hypermetabolic syndrome that occurs when the production of thyroid hormone is excessive. Hyperthyroidism affects about 2% of females and about 0.1% of males. The prevalence of hyperthyroidism in older patients varies between 0.5% and 2.3% but accounts for 10% to 15% of all thyrotoxic patients, depending on the population studied.

Graves' disease is the most common cause of hyperthyroidism. Toxic autonomous nodular goiters, both multinodular and uninodular, account for a large proportion of the remaining causes. Other causes of hyperthyroidism, including iatrogenic ones, are outlined in Table 49-5. Graves' disease is an autoimmune disorder characterized by one or more of the following features: hyperthyroidism, diffuse goiter, ophthalmopathy (exophthalmos), dermopathy (pretibial myxedema), and acropachy (thickening of fingers or toes). The production of excessive quantities of thyroid hormone is attributed to a circulating IgG or thyroid receptor antibody (TRAb), which has a TSH-like ability to stimulate hormone synthesis. The abnormal production of TRAb by plasma cells (differentiated B lymphocytes) results from a deficiency of suppressor T-cell lymphocytes. The peak incidence of Graves' disease occurs in the third or fourth decade of life, the duration of the disease is unknown, and its clinical course is characterized by remission and relapse.

The classic symptoms of hyperthyroidism, summarized in Table 49-6, mimic a hypermetabolic state and include nervousness, heat intolerance, palpitations, weight loss despite increased appetite, insomnia, proximal muscle weakness, frequent bowel movements, amenorrhea, and emotional lability. Often these symptoms are present for 3 to 12 months before the diagnosis is made. The typical symptoms often are absent in the older patient, producing a masked or "apathetic" picture. Because the clinical presentation of hyperthyroidism in the older patient is atypical, occult hyperthyroidism always must be considered, especially in patients with new or worsening cardiac findings (e.g., atrial fibrillation). Untreated hyperthyroidism can progress to thyroid storm, a life-threatening form of hyperthyroidism characterized by "exaggerated" symptoms of thyrotoxicosis and the acute onset of high fever (sine qua non). The diagnosis of hyperthyroidism is confirmed by a high serum concentration of free thyroxine and/or an undetectable TSH level. Positive thyroid antibodies confirm an autoimmune origin for the hyperthyroidism (e.g., Graves' disease).

Table 49-5 Causes of Hyperthyroidism

Graves' disease (toxic diffuse goiter)
Toxic uninodular goiter (Plummer's disease)
Toxic multinodular goiter
Nodular goiter with hyperthyroidism caused by exogenous iodine (Jod-Basedow)
Exogenous thyroid excess through self-administration (factitious hyperthyroidism)
Tumors (thyroid adenoma, follicular carcinoma, thyrotropin-secreting tumor of the pituitary, and hydatidiform mole with secretion of a thyroid-stimulating substance)
Iatrogenic (iodides, amiodarone, interferon-α)

Table 49-6 Clinical and Laboratory Findings of Hyperthyroidism

Symptoms

Heat intolerance
Weight loss common; or weight gain caused by $\uparrow$ appetite
Palpitations
Pedal edema
Diarrhea/frequent bowel movements
Amenorrhea/light menses
Tremor
Weakness, fatigue
Nervousness, irritability, insomnia

Physical Findings

Thinning of hair (fine)
Proptosis, lid lag, lid retraction, stare, chemosis, conjunctivitis, periorbital edema, loss of extraocular movements
Diffusely enlarged goiter, bruits, thrills
Wide pulse pressure
Pretibial myxedema
Plummer's nails[a]
Flushed, moist skin
Palmar erythema
Brisk DTRs

Laboratory Findings

$\uparrow$ TT$_4$
$\uparrow$ TT$_3$
$\uparrow$ FT$_4$I/FT$_4$
$\uparrow$ FT$_3$I
Suppressed TSH
$\oplus$ TRAb
$\oplus$ ATgA
$\oplus$ TPO
RAIU >50%
$\downarrow$ cholesterol
$\uparrow$ alkaline phosphatase
$\uparrow$ calcium
$\uparrow$ AST

[a]The fingernail separates from its matrix, but only 1 or 2 nails generally are affected. AST, aspartate aminotransferase; ATgA, antihydroglobulin antibody; DTRs, deep tendon reflexes; FT$_4$, free thyroxine; FT$_3$I, free triiodothyronine index; FT$_4$I, free thyroxine index; RAIU, radioactive iodine uptake; TPO, thyroperoxidase antibody; TRAb, thyroid-receptor antibodies; TSH, thyroid-stimulating hormone; TT$_3$, total triiodothyronine; TT$_4$, total thyroxine.

The primary options for treatment of hyperthyroidism are antithyroid drugs (thioamides), radioiodine, and surgery. All three treatments are effective, and the treatment of choice is influenced by the cause of the hyperthyroidism, the size of the goiter, ophthalmopathy, concomitant disorders (e.g., cardiac), likelihood of pregnancy, patient age, patient preference, and physician bias. Older patients and those with cardiac disease, ophthalmopathy, and hyperthyroidism secondary to a toxic multinodular goiter are treated best with radioactive iodine. Surgery is preferable if obstructive symptoms are present or concomitant malignancy is suspected. Pregnant patients can be managed with thioamides or surgery in the second trimester; radioactive iodine is absolutely contraindicated.

The thioamides are used as primary therapy for hyperthyroidism and as adjunctive short-term therapy to produce euthyroidism before surgery or radioactive iodine. The thioamides (e.g., methimazole [Tapazole], propylthiouracil [PTU]) primarily prevent hormone synthesis but do not affect existing stores of thyroid hormone. Therefore, hyperthyroid symptoms will continue for 4 to 6 weeks after beginning thioamide therapy, and initial treatment with β-blockers or iodides often is required for symptomatic relief. The onset of action of PTU is more rapid than methimazole because PTU has an additional mechanism of action, which is to inhibit the peripheral conversion of T_4 to T_3. Therefore, PTU is the thioamide of choice for thyroid storm. PTU also is the drug of choice during breast-feeding because it is not secreted in breast milk. Otherwise, methimazole is preferred over PTU to enhance compliance; it can be administered once daily, whereas PTU must be given two or three times daily. The duration of treatment is empiric, and thioamides generally are prescribed for 12 to 18 months in hopes of long-term spontaneous remission once the drug is discontinued. Although thioamides maintain euthyroidism, they do not change the natural course of the disease, and the likelihood of spontaneous remission, once treatment is discontinued, is poor. The expectation that the combination of thioamide and thyroxine therapy might increase the likelihood of remission has been disappointing. The major adverse effects from thioamides include skin rash, gastrointestinal (GI) complaints, agranulocytosis, and hepatitis. Cross-sensitivity between the thioamides is not complete, and the alternative drug can be used if rash or GI complaints do not resolve.

Nodular goiters, both multinodular and uninodular, are common thyroid problems. The estimated prevalence is 4% to 5% of the adult population. The origin of thyroid nodules is unknown, although TSH stimulation, iodine deficiency, goitrogens (e.g., iodides, lithium, amiodarone), and radiation exposure are contributory. The nodular goiter usually is found on routine physical examination in asymptomatic and euthyroid patients. However, patients can present with hyperthyroidism caused by autonomous functioning "hot" nodules, overt hypothyroidism, or obstructive symptoms of dysphagia and respiratory difficulty. Thyroid function tests, including TSH and free thyroxine levels, and antibodies should be obtained. Additional information can be obtained from radioactive iodine uptake, ultrasound, or magnetic resonance imaging.

Treatment options include surgery, radioactive iodine, thyroid replacement therapy if necessary to correct hypothyroidism, or TSH suppression therapy using levothyroxine dosages of 2.2 μg/kg per day. All goitrogens should be removed if possible. Thyroid suppression therapy can prevent further growth of a benign nodular goiter but is not effective in reducing or normalizing the goiter. The goal of thyroxine suppression therapy is a suppressed but detectable TSH level to prevent further gland stimulation. However, thyroid suppression therapy might not be indicated if the dangers from supraphysiologic dosages of thyroxine (e.g., osteoporosis and the potential for cardiac arrhythmias) exceed the benefits of nodular suppression.

Malignancy must be considered if there is recent growth in a "cold" single or dominant nodule, a history of thyroid irradiation, or a strong family history of medullary thyroid carcinoma. A fine-needle aspiration (FNA) of the thyroid nodule can document an underlying malignancy. The risk of malignancy in a toxic multinodular goiter is small, and definitive treatment with radioactive iodine is usually required to manage any hyperthyroid symptoms. Surgery is indicated if malignancy is highly suspected or if any obstructive or respiratory symptoms are present.

Following a total thyroidectomy for thyroid cancer, radioactive iodine ablation is usually given to remove any remaining thyroid tissue. This dosage is higher than the dosage required for treatment of Graves' disease. A yearly evaluation for detection of recurrence of some thyroid cancers requires the patient to be off thyroxine for 4 to 6 weeks so that a repeat radioactive uptake and scan can be completed. An elevated TSH level is also necessary to allow thyroglobulin levels, a tumor marker, to rise if any malignant tissue is present. Therefore, recurrent thyroid cancer is evidenced by either a positive finding on the scan or an elevation in thyroglobulin levels. The administration of recombinant human TSH (Thyrogen) may improve quality of life because comparable elevations in TSH occur without stopping levothyroxine therapy, permitting use of the radioactive scan and thyroglobulin levels.

THYROID FUNCTION TESTS

The principal laboratory tests recommended in the initial evaluation of thyroid disorders are the sensitive TSH and the free thyroxine (FT_4) levels.[1–3] If a direct measure of the free thyroxine level is not available, the estimated free thyroxine index (FT_4I) can provide comparable information. Measurement of only the total T_4 (TT_4) should not be used because it is less reliable than the FT_4 or FT_4I when alterations in thyroid-binding globulin or nonthyroidal illnesses exist. Positive thyroid antibodies identify an autoimmune thyroid disorder. Adjuncts to the above tests include the total T_3 (TT_3), free T_3 (FT_3), radioactive iodine uptake (RAIU) and scan, TRAb, and miscellaneous tests such as the FNA biopsy (Table 49-7).

Measurements of Free and Total Serum Hormone Levels

Free Thyroxine, Free Thyroxine Index, Free Triiodothyronine Index

Various laboratory methods (e.g., analog, ligand assays) are available to directly measure FT_4 levels. The FT_4 is the most reliable diagnostic test for the evaluation of hypothyroidism and hyperthyroidism when thyroid hormone binding abnormalities exist. In contrast, direct measurement of the free T_3 level is expensive, difficult, and unnecessary because the calculated FT_3 index (FT_3I) correlates well with the actual T_3 level. The FT_4I and the FT_3I are indirect estimates of the free T_4 and T_3 levels and are most helpful when TBG levels are abnormal. These indirect calculated values correlate favorably with the true thyroid status as derived from direct measurement of actual free hormone levels. Unfortunately, these indices do not correct for changes observed in patients with "euthyroid sick" nonthyroidal illnesses whose TBG binding affinity is altered. In these circumstances, the FT_4 and FT_3 are preferable. The FT_4I results are reported so that the clinician does not have to make calculations. In contrast, calculations are required to determine the FT_3I. The traditional method of estimating the FT_4I is to multiply the resin T_3 uptake (RT_3U)

Table 49-7 Common Thyroid Function Tests

Tests	Measures	Normals[a]	Assay Interference	Comments
Measurement of Circulating Hormone Levels				
FT_4	Direct measurement of free thyroxine	0.7–1.9 ng/dL (9–24 pmol/L)	No interference by alterations in TBG	Most accurate determination of FT_4 levels; might be higher than normal in patients on thyroxine replacement
FT_4I	Calculated free thyroxine index	T_4 uptake method: 6.5–12.5 $TT_4 \times RT_3U$ method: 1.3–3.9	Euthyroid sick syndrome (see Question 2)	Estimates direct FT_4 measurement; compensates for alterations in TBG
TT_4	Total free and bound T_4	5.0–12.0 mg/dL (64–154 mmol/L)	Alterations in TBG (see Table 49-1)	Specific and sensitive test if no alterations in TBG
TT_3	Total free and bound T_3	70–132 ng/dL (1.1–2.0 nmol/L)	Alterations in TBG levels; T_4 to T_3 (see Table 49-1). Euthyroid sick syndrome (see Question 2).	Useful in detecting early, relapsing, and T_3 toxicosis. Not useful in evaluation of hypothyroidism.
RT_3U	Indirect measure of saturation of TBG binding sites; does not measure either T_3 or T_4 levels directly	26–35%	Alterations in TBG levels (see Table 49-1)	Can be used to calculate FT_3I and FT_4I
Tests of Thyroid Gland Function				
RAIU	Gland's use of iodine after trace dose of either ^{123}I or ^{131}I	5 hr = 5–15% 24 hr = 15–35%	False decrease with excess iodide intake; false elevation with iodide deficiency	Useful in hyperthyroidism to determine RAI dose in Graves'. Does not provide information regarding hormone synthesis.
Scan	Gland size, shape, and tissue activity after ^{123}I or ^{99m}Tc	—	^{123}I scan blocked by antithyroid/thyroid medications	Useful in nodular disease to detect "cold" or "hot" areas
Test of Hypothalamic-Pituitary-Thyroid Axis				
TSH	Pituitary TSH level	0.5–4.7 mIU/L	Dopamine, glucocorticoids, metoclopramide, thyroid hormone, amiodarone (see Table 49-1)	Most sensitive index for hyperthyroidism, hypothyroidism, and replacement therapy
Tests of Autoimmunity				
ATgA	Antibodies to thyroglobulin	<8%	Nonthyroidal autoimmune disorders	Present in autoimmune thyroid disease; undetectable during remission
TPO	Thyroperoxidase antibodies	<100 IU/mL	Nonthyroidal autoimmune disorders	More sensitive of the two antibodies. Titers detectable even after remission.
TRAb	Thyroid receptor IgG antibody	Titers negative	—	Confirms Graves' disease; detects risk of neonatal Graves'
Miscellaneous				
Thyroglobulin	Colloid protein of normal thyroid gland	5–25 ng/dL	Goiters; inflammatory thyroid disease	Marker for recurrent thyroid cancer or metastases in thyroidectomized patients

[a]At University of California Laboratories.

ATgA, antithyroglobulin; FT_4, free thyroxine; FT_4I, free thyroxine index; IV, intravenous; RAIU, radioactive iodine uptake; RT_3U, resin triiodothyronine uptake; T_3, triiodothyronine; T_4, thyroxine; TBG, thyroxine-binding globulin; TPO, thyroperoxidase; TRAb, thyroid-receptor antibodies; TSH, thyroid-stimulating hormone; TT_3, total triiodothyronine; TT_4, total thyroxine.

by the TT_4. A newer method is to divide the TT_4 by the T_4 "uptake." The FT_3I can be calculated similarly using either method. It is important to identify which method (RT_3U or T_4 "uptake") is used to determine the free T_4 or T_3 index, because the normal values will be significantly different.

Total Thyroxine and Total Triiodothyronine

The total thyroxine (TT_4) and total triiodothyronine (TT_3) measure both free and bound (total) serum T_4 and T_3. Because the bound fraction is the major fraction measured, situations that change the hormone's affinity for TBG or the TBG level will influence the results. For example, falsely elevated levels of TT_4 and TT_3 are common in the euthyroid pregnant woman (see Question 4). In addition, the TT_3 often is low in older patients and in many acute and chronic nonthyroidal illnesses because the peripheral conversion of T_4 to T_3 is decreased (see Questions 2 and 3). Therefore, careful interpretation of these tests is necessary in situations that alter thyroid hormone binding, TBG levels, or T_4 to T_3 conversion (see Table 49-1). The TT_3 is particularly helpful in detecting early relapse of Graves' disease and in confirming the diagnosis of hyperthyroidism despite normal TT_4 levels. The TT_3 is not a good indicator of hypothyroidism because TT_3 can be normal.

Tests of the Hypothalamic-Pituitary-Thyroid Axis

Thyroid-Stimulating Hormone

The serum thyroid-stimulating hormone (TSH) or thyrotropin is the most sensitive test to evaluate thyroid function.[1-3] TSH secreted by the pituitary is elevated in early or subclinical hypothyroidism (when thyroid hormone levels appear normal) and when thyroid hormone replacement therapy is inadequate. TSH can be abnormal even if the FT_4 remains within the normal range because the TSH is specific for each person's physiologic set point. Therefore, low free hormone levels, even though values may still be within the normal range, stimulate the pituitary to synthesize increased amounts of TSH. Unfortunately, the test does not distinguish primary hypothyroidism (thyroid failure), which is characterized by elevated TSH levels, from secondary (pituitary or hypothalamus failure) hypothyroidism. In the latter instance, TSH levels may show low normal values. The TSH assay is capable of quantitating both the upper and lower limits of normal so that a suppressed TSH level is highly suggestive of hyperthyroidism or exogenous thyroid overreplacement. However, the TSH is not entirely specific for thyroid disease and can be abnormal in euthyroid patients with nonthyroidal illnesses and in patients receiving drugs that can interfere with TSH secretion. TSH secretion is suppressed physiologically by dopamine, which antagonizes the stimulatory effects of TRH. Therefore, dopaminergic agonists and antagonists can alter TSH secretion (see Question 5).

Tests of Gland Function

Radioactive Iodine Uptake

RAIU is a measure of iodine utilization by the gland and an indirect measure of hormone synthesis. It is elevated in hyperthyroidism and in early hypothyroidism when the failing gland is trying to increase hormone synthesis. A low or undetectable RAIU occurs in hypothyroidism, thyrotoxicosis facti-

tia, and subacute thyroiditis. Typically, RAIU is used to calculate the dose of radioactive iodine therapy for treatment of Graves' disease and to determine the activity of one or several nodules in a gland. The RAIU is not necessary to diagnose classic Graves' disease or hypothyroidism.

A tracer dose of ^{131}I is administered, and the radioactivity of the gland is measured at 5 and 24 hours after ingestion. It is necessary to measure both the 5- and 24-hour RAIU so that patients with rapid turnover of iodine will not be missed. In some hyperthyroid patients, the 5-hour uptake is elevated but the 24-hour uptake falls progressively to lower, even subnormal, levels, thereby producing spuriously normal results if only the 24-hour results were obtained.

The normal range of the RAIU (see Table 49-7) is affected by any condition that alters iodine intake. Therefore, iodine depletion caused by rigorous diuretic therapy or an iodine-deficient diet produces an increased uptake because of replenishment of depleted total iodide pools. Conversely, dilution of total body iodide pools with exogenous iodide sources (e.g., contrast dyes) produces a low RAIU.

Scan

A scan of the gland is performed simultaneously with the RAIU or after ingestion of technetium (^{99m}Tc) pertechnetate. The scan provides information concerning gland size and shape and identifies hypermetabolic ("hot") and hypometabolic ("cold") areas. The possibility of carcinoma must be considered if cold areas are present. A scan should be considered in the patient with nodular thyroid disease.

Tests of Autoimmunity

Thyroperoxidase and Antithyroglobulin Antibodies

Thyroperoxidase (TPO) and antithyroglobulin (ATgA) antibodies to the thyroid gland indicate an autoimmune process, although the nature of the problem is undetermined.[1,3] About 60% to 70% of patients with Graves' disease and 95% of patients with Hashimoto's thyroiditis have positive antibodies to both thyroid antigens. Positive antibodies alone do not indicate thyroid disease because 5% to 10% of asymptomatic patients, as well as patients with other nonthyroidal autoimmune disorders, have positive antibodies.

Clinically, the TPO is more specific than ATgA in assessing disease activity. Although both antibodies are elevated during acute flares of the disease, lower titers of TPO remain positive during quiescent periods of the disease, while ATgA levels revert to negative.

Thyroid-Receptor Antibodies

Thyroid receptor antibodies (TRAb) are IgG immunoglobulins that are present in virtually all patients with Graves' disease.[1,3] Like TSH, these immunoglobulins can stimulate the thyroid gland to produce thyroid hormones. High titers of TRAb are useful in diagnosing otherwise asymptomatic Graves' disease (i.e., opthalmopathy), in predicting the risk of relapse of Graves' disease after discontinuing medication, and in predicting the risk of neonatal hyperthyroidism in utero through transplacental passage of TRAb from the pregnant mother. Otherwise, TRAb measurement is expensive and offers no additional information in the patient with a typical Graves' disease presentation.

Clinical Application and Interpretation

Euthyroidism

1. R.K., an obese 42-year-old woman, is admitted to the hospital because of increasing fatigue, sluggishness, shortness of breath (SOB), and pitting edema of the legs during the past 3 weeks. Bilateral pleural effusions found on her chest radiograph indicate a worsening of her congestive heart failure (CHF). Her other medical problems include cirrhosis of the liver, diabetes, and chronic bronchitis, for which she takes glipizide 10 mg QD and Lugol's solution TID.

Pertinent physical findings include a palpable but normal-size thyroid, bibasilar rales, cardiomegaly, hepatomegaly, 4+ pitting edema, and normal deep tendon reflexes (DTRs). A diagnosis of worsening CHF secondary to hypothyroidism is suspected based on the following laboratory findings: cholesterol, 385 mg/dL (normal, <200); RAIU at 24 hours, 13% (normal, 15% to 35%); scan, normal-sized gland with homogenous uptake; TT_4, 1.4 μg/dL (normal, 5 to 12); TT_3, 22 ng/dL (normal, 70 to 132); TSH, 4 IU/mL (normal, 0.5 to 4.7); FT_4I, 3.5 (normal, 6.5 to 12.5); TPO, 30 IU/mL (normal, <100); ATgA, 3% (normal, <8%). Evaluate and explain R.K.'s thyroid status based on her clinical and laboratory findings.

[SI units: cholesterol, 9.96 mmol/L (normal, <5.2); TT_4, 18 nmol/L (normal, 64 to 154); FT_4I, 45 (normal, 84 to 161); TT_3, 0.3 nmol/L (normal, 1.1 to 2.0); TSH, 4 mIU/L (normal, 0.5 to 4.7)]

Although low-output failure can be a presenting sign of hypothyroidism, the normal TSH definitely indicates that R.K. is euthyroid despite the confusing results of her other thyroid function tests. The depressed RAIU is consistent with her history of iodide ingestion and dilution of total iodide pools. The low TT_4, TT_3, and FT_4I may be explained by her cirrhosis and "euthyroid sick" syndrome (see Question 2). The negative thyroid antibodies, the normal scan, and normal DTRs further substantiate the diagnosis of euthyroidism. In hypothyroidism a lower rate of cholesterol degradation can produce an elevated serum cholesterol level. However, because many extrathyroidal factors influence the serum concentration of cholesterol, this test is an imprecise reflection of thyroid status. In this case, the elevated cholesterol level is not related to hypothyroidism.

2. Assess the results and explain the significance of R.K.'s TT_4, FT_4I, and TT_3 values.

R.K.'s thyroid function test results are consistent with the "euthyroid sick" syndrome. Abnormal thyroid function tests commonly are found in euthyroid patients with various systemic diseases, including acute and chronic starvation, acute infections, acute psychiatric disorders, asymptomatic and symptomatic HIV disease, and chronic cardiac, pulmonary, renal, hepatic, and neoplastic diseases.[1,3,4–11] This euthyroid sick syndrome occurs in 37% to 70% of chronically ill or hospitalized patients and must be recognized. In general, the sicker the patient, the greater the degree of abnormal thyroid function findings, even though the patient has no thyroid disease.

Typical changes include a normal or low TT_4, a normal or low calculated FT_4I despite normal free T_4 and T_3 levels when directly measured, a normal or borderline-high compensatory TSH as patients recover from illness, a low total TT_3 (approximately 15 to 20 ng/dL), and a high reverse T_3 (rT_3). These findings are explained by alterations in the peripheral conversion of T_4 to T_3 and by complex changes in the hypothalamic-pituitary-thyroid relationships. The low serum T_3 levels and high inactive, rT_3 levels are caused by decreased activity of 5'-deiodinase, an enzyme that is necessary for the peripheral conversion of T_4 to T_3. Impaired protein synthesis of thyroid-binding prealbumin and an increase in the proportion of a lower-binding-capacity form of TBG can account for the low serum hormone levels, but the concomitant increase in the free hormone concentrations maintains a euthyroid state. Furthermore, circulating substances that inhibit the binding of T_4 and T_3 to the serum-binding proteins might be present.

Less common changes include a modestly elevated TT_4 and FT_4I in patients with acute viral hepatitis, psychiatric disorders, renal failure, and progression of HIV disease. The TT_3 usually is normal but can be low in critically ill patients. Modest elevations in hormonal binding affinity and increased synthesis of TBGs explain these findings.

Several studies have shown a strong inverse correlation between mortality and total serum T_4, T_3, and rT_3 levels.[7–9] Of 86 hospitalized, intensive care patients, 84% of those with a serum T_4 of <3 μg/dL died, whereas 85% of those with a serum T_4 of >5 μg/dL survived. In 331 patients with acute myocardial infarction, rT_3 levels >0.41 nmol/L were significantly associated with greater risk of death at 1 year. During recovery, TSH levels increase and serum hormone levels start to normalize. Therefore, a favorable outcome is associated with reversal of the hormone indices.

In summary, T_4 and T_3 measurements are of limited value in the diagnosis of thyroid dysfunction in patients with significant nonthyroid illness. A normal or near-normal TSH is necessary to establish euthyroidism in sick patients with nonthyroidal illness. The benefits of hormone replacement are unproven, and it can be dangerous.[10] In one trial, the mortality of patients with acute renal failure treated with thyroxine was 43% versus 13% in the control group.[11] Therefore, no thyroid hormone treatment is indicated at this time. Thyroxine therapy is not beneficial and, by inhibiting TSH, may be detrimental to normal thyroid recovery. The abnormal laboratory findings should reverse when R.K.'s nonthyroid illness is corrected. To confirm euthyroidism, the slightly elevated TSH should be replicated once R.K.'s medical condition improves.

3. J.R., a 45-year-old man, complains of fatigue, dry skin, and constipation. His other medical problems include alcoholism for 10 years, cirrhosis, grand mal seizures treated with phenytoin (Dilantin) 300 mg/day and phenobarbital 90 mg at night, and rheumatoid arthritis for which he takes aspirin 325 mg, 20 tablets/day.

The results of his thyroid function tests are TT_4, 4.2 μg/dL (normal, 5 to 12); FT_4, 0.6 ng/dL (normal, 0.7 to 1.9); and TSH, 2.5 IU/mL (normal, 0.5 to 4.7). How should these laboratory findings be interpreted? What factors are responsible for the observed changes?

[SI units: TT_4, 54 nmol/L (normal, 64 to 154); FT_4, 8 pmol/L (normal, 9 to 24); TSH, 2.5 mIU/L (normal, 0.5 to 4.7)]

Despite complaints that could be consistent with hypothyroidism (e.g., fatigue, dry skin, constipation) and findings of low serum hormone values, J.R. is euthyroid, as evidenced by the normal TSH level. Secondary hypothyroidism is unlikely at this age without a history of central nervous system (CNS) trauma or tumor. Some nonthyroidal factors could account for J.R.'s low TT_4 and FT_4 values.[4] Anti-inflammatory doses of salicylates >2 g/day and salicylate derivatives (i.e., Disalcid, salsalate) can displace thyroxine from both TBG and TBPA, causing these abnormal findings.[4,12,13] RT_3U values, if measured, are increased. Elevation in free T_4 levels and suppression of TSH below normal occur transiently (i.e., no longer than first 3 weeks of administration) but normalize with chronic administration. Cirrhosis, stress, severe infections, and hereditary factors can also decrease TBG and TBPA synthesis to produce similar TT_4 findings. A medication history for drugs such as androgens or glucocorticoids that can lower TBG levels and therefore TT_4 levels should be elicited (see Table 49-1).[4]

The anticonvulsants (phenytoin [Dilantin], phenobarbital, valproic acid [Depakene], carbamazepine [Tegretol]) and rifampin (Rimactane) can alter serum thyroid hormone levels.[4,14–17] A 40% to 60% reduction in total T_4 serum concentrations results from an increase in the metabolism (nondeiodination) of thyroxine and from hormone displacement in patients receiving chronic anticonvulsant therapy. Serum T_3 levels are normal or slightly decreased. In addition, therapeutic levels of phenytoin and carbamazepine interfere with the FT_4 assay, causing a 20% to 40% lower FT_4 than would be expected in euthyroid persons.[15] TSH levels remain normal and patients are euthyroid; however, those previously requiring thyroxine therapy might need a dosage increment to maintain euthyroidism.[18,19] Valproic acid is reported to have similar but less potent effects on thyroid function.[14,16] Rifampin, an enzyme inducer, can also increase T_4 requirements. Phenobarbital can increase T_4 uptake by the liver and increase the fecal excretion of thyroxine. Serum binding of thyroid hormones is unaffected by phenobarbital.

In summary, J.R. is taking several drugs that can further compromise the already low serum thyroxine levels resulting from his liver disease. The free thyroxine remains subnormal in euthyroid persons receiving phenytoin, but the normal TSH confirms euthyroidism.

4. S.T., a 23-year-old, sexually active woman whose only medication is birth control pills, comes to the clinic complaining of extreme nervousness, diaphoresis, and scanty menstrual periods. Although she appears healthy, the possibility of hyperthyroidism is considered on the basis of the following laboratory values: TT_4, 16 μg/dL (normal, 5 to 12); RT_3U, 23% (normal, 25 to 37); FT_4, 1.2 ng/dL (normal, 0.7 to 1.9); TSH, 1.2 IU/mL (normal, 0.5 to 4.7). Based on this information, what would be a reasonable assessment of S.T.'s thyroid status?

[SI units: TT_4, 206 nmol/L (normal, 64 to 154); FT_4, 16 pmol/L (normal, 9 to 24); TSH, 1.2 mIU/L (normal, 0.5 to 4.7)]

The normal FT_4, TSH, and calculated FT_4I confirm that S.T. is not hyperthyroid. The elevated TT_4 and the depressed resin uptake are consistent with increased TBG levels observed in patients with acute hepatitis; in pregnancy; and in persons taking estrogen, oral contraceptives, tamoxifen, raloxifene, heroin, or methadone.[4,20–24] Because TBG and therefore bound T_4 levels are increased by estrogens in S.T., total serum T_4 measurements are falsely elevated. Likewise, the RT_3U is decreased because of an absolute increase in the amount of thyroxine binding sites available. Thyroid function

tests should return to normal within 4 weeks after discontinuation of oral contraceptives. Progesterone-only oral contraceptives do not affect protein binding and therefore do not alter thyroid function tests.

Amiodarone

5. J.P., a 55-year-old woman, complains of 3 months of progressive tremors, dizziness, and ataxia. Two months ago, she had a silent myocardial infarction (MI) complicated by malignant ventricular ectopy that was responsive only to amiodarone (Cordarone) therapy. Her other medical problems include parkinsonism, insulin-dependent diabetes, and diabetic gastroparesis. Her current medications include amiodarone, insulin, metoclopramide (Reglan), bromocriptine (Parlodel), and levodopa/carbidopa (Sinemet). Physical examination of the thyroid was unremarkable. Thyroid function tests show TT_4, 14.5 μg/dL (normal, 5 to 12); FT_4 2.3 ng/dL (normal, 0.7 to 1.9); TSH, 3.8 IU/mL (normal, 0.5 to 4.7); TT_3 40 ng/dL (normal, 70 to 132); and TPO antibodies, 40 IU/L (normal, <100). How should J.P.'s laboratory values be interpreted?

[SI units: TT_4, 187 nmol/L (normal, 64 to 154); FT_4, 30 pmol/L (normal, 9 to 24); TSH, 3.8 mIU/L (normal, 0.5 to 4.7); TT_3, 0.63 nmol/L (normal, 1.1 to 2.0)]

Although the symptoms of tremors, dizziness, and weight loss are suggestive of hyperthyroidism, the low TT_3, negative antibodies, normal TSH, and normal thyroid examination make this diagnosis unlikely. Side effects of amiodarone could be responsible for J.P.'s symptoms. Her drug therapy could also explain her laboratory findings.

Amiodarone produces complex changes in thyroid function tests that are confusing if not properly interpreted.[25,26] Because amiodarone inhibits both the peripheral and pituitary conversion of T_4 to T_3, FT_4 levels are elevated above normal and TT_3 levels are subnormal in euthyroid patients. Transient elevations in TSH levels occur (usually <20 IU/mL) during the first few weeks of therapy but return to normal in approximately 3 months. If TSH levels do not normalize, then amiodarone-induced thyroid disease should be considered. Amiodarone can cause either hypothyroidism or hyperthyroidism in susceptible patients (see Question 54).

The other drugs J.P. is taking, bromocriptine, levodopa, and metoclopramide, also add to the diagnostic confusion. Although these drugs do not affect the actual circulating hormone levels, they affect the dopaminergic system that controls both TSH and TRH secretion.[2–4] Infusions of dopamine and dobutamine can decrease both TSH secretion and the TSH response to TRH in euthyroid and hypothyroid patients.[2–4,27] Therefore, dopamine agonists such as bromocriptine, cabergoline, and levodopa can blunt the normal TSH response.[2,4,28] Conversely, dopamine antagonists such as metoclopramide or domperidone can elevate TSH levels.[2,4] Fortunately, the alterations in TSH caused by these agents usually are not substantial enough to completely obscure the true thyroid abnormality.

HYPOTHYROIDISM

Clinical Presentation

6. M.W., a 70-kg, 23-year-old voice student, thinks that her neck has become "fatter" over the past 3 to 4 months. She has gained 20 lb, feels mentally sluggish, tires easily, and finds that she can no longer hit high notes. Physical examination reveals puffy facies, yellowish skin, delayed DTRs, and a firm, enlarged thyroid gland. Laboratory data include FT$_4$, 0.6 ng/dL (normal, 0.7 to 1.9); TSH, 60 IU/mL (normal, 0.5 to 4.7); TPO antibodies, 136 IU/L (normal, <100). Assess M.W.'s thyroid status based on her clinical and laboratory findings.

[SI units: FT$_4$, 8 pmol/L (normal, 9 to 24); TSH, 60 mIU/L (normal, 0.5 to 4.7)]

M.W. presents with many of the clinical features of hypothyroidism as presented in Table 49-3. These include weight gain, mental sluggishness, easy fatigability, lowering of the voice pitch, a puffy facies, a yellowish tint of the skin, delayed DTRs, and an enlarged thyroid. The diagnosis of hypothyroidism is confirmed by her laboratory findings of a low FT$_4$, an elevated TSH value, and positive antibodies.

A firm goiter, thyroid antibodies, and clinical symptoms of hypothyroidism strongly suggest Hashimoto's thyroiditis. She has no history of prior antithyroid drug use, surgery, or radioactive iodine treatment, which are common causes of iatrogenic hypothyroidism. She also is not taking any goitrogens or drugs known to cause hypothyroidism (see Table 49-2).

Treatment With Thyroid Hormones

Thyroid Hormone Products

7. What thyroid preparation should be used to treat M.W.'s hypothyroidism? Are differences, advantages, or disadvantages significant among the various generic and brand-name formulations of thyroid hormones?

The principal goals of thyroid hormone therapy are to attain and maintain a euthyroid state. Thyroid preparations (Table 49-8) are synthetic (levothyroxine, L-triiodothyronine [Cytomel], liotrix [Thyrolar]) or natural (desiccated thyroid). The latter come from animal tissues.

DESICCATED THYROID

Desiccated thyroid (USP) is derived from pork thyroid glands, although beef and sheep also are used. Today, starting patients on desiccated thyroid is not justified. The U.S. Pharmacopoeia (USP) requires only that desiccated thyroid contain 0.17% to 0.23% organic iodine by weight. These requirements do not seem stringent enough because potency may vary with changes in the proportion of the two active hormones (T$_3$ and T$_4$) or with changes in the amount of organic iodine present.[29,30] This variable potency seems to be particularly true of generic formulations compared with the biologically standardized Armour brand of desiccated thyroid. Inactive desiccated thyroid preparations that contain negligible amounts of T$_3$ and T$_4$ or even iodinated casein instead of active hormone have been identified in various brands sold in retail pharmacies and in over-the-counter products found in health food stores.[30-32] Likewise, preparations with greater-than-expected activity caused by an abnormally high T$_3$ content have resulted in thyrotoxicosis.

Allergic reactions to the animal protein are another concern. In addition, desiccated thyroid suffers from two problems inherent to all T$_3$-containing preparations. Because T$_3$ is absorbed more rapidly than T$_4$, supraphysiologic elevations in plasma T$_3$ levels occur after oral ingestion, which can produce mild thyrotoxic symptoms in some patients. FT$_4$ levels are low during T$_3$ administration and, if misinterpreted, can result in the erroneous administration of more hormone. These problems with T$_3$ are easily missed unless T$_3$ levels are routinely monitored. Because significant amounts of T$_4$ are converted to T$_3$ peripherally, oral administration of T$_3$ offers no advantage and is not usually needed. (See the section on triiodothyronine.)

Loss of tablet potency can occur from prolonged storage of desiccated thyroid preparations, but this instability is not as

Table 49-8 Thyroid Preparations

Drug/Dosage Forms	Composition	Dosage Equivalent	Comments
Thyroid USP (Armour) *Tab:* 0.25, 0.5, 1, 1.5, 2, 3, 4, and 5 gr	Desiccated hog, beef, or sheep thyroid gland. Standardized iodine content.	1 gr[a]	Unpredictable T$_4$:T$_3$ ratio; supraphysiologic elevations in T$_3$ levels might produce toxic symptoms; Armour brand preferred
L-thyroxine (Levoxyl, Synthroid, Unithroid, various) *Tab:* 0.025, 0.050, 0.075, 0.088, 0.112, 0.125, 0.137, 0.15, 0.175, 0.2, and 0.3 mg *Inj:* 200 and 500 µg	Synthetic T$_4$	60 µg[a]	Stable, predictable potency; well absorbed; more potent than desiccated thyroid. When changing from >2 gr desiccated thyroid to L-T$_4$, a lower dosage of L-T$_4$ might be needed to avoid toxicity. Weight should be considered in dosing (1.6–1.7 µg/kg/day).
L-triiodothyronine (Cytomel) *Tab:* 5, 25, and 50 µg *Inj:* 10 µg/mL (Triostat)	Synthetic T$_3$	25–37.5 µg	Complete absorption; requires multiple daily dosing; toxicity similar to all T$_3$-containing products; see desiccated thyroid comments
Liotrix (Thyrolar) *Tab:* 0.25, 0.5, 1, 2, and 3 gr	60 µg T$_4$:15 µg T$_3$ 50 µg T$_4$:12.5 µg T$_3$	Thyrolar-1	No need for liotrix because T$_4$ is converted to T$_3$ peripherally; expensive, stable, and predictable content

[a]60 mg (1 gr) of desiccated thyroid = 60 µg of T$_4$.[33]
gr, grain; Inj, injection; T$_3$, triiodothyronine; T$_4$, thyroxine; Tab, tablet.

important as once thought. Because the only apparent advantage of desiccated thyroid is its low cost, it should not be considered the drug of choice for replacement therapy. Patients maintained on desiccated thyroid should be encouraged to change to L-thyroxine (T_4). Although 60 mg (1 gr) of desiccated thyroid theoretically is equal in potency to 75 to 100 μg of T_4,[33] this equivalency may not hold true if the desiccated thyroid preparation is less active than its labeled content. The patient's weight also should be considered when switching therapy (see Question 8).

The synthetic thyroid preparations differ from one another in their relative potency, onset of action, and biologic half-life.

LEVOTHYROXINE OR L-THYROXINE

Levothyroxine is the thyroid replacement of choice.[34] Its advantages include stability, uniform potency, relatively low cost, and lack of an allergenic foreign protein content. The long half-life of 7 days permits once-a-day dosing and, if necessary, the creation of special convenience schedules, such as the omission of medication on weekends. The mean absorption of a commonly used branded preparation is 81%.[35] Spuriously low absorption values noted in earlier studies resulted from an overestimation of levothyroxine tablet content. Absorption is optimal on an empty stomach, at least 60 minutes before meals. Several medications can also impair levothyroxine absorption (see Question 15).

Concerns about generic and branded levothyroxine tablet stability and potency, bioavailability, and product interchangeability exist because levothyroxine preparations were grandfathered in by the 1938 Food, Drug, and Cosmetic Act.[34,37–41] To eliminate concerns about tablet potency and stability, the FDA required that all manufacturers of levothyroxine products submit a New Drug Application (NDA) by August 2001 or cease production. However, those manufacturers awaiting FDA approval would comply with a product distribution phase-down pending FDA approval. By August 14, 2003, all distribution would cease if the NDA were denied. At the end of 2002, several FDA-approved branded (Levoxyl, Synthroid, Unithroid) and generic (Levo-T, Mylan Pharmaceuticals, Novothyrox, ThyroTAB) levothyroxine preparations were available. Unithroid and the Mylan generic product are AB rated, while the others are BX rated. FDA approval for Levothroid (Forest) and generic tablets by Qualitest Pharmaceuticals were withheld. Pending definitive studies, the FDA does not consider any FDA-approved levothyroxine products interchangeable. Limited studies with pre-FDA-approved branded products suggest that these products might be interchangeable in most patients requiring thyroxine replacement.[42–44] One study has demonstrated bioequivalence for two generic products, Synthroid, and Levoxyl using the FDA bioequivalence criteria for oral products.[44]

TRIIODOTHYRONINE

Triiodothyronine (Cytomel) is not recommended for routine thyroid hormone replacement because of the problems identified earlier with T_3 administration (see the section on desiccated thyroid).[34] Nevertheless, studies with a limited number of patients concluded that replacement with the combination of T_4 and small doses of T_3 (i.e., substitution of 12.5 μg T_3 for 50 μg T_4) is preferable to T_4 alone in improving cognitive performance and mood changes.[45–47] However, further study is warranted in a larger study before this therapeutic concept can be embraced. Its use in coronary bypass surgery is controversial.[48]

Although T_3 is well absorbed, it has a relatively short half-life (1.5 days), necessitating multiple daily dosing to ensure a uniform response. Other disadvantages include higher expense and a greater potential for cardiotoxicity. Its primary use is for patients who require short-term hormone replacement therapy and those in whom T_4 conversion to T_3 might be impaired. T_3 therapy should be monitored using the TSH and TT_3 levels.

LIOTRIX

Liotrix (Thyrolar) is a combination of synthetic T_4 and T_3 in a physiologic ratio of 4:1. This preparation is subject to the same disadvantages common to all T_3-containing preparations. It also is stable and potent, but it is more expensive than other thyroid preparations. Because oral administration of T_3 is not needed, this is an obsolete and expensive preparation that is not recommended. Patients should be changed to an equivalent dosage of levothyroxine.

Thyroxine
DOSAGE

8. **What would you recommend as appropriate starting and maintenance dosages of thyroxine for M.W.?**

The maintenance dosage for M.W. can be estimated from her weight. Average replacement doses of 1.6 to 1.7 μg/kg per day (e.g., 100 to 125 mg) are sufficient in most patients to normalize the TSH.[34] Levothyroxine dosages that suppress TSH levels to below normal or undetectable levels (subclinical hyperthyroidism) should be avoided to prevent osteoporosis and cardiac toxicity.[34,49–53] Excessive levothyroxine can cause tachycardia, atrial arrhythmias, impaired ventricular relaxation, reduced exercise performance, and increased risk of cardiac mortality.[49] These considerations are especially important in older patients, who might require less thyroxine than their younger counterparts and who are particularly sensitive to minute changes in thyroxine doses (see Question 11). As patients age, the dosage should be evaluated yearly and decreased if necessary to maintain a normal TSH level.[51–55]

How rapidly thyroxine replacement can proceed depends on the likelihood of invoking cardiac toxicity in susceptible patients. Minute doses of T_4 (e.g., <75 μg) can increase heart rate, stroke volume, oxygen consumption, and cardiac workload before euthyroidism occurs. Because M.W. has no identifiable risk factors (see Question 21) for cardiotoxicity that require careful dosage titration (e.g., old age, cardiac disease, long duration of hypothyroidism), she can be started on an estimated replacement dose of 125 μg daily of L-thyroxine (70 kg $\times$ 1.7 μg/kg per day = 120 μg). Alternatively, a conservative approach would be to start with a dosage of 100 μg/day, check the FT_4 or FT_4I and TSH tests after 6 to 8 weeks of therapy, and if the TSH is still elevated without toxicity, increase the dosage to 125 μg/day. The appropriate replacement dose should normalize the TSH and FT_4 or FT_4I and reverse clinical symptoms of hypothyroidism. Generally, dosing adjustments should not exceed monthly increments of 12.5 to 25 μg/day.

MONITORING THERAPY

9. Two weeks after starting levothyroxine therapy, M.W. continues to complain of tiredness, fatigue, and difficulty singing despite excellent adherence. Thyroid function tests show a TT_4 of 4 µg/dL (normal, 5 to 12), an FT_4 of 0.5 ng/dL (normal, 0.7 to 1.9), and a TSH of 40 IU/mL (normal, 0.5 to 4.7). What therapeutic options are available? How should M.W.'s thyroid function tests be interpreted?

[SI units: TT_4, 52 nmol/L (normal, 64 to 154); FT_4, 6 pmol/L (normal, 9 to 24); TSH, 40 mIU/L (normal, 0.5 to 4.7)]

Clinical improvement in the signs and symptoms of hypothyroidism and normalization of laboratory parameters are appropriate therapeutic end points. If the replacement dose is sufficient, some correction of her symptoms should occur after 2 to 3 weeks, but maximal effects will not be evident for 4 to 6 weeks. Typically, improvement of anemia and hair and skin changes are delayed and require several months of treatment before resolution.[34]

In severely myxedematous patients, a transiently elevated T_4 level might occur at 6 weeks because thyroxine's metabolic clearance is decreased by the hypometabolic state of hypothyroidism.

FT_4 or FT_4I and TSH should be checked about 6 to 8 weeks after the initiation of therapy because T_4 has a half-life of 7 days, and three to four half-lives are needed to reach steady-state levels. Levels obtained before this time (as in M.W.) may be misleading and should be interpreted cautiously. No change in her levothyroxine dosage should be attempted at this time.

10. Eight weeks later, on a routine follow-up visit, M.W. feels well and claims to be back to her normal self. She denies any symptoms of hypothyroidism or hyperthyroidism. However, her thyroid function tests show a TT_4 of 14 µg/dL (normal, 5 to 12), a TT_3 of 50 ng/dL (normal 70 to 132), FT_4 of 1.9 ng/dL (normal, 0.7 to 1.9), and a TSH of 0.5 IU/mL (normal, 0.5 to 4.7). How should M.W.'s thyroid function tests be interpreted? What changes, if any, should be recommended in her therapeutic regimen?

[SI units: TT_4, 180 nmol/L (normal, 64 to 154); FT_4, 24 pmol/L (normal, 9 to 24); TT_3, 0.7 nmol/L (normal 1.1 to 2.0); TSH, 0.5 mIU/L (normal, 0.5 to 4.7)]

Patients treated with levothyroxine may develop an elevated TT_4 concentration and FT_4 without overt clinical signs of hyperthyroidism.[34,35] Despite these elevated levels, the patients are euthyroid, as evidenced by a low to normal TT_3 level, a decreased $T_3:T_4$ ratio, and a normal TSH. Because T_3 is not being released from the nonfunctioning thyroid gland, a higher concentration of T_4 is necessary to increase the amount of T_3 obtained from peripheral conversion.[54,55] Woeber reported that the mean free T_4 was significantly higher (16 pmol/L) and the mean free T_3 lower (4 pmol/L) in patients receiving levothyroxine than in those with thyroid disease not on levothyroxine (FT_4, 14 pmol/L; FT_3, 4.2 pmol/L).[54] As expected, patients receiving levothyroxine who had an elevated TT_4, an elevated TT_3, and an elevated $T_3:T_4$ ratio also had symptoms of hyperthyroidism. Thus, the $T_3:T_4$ ratio and TSH appear to be the best indicators of euthyroidism in patients treated with levothyroxine.

Another possibility is that the elevated thyroid levels may only be an artifact of the laboratory collection time. Before any changes in her dosing regimen are made, M.W. should be asked about the time she takes the drug and its relationship to the time of her blood draw. Random sampling of free thyroxine levels and TSH levels can be significantly different when compared with trough levels.[44,56] In one study, the free thyroxine level was 12% higher and the TSH level 19% lower when obtained from random samples compared with trough samples.[56] Transient elevations in free thyroxine levels were detected for 9 hours after ingestion of the oral levothyroxine.

In conclusion, if an elevated TT_4 and FT_4 are noted without any symptoms of thyrotoxicosis (as in M.W.), the dosage should not be decreased; rather, a trough TT_4, TT_3, and TSH should be obtained to evaluate excessive dosing. The repeat values should be in the normal range with the correct dosing. An excessively suppressed TSH confirms a dosage that is too high. In M.W., the lack of hyperthyroid symptoms suggests euthyroidism, and no changes in her therapeutic regimen should be attempted until the trough levels are available.

Triiodothyronine

11. C.B., a 65-year-old woman, complains of fatigue and vague muscle aches and pains, which she attributes to insufficient thyroid medication. On physical examination, the thyroid gland is palpable but not enlarged, and DTRs are 2+ and brisk. Her dose of triiodothyronine (Cytomel) was increased from 25 µg TID to 50 µg TID about 2 weeks ago based on the results of a recent FT_4 of 0.5 ng/dL (normal, 0.7 to 1.9). She denies taking any other medications. Is C.B.'s thyroid hormone replacement appropriate?

[SI units: FT_4, 6 pmol/L (normal, 9 to 24)]

As noted earlier, Cytomel is not the drug of choice for thyroid replacement. The use of levothyroxine would simplify her dosing regimen and facilitate monitoring.

The low FT_4 did not justify increasing C.B.'s dose of Cytomel. Because she is receiving T_3, the FT_4, which is a measure of free T_4, always will be low and will never reach normal levels. In fact, her vague complaints may be related to hyperthyroidism because she is receiving the equivalent of 0.2 to 0.3 mg of levothyroxine daily. TSH and TT_3 levels are most useful in monitoring patients receiving T_3 therapy. A TSH level should be obtained to evaluate her thyroid function. A suppressed TSH and an elevated TT_3 would indicate hyperthyroidism. It is important to remember that in an older patient, hyperthyroidism might not always produce symptoms because of an "apathetic" sympathetic system.

Levothyroxine should be initiated cautiously in older patients to avoid exacerbating any pre-existing arteriosclerotic heart disease that might be masked by the hypothyroidism (see Questions 20 and 21). In general, older patients require smaller replacement dosages (approximately ≤1.6 µg/kg per day of thyroxine) than their younger counterparts.[57–59] Dosages of ≤50 µg/day of T_4 are common in patients >60 years of age. However, this lower T_4 dosage is not universal for all older subjects.[59] Why older patients need lower dosages is unclear, but it has been suggested that the lower requirements result from an age-related decrease in thyroxine degradation rates. Because dosage requirements change with age, patients should be reassessed every year to determine whether the original dosage prescribed still is appropriate.

In C.B., who had been on T_3 without any evidence of cardiac toxicity, a less cautious approach in changing to thyroxine can be attempted. An empiric levothyroxine dosage of 68 μg/day (40 kg ×1.6 μg/kg per day) is an appropriate dosing end point for C.B. The Cytomel should be discontinued and T_4 initiated in a dosage of 50 μg/day; this dosage can be adjusted as needed based on C.B.'s symptoms and thyroid function tests. After T_3 therapy is discontinued, its effects will disappear over 3 to 5 days. In contrast, T_4 levels rise slowly over 4 to 5 days, so no overlap in T_3 administration is necessary to prevent hypothyroidism.

PARENTERAL DOSING

12. **G.F., a 70-year-old man with longstanding hypothyroidism, has been receiving L-thyroxine 0.2 mg/day. Currently, he is in the hospital with a stroke and paralysis that prohibits him from swallowing oral medications. His last thyroid function tests were normal. What is a reasonable method of administering thyroid hormone to G.F.?**

Because L-thyroxine has a half-life of 7 days, administration can be delayed for up to 1 week, assuming G.F. can resume oral intake at that time. However, if parenteral administration is required, L-thyroxine is available as an intramuscular (IM) or IV injection. The IV route is preferred because IM absorption may be slow and unpredictable, particularly if the circulation is compromised. Because the oral absorption of T_4 is approximately 80%,[35] parenteral doses should be decreased. Once IV levothyroxine replacement is successful, maintenance with a once-weekly IM injection is successful if oral ingestion is not feasible.[60]

IN PREGNANCY

13. **P.K. is a 35-year-old woman with Hashimoto's thyroiditis who is 6 weeks pregnant. Laboratory test results include TT_4, 5 μg/dL (normal, 5 to 12); RT_3U, 25% (normal, 25% to 37%); FT_4, 0.7 ng/dL (normal, 0.7 to 1.9). She takes all of her medications in the morning, which include L-thyroxine 0.1 mg/day and a prenatal vitamin enriched with iron and calcium. What dosing adjustments will be required because of P.K.'s pregnancy?**

[SI units: TT_4, 64 nmol/L (normal, 64 to 154); FT_4, 9 pmol/L (normal, 9 to 24)]

It is unclear whether women with primary hypothyroidism require a larger dosage of thyroxine during pregnancy.[61,62] Traditionally, a 20% to 50% increase in the prepregnancy thyroxine dosage was recommended to maintain euthyroidism. However, one recent theory is that pregnancy per se does not change thyroxine requirements. Rather, coadministration of iron- and calcium-containing prenatal vitamins, which decrease thyroxine absorption (see Question 15), may be primarily responsible for these increased needs. These dosage adjustments were recommended before these drug interactions were recognized. Often no clinical symptoms of hypothyroidism are evident, and the free thyroxine and the index are normal. The only evidence of increased thyroxine demands is an elevated TSH level (e.g., subclinical hypothyroidism).

Patients should be followed closely during pregnancy and the FT_4 and TSH levels should be evaluated monthly during the first trimester. If necessary, the thyroxine dosage should be adjusted to maintain a normal TSH and FT_4 or an FT_4I in the upper limits of normal. Because TBG is elevated, the TT_4

should be kept above the normal range; it is not the best indicator of adequate replacement.

Inadequately treated or undiagnosed maternal hypothyroidism can be detrimental to the developing fetus.[61–63] Abnormal fetal development secondary to poor placental maturation, spontaneous abortions, congenital defects, mental retardation, and an increased rate of stillbirths have been associated with maternal hypothyroidism. The IQ scores of children born to mothers with undiagnosed hypothyroidism during pregnancy averaged 7 points lower than children born to euthyroid mothers.[63] Because thyroid hormone does not cross the placenta in significant amounts, the effect of maternal hypothyroidism on the fetus (if it occurs) must be indirect. The risk of congenital hypothyroidism is small if maternal antibodies from Hashimoto's thyroiditis cross the fetal circulation. The infant's cord blood should be assayed at birth to ensure that TSH is normal and that the child is euthyroid. Screening all pregnant mothers for hypothyroidism to detect undiagnosed maternal hypothyroidism may be warranted.[64]

P.K.'s low TT_4 and RT_3U are of concern. The TT_4 should be much higher and the RT_3U lower because of pregnancy-associated increases in TBG. Most importantly, the calculated FT_4I of 1.25 and the FT_4 are somewhat low. The TSH level should be obtained and the daily dosage of T_4 should be increased to 125 μg after eliminating the possibility of patient nonadherence and drug interactions. Ingestion of the prenatal vitamins and thyroxine should be separated by at least 4 hours. The TSH should be repeated in 6 weeks, and the dosage should be adjusted as needed to keep the TSH in the normal range. After delivery, the dosage should be reduced to prepregnancy levels and the FT_4 and TSH rechecked to ensure euthyroidism.

Congenital Hypothyroidism

14. **P.K. delivered a healthy baby, T.K., at term without difficulty. T.K.'s postpartum screening serum T_4 level was 5 μg/dL (normal, 5 to 12) and TSH was 35 IU/mL (normal, 0.5 to 4.7). At home T.K. became lethargic, had a weak cry, sucked poorly, and failed to thrive. Assess the situation (include a treatment plan and prognosis). How is mental development affected?**

[SI units: T_4, 64 nmol/L (normal, 64 to 154); TSH, 15 mIU/L (normal, 0.5 to 4.7)]

T.K.'s symptoms are suggestive of congenital hypothyroidism, although in most infants the clinical signs and symptoms are so subtle and nonspecific that they are missed easily until the child is several months old. The early clinical findings include prolonged jaundice, skin mottling (cutis marmorata), lethargy, poor feeding, constipation, hypothermia, hoarse cry, large fontanels, distended abdomen, hypotonia, slow reflexes, and pig-like facies. Respiratory difficulties, delayed skeletal maturation, and choking (but not palpable goiter) may be present. These infants also are at risk for additional congenital defects or complications.[65–69] Mass neonatal screening programs have been successful in detecting congenital hypothyroidism within the first few weeks of life before clinical manifestations are apparent and before irreversible changes occur.

The postpartum low serum T_4 concentration and elevated TSH level (>20 IU/mL) in T.K. are of concern and should be verified. Transient hypothyroidism can result from intrauterine exposure to thioamides or excess iodides, or from transplacental passage of TRAb from the mother. Thyroid function tests often normalize without treatment in 3 to 6 months as the TRAb is cleared by the infant.[65,67] The diagnosis of hypothyroidism should be confirmed by a low serum T_4, a low free T_4, and an elevated TSH concentration during the next few weeks. In hypothyroid patients, serum T_3 concentrations often are in the normal range and are not helpful. Normal serum T_4 concentrations are higher in the first few weeks of life and gradually return to normal by 2 to 4 months of life. The FT_4I may also be elevated. Because of these confusing changes, thyroid serum levels should be compared with the normal range for the approximate postnatal age.

Thyroid hormones play a critical role in normal growth and development, particularly of the CNS, during the first 3 years of life. If untreated, dwarfism and irreversible mental retardation occur. T.K.'s normal mental (IQ) and physical development will be determined by the age at which treatment is started, the initial dosage of thyroxine, the serum thyroxine level attained during therapy, the adequacy with which treatment is maintained, and the cause and severity of the initial deficiency.[65–69]

Sodium levothyroxine is the preparation of choice for replacement. T_4 tablets can be crushed and mixed with breast milk or formula; suspensions are not stable and should not be used. T_3 also can be used, but this form is less desirable because its short half-life causes a greater fluctuation in plasma levels (see Table 49-8). The initial replacement dose of T_4 should raise the serum T_4 as rapidly as possible to minimize the consequences of hypothyroidism on cognitive function. A delay in starting therapy of even a few days has resulted in a poorer IQ outcome.[68,69] A minimum T_4 dosage of 10 to 15 $\mu g/kg$ per day is recommended to raise the serum T_4 to >10 $\mu g/dl$ (129 nmol/L) by 7 days. However, recent studies suggest that higher than previously recommended dosages of 12 to 17 $\mu g/kg/day$ might be more effective, but data on neurologic outcome are not yet available.[66,68] In the term healthy infant, full initial replacement T_4 doses are appropriate unless the infant has underlying heart disease or is extremely sensitive to the effects of thyroid hormones. In these infants, reduced doses of T_4 (approximately 25% to 33% of the recommended dose) can be started and increased gradually by similar increments until the therapeutic dose is achieved. The recommended replacement dose decreases with age and is shown in Tables 49-4 and 49-9.

Mental development and attainment of normal growth are not impaired if adequate thyroxine treatment is initiated before 3 months of age to achieve a serum thyroxine level >10 $\mu g/dL$ (129 nmol/L).[65–69] Newborns detected by screening programs who start therapy within the first 4 to 6 weeks of life

have mean IQs of 100 to 109, similar to the control populations. The mean IQ drops if treatment is delayed until 6 weeks and 3 months (mean IQ, 95), or until 3 and 6 months (mean IQ, 75). When treatment is not started until 6 months to 1 year of age, normal mental development is impaired despite subsequent treatment (mean IQ, 55). Higher IQs also were found in children who received dosages of thyroxine >10 $\mu g/kg$ per day compared to lower dosages and achieved a mean serum T_4 level >14 $\mu g/dL$ (181 nmol/L) in the first month of therapy.[66,68,69] Neurologic deficits also are more likely to occur in infants whose thyroid replacement is delayed or inadequate (as evidenced by a serum T_4 <8 $\mu g/dL$ [103 nmol/L] within 30 days of therapy and delayed suppression [18 to 24 months] of the TSH into the normal range). Additional risk factors for a low IQ and poor motor and speech skills despite adequate therapy include clinical signs of hypothyroidism during fetal life, more marked chemical hypothyroidism at birth (T_4 <2 $\mu g/dL$), thyroid aplasia, and retarded bone age.[65,67,69]

The goal of therapy is a T_4 in the upper normal range (e.g., 10 to 18 $\mu g/dL$ [129 to 232 nmol/L]) and/or an FT_4 of 2 to 5 ng/dL (27 to 64 pmol/L) during the first 2 weeks of therapy, and then a lower target thereafter: a T_4 of 10 to 16 $\mu g/dL$ (129 to 206 nmol/L) and/or an FT_4 of 1.6 to 2.2 ng/dL [20 to 30 pmol/L]). IQs are improved if TSH levels are normalized within the first month of therapy, but no later than 3 months.[66,68,69] Thyroid function tests should be routinely monitored 2 to 4 weeks after starting therapy, then every 1 to 2 months during the first year of life and every 2 to 3 months during the next 2 years of life. Although TSH suppression is the most reliable index of adequate replacement in older children, normalization of the TSH should not be used as the sole monitoring parameter in infants because the TSH may lag behind correction of the T_4 and/or FT_4 levels. Overtreatment should be avoided to prevent brain dysfunction, acceleration of bone age, and premature craniosynostosis. Normal growth and development also should be a treatment goal. Other clinical end points include an improvement in activity level, skin color, temperature, facial appearance, and reversal of other symptoms and signs of hypothyroidism.

Unresponsiveness to Thyroid Hormone

15. R.T., a 45-year-old woman, complains of weight gain, heavy menses, sluggishness, and cold intolerance. Her present medical problems include Hashimoto's thyroiditis, treated with desiccated thyroid 4 gr QD; hypercholesterolemia treated with cholestyramine (Questran) 4 g QID; anemia, treated with $FeSO_4$ 325 mg BID; menorrhagia treated with conjugated estrogens 1.25 mg QD; and a history of peptic ulcer disease, treated with antacids and sucralfate 1 g BID. She was recently started on calcium carbonate 1 g BID and raloxifene (Evista) 60 mg QD to protect her bones. Her laboratory data include a cholesterol serum concentration of 280 mg/dL (normal, <200), a TSH of 21 IU/mL (normal, 0.5 to 4.7), an FT_4 of 0.6 ng/dL (normal, 0.7 to 1.9), and positive ATgA and TPO antibodies. R.T. admits that she has increased her dosage of thyroid because she feels better on the higher dose. Why is R.T. apparently unresponsive to thyroid therapy?

[SI units: cholesterol, 7.2 nmol/L (normal, <5.2); FT_4, 8 pmol/L (normal, 9 to 24); TSH, 21 mIU/L (normal, 0.5 to 4.7)]

Table 49-9 T_4 Recommended Replacement Dose[a]

Age	Daily mg/kg T_4
3–6 mo	12–17
6–12 mo	5–7
1–10 yr	3–6
>10 yr	2–4

[a] T_4 = Thyroxine.

R.T.'s complaints and laboratory values confirm inadequate treatment of hypothyroidism despite thyroid therapy. Possible causes of therapeutic failure include noncompliance, error in diagnosis, poor absorption, inactive medication, rapid metabolism, and tissue resistance.[30-32,34,70,71] The last two factors are rare, and noncompliance and error in diagnosis do not appear to be reasonable explanations in R.T. The most likely explanations are poor bioavailability and/or an inactive preparation. The time of thyroxine administration with regard to her meals should be ascertained, because the bioavailability of thyroxine is improved when it is taken on an empty stomach.[34,36] Concomitant administration of soy protein supplements can also impair thyroxine absorption.[72] R.T.'s history does not include surgical bowel resection or GI disorders (e.g., steatorrhea, malabsorption) that can interfere with the enterohepatic circulation of orally administered thyroid and lead to excessive fecal loss.[71] Evidence for incomplete absorption of the hormone can be obtained by comparing R.T.'s response to oral and parenteral thyroxine.[70] Inactive desiccated thyroid preparations that contain small amounts of T_4 and T_3, or even iodinated casein instead of active hormone, have been identified.[30-32]

Thyroid bioavailability can also be compromised by the numerous medications that R.T. is taking. Estrogen therapy can also increase thyroxine requirements due to increases in TBG.[21] Cholestyramine, iron sulfate, antacids, sucralfate, calcium preparations, particularly the carbonate salt, and raloxifene can impair thyroid absorption if these medications are administered at the same time.[34,73-80] Other cholesterol-lowering agents (e.g., lovastatin) also might interfere with thyroid absorption.[76] R.T. should be questioned about the time she takes her thyroid medication. She should be instructed to take it on an empty stomach, and at least 12 hours apart from the raloxifene and 4 hours apart from the iron, calcium, and cholestyramine.[73-80] Aluminum-containing products (i.e., antacids, sucralfate) should be discontinued because separating the concurrent administration of thyroid and her aluminum-containing preparations does not consistently correct this interaction.[77,78] R.T. should be changed to an aluminum- and calcium-free antacid (e.g., Riopan) and, if necessary, an H_2-receptor antagonist. After R.T. has been instructed on the proper times of administration for her medications, her thyroid replacement should be changed to an appropriate dose of L-thyroxine (e.g., approximately 1.7 μg/kg per day). R.T.'s therapeutic response and thyroid function tests should be re-evaluated in 6 to 8 weeks.

16. Could R.T.'s hypothyroidism be responsible for her hypercholesterolemia?

Type IIa hypercholesterolemia is the most common lipid abnormality in patients with primary hypothyroidism.[81] Although the rate of cholesterol synthesis is normal in hypothyroid patients, the rate of cholesterol clearance is decreased. Similarly, slow removal of triglycerides may result in hyperlipidemia. Hypercholesterolemia frequently is observed before the appearance of clinical hypothyroidism. Treatment with thyroxine alone should lower the cholesterol levels if no other causes are contributing.

Myxedema Coma

Clinical Presentation

17. R.B., a 65-year-old, agitated woman who is an alcoholic, arrived at the emergency department complaining of chest pain unrelieved by nitroglycerin (NTG). Her medical problems include alcoholic cardiomyopathy, angina, and hypothyroidism. Although she has been advised repeatedly to take her thyroxine regularly, she continues to take it sporadically. An FT_4I drawn 4 months ago was 1.0 (normal, 6.5 to 12.5). Chlorpromazine (Thorazine) 25 mg IM and morphine sulfate 10 mg IM were given for the agitation. After the injection, the nurse noticed increased mental depression, lethargy, and shallow breathing. R.B.'s oral temperature was 34.5°C, and she exhibited chills and shakes. What is your assessment of R.B.'s subjective and objective data?

[SI units: FT_4I, 13 (normal, 84 to 161)]

R.B. has several symptoms consistent with myxedema coma.[82-84] Myxedema coma is the end stage of longstanding, uncorrected hypothyroidism. The classic features are hypothermia, delayed DTRs, and an altered sensorium that ranges from stupor to coma. Other predominant features include hypoxia, carbon dioxide retention, severe hypoglycemia, hyponatremia, and paranoid psychosis. Typical physical findings (see Table 49-3) include a puffy face and eyelids, a yellowish discoloration of the skin, and loss of the lateral eyebrows. Pleural and pericardial effusions and cardiomegaly may be present. Because myxedema coma frequently occurs in older women, it often is difficult to distinguish the signs and symptoms from dementia or other disease states, as illustrated by R.B. Precipitating factors include cold weather or hypothermia, stress (e.g., surgery, infection, trauma), coexisting disease states such as MI, diabetes, hypoglycemia, or fluid and electrolyte abnormalities (especially hyponatremia), and medications such as respiratory depressants and diuretics.

Chlorpromazine and morphine might be responsible for what appears to be impending myxedema coma in R.B. In severely myxedematous patients, respiratory depressants (anesthetics, narcotic analgesics, phenothiazines, sedative-hypnotics) alone or in combination with the hypothermic effects of the phenothiazines can aggravate the pre-existing hypothermia and carbon dioxide retention to precipitate myxedema coma.[82-84] Tranquilizers such as chlorpromazine should not be given; small doses of less depressive sedative-hypnotics such as the benzodiazepines should be used only when necessary. Myxedematous patients also are inherently sensitive to the respiratory depressant effects of narcotic analgesics, especially morphine. A dose as small as 10 mg may induce coma in a hypothyroid patient or cause death in a patient who already is comatose. If morphine is required, the dose should be decreased to one-third to one-half the usual analgesic dose and the respiratory rate should be monitored closely.

Treatment

18. What would be a reasonable therapeutic plan for the management of R.B.'s myxedema coma?

Emergency treatment of myxedema coma is directed toward thyroid replacement, maintenance of vital functions, and elimination of precipitating factors. Despite immediate and aggressive therapy with large replacement doses of thyroid, mortality rates of 60% to 70% are common.[82-84]

Which hormone preparation, T_4 or T_3, is the drug of choice in myxedema coma is controversial because no comparative trials have been conducted. Although T_3 is potentially more cardiotoxic, it has been recommended because its more rapid onset might reverse coma faster, and the peripheral conversion from T_4 to the biologically active T_3 might be inhibited in severe systemic disease.[83–87] T_4 alone, T_3 alone, and a combination of the two have all been successful in the treatment of myxedema coma. However, levothyroxine generally is regarded as the hormone of choice because of greater clinical experience with T_4 than with T_3. Also, mortality has occurred despite the higher T_3 levels achieved after T_3 administration.[88] T_3 might be considered after failure of T_4 or if systemic illness is concomitant (e.g., heart failure), in which failure of conversion from T_4 to T_3 is likely. Supraphysiologic elevations in T_3 levels occur only after oral administration but are not seen after IV T_3 infusion. Factors associated with a higher mortality 1 month after therapy include older age, cardiac complications, and T_4 replacement ≥ 500 μg/day or T_3 replacement ≥ 75 μg/day.[83]

L-thyroxine 400 to 500 μg should be given IV initially in patients <55 years of age without cardiac disease to saturate the TBG and raise the serum T_4 level to 6 to 7 μg/dL.[82–84,89] This initial dose can be adjusted based on the patient's weight and other restrictive factors (e.g., age, cardiac disease). The initial dosage for R.B. should be reduced to 300 μg/day to avoid worsening her angina. If the proper dosage is given, consciousness, restoration of vital signs, and decreased TSH levels should occur within 24 hours.

Maintenance doses should be titrated to the patient's clinical response. Because myxedema can impair oral absorption, the IV route is preferred to ensure adequate drug concentrations. Oral administration is permitted once GI function returns to normal. The smallest dosage (without untoward effects) administered should be 50 to 100 μg/day of T_4 or 10 to 15 μg of T_3 every 12 hours.[82–84,89]

Supportive measures include assisted ventilation, glucose for hypoglycemia, restriction of fluids for hyponatremia, and the use of blood or plasma expanders to prevent circulatory collapse and to maintain blood pressure. The use of blankets to treat R.B.'s hypothermia is not advised because vasodilation will occur and further compromise the cardiovascular components of shock. Although steroids have not been shown to be clearly beneficial in primary myxedema, they may be lifesaving in patients with hypopituitarism masquerading as myxedema coma. Because it is difficult to distinguish between primary and secondary myxedema, hydrocortisone 50 to 100 mg every 6 hours should be given empirically.[82,84]

Appropriate measures should be taken to relieve R.B.'s chest pain while ruling out the possibility of an MI. The use of a narcotic antagonist such as naloxone may be beneficial in this instance because it can reverse the effects of the morphine. Naloxone also can arouse comatose patients intoxicated with alcohol.

Hypothyroidism With Congestive Heart Failure

Clinical Presentation

19. E.B., a 45-year-old woman, is admitted with complaints of substantial substernal pressure and chest pain, SOB, dyspnea on exertion, and orthopnea. Other subjective and objective data suggest CHF complicated by MI. Significant past medical history reveals exertional angina and Graves' disease, which was treated with radioactive iodine (RAI) ablation 10 years ago. Symptoms have not recurred. Physical examination reveals cardiomegaly, diastolic hypertension, obesity, facial edema and puffiness, delayed DTRs, and nonpitting pretibial edema. Pertinent laboratory findings include FT_4, 0.4 ng/dL (normal, 0.7 to 1.9); TSH, 100 IU/mL (normal, 0.5 to 4.7); creatinine kinase, 300 units/L (normal, 32 to 267); aspartate aminotransferase (AST), 80 units/L (normal, 7 to 26); lactate dehydrogenase (LDH), 250 units/L (normal, 80 to 230); troponin, 0.3 ng/mL (normal, 0.3 to 1.5). A chest radiograph reveals cardiomegaly and pericardial effusions, and an electrocardiogram (ECG) shows bradycardia and flattened T waves with ST depression. Diuretics, nitrates, angiotensin II inhibitor, and digitalis are instituted. E.B.'s symptoms improve, but her cardiac abnormalities are not reversed. Why do these clinical findings suggest hypothyroidism?

[SI units: FT_4, 5 pmol/L (normal, 9 to 24); TSH, 100 mIU/L (normal, 0.5 to 4.7); creatinine kinase, 300 U/L (normal, 32 to 267); AST, 80 U/L (normal, 7 to 26); LDH, 250 U/L (normal, 80 to 230); troponin 0.3 g/L (normal, 0.3 to 1.5)]

E.B.'s abnormal thyroid function tests, symptoms, physical findings, and history of RAI therapy are consistent with severe hypothyroidism. "Myxedema heart" can be confused with low-output CHF because the symptoms are similar: cardiomegaly, dyspnea, edema, pericardial effusions, and an abnormal cardiogram.[82,84,90] Therefore, hypothyroidism should be excluded in all patients with new or worsening symptoms of cardiovascular disease (e.g., angina, arrhythmia). Although hypothyroidism alone rarely causes CHF, it can worsen an underlying cardiac condition. Rarely, ventricular arrhythmia, including torsades de pointes, can occur from a prolonged QT interval.[90]

Although E.B.'s enzyme elevations (i.e., AST, CK, LDH) are suggestive of an MI, they all may be moderately or significantly increased from chronic skeletal or cardiac muscle damage or from decreased enzyme clearance from hypothyroidism. The enzymes can be fractionated to determine their origin. The normal troponin level eliminates the possibility of an MI.

Treatment

20. What might be the effect of hypothyroidism on the cardiac treatment and status of E.B.?

If E.B.'s cardiac abnormalities are caused by hypothyroidism rather than organic disease, adequate doses of thyroxine will restore the heart size, normalize the diastolic blood pressure, reverse the ECG findings, and normalize the serum enzyme elevations within 2 to 4 weeks. However, improvement in myocardial function begins only at dosages of 50 to 75 μg/day of thyroxine, which may be tolerated poorly by cardiac patients.[90]

The relationship between the altered lipid metabolism of hypothyroidism and increased risk of atherosclerosis is controversial and poorly documented.[81] Interestingly, angina pectoris and MI are rather uncommon among hypothyroid patients. Theoretically, the hypometabolic state associated with hypothyroidism may protect the ischemic myocardium by reducing metabolic demands. However, hypothyroidism actually aggravates subendocardial ischemia during an acute MI by decreasing erythrocyte production of 2,3-diphosphoglycerate, which shifts the oxyhemoglobin dissociation curve to the left. This effect further diminishes oxygen delivery to already ischemic tissues. Angina might develop or worsen with the institution of thyroxine therapy,[91-93] so doses should be titrated carefully (see Question 21). Without organic disease, digitalis is ineffective and may even be harmful. Hypothyroid patients show an increased sensitivity to digitalis, and digitalis toxicity is possible unless the maintenance dose is decreased (see Question 26).[94,95] Nitrates may precipitate hypotension and/or syncope in hypothyroid patients because these patients have a low circulating blood volume and their response to vasodilation can be exaggerated. Furthermore, if β-blockers are required, the cardioselective β-blockers are preferred. The noncardioselective β-blockers have produced coronary spasm by exacerbating the increased norepinephrine levels and α-adrenergic tone found in hypothyroidism.

21. How aggressively should thyroid hormone therapy be initiated in a patient like E.B. who has angina? What is the hormone replacement of choice in patients with cardiac disease?

Patients with longstanding hypothyroidism, arteriosclerotic cardiac disease, or advanced age tend to be extremely sensitive to the cardiac effects of thyroid hormone. Initiation of normal or even subtherapeutic doses in these patients might produce severe angina, MI, cardiac failure, or sudden death. These effects underscore the need to replace thyroid cautiously, and sometimes suboptimally, to avoid cardiac toxicity.[91-93]

The angina and cardiac status should be controlled before initiating thyroxine therapy. In the patient with poorly controlled angina, cardiac catheterization is warranted to assess the coronary artery status before starting hormone therapy. Coronary bypass has been performed safely with minimal complications in the hypothyroid patient to control the angina and may allow institution of full replacement doses without cardiotoxicity.[96]

For E.B., 12.5 to 25 μg of T_4 should be initiated cautiously and increased as tolerated by similar increments of T_4 every 4 to 6 weeks until a therapeutic dosage is reached. The rapidity with which the increments can proceed is determined by how well each increased dose is tolerated. If cardiac toxicity occurs, therapy should be stopped immediately. Once symptoms resolve, therapy can be restarted using smaller dosage increments and longer intervals between dosage adjustments. If cardiac symptoms recur, further thyroxine therapy should be stopped pending cardiac evaluation. In some patients with severe cardiac sensitivity, complete euthyroidism might never be achieved. In these patients, the correct replacement dosage is a compromise between prevention of myxedema and avoidance of cardiac toxicity.[90,91] E.B.'s clinical status and ECG should be monitored closely during the titration period. Thyroxine should be discontinued or decreased at the first sign of cardiac deterioration. It is not necessary to monitor thyroid function tests (e.g., TSH or FT_4) during the titration period because the results will remain low until adequate replacement is achieved. Thyroid function tests should be obtained once maximally tolerated or estimated euthyroid dosages are achieved.

Some suggest that triiodothyronine (Cytomel) is the agent of choice in patients with cardiac abnormalities. The onset of action of T_3 is 1 to 3 days compared with 3 to 5 days for T_4. After therapy is withdrawn, the effects of T_3 dissipate in 3 to 5 days, while a period of 7 to 10 days is needed for T_4. Thus, if toxicity occurs, the effects of T_3 will disappear rapidly upon cessation of therapy, a theoretical advantage in the cardiac patient. Nevertheless, T_3 is not recommended because its greater potency requires finer and more difficult dosage titration to ensure smooth and uniform blood levels. Furthermore, the high serum T_3 levels that occur after oral administration might cause more cardiac toxicity, especially angina.

Subclinical Hypothyroidism

22. M.P., a healthy 53-year-old woman, comes in for her regular checkup. She denies any symptoms of hypothyroidism and feels well. She has no other medical problems, takes no medications, and has no known allergies. Her physical examination is within normal limits. Routine screening laboratory tests are normal except for an FT_4 of 1.2 ng/dL (normal, 0.7 to 1.9) and a TSH of 8 IU/mL (normal, 0.5 to 4.7). Does M.P. require thyroid treatment, based on her clinical presentation and laboratory findings?

[SI units: FT_4, 16 pmol/L (normal, 9 to 24); TSH, 8 mIU/L (normal, 0.5 to 4.7)]

M.P.'s free thyroid levels are normal, but her TSH level is elevated, indicating subclinical hypothyroidism. The prevalence of subclinical hypothyroidism ranges from 4% to 10% and increases to 26% in the elderly population, particularly women.[97-101] It is unclear whether subclinical hypothyroidism represents the early stages of thyroid failure. The estimated risk of developing overt hypothyroidism after 10 years in untreated patients by Kaplan-Meier curves was 0% for a TSH level of 4 to 6 mIU/L, 42.8% for a TSH level of 6 to 12 mIU/L, and 76.9% for a TSH level >12 mIU/L. This risk increased in patients with positive thyroid antibodies.[102] Because the most common clinical scenarios involve asymptomatic patients with TSH levels <10 mIU/L, negative thyroid antibodies, and no history of prior thyroid disease, routine thyroid screening has been recommended, particularly in elderly women.[98]

Mild symptoms of hypothyroidism, including psychiatric and cognitive abnormalities, are found in approximately 30% of patients with subclinical hypothyroidism, but the average TSH level usually exceeds 11 mIU/L. Cardiac dysfunction, including impaired left ventricular diastolic function at rest, systolic dysfunction with exercise, and an increased risk for atherosclerosis and MI, has been reported.[49,98-101] Other atypical and nonspecific signs and symptoms reflecting dysfunction of any part of the body may occur, primarily in the elderly. Failure to thrive, mental confusion, weight loss with poor appetite, incontinence, depression, inability to walk, carpal tunnel syndrome, deafness, ileus, anemia, hypercholesterolemia, and hyponatremia have been seen.[97-101]

Treatment of subclinical hypothyroidism with thyroxine is controversial because study results are conflicting. Potential benefits of treatment include (1) preventing progression to hypothyroidism; (2) improving the lipid profile and reducing cardiac risks; and (3) reversing symptoms of hypothyroidism. Patients with higher TSH levels (e.g., >10 mIU/L), a history of previously diagnosed thyroid disease, elevated lipid levels, or evidence of positive thyroid antibodies gained the most benefit from levothyroxine therapy.[49,101-103] Levothyroxine significantly reduced total cholesterol by 0.2 to 0.4 mmol/L (7.9

to 15.8 mg/dL) and low-density cholesterol concentrations by 0.33 mmol/L (10 mg/dL); serum HDL and triglyceride concentrations remain unchanged.[98,100,101,103] Improvement of elevated intraocular pressures, memory, mood, somatic complaints, and diastolic dysfunction also has been reported after thyroxine replacement.[51,100–103] However, in patients with mild TSH elevations (e.g., <10 mIU/L), well-designed studies showed no improvement in clinical symptoms of hypothyroidism with thyroxine supplementation.[97,98,100,101]

Treatment of older patients requires an assessment of the risks versus benefits of therapy. Thyroid therapy carries the risk of unmasking underlying cardiac disease in older patients. Nevertheless, thyroid replacement appears reasonable in asymptomatic patients with TSH levels >10 mIU/L and especially those with symptoms of mild hypothyroidism, laboratory abnormalities, or end-organ alterations.[97–103] Patients with asymptomatic subclinical hypothyroidism and a TSH level <10 mIU/L do not warrant immediate therapy.

Because M.P. is asymptomatic and has a TSH level <10 mIU/L, it is reasonable to delay therapy and recheck the TSH in a few months.

Hypopituitarism and T4 Replacement With a Normal TSH Level

23. J.P. is a 65-year-old woman who complains of fatigue, cold intolerance, dry skin, and weight gain for the past several months. Her thyroid examination and DTRs are within normal limits. A TSH level was 2.5 IU/mL (normal, 0.5 to 4.7). She denies taking any medications. J.P. is started empirically on a 3-month trial of levothyroxine. How should the TSH level be interpreted? Is thyroxine therapy indicated, based on her presenting findings?

[SI units: TSH 2.5 mIU/L (normal, 0.5 to 4.7)]

Despite complaints that could be consistent with hypothyroidism (e.g., fatigue, cold intolerance, dry skin, weight gain), the normal TSH level indicates that J.P. is euthyroid. However, since a diagnosis of hypopituitarism (i.e., TSH level could be normal or low) cannot be ruled out, an FT_4 level should be obtained; a low level would increase the likelihood of hypopituitarism. Some argue that hypopituitarism is underdiagnosed and would advocate adding FT_4 to the primary screening tests.[104]

If the FT_4 level is normal, indicating euthyroidism, then hypopituitarism is unlikely and levothyroxine therapy is not indicated. A randomized, double-blind, placebo-controlled crossover trial found that thyroxine supplementation in patients with hypothyroid symptoms and normal thyroid function tests was not more effective than placebo in improving cognitive function or psychological well-being despite changes in the TSH and FT_4 levels.[105,106]

In J.P., the thyroxine should be discontinued because there is no evidence of its efficacy in euthyroid individuals.

HYPERTHYROIDISM

Clinical Presentation

24. S.K., a 48-year-old woman, is admitted to the hospital for a possible MI. Her complaints include chest pain that is unrelieved by NTG, increasing SOB with exercise, nervousness, palpitations, muscle weakness, weight loss despite an increased appetite, and epistaxis; she also bruises easily. She has a history of deep venous thrombosis treated with warfarin (Coumadin) 5 mg/day; her last prothrombin time (PT) was 18 sec (normal, 10.5 to 12.1) and an International Normalized Ratio (INR) was 1.8 (normal, 1.0; therapeutic, 2.0 to 3.0). She has angina, treated with NTG 0.4 mg, and CHF, treated with digoxin (Lanoxin) 0.25 mg/day.

Physical examination reveals a thin, flushed, hyperkinetic, nervous woman. Blood pressure (BP) is 180/90 mm Hg; pulse is 130 beats/min, irregularly irregular; respiratory rate is 30 breaths/min; temperature is 37.5°C. Other pertinent findings include a lid lag with stare, proptosis with tearing, decreased visual acuity, a diffusely enlarged thyroid gland without nodules, a bruit in the left lobe of the thyroid, positive jugular venous distention (JVD), bibasilar rales, warm moist skin with multiple bruises, new-onset atrial fibrillation (AF), slight diarrhea, hepatomegaly, acropachy, 2+ pitting edema, a fine tremor, proximal muscle weakness, and irregular scant menses.

Laboratory data include FT_4, 2.9 ng/dL (normal, 0.7 to 1.9); TSH, <0.5 IU/mL (normal, 0.5 to 4.7); RAIU at 24 hours, 80% (normal, 15% to 35%); PT, 40 sec (normal, 10.5 to 12.1); INR, 4.8 (normal, 1.0; therapeutic, 2.0 to 3.0); TPO, 200 IU/mL (normal, <100); alkaline phosphatase, 200 units/L (normal, 41 to 133); total bilirubin, 1.1 mg/dL (normal, 0.1 to 1.2); AST, 60 units/L (normal, 7 to 26); alanine aminotransferase (ALT), 55 units/L (normal, 3 to 23). A scan shows a diffusely enlarged gland, three to four times normal size. What subjective and objective data are suggestive of hyperthyroidism in S.K.?

S.K. presents with many of the clinical and laboratory features[107] associated with an increased metabolic state resulting from excessive thyroxine (see Table 49-6). Her ocular symptoms are consistent with Graves' disease and include lid lag (lid falls behind the movement of the eye and a narrow white rim of sclera becomes visible between the upper lid and cornea, producing a "staring" appearance), ophthalmopathy (protrusion of the eyeball), and decreased visual acuity. The thyroid bruit, palpitations, exertional dyspnea, worsening CHF (JVD, bibasilar rales, edema, hepatomegaly), diarrhea, irregular scant menses, nervousness, tremor, muscle weakness, weight loss despite increased appetite, increased perspiration, and flushing of the skin are consistent with a hypermetabolic state. Although sinus tachycardia is the most common arrhythmia in hyperthyroidism, new-onset AF is the presenting symptom in 5% to 20% of patients with hyperthyroidism, particularly in those >70 years.[90,108] Together with S.K.'s symptoms, a diagnosis of Graves' disease is confirmed by an elevated FT_4 level, an undetectable TSH level, an increased RAIU, positive TPO antibodies, and a diffusely enlarged goiter. Her cardiac status and other medical problems are aggravated by the hyperthyroidism. (Table 49-5 lists the causes of hyperthyroidism.)

Hypoprothrombinemia

25. What factors contribute to S.K.'s hypoprothrombinemia? What effect could this have on her subsequent drug treatment?

The hypoprothrombinemia and bleeding observed in S.K. most likely are related to an exaggerated response to warfarin. This may be related to a decrease in the hepatic metabolism of warfarin (secondary to hepatic congestion), but it is more likely that S.K.'s findings are due to the combined effects of hyperthyroidism and warfarin on vitamin K–dependent clotting factors.

Warfarin Metabolism

Warfarin metabolism and the metabolism of vitamin K–dependent clotting factors can be altered by thyroid status. Net circulating levels of vitamin K–dependent clotting factors generally are not altered in hyperthyroid patients because both the synthesis and catabolism of these clotting factors are increased. However, an enhanced anticoagulant response occurs when the warfarin-induced decrease in clotting factor synthesis is combined with the hyperthyroidism-induced increase in clotting factor catabolism.[109,110] This may explain S.K.'s elevated prothrombin time, bruising, and history of epistaxis.

The opposite occurs in hypothyroidism, in which a decrease in both the metabolism and synthesis of clotting factors occurs. In hypothyroid patients, the response to oral anticoagulants is delayed because the clotting factors are eliminated more slowly.[109,110] Therefore, hyperthyroid patients need less warfarin, while hypothyroid patients require more warfarin to achieve the same hypoprothrombinemic response. The anticoagulant response to warfarin should be monitored carefully in patients with thyroid abnormalities and the dosage adjusted as the thyroid status changes.

Thioamide Effects

Because S.K.'s hyperthyroidism most likely will be treated with a thioamide, caution must be exercised. Treatment of hyperthyroid patients with thioamides, especially PTU, has been associated with hypoprothrombinemia, thrombocytopenia, and bleeding, albeit rarely.[111] These drugs can depress the bone marrow and the synthesis of clotting factors II, VII, III, IX, X, and XIII; vitamin K and prothrombin times may remain depressed for up to 2 months after discontinuation of therapy. These effects may be caused by a subclinical hepatic alteration in synthesis or hepatotoxicity (see Question 38).[112–114] Symptoms occur 2 weeks to 18 months after starting therapy. The bleeding is responsive to vitamin K or blood transfusions. (Also see Questions 31 and 32 for further discussion of treatment with thioamides.)

Response to Digoxin

26. After treatment with RAI, S.K.'s daily dose of digoxin was increased to 0.5 mg because of persistent AF and rapid ventricular response. Six weeks later, she returns with complaints of nausea and vomiting. The gland remains palpable but is decreased considerably in size. The ECG shows ST depression, atrioventricular (AV) block, and occasional bigeminy. Assess these subjective and objective data.

S.K.'s nausea and vomiting, together with the ECG changes of AV block and bigeminy, strongly suggest digitalis toxicity. Although a high dosage of digoxin is appropriate while a patient is thyrotoxic, continuation of this same dose as the hyperthyroidism resolves increases the likelihood of digitalis toxicity.[94,95]

27. Why was such a large dose of digoxin required initially? What other options can be used to control the ventricular rate?

The AF of hyperthyroidism often is resistant to digitalis. When euthyroid patients with AF were given digitalis before and after exogenous T_3 administration, the daily dose of digoxin required to maintain a ventricular rate of 70 was increased from 0.2 to 0.8 mg after T_3 administration.[115] Higher dosages of digoxin without side effects might be tolerated better by the hyperthyroid patient.[94,95,115] Nevertheless, the goal of digoxin therapy should be a higher target heart rate (i.e., 100 beats/min) than that achieved with digoxin in the euthyroid patient with AF to minimize cardiac toxicity. If additional rate control is required, β-blockers or calcium channel blockers (e.g., diltiazem or verapamil) can be added. Unless contraindicated by myocardial dysfunction or severe bronchospasm, β-blockers rather than calcium channel blockers are preferred because they are more effective in controlling the ventricular rate and are less likely to cause hypotension.

This apparent resistance to digitalis is attributed to intrinsic changes in myocardial function, to an increased volume of distribution for digoxin, and to an increased glomerular filtration of the glycoside.[94,95,115] Conversely, hypothyroid patients are inordinately sensitive to the effects of digitalis and require smaller doses to achieve a therapeutic response. Regardless of the mechanism, one should be aware that higher-than-normal doses might be required in patients with thyrotoxicosis and that the initial dosage should be reduced as the hyperthyroid state resolves.

Cardioversion

28. If the AF persists, when should cardioversion be attempted in S.K.? Is other treatment indicated?

Because S.K. received radioactive iodine 6 weeks ago, her thyroid function tests should be rechecked to determine her present thyroid status. Cardioversion, either medical or electrical, should not be attempted if she is still toxic because the success rate is low. AF spontaneously reverted to normal sinus rhythm (NSR) in 56% to 62% of patients within the first 3 to 4 months after control of the hyperthyroidism.[90,108] Spontaneous conversion is highly unlikely if the duration of the hyperthyroidism-induced AF exceeds 13 months or if the AF persists after 4 months of euthyroidism.[90,108] Older patients with or without underlying heart disorders (except CHF) also are less likely to spontaneously convert to NSR. Patients who meet these criteria are candidates for cardioversion at about the third or fourth month after achieving euthyroidism. Age and the duration of thyrotoxicosis are important determinants of successful cardioversion. Ninety percent of patients achieved NSR after cardioversion; of these, 57% and 48% maintained NSR at 10 and 14 years, respectively, of follow-up.[108]

S.K. should be maintained on warfarin because of a high prevalence of systemic embolization in thyrotoxic patients with AF.[90] Anticoagulation should be started when the AF is first diagnosed and continued until S.K. is euthyroid and in NSR. This is especially true for younger patients at low risk of bleeding with Coumadin. The risks versus benefits of anticoagulation should be weighed before therapy (see Chapter 16, Thrombosis). Because an increased sensitivity to warfarin is observed, close monitoring is warranted (see Question 25).

Thyrotoxicosis: Clinical Presentation

29. C.R., a 27-year-old woman, has a 3-month history of intermittent heat intolerance, sweats, tremor, and severe muscle weakness, which has limited her ability to climb stairs. Her weight has increased because of increased appetite. She also is bothered by the pounding of her heart and some minor difficulty in swallowing. There is a family history of thyroid disease, but she denies taking any thyroid medications or having had any radiation to her neck. C.R. previously received iodide drops with improvement in her symptoms, but her disease recurred despite continued administration. Her other medical problems include diabetes, which is controlled with diet, and osteoarthritis, which is treated with aspirin 2.5 g/day. She has a history of noncompliance with her clinic visits.

Pertinent physical findings include a BP of 180/90 mm Hg, a pulse of 110 beats/min, hyperreflexia, lid lag, and a diffusely enlarged thyroid gland that is about four times normal (about 100 g). Laboratory data include TT_4, 6 μg/dL (normal, 5 to 12); FT_4, 2 ng/dL (normal, 0.7 to 1.9); TSH, <0.01 IU/mL (normal, 0.5 to 4.7); TPO, 350 IU/mL (normal, <100); blood glucose, 350 mg/dL (normal, 60 to 115). Assess these subjective and objective data.

[SI units: TT_4, 77 nmol/L (normal, 64 to 154); FT_4, 28 pmol/L (normal, 9 to 24); TSH, <0.01 mIU/L (normal, 0.5 to 4.7); blood glucose, 19.4 mmol/L (normal, 3.3 to 6.4)]

C.R.'s clinical findings verify an autoimmune hyperthyroid state. However, the serum FT_4, is elevated only slightly and is disproportionately low relative to the severity of her symptoms, the undetectable TSH level, and her other laboratory findings. The low normal TT_4 could be explained by displacement of T_4 from TBG by aspirin (see Question 3). The possibility of a variant type of hyperthyroidism known as T_3 toxicosis should be considered. The clinical features include signs and symptoms of thyrotoxicosis, normal or borderline high FT_4, an undetectable TSH level, and elevated T_3 levels. The latter occurs through preferential secretion and peripheral conversion of T_4 to T_3. A T_3 level should be obtained to establish the diagnosis.

Asymptomatic elevations of T_3 levels often precede elevation of T_4 levels and the development of overt hyperthyroidism. T_3 toxicosis probably represents an early stage of classic T_4 toxicosis and is useful for early diagnosis or as an early indicator of relapse after discontinuation of thioamide therapy.

Iodides

30. Why were the iodide drops initially effective in improving C.R.'s symptoms and later ineffective? When are iodides indicated? What is their mechanism of action?

Iodides have several effects: they inhibit thyroid hormone release, they block iodotyrosine and iodothyronine synthesis by blocking organification, and they decrease the vascularity of the thyroid gland.[116] However, large doses may accentuate hyperthyroidism because they provide a significant increase in available substrate for hormone synthesis (see Question 54).[116,117]

The inhibitory effect of exogenous iodides on the intrathyroidal organification of iodides is known as the Wolff-Chaikoff effect. This is an inherent autoregulatory function of the normal gland to prevent excessive hormone synthesis in the event of a large iodide load. The Wolff-Chaikoff effect occurs when intrathyroidal concentrations of iodides reach a critical level, and this is not overcome by TSH stimulation. However, as illustrated by C.R., the gland can "escape" from this block even with continued iodide use. The gland escapes

by decreasing iodide transport or by leaking iodide. Both of these mechanisms decrease the critical intrathyroidal iodide level, thereby decreasing the block to organification. This effect is illustrated in C.R. Therefore, iodides should not be used as primary therapy for Graves' disease.

Conversely, some patients are responsive to iodide therapy, including (1) patients who already have high intrathyroidal iodine stores (i.e., "hot" nodules, Graves' disease); (2) patients with underlying defects in organic binding mechanisms (i.e., Hashimoto's); (3) patients who develop drug-induced thyroid disorders (see Questions 52 to 55); and (4) patients with Graves' disease made euthyroid with RAI or surgery and who are receiving no thyroid replacement.

These patients are so sensitive that small doses of iodide can elicit the Wolff-Chaikoff effect, resulting in either amelioration of hyperthyroid symptoms or precipitation of hypothyroidism.[116–118] For this reason, patients with recurrent hyperthyroidism after surgery or RAI often can be managed with iodides alone.

The most important pharmacologic effect of iodides is their ability to promptly inhibit thyroid hormone release when dosages of 6 mg/day are given.[116,118] The mechanism is unknown, but it is not related to the Wolff-Chaikoff effect, which may take several weeks to manifest. Unlike the Wolff-Chaikoff effect, this effect can be overcome partially by an increase in TSH secretion. Thus, the normal gland can escape in 7 to 14 days because inhibition of thyroid hormone release stimulates a reflex increase in TSH secretion. Because patients with hyperthyroidism experience an improvement in symptoms within 2 to 7 days of initiation of therapy, inhibition of hormone release must be the predominant mechanism of action for the iodides. This rapid onset is the reason iodides are used in the treatment of thyroid storm and as an ameliorative measure while awaiting the onset of the therapeutic effects of thioamides or RAI.

Large doses of iodides also are used 2 weeks before thyroid surgery to increase the firmness of the thyroid gland by decreasing its size, vascularity, and friability. Iodides facilitate a smoother, less complicated surgery and decrease postoperative complications by inducing a euthyroid state.[116]

Stable iodine can be administered orally either as an unpleasant-tasting Lugol's solution (5% iodine and 10% potassium iodide), containing 8 mg/drop of iodide, or as the more palatable saturated solution of potassium iodide (SSKI), containing 50 mg/drop of iodide. The minimum effective daily dose is 6 mg,[116] although larger doses (e.g., 5 to 10 drops QID of SSKI) are often administered.

The advantages of iodide therapy are that it is simple, inexpensive, and relatively nontoxic and involves no glandular destruction. Disadvantages include "escape," accentuation of thyrotoxicosis, allergic reactions, relapse after discontinuation of treatment, and subsequent interference with RAI if used before therapy.

Treatment Modalities

31. What are the advantages and disadvantages of the different treatment modalities available for C.R.?

The three major treatment modalities for Graves'-related hyperthyroidism are the thioamides, RAI, and surgery (Table 49-10).[107,119–124] In most cases, any of these three modalities

Table 49-10 Treatment for Hyperthyroidism

Modality	Drug/Dosage	Mechanism of Action	Toxicity	Indication
Primary Treatment				
Thioamides				
PTU 50 mg tab; rectal formulation can be made[175,176]	100–200 mg PO Q 6–8 hr (*max*: 1,200 mg/day) for 6–8 weeks or until euthyroid; then maintenance of 50–150 mg QD PO × 12–18 months	Blocks organification of hormone synthesis, blocks peripheral conversion of T_4 to T_3 (PTU only)	Skin rashes, GI symptoms, arthralgias, ↑ transaminases, hepatitis, agranulocytosis	DOC, thyroid storm, and breast-feeding
Methimazole (Tapazole) 5, 10 mg tab; rectal suppositories can be made[177]	Methimazole 30–40 mg PO QD or in 2 divided doses (*max*: 60 mg/day) for 6–8 wk or until euthyroid, then maintenance of 5–10 mg/day PO × 12–18 months	Similar to PTU except does not block conversion of T_4 to T_3	Similar to PTU; cholestatic jaundice, reports of aplasia cutis	Thioamide DOC because QD dosing and better compliance; not DOC in breast-feeding or thyroid storm
Surgery	Preoperative preparation with iodides, thioamides, ipodate, or propranolol before surgery; see specific operative agent	Subtotal or total thyroidectomy	Hypothyroidism, cosmetic scarring, hypoparathyroidism, risks of surgery, and anesthesia, vocal cord damage	Obstruction, choking, malignancy, pregnancy in second trimester, contraindication to RAI or thioamides
RAI	^{131}I radioactive isotope; 80–100 μCi/g thyroid tissue. Average dose, ≈10 mCi; pretreatment with corticosteroids indicated in patients with ophthalmopathy	Destruction of the gland	Hypothyroidism; worsening of ophthalmopathy; fear of radiation-induced leukemia; genetic damage; malignancy; rarely, radiation sickness	Adults, older patients who are poor surgical risks or have cardiac disease; patients with a history of prior thyroid surgery; contraindications to thioamide usage

Adjuncts to Primary Usage

Iodides

Drug	Dose	Mechanism	Adverse Effects	Comments
Iodinated contrast dye Ipodate (Oragrafin) Iopanoic acid (Telepaque) Na tyropanoate (Biopaque) Na diatrizoate (Hypaque)	0.5–1 g QD PO	Blocks T_4 to T_3 conversion; release of iodides to block hormone secretion from thyroid gland	Same as iodides	Alternative to thioamide for rapid control of hyperthyroidism, symptomatic relief of symptoms, adjuncts to surgery, thioamides, and possibly RAI; escape occurs with chronic usage

Iodides

| Lugol's solution 8 mg/drop (5% iodine, 10% potassium iodide; Saturated [SSKI] 50 mg/drop) | 5–10 drops TID PO for 10–14 days before surgery; minimum effective dose 6 mg/day | ↓ vascularity of gland and ↑ firmness; blocks release of thyroid hormone | Hypersensitivity reactions, skin rashes, mucous membrane ulcers, anaphylaxis, metallic taste, rhinorrhea, parotid and submaxillary swelling; fetal goiters and death | Preoperative preparation before surgery; thyroid storm, provides symptomatic relief of symptoms. *Do not use before RAI or chronically during pregnancy.* |

β-Blockers

| Propranolol or equivalent β-blocker. *Avoid* those with ISA | Propranolol 10–40 mg PO Q 6 hr or PRN to control HR <100 beats/min; IV 0.5–1 mg slowly | Blocks effects of thyroid hormone peripherally, no effect on underlying disease; blocks T_4 to T_3 conversion | Related to β-blockade: bradycardia, CHF, blocks hyperglycemic response to hypoglycemia, bronchospasm, CNS symptoms at high doses; fetal bradycardia | Symptomatic relief while awaiting onset of thioamides, RAI; preoperative preparation for surgery; thyroid storm |

Calcium channel blockers

| Calcium channel blockers | Diltiazem 120 mg TID–QID PO or verapamil 80–120 mg TID–QID PO PRN to control HR <100 beats/min | Blocks effects of thyroid hormone peripherally, no effect on underlying disease | Bradycardia, peripheral edema, CHF, headache, flushing, hypotension, dizziness | Alternative for symptomatic relief of hyperthyroid symptoms in patients who cannot tolerate β-blockers |

Corticosteroids

| Corticosteroids | Prednisone or equivalent corticosteroids 50–140 mg/day PO in divided doses; IV hydrocortisone 50–100 mg Q 6 hr or equivalent for thyroid storm | ↓ TRAb, suppression of inflammatory process; blocks T_4 to T_3 conversion | Complications of steroid therapy | Ophthalmopathy, thyroid storm (use IV steroid), pretibial myxedema, pretreatment before RAI therapy in patients with ophthalmopathy |

CHF, congestive heart failure; CNS, central nervous system; DOC, drug of choice; GI, gastrointestinal; HR, heart rate; ISA, intrinsic sympathomimetic activity; IV, intravenous; μCi, microcurie; mCi, millicurie; PTU, propylthiouracil; RAI, radioactive iodine; Tab, tablet.

can be used, and it is controversial which is the most effective therapy. Often the final decision is empiric, depending on the physician's available resources and the patient's desires. A review of treatment guidelines published by the major endocrine organizations showed that RAI is the most common treatment, while surgery is the least common.[120] Patients who are older and those with cardiac disease, concomitant ophthalmopathy, and hyperthyroidism caused by a toxic multinodular goiter are treated best with radioactive iodine. Surgery is the preferred therapy for pregnant women who are drug intolerant, when obstructive symptoms are present, or if malignancy is suspected.

Thioamides

The thioamides are the preferred treatment for children, pregnant women, and young adults with uncomplicated Graves' disease.[107,119–122] This is the only treatment that leaves the thyroid gland intact and does not carry the added risk of permanent hypothyroidism often associated with RAI or surgery.

Because the thyrotoxicosis of Graves' disease might be self-limiting, thioamides are used to control the symptoms until spontaneous remission occurs. Thioamides also should be given before treatment with RAI or surgery to deplete the gland of stored thyroid hormone, which prevents subsequent thyroid storm. Although hyperthyroidism from toxic nodules also will respond to thioamides, more definitive therapy (surgery or RAI) is needed because these other conditions do not undergo spontaneous remission.

Disadvantages of thioamide therapy include the numerous tablets required, patient compliance, possible drug toxicity, the long duration of treatment, and the low incidence of remission after discontinuation of therapy (see Questions 42 and 43).

The use of thioamides in C.R. has several potential drawbacks. Her relatively large gland and severe disease make the prognosis for spontaneous remission somewhat less favorable. A delay in the onset of thioamide's effect may be expected if intraglandular stores of thyroid have been increased by her prior iodide therapy. Furthermore, her noncompliance and difficulty swallowing may necessitate another means of treatment.

Surgery

Surgery is considered the treatment of choice[107,119,120,124,125] when (1) malignancy is suspected; (2) esophageal obstruction, evidenced by difficulty swallowing, is present; (3) respiratory difficulties are present; (4) contraindications to the use of thioamides (e.g., allergy) or radioactive iodine (e.g., pregnancy) exist; or (5) a large goiter is present that regresses poorly on RAI or thioamide therapy. Some argue that surgery is underused in the treatment of Graves' disease.[124] In a prospective, randomized trial comparing the three treatment options, surgery produced euthyroidism more quickly and was associated with a lower relapse rate than either RAI or thioamides.[125] If C.R.'s minor difficulty in swallowing persists because of poor regression of goiter size with drug therapy, then surgery is a reasonable alternative. If surgery is contemplated, C.R. must be brought to surgery in a euthyroid state to prevent rapid postoperative rises in T_4 levels and subsequent thyroid storm (see Question 50). Subtotal thyroidectomy is effective and successful in >90% of patients with Graves' dis-

ease. Subtotal thyroidectomy potentially avoids the predictable risk of hypothyroidism associated with total thyroidectomy; however, the risk of recurrent hyperthyroidism increases in proportion to the amount of residual thyroid tissue remaining.[119,124,125] Recurrent thyrotoxicosis following subtotal thyroidectomy should be treated with RAI because the incidence of surgical complications increases with a second surgery.

Surgical complication rates are low when the procedure is performed by an experienced, competent surgeon and when the patient is adequately prepared for surgery. The disadvantages of surgery are expense, hospitalization, hypothyroidism, the small risk of postoperative complications, and the patient's fear of surgery (see Question 40).[119,124,125]

Radioactive Iodine

RAI is the preferred treatment for (1) debilitated, cardiac, or older patients who are poor surgical candidates; (2) patients who fail to respond to drug therapy or who experience adverse drug reactions; and (3) patients who develop recurrent hyperthyroidism after surgery.[107,119–121,123]

Pregnancy is an absolute contraindication to RAI therapy. The use of RAI also has been restricted to adults over an arbitrary age of 20 to 35 years because it was feared that RAI could result in genetic damage or neoplasia. However, after >50 years of clinical experience with RAI, it generally is accepted as a safe and effective treatment.[121,123] There is no reported evidence of genetic damage after ^{131}I ingestion and the dose of radiation to the gonads is <3 rads, which is comparable to other radiographic diagnostic tests (e.g., barium enemas).[126] The incidence of leukemia or malignancy is no higher in recipients of ^{131}I than in thyrotoxic patients treated with drugs or surgery.[123]

Radioactive iodine is painless, effective, economical, and quick, but fear of radiation and the high incidence of hypothyroidism may deter its use. RAI could be used safely in this nonpregnant young patient. However, C.R.'s prior use of iodides has diluted her total iodide pools. Thus, it will be impossible to achieve therapeutic thyroid concentrations of RAI for as long as 3 to 6 months.

Iodinated Contrast Media

The radiographic iodinated contrast agents, oral iopanoic acid (Telepaque), sodium ipodate (Oragrafin), sodium tyropanoate (Biopaque), and diatrizoate sodium (Hypaque), are effective short-term antithyroid agents.[127] These iodinated agents inhibit the 5'monodeiodinase enzyme responsible for the pituitary and peripheral conversion of T_4 to T_3. They also inhibit thyroid hormone secretion directly or indirectly because of the iodine content. Each gram of the iodinated contrast agents contains 600 to 650 mg iodine. The onset of therapeutic effect is more rapid than that of the thioamides. Ipodate is the agent most commonly used, but its recent unavailability may increase the use of less well-studied iodinated agents. After administration of 0.5 to 1 g/day, a rapid decline in T_3 concentrations by 58% and T_4 levels by 20% occurred within 24 hours; the agent was more effective than 600 mg PTU, which decreases T_3 levels by only 23%.[128] Significant clinical improvement and maximal reductions of hormone levels were evident within 3 to 7 days. Ipodate and other contrast media are useful adjuncts to thioamides in the early treatment of severe hyperthyroidism. However, long-term use is not reasonable because the antithyroid effects are transient. Serum T_3 levels can return to baseline or hyperthyroid levels within 1 month despite continued administration; subsequent response to thioamides also might be impaired.[127–131] Thus, it is reasonable to consider these agents in severely thyrotoxic or storm patients who are allergic to thioamides and as part of a preoperative regimen. When used as sole therapy, loss of efficacy occurs after 2 to 12 weeks.[127–131] Iodinated contrast media also have been effective in the management of amiodarone-induced thyrotoxicosis (see Question 54).[131,132]

Treatment With Thioamides

Propylthiouracil Versus Methimazole

32. C.R. is started on PTU 200 mg Q 8 hr after a baseline FT_4I and TSH level have been obtained. Three weeks later, she angrily complains that her symptoms are worse and that the medication is not working; however, she reluctantly admits missing doses because of difficulty swallowing, nausea, vomiting, diarrhea, fatigue, a cough, and a sore throat. What are the advantages of using either PTU or methimazole in the treatment of hyperthyroidism?

Both thioamides are effective in treating hyperthyroidism. The antithyroid effectiveness of the thioamides primarily depends on their ability to block the organification of iodines, thereby inhibiting thyroid hormone synthesis.[121,122] Thyroid autoantibody synthesis also may be suppressed. In most hyperthyroid situations, methimazole should be considered the drug of choice rather than PTU because patient compliance and ease of administration are improved.

DOSING AND ADMINISTRATION

Methimazole is effective when administered initially as a single dose compared with the multiple-dose regimen required with PTU to achieve a euthyroid state.[121,122] Although a single-dose regimen of PTU has been tried acutely, it is most effective when given in divided doses (see Question 41). Compared to PTU, methimazole also is less expensive, requires daily ingestion of fewer numbers of tablets, and is not associated with a bitter tablet taste. However, PTU is preferred over methimazole in thyroid storm because, unlike methimazole, it also blocks the peripheral conversion of T_4 to T_3. Within 24 to 48 hours after PTU administration, a 25% to 40% reduction in peripheral T_3 production is seen, which contributes to PTU's therapeutic effectiveness. A significantly greater fall in T_3 concentration and the $T_3:T_4$ ratio can be demonstrated in hyperthyroid patients treated acutely with PTU and iodine than with methimazole and iodides. Lastly, PTU might be preferred over methimazole in pregnant or breast-feeding patients (see Question 44).

33. Why was the thioamide therapy ineffective in C.R.? Was the dose of PTU appropriate?

The inadequate response in C.R. suggests poor adherence to the thioamide dosing regimen or a delayed response caused by prior iodide loading of the gland.

The onset of action of the thioamides is slow because they block the synthesis rather than the release of thyroid hormone. Therefore, hormone secretion will continue until the glandular stores of hormone are depleted. If adequate doses were given, some improvement of clinical symptoms should be noted after 2 or 3 weeks.[122]

The dosage of PTU is appropriate. Thioamide dosing consists of two phases: initial therapy to achieve euthyroidism, and maintenance therapy to achieve remission. Initially, high blocking dosages of PTU (400 to 800 mg/day, depending on the severity of the toxicosis) should be given in three or four divided doses, as in C.R.[121,122] Rarely, dosages of 1,200 mg/day of PTU or its equivalent may be required in patients with severe disease or storm. Equipotent doses of methimazole (which is 10 times more potent than PTU on a mg-per-mg basis) also can be used. However, it usually is unnecessary to use >40 mg/day of methimazole to restore a euthyroid state.[119,121,122,133] Toxicity also is less common (see Questions 38 and 39). True resistance to thioamides is rare; thus, most cases of unresponsiveness are caused by poor patient compliance, as in C.R.

C.R.'s adherence also is hindered by the frequency of PTU administration. The serum half-life of PTU is short (1.5 hours), but it is the intrathyroidal drug concentrations that should determine the dosing intervals because they are most clearly related to the drug's antithyroid effects[122] (see Question 41). PTU must be dosed every 6 to 8 hours initially, or as frequently as every 4 hours in cases of severe hyperthyroidism and thyroid storm. In contrast, methimazole has a serum half-life of 6 to 8 hours, remains in the thyroid for 20 hours, and has a duration of activity of up to 40 hours.[122,134]

If C.R. is taking her PTU as directed, then an increase in the PTU dosage to 200 mg Q 6 hr is reasonable. However, noncompliance often is difficult to ascertain and is more likely when multiple daily doses are required. The best option for C.R. is to change to 30 to 40 mg of methimazole, given once daily to improve compliance, or divided into two doses to decrease GI distress. After methimazole is given for 4 to 6 weeks or until euthyroidism is achieved, the daily dosage can be reduced gradually by 25% to 30% monthly to a dosage that maintains euthyroidism, usually 5 to 10 mg/day of methimazole or 50 to 150 mg/day of PTU. If C.R. remains hyperthyroid despite adequate doses of thioamides, then the most likely reason is nonadherence.

MONITORING THERAPY

34. What additional objective baseline data should be obtained to monitor both the efficacy and toxicity of thioamides?

Before thioamides are administered, a baseline FT_4 and TSH should be obtained. A baseline white blood cell (WBC) count with differential also can help differentiate the leukopenia associated with hyperthyroidism from drug-induced leukopenia and/or agranulocytosis (see Question 39). Baseline liver function tests can assist in the evaluation of thioamide-induced hepatotoxicity (see Question 38). A repeat FT_4 and TSH should be obtained after 4 to 6 weeks on therapy and 4 to 6 weeks after any change in the dosing regimen. Once the patient is euthyroid on maintenance dosages, thyroid function tests can be obtained every 3 to 6 months.

DURATION OF THERAPY

35. How long should C.R. be continued on thioamide treatment?

Traditionally, thioamide therapy is continued for 1 to 2 years despite the lack of data regarding the optimal treatment period.[121,122] The goal of treatment is to control the symptoms of Graves' disease until spontaneous remission occurs. Graves' disease remits spontaneously in about 25% to 30% of patients.[135] Because it is unknown when or if remission will occur, it is understandable why the optimal duration of therapy is unclear. Short-term therapy (i.e., <6 months) has been advocated to save time and money and improve compliance since earlier studies suggested remission rates comparable to a longer course of therapy. However, short-term therapy is not recommended because longer follow-ups of patients receiving short-term therapy have noted remission rates comparable to those observed with spontaneous remission.[119,122]

Most data support a longer course of treatment of 12 to 18 months to achieve remission rates of approximately 60%.[119,136,137] Two prospective randomized trials found that extending treatment from 6 to 18 months was beneficial but that 42 months of therapy was not significantly better than 18 months.[136,137] However, one retrospective study of patients treated for >12 months observed remission rates of only 17.5%.[139] These conflicting results underscore the fact that determining the optimal treatment period is confounded by the large variability that exists with regard to spontaneous remission. Nevertheless, treatment periods of 1 to 2 years are justifiable in compliant patients. Therapy can be reinstituted if hyperthyroidism reappears shortly after therapy is discontinued. Thioamides also can be continued indefinitely if there are no side effects and treatment with either radioactive iodine or surgery is not desired. In C.R., this goal might not be achievable, given her history of noncompliance.

Precautions

36. Can thioamide therapy affect any of C.R.'s pre-existing medical conditions?

Thyrotoxicosis can activate or intensify diabetes, primarily by increasing the basal hepatic glucose production and the metabolism of insulin.[140] Therefore, effective therapy with thioamides may restore control of C.R.'s diabetes.

C.R.'s arthritis should not be affected by the PTU, although both PTU and methimazole are associated with the development of lupus erythematosus (LE), lupus-like syndromes, and vasculitis.[122,141] These adverse drug reactions are rare; the incidence is <0.1%. Lupus-like syndromes include skin ulcers, splenomegaly, migratory polyarthritis, pleuritis and pericarditis, periarteritis, and renal abnormalities. Serologic abnormalities also may occur with these connective tissue disorders and include hyperglobulinemia, positive LE preparations, and positive antinuclear antibodies. Recovery occurs with adequate steroid therapy and withdrawal of the thioamides. Because cross-reaction between methimazole and PTU is likely to occur, patients exhibiting these reactions should be treated with surgery or RAI. C.R.'s treatment should be monitored with this lupus-like adverse effect in mind, but the occurrence of this syndrome is so uncommon that a trouble-free course of therapy can be anticipated.

Adjunctive Therapy

37. What adjunctive therapy might help alleviate some of C.R.'s symptoms while awaiting the onset of thioamide's effects?

Iodides (see Question 30), β-adrenergic blocking agents without intrinsic sympathomimetic activity, or calcium channel blockers can be used acutely to ameliorate some of C.R.'s symptoms.[121,142] Iodinated contrast media (e.g., ipodate, iopanoic acid) also can be used (see Question 31). Because iodides previously were ineffective in C.R., a β-blocker should be tried.

β-Adrenergic blocking agents rapidly decrease the nervousness, palpitations, fatigue, weight loss, diaphoresis, heat intolerance, and tremor associated with thyrotoxicosis, probably because many of the signs and symptoms mimic sympathetic overactivity.[90,142] An increase in the number of β-adrenergic receptors rather than an elevation in catecholamine levels probably is responsible for this overactivity. Because the underlying disease process and thyroid hormone levels are not affected significantly by β-blockers, patients generally remain mildly symptomatic and fail to gain weight. For this reason, they should not be used as the sole treatment for thyrotoxicosis.

All β-blockers without intrinsic sympathetic activity (e.g., atenolol, metoprolol, propranolol) are effective in alleviating the hyperthyroid symptoms, but propranolol (Inderal) is the only β-blocker that inhibits peripheral conversion of T_4 to T_3.[142] Thyroid function tests generally are not affected except for a mild decrease in the T_3 level.

In summary, β-blockers are (1) effective adjuncts in the management of thyroid storm; (2) useful to prepare patients for surgery; and (3) useful in the short-term management of thyrotoxicosis during pregnancy.[121,124,142] Surprisingly, propranolol also improves many of the neuromuscular manifestations of hyperthyroidism, including thyrotoxic periodic paralysis.

Diltiazem or verapamil are effective alternatives when β-blockers are contraindicated.[143] Diltiazem 120 mg three or four times a day can be tried. The dihydropyridine calcium channel blockers are unlikely to be effective.

Because of C.R.'s history of diabetes, the effects of β-adrenergic blocking drugs in patients with diabetes must be considered (see Chapter 50, Diabetes Mellitus). If β-blockers are instituted, a cardioselective β-blocker would be a better choice. The appropriate dosage should be based on clinical and objective improvement of hyperthyroid symptoms, such as a reduction in heart rate. Metoprolol 25 to 50 mg BID can be started initially and the dosage titrated to maintain the heart rate at <90 beats/min. Otherwise, iodinated contrast media, diltiazem, or a retrial of iodides is warranted.

Adverse Effects

38. A pruritic area over the pretibial aspects of both legs as well as several maculopapular erythematous patches and abdominal tenderness were noticed during C.R.'s physical examination. Do these reactions require the discontinuation of her PTU?

THIOAMIDE RASH

Although C.R. may be experiencing a drug rash from PTU, pretibial myxedema or the dermopathy of Graves' disease also may be possibilities because of the location of the pruritic area. About 4% of patients with Graves' disease who exhibit infiltrative exophthalmos also have dermatologic changes. The skin is thickened, erythematous, and nonpitting because of mucopolysaccharide infiltration and accentuation of hair follicles. Pruritus or pain may be present. Treatment includes topical corticosteroids, control of the Graves' disease, and reassurance.

Both PTU and methimazole can produce a maculopapular pruritic rash in 5% to 6% of treated patients.[119,121,122] The rash can occur at any time but is more common early in therapy. If the rash is mild, drug therapy can be continued while the patient's symptoms are treated with an antihistamine and a topical steroid; such rashes generally subside spontaneously. Alternatively, another thioamide can be substituted because cross-sensitivity to this side effect is uncommon. If the rash is urticarial or is associated with other systemic manifestations of a drug reaction (e.g., fever, arthralgias), thioamides should be stopped and nondrug treatment considered.

HEPATITIS

C.R.'s symptoms of nausea, vomiting, diarrhea, fatigue, and abdominal tenderness require further evaluation. Her symptoms could be consistent with mild GI side effects from her PTU therapy or with impending thyroid storm from noncompliance (see Question 50). Taking the PTU after meals or changing to methimazole could improve medication intolerance and improve compliance. However, the possibility of drug-induced hepatitis should be considered. Typically, PTU-induced hepatotoxicity is hepatocellular in nature, but cholestasis, hepatic necrosis, and fulminant hepatic failures have been reported.[112,113,119] Transient elevations in transaminases occur in approximately 30% of asymptomatic patients within the first 2 months of PTU therapy and do not require drug discontinuation.[112] The liver enzymes usually normalize within 3 months of reducing the PTU to maintenance dosages despite drug continuation. However, PTU should be stopped immediately in patients with clinical symptoms of hepatitis to ensure complete recovery. The mechanism of PTU-induced hepatotoxicity appears to be autoimmune, because circulating autoantibodies and *in vitro* peripheral lymphocyte sensitization to PTU have been detected.[113] Overt hepatitis typically occurs during the first 2 months of PTU therapy and is not dose related. In contrast, methimazole typically produces a cholestatic jaundice picture and might be more common in older patients and in those receiving higher dosages (i.e., >40 mg/day).[113] In patients with thioamide-induced hepatitis, changing to the alternative thioamide is not recommended because fatalities have been reported upon rechallenge. In such patients, either radioactive therapy or surgery should be used.

The thyroid function tests, transaminases, and bilirubin should be checked in C.R. and the PTU stopped until these results are available. Routine monitoring of liver function tests is not recommended because patients can be asymptomatic. However, routine monitoring might be indicated in patients with a history of liver disease and risk factors for hepatitis (e.g., alcohol use). All patients receiving thioamides should be questioned closely during the first 2 months of therapy for symptoms of hepatitis, and hepatic function tests should be obtained if appropriate.

AGRANULOCYTOSIS

39. **Assess C.R.'s complaints of sore throat and cough.**

C.R.'s complaints should not be dismissed casually because they might indicate PTU-induced agranulocytosis.

Agranulocytosis (<500/mm³ of neutrophils) is the most severe adverse hematologic reaction associated with the thioamides and should be considered strongly in C.R.[119,122,144] In contrast, drug-induced leukopenia usually is transient, is not associated with impending agranulocytosis, and is not an indication to discontinue thioamide therapy. An accurate history should be obtained from C.R. The clinician should be alert particularly for a temperature of 101°F for 2 or more days, malaise, or other flu-like findings that appeared temporally with her sore throat. If subjective or objective data are consistent with agranulocytosis, the PTU should be discontinued immediately until the results of a repeat WBC count with a differential are obtained. Traditionally, routine serial determinations of WBC counts are not recommended for monitoring the development of agranulocytosis because the onset is so abrupt. Instead, patients should be instructed to immediately report rash, fever, sore throat, or any flu-like symptoms. However, one study suggested that weekly monitoring of the WBC count with a differential during the first 3 months of antithyroid therapy might identify asymptomatic patients with agranulocytosis before infection occurs.[144]

The prevalence of agranulocytosis is about 0.5% but ranges from 0.5% to 6%.[119,122,144] The risk factors for agranulocytosis are unknown. There is no predilection for either gender, and the reaction may be idiosyncratic or dose related. Some reports suggest that patients >40 years of age or those taking high dosages of methimazole (e.g., >40 mg/day) might be more susceptible than those on any dosage of PTU. Although controversial, patients receiving low dosages of methimazole (e.g., <40 mg/day) might be at less risk than those receiving high or conventional dosages of PTU.[119,122,144]

Agranulocytosis typically develops within the first 3 months of treatment, although it can occur at any time and as late as 12 months after starting thioamide therapy.[122] A delayed reaction is more common with methimazole therapy than with PTU. In 55 patients who developed agranulocytosis while taking thioamides, the duration of PTU therapy (17.7 ± 9.7 days) was significantly shorter than for methimazole therapy (36.9 ± 14.5 days).[144] The mechanism of thioamide-induced agranulocytosis is unknown. Both allergic-type (idiosyncratic) and toxic-type (dose-related) reactions have been suggested. An autoimmune reaction with circulating antineutrophil antibodies and lymphocyte sensitization to antithyroid drugs has been demonstrated.[145] Death usually results from overwhelming infection.

If agranulocytosis is diagnosed, the drug should be discontinued, the patient monitored for signs of infection, and antibiotics instituted if necessary. Data suggest that granulocyte colony-stimulating factor might help shorten the recovery period.[122,146] If the patient recovers, granulocytes begin to reappear in the periphery within a few days to 3 weeks; a normal granulocyte count occurs shortly thereafter.[144,146]

Although some cases of granulocytopenia have resolved with substitution or continuation of thioamides, the risks of drug rechallenge clearly outweigh the benefits, and other treatments should be instituted. Changing to an alternative thioamide also should be avoided because little is known regarding the cross-sensitivity between these agents.[122]

In summary, all patients receiving thioamide therapy should be well educated regarding the signs and symptoms of agranulocytosis. If these symptoms develop, they should be advised to contact their physician or pharmacist. If they cannot reach their own physician, patients should inform the emergency physician that they are taking thioamides, and a WBC count with differential should be obtained. Routine monitoring of a WBC and differential is not recommended until further studies justify that it is indicated and cost effective.

Preoperative Preparation

40. **C.R.'s PTU is discontinued because she developed agranulocytosis and hepatitis, and surgery is scheduled when her granulocyte level returns to normal. What thyroid preparation is needed for C.R. before thyroidectomy? What postoperative complications are associated with thyroidectomy?**

C.R. should be in a euthyroid state at the time of surgery to avoid precipitation of thyroid storm and morbidity. Generally, iodides (see Question 30), thioamides, or propranolol can be used.[121,122,124,142] The combination of iodides and propranolol may be more effective than either used alone. Propranolol used alone has been associated with thyroid crisis postoperatively and may be less effective than iodides in decreasing gland friability and vascularity.[142]

Iodinated contrast media (e.g., ipodate) can be used instead of iodides because iodides are released with its administration.[127] Several reports indicate that ipodate in combination with β-bockers and steroids provides rapid (5 days) and effective preoperative preparation. In a comparison of ipodate and Lugol's solution in 46 preoperative patients, those receiving ipodate required less preparation time and bled less during surgery (see Question 30).[147]

Because C.R. received only 1 week of thioamide therapy, it is likely that her gland still contains large stores of hormone; therefore, pretreatment is necessary.

In addition to the risks of anesthesia and surgery, postoperative complications include hypoparathyroidism, adhesions, laryngeal nerve damage, bleeding, infection, and poor wound healing. However, the surgery can be uneventful if it is performed by experienced surgeons.[124,125] Complications are also higher if a total rather than a subtotal thyroidectomy is performed, but there is a lower risk of recurrent hyperthyroidism.[119,124,125] Development of hypothyroidism, especially subclinical hypothyroidism, is greatest during the first year after surgery, with an insidious rise in incidence over the next 10 years. The incidence of permanent hypothyroidism varies from 6% to 75% and is related inversely to the amount of remnant tissue left behind.[119,124,125] Thyroid function tests should be monitored annually after surgery.

Single Daily Dosing

41. **J.R., a 23-year-old man newly diagnosed with Graves' disease, remains hyperthyroid after 6 weeks of PTU 200 mg TID. He admits he has trouble remembering to take it three times a day and desires a more simplified regimen. Could J.R. be placed on a single daily dose of PTU?**

A single daily dose of PTU should not be used as initial therapy because euthyroidism is achieved in only 39% to 68% of hyperthyroid patients using this approach.[119,122,148] However, once euthyroidism occurs, single daily doses of PTU are effective. In contrast, several clinical studies have documented that a single daily dose of methimazole is as effective as multiple daily doses in >90% of treated patients.[119,121,122] Although a low dosage of methimazole (10 to 15 mg QD) is effective in producing euthyroidism and produces fewer side effects than higher dosages, 30 to 40 mg/day of methimazole (or 40 mg of carbimazole) is recommended as the initial dosage because more patients achieve euthyroidism in 6 weeks than on the low-dosage regimen.[119,122,133]

Methimazole is the preferred agent for once-a-day dosing because of its longer intrathyroidal duration of action (40 hours).[122,134] However, as previously noted, PTU is preferable in toxic patients (i.e., thyroid storm) because it acts more rapidly. Despite its short plasma half-life of 4 to 6 hours, a single 30-mg dose of methimazole has a duration of action of 40 hours.[134] The duration of action of PTU is unknown, but it is shorter than methimazole. Apparently, the duration of action of the antithyroid agents correlates best with the size of the dose and the intrathyroidal concentration of the drug.

J.R. should be changed to 30 to 40 mg of methimazole given once daily. Thyroid function tests should be obtained after 4 to 6 weeks and the dosage reduced as necessary to maintain euthyroidism. An effective single daily dose regimen of methimazole should increase patient acceptance and adherence.

Remission and Addition of Thyroxine

42. **B.D., a 30-year-old woman, has been maintained on PTU 100 mg QD for >2 years. Her PTU has been discontinued twice in the past, and each time her hyperthyroidism recurred. She refuses either surgery or RAI therapy. Although she is clinically euthyroid on the PTU, her gland is larger than normal and has never decreased with therapy. Recent laboratory tests showed an FT$_4$ of 1.0 ng/dL (normal, 0.7 to 1.9) and a TSH level of 4.5 IU/mL (normal, 0.5 to 4.7). Levothyroxine 0.1 mg/day was initiated. Why was thyroxine added to B.D.'s PTU therapy?**

[SI units: FT$_4$, 14 pmol/L (normal, 9 to 24); TSH, 4.5 mIU/L (normal, 0.5 to 4.7)]

The addition of thyroxine to B.D.'s regimen might be helpful for several reasons. Thyroid supplements have been used with high-dose blocking regimens of thioamides to prevent hypothyroidism.[126] In this case, thyroxine might have been added to help decrease the size of the goiter caused by TSH stimulation. Stimulation of TSH secretion occurs if PTU's suppression of hormone synthesis is excessive. The normal FT$_4$ is of no value in supporting this assumption. However, the high normal TSH level suggests that TSH stimulation is contributing to the size of her goiter. The easiest solution to this problem is to decrease the maintenance dose of PTU; in patients for whom titration of the proper dose of PTU is difficult, the combination of T$_4$ and PTU is reasonable. Levothyroxine should be added in a dosage that maintains euthyroidism, normalizes the TSH level, and prevents further gland enlargement (e.g., 50 to 100 μg).

A major reason for adding thyroxine to her PTU therapy is to increase her chance of remission once thioamides are discontinued. Purportedly, TSH suppression with thyroxine decreases antigen release from the gland and thereby decreases TSH receptor antibody titers. Low or absent TSH receptor antibody titers are correlated with a higher likelihood of remission (see Question 43). In an encouraging study, the combination of levothyroxine and maintenance doses of thioamides given for 1 year, followed by an additional year of levothyroxine alone, significantly decreased the risk of relapse once thioamides were discontinued.[149] After patients were made euthyroid on 30 mg of methimazole for 6 months, the daily addition of 100 μg of thyroxine to 10 mg of methimazole resulted in a significant reduction in TSH receptor antibody titers compared with those who received methimazole alone. The thyroxine-treated patients demonstrated lower TSH levels and a lower rate of recurrence (1.7%) at 3 years after all therapy was discontinued than those receiving methimazole alone (recurrence rate, 34.7%). Unfortunately, several prospective studies evaluating the addition of thyroxine to thioamides have not validated these initial favorable results.[119,150–152] Support for this therapeutic approach has waned, and the addition of thyroxine to existing thioamide therapy is not recommended for this purpose.

43. **What subjective or objective data in B.D. would influence her remission rate and justify a longer course of thioamide therapy?**

Long-term remission rates achieved with the thioamides are disappointing. Remission rates within 6 years after discontinuing therapy average 50% (range, 14% to 75%),[119,122,136,138,150–152] although relapse rates are as high as 80%. The rate of permanent remission usually is <25% if the follow-up period is long enough.[119,138] Why some patients remain in remission while others relapse once thioamides are discontinued is unclear, although patients who remain euthyroid for >10 to 15 years after discontinuing therapy probably do so because of disease progression to Hashimoto's thyroiditis rather than as a direct result of treatment.[135] In other words, the natural course of Graves' hyperthyroidism might be eventual hypothyroidism regardless of the treatment modality used. Several factors have a limited role in predicting relapse and remission and have been used to guide therapy.

A longer duration of thioamide treatment (see Question 35) improved the remission rate by changing the basic underlying abnormality of Graves' disease.[119,122,135,136,138] Numerous studies show that titers of antithyroid receptor (TRAb) and antimicrosomal antibodies fall during therapy with the thioamides but are unchanged during therapy with placebo or β-blockers.[122,133,138] Patients with low or undetectable TRAb titers at the end of 12 to 24 months of thioamide therapy had a 45% chance of remission compared to a <10% chance of remission for those with higher TRAb titers within 1 to 5 years after completing therapy.[125,138,149,152,153] The best response was obtained in those with smaller goiters, those with less severe disease, and nonsmokers. A higher dosage of thioamides does not appear to improve the remission rate but causes a higher incidence of toxicity, including agranulocytosis, arthralgias, dermatitis, gastritis, and hepatotoxicity.[138]

Some clinical features might be predictive of a higher rate of remission and may help clinicians identify patients who deserve a longer trial of drug treatment before changing to RAI or surgery. These clinical features include smaller goiter, mild symptoms of short duration, a reduction in goiter size during treatment, nonsmokers, absence of ophthalmopathy, and undetectable or low TRAb levels.[122,138,153] Smokers should be advised to discontinue smoking to increase the chance of remission.

B.D.'s large goiter reduces her chance of remission with longer therapy. Thyroxine is unlikely to be effective and should not be considered (see Question 42). Although thioamide therapy can be continued indefinitely if well tolerated, surgery or radioactive iodine therapy seriously should be considered for B.D., who already has received PTU for >2 years. Alternative therapy is especially crucial if she plans to become pregnant within the next few years (see Question 44).

In Pregnancy

44. **N.N., a 32-year-old woman who is 3 months pregnant, is referred for management of her Graves' disease. What are the therapeutic ramifications of managing thyrotoxicosis during pregnancy?**

Hyperthyroidism develops in 0.02% to 1.4% of pregnant women and often precedes conception.[154] Symptoms of thyrotoxicosis typically are ameliorated during the second and third trimesters and exacerbated early in the postpartum period. Treatment is crucial to prevent damage to the fetus and to maintain the pregnancy. Radioactive iodine, chronic iodide therapy, and iodine-containing compounds are contraindicated during pregnancy because these will cross the placenta to produce fetal goiter and athyreosis.[118,154–156] As little as 12 mg/day of iodide has produced neonatal goiter and death. The long-term use of propranolol also should be avoided because it is associated with fetal respiratory depression, a small placenta, intrauterine growth retardation, impaired response to anoxia, and postnatal bradycardia and hypoglycemia.[154,155] However, if rapid control of hyperthyroidism is required, short-term use (<1 week) of propranolol or the iodides is safe.[154–156]

Either surgery or thioamide is the treatment of choice for hyperthyroidism in the pregnant patient. Surgery is safe during the second trimester with adequate preoperative preparation. During both other trimesters, thioamides are preferred because surgery can precipitate spontaneous abortion. Previously, PTU was considered the thioamide of choice because its higher protein binding minimized placental crossing. There were also anecdotal reports of methimazole-induced congenital scalp defects (e.g., aplasia cutis).[122,154,155,156,157] However, newer data show that thyroid hormone concentrations in fetal umbilical cord blood samples from mothers receiving either PTU or methimazole were not significantly different.[158] Furthermore, the risks of reversible aplasia cutis were not greater in women receiving methimazole (e.g., 2.7%) compared to PTU (e.g., 3.0%) or hyperthyroid controls (e.g., 6.0%)[157,159,160] Therefore, either PTU or methimazole can be safely used in pregnancy. (See Chapter 47, Teratogenicity and Drugs in Breast Milk.) Methimazole may be preferred because its longer half-life allows once-daily dosing.

Fetal hypothyroidism and goiter can develop when large doses of either thioamide are administered to the mother, even if the mother is still hyperthyroid.[154,155] Therefore, to avoid goiter and suppression of the fetal thyroid gland, which begins to function at about 12 to 14 weeks of gestation, any thioamide should be prescribed in the lowest effective doses that will maintain the mother's T_4 level in the upper ranges of normal. Control of maternal hyperthyroidism increases the risk of fetal hypothyroidism. The patient is initiated on maximum dosages of PTU (e.g., 450 mg/day in three divided doses) or methimazole (e.g., 20 to 30 mg given once daily) until control is achieved, and then the dosage is tapered to 50 to 150 mg/day of PTU or 5 to 15 mg/day of methimazole for the remainder of the pregnancy. Some patients can discontinue thioamides in the second half of pregnancy.[154] Such modest doses of thioamides provide satisfactory control of maternal hyperthyroidism and should not cause clinically evident thyroid dysfunction in the neonate. Patients requiring more than the maximum recommended thioamide dosages for control may need to consider the possibility of surgery in the second trimester.

Nevertheless, a small but significant reduction in neonatal serum thyroxine occurs even when small (100 to 200 mg) doses of PTU are administered during pregnancy to mothers with Graves' disease.[154,155,161] It is unclear whether this mild, transient reduction in serum thyroxine causes long-term impairment of mental development or is otherwise detrimental to the newborn. To date, no significant differences in intellectual development have been noted between children exposed to PTU or methimazole *in utero* and their unexposed siblings.[162–164] However, children exposed *in utero* to >300 mg/day of PTU had lower IQs.[162,163]

Although transient fetal or neonatal hypothyroidism does not appear to be a major threat to the baby, it is advisable to maintain the mother in a mildly hyperthyroid state.[154,155] Mild maternal hyperthyroidism seems to be well tolerated, but maternal hypothyroidism is poorly tolerated by both the mother and fetus (see Question 13). Laboratory indices should be maintained in the upper ranges of normal because normal thyroid function tests are suggestive of hypothyroidism during pregnancy (high TBG and TBPA levels).

It is not rational to add thyroid hormone to the mother's regimen to prevent fetal goiter or hypothyroidism because thyroid hormones do not reach the fetal circulation. Thyroid supplementation only complicates the treatment of maternal hyperthyroidism by increasing thioamide requirements, which can further compromise fetal thyroid hormone production.[154] If the mother has not been thyrotoxic throughout pregnancy, a normal infant can be expected. All pregnant patients with a history of, or active, autoimmune thyroid disease (i.e., Graves', Hashimoto's) should be screened during pregnancy for TRAb to evaluate the risk of neonatal hyperthyroidism.[154] Lastly, PTU is the drug of choice in the lactating mother.[122,154,155] Methimazole, propranolol, and iodides are secreted in breast milk and should be avoided[122,154] (see Chapter 47).

Treatment With RAI

Pretreatment

45. B.J., a 35-year-old woman, has newly diagnosed Graves' disease complicated by CHF and angina. After a few days of treatment with PTU 200 mg TID and Lugol's solution, 5 drops/day, B.J. received RAI therapy. Six months later, she is still symptomatic. Evaluate the influence of B.J.'s pretreatment therapy on the efficacy of her RAI therapy.

Patients with severe hyperthyroidism, patients with hyperthyroidism and cardiac disease, and those who are debilitated or older should receive antithyroid treatment before RAI therapy. The goal of pretreatment is to deplete stored thyroid hormone. This minimizes post-RAI hyperthyroidism (which oc-

curs during the first 10 days after ^{131}I administration) and thyroid storm, which is caused by leakage of hormones from the damaged thyroid gland.[121–123] Other patients with hyperthyroidism can be treated safely with RAI without pretherapy.

Lugol's solution or other iodides should not be given before RAI because iodides decrease the effectiveness of this therapy by decreasing the gland's uptake of RAI. This effect of iodides persists for several weeks. Iodides can be used for 1 to 7 days after RAI treatment if they are needed to rapidly control symptoms of hyperthyroidism.[123]

The thioamides can be used before RAI therapy to achieve a euthyroid state, but pretreatment with thioamides may lower the cure rate and increase the need for subsequent doses of RAI.[119,123,165–168] Purportedly, higher RAI failure rates occur with PTU than with methimazole due to the presence of the radioprotective sulfhydryl group in PTU.[165–168] To facilitate optimal uptake and retention of ^{131}I by the gland, PTU should be stopped at least 7 days before and methimazole at least 4 days before RAI administration.[119,165,166,168] If necessary, thioamides can be restarted after RAI administration without impairing its efficacy. β-Adrenergic blocking agents can be used before, during, and after RAI therapy without interfering with its uptake.

B.J. remains symptomatic because pretreatment with the PTU and iodides decreased the effectiveness of RAI therapy. Propranolol should be given to B.J. before RAI therapy to ameliorate symptoms of hyperthyroidism because she has received only a short course of thioamide. Iodides might be preferable to propranolol following RAI therapy if B.J.'s CHF worsens. For subsequent RAI doses, pretreatment with methimazole may be preferable to PTU since it can be stopped a few days prior to RAI therapy, thereby causing a shorter duration of hyperthyroidism.

Onset of Effects

46. B.J. still is symptomatic 2 weeks after a second dose of RAI. When can she expect to experience the therapeutic effects of RAI therapy?

Although some benefits from RAI therapy are evident within 1 month, a period of 8 to 12 weeks generally is required for maximal effects.[123] Euthyroidism or, more commonly, hypothyroidism occurs in approximately 80% to 90% of patients treated with a single nonablative dose of RAI; the remaining 10% to 20% become euthyroid or hypothyroid after two or more doses. This slow onset is a disadvantage, but symptomatic control can be obtained quickly by administration of a β-adrenergic blocking agent, iodinated contrast media, or iodides starting 1 to 14 days after the ^{131}I dose.[121,123,142] Iodides are less preferable if a second dose of RAI is necessary. Thioamides also can be given, although their therapeutic effects are delayed for 3 to 4 weeks.

At least 3 months should elapse before a second radioactive dose of iodide is administered, and most recommend waiting 6 months before repeating ^{131}I administration, unless the patient remains severely thyrotoxic. It is inadvisable to give a second dose before the major effects of the first dose have become apparent. Although the use of iodides before RAI in B.J. may have decreased the amount of ^{131}I retained by her thyroid, it still is advisable to wait at least 3 months before a second dose is given.

Iatrogenic Hypothyroidism

47. S.D., a 54-year-old woman, returns to the thyroid clinic after being lost to follow-up for 6 months. She initially received RAI 3 years ago but required a repeat dose of RAI 1 year ago for recurrence of hyperthyroidism. She currently has no other medical problems and is not taking any medications. She is a mildly obese, puffy-faced woman wearing several layers of clothing. She complains of fatigue and lack of energy. Her reflexes are delayed and her skin is cool and dry. What is a likely explanation for her symptoms?

S.D.'s clinical presentation and history are compatible with hypothyroidism secondary to RAI therapy. An FT_4 and a TSH level would confirm this diagnosis. Iatrogenic hypothyroidism is the major complication of ^{131}I therapy, although transient hypothyroidism may be seen in the first 3 to 6 weeks after RAI therapy.[123] The incidence of iatrogenic myxedema often is reported as 7% to 8%, but it increases at a constant rate of 2.5% per year.[123] The reported prevalence of this complication ranges from 26% to 70% after 1 to 14 years.[123,165]

The best predictor of eventual hypothyroidism is the dose of ^{131}I administered. Prevention of iatrogenic hypothyroidism is directed toward calculation of a dose that will produce neither recurrent hyperthyroidism nor hypothyroidism. Unfortunately, when lower doses of ^{131}I were used to avoid hypothyroidism, the cure rate was reduced but the incidence of hypothyroidism was unaffected. Thus, the appearance of iatrogenic hypothyroidism may be inevitable with time. However, hypothyroidism is managed easily and is an acceptable therapeutic end point. Because hypothyroidism after RAI therapy is latent and often insidious, patients should be made aware of this and monitored closely at monthly intervals for subsequent hypothyroidism. Awareness of a transient hypothyroidism soon after RAI therapy should minimize the institution of unnecessary hormone replacement.

Ophthalmopathy

Clinical Presentation

48. H.R., a 50-year-old man, first developed "large eyes with stare," weakness, diaphoresis, and thyroid enlargement in 1970. He was diagnosed with Graves' disease and treated with RAI with some regression of his eye symptoms. Although he is clinically euthyroid, physical examination reveals severe bilateral conjunctival edema and injection, proptosis of the right eye, incomplete lid closure, and decreased visual acuity. He complains of photophobia, tearing, and extreme irritation, which is worse after smoking cigarettes. What is the association of H.R.'s ocular changes with Graves' disease?

H.R. presents with symptoms consistent with the infiltrative ophthalmopathy of Graves' disease.[169] The eye signs of Graves' disease are the most striking abnormality of this disorder. Rarely, ophthalmopathy can occur without any evidence of hyperthyroidism. Fortunately, severe ophthalmopathy occurs in only 3% to 5% of patients, while 25% to 50% have some eye findings. Eye disease is more severe in older patients and in men than women. Smokers often have higher levels of TRAb and more severe ophthalmopathy.[170–173] The eye involvement can occur at any time and usually is bilateral. The ocular symptoms usually subside or remain stable once the patient is euthyroid; however, some cases will progress during the euthyroid period or following treatment of the hyperthyroidism (see Question 49).

It is unknown why the eye and its muscles are attacked in Graves' disease. Histologic examination reveals lymphocytic infiltration, increased mucopolysaccharide content, fat, and water in all retrobulbar tissue. Ocular symptoms include edema, chemosis, excessive lacrimation, photophobia, corneal protrusion (proptosis), scarring, ulceration, extraocular muscle paralysis with loss of eye movements, and blindness from retinal and optic nerve damage.

Management

49. Was previous treatment of H.R.'s hyperthyroidism appropriate? How should his current ocular symptoms be managed?

The optimal treatment of hyperthyroidism and its effect on the course of ophthalmopathy remain controversial.[169] Thioamides might improve eye symptoms through an immunosuppressive mechanism of action and control of the hyperthyroidism or exert a neutral effect.[169,172] However, many clinicians believe that gland ablation with RAI or surgical removal is preferable because it removes the antigen source and prevents progression of the ophthalmopathy.[123,124,169,172] However, several studies have confirmed development or worsening of eye symptoms immediately after RAI therapy.[123,173,174] One randomized study demonstrated that the concomitant use of 0.4 to 0.5 mg/kg of prednisone begun 2 to 3 days post-RAI and continued for a total of 3 months after RAI therapy in those with any degree of ocular involvement was well tolerated and prevented further deterioration of eye symptoms.[123,173,174] Regardless of the treatment used, control of the hyperthyroidism often improves most eye findings, except for proptosis.

In H.R., prednisone 40 to 60 mg/day should have been started after his RAI treatment and continued for 2 to 3 months until the eye symptoms improved.

Because the pathophysiology of the ophthalmopathy is unclear, treatment is limited to symptomatic and empiric measures once the patient is euthyroid.[169,171,172] H.R. also should be encouraged to stop smoking to prevent progression of the ophthalmopathy.[170]

Periorbital edema and chemosis are worse in the morning after being in the horizontal position; elevating the head of the bed, treatment with diuretics, and restricting salt may be helpful. Protective glasses can relieve photophobia and external irritation. Topical corticosteroid drops are effective in decreasing local irritation, but they should be used cautiously because they increase the risk of infection. Ocular irritants such as smoke and dust should be avoided. Bothersome symptoms (e.g., dry eye, redness, tearing) caused by eyelid retraction can be ameliorated with artificial tears and lubricants.[169,172] Incomplete lid closure predisposes the patient to corneal scarring and ulceration, so lubricant eyedrops should be applied several times daily and at night to keep the bulbs moist. Taping the eyelids shut at night helps prevent drying and scarring. Lateral surgical closure of the lids (tarsorrhaphy) may be required to improve lid closure.

When the ophthalmopathy is severe and progressive, an aggressive approach is necessary. Systemic corticosteroids can produce either dramatic or marginal results in the emergency treatment of progressive exophthalmos associated with decreasing visual acuity. Prednisone at dosages of 35 to 80 mg/day often is effective, although dosages as high as 100 to 140 mg/day may be necessary.[169,172] Pain, irritation, tearing, and other subjective complaints often respond within 24 hours of administration. Therapy for about 3 months is necessary for improvement of eye muscle and optic nerve function disturbances. Initial large doses should be tapered rapidly once the desired response is obtained to minimize adverse effects. Subconjunctival and retrobulbar injections of steroids are not as effective.

X-ray therapy to the orbit also relieves congestive and inflammatory symptoms.[169,172] The combination of orbital irradiation and systemic steroids may be required to achieve maximal benefits. Plasmapheresis and immunosuppressive agents, such as cyclophosphamide, azathioprine, cyclosporine, and methotrexate, also have been used with limited success in combination with steroids.[169,172]

When the above measures and thyroid ablation fail to arrest the progression of visual loss and exophthalmos, then surgical orbital decompression should be considered.

Thyroid Storm

Clinical Presentation

50. H.L., a 48-year-old woman, is admitted to the hospital with a 3-week history of fatigue, weakness, dyspnea on exertion, SOB, palpitations, and inability to keep food and liquids down. One year before admission, she began noticing a preference for cold weather and an increase in nervousness and emotional lability. After her husband died a few days ago, she experienced increased nausea and vomiting, irritability, insomnia, tremor, and a 104°F fever, which she attributed to an upper respiratory tract infection. She denies taking any current medication. Her laboratory data obtained on admission included an FT_4 of 4.65 ng/dL (normal, 0.7 to 1.9) and an undetectable TSH level. Assess H.L.'s subjective and objective data.

[SI unit: FT_4, 60 pmol/L (normal, 9 to 24)]

The presentation is consistent with thyroid storm, a lifethreatening medical emergency that might have been precipitated by the stress associated with the death of her husband. The clinical manifestations of thyroid storm[84] include the acute onset of high fever (*sine qua non*), tachycardia, tachypnea, and involvement of the following organ systems: cardiovascular (tachycardia, pulmonary edema, hypertension, and shock), CNS (tremor, emotional lability, confusion, psychosis, apathy, stupor, and coma), and GI (diarrhea, abdominal pain, nausea and vomiting, liver enlargement, jaundice, and nonspecific elevations of bilirubin and PT). Hyperglycemia was a clinical finding in 12 of 18 episodes.

Thyroid storm develops in about 2% to 8% of hyperthyroid patients. The pathogenesis of thyroid storm is not well understood, but the condition can be described as an "exaggerated" or decompensated form of thyrotoxicosis. The term *decompensated* implies failure of body systems to adequately resist the effects of thyrotoxicosis. It is not attributed solely to the release of massive quantities of hormones, which can occur after surgery or RAI therapy. Catecholamines also play an important role; the increased quantities of thyroid hormone in conjunction with increased sympathetic and adrenal output contribute to many of the manifestations of thyroid storm. Although thyroid hormones exert an independent effect, many of the symptoms of hyperthyroidism are ameliorated by catecholamine-blocking agents such as propranolol, reserpine, and guanethidine. Calcium channel blockers also are effective.

Treatment

51. What treatment plan (including route of administration) should be initiated promptly in H.L.?

Accurate, continuous, and immediate treatment can decrease the mortality of thyroid storm significantly. Mortality rates as low as 7% and survival rates as high as 50% are reported. Treatment of thyroid storm should be directed against four major areas discussed in the following sections (Table 49-11).[84]

DECREASE IN SYNTHESIS AND RELEASE OF HORMONES
High dosages of thioamides, preferably PTU 600 to 1,200 mg/day or methimazole 60 to 120 mg/day, should be given orally in divided doses. If H.L. cannot take oral doses, a rectal formulation of PTU (better bioavailability with enema than suppository) or methimazole, which is as effective as the oral route, can be administered.[175–177] No commercial parenteral preparation is available for either drug, limiting their use by the IV route. Unfortunately, extemporaneous preparation of an IV formulation using water-soluble methimazole is not possible because sterile methimazole no longer is available from the manufacturer. Theoretically, PTU is the thioamide of choice because it acts more rapidly than methimazole by blocking the peripheral conversion of T_4 to T_3, a dominant source of the hormone.

Iodides, which rapidly block further release of intraglandular stores of thyroxine, should be given at least 1 hour after thioamide administration. Given in this way, the substrate for hormone synthesis is not increased and thioamide's therapeutic effect is not blocked. The addition of iodides (e.g., iopanoic acid 1 g Q 8 hr for 24 hours, then 500 mg BID or Lugol's solution 15 to 30 drops/day orally) to the thioamides often ameliorates symptoms within 1 day.

REVERSAL OF THE PERIPHERAL EFFECTS OF HORMONES AND CATECHOLAMINES
β-Adrenergic blocking drugs are the preferred agents to decrease the tachycardia, agitation, tremulousness, and other symptoms of excessive adrenergic stimulation seen in thyroid storm. Propranolol is the β-blocker of choice because its clinical efficacy in storm is well documented and because it inhibits the peripheral conversion of T_4 to T_3.[84,142] Furthermore, propranolol is effective in patients refractory to reserpine and guanethidine. If rapid effects are necessary, propranolol 1 mg by slow IV push can be given every 5 minutes to lower the heart rate to 90 to 110 beats/min. A 5- to 10-mg/hour IV infusion can be given to maintain the desired heart rate. Otherwise, oral propranolol 40 mg every 6 hours can be given instead. The dose can be doubled every 12 hours until a therapeutic response is obtained.

Catecholamine-depleting agents, such as reserpine and guanethidine, have been used successfully in storm, but their use has been replaced by β-blockers. Reserpine in dosages of

Table 49-11   Treatment of Thyroid Storm

Drug	Dose	Comments
Thioamide	PTU 600–1200 mg/day Q 6 hr Methimazole 60–120 mg/day TID	No parenteral form available. Prepare rectal formulation of PTU if NPO. PTU theoretical DOC since it has a more rapid onset.
Iodides	Ipodate 1 g/day *or* Lugol's solution, 30 drops/day PO	Blocks release of hormone. Administer at least 1 hr after thioamides to avoid blocking action.
Propranolol	1 mg slow IV push Q 5 min until heart rate 90–110/min *Maintenance infusion:* 5–10 mg/hr *or* 40 mg PO Q 6 hr. Double dose Q 12 hr until therapeutic response achieved.	Used to ↓ symptoms of excess adrenergic stimulation (tachycardia, tremulousness, agitation). Preferred over reserpine and guanethidine.
Hydrocortisone	100–200 mg IV Q 6 hr	Used to combat hypoadrenalism. Actuely depresses T_3 levels.
Supportive therapy	Sedation, oxygen, glucose, hydration, antipyretics, antibiotics	—

DOC, drug of choice; NPO, nothing by mouth; FTU, propylthiouracil.

1 to 3 mg intramuscularly or IV every 8 hours or guanethidine 20 to 50 mg orally every 8 hours can be tried. IV reserpine is preferred over the intramuscular injection because absorption from intramuscular sites is poor, particularly if circulatory collapse is present.

SUPPORTIVE TREATMENT OF VITAL FUNCTIONS

This may include sedation, oxygen, IV glucose, vitamins, treatment of infections with antibiotics, digitalization to maintain the cardiac status, rehydration, and treatment of hyperpyrexia with cooling blankets, sponge baths, and the judicious use of antipyretics. Because hypoadrenalism often is suspected, hydrocortisone 100 to 200 mg should be given IV every 6 hours. Because pharmacologic doses of steroids acutely depress serum T_3 levels, a beneficial effect in storm, their routine use is recommended.[84]

ELIMINATION OF PRECIPITATING CAUSES OF STORM

Factors associated with the induction of thyroid storm include infection (most common), trauma, inadequate preparation before thyroidectomy, surgical operations, stress, diabetic acidosis, pregnancy, emboli, discontinuation or withdrawal of antithyroid medications, drug therapy, and RAI therapy.[84,123]

DRUG-INDUCED THYROID DISEASE

Lithium and Antidepressants

52. D.A., a 56-year-old man, complains of sluggishness, cold intolerance, fatigue, and a "run-down" feeling, which doctors attribute to the depressive phase of his bipolar affective illness. He previously had been well controlled with sertraline (Zoloft) 100 mg/day, but lithium carbonate (Eskalith) 900 mg/day was added 4 months ago because of unreasonable mirthfulness and uncontrollable gift-buying tendencies. Physical examination reveals a puffy face and a large goiter. What is a reasonable assessment of these subjective and objective data?

Thyroid function tests (i.e., TSH, FT_4) should be obtained to evaluate the possibility of lithium- and possibly sertraline-induced hypothyroidism and goiter.[178–181] If appropriate, thyroxine should be initiated. Although the incidence of goiter and hypothyroidism in the manic-depressive population is unknown, the incidence of baseline elevated TSH might be higher than in the general population; one study reported an incidence of 15%.[181]

The antithyroid effects of lithium were noted first in manic-depressive patients. The exact mechanism of lithium's antithyroid effect on the gland is unclear, although it is highly concentrated by the gland. Similar to the iodides, chronic lithium therapy inhibits the release of thyroid hormone from the gland. The fall in serum T_4 and T_3 hormone levels leads to a compensatory and transient increase in serum TSH levels until a new steady state is achieved.[179–181]

The incidence of subclinical hypothyroidism (i.e., increased TSH level) occurs in approximately 19% of patients on chronic lithium therapy.[181] Typically, the serum thyroid hormone levels decrease and the TSH levels increase during the first few months of treatment, returning to pretreatment levels after 1 year. In one study, TSH levels increased within 10 days after starting therapy. Normalization of the TSH level is less likely to occur in patients with pre-existing positive thyroid antibodies before lithium therapy. Induction of thyroid antibodies and increases in baseline antibody titers also occur after chronic lithium therapy. Because abnormal thyroid function tests can be transient, a longer period of observation is justified before starting thyroid hormone therapy in patients with subclinical hypothyroidism.

Lithium-induced goiter, with or without hypothyroidism, appears in a small percentage of the population after 5 months to 2 years of therapy.[179–181] Overt hypothyroidism develops most often during the first 2 years of treatment in women with a history of positive antibodies before lithium therapy. A direct goitrogenic effect of lithium might explain the occurrence of euthyroid goiter. The goiters respond to discontinuation of lithium or to suppression with thyroid hormone despite continuation of lithium therapy. Surgical removal of the goiter is required if there are local obstructive symptoms. In D.A.'s case, sertraline could be exerting an additive or synergistic antithyroid effect with lithium because antithyroid effects also have been associated with this drug.[178]

Most patients with lithium-induced thyroid abnormalities have a prior history of compromised thyroid function (e.g., Hashimoto's thyroiditis), positive thyroid antibodies before lithium therapy, or a strong family history of thyroid disease.[179–181] Therefore, baseline thyroid function tests (i.e., FT_4, TSH) and antibodies should be obtained before starting lithium therapy, and levels should be checked every 6 months thereafter or more frequently if clinically indicated. Patients also should be questioned about a positive history or family history for thyroid disease and the concurrent use of other, potentially goitrogenic medications (e.g., tricyclic antidepressants, iodides, iodinated expectorants).

53. A.B., a 66-year-old, otherwise healthy man, is admitted for evaluation of new-onset AF. His only other medical problem is a history of bipolar affective disorder treated with lithium for 1 year. However, A.B. discontinued the lithium 1 month before hospitalization without the knowledge of his physician. His laboratory studies are within normal limits except for a TT_3 of 380 ng/dL. What is the potential cause of A.B.'s AF?

[SI unit: TT_3, 6.0 nmol/L (normal, 1.1 to 2.0)]

AF may be the only manifestation of thyrotoxicosis in older patients.[52,53,90] Thyrotoxicosis is reported following lithium withdrawal, and A.B.'s AF most likely is the result of excessive thyroid hormone activity. Lithium's antithyroid action is substantial and is comparable to that of the thioamides; T_4 levels decline by 20% to 35%. Therefore, A.B.'s underlying hyperthyroidism probably has been unmasked by his discontinuation of the lithium. Rarely, lithium-induced thyrotoxicosis occurs.[182,183]

Although lithium is not considered the standard of care for hyperthyroidism, it is recommended as an adjunct to RAI therapy in patients allergic to conventional treatment modalities because it does not interfere with ^{131}I uptake. Furthermore, lithium can increase ^{131}I retention by decreasing its rate of elimination from the gland. The increased thyroidal half-life of ^{131}I by lithium is beneficial in localizing the dose of radiation to the gland and producing faster control of the hyperthyroidism.[184]

Because clinical experience with lithium in the treatment of thyrotoxicosis is limited and because it has such a narrow therapeutic index, its use should be restricted to situations when rapid suppression of thyroid hormone secretion is needed and thioamides, iodides, and ipodate are contraindicated. It should not be considered an alternative to thioamides, only an adjunct.

Iodides and Amiodarone

54. C.Y., a 54-year-old man with chronic obstructive airways disease (COAD), presents with a 6-month history of weakness, fatigue, tremor, heat intolerance, palpitations, and cardiac tachyarrhythmias, previously controlled for the last 2 years on amiodarone 400 mg/day. Physical examination reveals a 50-g multinodular gland, which C.Y. says has "been there forever." He denies any family history of thyroid disease or ingestion of any thyroid medication. He recently started to use an iodinated expectorant for his COAD. His current complaints began after an intravenous pyelogram (IVP). What might be responsible for C.Y.'s hyperthyroid symptoms?

The iodine load from the IVP, the iodinated expectorant, or the amiodarone could be responsible for C.Y.'s hyperthyroid symptoms.[25,26,116,117] Iodide-induced hyperthyroidism, known as the Jod-Basedow phenomenon, was described first in the 1800s when patients residing in iodide-deficient areas became toxic when given adequate iodide supplementation. Other reports have appeared since. Both T_3 toxicosis and classic T_4 toxicosis have occurred following iodide ingestion or injection of roentgenographic contrast media.

Although it is presumed that both iodide deficiency and a multinodular goiter, as in C.Y., are required to invoke the Jod-Basedow phenomenon, iodide-induced disease has been reported in patients residing in iodide-sufficient areas and in euthyroid patients with normal glands and no apparent risk factors (e.g., family history).[116,117]

Amiodarone can cause hypothyroidism or hyperthyroidism in susceptible patients because of its high iodine content.[25,26,116–118] Twelve milligrams (37%) of free iodine is released per 400-mg dose of amiodarone. Patients with multinodular goiters who lose the ability to turn off organification of iodide with increasing iodide loads (Wolff-Chaikoff effect) are most likely to develop iodide-induced thyrotoxicosis. Conversely, patients with positive antibodies or with underlying Hashimoto's thyroiditis who cannot escape from the Wolff-Chaikoff block are most likely to develop hypothyroidism.

Amiodarone-induced hypothyroidism may occur at any time during therapy and does not appear to be related to the cumulative dose. A normal FT_4 and a persistently elevated TSH (see Question 5) are consistent with amiodarone-induced hypothyroidism, which occurs in 6% to 10% of long-term users. The hypothyroidism responds readily to thyroxine therapy, and the amiodarone often can be continued.[25,26]

In contrast, the development of amiodarone-induced thyrotoxicosis occurs early and suddenly during therapy, so that routine monitoring of thyroid function tests often is not useful. Elevated hormone levels, an undetectable TSH level, and clinical symptoms consistent with hyperthyroidism are the best indicators of amiodarone-induced thyrotoxicosis, which occurs in 1% to 5% of long-term users. Worsening of tachyarrhythmias may be the first clinical clue to amiodarone-induced thyrotoxicosis.

Amiodarone-induced hyperthyroidism can be classified as either type I or type II.[25,26] Type I occurs in patients with underlying risk factors for thyroid disease (e.g., multinodular goiter) and is related to the iodine load. The formation of large amounts of preformed hormone from the massive iodine load produces a protracted course of hyperthyroidism, which is challenging to manage. Type II amiodarone-induced hyperthyroidism results from a direct destructive type of thyroiditis, causing excessive release of thyroid hormone into the systemic circulation. This occurs most often in patients with normal thyroid glands. Unique laboratory findings include a low radioactive iodine uptake and elevated interleukin-6 levels.

The management of amiodarone-induced thyrotoxicosis is complicated because it is not always possible to identify the type of hyperthyroidism. Stopping amiodarone alone does not immediately improve the hyperthyroidism because of the drug's long half-life (22 to 55 days) and its sequestration in fat. Radioactive iodine ablation is never appropriate because the high iodine load from amiodarone will suppress therapeutic uptake of the ^{131}I. The combination of methimazole and potassium perchlorate is the treatment of choice for type I hyperthyroidism.[25,26,116,117] The addition of corticosteroids to block T$_4$ to T$_3$ conversion is less effective because of amiodarone's already potent inhibitory effects on T$_4$ to T$_3$ conversion. However, in patients with type II hyperthyroidism, β-blockers, corticosteroids, and oral cholecystographic agents (e.g., sodium ipodate), rather than the aforementioned agents, are the most appropriate choices.[25,26,117,131,132] A total thyroidectomy can be effective by rapidly controlling the thyrotoxicosis, permitting continued therapy with amiodarone if necessary. Despite underlying cardiac disease in these patients, uneventful surgery and a low complication rate were observed if patients were treated before surgery with a short course of an oral cholecystographic agent.[132]

Large doses of iodides should be avoided in patients with nontoxic multinodular goiters who are predisposed to thyrotoxicosis (see Questions 5 and 30).

Interferon-α

55. **P.R., a 56-year-old woman, complains of hoarseness, fatigue, "slow movement," and forgetfulness. She is troubled by these new symptoms, which have worsened during the past few weeks. Her medical history includes persistent hepatitis C, which is responding to the combination of pegylated interferon-α injections and ribavirin. She notes that her mother had a history of Graves' disease treated with radioactive iodine ablation. Her medications include interferon-α and an over-the-counter dietary supplement, Cellasene, to reduce cellulite. On examination, facial edema, coarse skin, an enlarged thyroid gland without nodules, and delayed DTRs are noted. Thyroid function tests are pending. What might be responsible for her new complaints?**

The medications that P.R. is taking could be responsible for her complaints and physical findings, which are consistent with hypothyroidism. A detailed history of any other dietary and herbal supplements, especially those containing thyroid or iodine (e.g., kelp tablets), should be obtained. Cellasene, a dietary supplement promoted to reduce cellulite, contains a significant amount of iodine (e.g., 310 μg of iodine per capsule) and could cause thyroid illness in susceptible patients (see Questions 30 and 54).

Another possible cause for hypothyroidism could be the pegylated interferon-α injections that she has been receiving for the hepatitis C infection.[185–187] The prevalence of thyroid abnormalities observed with interferon-α ranges from 2.5% to 45.3%. Development or aggravation of pre-existing antithyroid antibodies is the most common abnormal finding. The presence of pre-existing antithyroid antibodies (seropositivity) before interferon-α therapy or its persistence at the end of therapy is a significant risk factor for the development of overt thyroid dysfunction. Other predisposing risk factors include female gender and Asian ethnicity.[186] The incidence of thyroid dysfunction was 46% in a seropositive group compared to 5.4% in the seronegative group.[186] Likewise, in a group of 114 patients with no pre-existing thyroid disease, those who were seropositive at the end of therapy had the highest risk of developing subclinical hypothyroidism 6.2 years later (odds ratio of 38.7).[187]

Hypothyroidism is more common (40% to 50% of patients) than hyperthyroidism (10% to 30%). There are two types of hyperthyroidism, a Graves'-like disorder and a hyperthyroid thyroiditis, similar to a type II amiodarone hyperthyroidism, which is due to a direct toxic effect of interferon on the gland. Approximately 20% of patients with a thyroiditis will first have transient symptoms of hyperthyroidism followed by hypothyroidism (biphasic thyroiditis).[188]

Fortunately, thyroid dysfunction appears to be transient in most patients, and treatment is not always necessary. Levothyroxine is required only if hypothyroid symptoms are bothersome; otherwise, therapy can be withheld because symptoms often resolve spontaneously within 2 to 3 months after stopping therapy. If thyroxine is begun, it should be stopped after 6 months to re-evaluate the need for continued thyroid replacement. Similarly, transient hyperthyroid laboratory indices do not require therapy with β-blockers unless the patient is symptomatic or laboratory values are dangerously elevated. Rarely, thyroid dysfunction is permanent, but it may take up to 17 months after stopping therapy for findings to resolve.

P.R. should be advised to stop taking the Cellasene and to avoid other iodide-containing herbal or dietary supplements. Once the laboratory values confirm hypothyroidism, thyroxine should be started concurrently with the interferon-α because of the severity of her symptoms. Once interferon therapy is completed, levothyroxine should be stopped to evaluate the need for continued replacement.

Iodide Prophylaxis for Radiation Emergencies

56. **J.M. is a healthy, 43-year-old Russian woman who lives near a nuclear reactor with her two young children. She has relatives living in Chernobyl who were exposed to the 1986 radiation fallout and developed various thyroid abnormalities, including cancer. J.M. would like to protect herself and her children. What prophylaxis and benefits, if any, might be indicated for J.M. in case of a nuclear accident?**

The most accurate data for irradiation-induced thyroid abnormalities come from the 1986 Chernobyl incident, where massive amounts of radioactive iodine was released into the environment, contaminating air, food, and water supplies. Significant increases in thyroid cancer were found, primarily in children, who received 5 centigrays or greater I^{131} exposures.[189]

The thyroid can be protected against radiation-induced thyroid cancer if potassium iodide (KI) is taken immediately before, coincident with, or possibly 3 to 4 hours after the radiation exposure.[190] Administration of KI 130 mg in adults and 65 mg in school-age children lasts approximately 24 hours and should be continued until the risk of exposure is over. Adolescents close to 70 kg should receive the full 130-mg dose; neonates should receive 16 mg. Repeat dosing is not recommended in pregnant women or neonates or during lactation unless there is ongoing contamination, because the risks of repeated KI administration (e.g., neonatal and fetal hypothyroidism) outweigh their protective benefits. In the aforementioned conditions, when repeated doses of KI are not advisable, and in those intolerant to KI, protective measures (e.g., sheltering, evacuation, and control of the food supply) should be implemented. Hypothyroidism can be managed with thyroxine supplementation. If repeat dosing is necessary during continued contamination, close monitoring for toxicity is recommended. Short-term administration of KI is safer in children than in adults.

Adverse effects include sialadenitis, GI disturbances, rash, and other allergic reactions, which are increased in patients with dermatitis herpetiformis and hypocomplementemic vasculitides. Hyperthyroidism, goiter, and hypothyroidism can occur, especially in adults with underlying thyroid disorders (see Question 54).

NODULES

"Hot" Nodule

57. N.S., a 20-year-old woman, noticed a "lump" in the right side of her neck. There is no history of irradiation and no family history of thyroid disease. She has no local symptoms and no symptoms suggestive of hypothyroidism or hyperthyroidism. The right lobe of the thyroid is occupied by a 3 × 3-cm firm, immovable nodule; the left lobe is barely palpable. All thyroid function tests are within normal limits, although the gland is not suppressible. A scan shows a large "hot" nodule occupying the right lobe and a nonexistent left lobe. How should N.S.'s single "hot" nodule, or Plummer's disease, be managed?

Hot nodule is a term used to describe a "hyperfunctioning" or iodine-concentrating area of the thyroid as shown on scan; it appears as an area of greater density than the rest of the gland. The hyperfunctioning autonomous nodule typically suppresses activity in the remainder of the gland, but it need not produce clinical or chemical evidence of hyperthyroidism and may remain unchanged for years. Some nodules may develop into toxic goiters, causing overt symptoms of toxicosis. Most hot nodules are benign; malignancies rarely are reported.[191]

Treatment of the hot nodule depends on the existing clinical situation. If it is suppressing the other lobe of the thyroid, is not causing toxic symptoms, and is the only source of thyroid production, the patient should be left alone and monitored closely for signs of toxicity. If the gland is not suppressed by the functioning hot nodule, then thyroid suppression therapy is indicated to avoid further nodule growth and stimulation by TSH.[191,192] A toxic hot nodule is best treated surgically or with RAI ablation. Because hot nodules do not spontaneously resolve, antithyroid drugs are not the treatment of choice. Because the normal thyroid tissue is suppressed, RAI is concentrated only by the hot nodule, sparing the suppressed tissue. After treatment, the suppressed tissue should begin functioning again.

"Cold" Nodule

58. P.L., a 29-year-old woman, is found to have a left thyroid nodule on routine physical examination. She has no history of neck irradiation, no family history of thyroid disease, and no symptoms suggestive of hypothyroidism or hyperthyroidism. A firm, nontender 1.0-cm nodule occupies the left lobe of the gland. Thyroid function tests are within normal limits. The scan shows a "cold" nodule and the echogram reveals a solid mass, ruling out the possibility of a cyst. The results of the FNA are pending. Antibodies are negative. What is the significance of a cold nodule, and how should it be managed?

A cold nodule is a "hypofunctioning" area of the thyroid that fails to collect radioiodine. It is depicted on the scan as a lighter or less dense area. The differential diagnosis includes Hashimoto's thyroiditis, benign adenomas, cysts, and malignant tumors. No antibodies and a solid mass as identified by echo rules out the possibility of a cyst or Hashimoto's thyroiditis. Most cold nodules turn out to be benign adenomas rather than cancers. The FNA can help distinguish a benign from a malignant nodule. However, a benign biopsy in a suspicious nodule or in a patient with risk factors for malignancy does not eliminate the possibility of malignancy. In these patients, surgery is recommended. The incidence of malignancy in a cold nodule varies between 10% and 20%.[191] A history of irradiation increases the likelihood of cancer in a nodule, and surgery is recommended in these instances.[199] The nature of the nodule is important. Fixation of the nodule to the strap muscles or the trachea, a hard bulging mass, any pain or tenderness, or voice hoarseness can indicate malignancy.

If the nodule is benign, then thyroxine suppressive therapy can be considered. However, only about 10% to 20% of nodules shrink with therapy.[193,194] Furthermore, levothyroxine may not actually shrink the nodule itself, but rather the surrounding thyroid tissue, making the nodule appear smaller. Spontaneous resolution of the nodule can also occur. The dangers of excessive levothyroxine therapy (e.g., osteoporosis, cardiac arrhythmias) exceed the benefits of benign nodule suppression.[50–52] Therefore, watchful waiting, with no therapy, is recommended.

Nontoxic Multinodular Goiter

59. G.D., a 35-year-old woman, is referred for a "goiter" discovered on routine physical examination. She denies any symptoms of hyperthyroidism or hypothyroidism or any history of irradiation. Her grandmother had hypothyroidism and a goiter. A large "lumpy, bumpy" gland is present, but she has no problems with breathing or swallowing. The FNA shows a benign lesion. The assessment is a nontoxic multinodular goiter. How should this be managed?

Nontoxic multinodular goiter is a common finding, occurring in about 5% of the population.[191,192] In low-risk patients, longstanding asymptomatic nodules that have not exhibited recent growth are likely to be benign and can be followed or excised surgically for cosmetic reasons. If the patient develops symptoms (swallowing or respiratory difficulty), surgery is the treatment of choice. Thyroxine suppression therapy to decrease TSH stimulation can be considered to prevent further growth if the patient has no cardiac contraindications. Observation with close follow-up is also an acceptable option. Thyroxine does not return the gland to normal size but prevents further goiter enlargement.[191,192] Some gland shrinkage should be noted 3 to 6 months following the initiation of thyroxine 0.1 to 0.2 mg/day to suppress the TSH to undetectable levels. If so, maintenance therapy can be continued. Patients should be carefully monitored for the development of hyperthyroidism. Most multinodular goiters contain autonomously functioning nodules that are independent of TSH control and could produce excessive thyroid hormone secretion spontaneously. If the nodules grow while the patient is receiving thyroxine therapy, rebiopsy or surgery should be considered. The dangers of long-term suppressive therapy include osteoporosis and cardiac changes.[50–52] Nodular responsiveness to thyroxine does not rule out malignancy.

Thyrotropin Alfa and Thyroid Cancer

60. J.R., a 28-year-old man, had a total thyroidectomy 2 years ago for follicular cancer. His TSH level is appropriately suppressed on 150 μg levothyroxine daily. He is hesitant to discontinue his levothyroxine so that an RAIU scan and thyroglobulin testing can be obtained to evaluate for tumor recurrence. His doctor has heard about a drug that will let J.R. stay on his levothyroxine and "feel functional" while carrying out these tests. What can you tell his physician about this medication?

Thyrotropin alfa (Thyrogen), a recombinant human TSH, is indicated as an adjunctive diagnostic tool for serum thyroglobulin testing with or without radioiodine imaging in the follow-up of patients with thyroid cancer. The evaluation for recurrence of some thyroid malignancies requires the withdrawal of thyroxine therapy for 4 to 6 weeks before the radioactive scanning and thyroglobulin test can be performed.

Elevations in the TSH level then permit detection of tumor recurrence, as evidenced by a rise in thyroglobulin or a positive finding on the RAIU scan. The development of hypothyroidism during this withdrawal period is often distressing to the patient. Thyrotropin alfa is intended to improve the quality of life in these patients by allowing these procedures to be undertaken without stopping the thyroxine. However, clinical trials show that when compared with the traditional method of thyroxine withdrawal, thyrotropin alfa failed to detect tumor recurrence in 16% of patients with localized disease and in 24% of patients with metastatic disease.[195]

Thyrotropin is generally well tolerated. Nausea and headaches were the most common adverse effects noted. Recombinant human TSH is available as 0.9-mg vial and is administered intramuscularly once daily for 2 days. Thyrotropin costs approximately $777 per vial and is covered under most health plans. Improved quality of life, avoidance of hypothyroidism, and increased patient productivity may offset the direct costs of thyrotropin. However, concerns exist about the efficacy of thyrotropin alfa to detect tumor recurrence compared with the current standard of practice, which is withdrawal of thyroxine therapy. Further studies are needed to identify its role in care.

REFERENCES

1. Demers LM, Spencer CA. Laboratory Medicine Practice Guidelines. Laboratory support for the diagnosis and monitoring of thyroid disease. Thyroid 2003;13:19.
2. Ross DS. Serum thyroid-stimulating hormone measurement for assessment of thyroid function and disease. Endocrinol Metab Clin North Am 2001;30:245.
3. Surks MI et al. ATA guidelines for use of laboratory tests in thyroid disorders. JAMA 1990;263:1529.
4. Surks MI, Sievert R. Drugs and thyroid function. N Engl J Med 1995;333:1688.
5. DeGroot LJ. Dangerous dogmas in medicine: the nonthyroidal illness syndrome. J Clin Endocrinol Metab 1999;84:151.
6. Chopra IJ. Clinical review 86: euthyroid sick syndrome: is it a misnomer? J Clin Endocrinol Metab 1997;82:329.
7. Camacho PM, Dwarkanathan AA. Sick euthyroid syndrome. What to do when thyroid function tests are abnormal in critically ill patients. Postgrad Med 1999;105:215.
8. Slag MF et al. Hypothyroxinemia in critically ill patients as a predictor of high mortality. JAMA 1981;245:43.
9. Friberg L et al. Association between increased levels of reverse triiodothyronine and mortality after acute myocardial infarction. Am J Med 2001;111:699.
10. Stathatos N et al. The controversy of the treatment of critically ill patients with thyroid hormone. Best Pract Res Clin Endocrinol Metab 2001;15:465.
11. Acker CG et al. A trial of thyroxine in acute renal failure. Kidney Int 2000;57:293.
12. Wang R et al. Salsalate administration: a potential pharmacological model of the sick euthyroid syndrome. J Clin Endocrinol Metab 1998;83:3095.
13. McDonnell RJ. Abnormal thyroid function test results in patients taking salsalate. JAMA 1992;267:1242.
14. Curran PG, Degroot LJ. The effect of hepatic enzyme-inducing drugs on thyroid hormones and the thyroid gland. Endocrinol Rev 1991;12:135.
15. Surks MI, DeFesi CR. Normal serum free thyroid hormone concentrations in patients treated with phenytoin or carbamazepine. A paradox resolved. JAMA 1996;275:1495.
16. Isojarvi JIT et al. Thyroid function in men taking carbamazepine, oxcarbazepine, or valproate for epilepsy. Epilepsia 2001;42:930.
17. Tiihonen M et al. Thyroid status of patients receiving long-term anticonvulsant therapy assessed by peripheral parameters: A placebo-controlled thyroxine therapy trial. Epilepsia 1995;36:1118.
18. Blackshear JL et al. Thyroxine replacement requirements in hypothyroid patients receiving phenytoin. Ann Intern Med 1983;99:341.
19. DeLuca F et al. Changes in thyroid function tests induced by 2 month carbamazepine treatment in L-thyroxine-substituted hypothyroid children. Eur J Paediatr 1986;145:77.
20. English TN et al. Abnormalities in thyroid function associated with chronic therapy with methadone. Clin Chem 1988;34:2202.
21. Arafah BM. Increased need for thyroxine in women with hypothyroidism during estrogen therapy. N Engl J Med 2001;344:1743.
22. Marqusee E et al. The effect of droloxifene and estrogen on thyroid function in postmenopausal women. J Clin Endocrinol Metab 2000;85:4407.
23. Hsu SHJ et al. Effect of long-term use of raloxifene, a selective estrogen receptor modulatory on thyroid function test profiles. Clin Chem 2001;10:1865.
24. Kostoglour-Athanassiou I et al. Thyroid function in postmenopausal women with breast cancer on tamoxifen. Eur J Gynaecol Oncol 1998;19:150.
25. Harjari KJ, Licata AA. Effects of amiodarone on thyroid function. Ann Intern Med 1997;126:63.
26. Martino E et al. The effects of amiodarone on the thyroid. Endocr Rev 2001;22:240.
27. Lee E et al. Effect of acute high-dose dobutamine administration on serum thyrotropin (TSH). Clin Endocrinol 1999;50:486.
28. Keogh MA, Wittert GA. Effect of cabergoline on thyroid function in hyperprolactinaemia [letter]. Clin Endocrinol 2002;57:699.
29. Rees-Jones RW, Larsen PR. Triiodothyronine and thyroxine content of desiccated thyroid tablets. Metabolism 1977;26:1213.
30. Rees-Jones RW et al. Hormonal content of thyroid replacement preparations. JAMA 1980;243:549.
31. Csako GA et al. Therapeutic potential of two over-the-counter thyroid hormone preparations. Drug Intell Clin Pharm 1990;24:26.
32. Sawin CT, London MH. "Natural" desiccated thyroid, a health food thyroid preparation. Arch Intern Med 1989;149:2117.
33. Sawin CT et al. A comparison of thyroxine and desiccated thyroid in patients with primary hypothyroidism. Metabolism 1978;27:1518.
34. Wiersinga WM. Thyroid hormone replacement therapy. Horm Res 2001;56(Suppl.1):74.
35. Fish LH et al. Replacement dose, metabolism, and bioavailability of levothyroxine in the treatment of hypothyroidism. N Engl J Med 1987;316:764.
36. Benvenga S et al. Delayed intestinal absorption of levothyroxine. Thyroid 1995;5:249.
37. Oppenheimer JH et al. A therapeutic controversy. Thyroid hormone treatment: when and what? J Clin Endocrinol Metab 1993;3:81.
38. Dong BJ et al. The nonequivalence of levothyroxine products [letter]. Drug Intell Clin Pharm 1986;20:77.
39. Stoffer SS, Szpunar WE. Potency of current levothyroxine preparations evaluated by high-performance liquid chromatography. Henry Ford Hosp Med J 1988;36:64.
40. Generic drugs. Med Lett Drugs Ther 1999;41:47.
41. Sawin CT et al. Oral thyroxine: variation in biologic action and tablet content. Ann Intern Med 1984;100:64.
42. Blouin RA et al. Biopharmaceutical comparison of two levothyroxine sodium preparations. Clin Pharm.1989;8:588.
43. Escalante DA et al. Assessment of interchangeability of two brands of levothyroxine preparations with a third-generation TSH assay. Am J Med.1995;98:374.
44. Dong BJ et al. Bioequivalence of generic and brand-name levothyroxine products in the treatment of hypothyroidism. JAMA 1997;277:1205.
45. Bunevicius R et al. Effects of thyroxine as compared with thyroxine plus triiodothyronine in patients with hypothyroidism. N Engl J Med 1999;340:424.

46. Bunevicius R, Prange AJ. Mental improvement after replacement therapy with thyroxine plus triiodothyronine: relationship to cause of hypothyroidism. Int J Neuropsychopharmacol 2000;3:167.

47. Bunevicius R et al. Thyroxine vs. thyroxine plus triiodothyronine in treatment of hypothyroidism after thyroidectomy for Graves' disease. Endocrine 2002;18:129.

48. Klemperer JD. Thyroid hormone and cardiac surgery. Thyroid 2002;12:517.

49. Biondi B et al. Effects of subclinical thyroid dysfunction on the heart. Ann Intern Med 2002; 137:904.

50. Greenspan SL, Greenspan FS. The effect of thyroid hormone on skeletal integrity. Ann Intern Med 1999;130:750.

51. Cooper DS. Subclinical thyroid disease: a clinician's perspective. Ann Intern Med.1998;129:135.

52. Sawin CT et al. Low serum thyrotropin concentrations as a risk factor for atrial fibrillation in older patients. N Engl J Med 1994;331:1249.

53. Marqusee E et al. Subclinical thyrotoxicosis. Endocrinol Metab Clin North Am 1998;27:37.

54. Woeber KA. Levothyroxine therapy and serum free thyroxine and free triiodothyronine concentrations. J Endocrinol Invest 2002;25:106.

55. Grund FM, Niewoehner CB. Hyperthyroxinemia in patients receiving thyroid replacement therapy. Arch Intern Med 1989;149:921.

56. Ain KB et al. Thyroid hormone levels affected by time of blood sampling in thyroxine-treated patients. Thyroid 1993;3:81.

57. Sawin CT et al. Aging and the thyroid. Decreased requirements for thyroid hormone in older hypothyroid patients. Am J Med 1983;75:206.

58. Davis FB et al. Estimation of a physiologic replacement dose of levothyroxine in elderly patients with hypothyroidism. Arch Intern Med 1984;144:1752.

59. Kabadi UM. Variability of L-thyroxine replacement dose in elderly patients with primary hypothyroidism. J Fam Pract 1987;24:473.

60. Grebe SKG et al. Treatment of hypothyroidism with once-weekly thyroxine. J Clin Endocrinol Metab 1997;82:870.

61. Brent GA. Maternal hypothyroidism: recognition and management. Thyroid 1999;9:661.

62. Chopra IJ, Baber K. Treatment of primary hypothyroidism during pregnancy: is there an increase in thyroxine dose requirement in pregnancy? Metabolism 2003;52:122.

63. Haddow JE et al. Maternal thyroid deficiency during pregnancy and subsequent neuropsychological development of the child. N Engl J Med 1999; 341:549.

64. Allan WC et al. Maternal thyroid deficiency and pregnancy complications: implications for population screening. J Med Screen 2000;7:127.

65. LaFranchi S. Congenital hypothyroidism: etiologies, diagnosis, and management. Thyroid 1999; 9:735.

66. Selva KA et al. Initial treatment dose of L-thyroxine in congenital hypothyroidism. J Pediatr 2002;141:786.

67. Rovet JF. Congenital hypothyroidism: long-term outcome. Thyroid 1999;9:741.

68. Salerno M et al. Effect of different starting doses of levothyroxine on growth and intellectual outcome at four years of age in congenital hypothyroidism. Thyroid 2002;12:45.

69. Bongers-Schokking JJ et al. Influence of timing and dose of thyroid hormone replacement on development in infants with congenital hypothyroidism. J Pediatr 2000;136:292.

70. Ain KB et al. Pseudomalabsorption of levothyroxine. JAMA 1991;266:2118.

71. Sherman SI, Malecha SE. Absorption and malabsorption of levothyroxine. Am J Ther 1995;2:814.

72. Bell DS, Ovalle F. Use of soy protein supplement and resultant need for increased dose of levothyroxine. Endocr Pract 2001;7:193.

73. Siraj ES et al. Raloxifene causing malabsorption of levothyroxine. Arch Intern Med 2003;163:1367.

74. Harmon SM, Seifert CF. Levothyroxine cholestyramine interaction reemphasized [letter]. Ann Intern Med 1991;115:658.

75. Campbell NRC et al. Ferrous sulfate reduces thyroxine efficacy in patients with hypothyroidism. Ann Intern Med 1992;117:1010.

76. Demke DM. Drug interaction between thyroxine and lovastatin [letter]. N Engl J Med 1989; 321:1341.

77. Sperber AD, Liel Y. Evidence for interference with the intestinal absorption of levothyroxine sodium by aluminum hydroxide. Arch Intern Med 1992;152:183.

78. Havrankova J, Lahaie R. Levothyroxine binding by sucralfate [letter]. Ann Intern Med 1992; 117:445.

79. Singh N et al. Effect of calcium carbonate on the absorption of levothyroxine. JAMA 2000;283:2822.

80. Singh N et al. The acute effect of calcium carbonate on the intestinal absorption of levothyroxine. Thyroid 2001;11:967.

81. Duntas LH. Thyroid disease and lipids. Thyroid 2002;12:287.

82. Nicoloff JT, LoPresti JS. Myxedema coma. A form of decompensated hypothyroidism. Endocrinol Metab Clin North Am 1993;22:279.

83. Yamamoto T et al. Factors associated with mortality of myxedema coma: report of eight cases and literature survey. Thyroid 1999;9:1167.

84. Ringel MD. Management of hypothyroidism and hyperthyroidism in the intensive care unit. Crit Care Clin 2001;17:59.

85. MacKerrow SD et al. Myxedema-associated cardiogenic shock treated with intravenous triiodothyronine. Ann Intern Med 1992;117:1014.

86. Pereira VG et al. Management of myxedema coma: report on three successfully treated cases with nasogastric or intravenous administration of triiodothyronine. J Endocrinol Invest 1982;5:331.

87. Ladenson PW et al. Rapid pituitary and peripheral tissue responses to intravenous L-triiodothyronine in hypothyroidism. J Clin Endocrinol Metab 1983;56:1252.

88. Hylander B, Rosenqvist U. Treatment of myxedema coma. Factors associated with fatal outcome. Acta Endocrinol (Copenhagen) 1985;108:65.

89. Ariot S et al. Myxoedema coma: response of thyroid hormones with oral and intravenous high-dose L-thyroxine treatment. Intensive Care Med 1991;17:16.

90. Klein I, Ojamaa K. Thyroid hormone and the cardiovascular system. N Engl J Med 2001;344:501.

91. Levine D. Compromise therapy in the patient with angina pectoris and hypothyroidism. Am J Med 1980;69:411.

92. Myerowitz PD. Diagnosis and management of the hypothyroid patient with chest pain. J Thorac Cardiovasc Surg 1983;86:57.

93. Kohno A, Hara Y. Severe myocardial ischemia following hormone replacement in two cases of hypothyroidism with normal coronary arteriogram. Endocrinol J 2001;48:565.

94. Lawrence JR et al. Digoxin kinetics in patients with thyroid dysfunction. Clin Pharmacol Ther.1977;22:7.

95. Doherty JE et al. Digoxin metabolism in hypo- and hyperthyroidism. Ann Intern Med 1966; 64:489.

96. Becker C. Hypothyroidism and atherosclerotic heart disease: pathogenesis, medical management and the role of coronary artery bypass surgery. Endocrinol Rev 1985;6:432.

97. Chu JW, Crapo LM. The treatment of subclinical hypothyroidism is seldom necessary. J Clin Endocrinol Metab 2001;86:4591.

98. Cooper DS. Subclinical hypothyroidism. N Engl J Med 2001;345:260.

99. McDermott MT, Ridgway EC. Subclinical hypothyroidism is mild thyroid failure and should be treated. J Clin Endocrinol Metab 2001;86:4585.

100. Kong WM et al. A 6-month randomized trial of thyroxine treatment in women with mild subclinical hypothyroidism. Am J Med 2002;112:348.

101. Meier C et al. TSH-controlled L-thyroxine therapy reduces cholesterol levels and clinical symptoms in subclinical hypothyroidism: a double blind placebo-controlled trial (Basel Thyroid Study). J Clin Endocrinol Metab 2001;86:4860.

102. Staub HG et al. Prospective study of the spontaneous course of subclinical hypothyroidism: prognostic value of thyrotropin, thyroid reserve, and thyroid antibodies. J Clin Endocrinol Metab 2002;87:3221.

103. Danese MD et al. Effect of thyroxine therapy on serum lipoproteins in patients with mild thyroid failure: a quantitative review of the literature. J Clin Endocrinol Metab 2000;85:2993.

104. Wardle CA et al. Pitfalls in the use of thyrotropin concentration as a first-line thyroid function test. Lancet 2001;357:1013.

105. Pollock MA et al. Thyroxine treatment in patients with symptoms of hypothyroidism but thyroid function tests within the reference range: randomised double-blind placebo-controlled crossover trial. Br Med J 2001;323:891.

106. Weetman AP. Thyroxine treatment in biochemically euthyroid but clinically hypothyroid individuals. Clin Endocrinol 2002;57:25.

107. Lazarus JH. Hyperthyroidism. Lancet 1997;349:339.

108. Shimizu T et al. Hyperthyroidism and the management of atrial fibrillation. Thyroid 2002; 12:489.

109. Loeliger EA et al. The biological disappearance rate of prothrombin factors VII, IX, X from plasma in hypo-, hyper-, and during fever. Thromb Diath Haemorrh 1964;10:267.

110. Hansten PD. Oral anticoagulants and drugs which alter thyroid function. Drug Intell Clin Pharm 1980;14:331.

111. Lipsky JJ, Gallego MO. Mechanism of thioamide antithyroid drug-associated hypoprothrombinemia. Drug Metabol Drug Interact 1988;6:317.

112. Liaw Y et al. Hepatic injury during propylthiouracil therapy in patients with hyperthyroidism: a cohort study. Ann Intern Med 1993;118:424.

113. Williams KV et al. Fifty years of experience with propylthiouracil-associated hepatotoxicity: what have we learned? J Clin Endocrinol Metab 1997;82:1727.

114. Woeber KA. Methimazole-induced hepatotoxicity. Endocr Pract 2002;8:222.

115. Frye RL, Braunwald E. Studies on digitalis III: the influence of triiodothyronine on digitalis requirement. Circulation 1961;23:376.

116. Burman KD, Wartoksky L. Iodine effects on the thyroid gland: biochemical and clinical. Rev Endocrinol Metab Disord 2000;1:19.

117. Roti E, Uberti ED. Iodine excess and hyperthyroidism. Thyroid 2001;11:493.

118. Markou K et al. Iodine-induced hypothyroidism. Thyroid 2001;11:501.

119. Leech NJ, Dayan CM. Controversies in the management of Graves' disease. Clin Endocrinol 1998;49:273.

120. Arbelle JE, Porath A. Practice guidelines for the detection and management of thyroid dysfunction. A comparative review of the recommendations. Clin Endocrinol 1999;51:11.

121. Gittoes NJ, Franklyn JA. Hyperthyroidism. Current treatment guidelines. Drugs 1998;55:543.

122. Cooper DS. Antithyroid drugs for the treatment of hyperthyroidism caused by Graves' disease. Endocrinol Metab Clin North Am 1998;27:225.

123. Kaplan MM et al. Treatment of hyperthyroidism with radioactive iodine. Endocrinol Metab Clin North Am 1998;27:205.

124. Alsanea O, Clark OH. Treatment of Graves' disease: the advantages of surgery. Endocrinol Metab Clin North Am 2000;29:321.

125. Torring O et al. Graves' hyperthyroidism: treatment with antithyroid drugs, surgery, or radioiodine: a prospective, randomized study. J Clin Endocrinol Metab 1996;81:2986.

126. Robertson J, Gorman CA. Gonadal radiation dose and its genetic significance in radioiodine therapy of hyperthyroidism. J Nucl Med 1976;17:826.

127. Fontanilla JC et al. The use of oral radiographic contrast agents in the management of hyperthyroidism. Thyroid 2001;22:561.

128. Wu SY et al. Comparison of sodium ipodate (Oragrafin) and propylthiouracil in early treatment of hyperthyroidism. J Clin Endocrinol Metab 1982;54:630.

129. Roti E et al. Sodium ipodate and methimazole in the long-term treatment of hyperthyroid Graves' disease. Metabolism 1993;42:403.

130. Martino E et al. Therapy of Graves' disease with sodium ipodate is associated with a high recurrence rate of hyperthyroidism. J Endocrinol Invest 1991;14:847.

131. Chopra IJ, Baber K. Use of oral cholecystographic agents in the treatment of amiodarone-induced hyperthyroidism. J Clin Endocrinol Metab 2001; 86:4707.

132. Bogazzi F et al. Preparation with iopanoic acid rapidly controls thyrotoxicosis in patients with amiodarone-induced thyrotoxicosis before thyroidectomy. Surgery 2002;132:1114.

133. Benke G et al. Response to methimazole in Graves' disease. Clin Endocrinol 1995;43:257.

134. Cooper DS et al. Methimazole pharmacology in man: studies using a newly developed radioimmunoassay for methimazole. J Clin Endocrinol Metab 1984;58:473.

135. McIver B, Morris JC. The pathogenesis of Graves' disease. Endocrinol Metab Clin North Am 1998;27:73.

136. Allannic H et al. Antithyroid drugs and Graves' disease: a prospective randomized evaluation of the efficacy of treatment duration. J Clin Endocrinol Metab 1990;70:675.

137. Maugendre D et al. Antithyroid drugs and Graves' disease: prospective randomized assessment of long-term treatment. Clin Endocrinol 1999; 50:127.

138. Orgiazzi J, Madec AM. Reduction of the risk of relapse after withdrawal of medical therapy for Graves' disease. Thyroid 2002;12:849.

139. Bolanos F et al. Remission of Graves' hyperthyroidism treated with methimazole. Rev Invest Clin 2002;54:307.

140. Nijs HG et al. Increased insulin action and clearance in hyperthyroid newly diagnosed IDDM patient. Restoration to normal with antithyroid treatment. Diabetes Care 1989;12:319.

141. Dolman KM et al. Vasculitis and antineutrophil cytoplasmic autoantibodies associated with propylthiouracil therapy. Lancet 1993;342:651.

142. Geffner DL, Hershman JM. Beta-adrenergic blockade for the treatment of hyperthyroidism. Am J Med 1992;93:61.

143. Milner MR et al. Double-blind crossover trial of diltiazem versus propranolol in the management of thyrotoxic symptoms. Pharmacotherapy 1990; 10:100.

144. Tajiri J et al. Antithyroid drug-induced agranulocytosis. The usefulness of routine white blood cell count monitoring. Arch Intern Med 1990;150:621.

145. Wall JR et al. In vitro immunosensitivity to propylthiouracil, methimazole, and carbimazole in patients with Graves' disease: a possible cause of antithyroid drug-induced agranulocytosis. J Clin Endocrinol Metab 1984;58:868.

146. Fukata S et al. Granulocyte colony-stimulating factor (G-CSF) does not improve recovery from antithyroid drug-induced agranulocytosis: a prospective study. Thyroid 1999;9:29.

147. Tomaski SM et al. Sodium ipodate (oragrafin) in the preoperative preparation of Graves' hyperthyroidism. Laryngoscope 1997;107:1066.

148. Greer MA et al. Treatment of hyperthyroidism with a single daily dose of propylthiouracil. N Engl J Med 1965;272:888.

149. Hashizume K et al. Administration of thyroxine in treated Graves' disease. Effects on the level of antibodies to thyroid-stimulating hormone receptors and on the risk of recurrence of hyperthyroidism. N Engl J Med 1991;324:947.

150. McIver B et al. Lack of effect of thyroxine in patients with Graves' hyperthyroidism who are treated with an antithyroid drug. N Engl J Med 1996;334:220.

151. Hoermann R et al. Relapse of Graves' disease after successful outcome of antithyroid drug therapy: results of a prospective randomized study on the use of levothyroxine. Thyroid 2002;12:1119.

152. Glinoer D et al. Effects of l-thyroxine administration, TSH-receptor antibodies and smoking on the risk of recurrence in Graves' hyperthyroidism treated with antithyroid drugs: a double-blind prospective randomized study. Eur J Endocrinol 2001;144:475.

153. Vitti P et al. Clinical features of patients with Graves' disease undergoing remission after antithyroid drug treatment. Thyroid 1997;3:369.

154. Masiukiewicz US, Burrow GN. Hyperthyroidism in pregnancy: diagnosis and treatment. Thyroid 1999;9:647.

155. Atkins P et al. Drug therapy for hyperthyroidism in pregnancy: safety issues for mother and fetus. Drug Safety 2000;23:229.

156. ACOG Practice Bulletin. Thyroid disease in pregnancy. Obstet Gynecol 2002;100:387.

157. Van Dijke CP et al. Methimazole, carbimazole, and congenital skin defects [letter]. Ann Intern Med 1987;106:60.

158. Momotani N et al. Effects of propylthiouracil and methimazole on fetal thyroid status in mothers with Graves' hyperthyroidism. J Clin Endocrinol Metab 1997;82:3633.

159. Momotani N et al. Maternal hyperthyroidism and congenital malformation in the offspring. Clin Endocrinol 1984;20:695.

160. Wing DA et al. A comparison of propylthiouracil versus methimazole in the treatment of hyperthyroidism in pregnancy. Am J Obstet Gynecol 1994;170:90.

161. Momotani N et al. Antithyroid drug therapy for Graves' disease during pregnancy. Optimal regimen for fetal thyroid status. N Engl J Med 1986; 315:24.

162. Eisenstein Z et al. Intellectual capacity of subjects exposed to methimazole or propylthiouracil in utero. Eur J Pediatr 1992;151:558.

163. Burrow GN et al. Intellectual development in children whose mothers received propylthiouracil during pregnancy. Yale J Biol Med 1978;51:151.

164. Messer MP et al. Antithyroid drug and Graves' disease in pregnancy: long-term effects on somatic growth, intellectual development and thyroid function of the offspring. Acta Endocrinol 1990;123:311.

165. Andrade V et al. The effect of methimazole pretreatment on the efficacy of radioactive iodine therapy in Graves' hyperthyroidism: one-year follow-up of a prospective randomized study. J Clin Endocrinol Metab 2001;86:3488.

166. Imseis RE et al. Pretreatment with propylthiouracil but not methimazole reduces the therapeutic efficacy of iodine-131 in hyperthyroidism. J Clin Endocrinol.Metab 1998;83:685.

167. Tuttle RM et al. Treatment with propylthiouracil before radioactive iodine therapy is associated with a higher treatment failure rate than therapy with radioactive iodine alone in Graves' disease. Thyroid 1995;5:243.

168. Braga M et al. The effect of methimazole on cure rates after radioiodine treatment for Graves' hyperthyroidism: a randomized clinical trial. Thyroid 2002;12:135.

169. Bartalena L et al. Management of Graves' ophthalmopathy: reality and perspectives. Endocrinol Rev 2000;21:168.

170. Vestergaard P. Smoking and thyroid disorders-a meta-analysis. Eur J Endocrinol. 2002;146:153.

171. Wiersinga WM, Bartalena L. Epidemiology and prevention of Graves' ophthalmopathy. Thyroid 2002;12:855.

172. Fatourechi V. Medical treatment of Graves' opthalmopathy. Ophthalmol Clin North Am 2000;13:683.

173. Bartalena L et al. Relation between therapy for hyperthyroidism and the course of Graves' ophthalmopathy. N Engl J Med 1998;338:73.

174. Marcocci C et al. Relationship between Graves' ophthalmopathy and type of treatment of Graves' hyperthyroidism. Thyroid 1992;2:171.

175. Jongjaroenprasert W et al. Rectal administration of propylthiouracil in hyperthyroid patients: comparison of suspension enema and suppository form. Thyroid 2002;12:627.

176. Yeung SCJ et al. Rectal administration of iodide and propylthiouracil in the treatment of thyroid storm. Thyroid 1995;5:403.

177. Nabil N et al. Methimazole: an alternative route of administration. J Clin Endocrinol Metab 1982; 54:180.

178. McCowen KC et al. Elevated serum thyrotropin in thyroxine treated patients with hypothyroidism given sertraline [letter]. N Engl J Med 1997; 337:1010.

179. Lazarus JH. The effects of lithium on thyroid and thyrotropin-releasing hormone. Thyroid 1998;8:909.

180. Bocchetta A et al. Ten-year follow-up of thyroid function in lithium patients. J Clin Psychopharmacol 2001;21:594.

181. Kleiner J et al. Lithium-induced subclinical hypothyroidism: review of the literature and guidelines for treatment. J Clin Psychiatr 1999;60:249.

182. Barclay ML et al. Lithium associated thyrotoxicosis: a report of 14 cases, with statistical analysis of incidence. Clin Endocrinol 1994;40:759.

183. Dang AH, Hershman JM. Lithium-associated thyroiditis. Endocrinol Pract 2002;8:232.

184. Bogazzi F et al. Treatment with lithium prevents serum thyroid hormone increase after thioamide withdrawal and radioiodine therapy in patients with Graves' disease. J Clin Endocrinol Metab 2002;87:4490.

185. Koh LK et al. Interferon-alpha induced thyroid dysfunction: three clinical presentations and a review of the literature. Thyroid 1997;7:891.

186. Dalgard O et al. Thyroid dysfunction during treatment of chronic hepatitis C with interferon alpha: no association with either interferon dosage or efficacy of therapy. J Intern Med 2002;251:400.

187. Carella C et al. Long-term outcome of interferon-α-induced thyroid autoimmunity and prognostic influence of thyroid autoantibody pattern at the end of treatment. J Clin Endocrinol Metab 2001;86:1925.

188. Wong V et al. Thyrotoxicosis induced by alpha-interferon therapy in chronic viral hepatitis. Clin Endocrinol 2002;56:793.

189. Becker DV et al. Childhood thyroid cancer following the Chernobyl accident: a status report. Endocrinol Metab Clin North Am 1996;25:197.

190. U.S. Department of Health and Human Services. Potassium iodide as a thyroid blocking agent in radiation emergencies. *http://www.fda.gov/cder/guidance/index.htm*

191. Meier CA. Thyroid nodules: pathogenesis, diagnosis, and treatment. Baillieres Best Pract Res Clin Endocrinol Metab 2000;14:559.

192. Gharib HG, Mazzaferri EL. Thyroxine suppressive therapy in patients with nodular thyroid disease. Ann Intern Med 1998;128:386.

193. Wemeau JL et al. Effects of thyroid-stimulating hormone suppression with levothyroxine in reducing the volume of solitary thyroid nodules and improving extranodular nonpalpable changes: a randomized, double-blind, placebo-controlled trial by the French Thyroid Research Group. J Clin Endocrinol Metab 2002;87:4928.

194. Castro MR et al. Effectiveness of thyroid hormone suppressive therapy in benign solitary thyroid nodules: a meta-analysis. J Clin Endocrinol Metab 2002;87:4154.

195. Richter B et al. Pharmacotherapy for thyroid nodules. A systematic review and meta-analysis. Endocrinol Metab Clin North Am 2002;31:699.

196. Ladenson PW et al. Comparison of administration of recombinant human thyrotropin with withdrawal of thyroid hormone for radioactive iodine scanning in patients with thyroid carcinoma. N Engl J Med 1997;337:888.

CHAPTER 50

Diabetes Mellitus

Betsy A. Carlisle, Lisa A. Kroon, Mary Anne Koda-Kimble

A worldwide epidemic of diabetes mellitus is looming. The Centers for Disease Control and Prevention (CDC) predicts the national incidence of diabetes will rise by 37.5% by the year 2025 and by 170% in developing countries over the next 30 years. Of particular concern is the alarming increase in the prevalence of type 2 diabetes in both adults and children. In 2002, an estimated 18.2 million people, or 6.3% of the United States population, had diabetes. Of these, 5.2 million or about one-third were undiagnosed.[1] But there is good news. Clinical studies have affirmed that type 2 diabetes can be delayed or prevented in high-risk populations and that good glycemic control and other interventions can slow the devastating complications of diabetes. Nevertheless, broad implementation of guidelines and goals established by the American Diabetes Association and others has been slow.[2,3]

Definition, Classification, and Epidemiology

Diabetes is a syndrome that is caused by a relative or an absolute lack of insulin. Clinically, it is characterized by symptomatic glucose intolerance as well as alterations in lipid and protein metabolism. Over the long term, these metabolic abnormalities, particularly hyperglycemia, contribute to the development of complications such as retinopathy, nephropathy, and neuropathy.

Clinically, etiologically, and genetically, diabetes is a heterogeneous group of disorders. Nevertheless, most cases of diabetes mellitus can be assigned to type 1 or type 2 diabetes (described below). The term gestational diabetes mellitus (GDM) is used to describe glucose intolerance that has its onset during pregnancy, and glucose intolerance that cannot be ascribed to causes consistent with these three classifications are addressed more specifically (e.g. specific genetic defects in insulin action; drug-induced diabetes; pancreatic disease). Subclinical glucose intolerance or "prediabetes" is identified as impaired glucose tolerance (IGT) or impaired fasting glucose (IFG).

Approximately 5% to 10% of the diagnosed diabetic population has type 1 diabetes, which results from autoimmune destruction of the pancreatic β-cells. At clinical presentation, these patients have little or no pancreatic reserve, have a tendency to develop ketoacidosis, and require exogenous insulin to sustain life. The incidence of type 1 diabetes peaks during puberty between 10 and 14 years of age, although the age at onset ranges from 9 months to 28 years. Approximately 7.4% of adults who are diagnosed with diabetes between 30 and 74 years of age have type 1 diabetes. In these individuals, the rate of pancreatic destruction seems to occur more slowly, leading to a later onset and less acute presentation[4,5] (Table 50-1).

Most people with diabetes have type 2 diabetes, a heterogeneous disorder that is characterized by obesity, β-cell dysfunction, resistance to insulin action, and increased hepatic glucose production. Both the incidence and prevalence of diabetes increase dramatically with age. For example, the prevalence of self-reported diabetes is 1.1% among persons 20 to 39 years of age and 12.6% among persons 65 to 74 years of age.[6] The prevalence of type 2 diabetes differs among ethnic populations. Relative to caucasians, the prevalence of diagnosed and undiagnosed type 2 diabetes is higher in African Americans (1.6 times), Mexican Americans (1.9 times), and Native Americans.[7] Growth in the aging population as well as greater racial and ethnic diversity are causing predicted increases in the prevalence of diagnosed diabetes from 4.2% to 5.2% of the population by 2020.[8]

Diabetes is a serious condition that places people at risk for greater morbidity and mortality relative to the nondiabetic population. For example, compared with the general population, the mortality rate for people with type 1 diabetes is 5 to 12 times higher, and for adults with type 2 diabetes, it is two times higher. Morbidity also is greater for people with diabetes and is primarily related to acute and chronic complications associated with the condition.[9]

Medical management of persons with a diagnosis of diabetes is costly. In 2002, the annual per capita health care expenditures for people with diabetes were approximately 2.4 times higher than those for individuals without diabetes. In one study[8], 19% of total health care costs in the United States was incurred by people with diabetes, even though they

Table 50-1 Type 1 and Type 2 Diabetes

Characteristics	Type 1	Type 2
Other names	Previously, type I; insulin-dependent diabetes mellitus (IDDM); juvenile-onset diabetes mellitus	Previously, type II; non–insulin-dependent diabetes mellitus (NIDDM); adult onset diabetes mellitus
Percentage of diabetic population	5–10%	90%
Age at onset	Usually <30 yr; peaks at 12–14 yr; rare before 6 mo; some adults develop type 1 during the fifth decade	Usually >40 yr, but increasing prevalence among obese children
Pancreatic function	Usually none, although some residual C-peptide can sometimes be detected at diagnosis, especially in adults	Insulin present in low, "normal," or high amounts
Pathogenesis	Associated with certain HLA types; presence of islet cell antibodies suggests autoimmune process	Defect in insulin secretion; tissue resistance to insulin; ↑ hepatic glucose output
Family history	Generally not strong	Strong
Obesity	Uncommon unless "overinsulinized" with exogenous insulin	Common (60–90%)
History of ketoacidosis	Often present	Rare, except in circumstances of unusual stress (e.g., infection)
Clinical presentation	Moderate to severe symptoms that generally progress relatively rapidly (days to weeks): polyuria, polydipsia, fatigue, weight loss, ketoacidosis	Mild polyuria, fatigue; often diagnosed on routine physical or dental examination
Treatment	Insulin Diet Exercise	Diet Exercise Oral antidiabetic agents (α-glucosidase inhibitors, biguanides, non-sulfonylurea insulin secretagogues, sulfonylureas, thiazolidinediones) Insulin

HLA, human leukocyte antigen.

represent only 4% of the population. Hospital costs, nursing home care, physician visits, and medicines made up the majority of these expenditures. Because many expenditures are related to treatment of long-term complications, considerable effort has been directed toward early diagnosis and metabolic control of patients with diabetes.

Carbohydrate Metabolism

An understanding of the signs and symptoms associated with diabetes is based on a knowledge of glucose metabolism and the metabolic effects of insulin in diabetic and nondiabetic subjects during the fed (postprandial) and fasting (postabsorptive) states.[10] Homeostatic mechanisms maintain plasma glucose concentrations between 55 and 140 mg/dL (3.1 to 7.8 mmol/L). A minimum concentration of 40 to 60 mg/dL (2.2 to 3.3 mmol/L) is required to provide adequate fuel for the central nervous system (CNS), which uses glucose as its primary energy source and is independent of insulin for glucose utilization. When blood glucose concentrations exceed the reabsorptive capacity of the kidneys (approximately 180 mg/dL), glucose spills into the urine resulting in a loss of calories and water. Muscle and fat also use glucose as a major source of energy, but these tissues require insulin for glucose uptake. If glucose is unavailable, these tissues are able to use other substrates such as amino acids and fatty acids for fuel.

Postprandial Glucose Metabolism in the Nondiabetic Individual

After food is ingested, blood glucose concentrations rise and stimulate insulin release. Insulin is the key to efficient glucose utilization. It promotes the uptake of glucose, fatty acids, and amino acids as well as their conversion to storage forms in most tissues. In muscle, insulin promotes the uptake of glucose and its storage as glycogen. It also stimulates the uptake of amino acids and their conversion to protein. In adipose tissue, glucose is converted to free fatty acids and stored as triglycerides. Insulin also prevents a breakdown of these triglycerides to free fatty acids, a form that may be transported to other tissues for utilization. The liver does not require insulin for glucose transport, but insulin facilitates the conversion of glucose to glycogen and free fatty acids. The latter are esterified to triglycerides, which are transported by very-low-density lipoproteins (VLDL) to adipose and muscle tissue.

Fasting Glucose Metabolism in the Nondiabetic Individual

As blood glucose concentrations drop toward normal during the fasting state, insulin release is inhibited. Simultaneously, a number of counter-regulatory hormones that oppose the effect of insulin and promote an increase in blood sugar are released (e.g., glucagon, epinephrine, growth hormone, glucocorticoids). As a result, several processes maintain a minimum blood glucose concentration for the CNS. Glycogen in the liver is broken down into glucose (glycogenolysis); amino acids are transported from muscle to liver, where they are converted to glucose through gluconeogenesis; uptake of glucose by insulin-dependent tissues is diminished to conserve glucose for the brain; and finally, triglycerides are broken down into free fatty acids, which are used as alternative fuel sources.

Type 1 Diabetes
Pathogenesis[11]

The loss of insulin secretion in type 1 diabetes mellitus results from autoimmune destruction of the insulin-producing β-cells in the pancreas, which is thought to be triggered by environmental factors, such as viruses or toxins, in genetically susceptible individuals. This form of diabetes is associated closely with histocompatibility antigens (HLA-DR3 or HLA-DR4) and the presence of circulating insulin and islet cell antibodies (ICAs). The capacity of normal pancreatic β-cells to secrete insulin far exceeds the normal amounts needed to control carbohydrate, fat, and protein metabolism. As a result, the clinical onset of type 1 diabetes is preceded by an extensive asymptomatic period during which β-cells are destroyed (Fig. 50-1). β-Cell destruction may occur rapidly but is more likely to take place over a period of weeks, months, or even years. The earliest detectable abnormality in insulin secretion is a progressive reduction of immediate or *first-phase* plasma insulin response. However, this initial impairment has few detrimental effects on overall glucose homeostasis, and plasma glucose concentrations remain normal. Most affected individuals have circulating antibodies to islet cells or to their own insulin at this stage of the disease. These represent markers of an ongoing autoimmune process that culminates in type 1 diabetes. Fasting hyperglycemia occurs when β-cell mass is reduced by 80% to 90%. Initially, only postprandial hyperglycemia occurs, but as insulin secretion becomes further compromised, progressive fasting hyperglycemia is seen.

On presentation, approximately 65% to 85% of patients have circulating antibodies directed against islet cells and 20% to 60% of patients have measurable antibodies directed

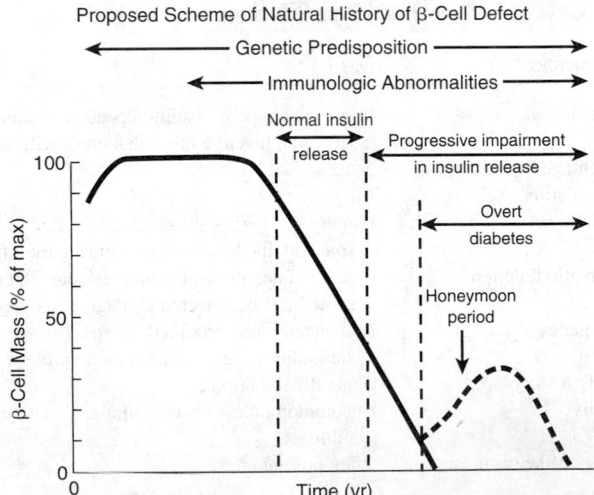

Timing of trigger in relation to immunologic abnormalities is unknown. Note that overt diabetes is not apparent until insulin secretory reserves are <10–20% of normal.

FIGURE 50-1 Pathogenesis of type 1 diabetes. In an individual with a genetic predisposition, an event (such as a virus or toxin) triggers autoimmune destruction of the pancreatic β-cells, probably over a period of several years. When the number of β-cells diminishes to approximately 250,000, the pancreas is unable to secrete sufficient insulin and intolerance to glucose ensues. At this point, a stressful event, such as a viral infection, can produce acute symptoms of hyperglycemia and ketoacidosis. Once the acute event has passed, the pancreas temporarily recovers, leading to a remission (honeymoon period). Continued destruction of the β-cell ultimately leads to an insulin-dependent state.

against insulin. Within 8 to 10 years following clinical presentation, β-cell loss is complete and insulin deficiency is absolute. Circulating ICAs can no longer be detected.

Clinical Presentation

Although the onset of type 1 diabetes appears to be abrupt, evidence now exists for an extended *preclinical period* that can precede obvious symptoms by several years. As insulin secretion becomes compromised, progressive fasting hyperglycemia occurs. When plasma glucose concentrations exceed the normal renal threshold of approximately 180 mg/dL (10 mmol/L), glucosuria results in an osmotic diuresis, producing the classic symptoms of polyuria with compensatory polydipsia. If symptoms are untreated, weight loss occurs as glucose calories are lost in the urine and body fat and protein stores are broken down owing to increased rates of lipolysis and proteolysis. Muscle begins to metabolize its own glycogen stores and fatty acids for fuel, and the liver begins to metabolize free fatty acids that are released in response to epinephrine and low insulin concentrations. An absolute lack of insulin may cause excessive mobilization of free fatty acids to the liver, where they are metabolized to ketones. This can result in ketonemia, ketonuria, and, ultimately, ketoacidosis. Patients present with complaints of fatigue, significant weight loss, polyuria, and polydipsia. A significant elevation in glycosylated hemoglobin confirms weeks or months of preceding hyperglycemia.

Because glucose provides an excellent medium for microorganisms, patients may present also with recurrent respiratory, vaginal, and other infections. Patients also may experience blurred vision secondary to osmotically induced changes in the lens of the eye. Treatment with insulin is essential to prevent severe dehydration, ketoacidosis, and death.

Honeymoon Period

Within days or weeks after the initial diagnosis, many patients with type 1 diabetes experience an apparent remission, which is reflected by decreased blood glucose concentrations and markedly decreased insulin requirements. This is called the *honeymoon period* because it may last for only a few weeks to months. Once hyperglycemia, metabolic acidosis, and ketosis resolve, endogenous insulin secretion recovers temporarily (see Fig. 50-1). Although the honeymoon period may last for up to a year, increasing exogenous insulin requirements are inevitable and should be anticipated. During this time, patients should be maintained on insulin even if the dose is very low, because interrupted treatment is associated with a greater incidence of resistance and allergy to insulin (see Question 25).

Type 2 Diabetes

Pathogenesis: Metabolic Syndrome (Insulin Resistance Syndrome, Syndrome X)

Impaired insulin secretion and resistance to the action of insulin, rather than an absolute insulin deficiency, characterize patients with type 2 diabetes. In the presence of insulin resistance, glucose utilization by tissues is impaired, hepatic glucose output or production is increased, and excess glucose accumulates in the circulation. This hyperglycemia stimulates the pancreas to produce more insulin in an effort to overcome the insulin resistance. The simultaneous elevation of both glucose and insulin is strongly suggestive of insulin resistance.

Type 2 diabetes is associated with a variety of disorders, including obesity, atherosclerosis, hyperlipidemia, and hypertension (Fig. 50-2). Dr. Gerald Reaven, who refers to this association as *syndrome X, insulin resistance syndrome, or metabolic syndrome,* proposed that either the insulin resistance itself, or the compensatory hyperinsulinemia that results from insulin resistance, may be the fundamental underlying pathophysiologic process responsible for the frequent occurrence of these conditions in the same patient.[12] However, the concept of a single defect explaining this cluster of disorders is the subject of considerable debate and research activity. Genetic as well as environmental factors such as central obesity, sedentary lifestyles, and ingestion of calorically dense foods contribute to the development of insulin resistance. Metabolic syndrome is common in the United States, and because it is highly correlated with cardiovascular events, the National Cholesterol Education Program (NCEP) has suggested criteria for its diagnosis and treatment to prevent cardiovascular events and diabetes.[13] The estimated prevalence of metabolic syndrome in adults >20 years old is >20% and >40% in adults 60 to 69 years of age.[14] Not all individuals with metabolic syndrome progress to IGT or diabetes, but those who do

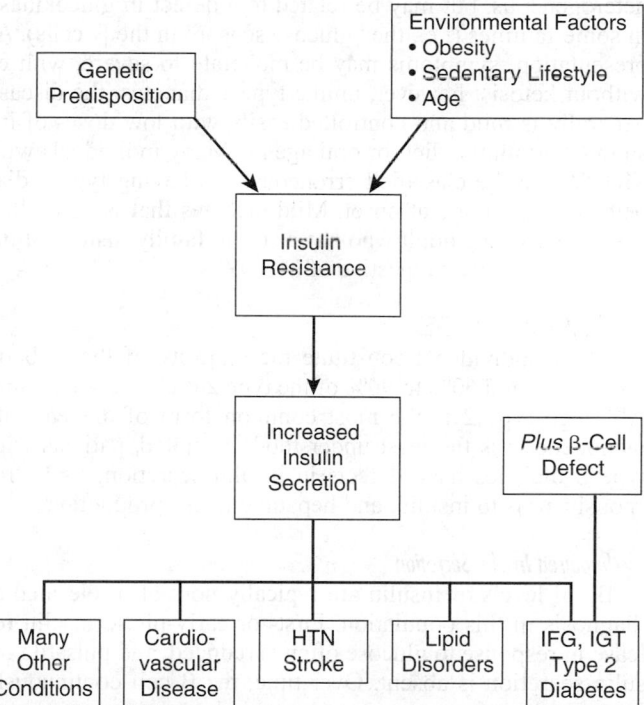

FIGURE 50-2 Metabolic syndrome (insulin resistance syndrome, syndrome X). Genetic and environmental factors (visceral obesity, sedentary lifestyle, aging) predispose some individuals to insulin resistance. To overcome the resistance, the pancreas secretes more insulin, leading to hyperinsulinemia. People with insulin resistance and hyperinsulinemia commonly develop a cluster of medical problems and biochemical abnormalities: cardiovascular disease, hypertension, dyslipidemia, hyperuricemia, and type 2 diabetes mellitus. Only those individuals who are further genetically predisposed to β-cell failure go on to develop impaired glucose tolerance and diabetes mellitus. Many people with type 2 diabetes already have evidence of cardiovascular disease at the time of diabetes diagnosis. The cause-and-effect-relationships between insulin resistance and/or hyperinsulinemia and these clinical conditions has not been clarified. See text for expanded discussion. DM, diabetes mellitus; HTN, hypertension; IFG, impaired fasting glucose; IGT, impaired glucose tolerance.

may be genetically predisposed to β-cell failure. People with type 2 diabetes have a stronger family history of diabetes than do those with type 1 diabetes. Circulating ICAs are absent, and there is no association with human lymphocyte antigen (HLA) types.[5,15]

Patients with type 2 diabetes exhibit varying degrees of tissue resistance to insulin, impaired insulin secretion, and increased basal hepatic glucose production. Subclassifications of these patients have been suggested based on weight, age of onset, and insulin levels. The most commonly used division of this class of diabetic patients is based on weight or age at diagnosis.

NONOBESE TYPE 2 DIABETES

This group comprises approximately 10% of the type 2 diabetic population. Typically, they develop a mild form of diabetes during childhood, adolescence, or as young adults (usually before age 25), and their insulin levels are low in response to a glucose challenge. Included in this group are patients who may actually have late-onset type 1 diabetes[16] or maturity-onset diabetes of the young (MODY).[5] This form of diabetes is associated with a strong family history that suggests an autosomal-dominant transmission. The underlying defect is heterogeneous, but may be related to a defect in glucokinase in some families (i.e., the "glucose sensor" in the β-cells). At presentation, symptoms may be moderate to severe, with or without ketosis; however, unlike type 1 diabetes, the disease generally is mild and controlled easily with low doses of insulin (<40 units), diet, or oral agents. Many individuals with MODY may be classified erroneously as having type 1 diabetes based on age at onset. Mild diabetes that is controlled easily in a young adult who has a strong family history of diabetes is strongly suggestive of MODY.

OBESE TYPE 2 DIABETES

Obese individuals constitute the majority of the diabetic population and 60% to 90% of the type 2 diabetic population. Although type 2 is the most common form of diabetes, its pathogenesis is the least understood. As noted, patients with type 2 diabetes have defects in insulin secretion, tissue responsiveness to insulin, and hepatic glucose production.[5]

Impaired Insulin Secretion

Basal levels of insulin are typically normal or elevated at diagnosis in this population. First- or early-phase insulin release in response to glucose often is reduced, and pulsatile insulin secretion is absent. Over time, the β cell continuously loses its ability to respond to elevated glucose concentrations, leading to increasing loss of glucose control. In a large cohort of newly diagnosed type 2 patients randomly assigned to various treatments, A_{1C} deteriorated at the rate of 0.2% to 0.3% per year.[22] In patients with severe hyperglycemia, the amount of insulin secreted in response to glucose is diminished (glucose toxicity).

Tissue Resistance

Most patients also exhibit decreased tissue responsiveness to insulin. Increasing evidence suggests that decreased peripheral glucose uptake and utilization in muscle is the primary site of insulin resistance and results in prolonged postprandial hyperglycemia. Resistance may be secondary to decreased numbers of insulin receptors on the cell surface, decreased affinity of receptors for insulin, or defects in insulin signaling and action that follows receptor binding. Defects in insulin signaling and action are referred to as *postreceptor* or *postbinding* defects and are likely to be the primary sites of insulin resistance. The precise nature of these defects is the focus of intense research.

Hepatic Glucose Production

Most people with type 2 diabetes also exhibit increased hepatic glucose production (glycogenolysis and gluconeogenesis), which is reflected by an elevated fasting plasma or blood glucose concentration. As noted previously, hepatic glucose production is the primary source of glucose in the fasting state. Because insulin normally suppresses hepatic glucose production, this phenomenon reflects decreased responsiveness of the liver to this action.

One can imagine the following scenario in a person genetically prone to insulin resistance and diabetes. Overeating stimulates secretion of large amounts of insulin. This hyperinsulinemia, in turn, promotes lipogenesis and downregulates, or decreases, the number of insulin receptors on the surface of the target organ. This leads to insulin resistance and, when the pancreas is unable to secrete sufficient insulin to overcome tissue resistance, hyperglycemia. High-glucose concentrations are toxic to the β-cells and peripheral tissues, leading to further deterioration of insulin secretion and resistance to insulin action. Thus, the obese patient with diabetes often is in a vicious cycle that can be broken only through decreased caloric intake, weight loss, and exercise.

Clinical Presentation

Type 2 diabetes is typically diagnosed incidentally during a routine physical examination or when the patient seeks attention for another complaint. This is because symptoms are so mild and their onset so gradual that they can easily be "explained away." When giving a history of their illness, people with type 2 diabetes acknowledge fatigue, polyuria, and polydipsia. Because these patients have sufficient insulin concentrations to prevent lipolysis, there is usually no history of ketosis except in situations of unusual stress (e.g., infections, trauma). Furthermore, weight loss is uncommon in these individuals because relatively high endogenous insulin levels promote lipogenesis. Commonly, macrovascular disease is evident at the time of diagnosis; occasionally, microvascular complications that suggest the presence of undiagnosed or subclinical diabetes for 7 to 10 years are evident as well. Because type 2 diabetes patients retain some pancreatic reserve at the time of diagnosis, they generally can be treated with diet, exercise, and oral antidiabetic medications for several years. Nevertheless, many eventually require insulin for control of their symptoms.

Gestational Diabetes Mellitus

Gestational diabetes mellitus (GDM) affects about 7% of all pregnancies and is defined as "any carbohydrate intolerance with onset or first recognition during pregnancy."[5,17] The onset of diabetes during pregnancy and its duration affect the prognosis for a good obstetric and perinatal outcome. See Chapter 46, Obstetrics.

Diagnosis

Diagnostic Criteria

In 1997, the diagnostic criteria for diabetes mellitus were modified by an Expert Committee of the American Diabetes Association (Table 50-2).[5,18] For nonpregnant individuals of any age, a diagnosis of diabetes can be made when one of the following is present:

1. Classic signs and symptoms of diabetes (polyuria, polydipsia, ketonuria, and rapid weight loss) combined with a random plasma glucose ≥200 mg/dL.
2. A fasting plasma glucose (FPG) ≥126 mg/dL.
3. Following a standard oral glucose challenge (75 g glucose for an adult or 1.75 g/kg for a child), the venous plasma glucose concentration is ≥200 mg/dL at 2 hours and >200 mg/dL at least one other time during the test (0.5, 1, 1.5 hours); this is the oral glucose tolerance test (OGTT).

The diagnosis must be confirmed on a subsequent day by any one of the aforementioned conditions in the absence of unequivocal hyperglycemia with acute metabolic complications.

Individuals with FPG values or OGTT values that are intermediate between normal and those considered diagnostic of diabetes are considered to have *IFG* or *IGT*. These individuals are not given the diagnosis of diabetes because of broad social, psychological, and economic implications. The categories of FPG values are as follows:

1. A normal FPG is <100 mg/dL. In 2003, this value was lowered from 110 mg/dL.[18]
2. An FPG 100–125 mg/dL is IFG.
3. An FPG ≥126 mg/dL indicates a *provisional* diagnosis of diabetes that must be confirmed, as described previously.

The corresponding categories when the OGTT is used for diagnosis are as follows:

1. A 2-hour postload glucose (2-hPG) <140 mg/dL indicates normal glucose tolerance.
2. A 2-hPG ≥140 mg/dL and <200 mg/dL indicates IGT.
3. A 2-hPG ≥200 mg/dL indicates a *provisional* diagnosis of diabetes, which must be confirmed by a second test.

Many factors can impair glucose tolerance or increase plasma glucose, and these must be excluded before a firm diagnosis of diabetes is made. For example, an individual who has not fasted for a minimum of 8 hours may have an elevated FPG; one who has fasted too long (>16 hours) or has ingested insufficient carbohydrates before testing may have an IGT. Patients who are tested for glucose tolerance during, or soon after, an acute illness (e.g., a myocardial infarction [MI]) may be misdiagnosed because of the presence of high concentrations of counter-regulatory hormones that increase glucose concentrations; glucose tolerance often returns to normal in these individuals. Pregnancy, many forms of stress, and lack of physical activity can affect the glucose tolerance similarly. Many drugs may alter glucose tolerance due to their effects on insulin release and tissue response to insulin, as well as through direct cytotoxic effects on the pancreas. These are discussed in more detail later in this chapter. Drugs and other chemicals also may falsely elevate the plasma glucose concentrations through interference with specific analytic methods.

Type 1 or Type 2 Diabetes Mellitus?

At times it may be difficult to classify patients as having type 1 or type 2 diabetes mellitus. Generally, if a patient is younger than 30 years of age, is lean, and has signs and symptoms of diabetes mellitus combined with an elevated FPG, type 1 diabetes is likely and the patient should be treated with insulin. Although the presence of moderate ketonuria with hyperglycemia in an otherwise unstressed patient strongly supports the diagnosis of type 1 diabetes, its absence is not of diagnostic value. However, relatively lean older adults initially presenting with what appears to be type 2 diabetes because they are responsive to oral agents or low doses of insulin may be discovered subsequently as having type 1 diabetes. The presence of antibodies to islet cell components may indicate the need for eventual insulin therapy.[16] Conversely, clinicians are beginning to observe more cases of type 2 diabetes in obese children.[19] Presently, 8% to 45% of children with newly diagnosed diabetes have type 2 disease. These clinical observations explain why the medical community is abandoning the terms *adult-onset diabetes, youth-onset diabetes,* and *non–insulin-dependent diabetes mellitus.*

Long-Term Complications and Their Relation to Glucose Control

The longer-term sequelae of diabetes account for most of the morbidity and mortality in the diabetic population. The management of selected complications of diabetes mellitus is considered later in this chapter. Here, we simply provide an

Table 50-2	Normal and Diabetic Plasma*a* Glucose Levels in mg/dL (mmol/L) for the Oral Glucose Tolerance Test		
	Fasting	*½, 1, 1½ hr*	*2 hr*
Normal	<100 (5.6)	<200 (11)	<140 (7.8)
Impaired glucose tolerance	<126 (7.0)	≥200 (11)	140–200 (7.8–11)
Impaired fasting glucose	100–125 (6.1–7.0)		
Diabetes (nonpregnant adult)	≥126 (7.0)	≥200 (11)	≥200 (11)

*a*Equivalent *venous whole blood* glucose concentrations are approximately 12% to 15% lower. *Arterial* samples are higher than venous samples postprandially because glucose has not yet been removed from peripheral tissues. *Capillary whole blood* samples contain a mixture of arterial and venous blood. Fasting levels will be equivalent to whole blood venous samples. One hour after a 100-g glucose load, capillary samples may be 30 to 40 mg/dL higher than venous samples.

overview of the types of complications that typically develop in people with type 1 and type 2 diabetes. Complications are typically assigned to macrovascular or microvascular complications. Diabetes mellitus is one of many risk factors for macrovascular disease (cardiovascular disease, stroke, peripheral vascular disease), but these risk factors tend to cluster in people prone to type 2 diabetes. As discussed more fully in subsequent sections, glucose toxicity appears to contribute most to the development and progression of microvascular complications, which include retinopathy, nephropathy, and neuropathy. However, epidemiologic studies also show a general relationship between degree of glucose control and risk for cardiovascular events.[20] Thus, the primary goal for both type 1 and type 2 diabetic individuals is to bring glucose concentrations as close to normal values as possible.

Results of the Diabetes Complications and Control Trial (DCCT) definitively established that intensive treatment of type 1 diabetes can prevent or slow the onset of long-term diabetes complications, including retinopathy, nephropathy, and neuropathy.[21] The DCCT was a multicenter, randomized study of 1,441 newly diagnosed type 1 diabetic patients ages 13 to 39 years that was designed to determine whether the complications of diabetes could be reduced or prevented with intensive insulin therapy aimed at achieving euglycemia. Patients were randomized to receive conventional or intensive insulin therapy and were followed for a mean of 6.5 years. Patients in the conventional treatment group received one to two insulin injections per day, performed daily blood glucose monitoring, and returned to clinic every 3 months. Patients in the intensive treatment group were initiated on insulin in the hospital. They were given three or more insulin injections per day or used an insulin pump. They performed blood glucose tests four or more times per day and had weekly to monthly clinic visits. A health care team provided extensive education and coaching to the intensively treated group throughout the study.

Intensive treatment reduced the risk of clinically meaningful retinopathy, nephropathy, and neuropathy by approximately 60%. Thus, patients treated with intensive therapy experienced a significant decrease in the incidence of long-term microvascular complications.

The effect of tight blood glucose control on the cardiovascular and microvascular complications of type 2 diabetes was addressed by the United Kingdom Prospective Diabetes Study (UKPDS).[22] Over a 10-year period, 3,867 newly diagnosed type 2 diabetics without complications were randomly assigned to an intensive treatment group using a sulfonylurea (glipizide, chlorpropamide, or glyburide) or insulin or metformin (if obese), or to a conventional treatment group using diet. The goal for the intensive treatment group was a FPG <108 mg/dL versus a FPG <270 mg/dL in the conventional treatment group. Drug therapy could be added in the diet-treated group if hyperglycemic symptoms occurred or to attain a FPG <270 mg/dL. Endpoints included diabetes-related complications, diabetes-related deaths, and all-cause mortality.

Hemoglobin A_{1c} (A_{1c}) values were 7.0% in the intensive treatment group versus 7.9% in the conventional group. There were no differences in A_{1c} values among the treatment arms in the intensive treatment group. By the end of the study, 80% of patients in the diet group required pharmacologic therapy to meet treatment goals, and investigators were unable to maintain the intensive treatment goal with monotherapy or a single daily dose of ultralente insulin. Consequently, many patients eventually were treated with combination therapy. Using an intent-to-treat analysis in the intensive treatment group, the risk of diabetes-related endpoints was 12% lower ($P < .0029$), diabetes-related death was 10% lower ($P < .34$), and all-cause mortality was 6% lower ($P < .44$) compared with conventional therapy. The risk of hypoglycemia and weight gain was significantly higher in the intensive treatment group. (*Note:* metformin analysis was the subject of a separate study.)

The overall microvascular complication rate was decreased by 25% in the intensive treatment group. Epidemiologic analysis of the data from UKPDS demonstrated a continuous relationship between the risks of microvascular complications and glycemia, such that for every percentage point reduction in A_{1c}, there was a 35% reduction in the risk of complications. Whether intensive therapy designed to attain sustained normoglycemia decreases the risk of macrovascular disease was less clear. In the UKPDS, a 16% reduction in the risk of combined fatal or nonfatal MI and sudden death was observed, which failed to reach statistical significance ($P = .052$). This issue is discussed more fully in Question 46.

Other studies support the use of a more comprehensive approach to preventing microvascular and macrovascular complications in patients with type 2 diabetes, especially since coronary heart disease is the leading cause of premature death in this group. In a UKPDS group substudy, tight blood control (<130/85 mm Hg) reduced the risk of stroke by 44% ($P = .013$) and microvascular endpoints by 37% ($P = .0092$).[22] The Steno group found that multifactorial intensive treatment of patients with type 2 diabetes and microalbuminura for a mean of 7.8 years reduced by 50% the risk of cardiovascular and microvascular events compared with patients treated conventionally according to Danish guidelines. Their interventions included lifestyle education and aggressive use of drugs to achieve a lower blood pressure, A_{1c}, and a normal lipid profile.[23] See Table 50-11 for the components of intensive insulin therapy.

Screening for Type 2 Diabetes

The ADA advises against routine screening for type 2 diabetes outside of the health care setting because of the low likelihood of follow-up care and testing in the case of both negative and positive results. The FPG is the preferred over the OGTT as a screening test based on cost and convenience. People age ≥45 years, particularly overweight individuals (BMI ≥25 kg/m²) should be tested every 3 years, but younger patients may be tested more frequently if they are overweight and have one or more other risk factors: family history of diabetes, sedentary lifestyle, ethnic predisposition, previous IFG or IGT, history of gestational diabetes or macrosomia, hypertension, dyslipidemia (high-density lipoprotein [HDL] cholesterol ≤35 mg/dL and triglycerides ≥250 mg/dL), history of polycystic ovary syndrome or vascular disease.[24]

Prevention of Type 1 and Type 2 Diabetes Mellitus

Because the clinical symptoms of type 1 diabetes mellitus are the overt expression of an insidious pathogenic process that begins years earlier, investigators are focusing attention on strategies that alter the natural history of the disease (see Fig. 50-1). First-degree relatives of individuals with type 1 diabetes mellitus have an increased risk for developing the diabetes and can be identified by the presence of immune markers that may herald the disease by many years.[25] This has led to attempts at immune intervention at the prediabetes stage with such drugs as nicotinamide and low doses of insulin, but neither was found to delay or prevent diabetes.[26–28] In contrast, treatment of newly diagnosed diabetes with agents that modify cytotoxic T-cells may slow pancreatic destruction and progression of diabetes.[29]

In addition to the 18.2 million people in the United States with diagnosed and undiagnosed type 2 diabetes, an additional 20.1 million Americans have prediabetes (IGT or IFG).[1] The annual risk of progression to type 2 diabetes mellitus in persons with IGT is 1% to 5%.[7] Persons at risk for IGT and who are eligible for further screening include those who are overweight, those who have a family history of diabetes, individuals who have a history of gestational diabetes or who have delivered a baby >9 lb, and those with a medical history of a high blood glucose test without a diagnosis of diabetes.

The Diabetes Prevention Program Research Group (DPP) studied people at high risk for developing diabetes to determine if lifestyle interventions or metformin would prevent or delay the onset of type 2 diabetes.[30] Subjects were at least 25 years old, overweight (BMI ≥24), and had a FPG of 95 to 125 mg/dL and a plasma glucose of 140 to 199 mg/dL 2 hours following a 75-g oral glucose tolerance test. Efforts were made to enroll a diverse population with regard to ethnicity, age, and history of gestational diabetes. Participants were randomly assigned to one of three interventions:

1. *Intensive lifestyle intervention:* This group received an intensive diet and exercise program (150 minutes/week) aimed at achieving and maintaining a 7% weight loss.
2. *Metformin 850 mg BID with standard diet and exercise:* The antihyperglycemic biguanide, metformin, was selected because it improves the metabolic abnormalities that accompany obesity and IGT.[31] This group also received standard advice regarding the benefits of a healthy diet and exercise.
3. *Standard therapy:* This group was given a placebo for metformin and received standard advice on the benefits of a healthy diet and exercise.

Results of the study were dramatic, leading to its early closure. Relative to the placebo group, the incidence of diabetes was reduced by 58% and 31% in the intensive lifestyle and metformin groups, respectively. The incidence rates for the three groups were 4.8, 7.8, and 11.0 cases per 100 person-years, respectively. A repeat oral glucose tolerance test was performed in the metformin group who had not developed diabetes 1 to 2 weeks after the drug had been discontinued to determine whether the drug simply masked diabetes through its antihyperglycemic effects. The incidence of diabetes was still reduced by 25% relative to the placebo group.[32] Other studies have confirmed the value of lifestyle intervention[33] and other drugs (acarbose, troglitazone) in the prevention of type 2 diabetes.[34,35]

Treatment

There are three major components to the treatment of diabetes: diet, drugs (insulin and oral hypoglycemic or antihy-

perglycemic agents), and exercise. Each of these components interacts with the others to the extent that no assessment and modification of one can be made without knowledge of the other two. Target blood glucose values for pregnant diabetics are very strict.

Medical Nutrition Therapy
PRINCIPLES
Medical nutrition therapy plays a crucial role in the therapy of all individuals with diabetes. Unfortunately, patient acceptance and adherence to diet is often poor, but revised recommendations that are evidence based and more flexible than previous approaches offer new opportunities to increase the effectiveness of nutrition therapy.[36]

Nutrition therapy is designed to help patients achieve appropriate metabolic and physiologic goals (e.g., glucose, lipids, blood pressure, proteinuria, weight), select healthy foods, and to take into consideration personal and cultural preferences. Appropriate levels and types of physical activity to achieve a healthier status are incorporated into the prescription.

NUTRITION THERAPY AND TYPE 1 DIABETES MELLITUS
For patients with type 1 diabetes taking fixed doses of insulin, a meal plan is designed to provide adequate carbohydrates timed to match the peak action of exogenously administered insulin. Regularly scheduled meals and snacks are required to prevent hypoglycemic reactions. Fortunately, newer insulins and insulin regimens provide much more flexibility in the amount and timing of food intake. Now, patients who are taught to "count carbohydrates" can inject rapid- or short-acting insulin doses designed to match their anticipated intake. Integration of food intake, physical activity, and insulin dose is critical and discussed extensively in the cases that follow.

NUTRITION THERAPY AND TYPE 2 DIABETES MELLITUS
For patients with type 2 diabetes, meal plans emphasize normalizing plasma glucose and lipid levels as well as maintaining a normal blood pressure (BP) to prevent or mitigate cardiovascular morbidity. Although weight loss reduces insulin resistance and improves glycemic control, traditional dietary strategies incorporating hypocaloric diets have not been effective in achieving long-term weight loss. A sustainable weight loss of 5% to 7% can be achieved within structured programs that emphasize lifestyle changes, physical activity, and food intake that modestly reduces caloric and fat intake. Tables 50-3 and 50-4 describe how to calculate the desirable body weight and estimate maintenance-calorie requirements for adults.

SPECIFIC NUTRITION COMPONENTS
Medical nutrition therapy is a critical component of diabetes care. For a more extensive discussion of the principles underlying nutrition therapy, the reader is directed to other sources.[36,37] A few key principles are briefly noted below because they are the common source of misunderstanding.

Carbohydrates and Artificial Sweeteners
Carbohydrates include sugar, starch, and fiber and they are liberally incorporated into the diet of a person with diabetes. In fact, the amount of dietary carbohydrate (CHO) is the main

Table 50-3   Estimating Ideal Body Weight[a]

1. Obtain height and weight.
2. Determine body frame (small, medium, or large).
3. Calculate ideal body weight:
   - Female: 100 lb (45 kg) for first 5 ft plus 5 lb (2.3 kg) for every inch over 5 ft
   - Male: 106 lb (48 kg) for first 5 ft plus 6 lb (2.7 kg) for each inch over 5 ft

Add 10% for large frame or subtract 10% for small frame

---

[a]The term *reasonable body weight* also is used. Reasonable body weight is defined as a weight that is achievable and maintainable for the patient, which may not be in the range considered desirable. Any weight loss, even 10 to 20 lb may dramatically improve glycemic control. Weight goals should always be individualized.
Adapted from reference 36.

Table 50-4   Determining Caloric Needs

1. Determine basal energy expenditure (BEE) using the Harris-Benedict equation[299]:
   - Female: $655 + (9.6 \times$ weight [kg]$) + (1.9 \times$ height [cm]$) - (4.7 \times$ age$)$
   - Male: $66 + (13.7 \times$ weight [kg]$) + (5 \times$ height [cm]$) - (6.8 \times$ age$)$
2. Select appropriate activity factor:
   - Sedentary: multiply by 1.3
   - Moderately active: multiply by 1.45
   - Heavily active: multiply by 1.6
3. Caloric needs = BEE × activity factor
4. For weight gain, add 500 calories to gain 1 lb/week. To lose weight, subtract 500 calories.

determinant of insulin demand and is commonly used to determine the pre-meal insulin dose. Furthermore, patients using fixed doses of insulin or oral hypoglycemic agents must eat meals containing consistent amounts of carbohydrate to avoid hypoglycemia. Avoiding "sugar" or *sucrose* does not prevent "sugar diabetes." Since isocaloric amounts of sucrose and starch produce the same degree glycemia, sucrose can be substituted for a portion of the total CHO intake and should be incorporated into an otherwise healthful diet.

Whole grains, fruits, and vegetables high in *fiber* are recommended for people with diabetes as they are for the general population. There is no evidence that larger amounts produce a differential metabolic benefit with regard to plasma glucose and lipid levels. *Nonnutritive sweeteners* (saccharin, aspartame, acesulfame potassium, sucralose) have been rigorously tested by the FDA for safety in people with diabetes and are safe at approved daily intakes. *Nutritive sweeteners* (sorbitol and fructose) produce lower postprandial glucose responses than sucrose, glucose, and starch. However, patients should be advised that when these sweeteners are used in foods labeled "dietetic," they still provide substantial calories. Furthermore, excessive intake of sorbitol-sweetened foods (e.g., 30 to 50 g/day) can induce an osmotic diarrhea, and excessive amounts of fructose can increase total and low-density lipoprotein (LDL) cholesterol.

Counting Carbohydrates

When patients are taught to estimate the grams of carbohydrate in a meal they are given the following guideline: One carbohydrate serving = 1 starch or 1 fruit or 1 milk = 15 g

carbohydrate. Patients vary with regard to their insulin:CHO ratio throughout time and throughout the day; however, a typical starting point is 1 unit/15 g CHO. Examples of one carbohydrate serving include 1 slice bread, ¼ bagel, ½ English muffin or hamburger bun, ¾ c dry cereal, ½ c cooked cereal, ½ c legumes, ⅓ c pasta or rice, ¼ large baked potato, 4 c popcorn, 1 small fruit, ½ fruit juice, 1 c milk, ½ c ice cream, 2 small cookies.

Fat

Cardiovascular disease is a major cause of morbidity and mortality in patients with diabetes. Therefore, a reduced fat diet (<30% of the total calories) with <10% of calories from saturated fats and <10% from polyunsaturated fats is recommended. The recommended cholesterol intake is <300 mg/day for patients with diabetes who have normal plasma cholesterol concentrations. For patients with elevated LDL cholesterol (≥100 mg/dL), <7% of total calories should be from saturated fat, and cholesterol intake should be restricted to <200 mg/day. These guidelines are consistent with those of the National Cholesterol Education Program.[13]

Protein

Data are insufficient to support special dietary protein recommendations for persons with diabetes if kidney function is normal. Generally, 15% to 20% of the daily caloric intake comes from animal and vegetable protein sources in the U.S. diet. This amount may be liberalized in pregnant and lactating women or in elderly people. With the onset of nephropathy, a lower protein intake of 0.8 g/kg per day is considered sufficiently restrictive.[36]

Sodium

The ADA has no particular restrictions on sodium intake, but recommends individualizing amounts based on the patient's sensitivity to salt and concurrent conditions such as hypertension or nephropathy. In general, sodium intake should be limited to <2,400 mg/day (or 6,000 mg NaCl).

Alcohol

The ADA's recommendation for alcohol is consistent with general recommendations of no more than two drinks per day for men or one drink/day for women. A drink is equivalent to 12 oz beer, 5 oz wine, or 1 oz distilled spirits. Nevertheless, its caloric contribution must be considered (1 alcoholic beverage = 2 fat exchanges), and it should always be taken with food to minimize its hypoglycemic effect. The effects of alcohol on glucose metabolism are addressed more fully later in this chapter.

Exercise

Exercise is a key factor in the treatment of diabetes, particularly in type 2 diabetes, because obesity and inactivity contribute to the development of glucose intolerance in genetically predisposed individuals. Regular exercise reduces cholesterol levels, lowers BP, augments weight-reduction diets, reduces the dose requirements or need for insulin or oral antidiabetic agents, enhances insulin sensitivity, and improves psychological well-being by reducing stress. Exercise increases glucose utilization, which is provided initially from the breakdown of muscle glycogen and, subsequently, from hepatic glycogenolysis and gluconeogenesis. These effects are mediated through norepinephrine, epinephrine, growth hormone, cortisol, and glucagon, along with the suppression of insulin secretion. In insulin-dependent diabetic patients, hyperglycemia, normoglycemia, or hypoglycemia can occur secondary to exercise depending on the degree of control, recent administration of insulin, and food intake. Exercise in patients taking insulin must be tempered by increased food intake, delayed administration of insulin, decreased doses of insulin, or a combination of these actions to minimize hypoglycemia (see Question 24).

In the type 2 diabetic population, plasma glucose concentrations usually decrease in response to exercise; symptomatic hypoglycemia is uncommon. Because diabetic individuals are predisposed to cardiovascular disease, attention has been focused on the metabolic response of the diabetic patient to exercise. In general, moderate, regular exercise is highly recommended for individuals with type 2 diabetes treated with diet and/or oral agents and encouraged in individuals taking insulin if special precautions are taken.

Pharmacologic Treatment

Insulin, along with diet, is crucial to the survival of individuals with type 1 diabetes and plays a major role in the therapy of people with type 2 diabetes when their symptoms cannot be controlled with diet or oral antidiabetic agents. Insulin also is used for patients with type 2 diabetes during periods of intercurrent illness or stress (e.g., surgery, pregnancy). The use of oral antidiabetic agents is reserved for the treatment of patients with type 2 diabetes whose symptoms cannot be controlled with diet and exercise alone. The clinical use of these agents and the complications associated with their use are discussed later in this chapter.

Pancreas and Islet Cell Transplants

Pancreas transplantation is the only available treatment for type 1 diabetes mellitus that induces an insulin-independent, normoglycemic state. Because it requires immunosuppression, it has been most widely used in uremic diabetic recipients of kidney transplant with a high success rate, particularly when performed simultaneously. As of October 2002, 14,000 pancreas transplantations had been performed in the United States. The 1-year graft survival rates (defined as total freedom from insulin therapy, normal fasting blood glucose concentrations, and normal or only slightly elevated A_{1C} values) are more than 80%.[38] Pancreas transplantation improves the quality of life, but there is little evidence that the development of microvascular or macrovascular complications are prevented or slowed. Furthermore, there is no evidence that pancreas transplantation prolongs life. The ADA considers pancreatic transplantation a viable option for diabetic patients with end-stage renal disease (ESRD) who must undergo kidney transplantation. However, pancreatic transplantation alone in a patient with diabetes mellitus remains controversial because the disadvantages of exogenous insulin therapy are replaced with risks of the transplantation procedure itself and the complications of immunosuppressive medications.[39]

Islet cell transplants have received increased attention with the success of the "Edmonton Protocol," which used a steroid-free immunosuppression regimen as well as other techniques. All patients achieved insulin independence after 1 year in contrast to a previous success rate of 8%. Many issues remain regarding islet cell transplantation, including availability of transplant material and assessment of long term outcomes.[40,41]

Overall Goals of Therapy

Specific therapeutic endpoints vary with different viewpoints on diabetic control and the methods used to monitor diabetic therapy (i.e., blood glucose and A_{1C}). These are discussed in appropriate sections of this chapter. However, some overall goals of therapy are agreed on by most diabetologists:

1. Try to keep patients free of symptoms associated with hyperglycemia (polyuria, polydipsia, weight loss, fatigue, recurrent infection, ketoacidosis) or hypoglycemia (hunger, anxiety, palpitations, sweatiness).
2. Strive for control at least equal to that achieved in the intensively treated patients in the DCCT. This may not be appropriate for all patients and must be based on sound clinical judgment. Target blood glucose goals may need to be adjusted for patients with frequent, severe hypoglycemia or hypoglycemia unawareness (see Questions 35 and 39). In addition, established renal insufficiency, proliferative retinopathy, severe neuropathy, and other advanced complications are not likely to be improved by tight glucose control.
3. Maintain normal growth and development in children. Adolescents were included in the DCCT; however, younger children were not. Intensive therapy is not recommended for children younger than 7 years of age and should be used cautiously in children ages 7 to 13 years old (see Questions 20 and 21).
4. Eliminate or minimize all other cardiovascular risk factors (obesity, hypertension, tobacco use, hyperlipidemia; Table 50-5).
5. Try to integrate the patient into the health care team through intensive education. The patient's knowledge and understanding of this disease can favorably influence its outcomes (see Table 50-16).

Table 50-5 American Diabetes Association Goals for Adults With Diabetes Mellitus[44]

Glycemic goals	
• A_{1C}	<7.0% (normal, 4–6%)[a]
• Preprandial plasma glucose	90–130 mg/dL (5.0–7.2 mmol/L)
[Blood glucose equivalent	80–120 mg/dL (4.4–6.7 mmol/L)]
• Postprandial plasma glucose	<180 mg/dL (<10.0 mmol/L)
[Blood glucose equivalent	<160 mg/dL (<8.9 mmol/L)]
Blood pressure	<130/80 mmHg
Lipids	
• LDL	<100 mg/dL <2.6 mol/L)
• Triglycerides	<150 mg/dL (<1.7 mmol/L)
• HDL	
Men	>40 mg/dL (>1.1 mmol/L)
Women	>50 mg/dL (>1.4 mmol/L)

Goals must be individualized to the patient. See Questions 2, 21, 46, 78, and 80 for broader discussion.
[a]More stringent goals (i.e., <6%) can be considered.

Methods of Monitoring Glycemic Control

In addition to monitoring signs and symptoms associated with hyperglycemia, hypoglycemia, and the long-term complications of diabetes, an ongoing assessment of metabolic control is an integral component of diabetes management. Ideally, self-monitored blood glucose (SMBG) results combined with laboratory measures of acute and chronic glycemia can be used to evaluate and adjust therapy. Several chemical measurements may be used by the patient and clinician to assess glycemic control directly or indirectly.[42]

Urine Ketone Testing

Urine ketone testing is recommended for patients with gestational and type 1 diabetes. Urine ketones should be evaluated when glucose concentrations consistently exceed 300 mg/dL (16.7 mmol/L) or during acute illness.[42] Persistently high glucose concentrations of this magnitude signal insulin deficiency that can, in turn, lead to lipolysis and ketoacidosis. A positive test may indicate impending or established ketoacidosis and demands a more extensive diagnostic workup. Testing also is recommended during pregnancy and if the patient has symptoms of ketoacidosis. Although there are generally no ketones in the urine, they may be present in people who are on extremely low caloric diets and in the first morning sample of women who are pregnant. Also, see discussions of sick day management and ketoacidosis in other sections of this chapter (Questions 31 and 40 through 46).

Plasma Glucose

FPG concentrations (normal FPG, 3.9 to 5.6 mmol/dL or 70 to 100 mg/dL) are commonly used to assess glycemic control in the fasting state because this is when glucose concentrations are most reproducible. FPG concentrations generally reflect glucose derived from hepatic glucose production because this is the primary source of glucose in the postabsorptive state. The FPG is the most frequent test performed by patients at home when self-monitoring. Postprandial glucose concentrations (1 to 2 hours after the start of the meal) also are used to assess glycemic control when fasting glucose concentrations are within normal limits or when there is a need to assess the effects of drugs on meal-related glycemia (e.g., lispro, α-glucosidase inhibitors). In nondiabetic individuals, glucose concentrations generally return to <140 mg/dL (7.8 mmol/L) within 2 hours after a meal. One to 2-hour postprandial concentrations primarily reflect the efficiency of insulin-mediated glucose uptake by peripheral tissue.

Because any glucose concentration can be affected by various factors (e.g., meals, medications, stress), measurement at a single point in time cannot be used to assess a patient's overall control. Most laboratories measure plasma glucose concentrations rather than whole blood because these values are not subject to changes in the hematocrit. Whole blood glucose concentrations are approximately 10% to 15% lower than plasma glucose concentrations because glucose is not distributed into hemoglobin. To convert plasma glucose concentrations (mg/dL) to whole blood glucose values (and vice versa), the following equation can be used:

- Whole blood glucose (mg/dL) = Plasma glucose (mg/dL) × 30.85

- To convert a glucose concentration in mg/dL to mmol/L, a factor of 18 is used:

Plasma glucose (mmol/L) = Plasma glucose (mg/dL) ÷ 18

Self-Monitored Blood Glucose

The advent of SMBG has made euglycemia, both preprandially and postprandially, an achievable goal (80 to 140 mg/dL). Patients and their health care providers are now able to assess directly the effects of drug doses, meals, exercise, and illness on daily blood glucose concentrations. With improved technology and decreasing costs, SMBG is the day-to-day monitoring test of choice for all patients with diabetes. However, SMBG remains expensive for some patients, is invasive, and is technique dependent. Furthermore, to achieve maximum benefit from SMBG, both the clinician and the patient must be motivated and willing to spend the time required to interpret the data and modify therapy to improve glycemic control. Based on the results of the DCCT and UKPDS, most persons with diabetes should attempt to achieve and maintain blood glucose levels as close to normal as is safely possible. This goal can realistically be achieved only by using SMBG. The frequency and timing of performing SMBG should be dictated by the individual's needs and goals. Selection and use of SMBG testing materials are discussed in Questions 10 and 11. Patients in whom blood glucose self-monitoring is particularly valuable include the following:

- *Patients with type 1 diabetes:* Frequent blood glucose measurements help the patient correlate meals, exercise, and insulin dose with blood glucose concentrations. This instant feedback gives the patient an increased sense of control and motivation, leading to improved glucose control.

- *Pregnant patients:* Infant morbidity and mortality are associated with the mother's overall glucose control. Using SMBG, the mother with diabetes who achieves normoglycemia before conception and throughout pregnancy, improves her chances of delivering a live, healthy infant.

- *Patients having difficulty recognizing hypoglycemia:* Over time, many patients with diabetes develop a sluggish counter-regulatory response to hypoglycemia whereby hypoglycemic symptoms are blunted or even absent. This is often referred to as *hypoglycemic unawareness.* Routine SMBG to detect asymptomatic hypoglycemia is essential in these individuals (see Question 39). In addition, acute anxiety attacks or signs and symptoms associated with a rapidly falling blood glucose concentration may mimic a true hypoglycemic reaction. This can be evaluated easily by measuring a fingerstick blood glucose concentration.

- *Patients who are using intensive insulin therapy:* Individuals who are on multiple daily doses of insulin or those using an insulin pump should use SMBG to evaluate the effectiveness of their insulin regimens and meal plans and to check for hypoglycemic or hyperglycemic reactions (see Question 11). Knowledge of preprandial, postprandial, bedtime, and nocturnal (e.g., 2 AM) blood glucose concentrations is essential in determining basal and preprandial insulin requirements.

Glycosylated Hemoglobin

Before the measurement of glycosylated hemoglobin, or A_{1C}, was available, clinicians could infer overall glycemic control only by extrapolating information from a series of fasting or random blood glucose measurements.[42] The introduction of the A_{1C} test has made possible an accurate assessment of glycemic control over a definite time period. A_{1C} is most commonly measured because it comprises the majority of glycosylated hemoglobin and is the least affected by recent fluctuations in blood glucose. A_{1C} measures the percentage of hemoglobin A that has been irreversibly glycosylated at the N-terminal amino group of the β-chain; the plasma glucose level and the life span of a red blood cell (RBC) (approximately 120 days) determine its value. Thus, A_{1C} is an indicator of glycemic control over the preceding 2 to 3 months. In patients without diabetes, A_{1C} comprises approximately 4% to 6% of the total hemoglobin. Values may be three times this level in patients with diabetes.

Each laboratory establishes its own normal values for A_{1C} because different components of hemoglobin A are measured by different assay methods. Because a 1% change in the glycosylated hemoglobin represents a 35-mg/dL change in the mean plasma glucose concentration, it is important to follow relative changes in A_{1C} values measured by a single laboratory. A movement to standardize methods to the DCCT values is underway.

The correlation between the A_{1C} level and mean plasma glucose levels are as follows[43,44]:

A_{1C} (%)	Mean plasma glucose	
	(mg/dL)	mmol/l
6	135	7.5
7	170	9.5
8	205	11.5
9	240	13.5
10	275	15.5
11	310	17.5
12	345	19.5

Alterations in RBC survival such as hemoglobinopathies, anemias, acute or chronic blood loss, and uremia may affect A_{1C} values, resulting in inaccurate indications of glycemic control. Antioxidants such as vitamins C and E also may interfere with the glycosylation process[45,46] (see Table 50-6).

A_{1C} can be measured without any special patient preparation (e.g., fasting) and generally is not subject to acute changes in insulin dosing, exercise, or diet. Normalization can indicate whether euglycemia has been achieved. However, A_{1C} does not replace the day-to-day monitoring of blood glucose concentrations, which is essential for evaluating acute changes in blood glucose concentrations. These values are needed to adjust the meal plan or medication doses.

CLINICAL USE

Currently, the A_{1C} value is used as an adjunct to assessing overall glycemic control in patients with diabetes. Often, it is used to verify clinical impressions related to glucose control and patient adherence. Some also have suggested the use of A_{1C} values for diabetes screening and diagnosis; however, until the test is standardized and more studies are completed, it cannot be recommended for these purposes. A_{1C} should be measured quarterly in patients who do not meet treatment goals, and at least semiannually in stable patients who are meeting treatment goals.

Table 50-6 **Factors Affecting A_{1C}**

Cause	Effect on A_{1C}
Alterations in RBC Survival	
Hemoglobinopathies	Decreased
Anemias	
Hemolytic	Decreased
Iron deficiency	Decreased[a]
Blood loss	Decreased
Assay Interference	
Uremia	Increased or no change[b,c]
Hemodialysis	No change[b]
Antioxidants	Decreased[d]

[a]For patients receiving iron replacement therapy. Normal levels would be expected in untreated patients.
[b]Interference seen in assays using high-pressure liquid chromatography (HPLC) and electroendosmosis. Affinity chromatography appears unaffected.
[c]Carbamylated hemoglobin equaling 0.063% of total hemoglobin is formed for every 1 mmol/L of serum urea.
[d]Reported with vitamins C (1 g/day) and E (1,200 mg/day). Possible mechanism is competitive inhibition of hemoglobin glycosylation.
A_{1C}, glycosylated hemoglobin; RBC, red blood cell.

Glycated Serum Protein, Glycated Serum Albumin, Fructosamine

Assays for glycated serum proteins (GSPs) reflect the extent of glycosylation of a variety of serum proteins, including glycated serum albumin (GSA).[42] The fructosamine assay is one of the most widely used methods to measure glycated proteins (normal, 2 to 2.8 mmol/L). Because the half-life of albumin is approximately 14 to 20 days, fructosamine provides an indication of glycemic control over a shorter time frame (1 to 2 weeks) than does the A_{1C}. The ADA does not consider measurement of fructosamine equivalent to that of A_{1C}, even though it correlates well with this value. Fructosamine levels may be useful as an adjunct to A_{1C} in determining whether a patient is improving or worsening in the short term (e.g., a patient on insulin therapy undergoing multiple dosage adjustments; for women with type 2 diabetes during pregnancy or gestational diabetes) or in patients with conditions such as hemolytic anemia in whom the A_{1C} test is inaccurate (Table 50-6). However, the exact role of GSP in monitoring glycemic control requires further study.

GLYCEMIC GOALS

The ADA recommendations for glycemic goals are summarized in Table 50-5.[44]

INSULIN

Insulin is a hormone secreted from the pancreatic β-cell in response to glucose and other stimulants (e.g., amino acids, free fatty acids, gastric hormones, parasympathetic stimulation, β-adrenergic stimulation).[47,48] The hormone is made up of two polypeptide chains (a 21–amino acid α chain and a 30–amino acid β chain), which are connected by two disulfide bonds (Fig. 50-3). Proinsulin, the precursor of insulin, is a single-chain, 86–amino acid polypeptide. In the storage granule of the β-cell, the connecting or C-peptide is cleaved from proinsulin to produce equimolar amounts of insulin and C-peptide. Thus, measurable C-peptide levels indicate the presence of endogenously produced insulin and functioning β-cells. Insulin is crucial to

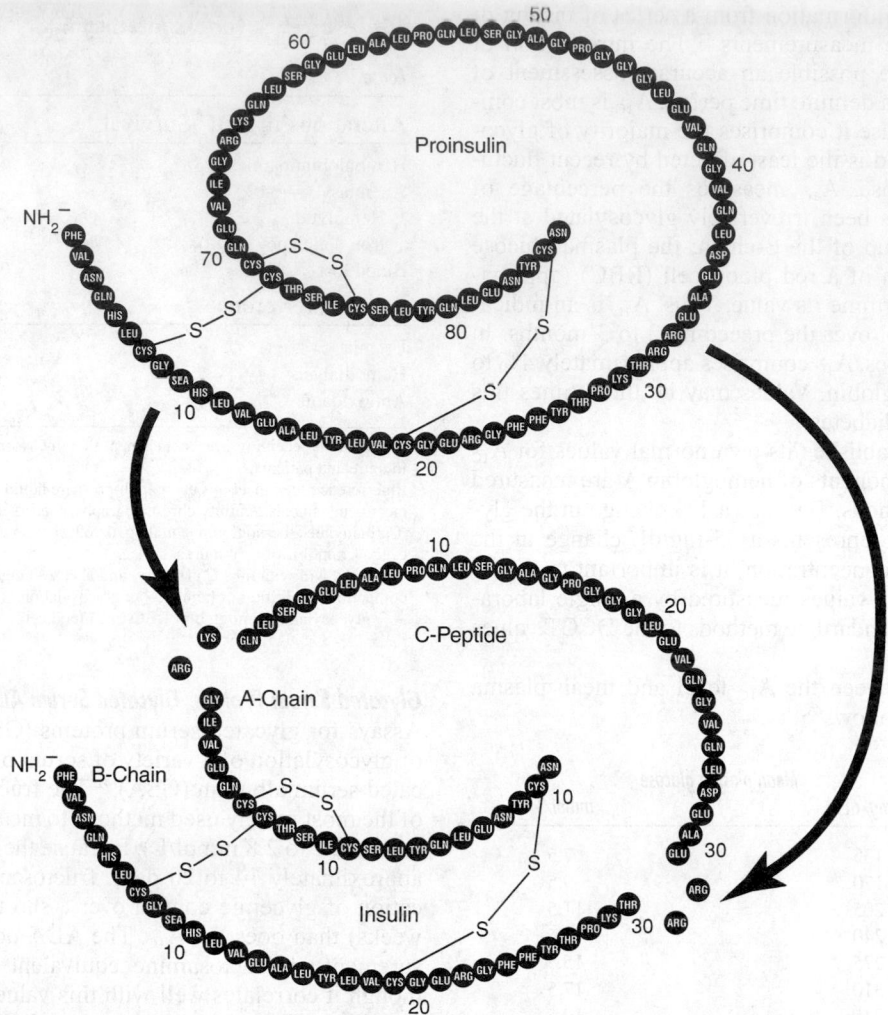

FIGURE 50-3 Proinsulin. Insulin is secreted from the pancreas as proinsulin. The connecting or C-peptide is cleaved to release the active insulin molecule. Thus, C-peptide levels are measured in study conditions to confirm the presence of a working pancreas. Insulin is a 51–amino acid protein made up of an A chain and a B chain connected by two disulfide bonds. (Reproduced with permission from reference 298.)

the survival of individuals with type 1 diabetes whose β-cells have been destroyed. It also plays a major role in the therapy of individuals with type 2 diabetes when their symptoms cannot be controlled with diet alone or oral antidiabetic agents. Insulin also is used in patients with type 2 diabetes during pregnancy or periods of intercurrent illness or stress (e.g., surgery).

Commercially available insulin products differ in their immunogenicity, physical and chemical properties, pharmacokinetics, and pharmacodynamics.

Immunogenicity

Modern manufacturing processes have virtually eliminated contaminants from current products, and most people now use human insulin. Consequently, immunologically mediated sequelae, such as lipodystrophy, hypersensitivity, and insulin resistance caused by "blocking" antibodies, are rare. When these events do occur, most are associated with beef or pork insulins. Beef (or mixed beef and pork insulin) products are more immunogenic than pork insulin. Pure beef products are no longer manufactured in the United States, and the produc-

tion of mixed beef–pork products was discontinued in 1998. Purified pork insulin is slightly more immunogenic than commercially available human insulin; however, the difference between these insulins is subtle. In most newly diagnosed diabetic patients, human insulin consistently produces less antibody response than purified pork insulin, albeit the difference often is slight and probably clinically unimportant.[49]

Physical and Chemical Properties

Regular insulin is a solution that can be administered by any parenteral route: intravenously, intramuscularly, and subcutaneously. Insulin lispro and insulin aspart, rapid-acting analogs, are also clear solutions approved by the U.S. Food and Drug Administration (FDA) for SC use. Insulin glargine, a long-acting insulin is a clear solution, but should not be administered intravenously because the product is designed to precipitate at physiologic pH. All other insulins (NPH, Lente, Ultralente) are suspensions in which regular insulin has been complexed or crystallized to extend their actions with protamine (e.g., NPH) and with varying amounts of zinc (e.g.,

Lente and Ultralente).[47] These insulins must be mixed well before administration and should never be administered intravenously. All insulin products have a neutral pH, except for insulin glargine, which has a pH of 4.0.

Pharmacokinetics: Absorption, Distribution, and Elimination

After SC injection, insulin is absorbed directly into the bloodstream, bypassing the lymphatic system. The rate-limiting step of insulin activity after SC administration is absorption of insulin from the injection site, which depends on the type of insulin administered, as well as a multitude of other factors. Although SC absorption generally follows a simple exponential course, it is highly irregular. Coefficients of variation for the time until 50% of the insulin dose is absorbed are approximately 25% within an individual and up to 50% among patients for all insulins studied.[50] A primary cause of this variation is attributed to changes in blood flow around the injection site.

Exogenous insulin is degraded at both renal and extrarenal (liver and muscle) sites. Degradation also takes place at the cellular level after internalization of the insulin-receptor complex. Approximately 30% to 80% of insulin is cleared from the systemic circulation by the kidneys, which have a larger role in clearing exogenously administered insulin. Endogenous insulin is secreted directly into the portal circulation and is primarily cleared by the liver in nondiabetic individuals (60%).[47] Insulin is filtered by glomerular capillaries, but >99% is reabsorbed by the proximal tubules. The insulin is then degraded in glomerular capillary cells and postglomerular peritubular cells.[51] Insulin pharmacokinetics are summarized in Table 50-7. (Also see Question 32.)

Pharmacodynamics

Clinically, the most important differences between insulin products relate to their onset and duration of activities. Current insulin products can be categorized as rapid or ultra-short-acting, short-acting, intermediate-acting, and long-acting. Products available in the United States are listed in Table 50-8, and the onset of action, peak effect, and durations of action of each insulin category are in listed Table 50-9. However, these data are derived primarily from studies in normal, healthy volunteers in the fasting state or in well-controlled patients with diabetes stabilized in a metabolic ward. In actuality, intersubject and intrasubject variations in response to insulin are substantial because an individual pattern of response to insulin can be affected by numerous factors (e.g., the formation of insulin hexamers, the presence of insulin-binding antibodies, dose, exercise, site of injection, massage of the injection site, ambient temperature, and interactions between insulins that have been mixed together).[52,50] (See Table 50-12 and Question 14.) Nevertheless, knowledge of when one might expect the various insulins to exert their effects is absolutely essential to the rational adjustment of insulin dosages.

Rapid-Acting Insulin (Ultra-Short-Acting Insulin)

INSULIN LISPRO

Insulin lispro [Lys(B28),Pro(B29)]-human insulin (Humalog, Eli Lilly) was the first available rapid-acting insulin analog and received FDA approval in 1996. The natural amino

Table 50-7	Insulin Pharmacokinetics
Clearance	
Total clearance	700–800 mL/min
Hepatic clearance	300–400 mL/min
Renal clearance	190–270 mL/min
IV Infusion	
Elimination follows multicompartment model	
Half-life for three compartments: 2.3–2.4 min, 14 min, 133 min	
Insulin action most closely corresponds to last compartment. Therefore, it is unnecessary to adjust the dose more frequently than Q 2 hr	
SC Administration of Regular Insulin[a]	
Intermittent Boluses	
Half-life (absorption, 70–120 min)	
Half-life (elimination, 53 min)	
SC Infusion	
Steady state achieved in 68 hr	
If infusion is discontinued, check for rise in glucose ketones after 2 or 3 hr. Because there is no SC pool, effects dissipate quickly	
SC Administration of Intermediate-Acting Insulins[a]	
NPH half-life (absorption) 12–19 hr	

[a]Insulin absorption varies by 25% within the same individual and 50% among individuals. See Table 50-12 for factors that influence absorption.
IV, intravenous; NPH, isophane insulin suspension; SC, subcutaneous.
Adapted from reference 50.

acid sequence of the insulin β-chain at positions 28 (proline) and 29 (lysine) is inverted to form lispro. This change results in an insulin molecule that more loosely self-associates into hexamers than does regular insulin. Consequently, the active monomeric form is more readily available, resulting in an onset of activity (15 minutes), peak action (30 to 90 minutes), and duration (3 to 4 hours) that more closely simulates physiologic insulin secretion relative to meals. Because it can be injected shortly before eating (0 to 15 minutes), lispro provides patients greater flexibility in lifestyle, lowers 2-hour postprandial blood glucose levels, and decreases risk for late postprandial and nocturnal hypoglycemia compared with regular insulin formulations.[53] Patients who use an insulin pump most often use a rapid-acting insulin instead of regular insulin. One randomized, two-way crossover open-label study compared lispro with regular insulin administered for 3 months by continuous SC insulin infusion.[54] Lispro resulted in A_{1C} values that were significantly lower than those produced by regular insulin (7.41% versus 7.65%). There were no differences in adverse events. Because lispro has a shorter duration of action than regular insulin, hyperglycemia and ketosis may occur more rapidly if insulin delivery is inadvertently interrupted.

INSULIN ASPART

Insulin aspart (NovoLog, Novo Nordisk), a rapid-acting insulin analog developed by Novo Nordisk, differs from human insulin by substitution of aspartic acid at B28. Insulin aspart controls postprandial glucose excursions similar to insulin lispro. Insulin aspart was approved by the FDA on June 7, 2000.

Table 50-8   Insulins Available in the United States

Type/Duration of Action	Animal Source/Manufacturing Process	Brand Name	Manufacturer
Rapid-Acting			
Insulin lispro	Recombinant DNA	Humalog	Lilly
Insulin aspart	Recombinant DNA	NovoLog	Novo Nordisk
Short-Acting			
Regular			
Purified	Pork	Regular Iletin II	Lilly
Human	Recombinant DNA	Humulin R	Lilly
		Novolin R[a]	Novo Nordisk
		Velosulin BR[b]	Novo Nordisk
Intermediate-Acting			
NPH (Isophane Insulin Suspension)			
Purified	Pork	Pork NPH Iletin II	Lilly
Human	Recombinant DNA	Humulin N	Lilly
		Novolin N[a]	Novo Nordisk
Lente (Insulin Zinc Suspension)			
Purified	Pork	Lente Iletin II (Pork)	Lilly
Human	Recombinant DNA	Humulin L	Lilly
		Novolin L[a]	Novo Nordisk
NPH/Regular Mixture (70%/30%)	Recombinant DNA	Humulin 70/30[a]	Lilly
Human insulin analog	Recombinant DNA	Novolin 70/30[a]	Novo Nordisk
Insulin Aspart Protamine/Insulin Aspart Mixture (70%/30%)		Novolog Mix 70/30	Novo Nordisk
			Lilly
Insulin Aspart	Recombinant DNA		
NPH/Regular Mixture (50%/50%)		Humulin 50/50	Lilly
Human insulin analog	Recombinant DNA		
Insulin NPL/Insulin Lispro Mixture (75%/25%)	Recombinant DNA	Humalog Mix75/25[a]	Lilly
Long-Acting			
Ultralente (Insulin Zn Suspension, Extended)			
Human	Recombinant DNA	Humulin U	Lilly
Insulin glargine			
Insulin analog	Recombinant DNA	Lantus	Aventis

[a]These products also are available in 1.5 and 3-mL cartridges for use in "pen" delivery devices (Novolin Pen and as prefilled pens).
[b]Phosphate buffered product. Used in insulin pumps.

Short-Acting Insulins

Regular insulin has an onset of action of 30 to 60 minutes, a peak effect at 1 to 5 hours, and a duration of action of 5 to 10 hours. The broad range in peak effect and duration reflects the many variables that affect insulin action (see Table 50-9). The 30- to 60-minute onset of action requires proper timing of premeal regular insulin, which is difficult for most patients.

Intermediate-Acting Insulins
NPH, Lente, and NPL

NPH (neutral protamine hagedorn or isophane) and Lente insulins are intermediate-acting insulins. Both have onsets of action at approximately 2 hours (1 to 3 hours), peak effects at approximately 6 to 14 hours, and durations of action of approximately 16 to 24 hours. Again, it must be emphasized that this pattern of response is at best a generalization. Patients

Table 50-9   Insulin Pharmacodynamics[a]

Insulin	Onset (hr)	Peak (hr)	Duration (hr)	Appearance
Insulin lispro	1/4	1/2–1 1/2	4–5	Clear
Insulin aspart	5–10 min	1–3	3–5	Clear
Regular	1/2–1	2–4	5–7	Clear
NPH	1–2	6–14	24%	Cloudy
Lente	1–3	6–14	24%	Cloudy
Ultralente[b]	6	18–24	36%	Cloudy
Insulin glargine	1.5	Flat	24	Clear[c]

[a]The onset, peak, and duration of insulin activity may vary considerably from times listed in this table. See text and Table 50-12.
[b]Human Ultralente may have a shorter duration of action. Some patients require twice-daily dosing.
[c]The only extended-duration insulin that is clear. Should not be mixed with other insulins or administered intravenously.

may have a variable pattern of response to both NPH and Lente insulins over time, and those on higher doses are likely to have a later peak and a longer duration of action than those who use lower doses an animal-source product (e.g., purified pork versus human insulin). Up to 80% of these day-to-day fluctuations in blood glucose responses can be accounted for by variation in the absorption of the intermediate-acting insulins.[50] NPL is a protamine-based insulin lispro formulation in which insulin lispro has been co-crystallized with protamine to produce an intermediate-acting insulin similar to NPH.[55] It is available as Humalog Mix 75/25, a premixed insulin formulation containing NPL and insulin lispro in a ratio of 75:25.

Long-Acting Insulins

Ultralente insulin is a long-acting insulin formulation. This insulin has a long onset of activity (4 to 6 hours), a delayed peak action (18 to 24 hours), and a prolonged duration of activity (24 to ≥36 hours). This time course of activity is not very useful in suppressing acute glucose challenges related to meals. However, when mimicking the physiologic release of insulin, long-acting insulin (used in combination regimens with frequent, rapid to short-acting insulin injections) is used to supply a low, "basal" level of insulin between meals (see Question 3 and Table 50-13). Unfortunately, Ultralente insulin often requires twice-daily administration to avoid a "peak action," provide 24-hour coverage, and achieve a smooth effect.

In April 2000, *insulin glargine* (Lantus, Aventis) was approved by the FDA "for once-daily SC administration in the treatment of adult and pediatric patients (≥6 years) with type 1 diabetes mellitus or adult patients with type 2 diabetes who require basal (long-acting) insulin for the control of hyperglycemia."

Insulin glargine is an insulin analog in which asparagine in position A21 is substituted with glycine and two arginines are added to the C-terminus of the β-chain. This change in the amino acid sequence causes a shift in the isoelectric point from pH 5.4 to 6.7, making it more soluble at an acidic pH.[56] Once injected, insulin glargine (which is a clear solution with a pH of 4.0) precipitates at physiologic pH forming a depot that releases insulin slowly over 24 hours. This results in delayed absorption and a less pronounced peak compared with NPH insulin.[57] Zinc is added to further prolong the duration of insulin glargine. In clinical trials of patients with type 1 and type 2 diabetes, once-daily injections of insulin glargine were as effective as NPH in lowering A_{1C} values with less nocturnal hypoglycemia.[58]

Insulin detemir (Novo Nordisk), a new basal insulin analog being developed, is expected to be available for use in 2004. Insulin detemir has a free fatty acid attached to the molecule, enabling it to bind to albumin in the subcutaneous tissue and bloodstream. This produces a slow and consistent rate of insulin release.

Premixed Insulin

Products that contain premixed NPH and regular insulin in fixed ratios of 70:30 and 50:50; NPL and insulin lispro in a fixed ratio of 75:25; and NPH and insulin aspart in a fixed ratio of 70:30 are available for patients who have difficulty measuring and mixing insulins. These insulins are compatible when mixed together and retain their individual pharmacodynamic profiles (see Question 14).

TREATMENT OF TYPE 1 DIABETES: CLINICAL USE OF INSULIN

Clinical Presentation of Type 1 Diabetes

1. The University Student Health Service refers to the Diabetic Clinic A.H., a slender, 18-year-old woman who was recently discharged from the hospital for severe dehydration and mild ketoacidosis (no records available). A fasting and a random plasma glucose ordered subsequently were 190 mg/dL (normal, 70 to 100) and 250 mg/dL (normal, 140 to <200). Approximately 4 weeks before she was hospitalized, A.H. had moved across the country to attend college—her first time away from home. In retrospect, she remembers that she had symptoms of polydipsia, nocturia (six times a night), fatigue, and a 12-lb weight loss over this period, which she attributed to the anxiety associated with her move away from home and adjustment to her new environment. Her medical history is remarkable for recurrent upper respiratory infections and three cases of vaginal moniliasis over the past 6 months. Her family history is negative for diabetes, and she takes no medications.

Physical examination is within normal limits. She weighs 50 kg and is 5'4" tall. Laboratory results are as follows: FPG, 280 mg/dL (normal, <110); A_{1C}, 14% (normal, 4 to 6%); trace urine ketones as measured by Keto-Diastix (negative). On the basis of the aforementioned history and laboratory findings, the presumptive diagnosis is type 1 diabetes. Which findings are consistent with this diagnosis in A.H.?

[SI units: FPG, 15.5 mmol/L (normal, <5.6); A_{1C}, 0.14 (normal, 0.04 to 0.06)]

A.H. meets several of the diagnostic criteria for diabetes. She has classic symptoms of the disease (polyuria, polydipsia, weight loss, glucosuria, fatigue, recurrent infections), a random plasma glucose > 200 mg/dL, and an FPG → 126 mg/dL on at least two occasions[5] (see Tables 50-1 and 50-2). The elevated A_{1C} also is consistent with diabetes mellitus. Features of A.H.'s history that are consistent with type 1 diabetes, in particular, include the relatively acute onset of symptoms in association with a major life event (moving away from home), ketones in the urine, negative family history, and a relatively young age at onset.

Treatment Goals

2. A.H. will be started on insulin therapy on this visit. What are the goals of therapy? Will normoglycemia prevent the development or progression of long-term complications?

In the early 1990s, most endocrinologists were leaning toward normoglycemia as an ideal goal of insulin therapy, although there was still some debate about the relation between hyperglycemia and the progression and development of long-term complications. As discussed in the introduction to this chapter, the results of the DCCT convincingly demonstrated that lowering blood glucose concentrations through intensive insulin therapy in persons with type 1 diabetes slows or prevents the development of microvascular complications.[21] Thus, the ADA now advocates "tight control," which it defines as "blood glucose levels equal to or better than those achieved in the intensively treated group in the DCCT trial."[59]

The original goal of intensive insulin therapy in the DCCT was to achieve glucose levels as close to the nondiabetic range as possible. However, even under ideal study conditions, the investigators were unable to achieve these ideal targets in the intensive insulin therapy group: the mean A_{1C} level was 7.2% (normal, 6%) and the mean blood glucose concentration was 155 mg/dL (normal, <100). Thus, intensive insulin therapy does not necessarily lead to the attainment of euglycemia, and most patients will require individualized glycemic goals.[44,59]

It is important to understand that intensive insulin therapy involves a *complete* program of diabetes management that includes a balanced meal plan, exercise, daily blood glucose self-monitoring, and insulin adjustments based on these factors (Table 50-10). Because the patient is the key member of the team, A.H. must be highly motivated and able to learn about the complex metabolic interplay between insulin and lifestyle.

In summary, A.H. is a newly diagnosed patient with type 1 diabetes who has not yet developed any signs or symptoms of long-term complications. Therefore, she is an ideal candidate for intensive insulin therapy and, if she is willing and motivated, normoglycemia with rare hypoglycemic reactions is a reasonable long-term goal. This goal should be achieved gradually over several months with intensive insulin therapy, diet, education, and strong clinical support. If A.H. is unwilling to pursue such a rigorous approach at this time or is unwilling to perform frequent blood glucose tests, a more conservative approach will have to be used. A desirable goal is an A_{1C} value as close to the normal range as possible with rare hypoglycemic reactions. Table 50-11 describes the ideal and acceptable metabolic goals for intensive insulin therapy.

Physiologic Insulin Therapy

3. What methods of insulin administration are available to achieve optimal glucose control?

Most methods of insulin delivery used in intensive insulin therapy are designed to mimic normal insulin secretion as closely as possible (thus the term "physiologic insulin therapy").[60] Problems with insulin delivery include factors that affect the SC absorption of insulin (Table 50-12). Before the development of the rapid-acting insulin analogs and insulin glargine as a basal insulin, insulins lacked pharmacodynamic profiles that allowed one to closely simulate the basal-bolus model (see text that follows). Some argue that euglycemia is not achievable unless insulin is administered directly into the portal vein or in a way that bypasses the peripheral circulation

initially, thereby mimicking its physiologic release into the portal circulation. Administering insulin subcutaneously or intravenously produces peripheral hyperinsulinemia and relatively low levels of insulin in the hepatic vein.

Clinicians now have more tools to mimic pancreatic release of the hormone. In the nondiabetic individual, the pancreas secretes boluses of insulin in response to snacks and meals. Between meals and throughout the night, the pancreas secretes small amounts of insulin that are sufficient to suppress lipolysis and hepatic glucose output (basal insulin). Two methods have been used to achieve a similar pattern of insulin release: (1) insulin pump therapy (previously referred to as "continuous SC infusion of insulin") (Fig. 50-4) and (2) multiple daily doses of insulin (see Question 4).

Insulin Pump Therapy

The use of an insulin pump is currently the most precise way to mimic normal insulin secretion. This consists of a battery-operated pump and a computer that can program the pump to deliver predetermined amounts of regular insulin, insulin lispro, or insulin aspart from a reservoir to a subcutaneously inserted catheter or needle (e.g., Medtronic MiniMed 508, Paradigm 512, Northridge, California and Animas IR 1000, Frazer, PA).[61,62] These systems are portable and designed to deliver various basal amounts of insulin throughout the day as well as meal-related boluses provided by regular insulin, insulin lispro, or insulin aspart. A bolus of regular insulin can be released by the patient 30 minutes before food ingestion. Insulin aspart is FDA approved for use in the insulin pump and approval of insulin lispro is pending.[61] If rapid-acting insulins are used, meal-related boluses are given 0 to 15 minutes before eating.

The preferred meal planning approach for patients using an insulin pump is carbohydrate counting. The "insulin to carbohydrate ratio" or how much carbohydrate is covered by 1 unit of insulin must be determined. This calculation can be based on the "500 Rule." The number 500 is divided by the total daily dose of insulin the patient is using to determine the insulin to carbohydrate ratio (see Question 17). The basal insulin infu-

---

Table 50-10 Components of Physiologic Insulin Therapy

Multicomponent insulin regimen of basal plus preprandial insulin doses

Balance of carbohydrate intake, exercise, and insulin dosage

Daily, multiple self-monitoring of blood glucose levels

Patient self-adjustment of carbohydrate intake and insulin dosage with use of supplemental rapid- or short-acting insulin according to a predetermined plan

Individualized target blood glucose and A_{1C} levels

Frequent contact between patient and diabetes team

Intensive patient education

Psychologic support

Regular objective assessment (as measured by A_{1C})

A_{1C}, glycosylated hemoglobin.
Modified from reference 76.

Table 50-11 Goals of Intensive Insulin Therapy[a]

Target Blood Glucose Values	Ideal[b] (mg/dL)	Acceptable[c] (mg/dL)	Pregnancy (mg/dL)
Fasting	70–120	70–140	60–90
Preprandial	70–105	70–130	60–105
1 hr postprandial	100–160	100–180	110–130
2 hr postprandial	80–120	80–150	90–120
2–4 AM	70–100	70–120	>60
A_{1C}	<6%	<7%	<6%
Urine ketones[e]	Absent	Rare	Rare

[a]Modified and extrapolated from references 21 and 65. Intensive insulin therapy is a complete therapeutic program of diabetes management and requires a team approach (see Table 50-10).
[b]Ideal values approximate those ssen in nondiabetic individuals and are included for illustrative purposes only.
[c]Acceptable values should be individualized to levels that are attainable without creating undue risk for hypoglycemia. These results are similar to the results achieved in the DCCT trial. These values may be inappropriate for patients with hypoglycemic unawareness, counter-regulatory insufficiency, angina pectoris, or other complicating features (see Table 50-15).
[d]A_{1C}, glycosylated hemoglobin. Normal values vary; normalize to laboratory.
[e]Does not apply to type 2 diabetes patients.

Table 50-12   Factors Altering Onset and Duration of Insulin Action

Factor	Comments
Route of Administration	Onset of action more rapid and duration of action shorter for IV>IM>SC[106,292,293]
	Intrapulmonary insulin has more rapid onset and shorter duration than SC insulin, resembling IV pharmacokinetics[50,294,295]
Factors Altering Clearance	
Renal function	Renal failure ↓ insulin clearance. May prolong and intensify action of exogenous and endogenous insulin
Insulin antibodies	IgG antibodies bind insulin as it is absorbed and release it slowly, thereby delaying and/or prolonging its effect[49]
Thyroid function	Hyperthyroidism ↑ clearance, but also ↑ insulin action, making control difficult. Patients stabilize as they become euthyroid[296]
Factors Altering SC Absorption	Factors that ↑ SC blood flow ↑ absorption rates of regular insulin. Effect on intermediate- and long-acting insulins minimal
Site of injection	Rate of absorption fastest from the abdomen, intermediate from the arm, and slowest from the thigh.[70] Less variation observed in type 2 patients. Less variation observed with lispro insulin
	Site Half-Life Absorption (min)
	Abdomen 87 ± 12
	Arm 141 ± 23
	Hip 153 ± 28
	Thigh 164 ± 15
Exercise of injected area	Strenuous exercise of an injected area within 1 hr of injection can ↑ absorption rate. Rate of absorption of regular insulin ↑, but little effect on intermediate-acting insulin[50,296]
Ambient temperature	Heat (e.g., hot weather, hot bath, sauna) ↑ absorption rate. Cold has opposite effect[47,50]
Local massage	Massaging injected area for 30 min substantially ↑ absorption rate of regular insulin as well as longer- acting insulins[296]
Smoking	Controversial. Vasoconstriction may ↓ absorption rate[50]
Jet injectors	Insulin absorption more rapid, probably secondary to ↑ surface area for absorption[297]
Lipohypertrophy	Insulin absorption is delayed from lipohypertrophic sites[72]
Insulin preparation	More soluble forms of insulin are absorbed more rapidly and have shorter durations of action (see Table 50-9 and text). Human insulin may have shorter action than animal insulin
Insulin mixtures	The short-acting properties of regular insulin may be lost if mixed with Lente insulins (see Question 14)
Insulin concentration	More dilute solutions (e.g., U-40, U-10) are absorbed more rapidly than more concentrated forms (U-100, U-500)[47]
Insulin dose	Lower doses are absorbed more rapidly and have a shorter duration of action than larger doses

IgG, immunoglobulin G; IM, intramuscular; IV, intravenous; SC, subcutaneous.

sion rate may be adjusted depending on the situation. Many patients find it advantageous to decrease the basal rate during the middle of the night when nocturnal hypoglycemia is most likely to occur. The basal rate also may be increased before awakening to avoid hyperglycemia due to the "dawn phenomenon"—adjustments that are not possible using conventional insulin regimens. Features of the current pump models include remote programming capabilities to administer or suspend insulin delivery; the capability to program multiple, patient-specific delivery patterns; a low-volume alert; an optional vibrate mode; and a child-block feature to restrict programming. The Health Care Financing Administration (HCFA) announced in September of 1999 that Medicare now covers insulin infusion pumps for eligible beneficiaries with type 1 diabetes. Factors to consider when choosing a pump include safety features, durability, ability of the manufacturer to provide service, availability of training, clinically desirable features and cosmetic attractiveness for the user.[61,63]

IMPLANTABLE INSULIN PUMPS

Remote-controlled implantable pumps that deliver insulin intravenously or intraperitoneally are under study.[64] Insulin is stored in a large reservoir that is surgically inserted subcutaneously into the abdomen or chest wall. Problems that have delayed development include expense, local erosion, infection, and catheter blockage. The Medtronic MiniMed 2007 implantable insulin pump is approved for sale in Europe;

however, it has not yet been cleared for marketing in the United States.

Multiple Daily Injections

4. **How can insulin injections be administered to A.H. in a way that mimics the physiologic release of insulin from the pancreas?**

Endocrinologists have developed a variety of insulin regimens that are intended to mimic the release of insulin from the pancreas.[65] Examples of these are displayed in Table 50-13 and illustrated in Figure 50-5. A total daily dose of insulin is estimated empirically (e.g., 0.5 U/kg per day) or according to guidelines similar to those listed in Table 50-14. The total daily dose of insulin then is split into several doses. In general, the basal dose comprises approximately 50% of the total daily dose.

A regimen that is becoming less commonly used involves injecting a mixture of intermediate-acting and regular insulin twice daily before breakfast and before dinner. (See Fig. 50-5A and Method 1 in Table 50-13.) The morning dose of regular insulin is intended to take care of the breakfast meal; the morning dose of NPH takes care of the noon meal and provides basal insulin throughout the day; the evening dose of regular insulin takes care of the evening meal; and the evening dose of NPH provides basal insulin levels during the night and takes care of any evening snack that is ingested. Because pa-

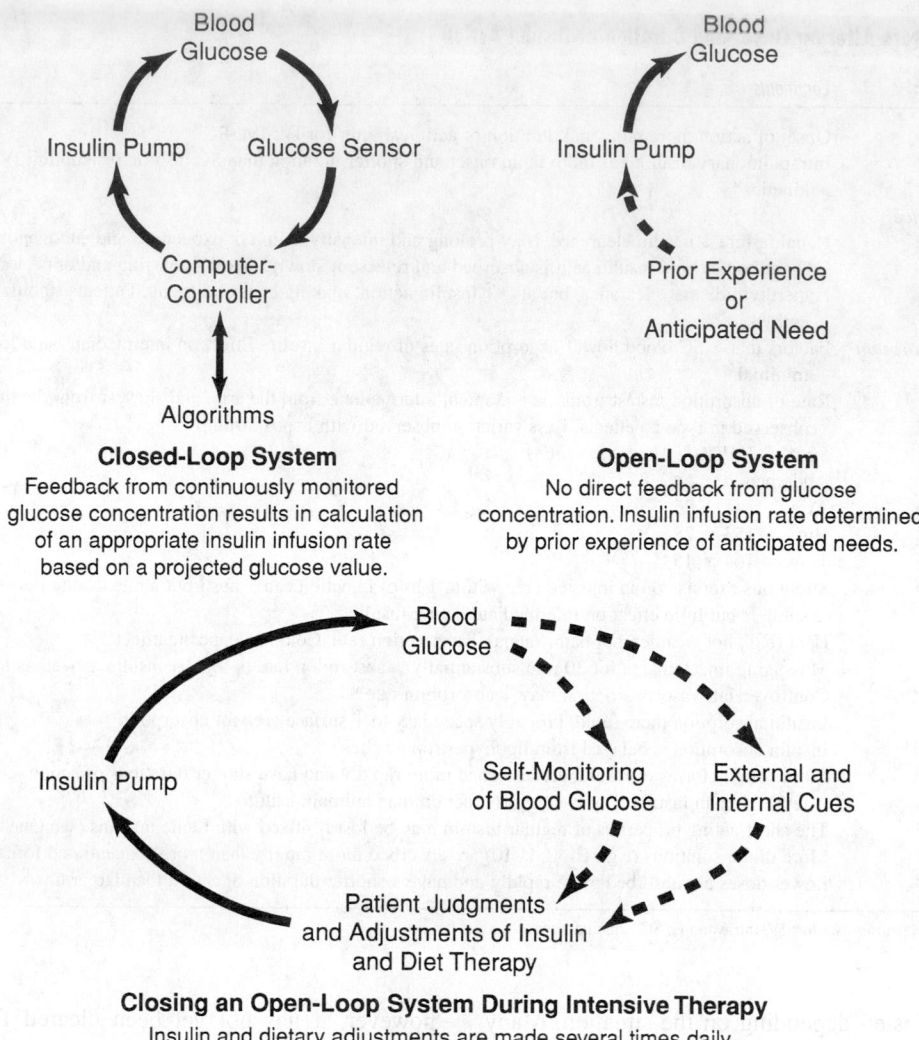

FIGURE 50-4 Insulin infusion pumps: comparison of closed-loop and open-loop systems. (Used with permission from reference 298.)

tients in the DCCT used three to four injections per day to achieve tight control, this twice-daily method of NPH and regular insulin administration is no longer considered "intensive insulin therapy." However, twice-daily regimens may be effective for a short period of time in newly diagnosed type 1 diabetic persons who are still producing a significant amount of insulin, such as A.H. Regular insulin is often replaced by insulin lispro or insulin aspart in this regimen, because they are both more rapid acting. However, because their duration of action is shorter than that of regular insulin, doses of NPH may have to be increased to minimize preprandial hyperglycemia.

Figure 50-5B depicts a variation of the aforementioned method. It is the same except that the evening dose of intermediate-acting insulin is given as a third injection at bedtime (see Method 2 in Table 50-13). This shifts the time of peak effect from approximately 2 to 3 AM to approximately 7 AM. By administering the intermediate-acting insulin at bedtime, nocturnal hypoglycemia is reduced and peak insulin activity occurs when the patient is more likely to be awake and ingesting food. This method may be useful for patients in whom noc-

turnal hypoglycemia and fasting hyperglycemia are particularly troublesome.

Figure 50-5C shows the theoretical effect provided by three equal doses of regular or insulin lispro (or insulin aspart) before meals and a dose of intermediate-acting insulin at bedtime to provide basal insulin levels during the night (see Methods 3 and 4 in Table 50-13). This regimen gives the patient more flexibility in both the timing and the size of meals. Although the regimen specifies equal doses, the carbohydrate content of the meal as well as preprandial blood glucose values ultimately determines these doses (see Questions 18 and 19). In some patients, inadequate basal insulin during the day results in preprandial hyperglycemia as the effects of insulin lispro, aspart or regular insulin wane.

An alternative that is gaining in popularity is the use of a long-acting insulin (Ultralente or insulin glargine) in the morning or evening to provide basal insulin levels throughout the day, along with doses of regular or insulin lispro or aspart before meals (see Fig. 50-5C). This method theoretically provides insulin in exactly the same way as the insulin pump (basal levels plus small boluses for meals and snacks). In do-

Table 50-13 Examples of Various Insulin Regimens

AM	Noon	PM	Bedtime	Comments
Method 1				
Reg/NPH	—	Reg/NPH	—	This regimen relies on the AM NPH or Lente to cover the noon meal
Reg/Lente		Reg/Lente		and to provide basal insulin during the day. The evening NPH or
Lispro/NPH		Lispro/NPH		Lente supplies basal insulin during the night. However, the evening
Lispro/Lente		Lispro/Lente		NPH has peak activity at ≈ 2–4 AM when plasma glucose is at a
Aspart/NPH		Aspart/NPH		physiologic nadir, predisposing the patient to nocturnal hypo-
Aspart/Lente		Aspart/Lente		glycemia. Empirically, some clinicians use a 1:2 ratio of Reg:NPH.
				If insulin lispro or insulin aspart is used, we recommend basing the
				dose on an empiric insulin unit:grams carbohydrate ratio of 1:15 ini-
				tially. See Table 50-14.
Method 2				
Reg/NPH	—	Reg	NPH	See notes for Method 1. By shifting the NPH or Lente dose to bed-
Reg/Lente		Reg	Lente	time, the peak action occurs in the early morning (5–7 am), when
Lispro/NPH		Lispro	NPH	the patient is awake and ready to eat. This also corresponds to the
Lispro/Lente		Lispro	Lente	dawn phenomenon, a natural rise in the plasma glucose from growth
Aspart/NPH		Aspart	NPH	hormone. See Method 1 comments for empirical doses.
Aspart/Lente		Aspart	Lente	
Method 3				
Reg	Reg	Reg	NPH	These methods provide premeal boluses of insulin. The evening dose
Reg	Reg	Reg	Lente	of NPH, Lente, ultralente, or insulin glargine provides basal levels at
Reg	Reg	Reg	Glargine	night to prevent lipolysis and suppress glycogenolysis and gluconeo-
Reg	Reg	Reg	Ultralente	genesis. Often, the intermediate- or long-acting insulins must be
				given twice daily to provide sufficient basal insulin throughout the
				day. When insulin glargine (Lantus) replaces two injections of NPH
				or Lente, the initial dose should be reduced by 20% from the previ-
				ous day's total daily dose of intermediate-acting insulin. See regi-
				mens for Method 4.
Method 4				
Lispro/NPH	Lispro	Lispro	NPH	Insulin lispro or insulin aspart is substituted for regular insulin in
Lispro/Lente	Lispro	Lispro	Lente	Method 3. Postprandial values are lower, but one may see prepran-
Lispro	Lispro	Lispro	Glargine	dial hyperglycemia because the duration of action is too brief to
Aspart/NPH	Aspart	Aspart	NPH	supply sufficient levels of basal insulin during the day. To address
Aspart/Lente	Aspart	Aspart	Lente	this issue, some clinicians are combining lispro with regular insulin
Aspart	Aspart	Aspart	Glargine	or very low doses of intermediate-acting insulin before meals (1
				unit/hr). When insulin lispro or insulin apart is used as the mealtime
				insulin, a minimum of two injections of intermediate-acting insulin
				is required. When insulin glargine (Lantus) replaces two injections
				of NPH or Lente, the initial dose should be reduced by 20% from
				the previous day's total daily dose of intermediate-acting insulin.
				See Method 6. Empirically, the lispro dose is based on the estimated
				CHO intake (1 unit/15 g). See Table 50-14.
Method 5				
Reg/Ultralente	Reg	Reg/Ultralente	—	Because human Ultralente has a relatively short duration of action, it
Lispro/Ultralente	Lispro or	Lispro/Ultralente		must be dosed twice daily to maintain smooth basal concentrations.
Aspart/Ultralente	Aspart	Aspart/Ultralente		However, because its onset is slow, a short-acting insulin must be
				given before the noon meal. Ultralente can be given at approxi-
				mately 50% of the total daily dose with half of the dose given be-
				fore breakfast and the other half given before dinner. Insulin
				glargine (Lantus), another long-acting insulin, cannot be mixed
				with other insulins because its pharmacodynamic profile could be
				altered. It may be given once daily.
Method 6				
Reg/Ultralente	Reg	Reg	NPH	Some patients achieve better control of fasting hyperglycemia by using
Lispro/Ultralente	Lispro or	Lispro	NPH	NPH at bedtime to target early-morning insulin resistance while
Aspart/Ultralente	Aspart	Aspart	NPH	continuing to take Ultralente each morning.

Reg, regular insulin.

ing so, it offers some of the same advantages of the pump in that it permits some degree of flexibility in the patient's lifestyle. For example, if a patient with diabetes chooses to skip a meal, he or she omits a premeal bolus; if the patient chooses to eat a larger meal than usual, he or she increases the premeal bolus. Similar dose adjustments can be made to accommodate snacks, exercise patterns, and acute illnesses. The excess zinc in Ultralente binds regular insulin, but not insulin lispro; therefore, regular and Ultralente insulins should be administered in separate syringes. Furthermore, to minimize the

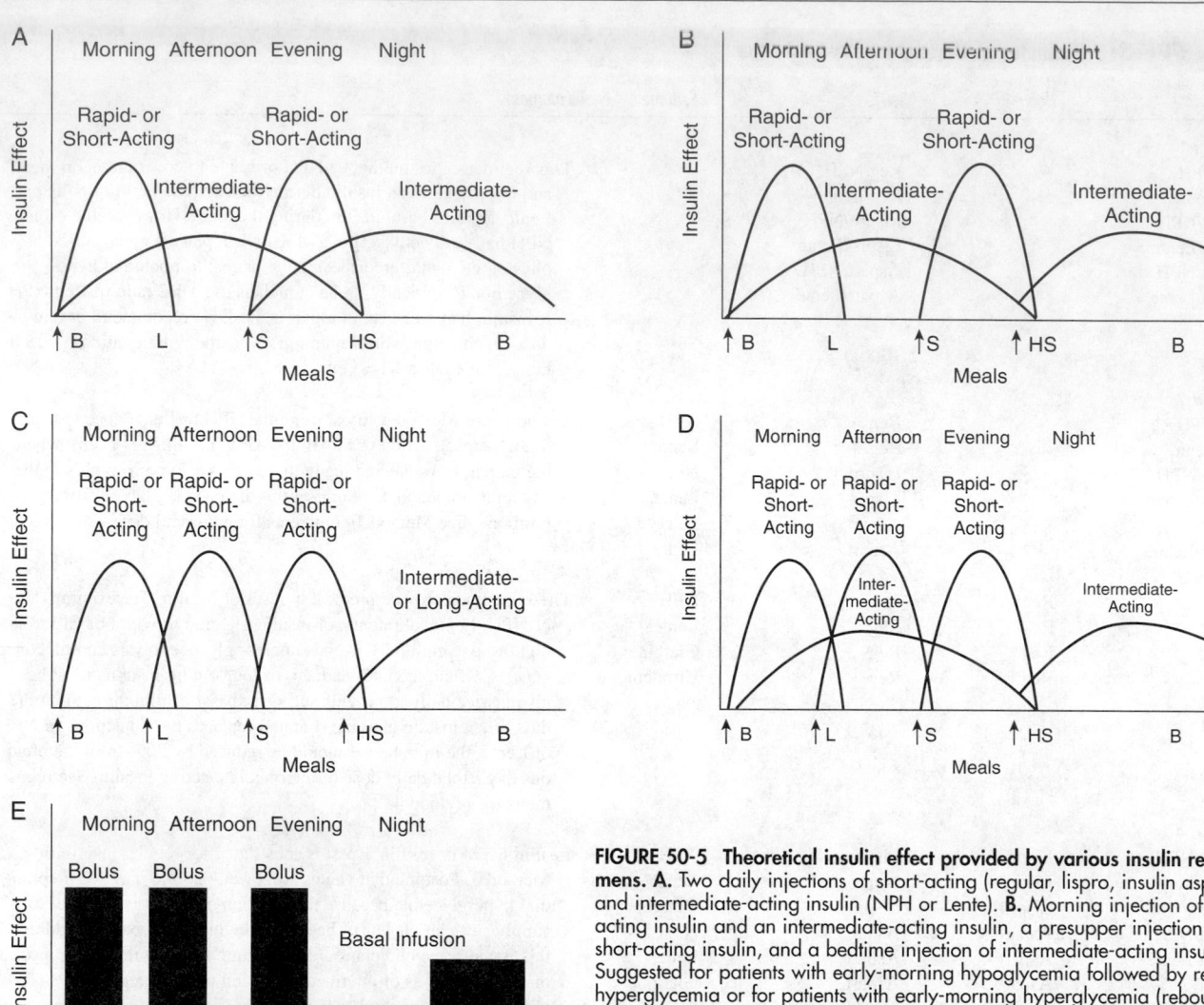

FIGURE 50-5 Theoretical insulin effect provided by various insulin regimens. A. Two daily injections of short-acting (regular, lispro, insulin aspart) and intermediate-acting insulin (NPH or Lente). **B.** Morning injection of short-acting insulin and an intermediate-acting insulin, a presupper injection of short-acting insulin, and a bedtime injection of intermediate-acting insulin. Suggested for patients with early-morning hypoglycemia followed by rebound hyperglycemia or for patients with early-morning hyperglycemia (rebound phenomenon). **C.** Preprandial injections of short-acting insulin and intermediate-acting insulin at bedtime. A long-acting insulin (insulin glargine) may be used in place of intermediate-acting insulin. **D.** Preprandial injections of short-acting insulin and intermediate-acting insulin at breakfast and bedtime. **E.** Continuous subcutaneous insulin infusion. B, breakfast; HS, bedtime snack; L, lunch; S, supper. *Arrows*, time of insulin injection (30 minutes before meals). (Adapted from reference 291.)

"peak" effects of Ultralente and to ensure 24-hour basal insulin levels, twice-daily administration may be needed. Insulin glargine appears to behave more like a true basal insulin because it lacks a "peak effect." It must, however, be injected separately.

5. **Should A.H. use an insulin pump or multiple insulin injections?**

Indications for intensive insulin therapy are listed in Table 50-15. As discussed previously, A.H. is an ideal candidate for intensive insulin therapy. She is newly diagnosed, has not yet developed the long-term complications of diabetes, and should derive the potential benefits of normoglycemia. Assuming A.H. will be able to comply with intensive insulin therapy, individualized target blood glucose levels that strive for the best level of glucose control possible without placing her at undue risk for hypoglycemia should be prescribed. She

must be willing to test her blood glucose concentrations four or more times daily and inject herself three to four times daily or learn about the use and care of an insulin pump. She also must be willing to keep detailed records and participate in an extensive education program that enables her to adjust her insulin doses based on blood glucose concentrations, physical activity, and the carbohydrate content of her snacks and meals.

Patients must be able to attain the above skills before they are considered viable users of an insulin pump. The ADA recommends that the use of insulin pumps be limited to highly motivated individuals under the guidance of a health care team trained and knowledgeable in their use. Pumps offer the patient flexibility with meal schedules and travel. Most studies have shown that pump therapy provides equivalent and sometimes better glycemic control than does intensive management with multiple injections.[61,66]

Table 50-14   Empiric Insulin Doses

Estimating Total Daily Insulin Requirements

These are initial doses only; they must be refined using SMBG results. Patients may be particularly resistant to insulin if their blood glucose concentrations are high (glucose toxicity); once glucose concentrations begin to drop, insulin requirements often decrease precipitously. The weight used is actual body weight. Insulin dose requirements can change dramatically over time depending on circumstances (e.g., a growth spurt, modest weight gain or loss, illness).

Type 1 Diabetes	
Initial dose	0.5–0.8 U/kg
Honeymoon phase	0.2–0.5 U/kg
With ketosis, during illness, during growth	1.0–1.5 U/kg
Type 2 Diabetes	
With insulin resistance	0.7–1.5 U/kg

Estimating Basal Insulin Requirements

These are empiric doses only and should be adjusted using appropriate SMBG results (fasting or premeal). Basal requirements vary throughout the day, often increasing during the early morning hours. The requirement also is influenced by the presence of endogenous insulin, the degree of insulin resistance, and body weight. The range is 0.3 to 1.4 U/hr.

   Approximately 50% of total daily dose
   Approximately 0.7 U/hr for a 70-kg person (154 lb)

Estimating Premeal Insulin Requirements

The "500 Rule" estimates the number of grams of carbohydrate (CHO) that will be covered by 1 unit of rapid-acing insulin.[56] The rule is modified to the "450 Rule" if using regular insulin.

   500/total daily dose of insulin (TDD) = number of grams covered
Example: For a patient using 50 units per day, 500/50 = 10. Therefore, 10 g carbohydrate would be covered by one unit of insulin lispro or insulin aspart. This equation works very well for type 1 patients in estimating their premeal insulin requirements. Because patients with type 2 diabetes have insulin resistance, the rule may underestimate their insulin requirements.

Determining the "Correction Factor"

Supplemental doses of rapid-acting insulin are administered to acutely lower glucose concentrations that exceed the target glucose concentration. These doses must be individualized for each patient and again are based on the degree of sensitivity to insulin action. For example, if the premeal or bedtime blood glucose target is 140 mg/dL and the patient's value is 190 mg/dL, additional units of insulin might be added to the premeal dose or an additional supplemental bedtime dose of lispro might be given. The correction factor determines how far the blood glucose drops per unit of insulin lispro or insulin aspart given and is known as the "1800 Rule".[65] For regular insulin, the rule is modified to the "1500 Rule". The equation is as follows:

   1800/TDD = point drop in blood glucose per unit of insulin
Example: If a patient uses 30 units of insulin per day, their correction factor (or insulin sensitivity) would be 1800/30 = 60 mg/dL. Therefore, the patient can expect a 60 mg/dL drop for every unit of rapid acting insulin administered. Patients with a higher sensitivity factor have lower insulin requirements. Individuals with a lower sensitivity factor (higher insulin requirements) typically achieve a smaller reduction in blood glucose per unit of insulin.

CHO, carbohydrate; SMBG, self-monitored blood glucose; TDD, total daily dose. Adapted from reference 60.

Table 50-15   Intensive Insulin Therapy: Indications and Precautions

Patient Selection Criteria

Type 1, otherwise healthy patients (older than 7 yr of age) who are highly motivated and compliant individuals. Must be willing to test blood glucose concentrations four times daily and inject three to four doses of insulin daily
Diabetic women who plan to conceive
Pregnant diabetic patients
Patients poorly controlled on conventional therapy (includes type 2 patients)
Technical ability to test blood glucose concentrations
Intellectual ability to interpret blood glucose concentrations and adjust insulin doses appropriately
Access to trained and skilled medical staff to direct treatment program and provide close supervision

Avoid or Use Cautiously in Patients Who Are Predisposed to Severe Hypoglycemic Reactions or in Whom Such Reactions Could Be Fatal

Patients with counter-regulatory insufficiency
Type 1 diabetes for ≥15 yr (not all patients)
β-Adrenergic blocker therapy
Autonomic insufficiency
Adrenal or pituitary insufficiency
Patients with coronary or cerebral vascular disease
(*Note:* Counter-regulatory hormones released in response to hypoglycemia may have adverse effects in these individuals)
Unreliable, noncompliant individuals, including those who abuse alcohol or drugs and those with psychiatric disorders

ing the insulin pump.[60,63] Since A.H. has just been diagnosed, she should be initiated on multiple daily doses of insulin at this time. Once she has acquired these skills, she may be considered for pump therapy.

Clinical Use of Insulin
Initiating Insulin Therapy

6. How should multiple-dose insulin therapy be initiated in A.H.?

There is no generally accepted approach to the initiation of multiple-dose insulin therapy in newly diagnosed patients. A conservative total daily dose of insulin is estimated empirically or according to guidelines similar to those listed in Table 50-14. Some endocrinologists prefer to begin with NPH, optimize the NPH doses, and then add rapid or short-acting insulin if needed later. The total daily dose of NPH is split initially into two doses: two-thirds in the morning and one-third before dinner. Others initiate the patient on mixed doses of NPH and regular insulin twice daily. On an outpatient basis, this latter approach may be somewhat impractical in that the patient will have to learn how to mix insulins in addition to several other skills on the first visit. One also should be aware that administration of two-thirds of the dose in the morning assumes consumption of two-thirds of the total daily carbohydrates at breakfast and lunch. This may not hold true for many patients.

Insulin glargine (Lantus) may also be used as a basal insulin with bolus doses of a rapid- or short-acting insulin (insulin lispro, insulin aspart, or regular) given with meals. Studies have suggested that the basal insulin profile obtained from

Insulin pumps are particularly useful in patients with frequent, unpredictable hypoglycemia or marked dawn phenomena (see Question 19). Others have described the methods by which insulin doses are established and altered in patients us-

glargine is superior to NPH or Ultralente with a reduction in the incidence of hypoglycemia.[67] However, the cost of insulin glargine, its availability on formularies, and its incompatibility with other insulins in the same syringe may cause some clinicians and patients to use NPH preferentially.

During the initial visit, A.H. needs to learn how to inject her insulin (see Question 9), how to test her blood glucose (see Table 50-17), how and when to test her urine for ketones, and how to recognize and treat hypoglycemia (see Table 50-25). She also needs to understand the importance of meal planning and the relationship between carbohydrate intake and insulin action. It is very important not to overwhelm A.H. with information on the first visit. One should be particularly sensitive to the psychological impact of this diagnosis on A.H., address her major concerns, and provide only the information that is absolutely essential before the next visit. Between visits, she should be assessed and provided information on an as-needed basis by phone. Table 50-16 lists important areas of patient education.

A reasonable first approach in A.H. is to provide a total daily dose of 24 units of NPH (approximately 0.5 U/kg) divided into two doses: 16 units 30 minutes before breakfast and 8 units 30 minutes before dinner. An alternative option would be to give a single daily dose of 24 units of insulin glargine, either at bedtime or in the morning. It should be noted that some physicians use more conservative doses initially to evaluate a patient's sensitivity to insulin. Furthermore, as the glucose concentration returns to normal, glucose toxicity will recede and the patient may require less insulin.

Selecting an Insulin Product

7. If the clinician decides to use an intermediate insulin initially, is there a preference between NPH or Lente insulin?

Table 50-16 Areas of Patient Education

Diabetes: Pathogenesis and the complications
Hyperglycemia: Signs and symptoms
Ketoacidosis: Signs and symptoms (see Table 50-26)
Hypoglycemia: Signs, symptoms, and treatment (see Table 50-25)
Exercise: Effect on blood glucose concentrations and insulin dose (see Table 50-23)
Diet: See text. Emphasis placed on carbohydrate counting because the carbohydrate is responsible for 90% of the rise in blood glucose following a meal.
Insulins:
    Injection technique
    Types of insulin
    Onset and peak actions
    Storage
    Stability (look for crystallization and precipitation)
Therapeutic Goals: A_{1C}, blood glucose, cholesterol, triglycerides, blood pressure
Self-Monitored Blood Glucose Testing: See Table 50-17
Interpretation of self-monitored blood glucose testing results
Foot Care: Inspect feet daily; wear well-fitted shoes; avoid self-care of ingrown toenails, corns, or athlete's foot; see a podiatrist
Sick Day Management: See Table 50-24
Cardiovascular Risk Factors: Tobacco use, high blood pressure, obesity, elevated cholesterol
Importance of annual ophthalmologic examinations; tests for microalbuminuria

Most clinicians use NPH and Lente insulins interchangeably. The onset of action, peak effect, and duration of action of these two insulins are basically the same, although Lente may have a slightly slower onset and slightly longer duration than NPH. Some have supported the use of Lente insulin because it does not contain protamine, a protein that is rarely antigenic. However, allergic reactions to both protamine and zinc (contained in Lente insulins) have been rare.[68]

The rapid onset of regular insulin is more likely to be retained when mixed with NPH than with Lente insulin, but lispro and aspart may be mixed with either (see Question 14). Because A.H. eventually will use a mixture of regular or rapid-acting insulin and intermediate-acting insulin, NPH insulin can be used initially.

Although purified pork insulin is still available, it is rarely used and patients should be initiated with human insulin. Pork insulin is slightly more antigenic and more expensive than human insulin.

Selecting an Insulin Syringe

8. What kind of insulin syringe should be prescribed for A.H.?

Insulin syringes are plastic, disposable syringes with needles that are very fine (28 to 30 gauge), sharp, and well lubricated to ease insertion. Needles and syringes have been improved so that insulin injections are relatively painless if proper technique is used. Less pain is associated with the smaller, 29- or 30-gauge needles. The "dead space" (air space at the hub of the needle) has been virtually eliminated so that mixing and measuring problems previously associated with its presence are no longer a concern. The lengths of needles are $^{5}/_{16}$, $^{3}/_{8}$, or $^{1}/_{2}$ inch. The shortest needle can be used for children or patients with little SC fat.[62]

Manufacturers produce 1-, 0.5-, and 0.3-mL syringes for U-100 insulin. For patients such as A.H., using <40 units of insulin per injection, the 0.5-mL (low-dose) syringe is preferred. Syringes with 0.3-mL capacities are recommended for pediatric and patients using <25 units of insulin per injection. The dose markings on the 0.3-mL and 0.5-mL syringe are much easier to read than the 1 mL syringe, allowing the patient to measure insulin more easily. Insulin syringes are available in 1-unit increments or $^{1}/_{2}$-unit increments (BD UltraFine II Short Needle Syringe, $^{1}/_{3}$ mL only).[62]

A 0.5 mL U-100 insulin syringe with a $^{1}/_{2}$ inch, 28- or 29-gauge needle should be prescribed for A.H. Cost and patient preference will govern the brand selected. Subjectively, patients can "feel" the difference between different brands, or they may prefer the "ease of bubble removal," physical characteristics, or packaging of one syringe over another.

Insulin pen and dosing devices (e.g., Innolet) are also available for injecting insulin. These devices are useful in patients with visual or dexterity problems in whom use of a vial and syringe method is difficult. Pens remove the need to withdraw insulin, and the insulin dose is dialed up on the device. Pen needles are available in 29, 30, and 31 gauge and $^{3}/_{16}$, $^{5}/_{16}$, or $^{1}/_{2}$ inch lengths.[62,69]

Measuring and Injecting Insulin

9. How should A.H. be instructed to measure and inject her NPH insulin?

AGITATION

All insulins, with the exception of regular, lispro, aspart, and glargine insulins, are suspensions and must be agitated before they are withdrawn from the vial. A new, unused vial of NPH or Lente insulin may require vigorous agitation to loosen the sediment, which may have become packed down with storage. The vial should be rolled between the palms of the hands to minimize foaming.

MEASUREMENT

First, A.H. should make sure her hands and the injection site are clean (it is not necessary to use alcohol to clean the site). She should withdraw the plunger to the level of insulin she intends to inject (16 units); then she should insert the needle into the vial and inject 16 units of air to prevent creation of a vacuum within the vial. The vial then should be inverted with the syringe inserted, and 16 units of NPH should be withdrawn. The bevel of the needle should be well below the surface of the insulin to avoid withdrawing air or bubbles into the syringe.

The barrel of the syringe should be held at eye level to check for air bubbles and to allow accurate placement of the plunger tip at the 16-unit mark. If bubbles are present, they should be removed by tapping the syringe gently to coax the bubbles to the top of the barrel, where they can be injected back into the insulin vial. To remove air bubbles in an insulin pen, prime the needle with 2-units of insulin before each use. Also, remove the needle from the pen device in between uses to prevent air bubbles from accumulating.

INJECTION

A.H. now should prepare an area for injection. Alcohol swabs may be used to clean the rubber stopper of the insulin vial. To inject the insulin subcutaneously, A.H. should be instructed to firmly pinch up the area to be injected (this creates a firm surface for the injection) and to quickly insert the needle perpendicularly (90-degree angle) into the center of this area. The syringe should be held toward the middle or back of the barrel, like a pencil. Anxious patients have a tendency to "choke" the hub of the syringe, and this prevents proper needle insertion. A 45-degree angle of injection may be used for infants and thin individuals who have little SC fat. The skin pinch should be released and the insulin injected.[69] Pressure should be applied at the site of injection for 5 to 8 seconds to prevent back leakage of the insulin as the needle is removed. The site should not be massaged, because this may accelerate the absorption and onset of action of insulin (see Table 50-12). When using an insulin pen, the needle should be embedded within the skin for about 5 seconds after depressing the plunger to ensure full delivery of the insulin dose.

Patients who are anxious about self-injection can be helped by applying an ice cube to the site before injection or by using an injection aid. However, injection aids are generally unnecessary once the patient realizes that injections are relatively pain free with proper technique.

ROTATING INJECTION SITES

Previously, patients were advised to rotate injection sites between the arms, thighs, abdomen, and buttocks (Fig. 50-6). However, differences in the rate of insulin absorption from these sites resulted in altered glucose control.[70] Now, the ADA

These drawings show areas of the body most suitable for insulin injections:

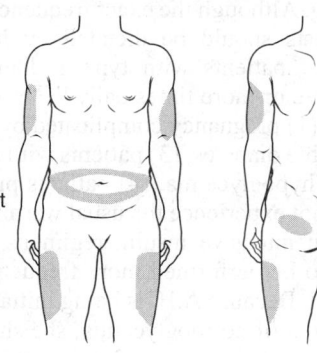

The actual point of injection should be varied each time within a chosen body area. Give injections at least one inch apart (Patients should consult with their physician or diabetes educator about which area is most appropriate for use.)

Insulin is injected in the subcutaneous tissue (between the skin and the muscle layer). If the skin is pinched up and the needle is pushed all the way in, the needle will reach the proper space under the skin.

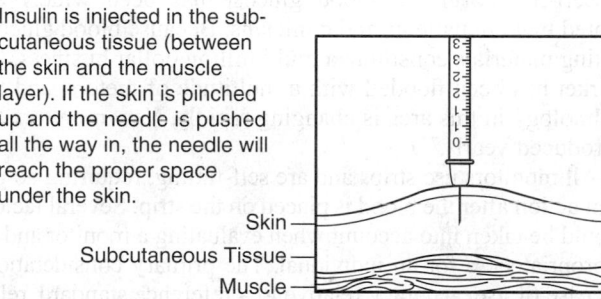

Skin —
Subcutaneous Tissue —
Muscle —

FIGURE 50-6 Selecting insulin injection sites. (Used with permission from reference 300.)

recommends that insulin injections be rotated within the same anatomic region to avoid this effect.[69,71] Some recommend insulin injections into the abdominal area because absorption from this site is least affected by exercise and the most predictable. Alternatively, A.H. can be instructed to rotate her morning injection within one region (e.g., the thigh) and her evening injection in another anatomic region. This minimizes the variables that can alter her response to insulin.

Rotating injection sites also was recommended at one time to avoid the lipodystrophic effect of insulin (lipohypertrophy and lipoatrophy); however, because insulin has been purified, these complications are less frequent and the importance of rotation is less critical. Nevertheless, repetitive use of the same site of injection may still result in lipohypertrophy and it does toughen the skin, making needle penetration more difficult. Furthermore, insulin absorption from lipohypertrophic sites can be slowed.[72]

Self-Monitored Blood Glucose

10. Should A.H. self-monitor her blood glucose? What types of home blood glucose monitoring tests are available, and what are the major differences between them? How accurate are results obtained from home blood glucose testing?

The advent of SMBG revolutionized the management of diabetes mellitus by providing a simple and portable method for periodic and repeated measurement of blood glucose in the ambulatory care setting. Based on the results of the DCCT, the ADA recommends that most individuals with diabetes should attempt to attain and achieve normoglycemia as safely as possible. For patients with type 1 diabetes, this can be achieved only by using SMBG; therefore, all treatment programs should include the routine use of daily glucose monitoring. Although the exact frequency and timing of blood glucose tests should be dictated by individualized patient goals, most patients with type 1 diabetes should perform SMBG three or more times daily.[42,73] SMBG is especially important in (1) pregnancy complicated by diabetes, (2) patients with unstable diabetes, (3) patients with a propensity to severe ketosis or hypoglycemia, (4) patients prone to hypoglycemia who may not experience the usual warning symptoms, and (5) patients on intensive insulin regimens. Glucose monitoring should also be performed more frequently whenever therapy is modified. Because A.H. is being initiated on insulin therapy with the goal of normoglycemia, she should self-monitor her blood glucose a minimum of three times per day.

Self-monitoring of blood glucose has been widely accepted by both patients and clinicians. Because blood glucose testing materials constitute a multimillion dollar business, the market has been flooded with a multitude of meters, and the technology in this area is changing rapidly. New monitors are introduced yearly.[73]

All monitors use strips and are self-timing, requiring no patient action after the blood is placed on the strip. Several factors should be taken into account when evaluating a monitor and its appropriateness for an individual. The primary considerations are ease of use, accuracy relative to a reference standard, reliability, insurance coverage and cost.[62,74] Convenience factors include meter size, volume of blood required for testing, site to obtain sample (e.g., finger versus alternate site such as forearm), capacity of the meter to store blood glucose values (memory) and manage data, testing time, size of read-out, general availability of strips, ability to turn off audible signals, and availability of technical support. Some devices are less reliable for use in anemic patients (e.g., renal transplant patients), and all function most reliably within certain temperature ranges (usually 60° to 95°F) and humidity (generally <90%) conditions. Strips are sensitive to light, moisture, and temperature extremes and must be stored and handled with care.

Several generic strips have become available (Quick Check, Biotel), offering patients an inexpensive solution to the cost of frequent monitoring if their insurance does not cover them. These strips are advertised as being compatible with several meters. However, few studies confirming their equivalency to brand name strips exist. One study found that brand name strips, which are calibrated to the machine by the manufacturer, were more accurate and precise than the generic strips.[75] (*Note:* Accuracy is a measure of agreement with a standard reference, and precision is a measure of variation between repeated tests.) If A.H. wants to try generic strips, she should compare her results with a laboratory determination to ensure that the strips are providing accurate results. Capillary values measured by the glucose meter are likely to be 10% to 15% lower than values measured by the laboratory unless the meter has already been calibrated to plasma levels. She also could compare results obtained from the generic strips with those of the brand name strips.

Patient education regarding testing procedures, the importance of recording results, and test times are critical. Ultimately, A.H. should be taught how to use blood glucose values to adjust her insulin dose, dietary intake, and exercise pattern (Table 50-17).

Used properly, available meters provide accurate, precise results that can be used by patients to manage their diabetes (see Table 50-17). However, several factors can affect the accuracy of meter results—most commonly, equipment malfunction and human error. Problems with a meter can be detected by performing a quality-control test once weekly and with each new vial of strips; human error can be minimized with adequate training. Table 50-18 lists factors that can affect results of SMBG test results. Anytime SMBG values are inconsistent with the patient's symptoms or A_{1C} values, sources of error should be evaluated (see Table 50-6). A.H.'s technique

---

Table 50-17   Self-Monitored Blood Glucose (SMBG) Testing: Areas of Patient Education

When and How Often to Test

Technique
How and when to calibrate the glucose monitor.
Review all "buttons" and their purposes. Identify battery case. Review cleaning procedures.
Preparation
1. Calibrate monitor/set code for batch of test strips.
2. Turn machine on.
3. Prepare all materials: tissue, strip, lancet.
4. Remember to close the lid of the strip container immediately. Strips exposed to air and moisture deteriorate rapidly.
5. Wash hands with warm water. *Dry thoroughly.* A wet finger causes blood to spread rather than form a drop. Milk the finger from the base to ensure an adequate flow of blood.
6. Lance the tip of the finger. Avoid the pads of the finger where nerves are concentrated.
7. Hold the finger *below* the heart with the lanced area pointing toward the floor.
8. Once a sufficient amount of blood is available, *quickly* apply blood to designated area of the test strip. Depending on the strip type, the blood sample is placed in an area on the surface of the strip or it is applied to the side of the strip where it is taken up by capillary action.

Record Results in a Log Book and Bring to All Clinician Visits. Include Relevant Information Regarding Diet or Exercise

How to Use Results to Achieve Normoglycemia

Table 50-18   Factors That Can Alter Self-Monitored Blood Glucose Test Results: Troubleshooting

Glucose monitor not coded for batch of test strips[a]
An inadequate amount of blood applied to test strip[b]
Dirty glucose monitor[a]
Low battery[a]
Test performed outside of temperature and humidity operating conditions[a]
Low[c] or high[b] hematocrit
Dehydration[b]
Hyperosmolar, nonketotic state[b]
Lipemia[a]
High levels of ascorbic acid or salicylates (rare)[b]

[a]Effect unpredictable.
[b]Values tend to be lower.
[c]Values tend to be higher.

should be reviewed periodically, because clinical decisions are based on the patient's blood glucose testing record.

Testing Frequency

11. **How often and when should A.H. be instructed to test her blood glucose concentrations?**

The objective of ongoing, frequent blood glucose testing is to determine whether normoglycemia is being achieved and to assess the action of specific insulin doses as well as the impact of meals, food, illness, or exercise on blood glucose levels. Ideally, patients should test their blood glucose concentration before meals, 90 to 120 minutes after meals to determine their "insulin to carbohydrate ratio," at bedtime, and occasionally, at 2 or 3 AM (i.e., eight times daily). However, most patients are unable to adhere to such a rigorous regimen. At the minimum, to determine her daily insulin requirements, A.H. should test her blood glucose concentrations six to eight times daily: before and after each meal and at bedtime. She also should set her alarm for 3 AM two or three times per week and test her blood glucose at that time. Blood glucose concentrations measured at these times more or less correspond to the peak action of short- and intermediate-acting insulins administered at various times of the day, enabling the clinician to evaluate the effect of various insulin components on meals and to identify nocturnal hypoglycemia. For example, the blood glucose measured before dinner reflects the action of A.H.'s morning dose of NPH on food she has eaten for breakfast and lunch, as well as hepatic glucose production between meals. Increasingly, patients who use carbohydrate counting with rapid-acting insulins are being advised to test 2-hour postprandial levels on initiating therapy to enhance proper dosage adjustment. (Table 50-19)

The importance of frequent blood glucose testing cannot be overemphasized. When blood glucose is tested less frequently than four times daily, glucose control deteriorates to baseline levels. This is because complete profiles are no longer available, and it is impossible to adjust insulin doses based on random blood glucose concentrations.[76] If patients refuse to test four times daily, they should be encouraged to test four times daily on representative days of the week or to test at different times of the day each day so that a weekly profile can be developed. A.H. also should be encouraged to test

her blood glucose concentration any time she is feeling unusual or to evaluate the effect of unusual circumstances on her blood glucose concentration (e.g., increased physical exercise, a large holiday meal, final examinations, a family crisis).

NONINVASIVE BLOOD GLUCOSE TESTING

Many patients refuse to perform SMBG or grow tired of self-testing because of the discomfort of the fingerstick. Thus, much research is being done in the area of noninvasive blood glucose testing. The GlucoWatch (Cygnus Inc., Redwood City, California) is a noninvasive, watchlike device that uses reverse iontophoresis to collect glucose samples through intact skin via interstitial fluid. The device allows users to monitor their glucose levels automatically, up to three times per hour for 12 hours. It has an alarm for low or high readings. The device is available by prescription only and restricted to adults 18 years of age or older or children 7 to 17 years of age with diabetes. Disadvantages include the necessity of daily calibration with a blood glucose meter, a long warm-up period (3 hours) and a high cost for the meter and strips.[77]

Using Blood Glucose Test Results to Evaluate Insulin Doses

12. **A.H. was instructed to inject herself twice daily with NPH insulin: 16 units before breakfast and 8 units before dinner. She was asked to test her blood glucose eight times daily (before and after meals and at bedtime), to record her results and other unusual events or symptoms during the day, and to bring her records to the clinic. A.H. was also instructed to keep a food diary and record the number of carbohydrates she ingested at each meal. The initial goal of therapy is to achieve preprandial blood glucose concentrations of <180 mg/dL and to eliminate symptoms of hyperglycemia. One week later, trends in her blood glucose concentrations were as follows:**

Time	Glucose Concentration (mg/dL)	mmol/L
7 AM	160–200	8.8–11.1
Noon	220–260	2.2–14.4
5 PM	130–180	7.2–10.0
11 PM	140–180	7.8–10.0

Occasional 3 AM tests averaged 160 mg/dL and A.H.'s urine is negative for ketones. She eats between two and four carbohydrate servings (30 to 60 g) per meal. Subjectively, A.H. feels a bit

---

Table 50-19	Interpreting Self-Monitored Blood Glucose Concentrations[a]	
Test Time	**Target Insulin Dose**	**Target Meal/Snack**
Prebreakfast (fasting)	Predinner/bedtime intermediate- or long-acting insulin	Bedtime snack
Prelunch	Prebreakfast regular insulin	Breakfast/midmorning snack
Predinner	Prebreakfast intermediate-acting insulin and/or prelunch regular insulin	Lunch/midafternoon snack
Bedtime	Predinner regular insulin	Dinner
2-hour postprandial	Premeal lispro insulin or insulin aspart	Preceding meal or snack
3 AM or later	Predinner intermediate-acting insulin	Dinner/bedtime snack

[a]Considerations: (1) Assumes a normal meal pattern. For patients who travel, have odd working or sleeping hours, or irregular meal patterns, these rules may not apply. (2) Assumes administration of regular insulin 30 to 60 minutes before meals or lispro insulin 0 to 15 minutes before meals and a normal pattern of insulin response (see Table 50-12 for factors that can alter insulin absorption and response). (3) If prebreakfast concentrations are high, rule out reactive hyperglycemia (Somogyi reaction or posthypoglycemic hyperglycemia). Consider contribution of dawn phenomenon as well. Whenever blood glucose concentrations are high, consider reactive hyperglycemia (excessive insulin doses). (4) Consider accuracy of reported test results: (a) Do they correlate with A$_{1c}$ and patient's signs and symptoms? (b) What is the patient's compliance? Could results be fabricated? (c) Is patient's technique appropriate? Check timing, adequate blood sample, machine, strips, and calibration (see Table 50-18). (d) Are insulin kinetics altered? (see Table 50-12) (e) Meals: consider content, quality, and regularity.

better, and her weight has stabilized, but she still urinates two to three times nightly. How would you interpret these results, and how should A.H.'s insulin dose be altered?

Health care providers should use the data obtained from self-monitoring to (1) set glycemic goals, (2) develop recommendations for pharmacologic therapy, (3) evaluate the effectiveness of pharmacologic therapy, (4) instruct patients to interpret and respond to blood glucose patterns, (5) evaluate the impact of dietary factors on glycemic control, (6) modify therapy during acute/intercurrent illness or whenever patients receive medications known to affect glycemic control, (7) modify the management plan in response to a change in activity levels, and (8) identify hypoglycemic unawareness.[42]

Before using A.H.'s blood glucose results to adjust her insulin dose, it is important to observe and reassess her testing technique. One also should determine whether there were any unusual circumstances in her life, diet, or exercise patterns over the past week that might have affected her response to insulin. Once these have been ruled out as confounding factors, one can begin making gross adjustments in A.H.'s insulin dose, realizing that fine-tuning will be impossible until a consistent diet and exercise pattern have been instituted.

Several principles must be kept in mind whenever blood glucose tests are used to adjust a patient's basic insulin dose (Table 50-20). Because many factors can alter a patient's response to insulin, it is important to use blood glucose concentration *trends* measured over a minimum of 3 days to adjust the basic insulin dose (i.e., the dose the patient will use every day). The only exception to this rule is the use of supplemental insulin doses to correct exceptionally high glucose concentrations after A.H. has acquired sophisticated insulin adjustment skills (see Questions 17 and 18). SMBG results should be evaluated in conjunction with other parameters such as A_{1C} and periodic laboratory blood glucose measurements.

The twice-daily dose of NPH is inadequately controlling A.H.'s symptoms and blood glucose concentrations. She is achieving some response in the late afternoon, but the delayed onset of NPH action and inadequate total daily dose have resulted in poor control of her blood glucose concentrations overall. The blood glucose concentration of 160 mg/dL at 3 AM indicates that rebound hyperglycemia is an unlikely cause of her high fasting levels (see Questions 15 and 18). As an initial step toward control, A.H.'s evening dose of NPH could be increased in an attempt to control her fasting hyperglycemia. However, this approach does not address A.H.'s elevated prelunch values.

Thus, if A.H. is capable and ready to learn how to mix short-acting and intermediate-acting insulins, the split-mix approach is preferred:

- Increase the total daily dose of insulin slightly because her overall control is poor, and hyperglycemia increases resistance to insulin action (e.g., 0.6 U/kg × 50 kg = 30 units).
- Split the dose of insulin so that approximately two-thirds (21 units) is administered in the morning and one-third (9 units) is administered in the evening.
- Provide a 2:1 ratio of NPH:regular or insulin lispro or aspart in the morning (14 U/7 U) and evening (6 U/3 U).

Table 50-20   Factors That Can Alter Blood Glucose Control

Diet

Insufficient calories (e.g., alcoholism, eating disorders, anorexia, nausea, and vomiting)
Overeating (e.g., during the holidays)
Irregularly spaced skipped or delayed meals
Dietary content (e.g., fiber, carbohydrate content)

Physical Activity

See Table 50-23 and Question 30

Stress

Infection
Surgery/trauma
Psychological

Drugs

See Tables 50-36 and 50-37 for information about medications that affect blood glucose levels

Hormonal Changes

Menstruation: glucose concentrations may increase premenstrually and return to normal postmenses
Pregnancy
Puberty: hyperglycemia probably related to high growth hormone levels

Gastroparesis

Delays gastric emptying time. Peak insulin action and meal-related glucose excursions may become mismatched

Altered Insulin Pharmacokinetics

See Table 50-12

Insulin Injection Technique

Measuring
Timing
Technique

Inactive Insulin

Outdated insulin
Improperly stored insulin (heat or cold)
Crystallized insulin

If this approach is used, it is essential that A.H. incorporate a bedtime snack into her diet and test her blood glucose concentrations periodically at 3 AM to ensure that she does not suffer from nocturnal hypoglycemia.

Mixing Insulins

13. A.H. is anxious to get her diabetes under control and agrees to mix the NPH and regular insulins. How should she be instructed to measure and withdraw this insulin mixture?

The procedure used to mix and withdraw NPH and regular insulin is basically the same as that described in Question 9. The major difference is that an adequate volume of air must be injected into the NPH vial *before* the regular or insulin lispro or aspart is measured and withdrawn. Also, regular insulin is measured and withdrawn into the insulin syringe *first* to avoid contamination of the vial of regular or aspart or lispro insulin with NPH. Contamination with NPH ultimately alters the NPH:regular insulin ratio that is administered. When patients withdraw NPH or Lente insulin first, the vial of regular insulin eventually becomes cloudy. In contrast, contamination of the NPH insulin with regular insulin probably is insignificant because the protamine contained in NPH can bind the regular insulin (see Question 14). The procedure A.H. should use to mix her insulins is described in the following section, using her morning dose as an example.

- After dispersing the NPH insulin suspension, inject 14 units of air into the NPH vial and withdraw the needle.
- Inject 7 units of air into the regular insulin vial, and withdraw the 7 units of insulin as described in Question 9.
- Insert the needle into the NPH vial, and pull the plunger down to the 21-unit mark (14 units of NPH plus 7 units of regular insulin).

Stability of Mixed Insulins

14. Will mixing NPH with regular insulin blunt the rapid action of regular insulin? How stable are other insulin mixtures? (See Table 50-21.)

REGULAR PLUS NPH

The onset and duration of action of regular and NPH insulin administered as a mixture are similar to those observed when the two insulins are administered by separate injection. The pharmacodynamic profiles of these insulins are retained in premixed preparations stored in vials or syringes for 3 months.[78,69] (See Table 50-21.) This is true even though protamine in NPH binds regular insulin in vitro.

REGULAR PLUS LENTE OR ULTRALENTE

In contrast to the regular–NPH mixtures, the rapid action of regular insulin is blunted significantly when premixed with Lente insulin. The excess zinc in Lente preparations binds the regular insulin, converting it to an intermediate-acting form. This effect is observed even when the two insulins are mixed just before injection; however, the clinical importance of this effect seems to be minimal.[69,79] Similar changes occur when regular insulin is mixed with Ultralente insulin.

RAPID-ACTING INSULIN PLUS NPH

Insulin lispro and aspart are compatible with human NPH insulin manufactured by Eli Lilly and Company (Humulin N) and NovoNordisk (Novolin N), respectively. However, relative to lispro and aspart alone, the absorption rate is slowed and the peak concentrations are blunted. The total bioavailability is unaltered. The manufacturers recommend mixing the two insulins just before administration, which should be scheduled 15 minutes before meals. The compatibility of lispro and aspart with other brands of human NPH insulin or animal source NPH is unknown.[69,80]

RAPID-ACTING INSULIN PLUS LANTUS

The long-acting Lantus must not be mixed with any other insulins. If Lantus is mixed or diluted with other insulins, its pH will be increased, which will affect its absorption kinetics. The onset of action and duration of effect may be altered unpredictably.[81]

RAPID-ACTING INSULIN PLUS ULTRALENTE

The insulin concentration-time curves for lispro and human Ultralente insulin (Humulin U) administered separately or in combination are virtually superimposable. Therefore, Ultralente insulin does not modify the pharmacokinetics of lispro. Although lispro–Lente mixtures have not been studied, one would anticipate similar results. Nevertheless, Lilly recommends mixing the two insulins just before injection.[80] No data are available regarding the stability of insulin aspart with crystalline insulin products; therefore, they should be avoided according to the manufacturer.

PHOSPHATE-BUFFERED REGULAR OR NPH PLUS LENTE OR ULTRALENTE

When phosphate-buffered insulins (e.g., NPH or Velosulin BR, Novo Nordisk) are mixed with Lente or Ultralente insulins, the phosphate binds with zinc and converts these insulin preparations into more rapid-acting forms.[69] This problem is not likely to be clinically encountered with Velosulin BR because it is generally reserved for use in insulin pumps.

Table 50-21	Compatibility of Insulin Mixtures	
Mixture	**Proportion**	**Comments**
Regular + NPH	Any proportion	The pharmacodynamic profiles of regular and NPH insulin are unchanged when premixed and
Regular + Lente	<1:1	stored in vials or syringes for up to 3 months. In contrast, the rapid action of regular insulin is significantly blunted when mixed with Lente or Ultralente insulin. The excess zinc in Lente preparations binds the regular insulin, converting it into an intermediate-acting form. When the two insulins are mixed just before injection, the clinical importance of this effect appears to be minimal.
Lispro + NPH	Any proportion	The absorption rate and peak concentration of lispro is blunted when mixed with NPH; however, total bioavailability is unaltered. The manufacturer recommends mixing the two insulins just before injection.
Lispro + Ultralente	Any proportion	Ultralente does not alter the pharmacokinetics of lispro.
Regular + normal saline	Any proportion	Use within 2–3 hours of preparation.
Regular + insulin diluting solution	Any proportion	Stable indefinitely.
Insulin glargine	Do not mix with other insulins	Pharmacodynamics could be modified.

INSULIN GLARGINE

Insulin glargine is a long-acting analog that is soluble at pH 4.0; it is designed to precipitate when injected into the neutral pH of subcutaneous tissue. Because all other insulin products have a pH of 7.0, it cannot be mixed with any of them.[81]

Evaluating Fasting Hyperglycemia

15. A.H. is instructed to inject 14 units NPH along with 7 units regular insulin before breakfast and 6 units NPH plus 3 units regular insulin before dinner. Two weeks later, she returns to the clinic with the following blood glucose trends:

Time	Glucose Concentration (mg/dL)	mmol/L
7 AM	140–180	7.8–10.0
Noon	120–140	6.7–7.8
5 PM	90–130	5.0–7.2
11 PM	90–120	5.0–6.7
3 AM	60–90	3.3–5.0

Subjectively, A.H. feels substantially better. Her energy level is beginning to return to normal and her nocturia has diminished, but she occasionally gets up one or two times nightly to urinate. A.H. has also noticed that nightmares or "sweats" sometimes awaken her. When this occurs, she generally has something to eat because she is "famished." She is able to get back to sleep but wakes up the next morning with a "splitting headache" and a "hung-over" feeling. A.H.'s weight remains the same, and she has begun to develop some consistency in her dietary patterns with the help of a dietitian. She is consuming two to three carbohydrate servings per meal and is feeling more comfortable in her ability to count carbohydrates. The A_{1c} from her last visit is 8.3%. The new goal is to achieve blood glucose concentrations <150 mg/dL preprandially. Evaluate A.H.'s blood glucose values. What are possible causes of A.H.'s fasting hyperglycemia?

A.H.'s prelunch, predinner, and bedtime blood glucose concentrations have improved considerably, indicating that her morning dose of regular insulin, morning dose of NPH, and evening dose of regular insulin are adequate (see Table 50-19). Her FPG concentration remains elevated, and her prelunch concentration could be improved. When evaluating morning hyperglycemia, several causes must be considered:

- An insufficient dose of evening NPH. If the evening dose of NPH is insufficient, hepatic glucose output during the fasting state will be excessive, thereby producing hyperglycemia.
- An insufficient duration of action of the evening dose of NPH (see following discussion).
- Reactive hyperglycemia in response to a nocturnal hypoglycemic episode (Somogyi effect).
- An excessive bedtime snack.
- The dawn phenomenon (see Question 19).

Somogyi Effect or Rebound Hyperglycemia

The presence of normoglycemia at bedtime, low blood glucose concentrations at 3 am, and symptoms of nocturnal hypoglycemia (nightmares, sweating, hunger, morning headache) in A.H. are consistent with a *rebound hyperglycemic reaction* in the morning (i.e., posthypoglycemic hyper-glycemia; Somogyi effect).[82] Theoretically, this effect occurs after any episode of severe hypoglycemia and is secondary to an excessive increase in glucose production by the liver that is activated by insulin counter-regulatory hormones such as cortisol, glucagon, epinephrine, and growth hormone.[83] The waning effects of the evening dose of NPH insulin also may contribute because insulin is needed to suppress hepatic glucose output during the fasting state. The existence of rebound hyperglycemia has been questioned.[84] However, as Gerich[85] points out, the studies' findings can be explained by the absence of counter-regulatory responses in some patients or hyperinsulinemia, which counteracts the effects of glucagon, epinephrine, and cortisol. Asymptomatic nocturnal hypoglycemia can occur in 33% of patients taking evening doses of insulin and may account for morning hyperglycemia in >10% of patients. Another potential consequence of nocturnal hypoglycemia is prolonged insulin resistance (perhaps a consequence of glucose toxicity), as signified by high postbreakfast glucose concentrations. By correcting the nocturnal hypoglycemia, normalization of A.H.'s fasting hyperglycemia also may be achieved. The following are therapeutic options:

- Decrease the evening dose of NPH by 2 to 3 units and have A.H. continue to monitor blood glucose concentrations at 3 AM.
- If A.H. is willing to give herself three injections of insulin, shift the evening injection of NPH (6 units) from predinner to bedtime. This preferred method effectively shifts the peak action of NPH to the early morning when she will be awake and decreases the risk of nocturnal hypoglycemia.[65,86] This peak action also corresponds to the dawn phenomenon (see Question 19) and the breakfast meal.
- If A.H. is willing to give herself three injections, another option is to change from NPH to insulin glargine (Lantus) as her basal insulin, since this product also is associated with less nocturnal hypoglycemia.[58,67,87] Decrease the daily dose of NPH by 20% and give 18 units of Lantus at bedtime or every morning, depending on A.H.'s preference. Remind A.H. that the dose of Lantus cannot be mixed with her Regular insulin.

Midmorning Hyperglycemia

16. Evaluate A.H.'s noon blood glucose concentration.

Midmorning hyperglycemia frequently represents the maximum glucose excursion in patients with diabetes and often is the most difficult to manage. The following are possible explanations for midmorning hyperglycemia:

- An insufficient dose of regular insulin before breakfast.
- Poor synchrony between meal intake and insulin action. This could be caused by administration of insulin just before or after meals or a delayed onset of action of regular insulin due to binding with intermediate-acting insulin or insulin-blocking antibodies.[49] The latter two explanations are unlikely in A.H. As discussed in Question 14, Lente insulin, but not NPH insulin, is more likely to delay the pharmacologic response to regular insulin. Because A.H. is a newly diagnosed patient with diabetes, it is unlikely that she has developed significant concentrations of insulin-blocking antibodies.

- An insufficient dose of evening NPH insulin to suppress hepatic glucose production (glycogenolysis and gluconeogenesis) during the fasting state or the dawn phenomenon (see Question 19).
- Excessive carbohydrate ingestion at breakfast.
- Increased peripheral resistance to insulin action caused by high fasting glucose levels (glucose toxicity).

When evaluating midmorning hyperglycemia, it is important to remember that the FPG concentration can contribute up to 50% of this plasma glucose excursion. Therefore, the primary approach to the control of hyperglycemia may be to normalize the fasting glucose concentration.

This should be the approach used for A.H. If control of her fasting hyperglycemia does not correct the midmorning hyperglycemia, the following interventions may be considered:

- Increase the dose of regular or insulin lispro or insulin aspart before breakfast.
- Inject the morning dose of regular insulin 45 to 60 minutes before breakfast in an attempt to match peak insulin concentrations with postmeal glucose excursions. If this maneuver is used, the patient should be warned of possible hypoglycemia before breakfast.
- Alter the carbohydrate content of the meals. This may include decreasing the amount of carbohydrate in the breakfast meal, changing the type of carbohydrate ingested, or adding fiber to that meal to minimize glucose excursions.

Preprandial Hypoglycemia —Use of Insulin Lispro and Aspart

17. **A.H. agrees to give herself three injections of insulin as follows: 14 units NPH/7 units regular insulin before breakfast; 3 units regular insulin before dinner; and 6 units NPH at bedtime. Two weeks later, she brings in her blood glucose concentration records:**

Time	Glucose Concentration (mg/dL)	mmol/L
7 AM	110–120	6.1–6.7
Noon	60–110	3.3–5.5
5 PM	90–110	5.0–6.1
11 PM	90–110	5.0–6.1
3 AM	80–110	4.2–6.1

A.H. feels that she is now "back to normal." She has no signs or symptoms of hyperglycemia, and her weight has remained stable. Occasionally, she becomes hypoglycemic before lunch, but this most often occurs when her lunch is delayed because of a busy work schedule. Evaluate A.H.'s blood glucose trends. What could be the cause of her prelunch hypoglycemia and how could she be managed? Is the use of insulin lispro an option? How should it be used?

A.H.'s blood glucose concentrations indicate that her basic insulin regimen is generally adequate to achieve the overall goal of preprandial blood glucose concentrations of <120 mg/dL. Note that correction of A.H.'s FPG concentration ultimately corrected her midmorning hyperglycemia. In fact, if one were to evaluate A.H.'s blood glucose concentrations from the previous visit, it is evident that the prebreakfast dose of regular insulin was working (see Question 15). That is, even though the absolute blood glucose concentration at midmorning was high, it was approximately 30 mg/dL less than the fasting glucose concentration of 160 mg/dL. This domino ef-

fect on blood glucose concentrations emphasizes the importance of correcting one blood glucose concentration at a time.

The hypoglycemia A.H. is experiencing before lunch could be caused by insufficient carbohydrate intake at breakfast, an excessive dose of regular insulin, or the relatively long duration of action of regular insulin. Thus, the problem could be resolved by augmenting A.H.'s breakfast meal, lowering the morning dose of regular insulin, or adding a midmorning snack. Another option is to use insulin lispro or aspart rather than regular insulin because its onset of action is more rapid than that of regular insulin. To calculate her insulin to carbohydrate ratio, divide the number 500 by her total daily dose of insulin (TDD):

$$500/30 = 17 \text{ g CHO per unit of insulin}$$

Since most single-servings of carbohydrate contain 15 grams, A.H. should use 1 unit for every 15 grams or single serving of carbohydrates she consumes at each meal. Insulin lispro or aspart are more conveniently administered just before a meal. However, A.H. must be warned to inject insulin lispro or aspart only if she will be eating within 15 minutes or so, because its onset of action is quite rapid. Because insulin lispro and aspart have a briefer duration of action than regular insulin, they cause fewer postprandial hypoglycemic episodes, although their effect on A_{1C} is comparable.[53,88]

Supplemental Insulin

18. **A.H. also notices that her preprandial blood glucose concentrations inexplicably exceed the new goal of 120 mg/dL on occasion. Sometimes they are as high as 200 mg/dL. Evaluate A.H.'s blood glucose trends. How should occasional preprandial glucose concentrations that exceed the desired goal of 120 mg/dL be managed?**

Once the basic dose of insulin has been established, one can begin to teach A.H. how to adjust her dose of insulin when preprandial blood glucose concentrations fall above or below the range of blood glucose concentrations that have been established as her goal of therapy (70 to 120 mg/dL). Two methods of supplementing doses of insulin can be used in this situation: compensatory insulin doses and anticipatory insulin doses[65] (Table 50-22).

Compensatory insulin doses are used to compensate for unusually high or low preprandial blood glucose concentrations. To re-emphasize, this assumes there are no unusual changes in the patient's overall diet or exercise patterns. Many clinicians favor insulin lispro or aspart over regular insulin because their action is brief and patients do not have to worry about residual effects 3 to 4 hours after its injection. This is particularly valuable when supplemental doses of insulin are needed at bedtime.

The patient's sensitivity to insulin, as reflected by his or her total daily dose on a unit/kg basis is a major determinant of any algorithm developed. Previously, it was advised that 1 to 2 units of supplemental insulin should be given for each 30 to 50 mg/dL elevation above the target level. However, this relationship was observed to apply only to a person of average size on average doses of insulin (i.e., the 70-kg patient on 50 U/day of insulin). A very small person on 10 U/day or a very obese individual with type 2 diabetes on 100 U/day has

Table 50-22   Guidelines for Dosing Insulin

Basic Insulin Dose

First adjust the basic insulin dose (i.e., the dose that the patient will be instructed to take daily). This assumes that diet and physical activity are stable. Set a reasonable goal initially. This may mean the upper limits of the acceptable concentrations may be high initially (e.g., <200 mg/dL). Move toward a more ideal goal slowly.

Only adjust insulin doses if a *pattern* of response is observed under stable diet and exercise circumstances. That is, the same response to insulin is observed for ≥3 days. It is important to verify the stability of diet and exercise. Consider adjusting these variables as well.

Unless all levels are >200 mg/dL, try to adjust one component of insulin therapy at a time.

Start with the insulin component affecting the fasting blood glucose concentration. This glucose level often is the most difficult to control and often affects all other glucose concentrations measured throughout the day.

Adjust the basic insulin dose by 1–2 U at a time. The amount prescribed is based on the individual patient's response to insulin. This can be determined by looking at the patient's total daily dose using the "500 Rule"(see the following, and Table 50-14).

Supplementary Insulin Doses

Once the basic dose of insulin has been established, supplemental doses of rapid- or short-acting insulin can be prescribed to correct *preprandial* hyperglycemia. For example, if the goal is 140 mg/dL, and the glucose value is 190 mg/dL, administer an additional unit of insulin lispro. Supplemental doses also can be used when the patient is ill (see Table 50-24).

Algorithms for supplemental doses are based on the patient's sensitivity to insulin using the "1500 or 1800 Rule" (see Table 50-14).

If premeal glucose concentrations are <60–70 mg/dL, the dose of lispro, aspart or regular insulin administered before the meal is ↓ 1–2 U; insulin administration is delayed until just before the meal; the meal should include an extra 15 g of glucose if the value is <50 mg/dL.

If supplemental doses before a given meal are required for ≥3 days, the basic insulin dose should be adjusted appropriately. For example, if a patient taking lispro before meals requires an extra 2 U before lunch for ≥3 days, 2 U should be added to the prebreakfast dose.

Anticipatory Insulin Doses

The basic insulin dose is increased or decreased based on the anticipated effects of diet or physical activity.

Increase lispro/aspart or regular insulin by 1 U for each additional 15 g of carbohydrate ingested (e.g., holiday meal) or decrease the usual dose by 1–2 U if the meal is smaller than usual (see Table 50-14).

See Table 50-23 for recommended insulin adjustments for exercise.

different responses to a given dose of insulin. An alternative method of estimating the drop in a person's blood glucose per unit of regular (or rapid-acting) insulin is the "1500 Rule."[60] The 1500 Rule was developed by Paul Davidson, MD, in Atlanta, Georgia, during the 1990s. The derived value is referred to as the "sensitivity factor":

$$1500/\text{Current Total Insulin Dose} = \text{Sensitivity Factor}$$
$$1500/30 = 50$$

Thus, 1 unit of regular insulin for A.H. will drop her blood glucose level by about 50 mg/dL. The 1500 Rule has proved to be a valuable way to initiate an algorithm for supplemental insulin. People with a lower sensitivity factor (higher insulin requirements) typically achieve a smaller reduction in blood glucose per unit of insulin compared with those with a higher sensitivity factor (lower insulin requirement). The rule has been modified to an "1800 Rule" for patients using insulin lispro or aspart because these insulins tend to drop the blood glucose level faster and farther.

Thus, an algorithm of 1 unit of regular insulin for every 50 mg/dL excursion above her goal of 120 mg/dL is a reasonable place to begin. If this dose of insulin is insufficient, one can increase the dose of insulin or decrease the blood glucose excursion required per unit of insulin dose. Supplementary insulin doses also are used for sick day management (see Question 31). The following is an example of an algorithm for A.H.:

Glucose Concentrations (mg/dL)	Regular Insulin
<80	1 unit less
80–120	Usual dose
120–170	1 unit extra
170–220	2 units extra
220–270	3 units extra
270–320*	4 units extra

*Check urine ketones. If urine ketones are positive and blood glucose concentrations remain >240 mg/dL for ≥12 hours, call the physician for directions.

Anticipatory insulin supplements are prescribed in anticipation of an immediate event that is likely to alter a patient's response to insulin. This includes an unusually large or small meal or exercise (see Table 50-22 and Question 30).

"Sliding scale" refers to an algorithmic method of adjusting doses of SC rapid- or short-acting insulin according to blood glucose test results. Sliding scales typically are used for hospitalized patients with diabetes whose insulin requirements may vary drastically because of stress (e.g., infections, surgery, and any acute illness), inactivity, or variable caloric intake (see Question 34). However, as previously noted, sliding scales also are used routinely by type 1 patients on intensive insulin therapy.

Typically, blood glucose concentrations are measured every 4 hours, and rapid or short-acting insulin is administered as prescribed. Sliding scales should be individualized to the patient's known sensitivity to insulin and adjusted according to his or her response. Generally, 1 to 2 units of lispro, aspart or regular insulin are administered for every 30 to 50 mg/dL above a predetermined target glucose concentration (e.g., 180 mg/dL) (see Tables 50-22 and 50-24). The principles applied in this case are similar to those used in establishing supplemental doses of insulin as previously described.

Dawn Phenomenon

19. R.D., a 37-year-old man, has had type 1 diabetes since age 14. Over the past 2 years, he has been very well controlled on the following insulin regimen: 20 units Lantus each morning with 3 to 4 units insulin lispro depending on carbohydrate intake before meals. On this regimen, his blood glucose concentrations for the past 2 weeks have been as follows:

Time	Glucose Concentration (mg/dL)	mmol/L
7 AM	140–170	7.8–9.4
Noon	100–120	5.5–6.7
5 PM	100–130	5.5–7.2
11 PM	115–140	6.4–7.8
3 AM	100–120	5.5–6.7

What are the likely causes of R.D.'s fasting hyperglycemia?

As discussed in Question 15, fasting hyperglycemia may be the result of insufficient doses of insulin in the evening, a decline in the effect of insulin over time, and, possibly, reactive hyperglycemia. In R.D.'s case, the dawn phenomenon also must be considered.[89] The *dawn phenomenon* is a rise in the blood glucose concentration that occurs between 4 and 8 AM after a physiologic nadir in the blood glucose concentration that occurs between midnight and 3 AM. This 30 to 40 mg/dL increase in the morning blood glucose concentration cannot be attributed to increases in counter-regulatory hormones secondary to an antecedent hypoglycemic event, but it may be secondary to rising growth hormone levels. This phenomenon is inconsistently observed in individuals with type 1 and type 2 diabetes as well as nondiabetic individuals; furthermore, it is inconsistently present from one day to the next.[90]

R.D.'s 3 AM blood glucose concentration indicates that posthypoglycemic hyperglycemia is an unlikely cause of his fasting hyperglycemia. Thus, the modest increase in his blood glucose concentration between 3 and 8 AM may be attributed to the waning effects of insulin or the dawn phenomenon. In both cases, an *increase* in R.D.'s daily dose of insulin glargine would be indicated. Another option would be to switch R.D. to an insulin pump. He has demonstrated a desire and ability for intensive management with multiple daily injections, frequent blood glucose monitoring, record-keeping skills, the ability to make appropriate insulin dose adjustments and accurate carbohydrate counting. The advantage to using a pump is the ability to program an increase in the basal infusion rate at approximately midnight. Because it takes 3 to 4 hours to observe a biologic response following a change in the infusion rate, the response would occur at approximately 3 to 4 AM, when the dawn phenomenon begins.[91]

Type 1 Diabetes in Children

Diagnosis and Clinical Presentation

20. J.C., a 7-year-old, 30-kg (95th percentile), 50" tall (90th percentile) girl, was brought to the emergency department (ED) by her parents because of nausea, vomiting, and a persistent "stomach ache" secondary to the flu. For the past week, J.C. had flulike symptoms, resulting in a 6-lb weight loss. Initial laboratory values revealed a blood glucose of 600 mg/dL, serum pH of 6.8 with bicarbonate level of 13 mEq/L, plasma ketone level of 5.2 mmol/L, and positive ketonuria. J.C. was diagnosed with diabetic ketoacidosis secondary to new-onset type 1 diabetes. In retrospect and on further questioning, J.C.'s parents realized that she probably had symptoms as early as 4 weeks before her hospitalization. While on a driving vacation, she drank large quantities of juice and had to stop hourly to urinate. She began experiencing enuresis, which her parents attributed to her increased fluid intake. What signs and symptoms are consistent with the diagnosis of type 1 diabetes in a child?

J.C.'s presentation is typical for a child newly diagnosed with diabetes who is brought in for medical attention because of severe symptoms related to the flu. An acute viral illness can trigger autoimmune destruction of the pancreas and abdominal pain, which may masquerade as gastroenteritis. Abdominal pain is a common presenting symptom of diabetic ketoacidosis (DKA).[92] J.C.'s weight loss probably represents fluid and caloric loss secondary to uncontrolled diabetes as well as decreased caloric intake from the flu.

As illustrated with J.C., the correct diagnosis of diabetes mellitus often is delayed in children because polyuria is incorrectly attributed to a urinary tract infection or enuresis; anorexia occurs rather than polyphagia; and symptoms of fatigue, irritability, weight loss, deterioration in school performance, and enuresis are attributed to "emotional" problems. A diagnosis of "failure to thrive" also may delay the diagnosis of diabetes in a young child, although this is not the case for J.C., who is above the 90th percentile in weight and height for children her age. The symptoms of polyuria are less obvious in an infant and are frequently missed until metabolic derangement has occurred. Unlike J.C., infants frequently present with severe dehydration and metabolic acidosis despite a negative history of diarrhea or significant vomiting.

Goals of Therapy

21. What are the goals of therapy for J.C.? Do the results of the DCCT apply to children such as J.C.?

The goals of therapy for children such as J.C. and adolescents with diabetes mellitus are as follows: (1) achieve normal growth and development, (2) obtain optimal glycemic control, (3) facilitate positive psychosocial adjustment to diabetes, and (4) prevent acute and chronic complications. Attainment of these goals requires a tremendous amount of support and education for the parents and can be best provided by a multidisciplinary team of professionals, including a physician, nurse educator, pharmacist, dietitian, and psychosocial expert.

Growth serves as an important clinical indication of overall general health and well-being in children with diabetes. Height and weight should be measured at each visit and plotted on standard growth grids. If, at the time of diagnosis, a child has fallen behind in height or weight, prompt and appropriate treatment should quickly return the child to the appropriate percentile and pattern of growth. An obese child should be encouraged to achieve a more appropriate percentile of weight gradually over a period of several months.

The DCCT demonstrated that intensive control reduced the incidence of long-term complications in patients 13 years of age or older; similar evidence in very young children is lacking. Thus, the ADA states: "glycemic goals may need to be modified to take into account the fact that most children younger than 6 or 7 years of age have a form of 'hypoglycemic unawareness,' in that they lack the cognitive capacity to recognize and respond to hypoglycemic symptoms and may be at greater risk for the sequelae of hypoglycemia."[93] J.C.'s pediatrician must strive for the best glucose control that she, her family circumstances, and currently available treatment regimens will permit.

Insulin Therapy

22. How should J.C. be started on insulin?

Because of considerable variability in sensitivity to insulin, treatment should commence with small doses of rapid- or short-acting insulin to avoid initial overtreatment. Even mild symptoms of hypoglycemia early in the course of therapy can frighten the patient and family and interfere with the effective use of insulin over the long term. Initial dosage requirements are 0.2 to 0.3U/kg per day. Most children eventually need 0.5 to 0.7 units/kg/day. Once the DKA has been treated with an insulin infusion, boluses of regular insulin, insulin lispro, or insulin aspart can be administered according to a sliding scale. The following day, most children can be treated with a mixture of regular or rapid-acting insulin (lispro or aspart) and intermediate insulin (Lente or NPH) or long-acting insulin (insulin glargine or Ultralente).

An alternative approach is to introduce twice-daily insulin injections using NPH or Lente. Based on a dose of 0.5 U/kg per day, 60% can be given before breakfast and 40% before the evening meal. For those children presenting with more substantial weight loss and appreciable ketonuria, regular insulin, insulin lispro, or insulin aspart equivalent to 0.25 U/kg per day can be added. However, younger children may be quite sensitive to regular insulin and require either minimal amounts or none at all. When very low doses are needed, dilution of insulin can be considered to increase the accuracy of measuring doses. Also, one might consider use of the BD Pen Mini that delivers 0.5 to 15 units of insulin in $\frac{1}{2}$-unit increments.

Clinical Note: J.C. was initially treated with twice-daily Humulin 70/30: 6 units every morning and 4 units each evening (0.5 U/kg per day). However, owing to frequent hypoglycemia occurring at 9 PM, her evening dose was changed to 4 units NPH at bedtime.

Injection Sites

23. Are the recommended sites of injection different for children? Does the age of the child play a factor?

Although many studies exist in adults investigating the rate of SC insulin absorption depending on the site and depth of injection, it is not clear whether these results are applicable to children. For infants with abundant SC tissue, injection sites are usually plentiful. For some toddlers who have lost their "baby fat," locating an appropriate site for injection can be difficult. Injecting insulin into the abdomen of children with minimal SC abdominal fat or in very young children may not be advisable. Rotation of injection sites between arms, thighs, and the upper-outer quadrant of the buttock or hip area, as well as the abdominal area in older children, is recommended. To achieve consistent absorption, insulin injections can be patterned; for example, using the arms for the morning injection and the thighs for the evening injection. Unfortunately, many children and teens consistently inject their insulin into a single area for convenience, accessibility, and comfort. This results in the development of fatty deposits and scar tissue due to insulin action at the local tissue level. Insulin absorption from these hypertrophied areas is generally poor and may make glycemic control quite variable. Spring-loaded injection devices may be helpful in reducing the child's fear of needles and easing access to difficult-to-reach injection sites.

Blood Glucose Monitoring

24. How often should J.C. monitor her blood glucose?

Immediately following diagnosis, blood glucose determinations should be obtained for J.C. before each meal and at bedtime. A minimum of three to four tests per day will con-

struct a useful profile of her daily fluctuations. Additional tests should be performed whenever J.C. experiences hypoglycemia or ketonuria or when she becomes acutely ill. These general recommendations must be individualized, however. For example, it may not be necessary for a child to test his or her blood glucose levels before lunch at school if there are no current problems with glucose control and performing the test is disruptive or makes the child feel "different." For infants, the earlobes and heel provide alternative blood sources for fingersticks. Enthusiasm for frequent blood glucose testing tends to wane with duration of diabetes. However, families who are instructed on managing diabetes on the basis of test results are better motivated to persevere with SMBG.

Honeymoon Period

25. Over the next 2 months, J.C.'s insulin requirements decreased to 2 units twice daily. Has her diabetes gone into remission?

Approximately 20% to 30% of individuals with type 1 diabetes go into a remission phase (honeymoon period) within days to weeks of their diagnosis.[94] During this time, which can last for weeks to months, C-peptide can be measured, indicating a return of pancreatic function; insulin requirements may diminish partially or completely. As illustrated by J.C., this presents clinically as markedly decreased insulin requirements to maintain normoglycemia. Although it is tempting to discontinue insulin, diabetes invariably recurs. To minimize the possibility of inducing insulin allergy secondary to intermittent insulin exposure and to avoid engendering a sense of false hope in J.C. that her disease has been cured, many clinicians continue insulin even if the doses are minuscule. J.C. should be followed closely for rising blood glucose concentrations.

Hypoglycemia

26. J.C.'s parents contacted the clinic to report that J.C. is having nightmares and is awakening in the middle of the night complaining of a headache and stomach pain. However, these symptoms resolve by noon the following day. Her current insulin regimen is NPH 4 units BID with regular insulin 2 units before breakfast and lunch. Could J.C. be experiencing nocturnal hypoglycemia? How do the symptoms of hypoglycemia differ in a child compared with an adult? How can the risk of hypoglycemia be minimized for J.C.?

J.C.'s parents are appropriately worried. Hypoglycemia is a serious and often life-threatening complication of diabetes management in children, and the risk of hypoglycemia increases with attempts to maintain meticulous control of blood glucose levels. Common causes of hypoglycemia include changes in meal amounts, late or skipped meals or snacks, exercise or unusual activity, and administration of excessive insulin. Because very young children may not be able to identify or express symptoms of hypoglycemia, caretakers must observe the child closely and identify symptoms or behaviors associated with a falling blood glucose. Symptoms of hypoglycemia may include crankiness, sudden crying, restless sleep, or nightmares as seen in J.C.

In a study of children and adolescents with type 1 diabetes treated with conventional insulin therapy, nocturnal hypoglycemia was observed in 47% and was asymptomatic in almost 50% of cases.[95] In an accompanying editorial, the common causes of hypoglycemia were reviewed, and parents were encouraged to offer snacks when bedtime glucose concentrations fall below 120 to 160 mg/dL, to test in the early morning hours when insulin levels may be peaking, to shift the evening dose of intermediate-acting insulin to bedtime, to avoid use of regular insulin at bedtime, and to consider using insulin lispro instead of regular insulin for the evening meal in particular.[96] The flat, prolonged time-action profile of insulin glargine may also be a solution to J.C.'s hypoglycemia.

J.C.'s parents should be instructed to test her blood glucose at bedtime and to provide a snack if glucose concentrations are less than 130 to 150 mg/dL (7.2 to 8.3 mmol/L). They should also test J.C. between 3 and 4 AM and whenever they suspect hypoglycemia, with the caveat that by the time they test, counter-regulatory hormones may be driving up plasma glucose concentrations. Treatment of hypoglycemia is addressed in Question 38.

27. J.C. was switched to a single daily dose of insulin glargine 6 units every morning and her nocturnal symptoms of hypoglycemia resolved. However, on a follow-up visit, her A₁C was 7.9% (normal, 4% to 6%) and her blood glucose concentrations at home ranged from 34 to 390 mg/dL (1.9 to 21.7 mmol/L). On occasion, J.C. refuses to eat after her prebreakfast or predinner injections of regular insulin, causing her parents to fear a hypoglycemic reaction. Why should insulin lispro or insulin aspart be substituted for regular insulin based on the aforementioned information?

Many patients find rapid-acting insulins more convenient because they can be injected 0 to 15 minutes before a meal so that little preplanning is involved. Because children often have erratic eating habits, an advantage of rapid-acting insulins over regular insulin is that they can also be injected immediately after a meal and the dose can be tailored to the amount of carbohydrate ingested. Thus, the risk of postmeal hypoglycemia and parental anxiety is lessened.

28. J.C. was prescribed the following regimen: Insulin glargine 6 units in the morning and lispro at breakfast and dinner according to the following algorithm:

0.5 unit if the blood glucose is <150 mg/dL (8.3 mmol/L)
1.0 unit if the blood glucose is 151 to 225 mg/dL (8.3 to 12.5 mmol/L)
1.5 units if blood glucose is >225 mg/dL (12.5 mmol/L)

The goal is to maintain J.C.'s blood glucose between 100 and 200 mg/dL (5.5 to 11.1 mmol/L). Her parents were advised to provide J.C. a 30-g carbohydrate snack at 10 PM if her bedtime glucose was <150 mg/dL. She returned to the clinic 3 days later with the following blood glucose values:

	8 AM	Noon	3 PM	6 PM	8 PM	10 PM
Day 1						
Lispro	1.0 unit			1.0 unit regular insulin		
Glargine	6.0 units					
Glucose (mg/dL)	159	46		196	292	184
Glucose (mmol/L)	8.8	2.6		10.9	16.2	10.0

	8 AM	Noon	3 PM	6 PM	8 PM	10 PM
Day 2						
Lispro	0.5 unit			0.5 unit		
Glargine	6.0 units					
Glucose (mg/dL)	165	215	191	131	142	208
Glucose (mmol/L)	9.2	11.9	10.6	7.3	7.9	11.5
Day 3						
Lispro	0.5 unit			0.5 unit		
Glargine	6.0 units					
Glucose (mg/dL)	83	159	147	109	99	193
Glucose (mmol/L)	4.6	8.8	8.2	6.1	5.5	10.8

After the first dose of 1.0 unit insulin lispro, J.C.'s blood glucose dropped to 46 mg/dL (2.6 mmol/L). That evening, J.C.'s parents gave her 1.0 unit regular insulin because they feared hypoglycemia secondary to insulin lispro. However, her 2-hour postprandial blood glucose concentration remained elevated at 292 mg/dL (16.2 mmol/L). The following day, after contacting the diabetes clinic, J.C.'s parents were instructed to decrease the lispro sliding scale by 0.5 unit at every glucose level. Explain these findings.

J.C. is clearly very sensitive to insulin and becomes more so as blood glucose concentrations come under control. An exaggerated but delayed response to insulin lispro occurred on the first day, which caused the parents to fear hypoglycemia from insulin lispro and they switched back to regular insulin before dinner. By decreasing the insulin lispro by 0.5 unit, good coverage is provided for her meals while the insulin glargine provides basal insulin. Furthermore, J.C.'s parents are less anxious because they are able to inject her lispro doses just after J.C. has eaten and adjust the dose based on the grams of carbohydrate J.C. consumes.

Using Insulin in Special Situations

Insulin Stability: Factors Altering Control

29. T.M., a 31-year-old farmer, has had type 1 diabetes for 20 years. He has been relatively well controlled on his current regimen of split-mixed doses of regular and NPH human insulin for some time. During the winter and spring seasons, his blood glucose concentrations have ranged from 90 to 140 mg/dL, and the A₁C measured at his last clinic visit 3 months ago was 7.5%. It is now August. For the past 2 months, T.M. has noticed that his diabetes is not under good control. His blood glucose concentrations vary widely from concentrations as low as 60 mg/dL (3.3 mmol/L) to as high as 240 mg/dL (13.3 mmol/L). He has no explanation for this. On inspection, his vial of regular insulin is cloudy and a white precipitate is clinging to the NPH vial, giving it a frosted appearance. Both vials are approximately one-third full. What factors may be contributing to T.M.'s poor glycemic control?

[SI units: blood glucose concentrations, 5.0 to 7.8 mmol/L; A₁C, 0.085 (normal, 0.04 to 0.06)]

Many factors may be contributing to T.M.'s poor control. These are discussed in the subsequent sections.

PHYSICAL CHANGES

Both of T.M.'s insulin vials have changed in appearance. T.M. should be instructed not to use his regular insulin if it is discolored; has become cloudy or thickened; or contains small, threadlike or other solid particles. As discussed in

Question 13, the cloudiness may be caused by contamination of regular insulin with NPH. If T.M. reuses his syringes, this also may be caused by the silicone oil that is used to coat needles of disposable syringes.[97] The silicone oil can denature the insulin, reducing its pharmacologic effect.

FLOCCULATION

Purified pork or human NPH can sometimes flocculate or crystallize onto the insulin bottle.[98] This results in a significant loss of potency, with insulin concentrations in the remaining suspensions varying from 6 to 64 U/mL (labeled 100 U/mL). This phenomenon can occur precipitously, generally after 3 to 6 weeks of use. Incorporation of additional zinc into these preparations during the manufacturing process has minimized this problem. Nevertheless, all patients should be warned to inspect their vials carefully before each injection and to discard or exchange them if they have crystallized (Fig. 50-7).

TEMPERATURE

Insulin is a fragile molecule that can be damaged by temperature extremes. Although all commercially available insulins are stable for at least 1 month at room temperature (68° to 75°F), manufacturers recommend that insulin be refrigerated and the ADA recommends avoiding temperature extremes (36° or 86°F).[69] In practice, most patients store vials currently in use at room temperature because injection of cold insulin is uncomfortable. The *United States Pharmacopeia* (USP) recommends that patients discard vials that have not been completely used in 1 month if they have been kept at room temperature.

The stability of insulin at temperatures of 75° to 100°F is unknown, but all insulins lose significant potency within 1 to 2 months at 100°F. T.M. lives in an area where temperatures frequently exceed 100°F during the summer months. Therefore, it is important that he not store his insulin in an automobile or in the sun, where it may be subject to deterioration. It also is of interest that many wholesale drug distributors and some mail order pharmacies do not take special packaging precautions when delivering insulins to pharmacies during the summer months. Thus, inadvertent exposure to high temperatures during these months may alter the potency and actions of insulins. Freezing apparently does not affect the potency of

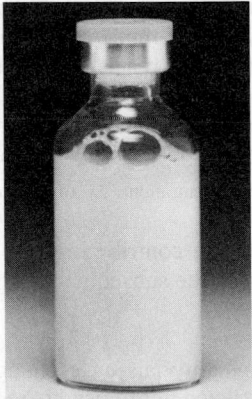

FIGURE 50-7 Insulin vial with crystallized insulin (photograph). (Used with permission from reference 298.)

insulin, but may cause aggregation of the precipitate. This could alter the absorption kinetics of the preparation.[99]

OTHER FACTORS ALTERING RESPONSE TO INSULIN

Many other factors may be altering T.M.'s response to insulin. The heat in the summer months may increase circulation to the injected site, thus increasing the onset and shortening the duration of action of his insulin. Exercise of the injected limb may affect insulin action similarly. During the summer months, farmers typically are more physically active and, as a consequence, require less insulin than usual. Other factors that can alter insulin action are listed in Tables 50-12 and 50-20.

When patients like T.M. observe that their insulin seems to work less well even when the product is well within the expiration date and there are no obvious physical changes, we recommend that they inject insulin from a fresh vial to assess whether insulin from the original vial has deteriorated. If the response remains the same, they should work with a clinician to identify other reasons for their decreased responsiveness to insulin.

Exercise and Insulin Requirements

30. J.S. is a 17-year-old, nonobese, patient with type 1 diabetes who was diagnosed at age 12. He currently is moderately well controlled on a single daily dose of Lantus 18 units at bedtime with 4 to 6 units of insulinaspart with meals (depending on carbohydrate intake). His A_{1C} is 7.8%, and his blood glucose levels before meals range from 150 to 190 mg/dL (8.3 to 10.5 mmol/L). Fasting blood glucose concentrations in the clinic range from 130 to 170 mg/dL (7.2 to 9.4 mmol/L). He has rare hypoglycemic reactions that are associated with skipped meals, and he generally is compliant with his prescribed meal plan. J.S. would like to begin a jogging program. What effect is jogging likely to have on his diabetic control? What precautions, if any, should he take?

[SI unit: A_{1C}, 0.10]

Exercise has varying effects on plasma glucose levels in patients, such as J.S., who are taking insulin. In the resting state, muscle derives approximately 10% of its metabolic requirement from glucose. In contrast, almost all of the muscle's metabolic requirements are derived from glucose during moderate to heavy exercise. Muscle glycogen stores are depleted quite rapidly, after which glucose is derived from the peripheral circulation. To meet the increased glucose demands, hepatic glycogenolysis and gluconeogenesis increase. This is mediated primarily through suppression of insulin secretion and increased secretion of counter-regulatory hormones such as glucagon. Low, permissive levels of insulin are required for glucose utilization by the muscle. In nondiabetic individuals, hepatic glucose output and peripheral utilization are balanced such that euglycemia is maintained during exercise.[100,101]

In a patient like J.S., exercise may cause hyperglycemia or hypoglycemia if he does not take proper precautions. If he is insulin deficient when he commences exercise, hepatic glucose output will be increased, but peripheral utilization will be decreased and hyperglycemia will ensue. Thus, patients like J.S. with type 1 diabetes should not exercise if their blood glucose concentrations exceed 250 and they have ketosis or if levels exceed 300 mg/dL (with or without ketosis), because these levels usually indicate insulin deficiency.[101]

Conversely, excess insulin will enhance peripheral utilization of glucose by muscle and suppress hepatic glucose output. Both can contribute to hypoglycemia. Hypoglycemia is more likely to occur in patients whose blood glucose concentrations are normal or low just before exercise. Thus, if J.S.'s blood glucose concentration is normal or low (<100 mg/dL) before he begins exercise, he should eat a carbohydrate snack (10 to 20 g) and have additional carbohydrates readily available during and after exercise.[101] He should delay his dose of lispro until after exercising and adjust the amount according to his postexercise blood glucose level.

It is less well appreciated that peripheral glucose utilization remains high after exercise has been discontinued. This is thought to be related to the replenishment of glycogen stores in the liver and muscle. Thus, if appropriate adjustments are not made in diet and insulin dose after exercise, hypoglycemia can occur 10 to 12 hours thereafter.[102]

For patients who inject insulin into their thighs, jogging may enhance insulin absorption. The absorption of regular insulin is increased when it is administered just before exercise (within 5 minutes), but it does not appear to be affected if injected 30 to 40 minutes before exercise. Absorption of the intermediate-acting or long-acting insulins is less likely to be augmented by exercise.[103] Some have suggested that insulin be injected at a site that is not exercised, for example, the abdomen, to minimize this effect.

In summary, J.S. should be encouraged to begin an exercise program. He should test his blood glucose concentrations before, during, and after exercise and adjust his insulin doses and food intake accordingly. In general, exercise should be avoided at times corresponding to peak insulin action, because high levels can suppress counter-regulatory hormones that stimulate hepatic glucose production (Table 50-23). Regular exercise may increase tissue sensitivity to insulin and eventually lower J.S.'s insulin requirements. Vigorous exercise is contraindicated in patients with retinal or vitreous hemorrhages because retinal detachment may occur.

In obese individuals with type 2 diabetes mellitus who are treated with diet, exercise is unlikely to cause hypoglycemia. An extremely low-calorie diet (<800 calories) that also is low in carbohydrates may decrease an individual's exercise endurance because muscle glycogen stores are not maintained.[100] Patients with type 2 diabetes who are treated with insulin secretagogues or insulin may become hypoglycemic if insulin levels are high enough to increase peripheral utilization of glucose and suppress hepatic glucose output. Thus, patients with type 2 diabetes who are normoglycemic before exercise also should consider increasing their carbohydrate intake.[104] Because patients with type 2 diabetes do not have an absolute lack of insulin, they are less likely to become hyperglycemic in response to exercise.

Sick Day Management

31. R.D., a 32-year-old woman with type 1 diabetes, has been well controlled on three daily doses of insulin for the past 6 months. However, 2 days ago, she began to develop signs and symptoms consistent with the flu. This has made her anorexic and nauseated and now she has begun to vomit; consequently, her food intake has been minimal. Because R.D. is not eating at this time, should she discontinue her insulin?

Insulin requirements always increase in the presence of an infection or acute illness, even if the food intake is diminished. Patients with type 1 diabetes, such as R.D., commonly decrease or eliminate insulin doses under these circumstances, and it is in just this setting that ketoacidosis occurs.

Therefore, R.D. should be instructed to maintain her usual dose of insulin and test her blood glucose concentration every 3 to 4 hours; the latter is particularly important if she has become nonadherent with her blood glucose testing. If blood glucose concentrations are above the usual range, supplemental doses of regular or insulin lispro or insulin aspart should be administered according to a prescribed algorithm based on her sensitivity factor. R.D. also should be instructed to test her urine for ketones if her blood glucose concentration is ≥300 mg/dL. She should call her physician if her blood glucose concentration remains >300 mg/dL after three supplemental insulin doses or if she begins to develop signs and symptoms related to ketoacidosis (polyuria, polydipsia, dehydration, ketonuria, and a fruity breath). (Also, see Question 40.) R.D. also should attempt to maintain her fluid, mineral, and carbohydrate intake with easily digested food and fluids (Table 50-24).[105]

Insulin Requirements in Renal Failure

32. M.B., a 32-year-old woman, has had type 1 diabetes for 15 years. Over the past 2 years, a gradual deterioration of her renal function—as reflected by increased proteinuria, serum creatinine (SrCr), and blood urea nitrogen (BUN) values—has been observed. What are the anticipated effects of decreased renal function on M.B.'s insulin requirements?

The effects of renal failure on insulin requirements are complex and, under various circumstances, insulin requirements may increase or decrease. The kidney is the most

---

Table 50-23   Exercise in Patients With Diabetes

1. Test blood glucose concentrations before, during, and after exercise.
2. For moderate exercise (e.g., bicycling or jogging for 30–45 min), ↓ the preceding dose of regular insulin by 30–50%. If glucose concentration is normal or low before exercise, supplement the diet with a snack containing 10–15 g of carbohydrate.
3. To avoid ↑ absorption of regular insulin by exercise, inject into the abdomen or exercise 30 min–1 hr after injection.
4. Individuals with low glycogen stores may be predisposed to the hypoglycemic effects of exercise. Examples include alcoholics, fasted individuals, or patients on extremely hypocaloric (<800 calories), low-carbohydrate (<10 g/day) diets.
5. Patients taking insulin are more susceptible to hypoglycemia than those taking sulfonylureas. Patients with type 2 diabetes mellitus treated with diet are unlikely to develop hypoglycemia.
6. Watch for postexercise hypoglycemia. Individuals who have been exercising during the day (e.g., skiing) should ↑ their carbohydrate intake and test their blood glucose concentration during the night to detect nocturnal hypoglycemia. Hypoglycemia can occur 8–15 after exercise.
7. If the glucose concentration is >240–300 mg/dL, the patient should not exercise. This indicates severe insulin deficiency. These patients are predisposed to hyperglycemia secondary to exercise.
8. Patients with severe proliferative retinopathy or retinal hemorrhage should avoid jarring exercise or exercise that involves moving the head below the waist.

Table 50-24 Sick Day Management

1. Continue taking your basic dose of insulin *even* if you are not eating well or have nausea or vomiting.
2. Test your blood glucose more frequently: every 3–4 hr.
3. If indicated, give yourself *supplemental* doses of lisproaspart or regular insulin: for example, 1–2 U for every 30–50 mg/dL over an agreed-upon target glucose concentration (e.g., 150 mg/dL). Supplemental doses must be individualized based on the patient's sensitivity to insulin (see Table 50-14).
4. Begin testing your urine for ketones, especially when glucose readings exceed 300 mg/dL.
5. Try to drink plenty of fluid (½ cup/hr for adults) and maintain your caloric intake (50 g carbohydrate Q 4 hr). Foods such as gelatin, noncarbonated soft drinks, crackers, soup, and soda may be used.
6. Call a physician if your blood glucose concentration remains >300 mg/dL or your urine ketones remain high after two or three supplemental doses of insulin.

important site of extrahepatic insulin metabolism and excretion. Renal clearance of insulin is 190 to 270 mL/minute, approximately two-thirds of hepatic clearance (320 to 400 mL/minute). In nondiabetic individuals, the liver extracts approximately 40% to 50% of insulin secreted endogenously before it reaches the peripheral circulation.[47,106] Because exogenous insulin is delivered directly to the periphery, the kidneys play a more important role in its elimination. Insulin is filtered by the glomerulus and reabsorbed in the proximal tubules, where it is destroyed enzymatically. The kidney also clears insulin from the peritubular circulation.[51,107] At that site, insulin can enhance the reabsorption of sodium, which may account for the edema occasionally observed following the initiation of insulin therapy in some individuals.

Diminished renal function can be accompanied by decreased clearance of endogenous and exogenous insulin, resulting in increased plasma concentrations of insulin. Therefore, M.B.'s insulin requirements may diminish as her renal disease progresses. Patients with moderate degrees of renal failure (glomerular filtration rate [GFR] >22.5 mL/minute) remove 39% of insulin from arterial plasma, similar to normal subjects. In contrast, patients with severe renal insufficiency (GFR <6 mL/minute) have a marked reduction in insulin removal from arterial plasma (9%).[108] Decreased insulin clearance in conjunction with the anorexia, nausea, and decreased food intake associated with uremia can lead to hypoglycemia in such individuals. In some patients with diabetes, particularly those with residual endogenous insulin secretion (type 2), glucose tolerance may normalize as renal function diminishes, eliminating the need for insulin.

In contrast, severe uremia is associated with glucose intolerance. This appears to be related to tissue resistance to insulin secondary to an unknown factor that can be removed by dialysis. Other factors that may alter blood glucose control in patients with renal failure include dialysis against glucose-containing dialysates and high-dose glucocorticoids in patients who have undergone renal transplantation.

As M.B.'s renal failure progresses through various stages of severity, many alterations in her insulin dose should be anticipated. During this time, M.B. should monitor her blood glucose concentrations closely and adjust her insulin according to an algorithm (see Table 50-22).

Traveling With Diabetes

33. J.R. is a 42-year-old woman with type 1 diabetes mellitus who has just taken a position that requires extensive overseas air travel. She is concerned about potential problems she may encounter managing her diabetes under these circumstances. What are some basic travel tips J.R. should consider?

J.R.'s predeparture preparations depend on the duration and destination of her trip. The following sections discuss basic considerations for diabetics when traveling.

SUPPLIES

J.R. should carry a plentiful back-up supply of insulin, syringes, blood-testing supplies (including an extra battery for her meter), and glucose tablets. She should double her anticipated insulin needs in case of loss, destruction, or unavailability of comparable products in foreign countries. For example, only U-40 insulin is available in some parts of the world. J.R.'s insulin supply should be insulated and separated in various bags she will carry with her. Most sources advise against carrying insulin in checked luggage, because its effectiveness might be altered by x-ray scanning or by freezing that could occur in the unpressurized baggage compartment. J.R. should take with her a brief medical history and a prescription for insulin for emergency situations.

IDENTIFICATION

J.R. should carry some identification, which alerts medical personnel or others to her diagnosis in emergency situations. This can take the form of a wallet card or a medical alert bracelet. In certain situations, she should consider informing key individuals of her diabetic condition (e.g., airline personnel, hotel managers, tour guides, traveling companions). She should review her insurance policy carefully so that she knows how to obtain care out of the country and bring along her policy and claim forms. Finally, she should provide friends or relatives with a detailed itinerary so that medical care can be summoned promptly if difficulties are encountered.

FOOT CARE

Shoes that are broken in and fit well are key if J.R. anticipates walking or standing for long periods. New shoes should not be worn longer than 1 hour to prevent blisters.

MEAL PLANNING

J.R. should try to maintain some regularity in her diet (time and amounts). When it is the custom to take the evening meal later than is usual in the United States, a late afternoon or early evening snack should be planned. To prevent hypoglycemia, J.R. should inform airline employees regarding the importance of serving her meal on time. To avoid unforeseen events (e.g., travel delays), J.R. should carry sufficient food and snacks with her on the plane and consider using insulin lispro or aspart as the prandial insulin if she is using intensive therapy. The rapid onset of these insulins will give her more flexibility in administering the insulin when she is certain the meal will be served. Anticipating the likely composition of her diet in a foreign country also will help her design a diet that maintains her pattern of carbohydrate and caloric intake.

INSULIN DOSES

If at all possible, J.R. should use insulin lispro or insulin aspart to cover meals and snacks, since these insulins provide maximum flexibility for unpredictable meal delays and food amounts. J.R. needs to adjust her basal insulin doses when she flies across several time zones to account for time lost or gained.[37] When traveling east, the insulin dose should be decreased proportionally for the time lost and a shorter day. Conversely, when traveling west, the basal insulin dose should be increased for the time gained and a longer day. The principle is to provide the same amount of basal insulin per hour. For example, if J.R. is using 10 units of NPH and is traveling from New York to London (a 5-hour difference), her dose would be reduced to 8 units. This is because she is receiving about 0.4 U/hr and she will be losing 5 hours as she crosses the time zones ($0.4 \times 5 = 2$ U). When she arrives in London and changes her watch, she may resume her NPH 10 units at the usual time of administration. When drawing up her insulin dose while on an airplane, J.R. should inject only half as much air into the vial; because the cabin pressure is lower than ground pressure, less pressure is needed inside the vial to balance the insulin she withdraws.

JET LAG

Because jet lag may be indistinguishable from symptoms of hypoglycemia or hyperglycemia, J.R. should test her blood glucose concentrations more frequently to better assess her symptoms.

Perioperative Management

34. A.G., a 27-year-old, 60-kg woman with a 15-year history of type 1 diabetes, was admitted to the hospital for an abdominal hysterectomy. Before admission, she has been well controlled on 24 units insulin glargine at bedtime and premeal doses of insulin aspart. A.G. will receive her usual doses of insulin plus supplemental doses of insulin according to a sliding scale. How should A.G.'s diabetes be managed perioperatively?

Perioperative management of a patient with diabetes is complex because so many variables can influence insulin requirements. Accordingly, common practice has been to aim for blood glucose concentrations in the range of 150 to 200 mg/dL. However, a study of ICU patients with hyperglycemia, in which liberal glucose control (blood glucose concentrations of 180 to 200 mg/dL) was compared with tight control (blood glucose concentrations of 80 to 110 mg/dL), has called this practice into question. Survival rate as well as incidence of systemic infection was significantly better in the tightly controlled group.[109] Another prospective randomized trial (DIGAMI trial) compared intensive insulin therapy (insulin glucose infusion for at least 24 hours followed by SC insulin four times daily for at least 3 months) in patients with diabetes after acute MI with standard therapy. Intensive insulin therapy improved long-term survival at one year and continued for 3.5 years, with an absolute risk reduction in mortality of 11%.[110] Thus, studies suggest that hyperglycemia is a risk factor for adverse outcomes in acutely ill patients, and treatment to maintain good glycemic control should be used.[111] Many approaches to the management of such patients have been suggested in the literature.[112,113] Most protocols include the use of intravenous regular insulin and 5% to 10% glucose. These include:

1. The administration of one-third to one-half the total daily dose as intermediate-acting insulin before surgery and postoperatively along with a 5% dextrose solution at a rate of 100 to 200 mL/hour. This is accompanied by supplemental rapid or short-acting insulin dosed subcutaneously according to blood glucose concentrations.

2. Administration of a combined insulin and glucose infusion at a fixed rate. A popular solution is 20 units of regular insulin and 20 mEq KCl in each liter of 5% dextrose in water administered at a rate of 100 mL/hour. The advantage of this approach is that if the glucose infusion is accidentally disconnected or obstructed, the insulin infusion will also be stopped. Thus, the risk of hypoglycemia is essentially eliminated. The disadvantage to this approach is that it eliminates the ability to change the delivery rate of one agent without changing the delivery rate of the other.

3. Administration of a separate continuous insulin infusion (usually 100 units of regular insulin in 100 mL normal saline) and glucose (usually dextrose 5% in water at 100 to 125 mL/hour) delivered by dedicated pumps to allow for independent adjustments of each. The infusion rate of each solution is determined by capillary blood glucose levels every 1 to 2 hours.

The last of these options seems most appropriate. It eliminates the uncertain pharmacokinetics of subcutaneously administered intermediate-acting insulin and, unlike option 2, acknowledges that glucose utilization and insulin response may be altered in such patients. Insulin infusion must be started at least 2 to 3 hours before the surgery to titrate to the desired level of glucose control. Other fluid and electrolyte requirements are administered through a separate line. To successfully monitor and regulate the insulin infusion regimen, accurate bedside measurement of blood glucose levels is mandatory. A representative protocol for an insulin-glucose infusion during the perioperative period is as follows:

Blood Glucose (mg/dL)	Insulin Infusion		D₅W infusion (mL/hr)
	mL/hr	U/hr	
<70*	0.5	0.5	150
71–100	1.0	1.0	125
101–150	1.5	1.5	100
151–200	2.0	2.0	100
201–250	3.0	3.0	100
251–300	4.0	4.0	75
>300	6.0	6.0	50

*Give 10 mL D5W IV and repeat blood glucose measurement 15 minutes later

Thus, A.G.'s usual dose of insulin should be discontinued, and she should be initiated on an insulin infusion that is adjusted according to an algorithm similar to the aforementioned suggestion. Throughout the perioperative period, she should receive a minimum of 100 g glucose daily to prevent starvation ketosis. If bedside measurements of glucose are impossible, any of the options suggested may be used.

Alternative Routes of Administration

35. W.C. is a 22-year-old male college student with type 1 diabetes, who is currently injecting multiple doses of insulin lispro throughout the day and insulin glargine at bedtime; however, he finds the traditional insulin injection process using vials and syringes time-consuming and cumbersome. He would like to find an easier, more convenient, and more discreet way to inject his insulin while at school. What insulin delivery devices are available for W.C.? What alternative routes of insulin delivery may be available for W.C. in the future?

PEN DEVICES AND PREFILLED SYRINGES

Pen devices and prefilled syringes eliminate the need to carry syringes and insulin vials separately. Insulin pens are available as prefilled pens, which are disposable, or reusable pens. Prefilled pens contain a built-in, single-use insulin cartridge. Each cartridge holds 150 to 300 units (1.5 to 3.0 mL) of insulin lispro, regular, insulin aspart, NPH, 70/30, Humalog Mix 75/25, or Novolog Mix 70/30. Prefilled pens are helpful for patients who have difficulty handling the cartridges in reusable pens or for patients with busy schedules who prefer not to have to change cartridges. However, prefilled pens are slightly more expensive than a durable, reusable pen, a factor that must be taken into account for W.C. With the reusable pen, the patient inserts an insulin cartridge into the pen's delivery chamber. This may allow greater flexibility for some patients, such as the ability to change the type of insulin injected without needing to purchase another pen if the insulin prescription changes. Although the pens are reusable, patients are advised to use a new disposable needle for each injection. These devices deliver doses up to 30 units (B-D) or 70 units (NovoPen 3) of insulin in 1-unit increments; the BD Pen Mini and NovoPen Junior deliver doses up to 15 and 35 units respectively in $\frac{1}{2}$-unit increments.[62]

The pens are particularly useful for patients with (1) regimens consisting of multiple daily doses of rapid- or short-acting insulin before meals and snacks (such as W.C.), (2) a fear of needles, (3) impaired hand dexterity, (4) hectic work/lifestyle or (5) for training alternate insulin administers (school nurse, siblings).

INSULIN PUMPS

Insulin pumps were discussed in Question 3 and have been reviewed elsewhere.[64]

INHALED INSULIN

Pulmonary administration of insulin is under aggressive investigation as a substitute for rapid- or short-acting insulins before meals (i.e., basal insulin must still be given by injection). Onset of action is more rapid than subcutaneous regular insulin (peak 5 to 60 minutes). Bioavailability of inhaled insulin is low compared with relative to subcutaneous insulin (8% to 25% depending on the study), but advances in delivery systems have enhanced the reproducibility of dose delivery.[114] The Cochrane Group completed a meta-analysis to "compare the efficacy, adverse effects and patient acceptability of inhaled versus injected insulin."[115] Six randomized controlled trials in which inhaled insulin was used to treat type 1 or type 2 diabetes met their criteria for inclusion. Inhaled insulin provided comparable glycemic control, and there was no difference in hypoglycemic events in five of the six studies. Patient satisfaction and quality of life measures were higher for inhaled insulin. Long-term consequences of this delivery route are yet unknown and questions have been raised with regard to its cost effectiveness and clinical outcomes.[116]

Adverse Effects of Insulin
Hypoglycemia

36. G.O., a 42-year-old, slightly overweight (5'11", 180 lb) man, has had a history of type 1 diabetes mellitus for 17 years. G.O.'s medical care was sporadic until 1 year ago when he referred himself to a diabetes clinic because he was beginning to develop pain and numbness in his feet. At that time, he was poorly controlled on a single daily dose of 45 units Humulin 70/30. He had not been testing his blood glucose concentrations, and his A_{1C} was 13%.

On physical examination, G.O. was found to have an elevated BP (160/94 mm Hg), background retinopathy, and decreased pedal pulses bilaterally. He had decreased sensation to vibration and monofilament testing in both feet. G.O. also complained of impotence and "shooting pains" in both legs. A spot collection for microalbuminuria was 450 μg of albumin/g creatinine (normal, 30–299 mg/g creatinine).

G.O. was treated with multiple daily doses of insulin. Over the last several months, he has been treated with the following regimen: 14 to 18 units insulin aspart /22 units Lente before breakfast; 14 to 18 units insulin aspart before lunch; 16 to 18 units insulin aspart before dinner; and 24 units Lente at bedtime. Blood glucose concentrations have been as follows:

Time	Glucose Concentration (mg/dL)
7 AM	60–320
Noon	140–280
5 PM	40–300

Over the past year, G.O.'s A_{1C} has decreased to 7.1%. Currently, he has approximately five hypoglycemic episodes per week, primarily in the late afternoon and evenings. These are characterized by intense hunger, sweating, palpitations, and (according to his wife) a short temper. He has found that he can avoid nocturnal hypoglycemia (night sweats, nightmares, and headaches) by eating a large bedtime snack. Over the past 3 months, he has gained 15 lb. Are G.O.'s signs and symptoms consistent with mild, moderate, or severe hypoglycemia? What are the causes?

[SI units: blood glucose 7 AM, 5.5 to 8.3 mmol/L; 12 PM, 15.5 mmol/L; 5 PM, 2.2 to 15.5 mmol/L; A_{1C}, 0.72]

G.O.'s case illustrates one of the major hazards of intensive insulin therapy: hypoglycemia. Hypoglycemia is a fact of life for patients with type 1 diabetes, virtually all of whom experience a hypoglycemic episode at one time or another. An estimated 4% of deaths related to type 1 diabetes are caused by hypoglycemia.[21,117,118]

Hypoglycemia is a blood glucose concentration of <60 mg/dL (<2.7 mmol/L), and its occurrence is potentially fatal if not promptly recognized and treated. However, the exact level at which a patient experiences symptoms is difficult to define. Clinical hypoglycemia is associated with typical autonomic (neurogenic) and neuroglycopenic symptoms relieved by the administration of a quickly-absorbed carbohydrate.

PATHOPHYSIOLOGY

Normal brain function depends on glucose, the exclusive fuel for cerebral metabolism. Because the brain is unable to synthesize or store glucose, it must be provided with a constant exogenous quantity via the brain's blood supply. As blood glucose concentrations fall, a series of physiologic responses occur to restore glucose levels. These responses create symptoms warning a patient to take corrective action by consuming carbohydrates. If these counter-regulatory responses fail to alert the patient and blood glucose concentrations fall below a critical level, cognitive function becomes impaired and confusion and coma may ensue.

In patients without diabetes, the peripheral responses to hypoglycemia are so efficient that clinically important hypoglycemia probably never occurs. As glucose levels fall between 50 and 60 mg/dL (2.7 to 3.3 mmol/L), a series of neuroendocrine events occur, raising the plasma glucose concentration back toward normal by increasing hepatic glucose output. The major hormone responsible for producing acute recovery from insulin-induced hypoglycemia is glucagon; however, epinephrine alone also can produce near-normal recovery. Rising levels of adrenergic and cholinergic hormones generate warning symptoms of hypoglycemia. When hypoglycemia is prolonged, growth hormone and cortisone play a greater role in producing recovery.

Patients with type 1 diabetes who maintain insulin depots throughout the day are predisposed to severe hypoglycemic reactions because deficiencies in the normal feedback system occur over time. Glucagon secretion becomes deficient within the first 2 to 5 years after diagnosis, and by ≥10 years, epinephrine secretion may become impaired. The latter defect leads to asymptomatic hypoglycemia or hypoglycemic unawareness (see Question 39).

Certain circumstances predispose patients with type 1 diabetes to severe hypoglycemia. These include (1) a defective counter-regulatory hormonal response to hypoglycemia (see Question 39), (2) medications such as β-blockers that diminish early warning signs of impending hypoglycemia, (3) intensive insulin therapy that can alter secretion of counter-regulatory hormones, (4) skipped meals or inadequate carbohydrate intake relative to the insulin dose, (5) physical activity, and (6) excessive alcohol intake (Table 50-25).

SYMPTOMS

The signs and symptoms associated with hypoglycemia vary in intensity according to the presence of cognitive deficits and the patient's ability to self-treat the reaction. They vary substantially from one patient to another. Symptoms are conventionally divided into two categories: neurogenic (or autonomic) and neuroglycopenic.[117]

Autonomic symptoms include sweating, intense hunger, palpitations, tremor, tingling, and anxiety. Epinephrine is thought to mediate many of the neurogenic responses to hypoglycemia.

Neuroglycopenic symptoms resulting from neuronal fuel deprivation (glucose) include difficulty concentrating; lethargy; confusion; agitation; weakness; and possibly, slurred speech, dizziness, and fainting. Profound behavioral changes, seizures, and coma are more severe manifestations of neuroglycopenia. Prolonged, severe neuroglycopenia ultimately results in death. Symptoms of mild, moderate, severe, and nocturnal hypoglycemia are as follows:

- *Mild hypoglycemia:* Symptoms include tremor, palpitations, sweating, and intense hunger. Diminished cerebral

---

Table 50-25 Hypoglycemia

Definition

Blood glucose concentration <60 mg/dL; patient may or may not be symptomatic. Blood glucose <40 mg/dL; patient generally symptomatic. Blood glucose <20 mg/dL can be associated with seizures and coma.

Signs and Symptoms

Blurred vision, sweaty palms, generalized sweating, tremulousness, hunger, confusion, anxiety, circumoral tingling and numbness. Patients vary with regard to their symptoms. Behavior can be confused with inebriation. Patients become combative and use poor judgment.
Nocturnal hypoglycemia: nightmares, restless sleep, profuse sweating, morning headache, morning "hangover." In one study, 80% of patients with nocturnal hypoglycemia had no symptoms.

Clinical Considerations

Irregular eating patterns
↑ Physical exercise
Gastroparesis = (delayed gastric emptying time)
Defective counter-regulatory responses
Excessive dose of sulfonylurea
Alcohol ingestion
Drugs

Treatment

10–20 g rapidly absorbed carbohydrate. Repeat in 15–20 min if glucose concentration remains <60 mg/dL or if patient is symptomatic. Follow with complex carbohydrate/protein snack if meal time is not imminent.
The following are examples of food sources that provide 15 g of carbohydrate:

Orange, grapefruit or apple juice; regular, nondiet soda	½ cup
Fat-free milk	1 cup
Grape juice, cranberry juice cocktail	⅓ cup
Sugar	1 T or 3 cubes
Lifesavers	5–6 pieces
Glucose tablets	3–4 tablets

If patient is unconscious the following measures should be initiated:
Glucagon 1 mg SC, IM, or IV (mean response time, 6.5 min)
Glucose 25 g IV (dextrose 50%, 50 mL) (mean response time, 4 min)

IM, intramuscular; IV, intravenous; SC, subcutaneous.

---

function is not present and patients are capable of self-treating mild reactions.

- *Moderate hypoglycemia:* Moderate hypoglycemic reactions include neuroglycopenic as well as autonomic symptoms: headache, mood changes, irritability, decreased attention, and drowsiness. Patients may require assistance in treating themselves because of the presence of impaired judgment or weakness. Symptoms are more severe, usually last longer, and often require a second dose of a simple carbohydrate.
- *Severe hypoglycemia:* Symptoms of severe hypoglycemia include unresponsiveness, unconsciousness, or convulsions. These reactions require assistance from another individual for appropriate treatment. Approximately 10% of patients treated with insulin develop at least one severe, disabling episode of hypoglycemia per year that requires emergency treatment with parenteral glucagon or IV glucose.[117]

• *Nocturnal hypoglycemia:* Tingling of the lips and tongue are common complaints of patients who develop nocturnal hypoglycemia. These patients also may complain of headache and difficulty arising in the morning, nightmares, or nocturnal diaphoresis.[117] Family members should be conscious of any unusual sounds or activity while the patient is sleeping.

G.O. has mild to moderate hypoglycemic reactions, which he is able to self-treat. These are likely due to overinsulinization.

Overinsulinization

37. **Evaluate G.O.'s overall control. What signs and symptoms in G.O. are consistent with overinsulinization? How should he be managed?**

The following is a list of signs and symptoms of overinsulinization in G.O.:

• A total daily insulin dose of 1.0 U/kg. This dose is unusually high for a patient with type 1 diabetes who should not be resistant to the action of insulin.
• Weight gain over the past several months. This is secondary to the anabolic effects of insulin as well as G.O.'s increased carbohydrate intake to match his high insulin doses or treatment of hypoglycemia.
• Frequent hypoglycemic reactions.
• An apparently "brittle" situation (i.e., blood glucose concentrations that fluctuate wildly between hypoglycemia and hyperglycemia). In G.O.'s case, high blood glucose concentrations may represent reactive hyperglycemia or overtreatment of hypoglycemic episodes.
• Near normal A_{1C} levels indicate mean blood glucose concentrations that must be within the normal range even though the patient has recorded numerous high blood glucose concentrations. Patients treated with intensive insulin therapy in the DCCT experienced hypoglycemic episodes three times more often than patients treated with standard insulin therapy.[21] A_{1C} levels were approximately 7.2%.

G.O. should be managed by gradually decreasing his insulin doses. Because most of his reactions are occurring in the late afternoon and evening, the morning dose of intermediate-acting insulin should be adjusted first. Changing his intermediate-acting insulin from Lente to insulin glargine also should be considered for two reasons: (1) the excess zinc in the Lente insulin may be converting some of the short-acting insulin to an intermediate-acting form (see Question 14), and (2) the Lente may be peaking in the late afternoon and evening. The total daily dose of intermediate-acting insulin should be reduced by 20% substituted with a single dose of long-acting insulin glargine in the morning or at bedtime.

G.O. also should begin testing his glucose concentrations at 2 or 3 AM, and he should be taught to treat his hypoglycemic episodes appropriately (see Question 38). If he is capable, an algorithm for adjusting his preprandial aspart insulin doses should be provided to minimize hypoglycemic and hyperglycemic reactions based on the "1800 Rule" or sensitivity factor (see Question 18). The equation is as follows:

1800/Current Total Daily Insulin Dose = Sensitivity Factor

The sensitivity factor for G.O. (using his new dose of Lantus plus aspart doses premeal) would be:

1800/84 = 21

Thus, for every unit G.O. injects, his blood sugar will drop approximately 21 mg/dL. To facilitate ease in understanding his sliding scale, this number can be rounded down to 20 mg/dL.

An example of an algorithm that may be appropriate for G.O. follows:

Glucose Concentrations (mg/dL)	Change Dose of insulin aspart by:
<60	–2 units
<80	–1 unit
80–100	No change
101–120	+1 unit
121–140	+2 units
141–160	+3 units
161–180	+4 units
181–200	+ 5 units
201–220	+ 6 units
221–240	+ 7 units

G.O. should be instructed to take insulin aspart immediately before each meal and adjust his dose according to the previous algorithm. It will be important that he record the actual dose he administers before each meal and bring the record to clinic so that his basic dose of insulin can be more finely tuned.

Treatment of Hypoglycemia

38. **How should G.O.'s hypoglycemic episodes be managed?**

As G.O. illustrates, many patients with diabetes are frightened of hypoglycemia and have a tendency to overtreat their reactions with, for example, large quantities of juice or several candy bars. This should be discouraged because overcorrection together with glucose generated by counter-regulatory hormones ultimately results in hyperglycemia.

The key to successful management of hypoglycemia is recognition and prevention. Because early warning symptoms of hypoglycemia vary from person to person, it is important that G.O. study and learn to recognize his earliest warning symptoms and to treat early. Patients generally can recall prodromal symptoms following recovery from a severe hypoglycemic reaction if they have not developed hypoglycemic unawareness (see Question 39). As a caveat, these authors occasionally have seen patients who "feel" hypoglycemic after their blood glucose concentrations have been normalized from very high levels with intensive insulin therapy. We encourage patients to test their blood glucose concentrations any time they "feel unusual" to verify a low blood glucose concentration before treatment. G.O. should treat his symptoms only if he is truly hypoglycemic.

A second component of prevention is determining its cause and taking preventive or corrective action. This entails assessment of his diet (did he skip or delay a meal or change its content?), exercise pattern, and time of insulin administration and dose (and accuracy of dose administered). If hypoglycemic reactions consistently occur at a certain time of day, he should determine whether this corresponds to the maximum effect of one of his insulin doses and reduce that insulin dose by 1 to 2 units. Alternatively, he can add a supplemental snack to that part of the day.

If a reaction occurs, G.O. should be instructed to treat it as follows (also see Table 50-25).

MILD HYPOGLYCEMIA

Most hypoglycemic reactions are managed readily with the equivalent of 10 to 20 g of glucose. (See Table 50-25 for examples of carbohydrate sources containing 15 g of glucose.) If the blood concentration remains low after 15 minutes, the patient should ingest another 10 to 20 g of carbohydrate. This quick-acting source of glucose should be followed by a small complex carbohydrate or protein snack (e.g., milk, peanut butter sandwich) to provide a continual source of glucose if a meal is not scheduled within the next 1 to 2 hours. An easy rule of thumb that can be used by patients is "15-15-15": 15 g of glucose followed by a second 15 g if the patient is still symptomatic after 15 minutes.

Glucose tablets are available and have the added benefit of being premeasured to prevent overtreatment of hypoglycemia. Glucose gels or small tubes of cake frosting are useful for children or patients who become uncooperative and combative when hypoglycemic.

MODERATE TO SEVERE HYPOGLYCEMIA

Glucagon can be injected by the SC or intramuscular (IM) route into the deltoid or anterior thigh region. The dose of glucagon recommended to treat moderate or severe hypoglycemia for a child younger than 5 years of age is 0.25 to 0.5 mg; for children 5 to 10 years of age, 0.5 to 1 mg; and for patients older than 10 years, 1 mg. Parents and spouses should be taught how to mix, draw up, and administer glucagon during emergency situations. Kits with prefilled syringes containing 1 mg glucagon are available. Patients who are given glucagon should be positioned so that their face is turned toward the floor to prevent aspiration in the event of vomiting. As soon as the patient awakens (10 to 25 minutes), he or she should be fed.

Intravenous Glucose

If glucagon is unavailable, the patient should be taken to the hospital's ED, where he or she can be treated with IV glucose (approximately 10 to 25 g administered as 20 to 50 mL of 50% dextrose over 1 to 3 minutes) in preference to glucagon. Following the bolus injection of glucose, IV glucose (5 to 10 g/hour) should be continued until the patient has gained consciousness and is able to eat.

Hypoglycemic Unawareness

39. M.M., a 35-year-old, 75-kg, unemployed man, has had type 1 diabetes since the age of 3. As a consequence of the diabetes, he has developed proliferative retinopathy and progressive diabetic nephropathy (current SrCr, 3.0 mg/dL). M.M. has an erratic lifestyle. Because he does not work, he often stays out late at night and sleeps late into the morning. His insulin is injected whenever he awakens, and his meals are irregularly spaced. Each time he comes to the clinic, he brings with him a complete log of glucose concentrations that range from 80 to 140 mg/dL. He has two to three severe hypoglycemic reactions a month that require emergency treatment with IV glucose. On several occasions, his blood glucose concentration has been 20 mg/dL. M.M.'s last A_{1C} was 10%. He says that he adheres to the following insulin regimen: 18 units NPH/11 units regular insulin before breakfast, 10 units regular insulin before lunch and dinner, and 14 units NPH at bedtime.

On this visit, M.M. comes with his girlfriend. He has a large gash on his nose that occurred 3 days ago when he lost consciousness at approximately 1:30 PM while pushing his stalled car. He was unable to eat lunch at the usual hour because he had problems with his car. Assess M.M.'s hypoglycemic reactions and blood glucose control. Should intensive insulin therapy be continued? How should he be managed?

[SI units: SrCr, 265 μmol/L; blood glucose, 4.4 to 7.8 mmol/L; A_{1C}, 0.10]

M.M. illustrates a patient with type 1 diabetes who has defective glucose counter-regulation and, as a result, is unable to counteract a hypoglycemic reaction effectively. He also is an example of a patient who should *not* be treated with intensive insulin therapy (see Table 50-15).[93]

M.M. clearly is unable to adhere to an intensive regimen. His lifestyle is erratic, he eats irregularly, and his reported blood glucose concentrations (80 to 140 mg/dL) do not correspond with his elevated A_{1C} value. This may indicate that M.M.'s technique is incorrect or that he simply fills in the log with fictitious numbers before he comes to the clinic. Irregular entries in different colored inks and blood stains usually indicate authentic records.

M.M. has developed advanced, long-term complications that are unlikely to be reversed by intensive insulin therapy. In fact, proliferative retinopathy may actually worsen with intensive insulin therapy initially.[21] In the DCCT study, severe hypoglycemic reactions were three times more common in patients treated with intensive insulin therapy, and nocturnal hypoglycemia accounted for 41% of the total hypoglycemic episodes.[21] In patients with defective counter-regulation, the risk of severe hypoglycemia may be 25 times higher than in patients with adequate counter-regulatory mechanisms treated with intensive insulin therapy.[117] M.M. is at great risk for death secondary to hypoglycemia.

As previously noted, the primary hormones that are secreted in response to a low blood glucose concentration are glucagon and epinephrine. In patients who have had type 1 diabetes for >2 to 5 years, a deficiency in glucagon secretion is a relatively consistent finding, and these patients must rely on epinephrine to reverse low blood glucose concentrations. Unfortunately, approximately 40% of patients with long-standing type 1 diabetes (8 to 15 years) have defective epinephrine secretion as well, and this may be related to the development of autonomic neuropathy. Patients whose diabetes is controlled closely with intensive insulin therapy also have reduced counter-regulatory hormone responses to hypoglycemia. As illustrated by M.M., patients with defective epinephrine secretory responses also lose the warning signs and symptoms of hypoglycemia. These patients are said to have "hypoglycemia unawareness" because they have no awareness of blood glucose concentrations <50 mg/dL. In these individuals, loss of consciousness, seizures, or irrational behavior may be the first objective signs of exceedingly low blood glucose concentrations. The glycemic threshold for symptoms also is lowered in patients on intensive insulin therapy whose glucose concentrations have been lowered to normal or near-normal levels.[117] Consequently, their hypoglycemic reactions may go unnoticed and untreated until they lose consciousness. M.M. should be managed as follows:

- Because his waking, sleeping, and eating patterns are highly irregular, M.M. should be treated with an insulin regimen that addresses his lifestyle. For example, he could be instructed to give himself insulin lispro or aspart just before he actually intends to eat. A dose of insulin glargine could be given before his first meal to supply a basal level of insulin between meals. Evening doses of NPH should be eliminated because of the danger of severe hypoglycemic reactions.

- Because M.M. has no warning symptoms for hypoglycemia, the importance of regular blood glucose testing should be emphasized. When blood glucose testing was reviewed with M.M., it was discovered that his eyesight was so poor that he was unable to distinguish between the right and wrong side of the glucose test strip. Furthermore, because he had lost his depth of field, he was unable to apply the drop of blood onto the test strip. To address this situation, M.M.'s girlfriend was taught how to perform blood glucose testing.

- M.M.'s girlfriend also was taught how to recognize and treat symptoms of hypoglycemia. Often, patients ignore early warning symptoms and progress to a point that they lose the judgment needed to treat the condition. If M.M. has not yet become combative, a "quick"-acting carbohydrate source should be offered. If he has lost consciousness, glucagon should be injected.

All of these maneuvers diminished the frequency of M.M.'s severe hypoglycemic reactions. On the whole, his blood glucose concentrations were maintained below 180 mg/dL, and he remained relatively free of hyperglycemic symptoms. M.M.'s A_{1C} using this insulin regimen was 8.0%.

DIABETIC KETOACIDOSIS

40. J.L., a 25-year-old, 60-kg woman with an 8-year history of type 1 diabetes, is moderately well controlled on 24 units Lantus plus pre-meal doses of insulin lispro. Her family brings her to the ED, where she complains of abdominal tenderness, nausea, and vomiting. According to her family, J.L. was well until 2 days ago when she awoke with nausea, vomiting, diarrhea, and chills. Because she was unable to eat, she omitted her usual morning dose of insulin. Her gastrointestinal (GI) symptoms progressed, and she was brought to the ED when she became lethargic.

Physical examination reveals an ill-appearing woman who is lethargic but responsive. Her temperature is 37°C. Skin turgor is poor, mucous membranes are dry, and her eyeballs are shrunken and soft. J.L.'s lungs are clear, but respirations are deep and her breath has a fruity odor. Cardiac examination is within normal limits.

In the supine position, J.L.'s pulse rate is 115 beats/min (normal, 60 to 100) and her BP is 105/60 mm Hg (normal, 85 to 130). In the upright position, her pulse increased to 140 beats/min, and her BP dropped to 85/40 mm Hg. There is mild, diffuse tenderness over her abdomen.

Laboratory results on admission disclosed the following: blood glucose, 750 mg/dL; sodium (Na), 148 mEq/L (normal, 135 to 147); potassium (K), 5.4 mEq/L (normal, 3.5 to 5.0); chlorine (Cl), 106 mEq/L (normal, 95 to 105); HCO_3, 6 mEq/L (normal, 22 to 28); SrCr, 2.0 mg/dL (normal, 0.6 to 1.2); hemoglobin (Hgh), 14.7 g/dL (normal, 11.5 to 15.5); hematocrit (Hct), 49% (normal, 33% to 43%); white blood cell (WBC) count, 15,000/mm³ (normal, 3,200 to 9,800) with 3% bands (normal, 3 to 5%), 70% polymorphonuclear neutrophils (normal, 54 to 62%), and 27% lymphocytes (normal, 25 to 33%); serum ketones were moderate at 1:10 dilution (normal, negative). The urinalysis showed 2% glucose (normal, 0); moderate ketones (normal, 0); pH, 5.5 (normal, 4.6 to 8); and a specific gravity of 1.029 (normal, 1.020 to 1.025); there were no WBCs, RBCs, bacteria, or casts. Arterial blood gas (ABG) results were as follows: pH, 7.05 (normal, 7.36 to 7.44); PCO_2, 20 mm Hg (normal, 35 to 45); PO_2, 120 mm Hg (normal, 90 to 100). What supports the diagnosis of DKA in J.L.?

[SI units: blood glucose, 41.6 mmol/L; Na, 148 mmol/L; K, 5.4 mmol/L; Cl, 106 mmol/L; HCO_3, 6 mmol/L; SrCr, 176.8 μmol/L; Hgb, 147 g/L; Hct, 0.49; WBC count, 15 × 10⁹/L with 0.03 bands; polymorphonuclear neutrophils, 0.70; lymphocytes, 0.27; PCO_2, 2.6 kPa; PO_2, 16.0 kPa]

The fact that J.L. has type 1 diabetes puts her at risk for developing ketoacidosis. An absolute or relative insulin deficiency promotes lipolysis and metabolism of free fatty acids to β-hydroxybutyrate, acetoacetic acid, and acetone in the liver. Excess glucagon enhances gluconeogenesis and impairs peripheral ketone utilization. Stress can contribute to the development of diabetic ketoacidosis (DKA) by stimulating release of insulin counter-regulatory hormones such as glucagon, catecholamines, glucocorticoids, and growth hormone. Common stress factors include infection, pregnancy, pancreatitis, trauma, hyperthyroidism, and acute MI.

J.L. presented with symptoms of nausea, vomiting, diarrhea, and chills, and these are suggestive of an acute viral gastroenteritis. Patients such as J.L. commonly discontinue their insulin in this setting, which further predisposes them to the development of DKA (see Question 31). Table 50-26 lists patient education points with regard to DKA.

As illustrated by J.L., patients with DKA present with moderate to high serum glucose concentrations secondary to decreased peripheral utilization and increased hepatic production (Table 50-27). This increases serum osmolality, which initially shifts fluid from the intracellular to the intravascular compartment. When glucose concentrations exceed the renal threshold, osmotic diuresis ensues and water, sodium, potassium, and other electrolytes are depleted. J.L. also has lost fluid and electrolytes from vomiting and diarrhea. Eventually, as losses exceed input, the patient becomes dehydrated (dry mucous membranes; dry skin; soft, shrunken eyeballs; increased hematocrit) and intravascular volume becomes depleted (orthostatic BP and pulse changes).

Evidence of excessive ketone production in J.L. includes ketonuria, ketonemia, and the characteristic fruity odor of acetone on the breath. Elevated levels of these organic acids increase the anion gap and decrease the pH and carbonate levels. The respiratory rate is increased to compensate for the metabolic acidosis leading to hypercapnia (see Table 50-26).[92,119]

Treatment

41. How should J.L. be treated?

Treatment of patients with DKA is aimed at correction of intravascular volume, dehydration, fluid and electrolyte losses, and hyperosmolarity (hyperglycemia) (Table 50-28).

Table 50-26 Diabetic Ketoacidosis (DKA): Patient Education

Definition: DKA occurs when the body has insufficient insulin.

Questions to Ask:

1. Has insulin use been discontinued or a dose skipped for any reason?
2. If an insulin pump is being used, is the tubing clogged or twisted? Has the catheter become dislodged?
3. Has the insulin being used lost its activity? Is the bottle of regular insulin cloudy? Does the bottle of NPH appear frosty?
4. Have insulin requirements increased due to illness or other forms of stress (infection, pregnancy, pancreatitis, trauma, hyperthyroidism, or myocardial infarction)?

What to Look For:

1. Signs and symptoms of hyperglycemia: thirst, excessive urination, fatigue, blurred vision, consistently elevated blood glucose concentrations (>300 mg/dL)
2. Signs of acidosis: fruity breath odor, deep and difficult breathing
3. Signs of dehydration: dry mouth; warm, dry skin; fatigue
4. Others: stomach pain, nausea, vomiting, loss of appetite

What to Do:

1. Review "Sick Day Management" (Table 50-24)
2. Test blood glucose four or more times daily
3. Test urine for ketones when blood glucose concentration is > 300 mg/dL
4. Drink plenty of fluids (water, clear soups)
5. Continue taking insulin dose
6. Contact physician immediately

Table 50-27 Common Laboratory Abnormalities in DKA

Glucose	> 250 mg/dL
Serum osmolarity	Variable, can be >320 in presence of coma
Sodium	Low, normal, or high[a]
Potassium	Normal or high
Ketones	Present in urine and blood
pH	Mild: 7.25–7.30
	Moderate: 7.00–7.24
	Severe: < 7.00
Bicarbonate	Mild: 15–18
	Moderate: 10–15
	Severe: <10
WBC count	15,000–40,000 cells/mm even without evidence of infection

[a]Total body sodium is always low.
DKA, diabetic ketoacidosis; WBC, white blood cell.

Fluids

Rapid correction of fluid loss is most crucial. The usual fluid deficit approximates 6 to 10 L or 10% of body weight in most patients with DKA. In the absence of cardiac compromise, hypernatremia or significant renal dysfunction, isotonic saline (0.9% NaCl) should be used.[92,119]

J.L. has evidence of significant dehydration and intravascular volume depletion. A rough calculation indicates that approximately 6 to 7 L will be needed (10% of body weight). Typically, fluids are replaced at the rate of 15 to 20 mL/kg/hr; during the first hour (~1 to 1.5 L in the average adult). The

Table 50-28 Management of Diabetic Ketoacidosis

Fluid Administration

Use normal saline unless patient has cardiac compromise, is hypernatremic (Na > 150 mEq/L), or has significant renal dysfunction
If perfusion is adequate (e.g., normal pulse and blood pressure, good skin turgor) and Na >150 mEq/L, use half normal saline.
Rate: 15–20 mL/kg body weight during first hour, then 4–14 mL/kg/hr

Insulin

Continuous IV infusion of regular insulin is preferred. Use IM route only if infusion is not available.
Loading Dose: 0.15 U/kg IV *or* 20 U IM
Maintenance Dose: 0.1 U/kg/hr IV *or* 5–10 U/hr IM
If no change in blood glucose level after 1 hr, double infusion rate.
Once blood glucose <250 mg/dL, reduce infusion rate and change fluid to 5% dextrose (do not stop insulin infusion).
When SC insulin can be initiated, administer dose 30 min before discontinuing IV infusion.

Potassium

Add 20–40 mEq to IV fluids except in patients with chronic renal failure, no urine output, or initial potassium level >5.5mEq/L.

Phosphate

Initiate if level <1 mg/dL. Use potassium phosphate salt, 20–30 mEq added to replacement fluid. Rarely needed.

Bicarbonate

Replacement is controversial and may be dangerous.
For adults with pH <6.9, 100 mmol sodium bicarbonate may be added to 400 mL sterile water and given at a rate of 200 mL/hr. For adults with pH of 6.9–7.0, 50 mmol sodium bicarbonate diluted in 200 mL sterile water can be infused at a rate of 200 mL/hr. No bicarbonate is necessary if pH >7.0.

subsequent choice for fluid replacement depends on the patient's state of hydration, serum electrolyte levels, and urinary output. In general, 0.45% NaCL infused at a rate of 4 to 14 mL/kg/hr is appropriate if the corrected serum sodium is normal or elevated. If the corrected serum sodium is low, 0.9% NaCl is preferred.[92,119] When serum glucose concentrations approach 250 to 300 mg/dL, solutions should be changed to 5% glucose in half-normal saline. Glucose is added to prevent hypoglycemia and cerebral edema that can occur if the osmolality is reduced too rapidly. The use of dextrose also allows for continued insulin administration that is required to resolve the ketoacidosis (see Question 42). These recommendations for fluid replacement must be adjusted in the elderly or those with compromised renal or myocardial function. In these patients, fluid administration must be titrated against central venous pressure.[92,119]

Sodium

Total body sodium usually is depleted by 7 to 10 mEq/kg of body weight in patients with DKA. In assessing serum sodium in these patients, it is important to remember that false low values (i.e., pseudohyponatremia) may be the result of hyperglycemia and hypertriglyceridemia. A corrected sodium value may be obtained by adding 1.6 to 2 mEq/L to the observed value for every 100 mg/dL glucose >200 mg/dL.[120] Sodium is replaced adequately with normal saline.[92,119]

Potassium

Potassium balance is altered markedly in patients with DKA because of combined urinary and GI losses. Invariably, total potassium is depleted; however, the serum potassium concentration may be high, normal, or low, depending on the degree of acidosis and volume contraction. Usual potassium deficits in this situation average 3 to 5 mEq/kg of body weight, although they may be as high as 10 mEq/kg.[92,119]

Thus, J.L. will need approximately 200 to 350 mEq of potassium to replenish her body stores, assuming her normal weight is 70 kg. In patients whose initial serum potassium concentrations are elevated (>5.5 mEq/L), potassium supplementation is withheld for the first hour or until serum levels begin to drop. An adequate urine output also should be established before potassium supplements are initiated; however, a low serum potassium (<3.3 mEq/L) in the face of pronounced acidosis suggests severe potassium depletion requiring early, aggressive therapy to prevent life-threatening hypokalemia during treatment. The latter can occur from dilution, continued urinary losses, correction of acidosis, and insulin-mediated cellular uptake. In these cases, initial IV solutions should contain KCl 20 to 30 mEq/L.

J.L.'s admission laboratory data reveal a slightly elevated SrCr (most likely prerenal azotemia). This, in conjunction with a high-normal serum potassium concentration, weighs in favor of withholding potassium until serum levels begin to decline and urine output increases. Potassium levels generally begin to decrease in 1 to 2 hours, but if the patient is given bicarbonate, a decline may occur more rapidly. Once potassium levels begin to fall, 20 to 40 mEq should be added to each liter of fluid (⅔ KCl and ⅓ KPO₄).

Phosphate

The need for phosphate in the treatment of DKA is controversial. Phosphate is lost as the result of increased tissue catabolism, impaired cellular uptake, and enhanced renal excretion. Like other electrolytes, serum levels initially may appear normal even though body stores are depleted. Profound hypophosphatemia can decrease cardiac output, alter mental status, and produce tissue hypoxia and hemolysis. Prospective, randomized studies have shown no particular advantage of phosphate therapy in the treatment of DKA.[92,119] In fact, overzealous replacement can result in hypomagnesemia or hypocalcemia. Nevertheless, if phosphate concentrations drop to 1 mg/dL or less, 20 to 30 mEq/L potassium phosphate can be added to the replacement fluids.

Insulin

42. What is an appropriate insulin dose and route of administration for J.L.?

Unless the episode of DKA is mild (pH = 7.25 to 7.30), regular insulin by continuous infusion is the treatment of choice. Once hypokalemia is excluded (K⁺ <3.3 mEq/L), an intravenous bolus of 0.15 units/kg followed by a continuous infusion at a dose of 0.1 unit/kg per hour should be administered. When the plasma glucose reaches 250 mg/dL, the insulin infusion may be decreased to 0.05 to 0.1 units/kg per hour. This is typically when the replacement fluid is changed to D₅W. At this point, the rate of insulin administration or the concentration of dextrose is adjusted to maintain the glucose value at around 250 mg/dL until the acidosis is resolved.[92,119]

Thus, for J.L., an IV bolus dose of 9 units followed by an infusion of 6 U/hour would be appropriate. The insulin should be infused separately from the fluids being used to replace volume so that its rate can be adjusted independently. A solution with an insulin concentration of 0.1 U/mL can be obtained by adding 50 units of regular insulin to 500 mL of normal saline. If a dose of 0.1 U/kg is used, the infusion rate is equivalent to the patient's weight in kg (in J.L., 60 mL/hour). If J.L.'s plasma glucose concentration remains unchanged after 2 hours, the infusion rate should be doubled. As noted previously, as the glucose concentration falls to 250 to 300 mg/dL, the insulin infusion rate should be decreased and a 5% dextrose solution should be instituted.

Sodium Bicarbonate

43. J.L. was treated with fluids, electrolytes, and insulin as discussed in previous questions. Laboratory and clinical data 4 hours after therapy are as follows: pH, 7.1; blood glucose, 400 mg/dL; K, 3.8 mEq/L; SrCr, 3.1 mg/dL; and serum ketones strongly positive at a 1:40 dilution. Her BP was 120/70 mm Hg with no orthostatic changes. Urine output over the last 3 hours has been 500 mL. Because serum ketones have increased, should J.L. receive more insulin? Should she receive bicarbonate therapy?

[SI units: blood glucose, 22 mmol/L; K, 3.8 mmol/L; SrCr, 274 μmol/L]

The assumption that ketosis is worse in J.L. is incorrect. In DKA, low levels of insulin and elevated glucagon levels promote the metabolism of free fatty acids in the liver to acetoacetate and β-hydroxybutyrate. The standard nitroprusside reaction test for ketones measures only acetoacetate, even though β-hydroxybutyrate is the more important ketone. The conversion of acetoacetic acid to β-hydroxybutyrate is coupled closely with the NADH:NAD ratio. If this ratio is high (as in the presence of alcohol) so much β-hydroxybutyrate may be formed that acetoacetate is virtually undetectable; thus, the absence of ketones in the serum does not rule out ketoacidosis.

Conversely, treatment with insulin begins to suppress lipolysis and fatty acid oxidation; NAD is regenerated shifting the reaction back in favor of acetoacetate.[92,119] Thus, even though there appears to be higher concentrations of ketones in the serum, J.L.'s declining blood glucose concentration, improved bicarbonate concentrations, and improved acid-base and cardiovascular responses indicate that she is responding appropriately. Therefore, no change in the insulin dose is indicated. It is important to emphasize that the glucose concentrations normalize before ketones (4 to 6 hours versus 6 to 12 hours) because the latter are metabolized more slowly. For this reason, it is important to continue insulin to maintain suppression of lipolysis until plasma and urine ketones have cleared.

The use of sodium bicarbonate in patients with DKA has been controversial.[92,119] Most investigators discourage its routine use, reserving it for patients with severe acidemia (pH <7.0) or those in clinical shock. Coma is correlated most closely to blood glucose concentrations (>700 mg/dL) and hyperosmolality (calculated osmolality >340 mOsm/kg).[92] In a randomized, prospective study, bicarbonate did not affect recovery in patients with severe DKA (arterial pH, 6.9 to 7.14).[121] Thus, even though J.L.'s acidosis seemed severe on admission (pH, 7.05; bicarbonate, 6 mEq/L; Kussmaul respirations), bicarbonate was not administered. It is apparent that with fluid and insulin therapy alone, her acidosis is beginning to improve.

44. **What is the expected course of DKA in J.L.?**

After 3 L of fluid and a constant insulin infusion of 6 U/hour for 3 hours, J.L.'s glucose concentration had dropped to 500 mg/dL and she had no orthostatic BP changes, reflecting recovery from her volume-depleted status. Potassium (40 mEq/L) was added to her fluids, which were administered at a reduced rate of 300 mL/hour.

Three hours later, the glucose concentration had dropped to 350 mg/dL and her pH had increased to 7.21. The serum potassium remained low-normal at 3.4 mEq/L, and serum sodium increased to 151 mEq/L. In view of these changes, the IV infusion fluid was changed to half-normal saline with 5% dextrose to which 40 mEq/L of potassium was added. The rate was slowed to 250 mL/hour, and the insulin infusion was decreased to 4 U/hour.

Four hours later (10 hours after admission), the blood glucose was 235 mg/dL and the serum potassium was 3.5 mEq/dL. The IV fluids were changed to 5% dextrose with 40 mEq/L of KCl, administered at a rate of 250 mL/hour, and the regular insulin infusion was decreased from 6 to 2 U/hour. J.L. continued to improve over the next 12 hours, and she began taking full oral liquids by the second hospital day. At that time, her IV infusion rate was decreased to 200 mL/hour but her insulin infusion was continued.

Approximately 24 hours after admission, J.L.'s blood glucose concentration was 175 mg/dL, potassium was 4.6 mEq/L, and sodium was 144 mEq/L. There were no ketones in the plasma. The urine contained 1% glucose and moderate amounts of ketones. IV fluids were discontinued and regular insulin was administered subcutaneously 1 hour before the insulin infusion was discontinued. J.L. continued to receive regular insulin subcutaneously every 4 hours according to a sliding scale (see Question 18). Thirty-six hours after admission, J.L. was given her usual dose of insulin glargine and insulin lispro and was sent home for follow-up in the clinic.

TREATMENT OF TYPE 2 DIABETES: ORAL ANTIDIABETIC AGENTS

This section of the chapter addresses the clinical pharmacology of agents used to treat type 2 diabetes. Although type 2 diabetes is the most common form of diabetes mellitus, it often is dismissed as "mild" diabetes or as a "touch of diabetes" and historically has been treated far less aggressively than type 1 diabetes mellitus. As described in the introduction, the medical community has now realized that type 2 diabetes is a serious condition that must be managed in the context of the metabolic syndrome. At the time of diagnosis, many people with type 2 diabetes already have evidence of macrovascular and microvascular disease. The UKPDS demonstrated that improved glycemic control will reduce the onset and progression of microvascular complications and blood pressure control will also reduce macrovascular complications. Thus, every effort to lower glucose concentrations toward normal values, control blood pressure, and lower cholesterol is important to delay the onset or slow the progression of these complications, improve the overall quality of the patient's life, and save the health care system millions of dollars in hospitalization costs to treat these complications. The importance of diet, exercise, and other lifestyle changes as cornerstones in treatment of people with type 2 diabetes cannot be overemphasized. Unfortunately, these measures alone usually are not successful in achieving control for the majority of patients, and drugs are eventually required.

Until 1995, only sulfonylureas and insulin were available to treat type 2 diabetes. Since then, metformin, α-glucosidase inhibitors (acarbose and miglitol), thiazolidinediones (rosiglitazone and pioglitazone), and nonsulfonylurea insulin secretagogues (repaglinide and nateglinide) have been approved by the FDA, and many other agents with differing mechanisms of action are in development. These agents give clinicians and patients more choice, but there is considerable confusion about which of these agents to use initially as monotherapy and how they should be used in combination with one another or with insulin. Patients with type 2 diabetes often are already taking several other drugs to treat their cardiovascular conditions, dyslipidemia, hypertension, depression, and other chronic illnesses that come with aging. This does not account for the many nutritional, herbal, homeopathic remedies and over-the-counter (OTC) medications patients often self-prescribe. Therefore, in our view, the aim should be the simplest, safest regimen that gives the patient the best glycemic control possible.

Figure 50-8 depicts the sources of hyperglycemia in people with type 2 diabetes and the primary site of action for each class of agents described subsequently. Tables 50-29, 50-30, and 50-31 summarize the pharmacokinetics, pharmacology, and drug interactions of the oral antidiabetic drugs. The clinical use of these agents in specific situations is illustrated by cases later in this chapter.

α-Glucosidase Inhibitors

Two oral agents for the treatment of type 2 diabetes mellitus belong to the α-glucosidase inhibitor class, acarbose (Precose) and miglitol (Glyset). Acarbose is available in Europe under the trade name Glucobay.

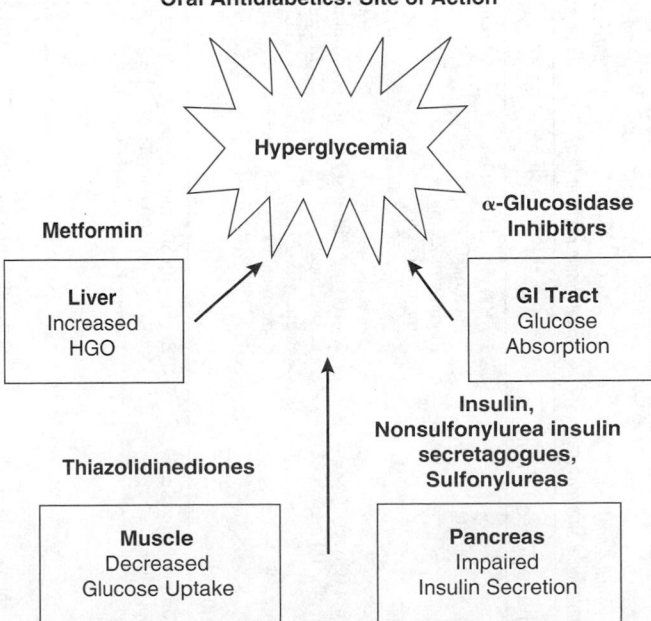

FIGURE 50-8 Sources of hyperglycemia in type 2 diabetes and site of action of oral antidiabetic agents. GI, gastrointestinal; HGO, hepatic glucose output.

Table 50-29 Oral Antidiabetic Pharmacokinetic Data[149,150]

Drug (Brand Name) Available Tablet Strengths (mg)	Typical Dosing Regimen (mg)	Usual Minimum and Maximum Total Daily Dose/How Divided	Mean Half-Life	Approximate Duration of Activity	Bioavailability Metabolism, and Excretion	Comments
α-Glucosidase Inhibitors						
Acarbose (Precose) 25, 50, 100 mg	25–100 mg with first bite of each meal. Begin with 25 mg; ↑ by 25 mg/meal every 4–8 weeks.	Minimum: 25 mg TID Maximum dose is 50 mg TID if <60 kg; 100 mg TID if >60 kg.	2.8 hr	Affects absorption of complex carbohydrates in a single meal	F = 0.5–1.7%; extensively metabolized by GI amylases to inactive products; 50% excreted unchanged in the feces	Titrate doses slowly to avoid GI effects
Miglitol (Glyset) 25, 50, 100 mg	25–100 mg with first bite of each meal. Begin with 25 mg; ↑ by 25 mg/meal every 4–8 weeks.	Minimum: 25 mg TID Maximum: 100 mg TID	2 hr	Affects absorption of complex carbohydrates in a single meal	Dose of 25 mg is completely absorbed; dose of 100 mg 50–70% absorbed; elimination by renal excretion as unchanged drug	
Biguanides						
Metformin (Glucophage) 500, 850 mg	Begin with 500 mg QD or BID; ↑ by 500 mg QD every 1–2 weeks.	0.5–2.5 g BID or TID	Plasma, 6.2 hr Whole blood, 17.6 hr	6–12 hr	F = 50–60%; excreted unchanged in urine	Avoid in patients with renal failure or those who could be predisposed to lactic acidosis (e.g., alcoholism, CHF, severe respiratory disorders, liver failure)
Metformin extended-release (Glucophage XR) 500 mg	500–1,000 mg QD with evening meal; ↑ by 500 mg every 1–2 weeks.	1,500–2,000 mg QD	As for metformin, but active drug is released slowly	24 hr	As for metformin	As for metformin
Nonsulfonylurea Insulin Secretagogues						
Repaglinide (Prandin) 0.5, 1, 2 mg	If A$_{1c}$ is <8% or if this is first drug, begin with 0.5 mg with each meal. For others, begin with 1–2 mg/meal.	0.5–4 mg with each meal (16 mg/day) TID–QID	1 hr	C$_{max}$ is at 1 hr; duration is approximately 2–3 hr	F = 56%; 92% metabolized to inactive products by the liver; 8% excreted as metabolites unchanged in the urine	Take only with meals. Skip dose if meal is skipped.
Netaglinide (Starlix) 60, 120 mg	120 mg TID 1–30 min before meals; 60 mg TID for patients with near-normal A$_{1c}$ at initiation.	60 or 120 mg TID	1.5 hr	Onset, 20 min; peak, 1 hr; duration, 2–4 hr	F = 73%; metabolized to inactive products (predominantly) that are excreted in the urine (83%) and feces (10%)	Skip dose if meal is skipped.
Combination Products						
Glipizide/metformin (Metaglip) 2.5/250 mg, 2.5/500 mg, 5/500 mg	Initial therapy: 2.5/250 mg QD 2nd line therapy: 2.5–5/500 mg BID; ↑ every 2 weeks	5/1,000–20/2,000 mg in two divided doses	See metformin and glyburide	See metformin and glyburide	See metformin and glyburide	See Glucovance
Glyburide/Metformin (Glucovance)[b] 1.25/500, 2.5/500 mg 5.0/500 mg	2.5/500 mg QD or BID; ↑ by 2.5/500 mg every 1–2 weeks.	7.5/1,500–10/2,000 mg in two to three divided doses with meals	See metformin	See metformin	See metformin and glyburide	Effect should be similar to the two agents given in combination. Minimum dose of 1,500 mg metformin is needed for effect. No need to exceed 10 mg glyburide
Metformin/rosiglitazone (Avandamet) 500/1 mg, 500/2 mg/500/4 mg	2/500 mg BID	4/1,000 mg–8/2,000 mg in two divided doses with meals	See metformin and rosiglitazone	See rosiglitazone	See metformin and rosiglitazone	Dose titration schedule is dependent on which drug is being adjusted.

Table 50-30 Comparative Pharmacology of Antidiabetic Agents

Agent Generic Name Brand Name Mechanism	FDA Indications	Efficacy	Adverse Effects	Comments
Insulin Replaces or augments endogenous insulin	Monotherapy; combined with any oral agent	↓ A$_{1c}$ 4 ↓ FPG∞ ↓ PPG∞ ↓ TG	Hypoglycemia, weight gain, lipodystrophy, local skin reactions.	Offers flexible dosing to match lifestyle and glucose concentrations. Rapid onset. Safe in pregnancy, renal failure, and liver dysfunction. Drug of choice when patients do not respond to oral agents.
Insulin-Augmenting Agents				
Nonsulfonylurea secretagogues Repaglinide (Prandin; NovoNorm) Netaglinide (Starlix) Stimulates insulin secretion.	Monotherapy; combined with metformin	↓ A$_{1c}$ 1.7% ↓ FPG 61 mg/dL ↓ PPG 48 mg/dL	Hypoglycemia, weight gain.	Take only with meals. If a meal is skipped, skip a dose. Flexible dosing with lifestyle. Safe in renal and liver failure. Rapid onset.
Sulfonylureas Various; see Table 50-29 Stimulates insulin secretion. May decrease hepatic glucose output and enhance peripheral glucose utilization.	Monotherapy; combined with metformin; combined with insulin (glimepiride)	↓ A$_{1c}$ 1.5–1.7% ↓ FPG 50–70 mg/dL ↓ PPG 92 mg/dL	Hypoglycemia, especially long-acting agents; weight gain (4–22 lb). Rash, hepatotoxicity, alcohol intolerance, and hyponatremia are rare.	Very effective agents, but cause hyperinsulinemia, which leads to hypoglycemia and weight gain. Some can be dosed once daily. Rapid onset of effect (1 week).
Delayers of Carbohydrate Absorption				
α-Glucosidase inhibitors Acarbose (Precose) Miglitol (Glyset) Slows absorption of complex carbohydrates.	Monotherapy; combined with SFUs	↓ A$_{1c}$ 0.5–1.0% ↓ FPG 20–30 mg/dL ↓ PPG 25–50 mg/dL	GI: flatulence, diarrhea. Elevations in LFTs seen in doses >50 mg TID of acarbose. Therefore, LFTs should be monitored every 3 months during the first year of therapy and periodically thereafter. Because miglitol is not metabolized, monitoring of LFTs is not required.	Titrate dose slowly to minimize GI effects. No hypoglycemia or weight gain. If used in combination with hypoglycemic agents, advise patients to treat hypoglycemia with glucose tablets because absorption is not inhibited as with sucrose.
Insulin Sensitizers				
Biguanides Metformin (Glucophage) ↓ Hepatic glucose output; ↑ peripheral glucose uptake	Monotherapy; combined with SFUs	↓ A$_{1c}$ 1.5–1.7% ↓ FPG 50–70 mg/dL ↓ PPG 83 mg/dL ↓ TG 10–20% ↓ Total cholesterol 5–10% ↑ HDL cholesterol (slight)	GI: cramping, diarrhea. Lactic acidosis (rare).	Titrate dose slowly to minimize GI effects. No hypoglycemia or weight gain; weight loss possible. Do not use in patients with renal or hepatic function or CHF requiring treatment.

Table 50-31   Pharmacokinetic Drug Interactions With Oral Antidiabetic Agents

Drugs	Comments

Pharmacokinetic Drug Interactions With Sulfonylureas

Drugs Increasing Sulfonylurea Effect

Drugs	Comments
Antacids	Enhanced glyburide absorption due to increased gastric pH. Avoid concomitant administration.
Chloramphenicol	↓ tolbutamide hepatic metabolism and ↑ t½ 2- to 3-fold. Possible prolongation of chlorpropamide t½.
Cimetidine	↓ tolbutamide hepatic metabolism by 17% in one study. Ranitidine had no effect.
Clofibrate	May displace sulfonylureas from proteins, ↓ insulin resistance, ↓ renal tubular secretion of chlorpropamide.
Doxepin	Mechanism unknown. Monitor for hypoglycemia.
Fluconazole	Increased plasma concentrations. Watch for hypoglycemia.
Gemfibrozil	Possibly due to protein displacement. May need to reduce dose of sulfonylurea.
Halofenate	Increases serum concentrations.
Heparin	Heparin may have significantly prolonged glipizide hypoglycemia in one unconvincing case report. Confirmation needed.
Methandrostenolone	Enhances hypoglycemic effect. Consider nandrolone and methenolone acetate.
Methyldopa	↑ mean tolbutamide t½ by 24% in one study.
Nonsteroidal anti-inflammatory drugs	Sulfinpyrazone and phenylbutazone ↓ tolbutamide hepatic metabolism and ↑ t½ 2- to 3-fold. Enhanced hypoglycemia secondary to acetohexamide (↓ renal excretion of active metabolite) and chlorpropamide also reported. Severe, fatal hypoglycemia can occur. Ibuprofen, naproxen, sulindac, and tolmetin do not affect sulfonylurea disposition.
Salicylates	Limited and indirect documentation (primarily in vitro) that salicylates may ↑ sulfonylurea activity through protein-binding displacement or inhibition of active renal tubular secretion.
Sulfonamide antimicrobials	Cotrimoxazole ↓ tolbutamide metabolism and t½ by 30% in one study. Severe hypoglycemia with glyburide and chlorpropamide reported rarely. Sulfisoxazole also rarely associated with tolbutamide- and chlorpropamide-induced severe hypoglycemia.
Warfarin	No evidence that warfarin affects sulfonylurea disposition; however, dicumarol ↑ tolbutamide (and possibly chlorpropamide) t½ 3- to 4-fold, probably by ↓ hepatic metabolism. Sulfonylureas do not appear to alter patient response to the anticoagulants. Warfarin response should be monitored if glyburide is initiated, discontinued, or changed in dosage.

Drugs Decreasing Sulfonylurea Effect

Drugs	Comments
Alcohol	Chronic ethanol use ↑ tolbutamide hepatic metabolism 2-fold. Conversely, short-term ethanol infusions ↓ tolbutamide clearance by 50%.
Rifampin	↑ tolbutamide and glyburide metabolism, thereby ↓ t½ and plasma drug concentrations.

Other Drugs

Drugs	Comments
Cyclosporine	May compete with glipizide for cytochrome P450 hydroxylation. Necessitated a 20–30% dosage reduction of cyclosporine in two case reports.
Phenytoin	Unknown effects on sulfonylureas; however, tolbutamide transiently ↑ free phenytoin concentrations through protein-binding displacement by approximately 45% in one study.

Pharmacokinetic Drug Interaction With Repaglinide

Drugs	Comments
Gemfibrozil	Significant ↑ in repaglinide blood levels (8-fold in AUC) due to reduced repaglinide metabolism; do not use concurrently.
Itraconazole/ketoconazole	↑ in repaglinide blood levels; do not use concurrently.

Pharmacokinetic Drug Interactions With Metformin

Drugs	Comments
Alcohol	Potentiates the effects of metformin on lactate metabolism. Patients should avoid excessive alcohol intake.
Cimetidine	Increase in peak metformin plasma concentrations. May necessitate a reduction in metformin dose. An alternate H_2 blocker is recommended.
Erythromycin	Severe cholestatic hepatitis reported when used in combination with chlorpropamide. Monitor liver enzymes and bilirubin or use alternate antibiotic.
Iodinated parenteral contrast dye	Can result in acute renal failure and metformin-induced lactic acidosis. Metformin should be withheld at least 48 hours before and 48 hours after the procedure. Reinstitute metformin only after renal function has been determined to be normal.

Pharmacokinetic Drug Interactions With α-Glucosidase Inhibitors

Drugs	Comments
Charcoal/digestive enzyme preparations	Intestinal adsorbents (e.g., charcoal) and digestive enzyme preparations (e.g., amylase, pancreatin) may reduce the effect of acarbose.
Digoxin	Serum digoxin concentrations may be reduced, decreasing the therapeutic effects.
Propranolol	Miglitol may significantly reduce the bioavailability of propranolol by 40%.
Ranitidine	Miglitol may significantly reduce the bioavailability of ranitidine by 60%.

Pharmacokinetic Drug Interactions With Thiazolidinediones (Pioglitazone)

Drugs	Comments
Ketoconazole	Ketoconazole appears to significantly inhibit the metabolism of pioglitazone. Glycemic control should be evaluated more frequently in patients taking these agents in combination.
Oral contraceptives	Pioglitazone reduces plasma concentrations of oral contraceptives containing ethinyl estradiol and norethindrone. Result is a possible loss of contraception. Watch for symptoms of estrogen deficiency (e.g., hot flushes) in women taking estrogen hormone-replacement therapy.

Mechanism of Action

The α-glucosidase inhibitors reversibly inhibit glucosidases present in the brush-border of the mucosa of the small intestine. These enzymes are responsible for the breakdown of complex polysaccharides and dissaccharides into absorbable glucose and other monosaccharides.

This results in delayed digestion of carbohydrates and subsequent glucose absorption with a lowering of postprandial blood glucose concentrations. This reduction occurs only when these agents are taken with a meal containing a complex carbohydrate.[122-124]

Pharmacokinetics

Acarbose is minimally absorbed from the GI tract; oral bioavailability of the parent compound is 0.5% to 1.7%. Acarbose is extensively metabolized by GI amylases to inactive metabolites. The elimination half-life for acarbose is 2.8 hours, although there may be a longer terminal half-life.[123,124] Unlike acarbose, miglitol is absorbed, does not undergo metabolism, and is excreted unchanged in the urine with an elimination half-life of 2 hours.

Adverse Effects

GASTROINTESTINAL EFFECTS

Flatulence, diarrhea, and abdominal pain are the most frequently reported adverse effects of α-glucosidase inhibitors, and in one placebo-controlled trial of acarbose, these complaints were experienced by 73.2%, 43.6%, and 25% of the subjects, respectively. Notably, many in the placebo group also complained of flatulence (39%), diarrhea (20.3%), and abdominal cramps or discomfort (8.8%).[125] These side effects, which are due to fermentation of unabsorbed carbohydrate in the small intestine, can be minimized by slowly titrating the dose of either agent. GI discomfort usually improves with continued therapy as induction of the α-glucosidase enzymes occurs in the distal jejunum and terminal ileum.

ELEVATED LIVER FUNCTION TESTS

In studies using doses of acarbose $\geq$300 mg/day, a transient increase in serum hepatic transaminases was reported.[126] The manufacturer recommends monitoring hepatic transaminases every 3 months for the first year of therapy and periodically therafter.[127] If elevations of serum transaminases occurs, the dose should be decreased or discontinued if elevations persist.[127] No incidents of hepatotoxicity have been reported to date with miglitol. Because miglitol is not metabolized, its lack of effect on hepatic function is expected.

Contraindications and Precautions[127,128]

GASTROINTESTINAL CONDITIONS

Because of their profound GI effects, acarbose and miglitol are not recommended for use in patients with malabsorption, inflammatory bowel disease, or intestinal obstruction.

RENAL IMPAIRMENT

Acarbose has not been studied in patients with severe renal impairment (SrCr >2.0 mg/dL) and should not be used in these patients.[127]

HYPOGLYCEMIA

Patients who use acarbose or miglitol in combination with other antidiabetic agents may develop hypoglycemia. These reactions should be treated with dextrose because acarbose may limit the availability of the disaccharide, sucrose (table sugar).

Drug Interactions

Because acarbose and miglitol delay carbohydrate passage through the bowel, they could influence the absorption kinetics of concomitantly administered drugs. Conversely, because their own absorption may be diminished by charcoal or digestive enzyme preparations, they should not be taken concomitantly with these agents. Acarbose and miglitol do not affect the absorption of glyburide in individuals with diabetes.[127,128] The bioavailability of digoxin can be reduced and may require dose adjustment. Miglitol decreases the bioavailability of ranitidine and propranolol by 60% and 40%, respectively.[128]

Efficacy

By delaying the absorption of glucose following ingestion of complex carbohydrates and disaccharides, the α-glucosidase inhibitors can lower postprandial plasma glucose concentrations in patients with type 2 diabetes by 25 to 50 mg/dL. FPG concentrations remain unchanged or are slightly lowered (20 to 30 mg/dL), but this effect may be related to decreased glucose toxicity, which improves insulin secretion and action. Mean A_{1C} values decline by 0.5% to 1%. Acarbose and miglitol have no effect on weight or lipid profiles.[122-125]

Dosage and Clinical Use

Acarbose can be used as monotherapy or in combination with a sulfonylurea, metformin or insulin.[127] Miglitol can be used as monotherapy or in combination with a sulfonylurea, and it has been studied in combination with insulin.[122,128,129] The recommended initial dose of either drug is 25 mg three times daily, taken at the beginning of each meal, although even lower doses have been used. The dosage can be gradually increased (e.g., 25 mg/meal) every 4 to 8 weeks to a maximum of 50 mg three times daily for individuals $\leq$60 kg, or 100 mg three times daily for individuals >60 kg. A maximum response is observed at 6 months.[125] Patients should be instructed to take the tablet at the start of each meal. Acarbose or miglitol can be used to treat patients with type 2 diabetes managed with diet and exercise whose A_{1C} levels are mildly elevated above the target value. They may also be used in combination with other oral antidiabetic agents and insulin, particularly when postprandial glucose concentrations are elevated. Also see Questions 51, 57 through 60, and 64.

Biguanides

Metformin (Glucophage) belongs to the biguanide class of oral hypoglycemic agents and has been available in the United States since 1995. Metformin became available generically in 2002. Phenformin, also a biguanide, was available in the United States until 1977 when the FDA, because of phenformin's association with fatal lactic acidosis, withdrew it. The clinical pharmacology of metformin has been extensively reviewed.[130-133]

Mechanism of Action

The biguanides are described more accurately as antihyperglycemic agents. Although they lower blood glucose concentrations in people with type 2 diabetes, they do not cause hypoglycemia in nondiabetic individuals. Unlike the oral sulfonylureas, the biguanides do not stimulate the release of insulin from the pancreas. The precise mechanisms by which metformin lowers blood glucose concentrations remain to be elucidated. There is evidence that metformin lowers FPG concentrations by decreasing gluconeogenesis and therefore hepatic glucose production. Metformin also seems to improve peripheral sensitivity to insulin, as illustrated by enhanced glucose disposal and clearance as well as a reduction in plasma insulin concentrations. Metformin also lowers plasma free fatty acid levels, and subsequent oxidation, which may contribute to its ability to reduce hepatic glucose production and increase insulin-mediated glucose disposal in the muscle.[134] In addition to its effects on FFAs, metformin produces small decrements (5% to 10%) in total cholesterol and triglycerides (10% to 20%). Small increments or no change in high-density cholesterol concentrations have been observed. These effects on lipid metabolism as well as many other effects on clotting factors, platelet function, and vascular function have generated interest in the potential favorable effects of metformin on cardiovascular disease and outcomes.[134] Unlike the sulfonylureas, TZDs and insulin, weight loss rather than weight gain is more likely to occur with metformin therapy (mean weight loss of 1.2 kg compared with 1.7 kg increase).[135]

Pharmacokinetics

Approximately 50% to 60% of metformin is absorbed from the small intestine. It is eliminated entirely by the kidney unchanged and has a plasma half-life of 6.2 hours and a whole blood half-life of 17.6 hours. It is not bound to plasma proteins.[136,137]

Adverse Effects
GASTROINTESTINAL EFFECTS

Transient side effects include diarrhea and other GI disturbances such as abdominal discomfort, metallic taste, nausea, and anorexia. Although these symptoms can be minimized by slowly titrating the dose, patients should be advised that they may experience GI side effects that are dose related and should subside with time; metformin should be taken with food to minimize GI disturbances. In a placebo-controlled trial, 5% of patients discontinued metformin because of side effects that were predominantly GI in nature. Relative to placebo, "digestive disturbances" occurred in 28% versus 15% of patients, and diarrhea was the most common complaint (15% versus 5%). Also see Question 53.

LACTIC ACIDOSIS

The risk of lactic acidosis secondary to metformin is 10 to 20 times lower than with phenformin.[133,138] Unlike phenformin, metformin is not metabolized, it does not inhibit peripheral glucose oxidation, and it does not enhance peripheral lactate production. However, it may decrease conversion of lactate to glucose (decreased gluconeogenesis) and increase lactate production in the gut and liver.[132,133,138] Consequently, metformin rarely has been associated with lactic acidosis. The few patients in whom this event has been reported had renal, liver, or cardiorespiratory contraindications to the use of biguanides. Patients should be warned to bring the following symptoms of lactic acidosis to the attention of their physician: weakness, malaise, myalgias, abdominal distress and heavy, labored breathing (see Question 66).

Contraindications and Precautions

Patients with renal impairment, hepatic disease, congestive heart failure (CHF) requiring pharmacologic treatment, acute or chronic metabolic acidosis or a history of lactic acidosis should be excluded from therapy. Metformin can accumulate in patients whose renal function is impaired, thus increasing the risk of lactic acidosis. Its use is not recommended in patients with decreased GFRs (<60 mL/minute) or elevated creatinine levels ($\geq$1.4 mg/dL for females or $\geq$1.5 mg/dL for males). Because even a temporary reduction in renal function could cause lactic acidosis in patients taking metformin, the manufacturer recommends withholding it after some radiologic procedures (see Drug Interactions). Other predisposing factors for lactic acidosis include the following: excessive alcohol ingestion, CHF, shock, hepatic failure, dehydration, sepsis or surgery. Because aging is associated with reduced renal function, metformin should be titrated to the minimum effective dose and renal function should be monitored regularly. A creatinine clearance (Cl_{Cr}) to ensure adequate renal function should be measured in patients over the age of 80 years, because these patients are more susceptible to developing lactic acidosis.[136]

Drug Interactions

- *Alcohol* potentiates the effect of metformin on lactate metabolism. Patients should be warned regarding excessive alcohol intake while taking metformin.
- *Cimetidine* increases peak metformin plasma concentrations by 60%, and use of an alternative H_2 blocker or a reduction in metformin dose is recommended.
- *Parenteral contrast studies* (e.g., pyelography or angiography) that use *iodinated materials* can result in acute renal failure and metformin-induced lactic acidosis. For patients requiring such a study, metformin should be withheld at the time of, or before, and 48 hours after the procedure. Metformin should be reinstituted only after renal function has been re-evaluated and determined to be normal.

Efficacy

As monotherapy, metformin can be expected to reduce the A_{1C} by 1.5% to 1.7% and the FPG by 50 to 70 mg/dL. In patients who have developed secondary failure to sulfonylureas, the addition of metformin can be expected to produce a similar or slightly greater improvement in the FPG and A_{1C}.[134]

Dosage and Clinical Use

Metformin is administered with meals to minimize its GI side effects. These disturbances also can be minimized by slowly increasing the dose (e.g., 500 mg once or twice daily initially, followed by weekly or biweekly increments of 500 mg daily). Metformin is dosed two to three times daily (500 to 1,000 mg per dose; maximum dose is 2,550 mg daily or 850 mg PO TID), unless an extended-release preparation is prescribed. Clinicians should obtain a SrCr and hepatic function tests at baseline and then annually. Metformin should not be used in patients older than 80 years unless a Cl_{Cr} demonstrates normal renal function. Patients are candidates for treatment if the Cl_{Cr} is >60 mL/minute.

Because metformin and the sulfonylureas are equally effective in reducing FPG concentrations, either can be used as initial therapy. Relative to the sulfonylureas, metformin has the advantage of decreasing hepatic glucose output, improving insulin resistance, reducing plasma insulin concentrations, and improving the lipid profile. It may produce some weight loss (or at least no weight gain) and rarely causes hypoglycemia when used alone. Thus, it is preferred as monotherapy in obese patients (also see Questions 52 through 54 and 58 through 60).

Nonsulfonylurea Insulin Secretagogues

Repaglinide (Prandin in the United States; NovoNorm in other countries) and nateglinide (Starlix) are nonsulfonylurea insulin secretagogues (i.e., stimulate insulin secretion); they belong to a class of agents referred to as meglitinides and amino acid derivatives, respectively. Repaglinide was approved by the FDA in December 1997 and nateglinide was approved in December 2000[139-141] (see Table 50-29).

Mechanism of Action

Like the sulfonylureas, these agents close the adenosine triphosphate (ATP)-sensitive potassium channels in the β-cell, which leads to cell membrane depolarization, an influx of Ca^{2+}, and secretion of insulin. Unlike the sulfonylureas, they have a rapid onset and shorter duration of action so that they are given with meals to enhance postprandial glucose utilization.

Pharmacokinetics

Repaglinide has a bioavailability of 56% and is rapidly absorbed and excreted.[142] Its C_{max} occurs at approximately 1 hour and its half-life is 1 hour. It is completely metabolized (CYP 3A4) by the liver to inactive products; 90% is excreted in the feces and 8% is excreted in urine. It is highly (>98%) protein bound (volume of distribution [Vd], 31 L).

Nateglinide has a bioavailability of 73% and is rapidly absorbed with a C_{max} occurring within 1 hour after dosing; its half-life is 1.5 hours. Nateglinide is metabolized (CYP2C9, 70% and CYP3A4, 30%) to less potent compounds, with 75% being excreted in the urine and 10% in the feces; 16% of nateglinide is excreted unchanged in the urine. It is highly (98%) protein bound, primarily to albumin and, to a lesser extent, to α_1 acid glycoprotein.

Adverse Effects

Mild hypoglycemia may occur, particularly if ingestion is not followed by food in an individual whose blood glucose concentrations are within the normal range. A weight gain of 0.9 to 3 kg compared with baseline has been observed.

Contraindications and Precautions

Because a functioning pancreas is required, these agents should not be used in people with type 1 diabetes. These agents should be cautiously used in patients with liver dysfunction. Nateglinide's clearance is not affected in patients with moderate-severe renal insufficiency, whereas the clearance of repaglinide is reduced in patients with severe renal insufficiency. Nevertheless, it may be used safely.[143]

Drug Interactions

When evaluated in clinical studies, repaglinide did not interact with digoxin, theophylline, or warfarin. Furthermore, cimetidine did not affect its metabolism. Drugs that induce the P450 system (e.g., rifampin) could theoretically decrease repaglinide's effects. Conversely, drugs that inhibit the P450 system (e.g., azole antifungal agents and macrolides) could enhance its effects. The latter concept was established when 3 days of treatment with gemfibrozil or itraconazole increased repaglinide's plasma concentration-time curve (AUC) by 28.6-fold and 8.1 fold, respectively. The combination increased the AUC by 70.4 fold.[144] New drug interaction warnings have been included in the package inserts for Lopid, Sporonax, and Prandin. Because hypoglycemia has been reported in patients taking the gemfibrozil/repaglinide combination, their use together is considered contraindicated.

Nateglinide is a potential inhibitor of CYP2C9. When evaluated in clinical studies, there were no clinically relevant interactions with nateglinide and glyburide, metformin, digoxin, diclofenac, or warfarin.

Efficacy

The efficacy of repaglinide is comparable to metformin and the sulfonylureas.[141] When used as monotherapy, the mean decrease in FPG, postprandial glucose, and the A_{1C} values were 61 mg/dL, 104 mg/dL, and 1.7%, respectively, compared with placebo (−31.0 mg/dL, −47.6 mg/dL, and −0.6 % compared with baseline). Newly diagnosed patients who have never been treated with oral agents and those whose A_{1C} is <8% respond more profoundly than poorly controlled individuals already on treatment. When repaglinide was added to metformin, the mean decline in FPG was approximately 40 mg/dL and the mean decrease in A_{1C} was 1.4% from baseline values.

Nateglinide as monotherapy results in a mean decrease in FPG and A_{1C} by 13.6 mg/dL and 0.7%, respectively, compared with placebo (−4.5 mg/dL and 0.5% compared with baseline).

Dosage and Clinical Use

Repaglinide and nateglinide are approved to treat people with type 2 diabetes as monotherapy or in combination with metformin; repaglinide is also approved for use with thiazolidinediones (TZDs).[141] Because they have the same mechanism of action as the sulfonylureas, combining these agents does not produce any additional benefit. When repaglinide is used as the initial treatment in patients who are "naive" to oral antidiabetic therapy or in patients with A_{1C} values <8%, the recommended starting dose is 0.5 mg with each meal. When used in patients who have failed sulfonylureas or in those with A_{1C} values >8%, the initial dose is 1 to 2 mg with each meal. Doses can be titrated weekly at a rate of 1 mg/meal to a maximum of 4 mg/dose or 16 mg/day. The recommended starting dose of nateglinide is 120 mg TID before meals; for patients close to their A_{1C} goal, a dose of 60 mg TID may be used. Doses should be taken 0 to 30 minutes before the meal, omitted if a meal is skipped and added if an extra meal is ingested (repaglinide only). Repaglinide should be initiated at a 0.5 mg dose in patients with severe renal dysfunction and should be titrated cautiously in patients with liver dysfunction.

Sulfonylureas

Until metformin and other antidiabetics became available in the United States, sulfonylureas were the first-line pharmacologic treatment for people with type 2 diabetes who had failed

LIVERPOOL
JOHN MOORES UNIVERSITY
AVRIL ROBARTS LRC
TEL. 0151 231 4022

diet and exercise therapy. Seven different sulfonylureas are available in the United States. The four *first-generation sulfonylureas* (acetohexamide [Dymelor], chlorpropamide [Diabinese], tolazamide [Tolinase], and tolbutamide [Orinase]) are considered equally effective despite differences in their pharmacokinetic properties and adverse effect profiles (see the following discussion and Table 50-29).

Glipizide (Glucotrol) and glyburide (DiaBeta, Micronase), two *second-generation sulfonylureas,* were first introduced into the United States in May 1984. Glimepiride (Amaryl) was approved for use in 1995. These agents are approximately 100 times more potent than the first-generation sulfonylureas on a milligram-for-milligram basis; however, there is no evidence that they are more effective clinically. They have a relatively favorable side-effect profile and have a duration of activity that requires no more than one or two daily doses. The basis on which specific agents are selected for patients is discussed in case studies that follow this introduction.

Mechanism of Action
PANCREATIC EFFECTS
Sulfonylureas stimulate the release of insulin from pancreatic β-cells and enhance β-cell sensitivity to glucose. A specific sulfonylurea receptor that is linked closely to the ATP-sensitive potassium ion channel has been identified on the β-cell, and sulfonylureas are believed to inhibit this potassium ion channel. As a result, they block the efflux of potassium and lower the membrane potential causing depolarization. The voltage-dependent calcium channels then open, increasing intracellular calcium concentration. The increased intracellular concentration of calcium ultimately stimulates insulin secretion.[47,145] Insulin levels tend to return to baseline values after a few months of continued sulfonylurea use.

EXTRAPANCREATIC EFFECTS
Sulfonylureas can normalize hepatic glucose production and partially reverse insulin resistance in the peripheral tissues of people with type 2 diabetes. Whether these "extrapancreatic" effects of the sulfonylureas are direct effects of these agents or are secondary to improved insulin release and lower glucose concentrations remains to be established. In any case, it is clear that tissues become more responsive to lower concentrations of endogenous insulin in type 2 patients treated with sulfonylureas.[146]

Pharmacokinetics
The biopharmaceutical and pharmacokinetic parameters of the sulfonylureas are summarized in the following text and in Table 50-29.[146,147] The duration of hypoglycemic activity is related to the half-life of these compounds only in very general terms and may correlate poorly in some cases. All sulfonylureas are highly protein bound (90% to 100%), mainly to albumin; however, binding characteristics vary among individual sulfonylureas. Food does not impair the extent of drug absorption but may delay the time to peak levels of some agents.

The relation between sulfonylurea doses and their blood glucose–lowering effect requires further study. One long-term study comparing glyburide and glipizide showed little or no improvement in glucose control at dosages ≥10 mg/day of either agent.[148] In single-dose and short-term studies with glipizide, an increased blood glucose–lowering effect was noted with up to 10 mg daily of glipizide.[149,150] In a placebo-controlled, double-blind study examining the effect of glipizide 10, 20, or 40 mg/day in patients with type 2 diabetes, the maximal insulin response and blood glucose–lowering effect was achieved with a glipizide dose of 10 mg/day.[150] These data suggest that sulfonylureas operate within a narrow range of plasma concentrations that may be achieved with low dosages of the drug. Therefore, there is a need to re-evaluate maximum recommended daily doses of 40 mg for glipizide and 20 mg for glyburide. Furthermore, addition of a second oral agent or insulin may be indicated for patients no longer responding to doses of glyburide or glipizide ≥10 mg.

Because of its variable renal excretion, long serum half-life, long duration of hypoglycemic activity, and adverse effects, chlorpropamide has fallen into disuse and should be avoided in the elderly or in patients with renal impairment (see Question 70).

Glipizide is an intermediate-acting second-generation agent with a half-life of 2 to 4 hours, but a duration of action of 12 to 24 hours. Many patients, especially those receiving small to intermediate daily doses of this drug (<20 mg), require only one dose per day. Glipizide is extensively metabolized by the liver to inactive products that are eliminated primarily by the kidney.[146,147] Food delays the rate of absorption of glipizide but not its bioavailability.[151] Administration 30 minutes before meals has been suggested, but this has been disputed by one study, which noted no acute effects of this drug in patients who had been taking it chronically with meals.[151] A sustained-release formulation of glipizide, Glucotrol XL, also is available.

Glyburide (or glibenclamide) is a longer-acting second-generation agent similar to glipizide. The half-life is approximately 1.5 to 4 hours following single-dose studies and up to 13.7 hours when chronically administered.[152] Nevertheless, as with glipizide, the duration of action can last for up to 24 hours in many patients, allowing single daily dosing with small to intermediate doses (<15 mg). Glyburide is metabolized completely by the liver to active metabolites, half of which are excreted in the urine and the remainder eliminated via the biliary tract.[153] Unlike glipizide, food does not delay the rate or extent of absorption of glyburide, and the time of ingestion relative to meals appears to be unimportant in patients on chronic therapy.[154] The micronized glyburide tablets (3 mg) are not bioequivalent to those of the conventionally formulated 5-mg tablets. Thus, patients switched from the conventional form to the micronized product must be retitrated.

Glimepiride is a long-acting second-generation sulfonylurea. The half-life of glimepiride is 9 hours, and its duration of action is 24 hours; thus, it can be given once daily. The absorption of glimepiride is unaffected by food, and its peak effect on plasma glucose concentrations is observed 2 to 3 hours after each dose. Glimepiride is completely metabolized by the liver, and its principal metabolite has 30% of the activity of the parent drug. Metabolites are excreted in feces and urine. Glimepiride is the first sulfonylurea approved by the FDA for concurrent use with insulin; however, any sulfonylurea can be used in combination therapy.[155–157]

Adverse Effects
The primary side effects of the sulfonylureas are hypoglycemia (particularly for those that are long-acting) and

weight gain (see Questions 69 and 74). Other adverse effects attributed to the sulfonylureas generally are so infrequent and mild that <2% of patients discontinue these agents because of them. In general, the type, incidence, and severity of reported side effects are similar for all the sulfonylureas. An important exception is chlorpropamide, which has several unique adverse effects (see following discussion). Adverse reactions to the sulfonylureas include GI symptoms (nausea, fullness, bloating that can be relieved if taken with meals), rare blood dyscrasias, allergic dermatologic reactions, hepatotoxicity, and hypothyroidism[158] (also see Questions 67 through 70 and 76).

A *disulfiram (Antabuse-like) reaction* occurs when patients take certain oral sulfonylurea drugs and drink ethanol. It is most frequently associated with chlorpropamide, occurring in approximately one-third of all patients receiving it. The flushing reaction seen so often with chlorpropamide is rare with other sulfonylureas.[158]

SYNDROME OF INAPPROPRIATE ANTIDIURETIC HORMONE SECRETION

Chlorpropamide, and to a much lesser extent, tolbutamide, may enhance the release of antidiuretic hormone (ADH) centrally, enhance the effect of ADH on the kidney, and override the inhibitory effects of waterloading on ADH release, resulting in syndrome of inappropriate antidiuretic hormone secretion.[146] This antidiuretic effect has been used clinically to treat diabetes insipidus.[159] In the UKPDS, the increase in blood pressure seen in patients on chlorpropamide was likely due to water retention.[22] In contrast to chlorpropamide and tolbutamide, glipizide, glyburide, tolazamide, and acetohexamide have a mild diuretic effect.

Contraindications and Precautions

Contraindications to the use of sulfonylureas include the following:

1. Type 1 diabetes
2. Pregnancy or breast-feeding, because these agents (except glyburide) can cross the placental barrier and can be excreted into breast milk
3. Documented hypersensitivity to sulfonylureas
4. Severe hepatic or renal dysfunction
5. Severe, acute intercurrent illness (e.g., infection, MI), surgery, or other stress that can unduly affect blood glucose control

Drug Interactions

Drug interactions with sulfonylureas have a pharmacodynamic or pharmacokinetic basis. Pharmacodynamic interactions occur with drugs that alter glucose tolerance intrinsically through their effects on insulin secretion, glucose production, and peripheral glucose utilization. These are discussed later in this chapter in sections addressing drug-induced hypoglycemia and hyperglycemia. Pharmacokinetic interactions occur when drugs alter the absorption, metabolism, elimination, or protein binding of the sulfonylureas.

Most of the reported pharmacokinetic drug interactions with the sulfonylureas involve chlorpropamide and tolbutamide, because these are the oldest agents and were once the most commonly prescribed and studied. However, because most of the clinically significant interactions occur with drugs that alter liver metabolism or urinary excretion, possible interactions with all of the sulfonylureas must be anticipated even though the outcomes may be quite different. For example, a drug that inhibits the hepatic metabolism of tolbutamide can increase its hypoglycemic activity; conversely, the same drug actually may diminish the hypoglycemic activity of acetohexamide by inhibiting formation of its active metabolite. This hypothesis has not been tested.

The second-generation sulfonylureas (glipizide, glyburide, and glimepiride) are dosed in milligram rather than gram quantities and thus seem to be less likely to interact with other drugs on a pharmacokinetic basis. Glipizide and glyburide also differ from the first-generation agents in that they are highly bound to albumin at nonionic rather than ionic sites.[146,147] On this basis, these agents are unlikely to interact with other highly protein-bound drugs, such as phenylbutazone, salicylates, or certain sulfonamide antibiotics that have been reported to enhance the effects of the first-generation sulfonylureas. However, these highly protein-bound drugs appear to interact with the sulfonylureas by altering their hepatic metabolism as well. Therefore, glipizide and glyburide should be used cautiously with drugs reported to interact with first-generation sulfonylureas. The many potential pharmacokinetic interactions reported with the sulfonylureas have been reviewed extensively, and only the more important or clinically significant interactions are included in Table 50-31.

Efficacy

Like metformin, the sulfonylureas decrease the A_{1C} by 1.5% to 1.7% and the FPG by 50% to 70%. In patients who have developed secondary failure to maximum doses of metformin, the addition of sulfonylureas will produce similar improvements in the A_{1C} and FPG, unless the disease has progressed and the pancreas is no longer able to respond appropriately.[47]

Dosage and Clinical Use

As monotherapy, the sulfonylureas are very effective and relatively safe; they are also relatively inexpensive and easy to titrate. Nevertheless, some clinicians favor use of metformin for initial therapy since it does not cause weight gain or hypoglycemia. The choice of agents is discussed more fully in the case studies that follow this section. The doses of the sulfonylureas are displayed in Table 50-29. As a general rule, one should begin with low doses and titrate upward every 1 to 2 weeks until the desired goal is achieved. Exceeding maximum doses is not likely to produce improvement, but may put the patient at risk for adverse effects (see Questions 55 through 60 and 74).

Thiazolidinediones

Rosiglitazone (Avandia, GlaxoSmithKline) and pioglitazone (Actos, Takeda Pharmaceuticals) were approved in 1999 and are the two available TZDs in the United States. Troglitazone (Rezulin) was FDA approved in 1997, but withdrawn from the market in March 2000 because of hepatoxicity.

Mechanism of Action

The TZDs are often referred to as *insulin sensitizers,* but the full nature of their effects remains incompletely understood. Clinically, these drugs decrease insulin resistance in muscle and liver, which enhances glucose utilization and decreases hepatic glucose output. The amelioration of insulin resistance reduces insulin, glucose, and free fatty acid levels, and has positive effects on lipid levels. (See Efficacy below.) Because TZDs enhance the effect of insulin, endogenous insulin must be present for them to exert their beneficial effects on glycemia. The precise molecular actions of these agents remain to be clarified; however, it is known that they bind to and activate a nuclear receptor (peroxisome proliferator–activated receptor–γ [PPAR-γ]), which is expressed in many insulin-sensitive tissues, primarily adipose tissue, but also skeletal muscle and liver tissue.[160] PPAR-γ regulates transcription of genes that influence glucose and lipid metabolism. For example PPAR-γ stimulation increases the transcription of GLUT-4, a glucose transporter that stimulates glucose uptake. It is thought that reduced expression of GLUT-4 contributes to the development of insulin resistance.

Furthermore, TZDs promote apoptosis of large adipocytes and increase the number of small adipose cells, which are more sensitive to insulin action. Insulin-dependent glucose uptake in adipose tissue is increased and lower rates of lipolysis, reduce free fatty acid levels, which further reduces insulin resistance in muscle and liver tissue.[160] The TZDs lower expression of tumor necrosis factor (TNF)-α, a cytokine produced by adipose tissue which may contribute to insulin resistance and fatty acid release.[160–162] Other effects of TZDs that may prove to be beneficial in patients with metabolic syndrome and type 2 diabetes include reduction of inflammatory mediators (e.g., plasminogen activator inhibitor type 1, C-reactive protein), inhibition of vascular smooth muscle cell proliferation, improved endothelial function, β-cell restoration, and lowered blood pressure.[161,163,164]

Pharmacokinetics

Rosiglitazone is completely absorbed, with peak plasma concentrations reached in approximately 1 hour; food does not alter its absorption. The plasma elimination half-life is 3 to 4 hours.[165] Rosiglitazone is extensively metabolized in the liver, mainly by CYP 2C8, and circulating metabolites are considerably less potent than the parent drug. Rosiglitazone is excreted two-thirds in urine and one-third in feces as conjugated metabolites.

Pioglitazone has a bioavailability of 83%, with peak plasma concentrations reached in approximately 1.5 hours; food does not alter its absorption.[161,166,167] Pioglitazone has a serum half-life of 3 to 7 hours and 16 to 24 hours for its metabolites. It is metabolized, mainly in the liver by CYP 3A4 and CYP 2C8, into two active metabolites. Approximately 15% to 30% of the dose is recovered in the urine as metabolites, with the remainder excreted into the bile either as unchanged drug or as metabolites.

Because the action of the TZDs relies on gene transcription and protein production, the onset and duration of action are unrelated to the plasma half-life. The onset of their effect occurs in 1 to 2 weeks, but maximum effects may not be seen for 8 to 12 weeks.[161,168]

The TZDs are primarily excreted via bile in the feces with small amounts excreted as metabolites in the urine; therefore, no dose adjustments are required in patients with renal failure. All of the TZDs are extensively bound to serum albumin.

Adverse Effects

HEPATOTOXICITY

Troglitazone, the first TZD to be approved by the FDA, was associated with idiosyncratic hepatoxocity leading to hepatic failure and death in some patients, which became apparent during postmarketing surveillance. During clinical trials, approximately 1.9% of troglitazone-treated patients experienced asymptomatic, reversible elevations in liver transaminase (alanine transaminase [ALT]) levels that were greater than three times the normal values (versus 0.6% of placebo-treated patients). In contrast, elevations in liver transaminase levels observed during pre-approval clinical trials for pioglitazone and rosiglitazone (0.26% and 0.2%, respectively) were similar to placebo (0.25% and 0.2%).[165,167] Two case reports of hepatotoxicity have been linked to rosiglitazone use; however, liver injury may have been caused by other factors.[169,170] A recent analysis of 13 clinical trials of rosiglitazone show no evidence of hepatotoxicity.[171] Monitoring of liver function tests (LFTs) is recommended at baseline, every 2 months for the first year of therapy, and periodically thereafter for pioglitazone and rosiglitazone (see Contraindications and Precautions).

HEMATOLOGIC EFFECTS

TZD therapy may result in small decreases in hemoglobin and hematocrit. Transient decreases in neutrophil counts occurred infrequently within the first 4 to 8 weeks of TZD therapy. Some have attributed these observations to a dilutional effect (this is discussed further in the following sections).[172]

VASCULAR AND CARDIOVASCULAR EFFECTS

Increases in plasma volume (6% to 7%) and peripheral edema (5% to 7%), possibly caused by an increased endothelial cell permeability, have been reported with the TZDs.[161,173] The incidence of peripheral edema is greatly increased when TZDs are used in combination with insulin (~15%).[167]

Although no CHF has been observed in the clinical trials, patients with New York Heart Association (NYHA) class III and class IV cardiac status have not been studied. Therefore, these agents should not be used in such patients, and caution is suggested in patients with milder CHF.[165,167] A small number of patients taking rosiglitazone and pioglitazone have experienced mild to moderate edema during clinical trials and in the postmarketing period. Thus, these agents should be used cautiously in patients with pre-existing edema. Six cases of TZD-associated CHF, marked peripheral edema and pulmonary edema were reported by Kermani and Garg,[174] who suggested that these agents be used cautiously in patients with chronic renal insufficiency and impaired cardiac function (e.g., left ventricular dysfunction).

WEIGHT GAIN

Dose-related weight gain has been seen with rosiglitazone and pioglitazone. The cause of weight gain is likely due to fluid retention and fat accumulation. The weight gain appears to be associated with an increase in peripheral adipose tissue along with a reduction in visceral adiposity.[174]

Contraindications and Precautions

• *Type 1 diabetes:* Because insulin is required for their action, TZDs should not be used in people with type 1 diabetes.

- *Pre-existing hepatic disease:* Pioglitazone and rosiglitazone should not be used in patients whose ALT is >2.5 times normal. TZDs should be discontinued if the ALT is >3 times normal, if serum bilirubin levels begin to rise or if the patient complains of any symptoms that could be attributed to hepatitis (e.g., fatigue, nausea, vomiting, abdominal pain, and dark urine).
- *Severe CHF* (NYHA classes III and IV): See previous discussion.
- *Premenopausal anovulatory women:* TZDs may cause resumption of ovulation and menstruation in women with polycystic ovarian syndrome, placing such patients at risk for an unwanted pregnancy. For the same reason, its use to stimulate ovulation in women with polycystic ovarian syndrome is under investigation.[168]
- *History of hypersensitivity to TZDs.*
- *Drugs metabolized by CYP 3A4:* See Drug Interactions in the next section for further details.

Drug Interactions

Pioglitazone induces the hepatic microsomal enzyme CYP 3A4, and this is the underlying mechanism for its established interactions with estrogens and terfenadine. Therefore, one should be alert for potential decreased effectiveness of other drugs metabolized by this enzyme, such as cyclosporine, tacrolimus, and 3-hydroxy-3-methyl-glutaryl-coenzyme A (HMG-CoA) reductase inhibitors. Rosiglitazone does not appear to inhibit any of the major CYP enzymes.

GLYBURIDE

Coadministration of glyburide with a TZD does not alter the pharmacokinetics of either drug, but may increase the patient's risk for hypoglycemia.

ORAL CONTRACEPTIVES

Troglitazone reduced plasma concentrations of oral contraceptives containing ethinyl estradiol and norethindrone by 30%. Although the pharmacokinetics of oral contraceptives when combined with pioglitazone have not been evaluated, the manufacturer cautions against their concomitant use. Because loss of contraceptive efficacy is possible, additional or alternative methods should be considered.[167] Although there have been no studies of interactions with estrogen replacement products used by postmenopausal women, one should be alert for recurring symptoms of estrogen deficiency. Rosiglitazone does not affect the pharmacokinetics of oral contraceptives, suggesting that rosiglitazone may not interact with other drugs metabolized by the CYP 3A4 isoenzyme.

Efficacy

The effects of TZDs on A_{1C} and FPG are intermediate between that of acarbose and the sulfonylureas or metformin.[47,163] When combined with other antidiabetic agents in a poorly controlled type 2 patient, one can expect to see an augmented effect on the A_{1C} (0.9% to 1.3% decrease with a sulfonylurea, 0.8% to 1.2% decrease with metformin, and 0.6% to 1.0% decrease with insulin)[165,167] (also see Question 58). When added to the therapy of a type 2 patient taking insulin, rosiglitazone and pioglitazone can enhance glycemic control while decreasing insulin requirements (see Questions 59 and 63).

Other potential benefits of the TZDs are their favorable, but variable, effects on lipids: pioglitazone decreases triglyceride levels by ~9% and both pioglitzaone and rosiglitazone increase HDL levels by ~15% to 20%.[161] Rosiglitazone has no effect on triglyceride levels, although free fatty acid levels are decreased by up to 22%.[161] Pioglitazone has little or no effect on LDL cholesterol levels, but rosiglitazone is associated with a 10% to 14% increase in these values.[165,167] This increase in LDL cholesterol may be due to a shift from smaller, dense particles to larger, more buoyant ones, which are less susceptible to oxidation.[161,163,175] Therapy with all of the TZDs has been associated with weight gain and, when used in combination with sulfonylureas or insulin, weight gain can be substantial (1.8 to 5.4 kg or 4 to 12 pounds).[165,167] Another interesting observation is that approximately 25% of individuals treated with TZDs are unresponsive. Although the reason is unknown, these individuals are less likely to be obese and have lower insulin and C-peptide levels, emphasizing the fact that the TZDs work only in individuals with endogenous insulin.[172]

Dosage and Clinical Use

A greater glucose-lowering effect has been observed when rosiglitazone is given as two divided doses rather than as a single daily dose. For monotherapy, a typical dose is 4 mg once daily or 2 mg twice daily, regardless of meals. If the response is inadequate, the dosage can be increased to 8 mg once daily or 4 mg twice daily. For combination therapy with a sulfonylurea, metformin, or insulin, rosiglitazone can be initiated at 4 mg once daily. Only doses of 8 mg have been studied in combination with metformin.[161,165]

For monotherapy with pioglitazone, the dose is 15 mg or 30 mg once daily with or without food, which can be increased to a maximum of 45 mg daily. For combination therapy with a sulfonylurea, metformin, or insulin, pioglitazone can be initiated at 15 or 30 mg once daily. No placebo-controlled clinical studies of >30 mg pioglitazone have been conducted to date with combination therapy.[167]

Although rosiglitazone and pioglitazone can be used as initial therapy for newly diagnosed type 2 diabetes, cost often limits their use to patients with contraindications to sulfonylureas or metformin or to those who cannot tolerate side effects associated with the other agents. All of the TZDs can be used in combination with other agents in uncontrolled type 2 diabetes patients (see Questions 50, 58, and 63).

TREATMENT OF PATIENTS WITH TYPE 2 DIABETES
Clinical Presentation

45. **L.H. is a 45-year-old moderately centrally obese (height, 5′5″; weight, 160 lb; BMI 26.6 kg/m²) Mexican-American woman, who was referred to the diabetes clinic when her gynecologist, who had been treating her for recurrent monilial infections, noted glucosuria on routine urinalysis. Subsequently, on two separate occasions she was found to have an FPG of 150 mg/dL and 167 mg/dL. L.H. denies any symptoms of polyphagia or polyuria, although lately she has been more thirsty than usual. She does complain of lethargy and often takes afternoon naps.**

L.H.'s other medical problems include mild hypertension, which is well controlled on lisinopril 20 mg/day, and recurrent monilial infections, which are treated with fluconazole. She has

given birth to four children (birth weights, 7, 8.5, 10, and 11 lb, respectively) and was told during her last pregnancy that she had "borderline diabetes." She currently works as a loan officer in a local bank and spends her weekends "catching up on her sleep" and reading. L.H. has been smoking one pack of cigarettes/day for 20 years and drinks an occasional glass of wine. Her family history is significant for a sister, aunt, and grandmother with type 2 diabetes; all have "weight problems." L.H.'s mother is alive and well at age 77; her father died of a heart attack at age 47.

Laboratory assessment reveals an FPG of 147 mg/dL (normal, 70 to 100); fasting plasma triglycerides of 400 mg/dL; and an A_{1C} of 9.2% (normal, 4% to 6%). All other values (including the complete blood count [CBC], electrolytes, liver function tests, and renal function tests) are within normal limits. L.H. is given the diagnosis of type 2 diabetes. What features in L.H.'s history and physical examination are consistent with this diagnosis?

[SI units: plasma glucose, 8.3, 9.3, and 8.1 mmol/L; plasma triglycerides, 6.77 mmol/L; A_{1C}, 0.09 (normal, 0.04 to 0.07)]

The features of L.H.'s history that are consistent with type 2 diabetes include an FPG concentration of $\geq$126 mg/dL on more than one occasion, an elevated A_{1C}, high BMI with central obesity, age greater than 40, family history of diabetes, and Mexican American descent. L.H. also has delivered large babies, which suggests that she may have had undiagnosed gestational diabetes, a condition that places women at high risk for subsequently developing type 2 diabetes. Diagnosis on routine examination and mild signs and symptoms of hyperglycemia (including increased thirst and lethargy), recurrent monilial infections, hypertriglyceridemia, and indications of cardiovascular disease (mild hypertension) also are typical in patients with type 2 diabetes (see Type 2 Diabetes and Table 50-1).

Treatment Goals

46. What should the goals of therapy be for L.H. and other patients with type 2 diabetes? Which biochemical indices should be monitored?

The beginning of this chapter discussed general goals of therapy for all people with diabetes, which include eliminating acute symptoms of hyperglycemia, avoiding hypoglycemia, reducing cardiovascular risk factors, and preventing or slowing the progression of both microvascular and macrovascular diabetic complications. The ADA recommends that otherwise healthy patients with type 2 diabetes strive to achieve the same biochemical goals as those recommended for people with type 1 diabetes[73,93] (see Tables 50-5 and 50-11).

The UKPDS was the longest and largest study of patients with type 2 diabetes. It conclusively demonstrated that improved blood glucose control reduces the risk of developing retinopathy, nephropathy, and potentially, neuropathy.[22] A 25% overall reduction in microvascular complication rate was observed in those patients receiving intensive therapy versus conventional therapy. An additional finding of the UKPDS was that aggressive control of BP also significantly reduced strokes, diabetes-related deaths, heart failure, microvascular complications, and vision loss.[176,177]

When determining treatment goals for L.H. and others with type 2 diabetes, the same individual characteristics should be considered as for type 1 diabetes, such as the patient's capacity to understand and carry out the treatment regimen, the patient's risk for severe hypoglycemia, and other patient-specific factors that may increase the risk or decrease the benefit of intensive treatment (e.g., advanced age, ESRD, advanced cardiovascular or cerebrovascular disease, or other coexisting diseases that may shorten life expectancy). Emphasis should be placed on assessment of all cardiovascular risk factors, including hypertension, tobacco use, dyslipidemia, and family history.

Macrovascular disease is the primary cause of death in this population, and its underlying pathogenesis may or may not be related to hyperglycemia per se. This is a subject of great complexity and controversy. Although the prevalence of cardiovascular morbidity and mortality correlates with A_{1C} levels in observational and epidemiologic studies, no prospective, randomized, controlled trials have established a relationship between macrovascular disease and the degree of glycemic control.[20,134] Whether intensive insulin therapy is appropriate for people with type 2 diabetes also has been questioned. Some have worried that hyperinsulinemia associated with intensive insulin therapy or the sulfonylureas actually could accelerate atherosclerosis or increase the risk of cardiovascular events. However, the UKPDS showed no increase in cardiovascular events or mortality in patients assigned to sulfonylurea or insulin therapy, despite their fasting plasma insulin levels being higher than those of the conventionally treated patients.[22] There is also concern that the counter-regulatory hormones that are released in response to hypoglycemia also could endanger those with existing cardiovascular disease. These views are summarized and analyzed by Colwell[178,179] and others,[180] who suggest taking a more aggressive stance toward glycemic control than that which has been previously practiced as well as attending to the reduction of all risk factors for cardiovascular disease (e.g., hypertension, dyslipidemia, platelet hyper-reactivity, microalbuminuria).

Most agree that glycemic goals for patients with type 2 diabetes must be individualized. For example, advanced age or significant cerebrovascular or coronary artery disease should be considered relative contraindications to intensive control in type 2 diabetes because of the serious consequences of hypoglycemia; however, many treatment options available today are associated with a very low risk of hypoglycemia.

Because L.H. is relatively young and has no symptoms of microvascular disease or neuropathy, every effort should be made to normalize her glucose concentrations to avoid these morbid events. Furthermore, a lipid panel should be ordered and steps taken to achieve normal LDL cholesterol, HDL cholesterol, and triglyceride levels. Often, triglyceride levels improve as blood glucose concentrations decline and the metabolic response to insulin improves. (Management of dyslipidemia is addressed more fully later in this chapter.)

Biochemical indices that should be followed to monitor L.H.'s response to therapy include fasting, postprandial and preprandial blood glucose concentrations, A_{1C} values, fasting triglyceride levels, and LDL and HDL cholesterol concentrations. Initial metabolic goals for L.H. should be an A_{1C} value of <7%, an FPG <130 mg/dL, a postprandial glucose concentration of <180 mg/dL, and triglyceride levels of <150 mg/dL.

Lifestyle Interventions

47. How should L.H. be managed initially?

Initial therapy of type 2 diabetes is aimed at lifestyle changes that will minimize insulin resistance and risk for cardiovascular disease. In L.H.'s case and in the case of other overweight (BMI 25.0 to 29.9) or obese (BMI 30.0 and above), type 2 individuals, this includes a lower-calorie, low-fat and cholesterol diet; regular exercise; smoking cessation (see Chapter 85, Tobacco Use and Dependence) and aggressive management of dyslipidemia and hypertension. Because obesity is associated with increased tissue resistance to endogenous insulin, L.H. should be strongly encouraged to decrease her caloric intake and lose weight. When signs and symptoms are mild, diet and exercise alone can correct glucose intolerance. SMBG monitoring should be encouraged and education that addresses the serious nature of diabetes mellitus and its long-term consequences also should begin. This is discussed in the previous sections, Medical Nutrition Therapy and Exercise, under Treatment (also see Table 50-16). Table 50-32 summarizes assessment and pharmacotherapy counseling points for patients with type 2 diabetes.

Self-Monitored Blood Glucose in Type 2 Diabetes

48. L.H. is interested in learning how to perform blood glucose testing. What are the advantages and disadvantages of SMBG tests? When and how often should L.H. be instructed to test her blood glucose concentrations?

Daily performance of SMBG is important for patients such as L.H. to assess the efficacy of therapy and guide adjustments in nutrition, exercise, and medications. Performing SMBG also helps to monitor for and prevent hypoglycemia. Disadvantages include cost of testing, inadequate understanding by both health care providers and patients regarding the benefits and proper use of SMBG results, patient psychological and physical discomfort associated with obtaining a blood sample, and the inconvenience of testing. However, with the current advances in meter technology and proper patient education, most of these potential barriers can be overcome.

The ADA recommends SMBG for all patients taking insulin, but its stance with regard to type 2 diabetics treated with diet or diet plus oral agents is less clear.[73] This is because several studies evaluating the effect of SMBG in people with type 2 diabetes have shown no effect on glycemic control.[181] Nevertheless, the ADA does suggest that the "optimal frequency and timing of SMBG for patients with type 2 diabetes is not known but should be sufficient to facilitate reaching glucose goals."[73] We often recommend SMBG for motivated type 2 patients who are learning to adjust their carbohydrate intake and want to measure how well medications and lifestyle changes are working to improve their glucose control. Initially, we may suggest testing four times daily before meals and at bedtime for 1 week so that the patient can observe his or her glucose profiles. Later, once the desired

A_{1C} has been achieved, we recommend a minimum of testing glucose concentrations twice daily, but at various times to evaluate fasting glucose concentrations, 2-hour postmeal concentrations, and preprandial concentrations. A study of type 2 patients treated with diet with or without oral agents, but not insulin, observed that 2-hour postlunch values (<150 mg/dL) and predinner values (<125 mg/dL) most closely correlated with A_{1C} values of <7%.[182] As emphasized by the ADA, intensive patient education regarding testing technique and interpretation are vital to the cost-effective use of this monitoring tool. The patient must be able to assess his or her glucose profile and institute lifestyle changes that can have a favorable effect.

Treatment: A Stepped-Care Approach

49. L.H. was quite motivated to improve her glucose control because her grandmother "lost a leg" to diabetes and her aunt is undergoing dialysis because "her kidneys have failed." She met with a dietitian who suggested an 1,800-calorie diet and 45 minute walks three times weekly. After 3 months, L.H. had lost 6 pounds. Although her FPG fell to 130 mg/dL (normal, 70 to 100), >50% of her postprandial blood glucose levels were often >180 mg/dL (normal, <140). Her A_{1C} is 8.0% (normal, 4% to 6%), and fasting triglyceride levels are now 260 mg/dL (normal, <150). Therapy is to be initiated with an oral antidiabetic medication. What factors should be considered when deciding on an agent?

Selecting an oral agent to treat type 2 diabetes has become more complex as new agents with unique mechanisms of action have been introduced into the market. As with all therapeutic decisions, clinicians must blend their knowledge of the drug (e.g., its efficacy, safety, dosing methods, and cost) with the unique characteristics of the patient (e.g., level of glycemic control, organ function, other concurrent diseases and medications, ability to adhere to complex medication regimens, health care coverage) when making a choice of drug products. We, like others, suggest a stepwise management approach to avoid unnecessarily complex therapy that may confuse the patient, increase drug costs, and complicate the clinician's ability to assess each medication's contribution to the overall therapeutic outcome[183-185] (Fig. 50-9).

After instituting appropriate lifestyle changes, we recommend monotherapy followed by combination therapy with two oral agents if therapeutic goals are not met. If patients fail therapy with two oral agents, one could move to triple oral therapy or treat with a single oral agent plus insulin. To avoid injections, many patients and caregivers opt for triple combination therapy (using oral agents with different mechanisms of action), but this is has not been studied extensively, with published studies consisting of small treatment groups.[186,187-189] One study compared triple oral therapy with insulin 70/30 Mix plus metformin in patients with type 2 diabetes poorly controlled on two oral agents.[190] Although both treatments were about equally effective in lowering A_{1C} and FPG values (1.77%; 55 mg/dL and 1.96%; 65 mg/dL, respectively), 10.2% of patients in the triple-therapy group were switched to the insulin plus metformin therapy because of inadequate response; however, these patients had higher A_{1C}

Table 50-32 Assessment and Counseling Points: Type 2 Diabetes

For All Patients

- Educate about symptoms of hyperglycemia, including frequent urination, excessive thirst, unexplained weight loss, fatigue, and recurrent infections, which signal inadequate control.
- Educate about symptoms of hypoglycemia, including hunger, anxiety, rapid heart rate, sweatiness, morning headaches, and restless sleep. Skipped meals can predispose to hypoglycemia. May occur when antidiabetic agents are used in combination.
- Encourage patients to follow blood glucose concentrations according to SMBG (self-monitoring of blood glucose). Review goals. Help patients interpret levels in context of diet, exercise, and drug therapy. Periodically review patients' technique for appropriate meter use.
- Reinforce principles of diet, exercise, and smoking cessation.
- Update medication profile. Include nonprescription medications, nutritional supplements, and alternative medicines. Review for drug–drug and drug–disease interactions.
- Review and reinforce ADA Standards of Care, including the following:
  - A_{1c} quarterly for patients poorly controlled; semiannually for stabilized patients. Review target values.
  - Annual lipid panel
  - Annual evaluation for microalbuminuria
  - Annual retinal examination by an ophthalmologist (Note: less frequent exams, every 2–3 years, may be considered in patients with a normal eye exam.)
  - Annual foot examinations (Note: Patients with history of previous lower extremity event should have monthly foot examinations.)
  - Blood pressure measurements every visit.

Sulfonylureas

- First Generation: Tolbutamide (Orinase), Chlorpropamide (Diabinese), Tolazamide (Tolinase), Acetohexamide (Dymelor)
- Second Generation: Glipizide (Glucotrol), Glyburide (Micronase, Glynase, DiaBeta), Glimepiride (Amaryl)
- This drug stimulates the release of insulin from the pancreas. The pancreas may not release insulin as rapidly as it should after one has eaten. The amount of insulin it releases may not be sufficient to lower blood glucose concentrations.
- Meals should not be skipped.
- Symptoms of hypoglycemia must be watched for.
- Weight gain is possible.

Repaglinide (Prandin), Nateglinide (Starlix)

- This drug stimulates the release of insulin from the pancreas. The pancreas may not release insulin as rapidly as it should after one has eaten. The amount of insulin it releases may not be sufficient to lower blood glucose concentrations.
- Dose should be taken up to 30 minutes before meals.
- Drug should not be taken if meal has been skipped.
- Symptoms of hypoglycemia must be watched for.
- Weight gain is possible.

Metformin (Glucophage)

- This drug decreases the production of glucose by the liver. The liver is probably producing more glucose than normal and this is contributing to high blood glucose levels.
- Initially, gastrointestinal discomfort or diarrhea may be experienced. This usually lessens with time and can be minimized if taken with food and if doses are gradually increased.

- Any change in general health should be brought to the attention of the clinician in charge of the patient's diabetes management. This applies particularly to problems affecting the heart, lungs, kidneys, or liver. Unusual symptoms to be reported to the clinician include the following: severe fatigue, unexpected stomach discomfort, dizziness, shortness of breath, unexpected fluid retention, or sudden development of a slow or irregular heartbeat.
- The drug may have to be discontinued temporarily if a special x-ray examination or radiologic procedure is needed. Under these circumstances, the radiologist or general physician must be reminded that metformin is being taken.

Thiazolidinediones (Rosiglitazone [Avandia], Pioglitazone [Actos])

- These drugs improve the ability of the muscle to respond to insulin. Insulin allows the muscle to take in glucose from meals and store it for future use.
- Drug should be taken once daily or twice daily with or without food.
- Rarely, rosiglitazone has been associated with liver problems. Blood tests should be checked for liver function every 2 months as directed by the clinician. Any unusual symptoms of fatigue, gastrointestinal distress, or increased abdominal girth should be reported to the clinician.
- Menstrual periods may resume and pregnancy may occur. (For patients with polycystic ovarian syndrome only.)
- A birth control pill with higher amounts of estrogen may be required. A physician should be consulted. (For patients taking low-dose oral contraceptives.)
- Any reappearance of menopausal symptoms, such as hot flushes, should be reported to the doctor. (For patients taking estrogen replacement therapy.)

α-Glucosidase Inhibitors (Acarbose [Precose], Miglitol [Glyset])

- These drugs slow the absorption of sugars and starches from the intestines. They do so by blocking the breakdown of these foods.
- Each dose should be taken with the first bite of each meal.
- When these drugs are begun, gas and soft stools or diarrhea may be experienced. This lessens with time and can be minimized by increasing the dose gradually as prescribed.
- Acarbose or miglitol by themselves do not cause hypoglycemia, but low blood glucose levels can occur if they are used in combination with other antidiabetic agents. Commercially available glucose tablets should be used to treat low blood sugar reactions because other carbohydrate sources, such as those containing sucrose or fructose, may not be absorbed quickly if acarbose or miglitol is being taken.

Insulin

- This drug is used to supplement the insulin secreted by the pancreas.
- Rapid- and short-acting insulins are designed to help cells utilize glucose from meals about to be eaten. Insulin lispro or insulin aspart should be given 15 minutes before a meal. Eating should not be delayed. Regular insulin generally is given 30 minutes before the meal.
- NPH (or Lente) insulin can last for 12–24 hours depending on the dose being used. This insulin is primarily used to maintain low levels of insulin between meals. This insulin decreases glucose production by the liver.
- Insulin glargine is used as a basal insulin. It cannot be mixed with other insulins in the same syringe.

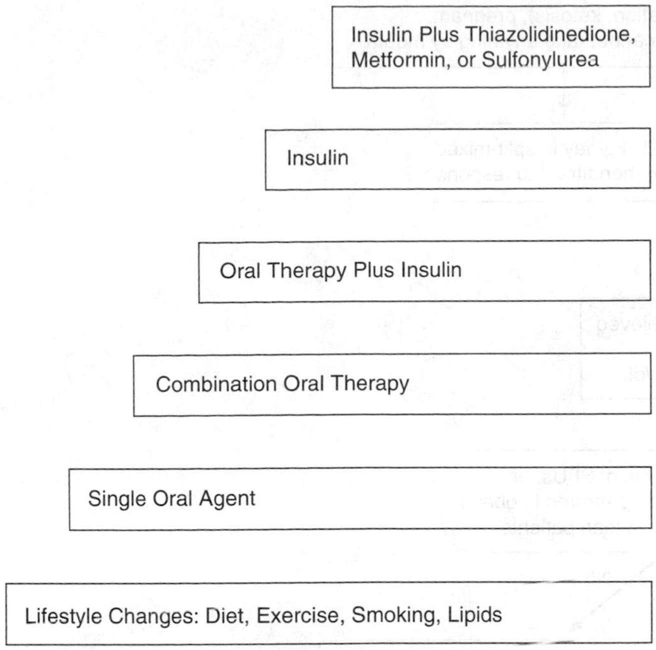

FIGURE 50-9 A stepped-care approach to treating type 2 diabetes mellitus. See Question 49 for discussion.

levels (ave: 10.6%) at baseline. The cost of triple therapy (drug cost plus LFT monitoring for the TZDs) was higher.

In summary, if two oral agents in combination do not work, one could try a different combination or triple oral therapy. However, it is likely that a bedtime dose of insulin in combination with the oral agents (e.g., a sulfonylurea, metformin, or TZD) will be needed. The combined use of insulin plus oral therapy was once considered a bridge to insulin monotherapy. However, a substudy of the UKPDS demonstrated that the early addition of insulin to patients with inadequate responses to oral sulfonylureas (FPG >108) improved glycemic control over insulin therapy alone over an average follow-up period of 6 years. Furthermore, the group on combined therapy suffered 50% more episodes of major hypoglycemia; weight gain was comparable.[191] If this fails, the patient is treated with insulin monotherapy. For patients who are gaining weight because they require large insulin doses, TZDs or metformin can be added to achieve control with lower doses in insulin.

Type 2 diabetes is a progressive condition, which is highly likely to require drug therapy. In the UKPDS, only 16% and 19% of the subjects achieved an FPG <108 and A_{1C} <7%, respectively, after 3 years of dietary therapy.[192] By 9 years, only 9% were able to maintain their glycemic goals using diet therapy alone.[192] We have developed a simple algorithm to aid the clinician in selecting drug therapy for a patient with type 2 diabetes who has not adequately responded to lifestyle interventions (Fig. 50-10). Although the UKPDS demonstrated that the sulfonylureas, metformin, and insulin reduce glucose with equal effectiveness (TZDs were not studied),[22,193] important factors come into play when selecting a drug for a patient. The algorithm is based on the patient's underlying pathogenesis, degree of current glycemic control, and pre-existing conditions that could predispose the patient to adverse effects of a drug. The pathogenic features are deduced from the patient's body weight. If the patient is obese, it is presumed there is an element of insulin resistance and increased hepatic glucose output. If the patient is lean, he or she is presumed to be insulin deficient.

In the case of insulin resistance in an obese patient, for example, metformin, which decreases hepatic glucose output and insulin resistance (indirectly) without causing weight gain might be preferred if there are no contraindications to its use. One must always keep in mind that the primary goal is to normalize glucose concentrations, because hyperglycemia has been most closely correlated to the development of long-term complications. Thus, agents that may cause weight gain (e.g., sulfonylureas) are still very effective.

Another feature that determines choice of agent is the degree of current control. If, for example, the patient's A_{1C} value is 2% to 3% higher than the target level, it will not make sense to use an agent that only modestly lowers this level. Finally, it is important to evaluate the patient's renal, liver, cardiovascular, and GI function before prescribing a specific agent, because these conditions could predispose the patient to adverse effects. Table 50-29 compares and contrasts the efficacy, advantages, and disadvantages of antidiabetic agents used to treat type 2 diabetic patients and can be used in conjunction with the basic algorithm to select drugs for a specific patient. Table 50-32 summarizes treatment of type 2 diabetes under special circumstances.

Several new combination products that combine two oral agents into one medication are available (see Table 50-29). Although these products are approved as first-line therapy (thus skipping the monotherapy step), we recommend that they be reserved for use in patients whose medication regimens must be simplified to enhance adherence.

Clinical Use of Oral Agents
Selecting an Oral Agent

50. Which of the oral agents would you recommend for L.H. at this time?

L.H. is a typical overweight type 2 patient with early evidence of cardiovascular disease (mild hypertension), but with no evidence of microvascular complications. Her liver, renal, and GI functions are normal. Finally, she has achieved improved control with diet and exercise as evidenced by an improved A_{1C}, FPG, and triglyceride concentration. However, her postprandial glucose and A_{1C} values continue to exceed target levels (<180 mg/dL and <7%, respectively).

Patients like L.H. with moderate to severe type 2 diabetes have varying degrees of β-cell dysfunction and tissue resistance to insulin. In these individuals, pulsatile insulin secretion and first-phase insulin release are absent, and the pancreas is "blind" or unresponsive to high glucose concentrations (glucotoxicity). Because target tissues are less responsive to insulin, hepatic glucose output typically is increased and patients may require higher concentrations of insulin to achieve the same degree of peripheral glucose utilization observed in people without diabetes mellitus. At this stage, all classes of oral antidiabetic agents and insulin are likely to work equally well, although insulin causes more weight gain and hypoglycemia than the oral agents.[22,193] Therefore, the mode of therapy selected depends on patient and prescriber preference.

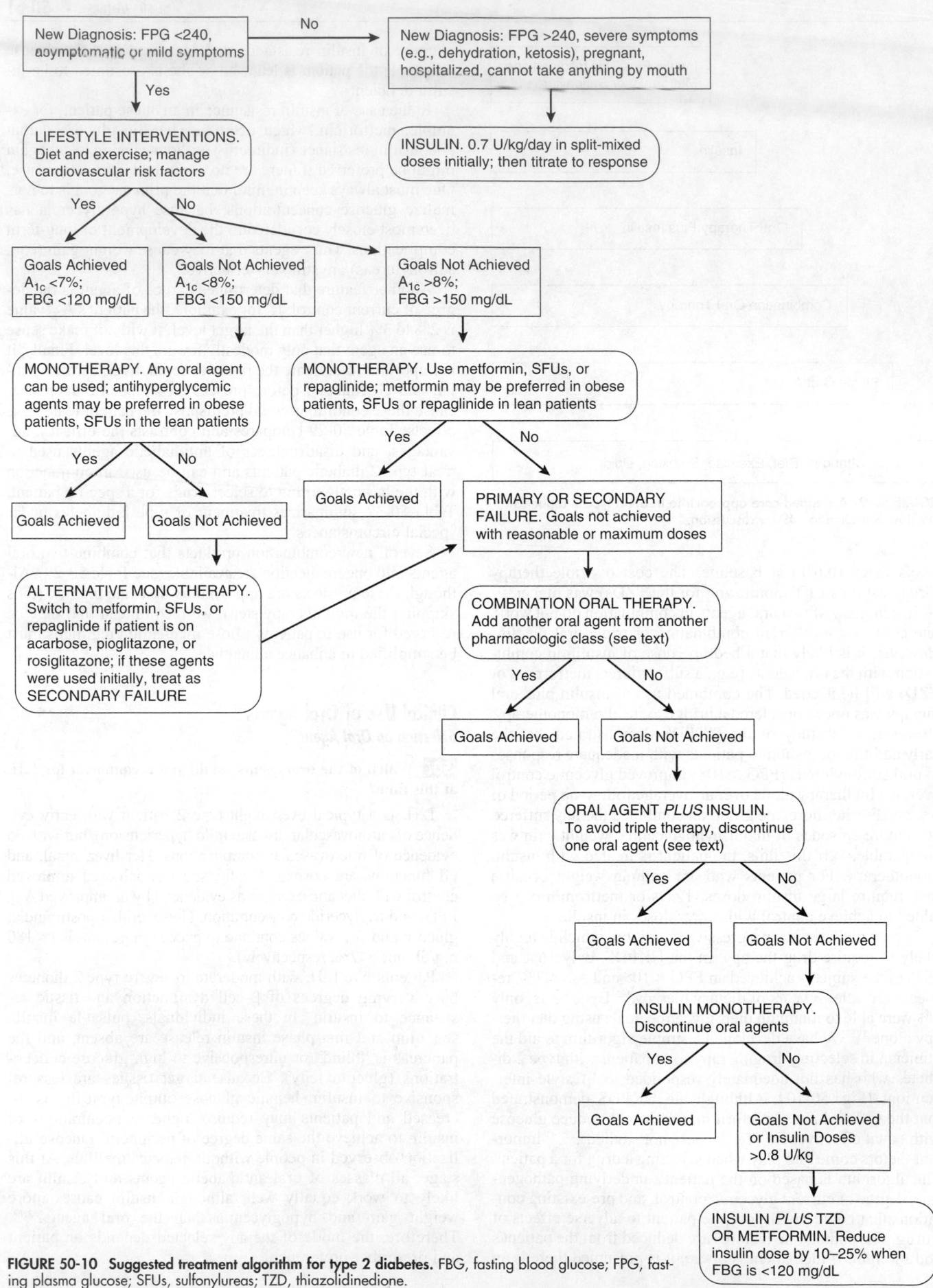

FIGURE 50-10 Suggested treatment algorithm for type 2 diabetes. FBG, fasting blood glucose; FPG, fasting plasma glucose; SFUs, sulfonylureas; TZD, thiazolidinedione.

Because L.H. is overweight, the algorithm suggests the use of agents that lower the blood glucose without causing weight gain. Thus, acarbose and metformin are favored. A TZD may also be considered even though it can cause weight gain, since the pattern of weight gain induced by this agent (reduction in visceral adipose tissue) is metabolically beneficial.

Often, *acarbose* is eliminated from consideration because slow titration is required to minimize GI effects; anecdotally, however, people of Mexican-American origin, such as L.H., seem less susceptible to flatulence and diarrhea. Also, because acarbose has less dramatic effects on the FPG (20 to 30 mg/dL decrease) and A_{1C} (0.5% to 1.0% decrease) than the other agents, biochemical goals are less likely to be achieved in patients whose A_{1C} is ≥8.5%. However, acarbose can be considered in L.H. because her poor control is characterized by postprandial hyperglycemia as well as an FPG and A_{1C} that are nearing the goals established for her.

Metformin is favored as a first-choice agent for obese, type 2 diabetic patients by many endocrinologists because it is as effective as the sulfonylureas but does not cause hypoglycemia or weight gain (see Table 50-30). However, multiple daily dosing is required initially, and its dose also must be titrated to minimize GI effects. After the dose is established, it is possible to use a long-acting product that can be dosed once daily. Renal function tests should be evaluated before the drug is initiated. L.H. does not have any contraindications (renal, liver, hepatic dysfunction, binge alcohol use) to the use of metformin that could predispose her to its most significant side effect, lactic acidosis (see Question 66).

Rosiglitazone or *pioglitazone* also can be used as monotherapy and, like metformin, neither is likely to cause hypoglycemia, but weight gain is possible. Their effects on FPG and A_{1C} are intermediate between those of acarbose and metformin or the sulfonylureas, so that it is likely that the goals established for L.H. could be achieved with either agent as monotherapy. Side effects are rare, and both can be given as a single daily dose, which is appealing for patients on multiple-drug therapy. LFTs must be evaluated at baseline and bimonthly thereafter for the first year of therapy for rosiglitazone or pioglitazone, which can be difficult for patients to adhere to and adds to the cost of therapy. The TZDs remain the most expensive of the antidiabetic agents.[190]

Finally, one should not forget that until the newer agents became available, *sulfonylureas* were used quite successfully to treat obese patients with type 2 diabetes. These agents are relatively trouble free with regard to side effects (weight gain and occasional hypoglycemia), and many can be dosed once daily. They are very effective and many are now available in generic form, making them quite affordable when cost is a primary consideration (see Table 50-30).

Based on this discussion, we favor the use of metformin (see Question 52) or acarbose in L.H.

Acarbose

51. If acarbose is used, how should it be prescribed? How should L.H. be counseled and monitored?

Acarbose should be taken with each meal to delay and slow the absorption of complex carbohydrates. However, because many patients experience bothersome flatulence, bloating, diarrhea, and abdominal pain initially, one should begin with 25 mg three times daily and then titrate upward by doubling the dose every 4 to 8 weeks. This titration minimizes GI effects, which dissipate with time. Alternatively, a dose of 25 mg once a day (with an evening meal over the weekend when unexpected effects are least likely to interfere with a work schedule) can be initiated. As one can see, it could take approximately 3 to 4 months to titrate L.H. to the maximum dose. Thus, she should be advanced as quickly as possible based on her tolerance to the GI effects, because some individuals tolerate the drug quite well.

L.H. should be instructed to take acarbose with the first bite of each meal, because its mechanism of action is to delay the absorption of carbohydrates. The nature of acarbose's GI side effects should be explained in the context of teaching her how to gradually increase her dose. She should continue to perform SMBG as described in Question 48 because her final dose will be determined by her glycemic control as well as the highest dose she is able to tolerate. She should also be advised to avoid products such as Beano, which are designed to minimize flatulence, because they contain carbohydrate-splitting enzymes and may decrease the effectiveness of the drug.

Metformin

52. N.H. is a 46-year-old, obese (BMI 28 kg/m²) man with a history of hypertension, peripheral vascular disease, recurrent deep venous thrombosis, and hyperlipidemia. He presents with complaints of fatigue and nocturia. N.H. has smoked 2 packs of cigarettes/day for 15 years and has a strong family history of CHD. A random plasma glucose >200 mg/dL on two occasions (248 and 207 mg/dL) an FPG of 150 mg/dL (normal, <126 mg/dL) and an A_{1C} of 9.2% (normal, 4% to 6%) an FPG of 150 mg/dL confirms the diagnosis of type 2 diabetes. Current medications include enalapril and lovastatin and tests of liver and renal function are within normal limits. A 1-month trial of diet and exercise has little effect on N.H.'s glucose concentrations. Why would metformin or a TZD be the initial drugs of choice for N.H.?

We would not select sulfonylureas or insulin as initial drugs of choice for N.H. because they do not exert a favorable effect on plasma lipids and generally are associated with weight gain. We acknowledge that some sulfonylureas remain the least expensive oral antidiabetic agents, and this may be an important factor in the initial selection of therapy for some patients. Although sulfonylureas or insulin decrease blood glucose concentrations in patients like N.H., they do so by increasing insulin concentrations. Patients such as N.H. are likely to have β-cell dysfunction, as evidenced by poor first-phase insulin release; however, in the early stages of type 2 diabetes, they also are likely to exhibit high insulin concentrations, which suggests resistance of peripheral tissues to insulin action. This can be overcome by increasing insulin levels, but hyperinsulinemia promotes fuel storage and often is accompanied by hunger, occasional hypoglycemia, and weight gain. Interestingly, research suggests that the sulfonylureas may close ATP-sensitive potassium channels in cardiac tissue, similar to their action at the β-cell. In the heart, this effect could limit circulation to an ischemic area.[128,178] The availability of antihyperglycemic agents such as acarbose, metformin, and TZDs provides alternatives for patients like N.H., who possess the characteristics of the insulin resistance or metabolic syndrome (see Pathogenesis).

In light of N.H.'s A_{1C} value (9.2%), acarbose as monotherapy would not be sufficient to attain near-normal plasma glucose concentrations. Rosiglitazone or pioglitazone improve peripheral target tissue responses to insulin and lipid profiles. However, they are considerably more expensive than metformin, which is available generically, and their efficacy as monotherapy is somewhat less. However, N.H. is taking several other medications and may prefer the convenience of a single-daily-dose therapy.

Metformin appears to lower blood glucose concentrations by decreasing hepatic glucose production. It also has beneficial effects on plasma lipid concentrations and promotes weight loss or at least prevents weight gain. N.H. has no risk factors for lactic acidosis (e.g., renal, liver, or cardiorespiratory disease) that would be contraindications for the use of metformin. Because N.H. exhibits the typical features of insulin resistance syndrome and has no contraindications for its use, metformin would be the initial drug of choice.

TITRATING METFORMIN DOSES

53. N.H. is started on metformin 500 mg BID with food and instructed to increase his dosage to 500 mg TID after 1 week. Two days later, he phones the clinic complaining of nausea and diarrhea. He admits to taking his doses on an empty stomach. How should N.H.'s symptoms be addressed?

GI disturbances such as diarrhea, bloating, anorexia, abdominal discomfort, nausea, and metallic taste often dissipate with time and can be minimized by initiating metformin in a single, 500- or 850-mg dose at breakfast or with the patient's largest meal of the day. The dosage should be *slowly* increased (e.g., 500 mg/day every 2 weeks) until the appropriate clinical effect is achieved or the patient is taking the maximum dose (1,000 mg twice daily or 850 mg three times a day). Therefore, N.H.'s metformin dose should be reduced to 500 mg daily with a meal, and he should be titrated more slowly over a period of several weeks to 500 mg three times a day or higher as tolerated. Metformin is typically dosed two to three times daily (the long-acting formulation is dosed once daily with dinner).

MONITORING METFORMIN THERAPY

54. How should metformin therapy be monitored in N.H.?

As is standard with other agents, N.H. should be encouraged to perform SMBG and have an A_{1C} test performed quarterly until he achieves consistent values of <7%. Additional evidence of metformin's therapeutic benefits may include an improved lipid profile and some weight loss. Initially, it is important to follow GI problems and, although lactic acidosis is unlikely, N.H. should be warned to bring to the attention of his physician any sudden symptoms of shortness of breath, weakness, and malaise. A baseline SrCr, LFTs, and CBC should be obtained for N.H. and repeated yearly.

Sulfonylureas

55. After 3 weeks, N.H. returns to the clinic complaining vigorously about unrelenting "stomach pain" and diarrhea. He continues to take metformin 500 mg BID with food and has even tried antacids, which fail to relieve the pain. His blood glucose records suggest that the metformin is beginning to work well (fasting, 130 to 160 mg/dL; pre-lunch and pre-dinner, 150 to 180 mg/dL), but N.H. wants to switch to another agent—preferably

something that can be taken once daily. Rosiglitazone is suggested, but N.H.'s health insurance does not include drug benefits and it would be prohibitively expensive. Everyone agrees that the sulfonylureas should be tried. Which agents could be used? How should they be dosed?

Patients who are most likely to respond favorably to oral sulfonylureas include those who are older than 40 years of age, have been diagnosed within the last 5 years, are within 110% to 160% of IBW, and have an FPG of <200 mg/dL. If patients have been treated with insulin, those whose requirements are <40 U/day (indicating endogenous pancreatic reserve) are most likely to respond.[145,146] N.H. fulfills these criteria and does not have any contraindications to sulfonylurea use (see Oral Antidiabetic Agents). Approximately two-thirds to three-fourths of the patients who meet all of the previously specified criteria will achieve satisfactory control initially. The remainder (16% to 36%) fail to respond to a 1-month trial of maximum therapeutic doses and are considered primary failures.[145,146]

There is little evidence that any particular oral sulfonylurea is more effective than another in properly selected patients with type 2 diabetes. However, as previously discussed, there are differences in duration of action and side effects that should be considered in the selection of these agents. (See Tables 50-29 and 50-30 and the section on Oral Antidiabetic Agents.)

We recommend against the routine use of chlorpropamide and acetohexamide because of their side effects and accumulation in people with renal dysfunction. Tolbutamide is a safe option in patients with renal dysfunction since it is converted to inactive metabolites; a disadvantage is that is must be dosed two to three times daily. Of the first-generation agents, tolazamide has several advantages. It has an intermediate activity so that control usually can be achieved with one dose and, in some cases, two doses per day. However, its duration of action is not so prolonged that accumulation is likely to result in severe hypoglycemic episodes. However, one should be cautious of its use in patients with Cl_{Cr} of <30 mL/minute, because its metabolites are mildly active.[194]

Glimepiride, glipizide, and glyburide are second-generation agents. Glipizide is metabolized to inactive products and has an intermediate duration of action. As with tolazamide, many patients can be controlled on single daily doses, but twice-daily doses are recommended for patients who require >15 mg. Because glyburide has a longer duration of action, it is associated more frequently with severe, prolonged hypoglycemia than is glipizide. For this reason, it should be used cautiously in frail, elderly individuals or in those who, for any reason, are predisposed to hypoglycemia (see Questions 69 and 74). Glimepiride can be dosed once daily and may be associated with a slightly lower incidence of hypoglycemia than glyburide.

For N.H., tolazamide, glimepiride, glipizide, or glyburide would be the agents of choice because they are reasonably safe, can be dosed once daily, and are relatively inexpensive. He should be initiated on low dosages (e.g., 100 to 250 g tolazamide; 1 to 2 mg glimepiride; 5 mg glipizide; or 1.25 to 2.5 mg glyburide) once daily. Every 1 to 2 weeks, the dosage can be increased until the therapeutic goals are achieved or maximum doses of these agents have been reached (see Table

50-29). The manufacturers of tolazamide, glipizide, and glyburide recommend twice-daily dosing of these agents once a specified dose has been exceeded; whether this actually is necessary has not been documented. Many clinicians recommend taking these agents 30 minutes before meals so that the onset of action more closely matches food absorption[146]; this may be less important in patients taking these agents chronically, particularly for the intermediate- and longer-acting agents.[154,195] If GI intolerance occurs, these agents should be taken with food.

Clinical Note: N.H. was successfully treated with diet, exercise, and relatively low doses of glyburide (5 mg daily). Within 4 months, his A_{1C} dropped to 7.3% and his SMBG results ranged from 120 to 160 mg/dL. By decreasing dietary fat and exercising more regularly, he was able to lose 10 pounds. It is likely that the modest weight loss as well as his improved glucose concentrations reduced insulin resistance, thereby improving tissue responsiveness to his endogenous insulin. N.H. enrolled in a smoking cessation program, but has been unable to quit smoking completely (see Chapter 85, Tobacco Use and Dependence).

Secondary Failure to Oral Agents
Pathogenesis
SECONDARY FAILURE TO ORAL SULFONYLUREAS

56. **Q.R. is a 68-year-old, 5'1", 140-lb (BMI 26.4 kg/m²) Japanese woman with an 8-year history of type 2 diabetes that has been treated with diet, exercise, and a variety of "pills." According to clinic records, she was moderately controlled (FPG, 130 to 160 mg/dL; A_{1C}, 7.5% to 8.5%) for 5 years with a succession of oral sulfonylureas—most recently, glipizide. Recent chart notes indicate that Q.R.'s chief complaints have included loss of appetite and fatigue. She has lost 15 lb over the past year, and her A_{1C} has been increasing at each visit (from 8.5% 1 year ago to 11% currently). The dose of glipizide also has been increased from 10 mg daily 1 year ago to 20 mg twice daily for the past 6 months. Other medical problems include hypertension managed with hydrochlorothiazide 25 mg daily and mild peripheral neuropathy managed with naproxen 500 mg twice daily.**

At this clinic visit Q.R., who is well known to you, seems particularly listless and flat in her affect. Her blood glucose records, which are typically meticulous, are incomplete. Blood glucose values consistently exceed 200 mg/dL and range from 202 to 340 mg/dL. While taking her history, you discover that her husband passed away last year and that one of her adult children has recently been diagnosed with a terminal illness. What factors may be contributing to Q.R.'s poor glucose control?

Several factors may be contributing to Q.R.'s deteriorating blood glucose control and apparent lack of responsiveness to the oral sulfonylureas over the past year (as evidenced by her elevated blood glucose and A_{1C}, listlessness, and weight loss). Secondary failure to the sulfonylurea therapy is fairly common and occurs at a rate of approximately 5% to 10% per year in patients who initially are well controlled on these agents, as was Q.R.[145,146] Secondary failure is characterized by progressively poor glucose control that occurs after a 1-month to a several-year period of good response. The cause of secondary failure is unknown, but it may be related to progressive pancreatic failure; poor compliance with diet, exercise, or medications; and exogenous diabetogenic factors such as obesity, illness, or drugs. (See Table 50-36. Drug-induced hyperglycemia is addressed later in this chapter.)

The UKPDS confirmed that secondary failure represents a natural progression of type 2 diabetes. The investigators found secondary failure occurred at the same rate regardless of the initial treatment selected: glyburide, chlorpropamide, metformin, or ultralente insulin. In all the monotherapy treatment groups, patients required additional therapies over the study duration.[192] At 3 years, <55% of patients randomized to single pharmacologic therapy could maintain an A_{1C} <7% and by 9 years this dropped to ~25% of patients. This is likely due to the natural progression of type 2 diabetes in which β-cell function declines with increased duration of disease. Also, when the blood glucose becomes very elevated, (FPG >250 to 300 mg/dL; preprandial glucose concentrations ≥200 mg/dL), the pancreas's ability to secrete insulin is diminished and postreceptor (postbinding) defects in insulin activity become more important. Postreceptor defects are characterized by a reduced responsiveness of tissues to any level of insulin. If glucose concentrations can be normalized, postreceptor defects and pancreatic responsiveness to glucose can be improved. This may be related to the hypothesis that high glucose concentrations in and of themselves may be toxic to the β-cells and peripheral tissues (glucotoxicity).[196]

Q.R.'s deteriorating control on maximum doses of glipizide after 5 years of reasonable response fits the definition of secondary failure. However, the stress and depression arising out of her life situation have no doubt contributed to her poor control. The latter may have led to a change in her usual compliance with diet, exercise, and medications and should resolve with time and appropriate management. Although hyperglycemia has been attributed to hydrochlorothiazide, the dose prescribed for Q.R. has few adverse metabolic effects.

Managing Secondary Failure

57. **How should Q.R. be managed? Should she be switched from oral sulfonylureas to metformin?**

Q.R. is exhibiting symptoms of depression (e.g., listlessness and flat affect). Her depression likely started after her husband's death. Every effort must be made to address Q.R.'s depression because it is unlikely that she will be able to effectively implement more aggressive treatment of her diabetes until her situation is improved. Resources that may be used include her family, a therapist, and a social worker.

Treatment of secondary sulfonylurea failure includes identifying and correcting any diabetogenic factors and altering her drug therapy. When secondary failure to any oral agent occurs, one should always *add* another agent rather than switch to another. This is supported by a study that evaluated the effect of metformin alone in a population of patients who had failed oral sulfonylureas and the effect of metformin plus the sulfonylureas. Substitution of metformin for glyburide did not produce any significant change in glycemic control, but the addition of metformin to glyburide therapy substantially improved glucose concentrations.[197] Although many combinations of oral antidiabetic agents can be used, it makes more sense to maintain the current agent and add another rather than to change to two new medications. Options for Q.R. include the following:

- Adding metformin to the sulfonylurea
- Adding acarbose to the sulfonylurea
- Adding rosiglitazone or pioglitazone to the sulfonylurea

One also could introduce insulin therapy at this time, but it is an unreasonably complicated intervention under the circumstances. These options include the following:

- Adding an evening dose of insulin to the sulfonylurea
- Switching to insulin monotherapy

In summary, patients such as Q.R. who are unresponsive to maximum doses of sulfonylureas are unlikely to respond to monotherapy with metformin. Furthermore, metformin alone is unlikely to be effective in patients whose glycemic control has deteriorated so severely that pancreatic reserve is lost and resistance to insulin action is high (e.g., FPG >240 mg/dL). Thus, Q.R. should not be switched to metformin in lieu of glipizide; rather, combination therapy should be instituted.

Combination Oral Antidiabetic Therapy

58. As anticipated, Q.R. refuses to consider insulin therapy at this time. Which combination of oral agents is preferred?

When agents from different antidiabetic classes are combined, their effects are essentially additive. At dosages approved for use in the United States, acarbose has been used successfully in combination with both sulfonylureas and metformin,[122,125] lowering the A_{1C} by approximately 1%. However, an agent that can be titrated more quickly than acarbose and one that is more likely to have a profound effect on blood glucose concentrations should be used in Q.R.

Pioglitazone and rosiglitazone are approved for use in combination with sulfonylureas. When pioglitazone was added to sulfonylurea therapy, an improvement in both the FPG and A_{1C} was observed: 39 to 58 mg/dL and 0.9 to 1.3%, respectively, depending on the dose of pioglitazone used (15 or 30 mg daily). Pioglitazone 30 mg added to metformin monotherapy reduced the FPG by a mean of 38 mg/dL and the A_{1C} by 0.8%.[167] When rosiglitazone (2 mg BID) was added to a sulfonylurea, the A_{1C} and FPG were reduced 1.0% and 44 mg/dL, respectively, compared with the sulfonylurea alone. Rosiglitazone 4 mg daily added to metformin reduced A_{1C} and FPG by 1.0% and 40 mg/dL, respectively, compared with metformin alone.[165,198]

Metformin also has been used successfully in combination with the sulfonylureas when primary or secondary failure occurs. The combination lowers fasting glucose concentrations approximately 80 mg/dL and A_{1C} values by 2% when metformin is given in full dose (2,500 mg/day in three divided doses).[197]

In the later stages of the UKPDS, 537 obese and nonobese patients who failed sulfonylurea monotherapy were randomly assigned to continue sulfonylurea monotherapy or to have metformin added. An intention-to-treat analysis of this substudy showed that those patients assigned to combined metformin–sulfonylurea therapy had a 96% increase in diabetes-related deaths P <.039) and a 60% increase in all-cause

deaths ($P < .041$) compared with those patients continued on sulfonylurea monotherapy.[193] However, owing to the lack of a placebo control and the inability to use masking, these detrimental effects have been questioned. The ADA currently does not recommend any change in the current guidelines for the use of combination metformin–sulfonylurea therapy until a new, appropriately designed, randomized placebo-controlled trial can delineate some specific mechanism of adverse interaction between the two drugs.

Although Q.R. has recently lost weight, she remains overweight. Thus, glipizide should be maintained and metformin added. However, because studies have suggested that maximum metabolic effects are observed at glipizide doses of 10 mg daily,[150] Q.R.'s dose can be decreased to this dose while metformin doses are slowly increased as described in Question 53.

Combination Oral Antidiabetic and Insulin Therapy

59. Q.R. tolerated slow titration of metformin to a maximum dose of 850 mg three times daily, while maintaining a dose of glipizide 10 mg daily. This improved her FPG and A_{1C} modestly for approximately 6 months (FPG, 170 to 200 mg/dL; A_{1C}, 7.6%). Acarbose was added to her therapy, but she was discomforted by its GI side effects. However, she remained symptomatic and finally agreed to consider insulin therapy. Why would it be reasonable to use insulin in combination with an oral antidiabetic agent for Q.R.?

When a combination of oral agents fails, it is tempting to add yet another agent, but as discussed previously, the use of three oral agents in combination has not been extensively studied. Instead, we recommend reversion to a single agent in combination with a single dose of an intermediate- or long-acting insulin, or insulin monotherapy if fasting glucose concentrations suggest severe insulin deficiency (e.g., FPG >200 mg/dL).

The combined use of insulin with a variety of oral agents has been evaluated, but the studies differ in their design. In some studies, single doses of an intermediate- or long-acting insulin are added to a single oral antidiabetic agent in patients who have developed secondary failure. In others, oral agents are instituted in poorly controlled patients taking high doses of insulin (e.g., >70 U/day). The primary outcomes that have been evaluated include measures of glycemic control (e.g., A_{1C}, FPG) and the extent to which insulin doses have been decreased. Thus, the combined use of insulin and oral agents can be considered at both Step 4 and Step 6 in the proposed algorithm (see Fig. 50-9). This therapeutic approach also might be used as an intermediate step when evaluating whether patients on relatively low total-daily doses of insulin could be managed with oral antidiabetic therapy.[199]

60. How should insulin be combined with oral agents, and is this combination more effective than insulin alone?

Insulin Plus Sulfonylureas

Several investigators have explored the beneficial effects of sulfonylureas used in combination with insulin, and the results of their work have been subjected to critical reviews and meta-analyses.[200–203] Placebo-controlled and uncontrolled studies indicate that in some patients with type 2 diabetes who have failed monotherapy with a sulfonylurea or insulin, the combination of a sulfonylurea plus insulin may improve FPG concentrations and A_{1C} values modestly (40 to 50 mg/dL and 1 to 2%, respectively). This may or may not be accompanied by a modest decrease in insulin requirement (approximately 25%). Because many patients treated in these studies were not optimally controlled on insulin before combination therapy was instituted, it is impossible to tell whether combination therapy was more effective than intensive insulin regimens. Other potential drawbacks of combination therapy include increased costs, complex therapeutic regimens, and a higher risk for hypoglycemic reactions.

A popular regimen is bedtime insulin, daytime sulfonylurea (BIDS therapy), although one short-term study (3 months) suggests that morning insulin and insulin alone work equally well.[204] Investigators compared the effectiveness of the following insulin regimens: (1) oral hypoglycemic therapy plus NPH given in the evening, (2) oral hypoglycemic therapy plus NPH given in the morning, (3) NPH and regular insulin (2:1 ratio) given twice daily, (4) regular insulin before meals and NPH at bedtime, and (5) continued oral hypoglycemic drug therapy (the control group). All treatment regimens were equally effective in achieving glycemic control; however, the addition of NPH at bedtime was associated with less weight gain and hyperinsulinemia. A meta-analysis of similar trials confirmed that combination therapy with insulin and sulfonylurea may be more appropriate than insulin monotherapy in type 2 diabetes patients who have developed primary or secondary failure.[201] Insulin glargine can also been used with a sulfonylurea.[205,206]

Insulin Plus Metformin

The combined use of insulin and metformin has not been studied extensively, but when metformin is added to insulin therapy or vice versa, measures of glycemic control improve and insulin requirements decrease. In a double-blind, placebo-controlled study of 50 obese patients with type 2 diabetes poorly controlled with insulin monotherapy, metformin (850 mg twice daily) or placebo was added to insulin for 6 months. Metformin significantly improved all glycemic indices (A_{1C} decreased 1.8%; mean plasma glucose decreased 74 mg/dL versus no change in the placebo group) and decreased mean insulin requirements by 25%. Cholesterol and triglyceride levels also were improved, especially in the 14 subjects who responded particularly well to metformin. Those subjects who did not respond as well (13) had higher mean plasma glucose concentrations (>180 mg/dL).[207]

Although metformin is an antihyperglycemic agent, one must be alert for increased susceptibility to hypoglycemia when it is used in combination with insulin. Studies seem to confirm potential advantages of metformin over sulfonylureas when used in combination with insulin. These include its favorable effects on the lipid profile, insulin concentrations, and lack of weight gain. The risk for hypoglycemia may also be lower with metformin.[193,208,209]

Insulin Plus TZD

In a randomized, placebo-controlled study, 566 type 2 diabetic patients treated with insulin (mean insulin dose, 60.5 U/day) were randomized to treatment with 15 or 30 mg pioglitazone or placebo in addition to their insulin. Treatment with pioglitazone plus insulin reduced A_{1C} values by 1.0% for the 15-mg dose and 1.3% for the 30-mg dose compared with baseline; FPG values decreased 34.5 mg/dL and 48.0 mg/dL for the 15 mg and 30 mg dose respectively.[210]

Insulin Plus an α-Glucosidase Inhibitor

The addition of acarbose or miglitol to insulin therapy has modest effects on measures of glycemia and insulin requirements. In a multicenter, randomized, double-blind, placebo-controlled trial, 219 men and women with type 2 diabetes treated with insulin received 24 weeks of treatment with acarbose or placebo. Patients were initiated on acarbose 50 mg three times daily, and doses were increased at 6-week intervals to 300 mg three times daily. Compared with the placebo group, the A_{1C} decreased by 0.4% and daily insulin requirements decreased by 8.3% in the acarbose group ($P < .0001$).[126] A similar improvement in A_{1C} was observed in another controlled trial in which people with insulin-treated type 2 diabetes received acarbose (150 to 600 mg) for 1 year.[125] A 6-month, double-blind, placebo-controlled trial in 117 subjects with type 2 diabetes treated with insulin demonstrated a 1.3% reduction in A_{1C} values with the addition of miglitol 100 mg three times daily versus placebo.

In Q.R.'s case, it makes the most sense to discontinue the sulfonylurea and to add a single dose of intermediate-acting insulin to metformin therapy (see subsequent discussion). Advantages attributed to adding insulin to an oral agent as the "next step" after failure, as opposed to using insulin alone, include the following[206,211,212]:

- Lower insulin dosages can be used, and this minimizes weight gain and hypoglycemia.
- Simpler, single dose insulin regimens are possible (versus monotherapy with insulin).
- Lowering the fasting glucose concentrations improves glucose control throughout the day because glucose excursions related to meals are layered over lower values. Furthermore, lower glucose values improve β-cell responsiveness to glucose and enhance tissue responsiveness to insulin action.
- Use of the insulin sensitizers may enhance the effect of exogenous insulin while minimizing weight gain and hyperinsulinemia. They also may have beneficial effects on lipid profiles and other cardiovascular defects.

Therefore, glipizide should be discontinued and metformin maintained; Q.R. should be started on 5 to 10 units of NPH, Lente, ultralente, or insulin glargine at bedtime. This dose is based on empiric use of insulin in a variety of studies (0.1 to 0.35 U/kg)[213] and a conservative estimate for basal insulin of approximately 0.5 U/hour (Q.R. weighs 140 pounds, or 64 kg). The dose also takes into account the possibility that Q.R. is secreting some basal insulin of her own and will have some residual stimulation of insulin secretion by glipizide. The NPH dose should be adjusted upward weekly in 5-unit increments (depending on individual response to insulin) until a desirable FPG concentration is obtained (preferably <126 mg/dL). If there is no improvement in glycemic control after 3 months, Q.R. should be converted to multiple daily insulin injections (see Question 61).

An alternative for Q.R. is to discontinue all oral agents and begin insulin monotherapy using methods similar to those described for type 1 patients. This option also is rational based on the observation that patients like Q.R. are likely to require insulin therapy because of progressive β-cell failure. Furthermore, insulin monotherapy may be less expensive and easier to assess than combination oral + insulin therapy. Nevertheless, many clinicians use single doses of insulin in combination with oral agents as a bridge to eventual insulin monotherapy, especially for those patients unwilling to adhere to multiple daily insulin injections.

Insulin Monotherapy in Patients With Type 2 Diabetes
Insulin Regimens

61. Q.R.'s NPH insulin dose was eventually titrated to 25 units at bedtime. In combination with metformin 850 mg three times daily, her fasting glucose levels fell to the 120s and 130s on most occasions; her A_{1C} dropped to 7.5%. However, after 1 year, she began to note a gradual rise in glucose concentrations throughout the day. This resulted in a further increase in her bedtime NPH to 40 units (0.62 U/kg). Currently, her morning glucose concentrations are 140 to 160 mg/dL, and glucose concentrations measured before or after meals range between 170 and 200 mg/dL. A recent A_{1C} value was 8.8%. For the past 6 months or so, Q.R. has noted increasing fatigue, bouts of blurred vision, and recurrence of her monilial infections. How should she be managed now?

The next step in managing Q.R.'s diabetes is to institute insulin monotherapy. Because people with type 2 diabetes retain some pancreatic function, it often is possible to achieve an acceptable level of control with once- or twice-daily doses of intermediate- or long-acting insulin in combination with rapid to short-acting insulins. Unfortunately, large doses of insulin (0.7 to 1.0 U/kg per day) often are needed because these patients are resistant to its action. Thus, weight gain and the potential for hypoglycemia accompany glycemic control. Furthermore, it may be difficult to achieve acceptable glycemic control with insulin in a "real-world" situation. Studies of patients with type 2 diabetes who were cared for within a health maintenance organization suggest that patients managed with insulin use more medical resources than do patients treated with oral agents—at least within the 2 years of study. A_{1C} values declined by a mean of 0.9% at 1 year, but only 40% achieved an A_{1C} <8%.[214] Whether insulin therapy will translate into long-term cost savings in the care of people with type 2 diabetes by delaying the onset and progression of complications remains an unanswered question.[215]

Typically, type 2 diabetes patients are initiated on twice-daily doses of split-mixed insulin. Like type 1 patients, people with severe type 2 disease may require regular insulin, insulin lispro or insulin aspart before meals to minimize postprandial excursions. Insulin lispro has been shown to decrease postprandial glucose concentrations to a greater extent than regular insulin (30% lower at 1 hour and 53% lower at 2 hours) and was associated with a lower rate of hypoglycemia, particularly between midnight and 6 AM (36%). However, A_{1C} levels were not significantly different after 6 months.[216] A similar response with insulin aspart would be expected. One should be aware that when high doses of insulin are used, patients have difficulty losing weight. This is secondary to the anabolic effects of insulin and the hunger that can occur in association with hypoglycemia. There also is concern about the potential atherogenic consequences of chronically elevated

insulin levels, but this has not been established.[217,218] In patients like Q.R., lowering glucose concentrations is the first priority.

As described in Question 6, which address initiation of insulin therapy in type 1 patients, one could begin with a conservative total daily dose of 0.5 U/kg per day as NPH and regular insulin split into two doses (two-thirds in the morning and one-third in the evening). However, Q.R. is already using 0.62 U/kg per day. Therefore, this dose should be split (e.g., 18 units NPH/10 units regular insulin in the morning and 6 units NPH/6 units regular insulin in the evening) and the effects evaluated through more frequent SMBG. Q.R. should be instructed to inject the regular/NPH insulin mixture 30 minutes before breakfast and dinner. If she were to use a premixed insulin with either insulin aspart or lispro, she would need to inject the insulin immediately before eating (within 15 minutes of eating).

Premixed Insulins

62. Q.R. has difficulty mixing her NPH and regular insulins. Even with repeated education, she continues to make dosing errors and her vial of regular insulin is consistently clouded. Her current insulin regimen is as follows: NPH 20 U/regular insulin 10 U in the morning and NPH 6 U/regular insulin 10 U in the evening. What are options for Q.R.?

Several options are available for individuals who have difficulty mixing NPH and short-acting insulins. The first is to prescribe a fixed, mixed dose of NPH and regular insulin. In the United States, fixed mixtures of NPH and regular insulin in a 70:30 ratio and a 50:50 ratio are available (see Table 50-8). In Europe, many other fixed ratios are available. Commercial combinations of the rapid-acting insulins plus an intermediate-acting insulin also are available: Humalog Mix 75/25 (a mixture of insulin lispro plus NPL- neutral protamine lispro) and Novolog Mix 70/30 (a mixture of insulin aspart plus NPH). The biggest advantage of premixed insulins is convenience, especially for patients who administer their injections away from home. Another important advantage is accuracy. As Q.R. illustrates, a large percentage of patients make errors in measuring and mixing insulin, especially the elderly. Ideally, the ratio of NPH and prandial insulin should be individualized for each patient. Practically, however, there are occasional patients in whom the fixed, mixed products must be used to provide both the rapid-acting action of regular, insulin lispro, or aspart insulin and the more prolonged action of NPH. The onset and duration of action of these fixed mixtures is identical with that achieved when the prandial insulin and NPH in the same doses are administered by separate injection. In addition, it is now possible to purchase prefilled syringes containing these fixed mixtures. Currently, Q.R.'s evening dose of insulin exceeds the 70:30 ratio of the premixed insulin as well as the 50:50 ratio. Therefore, if Q.R. is eligible for visiting nursing services or if she lives with someone who can be taught how to mix insulins, several syringes can be predrawn for her and placed in the refrigerator. Insulin stored in this way is stable for up to 3 months.[78]

Insulin Plus Oral Antidiabetic Agents

63. Q.R.'s daughter was instructed on how to predraw insulin syringes for her mother. Over a period of 2 months, Q.R.'s glycemic control has steadily improved with multiple insulin adjustments. Her current dose is 36 units NPH/12 units regular insulin in the morning, and 10 units NPH/18 units regular insulin before dinner. She now performs SMBG; fasting blood glucose concentrations range from 140 to 160 mg/dL; however, preprandial blood glucose concentrations range from 120 to 200 mg/dL. Also, despite earnest attempts to comply with her meal plans, Q.R. has gained 12 lb since beginning insulin monotherapy. What are therapeutic options for Q.R.? Is it rational to add an insulin sensitizing drug to Q.R.'s therapy?

Q.R.'s glycemic control remains unsatisfactory despite a very high total-daily dose of insulin (1.1 U/kg per day). Furthermore, these high insulin doses are contributing to her weight gain. If Q.R. is motivated and able, one option is to "intensify" her insulin therapy. By providing doses more physiologically, it may be possible to decrease her total daily dose. For example, one could consider augmenting Q.R.'s endogenous insulin with small boluses of insulin lispro or aspart with each meal (e.g., 5 to 7 units or 0.1 U/kg) accompanied by lower doses of NPH or Ultralente (e.g., 0.35 U/kg per day) split equally into 12 units in the morning and at bedtime or a single dose of insulin glargine to provide higher basal levels. This is based on a total-daily-insulin requirement of approximately 0.7 U/kg per day, with the basal dose comprising 50% of the total dose. Insulin lispro and aspart doses would be adjusted based on 2-hour postprandial levels (100 to 140 mg/dL), and carbohydrate intake and NPH doses would be based on glucose concentrations measured before dinner (morning NPH) and in the morning (bedtime NPH).[216] Many other insulin regimens could be used, but it often is possible to avoid periods of hyperinsulinemia and minimize insulin dose requirements by use of this strategy.

A second option is to simplify Q.R.'s insulin regimen by continuing her present mixed doses of NPH and regular insulin (see following discussion) and to try improving control with lower doses by adding pioglitazone 15 or 30 mg once daily or rosiglitazone 4 mg once daily. When FPG concentrations reach ≤120 mg/dL, insulin doses should be decreased by 10% to 25%. One should be aware that TZD's onset of action occurs gradually and that maximum effects may not be observed for 6 to 8 weeks. The primary objective of therapy is to achieve metabolic control. Another option would be to reinstitute metformin. Weight loss is a secondary objective and may be impossible to achieve.

Reusing Insulin Syringes

64. A.M., a 45-year-old woman with type 2 diabetes, has been using insulin 20 units NPH for the past 5 years. In the course of her visit, she discloses that she reuses her disposable insulin syringes three to four times before discarding them. Is this practice safe?

Those who work with patients with diabetes know that they are extremely resourceful in cutting their health care costs. A frequently encountered practice is the reuse of disposable syringes. In a survey of 254 adult insulin users, 45% reused their syringes for an average of four days, 16% refrigerated their syringes between uses, and 35% wiped their needles with alcohol. Dullness was the major reason for changing to a new syringe. Borders and colleagues examined approximately 2,800 injection sites, and no infection was noted.[219]

The ADA does not encourage the reuse of syringes, but offers guidelines for patients who choose to do so. They recommend that patients inspect injection sites for redness or swelling and to discard syringes into puncture-resistant, disposable containers if they are dull, bent, or have come in contact with surfaces other than the skin. Some of the smaller 30- and 31-gauge needles seem particularly susceptible to bending and can form hooks. They do not recommend refrigeration or wiping the needle with alcohol between uses, only recapping. Patients who reuse their syringes should inspect their skin for signs of infection.[69]

Cardiovascular Effects

65. J.A. a 47-year-old man was diagnosed with type 2 diabetes when he developed "very high blood sugars in the 300s" while being treated for a foot infection. He states he has had "borderline diabetes" for >10 years. Other medical problems include hypertension and mild CHF, which is currently well controlled on benazepril (10 mg daily), furosemide (40 mg daily), and digoxin (0.25 mg daily). For the past 3 months, he has adhered to a low-fat diet and exercise program and has managed to lose 10 pounds (J.A. is currently 5`9" tall and weighs 190 pounds; BMI 28.1 kg/m²). FPG concentrations measured over the past 2 months were 160 mg/dL and 145 mg/dL. Liver and renal function tests are within normal limits. How will J.A.'s cardiovascular history affect the choice of oral agents? The package insert for all sulfonylureas includes a special warning on increased risk of cardiovascular mortality. What is the basis of this warning? Are sulfonylureas contraindicated in patients such as J.A. with a history of cardiovascular disease?

Because J.A.'s CHF is under treatment, the use of metformin is not recommended. This is because when metformin-associated cases of lactic acidosis were analyzed, virtually all patients had concurrent conditions that predisposed them to this potentially fatal condition. One of these was clinically significant CHF, a condition that could decrease circulation to the periphery, thereby predisposing the patient to anaerobic metabolism.[220,221] Although TZDs should not be used in patients with NYHA class III or IV heart failure, practitioners often avoid their use altogether in patients with heart failure because of a concern for CHF exacerbation (see question 66).

Sulfonylureas are not contraindicated in individuals with a history of cardiovascular disease. However, the FDA required all manufacturers of sulfonylureas to include in their package inserts a special "black box" warning prescribers of an increased risk for cardiovascular mortality. This was based on an unexpected finding of the University Group Diabetes Program (UGDP) study in 1970. This was a cooperative, prospective study to evaluate the effectiveness of antidiabetic therapy in preventing vascular and other late complications of diabetes in mild type 2 diabetic patients. Unexpectedly, twice as many cardiovascular deaths occurred in the tolbutamide-treated group than in the placebo- and insulin-treated groups.[222]

After publication of the UGDP results, a great controversy regarding the study's validity and clinical implications appeared in both the professional and lay press; these are summarized elsewhere.[223] Growing evidence that normalization of glucose concentrations may in fact delay long-term complications, and the failure of others to find higher cardiovascular mortality,[224] has diminished any cardiovascular concerns with sulfonylureas. Of note, the UKPDS found no increase in the rates of MI or diabetes-related deaths when participants treated intensively with a sulfonylurea were compared with those treated conventionally.[22]

Thus, current evidence indicates that the benefits of sulfonylureas far outweigh their risks in type 2 diabetic patients with cardiovascular disease. On this basis, their use is not contraindicated.

Lactic Acidosis

66. M.R. is a 76-year-old, 5'11", 150-lb man (BMI 20.9 kg/m²) with type 2 diabetes who was hospitalized when his son found him in a "near-unconscious state." According to his son, M.R.'s diabetes had been adequately managed with glipizide 10 mg BID and acarbose 100 mg TID with each meal until approximately 2 months ago, when M.R. was hospitalized for pneumonia. Because M.R. lived alone and adamantly refused to take "shots," he was discharged on metformin, which was to be added to his other medications. A review of the hospital records revealed an SrCr of 1.4 mg/dL and several random blood glucose concentrations >190 mg/dL. He also has a history of chronic obstructive pulmonary disease (COPD). His current dose of metformin is 850 mg TID with meals.

On physical examination, the patient was oriented, but appeared acutely ill. Temperature, pulse, and BP were within normal limits. The respiratory rate was 32 breaths/min. Significant laboratory values included the following: Na, 140 mEq/L; K, 6.2 mEq/L (normal, 3.5 to 5); Cl, 103 mEq/L (normal, 95 to 105); HCO_3, 5 mEq/L (normal, 22 to 28); arterial pH, 6.8 (normal, 7.36 to 7.42); SrCr 3.2 mg/dL (normal, 0.7 to 1.4); blood glucose, 130 mg/dL; serum acetones, negative; serum lactate, 12.3 mmol/L (normal, 0.7 to 2.0); and serum pyruvate, 0.49 mmol/L (normal, 0.05 to 0.08).

A diagnosis of lactic acidosis was made. What signs and symptoms are consistent with this diagnosis? What is the relation between metformin and lactic acidosis, and what are the predisposing factors?

The most notorious side effect associated with metformin—though extremely rare—is lactic acidosis. Lactic acidosis is a metabolic acidosis characterized by a significant reduction in the arterial pH and an accumulation of serum lactate, a product of anaerobic metabolism. It is a condition that is highly lethal (50% mortality) and resistant to therapy. Lactic acidosis occurs when there is an increased production of or decreased utilization of lactate. Decreased utilization of lactate occurs when tissues are unable to oxidize lactate to pyruvate (these two substances are normally present in the serum in a ratio of 10:1). Metformin might predispose a patient to lactic acidosis by augmenting anaerobic metabolism or by decreasing the kidney's ability to handle an acid load. Other factors that might contribute to lactic acidosis include severe cardiac or pulmonary disease (anoxia, increased lactate production), septic shock, renal dysfunction (retention of metformin and lactate), and excessive alcohol intake (increased lactate production and decreased utilization).

Signs and symptoms generally are acute in onset and commonly include nausea, vomiting, diarrhea, and hyperventilation. Hypovolemia, hypotension, confusion, and coma also may occur; death is usually secondary to cardiovascular collapse.

As illustrated by M.R., typical laboratory findings include a low serum bicarbonate and PCO_2; a low arterial pH; an elevated potassium; a normal or low serum chloride; elevated lactate and pyruvate levels; an increased L:P ratio; and an anion gap of ≥30 mEq/L.

Treatment is empiric and includes the following: correction of any underlying cause of anoxia and elimination of factors predisposing to lactic acidosis, large doses of sodium bicarbonate with frequent arterial pH determinations, hemodialysis, and glucose plus insulin infusion. The latter are administered in an attempt to improve the metabolic utilization of lactate and pyruvate.[138,225]

Although metformin rarely is associated with lactic acidosis, the manufacturer and the FDA have taken extreme measures to prevent its improper use because another biguanide, phenformin, which induced this life-threatening condition was removed from the market in 1977.[211] The estimated rate of phenformin-induced lactic acidosis was 0.25 to four cases per 1,000 users versus five to nine cases per 100,000 users for metformin.[220,226,227] A group of clinicians from the FDA summarized 47 confirmed cases of metformin-related lactic acidosis (lactate levels ≥5 mmol/L) that had been reported to the FDA between May 1995 and June 1996.[227] Unfortunately, the condition continues to be resistant to treatment in that there was a 43% mortality rate. Importantly, 43 of the 47 cases (91%) had concurrent conditions that predisposed them to lactic acidosis. These included cardiac disease (64%), decreased renal function (28%), and chronic pulmonary disease (6%). Several patients (17%) were over the age of 80 years and may have had decreased renal function despite normal SrCr concentrations. Interestingly, 38% of the patients had CHF, and those who died were more likely to be under treatment with digoxin and furosemide. The mean daily dose of metformin was well within the therapeutic range and was not higher in the group that succumbed (1,259 ± 648 mg in the group that died and 1,349 ± 598 mg in the group that survived).

As a consequence of this analysis, the manufacturer has changed its labeling to warn against the use of metformin in individuals who are being treated for CHF. Furthermore, metformin should not be initiated in patients over 80 years old unless a Cl_{Cr} evaluation confirms normal renal function. The drug should not be used when patients are in sepsis.[136]

Unfortunately, studies assessing the appropriate use of metformin (according to the manufacturer's recommendations) reveal that metformin is frequently used in patients in whom it is contraindicated.[228–231] A retrospective cohort study of 1,847 patients found that 24.5% of patients who received metformin had conditions for which it was contraindicated (21.0% had CHF and were receiving loop diuretics, and 4.8% had renal impairment).[228] Medicare patients hospitalized with the primary diagnosis of heart failure and concomitant diabetes were assessed for metformin and TZD use, both of which are contraindicated in this situation.[231] Between 1998 and 1999, 7.1% and 7.2% of patients were treated with metformin and a TZD, respectively, at discharge; these numbers increased between 2000 and 2001 to 11.2% and 16.1%. In patients with renal dysfunction (SrCr 1.5 mg/dL or higher), metformin was used in 9.3% and 15.2% of patients in 1998–1999 and 2000–2001, respectively. See Question 65 for discussion of TZDs and heart failure. Clinicians need to carefully assess patients for contraindications before initiating oral agents.

M.R.'s pulmonary disease may have caused an anoxic state, which predisposed him to lactic acidosis. Furthermore, even though his SrCr was <1.5 mg/dL, this value may not have reflected normal renal function in this elderly gentleman.[232] Finally, dehydration caused by extensive vomiting and diarrhea has caused prerenal failure that is likely contributing to the acidosis.

Clinical Note: M.R. recovered following aggressive treatment with fluids and sodium bicarbonate. Metformin was discontinued and he was managed with insulin.

Hypoglycemia

67. C.A., a 68-year-old woman who has had a 20-year history of type 2 diabetes and a 5-year history of mild renal failure (SrCr, 1.5 mg/dL; BUN, 30 mg/dL), is admitted to the hospital in a coma. According to her daughter, C.A.'s diabetes has been well controlled over the past several months with glyburide 10 mg BID. She took her last dose approximately 5 hours before admission. Three days before admission C.A. developed anorexia, nausea, and vomiting in association with the flu and became progressively lethargic. Laboratory results on admission are as follows: plasma glucose, 20 mg/dL (normal, 70 to 140); SrCr, 3.0 mg/dL (normal, 0.6 to 1.2); and BUN, 80 mg/dL (normal, 7 to 20). What is C.A.'s diagnosis? Were there any predisposing factors?

[SI units: SrCr, 132.6 and 265.2 μmol/L; BUN, 10.7 and 28.6 mmol/L; plasma glucose, 1.1 mmol/L]

C.A. has developed a case of severe hypoglycemia secondary to glyburide. Hypoglycemia is the most common (incidence, 2.4 of 100 patients per year) and potentially severe (4% to 7% mortality) adverse effect of the sulfonylureas. The incidence and severity of this effect increase with the duration of action and potency of the agents. Thus, the incidence of severe, prolonged hypoglycemia secondary to chlorpropamide and glyburide is approximately two times higher than that for glipizide and approximately five times higher than that for tolbutamide.[145,146,233] As discussed in the section on drug-induced hypoglycemia later in this chapter, the sulfonylureas account for almost all cases of drug-induced hypoglycemia in individuals older than age 60.

Most sulfonylurea-induced hypoglycemia occurs in patients who are predisposed to hypoglycemia in some way, and C.A. is no exception. She is an elderly woman with renal impairment who was on relatively high doses of an agent, a portion of which is excreted unchanged in the urine. Even in the face of decreased carbohydrate intake (anorexia and vomiting), she continued to take her usual dose of glyburide. Even though the stress of illness most often raises glucose levels, the decreased intake and vomiting probably led to dehydration and further compromised renal function.

Because glyburide and chlorpropamide have a long duration of action, hypoglycemia induced by these agents may last for several hours, or days in the case of chlorpropamide. Therefore, patients such as C.A. must be hospitalized and treated with continuous glucose infusions until oral intake resumes. Otherwise, severe hypoglycemia may recur.

Use of Oral Antidiabetic Agents in Special Situations
Renal Dysfunction

68. Glyburide was withheld and C.A.'s kidney function stabilized with fluid replacement (Cl$_{Cr}$ = 35 mL/min). Because she lives alone, has impaired eyesight secondary to cataracts, and has severe arthritis, insulin treatment is impractical. Oral agents are to be continued. Which agents should be avoided? Which agents could be used?

[SI unit: Cl$_{Cr}$, 5.83 mL/sec]

Once C.A.'s plasma glucose concentrations and renal function have stabilized, reinstitution of antidiabetic therapy must be considered. Sulfonylurea compounds that are metabolized to active products that depend on the kidney for elimination (e.g., acetohexamide, chlorpropamide glyburide, and tolazamide) should be avoided in the elderly and in patients with decreased renal function. Sulfonylureas that are completely metabolized to inactive or weakly active products may be used (i.e., glipizide, glimeperide, or tolbutamide). Although glyburide is unlikely to accumulate in patients with a Cl$_{Cr}$ >30 mL/minute, it should not be used in C.A. because in her, it caused a severe hypoglycemic reaction. Furthermore, even patients who are not taking sulfonylureas are more likely to experience hypoglycemic reactions if they have renal insufficiency; therefore, any oral hypoglycemic agent should be initiated at a low dose and titrated slowly (Table 50-33). C.A. should be instructed to eat regularly, because skipped meals may result in recurrent hypoglycemia.[147,234]

Metformin is contraindicated in C.A. because her renal function is abnormal (see Question 66). Decreased renal function can result in accumulation of metformin, which can, in turn, predispose her to lactic acidosis.

The TZDs are primarily metabolized by the liver and are not contraindicated in patients with mild renal failure. The use of rosiglitazone or pioglitazone, beginning with low doses, could be considered as can acarbose, which is poorly absorbed from the GI tract. None of these agents cause hypoglycemia when used as monotherapy.

Hepatic Dysfunction

69. B.R., a 60-year-old man with cirrhosis of the liver, is found to have type 2 diabetes. Glipizide 10 mg QD is initiated. How will B.R.'s liver function affect the disposition of glipizide and his response to this agent?

Because hepatic metabolism is the primary route of elimination for most sulfonylureas, including glipizide, patients with hepatic disease should be expected to have an exaggerated response to those drugs metabolized to less active products.

Tolbutamide is the sulfonylurea that has been studied most extensively with respect to liver disease. In a double-blind, placebo-controlled trial of 50 cirrhotic patients, hypoglycemia was a complication in 20% of the tolbutamide-treated group.[235] Tolbutamide's elimination half-life in subjects with cirrhosis has been reported to be increased or unaltered in different studies.[236] A complicating factor is that alcohol can induce hepatic enzymes, markedly increasing tolbutamide metabolism in alcoholic patients with cirrhosis.

Liver disease can be a separate predisposing factor for severe, prolonged hypoglycemia because glycogenolysis and gluconeogenesis are impaired; thus, sulfonylureas are relatively contraindicated for cirrhotic patients. If they are used, shorter-acting agents are preferred and small initial doses should be used. For B.R., glipizide could be initiated at a dose no greater than 2.5 mg/day and increased if needed by 2.5-mg increments

Table 50-33   Treating Type 2 Diabetes Under Special Circumstances

Circumstance	Avoid	Consider
Patients with decreased renal function	Acarbose[a] Acetohexamide Chlorpropamide Glyburide Metformin	Glipizide Glimepiride Tolazamide or tolbutamide Insulin Repaglinide/nateglinide Thiazolidinediones
Patients with impaired liver function	Acarbose[a] Acetohexamide Chlorpropamide Metformin Thiazolidinediones ? Glyburide	Insulin Repaglinide[b] Miglitol
Patients who are obese or gaining excessive weight	Insulin[c] Sulfonylureas Repaglinide ? Thiazolidinediones[d]	Acarbose Miglitol Metformin
Patients experiencing hypoglycemia due to irregular eating patterns	Insulin Long-acting sulfonylureas	Acarbose Metformin Repaglinide/nateglinide Thiazolidinediones

[a]This is a labeled recommendation. Although very little acarbose is absorbed into the systemic circulation, the small amount available relies on the kidneys for elimination. This accumulation and doses ≥300 mg daily rarely have been associated with elevated liver enzymes. Plasma concentrations of miglitol in renally impaired volunteers were proportionally increased relative to the degree of renal dysfunction.
[b]The manufacturer recommends more cautious dose titration in these cases.
[c]This recommendation presumes that the patient can be controlled on oral agents. Often by the time insulin is required in type 2 diabetes, pancreatic function may have deteriorated considerably.
[d]Rosiglitazone is associated with mild weight gain (1.2 to 3.5 kg) and pioglitazone has been associated with mild to moderate weight gain (2 to 8 kg).

at no less than weekly intervals. Another option is low doses of repaglinide (0.5 mg) or nateglinide (60 mg) with meals.

Diabetes in the Elderly
Clinical Presentation

70. J.M. is a frail, 82-year-old, unresponsive man, who is brought to the ED. According to J.M.'s family, he has become increasingly confused, dizzy, and lethargic, with a recent weight loss of 10 lb. J.M. lives by himself and has been generally healthy with the exception of mild to moderate COPD and arthritis. Fasting serum chemistry reveals the following: Na, 128 mEq/L (normal, 135 to 145); glucose, 798 mg/dL (normal, 70 to 100); and serum osmolality, 374 mOsm/L (normal, 280 to 295 mOsm/kg H$_2$O). His serum is negative for ketones. On physical examination, J.M. has poor skin turgor and dry mucous membranes and is responsive only to deep pain. His BP is 90/60 mm Hg with a pulse of 96 beats/min. He is noted to have rales at the left lower base of his lung, and a chest radiograph confirms pneumonia. Despite aggressive fluid replacement, J.M.'s blood glucose remains consistently >250 mg/dL and his A$_{1C}$ is 11% (normal, ≤6%). J.M. presents with very high glucose concentrations, but has no history of diabetes mellitus. What special factors contribute to a late and atypical presentation of diabetes in the elderly?

[SI units: Na, 128 mmol/L (normal, 135 to 145); glucose, 44.3 and >13.9 mmol/L (normal, 3.9 to 6.1); serum osmolality, 374 mmol/kg; A$_{1C}$, 0.11]

Diabetes in the elderly commonly is underdiagnosed and undertreated because it often presents atypically.[237–239] Classic symptoms associated with diabetes mellitus may be masked by other illnesses, may be entirely absent, or may be explained away by the normal aging process. For example, polyuria is minimized by higher renal thresholds for glucose or may be confounded by urinary incontinence or "prostate problems." Thirst is commonly blunted in elderly persons, increasing their risk of dehydration and electrolyte imbalance. Hunger can be altered by medications or depression. Fatigue often is discounted as "part of getting old," and weight loss, though sometimes profound, may be so gradual that it goes unnoticed for months to years. (See Table 50-34 for a comparison of presenting symptoms for diabetes mellitus in elderly patients compared with younger patients.)

Hyperosmolar Hyperglycemic State

71. J.M. is diagnosed with hyperosmolar hyperglycemic state (HHS). Why are the elderly predisposed to this condition and what signs and symptoms are consistent with this diagnosis?

HHS is a condition characterized by extremely elevated plasma glucose concentrations (>600 mg/mL) and high serum osmolality (>330 mOsm/L) without ketoacidosis. Because patients with type 2 diabetes have some residual insulin pro-

Table 50-34   Presentation of Diabetes Mellitus in Elderly Patients Compared With Younger Patients

Metabolic Abnormality	Symptoms in Young Patients	Symptoms in Elderly Patients
Serum osmolality	Polydipsia	Dehydration, confusion, delirium
Glycosuria	Polyuria	Incontinence
Catabolic state due to insulin deficiency	Polyphagia	Weight loss, anorexia

duction, they are usually protected against excessive lipolysis and ketone production. Measurements of serum ketones and blood pH differentiate this condition from DKA (see Question 40). The condition occurs when urinary fluid and electrolyte losses secondary to glucosuria are inadequately replaced by oral fluid intake.[92,240]

HHS primarily occurs in the elderly because several situations predispose this population to hypodipsia. These include an inability to recognize thirst,[241] an inability to ask for fluids (e.g., dementia, sedation, intubation), and an inability to get fluids on demand (e.g., physical disabilities or restraints). Infections or other acute illnesses (e.g., MI, GI bleeding, pancreatitis) that exacerbate diabetes can interact with the hyperosmolar diuresis and hypodipsia to produce severe dehydration and hyperglycemia. Drugs that increase plasma glucose concentrations (e.g., glucocorticoids), increase diuresis, or decrease mentation also can contribute to this unfortunate situation.

J.M. presents with several symptoms of HHS dehydration, including osmolality >320 mOsm, plasma glucose >600 mg/dL, decreased skin turgor, hypotension, and the absence of serum ketones. His pneumonia was probably the precipitating factor. The mortality rate for this disorder is 3% in patients younger than 50 years of age; it increases to 30% for those older than 50.[242] Treatment involves rapid IV hydration, replacing half of the water deficit in the first 5 hours using 1 L/hour of normal saline. The administration rate is then reduced to 250 to 500 mL/hour until adequate hydration has been established.[92,240] Insulin may be given simultaneously, if indicated, to correct the hyperglycemia more rapidly. Rehydration has been sufficient to correct J.M.'s metabolic imbalance, allowing his diabetes control to be addressed now.

Goals of Therapy

72. What are the goals of therapy for J.M.?

It is widely recognized that strict glycemic control is associated with an increased incidence of hypoglycemia.[21] In the elderly patient with age-related autonomic dysfunction, hypoglycemia may present without the usual premonitory symptoms and can result in severe adverse effects such as angina, seizures, stroke, or MI. Therefore, the general tendency when treating elderly diabetic patients is to aim for slightly more liberal outcome objectives.

The basic principles of management are to maintain J.M.'s fasting blood glucose between 100 and 140 mg/dL with postprandial glucose values <180 mg/dL, while avoiding hypoglycemia. An A_{1C} goal of 8% would be appropriate in this frail patient.[243]

Diet and Exercise

73. How should diet and exercise recommendations be modified for elderly diabetic patients such as J.M.?

NUTRITION

Because most elderly patients have type 2 diabetes, nutrition and exercise programs are the initial steps in therapy. In 2001, the prevalence of obesity in the United States was 20.9%.[244] Elderly persons between the ages of 60 and 69 had a 25.3% prevalence of obesity and people at 70 and older had a prevalence of 17.1%. Older people with diabetes, especially those in a long-term care facility, have a tendency to be underweight rather than overweight.[36] Therefore, caution should

be used when considering a weight loss diet, since this could cause malnutrition or dehydration. The use of calorie-restricted diets in the elderly must ensure that the extent of weight loss is limited and that most weight loss primarily comes from adipose or fat stores, not from protein or muscle stores. Weight reduction is recommended in elderly persons over the age of 70 only if the patient is ≥20% overweight.

Several factors can adversely affect proper nutrition in the elderly. They include an impaired ability to shop for and prepare food, limited finances, an age-related decline in taste perceptions, and coexisting illnesses. Ill-fitting dentures, difficulty in chewing and swallowing, and lack of companionship during meals also can contribute to malnutrition.

A decrease in the proportion of saturated fat to <10% of calories, as recommended in the ADA medical nutrition therapy, may not be appropriate if malnutrition is present. Other considerations include individual food preferences, ethnic background, and physical and functional limitations that may affect adherence to specific dietary advice.

High-fiber diets may lower blood glucose and improve plasma lipids. However, high-fiber diets in frail, elderly patients, particularly those who are bedridden, should be used cautiously because they can be constipating and result in fecal impaction. Ambulatory patients, on the other hand, generally benefit from increased dietary fiber. Because many elderly patients are malnourished, a daily multiple-vitamin preparation containing the recommended daily allowance of each vitamin should be prescribed. Adequate calcium intake (at least 1,200 mg daily) should be assessed and supplemented if required.[36]

EXERCISE

Exercise in the elderly provides all the benefits derived by younger individuals. It increases well-being and glucose stability and may decrease a propensity to fall. Exercise also improves BP, the lipid profile, hypercoagulability, and bone density. For patients with arthritis, aquatic exercise may be substituted. Before such an exercise program is initiated, careful evaluation is mandatory to avoid myocardial ischemia or the acceleration of retinopathy.[101]

Selecting an Oral Antidiabetic Agent in the Elderly

74. Why is it important to institute drug therapy to treat J.M.'s diabetes? What considerations should be made in selecting an initial treatment regimen?

As in all patients with diabetes mellitus, poor glycemic control increases the risk of long-term complications. Although it is tempting to minimize the importance of glycemic control because these complications take so long to develop, patients such as J.M. may have had unrecognized hyperglycemia for many years before clinical diagnosis. Thus, many have already begun to develop complications. Furthermore, as life expectancy increases one can expect that these individuals will live long enough to experience morbidity related to diabetes if they are not treated. Therefore, pharmacologic treatment should be strongly considered in J.M. and most elderly patients whether or not they are symptomatic.[245]

The general approach to treating an elderly patient with type 2 diabetes is basically the same as described in Questions 50 and 52. The initial choice of an antidiabetic agent should be based on the severity of hyperglycemia. Other considerations include body weight, coexisting diseases, and cost of the agent. Patients with IFG (FPG >100, but <126 mg/dL) should be treated with diet and exercise tailored to their individual capabilities. For patients with diabetes (FPG ≥126 mg/dL or 2-hour postprandial blood glucose >200 mg/dL), acarbose, nateglinide or repaglinide, or a TZD are all appropriate options. Sulfonylurea-induced hypoglycemia is a concern in these patients. However, if inability to adhere to the multiple-daily regimen is problematic, a sulfonylurea would be an appropriate alternative agent. In J.M.'s case, metformin should probably be avoided because he has COPD. Also, he is older than age 80 and requires a Cl_{Cr} to assess his kidney function, because renal function calculated using the SrCr is often overestimated in elderly individuals with reduced muscle mass. There is a strong relationship between the pharmacokinetics of metformin and both kidney function and age. In healthy elderly patients, renal clearance of metformin was 35% to 40% lower than respective values for healthy young individuals.[137] Finally, the favorable effect metformin has on weight is irrelevant in J.M. Thus, although the efficacy of metformin is comparable to that of sulfonylureas, it is not the agent of first choice for elderly patients such as J.M.[243]

Patients with FPG >300 mg/dL and no overt stress should be considered insulin deficient and started on insulin therapy.

Selecting a Sulfonylurea

75. **Because his FPG concentrations remain 200 to 250 mg/dL, the decision is made to start J.M. on a sulfonylurea. What factors should be considered in selecting a sulfonylurea for J.M.?**

There are several age-associated problems with the use of oral hypoglycemic agents. Hepatic blood flow and oxidative metabolism are decreased with aging, resulting in prolonged half-lives of hepatically metabolized drugs. Serum albumin is reduced in the elderly, and this affects the highly protein-bound first-generation sulfonylureas, resulting in increased serum levels of free drug.[246] Response to hypoglycemic counter-regulatory hormones is diminished in the elderly, predisposing them to prolonged hypoglycemia. Decreased renal function and mass that occurs with aging decreases the clearance and increases the half-lives of oral agents excreted renally, specifically acetohexamide, chlorpropamide, and glyburide. Chlorpropamide should not be used in the elderly population owing to its long half-life (≥35 hours) and high incidence of hypoglycemia and hyponatremia.[246] Of the second-generation agents, glipizide is preferred over glyburide in frail, elderly patients like J.M. This is because its duration of action is shorter than that of glyburide and it is metabolized to inactive products. Consequently, it is 50% less likely to cause severe and prolonged hypoglycemia in the elderly population.[145,247] This is a concern because several factors predispose the elderly to drug-induced hypoglycemia. These include anorexia, irregular or inadequate food intake, and other factors affecting nutrition (see Question 73). Tolbutamide (which is converted to inactive metabolites), glimepiride (which has been studied in renal insufficiency), and repaglinide[143] and nateglinide (which are very short-acting) are also appropriate options.

Maturity-Onset Diabetes of the Young

76. **B.L. is a 34-year-old, slender (5'6", 120 lb, BMI 19.4 kg/m²) woman who developed diabetes at the age of 23. Until recently, her diabetes was very well controlled (A_{1C}, 6% to 7%) on glipizide 5 mg daily. Approximately 3 months ago, her physician dis-**

continued glipizide and began treating her with very low doses of insulin (7 units of 70/30 insulin twice daily) when she announced her intention to become pregnant. However, she is experiencing frequent hypoglycemic reactions and would like to switch back to glipizide. B.L. has no other medical problems, and her physical examination is within normal limits. B.L.'s mother (onset at age 32) and younger sister (onset at age 25) also have diabetes and are well controlled on oral agents. Assess B.L.'s diabetes. How should she be managed?**

It is quite likely that B.L. has a relatively rare form of diabetes often referred to as *maturity-onset diabetes of the young* (MODY).[248] Typically, the patient is normal weight, has a strong family history of diabetes, and is diagnosed during his or her young-adult years.[249] Unlike obese patients with type 2 diabetes, tissue sensitivity to insulin action is normal, but insulin secretion in response to glucose is defective. Consequently, patients such as B.L. respond to oral sulfonylureas and low doses of insulin. The physician's decision to treat B.L. with insulin is rational because she intends to conceive and oral sulfonylureas cross the placental barrier; however, it appears as though her dose and regimen will have to be adjusted.

Complications

Note to the reader: A thorough and extensive discussion addressing the clinical presentation of diabetic complications is beyond the scope of this chapter. Thus, the following cases and responses are presented only to give the beginning clinician a flavor of the presentation of some of the most common complications and a general approach to their treatment. Also see Chapters 14, Essential Hypertension, and 32, Chronic Kidney Disease.

77. **L.S. is a 46-year-old, obese man with an 8-year history of type 2 diabetes. His current problems include a BP of 155/103 mm Hg (documented on two occasions), blurry vision, and sexual impotence, which he now admits has troubled him for the last few years. Physical examination reveals decreased pedal pulses bilaterally, loss of sensation to monofilament testing, and evidence of an amputated toe on the right foot. His laboratory values are as follows: FPG, 170 mg/dL (normal, 70 to 100); A_{1C}, 7.8% (normal, 4 to 6%); fasting cholesterol, 240 mg/dL; and triglycerides, 160 mg/dL. L.S. has normal electrolyte values and microalbuminuria (180 µg/g creatinine). His only medication is glipizide 10 mg/day. Describe the pathogenesis of hypertension in patients such as L.S. Why is it important to treat L.S.'s hypertension?**

[SI units: FPG, 9.4 mmol/L; fasting cholesterol, 13.3 mmol/L; triglycerides, 8.9 mmol/L]

Hypertension

Hypertension is the main determinant of life expectancy and complications in diabetic patients and determines the evolution of diabetic nephropathy and retinopathy, in particular. Patients with type 1 diabetes usually are normotensive in the absence of nephropathy, but blood pressures rise 1 to 2 years after the onset of incipient nephropathy as indicated by microalbuminuria (see Question 79). Thus, hypertension in a patient with type 1 diabetes usually is of renal parenchymal origin. The relation between hypertension and type 2 diabetes is more complex and not as closely correlated to nephropathy. In type 2 diabetes, hypertension is often part of the metabolic syndrome of insulin resistance. Hypertension may be present for years or decades in these patients before overt diabetes mellitus is demonstrable. Hyperinsulinemia may contribute to the pathogenesis of hypertension by decreasing renal excretion of sodium, stimulating activity of and tissue response to the sympathetic nervous system, and increasing peripheral vascular resistance through vascular hypertrophy.

Aggressive management of hypertension (<130/80 mm Hg) reduces the progression of both macrovascular and microvascular complications and is essential in L.S.[176,177,250,251] In the UKPDS, a 5-mm Hg reduction in mean diastolic blood pressure produced a 37% reduction in microvascular complications.[176,177] Many patients require two or three medications to achieved the target blood pressure goal of <130/80 mm Hg. Weight reduction and exercise decrease insulin resistance (and therefore hyperinsulinemia) and will be additive to medications in lowering the BP. Dietary sodium restriction addresses the increased total body sodium found in these patients secondary to increased sodium retention.

78. **What must be considered in selecting an antihypertensive agent for L.S.?**

Since numerous studies have documented the effectiveness of ACE inhibitors and angiotensin-receptor blockers (ARBs) in retarding the development and progression of nephropathy,

these agents are appropriate as initial therapy for the management of hypertension in patients with diabetes. The choice of a second agent for the management of hypertension in persons with diabetes is more controversial. Data support the benefits of β-blockers. No difference was discerned between patients randomized to atenolol or captopril as initial therapy in the UKPDS.[177] Owing to the high prevalence of CHD in people with diabetes, a β-blocker is preferred as second-line therapy in most patients. Thiazide diuretics are also associated with clear treatment benefits and improved outcomes for patients with diabetes. For African-American patients, diuretic therapy may be a better choice as a second-line agent. Certainly, if either the first- or second-line therapies fail to achieve a BP < 130/80 mm Hg, then all three agents should be used in combination. Other agents, such as calcium channel blockers, peripheral vasodilators, and centrally acting agents have somewhat less desirable effects with respect to diabetes and are not preferred over ACE inhibitors, ARBs, β-blockers, and diuretics. The management of hypertension in people with diabetes is discussed in Chapter 14, Essential Hypertension. Adverse effects of antihypertensive agents of particular importance to patients with diabetes are summarized in Table 50-35.

Table 50-35   Antihypertensive Agents: Important Adverse Effects in Patients with Diabetes

Drug	Blood Glucose	Lipid Profile	Impotence	Insulin Sensitivity	Proteinuria	Comments
First-Line Antihypertensive Agents[a]						
ACE inhibitors	↑	Neutral	Rare	↑	↓	May cause hyperkalemia in patients with impaired renal function
ARBS (angiotensin receptor blockers)	↑	Neutral	Rare	↑	↑	May cause less cough than ACE inhibitors
Second-Line Antihypertensive Agents[b]						
β-Adrenergic blockers	↑↓	↑ TG ↓ HDL	+	↓	↓	Can prolong and mask hypoglycemic symptoms (most important in patients on insulin and with long-term type 1 DM). Response to counter-regulatory hormones may be exaggerated due to unopposed α-effects (e.g., arrhythmias, hypertension). Cardioselective agents may be preferable. Hyperosmolar nonketotic coma may occur in patients with endogenous insulin. Unopposed α-effects may ↓ peripheral circulation
Thiazide diuretics	↑	↑ Chol ↑ TG	+	↓	↓	Commonly used in low doses. Hypokalemia can ↓ insulin secretion, cause tissue resistance, and promote arrhythmias. Diabetogenic effects most prevalent in type 2 DM. To minimize metabolic effects, do not exceed 25 mg/day HCTZ or use indapamide 2.5 mg/dL
Third-Line Antihypertensive Agents						
Calcium channel blockers	None	Neutral	Rare	No effect	Variable	Nifedipine potentially may worsen proteinuria
α-Adrenergic blockers	None or ↑	↓ LDL-C ↑ HDL-C ↓ TG	Rare	↑	Unknown	First-dose hypotension
Central adrenergic inhibitors	None	None	++	No effect	No effect	Sedation, depression, dry mouth, sodium retention, orthostasis
Peripheral adrenergic inhibitors	None	None	+++	No effect	No effect	Orthostasis; sodium retention usually requires addition of thiazides
Vasodilators	None	None	Rare	No effect	No effect	Tachycardia and sodium retention require addition of thiazide and β-blocker

[a]These agents are preferred because they have minimal adverse metabolite effects. Agents are listed in general order of use; individualize selection to patient needs.
[b]These agents are not contraindicated, but are not preferred because of adverse effects on glucose and lipid metabolism or sexual function.
ACE inhibitors, angiotensin-converting enzyme inhibitors; Chol, cholesterol; DM, diabetes mellitus; HCTZ, hydrochlorothiazide; HDL-C, high-density lipoprotein cholesterol; LDL-C, low-density lipoprotein cholesterol; TG, triglycerides.

Nephropathy

Thickening of the glomerular capillary basement membranes is the hallmark of diabetic nephropathy. Diffuse deposition of basement membrane–like material expands the mesangium. This process narrows the capillary lumina, impedes blood flow, and thereby reduces the filtering surface area in the glomerulus. Hyperglycemia causes intraglomerular hypertension and renal hyperfiltration. Hyperfiltration then is followed by microalbuminuria with minimal glomerulosclerosis, which still is potentially reversible. If appropriate therapy is not initiated, overt proteinuria occurs and the patient usually progresses to nephrotic syndrome. Progression of diabetic renal disease can be accelerated in the presence of hypertension, proteinuria,[252] and diabetic retinopathy (another microvascular complication). Lipid abnormalities also may contribute to the progression of glomerulosclerosis.

SCREENING AND CONFIRMATION OF MICROALBUMINURIA

Microalbuminuria is defined as a urinary albumin excretion (UAE) of 20 μg/minute or >30 mg/24 hours or 30 mg albumin/g creatine during a random urine collection. Because of day-to-day variability in albumin excretion, at least two of three urine samples collected in a 3- to 6-month period need to have elevated levels before the designation of microalbuminuria.[5,73,253]

Microalbuminuria rarely occurs in type 1 patients who are younger than 14 years of age or in those diagnosed for <5 years. Therefore, patients with type 1 diabetes should be screened for microalbuminuria annually after 5 years of diabetes or at the onset of puberty. Patients with type 2 diabetes should be screened annually from the time of diagnosis. The development of hypertension, or any increase in the concentration of SrCr, and retinopathy are indications for more frequent screening for microalbuminuria. Measurement of the albumin:creatinine ratio from a random spot urine collection (preferably the first-void or morning sample) is the preferred laboratory test for assessing microalbuminuria. Urine albumin concentrations can be falsely elevated by exercise, excessive protein intake, uncontrolled diabetes, uncontrolled hypertension, and urinary tract infection. Therefore, screening should be delayed if a patient has one of these conditions.

After the diagnosis of albuminuria, and initiation of an ACE inhibitor or ARB, the role of annual microalbinura assessment is not well established.[253] However, we recommend continued monitoring to assess response to therapy and progression of disease.

79. **What is the significance of the presence of albumin in L.S.'s urine? How should it be managed?**

Diabetic nephropathy, characterized by nephrotic syndrome and azotemia, accounts for 35% of all patients with ESRD. It is a major cause of death in patients with type 1 diabetes and is an increasing source of morbidity in type 2 diabetic individuals.[253,254] L.S. has microalbuminuria (180 mg albumin/g creatine). Depending on the method of measurement, macroalbuminuria, or overt nephropathy, is defined as >300 mg/g creatinine, >200 μg /min, or >300 mg/24-hour collection. Management includes early detection through screening for microalbuminuria; tight glucose control; ACE inhibitors and ARBs for patients with microalbuminuria (to slow progression); aggressive management of hypertension, which can accelerate deterioration of renal function; aggressive management of dyslipidemia; and smoking cessation.[252] A thorough discussion on the management of diabetic nephropathy and ESRD is discussed in Chapter 32, Chronic Kidney Disease.

Cardiovascular Disease

80. **L.S. is treated with lisinopril 20 mg daily, which controls his BP and improves his microalbuminuria. His dose of glipizide is titrated to 10 mg daily. Recent laboratory values include an FPG of 130 mg/dL, A$_{1C}$ of 6.0% (normal, 4% to 6%), a triglyceride level of 450 mg/dL (normal, <150 mg/dL), total cholesterol of 160 mg/dL (normal, < 200 mg/dL), and HDL cholesterol of 20 mg/dL (normal, >40 mg/dL). How does the risk of heart disease for patients such as L.S. compare with persons without diabetes? What is the pathogenesis of CHD in persons with diabetes?**

[SI units: FPG, 7.2 mmol/L; A$_{1C}$, 0.07; triglycerides, 7.34 mmol/L; total cholesterol, 8.9 mmol/L; HDL, 0.52 mmol/L]

CHD is the leading cause of premature death in the type 2 population and accounts for 50% of the deaths in people with diabetes. Renal complications of type 1 diabetes were previously the principal cause of death; however, with the advent of dialysis and renal transplantation, cardiovascular complications have become the principal cause of morbidity and mortality. Relative to nondiabetic individuals, those with diabetes are two to three times more likely to develop CHD, and their risk of death following an MI also is two to three times higher than their nondiabetic counterparts. Women with diabetes, regardless of their age or menopausal status, have equal risk for CHD to that of nondiabetic men. These sobering figures point to the importance of minimizing or eliminating all other preventable risk factors for cardiovascular disease in patients with diabetes (i.e., tobacco use, hypertension, hypercholesterolemia, obesity) through the prescription of exercise, diet, and appropriate medications.[255]

PATHOGENESIS

The pathogenesis of cardiovascular disease in people with diabetes is complex. The metabolic syndrome with its attendant cardiovascular risk factors, dyslipidemia, inflammation, and hemostatic abnormalities are only some of the mechanisms under study.[13,256]

The most common lipid abnormality in type 2 diabetes is hypertriglyceridemia (>150 mg/dL) with low levels of HDL cholesterol (< 40 mg/dL in males or < 50 mg/dL in females), similar to the lipid profile seen in L.S.[257,258] Poor control of type 1 diabetes also is associated with elevated LDL cholesterol levels as well as hypertriglyceridemia.[258] All of these lipid abnormalities contribute to the risk for cardiovascular disease.

Although primary prevention trials specifically evaluating lipid lowering in persons with diabetes have not been performed, two subgroup analyses of large-scale secondary prevention trials have been performed. In the Scandinavian Simvastatin Survival Study (4S Study), which was a multicenter, randomized, placebo-controlled trial, 202 of the 4,444 subjects had diabetes.[259] Subjects were randomized to simvastatin versus placebo. The risk reduction of CHD in diabetic subjects receiving treatment was 55% versus 32% in nondiabetic subjects. Another secondary prevention trial, the Cholesterol and Current Events (CARE) Study, examined the effects of treatment with 40 mg daily of pravastatin versus placebo in

586 patients with diabetes.[260,261] Treatment was associated with a 25% decrease in major CHD events, similar to a 23% decrease in nondiabetic subjects. These studies demonstrate the key role of LDL cholesterol in the genesis and progression of atherosclerosis. Another important finding is the 2.5-fold higher CHD risk observed in diabetic subjects versus nondiabetic subjects, indicating that diabetic subjects with a history of prior MI are at a very high risk for future disease.

Adults with diabetes should be screened annually for serum lipoprotein levels, including triglycerides, total cholesterol, LDL cholesterol, and HDL cholesterol. A total cholesterol level of <200 mg/dL, triglyceride level <150 mg/dL, and LDL cholesterol levels maintained at ≤100 mg/dL are acceptable. In almost all instances, a statin should be used in patients with diabetes. The ADA now recommends statin therapy in patients over the age of 40 with a TC ≥135 mg/dL regardless of baseline LDL levels.[257] For those patients with diabetes and known atherosclerotic coronary artery disease, a statin is overwhelmingly indicated.[257]

Dyslipidemia

81. Should L.S. be treated with drug therapy for his dyslipidemia?

Diet and exercise are cornerstones in the management of dyslipidemia in patients such as L.S. Weight loss is associated with improvements in insulin sensitivity and glucose control, as well as a reduction in triglycerides, total cholesterol, and LDL cholesterol. Physical activity enhances weight loss and increases HDL cholesterol levels. Thus, L.S.'s diet and exercise habits should be reassessed and instruction in both reinforced as appropriate. Blood glucose concentrations should be optimally controlled with diet, exercise, and oral agents or insulin when indicated. However, the attainment of diabetes control in patients with type 2 diabetes does not necessarily correct lipid abnormalities, as seen in L.S. Because insulin resistance may be the underlying cause of elevated lipids in these patients, efforts should be devoted to reversing insulin resistance as well. Because L.S.'s FPG and A_{1C} values indicate that he has achieved diabetes control, a lipid-lowering agent is warranted if he does not respond to lifestyle modifications.

BILE ACID SEQUESTRANTS

Bile acid sequestrants primarily lower total and LDL cholesterol levels with little effect on HDL cholesterol. These agents can elevate triglyceride levels and may be problematic as monotherapy for patients such as L.S. with mild to moderate hypertriglyceridemia. Low doses of bile acid sequestrants may be useful as adjunctive therapy when combined with a fibric acid derivative or an HMG Co-A reductase inhibitor.

FIBRIC ACID DERIVATIVES

Gemfibrozil and fenofibrate are the fibric acid derivatives currently available in the United States. These drugs activate lipoprotein lipase, which reduces triglycerides and increases HDL cholesterol. They exert a variable but generally modest LDL cholesterol–lowering effect. Gemfibrozil or fenofibrate may be useful in patients like L.S. whose dyslipidemia is predominantly characterized by hypertriglyceridemia. Gemfibrozil should not be used in combination with repaglinide (see Table 50-31).

HMG-COA REDUCTASE INHIBITORS

Simvastatin, pravastatin, lovastatin, fluvastatin, atorvastatin, and rosuvastatin inhibit HMG-CoA reductase, a key regulatory enzyme for cholesterol biosynthesis. As a result, hepatic cholesterol synthesis declines, surface LDL particle receptors increase, and LDL cholesterol clearance increases. The statins' lipid effects are dose-dependent. Rosuvastatin and higher doses of atorvastatin and simvastatin can have a substantial effect on triglycerides, which is helpful in patients with elevations in both LDL cholesterol and triglycerides. They raise HDL cholesterol slightly.

NIACIN

Niacin effectively lowers LDL cholesterol. However, it has a dose-dependent effect in increasing plasma glucose. Although precise mechanisms by which this occurs are unknown, it may be due to accentuation of insulin resistance. Therefore, niacin's use as first-line therapy for dyslipidemia in people with diabetes is not recommended.[257] While two studies have demonstrated a minimal glycemic effect (increases in blood glucose by 9 mg/dL and A_{1C} 0.3%), practitioners still reserve its use as third-line therapy when combination therapy is indicated.[262,263]

Because hypertriglyceridemia is the main abnormality in L.S.'s lipid profile, gemfibrozil in a dose of 600 mg twice daily or fenofibrate 67 mg daily can be used to attain a triglyceride level of <200 mg/dL. Also see Chapter 13, Dyslipidemias, and reviews on this subject.[257]

Retinopathy

82. L.S. is referred to the ophthalmologist for his persistent complaints of vision problems despite improvement in his glycemic control. He is diagnosed with mild background retinopathy. Should L.S. be concerned?

Ocular disorders related to diabetes are the leading cause of new cases of legal blindness in Americans. Patients with diabetes may experience blurred vision associated with poor glycemic control, but retinopathy, senile-type cataracts, and glaucoma are the complications that threaten sight. Diabetic retinopathy appears as early as 3 years after diagnosis and is evident in 90% of type 1 diabetic individuals after 15 years. Comparable figures for patients with type 2 diabetes treated with insulin and type 2 patients treated with diet and oral agents are 80% and 55%, respectively. Proliferative retinopathy is less prevalent, but nevertheless is present in 30% of people with type 1 diabetes and in 10 to 15% of insulin-treated patients with type 2 diabetes who have had diabetes for ≥15 years.[7,9,264,265]

Patients with type 1 diabetes should have a dilated retinal examination within 3 to 5 years of diagnosis; evaluation is not necessary before 10 years of age. Patients with type 2 diabetes should have a comprehensive eye examination soon after diagnosis. The ADA recommends annual comprehensive eye examinations.[5,73,265] Less frequent eye exams (every 2-3 years) can be considered inpatients with normal exams based on the advice of an ophthalmologist.[265]

Current theories addressing the possible causes of this complication have been thoroughly reviewed.[264] Microvascular disease characterized by thickening of the capillary membrane may be the underlying lesion for two forms of retinopathy. The first and most common presentation is a nonproliferative retinopathy characterized by microaneurysms that may progress to hard yellow exudates, signifying chronic leakage, retinal edema, and punctate hemorrhage. This form of retinopathy may be associated with loss of central vision, but generally is associated with an excellent visual prognosis. Focal laser photocoagulation of the retina in patients with nonproliferative diabetic retinopathy and macular edema decreases the likelihood of visual loss by 50%.

A second, less common presentation is proliferative retinopathy. This form is characterized by neovascularization (presumably due to retinal hypoxia) and occurs in approximately 45% of people with type 1 diabetes and in 15% of people with type 2 diabetes who have had the disease for 15 years. Neovascularization ultimately leads to fibrosis, vitreous hemorrhage, and retinal detachment. Photocoagulation therapy may arrest progression and decrease loss of vision associated with neovascularization.[264] Because hypertension, smoking, uremia, and hyperglycemia may lead to more rapid progression of the retinopathy, every effort should be made to eliminate these risk factors for L.S.

Autonomic Neuropathy: Gastroparesis

83. H.D. is a 36-year-old man with a 20-year history of type 1 diabetes. He is in poor glycemic control (A$_{1C}$, 12%) and complains of frequent, severe hypoglycemic reactions that don't make sense. According to H.D., "I have insulin reactions right after I eat, but later on, my glucose concentrations are sky high." H.D. presents to the diabetes clinic with a 2-month history of nausea, postprandial fullness, and occasional vomiting, all of which are unrelieved by antacids. H.D. also has peripheral neuropathy involving both his hands and feet and manifestations of autonomic neuropathy (impotence and orthostatic hypotension). An upper GI series was ordered to rule out peptic ulcer disease and reflux esophagitis, but the preliminary diagnosis was diabetic gastroparesis. What is the cause of diabetic gastroparesis? How should H.D. be treated?

Autonomic neuropathy may present as gastroparesis with the feeling of fullness and nausea, urinary retention, impotence in men (manifested as retrograde ejaculation or an inability to attain an erection), postural hypotension, tachycardia, and diarrhea with incontinence of stool.[266] The presence of autonomic insufficiency may have profound effects on the patient's response to vasodilating drugs and ability to counteract hypoglycemia.[267]

Impaired diabetic control with "unexplained" hypoglycemia may result from the disrupted delivery of food to the intestine; that is, glucose delivery does not correspond with prandial insulin action. Many patients with diabetic gastroparesis, like H.D., have had diabetes for many years and also have evidence of peripheral and autonomic neuropathies.

Conventional antiemetic therapy is usually not helpful in the treatment of gastroparesis. Prokinetic agents, such as metoclopramide, are considered first-line therapy. *Metoclopramide* increases gut motility through indirect cholinergic stimulation of the gut muscle. However, symptomatic improvement does not always correlate with improved gastric emptying, which implies that the effectiveness of metoclopramide also is due to its centrally mediated antiemetic activity. A usual starting dose of metoclopramide is 10 mg orally four times daily, 30 minutes before meals and at bedtime. Although treatment may not eliminate all symptoms, it should minimize most of the patient's complaints. If oral therapy is ineffective for H.D., metoclopramide may be effective in extemporaneously compounded suppository form. Other pharmacotherapeutic interventions include domperidone (not available in the United States), cisapride (withdrawn from the U.S. market), erythromycin, and cholinergic agonists.[268] They are reviewed by Vinik and colleagues.[267]

Peripheral Neuropathy

84. Six months after institution of metoclopramide 10 mg QID and several insulin adjustments, H.D.'s GI symptoms have been alleviated, and his diabetes is now reasonably well controlled as evidenced by elimination of hypoglycemic episodes and a recent A$_{1C}$ of 7.5% (normal, 4% to 6%). However, H.D. has been complaining of increasing bilateral foot and leg pain, which he describes as a burning or aching sensation. An examination of his feet reveals cool extremities with absent pulses and loss of monofilament sensation. Outline appropriate steps that can be taken to alleviate H.D.'s peripheral neuropathy.

Diabetic neuropathy may be a consequence of metabolic disturbances in the neurons, microangiopathy affecting the capillary supply to neurons, or an autoimmune process. It affects 60% to 70% of the diabetic population and has a broad spectrum of presentation. Clinically, it most commonly presents as a diffuse symmetric sensorimotor syndrome, as carpal tunnel syndrome, or as autonomic neuropathy. Symptomatic diabetic peripheral neuropathy (DPN) occurs in 25% of patients with diabetes. It is characterized by paresthesia and pain in the lower extremities that may be mild or severe and unrelenting; decreased sensation to monofilament testing; decreased ankle and knee jerks; and decreased nerve conduction velocity. The decreased sensation associated with peripheral neuropathy contributes to the progression of foot injuries and infections that may go unnoticed by the patient until they are severe.[269,270] The management of diabetic neuropathies has been reviewed.[271]

SIMPLE ANALGESICS

Painful neuropathy may respond to simple analgesics (e.g., acetaminophen) or nonsteroidal anti-inflammatory drugs (NSAIDs). The analgesic selected should be based on the patient's history of responsiveness to these agents as well as their duration of action and side-effect profiles. Side effects include GI upset and bleeding, and renal and hepatic toxicity.

TRICYCLIC ANTIDEPRESSANTS

For painful neuropathy that becomes incapacitating and is unrelieved by simple analgesics, tricyclic antidepressants (TCAs) can be effective and are the most thoroughly studied. TCAs relieve pain by inhibiting re-uptake of serotonin and norepinephrine; by a quinidine-like local analgesic effect; or by other, as yet unexplained, mechanisms. Amitriptyline and imipramine are the most commonly prescribed TCAs because of their favorable effects on DPN. Daily doses that have been used have been low to moderate (25 to 150 mg), and the onset of analgesia is evident in 1 to 4 weeks; usually doses of 75 to 150 mg daily are required for adequate pain relief. To minimize side effects, attempts should be made to use antidepressants alone.

85. Amitriptyline (Elavil) 25 mg at bedtime was begun in H.D. with the dose titrated to 100 mg at bedtime over 1 month. H.D. experienced moderate relief of pain, and both his psychological and somatic complaints of depression lessened dramatically. However, H.D. also experienced intolerable constipation, dry mouth, and urinary hesitancy. Attempts to taper the dose of amitriptyline while maintaining pain relief were unsuccessful. What other drugs are effective for treating DPN?

Most of the adverse effects of psychotropic drug therapy (sedation, anticholinergic effects, extrapyramidal reactions, cardiovascular effects) are dose related except for tardive dyskinesia. Patients with autonomic neuropathy and the elderly are at increased risk for complications. Since desipramine and nortriptyline are less likely to cause sedation, anticholinergic side effects, and orthostatic hypotension, we recommend their preferential use over amitriptyline.

ANTICONVULSANTS
Carbamazepine
For cases of extremely painful DPN resistant to simple analgesics and TCAs, carbamazepine can be tried. Doses have varied from 100 mg three times daily to 200 mg four times daily. Dizziness and drowsiness are common but often transient, and GI disturbances or dermatologic reactions are observed in 5% to 10% of patients. Carbamazepine is now rarely used because of its side effects. Phenytoin (Dilantin) generally is not of value in the treatment of diabetic neuropathy because toxicity (such as nystagmus, ataxia, and sedation) often develops before a therapeutic effect is seen. Furthermore, phenytoin potentially decreases insulin secretion in type 2 patients.

Gabapentin
Gabapentin's exact mechanism of action in treating neuropathic pain is not known, but it may be through its modulation of calcium channels.[272] A randomized, double-blind, placebo-controlled 8-week trial evaluated the use of gabapentin in 165 patients with painful diabetic neuropathy.[273] Gabapentin was titrated from 900 mg daily (divided TID) in the first week up to 3,600 mg daily (divided TID) to assess its efficacy and tolerability. Gabapentin significantly improved pain compared to placebo. Although gabapentin was associated with more dizziness and somnolence, only 2 of the 84 patients treated with gabapentin withdrew because of side effects. Backonja[272] reviewed data from five clinical trials of gabapentin and recommends a starting dose of gabapentin of 900 mg daily (300 mg on the first day, 600 mg on the second day, and 900 mg daily on the third day taken in three divided doses); the dose should be titrated to 1,800 to 3,600 mg/day for effective relief of neuropathic pain. An advantage of gabapentin is its lack of significant drug interactions.

Other Anticonvulsants
Lamotrigine and topiramate are newer anticonvulsants that have been found to be effective in painful diabetic neuropathy.[165,274,275] Lamotrigine can be started at 25 to 50 mg daily and titrated by 50-mg increments to 400 mg daily; patients should be closely monitored for rash. Topiramate can be started at 25 mg daily and increased in 25-mg increments to 400 mg day (taken in two to three divided doses).

OTHER AGENTS
Another analgesic, tramadol, which binds to μ-opioid receptors and weakly inhibits norepinephrine and serotonin uptake, has been shown to be effective in DPN.[276,277] Patients can be started on 50 mg daily and titrated in 50-mg increments to 400 mg daily. In one clinical trial, an average dose of 210 mg of tramadol was found to be significantly more effective than placebo in treating painful diabetic neuropathy.[276]

The antiarrhythmics, mexiletine and lidocaine, can be beneficial in the treatment of resistant neuropathy.[278] However, because of inconsistent therapeutic benefits and an increased risk of side effects, these agents are reserved for cases that cannot be treated successfully with other, less toxic agents. The use of clonidine (Catapres) also has been studied for the treatment of DPN because peripheral vasodilation may decrease neuronal ischemia. In two controlled studies, transdermal clonidine resulted in relief of painful diabetic neuropathy in a subpopulation of patients.[271]

Topical application of 0.075% capsaicin (Zostrix), the active ingredient in hot peppers, is used to treat postherpetic neuralgia and has been recommended for diabetic neuropathy. This nonprescription preparation enhances the release and prevents the reaccumulation of substance P in nerve terminals of type-C nociceptive fibers. In this way, it impedes the conduction and transmission of peripheral pain impulses. Because capsaicin acts to deplete substance P from nerve fiber terminals, initial high levels are released from the fibers, resulting in a burning and stinging sensation. H.D. should be advised that benefit from capsaicin may not occur for several weeks. Patients should use gloves or an applicator to apply capsaicin and avoid contact with the eyes or mucous membranes. Capsaicin may be useful in diabetic patients intolerant of oral medications.[271]

The treatment of DPN continues to center on providing symptomatic relief. The use of gabapentin or TCAs continues to provide the best analgesic effect. A variety of other medications may provide relief in refractory patients.

86. Can anything be done for H.D.'s peripheral vascular disease?

Peripheral vascular disease or peripheral arterial disease (PAD) presents as diminished or absent foot pulses (35%), intermittent claudication (24% to 35%), skin ulcers, gangrene, or amputation. People with diabetes are 2 to 10 times more likely to develop symptoms of PAD than those without diabetes, and half of all nontraumatic amputations in the United States are performed in patients with diabetes. In one study that followed up type 2 patients for 7 years, 5.5% had an amputation. The prevalence of this condition increases with age, duration of diabetes, and the presence of risk factors such as hypertension or smoking.[269,279]

Signs and symptoms of PAD include leg pain, which is relieved by rest; cold feet; nocturnal leg pain, which is relieved by dangling the feet over the bed or walking; absent pulses; loss of hair on the foot and toes; and gangrene. Treatment of this condition includes elimination and treatment of risk factors such as smoking, dyslipidemia, hypertension, and hyperglycemia; antiplatelet therapy; exercise, the mainstay of therapy; and revascularization and surgery.[279] H.D. should be thoroughly educated regarding proper foot care and have frequent foot examinations.[280,281]

87. **Should L.S. be started on aspirin therapy?**

L.S. has several cardiovascular risk factors (microalbuminuria, dyslipidemia, hyptertension, obesity, and age) and should be started on aspirin therapy as primary prevention. The ADA recommends aspirin therapy as secondary prevention in patients with a history of MI, vascular bypass procedure, PVD, stroke or transient ischemic attack, claudication, and/or angina.[282] Primary prevention is indicated in individuals over 40 years of age or who have additional risk factors (a family history of CHD, smoking, hypertension, albuminuria, dyslipidemia). L.S. should take an enteric-coated aspirin, 81 mg daily.

DRUG-INDUCED ALTERATIONS IN GLUCOSE HOMEOSTASIS

Persons with diabetes are likely to take more drugs over their lifetime than any other group of patients. Patients with type 2 diabetes present with a constellation of chronic conditions, including hypertension, dyslipidemia, and cardiovascular disease, all of which are amenable to drug therapy. Drugs to manage depression, intermittent infections, obesity, and neurologic and ophthalmologic conditions also are commonly prescribed. Because we know that the actions of drugs are complex, and that for every desired effect there are several other unwanted effects, each time a drug is added to the regimen of someone with diabetes, it is important to assess the patient's situation to determine whether a potential exists for a drug–drug interaction or if the benefit of the newly prescribed drug is likely to outweigh its risks.

Representative drugs or drug classes that have been reported to cause or exacerbate hyperglycemia and hypoglycemia are listed in Tables 50-36 and 50-37, respectively. The subject has been reviewed by others.[283,284]

Drug-Induced Hyperglycemia
Corticosteroids

88. **A.L., a 37-year-old obese woman with systemic lupus erythematosus (SLE), has been taking 60 mg/day of prednisone for 6 months. During this period, her weight has increased by 30 lb and she has developed glycosuria. She was referred to the diabetes clinic, where her FPG was found to be 190 mg/dL; there was 1% glucose in her urine and no ketones. Physical examination shows a 5′2″, 150-lb, depressed woman with truncal obesity and an acneiform rash. Her mother and one sister have diabetes mellitus. How do corticosteroids contribute to diabetes mellitus? How should A.L. be treated?**

The term *steroid diabetes* was first used to describe the hyperglycemia and glycosuria seen in patients with Cushing's syndrome. Now it is associated more commonly with exogenously administered glucocorticoids and has been a side effect of parenteral, oral, and even topical therapy.[285] Corticosteroids are one of the most common drug groups that unmask latent diabetes or aggravate pre-existing disease, and they may produce hyperglycemia and overt diabetes in individuals who are not otherwise predisposed.

Corticosteroids increase hepatic gluconeogenesis and decrease tissue responsiveness to insulin. Although steroid-induced diabetes generally is mild and rarely associated with

ketonemia, a wide spectrum of severity may be encountered—from asymptomatic, abnormal glucose tolerance tests to difficult-to-control, insulin-requiring disease. The onset of glucose tolerance can occur within hours to days or after months to years of chronic therapy. The effect generally is considered dose dependent and usually is reversible upon discontinuation of the drug; reversal may take several months.[283,286]

A.L. exhibits many symptoms that can be attributed to supraphysiologic doses of corticosteroids: truncal obesity, depression, an acneiform rash, and diabetes. Mild diabetes in obese individuals, as in A.L.'s case, sometimes can be controlled by diet, but may require treatment with antidiabetic medications. A person with diabetes prior to glucocorticoid use, whose condition is aggravated by use of a glucocorticoid, should modify treatment appropriately to restore glycemic control. It is important to anticipate the need to modify insulin or oral antidiabetic therapy as corticosteroid doses are increased or decreased.

Sympathomimetics

89. **R.C., a 41-year-old man with type 1 diabetes, is well controlled on split doses of regular and NPH insulin and has been taking pseudoephedrine 30 mg QID for 7 days and Robitussin DM 10 mL QID (which contains 2.92 gm/5 mL sugar) for a cold. Recently, glucose concentrations have been higher than usual. Can pseudoephedrine or the cough preparation be the cause of his poor glycemic control? Discuss the use of sympathomimetics and cough preparations in patients with diabetes.**

OTC drug products, such as decongestants and diet aids, which contain sympathomimetics carry warning labels that caution against their use in patients with diabetes. Standard sugar- and ethanol-containing cough preparations also carry such warning labels. However, clinically significant drug-induced glucose intolerance probably is very infrequent. It is well established that parenterally administered epinephrine increases blood glucose concentrations secondary to increased glycogenolysis and gluconeogenesis. Other sympathomimetics generally do not have as potent an effect on blood glucose as epinephrine, and their use usually does not pose a practical problem in diabetic patients. Nevertheless, therapeutic to high oral doses of phenylephrine caused hyperglycemia and acetonuria in three nondiabetic children.[287,288] Furthermore, the effects of sympathomimetics on BP must be considered in many patients with diabetes. Therefore, we recommend antihistamines or occasional use of nasal sprays for severe congestion.

In summary, pseudoephedrine or the cough preparation may be aggravating R.C.'s diabetic control, although at these low to normal therapeutic doses it is quite unlikely. The stress related to R.C.'s underlying cold is more likely to be impairing his glucose tolerance than these low doses of sympathomimetic agents or the small amounts of sugar contained in the cough syrup.

Drug-Induced Hypoglycemia
Ethanol

90. **C.F., a 22-year-old woman with newly diagnosed type 1 diabetes, enjoys a glass or two of wine with her evening meal. What effect does alcohol have on a patient with diabetes, particularly**

Table 50-36   Drugs That Can Increase Blood Glucose Levels[a,b]

Drug/Class Name	Clinical Significance[c]	Comments
Asparaginase	++	Generally resolves during or after asparaginase therapy is completed. Concomitant corticosteroids may increase the incidence and severity of glucose intolerance.
Atypical antipsychotic agents	+++	Cause hyperglycemia and new-onset type 2 diabetes (reported with olanzepine and clozapine)
β_2-Agonists	++	Can induce maternal hyperglycemia when used as a tocolytic. For effect on infants, see Table 50-37.
β-Adrenergic blockers	++	Alternative antihypertensive therapy preferred, unless the benefits outweigh the risks (i.e., prevention of second myocardial infarction). Cardioselective α-blockers may cause fewer adverse effects than non-selective agents.
Calcitonin	+	Few case reports.
Calcium antagonists	+	Do not appear to cause clinically significant long-term adverse effects on carbohydrate metabolism.
Carbamazepine	+	One known case report.
Cimetidine	+	Few case reports.
Corticosteroids	+++	Glucose intolerance can occur within hours to days or after months of chronic therapy. The adverse effect generally is considered dose dependent and reversible upon discontinuation; the reversal may take several months.
Cyclosporine	++	May cause hyperglycemia and require insulin therapy during long-term therapy, whether or not concomitant corticosteroids are part of the immunosuppressant regimen.
Diazoxide	+++	Causes hyperglycemia predictably in most patients. Oral formulation used as therapeutic glucose-elevating agent.
Didanosine	+	Hyperglycemia without pancreatitis possible.
Diuretics	+++	All classes of diuretics, and in particular thiazides, have been reported to cause diabetes mellitus or worsen glucose control in people with diabetes; some may tolerate low doses (25 mg hydrochlorothiazide equivalent).
Encainide	+	Two known reports in the biomedical literature.
Imipramine	+	Few case reports.
Isoniazid	+	Few case reports.
Lithium	+	Conflicting data in the biomedical literature.
Marijuana	++	One case required 3-fold increase in insulin dose; another developed diabetic ketoacidosis after ingesting large amounts orally. δ-9-tetrahydrocannabinol impaired glucose tolerance in six subjects (6 mg IV).
Megestrol acetate	+	Few case reports.
Nicotinic acid	++	Alternative agents for hyperlipidemia preferred for people with diabetes. See Question 81.
Oral contraceptives	++	Appears to occur less frequently with an estrogen dose <50 μg.
Pentamidine	+++	Diabetes mellitus may occur days after initiation of therapy, but more often is delayed by several weeks or even months. Initially, pentamidine may cause hypoglycemia (see Table 50-37).
Phenothiazines	+	Many case reports, most involving chlorpromazine. Controlled studies lacking.
Phenytoin	++	Predisposed individuals (family history, underlying insulin resistance, high doses) may develop hyperglycemia. Overall incidence very small.
Pravastatin	+	One known case report.
Protease inhibitors	+++	Many cases of new-onset diabetes or worsening diabetes reported to the FDA. Some cases required hospitalization and were irreversible. Related to lipodystrophy and insulin resistance.
Rifampin	+	Few case reports.
Sympathomimetics	++	Clinically significant hyperglycemia infrequent, especially at usual doses.
Tacrolimus	++	May cause hyperglycemia and require insulin therapy during long-term therapy, whether or not concomitant corticosteroids are part of the immunosuppressant regimen.
Thyroid hormones	+	Adverse effect at excessive doses.

[a]The authors acknowledge Joanne M. Yasuda, Pharm D, who updated this table using primary references.
[b]This table does not include the many drugs that interact with the drugs used to treat diabetes (e.g., sulfonylureas).
[c]Clinical significance:
+ Clinical significance possible. Limited or conflicting reports or studies.
++ Clinically significant. Primarily important under certain conditions.
+++ Clinically significant effect of substantial prevalence and/or magnitude.
Adapted from reference 284.

one using insulin? Is alcohol contraindicated in C.F. or any person with diabetes?

Clinicians often are reluctant to permit the use of alcoholic beverages in patients with diabetes. However, barring contraindications that are similar in the nondiabetic and diabetic alike (e.g., alcoholism, hypertriglyceridemia, gastritis, pancreatitis, pregnancy), a person with diabetes can safely enjoy a moderate alcohol intake as long as certain precautions are taken. For an in-depth discussion, the reader is referred to two comprehensive reviews of alcohol and diabetes, parts of which are summarized in the following list.[289,290]

Table 50-37 **Drugs That Can Decrease Blood Glucose Levels**[a,b]

Drug/Class Name	Clinical Significance[c]	Comments
Anabolic steroids	+	Complex metabolic effects. Only certain steroids studied.
Angiotensin-converting enzyme (ACE) inhibitors	+	May increase peripheral sensitivity to insulin effects. Two case reports and one case-control study.
β-Adrenergic blockers	++	β-Blockers may prolong and mask the symptoms of hypoglycemia. Cardioselective β-blockers may cause less adverse effects than nonselective agents.
β$_2$-Agonists	++	Can induce hypoglycemia in the infants of mothers who received these agents for tocolysis. For effect on mother, see Table 50-36.
Disopyramide	++	Elderly patients with liver and/or renal impairment appear to be the most susceptible to this serious adverse effect.
Ethanol	+++	Most often occurs in individuals chronically drinking large amounts of ethanol. The adverse effect can follow binge drinking and even moderate alcohol intake in fasting individuals. Symptoms of hypoglycemia may be mistaken for intoxication.
Insulin	+++	Injectable solution or suspension used therapeutically to decrease glucose levels in people with diabetes.
Pentamidine	+++	Usually occurs several days to 2 weeks following initiation of therapy. It can be sudden, recurrent, and life-threatening. Pentamidine also may cause hyperglycemia (see Table 50-36).
Quinine/quinidine	++	Quinine 600–800 mg Q 8 hours for malaria may induce hypoglycemia in 10% of patients. Doses of 300 mg for leg cramps produce hypoglycemia infrequently.
Salicylates	++	Occurs with salicylate intoxication or anti-inflammatory doses (4–6 g/day in adults). Low doses unlikely to cause this adverse effect.
Sulfonamides	+	Rare reaction with renal failure and/or high doses.
Sulfonylureas	+++	Oral hypoglycemic agents used therapeutically to decrease glucose levels in people with type 2 diabetes.

[a]The authors acknowledge Joanne M. Yasuda, Pharm D, who updated this table using primary references.
[b]This table does not include the many drugs that interact with the drugs used to treat diabetes (e.g., sulfonylureas).
[c]Clinical significance:
+ Clinical significance possible. Limited or conflicting reports or studies.
++ Clinically significant. Primarily important under certain conditions.
+++ Clinically significant effect of substantial prevalence and/or magnitude.
Adapted from reference 233.

- Drink in moderation. The ADA defines this as a daily intake of one drink for adult women and two drinks for adult men (5 oz wine, 12 oz beer, 1.5 oz distilled liquor). The patient should be aware of his or her own sensitivity to the intoxicating effects of ethanol and adjust consumption downward, if needed. This is particularly important for insulin-dependent patients. When having a drink, be sure to have it with a meal.
- Avoid drinks that contain large amounts of sugar, such as liqueurs, sweet wines, and sugar-containing mixes. Instead, consider dry wines, light beers, and distilled spirits. Not only does the simple sugar content add an additional source of glucose and calories to the diet, but ethanol ingested with simple sugar–containing mixers enhances reactive hyperglycemia.
- Remember to count the calories in alcohol (calories = [0.8] × [proof] × [oz]); substitute 1 oz of alcohol for two fat exchanges.
- Be aware that the symptoms of alcohol intoxication and hypoglycemia are similar. If hypoglycemia is mistaken for intoxication by others, appropriate and potentially life-saving treatment can be delayed.
- Be aware of alcohol–sulfonylurea drug interactions, specifically the alcohol-induced enzyme induction of tolbutamide metabolism and the chlorpropamide–alcohol flush reaction.

REFERENCES

1. Centers for Disease Control and Prevention. National diabetes fact sheet: general information and national estimates on diabetes in the United States, 2003. Atlanta, GA: U.S. Department of Health and Human Services, Centers for Disease Control and Prevention, 2003.
2. Bouldin MJ et al. Quality of care in diabetes: understanding the guidelines. Am J Med Sci 2002; 324:196.
3. Nathan DM et al. Glycemic control in diabetes mellitus: have changes in therapy made a difference? Am J Med 1996;100:157.
4. LaPorte RE et al. Prevalence and incidence of insulin-dependent diabetes. In: Harris MI et al, eds. Diabetes in America. Vol. NIH Publication No. 95-

1468. 2nd Ed. Bethesda, MD: National Institutes of Health, 1995:37.
5. American Diabetes Association (ADA). Report of the expert committee on the diagnosis and classification of diabetes mellitus. Diabetes Care 2004; 27(Suppl 1):S5.
6. Kenny SJ et al. Prevalence and incidence of non-insulin-dependent diabetes. In: Harris M, ed. Diabetes in America, 2nd Ed. Bethesda, MD: NIH Publication No. 95-1468, 1995:47.
7. Harris MI et al. Prevalence of diabetes, impaired fasting glucose, and impaired glucose tolerance in U.S. adults. The Third National Health and Nutrition Examination Survey, 1988-1994. Diabetes Care 1998;21:518.

8. Hogan P et al. Economic costs of diabetes in the US in 2002. Diabetes Care 2003;26:917.
9. Harris MI. Summary. In: Harris M et al, eds. Diabetes in America. Vol. NIH Publication No. 95-1468. 2nd Ed. Bethesda, MD: National Institutes of Health, 1995:1.
10. Shulman GI et al. Integrated fuel metabolism. In: Porte D, Jr, Sherwin R, eds. Ellenberg's and Rifkin's Diabetes Mellitus. 5th edition ed. Stamford, CT: Appleton & Lange, 1997:1.
11. Palmer J, Lernmark A. Pathophysiology of type 1. In: Porte D, Jr, Sherwin R, eds. Ellenberg's and Rifkin's Diabetes Mellitus, 5th Ed. Stamford, CT: Appleton & Lange, 1997:455.

12. Reaven GM. Pathophysiology of insulin resistance in human disease. Physiol Rev 1995;75:473.

13. Executive Summary of The Third Report of The National Cholesterol Education Program (NCEP) Expert Panel on Detection, Evaluation, And Treatment of High Blood Cholesterol In Adults (Adult Treatment Panel III). JAMA 2001;285:2486.

14. Ford ES et al. Prevalence of the metabolic syndrome among US adults: findings from the third National Health and Nutrition Examination Survey. JAMA 2002;287:356.

15. Kahn S, Porte D, Jr. The pathophysiology of type II (noninsulin-dependent) diabetes mellitus: implications for treatment. In: Porte D, Jr, Sherwin R, eds. Ellenberg's and Rifkin's Diabetes Mellitus, 5th Ed. Stamford, CT: Appleton & Lange, 1997:487.

16. Turner R et al. UKPDS 25: autoantibodies to islet-cell cytoplasm and glutamic acid decarboxylase for prediction of insulin requirement in type 2 diabetes. UK Prospective Diabetes Study Group. Lancet 1997;350:1288.

17. American Diabetes Association (ADA) Position Statement. Gestational Diabetes Mellitus. Diabetes Care 2004;27(Suppl 1):S88.

18. ADA. The Expert Committee on the Diagnosis and Classification of Diabetes Mellitus: follow-up report on the diagnosis of diabetes mellitus. Diabetes Care 2003;26:3160.

19. Goran MI et al. Obesity and risk of type 2 diabetes and cardiovascular disease in children and adolescents. J Clin Endocrinol Metab 2003;88:1417.

20. Stratton IM et al. Association of glycaemia with macrovascular and microvascular complications of type 2 diabetes (UKPDS 35): prospective observational study. Br Med J 2000;321:405.

21. The effect of intensive treatment of diabetes on the development and progression of long-term complications in insulin-dependent diabetes mellitus. The Diabetes Control and Complications Trial Research Group. N Engl J Med 1993;329:977.

22. Intensive blood-glucose control with sulphonylureas or insulin compared with conventional treatment and risk of complications in patients with type 2 diabetes (UKPDS 33). UK Prospective Diabetes Study (UKPDS) Group. Lancet 1998;352:837

23. Gaede PH et al. [The Steno-2 study. Intensive multifactorial intervention reduces the occurrence of cardiovascular disease in patients with type 2 diabetes]. Ugeskr Laeger 2003;165:2658.

24. ADA. American Diabetes Association Position Statement. Screening for type 2 diabetes. Diabetes Care 2004;27(Suppl 1):S11.

25. Kakka R, Koda-Kimble MA. Can insulin therapy delay or prevent insulin-dependent diabetes mellitus? Pharmacotherapy 1997;17:38.

26. Schatz DA, Bingley PJ. Update on major trials for the prevention of type 1 diabetes mellitus: the American Diabetes Prevention Trial (DPT-1) and the European Nicotinamide Diabetes Intervention Trial (ENDIT). J Pediatr Endocrinol Metab 2001;14(Suppl 1):619.

27. Effects of insulin in relatives of patients with type 1 diabetes mellitus. N Engl J Med 2002;346:1685.

28. Gale EA. Intervening before the onset of Type 1 diabetes: baseline data from the European Nicotinamide Diabetes Intervention Trial (ENDIT). Diabetologia 2003;46:339.

29. Herold KC et al. Anti-CD3 monoclonal antibody in new-onset type 1 diabetes mellitus. N Engl J Med 2002;346:1692.

30. Knowler WC et al. Reduction in the incidence of type 2 diabetes with lifestyle intervention or metformin. N Engl J Med 2002;346:393.

31. Fontbonne A et al. The effect of metformin on the metabolic abnormalities associated with upper-body fat distribution. BIGPRO Study Group. Diabetes Care 1996;19:920.

32. Effects of withdrawal from metformin on the development of diabetes in the diabetes prevention program. Diabetes Care 2003;26:977.

33. Tuomilehto J et al. Prevention of type 2 diabetes mellitus by changes in lifestyle among subjects with impaired glucose tolerance. N Engl J Med 2001;344:1343.

34. Chiasson JL et al. Acarbose for prevention of type 2 diabetes mellitus: the STOP-NIDDM randomised trial. Lancet 2002;359:2072.

35. Buchanan TA et al. Preservation of pancreatic beta-cell function and prevention of type 2 diabetes by pharmacological treatment of insulin resistance in high-risk hispanic women. Diabetes 2002;51:2796.

36. Franz MJ et al. Nutrition principles and recommendations in diabetes. Diabetes Care 2004;27(Suppl 1):S36.

37. Franz MJ. Medical Nutrition Therapy. In: Franz MJ, ed. Diabetes Management Therapies, 4th Ed. Chicago: American Association of Diabetes Educators, 2001:3.

38. Gruessner AC, Sutherland DE. Pancreas transplant outcomes for United States (US) and non-US cases as reported to the United Network for Organ Sharing (UNOS) and the International Pancreas Transplant Registry (IPTR) as of October 2002. Clin Transpl 2002:41.

39. Robertson RP et al. Pancreas transplantation for patients with type 1 diabetes. Diabetes Care 2004;27(Suppl 1):S105.

40. Shapiro AM et al. Islet transplantation in seven patients with type 1 diabetes mellitus using a glucocorticoid-free immunosuppressive regimen. N Engl J Med 2000;343:230.

41. Oberholzer J et al. Current status of islet cell transplantation. Adv Surg 2003;37:253.

42. Goldstein DE et al. American Diabetes Association Position Statement. Tests of glycemia in diabetes. Diabetes Care 2004;27(Suppl 1):S91.

43. Rohlfing CL et al. Defining the relationship between plasma glucose and HbA(1c): analysis of glucose profiles and HbA(1c) in the Diabetes Control and Complications Trial. Diabetes Care 2002;25:275.

44. ADA. Standards of medical care for patients with diabetes mellitus. Diabetes Care 2004;(27 Suppl 1):S15.

45. Ceriello A et al. Vitamin E reduction of protein glycosylation in diabetes. New prospect for prevention of diabetic complications? Diabetes Care 1991;14:68.

46. Davie SJ et al. Effect of vitamin C on glycosylation of proteins. Diabetes 1992;41:167.

47. Nolte MS, Karam, J.H. Pancreatic Hormones & Antidiabetic Drugs. In: Katzung B, ed. Basic and Clinical Pharmacology, 8th Ed. New York: Lange Medical Books/McGraw Hill, 2001:711.

48. DeFelippes M et al. Insulin Chemistry and Pharmacokinetics. In: Porte DS, RS, Baron A, eds. Ellenberg and Rifkin's Diabetes Mellitus, 6th Ed. New York: McGraw-Hill, 2003:481.

49. Van Haeften TW. Clinical significance of insulin antibodies in insulin-treated diabetic patients. Diabetes Care 1989;12:641.

50. Binder C, Brange J. Insulin chemistry and pharmacokinetics. In: Porte D, Jr, Sherwin R, eds. Ellenberg's and Rifkin's Diabetes Mellitus, 5th Ed. Stamford, CT: Appleton & Lange, 1997:689.

51. Rabkin R et al. The renal metabolism of insulin. Diabetologia 1984;27:351.

52. Burge MR, Schade DS. Insulins. Endocrinol Metab Clin North Am 1997;26:575.

53. Holleman F et al. Reduced frequency of severe hypoglycemia and coma in well-controlled IDDM patients treated with insulin lispro. The Benelux-UK Insulin Lispro Study Group. Diabetes Care 1997;20:1827.

54. Raskin P et al. A comparison of insulin lispro and buffered regular human insulin administered via continuous subcutaneous insulin infusion pump. J Diabetes Complications 2001;15:295.

55. Heise T et al. Time-action profiles of novel premixed preparations of insulin lispro and NPL insulin. Diabetes Care 1998;21:800.

56. Bolli GB, Owens DR. Insulin glargine. Lancet 2000;356:443.

57. Lepore M et al. Pharmacokinetics and pharmacodynamics of subcutaneous injection of long-acting human insulin analog glargine, NPH insulin, and ultralente human insulin and continuous subcutaneous infusion of insulin lispro. Diabetes 2000;49:2142.

58. Dunn CJ et al. Insulin glargine: an updated review of its use in the management of diabetes mellitus. Drugs 2003;63:1743.

59. American Diabetes Association (ADA) Position Statement. Implications of the Diabetes Control and Complications Trial. Diabetes Care 2003;24(Suppl 1):S28.

60. Walsh J, Roberts R. Pumping Insulin, 3nd Ed. San Diego, CA: Torrey Pine Press, 2000.

61. ADA. American Diabetes Association Position Statement. Continuous subcutaneous insulin infusion. Diabetes Care 2004;27(Suppl 1):S110.

62. ADA. Resource Guide. Diabetes Forecast 2003; January.

63. Pickup J, Keen H. Continuous subcutaneous insulin infusion at 25 years: evidence base for the expanding use of insulin pump therapy in type 1 diabetes. Diabetes Care 2002;25:593.

64. Saudek CD. Novel forms of insulin delivery. Endocrinol Metab Clin North Am 1997;26:599.

65. Hirsch IB. Implementation of intensive insulin therapy for IDDM. Diabetes Review 1995;3:288.

66. Lenhard MJ, Reeves GD. Continuous subcutaneous insulin infusion: a comprehensive review of insulin pump therapy. Arch Intern Med 2001;161:2293.

67. Ratner RE et al. Less hypoglycemia with insulin glargine in intensive insulin therapy for type 1 diabetes. U.S. Study Group of Insulin Glargine in Type 1 Diabetes. Diabetes Care 2000;23:639.

68. Gin H, Aubertin J. Generalized allergy due to zinc and protamine in insulin preparation treated with insulin pump. Diabetes Care 1987;10:789.

69. ADA. American Diabetes Association Position Statement. Insulin administration. Diabetes Care 2004;27(Suppl 1):S106.

70. Koivisto VA, Felig P. Alterations in insulin absorption and in blood glucose control associated with varying insulin injection sites in diabetic patients. Ann Intern Med 1980;92:59.

71. American Diabetes Association (ADA). Insulin administration. Diabetes Care 2004;27(Suppl 1):S121.

72. Young RJ et al. Diabetic lipohypertrophy delays insulin absorption. Diabetes Care 1984;7:479.

73. ADA. American Diabetes Association Position Statement. Standards of medical care for patients with diabetes mellitus. Diabetes Care 2004;27(Suppl 1):S15.

74. Anon. Bringing medicine home: self-test kits monitor your health. Consumer Reports, October 1996.

75. Lenhard MJ et al. A comparison between alternative and trade name glucose test strips. Diabetes Care 1995;18:686.

76. Skyler JS. Tactics for type I diabetes. Endocrinol Metab Clin North Am 1997;26:647.

77. Glucowatch Biographer: a noninvasive glucose monitoring device. Med Lett Drugs Ther 2001;43:42.

78. Peters AL, Davidson MB. Effect of storage on action of NPH and regular insulin mixtures. Diabetes Care 1987;10:799.

79. Tunbridge FK et al. Double-blind crossover trial of isophane (NPH)- and lente-based insulin regimens. Diabetes Care 1989;12:115.

80. Eli Lilly and Company. Humalog Package Insert. May 2002.

81. Aventis Pharmaceuticals Inc. Lantus Package Insert. May 2003.

82. Perriello G et al. The effect of asymptomatic nocturnal hypoglycemia on glycemic control in diabetes mellitus. N Engl J Med 1988;319:1233.

83. Shade DS, Burge, MR. Britle Diabetes: Pathogenesis and Therapy. In: Porte DS, RS, ed. Ellenberg & Rifkin's Diabetes Mellitus, 5th Ed. Stamford, CT: Appleton & Lange, 1997:789.

84. Tordjman KM et al. Failure of nocturnal hypoglycemia to cause fasting hyperglycemia in patients with insulin-dependent diabetes mellitus. N Engl J Med 1987;317:1552.

85. Gerich JE. Lilly lecture 1988. Glucose counterregulation and its impact on diabetes mellitus. Diabetes 1988;37:1608.

86. Fanelli CG et al. Administration of neutral protamine Hagedorn insulin at bedtime versus with

dinner in type 1 diabetes mellitus to avoid nocturnal hypoglycemia and improve control. A randomized, controlled trial. Ann Intern Med 2002; 136:504.

87. Riddle MC et al. The Treat-to-Target Trial: Randomized addition of glargine or human NPH insulin to oral therapy of type 2 diabetic patients. Diabetes Care 2003;26:3080.

88. Torlone E et al. Effects of the short-acting insulin analog [Lys(B28),Pro(B29)] on postprandial blood glucose control in IDDM. Diabetes Care 1996;19:945.

89. Campbell PJ et al. Pathogenesis of the dawn phenomenon in patients with insulin-dependent diabetes mellitus. Accelerated glucose production and impaired glucose utilization due to nocturnal surges in growth hormone secretion. N Engl J Med 1985;312:1473.

90. Bolli GB, Gerich JE. The "dawn phenomenon"—a common occurrence in both non-insulin-dependent and insulin-dependent diabetes mellitus. N Engl J Med 1984;310:746.

91. Zinman B et al. Insulin lispro in CSII: results of a double-blind crossover study. Diabetes 1997; 46:440.

92. ADA. American Diabetes Association Position Statement. Hyperglycemic Crises in Diabetes. Diabetes Care 2004;27:S94.

93. ADA. American Diabetes Association Position Statement. Implications of the Diabetes Control and Complications Trial. Diabetes Care 2003; 24(Suppl 1):S25.

94. Agner T et al. Remission in IDDM: prospective study of basal C-peptide and insulin dose in 268 consecutive patients. Diabetes Care 1987;10:164.

95. Beregszaszi M et al. Nocturnal hypoglycemia in children and adolescents with insulin-dependent diabetes mellitus: prevalence and risk factors. J Pediatr 1997;131:27.

96. Santiago JV. Nocturnal hypoglycemia in children with diabetes: an important problem revisited. J Pediatr 1997;131:2.

97. Bernstein RK. Clouding and deactivation of clear (regular) human insulin: association with silicone oil from disposable syringes? Diabetes Care 1987;10:786.

98. Benson EA et al. Flocculated humulin N insulin. N Engl J Med 1987;316:1026.

99. Storvick WO, Henry HJ. Effect of storage temperature on stability of commercial insulin preparations. Diabetes 1968;17:499.

100. Qing Shi Z et al. Metabolic implications of exercise and physical fitness in physiology and diabetes. In: Porte D, Jr, Sherwin R, eds. Ellenberg's and Rifkin's Diabetes Mellitus, 5th Ed. Stamford, CT: Appleton & Lange, 1997:653.

101. Zinman B et al. Physical activity/exercise and diabetes mellitus. Diabetes Care 2003;26(Suppl 1):S73.

102. MacDonald MJ. Postexercise late-onset hypoglycemia in insulin-dependent diabetic patients. Diabetes Care 1987;10:584.

103. Koivisto VA, Felig P. Effects of leg exercise on insulin absorption in diabetic patients. N Engl J Med 1978;298:79.

104. Kemmer FW et al. Mechanism of exercise-induced hypoglycemia during sulfonylurea treatment. Diabetes 1987;36:1178.

105. ADA. Medical Management of Insulin-Dependent (Type I) Diabetes Mellitus, 3rd Ed. Alexandria, VA: American Diabetes Association, 1998.

106. Turnheim K. Basic aspects of insulin pharmacokinetics. In: Brunetti P, Waldhausl W, eds. Advanced Models for the Therapy of Insulin-Dependent Diabetes. New York: Raven Press, 1987:91.

107. Rubenstein AH, Spitz I. Role of the kidney in insulin metabolism and excretion. Diabetes 1968;17:161.

108. Rabkin R et al. Effect of renal disease on renal uptake and excretion of insulin in man. N Engl J Med 1970;282:182.

109. van den Berghe G et al. Intensive insulin therapy in the critically ill patients. N Engl J Med 2001; 345:1359.

110. Malmberg K. Prospective randomised study of intensive insulin treatment on long term survival after acute myocardial infarction in patients with diabetes mellitus. DIGAMI (Diabetes Mellitus, Insulin Glucose Infusion in Acute Myocardial Infarction) Study Group. Bmj. 1997;314:1512.

111. Montori VM et al. Hyperglycemia in acutely ill patients. JAMA 2002;288:2167.

112. Hirsch IB, McGill JB. Role of insulin in management of surgical patients with diabetes mellitus. Diabetes Care 1990;13:980.

113. Gavin LA. Perioperative management of the diabetic patient. Endocrinol Metab Clin North Am 1992;21:457.

114. Patton JS et al. Inhaled insulin. Adv Drug Deliv Rev 1999;35:235.

115. Royle P et al. Inhaled insulin in diabetes mellitus. Cochrane Database Syst Rev 2003:CD003890.

116. Nathan DM. Inhaled insulin for type 2 diabetes: solution or distraction? Ann Intern Med 2001; 134:242.

117. Cryer PE, Gerich J. Hypoglycemia in insulin-dependent diabetes mellitus: interplay of insulin excess and compromised glucose regulation. In: Porte D, Jr, et al, eds. Ellenberg's and Rifkin's Diabetes Mellitus, 6th Ed. New York: McGraw-Hill, 2003:523.

118. Pramming S et al. Symptomatic hypoglycaemia in 411 type 1 diabetic patients. Diabet Med 1991;8:217.

119. Ennis E et al. Diabetic Ketoacidosis. In: Porte D, Jr, Sherwin R, eds. Ellenberg's and Rifkin's Diabetes Mellitus, 5th Ed. Stamford, CT: Appleton & Lange, 1997:827.

120. Hillier TA et al. Hyponatremia: evaluating the correction factor for hyperglycemia. Am J Med 1999; 106:399.

121. Viallon A et al. Does bicarbonate therapy improve the management of severe diabetic ketoacidosis? Crit Care Med 1999;27:2690.

122. Lebovitz HE. alpha-Glucosidase inhibitors. Endocrinol Metab Clin North Am 1997;26:539.

123. Martin AE, Montgomery PA. Acarbose: an alpha-glucosidase inhibitor. Am J Health Syst Pharm 1996;53:2277;quiz 2336.

124. Yee HS, Fong NT. A review of the safety and efficacy of acarbose in diabetes mellitus. Pharmacotherapy 1996;16:792.

125. Chiasson JL et al. The efficacy of acarbose in the treatment of patients with non-insulin-dependent diabetes mellitus. A multicenter controlled clinical trial. Ann Intern Med 1994;121:928.

126. Coniff RF et al. Reduction of glycosylated hemoglobin and postprandial hyperglycemia by acarbose in patients with NIDDM. A placebo-controlled dose-comparison study. Diabetes Care 1995;18:817.

127. Bayer Corporation. Precose Package Insert. May 2003.

128. Pharmacia & Upjohn Company. Glyset Package Insert. July 2003.

129. Mitrakou A et al. Long-term effectiveness of a new alpha-glucosidase inhibitor (BAY m1099-miglitol) in insulin-treated type 2 diabetes mellitus. Diabet Med 1998;15:657.

130. Klepser TB, Kelly MW. Metformin hydrochloride: an antihyperglycemic agent. Am J Health Syst Pharm 1997;54:893.

131. Wildasin EM et al. Metformin, a promising oral antihyperglycemic for the treatment of noninsulin-dependent diabetes mellitus. Pharmacotherapy 1997;17:62.

132. Bell PM, Hadden DR. Metformin. Endocrinol Metab Clin North Am 1997;26:523.

133. Bailey CJ, Turner RC. Metformin. N Engl J Med 1996;334:574.

134. Kirpichnikov D et al. Metformin: an update. Ann Intern Med 2002;137:25.

135. UKPDS 28: a randomized trial of efficacy of early addition of metformin in sulfonylurea-treated type 2 diabetes. U.K. Prospective Diabetes Study Group. Diabetes Care 1998;21:87.

136. Bristol-Myers, Squibb Company. Glucophage Package Insert. April 2003.

137. Sambol NC et al. Kidney function and age are both predictors of pharmacokinetics of metformin. J Clin Pharmacol 1995;35:1094.

138. Gan SC et al. Biguanide associated lactic acidosis. Case report and review of the literature. Arch Intern Med 1992;152:2333.

139. Novartis Pharmaceuticals Corporation. Starlix Package Insert. November 2002.

140. Novo Nordisk Pharmaceuticals, Inc. Prandin Package Insert. October 2002.

141. Culy CR, Jarvis B. Repaglinide: a review of its therapeutic use in type 2 diabetes mellitus. Drugs 2001;61:1625.

142. Hatorp V. Clinical pharmacokinetics and pharmacodynamics of repaglinide. Clin Pharmacokinet 2002;41:471.

143. Hasslacher C. Safety and efficacy of repaglinide in type 2 diabetic patients with and without impaired renal function. Diabetes Care 2003;26:886.

144. Niemi M et al. Effects of gemfibrozil, itraconazole, and their combination on the pharmacokinetics and pharmacodynamics of repaglinide: potentially hazardous interaction between gemfibrozil and repaglinide. Diabetologia 2003;46:347.

145. Zimmerman BR. Sulfonylureas. Endocrinol Metab Clin North Am 1997;26:511.

146. Groop LC. Sulfonylureas in NIDDM. Diabetes Care 1992;15:737.

147. Marchetti P, Navalesi R. Pharmacokinetic-pharmacodynamic relationships of oral hypoglycaemic agents. An update. Clin Pharmacokinet 1989;16:100.

148. Groop LC et al. Effect of sulphonylurea on glucose-stimulated insulin secretion in healthy and non-insulin dependent diabetic subjects: a dose-response study. Acta Diabetol 1991;28:162.

149. Wahlin-Boll E et al. Impaired effect of sulfonylurea following increased dosage. Eur J Clin Pharmacol 1982;22:21.

150. Stenman S et al. What is the benefit of increasing the sulfonylurea dose? Ann Intern Med 1993; 118:169.

151. Wahlin-Boll E et al. Bioavailability, pharmacokinetics and effects of glipizide in type 2 diabetics. Clin Pharmacokinet 1982;7:363.

152. Jaber LA et al. Comparison of pharmacokinetics and pharmacodynamics of short- and long-term glyburide therapy in NIDDM. Diabetes Care 1994;17:1300.

153. Feldman JM. Glyburide: a second-generation sulfonylurea hypoglycemic agent. History, chemistry, metabolism, pharmacokinetics, clinical use and adverse effects. Pharmacotherapy 1985;5:43.

154. Faber OK et al. Acute actions of sulfonylurea drugs during long-term treatment of NIDDM. Diabetes Care 1990;13(Suppl 3):26.

155. Sonnenberg GE et al. Short-term comparison of once- versus twice-daily administration of glimepiride in patients with non-insulin-dependent diabetes mellitus. Ann Pharmacother 1997; 31:671.

156. Rosenkranz B. Pharmacokinetic basis for the safety of glimepiride in risk groups of NIDDM patients. Horm Metab Res 1996;28:434.

157. Draeger KE et al. Long-term treatment of type 2 diabetic patients with the new oral antidiabetic agent glimepiride (Amaryl): a double-blind comparison with glibenclamide. Horm Metab Res 1996;28:419.

158. Koda-Kimble MA, Rotblatt M. Diabetes mellitus. In: Young L, Koda-Kimble MA, eds. Applied Therapeutics. The Clinical Use of Drugs, 4th Ed. Vancouver, WA: Applied Therapeutics, 1988:1663.

159. Earley LE. Chlorpropamide antidiuresis. N Engl J Med 1971;284:103.

160. Spiegelman BM. PPAR-gamma: adipogenic regulator and thiazolidinedione receptor. Diabetes 1998;47:507.

161. Mudaliar S, Henry RR. New oral therapies for type 2 diabetes mellitus: The glitazones or insulin sensitizers. Annu Rev Med 2001;52:239.

162. Malinowski JM, Bolesta S. Rosiglitazone in the treatment of type 2 diabetes mellitus: a critical review. Clin Ther 2000;22:1151;discussion 1149.

163. Inzucchi SE. Oral antihyperglycemic therapy for type 2 diabetes: scientific review. JAMA 2002; 287:360.

164. Satoh N et al. Antiatherogenic effect of pioglitazone in type 2 diabetic patients irrespective of the responsiveness to its antidiabetic effect. Diabetes Care 2003;26:2493.

165. GlaxoSmithKline. Avandia Package Insert. March 2003.

166. Hanefeld M. Pharmacokinetics and clinical efficacy of pioglitazone. Int J Clin Pract Suppl 2001:19.

167. Takeda Pharmaceuticals America, Inc. and Eli Lilly and Company. Actos Package Insert. July 2002.

168. Saltiel AR, Olefsky JM. Thiazolidinediones in the treatment of insulin resistance and type II diabetes. Diabetes 1996;45:1661.

169. Al-Salman J et al. Hepatocellular injury in a patient receiving rosiglitazone. A case report. Ann Intern Med 2000;132:121.

170. Forman LM et al. Hepatic failure in a patient taking rosiglitazone. Ann Intern Med 2000;132:118.

171. Lebovitz HE et al. Evaluation of liver function in type 2 diabetic patients during clinical trials: evidence that rosiglitazone does not cause hepatic dysfunction. Diabetes Care 2002;25:815.

172. Henry RR. Thiazolidinediones. Endocrinol Metab Clin North Am 1997;26:553.

173. Niemeyer NV, Janney LM. Thiazolidinedione-induced edema. Pharmacotherapy. 2002;22:924.

174. Kelly IE et al. Effects of a thiazolidinedione compound on body fat and fat distribution of patients with type 2 diabetes. Diabetes Care 1999;22:288.

175. Winkler K et al. Pioglitazone reduces atherogenic dense LDL particles in nondiabetic patients with arterial hypertension: a double-blind, placebo-controlled study. Diabetes Care 2003;26:2588.

176. Tight blood pressure control and risk of macrovascular and microvascular complications in type 2 diabetes: UKPDS 38. UK Prospective Diabetes Study Group. Br Med J 1998;317:703.

177. Efficacy of atenolol and captopril in reducing risk of macrovascular and microvascular complications in type 2 diabetes: UKPDS 39. UK Prospective Diabetes Study Group. Br Med J 1998; 317:713.

178. Colwell JA. DCCT findings. Applicability and implications for NIDDM. Diabetes Res 1994:277.

179. Colwell JA. Should we use intensive insulin therapy after oral agent failure in type II diabetes? Diabetes Care 1996;19:896.

180. Henry RR, Genuth S. Forum One: Current recommendations about intensification of metabolic control in non-insulin-dependent diabetes mellitus. Ann Intern Med 1996;124:175.

181. Faas A et al. The efficacy of self-monitoring of blood glucose in NIDDM subjects. A criteria-based literature review. Diabetes Care 1997;20:1482.

182. Avignon A et al. Nonfasting plasma glucose is a better marker of diabetic control than fasting plasma glucose in type 2 diabetes. Diabetes Care 1997;20:1822.

183. Lebovitz HE. Stepwise and combination drug therapy for the treatment of NIDDM. Diabetes Care 1994;17:1542.

184. American Diabetes Association (ADA). The pharmacological treatment of hyperglycemia in NIDDM. Diabetes Care 1996;19(Suppl):54.

185. Nathan DM. Clinical practice. Initial management of glycemia in type 2 diabetes mellitus. N Engl J Med 2002;347:1342.

186. Charpentier G. Oral combination therapy for type 2 diabetes. Diabetes Metab Res Rev 2002; 18(Suppl 3):S70.

187. Gavin LA et al. Troglitazone add-on therapy to a combination of sulfonylureas plus metformin achieved and sustained effective diabetes control. Endocr Pract 2000;6:305.

188. Bell DS, Ovalle F. Long-term efficacy of triple oral therapy for type 2 diabetes mellitus. Endocr Pract 2002;8:271.

189. Kaye TB. Triple oral antidiabetic therapy. J Diabetes Complications 1998;12:311.

190. Schwartz S et al. Insulin 70/30 mix plus metformin versus triple oral therapy in the treatment of type 2 diabetes after failure of two oral drugs: efficacy, safety, and cost analysis. Diabetes Care 2003;26:2238.

191. Wright A et al. Sulfonylurea inadequacy: efficacy of addition of insulin over 6 years in patients with type 2 diabetes in the U.K. Prospective Diabetes Study (UKPDS 57). Diabetes Care 2002;25:330.

192. Turner R et al. United Kingdom Prospective Diabetes Study 17: a 9-year update of a randomized, controlled trial on the effect of improved metabolic control on complications in non-insulin-dependent diabetes mellitus. Ann Intern Med 1996;124:136–145.

193. Effect of intensive blood-glucose control with metformin on complications in overweight patients with type 2 diabetes (UKPDS 34). UK Prospective Diabetes Study (UKPDS) Group. Lancet 1998;352:854.

194. Melander A et al. Sulfonylureas. Why, which, and how? Diabetes Care 1990;13(Suppl 3):18.

195. Kradjan WA et al. Pharmacokinetics and pharmacodynamics of glipizide after once-daily and divided doses. Pharmacotherapy 1995;15:465.

196. Leahy JL. Natural history of beta-cell dysfunction in NIDDM. Diabetes Care 1990;13:992.

197. DeFronzo RA, Goodman AM. Efficacy of metformin in patients with non-insulin-dependent diabetes mellitus. The Multicenter Metformin Study Group. N Engl J Med 1995;333:541.

198. Fonseca V et al. Effect of metformin and rosiglitazone combination therapy in patients with type 2 diabetes mellitus: a randomized controlled trial. JAMA 2000;283:1695-1702.

199. Bell D, Mayo M. Outcome of metformin-facilitated reinitiation of oral diabetic therapy in insulin-treated patients with non-insulin-dependent diabetes mellitus. Endocrine Practice 1997:73.

200. White J. Combination oral agent/insulin therapy in patients with type II diabetes mellitus. Clin Diabetes 1997:102.

201. Johnson JL et al. Efficacy of insulin and sulfonylurea combination therapy in type II diabetes. A meta-analysis of the randomized placebo-controlled trials. Arch Intern Med 1996;156:259.

202. Yki-Jarvinen H. Combination therapies with insulin in type 2 diabetes. Diabetes Care 2001;24:758.

203. Yki-Jarvinen H. Combination therapy with insulin and oral agents: optimizing glycemic control in patients with type 2 diabetes mellitus. Diabetes Metab Res Rev 2002;18(Suppl 3):S77.

204. Yki-Jarvinen H et al. Comparison of insulin regimens in patients with non-insulin-dependent diabetes mellitus. N Engl J Med 1992;327:1426.

205. Fritsche A et al. Glimepiride combined with morning insulin glargine, bedtime neutral protamine hagedorn insulin, or bedtime insulin glargine in patients with type 2 diabetes. A randomized, controlled trial. Ann Intern Med 2003;138:952.

206. DeWitt DE, Hirsch IB. Outpatient insulin therapy in type 1 and type 2 diabetes mellitus: scientific review. JAMA 2003;289:2254.

207. Giugliano D et al. Metformin for obese, insulin-treated diabetic patients: improvement in glycaemic control and reduction of metabolic risk factors. Eur J Clin Pharmacol 1993;44:107.

208. McNulty et al. Comparison of metformin and sulfonylurea (glicazide) in combination with daily NPH insulin in type 2 diabetic patients inadequately controlled on maximal oral therapy [Abstract #0622]. Diabetes 1997:161A.

209. Yki-Jarvinen H et al. Comparison of bedtime insulin regimens in patients with type 2 diabetes mellitus. A randomized, controlled trial. Ann Intern Med 1999;130:389.

210. Rosenstock J et al. Efficacy and safety of pioglitazone in type 2 diabetes: a randomised, placebo-controlled study in patients receiving stable insulin therapy. Int J Clin Pract 2002;56:251.

211. Riddle MC. Tactics for type II diabetes. Endocrinol Metab Clin North Am 1997;26:659.

212. Genuth S. Management of the adult onset diabetic with sulfonylurea drug failure. Endocrinol Metab Clin North Am 1992;21:351.

213. DeWitt DE, Dugdale DC. Using new insulin strategies in the outpatient treatment of diabetes: clinical applications. JAMA 2003;289:2265.

214. Hayward RA et al. Starting insulin therapy in patients with type 2 diabetes: effectiveness, complications, and resource utilization. JAMA 1997; 278:1663.

215. Colwell JA. Controlling type 2 diabetes: are the benefits worth the costs? JAMA 1997;278:1700.

216. Anderson JH, Jr, et al. Mealtime treatment with insulin analog improves postprandial hyperglycemia and hypoglycemia in patients with non-insulin-dependent diabetes mellitus. Multicenter Insulin Lispro Study Group. Arch Intern Med 1997;157:1249.

217. Despres JP et al. Hyperinsulinemia as an independent risk factor for ischemic heart disease. N Engl J Med 1996;334:952.

218. Wingard DL et al. Is insulin really a heart disease risk factor. Diabetes Care 1995;18:1299.

219. Borders LM et al. Traditional insulin-use practices and the incidence of bacterial contamination and infection. Diabetes Care 1984;7:121.

220. Misbin RI et al. Lactic acidosis in patients with diabetes treated with metformin. N Engl J Med 1998;338:265.

221. Cusi K, DeFronzo R. Metformin: a review of its metabolic effects. Diabetes Review 1998;6:89.

222. University Group Diabetes Program: a study of the effects of hypoglycemic agents on vascular complications in patients with adult-onset diabetes I. Design, methods, and baseline results. Diabetes 1970:747.

223. Kilo C et al. The Achilles heel of the University Group Diabetes Program. JAMA 1980;243:450.

224. Sartor G et al. Ten-year follow-up of subjects with impaired glucose tolerance: prevention of diabetes by tolbutamide and diet regulation. Diabetes 1980;29:41.

225. Misbin RI. Phenformin-associated lactic acidosis; pathogenesis and treatment. Ann Intern Med 1977;87:591.

226. Phenformin: removal from the general market. FDA Drug Bull 1977;Aug:19.

227. Stang M et al. Incidence of lactic acidosis in metformin users. Diabetes Care 1999;22:925.

228. Emslie-Smith AM et al. Contraindications to metformin therapy in patients with Type 2 diabetes—a population-based study of adherence to prescribing guidelines. Diabet Med 2001;18:483.

229. Calabrese AT et al. Evaluation of prescribing practices: risk of lactic acidosis with metformin therapy. Arch Intern Med 2002;162:434.

230. Horlen C et al. Frequency of inappropriate metformin prescriptions. JAMA 2002;287:2504.

231. Masoudi FA et al. Metformin and thiazolidinedione use in Medicare patients with heart failure. JAMA 2003;290:81.

232. Swedko PJ et al. Serum creatinine is an inadequate screening test for renal failure in elderly patients. Arch Intern Med 2003;163:356.

233. Seltzer HS. Drug-induced hypoglycemia. A review of 1418 cases. Endocrinol Metab Clin North Am 1989;18:163.

234. Pearson JG et al. Pharmacokinetic disposition of 14C-glyburide in patients with varying renal function. Clin Pharmacol Ther 1986;39:318.

235. Gulati P et al. A double-blind trial of tolbutamide in cirrhosis of the liver. Am J Dig Dis 1967:42.

236. Ueda H et al. Disappearance rate of the tolbutamide in normal subjects and in diabetes mellitus, liver cirrhosis, and renal disease. Diabetes 1963:414.

237. Gambert SR. Atypical presentation of diabetes mellitus in the elderly. Clin Geriatr Med 1990;6:721.

238. Morley JE, Perry HM, 3rd. The management of diabetes mellitus in older individuals. Drugs 1991; 41:548.

239. Carlisle B. Diabetes in the elderly: factors to consider. Pharm Times 1992:130.

240. Matz R. Hyperosmolar Hyperosmolar Syndrome. In: Porte D, Jr, et al, eds. Ellenberg's and Rifkin's Diabetes Mellitus, 6th Ed. New York: McGraw-Hill, 2003:587.

241. Silver AJ, Morley JE. Role of the opioid system in the hypodipsia associated with aging. J Am Geriatr Soc 1992;40:556.

242. Morley JE. Diabetes mellitus in elderly patients. Is it different? Am J Med 1987;83:533.

243. Brown AF et al. Guidelines for improving the care of the older person with diabetes mellitus. J Am Geriatr Soc 2003;51:S265.

244. Mokdad AH et al. Prevalence of obesity, diabetes, and obesity-related health risk factors, 2001. JAMA 2003;289:76.

245. Hogikyan R, Halter J. Aging and Diabetes. In: Porte DS, RS, Baron A, eds. Ellenberg and Rifkin's Diabetes Mellitus, 6th Ed. New York: McGraw Hill, 2003:415.

246. Greenblatt DJ. Reduced serum albumin concentration in the elderly: a report from the Boston Collaborative Drug Surveillance Program. J Am Geriatr Soc 1979;27:20.

247. Shorr RI et al. Individual sulfonylureas and serious hypoglycemia in older people. J Am Geriatr Soc 1996;44:751.

248. Fajans S. Classification and diagnosis of diabetes. In: Porte D, Jr, Sherwin R, eds. Ellenberg's and Rifkin's Diabetes Mellitus, 5th Ed. Stamford, CT: Appleton & Lange, 1997:357.

249. Fajans SS et al. Molecular mechanisms and clinical pathophysiology of maturity-onset diabetes of the young. N Engl J Med 2001;345:971.

250. Arauz-Pacheco C et al. Hypertension management in adults with diabetes. Diabetes Care 2004;27(Suppl 1):S65.

251. Cooper ME, Johnston CI. Optimizing treatment of hypertension in patients with diabetes. JAMA 2000;283:3177.

252. Remuzzi G et al. Clinical practice. Nephropathy in patients with type 2 diabetes. N Engl J Med 2002;346:1145.

253. ADA Position Statement. Nephropathy in Diabetes. Diabetes Care 2004;27(Suppl 1):S79.

254. Ritz E, Orth SR. Nephropathy in patients with type 2 diabetes mellitus. N Engl J Med 1999;341:1127.

255. Lteif AA et al. Diabetes and heart disease an evidence-driven guide to risk factors management in diabetes. Cardiol Rev 2003;11:262.

256. Young L, Chyun D. Heart Disease in Patients with Diabetes. In: Porte DS, RS, Baron A, eds. Ellenberg and Rifkin's Diabetes Mellitus, 6th Ed. New York: McGraw-Hill, 2003:823.

257. Haffner SM. Dyslipidemia Management in adults with diabetes. Diabetes Care 2004;27(Suppl 1:S68.

258. Consensus development conference on the diagnosis of coronary heart disease in people with diabetes: 10-11 February 1998, Miami, Florida. American Diabetes Association. Diabetes Care 1998;21:1551.

259. Haffner SM et al. Reduced coronary events in simvastatin-treated patients with coronary heart disease and diabetes or impaired fasting glucose levels: subgroup analyses in the Scandinavian Simvastatin Survival Study. Arch Intern Med 1999;159:2661.

260. Sacks FM et al. The effect of pravastatin on coronary events after myocardial infarction in patients with average cholesterol levels. Cholesterol and Recurrent Events Trial investigators. N Engl J Med 1996;335:1001.

261. Goldberg RB et al. Cardiovascular events and their reduction with pravastatin in diabetic and glucose-intolerant myocardial infarction survivors with average cholesterol levels: subgroup analyses in the cholesterol and recurrent events (CARE) trial. The Care Investigators. Circulation 1998;98:2513.

262. Elam MB et al. Effect of niacin on lipid and lipoprotein levels and glycemic control in patients with diabetes and peripheral arterial disease: the ADMIT study: A randomized trial. Arterial Disease Multiple Intervention Trial. JAMA 2000;284:1263.

263. Grundy SM et al. Efficacy, safety, and tolerability of once-daily niacin for the treatment of dyslipidemia associated with type 2 diabetes: results of the assessment of diabetes control and evaluation of the efficacy of niaspan trial. Arch Intern Med 2002;162:1568.

264. Aiello LP et al. Diabetic retinopathy. Diabetes Care 1998;21:143.

265. Fong DS et al. Diabetic retinopathy. Diabetes Care 2004;27(Suppl 1):S84.

266. Vinik A et al. Recent advance in the diagnosis and treatment of diabetic neuropathy. Endocrinologist 1996:443.

267. Vinik A et al. Gastrointestinal, genitourinary, and neurovascular disturnbances in diabetes. Diabetes Review 1999:358.

268. Patterson D et al. A double-blind multicenter comparison of domperidone and metoclopramide in the treatment of diabetic patients with symptoms of gastroparesis. Am J Gastroenterol 1999;94:1230.

269. Boulton AJ et al. Guidelines for the diagnosis and outpatient management of diabetic peripheral neuropathy. Diabet Med 1998;15:508.

270. Malik R. Pathology and pathogenesis of diabetic neuropathy. Diabetes Review 1999:253.

271. Boulton AJ. Current and emerging treatment of diabetic neuropathies. Diabetes Review 1999:379.

272. Backonja M, Glanzman RL. Gabapentin dosing for neuropathic pain: evidence from randomized, placebo-controlled clinical trials. Clin Ther 2003;25:81.

273. Backonja M et al. Gabapentin for the symptomatic treatment of painful neuropathy in patients with diabetes mellitus: a randomized controlled trial. JAMA 1998;280:1831.

274. Eisenberg E et al. Lamotrigine reduces painful diabetic neuropathy: a randomized, controlled study. Neurology 2001;57:505.

275. Kline KM et al. Painful diabetic peripheral neuropathy relieved with use of oral topiramate. South Med J 2003;96:602.

276. Harati Y et al. Double-blind randomized trial of tramadol for the treatment of the pain of diabetic neuropathy. Neurology 1998;50:1842.

277. Harati Y et al. Maintenance of the long-term effectiveness of tramadol in treatment of the pain of diabetic neuropathy. J Diabetes Complications 2000;14:65

278. Mendell JR, Sahenk Z. Clinical practice. Painful sensory neuropathy. N Engl J Med 2003;348:1243.

279. Luscher TF et al. Diabetes and vascular disease: pathophysiology, clinical consequences, and medical therapy: Part II. Circulation 2003;108:1655.

280. Mayfield JA et al. Preventive foot care in diabetes. Diabetes Care 2004;27(Suppl 1):S63.

281. Shilling F. Foot care in patients with diabetes. Nurs Stand 2003;17:61, 66, 68.

282. ADA Position Statement. Aspirin Therapy in Diabetes. Diabetes Care 2004;27(Suppl 1):S72.

283. McMahon M et al. Effects of glucocorticoids on carbohydrate metabolism. Diabetes Metab Rev 1988;4:17.

284. Bressler P, DeFronzo RA. Drugs and diabetes. Diabetes Review 1994:53.

285. Gomez EC, Frost P. Induction of glycosuria and hyperglycemia by topical corticosteroid therapy. Arch Dermatol 1976;112:1559.

286. Davies D, ed. Textbook of Adverse Drug Reactions, 3rd Ed. Oxford: Oxford University Press, 1985.

287. Baker L et al. Hyperglycemia and acetonuria simulating diabetes. Phenylephrine associated hyperglycemia and acetonuria simulating diabetes mellitus. Am J Dis Child 1966;111:59.

288. Porte D, Jr. Sympathetic regulation of insulin secretion. Its relation to diabetes mellitus. Arch Intern Med 1969;123:252.

289. McDonald J. Alcohol and diabetes. Diabetes Care 1980;3:629.

290. Franz MJ. Diabetes mellitus: considerations in the development of guidelines for the occasional use of alcohol. J Am Diet Assoc 1983;83:147.

291. Farkas-Hirsch R. Intensive Diabetes Management. Alexandria, VA: American Diabetes Association, Inc., 1995:57.

292. Vaag A et al. Variation in absorption of NPH insulin due to intramuscular injection. Diabetes Care 1990;13:74.

293. Thow JC et al. Effect of raising injection-site skin temperature on isophane (NPH) insulin crystal dissociation. Diabetes Care 1989;12:432.

294. Salzman R et al. Intranasal aerosolized insulin. Mixed-meal studies and long-term use in type I diabetes. N Engl J Med 1985;312:1078.

295. Frauman AG et al. Long-term use of intranasal insulin in insulin-dependent diabetic patients. Diabetes Care 1987;10:573.

296. Koivisto VA. Various influences on insulin absorption. Neth J Med 1985;28(Suppl 1):25.

297. Selam JL, Charles MA. Devices for insulin administration. Diabetes Care 1990;13:955.

298. Eli Lilly & Company. Originally in Galloway JA et al, eds. Diabetes Mellitus, 9th Ed. Indianapolis, IN :Eli Lilly & Company, 1988.

299. ADA. Nutrition recommendations and principles for people with diabetes mellitus. Diabetes Care 2001:24(Suppl 1):S44.

300. How to inject your insulin. Patient education pamphlet #000-180pl Novo Nordisk Pharmaceuticals Inc., 1995.

EYE DISORDERS

Eye Disorders

Steven R. Abel, Suellyn J. Sorensen

Understanding primary ocular disorders requires some knowledge of ocular anatomy and physiology. Vaughan provides a comprehensive discussion in his text.[1] The following review will assist the practitioner in understanding conditions covered in this chapter.

OCULAR ANATOMY AND PHYSIOLOGY

The eyeball is approximately 1 inch wide and is highly complex. It is housed in the orbital cavity, which is formed by two bony orbits that serve as sockets that are lined with fat to pro-

tect the eyeball. Six ocular muscles allow for movement of the eyeball (Fig. 51-1).

The outer coat of the eye is made up of the sclera, conjunctiva, and cornea. The sclera is the white, dense, fibrous protective coating. A thin layer of loose connective tissue, the episclera, which contains blood vessels that nourish the sclera, covers it. The conjunctiva is a mucous membrane that covers the anterior portion of the eye and lines the eyelids. The cornea is the transparent, avascular tissue that functions as a refractive and protective window membrane through which light rays pass en route to the retina. The

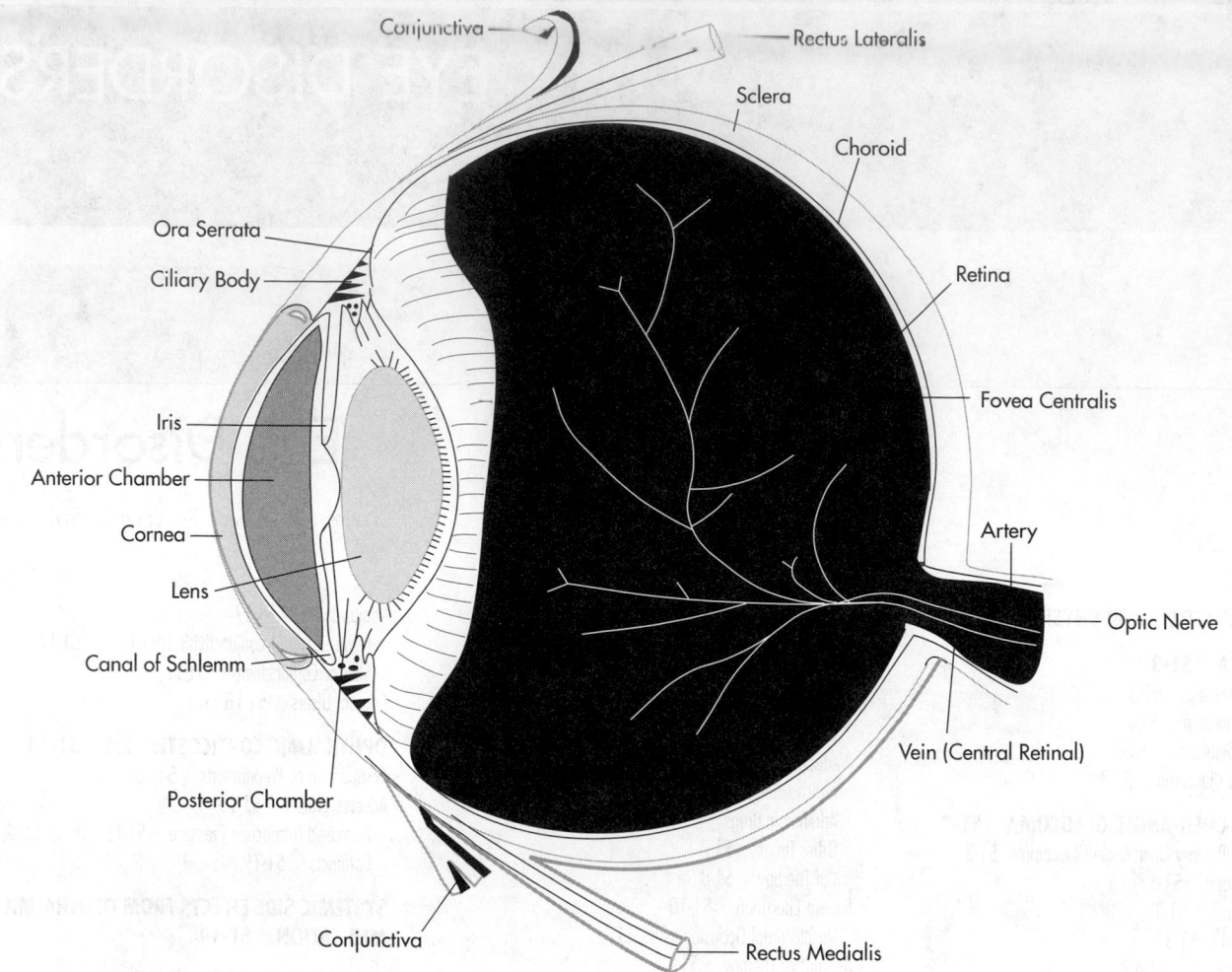

FIGURE 51-1 Anatomy of the human eye. (Adapted from artwork courtesy of Burroughs Wellcome.)

corneal epithelium and endothelium are lipophilic, and the centrally located stroma is hydrophilic. These three corneal layers are particularly important because they affect drug penetration through the cornea. The best penetration through the intact cornea is accomplished with biphasic preparations or those that are both fat- and water-soluble.

The choroid, ciliary body, and iris are known collectively as the uveal tract. The iris is a colored, circular membrane suspended between the cornea and the crystalline lens. It controls the amount of light that enters the eye. The choroid lies between the sclera and retina. It is largely made up of blood vessels, which nourish the retina. The ciliary body is adherent to the sclera and contains the ciliary muscle and ciliary processes. The ciliary muscle contracts and relaxes the zonular fibers, which hold the crystalline lens in place. The ciliary processes are responsible for the secretion of aqueous humor, a clear liquid that occupies the anterior chamber. The anterior chamber is bounded anteriorly by the cornea and posteriorly by the iris; the posterior chamber lies between the posterior iris and the crystalline lens.

The inner segment of the eye contains the retina with the optic nerve. The retina contains all sensory receptors for light transmission. The optic nerve transmits visual impulses from the retina to the brain.

The crystalline lens, aqueous humor, and vitreous assist the cornea with the process of refraction. The lens has an inner nucleus, which is surrounded by the cortex. An outer capsule, in turn, envelops this. Disorders involving the aqueous humor are discussed in the section on glaucoma. The primary function of the vitreous is to maintain the shape of the eye.

The eyelids and eyelashes are the outermost means of protection for the eye. The eyelids contain various sebaceous and sweat glands, which may become infected or inflamed, contributing to many ocular disorders.

The eye is innervated by both the sympathetic and parasympathetic nervous systems. Parasympathetic fibers originating from the oculomotor nerve in the brain innervate the ciliary muscle and sphincter pupillae muscle, which constricts the pupil. Therefore, parasympathomimetic (cholinergic) agents cause miosis (pupillary contraction), and parasympatholytic (anticholinergic) agents cause mydriasis (pupillary dilation) and cycloplegia. Cycloplegia is paralysis of the ciliary muscle and zonules that results in decreased accommodation (adjustment of the lens curvature for various distances) and blurred vision. Tear secretion by the lacrimal glands also is a parasympathetic function.

Sympathetic fibers from the superior cervical ganglion in the spinal cord innervate the dilator pupillae muscle, the

EYE DISORDERS · **51-3**

blood vessels of the ciliary body, the episclera, and the extraocular muscles. Sympathomimetics cause mydriasis without affecting accommodation. The exact role of the sympathetic nervous system in glaucoma and its treatment is not understood fully.

GLAUCOMA

Glaucoma is a leading cause of blindness worldwide. It consists of progressive irreversible optic nerve damage resulting in visual field loss. Glaucoma is not always associated with an elevation in intraocular pressure (IOP). However, elevated IOPs are a risk factor for the development of glaucoma. The higher the IOP, the greater the risk for developing glaucoma. Other risk factors include increasing age, African-American race, family history, thinner central corneas, and larger vertical cup–disk ratios. An estimated 2% of all individuals older than 40 have glaucoma. However, it may occur in other age groups, including children.[1,2]

Intraocular Pressure

IOP is influenced by the production of aqueous humor by the ciliary processes and the outflow of aqueous humor through the trabecular meshwork. Applanation tonometry is used to measure the IOP and is based on the pressure required to flatten a small area of the central cornea. Generally, an IOP of 10 to 20 mm Hg is considered normal. An IOP of 22 mm Hg or higher should arouse suspicion of glaucoma, although a more rare form of glaucoma is associated with a low IOP.

Ocular Hypertension

Ocular hypertension has been defined as an IOP greater than 21 mm Hg, normal visual fields, normal optic discs, open angles, and the absence of any ocular disease contributing to the elevation of IOP. Only a small percentage of patients with ocular hypertension develop open-angle glaucoma. A pathologic cupping of the optic nerve occurs with glaucoma so that diagnosis often can be made by inspection of the optic disc with an ophthalmoscope. Other provocative and confirmatory tests for open-angle glaucoma include tonography and a water-drinking test, but these are used rarely.

Open-Angle Glaucoma

Open-angle glaucoma occurs in about 0.4% to 0.7% of people older than 40 and in 2% to 3% of people older than 70.[1] In primary open-angle glaucoma (POAG), aqueous humor outflow from the anterior chamber is constantly subnormal primarily because of a degenerative process in the trabecular meshwork. The IOP may vary in the course of a day from normal to significantly elevated pressures.[1] The decreased outflow appears to be caused by degenerative changes in outflow channels, such as the trabecular meshwork and Schlemm's canal and tends to worsen with the passage of time.[1] In rare cases, the outflow is normal even during a phase of elevated IOP, and the elevation appears to be to the result of hypersecretion of aqueous humor.[1]

The onset of POAG usually is gradual and asymptomatic. A defect in the visual field examination may be present in early glaucoma, but loss of peripheral vision usually is not seen until late in the course of the disease. Visual field defects correlate well with changes in the optic disc and help differentiate glaucoma from ocular hypertension in patients with increased IOP. Studies indicate that patients with normal visual fields and an IOP between 22 and 30 mm Hg have no greater than a 5% likelihood of developing visual field loss over periods of up to 10 years.[1]

Angle-Closure Glaucoma

Examination of the anterior chamber angle by gonioscopy, using a corneal contact lens, magnifying device (e.g., a slit-lamp microscope), and light source, assists in differentiating between open-angle glaucoma and angle-closure glaucoma. Angle-closure glaucoma accounts for approximately 5% of all primary glaucoma. In angle-closure glaucoma, there is no abnormal resistance to aqueous humor outflow. The sole cause of the elevated IOP is closure of the anterior chamber angle.[1]

Angle-closure glaucoma, a medical emergency, usually presents as an acute attack with a rapid increase in IOP, blurring or sudden loss of vision, appearance of haloes around lights, and pain that is often severe. Patients predisposed to angle-closure glaucoma should not have their pupils dilated during an ophthalmic examination and should be educated regarding the signs and symptoms of angle closure. Acute attacks may terminate without treatment, but if the IOP remains high, irreparable damage to the optic nerve may occur.[1] In chronic angle closure, the closure is gradual and the patient may be asymptomatic until the glaucoma is in an advanced state.[1] Permanent medical management of acute or chronic angle closure is difficult, and surgical procedures, such as peripheral iridectomies, often are required to improve the prognosis.

PRIMARY OPEN-ANGLE GLAUCOMA
Therapeutic Agents for Treatment of Primary Open-Angle Glaucoma
Initial Therapy
β-BLOCKERS

All of the ocular β-blockers (timolol, levobunolol, metipranolol, carteolol, betaxolol) have the same basic mechanism of action. Ophthalmic β-blockers block the β-adrenergic receptors in the ciliary epithelium of the eye and lower IOP by decreasing aqueous humor production. Some studies have demonstrated a slight effect on the facility of outflow, but this does not seem to be significant.[3,4]

Timolol (Timoptic)

Timolol, a nonselective β_1- and β_2-adrenergic antagonist, is the most commonly prescribed glaucoma medication. It was the first ocular β-blocker marketed; therefore, all of the newer ophthalmic β-blockers are compared with timolol for safety and effectiveness. Concentrations or dosages exceeding one drop of timolol 0.5% BID do not produce further significant decreases in IOP.[5] Therapy usually is initiated with a 0.25% solution administered as one drop BID. Monocular administration of timolol has resulted in equal bilateral IOP reduction and may reduce the cost of therapy and side effects in some patients.[6] An escape phenomenon, or tachyphylaxis, can occur with timolol.

If a patient has a large initial decrease in IOP, the IOP often stabilizes at a lesser reduction in approximately 4 to 6 weeks.[7,8] Timolol is safe and effective in both adult and pediatric patients.[9,10] Timolol is at least as effective as pilocarpine and epinephrine and may be more efficacious in diurnal IOP control.[11,12]

Timolol has been associated with a reduction of resting pulse rate and worsening of congestive heart failure (CHF), although the change in pulse rate generally is slight (5 to 8 beats/minute).[13,14] Pulmonary effects such as dyspnea, airway obstruction, and pulmonary failure also have occurred.[15,16] Timolol can produce corneal anesthesia after chronic administration in susceptible individuals.[17,18] Uveitis has been reported in patients receiving ophthalmic timolol; however, a cause-and-effect relationship has not been established.[19,20]

Systemic absorption of timolol has been studied in rabbits and humans after topical administration.[21,22] Plasma levels of timolol were not detected in most human subjects after topical administration, but a level of 9.6 ng/mL was detected in one subject.[22] In 10 patients older than 60 years of age receiving chronic topical timolol therapy, the baseline mean plasma timolol level was 0.34 ng/mL and increased to 1.34 ng/mL 1 hour after administration of one drop of 0.5% timolol.[23] With punctal occlusion, the mean 1-hour plasma timolol level decreased to 0.9 ng/mL.

The β-blocking plasma concentration of timolol has been estimated to be about 5 to 10 ng/mL.[8] Although systemic absorption after topical administration does not appear to be significant in most cases, care should be taken when timolol is used in patients with sinus bradycardia, CHF (see Chapter 19, Heart Failure), or pulmonary disease. Systemic side effects may be exaggerated in the elderly secondary to inadvertent overdosing associated with poor administration technique (see Question 3).

A breast milk sample from a nursing mother was obtained 1½ hours after administration of one drop of 0.5% topical timolol.[24] The drug level in the breast milk was 5.6 ng/mL versus a concomitant plasma concentration of 0.93 ng/mL. Therefore, timolol should be used cautiously in nursing mothers.

Timoptic XE

Timoptic XE is a timolol ophthalmic gel-forming solution that is administered once daily. The ophthalmic vehicle, gellan gum (Gelrite), is a solution that forms a clear gel in the presence of mono or divalent cations.[25] This ion-activated gelation prolongs precorneal residence time and increases ocular bioavailability, allowing timolol to be administered once daily.[25] A 24-week study compared Timoptic XE 0.5% once daily with Timoptic solution 0.5% twice daily and found both formulations to be equally effective in lowering IOP.[26]

Levobunolol (Betagan)

Levobunolol, another nonselective β-adrenergic antagonist, can decrease IOP on average about 9 mm Hg with either the 0.5% or 1% solutions and is approved for both QD or BID administration.[27,28] When levobunolol 0.5% QD was compared with BID administration, both regimens reduced IOP similarly.[29] When levobunolol 0.5% and 1% BID was compared with timolol 0.5% BID, ocular hypotensive effects, incidence of adverse reactions, and slight to significant decreases in heart rate were noted for both agents.[30,31] In one 3-month study, levobunolol QD was more effective than timolol at various concentrations[32]; however, in another study both timolol 0.25% and levobunolol 0.25% QD were equally effective.[33] Levobunolol can be more expensive than timolol (depending on negotiated contract purchase prices) whether it is administered once or twice daily.[34]

Metipranolol (Optipranolol)

Another nonselective β-blocking agent, metipranolol 0.1% to 0.6%, is comparable to timolol 0.25% to 0.5% in reducing IOP in patients with open-angle glaucoma.[35,36] Single-dose metipranolol 0.1% and 0.3% and timolol 0.25% did not significantly change resting heart rate or the resting or exercise mean blood pressure,[37] but timolol significantly reduced exercise tachycardia. Metipranolol 0.6% and levobunolol 0.5% BID reduced IOP by about 7 mm Hg (29%), and neither significantly reduced heart rate or blood pressure[38] Metipranolol is associated with a greater incidence of stinging or burning upon administration than other ophthalmic β-blockers. Topical metipranolol appears to offer no advantage over timolol or levobunolol in the treatment of glaucoma.

Like timolol, metipranolol produces corneal anesthesia, which occurs within 1 minute of instillation and returns to baseline after 10 minutes.[18] Metipranolol has been withdrawn from clinical use in the United Kingdom because it has been associated with granulomatous anterior uveitis. Although this adverse effect was initially attributed to its irradiated plastic containers,[39] metipranolol subsequently was deemed to be the responsible agent for these inflammatory reactions.[40] A significant secondary elevation (57.6%) in IOP occurred in patients with metipranolol-associated adverse reactions.[41] Although metipranolol may be cost-effective, its higher association with ocular burning and stinging and granulomatous anterior uveitis limit its use.

Carteolol (Ocupress)

Carteolol is a nonselective β-blocking agent with partial β-agonist activity, which theoretically should minimize the bronchospastic, bradycardic, and hypotensive effects associated with other ocular β-blockers.[42] When the cardiovascular and pulmonary function effects of carteolol were compared with timolol, no clinical difference was noted. Carteolol 1% and timolol 0.25% administered BID are equally effective in reducing IOP.[43–45]

Betaxolol (Betoptic)

In contrast to all the other β-blocker ophthalmic products, betaxolol is a selective β₁-adrenergic blocker. Betaxolol 0.125% to 0.5% can reduce IOP up to 35%.[46] In comparative studies, betaxolol 0.5% and timolol 0.5% BID decreased IOP with similar side-effect profiles including slight, but insignificant, decreases in systolic and diastolic blood pressure (BP).[46–48] In these studies, timolol was slightly, but not significantly, more effective in decreasing IOP, with fewer patients requiring adjunctive therapy for adequate IOP control. In another study, timolol 0.25% and 0.5% consistently and significantly decreased median IOP more than comparable doses of betaxolol and more of the betaxolol-treated patients required adjunctive therapy.[49]

α₂-ADRENERGIC AGONISTS

Apraclonidine (Iopidine) and brimonidine (Alphagan) are selective α₂-adrenergic agonists similar to clonidine. Apraclonidine is less lipophilic than clonidine and brimonidine; does not cross the blood-brain barrier as readily; and, theoretically, has less systemic side effects (e.g., hypotension, decreased pulse, dry mouth). Brimonidine is more highly selective for α₂-adrenergic receptors than clonidine or apraclonidine and theoretically should be associated with less ocular side effects. α₂-Adrenergic agonists appear to lower IOP by decreasing the production of aqueous humor and by increasing uveoscleral outflow.[88]

Brimonidine is an alternative first-line agent in the treatment of POAG. It may also be used as adjunctive therapy in patients not responding to other agents. Apraclonidine 1% is indicated to control or prevent postsurgical elevations in IOP after argon laser trabeculoplasty or iridotomy. The 0.5% apraclonidine solution is indicated for short-term adjunctive therapy in patients on maximally tolerated medical therapy. Long-term IOP control should be monitored closely in patients on α₂-adrenergic agonists because tachyphylaxis can occur. Common ocular side effects include burning, stinging, blurring, conjunctival follicles, and an allergic-like reaction consisting of hyperemia, pruritus, edema of the lid and conjunctiva, and foreign body sensation. Although, ocular side effects are less common with brimonidine than with apraclonidine, systemic side effects (e.g., dry nose and mouth, mild hypotension, decreased pulse, and lethargy) are more common with brimonidine. α₂-Adrenergic agonists should be used with caution in patients with cardiovascular disease, orthostatic hypotension, depression, and renal or hepatic dysfunction.[88,89] Brimondine is now available with purite as a preservative which facilitates drug delivery into the eye allowing use of a lower drug concentration.

The IOP-reduction effects (peak and trough) of brimonidine 0.2% BID is 14% to 28%. Although the approved dosing schedule of brimonidine is TID, brimonidine 0.2% BID lowers IOP comparably to timolol 0.5% BID, and both are slightly better than betaxolol 0.25% BID.[50,54,89] The IOP-lowering effect of brimonidine also may be comparable to that of latanoprost; however, conflicting efficacy and tolerability results in clinical studies may be related to differences in study design.[51] The combination of brimonidine and timolol are equally tolerable and effective as the combination of dorzolamide and timolol.[52] Brimonidine does have a role as adjunctive therapy in the treatment of glaucoma; however, the effect of combination therapy is usually less than the sum of both drugs when used individually.

TOPICAL CARBONIC ANHYDRASE INHIBITORS

Carbonic anhydrase occurs in high concentrations in the ciliary processes and retina of the eye. Carbonic anhydrase inhibitors (CAIs) lower IOP is by decreasing bicarbonate production and, therefore, the flow of bicarbonate, sodium, and water into the posterior chamber of the eye resulting in a 40% to 60% decrease in aqueous humor secretion.

Although CAIs have been used orally for many years in the treatment of elevated IOPs, they rarely were used because of significant side effects. The introduction of the safer topical ophthalmic CAIs, dorzolamide (Trusopt) and brinzolamide (Azopt), has increased the use of this medication class.

Topical CAIs are excellent alternatives to β-blockers in the initial management of elevated IOPs, and are effective as adjunctive agents. Brinzolamide 1% TID reduces IOP comparably to that achieved with dorzolamide 2% TID and to betaxolol 0.5% BID, but slightly less than timolol 0.5% BID. The IOP-reduction effects (peak and trough) of dorzolamide 2% TID is 16% to 25%. Brinzolamide and dorzolamide are approved for TID dosing; however, BID dosing may be adequate. As mentioned above, dorzolamide provides additional IOP-lowering effects when added to existing β-blocker therapy.[53,55] The combined use of topical dorzolamide and oral acetazolamide does not result in additive effects and may increase the risk of toxicity. Therefore, the concomitant use of topical and oral CAIs is not advised.[56–58]

The topical CAIs are well tolerated with few systemic side effects. The most common adverse effects reported with dorzolamide are ocular burning, stinging, discomfort and allergic reactions, bitter taste, and superficial punctate keratitis. Brinzolamide causes less burning and stinging of the eyes than dorzolamide because its pH more closely resembles that of human tears. Dorzolamide and brinzolamide are sulfonamides and may cause the same types of adverse reactions attributable to sulfonamides. These drugs should not be used in patients with renal or hepatic impairment.

PROSTAGLANDIN ANALOGS

Latanoprost (Xalatan), travoprost (Travatan), bimatoprost (Lumigan), and unoprostone (Rescula) are all prostaglandin analogs. Latanoprost and travoprost are analogs of prostaglandin F_α and they lower intraocular pressure by serving as selective prostaglandin F_{2α} receptor agonists. Bimatoprost is a synthetic prostamide analog and unoprostone is a docosanoid, which is an omega-3 polyunsaturated fatty acid analog of a derivative of docosahexaenoic acid. The prostaglandin analogs increase uveoscleral outflow of aqueous humor and thereby decrease IOP.[59]

Latanoprost

Latanoprost (Xalatan) is approved for the initial treatment of POAG or ocular hypertension.[60] When administered once daily in the evening, latanoprost is at least as effective as timolol in decreasing IOP. When the effectiveness of latanoprost 0.005% QD was compared with timolol 0.5% BID, the IOP-lowering effects of latanoprost were superior to timolol.[61,62] In addition, the nocturnal control of IOP was better with latanoprost than with timolol. Latanoprost 0.005% should be dosed once daily in the evening because the IOP-lowering effects of latanoprost may actually be inferior when administered more frequently.

Minimal systemic side effects are seen with latanoprost, but local reactions that are relatively common include iris pigmentation that may be permanent; eyelid skin darkening; eyelash lengthening, thickening, pigmentation, and misdirected growth; conjunctival hyperemia; ocular irritation; and superficial punctate keratitis. Latanoprost causes a gradual increase in the amount of brown pigment in the iris by increasing the melanin content in the stromal melanocytes of the iris. This pigment change occurs in 7% to 22% of patients and is most noticeable in those with green-brown, blue/gray-brown, or yellow-brown eyes.[60,61] Latanoprost has maintained effective IOP lowering effects for up to 2 years in clinical studies and adverse consequences of increased iris pigmentation were not evident. The onset of noticeable increased iris pigmentation usually occurred within the first year of treatment and continued to be present throughout the 5 years of one study. The nature or severity of adverse events were not affected by the increased iris pigmentation; however, effects of increased pigmentation beyond 5 years are unknown.

Latanoprost has additive effects when administered with timolol, dorzolamide, acetazolamide, α_2-adrenergic agonists, and dipivefrin. The additional IOP-lowering effects of latanoprost when added to existing therapy ranges from 2.9 to 6.1 mm Hg. Therefore, latanoprost is a rational choice when selecting adjunctive therapy in patients who are unresponsive to other agents. The adjunctive IOP-lowering effects of latanoprost are comparable to those of brimonidine (at least a 15% reduction in IOP) in patients uncontrolled on β-blockers; however, brimonidine was better tolerated with fewer adverse quality of life effects. Watery or teary eyes and cold hands and feet were reported more frequently in latanoprost-treated patients.[63] The excellent effects seen with mono- and adjunctive therapy, the relative tolerability and once-daily administration makes latanoprost an important treatment option in POAG and ocular hypertension.[62,64–66]

Travoprost

Travoprost (Travatan) is FDA approved for the reduction of elevated IOP in patients who are intolerant to other agents. The lack of long-term safety data relating to the increased iris pigmentation with the newer prostaglandin analogs prevented the FDA from granting an initial therapy indication. Travoprost is used as a first-line agent in clinical practice because it is more effective than timolol and at least as effective as latanoprost. The mean IOP reduction with travoprost in African-American patients was 1.8 mm Hg greater than in non–African-American patients. It is not yet known whether this difference is because of race or darker iris pigmentation. This finding can be clinically significant because African Americans have a high incidence of glaucoma. Travoprost, as adjunctive therapy to timolol in patients not responding adequately to timolol alone, reduced IOP an additional 6 to 7 mm Hg. The side-effect profile of travoprost is similar to latanoprost including increased iris pigmentation and eyelash changes.[67–69]

Bimatoprost

Like travoprost, bimatoprost (Lumigan) QD and BID achieved lower target IOPs than did timolol BID. Bimatoprost BID, however, was less effective than bimatoprost QD. Iris pigmentation changed in 1.1% of bimatoprost-treated patients. In a 6-month randomized multicenter study, bimatoprost once a day lowered IOP more effectively than latanoprost once a day. Side effects were similar between treatment groups; however, conjunctiva hyperemia was more common ($P < .001$) in bimatoprost treated patients. Overall, the side effect profile of bimatoprost appears to be similar to latanoprost and travoprost.[70–72]

Unoprostone

Unoprostone (Rescula) 0.15% is approved as a twice-daily topical medication for the treatment of POAG or ocular hypertension in patients who do not tolerate or respond to other agents. When compared with timolol BID and latanoprost QD, the IOP-lowering effects of unoprostone were slightly less than timolol and significantly less than latanoprost. Iris and eyelid hyperpigmentation from unoprostone have been reported infrequently. Some attribute the paucity of these adverse events to the short-term nature of the studies; the predominately brown eyes of patients enrolled in these studies, and the low affinity of unoprostone for the prostaglandin $F_{2\alpha}$ receptor. Unoprostone may have a limited role in clinical use compared with other prostaglandin analogs because of its lower effectiveness and BID administration.[73–76]

PILOCARPINE

Pilocarpine (IsoptoCarpine) historically was an initial treatment of choice, but with the introduction and widespread use of newer agents, pilocarpine has fallen out of favor as an initial treatment. Therapy usually is begun using lower concentrations (0.5% to 1%), such as one drop QID. Pilocarpine is a direct-acting cholinergic (parasympathomimetic) that causes contraction of ciliary muscle fibers attached to the trabecular meshwork and scleral spur. This opens the trabecular meshwork to enhance aqueous humor outflow. There also may be a direct effect on the trabecular meshwork. Pilocarpine causes miosis by contraction of the iris sphincter muscle, but the miosis is not related to the decrease in IOP.

EPINEPHRINE

Epinephrine (Glaucon, Eppy/N, Epitrate) is a sympathomimetic that stimulates both α- and β-receptors. The β-adrenergic stimulation is responsible for increasing aqueous humor outflow and is the probable basis of epinephrine's ability to lower IOP.[77,78] In contrast, the β-adrenergic blockers decrease aqueous humor production. The α-adrenergic effect of epinephrine predominantly decreases the inflow of aqueous humor, which is not as significant as the increase in aqueous humor outflow.[77,78] When used alone, epinephrine produces a 30% to 35% decrease in the rate of aqueous humor production, whereas use in conjunction with CAIs may produce a 65% to 70% decrease. As with timolol, patients in whom systemic effects could potentiate pre-existing problems should be monitored closely. Dipivefrin is an epinephrine prodrug that is better tolerated and absorbed than epinephrine. It is usually the preferred product when agents from this class are indicated. Dipivefrin or epinephrine are often used in younger patients or patients with cataracts in which miosis and the resultant decreased vision from cholinergic agents are a problem. Both are second-line drugs in the therapy of POAG and are used most often as second agents in combination regimens rather than as monotherapy.

CARBACHOL

Carbachol (IsoptoCarbachol) is reserved as a third-line agent in patients who are unresponsive or intolerant to initial medications. In addition to having direct cholinergic effects, carbachol is more resistant to cholinesterase than pilocarpine. Added benefits include increased release of acetylcholine from parasympathetic nerve terminals and a weak anticholinesterase effect. Carbachol is administered three times a day.

ANTICHOLINESTERASE AGENTS

If control of IOP is not achieved with optimal use of other topical monotherapy and combination therapy agents, then anticholinesterase agents may be prescribed as a last topical therapy option. Anticholinesterase agents inhibit the enzyme cholinesterase, thereby increasing the amount of acetylcholine and its naturally occurring cholinergic effects.

Echothiophate Iodide

Phospholine iodide (Phospholine Iodide) is an irreversible cholinesterase inhibitor that primarily inactivates pseudocholinesterase and secondarily inhibits true cholinesterase. Echothiophate iodide is the most widely used cholinesterase inhibitor for open-angle glaucoma and can be used if maximal doses of other agents and combination therapy are ineffective. Echothiophate iodide has a long duration of action that affords good control of IOP; however, miosis and myopia are significant side effects. Concentrations higher than 0.06% are associated with a significant increase in subjective complaints (e.g., brow ache).[79]

Combination Therapy

In general, drugs with different pharmacologic actions have at least partially additive effects in lowering IOP in the treatment of glaucoma. Drugs with similar pharmacologic actions (i.e., from the same pharmacologic class) should not be combined because dose-related adverse effects are more likely and the incremental increase in benefits is likely to be more modest.

Timolol and other β-adrenergic blocking drugs have additive IOP-lowering effects when used in combination with epinephrine,[80] dipivefrin,[80,81] miotics, prostaglandin analogs,[63,74] α₂-agonists,[82] and CAIs.[83–85] More specifically, for example, the IOP-lowering effect is greater when timolol is used in combination with pilocarpine,[62,86] dorzolamide,[86] brimonidine,[63,82,87] and travoprost.[62,67] Likewise, for example, latanoprost has additive effects when administered with timolol,[62,67] dorzolamide,[64,65] α₂-adrenergic agonists,[63,64,87] and dipivefrin.[62,64–66] Other combinations of drugs also provide additive effects when used in combination for the management of increased intraocular pressure.

Predisposing Factors

1. M.H., a 52-year-old African-American woman with brown eyes, presented for routine ophthalmic examination. Visual acuity without correction was 20/40 OD (right eye) and 20/80 OS (left eye). Tonometry measured an IOP of 36 mm Hg OU (both eyes). Ophthalmoscopy revealed physiologic cupping of the optic discs OU, and visual field examination revealed a nerve fiber bundle defect consistent with glaucoma. Pupils were normal OU, and gonioscopy indicated that anterior chamber angles were open OU. There were no signs of cataract formation. M.H. related a positive family history for glaucoma and presently is being treated for hypertension, CHF, and asthma. Her medications include the following:

Amitriptyline	75 mg QHS
Chlorpheniramine	4 mg Q 6 hr PRN
Digoxin	0.25 mg QD
Furosemide	40 mg BID
Nitroglycerin	1/150 g SL PRN
Theophylline SR	300 mg Q 12 hr

Findings on examination indicate that M.H. has POAG. What other factors may predispose M.H. to an increased IOP?

POAG is thought to be determined genetically, and M.H. has a positive family history. The disease is more prevalent and aggressive in African Americans.[1] In addition, she is taking several medications that have been associated with increases in IOP.

Anticholinergic Drugs

Most reports dealing with drug-induced increases in IOP center around precipitation of angle-closure glaucoma by topical mydriatic/cycloplegic agents (anticholinergics). In patients with open-angle glaucoma, topical anticholinergics can significantly increase resistance to aqueous humor outflow and elevate IOP while the anterior chamber remains grossly open.[2] As part of any routine ophthalmic examination, the pupils are dilated with a mydriatic/cycloplegic (unless otherwise contraindicated). The IOP is always measured before this procedure, so the use of these agents would not have influenced the IOP readings in M.H.

If systemic anticholinergic agents are administered in doses sufficient to cause pupillary dilation, the risk of precipitating angle-closure increases. However, it is unlikely that these agents will aggravate open-angle glaucoma unless the amount reaching the eye is sufficient to cause cycloplegia.[2] Although literature documentation of POAG exacerbation by these agents is scarce, medications with anticholinergic side effects (antihistamines, benzodiazepines, disopyramide, phenothiazines, tricyclic antidepressants) should be considered. M.H. is receiving chlorpheniramine as needed (PRN) and amitriptyline at bedtime (HS), but her pupil examination is normal with no evidence of mydriasis or cycloplegia. Therefore, it is highly unlikely that these medications contributed to her increased IOP.

Adrenergic Drugs

Adrenergic agents, such as central nervous system (CNS) stimulants, vasoconstrictors, appetite suppressants, and bronchodilators, may produce minimal pupillary dilation. These have no proven adverse influences on IOP in patients with either normal eyes or eyes with open-angle glaucoma. Consequently, the use of theophylline in M.H. is also an unlikely source of the increased IOP.

Other Drugs

No conclusive evidence for the production of angle-closure glaucoma by vasodilators has ever been published, although slight increases in IOP have been reported. Use of nitroglycerin (NTG) as needed in M.H. is not a cause for concern. There have been isolated reports of other medications causing mydriasis in glaucoma patients. These include muscle relaxants (carisoprodol), monoamine oxidase inhibitors, fenfluramine, ganglionic blocking agents, salicylates, oral contraceptives, and chlorpropamide (Diabinese). Succinylcholine, ketamine, and caffeine have been associated with increases in IOP. α-Chymotrypsin has been reported to increase IOP in patients who have received the medication during operative procedures; these patients' outflow channels probably were obstructed by debris generated from use of the enzyme.[51] Corticosteroid-induced IOP elevation is discussed in Question 13. If M.H. require administration of any other medications associated with increases in IOP, potential adverse effects may be avoided by routine follow-up.

Initial Therapy

2. **What is the best initial therapeutic treatment in M.H.?**

Topical β-blockers are the initial agents of choice in the treatment of POAG (Fig. 51-2). β-Blockers are used most fre-

quently in the treatment of POAG. Their efficacy is well documented in numerous studies, and side effects are well characterized. Brimonidine (Alphagan), topical CAIs, and prostaglandin analogs are alternative first-line agents (Table 51-1 lists the topical agents commonly used in the treatment of primary open angle glaucoma).

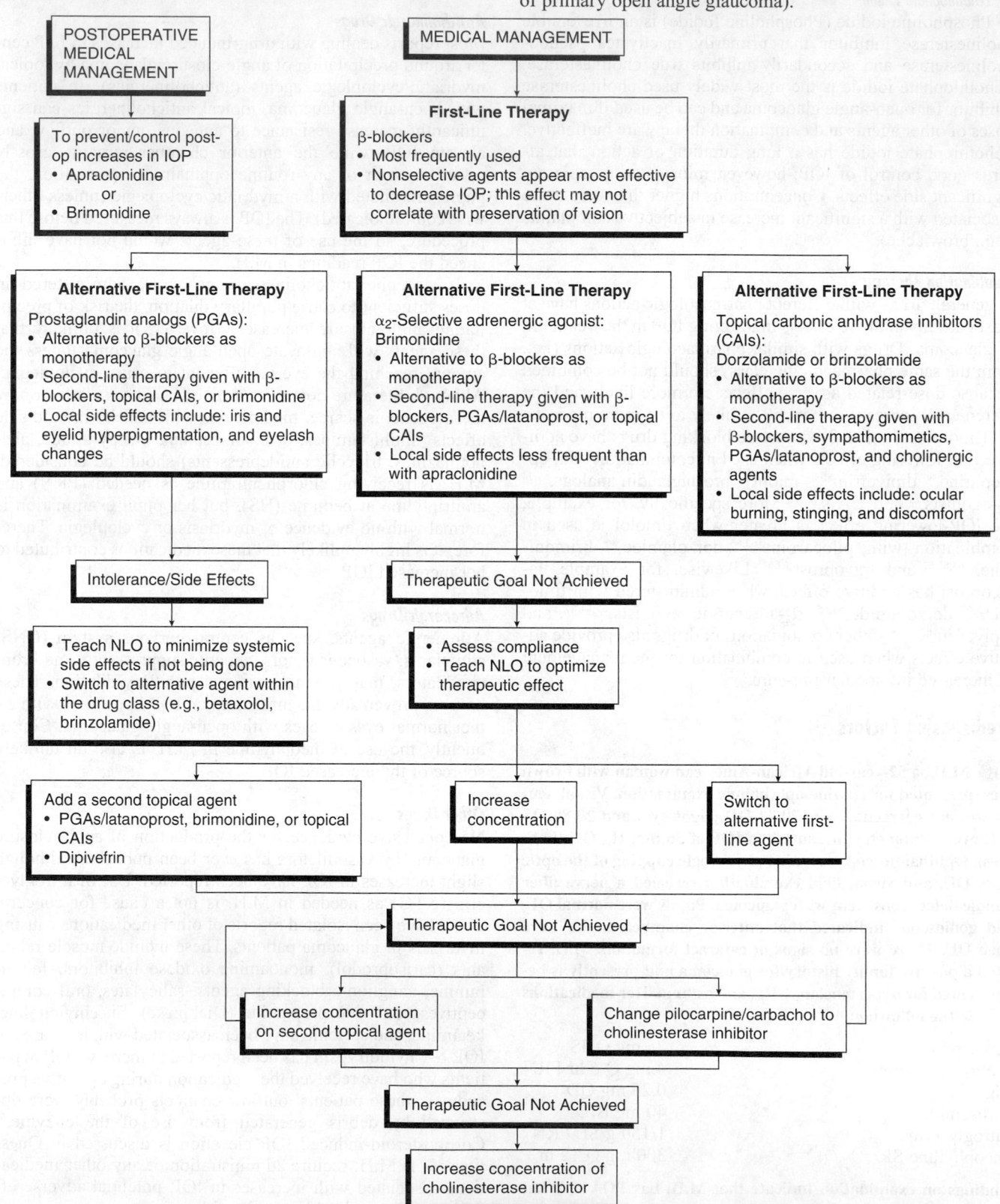

FIGURE 51-2 Medical management of glaucoma. IOP, intraocular pressure; NLO, nasolacrimal occlusion.

Table 51-1 Common Topical Agents Used in the Treatment of Open-Angle Glaucoma

Generic	Mechanism	Strength	Usual Dosage	Comments
β-Blockers				
Betaxolol (Betoptic [solution],	Sympatholytic	0.25% (suspension)	1 drop BID	Effective with few associated ocular side effects. BID dosage enhances compliance. May be the ocular β-blocker of choice in patients with pre-existing CHF or pulmonary disease, because of β_1 specificity. Patient response may be less than that seen with timolol.
Betoptic S [suspension])	Sympatholytic	0.5% (solution)		
Carteolol (Ocupress)	Sympatholytic	1%	1 drop BID	Effective with few associated side effects. BID dosage enhances compliance. Use with caution in patients with pre-existing CHF or pulmonary disease.
Levobunolol (Betagan)	Sympatholytic	0.25–0.5%	1 drop QD–BID	Effective with few associated ocular side effects. QD–BID dosage enhances compliance. Use with caution in patients with pre-existing CHF or pulmonary disease.
Metipranolol (OptiPranolol)	Sympatholytic	0.3%	1 drop BID	Effective with few associated side effects. BID dosage enhances compliance. Use with caution in patients with pre-existing CHF or pulmonary disease.
Timolol (Timoptic)		0.25–0.5%	1 drop BID	Effective with few associated ocular side effects. BID dosage enhances compliance. Use with caution in patients with pre-existing CHF or pulmonary disease. Proven long-term effectiveness, with well-defined side effect profile.
Timoptic XE	Sympatholytic	0.25–0.5%	1 drop QD	New once-daily timolol formulation. The ophthalmic vehicle, gellan gum (Gelrite), prolongs precorneal residence time and ↑ ocular bioavailability, allowing QD administration.
α₂-Selective Adrenergic Agonists				
Apraclonidine (Iopidine)	Sympathomimetic	0.5–1%	1 drop preop and postop or 1 drop BID–TID	May be used preop and postop for the prevention of increased IOP after anterior-segment laser procedures. Use of NLO minimizes systemic side effects and allows for BID dosing. Does not penetrate the blood-brain barrier; therefore, negligible systemic hypotension. Local adverse effects fairly common. Tachyphylaxis may be observed.
Brimonidine (Alphagan)	Sympathomimetic	0.2%	1 BID–TID	Effective long-term monotherapy or adjunctive therapy. Use of NLO minimizes systemic side effects and allows for BID dosing. Penetrates the blood-brain barrier; therefore, may cause mild systemic hypotension, and lethargy. Local adverse effects less common than with apraclonidine.
Topical Carbonic Anhydrase Inhibitor				
Brinzolamide (Azopt)	Decreased aqueous humor production	1%	1 drop TID	Effective long-term monotherapy or adjunctive therapy. Well tolerated with few systemic side effects. Less burning and stinging compared to dorzolamide.
Dorzolamide (Trusopt)	Decreased aqueous humor production	2%	1 drop TID	Effective long-term monotherapy or adjunctive therapy. Well tolerated with few systemic side effects.
Prostaglandin Analogs				
Latanoprost (Xalatan)	Prostaglandin F$_{2\alpha}$ agonist	0.005%	1 drop QHS	BID dosing may be less effective than QHS dosing. May cause increased pigmentation of the iris. Systemic side effects are rare but may cause muscle, joint, back pain and skin rash. Effective monotherapy or adjunctive therapy. May cause increased pigmentation of the iris and eyelid. Store unopened bottles in refrigerator. Opened bottles may be stored at room temperature up to 6 weeks.
Travoprost (Travatan)	Prostaglandin F$_{2\alpha}$ agonist	0.004%	1 drop QHS	BID dosing may be less effective than QHS dosing. May cause increased pigmentation of the iris and eyelid. Systemic side effects are rare but may include colds and upper tract infections. Effective monotherapy or adjunctive therapy with timolol. May be more effective than timolol and latanoprost and more effective in African Americans
Bimatoprost (Lumigan)	Prostamide	0.03%	1 drop QHS	BID dosing may be less effective than QHS dosing. May cause increased pigmentation of the iris and eyelid. Systemic side effects are rare but include colds and upper respiratory tract infections and headache. May be more effective than timolol and latanoprost.

continued

Table 51-1   Common Topical Agents Used in the Treatment of Open-Angle Glaucoma—cont'd

Generic	Mechanism	Strength	Usual Dosage	Comments
Prostaglandin Analogs—cont'd				
Unoprostone (Rescula)	Docosanoid	0.15%	1 drop BID	Increased pigmentation of the iris and eyelid are rare. Systemic side effects are rare but include flulike symptoms, cough, and back pain. May be less effective than timolol and latanoprost.
Miotics				
Pilocarpine (Isopto-Carpine)	Parasympath-omimetic	0.25–10% 4% (ointment) 20–40 µg/hr (Ocusert)	1–2 drops TID–QID ½ inch in cul-de-sac QD Weekly	Long-term proven effectiveness. Little rationale for use of concentrations >4% or administration more frequently than Q 4 hr. Side effects of miosis with decreased vision and brow ache are common sources of patient complaints. Once-daily administration of ointment may ↑ compliance. Effectiveness over 24 hr should be assessed in patients receiving the ointment. Ointment may cause a visual haze and blurred vision.
Carbachol (Isopto-Carbachol)	Parasympath-omimetic	0.75–3%	1–2 drops TID–QID	Used in patients allergic to or intolerant of other miotics. May be used as frequently as Q 4 hr. Corneal penetration is enhanced by benzalkonium chloride in commercial preparations. Side effects are similar to those of pilocarpine.
Echothiophate Iodide (Phospholine Iodide)	Anticholinesterase	0.03–0.25%	1 drop BID	Most used anticholinesterase agent. Long duration, although usually dosed BID, which enhances compliance. Available as powder + diluent, following reconstitution stable 30 days room temp, 6 months refrigerated. Side effects similar to those of pilocarpine, especially in concentrations >0.06%. ↑ cataract formation has been associated with its use.
Mydriatics				
Epinephrine (Glaucon, Eppy/N, Epitrate)	Sympathomimetic	0.25–2%	1 drop BID	Good response often seen with use of lower concentrations (0.5–1%). Bitartrate salt contains ½ labeled strength in epinephrine-free base equivalent. BID dosage enhances compliance. Cosmetic complaints associated with use include hyperemia and pigment deposits on the cornea and conjunctiva. Not recommended for use in aphakic patients because of 20–30% incidence of cystoid macular edema.
Dipivefrin (Propine)	Sympathomimetic	0.1%	1 drop BID	Prodrug of epinephrine associated with ↑ in systemic side effects if absorbed. BID dosage enhances compliance.

CHF, congestive heart failure; NLO, nasolacrimal occlusion.

M.H. should not be initiated on timolol or other nonselective β-adrenergic blockers because of her history of asthma (the indications and use of β-blockers for patients with heart failure are described in Chapter 19, Heart Failure). Betaxolol, a β₁-adrenergic blocker, is better tolerated than the nonselective β-adrenergic blocker, timolol, in patients with reactive airway disease and should be considered for use when topical β-blocker therapy is indicated in patients such as M.H.[46–48] Betaxolol 0.25% suspension BID would be reasonable for the initial treatment of M.H.'s glaucoma. Adverse pulmonary and cardiac side effects can occur with betaxolol: M.H. should be followed up closely. Although ocular burning and stinging have been associated more frequently with betaxolol and metipranolol than with other topical β-blockers, the 0.25% suspension is better tolerated than the 0.5% solution and is as effective.[49] Brimonidine, a topical CAI, or a prostaglandin analog such as latanoprost are acceptable alternatives to betaxolol as initial therapy. Although brimonidine, topical CAIs, and latanoprost may not exacerbate her asthma or CHF, they may cause local side effects and brimonidine may cause systemic hypotension and lethargy.

Patient Education

3. Betaxolol 0.25% suspension, one to two drops OU BID, is ordered for M.H. How should M.H. be instructed regarding proper use of her betaxolol and expected therapeutic side effects?

The clinician should instruct M.H. to hold the inverted betaxolol bottle between her thumb and middle finger and to rest this hand on her forehead to minimize the risk of inadvertent eye injury caused by sudden unexpected movement of the hand. The index finger is left free to depress the bottom of the container, releasing one drop for the dose. With a little practice, this technique is easy to master. The lower eyelid should be drawn downward with the index finger of the opposite hand or pinched between the thumb and index finger to form a pouch. The patient should look up and administer the drug into the pouch of the eye.

Patients must be encouraged to continue regular use of their medications for effective treatment of glaucoma. Chronic glaucoma is a silent disease and often not associated with symptoms; therefore, the continuation of therapy should be encouraged continuously in patients, especially when side effects to drug therapy can be encountered. Betaxolol is best administered every 12 hours because this schedule of administration is consistent with its duration of action (see Table 51-1).

Systemic side effects are rare with betaxolol but include bradycardia, heart block, CHF, pulmonary distress, and CNS side effects. M.H. should report any of these side effects to her physician.

Nasolacrimal Occlusion

4. **How much would occlusion of the nasolacrimal ducts (punctal occlusion) by M.H. influence systemic absorption or alter the therapeutic effects of betaxolol?**

Nasolacrimal, or punctal, occlusion is a technique that can decrease the amount of drug absorbed systemically.[90] Occlusion of the puncta (through the application of slight pressure with the finger to the inner corner of the eye closest to the nose for 3 to 5 minutes during and after drug instillation) may minimize systemic absorption of ophthalmic medications (e.g., betaxolol) and decrease the incidence of side effects and improve medication effectiveness.[90–92] When a single drop of ophthalmic timolol 0.5% was instilled into the eyes of patients at various times before cataract surgery and the nasolacrimal duct occluded for 5 minutes, drug levels in the aqueous humor were significantly greater in patients who had their nasolacrimal ducts occluded than those who did not.[91] The average measured maximum aqueous humor timolol concentration of 1.66 μg/mL in the occlusion group was significantly greater than 0.85 μg/mL in the nonocclusion group. The area under the curve was 1.7 times greater in patients who used the technique of nasolacrimal occlusion, and the duration of action was prolonged.[91]

Nasolacrimal occlusion is effective and can maximize drug benefits because a lower concentration of an ophthalmic formulation can be used and the dose administered less frequently. Pilocarpine 1% and 2% significantly decreased IOP at 6, 8, and 12 hours after instillation when the technique of nasolacrimal occlusion was applied.[90] Similarly, carbachol 1.5%, 3%, and the combination of carbachol 1.5% with timolol 0.25% Q 12 hr also were maximally beneficial with nasolacrimal occlusion.[90] Timolol reduced IOP by 15% and maintained this reduction of IOP at 24 hours in 92% of patients when nasolacrimal occlusion was used; in comparison, only 55% achieved comparable IOP reductions when nasolacrimal ducts were not occluded.[90] When nasolacrimal occlusion is used, pilocarpine 2% and carbachol 1.5% can be administered Q 12 hr, rather than the usual TID-QID regimens needed when the technique of nasolacrimal occlusion is not applied.[90] The Q 12 hr regimen of treatment then can be adjusted according to the patient's response. Timolol can be administered every 24 hours if the nasolacrimal occlusion technique is used.[90] If nasolacrimal occlusion is used consistently and properly, maximal drug effect can be achieved with a reduced frequency of administration and at about half of the drug concentrations typically used. Nasolacrimal occlusion should be incorporated into patient counseling for instillation of all eye drops.[90]

Alternative Therapy

5. **Two weeks after initiation of therapy, M.H. returns to clinic for a follow-up evaluation. Her IOP measures 32 mm Hg OD and 30 mm Hg OS. She denies noncompliance and has no complaints**

of intolerable side effects. How should therapy be altered? Are there alternative dosage forms or drugs that can be used?

Betaxolol may not be as effective as other ocular β-blockers. Therefore, adjunctive therapy may be required. However, M.H. should be evaluated to determine whether she has been using the technique of nasolacrimal occlusion. If not, M.H. should be again instructed on the technique of nasolacrimal occlusion and the importance of this technique in achieving the maximum therapeutic effect of her therapy (see previous question).

After the initiation of therapy, patients should be seen for a follow-up evaluation within about 2 weeks. If M.H. has been adherent to therapy and has been occluding her nasolacrimal ducts, a new course of action is needed because her intraocular pressure still is elevated. When the goal of therapy has not been achieved, the drug concentration of the ophthalmic formulation can be increased; adjunctive therapy can be initiated (e.g., brimonidine, a topical CAI, latanoprost/travoprost), or an alternative first-line agent can be selected. Patients who are experiencing unstable reductions of IOP should be followed up at 1- to 3-month intervals. Stable patients usually are evaluated every 6 months.

Adverse Effects

6. **Several weeks later, dorzolamide 2% solution, one drop OU BID is added to M.H.'s betaxolol therapy. Two weeks later, M.H. returns for a follow-up evaluation and complains of bilateral stinging and foreign body sensation. Her IOP measures 30 mm Hg OD and 29 mm Hg OS. What are the possible causes of her side effects and poor response to therapy?**

The exposure of dorzolamide to the outside environment may result in the aggregation of dry white granules on the tip of the dorzolamide bottle. These granules may drop into a patient's eyes when instilling the medication, leading to local side effects such as stinging and foreign body sensation. Such foreign bodies may cause enough discomfort to induce noncompliance, resulting in a poor response to therapy. M.H. should be questioned about the presence of dry white granules on the tip of her dorzolamide bottle.[93]

These complaints may also be a side effect from the medications, regardless of the granule presence. Ocular burning, stinging, and discomfort were reported in one-third of patients in dorzolamide clinical trials. M.H.'s administration technique should also be assessed to determine whether she is administering the two drugs at least 5 to 10 minutes apart so that the first drug is not washed away by the second drug. This should be a consideration when assessing her response to therapy.[5]

7. **After further discussions with M.H., it is determined that she has not been adherent to her dorzolamide therapy because of intolerable side effects. The dozolamide is discontinued and replaced with travoprost 0.004% one drop OU Q hs. Why might this drug selection be especially appropriate for M.H.? What patient education information should be provided to M.H. about travoprost side effects?**

Prostaglandin analogs are alternative first-line agents and are indicated in patients who are not responding or having intolerable side effects from other medications. Travoprost is an ideal choice for M.H. because in a clinical trial, African Americans had a greater response to travoprost.[67] M.H. still needs to be informed about the potential for hyperpigmentation of the iris, which may be permanent. She also needs to be educated on the possibility of eyelid skin darkening and increased thickness, length, and pigmentation of her eyelashes, which all may be reversible. These side effects may not be as cosmetically concerning to M.H. because she has brown eyes and will be instilling travoprost eye drops into both eyes.

ANGLE-CLOSURE GLAUCOMA
Treatment

8. D.H., a 72-year-old man, presents to the emergency department (ED) with an intensely red right eye, a "steamy" appearing cornea, complaints of haloes around lights, and extreme pain. A diagnosis of acute angle-closure glaucoma is made. How should D.H. be managed?

D.H. should be seen by an ophthalmologist because acute angle-closure glaucoma is a medical emergency. Medical treatment usually consists of pilocarpine 2% to 4%, one drop every 5 minutes for four to six administrations. It is recommended that the puncta be covered during administration to decrease the possibility of systemic absorption. Stronger miotics are contraindicated because they may potentiate angle closure. Topical timolol also has been used in acute angle-closure glaucoma, commonly in combination with pilocarpine.

Hyperosmotic Agents

Hyperosmotic agents act by creating an osmotic gradient between the plasma and ocular fluids.[94] Agents that are confined to the extracellular fluid space (e.g., mannitol) provide a greater effect on blood osmolality at the same dosage than do agents distributed in total body water.[94] Intravenously administered drugs provide a faster, somewhat greater effect than oral agents. Palatability may be a problem with oral agents and can be improved by serving these agents over crushed ice or with lemon juice or cola flavoring.

Orally, 50% glycerin is the usual drug of choice and is administered in dosages of 1 to 1.5 g/kg.[95] Isosorbide is an alternative, especially in diabetic patients because it is not metabolized to provide calories.[96] Ethyl alcohol (2 to 3 mL/kg) has been proved effective and may be helpful in emergency situations when other agents are unavailable.[97] Parenterally, mannitol is the drug of choice. It is administered in doses of 1 to 2 g/kg, is not metabolized to provide calories, and may be used in patients with renal failure.[98,99]

Primary side effects of hyperosmotic agents include headache, nausea, vomiting, diuresis, and dehydration. It is important that the patient not be allowed to drink because this will counteract the osmotic effects of these agents. Precipitation of pulmonary edema and CHF have been reported with hyperosmotic agents, and an allergic reaction has been reported with mannitol.[99,100]

Acetazolamide (Diamox) 500 mg intravenously is often administered in addition to hyperosmotic agents (Tables 51-2 and 51-3).

OCULAR SIDE EFFECTS OF DRUGS

9. B.C., a 58-year-old man, has a history of hypertension managed with hydrochlorothiazide 25 mg/day. He takes amiodarone 800 mg/day for cardiac arrhythmia, and chlorpheniramine 12 mg BID PRN for allergies. Four weeks ago, risperidone 1 mg BID was added to his medication regimen. He complains of occasional blurred vision. Could these symptoms be related to his medications?

All the drugs that B.C. is taking have been associated with ocular side effects. Thiazide diuretics have been associated

Table 51-2 CAIs Used in Treatment of Glaucoma

Agent	Strength	Onset (min)	Peak (hr)	Duration (hr)	Usual Dose
Acetazolamide injection	500 mg	5–10		2	500 mg
Acetazolamide tablets	125 mg 250 mg	120	4	6–8	250 mg QID
Acetazolamide sequels	500 mg	120	8–18	22–30	500 mg BID
Dichlorphenamide	50 mg	30	2–4	6–12	50 mg TID
Ethoxyzolamide	125 mg	90	3–4	7	125 mg QID
Methazolamide	50 mg	120	4–8	10–12	50 mg TID

CAIs, carbonic anhydrase inhibitors.

Table 51-3 Hyperosmotic Agents

Generic	Mode of Administration	Strength	Onset	Peak	Duration	Dose	Ocular Penetration	Distribution
Urea	IV	30%	30–45 min (at 90–120 drops/min)	1 hr	5–6 hr	1–1.5 g/kg	Good	TBW
Mannitol	IV	5%, 10%, 15%, 20%	30–60 min	1 hr	6–8 hr	1–2 g/kg	Very poor	E
Glycerin	PO	50%	10–30 min	30 min	4–5 hr	1–1.5 g/kg	Poor	E
Isosorbide	PO	45%	10–30 min	1 hr	5 hr	1.5–2 g/kg	Good	TBW
Sodium ascorbate	IV	20%	70 min	1–2 hr	2 hr	2–5 mL/kg	Good	TBW
Ethyl alcohol	PO	50%				2–3 mL/kg	Good	TBW

E, Extracellular water; TBW, total body water.

with acute myopia that may last from 24 to 48 hours.[101,102] However, hydrochlorothiazide is an unlikely cause of B.C.'s blurred vision considering its recent onset.

Amiodarone can cause keratopathy, but it is asymptomatic.[103,104] A high percentage of patients who receive this drug develop microdeposits within the corneal epithelium that resemble the verticillate keratopathy induced by chloroquine.[103] These corneal deposits are bilateral, dose and duration related, reversible, and unassociated with visual symptoms.

Risperidone has been associated with disturbances of accommodation and blurred vision.[104,105]

B.C. may be one of the approximately 1% of the population who experiences blurred vision with chlorpheniramine. This effect has been seen in patients receiving 12 to 14 mg/day.[100,101]

Table 51-4 outlines some of the more common ocular side effects associated with systemic medications. Each case should be evaluated individually and alternative therapy considered in intolerant patients.

Table 51-4 Ocular Side Effects of Systemic Medications

Drug Class	Effect(s)	Clinical Remarks
Analgesics		
Ibuprofen	Reduced vision	Rare; blurred vision reported in patients taking from four 200 mg tablets/wk to six tablets/day; changes in color vision rarely reported[159]
Narcotics, including pentazocine	Miosis	Miosis often with morphine in normal doses; slight with other agents; effect secondary to CNS action on the pupilloconstrictor center[101,102]
	Tearing Irregular pupils Paresis of accommodation Diplopia	Effects associated with narcotic withdrawal[101,102]
Antiarrhythmics		
Amiodarone	Keratopathy	Dose and duration related; resembles chloroquine keratopathy. Corneal deposits are bilateral, reversible, and unassociated with visual symptoms. Patients taking 100–200 mg/day have only minimal deposits. Deposits occur in almost 100% of patients receiving 400 mg/day.[101–104]
"	Cataracts	Previously reported as insignificant, anterior subcapsular lens opacities have been associated with amiodarone therapy. Rarely, such opacities may progress, increasing in density and in the diffuse distribution of the deposits, ultimately covering an area somewhat larger than the undilated pupil's aperture. The mechanism for this effect is unclear, but like chlorpromazine, amiodarone is a photosensitizing agent. Given that the lens changes are limited largely to the pupillary aperture, light exposure may result in the lens changes.[187]
Anticholinergics		
Atropine Dicyclomine Glycopyrrolate Propantheline Scopolamine Trihexyphenidyl	Mydriasis Cycloplegia ↓ accommodation Photophobia	Systemic and transdermal anticholinergic agents may cause mydriasis and, less frequently, cycloplegia. Mydriasis may precipitate angle-closure glaucoma. Photophobia is related to the mydriasis. Accommodation for near objects.[101,102,160]
Anticonvulsants		
Carbamazepine	Diplopia Blurred vision	Ocular adverse reactions when dosage >1–2 g/day; disappear when dosage is reduced.[101]
Phenytoin	Nystagmus Cataracts	Nystagmus in patients with high blood levels (>20 μg/mL); rarely occurs with other hydantoins. Cataracts may occur rarely with prolonged therapy.[101,102,161]
Topiramate	Acute myopia Secondary angle closure glaucoma	Twenty-three case reports; 22 in adults, 1 in pediatrics. Usually occurs within first month of therapy.[185]
Trimethadione	Visual glare	A prolonged glare or dazzle occurs when eyes are exposed to light. The glare is reversible, occurs at the retinal level, and is more common in adolescents and adults; rarely in young children.[101,102]
Anesthetics		
Propofol	Inability to open eyes	6 of 50 patients undergoing ENT procedures using standardized anesthesia with propofol were unable to open their eyes either spontaneously or in response to verbal commands. This effect lasted from 3–20 min after the end of anesthetic administration. Two patients showed complete loss of ocular motility. This was a transient, myasthenic-like weakness.[162]
Antidepressants		
Tricyclic antidepressants (TCAs)		Mydriasis is most common ocular side effect of TCAs. Cycloplegia is rare. Reports of precipitation of angle-closure glaucoma.[101,102]

continued

Table 51-4   Ocular Side Effects of Systemic Medications—cont'd

Drug Class	Effect(s)	Clinical Remarks
Antidepressants—cont'd		
Fluoxetine	Mydriasis Cycloplegia Eye tics	Administration of fluoxetine 20–40 mg/day has been associated with paroxysmal contractions of the muscles around the lateral aspect of the eye. This effect occurred 3–4 wk after initiation of fluoxetine therapy and resolved within 2 wk of discontinuation.[163]
Antihistamines		
Chlorpheniramine	Blurred vision Mydriasis ↓ lacrimal secretions	Blurred vision occurs rarely (≈ 1% of patients taking 12–14 mg/day).[101,102] Rare[101,102]
Antihypertensives		
Clonidine	Miosis Dry itchy eyes	Miosis is seen in overdose.[102] Rare[102]
Diazoxide	Lacrimation	About 20% experience lacrimation, which may continue after drug is discontinued.[101]
Guanethidine	Miosis Ptosis Conjunctivitis Blurred vision	Sporadically documented. One study reported a 17% incidence of blurred vision in patients taking guanethidine 70 mg/day.[101,102]
Reserpine	Miosis Conjunctivitis	Miosis is slight, but can last up to 1 wk after a single dose[101,102] Common, secondary to dilation of conjunctival blood vessels[101,102]
Anti-Infectives		
Amantadine	Corneal lesions	Diffuse, white punctate subepithelial corneal opacities have been reported, occasionally associated with superficial punctate keratitis. Onset has been 1–2 wk after initiation of therapy with dosages of 200–400 mg/day. Resolves with drug discontinuation.[164]
Chloramphenicol	Optic neuritis	Rare unless a total dose of 100 g and duration >6 wk are exceeded. Vision usually improves after the drug is discontinued.[101,102]
Chloroquine	Corneal deposits	Some patients using ordinary doses may develop corneal deposits in a few months. The deposits are visible with use of a biomicroscope, appear as white-yellow in color, but are of no consequence.[101,102]
	Retinopathy (macular degeneration)	Serious retinopathy when total dose >100 g. Usually develops after 1–3 yr; can occur in 6 mo. Visual loss may be peripheral, with progression to central vision loss and disturbance of color vision. Rarely, effects such as blurred vision are seen earlier when larger doses (500–700 mg/day) are used. Macular changes may progress after drug is discontinued. These agents concentrate in pigmented tissue.[101,102]
Ethambutol	Retrobulbar neuritis	At dosages of 15 mg/kg/day, virtually void of ocular side effects. Such effects are rare at dosages of 25 mg/kg/day for a duration of a few months. Patients treated for prolonged periods should have routine visual examinations including visual fields. Most effects are reversible after the drug is discontinued.[101,102]
Gentamicin	Pseudotumor cerebri	Rare, but has been well documented with secondary papilledema and visual loss[101,102]
Isoniazid	Optic neuritis	Prevalence not well defined, but appears to be significantly less than peripheral neuritis. Evaluation difficult because most patients malnourished, chronic alcoholics, or receiving multiple medications. Pre-existing eye disease does not appear to be a predisposing factor.[101,102]
Nalidixic acid	Visual sensations	Most common ocular side effect. Main feature a brightly colored appearance of objects; occurs soon after the drug is taken. Although quinolone antibiotics are nalidixic acid derivatives, they have rarely been associated with these ocular side effects.[101,102]
	Visual loss	Temporary effect (30 min–3 days.)
	Papilledema	Primarily in infants and young children and secondary to intracranial pressure; reversible upon withdrawal of the drug.
Sulfonamides	Myopia	Acute and reversible; most common ocular side effect.[101,102]
	Conjunctivitis	Primarily with topical sulfathiazole, 4% incidence between the fifth and ninth days of therapy.[101,102]
	Optic neuritis	Even in low dosages. Usually reversible with complete recovery of vision.[101,102]
	Photosensitivity	Associated with use of sulfisoxazole lid margin therapy.[165,166]
Tetracyclines	Myopia	Appears to be acute, transient, and rare.[101,102]
	Papilledema	More common in children and infants than adults; rare.[101,102]
Voriconazole	Altered visual perception Blurred vision	May be associated with higher doses or plasma concentrations.[186]

Table 51-4   Ocular Side Effects of Systemic Medications—cont'd

Drug Class	Effect(s)	Clinical Remarks
Anti-Inflammatory Agents (also see Analgesics; Corticosteroids)		
Gold	Corneal Conjunctival deposits	Deposition in the conjunctiva and superficial cornea more common than in the lens or deep cornea. Incidence in cornea of 40–80% in total doses of 1.5 g; visual acuity is unaffected. One reported case after oral therapy.[101]
Indomethacin	↓ vision	Rare; also changes in color vision have been rarely reported. [101,102]
Phenylbutazone	↓ vision	Most common ocular side effect with this drug may be caused by lens hydration. [101,102]
	Conjunctivitis Retinal hemorrhage	Occurs less often than vision. The conjunctivitis may be associated with development of Stevens-Johnson syndrome or an allergic reaction.[101,102]
Antilipemic Agents		
Lovastatin	Cataracts	The crystalline lenses of hypercholesteremic patients were assessed before and after 48 wk of treatment with lovastatin 20–80 mg/day. Statistical analyses of the distribution of cortical, nuclear, and subcapsular opacities at 48 weeks showed no significant differences between placebo-treated and lovastatin-treated groups. Visual acuity assessments also were not significantly different among the groups.[167]
Antineoplastic Agents		
Busulfan	Cataracts	Reported with high dosages. [101,102]
Carmustine	Arterial narrowing Nerve fiber-layer infarcts Intraretinal hemorrhages	These ocular side effects are not well established. Evidence of delayed bilateral ocular toxicity developed in 2 of 50 patients treated with high-dose IV carmustine (800 mg/ m²). Symptoms of ocular toxicity became evident 4 wk after IV treatment. Evidence of delayed ocular toxicity (mean onset 6 wk) ipsilateral to the site of infusion developed in 7 of 10 patients treated with intra-arterial carotid doses of carmustine to a cumulative minimum of 450 mg/m² in two treatments.[168]
Cytarabine	Keratoconjunctivitis Ocular burning Photophobia Blurred vision	Corneal toxicity and conjunctivitis have been reported with high-dose (3 g/m²) therapy.[169,170]
Doxorubicin	Conjunctivitis Excessive tearing	May last for several days after treatment[101,102]
Fluorouracil	Ocular irritation Lacrimation	Reversible and seldom interfere with continued therapy. [101,102]
Tamoxifen	Corneal opacities ↓ vision Retinopathy	Generally occur in patients taking higher than normal doses for 12–18 mo[90]
Vinca alkaloids (especially vincristine)	Extraocular muscle paresis (EMP) Ptosis	The onset of EMP or paralysis may be seen as early as 2 wk. Dose related. Most recover fully when drug is discontinued. [101,102]
Barbiturates	Miosis Mydriasis Disturbances in ocular movement Ptosis	Most significant ocular side effects occur in chronic users or in toxic states. Pupillary responses are variable; miosis seen most frequently except in toxicity when mydriasis predominates. Nystagmus and weakness in extraocular muscles may be seen. Chronic abusers have a characteristic ptosis. [101,102]
Calcium channel blockers	Blurred vision Transient blindness	Primarily blurred vision; transient blindness at peak concentrations has been observed in several patients.[121]
Corticosteroids	Cataracts	Posterior subcapsular cataracts have been associated with systemic corticosteroids. ↑ in patients who have received >15 mg/day of prednisone or its equivalent daily for periods >1 yr. [101,102] Rare reports of bilateral posterior subcapsular cataracts associated with nasal aerosol or inhalation of beclomethasone dipropionate have been received. Most patients had received therapy for >5 yr, often in higher than the recommended dosage. About 40% of patients also were receiving systemic corticosteroids.[188] (Also see Question 14.)
	↑ intraocular pressure	More common with topical corticosteroids than with systemic therapy. Of little consequence in patients without pre-existing glaucoma. Glaucoma patients should be monitored routinely if receiving systemic corticosteroids. [101,102] (See Question 13.)
	Papilledema	Intracranial hypertension or pseudotumor cerebri from systemic corticosteroids has been well documented. The incidence appears to be greater in children than in adults; primarily associated with chronic therapy.
Digitalis	Altered color vision, visual acuity	Changes in color vision. A glare phenomenon, and a snowy appearance in objects have been associated primarily with digitalis intoxication. In a small number of cases, reversible reduction in visual acuity has been noted. Also associated with changes in the visual fields.[101,102]
	↓ intraocular pressure	Digitalis derivatives can intraocular pressure, but clinical use for glaucoma is not practical because the therapeutic systemic dose for this effect is very near the toxic dose. [101,102]

continued

Table 51-4   Ocular Side Effects of Systemic Medications—cont'd

Drug Class	Effect(s)	Clinical Remarks
Diuretics		
Carbonic anhydrase inhibitors Thiazides	Myopia	Acute myopia that may last from 24–48 hr. Probably caused by an in the anteroposterior diameter of the lens, which may be reversible even if drug use is continued.[101,102]
Estrogens		
Clomiphene	Blurred vision Mydriasis Visual field changes Visual sensations	5–10% experience ocular side effects. Blurred vision is the most common effect, although visual sensations such as flashing lights, distortion of images, and various colored lights (primarily silver) may occur.[101,102]
Oral contraceptives (OCs)	Optic neuritis Pseudotumor cerebri Retrobulbar neuritis	Quite rare. In patients with retinal vascular abnormalities, use of OCs is questionable. Numerous other possible ocular side effects are associated with these agents, and further documentation is required.[101,102]
Hypouricemics		
Allopurinol	Cataracts	Conflicting reports have suggested allopurinol may be associated with anterior and posterior lens capsule changes and with anterior subcapsular vacuoles; 42 cases of cataracts have been reported; these have been observed primarily in age groups in whom normal lens aging changes would not be expected. No cause-and-effect relationship has been proven.[101,171,188–190]
Immune Modulators		
Interleukin-2	Visual deficits	Interleukin-2 visual complications have occurred during the first or second treatment cycle, usually within 5–6 days of initiation of therapy. Ocular symptoms included diplopia, binocular negative scotomata (isolated areas of varying size and shape in which vision is absent or depressed. These are not perceived ordinarily but would be apparent upon completion of a visual field examination), and palinopsia (abnormal recurring visual imagery). In most cases, treatment was continued for the entire planned duration of therapy. Symptoms resolved after discontinuation.[172]
Phenothiazines		
Chlorpromazine	Deposits on the lens	Rare when total dose <0.5 kg. Visible after a total dose of 1 kg in most cases; incidence may ↑ to 90% after ≥2.5 kg. Usually, deposits do not affect vision appreciably. The cornea and conjunctiva may be affected after the lens shows pigment changes.[101,102]
	Retinal pigment deposits	The number of reported cases is small; further documentation is necessary.[101,102]
Thioridazine	Pigmentary retinopathy	Primarily associated with maximal daily dosages or average doses .1,000 mg. Daily dosages up to 600 mg are relatively safe; 600–800 mg is uncertain, but rarely suspect. If .800 mg/day is used, periodic ophthalmoscopic examinations may uncover problems before visual acuity is compromised.[101,102]
Therapy for Erectile Dysfunction		
Sildenafil Tadalafil Vardenafil	Disturbance of color vision Increased brightness Blurred vision	Color vision alterations are mild to moderate. Blurred vision does not impair visual acuity. Visual alterations usually subside within 4 hr after the dose.[173,189,190]

CNS, central nervous system; ENT, ear, nose, and throat.

OCULAR EMERGENCIES
Chemical Burns

10. **S.J., a 24-year-old construction worker, has splashed an unidentified chemical in his eyes and enters a nearby pharmacy complaining of burning in both eyes. Should the pharmacist attempt to treat S.J. or refer him to the ED?**

Chemical burns require immediate attention. The immediate treatment is copious irrigation using the most accessible source of water (e.g., shower, faucet, drinking fountain, hose, bathtub). After at least 5 minutes of initial irrigation, S.J. should be taken immediately to the ED. A water-soaked towel or cloth should be kept on his eyes during transport.

Other Ocular Emergencies

Health care professionals often are approached by patients with acute ocular problems. Before briefly reviewing these conditions, it is necessary to stress that patients should be referred to an ophthalmologist if the practitioner has even the slightest doubt regarding proper therapy. It generally is difficult to effectively evaluate the severity of ocular disorders without the benefit of training or a thorough ophthalmologic workup.

In addition to chemical burns, there are other cases that can be considered ocular emergencies requiring immediate treatment.[1] Included in this listing is corneal trauma from abrasion or foreign bodies. Often, the patient complains of a gritty, scratchy feeling and is aware of a foreign body's presence. Patients with corneal ulcers also should see an ophthalmologist immediately. The corneal tissue is an excellent culture medium for bacteria such as *Pseudomonas aeruginosa,* and therapy should be initiated as soon as possible to avoid corneal perforation and possible loss of the eye.[1]

Generally, cases of conjunctivitis are not emergency situations, with the exception of gonococcal conjunctivitis. In suspected cases, the patient should see an ophthalmologist to avoid potential corneal perforation.[1] Patients with symptoms of red, tender, swollen eyelids with exophthalmos and mild pain may be suffering from orbital cellulitis or endophthalmitis, which require immediate treatment with systemic antibiotics.

Signs and symptoms of acute angle-closure glaucoma, an ocular emergency, are reviewed in Question 8. Severe iritis causes extreme pain and photophobia, and patients should be referred for prompt treatment. Vision loss, whether sudden, complete, or transient, or flashes of light may signify various potentially damaging ocular disorders, including retinal artery occlusion, optic neuritis, amaurosis fugax, or retinal detachment. An ophthalmologist should evaluate the patient as soon as possible. Referral also is recommended for patients with blurred vision, pupil disorders, diplopia, nystagmus, or ocular hemorrhage.

COMMON OCULAR DISORDERS
Stye (Hordeolum)

Sties are infections of the hair follicles or sebaceous glands of the eyelids. The most common infecting organism is *Staphylococcus aureus.* Treatment consists of hot, moist compresses and topical antibiotics (e.g., sulfacetamide). Over-the-counter products should not be recommended. Sties that do not respond to warm compresses within a few days should be evaluated by an ophthalmologist.

Conjunctivitis

Conjunctivitis is a common external eye problem that involves inflammation of the conjunctiva. The symptoms are a diffusely reddened eye with purulent or serous discharge accompanied by itching, smarting, stinging, or a scratching, and foreign-body sensation. Patients with pain, decreased vision, unequal distribution of redness, irregular pupils, or opacity should be referred immediately to an ophthalmologist because these are signs of more serious eye disease.

Conjunctivitis can be bacterial, fungal, parasitic, viral, or allergic in origin. Most cases of bacterial conjunctivitis are caused by *S. aureus, S. pneumococcus* (in temperate climates), or *Haemophilus aegyptius* (in warm climates), although a number of other organisms may be responsible. The infection usually starts in one eye and is spread to the other by the hands. It also may be spread to other persons. Unlike bacterial conjunctivitis, corneal infections can obliterate vision rapidly; therefore, accurate diagnosis is important.

Acute Bacterial Conjunctivitis (Pink-Eye)

11. **L.T. is a 6-year-old boy with diffuse bilateral conjunctival redness that has been present for 2 days. A crusting discharge is deposited on his lashes and the corners of his eyes. His vision is** normal, and his pupils are round and equal. The diagnosis of acute bacterial conjunctivitis is made, and sodium sulfacetamide 10% ophthalmic drops, two drops OU Q 2 hr while awake, are prescribed. What other measures should be used? What instructions should his caregivers receive?

Although treatment of typical bacterial conjunctivitis such as this is empirical, a culture should be obtained. Other ophthalmic antibiotic drops or ointments, such as neomycin-polymyxin-B-gramicidin combination (Neosporin), also are used in these situations. Although other antimicrobials such as the ocular quinolones may be used for bacterial conjunctivitis, these agents should be reserved as second-line therapies because of cost and the potential development of resistance. Proper management of this infection also includes mechanical cleaning of the eyelids and hygienic measures that prevent spreading the infection to other children. The deposits should be removed as often as possible with moist cotton swabs or cotton-tipped applicators. A mild baby shampoo can be used to moisten the applicator. Firm adherent crusts may be softened with warm, moist compresses. Because this material is infectious, it should be disposed of in a sanitary fashion. The common use of washcloths by several individuals will spread bacterial conjunctivitis.

Allergic Conjunctivitis

12. **N.V., a 10-year-old girl, has had redness OU accompanied by "hay fever" for the past 2 months (June and July). There is no crusting on her eyelids, and her vision is normal; she rubs her eyes often because they itch. What treatment is best for N.V.'s allergic conjunctivitis?**

Topical vasoconstrictors (e.g., naphazoline, tetrahydrozoline) with or without antihistamines (e.g., antazoline, pheniramine) may be used to treat hyperemia, but they should not be used excessively because rebound congestion may occur secondary to the vasoconstrictors. Antihistamine tablets or syrup will give considerable but temporary relief. Several ophthalmic histamine H_1-receptor antagonists are effective in the treatment of allergic conjunctivitis. Levocabastine 0.05% is administered BID–QID, olopatadine 0.1% BID (separating doses by 6 to 8 hours), emedastine 0.05% QID, and ketotifen 0.025% BID–QID.[106–108] Ketotifen, olopatadine, and azelastine exhibit both antihistamine and mast cell stabilizing effects. Olapatidine inhibits the release of other mast cell inflammatory mediators such as tryptase and prostaglandin. Ketotifen and azelastine suppress the release of mediators from cells involved in hypersensitivity reactions and decrease chemotaxis and activation of eosinophils. Azelastine inhibits other mediators involved in allergic reactions such as leukotrienes and platelet activating. Emedastine was more efficacious than levocabastine when used BID for 6 weeks in adult and pediatric patients with seasonal allergic conjunctivitis.[109] Olopatadine provided superior efficacy and a more rapid resolution of the signs and symptoms of allergic conjunctivitis when compared with ketotifen in a small trial involving adult patients.[110] Azelastine has a slightly quicker onset of therapeutic effect when compared to olopatadine and placebo.[111] Information to date is insufficient to definitely recommend one of these products as superior to the others. The ideal treatment would be removal of the allergen, but this usually is impossible when the conjunctivitis is secondary to seasonal allergies. Topical corticosteroids provide dramatic relief, but their use must be limited because of potential adverse effects (see Ophthalmic Corticosteroids).

Sodium cromoglycate, a drug that inhibits the release of histamine in response to antigen, may be effective as an alternative for patients who fail to respond to more conservative measures. Lodoxamide, pemirolast, and nedocromil have a similar mechanism of action to sodium cromoglycate, but these agents also decrease chemotaxis and activation of eosinophils. Comparative studies have documented that lodoxamide tromethamine 0.1% is at least as effective as sodium cromoglycate 2% to 4% in treating allergic ocular disorders, including vernal keratoconjunctivitis.[112,113] Patients in these studies demonstrated more rapid and greater response when treated with lodoxamide, one drop QID. Nedocromil and olopatadine administered BID were compared in a 2-week crossover study involving 28 patients aged 7 years and older.[113,114] There was a tendency toward greater patient acceptance of nedocromil, but treatment outcomes were essentially equal.

Corneal Ulcers

13. T.S. presents with a diagnosis of bacterial corneal ulcer OD and prescriptions for "fortified gentamicin" and cefazolin eye drops, which are not commercially available. What is the rationale for this therapy?

The initial choice of therapy for bacterial corneal ulcers commonly is based on Gram's stain and clinical impression of the severity of the ulcer. Single or combination antimicrobial therapy may be prescribed. Although commercial antimicrobial products are available, some believe that the antimicrobial concentrations that these products contain are too low to effectively treat bacterial corneal ulcers.[115,116]

Topical antimicrobials for the treatment of bacterial corneal ulcers may be prepared from parenteral antimicrobials or by the addition of parenteral antimicrobials to "fortify" commercially available products. Commonly prescribed products include bacitracin 5,000 to 10,000 U/mL, cefazolin 33 to 100 mg/mL, gentamicin or tobramycin 9.1 to 13.6 mg/mL, and vancomycin 25 to 50 mg/mL. Fortified gentamicin usually is prepared by adding 80 mg of parenteral gentamicin to the commercially available gentamicin ophthalmic

solution. The final concentration of this solution is 13.6 mg/mL. Cefazolin ophthalmic solution is prepared by reconstituting 500 mg parenteral cefazolin with 2 mL sterile normal saline. Two milliliters of artificial tears solution are removed from a commercially available 15-mL bottle and replaced with the 2-mL reconstituted cefazolin solution. This results in a final cefazolin concentration of 33 mg/mL. Comprehensive guidelines for preparation of such products are included in the book *Extemporaneous Ophthalmic Preparations*. Therapy initially may be administered as frequently as every 15 to 30 minutes with extension of intervals as the ulcer resolves.[117,118]

OPHTHALMIC CORTICOSTEROIDS
Comparison of Preparations

The various topical ophthalmic corticosteroid preparations are described in Table 51-5. The salt form affects the ability of the preparation to penetrate the cornea; biphasic salts penetrate the intact cornea better than water-soluble salts. However, ability to penetrate the cornea does not indicate increased therapeutic effectiveness. Prednisolone acetate 1% and fluorometholone acetate 0.1% have the best anti-inflammatory effects.[117–120]

Adverse Effects
Increased Intraocular Pressure

14. L.P. has been treated with topical prednisolone acetate 1%, one drop OU QID for 8 weeks. Before therapy, IOP measured 16 mm Hg OU, but on the last follow-up visit, readings were 26 mm Hg OD and 22 mm Hg OS. Assess these observations.

L.P.'s elevated IOP could be related to topical steroid therapy. In one study, the ophthalmic administration of corticosteroid preparations (Table 51-6) increased intraocular pressure in three genetically distinct subgroups.[121,122] Fluorometholone acetate increased IOP of ≥10 mm Hg in known steroid responders in 29.5 days (median), whereas dexamethasone did the same in 22.7 days (median).[123] In a retrospective follow-up, 13% of high-corticosteroid responders developed POAG and 63.8% developed ocular hypertension. No low responders developed POAG, and only 2.4% developed ocular hypertension.[123] Although corticosteroid-induced increases in IOP are associated most frequently with topical ophthalmic

---

Table 51-5 Ophthalmic Corticosteroids

Low Potency	Intermediate Potency	High Potency
Dexamethasone 0.05% (Decadron Phosphate)	Clobetasone 0.1%[a]	Clobetasone 0.5%[a]
Dexamethasone 0.1% (Decadron Phosphate)	Dexamethasone Alcohol 0.1% (Maxidex)	Fluorometholone Acetate 0.1% (Flarex)
Medrysone 1% (HMS)	Fluorometholone 0.1% (FML)	Prednisolone Acetate 1% (Pred Forte)
	Fluorometholone 0.25% (FML Forte)	Rimexolone 1% (Vexol)
	Loteprednol 0.2% (Lotemax)	
	Loteprednol 0.5% (Alrex)	
	Prednisolone Acetate 0.12% (Pred Mild)	
	Prednisolone Sodium Phosphate 0.125% (Inflamase Mild)	
	Prednisolone Sodium Phosphate 1% (Inflamase Forte)	

[a]Not commercially available in the United States.

Table 51-6 Intraocular Pressure Response to Topical Steroids in Random Populations

Author	Parameter of Response	No. of Subjects	Low	Medium	High	Mean
Armalay[121]	↑ of pressure in eye medicated with 0.1% dexamethasone	80	≤5 mm Hg 66%	6–15 mm Hg 29%	≥16 mm Hg 5%	5.5 mm Hg
Becker et al.[122]	Final pressure in eye medicated for 6 wk with 0.1% betamethasone	50	≤19 mm Hg 70%	20–30 mm Hg 26%	≥32 mm Hg 4%	17.0 mm Hg
	Time to maximum response		2 wk	4 wk	4 wk	

preparations, systemic corticosteroids may cause a similar response, although the magnitude is somewhat less.[124]

Topical corticosteroids exert their effects by decreasing aqueous humor outflow, whereas systemic corticosteroids may increase aqueous humor production.[124] The effects on IOP apparently are unrelated to the corticosteroid's ability to penetrate the cornea. Dexamethasone has been associated with the greatest IOP increase.[125] Fluorometholone, medrysone, rimexolone, and loteprednol have been associated with lower, although sometimes significant, increases in IOP.[126,127–129] The pressure response often is reversible when the offending agent is discontinued. In subjects with prolonged IOP elevation, glaucomatous field defects are more likely to develop in corticosteroid-responsive patients.[130]

Cataracts

15. G.A., who had asthma, has been taking prednisone 10 mg/day for 1 year. A routine ophthalmic examination revealed early cataract formation. Why could this be related to the prednisone?

Systemic and topical ophthalmic corticosteroids have been associated with the development of cataracts. About 23% of patients treated with 10 to 16 mg/day of prednisone orally (or its equivalent dose) for 1 year or more developed posterior subcapsular cataracts (PSC).[131,132] The estimated occurrence of PSC in patients treated with more than 16 mg/day of prednisone for more than a year increased to more than 70% over the same time period. Patients receiving <10 mg/day prednisone or its equivalent are unlikely to develop PSC, although some contend that the concept of a "safe" dosage should be abandoned because of variable patient sensitivity to this side effect.[133] As illustrated by G.A., the cataracts cause few subjective complaints and little measurable decrease in visual acuity. Although systemic corticosteroids primarily are implicated, use of topical corticosteroids also has been associated with PSC formation.[134] Patients treated with alternate-day dosing of oral corticosteroids may be at lower risk for PSC formation.[135] Any patient receiving long-term corticosteroids should receive routine ophthalmic follow-up.

SYSTEMIC SIDE EFFECTS FROM OPHTHALMIC MEDICATION

16. J.F., a 62-year-old woman, received one drop of phenylephrine 10% in each eye to dilate the pupils. Shortly after administration, her BP increased to 210/130 mm Hg for 5 minutes, and she became confused. How common is this type of reaction in patients receiving topical phenylephrine? What other topical ophthalmic medications been associated with systemic effects?

One group of investigators reported 33 cases of possible adverse effects associated with topical phenylephrine 10%.[136] However, when phenylephrine 10% or tropicamide (Mydriacyl) 1% was administered to 150 patients in a double-blind study, no statistically significant differences between experimental and control groups with respect to BP or pulse rate were observed.[137] Care should be taken when phenylephrine 10% is administered in patients with hypertension or cardiac abnormalities in whom systemic absorption could be hazardous. No similar reports have been associated with topical use of phenylephrine 2.5%.

In addition to the systemic effects from topical administration of cholinergic agents, epinephrine, and timolol that have been described earlier, topical atropine, cyclopentolate (Cyclogyl), and scopolamine have been associated with psychosis.[138–140] There also have been reports of death associated with topical atropine.[141] Ataxia has been seen with use of homatropine, whereas only a single report of unconsciousness has been associated with the use of tropicamide.[141,142]

Topical chloramphenicol-polymyxin-B sulfate ophthalmic ointment has been associated with bone marrow aplasia after intermittent use for 4 months.[143] A cushingoid reaction has been reported in a 30-month-old baby girl treated with dexamethasone alcohol (Maxidex) four times a day in both eyes for 14 months.[144]

OCULAR NONSTEROIDAL ANTI-INFLAMMATORY DRUGS

17. W.A. is scheduled to undergo cataract extraction with implantation of an intraocular lens. Preoperative orders include administration of flurbiprofen 0.03% to inhibit intraoperative miosis. The formulary includes only diclofenac 0.1%. Is this a suitable alternative to flurbiprofen?

Within the eye, prostaglandins produce various effects including miosis, increased vascular permeability of the blood-ocular barrier, conjunctival hyperemia, and changes in IOP.[142] Ocular instillation of nonsteroidal anti-inflammatory drugs (NSAIDs) provides ocular tissue levels adequate to inhibit prostaglandin synthesis and reduce these prostaglandin-mediated ocular effects.[145] Commercially available ocular NSAIDs include the phenylacetic acid derivative, diclofenac, and the phenylalkanoic acids flurbiprofen and ketorolac (Table 51-7). These agents are well tolerated, but there is transient burning and stinging upon installation. Although the ocular NSAIDs share a similar mechanism of action, there is considerable variability in their studied and approved indica-

Table 51-7   Ocular Nonsteroidal Anti-Inflammatory Drugs

Indication	Drug/Approval Status for Indication	Dosage(s)
Inhibition of intraoperative miosis	Diclofenac 0.1% (Voltaren, U)[174]	3 reported regimens; 1 drop Q 15–30 min for 4 doses; 1 drop TID for 2 pre-operative days; 1 drop at 2 hr, 1 hr, and 15 min before surgery
	Flurbiprofen 0.03% (Ocufen, A)[175]	1 drop Q 30 min for 2 hr before surgery
	Ketorolac 0.5% (Acular, U)	1 drop Q 15 min beginning 1 hr before surgery
Anti-inflammatory postcataract surgery	Diclofenac 0.1% (A)[172,176]	1 drop BID–QID, including 24 hr preoperative administration
	Flurbiprofen 0.03% (U)	1 drop 4–5 times daily
	Ketorolac 0.5% (A)[177]	1 drop TID, including 24 hr preoperative administration
Prevention/treatment of cystoid macular edema	Diclofenac 0.1% (U)[178]	2 drops 5 times preoperatively followed by 1 drop 3–5 times daily
	Ketorolac 0.5% (U)[177,179]	1 drop TID–QID, including 24 hr preoperative administration
Ocular inflammatory conditions (iritis, iridocyclitis, episcleritis)	Diclofenac 0.1% (U) Diclofenac 0.1% (U)	1 drop QID
Seasonal allergic/vernal conjunctivitis		1 drop Q 2 hr for 48 hr; then QID
	Ketorolac 0.5% (A)[183,184]	1 drop QID

A, approved use; U, unapproved use.

tions. Published data suggest that minor clinical differences, which probably are insignificant, exist among these agents. Accordingly, diclofenac and ketorolac are likely to be acceptable alternatives to flurbiprofen, despite the lack of an approved indication for inhibition of intraoperative miosis. Table 51-7 provides an overview of commercially available ocular NSAIDs.

OCULAR HERPES SIMPLEX VIRUS INFECTIONS
Treatment

18. P.B., a 34-year-old man, presents with a 2-week history of a red, irritated left eye with watery discharge. Recently, vision in his left eye became blurred, and he complained of light sensitivity. A slit-lamp examination with rose Bengal stain revealed a multibranched corneal epithelial defect. This dendritic ulcer is the hallmark of ocular herpes simplex (type I) infection. What is the therapy of choice?

Approximately 300,000 to 500,000 cases of corneal herpes develop each year.[146] Before 1962, the standard form of therapy for epithelial herpetic keratitis was debridement in which the margins of the corneal ulcers are scraped to remove the virus-laden cells.

Idoxuridine
In 1962, the antimetabolite idoxuridine (Stoxil) was marketed. Idoxuridine (IDU) is structurally similar to thymidine and alters DNA synthesis of the herpes simplex virus (HSV). IDU is applied topically to the eye in the form of a 0.1% solution or 0.5% ointment.

Because continued presence of the antimetabolite IDU is necessary to inhibit multiplication of HSV, the recommended dosage is one drop of solution in each infected eye every hour during the day and every 2 hours throughout the night until improvement is confirmed by ophthalmic examination. The dosage then may be reduced to one drop every 2 hours during the day and every 4 hours throughout the night. IDU therapy should be continued for 3 to 5 days after healing is complete to prevent recurrence of the infection. Alternatively, IDU ointment may be applied four to five times daily as single-agent therapy or as a nighttime medication when the solution is used during the day.

Idoxuridine therapy is efficacious: approximately 80% to 85% of initial dendritic ulcers resolve within 2 weeks.[147] Because IDU does not penetrate well into and through the cornea, it has no proven effectiveness in the treatment of herpetic iritis or stromal keratitis.

Patients occasionally experience ocular irritation, pain, inflammation, and photophobia after topical administration of IDU. A temporary visual haze may occur in patients using the ointment form, as would be expected from the use of any ocular ointment. IDU therapy also may cause contact dermatitis, punctate epithelial keratopathy, follicular conjunctivitis, and thickening of the lid margins associated with stenosis of the lacrimal canaliculi. IDU's major disadvantage may be that it also is incorporated into host DNA, thus inhibiting the replication of normal, noninfected cells. This nonselectivity actually could delay healing of the dendritic lesions as normal cells may regenerate at a slower rate. The emergence of IDU-resistant strains, the potential for toxicity, and the inability of IDU to prevent recurrence of latent infection led to the search for more effective and less toxic antiherpetic agents.

Vidarabine
Vidarabine (Vira-A) was the second clinically useful drug to be developed for use against ocular HSV infections. Its exact mechanism of antiviral activity has not been determined, although the primary effect, like that of IDU, appears to be inhibition of DNA synthesis.[148] Vidarabine is similar to IDU with respect to its effect on epithelial herpes keratitis.

Vidarabine is available as a 3% ophthalmic ointment for administration into the conjunctival sac. Approximately one-half inch of ointment should be applied five times daily (at 3-hour intervals) until re-epithelialization has occurred. An additional 7 days of treatment at reduced dosages (e.g., twice daily) is advised to prevent recurrence of the infection.

Adverse reactions associated with topical vidarabine are similar to those described for IDU, including increased lacrimation, foreign-body sensation, burning, and ocular irritation. Vidarabine appears to interfere less with the growth of normal cells as the corneal epithelium heals. Vidarabine has proved especially beneficial in patients who are hypersensitive to IDU or who are infected with IDU-resistant viral strains.

Trifluridine

At present, trifluridine is the drug of choice for the treatment of ocular herpes.[149] In vitro, trifluridine's mechanism of action is similar to that of IDU. Trifluridine also inhibits thymidylate synthase, an enzyme required for DNA synthesis. The actual in vivo antiviral effects of trifluridine have not been determined.

Trifluridine is available as a 1% ophthalmic solution. One drop should be instilled into the affected eye every 2 hours while awake with a maximum daily dose of nine drops. Following re-epithelialization, application of trifluridine should be continued for an additional 7 days at a reduced dosage of one drop every 4 hours while awake with a minimum of five drops daily. Continuous administration for periods exceeding 21 days is not recommended because of potential ocular toxicity.

Clinical trials have proved trifluridine to be more effective than IDU and vidarabine. Approximately 96% of treated herpetic corneal ulcers are healed within 2 weeks.[150] Therapeutic levels of trifluridine can be found in the aqueous humor after topical administration of a 1% solution, enhancing its possible effectiveness in the treatment of stromal keratitis and uveitis.[149] Other advantages of trifluridine include its effectiveness in treating HSV infections resistant to IDU and/or vidarabine and its lack of cross-toxicity or allergenicity with these agents.[150]

Despite the apparent superiority of trifluridine over its antiviral predecessors, it is not without disadvantages. Trifluridine is activated by noninfected corneal cells and is incorporated into cellular as well as viral DNA. Punctate lesions in the corneal epithelium are clinical manifestations of trifluridine cytotoxicity.[151] Yet these effects seem to occur less often than with IDU and vidarabine.

Acyclovir

In vitro studies (plaque inhibition assays) have found acyclovir to have 5 to 10 times the activity of IDU and trifluridine and more than 100 times the activity of vidarabine against several strains of type I and type II HSV.[152] In experimental (rabbit) herpes simplex keratitis, 3% acyclovir ointment was significantly more effective than 0.5% IDU, and 3% vidarabine ointments in healing established herpes epithelial ulcerations at a faster rate and in eliminating the virus.[153] Rabbit ocular models were used because of their similarity to human eyes. Other rabbit studies have shown similarities in the activities of acyclovir, IDU, vidarabine, and trifluridine in therapy of superficial dendritic ulcers.[146,154,155] As with rabbit models, ulcerative corneal epithelial lesions in humans appear to respond similarly to acyclovir, IDU, and trifluridine, with no statistically significant differences evident in most studies.[156] Acyclovir's apparent superiority lies in its lack of toxicity to normal host cells. Administered systemically, acyclovir shows promise in the management of latent herpes viral infections.[147] Based on its high degree of viral specificity and apparent lack of toxicity, acyclovir presents a potentially important addition to currently available ocular antiviral arsenal. However, because no ophthalmic preparation is available, trifluridine remains the drug of choice. (For more information on acyclovir and acyclovir resistance, see Chapter 70, Opportunistic Infections in HIV-Infected Patients, and Chapter 72, Viral Infections.)

Other Drugs

Ganciclovir 0.05% and 0.15% gel has been shown to be equivalent to 3% acyclovir ointment in the treatment of superficial herpes simplex keratitis.[157] Cidofovir 1% ointment administered twice a day was equivalent to trifluridine administered five times daily in the rabbit model.[158] Cidofovir was more efficacious than 3% penciclovir ointment administered two or four times a day.[158] The potential for less frequent administration of cidofovir should be further evaluated.

REFERENCES

1. Vaughan D et al. General ophthalmology, 15th Ed. Stamford, CT: Appleton & Lange, 1999.
2. Gordon MO et al. The ocular hypertension treatment study: baseline factors that predict the onset of primary open-angle glaucoma. Arch Ophthalmol. 2002;120:714.
3. Zimmerman T et al. Timolol and facility of outflow. Invest Ophthalmol Vis Sci 1977;16:623.
4. Sonntag JR et al. Effect of timolol therapy on outflow facility. Invest Ophthalmol Vis Sci 1978; 17:293.
5. Zimmerman TJ et al. Timolol: dose response and duration of action. Arch Ophthalmol 1977;95:605.
6. Kwitko GM et al. Bilateral effects of long-term monocular timolol therapy. Am J Ophthalmol 1987; 104:591.
7. Boger WP et al. Long-term experience with timolol ophthalmic solution in patients with open-angle glaucoma. Ophthalmology 1978;85:259.

8. Heel RC et al. Timolol: a review of its therapeutic efficacy in the topical treatment of glaucoma. Drugs 1979;17:38.
9. Goethals M. Ten-year follow-up of timolol-treated open-angle glaucoma (summary). Surv Ophthalmol 1989;33:S463.
10. Zimmerman TJ et al. Safety and efficacy of timolol in pediatric glaucoma. Surv Ophthalmol 1983; 28:262.
11. Boger WP et al. Clinical trials comparing timolol ophthalmic solution to pilocarpine in open-angle glaucoma. Am J Ophthalmol 1978;86:8.
12. Moss AP et al. A comparison of the effects of timolol and epinephrine on intraocular pressure. Am J Ophthalmol 1978;86:489.
13. Britman NA. Cardiac effects of topical timolol. N Engl J Med 1979;300:566.
14. Kim JW et al. Timolol-induced bradycardia. Anesth Analg 1980;59:301.

15. McMahon CD et al. Adverse effects experienced by patients taking timolol. Am J Ophthalmol 1979; 88:736.
16. Jones FC et al. Exacerbation of asthma by timolol. N Engl J Med 1979;301:270.
17. Van Buskirk EM. Corneal anesthesia after timolol maleate therapy. Am J Ophthalmol 1979;88:739.
18. Draeger J, Winter R. The local anaesthetic action of metipranolol versus timolol in patients with healthy eyes. In: Merte, HJ ed. Metipranolol. New York: Springer-Verlag Wien 1983:76.
19. Akingbehin T, Villada JR. Metipranolol-associated granulomatous anterior uveitis. Br J Ophthalmol 1991;75:519.
20. Zimmerman TJ et al. Side effects of timolol. Surv Ophthalmol 1983;28(Suppl):243.
21. Schmitt CJ et al. Penetration of timolol into the rabbit eye. Arch Ophthalmol 1980;98:547.

22. Afffrime MD et al. Dynamics and kinetics of ophthalmic timolol. Clin Pharmacol Ther 1980;27:471.

23. Passo MS et al. Plasma timolol in glaucoma patients. Ophthalmology 1984;91:1361.

24. Lustgarten JS, Podos SM. Topical timolol and the nursing mother. Arch Ophthalmol 1983;101:1381.

25. Rozier A et al. Gelrite: a novel, ion-activated, in situ gelling polymer for ophthalmic vehicles. Effect on bioavailability of timolol. Int J Pharm 1989;57:163.

26. Shedden AH et al. Multiclinic, double-masked study of 0.5% Timoptic-XE once daily versus 0.5% Timoptic twice daily. Ophthalmology 1993;100:111.

27. Partamian LG et al. A dose-response study of the effect of levobunolol on ocular hypertension. Am J Ophthalmol 1983;95:229.

28. Bensinger RE et al. Levobunolol: a three-month efficacy study in the treatment of glaucoma and ocular hypertension. Arch Ophthalmol 1985;103:375.

29. Rakofsky SI et al. A comparison of the ocular hypotensive efficacy of once-daily and twice-daily levobunolol treatment. Ophthalmology 1989;96:8.

30. Berson FG. Levobunolol compared with timolol for the long-term control of elevated intraocular pressure. Arch Ophthalmol 1985;103:379.

31. Berson FG et al. Levobunolol: a beta-adrenoreceptor antagonist effective in the long-term treatment of glaucoma. Ophthalmology 1985;92:1271.

32. Wandel T et al. Glaucoma treatment with once-daily levobunolol. Am J Ophthalmol 1986;101:298.

33. Silverstone D et al. Evaluation of once-daily levobunolol 0.25% and timolol 0.25% therapy for increased pressure. Am J Ophthalmol 1991;112: 56.

34. Ball SF, Scheider E. Cost of β-adrenergic receptor blocking agents for ocular hypertension. Arch Ophthalmol 1992;110:654.

35. Battershill PE, Sorkin EM. Ocular metipranolol: a preliminary review of its pharmacodynamic and pharmacokinetic properties, and therapeutic efficacy in glaucoma and ocular hypertension. Drugs 1988;36:601.

36. Mills KB, Wright G. A blind randomized crossover trial comparing metipranolol 0.3% with timolol 0.25% in open-angle glaucoma: a pilot study. Br J Ophthalmol 1986;70:39.

37. Bacon PJ et al. Cardiovascular responses to metipranolol and timolol eyedrops in healthy volunteers. Br J Clin Pharmacol 1989;27:1.

38. Krieglstein GK et al. Levobunolol and metipranolol: comparative ocular hypotensive efficacy, safety, and comfort. Br J Ophthalmol 1987;71:250.

39. Anon. Dr. Mann on metipranolol difference. Scrip 1991;1601:26.

40. Akingbehin T et al. Metipranolol-induced adverse reactions: I. The rechallenge study. Eye 1992; 6:277.

41. Akingbehin T, Villada JR. Metipranolol-induced adverse reactions: II. Loss of intraocular pressure control. Eye 1992;6:280.

42. James IM. Pharmacologic effects of beta-blocking agents used in the management of glaucoma. Surv Ophthalmol 1989;33(Suppl):453.

43. Scoville B et al. A double-masked comparison of carteolol and timolol in ocular hypertension. Am J Ophthalmol 1988;105:150.

44. Stewart WC et al. A 3-month comparison of 1% and 2% carteolol and 0.5% timolol in open-angle glaucoma. Graefes Arch Clin Exp Ophthalmol 1991;229:258.

45. Brazier DJ, Smith SE. Ocular and cardiovascular response to topical carteolol 2% and timolol 0.5% in healthy volunteers. Br J Ophthalmol 1988; 72:101.

46. Levy NS et al. A controlled comparison of betaxolol and timolol with long-term evaluation of safety and efficacy. Glaucoma 1985;7:54.

47. Berry DP et al. Betaxolol and timolol: a comparison of efficacy and side effects. Arch Ophthalmol 1984;102:42.

48. Stewart RH et al. Betaxolol vs. timolol: a six-month double-blind comparison. Arch Ophthalmol 1986;104:46.

49. Allen RC et al. A double-masked comparison of betaxolol vs. timolol in the treatment of open-angle glaucoma. Am J Ophthalmol 1986;101:535.

50. Meland S et al. Ongoing clinical assessment of the safety profile and efficacy of brimonidine compared with timolol: year-three results. Brimonidine Study Group II. Clin Ther 2000;22:103–111.

51. DuBiner HB et al. A comparison of the efficacy and tolerability of brimonidine and latanoprost in adults with open-angle glaucoma or ocular hypertension: a three-month, multicenter, randomized, double-masked, parallel-group trial. Clin Ther 2001; 23:1969.

52. Sall KN et al. Dorzolamide/timolol combination verses concomitant administration of brimonidine and timolol: six-month comparison of efficacy and tolerability. Ophthalmology 2003;110:615.

53. Strahlman E et al. A double-masked, randomized 1-year study comparing dorzolamide, timolol, and betaxolol. Arch Ophthalmol 1995;113:1009.

54. Serle JB et al. A comparison of the safety and efficacy of twice daily brimonidine 0.2% versus betaxolol 0.25% in subjects with elevated intraocular pressure. Surv Ophthalmol 1996;41:S39.

55. Wayman L et al. Comparison of dorzolamide and timolol as suppressors of aqueous humor flow in humans. Arch Ophthalmol 1997;115:1368.

56. Alcon Laboratories, Inc. Azopt package insert. Fort Worth, TX. 1998.

57. Merck & Co., Inc. Trusopt package insert. West Point, PA, 2001 October.

58. Rosenburg LF et al. Combination of systemic acetazolamide and topical dorzolamide in reducing intraocular pressure and aqueous humor formation. Ophthalmology 1998;105:88.

59. Alexander CL et al. Prostaglandin analog treatment of glaucoma and ocular hypertension. Ann Pharmacother 2002;36:504-11.

60. Pharmacia and Upjohn Company. Xalatan package insert. Kalamazoo, MI, 2003 February.

61. Camras CB et al. Latanoprost treatment for glaucoma: effects of treating for 1 year and of switching from timolol. United States Latanoprost Study Group. Am J Ophthalmol 1998;126:390.

62. Bucci MG. Intraocular pressure-lowering effects of latanoprost monotherapy versus latanoprost or pilocarpine in combination with timolol: a randomized, observer-masked multicenter study in patients with open-angle glaucoma. Italian Latanoprost Study Group. J Glaucoma 1999;8:24.

63. Simmons ST et al. Three-month comparison of brimonidine and latanoprost as adjunctive therapy in glaucoma and ocular hypertension patients uncontrolled on beta-blockers: tolerance and peak intraocular pressure lowering. Ophthalmology 2002; 109:307.

64. Hoyng PF et al. The additive intraocular pressure-lowering effects of latanoprost in combined therapy with other ocular hypotensive agents. Surv Ophthalmol 1997;41:S93.

65. Kimal Arici M, Topalkara A, Guler C. Additive effect of latanoprost and dorzolamide in patients with elevated intraocular pressure. Int Ophthalmol 1998; 22:37.

66. Smith SL et al. The use of latanoprost 0.005% once daily and its effects on intraocular pressure as primary or adjunctive therapy. J Ocular Pharm Ther 1999;15:29.

67. Netland PA et al. Travoprost compared with latanoprost and timolol in patients with open-angle glaucoma or ocular hypertension. Am J Ophthalmol 2001;132:472.

68. Goldberg I et al. Comparison of topical travoprost eye drops given once daily and timolol 0.5% given twice daily in patients with open-angle glaucoma or ocular hypertension. J Glaucoma 2001;10:414.

69. Alcon Pharmaceuticals. Travatan package insert. Fort Worth, Texas, 2001.

70. Sherwood M et al. Six-month comparison of bimatoprost once-daily and twice daily with timolol twice daily in patients with elevated intraocular pressure. Surv Ophthalmol 2001;45(Suppl 4):S361.

71. Noecker RS et al. A six-month randomized clinical trial comparing the intraocular pressure-lowering of bimatoprost and latanoprost in patients with ocular hypertension or glaucoma. Am J Ophthalmol 2003;135:55.

72. Allergan. Lumigan package insert. Irvine, CA; 2001 November.

73. Alexander CL et al. Prostaglandin analog treatment of glaucoma and ocular hypertension. Ann Pharmacother 2002;36:504.

74. Nordmann JP et al. A double-masked randomized comparison of the efficacy and safety of unoprostone and timolol and betaxolol in patients with primary open-angle glaucoma including pseudoexfoliation glaucoma or ocular hypertension. Am J Ophthalmol 2002;133;1.

75. Susanna R Jr et al. A double-masked, randomized clinical trial comparing latanoprost and unoprostone in patients with open-angle glaucoma or ocular hypertension. Ophthalmology 2001;108;259.

76. Novartis Ophthalmics. Rescula Package insert. Duluth, GA; 2001 February.

77. Polansky JR. Beta-adrenergic therapy for glaucoma. Int Ophthalmol Clin 1990;20:219.

78. Allen RC, Epstein DL. Additive effect of betaxolol and epinephrine in primary open angle glaucoma. Arch Ophthalmol 1986;104:1178.

79. Harris LS. Dose response analysis of echothriphate iodide. Arch Ophthalmol 1971;86:502.

80. Keates EU, Stone RA. Safety and effectiveness of concomitant administration of dipivefrin and timolol. Am J Ophthalmol 1981;91:243.

81. Cebon L et al. Experience with dipivalyl epinephrine: its effectiveness alone or in combination and its side effects. Aust J Ophthalmol 1983;11:159.

82. Yuksel N et al. The short-term effect of adding brimonidine 0.2% to timolol treatment in patients with open-angle glaucoma. Ophthalmologica 1999; 213:228.

83. VanBuskirk EM et al. Betaxolol in patients with glaucoma and asthma. Am J Ophthalmol 1986; 101:531.

84. Sorensen SJ, Abel SR. Comparison of the ocular beta-blockers. Ann Pharmacother 1996;30:43.

85. Berson FG, Epstein DL. Separate and combined effects of timolol maleate and acetazolamide in open-angle glaucoma. Am J Ophthalmol 1981; 92:788.

86. Strahlman ER et al. The use of dorzolamide and pilocarpine as adjunctive therapy to timolol in patients with elevated intraocular pressure. Ophthalmology 1996;103:1283.

87. thoe Schwartzenberg GW, Buys YM. Efficacy of brimonidine 0.2% as adjunctive therapy for patients with glaucoma inadequately controlled with otherwise maximal medical therapy. Ophthalmol 1999; 106:1616.

88. Toris CB et al. Effects of brimonidine on aqueous humor dynamics in human eyes. Arch Ophthalmol 1995;113:1514.

89. Allergan. Alphagan package insert. Irvine, CA, 2002.

90. Zimmerman TJ et al. Therapeutic index of pilocarpine, carbachol, and timolol with nasolacrimal occlusion. Am J Ophthalmol 1992;114:1.

91. Ellis PP et al. Effect of nasolacrimal occlusion on timolol concentrations in the aqueous humor of the human eye. J Pharm Sci 1992;81:219.

92. Urtti A, Salminen L. Minimizing systemic absorption of topically administered ophthalmic drugs. Surv Ophthalmol 1993;37:435.

93. Zambarakji HJ, Spencer AF, Vernon SA. An unusual side effect of dorzolamide. Eye 1997;11:418.

94. Galin MA et al. Ophthalmological use of osmotic therapy. Am J Ophthalmol 1966;62:629.

95. Drance SM. Effect of oral glycerol on intraocular pressure in normal and glaucomatous eyes. Arch Ophthalmol 1964;72:491.

96. Becker B et al. Isosorbide: an oral hyperosmotic agent. Arch Ophthalmol 1967;78:147.

97. Obstbaum SA et al. Low-dose oral alcohol and intraocular pressure. Am J Ophthalmol 1973;76:926.

98. Adams RE et al. Ocular hypotensive effect of intravenously administered mannitol. Arch Ophthalmol 1963;69:55.

99. D'Alena P et al. Adverse effects after glycerol orally and mannitol parenterally. Arch Ophthalmol 1966;75:201.

100. Spaeth GL et al. Anaphylactic reaction to mannitol. Arch Ophthalmol 1967;78:583.

101. Fraunfelder FT. Drug-Induced Ocular Side Effects and Drug Interactions. Philadelphia: Lea & Febiger, 1976.

102. Grant WM. Toxicology of the Eye, 2nd ed. Springfield, IL: Charles C Thomas, 1974.

103. D'Amico DJ et al. Amiodarone keratopathy: drug-induced lipid storage disease. Arch Ophthalmol 1981;99:257.

104. Kaplan LJ, Cappaert WE. Amiodarone keratopathy: correlation to dosage and duration. Arch Ophthalmol. 1982;100:601.

105. Risperidone package insert, Risperdal, Janssen-US, November 1997.

106. Abelson MB, Spitalny L. Combined analysis of two studies using the conjunctival allergen challenge model to evaluate olopatadine hydrochloride, a new ophthalmic antiallergic agent with dual activity. Am J Ophthalmol 1998;125:797.

107. Alcon Laboratories. Emadine package insert. Fort Worth, TX, 1999 August.

108. CIBA Vision. Zaditor package insert. Duluth, GA, 1999 July.

109. Yanni JM et al. Preclinical efficacy of emedastine, a potent selective histamine H1 antagonist for topical ocular use. J Ocular Pharmacol 1994;10:665.

110. Aguilar A. Comparative study of clinical efficacy and tolerance in seasonal allergic conjunctivitis management with 0.1% olopatadine hydrochloride versus ketotifen fumarate. Acta Ophthalmol Scand Suppl. 2000;(230):52.

111. Spangler SL et al. Evaluation of the efficacy of olopatadine hydrochloride 0.1% ophthalmic solution and azelastine hydrochloride 0.05% ophthalmic solution in the conjunctival allergen challenge model. Clin Ther 2001;23;1272.

112. Caldwell DR et al. Efficacy and safety of lodoxamide 0.1% vs cromolyn sodium 4% in patients with vernal keratoconjunctivitis. Am J Ophthalmol 1992;113:632.

113. Fahy GT et al. Randomized double-masked trial of lodoxamide and sodium cromoglycate in allergic eye disease. A multicentre study. Eur J Ophthalmol 1992;2:144.

114. Butrus S et al. Comparison of the clinical efficacy and comfort of olopatadine hydrochloride 0.1% ophthalmic solution and nedocromil sodium 2% solution in the human conjunctival allergen challenge model. Clin Ther 2000;22:1462.

115. Baum JL. Initial therapy of suspected microbial corneal ulcers: antibiotic therapy based on prevalence of organisms. Surv Ophthalmol 1979;24:97.

116. Jones DB. Initial therapy of suspected microbial corneal ulcers: specific antibiotic therapy based on corneal smears. Surv Ophthalmol 1979;24:97.

117. Leibowitz H et al. Bioavailability and effectiveness of topically administered corticosteroids. Trans Am Acad Ophthalmol Otolaryngol 1975;79:78.

118. Leibowitz H et al. Anti-inflammatory effectiveness in the cornea of topically administered prednisolone. Invest Ophthalmol Vis Sci 1974;13:757.

119. Kupferman A et al. Therapeutic effectiveness of fluorometholone in inflammatory keratitis. Arch Ophthalmol 1975;93:1011.

120. Leibowitz HM et al. Comparative anti-inflammatory efficacy of topical corticosteroids with low glaucoma-inducing potential. Arch Ophthalmol 1992;110:118.

121. Armalay MF. Statistical attributes of the steroid hypertensive response in the clinically normal eye. Invest Ophthalmol 1965;4:187.

122. Becker B et al. Glaucoma and corticosteroid provocative testing. Arch Ophthalmol 1965,74.621.

123. Lewis JM et al. Intraocular pressure response to topical dexamethasone as a predictor for the development of primary open-angle glaucoma. Am J Ophthalmol 1988;106:607.

124. Godel V et al. Systemic steroids and ocular fluid dynamics II: systemic versus topical steroids. Acta Ophthalmol (Copenh) 1972;50:664.

125. Cantrill HL et al. Comparison of in vitro potency of corticosteroids with ability to raise intraocular pressure. Am J Ophthalmol 1975;79:1012.

126. Stewart RH, Smith JP, Rosenthal AL. Ocular pressure response to fluorometholone acetate and dexamethasone phosphate. Curr Eye Res 1984;3:835.

127. Stewart RH et al. Intraocular pressure response to topically administered fluorometholone. Arch Ophthalmol 1979;97:2139.

128. Leibowitz HM et al. Intraocular-pressure raising potential of 1.0% rimexolone in patients responding to corticosteroids. Arch Ophthalmol 1996; 114:933.

129. Dell SJ et al. A controlled evaluation of the efficacy and safety of loteprednol etabonate in the prophylactic treatment of seasonal allergic conjunctivitis. Am J Ophthalmol 1997;123:791.

130. Kitazawa Y, Horie T. The prognosis of corticosteroid-responsive individuals. Arch Ophthalmol 1981;99:819.

131. Oglesby RB et al. Cataracts in rheumatoid arthritis patients treated with corticosteroids: description and differential diagnosis. Arch Ophthalmol 1961;66:519.

132. Oglesby RB et al. Cataracts in patients with rheumatic diseases treated with corticosteroids: further observations. Arch Ophthalmol 1961;66:625.

133. Skalka HW, Prchal JT. Effect of corticosteroids on cataract formation. Arch Ophthalmol 1980;98:1773.

134. Yablonski MF et al. Cataracts induced by topical dexamethasone in diabetics. Arch Ophthalmol 1975;94:474.

135. Sevel D et al. Lenticular complications of long-term steroid therapy in children with asthma and eczema. J Allergy Clin Immunol 1977;60:215.

136. Fraunfelder FT et al. Possible adverse effects from topical ocular 10% phenylephrine. Am J Ophthalmol 1978;85:447.

137. Brown MN et al. Lack of side effects from topically administered 10% phenylephrine eye drops: a controlled study. Arch Ophthalmol 1980;98:487.

138. Morton HG. Atropine intoxication: its manifestations in infants and children. J Pediatr 1939; 14:755.

139. Marks HH. Psychotogenic properties of cyclopentolate. JAMA 1963;186:430.

140. Freund M et al. Toxic effects of scopolamine eye drops. Am J Ophthalmol 1970;70:637.

141. Hoefnagel D. Toxic effects of atropine and homatropine eye drops in children. N Engl J Med 1961;264:168.

142. Wahl JW. Systemic reaction to tropicamide. Arch Ophthalmol 1969;82:320.

143. Abrams SM et al. Marrow aplasia following topical application of chloramphenicol eye ointment. Arch Intern Med 1980;140:576.

144. Musson K. Cushingoid status: induced by topical steroid medication. J Pediatr Ophthalmol Strabismus 1968;5:33.

145. Flach AJ. Cyclo-oxygenase inhibitors in ophthalmology. Surv Ophthalmol 1992;36:259.

146. Kaufman HE. Herpetic keratitis. Invest Ophthalmol Vis Sci 1978;17:941.

147. Kaufman HE. Antimetabolite drug therapy in herpes simplex. Ophthalmology 1980;87:135.

148. Bauer DJ et al. Treatment of experimental herpes simplex keratitis with acycloguanosine. Br J Ophthalmol 1979;63:429.

149. Kaufman HE. Antiviral update. Ophth AAO 1979;86:131.

150. Pavan-Langston DR, Foster CS. Trifluorothymidine and idoxuridine therapy of ocular herpes. Am J Ophthalmol 1977;84:818.

151. McGill J et al. Some aspects of the clinical use of trifluorothymidine in the treatment of herpetic ulceration of the cornea. Trans Ophthalmol Soc U K 1974;94:342.

152. Collins P, Bauer DJ. The activity in vitro against herpes virus of 9-(2-hydroxyethoxymethyl) guanine (acycloguanosine), a new antiviral agent. J Antimicrob Chemother 1979;5:431.

153. Pavan-Langston DR et al. Acyclic antimetabolite therapy of experimental herpes simplex keratitis. Am J Ophthalmol 1978;86:618.

154. Falcon MG, Jones BR. Acycloguanosine: antiviral activity in the rabbit cornea. Br J Ophthalmol 1979;63:422.

155. Shiota J et al. Efficacy of acycloguanosine against herpetic ulcers in rabbit cornea. Br J Ophthalmol 1979;63:425.

156. Coster DJ et al. A comparison of acyclovir and idoxuridine as treatment for ulcerative herpetic keratitis. Br J Ophthalmol 1980;64:763.

157. Colin J et al. Ganciclovir ophthalmic gel in the treatment of herpes simplex keratitis. Cornea 1997;16:393.

158. Kaufman HE et al. Trifluridine, cidofovir, and penciclovir in the treatment of experimental herpetic keratitis. Arch Ophthalmol 1998;116:777.

159. Nicastro NJ. Visual disturbances associated with over-the-counter ibuprofen in three patients. Ann Ophthalmol 1989;29:447.

160. Hamill MB et al. Transdermal scopolamine delivery system and acute angle-closure glaucoma. Ann Ophthalmol. 1983;1:1011.

161. Bar S et al. Presenile cataracts in phenytoin-treated epileptic patients. Arch Ophthalmol 1983; 101:422.

162. Marsch SCU, Schaefer HG. Problems with eye opening after propofol anesthesia. Anesth Analg 1990;70:115.

163. Cunningham M et al. Eye tics and subjective hearing impairment during fluoxetine therapy. Am J Psychiatry 1990;147:947.

164. Fraunfelder FT, Meyer SM. Amantadine and corneal deposits. Am J Ophthalmol 1990;110:96.

165. Flach A. Photosensitivity to sulfisoxazole ointment. Arch Ophthalmol 1981;99:609.

166. Flach AJ et al. Photosensitivity to topically applied sulfisoxazole ointment. Arch Ophthalmol 1982;100:1286.

167. Laties AM et al. Expanded clinical evaluation of lovastatin (EXCEL) study results II. Assessment of the human lens after 48 weeks of treatment with lovastatin. Am J Cardiol 1991;67:447.

168. Shingleton BJ et al. Ocular toxicity associated with high-dose carmustine. Arch Ophthalmol 1981;100:1766.

169. Hopen G et al. Corneal toxicity with systemic cytarabine. Am J Ophthalmol 1981;91:500.

170. Smollen KW et al. Non-hematologic toxicities from high-dose cytarabine: analysis of seven patients and development of a monitoring guide. PharmFax 1984;13:4.

171. Jick H, Brandt DE. Allopurinol and cataracts. Am J Ophthalmol 1984;98:355.

172. Friedman DI et al. Neuro-ophthalmic complications of interleukin 2 therapy. Arch Ophthalmol 1991;109:1679.

173. Pfizer, Inc. Viagra Package Insert. New York, NY, 1999 June.

174. Goa KL, Chrisp P. Ocular diclofenac: a review of its pharmacology and clinical use in cataract surgery, and potential in other inflammatory ocular conditions. Drugs Aging 1992;2:473.

175. Allergan America. Ocufen package insert. Hormigueros, PR, 1992.

176. CIBA Vision Ophthalmics. Voltaren Ophthalmic package insert. Atlanta, GA, 1991 August.

177. Flach AJ et al. The effect of ketorolac tromethamine solution in reducing postoperative inflammation after cataract extraction and intraocular lens implantation. Ophthalmology 1988;95: 1279.

178. Flach AJ et al. Prophylaxis of aphakic cystoid macular edema without corticosteroids. Ophthalmology 1990;97:1253.

179. Flach AJ et al. Improvement in visual acuity in chronic aphakic and pseudophakic cystoid macular edema after treatment with topical 0.5% ketorolac tromethamine. Am J Ophthalmol 1991; 112:514.

180. Tinkelman DG et al. Double-masked, paired-comparison clinical study of ketorolac tromethamine 0.5% ophthalmic solution compared with placebo eyedrops in the treatment of seasonal allergic conjunctivitis. Surv Ophthalmol 1993;38(Suppl):133.

181. Flach AJ et al. Effectiveness of ketorolac tromethamine 0.5% ophthalmic solution for chronic aphakic and pseudophakic cystoid macular edema. Am J Ophthalmol 1987;103:479.

182. Flach AJ et al. Improvement in visual acuity in chronic aphakic and pseudophakic cystoid macular edema after treatment with topical 0.5% ketorolac tromethamine. Am J Ophthalmol 1991; 112:514.

183. Tinkelman DG et al. Double-masked, paired-comparison clinical study of ketorolac tromethamine 0.5% ophthalmic solution compared with placebo eyedrops in the treatment of seasonal allergic conjunctivitis. Surv Ophthalmol 1993;38(Suppl):133.

184. Ballas Z et al. Clinical evaluation of ketorolac tromethamine 0.5% ophthalmic solution for the treatment of seasonal allergic conjunctivitis. Surv Ophthalmol 1993;38(Suppl):141.

185. Ortho McNeil Pharmaceuticals Inc. Topamax package insert. Raritan, NJ. 2003 December.

186. Pfizer Roerig Pharmaceuticals. VFEND package insert. New York, New York. 2003 December.

187. Flach AJ, Bolan BJ. Amiodarone-induced lens opacities: an 8-year follow-up study. Arch Ophthalmol 1996;108:1668.

188. Franufelder FT, Meyer SM. Posterior subcapsular cataracts associated with nasal or inhalation corticosteriods. Am J Ophthalmol 1990;109:489

189. EliLilly & Company. Cialis package insert. Indianapolis, IN. 2003 November.

190. Bayer Health Care. Levitra Package insert. West Haven, CT. 2003 August.

CHAPTER 52

Headache

Brian K. Alldredge

Clinical features and drug therapy of the common headache syndromes are presented in this chapter. Proposed pathophysiologic features of the major headache types also are presented to provide the reader with an understanding of the rationale for current and future therapies.

Prevalence

In the United States, migraine headache affects approximately 23 million persons, and 11 million experience significant headache-related disability.[1] Headache is the fourth most common symptom reported at outpatient medical visits,[2] and the associated economic costs in America are estimated to be between $1 billion and $17 billion dollars annually.[3] Overall, the prevalence of headache is highest in adolescence and early adulthood and declines with age through the elderly years.[4,5] Despite numerous potential causes of headaches, more than 90% of patients with a chief complaint of continuous or sporadically recurring headaches are eventually diagnosed as having either tension-type or migraine headache.[6]

Classification

Headache is a symptom that can be caused by many disorders. For example, head pain can result from traction, displacement, or inflammation of pain-sensitive structures within the head, or it can be due to disorders of extracranial structures such as the eyes, ears, or sinuses. For diagnostic and therapeutic purposes, it is useful to categorize headache into one of two major types (*primary* and *secondary*) on the basis of the underlying etiology. *Primary headache disorders* are characterized by the lack of an identifiable and treatable underlying cause. Migraine, tension-type, and cluster headaches are examples of primary headache disorders. *Secondary headache disorders* are those associated with a variety of organic causes such as trauma, cerebrovascular malformations, and brain tumors. Depending on the cause, headache may manifest in a variety of ways or may be accompanied by other associated signs or symptoms. A comprehensive classification scheme of the different types of headaches, modified from the International Headache Society (IHS) is shown in Table 52-1.[7] Readers are referred to the IHS classification report for the comprehensive headache classification scheme and a detailed description of the specific diagnostic features of each headache type. This classification scheme is useful for grouping headaches with similar clinical features or etiologies. Headache must be accurately evaluated and classified because this symptom may reflect an ominous problem such as the presence of a brain tumor or a much more benign process such as muscle tension. Moreover, effective intervention depends on a correct diagnosis.

Primary Headache Disorders
MIGRAINE HEADACHES

Migraine headaches usually develop over a period of minutes to hours, progressing from a dull ache to a more intense pulsating pain that worsens with each pulse. The headache usually begins in the frontotemporal region and may radiate to the occiput and neck; it may occur unilaterally or bilaterally. Migraine headaches often are accompanied by nausea and vomiting and may last for up to 72 hours. These headaches usually are alleviated by relaxation in a dark room and sleep. Migraine is more common in females than males. Migraine headaches are divided into those with and without an aura. The term, *aura,* refers to the complex of focal neurologic symptoms (e.g., alterations in vision or sensation) that initiate or accompany a migraine attack. Migraine may be precipitated by a variety of dietary, pharmacologic, hormonal, or environmental factors.

Table 52-1 Classification of Headache[7]

Migraine

Migraine without aura
Migraine with aura
Complicated migraine (see Table 52-2)

Tension-Type Headache

Episodic tension-type headache
Chronic tension-type headache

Cluster Headache

Episodic cluster headache
Chronic cluster headache

Miscellaneous Headaches Unassociated with Structural Lesion (e.g., cold stimulus headache, benign exertional headache)

Headache Associated with Head Trauma

Acute post-traumatic headache
Chronic post-traumatic headache

Headache Associated with Vascular Disorders

Acute ischemic cerebrovascular disease (TIA or stroke)
Intracranial hematoma
Subarachnoid hemorrhage
Unruptured vascular malformation
Arteritis
Carotid or vertebral artery pain
Venous thrombosis
Arterial hypertension

Headache Associated with Nonvascular Intracranial Disorder (e.g., high or low CSF pressure, intracranial infection, or neoplasm)

Headache Associated with Substances or their Withdrawal (e.g., withdrawal from alcohol, caffeine, ergotamine, narcotics; also see Table 52-3).

Headache Associated with Noncephalic Infection (e.g., viral or bacterial infection)

Headache Associated with Metabolic Disorder (e.g., hypoxia, hypercapnia, hypoglycemia, dialysis)

Headache or Facial Pain Associated with Disorder of Cranium, Neck, Eyes, Ears, Nose, Sinuses, Teeth, Mouth, or Other Facial or Cranial Structures (e.g., cervical spine, acute glaucoma, refractive errors, acute sinus headache)

Cranial Neuralgias, Nerve Trunk Pain and Deafferentation Pain (e.g., compression, demyelination, infarction, or inflammation of cranial nerves)

Headache Not Classifiable

CSF, cerebrospinal fluid; TIA, transient ischemic attacks.

CLUSTER HEADACHES

Cluster headaches derive their name from a characteristic pattern of recurrent headaches that are separated by periods of remission that last from months to even years. During those periods when clusters of headaches are experienced, the headaches usually occur at least once daily. The headache generally is unilateral, occurs behind the eye, reaches maximal intensity over several minutes, and lasts for less than 3 hours. Unilateral lacrimation, rhinorrhea, and facial flushing may accompany the cluster headache. During cluster periods, headache is commonly precipitated by alcohol, naps, and vasodilating drugs. In contrast to migraine headaches, cluster headaches are more common in males than females.

TENSION-TYPE HEADACHES

A dull, persistent headache, occurring bilaterally in a hatband distribution around the head is characteristic of tension-type headaches. The headache is usually not debilitating and may fluctuate in intensity throughout the day. Tension-type headaches often occur during or after stress, but chronic tension-type headaches may persist for months even in the absence of recognizable stress. Skeletal muscle overcontraction, depression, and occasionally nausea may accompany the headache. Prodrome neurologic symptoms do not occur in association with tension-type headache. More detailed descriptions of migraine, cluster, and tension-type headaches appear in following sections of this chapter.

Secondary Headache Disorders

In addition to migraine, cluster, and tension-type headaches, patients may also experience headache associated with head trauma, vascular disorders, central nervous system (CNS) infection (including HIV), or metabolic disorders. More than 300 disorders capable of producing headache have been identified.[8] Examples of secondary headache disorders are given in Table 52-1.

The length of time that a patient has experienced headaches provides highly useful information for assessing the nature and etiology of the headaches. A new severe headache in a patient without a previous history is the most useful single piece of information for identifying potentially destructive intracranial or extracranial causes of headache. Such headaches may develop suddenly, over a period of hours to days (acute headache), or more gradually over days to months (subacute headache).

Acute Headaches

Acute headaches can be symptomatic of subarachnoid hemorrhage, stroke, meningitis, or intracranial mass lesion (e.g., brain tumor, hematoma, abscess). The headache that accompanies subarachnoid hemorrhage is typically severe (often described by the patient as the "worst headache of my life") and may occur in conjunction with alteration of mental status and focal neurologic signs. The headache of meningitis is usually bilateral and develops gradually over hours to days; symptoms such as fever, photophobia, and positive meningeal (Kernig's and Brudzinski's) signs often accompany the meningeal headache. Although the acute onset of headache associated with coughing, sneezing, straining, or change in head position is commonly thought to indicate a cranial mass lesion with cerebrospinal fluid (CSF) pathway obstruction,

several varieties of exertional headache are benign (see Table 52-1).

Subacute Headaches

Subacute headaches may be a sign of increased intracranial pressure, intracranial mass lesion, temporal arteritis, sinusitis, or trigeminal neuralgia (i.e., tic douloureux). Trigeminal neuralgia usually occurs after the age of 40 and is more common in women than men. The pain usually occurs along the second or third divisions of the trigeminal (facial) nerve and lasts only moments. Trigeminal neuralgia is characterized by sudden, intense pain that recurs paroxysmally, often in response to triggers such as talking, chewing, or shaving.

The clinical manifestations of headache, as described previously, focus on the onset, frequency, duration, site, gender of the patient, distribution, and other unique characteristics of the head pain. A comprehensive medical history and physical examination of the patient often provide sufficient information to make an adequate assessment of a patient's headache complaint, and may enable the practitioner to rule out headache as a manifestation of more serious illness. Physical examination of the patient suffering from the common, benign forms of headache (e.g., migraine, cluster, and tension-type headaches) is usually normal. When the medical history of the patient is suggestive of a secondary cause of headache, a more extensive evaluation with referral to or consultation by a neurologist is necessary.

Pathophysiology

Intracranially, only a limited number of structures are sensitive to pain. The most important pain-sensitive structures within the cranium are the proximal portions of the cerebral arteries, large veins, and the venous sinuses.[9] Headache may result from dilation, distention, or traction of the large intracranial vessels. The brain itself is insensitive to pain. Referred pain from inflammation of frontal or maxillary sinuses or refractive errors of the eye are potential, although over-diagnosed, causes of headache.[10] Scalp arteries and muscles are also capable of registering pain and have been implicated in the pathophysiology of migraine and tension-type headache. Extracranially, most of the structures outside the skull (e.g., periosteum, eye, ear, teeth, skin, deeper tissues) have pain afferents. In general, pain can be produced by activation of peripheral pain receptors (nociceptors), injury to CNS or peripheral nervous system, or displacement of the pain-sensitive structures mentioned earlier.

Historically, the primary headache disorders have been thought to be related either to vascular disturbances (migraine and cluster headache) or muscular tension (tension-type headache). However, clinical and experimental evidence no[w] suggests that these headaches have their origin in an underly]ing disturbance in brain function.[11] Evidence in this reg[ard] particularly strong for migraine and cluster headach[es] authors now hold the opinion that these clinically primary headache syndromes represent variabl[e] tions of a common pathogenetic phenomeno[n] neural innervation of the cranial circulati[on] mechanisms that lead to primary headac[he] identified. However, a *neurovascular* proposed in which headache is trigg[ered] central pain processing pathways (the trigeminocervical complex) leading to the release of potent neuropeptides (calcitonin gene–related peptide [CGRP], substance P, and neurokinin A) and subsequent vasodilation.[12] Serotonin, a vasoactive neurotransmitter released by brainstem nuclei of the trigeminovascular system, likely plays a role in migraine pathogenesis.[13] Furthermore, drugs that alter serotonergic function are highly effective for the symptomatic treatment of migraine and cluster headache.

Drug Therapy

Drug therapy for headache is divided into two major categories: (1) abortive therapy to provide relief during an acute headache attack and (2) prophylactic therapy to prevent or reduce the severity of recurrent headaches. Most people with infrequent tension-type headaches self-medicate with over-the-counter (OTC) analgesics to abort the acute event and do not require prophylactic therapy. By contrast, migraine and cluster headache sufferers who experience frequent headaches and who respond poorly to abortive measures are good candidates for preventive therapy.

Although analgesics are often useful for the treatment of episodic tension-type headaches, most patients with migraine and all patients with cluster headaches require other abortive measures. Until recently, ergot alkaloids (e.g., ergotamine and dihydroergotamine) were the most commonly prescribed agents for relief of migraine and cluster headaches. Now, the triptan class of agents (e.g., sumatriptan, zolmitriptan, naratriptan, rizatriptan, almotriptan, frovatriptan and eletriptan) is often preferred because of their favorable efficacy and tolerable adverse effect profiles.[14] However, the greater expense of the triptans limits the availability of these drugs for some patients.

Antidepressant agents (e.g., amitriptyline) are useful for prophylactic treatment of migraine and tension-type headaches. Because many patients suffer from mixed headache types, these agents can be useful for patients who might otherwise require preventive polytherapy. Other agents useful for migraine headache prophylaxis include beta-blocking agents (e.g., propranolol), valproate, calcium channel blocking agents (particularly verapamil), and nonsteroidal anti-inflammatory drugs (NSAIDs). Among the agents effective for prophylaxis against episode cluster headaches, verapamil, corticosteroids (e.g., prednisone) and lithium are usually preferred.

MIGRAINE HEADACHE

The word *migraine* comes from the Greek "hemicrania" and historically was used to describe unilateral headaches with associated symptoms. More recently, the IHS described migraine as follows. Migraine is an "idiopathic, recurring headache disorder manifesting in attacks lasting 4 to 72 hours. Typical characteristics of [migraine] headache are unilateral location, pulsating quality, moderate or severe intensity, aggravation by routine physical activity, and association with nausea, photo- and phonophobia."[7] Migraine headaches are classified according to the presence or absence of aura symptoms. Most persons who suffer from migraine do not experience aura symptoms. In patients with aura, visual symp-

toms are most common. Complicated migraine is a less common type of migraine in which the neurologic symptoms are more pronounced or disabling; in some cases the aura symptoms may outlast the headache itself. Table 52-2 outlines the predominant types of complicated migraine. Although patients with persistent symptoms should be thoroughly evaluated by a neurologist, permanent neurologic sequelae after migraine are rare even for patients with complicated migraine.

Pathophysiology

Past theories of pathogenesis have focused on alterations in cranial vessel diameter and blood flow as the primary cause of migraine. In this "vascular hypothesis," it was thought that focal neurologic symptoms preceding or accompanying the headache were caused by vasoconstriction and reduction in cerebral blood flow. The headache was thought to be caused by a compensatory vasodilation with displacement of pain-sensitive intracranial structures. Although blood flow is decreased during the aura of migraine,[15] other observations do not support the vascular hypothesis. The headache phase of migraine with aura has been shown to begin while blood flow is reduced,[15] and migraine without aura is not associated with alterations in regional cerebral blood flow.[16] Furthermore, the therapeutic effect of sumatriptan, a drug highly specific for neurovascular headaches, is not temporally related to its vasoconstrictive effect.[17] More recent evidence suggests that the pain of migraine is generated centrally and involves episodic dysfunction of neural structures that control the cranial circulation (the *trigeminovascular system*). The availability of functional brain imaging has had a dramatic effect on the ability to visualize the pathophysiologic events of a migraine attack.[12] The trigeminovascular system consists of neurons, originating in the trigeminal ganglion, which innervate the cerebral circulation. Several potent vasodilator neuropeptides are contained within these trigeminal neurons, including calcitonin gene-related peptide, substance P, and neurokinin A.

Table 52-2 Types of Complicated Migraine[7]
Migraine with Prolonged Aura
Aura symptoms lasting >60 min but <1 wk
Familial Hemiplegic Migraine
Aura with hemiparesis; identical attacks in a first-degree relative
Basilar Migraine
Aura symptoms arising from brainstem or occipital lobes (e.g., dysarthria, vertigo, ataxia, decreased level of consciousness)
Ophthalmoplegic Migraine
Paresis of one or more ocular cranial nerves
Retinal Migraine
Aura symptoms with monocular scotoma or blindness lasting <1 hr
Status Migrainosus
Migraine headache lasting >72 hr despite treatment
Migrainous Infarction
Aura symptoms lasting longer than 7 days

In animals, stimulation of the trigeminal ganglion significantly alters regional brain blood flow.[12] Stimulation of the trigeminal ganglion in humans causes facial flushing, an increase in facial temperature,[18] and increases in extracerebral venous concentrations of calcitonin gene-related peptide and substance P.[19] The specific events leading to trigeminovascular dysfunction in migraine are unknown. However, evidence from positron emission tomography (PET) scanning (a technique to measure regional cerebral blood flow as an index of neuronal activity) suggests that episodic dysfunction of the brainstem, with corresponding effects on the trigeminal system, are involved. Using PET, Weiller and colleagues[20] found activation of the brainstem (periaqueductal gray, dorsal raphe nucleus, and locus ceruleus) at the onset of migraine headaches in nine patients. This area may represent an endogenous "migraine generator." Sporadic dysfunction of the nociceptive system (periaqueductal gray and dorsal raphe nucleus) and the neural control of cerebral blood flow (dorsal raphe nucleus and locus ceruleus) is hypothesized to trigger migraine headache via their effects on the trigeminovascular system. Further support for a trigeminovascular mechanism for migraine comes from studies that demonstrate inhibition of trigeminal neurons and associated nociceptive responses by various antimigraine drugs such as dihydroergotamine,[21] rizatriptan,[22] and zolmitriptan.[23] Abnormalities in serotonin (5-HT) activity are also thought to play a role in migraine headache. Plasma 5-HT levels decrease by nearly half during a migraine attack,[24] with a corresponding rise in the urinary excretion of 5-hydroxyindoleacetic acid,[25] the primary metabolite of 5-HT. Also, reserpine, a drug that depletes 5-HT from body stores, has been found to induce a stereotypical headache in migraineurs and a dull discomfort in patients not prone to migraine.[24,26] An intravenous (IV) injection of 5-HT effectively relieved both reserpine-induced and spontaneous migraine headache.[24,26] The therapeutic effects of drugs that stimulate 5-HT_1 receptors (e.g., dihydroergotamine, sumatriptan), antagonize 5-HT_2 receptors (e.g., methysergide, cyproheptadine), prevent 5-HT reuptake (e.g., amitriptyline) or release (e.g., calcium channel blockers), or inhibit brainstem serotonergic raphe neurons (e.g., valproate) all lend support to the hypothesis that 5-HT is an important mediator of migraine. Furthermore, brainstem nuclei activated during migraine have high densities of serotonergic neurons. Specific 5-HT receptor subtypes, 5-HT_{1B} and 5-HT_{1D}, are largely distributed in blood vessels[27] and nerves,[28] respectively. These same 5-HT receptor subtypes are the targets of antimigraine drugs such as the triptans and ergot alkaloids.

Genetics

A familial predisposition for migraine has been well recognized, although not until recent advances in gene mapping techniques has the genetic basis of a specific migraine disorder been discovered. The first identified migraine gene was found among several unrelated families with familial hemiplegic migraine. The mutations involved a gene encoding the α_1 subunit of a voltage-gated P/Q-type neuronal calcium channel.[29] The relevance of this discovery to other migrainous disorders is unknown, but it suggests that some forms of migraine may be fundamentally related to other episodic disorders of neurologic dysfunction known as "channelopathies."[11] Recently, genomewide linkage analysis in families with migraine (both with and without aura) have identified susceptibility loci on chromosomes 4 and 14.[30,31] An improved understanding of the genetics of migraine is likely to improve our understanding of the pathophysiology of the disorder as well as to hold promise for the identification of homogenous subgroups of patients in whom targeted drug (or other) interventions are likely to be highly effective.

In summary, the pathophysiology of migraine probably involves dysfunction of the trigeminal neurons that provide sensory innervation and modulate blood flow for intracranial blood vessels. The endogenous stimulus causing this dysfunction may arise from a "migraine generator" in the brainstem. Disturbances in 5-HT activity are also probably involved and it is this feature that serves as the target for many migraine-specific therapies.

Signs and Symptoms
Migraine With and Without Aura

1. K.L., a 29-year-old woman, presents to the clinic with a 5-month history of left-sided pulsatile head pain recurring on a weekly basis. Her headaches are usually preceded by unformed flashes of light bilaterally and a sensation of light-headedness. The ensuing pain is always unilateral and is commonly associated with nausea, vomiting, and photophobia. The headache is not relieved by two tablets of either aspirin 325 mg or ibuprofen 200 mg and generally lasts all day unless she is able to lie in a dark room and sleep. The headaches usually interfere with her ability to continue work. K.L. is unable to identify any external factors that precipitate a migraine attack. Both K.L.'s mother and grandmother also were affected by migraine headaches. Medical history is unremarkable, and K.L. denies any other medical problems. Current medications include only the OTC analgesics for headache and the contraceptive, Ortho-Novum 7/7/7. General physical and neurologic examinations are within normal limits. What subjective and objective data from the above description are consistent with a diagnosis of migraine with aura?

Given K.L.'s headache description, normal physical examination, and age of onset, she is most likely suffering from migraine with aura; a benign, though often disabling, disorder.

Approximately 17% of females and 6% of males in the United States suffer from migraine headaches,[1] and the incidence and prevalence of migraine has increased in recent decades.[32,33] The typical age of onset of migraine headaches is 15 to 35 years; after the age of 50, the onset of new migraine headaches is less common and is suggestive of a secondary cause. Although influenced by physiologic and environmental factors, migraine headaches occur more frequently among first-degree relatives, suggesting a genetic basis for this disorder.[33] K.L.'s gender (female), age (29 years), and positive family history are compatible with these aspects of migraine.

In the assessment of headache, the site or location of the pain, the quality of the pain, the duration and time course of the pain, and the conditions that provoke or palliate the pain should be considered.

The site or location of head pain can provide the clinician with clues as to the potential for secondary causes (e.g., lesions in the frontal sinuses, eyes, ears, teeth, or cerebral arteries). However, pain often is referred from other regions and the location of pain can provide misleading information.

Thus, the site of head pain need not be related to the apparent site of the focal neurologic symptoms that accompany migraine with aura. Head pain may be either unilateral or bilateral, and the pain need not recur on the same side if unilateral. In fact, 50% of patients with unilateral headache report that either side of the head may be affected during any individual migraine attack.[34]

The quality of migraine head pain usually begins as a dull ache that intensifies over a period of minutes or hours to a throbbing headache, which worsens with each arterial pulse. If untreated, the headache lasts from several hours to as long as 3 days or until the patient goes to sleep. The pain usually is intense enough to interfere with daily activities. Although migraine headaches seldom occur more often than once every few weeks, there is great interpatient variability in the frequency of occurrence. A patient may experience only several migraines in a lifetime, whereas others may suffer several headaches weekly on a chronic basis. K.L., like half of all patients with migraine, describes headaches that recur between one to four times monthly.[34] In this patient, the quality of the pain (i.e., interferes with K.L.'s ability to continue work); the duration and the time course of the pain (i.e., usually lasts all day); and the conditions that palliate the pain (i.e., lie in a dark room and sleep) are all compatible with the description of migraine headaches.

Aura symptoms are focal neurologic features that precede or accompany the headache in up to 30% of migraine sufferers.[35] When they precede the headache, aura symptoms usually begin 10 minutes to 1 hour before the onset of head pain. Light-headedness and photopsia (unformed flashes of light) are frequently reported and were described by K.L. before the onset of her head pain. Visual disturbances, such as scotoma (an isolated area within the visual field where vision is absent), occur in 30% of migraine patients.[35] At times, the scotoma is preceded only by a sensation that something is wrong with vision that cannot be more specifically characterized. At other times, the scotoma may be preceded by other visual distortions (e.g., the "halves of peoples' faces were vertically displaced in such a way that one eye appeared to be 1 or 2 centimeters lower than the other").[36] When scotomata are surrounded by a shiny pattern, they are termed *scintillating scotomata*. These scintillating scotomata can have "the visual quality of images in the kaleidoscopes we looked into as children, with the difference that the scotoma are silvery instead of multicolored as in the toy."[36] Other neurologic symptoms of cortical origin (e.g., paresthesias, temporal lobe symptoms) occur less commonly in patients who suffer from migraine with aura. K.L.'s physical and neurologic examinations were within normal limits. The nausea and vomiting that were experienced by K.L. accompany migraine headaches (with or without aura) in 90% of patients. Vomiting is occasionally followed by a gradual resolution of migraine symptoms. Diarrhea may also occur.

In summary, K.L.'s history and relative lack of important physical findings are compatible with a diagnosis of migraine with aura.

Diagnostic Tests

2. What further laboratory or diagnostic tests should be ordered for K.L.?

Headaches are common medical complaints and evaluation of these headaches with sophisticated diagnostic procedures (e.g., computed tomography [CT], magnetic resonance imaging [MRI] scans) are generally unnecessary in the uncomplicated migraine patient. Because K.L.'s headaches are not of recent origin, not progressive, and unassociated with traumatic injury or persistent neurologic deficits, CT or MRI scanning procedures should be unnecessary. Her headaches are unaccompanied by fever or nuchal rigidity, and she does not present with headache described as being "the worst headache of my life." Therefore, a lumbar puncture would not likely be of diagnostic value because meningitis or subarachnoid hemorrhage is unlikely. The signs and symptoms experienced by K.L., as described in the answer to Question 1, are typical of migraine with aura. The most important diagnostic evaluations of patients presenting with headache should be based on a thorough medical history and physical examination. The role of costly or invasive diagnostic procedures is limited to their usefulness in detecting other more serious disorders that may manifest as migrainous headache.

Therapeutic Considerations

3. What should be the general approach to the treatment of K.L.'s headache attacks?

The concept that moderate to severe headaches can be classified into distinct types with unrelated pathophysiologic features is probably incorrect. Patients commonly complain of more than one type of headache or report symptoms or recurrence patterns that are inconsistent with a single diagnosis. Because the selection of therapy is based primarily on the characteristics of headache gathered from the history, the practitioner needs to be flexible in the choice of treatments when the features do not fit within classic definitions. Even for patients with well-defined headache types, specific therapies may alleviate pain in only 50% to 80% of patients. Still, with careful monitoring of therapeutic response and optimization of effective treatments, patients with a wide variety of headache complaints can be successfully managed with relatively few drugs.

Abortive Therapy

The general approach to treatment of acute migraine headache attacks is one of pharmacotherapy aimed at relieving migraine headache pain and associated symptoms. Such a treatment plan may include (1) 5-HT receptor agonists (e.g., triptans or ergot derivatives), (2) analgesics, (3) sedatives, and (4) antiemetic drug therapy, depending on the exact nature of the patient's complaint. The selection of a specific treatment should be based on the level of disability and associated symptoms such as nausea and vomiting. This "stratified care" approach is preferred over a "step care" approach that may begin with agents that are likely to be ineffective for the patient's headache.[37] This latter approach, when applied to all patients regardless of headache severity, only serves to delay effective therapy in many people.[38]

Aggravating Factors

Clinicians should always search for factors that might precipitate migraine attacks in their patients before initiating drug therapy. Although K.L. could not associate her migraine attacks with any external events, the factors listed in Table 52-3 should be discussed with her in hopes that their elimination or avoidance may improve her headaches. However, complete relief, even in patients who can clearly identify such precipitants, is unlikely.

ORAL CONTRACEPTIVES

4. K.L. recalls being told by her gynecologist that headaches are a possible side effect of oral contraceptive use. She initially started oral contraceptives 2 years ago and did not associate the medication with the recent onset of migraine attacks. Why should the discontinuation of Ortho-Novum 7/7/7 be considered in K.L.?

Oral contraceptives may either worsen or precipitate migraine attacks in women without a previous history of this problem.[39] Although headaches usually arise within the first few months of oral contraceptive use, headaches developing after several years have been described.[40] The adverse effect of oral contraceptives on migraine headaches is likely related to the estrogen content. The use of a lower-potency estrogen product decreases the frequency of migraine attacks in some women. Migraine with aura is an independent risk factor for stroke in women, with the highest risk found among those younger than 45 years of age.[41] No consistent increased risk for stroke has been found among men, women older than 45 years old, and women who have migraine without aura.[39] Use of oral contraceptives increases the risk of stroke even further. Adjusted odds ratios for stroke risk in women with migraine are 4 for oral contraceptives containing >50 μg estrogen and 2 for oral contraceptives containing <50 μg estrogen.[39] K.L. should be counseled about her increased risk for stroke and the options for alternative birth control methods. She can then make an informed decision regarding whether or not to continue oral contraceptives. When oral contraceptives are discontinued, 30% to 40% of women[42] notice an improvement in their headaches, although several months may elapse before a benefit is realized.[43] If K.L. elects to discontinue oral contraceptives an alternative form of birth control should be recommended, and the frequency of her headaches should be monitored to detect an improvement in this problem.

Abortive Therapy
Triptans (5-HT$_{1B/1D}$ Receptor Agonists)

5. What would be an appropriate drug of first choice for the treatment of K.L.'s acute headaches?

Agents in the triptan class (sumatriptan, zolmitriptan, naratriptan, rizatriptan, almotriptan, frovatriptan and eletriptan) are effective and well tolerated relative to other agents used for the abortive treatment of acute migraine headaches. Consequently, triptans are appropriate initial therapy for patients with moderate to severe migraine headaches who have no contraindications to their use. Introduction of these agents has had a dramatic effect on the successful relief of disabling headache in many patients. Before this, ergot alkaloids (e.g., ergotamine tartrate) were the preferred agents for migraine headaches when non-narcotic analgesics were ineffective.

Unlike ergotamine, which needs to be taken at the earliest sign of a migraine attack for maximal benefit, the triptans are effective when given 4 hours or longer after the onset of headache.[44] However, they are more expensive than ergotamine. For this reason, some prescribers and health plans reserve the triptans for patients who are unresponsive or intolerant to less expensive alternatives (e.g., ergotamine, NSAIDs). Pharmacoeconomic studies have suggested an advantage of triptan agents over nontriptan medications when costs are considered from a societal perspective (i.e., take into account lost work productivity in addition to health care costs).[45]

Unlike the ergot alkaloids, which stimulate serotonergic, dopaminergic, and noradrenergic receptors, the triptans have selective agonist activity at 5-HT$_{1B/1D}$ subtype receptors. This feature is likely responsible for the improved tolerability profile for these agents. There are three proposed mechanisms for the effectiveness of the triptans in acute migraine headache: (1) reducing the excitability of neurons in the trigeminovascular system via stimulation of brainstem 5-HT$_{1B/1D}$ receptors, (2) attenuating the release of neuropeptides with inflammatory and vasodilating properties (e.g., CGRP, substance P, and neurokinin A) via a presynaptic 5-HT$_{1D}$ receptor effect, and (3) vasoconstriction of cerebral and extracerebral vessels by stimulation of vascular 5-HT$_{1B}$ receptors.[35] The coronary vasculature also contains 5-HT$_{1B}$ receptors; thus, these agents have the potential to cause coronary artery vasoconstriction. For this reason, patients with coronary artery disease and uncontrolled hypertension were excluded from premarketing clinical trials, and the triptans are contraindicated in these patients. Sumatriptan (Imitrex) was the first triptan approved for use, and it is the prototype against which the other "second-generation" triptans are compared. Table 52-4 compares the triptans with regard to selected clinical and pharmacokinetic features.

SUMATRIPTAN

Sumatriptan (Imitrex) is a structural analog of 5-HT that was introduced in 1993 for the abortive treatment of migraine

Table 52-3 Factors That May Precipitate Migraine Headache

Stress
Emotion
Glare
Hypoglycemia
Altered sleep pattern
Menses
Exercise
Alcohol
Carbon monoxide
Excess caffeine use or withdrawal
Foods containing:
  MSG (e.g., Chinese food, canned soups, seasonings)
  Tyramine (e.g., red wine, ripened cheeses)
  Nitrites (e.g., cured meat products)
  Phenylethylamine (e.g., chocolate, cheese)
Aspartame (e.g., artificial sweeteners, diet sodas)
Drugs
Excess use or withdrawal (ergots, triptans, analgesics)
  Estrogens (e.g., oral contraceptives)
  Cocaine
  Nitroglycerin

MSG, monosodium glutamate.

Table 52-4 Clinical and Pharmacokinetic Features of the Triptans for Acute Migraine Headache[60]

Drug	Route	Bioavailability (%)	T-max (hr)	Half-Life (hr)	Response Rate at 2 hr (%)	HA Recurrence Within 24–48 hr (%)	Dose/Attack (mg)	Maximum Dose in 24 hr (mg)
Sumatriptan (Imitrex)	PO	14	1.2–2.3	2	50–69	25–41	25–100	200
	IN	—	1–1.5	2	62–78	10–40	20–40	40
	SC	96	0.2	2	63–82	10–40	6–12	12
Zolmitriptan (Zomig)	PO	40–46	1.5	2.5–3	62–67	22–37	2.5–10	10
	IN	100	3	2.5–3	69	—	5–10	10
Naratriptan (Amerge)	PO	60–70	3–5	6	43–49	17–28	1–5	5
Rizatriptan (Maxalt)	PO	40–45	1.3	1.8	60–77	35–47	5–20	30
Almotriptan (Axert)	PO	70	1–3	3–4	55–65	18–30	6.25–25	25
Frovatriptan (Frova)	PO	20–30	2–4	2.6	37–46	7–25	2.5–5	7.5
Eletriptan (Relpax)	PO	50	2	4	47–65	6–34	20–40	80

HA, headache; IN, intranasal; PO, oral; SC, subcutaneous.
Adapted from reference 60.

headache (Fig. 52-1). Available formulations include an injection pen device for subcutaneous self-administration, oral tablets, and a nasal spray. All of these formulations (including a rectal formulation not available in the United States) reduce the severity of migraine headache and improve associated symptoms such as nausea, vomiting, photophobia, and phonophobia.[45] The choice of dosage form depends on the intensity of the headache and the presence of severe nausea. For patients who are nauseated and prone to vomit during an acute attack, the subcutaneous and intranasal dosage forms are preferred. Both formulations have a rapid onset of effect. Reduction in headache intensity is reported within 10 minutes after subcutaneous injection and within 15 minutes after administration of the nasal spray.[46] Clinical response is delayed after oral administration of sumatriptan tablets,[46] but this dosage form is more convenient and preferred by many patients. During migraine attacks, the gastrointestinal absorption of many drugs is delayed.[47] This may contribute to the faster onset of action of the nonoral dosage forms of sumatriptan and other drugs.

The efficacy of the triptans has been evaluated using the primary endpoint of headache response (reduction in headache intensity to mild pain or no pain) at 2 hours. Response rates for sumatriptan vary from 50% to 82% (see Table 52-4).

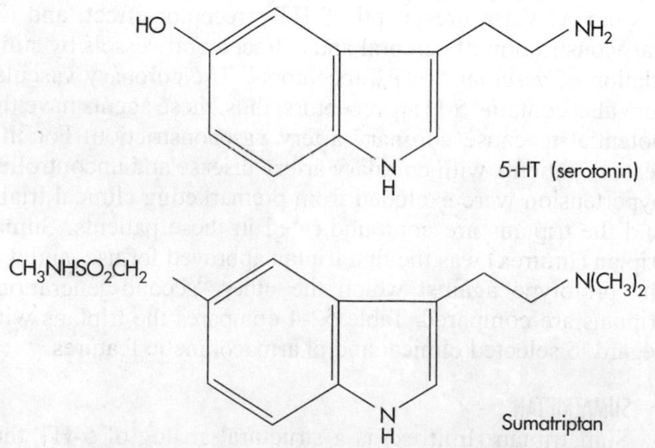

FIGURE 52-1 Structures of 5-HT (serotonin) and sumatriptan.

Subcutaneous injection is associated with higher response rates than non-parenteral routes of administration. Comparative trials with other antimigraine therapies also support the efficacy of sumatriptan. Subcutaneous sumatriptan is more effective and faster acting than dihydroergotamine (DHE) nasal spray.[48] When compared with subcutaneous DHE, subcutaneous sumatriptan is more effective at 1 and 2 hours, but the two treatments are equally effective at 3 and 4 hours.[49] In this trial, headache recurrence rates at 24 hours favored subcutaneous DHE.[49] Studies of oral sumatriptan show this treatment is more effective than both ergotamine 2 mg with caffeine 200 mg[50] and aspirin 900 mg plus metoclopramide 10 mg.[51]

Adverse Effects

Sumatriptan is usually well tolerated, and this feature offers a significant advantage over ergot alkaloids in many patients. After oral administration, the most common adverse effects of sumatriptan include nausea and vomiting (which could be related to the migraine itself), malaise, and dizziness. Intranasal sumatriptan is associated with a bitter, unpleasant taste in most patients. Adverse effects following subcutaneous sumatriptan are more common and more uncomfortable than those following oral or intranasal administration. The most common adverse events after subcutaneous administration are mild pain or redness at the site of injection.[52] These injection site reactions occur in 40% of patients and usually resolve within 60 minutes.[52] Symptoms of chest pressure or tightness (sometimes extending to the throat) have been reported in 3% to 5% of patients treated with oral or subcutaneous sumatriptan in controlled trials.[52] However, a questionnaire-based study of 453 users of sumatriptan found a much higher incidence—42% of subcutaneous sumatriptan users and 26% of oral sumatriptan users reported chest symptoms in almost all of their sumatriptan-treated migraine attacks.[53] These symptoms are usually mild, resolve within 2 hours, and are unrelated to cardiac ischemia. However, they are uncomfortable enough that 7% to 12% of patients discontinue the drug based on these symptoms.[53] Although chest symptoms are rarely serious, sumatriptan has been associated with vascular events, including coronary vasospasm,[54] angina,[55] myocardial infarction,[56] and stroke.[57] These adverse events usually occur in patients with coronary artery disease or significant risk factors. However, myocardial infarction was reported in one otherwise healthy young woman after sumatriptan.[58] Because of potential vasoconstrictive effects, sumatriptan should not be used in patients with uncontrolled hypertension, peripheral or cerebral vascular disease, coronary artery disease, previous myocardial infarction, Prinzmetal's angina, or coronary vasospasm. For patients with risk factors of coronary artery disease but who are otherwise deemed appropriate for sumatriptan, the first dose should be administered in a physician's office or an area in which medical support in available.

Headache Recurrence

Another complication of sumatriptan use is recurrent migraine headache. In 25% to 40% of patients, migraine headache recurs within 24 hours after initial successful treatment with sumatriptan.[59] This phenomenon may be related to the short half-life of the drug, and the recurrent headache often responds to a repeat dose of sumatriptan.[60]

Drug Interactions

Although few drug interactions have been reported with sumatriptan, concomitant use with ergot alkaloids, lithium, serotonin-specific reuptake inhibitors (SSRIs), other triptans, and monoamine oxidase (MAO) inhibitors is not recommended because of the potential for precipitating the serotonin syndrome.[45] However, several reports describe the safe use of sumatriptan in conjunction with MAO-B inhibitors, SSRIs, and lithium, and clinical evidence of adverse effects is minimal.[61-63] The potential risks and benefits should be considered when these therapies are used in combination.

Dosing

The recommended dosage of sumatriptan varies according to the route of administration. The initial dose of subcutaneous sumatriptan is 6 mg. If there is no relief within 1 hour, the dose can be repeated. Initial doses of oral and intranasal sumatriptan are 25 to 100 mg and 5 to 20 mg, respectively. These doses may be repeated if there is no relief within 2 hours. When migraine headache recurs after an initial positive response, a repeat dose is often effective. However, the maximum doses in a 24-hour period listed in Table 52-4 should not be exceeded.

SECOND-GENERATION TRIPTANS (ZOLMITRIPTAN, NARATRIPTAN, RIZATRIPTAN, ALMOTRIPTAN, FROVATRIPTAN, ELETRIPTAN)

Since the introduction of sumatriptan, several second-generation triptan agents have been approved for the acute treatment of migraine. In general, these agents have similar pharmacologic features (all are 5-HT$_{1B/1D}$ receptor agonists), and improved oral bioavailability over sumatriptan. Although these agents have similar pharmacologic effects on 5-HT receptors, patients who fail to respond to one triptan may respond to another agent in this class. Like sumatriptan, second-generation triptans also have potential vasoconstrictive effects on coronary arteries. The pharmacokinetic and clinical effects of the second-generation triptans are shown in Table 52-4.

All second-generation triptans have been shown to be superior to placebo for acute migraine relief. Fewer studies compare one agent to another. A recent meta-analysis of 53 controlled clinical trials compared the second-generation triptans with sumatriptan 100 mg orally with regard to efficacy, consistency

of relief, and tolerability.[44,64] Rizatriptan (Maxalt) eletriptan (Relpax) 80 mg were significantly more than sumatriptan 100 mg in headache response at 2 hour triptan (Amerge) 2.5 mg, eletriptan 20 mg and frovat (Frova) 2.5 were significantly less effective. Agents were compared with regard to the percentage of patients with sus tained freedom from headache (i.e., no pain at 2 hours, no requirement for rescue medication, and no headache recurrence within 24 hours). Compared with sumatriptan 100 mg, response rates were higher for rizatriptan 10 mg, eletriptan 80 mg and almotriptan (Axert) 12.5 mg, and lower for eletriptan 20 mg. The consistency of therapeutic effect across multiple attacks was also compared. Rizatriptan 10 mg provided more consistent relief than sumatriptan 100 mg. Differences between the triptans in tolerability were generally small. However, the adverse effect rates of naratriptan 2.5 mg and almotriptan 12.5 mg were lower than that for sumatriptan 100 mg.[44,64] Although comparison of drugs based on results from different trials may not be reliable, the results of head-to-head comparison studies were consistent with those from single triptan studies when results were pooled for meta-analysis.[64]

Drug Interactions

The metabolism of rizatriptan and zolmitriptan (Zomig) is reduced by MAO inhibitors (particularly MAO-A inhibitors). Thus, like sumatriptan, rizatriptan and zolmitriptan should be avoided in patients taking MAO inhibitors. Propranolol reduces the metabolic clearance of frovatriptan, zolmitriptan, rizatriptan and eletriptan to varying extents. The clinical significance of these interactions is unknown but increased exposure to these triptans should be considered in patients concomitantly receiving propranolol. Inhibitors of CYP3A4 reduce the clearance of almotriptan and eletriptan. For almotriptan, increased exposure to triptans should be anticipated, however no specific dosing adjustments are proposed. The interaction between eletriptan and CYP3A4 inhibitors is more significant, and particular precautions are necessary. Eletriptan should not be used within 72 hours of treatment with potent CYP3A4 inhibitors (e.g., ketoconazole, itraconazole, nefazodone, trolenadomycin, clarithromycin, ritonavir and nelfinavir). As with sumatriptan, there is potential concern regarding the coadministration of second generation triptans and SSRIs. Weakness, hyperreflexia and incoordination have been reported when 5-HT$_{1B/1D}$ agonists are administered to patients taking SSRIs. These potential adverse effects should be considered in patients who require both classes of medication.

Precautions regarding the use of second generation triptans in patients with known or suspected cardiovascular disease are similar to those for sumatriptan and should be strictly followed (see Sumatriptan, Adverse Effects).

All second-generation triptans are available as oral tablets. Rizatriptan and zolmitriptan are also available as oral disintegrating tablets that are placed on the tongue where they dissolve and are swallowed with saliva. Patients who receive these formulations (Maxalt-MLT, Zomig-ZMT) should be told to handle the tablet with dry hands. Zolmitriptan is al available as a nasal spray.

K.L.'s migraine headaches are of moderate to sev sity (her activities of daily living are negatively do not respond to moderate doses of aspirin

Triptans (including sumatriptan and second-generation agents) are appropriate initial antimigraine agents for patients such as K.L. Although her headaches are frequently associated with nausea and vomiting, it is not clear whether these symptoms occur soon after the onset of the attack or whether they evolve gradually as the migraine progresses. If vomiting occurs early, a nonoral route of administration should be considered. Subcutaneous or intranasal sumatriptan are appropriate therapy options. If K.L.'s migraines evolve gradually after the onset of her aura symptoms, then an oral triptan may provide sufficiently rapid relief to be effective. Most patients prefer the convenience of oral dosing. The initial choice of a triptan for oral administration can be made based on cost, pharmacokinetic features and familiarity of the prescriber.

6. Ortho-Novum 7/7/7 was discontinued, and K.L. was fitted for a diaphragm and given instructions on its proper use. She was also given a prescription for sumatriptan 50 mg and told to take one tablet at the onset of her aura symptoms. At her follow-up clinic visit 2 months later, K.L. reported inconsistent relief from migraine headache with sumatriptan. She experienced six headaches over the past 2 months. The first attack responded to a single dose of sumatriptan 50 mg. The next three migraine attacks failed to respond to the first dose, but responded when she took another 50-mg tablet of sumatriptan 2 hours after the first. However, K.L. is concerned that she is becoming "tolerant" to this medication and has been hesitant to take more than one tablet of sumatriptan for subsequent migraines. Is tolerance a concern with the triptan agents? Should K.L. be changed to another triptan for acute relief of her migraine headaches?

Although there can be some inconsistency in response when triptans are used to treat multiple migraine attacks, the gradual development of tolerance in patients who experience an initial favorable effect is uncommon and not expected. Patients who experience relief after treatment of several migraines with the same dose of a triptan usually continue to experience similar relief over long periods of time.[53] Thus, K.L. need not avoid taking sumatriptan (at an effective dosage) because of concerns regarding headache tolerance. In those instances when K.L. experienced adequate relief of her migraine attacks, she usually required two doses of sumatriptan 50 mg. Given this response pattern, she should be encouraged to take 100 mg of sumatriptan at the onset of her migraines in the future. Potential adverse effects should again be discussed with K.L., and she should be informed that these side effects might be more significant with the higher initial dose. However, most patients who tolerate an initial dose of sumatriptan 50 mg are able to tolerate 100 mg as well. At this time, there is no need to consider an alternate triptan for K.L.. However, if she is intolerant of sumatriptan 100 mg, then alternate agents such as naratriptan or almotriptan could be considered. However, naratriptan generally has a slower onset of effect than other triptans, and this may be a disadvantage for K.L. If, at a future visit, K.L. is not obtaining adequate relief from sumatriptan 100 mg (followed by an additional dose at 2 hours), then rizatriptan 10 mg should be considered as initial treatment for her migraines. Although eletriptan 80 mg also was superior to sumatriptan 100 mg for migraine response at 2 hours in the meta-analysis discussed above, this dose of eletriptan is higher than that recommended by the manufacturer for initial treatment.[44]

Ergotamine Tartrate

7. What is the role of ergotamine tartrate in the acute treatment of migraine headaches?

Ergotamine tartrate (Bellergal-S, Cafergot) has been used since 1925 for the acute treatment of migraine headaches. Before the availability of agents in the triptan class, ergotamine was widely considered the drug of choice when non-narcotic analgesics were ineffective. The major advantages of this agent are low cost and long history of experience with its use. However, adverse effects of ergotamine are common and potentially serious, particularly when the drug is used in excessive doses or for prolonged periods.[42] Furthermore, the strength and quality of evidence for ergotamine in acute migraine therapy is less than that for the triptans.[38] For these reasons, triptans are often preferred as initial therapy. About 50% to 70% of migraine sufferers benefit from ergotamine given during an acute attack.[65] Ergotamine is highly specific for migraine and cluster headaches; only occasionally are other types of headaches affected by this drug.

Ergotamine and other ergot derivatives (e.g., dihydroergotamine [DHE]) have numerous pharmacologic effects. However, their precise mechanism of action in migraine is unknown. These drugs are agonists at numerous 5-HT$_1$ receptor subtypes (5-HT$_{1A}$, 5-HT$_{1B}$, 5-HT$_{1D}$, 5-HT$_{1F}$), 5-HT$_2$, adrenergic, and dopaminergic receptors.[42] Ergotamine has both venous and arterial vasoconstrictive effects. Although it has been presumed that ergot alkaloids relieve migraine by their cerebral vasoconstrictive effects, experimental evidence does not support this as the sole mechanism.[66] Ergotamine and dihydroergotamine block inflammation of the trigeminal neurovascular system, presumably by inhibiting the release of the neuropeptides discussed above (see Pathophysiology). This action, possibly mediated by 5-HT receptor effects, may be responsible for both the pain-relieving and vasoconstrictive effects of the ergot alkaloids.

Ergotamine should be given at the first sign of a migraine attack in a dosage that is effective and acceptable to the patient. If administration is delayed until the headache is firmly established, ergotamine is rarely effective and other therapies (e.g., DHE, triptans, or narcotic analgesics) are usually required.

CAFFEINE

8. Why is caffeine added to some ergotamine products (e.g., Cafergot)?

Caffeine is combined with ergotamine in several preparations and was originally added to potentiate the vasoconstrictive properties of ergotamine.[67] Subsequent studies have shown that caffeine improves intestinal ergotamine absorption[68] and potentiates the pain relief properties of analgesics.[69] However, it should be kept in mind that caffeine's stimulant effect may prevent the sleep, which is beneficial to many migraine sufferers.

9. How do different ergotamine dosage forms compare with each other? What is the usual dosage of ergotamine for acute migraine?

ROUTE OF ADMINISTRATION

Ergotamine tartrate is available for oral, sublingual, rectal, or parenteral use. The rate and extent of drug absorption are erratic following oral, sublingual, and rectal administration. The rectal and sublingual routes of administration bypass the portal circulation, avoid first-pass metabolism, and are more bioavailable than the oral route of administration. However, documentation of improved efficacy is lacking.[70,71] A metered-dose inhaler containing ergotamine tartrate was previously marketed in the United States, but this product has been withdrawn.

When ergotamine is prescribed, the sublingual preparation is often preferred because it is convenient to use and has a faster onset of action than oral ergotamine.[72] Acute migraine attacks also are associated with decreased gastric motility.[73] This phenomenon is presumably responsible for the impaired oral absorption of aspirin and ergotamine when given during an acute migraine attack.[47,74] Delayed drug absorption during a migraine attack occurs independent of associated nausea or vomiting and is primarily related to headache severity.[75] In patients who do not respond to oral or sublingual dosage forms, a trial with ergotamine rectal suppositories may be successful.[75] Some studies report higher rates of success with rectal administration of ergotamine (i.e., about 70%) than with the oral or sublingual routes of administration (about 50% to 60% effective).[76] This difference may be due to improved bioavailability of ergotamine when administered rectally.[77] The usual ergotamine dosage (when given by either oral, sublingual, or rectal routes) is 1 to 4 mg given immediately and followed by 1 to 2 mg at 30-minute intervals to a maximum of 6 mg/attack or 10 mg/week. Also, the use of ergotamine should be limited to no more than twice per week to reduce the risk of chronic ergot-related adverse effects (see Question 11).[42]

CONTRAINDICATIONS

10. **What are the contraindications to the use of an ergotamine-containing product?**

Contraindications to the use of ergot alkaloids include cardiac, peripheral, and cerebral vascular disease; sepsis; liver and kidney disease; pregnancy; breast-feeding; and concomitant use of triacetyloleandomycin or erythromycin.[65] The latter drugs can inhibit the metabolism of ergotamine and may potentiate the toxicity of this agent.[78] The vasoconstrictive effects of ergotamine can be particularly harmful to the patient with these pre-existing conditions. Some sources cite hypertension as a contraindication to ergotamine use, but this is controversial. The usual therapeutic doses of ergotamine used for migraine therapy have minimal effects on blood pressure, and hypertension need not be a strict contraindication to its occasional use.[79]

Concerns about using ergotamine during the aura of migraine when focal neurologic deficits may be due to cerebral ischemia have not been validated. Human studies have found no alteration in regional cerebral blood flow after parenteral administration of either ergotamine or dihydroergotamine and their use during the prodrome is not contraindicated.[66,80,81] Occasionally, patients experience a prolonged aura or more prominent neurologic symptoms with ergotamine use. In these individuals, ergotamine use should not be continued.[42]

ADVERSE EFFECTS

11. **What adverse effects should be monitored for in patients who receive ergotamine?**

Gastrointestinal (GI) disturbances can be a limiting factor to the use of ergotamine for headache therapy. Nausea, vomiting, and anorexia are common, dose-dependent ergotamine adverse effects, which may worsen the GI symptoms that commonly accompany acute migraine headaches. These GI symptoms after ergotamine use are likely the result of central dopamine receptor agonism at the chemoreceptor trigger zone. Because these effects are centrally mediated, they can occur after administration of ergotamine by any bioavailable route. Patients are reluctant to continue therapy if their initial experience with the medication has been unpleasant. Therefore, patients should be educated as to the potential for this adverse effect.

Clinicians can also take measures to minimize migraine-associated and ergotamine-induced GI upset. One useful technique is to determine the smallest dose of ergotamine that will elicit GI distress in a patient during a headache-free interval. For example, if the suppository form of ergotamine is being used, the patient can be instructed to insert one-fourth of a suppository at hourly intervals until nausea develops. The total dosage is then reduced by one-fourth of a suppository and used as the initial dose for subsequent migraine attacks.[79] The same technique can be used for patients using oral or sublingual ergotamine by splitting the tablets in half.

The peripheral vasoconstrictive effects of ergotamine most commonly involve the lower extremities and are often characterized by coldness, decreased distal pulses, and a tingling sensation. Continuous paresthesias, limb pain, venous thrombosis, or gangrene necessitating amputation are more severe consequences of ergotamine therapy.[82] Although some of these symptoms may occur with therapeutic doses in hypersensitive individuals, they are most commonly associated with overdose or excessive therapeutic use of ergotamine. Beta-adrenergic receptor blocking agents, commonly used in migraine prophylaxis, occasionally can potentiate the vasoconstrictive effects of ergotamine.[83,84] Their concomitant use is not contraindicated, but patients should be closely monitored for the signs and symptoms of peripheral vasoconstriction.

Rebound headache after discontinuation of long-term, daily ergotamine use is another common adverse effect. These rebound headaches respond to larger ergotamine doses, but ultimately the headaches become more frequent and other symptoms of ergotamine overuse become apparent (e.g., symptoms of peripheral vascular insufficiency). This cycle of overmedication and resultant headaches can render patients refractory to other forms of headache treatment.[85]

ANTIEMETICS

12. **What is the role of antiemetic therapy for the outpatient treatment of migraine-associated nausea and vomiting?**

In most patients, triptan agents provide effective relief of migraine-associated nausea. Therefore, specific antiemetic therapy usually is not required. However, as mentioned above, persistent nausea is more common in patients who use ergotamine for acute migraine therapy. In these patients, and in triptan-treated patients who experience incomplete nausea relief, adjunctive antiemetic therapy should be considered. Phenothiazine antiemetics can provide symptomatic relief from nausea; however, they can also reduce GI motility and further impair absorption of medication taken orally.[86] Metoclopra

(Reglan) is the anticmetic of choice in migraine.[87] The recommended dose is 10 mg taken orally as soon as possible. Although the drug has no direct antimigraine effect,[88] it does provide symptomatic relief from nausea and vomiting while enhancing the oral absorption of medications taken during the migraine attack.[86] Unfortunately, metoclopramide is not available in a suppository dosage form.

13. In addition to the triptans and ergotamine tartrate, what other abortive agents are available for outpatient treatment of acute migraine headache?

In the stratified care approach, isometheptene compound, NSAIDs, and combination analgesics are reasonable treatment options for patients with mild-to-moderate migraine headaches or those with severe attacks that have responded to these agents in the past.[38] Dihydroergotamine nasal spray is indicated for moderate-to-severe migraine headache.[38]

Isometheptene Compound

Isometheptene, a sympathomimetic amine, is combined with acetaminophen and a sedative (dichloralphenazone) in the product of Midrin. This combination is as effective as oral ergotamine in the treatment of acute migraine headaches[89,90] and, in many patients, better tolerated. Although the contraindications to Midrin are similar to those of ergotamine, severe adverse effects are less common. Patients unresponsive to ergotamine products occasionally respond to Midrin. In patients with mild to moderate migraine, isometheptene compound provides comparable relief to sumatriptan 25 mg given orally.[91] The usual dosage of Midrin is two capsules taken immediately followed by one additional capsule every hour until the headache is relieved. Subsequent migraine attacks can be managed by administering the same total dose of Midrin that was effective in treating the previous headache, but no more than five Midrin capsules should be taken within a 12-hour period.[89]

Nonsteroidal Anti-Inflammatory Drugs and Combination Analgesics

Many NSAIDs and combination analgesics containing caffeine have been shown to be effective for the acute treatment of migraine headache.[92] Significant clinical benefit in double-blind, placebo-controlled trials has been shown for aspirin, ibuprofen, naproxen sodium, and combination analgesics containing acetaminophen, aspirin, and caffeine.[38] Selected NSAIDs (e.g., naproxen sodium, ketoprofen, diclofenac potassium) are as effective as ergotamine[93–95] or sumatriptan[93] in the relief of migraine headache. However, consistent differences among NSAIDs in migraine therapy have not been demonstrated. If NSAIDs are to be used in the abortive treatment of migraine, the concomitant administration of metoclopramide can enhance their absorption, providing more effective and rapid pain relief.[47,96]

Dihydroergotamine Nasal Spray

A nasal spray formulation of dihydroergotamine (DHE) (Migranal) has become available for abortive therapy of migraine. Previously, this agent was available for parenteral use only and was usually restricted to use in clinic and emergency department (ED) settings (see Intractable Migraine). DHE is less likely than ergotamine to cause severe nausea and vomiting, and it is a less potent arterial vasoconstrictor.[97] In clinical trials, DHE nasal spray is more effective than placebo in relieving pain (beginning as early as 30 minutes after treatment) and reducing post-treatment nausea.[98–100] In an unpublished, active control trial, DHE nasal spray was equally effective and better tolerated than an ergotamine/caffeine combination product (Cafergot).[101] Patients given this treatment should self-administer one spray (1 mg) into each nostril followed in 15 minutes by an additional spray in each nostril for a total of four sprays (4 mg). DHE nasal spray is reasonable to consider as an initial agent for moderate to severe migraine headache.[38]

Intractable Migraine

14. K.L. used sumatriptan 100 mg PO for her next two migraine headache attacks and obtained good relief. K.L. experienced another headache with severe nausea. She took sumatriptan 100 mg PO but vomited immediately thereafter, and the headache continued to worsen throughout the day until she could no longer work. K.L. was taken to the ED by a friend. The diagnosis of intractable migraine was made. How should K.L. be treated?

Dihydroergotamine

Intractable migraine with associated vomiting usually requires parenteral therapy with ergot derivatives, sumatriptan, or potent narcotic analgesics. DHE-45, 1 mg subcutaneously[102] or intramuscularly[103] or 0.75 mg intravenously,[104] is particularly effective in the treatment of acute and intractable migraine headaches and thereby reduces the necessity for narcotic analgesics. If ineffective, a second dose of DHE should be administered 30 to 45 minutes later. An IV antiemetic (prochlorperazine 5 to 10 mg or metoclopramide 10 mg) should be administered 15 to 30 minutes before DHE to minimize the GI side effects of this agent. Intramuscular administration of ergotamine tartrate 0.5 mg is also effective, but ergot-related side effects are more severe with ergotamine tartrate than with DHE. Ergotamine tartrate administered by the oral, sublingual, or rectal routes is unlikely to be effective in this setting.

Sumatriptan

Sumatriptan 6 mg subcutaneously is also effective for the treatment of established migraine.[53] If the first injection does not provide relief at 1 hour, a second injection may be administered. However, the daily dosage should not exceed 12 mg. Sumatriptan should not be administered within 24 hours of ergot alkaloids because of the potential for prolonged vasospastic reactions.

Prochlorperazine

Prochlorperazine (Compazine) is an antiemetic agent often used as an adjunct for patients with migraine-associated nausea and vomiting. However, when given by IV route prochlorperazine is also a nonspecific yet highly effective agent for aborting intractable migraine.[38] In randomized, controlled trials, prochlorperazine 10 mg IV was more effective than placebo, IV metoclopramide, IV ketorolac, and IV valproate for the treatment of acute migraine in the emergency department.[105–107]

Chlorpromazine

Like prochlorperazine, chlorpromazine (Thorazine) given parenterally has both antimigraine and antiemetic properties and has gained increased acceptance in EDs as a pharmacologic alternative to potent narcotic analgesics such as meperidine. In a double-blind, controlled trial, IV chlorpromazine (0.1 mg/kg) provided more effective pain relief from intractable migraine than meperidine (0.4 mg/kg) plus dimenhydrinate.[108] Chlorpromazine 1 mg/kg intramuscularly has also been shown to relieve migraine headache more effectively than placebo.[109]

Narcotic Analgesics

Parenteral narcotic analgesics also effectively relieve intractable migraine headache pain, but they should generally be reserved for second- or third-line therapy after patients have failed to respond to parenteral sumatriptan, DHE, prochlorperazine or chlorpromazine. ED treatment of headache with narcotics is a common antecedent to iatrogenic drug addiction.[110] In some EDs that deal with a large number of drug-seeking patients, the use of synthetic narcotic agonist/antagonists (e.g., butorphanol, nalbuphine) has been advocated for treatment of intractable migraine.[111,112] Butorphanol is also available as a nasal spray for self-administration during migraine headache. Although this product was initially thought to have a low addiction liability, subsequent experience suggests that the product is often misused or diverted for misuse purposes.[113] Patients receiving this medication should be monitored for excessive use. In a comparison with intramuscular butorphanol and intramuscular meperidine plus hydroxyzine, the superiority of IV DHE plus metoclopramide was clearly demonstrated.[111]

In general, narcotic analgesics can be highly effective therapies for acute and intractable migraine. However, these agents often cause or exacerbate nausea and vomiting. Also, excessive use should be monitored closely because of the risk of addiction and dependence. Alternative symptomatic therapies should be pursued for those patients who require frequent use of narcotic analgesics (usually defined as two or more treatments per week).[44]

Corticosteroids

Prednisone 40 to 60 mg orally for 3 to 5 days or dexamethasone 4 to 16 mg intramuscularly may be used as alternative treatments for intractable migraine and presumably work by suppressing the sterile perivascular inflammation of resistant headache.[114] Table 52-5 summarizes the agents commonly used for the treatment of acute migraine headaches.

Table 52-5 Drug Treatment of Acute Migraine Headache[a]

Drug	Route	Dose	Contraindications	Adverse Effects	Comments
Sumatriptan (Imitrex)	PO, IN, SC	6 mg SC stat; may repeat in 1 hr	Ischemic heart disease, within 24 hr of ergot alkaloids	Heavy sensation in head or chest, tingling, pain at injection site	First-line therapy for moderate-to-severe headaches; SC for intractable migraine
Ibuprofen (Motrin) or other NSAIDs	PO	400–800 mg	Aspirin or NSAID-related bronchospasm	N, V, bleeding, renal dysfunction	First-line therapy for mild-to-moderate headaches
Dihydroergotamine (Migranal)	IN, IM, IV	2 mg IN stat; repeat in 15 min	See Ergotamine	Rhinitis, dizziness, N, V	For moderate-to-severe headaches; parenteral use for intractable migraine
Ergotamine tartrate (Cafergot, Ergostat)	PO, SL, PR	1–4 mg stat, then 1–2 mg Q 30 min to max of 6 mg/attack or 10 mg/wk	CV disease, sepsis, liver or kidney disease, arterial insufficiency, pregnancy, breast feeding, concomitant macrolide use	N, V, anorexia, limb paresthesias or pain	Use at HA onset for max effect; ↓ N and V by using smallest effective dose
Isometheptene/ dichloralphenazone/ acetaminophen (Midrin)	PO	2 cap stat, then 1 cap Q hr to max 5 cap/12 hr	See Ergotamine tartrate; avoid in patients taking MAOIs	N, V, dizziness, drowsiness	As effective as ergotamine tartrate
Prochlorperazine (Compazine)	IM, IV	10 mg stat	CV disease	Extrapyramidal reactions, sedation, dizziness	IV/IM for adjunctive antiemetic therapy; IV for antimigraine effect in intractable migraine
Chlorpromazine (Thorazine)	IM	1 mg/kg	CV disease, history of seizures	Extrapyramidal reactions, sedation, hypotension	For intractable migraine; also has antiemetic properties
Morphine (or meperidine)	IM	5–10 mg	↑ ICP or head trauma with funduscopic changes	Sedation, hypoventilation	For intractable migraine
Metoclopramide (Reglan)	PO, IM	10 mg stat	GI hemorrhage or obstruction; pheochromocytoma	Extrapyramidal reactions, sedation, restlessness	For adjunctive antiemetic therapy; prochlorperazine also effective

[a]See text for references and additional details. See Table 52-4 for additional information on sumatriptan and other triptan agents.
CV, cardiovascular; GI, gastrointestinal; HA, headache; ICP, intracranial pressure; IM, intramuscular; IN, intranasal; MAOIs, monoamine oxidase inhibitors; N, nausea; NSAID, nonsteroidal anti-inflammatory drug; PO, oral; PR, rectal; SC, subcutaneous; SL, sublingual; V, vomiting.

Appropriate treatments for K.L.'s current headache include DHE (by subcutaneous, intramuscular, or IV route), subcutaneous sumatriptan, or intravenous prochlorperazine. Each of these treatments has proved effective in at least two double-blind trials.[44] Although ergot alkaloids should not be administered within 24 hours of sumatriptan, K.L. vomited immediately after taking sumatriptan and it is unlikely that she absorbed the drug. Thus, DHE is not contraindicated. Since K.L. has responded to oral sumatriptan in the past, subcutaneous administration of this drug would be appropriate initial therapy at this time. Adjunctive therapy with prochlorperazine (5 mg intramuscularly or intravenously) would provide relief from nausea and vomiting, and may also contribute to a reduction in headache severity. If K.L.'s headache persists after 6 mg subcutaneous sumatriptan, a second injection can be given 1 hour after the first.

Prophylactic Therapy

15. K.L. returns to the clinic 6 weeks later for follow-up. Her current medications include oral sumatriptan and acetaminophen with codeine. Acetaminophen with codeine 30 mg (#20) was prescribed by the ED physician who treated her single episode of intractable migraine. Since that episode, about 75% of her headaches have responded to sumatriptan 100 mg orally. The remainder of her attacks have been aborted with two acetaminophen with codeine tablets and rest. Her concern is that these resistant headaches occur as often as once or twice monthly and necessitate her taking the rest of the day off from work. K.L. reports no adverse effects from sumatriptan.

K.L.'s primary care physician wants to initiate treatment to reduce the frequency and severity of K.L.'s migraine attacks and chooses propranolol as the initial agent. When should prophylactic therapy of migraine be considered? Is propranolol a reasonable choice for K.L.?

Criteria for Use

K.L.'s present drug regimen is effectively aborting about 75% of her migraine attacks. The frequency of her disabling, drug-resistant headaches, however, is sufficient to warrant additional therapy that is directed toward preventing migraine attacks. Prophylactic migraine treatment not only reduces the frequency of migraine attacks, but also may reduce the severity of ensuing headaches, render them more responsive to abortive measures, or reduce the duration of headaches. The usual criteria for migraine prophylaxis are (1) headaches that impact a patient's life despite the use of abortive treatments (e.g., twice monthly or more), (2) headaches occurring so frequently that acute medications are overused, (3) disabling headaches that are unresponsive to abortive treatments, (4) patients in whom abortive agents are contraindicated, and (5) headaches that present a significant risk for future morbidity or mortality (e.g., hemiplegic migraine, migraine with prolonged aura, basilar migraine, or migraines associated with stroke).[115] Given the frequency with which K.L. continues to experience migraine headaches and the detrimental effect they have on her job performance, prophylactic migraine therapy is warranted.

Various prophylactic agents have been advocated to reduce the frequency and severity of migraine headaches. For many of these drugs, it is difficult to make an adequate assessment of relative efficacy based on the available literature. Therapeutic trials often are not optimally designed to establish the relative usefulness of a given drug relative to other prophylactic agents. For example, the efficacy of newer therapies may be repeatedly compared with placebo rather than with other agents whose effectiveness is well documented, whose dosages are often suboptimal, or whose duration of therapy may be insufficient to document maximal efficacy. Ideally, the evaluation of migraine drug therapy should be based on double-blind, controlled, crossover trials with optimal dosage titration (to effect, toxicity, or established maximum dosing recommendations) and with sufficient wash-out periods to minimize ambiguous results. Many prophylactic therapy recommendations are not so well grounded. Recently, a structured, evidence-based guideline for prophylactic treatment of migraine headache was published.[115,116] Recommendations given below are based on these guidelines, which represent a synthesis of the results from published trials and expert opinion. Generally, the preferred agents for prophylaxis of migraine headache are propranolol, timolol, amitriptyline, and valproate (including divalproex sodium). The use of these agents is supported by multiple randomized controlled trials and mild-to-moderate adverse effects. Other agents discussed below either have less evidence basis for a strong recommendation (i.e., few or no randomized controlled trials), or have been associated with significant adverse effects that limit their usefulness. In the United States, the only agents approved by the FDA for migraine prophylaxis are propranolol, timolol, valproate and methysergide. Table 52-6 contains a list of the more well-established drugs used for migraine headache prophylaxis.

Propranolol

K.L.'s primary care physician has chose propranolol for prophylactic therapy of migraine. This is an appropriate choice. Propranolol (Inderal) is a first-line agent for migraine prophylaxis because of its safety, efficacy, favorable adverse effect profile, and the large number of studies that support its effectiveness.[117,118] Although the effectiveness of propranolol in the prophylaxis of migraine is well established, not all individuals respond to this treatment.[118–124] When propranolol is used, approximately 50% to 80% of patients obtain complete or partial relief from migraine attacks[118,124,125]; most patients who initially respond to propranolol continue to benefit without any evidence of drug tolerance.[124]

The mechanism by which propranolol exerts its antimigraine effects is unknown. It was generally assumed, without evidence to support the hypothesis, that β-receptor blockade prevented the vasodilatory phase of migraine; however, propranolol has no significant effect on cerebral blood flow.[126] The mechanism of action may be related to the drug's effects on the serotonergic system.[127,128] Propranolol has a high affinity for serotonin receptors[128] and has been shown to inhibit platelet uptake of serotonin in vivo and in vitro.[129]

Other β-adrenergic blocking drugs such as timolol[134] and the cardioselective agents, metoprolol[130] and atenolol,[131,132] appear to be as efficacious as propranolol in double-blind, crossover trials. However, besides propranolol, timolol is the only β-blocker with FDA approval for this indication. Atenolol is an appropriate therapeutic alternative for patients who cannot tolerate propranolol's CNS adverse effects. The lack of efficacy

Table 52-6   Drugs Useful for Migraine Headache Prophylaxis[a]

Drug	Dose	Dosage Forms/Strengths	Effectiveness	Comments
Propranolol (Inderal)	20 mg BID–TID; gradually ↑ dose at weekly intervals to effect or max of 320 mg/day	Tab: 10, 20, 40, 60, 80, 90 mg ER Cap: 60, 80, 120, 160 mg	50–80% obtain complete or partial relief; comparable to methysergide	First line therapy; atenolol, metoprolol, and timolol also effective
Amitriptyline (Elavil)	10–25 mg HS; ↑ by 10–25 mg/day at weekly intervals to max 150 mg/day; most should benefit from 50–75 mg/day	Tab: 10, 25, 50, 75, 100, 150 mg	Effectiveness comparable to propranolol and methysergide	First line therapy effective for prophylaxis of migraine and tension-type headache
Valproate (Depakote)	250 mg BID; ↑ by 250 mg/day at weekly intervals to effect or adverse effects; most should benefit from 1,000–2,000 mg/day	Cap[b]: 250 mg DR Tab[c]: 125, 250, 500 mg ER Tab: 250,500 mg SCaps: 125 mg	50% obtain complete or partial relief	First line therapy
Verapamil (Isoptin, Calan)	80 mg TID. If needed, ↑ dose gradually to max of 480 mg/day	Tabs: 40, 80, 120 mg ER Cap: 120, 240 mg ER Tab: 180, 240 mg	50% obtain complete or partial relief	Second line therapy Delay of 1–2 months for maximal effect; efficacy of nifedipine and diltiazem questionable
Methysergide (Sansert)	2–8 mg/day in 3–4 divided daily doses to be taken with food	Tab: 2 mg	60–70% obtain complete or partial relief	Use limited by propensity for frequent and sometimes severe adverse effects; drug holidays should be planned every 6 mo. Rarely used
Naproxen sodium	550 mg BID	Tab: 220, 275, 550 mg	30% obtain complete or partial relief	Second line therapy Modest efficacy; effective for menstrual migraine; naproxen, flurbiprofen, ketoprofen, mefenamic acid also effective

[a]See text for references and additional details.
[b]Valproic acid capsules.
[c]Divalproex sodium delayed-release tablets.
Cap, capsules; DR, delayed release; ER, extended release; SCap, sprinkle capsules containing coated particles; Tab, tablets.

demonstrated for pindolol,[133] acebutolol,[134] alprenolol,[135] and oxprenolol[136] may be related to their intrinsic sympathomimetic activity, and these agents should not be used.

DOSING

16. **What dose of propranolol should be prescribed for K.L.? When can she expect a response?**

Propranolol 80 to 240 mg/day in two to four divided doses is effective in the prophylaxis of migraine headaches.[115,118] Because the dosage range is wide, propranolol therapy should be initiated with 20 mg two or three times a day; this dose can be increased gradually at weekly intervals according to patient tolerability or to a maximum of 320 mg/day.[117] Once the daily dosage of propranolol required to control headaches is established, patient adherence may be improved by changing to a long-acting oral dosage form (e.g., Inderal LA). Although the usual dosage for migraine prophylaxis is 80 to 240 mg/day, up to 30% of patients prophylactically treated with propranolol would not have benefited in one clinical study of 865 patients if the propranolol dosage had not been titrated to a maximum of 320 mg/day.[125] Most propranolol responders will experience relief within 4 to 6 weeks of beginning ther-

apy.[79] However, in unusual circumstances, 3 to 6 months may be required before maximal benefit is realized.[125] Tolerance to the antimigraine effects of propranolol over long-term therapy does not occur.[124]

Because propranolol is highly effective and well tolerated in most patients, it is an appropriate prophylactic agent for K.L. She has no pre-existing disease states that would prohibit its use. K.L. should be started at a low dosage with gradual titration to either therapeutic response, side effects, or a maximum dose of 320 mg/day. Six weeks or longer may be required before optimal results are achieved.

Methysergide

17. **G.W., a 46-year-old man with an 11-year history of migraine without aura, comes to a clinic with a complaint of epigastric distress for the past 2 days. Current medications include Fiorinal (aspirin 325 mg, butalbital 50 mg, caffeine 40 mg) two capsules PO at headache onset, methysergide (Sansert) 2 mg PO TID, salmeterol inhaler 1 puff every 12 hours, fluticasone (44 μg/puff) 2 puffs every 12 hours, albuterol metered-dose inhaler 2 puffs as needed for shortness of breath, and Theo-Dur 300 mg PO BID. G.W.'s headaches are notable for bilateral, throbbing,**

temporal head pain and the absence of associated GI or focal neurologic symptoms. Migraine prophylaxis with methysergide has reduced his headache frequency from three headaches monthly to about one headache every 2 to 3 months. A review of G.W.'s medical record reveals that methysergide therapy was initiated 2 years ago and that a drug holiday was not taken. Past medical history includes asthma since adolescence, with frequent ED visits for exacerbation of symptoms and a 3-year history of painful lower extremity peripheral vascular disease (PVD). Why is methysergide an inappropriate alternative to propranolol prophylaxis of migraine in this asthmatic patient with PVD?

Methysergide, a semisynthetic ergot alkaloid with 5-HT$_2$-receptor antagonist properties, is one of the most effective agents for migraine prophylaxis;[137] in past decades, it was the standard by which newer therapies were often judged. However, its use is limited by a propensity for frequent, and sometimes severe, side effects. For this reason, methysergide is considered a fourth-line agent for migraine prophylaxis.[115]

Within the usual dosage range of 2 to 8 mg in three to four daily divided doses, as many as 40% of patients treated with methysergide will experience side effects. Adverse effects are severe enough to require discontinuation in 10% of patients.

CONTRAINDICATIONS

Like other ergot alkaloids, methysergide has peripheral vasoconstrictive properties that may preclude its use in some patients. Contraindications to methysergide use include PVD, coronary artery disease, thrombophlebitis, and pregnancy. Even when such precautions are kept in mind, some patients experience side effects attributable to the drug's vasoconstrictive properties (e.g., coldness, numbness, and tingling of the extremities or even anginal pain).

Given G.W.'s history of PVD, methysergide is not an appropriate agent for migraine prophylaxis. Although he had a history of PVD before methysergide was initiated, the continued use of this drug may have aggravated his condition. G.W.'s methysergide should be tapered immediately and an alternative treatment regimen initiated.

ADVERSE EFFECTS

18. In addition to G.W.'s history of PVD, what is another reason for discontinuing his methysergide therapy, and how should it be tapered?

Retroperitoneal, endocardial, and pleuropulmonary fibrosis are severe complications of methysergide. Fibrosis has developed after 7 to 79 months of methysergide therapy and has been associated with dosages in excess of 8 mg/day.[79] Because most fibrotic complications have been reported following long-term, uninterrupted use of methysergide,[138] drug-free holidays of 3 to 4 weeks are recommended after each 6-month treatment period to minimize this risk. However, the discontinuation of methysergide should be gradual to avoid the rebound vascular headache that can occur after abrupt discontinuation. Patients receiving long-term therapy should be counseled to report any flank pain, dysuria, or chest pain to their physician. During each patient visit, cardiac auscultation should be performed. An IV pyelogram and chest radiograph also should be obtained after 6 months of therapy to monitor for the development of fibrosis. When the therapeutic benefits of methysergide become evident (approximately 3 to 4 weeks

after initiation of therapy), the dose of this drug should be reduced to the minimum effective amount.[79]

Because G.W. has received methysergide continuously for 2 years without a drug holiday, he is at risk for developing methysergide fibrosis. The methysergide should be discontinued in G.W. because of the risk of drug-induced fibrosis and because of his history of PVD. His methysergide therapy should be gradually tapered to discontinuation over a 3-week period to avoid migraine headache rebound. Subsequently, another form of prophylactic therapy should be initiated for G.W.

19. G.W. has been experiencing nausea for the past 2 days. What is one approach to resolving these GI complaints?

GI distress is the most common side effect to methysergide therapy. However, the discomfort is usually mild and disappears within the first several days to weeks of therapy. GI distress can be minimized by administering methysergide doses with food and by avoiding rapid increases in dose. Because G.W. has received methysergide therapy for 2 years and his GI complaints appear to be of recent origin, other potential causes for GI distress should be investigated. Methysergide can also activate latent peptic ulcer disease,[139] presumably by increasing gastric acid secretion.[140] However, G.W. has no known history of ulcer disease and his GI complaint does not specifically suggest this complication.

G.W.'s GI distress may be the result of gastritis or peptic ulcer disease caused by the aspirin component in Fiorinal (G.W. receives 650 mg aspirin with each two capsule Fiorinal dose). The nausea also could be due to theophylline toxicity. These potential causes of G.W.'s nausea should be evaluated. A laboratory determination of G.W.'s hemoglobin (Hgb) concentration and evaluation of his stools for occult blood would be helpful in assessing aspirin-induced gastritis with blood loss. A serum theophylline concentration also should be obtained. A more detailed history that focuses on the relation between nausea and medication use or other concurrent illness may also provide useful information for assessing G.W.'s GI distress.

20. What drug should be prescribed in place of methysergide to prevent G.W.'s migraine attacks?

Along with propranolol, amitriptyline and valproate are effective first-line therapies for prevention of migraine headache. The effectiveness of these agents is supported by randomized controlled trials, and adverse effects are generally mild-to-moderate in severity.

Amitriptyline

Amitriptyline (Elavil) is effective for prevention of both migraine and tension-type headaches. It may be the drug of choice for patients whose symptoms suggest features of both headache types (i.e., mixed tension-type/migraine headaches), and for those with coexisting depression. Along with propranolol and valproate, amitriptyline is considered a first-line therapy for migraine prophylaxis.[115]

In a double-blind, placebo-controlled, cross-over study, amitriptyline was as effective as propranolol.[141] It also was as effective as methysergide based on comparative results from previous studies.[142] The mechanism of amitriptyline's antimigraine effect is independent of its antidepressant activity[141,143] and may be related to its ability to block the reuptake of serotonin at central sites.[144] However, other antidepressant agents that block 5-HT reuptake (e.g., clomipramine) have been ineffective for migraine prophylaxis.[145] Amitriptyline and other antidepressants have been reported to down-regulate 5-HT receptors, although this effect has been inconsistent in published reports.[146]

DOSING

The initial dose of amitriptyline is 10 to 25 mg at bedtime. This nightly dose can be increased at weekly intervals by 10 to 25 mg until the maximum dose of 150 mg/day is reached. Most patients achieve optimal benefit from 50 to 75 mg/day of amitriptyline; doses greater than 150 mg/day are unlikely to produce better results.[79] Two-thirds of patients note a decrease in the number of headaches within 7 days of starting amitriptyline therapy, but a 6-week trial is warranted before the drug should be considered ineffective.[142,143]

No other antidepressant agents have been studied as extensively as amitriptyline for migraine prophylaxis and their efficacy remains unproven. Fluoxetine (Prozac) was effective in one small trial.[147] However, the favorable results were not reproduced in a larger, subsequent study.[148] A study of amitriptyline 25 mg/day and fluvoxamine 50 mg/day demonstrated reductions in headache frequency for both drugs when pretreatment and post-treatment periods were compared.[149]

Valproate

The antiepileptic drug valproate (and divalproex sodium, Depakote) is also approved for the prevention of migraine headaches and is useful as a first-line agent in this regard.[115,150] In a randomized, double-blind, parallel treatment comparison of valproate (titrated to trough serum concentrations of 70 to 120 μg/mL) and placebo, 48% of valproate-treated patients had a 50% or greater reduction in the frequency of migraine.[151] In a single-blind comparison of valproate and propranolol, both agents were equally effective as prophylaxis for migraine without aura.[152]

DOSING

The initial dose of valproate is 250 mg PO BID. The dose can be increased in 250- to 500-mg/day increments at weekly intervals. The usual range of effective doses is 500 to 1,500 mg/day. Serum levels of valproate may be useful to monitor therapy; however, a clear relation between concentration and antimigraine effect has not been established. Enteric-coated products (e.g., Depakote) are preferred over immediate release products (e.g., Depakene) to minimize gastrointestinal upset. An extended-release dosage form (Depakote ER) is approved for once-daily dosing and may be useful to improve medication adherence.

Either amitriptyline or valproate would be reasonable choices for prevention of migraine headaches in G.W. Although direct comparative trials have not been performed, these agents appear to be equally effective. Thus, the choice can be made on the basis of the adverse effect profile of these agents. The most common adverse effects of amitriptyline include dry mouth, reflex tachycardia, blurred vision, weight gain, and difficulty with cognition. The most common adverse effects of valproate include nausea, alopecia, tremor, and weight gain. The adverse effect profiles of each agent should

be discussed with G.W., and, on the basis of his preference, a choice between these agents should be made.

21. S.A. is a 31-year old woman with a 4-year history of disabling migraine headaches (with aura) occurring two to three times weekly. She is currently using zolmitriptan (Zomig) 5 mg for abortive therapy, and the clinic physician is concerned about overuse of this agent. Medical history includes bipolar affective disorder and a history of polydrug abuse. S.A. has failed prophylactic therapy with propranolol (ineffective) and valproate (modestly effective, but caused unacceptable weight gain). She is currently taking lithium for her bipolar disorder, and her serum levels have been stable at 0.8 mEq/L. Her physician wishes to avoid antidepressants because of her psychiatric history. What other prophylactic therapies are available?

Nonsteroidal Anti-Inflammatory Drugs

In addition to being effective as symptomatic therapy for migraine, selected NSAIDs are also effective as prophylactic agents. However, their effectiveness as preventive therapy is considered to be modest compared with the first-line agents, propranolol, amitriptyline, and valproate.[115] The rationale for their use is that inhibition of prostaglandin and leukotriene synthesis might inhibit the neurogenic inflammation of migraine. However, their actual mechanism of action is unknown. Placebo-controlled trials have documented the effectiveness of naproxen,[153] naproxen sodium,[154,155] ketoprofen,[156] flurbiprofen,[157] and mefenamic acid.[158]A comparative study of naproxen sodium 1,100 mg/day and propranolol 120 mg/day found a trend favoring propranolol, although the difference in response between the two treatments was not significant.[159] Given the favorable trend toward propranolol and the use of a suboptimal dose of the drug in this trial, it is unlikely that naproxen sodium is a superior agent for migraine prophylaxis. The NSAIDs mentioned above may be effective as short-term therapy for menstruation-associated migraine.[115]

Calcium Channel Blockers
VERAPAMIL

Calcium channel blockers influence the final common pathway of vascular reactivity by altering calcium flux across smooth muscle. Hormone and neurotransmitter secretion are also calcium-dependent processes that can be altered by calcium channel blockers.[160] Whether the efficacy of calcium antagonists in migraine therapy is due to their vasoactive properties, modulation of neurotransmitter release, or a serotonergic effect is unknown.

Verapamil (Isoptin, Calan, Verelan) is the calcium channel blocker of choice for preventive migraine therapy because it is effective and has been most extensively studied in randomized controlled trials. Most patients respond to verapamil at doses of 240 to 320 mg/day. Therefore, treatment can be initiated with an 80-mg dose three times a day and increased to 80 mg four times a day after 1 week. Observable benefits from this treatment may not be apparent for 3 to 8 weeks; as a result, verapamil should be continued for at least 2 months to properly evaluate response to therapy. This is one of the limiting properties of calcium channel antagonists. If an adequate response is not achieved in this interval, the verapamil dose can be increased weekly by increments of 80 mg to a maximum of 480 mg/day. Sustained-release (SR) formulations

(Calan SR, Isoptin SR) and extended-release formulations (Covera-HS, Verelan) of verapamil, are available and are often useful in improving patient adherence with long-term therapy. Headache frequency, intensity, and duration are reduced in 50% of patients treated with verapamil.[161–163] Patients who suffer from migraine with or without aura respond equally well.[161,162] Verapamil may be particularly effective for patients with a prolonged or atypical migraine aura.[116] Although there are few comparative studies, most practitioners consider the benefits of calcium channel blockers to be modest relative to β-blockers, valproate, and amitriptyline. For this reason, verapamil is usually considered when these agents fail or are contraindicated.[8,117]

NIFEDIPINE, DILTIAZEM AND NIMODIPINE

Nifedipine (Procardia) and diltiazem (Cardizem) are other calcium antagonists that have been used to treat migraine.[164–166] Although preliminary experience suggested that nifedipine was effective, a double-blind, crossover study found nifedipine to be no more effective than placebo for preventing migraine headaches with aura. This study was designed to detect a 50% reduction in migraine frequency during treatment.[167] The effectiveness of diltiazem is based on two open-label studies with no control treatment.[166,168] As yet, no placebo-controlled, crossover studies have been reported. On the basis of current evidence, neither nifedipine nor diltiazem can be recommended for prophylaxis of migraine headache until other, better-established therapies (see Table 52-6) have been adequately tried and yielded unsatisfactory results.

Nimodipine (Nimotop) is a calcium antagonist with marked selectivity for the cerebral vasculature.[169] The drug is approved only to improve neurologic deficits after aneurysmal subarachnoid hemorrhage. Results from double-blind, placebo-controlled trials have been inconsistent in showing a benefit of nimodipine for preventing migraine headaches.[170–173] In most studies, the dose of oral nimodipine was 40 mg given three times daily.[171–173] Unfortunately, no adequate studies are available that compare nimodipine to other first-line preventative therapies. In light of the inconsistent results from placebo-controlled trials and the high cost of this drug, nimodipine appears to have little utility as a prophylactic agent.

Other Prophylactic Therapies

Some of the less established therapies occasionally recommended for migraine prophylaxis are listed in Table 52-7.[79,115,174–177] Evaluative reports for some of these agents do not meet the criteria for establishing a clear benefit in migraine. In general, a significant reduction of headache frequency in 50% of patients should be demonstrated before a drug can be said to be more effective than placebo. Placebo response rates for migraine and other painful conditions range from 30% to 50%[10,178,179] and may be maintained over several months.[179] This significant effect should also be considered when evaluating studies of migraine therapy.

On the basis of efficacy, either NSAIDs (i.e., naproxen, naproxen sodium, flurbiprofen, ketoprofen or mefenamic acid) or verapamil could be considered for prophylactic therapy to reduce the frequency of S.A.'s migraine headaches. However, NSAIDs are likely to interact with her lithium therapy, resulting in an increase in serum concentration and risk for adverse effects. For this reason, NSAIDs are best avoided at this time. S.A. should be started on verapamil 80 mg three times a day with gradual dosage titration to side effects, cessation of migraine attacks, or a maximum dose of 480 mg/day. She should be counseled regarding the possible occurrence of constipation and the appropriate management of this common side effect of verapamil. A 2-month trial may be necessary to demonstrate optimal therapeutic effect. Prophylactic therapy for migraine should be continued for 3 to 6 months. If a satisfactory response is achieved, the prophylactic agent should be gradually discontinued over several weeks to assess the continued need for this mode of therapy.

Analgesic Overuse

22. L.D. is a 39-year-old woman with a 7-year history of migraine (without aura) and tension-type headache who comes to clinic requesting a refill of her Fiorinal (aspirin, butalbital, and caffeine) and acetaminophen with codeine (30 mg). She reports an increase in the frequency of both her "throbbing" and "dull, pressure-sensation" headaches over the past year, and lately she has had difficulty distinguishing the two types. Over the past 2 months, she has had only 5 days with no headache, and she has been much less productive in her work as a magazine editor. A

Table 52-7 Other Drugs for Migraine Headache Prophylaxis[a]

Drug	Dose/Day (Oral)	Comments
Clonidine	0.1–0.2 mg BID–TID	No benefit found in some studies
Cyproheptadine	4–8 mg TID–QID (adults)	Particularly useful for migraine in children
Ergonovine maleate	0.2 mg TID–QID during menses or continuously	Effective for menstrual migraine and when other prophylactic agents contraindicated; recommended by some authors as a first-line prophylactic agent
Feverfew	Variable	Demonstrated effective in randomized, controlled trial though additional study needed
Phenelzine	15 mg TID–QID	Caution when used simultaneously with antidepressants and β-blockers
Phenytoin	200–400 mg QD	Benefits in children and adults established by uncontrolled studies
Riboflavin	400 mg QD	Demonstrated effective in a randomized, controlled trial though additional study needed
Topiramate	25–325 mg/day (given BID)	Effective in one of two randomized controlled trials
Gabapentin	900–2400 mg/day (given TID)	Effective in one randomized controlled trial

review of her medication refill records indicates that she has had four refills of Fiorinal (#30) and three refills of acetaminophen with codeine (#20) in the past 2 months and that her use of these drugs has increased over the past year. During the visit, she also indicates that she uses OTC acetaminophen and naproxen sodium on an "as-needed" basis. Although L.D. had experienced relief of mild headaches in the past with the use of OTC analgesics, these medications no longer reduce the intensity of her pain. What is the potential role of analgesic overuse in the worsening of L.D.'s headaches? How should her condition be managed?

Narcotics, NSAIDs, and other analgesics can be very effective for the treatment of infrequent, episodic migraine and other headache types. However, the use of these agents in patients with frequent headaches should be undertaken with caution. Analgesic overuse is common in these patients and associated with a gradual worsening of the headache symptoms. Any type of headache syndrome (e.g., migraine, tension-type, and other headaches) can be worsened by analgesic overuse.[180] This exacerbation is termed *analgesic-induced headache* (also, *analgesic rebound headache*) and is characterized by an increase in the use of analgesics, development of tolerance to the pain-relieving effect of these drugs, an increase in headache intensity, and an increase in headache frequency. In severe circumstances, a pattern of chronic daily headache can emerge. These chronic daily headaches often have features of both migraine and tension-type headaches.[181] The mechanism of analgesic rebound headache is unknown. However, alterations in serotonergic transmission are suspected.[182,183] L.D. displays many of the features of analgesic-induced headache. She reports an increase in the frequency of headaches to a near-daily pattern and she is no longer able to distinguish between migrainous and tension-type headaches. Furthermore, the exacerbation of her headaches appears to coincide with the escalating use of analgesics. L.D. should be questioned carefully to determine the total amount of acetaminophen, naproxen sodium, and aspirin that she consumes daily and weekly. Daily users of analgesics are at increased risk for chronic renal disease, chronic liver disease, and acute GI bleeding.[183–185] Laboratory tests should be ordered to assess L.D.'s renal and hepatic function, and she should be questioned regarding the occurrence of GI discomfort, acute bleeding, or a change in her stool color.

In general, patients who receive analgesics for headache treatment should be counseled to restrict their use of these agents to no more than twice per week.[44] However, in patients with analgesic-induced headache, a reduction in the use of these drugs will likely worsen their headache condition. The management of analgesic-induced headache is a challenge to clinicians and the patients who suffer from them. These headaches are often unresponsive to the usual abortive and prophylactic therapy measures discussed in earlier sections of this chapter. Successful management requires gradual withdrawal from the overused drugs. This process can be protracted and made even more difficult when barbiturate, codeine, or ergotamine-containing drugs are involved.[181] Withdrawal can usually be accomplished on an outpatient basis although in some patients, inpatient detoxification is required. Once the frequency and quantity of analgesic use by

L.D. have been adequately quantified, a process of gradual drug removal should be initiated. Medications taken on an infrequent basis (e.g., fewer than two times per week) can be abruptly stopped. For medications currently taken on a daily basis, L.D. should be counseled to reduce the medication by one tablet per day at 3-day intervals.[181] She should be informed that her headaches may worsen during this period but that symptoms will gradually improve as she proceeds through the detoxification process.

L.D.'s use of acetaminophen with codeine does not appear to be frequent enough to place her at risk for the development of opiate withdrawal symptoms. However, she should be counseled to report symptoms such as anxiety, tremulousness, insomnia, or diarrhea. If these symptoms occur, the rate of drug withdrawal should be reduced. Some clinicians prescribe a tricyclic antidepressant such as amitriptyline during the withdrawal period.[181] These agents can be useful for their central pain-relieving properties, antidepressant effects, and for their effect as preventative therapy for both migraine and tension-type headaches. Even if a tricyclic antidepressant is not prescribed during the withdrawal period, L.D. should be considered as a candidate for prophylactic headache therapy once analgesic withdrawal has been accomplished. If prophylaxis of both migraine and tension-type headache is necessary, amitriptyline would be an appropriate choice for L.D. After withdrawal is complete, L.D. should be educated regarding the future risk of analgesic-induced headache. A medication other than the withdrawn drugs should be prescribed for treatment of her acute attacks. For example, a triptan agent may be useful for abortive treatment of her migraine headaches. An NSAID may be considered for acute treatment of her tension-type headaches. L.D. must clearly understand that these agents should not be used more than twice per week, and her use of all abortive or symptomatic therapies should be monitored closely.

In extreme circumstances, analgesic abuse can precipitate chronic daily headache. In addition, analgesic abuse is a common cause of failure of the usual abortive treatment measures (e.g., sumatriptan and ergotamine). Successful abortive and prophylactic treatment of migraine headache in patients with a history of analgesic overuse necessitates detoxification from the abused agents.[186] Headaches often worsen during the withdrawal period, but within several weeks the headache characteristics return to baseline and responsiveness to traditional pharmacotherapy is restored. To minimize the risk of analgesic abuse and rebound headaches, patients should restrict their use of these agents to no more than twice per week.[44]

CLUSTER HEADACHE

Cluster headache is a relatively infrequent headache disorder (estimated prevalence 0.07 to 0.4%) that derives its name from the characteristic pattern of headache recurrence—headaches tend to occur nightly over a relatively short period of time (i.e., several weeks or months), followed by a long period of complete remission.[187] Cluster headaches occur more commonly in males than females. There may be a seasonal predilection to cluster attacks with the spring and fall being common times for headache recurrence. Headaches are usually of short duration and present as severe, unrelenting, unilateral pain occurring behind the eye with radiation to the territory of the ipsilateral trigeminal nerve (temple, cheek, or gum).

The different clinical characteristics between cluster and migraine headaches (e.g., sex ratio, periodicity of attacks, duration of headaches, aura symptoms) suggest that these two types of vascular headaches are different clinical entities.[188]

Pathophysiology

The pathophysiology of cluster headache is undetermined. As in migraine, vascular, neurogenic, metabolic, and humoral factors have been proposed to play a role in cluster headache pathogenesis. Precipitation of headaches during a cluster period by vasodilators and response to vasoconstrictors suggests an underlying vascular component. During a cluster headache, thermography shows increased periorbital heat emission ipsilateral to the head pain.[189] Also, patients commonly report flushing in the same area, and these observations suggest that extracranial vasodilation occurs in cluster headache. However, intracranial blood flow studies fail to show consistent changes during a cluster attack,[190–192] and the alterations in extracranial blood flow follow the onset of head pain,[193] suggesting that vasodilation occurs in response to some other initiating stimulus. Abnormal plasma levels of melatonin, growth hormone, testosterone, and prolactin have been reported in patients with cluster headache. These findings, along with the cyclic recurrence pattern of the disorder suggest a disturbance in hypothalamic function.[194]

Observations that suggest a neural component to cluster headache include the occurrence of headache in the distribution of the trigeminal nerve, accompanying autonomic symptoms, and the fact that headache precedes extracranial vasodilation. Stimulation of the trigeminal nerve results in the release of substance P and vasoactive polypeptides, vasodilation, and pain.[195] These features implicate the trigeminovascular system in cluster headache pathogenesis. However, a coherent theory to explain the symptoms, periodicity, and circadian regularity of cluster headaches remains elusive.

In recent years, the role of heredity in cluster headache has been appreciated.[187] Cluster headache has been reported in monozygotic twins,[196] and first-degree relatives of individuals with cluster headache have a 14-fold higher risk of also having cluster headaches.[197] However, a specific genetic basis for the disorder remains elusive.[198]

Signs and Symptoms

23. R.H. is a 31-year-old man with a 3-year history of episodic cluster headache. He has been headache free for the past year but today states that the headaches are returning in their characteristic fashion. He reports abrupt onset of right-sided retro-orbital pain with occasional superimposed knifelike "jabs" that increase in intensity over several minutes to a severe, unrelenting pain lasting about 90 minutes. The headache then gradually subsides. Associated symptoms include right-sided lacrimation, conjunctival injection, and rhinorrhea. He denies any premonition of ensuing headache or GI upset during the attacks. Physical examination during a cluster headache shows right eyelid droop and pupillary miosis. R.H.'s cluster periods characteristically last about 2 months and usually recur once or twice yearly. The first headache of the current bout awoke him from a short nap. R.H. expects to suffer one or two such headaches daily because this has been the usual pattern during each cluster period. Previous cluster headaches have been symptomatically treated with aspirin and codeine 30 mg. However, R.H. reports only modest relief with this treatment approach.

R.H.'s medical history is unremarkable. He does not use tobacco but admits to occasional social drinking. What subjective and objective evidence in this case is consistent with a diagnosis of cluster headaches?

R.H.'s gender, age of onset, quality and intensity of headache pain, periodicity of headache attacks, and associated symptoms all support the diagnosis of cluster headaches.

Cluster headaches affect men more commonly than women by a ratio of 5:1,[189,199] and have their usual onset between the second and fourth decades of life.[199] R.H.'s gender (male) and age of onset (28 years) are compatible with these aspects of cluster headaches.

Recurrent cluster headaches are usually severe and throbbing and affect the same side of the head. Occasionally, cluster headaches may involve the entire hemicranium. The pain starts abruptly, often waking the patient from sleep, reaches maximum intensity over 5 to 15 minutes, and usually lasts 45 to 60 minutes.[189] Unlike migraine, cluster headache is not preceded by an aura. Thus, patients have no warning before onset of head pain. Cluster periods often last from 2 to 3 months and recur once or twice yearly.[189] Patients suffering from chronic cluster headaches have bouts that last 12 months or longer. R.H.'s headache quality (severe, unrelenting pain), site (unilateral), evolution and resolution pattern (worsens over several minutes and resolves within 90 minutes), and periodicity of attacks (one or two headaches occurring daily for about 2 months followed by a period of remission that lasts about 1 year) are all compatible with the usual character of cluster headaches.

Associated features may include ipsilateral lacrimation, injected conjunctiva, and rhinorrhea or blocked nasal passage. A partial Horner's syndrome (ptosis with miosis) occurs in one-third of patients and is often the only abnormal physical finding during a cluster headache. Nausea, vomiting, and focal neurologic symptoms are often absent. Associated symptoms reported by R.H. during headache attacks (e.g., lacrimation, rhinorrhea, conjunctival injection) and the absence of GI or neurologic disturbances are also compatible with the diagnosis of cluster headaches.

During a cluster period, headaches may be precipitated by alcohol (even in small amounts), vasodilators, stress, warm weather, missed meals, and excessive sleep. Therefore, during the current cluster period, R.H. should be counseled to avoid all alcohol and daytime naps.

Abortive Therapy

24. What abortive measures are available for symptomatic treatment of individual headaches during R.H.'s current cluster period?

The treatments of choice for abortive treatment of cluster headaches are sumatriptan by subcutaneous injection and oxygen inhalation.[187,198] The expense and inconvenience of having oxygen inhalation apparatus close at hand limit the usefulness of this treatment for many patients. A recent community-based study found that most patients suffering from cluster headaches do not receive optimal treatment for their condition.[200] Table 52-8 is a summary of drugs commonly used for the acute treatment of cluster headache.

Sumatriptan

Sumatriptan 6 mg subcutaneously has been shown to effectively relieve cluster headache in randomized, double-blind, placebo-controlled trials. Cluster headaches are reduced in severity in 74% of attacks within 15 minutes, compared with 26% of attacks treated with placebo.[187] An additional injection of 6 mg does not appear to give additional headache relief.[201] However, in patients who experience a recurrent headache after initial relief with sumatriptan, a second injection is often useful.[194] Sumatriptan should not be used more often than twice daily during cluster bouts. For patients who experience more than two attacks per day, adjunctive therapy with oxygen inhalation should be considered.[187]

Intranasal and oral sumatriptan have also been evaluated in patients with cluster headache. A randomized, open-label comparison of sumatriptan by intranasal (20 mg) and subcutaneous (6 mg) routes found a much higher response with the injectable form of the drug at 15 minutes post-treatment (94% versus 13%, respectively). Patients included in this study indicated a clear preference for the subcutaneous dosage form.[202] Oral sumatriptan (100 mg three times a day) was studied as a prophylactic agent during cluster headache bouts and found to be ineffective.[203]

Oxygen

Oxygen inhalation is preferred not only for in-hospital treatment of cluster headache but also for use by some patients at home or at work. Oxygen is also useful for patients with frequent cluster headaches who would otherwise exceed maximum dosing restrictions of sumatriptan.[187] The benefits of oxygen inhalation at 7 L/minute for 15 minutes, are superior to placebo[204] and equal to those of ergotamine[205] in relieving cluster headaches. In addition, oxygen is very fast-acting, with most patients experiencing headache relief within 7 minutes of beginning inhalation.[205] The mechanism of oxygen's effect is unknown but may be related to a direct vasoconstrictive action.[187]

Ergotamine Tartrate

Inhalational, sublingual, and parenteral routes of ergotamine administration have a rapid onset of action and are effective for aborting acute cluster headaches.[206] Ergotamine by inhalation or sublingual administration is effective in 70% to 80% of patients,[207,208] and traditionally these routes of administration have been preferred. Unfortunately, no inhaled ergotamine product is currently marketed in the United States, and the product is likely to remain unavailable. Ergotamine tartrate 2 mg given rectally also can be effective if given early in the attack.[207] Ergotamine tartrate 0.5 mg and DHE 1 mg given intramuscularly are equally effective; DHE is better tolerated and less likely to cause vasoconstrictive adverse effects.[207]

Other Therapeutic Interventions

Cluster headaches also can be relieved by less commonly used therapeutic interventions such as intranasal capsaicin,[209] dexamethasone 8 mg orally,[194] methoxyflurane inhalation (10 to 15 drops applied to a handkerchief and inhaled for several seconds),[79] somatostatin IV infusion (25 μg/ minute for 20 minutes),[210] and local anesthesia with either intranasal application of 1 mL of 4% lidocaine hydrochloride[211] or 0.3 mL of

---

Table 52-8 Drugs Commonly Used for Acute Treatment of Cluster Headache[a]

Drug	Route	Dose	Contraindications	Adverse Effects	Comments
Sumatriptan (Imitrex)	SC	6 mg at HA onset	Ischemic heart disease, within 24 hr of ergot alkaloids	Heavy sensation in head or chest, tingling, pain at injection site	Not an FDA-approved indication; costly but well tolerated
Oxygen	Inhalation	7 L/min for 15 min	—	—	Fast onset of effect; equally effective as ergotamine tartrate
Ergotamine tartrate (Ergostat, Cafergot)	SL, PR	1–2 mg at HA onset; may repeat in 5 min (SL only); do not exceed 6 mg/attack or 10 mg/wk	CV disease, sepsis, liver or kidney disease, arterial insufficiency, pregnancy, breast feeding, concomitant macrolide use	N, V, anorexia, limb paresthesias or pain	SL ergotamine may have faster onset of effect; ↓ N and V by using smallest effective dose
DHE-45	SC, IM, IV	1 mg (SC, IM) or 0.75 mg (IV) stat; may repeat in 45 min	CV disease, sepsis, liver or kidney disease, arterial insufficiency, pregnancy, breast feeding	N, V, limb paresthesias or pain	More effective and faster onset than SL or PR ergotamine. Premedicate with antiemetic (e.g., metoclopramide or prochlorperazine)

[a]See text for references and additional details.

CV, cardiovascular; HA, headache; IM, intramuscular; IV, intravenous; N, nausea, PR, rectal; SC, subcutaneous; SL, sublingual; V, vomiting.

a 5% to 10% solution of cocaine hydrochloride[212] to the ipsilateral sphenopalatine fossa.

Orally administered narcotic analgesics are usually ineffective in cluster headache,[189] and R.H. has suffered several cluster periods with inadequate therapy. Improved response can be expected with the use of a more effective agent that has a faster onset of action. Reasonable options for the acute treatment of R.H.'s acute cluster headaches include subcutaneous sumatriptan or oxygen inhalation. The success rate with each of these therapies is high. For many patients, oxygen is a less convenient therapy since the equipment is not easily portable and the patient must sit still during the treatment. The choice can be made on the basis of patient preference or cost.

Prophylactic Therapy

25. **What therapeutic agents are available for headache prophylaxis during an active cluster period?**

Pharmacotherapy aimed at preventing cluster headaches during an active period should be considered if symptomatic therapy is ineffective, intolerable, or if headaches occur more frequently than twice daily. Table 52-9 contains a list of available drugs for cluster headache prophylaxis.

Verapamil

Verapamil is effective for the prevention of cluster headaches,[165,213,214] and many authors now considered this agent to be the prophylactic agent of choice.[187,189] The usual effective daily dose is 240 to 480 mg/day and approximately two-thirds of patients have a 50% or greater reduction in headache frequency. Verapamil can be combined with lithium for prophylaxis in patients with chronic cluster headaches.[187]

Prednisone

Prednisone 40 to 80 mg daily provides relief from episodic cluster headache in 50% to 75% of patients[215,216] and is superior to methysergide in both episodic and chronic cluster types.[216] Prednisone also has a faster onset of action than many other agents used for cluster headache prophylaxis. The beneficial effect is usually evident within 48 hours of initiating treatment.[79] Corticosteroids are best used for short bouts of cluster headaches (1 to 2 months or less) because of the side effects associated with prolonged use.

Ergotamine

Ergotamine's use as a prophylactic agent is particularly attractive when headache recurrence follows a predictable pattern (e.g., nocturnal attacks). Prophylactic administration at bedtime or at least 30 minutes before the anticipated headache often will prevent the attack.[189]

Methysergide

Methysergide is effective in 65% to 70% of patients with episodic cluster headache and can be used for cluster periods of less than 3 months' duration without the same degree of concern for fibrotic complications because of the anticipated shorter period of drug exposure.[207,216] A limitation to the use of methysergide as the sole prophylactic agent for cluster headache is the delay in symptomatic response, which may be up to 2 weeks in some patients. Chronic cluster headache re-

Table 52-9 Drugs for Prophylaxis of Cluster Headache[a]

Drug	Dose/Day	Route	Comments
Ergotamine tartrate (Cafergot, Ergostat)	0.25–0.5 mg BID–TID 5 days/wk 1–2 mg BID or HS for nocturnal HA; max 12 mg/wk	SC, PO, SL, PR	Effective when given 30 min before anticipated cluster HA
Indomethacin (Indocin)	50 mg TID	PO	Effective for chronic cluster HA
Lithium carbonate	600–1,500 mg	PO	Effective for chronic cluster HA; effective in 80% of patients
Melatonin	10 mg QD	PO	Efficacy demonstrated in 1 randomized controlled trial; patients with chronic cluster headache did not respond
Methylergonovine maleate	0.2 mg TID–QID	PO	Effective in 75% of patients in one retrospective study
Methysergide (Sansert)	2 mg TID–QID	PO	Effective in 65–70% of patients with episodic cluster HA; less effective for chronic cluster HA
Prednisone	40 mg QID × 2 days, then taper by 5 mg/day to maintenance dose of 15–30 mg QID	PO	A first-line agent for episodic cluster HA; more effective and faster-acting than methysergide; benefits usually within 48 hr; best for short bouts of cluster HA because of long-term adverse effects
Triamcinolone (Aristocort)	4–8 mg QID	PO	May be useful in patients unresponsive to prednisone
Valproate (Depakote)	600–2000 mg/day divided TID–QID	PO	Effective in 73% of patients in 1 open trial
Verapamil (Isoptin, Calan)	240–480 mg/day divided TID–QID	PO	Drug of choice for prophylaxis

[a]See text for references and additional details.
HA, headache; PO, oral; PR, rectal; SC, subcutaneous; SL, sublingual.

sponds less dramatically to methysergide and other agents (e.g., lithium) are preferred.[207]

Lithium Carbonate

Lithium carbonate is effective in preventing episodic and chronic cluster headache.[207,217,218] Benefits from lithium prophylaxis are observable 1 to 2 weeks after initiation of therapy[79,217,218] and are maintained with long-term use.[219] Lithium serum levels associated with efficacy in cluster headache prophylaxis are usually between 0.6 and 1.2 mEq/L.[189] However, lower levels (0.3 to 0.8 mEq/L) may also be effective.[187] Adverse effects from long-term lithium use (e.g., renal toxicity) are discussed in Chapter 80, Mood Disorders II: Bipolar Disorders.

Other Therapies

Valproate has not been adequately studied, but one open trial reported that 73% of patients with cluster headache responded to this treatment.[220] In a recent pilot study, melatonin was superior to placebo for prophylaxis of cluster headache.[221] β-Blockers, antidepressants, and carbamazepine have no proven usefulness in the treatment of cluster headaches.[79]

R.H. should be evaluated at his next clinic visit for response to abortive sumatriptan or oxygen therapy. Prompt consideration should be given to the aforementioned additional treatments if suppression of headaches during the cluster period is warranted. In general, after response to a prophylactic agent has been established and maintained for at least 2 weeks, attempts can be made to discontinue the drug. Treatment should be reinstituted if headaches recur.

TENSION-TYPE HEADACHE

Tension-type headache is the most common headache type with a lifetime prevalence of 88% in women and 69% in men.[222] In a population-based study, the 1-year prevalence of tension-type headache was 38%. Highest prevalence rates were found in women between 30 and 39 years of age and, in both sexes, those with higher education levels.[223] Tension-type headaches (previously known as *tension* or *muscle contraction* headaches) are usually characterized by a dull aching sensation bilaterally that occurs in a hatband distribution around the head. The pain is usually mild to moderate in severity and has a nonpulsating quality.[224] Tension-type headaches are not associated with aura symptoms, nor are they accompanied by nausea, vomiting, or photophobia. The headache is usually not of sufficient intensity to interfere with daily activities but may be a nuisance by virtue of its persistent nature. Headache frequency varies widely between patients. Chronic tension-type headache occurs in approximately 2% of the population (1-year prevalence rate) and sufferers may have headache continuously for months or even years.[223]

Pathophysiology

The throbbing pain associated with migraine headaches is not characteristic of tension-type headaches, although it may occur in 25% of tension-type headache sufferers when the pain becomes severe.[79] Such patients may be diagnosed more appropriately as having a mixed tension-type/migraine headache disorder.[225] Indeed, in recent years the traditional boundaries

distinguishing migraine from tension-type headaches have become less clear. Headache features such as neck muscle contraction and precipitation by stress were previously thought to be specific for tension-type headaches but are now recognized to occur in migraine as well.

For many years, excessive muscle contraction with constriction of pain-sensitive extracranial structures was thought to be the cause of tension-type headache.[226] More recent evidence shows no correlation between muscle contraction and the presence of tension-type headache.[227] Abnormal vascular reactivity was also thought to play a role in tension-type headache, but temporal muscle blood flow is unaltered compared with controls.[227] Platelet 5-HT content is lower in patients with chronic tension-type headache suggesting that migraine and tension-type headaches share some pathophysiologic features.[224]

Tension-type headaches also may be associated with depression,[225] repressed hostility, or resentment.[228] However, these psychological associations may be the result of the chronic pain syndrome rather than a cause or feature of the headache disorder. Patients with recurrent tension-type headaches probably do not experience more frequent stressful events, but may use less effective coping strategies in stressful situations.[229]

General Management and Abortive Therapy

26. K.B., a 27-year-old female financial analyst, presents to her general practitioner with a complaint of recurring headaches that worsened when she started her current job. Before this time, she had experienced infrequent headaches, which she associated with periods of stress. The headaches would occur three to four times yearly, were of a constant, dull, or "pressing" character and were present around the entire head. Recently, headaches of similar character have been occurring about one to two times weekly, usually toward the end of her work day. The pain usually lasts the rest of the day but varies in intensity. Occasionally, a headache is present when she wakes up in the morning as well. K.B. denies GI and aura symptoms associated with her headaches. She has noticed that relaxation and alcohol ingestion seem to relieve these headaches, but aspirin and acetaminophen have been ineffective. Her blood pressure is 120/74 mm Hg; her physical and neurologic examinations are completely normal. What measures should be taken to relieve K.B.'s headaches? What is an appropriate goal for treatment?

As in the treatment of other chronic headache disorders, a cure for recurrent tension-type headache is unlikely. K.B. should clearly understand that the goal of treatment is a reduction in the frequency and severity of headache. Drug therapy and relaxation techniques are the primary means by which tension-type headaches are treated.

Analgesics

Analgesics are the drugs of choice for treatment of acute tension headache attacks.[224] The initial choice of an analgesic should be based on the severity of the pain. Acetaminophen, aspirin, and NSAIDs are often effective, although their benefits may be short lived. Acetaminophen 1,000 mg provides equal relief from moderately severe tension-type headache when compared with 650 mg aspirin; both are superior to placebo.[230] Ibuprofen is as effective as aspirin for relief from tension headache discomfort, and side effects with both 400 and 800 mg ibuprofen are less common than with aspirin.[231] Ibuprofen 400 mg is superior to acetaminophen 1,000 mg for relief of tension-type headache pain.[232] Naproxen sodium 550 mg is more effective than placebo and acetaminophen 650 mg for relieving the pain of tension-type headache.[224] The potency of some analgesics may be enhanced by combination with an antihistamine (e.g., doxylamine).[233] Because the relative potencies of non-narcotic analgesics are equivalent, the choice between agents should be guided by cost and patient preference.

Sedatives (e.g., butalbital),[79] anxiolytics (e.g., meprobamate,[234] diazepam[235]), and skeletal muscle relaxants (e.g., orphenadrine) have also been used to treat tension-type headache and occasionally, patients respond to their concomitant use when an analgesic alone affords insufficient relief.

Nondrug Techniques

Nondrug techniques such as massage, hot baths, acupuncture, and various relaxation methods can provide relief from tension headache and are often effective adjuncts to drug therapy.[236] The literature both supports and refutes the effectiveness of acupuncture,[10,237] EMG (electromyography) biofeedback,[238–240] and other relaxation techniques in the therapy of tension-type headache. The utility of biofeedback and other relaxation techniques is based on the premise that voluntary control of muscle contraction could benefit the headache sufferer. These techniques are most successful in young, episodic headache sufferers who are motivated to apply the techniques as instructed.[241] A randomized, controlled trial of spinal manipulation for the treatment of tension-type headache failed to demonstrate a benefit of this approach.[242]

An NSAID (e.g., ibuprofen or naproxen) would be an appropriate recommendation for therapy of K.B.'s tension-type headaches because of her previous inadequate responses to aspirin and acetaminophen. Drug use should be carefully monitored because analgesic abuse in patients with frequently recurring tension headache is a primary factor in the perpetuation of chronic pain syndromes.[243]

Prophylactic Therapy

27. **Ibuprofen 400 mg Q 4 to 6 hours as needed for headache was prescribed for acute relief of K.B.'s recurrent tension-type headaches. At her next scheduled follow-up visit, K.B. reported moderate relief with ibuprofen but complained of GI upset with each dose, even when taken with food. Because headaches have** been occurring more frequently, her use of ibuprofen has also increased. **What prophylactic agents are available for continuous suppression of K.B.'s tension-type headaches?**

Antidepressants are the most useful group of agents in the prophylaxis of tension-type and mixed-type headaches. Amitriptyline (Elavil) is considered the drug of choice because it is most effective[244,245]; 65% of patients improved by more than 50% and 25% became headache-free in an early report.[225] The effective daily dose of amitriptyline for most patients is 10 to 75 mg,[244] although up to 300 mg/day may be required.[79] Response to amitriptyline does not require a history of depressive symptoms, and benefit to the tension-type headache sufferer is usually evident within 2 to 10 days.[79] Amitriptyline should be initiated at a dose of 10 to 25 mg/day at bedtime and increased gradually as needed to allow for the development of tolerance to the sedative and anticholinergic side effects of this drug. About 7% of patients discontinue amitriptyline because of side effects.[10] Although there is less experience with their use, doxepin (Sinequan),[246] imipramine (Tofranil),[6,225] maprotiline (Ludiomil),[247] and protriptyline (Vivactil)[248] are also effective in tension-type headache prophylaxis. Like amitriptyline, these agents have significant anticholinergic activity. If an agent with less anticholinergic activity is desired, desipramine (Norpramin) may be used. Although fluoxetine has been suggested as an alternative for the treatment of tension-type headache,[249] its effectiveness has not been established in a randomized, controlled trial. A randomized placebo-controlled trial comparing citalopram (an SSRI) with amitriptyline found that citalopram was not effective for prophylaxis of chronic tension-type headache.[250] At this time, SSRI antidepressants are not recommended for tension-type headache prophylaxis.[244] Given K.B.'s increasing frequency of tension-type headache and her intolerance to moderate doses of ibuprofen, prophylactic treatment with amitriptyline would be appropriate. A starting dose of amitriptyline 10 mg nightly, increasing by 10 to 25 mg at 1-week intervals to a maintenance dose of 50 mg/day should be prescribed, at which time headache response can be assessed and the dose increased or decreased as necessary. If effective, amitriptyline should be continued for 3 to 4 months before gradually decreasing the dose until the drug is completely discontinued. Therapy should be reinstituted if headaches return.

Because the dividing line between migraine and tension-type headache is often vague, the entire range of migraine drugs may be tried in refractory cases of tension-type headache or when symptoms suggest a mixed tension-type/migraine headache disorder.

REFERENCES

1. Stewart WF et al. Prevalence of migraine headache in the United States. Relation to age, income, race, and other sociodemographic factors. JAMA 1992;267:64.
2. Kroenke K, Mangelsdorff AD. Common symptoms in ambulatory care: incidence, evaluation, therapy, and outcome. Am J Med 1989;86:262.
3. Stang PE, Osterhaus JT. Impact of migraine in the United States: data from the National Health Interview Survey. Headache 1993;33:29.
4. Cook NR et al. Correlates of headache in a population-based cohort of elderly. Arch Neurol 1989;46:1338.
5. Linet MS et al. An epidemiologic study of headache among adolescents and young adults. JAMA 1989;261:2211.
6. Lance JW et al. Investigations into the mechanism and treatment of chronic headache. Med J Aust 1965;2:909.
7. Classification and diagnostic criteria for headache disorders, cranial neuralgias and facial pain. Headache Classification Committee of the International Headache Society. Cephalalgia 1988;8(Suppl 7):1.
8. Saper JR. Headache disorders. Med Clin North Am 1999;83:663.
9. Ray B, Wolff HG. Experimental studies on headache. Pain sensitive structures of the head and their significance in headache. Arch Surg 1940; 41:813.
10. Lance JW. Mechanism and Management of Headache, 4th Ed. London: Butterworths Scientific, 1982
11. Welch KM. Current opinions in headache pathogenesis: introduction and synthesis. Curr Opin Neurol 1998;11:193.
12. May A, Goadsby PJ. The trigeminovascular system in humans: pathophysiologic implications for primary headache syndromes of the neural influences

on the cerebral circulation. J Cereb Blood Flow Metab 1999;19:115.

13. Silberstein SD. Serotonin (5-HT) and migraine. Headache 1994;34:408.

14. Goadsby PJ. Mechanisms and management of headache. J R Coll Physicians Lond 1999;33:228.

15. Olesen J et al. Timing and topography of cerebral blood flow, aura, and headache during migraine attacks. Ann Neurol 1990;28:791.

16. Olesen J et al. The common migraine attack may not be initiated by cerebral ischaemia. Lancet 1981;2:438.

17. Limmroth V et al. Changes in cerebral blood flow velocity after treatment with sumatriptan or placebo and implications for the pathophysiology of migraine. J Neurol Sci 1996;138:60.

18. Drummond PD et al. Facial flushing after thermocoagulation of the Gasserian ganglion. J Neurol Neurosurg Psychiatry 1983;46:611.

19. Goadsby PJ et al. Release of vasoactive peptides in the extracerebral circulation of humans and the cat during activation of the trigeminovascular system. Ann Neurol 1988;23:193.

20. Weiller C et al. Brain stem activation in spontaneous human migraine attacks. Nat Med 1995;1:658.

21. Hoskin KL et al. Central activation of the trigeminovascular pathway in the cat is inhibited by dihydroergotamine. A c-Fos and electrophysiological study. Brain 1996;119(Pt 1):249.

22. Cumberbatch M et al. Rizatriptan inhibits central trigeminal nociceptive responses in an electrophysiological assay in the anaesthetized rat [Abstract]. In: Elesen J, Edvinsson L, eds. Messenger Molecules in Headache Pathogenesis: Monoamines, Neuropeptides, Purines and Nitric Oxide. Proceedings of the 7th International headache research seminar. Copenhagen, 1996:18.

23. Goadsby PJ, Hoskin KL. Inhibition of trigeminal neurons by intravenous administration of the serotonin (5HT)1B/D receptor agonist zolmitriptan (311C90): are brain stem sites therapeutic target in migraine? Pain 1996;67:355.

24. Anthony M et al. Plasma serotonin in migraine and stress. Arch Neurol 1967;16:544.

25. Curran DA et al. Total plasma serotonin, 5-hydroxyindoleacetic acid and p-hydroxy-m-methoxymandelic acid excretion in normal and migrainous subjects. Brain 1965;88:997.

26. Kimball RW et al. Effect of serotonin in migraine patients. Neurology 1960;10:107.

27. Hamel E et al. Expression of mRNA for the serotonin 5-hydroxytryptamine1D beta receptor subtype in human and bovine cerebral arteries. Mol Pharmacol 1993;44:242.

28. Rebeck GW et al. Selective 5-HT1D alpha serotonin receptor gene expression in trigeminal ganglia: implications for antimigraine drug development. Proc Natl Acad Sci U S A 1994;91:3666.

29. Ophoff RA et al. Familial hemiplegic migraine and episodic ataxia type-2 are caused by mutations in the Ca2+ channel gene CACNL1A4. Cell 1996;87:543.

30. Wessman M et al. A susceptibility locus for migraine with aura, on chromosome 4q24. Am J Hum Genet 2002;70:652.

31. Soragna D et al. A locus for migraine without aura maps on chromosome 14q21.2-q22.3. Am J Hum Genet 2003;72:161.

32. Rozen TD et al. Increasing incidence of medically recognized migraine headache in a United States population. Neurology 1999;53:1468.

33. Russell MB et al. Familial occurrence of migraine without aura and migraine with aura. Neurology 1993;43:1369.

34. Selby G, Lance JW. Observations on 500 cases of migraine and allied vascular headache. J Neurol Neurosurg Psychiatry 1960;23:23.

35. Ferrari MD. Migraine. Lancet 1998;351:1043.

36. Creditor MC. Me and migraine. N Engl J Med 1982;307:1029.

37. Lipton RB et al. Stratified care vs step care strategies for migraine: the Disability in Strategies of Care (DISC) Study: A randomized trial. JAMA 2000;284:2599.

38. Silberstein SD. Practice parameter: evidence-based guidelines for migraine headache (an evidence-based review): report of the Quality Standards Subcommittee of the American Academy of Neurology. Neurology 2000;55:754.

39. Becker WJ. Use of oral contraceptives in patients with migraine. Neurology 1999;53:S19.

40. Ryan RE. A controlled study of the effect of oral contraceptives on migraine. Headache 1978;17:250.

41. Tzourio C et al. Case-control study of migraine and risk of ischaemic stroke in young women. Br Med J 1995;310:830.

42. Silberstein SD, Young WB. Safety and efficacy of ergotamine tartrate and dihydroergotamine in the treatment of migraine and status migrainosus. Working Panel of the Headache and Facial Pain Section of the American Academy of Neurology. Neurology 1995;45:577.

43. Bousser MG, Massiou H. Migraine in the reproductive cycle. In: Olesen J et al., eds. The Headaches. New York: Raven Press, 1993:313.

44. Goadsby PJ et al. Migraine—current understanding and treatment. N Engl J Med 2002;346:257.

45. Perry CM, Markham A. Sumatriptan. An updated review of its use in migraine. Drugs 1998;55:889.

46. O'Quinn S et al. Sumatriptan injection and nasal spray: onset of efficacy in the acute treatment of migraine [Abstract]. Neurology 1998;50:A264.

47. Volans GN. Absorption of effervescent aspirin during migraine. Br Med J 1974;4:265.

48. Touchon J et al. A comparison of subcutaneous sumatriptan and dihydroergotamine nasal spray in the acute treatment of migraine. Neurology 1996;47:361.

49. Winner P et al. A double-blind study of subcutaneous dihydroergotamine vs subcutaneous sumatriptan in the treatment of acute migraine. Arch Neurol 1996;53:180.

50. A randomized, double-blind comparison of sumatriptan and Cafergot in the acute treatment of migraine. The Multinational Oral Sumatriptan and Cafergot Comparative Study Group. Eur Neurol 1991;31:314.

51. A study to compare oral sumatriptan with oral aspirin plus oral metoclopramide in the acute treatment of migraine. The Oral Sumatriptan and Aspirin plus Metoclopramide Comparative Study Group. Eur Neurol 1992;32:177.

52. Brown EG et al. The safety and tolerability of sumatriptan: an overview. Eur Neurol 1991;31:339.

53. Visser WH et al. Sumatriptan in clinical practice: a 2-year review of 453 migraine patients. Neurology 1996;47:46.

54. Lippolis A et al. [Coronary vasospasm secondary to subcutaneous administration of sumatriptan]. G Ital Cardiol 1994;24:883.

55. Walton-Shirley M et al. Unstable angina pectoris associated with Imitrex therapy. Cathet Cardiovasc Diagn 1995;34:188.

56. Mueller L et al. Vasospasm-induced myocardial infarction with sumatriptan. Headache 1996;36:329.

57. Cavazos JE et al. Sumatriptan-induced stroke in sagittal sinus thrombosis. Lancet 1994;343:1105.

58. Ottervanger JP et al. Transmural myocardial infarction with sumatriptan. Lancet 1993;341:861.

59. Saxena P, Tfelt-Hansen P. Sumatriptan. In: Olesen J, ed. The Headaches. New York: Raven Press, 1993:329.

60. Geraud G et al. Migraine headache recurrence: relationship to clinical, pharmacological, and pharmacokinetic properties of triptans. Headache 2003;43:376.

61. Diamond S. The use of sumatriptan in patients on monoamine oxidase inhibitors. Neurology 1995;45:1039.

62. Blier P, Bergeron R. The safety of concomitant use of sumatriptan and antidepressant treatments. J Clin Psychopharmacol 1995;15:106.

63. Gardner DM, Lynd LD. Sumatriptan contraindications and the serotonin syndrome. Ann Pharmacother 1998;32:33.

64. Ferrari MD et al. Oral triptans (serotonin 5-HT(1B/1D) agonists) in acute migraine treatment: a meta-analysis of 53 trials. Lancet 2001;358:1668.

65. Tfelt-Hansen P, Johnson ES. Ergotamine. In: Olesen J et al, eds. The Headaches. New York: Raven Press, 1993:313.

66. Hachinski V et al. Ergotamine and cerebral blood flow. Stroke 1978;9:594.

67. Moyer JH et al. The effect of theophylline with ethylenediamine (aminophylline) and caffeine on cerebral hemodynamics and cerebrospinal fluid pressure in patients with hypertensive headaches. Am J Med Sci 1952;224:377.

68. Schmidt R, Fanchamps A. Effect of caffeine on intestinal absorption of ergotamine in man. Eur J Clin Pharmacol 1974;7:213.

69. Laska EM et al. Caffeine as an analgesic adjuvant. JAMA 1984;251:1711.

70. Sutherland JM et al. Buccal absorption of ergotamine. J Neurol Neurosurg Psychiatry 1974;37:1116.

71. Tfelt-Hansen P et al. Clinical pharmacology of ergotamine studied with a high performance liquid chromatographic method. In: Rose FC, ed. Advances in Migraine Research and Therapy. New York: Raven Press, 1982:173.

72. Crooks J et al. Clinical Trial of Inhaled Ergotamine Tartrate in Migraine. Br Med J 1964;5377:221.

73. Carstairs LS. Headache and gastric emptying time. Proc R Soc Med 1958;51:790.

74. Orton D. Ergotamine tartrate levels in migraine, ergotamine tartrate overdose, and normal subjects using a rasioimmunoassay. Proceedings of the Migraine Trust International Symposium. London, 1976

75. Raskin NH. Acute and prophylactic treatment of migraine: practical approaches and pharmacologic rationale. Neurology 1993;43:S39.

76. Saper J. Headache Disorders: Current Concepts and Treatment Strategies. Littleton, MA: Wright-PSG Publishers, 1983

77. Ala-Hurula V et al. Systemic availability of ergotamine tartrate after oral, rectal and intramuscular administration. Eur J Clin Pharmacol 1979;15:51.

78. Krupp P, Haas G. Effects indesirables et interactions medicamenteuse des alcaloides de l'ergot de seigle. J Pharmacol 1979;10:401.

79. Raskin NH. Headache, 2nd Ed. New York: Churchill Livingstone, 1988

80. Andersen AR et al. The effect of ergotamine and dihydroergotamine on cerebral blood flow in man. Stroke 1987;18:120.

81. Edmeads J. Ergotamine and the cerebral circulation. Hemicrania 1976;7:6.

82. Blau JN et al. Ergotamine tartrate overdosage. Br Med J 1979;1:265.

83. Baumrucker JF. Drug interaction—propranolol and cafergot. N Engl J Med 1973;288:916.

84. Venter CP et al. Severe peripheral ischaemia during concomitant use of beta blockers and ergot alkaloids. Br Med J (Clin Res Ed) 1984;289:288.

85. Saper JR, Jones JM. Ergotamine tartrate dependency: features and possible mechanisms. Clin Neuropharmacol 1986;9:244.

86. Tokola RA. The effect of metoclopramide and prochlorperazine on the absorption of effervescent paracetamol in migraine. Cephalalgia 1988;8:139.

87. Tfelt-Hansen P, Johnson ES. Antiemetic and prokinetic drugs. In: Olesen J, ed. The Headaches. New York: Raven Press, 1993:343.

88. Tfelt-Hansen P et al. A double blind study of metoclopramide in the treatment of migraine attacks. J Neurol Neurosurg Psychiatry 1980;43:369.

89. Diamond S. Treatment of migraine with isometheptene, acetaminophen, and dichloralphenazone combination: a double-blind, crossover trial. Headache 1976;15:282.

90. Yuill GM et al. A double-blind crossover trial of isometheptene mucate compound and ergotamine in migraine. Br J Clin Pract 1972;26:76.

91. Freitag FG et al. Comparative study of a combination of isometheptene mucate, dichloralphenazone with acetaminophen and sumatriptan succinate in the treatment of migraine. Headache 2001;41:391.

92. Deleu D et al. Symptomatic and prophylactic treatment of migraine: a critical reappraisal. Clin Neuropharmacol 1998;21:267.

93. McNeely W, Goa KL. Diclofenac-potassium in migraine: a review. Drugs 1999;57:991.

94. Pradalier A et al. Acute migraine attack therapy: comparison of naproxen sodium and an ergotamine tartrate compound. Cephalalgia 1985;5:107.

95. Kangasniemi P, Kaaja R. Ketoprofen and ergotamine in acute migraine. J Intern Med 1992;231:551.

96. Volans GN. Migraine and drug absorption. Clin Pharmacokinet 1978;3:313.

97. Goldstein J. Ergot pharmacology and alternative delivery systems for ergotamine derivatives. Neurology 1992;42:45.

98. Ziegler D et al. Dihydroergotamine nasal spray for the acute treatment of migraine. Neurology 1994;44:447.

99. Efficacy, safety, and tolerability of dihydroergotamine nasal spray as monotherapy in the treatment of acute migraine. Dihydroergotamine Nasal Spray Multicenter Investigators. Headache 1995;35:177.

100. Gallagher RM. Acute treatment of migraine with dihydroergotamine nasal spray. Dihydroergotamine Working Group. Arch Neurol 1996;53:1285.

101. Hirt D. A comparison of DHE nasal spray and Cafegot in acute migraine [Abstract]. Cephalalgia 1989;9[Suppl 10]:410.

102. Klapper JA, Stanton J. Clinical experience with patient administered subcutaneous dihydroergotamine mesylate in refractory headaches. Headache 1992;32:21.

103. Saadah HA. Abortive headache therapy with intramuscular dihydroergotamine. Headache 1992;32:18.

104. Callaham M, Raskin N. A controlled study of dihydroergotamine in the treatment of acute migraine headache. Headache 1986;26:168.

105. Coppola M et al. Randomized, placebo-controlled evaluation of prochlorperazine versus metoclopramide for emergency department treatment of migraine headache. Ann Emerg Med 1995;26:541.

106. Seim MB et al. Intravenous ketorolac vs intravenous prochlorperazine for the treatment of migraine headaches. Acad Emerg Med 1998;5:573.

107. Tanen DA et al. Intravenous sodium valproate versus prochlorperazine for the emergency department treatment of acute migraine headaches: a prospective, randomized, double-blind trial. Ann Emerg Med 2003;41:847.

108. Lane PL et al. Comparative efficacy of chlorpromazine and meperidine with dimenhydrinate in migraine headache. Ann Emerg Med 1989;18:360.

109. McEwen JI et al. Treatment of migraine with intramuscular chlorpromazine. Ann Emerg Med 1987;16:758.

110. Lane PL, Ross R. Intravenous chlorpromazine—preliminary results in acute migraine. Headache 1985;25:302.

111. Belgrade MJ et al. Comparison of single-dose meperidine, butorphanol, and dihydroergotamine in the treatment of vascular headache. Neurology 1989;39:590.

112. Tek D, Mellon M. The effectiveness of nalbuphine and hydroxyzine for the emergency treatment of severe headache. Ann Emerg Med 1987;16:308.

113. Fisher MA, Glass S. Butorphanol (Stadol): a study in problems of current drug information and control. Neurology 1997;48:1156.

114. Rapoport AM, Silberstein SD. Emergency treatment of headache. Neurology 1992;42:43.

115. Silberstein SD, Freitag FG. Preventative treatment of migraine. Neurology 2003;60(Suppl 2):S38.

116. Ramadan NM et al. Evidence-based guidelines for migraine headache in the primary care setting: pharmacological management for prevention of migraine. www.aan.com 2000.

117. Tfelt-Hansen P. Prophylactic pharmacotherapy of migraine. Some practical guidelines. Neurol Clin 1997;15:153.

118. Holroyd KA et al. Propranolol in the management of recurrent migraine: a meta-analytic review. Headache 1991;31:333.

119. Weber RB, Reinmuth OM. The treatment of migraine with propranolol. Neurology 1972;22:366.

120. Wideroe TE, Vigander T. Propranolol in the treatment of migraine. Br Med J 1974;2:699.

121. Diamond S, Medina JL. Double blind study of propranolol for migraine prophylaxis. Headache 1976;16:24.

122. Forssman B et al. Propranolol for migraine prophylaxis. Headache 1976;16:238.

123. Stensrud P, Sjaastad O. Short-term clinical trial of phopranolol in racemic form (Inderal), D-propranolol and placebo in migraine. Acta Neurol Scand 1976;53:229.

124. Diamond S et al. Long-term study of propranolol in the treatment of migraine. Headache 1982;22:268.

125. Rosen JA. Observations on the efficacy of propranolol for the prophylaxis of migraine. Ann Neurol 1983;13:92.

126. Olesen J et al. Isoproterenol and propranolol: ability to cross the blood-brain barrier and effects on cerebral circulation in man. Stroke 1978;9:344.

127. Middlemiss D. Direct evidence for an interaction of beta-adrenergic blockers with the 5-HT receptor. Nature 1977;267:289.

128. Hiner BC et al. Antimigraine drug interactions with 5-hydroxytryptamine1A receptors. Ann Neurol 1986;19:511.

129. Lingjaerde O. Platelet uptake and storage of serotonin. In: Essman W, ed. Serotonin in Health and Disease. New York: Spectrum, 1977:139.

130. Olsson JE et al. Metoprolol and propranolol in migraine prophylaxis: a double-blind multicentre study. Acta Neurol Scand 1984;70:160.

131. Stensrud P, Sjaastad O. Comparative trial of Tenormin (atenolol) and Inderal (propranolol) in migraine. Headache 1980;20:204.

132. Forssman B et al. Atenolol for migraine prophylaxis. Headache 1983;23:188.

133. Sjaastad O, Stensrud P. Clinical trial of a beta-receptor blocking agent (LB 46) in migraine prophylaxis. Acta Neurol Scand 1972;48:124.

134. Nanda RN et al. A double blind trial of acebutolol for migraine prophylaxis. Headache 1978;18:20.

135. Ekbom K. Alprenolol for migraine prophylaxis. Headache 1975;15:129.

136. Ekbom K, Zetterman M. Oxprenolol in the treatment of migraine. Acta Neurol Scand 1977;56:181.

137. Curran DA, Lance JW. Clinical Trial of Methysergide and Other Preparations in the Management of Migraine. J Neurol Neurosurg Psychiatry 1964;27:463.

138. Graham JR et al. Inflammatory fibrosis associated with methysergide therapy. Res Clin Stud Headache 1967;1:123.

139. Curran DA et al. Methysergide. Res Clin Stud Headache 1967;1:74.

140. Caldara R et al. Effect of two antiserotoninergic drugs, methysergide and metergoline, on gastric acid secretion and gastrin release in healthy man. Eur J Clin Pharmacol 1980;17:13.

141. Ziegler DK et al. Migraine prophylaxis. A comparison of propranolol and amitriptyline. Arch Neurol 1987;44:486.

142. Couch JR, Hassanein RS. Amitriptyline in migraine prophylaxis. Arch Neurol 1979;36:695.

143. Couch JR et al. Amitriptyline in the prophylaxis of migraine. Effectiveness and relationship of antimigraine and antidepressant effects. Neurology 1976;26:121.

144. Pringsheim T et al. Selective decrease in serotonin synthesis rate in rat brainstem raphe nuclei following chronic administration of low doses of amitriptyline: an effect compatible with an antimigraine effect. Cephalalgia 2003;23:367.

145. Langohr HD et al. Clomipramine and metoprolol in migraine prophylaxis—a double-blind crossover study. Headache 1985;25:107.

146. Heninger G, Charney D. Mechanism of action of antidepressant treatments: implications for the etiology and treatment of depressive disorders. In: Meltzer H, ed. Psychopharmacology: The Third Generation of Progress. New York: Raven Press, 1987:535.

147. Adly C et al. Fluoxetine prophylaxis of migraine. Headache 1992;32:101.

148. Saper JR et al. Double-blind trial of fluoxetine: chronic daily headache and migraine. Headache 1994;34:497.

149. Bank J. A comparative study of amitriptyline and fluvoxamine in migraine prophylaxis. Headache 1994;34:476.

150. Hering R, Kuritzky A. Sodium valproate in the prophylactic treatment of migraine: a double-blind study versus placebo. Cephalalgia 1992;12:81.

151. Mathew NT et al. Migraine prophylaxis with divalproex. Arch Neurol 1995;52:281.

152. Kaniecki RG. A comparison of divalproex with propranolol and placebo for the prophylaxis of migraine without aura. Arch Neurol 1997;54:1141.

153. Lindegaard KF et al. Naproxen in the prevention of migraine attacks. A double-blind placebo-controlled cross-over study. Headache 1980;20:96.

154. Bellavance AJ, Meloche JP. A comparative study of naproxen sodium, pizotyline and placebo in migraine prophylaxis. Headache 1990;30:710.

155. Sances G et al. Naproxen sodium in menstrual migraine prophylaxis: a double-blind placebo controlled study. Headache 1990;30:705.

156. Stensrud P, Sjaastad O. Clinical trial of a new anti-bradykinin, anti-inflammatory drug, ketoprofen (19.583 r.p.) in migraine prophylaxis. Headache 1974;14:96.

157. Solomon GD, Kunkel RS. Flurbiprofen in the prophylaxis of migraine. Cleve Clin J Med 1993;60:43.

158. Johnson RH et al. Comparison of mefenamic acid and propranolol with placebo in migraine prophylaxis. Acta Neurol Scand 1986;73:490.

159. Sargent J et al. A comparison of naproxen sodium to propranolol hydrochloride and a placebo control for the prophylaxis of migraine headache. Headache 1985;25:320.

160. Reuter H. Calcium channel modulation by neurotransmitters, enzymes and drugs. Nature 1983;301:569.

161. Markley HG et al. Verapamil in prophylactic therapy of migraine. Neurology 1984;34:973.

162. Solomon GD et al. Verapamil prophylaxis of migraine. A double-blind, placebo-controlled study. JAMA 1983;250:2500.

163. Solomon GD. Comparative efficacy of calcium antagonist drugs in the prophylaxis of migraine. Headache 1985;25:368.

164. Meyer JS et al. Migraine and cluster headache treatment with calcium antagonists supports a vascular pathogenesis. Headache 1985;25:358.

165. Meyer JS, Hardenberg J. Clinical effectiveness of calcium entry blockers in prophylactic treatment of migraine and cluster headaches. Headache 1983;23:266.

166. Smith R, Schwartz A. Diltiazem prophylaxis in refractory migraine. N Engl J Med 1984;310:1327.

167. McArthur JC et al. Nifedipine in the prophylaxis of classic migraine: a crossover, double-masked, placebo-controlled study of headache frequency and side effects. Neurology 1989;39:284.

168. Riopelle R, McCans J. A pilot study of the calcium antagonist diltiazem in migraine syndrome prophylaxis. J Can Sci Neurol 1982;9:269.

169. Flaim S. Comparative pharmacology of calcium blockers based on studies of vascular smooth muscle. In: Flaim S, Zelig R, eds. Calcium Blockers: Mechanism of Action and Clinical Applications. Baltimore: Urban & Schwarzenberg, 1982:155.

170. Havanka-Kanniainen H et al. Efficacy of nimodipine in the prophylaxis of migraine. Cephalalgia 1985;5:39.

171. Gelmers HJ. Nimodipine, a new calcium antagonist, in the prophylactic treatment of migraine. Headache 1983;23:106.

172. Stewart DJ et al. Effect of prophylactic administration of nimodipine in patients with migraine. Headache 1988;28:260.

173. Ansell E et al. Nimodipine in migraine prophylaxis. Cephalalgia 1988;8:269.

174. Stensrud P, Sjaastad O. Clonidine (Catapresan)-double-blind study after long-term treatment with the drug in migraine. Acta Neurol Scand 1976; 53:233.

175. Vogler BK et al. Feverfew as a preventive treatment for migraine: a systematic review. Cephalalgia 1998;18:704.

176. Anthony M, Lance JW. Monoamine oxidase inhibition in the treatment of migraine. Arch Neurol 1969;21:263.

177. Schoenen J et al. Effectiveness of high-dose riboflavin in migraine prophylaxis. A randomized controlled trial. Neurology 1998;50:466.

178. Beecher HK. The powerful placebo. J Am Med Assoc 1955;159:1602.

179. Couch JR et al. The long-term effect of placebo on migraine [Abstract]. Neurology 1987;27(Suppl 1):238.

180. Sandrini G et al. An epidemiological approach to the nosography of chronic daily headache. Cephalalgia 1993;13(Suppl 12):72.

181. Martignoni E, Solomon S. The complex chronic headache: mixed headache and drug overuse. In: Olesen J et al, eds. The Headaches. New York: Raven Press, 1993:849.

182. Srikiatkhachorn A, Anthony M. Serotonin receptor adaptation in patients with analgesic-induced headache. Cephalalgia 1996;16:419.

183. Sandler DP et al. Analgesic use and chronic renal disease. N Engl J Med 1989;320:1238.

184. McGoldrick MD, Bailie GR. Nonnarcotic analgesics: prevalence and estimated economic impact of toxicities. Ann Pharmacother 1997;31:221.

185. Tolman KG. Hepatotoxicity of non-narcotic analgesics. Am J Med 1998;105:13S.

186. Hering R, Steiner TJ. Abrupt outpatient withdrawal of medication in analgesic-abusing migraineurs. Lancet 1991;337:1442.

187. Ekbom K, Hardebo JE. Cluster headache: aetiology, diagnosis and management. Drugs 2002; 62:61.

188. Ekbom K. A clinical comparison of cluster headache and migraine. Acta Neurol Scand 1970:Suppl 41:1.

189. Mathew NT. Cluster headache. Neurology 1992; 42:22.

190. Sakai F, Meyer JS. Regional cerebral hemodynamics during migraine and cluster headaches measured by the 133Xe inhalation method. Headache 1978;18:122.

191. Sakai F, Meyer JS. Abnormal cerebrovascular reactivity in patients with migraine and cluster headache. Headache 1979;19:257.

192. Krabbe AA et al. Tomographic determination of cerebral blood flow during attacks of cluster headache. Cephalalgia 1984;4:17.

193. Drummond PD, Lance JW. Thermographic changes in cluster headache. Neurology 1984;34:1292.

194. Mendizabal JE et al. Cluster headache: Horton's cephalalgia revisited. South Med J 1998;91:606.

195. Buzzi M et al. Morphological effects of electrical trigeminal ganglion stimulation on intra and extracranial vessels [Abstract]. Soc Neurosci 1990;16:591.

196. Sjaastad O et al. Cluster headache in identical twins. Headache 1993;33:214.

197. Russell MB et al. Familial occurrence of cluster headache. J Neurol Neurosurg Psychiatry 1995;58:341.

198. May A, Leone M. Update on cluster headache. Curr Opin Neurol 2003;16:333.

199. Manzoni GC et al. Lithium carbonate in cluster headache: assessment of its short- and long-term therapeutic efficacy. Cephalalgia 1983;3:109.

200. Riess CM et al. Episodic cluster headache in a community: clinical features and treatment. Can J Neurol Sci 1998;25:141.

201. Ekbom K, Sakai F. Tension-type headache, cluster headache and miscellaneous headaches; management. In: Olesen J, ed. The Headaches. New York: Raven Press, 1993:591.

202. Hardebo JE, Dahlof C. Sumatriptan nasal spray (20 mg/dose) in the acute treatment of cluster headache. Cephalalgia 1998;18:487.

203. Monstad I et al. Preemptive oral treatment with sumatriptan during a cluster period. Headache 1995;35:607.

204. Fogan L. Treatment of cluster headache. A double-blind comparison of oxygen v air inhalation. Arch Neurol 1985;42:362.

205. Kudrow L. Response of cluster headache attacks to oxygen inhalation. Headache 1981;21:1.

206. Ekbom K et al. Optimal routes of administration of ergotamine tartrate in cluster headache patients. A pharmacokinetic study. Cephalalgia 1983;3:15.

207. Kudrow L. Cluster Headache: Mechanisms and Management. Oxford: Oxford University Press, 1980.

208. Graham JR et al. Aerosol ergotamine tartrate for migraine and Horton's syndrome. N Engl J Med 1960;263:802.

209. Marks DR et al. A double-blind placebo-controlled trial of intranasal capsaicin for cluster headache. Cephalalgia 1993;13:114.

210. Sicuteri F et al. Pain relief by somatostatin in attacks of cluster headache. Pain 1984;18:359.

211. Kittrelle JP et al. Cluster headache. Local anesthetic abortive agents. Arch Neurol 1985;42:496.

212. Barre F. Cocaine as an abortive agent in cluster headache. Headache 1982;22:69.

213. de Carolis P et al. Nimodipine in episodic cluster headache: results and methodological considerations. Headache 1987;27:397.

214. Meyer JS et al. Clinical and hemodynamic effects during treatment of vascular headaches with verapamil. Headache 1984;24:313.

215. Couch JR, Jr., Ziegler DK. Prednisone therapy for cluster headache. Headache 1978;18:219.

216. Kudrow L. Comparative results of prednisone, methysergide, and lithium therapy in cluster headache. In: Greene R, ed. Current Concepts in Migraine Research. New York: Raven Press, 1978:159.

217. Damasio H, Lyon L. Lithium carbonate in the treatment of cluster headaches. J Neurol 1980; 224:1.

218. Ekbom K. Lithium for cluster headache: review of the literature and preliminary results of long-term treatment. Headache 1981;21:132.

219. Savoldi F et al. Lithium salts in cluster headache treatment. Cephalalgia 1983;3(Suppl 1):79.

220. Hering R, Kuritzky A. Sodium valproate in the treatment of cluster headache: an open clinical trial. Cephalalgia 1989;9:195.

221. Leone M et al. Melatonin versus placebo in the prophylaxis of cluster headache: a double-blind pilot study with parallel groups. Cephalalgia 1996;16:494.

222. Rasmussen BK et al. Epidemiology of headache in a general population—a prevalence study. J Clin Epidemiol 1991;44:1147.

223. Schwartz BS et al. Epidemiology of tension-type headache. JAMA 1998;279:381.

224. Silberstein SD. Tension-type and chronic daily headache. Neurology 1993;43:1644.

225. Lance JW, Curran DA. Treatment of chronic tension headache. Lancet 1964;42:1236.

226. Tunis MM, Wolff HG. Studies on headache; cranial artery vasoconstriction and muscle contraction headache. AMA Arch Neurol Psychiatry 1954;71:425.

227. Langemark M et al. Temporal muscle blood flow in chronic tension-type headache. Arch Neurol 1990;47:654.

228. Kolb LC. Psychiatric aspects of the treatment of headache. Neurology 1963;2:34.

229. Holm JE et al. The role of stress in recurrent tension headache. Headache 1986;26:160.

230. Peters BH et al. Comparison of 650 mg aspirin and 1,000 mg acetaminophen with each other, and with placebo in moderately severe headache. Am J Med 1983;74:36.

231. Diamond S. Ibuprofen versus aspirin and placebo in the treatment of muscle contraction headache. Headache 1983;23:206.

232. Schachtel BP et al. Nonprescription ibuprofen and acetaminophen in the treatment of tension-type headache. J Clin Pharmacol 1996;36:1120.

233. Gawel MJ et al. Evaluation of analgesic agents in recurring headache compared with other clinical pain models. Clin Pharmacol Ther 1990;47:504.

234. Friedman AP. The treatment of chronic headache with meprobamate. Ann N Y Acad Sci 1957; 67:822.

235. Weber MB. The treatment of muscle contraction headaches with diazepam. Curr Ther Res Clin Exp 1973;15:210.

236. Jay GW et al. The effectiveness of physical therapy in the treatment of chronic daily headaches. Headache 1989;29:156.

237. Hansen PE, Hansen JH. Acupuncture treatment of chronic tension headache—a controlled crossover trial. Cephalalgia 1985;5:137.

238. Nuechterlein KH, Holroyd JC. Biofeedback in the treatment of tension headache. Current status. Arch Gen Psychiatry 1980;37:866.

239. Bakal DA, Kaganov JA. Muscle contraction and migraine headache: psychophysiologic comparison. Headache 1977;17:208.

240. Andrasik F, Holroyd KA. Specific and nonspecific effects in the biofeedback treatment of tension headache: 3-year follow-up. J Consult Clin Psychol 1983;51:634.

241. Solbach P et al. An analysis of home practice patterns for non-drug headache treatments. Headache 1989;29:528.

242. Bove G, Nilsson N. Spinal manipulation in the treatment of episodic tension-type headache: a randomized controlled trial. JAMA 1998;280: 1576.

243. Black RG. The chronic pain syndrome. Surg Clin North Am 1975;55:999.

244. Jensen R, Olesen J. Tension-type headache: an update on mechanisms and treatment. Curr Opin Neurol 2000;13:285.

245. Diamond S, Baltes BJ. Chronic tension headache—treated with amitriptyline—a double-blind study. Headache 1971;11:110.

246. Morland TJ et al. Doxepin in the prophylactic treatment of mixed 'vascular' and tension headache. Headache 1979;19:382.

247. Fogelholm R, Murros K. Maprotiline in chronic tension headache: a double-blind cross-over study. Headache 1985;25:273.

248. Diamond S. Management of headaches. Focus on new strategies. Postgrad Med 1990;87:189.

249. Diamond S, Freitag FG. The use of fluoxetine in the treatment of headache. Clin J Pain 1989;5:200.

250. Bendtsen L et al. A non-selective (amitriptyline), but not a selective (citalopram), serotonin reuptake inhibitor is effective in the prophylactic treatment of chronic tension-type headache. J Neurol Neurosurg Psychiatry 1996;61:285.

CHAPTER 53

Parkinson's Disease

Michael E. Ernst, Mildred D. Gottwald, Barry E. Gidal

Incidence, Prevalence, and Epidemiology

Parkinson's disease (PD), like epilepsy and migraine headache, is a neurologic disorder in which drug therapy plays a central role. PD is a chronic, progressive disorder of motor function primarily of middle to late life. Although first described as the "shaking palsy" by James Parkinson in 1817, it was not until recently that major breakthroughs in understanding the disorder's neurochemistry and pathophysiology have led to more effective drug therapies.[1] Most cases of PD are of unknown cause, referred to as idiopathic parkinsonism; however, a parkinsonian syndrome has been associated with viral encephalitis, neurotoxins, and neuroleptic drugs.[1] In addition, other neurologic disorders such as benign essential tremor and progressive supranuclear palsy have symptoms similar to PD as part of their clinical presentation. Unless otherwise stated, all references to PD in this chapter refer to the idiopathic type.

The age at onset of PD is variable, usually between 50 and 80 years.[2,3] In a retrospective study of 802 patients, a mean age at onset of 55 years was noted; in two thirds of patients the disease began between the ages of 50 to 69 years. Men and women are affected equally.[2,3] The prevalence of PD is about 100 cases per 100,000 population, and the incidence is estimated at 20 cases per 100,000 people annually.[3,4] An estimated 1 million Americans, or 1% of the population age >65, have PD.[3] Although the progression of the disease is highly variable, the symptoms of PD may progress over time such that within 10 to 20 years total immobility can result despite drug treatment.[5,6] The patient's age at the time of onset of clinically recognizable disease may significantly influence the rate of disease progression. A more rapid rate of progression has been observed in elderly patients and may be associated with a greater degree of motor disability. Since the introduction of levodopa, mortality rates for patients with PD have decreased, approaching those of the general population.[3,7] Mortality data derived from the DATATOP trial demonstrate an overall death rate of 17.1% over the 8-year observation period (2.1% per year), a rate somewhat lower than that expected for U.S. age-matched control subjects.[8] Death usually is not caused by the disease itself, but rather by complications related to immobility (e.g., aspiration pneumonia, cardiovascular and cerebrovascular disease).[2,6]

Several organizations provide services for persons with PD and their families. Valuable information in the form of

Internet monographs, books, newsletters, videos, and audiotapes in addition to information about local support groups is available from the organizations listed in Table 53-1.

Etiology

Many theories have been advanced regarding the origin of PD. Environmental factors and genetic predisposition have been discussed most frequently. Environmental factors have been implicated since it was discovered that many patients developed a parkinsonian syndrome following the epidemic of encephalitis lethargica in the United States between 1919 and the early 1930s.[1] Attempts to isolate a virus as a causative agent of the disease have been unsuccessful. Renewed interest in environmental factors resurfaced with the discovery that ingestion of a meperidine analog, 1-methyl-4-phenyl-1,2,3,6-tetrahydropyridine (MPTP), causes irreversible parkinsonism.[9] It also is now recognized that the byproducts of dopamine metabolism (e.g., hydrogen peroxide) can lead to the production of free radicals that cause peroxidation of cell membranes and ultimately cell death. Thus, the most attractive hypothesis at present is that exposure to an environmental contaminant resembling MPTP (or possibly MPTP itself) superimposed on the normal loss of nigrostriatal dopamine, which occurs with the aging process, may result in the clinical manifestations of PD.[10,11]

Table 53-1 Service Organizations for Patients with Parkinson's Disease

American Parkinson Disease Association, Inc.
1250 Hylan Boulevard, Suite 4B
Staten Island, NY 10305
1-800-223-2732
Website: http://www.apdaparkinson.com

National Parkinson Foundation, Inc.
1501 NW Ninth Avenue NW, Bob Hope Road
Miami, FL 33136-1494
1-800-327-4545
Website: http://www.parkinson.org

The Parkinson's Disease Foundation
William Black Medical Building
710 West 158 Street
New York, NY 10032
1-800-457-6676
Website: http://www.pdf.org

Parkinson's Action Network
300 North Lee Street
Alexandria, VA 22314
1-800-850-4726
Website: http://www.parkinsonaction.org

WE MOVE
204 West 84th Street
New York, NY 10024
1-800-437-6682
Website: http://www.wemove.org

The issue of genetic predisposition as a risk factor for PD is controversial. Although studies of identical twins have shown a low concordance rate for acquiring the disease,[12] recent studies have refueled the interest in a genetic predisposition. Researchers have isolated a gene for a rare autosomal dominant familial form of PD caused by a mutation of the α-synuclein gene.[13,14] Demographic studies have also suggested that a racial link may be involved, because a higher incidence of the disease has been found in North America and Europe compared with China or Japan.[15] In addition, a deficit in the mitochondrial respiratory chain, as evidenced by decreased complex I activity in the parkinsonian brain, has been identified and is being actively pursued as a primary mechanism for increased neuronal vulnerability.[16]

Pathophysiology

PD is a disorder of the extrapyramidal system of the brain involving the basal ganglia.[17-19] The extrapyramidal system is involved with maintaining posture and muscle tone and with regulating voluntary smooth motor activity. For reasons not understood, melanin-containing cells within the substantia nigra are lost in PD.[17] The pigmented neurons within the substantia nigra have dopaminergic fibers that project into the neostriatum and globus pallidus. Together, the substantia nigra, neostriatum, and globus pallidus make up the basal ganglia. In PD, dopamine (the inhibitory neurotransmitter) is progressively lost in the nigrostriatal tracts, and acetylcholine (the excitatory neurotransmitter) is relatively increased.[17-19]

The pathologic hallmark of PD is Lewy bodies, or intraneuronal inclusion bodies within the dopaminergic cells of the substantia nigra.[4,6] It is generally believed that a 70% to 80% loss of nigral neurons must occur before PD becomes clinically recognizable.[20] Current evidence suggests that a substantial preclinical or latent phase of PD exists (approximately 5 to 20 years) before this critical threshold of nigral cell loss occurs.[21,22] The imbalance between dopamine and acetylcholine is primarily responsible for the manifestations of the disease, and drug therapy is directed toward correcting this imbalance.[23,24]

Overview of Drug Therapy

Since the salient pathophysiologic feature of PD is the progressive loss of dopamine from the nigrostriatal tracts in the brain, drug therapy for the disease is aimed primarily at replenishing the supply of dopamine. This is accomplished through one, or a combination, of the following methods: (1) administering exogenous dopamine in the form of a precursor, levodopa; (2) stimulating dopamine receptors within the corpus striatum through the use of dopamine agonists (e.g., pramipexole, ropinirole); or (3) inhibiting the major metabolic pathways within the brain that are responsible for the degradation of levodopa and its metabolites. This latter effect is achieved through the use of aromatic L-amino acid decarboxylase inhibitors (e.g., carbidopa) and/or catechol-O-methyltransferase-inhibitors (e.g., entacapone). Additional therapies designed to provide neuroprotection (e.g., selegiline) or counterbalance the negative effects of the relative increase in acetylcholine activity (e.g., use of anticholinergics to treat Parkinson's-associated tremor) are also occasionally employed.

In many instances, the limitations of the medications used to treat PD lead to additional problems that make treatment of the disease quite difficult. Many PD sufferers experience response fluctuations described as an "on-off" effect, where mobility ranges from a fluid and unencumbered state to "freezing," or almost complete immobility. These changes can be abrupt, similar to the turning of a switch, and can last from several minutes to hours. A second common motor complication associated with drug therapy is the "wearing off" or "end-of-dose deterioration" effect. This refers to a transition from mobility to immobility that occurs near the end of the levodopa dosing interval and is related to the short half-life of the drug (approximately 1.5 hours). Unfortunately, attempts to adjust the frequency of dosing or strength of dopaminergic medications to increase the "on" time and/or reduce the "wearing off" effects often result in an overstimulation of dopamine receptors, leading to dyskinesias and other uncontrollable choreiform movements.

PD is a debilitating disease that affects both physical and mental functions of the body. Despite our best treatment efforts to restore dopaminergic function and preserve dopamine production, the disease will invariably progress. Therefore, supportive drug treatment of the complications of the disease is also necessary. These complications include neuropsychiatric problems (cognitive impairment and dementia, hallucinations and delirium, depression, agitation, anxiety), autonomic dysfunction (constipation, urinary problems, sexual problems, orthostasis, thermoregulatory imbalances), falls, and sleep disorders (insomnia/sleep fragmentation, nightmares, restless leg syndrome).

CLINICAL PRESENTATION

1. **L.M., a 55-year-old, right-handed male artist, presents to the neurology clinic complaining of difficulty painting because of unsteadiness in his right hand. He also complains of increasing difficulty getting out of chairs and tightness in his arms and legs. His wife claims that he has become more "forgetful" lately, and L.M. admits that his memory does not seem to be as sharp. His past medical history is significant for depression for the past year, gout (currently requiring no treatment), constipation, and benign prostatic hypertrophy. On physical examination, L.M. is noted to be a well-developed, well-nourished man who displays a notable lack of normal changes in facial expression and speaks in a soft, monotone voice. A strong body odor is noted. Examination of his extremities reveals a slight "ratchet-like" rigidity in both arms and legs, and a mild resting tremor is present in his right hand. His gait is slow but otherwise normal, with a slightly bent posture. His balance is determined to be normal, with no retropulsion or loss of righting reflexes after physical threat. His genitourinary examination is remarkable only for prostatic enlargement. The remainder of L.M.'s physical examination and laboratory studies are within normal limits. What signs and symptoms suggestive of PD are present in L.M.? Which of these symptoms are among the classic symptoms for diagnosing PD and which are considered "associated" symptoms? How can the associated symptoms of PD be managed in L.M.?**

Establishing the diagnosis of PD is based entirely on clinical symptoms.[25-27] The four classic features of PD—tremor, rigidity, bradykinesia, and postural disturbances—are easily recognized. Tremor, which is most often the first symptom observed, is usually unilateral on initial presentation. Frequently,

the tremor is of a "pill-rolling" type involving the thumb and index finger, is present at rest, worsens under fatigue or stress, and is absent with purposeful movement or when asleep.[2,26,27] Muscular rigidity resulting from increased muscle tone often manifests as a "cogwheel" or "ratchet" (catch-release) type of motion when an extremity is moved passively. It is caused by the action of opposing muscle groups.[2,26,27] Bradykinesia, or a poverty of spontaneous movements, often is evidenced by a "masked facies," or blank stare and is associated with reduced eye blinking.[2,26,27] As the disease progresses, difficulty initiating and terminating steps results in a hurried or festinating gait; the posture becomes stooped (simian posture), and postural reflexes are impaired.[2,26,27] Symptoms that were unilateral on initial presentation often become bilateral and more severe as the disease progresses.[6,28] Although unilateral tremor (frequently on the right side) is one of the most common initial presenting symptoms, approximately 30% of patients with idiopathic PD do not present with tremor.[28] Therefore, all four symptoms do not need to be present to make the diagnosis of PD.[27,28]

Drugs with strong antidopaminergic activity (e.g., neuroleptics, prochlorperazine, and metoclopramide) may cause a state of drug-induced parkinsonism that mimics idiopathic PD. It is important to rule out these drugs as a cause of symptoms before the diagnosis of PD is established. To confirm the diagnosis of PD, a therapeutic trial of levodopa may be employed. A resulting improvement in motor and/or cognitive function in response to levodopa therapy suggests the diagnosis of idiopathic PD. However, patients with the tremor-predominant form of the disease may not respond to levodopa, especially in the early stages of the disease.[28] Furthermore, some experts recommend against using the "levodopa challenge test" (administration of levodopa to aid in diagnosis) because animal studies suggest that even single doses of levodopa may prime the basal ganglia for the subsequent development of dyskinesia.[28]

L.M. presents with many of the classic symptoms of PD. A noticeable unilateral resting tremor is present along with decreased manual dexterity, as evidenced by his difficulty handling a paintbrush. Rigidity ("ratcheting" of the arms), bradykinesia (slowness of movement), and a mask-like facial expression also are present. Although he has a partially stooped posture, it is difficult to attribute this entirely to the disease because postural changes commonly occur with advancing age, and on physical examination his balance was normal.[27] Because his symptoms are causing functional impairment, L.M. will require treatment with an antiparkinsonian medication to alleviate his symptoms of bradykinesia and rigidity.

Numerous features are associated with parkinsonism. Handwriting abnormalities occur frequently, particularly micrographia, a symptom of bradykinesia.[2,26,27] Because L.M. is an artist, this abnormality would be particularly troublesome. He also is showing signs of autonomic nervous system dysfunction, such as drooling (sialorrhea), seborrhea, and constipation, all of which can be particularly embarrassing to the patient. Drooling also may be a consequence of impaired swallowing.[28] The foul body odor exhibited by L.M. could be ascribed to excess sebum production. L.M.'s seborrhea may be treated with coal tar or selenium-based shampoos twice weekly, topical hydrocortisone, or topical ketoconazole.[28]

His constipation should be managed first by evaluating his diet and exercise level, by stopping all medications such as anticholinergics (including over-the-counter cold and sleep medications) that may exacerbate constipation, and by trying a stool softener such as sodium or calcium docusate. In the past, cisapride, a prokinetic agent, was tried, but this agent is no longer available.[29] In more severe cases, lactulose, mild laxatives, or enemas may be required.

L.M. should also be evaluated for other manifestations of dysautonomia, including urinary problems, increased sweating, orthostatic hypotension, erectile dysfunction, pain or dysesthesias, and problems swallowing. L.M. has benign prostatic hypertrophy; therefore, a urologic workup may be necessary. He also should be counseled to avoid anticholinergic agents that may exacerbate this problem. Anticholinergic agents also should not be used to treat his hypersalivation, but he should be referred to a speech and swallowing expert because dysphagia may result in impaired absorption and lead to aspiration.[28,30] A soft diet may be indicated. L.M.'s soft, mumbled, or monotone voice is also consistent with the disease and is often one of the first symptoms noted.[2,30] Speech therapy is often beneficial for managing this problem.

Psychiatric disturbances such as nervousness, anxiety, and depression also may occur.[28,31] L.M. has a history of depression that could be attributable to PD. Finally, the prevalence of cognitive decline and dementia among parkinsonian patients ranges from 10% to 30% and may be associated with a more rapid progression of disease-related disability. Many neurologists consider dementia part of the clinical syndrome of PD in a small subgroup of patients.[28,32] The development of hallucinations in Parkinson's patients with dementia is a poor prognostic sign.[33] The "forgetfulness" and decreased memory described by L.M. could be early signs of dementia and warrant close observation.

Staging of Parkinson's Disease

2. **What are the stages of PD? In what stage of the disease is L.M.?**

The symptomatology and progression of symptoms among parkinsonian patients is tremendously variable. To assess the degree of disability and determine the rate of disease progression relative to treatment, various scales have been developed.

The most common of these is the Hoehn and Yahr scale (Table 53-2).[2] In general, patients in stages I and II of PD have mild disease that does not interfere with activities of daily living or work and usually requires minimal or no treatment. In stage III disease, daily activities are restricted and employment may be significantly affected unless effective treatment is initiated. These patients are usually managed with low doses of dopamine agonists or levodopa/carbidopa (Table 53-3). With further disease progression, patients already receiving levodopa/carbidopa may benefit from the addition of a dopamine agonist or a catechol-O-methyltransferase (COMT) inhibitor if not already added. For patients receiving a dopamine agonist as their initial therapy, levodopa/carbidopa may be added, followed by the addition of a COMT inhibitor if symptoms persist.[28,34]

In choosing when to treat the symptoms of PD and which therapy to use, care must be exercised not to generalize, but rather to approach each patient individually. Although no consensus has been reached about when to initiate symptomatic treatment, most health care professionals agree that treatment should begin when the patient begins to experience functional impairment as defined by (1) employment status; (2) whether the dominant side is affected; and (3) bradykinesia or rigidity. Individual patient preferences also should be considered. For example, a neurosurgeon's practice may be severely impaired

Table 53-2 Staging of Disability in Parkinson's Disease

Stage I	Unilateral involvement only; minimal or no functional impairment
Stage II	Bilateral involvement, without impairment of balance
Stage III	Evidence of postural imbalance; some restriction in activities; capable of leading independent life; mild to moderate disability
Stage IV	Severely disabled, cannot walk and stand unassisted; significantly incapacitated
Stage V	Restricted to bed or wheelchair unless aided

From reference 2.

Table 53-3 Medications Used for the Treatment of Parkinson's Disease

Generic (Trade) Name	Dosage Unit	Titration Schedule	Usual Daily Dose	Adverse Effects
Amantadine (Symmetrel)	100-mg capsule Liquid: 50 mg/5 mL	100 mg QD; increased by 100 mg 1–2 wk	100–300 mg	Orthostatic hypotension, insomnia, depression, hallucinations, livedo reticularis, xerostomia
Anticholinergic Agents				
Benztropine (Cogentin)	0.5-, 1-, and 2-mg tablets Injection: 2 mL (1 mg/mL)	0.5 mg/day increased by 0.5 mg Q 3–5 days	1–3 mg QD to BID	Constipation, xerostomia, dry skin, dysphagia, confusion, memory impairment
Procyclidine (Kemadrin)	5-mg tablet	0.75 mg TID increased by 2.5 mg Q 3–4 days up to 20 mg	2.5–5 mg TID to QID	Constipation, xerostomia, dry skin, dysphagia, confusion, memory impairment
Trihexyphenidyl (Artane)	2- and 5-mg tablets Liquid: 2 mg/5 mL	1–2 mg/day increased by 1–2 mg Q 3–5 days	6–15 mg divided TID to BID	Constipation, xerostomia, dry skin, dysphagia, confusion, memory impairment

Table 53-3 Medications Used for the Treatment of Parkinson's Disease—cont'd

Generic (Trade) Name	Dosage Unit	Titration Schedule	Usual Daily Dose	Adverse Effects
Antihistamines				
Diphenhydramine (Benadryl)	25-, 50-mg capsules Liquid: 12.5 mg/5 mL Injection: 50 mg/mL 100-mg tablet	As tolerated up to 50 mg QID	25–50 mg TID to QID	Slight to moderate drowsiness; thickening of bronchial secretions; changes in appetite; headache, xerostomia
Orphenadrine (Norflex)	Injection: 30 mg/mL	As tolerated up to 100 mg BID	Oral: 100 mg BID Injection: 60 mg Q 12 hr	Drowsiness, blurred vision, rash, nausea, vomiting, decreased urination, facial flushing, tachycardia
Dopamine Replacement				
Carbidopa-Levodopa (Regular) (Sinemet)	10/100, 25/100, and 25/200 tablets	25/100 BID, increased by 25/100 weekly to effect and as tolerated	30/300 to 150/ 1,500 divided TID to QID	Nausea, orthostatic hypotension, confusion, dizziness, hallucinations, dyskinesias, blepharospasm
Carbidopa-Levodopa (CR) (Sinemet CR)	25/100 and 50/200 tablets	25/100 BID (spaced at least 6 hr apart), increased Q 3–7 days	50/200 to 500/ 2,000 divided QID	Same as regular Sinemet
Dopamine Agonists				
Bromocriptine (Parlodel)	2.5-mg tablet, 5-mg capsule	1.25 HS, titrate slowly as tolerated over 4–6 weeks	10–40 mg divided TID	Orthostatic hypotension, confusion, dizziness, hallucinations, nausea, leg cramps
Pergolide (Permax)	0.05-, 0.25-, and 1-mg tablets	0.05 mg HS titrate slowly as tolerated over 4–6 weeks	1–4 mg divided TID	Orthostatic hypotension, confusion, dizziness, hallucinations, nausea, leg cramps
Pramipexole (Mirapex)	0.125-, 0.25-, 0.50-, 1-, 1.5-mg tablets	0.375 divided TID; titrate weekly by 0.125–0.25 mg/dose	1.5–4.5 mg divided TID	Orthostatic hypotension, confusion, dizziness, hallucinations, nausea, somnolence
Ropinirole (Requip)	0.25-, 0.5-, 1-, 2-, 4-, 5-mg tablet	Titrate weekly by 0.25 mg/dose	3–12 mg divided TID	Orthostatic hypotension, confusion, dizziness, hallucinations, nausea, somnolence
COMT Inhibitors				
Entacapone (Comtan)	200-mg tablet	One tablet with each administration of levodopa/ carbidopa, up to 8 tablets daily	3–8 tablets daily	Diarrhea, dyskinesias, abdominal pain, urine discoloration
Tolcapone (Tasmar)	100-, 200-mg tablet	100–200 mg TID	300–600 mg divided TID	Diarrhea, dyskinesias, abdominal pain, urine discoloration, hepatotoxicity
MAO-B Inhibitor				
Selegiline (Eldepryl)	5-mg tablet, capsule	5 mg am; may increase to 5 mg BID	5–10 mg (take 5 mg with breakfast and 5 mg with lunch)	Insomnia, dizziness, nausea, vomiting, xerostomia, dyskinesias, mood changes

COMT, catechol-O-methyltransferase.

by even a mild tremor, and early treatment may be beneficial. Judging by the symptoms L.M. is displaying, he would likely benefit from immediate treatment. His symptoms are unilateral but are occurring on his dominant side and are interfering with his ability to paint, thus affecting his livelihood. He is also showing signs of rigidity and bradykinesia but can otherwise live independently.

With advanced-stage disease (III to IV), most patients require levodopa therapy (with a peripheral decarboxylase inhibitor such as carbidopa [Sinemet]) and often in combination with a COMT inhibitor such as entacapone or a dopamine agonist such as bromocriptine (Parlodel), pergolide (Permax), pramipexole (Mirapex), or ropinirole (Requip). In some cases, selegiline (Eldepryl) or amantadine may provide further symptomatic relief. Patients with end-stage disease (stage V) are severely incapacitated and, because of extended disease progression, often do not respond well to drug therapy.

TREATMENT

An algorithm for the management of patients with PD is presented in Figure 53-1. No cure is known for PD; therefore, treatment is symptomatic only. The long-term, individualized treatment plan is usually characterized by frequent dosage adjustments over time because of the chronic and progressive nature of this disease. Although most of this chapter is de-

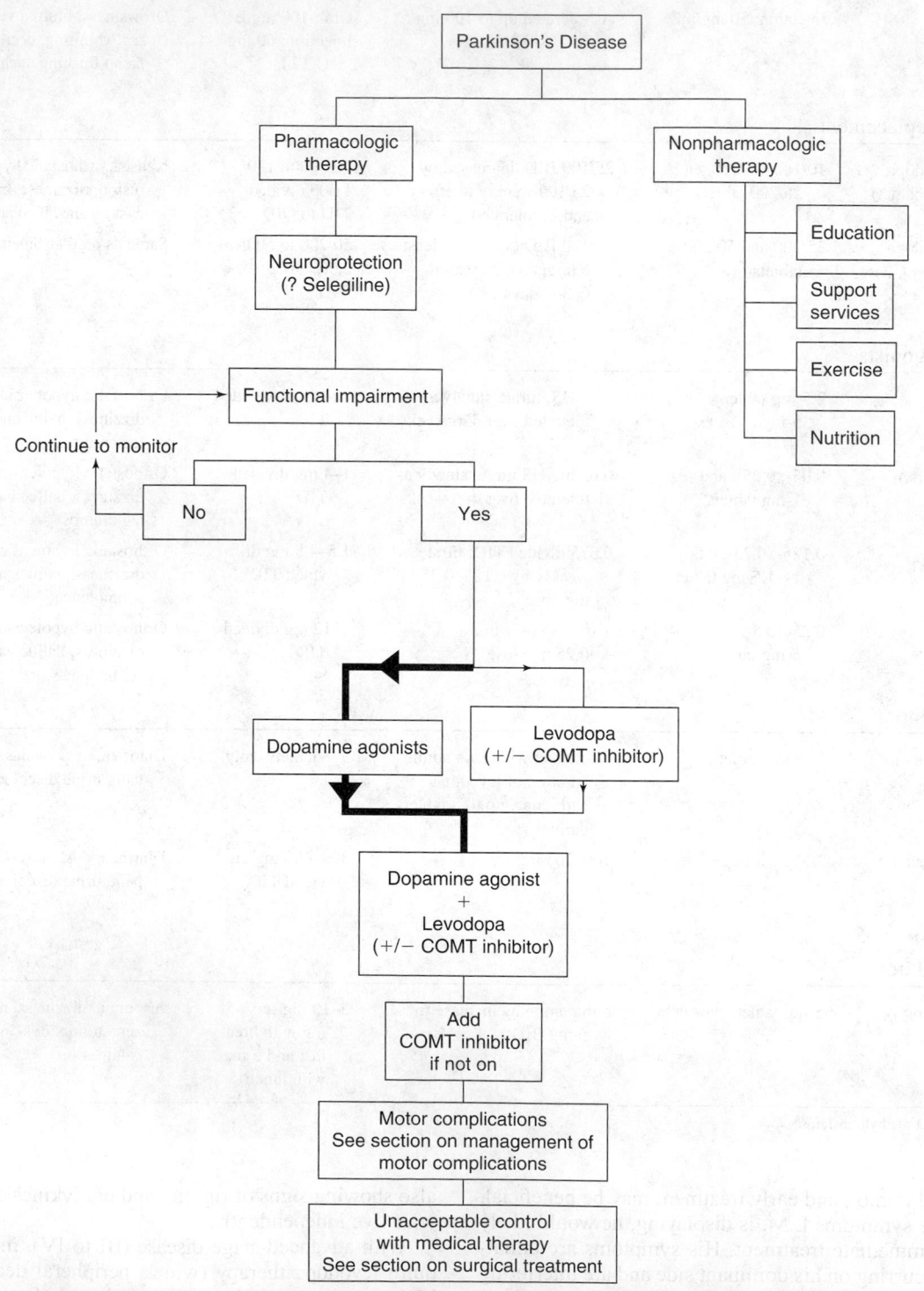

FIGURE 53-1. Treatment algorithm for the management of Parkinson's disease. (Reprinted with permission from Olanow CW et al. Neurology 2001;56[Suppl 5]:S1–88.)

voted to the drug therapy of PD, the importance of supportive care cannot be overemphasized. Exercise, physiotherapy, and good nutritional support can be beneficial at the earlier stages to improve mobility, increase strength, and enhance well-being and mood.[28] Speech therapy may be helpful, and psychological support is often necessary in dealing with depression and other related problems.[30] Newly diagnosed patients need to be educated about what to expect from the disease and the various forms of treatment available. In addition, enlisting the support of family members is vital in establishing an overall effective therapeutic plan.

Dopamine Agonists

Initial Therapy

3. The decision is made to begin therapy for L.M. Should therapy be initiated with a dopamine agonist or levodopa?

Levodopa, without question, has revolutionized the treatment of PD. However, declining efficacy and response fluctuations encountered with long-term levodopa therapy, as well as a high frequency of undesirable side effects, prompted investigators to search for agents that could directly stimulate dopamine receptors. This led to the discovery of the dopamine agonists (Fig. 53-2).[28]

The dopamine agonists work by directly stimulating postsynaptic dopamine receptors within the corpus striatum.[34,35] There are two families of dopamine receptors, D_1 and D_2. The D_1 family includes the D_1 and D_5 dopamine subtype receptors and the D_2 family includes D_2, D_3, and D_4 dopamine subtype receptors. Stimulation of D_2 receptors is largely responsible for improving rigidity and bradykinesia, whereas the precise role of the D_1 receptors remains uncertain.[34,35] Although the dopamine agonists differ slightly from each other in terms of their affinities for dopamine receptors (Table 53-4), these agents produce essentially the same clinical effects when used to treat PD.[28,36–38]

Dopamine agonists have a number of potential advantages over levodopa. Since dopamine agonists act directly on dopamine receptors, they do not require metabolic conversion to an active product and therefore act independently of degenerating dopaminergic neurons.[28] Unlike levodopa, circulating plasma amino acids do not compete with dopamine agonists for absorption and transport into the brain. Dopamine agonists have a longer half-life than levodopa formulations, reducing the need for multiple daily dosing. In contrast to levodopa, dopamine agonists do not undergo oxidative metabolism and do not result in the generation of free radicals and associated oxidative stress. Finally, initial therapy with

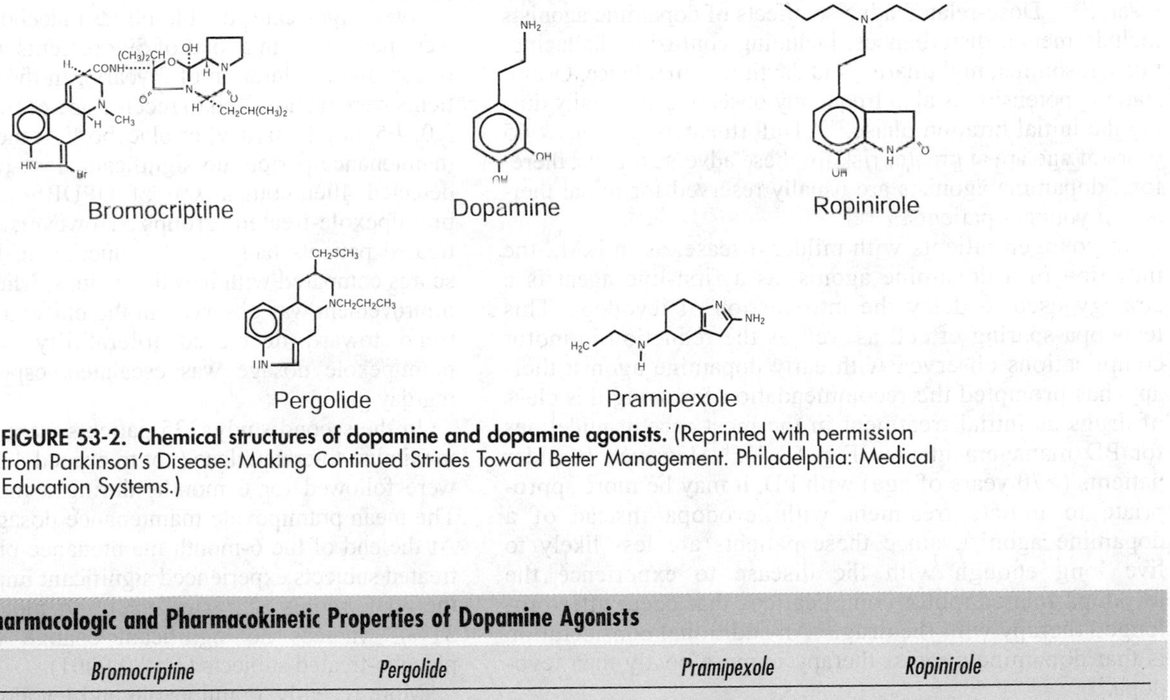

Bromocriptine   Dopamine   Ropinirole

Pergolide   Pramipexole

FIGURE 53-2. Chemical structures of dopamine and dopamine agonists. (Reprinted with permission from Parkinson's Disease: Making Continued Strides Toward Better Management. Philadelphia: Medical Education Systems.)

Table 53-4 Pharmacologic and Pharmacokinetic Properties of Dopamine Agonists

	Bromocriptine	Pergolide	Pramipexole	Ropinirole
Type of compound	Ergot derivative	Ergot derivative	Nonergoline	Nonergoline
Receptor specificity	D_2, D_1,[a] α1, α2, 5-HT	D_2, D_1, α1, α2, 5-HT, β	D_2, D_3, D_4, α2	D_2, D_3, D_4
Bioavailability	8%	20%	>90%	55% (first-pass metabolism)
T_{max} (min)	70–100	60–120	60–180	90
Protein binding	90–96%	90%	15%	40%
Elimination route	Metabolic (hepatic)	Metabolic (hepatic)	Renal	Metabolic (hepatic)
Half-life (hr)	3–8	27	8–12	6

[a]Antagonist.

dopamine agonists is associated with fewer motor complications (intractable symptoms of advanced disease) in comparison with levodopa.

Dopamine agonists were introduced in the 1970s for use in patients experiencing motor fluctuations with levodopa.[28,36] However, considerable interest existed in using this class of drugs earlier in the course of the disease in an attempt to delay the progression of symptoms and the need for levodopa.[28] Because of their ability to bind to presynaptic dopamine autoreceptors, they may have a role in neuroprotection by regulating dopamine synthesis, release, and turnover by feedback inhibition.[38] The dopamine agonists in present use that are derived from the ergoline class of ergot alkaloids include bromocriptine, pergolide, and cabergoline.[38–40] Although cabergoline is widely used in Europe, it is approved in the United States only for use in treating hyperprolactinemia. Two newer nonergoline dopamine agonists, pramipexole and ropinirole, are now marketed in the United States with a Food and Drug Administration (FDA)-approved indication for the treatment of idiopathic, early-stage PD as monotherapy, or as an adjunct to levodopa in patients with advanced disease.[28,36,38–40]

As a class, dopamine agonists provide adequate control of symptoms when given as monotherapy in up to 80% of patients with early-stage disease. These benefits are sustained for 3 years or more in most patients.[41] However, with progression of the disease, levodopa rescue therapy is often necessary.[38–40] Dose-related adverse effects of dopamine agonists include mental disturbances, including confusion, hallucinations, insomnia, nightmares, and daytime somnolence. Orthostatic hypotension is also frequently observed, especially during the initial titration phase.[28,36] Unfortunately, patients >65 years of age are at greater risk for these adverse effects; therefore, dopamine agonists are usually reserved for initial therapy in younger patients.[36,38]

In younger patients with milder disease, as in L.M., the initiation of a dopamine agonist as a first-line agent is a strategy used to delay the introduction of levodopa. This levodopa-sparing effect, as well as the reduction in motor complications observed with early dopamine agonist therapy, has prompted the recommendation for using this class of drugs as initial treatment in the most recent guidelines for PD management (see Fig. 53-1).[28] However, in older patients (>70 years of age) with PD, it may be more appropriate to initiate treatment with levodopa instead of a dopamine agonist, since these patients are less likely to live long enough with the disease to experience the levodopa-related motor complications that occur after prolonged therapy with the drug.[28] An additional consideration is that dopamine agonist therapy is more costly than levodopa.[42]

In the case of L.M., his relatively young age (<70 years old) and mild disease make him a good candidate for initial therapy with a dopamine agonist. L.M. will certainly require levodopa therapy later, when he reaches more advanced stages of the disease. By initiating therapy first with a dopamine agonist, rescue levodopa therapy can likely be started at smaller doses, and the onset of motor complications that often occur with escalating doses and extended therapy with levodopa may be delayed.[28,36,42]

Pramipexole

4. L.M. is to be started on pramipexole. How effective is pramipexole in the treatment of PD?

EFFICACY

Pramipexole (Mirapex) is a synthetic nonergot aminobenzothiazole derivative and a full agonist at D_2 receptors.[35,43] Pramipexole binds with a sevenfold higher affinity to D_3 than D_2 receptors.[43] The clinical significance of this effect is unknown. Unlike other dopamine agonists, pramipexole is primarily eliminated unchanged via the kidneys; therefore, no significant interactions occur with drugs undergoing hepatic biotransformation via oxidative pathways.[44]

The efficacy of pramipexole was first evaluated in two populations of patients: (1) de novo patients with early-stage PD receiving pramipexole as monotherapy[45–48] and (2) patients with advanced-stage disease receiving pramipexole as an adjunct to levodopa therapy.[49,50] These trials were multicenter, placebo-controlled, parallel-group studies, and the primary outcome measures included improvement in activities of daily living (ADLs, part II) and motor function scores (part III) as measured by the Unified Parkinson's Disease Rating Scale (UPDRS).[51] Each evaluation on the UPDRS is rated on a scale of 0 (normal) to 4 (can barely perform). Lower scores on the UPDRS after treatment indicate an improvement in overall performance.

Two large-scale, double-blind, placebo-controlled studies were performed in a total of 599 patients with early-stage PD (mean disease duration of 2 years). In the first study, 264 patients were randomized to receive one of four fixed doses (1.5, 3.0, 4.5, or 6.0 mg/day) or placebo.[47] At the end of the 4-week maintenance period, no significant dose-response effect was detected after comparison of UPDRS scores for the four pramipexole-treated groups. However, the pramipexole-treated patients had a 20% reduction in their total UPDRS scores compared with baseline values, whereas no significant improvement was observed in the placebo-treated patients. A trend toward decreased tolerability was noted as the pramipexole dosage was escalated, especially in the 6.0-mg/day group.

In the second study, 335 patients were titrated up to their maximum tolerated dose (not to exceed 4.5 mg/day) and then were followed for 6 months during a maintenance phase.[48] The mean pramipexole maintenance dosage was 3.8 mg/day. At the end of the 6-month maintenance phase, pramipexole-treated subjects experienced significant improvements in both the ADL scores (22% to 29%) and motor scores (25% to 31%), whereas no significant change was noted in the placebo-treated subjects ($P < 0.0001$).

More recently, pramipexole and levodopa were compared in a randomized controlled trial as initial treatment of early PD.[52] The purpose of this study was to evaluate the risk for development of motor complications with the two therapies. Three hundred one untreated patients with early PD were randomized to receive either pramipexole 0.5 mg three times daily or carbidopa/levodopa 25/100 mg three times daily. Doses could be escalated during the first 10 weeks of the study, following which open-label levodopa was permitted if necessary. The primary end point was the time to the first occurrence of wearing off, dyskinesias, or on-off motor fluctuations. After a mean follow-up of 24 months, patients in the pramipexole group were receiving a mean daily dose of 2.78 mg pramipexole and 264 mg of supplemental levodopa, while patients in the levodopa group were receiving a mean total of 509 mg levodopa per day. Fewer pramipexole-treated patients reached the primary end point (28% versus 51%; $P < 0.001$) than the patients initially randomized to levodopa therapy. Dyskinesias were noted in only 10% of pramipexole-treated patients compared to 31% of levodopa-treated patients ($P < 0.001$), and fewer wearing-off effects were reported with pramipexole (24% versus 38%; $P = 0.01$).

While dopamine agonists such as pramipexole have demonstrated efficacy as monotherapy, they are also effective as adjuncts to levodopa therapy. The effectiveness of pramipexole as an adjunct to levodopa therapy was evaluated in one large multicenter, placebo-controlled study of 360 patients with a mean disease duration of 9 years and an average duration of levodopa therapy of 8 years.[50] Patients were titrated gradually to their maximum effective dosage as tolerated and not to exceed 4.5 mg/day in three divided doses. At the end of a 6-month maintenance period, the pramipexole-treated patients had a 22% improvement in their ADLs ($P < 0.0001$) and a 25% improvement in their motor scores ($P < 0.01$) compared with baseline values. Pramipexole-treated patients also had a 31% improvement in the mean "off" time, compared with a 7% improvement in the placebo-treated group ($P < 0.0006$). Levodopa dose reduction was permitted for increased dyskinesias or hallucinations and occurred in 76% of the pramipexole group compared with 54% in the placebo group. The total daily levodopa dose was decreased by 27% in the pramipexole-treated subjects compared with 5% in the placebo group.

DOSING

5. What is the most effective way to dose pramipexole?

Pramipexole should always be initiated at a low dosage and gradually titrated to the maximum effective dose, as tolerated. This approach minimizes adverse effects that may result in noncompliance or discontinuation of the drug. In clinical trials, the maximum effective dose was variable and correlated with disease severity and tolerability. However, one fixed-dose study in early PD showed that most patients responded maximally at a dosage of 0.5 mg three times daily.[47] In patients with advanced-stage disease, an average of 3.4 mg/day is usually required to reach the maximum effect of pramipexole.[50] Studies have shown that pramipexole is nearly equipotent with pergolide, about tenfold more potent than bromocriptine, and about threefold more potent than ropinirole.[38]

L.M. has normal renal function and therefore should be started at an initial dosage of 0.125 mg three times daily for 5 to 7 days. At week 2, the dosage should be increased to 0.250 mg three times daily. Thereafter, his dosage may be increased weekly by 0.25 mg/dose (0.75 mg/day) as tolerated and up to the maximum effective dose, not to exceed 1.5 mg three times daily.[44] The titration period usually takes about 4 to 7 weeks, depending on the optimal maintenance dose.

Patients with a creatinine clearance of <60 mL/min should be dosed less frequently than those with normal renal func-

tion.[44] Patients with a creatinine clearance of 35 to 59 mL/min should receive a starting dose of 0.125 mg twice daily up to a maximum dose of 1.5 mg twice daily; patients with a creatinine clearance of 15 to 34 mL/min should receive a starting dose of 0.125 mg daily up to a maximum dose of 1.5 mg daily. Pramipexole has not been studied in patients with a creatinine clearance of <15 mL/min or those receiving hemodialysis.

ADVERSE EFFECTS

6. What are the adverse effects of pramipexole? How can these be managed?

Because pramipexole is approved for use as both monotherapy in early-stage disease and as adjunctive therapy in advanced-stage disease, the adverse events have been evaluated as a function of disease stage.[44] In studies of patients with early-stage disease, the most common adverse effects were nausea (28%), dizziness (25%), somnolence (22%), insomnia (17%), constipation (14%), asthenia (14%), and hallucinations (9%).[44-48] Nausea, with or without vomiting, can be a significant problem, particularly with higher doses.[44] Administering pramipexole with food may partially alleviate this problem. With continued use, many patients develop tolerance to the gastrointestinal side effects of pramipexole. Mental changes were the most common reason for discontinuation of pramipexole in both patient populations. Patients >65 years of age are threefold more likely to experience pramipexole-induced hallucinations.[36] The incidence of orthostatic hypotension was relatively low (1%) and may in part reflect the exclusion of patients with underlying cardiovascular disease from studies.[44]

In advanced-stage disease, the most common adverse events were orthostatic hypotension (54%), dyskinesias (47%), insomnia (27%), confusion (10%), and hallucinations (17%).[44,50] As expected, in patients with advanced-stage disease, the most common reasons for discontinuing pramipexole were mental disturbances (nightmares, confusion, hallucinations, insomnia) and orthostatic hypotension.

Dyskinesias experienced when pramipexole is used in combination with levodopa in advanced-stage disease may be managed by first lowering the daily dose of levodopa. If unsuccessful, the pramipexole dose may be lowered; however, parkinsonian symptoms may worsen.

Excessive daytime somnolence during ADLs, including driving, has been reported with pramipexole and has resulted in accidents.[53,54] Affected patients have not always reported warning signs before falling asleep and believed they were alert immediately prior to the event. Labeling for the drug has since been changed to warn that patients should be alerted to the possibility of falling asleep while engaged in ADLs. Patients should be advised to refrain from driving or engaging in other potentially dangerous activities until they have gained sufficient experience with pramipexole to determine whether it will hinder their mental and/or motor performance. Caution should be advised when patients are taking other sedating medications or alcohol in combination with pramipexole. If excessive daytime somnolence does occur, patients should be advised to contact their physician.

Although L.M. is <65 years of age, he is experiencing memory difficulty and may be at increased risk for visual hallucinations and cognitive problems from dopamine agonist therapy. Occurrence or exacerbation of these problems should be monitored closely. He also should be evaluated for postural hypotension before initiation of pramipexole and counseled to report dizziness or unsteadiness, because this may lead to falls. He should also be reassured that these effects may subside with time and that he should not drive or operate complex machinery until he can assess the drug's effect on his mental status. L.M. should be counseled about the possibility of excessive, and potentially unpredictable, daytime somnolence as pramipexole is introduced. Appropriate precautions should be discussed with both the patient and his spouse.

7. **How do ropinirole, bromocriptine, and pergolide compare to pramipexole?**

Ropinirole

Ropinirole is a synthetic nonergoline aminoindolone and a full dopamine agonist with selectivity for D_2 receptors, but like pramipexole it has no significant affinity for D_1 receptors.[55] Although the drug is pharmacologically similar to pramipexole, it has some distinct pharmacokinetic properties, as shown in Table 53-4. Unlike pramipexole, which is primarily eliminated by renal excretion, ropinirole is metabolized by the cytochrome P450 (primarily CYP1A2) oxidative pathway and undergoes significant first-pass hepatic metabolism.[56]

EFFICACY

Like pramipexole, ropinirole has been approved for use as monotherapy in early-stage idiopathic PD and as an adjunct to levodopa therapy in patients with advanced-stage disease.[57]

The efficacy of ropinirole as early monotherapy in de novo patients was evaluated in three randomized, double-blind, multicenter, parallel group studies.[41,58,59] One study was placebo-controlled,[58] another study compared ropinirole to bromocriptine,[59] and the third study compared initial therapy with ropinirole versus levodopa in early PD.[41] After 6 months of maintenance therapy with ropinirole, all three studies showed a significant improvement in UPDRS motor scores compared with baseline values (20% to 30%). In the placebo-controlled study, ropinirole-treated patients had a 24% reduction in their UPDRS motor scores compared with their baseline values, whereas the placebo-treated patients decreased their scores by only 3%.[58]

In the second study comparing the effectiveness of ropinirole to bromocriptine, a significantly greater number of ropinirole-treated patients (58%) experienced a 30% reduction in their UPDRS scores compared with bromocriptine-treated patients (43%).[59] This study also stratified patients for selegiline use, and without selegiline, the ropinirole-treated subjects significantly improved their motor scores to a greater extent than the bromocriptine-treated subjects (34% versus 20%). However, with selegiline, no significant difference was found in the responder rate for the two study groups, as measured by a 30% reduction in their UPDRS motor scores.

A 6-month interim analysis of the third study, which compared the efficacy of ropinirole (mean dosage, 9 mg/day) with levodopa (mean dosage, 464 mg/day), reported that the levodopa-treated patients had a 44% improvement in their UPDRS motor scores compared with a 32% improvement in the ropinirole-treated patients.[41] However, when the two treatments were stratified for disease stage, the two treatments were equally effective in patients with mild PD. Open-label levodopa supplementation was available for patients in both groups at the discretion of the investigators.

After 5 years of follow-up, ropinirole-treated patients had a reduced risk for developing dyskinesias compared to initial therapy with levodopa.[60] At the end of the study, the mean daily dose of ropinirole was 16.5 mg plus 427 mg of open-label levodopa, compared to a mean daily dose of 753 mg of levodopa for the levodopa group. Sixty-six percent of patients in the ropinirole group required open-label levodopa supplementation compared to 36% in the levodopa group. Dyskinesias developed in 20% of the ropinirole-treated patients compared to 45% of the levodopa-treated patients (hazard ratio for remaining free of dyskinesia in the ropinirole group, compared with the levodopa group, 2.82; $P < 0.001$). This difference between the two groups was not dependent on whether the patient received open-label levodopa supplementation. For ropinirole-treated patients who were able to remain on monotherapy without open-label levodopa supplementation, only 5% developed dyskinesia, compared to 36% of those receiving levodopa monotherapy.

Ropinirole has also shown efficacy in improving motor scores when added to levodopa therapy in patients with advanced-stage disease.[61] In a multicenter, double-blind, randomized parallel-group study, ropinirole-treated patients experienced an average time spent "off" that was decreased by 1.9 hours daily. In ropinirole-treated patients, the total daily levodopa dose was decreased by an average of 19%. Twenty-eight percent of patients experienced at least a 35% reduction in both time spent "off" and in their levodopa dose, compared with 13% of the placebo-treated patients. After 1 year of treatment, 47.5% of patients (n = 865) continued treatment with ropinirole as an adjunct to levodopa therapy in advanced-stage disease.

DOSING

Ropinirole should be initiated at a dosage of 0.25 mg three times daily with gradual titration in weekly increments of 0.25 mg per dose over 4 to 6 weeks.[28] Clinical response to ropinirole is usually observed at a daily dose of 9 to 12 mg given in three divided doses.

ADVERSE EFFECTS

The adverse effects associated with ropinirole are similar to those observed with other dopamine agonists. In patients receiving ropinirole as monotherapy for mild PD, nausea (44.3%), dizziness (24%), and somnolence (24.9%) were the most frequently reported adverse effects.[41,58,59,62] The most common reason for discontinuation was nausea (4.7%). Hallucinations occurred with a frequency of 7.9% but accounted for only 2% of discontinuations. Postural hypotension occurred in 6.9% of patients compared with 3.9% in the placebo-treated group. Patients receiving ropinirole should be advised of the potential for experiencing excessive daytime somnolence, similar to pramipexole.

As adjunctive therapy in advanced-stage disease, the most commonly reported adverse effects were dyskinesias (26.3%), nausea (25.6%), dizziness (18.7%), aggravated PD (16.4%), somnolence (11.4%), hallucinations (11.2%), and postural hypotension (10.8%).[61,62]

Bromocriptine

Bromocriptine (Parlodel) is a semisynthetic ergot alkaloid that was initially approved for use as a prolactin inhibitor for conditions such as amenorrhea, galactorrhea, and infertility.[63–66] It has been used to treat parkinsonism since the early 1970s. Bromocriptine is an agonist at D_1 and D_2 receptors. Like other dopamine agonists, its therapeutic effect is primarily related to its ability to stimulate postsynaptic D_2 receptors.[63]

EFFICACY

Numerous investigators have studied bromocriptine in PD.[67–79] In patients with moderate to severe parkinsonism maintained on levodopa, 75% improved clinically.[50,67,68] Improvement in response fluctuations (primarily end-of-dose deterioration) also occurred in approximately 60% of cases.

Among patients with mild to moderate disease who received lower doses of bromocriptine as monotherapy, approximately 60% had an improvement in disability.[72–74] Patients with response oscillations also experienced substantial improvement. Declining efficacy was seen with early de novo bromocriptine therapy, such that by 2 years many patients required the addition of levodopa for optimal results.[68,73,74]

An open-label randomized trial comparing levodopa (with benserazide, a decarboxylase inhibitor), levodopa with selegiline, and bromocriptine in 262 patients with early, mild PD found that all three treatments reduced parkinsonian disability.[76] However, a significant trend for greater efficacy in the levodopa-treated groups was noted. Also, more patients receiving bromocriptine experienced gastrointestinal and psychiatric disturbances, which resulted in a higher withdrawal rate from the study (about 30%).

The effectiveness of bromocriptine in treating patients with advanced PD (n = 246) was compared with pramipexole in a multicenter, double-blind, randomized placebo-controlled study.[80] The average maintenance dosage for pramipexole was 3.4 mg/day, and the average maintenance dosage for bromocriptine was 22.4 mg/day. Six months after receiving the maximum tolerated doses of each study drug, patients were evaluated for improvements in ADLs (UPDRS part II) and motor scores (UPDRS part III). Both pramipexole- and bromocriptine-treated patients improved significantly ($P < 0.01$) relative to placebo-treated patients in their ADL scores (27%, 14%, and 4.8%, respectively) and in their motor scores (35%, 24%, and 5.7%, respectively). However, only the pramipexole group showed a significant reduction in time spent "off" (15%). Pramipexole and bromocriptine were tolerated equally.

DOSING

8. What is the most effective way to dose bromocriptine?

Results from studies using low dosages (<30 mg/day) of bromocriptine alone versus those using high dosages (usually 30 to 80 mg/day) alone showed improvement in 58% versus 62% of patients, respectively.[63] Side effects leading to discontinuation of therapy were encountered in 9% and 27% of patients in the low- and high-dosage groups, respectively. Similarly, 71% of patients given low-dose bromocriptine with levodopa improved, compared with 58% of those given high-dose therapy together with levodopa.[63] Adverse effects causing discontinuation of therapy were observed in 26% of the low-dose patients and 32% of the high-dose patients when combined with levodopa. Although these results seem to favor the use of lower doses, patients receiving higher doses often had the disease for a longer duration and tended to have more advanced symptoms.[63] Thus, the dose required for optimal therapeutic response is most likely a function of the severity of illness.[65] Therefore, the goal of bromocriptine therapy is to keep the dose as low as possible, while recognizing that as the disease progresses, higher doses may be required. Consequently this will increase the costs of therapy and the risk for adverse effects.

The best approach to dosing bromocriptine is to start low and slowly titrate upward. Therapy should be initiated at 1.25 mg/day at bedtime and increased by 2.5 mg every 2 to 4 weeks. It may take months to achieve optimal results.[71–73]

ADVERSE EFFECTS

As with other dopamine agonists, the most commonly experienced adverse effects are mental changes, occurring in up to 40% of patients.[50] Most notable of these mental effects are visual hallucinations, but confusion, paranoid delusions, and mania are all associated with bromocriptine use and may persist for weeks after the drug is discontinued.[81] As with levodopa, mental effects are more pronounced in patients with underlying psychiatric disturbances.[50,81]

Orthostatic hypotension with dizziness is the next most common side effect.[50,81] Administering the first bromocriptine dose at bedtime may minimize symptoms of orthostasis in patients who are susceptible to this adverse effect. Nausea, with or without vomiting, can be a significant problem, particularly with higher doses. Although the nausea with bromocriptine is less severe than that associated with levodopa given alone, it is more severe than with levodopa combined with carbidopa.[71,81] Administering bromocriptine with food may partially alleviate this problem. With continued use, many patients develop tolerance to the hypotensive and gastrointestinal side effects of bromocriptine.

Ergot-related peripheral vascular effects are uncommonly associated with bromocriptine (<5% of patients). These vascular adverse effects include digital vasospasm, Raynaud's phenomenon, and angina; all are usually reversible with discontinuation of therapy.[50,81] Erythromelalgia, an unusual vascular complaint characterized by redness, warmth, tenderness, and edema of the legs, occurs uncommonly in patients taking bromocriptine. This side effect may improve with a decrease in dose and reverses when the drug is stopped.[81]

Dyskinesias have been reported in up to 80% of patients receiving bromocriptine for the treatment of parkinsonism. These abnormal involuntary movements are similar to those seen with levodopa and include orofacial dyskinesias, facial grimacing, and choreic movements of the trunk and limbs.[81] Because this adverse effect is not as common in patients receiving this drug for the treatment of other disorders, it is unclear whether the dyskinesias are primarily attributed to disease progression or failure to optimize concomitantly administered levodopa. When bromocriptine is added as an adjunct to levodopa, consideration should be given to lowering the levodopa dosage. The timing and magnitude of levodopa dose adjustments should be guided by clinical response.

Finally, in rare instances, bromocriptine has been associated with pleuropulmonary fibrosis, similar to that seen with methysergide, another ergot alkaloid.[81] Chest radiographs should be checked on all bromocriptine-treated patients who have an abnormal pulmonary examination. Hypertension, seizures, fatal cerebrovascular accident (stroke), and acute myocardial infarction have occurred rarely in women receiving bromocriptine for postpartum lactation.

Pergolide

Pergolide is a synthetic ergoline derivative with pharmacologic properties differing from pramipexole (see Table 53-4 and Fig. 53-2).[35,64,82] Pergolide exerts an antiparkinsonian effect through direct stimulation of both D_1 and D_2 postsynaptic receptors.[37,82] Pergolide is more potent and longer acting than ropinirole or bromocriptine.

EFFICACY

In open trials, the addition of pergolide improves parkinsonian disability in up to 75% of patients with advanced PD who no longer respond satisfactorily to levodopa.[82] In double-blind, placebo-controlled trials, a significant placebo effect has been observed, but pergolide was associated with improvements greater than could be attributed to placebo alone.[82,83] Pergolide has been compared with bromocriptine in patients with advanced parkinsonism in a randomized, double-blind trial, with the two treatments providing similar results.[84] These studies indicate that like bromocriptine, pergolide is an effective adjunctive agent in patients taking long-term levodopa. Improvements induced by pergolide are greatest at 1 month and begin to decline after 6 months of therapy. By the second year of therapy, most patients on pergolide fail to show improvement over pretreatment values.[82,83,85] Early responders to pergolide tend to experience more prolonged benefit with the drug.[83] Small numbers of patients given pergolide as monotherapy showed some minor improvements; however, these were inferior to those obtained with levodopa.[83,86]

A major advantage of pergolide relative to other dopamine agonists is its ability to improve response fluctuations in levodopa-treated patients. This benefit of pergolide directly relates to its potency and prolonged duration of action.[83,86,88] Improvements in "end-of-dose" deterioration respond more favorably than the "on-off" phenomenon.[83,86] A mean improvement of 120% in the number of hours the patients were "on" has been observed from various trials performed to date.[86] Pergolide also can improve disability during "off" periods.[83,85–88] As a result, its long duration of action may make it especially advantageous for managing cases of early morning akinesia if the dose is taken at bedtime. This property could be of benefit to L.M., who suffers from this effect. Finally, a few studies suggest that pergolide can be efficacious in up to 50% of patients showing unresponsiveness, decreased responsiveness over time, or intolerance to bromocriptine.[82,89]

DOSING

Therapy with pergolide should be started with 0.05 to 0.1 mg/day given at bedtime and slowly increased by 0.05- to 0.15-mg increments every third day to a maximum of 6 mg/day. Most patients respond to dosages between 2 and 4 mg/day, with a few requiring dosages as high as 10 mg/day. A daily dose ratio for bromocriptine to pergolide of 13:1 has been suggested from comparative studies.[38]

ADVERSE EFFECTS

The adverse effects of pergolide are similar to those of bromocriptine.[37] Although in some studies up to 40% of patients had to discontinue pergolide therapy because of unacceptable side effects, this estimate is probably high, and other evidence suggests that only about 25% of patients are intolerant to this drug.[82] As with bromocriptine, the higher incidence of side effects may be the result of escalating the dose too rapidly, inappropriate management of concomitant levodopa, or severity of the disease.

The incidence of mental changes with pergolide appears to be similar to other dopamine agonists.[82] Nausea and vomiting occur, particularly upon initiation of therapy, and may lessen with time. Orthostasis and other cardiovascular effects may be more frequent with pergolide than with other dopamine agonists.[86] Cardiac arrhythmias were a concern in the early period of clinical trials, but well-designed studies using careful cardiac monitoring techniques have found no significant arrhythmogenic properties in patients without underlying cardiac problems.[90] However, pergolide can cause mild bradycardia, and angina has been seen in 2% to 13% of patients in some trials.[82] Therefore, pergolide should be administered cautiously in patients with cardiac arrhythmias or angina. If dyskinesias worsen when pergolide is added to levodopa, the levodopa dose should be decreased if tolerated.[82,83,86] Finally, peripheral vascular side effects also occur with pergolide, and erythromelalgia has been reported.[82]

Levodopa

9. L.M. has responded well to pramipexole 1.0 mg TID for the past 18 months, with an increased ability to paint and carry out ADLs. However, over the past few weeks, he has noticed a gradual worsening in his symptoms and once again is having difficulty holding a paintbrush. He currently complains of feeling more "tied up," he has more difficulty getting out of a chair, and his posture is slightly more stooped. Otherwise, he can carry out most of his ADLs without a lot of difficulty. Should levodopa be considered for the treatment of L.M.'s PD at this time?

For patients with advancing PD, levodopa remains the mainstay of treatment. Nearly all patients will eventually require treatment with the drug, regardless of initial therapy. Since PD is characterized by absence of dopamine in the brain, the most rational approach to treatment is to replenish the depleted dopamine. However, dopamine itself does not cross the blood–brain barrier. In high doses, levodopa, a dopamine precursor with no known pharmacologic action of its own, penetrates into the brain, where it is converted by aromatic L-amino acid decarboxylase to dopamine.[91] Early trials by Cotzias[91,92] and Barbeau[93] demonstrating significant (often dramatic) improvement in the classic features of the disease soon led to further studies, which clearly established levodopa as the drug of choice for long-term treatment of PD.[36,94] Although levodopa/carbidopa is the most effective therapy for treating the rigidity and bradykinesia of PD, like other dopaminergic agents, it does not effectively improve postural instability, dementia, autonomic dysfunction, or "freezing," an extreme type of akinesia that often occurs in advanced-stage disease.[95]

Efficacy

Levodopa provides clinically meaningful benefits in nearly all patients with pathologically confirmed PD.[28] In an early open trial involving 86 patients, 79% experienced 50% improvement in all their symptoms when given an average levodopa dosage of 4.8 g/day.[93] Only 8 of the 79 patients (10%) failed therapy, two of these because of side effects.[93] Similar findings were reported in another study of 100 patients.[94] A dramatic improvement (>75%) in bradykinesia, rigidity, and tremor was observed in 33 patients.[94]

Sinemet: Advantages and Disadvantages

10. **What are the advantages and disadvantages of Sinemet over levodopa alone?**

Although levodopa is highly effective, its use is not without problems. High doses are required because significant amounts are peripherally (extracerebrally) metabolized to dopamine by the enzyme aromatic L-amino acid (dopa) decarboxylase. These high doses result in many undesirable side effects such as nausea, vomiting, and anorexia (50% of patients); postural hypotension (30% of patients); and cardiac arrhythmias (10% of patients).[93–95] In addition, mental disturbances (see Question 15) are encountered in 15% of patients, and abnormal involuntary movements (dyskinesias) can be seen in up to 55% of patients during the first 6 months of levodopa treatment.[93–96]

By combining levodopa with a dopa decarboxylase inhibitor that does not penetrate the blood–brain barrier, a decrease in the peripheral conversion of levodopa to dopamine can be achieved, while the desired conversion within the basal ganglia remains unaffected (Fig. 53-3).[97] The two peripheral decarboxylase inhibitors in clinical use are benserazide (unavailable in the United States) and carbidopa (Lodosyn).[28] Sinemet is the fixed combination of carbidopa and levodopa and is available in ratios of 1:4 (Sinemet 25/100) and 1:10 (Sinemet 10/100 and 25/250).[28] A controlled-release product (Sinemet CR) is available in a ratio of 25/100 and 50/200.

Combining levodopa with carbidopa enhances the amount of dopamine available to the brain and thereby allows the dose of levodopa to be decreased by 80%.[98] This combination also shortens by several weeks the time needed to increase the levodopa dose to achieve maximal effects because carbidopa substantially decreases levodopa-induced nausea and vomiting.[28,95]

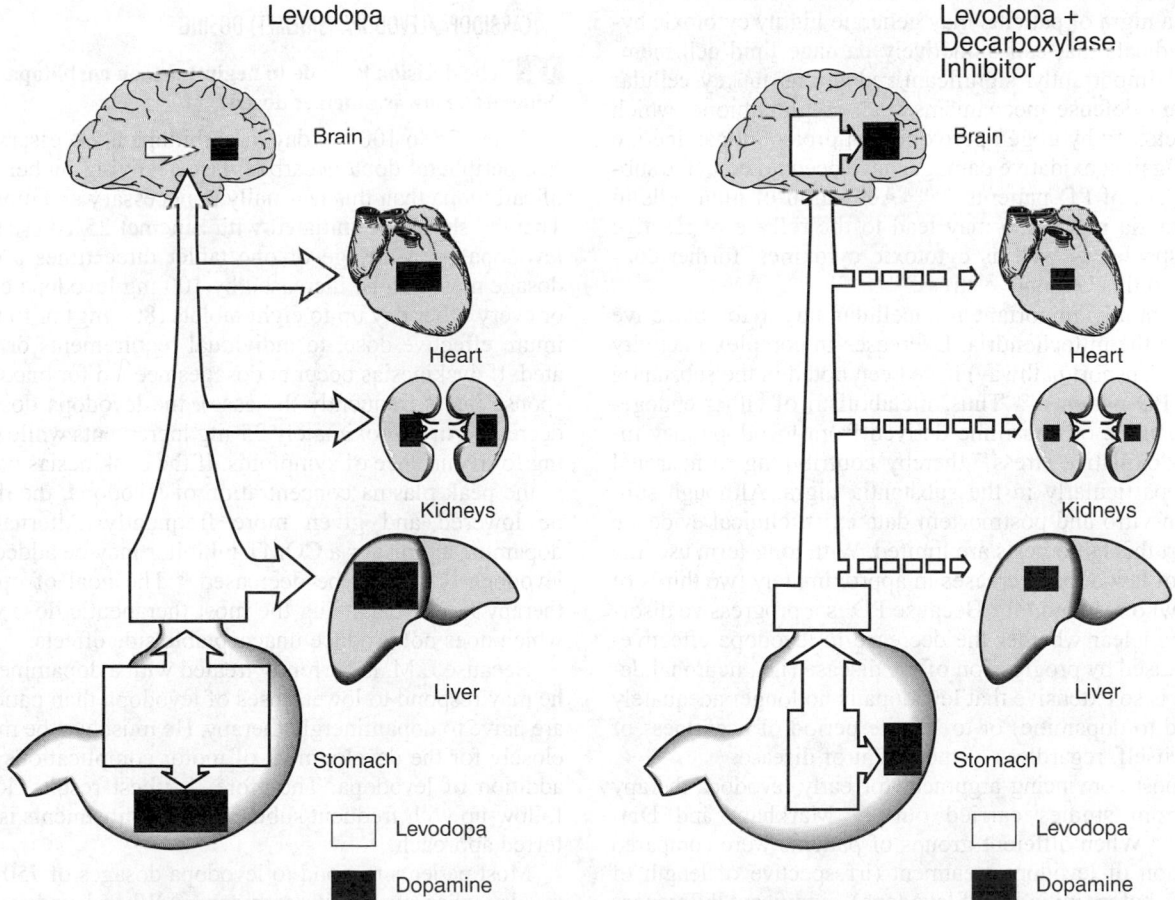

FIGURE 53-3. Peripheral decarboxylation of levodopa when given alone (*left*) and with a peripheral decarboxylase inhibitor (*right*). When combined with a decarboxylase inhibitor, less drug is required and more levodopa reaches the brain. (Reproduced with permission from Pinder RM et al. Levodopa and decarboxylase inhibitors: a review of their clinical pharmacology and use in the treatment of parkinsonism. Drugs 1976;11:329.)

Cardiac arrhythmias are lessened and postural hypotension may be slightly improved.[95] Although the therapeutic effects of levodopa occur sooner with coadministration of carbidopa, a disadvantage of the combination is the risk for earlier development of dyskinesias.[97] Sinemet is more expensive than levodopa by itself. However, the advantages of Sinemet far outweigh the disadvantages, such that nearly all patients are given this form of treatment rather than levodopa alone.

INITIATION OF THERAPY

11. **L.M. does not appear to have severe disability at this time. Should he be started on levodopa therapy now, or should it be reserved for a later date, when symptoms are more severe?**

The question of when to begin levodopa remains a controversial issue in the treatment of PD. Despite initial hopes to the contrary, levodopa therapy does not alter the progression of the disease.[99–101] In fact, it has been suggested that chronic levodopa therapy may actually accelerate the neurodegenerative process through formation of free radicals via dopamine metabolism.[101,102] The autoxidation of dopamine can generate potentially toxic species such as neuromelanin and semiquinones. Metabolism of dopamine by monoamine oxidase (MAO) leads to the generation of hydrogen peroxide, which can then react with ferrous iron. Elevated iron levels in the substantia nigra of patients may generate highly cytotoxic hydroxyl radicals that can oxidatively damage lipid cell membranes.[103] Importantly, significant reductions in key cellular antioxidant defense mechanisms such as glutathione, which acts to detoxify hydrogen peroxide and protect dopaminergic neurons against oxidative damage, have been noted in the substantia nigra of PD patients.[104,105] Activation of glial cells in the substantia nigra also may lead to the release of reactive oxygen species as well as cytotoxic cytokines, further contributing to this "oxidative stress."[103]

A potentially important intracellular target for oxidative damage is the mitochondria. Decreases in complex I activity (electron transport pathway) have been noted in the substantia nigra of PD patients.[106] Thus, metabolism of either endogenous dopamine or dopamine derived from levodopa may induce an "oxidative stress," thereby contributing to neuronal damage, particularly in the substantia nigra. Although substantial in vitro and postmortem data exist, clinical evidence to support this hypothesis are limited. With long-term use, the efficacy of levodopa decreases in approximately two thirds of patients who respond.[95,100] Because PD is a progressive disorder, it is unclear whether the decrease in levodopa effectiveness is caused by progression of the disease (i.e., neuronal destruction is so extensive that levodopa is no longer adequately converted to dopamine) or to a finite period of usefulness of the drug itself, regardless of the extent of disease.

The most convincing argument for early levodopa therapy comes from studies carried out by Markham and Diamond.[107,108] When different groups of patients were compared for duration of levodopa treatment (irrespective of length of symptoms before initiation of levodopa), significant differences were observed between the groups in terms of disability scores (i.e., subjects with the shortest symptom duration were the least disabled). Conversely, when the subjects were matched for duration of symptoms (irrespective of treatment duration), similar disability scores were found for the groups. These results strongly implicate duration of disease, rather than duration of

therapy, as the reason for loss of levodopa efficacy. As the disease progresses, dopamine terminals are lost and the capacity to store dopamine presynaptically is diminished.[109,110] This can impair buffering of the rising and falling concentrations of levodopa. Consequently, dopamine receptors are subject to intermittent or phasic stimulation rather than by physiologic tonic stimulation. Furthermore, continuous dopaminergic stimulation with either intravenously administered levodopa or a long-acting dopamine agonist (cabergoline) has been shown to improve the motor fluctuations observed with shorter-acting dopaminergic agents.[111] Long-term levodopa therapy itself may lead to motor fluctuations ("on-off" and "wearing off" effects) in a substantial number of patients; thus, delaying the initiation of therapy may delay the onset of these problems.[100]

Given these considerations, the optimal time to initiate levodopa therapy must be individualized.[28] Most neurologists agree that there is little reason to start levodopa until the patient is clearly bothered (socially, vocationally, or otherwise) by the disease. Before levodopa is started, patients must fully understand the nature of the disease and what to expect with long-term therapy. L.M. should be seriously considered for levodopa therapy because his disease has progressed enough to threaten his job performance, and his symptoms have progressed despite therapy with a dopamine agonist.

CARBIDOPA/LEVODOPA (SINEMET) DOSING

12. **The decision is made to begin L.M. on carbidopa/levodopa (Sinemet). How is Sinemet dosed?**

About 75 to 100 mg/day of carbidopa is necessary to saturate peripheral dopa decarboxylase.[28] Giving higher amounts of carbidopa than this is usually unnecessary and more costly. Therapy should be initiated with Sinemet 25/100 (carbidopa/levodopa) at a dosage of one tablet three times a day. The dosage may then be increased by 100 mg levodopa every day or every other day up to eight tablets (800 mg) or to the maximum effective dose, to individual requirements or as tolerated. If dyskinesias occur at dosages needed for maximum response (as is frequently the case), the levodopa dose can be decreased in approximately 25-mg increments while monitoring for recurrence of symptoms. If the dyskinesias occur only at the peak plasma concentration of levodopa, the dose may be lowered and given more frequently. Alternatively, a dopamine agonist or a COMT inhibitor may be added and the levodopa dose may be decreased.[28] The goal of optimizing therapy lies in balancing the most therapeutic dose with that which does not produce unacceptable side effects.

Because L.M. is currently treated with a dopamine agonist, he may respond to lower doses of levodopa than patients who are naive to dopaminergic therapy. He must also be monitored closely for the development of motor complications with the addition of levodopa. Therefore, for best results, long-term follow-up with frequent subtle dosage adjustments is the preferred approach.

Most patients respond to levodopa dosages of 750 to 1,000 mg/day when given with carbidopa.[28] When levodopa dosages exceed 750 mg/day, patients such as L.M. can be switched from the 1:4 ratio of carbidopa/levodopa to the 1:10 ratio to prevent providing excessive amounts of decarboxylase inhibitor. For example, if L.M. needed 800 mg of levodopa per day, two Sinemet 10/100 tablets four times daily could be given. If L.M. had not been initially treated with a dopamine agonist, some clinicians would consider adding a dopamine agonist after the daily levodopa dose has been increased to >600 mg because dopamine agonists directly stimulate dopamine receptors, have longer half-lives, and result in a lower incidence of dyskinesias, thus providing a smoother dopaminergic response.[28,36] A more recent approach that is considered as the effect of levodopa begins to "wear off" at the end of a dosing interval is the addition of a COMT inhibitor such as entacapone or tolcapone.

LEVODOPA RESPONSE FLUCTUATIONS

13. **L.M. had a dramatic improvement in all of his parkinsonian symptoms with the initiation of levodopa therapy after being maintained on 25/250 regular Sinemet five times a day. After 6 months of treatment, he began to experience dyskinesias. These usually occurred 1 to 2 hours after a dose and were manifested by facial grimacing, lip smacking, tongue protrusion, and rocking of the trunk. These dyskinetic effects were lessened by decreasing his pramipexole dose to 0.5 mg TID and gradually decreasing his dosage of Sinemet to 25/250 QID, but they have not totally cleared.**

After 3 years of levodopa therapy, more serious problems have begun to emerge. In the mornings, L.M. often experiences immobility. Nearly every day, he has periods (lasting for a few minutes) in which he cannot move, followed by a sudden switch to a fluid-like state, often associated with dyskinetic activity. He continues to take Sinemet (25/250) four times daily but gains symptomatic relief only for about 3 to 4 hours after a dose. Also, the response to a given dose varies and is often less in the afternoon. At times he becomes "frozen," particularly when he needs to board an elevator or is required to move quickly. What are possible explanations for these alterations in clinical response?

For most patients, the initial response to levodopa is favorable, and this early phase is called the "honeymoon period." Although variable, the honeymoon period may last for up to 5 years. However, after an initial period of stability, 50% to 90% of patients with PD will experience motor complications after receiving levodopa for 5 or more years.[28] In attempting to describe response fluctuations, it is important to separate those effects attributable to the disease and those attributable to the drug. Levodopa-induced dyskinesias often appear concurrently with the development of motor fluctuations.[28,112] Reducing the levodopa dosage will often reverse these symptoms. Unfortunately, the reduction in levodopa dosage usually results in deterioration in the control of the disease.

Because levodopa is a short-acting agent with an elimination half-life of about 1.5 hours, much of the effect from the evening dose has dissipated by morning.[98] For this reason, it is not surprising that L.M. is experiencing a period of immobility on arising. This is alleviated in most patients shortly after taking the morning dose.[109,113]

Two of the more common response fluctuations are the true "on-off" effect and the "wearing off," or "end-of-dose deterioration" effect.[109,112] The true "on-off" effect is described as random fluctuations from mobility to the parkinsonian state, which appears suddenly as if a switch has been turned. These fluctuations can last from minutes to hours and increase in frequency and intensity with time. Although most patients prefer to be "on" with dyskinesias rather than "off" with akinesis, dyskinesias in some patients can be more disabling than the parkinsonism.[28] Early in the course of disease, it is usually possible to adjust the amount and timing of the doses of levodopa to control parkinsonian symptoms without inducing

dyskinesias; however, as the disease advances and the therapeutic window narrows, cycling between "on" periods complicated by dyskinesia and "off" periods with resulting immobility is common.[28]

Eventually, despite adjustments in levodopa dosage, many patients with end-stage PD experience either mobility with severe dyskinesias or complete immobility.[114,115] In most patients this effect bears no clear-cut relation to the timing of the dose or levodopa serum levels.[116-118] The "wearing off" or "end-of-dose" effect is a more predictable effect that occurs at the latter part of the dosing interval following a period of relief; it can be improved by various means such as shortening the dosing interval or by adjunctive dopamine agonist or COMT inhibitor therapy.

The explanations for these motor responses are not entirely clear, but incomplete delivery of dopamine to central receptors is at least partially responsible. Variations in the rate and extent of levodopa absorption; dietary substrates (e.g., large neutral amino acids), which compete with cerebral transport mechanisms; and competition for receptor binding by levodopa metabolites can explain these variable responses to levodopa.[112,116] Furthermore, early in the course of the disease, sufficient dopaminergic neurons remain that can store dopamine derived from levodopa administration and release it in a more physiologic manner. These neurons act as a buffer against fluctuating levodopa concentrations. With disease progression, the buffering capacity of these neurons is diminished and motor response becomes more dependent on fluctuations in synaptic dopamine concentrations.[109,110,116,117]

CONTROLLED-RELEASE SINEMET

14. **L.M. is to be converted from immediate-release Sinemet to Sinemet CR because of his continuing motor fluctuations. How useful is controlled-release Sinemet in improving levodopa response fluctuations? How should L.M.'s immediate-release Sinemet be converted to Sinemet CR?**

The ability to partially alleviate response fluctuations by using continuous infusions of levodopa has prompted the development of slow-release carbidopa/levodopa formulations in attempts to ensure a smoother, more sustained delivery of drug.[119] Sinemet CR contains 25 mg carbidopa and 100 mg levodopa or 50 mg carbidopa and 200 mg levodopa in an erodible polymer matrix that retards dissolution in gastric fluids. By gradually dissolving, Sinemet CR may provide a more gradual absorption of levodopa and more sustained plasma concentrations of levodopa compared with standard Sinemet.[119] The end-of-dose deterioration ("wearing off") effect may be improved by the slower rate of plasma levodopa decline. Because of the sustained-release properties of Sinemet CR, the dosing interval can be extended and the number of doses per day can be decreased. However, the delay in reaching maximum effect (by 1 to 1.5 hours) is often problematic in the morning and may be unacceptable to L.M. because he is experiencing morning immobility. To manage this, he can either take the morning dose of Sinemet CR 1 hour before arising, or he can supplement the regimen with a dose of the immediate-release product in the morning. Also, with repeated dosing of Sinemet CR, levodopa can accumulate, resulting in dyskinesias later in the day in some cases. Furthermore, controlled-release Sinemet is more expensive than standard Sinemet.[28,119,120]

The bioavailability of controlled-release Sinemet is about 30% less than immediate-release Sinemet. Patients converted from standard Sinemet should receive a dose of Sinemet CR that will provide 10% more levodopa, then the dose should be titrated upward to clinical reponse.[28] Accordingly, L.M.'s dosage of Sinemet CR should be increased to offset the relative decrease in bioavailability. L.M. should be advised that his dose will initially be raised by about 10% (100 mg), and it may need to be raised further, depending on his response to the new medication. He should also be advised not to crush or chew Sinemet CR. Standard Sinemet 25/100 can be added in the morning as a strategy for providing a quicker onset, thus reducing morning rigidity. Sinemet CR 50/200 should be administered four times daily, spaced 5 hours apart.[28] Treatment with Sinemet CR also might improve L.M.'s sleeping patterns by decreasing the frequency of nocturnal awakenings. Sinemet CR dosages for L.M. should not be adjusted more frequently than every 3 to 5 days to allow for the full clinical effect of this formulation.

Clinical response to L.M.'s levodopa therapy may be improved by modifying dietary protein ingestion.[28,121] Levodopa is actively transported across the blood–brain barrier by a large neutral amino acid transport system. This transport system also facilitates the blood-to-brain transport of amino acids such as L-leucine, L-isoleucine, L-valine, and L-phenylalanine. Levodopa and these neutral amino acids compete for transport mechanisms, and high plasma concentrations of these amino acids can decrease brain concentrations of levodopa.[121,122] Overall reduction or redistribution of the total daily dietary protein intake (i.e., having L.M. consume most of his dietary protein at the evening meal) may improve levodopa response fluctuations.[122] Patients are generally instructed to take immediate-release Sinemet 30 minutes before or 60 minutes after meals for maximal effect. This relationship of dosing around mealtime is less important with the controlled-release formulation. Nevertheless, Sinemet CR should be taken at about the same time each day to facilitate compliance.

Other means for improving levodopa response fluctuations include the use of adjunctive agents such as the dopamine agonists, COMT inhibitors, and in some cases selegiline. In severe cases, continuous duodenal infusion of levodopa or administration of liquid levodopa has been useful in managing motor fluctuations ("wearing off," unpredictable "on" and "off" times, and dyskinesias).[123,124] Liquid levodopa is administered by crushing 10 immediate-release 25/100 tablets and dissolving them in 1 L of tap water, ginger ale, juice, or lemon-lime soda (final concentration is 1 mg/L levodopa). Vitamin C (four 500-mg tablets or 2 g of powder) should be added as a preservative and the mixture shaken well. This provides a solution that is stable for 24 hours at room temperature or 3 days refrigerated. Although this is an effective means for achieving fine titration increments and managing dyskinesias, the duration of effect is extremely short (60 to 90 minutes), and frequent administration is needed.[28,124]

If L.M. prefers not to convert to Sinemet CR, his condition may be improved by taking his daily doses of immediate-release Sinemet at shorter dosing intervals while avoiding substantial increases in the daily dosage, which could worsen his dyskinesias. Taking his morning dose before arising from bed may help with early morning problems and prevent other response fluctuations.

Adverse Effects: Mental Changes

15. L.M. has become notably more depressed, often feeling helpless and hopeless. At times he does not even feel like getting out of bed in the morning, and he does not have much of an appetite. He feels increasingly confused at times and has trouble remembering things that recently happened. In addition to these complaints, L.M. reports that he occasionally has vivid dreams and visual hallucinations. To what extent is levodopa contributing to these mental problems? How should they be managed?

Several psychiatric side effects have been associated with levodopa therapy. These include confusion, depression, restlessness and overactivity, psychosis, hypomania, and vivid dreams.[125] Mental side effects occur in approximately 20% of patients receiving levodopa, but the incidences vary. In one early study, confusion, hallucinations, or vivid dreams occurred in 16% and depression in 11% of 80 patients treated with levodopa.[93] Another group encountered mental changes in 51% of patients given levodopa for 5 years.[126] The combination of levodopa and a decarboxylase inhibitor has little effect on the incidence of mental disturbances.[127] Patients predisposed to levodopa-induced mental disturbances include those with underlying or pre-existing psychiatric disorders and those receiving high doses for prolonged periods.[125]

An organic confusional state with disorientation, which may progress to toxic delirium, is the most commonly observed mental side effect.[125] This side effect can be exacerbated by concurrent anticholinergic or amantadine therapy. Because of its ability to improve disease symptoms and profoundly affect neurologic function, levodopa often produces an elevation in mood, but this is not always the case. Depression, often out of proportion to the degree of neurologic impairment, is another commonly observed finding and may precede motor dysfunction.[125] This disorder may be linked to a decrease in serotonin metabolism, as evidenced by decreased 5-hydroxyindoleacetic acid (5-HIAA) concentrations in the cerebrospinal fluid of depressed PD patients.[128]

Although a few patients like L.M. may experience depression, some receiving levodopa experience psychomotor excitation.[125] Symptoms associated with psychomotor activation include overactivity, restlessness, and agitation. Similarly, hypomania has been reported in up to 8% of patients and is characterized by grandiose thinking, flight of ideas, tangential thinking, and poor social judgment. Normal sexual activity often is restored with improved motor function; however, hypersexuality and libido are increased in about 1% of levodopa-treated patients.[125] Hypersexuality is most likely an associated feature of levodopa-induced hypomania. Psychotic behavior, often in the form of paranoid delusions and visual or olfactory hallucinations, is seen less frequently.[125]

From the symptoms described by L.M., several levodopa-associated mental disturbances are likely present. He has a predisposition for these particular side effects because he presented with underlying depression, confusion, and disturbances of cognition. In general, most of the mental disturbances are dose related and can be lessened by reducing the dosage of levodopa. In patients such as L.M who are concurrently receiving levodopa and a dopamine agonist, the dosage reduction should be attempted first with levodopa. If symptoms do not improve, a reduction in the dosage of the dopamine agonist may also be warranted. However, these dosage reductions may be impractical for L.M. because a return of parkinsonian symptoms is likely, and the benefits of levodopa therapy may outweigh the risk for mental disturbances.

In some cases, depression in PD patients can be treated successfully with antidepressant drugs.[28,129] Care must be exercised, however, because several drugs, including the tricyclic antidepressants, may interact adversely with levodopa (Table 53-5).[130-136] Hypertensive crisis has been reported with levodopa and imipramine, particularly when an insufficient

Table 53-5   Levodopa Drug Interactions[a]

Drug	Interaction	Mechanism	Comments
Anticholinergics	↓ levodopa effect	↓ gastric emptying, thus ↑ degradation of levodopa in gut, and ↓ amount absorbed	Watch for ↓ levodopa effect when anticholinergics used in doses sufficient to ↓ GI motility. When anticholinergic therapy discontinued in a levodopa patient, watch for signs of levodopa toxicity. Anticholinergics can relieve symptoms of parkinsonism and might offset the reduction of levodopa bioavailability. Overall, interaction of minor significance.
Benzodiazepines	↓ levodopa effect	Mechanism unknown	Use together with caution; discontinue if interaction observed.
Ferrous sulfate	↓ levodopa oral absorption by 50%	Formation of chelation complex	Avoid concomitant administration.
Food	↓ levodopa effect	Large, neutral amino acids compete with levodopa for intestinal absorption	Although levodopa usually taken with meals to slow absorption and ↓ central emetic effect, high-protein diets should be avoided.
MAOIs (e.g., phenelzine, tranylcypromine)	Hypertensive crisis	↑ peripheral dopamine and norepinephrine	Avoid using together; selegiline and levodopa used successfully together. Carbidopa might minimize hypertensive reaction to levodopa in patients receiving an MAOI.
Methyldopa	↑ or ↓ levodopa effect	Acts as central and peripheral decarboxylase inhibitor	Observe for response, may need to switch to another antihypertensive.
Metoclopramide	↓ levodopa effect	Central dopamine blockade	Avoid using together; domperidone; a peripheral dopamine blocking antiemetic preferred.[b]
Moclobemide	↑ adverse effects (e.g., nausea, headache)	Not established	Although MAO-B is more important than MAO-A in the metabolism of dopamine, an MAO-A inhibitor such as moclobemide may have some effect on dopamine response.
Neuroleptics (e.g., butyrophenones, phenothiazines)	↓ levodopa effect	Central blockade of dopamine neurotransmission	Important interaction; avoid using these drugs together.
Papaverine	↓ levodopa effect	Unknown; might block dopamine receptors	Should be avoided. Therapeutic response to levodopa returns 5–10 days after papaverine discontinued.
Phenytoin	↓ levodopa effect	Mechanism unknown	Avoid using together if possible.
Pyridoxine	↓ levodopa effect	↑ peripheral decarboxylation of levodopa	Not observed when levodopa given with carbidopa
Reserpine	↓ levodopa effect	Central dopamine depletion	Clinical evidence lacking; best to avoid if possible
Tacrine	↓ levodopa effect	↑ central cholinergic activity	Try to avoid combination. Doses of tacrine and/or antiparkinsonian drugs may need to be adjusted if used concomitantly.
TCAs	↓ levodopa effect	↑ levodopa degradation in gut because of delayed emptying	TCAs and levodopa have been used successfully together; use with caution.

[a]For more information regarding these and other levodopa drug interactions, see Hansten PD, Horn JR. Drug Interactions & Updates Quarterly. St. Louis: Facts and Comparisons, 2001.
[b]Not available in the United States.
MAO-A, monoamine oxidase A; MAO-B, monoamine oxidase B; MAOI, monoamine oxidase inhibitor; TCAs, tricyclic antidepressants.

amount of carbidopa is administered.[130] The tricyclic antidepressants also possess significant anticholinergic properties that may delay gastric emptying, exacerbate orthostatic hypotension, and increase levodopa degradation in the gut.[132,133] In addition, these properties may result in additive toxicity in patients concomitantly receiving anticholinergic agents or in patients like L.M. who have conditions that can be exacerbated by anticholinergic therapy. Nonselective MAO inhibitors such as phenelzine (Nardil) and tranylcypromine (Parnate) are used to treat certain types of depressive disorders; however, these should be avoided in patients taking levodopa because hypertensive crisis is a significant risk.[134] Selegiline selectively binds to MAO-B receptors in the central nervous system and does not cause a hypertensive reaction.[137]

Since depression is related to serotonin metabolism, other classes of antidepressants that act specifically on serotonergic mechanisms such as fluoxetine (Prozac), sertraline (Zoloft), paroxetine (Paxil), nefazodone (Serzone), or trazodone (Desyrel) can be used to treat depression in PD patients.[129] However, selective serotonin reuptake inhibitors (SSRIs) such as fluoxetine can be activating. While this may be beneficial in patients who are apathetic or withdrawn, it may worsen symptoms in agitated patients.[28] Fluoxetine also has a prolonged elimination half-life and is metabolized to an active metabolite, which can increase the risk for side effects even after the drug is withdrawn. It is reasonable to start L.M. on an SSRI at the lowest dose and gradually titrate to effect. He should be observed carefully for adverse effects or changes in parkinsonian symptoms, including development of extrapyramidal symptoms, as well as any signs of psychomotor agitation.[138]

Visual hallucinations of PD are not usually bothersome to the patient and may be managed by offering reassurance, adjusting the levodopa dose, and eliminating any contributory agents other than levodopa (e.g., amantadine, anticholinergic agents, selegiline, antispasmodics, or tricyclic antidepressants).[28,129] However, if L.M.'s hallucinations worsen or become problematic, a trial of low-dose clozapine (12.5 mg at bedtime) may be initiated.[28,129] Clozapine is unique among antipsychotic drugs because it does not block striatal D_2 receptors or worsen parkinsonian symptoms.[139,140] However, L.M. must be monitored for adverse effects such as orthostatic hypotension and agranulocytosis as measured by weekly complete blood counts with differential for the first 6 months of therapy and every 2 weeks thereafter. A disadvantage of this approach in L.M. is that clozapine frequently causes sialorrhea, and for L.M. this is a pre-existing condition. Alternatively, newer selective neuroleptics such as olanzapine or quetiapine may be tried, as they may have less propensity for causing agranulocytosis.

16. To what extent is levodopa contributing to the nausea L.M. is experiencing, and what can be done to manage it?

Although carbidopa is concomitantly administered with levodopa to reduce the incidence of peripheral side effects, nausea, vomiting, and anorexia occur frequently. Usually 75 to 100 mg of carbidopa is required to completely inhibit peripheral decarboxylases; however, some patients may benefit from additional doses of carbidopa (Lodosyn) administered 25 mg three times daily. Alternatively, domperidone is a peripheral dopamine receptor antagonist with antiemetic properties that cannot penetrate the blood–brain barrier, and it has been effective when administered at a dosage of 20 to 30 mg 30 minutes before each levodopa dose.[28,141] Unfortunately, this drug is not yet available in the United States.

Drug Holiday

17. What is the current status of "drug holidays" in the management of PD?

The concept of a drug holiday in PD was prompted by observations of improved response in patients whose levodopa therapy was temporarily discontinued while they were undergoing surgical procedures or for other reasons.[142] Defined as a brief period of drug withdrawal, the drug holiday has been attempted in the past as a means of improving response and minimizing side effects in patients on long-term levodopa therapy.[142–144] Theoretically, long-term levodopa downregulates dopamine receptors.[116,142] The drug holiday is believed to exert a beneficial effect by allowing striatal dopamine receptors to be resensitized.[142] Although some studies have demonstrated a temporary benefit, other studies show no improvement in motor performance or the side effect profile at 6 months and 1 year following a 10-day period of levodopa withdrawal.[143–145]

Drug holidays can pose substantial risks because the immobility experienced by patients during the withdrawal period can have devastating psychological and physiologic consequences. Drug holidays require hospitalization and careful observation for complications of immobility such as deep venous thrombosis, aspiration pneumonia, and decubitus ulcer formation.[142,144] Also, potentially fatal hyperpyrexic reactions have been reported.[146] Because of the serious complications and the lack of sustained improvement, a drug holiday should not be considered for L.M.

Interference With Laboratory Tests

18. L.M. returned to the neurology clinic for his routine follow-up visit and had a panel of laboratory tests performed. Laboratory results are electrolytes (sodium, potassium, chloride, CO_2), within normal limits; blood urea nitrogen (BUN), 22 mg/dL; creatinine, 0.9 mg/dL; complete blood count (hemoglobin, hematocrit, white blood cell count), within normal limits. Other values included uric acid, 8.0 mg/dL; aspartate aminotransferase (AST), 15 IU; alanine aminotransferase (ALT), 35 IU; alkaline phosphatase, 190 mg/dL; fasting glucose, 190 mg/dL, with "trace" glucose and 1+ ketones on urinalysis. Which of these laboratory results may be affected by levodopa therapy?

[SI units: uric acid, 475.84 mmol/L; AST, 15 U/L; ALT, 19 U/L; glucose, 10.55 mmol/L]

Several of the laboratory abnormalities displayed by L.M. may be related to levodopa therapy. Levodopa has been associated with asymptomatic elevations in serum uric acid levels that are believed to be caused by interfering substances produced by levodopa metabolism (DOPAC), creating false elevations when determined by the colorimetric method.[147,148] Elevations do not occur when the uricase method is used.[147] Gout was reported in two patients receiving levodopa who had no apparent history of the disease, but the relationship between levodopa and gout is unclear. However, given his history of gout, L.M. should be watched for signs and symptoms of an acute gouty attack.

Mild elevations in BUN have been observed and may improve with hydration.[93] Elevations in AST, ALT, lactate dehydrogenase, bilirubin, and alkaline phosphatase all have been reported.[93] However, the AST, ALT, and alkaline phosphatase levels reported for L.M. are within normal limits. Levodopa can increase fasting blood sugar and may decrease glucose tolerance, but a direct correlation between levodopa and diabetes has not been established.[149] False-positive "trace" readings have been seen without glucosuria when urine is tested by the copper reductase method (Clinitest), and false-negative readings with glucosuria can occur with the glucose oxidase method (Clinistix, Tes-Tape).[150,151] False-negative readings with Tes-Tape can be averted by holding the tape vertically and reading the uppermost region of the strip.[150,151] Finally, false-positive readings for urine ketones may result with the Ketostix and Labstix testing methods.[152]

Catechol-O-Methyltransferase Inhibitors

Although levodopa has been the mainstay of symptomatic treatment of PD for almost 30 years, the increased incidence of motor complications and mental disturbances that occur after prolonged therapy has prompted researchers to develop strategies other than replenishment of dopamine. One of these strategies is to prevent the peripheral degradation of levodopa by metabolizing enzymes.[153,154] Continuous dopaminergic stimulation with long-acting dopamine agonists such as cabergoline, continuous IV infusions of levodopa, and apomorphine reduced motor fluctuations in the advanced stages of PD.[110,111,117,118] Therefore, agents that promote tonic or continuous stimulation rather than intermittent or phasic stimulation of levodopa receptors may act similarly. Carbidopa, an inhibitor of aromatic L-amino acid decarboxylase (AAD),

prevents the peripheral conversion of levodopa to dopamine. With AAD inhibitors such as carbidopa or benserazide, the conversion of levodopa to 3-O-methyldopa (3-OMD) by COMT becomes a major metabolic pathway and is increased.[155] The metabolite 3-OMD lacks antiparkinsonian activity and may compete with levodopa for transport into the circulation and brain.

COMT is an enzyme found in many body tissues, especially the liver, kidney, and intestines.[154,155] Most of the enzyme exists as a soluble protein and a small percentage is membrane bound. COMT, which catalyzes the transfer of a methyl group of S-adenosyl-L-methionine to a phenolic group of the catechol, is responsible for the biotransformation of many catechols and hydroxylated metabolites.[156]

Mechanism of Action

Entacapone and tolcapone are selective, reversible, and potent COMT inhibitors that increase the amount of levodopa available for transport across the blood–brain barrier (Fig. 53-4).[157-159] This effect improves and prolongs the response to levodopa as measured by an increase in the amount of time spent "on" and a decrease in the daily levodopa dosage.[155] The pharmacologic and pharmacokinetic effects of entacapone and tolcapone are compared in Table 53-6.

Entacapone

19. Six months after switching to extended release levodopa, L.M. reports that his dyskinetic activity has lessened, but he is having periods (lasting a few minutes) in which he cannot move. He continues to take pramipexole 0.5 mg TID, Sinemet CR QID (Sinemet 50/200), and immediate-release levodopa/carbidopa 25/100 QD, but "even on a good day" gains symptomatic relief

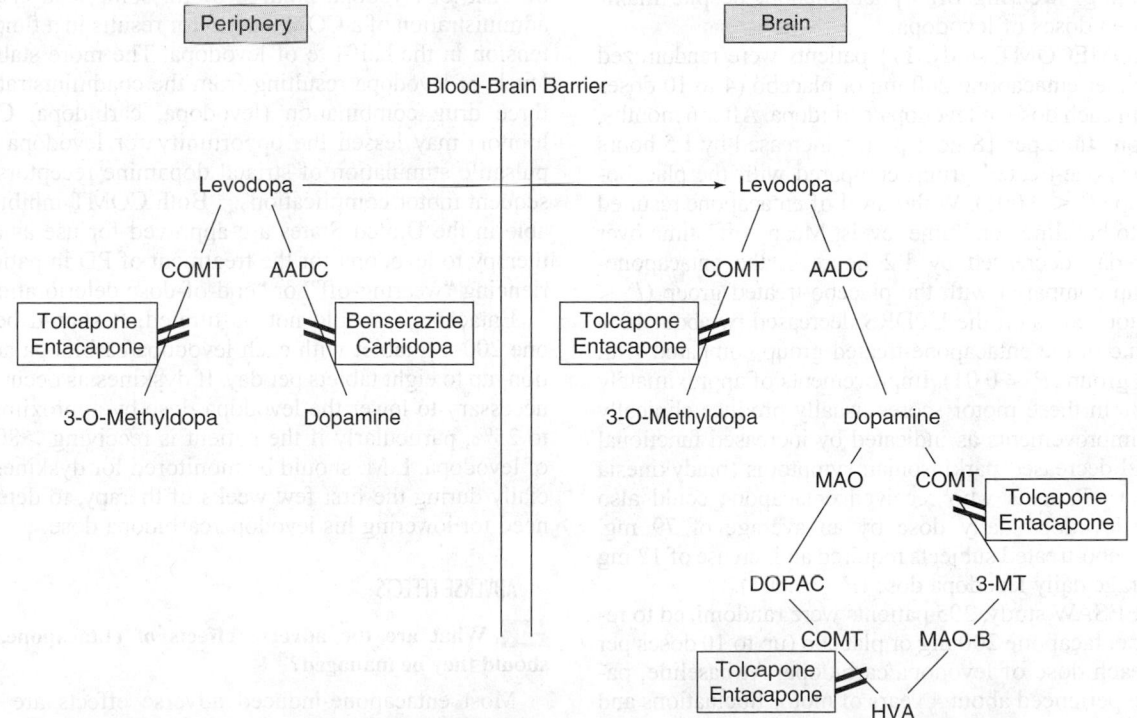

FIGURE 53-4. Levodopa metabolism in the human body. COMT, catechol-O-methyltransferase; AADC, aromatic amino acid decarboxylase; DOPAC, dihydroxyphenylacetic acid; 3-MT, 3-methoxytyramine; MAO, monoamine oxidase.

Table 53-6   Pharmacologic and Pharmacokinetic Properties of Catechol-O-Methyltransferase Inhibitors

	Tolcapone	Entacapone
Bioavailability	65%	30–46%
T_{max} (hr)	2.0	0.7–1.2
Protein binding	99.9%	98%
Metabolism	Glucuronidation; CYP 3A4, 2A6 Acetylation; methylated by COMT	Glucuronidation
Half-life (hr)	2–3	1.6–3.4
Time to reverse COMT inhibition (hr)	16–24	4–8
Maximum COMT inhibition at 200-mg dose	80–90%	60%
Increase in levodopa AUC	100%	30–45%
Increase in levodopa half-life	75%	60–75%
Dosing method	TID, spaced 6 hr apart	With every administration of levodopa

COMT, catechol-O-methyltransferase.

for only about 2 to 3 hours following a dose. Also, he reports continued visual hallucinations and nightmares. The decision is made to gradually discontinue pramipexole and to initiate entacapone therapy. How effective is entacapone for improving the symptoms of PD?

EFFICACY

The efficacy and safety of entacapone as an adjunct to levodopa therapy have been studied in two long-term phase III trials. The NOMECOMT study was conducted in the Nordic countries;[160] the Safety and Efficacy Study of Entacapone Assessing Wearing Off (SEESAW) study[161] was conducted in North America. Both trials were multicenter, randomized, double-blind, placebo-controlled, parallel-group studies. Subjects for both studies had idiopathic PD with motor fluctuations, including "wearing off" phenomenon, despite maximum tolerated doses of levodopa.

In the NOMECOMT study, 171 patients were randomized to receive either entacapone 200 mg or placebo (4 to 10 doses per day) with each dose of levodopa/carbidopa. After 6 months, the mean "on" time per 18-hour period increased by 1.5 hours in the entacapone-treated group compared with the placebo-treated group ($P < 0.001$). Withdrawal of entacapone resulted in a return to baseline "on" time levels. Mean "off" time over an 18-hour day decreased by 1.2 hours in the entacapone-treated group compared with the placebo-treated group ($P < 0.001$). Motor scores on the UPDRS decreased by about 10% from baseline in the entacapone-treated group compared with the placebo group ($P < 0.01$). Improvements of approximately 10% to 20% in these motor scores usually produce clinically significant improvements as indicated by increased functional capacity and decreased parkinsonian symptoms (bradykinesia and rigidity).[28] Patients who received entacapone could also lower their levodopa daily dose by an average of 79 mg, whereas placebo-treated subjects required an increase of 12 mg in their average daily levodopa dose ($P < 0.001$).

In the SEESAW study, 205 patients were randomized to receive either entacapone 200 mg or placebo (up to 10 doses per day) with each dose of levodopa/carbidopa. At baseline, patients had experienced about 4 years of motor fluctuations and had been taking levodopa for about 9 years. Approximately 80% of the study subjects continued to take other antiparkinsonian therapies, including anticholinergic agents, selegiline,

dopamine agonists, and amantadine. Compared with placebo over 8 to 24 weeks, daily "on" time increased by about 1 hour ($P < 0.05$), with the greatest improvements observed in those who had a smaller percentage of "on" time at baseline. Entacapone-treated patients also had about a 10% reduction in their total UPDRS scores, and they could decrease their daily levodopa dose by about 100 mg (13%).

DOSING

20. When should entacapone be initiated, and what is the most effective method for dosing the drug?

No studies have yet examined the effect of early initiation of a COMT inhibitor from the time levodopa is first introduced. This strategy has been proposed as a way of reducing the risk for levodopa-induced motor complications, since the administration of a COMT inhibitor results in a functional extension in the half-life of levodopa. The more stable plasma levels of levodopa resulting from the coadministration of the three drug combination (levodopa, carbidopa, COMT inhibitor) may lessen the opportunity for levodopa to induce pulsatile stimulation of striatal dopamine receptors and consequent motor complications.[28] Both COMT inhibitors available in the United States are approved for use as adjunctive therapy to levodopa for the treatment of PD in patients experiencing "wearing-off" or "end-of-dose deterioration."

Entacapone should not be titrated. It should be given as one 200-mg tablet with each levodopa/carbidopa administration, up to eight tablets per day. If dyskinesias occur, it may be necessary to lower the levodopa dose by approximately 10% to 25%, particularly if the patient is receiving >800 mg/day of levodopa. L.M. should be monitored for dyskinesias, especially during the first few weeks of therapy, to determine the need for lowering his levodopa/carbidopa dose.

ADVERSE EFFECTS

21. What are the adverse effects of entacapone, and how should they be managed?

Most entacapone-induced adverse effects are consistent with increased levodopa exposure. They include dyskinesias (50% to 60%), nausea (15% to 20%), dizziness (10% to 25%), and hallucinations (1% to 14%).[160,161] Reducing the levodopa dosage by 10% to 15% as a strategy for circumventing these effects was successful in about one third of patients experiencing dyskinesias. One study evaluated the incidence of dyskinesias compared with baseline frequency and found an increase of 8% in the entacapone-treated group.[160] Adverse effects related to entacapone include urine discoloration (11% to 40%), abdominal pain (6%), and diarrhea (10%).[160,161] Urine discoloration (brownish-orange) is attributed to the color of entacapone and its metabolites and is considered benign, but patients should be counseled regarding this effect to avoid undue concern. The most common reason for withdrawal from clinical studies and discontinuation of therapy was severe diarrhea (2.5%). One of the 406 patients studied in both studies cited experienced an elevation in liver transaminases. No monitoring of liver function tests is required during entacapone therapy.

Tolcapone

22. How does tolcapone compare to entacapone for treating the symptoms of PD?

Tolcapone, like entacapone, is a dose-dependent reversible inhibitor of COMT.[162] The pharmacologic effects of tolcapone are similar to those of entacapone, with several differences (see Table 53-6). Tolcapone is slightly more potent and has a longer duration of action.[163,164] Unlike entacapone, which is usually given with every administration of levodopa/carbidopa (up to eight tablets per day), tolcapone is dosed three times daily,. No studies have directly compared the efficacy of entacapone and tolcapone. Clinical studies and postmarketing experience data gathered so far indicate that entacapone has a lower incidence of hepatotoxicity and diarrhea than tolcapone.[160,161,165]

EFFICACY

The efficacy of tolcapone has been studied in patients with and without response fluctuations, such as "wearing off" despite maximum tolerated doses of levodopa.[166–168] Two large multicenter, randomized, double-blind, placebo-controlled studies in the United States and Europe have evaluated the efficacy of tolcapone in patients with motor fluctuations, including "on-off" and "wearing off" effects.[166,167] These studies showed that after 3 months of treatment, those in the tolcapone-treated group gained an additional 1 to 2 hours of "on" time relative to the placebo-treated group and could reduce their levodopa dose by about 20% to 30%. Another trial evaluated the efficacy of tolcapone in 298 patients on levodopa therapy who had not yet developed motor fluctuations.[168] After 6 months of treatment, tolcapone produced a 20% improvement in the UPDRS scores for ADLs. In addition, the mean total daily dose of levodopa decreased by 20 to 30 mg in the tolcapone-treated group, whereas the placebo-treated group had a mean increase of 50 mg.[168]

DOSING

23. What is the most effective method for dosing tolcapone?

Tolcapone is indicated as an adjunct to levodopa therapy; it has no significant antiparkinsonian effect when administered as monotherapy. Tolcapone does not require a titration phase and is initiated at a dosage of 100 to 200 mg three times

daily, with doses spaced at least 6 hours apart.[165] Although food reduces the bioavailability of tolcapone by 10% to 20%, this effect is unlikely to be clinically significant; therefore, tolcapone may be administered without regard to meals.[165] Because tolcapone reduces levodopa metabolism, reduction of the levodopa dosage should be considered when initiating tolcapone therapy. In clinical trials, the dosage of levodopa was reduced by 25% to 30% in approximately 70% of patients with dyskinesias before tolcapone therapy was begun.[165–168]

ADVERSE EFFECTS

24. What are the adverse effects of tolcapone, and how should they be managed? How should tolcapone therapy be monitored?

The adverse effects of tolcapone are consistent with increased levodopa exposure and include worsening of dyskinesias (40% to 50%), nausea (30% to 35%), sleep disorders (15%), dystonia (20%), anorexia (20%), somnolence (15%), hallucinations (10%), and postural hypotension (17%).[165] Reducing the levodopa dosage is a strategy for circumventing these effects. Urine discoloration (brownish-orange) also occurs and is attributed to the color of tolcapone and its metabolites. Additional tolcapone-related adverse effects include headache, abdominal pain, and diarrhea (17%).[165] Severe diarrhea is the most common reason for withdrawal from therapy (3% to 4%), and hospitalization occurred in 1.7% of patients receiving the 200-mg, three-times-daily dose. The onset of diarrhea may be delayed by up to 3 months after initiation of therapy.[165]

In clinical trials, patients receiving tolcapone 200 mg three times daily were more likely to develop elevations of AST and ALT.[165–168] Subsequently, rare cases of severe and potentially fatal hepatotoxicity have been reported.[165,169] Consequently, tolcapone should not be given to patients with underlying liver disease, and its use should be discontinued if a satisfactory response has not been achieved within 3 weeks. Liver function tests should be monitored at baseline, every 2 weeks during the first year of therapy, every 4 weeks during the next 6 months of therapy, and every 8 weeks thereafter.[165] The drug should be immediately discontinued if liver function tests exceed the normal values. Before tolcapone therapy is initiated, a written informed consent should be obtained (as advised by the manufacturer in the product labeling). The patient should be educated about the importance of compliance with liver function testing to avoid irreversible liver injury. Because of the potential for liver toxicity, the use of tolcapone has been severely restricted, and entacapone should be the COMT inhibitor of choice.

Monoamine Oxidase-B Inhibitors

Selegiline

25. What type of antiparkinsonian drug is selegiline, and what place does it have in the treatment of PD?

MECHANISM OF ACTION

Selegiline (also referred to as deprenyl) is an MAO inhibitor that irreversibly inhibits MAO type B (MAO-B).[28,170] Two types of MAO enzymes are present: type A (MAO-A) oxidatively deaminates catecholamines such as serotonin, norepinephrine, and tyramine, and MAO-B, among other actions, is responsible for the metabolism of dopamine.[28,170] Within the brain, approximately 80% of MAO activity is attributable to MAO-B.[170] The antiparkinsonian activity of selegiline presumably lies in its ability to act centrally to prevent the destruction of endogenous and exogenously administered dopamine.[170] Because selegiline selectively binds to MAO-B, it does not, in usual doses, produce a hypertensive reaction ("cheese effect") with dietary tyramine or other catecholamines.[170]

EFFICACY

Selegiline has been studied in PD since 1975. Although results have been variable, it can improve the "wearing off" effect of levodopa in 50% to 70% of patients and may allow as much as a 30% reduction in the total daily dose of levodopa.[171,172] The "on-off" effect is less responsive to the addition of selegiline.[171,172] Modest symptomatic improvement is seen when selegiline is used alone in early forms of the disease. Data from the Deprenyl and Tocopherol Antioxidative Therapy of Parkinsonism (DATATOP) study extension trials have been useful in delineating the role of this agent. Overall, the benefits of selegiline are only modest, and tolerance to the beneficial effects is seen with long-term use.

Selegiline is well tolerated by most patients, provided it is not given late in the evening, when excess stimulation from metabolites (L-methamphetamine and L-amphetamine) can cause insomnia and other psychiatric side effects.[170] Importantly, the potency of the L-amphetamine metabolites of selegiline is only one-tenth that of the d-isomeric form found in commercial amphetamine products (e.g., dextroamphetamine); the administered form of selegiline is the L-isomer. The usual dosage of selegiline is 10 mg/day given in 5-mg doses in the morning and early afternoon.[170]

USE TO SLOW DISEASE PROGRESSION

26. Can selegiline slow the progression of L.M.'s PD?

Attention initially focused on the potential of selegiline as an agent that could conceivably slow the progression of PD.[10,11,170,173–177] Birkmayer[173] was the first to suggest that the addition of selegiline to levodopa therapy leads to increased life expectancy; however, the data supporting this assertion were uncontrolled and retrospective in nature.

With the discovery of parkinsonism developing in addicts who injected L-methyl-4-phenyl-1,2,3,6-tetrahydropyridine (MPTP), a synthetic meperidine analog, exciting new information regarding the pathophysiology and potential for new forms of treatment began to emerge.[10,174] With the isolation and identification of this compound came the development of superior animal models in which it was found that the neurotoxicity associated with MPTP is not caused by MPTP itself, but rather the oxidized product, L-methyl-4- phenylpyridinium ion (MPP), a compound that can persist for long periods in the brain.[174] The conversion of MPTP to its neurotoxic metabolite MPP is a two-step process mediated in part by MAO-B.[174,175] Inhibition of MAO-B can inhibit the oxidative conversion of dopamine to potentially reactive peroxides. In animals, pretreatment with selegiline protects against neuronal damage following the administration of MPTP.[176]

If PD is caused by an environmental toxin similar to MPTP (or perhaps MPTP itself), then it is reasonable to hypothesize

that treatment with MAO-B inhibitors, such as selegiline, might retard neuronal degeneration. Furthermore, as the brain dopamine content declines in parkinsonian patients, a compensatory increase in dopamine generation and metabolism by remaining neurons generates free radicals that also are capable of causing neuronal damage.[11,177] Antioxidative therapy aimed at decreasing the activity of these free radicals also may prove to be beneficial. At present, the only well-documented data regarding the value of antioxidants are from the following descriptions of DATATOP studies.

The DATATOP study was initiated by the Parkinson Study Group to test the hypothesis that the combined use of both an MAO-B inhibitor (selegiline) and an antioxidant (α-tocopherol) early in the course of the disease may slow disease progression.[177–180] The principal outcome measure was the length of time that patients could be sustained without levodopa therapy (an indication of disease progression). Results of this study demonstrated that early treatment with selegiline 10 mg/day delayed the need to start levodopa therapy by approximately 9 months compared with patients given placebo.[178] However, long-term observation demonstrated that the benefits of selegiline diminished over time.

During an additional year of observation, patients originally randomized to selegiline tended to reach the end point of disability more quickly than did those not assigned to receive selegiline. Initial selegiline treatment also did not alter the development of levodopa adverse effects such as dyskinesias and "wearing-off" and "on-off" phenomena. In other words, early treatment with this agent did not produce a sustained benefit.[179] In addition, no evidence indicates that selegiline administration can alter the cognitive decline noted in PD patients. No conclusive data support the notion that selegiline possesses neuroprotective properties that may slow disease progression. More likely, the DATATOP study results reflect modest early symptomatic benefit from the drug.

Regardless of the exact mechanism, results from the DATATOP study suggest that the early use of selegiline can delay the need for levodopa therapy in patients with untreated disease, perhaps by retarding disease progression. This delay in the need to initiate levodopa therapy may be clinically relevant and important to many patients. Conceivably, to be effective as a neuroprotective agent, therapy with selegiline may need to be introduced *before* the onset of clinically recognizable disease. As discussed previously, significant reductions in nigrostriatal dopaminergic neurons occur before the development of parkinsonian symptoms, and this latent period may last for years. Advances in the early diagnosis of PD may facilitate future investigations in neuroprotective therapy.

In summary, there is no convincing evidence that selegiline offers neuroprotection in patients with PD.[28,42] Until more information becomes available, selegiline should be considered only for supportive therapy in L.M. Its efficacy in reducing the "wearing off" effect is modest at best, and selegiline is not effective in controlling the "on-off" effect that L.M. has been experiencing. Thus, for L.M., selegiline does not appear to offer any advantages at this time.

27. Does selegiline administration lead to increased mortality?

Early observations of decreased mortality in PD patients receiving selegiline were reported by Birkmayer and associates.[173] More recently, long-term mortality has been evaluated in the DATATOP study group. After an average of 8 years of observation, an annual mortality rate of 2.1% per year was observed, a rate comparable to what would be expected for age-matched controls.[180] Other intervention trials evaluating selegiline have also suggested that although this agent does not extend life expectancy in PD patients, there was no evidence of increased mortality.[181] In contrast, the U.K. Parkinson's Disease Research Group reported an increased mortality in patients receiving the combination of levodopa and selegiline compared with those receiving levodopa monotherapy.[182] However, these findings remain unexplained, and concerns regarding patient demographics and study methodology must temper the conclusions derived from this trial. Based on the available data, selegiline treatment in patients with early PD does not appear to extend life expectancy, nor are data compelling enough to suggest that it increases mortality.

Anticholinergics

28. Do anticholinergic drugs provide any benefit in the treatment of PD?

Anticholinergic drugs have been used to treat PD since 1867, when it was discovered that symptoms were improved by the belladonna derivative hyoscyamine sulfate (scopolamine).[28] These drugs remained the mainstay of treatment until the late 1960s, when amantadine and levodopa were introduced. Because of their undesirable side effect profile and poor efficacy, anticholinergic agents have been abandoned as first-line agents.

In PD, the loss of dopamine-producing neurons results in a loss of the balance that normally exists between acetylcholine and dopamine-mediated neurotransmission. The anticholinergic agents work by blocking the excitatory neurotransmitter acetylcholine in the striatum, thereby minimizing the effect of the relative increase in cholinergic sensitivity. This form of therapy is usually reserved for the treatment of resting tremor early in the disease, particularly in younger patients with preserved cognitive function. Anticholinergic agents are considered less effective than levodopa/carbidopa or dopamine agonists for the treatment of bradykinesia and rigidity.[28] Overall, only a mild improvement in symptoms can be expected with anticholinergic therapy, and the risk for side effects would probably outweigh any benefit in L.M.[28,36]

Comparison of Agents

29. What are the most commonly used anticholinergic agents in PD? How are they administered?

The anticholinergic drugs of most value in PD are the synthetic agents that are more centrally selective than atropine and scopolamine (see Table 53-3).[28] The most commonly used anticholinergic drugs are trihexyphenidyl and benztropine. The antihistamines diphenhydramine, orphenadrine, phenothiazine, and ethopropazine have significant anticholinergic properties and are useful antiparkinsonian agents.

Although no single agent has been proven superior to another, patients who do not respond to one anticholinergic agent may respond to another. Many neurologists prefer one agent to another simply on the basis of having more experience with a particular drug. Benztropine, biperiden, and diphenhydramine are available in an injectable form, but the oral route is preferred unless the patient cannot take anything by mouth.

The dosage ranges of the anticholinergic agents are listed in Table 53-3. Therapy should be initiated with small doses and increased slowly as tolerated.[28] A response should be evident within days after starting therapy. Anticholinergic agents never should be abruptly discontinued because this has led to "withdrawal" reactions, characterized by an immediate worsening of parkinsonian symptoms in several patients.[28]

Adverse Effects

30. What are the adverse effects of anticholinergic agents? How might these affect the decision of whether to use one in L.M.?

Anticholinergic drugs produce both peripherally and centrally mediated side effects. Peripheral side effects such as dry mouth, blurred vision, constipation, and urinary retention are common and bothersome.[28] Anticholinergic agents can increase intraocular pressure and should be avoided in patients with angle-closure glaucoma. The central nervous system side effects of confusion, impairment of recent memory, hallucinations, and delusions are usually the most disturbing.[28] PD patients are more prone to the side effects of these drugs because of their older age, intercurrent illnesses, and impaired cognition.[28] If a patient experiences significant central nervous system side effects, the anticholinergic drug should be used in lower doses or discontinued.

Given his history and clinical presentation, L.M. probably should not be given an anticholinergic drug. He originally presented with signs of intellectual impairment and subsequently developed hallucinations. These symptoms may worsen on anticholinergic therapy. L.M. also has prostatic hyperplasia that could result in urinary retention if exacerbated by anticholinergic drugs. The mydriasis and cycloplegia associated with these drugs could interfere with his ability to paint. Finally, anticholinergic drugs also could aggravate his constipation.

Amantadine

31. How does amantadine work in PD, and what place does it have in treatment of the disease?

Amantadine, an antiviral agent, was discovered serendipitously to have antiparkinsonian activity when a patient given the drug for influenza experienced a remission in her tremor, rigidity, and bradykinesia.[183] Shortly thereafter, clinical trials documented its effectiveness when used alone and in combination with levodopa to treat mild forms of PD.[184–186]

Mechanism of Action

The precise mechanism of action of amantadine for PD treatment is not entirely understood, but it probably augments dopamine release from presynaptic nerve terminals and possibly inhibits dopamine reuptake into storage granules.[187] Others have suggested an anticholinergic mechanism of action because certain anticholinergic-type side effects are caused by the drug.[184] Recently, amantadine has been found to be an antagonist at N-methyl-D-aspartate (NMDA) receptors; therefore, it may block glutamate transmission and display antidyskinetic effects.[188] This finding has been corroborated in studies of PD patients.[185,189]

Efficacy

When 351 PD patients at various stages of the disease were treated with amantadine 200 mg/day for 60 days, an overall positive response was noted in 64% of the patients.[184] Patients receiving levodopa were more likely to respond than those who took amantadine alone (78% versus 48%, respectively). About half of the patients experienced a loss of efficacy 30 to 60 days after therapy was initiated.[184] A double-blind, placebo-controlled crossover study of 14 patients with advanced PD found that amantadine given as an adjunct to levodopa significantly reduced motor fluctuations.[185]

Amantadine improves all of the symptoms of parkinsonian disability in about 50% of patients, usually within days after starting therapy; however, a substantial number of patients develop tachyphylaxis within 1 to 3 months. Temporary withdrawal, discontinuation, and subsequent reinstitution of amantadine at a later date can be beneficial in some patients.[186] Although amantadine has enjoyed more widespread use in the past for PD, experts now agree that its use is limited by its potential for neuropsychiatric side effects, and more studies are necessary to delineate any role the drug may have in the management of levodopa-induced dyskinesias.[28]

32. How is therapy with amantadine initiated?

Initiation of Therapy

Amantadine should be started with one 100-mg capsule taken with breakfast; an additional 100-mg capsule can be taken with lunch 5 to 7 days after the initiation of the drug.[184] The dosage can be increased to a maximum of 300 mg/day; however, doses >200 mg/day are rarely necessary and pose a greater risk of adverse effects. The second dose is best taken in the early afternoon to minimize the likelihood of insomnia. Amantadine also is available in a liquid preparation, which is advantageous for patients with dysphagia. The liquid formulation allows more subtle dosage adjustments, but such adjustments are rarely necessary.

Amantadine is renally excreted and the dosage needs to be reduced in patients with renal impairment (Table 53-7).[190,191] Because the elimination half-life is about 7 days in patients with end-stage renal disease, a loading dose of 200 mg on the first day of therapy is recommended for patients with significant renal impairment.[191] Insignificant amounts of amantadine are removed by hemodialysis.[191] Baseline blood urea nitrogen

Table 53-7 Amantadine Dosing Guidelines in Renal Impairment

Creatinine Clearance (mL/min/1.73 m²)	Suggested Maintenance Regimen
>80	100 mg BID
60	200 mg/100 mg alternate days
50	100 mg/day
40	100 mg/day
30	200 mg TIW[a]
20	100 mg TIW
10	200 mg/100 mg alternating Q 7 days[b]

[a]Loading dose of 200 mg recommended on the first day for creatinine clearance, 30 mL/min.
[b]Includes patients maintained on thrice-weekly hemodialysis.

and serum creatinine concentrations should be evaluated before therapy is initiated and periodically (e.g., every 3 months) thereafter.

33. What side effects are reported with amantadine?

Adverse Effects

Side effects of amantadine mainly involve the gastrointestinal, cardiovascular, and central nervous systems. In one large-scale study, at least one side effect was experienced by 15% of patients, while 9% had two or more adverse effects.[184] Amantadine was discontinued because of side effects in only 5% of patients. Neuropsychiatric complaints are seen most frequently and include dizziness, confusion, disorientation, depression, nervousness, irritability, insomnia, nightmares, and hallucinations.[95,184,185] Convulsions have been observed on rare occasions with high dosages (>800 mg/day), particularly in patients with renal impairment.[95] Amantadine does have some anticholinergic properties, and patients concomitantly receiving anticholinergic agents appear to experience more prominent central nervous system side effects.[95,184,185] Dry mouth, nausea, vomiting, cramps, diarrhea, and constipation are less frequently encountered. Amantadine can cause mild elevations in blood urea nitrogen and alkaline phosphatase, which are believed not to be clinically important.[95,191] Patients receiving amantadine should be monitored carefully for gastrointestinal and central nervous system complaints. The gastrointestinal side effects can be managed by taking the drug with food.

Livedo reticularis is a rose-colored mottling of the skin, usually involving the lower extremities (but can involve the upper extremities as well), that occurs in up to 80% of patients receiving amantadine.[95,185,186,190] It can be observed as early as 2 weeks after initiating amantadine therapy and persists until therapy is discontinued, often intensifying to a blackish-purple color.[185] It is more commonly observed in women taking higher dosages (>200 mg/day) and is worse on standing and in colder climates.[95,185] Livedo reticularis is believed to be caused by local release of catecholamines, which cause vasoconstriction and alter the permeability of cutaneous blood vessels.[190] The consequences of livedo reticularis are entirely cosmetic; therefore, discontinuation of therapy is unnecessary.

Ankle edema occurs in up to 10% of patients, usually in association with livedo reticularis, and may contribute to congestive heart failure and related problems.[95] Elevation of the legs, diuretic therapy, and dosage reduction often alleviate the edema.

Antioxidant Therapy/Supplements

34. What antioxidants or supplements that have been evaluated in the treatment of PD?

If free radical generation is important in the pathophysiology of PD, then adjunctive therapy with antioxidant drugs early in the course of disease may offer some benefit.[192] The most comprehensive evaluation of antioxidant therapy for PD has come from the DATATOP study.[177,178,193] In this study, patients were assigned to one of four treatment regimens: α-tocopherol (2,000 IU/day) and selegiline placebo, selegiline 10 mg/day and α-tocopherol placebo, selegiline and α-tocopherol active treatments, or placebos. After approximately 14 months of follow-up, the results indicated that although selegiline had an initial beneficial effect (as previously described), significant additional benefit derived from α-tocopherol therapy was not observed.[193] Thus, despite the theoretical benefit, clinical data are lacking to support the routine use of α-tocopherol.

Coenzyme Q10 is an antioxidant involved in the mitochondrial electron transport chain that has been shown to have reduced activity in PD patients.[194] The finding that MPTP can induce parkinsonism through inhibition of complex I in the mitochondrial electron transport chain, resulting in injury of nigral dopaminergic neurons, led investigators to evaluate whether supplementation with coenzyme Q10 could restore dysfunctional mitochondria. In a randomized, placebo-controlled trial, 80 patients with early untreated PD were randomly assigned to placebo or coenzyme Q10 at dosages of 300, 600, or 1,200 mg/day in four divided doses.[195] Subjects were followed for up to 16 months or until therapy with levodopa was required. The primary outcome variable was a change in total score on the UPDRS from baseline to the last visit. Total UPDRS scores increased (indicating worsening of symptoms) to a greater extent in placebo-treated patients than in coenzyme Q10–treated patients (+11.99 for placebo, +8.81 for 300 mg/day, +10.82 for 600 mg/day, and +6.69 for 1200 mg/day). These results indicated a linear trend between coenzyme Q10 dosage and changes in UPDRS scores. However, time to requirement of levodopa was not different among the groups. Side effects of coenzyme Q10 were minimal and not different than placebo.

Although it is too early to recommend routine use of coenzyme Q10, the results from this study appear promising and support a possible role of mitochondrial dysfunction in the pathogenesis of PD. A similar model of restoration of dysfunctional mitochondria has been proposed with glutathione supplementation, and studies are ongoing to assess its efficacy.[196] Future studies are needed to delineate the role of coenzyme Q10 and/or other antioxidants and supplements in the therapy of PD.

Adjunctive Treatment of Parkinsonian Tremor

35. L.M. has gained additional improvement in rigidity, bradykinesia, and posture, as well as improvement in the "on-off" and "wearing off" effects, with the combination of Sinemet (carbidopa/levodopa) and entacapone. He has experienced little if any improvement in his tremor, which is one of the most debilitating symptoms of his disease. What are other therapies for severe parkinsonian tremor?

Parkinsonian tremor is often less responsive to dopaminergic therapy than other symptoms. There can be considerable interpatient variability in the frequency and amplitude of parkinsonian tremor. Tremor can be worsened by peripheral factors such as catecholamine release, often in association with stress or anxiety, as well as central factors inherent to the disease.[197]

β-Adrenergic Blockers
Adjunctive therapy with β-adrenergic blockers in double-blind, placebo-controlled trials improves parkinsonian tremor in approximately 50% of patients.[197,198] An early study of propranolol (Inderal) showed subjective and objective improve-

ment in the severity of tremor of 54% in resting tremor, 32% in postural tremor, and 54% in intention tremor at a maximum dosage of 240 mg/day.[197] Nadolol (Corgard) treatment did not affect the frequency but significantly reduced the amplitude of tremor in the patients studied.[198] These results suggest that β-blocker therapy can be safe and effective in selected patients with debilitating tremor.

L.M. may benefit from a trial of a β-blocker for his tremor. Nadolol would be the preferred choice because it is less lipophilic than propranolol and does not cross the blood–brain barrier; thus, it is less likely to cause central nervous system side effects such as depression, which has been a problem for L.M.[198] Also, nadolol can be dosed once daily because it has a longer half-life than propranolol. L.M. is already taking several medications at frequent intervals over the course of a day; therefore, the simplicity of giving the drug once daily has appeal. Therapy can be initiated at 40 to 60 mg/day and increased weekly to a maximum of 320 mg/day. The dosage should be reduced if bradycardia or hypotension is encountered.

Clozapine
Several reports suggest a beneficial effect of the neuroleptic clozapine (Clozaril) on parkinsonian symptoms.[199–201] Although the precise mechanisms are not well understood, low doses of clozapine can reduce the severity of levodopa-related dyskinesias,[200] improve resting tremor, and modulate the severity of levodopa-induced motor fluctuations (i.e., "on-off").[199] Given the potential for serious toxicity (agranulocytosis) to clozapine, and the preliminary nature of these findings, indiscriminate use of adjunctive clozapine should be discouraged until more data are available.

Surgery
Surgery has played a role in the management of PD, particularly in patients who cannot achieve a satisfactory response to available medications (see Fig. 53-1). Before the introduction of levodopa, PD was primarily viewed as a surgically treated condition. With the availability of effective drug therapies, the importance of surgical intervention lessened.[202–208] Posteroventral pallidotomy is an effective method for reducing dyskinesias on the contralateral side and may permit the use of higher dosages of levodopa for managing rigidity and bradykinesia.[203,204] One of its disadvantages is the need to make a lesion near the optic tract; however, studies have shown significant improvements in rigidity and bradykinesia and also relief from tremor following posteroventral pallidotomy. The risks of pallidotomy include visual loss, weakness, including paralysis, and hemorrhage that can cause stroke and speech difficulty.

In patients with mild forms of parkinsonism in which bradykinesia and gait disturbances are absent, symptoms of debilitating tremor and rigidity can benefit from stereotaxic thalamotomy. This intervention has eliminated contralateral tremor in 80% of patients, and improvement has been sustained for up to 10 years.[204,205] A disadvantage of both pallidotomy and thalamotomy is the need to make an irreversible lesion in the basal ganglia that may limit the effectiveness of newer procedures as they become available.

Deep brain stimulation (DBS) is a method that uses an implanted electrode in the brain with a lead connected to a subcutaneously implanted pacemaker.[206,207] This permits delivery of a high-frequency stimulation to the desired target. DBS of the globus pallidus not only improves the symptoms of PD but also reduces dyskinesias, thus permitting the use of increased levodopa dosages. Its other advantages include (1) no need for an irreversible brain lesion; (2) possibility of low-risk bilateral procedures; and (3) flexibility for altering the target site and program stimulation parameters. However, DBS is a relatively new and expensive procedure that is not widely available. Stimulation of the subthalamic nucleus and the internal segment of the globus pallidus both have been shown to improve motor signs of PD. Additional research may refine the target areas for optimal stimulation.

Attention also has been directed toward surgical treatment of PD by transplanting fetal dopaminergic neurons directly into dopamine-depleted regions of the basal ganglia in the hopes of providing a localized infusion of dopamine from these cells.[207,208] The observed benefits from this procedure have included improved motor response while lowering the incidence and severity of dyskinesias.[207] Research efforts also include transplanting genetically engineered cell lines such as those capable of overexpressing tyrosine hydroxylase or neurotrophic factors. However, all of these methods are considered experimental and are not yet available.[207]

Other Treatment Considerations in PD

Dementia

36. As L.M.'s disease has progressed, he has become increasingly demented. He scored 16 (below normal) on his most recent Mini-Mental Status Examination, and his family describes periodic episodes of hostility and defiance toward others. Subsequent neuropsychiatric testing confirmed dementia, probably of subcortical origin. His physician recommended that he avoid driving and receive 24-hour supervision, along with participation in structured leisure activities. In addition, L.M. has become increasingly reliant on family members for help in performing ADLs. He now attends adult day care three times per week for 4 hours to help relieve his wife's caregiver burden. How should L.M.'s progressive cognitive decline be managed?

Cognitive impairment, manifested by bradyphrenia (slowed mental processes), altered executive functions, memory loss, decreased attention span, or inappropriate behavior, is common in patients with PD. The prevalence of dementia in patients with PD increases with age and duration of disease and is approximately 6- to 12-fold greater than in age-matched controls.[28] Successful management of cognitive impairment in PD patients requires first that all potentially reversible causes or contributing factors be addressed. These include treating infections, dehydration, and metabolic abnormalities, as well as eliminating unnecessary medications (particularly anticholinergics, sedatives, anxiolytics) that can exacerbate dementia or delirium.

There is limited experience with anticholinesterase inhibitors such as donepezil (Aricept) for treating cognitive impairment in PD, but preliminary studies suggest that some improvement may occur.[209–211] L.M. may benefit from a trial of donepezil, but this medication is very expensive, and he must be monitored closely for signs of deterioration of motor function. Most importantly, adequate supportive home care for L.M. should be ensured. As he becomes increasingly dependent on family members for assistance with ADLs, the increased needs of the caregiver(s) should also be considered. In L.M.'s case, he attends adult day care three times weekly, which should provide a structured, supervised environment for interaction with others, as well as providing a rest period for his caregiver. When severe, dementia is a leading cause of nursing home placement for PD patients.[28]

Depression

Depression occurs frequently in PD patients. However, the physical appearance of the patient may make it difficult to determine whether the symptoms are attributed to depression or to the PD.[28] Patients manifesting symptoms of hypomimia (facial masking), hypophonia (weak voice), psychomotor retardation, and a stooped posture may be incorrectly diagnosed with depression if these features are solely the result of the PD. In contrast, depression in patients with loss of energy, decreased appetite, reduced libido, and insomnia may go unrecognized, as the symptoms are often attributed to the PD.[28]

Treatment of the depressed patient should first focus on providing adequate treatment of the symptoms of the PD through restoring mobility and independence, particularly in patients whose depression can be attributed to lengthy "off" periods. SSRIs are the treatment of choice for prolonged bouts of depression (see Question 15), although other classes of antidepressants such as tricyclic antidepressants are also effective. Therapy should be started at the lowest dose and gradually titrated to effect. Regardless of the choice of antidepressant agent, patients should be monitored closely for side effects, particularly anticholinergic symptoms with tricyclic antidepressants, and for any adverse effects on mobility. Psychotherapy should also be considered. Lastly, electroconvulsive therapy may be beneficial if medications fail.

Psychomotor Agitation

The incidence of hallucinations and delirium increases with age and cognitive impairment in PD patients. These symptoms are often caused or exacerbated by medications.[28] Symptoms are often more pronounced at night (the "sundowning" effect), and hallucinations are typically visual. As with managing cognitive impairment, it is important to eliminate or minimize any potential causative factors, particularly anticholinergic medications, that could be contributing to the hallucinations or delirium. In some patients, reducing the dose of levodopa improves mental function while also providing satisfactory control of motor features (see Question 15). If it is not possible to achieve a balance between preserving motor control and decreasing neuropsychiatric symptoms through reduction in levodopa dosage, neuroleptics may be considered.

Older antipsychotic medications such as haloperidol, perphenazine, and chlorpromazine block striatal dopamine D_2 receptors and may exacerbate parkinsonian symptoms. Therefore, these agents are not recommended.[28] Newer "atypical" antipsychotics are more selective for limbic and cortical D_3, D_4, D_5 receptors, have minimal activity at D_2 receptors, and show promise in controlling symptoms without worsening parkinsonism. Of these agents, clozapine is the best studied in patients with PD. However, its use is limited by the need for frequent monitoring of white blood cell counts (see Question 15). Other newer agents, particularly quetiapine (Seroquel), appear promising and have controlled psychosis without worsening parkinsonism. Risperdal (Risperdal) and olanzapine (Zyprexa) have also been studied, but high doses of olanzapine have worsened parkinsonism, and both agents were inferior to clozapine in clinical trials in PD patients.[212–215]

Agitation, characterized by restlessness, irritability, apprehension, and/or dysphoria, occurs commonly in patients with PD.[28] These symptoms often occur during "off" periods and may be a manifestation of underlying anxiety. Treatment should begin by ensuring optimal control of motor fluctuations, followed by discontinuation or reduction in dosage of any antiparkinsonian drugs, particularly anticholinergics, that might exacerbate the symptoms. Short-term use of short-acting benzodiazepines, such as lorazepam or alprazolam, may also provide relief.[28]

Autonomic Dysfunction
Patients with PD also experience symptoms of dysautonomia, including orthostasis, erectile dysfunction, constipation, nocturia, sensory disturbances, dysphagia, seborrhea, and thermoregulatory imbalances.[28] Management of these symptoms is generally supportive, and appropriate medical interventions similar to those used in other geriatric patients can be employed to treat these symptoms whenever encountered.

Falls
Patients with PD and their caregivers should be counseled on the prevention of falls, since they can result in serious morbidity and mortality. Falls generally result from one of several factors, including postural instability, freezing and festination, levodopa-induced dyskinesia, symptomatic orthostatic hypotension, coexisting neurologic or other medical disorders, and environmental factors.[28] Prevention remains the best strategy and includes environmental precautions, such as proper lighting, use of handrails, removing tripping hazards, and incorporating physical and occupational therapy. Reversible causes of postural or gait instability should be addressed whenever suspected.

Sleep Disorders
The sleep disorders often experienced by elderly persons are accentuated in PD patients.[28] Insomnia, sleep fragmentation due to PD symptoms, restless legs syndrome, and nightmares are common. When sleep dysfunction can be directly attributed to PD symptoms such as akinesia, tremor, dyskinesia, or nightmares, dosage adjustment of dopaminergic medications is indicated. Proper sleep hygiene should be encouraged. Similar to dysautonomia, management of sleep disorders that are not directly attributable to PD symptoms can be managed supportively, similarly to other geriatric patients.

Levodopa Treatment Failure

37. J.B., an 80-year-old retired pharmacist, presents to his doctor complaining of a tremor in both hands. He was begun on Sinemet 25/100 TID, and this dosage was gradually increased to 100 mg carbidopa/1,000 mg levodopa per day with little if any improvement in his symptoms. J.B. has a long history of adult-onset diabetes controlled by diet and diabetic gastroparesis managed with oral metoclopramide 10 mg TID. He has been feeling "run down" lately and started taking ferrous sulfate to increase his energy. J.B. also is anxious at times and takes oral diazepam 5 mg Q 6 hr PRN. Otherwise, J.B. is healthy, except that he occasionally forgets things. His family history is significant for diabetes and his father also suffered from "tremors." What is the explanation for J.B.'s lack of response to levodopa therapy?

Misdiagnosis
As previously discussed, most PD patients show at least a partial response to levodopa when given in therapeutic doses. In fact, the response to levodopa is so predictable that many neurologists consider a lack of response strong evidence that the patient may have a neurologic disorder other than PD.[28] Because the diagnosis of PD usually is made entirely on clinical grounds, it is possible that J.B. does not have the disease. He may have another disorder with similar clinical features such as benign essential tremor.[25,26,28] Although a further diagnostic workup is warranted, this diagnosis is supported by the bilateral nature of his tremors, along with a significant family history of tremor.[4]

Another important reason for levodopa failure is inadequate dosage.[28] Most patients respond to levodopa dosages of 1,000 mg/day when given as Sinemet; however, the response to levodopa in PD patients is highly variable, with some patients requiring much higher doses.[28] Many elderly patients take numerous medications and some, like J.B., have difficulty with memory; thus, compliance may be a significant problem.

Drug Interactions
Many drugs can interact with levodopa to decrease its effectiveness (see Table 53-5).[130–136] Several drugs possess central dopamine blocking properties that can interfere with the dopaminergic effects of levodopa. Most notable of these are the neuroleptic drugs such as the phenothiazines (e.g., chlorpromazine, fluphenazine, and the antiemetic prochlorperazine), the butyrophenones (e.g., haloperidol), and the thioxanthenes (e.g., thiothixene).[216] Antihypertensive medications such as reserpine and methyldopa are known to decrease levodopa response.[217] Metoclopramide, an agent used to treat diabetic gastroparesis and nausea, can produce central dopamine blockade, leading to a decreased levodopa effect.[218] J.B. is receiving metoclopramide; if possible, it should be discontinued. Domperidone, an antiemetic similar to metoclopramide (not yet available in the United States), does not cross the blood–brain barrier and thus does not adversely interact with levodopa.[141]

Before the combination of levodopa with carbidopa was available, a significant interaction existed between pyridoxine (vitamin B6) and levodopa.[131] Pyridoxine, as a cofactor for the enzyme dopa decarboxylase, can increase the peripheral metabolism of levodopa, leaving less drug available for penetration into the brain.[131] This interaction is of little significance when levodopa is combined with a peripheral decarboxylase inhibitor. A study in healthy volunteers showed that ferrous sulfate 325 mg can decrease levodopa absorption by a factor of 50% through chelation of iron by levodopa.[136] Thus, unless necessary, iron therapy should be discontinued in J.B. Other agents that can decrease levodopa's effect include phenytoin and the benzodiazepines.[135,219] J.B. is taking diazepam for anxiety. A careful drug history should be taken to assess how often he is taking this drug. If he requires regular intake to relieve anxiety, an alternative agent should be substituted.

Finally, many patients show a response to levodopa but cannot take the drug chronically because of intolerable side effects.[109,115,125] Every effort should be made to minimize the levodopa dose while maximizing clinical response. Often this can be achieved through the use of adjunctive agents (as discussed above), which often allow a substantial reduction in levodopa dose and, subsequently, improved tolerance.

The key to successful management of the patient with PD requires a thorough knowledge of the various treatment modalities available, coupled with an individualized approach that takes into account the needs and concerns of the patient.[28,36]

REFERENCES

1. Duvoisin R. History of parkinsonism. Pharmacol Ther 1987;32:1.
2. Hoehn MM, Yahr MD. Parkinsonism: onset, progression, and mortality. Neurology 1967;17:427.
3. Rajput AH et al. Epidemiology of parkinsonism: incidence, classification, and mortality. Ann Neurol 1984;16:27.
4. Tanner CM, Goldman SM. Epidemiology of Parkinson's disease. Neurol Clin 1996;14:317.
5. Mitchell SL et al. The epidemiology, clinical characteristics and natural history of older nursing home residents with a diagnosis of Parkinson's disease. J Am Geriatr Soc 1996;44:394.
6. Hoehn MMM. The natural history of Parkinson's disease in the pre-levodopa and post-levodopa eras. Neurol Clin 1992;10:331.
7. Joseph C et al. Levodopa in Parkinson disease: a long-term appraisal of mortality. Ann Neurol 1978;3:116.
8. The Parkinson Study Group. Mortality in DATATOP, a multicenter trial in early Parkinson's disease. Ann Neurol 1998;43:318.
9. Ballard PA et al. Permanent human parkinsonism due to L-methyl-4-phenyl- 1,2,3,6-tetrahydropyridine (MPTP): seven cases. Neurology 1985;35:949.
10. Langston JW. MPTP: insights into the etiology of Parkinson's disease. Eur Neurol 1987;26(Suppl 1):2.
11. Tanner CM. The role of environmental toxins in the etiology of Parkinson's disease. Trends Neurosci 1989;12:49.
12. Ward CD et al. Parkinson's disease in 65 pairs of twins and in a set of quadruplets. Neurology 1983;33:815.
13. Golbe LI. The genetics of Parkinson's disease: a reconsideration. Neurology 1990;40(Suppl 3):7.
14. Polymeropoulos MH et al. Mutation in the α-synuclein gene identified in families with Parkinson's disease. Science 1997;276:2045.
15. Zhang Z-X, Roman GC. Worldwide occurrence of Parkinson's disease: an updated review. Neuroepidemiology 1993;12:195.
16. Schapira AHV et al. Mitochondrial complex I deficiency in Parkinson's disease. J Neurochem 1990;54:823.
17. Mann DMA, Yates PO. Pathogenesis of Parkinson's disease. Arch Neurol 1982;39:545.
18. Hornykiewicz O. Biochemical aspects of Parkinson's disease. Neurology 1998;51(Suppl 2):S2.
19. Young AB. Penney JB. Biochemical and functional organization of the basal ganglia. In: Jankovich J, Tolosa E, eds. Parkinson's Disease and Movement Disorders. Baltimore: Williams & Wilkins, 1993:77.
20. Bernheimer H et al. Brain dopamine and syndromes of Parkinson and Huntington. Clinical, morphological and neurochemical correlations. J Neurol Sci 1973;20:415.
21. Vingerhoets FJG et al. Longitudinal fluorodopa positron emission tomographic studies: the evolution of idiopathic parkinsonism. Ann Neurol 1994;36:759.
22. Moorish PK et al. An [18F] dopa-PET and clinical study of the rate of progression of Parkinson's disease. Brain 1996;119:585.
23. Jenner P. The rationale of the use of dopamine agonists in Parkinson's disease. Neurology 1995;45(Suppl 3):S6.
24. De Yebenes JG, Gomez MAM. Dopamine systems in the mammalian brain. In: Jankovich J, Tolosa E, eds. Parkinson's Disease and Movement Disorders. Baltimore: Williams & Wilkins, 1993:13.
25. Stacy M, Jankovich J. Differential diagnosis in Parkinson's disease and the parkinsonism plus syndromes. Neurol Clin 1992;01:341.
26. Delwaide PJ, Gonce M. Pathophysiology of Parkinson's signs. In: Jankovich J, Tolosa E, eds. Parkinson's Disease and Movement Disorders. Baltimore: Williams & Wilkins, 1993:77.
27. Hughes AJ et al. What features improve the accuracy of clinical diagnosis in Parkinson's disease: a clinicopathologic study. Neurology 1992;42:1142.
28. Olanow CW et al. An algorithm (decision tree) for the management of Parkinson's disease: treatment guidelines. Neurology 2001;56(Suppl 5):S1.
29. Jost WH, Schimrigk K. Cisapride treatment of constipation in Parkinson's disease. Move Disord 1993;8:339.
30. Critchley EMR. Speech disorders in parkinsonism: a review. J Neurol Neurosurg Psychiatry 1981; 44:751.
31. Dooneief G et al. An estimate of the incidence of depression in idiopathic Parkinson's disease. Arch Neurol 1993;49:305.
32. Mayeux R et al. An estimate of the incidence of dementia in idiopathic Parkinson's disease. Neurology 1990;40:1513.
33. Goetz CG, Strebbins GT. Mortality and hallucinations in nursing home patients with advanced Parkinson's disease. Neurology 1995;45:669.
34. Palacios JM et al. Brain dopamine receptors: characterization, distribution, and alteration in disease. In: Jankovich J, Tolosa E, eds. Parkinson's Disease and Movement Disorders. Baltimore: Williams & Wilkins, 1993:35.
35. Piercy MF et al. Functional roles for dopamine-receptor subtypes. Clin Neuropharmacol 1995;18:34.
36. Stern MB. Contemporary approaches to the pharmacotherapeutic management of Parkinson's disease: an overview. Neurology 1998;49(Suppl 1):S2.
37. Uitti RJ, Ahlskog JE. Comparative review of dopamine receptor agonists in Parkinson's disease. Drugs 1996;5:369.
38. Watts RL. The role of dopamine agonists in early Parkinson's disease. Neurology 1997;49(Suppl 1):S2.
39. Tolosa ET et al. History of levodopa and dopamine agonists in Parkinson's disease treatment. Neurology 1998;50(Suppl 6):S2.
40. Rabey JM. Second-generation dopamine agonists: pros and cons. J Neural Transm 1995;45(Suppl):213.
41. Rascol O et al. Ropinirole in the treatment of early Parkinson's disease: a 6-month interim report of a 5-year levodopa-controlled study. Move Disord 1998;13:39.
42. Miyasaki JM et al. Practice parameter: initiation of treatment for Parkinson's disease: an evidence-based review. Report of the Quality Standards Subcommittee of the American Academy of Neurology. Neurology 2002;58:11.
43. Mierau J et al. Pramipexole binding and activation of cloned and expressed dopamine D_2, D_3 and D_4 receptors. Eur J Pharmacol 1995;290:26.
44. Mirapex (Pramipexole) Package Insert, Kalamazoo, MI: Pharmacia Upjohn, 1997.
45. Dooley M, Markham A. Pramipexole. A review of its use in the management of early and advanced Parkinson's disease. Drugs Aging 1998;6:495.
46. Hubble JP et al. Pramipexole in patients with early Parkinson's disease. Clin Neuropharmacol 1995; 18:338.
47. Parkinson Study Group. Safety and efficacy of pramipexole in early Parkinson's disease. A randomized dose-ranging study. JAMA 1997;278:125.
48. Shannon KM et al. Efficacy of pramipexole, a novel dopamine agonist, as monotherapy in mild to moderate Parkinson's disease. The Pramipexole Study Group. Neurology 1997;49:724.
49. Molho ES et al. The use of pramipexole, a novel dopamine agonist, in advanced Parkinson's disease. J Neural Transm 1995;45(Suppl):225.
50. Lieberman A et al. Clinical evaluation of pramipexole in advanced Parkinson's disease: results of a double-blind, placebo-controlled, parallel-group study. Neurology 1997;49:162.
51. Fahn S et al. Unified Parkinson's Disease Rating Scale. In: Fahn S et al, eds. Recent Developments in Parkinson's Disease, Vol. II. Macmillan Health Care Information, Florham Park, 1987:153.
52. Parkinson Study Group. Pramipexole vs. levodopa as initial treatment for Parkinson disease: a randomized controlled trial. JAMA 2000;284:1931.
53. Frucht S et al. Falling asleep at the wheel: motor vehicle mishaps in persons taking pramipexole and ropinirole. Neurology 1999;52:1908.
54. Boehringer Ingelheim Pharmaceuticals. Dear Health Care Professional advisory letter, Sept. 21, 1999.
55. Tulloch IF. Pharmacologic profile of ropinirole: a nonergoline dopamine agonist. Neurology 1997; 49(Suppl 1):S58.
56. Bloomer JC et al. In vitro identification of the P450 enzymes responsible for the metabolism of ropinirole. Drug Metab Disp 1997;25:840.
57. Montastruc JL et al. Current status of dopamine agonists in Parkinson's disease management. Drugs 1993;46:384.
58. Adler CH et al. Ropinirole for the treatment of early Parkinson's disease. Neurology 1997;49:393.
59. Korczyn AD et al. Ropinirole versus bromocriptine in the treatment of early Parkinson's disease: a 6-month interim report of a 3-year study. Move Disord 1998;13:46.
60. Rascol O et al. A five-year study of the incidence of dyskinesia in patients with early Parkinson's disease who were treated with ropinirole or levodopa. N Engl J Med 2000;342:1484.
61. Lieberman A et al. A multicenter trial of ropinirole as adjunct treatment for Parkinson's disease. Neurology 1998;51:1057.
62. Schrag AE et al. The safety of ropinirole, a selective nonergoline dopamine agonist, in patients with Parkinson's disease. Clin Neuropharmacol 1998; 21:169.
63. Lieberman AN, Goldstein M. Bromocriptine in Parkinson disease. Pharmacol Rev 1985;37:217.
64. Piccoli F, Ruiggeri RM. Dopamine agonists in the treatment of Parkinson's disease: a review. J Neural Transm 1995;45(Suppl):187.
65. Beramasco B et al. Long-term bromocriptine treatment of de novo patients with Parkinson's disease. A seven-year follow-up. Acta Neurol Scand 1990;81:383.
66. Calne DB et al. Long-term treatment of parkinsonism with bromocriptine. Lancet 1978;1:735.
67. Lieberman AN et al. Bromocriptine in Parkinson disease: further studies. Neurology 1979;29: 363.
68. Kartzinel R, Calne DB. Studies with bromocriptine, Part 1. "On-off" phenomena. Neurology 1976; 26:508.

69. Kartzinel R et al. Studies with bromocriptine, Part 2. Double-blind comparison with levodopa in idiopathic parkinsonism. Neurology 1976;26:511.

70. Lees AJ, Stern GM. Sustained bromocriptine therapy in previously untreated patients with Parkinson's disease. J Neurol Neurosurg Psychiatry 1981;44:1020.

71. Tolosa E et al. Low-dose bromocriptine in the early phases of Parkinson's disease. Clin Neuropharmacol 1987;10:169.

72. Teychenne PF et al. Bromocriptine: low-dose therapy in Parkinson disease. Neurology 1982;32:577.

73. Staal-Schreinemachers AL et al. Low-dose bromocriptine therapy in Parkinson's disease: double-blind, placebo-controlled study. Neurology 1986;36:291.

74. Grimes JD, Delgado MR. Bromocriptine: problems with low-dose de novo therapy in Parkinson's disease. Clin Neuropharmacol 1985;8:73.

75. Larsen TA et al. Severity of Parkinson's disease and the dosage of bromocriptine. Neurology 1984; 34:795.

76. Parkinson's Disease Research Group in the United Kingdom. Comparisons of therapeutic effects of levodopa, levodopa and selegiline, and bromocriptine in patients with early, mild Parkinson's disease: three-year interim report. Br Med J 1993;307:469.

77. Rinne UK. Early combination of bromocriptine and levodopa in the treatment of Parkinson's disease: a 5-year follow-up. Neurology 1987;37:826.

78. Olsson JE, European Multicenter Trial Group. Bromocriptine and levodopa in early combination in Parkinson's disease. Adv Neurol 1990;53:421.

79. Parkes JD. Bromocriptine in the treatment of parkinsonism. Drugs 1979;17:365.

80. Guttman M et al. Double-blind comparison of pramipexole and bromocriptine treatment with placebo in advanced Parkinson's disease. Neurology 1997;49:1060.

81. Rajput AH. Adverse effects of ergot-derivative dopamine agonists. In: Olanow CW, Obeso JA, eds. Dopamine Agonists in Early Parkinson's Disease. Kent: Wells Medical, 1997:209.

82. Langtry HD, Clissold SP. Pergolide. A review of its pharmacological properties and therapeutic potential in Parkinson's disease. Drugs 1990;39:491.

83. Ahlskog JE, Muenter MD. Treatment of Parkinson's disease with pergolide: a double-blind study. Mayo Clin Proc 1988;63:969.

84. LeWitt PA et al. Comparison of pergolide and bromocriptine therapy in parkinsonism. Neurology 1983;33:1009.

85. Goetz CG et al. Chronic agonist therapy for Parkinson's disease: a 5-year study of bromocriptine and pergolide. Neurology 1985;35:749.

86. Lieberman AN et al. Further studies with pergolide in Parkinson disease. Neurology 1982;32:1181.

87. Ahlskog JE, Muenter MD. Pergolide: long-term use in Parkinson's disease. Mayo Clin Proc 1988;63:979.

88. Goetz CG et al. Chronic agonist therapy of Parkinson's disease: a 5-year study of bromocriptine and pergolide. Neurology 1985;35:749.

89. Factor SA et al. Parkinson's disease: an open label trial of pergolide in patients failing bromocriptine therapy. J Neurol Neurosurg Psychiatry 1988;51:529.

90. Kurlan R et al. Double-blind assessment of potential pergolide-induced cardiotoxicity. Neurology 1986;36:993.

91. Cotzias GC et al. Aromatic amino acids and modification of parkinsonism. N Engl J Med 1967; 267:374.

92. Cotzias GC et al. Modification of parkinsonism—chronic treatment with L-dopa. N Engl J Med 1969;280:337.

93. Barbeau A. L-dopa therapy in Parkinson's disease. Can Med Assoc J 1969;101:791.

94. McDowell F et al. Treatment of Parkinson's syndrome with L-dihydroxyphenyl-alanine (levodopa). Ann Intern Med 1970;72:29.

95. Parkes JD. Adverse effects of antiparkinsonian drugs. Drugs 1981;21:341.

96. Riley DE, Lang AE. The spectrum of levodopa-related fluctuations in Parkinson's disease. Neurology 1993;43:1459.

97. Papavasiliou PS et al. Levodopa in parkinsonism: potentiation of central effects with a peripheral inhibitor. N Engl J Med 1972;285:8.

98. Nutt JC, Fellman JH. Pharmacokinetics of levodopa. Clin Neuropharmacol 1984;7:35.

99. Markham CH, Diamond SG. Modification of Parkinson's disease by long-term levodopa treatment. Arch Neurol 1986;43:405.

100. Fahn S, Bressman SB. Should levodopa therapy for parkinsonism be started early or late? Evidence against early treatment. Can J Neurol Sci 1984;11(Suppl):200.

101. Melamed E. Initiation of levodopa therapy in parkinsonian patients should be delayed until advanced stages of the disease. Arch Neurol 1986; 43:402.

102. Olanow CW. An introduction to the free radical hypothesis in Parkinson's disease. Ann Neurol 1992;32:S2.

103. Jenner P, Olanow W. Understanding cell death in Parkinson's disease. Ann Neurol 1998;44(Suppl 1):72.

104. Sian J et al. Alterations in glutathione levels in Parkinson's disease and other neurodegenerative disorders affecting basal ganglia. Ann Neurol 1994;36:348.

105. Nakamura K et al. The role of glutathione depletion in dopaminergic neuronal survival. J Neurochem 1997;69:1850.

106. Yoshino MY et al. Mitochondrial dysfunction in Parkinson's disease. Ann Neurol 1998;(Suppl 1):99.

107. Markham CH, Diamond SG. Evidence to support early levodopa therapy in Parkinson's disease. Neurology 1981;31:125.

108. Markham CH, Diamond SG. Long-term follow-up of early dopa treatment in Parkinson's disease. Ann Neurol 1986;19:365.

109. Obeso JA et al. Complications with chronic levodopa therapy in Parkinson's disease. In: Olanow CW, Obeso JA, eds. Dopamine Agonists in Early Parkinson's Disease. Kent: Wells Medical Limited, 1997:11.

110. Stocchi F et al. Motor fluctuations in levodopa treatment: clinical pharmacology. Eur Neurol 1996;36(Suppl 1):38.

111. Rinne UK et al. Early treatment of Parkinson's disease delays the onset of motor complications. Drugs 1998(Suppl 1):23.

112. Wooten GF. Progress in understanding the pathophysiology of treatment-related fluctuations in Parkinson's disease. Ann Neurol 1988;24:363.

113. Nutt JG, Holford NHG. The response to levodopa in Parkinson's disease: imposing pharmacological law and order. Ann Neurol 1996;39:561.

114. Luquin MR et al. Levodopa-induced dyskinesias in Parkinson's disease: clinical and pharmacological classification. Move Disord 1992;7:117.

115. Nutt JG. Levodopa-induced dyskinesia: review, observations, and speculations. Neurology 1990; 40:340.

116. Harder S et al. Concentration–effect relationship of levodopa in patients with Parkinson's disease. Clin Pharmacokinet 1995;29:243.

117. Mouradian MM et al. Motor fluctuations and Parkinson's disease: pathogenetic and therapeutic studies. Ann Neurol 1987;22:475.

118. Mouradian MM et al. Motor fluctuations in Parkinson's disease: central pathophysiology mechanisms, Part II. Ann Neurol 1988;24:372.

119. LeWitt PA. Clinical studies with and pharmacokinetic considerations of sustained-release levodopa. Neurology 1992;42(Suppl 1):29.

120. Block G et al. Comparison of immediate-release and controlled-release carbidopa/levodopa in Parkinson's disease. A multicenter 5-year study. The CR First Study Group. Eur Neurol 1997;37:23.

121. Alexander GM et al. Effect of plasma levels of larger neutral amino acids and degree of parkinsonism on the blood-to-brain transport of levodopa in naive and MPTP parkinsonian monkeys. Neurology 1994;44:1491.

122. Braco F et al. Protein redistribution diet and antiparkinsonian response to levodopa. Eur Neurol 1991;31:68.

123. Kurth MC et al. Double-blind, placebo-controlled, crossover study of duodenal infusion of levodopa/carbidopa in Parkinson's disease patients with "on-off" fluctuations. Neurology 1993;43: 1698.

124. Pappert E et al. Liquid levodopa/carbidopa produces significant improvement in motor function without dyskinesia exacerbation. Neurology 1996;47:1493.

125. Goodwin FK. Psychiatric side effects of levodopa in man. JAMA 1971;218:1915.

126. Sweet RD, McDowell FH. Five years' treatment of Parkinson's disease with levodopa. Ann Intern Med 1975;83:456.

127. Koller WC et al. Levodopa therapy in Parkinson's disease. Neurology 1990;40(Suppl 3):S40.

128. Mayeux R et al. Altered serotonin metabolism in depressed patients with Parkinson's disease. Neurology 1984;34:642.

129. Waters CH. Managing the late complications of Parkinson's disease. Neurology 1997;49(Suppl 1):S49.

130. Edwards M. Adverse interaction of levodopa with tricyclic antidepressants. Practitioner 1982;226: 1447.

131. Leon AS et al. Pyridoxine antagonism of levodopa in parkinsonism. JAMA 1971;218:1924.

132. Algeri S et al. Effect of anticholinergic drugs on gastrointestinal absorption of L-dopa in rats and man. Eur J Pharmacol 1976;35:293.

133. Morgan JP et al. Imipramine-mediated interference with levodopa absorption from the gastrointestinal tract in man. Neurology 1975;25:1029.

134. Hunter KR et al. Monoamine oxidase inhibitors and L-dopa. Br Med J 1970;3:388.

135. Yosselson-Superstine S, Lipman AG. Chlordiazepoxide interaction with levodopa. Ann Intern Med 1982;96:259.

136. Campbell NRC, Hasinoff B. Ferrous sulfate reduces levodopa bioavailability: chelation as a possible mechanism. Clin Pharmacol Ther 1989;45: 220.

137. Youdim MBH. Pharmacology of MAO-B inhibitors: mode of action of (-) deprenyl in Parkinson's disease. J Neural Transm 1986;22(Suppl):91.

138. Leo RJ. Movement disorders associated with the serotonin selective reuptake inhibitors. J Clin Psychol 1996;57:449.

139. Musser WS, Akil M. Clozapine as a treatment for psychosis in Parkinson's disease: a review. J Neuropsychiatry Clin Neurosci 1996;8:1.

140. Factor SA, Friedman JH. The emerging role of clozapine in the treatment of movement disorders. Move Disord 1997;12:483.

141. Barone JA. Domperidone: mechanism of action and clinical use. Hosp Pharm 1998;33:191.

142. Kofman OS. Are levodopa "drug holidays" justified? Can J Neurol Sci 1984;11(Suppl):206.

143. Weiner WJ et al. Drug holiday and management of Parkinson disease. Neurology 1980;30:1257.

144. Goetz CG et al. Drug holiday in the management of Parkinson disease. Clin Neuropharmacol 1982;5:351.

145. Mayeux R et al. Reappraisal of temporary levodopa withdrawal ("drug holiday") in Parkinson's disease. N Engl J Med 1985;313:724.

146. Maesner JE. Transient levodopa withdrawal in Parkinson's disease. Clin Pharm 1987;6:22.

147. Cawein MJ. False rise in serum uric acid after L-dopa. N Engl J Med 1969;281:1489.

148. Honda H, Gindin A. Gout while receiving levodopa for parkinsonism. JAMA 1972;219:55.

149. Sirtori CR et al. Metabolic responses to acute and chronic L-dopa administration in patients with parkinsonism. N Engl J Med 1972;287:729.

150. Rotblatt MD, Koda-Kimble MA. Review of drug interference with urine glucose tests. Diabetes Care 1987;10:103.

151. Feldman JM, Lebovitz HE. Levodopa and tests for urinary glucose. N Engl J Med 1970;283:1053.

152. Cawein MJ et al. Levodopa and tests for ketonuria. N Engl J Med 1970;283:659.

153. Mannisto PT et al. Characteristics of catechol-O-methyltransferase (COMT) and properties of

selective COMT inhibitors. Prog Drug Res 1992;39:291.

154. Kaakola S et al. General properties and clinical possibilities of new selective inhibitors of catechol-O-methyltransferase. Gen Pharmacol 1994; 25:813.

155. Bonifati V, Meco G. New, selective catechol-O-methyltransferase inhibitors as therapeutic agents in Parkinson's disease. Pharmacol Ther 1999; 81:1.

156. Backstrom R et al. Synthesis of some novel potent and selective catechol-O-methyltransferase inhibitors. J Med Chem 1989;32:841.

157. Cederbaum JM, Olanow CW. Aspects of levodopa pharmacokinetics and pharmacodynamics: bases of the modification of drug response during chronic treatment of Parkinson's disease. In: Olanow CW, Lieberman AN, eds. The Scientific Basis for the Treatment of Parkinson's Disease. Park Ridge: The Parthenon Publishing Group, 1992:113.

158. De Santi C et al. Catechol-O-methyltransferase: variation in enzyme activity and inhibition by entacapone and tolcapone. Eur J Pharmacol 1998;54:215.

159. Keranen T et al. Inhibition of soluble catechol-O-methyltransferase and single-dose pharmacokinetics after oral and intravenous administration of entacapone. Eur J Pharmacol 1994;46:151.

160. Rinne UK et al. Entacapone enhances the response to levodopa in parkinsonian patients with motor fluctuations. Neurology 1998;51:1309.

161. Parkinson Study Group. Entacapone improves motor fluctuations in levodopa-treated Parkinson's disease patients. Ann Neurol 1997;42:747.

162. Micek ST, Ernst ME. Tolcapone: a novel approach to Parkinson's disease. Am J Health Syst Pharm 1999;56:2195.

163. Dingemanse J et al. Integrated pharmacokinetics and pharmacodynamics of the novel catechol-O-methyltransferase inhibitor tolcapone during first administration to humans. Clin Pharmacol Ther 1995;57:508.

164. Jorga KM et al. Effect of liver impairment on the pharmacokinetics of tolcapone and its metabolites. Clin Pharmacol Ther 1998;63:646.

165. Roche Laboratories. Tasmar (Tolcapone) Package Insert. Nutley, NJ, Nov. 1998.

166. Kurth MC et al. Tolcapone improves motor function and reduces levodopa requirement in patients with Parkinson's disease experiencing motor fluctuations: a multicenter, double-blind, randomized, placebo-controlled trial. Neurology 1997;48:81.

167. Rajput AH et al. Tolcapone improves motors function in parkinsonian patients with the "wearing-off" phenomenon: a double-blind, placebo-controlled, multicenter trial. Neurology 1997;49:1066.

168. Waters CH. Tolcapone in stable Parkinson's disease: efficacy and safety of long-term treatment. The Tolcapone Stable Study Group. Neurology 1997;49:665.

169. Assal F et al. Tolcapone and fulminant hepatitis. Lancet 1998;352:958.

170. Tetrud JW, Langston JW. The effect of deprenyl (selegiline) on the natural history of Parkinson's disease. Science 1989;245:519.

171. Golbe LI. Deprenyl as symptomatic therapy in Parkinson's disease. Clin Neuropharmacol 1988;11:387.

172. Elizam TS et al. Selegiline as an adjunct to conventional levodopa therapy in Parkinson's disease. Arch Neurol 1989;46:1280.

173. Birkmayer W et al. Increased life expectancy resulting from addition of L-deprenyl to Madopar treatment in Parkinson's disease: a long-term study. J Neural Transm 1985;64:113.

174. Snyder SH, D'Amato RJ. MPTP: a neurotoxin relevant to the pathophysiology of Parkinson's disease. Neurology 1986;36:250.

175. Markey SP et al. Intraneuronal generation of a pyridinium metabolite may cause drug-induced parkinsonism. Nature 1984;311:464.

176. Heikkila TE et al. Protection against the dopaminergic neurotoxicity of L-methyl-4-phenyl-1,2,5,6-tetrahydropyridine by monoamine oxidase inhibitors. Nature 1984;311:467.

177. Parkinson Study Group. DATATOP: a multicenter controlled clinical trial in early Parkinson's disease. Arch Neurol 1989;46:1052.

178. Parkinson Study Group. Effect of deprenyl on the progression of disability in early Parkinson's disease. N Engl J Med 1989;321:1364.

179. Parkinson Study Group. Impact of deprenyl and tocopherol treatment on Parkinson's disease in DATATOP subjects not requiring levodopa. Ann Neurol 1996;39:29.

180. Parkinson Study Group. Mortality in DATATOP: a multicenter trial in Parkinson's disease. Ann Neurol 1998;43:318.

181. Olanow CW et al. Selegiline and mortality in Parkinson's disease. Ann Neurol 1996;40:841.

182. Lees AJ. Parkinson's Disease Research Group of the United Kingdom. Comparison of the therapeutic effects and mortality data of levodopa combined with selegiline in patients with early, mild Parkinson's disease. Br Med J 1995;311:1602.

183. Schwab RS et al. Amantadine in the treatment of Parkinson's disease. JAMA 1969;208:1168.

184. Schwab RS et al. Amantadine in Parkinson's disease. JAMA 1972;222:792.

185. Verhagen ML et al. Amantadine as treatment for dyskinesias and motor fluctuations in Parkinson's disease. Neurology 1998;50:1323.

186. Fahn S, Isgreen WP. Long-term evaluation of amantadine and levodopa combination in parkinsonism by double-blind crossover analyses. Neurology 1975;25:695.

187. Bailey EV, Stone TW. The mechanism of action of amantadine in parkinsonism: a review. Arch Intl Pharmacodyn Ther 1975;216:246.

188. Greenamayre JT, O'Brien CF. N-methyl-D-aspartate antagonists in the treatment of Parkinson's disease. Arch Neurol 1991;48:977.

189. Metman LV et al. Amantadine for levodopa-induced dyskinesias: a 1-year follow-up study. Arch Neurol 1999;56:1383.

190. Kulisevsky J, Tolosa E. Amantadine in Parkinson's disease. In: Koller WC, Paulson G, eds. Therapy of Parkinson's Disease. New York: Marcel Dekker, 1990:143.

191. Aoki FY, Sitar DS. Clinical pharmacokinetics of amantadine hydrochloride. Clin Pharmacokinetics 1988;14:35.

192. Dexter D et al. Alpha-tocopherol levels in brain are not altered in Parkinson's disease. Ann Neurol 1992;32:591.

193. Parkinson Study Group. Effects of tocopherol and deprenyl on the progression of disability in early Parkinson's disease. N Engl J Med 1993;328:176.

194. Shults CW et al. Coenzyme Q10 levels correlate with the activities of complexes I and II/III in mitochondria from parkinsonian and non-parkinsonian subjects. Ann Neurol 1997;42:261.

195. Shults CW et al. Effects of coenzyme Q10 in early Parkinson's disease: evidence of slowing of the functional decline. Arch Intern Med 2002;59:1541.

196. Schulz JB et al. Glutathione, oxidative stress and neurodegeneration. Eur J Biochem 2000;267:4904.

197. Owen DAL, Marsden CD. Effect of adrenergic beta-blockade on parkinsonian tremor. Lancet 1965;2:1259.

198. Foster NL et al. Peripheral beta-adrenergic blockade treatment of parkinsonian tremor. Ann Neurol 1984;16:505.

199. Friedman JH et al. Clozapine responsive tremor in Parkinson's disease. Move Disord 1990;5:225.

200. Bennet JP et al. Suppression of dyskinesias in advanced Parkinson's disease: part II. Increasing clozapine doses suppress dyskinesias and improve Parkinson's symptoms. Neurology 1993;43:1551.

201. Arevalo GJ, Gershank OS. Modulatory effect of clozapine on levodopa response in Parkinson's disease: a preliminary study. Move Disord 1993;8:349.

202. Iacono RP et al. The results, indications and physiology of posteroventral pallidotomy for patients with Parkinson's disease. Neurosurgery 1995;36:1118.

203. Lang AE et al. Posteroventral medial pallidotomy in advanced Parkinson's disease. N Engl J Med 1997;337:1036.

204. Jankovic J et al. Outcome after stereotactic thalamotomy for parkinsonian, essential and other types of tremor. Neurosurgery 1995;37:680.

205. Kelly PJ, Gillingham FJ. The long-term results of stereotaxic surgery and L-dopa therapy in patients with Parkinson's disease. J Neurosurg 1980; 53:332.

206. Olanow CW et al. Deep brain stimulation of the subthalamic nucleus for Parkinson's disease. Move Disord 1996;11:598.

207. Pollak P et al. New surgical treatment strategies. Eur Neurol 1996;36:396.

208. Ahlskog JE. Cerebral transplantation for Parkinson's disease: current progress and future prospects. Mayo Clin Proc 1993;68:578.

209. Aarsland D et al. Donepezil for cognitive impairment in Parkinson's disease: a randomized controlled study. J Neurol Neurosurg Psychiatry 2002;72:708.

210. Bergman J et al. Successful use of donepezil for the treatment of psychotic symptoms in patients with Parkinson's disease. Clin Neuropharmacol 2002;25:107.

211. Fabbrini G et al. Donepezil in the treatment of hallucinations and delusions in Parkinson's disease. Neurol Sci 2002;23:41.

212. Fernandez HH et al. Quetiapine for the treatment of drug-induced psychosis in Parkinson's disease. Mov Disord 1999;14:484.

213. Wolters EC et al. Olanzapine in the treatment of dopaminomimetic psychosis in patients with Parkinson's disease. Neurology 1996;47:1085.

214. Goetz CG et al. Olanzapine and clozapine: comparative effects on motor function in hallucinating Parkinson's disease patients. Neurology 2000; 55:789.

215. Rich SS et al. Risperidone versus clozapine in the treatment of psychosis in six patients with Parkinson's disease and other akinetic-rigid syndromes. J Clin Psychol 1995;56:556.

216. Tarsy D. Neuroleptic-induced extrapyramidal reactions: classification, description, and diagnosis. Clin Neuropharmacol 1983;6(Suppl 1):S9.

217. Strang RR. Parkinsonism occurring during methyldopa therapy. Can Med Assoc J 1966; 95:928.

218. Yamamoto M et al. Metoclopramide-induced parkinsonism. Clin Neuropharmacol 1987;10:287.

219. Mendez JS et al. Diphenylhydantoin blocking of levodopa effects. Arch Neurol 1975;32:44.

CHAPTER 54

Seizure Disorders

James W. McAuley, Rex S. Lott

Incidence, Prevalence, and Epidemiology

Approximately 10% of the population will experience a seizure at some time. Up to 30% of all seizures are caused by central nervous system (CNS) disorders or insults (e.g., meningitis, trauma, tumors, and exposure to toxins); these seizures may become recurrent and require chronic treatment with antiepileptic drugs (AEDs). Reversible conditions such as alcohol withdrawal, fever, and metabolic disturbances may cause isolated seizures that usually do not require long-term AED therapy. Between 0.5% and 1% of the U.S. population has recurrent epileptic seizures.[1]

Terminology, Classification, and Diagnosis of Epilepsies

Classification of Seizures and Epilepsies

An epileptic seizure is the "clinical manifestation presumed to result from an abnormal and excessive discharge of a set of neurons in the brain. The clinical manifestation consists of sudden and transitory abnormal phenomena that may include alterations of consciousness, motor, sensory, autonomic, or psychic events perceived by the patient or observer."[2] Epilepsy is a "condition characterized by recurrent (≥2) epileptic seizures, unprovoked by any immediate identified cause."[2] The nomenclature associated with epilepsy and epileptic seizures has been revised.[1,3,4] The current International Classification of Epileptic Seizures is shown in Table 54-1. Older terms such as "grand mal" and "petit mal" should not be used, as this may create confusion in the clinical setting. For example, it is common for patients or caregivers to identify any seizure other than a generalized tonic-clonic seizure as a "petit mal" seizure. This labeling may result in the selection of an inappropriate medication.

Generalized tonic-clonic (grand mal) seizures are a common seizure type in which the patient loses consciousness and falls at the onset. Simultaneously, tonic muscle spasms begin and may be accompanied by a cry that results from air being forced through the larynx. A period of bilateral, repetitive clonic movements follows. After the clonic phase, patients return to consciousness but remain lethargic and may be confused for varying periods of time (postictal state). Urinary incontinence is common. Primary generalized tonic-clonic seizures affect both cerebral hemispheres from the outset. Secondarily generalized tonic-clonic seizures begin as either simple or complex partial seizures. The aura described by some patients before a generalized tonic-clonic seizure actually represents an initial partial seizure that spreads to become a secondarily generalized seizure. Identification of secondarily generalized tonic-clonic seizures is important because some AEDs are more effective at controlling primary generalized seizures than secondarily generalized seizures, and partial seizures are often more difficult to control with currently available AEDs.[5–7]

Absence (petit mal) seizures occur primarily in children and often remit during puberty; affected patients may develop a second type of seizure. Absence seizures consist of a brief loss of consciousness. Simple (typical) absence seizures are not accompanied by motor symptoms; automatisms, muscle twitching, myoclonic jerking, or autonomic manifestations may accompany atypical (complex) absence seizures. Although consciousness is lost, patients do not fall during absence seizures. Patients are unaware of their surroundings and will have no recall of events during the seizure. Consciousness returns immediately when the seizure ends, and postictal confusion is absent. Differentiation of atypical absence seizures from complex partial seizures may be difficult if only observation of episodes is available; identification of a focal abnormality by an electroencephalogram (EEG) often is necessary to identify complex partial seizures. This distinction is important for the proper selection of AEDs.

Also known as "auras," simple partial (focal motor or sensory) seizures are localized in a single cerebral hemisphere or portion of a hemisphere. No loss of consciousness is experienced. Various motor, sensory, or psychic manifestations may occur. A single part of the body may twitch, or the patient may experience only an unusual sensory experience.

Complex partial (psychomotor or temporal lobe) seizures result from the spread of focal discharges to involve a larger area. Consciousness is impaired and patients may exhibit complex but inappropriate behavior (automatisms) such as lip smacking, picking at clothing, or aimless wandering. A period of brief postictal lethargy or confusion is common.

Epileptic Syndromes

Seizures can be classified based on seizure type as shown in Table 54-1, or they can be described as epileptic syndromes that may include cause (if known), precipitating factors, age of onset, characteristic EEG patterns, severity, chronicity, family history, and prognosis. Accurate diagnosis of an epileptic syndrome often guides the clinician regarding the need for drug therapy, the choice of appropriate medication, and the likelihood of successful treatment.[1,4,8,9] Many epileptic syndromes have been defined, and a complete listing is beyond the scope of this chapter. However, several are of interest with respect to pharmacotherapy (Table 54-2).[9]

Table 54-1   International Classification of Epileptic Seizures

Partial Seizure (Local or Focal)

Simple Partial Seizures (Without Impairment of Consciousness)

    Motor symptoms
    Special sensory or somatosensory symptoms
    Autonomic symptoms
    Psychic symptoms

Complex[a] Partial Seizures (with Impairment of Consciousness)

    Progressing to impairment of consciousness
      With no other features
      With features as in simple partial seizures
      With automatisms
    With impaired consciousness at onset
      With no other features
      With features as in simple partial seizures
      With automatisms

Partial Seizures That Evolve to Generalized Seizures

    Simple partial seizures evolving to generalized seizures
    Complex partial seizures evolving to generalized seizures
    Simple partial seizures evolving to complex partial seizures to generalized seizures

Generalized Seizures (Convulsive or Nonconvulsive)

Absence Seizures

    Typical seizures (impaired consciousness only)
    Atypical absence seizures

Myoclonic Seizures

Clonic Seizures

Tonic Seizures

Tonic-Clonic Seizures

Atonic (Astatic or Akinetic) Seizures

Unclassified Epileptic Seizures

    All seizures that cannot be classified because of inadequate or incomplete data and some that cannot be classified in previously described categories

[a]Complex implies organized, high-level activity.
From references 1, 3, and 4.

Table 54-2 Selected Epileptic Syndromes

Syndrome	Seizure Patterns and Characteristics	Preferred AED Therapy	Comments
Juvenile myoclonic epilepsy	Myoclonic seizures often precede generalized tonic-clonic seizures. Myoclonic and generalized tonic-clonic episodes upon awakening. Absence seizures also common. ↓ sleep, fatigue, and alcohol commonly precipitate seizures.	Valproic acid. Phenytoin or carbamazepine as adjuncts to valproate in resistant cases. Carbamazepine reported to exacerbate seizures in some patients.	5–10% of all epilepsies; 85-90% response to valproate. Lifelong therapy usually needed. High relapse rate with attempts to discontinue AED therapy.
Lennox-Gastaut syndrome	Generalized seizures: atypical absence, atonic/akinetic, myoclonic, and tonic most common. Abnormal interictal EEG with slow spike-wave pattern. Cognitive dysfunction and mental retardation. Status epilepticus common.	Valproic acid, benzodiazepines, lamotrigine. Topiramate may be effective. Felbamate also may be effective, but potential hematologic toxicity limits use. Poorly responsive to AEDs.	Oversedation with aggressive AED trials may ↑ seizure frequency. Tolerance to benzodiazepines limits their usefulness.
Childhood absence epilepsy (true petit mal)	Typical absences often in clusters of multiple seizures (pyknolepsy). Tonic-clonic seizures in ≈40%. Onset usually between ages 4 and 8. Significant genetic component. EEG shows classic 3-Hz spike-wave pattern.	Ethosuximide or valproic acid	80–90% response rate to AED therapy. Good prognosis for remission. Tonic-clonic seizures may persist.
Reflex epilepsy	Tonic-clonic seizures most common. Induced by flicker or patterns (photosensitivity) most commonly. Reading also may precipitate partial seizures affecting the jaw, which may generalize. Some cases involve precipitation of underlying seizures; some seem primary.	AED specific to underlying seizures. Avoidance of precipitating stimuli when possible. Valproic acid usually effective for cases of spontaneous seizures precipitated by photosensitivity.	Relatively rare; seizures may be precipitated by television or video games
Temporal lobe epilepsy	Complex partial seizures with automatisms. Simple partial seizures (auras) common; secondary generalized seizures occur in 50%.	Carbamazepine, phenytoin, valproic acid, gabapentin, lamotrigine, topiramate, tiagabine, levetiracetam, oxcarbazepine, zonisamide	Often incompletely controlled with current AEDs. Emotional stress may precipitate seizures; psychiatric disorders seen with temporal lobe epilepsy; surgical resection can be effective when patient is identified as a good surgical candidate.

AED, antiepileptic drug; EEG, electroencephalogram.
From references 9–14.

Juvenile myoclonic epilepsy is an hereditary disorder characterized by generalized tonic-clonic seizures (frequently occurring upon awakening or precipitated by sleep deprivation or alcohol intake), mild myoclonic seizures, which are most prominent in the morning, and occasionally absence seizures. The EEG pattern is characteristic and is distinct from patterns typically seen in absence epilepsy. Juvenile myoclonic epilepsy responds extremely well to several AEDs; valproate is usually preferred. Despite the excellent response to medication, discontinuation of AED treatment usually is unsuccessful, and lifelong therapy is required.[12,15]

Lennox-Gastaut syndrome involves mixed seizures (tonic, generalized tonic-clonic, partial seizures, atypical absence, and frequent atonic seizures) that begin early in life; the syndrome almost always is associated with brain damage, mental retardation, and other developmental disabilities. The EEG pattern is distinct from patterns seen with other seizure disorders. Seizures associated with Lennox-Gastaut syndrome often are refractory to AED therapy, and affected children often must wear helmets to minimize injuries associated with almost daily falls from atonic seizures. Patients suffer frequent episodes of status epilepticus and often are stuporous because of recurrent seizure activity. In addition, chronic intoxication with AEDs is a risk because of attempts to control refractory seizures with multiple medications.[13] Characteristics of other selected epilepsy syndromes are described in Table 54-2.

Diagnosis

Optimal treatment of seizure disorders requires accurate classification (diagnosis) of seizure type and appropriate choice and use of medications. Seizure classification may be straightforward if an adequate history and description of the clinical seizure are available. Physicians often do not observe patients' seizures; thus, family members, teachers, nurses, and others who have frequent direct contact with patients should learn to accurately observe and objectively describe and record these events. The onset, duration, and characteristics of a seizure should be described as completely as possible. Several aspects of the events surrounding a seizure may be especially significant: the patient's behavior before the seizure (e.g., did the patient complain of feeling ill or describe an unusual sensation?), deviation of the eyes or head to one side or localization of convulsive activity to one portion of the body, impaired consciousness, loss of continence, and the patient's behavior after the seizure (e.g., was there any postictal confusion?). In addition, it is helpful if the observer can record the length of the event and how long it took for the patient to return to baseline. The patient and/or caregivers should have a seizure calendar or diary to record events. Those who observe a seizure should not try to label the seizure but should be encouraged to describe the event fully and objectively.

Accurate seizure diagnosis and identification of the type of epilepsy or epileptic syndrome also depend on neurologic examination, medical history, and diagnostic techniques such as EEG, computed tomography (CT), and magnetic resonance imaging (MRI). The EEG often is critical for identifying specific seizure types. CT scanning is often used to assess newly diagnosed patients, but MRI is preferred. MRI may locate brain lesions or anatomic defects that are missed by conventional radiographs or CT scans.[16]

Treatment

Early control of epileptic seizures is important because it allows normalization of the patient's lives and prevents acute physical harm and long-term morbidity associated with recurrent seizures. In addition, early control of tonic-clonic seizures is associated with a reduced likelihood of seizure recurrence.[17] Early control of epileptic seizures also correlates with successful discontinuation of AED treatment after long-term seizure control.[18–20]

Nonpharmacologic Treatment of Epilepsy

Alternatives or adjuncts to pharmacotherapy may be important in some patients. Surgery has become recognized as an extremely useful form of treatment in selected patients. Depending on the epileptic syndrome and procedure performed, up to 90% of patients treated surgically may improve or become seizure free. A study of 80 patients with medically refractory temporal lobe epilepsy randomized to either surgery or continued medical treatment showed that after 1 year, patients were more likely to be seizure free after surgery.[21] Surgery is advocated as early therapy for some patients with specific epileptic syndromes such as Lennox-Gastaut syndrome or mesial temporal lobe epilepsy. Early surgical intervention may prevent or lessen the neurologic deterioration and developmental delay often associated with these forms of epilepsy.

Dietary modification may be used for patients who cannot tolerate AEDs or to treat seizures that are not completely responsive to AEDs. In most circumstances, dietary modification consists of a ketogenic diet; this low-carbohydrate, high-fat diet results in persistent ketosis, which is believed to play a major role in the therapeutic effect. Ketogenic diets are most commonly used and seem to be most beneficial in children; they are also used as adjuncts to ongoing AED treatment.[22,23]

The U.S. Food and Drug Administration (FDA) has approved the use of a vagus nerve stimulator for treatment of intractable partial seizures. This device uses electrodes attached around the left branch of the vagus nerve. The electrodes are attached to a programmable stimulator that delivers stimuli on a regular cycling basis; patients can also use "on demand" stimulation at the onset of seizures by placing a magnet next to the subcutaneously implanted stimulator. Approximately 30% to 40% of patients who are treated have a positive response ($\geq$50% reduction in seizures).[24] The primary side effect of this device is hoarseness during stimulation; infrequently, this is accompanied by left vocal cord paralysis.

AVOIDANCE OF POTENTIAL SEIZURE PRECIPITANTS

It is impossible to generalize about environmental and lifestyle precipitants of seizure activity in persons with epilepsy. Individual patients or caregivers may identify specific circumstances, such as stress, sleep deprivation, or ingestion of excessive amounts of caffeine or alcohol, that increase the likelihood of a seizure. Some women experience an increase in the frequency and/or severity of seizures around the time of menstruation or ovulation. Patients with seizure disorders should avoid any activities that seem to precipitate seizures; as always, the goal is complete seizure control with as little alteration in quality of life as possible.

Antiepileptic Drug Therapy

Seizure disorders most often are treated with pharmacotherapy. Therefore, patient education regarding medications and consultation among health care professionals regarding the optimal use of AEDs are essential to quality patient care. Optimal AED therapy completely controls seizures in 60% to 95% of patients.[8,25–27] Optimization of drug therapy depends on several factors; the choice of appropriate AED, individualization of dosing, and compliance are perhaps the most important.

CHOICE OF AED

Many AEDs have a relatively narrow spectrum of efficacy; therefore, choice of appropriate drug therapy for a specific patient depends on accurate classification of seizures and, if possible, diagnosis of epileptic syndrome. In addition, the risks of side effects and potential toxicity must be considered when selecting an AED. Preferred drugs for specific types of seizures and common epileptic syndromes are listed in Tables 54-2 and 54-3. Although certain drugs are preferred, the identification of the most effective drug for a particular patient may be a process of trial and error; trials of several medications may be necessary before therapeutic success is achieved. The expert consensus method was used to analyze expert opinion on treatment of three epilepsy syndromes and status epilepticus.[31] The experts recommended monotherapy first, followed by a second monotherapy agent if the first failed. If the second monotherapy failed, the experts were not in agreement on whether to try a third monotherapy agent or two therapies. The experts recommended epilepsy surgery evaluation after the third failed step for patients with symptomatic localization-related epilepsies.

THERAPEUTIC END POINTS

The individual patient's response to AED treatment (i.e., seizure frequency and severity, presence and severity of symptoms of dose-related toxicity) must be the major focus for assessment of therapy. In general, the goal of AED treatment is administration of sufficient medication to completely prevent seizures without producing significant dose-related side effects. Careful titration of doses to achieve seizure control is the mainstay of optimization of therapy. Realistically, this goal may be compromised for many patients; it may not be possible to completely prevent seizures without producing intolerable adverse effects. Thus, the therapeutic end points actually achieved will vary among patients; optimization of AED therapy for a specific person depends largely on individualization of the drug therapy regimen to his or her needs and lifestyle. It is rarely optimal to administer "standard" or "usual" doses of an AED to a patient or to adjust doses to achieve a "therapeutic blood level" without paying due consideration to the effect

Table 54-3 Antiepileptic Drugs Useful for Various Seizure Types[a]

Primary Generalized Tonic-Clonic	Secondarily Generalized Tonic-Clonic	Simple or Complex Partial	Absence	Myoclonic, Atonic/Akinetic
Most Effective With Least Toxicity				
Valproate	Carbamazepine	Carbamazepine	Ethosuximide	Valproate
Phenytoin	Oxcarbazepine	Oxcarbazepine	Valproate	Clonazepam
Carbamazepine	Phenytoin	Phenytoin		Lamotrigine[b]
(Lamotrigine)[b]	Valproate	Valproate		(Topiramate)[b]
(Oxcarbazepine)[b]	(Gabapentin)[b]	Lamotrigine		
(Topiramate)[b]	(Lamotrigine)[b]	(Gabapentin)[b]		
(Zonisamide)[b]	(Topiramate)[b]	(Levetiracetam)[b]		
	(Tiagabine)[b]	(Topiramate)[b]		
	(Zonisamide)[b]	(Tiagabine)[b]		
	(Levetiracetam)[b]	(Zonisamide)[b]		
Effective, But Often Cause Unacceptable Toxicity				
Phenobarbital	Phenobarbital	Clorazepate	Clonazepam	(Felbamate)[c]
Primidone	Primidone	Phenobarbital	Trimethadione	
(Felbamate)[c]	(Felbamate)[c]	Primidone		
		(Felbamate)[c]		
Of Little Value				
Ethosuximide	Ethosuximide	Ethosuximide	Phenytoin	
Trimethadione	Trimethadione	Trimethadione	Carbamazepine	
			Phenobarbital	
			Primidone	

[a]Drugs are listed in general order of preference within each category. Recommendations by various authorities may differ, especially regarding the relative place of valproate and the role of phenytoin as a first-line AED. Many authorities now discourage the use of phenobarbital and primidone.
[b]The place of gabapentin, lamotrigine, oxcarbazepine, levetiracetam, topiramate, tiagabine, and zonisamide is yet to be determined. They are placed on this table only to indicate the types of seizures for which they appear to be effective. Much more clinical experience is needed before their roles as possible primary AEDs are clarified.
[c]The place of felbamate is yet to be determined. It is placed on this table only to indicate the types of seizures for which it appears to be effective. Felbamate has been associated with aplastic anemia and hepatic failure; until a possible causative role is clarified, felbamate cannot be recommended for treatment of epilepsy unless all other, potentially less toxic treatment options have been exhausted.
From references 26 and 28–30.

of the dose or serum concentration on the patient's condition and quality of life. As with many chronic conditions requiring maintenance drug therapy, patient participation in developing and evaluating a therapeutic plan is extremely important. Patients should be educated regarding the expected positive and negative effects of their AED therapy, and they must be encouraged to communicate with their health care provider regarding their responses to prescribed AEDs.

SERUM DRUG CONCENTRATIONS

Relation to Dosage. Wide availability of AED serum concentration determinations has had a significant impact on the treatment of seizure disorders. The correlation between the administered maintenance dose of an AED and the resulting steady-state serum concentration is poor. Administration of "usual therapeutic doses," even when calculated on the basis of body weight, is equally likely to produce subtherapeutic, therapeutic, or potentially intoxicating serum concentrations. Interindividual variation in hepatic metabolic capacity probably accounts for most of this variability. For some AEDs, the correlation between serum concentrations and both therapeutic response and toxic symptoms is better.

Relation to Clinical Response. Proper use and interpretation of AED serum concentrations is important for optimizing treatment regimens in epilepsy.[32, 33] An individual patient's clinical response to AED treatment (i.e., seizure frequency and severity, symptoms of dose-related toxicity) must be the major focus for assessment of therapy. Neither therapeutic effects nor toxic symptoms are "all or none"; in most situations, there are gradations of efficacy and toxicity. Dosage increases and titration to AED serum concentrations within and occasionally above the "therapeutic range" may significantly improve therapeutic responses without producing significant toxicity.[33] Individual patients often differ dramatically in their response to a particular serum drug concentration; therefore, "therapeutic" serum concentrations should be considered only as guidelines for treatment. Seizure type and other clinical variables, such as how many seizures occur before control is achieved, may significantly influence the serum drug concentrations required for seizure control. For example, complete control of simple or complex partial seizures requires serum concentrations of carbamazepine (Tegretol) 27% higher than those needed for complete control of generalized tonic-clonic seizures; corresponding figures for phenytoin (Dilantin) and phenobarbital were 64% and 11%, respectively.[5,6] Likewise, many patients may be controlled with serum drug concentrations below the usual "therapeutic" range.[34] In these patients, dosage adjustment to increase the serum drug concentration is not warranted.

Indications for Use. Measurement of serum drug concentrations often provides clinically useful information in the following situations:

- Uncontrolled seizures despite administration of greater-than-average doses: Serum concentrations of AEDs may help distinguish drug resistance from subtherapeutic drug concentrations caused by malabsorption, noncompliance, or rapid metabolism.
- Seizure recurrence in a previously controlled patient: This often is due to noncompliance with the prescribed medication regimen.

- Documentation of intoxication: In patients who develop signs or symptoms of dose-related AED toxicity, documentation of the dose and serum concentration of the responsible drug is helpful.
- Assessment of patient compliance: Although monitoring AED serum concentrations can be used to assess patient compliance with therapy, conclusions must be based on comparisons with previous steady-state serum concentrations that reflected reliable intake of a given dose of AED.
- Documentation of desired results from a dose change or other therapeutic maneuver (e.g., administration of a loading dose): When patients are receiving multiple AEDs, serum concentrations of all drugs should be measured following a change in the dose of one drug because changes in the serum concentration of one drug frequently change the pharmacokinetic disposition of other drugs.
- When precise dosage changes are required: On occasion, small changes in the dose of a drug (e.g., phenytoin) may result in large changes in both the serum concentration and clinical response. In addition, cautious titration of dosage and serum concentration may be necessary to avoid intoxication. Knowledge of the serum drug concentration before the dosage change may allow the clinician to select a more appropriate new maintenance dose.

Frequent, "routine" determinations of serum AED concentrations are costly and not warranted for patients whose clinical status is stable. Clinicians may tend to focus attention on normal variability in serum concentrations rather than on the patient's clinical status; as a result, unnecessary dosage adjustments may be made to make serum concentrations fit the "normal range." A plan of action for what the clinician is going to do with the information once it is obtained should be in place before obtaining the sample. Therefore, the results of individual serum concentration determinations must be evaluated carefully to decide whether a significant, clinically meaningful change has occurred.[35]

Interpretation of Serum Concentrations. Several factors may alter the relationship between AED serum concentration and the patient's response to the drug. Whenever a change in serum concentration is apparent, pharmacokinetic factors (Table 54-4) should be considered (along with the patient's clinical status) before a decision is made to adjust the AED dosage. Laboratory variability may cause minor fluctuations in reported AED serum concentrations. Under the best conditions, reported values for serum concentrations may be within ±10% of "true" values.[36,37] Therefore, the magnitude of any apparent change must be considered. Therapeutic ranges are not well established for some drugs (e.g., valproate and the newer AEDs such as lamotrigine, topiramate, and tiagabine). Published "therapeutic ranges" may have been determined in small numbers of patients or may more accurately represent "average serum concentrations" at "usual doses." As an example, many clinicians now agree that "pushing" valproate serum concentrations up to 150 to 200 μg/mL may be beneficial for some patients; these higher concentrations are not consistently associated with specific toxicity symptoms.[38–41] Nevertheless, most laboratories report 50 to 100 g/mL as a "therapeutic range" for valproate. Inappropriate sample timing may result in inconsistent and clinically meaningless changes in AED

Table 54-4 Pharmacokinetic Properties of Antiepileptic Drugs

Drug	Oral Absorption	Half-Life (hr)	Time to Steady State[a]	Dosage Schedule	Usual Therapeutic Serum Concentration	Plasma Protein Binding	Volume of Distribution (L/kg)
Carbamazepine	90–100%	Chronic: 5–25	2–4 days	BID to TID	5–12+ µg/mL	75% (50–90)	0.8–1.6
Ethosuximide	90–100%	Pediatric: 30	5–10 days	QD (BID)	40–100 µg/mL	0%	0.7
		Adult: 60					
Gabapentin	40–60%; ↓ with ↑ dose	Normal renal function: 5–9; ↑ with ↓ renal function	Normal renal function: 1–.5 days	TID to QID (Q 6–8 hr)	>2 µg/mL (proposed)	0%	≈0.8
Lamotrigine	90–100%	Monotherapy: 24–29 Enzyme inducers: 15 Enzyme inhibitor (VPA): 59	4–9 days	BID	4–18 µg/mL (proposed)	55%	0.9–1.2
Levetiracetam	100%	Normal renal function: 6–8; ↑ with ↓ renal function	Normal renal function: 1–1.5 days	BID	Not determined	<10%	≈0.7
Oxcarbazepine	100%	8–13	2–3 days	BID to TID	Not determined	40%	—
Phenobarbital	90–100%	2–4 days	8–16 days	QD	15–40 µg/mL	50%	0.5–0.6
Phenytoin	90–100%	Varies with dose	5–30+ days	QD to BID	10–20 µg/mL	95%	0.5–0.7
Primidone	90–100%	3–12	12–48 hr	BID to TID	5–15 µg/mL (15–40 µg/mL for derived phenobarbital)	<50%	0.4–1.1
Tiagabine	90%	Monotherapy: 7–9 Enzyme inducers: 4–7	1–2 days	BID to QID	Not determined	96%	1.1
Topiramate	≥80%	12–24	3–4 days	BID	Not determined	10–15%	0.7
Valproate	100%	10–16	2–3 days	BID to QID	50–150+ µg/mL	90+%	0.09–0.17
Zonisamide	≈80%	Monotherapy: ≈60 Enzyme inducers: 27–36	2 wk	QD to BID	Not determined	50–60%	1.3

[a]Based on four half-lives. This lag time should allow determination of steady-state serum concentrations within limits of most assay sensitivities.
VPA, valproic acid.

serum concentrations.[32] Generally, serum concentrations of AEDs should not be measured until a minimum of four to five half-lives have elapsed since initiation of therapy or a dosage change. Blood samples should be obtained in the morning, before any doses of the AED have been taken; this practice provides reproducible, postabsorptive (i.e., "trough") serum concentrations. On occasion, especially for rapidly absorbed drugs with short half-lives (e.g., valproate), determination of peak serum concentrations may help assess possible toxic symptoms. Interindividual variability in response to a given serum concentration of medication is common. Excellent therapeutic response or even symptoms of intoxication may be associated with AED serum concentrations that are classified as "subtherapeutic."[42] Active metabolites of AEDs usually are not measured when serum concentrations are determined.[37,43] Alterations in the relative proportion of parent drug and active metabolite may result in an apparent alteration in the relationship between the serum concentration of the parent drug and the patient's response. Binding to serum proteins is significant for some AEDs (e.g., phenytoin, valproate). Changes in protein binding may result from drug interaction, renal failure, pregnancy, or changes in nutritional status. These changes may alter the usual relationship between the measured total drug concentration (bound and unbound to plasma proteins) and the unbound (pharmacologically active) drug concentration. This change may not be apparent when only total serum concentrations are measured. Determination of serum concentrations of free (i.e., unbound) AEDs is available from many commercial laboratories; these determinations are expensive and results may not be available for several days. If significant changes in protein binding are suspected, measurement of free concentrations of AEDs may provide additional information useful for adjustment of doses or interpretation of the patient's symptoms.[36,37,43]

MONOTHERAPY VERSUS POLYTHERAPY

Historically, seizure disorders were often treated with multiple AEDs (polytherapy). A second, third, or even fourth drug was added when seizures were incompletely controlled with a single AED. Evaluation of the effectiveness of polytherapy in recent years has shown little advantage for most patients. Use of a single drug at optimal tolerated serum concentrations produces excellent therapeutic results and minimal side effects in up to 80% of patients. Addition of a second AED significantly improves seizure control in only 10% to 20% of patients.[44,45] Reduction or elimination of existing polytherapy in patients with longstanding seizure disorders often lessens or eliminates cognitive impairment and other side effects: seizure control actually may improve.[44,46–49]

Most experts advocate the use of monotherapy (i.e., use of a single AED) whenever possible. Successful monotherapy may require higher-than-usual AED doses that may produce serum concentrations above the upper limit of the "usual therapeutic range."[26,50] Addition of a second drug may be necessary in some patients; however, polytherapy should be reserved for patients with multiple seizure types or for patients in whom first-line AEDs have failed to control seizures when titrated to maximum tolerated doses.[26,47]

Use of polytherapy creates several disadvantages that must be weighed against possible benefits. Seizure control may not significantly improve; in fact, these authors' experience and information from studies in which patients were converted from polytherapy to monotherapy indicate that even with use of an optimal AED, seizure control may be worsened in some patients by polytherapy regimens.[49] Patient expenses for medications and for increased laboratory monitoring may increase significantly with polytherapy. In addition, drug interactions among AEDs may complicate assessment of the patient's response and serum concentrations. Patient compliance often is worsened when multiple medications are prescribed, and adverse effects often increase because the side effects of many of these drugs are additive.

Although AED monotherapy is preferred whenever feasible, the recent introduction of several new AEDs has increased the use of polytherapy.[50] Owing to limitations on the patient populations used for clinical trials of new drugs (i.e., patients with seizure disorders not completely controlled by previous medications), most new AEDs are labeled only for use as add-on therapy. Though reports exist on the efficacy of the new AEDs as monotherapy,[51–54] only lamotrigine, oxcarbazepine, and felbamate have an FDA-approved indication for monotherapy. Lamotrigine is indicated for conversion to monotherapy in adults with partial seizures who are receiving treatment with a single enzyme-inducing AED.[55] Felbamate should be considered (as monotherapy or polytherapy) only when other AEDs have failed. Other AEDs will undoubtedly follow with monotherapy indications. At present, though, data concerning the use of these new drugs as single agents are limited. Therefore, patients treated with these drugs most often receive another AED and require monitoring for possible drug interactions and additive adverse effects.

DURATION OF THERAPY AND DISCONTINUATION OF ANTIEPILEPTIC DRUGS

A diagnosis of epilepsy may no longer necessitate lifelong drug therapy. Several long-term studies have examined the prognosis of epilepsy following drug discontinuation; AED therapy may be successfully withdrawn from some patients after a seizure-free period of 2 to 5 years.[18–20] Seizures recurred in only 12% to 36% of patients who were followed for up to 23 years after AED withdrawal. Therefore, many patients whose epilepsy is completely controlled with medication can stop therapy after a seizure-free period of at least 2 years.

Discontinuation of medications is advantageous for economic, medical, and psychosocial reasons. Costs associated with physician visits, serum concentration determinations, and the medications themselves are eliminated. The risk of adverse effects from long-term medication use is eliminated, and patients can expect fewer lifestyle restrictions. However, attempts to withdraw AED therapy are associated with risks: reappearance of seizure activity may result in status epilepticus, loss of driving privileges, employment difficulties, or physical injury.

Risk factors for seizure recurrence following discontinuation of AEDs have been identified in observational studies; unfortunately, there is not complete agreement between studies regarding the nature and importance of specific risk factors. Opinions and data also differ regarding the optimal duration of the seizure-free period before discontinuation of AEDs is attempted. Nevertheless, at least some consensus has been reached regarding certain factors that may predict a higher risk of seizure recurrence (Table 54-5).[18–20,56,57]

Table 54-5 Risk Factors Possibly Predicting Seizure Recurrence Following AED Withdrawal

- <2 yr seizure free before withdrawal
- Onset of seizures after age 12
- History of atypical febrile seizures
- Family history of seizures
- >2–6 yr before seizures controlled
- Large number of seizures (>30) before control or total of >100 seizures
- Partial seizures (simple or complex)
- History of absence seizures
- Abnormal EEG persisting throughout treatment
- Slowing on EEG before medication withdrawal
- Organic neurologic disorder
- Moderate to severe mental retardation
- Withdrawal of valproate or phenytoin (higher rate of recurrence than withdrawal of other AEDs)

AED, antiepileptic drug; EEG, electroencephalogram.
From references 18–20, 56, and 57.

In nonemergency situations, AEDs should be withdrawn slowly; if a patient receives multiple drugs, each drug should be withdrawn separately. Too-rapid withdrawal may result in status epilepticus. Clinical studies of AED discontinuation usually used a 2- to 3-month withdrawal schedule for each drug. The optimal rate of withdrawal of AEDs has not been identified. One study compared withdrawal of individual drugs over a 6-week and a 9-month period and found no difference in seizure recurrence between the groups.[58] Another study compared seizure frequencies in patients withdrawn from carbamazepine rapidly (over 4 days) and in patients withdrawn more slowly (over 10 days).[59] Significantly more generalized tonic-clonic seizures occurred when carbamazepine was withdrawn rapidly; complex partial seizures, however, did not occur at a higher rate with rapid withdrawal. Therefore, withdrawal of each AED over at least 6 weeks would seem to be a safe approach. Gradual withdrawal is recommended even for medications such as phenobarbital that have long half-lives and should theoretically be "self-tapering." In these authors' experience, gradual reduction of medications such as phenobarbital is associated with a significantly higher success rate. Appearance of seizures during medication withdrawal is not necessarily an indication for reinstitution of maintenance therapy; many patients who experience seizures during drug withdrawal remain seizure free after complete withdrawal.[60] At least some seizures that occur during withdrawal may result from the withdrawal process itself or from other causes such as infection and are not related to reappearance of the underlying seizure disorder.[49]

CLINICAL ASSESSMENT AND TREATMENT OF SEIZURE DISORDERS

Complex Partial Seizures With Secondary Generalization

Diagnosis

1. A.R. is a 14-year-old, 40-kg, female high school student. A.R. had three febrile seizures when she was 3 years old. She received phenobarbital prophylaxis "off and on," according to her parents, for about 6 months following her second febrile seizure. Since then, she had no reported seizures until 24 hours before admission. At that time she had a "convulsion" shortly after arriving at school in the morning. A teacher who witnessed the episode describes her as behaving "oddly" before the seizure. She abruptly got up from her desk and began to walk clumsily toward the door; she bumped into several desks and did not respond to the teacher's attempts to redirect her back to her seat. After approximately 1 minute of this behavior, she fell to the floor and experienced an apparent generalized tonic-clonic seizure that lasted approximately 90 seconds. During the episode, she was incontinent of urine and was described as "turning kind of blue." Following this episode, A.R. was transported to the hospital.

On arrival at the hospital, A.R. appeared drowsy and confused. Laboratory studies—a complete blood count (CBC), serum glucose, electrolytes, drug/alcohol screen, and lumbar puncture—were normal. Physical examination and a complete neurologic evaluation were normal. An EEG showed diffuse slowing with focal epileptiform discharges in the left temporal area; it was interpreted as abnormal. There was no history of recent illness or injury, although A.R. had stayed up late several nights recently studying for an examination.

A second seizure occurs in the hospital. The nursing staff's description of the episode is similar to that provided by the observers at school. After recovery from each episode, A.R. has no memory of events during the seizures; she only remembers a "funny feeling" in her stomach and a "buzzing" in her head before she lost consciousness. She describes having these feelings "a couple of times" in the past; she attributed them to "just getting dizzy" and had not reported them to her parents. After these previous episodes, A.R. described feeling "mixed up" and groggy for a few minutes. What subjective and objective features of A.R.'s seizures are consistent with a diagnosis of complex partial seizures with secondary generalization?

A.R.'s clinical pattern of observed seizure activity (an apparent aura preceding her generalized tonic-clonic seizures), her history of apparent complex partial seizures not accompanied by generalized seizures, and the findings of focal abnormal activity on EEG are all typical of this diagnosis. Postictal confusion and grogginess are also common after both generalized tonic-clonic and complex partial seizures. Her unusual or inappropriate behavior represents a complex partial seizure that subsequently generalized. The clinical features, accompanied by her EEG findings, also help rule out possible atypical absence seizures; atypical absence seizures may be confused with complex partial epileptic syndromes based on only clinical presentation. In both syndromes, patients may briefly appear to lose contact with their surroundings and display automatisms and mild clonic movements during seizure activity. In A.R.'s case, the EEG and the generalized tonic-clonic seizures during her episodes would rule out atypical absence as a likely possibility.

Decision to Use Antiepileptic Drug Therapy

2. What factors should be considered in a decision to treat A.R.'s seizures with AED therapy?

Once a diagnosis of epileptic seizures is established, the decision to treat the patient with medication is based on the likelihood of recurrence. The need for AED therapy after a single seizure is controversial; however, recurrence of generalized tonic-clonic seizures is less likely if AED therapy is initiated after the first generalized tonic-clonic seizure.[17] Therefore, at least for this one specific seizure type, early use of AEDs is supported. Whether this information applies to other types of seizures is not known. Clinical wisdom, however, holds that "seizures beget seizures," and most experts advocate early treatment of epileptic seizures (i.e., after a first or second unprovoked seizure).

In A.R.'s case, the potential benefits of immediate introduction of AED therapy appear to outweigh potential risks. She experienced complex partial seizures followed by secondarily generalized tonic-clonic seizures. Recurrences of seizure activity are likely to result in physical injury, social embarrassment, and interference with her participation in activities typical of a person her age. If her seizures are not controlled, she faces future limitation of her driving privileges and may face barriers to employment. Although AED therapy is associated with risks, they probably are outweighed by the potential benefits.

Choice of Antiepileptic Drug

3. Discuss the AEDs commonly used for A.R.'s seizure type. Based on the subjective and objective data available, recommend a first-choice AED for A.R. and a plan for initial dosing of this medication.

Phenytoin and carbamazepine are currently considered first-choice AEDs for complex partial seizures with secondarily generalized tonic-clonic seizures (see Table 54-3).[28,29,45] Valproate (Depakene/Depakote) is effective for treating both generalized and complex partial seizures.[63] Although valproate is used most often as a second-line agent for treatment of partial seizures, its usefulness is widely recognized, and it is approved by the FDA for this indication. Clorazepate (Tranxene) is useful primarily in situations in which an adjunctive medication is required because of incomplete response to primary drugs, but its usefulness is limited by the common development of tolerance and by its prominent sedative effects.[64] Phenobarbital and primidone (Mysoline) are less commonly used. Although both drugs are effective, the rate of side effects is high and long-term adherence to therapy is difficult.[28]

Felbamate (Felbatol), gabapentin (Neurontin), lamotrigine (Lamictal), topiramate (Topamax), tiagabine (Gabitril), levetiracetam (Keppra), oxcarbazepine (Trileptal), and zonisamide (Zonegran) are effective for control of partial seizures with or without secondary generalization. Most experience with these drugs was obtained when they were used as adjunctive agents in addition to other drugs when previous therapies were unsuccessful. Initial clinical trials with these newer medications indicate that several of them may be useful as single agents. As mentioned previously, lamotrigine and oxcarbazepine have monotherapy indications. Most of these more recent medications appear to be safe and are usually well tolerated. The usefulness of felbamate is, however, limited owing to its potential for serious hematologic and hepatic toxicity (see later discussion).

Carbamazepine has several advantages over phenytoin that make it a preferred first-choice agent in the opinion of many clinicians. Carbamazepine is less sedating than phenytoin for many patients. It also is not associated with dysmorphic effects such as hirsutism, acne, gingival hyperplasia, and coarsening of facial features. Carbamazepine's pharmacokinetic profile also makes dosage adjustment easier. In A.R.'s case, the lack of cosmetic side effects may be especially significant because she may be taking medication for many years. In addition, reduced sedation may be important with respect to her school performance. Moreover, in recent years, the relative cognitive effects of AEDs have become a focus.[65] Initial studies comparing the cognitive effects of phenytoin and carbamazepine found a significantly higher rate of cognitive impairment with phenytoin therapy as measured by neuropsychological tests of motor performance, learning, attention, and memory.[66] Based on these studies and clinical observation, phenytoin has gained a reputation for causing significant impairment of function. More recent studies and reanalysis of data from the initial studies have revealed that much of the cognitive impairment attributed to phenytoin could be explained by elevations in phenytoin serum concentrations and overemphasis on neuropsychological tests involving motor function.[67–69] The actual differences between these two drugs usually are subtle and difficult to detect; nevertheless, many clinicians and patients prefer carbamazepine to phenytoin because of its presumed lesser effects on cognition and motor function.

Carbamazepine Therapy
INITIATION AND DOSAGE

Initiation of treatment with full therapeutic maintenance doses of carbamazepine often causes excessive side effects such as nausea, vomiting, diplopia, and significant sedation. Therefore, carbamazepine therapy should be initiated gradually and patients should be allowed time to acclimate to the effects of the drug. Final dosing requirements are difficult to anticipate in individual patients. A reasonable starting dosage of carbamazepine for A.R. would be 100 mg twice a day; her dosage could be increased by 100 to 200 mg/day every 7 to 14 days. The rapidity of increases will depend on A.R.'s tolerance for the drug and the frequency of seizures. Serum concentrations of carbamazepine may be helpful in assessing the adequacy of dosage after A.R. is receiving usual therapeutic doses of the drug. Reasonable target serum concentrations of carbamazepine would be approximately 6 to 8 μg/mL.[6,33,37]

HEMATOLOGIC TOXICITY

4. Carbamazepine has been associated with hematologic and hepatic toxicities. What is the incidence and significance of these toxicities? How should A.R. be monitored for them?

Aplastic anemia and agranulocytosis have occurred in association with carbamazepine therapy.[70] Several cases have been fatal; however, most cases occurred in older patients treated for trigeminal neuralgia. Many patients were receiving other medications, and occasionally the reports were incomplete; thus, assessment of a causal role for carbamazepine is difficult.[71] Severe blood dyscrasias from carbamazepine seem rare (estimated prevalence of <1/50,000) and have predominantly occurred in nonepileptic patients. The lack of severe hematologic toxicity in various published series and clinical trials in patients with epilepsy has been notable.[72,73]

Leukopenia is relatively common in patients taking carbamazepine. It is usually mild and often reverses despite continued administration of the drug.[72,74] Total leukocyte counts may fall to <4,000 cells/mm³ in some patients, but differentials and platelet and erythrocyte counts remain normal. Symptoms (e.g., fever, sore throat) that might suggest early stages of agranulocytosis do not occur. No information supports a dose–toxicity relationship for carbamazepine-associated hematologic disorders, and this reaction is idiosyncratic.

Routine Hematologic Testing. Laboratory monitoring of A.R.'s hematologic status is recommended during carbamazepine therapy. The likelihood of early detection of aplastic anemia or agranulocytosis through frequent blood counts is low, however, and such monitoring is costly.[72,75] Because hematologic toxicity from carbamazepine primarily occurs early in therapy, CBCs can be obtained before therapy and at monthly intervals during the first 2 to 3 months of therapy; thereafter, a yearly or every-other-year CBC, white blood cell (WBC) count with differential, and platelet count should be sufficient.

HEPATOTOXICITY

Carbamazepine-related liver damage appears to be extremely rare despite frequent mention as a potential problem and strong warnings in the package insert.[76,77] Hepatic adverse reactions are believed to be idiosyncratic or immunologically based. Aggressive laboratory monitoring of liver function tests (LFTs) probably is unnecessary.[75] Alkaline phosphatase and γ-glutamyl-transferase (GGT) concentrations often are elevated in patients taking carbamazepine (and other AEDs). This is believed to result from hepatic enzyme induction and is not necessarily evidence for hepatic disease.[78]

In summary, hepatic and hematologic toxicities of carbamazepine are rare. Although potentially serious, they are best monitored on clinical grounds rather than by ongoing, intensive laboratory testing. Patients, families, and/or caregivers should be aware that the appearance of unusual symptoms (e.g., jaundice, abdominal pain, excessive bruising/bleeding, or sudden onset of severe sore throat with fever) should be reported to a health care professional. Baseline (pretreatment) determination of A.R.'s hepatic and hematologic status, possibly followed by monthly follow-up testing for 2 to 3 months, probably will be sufficient.[73,75] Thereafter, a CBC and a liver function battery should probably be evaluated only every 1 to 2 years, unless signs or symptoms of hepatic or hematologic disorders are observed.

PHARMACOKINETICS AND AUTOINDUCTION OF METABOLISM

5. Over the following 6 weeks, A.R.'s carbamazepine dosage was gradually increased to 400 mg BID (20 mg/kg per day). Until the last dose increase, she had been experiencing one or two complex partial seizures weekly; she had had only one generalized tonic-clonic seizure since her hospitalization. One week following the increase to 20 mg/kg per day, her serum carbamazepine concentration was 9 μg/mL just before her first dose of the day. No seizures occurred for 4 weeks, and she tolerated the medication well. Subsequently, she again began experiencing one seizure weekly. A repeated measurement of her trough serum carbamazepine concentration was 6 μg/mL. How might this change in serum concentration and recurrence of seizure activity be explained?

Several factors may account for this change. One should always consider the possibility of poor compliance with the medication regimen when serum concentrations and/or clinical response change unexpectedly. This should be investigated, and A.R. and her family should be educated regarding the importance of regular medication intake if necessary.

The observed changes in A.R.'s carbamazepine serum concentrations also are characteristic of this drug's pharmacokinetic behavior. Carbamazepine is a potent inducer of hepatic cytochrome P450 (CYP3A4). The drug is also a substrate for this enzyme. As a result, carbamazepine not only stimulates the metabolism of other CYP3A4 substrates but also induces its own metabolism by autoinduction. Carbamazepine's half-life following single acute doses is approximately 35 hours; with chronic dosing, its half-life decreases to 15 to 25 hours. This induction of metabolism may be enhanced by combined administration of carbamazepine and other enzyme-inducing AEDs; with polytherapy, carbamazepine's half-life may be as short as 6 to 10 hours.[37] This increase in clearance necessitates increased doses and/or increased frequency of carbamazepine administration. Autoinduction of carbamazepine metabolism appears to be related to dose or serum concentration. Approximately 1 month may be required for the autoinduction process to reach completion after each increase in carbamazepine dose.[79]

Assuming that compliance was not the main problem, A.R.'s carbamazepine dose should be increased. The drug's pharmacokinetics are generally linear with respect to acute dosage changes.[80] A 50% increase in dosage to 1,200 mg/day should re-establish seizure control with a serum concentration of approximately 9 μg/mL. Some decrease in this concentration should be anticipated after autoinduction has reached completion; depending on A.R.'s clinical status, further increases in dosage may be necessary.

BIOEQUIVALENCE OF GENERIC DOSAGE FORMS AND EFFECTS OF STORAGE ON BIOEQUIVALENCE

6. A.R.'s dosage was increased to 600 mg BID. Four weeks later, she was still experiencing approximately one complex partial seizure weekly. A repeat trough serum carbamazepine concentration was 6.5 μg/mL. Upon questioning, A.R. denied missing doses of medication, and a tablet count confirmed apparently accurate drug intake. A.R. relates that she experiences some mild nausea following her doses, but she has not vomited. It is noted that her pharmacist has begun substituting generic carbamazepine tablets for the Tegretol that was previously dispensed. What role, if any, might this change in carbamazepine tablet brand have played in the failure of A.R.'s serum concentrations to increase as expected? What other factors might be considered in explaining this situation?

Several manufacturers market generic carbamazepine tablets. Bioavailability data supplied by the manufacturers are based on single-dose or short multiple-dose studies in normal healthy subjects. Therefore, it is impossible to completely predict the results of a change from Tegretol to generic carbamazepine for maintenance therapy in an individual patient.[81] Bioavailability data and the author's (R.L.) experience with institutionalized patients with severe seizure disorders suggest that the generic carbamazepine preparations currently on the market may be substituted for Tegretol with little need for dosage adjustment. Nevertheless, significant differences in dissolution rates and absorption characteristics between generic carbamazepine and Tegretol have been reported.[43,82] In A.R.'s case, substitution of generic carbamazepine may be a possible cause for the lower-than-expected serum concentrations. Readjustment of her dose to gain seizure control and consistent use of one manufacturer's product might alleviate this problem.

Another factor may be partly responsible for the failure of A.R.'s serum concentrations to increase. Carbamazepine absorption appears somewhat capacity limited; as larger single doses are administered, smaller fractions of the administered dose may be absorbed.[83] Twice-daily administration of carbamazepine, when relatively large doses must be used, may be reducing A.R.'s capacity to absorb the drug. Changing to a three-times-daily or even four-times-daily dosing schedule with immediate-release carbamazepine tablets may result in improved absorption, increased serum concentrations, and improved clinical response. In addition, A.R.'s transient nausea also may improve because this side effect may be caused by direct irritation from the large quantities of carbamazepine ingested or by elevated peak serum concentrations of the drug.

Two extended-release forms of carbamazepine have recently become available, Tegretol XR and Carbatrol, and may be an alternative for A.R. Tegretol XR employs an "osmotic pump" type (Oros tablet) of extended release, and Carbatrol uses immediate-, extended-, and enteric-release beads in a capsule. These formulations allow more reliable absorption of drug when administered on a twice-daily dosing schedule. Many patients can better tolerate carbamazepine when these forms are used because large fluctuations in plasma concentrations are avoided. Use of Tegretol XR to avoid three-times-daily or four-times-daily dosing schedules has been shown to increase compliance for many patients.[84] It is important to counsel the patient on the fact that the empty Oros tablet shell from the Tegretol XR dose does not dissolve as it passes through the gastrointestinal (GI) tract, and it may be visible in the stool. The patient needs to understand that the carbamazepine has been absorbed, and that this is an empty shell. Tegretol XR tablets lose their extended-release properties when broken or crushed; Carbatrol beads may be emptied onto food or administered via feeding tube.[85]

In conclusion, it is impossible to identify a single cause for the unexpected serum concentration results in A.R. Use of a generic substitute for Tegretol and capacity-limited absorption may be playing roles. Poor compliance cannot be completely ruled out despite accurate tablet counts, especially when the medication causes the patient physical discomfort. Patients may go to elaborate lengths to conceal inaccurate drug intake. While multiple daily dosing regimens may make patient compliance more difficult, changing A.R.'s regimen to a three- or even four-times-daily schedule may reduce nausea and improve absorption. The use of Tegretol XR or Carbatrol may also relieve nausea and improve absorption while allowing A.R. to continue using a twice-daily dosing schedule.

CARBAMAZEPINE INTOXICATION AND CARBAMAZEPINE-INDUCED HYPONATREMIA

7. **A.R.'s carbamazepine regimen was changed to 400 mg TID and her seizure frequency decreased to approximately one every 2 to 3 months. She continued to receive the same generic** carbamazepine product. Steady-state trough serum concentrations were consistently reported as 10 to 11 μg/mL. She was not experiencing any significant side effects other than occasional mild nausea following doses; this was prevented if she took her medication with food. Following a generalized tonic-clonic seizure, her physician decided to increase her carbamazepine dosage to 1,600 mg/day (400 mg am, 400 mg noon, 400 mg late afternoon, and 400 mg HS) in an attempt to further control her seizures. Ten days after the dosage increase, A.R. began complaining of nausea, double vision, dizziness, a mildly unsteady gait, and inability to concentrate. Discuss the possible explanations for A.R.'s new symptoms. What further information should be obtained to assess this situation?

The carbamazepine intoxication syndrome is not as well defined nor as closely correlated with serum concentrations as intoxication with other AEDs such as phenytoin. Therefore, carbamazepine intoxication is defined primarily by symptoms; serum concentrations may not help in its confirmation.[33,73] A.R.'s current complaints are similar to those commonly associated with elevated serum carbamazepine concentrations; the same symptoms may, however, occur at much lower concentrations. GI intolerance (e.g., A.R.'s nausea) may occur at low doses and limit therapy despite "subtherapeutic" serum concentrations. Determination of a carbamazepine serum concentration would be helpful at this time to document the concentrations that produce symptoms of intoxication in A.R.

Carbamazepine also may cause "paradoxical intoxication" at serum concentrations of ≥ 20 μg/mL (usually seen in the setting of acute overdose). This condition is characterized by increased seizure frequency and is similar to the paradoxical intoxication occasionally seen with significantly elevated serum concentrations of phenytoin.[73] Accumulation of carbamazepine's active metabolite, carbamazepine-10,11-epoxide (CBZ-E), also may result in increased seizure activity without other symptoms of intoxication in some patients despite usual serum concentrations of the parent compound.[86] This is most likely to occur in patients receiving other drugs (usually AEDs such as valproate and felbamate) that inhibit the metabolism of CBZ-E. Mental retardation also may be a predisposing factor for this form of intoxication. Although A.R. does not seem especially predisposed to this adverse reaction to carbamazepine and CBZ-E, her recent dosage increase may have resulted in a significant elevation in CBZ-E serum concentrations; measurement of CBZ-E concentrations is indicated as part of the laboratory assessment of her present condition.

In addition, A.R. should be questioned about overcompliance and any new medicines (over-the-counter, prescription, or alternative) that may have been added to her current drug regimen for acute or chronic dosing purposes.

Hyponatremia associated with syndrome of inappropriate antidiuretic hormone (SIADH) also should be evaluated as a possible cause of A.R.'s symptoms. SIADH, which is less likely to occur in children, is a well-documented but uncommon adverse reaction to carbamazepine.[73] Symptoms associated with water intoxication can resemble those exhibited by A.R. Affected patients usually complain of headache, nausea, vomiting, and dizziness; in more severe cases, confusion and increased seizure activity may occur. This symptom pattern may be mistakenly attributed to carbamazepine intoxication.

The mechanism by which carbamazepine produces hyponatremia is unclear. It was believed that the drug stimulates the release of antidiuretic hormone (ADH) from the pituitary, but this mechanism has been questioned. Carbamazepine may act directly on the kidney to increase sodium loss, or it may cause resetting of osmoreceptors.[87,88] Although this effect is predictable enough for carbamazepine to be used in the treatment of some forms of diabetes insipidus, clinically significant water intoxication in patients treated with carbamazepine is uncommon. Nevertheless, laboratory monitoring often reveals depression of serum sodium concentrations in many patients receiving this drug. The effect of carbamazepine on ADH probably depends on serum concentration.[89]

SIADH may be less common in patients who receive both phenytoin and carbamazepine; phenytoin appears to counteract the antidiuretic effect of carbamazepine in some, but not all, affected patients.[89,90] This may result from either inhibition of ADH release or stimulation of carbamazepine metabolism by phenytoin; the relative contribution of each effect has not been determined. A.R.'s serum electrolytes should be measured to evaluate the possible role of hyponatremia in causing her current symptoms.

When significant SIADH related to carbamazepine therapy is identified, the condition usually can be treated by dosage reduction and mild fluid restriction. Discontinuation of carbamazepine and substitution of an alternative AED may be necessary in some patients. Demeclocycline (Declomycin) has been used successfully to manage some cases of carbamazepine-induced SIADH.[87] Demeclocycline inhibits activation of ADH-sensitive adenyl cyclase in the distal renal tubules and collecting ducts. Some patients may respond positively to increased sodium intake.[88]

8. A.R.'s serum concentrations of carbamazepine and CBZ-E were 14 μg/mL and 3.1 μg/mL (usual range, 0.4 to 4.0 μg/mL), respectively. Other laboratory values included serum sodium (Na), 130 mEq/L (normal, 136 to 145); chloride (Cl), 94 mEq/L (normal, 90 to 110); potassium (K), 3.8 mEq/L (normal, 3.5 to 5.0); blood urea nitrogen (BUN), 9 mg/dL (normal, 10 to 20); albumin, 3.2 g/dL (normal, 3.5 to 5.0). A CBC and a 12-panel chemistry screen were otherwise normal. On the basis of the subjective and objective information available, recommend a plan for management of A.R.'s condition.

[SI units: Na 130 mmol/L (normal, 136 to 145); Cl 94 mmol/L (normal, 90 to 110); K 3.8 mmol/L (normal, 3.5 to 5.0); BUN 3.21 mmol/L of urea (normal, 3.6 to 7.1); albumin 32 g/L (normal, 35 to 50)]

Although A.R.'s serum sodium concentration is somewhat low, it is not sufficiently reduced to account for her symptoms. Significant symptoms usually are not seen until serum sodium concentrations are <120 to 125 mEq/L. The temporal relationship between A.R.'s symptom onset and dosage increase and the elevated carbamazepine serum concentration suggest CNS intoxication from carbamazepine as the cause of her symptoms. Neither the serum concentration of CBZ-E nor the ratio of CBZ-E to carbamazepine serum concentrations is unusually elevated; however, CBZ-E may be contributing to A.R.'s apparent intoxication syndrome by exerting additive effects with those of carbamazepine. A.R.'s carbamazepine dosage regimen should be adjusted. The pattern of her symptoms, however, also should be evaluated before a decision is made to reduce the total daily dose. If the symptoms occur 2 to 4 hours after dosing, it may be possible to alleviate them by altering the pattern of dosing or changing the carbamazepine dosage form to an extended-release form.[73,91] Transient intoxication associated with peak serum concentrations is relatively common with carbamazepine. If A.R.'s symptoms do not coincide with expected times of peak drug absorption, then reducing her total daily dose to an intermediate level of 1,400 mg may relieve her intoxication while still producing improved seizure control. No additional alteration in A.R.'s regimen is necessary to control her reduced serum sodium concentration. Should her daily dose of carbamazepine be reduced, this change will minimize the effect of the drug on her water excretion.

Treatment Failure and Alternative Antiepileptic Drugs

9. R.H., a 17-year-old, 53-kg girl, has experienced simple partial seizures, complex partial seizures, and secondarily generalized tonic-clonic seizures for the past 2 years. She could not tolerate treatment with phenytoin (severe gingival hyperplasia, hypertrichosis, and mental "dullness") or valproate (persistent GI distress, tremor, and a weight gain of 8 kg). In addition, neither phenytoin nor valproate was dramatically effective for reduction of her seizures at tolerable serum concentrations. She currently receives carbamazepine 600 mg TID. Over the past 3 months, while being treated with carbamazepine, she has had approximately five simple partial seizures, three complex partial seizures, and one generalized tonic-clonic seizure following a complex partial seizure episode. This represents an approximate 30% reduction in her frequency of seizures. She tolerates her present dose of carbamazepine but has experienced significant drowsiness, GI upset, and mental confusion at higher doses. Her most recent serum concentration of carbamazepine was 14 μg/mL. What are possible therapeutic options for R.H.? Evaluate the newer AEDs and their possible usefulness for R.H.

R.H. is exhibiting a partial response to maximally tolerated doses of carbamazepine. An alteration in her current AED regimen appears to be indicated. She cannot tolerate other preferred medications because of side effects. Valproate is effective for control of partial seizures and is considered a useful alternative to first-choice medications such as carbamazepine and phenytoin.[63] R.H.'s prominent CNS side effects (e.g., persistent drowsiness) with other AEDs would make many clinicians reluctant to consider medications such as phenobarbital, primidone, clorazepate, or clonazepam as either alternatives or adjunctive agents to her current carbamazepine regimen. Use of one of the newer AEDs as adjunctive medication may be of value for R.H.

Eight new AEDs have been marketed in the United States since 1993 for maintenance treatment of seizure disorders: felbamate (Felbatol), gabapentin (Neurontin), lamotrigine (Lamictal), levetiracetam (Keppra), oxcarbazepine (Trileptal), topiramate (Topamax), tiagabine (Gabitril), and zonisamide (Zonegran) (Table 54-6).[92–103] These newer or second-generation AEDs are approved as "add-on" or adjunctive treatment of partial seizures with or without secondary generalization. Oxcarbazepine is approved as monotherapy or add-on therapy for partial seizures in adults and as add-on therapy in children >4 years of age. New AEDs, such as these eight agents, are primarily evaluated as "add-on" medications. Clinical trials are most often carried out in patients with partial seizures

Table 54-6 Drugs Used for the Treatment of Partial and Generalized Tonic-Clonic Seizures

AED	Regimen	Adverse Effects	Comments
Carbamazepine (Tegretol) (Tegretol XR) (Cabatrol)	Initial 200 mg BID (adults) or 100 mg BID (children) and ↑ weekly until therapeutic response or target serum concentrations. Usual maintenance doses 7–15 mg/kg/day in adults; 10–40 mg/kg/day in children.	GI upset, sedation, visual disturbance may limit dosage. Severe blood dyscrasias extremely rare (<1/50,000). Mild leukopenia more common. Laboratory monitoring of little value. Hepatotoxicity rare. May cause SIADH.	Usually little sedation and minimal interference with cognitive function or behavior. Preferred by most for partial or secondarily generalized seizures. Tegretol-XR or Carbatrol may allow less frequent dosing with fewer peak serum concentration–related side effects. These extended-release preparations may also facilitate compliance.
Phenytoin (Dilantin) (Phenytek)	Initiate at maintenance dose of 4–5 mg/kg/day (300–400 mg/day). Titrate on basis of clinical response and target serum concentration. 3–4 weeks between dose ↑ recommended because of potentially slow accumulation.	Nystagmus, ataxia, sedation, mental changes usually predictable from serum concentrations. Gum hyperplasia, hirsutism common. Osteomalacia uncommon. Seizure frequency may ↑ with significantly ↑ serum concentrations. Peripheral neuropathy, pseudolymphoma, hypersensitivity with liver damage rare.	Clearance and $t_{1/2}$ change with dose. Small ↑ in dose (30 mg capsule dosage form) recommended as therapeutic range approached. Suspension and chewable tablets contain free-acid form of phenytoin; capsules contain sodium phenytoin (converts to 92% of free-acid form). Cautious use of suspension; dose measurement and potential mixing difficulties. IM administration not recommended. Potential precipitation in IV solutions. Dilute in small volume of normal saline and administer IV using 0.45–0.22 micron filter. Administer IV at <50 mg/min. Fosphenytoin (Cerebyx) recommended for IM and IV use. Can be diluted for IV infusion in saline or dextrose-containing fluids. Can be administered at up to 150 mg PE/minute IV. Lower rate of injection site complications.
Valproate (Depakene, Depakote)	See Table 52-7.		
Phenobarbital	Initial 1 mg/kg/day; titrate to therapeutic response or target serum concentration. 2–3 weeks between dose ↑.	Sedation (chronic), behavior disturbances common, especially in children. Possibly impairs learning and intellectual performance. Osteomalacia uncommon.	Considered outmoded for antiepileptic therapy in most patients. Questionable benefit for prophylaxis of febrile seizures; adverse effects outweigh benefits. IV use for refractory status epilepticus. 10–20 mg/kg IV at <100 mg/min; caution when used with diazepam for status epilepticus because of additive cardiovascular and respiratory depression.
Primidone (Mysoline)	Initial 5–15 mg/kg/day; then titrate to therapeutic response or target serum concentration. 2–3 weeks between dose ↑.	Sedation, ataxia, GI toxicity common with initial therapy. Essentially similar profile to phenobarbital.	Considered outmoded for antiepileptic therapy in most patients. Most antiepileptic effects from phenobarbital as metabolite. Expensive with less favorable side effect profile.
Gabapentin (Neurontin)	Initial 300 mg/day with titration to 900–1,800 mg/day over 1–2 wk. Up to 2,400 mg/day or higher may be needed for some patients. Owing to short $t_{1/2}$, TID or QID dosing recommended.	Sedation, dizziness, and ataxia relatively common with initiation of therapy. Gabapentin therapy usually not associated with prominent side effects.	Primarily excreted unchanged by kidneys. No significant interactions with other AEDs or other drugs identified to date. Absorption may be dose dependent; fraction absorbed ↓ as size of individual dose ↑.

Drug	Dosing	Side Effects	Interactions
Lamotrigine (Lamictal)	*When added to enzyme inducers alone:* Initiate at 50 mg QD HS. May start at 50 mg BID. Daily dose can be ↑ by 50–100 mg Q 7–14 days. Usual maintenance doses of 400–500 mg/day. Doses up to 700 mg/day have been used. BID dosing may be necessary with enzyme inducer cotherapy. *When added to valproate alone:* Initiate at 25 mg QOD HS. Daily dose can be ↑ by 25 mg Q 14 days. Usual maintenance doses of 100–200 mg/day. *When added to valproate and enzyme inducers:* Initiate at 25 mg QOD HS. Daily dose can be ↑ by 25 mg Q 14 days. Usual daily doses of 100–200 mg/day.	Dizziness, diplopia, sedation, ataxia, and blurred vision. Common with initiation of therapy; limit speed of titration. Rash in ≈10% of treated patients; more common with coadministration with valproate and rapid dose escalation.	Significant ↑ in clearance of lamotrigine when coadministered with enzyme inducer such as carbamazepine. Significant ↓ in clearance when coadministered with valproate; valproate appears to inhibit metabolism of lamotrigine. ↑ CNS side effects when lamotrigine is used with carbamazepine. Slow, gradual titration of dose may reduce risk of skin rash.
Tiagabine (Gabitril)	Initial 4 mg/day, ↑ by 4 mg/day at 7 days. Then ↑ daily dose by 4–8 mg Q wk. Maximum recommended dose of 32 mg/day in adolescents or 56 mg/day in adults. BID to QID dosing recommended.	Drowsiness, nervousness, difficulty with concentration or attention, tremor. Nonspecific dizziness described by some patients.	Increase clearance when given with enzyme inducers. TID or QID doses probably needed. Potential for protein-binding displacement interactions with other highly protein bound drugs (e.g., valproate). Significance of protein-binding displacement not known at present. Substrate for CYP 3A.
Topiramate (Topamax)	Initial 50 mg HS. ↑ daily dose by 50 mg Q 7 days. 200–400 mg/day recommended as target dosage range. Larger daily doses associated with increased CNS side effects without improved seizure control. BID dosing recommended.	Sedation, dizziness, difficulty concentrating, confusion. May be dose related. Possible weight loss. Weak carbonic anhydrase (CA) inhibitor; may cause or predispose to kidney stones; CA inhibition also possibly related to paresthesias in up to 15%.	Approximately 70% renal elimination. Phenytoin and carbamazepine may reduce topiramate plasma concentrations and potentially increase dosage requirements. Topiramate may cause small ↑ in phenytoin plasma concentration and small ↓ in valproate concentrations. May ↓ effect of oral contraceptives.
Levetiracetam (Keppra)	Initial 250–500 mg BID. ↑ by 500–1000 mg/day Q 2 weeks. Usual maximum dose is 3,000 mg/day. Doses up to 4,000 mg/day have been used. BID dosing recommended.	Somnolence, dizziness, asthenia are commonly reported. Minor viral illnesses ("infection") may be more common with levetiracetam therapy; not associated with changes in WBC. Behavioral symptoms (agitation, emotional lability, hostility, depression, and depersonalization) reported.	No hepatic (CYP450 or UGT) metabolism. 66% excreted unchanged in urine. Less than 10% protein bound. No significant drug interactions reported. Apparently unique mechanism of antiepileptic action may make levetiracetam a logical choice for combination with other drugs.

Continued

Table 54-6   Drugs Used for the Treatment of partial and Generalized Tonic-Clonic Seizures—cont'd

AED	Regimen	Adverse Effects	Comments
Oxcarbazepine (Trileptal)	*Monotherapy:* Initial 300 mg BID. ↑ weekly up to 1,200 mg/day. *Adjunctive therapy:* Initial 300 mg BID. ↑ weekly up to 1,200 mg/day. Can go up to 2,400 mg/day.	Dizziness, somnolence, diplopia, fatigue, nausea, vomiting, dyspepsia, ataxia, abnormal vision, tremor, and abnormal gait are commonly reported. Hyponatremia is described with the administration of this drug; most cases asymptomatic, more common in elderly. A 25% cross-sensitivity has been reported between oxcarbazepine and carbamazepine.	Parent is a prodrug; the monohydroxy derivative (MHD) is the active component. It is readily converted to MHD via omnipresent cytosolic enzymes. Lacks autoinduction properties. Many years of experience with this drug in Europe.
Zonisamide (Zonegran)	Initial 100 mg QD. ↑ by 100 mg/day Q 2 weeks. General 200 to 400 mg/day; maximum 600 mg/day.	Somnolence, nausea, ataxia, dizziness, headache, and anorexia are common. Also reported are confusion, memory impairment, psychosis, diplopia, nystagmus, tremor, paresthesias, anemia and leukopenia, vomiting, weight loss, and nephrolithiasis. Serious skin eruptions, oligohidrosis, and hyperthermia have also occurred.	Broad spectrum, long $t_{1/2}$. 35% of dose is excreted unchanged in the urine. Advise patients to drink plenty of fluids. Many years of experience with this drug in Korea and Japan.

AEDs, antiepileptic drugs; CNS, central nervous system; GI, gastrointestinal; PE, phenytoin sodium equivalent; SIADH, syndrome of inappropriate antidiuretic hormone secretion; $t_{1/2}$, half-life; WBC, white blood cell count.

refractory to standard AEDs. Therefore, upon initial release of these medications for general use, they are likely to carry FDA-approved labeling only for treatment of partial seizures as adjunctive therapy. Lamotrigine has an FDA-approved indication for monotherapy. It is indicated for conversion to monotherapy in adults with partial seizures who are taking a single enzyme-inducing AED. Felbamate and lamotrigine have been evaluated intensively in controlled trials for treatment of seizures associated with Lennox-Gastaut syndrome and both are effective;[104,105] experience with topiramate suggests that this drug also may be effective in this syndrome.[106] Although reports exist on the efficacy of gabapentin, lamotrigine, topiramate, tiagabine, and levetiracetam when used as monotherapy,[51–55,107] only lamotrigine, felbamate, and oxcarbazepine have an FDA-approved indication for monotherapy. Other AEDs will undoubtedly follow with monotherapy indications. Animal screening tests and limited clinical reports suggest a broad spectrum of efficacy for felbamate, lamotrigine, topiramate, and zonisamide;[92,108–110,117] these drugs may prove useful in other seizure types such as absence.

SIDE EFFECTS

Common side effects for the newer AEDs are described in Table 54-6. Most of the newer AEDs are less sedating than older medications such as phenobarbital or phenytoin. Felbamate causes insomnia and irritability in a significant proportion of treated patients. Other side effects that may be prominent during felbamate therapy include headaches, insomnia, weight loss, and GI effects such as nausea, vomiting, and anorexia. Felbamate's usefulness is seriously limited by its association with aplastic anemia and hepatic failure. Some cases of felbamate-associated aplastic anemia and hepatotoxicity were fatal. A conservative, preliminary estimate of the occurrence rate is 1 case per 2,000 to 5,000 patients treated.[111] Too few cases of hepatic failure associated with felbamate therapy have been reported to allow conclusions to be drawn regarding characteristics of this potential adverse effect and risk factors for its development. Routine hematologic studies and LFTs should be performed and patients and their families should be fully informed of the potential risks. Written consent is recommended. Patients must be educated about the symptoms of hematologic and hepatic toxicity. Because of the relationship between felbamate therapy and aplastic anemia and hepatic failure, the place of felbamate in the treatment of epilepsy is uncertain.

Topiramate may cause cognitive disturbances, lethargy, and impaired mental concentration when given in large daily doses or when the dosage is titrated aggressively.[112] Topiramate has caused nephrolithiasis in approximately 1.5% of treated patients. This adverse effect is believed to be related to inhibition of carbonic anhydrase by topiramate, with resulting increased urinary pH and decreased citrate excretion. Topiramate may also cause dose-related weight loss.

Gabapentin, tiagabine, and levetiracetam to date have not been associated with serious side effects; in clinical use, tiagabine has caused nonspecific dizziness relatively frequently.[103,113,114]

The most serious side effect associated with lamotrigine has been skin rash. Rashes occur in approximately 10% of treated patients, usually in the first 8 weeks.[115] Rashes leading to hospitalization occurred in 1 of 300 adults and 1 of 100 children. Widespread, maculopapular rashes usually appear and may progress to erythema multiforme or toxic epidermal necrolysis. Lamotrigine-related rashes may resolve rapidly when lamotrigine is discontinued. Coadministration of valproate with lamotrigine may increase the likelihood of dermatologic reactions; it is partly for this reason that more conservative dosage titration and lower maintenance doses of lamotrigine are recommended for patients receiving concomitant valproate. Higher starting doses and more rapid dose escalation than those recommended by the manufacturer also increase the risk of skin rash.

Oxcarbazepine, a keto-derivative of carbamazepine, is essentially a prodrug for the monohydroxy active metabolite.[116] Oxcarbazepine probably causes less frequent, less severe adverse effects compared with carbamazepine. It may be better tolerated than carbamazepine by some patients because it is not converted to the 10,11-epoxide metabolite. The most commonly reported side effects in clinical trials include ataxia, dizziness, fatigue, nausea, somnolence, and diplopia. Hyponatremia has been reported, which suggests the need for periodic monitoring of serum sodium levels.

Zonisamide, developed in Japan, is a potent broad-spectrum AED tested in both animal models of epilepsy and patients with epilepsy.[117] Zonisamide is a sulfonamide derivative and thus is contraindicated in patients allergic to sulfonamides. The most commonly reported adverse events include ataxia, somnolence, agitation, and anorexia. Kidney stones have developed in 3% to 4% of patients, some of whom had a family history of nephrolithiasis.

PHARMACOKINETICS

The newer AEDs have somewhat different pharmacokinetic profiles from those of older agents. They also differ in their tendency to interact with other AEDs. Gabapentin is excreted entirely by the kidneys as unchanged drug and is not significantly bound to serum protein. Gabapentin has a relatively short half-life and should be administered three times daily.[118]

Topiramate has a half-life of approximately 20 hours, which allows twice-daily administration. It is only partially excreted by hepatic metabolism; approximately 70% of the drug is excreted unchanged by the kidneys. Topiramate is minimally protein bound (approximately 10% to 15%). When topiramate is coadministered with enzyme-inducing agents such as carbamazepine, hepatic metabolism is increased and topiramate clearance is increased. This interaction may necessitate titration to somewhat higher doses when topiramate is used with enzyme-inducing drugs. Inconsistently, topiramate may cause a small and often nonsignificant decrease in phenytoin plasma concentrations.

Tiagabine has a relatively short half-life (4 to 7 hours). It should be administered at least twice daily.[119] Concurrently administered enzyme-inducing AEDs may reduce tiagabine's half-life to 2 to 3 hours and necessitate use of larger daily doses and, possibly, more frequent dosing intervals. Tiagabine is highly protein bound (96%), and it is displaced from protein binding sites by valproate, salicylate, and naproxen. The clinical significance of these protein-binding interactions is unknown.

Felbamate undergoes both hepatic metabolism and renal excretion as unchanged drug. Phenytoin and carbamazepine induce the hepatic metabolism of felbamate and lower steady-state felbamate concentrations.[92] Interactions between felbamate and other AEDs may make therapeutic monitoring difficult. Felbamate reduces the clearance of phenytoin, valproate, and probably phenobarbital; it also reduces the clearance of CBZ-E while apparently increasing the conversion of carbamazepine to the epoxide metabolite.[120,121] Clinically, this latter effect may create a somewhat paradoxical situation: patients may experience symptoms of carbamazepine intoxication (including increased seizure activity)[86] with carbamazepine serum concentrations lower than those found before the addition of felbamate. CBZ-E serum concentrations are often elevated in these situations.

Lamotrigine is primarily eliminated by hepatic glucuronidation and excretion of metabolites in the urine. Other AEDs such as carbamazepine and phenytoin induce lamotrigine's hepatic metabolism. When lamotrigine is coadministered with enzyme-inducing drugs, its half-life decreases from approximately 24 hours to 15 hours. Valproate inhibits lamotrigine metabolism, causing increases in half-life and serum concentrations.[122,123] Patients treated with both lamotrigine and carbamazepine may experience more nausea, drowsiness, and ataxia. Although this interaction has been attributed to lamotrigine-induced increases in serum concentrations of CBZ-E in some patients,[124] lamotrigine does not consistently produce increases in this metabolite. It appears more likely that this interaction represents a pharmacodynamic interaction between lamotrigine and carbamazepine.[125]

Levetiracetam has a short half-life and is eliminated primarily by renal mechanisms. Dosage reductions are warranted for patients with renal impairment (creatinine clearance <80 mL/min). It appears to have a low potential for interactions with other drugs.[126]

Zonisamide has a long half-life and low protein binding. It is eliminated by both liver metabolism and renal excretion. The average half-life of zonisamide is 63 hours, but there is wide interpatient variation. Serum levels of zonisamide have been shown to be reduced by enzyme-inducing AEDs.[117]

Oxcarbazepine is a prodrug that is converted to the monohydroxy derivative (MHD), its primary active metabolite. It may cause less hepatic enzyme induction than carbamazepine and may therefore be less likely to interact with other medications. However, oxcarbazepine does increase the metabolism of oral contraceptive hormones.[127] Because oxcarbazepine probably has a similar mechanism of action to that of carbamazepine, it is unlikely that it would offer significant benefits to R.H. because she has not responded to maximum tolerated doses of carbamazepine.[116]

On the basis of efficacy and side effect characteristics, gabapentin, lamotrigine, topiramate, tiagabine, levetiracetam, or zonisamide could be considered for use as adjunctive therapy for R.H. In young, active patients such as R.H., sedation might prove to be a problem; however, it is not clear that any of these drugs predictably causes more initial or long-term sedation. The short half-lives of gabapentin and tiagabine and the associated need for R.H. to take several doses during the day might decrease her compliance with treatment. Therefore, topiramate, lamotrigine, levetiracetam, or zonisamide would be reasonable choices on the basis of convenience.

POTENTIAL THERAPIES

Other AEDs that may become available in the near future include pregabalin, remacemide, rufinamide, and harkos-

eride.[128] These drugs may become alternatives or adjuncts to established and newer medications for treatment of partial-onset seizures.

With advancing technology and knowledge about genes and brain networks, better imaging of seizure origin sites, and more, future treatment strategies should move from controlling symptoms of epilepsy with AEDs to prevention and cure.[129] For AED-resistant epilepsy, there is much research examining the role of multidrug transporters (e.g., P-glycoprotein) in the blood–brain barrier. These may act as a defense mechanism by limiting the accumulation of AEDs in the brain.[130]

Lamotrigine Therapy
INITIATION AND DOSAGE TITRATION

10. **R.H. is to be started on lamotrigine as adjunctive therapy to her carbamazepine. Outline a treatment plan for initiating and monitoring therapy for R.H. What should R.H. and her family be told about this medication and how to use it?**

Lamotrigine therapy (also see Question 9) should be initiated in RH with slow upward dosage titration to minimize early sedative effects and reduce the likelihood of skin rash. An initial dosage of 50 mg/day given at bedtime is recommended; the daily dose can be increased by 50 mg every 1 to 2 weeks. Usual maintenance dosages of lamotrigine are approximately 300 to 500 mg/day, although there is some experience with dosages of up to 700 mg/day. A patient's ability to tolerate this medication ultimately determines dosage limitations. Onset of side effects such as nausea, diplopia, ataxia, and dizziness may prevent further dosage increases. Lower initial dosages (25 mg every other day) with more conservative increases (i.e., by 25 mg/day every 2 weeks) have been recommended for patients who are receiving valproate when lamotrigine is added. Valproate's inhibition of lamotrigine metabolism results in significantly lower lamotrigine dosage requirements; side effects appear to be much more common with lamotrigine doses >200 mg when it is administered with valproate.

Because R.H. is currently receiving carbamazepine, induction of liver enzymes is likely to increase her dosage requirements for lamotrigine and allow a less conservative dosage titration. An initial dosage of 50 mg/day (at bedtime), with increases of 50 mg/day every 1 to 2 weeks, should be recommended. A twice-daily schedule is recommended for maintenance therapy. She should be told that she may feel drowsy and possibly experience headache and upset stomach, but that these side effects usually disappear with ongoing therapy. R.H. should contact her physician or other health care professional if severe side effects occur that make it difficult to take the medication; this is especially important if she develops a skin rash.

SIDE EFFECTS AND POSSIBLE INTERACTION WITH CARBAMAZEPINE

11. **Two days after her dosage of lamotrigine was increased to 300 mg/day (12 weeks after beginning therapy), R.H. noticed that her vision was blurring; she also complained of feeling dizzy and having difficulty maintaining her balance. Previously she had experienced only mild, occasional nausea. She had continued to experience seizures at approximately the same frequency**

she had before the initiation of lamotrigine. Her physician had encouraged her to continue taking the medication and explained that it would take time to increase the dose to possibly effective levels. Serum concentrations of carbamazepine and CBZ-E were 13.5 μg/mL and 3.1 μg/mL, respectively. Do these new side effects represent treatment failure with lamotrigine? If not, how might these new side effects be managed?

R.H.'s seizure disorder may be unresponsive to lamotrigine therapy, and her side effects may limit further dosage increases. Her current side effects, on clinical grounds, might represent carbamazepine intoxication, lamotrigine side effects, or an interaction between these two medications. Because R.H. tolerated the same carbamazepine serum concentration previously, carbamazepine "intoxication" seems a less likely cause. Assessing the role of lamotrigine as a single agent is difficult. Obtaining a lamotrigine serum concentration to aid in assessing her situation is not likely to be helpful. A usual "therapeutic range" for lamotrigine serum concentrations has not been established. Clinical studies have failed to demonstrate a significant correlation between lamotrigine serum concentrations and either therapeutic or adverse responses.[131,132] Her symptoms may also be related to the apparent pharmacodynamic interaction between lamotrigine and carbamazepine reported by some authors.[125] The effects experienced by some patients taking both drugs can be relieved by reducing the carbamazepine dosage. Subsequently, it may be possible to further increase her lamotrigine dosage to improve seizure control. This situation also should be assessed and possibly managed by empirically decreasing R.H.'s carbamazepine dosage by 200 to 400 mg/day and observing the effect on her symptoms.

Levetiracetam Therapy
INITIATION AND DOSAGE TITRATION

12. R.H.'s carbamazepine dosage was reduced to 1,400 mg/day. After 5 days, her symptoms persisted and her seizure frequency appeared to be increasing. The clinician decides to abandon lamotrigine therapy and institute treatment with levetiracetam. Recommend a plan for initiating R.H.'s levetiracetam treatment.

R.H. previously tolerated and had a better therapeutic response to a higher carbamazepine dose. Therefore, the dosage of carbamazepine should be returned to 1,800 mg/day before levetiracetam therapy is initiated. Little specific information is available to help determine how lamotrigine can be safely discontinued. As a general rule, rapid discontinuation of AEDs is not recommended in other than emergency situations. Therefore, immediate reduction of R.H.'s lamotrigine dosage to 200 mg/day would seem reasonable. This dosage could then be reduced by 50 to 100 mg every week until lamotrigine was discontinued.

Levetiracetam treatment (also see Question 9) can be instituted immediately for R.H. Levetiracetam does not interact with other AEDs, and R.H. is continuing to have seizures. Therefore, discontinuing lamotrigine during initiation of levetiracetam should not create difficulties in assessing R.H.'s response. Levetiracetam should be initiated at a dosage of 250 to 500 mg two times daily.[103,126] Although the manufacturer recommends initiating treatment at 500 mg twice daily, patients may better tolerate lower initial doses and more gradual

titration.[126] R.H.'s daily levetiracetam dose can be increased by 500 to 1,000 mg every 2 or 3 weeks, according to her tolerance of side effects and her change in seizure frequency. While the drug reaches steady state quickly, allowing at least 2 weeks for observation before dosage increases may improve patient tolerability and allow for a more thorough evaluation of therapeutic response. At present, the relationship between serum concentrations of levetiracetam and therapeutic response or symptoms of intoxication is not well defined. Therefore, R.H.'s dose should be titrated to the maximum tolerated levels required to control her seizures. There is limited published experience with levetiracetam dosages as high as 4,000 mg/day.

PATIENT EDUCATION

R.H. should be informed that with levetiracetam she may experience side effects similar to those she had with lamotrigine, but that they are less likely and should be temporary. A great deal of reassurance and encouragement may need to be given along with this information to help ensure that R.H. adheres to her treatment regimen. Many patients become discouraged when multiple trials of medication are necessary and side effects are prominent. They may express feelings of being "guinea pigs" and may become uncooperative with the therapeutic plan.

Phenytoin Therapy
INITIATION AND DOSAGE

13. J.N., an 18-year-old, 88-kg male college student, was diagnosed with epilepsy. He experiences generalized tonic-clonic seizures that last approximately 2 minutes approximately three times monthly. J.N. describes a "churning" feeling in his abdomen before his seizures; this is followed by involuntary right-sided jerking of his upper extremities, during which J.N. is awake and aware of his surroundings. His seizures have been observed and described well both by his family and by nursing staff who cared for him during a brief hospitalization following his first seizure. An EEG showed diffuse slowing with focal epileptiform discharges in the left temporal area; it was interpreted as abnormal. No correctable cause for his seizure disorder was identified despite a thorough workup. He has no other medical conditions and takes no routine medications. He was treated initially with carbamazepine up to 600 mg/day. He could not tolerate the medication because of nausea and diplopia despite serum concentrations of only 5 μg/mL. His physician has elected to implement a therapeutic trial of phenytoin for J.N. Recommend an initial dosage. What information should be provided to J.N. about his new medication?

Selecting a nontoxic, therapeutic dose of any drug is difficult without having information about the drug's disposition in the individual patient (i.e., prior dosages and resulting steady-state serum concentrations and clinical response). Although "average" dosages and resulting serum concentrations often are quoted, interpatient variability is significant. Phenytoin serum concentrations of ≥10 μg/mL are achieved in many adults receiving a daily dose of 4 to 5 mg/kg of phenytoin; however, either subtherapeutic or potentially toxic concentrations also may occur in significant numbers.[133] Therefore, careful monitoring of patient response is necessary to ensure effective, nontoxic therapy. An initial dosage of 400 mg/day would be appropriate for J.N. This represents a dosage of approximately 4.5 mg/kg per day. To avoid patient non-compliance because of transient side effects, J.N. could be instructed to take 100 mg in the morning and 200 mg 12 hours later for 1 week. If he can tolerate this regimen, he could then take 200 mg every 12 hours.

PATIENT EDUCATION

In addition to the name and strength of the medication and instructions for when and how it should be taken, J.N. should be informed that he may experience initial mild sedation from phenytoin. He should be cautioned that symptoms such as blurred or double vision, dysarthria ("thick" tongue), dizziness, or staggering may indicate that his dosage is too high; he should be instructed to notify his physician, pharmacist, or other health care professional of these symptoms. It is also a good idea to inform patients, at the beginning of therapy, that adjustments of medication dosage and possibly medication changes may be necessary before the medication regimen is stabilized.

ACCUMULATION PHARMACOKINETICS

14. **What are the characteristics of phenytoin accumulation pharmacokinetics?**

Phenytoin exhibits dose-dependent (Michaelis-Menten or capacity-limited) pharmacokinetics; therefore, the usual pharmacokinetic concepts of "clearance" and "half-life" are meaningless. The apparent half-life of phenytoin changes with the dose and serum concentration. Thus, the time required to reach a new steady state after alteration in dosage is difficult to predict because it depends on the dosage itself and the patient's pharmacokinetic parameters, V_{max} and K_m.[133] V_{max} is a kinetic constant representing the maximum rate of phenytoin elimination from the body. K_m is the Michaelis constant, the serum concentration at which the rate of elimination is 50% of V_{max}. Values for these parameters vary widely among patients; as a result, patterns of phenytoin accumulation and the time required to achieve steady state also are variable.

Many clinicians assume that phenytoin's apparent half-life is approximately 24 hours, and they wait 5 to 7 days before assessing the patient's clinical response and measuring serum phenytoin concentrations. Both clinical studies[134] and model simulations[138] using observed values for K_m and V_{max} indicate that up to 30 days may be required for serum concentrations to reach 90% of the steady state resulting from a dosage of 4 mg/kg per day. Occasionally, such a dose may exceed a patient's V_{max}; the result is extremely high serum phenytoin concentrations, with probable intoxication. If doses sufficient to produce steady-state serum concentrations of 10 to 15 µg/mL are given, 5 to 30 days may be required to achieve 90% of these concentrations.[133,135] One should not assume that steady state has been reached unless widely spaced, serial serum concentrations indicate that accumulation has ceased. Alterations in phenytoin dosage before steady state has been reached may result in significant fluctuations in serum concentrations and the patient's clinical status. In this author's experience (R.L.), such situations occur frequently and result in unnecessary confusion and expense. As always, serum concentrations in J.N. must be interpreted in the context of his clinical response.

ORAL LOADING DOSES

15. **Would a loading dose be of value for J.N. to reduce the potential delay in achieving a "therapeutic" serum concentration of phenytoin? How large a loading dose should be used, and how should it be administered?**

Administration of a loading dose would allow therapeutic serum concentrations of phenytoin to be achieved more rapidly, and more rapid control of J.N.'s seizure activity also would result. Because he is active and pursuing an education, more rapid seizure control may be a significant therapeutic goal. Studies of oral phenytoin loading indicate that doses of approximately 18 mg/kg will achieve serum concentrations approaching the usual therapeutic range after approximately 8 hours in most patients.[136,137] Oral loading doses appear to be better tolerated when administered in divided doses over 4 or more hours. GI upset appears to be the most common side effect related to this procedure. Cardiac side effects (e.g., sinus bradycardia, shortened PR intervals) have been observed rarely; they were not related to serum phenytoin concentrations, and their significance is uncertain.[138]

Oral phenytoin absorption after large doses is unpredictably slow, and it may be less complete than after smaller doses.[139] Although potentially therapeutic serum concentrations usually are seen after approximately 8 hours, peak concentrations may not occur for up to 60 hours after administration of large single doses.[133,138,139] Record and coworkers estimated that 18 mg/kg given in three doses over 6 hours would produce serum concentrations of 13 to 20 µg/mL 12 hours after completion of loading.[140] No rigorous clinical evaluations of this recommendation are available, although these suggested doses compare well with intravenous (IV) loading regimens. IV loading doses of 18 mg/kg will maintain phenytoin serum concentrations >10 µg/mL for 24 hours.[141]

Although administration of an oral loading dose to J.N. is pharmacokinetically sound and has certain therapeutic advantages, practical difficulties in monitoring an ambulatory patient for potential complications may indicate caution in recommending such a procedure. In addition, because J.N. had difficulty tolerating carbamazepine, it may be difficult to justify exposing him to the potential neurologic side effects of a phenytoin loading dose. A more practical approach with a lower risk of complications involves giving 1.5 to 2 times the prescribed maintenance dose for the first 2 or 3 days of treatment. Serum phenytoin concentrations should be checked on the day after completion of such a "miniloading" and weekly thereafter.

PHENYTOIN INTOXICATION

16. **J.N. was given phenytoin 200 mg am and 400 mg pm for 3 days. A phenytoin serum concentration drawn the morning of the fourth day was 12 µg/mL. No seizures had occurred, and J.N. experienced no side effects other than mild morning sedation. He was then instructed to take only 400 mg HS. One week later, his phenytoin concentration was 18 µg/mL. Mild nystagmus on far lateral gaze was noted, but J.N. had no subjective complaints and remained seizure-free. After 3 weeks, J.N. complained of double vision and feeling "drunk" and "unsteady." Significant nystagmus was present. His phenytoin concentration was 24 µg/mL. How should J.N.'s phenytoin dosage be altered?**

J.N.'s signs and symptoms in conjunction with the phenytoin serum concentration indicate mild phenytoin intoxication. Dosage reduction is indicated. Because there is no indication that steady state has been achieved, techniques for estimating J.N.'s V_{max} and K_m cannot be readily employed; the size of any dose reduction must be determined empirically.

Reducing J.N.'s dosage to 360 or 330 mg/day would be reasonable. This dosage reduction can be accomplished using 30-mg phenytoin capsules along with the usual 100-mg capsules. A larger reduction may result in a dramatic fall in serum concentrations, with some risk of loss of seizure control. Many clinicians also would have J.N. omit one day's dose of phenytoin before beginning the new maintenance dosage. This would accelerate the decline in phenytoin serum levels. Following this dosage change, clinical response and serum concentrations should be monitored closely. The new maintenance dose may still be excessive; if J.N.'s V_{max} for phenytoin is low, continued accumulation of drug may occur and serum concentrations may continue to increase despite the dosage reduction.[133]

BIOEQUIVALENCE OF DOSAGE FORMS

17. S.D. is a 24-year-old, male state hospital patient with a history of complex partial and secondarily generalized tonic-clonic seizures. On his current phenytoin dosage of 300 mg/day, his serum phenytoin concentrations have ranged from 3.2 to 13.5 μg/mL. Control of his seizures also fluctuates widely, correlating well with plasma concentrations of phenytoin. Nurses suspect S.D. of "cheeking" his phenytoin capsules, and his phenytoin has been changed to a suspension form to reduce this behavior. Discuss differences in bioavailability and biopharmaceutics among oral phenytoin dosage forms. Based on these differences, what would be an appropriate dosage of phenytoin suspension for S.D.?

Surreptitious refusal to take medications is a common problem in psychiatric patients. In addition, elderly, physically handicapped, or pediatric patients may have difficulty swallowing capsules. In these situations, phenytoin suspension is potentially useful.

No significant differences in bioavailability between phenytoin (i.e., Dilantin, Pfizer) suspension and capsules are reported; in addition, chewable phenytoin tablets (i.e., Dilantin Infatabs) are equally well absorbed.[133] The suspension and chewable tablets, however, contain phenytoin free acid; capsules contain sodium phenytoin. Unlike many drugs, phenytoin products are labeled with their contents listed as either phenytoin acid or sodium phenytoin rather than in terms of active drug. Therefore, phenytoin capsule products contain only 92% of the labeled content as phenytoin acid (i.e., a 100-mg sodium phenytoin capsule contains only 92 mg of phenytoin acid). Because small changes in dosage may result in dramatic changes in phenytoin serum concentrations and clinical response, this difference in phenytoin content should be considered when dosage forms are changed.[142]

If it is assumed that 300 mg of phenytoin capsules is a therapeutic daily dose for S.D., an appropriate daily dose of phenytoin suspension would be approximately 92% of 300 mg, or 275 mg (11 mL of the adult phenytoin suspension containing 125 mg/5 mL).

PATIENT EDUCATION

18. What special instructions should be provided to S.D. or the nursing staff to ensure proper, efficacious administration of this medication?

In the author's experience (R.L.), use of phenytoin suspension often results in unstable phenytoin serum concentrations and seizure control. This instability has been attributed to rapid settling of suspension between doses; however, significant between-dose or long-term settling does not appear to explain the clinical instability in patients receiving this dosage form. More likely, observed fluctuations in patient status result from inconsistent or improper dose measurement.[143,144] An accurate dose measuring device such as an oral syringe should be provided with phenytoin suspension. Patients or caregivers should be informed of the importance of accurate measurement and discouraged from using household measures such as "teaspoons." The person measuring the dose should be instructed to thoroughly shake the container before measuring each dose. Crushed chewable phenytoin tablets may provide better clinical stability and acceptable ease of administration if the use of phenytoin suspension is being considered.

EXTENDED-RELEASE DOSAGE FORMS AND GENERIC PREPARATIONS

19. Is there any need to alter the frequency of phenytoin administration when phenytoin suspension is used for S.D.?

The FDA requires phenytoin capsule preparations to be labeled as either "prompt" or "extended" on the basis of their rates of dissolution and absorption. Only extended phenytoin products are recommended for once-daily dosing. Presumably, the use of rapidly absorbed preparations as single daily doses will result in wide fluctuation of phenytoin serum concentrations between doses and will cause either loss of seizure control or toxicity.

Published documentation of significant differences in phenytoin serum concentrations and clinical response resulting from the use of rapidly versus slowly absorbed preparations during maintenance therapy is lacking.[145] A single-dose study in normal volunteers compared the absorption characteristics and bioavailability of phenytoin extended-release capsules and phenytoin suspension.[146] Differences in bioavailability or pharmacokinetics between the two dosage forms were not significant, and once-daily administration of properly measured phenytoin suspension is feasible on the basis of pharmacokinetic characteristics. Most studies on the feasibility of single daily phenytoin doses have used Dilantin Kapseals.[147,148] The likely effects of absorption rate and dosing interval on steady-state phenytoin serum concentration have been examined using a Michaelis-Menten pharmacokinetic model.[149] Predicted fluctuations resulting from the use of rapidly absorbed products administered once daily are not likely to be clinically significant unless the patient requires a high daily dose or has a low therapeutic index. Although the rate of phenytoin absorption does not appear to be of major clinical significance to therapy, the extent of absorption (relative bioavailability) may dramatically affect steady-state serum concentrations and clinical response. Dose-dependent pharmacokinetics magnify the effects of even minor changes in bioavailability or variations in drug content between dosage forms.[150] Therefore, the clinical significance of differences in absorption rates for oral phenytoin preparations is yet to be determined, but it appears to be minor.[145,149,151] If fluctuations in serum concentrations are of concern, use of a twice-daily dosing schedule should alleviate any potential problems.

Two forms of extended phenytoin capsules are available. Although these preparations may be bioequivalent to Dilantin Kapseals, there may be instances in which significant alterations in absorption can occur. Differences in bioavailability between the Mylan formulation of extended phenytoin capsules and the Dilantin Kapseals product were recently shown following single-dose administration to healthy volunteers. When administered with a high-fat meal, bioavailability of the Mylan product was 13% lower than that observed with Dilantin Kapseals. The authors estimated that this would result in a median 37% decrease in plasma phenytoin concentrations if patients routinely took their phenytoin with a high-fat meal and were switched from Dilantin Kapseals to Mylan extended phenytoin. Conversely, a switch from Dilantin Kapseals to Mylan extended phenytoin capsules (under the same dietary conditions) was estimated to result in a 102% increase in plasma phenytoin concentrations.[151a] Thus, patients taking the Mylan product should be counseled to avoid taking this medication with food.

Recently a new form of extended sodium phenytoin capsules, Phenytek, was approved. Only the manufacturer's bioavailability data are available for this preparation; there have been no clinical studies evaluating outcomes in patients in whom this generic preparation was used to replace Dilantin. The manufacturer's data appear to support equivalent absorption profiles and bioavailability for Phenytek compared to Dilantin when administered on an empty stomach or with food. Area under the plasma concentration–time curve (AUC) for the new generic preparation is approximately 6% smaller following administration of 300-mg doses with food. Because of phenytoin's dose-dependent pharmacokinetics, this difference could be clinically significant. Resolution of this question will require outcome studies in patients. The new preparation is available only as 200-mg and 300-mg capsules. Capsules contain either two or three erodible-matrix tablets.

S.D. can probably be adequately managed with administration of his phenytoin suspension as a single daily dose. His clinical response should be monitored to detect significant effects of the suspension or dosage schedule on seizure control.

INTRAMUSCULAR PHENYTOIN AND FOSPHENYTOIN (PHENYTOIN PRODRUG)

20. S.D. has been stabilized on 275 mg/day of phenytoin suspension. Serum drug concentrations are stable at 10 to 12 μg/mL, and he has had no seizures for 2 months. S.D. has been transferred to the acute medical unit following a 2-day history of anorexia, nausea, occasional vomiting, and abdominal pain accompanied by diarrhea. He is now "nothing per os" (NPO). Intramuscular (IM) fosphenytoin, 275 mg (PE) per day, has been ordered. Discuss the use of IM fosphenytoin, and devise a dosage regimen for S.D.

S.D. is a candidate for parenteral administration of his AED. If placement of an IV line for fluid administration is not planned, then IM administration is probably an acceptable approach to treatment. Previously, sodium phenytoin (Dilantin) injection was the only parenteral preparation available for re-

placement of oral phenytoin. Fosphenytoin sodium (Cerebyx) injection is available, and Dilantin injection has been discontinued. Generic preparations of sodium phenytoin injection are still available. IM administration of phenytoin is not recommended. Injectable phenytoin is highly alkaline (pH 12) and extremely irritating to tissue. Following IM injection, the drug may precipitate at the injection site because of the change in pH. As a result, phenytoin crystals form a repository or depot from which the drug is slowly absorbed.[152–154] There may be injection site discomfort, although severe muscle damage does not seem to occur.[154]

Fosphenytoin, a phosphate ester prodrug of phenytoin, is highly water soluble. Its solubility allows this preparation to be administered parenterally without the need for solubilization using propylene glycol or the adjustment of pH to nonphysiologic levels. Therefore, fosphenytoin may be administered either IM or IV with less risk of tissue damage and venous irritation than with parenteral administration of phenytoin.[155–157] (See Questions 49 to 51 for discussion of IV administration of phenytoin and fosphenytoin.) After administration, the prodrug is rapidly absorbed and converted to phenytoin by phosphatase enzymes. Ultimately, the bioavailability of phenytoin from IM fosphenytoin administration is 100%.

Fosphenytoin is available as a solution containing 50 mg PE/mL, where PE equals phenytoin sodium equivalents. By labeling fosphenytoin this way, no dosing adjustments are necessary when converting from phenytoin sodium to fosphenytoin or vice versa. Although the prescriber ordered 275 mg PE, S.D. may be underdosed. His dosage of phenytoin suspension is providing the equivalent of 300 mg/day of sodium phenytoin. He should receive a 300-mg dose of fosphenytoin daily to fully replace his current dosage of phenytoin suspension.[157]

Assuming that S.D. will be given 300 mg PE of fosphenytoin daily, he will require a total of 6 mL of this injection given IM. This medication is well tolerated when it is given IM, and S.D.'s full daily dose can probably be given in a single injection site without causing excessive discomfort. Some clinicians report administering IM injections of fosphenytoin as large as 20 mL in a single site without adverse consequences or serious discomfort.[158] It is also possible to divide his daily dosage into two injections given in two different sites, although many patients prefer to receive fewer injections.

ADVERSE EFFECTS

21. M.N., a 10-year-old boy receiving 150 mg/day of phenytoin as chewable tablets, is to be fitted with orthodontic braces. He exhibits moderate gingival hyperplasia resulting in difficulty maintaining oral hygiene and halitosis. Discuss phenytoin-related gingival hyperplasia and management techniques that may be helpful for M.N.

Gingival Hyperplasia. Gum hyperplasia related to phenytoin is common and troublesome. Prevalence is estimated at up to 90%,[159] depending on the rating system used and the degree of gum change rated as hyperplastic. A realistic prevalence estimate is probably 40% to 50% of treated patients.[160] Prevalence and incidence rates, however, are misleading because the occurrence and severity of hyperplasia are related to the dose and serum concentration of phenytoin.[160,161] Gingival hyperplasia is of obvious cosmetic importance. Also, as in M.N., formation of pockets of tissue leads to difficulties with oral hygiene, and severe halitosis may result.

The mechanism of phenytoin-induced gingival hyperplasia is not well understood. The drug is excreted in saliva and saliva phenytoin concentrations and hyperplasia are correlated; however, this correlation may simply reflect higher serum concentrations producing a greater pharmacologic effect. Phenytoin may stimulate gingival mast cells to release heparin and other mediators. These mediators may encourage the synthesis of excessive amounts of new connective tissue by fibroblasts. Local irritation caused by dental plaque and food particles may further stimulate this process. Some patients may be predisposed to gum hyperplasia because they accumulate higher concentrations of phenytoin in gum tissue.[160,161]

There are three approaches to the treatment of existing hyperplasia[161]: (1) dosage reduction or replacement of phenytoin with an alternative AED, if possible, will permit partial or complete reversal of hyperplasia; (2) surgical gingivectomy will correct the problem temporarily, but hyperplasia eventually recurs; and (3) oral physiotherapy (periodontal treatment) eliminates local irritants and maintains oral hygiene. Because M.N. is to be fitted with braces, oral hygiene will be further complicated. Some form of treatment for existing hyperplasia and prevention of further tissue enlargement is important. Assuming that phenytoin is producing adequate seizure control, a combination of gingivectomy and follow-up periodontal treatment may be the best approach.

Theoretically, the use of chewable phenytoin tablets in M.N. may aggravate hyperplasia. Exposure of the gingiva to high localized concentrations of phenytoin may result from braces holding tablet fragments in close physical contact with gum tissue. The significance of this relationship, however, is questionable. If M.N. can swallow capsules, a change to this dosage form may be beneficial and is usually less expensive. The most appropriate dosage of phenytoin sodium capsules for M.N. would be 160 mg/day. If chewable tablets are used, having M.N. rinse and swallow after each dose may eliminate problems. Use of phenytoin suspension also may be a useful option. Drug particles, however, may still be retained by the braces, and maintenance of uniform dosage may be more difficult.

Oral hygiene programs appear to reduce the degree and severity of gingival hyperplasia when they are initiated before phenytoin therapy is started.[161] Patients who are beginning phenytoin therapy should be educated about the role of oral hygiene in diminishing this side effect. The use of dental floss, gum stimulators, and Water Pik-type appliances may be beneficial adjuncts to other oral hygiene techniques.

22. G.R. is a 53-year-old man with primary generalized epilepsy characterized by occasional tonic-clonic seizures. His dosage of phenytoin was recently reduced from 400 mg/day to 360 mg/day because of symptoms of phenytoin intoxication. G.R.'s serum phenytoin concentration was 32 μg/mL. The neurologic evaluation was otherwise negative. After the daily dose of phenytoin was reduced to 360 mg, his symptoms of intoxication (confusion and ataxia) decreased significantly. No seizures occurred during the following 8 weeks. He continued to complain of being mildly "unsteady" on his feet. Nystagmus on far lateral gaze was present. The serum phenytoin concentration was decreased to 24 μg/mL. Because G.R.'s seizures are apparently under complete control, is there any problem maintaining him on mildly intoxicating doses of phenytoin? Does prolonged intoxication with phenytoin increase the likelihood of permanent neurologic impairment?

Neurotoxicity. Patients chronically maintained on intoxicating doses of phenytoin appear to be at some risk for developing irreversible cerebellar damage or peripheral neuropathy. Cerebellar degeneration, resulting in symptoms such as dysarthria, ataxic gait, intention tremor, and muscular hypotonia, is of particular concern; this complication has been observed following episodes of acute phenytoin intoxication.[162,163] Generalized seizures also may cause cerebellar degeneration secondary to hypoxia. For this reason, the relative importance of phenytoin in the development of this condition is controversial. Nevertheless, several cases involved patients without hypoxic seizures.[163,164]

Symptomatic phenytoin-related peripheral neuropathy is rare, although electrophysiologic evidence of impaired neuronal conduction may be found in many patients.[162,165] Symptomatic patients may complain of paresthesias, muscle weakness, and occasional muscle wasting. Knee and ankle tendon reflexes are absent in 18% of patients on long-term phenytoin therapy; the upper limbs are affected rarely. Although areflexia may be irreversible,[166] electrophysiologic abnormalities may be closely related to excessive serum phenytoin concentrations and are reversible following dosage reduction or discontinuation.[164]

In G.R., the general discomfort of mild phenytoin intoxication and the potential for producing cerebellar degeneration would appear to dictate an alteration in therapy. The phenytoin dosage should be reduced to 330 mg/day because this dosage may produce adequate seizure control without toxic symptoms. Should seizures recur at this lower dosage, it may be advisable to attempt to treat G.R. with an alternative AED.

INTERACTION WITH VALPROATE

23. G.R.'s phenytoin dosage was reduced to 330 mg/day. Over the following 6 weeks, his serum phenytoin concentrations decreased to 18 μg/mL and neurotoxic symptoms were completely reversed. G.R. has once again begun to experience generalized tonic-clonic seizures twice monthly. His seizures appear to be primarily generalized from their onset; no aura accompanies the seizures, and no focal changes are evident on the EEG. His physician decided to initiate treatment with divalproex (Depakote). The therapeutic goal is to titrate divalproex to achieve seizure control and subsequently discontinue phenytoin. Divalproex was started at 250 mg TID and over 3 weeks was increased to 1,000 mg BID. At the next office visit, G.R. complained again of feeling "unsteady" on his feet. Nystagmus on far lateral gaze was again noted. Serum concentrations of valproic acid and phenytoin were 62 μg/mL and 15 μg/mL, respectively. A complete laboratory screening battery showed no abnormalities other than a serum albumin concentration of 3.0 g/dL. How might the interaction between valproate (divalproex) and phenytoin have caused these symptoms? How should this interaction be managed?

[SI unit: serum albumin, 30 g/L]

The interaction between valproate and phenytoin is often troublesome because clinical manifestations of the interaction may not correlate with serum drug concentrations. Valproate potentially has two effects on phenytoin's pharmacokinetic disposition; the clinical results of this interaction vary among patients, depending on the magnitude of each effect and the patient's ability to metabolize phenytoin. Valproate displaces phenytoin from binding sites on serum albumin, causing an increase in the free fraction of phenytoin. For some patients, there is no net clinical effect of this displacement because the metabolism of phenytoin increases and free serum concentrations of phenytoin return to their predisplacement levels. Under these circumstances, the total serum phenytoin concentration would be reduced while the free fraction would remain elevated. If a patient's serum concentration of phenytoin is high enough to approach saturation of metabolic enzymes, the increase in metabolism of unbound phenytoin may not occur. As a result, unbound concentrations of phenytoin may remain elevated, and total serum phenytoin concentrations may change only slightly or may even increase. Valproate also is capable of inhibiting the metabolism of several drugs, including phenytoin. This effect may cause an increase in both unbound and total serum phenytoin concentrations.[167–169] Because of the complexity of the mechanisms involved in this interaction, prediction of the clinical or pharmacokinetic effect of addition of valproate to phenytoin therapy is extremely difficult. Clinicians should be aware that a significant, persistent increase in the serum concentration of unbound, pharmacologically active phenytoin is possible. The clinical status of the patient must be monitored carefully; determination of free (unbound) serum phenytoin concentrations may provide information helpful in assessing the reasons for any changes observed in the patient's clinical status. Most clinical laboratories can provide analysis of free serum phenytoin concentrations, although samples may need to be sent to an outside reference laboratory, resulting in a delay of several days before results are available. These tests are typically more expensive also.

In G.R.'s case, the addition of valproate probably has caused unbound phenytoin serum concentrations to increase significantly. This interaction usually is not observed unless serum valproate concentrations approach 100 μg/mL. G.R.'s reduced serum albumin level may account for this interaction. With a reduced serum albumin concentration, binding sites for phenytoin and valproate are already limited; therefore, displacement interactions such as this are more likely to occur. G.R.'s symptoms are identical to those he exhibited previously while intoxicated on phenytoin; they are not characteristic of symptoms associated with initiation of valproate therapy. The elevation in the unbound serum phenytoin concentration has the same effect as an increase in his phenytoin dose. G.R.'s total phenytoin serum concentration of 15 μg/mL is misleading because it does not reflect the increased free fraction and free concentration of phenytoin. A free phenytoin serum concentration should be determined to help assess this situation. Because laboratory test results may be delayed, G.R.'s phenytoin dose should be reduced empirically to alleviate his toxicity. A reduction of at least 30 mg/day in G.R.'s dosage would be appropriate.

24. G.R.'s phenytoin dose was held for 1 day and then reduced to 300 mg/day. Within 3 days his symptoms had improved significantly. The serum concentration of free phenytoin was reported as 2.4 μg/mL (usual therapeutic range, 1.0 to 2.0 μg/mL). Because G.R. remained seizure-free, his phenytoin dosage was reduced by 30 to 40 mg/day every week in an effort to eliminate phenytoin and employ divalproex monotherapy. What effect is discontinuation of phenytoin likely to have on G.R.'s valproate serum concentrations and his clinical response? How should G.R. be monitored during this reduction?

The interaction between phenytoin and valproate also involves stimulation of valproate metabolism. Induction of hepatic metabolic enzymes by phenytoin may significantly increase the clearance of valproate.[170] During concomitant therapy, larger doses of valproate will be required to achieve effective seizure control. Upon discontinuation of an enzyme inducer such as phenytoin, valproate serum concentrations may increase significantly as clearance decreases. In this author's experience (R.L.), discontinuation of phenytoin (and other enzyme-inducing drugs such as carbamazepine) is not always associated with a gradual stepwise increase in valproate serum concentrations. Instead, valproate concentrations may increase only slightly until phenytoin is discontinued completely. Subsequently, there may be a striking increase in valproate concentrations as hepatic metabolism returns to a noninduced state. G.R. should be monitored for clinical signs and symptoms that may indicate excessive serum valproate concentrations (see later discussion). Although elevated valproate serum concentrations do not always indicate intoxication, they may be useful as guidelines for reduction of G.R.'s divalproex dose. If his seizures remain well controlled, the dosage of divalproex can be reduced to the lowest level necessary. G.R. should be instructed to report any signs or symptoms possibly caused by excessive valproate serum concentrations (e.g., GI symptoms such as nausea, tremor, or drowsiness).[171]

Absence Seizures

Choice of Medication and Initiation of Ethosuximide Therapy

25. T.D., a 7-year-old, 25-kg girl, is reported by her teacher to have three or four episodes of "staring" daily. Each spell lasts 5 to 10 seconds. There are no convulsive movements, although her eyelids appear to flutter during the episodes. She is fully alert afterward. T.D.'s school performance is somewhat below average, despite an IQ of 125. An EEG shows 3-second spike-wave activity. Typical absence epilepsy is diagnosed. A physical examination and laboratory evaluation are normal, and no other positive findings are evident on the neurologic examination. What drug should be prescribed for T.D., and how should therapy with this drug be initiated?

Only a few drugs are routinely used for treatment of absence epilepsy (see Tables 54-2 and 54-7). At present, ethosuximide (Zarontin) and valproate are the primary drugs available in the United States. Both drugs are equally effective against absence seizures. Trimethadione (Tridione) was formerly used, but it is less effective and is associated with a high rate of neurologic side effects and a risk of hematologic toxicity.[172] At present, most authorities consider ethosuximide the drug of first choice for treatment of absence seizures. Controlled trials have demonstrated its efficacy, and it is potentially less toxic than valproate. In comparison to ethosux-

Table 54-7   **Common Drugs for the Treatment of Absence Seizures**

AED	Regimen	Adverse Effects	Comments
Valproate (Depakene, Depakote, Depakote ER)	Initial 5–10 mg/kg/day (sprinkle caps or syrup); then ↑ by 5–10 mg/kg/day weekly to therapeutic effect or target serum concentration. Manufacturer's recommended usual maximum dose of 60 mg/kg/day often must be exceeded clinically (especially for patients receiving enzyme-inducing AEDs) to achieve optimal clinical results. QD dosing recommended for extended-release (ER) product; doses should be 8–20% higher than non-ER products.	GI upset, appetite stimulation, and weight gain common. Serious hepatotoxicity extremely rare with monotherapy and in patients >2 yr old.	Enteric-coated tablets or capsules preferred oral dosage forms because of ↓ GI toxicity. Time to peak serum concentrations delayed for 3–8 hr with enteric coating; longer delay if given with food; serum concentrations must be interpreted carefully. Also effective against primarily generalized tonic-clonic seizures.
Ethosuximide (Zarontin)	Initial 20 mg/kg/day or 250 mg QD or BID; then ↑ by 250 mg/day Q 2 wk to therapeutic effect or target serum concentration	GI upset and sedation common with large single dose, especially on initiation of therapy. Daily divided doses may be necessary despite long $t_{1/2}$. Leukopenia (mild, transient) in up to 7%; serious hematologic toxicity extremely rare.	Parents/patient should be informed that GI effects and sedation may occur but tolerance usually develops. No good evidence that ethosuximide precipitates tonic-clonic seizures. Up to 50% of patients with absence may develop tonic-clonic seizures independent of ethosuximide.

AED, antiepileptic drug; GI, gastrointestinal.

imide, valproate is more likely to cause significant nausea and initial drowsiness, it is more expensive than ethosuximide, and it is more likely to interact with other AEDs. Valproate usually is reserved for patients whose absence seizures do not respond to ethosuximide.[173] Clonazepam (Klonopin), a benzodiazepine, often is effective for control of absence seizures. Therapy with this drug is limited by prominent CNS side effects (sedation, ataxia, and mood changes) and development of tolerance to its antiepileptic effect after long-term use.[174] Most authorities consider clonazepam a third-choice drug for treatment of absence seizures.

Ethosuximide therapy should be initiated for T.D. at a dosage of 15 to 20 mg/kg per day or 250 mg twice daily. The daily dose can be increased by 250 mg every 10 to 14 days as necessary to control seizures. Because the average half-life of ethosuximide in children is ≥30 hours, a delay of 10 to 14 days between dosage increments allows approximately 7 days for achievement of steady state and 7 days for assessment of response.[37]

PATIENT/CAREGIVER EDUCATION

Educating T.D. and her parents regarding the importance of regular administration of the drug is extremely helpful in ensuring successful therapy. Noncompliance is common in patients taking AEDs, and rapid discontinuation of these drugs (often secondary to noncompliance) may precipitate status epilepticus. The concept that medication controls rather than cures the seizure disorder should be strongly reinforced. It is also critical to inform both the parents and T.D. that a therapeutic response may not occur immediately and that dosage adjustments may be necessary to establish an effective dose with minimal side effects.

THERAPEUTIC MONITORING

26. **What subjective or objective clinical data should be monitored in T.D. for evidence of ethosuximide's therapeutic and adverse effects?**

Serum concentrations of 40 to 100 µg/mL of ethosuximide are considered necessary for therapeutic benefits; however, a clearly defined toxicity syndrome does not seem to develop when ethosuximide serum concentrations exceed 100 µg/mL. Thus, a gradual and cautious increase in the dose of ethosuximide when serum concentrations are already beyond the upper limits of the "usual therapeutic range" may allow further response in resistant patients. Although ethosuximide traditionally is administered in divided doses, its long half-life allows successful use of single daily doses for many patients. Clinicians should be alert to acute side effects of nausea and vomiting that are associated with large single doses of ethosuximide; should these occur, divided daily doses may be necessary.[37]

Laboratory monitoring for idiosyncratic hematologic toxicity from ethosuximide often is recommended. Ethosuximide causes neutropenia in approximately 7% of patients. Although this reaction often is transient even if the drug is continued, rare patients may develop fatal pancytopenia. Presumably, early detection of neutropenia by means of periodic CBCs will allow discontinuation of the drug and potential reversal of this adverse effect.[175] These hematologic reactions, however, can occur unpredictably at any time during therapy and often are missed by routine laboratory monitoring. Patient/caregiver education regarding signs and symptoms associated with leukopenia and pancytopenia (e.g., sudden onset of severe sore throat with oral lesions, easy bruisability, increased bleeding tendency) and instructions to consult the physician if these symptoms occur may be more important than laboratory monitoring.[75]

T.D.'s parents should be informed that nausea or sedation may occur with initiation of ethosuximide. Tolerance to these effects usually develops, although temporary dose reductions may be necessary. Subtle degrees of sedation may persist throughout therapy and may not be recognized until the drug has been discontinued and alertness improves.

Generalized Tonic-Clonic Seizures Accompanying Absence Seizures

27. Three months later, T.D.'s absence spells have been reduced to a frequency of one every 2 weeks with an ethosuximide dosage of 750 mg/day and a serum concentration of 85 μg/mL. Her initial drowsiness has almost disappeared, and nausea was alleviated by administering doses with food. She has, however, experienced two tonic-clonic convulsions in the past month. Both seizures were witnessed by her parents and were well described: no auras or signs of focal seizure activity were apparent, and each episode lasted 3 to 4 minutes and apparently consisted of typical tonic-clonic activity. T.D. was incontinent of urine on both occasions, and postictal confusion and drowsiness was significant. Physical examination and laboratory testing showed no abnormalities. A repeat EEG continued to show infrequent 3-second spikes and waves; no abnormal focal discharges were noted. What is the relationship between T.D.'s tonic-clonic seizures and ethosuximide therapy?

It is commonly believed, and often stated in the literature, that ethosuximide may precipitate or worsen tonic-clonic seizures; however, this effect has not been clearly demonstrated. As many as 50% of patients who initially present with absence seizures also develop tonic-clonic seizures.[176] In the past, it was common practice to add phenobarbital or phenytoin to ethosuximide therapy to prevent this. Livingston and associates[177] found that 80.5% of their patients treated with a drug specific for absence spells developed "grand mal" seizures, while only 36% did so while receiving combined therapy. On the other hand, Browne and Mirsky[176] pointed out that a child with absence seizures who has not yet had a tonic-clonic seizure has only a 25% chance of doing so in the future. In addition, routine use of drugs for prophylaxis of tonic-clonic seizures may increase the risk of toxicity and potentially reduce compliance with medication regimens. Sedative drugs, especially phenobarbital, actually may aggravate absence seizures in some patients.[178]

In summary, subsequent generalized tonic-clonic seizures are common in patients who initially develop absence spells.

It is not possible to assess the causative role of ethosuximide for this development in T.D.

Assessment Regarding Need for Alteration in Antiepileptic Drug Therapy and Choice of Alternative Antiepileptic Drug

28. What alterations are indicated in T.D.'s drug therapy because of the appearance of generalized tonic-clonic seizures?

Drug therapy for prevention of further tonic-clonic seizures would seem indicated at this time. Phenobarbital, phenytoin, carbamazepine, or valproate might be considered for use in T.D. Owing to her age and sex, many clinicians would avoid using phenytoin because of its dysmorphic and cosmetic side effects. Phenobarbital may cause sedation and behavioral disturbances (see below) and may aggravate coexisting absence seizures. Carbamazepine is now considered by many experts to be the drug of first choice for secondarily generalized tonic-clonic seizures and some cases of primary tonic-clonic seizures in children. It lacks many of the troublesome, common side effects associated with phenobarbital and phenytoin; in young children with primary generalized tonic-clonic seizures, carbamazepine may be preferred over valproate because it is less likely to induce serious hepatotoxicity.[1] Carbamazepine, however, is not effective for control of absence seizures. Therefore, it is likely that both ethosuximide and carbamazepine would be needed by T.D. Carbamazepine also has been occasionally associated with exacerbation of seizures (including atonic, myoclonic, and absence seizures) in children with mixed seizure disorders who exhibit bilaterally synchronous 2.5- to 3-cycle-per-second discharges on the EEG.[179,180] The need for polytherapy and the possible risk of seizure exacerbation make carbamazepine a less attractive treatment option for T.D.

Valproate is effective for controlling both absence and primary generalized tonic-clonic seizures.[26,29] In T.D., the difference in potential efficacy for tonic-clonic seizures between carbamazepine and valproate may be significant. She appears to have primary generalized tonic-clonic convulsions; focal signs (e.g., unilateral or single limb involvement) were not observed by the parents, and focal discharges (e.g., isolated abnormal electrical activity localized to one portion of the brain) were not found on the EEG. Although neither observation completely rules out secondarily generalized tonic-clonic seizures, the likelihood seems low. Therefore, valproate may offer some advantages over carbamazepine in terms of efficacy. In addition, both of T.D.'s seizure types potentially could be controlled with a single medication.

Valproate Therapy
INITIATION AND DOSAGE

29. T.D.'s physician elects to use valproate. The therapeutic goal is control of her seizures with valproate alone. What procedure should be followed regarding discontinuation of ethosuximide and initiation of valproate?

Techniques used by clinicians to substitute one AED for another depend largely on experience and judgment. Generally, it is best to attain potentially therapeutic doses per serum concentrations of a new medication before attempting to discontinue the previous drug. Ethosuximide has a relatively long half-life, while valproate's half-life is short. Therefore, if necessary, steady-state serum concentrations of valproate can be established and evaluated rapidly; evaluation of the effect of decreases in the ethosuximide dosage must await the prolonged elimination of this drug. Once a desired valproate dose has been achieved, the ethosuximide dosage can be reduced gradually by 250 mg/day every 2 to 4 weeks.

Valproate should be initiated at 125 mg twice daily. Valproic acid syrup or divalproex sodium (Depakote tablets or Depakote Sprinkle capsules) can be used. Divalproex often is preferred because it is enteric coated and causes fewer GI side effects than plain valproic acid. T.D.'s starting dosage of approximately 8 mg/kg per day is more conservative than that recommended by the manufacturer; lower initial doses are less likely to cause acute side effects (e.g., drowsiness and GI upset). Weekly dosage increases of 5 to 10 mg/kg per day of valproate usually are well tolerated and would be appropriate for T.D. More rapid increases may be desirable if tonic-clonic seizures are occurring frequently. The maximum recommended dosage of valproate is 60 mg/kg per day. Many patients, especially those receiving enzyme-inducing drugs (e.g., carbamazepine or phenytoin), require higher-than-recommended doses to achieve adequate clinical effect; other patients may respond at much lower doses. Valproate can be titrated in T.D. to produce a "target" serum concentration of approximately 75 µg/mL. As ethosuximide is withdrawn, the valproate dose can be further adjusted on the basis of seizure frequency and side effects.

DOSAGE FORMS

30. Three months later, T.D. has been taking sodium valproate syrup, 250 mg TID, for 3 weeks. Ethosuximide was discontinued 2 weeks ago; at that time, a valproate serum level just before her morning dose was 68 µg/mL. She has not experienced generalized tonic-clonic seizures for 6 weeks but continues to have an absence spell every 2 to 3 weeks. T.D. complains of nausea, epigastric burning pain, and occasional vomiting lasting approximately 1 hour following her doses of valproate. All recent laboratory tests were within normal limits. Administration of the drug with meals is only partially helpful. What alterations can be made in T.D.'s dosing regimen to relieve these symptoms and possibly improve seizure control?

T.D. appears to be a candidate for the use of divalproex (Depakote), an enteric-coated preparation of a complex salt of valproic acid. Capsules containing enteric-coated beads of divalproex (Depakote Sprinkles 125 mg) also are available; the capsule contents can be dispersed in food for administration to children or others who have difficulty swallowing tablets or capsules. In addition, use of the "cap" end of the capsule to measure half of the contents can approximate doses of 62.5 mg. Syrup forms of valproate probably should be avoided unless extremely small doses are required (e.g., infants) or patients cannot swallow. Valproate syrup has an unpleasant taste, and its rapid absorption increases the likelihood of acute, dose-related side effects such as nausea. Patients with feeding tubes in place may be given opened Depakote Sprinkles through their feeding tubes; however, patients with certain types of feeding gastrostomies should be assessed frequently for possible leakage at the insertion point. This complication may occur because of adherence of undissolved medication beads to the exterior of the feeding tube.

This complication seems more likely when the sprinkle formulation is administered through "button"-type gastrostomy feeding tubes; use of divalproex sprinkles should be avoided in such patients.[181] The beads contained in Depakote Sprinkles may also clog the lumen of smaller-bore feeding tubes.

Administration of divalproex tablets results in delayed rather than prolonged absorption of valproate; therefore, these tablets are not a sustained-release product formulation. When patients are switched from nonenteric-coated formulations to divalproex tablets, the frequency of administration should not be decreased. The sprinkle formulation, owing to the numerous enteric-coated beads, acts as a sustained-release dosage form and may be administered less frequently without producing unacceptable fluctuations in serum concentrations. The FDA has just approved divalproex sodium extended release (Depakote ER) for the treatment of epilepsy. It is a once-daily formulation of Depakote. Bioavailability data and widespread clinical experience indicate that all older dosage forms of valproate are completely absorbed; therefore, dosage forms can be interconverted at the same total daily dose of medication.[182,183] Depakote ER, however, is not bioequivalent to other dosage forms of valproate.[184] When equal doses are administered, Depakote ER achieves plasma concentrations that are approximately 89% of those produced by other valproate dosage forms. Accordingly, when patients are converted to Depakote ER from other forms of valproate, the manufacturer recommends an increase of 8% to 20% in the administered dose. Therefore, T.D.'s valproate syrup should be replaced with an equal daily dose of divalproex tablets. Divalproex should be administered on a three-times-daily dosing schedule. As an alternative, T.D. could be given 1,000 mg of Depakote ER once daily. The results of this change should be apparent within approximately 1 week. By that time, significant relief from GI side effects should have occurred. It may then be possible to increase the dose of divalproex in an effort to improve control of both absence and generalized tonic-clonic seizures.

PHARMACOKINETICS AND SERUM CONCENTRATION MONITORING

31. Two weeks later, T.D. returns for follow-up. Her GI symptoms have almost completely disappeared. She has been taking divalproex 250 mg with breakfast and lunch and 375 mg with a bedtime snack for the past week. She has had no seizures in the past 2 weeks and complains of no side effects. A valproate serum level before her morning dose today was 117 µg/mL (considerably higher than her previous valproate level of 68 µg/mL). The laboratory reports that duplicate determinations of this level agreed within 5 µg/mL. T.D. denies taking her medication incorrectly; her parents support this, and the tablet count in her prescription bottle is correct. She has taken no other drugs except a multivitamin. How can this disproportionate increase in her valproate serum concentration be explained, and what is its clinical significance? Does valproate exhibit dose-dependent pharmacokinetics?

Changes in valproate serum concentrations of this nature are, in this author's experience (R.L.), relatively common with divalproex. They are probably not the result of saturable, dose-dependent metabolism as is seen with phenytoin; instead, these changes are more readily explained by the absorption characteristics of divalproex tablets. Peak serum concentrations of valproate after administration of divalproex may be delayed for 3 to 8 hours, and administration of food may further delay absorption.[185] In addition, diurnal fluctuation in both the rate and extent of absorption of divalproex may be significant. Absorption may be reduced by approximately one third and peak plasma concentrations may be delayed for up to 12 hours for divalproex doses administered in the evening.[43] Twelve to 15 hours probably elapsed between the administration of T.D.'s last dose and blood sampling; therefore, the currently reported blood level may more closely approximate a peak concentration. Previous blood levels, determined while she was receiving rapidly absorbed valproate syrup, are more likely to have been trough concentrations. T.D.'s compliance with her prescribed dosage regimen also may have increased because of the change in dosage form and reduced side effects; her previous serum concentrations may not have reflected administration of the prescribed dose.

Other pharmacokinetic factors may have moderated this unusual increase in valproate concentrations. Fluctuation in these concentrations throughout the day in a pattern that does not reflect the timing of doses is inherent.[186] This fluctuation may be partially related to changes in serum concentrations of endogenous fatty acids. Fatty acids displace valproate from protein-binding sites.[38] Valproate's hepatic clearance is restrictive (i.e., valproate has a low extraction ratio and its clearance is limited by the free fraction of drug in blood); therefore, protein-binding displacement increases plasma concentration of free drug and clearance. As a result, total serum concentrations decrease. Valproate also exhibits dose dependency in its binding to serum proteins. As concentrations approach 70 to 80 μg/mL, binding sites on albumin molecules become saturated, and the free fraction of drug in plasma increases.[37,182] This effect also increases valproate clearance and reduces total serum concentrations. Both of these effects may actually "dampen" the apparent increase in plasma concentrations seen in T.D. When one also considers the poorly established "therapeutic range" for this drug, it becomes apparent that monitoring serum concentrations is a less useful tool in valproate therapy than with other AEDs.[38,182]

The clinical significance of T.D.'s elevated valproate serum concentrations is minimal. She is not experiencing any symptoms suggestive of valproate toxicity, and it is too soon following the dosage increase to assess the effect of this change on her seizure frequency. Therefore, alteration in her drug therapy is unnecessary at present and might only confuse evaluation of her response to this drug. She should be observed for an additional 4 to 6 weeks to evaluate seizure frequency before further alterations in her dosing regimen are considered. These apparently elevated valproate levels should not discourage further increases in her dosage as long as she is tolerating the medication and such increases are justified on the basis of seizure frequency. This case illustrates what can happen if too much attention is paid to serum concentrations.

HEPATOTOXICITY

32. Two months later, T.D. is taking 500 mg of divalproex BID with meals. She has had no absence spells for 5 weeks and no generalized tonic-clonic seizures for 10 weeks. Yesterday her valproate plasma concentration was 132 μg/mL. In addition, her alanine aminotransferase (ALT) was 32 IU/mL (normal, 6 to 14)

and her aspartate aminotransferase (AST) was 41 IU/mL (normal, 7 to 17). All other laboratory tests (bilirubin, alkaline phosphatase, lactate dehydrogenase [LDH], prothrombin time, and serum albumin) were normal. T.D.'s LFTs have been monitored monthly since she began taking valproate, and they were previously normal. Physical examination was negative for scleral icterus, abdominal pain, or other signs of liver disease. Discuss these laboratory abnormalities and physical findings in relation to possible valproate-induced hepatotoxicity in T.D.

Liver damage related to valproate therapy appears to be caused by accumulation of directly hepatotoxic metabolites of valproate (probably 4-en-valproate) in certain patients.[187,188] These metabolites may be formed in larger quantities in patients who also receive enzyme-inducing drugs such as phenobarbital. Most cases of fatal hepatotoxicity have occurred in young (<2 years old) patients with neurologic and metabolic abnormalities who also suffered from severe, difficult-to-control seizures and who were taking multiple AEDs.[187–192] Liver damage occurs early in therapy and symptomatically resembles fulminant hepatitis with hepatic failure. Patients may experience vomiting, drowsiness, lethargy, anorexia, edema, and jaundice; these symptoms often precede laboratory evidence of hepatic damage. Liver biopsies in affected patients show evidence of hepatic necrosis and steatosis. Laboratory findings consist of dramatic elevations of AST, total bilirubin, and serum ammonia; coagulation disturbances accompanied by prolonged prothrombin times, low fibrinogen concentrations, and thrombocytopenia also may be observed. Death results from hepatic failure or a Reye's-like syndrome.[188,190,193]

Asymptomatic elevations in liver enzymes (such as those found in T.D.) occur commonly during the first 6 months of treatment with valproate and usually are not associated with severe or potentially fatal valproate-induced hepatotoxicity. These changes in aminotransferase usually disappear without alteration in therapy; in some cases, temporary dosage reduction is followed by normalization of laboratory tests within 4 to 6 weeks.[188,190] Without systemic symptoms or other signs of significant liver damage, it is unlikely that the laboratory abnormalities observed in T.D. represent severe liver toxicity from valproate. Because T.D. is responding well to valproate therapy, no change in therapy is warranted at this time. Laboratory testing probably can be repeated in 4 to 6 weeks. T.D. and her family should be educated regarding the possible signs and symptoms of valproate-induced liver damage and instructed to consult their physician if these symptoms are noted.

Routine Liver Function Tests

33. What is the usefulness of routinely monitoring LFTs in patients receiving valproate?

Serious hepatotoxicity related to valproate therapy is extremely rare. Dreifuss and others[190,191] estimated that <0.002% of valproate-treated patients developed fatal hepatotoxicity between 1985 and 1986. This compares with an incidence of 0.01% between 1978 and 1984.[189] The lower recent incidence (despite much wider use of valproate) is attributed to increased valproate monotherapy and reduced use of this drug in high-risk patients such as the very young (see Table 54-7). Most cases of fatal hepatotoxicity occur in children <10 years of age. In children <2 years old who receive AED polytherapy, the incidence of this complication is 1 in 500 to 1 in 800. Because asymptomatic, apparently benign elevations in liver enzymes are common early in therapy with valproate and symptoms of liver damage often precede laboratory changes, frequent LFTs during early valproate therapy are unlikely to detect serious hepatotoxicity.[75,188–190,194] In addition, this type of laboratory monitoring adds significant cost while providing little benefit for patients. Education of caregivers and/or patients regarding potential symptoms of hepatotoxicity, with careful observation and follow-up by health care professionals, is recommended as the most effective method for monitoring for this drug-induced illness.

Especially careful monitoring should be provided for predisposed patients (i.e., very young children with associated neurologic abnormalities and/or those receiving polytherapy). In predisposed patients, significant increases in LFTs that are noted early in therapy may be clinically significant. At the onset of symptoms suggesting this condition, laboratory testing may help confirm its presence. Practitioners who feel compelled to perform frequent laboratory testing for liver dysfunction on the basis of manufacturer's package insert recommendations should be cautious not to overinterpret common, transient, and apparently benign elevations in aminotransferases or ammonia levels.

Acute Repetitive ("Cluster") Seizures

Rectal Diazepam Gel

34. B.N., a 7-year-old, 28-kg boy, has had seizures since age 3 months. He suffered anoxia at birth. His seizures usually involve initial confusion and disorientation, shortly followed by generalized tonic-clonic convulsive activity. Despite treatment with carbamazepine at maximum tolerated doses and serum concentrations (300 mg TID; 9 to 11 μg/mL), he continues to have approximately two seizures monthly. Recent trials of topiramate and tiagabine as additions to his carbamazepine were unsuccessful and caused intolerable sedation and lethargy. During the past year, he has been admitted to the emergency department (ED) five times because of seizure "flurries" consisting of three to six seizures occurring over a period of 12 hours or less. While he regains consciousness between these "flurry" seizures, he becomes lethargic. During ED admissions, IV diazepam was administered. This was rapidly successful in terminating seizure activity. B.N.'s mother relates that she usually can identify the onset of seizure flurries; B.N.'s behavior changes and he becomes "clinging" and "whiny" and hyperactive. She also indicates that the initial seizure in a flurry is different from B.N.'s typical episodes. Before the onset of generalized seizure activity, he experiences much briefer periods of confusion. In addition, the generalized seizures are longer and more severe (often with dramatic cyanosis) at the beginning of a "flurry."

Why is prophylactic or abortive therapy for B.N.'s seizure flurries indicated? What factors about B.N. predict successful use of such treatment, and how can it be administered?

B.N.'s relatively frequent flurries or clusters of seizures are causing him and his family significant difficulty. Frequent ED visits are expensive and frightening for many patients and their families. B.N. continues to experience seizure flurries despite carbamazepine therapy. He responds well to IV diazepam and has a caregiver who can identify the onset of seizure clusters. His seizure clusters appear to be distinct from the other seizures that he experiences. All of these factors indicate that a trial of home-administered treatment to abort these cluster episodes is likely to be helpful and should be initiated.

Rectal diazepam gel (Diastat) is available for home administration to patients with acute episodes of repetitive seizure activity.[195] For several years, clinicians have been prescribing rectal administration of diazepam injection for this indication. When diazepam gel is administered rectally, it is absorbed relatively rapidly (peak plasma concentrations occur in approximately 1.5 hours),[196] and it is often effective in terminating cluster seizures within 15 minutes or less. Use of diazepam rectal gel is recommended only when caregivers can recognize the onset of cluster seizures, which are different from a patient's usual seizure activity, and when the caregivers can be trained to administer the preparation safely and to monitor the patient's response (e.g., respiratory status) following administration. Caregivers should be informed that this preparation is not for PRN use with every seizure; it should be used only for identifiable cluster seizures or prolonged seizures. Home use of rectal diazepam may result in significant reduction in the costs of treating these events and may decrease ED visits.[197]

B.N.'s mother should administer rectal diazepam gel at the onset of identifiable cluster seizure activity. A dose of approximately 0.3 mg/kg (10 mg) should be given and repeated, if necessary, within 4 to 12 hours of the first dose. B.N.'s mother should be counseled on the administration of this product and given the patient package insert, which gives complete instructions for the administration of rectal diazepam. She should also be instructed to use the form included with the insert to document B.N.'s response to the medication. After administration, B.N. should be monitored for at least 4 hours to ensure that no respiratory depression or other adverse side effects are occurring and to assess the effect of the medication on his seizures. The most common adverse effect seen with rectal diazepam is somnolence, occasionally accompanied by dizziness and ataxia. Respiratory depression is very uncommon.

Febrile Seizures

Incidence and Classification

35. J.J., a 14-month-old girl, is brought to the ED after having a generalized tonic-clonic convulsion lasting approximately 10 minutes. The episode occurred in association with an upper respiratory infection. Upon arrival in the ED, her temperature was 39.5°C rectally. She was alert at that time; all laboratory and neurologic findings, including lumbar puncture, were normal. J.J. has no history of neurologic abnormality. Her 7-year-old brother suffers from both absence and generalized tonic-clonic seizures. What is the relationship between febrile seizures and epilepsy? How may J.J.'s convulsion be classified on the basis of the data available?

Up to 5% of children have a febrile seizure between 6 months and 6 years of age.[198] Simple febrile seizures occur with a fever of ≥38°C in previously normal children <5 years of age. They last <15 minutes and have no focal features. The associated seizure does not arise from CNS pathology. Complex febrile seizures show focal characteristics or are prolonged. The child may or may not have previous neurologic abnormalities. Febrile status epilepticus consists of continuous or serial tonic-clonic seizures lasting >30 minutes without return of consciousness. Seizures with fever occur in association with febrile illnesses and may be of any type or duration. The previous neurologic status of the patient may or may not have been normal. This category is most commonly used to classify symptomatic seizures associated with neurologic conditions such as meningitis. The risk of occurrence of afebrile seizures following one or more febrile seizures is two to three times greater than in the general population. A family history of afebrile seizures, a complicated initial seizure, and pre-existing neurologic abnormality are risk factors associated with the later development of chronic epilepsy.[199]

J.J.'s seizure appears to be a typical simple febrile seizure that developed in association with her upper respiratory tract infection. The lack of previous neurologic abnormality and normal findings on lumbar puncture and laboratory evaluation help confirm this assessment.

Treatment of Acute Seizure

36. How should J.J.'s febrile seizures be treated?

Because J.J. is not having a seizure at present, immediate antiepileptic therapy is not required. Nevertheless, measures to reduce her elevated temperature should be initiated immediately to reduce the risk of further seizures. Acetaminophen and tepid sponge baths usually are helpful.

If patients experience prolonged or repeated febrile seizures, either phenobarbital or diazepam may be administered.[199] If long-term prophylactic treatment for febrile seizures is anticipated, phenobarbital may be preferred for acute treatment.

Prophylaxis and Choice of Antiepileptic Drug

37. On the basis of the subjective and objective data available for J.J., is AED therapy indicated on a long-term basis? What are the benefits and risks of AED prophylaxis for febrile seizures?

Long-term treatment of simple febrile seizures remains controversial. Up to 54% of affected patients will have recurrent febrile seizures. The risk of recurrence is even higher when the first episode occurs before 13 months of age. Although recurrent, multiple, or severe febrile seizures have been believed to cause temporal lobe lesions that result in complex partial (temporal lobe) epilepsy, data available from epidemiologic studies do not support this belief.[198] The efficacy of prophylactic AEDs for prevention of chronic epilepsy following febrile seizures has not been evaluated.[200] Thus, the primary potential benefit of long-term AED therapy would be prevention of recurrent febrile seizures.

A National Institutes of Health (NIH) Consensus Development Conference in 1980 recommended that prophylactic medication after a first febrile seizure be considered when one of the following risk factors was present: (1) focal or prolonged seizures; (2) neurologic abnormalities; (3) afebrile seizures in a first-degree relative; (4) age <1 year; and (5) multiple febrile seizures occurring within 24 hours.[201] A reanalysis of published studies has, however, questioned these recommendations, because the NIH Consensus Statement risk

factors were not strong predictors of febrile seizure recurrence.[200] Only early age (<1 year) at first febrile seizure and a family history of febrile seizures reliably predicted a significant increase in the risk of repeat febrile seizures. AED prophylaxis should be considered only when multiple risk factors or other medical conditions that place the patient at special risk are present. Complex febrile seizures or febrile status epilepticus should be treated with chronic AED therapy because these episodes represent significant neurologic dysfunction, even though they do not necessarily increase the risk of febrile seizure recurrence.[199,200]

The efficacy and risk–benefit profile of AED prophylaxis for febrile seizures also have been questioned.[202] A reanalysis of published British trials of both valproate and phenobarbital for febrile seizure prophylaxis found that neither drug was reliably effective.[203] Although phenobarbital has been considered at least partially effective, the high rate of side effects (40%) preclude recommending its use. When the effects on intelligence of phenobarbital versus placebo prophylaxis for febrile seizures in young children were compared against NIH Consensus Statement risk factors for recurrence, IQ scores were significantly lower in children treated with phenobarbital.[204] This effect persisted for at least 6 months after discontinuation of drug therapy. In addition, reduction in the recurrence rate of febrile seizures in children treated with phenobarbital was not statistically significant. However, approximately one third of those patients who experienced recurrent febrile seizures were noncompliant with phenobarbital therapy. This study's design and findings have been criticized on the basis of patient selection and "crossing over" of patients from the control group to the study group.[205]

Recently, a report was published on the retesting of many of the original toddler-aged children whose IQ was lower after receiving phenobarbital for febrile seizures compared with placebo.[206] Upon retesting 3 to 5 years later of the now school-age children, the phenobarbital group scored significantly lower than the placebo group on the Wide Range Achievement Test reading achievement standard score. Their IQs were lower by 3.71 points, but this mean difference was not statistically different from the placebo group. The authors concluded that phenobarbital has a long-term adverse cognitive consequence on developmental skills and no beneficial effect on seizure recurrence.

AED prophylaxis for febrile seizures is probably not warranted for J.J., even though she is at risk for both development of epilepsy and recurrence of febrile seizures. No evidence supports that medication will significantly affect her later development of epilepsy. Phenobarbital and valproate are the only AEDs that have been considered useful for febrile seizure prophylaxis, and even their efficacy is being seriously questioned. Phenobarbital's use for this purpose is difficult to justify when one considers the risk of learning impairment. In addition, phenobarbital therapy is associated with hyperactivity and behavioral disturbance in up to 75% of children receiving the drug.[65,207,208]

J.J.'s age places her at higher risk of valproate-related hepatotoxicity, and this risk probably outweighs any potential benefit from treatment with this drug. Close medical follow-up of J.J. is warranted. In addition, her parents should be instructed to institute antipyretic measures (i.e., acetaminophen and tepid sponge baths) at the onset of any febrile illness.

Many febrile seizures occur early in the course of an illness before fever is detected[199]; nevertheless, vigilance by her parents and early antipyretic therapy may help prevent further febrile seizures. The intermittent administration of oral diazepam (Valium) at the onset of a febrile illness also can be of value. A dosage of 0.33 mg/kg orally given every 8 hours appears to be effective in reducing the recurrence rate of febrile seizures.[209] Diazepam should be initiated as soon as a febrile illness appears and continued until J.J. has been afebrile for 24 hours. Side effects are common when diazepam is used in this manner; approximately one third of patients will experience ataxia, lethargy, or irritability. These and other common CNS side effects such as dysarthria and insomnia may confuse assessment of the condition of children with febrile illnesses.

Seizures Secondary to Toxic Exposures: Nerve Gas

38. How likely are seizures to result from exposure to chemical warfare agents such as sarin nerve gas, and how are these seizures treated?

Nerve agents that may be used in chemical warfare or terrorist attacks can cause seizures. These agents include tabun (synonym, GA), sarin (GB), soman (GD), and VX. At normal environmental temperatures, all of these agents except VX are volatile and therefore become "nerve gases." VX is a viscous liquid. Nerve agents are both lipophilic and hydrophilic and therefore can rapidly penetrate clothing, skin, and mucous membranes and be absorbed systemically.[61,62] Nerve agents are closely related to organophosphate insecticides, and their toxic effects result from their actions as acetylcholinesterase (AChE) inhibitors. The toxins bind to the active site of AchE and prevent hydrolysis of acetylcholine (ACh). Excessive quantities of ACh then accumulate, causing excessive stimulation of muscarinic and nicotinic receptors. Manifestations of nerve agent exposure can be broadly described as muscarinic (ophthalmic symptoms such as miosis, lacrimation, and blurred vision; respiratory symptoms such as severe rhinorrhea, wheezing, and dyspnea; cardiovascular symptoms such as bradydysrhythmia, A-V block and hypotension; and GI symptoms such as salivation, nausea, vomiting, and severe diarrhea), nicotinic (cardiovascular symptoms such as tachydysrhythmia and hypertension; fasciculation of voluntary muscles; and metabolic symptoms such as hyperglycemia, metabolic acidosis, and hypokalemia), and CNS symptoms (anxiety, agitation, vertigo, ataxia, central respiratory depression, convulsions, and coma). The likelihood and the severity of CNS toxicity and/or seizures will depend on the amount of nerve agent and the route of exposure. CNS symptoms are associated with severe exposure to nerve agents. When seizures occur, they are usually generalized; the exact mechanism of seizure induction by these agents has not been identified.[62]

Following exposure to nerve agents, early treatment with antidotes may prevent severe toxic manifestations. Large doses of IM atropine (2 to 6 mg) should be given; dosing is based on respiratory symptoms. Therapeutic end points are drying of respiratory secretions and relief of dyspnea.[61,62] Pralidoxime (Protopam) is an AChE reactivator. This antidote binds nerve agents and removes them from binding sites on AChE. Pralidoxime is useful only if given before the bond between the nerve agent and AChE becomes permanent. This time interval varies from minutes to hours, depending on the nerve agent.[62a] Pralidoxime is a quaternary agent, and it is not clear to what extent it enters the CNS. The effects of pralidoxime are most dramatically seen on skeletal muscle symptoms. Pralidoxime should be given along with the antimuscarinic agent atropine.

There are few published data regarding the use of anticonvulsant drugs for treatment of nerve agent exposure. It is claimed that early administration of 10 mg IM diazepam may prevent permanent CNS damage in patients with severe nerve agent toxicity.[61] In situations of severe exposure with CNS manifestations and seizures, use of a more rapidly absorbed IM agent such as lorazepam would be expected to produce a more rapid and reliable response; IV administration of diazepam or lorazepam, if feasible, would be more likely to rapidly control seizure activity. If necessary, rectal administration of diazepam gel would be an option (see Question 34).

ANTIEPILEPTIC DRUG INTERACTIONS AND ADVERSE EFFECTS

Carbamazepine–Erythromycin Interaction

39. J.N., a 17-year-old boy, is treated with carbamazepine 600 mg/day for complex partial seizures. His seizures are well controlled with serum carbamazepine concentrations of 8 μg/mL. He developed an upper respiratory infection, assessed as probable streptococcal pharyngitis. Because J.N. is allergic to penicillin, erythromycin 333 mg TID with meals for 10 days was prescribed. Four days after beginning erythromycin therapy, J.N. complains that although his upper respiratory symptoms are improving, he is constantly drowsy and is experiencing dizziness and double vision. He also complains of nausea and has vomited once this morning. He receives no other routine medication, although he did take approximately five doses of two tablets of Extra-Strength Tylenol (acetaminophen 500 mg/tablet) during the initial stage of his current illness for fever and general discomfort. What is the relationship between J.N.'s symptoms and the potential interaction between carbamazepine and erythromycin? How might this interaction be further assessed and managed at this point?

Inhibition of CYP3A4 by erythromycin may result in dramatic elevations in carbamazepine serum concentrations and precipitation of intoxication.[210,211] J.N.'s symptoms are consistent with carbamazepine toxicity, although erythromycin therapy may be contributing to his GI symptoms. Although dramatic elevation of carbamazepine serum concentrations is not consistently seen, susceptible patients may exhibit a twofold increase in serum levels. Determination of a carbamazepine serum concentration is indicated to help confirm probable toxicity and assess the magnitude of the interaction. Erythromycin is believed to inhibit metabolic conversion of carbamazepine to its epoxide metabolite, with a resulting decrease in carbamazepine clearance. This potential interaction is commonly encountered and represents a significant risk factor for precipitation of carbamazepine intoxication.

Management of this interaction at this point is somewhat difficult; prevention of the interaction by avoiding the use of erythromycin whenever possible is usually the best clinical strategy. Because J.N. is allergic to penicillin, alternatives to erythromycin for treatment of his presumed streptococcal infection are limited. Replacement of erythromycin with clindamycin should provide adequate antibiotic therapy with no risk of further interaction with carbamazepine. One or two doses of carbamazepine could be held to allow carbamazepine serum concentrations to decrease to pre-erythromycin levels and correct J.N.'s present intoxication. An alternative approach would be to reduce J.N.'s carbamazepine dose, based on his present serum level, for the duration of erythromycin therapy. This approach may be more difficult to manage; the time required for erythromycin-induced metabolic inhibition to subside when the antibiotic is stopped is unpredictable. With either approach to management of this interaction, J.N.'s clinical status will need to be monitored carefully. Further adjustment of carbamazepine dosage may be required, and repeat serum level determinations may be helpful.

Valproate–Carbamazepine Interaction

40. D.H., a 21-year-old, 84-kg man, was taking carbamazepine 1,400 mg/day (600 mg Q am and 800 mg HS) for treatment of generalized tonic-clonic seizures. Despite carbamazepine serum concentrations of 14 μg/mL, he continued to have a seizure every 6 to 8 weeks. Higher serum levels have been associated with toxicity symptoms. Valproate (divalproex) was recently added and gradually increased to a dosage of 1,000 mg TID; the therapeutic goal is replacement of carbamazepine with valproate. At this dose, D.H. again experienced symptoms of carbamazepine intoxication (double vision, unsteady gait, and drowsiness), although his carbamazepine serum concentration was 12 μg/mL. Valproate serum levels were 40 μg/mL and 43 μg/mL on two occasions. D.H. has continued to experience seizures at his previous rate. He appears to be compliant with his prescribed medication regimen. How can D.H.'s symptoms and low valproate levels be explained on the basis of an interaction between his two AEDs?

Difficulty in achieving serum valproate concentrations adequate for improvement in seizure control frequently is encountered in patients who receive concomitant therapy with potent enzyme inducers such as carbamazepine. Clinicians frequently note that it is difficult to administer doses of valproate large enough to achieve desired serum levels under these circumstances.[37,169] Serum concentrations of valproate in patients receiving carbamazepine may be only approximately 50% of those expected on the basis of single-dose valproate pharmacokinetic studies.

D.H.'s symptoms of carbamazepine intoxication at plasma levels that were previously tolerated suggest possible accumulation of CBZ-E (also see Question 42). Valproate may inhibit epoxide hydrolase and cause accumulation of CBZ-E sufficient to exert significant pharmacologic effects, including intoxication. This author (R.L.) has observed a patient receiving both valproate and carbamazepine who developed serum concentrations of CBZ-E equal to the concentration of carbamazepine itself (both compounds were measured at approximately 12 μg/mL) and experienced significant intoxication. Determination of the serum concentration of carbamazepine and its epoxide should help confirm the clinical impression. Unfortunately, the assay for CBZ-E is not readily available in many clinical laboratories.

41. What recommendations can be made for alteration in D.H.'s drug therapy regimen to alleviate the effects of this drug interaction and enhance his therapeutic response to the medication?

On clinical/empirical grounds, D.H.'s dosage of carbamazepine should be reduced; this would seem especially appropriate because the therapeutic goal was replacement of carbamazepine with valproate. Dosage reduction will result in a decrease in serum concentrations of both carbamazepine and CBZ-E and improvement in symptoms of intoxication. An initial decrease of 10% to 20% (200 mg) of D.H.'s daily carbamazepine dose would be reasonable. Subsequently, his carbamazepine dose can be tapered using reductions of 200 mg every 1 to 2 weeks. During tapering of carbamazepine, D.H. should be monitored carefully for increased seizure activity.

Valproate-Related Thrombocytopenia

42. D.H.'s symptoms improved significantly within 3 days of reduction of his carbamazepine dosage to 1,200 mg/day. A CBZ-E serum concentration was not determined. His carbamazepine dosage was reduced by 200 mg/day in weekly steps, with no increase in seizure activity. A serum valproate concentration after his carbamazepine dosage reached 600 mg/day was 53 μg/mL. At that time he had not had a seizure in approximately 6 weeks. A serum valproate concentration was repeated when his carbamazepine dosage reached 200 mg/day and was 58 μg/mL. Three weeks following discontinuation of carbamazepine, D.H. noted the onset of tremor affecting his hands and a "fuzzy sensation in my head" accompanied by difficulty concentrating on tasks. His serum valproate concentration was 126 μg/mL. In addition, a CBC showed a platelet count of 60,000/mm³ cells; no other abnormalities were seen. No bleeding tendencies were noted, and D.H. denied easy bruisability or unusual bleeding. Previous CBCs had been normal. Is this pattern of increase in valproate serum concentrations consistent with the loss of carbamazepine-related enzyme induction? What is the relationship between D.H.'s new symptoms, his reduced platelet count, and the elevation in his valproate serum concentration?

[SI unit: 60×10^9/L]

D.H.'s valproate serum concentrations were expected to increase with "de-induction" of hepatic microsomal enzymes while carbamazepine was being discontinued. The pattern and timing of de-induction are not consistently predictable. While one might anticipate a somewhat linear increase in valproate concentrations as enzyme inducers such as carbamazepine are gradually reduced, it is not unusual for valproate levels to remain relatively constant until 1 to 2 weeks after discontinuation of enzyme inducers.[169] Therefore, patients should be monitored for signs or symptoms of possible valproate intoxication during and for several weeks after such a discontinuation process; clinicians and patients should be aware that dosage adjustment may not be required until the enzyme-inducing drug has been completely discontinued. The magnitude of the increase observed in D.H. is somewhat unusual, although this author (R.L.) has observed similar patterns in patients.

D.H.'s new symptoms appear to be consistent with mild to moderate intoxication with valproate. Tremor is a relatively common side effect of valproate that is likely to appear as serum concentrations exceed approximately 80 μg/mL.[37] This side effect may be troublesome for some patients because the tremor is usually an intention tremor, which worsens with physical activity. In most patients, dose reduction will improve or eliminate tremor. Some investigators have counteracted this side effect with propranolol therapy in doses similar to those used to treat essential tremor.[171] The neurologic symptoms exhibited by D.H. also are typically seen with valproate intoxication. All of these symptoms are reversible with dosage reduction.

Reductions in platelet counts are not rare in valproate-treated patients. Significant thrombocytopenia with bleeding manifestations is extremely uncommon, although measurable changes in platelet function may occur.[212,213] The mechanism underlying thrombocytopenia is not known; there is evidence for both a dose- or serum concentration–related effect[213] and an immunologic mechanism.[214] Affected patients usually can be continued on valproate therapy at reduced doses without adverse effects. The author (R.L.) has observed two patients who developed significant valproate-related thrombocytopenia without bleeding complications; both cases were associated with dramatic increases in valproate serum concentrations following discontinuation of enzyme-inducing drugs. In one of these patients, the relationship between valproate serum concentrations and platelet counts appeared to be significant.

Both the neurologic symptoms and thrombocytopenia exhibited by D.H. probably can be corrected by reducing his dose of divalproex. The magnitude of dose reduction will need to be determined by titration using remission of symptoms and normalization of his platelet count as end points. Periodically rechecking valproate serum concentrations will help establish a safe upper limit dose and serum levels for D.H. Ongoing monitoring also will be important for several weeks as the process of de-induction of hepatic enzymes may not yet be complete. Further dose reductions may be necessary as this process reaches completion and D.H.'s valproate clearance gradually decreases. Reduction of D.H.'s dosage to 2,000 mg/day should approximate serum concentrations between those that were previously subtherapeutic and those that are causing his current adverse effects.

Skin Rash: Hypersensitivity Reactions to Antiepileptic Drugs

43. R.S., a 34-year-old man, has been taking phenytoin 200 mg BID for the past 7 weeks to control complex partial and secondarily generalized tonic-clonic seizures. Seizures began approximately 4 months ago following surgical evacuation of a subdural hematoma. Today he appeared at the walk-in clinic and complained of an "itchy rash" that had begun 2 days ago. He described "feeling lousy" for the past week. On examination he is febrile (38.5°C orally). A maculopapular, scaly, erythematous rash covered his upper extremities and torso, and the mucous membranes of his mouth appeared to be mildly inflamed. Cervical lymphadenopathy was noted, and the liver was found to be enlarged and tender. R.S. also related that his urine had become very dark in the past 2 days and that his stools were light-colored. What is the significance of R.S.'s skin rash and other signs and symptoms? Are these likely to be related to his phenytoin therapy?

Skin rash is a relatively common (2% to 3% of patients) side effect related to AED therapy. It is most commonly associated with phenytoin, lamotrigine, carbamazepine, and phenobarbital. Most cases are relatively mild, but severely affected patients may develop Stevens-Johnson syndrome and/or a systemic hypersensitivity syndrome accompanied by severe hepatic damage. In R.S.'s case, signs and symptoms suggesting hepatic involvement accompany the skin rash. Fever, lymphadenopathy, and apparent inflammation of mucous membranes also suggest a possible hypersensitivity reaction to phenytoin with multisystem involvement and the potential for progression to Stevens-Johnson syndrome. Viral infection (e.g., hepatitis, influenza, infectious mononucleosis) should be considered and ruled out as a possible cause of R.S.'s symptoms before they are attributed to phenytoin therapy.[159,215–218]

Phenytoin hypersensitivity syndrome is most commonly seen in adults and is more likely to affect African Americans.[216] Typically, patients with this syndrome present with complaints of fever, skin rash, and lymphadenopathy during the first 2 months of phenytoin therapy. Hepatomegaly, splenomegaly, jaundice, and bleeding manifestations such as petechial hemorrhage also are relatively common. Laboratory manifestations usually include leukocytosis with eosinophilia, elevated serum bilirubin, and elevated AST and ALT. When a phenytoin hypersensitivity reaction includes significant hepatotoxicity, fatality may occur in as many as 38% of affected patients.[215]

There appears to be a high likelihood that R.S. has developed a severe reaction to phenytoin; the clinical manifestations and the timing of their appearance are typical of this reaction. Phenytoin should be discontinued immediately pending diagnostic clarification (i.e., evaluation for other possible causes of his symptoms such as viral illness). R.S. should be hospitalized for further diagnostic evaluation and treatment. Treatment of phenytoin-related hypersensitivity and hepatotoxicity is symptomatic and supportive. Intensive therapy with corticosteroids has commonly been used, although little objective evidence exists for beneficial effects of this treatment. Potential complications of this reaction include sepsis and hepatic failure; these conditions should be treated specifically.

44. R.S. was hospitalized and treated with oral prednisone and topical corticosteroids. Other potential causes for his condition were ruled out, and his signs and symptoms were attributed to phenytoin hypersensitivity. His fever resolved within 5 days; the skin rash became exfoliative but resolved without infectious complications. Laboratory parameters began to normalize after 10 days. While he was hospitalized, R.S. experienced three episodes of generalized seizure activity that were treated with acute administration of IV lorazepam. R.S. was afebrile at the time these episodes occurred. What information regarding the pathogenesis of phenytoin hypersensitivity and hepatotoxicity can be used to guide selection of an alternative AED for R.S.?

Further administration of phenytoin to R.S. is contraindicated on the basis of his history of a severe hypersensitivity reaction to this drug. Readministration of phenytoin is likely to result in rapid recurrence of severe symptoms of this syndrome. Although the mechanism of this reaction is not fully understood, research implicates reactive epoxide metabolites (arene oxides) of phenytoin (and other chemically similar AEDs) as possible causative agents for hypersensitivity reactions. Affected patients purportedly are predisposed genetically to the development of hypersensitivity, possibly because a relative deficiency of epoxide hydrolase enzymes allows the accumulation of toxic concentrations of reactive epoxide metabolites, which are believed to exert a direct cytotoxic effect and/or to interact with cellular macromolecules, thereby functioning as haptenes that stimulate an immunologic reaction.[219,220] Carbamazepine, phenytoin, and phenobarbital all are metabolized by similar pathways and converted to reactive arene oxides. It is hypothesized that carbamazepine-induced liver damage also may result from the effects of accumulation of reactive epoxide metabolites; these reactive metabolites are different from the 10,11-epoxide metabolite that accumulates during carbamazepine therapy. For this reason, these drugs potentially cross-react in susceptible patients. Cases of apparent cross-reactivity between phenytoin and phenobarbital or carbamazepine have been documented.[221–223] In addition, both carbamazepine and phenobarbital may produce hypersensitivity reactions similar to those seen with phenytoin. This potential for cross-reactivity should be considered when an alternative AED is selected for R.S.

Valproate has been suggested as the preferred alternative AED for patients who have developed hypersensitivity reactions to phenytoin.[222] Valproate is not metabolized to arene oxides and also is chemically dissimilar to all other AEDs. Because valproate often shows good efficacy for complex partial seizures with secondary generalization, it would seem to be a safe and potentially effective alternative AED for R.S. Of the newer AEDs, lamotrigine should probably be avoided in R.S. because of its likelihood of causing skin rash and apparent hypersensitivity reactions. Topiramate, tiagabine, levetiracetam, or zonisamide could be considered as alternative medications for R.S., although experience with these medications is still limited.

WOMEN'S ISSUES IN EPILEPSY

Although epilepsy affects men and women equally, there are many health issues of specific importance to women, such as contraceptive interactions with AEDs, teratogenicity, pharmacokinetic changes during pregnancy, breast-feeding, menstrual cycle influences on seizure activity (catamenial epilepsy), AED impact on bone, and sexual dysfunction.[224] There is much to be done to educate both health care professionals and patients about the many complex issues facing women with epilepsy.

For women of child-bearing potential, prepregnancy planning and counseling are important, since significant AED exposure of the fetus often occurs by the time the pregnancy is confirmed. This is especially important because of the potential for unplanned pregnancies from the AED–contraceptive drug interactions. Prepregnancy counseling also should include the importance of folic acid supplementation and medication adherence. Patients should be informed about the risk of teratogenicity and the importance of prenatal care.

Though complete seizure control is desirable for all patients with epilepsy, it is especially favorable for a woman's seizures to be well controlled before conception. Monotherapy is preferred whenever possible, since the relative risk of birth defects dramatically increases with AED polytherapy.[225,226] Monotherapy also improves patient compliance, as does having a better understanding of birth defects caused by AEDs. The AED should be given at the lowest effective dose to reduce the possibility of birth defects.[227] The gradual discontinuation of AEDs may be considered if a woman has been seizure-free for ≥ 2 years.

Antiepileptic Drug–Oral Contraceptive Interaction

45. **P.Z., a 26-year-old woman, experiences complex partial and secondarily generalized tonic-clonic seizures. She is taking phenytoin 400 mg/day, carbamazepine 800 mg/day, and divalproex 2,000 mg/day. She reports having two or three partial seizures and one generalized seizure every 3 to 4 months. Despite treatment with Lo/Ovral (norgestrel 0.3 mg with ethinyl estradiol 30 μg), she has just learned she is pregnant. Her last menstrual period was 6 weeks ago. What is the relationship between P.Z.'s apparent contraceptive failure and her anticonvulsant therapy?**

There have been several reports of reduced efficacy of oral contraceptives in patients receiving various AEDs.[228,229] These reports describe both breakthrough bleeding and pregnancy. Phenobarbital, phenytoin, carbamazepine, oxcarbazepine, and felbamate have been shown to increase the metabolism of ethynylestradiol and progestogens.[230] This effect is not associated with valproate, lamotrigine, gabapentin, tiagabine, or levetiracetam.[224] Topiramate in polytherapy and at high dosages (200 to 800 mg/day) appears to have a mild though measurable effect on oral contraceptive pharmacokinetics; apparent clearance of the estrogen component of combined oral contraceptives is increased in patients taking topiramate.[231] In a more recent study with topiramate monotherapy in lower dosages (50 to 200 mg/day), there was a lesser impact on the pharmacokinetics of the oral contraceptive.[232] At present, studies with zonisamide are not available to evaluate the potential interaction with oral contraceptives. Some AEDs also stimulate synthesis of sex hormone binding globulin (SHBG).[233] Increased binding of steroid contraceptive hormones to SHBG would result in lower concentrations of unbound, biologically active hormones and reduced contraceptive efficacy. The effects of newer AEDs (lamotrigine, felbamate, gabapentin, tiagabine, topiramate, levetiracetam, oxcarbazepine, and zonisamide) on concentrations of SHBG have not been determined.

A lack of contraceptive efficacy may present as irregular or breakthrough menstrual bleeding. However, decreased efficacy is not always associated with breakthrough bleeding. Oral contraceptive doses can be increased to compensate for the effect of an AED, though most physicians do not increase the dose.[234] Estrogens also may exacerbate seizures in some women.[235] Women >35 years old or those who smoke must consider the risk of thromboembolic complications associated with higher doses of contraceptives. A second contraceptive method (e.g., condoms, intrauterine devices, or spermicide) is recommended to avoid contraceptive failure.[224] Tubal ligation is also an alternative.

Assuming P.Z. was taking her contraceptive pills on a regular basis, it is possible that her enzyme-inducing AEDs are responsible for their failure. Patients receiving AEDs should be prospectively informed that this interaction may occur and advised concerning the use of alternative contraceptives (see Chapter 45, Contraception).

Teratogenicity

46. What are the risks of teratogenic effects from P.Z.'s medications? What steps might be taken to minimize these risks?

P.Z.'s child is at a relatively high risk of congenital malformations because of exposure to several potentially teratogenic drugs: estrogen/progestin combination oral contraceptives, valproate, phenytoin, and carbamazepine (also see Chapter 47, Teratogenicity and Drugs in Breast Milk).

Many AEDs have teratogenic effects.[236] Animal data regarding the teratogenic potential of lamotrigine, felbamate, gabapentin, topiramate, tiagabine, levetiracetam, oxcarbazepine, and zonisamide are encouraging, but conclusions regarding the teratogenic potential of these recently marketed AEDs cannot be made because of limited experience in pregnant women. Carbamazepine was previously believed to have a lower risk of teratogenicity than other AEDs; however, both the pattern and risk of malformations secondary to carbamazepine are comparable to those associated with phenytoin.[237] Controversy has been significantly reduced regarding the relative contributions of parental epilepsy itself, genetic influences, and drug therapy since recent data showed that the infants of women with epilepsy but not on AEDs had fewer abnormalities compared to those born to women with epilepsy on AEDs.[238] The risk of major congenital malformations (e.g., facial clefts, cardiac septal defects) in children exposed to AEDs in utero may be as high as two to three times the baseline risk in the general population.[239] However, syndromes consisting of multiple, often minor abnormalities associated with prenatal exposure to AEDs appear to exist, and these syndromes may be more common than one would expect on the basis of relative risk figures developed for isolated major malformations. In addition, maternal epilepsy increases the risk of complications of pregnancy, prenatal or postnatal infant mortality, premature birth, low infant birth weight, and symptoms of withdrawal from AEDs.

Most AEDs, with the exception of valproate, are believed to exert their teratogenic effects (and possibly other adverse effects such as hepatotoxicity) partly via reactive epoxide metabolites.[239] Enhancement of the formation of these metabolites via hepatic enzyme induction (e.g., by carbamazepine or phenobarbital) or inhibition of their breakdown (e.g., through inhibition of epoxide hydrolase by valproate) would increase the risk of teratogenicity. Combined administration of enzyme inducers and valproate (specifically the combination of carbamazepine, phenobarbital, and valproate with or without phenytoin) is associated with an especially high risk of teratogenicity.[240] In addition, each of the present major AEDs has been associated with production of congenital malformations when administered alone. Valproate and phenytoin (and possibly other AEDs) also appear to interfere with folic acid metabolism; this effect may be responsible for a portion of the congenital malformations observed with these drugs.[239]

It may be possible to minimize drug-related risks in the pregnant patient with epilepsy and her child.[224,236] If feasible, before conception, seizure control should be optimized using the AED of first choice for the prospective mother's seizure type or epilepsy syndrome. Monotherapy at the lowest effective dose is the goal. Maintenance of adequate folic acid stores before conception and during fetal organogenesis is also important. Folic acid supplementation can reduce the risk of congenital neural tube malformations in infants at risk who are born to women without epilepsy, but folate supplementation does not reliably reduce the teratogenic effects of AEDs. Nevertheless, supplementation of folic acid (and ensuring adequate folate levels) is recommended. Because about half of pregnancies are unplanned and not evident until weeks after conception, folate supplementation should be routinely given to women of child-bearing age with epilepsy. No study has been conducted to determine the optimal dose of folic acid supplementation in patients taking AEDs. There is much discussion on this topic by clinicians, but the current practices are not evidence-based. Even though this is the case, P.Z. should start taking 4 mg of folic acid supplementation each day.

Physiologic changes in pregnant women may affect the pharmacokinetics of AEDs.[224] Absorption may be influenced by nausea and vomiting. The binding capacity of albumin is decreased during pregnancy, resulting in decreased protein binding for highly bound drugs. Unbound fractions of phenobarbital, phenytoin, and valproate increase with decreased concentrations of albumin.[241–243] For drugs predominately metabolized by the liver with a restrictive clearance (e.g., carbamazepine and valproate), a decreased protein binding without changes in intrinsic clearance should result in a decrease in total drug concentrations; unbound drug concentrations should remain unchanged. For drugs with both increased hepatic metabolism and decreased protein binding (e.g., phenytoin and phenobarbital), both total and unbound plasma concentrations decrease, but not necessarily proportionately. Hepatic metabolism and renal function both increase during pregnancy.

During pregnancy, serum levels of AEDs (including free serum levels for highly protein-bound drugs) should be monitored. Dosage adjustments may aid in preventing the increased seizure frequency seen in approximately 25% of pregnant women with epilepsy. Because falls and anoxia associated with uncontrolled seizure activity may increase the risk to the unborn baby, P.Z. should be educated on the value of compliance with her AED regimen to prevent further seizure activity.

In P.Z., one can presume that significant exposure of the fetus to any teratogenic influence of AEDs has already occurred. Optimization of seizure control is a primary concern for this woman. Any major alterations in P.Z.'s AED regimen should be made cautiously to avoid precipitating seizures. In addition, she should be instructed to contact the AED pregnancy registry at Massachusetts General Hospital (1-888-233-2334). Information provided to the registry will aid in the ongoing monitoring of outcomes of babies born to mothers taking AEDs. Recently, reports from this registry have provided risk information on two of the older AEDs (phenobarbital and valproate). In utero exposure to either of these AEDs in monotherapy caused a fivefold increased incidence of major birth defects compared to controls.

Vitamin K Supplementation

Babies born to women with epilepsy who are taking enzyme-inducing AEDs are at risk of hemorrhage due to decreased vitamin K–dependent clotting factors. Women taking carbamazepine, phenobarbital, primidone, and/or phenytoin should receive vitamin K 20 mg every day from 36 weeks of gestation until delivery, and babies should also receive vitamin K 1 mg IM at birth.[244]

Breast-Feeding

In a lactating woman who is taking medications, the risk of drug exposure to the infant needs to be weighed against the benefits of breast-feeding.[245] All drugs transfer into milk to some extent. A drug in the mother's blood distributes into breast milk by simple diffusion. The extent of protein binding of the drug is the most important predictor of drug passage into milk.[246,247] For many drugs, the milk to plasma ratio (M/P) has been determined. For the AEDs, there is a large intersubject variability in this ratio, presumably due to a difference in volume and composition of the milk, and the ratio is not useful for predicting infant AED exposure. There have been two recent reviews on AEDs and breast-feeding.[248,249] For the majority of the first-generation AEDs (carbamazepine, phenytoin, valproic acid), breast-feeding results in negligible plasma concentrations in the infants. For the second-generation AEDs, breast-feeding should be done cautiously and the infant should be monitored for excess AED plasma concentrations and toxicity, if possible. This information should be presented to P.Z. in an appropriate manner. Once she delivers her baby, a re-evaluation and optimization of P.Z.'s AED therapy should occur.

STATUS EPILEPTICUS

Characteristics and Pathophysiology

47. V.S., a 22-year-old, 85-kg man, was recently diagnosed as having idiopathic epilepsy. For the past 3 months, he has been treated with 600 mg/day of carbamazepine, which completely eliminated his generalized tonic-clonic seizures. His steady-state carbamazepine serum concentration was 10 μg/mL. While at his parents' home, he had two tonic-clonic seizures, each lasting 3 to 4 minutes. On arrival at the hospital (approximately 30 minutes after the first seizure began), he was noted to be only semiconscious. His blood pressure was 197/104 mm Hg, his pulse was 124 beats/min, respirations were 23 breaths/min, and his body temperature was 37.5°C rectally. Shortly after his arrival, another generalized tonic-clonic seizure began. How does V.S.'s current condition meet accepted diagnostic criteria for status epilepticus? What risks are associated with status epilepticus?

Status epilepticus (SE) exists if there is "more than 30 minutes of (1) continuous seizure activity or (2) two or more sequential seizures without full recovery of consciousness between seizures."[250] Because V.S. has had three seizures within slightly more than 30 minutes and remains unconscious, his present condition meets this definition. V.S. is experiencing generalized convulsive SE; this is the most common type and is associated with the greatest risk of physical and neurologic damage. SE also may be characterized by nonconvulsive seizures that produce a persistent state of impaired consciousness or by partial seizures (motor or sensory) that may not interfere with consciousness.

Uncontrolled convulsive SE may cause severe metabolic and hemodynamic alterations. V.S.'s vital signs (tachycardia, elevated blood pressure, increased respiratory rate, and elevated body temperature) are typical for a patient in SE. Prolonged, severe muscle contractions and CNS dysfunction from uncontrolled seizure discharges result in hyperthermia, cardiorespiratory collapse, myoglobinuria, renal failure, and neurologic damage. Neurologic damage also may occur with nonconvulsive SE; the neurologic sequelae of SE are related to the excessive electrical activity and resulting alterations in brain metabolism. When seizure activity persists longer than approximately 30 minutes, failure of mechanisms that regulate cerebral blood flow is more likely; this failure accompanies dramatic increases in brain metabolism and demand for glucose and oxygen. Failure to meet the metabolic demands of brain tissue results in accumulation of lactate and necrosis. Peripherally, lactate accumulates and serum glucose and electrolytes are altered. After 30 minutes of seizure activity, the body often fails to compensate for increased metabolic demands, and cardiovascular collapse may occur.[251,252] For these reasons, SE is considered a medical emergency that requires immediate treatment to prevent or lessen both physical and neurologic damage. Mortality in adults with SE may be as high as 30%[250]; fatal outcome is often the result of the injury or condition that precipitated SE (e.g., cardiopulmonary arrest, stroke). Long-term neurologic consequences of severe SE may include cognitive impairment, memory loss, and worsening of seizure disorders. However, the effect of SE on cognitive function is not clearly established; cognitive impairment may result from the neurologic disorder underlying SE rather than from SE itself.[253]

General Treatment Measures and Antiepileptic Drug Therapy

48. Describe a general treatment plan for V.S.'s episode of status epilepticus.

The immediate therapeutic concern in V.S. is to ensure ventilation and terminate current seizure activity. If possible, an airway should be placed; however, this may not be possible while he is convulsing. Objects (e.g., spoons, tongue blades) should never be forced into the mouth of a seizing patient. If airway placement is impossible, V.S. should be positioned on his side to allow drainage of saliva and mucus from the mouth and prevent aspiration. An IV line should be established using normal saline, and blood should be obtained for serum chemistries (especially glucose and electrolytes), AED serum concentrations, and toxicology screens. Thiamine 100 mg or vitamin B complex should be given IV. This should be followed by 25 g of glucose (50 mL of 50% dextrose solution) by IV push; these measures will correct any hypoglycemia, which may be responsible for SE. Glucose administration should be preceded by IV thiamine 100 mg or vitamin B complex to prevent Wernicke's encephalopathy.[250]

IV administration of rapidly effective anticonvulsant medication should begin as soon as possible to terminate V.S.'s seizure activity. IM or rectal administration of medication is not recommended in the initial treatment of this condition unless IV access is impossible.[250] IM medications are unlikely to be absorbed rapidly enough to achieve the CNS concentrations needed to terminate status seizures.

49. **Which anticonvulsants are available for IV administration? Evaluate the available drugs and recommend a drug, dosage, and regimen for initial treatment of status epilepticus in V.S.**

Lorazepam (Ativan), diazepam (Valium), phenytoin (Dilantin), and fosphenytoin (Cerebyx) are the agents most commonly employed as IV therapy in the initial treatment of SE.[254] IV sodium valproate (Depacon) is now available, but it is not indicated for use in SE. Although the manufacturer only recommends Depacon be administered slowly (≤20 mg/min), it has been shown to be administered safely at higher doses and rates.[255] Currently, IV valproate is indicated only as a replacement for oral valproate for patients who cannot use oral dosage forms. IV phenobarbital is usually reserved for use in cases of SE that do not respond to benzodiazepines and phenytoin. Phenytoin and fosphenytoin are indicated for treatment of SE, but owing to limitations on their rates of infusion, the onset of their peak effect may be delayed. Therefore, phenytoin or fosphenytoin is usually used following initial treatment with lorazepam or diazepam.

A recently completed trial studied four IV regimens for generalized convulsive SE.[256] The trial evaluated diazepam (0.15 mg/kg) followed by phenytoin (18 mg/kg), lorazepam (0.1 mg/kg) alone, phenobarbital (15 mg/kg) alone, and phenytoin (18 mg/kg) alone. For initial IV treatment of overt generalized SE, lorazepam was more effective than phenytoin, and although lorazepam was as effective as the other two regimens, it was easier to use.

IV administration of either diazepam or lorazepam is usually effective for rapid termination of seizure activity in SE.[257] Owing to diazepam's higher lipid solubility, it redistributes from the CNS to peripheral tissues rapidly after administration; this results in a short duration of action (<60 minutes).[258] Lorazepam's lower lipid solubility prevents rapid redistribution and accounts for its longer duration of action.[258] Lorazepam may be effective for up to 72 hours.[259,260] Owing to this longer duration, lorazepam is now the preferred benzodiazepine for immediate treatment of SE in many centers.[250] Repeated doses of lorazepam have been associated with development of tachyphylaxis, and lorazepam may be less effective for patients who have received chronic maintenance doses of benzodiazepines.[261,262] At adequate doses, the onsets of antiepileptic activity and efficacy of lorazepam and diazepam are equal.[257]

Either 0.1 mg/kg of lorazepam at 2 mg/min or 0.2 mg/kg of diazepam at 5 mg/min by IV is administered to stop SE.[250] Lorazepam may cause significant venous irritation, and the manufacturer recommends dilution with an equal volume of normal saline solution or water for injection before IV administration. Doses of either lorazepam or diazepam should be repeated after 5 to 10 minutes if seizure activity has not stopped. The efficacy of either drug depends on rapid achievement of high serum/CNS concentrations. Although both diazepam and lorazepam may be administered IM, this route should not be used for treatment of SE[250] because it is unlikely that either drug would achieve serum concentrations necessary for termination of seizure activity when thus administered. This is especially true for diazepam, which is absorbed slowly and erratically from IM gluteal injection sites.[258] Both lorazepam and diazepam are relatively safe drugs. Their primary adverse effects are sedation, hypotension, and respiratory arrest.[258] These side effects are usually short-lived and, when adequate facilities are available for assisted ventilation and administration of fluids, they usually can be managed without major risk to the patient. Respiratory depression occurs most commonly in patients who receive multiple IV medications for control of SE.

Intravenous Phenytoin and Fosphenytoin

50. **V.S. was given lorazepam 8 mg IV. Seizure activity ceased 5 minutes after the injection was completed. What drug should be administered to V.S. for prolonged control of seizures? Recommend a dose, route, and method of administration.**

Continued effective seizure control is important for patients who experience SE. In the past, when diazepam was the benzodiazepine predominantly used for immediate control of SE, a long-acting AED such as phenytoin was routinely administered at the same time to ensure continued suppression of seizure activity. Routine use of phenytoin has been somewhat de-emphasized with increased use of lorazepam[250]; lorazepam's apparent longer duration of effect may make routine use of IV phenytoin less necessary. Nevertheless, phenytoin is still used in conjunction with both lorazepam and diazepam by many centers.

The availability of fosphenytoin (Cerebyx) for IV administration has provided an additional option for administration of phenytoin in the treatment of SE. Use of this phenytoin prodrug allows more rapid administration of large IV loading doses of phenytoin with less risk of injection site complications and potentially fewer cardiovascular adverse effects. Fosphenytoin itself is inactive; its only therapeutic effect results from its conversion to phenytoin.[156,157] Because fosphenytoin is more expensive, many facilities have been reluctant to place this product on their formularies. However, preliminary pharmacoeconomic studies seem to indicate that although it is initially more expensive, fosphenytoin may be a more economical preparation because it causes fewer adverse effects than phenytoin.[263] Generic formulations of injectable sodium phenytoin are still available; nevertheless, when the safety profile of fosphenytoin is considered, fosphenytoin may ultimately replace parenteral sodium phenytoin injection.

Phenytoin (administered as either sodium phenytoin injection or as sodium fosphenytoin injection) is considered the long-acting anticonvulsant of choice for most patients with generalized convulsive SE.[254] Extensive clinical experience with the use of IV loading doses of phenytoin has established its efficacy and general safety. Phenytoin causes much less sedation and respiratory depression than drugs such as phenobarbital when it is used in conjunction with IV benzodiazepines.[250] V.S.'s maintenance carbamazepine therapy produced moderate serum concentrations and was previously effective. Without obvious precipitating factors such as head trauma, CNS infection, or drug/alcohol abuse, SE, in a patient with a history of epilepsy, most commonly results from poor compliance with maintenance medication. Therefore, IV use of either phenytoin or fosphenytoin is a good choice for re-establishing effective AED therapy for V.S. SE is uncommonly the first presentation of idiopathic epilepsy.

LOADING DOSE

Although V.S. presumably has existing serum concentrations of carbamazepine, he should be given an IV loading dose of either phenytoin or fosphenytoin. A dose of phenytoin (20 mg/kg IV at 50 mg/min) or fosphenytoin (20 mg/kg PE IV at 150 mg/min) is recommended. Serum phenytoin concentrations should remain >10 µg/mL for approximately 24 hours; this will allow time for determination of V.S.'s serum carbamazepine concentration and estimation of an appropriate maintenance dose of oral carbamazepine. In this setting, the use of IV phenytoin/fosphenytoin is a temporary measure. V.S.'s previously positive response to carbamazepine indicates that he should continue to receive this drug as oral maintenance medication.

IV phenytoin can be administered by direct injection into a running IV line. The rate of administration should be no faster than 50 mg/min to minimize the risk of hypotension and acute cardiac arrhythmias. Cardiovascular status (blood pressure, electrocardiogram) should be monitored closely during administration. Hypotension or electrocardiographic abnormalities usually reverse if the administration of phenytoin is slowed or stopped temporarily. If fosphenytoin is administered, it can be given by either direct IV injection or, after dilution in any suitable IV solution, by infusion at up to 150 mg PE per minute.[156] Absence of propylene glycol as a diluent renders fosphenytoin potentially less likely than phenytoin to cause cardiovascular adverse effects; however, clear documentation of this effect is lacking. Electrocardiographic and blood pressure monitoring is recommended when this drug is given IV. Pruritus and paresthesias, usually localized to the face and groin, are relatively common side effects during IV fosphenytoin administration. These sensations are not allergic reactions to the medication. Their occurrence is related to the administration rate, and they are reversible with temporary discontinuation or slowing of the injection.[156] These side effects are thought to be related to the phosphate component of fosphenytoin.

INTRAVENOUS INFUSION

51. V.S.'s physician is reluctant to administer this dose of either phenytoin or fosphenytoin by direct IV injection. What are the guidelines for administration of phenytoin and fosphenytoin by IV infusion?

Practical difficulties associated with administration of phenytoin by direct IV push undoubtedly have contributed to its low usage rate. In many hospitals or other facilities, direct IV injections must be administered by a physician, and many physicians would be unwilling to commit the 30 to 45 minutes necessary to administer V.S.'s loading dose at a safe rate. In addition, the rate of direct IV administration is difficult to control, and too-rapid administration resulting in cardiac toxicity is a risk. Although fosphenytoin can be given at a faster injection rate with a lower risk of complications, direct IV administration of this drug still presents practical difficulties.

The compatibility of phenytoin injection with IV solutions has been controversial. Phenytoin's chemical properties (weakly acidic with a pKa of 8 and low water solubility) require that the commercial injectable dosage form of sodium phenytoin be dissolved in a mixture of 40% propylene glycol and 10% alcohol; the pH of the final product is adjusted to approximately 12 with sodium hydroxide. Addition of the preparation to IV fluids dilutes the drug's solvent system and reduces pH. A possible result would be precipitation of free phenytoin. However, several studies indicate that phenytoin may be diluted, preferably in small total volumes, with saline solution.[264,265] Despite the formation of crystals in many solutions, measured phenytoin concentrations are essentially identical to those predicted. Thus, dilution of the required volume of phenytoin injection in approximately 100 to 500 mL of 0.45% or 0.9% saline should provide an appropriate solution for IV administration. An in-line filter of 0.45 to 0.22 micron pore size may be used to prevent the infusion of crystals.[264] The administration rate should be no faster than 50 mg/min. This method of administration is both safe and effective when the infusion rate is monitored carefully. Burning pain at the IV infusion site, hypotension, and cardiac arrhythmias may occur during the infusion and appear to be related to the infusion rate. Either slowing or temporarily stopping the infusion may relieve these side effects.[266,267] IV administration of phenytoin is also associated with phlebitis; extravasation has resulted in chemical cellulitis and tissue necrosis.[268]

IV infusion of fosphenytoin is less troublesome. Fosphenytoin is compatible with virtually all IV fluids because of its high water solubility and the lower pH required to maintain the drug in solution. Hypotension may occur during fosphenytoin infusion, and cardiovascular status should still be monitored closely. Fosphenytoin should not be infused at a rate >150 mg PE per minute. Injection site complications and phlebitis are significantly less likely with administration of fosphenytoin.[155]

Maintenance Therapy

52. Following administration of IV phenytoin, no further seizures occurred. The laboratory reported that serum chemistries were all normal. The carbamazepine serum concentration was 5 µg/mL on admission. A serum phenytoin concentration determined 1 hour after administration of the IV loading dose was 24 µg/mL. How should V.S.'s maintenance therapy with anticonvulsants be altered?

The reduced serum concentration of carbamazepine appears to confirm the role of noncompliance in this episode of SE. As V.S. was previously well controlled on 600 mg/day, this also would be a reasonable maintenance dosage at this time. Administration of maintenance doses should be resumed as soon as V.S. can take oral medication. V.S. should be counseled regarding the importance of taking his medication according to directions.

Alternative Therapies for Refractory Status Epilepticus

53. What other medications are useful for treatment of SE that does not respond to benzodiazepines and/or phenytoin?

Phenobarbital may be useful for treatment of SE if the patient cannot tolerate phenytoin or when seizures continue following administration of appropriate loading doses of phenytoin. Patients who receive phenobarbital after being treated with IV benzodiazepines should be monitored closely for respiratory depression because this effect may be additive. Equipment and personnel to provide ventilatory assistance should be available.[250] Administration of IV phenobarbital may cause hypotension, which may necessitate discontinuation of the drug or the use of pressor agents. An initial dose of 20 mg/kg given IV at a rate no faster than 100 mg/min is recommended.[250] IM administration of phenobarbital results in slow absorption, and this route of administration is not recommended for treatment of SE.

Pentobarbital or other anesthetic barbiturates are administered for treatment of SE that has not responded to more conservative measures, including phenobarbital. Significant respiratory depression is expected with this therapy; patients will require intubation and mechanical ventilation. In addition, vasopressors such as dopamine or dobutamine may be required to control hypotension. Constant EEG monitoring also is required to assess the effect of the drug.

Pentobarbital is given as a loading dose of 5 mg/kg IV and is followed by an IV infusion of 0.5 to 3 mg/kg per hour.[250] The dose and infusion rate are adjusted to produce either a flat or a burst-suppression EEG pattern.[269] Most protocols for pentobarbital coma recommend attempts at gradually reducing the dose of medication after 12 to 24 hours of treatment. If clinical or EEG seizure activity recurs, the dose is increased again to produce continued EEG suppression. Pentobarbital coma may be continued for several days in some patients.

Several other drugs have been used for treatment of refractory SE, but experience with these agents is somewhat limited. Midazolam (Versed), a short-acting anesthetic benzodiazepine, has been used by IV infusion.[270–272] Valproate has been used for treatment of refractory SE. Because no parenteral form of this drug has been available until recently, the syrup form has been administered either rectally or via nasogastric tube. At present, information regarding the IV use of valproate for SE is largely anecdotal.[273] Other drugs that have been used for refractory SE include lidocaine (Xylocaine), general anesthetics (halothane or isoflurane), and propofol.[254]

REFERENCES

1. Scheuer ML, Pedley TA. The evaluation and treatment of seizures. N Engl J Med 1990;323:1468.
2. Commission on Epidemiology and Prognosis, International League Against Epilepsy. Guidelines for epidemiologic studies on epilepsy. Epilepsia 1993;34:592.
3. Commission on Classification and Terminology of the International League Against Epilepsy. Proposal for revised clinical and electroencephalographic classification of epileptic seizures. Epilepsia 1981;22:489.
4. Penry JK, ed. Epilepsy: Diagnosis, Management, Quality of Life. New York: Raven Press, 1986:4.
5. Schmidt D, Haenel F. Therapeutic plasma levels of phenytoin, phenobarbital, and carbamazepine: individual variation in relation to seizure frequency and type. Neurology 1984;34:1252.
6. Schmidt D et al. The influence of seizure type on the efficacy of plasma concentrations of phenytoin, phenobarbital, and carbamazepine. Arch Neurol 1986;43:263.
7. Mattson RH et al. Prognosis for total control of complex partial and secondarily generalized tonic clonic seizures. Neurology 1996;47:68.
8. Dreifuss FE. Classification of epileptic seizures and the epilepsies. Pediatr Clin North Am 1989;36:265.
9. Dreifuss FE. The epilepsies: clinical implications of the international classification. Epilepsia 1990;31(Suppl 3):S3.
10. Kotagal P. Complex partial seizures. In: Wyllie E, ed. The Treatment of Epilepsy: Principles and Practice, 3rd ed. Philadelphia: Lippincott Williams & Wilkins, 2001:309.
11. Berkovic SF, Benbadis S. Absence seizures. In: Wyllie E, ed. The Treatment of Epilepsy: Principles and Practice, 3rd ed. Philadelphia: Lippincott Williams & Wilkins, 2001:357.
12. Serratosa JM. Juvenile myoclonic epilepsy. In: Wyllie E, ed. The Treatment of Epilepsy: Principles and Practice, 3rd ed. Philadelphia: Lippincott Williams & Wilkins, 2001:491.
13. Farrell K. Secondary generalized epilepsy and Lennox-Gastaut syndrome. In: Wyllie E, ed. The Treatment of Epilepsy: Principles and Practice, 3rd ed. Philadelphia: Lippincott Williams & Wilkins, 2001:525.
14. Zifkin BG, Andermann F. Epilepsy with reflex seizures. In: Wyllie E, ed. The Treatment of Epilepsy: Principles and Practice, 3rd ed. Philadelphia: Lippincott Williams & Wilkins, 2001:537.
15. Asconape J, Penry JK. Some clinical and EEG aspects of benign juvenile myoclonic epilepsy. Epilepsia 1984;25:108.
16. Holmes GL. Electroencephalographic and neuroradiologic evaluation of children with epilepsy. Pediatr Clin North Am 1989;36:395.
17. First Seizure Trial Group. Randomized clinical trial on the efficacy of antiepileptic drugs in reducing the risk of relapse after a first unprovoked tonic-clonic seizure. Neurology 1993;43:478.
18. Berg AT et al. Discontinuing antiepileptic drugs. In: Engel J, Pedley TA, eds. Epilepsy: A Comprehensive Textbook. Philadelphia: Lippincott-Raven, 1998:1275.
19. Callaghan N et al. Withdrawal of anticonvulsant drugs in patients free of seizures for two years: a prospective study. N Engl J Med 1988;318:942.
20. Mauleardi M et al. Outcome after discontinuation of antiepileptic drug therapy in children with epilepsy. Epilepsia 1989;30:582.
21. Wiebe S et al. A randomized, controlled trial of surgery for temporal-lobe epilepsy. N Engl J Med 2001;345:311.
22. Bainbridge JL et al. The ketogenic diet. Pharmacotherapy 1999;19:782.
23. Hassan AM et al. Ketogenic diet in the treatment of refractory epilepsy in childhood. Pediatr Neurol 1999;21:548.
24. Fisher RS, Handforth A. Reassessment: vagus nerve stimulation for epilepsy: a report of the Therapeutics and Technology Assessment Subcommittee of the American Academy of Neurology. Neurology 1999;53:666.
25. Reynolds EH. Early treatment and prognosis of epilepsy. Epilepsia 1987;28:97.
26. Pellock JM. Efficacy and adverse effects of antiepileptic drugs. Pediatr Clin North Am 1989;36:435.
27. Devinsky O. Patients with refractory seizures. N Engl J Med 1999;340:1565.
28. Mattson RH et al. Comparison of carbamazepine, phenobarbital, phenytoin, and primidone in partial and secondarily generalized tonic-clonic seizures. N Engl J Med 1985;313:145.
29. Mattson RH et al. A comparison of valproate with carbamazepine for the treatment of complex partial seizures and secondarily generalized tonic-clonic seizures in adults. N Engl J Med 1992;327:765.
30. Fisch BJ, Olejniczak PW. Generalized tonic-clonic seizures. In: Wyllie E, ed. The Treatment of Epilepsy: Principles and Practice, 3rd ed. Philadelphia: Lippincott Williams & Wilkins, 2001:369.
31. Karceski S et al. The expert consensus guideline series: the treatment of epilepsy. Epilepsy Behav 2001;2:A1.
32. Schoenenberger RA et al. Appropriateness of antiepileptic drug level monitoring. JAMA 1995;274:1622.
33. Choonara IA, Rane A. Therapeutic drug monitoring of anticonvulsants: state of the art. Clin Pharmacokinet 1990;18:318.
34. Hayes G, Kootsikas ME. Reassessing the lower end of the phenytoin therapeutic range: a review of the literature. Ann Pharmacother 1993;27:1389.
35. Commission on Antiepileptic Drugs, International League Against Epilepsy. Guidelines for therapeutic monitoring on antiepileptic drugs. Epilepsia 1993;34:585.
36. Tozer TN, Winter ME. Phenytoin. In: Evans WE et al, eds. Applied Pharmacokinetics: Principles of Therapeutic Drug Monitoring, 3rd ed. Vancouver: Applied Therapeutics, 1992:25.
37. Levy RH et al. Carbamazepine, valproic acid, phenobarbital, and ethosuximide. In: Evans WE et al, eds. Applied Pharmacokinetics: Principles of Therapeutic Drug Monitoring, 3rd ed. Vancouver: Applied Therapeutics, 1992:26.
38. Chadwick DW. Concentration-effect relationships of valproic acid. Clin Pharmacokinet 1985;10:155.
39. Bourgeois BFD. Valproic acid: clinical efficacy and use in epilepsy. In: Levy RH et al, eds. Antiepileptic Drugs, 5th ed. Philadelphia: Lippincott Williams & Wilkins, 2002:808.
40. Ohtsuka Y et al. Treatment of intractable childhood epilepsy with high-dose valproate. Epilepsia 1992;33:158.
41. Hurst DL. Expanded therapeutic range of valproate. Pediatr Neurol 1987;3:342.
42. Woo E et al. If a well-stabilized epileptic patient has a subtherapeutic antiepileptic drug level, should the dose be increased? A randomized prospective study. Epilepsia 1988;29:129.
43. Cloyd JC. Pharmacokinetic pitfalls of present antiepileptic medications. Epilepsia 1991;32(Suppl 5):S53.
44. Schmidt D. Reduction of two-drug therapy in intractable epilepsy. Epilepsia 1983;24:368.
45. Smith DB et al. Results of a nationwide Veterans Administration Cooperative Study comparing the efficacy and toxicity of carbamazepine, phenobarbital, phenytoin, and primidone. Epilepsia 1987;28(Suppl 3):S50.
46. Thompson PJ, Trimble MR. Anticonvulsant drugs and cognitive functions. Epilepsia 1982;23:531.
47. Albright P, Bruni J. Reduction of polypharmacy in epileptic patients. Arch Neurol 1985;42:797.
48. Prevey ML et al. Improvement in cognitive functioning and mood state after conversion to valproate monotherapy. Neurology 1989;39:1640.

49. Mirza WU et al. Results of antiepileptic drug reduction in patients with multiple handicaps and epilepsy. Drug Invest 1993;5:320.

50. Guberman A. Monotherapy or polytherapy for epilepsy? Can J Neurol Sci 1998;25:S3.

51. Chadwick DW et al. A double-blind trial of gabapentin monotherapy for newly diagnosed partial seizures. International Gabapentin Monotherapy Study Group 945-77. Neurology 1998;51:1282.

52. Devinsky O et al. Efficacy of felbamate monotherapy in patients undergoing presurgical evaluation of partial seizures. Epilepsy Res 1995;20:241.

53. Sachdeo RC et al. Topiramate monotherapy for partial seizures. Epilepsia 1997;38:294.

54. Schacter SC. Tiagabine monotherapy in the treatment of partial epilepsy. Epilepsia 1995;36:S2.

55. Gilliam F et al. An active-control trial of lamotrigine monotherapy for partial seizures. Neurology 1998;51:1018.

56. Shinnar S et al. Discontinuing antiepileptic drugs in children with epilepsy: a prospective study. Ann Neurol 1994;35:534.

57. Berg AT, Shinnar S. Relapse following discontinuation of antiepileptic drugs: a meta-analysis. Neurology 1994;44:601.

58. Tennison M et al. Discontinuing antiepileptic drugs in children: a comparison of a six-week and a nine-month taper period. N Engl J Med 1994;330:1407.

59. Malow BA et al. Carbamazepine withdrawal: effects of taper rate on seizure frequency. Neurology 1993;43:2280.

60. Todt H. The late prognosis of epilepsy in childhood: results of a prospective follow-up study. Epilepsia 1984;25:137.

61. Prevention and treatment of injury from chemical warfare agents. Med Letter Drugs Therapeutics 2002;44:1.

62. Holstege CP et al. Chemical warfare: Nerve agent poisoning. Crit Care Clin 1997;13:923.

62a. Leikin JB et al. A review of nerve agent exposure for the critical care physician. Crit Care Med 2002;30:2346.

63. Beydoun A et al. Safety and efficacy of divalproex sodium monotherapy in partial epilepsy: a double-blind, concentration-response design clinical trial. Neurology 1997;48:182.

64. Wilensky AJ. Benzodiazepines: clorazepate. In: Levy RH et al, eds. Antiepileptic Drugs, 4th ed. New York: Raven Press, 1995:751.

65. Meador KJ. Cognitive effects of epilepsy and of antiepileptic medications. In: Wyllie E, ed. The Treatment of Epilepsy: Principles and Practice, 3rd ed. Philadelphia: Lippincott Williams & Wilkins, 2001:1215.

66. Dodrill CB, Troupin AS. Psychotropic effects of carbamazepine in epilepsy: a double-blind comparison with phenytoin. Neurology 1977;27:1023.

67. Dodrill CB, Troupin AS. Neuropsychological effects of carbamazepine and phenytoin: a reanalysis. Neurology 1991;41:141.

68. Meador KJ et al. Comparative cognitive effects of carbamazepine and phenytoin in healthy adults. Neurology 1991;41:1537.

69. Aldenkamp AP et al. Withdrawal of antiepileptic medication in children: effects on cognitive function: the multicenter Holmfrid study. Neurology 1993;43:41.

70. Franceschi M et al. Fatal aplastic anemia in a patient treated with carbamazepine. Epilepsia 1988;29:582.

71. Pisciotta AV. Carbamazepine: hematological toxicity. In: Woodbury DM et al, eds. Antiepileptic Drugs, 2nd ed. New York: Raven Press, 1982:533.

72. Pellock JM. Carbamazepine side effects in children and adults. Epilepsia 1987;28(Suppl 3):S64.

73. Holmes GL. Carbamazepine: adverse effects. In: Levy RH et al, eds. Antiepileptic Drugs, 5th ed. Philadelphia: Lippincott Williams & Wilkins, 2002:285.

74. Graves NM, Bodor MC. Carbamazepine-induced leukopenia. Drug Therapy 1989;August:56.

75. Camfield C et al. Asymptomatic children with epilepsy: little benefit from screening for anticonvulsant-induced liver, blood, or renal damage. Neurology 1986;36:838.

76. Horowitz S et al. Hepatotoxic reactions associated with carbamazepine therapy. Epilepsia 1988;29:149.

77. Hadzic N et al. Acute liver failure induced by carbamazepine. Arch Dis Child 1990;65:315.

78. Livingston S et al. Carbamazepine (Tegretol) in epilepsy: nine-year follow-up study with special emphasis on untoward reactions. Dis Nerv System 1974;35:103.

79. Tomson T et al. Relationship of intraindividual dose to plasma concentration of carbamazepine: indication of dose-dependent induction of metabolism. Ther Drug Monit 1989;11:533.

80. Sanchez A et al. Steady-state carbamazepine concentration-dose ratio in epileptic patients. Clin Pharmacokinet 1986;11:41.

81. Oles KS, Gal P. Bioequivalency revisited: Epitol versus Tegretol. Neurology 1993;43:2435.

82. Gilman JT et al. Carbamazepine toxicity resulting from generic substitution. Neurology 1993;43:2696.

83. Spina E. Carbamazepine: chemistry, biotransformation, and pharmacokinetics. In: Levy RH et al, eds. Antiepileptic Drugs, 5th ed. Philadelphia: Lippincott Williams & Wilkins, 2002:236.

84. The Tegretol Oros Osmotic Release Delivery System Study Group. Double-blind crossover comparison of Tegretol-XR and Tegretol in patients with epilepsy. Neurology 1995;45:1703.

85. Riss JR et al. Administration of Carbatrol to children with feeding tubes. Pediatr Neurol 2002;27:193.

86. So EL et al. Seizure exacerbation and status epilepticus related to carbamazepine-10,11-epoxide. Ann Neurol 1994;35:743.

87. Ringel RA, Brick JF. Perspective on carbamazepine-induced water intoxication: reversal by demeclocycline. Neurology 1986;36:1506.

88. Ramsay RE, Slater JD. Effects of antiepileptic drugs on hormones. Epilepsia 1991;32(Suppl 5):S60.

89. Lahr MB. Hyponatremia during carbamazepine therapy. Clin Pharmacol Ther 1985;37:693.

90. Perucca E, Richens A. Water intoxication produced by carbamazepine and its reversal by phenytoin. Br J Clin Pharmacol 1980;9:302P.

91. Hoppener RJ et al. Correlation between daily fluctuations of carbamazepine serum levels and intermittent side effects. Epilepsia 1980;21:341.

92. Graves NM. Felbamate. Ann Pharmacother 1993;27:1073.

93. Sachdeo R et al. Felbamate monotherapy: controlled trial in patients with partial onset seizures. Ann Neurol 1992;32:386.

94. US Gabapentin Study Group No. 5. Gabapentin as add-on therapy in refractory partial epilepsy: a double-blind, placebo-controlled, parallel-group study. Neurology 1993;43:2292.

95. US Gabapentin Study Group. The long-term safety and efficacy of gabapentin (Neurontin) as add-on therapy in drug-resistant partial epilepsy. Epilepsy Res 1994;18:67.

96. UK Gabapentin Study Group. Gabapentin in partial epilepsy. Lancet 1990;335:1114.

97. Matsuo F et al. Placebo-controlled study of the efficacy and safety of lamotrigine in patients with partial seizures. Neurology 1993;43:2284.

98. Messenheimer J et al. Lamotrigine therapy for partial seizures: a multicenter, placebo-controlled, double-blind, cross-over trial. Epilepsia 1994;35:113.

99. Sachdeo RC et al. Tiagabine therapy for complex partial seizures. A dose-frequency study. Arch Neurol 1997;54:595.

100. Ben-Menachem E et al. Double-blind, placebo-controlled trial of topiramate as add-on therapy in patients with refractory partial seizures. Epilepsia 1996;37:539.

101. Sharief M et al. Double-blind, placebo-controlled study of topiramate in patients with refractory partial epilepsy. Epilepsy Res 1996;25:217.

102. Faught E. Efficacy of topiramate as adjunctive therapy in refractory partial seizures: United States trial experience. Epilepsia 1997;38 (Suppl 1):S24.

103. McAuley JW et al. Newer therapies in the drug treatment of epilepsy. Ann Pharmacother 2002;36:119.

104. The Felbamate Study Group in Lennox-Gastaut Syndrome. Efficacy of felbamate in childhood epileptic encephalopathy (Lennox-Gastaut syndrome). N Engl J Med 1993;328:29.

105. Motte J et al. Lamotrigine for generalized seizures associated with the Lennox-Gastaut syndrome. Lamictal Lennox-Gastaut Study Group. N Engl J Med 1997;337:1807.

106. Sachdeo RC et al. A double-blind, randomized trial of topiramate in Lennox-Gastaut syndrome. Topiramate YL Study Group. Neurology 1999;52:1882.

107. Alsaadi TM et al. Levetiracetam monotherapy for adults with localization-related epilepsy. Epil Behav 2002;3:471.

108. White HS. Clinical significance of animal seizure models and mechanism of action studies of potential antiepileptic drugs. Epilepsia 1997;38 (Suppl 1):S9.

109. Fitton A, Goa KL. Lamotrigine: an update of its pharmacology and therapeutic use in epilepsy. Drugs 1995;50:691.

110. Sachdeo RC. Topiramate. Clinical profile in epilepsy. Clin Pharmacokinet 1998;34:335.

111. Pellock JM, Brodie MJ. Felbamate: 1997 update. Epilepsia 1997;38:1261.

112. Jones MW. Topiramate: safety and tolerability. Can J Neurol Sci 1998;25:S13.

113. McLean MJ et al. Safety and tolerability of gabapentin as adjunctive therapy in a large, multicenter study. Epilepsia 1999;40:965.

114. Leppik IE et al. Safety of tiagabine: summary of 53 trials. Epilepsy Res 1999;33:235.

115. Guberman AH et al. Lamotrigine-associated rash: risk/benefit considerations in adults and children. Epilepsia 1999;40:985.

116. Tecoma ES. Oxcarbazepine. Epilepsia 1999;40 (Suppl 5):S37.

117. Oommen KJ, Mathews S. Zonisamide: a new antiepileptic drug. Clin Neuropharmacol 1999;22:192.

118. Goa KL, Sorkin EM. Gabapentin: a review of its pharmacological properties and clinical potential in epilepsy. Drugs 1993;46:409.

119. Luer MS, Rhoney DH. Tiagabine: a novel antiepileptic drug. Ann Pharmacother 1998;32:1173.

120. Sachdeo R et al. Coadministration of phenytoin and felbamate: evidence of additional phenytoin dose-reduction requirements based on pharmacokinetics and tolerability with increasing doses of felbamate. Epilepsia 1999;40:1122.

121. Albani F et al. Effect of felbamate on plasma levels of carbamazepine and its metabolites. Epilepsia 1991;32:130.

122. Yuen AWC et al. Sodium valproate acutely inhibits lamotrigine metabolism. Br J Clin Pharmacol 1992;33:511.

123. Anderson GD et al. Bidirectional interaction of valproate and lamotrigine in healthy subjects. Clin Pharmacol Ther 1996;60:145.

124. Warner T et al. Lamotrigine-induced carbamazepine toxicity: an interaction with carbamazepine-10,11-epoxide. Epilepsy Res 1992;11:147.

125. Besag FM et al. Carbamazepine toxicity with lamotrigine: pharmacokinetic or pharmacodynamic interaction? Epilepsia 1998;39:183.

126. Welty TE et al. Levetiracetam: A different approach to the pharmacotherapy of epilepsy. Ann Pharmacother 2002;36:296.

127. Fattore C et al. Induction of ethynylestradiol and levonorgestrel metabolism by oxcarbazepine in healthy women. Epilepsia 1999;40:783.

128. Bialer M et al. Progress report on new antiepileptic drugs: a summary of the Fifth Eilat Conference (EILAT V). Epilepsy Res 2001;43:11.

129. Jacobs MP et al. Future directions for epilepsy research. Neurology 2001 13;57:1536.
130. Loscher W, Potschka H. Role of multidrug transporters in pharmacoresistance to antiepileptic drugs. J Pharmacol Exp Ther 2002;301:7.
131. Fitton A, Goa KL. Lamotrigine: an update of its pharmacology and therapeutic use in epilepsy. Drugs 1995;50:691.
132. Kilpatrick ES et al. Concentration-effect and concentration-toxicity relations with lamotrigine: a prospective study. Epilepsia 1996;37:534.
133. Tozer TN, Winter ME. Phenytoin. In: Evans WE et al, eds. Applied Pharmacokinetics: Principles of Therapeutic Drug Monitoring, 3rd ed. Vancouver: Applied Therapeutics, 1992:25.
134. Allen JP et al. Phenytoin cumulation kinetics. Clin Pharmacol Ther 1979;26:445.
135. Ludden TM et al. Rate of phenytoin accumulation in man: a simulation study. J Pharmacokinetics Biopharm 1978;6:399.
136. Osborn HH et al. Single-dose oral phenytoin loading. Ann Emerg Med 1987;16:407.
137. Goff DA et al. Absorption characteristics of three phenytoin sodium products after administration of oral loading doses. Clin Pharm 1984;3:634.
138. Evans RP et al. Phenytoin toxicity and blood levels after a large oral dose. Am J Hosp Pharm 1980;37:232.
139. Jung D et al. Effect of dose on phenytoin absorption. Clin Pharmacol Ther 1980;28:479.
140. Record KE et al. Oral phenytoin loading in adults: rapid achievement of therapeutic plasma levels. Ann Neurol 1979;5:268.
141. Cranford RE et al. Intravenous phenytoin: clinical and pharmacokinetic aspects. Neurology 1978;28:874.
142. Ludden TM et al. Sensitivity analysis of the effect of bioavailability or dosage form content on mean steady state phenytoin concentration. Ther Drug Monitoring 1991;13:120.
143. Sarkar MA et al. The effects of storage and shaking on the settling properties of phenytoin suspension. Neurology 1989;39:207.
144. Rankine DA, Sadler RM. Phenytoin suspension [letter]. Neurology 1989;39:1644.
145. Sawchuk RJ et al. Rapid and slow release phenytoin in epileptic patients at steady state: comparative plasma levels and toxicity. J Pharmacokinet Biopharm 1982;10:365.
146. Fitzsimmons WE et al. Single dose comparison of the relative bioavailability of phenytoin suspension and extended capsules. Epilepsia 1986;27:464.
147. Haerer AF, Buchanan RA. Effectiveness of single daily doses of diphenylhydantoin. Neurology 1972;22:1021
148. Cooks DA et al. Control of epilepsy with a single daily dose of phenytoin sodium. Br J Clin Pharmacol 1975;2:449.
149. Sawchuk RJ et al. Steady-state plasma concentrations as a function of the absorption rate and dosing interval for drugs exhibiting concentration-dependent clearance: consequences for phenytoin therapy. J Pharmacokinet Biopharm 1979;7:543.
150. Mikati M et al. Double-blind randomized study comparing brand-name and generic phenytoin monotherapy. Epilepsia 1992;33:359.
151. Tindula PJ et al. Generic phenytoin versus Dilantin for once-a-day dosing. Am J Hosp Pharm 1981;38: 1114.
151a. Wilder BJ et al. Effect of food on absorption of Dilantin Kapseals and Mylan extended phenytoin sodium capsules. Neurology 2001;57:582.
152. Kostenbauder HB et al. Bioavailability and single-dose pharmacokinetics of intramuscular phenytoin. Clin Pharmacol Ther 1975;18:449.
153. Serrano EE et al. Plasma diphenylhydantoin values after oral and intramuscular administration of diphenylhydantoin. Neurology 1973;23:311.
154. Serrano EE et al. Intramuscular administration of diphenylhydantoin: histologic follow-up studies. Arch Neurol 1974;31:276.

155. Jamerson BD et al. Venous irritation related to intravenous administration of phenytoin versus fosphenytoin. Pharmacotherapy 1994;14:47.
156. Fischer JH et al. Fosphenytoin: clinical pharmacokinetics and comparative advantages in the acute treatment of seizures. Clin Pharmacokinet 2003;42:33.
157. Boucher BA. Fosphenytoin: a novel phenytoin prodrug. Pharmacotherapy 1996;16:777.
158. Ramsay RE et al. Intramuscular fosphenytoin (Cerebyx) in patients requiring a loading dose of phenytoin. Epilepsy Res 1997;28:181.
159. Silverman AK et al. Cutaneous and immunologic reactions to phenytoin. J Am Acad Dermatol 1988;18:721.
160. Butler RT et al. Drug-induced gingival hyperplasia: phenytoin, cyclosporine, and nifedipine. J Am Dent Assoc 1987;114:56.
161. Stinnett E et al. New developments in understanding phenytoin-induced gingival hyperplasia. J Am Dent Assoc 1987;114:814.
162. Bruni J. Phenytoin: adverse effects. In: Levy RH et al, eds. Antiepileptic Drugs, 5th ed. Philadelphia: Lippincott Williams & Wilkins, 2002:605.
163. Kuruvilla T, Bharucha NE. Cerebellar atrophy after acute phenytoin intoxication. Epilepsia 1997;38:500.
164. Rapport RL et al. Phenytoin-related cerebellar degeneration without seizures. Ann Neurol 1977;2:437.
165. So EL, Penry JK. Adverse effects of phenytoin on peripheral nerves and neuromuscular junction: a review. Epilepsia 1981;22:467.
166. Lovelace RE, Horwitz SJ. Peripheral neuropathy in long-term diphenylhydantoin therapy. Arch Neurol 1968;18:69.
167. Ragueneau-Majlessi I et al. Phenytoin: interactions with other drugs. In: Levy RH et al, eds. Antiepileptic Drugs, 5th ed. Philadelphia: Lippincott Williams & Wilkins, 2002:581.
168. May T, Rambeck B. Fluctuations of unbound and total phenytoin concentrations during the day in epileptic patients on valproic acid comedication. Ther Drug Monitoring 1990;12:124.
169. Scheyer RD. Valproate: drug interactions. In: Levy RH et al, eds. Antiepileptic Drugs, 5th ed. Philadelphia: Lippincott Williams & Wilkins, 2002:801.
170. Anderson GD. A mechanistic approach to antiepileptic drug interactions. Ann Pharmacother 1998;32:554.
171. Genton P, Gelisse P. Valproate: adverse effects. In: Levy RH et al, eds. Antiepileptic Drugs, 5th ed. Philadelphia: Lippincott Williams & Wilkins;2002:837.
172. Pellock JM, Coulter DA. Trimethadione. In: Levy RH et al, eds. Antiepileptic Drugs, 4th ed. New York: Raven Press, 1995:689.
173. Mattson RH. Antiepileptic drug monotherapy in adults: selection and use in new-onset epilepsy. In: Levy RH et al, eds. Antiepileptic Drugs, 5th ed. Philadelphia: Lippincott Williams & Wilkins, 2002:72.
174. Sato S, Malow B. Benzodiazepines: clonazepam. In: Levy RH et al, eds. Antiepileptic Drugs, 4th ed. New York: Raven Press, 1995:725.
175. Glauser TA. Succinimides: adverse effects. In: Levy RH et al, eds. Antiepileptic Drugs, 5th ed. Philadelphia: Lippincott Williams & Wilkins, 2002:658.
176. Browne TR, Mirsky AF. Absence (petit mal) seizures. In: Browne TR, Feldman RG, eds. Epilepsy: Diagnosis and Management. Boston: Little Brown, 1983:61.
177. Livingston S et al. Petit mal epilepsy: results of a prolonged follow-up study of 117 patients. JAMA 1965;194:227.
178. Penry JK et al. Refractiveness of absence seizures and phenobarbital. Neurology 1981;31:158.
179. Snead OC, Hosey LC. Exacerbation of seizures in children by carbamazepine. N Engl J Med 1985;313:916.

180. Shields WD, Saslow E. Myoclonic, atonic and absence seizures following institution of carbamazepine therapy in children. Neurology 1983;33:1487.
181. Jones-Saete C et al. External leakage from feeding gastrostomies in patients receiving valproate sprinkle. Epilepsia 1992;33:692.
182. Zaccara G et al. Clinical pharmacokinetics of valproic acid, 1988. Clin Pharmacokinet 1988; 15:367.
183. Cloyd JC et al. Comparison of sprinkle versus syrup formulations of valproate for bioavailability, tolerance, and preference. J Pediatr 1992;120:634.
184. Dutta S et al. Comparison of the bioavailability of unequal doses of divalproex sodium extended-release formulation relative to the delayed-release formulation in healthy volunteers. Epilepsy Res 2002;49:1.
185. Fischer JH et al. Effect of food on the serum concentration profile of enteric-coated valproic acid. Neurology 1988;38:1319.
186. Bauer LA et al. Valproic acid clearance: unbound fraction and diurnal variation in young and elderly adults. Clin Pharmacol Ther 1985;37:697.
187. Tennison MB et al. Valproate metabolites and hepatotoxicity in an epileptic population. Epilepsia 1988;29:543.
188. Eadie MJ et al. Valproate-associated hepatotoxicity and its biochemical mechanisms. Med Toxicol 1988;3:85.
189. Dreifuss FE et al. Valproic acid hepatic fatalities: a retrospective review. Neurology 1987;37:379.
190. Dreifuss FE et al. Valproic acid hepatic fatalities. II. US experience since 1984. Neurology 1989;39:201.
191. Dreifuss FE. Valproic acid hepatic fatalities: revised table [letter]. Neurology 1989;39:1558.
192. Scheffner E et al. Fatal liver failure in 16 children with valproate therapy. Epilepsia 1988;29:530.
193. Willmore LJ. Clinical manifestations of valproate hepatotoxicity. In: Levy RH, Penry JK, eds. Idiosyncratic Reactions to Valproate: Clinical Risk Patterns and Mechanisms of Toxicity. New York: Raven Press, 1991:3.
194. Willmore LJ et al. Valproate toxicity: risk-screening strategies. J Child Neurol 1991;6:3.
195. Kriel RL et al. Rectal diazepam gel for treatment of acute repetitive seizures. The North American Diastat Study Group. Pediatr Neurol 1999;20:282.
196. Cloyd JC et al. A single-blind, crossover comparison of the pharmacokinetics and cognitive effects of a new diazepam rectal gel with intravenous diazepam. Epilepsia 1998;39:520.
197. Kriel RL et al. Home use of rectal diazepam for cluster and prolonged seizures: efficacy, adverse reactions, quality of life, and cost analysis. Pediatr Neurol 1991;7:13.
198. Sofijanov N et al. Febrile convulsions and later development of epilepsy. Am J Dis Child 1983;137:123.
199. Duchowny M. Febrile seizures. In: Wyllie E, ed. The Treatment of Epilepsy: Principles and Practice, 3rd ed. Philadelphia: Lippincott Williams & Wilkins, 2001:601.
200. Berg AT et al. Predictors of recurrent febrile seizures: a metaanalytic review. J Pediatr 1990;116:329.
201. Freeman JM. Febrile seizures: a consensus of their significance, evaluation, and treatment. Pediatrics 1980;66:1009.
202. Fischbein CA et al. Diazepam to prevent febrile seizures [letter]. N Engl J Med 1993;329:2033.
203. Newton RW. Randomized controlled trials of phenobarbitone and valproate in febrile convulsions. Arch Dis Child 1988;63:1189.
204. Farwell JR et al. Phenobarbital for febrile seizures: effects on intelligence and on seizure recurrence. N Engl J Med 1990;322:364.
205. Holmes GL et al. Panel discussion. Epilepsia 1991;32(Suppl 5):S80.
206. Sulzbacher S et al. Late cognitive effects of early treatment with phenobarbital. Clin Pediatr 1999;38:387.

207. Committee on Drugs. Behavioral and cognitive effects of anticonvulsant therapy. Pediatrics 1985;76:644.

208. Hanzel TE et al. A case of phenobarbital exacerbation of a preexisting maladaptive behavior partially suppressed by chlorpromazine and misinterpreted as chlorpromazine efficacy. Res Dev Disabil 1992;13:381.

209. Rosman NP et al. A controlled trial of diazepam administered during febrile illnesses to prevent recurrence of febrile seizures. N Engl J Med 1993;329:79.

210. Wroblewski BA et al. Carbamazepine–erythromycin interaction: case studies and clinical significance. JAMA 1986;255:1165.

211. Miles MV, Tennison MB. Erythromycin effects on multiple-dose carbamazepine pharmacokinetics. Ther Drug Monit 1989;11:47.

212. Blackburn SC et al. Antiepileptics and blood dyscrasias: a cohort study. Pharmacotherapy 1998;18:1277.

213. Gidal B et al. Valproate-mediated disturbances of hemostasis: relationship to dose and plasma concentration. Neurology 1994;44:1418.

214. Barr RD et al. Valproic acid and immune thrombocytopenia. Arch Dis Childhood 1982;57:681.

215. Dreifuss FE, Langer DH. Hepatic considerations in the use of antiepileptic drugs. Epilepsia 1987;28(Suppl 2):S23.

216. Smythe MA, Umstead GS. Phenytoin hepatotoxicity: a review of the literature. DICP 1989;23:13.

217. Howard PA et al. Phenytoin hypersensitivity syndrome: a case report. DICP 1991;25:929.

218. Pelekanos J et al. Allergic rash due to antiepileptic drugs: clinical features and management. Epilepsia 1991;32:554.

219. Shear NH, Spielberg SP. Anticonvulsant hypersensitivity syndrome: in vitro assessment of risk. J Clin Invest 1988;82:1826.

220. Pirmohamed M et al. Detection of an autoantibody directed against human liver microsomal protein in a patient with carbamazepine hypersensitivity. Br J Clin Pharmacol 1992;33:183.

221. Engel JN et al. Phenytoin hypersensitivity: a case of severe acute rhabdomyolysis. Am J Med 1986;81:928.

222. Reents SB et al. Phenytoin-carbamazepine cross-sensitivity. DICP 1989;23:235.

223. Ettinger AB et al. Use of ethotoin in phenytoin-related hypersensitivity reactions. J Epilepsy 1993;6:29.

224. McAuley JW, Anderson GA. Treatment of epilepsy in women of reproductive age: pharmacokinetic considerations. Clin Pharmacokin 2002;41:559.

225. Dansky LV. The teratogenic effects of epilepsy and anticonvulsant drugs. In: Hopkins A et al, eds. Epilepsy. New York: Demos; 1995:535.

226. Yerby MS et al. Antiepileptics and the development of congenital anomalies. Neurology 1992;42 (Suppl 5):132.

227. Delgado-Escueta AV, Janz D. Consensus guidelines: preconception counseling, management, and care of the pregnant woman with epilepsy. Neurology 1992;42(Suppl 5):149.

228. Mattson RH et al. Use of oral contraceptives by women with epilepsy. JAMA 1986;256:238.

229. Back DJ et al. Evaluation of Committee on Safety of Medicines yellow card reports on oral contraceptive-drug interactions with anticonvulsants and antibiotics. Br J Clin Pharmacol 1988;25:527.

230. Crawford P. Interactions between antiepileptic drugs and hormonal contraception. CNS Drugs 2002;16:263

231. Rosenfeld WE et al. Effect of topiramate on the pharmacokinetics of an oral contraceptive containing norethindrone and ethinyl estradiol in patients with epilepsy. Epilepsia 1997;38:317.

232. Doose DR. Oral contraceptive–AED interactions: no effect of topiramate as monotherapy at clinically effective dosages of 200 mg or less. Epilepsia 2002;43(Suppl 7):205.

233. Stoffel-Wagner B et al. Serum sex hormones are altered in patients with chronic temporal lobe epilepsy receiving anticonvulsant medication. Epilepsia 1998;39:1164.

234. Krauss GL et al. Antiepileptic medication and oral contraceptive interactions: a national survey of neurologists and obstetricians. Neurology 1996;46:1534.

235. Morrell MJ. Catamenial epilepsy and issues of fertility, sexuality, and reproduction. In: Wyllie E, ed. The Treatment of Epilepsy: Principles and Practice, 3rd ed. Philadelphia: Lippincott Williams & Wilkins, 2001:671.

236. Zahn CA et al. Management issues for women with epilepsy: a review of the literature. Neurology 1998;51:949.

237. Jones KL et al. Pattern of malformations in the children of women treated with carbamazepine during pregnancy. N Engl J Med 1989;320:1661.

238. Holmes LB et al. The teratogenicity of anticonvulsant drugs. N Engl J Med 2001;344:1132.

239. Yerby MS, Collins SD. Teratogenicity of antiepileptic drugs. In: Engel J, Pedley TA, eds. Epilepsy: A Comprehensive Textbook. Philadelphia, Lippincott-Raven, 1998:1195.

240. Kaneko S et al. Teratogenicity of antiepileptic drugs: analysis of possible risk factors. Epilepsia 1988;29:459.

241. Perucca E, Crema A. Plasma protein binding of drugs in pregnancy. Clin Pharmacokinet 1982;7:336.

242. Chen SS et al. Serum protein binding and free concentration of phenytoin and phenobarbitone in pregnancy. Br J Clin Pharmacol 1982;13:547.

243. Patel IH, Levy RH. Valproic acid binding to human serum albumin and determination of free fractions in the presence of anticonvulsants and free fatty acids. Epilepsia 1979;20:85.

244. Thorp JA et al. Current concepts and controversies in the use of vitamin K. Drugs 1995;49:376.

245. American Academy of Pediatrics Committee on Drugs. The transfer of drugs and other chemicals into human milk. Pediatrics 1994;93:137.

246. Begg EJ et al. Prospective evaluation of a model for the prediction of milk:plasma drug concentrations from physiochemical characteristics. Br J Clin Pharmacol 1992;33:501.

247. Notarianni LJ et al. An in vitro technique for the rapid determination of drug entry into breast milk. Br J Clin Pharmacol 1995;40:333.

248. Hagg S, Spigset O. Anticonvulsant use during lactation. Drug Saf 2000;22:425.

249. Bar-Oz B et al. Anticonvulsants and breast-feeding: A critical review. Pediatr Drugs 2000;2:113.

250. Dodson WE et al. Treatment of convulsive status epilepticus: recommendations of the Epilepsy Foundation of America's Working Group on Status Epilepticus. JAMA 1993;270:854.

251. Wasterlain CG et al. Pathophysiologic mechanisms of brain damage from status epilepticus. Epilepsia 1993;34(Suppl 1):S37.

252. Lothman E. The biochemical basis and pathophysiology of status epilepticus. Neurology 1990;40(Suppl 2):13.

253. Dodrill CB, Wilensky AJ. Intellectual impairment as an outcome of status epilepticus. Neurology 1990;40.

254. Lowenstein DH, Alldredge BK. Status epilepticus. N Engl J Med 1998;338:970.

255. Ramsay RE et al. Safety and tolerance of rapidly infused Depacon. A randomized trial in subjects with epilepsy. Epilepsy Res 2003;52:189

256. Treiman DM et al. A comparison of four treatments for generalized convulsive status epilepticus. Veterans Affairs Status Epilepticus Cooperative Study Group. N Engl J Med 1998;339:792.

257. Leppik IE et al. Double-blind study of lorazepam and diazepam for status epilepticus. JAMA 1983;249:1452.

258. Rey E et al. Pharmacokinetic optimization of benzodiazepine therapy for status epilepticus. Focus on delivery routes. Clin Pharmacokinet 1999;36:409.

259. Levy RJ, Krall RL. Treatment of status epilepticus with lorazepam. Arch Neurol 1984;41:605.

260. Lacey DJ et al. Lorazepam therapy of status epilepticus in children and adolescents. J Pediatr 1986;108:771.

261. Treiman DM. The role of benzodiazepines in the management of status epilepticus. Neurology 1990;40(Suppl 2):32.

262. Crawford TO et al. Lorazepam in childhood status epilepticus and serial seizures: effectiveness and tachyphylaxis. Neurology 1987;37:190.

263. Armstrong EP et al. Phenytoin and fosphenytoin: a model of cost and clinical outcomes. Pharmacotherapy 1999;19:844.

264. Cloyd JC et al. Concentration-time profile of phenytoin after admixture with small volumes of intravenous fluids. Am J Hosp Pharm 1978;35:45.

265. Salem RB et al. Investigation of the crystallization of phenytoin in normal saline. Am J Hosp Pharm 1980;14:605.

266. DelaCruz FG et al. Efficacy of individualized phenytoin sodium loading doses administered by intravenous infusion. Clin Pharm 1988;7:219.

267. Vozeh S et al. Intravenous phenytoin loading in patients after neurosurgery and in status epilepticus: a population pharmacokinetic study. Clin Pharmacokinet 1988;14:122.

268. Spengler RF et al. Severe soft-tissue injury following intravenous infusion of phenytoin. Patient and drug administration risk factors. Arch Intern Med 1988;148:1329.

269. Yaffe K, Lowenstein DH. Prognostic factors of pentobarbital therapy for refractory generalized status epilepticus. Neurology 1993;43:895.

270. Lal-Koul R et al. Continuous midazolam infusion as treatment of status epilepticus. Arch Dis Child 1997;76:445.

271. Denzel D, Burstein AH. Midazolam in re-fractory status epilepticus. Ann Pharmacother 1996;30:1481.

272. Lowenstein DH, Parent DM. Treatment of refractory generalized status epilepticus with continuous infusion of midazolam. Neurology 1994;44:1837.

273. Hovinga CA et al. Use of intravenous valproate in three pediatric patients with nonconvulsive or convulsive status epilepticus. Ann Pharmacother 1999;33:579.

CHAPTER 55

Cerebrovascular Disorders

Timothy E. Welty

Definitions

Cerebrovascular Disease

Cerebrovascular disease is a broad term encompassing many disorders of the blood vessels of the central nervous system (CNS). These disorders result from either inadequate blood flow to the brain (i.e., cerebral ischemia) with subsequent infarction of the involved portion of the CNS or from hemorrhages into the parenchyma or subarachnoid space of the CNS and subsequent neurologic dysfunction.

Transient Ischemic Attack

A transient ischemic attack (TIA) describes the clinical condition in which a patient experiences a temporary focal neurologic deficit such as slurred speech, aphasia, weakness or paralysis of a limb, or blindness. These symptoms appear rapidly and are temporary, lasting <24 hours (usually only 2 to 15 minutes). The exact clinical presentation depends on the portion of the cerebrovascular tree (e.g., carotid artery, vertebrobasilar artery, or both) affected by diminished or absent blood flow. TIAs frequently result from small clots breaking away from larger, distant blood clots. These emboli are then dissolved by the fibrinolytic system, allowing re-establishment of blood flow and return of neurologic function.

Cerebral Infarction

A cerebral infarction is a permanent neurologic disorder characterized by symptoms similar to a TIA. The patient with a cerebral infarction presents with neurological deficits caused by the death of neurons in a focal area of the brain. The two primary causes of infarction and persistent ischemia are atherosclerosis of cerebral blood vessel or an embolus to cerebral arteries from a distant clot. Cerebral infarctions can present in three forms: stable, improving, or progressing. A *stable infarction* describes the condition when the neurologic deficit is permanent, will not improve, and will not deteriorate. An *improving infarction* is marked by return of previously lost neurologic function over several days or weeks. Finally, a *progressing infarction* is one in which the patient's neurologic status continues to deteriorate following the initial onset of focal deficits.

Cerebral Hemorrhage

Cerebral hemorrhage is a cerebrovascular disorder that involves escape of blood from blood vessels into the brain and its surrounding structures. The leakage of blood causes clinical symptoms similar to those associated with a TIA or infarction. The neurologic damage that is associated with TIAs or cerebral infarction results from the lack of blood flow to a given portion of the brain. In a cerebral hemorrhage, the initial neurologic deficits are due to the direct irritant effects of blood that is in direct contact with brain tissue. Primary causes of a cerebral hemorrhage include cerebral artery aneurysm, arteriovenous malformation, hypertensive hemorrhage, and trauma.

The terms *apoplexy, stroke,* and *paralytic stroke* are commonly used by lay persons to describe a sudden neurologic affliction that usually is related to the cerebral blood supply. The term *stroke* is used to describe a cerebral vascular event when neurologic deficits persist for at least 24 hours.

Epidemiology

Annually, approximately 700,000 individuals in the United States experience a cerebral infarction, and approximately 150,000 will die as a result of the neurologic destruction.[1] Of the 700,000 strokes annually, 500,000 are first-ever strokes and 200,000 are recurrent events. Cerebrovascular disease is the third most common cause of death in adults and is one of the more commonly encountered causes of neurologic dysfunction.[2] Nevertheless, this represents a dramatic decrease in the mortality rate of ischemic stroke from 88.8 per 100,000 population in 1950 to 60.8 per 100,000 in 2000.[1,3] The incidence of first-ever stroke is significantly greater among blacks (323 per 100,000 population per year for men and 260 per 100,000 for women) compared with whites (167 per 100,000 population per year for men and 138 per 100,000 for women).[1] There are also important racial differences in mortality rates for ischemic stroke. The mortality rate for black men is 87.1 per 100,000 and 78.1 per 100,000 for black women, whereas the mortality rate for white men is 58.6 per 100,000 and 57.8 per 100,000 for white women. In 1999 the mortality rate was 40.0 per 100,000, 39.7 per 100,000, and 52.4 per 100,000 for Hispanics, American Indians/Alaska Natives, and Asian/Pacific Islanders, respectively.[1] The precise reasons for these differences are unclear, but genetic, geographic, dietary, and cultural factors have been speculated.[3] In addition, the incidence of risk factors for stroke such as hypertension, diabetes, and hypercholesterolemia differ between racial groups.[1,2]

Atherothrombotic disease of the cerebrovasculature is responsible for approximately 61% of cerebral ischemic events and infarctions. Disease of penetrating arteries that are responsible for oxygenation and nutrition of the CNS account for another 20%; thromboembolic causes (e.g., atrial fibrillation) account for 24%; and the remaining 5% are due to unusual causes such as infection or inflammation of arteries.[1]

There is a strong relationship between the occurrence of TIA and an increased risk for subsequent cerebral infarction; however, the precise incidence of this risk is unclear. Studies of TIAs associated with carotid artery stenosis have shown that 4% to 8% of patients each year will experience a subsequent cerebral infarction.[4]

Definite risk factors for cerebral infarction are listed in Table 55-1. A key element in the prevention of stroke is the elimination or control of risk factors.[5–8] The control of risk factors is of primary importance in managing a patient with a TIA or cerebral infarction.

Hemorrhage into the brain accounts for 12% of all strokes in North America.[1] Hypertensive hemorrhage is the most common cause of intracerebral hemorrhages (ICHs), with 46% of ICHs resulting from hypertension.[9] Subarachnoid hemorrhage occurs in approximately 26,000 individuals annually and the mortality rate is approximately 50%. Patients with subarachnoid hemorrhage are usually 20 to 70 years old, and 20% to 50% of the survivors suffer permanent neurologic deficits. Most neurologic deficits are not caused by the original hemorrhage, but rather by complications of rebleeding, hydrocephalus, or problems from delayed cerebral ischemia. A less common cause of ICH is an arteriovenous malformation (AVM), which is a clump of arteries and veins that are intertwined, resulting in weakened blood vessel walls. AVMs usually result from a congenital defect or trauma.

Pathophysiology
Thrombotic Events

Usually, the neurologic sequelae of cerebral ischemia or infarction directly result from an embolic or thrombotic source. A clot may form in the heart, along the wall of a major blood vessel (e.g., aorta, carotid, or basilar artery), or in small arteries penetrating deep into the brain. If the clot is located near the infarction, it is considered to be a thrombus; however, when the clot has migrated to the brain from a distant source, it is considered an embolus. Either can diminish or block blood flow to the affected area of the brain.

Table 55-1   Definite Risk Factors for Stroke

Modifiable	Potentially Modifiable	Nonmodifiable
Hypertension	Diabetes mellitus	Genetics
Cigarette smoking	Hyperhomocysteinemia	Age
Hyperlipidemia (total cholesterol > 240 mg/dL [6.21 mmol/L])	Left ventricular hypertrophy	Males
	Obesity	Race
Transient ischemic attack	Coagulopathies/hypercoagulable states (e.g., protein C deficiency, protein S deficiency, antithrombin III deficiency)	Ethnicity
Asymptomatic carotid stenosis		
Dilated cardiomyopathy	Migraine headaches	
Alcohol consumption (>5 drinks/day)	Antiphospholipid antibodies	
Drug abuse (e.g., cocaine, amphetamines)		
Physical inactivity		
Heart disease		
Atrial fibrillation		
Infective endocarditis		
Mitral stenosis and other valvular disease		
Recent myocardial infarction		

Clots, both embolic and thrombotic, affecting the cerebral vasculature are typically arterial in origin. These are fibrin clots, also known as *white thrombi,* which evolve from a complex series of events (Fig. 55-1). Tissue injury or turbulent blood flow cause the release of adenosine diphosphate (ADP), thrombin, epinephrine, and a variety of other substances to stimulate platelet migration. Exposure of collagen and other subendothelial surfaces of the blood vessel wall cause adhesion of platelets to the damaged vessel wall. Additional granular release of ADP causes increased adhesion of platelets and the formation of platelet aggregates.

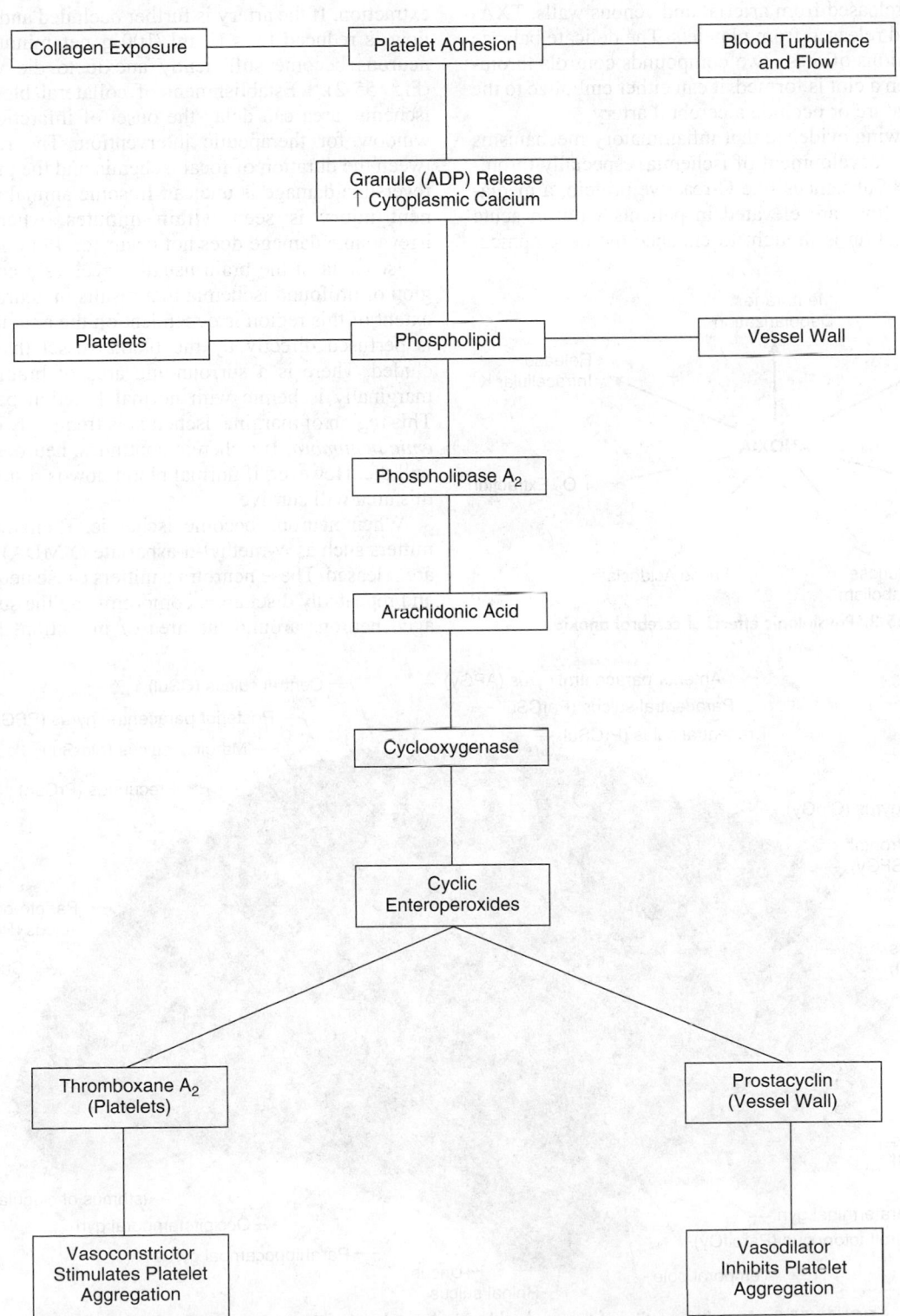

FIGURE 55-1. Arachidonic acid cascade and platelet plug formation.

As platelets adhere and aggregate, phospholipase is activated, leading to the splitting of arachidonic acid from platelet membrane phospholipid. This begins a cascade of events ultimately ending in the formation of thromboxane A_2 (TXA_2) and prostacyclin. Prostacyclin inhibits platelet aggregation and is a powerful vasodilator, whereas TXA_2 is a potent inducer of platelet release and aggregation. Prostacyclin is formed in and released from arterial and venous walls. TXA_2 is formed in and released from platelets. The delicate balance between the actions of these two compounds controls thrombogenesis. When a clot is formed, it can either embolize to the cerebral vasculature or occlude a cerebral artery.

There is growing evidence that inflammatory mechanisms contribute to the development of ischemia, especially thrombotic lesions.[8,10] Substances like C-reactive protein, a mediator of inflammation, are elevated in patients with an acute stroke. Inflammation is thought to enhance the development of thrombotic lesions and result in sudden, intermittent occlusion of blood vessels.

Cerebral blood flow in the normal adult brain is 30 to 70 mL/100 g per minute. When a thrombotic or embolic clot partially occludes a cerebral artery, causing blood flow to be <20 mL/100 g per minute, various compensatory mechanisms are activated. These include vasodilation and increased oxygen extraction. If the artery is further occluded and cerebral blood flow is reduced to <12 mL/100 g per minute, the affected neurons become sufficiently anoxic to die within minutes (Fig. 55-2).[11] Establishment of collateral blood flow to the ischemic area can delay the onset of infarction, providing a window for therapeutic intervention. The relationship between the duration of focal ischemia and the production of irreversible damage is unclear. In some animal models permanent injury is seen within minutes, whereas in others irreversible damage does not occur for 4 to 6 hours.

Ischemia in the brain usually involves a core or focal region of profound ischemia that results in neuronal death. The extent of this region is dependent on the amount of brain that is perfused directly by the blood vessel that becomes occluded. There is a surrounding area of brain that becomes marginally ischemic with normal function being disrupted. This region of marginal ischemia is frequently called the *ischemic penumbra*. If ischemia continues, neurons in this region will die. However, if normal blood flow is restored neurons in this area will survive.

When neurons become ischemic, excitatory neurotransmitters such as *N*-methyl-d-aspartate (NMDA) and glutamate are released. These neurotransmitters cause neurons to rapidly and repeatedly discharge, compromising the survival of damaged neurons around the area of infarction. Increased neu-

FIGURE 55-2. Physiologic effects of cerebral anoxia.

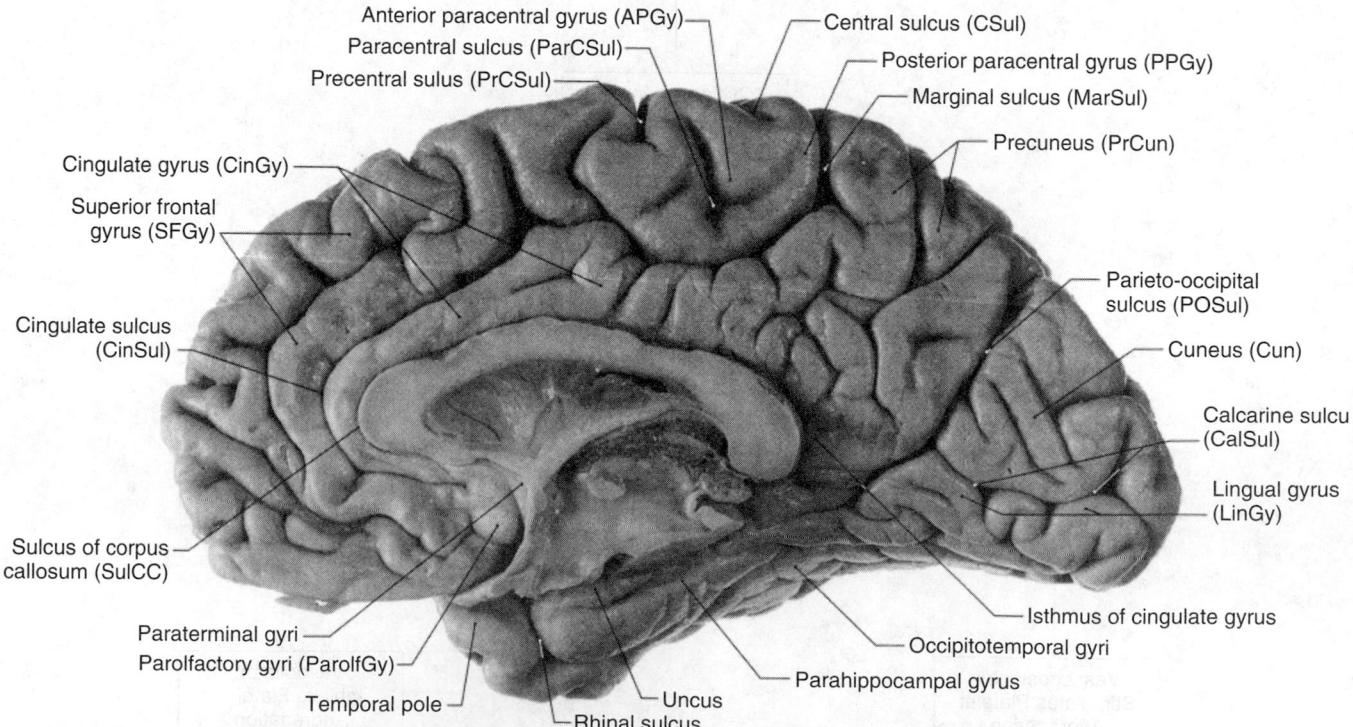

FIGURE 55-3. A sagittal section of the cerebral hemisphere showing the major anatomic landmarks.
(Adapted with permission from Haines DE. Neuroanatomy: An Atlas of Structures, Sections, and Systems. 5th Ed. Baltimore: Lippincott Williams & Wilkins, 2000.)

ronal activity results in extreme metabolic demands, disrupts neuronal homeostasis, and synergistically increases the effects of hypoxia. Especially vulnerable to ischemic effects are neurons in the middle layers of the cerebral cortex; portions of the hippocampus (CA-1 and subiculum regions), a structure running parallel to the parahippocampal gyrus; and Purkinje cells in the cerebellum (Fig. 55-3).[12]

Ischemia leads to rapid intracellular influx of calcium. Both voltage-dependent and chemical-dependent calcium channels are unable to act as a gate to prevent calcium influx. Intracellular stores of calcium ions also are disrupted, causing release of calcium into the cytoplasm. Increased concentration of calcium ions enhances phospholipase and protease activity and increased reactive metabolites, such as $\cdot O_2$, $\cdot OH$, and nitric oxide (Fig. 55-4). This eventually causes neuronal death.[11,12] In addition, lipolysis of cell membranes occurs in the presence of an accumulation of neurotoxic free radicals.

Immediate therapeutic intervention is needed to limit and prevent permanent neurologic damage from these rapidly occurring events.

Intracerebral Hemorrhage

Cerebral aneurysms, AVMs, hypertension, and adverse drug reactions are the primary causes of ICH. One type of ICH, subarachnoid hemorrhage, can result from weakened blood vessel walls (i.e., aneurysms) caused by congenital defects, trauma, infection, and hypertension. Blood slowly leaks from the involved vessel or the aneurysm may rupture suddenly. In this type of hemorrhage, blood typically is released into the subarachnoid space and, depending on the severity of the hemorrhage, into the ventricles of the brain. Direct contact of blood with brain tissue irritates and damages brain cells. Rebleeding, hydrocephalus, and delayed cerebral ischemia frequently occur after the aneurysm first ruptures, further worsening the patient's neurologic function.

AVMs due to congenital causes or traumatic injury, and uncontrolled hypertension also can cause devastating intracerebral bleeding. In these patients, blood is usually released directly into the brain parenchyma. In more severe cases blood is released into the surrounding brain structures. ICHs can be the result of adverse reactions to drugs, such as anticoagulants, thrombolytics, and sympathomimetics.

General Treatment Principles

Rapid recognition of stroke symptoms and immediate initiation of treatment are essential to the management of ischemic or hemorrhagic stroke. Appropriate pharmacotherapy of cerebrovascular disease requires a precise diagnosis. It is vital to differentiate between an ischemic stroke and a hemorrhagic stroke, because an inaccurate diagnosis can lead to the use of drugs that may cause severe morbidity or mortality. Interventions to prevent and treat ischemic strokes are directed at reducing risk factors, eliminating or modifying the underlying pathologic process, reducing secondary brain damage, and rehabilitation.

Treatments for ischemic stroke and hemorrhagic stroke vary. In ischemic stroke, treatment involves acute management, chronic management of the effects of the stroke, and prevention of further events. In acute management, the only effective treatment is the use of tPA in combination with supportive measures. Chronic management of the effects of a stroke focus primarily on treating depression, spasticity, possible neurogenic bowel or bladder, and self-care issues. Antiplatelet agents, especially, aspirin, clopidogrel, and aspirin/dipyridamole combination, form the cornerstone of prevention.

In hemorrhagic stroke, the emphasis of treatment is on supportive therapy to maximize neurological function, prevention of further hemorrhagic events, and management of complications. This involves wise management of blood pressure, pulmonary function, fluid and electrolytes, and elimination of drugs that inhibit coagulation. There are no proven direct therapies for hemorrhagic events.

TRANSIENT ISCHEMIC ATTACKS
Clinical Presentation

1. J.S., a 55-year-old, 5'6" tall, 85-kg man, experienced a rapidly progressive paralysis of his right arm and slurred speech yesterday. These symptoms lasted for 15 to 20 minutes and resolved rapidly. His neurologic examination is entirely normal, and he denies any feeling of weakness. He smokes 2 packs of cigarettes daily and drinks 3 to 6 cans of beer each evening. His physical examination is entirely normal except for a left carotid

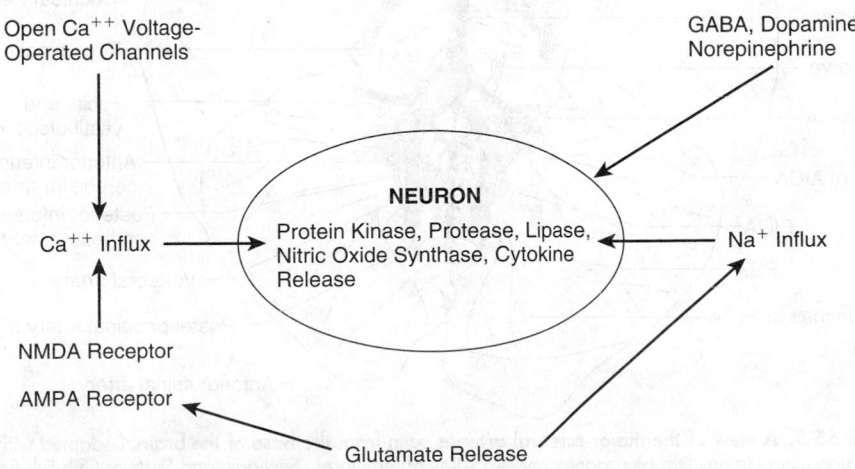

FIGURE 55-4. The effects of membrane depolarization.

bruit, which was first noted 2 years ago. His blood pressure (BP) is 165/100 mm Hg, and he has a long history of hypertension. His hemoglobin (Hgb) is 16.5 g/dL (normal, 12 to 16 g/dL), his hematocrit (Hct) is 51% (normal, 42% to 52%), and his total serum cholesterol concentration is 275 mg/dL (normal, <200 mg/dL). A Doppler examination of his carotid arteries shows a 90% stenosis on the left and a 40% stenosis on the right. What subjective and objective data in J.S.'s history are consistent with a TIA?

[SI units: Hgb, 165 g/L (normal, 120 to 160); Hct, 0.51 (normal, 0.42 to 0.52); cholesterol, 7.11 mmol/L]

A TIA can present with any type of neurologic symptoms. The presentation is determined entirely by the location of the involved arteries and the portion of the brain that they supply (Fig. 55-5). For example, if the affected artery provides circulation to the motor area in the left hemisphere of the brain, the expected result would be impairment of muscle strength on the right side of the body. Symptoms of TIA may include paresis or paralysis of one or more limbs, paraesthesia, slurred speech, blurred vision, blindness (amaurosis fugax), facial droop, dizziness, or difficulty in swallowing (Table 55-2). Patients rarely lose consciousness. Symptoms always resolve within 24 hours, and there is no residual focal neurologic deficit. Most often, the neurologic deficits last for only 2 to 15 minutes, and neurologic function rapidly returns to normal.

J.S.'s rapid onset of right arm paralysis and slurred speech suggest involvement of the left cerebral cortex. The 15- to 20-minute duration of these symptoms and the entirely normal neurologic examination on the day after these symptoms also are compatible with a TIA. The left carotid bruit heard on physical examination suggests a left-sided process.

Right-sided neurologic deficits generally suggest a left-sided cerebral lesion because motor and sensory neuronal tracts cross over in the midbrain. Thus, the left hemisphere of the cerebral cortex controls the right or contralateral side of the body. CNS lesions occurring below the midbrain will cause ipsilateral neurologic deficits. Therefore, J.S.'s right arm paralysis suggests a left-sided cerebral lesion above the midbrain.

Risk Factors

2. How can risk factors for J.S. be limited to prevent another TIA?

J.S. has several modifiable and nonmodifiable risk factors for TIA and ischemic stroke (see Table 55-1): a smoking history, excessive alcohol consumption, obesity, older age, male gender, hypercholesterolemia, and hypertension. He should be instructed and counseled to change his lifestyle by discontinuing his smoking, limiting his alcohol consumption, reduc-

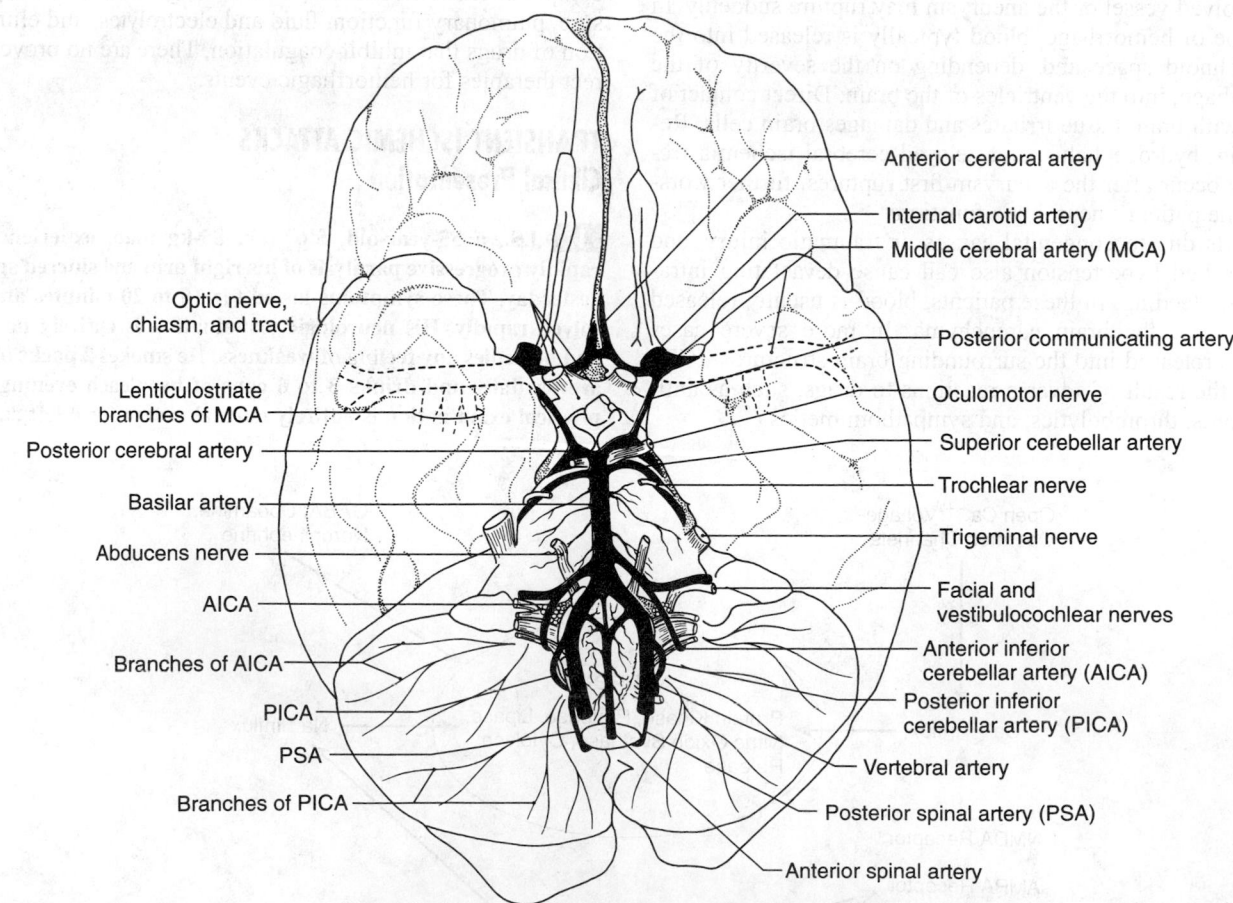

Anterior cerebral artery
Internal carotid artery
Middle cerebral artery (MCA)
Posterior communicating artery
Oculomotor nerve
Superior cerebellar artery
Trochlear nerve
Trigeminal nerve
Facial and vestibulocochlear nerves
Anterior inferior cerebellar artery (AICA)
Posterior inferior cerebellar artery (PICA)
Vertebral artery
Posterior spinal artery (PSA)
Anterior spinal artery

Optic nerve, chiasm, and tract
Lenticulostriate branches of MCA
Posterior cerebral artery
Basilar artery
Abducens nerve
AICA
Branches of AICA
PICA
PSA
Branches of PICA

FIGURE 55-5. A view of the major cerebral arteries seen from the base of the brain. (Adapted with permission from Haines DE. Neuroanatomy: An Atlas of Structures, Sections, and Systems. 5th Ed. Baltimore: Lippincott Williams & Wilkins, 2000.)

Table 55-2 Symptoms Associated With Transient Ischemic Attacks

Symptom	Right Carotid	Left Carotid	Vertebrobasilar
Aphasia	Possible	Yes	No
Ataxia	No	No	Yes
Blindness	Right	Left	Right or left side
Clumsiness	Yes	Yes	Yes
Diplopia	No	No	Yes
Dysarthria	Yes	Yes	No
Paralysis	Left side	Right side	Any limb
Paresthesia	Left side	Right side	Any limb
Vertigo	No	No	Yes

ing his weight, and increasing his physical exercise. Hypoxia and hypercarbia induced by cigarette smoking may have caused his increased hematocrit, and his high serum cholesterol and obesity suggest the need for dietary changes. A smoking cessation program, substance abuse program, and consultation with a dietitian should be useful in reducing his risk factors. Aggressive reduction of risk factors is the primary method to reduce the recurrence risk of a TIA.[13]

Because approximately 70% of strokes result from uncontrolled hypertension, blood pressure control is vital for stroke prevention; an increased risk for stroke is associated with both systolic and diastolic hypertension.[14,15] The goals of antihypertensive therapy should be at least a systolic blood pressure <140 mm Hg and a diastolic pressure <90 mm Hg.[16,17] Since the 1960s, the control of hypertension has been shown repeatedly to decrease the risk of stroke and has proved to be of significant pharmacoeconomic benefit.[18]

Thus, continued management of J.S.'s hypertension is imperative. His blood pressure should be reduced gradually. A sudden or dramatic decrease in blood pressure could compromise cerebral perfusion and result in a decreased level of consciousness or infarction. The degree of his carotid artery stenosis will contribute to the problem of decreased perfusion if the blood pressure is decreased rapidly. A mild degree of hypertension may be temporarily acceptable because of the extent of carotid stenosis. Initiation of hydrochlorothiazide at a dosage of 12.5 mg/day or an angiotensin-converting enzyme inhibitor should be considered.

Reduction of serum cholesterol is important for J.S. Several placebo controlled studies have shown that HMG-CoA reductase inhibitors significantly reduce the risk of stroke and TIA.[19–23] For example, individuals with coronary disease who received pravastatin had a 20% to 40% reduction in the risk of stroke. A study of atorvastatin showed similar risk reductions.[24] These findings are reinforced by two meta-analyses that reported a 25% to 32% reduction in the risk of stroke.[25,26] These data differ from previous studies of other cholesterol-lowering therapies. A meta-analysis of other lipid lowering treatments failed to demonstrate benefit in the reduction of risk for stroke.[27] Outcomes from studies of other lipid-lowering agents suggest that other factors are involved in the effectiveness of HMG-CoA reductase inhibitors in reducing the risk of stroke. It is known that HMG-CoA reductase inhibitors have anti-inflammatory activity that may influence the development of atherosclerotic plaques and cerebral ischemic processes.[28–30] Based on these data, J.S. should receive a

HMG-CoA reductase inhibitor. Pravastatin 40 mg daily may be the preferred agent, because there are extensive data supporting its use. Typically, the treatment goals in patients with known vascular disease are total cholesterol <200 mg/dL (5.18 mmol/L), HDL >40 mg/dL (1.04 mmol/L), and LDL <130 mg/dL (3.37 mmol/L). One recent meta-analysis suggested a goal of total cholesterol <232 mg/dL (6.90 mmol/L).

Treatment
Goals of Therapy

3. What are the initial and long-term goals in treating J.S.?

The immediate goal is to re-establish adequate blood flow in his diseased cerebral vessels. Longer-range objectives are to prevent reocclusion, decrease the risk of future symptomatic TIAs, and ultimately, prevent a cerebral infarction.[31]

Surgical Interventions

4. What nonpharmacologic interventions might be available to prevent another TIA? What would be the best choice for J.S.?

Various surgical interventions are available to prevent TIA or infarction. These are designed to either remove the source for an embolism or improve circulation to ischemic areas of the brain.

CAROTID ENDARTERECTOMY

Carotid endarterectomy (CEA) is a common surgical procedure for correcting atheromatous lesions responsible for causing a TIA. In this procedure, the carotid artery is surgically exposed, and the atheromatous plaque is excised. Balloon angioplasty and placement of stents also can improve blood flow through a stenosed artery. During this procedure, a catheter with a small, deflated balloon is placed in the stenosed artery and the atherosclerotic lesion is pressed into the arterial wall when the balloon is inflated. A small, plastic tube stent is placed in the artery to prevent the vessel from collapsing at the site of the lesion.

CEA is most effective for patients with an ulcerated lesion or stenotic clot that occludes >70% of blood flow in the carotid artery and who experience symptoms of a TIA or stroke. Use of CEA in these patients may result in a 60% reduction in stroke risk over the subsequent 2 years.[32] Of six to eight patients treated with CEA, one stroke will be prevented within 2 years.[33] The use of CEA in other patient groups must be balanced with the risk of the procedure and life expectancy.[34] CEA may prove beneficial in patients with 60% stenosis of the carotid artery and no symptoms, those with a life expectancy of at least 5 years, and those with a less than <3% risk from CEA surgery. In other patients, the benefits of CEA are questionable. Generally, CEA is not indicated in patients who have permanent neurologic deficits or total occlusion of the carotid artery.[34]

J.S. should undergo CEA for his left carotid lesion as soon as possible. The lesion on the right should be monitored closely for continued progression. If further TIAs occur or the right carotid stenosis is >60%, he should have a CEA performed on the right carotid artery.

Drug Therapy
ASPIRIN

5. What role does aspirin have in preventing the occurrence of ischemic stroke in patients who have experienced a TIA?

Because platelets play a key role in the formation of atheromatous clots (see Fig. 55-1), various antiplatelet drugs, such as aspirin, sulfinpyrazone, dipyridamole, ticlopidine, and clopidogrel have been tried to prevent ischemic strokes. These agents generally work by either preventing the formation of TXA_2 or increasing the concentration of prostacyclin. These actions seek to re-establish the proper balance between these two substances, thus preventing the adhesion and aggregation of platelets (Table 55-3).

Because of its wide availability and well-understood actions on platelet function, aspirin has been the most widely tested agent for use in preventing TIA and ischemic stroke. Aspirin primarily acts by irreversibly inactivating platelet cyclooxygenase. Inactivation of cyclooxygenase decreases platelet aggregation, prevents release of vasoactive substances, and prolongs the bleeding time. These changes are due to suppression of TXA_2 synthesis by cyclooxygenase. Because binding of cyclooxygenase by the acetyl component of acetylsalicylic acid ([ASA] aspirin) is irreversible and the platelet cannot synthesize new protein, platelet function is altered for the duration of the platelet's life, usually 5 to 7 days. Aspirin's ability to prevent clot formation and subsequent embolic or thrombotic events also can be attributed to an inhibition of TXA_2 vasoconstriction, activation of fibrinolysis, inhibition of synthesis of vitamin K–dependent clotting factors, and inhibition of lipoxygenase pathways.

In addition to its action on platelet cyclooxygenase, high concentrations of aspirin also inhibit prostacyclin synthesis in the walls of blood vessels. Because prostacyclin inhibits platelet aggregation, depletion of prostacyclin could result in an undesirable increase in aggregation of platelets. However, depletion of prostacyclin is not prolonged because the vascular endothelium is able to synthesize new enzymes. Higher dosages of aspirin (1.3 g/day) also may decrease vascular plasminogen activator, thereby enhancing thrombus formation.[35] Therefore, aspirin should be dosed carefully.

At least 15 randomized trials, with 7 being placebo-controlled, have studied aspirin alone or in combination with other antiplatelet drugs in the prevention of vascular events.[36–41] Patients were enrolled in these studies for as long as 5 years after experiencing a vascular event (i.e., TIA, stroke, unstable angina, or myocardial infarction). Follow-up periods lasted from 1 to 6 years. The incidence of ischemic stroke or TIA ranged from 7% to 23%: the aspirin-treated patients experienced an average 22% decrease in relative risk of a stroke compared with those receiving placebo. Of these 15 trials, only 4 reported no statistically significant benefit with aspirin, and these 4 studies involved small numbers of patients.

In 10 trials that considered only TIA or stroke patients, there was a 24% relative risk reduction in the incidence of nonfatal stroke associated with the use of aspirin. A statistically significant benefit from aspirin was demonstrated in all but two of these studies. When considered in total, it is conclusive that aspirin reduces the risk of stroke and death for patients who have experienced a previous TIA or stroke. Although this fact has been firmly established, questions about the optimal dose, gender differences, and its efficacy relative to clopidogrel and the combination of aspirin with dipyridamole have been debated.

In initial studies of aspirin in stroke prevention, the positive effects were seen primarily in men. However, the European Stroke Prevention Study and a French study included an equal balance of men and women.[36,42] In both studies, the risk reduction rate was equal for men and women, indicating that the benefit of aspirin in stroke prevention extends to both sexes.

Aspirin also has been used for prevention of restenosis following CEA. Over the first year after CEA, 25% of patients will redevelop a stenotic lesion, with more than half of these causing a >50% reduction in carotid blood flow.[43] Stent placement is useful in preventing restenosis. Initial studies indicated that combination therapy with aspirin 325 mg/day and dipyridamole 75 mg three times a day would decrease the rate of restenosis. However, a subsequent randomized, placebo-controlled study using this regimen in post-CEA patients did not substantiate the earlier findings.[44] A combination of clopi-

Table 55-3	Drugs for Preventing Transient Ischemic Attacks and Ischemic Stroke		
Drug	*Action*	*Dose*	*Adverse Effects*
Aspirin	Antiplatelet	50–1,300 mg/day	Diarrhea, gastric ulcer, GI upset
Dipyridamole	Antiplatelet (use in combination with aspirin)	200 mg sustained release twice daily	GI upset
Ticlopidine	Antiplatelet	500 mg/day	Diarrhea, neutropenia, rash
Clopidogrel	Antiplatelet	75 mg/day	Thrombocytopenia, neutropenia
Warfarin	Anticoagulant	Titrate to INR 2–3	Bleeding, bruising, petechiae

GI, gastrointestinal; INR, international normalized ratio.

dogrel with aspirin has been shown to reduce postoperative ischemic events.[45] Stents impregnated with anticoagulants are being evaluated.

6. If J.S. had been taking aspirin regularly before this event, would he have been at a lower risk for developing a TIA or stroke?

The data for primary prevention (i.e., prophylactic treatment in previously asymptomatic individuals) are controversial. In a study of 22,071 male physicians who took 325 mg of aspirin or placebo every other day for 5 years, there was not a reduced incidence of stroke.[46] This group of individuals who had no previous history of cerebrovascular disease experienced 217 strokes, 119 in the aspirin group and 98 in the placebo group. In addition, there was an increased risk of cerebrovascular events due to hemorrhage in the aspirin group.

Additional studies supporting the use of aspirin in previously asymptomatic patients are lacking. A recent study considered the role of aspirin for primary stroke prevention in women.[41] Women who took one to six aspirin per week had a slightly reduced risk of stroke and a lower risk of large-artery occlusive disease (relative risk, 59%; 95% confidence interval, 0.29 to 0.85, $P = 0.01$). An increased risk of stroke was seen in women who took >7 aspirin weekly and an excess risk of subarachnoid hemorrhage was seen for those taking >15 aspirin a week. Chen and colleagues reported a meta-analysis of 40,000 patients randomly assigned to aspirin and found a reduction from 47% to 45.8% in death and disability due to stroke.[47] Using aspirin for the primary prevention of stroke remains controversial and decisions regarding this indication are at the discretion of the clinician.

7. What dosage of aspirin should be used for J.S.?

Dosages of aspirin used in clinical trials have ranged from 30 to 1,500 mg/day. In a meta-analysis of placebo-controlled studies comparing 900 to 1,500 mg/day of aspirin with similar studies of 300 to 325 mg/day, there was a 23% reduction in the risk of cerebrovascular events for patients receiving 900 to 1,500 mg/day and a 24% reduction in risk for patients receiving 300 to 325 mg/day.[38] More direct studies of aspirin dosing have been attempted and have produced conflicting results. A Dutch trial in 3,131 patients showed a 14.7% frequency of nonfatal stroke or nonfatal myocardial infarction in patients receiving 30 mg of aspirin a day and a 15.2% frequency in patients receiving 283 mg of aspirin a day, a nonsignificant difference between these two doses.[48] The Swedish Aspirin Low-Dose Trial (SALT) showed an 18% reduction in stroke in patients taking 75 mg of aspirin daily compared with placebo.[49] Helgason and colleagues compared the effects of 325, 650, 975, and 1,300 mg of aspirin a day in stroke patients.[50] Platelet aggregation studies were performed to determine the effects of aspirin. Complete suppression of aggregation at a daily dose of 325 mg was achieved in 85 of 107 patients. An additional five patients responded at 650 mg/day, and only one more responded at 975 mg/day. There was no further response at 1,300 mg.

A meta-analysis of all published trials of antiplatelet agents did show that aspirin doses of 75 to 325 mg/day were effective in preventing stroke.[51] These findings are corroborated by another meta-analysis showing that aspirin of 50 to 1,500 mg/day produced similar risk reductions of 15%.[52]

The recommended dose for aspirin is 50 to 975 mg/day. The goal is to use the lowest effective aspirin dosage thereby limiting the risk of gastrointestinal (GI) adverse effects. J.S. should start taking aspirin at a dosage of 50 to 75 mg/day. In the United States, a dose of 81 mg enteric-coated aspirin is usually started.

DIPYRIDAMOLE

8. Should dipyridamole be used alone or in combination with aspirin for J.S.?

Two pharmacologic actions of dipyridamole prompted investigations into its use in preventing TIAs and ischemic stroke. Dipyridamole weakly inhibits platelet aggregation and platelet phosphodiesterase. In addition, increased platelet survival has been noted after administration of dipyridamole in patients and animals suffering from platelet consumptive disorders. Dipyridamole also has potential vasodilating properties through its inhibition of adenosine uptake in vascular smooth muscle.

The Second European Stroke Prevention Study enrolled patients who had experienced a previous stroke or TIA and found that aspirin combined with dipyridamole was more effective than placebo, dipyridamole alone, and aspirin alone.[53] A sustained-release formulation of dipyridamole was used for this study. A 37% relative-risk reduction was found for the combination treatment, and a 23% relative risk reduction was found for aspirin alone. The dipyridamole dose for this study was 200 mg twice daily, and the aspirin dose was 25 mg twice daily. Absolute risk reduction was approximately 1.5% annually. Headache occurred more frequently in patients receiving dipyridamole alone or in combination with aspirin. Bleeding complications were less frequent in patients receiving dipyridamole compared with aspirin alone. As a result of these findings, a combination product of aspirin and dipyridamole is available. The combination of sustained-release dipyridamole and aspirin is an acceptable alternative for secondary prevention of stroke when initial secondary prevention has failed.

TICLOPIDINE

9. What are the risks and benefits of using ticlopidine instead of aspirin in J.S.?

Ticlopidine (Ticlid) is an antiplatelet agent approved only for the prevention of TIA and stroke for patients with a prior cerebral thrombotic event. By inhibiting ADP-induced platelet aggregation, its activity differs from aspirin.

A randomized, double-blind, placebo-controlled, multicenter trial, the Canadian American Ticlopidine Study (CATS), shows that ticlopidine significantly reduces the risk of stroke.[54] A risk reduction of 30.2% for all vascular events and a 33.5% reduction for stroke was observed. At all evaluation points, the number of vascular events was significantly less in the ticlopidine group for men and women.

The Ticlopidine Aspirin Stroke Study Group (TASS), a triple-blind (patients, physicians, and study sponsor were unaware of the randomization), multicenter study, evaluated 3,069 patients who received either 500 mg/day of ticlopidine or 1,300 mg/day of aspirin.[55] Stroke occurred in 172 patients taking ticlopidine and in 212 patients taking aspirin. Ticlopidine reduced the risk of stroke by 21% and the risk of all events by 12% compared with aspirin.

One subgroup analysis from the TASS yielded interesting findings regarding the efficacy of ticlopidine in non-white patients.[56] Over 1 year, 5.5% of non-white patients who received ticlopidine suffered a nonfatal stroke or death from any cause, compared with 10.6% of 291 non-white, aspirin-treated patients. This represents a 48.1% risk reduction associated with ticlopidine relative to aspirin in non-white patients. Another important finding in this subgroup analysis is that none of the neutropenia events occurred in non-white patients. However, a randomized study of aspirin and ticlopidine in black patients failed to substantiate this finding.[57]

Ticlopidine is associated with hematologic disturbances. Neutropenia developed in 1 to 2% of patients on ticlopidine in both the CATS and TASS studies. Severe neutropenia (absolute neutrophil count [ANC] <450/mm^3) usually appears in the first 3 months of therapy and is reversible when the drug is discontinued. One episode of neutropenia-associated infection was reported in the CATS study. In the TASS group, mild to moderate neutropenia (ANC, 450 to 1,200/mm^3) was reported, but ticlopidine was not discontinued in these patients. Because of the rather high potential for this adverse reaction, a complete blood count should be performed at baseline and every 2 weeks for the first 3 months of therapy. Additional data have shown that severe bone marrow depression is fatal in 16% of patients who develop this complication.[58] Thrombotic thrombocytopenia purpura has also been associated with ticlopidine and proved fatal in 33% of 60 patients.[59]

Ticlopidine is more effective in the secondary prevention of stroke and less likely to cause GI bleeding when compared with aspirin. Hematologic complications and the marked increased cost associated with ticlopidine (both for the drug itself and for laboratory monitoring) limit its use. Ticlopidine should be used only after a patient's condition has failed to respond to aspirin, aspirin combined with dipyridamole, and clopidogrel.

CLOPIDOGREL

10. Is clopidogrel a reasonable alternative for J.S.?

Clopidogrel (Plavix) is chemically related to ticlopidine and works by inhibiting platelet aggregation induced by ADP. A randomized, double-blind, international trial (Clopidogrel versus Aspirin in Patients at Risk of Ischaemic Events [CAPRIE]) compared clopidogrel 75 mg/day with aspirin 325 mg/day.[60] Patients enrolled in the study had a history of atherosclerotic vascular disease manifested by recent ischemic stroke, myocardial infarction, or symptomatic peripheral vascular disease. Using intention-to-treat analysis, a 5.3% risk of an event in patients receiving clopidogrel and a 5.83% risk in patients receiving aspirin was observed. This represents a statistically significant relative risk reduction of 8.7%, favoring clopidogrel. On-treatment analysis showed a relative risk reduction of 9.4%, again in favor of clopidogrel. For patients whose primary condition for entry into CAPRIE was stroke, the relative risk reduction was 7.3%, however this difference was not statistically significant. Patients receiving clopidogrel more frequently experienced rash and diarrhea compared with those receiving aspirin. Patients receiving aspirin were more frequently affected by upper GI distress, intracranial hemorrhage, and GI hemorrhage. Significant reductions in neutrophils occurred in 0.10% of patients on clopidogrel and in 0.17% of patients on aspirin.

Results of the CAPRIE study indicate that clopidogrel is at least as effective and safe as aspirin in preventing all vascular events. Clopidogrel is considered to be an alternative in initial, secondary prevention of stroke.

WARFARIN/ANTICOAGULANTS

11. Is an anticoagulant such as warfarin an alternative instead of aspirin for a patient such as J.S.? What situations make anticoagulants more desirable?

Original studies using warfarin for stroke prophylaxis were performed before the development of modern study methodologies and did not show a significant benefit. The results of these studies are confounded by the high levels of anticoagulation, poor management of hypertension, and the lack of computed tomography (CT) imaging to distinguish hemorrhagic from ischemic strokes. Such inadequacies make these trials useless in evaluating the role of warfarin in stroke prophylaxis.

Two large randomized trials have compared oral anticoagulants to aspirin in the secondary prevention of stroke and TIA. In one study, aspirin 30 mg daily was compared to oral anticoagulants in doses adjusted to maintain an International Normalized Ratio (INR) between 3.0 to 4.5.[61] This study was terminated early when the mortality rate in the anticoagulant group was double the rate in the aspirin group. The increase in mortality was attributed to major bleeding events. In this study there was no difference between anticoagulants and aspirin in the frequency of stroke. A second study compared warfarin, dosed to maintain the INR between 1.4 to 2.8, and aspirin 325 mg daily.[62] Results from this study did not demonstrate a significant difference between aspirin and warfarin with regard to the prevention of stroke or major hemorrhagic events. However, minor hemorrhages were significantly more frequent among patients receiving warfarin. These studies show that warfarin is comparable to aspirin in preventing strokes, but warfarin should be dosed to keep the INR <2.8.

Certain subgroups of patients may benefit from anticoagulant treatment for stroke prevention. For example, anticoagulants may be indicated when the affected region of the brain is the pons or medulla because the consequences of further events in this region would be devastating for the individual; in patients with cervical artery dissection, antiphospholipid antibody syndrome, coagulation factor deficiencies; and in those who have previously had a myocardial infarction.[63] Thus, J.S. should not be anticoagulated unless he has recurrent TIAs while taking aspirin, clopidogrel, or ticlopidine as prescribed.[64]

Although oral anticoagulants are not considered safe for initial, secondary prevention of stroke, a major exception is for patients with atrial fibrillation. These individuals are at risk for an embolic event arising from clot formation in the atrium of the heart. Numerous studies have clearly shown that warfarin prevents embolic cerebrovascular events for patients with nonvalvular atrial fibrillation.[65–69] In these studies, the warfarin dose was adjusted to maintain a prothrombin time INR of 1.5 to 4.5. The Stroke Prevention in Atrial Fibrillation (SPAF) trial included aspirin combined with warfarin in one study arm and indicated that some benefit may be derived by combining antiplatelet agents with anticoagulants.[65] Because this study was not designed to answer this question, a follow-up study was performed and showed no difference between warfarin and aspirin in preventing stroke in atrial fibrillation.[69] A meta-analysis of the studies using warfarin or aspirin in atrial fibrillation failed to demonstrate any benefit from aspirin.[70] Additional work needs to be done on a comparison of warfarin and aspirin for prevention of stroke in atrial fibrillation.

Besides embolic events in patients with atrial fibrillation, there is growing evidence that emboli can originate from complex atherosclerotic plaques in the aorta.[71] In addition, a patent foramen ovale may permit a venous thrombus to pass from right to left in the heart, allowing it to migrate to the cerebrovasculature, resulting in a stroke.[64] A meta-analysis of five retrospective studies suggest that anticoagulation with warfarin is superior to antiplatelet therapy in preventing stroke from a patent foramen ovale.[72]

J.S. is clearly at risk for additional TIAs or an ischemic stroke. The most important step in reducing this risk is to change his lifestyle. However, because J.S. has experienced a TIA, he also should be placed on an antiplatelet agent. Aspirin, dipyridamole combined with aspirin, or clopidogrel are acceptable alternatives for J.S. Warfarin is not an acceptable alternative in J.S. for initial, secondary prevention of TIA or stroke. Considering the overall costs of therapy and that he does not have any definite contraindications to aspirin, J.S. should be started on aspirin 81 mg/day. Clopidogrel or a combination of aspirin and dipyridamole can be used if J.S. is unable to tolerate aspirin or he continues to have TIA or a stroke while taking aspirin (Table 55-3).

Aspirin; Patient Education

12. The physician decides to begin J.S. on aspirin 81 mg/day. How should he be counseled on the use of aspirin? Should J.S. be advised to discontinue aspirin before surgical and dental procedures?

Even low dosages of aspirin may cause gastric erosions and gastric ulcers. J.S. should be instructed to take aspirin with the largest meal of the day, inform his physician of any epigastric pain, and seek medical attention at the first sign of any gastric bleeding (e.g., dark stools). Enteric-coated aspirin may cause less gastric upset than uncoated aspirin formulations.

J.S. should inform all of his healthcare providers, especially his physicians, pharmacist, and dentist, that he is taking aspirin daily. The decision to discontinue aspirin is at the discretion of his physician or dentist. This decision is based on the possibility of bleeding complications from the procedure and the risk of J.S. having a TIA while off aspirin. If aspirin is to be temporarily discontinued, it should be stopped at least 5 to 7 days before the procedure and restarted several days after the procedure.

CEREBRAL INFARCTION AND ISCHEMIC STROKE
Clinical Presentation and Diagnostic Tests

13. P.C., a 65-year-old man, is admitted through the emergency department (ED) after collapsing to the ground and experiencing a brief loss of consciousness. He regained consciousness

by the time he arrived in the ED, 1 hour after the initial event. Both right extremities are flaccid. He is unable to speak but is capable of understanding instructions (i.e., expressive aphasia). Gross ophthalmologic examination indicates right-sided neglect (inability of his eyes to track to the right or acknowledge the right side of his body). His BP is 175/105 mm Hg; other vital signs are normal. Laboratory studies are all within normal limits. By the next day, his neurologic status is unchanged and he is diagnosed as having an ischemic stroke. What diagnostic tests and evaluations will be helpful in guiding P.C.'s therapy?

A careful diagnosis of ischemic stroke is key to guiding further therapy. Because hemorrhagic or ischemic cerebrovascular events cause similar symptoms, the etiology of the altered neurologic status must be determined. Therapy must not be initiated until an accurate diagnosis is made.

Basic laboratory and diagnostic tests should be performed to exclude noncerebrovascular causes, such as metabolic or toxicologic derangement, or infections for the neurologic compromise that P.C. has experienced. These tests include a routine serum chemistry profile (electrolytes, blood urea nitrogen [BUN], serum creatinine [SrCr], hepatic enzymes, calcium, phosphorus, magnesium, albumin), complete blood count, and toxicology screen. Coagulation studies, including a prothrombin time with INR and partial thromboplastin time (PTT), should be performed to provide baseline values for potential anticoagulation or thrombolytic therapy. In addition, a thorough physical, neurologic, and mental status examination should be performed. The neurologic examination will allow a localization of the lesion in the CNS. In addition to providing important information for diagnosis of the neurologic compromise, these tests will provide baseline data for ongoing assessment of P.C.'s progress and recovery.

However, the etiology of a stroke is difficult to discern based solely on a physical and neurologic examination. As a result, CT or magnetic resonance imaging (MRI) is imperative in the evaluation of these patients. An MRI is preferred to a CT due to its superior tissue contrast, ability to obtain images in multiple planes, absence of artifacts caused by bone, vascular imaging capabilities, absence of ionizing radiation, and safer contrast medium. Another advantage of the MRI is that a magnetic resonance angiogram can also be performed, allowing visualization of the cerebrovasculature and possible identification of the precise location of the thrombus or embolus. Within the first 24 hours of an ischemic stroke, an MRI is clearly more sensitive than a CT. However, an MRI is not reliable within the first 8 hours. After 48 hours, the MRI and CT are equally effective in detecting ischemic infarcts. The primary disadvantage of the MRI is that it is more sensitive to artifacts and less practical in unstable patients. In addition, a CT is often the only imaging test available and is acceptable in emergencies.

P.C. must have either a CT or an MRI before initiation of anticoagulation, thrombolytic agents, or other therapies that may increase his risk of bleeding. A follow-up CT or MRI in 5 to 7 days is useful to determine the extent of neurologic damage resulting from the ischemic stroke.

Positron emission tomography (PET) scanning of the CNS can be used to demonstrate the ischemic changes associated with a stroke. A PET image displays areas of cerebral hypometabolism following administration of a specially labeled metabolic substrate such as glucose. A PET image of the CNS has the capability of picturing the primary region of the stroke, the marginally ischemic region (penumbra) surrounding the infarction, and secondary metabolic changes in areas of the CNS that are distant from the primary infarction, but connected through neuronal pathways.

Angiographic, Doppler, or sonographic examination of the cerebral vasculature may be helpful in identifying the location of the vascular lesion. These tests usually are performed after the patient has been stabilized. A lumbar puncture with collection of cerebrospinal fluid (CSF) for evaluation may be helpful in identifying the presence of blood in the CNS. In the presence of suspected increased intracranial pressure, a lumbar puncture must be avoided because of the potential for tentorial herniation. Tentorial herniation occurs when the ventral half of the midbrain (i.e., the cerebral peduncles) pass through the tentorial notch (i.e., a portion of the dura mater that provides support for the occipital lobe and covers the cerebellum). This causes pressure on blood vessels that supply the cerebral cortex, resulting in restricted blood flow.

Treatment

14. What general treatment interventions should be made for P.C.?

In addition to the general supportive therapy needed for a hospitalized patient, several issues are important to the proper management of a stroke patient. Careful attention should be given to fluid and electrolyte control. Excessive hydration or inadequate sodium supplementation may result in hyponatremia, thereby forcing fluid into neurons to further increase the damage from ischemia. In addition, hyponatremia can produce seizures, which increases the metabolic demand on compromised neurons. Thus, it is advisable to initiate fluid therapy with a solution containing at least 0.45% saline and preferably 0.9% saline.

Another metabolic parameter that must be followed carefully is the serum glucose concentration, because hyperglycemia may adversely affect ischemic infarction outcomes. A review of multiple studies on the effects of hyperglycemia in acute stroke concluded that hyperglycemia results in poor outcomes and increased mortality.[73] If hyperglycemia is detected, appropriate insulin therapy should be initiated to keep the serum glucose concentration <155 mg/dL as much as possible.

Caution should be exercised in the acute management of P.C.'s blood pressure. Decreasing the blood pressure too rapidly will compromise cerebral blood flow and expand the region of ischemia and infarction, whereas hypertension will place him at a greater risk for cerebral hemorrhage, especially if a thrombolytic agent is used. However, a study comparing treated and untreated patients who were hypertensive in association with an acute stroke failed to demonstrate any difference in outcomes between the groups.[74] The goal should be to maintain a systolic pressure of <160 mm Hg and diastolic pressure of <100 mm Hg using a parenteral β-blocker or nitroprusside, if necessary. If there is a clinical deterioration of neurologic function associated with the reduction of blood pressure, the infusion rate of the antihypertensive agent should be slowed or the drug discontinued. Maintenance

antihypertensive therapy can then be initiated using an oral agent such as a calcium channel antagonist or angiotensin-converting enzyme inhibitor.

The general daily needs of the patient should be assessed and provided on an as-needed basis. These include nutrition, urination, defecation, and prevention of decubitus ulcers. Neurologic deficits will compromise the ability of many patients to adequately meet these needs, increasing the necessity for medical assistance.

Two interventions that have been shown to improve outcomes of ischemic stroke are reducing the time to treatment of stroke and admitting patients to specialized stroke care units. Reduction of the time to treatment permits the use of interventions shown only to work within the first 2 hours of a stroke.[75] Pharmacists can assist in this process by educating patients on the signs and symptoms of stroke and ensuring that medications for emergent treatment of stroke are readily available and accessible to emergency medical personnel. In addition, Indredavik and colleagues have shown that stroke care units significantly improve long-term survival and functionality of patients after a stroke.[76]

15. Should anticoagulation or antiplatelet agents be used acutely in P.C.?

Several studies have evaluated the use of anticoagulants and antiplatelet agents in the treatment of acute strokes. However, most of these studies are poorly designed or underpowered to determine the efficacy of these agents. Despite these problems with published studies, many physicians prefer to use anticoagulants or antiplatelets in the management of patients with acute stroke.

Heparin

Duke and colleagues compared intravenous heparin to placebo in patients with acute partially stable stroke.[77] In this double-blind study, heparin doses were adjusted to maintain the PTT at 1.5 to 2 times control and continued for 7 days. There were no significant differences in death at 7 days, and no differences in functional ability were observed to 1 year following the stroke. At 1 year there was a significantly greater mortality rate in heparin-treated patients. The International Stroke Trial compared aspirin, subcutaneous heparin (5,000 IU or 12,500 IU twice daily), both and neither treatments for patients with acute ischemic stroke.[78] There was no reduction of mortality or morbidity for patients receiving either dose of heparin. Neither of these studies demonstrated benefit from heparin in preventing early stroke recurrence. Additionally, there was no relationship between location of the stroke and response to heparin in either the study by Duke or IST.

Heparinoids

Low-molecular-weight heparins and heparinoids have been evaluated in several studies for acute stroke. Two doses of nadroparin were compared to placebo in one randomized, double blind, placebo controlled trial.[79] There were no differences in death rates or functional ability at 3 months between the 3 treatment arms. However, at 6 months patients receiving high-dose nadroparin (i.e., 4100 anti-Xa IU twice daily) had improved function. A large randomized, placebo controlled trial of dose-adjusted danaparoid, a low-molecular-weight heparinoid, did not demonstrate improvement in danaproid treated patients.[80] In addition, no improvements were observed in studies of dalteparin and certoparin.[81,82] Similar to heparin, low-molecular-weight heparins and heparinoids did not prevent early, recurrent strokes. There was no relationship between type of stroke and response to these agents.

Aspirin

One study evaluated early administration of aspirin in acute stroke. The Chinese Acute Stroke Trial (CAST) compared 160 mg/day of aspirin administered within 48 hours of the onset of stroke symptoms to placebo.[83] Patients who received aspirin had reduced early mortality rates, but there was no difference in the primary endpoint of death or dependency at discharge from the hospital. The IST and the Multicenter Acute Stroke Trial-Italy studies included aspirin arms in their study design. Neither of these studies demonstrated benefit with aspirin.[78,84] When data from the CAST and IST studies are combined, a slight beneficial effect of aspirin is seen with regard to reducing the risk of early stroke recurrence.

Glycoprotein IIb/IIIa Inhibitors

Platelet glycoprotein IIb/IIIa inhibitors have also been studied in acute stroke. A placebo controlled Phase II trial of abciximab given within 24 hours of acute stroke showed a trend toward improved functionality in abciximab-treated patients, but the study was not powered to show significance for this outcome.[85] In another placebo controlled, Phase II study of patients with acute stroke the direct thrombin inhibitor, argatroban, was associated with statistically significant improvements in neurologic symptoms and daily living activities.[86] The number of patients enrolled in this study was small, but the results show promise. Larger trials are needed to confirm this result.

Ancrod

Derived from the venom of the Malayan pit viper snake, ancrod cleaves fibrinogen in a way similar to thrombin. This produces a circulating soluble ancrod-fibrin complex that is not cross-linked and may stimulate tissue plasminogen activator (tPA) activation from vascular endothelium. Ancrod leads to fibrinolysis soon after its administration and is rarely associated with significant bleeding complications. This low risk of hemorrhagic complications makes ancrod especially attractive for use in ischemic stroke.

The Stroke Treatment with Ancrod Trial (STAT) compared a continuous 72-hour infusion of ancrod dosed to decrease fibrinogen levels to 1.18 to 2.03 μmol/L to receive placebo.[87] This infusion was followed by 1-hour infusions at approximately 96 and 120 hours after treatment was started. Ancrod infusion rates of 0.167, 0.125, and 0.082 IU/kg per hour were used based on pretreatment fibrinogen concentrations. Significantly more patients treated with ancrod achieved favorable functional status and had fewer disabilities. There was no difference in mortality rates between ancrod and placebo. Ancrod was associated with significantly more asymptomatic ICHs and a trend toward more symptomatic hemorrhages. This study shows that successful use of ancrod depends on achieving controlled defibrinogenation.

Deep vein thrombosis and pulmonary embolism are common complications in patients following a stroke. The incidence of deep vein thrombosis (DVT) and pulmonary embolus (PE) were reduced in most studies where patients received heparin, low-molecular-weight heparins, or heparinoids.[88]

While there is considerable evidence to support the use of selected antithrombotic agents in the treatment of acute ischemic stroke, there is still controversy regarding the optimal choice of agents and patients for whom these treatments are most appropriate. A recent systematic review of the literature in this area resulted in the following recommendations[88]:

1. Aspirin 160 to 325 mg daily should be initiated within 48 hours of the onset of stroke symptoms.
2. Heparin, low-molecular-weight heparins, and heparinoids may be considered for prevention of DVT and PE. Use of these agents must be weighed against the risk of hemorrhagic complications.
3. Fixed dose heparin may have some early benefit in the treatment of acute stroke, but this benefit is negated by an increased risk of hemorrhage.
4. Dose-adjusted heparin is associated with increased bleeding complications and is not recommended.
5. Low-molecular-weight heparins and heparinoids at high doses have not been associated with benefit or harm in patients with acute stroke.
6. Intravenous heparin, high-dose low-molecular-weight heparins, or heparinoids are not recommended for any subgroup or specific type of stroke.

On the basis of these recommendations, P.C. should receive 160 to 325 mg daily of aspirin to be started within 2 days of admission for his stroke. Use of other anticoagulants is not recommended.

Thrombolytics

16. **Would thrombolytic agents be useful to treat P.C.'s acute ischemic stroke?**

The critical primary event in a thromboembolic stroke is the development of an acute thrombus. Prospective cerebral angiography has demonstrated an arterial occlusion corresponding to the area of acute neurologic deficit in >90% of cases.[89] Occlusion of cerebral arteries does not cause complete ischemia because collateral circulation from other arterial sources provides unstable and incomplete circulation to the ischemic region of the brain.[90] When blood flow is sustained in the range of 10 to 18 mL/100 g per minute, irreversible cellular damage may occur. Thrombolytic agents can reestablish blood flow to ischemic regions of the brain.

Blood flow must be restored quickly after the event. Experimental studies in dogs and cats have shown that when blood flow is restored within 2 to 3 hours, neurologic deficits are prevented.[91,92] Occlusions lasting 3 to 7 hours produce permanent neurologic damage but are far less severe than those associated with a sustained occlusion. Based on these studies, it appears that rapid administration of a thrombolytic agent to a patient experiencing an acute ischemic stroke is required to minimize the neurologic damage.

A number of early studies using various thrombolytic agents were performed before CT scanning was available. Because ischemic and hemorrhagic strokes were difficult to differentiate, the findings of these studies are confusing. In these studies, many patients had significant neurological improvements, but there were high mortality rates. The mortality rates discouraged additional investigations.

Since CT scans have become widely available, there has been renewed interest in the use of thrombolytic agents, particularly in tPA. A total of five large, placebo-controlled trials using either tPA or streptokinase for acute stroke have been published. In three studies, streptokinase was used as the thrombolytic and all of these studies were terminated early due to high rates of mortality and intracranial hemorrhage associated with streptokinase.[84,93,94] Studies with tPA demonstrate some benefit associated its use.[95,96]

The three aforementioned streptokinase trials were the Multicentre Acute Stroke Trial-Italy (MAST-I), the Multicenter Acute Stroke Trial-Europe (MAST-E), and the Australian Streptokinase Trial (ASK). These trials clearly demonstrate that streptokinase is associated with increased mortality and disability. In the MAST-E and MAST-I trials the rates of intracranial hemorrhage ranged from 6% to 17% for patients receiving streptokinase compared with 0.6% to 3% for patients receiving placebo. In all three trials the mortality rates were significantly greater for patients receiving streptokinase. Streptokinase should not be used for P.C.

The National Institute of Neurological Disorders and Stroke (NINDS) tPA trial and the European Cooperative Acute Stroke Study (ECASS) used different doses, inclusion criteria, and treatment protocols. Both trials showed the benefit of tPA in at least some outcome parameters. In the NINDS tPA study, patients were enrolled using strict inclusion and exclusion criteria (Table 55-4). All patients were within 3 hours of symptom onset and had to undergo a CT scan before enrollment. When enrolled, patients received either tPA 0.9 mg/kg (maximum dose, 90 mg), with 10% of the dose given as a bolus over 1 minute and the remainder infused over 60 minutes, or placebo. Patients were divided into two groups for the purpose of analysis. One group consisted of 291 patients whose early neurologic recovery was assessed 24 hours after enrollment. The second group of 333 patients had neurologic outcomes evaluated at 3 months. In the first group, there was no difference in positive responses between patients receiving tPA or placebo. However, a secondary analysis showed that National Institutes of Health Stroke Scale scores were significantly greater at 24 hours for patients receiving tPA. Results

in the second group were also favorable for tPA. At 3 months, patients who received tPA were 30% more likely to have minimal or no disability and there was an 11% to 13% absolute increase in the number of patients with excellent outcomes. There was a corresponding decrease in the number of patients with severe neurologic impairment or death at 3 months. Improvements associated with tPA were seen across age groups, stroke subtypes, stroke severity, and status of aspirin use before the stroke. Intracranial hemorrhage occurred more frequently among patients receiving tPA (6.4%) than in patients receiving placebo (0.6%). Despite the increased incidence of ICH, outcomes remained better for patients receiving tPA.

For the ECASS I trial, patients with onset of stroke were enrolled within 6 hours of the onset of symptoms.[96] The treatment protocol consisted of IV tPA 1.1 mg/kg (maximum, 100 mg) or placebo. Using intention-to-treat analysis, there was no difference in the primary outcome measures of functionality at 3 months. However, with target population analysis, there was a significant difference favoring tPA. Of tPA-treated patients, 41% had minimal or no disability compared with 29% of placebo-treated patients. A variety of secondary outcome measures favored tPA. There was no difference in 30-day mortality rates, but 19.8% of tPA-treated patients had major parenchymal hemorrhages compared with 6.5% of placebo-treated patients. A more recent trial, ECASS II, used a tPA dose of 0.9 mg/kg and was designed to replicate the NINDS trial.[97] However, patients were enrolled up to 6 hours after the onset of stroke symptoms. This study found no difference between tPA and placebo. Too few patients were enrolled with stroke symptoms <3 hours to reliably evaluate the influence of this variable on outcome.

Time from onset of stroke symptoms to treatment with tPA is an important variable. The Alteplase Thrombolysis for Acute Ischemic Stroke (ATLANTIS) trial compared tPA started 3 to 5 hours after the onset of stroke symptoms with placebo.[98] The study found no significant benefit for tPA in this group of patients and a significant increase in the number of symptomatic and fatal ICHs with tPA.

The Cochrane Stroke Review Group performed a meta-analysis of 17 thrombolytic trials.[99] In this analysis, thrombolytic therapy was associated with an excess of early deaths (odds ratio, 1.85; 95% confidence interval, 1.48 to 2.32) and early symp-

Table 55-4	Criteria for Alteplase Use in Treatment of Acute Stroke	

Inclusion Criteria	Exclusion Criteria
18 years of age or older	Minor or rapidly improving symptoms
Clinical diagnosis of stroke with clinically meaningful neurologic deficit	CT signs of intracranial hemorrhage
Clearly defined onset within 180 min before treatment	History of intracranial hemorrhage
Baseline CT with no evidence of intracranial hemorrhage	Seizure at onset of stroke
	Stroke or serious head injury within 3 months
	Major surgery or serious trauma within 2 weeks
	GI or urinary tract hemorrhage within 3 weeks
	Systolic BP >185 mm Hg, diastolic BP >110 mm Hg
	Aggressive treatment to lower BP
	Glucose 400 mg/dL
	Symptoms of subarachnoid hemorrhage

BP, blood pressure; CT, computed tomography; GI, gastrointestinal.

tomatic hemorrhages (odds ratio, 3.53; 95% confidence interval, 2.79 to 4.45). However, thrombolytic therapy initiated within 6 hours of symptom onset reduced the proportion of patients who were dead or dependent at the end of follow-up (odds ratio, 0.83; 95% confidence interval, 0.73 to 0.94). Similar results were obtained when the analysis included patients treated within 3 hours of symptom onset (odds ratio, 0.58; 95% confidence interval, 0.46 to 0.74). About half of the data included in these analyses came from trials of tPA and the results support the use of tPA in the treatment of acute ischemic stroke.

Thrombolytic therapy appeared to reduce death and neurologic deficits when treatment was initiated within 6 hours of symptom onset (odds ratio, 0.83; 95% confidence interval, 0.73 to 0.94) and within 3 hours of symptom onset (odds ratio, 0.58; 95% confidence interval, 0.46 to 0.74). This analysis substantiates the use of tPA in the treatment of ischemic stroke.

Several studies have reported the use of intra-arterial thrombolytic therapy. In one trial, patients were randomized to receive either 6 mg of recombinant prourokinase or placebo over 120 minutes.[100] All patients received IV heparin. Patients who were randomized received treatment at a median of 5.5 hours from symptom onset. Recanalization was significantly greater in the prourokinase group. However, hemorrhagic transformation occurred in 15.4% of prourokinase-treated patients compared with 7.1% of placebo-treated patients. Hemorrhage frequencies and recanalization rates were influenced by heparin dose. A second trial has confirmed these findings, showing significantly improved outcomes with intra-arterial prourokinase, despite increased intracranial hemorrhage.[101] Although useful in major medical centers, intra-arterial prourokinase presents major technical obstacles that limit its use in most emergency departments.

The only study that has clearly shown benefit associated with systemic tPA use for acute stroke is the NINDS tPA trial. If tPA is to be used for acute stroke, the NINDS inclusion and exclusion criteria and treatment protocol should be used.

Because P.C. presented to the ED within 1 hour of the onset of his stroke symptoms, he is a candidate for tPA therapy in accordance with the NINDS study protocol. A thorough history and CT scan must be performed before initiation of tPA to ensure compliance with inclusion and exclusion criteria.

Preservation of Central Nervous System Function

Preservation of marginally ischemic regions of the brain is an active area of investigation. Hemodilution, corticosteroids, calcium channel blockers, 21-aminosteroids, NMDA receptor antagonists, lubeluzole, citicoline, anti–intercellular adhesion molecule (ICAM)-1 antibody, clomethiazole, fosphenytoin, piracetam, ebselen, and ganglioside GM-1 are therapeutic interventions that have been studied to retain CNS function in the ischemic penumbra. None of these interventions has been clearly shown to preserve neurologic function. Because the events leading to neuronal death involve numerous pathways, it is possible that a combination of some of these agents will prove to be most effective.

Hemodilution

17. What is the rationale for hemodilution therapy in ischemic stroke? Should this therapeutic approach be recommended for P.C.?

Based on a direct relationship between a lowered hematocrit and decreased blood viscosity, various colloid and crystalloid solutions have been administered to ischemic stroke patients. Initial studies indicated that volume expansion might be useful, but larger trials have not supported the original findings.[102,103] A more recent trial failed to show any benefit from hemodilution, but found this practice to be as safe as regular hydration therapy.[104] These conflicting results can be attributed to late initiation of therapy, varying protocols for hemodilution and hypervolemia, different goals for reduction of the hematocrit, and the possibility that only specific subgroups of patients might benefit. Hemodilution remains a questionable practice in ischemic stroke and is not to be recommended in P.C.'s management.

A typical hemodilution regimen would use albumin or plasma-protein fraction to decrease the hematocrit to 30% to 35% or to maintain a pulmonary capillary wedge pressure of 14 to 18 mm Hg. Hetastarch is relatively contraindicated due to the possibility of hemorrhage associated with its use.

Corticosteroids

18. Should corticosteroids be used in P.C.?

Corticosteroids have been used to treat stroke on the theory that decreasing edema and swelling of the brain will increase cerebral blood flow to ischemic regions. Dexamethasone (4 to 20 mg every 6 hours) was commonly used because it has substantial anti-inflammatory effects without mineralocorticoid activity; however, multiple studies have shown that corticosteroids are ineffective in treating cerebral infarction or hemorrhagic stroke.[105–110] The lack of efficacy of steroids might be explained by inflammation of dead neurons rather than in marginally ischemic neurons. The use of corticosteroids is relatively contraindicated in these patients because of possible increases in morbidity and mortality.[105] Although corticosteroids are ineffective in the treatment of cerebral infarction or hemorrhagic stroke, they clearly are effective in acute cases of spinal cord injuries and some space-occupying tumors of the brain.

Calcium Channel Blockers

19. What is the rationale for using calcium channel blockers in ischemic stroke? Are they indicated for use in P.C.?

Studies of the pathophysiologic responses of the CNS to ischemia have demonstrated that calcium influx into neurons coincides with much of the cellular destruction associated with ischemia. Because calcium influx into the neuron is modulated by both voltage-dependent channels and neurotransmitter-dependent channels, calcium channel blockers that penetrate the CNS could be useful for limiting the neurologic damage associated with an ischemic stroke. In addition, the calcium channel blockers have been shown to increase blood flow into ischemic regions of the brain.

Initial studies of nimodipine for ischemic stroke indicated that treatment positively improved outcomes. However, subsequent studies have not substantiated these findings. In one study of 186 patients, there was an 8.6% mortality rate in the nimodipine-treated group compared with a 20.4% mortality rate in the placebo-treated group.[111] Stratification according to gender indicated a significant difference in males but not in females. Using a standardized evaluation scale, neurologic outcomes were assessed by the investigators; significant improvements occurred in the nimodipine group. Nimodipine doses of 30 mg orally every 6 hours for 28 days were used in this trial.

Eight other studies failed to substantiate this first study. A study group in the United Kingdom evaluated nimodipine 120 mg/day in a double blind, randomized trial.[112] Based on two stroke rating scales and mortality rates, there was no difference between nimodipine and placebo. Another randomized, double blind, placebo- controlled study of nimodipine (120 mg/day for 21 days) showed no improvement with nimodipine.[113] A meta-analysis of nimodipine use in 3,719 patients showed a benefit only for patients who were treated with 30 mg every 6 hours beginning within 12 hours of symptom onset.[114] A more recent systematic review came to a similar conclusion and effectively ruled out a clinically significant benefit of calcium channel blockers in acute ischemic stroke.[115]

The precise place of calcium channel blockers in the management of acute ischemic stroke is uncertain, but clinical trials do not hold much promise of their efficacy. An important key to their use may be early initiation of therapy (i.e., within 6 to 8 hours following the stroke). Calcium channel blockers are not indicated in P.C. Their use in subarachnoid hemorrhage is discussed in question 27.

20. **What other neuroprotective agents might be useful in ischemic stroke? Would P.C. be a candidate for any of them?**

Numerous agents have been investigated as neuroprotective agents in acute stroke. None of these drugs have been shown to be effective in improving outcomes.[116] Reasons for lack of effect include the complexity of pathology of ischemic damage, inappropriate outcome measures, and occurrence of dose-limiting adverse effects. At this time, no neuroprotective pharmacotherapeutic interventions have been shown to be effective in acute stroke.

Stroke Education

21. **What information and instruction should be given to P.C. regarding future stroke symptoms?**

Early treatment of acute stroke with available or investigational drugs appears to be the most important factor in determining optimal outcome. Nearly every clinical trial demonstrating some benefit of pharmacotherapy for acute stroke has shown the greatest effect for patients who have been treated within a few hours of the onset of stroke symptoms. Immediate detection of stroke symptoms and initiation of treatment are imperative. The primary rate-limiting step in diagnosis and provision of medical care is recognition by the patient of stroke symptoms. Every patient who is at increased risk of stroke should be carefully instructed to seek emergent medical attention if they experience any weakness or paralysis, speech impairment, numbness, blurred vision or sudden loss of vision, or altered level of consciousness. These symptoms should be handled with the same urgency as the symptoms of a myocardial infarction. The pharmacist should ensure that P.C. and his caregivers know the symptoms of stroke and understand what to do when they occur.

Complications

22. **What complications associated with stroke might P.C. experience?**

Agitation, delirium, stupor, coma, cerebral edema, or increased intracranial pressure are other symptoms that can be associated with ischemic stroke. These symptoms correlate with the specific blood vessels that are affected, and the development of these complications in P.C. would depend on the progression of his stroke.

Seizures may occur in up to 20% of stroke patients. Pneumonia, pulmonary edema, cardiac arrest, deep vein thrombosis, and arrhythmias commonly are associated with ischemic stroke and should be managed as they occur. In P.C., these may occur soon after his stroke or be related to a rapidly developing neurologic event such as further infarction, hemorrhage, or severe cerebral edema. Pneumonia or deep venous thrombosis are related primarily to inactivity, and the risk of these events will increase the longer P.C. remains immobile.

Stroke patients frequently experience psychologic reactions. The most common psychiatric complication is depression, occurring in 30% to 50% of patients.[117] The severity of depression varies from mild to major depressive episodes. If the depression interferes with recovery and the rehabilitative process, it should be managed with the use of a selective serotonin reuptake inhibitor (SSRI) or nortriptyline. Severe psychomotor depression may respond to CNS stimulants, such as methylphenidate or dextroamphetamine. Because of P.C.'s hypertension, stimulants only should be used with careful blood pressure monitoring.

Prognosis

23. **After 7 days in the hospital, P.C.'s neurologic status is stabilized. Will further neurologic improvements be realized?**

Neurologic deficits in stroke patients are not considered stable or fixed until at least 8 to 12 months have elapsed. During this time, neurologic function may return, but rarely to normal. The prognosis following ischemic stroke depends on a variety of factors including age, hypertension, coma, cardiopulmonary complications, hypoxia, and neurogenic hyperventilation. However, infarction of the middle cerebral artery is associated with a poor chance for recovery. Therefore, it is possible that P.C. will experience further neurologic improvement.

Rehabilitation

24. **As P.C. enters rehabilitation, what interventions will aid his recovery?**

Rehabilitation for P.C. is directed at managing daily functions and enhancing existing neurologic function. Considerations for daily functions include activities of daily living and bowel and bladder management through balanced pharmacologic interventions. Efforts should be made to allow P.C. to function independently with activities of daily living and manage the psychologic effects of stroke. Enhancement of current neurologic function and minimizing depression includes elimination of drugs that may compromise P.C.'s memory and mental function. These include benzodiazepines, major tranquilizers, and sedating antiepileptic drugs.

Spasticity of the affected limb may present a problem for P.C. Because spasticity often is localized to a single limb after ischemic stroke, it frequently responds to regional motor nerve blocks with botulinum toxin. Aggressive physical therapy also is essential to the management of spasticity. Systemic antispasticity agents such as diazepam, baclofen, or dantrolene sodium are not used routinely because of the risk for toxicity. They are used only when spasticity involves multiple parts of the body or is unresponsive to other therapies.

Other less common impediments to P.C.'s recovery include decubitus ulcers, hypercalcemia, and heterotopic ossification (e.g., the laying down and calcification of a bone matrix in muscle surrounding major joints). Prevention through meticulous skin care is the key to the management of pressure ulcers. Mobilizing P.C. as soon as possible after the stroke can prevent hypercalcemia and heterotopic ossification. If necessary, these complications may be treated with etidronate (Didronel).

SUBARACHNOID HEMORRHAGE
Clinical Presentation and Treatment

25. **R.A., a 65-year-old woman, suddenly collapsed in the bathroom of her home. An ambulance was immediately called, and on arrival at the ED she had regained consciousness. She complained of a severe headache and kept dropping off to sleep during the examination. Nuchal rigidity (i.e., a stiff and painful neck when flexed) and mild mental confusion with regard to place also were observed. A CT scan demonstrated blood in the subarachnoid space and in her ventricles. A cerebral angiogram demonstrated a posterior communicating artery aneurysm. Electrolytes, coagulation studies, and blood counts were within normal limits. What pharmacotherapy is used for subarachnoid hemorrhage?**

R.A.'s neurologic symptoms and the appearance of blood on her CT scan are consistent with a diagnosis of subarachnoid hemorrhage. Unfortunately, there are no direct pharmacotherapeutic interventions that are effective for subarachnoid hemorrhage. Surgical repair and clipping of the aneurysm is the definitive intervention. Pharmacotherapy is directed at preventing or managing complications of SAH.

Complications

26. **R.A.'s neurologic status deteriorated approximately 3 days after admission. What complications may be responsible for these changes?**

Following the initial hemorrhagic event, there are three major complications that usually are responsible for neurologic changes (Table 55-5). *Rebleeding* from an aneurysm occurs in 20% of patients, usually within the first 48 hours after the initial event. In some cases, rebleeding can happen as long as 14 days later. From 24 hours to weeks after the hemorrhage, *hydrocephalus* (i.e., accumulation of CSF within the ventricular system of the brain) may be caused by blood interrupting CSF flow through the ventricles and reabsorption of CSF through the arachnoid villa. Another 20% to 40% of patients will develop *delayed cerebral ischemia,* usually within 5 to 12 days following the initial hemorrhage. Delayed ischemia caused by vasospasm of the cerebral vessels is evidenced by development of new neurologic deficits and confirmed by a cerebral angiogram. At least half of these individuals will die or experience permanent neurologic damage. Approximately 5% to 15% of patients have seizures.

27. **How should each of these complications (rebleeding, hydrocephalus, vasospasm, and seizures) be managed in R.A.? Are calcium channel blockers more effective in treating subarachnoid hemorrhage than ischemic stroke?**

Rebleeding

Surgical clipping of the aneurysm is the best method to prevent rebleeding. If early surgery is contraindicated or unavailable, antifibrinolytic therapy with epsilon aminocaproic acid (EACA) may be instituted. EACA blocks the activation of plasminogen and inhibits the action of plasmin on the fibrin clot. EACA enhances hemostasis when fibrinolysis contributes to bleeding and stabilizes the clot that has formed around the ruptured aneurysm. The incidence of rebleeding is decreased from 20-30% to 10-15% by EACA.[118,119] However, delayed cerebral ischemia occurs more frequently in patients receiving EACA.[118] It is unclear whether this is a direct effect of EACA or whether more individuals survive to experience delayed cerebral ischemia. EACA usually is given as a 5-g IV bolus followed by a continuous infusion of 1 to 2 g/hour. Dosages can be adjusted to maintain serum concentrations of 200 to 400 mg/mL. R.A. may benefit from receiving EACA as soon as a subarachnoid hemorrhage is diagnosed, and it should be continued until surgical clipping can be performed or for at least 2 weeks after the initial hemorrhage. It is preferable to surgically repair the aneurysm as soon as possible after R.A. is admitted to the hospital.

Hydrocephalus

The only effective treatment for hydrocephalus is surgical intervention. If a CT scan demonstrates hydrocephalus, a

Table 55-5	Therapy for Subarachnoid Hemorrhage Complications	
Rebleeding	*Hydrocephalus*	*Delayed Ischemia*
Surgical clip	Ventricular drain	Nimodipine 60 mg Q 4 hr for 21 days
Aminocaproic acid 5 g loading dose and 1 to 2 g/hr	Ventricular-peritoneal shunt	Hypervolemia
		PCWP 12–15 mm Hg
		Hypertension
		Systolic BP 170–220 mm Hg

BP, blood pressure; PCWP, pulmonary capillary wedge pressure.

ventricular drain should be surgically placed after the aneurysm has been clipped. When hydrocephalus becomes a chronic problem, the drain can be replaced with a permanent ventriculoperitoneal shunt.

Ventriculitis is a common complication of a ventricular drain and is most likely caused by staphylococci or Gram-negative bacteria. Antibiotic therapy for this complication should consist of an IV agent (e.g., chloramphenicol, ceftri-axone, ampicillin, penicillin, vancomycin, ceftazidime, ce-furoxime, nafcillin, and rifampin) that readily crosses the blood–brain barrier with inflamed meninges. Alternatively, gentamicin and vancomycin can be instilled through the ventricular drains directly to the site of infection.[120] The antibiotic solution is prepared using a preservative-free sterile powder for injection. Gentamicin 4 to 8 mg or vancomycin 5 to 20 mg is instilled once a day. Systemic and intraventricular antibiotics should be continued until three consecutive CSF cultures are free of bacterial growth.

Delayed Cerebral Ischemia (Vasospasm)

The occurrence of delayed cerebral ischemia probably is due to vasospasm of the cerebral blood vessels. Current therapy for delayed ischemia is not optimal and is rather confusing. Volume expansion with normal saline or plasma protein fraction usually is initiated when focal neurologic changes develop, with the goal of maintaining a pulmonary capillary wedge pressure of 15 to 20 mm Hg.[121–124] Some clinicians may institute hypervolemia therapy in anticipation of delayed cerebral ischemia. If the neurologic deficits are not reversed with hypervolemia, systolic blood pressure can be increased to as high as 200 to 220 mm Hg using dopamine or norepinephrine. A high systolic pressure allows the brain to redirect flow to ischemic areas, and such therapy is often continued for 7 to 14 days.

CALCIUM CHANNEL BLOCKERS
Nimodipine

Nimodipine also is indicated for the prevention of delayed cerebral ischemia for patients with a subarachnoid hemorrhage. Its mechanisms of action may include preventing cerebral vasospasm that is responsible for delayed ischemia, inhibiting calcium influx into ischemic neurons, or re-establishing cerebrovascular autoregulation (i.e., the ability of the brain to control blood flow in accordance with metabolic needs).

Nimodipine has been administered in clinical studies intravenously, orally, or topically (i.e., direct application to the brain's surface and the cerebral vasculature during surgery). Several studies of nimodipine in subarachnoid hemorrhage have used oral formulations. In these studies, a total of 1,038 patients were given nimodipine prophylactically according to double-blind, placebo-controlled, randomized protocols.[125–128] Angiographic improvement was not significantly different in patients treated with nimodipine or placebo, but neurologic outcomes improved significantly in nimodipine-treated patients who presented with a mild to moderately severe subarachnoid hemorrhage. In another study, nimodipine significantly benefited patients with severe hemorrhage. Nimodipine 60 to 90 mg every 4 hours for 21 days was initiated within the first 96 hours after the original subarachnoid hemorrhage in these patients. No trial has compared the efficacy of nimodipine with hypervolemia therapy and interventions to increase systolic blood pressure. Nimodipine's approved dose is 60 mg orally every 6 hours.

R.A. should receive nimodipine 60 mg orally every 4 hours for 21 days because she was diagnosed within several hours of her subarachnoid hemorrhage.

Seizures
PHENYTOIN

Seizures occur in approximately 9% of patients experiencing a subarachnoid hemorrhage. Only two factors associated with subarachnoid hemorrhage have been identified as predictive of seizures: rebleeding or large amounts of cisternal blood on CT scan.

Phenytoin often is used for seizure prophylaxis. However, no trials have investigated the efficacy of phenytoin in preventing seizure in patients with subarachnoid hemorrhage. The usual dose of phenytoin is 15 to 20 mg/kg administered as an IV bolus at a rate <50 mg/min. A maintenance dose of 5 to 7 mg/kg per day either orally or intravenously is titrated to maintain steady-state serum concentrations of 10 to 20 mg/mL. Alternatively, fosphenytoin, a phenytoin prodrug, can be administered intravenously or intramuscularly at a loading dose of 15 to 20 mg phenytoin equivalents (PE)/kg and a maintenance dose of 5 to 7 mg PE/kg per day. Infusion rates of fosphenytoin should be <150 mg PE/min. Maintenance phenytoin usually is continued for 1 to 2 years or longer if the patient experiences seizures. Because there is a 5% to 20% risk of seizures for R.A., she should receive phenytoin prophylactically. Carbamazepine is an acceptable alternative, but a parenteral form of the drug is unavailable.

REFERENCES

1. American Heart Association. Heart Disease and Stroke Statistics-2003 update. Available at: http://www.americanheart.org/downloadable/heart/1046120785214200HDSStatsBook.pdf.
2. Fang J et al. Trend of stroke hospitalization, United States, 1988-1997. Stroke 2001;32:2221.
3. Howard G et al. Decline in US stroke mortality an analysis of temporal patterns by sex, race, and geographic region. Stroke 2001;32:2213.
4. Brust JCM. Transient ischemic attacks: natural history and anticoagulation. Neurology 1977;27:701.
5. Straus SE et al. New evidence for stroke prevention. JAMA 2002;288:1388.
6. Chaturvedi S et al. Ischemic stroke prevention. Curr Treat Options Neurol 1999;1:113.
7. MacWalter RS et al. A benefit-risk assessment of agents used in the secondary prevention of stroke. Drug Saf 2002;25:943.
8. Gorelick PB. Stroke prevention therapy beyond antithrombotics: unifying mechanisms in ischemic stroke pathogenesis and implications for therapy. Stroke 2002;33:862.
9. Woo D et al. Genetic and environmental risk factors for intracerebral hemorrhage: preliminary results of a population-based study. Stroke 2002;33:1190.
10. Zebrack JS et al. Role of inflammation in cardiovascular disease: how to use C-reactive protein in clinical practice. Prog Cardiovasc Nurs 2002;17:174.
11. Astrup J. Cortical evoked potential and extracellular K+ and H+ at critical levels of brain ischemia. Stroke 1977;8:51.
12. Hickenbottom SL et al. Neuroprotective therapy. Semin Neurol 1998;18:485.
13. Goldstein LB et al. Primary prevention of ischemic stroke a statement for healthcare professionals from the Stroke Council of the American Heart Association. Circulation 2001;103:163.

14. Prospective Studies Collaboration. Cholesterol, diastolic blood pressure, and stroke:13,000 strokes in 450,000 people in 45 prospective cohorts. Lancet 1995;346:1647.

15. Dunbalin DW et al. Preventing stroke by the modification of risk factors. Stroke 1990;21(Suppl IV):IV-36.

16. Du X et al. Case control study of stroke and the quality of hypertension control in north west England. Br Med J 1997;14:272.

17. National Institutes of Health. The seventh report of the Joint National Committee on prevention, detection, evaluation, and treatment of high blood pressure (JNC) 2003. Available at http://www.nhlbi.nih.gov/guidelines/hypertension/.

18. Murray CJ et al. Effectiveness and costs of interventions to lower systolic blood pressure and cholesterol: a global and regional analysis on reduction of cardiovascular-disease risk. Lancet 2003;361:717.

19. Plehn JF et al. Reduction of stroke incidence after myocardial infarction with pravastatin the Cholesterol and Recurrent Events (CARE) study. Circulation 1999;99:216.

20. The Long-Term Intervention with Pravastatin in Ischaemic Disease (LIPID) Study Group. Prevention of cardiovascular events and death with pravastatin in patients with coronary heart disease and a broad range of initial cholesterol levels. N Engl J Med 1998;339:1349.

21. White HD et al. Pravastatin therapy and the risk of stroke. N Engl J Med 2000;343:317.

22. Shepherd J et al. Pravastatin in elderly individuals at risk of vascular disease (PROSPER): a randomized controlled trial. Lancet 2002;360:1623.

23. Hunt D et al. Benefits of pravastatin on cardiovascular events and mortality in older patients with coronary heart disease are equal to or exceed those seen in younger patients: results from the LIPID trial. Ann Intern Med 2001;134.931.

24. Sever PS et al. Prevention of coronary and stroke events with atorvastatin in hypertensive patients who have average or lower-than-average cholesterol concentrations, in the Anglo-Scandinavian Cardiac Outcomes Trial—Lipid Lowering Arm (ASCOT-LLA): a multicentre randomised controlled trial. Lancet 2003;361.1149.

25. Byington RP et al. Reduction of stroke events with pravastatin The Prospective Pravastatin Pooling (PPP) Project. Circulation 2001;103:387.

26. Ross SD et al. Clinical outcomes in statin treatment trials a meta-analysis. Arch Intern Med 1999;159:1793.

27. Atkins D et al. Cholesterol reduction and the risk for stroke in men: a meta-analysis of randomized controlled clinical trials. Ann Intern Med 1993;119:136.

28. Blake GJ et al. Projected life-expectancy gains with statin therapy for individuals with elevated C-reactive protein levels. J Am Coll Cardiol 2002;40:49.

29. Vaughan CJ et al. Do statis afford neuroprotection in patients with cerebral ischaemia and stroke? CNS Drugs 2001;15:589.

30. Gil-Núñez AC et al. Advantages of lipid-lowering therapy in cerebral ischemia: role of HMG-CoA reductase inhibitors. Cerebrovasc Dis 2001;11(Suppl 1):85.

31. Albers GW et al. Supplement to the guidelines for the management of transient ischemic attacks a statement from the Ad Hoc Committee on Guidelines for the Management of Transient Ischemic Attacks, Stroke Council, American Heart Association. Circulation 1999;30:2502.

32. North American Symptomatic Carotid Endarterectomy Trial Collaborators. Beneficial effect of carotid endarterectomy in symptomatic patients with high-grade stenosis. N Engl J Med 1991; 325:445.

33. Barnett HJM et al. Prevention of ischemic stroke. Br Med J 1999;318:1539.

34. Biller J et al. Guidelines for carotid endarterectomy a statement for healthcare professionals from a special writing group of the Stroke Council, American Heart Association. Circulation 1998;97:501.

35. Levin RI et al. Aspirin inhibits vascular plasminogen activity in vivo. J Clin Invest 1984;74:571.

36. Bousser MG et al. "AICLA" controlled trial of aspiring and dipyridamole in the secondary prevention of Atherothrombotic cerebral ischemia. Stroke 1983;14:5.

37. Sorenson PS et al. Acetylsalicylic acid in the prevention of stroke in patients with reversible cerebral ischemic attacks. A Danish Cooperative Study. Stroke 1983;14:15.

38. Antiplatelet Trialists' Collaboration. Secondary prevention of vascular disease by prolonged antiplatelet treatment. Br Med J (Clin Res Ed) 1988; 290:320.

39. Swedish Cooperative Study. High-dose acetylsalicylic acid after cerebral infarction. Stroke 1987;18:325.

40. UK-TIA Study Group. The United Kingdom transient ischemic attack (UK-TIA) aspirin trial: final results. J Neurol Neurosurg Psychiatry 1991;54:1044.

41. Hiroyasu I et al. Prospective study of aspirin use and risk of stroke in women. Stroke 1999;30:1764.

42. Sivenius J et al. Antiplatelet therapy is effective in the prevention of stroke or death in women: subgroup analysis of the European Stroke Prevention Study (ESPS). Acta Neurol Scand 1991;84:286.

43. Bernstein EF et al. Life expectancy and late stroke following carotid endarterectomy. Ann Surg 1983;198:80.

44. Harker LA et al. Failure of aspirin plus dipyridamole to prevent restenosis after carotid endarterectomy. Ann Intern Med 1992;116:731.

45. Bhatt DL et al. Dual antiplatelet therapy with clopidogrel and aspirin after carotid artery stenting. J Invasive Cardiol 2001;13:767.

46. Steering Committee of the Physicians' Health Study Research Group. Final report on the aspirin component of the ongoing physicians' health study. N Engl J Med 1989;321:129.

47. Chen ZM et al. Indications for early aspirin use in acute ischemic stroke: a combined analysis of 40 000 randomized patients from the Chinese acute stroke trial and the international stroke trial. On behalf of the CAST and IST collaborative groups. Stroke 2000;31:1240.

48. The Dutch TIA Trial Study Group. A comparison of two doses of aspirin (30 mg versus 283 mg a day) in patients after a transient ischemic attack or minor ischemic stroke. N Engl J Med 1991;325:1261.

49. The SALT Collaborative. Swedish aspirin low-dose trial (SALT) of 75 mg aspirin as secondary prophylaxis after cerebrovascular ischemic events. Lancet 1991;338:1345.

50. Helgason CM et al. Aspirin response and failure in cerebral infarction. Stroke 1993;24:345.

51. Antiplatelet Trialists' Collaboration. Collaborative overview of randomized trials of antiplatelet therapyI: prevention of death, myocardial infarction, and stroke by antiplatelet therapy in various categories of patients. Br Med J 1994;308:83.

52. Johnson ES et al. A meta-regression analysis of dose-response effect of aspirin in stroke. Arch Intern Med 1999;159:1258.

53. Diener HC et al. European stroke prevention study 2. dipyridamole and acetylsalicylic acid in the secondary prevention of stroke. J Neurol Sci 1996;143:1.

54. Gent M et al. The Canadian-American ticlopidine study (CATS) in thromboembolic stroke. Lancet 1989;2:1215.

55. Hass WK et al. A randomized trial comparing ticlopidine hydrochloride with aspirin for the prevention of stroke in high risk patients. N Engl J Med 1989;321:501.

56. Weisburg LA et al. The efficacy and safety of ticlopidine and aspirin in non-whites: analysis of a patient subgroup from the ticlopidine aspirin stroke study. Neurology 1993;43:27.

57. Gorelick PB, et al. Aspirin and ticlopidine for prevention of recurrent stroke in black patients: a randomized trial, JAMA 2003;289:3005.

58. Barnett HJM et al. Prevention of ischemic stroke [letter]. N Engl J Med 1995;333:460.

59. Bennett CL, et al. Thrombotic thrombocytopenia purpura associated with ticlopidine. Ann Intern Med 1998;128:541.

60. CAPRIE Steering Committee. A randomized, blinded, trial of clopidogrel versus aspirin in patients at risk of ischaemic events (CAPRIE). Lancet 1996;348:1329.

61. The Stroke Prevention in Reversible Ischemia Trial (SPIRIT) Study Group. A randomized trial of anticoagulants versus aspirin after cerebral ischemia of presumed arterial origin. Ann Neurol 1997;42:857.

62. Mohr JP et al. A comparison of warfarin and aspirin for the prevention of recurrent ischemic stroke. N Engl J Med 2001;345:1444.

63. Powers WJ. Oral anticoagulant therapy for the prevention of stroke. N Engl J Med 2001;345:1493.

64. Albers GW et al. Antithrombotic and thrombolytic therapy for ischemic stroke. Circulation 2001; 119(Suppl):300S.

65. Stroke Prevention in Atrial Fibrillation Study Group Investigators. The Stroke Prevention in Atrial Fibrillation Study: patient characteristics and final results. Circulation 1991;84:527.

66. Peterson P et al. Placebo-controlled, randomized trial of warfarin and aspirin for prevention of thromboembolic complications in chronic atrial fibrillation: the Copenhagen AFASAK study. Lancet 1989;1:175.

67. The Boston Area Anticoagulation Trial for Atrial Fibrillation Investigators. The effect of low-dose warfarin on the risk of stroke in patients with non-rheumatic atrial fibrillation. N Engl J Med 1990; 323:1505.

68. Connolly SJ et al. Canadian atrial fibrillation anticoagulation (CAFA) study. J Am Coll Cardiol 1991;18:349.

69. Stroke Prevention in Atrial Fibrillation Investigators. Warfarin versus aspirin for prevention of thromboembolism in atrial fibrillation: Stroke Prevention in Atrial Fibrillation II study. Lancet 1994;343:687.

70. Atrial Fibrillation Investigators. Risk factors for stroke and efficacy of antithrombotic in atrial fibrillation. Arch Intern Med 1994;154:1449.

71. Ferrari E et al. Atherosclerosis of the thoracic aorta and aortic debris as a marker of poor prognosis: benefit of oral anticoagulants. J Am Coll Cardiol 1999;33:1317.

72. Orgera MA et al. Secondary prevention of cerebral ischemia in patent foramen ovale: systematic review and meta-analysis. South Med J 2001; 94:699.

73. Kagansky N et al. The role of hyperglycemia in acute stroke. Arch Neurol 2001;58:1209.

74. Brott T et al. Hypertension and its treatment in the NINDS rt-PA stroke trial. Stroke 1998;29:1504.

75. Tilley BC et al. Total quality improvement method for reduction of delays between emergency department admission and treatment of ischemic stroke. Arch Neurol 1997;54:1466.

76. Indredavik B et al. Stroke unit care improved survival and function for 5 years after an acute stroke. Stroke 1997;28:1861.

77. Duke RJ et al. Intravenous heparin for the prevention of stroke progression in acute partial stable stroke. Ann Intern Med 1986;105:825.

78. International Stroke Trial Collaboration Group. The International Stroke Trial (IST): a randomized trial of aspirin, subcutaneous heparin, both or neither among 19435 patients with acute stroke. Lancet 1997;349:1569.

79. Kay R et al. Low molecular weight heparin for the treatment of acute ischemic stroke. N Engl J Med 1995;333:1588.

80. The Publications Committee for the Trial of ORG 10172 in Acute Stroke Treatment (TOAST) Investigators. Low molecular weight heparinoid, ORG 10172 (danaparoid), and outcome after acute ischemic stroke: a randomized controlled trial. JAMA 1998;279:1265.

81. Berge E et al. Low molecular-weight heparin versus aspirin in patients with acute ischaemic stroke and atrial fibrillation: a double-blind randomised study. HAEST Study Group. Heparin in Acute Embolic Stroke Trial. Lancet 2000;355:1205.

82. Diener HC et al. Treatment of acute ischemic stroke with the low-molecular-weight heparin certoparin: results of the TOPAS trial. Therapy of Patients With Acute Stroke (TOPAS) Investigators. Stroke 2001;32:22.

83. CAST (Chinese Acute Stroke Trial) Collaboration Group. CAST: randomized placebo-controlled trial of early aspirin use in 20,000 patients with acute ischaemic stroke. Lancet 1997;349:1641.

84. Multicentre Acute Stroke Trial-Italy (MAST-I) Group. Randomised controlled trial of streptokinase, aspirin, and combination of both in treatment of acute ischaemic stroke. Lancet 1995;346:1509.

85. The Abciximab in Ischemic Stroke Investigators. Abciximab in acute ischemic stroke: a randomized, double-blind, placebo-controlled, dose-escalation study. The Abciximab in Ischemic Stroke Investigators. Stroke 2000;31:601.

86. Kobayashi S et al. Effect of the thrombin inhibitor argatroban in acute cerebral thrombosis. Semin Thromb Hemost 1997;23:531.

87. Sherman DG et al. Intravenous ancrod for treatment of acute ischemic stroke: the STAT study: a randomized controlled trial. JAMA 2000;283:2395.

88. Coull BM et al. Anticoagulants and antiplatelet agents in acute ischemic stroke report of the Joint Stroke Guideline Development Committee of the American Academy of Neurology and the American Stroke Association (a division of the American Heart Association). Neurology 59;2002:13.

89. Solis OJ et al. Cerebral angiography in acute cerebral infarction. Rev Interam Radiol 1977;2:19.

90. Symon L et al. The concept of thresholds of ischaemia in relation to brin structure and function. J Clin Pathol Suppl (R Coll Pathol) 1977;30(Suppl II):149.

91. Sharbrough FW et al. Correlation of continuous electroencephalograms with cerebral blood flow measurements during carotid endarterectomy. Stroke 1973;4:674.

92. Sundt TM Jr et al. Restoration of middle cerebral artery flow in experimental infarction. J Neurosurg 1969;31:311.

93. The Multicenter Acute Stroke Trial-Europe Study Group. Thrombolytic therapy with streptokinase in acute ischemic stroke. N Engl J Med 1996; 335:145.

94. Donnan GA et al. Streptokinase for acute ischemic stroke with relationship to time of administration. JAMA 1996;276:961.

95. The National Institute of Neurological Disorders and Stroke rt-PA Stroke Study Group. Tissue plasminogen activator for acute ischemic stroke. N Engl J Med 1995;333:1581.

96. Hacke W et al. Intravenous thrombolysis with recombinant tissue plasminogen activator for acute hemispheric stroke. JAMA 1995;274:1017.

97. Hacke W et al. Randomised double-blind placebo-controlled trial of thrombolytic therapy with intravenous alteplase in acute ischemic stroke. Lancet 1998;352:1245.

98. Clark WM et al. Recombinant tissue-type plasminogen activator (alteplase) for ischemic stroke 3 to 5 hours after symptom onset. JAMA 1999; 282:2019.

99. Wardlaw JM et al., Thrombolysis for acute ischaemic stroke (Cochrane review). In: The Cochrane Library, Issue 2, 2003. Oxford: Update Software.

100. Del Zoppo GJ et al. PROACT: a phase II randomized trial of recombinant pro-urokinase by direct arterial delivery in acute middle cerebral artery stroke. Stroke 1998;29:4.

101. Furlan A et al. Intra-arterial prourokinase for acute ischemic stroke. JAMA 1999;282:2003.

102. Scandinavian Stroke Study Group. Multicenter trial of hemodilution in acute ischemic stroke. Stroke 1987;18:691.

103. Strand T et al. A randomized controlled trial of hemodilution therapy in acute ischemic stroke. Stroke 1984;15:980.

104. Aichner FT et al. Hypervolemic hemodilution in acute ischemic stroke. Stroke 1998;29:743.

105. Bauer RB et al. Dexamethasone as treatment in cerebrovascular disease. A controlled study in acute cerebral infarction. Stroke 1973;4:547.

106. Norris JW. Steroid therapy in acute cerebral infarction. Arch Neurol 1976;33:69.

107. Dyken M et al. Evaluation of cortisone in the treatment of cerebral infarction. JAMA 1956;162:1531.

108. Mulley G et al. Dexamethasone in acute stroke. Br Med J 1978;2:994.

109. Norris JW et al. High-dose steroid treatment in cerebral infarction. Br Med J (Clin Res) 1986; 292:21.

110. Poungvarin N et al. Effects of dexamethasone in primary supratentorial intracerebral hemorrhage. N Engl J Med 1987;315:1229.

111. Gelmers HJ et al. A controlled trial of nimodipine in acute ischemic stroke. N Engl J Med 1988; 318:203.

112. TRUST Study Group. Randomized, double-blind, placebo-controlled trial of nimodipine in acute stroke. Lancet 1990;336:1205.

113. Kaster M et al. A randomized, double-blind, placebo-controlled trial of nimodipine in acute ischemic stroke. Stroke 1994;25:1348.

114. Mohr J et al. Meta-analysis of oral nimodipine in acute ischemic stroke. Cerebrovasc Dis 1994; 4:197.

115. Horn J et al. Calcium antagonists for ischemic stroke: a systematic review. Stroke 2001;32:570.

116. Ovbiagele B et al. Neuroprotective agents for the treatment of acute ischemic stroke. Curr Neurol Neurosci Rep 2003;3:9.

117. Robinson RG. Treatment issues in poststroke depression. Depress Anxiety 1998;8:85.

118. Vermeulen M et al. Antifibrinolytic treatment in subarachnoid hemorrhage. N Engl J Med 1984; 311:432.

119. Adams HP et al. Antifibrinolytic therapy in patients with aneurysmal subarachnoid hemorrhage: a report of the cooperative aneurysmal study. Arch Neurol 1981;38:25.

120. Baystone R et al. Intraventricular vancomycin in the treatment of ventriculitis associated with cerebrospinal fluid shunting and drainage. J Neurol Neurosurg Psychiatry 1987;50:1419.

121. Kassell NJ et al. Treatment of ischemic deficits from vasospasms with intravascular volume expansion and induced arterial hypertension. Neurosurgery 1982;11:337.

122. Kosnik EJ et al. Postoperative hypertension in the management of patients with intracranial arterial hypertension. J Neurosurg 1976;45:148.

123. Awad IA et al. Clinical vasospasm after subarachnoid hemorrhage: response to hypervolemic hemodilution and arterial hypertension. Stroke 1987;18:365.

124. Otsubo H et al. Normovolemic induced hypertension therapy for cerebral vasospasm after subarachnoid hemorrhage. Acta Neurochi (Wien) 1990;103:18.

125. Allen GS et al. Cerebral arterial spasm-a controlled trial of nimodipine in patients with subarachnoid hemorrhage. N Engl J Med 1983; 308:619.

126. Petruk KC et al. Nimodipine treatment in poor-grade aneurysm patients-results of a multicenter double-blind placebo-controlled trial. J Neurosurg 1988;68:505.

127. Phillippon J et al. Prevention of vasospasm in subarachnoid hemorrhage: a controlled study with nimodipine. Acta Neurochir (Wien) 1986;82:110.

128. Pickard JD et al. Effect of oral nimodipine on cerebral infarction and outcome after subarachnoid hemorrhage: British Aneurysm Nimodipine Trial. Br Med J (Clin Res Ed) 1989;289:636.

INFECTIOUS DISORDERS

B. Joseph Guglielmo
SECTION EDITOR

CHAPTER **56**

Principles of Infectious Diseases

B. Joseph Guglielmo

APPROACHING THE PROBLEM

The proper selection of antimicrobial therapy is based on several factors. However, before initiating therapy, it is important first to clearly establish the presence of an infectious process because several disease states (e.g., malignancy, autoimmune disease) and drugs can mimic infection. Once infection has been documented, the most likely site of infection must be identified. Signs and symptoms (e.g., erythema associated with cellulitis) direct the clinician to the likely source. Because certain pathogens are known to be associated with a specific site of infection, therapy often can be directed against these organisms. Additional laboratory tests, including the Gram's stain, serology, and antimicrobial susceptibility testing, generally identify the primary pathogen. Although several antimicrobials potentially can be considered, their spectrum of activity, clinical efficacy, adverse effect profile, pharmacokinetic disposition, and cost considerations ultimately guide the choice of therapy. Once an agent has been selected, the dosage must be based on the size of the patient, site of infection, route of elimination, and other factors.

ESTABLISHING THE PRESENCE OF AN INFECTION

1. **R.G., a 63-year-old man in the intensive care unit, underwent emergency resection of his large bowel. He has been intubated throughout his postoperative course. On day 20 of his hospital stay, R.G. suddenly becomes confused; his blood pressure (BP) drops to 70/30 mm Hg, with a heart rate of 130 beats/min. His extremities are cold to the touch, and he presents with circumoral pallor. His temperature increases to 40°C (axillary) and his respiratory rate is 24 breaths/min. Copious amounts of yellow-green secretions are suctioned from his endotracheal tube.**

Physical examination reveals sinus tachycardia with no rubs or murmurs. Rhonchi with decreased breath sounds are observed on auscultation. The abdomen is distended and R.G. complains of new abdominal pain. No bowel sounds can be heard and the stool is guaiac positive. Urine output from the Foley catheter has been 10 mL/hr for the past 2 hours. Erythema is noted around the central venous catheter.

A chest radiograph reveals bilateral lower lobe infiltrates, and urinalysis reveals >50 white blood cells/high-power field

(WBCs/HPF), few casts, and a specific gravity of 1.015. Blood, tracheal aspirate, and urine cultures are pending. Other laboratory values include sodium (Na), 131 mEq/L (normal, 135 to 147); potassium (K), 4.1 mEq/L (normal, 3.5 to 5); chloride (Cl), 110 mEq/L (normal, 95 to 105); CO_2, 16 mEq/L; blood urea nitrogen (BUN), 58 mg/dL (normal, 8 to 18); creatinine, 3.8 mg/dL (increased from 0.9 mg/dL at admission) (normal, 0.6 to 1.2); glucose 320 mg/dL (normal, 70 to 110); serum albumin, 2.1 g/dL (normal, 4 to 6); hemoglobin (Hgb), 10.3 g/dL; hematocrit (Hct), 33% (normal, 39% to 49% [males]); WBC count, 15,600/mm³ with bands present; platelets, 40,000/mm³ (normal, 130,000 to 400,000); prothrombin time (PT), 18 seconds (normal, 10 to 12); erythrocyte sedimentation rate (ESR), 65 mm/hr (normal, 0 to 20). Which of R.G.'s signs and symptoms are consistent with infection?

[SI units: Na, 131 mmol/L; K, 4.1 mmol/L; Cl, 110 mmol/L; CO_2, 16 mmol/L; BUN, 20.71 mmol/L of urea; creatinine, 335.92 and 7.56 mmol/L, respectively; glucose, 17.76 mmol/L; albumin, 235.62 mmol/L; Hgb, 103 g/L; Hct, 0.33; WBC, 15.6 ×10⁹; platelets, 40 ×10⁹; ESR 65 mm/hr]

R.G. has numerous signs and symptoms consistent with an infectious process. He has both an increased WBC count (15,600/mm³) and a "shift to the left" (bands are present on the differential). An increased WBC count commonly is observed with infection, particularly with bacterial pathogens. The WBC differential in patients with a bacterial infection often demonstrates a shift to the left (i.e., presence of immature neutrophils), suggesting that the bone marrow is responding to an infectious insult. However, infection is not always associated with leukocytosis. Overwhelming sepsis can cause a decreased WBC count; some patients become neutropenic secondary to infection. In less acute infection (e.g., subacute bacterial endocarditis, abscesses), the WBC count may remain within the normal range. Because the abscess is a localized lesion, less bone marrow response would be anticipated; thus, the WBC count may not increase in these patients.

R.G.'s temperature is 40°C by axillary measurement. Fever is a common manifestation of infection, with oral temperatures generally >38°C. Oral and axillary temperatures tend to be approximately 0.4°C lower compared with rectal measurement.[1] As a result, R.G.'s temperature would be expected to be 40.4°C if his temperature had been taken rectally. In general, rectal measurement of temperature is a more reliable determination of fever. Some patients with overwhelming infection, however, may present with hypothermia and temperatures <36°C. Furthermore, patients with localized infections (e.g., uncomplicated urinary tract infection, chronic abscesses) may be afebrile.

The bilateral lower lobe infiltrates on R.G.'s chest radiograph, the presence of copious amounts of yellow-green secretions from his endotracheal tube, and the erythema surrounding his central venous catheter also are compatible with an infectious process. Furthermore, R.G. has the following signs and symptoms that also are consistent with sepsis.

ESTABLISHING THE SEVERITY OF AN INFECTION

2. What signs and symptoms manifested by R.G. are consistent with a serious systemic infection?

The term *sepsis* is used to describe a poorly defined syndrome; however, sepsis generally suggests more systemic infection associated with the presence of pathogenic microorganisms or their toxins in the blood. A uniform system for defining the spectrum of disorders associated with sepsis has been established.[2]

The pathogenesis of sepsis is complex (Fig. 56-1) and only partially understood.[2-4] Gram-negative aerobes produce endo-

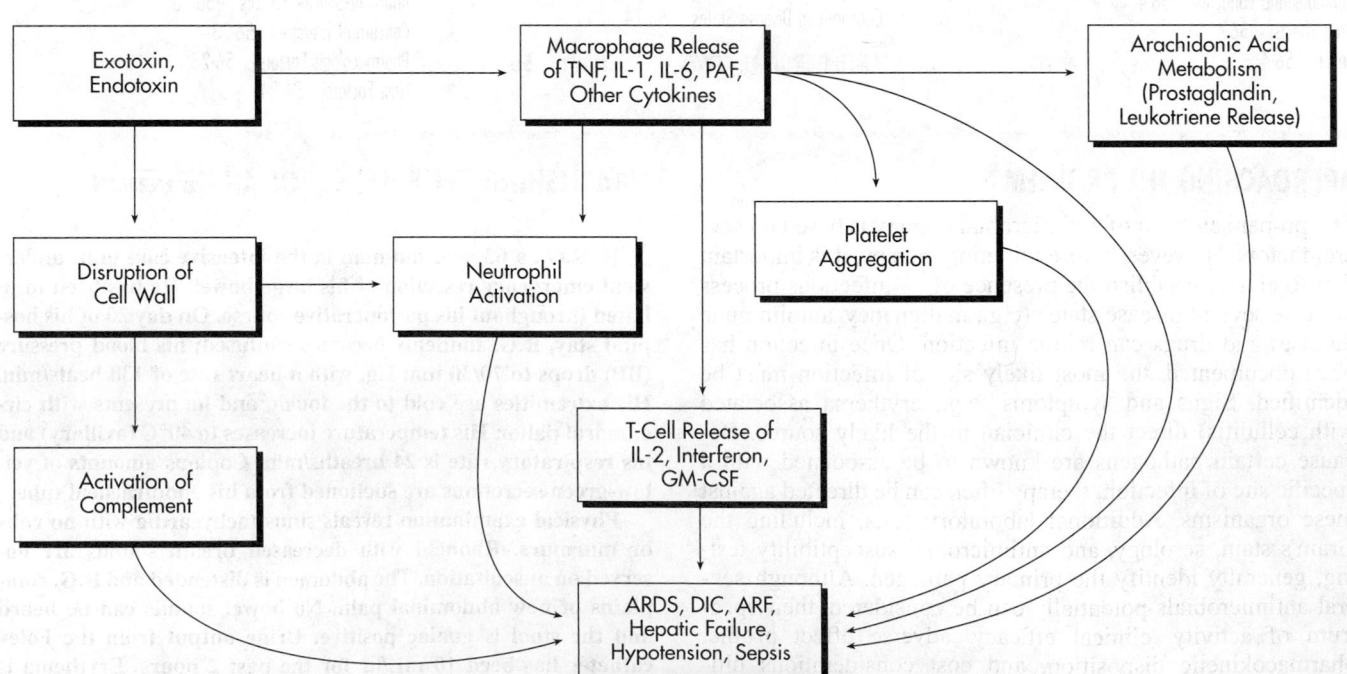

FIGURE 56-1. The sepsis cascade. ARDS, acute respiratory distress syndrome; ARF, acute renal failure; DIC, disseminated intravascular coagulation; GM-CSF, granulocyte–macrophage colony-stimulating factor; IL-1, interleukin-1; IL-6, interleukin-6; PAF, platelet activating factor; TNF, tumor necrosis factor.

toxin that results in a cascade of endogenous mediator release, including tumor necrosis factor (TNF), interleukin-1 (IL-1) and interleukin-6 (IL-6), platelet activating factor (PAF), and various other substances, from mononuclear phagocytes and other cells. Although this initial stimulus commonly is associated with Gram-negative endotoxin, other substances, including Gram-positive exotoxin and fungal cell wall constituents, also may be associated with cytokine release. After release of TNF, IL-1, and PAF, arachidonic acid is metabolized to form leukotrienes, thromboxane A_2, and prostaglandins, particularly prostaglandin E_2 and prostaglandin I_2. IL-1 and IL-6 activate the T cells to produce interferon, IL-2, IL-4, and granulocyte–macrophage colony-stimulating factor (GM-CSF). Increased endothelial permeability ensues. Subsequently, the endothelium releases two hemodynamically active substances: endothelium-derived relaxing factor (EDRF) and endothelin-1. Activation of the complement cascade (fragments C3a and C5a) follows with additional vascular abnormalities and neutrophil activation. Other potentially important agents in this cascade include adhesion molecules, kinins, thrombin, myocardial depressant substance, β-endorphin, and heat shock protein. The net result of this cascade is several hemodynamic, renal, acid–base, and other disorders. More recently, sepsis has been suggested to be primarily a disorder due to uncontrolled inflammation and coagulation.[4]

Hemodynamic Changes

Critically ill patients often have central intravenous (IV) lines in place for measuring cardiac output and systemic vascular resistance (SVR). A normal SVR of 800 to 1,200 dyne·sec·cm^{-5} may fall to 500 to 600 dyne·sec·cm^{-5} with septic shock because of intense vasodilation. In response to this vasodilation, the heart reflexively increases cardiac output from its normal 4 to 6 L/min to as much as 11 to 12 L/min in septic patients. This increase in cardiac output primarily is due to an increased heart rate; stroke volume is unchanged or decreased because of the hypovolemic state. Although the heart rate is increased on the basis of reflex tachycardia, a chronotropic response also takes place as a result of stress-induced catecholamine release (norepinephrine, epinephrine). Thus, the cardiac output increases in response to arterial vasodilation; however, this increase generally is insufficient to overcome the vasodilatory state, and hypotension ensues. In overwhelming septic shock, myocardial depression results in a decreased cardiac output. The combination of decreased cardiac output and decreased SVR result in hypotension unresponsive to pressors and IV fluids. R.G. has hemodynamic evidence of septic shock. He is hypotensive (BP 70/30 mm Hg) and tachycardic (130 beats/min), presumably in response to significant vasodilation and catecholamine release.

Although vasodilation commonly occurs in sepsis, hemodynamic changes are not equal throughout the vasculature. Some vascular beds constrict, resulting in maldistribution of blood flow. Significant amounts of blood are shunted away from the kidneys, mesentery, and extremities.

Normal urine output of approximately 0.5 to 1.0 mL/kg per hour (30 to 70 mL/hour for a 70-kg patient) can decrease to <20 mL/hour in sepsis. The urine output for R.G. has decreased to 10 mL/hour, consistent with sepsis-induced perfusion abnormalities. Decreased blood flow to the kidney as well

as mediator-induced microvascular failure can cause acute tubular necrosis (ATN). R.G.'s uremia (BUN 58 mg/dL) and increased serum creatinine concentration (3.8 mg/dL) are consistent with decreased renal perfusion secondary to sepsis. When sepsis has progressed to septic shock, blood flow to most major organs is decreased. Decreased blood flow to the liver may result in "shock liver," in which liver function tests, including alanine aminotransferase (ALT), aspartate aminotransferase (AST), and alkaline phosphatase, become elevated. The liver function tests for R.G. are not available; however, his serum albumin concentration is low (2.1 g/dL) and his PT of 18 seconds is prolonged. Decreased blood flow to the musculature classically is characterized by cool extremities, and decreased blood flow to the brain can result in decreased mentation. R.G. is confused, his extremities are cold, and the area around his mouth appears pale. All these signs and symptoms provide strong evidence that he is in septic shock.

Cellular Changes

The sepsis syndrome is associated with significant abnormalities in cellular metabolism. Glucose intolerance commonly is observed in sepsis, and patients with previously normal blood glucose levels may experience sudden increases in blood sugar. In some cases, an increase in glucose is one of the first signs of an infectious process. R.G.'s increased blood glucose concentration (320 mg/dL) is, therefore, consistent with sepsis. Another sensitive indicator of sepsis-associated inflammation is the ESR, a nonspecific test that is commonly elevated in various inflammatory states, including infection. The ESR can be used to determine the progression of infection; currently, R.G.'s ESR is elevated at 65 mm/hour. With appropriate management of infection, the ESR would be expected to decrease; inadequate treatment would be associated with persistent elevation of the ESR.

Respiratory Changes

Production of organic acids, such as lactate, increased glycolysis, decreased fractional extraction of oxygen, and abnormal delivery-dependent oxygen consumption are observed.[4] This increase in lactic acid results in metabolic acidosis, with accompanying decreased serum bicarbonate levels. The lungs normally respond in a compensatory manner with an increased respiratory rate (tachypnea), resulting in an increased elimination of arterial carbon dioxide. R.G.'s acid–base status is consistent with sepsis-associated metabolic acidosis (CO_2 16 mEq/L) and compensatory respiratory alkalosis (respiratory rate 24/min).

While not currently present in R.G., a late complication of the above-mentioned sepsis cascade is acute respiratory distress syndrome (ARDS). ARDS initially was described as noncardiogenic pulmonary edema with severe hypoxemia caused by right-to-left intrapulmonary shunting resulting from atelectasis and edema-filled alveoli. The primary pathophysiology of ARDS is a breakdown in the natural integrity of the alveolar capillary network in the lung.[5] In the early phase of ARDS, patients have severe alveolar edema with large numbers of inflammatory cells, primarily neutrophils. The chronic phase of ARDS (10 to 14 days after development of the syndrome) is associated with significant lung destruction. Emphysema, pulmonary vascular obliteration, and fibrosis commonly are observed. Severe ARDS is associated with arterial oxygen level/fraction of inspired oxygen (PaO_2/FiO_2) ratios of <100, low lung compliance, a need for high positive end-expiratory pressure (PEEP), and other respiratory maneuvers. At present the treatment for this syndrome primarily is supportive, including mechanical ventilation, high inspired oxygen, and PEEP. If patients fail to show improved gas exchange by day 7, the mortality associated with ARDS is high (>80%).[6] While R.G. currently does not have ARDS, the severity of his septic episode strongly suggests he may develop this complication in the next few days.

Hematologic Changes

Disseminated intravascular coagulation (DIC) is a well-recognized sequela of sepsis. Huge quantities of clotting factors and platelets are consumed in DIC as widespread clotting takes place throughout the circulatory system. As a result, the PT and the activated partial thromboplastin time (aPTT) are prolonged and the platelet count commonly is decreased in sepsis. Decreased fibrinogen levels and increased fibrin split products generally are diagnostic for DIC. The PT of 18 seconds and the decreased platelet count of 40,000/mm³ in R.G. are consistent with sepsis-induced DIC.

Neurologic Changes

Central nervous system (CNS) changes, including lethargy, disorientation, confusion, and psychosis, predominate in sepsis. Altered mental status is well recognized as a symptom associated with infections of the CNS, such as meningitis and brain abscess. However, these changes also are common with other sites of sepsis. On day 20 of his hospital stay, R.G. suddenly became confused, his BP dropped, and his heart rate increased. Thus, R.G.'s CNS effects as well as his hematologic, respiratory, hemodynamic, and cellular effects all provide substantial evidence of septic shock.

PROBLEMS IN THE DIAGNOSIS OF AN INFECTION

3. his past medical history, R.G. is noted to have a history of temporal arteritis and seizures chronically treated with corticosteroids and phenytoin. Perioperative "stress doses" of hydrocortisone recently were administered because of his surgical procedure. What medications or disease states confuse the diagnosis of infection?

Confabulating Variables

Various factors, including major surgery, acute myocardial infarction, and initiation of corticosteroid therapy are associated with an increased WBC count. However, unlike infection, a shift to the left does not occur with these disease states. In R.G. the stress dose of hydrocortisone and his recent surgical procedure might have contributed to the increased WBC count. The presence of bands in R.G., however, strongly suggests an infectious process.

Drug Effects

The ability of corticosteroids to mimic or mask infection is noteworthy. Corticosteroids are associated with an increased WBC count and glucose intolerance when therapy is initiated or when doses are increased. Furthermore, some patients experience corticosteroid-induced mental status changes that may complicate the diagnosis of a septic infection. Although corticosteroids mimic infection, they also have the ability to mask infection. Bowel perforation in a patient with ulcerative colitis would result in significant peritoneal contamination. However, concomitant corticosteroids, because of their potent anti-inflammatory effects, may reduce the classic findings of peritonitis. Furthermore, corticosteroids can reduce and sometimes ablate the febrile response. Thus, these corticosteroid-treated patients may be asymptomatic but at great risk for Gram-negative septic shock.

Another example of the influence of corticosteroids on the diagnosis of infection relates to neurosurgical procedures. Dexamethasone is a corticosteroid commonly used to reduce the inflammation and swelling associated with neurosurgical procedures. Certain neurosurgical procedures are associated with significant trauma to the meninges; however, the patient often is asymptomatic while receiving high-dose dexamethasone. When the dexamethasone dose is decreased, the patient subsequently may experience classic meningismus, including stiff neck, photophobia, and headache. The lumbar puncture may demonstrate cloudy cerebrospinal fluid (CSF), an elevated WBC count, high CSF protein, and low CSF glucose. Although the signs and symptoms are consistent with infectious meningitis, this disease state is considered aseptic meningitis (i.e., inflammation of the meninges without an infectious origin).[7] Certain drugs may cause aseptic meningitis, including OKT3,[8] nonsteroidal anti-inflammatory agents, and sulfonamides.

Fever

Fever also is consistent with autoimmune diseases, such as lupus erythematosus and temporal arteritis.[9,10] Neoplasms, such as leukemia and lymphoma, also may present with low-grade fevers, similar to those observed in an infectious process. One evaluation of fever of unknown origin (FUO) in community hospitals demonstrated a 25% incidence of FUO caused by cancer.[10] Other diseases associated with fever include sarcoidosis, chronic liver disease, and familial Mediterranean fever. Acute myocardial infarction, pulmonary embolism, and postoperative pulmonary atelectasis are commonly associated with an elevated temperature. Factitious fever or self-induced disease must be considered in certain patients. After infection, autoimmune disease, and malignancy have been ruled out, drug fever should be considered. Drugs, including certain antimicrobials (e.g., amphotericin B) and phenytoin, have been associated with drug fever. Drug fever generally occurs after 7 to 10 days of therapy and resolves within 48 hours of the drug's discontinuation.[11] Some clinicians claim that patients with drug fever generally feel "well" and are unaware of their fever. Rechallenge with the offending agent usually results in recurrence of fever within hours of administration. However, drug fever should be considered a diagnosis of exclusion and should be considered only after eliminating the presence of other disease states (also see Chapter 4, Anaphylaxis and Drug Allergies).

Neoplasms may be radiographically indistinguishable from an abscess. An example of this dilemma is the differential diagnosis of toxoplasmosis versus lymphoma in HIV patients with brain lesions documented by a computed axial tomography scan. One method for diagnosis is to use empiric therapy against *Toxoplasma gondii*. If the lesions are unresponsive to therapy, the presumptive diagnosis of malignancy can be made.

In summary, R.G. has an autoimmune disease, temporal arteritis, that has been associated with fever. Similarly, his corticosteroid administration and phenytoin use may confound the diagnosis of infection. His other signs and symptoms, however, strongly suggest that R.G.'s problems are of an infectious origin.

ESTABLISHING THE SITE OF THE INFECTION

4. What are the most likely sources of R.G.'s infection?

Independent of the presumed site of infection, a blood culture should be drawn to demonstrate the presence of bacteremia. After blood cultures are sampled, a thorough physical examination generally documents the source of infection. Urosepsis, the most common cause of nosocomial infection, may be associated with dysuria, flank pain, and abnormal urinalysis.[12] Tachypnea, increased sputum production, altered

chest radiograph, and hypoxemia may direct the clinician toward a pulmonary source. Evidence for an infected IV line would include pain, erythema, and purulent discharge around the IV catheter. Other potential sites of infection include the peritoneum, pelvis, bone, and CNS.

R.G. is demonstrating several possible sites of infection. The copious production of yellow-green sputum, tachypnea, and the altered chest radiograph suggest the presence of pneumonia. The abdominal pain, absent bowel sounds, and recent surgical procedure, however, require evaluation for an intra-abdominal source.[13] Lastly, the abnormal urinalysis (>50 WBC/HPF) and the erythema around the central venous catheter suggest other sites of infection.

DETERMINING LIKELY PATHOGENS

5. What are the most likely pathogens associated with R.G.'s infection(s)?

R.G. has several possible sources of infection. The suspected pathogens depend on the presumed site of infection. Table 56-1 provides a classification of infectious organisms

---

Table 56-1 Classification of Infectious Organisms

1. Bacteria

Aerobic

Gram-Positive
Cocci
  Streptococci: pneumococcus, viridans streptococci; group A streptococci
  Enterococcus
  Staphylococci: *Staphylococcus aureus, Staphylococcus epidermidis*
Rods (bacilli)
  Corynebacterium
  Listeria
Gram-Negative
Cocci
  Moraxella
  Neisseria (Neisseria meningitides, Neisseria gonorrhoeae)
Rods (bacilli)
  Enterobacteriaceae (*Escherichia coli, Klebsiella, Enterobacter, Citrobacter, Proteus, Serratia, Salmonella, Shigella, Morganella, Providencia*)
  Campylobacter
  Pseudomonas
  Helicobacter
  Haemophilus (coccobacilli morphology)
  Legionella

Anaerobic

Gram-Positive
Cocci
  Peptococcus
  Peptostreptococcus
Rods (bacilli)
  Clostridia (*Clostridium perfringens, Clostridium tetani, Clostridium difficile*)
  Propionibacterium acnes

Gram-Negative
Cocci
None
Rods (bacilli)
  Bacteroides (*Bacteroides fragilis, Bacteroides melaninogenicus*)
  Fusobacterium
  Prevotella

2. Fungi

Aspergillus, Candida, Coccidioides, Cryptococcus, Histoplasma, Mucor, Tinea, Trichophyton

3. Viruses

Influenza, hepatitis A, B, C, D, E; human immunodeficiency virus; rubella; herpes; cytomegalovirus; respiratory syncytial virus; Epstein-Barr virus, SARS virus

4. Chlamydiae

Chlamydia trachomatis
Chlamydia psittaci
Chlamydia pneumoniae (TWAR)
LGV ([lymphogranuloma venereum] disease caused by *Chlamydia trachomatis* of immunotype L1-L3)

5. Rickettsiae

Rocky Mountain spotted fever, Q fever
Ureaplasma

6. Mycoplasmas

Mycoplasma pneumoniae, Mycoplasma hominis

7. Spirochetes

Treponema pallidum, Borrelia burgdorferi (Lyme disease)

8. Mycobacteria

Mycobacterium tuberculosis
Mycobacterium avium intracellulare

(e.g., Gram-positive, Gram-negative, aerobic, anaerobic), and Table 56-2 lists the most likely organisms associated with sites of infection. Determining the most likely infectious agent depends not only on the site of infection but also on host factors. For example, bacterial pneumonia may be caused by various pathogens, including *Streptococcus pneumoniae*, Enterobacteriaceae, and atypical pathogens (e.g., *Legionella pneumophila*).[14] Empiric antimicrobial therapy directed against all the above organisms, however, is unnecessary. Several host factors must be evaluated to streamline therapy against the most likely pathogens. If the pneumonia is community acquired, *S. pneumoniae*, *Haemophilus influenzae*, *Moraxella catarrhalis*, and "atypical" bacterial pathogens may predominate.[15] However, in nosocomial (hospital, nursing home) pneumonia, Gram-negative enterics (e.g., *Escherichia coli*, *Klebsiella* species, *Enterobacter* species, and

---

Table 56-2   Site of Infection: Suspected Organisms

Site/Type of Infection	Suspected Organisms
1. Respiratory	
Pharyngitis	Viral, group A streptococci
Bronchitis, otitis	Viral, *Haemophilus influenzae*, *Streptococcus pneumoniae*, *Moraxella catarrhalis*
Acute sinusitis	Viral, *Streptococcus pneumoniae*, *Haemophilus influenzae*, *Moraxella catarrhalis*
Chronic sinusitis	*Anaerobes*, *Staphylococcus aureus* (as well as suspected organisms associated with acute sinusitis)
Epiglottitis	*Haemophilus influenzae*
Pneumonia	
Community-Acquired	
Normal host	*Streptococcus pneumoniae*, viral, mycoplasma
Aspiration	Normal aerobic and anaerobic mouth flora
Pediatrics	*Streptococcus pneumoniae*, *Haemophilus influenzae*
COAD	*Streptococcus pneumoniae*, *Haemophilus influenzae*, *Legionella*, *Chlamydia*, *Mycoplasma*
Alcoholic	*Streptococcus pneumoniae*, *Klebsiella*
Hospital-Acquired	
Aspiration	Mouth anaerobes, aerobic Gram-negative rods, *Staphylococcus aureus*
Neutropenic	Fungi, aerobic Gram-negative rods, *Staphylococcus aureus*
HIV	Fungi, *Pneumocystis*, *Legionella*, *Nocardia*, *Streptococcus pneumoniae*, *Pseudomonas*
2. Urinary Tract	
Community-Acquired	*Escherichia coli*, other Gram-negative rods, *Staphylococcus aureus*, *Staphylococcus epidermidis*, enterococci
Hospital-Acquired	Resistant aerobic Gram-negative rods, enterococci
3. Skin/Soft Tissue	
Cellulitis	Group A streptococci, *Staphylococcus aureus*
IV catheter site	*Staphylococcus aureus*, *Staphylococcus epidermidis*
Surgical wound	*Staphylococcus aureus*, Gram-negative rods
Diabetic ulcer	*Staphylococcus aureus*, Gram-negative aerobic rods, anaerobes
Furuncle	*Staphylococcus aureus*
4. Intra-Abdominal	*Bacteroides fragilis*, *Escherichia coli*, other aerobic Gram-negative rods, enterococci
5. Gastroenteritis	*Salmonella*, *Shigella*, *Helicobacter*, *Campylobacter*, *Clostridium difficile*, amoeba, Giardia, viral, enterotoxigenic-hemorrhagic *Escherichia coli*
6. Endocarditis	
Pre-existing valvular disease	*Streptococcus viridans*
IV drug abuser	*Staphylococcus aureus*, aerobic Gram-negative rods, enterococci, fungi
Prosthetic valve	*Staphylococcus epidermidis*
7. Osteomyelitis/Septic Arthritis	*Staphylococcus aureus*, aerobic Gram-negative rods
8. Meningitis	
<2 months	*Escherichia coli*, group B streptococci, *Listeria*
2 months–12 years	*Streptococcus pneumoniae*, *Neisseria meningitides*, *Haemophilus influenzae*
Adults	*Streptococcus pneumoniae*, *Neisseria meningitides*
Hospital-acquired	*Streptococcus pneumoniae*, *Neisseria meningitides*, aerobic Gram-negative rods
Postneurosurgery	*Staphylococcus aureus*, aerobic Gram-negative rods

COAD, chronic obstructive airways disease; IV, intravenous.

Pseudomonas aeruginosa) become more significant pathogens. If the pneumonia is a result of a gastric aspiration, mouth anaerobes should probably be covered empirically. In nosocomial pneumonia, knowledge of the hospital-specific flora is important. If *E. coli* is the most commonly isolated pathogen at a given institution, antimicrobials, such as first- or second-generation cephalosporins, can be used. If *P. aeruginosa* or *Enterobacter cloacae* predominates, then alternative, broader-spectrum therapy is necessary. A thorough evaluation of antimicrobial exposure also is necessary. Recent use of antimicrobials is more likely to result in infection due to resistant Gram-negative organisms.

The patient's age is also an important determinant in the epidemiology of infection. For example, meningitis in a neonate is commonly caused by group B streptococci, *E. coli,* and *Listeria monocytogenes,* whereas these bacteria are uncommon pathogens in normal adults. The presence of concomitant diseases, such as chronic obstructive airways disease (COAD) or alcohol and IV drug abuse, also can help determine the pathogen. For example, patients with COAD-associated pneumonia are more likely to be infected by *S. pneumoniae, H. influenzae,* and *M. catarrhalis.* Chronic alcoholics are more likely to have infection caused by enteric Gram-negative pathogens, such as *Klebsiella* species, compared with normal patients.

Immune status is an important predictor of likely pathogens. HIV-positive patients or those receiving cyclosporine and corticosteroids have lymphocyte deficiency–associated infections, including those caused by cytomegalovirus, *Pneumocystis carinii,* atypical mycobacteria, and *Cryptococcus neoformans.* Patients with leukemia and neutropenia are at risk for infection caused by aerobic Gram-negative bacilli, including *P. aeruginosa* and fungi.

In R.G., the abdomen, respiratory tract, urinary tract, and IV catheter are all potential sites of infection. Intra-abdominal infection is likely caused by Gram-negative enterics and *Bacteroides fragilis;* nosocomial urinary tract infection is usually secondary to aerobic Gram-negative rods. R.G.'s pneumonia possibly is caused by Gram-negative bacilli, staphylococci, and various other organisms. Furthermore, his use of corticosteroids may predispose him to infection due to more opportunistic organisms, including *Legionella, P. carinii,* and fungi. Lastly, his IV catheter infection suggests infection caused by staphylococci, including *Staphylococcus epidermidis* and *Staphylococcus aureus.*

MICROBIOLOGIC TESTS AND SUSCEPTIBILITY OF ORGANISMS

6. A Gram's stain of R.G.'s tracheal aspirate shows Gram-negative bacilli. What tests may assist with the identification of the pathogen(s)?

Once the site of infection has been determined and host defense and other epidemiologic factors have been evaluated, additional tests can be performed to identify the pathogen. Some tests that provide immediate information to guide selection of the initial antimicrobial regimen can be performed. The Gram's stain uses crystal violet solution and iodine, which results in bacteria staining Gram positive or Gram negative; some organisms are Gram variable. In addition, the shape of the organism (cocci, bacilli) is readily apparent with the use of the Gram's stain. Streptococci and staphylococci are Gram-positive cocci, whereas *E. coli, E. cloacae,* and *P. aeruginosa* appear as Gram-negative bacilli (see Table 56-1).[16] If the Gram's stain of the tracheal aspirate demonstrates Gram-positive cocci in clusters, empiric antistaphylococcal therapy is indicated. In contrast, if the Gram's stain shows Gram-negative rods, antimicrobials with activity against these pathogens are indicated.

Similar to the Gram's stain in bacterial infection, the India ink and potassium hydroxide (KOH) stains are helpful in the identification of certain fungi. The acid-fast bacilli (AFB) stain is critical in the diagnosis of infection caused by *Mycobacterium tuberculosis* or atypical mycobacteria.

In R.G., the Gram's stain suggests that antimicrobials active against Gram-negative bacilli should be used. Table 56-3 provides a classification of antibacterials (e.g., different generations of cephalosporins). Tables 56-4, 56-5, and 56-6 list in vitro susceptibilities of aerobic Gram-positive organisms, Gram-negative aerobes, and anaerobic organisms, respectively.

Culture and Susceptibility Testing

Culture and susceptibility testing provides final identification of the pathogen, as well as information regarding the effectiveness of various antimicrobials. Although these tests provide more information than the Gram's stain, they generally require 18 to 24 hours to complete. After the pathogen has been identified, Table 56-7 can be used in conjunction with an institution's specific susceptibility studies to select the most appropriate antimicrobial.

Disk Diffusion

The most widely used tests for bacterial susceptibility are the disk diffusion and the broth dilution methods. The disk diffusion (Kirby-Bauer) technique uses an agar plate on which an inoculum of the organism is placed. After inoculation, several antimicrobial-laden disks are placed on the plate, and evidence of bacterial growth is observed after 18 to 24 hours. If the antimicrobial is active against the pathogen, a zone of growth inhibition is observed around the disk. Based on guidelines provided by the National Committee for Clinical Laboratory Standards (NCCLS), the diameter of inhibition is reported as susceptible, intermediate, or resistant.

Broth Dilution

The broth dilution method involves placing a bacterial inoculum into several tubes or wells filled with broth. Serial dilutions of antimicrobials (e.g., nafcillin 0.5, 1.0, and 2.0 µg/mL) are placed in the respective wells. After bacteria are allowed to incubate for 18 to 24 hours, the wells are examined for bacterial growth. If the well is cloudy, bacterial growth has occurred, suggesting resistance to the antimicrobial at that concentration. As an example, if bacterial growth is observed with *S. aureus* at 0.5 µg/mL of nafcillin but not at 1.0 µg/mL, then 1.0 µg/mL would be considered the minimum inhibitory concentration (MIC) for nafcillin against *S. aureus.*

Similar to the disk diffusion method, the NCCLS provides guidelines[17] that also take into account the pharmacokinetic characteristics of an antimicrobial to determine whether the

Table 56-3   Classification of Antibacterials

β-Lactam Antibiotics

Cephalosporins

First-Generation
Cefadroxil (Duricef)
Cefazolin (Ancef)
Cephalexin (Keflex)
Cephalothin (Keflin)
Cephapirin (Cefadyl)
Cephradine (Anspor)
Second-Generation
Cefaclor (Ceclor)
Cefamandole (Mandol)
Cefmetazole (Zefazone)
Cefonicid (Monocid)
Ceforanide (Precef)
Cefotetan (Cefotan)
Cefoxitin (Mefoxin)
Cefprozil (Cefzil)
Cefuroxime (Zinacef)
Cefuroxime axetil (Ceftin)
Third-Generation
Cefdinir (Omnicef)
Cefditoren (Spectracef)
Cefixime (Suprax)
Cefoperazone (Cefobid)
Cefotaxime (Claforan)
Cefpodoxime proxetil (Vantin)
Ceftazidime (Fortaz)
Ceftibuten (Cedax)
Ceftizoxime (Cefizox)
Ceftriaxone (Rocephin)
Fourth-Generation
Cefepime (Maxipime)

Carbacephems

Loracarbef (Lorabid)

Monobactams

Aztreonam (Azactam)

Penems

Ertapenem (Invanz)
Imipenem (Primaxin)
Meropenem (Merem)

Penicillins

Natural Penicillins
Penicillin G
Penicillin V
Aminopenicillins
Ampicillin (Omnipen)
Amoxicillin (Amoxil)
Bacampicillin (Spectrobid)

β-Lactam Antibiotics

Penicillinase-Resistant Penicillins
Isoxazolyl penicillins (dicloxacillin, oxacillin, cloxacillin)
Nafcillin (Unipen)
Carboxypenicillins
Carbenicillin (Geocillin)
Ticarcillin (Ticar)
Ureidopenicillins
Piperacillin (Pipracil)
Combination with β-Lactamase Inhibitors
Augmentin (amoxicillin plus clavulanic acid)
Timentin (ticarcillin plus clavulanic acid)
Unasyn (ampicillin plus sulbactam)
Zosyn (piperacillin plus tazobactam)

Aminoglycosides

Amikacin (Amikin)
Gentamicin (Garamycin)
Neomycin (Mycifradin)
Netilmicin (Netromycin)
Streptomycin
Tobramycin (Nebcin)

Protein Synthesis Inhibitors

Azithromycin (Zithromax)
Clarithromycin (Biaxin)
Clindamycin (Cleocin)
Chloramphenicol (Chloromycetin)
Dalfopristin/Quinupristin (Synercid)
Dirithromycin (Dynabac)
Erythromycin (Erythrocin)
Linezolid (Zyvox)
Telithromycin (Ketek)
Tetracyclines (doxycycline, minocycline, tetracycline)

Folate Inhibitors

Sulfadiazine
Sulfadoxine (Fansidar)
Trimethoprim (Trimpex)
Trimethoprim-sulfamethoxazole (Bactrim, Septra)

Quinolones

Ciprofloxacin (Cipro)
Gatifloxacin (Tequin)
Gemifloxacin (Factive)
Levofloxacin (Levoquin)
Moxifloxacin (Avelox)
Norfloxacin (Noroxin)
Ofloxacin (Floxin)
Trovafloxacin (Trovan)

Daptomycin (Cidecin)

Vancomycin (Vancocin)

Metronidazole (Flagyl)

MIC should be reported as susceptible, moderately susceptible, or resistant. MIC interpretations are specific to both the organism and the antimicrobial. For example, ciprofloxacin achieves serum concentrations of 1 to 4 μg/mL and ceftriaxone achieves peak serum concentrations of 100 to 150 μg/mL; an MIC of 4 μg/mL for *E. coli* would be interpreted as resistant to ciprofloxacin and susceptible to ceftriaxone.

Although these tests provide an accurate assessment of in vitro susceptibility, the time delay (18 to 24 hours) can hinder streamlining of therapy. An alternative efficient but more ex-

Table 56-4   In Vitro Antimicrobial Susceptibility: Aerobic Gram-Positive Cocci

Drugs	Staphylococcus aureus	Staphylococcus aureus (MR)	Staphylococcus epidermidis	Staphylococcus epidermidis (MR)	Streptococci[a]	Enterococci[b]	Pneumococci
Ampicillin	+	−	+	−	++++	++	+++
Augmentin	++++	+	++++	−	++++	++	++++
Aztreonam	−	−	−	−	−	−	−
Cefazolin	++++	−	++++	−	++++	−	++
Cefepime	++++	−	++++	−	++++	−	+++
Cefoxitin/Cefotetan	++	−	++	−	++	−	+
Cefuroxime	++++	−	++++	−	++++	−	+++
Ciprofloxacin[c]	+++	++	+++	++	+	+	++
Clindamycin	++++	+	++++	+	+++	−	+++
Cotrimoxazole	++++	+++	++	+	++	+	+
Daptomycin[f]	++++	++++	++++	++++	++++	++++	++++
Erythromycin (azithromycin/ clarithromycin)	++	−	+	−	+++	−	++
Imipenem	++++	−	++++	−	++++	++	+++
Levofloxacin (gatifloxacin, gemifloxacin, moxifloxacin)	++++	++	+++	++	+++	++	++++
Linezolid[f]	++++	++++	++++	++++	++++	++++	++++
Nafcillin	++++	−	++++	−	++++	−	++
Penicillin	+	−	+	−	++++	++	+++
Quinupristin/dalfopristin[d,f]	++++	++++	++++	++++	++++	++++	++++
TGC[e]	+++	−	++	−	++++	−	+++
Ticarcillin	+	−	+	−	++++	+	+
Timentin	++++	−	++++	−	++++	+	+
Unasyn	++++	−	++++	−	++++	++	+++
Vancomycin	++++	++++	++++	++++	++++	+++	++++
Zosyn	++++	−	++++	−	++++	++	+++

[a]Nonpneumococcal streptococci.

[b]Usually requires combination therapy (e.g., ampicillin and an aminoglycoside) for serious infection.

[c]Levofloxacin (gatifloxacin, gemifloxacin, moxifloxacin) is more active than ciprofloxacin against staphylococci and streptococci.

[d]Active against *E. faecium* but unpredictable against *E. faecalis*.

[e]TGC = cefotaxime, ceftizoxime, ceftriaxone, cefoperazone. Ceftazidime has comparatively inferior antistaphylococcal and antipneumococcal activity. Cefotaxime and ceftriaxone are the most reliable cephalosporins versus *S. pneumoniae*.

[f]Active versus vancomycin-resistant *Enterococcus faecium*.

MR, methicillin resistant.

pensive MIC test is the E test, which uses an antibiotic-laden plastic strip with increasing concentration of a specific antimicrobial from one end to the other. The strip is placed on an agar plate with the actively growing pathogen. Inhibition of growth observed at specific marks on the strip coincide with the MIC of the organism. Numerous studies have confirmed that the E test is as effective as traditional susceptibility testing. Some rapid diagnosis culture and susceptibility tests may provide similar information within hours, potentially resulting in more rapid selection of appropriate antimicrobial therapy.

Although susceptibility testing is relatively well standardized for aerobic Gram-negative and Gram-positive organisms, its utility continues to evolve for anaerobes[18] and fungi.[19] In general, despite improvements in the standardization of testing in anaerobes and fungi, most institutions do not routinely perform susceptibility testing for anaerobes or fungi.

The consensus of the NCCLS and other experts is that anaerobic isolates from blood, bone, and joint sources, brain abscesses, empyemic fluid, and other body fluids that are normally sterile should be considered for susceptibility testing. Isolates from other sources should be considered for testing only if the physician believes the test is clearly indicated in the given patient.[18] Although progress has been made in developing a standardized test for determining fungal susceptibility, the primary emphasis has been on the susceptibility of *Candida* species and other yeasts to azoles in oropharyngeal candidiasis. Standardized susceptibility testing for molds recently has been established by the NCCLS.[19]

The MIC is the minimum concentration at which an antimicrobial inhibits the growth of the organism; the test does not provide information regarding whether the organism is actually killed. In some disease states (e.g., endocarditis, meningitis), bactericidal therapy may be necessary. The minimum bactericidal concentration (MBC) is the test that can be used to determine the killing activity associated with an antimicrobial. The MBC is determined by taking an aliquot from each clear MIC tube for subculture onto agar plates. The concentration at which no significant bacterial growth is observed on these plates is considered the MBC.

The serum bactericidal test (SBT) occasionally is used as an in vivo test of antimicrobial activity.[20] The test may have utility in assessing the treatment of more severe infections,

Table 56-5   In Vitro Antimicrobial Susceptibility: Gram-Negative Aerobes

Drugs	Escherichia coli	Klebsiella pneumoniae	Enterobacter cloacae	Proteus mirabilis	Serratia marcescens	Pseudomonas aeruginosa	Haemophilus influenzae	Haemophilus influenzae[b]
Ampicillin	++	—	—	+++	—	—	++++	
Augmentin	+++	++	—	++++	—	—	++++	++++
Aztreonam	++++	++++	+	++++	++++	++++	++++	++++
Cefazolin	+++	+++	—	++++	—	—	+	—
Cefepime	++++	++++	+++	++++	++++	++++	++++	++++
Cefoperazone	+++	+++	+	++++	++++	++	++++	++++
Ceftazidime	++++	++++	+	++++	++++	++++	++++	++++
Cefuroxime	+++	+++	—	++++	+	—	++++	++++
Cotrimoxazole	++	+++	+++	++++	+++	—	++++	++++
Ertepenem	++++	++++	++++	++++	++++	+	++++	++++
Gentamicin	++++	++++	++++	++++	++++	+++	++	++
Imipenem/ Meropenem	++++	++++	++++	+++	++++	++++	++++	++++
Piperacillin	++	+++	+	+++	+++	++++	+++	—
Quinolones	+++	++++	+++	++++	++++	++	++++	++++
TGC	++++	++++	+	++++	++++	+	++++	++++
Ticarcillin	++	+	+	+++	+++	+++	+++	—
Timentin	+++	++	+	++++	+++	+++	++++	++++
Tobramycin	++++	++++	++++	++++	+++	++++	++	++
Unasyn	+++	+++	—	++++	++	—	++++	++++
Zosyn	++++	++++	++	++++	++++	++++	++++	++++

TGC, Cefataxime, ceftizoxime, ceftriaxone.
[b]β-Lactamase-producing strains.

Table 56-6   Antimicrobial Susceptibility: Anaerobes

Drugs	Bacteroides fragilis	Peptococcus	Peptostreptococcus	Clostridia
Ampicillin	+	++++	++++	+++
Aztreonam	—	—	—	—
Cefazolin	—	+++	+++	—
Cefepime	+	+++	+++	+
Cefotaxime	++	+++	+++	+
Cefoxitin	+++	+++	++++	+
Ceftazidime	—	+	+	+
Ceftizoxime	+++	+++	+++	+
Ciprofloxacin	+	+	+	+
Clindamycin	+++	++++	++++	++
Moxifloxacin	+++	+++	+++	++
Imipenem (Ertapenem/Meropenem)	++++	++++	++++	++
Metronidazole	++++	+++	++	+++
Penicillin	+	++++	++++	++++
Timentin	++++	+++	+++	+++
Unasyn	++++	++++	++++	++++
Vancomycin	—	+++	+++	+++
Zosyn	++++	++++	+++	+++

such as endocarditis (see Chapter 59, Endocarditis) and osteomyelitis. A blood sample taken from a patient receiving an antibiotic is serially diluted using Mueller-Hinton broth (e.g., 1:2, 1:4, 1:8, 1:16) and then inoculated with the infecting organism. After 18 to 24 hours the samples are visually inspected for evidence of bacterial growth. If no growth is observed at dilutions of 1:8 and 1:16 but growth is seen at 1:32 and above, the serum is considered inhibitory at 1:16. Similar to the MIC methodology, the clear tubes define the inhibitory titers; however, it is unknown whether bactericidal concentrations have been achieved. As a result, aliquots of each of the clear tubes are plated onto agar. If significant bacterial growth

Table 56-7 Antimicrobials of Choice in the Treatment of Bacterial Infection

Organism	Drug of Choice	Alternatives	Comments
Aerobes			
Gram-Positive Cocci			
Streptococcus pyogenes (Group A streptococci)	Penicillin	Clindamycin, macrolide, cephalosporin	Clindamycin is the most reliable alternative for penicillin-allergic patients.
Streptococcus pneumoniae	Penicillin, amoxicillin	Macrolide, cephalosporin, doxycycline	Although the incidence of penicillin nonsusceptible pneumococci continues to increase, high-dose penicillin or amoxicillin is active against most of these isolates. Penicillin-resistant pneumococci commonly demonstrate resistance to other agents, including erythromycin, tetracyclines, and cephalosporins. Antipneumococcal quinolones (gatifloxacin, gemifloxacin, levofloxacin, moxifloxacin), ceftriaxone, cefotaxime, and telithromycin are options for treatment of high-level penicillin-resistant isolates.
Enterococcus faecalis	Ampicillin ± gentamicin	Vancomycin ± gentamicin; daptomycin, linezolid	Most commonly isolated enterococcus (80–85%). Most reliable antienterococcal agents are ampicillin (penicillin, piperacillin), vancomycin, daptomycin and linezolid. Monotherapy generally inhibits but does not kill the enterococcus. Daptomycin is unique in its bactericidal activity against Enterococci. Aminoglycosides must be added to ampicillin or vancomycin to provide bactericidal activity. Ampicillin resistance and high-level aminoglycoside resistance takes place commonly.
Enterococcus faecium	Vancomycin ± gentamicin	Daptomycin, dalfopristin/quinupristin (D/Q), linezolid	Second most common enterococcal organism (10–20%) and is more likely than *E. faecalis* to be resistant to multiple antimicrobials. Most reliable agents are daptomycin, D/Q and linezolid. Monotherapy generally inhibits but does not kill the enterococcus. Aminoglycosides must be added to cell wall active agents to provide bactericidal activity. Ampicillin and vancomycin resistance is common. Daptomycin, D/Q, and linezolid are drugs of choice for vancomycin-resistant isolates.
Staphylococcus aureus	Nafcillin	Cefazolin, vancomycin, clindamycin, trimethoprim-sulfamethoxazole	≈ 10–15% of isolates inhibited by penicillin. Most isolates susceptible to nafcillin, cephalosporins, trimethoprim-sulfamethoxazole, and clindamycin. First-generation cephalosporins are equal to nafcillin. Most second- and third-generation cephalosporins adequate in the treatment of infection (exceptions include ceftazidime and cefonicid). Methicillin-resistant *S. aureus* must be treated with vancomycin; however, trimethoprim-sulfamethoxazole, daptomycin, D/Q, linezolid, or minocycline can be used.
(Nafcillin-resistant)	Vancomycin	Linezolid, trimethoprim-sulfamethoxazole, minocycline, daptomycin	

Table 56-7 Antimicrobials of Choice in the Treatment of Bacterial Infection—cont'd

Organism	Drug of Choice	Alternatives	Comments
Staphylococcus epidermidis (Nafcillin-resistant)	Nafcillin Vancomycin	Cefazolin, vancomycin, clindamycin Daptomycin, linezolid, D/Q	Most isolates are β-lactam-, clindamycin-, and trimethoprim-sulfamethoxazole-resistant. Most reliable agents are vancomycin, daptomycin, D/Q, and linezolid. Rifampin active and can be used in conjunction with other agents; however, monotherapy with rifampin is associated with development of resistance.
Gram-Positive Bacilli			
Diphtheroids	Penicillin	Cephalosporin	
Corynebacterium jeikeium	Vancomycin	Erythromycin, quinolone	
Listeria monocytogenes	Ampicillin (± gentamicin)	Trimethoprim-sulfamethoxazole	
Gram-Negative Cocci			
Moraxella catarrhalis	Trimethoprim-sulfamethoxazole	Amoxicillin-clavulanic acid, erythromycin, doxycycline, second- or third-generation cephalosporin	
Neisseria gonorrhoeae	Quinolone, cefixime	Ceftriaxone	
Neisseria meningitides	Penicillin	Third-generation cephalosporin	
Gram-Negative Bacilli			
Campylobacter fetus	Imipenem	Gentamicin	
Campylobacter jejuni	Quinolone, erythromycin	Tetracycline, amoxicillin-clavulanic acid	
Enterobacter	Trimethoprim-sulfamethoxazole	Quinolone, imipenem, aminoglycoside	Not predictably inhibited by most cephalosporins. Imipenem, quinolones, trimethoprim-sulfamethoxazole, cefepime, and amino-glycosides are most active agents.
Escherichia coli	Third-generation cephalosporin	First- or second-generation cephalosporin, gentamicin	
Haemophilus influenzae	Third-generation cephalosporin	β-lactamase inhibitor combinations, second-generation cephalosporin, trimethoprim-sulfamethoxazole	
Helicobacter pylori	Amoxicillin + clarithromycin + omeprazole	Tetracycline + metronidazole + bismuth subsalicylate	
Klebsiella pneumoniae	Third-generation cephalosporin	First- or second-generation cephalosporin, gentamicin, trimethoprim-sulfamethoxazole	
Legionella	Fluoroquinolone	Erythromycin ± rifampin, doxycycline	
Proteus mirabilis	Ampicillin	First-generation cephalosporin, trimethoprim-sulfamethoxazole	
Other *Proteus*	Third-generation cephalosporin	β-Lactamase inhibitor combination, aminoglycoside, trimethoprim-sulfamethoxazole	

Organism	Drug of choice	Alternative agents	Comments
Pseudomonas aeruginosa	Antipseudomonal penicillin (or ceftazidime) ± aminoglycoside (or quinolone)	Quinolone or imipenem ± aminoglycoside	Most active agents include aminoglycosides, imipenem, meropenem, ceftazidime, cefepime, aztreonam and the extended-spectrum penicillins. Monotherapy is adequate for most pseudomonal infections.
Salmonella typhi	Quinolone	Ceftriaxone	
Serratia marcescens	Third-generation cephalosporin	Trimethoprim-sulfamethoxazole, aminoglycoside	
Shigella	Quinolone	Trimethoprim-sulfamethoxazole, ampicillin	
Stenotrophomonas maltophilia	Trimethoprim-sulfamethoxazole	Ceftazidime, minocycline, β-lactamase inhibitor combination (Timentin)	

Anaerobes

Organism	Drug of choice	Alternative agents	Comments
Bacteroides fragilis	Metronidazole	β-lactamase inhibitor combinations, penems	Most active agents (95–100%) include metronidazole, the β-lactamase inhibitor combinations (ampicillin-sulbactam, piperacillin-tazobactam, ticarcillin-clavulanic acid), and penems. Clindamycin, cefoxitin, cefotetan, cefmetazole, ceftizoxime, and the antipseudomonal penicillins (piperacillin, mezlocillin) have good activity but not to the degree of metronidazole. Aminoglycosides and aztreonam are inactive.
Clostridia difficile	Metronidazole	Vancomycin	
Fusobacterium	Penicillin	Metronidazole, clindamycin	

Other Oropharyngeal

Organism	Drug of choice	Alternative agents	Comments
Prevotella	β-lactamase inhibitor combination	Metronidazole, clindamycin	
Peptostreptococcus	Penicillin	Clindamycin, cephalosporin	Most β-lactams active (exceptions include aztreonam, nafcillin, ceftazidime).

Other

Actinomycetes

Organism	Drug of choice	Alternative agents
Actinomyces israelii	Penicillin	Tetracyclines
Nocardia	Trimethoprim-sulfamethoxazole	Amikacin, minocycline, imipenem

Chlamydiae

Organism	Drug of choice	Alternative agents
Chlamydia trachomatis	Doxycycline	Erythromycin, azithromycin
Chlamydia pneumoniae	Doxycycline	Erythromycin, azithromycin, clarithromycin

Mycoplasma

Organism	Drug of choice	Alternative agents
Mycoplasma pneumoniae	Erythromycin, doxycycline	Azithromycin, clarithromycin

Spirochetes

Organism	Drug of choice	Alternative agents
Borrelia burgdorferi	Doxycycline	Ampicillin, second- or third-generation cephalosporin
Treponema pallidum	Penicillin	Doxycycline

is observed at 1:16 but not at 1:8 or less, the serum is considered bactericidal at 1:8. The NCCLS considers as appropriate "peak" SBTs of 1:8 to 1:16 and "trough" SBTs of 1:4 to 1:8. Although the SBT provides an in vivo test of antibacterial activity, the practical utility of the test is limited.

DETERMINATION OF ISOLATE PATHOGENICITY

7. *Serratia marcescens* grows from a culture of R.G.'s tracheal aspirate, and the decision to treat this organism is based on whether the isolate is a true pathogen. How does one determine the difference between true bacterial infection and colonization or contamination?

A positive culture may represent colonization, contamination, or infection. Colonization indicates that bacteria are present at the site but are not actively causing infection. Poor sampling techniques or inappropriate handling of specimens can result in contamination. Infection, colonization, and contamination might all be applicable to R.G. If a suction catheter was used for a sample of R.G.'s tracheal aspirate, the infecting organism likely would be cultured; however, other flora present in the oropharynx (but not associated with infection) would also appear in the culture medium (colonization). Furthermore, if the sample is not handled aseptically by the clinician or the microbiology laboratory, bacterial contamination is possible.

In summary, culture results do not necessarily identify only the actual pathogens. In R.G., the *Serratia* may be a pathogen, contaminant, or colonizer. Nevertheless, considering the severity of R.G.'s illness, treatment directed against this pathogen is necessary.

ANTIMICROBIAL TOXICITIES

8. In light of the positive culture for *Serratia*, his increased respiratory secretions, and a worsening chest radiograph, R.G.'s lungs are considered the primary source of infection. In this case, the *S. marcescens* is susceptible to ciprofloxacin; therefore, ciprofloxacin 400 mg IV Q 12 hr is prescribed. Erythromycin 1.0 g IV Q 6 hr is added to provide empiric coverage against atypical pathogens such as *Legionella*. Upon review of R.G.'s medical record, gastric intolerance to both ciprofloxacin and erythromycin is noted. What steps should be taken to facilitate the safe use of these agents?

Adverse Effects and Toxicities

Before therapy is started, it is important to elicit an accurate drug and allergy history. When "allergy" has been reported by the patient, it is necessary to determine whether the reaction was intolerance, toxicity, or true allergy (see Chapter 4). Table 56-8 lists the most common adverse effects and toxicities associated with antimicrobial therapy. For example, gastric intolerance caused by oral erythromycin is common; however, this adverse effect does not represent an allergic manifestation or toxicity caused by the drug. As a result, if IV erythromycin were necessary to treat presumed *Legionella* pneumonitis, the drug could be used. True toxicity (e.g., hearing loss) has been associated with erythromycin with dosages >2 g/day, especially in the presence of concomitant renal or hepatic failure.[21] Because R.G. has an increased serum creatinine concentra-

tion and is receiving 4 g/day, he is at higher risk for erythromycin toxicity. Erythromycin-induced ototoxicity differs from the gastrointestinal (GI) side effects in that the effects on the ear are dose related. Thus, lower dosages of erythromycin could be used in a patient at high risk for ototoxicity or with a past history of auditory problems. On the other hand, if the patient had experienced a true severe allergic reaction (e.g., bronchospasm or anaphylaxis), then the drug would be contraindicated. Ciprofloxacin provides adequate coverage of *Legionella*. Considering the previous intolerance to erythromycin and the duplication in coverage, the erythromycin should be discontinued and the patient should receive quinolone monotherapy.

Concomitant Disease States

Concomitant disease states also should be considered in the selection of therapy. Older patients with hearing deficits are poor candidates for potentially ototoxic aminoglycoside therapy. Diabetics or patients with kidney transplants may be better treated with IV fluconazole than nephrotoxic amphotericin B in candidemia. Patients with a pre-existing seizure history should not receive imipenem if less toxic therapy can be used. In summary, the toxicologic profile must be taken into account in the selection of antimicrobial therapy. If properly dosed, erythromycin and ciprofloxacin can be safely prescribed in R.G.

ANTIMICROBIAL COSTS OF THERAPY

9. What factors should be included in calculating the cost of R.G.'s ciprofloxacin therapy?

The true cost of antimicrobial therapy is difficult to quantitate.[22] Although acquisition cost traditionally has been the primary factor in the overall cost of therapy, drug administration labor costs (i.e., nursing and pharmacy) and the use of IV sets, piggyback bags, and infusion control devices must be included in the analysis. As a result, a drug that must be administered several times daily, such as penicillin, will incur increased administration costs compared with one that requires once-a-day dosing.

Some drugs, such as aminoglycosides, are associated with increased laboratory costs (e.g., aminoglycoside serum concentrations, serum creatinine, audiometry) that are not required for other agents,[23] such as the third-generation cephalosporins and quinolones. Similarly, drugs with a high potential for misuse or toxicity may be associated with increased costs because of monitoring (e.g., drug use evaluation, pharmacokinetic monitoring). Although ciprofloxacin would be expected to be associated with relatively few laboratory costs, its broad spectrum of activity[24] and potential for misuse might result in increased monitoring costs.

Costs that are difficult to quantitate include the cost of failure of therapy and the cost of antimicrobial toxicity. Ineffective or toxic therapy can prolong hospitalization and may require expensive interventions, such as hemodialysis,[23] mechanical ventilation, and intensive care unit admission. The net effect of these latter costs can be significantly greater than the acquisition and administration costs of antimicrobial therapy.

Table 56-8   Antibiotic Adverse Effects and Toxicities

Antibiotic	Side Effects	Comments
β-Lactams, (penicillin, cephalosporins, monobactams, penems)	*Allergic:* anaphylaxis, urticaria, serum sickness, rash, fever	Many patients will have "ampicillin rash" with no cross-reactivity with any other penicillins. Most common in patients with mononucleosis or those receiving allopurinol. Likelihood of IgE-mediated cross-reactivity between penicillins and cephalosporins ≈3–7%. More extensive cross-reactivity between penicillins and imipenem. No IgE cross-reactivity between aztreonam and penicillins.
	Diarrhea	Particularly common with ampicillin, Augmentin, ceftriaxone, and cefoperazone. Antibiotic-associated colitis can occur with most antimicrobials
	Hematologic: anemia, thrombocytopenia, antiplatelet activity, hypothrombinemia	Hemolytic anemia more common with higher doses. Antiplatelet activity (inhibition of platelet aggregation) most common with the antipseudomonal penicillins and high serum levels of other β-lactams. Hypothrombinemia more often associated with those cephalosporins with the methyltetrazolethiol side chain (cefamandole, cefotetan, cefoperazone, cefmetazole). Reaction preventable and reversible with vitamin K.
	Hepatitis/biliary	Most common with oxacillin. Biliary sludging and stones reported with ceftriaxone.
	Phlebitis	
	Seizure activity	Associated with high levels of β-lactams, particularly penicillins and imipenem
	Potassium load	Penicillin G (K⁺)
	Sodium load	Ticarcillin, ticarcillin-clavulanic acid
	Nephritis	Most common with methicillin; however, occasionally reported for most other β-lactams
	Neutropenia	Nafcillin
	Disulfiram reaction	Associated with cephalosporins with methyltetrazolethiol side chain (cefamandole, cefotetan, cefoperazone, cefmetazole)
	Hypotension, nausea	Associared with fast infusion of imipenem
Aminoglycosides (gentamicin, tobramycin, amikacin, netilmicin)	Nephrotoxicity	Averages 10–15% incidence. Generally reversible, usually occurs after 5–7 days of therapy. *Risk factors:* dehydration, age, dose, duration, concurrent nephrotoxins, liver disease.
	Ototoxicity	1–5% incidence, often irreversible. Both cochlear and/or vestibular toxicity occur.
	Neuromuscular paralysis	Rare, most common with large doses administered via intraperitoneal instillation or in patients with myasthenia gravis
Macrolides (erythromycin, azithromycin, clarithromycin)	Nausea, vomiting, "burning" stomach	Oral administration. Azithromycin and clarithromycin associated with less nausea than erythromycin.
	Cholestatic jaundice	Reported for all erythromycin salts, most common with estolate
	Ototoxicity	Most common with high doses in patients with renal and/or hepatic failure
Clindamycin	Diarrhea	Most common adverse effect. High association with antibiotic-associated colitis.
Tetracyclines	Allergic	
	Photosensitivity	
	Teeth/bone deposition and discoloration	Avoid in pediatrics, pregnancy, and breast-feeding.
	GI	Upper GI predominates.
	Hepatitis	Primarily in pregnancy or the elderly
	Renal (azotemia)	Tetracyclines have antianabolic effect and should be avoided in patients with ↓ renal function. Less problematic with doxycycline.
	Vestibular	Associated with minocycline, particularly high doses

continued

Table 56-8 Antibiotic Adverse Effects and Toxicities—cont'd

Antibiotic	Side Effects	Comments
Vancomycin	Ototoxicity	Only with receipt of concomitant ototoxins such as aminoglycosides or macrolides
	Nephrotoxicity	Little to no nephrotoxicity. May ↑ nephrotoxicity of aminoglycosides.
	Hypotension, flushing	Associated with rapid infusion of vancomycin. More common with increased doses.
	Phlebitis	Needs large volume dilution
Dalfopristin/Quinupristin (D/Q)	Phlebitis	Generally requires central line administration
	Myalgia	Moderate to severe in many patients
	Increased bilirubin	
Daptomycin	Myalgia	Primarily at high doses and reversible
Linezolid	Thrombocytopenia, neutropenia, anemia, MAO inhibition, tongue discoloration	
Sulfonamides	GI	Nausea, diarrhea
	Hepatic	Cholestatic hepatitis, ↑ incidence in HIV.
	Rash	Exfoliative dermatitis, Stevens-Johnson syndrome. More common in HIV.
	Bone marrow	Neutropenia, thrombocytopenia. More common in HIV.
	Kernicterus	Caused by ↑ unbound drug in the neonate. Premature liver cannot conjugate bilirubin. Sulfonamide displaces bilirubin from protein, resulting in excessive free bilirubin and kernicterus
Chloramphenicol	Anemia	Idiosyncratic irreversible aplastic anemia (rare). Reversible dose-related anemia
	Gray syndrome	Caused by inability of neonates to conjugate chloramphenicol
Quinolones	GI	Nausea, vomiting, diarrhea
	Prolonged QT	Moxifloxacin; possibly all quinolones as a class
	Drug interactions	↓ oral bioavailability with multivalent cations
	CNS	Altered mental status, confusion, seizures
	Cartilage toxicity	Toxic in animal model. Avoid in children; however, appears safe in cystic fibrosis
	Tendonitis/tendon rupture	Common in elderly, renal failure, concomitant glucocorticoids
Antifungals		
Amphotericin B	Nephrotoxicity	Common. May depend on patient Na load. ↓ dose or QOD dosing may result in improvement of renal function. Caution with concomitant nephrotoxins (e.g., aminoglycosides, cyclosporine).
	Hypokalemia	Predictable. Probably caused by renal tubular excretion of potassium. More common in patients receiving concomitant ticarcillin, piperacillin.
	Hypomagnesemia	Less commonly observed than hypokalemia
	Anemia	Long-term adverse effect. Similar to anemia of chronic disease.
Caspofungin	Mild LFT increase with concomitant cyclosporine	
Flucytosine	Neutropenia, thrombocytopenia	Secondary to metabolism of flucytosine to fluorouracil. More commonly observed with flucytosine levels >100 µg/mL. More common in HIV patients.
	Hepatitis	Usually moderate ↑ in LFTs. Rarely clinical hepatitis.

Drug	Adverse effect	Comments
Ketoconazole (fluconazole, itraconazole, voriconazole)	Drug interactions	↓ oral bioavailability of ketoconazole tablet, and itraconazole capsules with ↑ gastric pH
	Hepatitis	Ranges from mild ↑ in LFTs to occasional fatal hepatitis. More common with high-dose ketoconazole (>400 mg/day). Less common with other azoles.
	Gynecomastia, ↓ libido	
	Visual disturbance	Unique to voriconazole, particularly first week of therapy
Antivirals		
Abacavir	Hypersensitivity	Occurs in 3% of patients and includes fever, GI, malaise, rash. Repeated administration associated with severe reactions, including hypotension, respiratory distress.
Acyclovir	Phlebitis	Caused by poor solubility of IV preparation. Reported in 1–20% of cases.
	Renal failure	Low solubility of acyclovir associated with renal failure. Dehydrated patients, as well as rapid infusions, predispose to toxicity. 1% incidence in AIDS. ↑ incidence in AIDS with dose in >10 mg/kg/day.
Delavirdine (efavirenz, nevirapine)	CNS	
	Rash	
	Headache, insomnia, dizziness, nausea	
	Hepatitis	Primarily with initiation of therapy with efavirenz
		Primarily with nevirapine
Didanosine (ddI)	Pancreatitis	Fatalities reported
	Peripheral neuropathy	Dose related
Emtricitabine	Hyperpigmentation	
Foscarnet	Nephrotoxicity	Occurs in up to 60% of patients. May be prevented with normal saline bolus before dose. Frequent monitoring of renal function imperative.
	Mineral and electrolyte abnormalities	↑ and ↓ calcium/phosphate may be observed. Hypocalcemia, hypo- and hyperphosphatemia, hypomagnesemia, hypokalemia. ↑ risk of cardiomyopathy and seizures.
	Anemia	Anemia in 33%; usually manageable with transfusions and discontinuation of foscarnet
Ganciclovir	Nausea, vomiting	
	Neutropenia, thrombocytopenia	↑ incidence in AIDS. ↑ incidence with doses in excess of 10 mg/kg/day.
	Hepatitis	Usually mild to moderate ↑ in LFTs
Indinavir (amprenavir, atazanavir, lopinavir, nelfinavir, ritonavir, saquinavir)	Nausea, diarrhea, ↑ LFTs, hyperglycemia, fat wasting and redistribution, hyperlipidemia	
	Paresthesia	Ritonavir
	Nephrolithiasis	Indinavir
	Hyperbilirubinemia	Atazanavir
		Adverse effects are uncommon
Lamivudine (3TC)	Nausea	
Oseltamivir		
Stavudine (D4T)	Peripheral neuropathy, lipodystrophy	
Tenofovir	Rare nephrotoxicity	
Zalcitabine (ddC)	Peripheral neuropathy	Dose related, delayed, often severe
Zidovudine (AZT)	Anemia, neutropenia	Anemia at 2–4 wk occasionally with ↑ MCV. Neutropenia appears later (6–8 wk).
	General	Severe headache, nausea, insomnia, myalgia, lethargy

CNS, central nervous system; GI, gastrointestinal; IV, intravenous; LFTs, liver function tests; MCV, mean corpuscular volume; Na, sodium.

In summary, determining the true cost of antimicrobial therapy, including ciprofloxacin, is complex. Acquisition cost, IV bags, infusion controllers, and labor must be incorporated into the analysis. Although they are difficult to estimate, other costs, including antibiotic toxicity and failure of therapy, also should be included.

ROUTE OF ADMINISTRATION

10. Oral ciprofloxacin was considered for the treatment of R.G.'s presumed *Serratia* pneumonia, but the IV route was prescribed. Why is the oral administration of ciprofloxacin reasonable (or unreasonable) in R.G.?

The proper route of antibiotic administration depends on many factors, including the severity of infection, bioavailability, and other patient factors. In patients who appear "septic," blood flow often is shunted away from the mesentery and extremities, resulting in unreliable bioavailability from the GI tract or muscles. Therefore, hemodynamically unstable patients should receive antimicrobials by the IV route to ensure therapeutic antimicrobial levels. Furthermore, some drug interactions can result in subtherapeutic serum concentrations (e.g., reduced bioavailability associated with concomitant quinolone and antacid administration and the decreased absorption of ketoconazole or itraconazole with concurrent H_2-blocker therapy).

R.G. is clinically septic with a possible *Serratia* pneumonia. Considering his unstable state, the bioavailability of oral ciprofloxacin cannot be guaranteed; thus, he should be treated with IV antimicrobials.

ANTIMICROBIAL DOSING

11. What dose of IV ciprofloxacin should be given to R.G.? What factors must be taken into account in determining a proper antimicrobial dose?

The choice of dosing regimen is based on many factors. Table 56-9 provides a guide for the dosing of more commonly administered antimicrobials. Selection of the appropriate dosage should be based on information that documents the

Table 56-9 UCSF/Mt. Zion Medical Center Adult Antimicrobial Dosing Guidelines#

Approved by the Antibiotic Advisory Subcommittee (3/13/91) and the Pharmacy and Therapeutics Committee (4/11/91) Rev 4/03

Drug	CrCl >50 mL/min	CrCl 10–50 mL/min	CrCl <10 mL/min (ESRD not on HD)
Acyclovir	*Herpes simplex infections* 5 mg/kg per dose Q 8 hr	5 mg/kg per dose Q 12–24 hr	2.5 mg/kg Q 24 hr
	HSV encephalitis/Herpes zoster 10 mg/kg per dose Q 8 hr	10 mg/kg per dose Q 12–24 hr	5 mg/kg Q 24 hr
Amphotericin B	0.3–1.0 mg/kg	No change	No change
Dosage reductions in renal disease are not necessary. However, due to the nephrotoxic potential of the drug, reducing the dose or holding the drug in the setting of a rising serum creatinine may be warranted.			
Ampicillin	1–2 g Q 4–6 hr	1–1.5 g Q 6 hr	1 g Q 8–12 hr
Cefazolin	1–2 g Q 8 hr	1–2 g Q 12 hr	0.5–1.0 g Q 24 hr
Caspofungin	LD = 70 mg × 1, then 50 mg Q 24 hr	No change	No change
Cefepime	≥60 mL/min 1–2 g Q 12 hr Febrile neutropenia: 2 g Q 8 hr	30–60 mL/min 10–30 mL/min 1–2 g Q 24 hr 0.5–1 g Q 24 hr	0.25–0.5 g Q 24 hr
Ceftazidime	1–2 g Q 8 hr	1–2 g Q 12–24 hr	0.5 g Q 24 hr
Ceftriaxone	1 g Q 24 hr Meningitis: 2 g Q 12 hr	No change Endocarditis & osteomyelitis: 2 g Q 24 hr	No change
Cefuroxime	0.75–1.5 g Q 8 hr	0.75–1.5 g Q 12–24 hr	0.5 g Q 24 hr
Ciprofloxacin	400 mg Q 12 hr*	30–50 mL/min No change No change	10–30 mL/min 200–400 mg Q 12 hr 250–500 mg Q 12 hr (PO) 500–750 mg Q 12 hr (PO)	200 mg Q 12 hr 250 mg Q 12 hr (PO)
The use of Q 12 hr dosing intervals is recommended in ESRD due to the variability in half-life data observed in anephric patients. *Note: higher doses and/or increased frequency may be necessary in the treatment of serious pseudomonal infections.			
Clindamycin	600–900 mg Q 8 hr	No change	No change
Ethambutol	15 mg/kg QD	7.5–10 mg/kg QD	5 mg/kg QD
Fluconazole	100–400 mg Q 24 hr	50–200 mg Q 24 hr	50–100 mg Q 24 hr
Flucytosine (PO)	12.5–37.5 mg/kg per dose Q 6 hr	25–50 mL/min 10–25 mL/min 12.5–37.5 mg/kg 12.5–37.5 mg/kg Q 12 hr Q 24 hr	12.5–25 mg/kg Q 24 hr
Steady-state serum 5-FC level measurements are difficult to obtain. However, they may be useful in guiding dosing of 5-FC in anuria. Bone marrow suppression has been associated with 2-hour postdose 5-FC peaks of ≥100 mg/L.			

**Table 56-9 UCSF/Mt. Zion Medical Center
Adult Antimicrobial Dosing Guidelines[#]**

Drug	CrCl >50 mL/min		CrCl 10–50 mL/min		CrCl <10 mL/min (ESRD not on HD)
Ganciclovir	≥ 80 mL/min 5 mg/kg per dose Q 12 hr	50–79 mL/min 2.5 mg/kg per dose Q 12 hr	1.25–2.5 mg/kg Q 12–24 hr		1.25 mg/kg Q 24 hr
Gentamicin	≥60 mL/min 5 mg/kg per dose Q 24 hr		See below		See below

The total daily dose of gentamicin can be administered as a single daily dose in patients with normal renal function (CrCl ≥60 mL/min). Patients with decreased renal function or abnormal body composition should have their doses adjusted according to the recommendations below. All patients who are anticipated to receive aminoglycosides for ≥7 days should be monitored with gentamicin levels. Peak levels are not useful with this dosing regimen; however, trough levels are recommended and in most cases will be nondetectable.

			40–60 mL/min 1.2–1.5 mg/kg Q 12 hr	20–40 mL/min 1.2–1.5 mg/kg Q 12–24 hr	<20 mL/min 2 mg/kg loading dose (Consult pharmacy for maintenance dose)

With traditional dosing of gentamicin, peak (5–8 mg/L) and trough (<2 mg/L) levels are recommended in patients anticipated to receive aminoglycosides for ≥7 days for severe Gram-negative infection. Lower doses (1 mg/kg per dose Q 8 hr) are suggested when aminoglycosides are used synergistically in Gram-positive infections. Those patients with CrCl <60 mL/min, obesity, or increased fluid volume should be monitored with serum gentamicin levels.

Drug	CrCl >50 mL/min		CrCl 10–50 mL/min		CrCl <10 mL/min (ESRD not on HD)
Imipenem	500 mg Q 6–8 hr; max, 50 mg/kg per day		500 mg Q 8 hr		<20 mL/min 250–500 mg Q 12 hr (or consider meropenem)
Isoniazid	300 mg QD		No change		No change
Levofloxacin	250–500 mg Q 24 hr		LD = 500 mg ×1, then 250 mg Q 24 hr		LD = 500 mg ×1, then 250 mg Q 48 hr
Meropenem	0.5–1 g Q 8 hr Meningitis: 2 g Q 8 hr		25–50 mL/min 0.5–1 g Q 12 hr	10–25 mL/min 0.5 g Q 12 hr	0.5 g Q 24 hr
Metronidazole	500 mg Q 8 hr		500 mg Q 8 hr		500 mg Q 12 hr; metabolites accumulate in ESRD
Nafcillin	1–2 g Q 4–6 hr		No change		No change
Penicillin G	2–3 MU Q 4–6 hr		1–2 MU Q 4–6 hr		1 MU Q 6 hr
Piperacillin/Tazobactam (Zosyn)	3.375–4.5 g Q 6–8 hr Pseudomonas: 4.5 g Q 6 hr for ClCr >20 mL/min		3.375–4.5 g Q 6–8 hr		2.25–3.375 g Q 8 hr
Pyrazinamide	20–25 mg/kg per day		No change		No change
Rifampin	600 mg QD		No change		No change
Ticarcillin/Clav (Timentin)	≥60 mL/min 3.1 g Q 4–6 hr		30–59 mL/min 3.1 g Q 8 hr	10–29 mL/min 2–3.1 g Q 8–12 hr	2 g Q 12 hr
Tobramycin	See Gentamicin		See Gentamicin		See Gentamicin
TMP-SMX	Systemic GNR infections 10 mg TMP/kg per day divided Q 6–12 hr		5–7.5 mg TMP/kg per day divided Q 12–24 hr		2.5–5.0 mg TMP/kg Q 24 hr
	Pneumocystis carinii pneumonia 15–20 mg TMP/kg per day divided Q 6–12 hr		10–15 mg TMP/kg per day divided Q 12–24 hr		5–10 mg TMP/kg Q 24 hr
Voriconazole	LD = 400 mg Q 12 hr ×1 day, then 200 mg Q 12 hr (PO)		No change		No change

PO should be used when possible, as oral bioavailability >95%. IV dose: LD = 6 mg/kg per dose Q 12 hr ×1 day, then 4 mg/kg per dose Q 12 h. The use of IV should be avoided in patients with CrCl <50 mL/min due to the accumulation of the IV vehicle and is contraindicated in ESRD.

Vancomycin	>60 mL/min 10–15 mg/kg Q 12 hr	40–60 mL/min 10–15 mg/kg Q 12–24 hr	20–40 mL/min 10–15 mg/kg Q 24–48 hr	10–20 mL/min 10–15 mg/kg Q 48–72 hr	≤10 mL/min 10–15 mg/kg Q 4–7 days

Vancomycin dosing should be guided by serum level measurements in patients with decreased renal function or abnormal body composition. Peak levels are not recommended. Trough levels (≤30 min before next dose) should be 5–15 mg/L.

[a]Doses are those recommended for systemic infections commonly treated with these agents.
• Infections involving the urinary tract may require lower doses.
• Infections involving the central nervous system may require higher doses.
Estimate of Renal Function using Cockcroft and Gault equation:

$$\text{CrCl (mL/min)} = \frac{(140 - \text{age}) * \text{Wt (kg)}}{72 * \text{SCr (mg/dL)}} \quad \text{(for females multiply by 0.85)}$$

efficacy of the dosage in the treatment of infection. Patient-specific factors, including weight, site of infection, and route of elimination, also must be considered in the selection of dosage. The weight of the patient is important, particularly for agents with a low therapeutic index (e.g., aminoglycosides, vancomycin, flucytosine); these drugs should be dosed on a mg/kg per day basis. Other agents with a more favorable adverse effect profile, such as cephalosporins, are less likely to require weight-specific dosing.

Site of Infection

The site of infection also results in differing dosage requirements. An uncomplicated urinary tract infection requires low antimicrobial doses because of the high urinary drug concentrations that are achieved. In contrast, a more serious systemic infection, such as pyelonephritis, requires increased antimicrobial dosages to achieve therapeutic drug levels in tissue and in serum.

Anatomic and Physiologic Barriers

Anatomic and physiologic barriers also must be considered in evaluating a dosing regimen. For example, penetration into the CNS necessitates high doses to ensure adequate antimicrobial concentrations at the site of infection.[25] Vitreous humor[26] and the prostate gland[27] are additional sites in which therapeutic antimicrobial concentrations are more difficult to achieve.

Route of Elimination

Route of elimination must also be considered in the dosage calculation. In general, antimicrobials are eliminated via the kidney or nonrenally (metabolic/biliary). Renal function can be estimated via 24-hour urine collection or with equations such as the Cockcroft and Gault equation[28]:

$$\text{Creatinine clearance} = ([140 - \text{age}] * [\text{weight in kg}])/(72 * \text{SrCr})$$

Several anti-infectives are eliminated renally (Table 56-10). Most β-lactams are eliminated by the kidney. Ceftriaxone, cefoperazone, most antistaphylococcal penicillins (e.g., nafcillin, oxacillin, dicloxacillin), and most extended-spectrum penicillins (e.g., piperacillin) are eliminated both renally and nonrenally. Aminoglycosides, vancomycin, acyclovir, and ganciclovir are cleared extensively by the kidney. Thus, dosage adjustment is recommended for these drugs in patients with renal failure (see Table 56-9 and Fig. 56-2). Azithro-

---

Table 56-10   UCSF Medical Center

ADULT ANTIMICROBIAL DOSING CARD FOR CONTINUOUS RENAL REPLACEMENT THERAPY (CRRT) AND HEMODIALYSIS (HD)[A]
Department of Clinical Pharmacy, Division of Infectious Diseases and
Division of Nephrology University of California,
San Francisco Medical Center (6/03)

CRRT: This assumes an ultrafiltration (UF) rate of 2 L/h with continuous venous-venous hemofiltration (CVVH) and an UF rate of 1 L/h and dialysate flow rate of 1 L/h with continuous veno-venous hemodiafiltration (CVVHDF) and residual native GFR <10 mL/min

Drug	CRRT	HD
Acyclovir	**Herpes simplex infections** 2.5–5.0 mg/kg Q 24 hr **HSV Encephalitis/** **Herpes Zoster** 5–7.5 mg/kg Q 24 hr	**Herpes simplex infections** 2.5 mg/kg Q 24 hr and post HD **HSV Encephalitis/** **Herpes Zoster** 5 mg/kg Q 24 hr and post HD
Ampicillin	1 g Q 6 hr	1 g Q 12 hr
Ampicillin/Sul (Unasyn)	1.5 g Q 6 hr	1.5 g Q 12 hr
Cefazolin	1 g Q 12 hr	2 g post HD only
Cefepime	2 g Q 12 hr	2 g post HD only
Cefotetan	1 g Q 12 hr	2 g post HD only
Ceftazidime	2 g Q 12 hr	1 g post HD
Ciprofloxacin	400 mg IV Q 12 hr	200 mg IV Q12 hr or 250 mg PO Q 12 hr
Fluconazole	400 mg PO Q 24 hr	200 mg PO post HD only
Ganciclovir	2.5–5.0 mg/kg Q 24 hr	1.25 mg/kg post HD only
Gentamicin	Gram-negative infections: 2 mg/kg loading dose *then* 1.5 mg/kg Q 24 hr Monitoring of serum levels is recommended; trough <2 µg/mL	Gram-negative infections: 2 mg/kg loading dose *then* 1 mg/kg post HD Monitoring of serum levels is recommended; trough <2 µg/mL
Imipenem	500 mg Q 8 hr	250 mg Q 12 hr

Table 56-10   UCSF Medical Center—cont'd

Drug	CRRT	HD
Levofloxacin	500 mg loading dose _then_ 250 mg IV/PO Q 24 hr	500 mg loading dose _then_ 250 mg IV/PO Q 48 hr
Meropenem	1 g Q 12 hr	500 mg Q 24 hr and post HD
Penicillin G	2 MU Q 46 hr	1 MU Q 6 hr
Piperacillin/Tazobactam (Zosyn)	3.375 g Q 6 hr or 4.5 g Q 8 hr	2.25 g Q 8 hr
Ticarcillin/Clav (Timentin)	3.1 g Q 8 hr	2 g Q 12 hr
Tobramycin	Gram-negative infections: 2 mg/kg loading dose _then_ 1.5 mg/kg Q 24 hr Monitoring of serum levels is recommended; trough <2 μg/mL	Gram-negative infections: 2 mg/kg loading dose _then_ 1 mg/kg post HD Monitoring of serum levels is recommended; trough <2 μg/mL
TMP-SMX	5–7.5 mg TMP/kg per day divided Q 12–24 hr	2.5–5.0 mg TMP/kg Q 24 hr
Vancomycin	7.5–15 mg/kg Q 24 hr Monitoring of serum levels is recommended; trough 10–15 mg/mL	Loading dose 15–20 mg/kg _then_ 500 mg post HD only Monitoring of serum levels is recommended; trough 10–15 mg/mL
Voriconazole	**ORAL** formulation should be administered when possible, as oral bioavailability >95%. The use of IV should be avoided in patients with CrCl <50 mL/min due to the accumulation of the IV vehicle (cyclodextran) and is contraindicated in ESRD. LD: 400 mg PO Q 12 hr ×2 doses only [≥40 kg] MD: 200 mg PO Q 12 hr [≥40 kg]	

STANDARD DOSING for the following:
Amphotericin B, Caspofungin, Ceftriaxone, Clindamycin, Erythromycin, Metronidazole, Nafcillin
Please refer to Table 57-9 for additional information.
[a]Recommended doses are for critically ill patients with serious systemic infection. Lower doses may be used for less serious infections.

hepatic function is more difficult to evaluate. No standard liver function test (AST, ALT, alkaline phosphatase) has been demonstrated to correlate well with hepatic drug clearance. Some tests, such as PT and albumin, are markers of hepatic function, but even these tests do not clearly predict drug clearance. Patients receiving hemodialysis or continuous hemofiltration provide additional dosing challenges. Table 56-10 provides dosing recommendations in patients receiving hemodialysis or continuous hemofiltration.

Patient Age

Most dosing information has been derived from a young, relatively healthy patient population, so total drug clearance for several antimicrobials may be decreased in neonatal and geriatric patients. As a result, the age of the patient may be an important factor in the selection of a proper dose.

Fever and Inoculum Effect

The impact of other factors on the selection of an antimicrobial dose is less clear. Fever increases and decreases blood flow to mesenteric, hepatic, and renal organ systems[29] and can either increase or decrease drug clearance. Inoculum effect also may be a factor in the selection of a dosing regimen because it is associated with an increase in the MIC of the

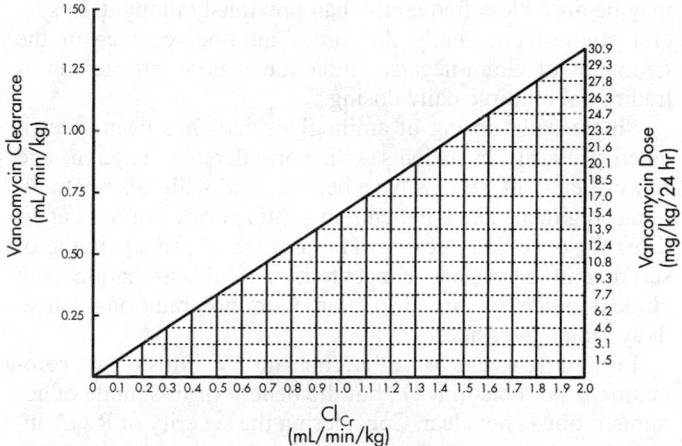

FIGURE 56-2. Reduced dosage nomogram for vancomycin in patients with impaired renal function as derived by Moellering et al. Cl_{cr}, creatinine clearance. (Reprinted with permission from Ann Intern Med 1981;94:343.)

mycin, clindamycin, and metronidazole are metabolized primarily by the liver and as a result do not accumulate appreciably in end-stage renal disease.

Although renal function can be approximated with the use of the Cockcroft and Gault equation (or a similar equation),

organism in response to increasing bacterial concentrations.[30] For example, piperacillin may demonstrate an MIC of 8.0 μg/mL against *P. aeruginosa* at a concentration of 10^5 colony-forming units/mL (CFU/mL); however, at 10^9 CFU/mL, the minimum inhibitory concentration may increase to 32 to 64 μg/mL. This phenomenon is well recognized, particularly with β-lactamase–producing bacteria treated with β-lactam antimicrobials. The more β-lactamase stabilizes the antimicrobial, the less the influence of inoculum effect. Aminoglycosides, quinolones, and imipenem appear to be less affected by the inoculum effect than β-lactams. The inoculum effect probably is most relevant in the treatment of a bacterial abscess, in which extremely high concentrations of bacteria would be expected. As a result, antimicrobials that are more susceptible to the inoculum effect may require increased drug dosages for optimal outcome in the treatment of abscesses.

In summary, R.G. normally would be given an IV dosage of ciprofloxacin at 400 mg Q 12 hr. However, his reduced renal function suggests that his dosage should be decreased to 200 to 300 mg Q 12 hr.

PHARMACOKINETICS/PHARMACODYNAMICS

12. R.G.'s respiratory status remains unchanged; thus, the ciprofloxacin is discontinued and cefotaxime and gentamicin are started empirically. The use of a constant IV infusion of cefotaxime is being considered in R.G. In addition, the use of single daily dosing of gentamicin is being discussed. What is the rationale for these approaches, and would either be advantageous for R.G.?

The in vivo bactericidal activities of β-lactams such as cefotaxime show minimal enhancement with increasing drug concentrations. Activity appears to correlate better with the duration of exposure to β-lactam levels above the MIC than with the magnitude of drug concentration.[31] The animal model suggests that β-lactam antimicrobials should be dosed such that their serum levels always exceed the MIC of the pathogen.[32] This observation appears to be most important in the neutropenic model, in which the use of a constant infusion more reliably inhibits bacterial growth compared with traditional intermittent dosing. An additional benefit of the use of constant infusions of β-lactams is that smaller daily doses appear to be as effective as higher doses administered intermittently. However, other than this latter outcome, it is unclear whether constant infusions have any distinct advantages or disadvantages compared with usual dosing of β-lactams. The efficacy of quinolone antimicrobials appears to correlate with the peak plasma concentration to MIC ratio or area-under-the-curve to MIC ratio.[33] Possibly ciprofloxacin was underdosed in this patient, contributing to the therapeutic failure, particularly if the MIC was in the upper range of susceptibility for this agent.

Aminoglycosides traditionally have been administered Q 8 to 12 hr to achieve peak serum gentamicin levels of 5 to 8 μg/mL to ensure efficacy in the treatment of serious Gram-negative infection.[34,35] Gentamicin troughs of >2 μg/mL have been associated with an increased risk for nephrotoxicity.[35,36] These studies attempting to correlate efficacy and toxicity with serum levels and the association of peaks or troughs with clinical outcomes have been questioned.[37] Vancomycin peaks generally have been recommended to be <50 μg/mL and

troughs 5 to 10 μg/mL[38,39]; however, the validity of these recommendations has also been questioned.[40]

Several antimicrobials (e.g., aminoglycosides) have been associated with a pharmacodynamic phenomenon known as a postantibiotic effect (PAE). PAE is delayed regrowth of bacteria following exposure to an antibiotic[41,42] (i.e., continued suppression of normal growth in the absence of antibiotic levels above the MIC of the organism). As an example, if *P. aeruginosa* is cultured in broth, it will multiply to a concentration of 10^9 CFU/mL. If piperacillin is added in a concentration above the MIC for the organism, a reduction in the bacterial concentration is observed. When piperacillin is removed from the broth, immediate bacterial growth takes place. Some clinicians suggest that β-lactam antibiotics always must be present in concentrations above the MIC because of this growth pattern. If the above experiment is repeated with gentamicin, a reduction in bacterial CFUs is observed. In contrast with β-lactam antibiotics, if the gentamicin is removed from the system, a lag period of 2 to 6 hours takes place before characteristic bacterial growth occurs. This lag period is defined as the PAE. A PAE also has been observed with quinolones and imipenem against Gram-negative organisms. While most β-lactam antibiotics, such as antipseudomonal penicillins or cephalosporins, do not exhibit PAE with Gram-negative organisms, PAE has been demonstrated with Gram-positive pathogens such as *S. aureus*.

Once-Daily Dosing of Aminoglycosides

As a result of PAE and other pharmacodynamic factors, certain antimicrobials may be dosed less frequently. The greatest clinical experience has been with the aminoglycosides in the treatment of Gram-negative infection.[43,44] Earlier data suggested that the maximal aminoglycoside peak level:MIC ratio correlates well with clinical response. Thus, the higher the achievable peak, the greater likelihood of a favorable outcome. As a result of PAE, it is possible that aminoglycosides may be dosed less frequently than previously thought. In several studies, once-daily dosing of aminoglycosides in the treatment of Gram-negative infection was as efficacious as traditional multiple daily dosing.[45]

Single daily dosing of aminoglycosides has been investigated primarily in patients with normal renal function, and few critically ill patients have been treated with this nontraditional regimen. Thus, patients in septic shock are not candidates for once-daily dosing. The utility and proper timing of serum aminoglycoside concentrations and association with clinical outcomes are debatable with nontraditional once-daily aminoglycosides.

In summary, the use of a constant IV infusion of cefotaxime is possible in R.G., but the benefit of this mode of administration is not clear. Considering the severity of R.G.'s infection and his elevated creatinine level, he is not a candidate for single daily dosing of aminoglycosides (i.e., 5 to 6 mg/kg Q 24 hr). Independent of the aminoglycoside-associated PAE, his current renal function requires a reduced gentamicin dose to treat his infection.

Antimicrobial Protein Binding

13. Ceftriaxone (Rocephin), rather than cefotaxime (Claforan), is being considered for the treatment of R.G.'s infection. Ceftriaxone is more highly protein bound than cefotaxime. Why is protein binding important in the selection of therapy?

Free (i.e., unbound) rather than total drug levels are best correlated with antimicrobial activity,[46] and the degree of protein binding may have important clinical consequences in some patients. Chambers and associates[47] reported treatment failures with the highly protein-bound cefonicid (98% protein bound) in patients with endocarditis caused by *S. aureus*. Despite achievable serum drug concentrations well above the MIC of the organism, breakthrough bacteremia occurred in three of four patients. However, while total drug concentrations greatly exceeded the MIC of the pathogen, free concentrations were consistently below the level necessary to inhibit bacterial growth. Similar experiences have been reported with teicoplanin (98% protein bound).[48] Thus, clinical cure appears to be more likely if unbound antibiotic concentrations exceed the MIC of the infecting organism. Although ceftriaxone is 85% to 90% protein bound, the free concentrations probably remain far above the MIC of the *Serratia*. Therefore, protein-binding considerations are unlikely to be important in the treatment of R.G.'s infection.

ANTIMICROBIAL FAILURE

Antibiotic-Specific Factors

14. Despite "appropriate" treatment, R.G. is unresponsive to antimicrobial therapy. What antibiotic-specific factors may contribute to "antimicrobial failure"?

Antimicrobials may fail for various reasons, including patient-specific host factors, drug/dosage selection, and concomitant disease states. One of the most common reasons for antimicrobial failure is drug resistance.[49–51] Several clinically important pathogens have been associated with emergence of resistance over the past decade, including *M. tuberculosis*,[52] enterococci,[53] Gram-negative rods,[54] *S. aureus*,[55] *S. pneumoniae*,[56] and others. Of particular concern is the isolation of glycopeptide-resistant *S. aureus*[55] and vancomycin-tolerant pneumococci.[57] Considering the common prevalence of these two Gram-positive pathogens and the role of vancomycin as the last-line therapy for these organisms, these findings are worrisome. Development of resistance, although less common than initial resistance, may also account for failure to respond to therapy. Cephalosporin-susceptible *E. cloacae* may appear to be susceptible to a cephalosporin; however, β-lactamase production can result in development of resistance to the agent.[51]

Superinfection also may play a role in the unsuccessful treatment of infection.

Superinfection is isolation of a new pathogen resistant to the previous antimicrobial regimen. If R.G.'s ceftriaxone-treated *Serratia* pneumonia subsequently worsens and a tracheal aspirate is positive for *P. aeruginosa,* then superinfection has occurred.

Concurrent Therapy

Most infections can be treated with monotherapy (e.g., an *E. coli* wound infection is treatable with a cephalosporin). However, some infections require two-drug therapy, including enterococcal endocarditis and certain *P. aeruginosa* infec-

tions. Hilf and colleagues[59] studied 200 consecutive patients with *P. aeruginosa* bacteremia and demonstrated a 47% mortality in those receiving monotherapy (antipseudomonal β-lactam or aminoglycoside) versus 27% in those in whom two-drug therapy was used. Thus, monotherapy can contribute to antimicrobial failure in certain infections.

In contrast to these findings, most current investigations do not support the use of two drugs over monotherapy in the treatment of serious Gram-negative infection.[60–62] An exception to this rule is bacteremia caused by *P. aeruginosa* in neutropenic patients.[62]

If two antimicrobials are used in the treatment of infection, one of three sequelae will result: indifference, synergism, or antagonism.[63] Indifference occurs when the antimicrobial effect of drug A plus that of drug B equals the anticipated sum activity of drug A plus Drug B. While numerous definitions exist, synergism generally occurs when the addition of drug A to drug B results in a total antibiotic activity greater than the expected sum of the two agents. Antagonism occurs if the addition of drug A to drug B results in a combined activity less than the sum of drug A plus drug B. An example of antagonism is the combination of imipenem with a less β-lactamase stable β-lactam, such as piperacillin.[64] Certain organisms, including *P. aeruginosa* and *E. cloacae,* can be induced to produce β-lactamases.[51] If *P. aeruginosa* is exposed to imipenem and piperacillin, the large amount of generated β-lactamase degrades and inactivates piperacillin, and antagonism has resulted. Antagonism is not unique to antibacterials; itraconazole may antagonize amphotericin B in the treatment of certain infections.[65]

Pharmacologic Factors

15. What pharmacologic or pharmaceutic factors may be implicated in failure of therapy?

Subtherapeutic dosing regimens are common, especially for agents with a low therapeutic index, such as the aminoglycosides. For example, a serious Gram-negative pneumonitis may not respond to therapy if the achievable peak gentamicin serum levels are only 3 to 4 μg/mL.[34] Considering that only 20% to 30% of the aminoglycoside penetrates into bronchial secretions, only 0.5 to 1.0 μg/mL may exist at the site of infection,[66] a level that may be inadequate to treat pneumonia. As another example, the use of an aminoglycoside loading dose is particularly important in patients with renal failure because it may otherwise take several days before a therapeutic level is achieved. Yet another reason for subtherapeutic levels is reduced oral absorption secondary to drug interactions (e.g., ciprofloxacin with antacids or sucralfate).

The site of infection also contributes to antimicrobial failure. Most antimicrobials concentrate in the urine, resulting in therapeutic levels even with low doses. However, in some infections, such as meningitis, prostatitis, and endophthalmitis, antimicrobial penetration to the site of infection may be inadequate. Agents that have been proven to penetrate into these infected sites are required for a favorable outcome.

Another potential reason for antimicrobial failure is inadequate duration of therapy. A woman with a first-time uncomplicated cystitis may respond adequately to a single dose of an antibiotic. However, patients with recurrent urinary tract infections are not candidates for this therapy, and failure would be expected with the use of a single dose in these patients.

Host Factors

16. What host factors may contribute to the failure of antimicrobial therapy?

Several host factors may limit the ability of an antibiotic to cure infection. Infection of prosthetic material (e.g., IV catheters, prosthetic hip replacement, mechanical cardiac valves, and vascular grafts) is difficult to eradicate without removal of the hardware. In most cases, surgical intervention is necessary. To adequately treat R.G.'s IV catheter infection, removal of his central line probably would be required. Similar to removal of prostheses, large undrained abscesses are difficult, if not impossible, to treat with antimicrobial therapy.

These infections generally require surgical drainage for successful outcome.

Diabetic foot ulcer cellulitis may not respond adequately to antimicrobial therapy. Reasons for antimicrobial failure in patients with diabetes include poor wound healing as well as significant peripheral vascular disease that reduces the delivery of antibiotics to the site of infection.

Immune status, particularly neutropenia or lymphocytopenia, also affects the outcome in the treatment of infection. Profoundly neutropenic patients with disseminated *Aspergillus* infections are unlikely to respond to amphotericin B therapy. Similarly, patients with AIDS who have low CD4 lymphocyte counts cannot eradicate various infections, including cytomegalovirus, atypical mycobacteria, and cryptococci.

Once these factors have been eliminated as causes for antimicrobial failure, noninfectious sources must be ruled out. As discussed previously, malignancy, autoimmune disease, drug fever, and other diseases must be evaluated.

REFERENCES

1. Cranston WI et al. Oral, rectal and esophageal temperatures and some factors affecting them in man. J Physiol 1954;126:347.
2. Bone RC et al. Definitions for sepsis and organ failure and guidelines for the use of innovative therapies in sepsis. Chest 1992;101:1644.
3. Nystrom P-O. The systemic inflammatory response syndrome: definitions and aetiology. J Antimicrob Chemother 1998;41(Suppl A):1.
4. Hotchkiss RS et al. The pathophysiology and treatment of sepsis. N Engl J Med 2003;348:138.
5. Kollef MH, Schuster DP. The acute respiratory distress syndrome. N Engl J Med 1995;332:27.
6. Headley AS et al. Infections and the inflammatory response in acute respiratory distress syndrome. Chest 1997;111:1306.
7. Forgacs P et al. Characterization of chemical meningitis after neurological surgery. Clin Infect Dis 2001;32:179.
8. Hasbun R. The acute aseptic meningitis syndrome. Curr Infect Dis Rep 2000;2:345.
9. Vanderschueren S et al. From prolonged febrile illness to fever of unknown origin: the challenge continues. Arch Intern Med 2003;163:1033.
10. Mourad O et al. A comprehensive evidence-based approach to fever of unknown origin. Arch Inten Med 2003;163:545.
11. Lipsky BA, Hirschmann JV. Drug fever. JAMA 1981;245:851.
12. Bent S et al. Does this woman have an acute uncomplicated urinary tract infection? JAMA 2002;287:2701.
13. Podnos YD et al. Intra-abdominal sepsis in elderly persons. Clin Infect Dis 2002;35:62.
14. Benin AL et al. Trends in legionnaires' disease, 1980–1998: declining mortality and new patterns of diagnosis. Clin Infect Dis 2002;35:1039.
15. Bartlett JG et al. Practice guidelines for the management of community-acquired pneumonia in adults. Clin Infect Dis 2000;31:347.
16. Mandell GL et al, eds. Principles and Practice of Infectious Diseases, 5th ed. Churchill Livingstone, 2000.
17. Jones RN. Method preferences and test accuracy of antimicrobial susceptibility testing: updates from the College of Amercian Pathologists Microbiology Surveys Program. Arch Pathol Lab Med 2001;125:1285.
18. Hecht DW. Evolution of anaerobe susceptibility testing in the United States. Clin Infect Dis 2002;35(Suppl 1):S28.
19. Rex JH et al. Has antifungal susceptibility testing come of age? Clin Infect Dis 2002;35:982.

20. Wolfson JS, Swartz MN. Serum bactericidal activity as a monitor of antibiotic therapy. N Engl J Med 1985;312:968.
21. Haydon RC et al. Erythromycin ototoxicity: analysis and conclusions based on 22 case reports. Otolaryngol Head Neck Surg 1984;92:678.
22. Guglielmo BJ, Brooks GF. Antimicrobial therapy. Cost-benefit considerations. Drugs 1989;38:473.
23. Eisenberg JM et al. What is the cost of nephrotoxicity associated with aminoglycosides? Ann Intern Med 1987;107:900.
24. Blondeau JM et al. In vitro susceptibility of 1982 respiratory tract pathogens and 1921 urinary tract pathogens against 19 antimicrobial agents: a Canadian multicentre study. J Antimicrob Chemother 1999;43(Suppl A):1.
25. Lutsar I et al. Antibiotic pharmacodynamics in cerebrospinal fluid. Clin Infect Dis 1998;27:1117.
26. Papastamelos AG et al. Antibacterial agents in infections of the central nervous system and eye. Infect Dis Clin North Am 1995;9:615.
27. Schaeffer AJ et al. Overview summary statement. Diagnosis and management of chronic prostatitis/chronic pelvic pain syndrome (CP/CPPS). Urology 2002;60(6 Suppl):1.
28. Cockcroft DW, Gault MH. Prediction of creatinine clearance from serum creatinine. Nephron 1976;16:31.
29. Mackowiak PA. Influence of fever on pharmacokinetics. Rev Infect Dis 1989;11:804.
30. Brook I. Inoculum effect. Rev Infect Dis 1989;11:361.
31. Craig WA. Pharmacokinetic/pharmacodynamic parameters: rationale for antibacterial dosing of mice and men. Clin Infect Dis 1998;26:1.
32. Roosendaal R et al. Continuous infusion versus intermittent administration of ceftazidime in experimental *Klebsiella pneumoniae* pneumonia in normal and leukopenic rats. Antimicrob Agents Chemother 1986;30:403.
33. Preston SL et al. Pharmacodynamics of levofloxacin. A new paradigm for early clinical trials. JAMA 1998;279:125.
34. Moore RD et al. Association of aminoglycoside levels with therapeutic outcome in gram-negative pneumonia. Am J Med 1984;77:657.
35. Mattie H. Determinants of efficacy and toxicity of aminoglycosides. J Antimicrob Chemother 1989;24:281.
36. Matske GR et al. Controlled comparison of gentamicin and tobramycin nephrotoxicity. Am J Nephrol 1983;3:11.

37. McCormack JP, Jewesson PJ. A critical reevaluation of the "therapeutic range" of aminoglycosides. Clin Infect Dis 1992;14:320.
38. Begg EG et al. The therapeutic monitoring of antimicrobial agents. Br J Clin Pharmacol 2001;52(Suppl 1):35S.
39. MacGowan AP. Pharmacodynamics, pharmacokinetics, and therapeutic drug monitoring of glycopeptides. Ther Drug Monit 1998;20:473.
40. Cantu TG et al. Serum vancomycin concentrations: reappraisal of their clinical value. Clin Infect Dis 1994;18:533.
41. MacKenzie FM, Gould IM. The post-antibiotic effect. J Antimicrob Chemother 1993;32:519.
42. Andes DA et al. Animal model pharmacokinetics and pharmacodynamics: a critical review. Intl J Antimicrob Agents 2002;19:261.
43. Hatala R et al. Single daily dosing of aminoglycosides in immunocompromised adults: a systematic review. Clin Infect Dis 1997;24:810.
44. Ferriols-Lisart R. Effectiveness and safety of once-daily aminoglycosides: a meta-analysis. Am J Health Syst Pharm 1996;53:1141.
45. McCormack JP. An emotional-based medicine approach to monitoring once-daily aminoglycosides. Pharmacother 2000;20:1524.
46. Lam YWF et al. Effect of protein binding on serum bactericidal activities of ceftazidime and cefoperazone in healthy volunteers. Antimicrob Agents Chemother 1988;32:298.
47. Chambers HF et al. Failure of a once-daily regimen of cefonicid for treatment of endocarditis due to *Staphylococcus aureus*. Rev Infect Dis 1984;6(Suppl 4):S870.
48. Greenberg RN. Treatment of bone, joint, and vascular-access-associated gram-positive bacterial infections with teicoplanin. Antimicrob Agents Chemother 1990;34:2392.
49. Finch RG. Antibiotic resistance. J Antimicrob Chemother 1998;42:125.
50. Phillips I. The subtleties of antibiotic resistance. J Antimicrob Chemother 1998;42:5.
51. Acar JF, Goldstein FW. Consequences of increasing resistance to antimicrobial agents. Clin Infect Dis 1998;27(Suppl 1):S125.
52. Small PM et al. Management of tuberculosis in the United States. N Engl J Med 2001;345:189.
53. Effects of antibiotics on nosocomial epidemiology of vancomycin-resistant enterococci. Antimicrob Agents Chemother 2002;46:1619.
54. Neuhauser MM et al. Antibiotic resistance among gram-negative bacilli in US intensive care units:

implications for fluoroquinolone use. JAMA 2003;289:885.

55. Chang S et al. Infection with vancomycin-resistant *Staphylococcus aureus* containing the vanA resistance gene. N Engl J Med 2003;348:1342.

56. Butler JC, Cetron MS. Pneumococcal drug resistance: the new "special enemy of old age." Clin Infect Dis 1999;28:730.

57. Novak R et al. Emergence of vancomycin tolerance in *Streptococcus pneumoniae*. Nature 1999; 399:590.

58. Chow JW et al. Enterobacter bacteremia: clinical features and emergence of antibiotic resistance during therapy. Ann Intern Med 1991;115:585.

59. Hilf M et al. Antibiotic therapy for *Pseudomonas aeruginosa* bacteremia: outcome correlations in a prospective study of 200 patients. Am J Med 1989;87:540.

60. Vidal F et al. Epidemiology and outcome of *Pseudomonas aeruginosa* bacteremia, with special emphasis on the influence of antibiotic treatment. Arch Intern Med 1996;156:2121.

61. Siegman-Igra Y et al. Pseudomonas aeruginosa bacteremia: an analysis of 123 episodes, with particular emphasis on the effect of antibiotic therapy. Intl J Infect Dis 1998;2:211.

62. Leibovici L et al. Monotherapy versus β-lactam-aminoglycoside combination treatment for gram-negative bacteremia: a prospective, observational study. Antimicrob Agents Chemother 1997;41: 1127.

63. Fantin B, Carbon C. In vivo antibiotic synergism: contribution of animal models. Antimicrob Agents Chemother 1992;36:907.

64. Bertram MA, Young LS. Imipenem antagonism of the in vitro activity of piperacillin against *Pseudomonas aeruginosa*. Antimicrob Agents Chemother 1984;26:272.

65. Sugar AM, Liu X-P. Interactions of itraconazole with amphotericin B in the treatment of murine invasive candidiasis. J Infect Dis 1998;177:1660.

66. Bergogne-Berezin E. New concepts in the pulmonary disposition of antibiotics. Pulm Pharmacol 1995;8:65.

CHAPTER 57

Antimicrobial Prophylaxis for Surgical Procedures

Daniel J. G. Thirion, B. Joseph Guglielmo

Prophylactic antibiotics are widely used in surgical procedures and account for substantial antibiotic use in many hospitals.[1] The purpose of surgical antibiotic prophylaxis is to reduce the prevalence of postoperative wound infection (about 5% of surgical cases overall) at or around the surgical site.[2] Such surgical site infections reportedly extend the duration of hospitalization by at least 1 week, at an annual cost of more than $1.5 billion nationwide.[3-5] By preventing surgical site infections, prophylactic antimicrobial agents have the potential to decrease patient morbidity and hospitalization costs for many surgical procedures that pose significant risk of infection (e.g., appendectomy); however, the benefits of prophylaxis are controversial, and prophylaxis is not justified for some surgical procedures (e.g., urologic operations in patients with sterile urine).[6] Consequently, the inappropriate or indiscriminate use of prophylactic antibiotics can increase the risk of drug toxicity, selection of resistant organisms, and costs.

RISK FACTORS FOR INFECTION

The development of postoperative site infection is related to the degree of bacterial contamination during surgery, the virulence of the infecting organism, and host defenses. Risk factors for postoperative site infection can be classified according to operative and environmental factors, and patient characteristics.[7]

Bacterial contamination may occur from exogenous sources (e.g., the operative team, instruments, airborne organisms) or from endogenous sources (e.g., the patient's microflora of the skin, respiratory, genitourinary, or gastrointestinal [GI] tract).[7,8] Infection control procedures to minimize all sources of bacterial contamination, including patient and surgical team preparation, operative technique, and incision care, are compiled in Centers for Disease Control and Prevention guidelines for surgical site infection.[7]

The risk of postoperative site infection is affected by host factors such as extremes of age, obesity, cigarette smoking, malnutrition, and comorbid states, including diabetes mellitus, remote infection, colonization with microorganisms, and immunosuppressive therapy.[8,9] In addition, the longer the preoperative hospital stay and the surgical procedure, the greater the likelihood of developing a postoperative wound infection, presumably as a result of nosocomial bacterial acquisition in the former and the greater amount of bacterial contamination occurring over time in the latter.[8]

Another major risk factor for infection is the skill of the surgeon. In one study,[10] postoperative wound infection rates were related inversely to the frequency of performing a surgical procedure; thus, hospitals with the highest frequency of surgical procedures have the lowest incidence of postoperative infection.

Based on these risk factors for infection, the decision as to whether a given patient should receive antimicrobial prophylaxis is multifactorial. Many experts recommend that antimicrobial prophylaxis should be given for surgical procedures with a high rate of infection, procedures involving the implantation of prosthetic materials, or procedures in which an infection would have catastrophic consequences.[9,11] A widely used surgical wound classification system to assist in this decision-making process follows.

CLASSIFICATION OF SURGICAL WOUNDS

From 1960 to 1964, the National Academy of Sciences National Research Council conducted a landmark study of surgical wound infections and formulated a widely used standard classification of surgical wounds based on the risk of intraoperative bacterial contamination (Table 57-1).[8] Current recommendations for surgical prophylaxis pertain to clean surgeries involving implantation of prosthetic material, clean-contaminated surgeries, and select contaminated wounds. Antimicrobial therapy for most contaminated and all dirty surgeries in which infection already is established is considered treatment instead of prophylaxis and is not discussed further in this chapter. Table 57-2 lists suspected pathogens and recommendations for site-specific prophylactic antimicrobial regimens; a detailed examination of clinical trials supporting these recommendations is presented elsewhere.[6]

Table 57-1   National Research Council Wound Classification

Classification	Criteria	Infection Rate (%)
Clean	No acute inflammation or entry into GI, respiratory, GU, or biliary tracts; no break in aseptic technique occurs; wounds primarily closed	<5
Clean-contaminated	Elective, controlled opening of GI, respiratory, biliary, or GU tracts without significant spillage; clean wounds with major break in sterile technique	<10
Contaminated	Penetrating trauma (<4 hr old); major technique break or major spillage from GI tract; acute, nonpurulent inflammation	15–20
Dirty	Penetrating trauma (>4 hr old); purulence or abscess (active infectious process); preoperative perforation of viscera	30–40

GI, gastrointestinal; GU, genitourinary.
From references 3 and 8.

Table 57-2   Suggested Prophylactic Antimicrobial Regimens for Surgical Procedures

Procedure	Predominant Organism(s)	Antibiotic Regimen (Alternative)	Adult Preoperative IV Dose (Alternative)
Clean			
Cardiac (all with sternotomy, cardiopulmonary bypass)	*Staphylococcus aureus, Staphylococcus epidermidis*	Cefazolin (Vancomycin)	1 g (1 g)
Vascular (aortic resection, groin incision, prosthesis)	*S. aureus, S. epidermidis*, Gram-negative enterics	Cefazolin (Vancomycin)	1 g (1 g)
Orthopedic (total joint replacement, internal fixation of fractures)	*S. aureus, S. epidermidis*	Cefazolin (Vancomycin)	1 g (1 g)
Neurosurgery	*S. aureus, S. epidermidis*	Cefazolin (Vancomycin)	1 g (1 g)
Clean-Contaminated			
Head and neck	*S. aureus*, oral anaerobes, streptococci	Cefazolin (Clindamycin ± gentamicin)	2 g (600 mg clindamycin ± 1.5 mg/kg gentamicin)
Gastroduodenal (only for procedures entering stomach)	Gram-negative enterics, *S. aureus*, mouth flora	Cefazolin	1 g
Colorectal	Gram-negative enterics, anaerobes (*Bacteroides fragilis*)	Oral neomycin–erythromycin base (IV Cefoxitin or cefotetan)	1 g each at 1 PM, 2 PM, and 11 PM day before surgery (1 g of either)
Appendectomy (uncomplicated)	Gram-negative enterics, anaerobes (*B. fragilis*)	Cefoxitin or cefotetan	1–2 g
Biliary tract (only for high-risk procedures)	Gram-negative enterics, *Enterococcus faecalis, Clostridia*	Cefazolin	1 g
Cesarean section	Group B streptococci, enterococci, anaerobes, Gram-negative enterics	Cefazolin	2 g after umbilical cord clamped
Hysterectomy	Group B streptococci, enterococci, anaerobes, Gram-negative enterics	Cefazolin, cefoxitin, or cefotetan	1 g
Genitourinary (only for high-risk procedures)	Gram-negative enterics, enterococci	Ciprofloxacin	400 mg

PRINCIPLES OF SURGICAL ANTIMICROBIAL PROPHYLAXIS

Decision to Use Antimicrobial Prophylaxis

1. M.R., a 72-year-old woman, is admitted to the hospital with severe abdominal pain, nausea and vomiting, and temperature of 39.3°C. A diagnosis of acute cholecystitis is made, and M.R. is scheduled for biliary tract surgery (cholecystectomy). Why is antimicrobial prophylaxis warranted for M.R.?

Biliary tract surgery is considered a clean-contaminated procedure and therefore carries a risk of surgical wound infection approaching 10% (see Tables 57-1 and 57-2). Prophylaxis for biliary tract surgery is limited to "high-risk" procedures, which include obesity, age >70 years, diabetes mellitus, acute cholecystitis, obstructive jaundice, or common duct stones.[6,9,12] Thus, prophylaxis is warranted in M.R., who falls into at least two high risk categories (age >70 years and acute cholecystitis).

2. An order for cefazolin 1 g IV on call to the operating room (OR) is written for M.R. Why is this an appropriate (or inappropriate) antibiotic selection?

The selected prophylactic agent should be directed against likely infecting organisms (see Table 57-2) but need not eradicate every potential pathogen. Cefazolin has been proven effective for most surgical procedures, including biliary tract surgery, given that the goal of prophylaxis is to decrease bacterial counts below critical levels necessary to cause infection. Broad-spectrum agents such as third-generation cephalosporins should be avoided for prophylaxis because they are no more effective than cefazolin and may alter microbial flora, increasing the emergence of microbial resistance to these otherwise valuable agents.

Timing of Antimicrobial Administration

3. Why is the administration time for this antimicrobial appropriate (or inappropriate) for M.R.?

Classic animal studies conducted by Burke[13] and others[14] clearly demonstrated the need for therapeutic antibiotic concentrations in the bloodstream and in vulnerable tissue at the time of wound contamination. Bacteria were most likely to enter the tissue beginning with the initial surgical incision and continuing until the wound was closed; antibiotics administered >3 hours after bacterial contamination were ineffective in minimizing the development of wound infection.[13,14] This 2- to 3-hour period after the surgical incision was deemed the "effective" or "decisive" period for prophylaxis, when the animal wound was most susceptible to the beneficial effects of the antibiotic. This decisive period for administration of prophylactic antibiotics has been confirmed in humans.[15,16]

For maximal efficacy, an antibiotic should be present in therapeutic concentrations at the incision site as early as possible during the decisive period and continuing until the wound is closed. Because an antibiotic administered postoperatively cannot achieve therapeutic concentrations during the decisive period, such timing of surgical "prophylaxis" is of no benefit in preventing postoperative wound infections, and in-

fection rates are similar to those in patients who receive no antibiotics.[16] An exception in which post-incision administration sometimes is justified is in cesarean sections, because the incidence of post-cesarean endometritis is decreased significantly by postoperative administration of antibiotics.[6]

Based on these study results, prophylactic antibiotics should be administered before the surgical procedure in the OR before the induction of anesthesia.[7] Prophylactic antibiotics are most effective when given during the 2-hour period before the surgical incision is made, and rates of infection increase significantly if antibiotics are administered >2 hours preoperatively or any time postoperatively.[17]

The "on call" prescribing practice for surgical prophylaxis, as with M.R., has fallen into disfavor because the time between antibiotic administration and the actual incision may exceed 2 hours and therefore may result in subtherapeutic antibiotic concentrations during the decisive period.[18,19] M.R.'s cefazolin should be ordered preoperatively and should be administered in the operating room no earlier than 2 hours before the operative procedure.

4. Will M.R. require a second dose of cefazolin during the surgical procedure?

The duration of the surgical procedure and the half-life of the administered antibiotic should be considered when determining whether an additional dose is necessary to maintain adequate antibiotic concentrations at the operative site. Studies have indicated an inverse relationship between the efficacy of short-acting antibiotics and the duration of the surgical procedure; as operative time increases, so does the incidence of postoperative infection.[20,21] Cefazolin, with a half-life of approximately 1.8 hours, is effective in a single preoperative dose for most surgical procedures. For procedures lasting >3 hours, additional intraoperative doses should be administered every 3 to 8 hours during the procedure,[9,22] especially if an antibiotic with a short half-life, such as cefoxitin, has been administered. M.R. should require an additional intraoperative cefazolin dose only if the surgical procedure is prolonged (>3 hours).

Route of Administration

5. G.B., a 55-year-old woman recently diagnosed with carcinoma of the large bowel, is admitted to the hospital for an elective colorectal surgical resection; the surgery is expected to last ≥5 hours. Physical examination reveals a cachectic woman with a 9-kg weight loss over the previous 3 months (current weight, 60 kg). Increased frequency of bowel movements and chronic fatigue are noted; all other systems are normal. Laboratory data include hemoglobin (Hgb), 10.4 g/dL (normal, 11.5 to 15.5); hematocrit (Hct), 29.7% (normal, 33% to 43%); and prothrombin time (PT), 15 seconds (normal, 11 to 13). Stool guaiac is positive. Vital signs are within normal limits. G.B. is taking no medications and has no history of drug allergies. The following orders are written to begin at home on the day before surgery: (1) Clear liquid diet; (2) Mechanical bowel cleansing with polyethylene glycol-electrolyte lavage solution (CoLYTE, GoLYTELY); (3) Neomycin sulfate 1 g and erythromycin 1 g PO at 1 PM, 2 PM, and 11 PM. Comment on the appropriateness of the oral route of administration of antibiotic prophylaxis for G.B.

[SI units: Hgb, 104 g/L; Hct, 0.297]

In general, oral administration of surgical antimicrobial prophylaxis is not recommended because of unreliable or poor absorption of oral agents in the anesthetized bowel. Oral agents, however, function effectively as GI decontaminants because high intraluminal drug concentrations are sufficient to decrease bacterial counts.[23] The concentration of bacteria in the colon may approach 10^{13} bacteria/mm^3 and colorectal procedures, such as the one G.B. will undergo, carry a relatively high risk of postoperative infection. Antimicrobial regimens with activity against the mixture of aerobic and anaerobic bacteria that make up the fecal flora (*Escherichia coli* and other Enterobacteriaceae and *Bacteroides fragilis*) are effective in preventing postoperative wound infections.[24,25]

The most widely used oral antimicrobial regimen directed against the fecal flora is 1 g each of the nonabsorbable antibiotics neomycin sulfate (for Gram-negative aerobes) and erythromycin base (for anaerobes), given 1 day before surgery at the times indicated for G.B.[16,25] Mechanical bowel cleansing, such as with polyethylene glycol-electrolyte lavage solution, must precede this regimen; the purpose of such bowel purging is to evacuate the colonic contents as completely as possible to decrease colonic bacterial counts. Effective oral alternatives to neomycin plus erythromycin include metronidazole with or without neomycin or with kanamycin, or kanamycin plus erythromycin[24,26]; however, clinical situations warranting the use of such alternatives over the well-established neomycin–erythromycin regimen are practically nonexistent. Thus, the regimen selected for G.B. is highly appropriate.

6. **The surgical resident has canceled the oral neomycin–erythromycin bowel regimen for G.B. Instead, he orders cefoxitin (Mefoxin) 1 g IV preoperatively. Why is (or is not) this change in therapy an effective and rational choice for G.B.?**

Numerous parenteral regimens, specifically with agents that possess both aerobic and anaerobic activity, are effective as surgical prophylaxis in colorectal procedures.[24] The second-generation cephalosporins with significant anaerobic activity (e.g., cefoxitin, cefotetan) are superior to first-generation cephalosporins, which lack sufficient anaerobic activity.[27,28] At present, it is not clear whether oral antimicrobial prophylaxis is superior to parenteral therapy in the prevention of infection after colorectal surgery.[29]

Thus, although both intravenous (IV) and oral regimens are effective for prophylaxis before colorectal surgery, the parenteral route of administration, selected because of physician preference, may be less effective.[9] Furthermore, the cefoxitin order for G.B. would be unacceptable if the surgery lasts >3.5 hours (the relatively short half-life of cefoxitin could render G.B. antibiotic-free and predispose her to infection).[30] For prolonged procedures (>3 hours) such as anticipated for G.B., an alternative agent with a longer half-life (e.g., cefotetan) or a second dose of cefoxitin should be administered. However, cefotetan may be a poor choice for G.B. because of its propensity to cause hypoprothrombinemia with or without associated bleeding episodes. This effect is attributed in part to the N-methylthiotetrazole side chain in the chemical structure of cefotetan. G.B. currently has an increased prothrombin time, so it would be prudent to avoid cefotetan. Thus, for G.B., the importance and efficacy of established oral prophylactic regimens (plus bowel cleansing) should be stressed to the resident.

7. **The surgical resident has reconsidered the cefoxitin order and decided to prescribe both the oral and parenteral prophylactic regimens for G.B. Will the combination significantly reduce the rate of postoperative wound infection compared with either regimen administered singly?**

Although the coadministration of both oral and parenteral prophylactic regimens occurs commonly in practice (88% of one survey's respondents),[31] data in support of this practice are inadequate,[29] presumably because a study of large numbers of patients would be required to document a further decrease in already low infection rates (approximately 5% to 10%).[32] Colorectal surgical procedures, however, are associated with a higher infection rate (than colonic procedures), and an oral plus parenteral antimicrobial prophylaxis combination is superior to orally administered regimens alone in reducing infection rates.[30] As a result, a combination of oral and parenteral antimicrobial prophylaxis is recommended for colorectal surgery.[9]

Thus, evidence is conflicting for combination oral plus parenteral therapy for colon surgery prophylaxis in G.B., although the standard of practice often dictates its use.[31]

Duration of Administration

8. **L.G., a 28-year-old man with a history of rheumatic heart disease, has a 12-year history of a heart murmur consistent with mild mitral stenosis and mitral regurgitation. Over the past 4 months his murmur has become much more prominent. In addition, he has developed severe dyspnea with light physical activity and 3+ pitting edema over both lower legs. Physical examination is notable for coarse rales and an S_3 gallop. For the past 6 weeks he has been maintained on digoxin and diuretics without significant relief of his shortness of breath (SOB). The cardiothoracic surgeon recommends mitral valve replacement and orders the following surgical antibiotic prophylaxis regimen: cefazolin 1 g IV preoperatively, then Q 8 hr for 48 hours. Why is cefazolin the most appropriate antimicrobial for L.G.? Why was prophylaxis ordered for only 48 hours?**

Although the incidence of postoperative wound infection for cardiothoracic procedures is low (<5%), the devastating consequences of a postoperative endocarditis (following valve replacement) and mediastinitis or sternal osteomyelitis (following sternotomy) warrant careful antimicrobial prophylaxis.[33–46] Organisms of concern for cardiothoracic surgery include *Staphylococcus aureus* and *Staphylococcus epidermidis* (see Table 57-2); based on these potential pathogens, successful prophylactic regimens include cefazolin (Ancef), cefamandole (Mandol), and cefuroxime (Zinacef). When cefazolin has been compared with cefuroxime or cefamandole, a statistical trend in favor of the second-generation cephalosporins has been noted, and collective wound infection rates were slightly higher in the cefazolin group.[35–37] In contrast, a comparison of prophylactic cefazolin and cefuroxime in patients undergoing open heart surgery noted a significantly greater incidence of sternal wound infection and mediastinitis in the cefuroxime group.[38] Furthermore, equal efficacy between the two agents was noted in yet another study.[39] In conclusion, cefazolin probably is at least as effective as second-generation cephalosporins; therefore, the choice of agent should be based on an institution's antimicrobial susceptibility and cost data. Hospital-specific antimicrobial resistance patterns are especially important in determining the incidence of methicillin-resistant *S. aureus* (MRSA) or methicillin-resistant *S. epidermidis* (MRSE); vancomycin is the drug of choice for prophylaxis of such organisms.

Meta-analyses of the use of prophylactic antibiotics in cardiac surgery demonstrated no significant differences in the rate of surgical site infection between first- and second-generation cephalosporins.[40,46] Thus, the cefazolin prophylaxis selected for L.G. is acceptable, provided MRSA and MRSE are not of concern in this institution.

With regard to duration, the shortest effective prophylactic course of antibiotics should be used (i.e., single dose preoperatively or not more than 24 hours postoperatively for most procedures).[45] Single-dose prophylaxis, a viable option for many surgical procedures (see Question 9), is controversial for cardiac procedures.[33] In practice, cardiothoracic antimicrobial prophylaxis often is continued 48 hours after surgery,[9] as in L.G. There is no benefit to prolonging prophylaxis to >48 hours, and such use should be discouraged. The duration of antimicrobial prophylaxis ordered for L.G. is appropriate.

9. G.J., a 27-year-old woman, is admitted to the obstetrics unit at term with her first pregnancy. She is scheduled for a cesarean section because the baby is breech. Cefazolin 1 g IV to be administered after the cord is clamped and Q 8 hr for 24 hours is ordered. Why is this surgical prophylaxis inappropriate?

As noted previously, the shortest effective duration of prophylaxis is desired. In the past, 5- or 6-day antimicrobial regimens were used for cesarean section, but 24-hour regimens have since been proven as effective as these longer regimens.[47,48] Faro and colleagues demonstrated that a single 2-g dose of cefazolin was superior to either a single 1-g dose or to a three-dose, 1-g prophylactic regimen.[48] Others have noted similar results (i.e., a single cefazolin dose administered after the umbilical cord is clamped seems to be sufficient in preventing postoperative wound infections in cesarean section).[49–51] Single-dose prophylaxis is less costly[52] and minimizes the development of bacterial resistance.[53] Thus, G.J. should receive a single 2-g dose of cefazolin after the cord has been clamped, without the three additional doses.

Single-dose prophylaxis also is effective in a variety of GI tract, orthopedic, and gynecologic procedures.[21] A single dose of an antibiotic with a short half-life, however, may provide insufficient antimicrobial coverage during a prolonged surgical procedure, and repeated intraoperative dosing or selection of an agent with a longer half-life is recommended when the duration of surgery is long.

Signs of Wound Infection

10. G.J. is discharged on the fifth hospital day and instructed to observe her incision site carefully for signs of infection. What are the typical signs of site infection? What is the typical time course for signs of site infection to become manifest?

Most surgical site infections involve the incision site. Typically, an infected incision site wound is red, inflamed, and purulent. The purulent drainage should be cultured to identify the causative pathogen and to direct antimicrobial therapy. Empiric therapy directed against the most likely pathogens

should be instituted while awaiting culture and sensitivity test results. Although most incision site infections are clinically apparent shortly after surgery (within 30 days), some deep-seated infections present indolently over weeks to months, by which time an abscess may have developed.[8] When implants are involved, infections occurring up to a year after surgery may be related to the operation.[54]

Selection of an Antimicrobial Agent

11. L.T., a 46-year-old woman, has a recent history of abnormal uterine bleeding and vaginal discharge. Endometrial biopsy is positive for squamous cell carcinoma. Invasive disease is not evident. The diagnosis is carcinoma in situ, and a vaginal hysterectomy is scheduled. What would be a good surgical prophylaxis antimicrobial regimen for L.T.?

The selection of a prophylactic regimen should incorporate such factors as the agent's microbiologic activity against the most likely potential pathogens encountered during the surgical procedure (see Table 57-2), pharmacokinetic characteristics (e.g., half-life), inherent toxicity, potential to promote the emergence of resistant strains of bacteria, and cost.

The usefulness of antimicrobial prophylaxis in vaginal hysterectomies is well established and is directed against vaginal microflora, including Gram-positive and Gram-negative aerobes and anaerobes (see Table 57-2). The narrowest-spectrum agent that is efficacious is desired, given that the goal of prophylaxis is not to eradicate every potential pathogen, but to reduce bacterial counts below a critical level necessary to cause infection. Cefazolin has been proven to be an effective prophylactic agent for vaginal hysterectomy when compared with broad-spectrum agents such as ceftriaxone (Rocephin).[55] This indicates that a broader-spectrum agent with anaerobic activity (which cefazolin lacks) is unwarranted.

Similar to vaginal hysterectomy, cefazolin and numerous agents have been documented to reduce the incidence of postoperative surgical infection via the abdominal approach.[56,57] However, as with vaginal hysterectomy, most trials have not documented significant differences between first- and second-generation cephalosporins.[56] In contrast, Hemsell and associates observed a significantly higher incidence of major postoperative surgical infection in patients receiving the first-generation agent cefazolin when compared with cefotetan.[58] As a result of this controversy, the American College of Obstetricians and Gynecologists has recommended first-, second-, or third-generation cephalosporins for prophylaxis in these procedures.[59] Cefazolin exhibits a favorable toxicity profile and has a relatively long half-life (approximately 1.8 hours) such that a single dose has proven prophylactic efficacy.[55] Cefazolin also is considerably less expensive than broader-spectrum agents. Although it has a broader spectrum of coverage, a single dose of cefotetan would also be an appropriate choice for this patient.

12. Because cefotetan has an increased spectrum of activity against the anaerobe *B. fragilis*, it is being considered as an alternative to cefazolin prophylaxis for L.T. Comment on the appropriateness of this proposed change in prophylaxis.

The second- and third-generation cephalosporins generally are not more effective than the first-generation cephalosporins for surgical prophylaxis in vaginal hysterectomy or gastroduodenal, biliary, and clean surgical procedures.[6] One clear exception to these findings is in the prevention of infection after colorectal procedures and perhaps hysterectomy. Several investigations have documented the failure of first-generation agents when used as prophylaxis in colorectal procedures, probably a consequence of their weak anaerobic coverage.[27,28] As stated previously, second- and third-generation agents generally are no more efficacious than cefazolin and should not be used for surgical prophylaxis in most procedures. However, cefotetan would be a reasonable choice in colorectal surgery or hysterectomy. Considering that this patient is undergoing a hysterectomy, either cefazolin or cefotetan is appropriate.

13. S.N., a 57-year-old woman with rheumatoid arthritis and degenerative joint disease, has been admitted for total hip arthroplasty. She has an allergy to penicillin. What should be prescribed for S.N. for surgical prophylaxis?

Cefazolin is the preferred prophylactic agent for most clean procedures, including cardiac, vascular, and orthopedic procedures[6] (see Table 57-2). Although the risk of cefazolin cross-allergenicity to penicillin is minimal, S.N. experienced a significant penicillin allergy (hives, SOB); therefore, an alternative prophylactic agent definitely is appropriate. The organisms most likely to cause postoperative infection after total hip replacement are *S. aureus* and *S. epidermidis* (see Table 57-2). Nafcillin, cefazolin, and vancomycin possess excellent activity against *S. aureus,* however, the β-lactams have only marginal activity against *S. epidermidis*. Regardless, nafcillin clearly must be avoided because of the penicillin allergy. Thus, the preferred agent for S. N. is vancomycin.

Preoperative vancomycin 1 g should be administered IV slowly, over at least 60 minutes. This slow rate of infusion is necessary to reduce the risk of infusion-related hypotension, which poses a particular danger during anesthesia induction and has been reported to cause cardiac arrest.[60]

14. B.K., an 18-year-old woman, complains of severe acute abdominal pain and nausea; the pain is localized to the periumbilical region. B.K. has a temperature of 39.5°C. After initial examination by her pediatrician, she is admitted to hospital with presumed appendicitis and an exploratory laparotomy is scheduled. What surgical antimicrobial prophylaxis should be ordered for B.K.?

As with colorectal surgery, the most likely infecting organisms in appendectomy are *Bacteroides* species and Gram-negative enterics (see Table 57-2). Upon surgical inspection, if the appendix appears normal (uninflamed, without perforation), then antimicrobial prophylaxis is unnecessary.[61] If the appendix is inflamed without perforation, a single preoperative antibiotic dose is necessary. If the appendix is perforated or gangrenous (complicated), infection is already established and postoperative treatment is warranted. Unfortunately, the status of the appendix cannot be determined before surgery; therefore, all patients should receive at least one dose of an appropriate antibiotic preoperatively. After surgical inspection

of the appendix, the need for postoperative antibiotic therapy can be determined.

Based on the pathogens likely to be encountered, an antimicrobial agent with both aerobic and anaerobic activity is desired for surgical prophylaxis in this situation. Consequently, cefoxitin (Mefoxin), cefotetan (Cefotan), ceftizoxime (Cefizox), or cefotaxime (Claforan) are acceptable choices for prophylaxis.[62,63]

Risks of Indiscriminate Antimicrobial Use

15. Upon surgical exploration, B.K. was found to have uncomplicated (nonperforated, nongangrenous) appendicitis; however, cefoxitin therapy was continued for 3 days for unclear reasons. What are the risks of indiscriminate use of antimicrobials for surgical prophylaxis?

The risks of indiscriminate use of antimicrobials to a given patient include the potential for adverse effects and superinfection. The administration of any β-lactam agent poses the risk of a hypersensitivity reaction, and many antibiotics, including cefoxitin, such as in B.K., are known to predispose patients to *Clostridium difficile*–associated disease. In addition, widespread or prolonged use of antimicrobial agents increases the potential for the development or selection of resistant organisms in a given patient or other patients who may acquire a pathogen nosocomially.[64]

OPTIMIZING SURGICAL ANTIMICROBIAL PROPHYLAXIS

Antibiotic control strategies have improved the appropriate use of antimicrobial agents for surgical prophylaxis. The implementation of an automatic stop-order policy for surgical prophylaxis has reduced the duration of antimicrobial prophylaxis dramatically. These stop-order policies can be printed directly onto an antibiotic order form.[65,66] In one early study, the creation of an antibiotic order form with an automatic stop order after 2 days of surgical prophylaxis reduced the mean duration of surgical prophylaxis from 4.9 to 2.9 days.[65] One study noted that the duration of surgical prophylaxis exceeded the recommended 24 hours in only 4% to 18% of cases.[66] Both examples demonstrate significant improvement in the use of antimicrobial prophylaxis.

In collaboration with other health care providers, the pharmacy department of health care organizations is responsible for optimizing the timing, choice, and duration of antimicrobial surgical prophylaxis.[67–69] In one program, computer-assisted monitoring of the duration of surgical prophylaxis helped identify and automatically discontinue inappropriately long courses of surgical antimicrobial prophylaxis, significantly reduced the average number of antibiotic doses administered, and generated reduced costs without jeopardizing clinical outcomes.[68] Similar cost savings can be achieved by orchestrating changes within an institution aimed at reducing the duration and frequency of prophylactic surgical antibiotic administration.[67]

REFERENCES

1. Shapiro M et al. Use of antimicrobial drugs in general hospitals: patterns of prophylaxis. N Engl J Med 1979;301:351.
2. Cruse PJE et al. The epidemiology of wound infection: a 10-year prospective study of 62,939 wounds. Surg Clin North Am 1980;60:27.
3. Haley RW et al. Extra charges and prolongation of stay attributable to nosocomial infections: a prospective interhospital comparison. Am J Med 1981;70:51.
4. Wenzel RP. Preoperative antibiotic prophylaxis. N Engl J Med 1992;326:337.
5. Kirkland KB et al. The impact of surgical-site infections in the 1990s: attributable mortality, excess length of hospitalization, and extra costs. Infect Control Hosp Epidemiol 1999;20:725.
6. Anon. Antimicrobial prophylaxis in surgery. Med Letter 2001;43:92.
7. Mangram AJ et al. Guideline for prevention of surgical site infection, 1999. Hospital Infection Control Practices Advisory Committee. Infect Control Hosp Epidemiol 1999;20:250.
8. Ad Hoc Committee of the Committee on Trauma, Division of Medical Sciences. National Academy of Sciences/National Research Council. Postoperative wound infections: the influence of ultraviolet irradiation of the operating room and various other factors. Ann Surg 1964;160(Suppl 2):1.
9. American Society of Health-System Pharmacists. ASHP Therapeutic Guidelines on Antimicrobial Prophylaxis in Surgery. Am J Health-Syst Pharm 1999;56:1839.
10. Farber BF et al. Relation between surgical volume and incidence of postoperative wound infection. N Engl J Med 1981;305:200.
11. Lewis RT. Antibiotic prophylaxis in surgery. Can J Surg 1981;24:561.
12. Grant MD et al. Single-dose cephalosporin prophylaxis in high-risk patients undergoing surgical treatment of the biliary tract. Surg Gynecol Obstet 1992;174:347.
13. Burke JF. Effective period of preventive antibiotic action in experimental incisions and dermal lesions. Surgery 1961;50:161.
14. Miles AA et al. The value and duration of defence reactions of the skin to the primary lodgement of bacteria. Br J Exp Pathol 1957;38:79.
15. Polk HC et al. Postoperative wound infection: a prospective study of determinant factors and prevention. Surgery 1969;66:97.
16. Stone HH et al. Antibiotic prophylaxis in gastric, biliary and colonic surgery. Ann Surg 1976;184:443.
17. Classen DC et al. The timing of prophylactic administration of antibiotics and the risk of surgical-wound infection. N Engl J Med 1992;326:281.
18. Nix DE et al. Cephalosporins for surgical prophylaxis: computer projections of intraoperative availability. South Med J 1985;78:962.
19. Galanduik S et al. Re-emphasis of priorities in surgical antibiotic prophylaxis. Surg Gynecol Obstet 1989;169:219.
20. Shapiro M et al. Risk factors for infection at the operative site after abdominal or vaginal hysterectomy. N Engl J Med 1982;307:1661.
21. DiPiro JT et al. Single dose systemic antibiotic prophylaxis of surgical wound infections. Am J Surg 1986;152:552.
22. Scher KS. Studies on the duration of antibiotic administration for surgical prophylaxis. Am Surg 1997;63:59.
23. Bartlett JG et al. Veterans Administration Cooperative Study on bowel preparation for elective colorectal operations. Ann Surg 1978;188:249.
24. Guglielmo BJ et al. Antibiotic prophylaxis in surgical procedures: a critical analysis of the literature. Arch Surg 1983;118:943.

25. Nichols RL et al. Effect of preoperative neomycin–erythromycin intestinal preparation on the incidence of infectious complications following colon surgery. Ann Surg 1973;178:453.
26. DiPiro JT et al. Antimicrobial prophylaxis in surgery. Part 1. Am J Hosp Pharm 1981;38:320.
27. Lewis RT. Are first-generation cephalosporins effective for antibiotic prophylaxis in elective surgery of the colon? Can J Surg 1983;26:504.
28. Condon RE et al. Preoperative prophylactic cephalothin fails to control septic complications of colorectal operations: results of a controlled clinical trial. Am J Surg 1979;137:68.
29. Song F, Glenny AM. Antimicrobial prophylaxis in colorectal surgery: a systematic review of randomised controlled trials. Health Technol Assessment 1998;2(7).
30. Coppa G et al. Factors involved in antibiotic selection in elective colon and rectal surgery. Surgery 1988;104:853.
31. Solla J et al. Preoperative bowel preparation: a survey of colon and rectal surgeons. Dis Colon Rectum 1990;33:154.
32. Condon RE et al. Efficacy of oral and systemic antibiotic prophylaxis in colorectal operations. Arch Surg 1983;118:496.
33. Ariano RE et al. Antimicrobial prophylaxis in coronary bypass surgery: a critical appraisal. DICP 1991;25:478.
34. Gelfond MS et al. Cefamandole versus cefonicid prophylaxis in cardiovascular surgery: A prospective study. Ann Thorac Surg 1990;49:435.
35. Slama T et al. Randomized comparison of cefamandole, cefazolin and cefuroxime prophylaxis in open-heart surgery. Antimicrob Agents Chemother 1986;29:744.
36. Kaiser A et al. Efficacy of cefazolin, cefamandole, and gentamicin as prophylactic agents in cardiac surgery. Ann Surg 1987;206:791.
37. Geroulanos S et al. Antimicrobial prophylaxis in cardiovascular surgery. Thorac Cardiovasc Surg 1987;35:199.
38. Doebbeling B et al. Cardiovascular surgery prophylaxis: a randomized, controlled comparison of cefazolin and cefuroxime. J Thorac Cardiovasc Surg 1990;99:981.
39. Conklin C et al. Determinants of wound infection incidence after isolated coronary artery bypass surgery in patients randomized to receive prophylactic cefuroxime or cefazolin. Ann Thorac Surg 1988;46:172.
40. Kreter B, Woods M. Antibiotic prophylaxis for cardiothoracic operations. Meta-analysis of thirty years of clinical trials. J Thorac Cardiovasc Surg 1992;104:590.
41. Townsend TR et al. Clinical trial of cefamandole, cefazolin, and cefuroxime for antibiotic prophylaxis in cardiac operations. J Thorac Cardiovasc Surg 1993;106:664.
42. Curtis JJ et al. Randomized, prospective comparison of first- and second-generation cephalosporins as infection prophylaxis for cardiac surgery. Am J Surg 1993;166:734.
43. Goldmann DA et al. Cephalothin prophylaxis in cardiac valve surgery. A prospective, double-blind comparison of two-day and six-day regimens. J Thorac Cardiovasc Surg 1977;73:470.
44. Da Costa A et al. Antibiotic prophylaxis for permanent pacemaker implantation. Circulation 1998;97:1796
45. Bucknell SJ et al. Single-versus multiple-dose antibiotics prophylaxis for cardiac surgery. Aust NZ J Surg 2000;70:409.
46. Kriaras I et al. Evolution of antimicrobial prophylaxis in cardiovascular surgery. Eur J Cardiothorac Surg 2000;18:440.

47. D'Angelo LJ et al. Short-versus long course prophylactic antibiotic treatment in cesarean section patients. Obstet Gynecol 1980;55:583.
48. Faro S et al. Antibiotic prophylaxis: is there a difference? Am J Obstet Gynecol 1990;162:900.
49. Jacobi P et al. Single-dose cefazolin prophylaxis for cesarean section. Am J Obstet Gynecol 1988;158:1049.
50. Crombleholme WR. Use of prophylactic antibiotics in obstetrics and gynecology. Clin Obstet Gynecol 1988;31:466.
51. Chelmow D et al. Prophylactic use of antibiotics for nonlaboring patients undergoing cesarean delivery with intact membranes: a meta-analysis. Am J Obstet Gynecol 2001;184:656.
52. Smith KS et al. Multidisciplinary program for promoting single prophylactic doses of cefazolin in obstetrical and gynecological surgical procedures. Am J Hosp Pharm 1988;45:1338.
53. Kaiser AB. Antimicrobial prophylaxis in surgery. N Engl J Med 1986;315:1129.
54. Horan TC et al. CDC definitions of nosocomial surgical site infections, 1992: a modification of CDC definitions of surgical wound infections. Am J Infect Control 1992;20:271.
55. Hemsell D et al. Ceftriaxone or cefazolin prophylaxis for the prevention of infection after vaginal hysterectomy. Am J Surg 1984;148(4A):22.
56. Mittendorf et al. Avoiding serious infections associated with abdominal hysterectomy: a meta-analysis of antibiotic prophylaxis. Am J Obstet Gynecol 1993;169:1119.
57. Kamat AA et al. Wound infection in gynecologic surgery. Infect Dis Obstet Gynecol 2000;8:230.
58. Hemsell DL et al. Cefazolin is inferior to cefotetan as single-dose prophylaxis for women undergoing elective total abdominal hysterectomy. Clin Infect Dis 1995;20:677.
59. American College of Obstetricians and Gynecologists (ACOG). Antibiotics and gynecologic infections. ACOG Educational Bulletin 1997;237;1.
60. Dajee H et al. Profound hypotension from rapid vancomycin administration during cardiac operation. J Thorac Cardiovasc Surg 1984;87:145.
61. Górecki WJ, Grochowski JA. Are antibiotics necessary in nonperforated appendicitis in children? A double-blind randomized controlled trial. Med Sci Monit 2001;7:289.
62. Liberman MA et al. Single-dose cefotetan or cefoxitin versus multiple-dose cefoxitin as prophylaxis in patients undergoing appendectomy for acute nonperforating appendicitis. J Am Coll Surg 1995;180:77.
63. Salam IM et al. A randomized prospective study of cefoxitin versus piperacillin in appendectomy. J Hosp Infect 1994;26:133.
64. Moellering RC. Interaction between antimicrobial consumption and selection of resistant bacterial strains. Scand J Infect Dis 1990;(Suppl 70):18.
65. Durbin WA et al. Improved antibiotic usage following introduction of a novel prescription system. JAMA 1981;246:1796.
66. Lipsy RJ et al. Design, implementation, and use of a new antimicrobial order form: a descriptive report. Ann Pharmacother 1993;27:856.
67. Peterson CD et al. Reducing prophylactic antibiotic costs in cardiovascular surgery: the role of the clinical pharmacist. DICP 1985;19:134.
68. Evans RS et al. Reducing the duration of prophylactic antibiotic use through computer monitoring of surgical patients. DICP Ann Pharmacother 1990;24:351.
69. Michael KA et al. Impact of a pharmacist/physician cooperative target drug monitoring program on prophylactic antibiotic prescribing in obstetrics and gynecology. Hosp Pharm 1992;27:213.

CHAPTER 58

Central Nervous System Infections

Vicky Dudas

The pharmacotherapy of central nervous system (CNS) infections presents a tremendous challenge to the clinician. CNS infections often are caused by virulent pathogens. These infections occur in an area of the body in which antibiotic penetration often is limited and where host defenses are absent or inadequate. Thus, morbidity and mortality from infections of the CNS remain high despite the availability of highly potent, bactericidal antibiotics. In a review of 493 adult patients treated for bacterial meningitis at the Massachusetts General Hospital between 1962 and 1988, the mortality rates were 25% and 35% for community-acquired and hospital-acquired cases, respectively.[1] The overall case fatality rate of 25% did not change significantly over the 27-year period of the study. Although eradication of bacteria is essential, it is only one of the variables that affect mortality from CNS infections. In an attempt to improve morbidity and mortality statistics, the pathophysiologic mechanisms of CNS infections continue to be further scrutinized.[2-4] In addition, the beneficial effects of corticosteroids in bacterial meningitis continue to be evaluated.[5]

A number of infectious processes can occur within the CNS (e.g., meningitis, encephalitis, meningoencephalitis, brain abscess, subdural empyema, and epidural abscess).[6,7] In addition, prosthetic devices placed into the CNS (e.g., cerebrospinal fluid [CSF] shunts for management of hydrocephalus) often are complicated by infection.[8] Many etiologic agents are capable of inducing CNS infections, including bacteria, viruses, fungi, and certain parasites. This chapter focuses primarily on bacterial infections of the CNS, with an emphasis on the pharmacotherapy of bacterial meningitis and brain abscess. (Also see Chapter 69, Pharmacotherapy of Human Immunodeficiency Virus Infection, and Chapter 70, Opportunistic Infection in HIV-Infected Patients, for presentations pertaining to CNS infections in these populations.)

REVIEW OF CENTRAL NERVOUS SYSTEM

Anatomy and Physiology

Meninges
Proper therapy of CNS infections first requires an understanding of the anatomic and physiologic characteristics of this region. The brain and spinal cord are ensheathed by a protective covering known as the meninges and suspended in CSF, which acts as a "shock absorber" to outside trauma.[9,10]

The meninges consist of three layers of fibrous tissue: the *pia mater, arachnoid,* and *dura mater.* The pia mater, the innermost layer of the meninges, is a thin, delicate membrane that closely adheres to the contours of the brain. Separating the pia mater from the more loosely enclosed arachnoid membrane is the subarachnoid space, where the CSF resides. The pia mater and arachnoid, known collectively as the leptomeninges, lie interior to the dura mater, a tough outer membrane that adheres to the periosteum and vertebral column.[9,11] *Meningitis* is a term describing inflammation (often the result of infection) of the subarachnoid space, whereas *subdural empyema* refers to a collection of purulent material (pus) in the region separating the dura and arachnoid.[7,9] Abscesses also can form outside the dural space (epidural abscess), often with devastating consequences.[7]

Cerebrospinal Fluid

CSF is produced and secreted by the choroid plexus in the lateral ventricles and, to a lesser extent, by the choroid plexuses within the third and fourth ventricles.[10,12] The choroid plexus is histologically similar to the renal tubules and removes organic acids (including penicillins) from the CSF via active transport mechanisms. These transport processes can be inhibited by probenecid (Benemid) administration.[12] CSF flows unidirectionally from the lateral ventricles through the foramina of the third and fourth ventricles into the subarachnoid space, then over the cerebral hemispheres and downward into the spinal canal. CSF is absorbed through villous projections (arachnoid villi) into veins, primarily the cerebral venous sinuses.[10,12] About 550 mL/day of CSF is produced, with complete exchange occurring every 3 to 4 hours.[10,12] The flow of CSF is unidirectional from the ventricles to the intralumbar space. Therefore, intrathecal injection of antibiotics results in little, if any, antibiotic reaching the cerebral ventricles.[13,14] This unidirectional flow of CSF presents a problem because ventriculitis commonly occurs in conjunction with bacterial meningitis. Direct intraventricular instillation of antibiotics, usually by means of a reservoir, is preferable in the setting of ventriculitis (see Question 22).[13,14]

In adults, children, and infants the volume of CSF is approximately 150 mL, 60 to 100 mL, and 40 to 60 mL, respectively.[10,12] Knowledge of approximate CSF volume facilitates estimation of the CSF concentration of a drug subsequent to intrathecal administration. For example, administration of gentamicin 5 mg (5,000 µg) intrathecally should result in a CSF concentration of roughly 33 µg/mL in an adult shortly after administration.

The composition of CSF differs from other physiologic fluids. The pH of CSF is slightly acidic (normal pH, 7.3), and with the exception of chloride ion, electrolyte concentrations are slightly less than those in serum.[10,12] Under normal conditions, the protein concentration in CSF is <50 mg/dL, CSF glucose values are approximately 60% those of plasma, and few if any white blood cells (WBCs) are present (<5 cells/mm³).[10,12] When the meninges become inflamed (i.e., in meningitis), the composition of the CSF is altered. In particular, the protein concentration in the CSF increases, and the glucose concentration in the CSF usually declines with meningitis. Therefore, careful evaluation of CSF chemistries is useful when establishing a diagnosis of meningitis.

Blood–Brain Barrier

The blood–brain barrier plays a crucial role in protecting the brain and maintaining homeostasis within the CNS.[10,15,16] There actually are two distinct barriers that exist within the brain: the blood–CSF barrier and the blood–brain barrier.[15,16] The blood–CSF barrier is located in the choroid plexus and circumventricular organs (e.g., area postrema) and is characterized morphologically by fenestrated (porous) capillaries (Fig. 58-1).[15] This arrangement allows proteins and other molecules (including antibiotics) to pass freely into the immediate interstitial space. Diffusion of substances into the CSF is restricted by tightly fused ependymal cells lining the ventricular side of the choroid plexus (see Fig. 58-1).[15] Cerebral capillary endothelial cells make up the blood–brain barrier, which separates blood from the interstitial fluid of the brain. Unlike capillaries in other areas of the body, the capillary endothelia of the brain are packed closely together, forming tight junctions that in effect produce a barrier physiologically similar to a continuous lipid bilayer.[15] The surface area of the blood–brain barrier is >5,000 times greater than that of the blood–CSF barrier; thus, the blood–brain barrier plays a more important role in protecting the brain and regulating its chemical composition.[12,15] Many antimicrobials traverse the

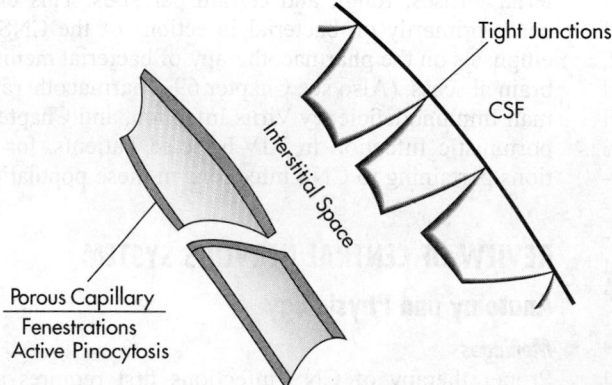
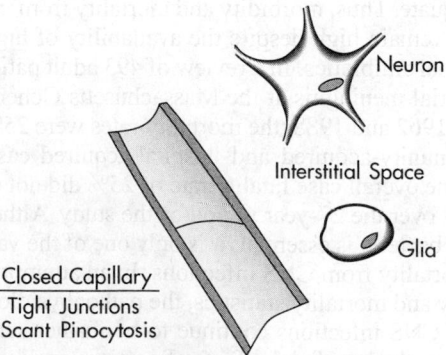

A. Capillary Surface Area = 1

Porous Capillary
Fenestrations
Active Pinocytosis

Tight Junctions

CSF

Interstitial Space

B. Capillary Surface Area = 5,000

Closed Capillary
Tight Junctions
Scant Pinocytosis

Neuron

Interstitial Space

Glia

FIGURE 58-1. The two membrane barrier systems in the central nervous system: the blood–CSF barrier (left) and the blood–brain barrier. (Reproduced with permission from reference 15.)

blood–brain barrier with difficulty, particularly agents having low lipid solubility (see the following discussion).[16]

MENINGITIS

Meningitis is the most common type of CNS infection. The signs and symptoms associated with bacterial meningitis usually are acute in onset, evolving over a few hours.[6] Prompt recognition and early institution of therapy are essential to ensuring beneficial outcomes. In contrast, a diverse group of infectious (e.g., viruses, fungi, and mycobacteria) and noninfectious (e.g., chemical irritants) agents produce a meningitic picture often of a less acute or chronic nature.[17] On occasion, such "aseptic" causes can produce signs and symptoms nearly indistinguishable from those of acute bacterial meningitis.[6,17] Drugs that can induce aseptic meningitis include trimethoprim-sulfamethoxazole (TMP-SMX), the antirejection monoclonal antibody muromonab (OKT3), azathioprine, and nonsteroidal anti-inflammatory drugs (NSAIDs) such as ibuprofen, naproxen, and sulindac.[18]

Microbiology

The bacterial etiologies of meningitis correlate very well with age and underlying conditions such as head trauma or recent neurosurgery (Table 58-1).[19–21] Generally, meningitis is a disease of the very young and very old: most cases occur in children <2 years of age and in elderly adults.[19,20]

Table 58-1   Microbiology of Bacterial Meningitis

Age Group or Predisposing Condition	Most Likely Organisms[a]
Neonates (<2 mo)	Group B streptococcus (*S. agalactiae*), *E. coli*, and other Gram-negative bacilli (*Klebsiella, Serratia* species), *L. monocytogenes*
Infants and children (2 mo–10 yr)	*H. influenzae,[b] S. pneumoniae, N. meningitidis*
Children and adults (>10–30 yr)	*N. meningitidis, S. pneumoniae*
Adults (30–60 yr)	*S. pneumoniae, N. meningitidis*
Elderly (>60 yr)	*S. pneumoniae, N. meningitidis, E. coli, Klebsiella* species, and other Gram-negative bacilli, *L. monocytogenes*
Postneurosurgical	*S. aureus,* Gram-negative bacilli (e.g., *E. coli, Klebsiella* species), *S. epidermidis[c]*
Closed head trauma	*S. pneumoniae, H. influenzae*
Open head trauma	*S. aureus,* Gram-negative bacilli (e.g., *E. coli, Klebsiella* species)

[a]Organisms listed in descending order of frequency.
[b]Need to consider this pathogen only in children not vaccinated with Hib.
[c]Most commonly seen in association with prosthetic devices (e.g., cerebrospinal fluid shunts).

Neonates (infants <2 months) are at an especially high risk of developing meningitis. Meningitis in neonates most often is caused by group B streptococci (*Streptococcus agalactiae*) or coliform organisms such as *Escherichia coli*.[19,20,22] These highly virulent pathogens usually are acquired during passage through the birth canal or from the hospital environment and are associated with significant morbidity and mortality, particularly in premature infants.[19,20,22] Case fatality rates of over 20% and 30% have been reported for meningitis due to group B streptococci and Gram-negative bacilli, respectively.[19] *Listeria monocytogenes* is another important and often overlooked pathogen in neonates.[19,20,23] Because *L. monocytogenes* is resistant to many antimicrobial agents, including third-generation cephalosporins, selection of initial (empiric) therapy in neonates must be approached with this pathogen in mind.[23]

Infants >1 month of age and children <4 years of age are at the highest risk for meningitis. There have been dramatic changes in the epidemiology of bacterial meningitis in this age group over the past several years. Historically, in this age group, the disease was caused predominantly by three pathogens: *Haemophilus influenzae, Streptococcus pneumoniae,* and *Neisseria meningitidis.*[19,20] Up to 45% of all cases of meningitis in the United States before 1985 were caused by *H. influenzae* type b (Hib).[20] However, from 1987 through 1997, Hib meningitis cases in children <5 years of age decreased by 97%.[24,25] This reduction in *H. influenzae*–induced meningitis correlates with the widespread vaccination of children against invasive *H. influenzae* disease with the Hib polysaccharide–protein conjugate vaccines. Invasive *H. influenzae* infection now is considered a vaccine-preventable disease in the United States as well as in other countries, highlighting the importance of vaccinating children against Hib invasive disease.[26,27] Further follow-up from 1998 to 2000 indicates that the incidence of Hib has remained extremely low. One of the national health objectives in *Healthy People 2010* is to reduce the incidence of Hib to zero.[27] In addition, widespread vaccination has caused a shift in the age distribution of bacterial meningitis. Before the Hib vaccine was available, more than two thirds of cases occurred in children <5 years of age. With the dramatic reduction of Hib cases in this age group, the majority of cases now are observed in adults.[26,27]

In adults and children who have received the conjugated Hib vaccine, community-acquired meningitis most often is caused by *S. pneumoniae* (the pneumococcus) and *N. meningitidis* (the meningococcus).[4,19,20] Meningococci more commonly are implicated in individuals ages 5 to 30 years, whereas pneumococci are the predominant pathogens in adults >30 years of age.[19] In the past several years, meningococcal meningitis has been occurring in clusters within the general population with increased frequency. The observed clusters, defined as two or more cases of the same serogroup that are closer in time/space than expected, usually occur in secondary schools or university settings.[27]

Traditionally, pneumococci and meningococci have been highly susceptible to penicillin G (minimum inhibitory concentration [MIC] <0.1 µg/mL). Pneumococcal strains showing intermediate penicillin resistance (MIC 0.1 to 1.0 µg/mL) and high resistance (MIC ≥2.0 µg/mL), however, are a problem in many areas of the world, including the United States. Penicillin-resistant pneumococci are of particular concern in relation to meningitis since there is the additional challenge of delivering adequate levels to the site of infection, the CSF.[2,28] Optimal therapy for resistant pneumococci is controversial and is discussed in greater detail in Question 15.

The elderly also are prone to developing meningitis, and the infection-related mortality in this population often is higher than in other age groups.[19,20,29] For example, the case-fatality rate for pneumococcal meningitis is 5% in children <5 years of age but 31% in the elderly.[20] Patients of advanced age are most susceptible to meningitis from pneumococci and meningococci. However, enteric Gram-negative bacilli (e.g., *E. coli*, *Klebsiella pneumoniae*) also are occasionally isolated.[19,20,29] Furthermore, *L. monocytogenes* is a problem pathogen in the elderly, especially in immunocompromised patients.[19,20,23,29,30]

Meningitis after neurosurgical procedures or open trauma to the head most often is caused by enteric Gram-negative bacilli (predominantly *E. coli* and *K. pneumoniae*) and to a lesser extent staphylococci, particularly *Staphylococcus aureus*.[1,21,30] Meningitis that occurs after neurosurgery is occasionally caused by resistant pathogens such as *Enterobacter* species and *Pseudomonas aeruginosa*, often with devastating consequences.[21,31–33] In addition, patients requiring ventriculostomy or placement of CSF shunts can develop infections of these prosthetic devices by coagulase-negative staphylococci (e.g., *S. epidermidis*) or diphtheroids.[8,21] Closed head trauma, particularly when associated with CSF rhinorrhea or otorrhea, can lead to pneumococcal meningitis or, to a lesser extent, *H. influenzae* meningitis.[21]

Pathogenesis and Pathophysiology

The steps leading to the development of meningitis and the underlying pathophysiologic processes involved have become more clearly understood in the past few years.[2,4] In general, meningitis can develop from *hematogenous* spread of organisms (the most common mechanism), by *contiguous* spread from a parameningeal focus (e.g., sinusitis or otitis media), or by direct bacterial *inoculation*, as occurs with head trauma or neurosurgery.

The list of pathogens causing bacterial meningitis is relatively short because only bacteria possessing certain virulence factors are capable of invading the meninges. Specifically, the presence of a polysaccharide capsule and other cell surface structures (e.g., pili) are necessary for bacteria to evade host defenses and gain entry into the subarachnoid space.[2–4] Once in the CSF, virulence factors contained within the cell wall (e.g., lipopolysaccharide or endotoxin in the case of *H. influenzae*) initiate a complex cascade of events culminating in neurologic damage.[2,3] These cell wall substances trigger the release of various cytokines, which act as mediators of the inflammatory response.[2–4]

Colonization of mucosal surfaces is a necessary first step in the pathogenesis of meningitis (Fig. 58-2).[3,4] The polysaccharide capsule and pili or fimbriae on the bacterial cell surface allow attachment to oropharyngeal or nasopharyngeal mucosa.[2–4] Secretion of protease enzymes that neutralize the protective activity of mucosal IgA and intrinsic resistance to ciliary clearance mechanisms allow meningeal pathogens to adhere to and penetrate through the epithelial surface and enter the intravascular space.[3] The presence of a capsule prevents binding by the alternative complement pathway and

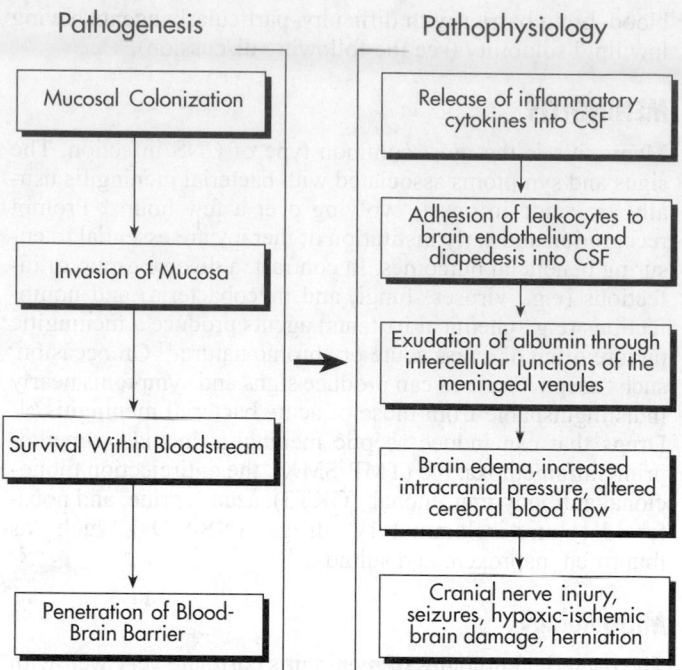

Pathogenesis | Pathophysiology

Pathogenesis:
- Mucosal Colonization
- Invasion of Mucosa
- Survival Within Bloodstream
- Penetration of Blood-Brain Barrier

Pathophysiology:
- Release of inflammatory cytokines into CSF
- Adhesion of leukocytes to brain endothelium and diapedesis into CSF
- Exudation of albumin through intercellular junctions of the meningeal venules
- Brain edema, increased intracranial pressure, altered cerebral blood flow
- Cranial nerve injury, seizures, hypoxic-ischemic brain damage, herniation

FIGURE 58-2. Summary of the pathogenesis and pathophysiology of bacterial meningitis. (Adapted from references 2 and 3.)

prolongs survival within the bloodstream.[3,4] Eventually, organisms multiply to sufficient numbers that allow invasion of the blood–brain barrier. The exact mechanism by which bacteria invade the blood–brain barrier is not well understood. However, bacteria probably adhere to cerebral capillary endothelia or perhaps the epithelium of the choroid plexus.[3,4]

Once bacteria gain entry into the CSF, host defenses are inadequate to contain the infection, and bacteria replicate rapidly. Humoral immunity (both complement and immunoglobulin) essentially is absent within the CSF.[2–4] In addition, opsonic activity in CSF is negligible, and although leukocytosis ensues shortly after bacterial invasion, phagocytosis also is inefficient.[3,4] Therefore, this relative immunodeficiency state necessitates the initiation of bactericidal therapy.[2]

Inflammation of the meninges is initiated by contents within the bacterial cell wall.[2–4] Specifically, Gram-negative bacteria possess lipopolysaccharide, or endotoxin, and Gram-positive bacteria contain teichoic acid in their cell walls. Release of lipopolysaccharide (or teichoic acid) induces the production and secretion of inflammatory cytokines such as interleukin-1 (IL-1), interleukin-6 (IL-6), prostaglandin E_2, and tumor necrosis factor (TNF) from astrocytes, endothelial cells, and circulating monocytes.[3,4] These cytokines play an essential role in promoting the adherence of leukocytes to cerebral capillary endothelial cells, and they also facilitate the migration of leukocytes into the CSF.[2,3] Upon attachment to brain endothelium, leukocytes release toxic oxygen products that damage endothelial cells. This increases pinocytotic activity, widens tight junctions, and eventually increases blood–brain barrier permeability (see Fig. 58-2).[2–4]

Inflammation of the blood–brain barrier allows the influx of albumin and, consequently, vasogenic cerebral edema.[2,3] The brain edema combined with obstruction of CSF outflow increases intracranial pressure and alters cerebral blood flow.[3] Altered cerebral blood flow is a problem because it often is coupled with a loss of cerebrovascular autoregulation. Hyperperfusion or hypoperfusion of the brain secondary to increases or decreases in systemic blood pressure, respectively, ultimately can result in neuronal injury, cerebral ischemia, and irreversible brain damage.[3] The use of adjunctive corticosteroids in certain patient populations can substantially reduce inflammation and the subsequent neurologic sequelae of meningitis.[2,5]

The inflammatory response in meningitis also can be aggravated by some antibiotics, notably the penicillins and cephalosporins.[2,33] When the β-lactam antibiotics lyse bacterial cell walls, large amounts of cell wall products are liberated early in the course of disease, and these contents of bacterial cell walls amplify the inflammatory response.[33] The long-term benefits of β-lactam therapy far outweigh such transient detrimental effects. However, the use of less rapidly bacteriolytic agents may be theoretically advantageous.[2] The proinflammatory effect of β-lactam antibiotics is attenuated by concomitant corticosteroid therapy.[2,5]

Neurologic sequelae develop in one third to one half of patients with bacterial meningitis.[34–36] The type and severity of neurologic complications vary with the specific infecting organism, the severity of the infection, and the susceptibility of the host. In children, pneumococcal meningitis carries the highest risk of permanent neurologic sequelae, particularly sensorineural hearing loss.[6,36] In a long-term prospective study of 185 children with acute bacterial meningitis, permanent hearing loss occurred in 6%, 10.5%, and 31% of children with meningitis due to *H. influenzae, N. meningitidis,* and *S. pneumoniae,* respectively.[36] Although seizures are fairly common upon initial presentation, long-term epilepsy occurs in approximately 7% of patients.[34] Other important long-term complications include spastic paraparesis, behavioral disorders, and learning deficits.[34]

Diagnosis and Clinical Features

Clinical and Laboratory Features of Bacterial Meningitis

1. S.C., a 5-year-old boy, is brought to the emergency department (ED) by his mother, who says her son has a temperature of 102°F, is irritable and lethargic, and has a rash. S.C. was in his usual state of good health until last night, when he awoke crying. When she went to investigate, her son began to stiffen up and rock back and forth in his bed. Because he was unarousable, S.C.'s mother rushed him to the hospital. S.C.'s medical history is noncontributory except for an allergy to amoxicillin described as a skin rash. S.C., his mother and father, and his 7-year-old brother recently moved to the United States. S.C.'s vaccination history currently is unknown. S.C. and his brother currently attend a community day care center.

Upon physical examination, S.C. was in marked distress, with a temperature of 40°C, blood pressure (BP) of 90/60 mm Hg, and a respiratory rate of 32 breaths/min. His weight upon admission was 20 kg. Neurologic examination showed evidence of nuchal rigidity; he was lethargic and difficult to arouse. Brudzinski's and Kernig's signs were positive. On head, eyes, ears, nose, and throat examination, S.C. demonstrated photophobia (he squinted severely when the examiner shined a light in his eyes), but there was no evidence of papilledema. A petechial rash was visible on his extremities. The remainder of S.C.'s examination was essentially normal.

Blood drawn for laboratory tests revealed sodium (Na), 128 mEq/L (normal, 135 to 145); potassium (K), 3.2 mEq/L (normal, 3.5 to 5); chloride (Cl), 100 mEq/L (normal, 95 to 105); bicarbonate (HCO_3), 25 mEq/L (normal, 22 to 28); blood urea nitrogen (BUN), 16 mg/dL (normal, 8 to 18); serum creatinine (SrCr), 0.6 mg/dL (normal, 0.6 to 1.2); and serum glucose, 80 mg/dL (normal, 70 to 110). The WBC count was 18,000 cells/mm³ with 95% polymorphonuclear cells (PMN) (normal, 54% to 62%); the hemoglobin (Hgb), hematocrit (Hct), and platelet count all were within normal limits.

What clinical and laboratory features does S.C. display that are suggestive of meningitis?

[SI units: Na, 128 mmol/L; K, 3.2 mmol/L; Cl, 100 mmol/L; 25, mmol/L; BUN, 5.7 mmol/L; SrCr, 53.04 μmol/L; serum glucose, 4.44 mmol/L; WBC count, 18×10^9/L]

S.C.'s presentation contains many features typical of acute bacterial meningitis. For example, the boy was in good health until he awoke at night confused and disoriented. When symptoms present abruptly and evolve quickly over a period of several hours, an acute bacterial process is a strong possibility.[37,38] S.C. has several predisposing factors for the development of meningitis: young age, an unknown vaccination history, and day care exposure.[1,35]

The clinical features of bacterial meningitis are summarized in Table 58-2.[1,6,21,37,38] The most common symptoms include the triad of fever, stiff neck (nuchal rigidity), and altered mental status.[1,6,37] When all three of these features are present, as is S.C.'s case, meningitis should be strongly suspected. Other less common signs and symptoms include headache, photophobia (unusual intolerance to light), and focal neurologic deficits, including cranial nerve palsies.[1,6,37,38] A positive Brudzinski's sign (reflex flexion of the hips and knees produced upon flexion of the neck when lying in the recumbent position), and Kernig's sign (pain upon extension of the hamstrings when lying supine with the thighs perpendicular to the trunk) provide physical evidence of meningeal irritation.[39] Brudzinski's and Kernig's signs both were positive in S.C. Seizures occur on initial presentation in 15% to 30% of patients and may be focal or generalized.[1,6,34] The presence of seizures or a severely depressed mental status (i.e., obtundation or coma) generally is associated with a poorer prognosis.[1,6,34] Headache, nausea, vomiting, photophobia, and papilledema upon eye examination all suggest increased intracranial pressure.[6,37,38] When these symptoms or focal neurologic deficits are present, a computed tomographic (CT)

Table 58-2	**Signs and Symptoms of Acute Bacterial Meningitis**
Fever	Anorexia
Nuchal rigidity (stiff neck)	Headache
Altered mental status	Photophobia
Seizures	Nausea and vomiting
Brudzinski's sign[a]	Focal neurologic deficits
Kernig's sign[a]	Septic shock
Irritability[b]	

[a]See text for description of sign.
[b]Symptoms seen in infants with meningitis.

scan is recommended before lumbar puncture to rule out an intracranial mass.[6,37,38] Although controversial, brain herniation may occur when lumbar puncture is performed in such patients because of the pressure changes induced within the cranial vault.[40]

As is clearly evident, S.C. has many of the clinical features associated with acute bacterial meningitis. High fever, stiff neck, altered mentation, photophobia, and positive Kernig's and Brudzinski's signs all are consistent with bacterial meningitis. Furthermore, the low blood pressure (hypotension) and increased respiratory rate are characteristic findings in severe, life-threatening types of bacterial infection (e.g., septic shock, meningitis) and are likely the result of endotoxin release.

The signs and symptoms of meningitis in the very young and very old differ from those in older children and adults.[6,22,29,35] In neonates, signs of meningeal irritation may be absent; fever, irritability, and poor feeding are often the only symptoms manifested.[6,22] Fullness of the fontanel in infants also may reflect the increased intracranial pressure that occurs with meningitis.[6,36] Because S.C. is 5 years old, accurate assessment of his mental status is challenging. Irritability (crying), as was manifested by S.C., is an important finding that suggests an altered mental status.

In elderly patients, many of the classic signs of meningeal irritation are absent as well, and the disease presentation can be subtler.[6,29,37] Therefore, given the grave consequences of a misdiagnosis, clinicians caring for infants and elderly patients must have a particularly high index of suspicion for meningitis.

Laboratory evaluation of meningitis should include serum chemistries and a hemogram as well as a detailed examination of the CSF.[6,12,37] The peripheral WBC count often is markedly elevated in acute bacterial meningitis, usually with a left shift evident on the differential. However, this finding is nonspecific and occurs in many acute inflammatory and infectious diseases. S.C. has a marked leukocytosis with a predominance of polymorphonuclear cells on the differential. A low serum sodium value, which is present in S.C., reflects the syndrome of inappropriate secretion of antidiuretic hormone (SIADH), a frequent complication of acute bacterial meningitis.[4,6] SIADH is an important finding in meningitis because it worsens cerebral edema.[4,6]

The abrupt onset of S.C.'s clinical symptoms is consistent with an acute bacterial process rather than a fungal or viral etiology. Given his age (5 years) and the community-acquired nature of the infection, the most likely pathogens for his meningitis are *H. influenzae, N. meningitidis,* and *S. pneumoniae.* The presence of maculopapular lesions argues for *N. meningitis* as the causative pathogen because this is a common finding in cases of meningococcemia or meningococcal meningitis.[3] To make an accurate clinical and microbiologic diagnosis in S.C., it is necessary to obtain CSF for analysis. Thus, a lumbar puncture is required as soon as possible.

Cerebrospinal Fluid Examination

2. The resident in the ED performs a lumbar puncture, which yielded the following: opening pressure, 300 mm CSF (normal, <20); CSF glucose, 20 mg/dL (normal, 60% of plasma glucose); protein, 250 mg/dL (normal, <50); WBC count, 1,200 cells/mm³ (normal, <5), with 90% PMNs, 4% monohistiocytes, and 6% lymphocytes. The CSF red blood cell (RBC) count was 50/mm³. A stat Gram's stain of CSF revealed numerous WBCs but no organisms. CSF, blood, and urine cultures are pending. What CSF findings in S.C. are consistent with a diagnosis of bacterial meningitis?

[SI units: CSF glucose, 1.1 mmol/L; protein, 2.5 g/L; WBC count, 1,200 × 10⁶ cells/L; RBC count, 5 × 10⁶/L]

Careful examination of the CSF is essential to confirm the diagnosis of meningitis.[10] Table 58-3 compares the typical findings in CSF obtained from patients with acute bacterial meningitis with those seen with fungal or viral etiologies.[6,17,37] In acute bacterial meningitis, the CSF is purulent, containing numerous WBCs (usually >500 cells/mm³) with a predominance of PMNs, and often is turbid.[12,37] CSF protein nearly always is elevated, usually >100 mg/dL, and the CSF glucose concentration is low, either <50 mg/dL or <50% of a simultaneously obtained serum glucose value.[10,13] In contrast, CSF obtained in viral and fungal cases of meningitis usually is clear and characterized by a much lower WBC count (<100 cells/mm³), with a mononuclear or lymphocyte predominance.[17,37] Although the CSF protein concentration often is elevated, it may be normal.[17] A variable effect is observed with CSF glucose.[17]

Microbiologic Evaluation

Microbiologic evaluation should include examination of CSF by Gram's stain and culture as well as cultures obtained from other potential sites of infection (e.g., blood, sputum, urine).[6,37] Gram's stain of the CSF is positive in >50% of acute bacterial meningitis cases and is an extremely useful test to help direct initial (empiric) antimicrobial therapy.[6,10,37] The presence of organisms on smear is indicative of a high bacterial inoculum (i.e., inoculum >10⁵ colony-forming units/mL) and is associated with more fulminant disease.[2] The absence of organisms on Gram's stain by no means rules out infection but does make selection of empiric therapy more difficult.

S.C. has a negative Gram's stain, which may be the result of previous antibiotic therapy or the early detection of disease. Given the negative CSF Gram's stain result, S.C. must receive antibacterial therapy broad enough to cover all pathogens associated with meningitis in his age group until the results from his CSF culture are available (usually within 24 to 48 hours). The CSF culture nearly always is positive in purulent meningitis, and the presence of any organism in this normally sterile fluid must always be taken seriously.[6,37,41] In a few instances, particularly when prior antibiotic therapy has been given, CSF cultures are negative in a patient who clearly appears to have meningitis.[10,35,41] In this setting, newer diagnostic tests such as latex particle agglutination that reliably detect

Table 58-3 CSF Findings in Various Types of Meningitis

Microbial Etiology	WBC Count (cells/min³)	Predominant Cell Type	Protein	Glucose
Bacterial	>500	PMN	Elevated	↓
Fungal	10–500	MN	Elevated	Variable
Viral	10–200	PMN or MN	Variable	Normal

CSF, cerebrospinal fluid; MN, mononuclear cells; PMN, polymorphonuclear neutrophils; WBC, white blood cell.

antigens of *H. influenzae, S. pneumoniae, N. meningitidis, E. coli* (K-1 capsular antigen), and group B streptococci in CSF are available. Latex particle agglutination should be considered for S.C., especially if his cultures fail to yield any growth. Finally, results from cultures of other sites such as the blood, urine, and sputum (when appropriate) can yield very useful microbiologic information.[37,41]

The CSF findings in S.C. also strongly support the diagnosis of bacterial meningitis. He has a markedly elevated opening CSF pressure, CSF leukocytosis (with a predominance of PMNs), an elevated CSF protein concentration, and a depressed CSF glucose value. A small number of RBCs are present in the CSF, which suggests contamination with peripheral blood caused by the traumatic nature of the lumbar puncture. Precise identification of the offending organism is not possible until CSF culture results are available.

Treatment Principles

Prompt institution of appropriate antimicrobial therapy is essential when treating meningitis.[37] When choosing antimicrobial therapy, a number of factors must be considered. First, the antibiotics selected must penetrate adequately into the CSF.[13,16,42] In addition, the regimen chosen must have potent activity against known or suspected pathogens and exert a bactericidal effect.[16,42–44]

Antimicrobial Penetration Into the Cerebrospinal Fluid

In cases of purulent meningitis, the amount of bacteria in the CSF often is much higher than the standard inoculum (approximately 10^5 colony-forming units per milliliter) used in routine antimicrobial susceptibility testing.[16,43] As a result, extrapolation of in vitro sensitivity results to clinical efficacy is difficult, particularly for antimicrobials susceptible to an inoculum effect (i.e., an increase in the MIC with an increase in inoculum size). Cefuroxime (Zinacef), for example, is affected by an inoculum effect against *H. influenzae,* and extended-spectrum penicillins (e.g., piperacillin and mezlocillin) are affected similarly by enteric Gram-negative bacilli.[16,45] In addition, some antimicrobials (e.g., aminoglycosides, fluoroquinolones) have reduced bactericidal activity in the acidic milieu of purulent CSF.[16,42,46,47] For example, gentamicin has a minimum bactericidal concentration (MBC) of 1 µg/mL against *E. coli* at a pH of 7.35, and a decrease in the pH to 7.0 results in an eightfold increase in MBC.[47] This may partially explain why aminoglycoside therapy for Gram-negative bacillary meningitis is suboptimal, even when direct intrathecal therapy is given.[30,33] The ability of antimicrobials to penetrate into CSF is affected by lipid solubility, degree of ionization, molecular weight, protein binding, and susceptibility to active transport systems operative within the choroid plexus.[13,16,43,48] In general, the penetration of most antibiotics into the CSF is increased when the meninges are inflamed. Although the optimal degree of CSF penetration has not been elucidated entirely, experiments in the rabbit meningitis model indicate that bactericidal effects are maximal when CSF antibiotic concentrations exceed the MBC of the infecting pathogen by 10- to 30-fold.[16,42,44] The degree of antimicrobial penetration is most commonly reported as CSF/serum concentration in the literature.[44] Table 58-4 summarizes the CSF penetration characteristics of various antimicrobials dur-

Table 58-4	CSF Penetration Characteristics of Various Antimicrobials
Very Good[a]	
Chloramphenicol, metronidazole, TMP-SMX	
Good[b]	
Penicillins: Penicillin G, ampicillin, mezlocillin, nafcillin, piperacillin, ticarcillin	
Other β-lactams: Aztreonam, clavulanic acid, imipenem, meropenem, sulbactam	
Cephalosporins: Cefepime, cefotaxime, cefazidime, ceftizoxime, ceftriaxone, cefuroxime	
Fluoroquinolones: Ciprofloxacin	
Other agents: Rifampin	
Fair to Poor[c]	
Aminoglycosides: Amikacin, gentamicin, tobramycin	
Other agents: Azithromycin, clarithromycin, clindamycin, erythromycin, vancomycin	

[a]Penetrate CSF well regardless of meningeal inflammation.
[b]Adequate CSF penetration achieved when the meninges are inflamed.
[c]Penetration often inadequate even when the meninges are inflamed.
CSF, cerebrospinal fluid; TMP-SMX, trimethoprim-sulfamethoxazole.

ing acute bacterial meningitis.[13,14,42,44,49] Chloramphenicol, metronidazole, and trimethoprim are highly lipophilic compounds and penetrate into the CSF extremely well, achieving high concentrations even when meningeal inflammation is absent.[13,42,50] Rifampin also has good CSF penetration; because of this, it often is combined with vancomycin to treat coagulase-negative staphylococcal infections in the CNS.[8,42,50] Because β-lactams and aminoglycosides usually are ionized at physiologic pH, they are more polar and do not penetrate into the CSF as well. β-Lactams penetrate poorly when the meninges are intact, but when the meninges are inflamed, most penicillins and the third-generation cephalosporins achieve CSF concentrations sufficient to treat meningitis (approximately 10% to 30% of simultaneously obtained serum concentrations).[13,42,48–50] An additional factor working against maintenance of therapeutic concentrations of β-lactams in the CSF is the active transport system of the choroid plexus, which pumps these organic acids out of the CSF.[16] Carbapenems, namely meropenem, attain CSF levels that are 10% to 40% of serum levels.[44]

The aminoglycosides have a low therapeutic index, and adequate CSF concentrations are difficult to achieve with intravenous (IV) dosing alone without risking significant toxicity.[14,42] Furthermore, the acidic nature of purulent CSF reduces the antimicrobial activity of the aminoglycosides.[47] Thus, when aminoglycoside therapy is initiated for adults with CNS infections, concomitant intrathecal therapy is required.[14,51] Direct instillation of aminoglycosides into the ventricles is preferred, but this approach requires the surgical insertion of a reservoir (e.g., Ommaya reservoir), which often is not possible, particularly in the early stages of bacterial meningitis.[16,42] Thus, at the very least, patients requiring aminoglycosides for meningitis should receive daily intralumbar injections until clinical improvement is seen and CSF cultures are sterilized.[14,16]

The degree of serum protein binding correlates well with the extent of CSF penetration.[16,48] Cefoperazone and ceftriaxone are highly bound to serum proteins and thus are more confined to the intravascular space and not as readily available for CSF penetration as cefotaxime and ceftazidime, which are protein bound to a lesser extent. Although cefoperazone penetrates the CSF inconsistently and is best avoided in meningitis,[49] ceftriaxone achieves sustained, reliable bactericidal activity within the CSF despite its high protein binding.[42,49] Ceftriaxone has been used successfully to treat meningitis in both children and adults for many years.[5,49,52]

Vancomycin and polymyxin B do not diffuse well across the blood–CSF barrier, primarily because of their large molecular size.[13,16,42,50] Therapeutic concentrations in the CSF (up to 22% of serum concentrations) are attained with systemic vancomycin therapy when the meninges are inflamed. However, in selected circumstances, concomitant intralumbar or intraventricular therapy also may be necessary.[8,42] The commonly prescribed antimicrobials, clindamycin and erythromycin, penetrate the CSF poorly,[13,42,50] and they have limited usefulness because of their bacteriostatic mode of action.

Finally, fluoroquinolones, such as ciprofloxacin and ofloxacin, penetrate reasonably well into the CSF on a percentage basis (approximately 20% to 30%); however, the concentrations attained are fairly low (≤ 1 μg/mL) when standard doses are administered.[42,46] Given the potential neurotoxicity and the limited amount of clinical data, the quinolones have limited use in treating meningitis.

Empiric Therapy for Childhood Meningitis

3. A detailed medication and vaccination history reveals that S.C. and his brother appropriately received vaccination for Hib when they were 2 months of age. What constitutes appropriate empiric therapy for childhood meningitis? Which antibiotic would be appropriate for S.C.? What dose and route of administration should be used?

Because results from culture and sensitivity testing of CSF will not be available for >24 hours, empiric therapy must be instituted promptly to provide coverage of potential pathogens. The initial antimicrobial regimen should take into consideration the patient's age, any predisposing conditions that might make the patient vulnerable to increased morbidity and mortality, results from the CSF Gram's stain, history of allergy, and the presence of organ dysfunction. Table 58-5 gives recommendations for empiric antimicrobial therapy for acute bacterial meningitis.[4,6,20,37,38,51–53]

S.C. is 5 years old and has a negative CSF Gram's stain. Therefore, therapy with a third-generation cephalosporin, such as ceftriaxone (Rocephin) or cefotaxime (Claforan), is preferred. Either of these two agents will provide excellent coverage of the most likely pathogens in this age group (*S. pneumoniae* and *N. meningitidis*).[19,20,53] Of these two pathogens, S.C.'s rash suggests that *N. meningitidis* is likely.[37] *H. influenzae* is not very likely because he was vaccinated against Hib. Thus, initiation of ceftriaxone would be appropriate for S.C. at this time.

Use of a cephalosporin in this case is appropriate even though S.C. may be allergic to amoxicillin (history of skin rash). Patients with penicillin allergy carry a 5% to 12% risk of cross-reactivity when cephalosporins are prescribed.[54] In this setting, the type of reaction to penicillin is important to consider.[54] Patients with a history of accelerated hypersensitivity reactions (e.g., hives, shortness of breath [SOB], or anaphylaxis) to penicillins should not be given cephalosporins because the risk of cross-reactivity is too high. Conversely, a benign skin rash would not contraindicate use of a cephalosporin. If S.C. had experienced an accelerated reaction to penicillin, vancomycin plus aztreonam would be the best alternative choice (see Table 58-5).[4,6,53]

Dosing Considerations

In general, therapy of meningitis requires the use of high dosages of antimicrobials administered by the IV route. Table 58-6 lists the recommended dosing regimens for the treatment of CNS infections.[4,6,8,14,51,53,55]

S.C. should receive ceftriaxone in a dosage of 100 mg/kg per day given in one or two doses.[6,52,53] A ceftriaxone regimen of 1,000 mg IV Q 12 hr is reasonable for S.C. The elimination half-life of ceftriaxone is long (usually 6 to 8 hours), and once-daily dosing is feasible. However, many clinicians prefer to administer ceftriaxone on a twice-daily schedule[4,53] because most published trials used the twice-daily regimen and such a schedule reduces the potential for prolonged periods of subtherapeutic CSF concentrations if a dose is delayed or missed.[4] Nevertheless, the U.S. Food and Drug Administration (FDA) has approved use of the once-daily dosing regimen of ceftriaxone for treatment of pediatric meningitis.[56]

Adjunctive Corticosteroid Therapy

4. What is the rationale for adjunctive corticosteroid therapy in acute bacterial meningitis, and would it be appropriate for S.C.? How should dexamethasone be dosed and monitored for S.C.?

Table 58-5 Empiric Therapy for Bacterial Meningitis

Age Group or Predisposing Condition	Recommended Therapy	Alternative Therapy
Neonates (<2 mo)	Ampicillin and cefotaxime	Ampicillin and gentamicin
Infants and children (2 mo–10 yr)	Cefotaxime or ceftriaxone + vancomycin	Cefotaxime or ceftriaxone + rifampin
Older children and adults (10–60 yr)	Cefotaxime or ceftriaxone + vancomycin	Cefotaxime or ceftriaxone + rifampin
Elderly (>60 yr)	Ampicillin, cefotaxime, and vancomycin	Ampicillin, cefotaxime, and rifampin
Postneurosurgical	Nafcillin and ceftazidime or cefepime ± gentamicin	Vancomycin and ceftazadime or cefepime ± gentamicin
Open head trauma	Vancomycin and cefotaxime or ceftriaxone	Natcillin and cefotaxime

Table 58-6   Suggested Antibiotic Dosing Regimens for Treatment of Central Nervous System Infections

	Daily Dose[a]			Dosing Interval (hr)	
Antibiotic	Neonates[b]	Children	Adults	Neonates	Children/Adults
Penicillins					
Ampicillin	100–200 mg/kg	200–300 mg/kg	12 g	8–12	4–6
Nafcillin	100–150 mg/kg	150–200 mg/kg	12 g	8–12	4–6
Penicillin G	0.1–0.2 million units/kg	0.15–0.2 million units/kg	20–24 million units	8–12	4–6
Meropenem	20 mg/kg	120 mg/kg	6 g	8–12	8
Cephalosporins					
Cefotaxime	100–150 mg/kg	200–300 mg/kg	12 g	9–12	4–6
Ceftizoxime	100–150 mg/kg	200 mg/kg	12 g	8–12	6–8
Ceftriaxone	NR	100 mg/kg	4 g	—	12–24
Cefazidime	100–150 mg/kg	150–200 mg/kg	8–12 g	8–12	6–8
Cefepime	NR	150 mg/kg	6 g	—	8
Aminoglycosides					
Gentamicin	5–7.5 mg/kg[d,e]	—	5–6 mg/kg[d,e]	12	8–12
Tobramycin	5–7.5 mg/kg[d,e]	—	5–6 mg/kg[d,e]	12	8–12
Amikacin	15–30 mg/kg[d,e]	—	15–25 mg/kg[d,e]	12	8–12
Chloramphenicol	NR	75–100 mg/kg	4–6 g	—	6
Metronidazole	—	30 mg/kg	1.5–2 g	—	6–8
TMP-SMX	—	12–15 mg/kg[f]	12–15 mg/kg[f]	—	8
Vancomycin	20–30 mg/kg	40–60 mg/kg[g]	2–3 g[g] or 20–30 mg/kg[g]	12	8–12

[a]Recommended daily dose when renal and hepatic function are normal.
[b]Infants <1 month old; lower end of dosage range applies to neonates ≤7 days old.
[c]Concurrent intraventricular doses of 5–10 mg (gentamicin, tobramycin), or 20 mg (amikacin) often required when treating Gram-negative bacillary meningitis.
[d]Dose should be individualized based upon serum level monitoring.
[e]Concurrent intraventricular therapy not recommended for neonatal meningitis.
[f]Dose is based upon the trimethoprim component.
[g]Concurrent intraventricular doses of 5–20 mg recommended if response to intravenous therapy is inadequate.

Corticosteroids, particularly dexamethasone, can reduce cerebral edema and lower intracranial pressure.[57] However, before 1988, studies that evaluated the efficacy of corticosteroids in bacterial meningitis failed to demonstrate any beneficial effects.[58,59] These studies were not designed very well, and importantly, hearing loss was not a routinely monitored complication. Given the recent elucidation of the pathophysiologic mechanisms of meningeal inflammation and the important role of cytokine mediators in this process, attention has been refocused on adjunctive corticosteroid therapy for meningitis.

The rationale for steroid therapy in meningitis stems from the fact that steroids reduce the synthesis and release of the proinflammatory cytokines TNF-α and IL-1β from monocytes and astrocytes.[3–5] These two cytokines play a central role in initiating the cascade of events that lead to neuronal tissue damage and neurologic sequelae. Early use of steroids now has been shown in several studies to reduce neurologic complications, particularly sensorineural hearing loss.[5,60–63]

Despite these studies, controversy remains regarding the efficacy and safety of adjunctive dexamethasone therapy in the treatment of bacterial meningitis. Several prospective placebo-controlled randomized trials have demonstrated that adjunctive dexamethasone therapy significantly reduces audiologic and neurologic sequelae in children >2 months of age. However, *H. influenzae* was the causative pathogen in the majority of these meningitis cases, whereas the number of children with streptococcal and meningococcal meningitis in these trials was small.[5,60–64] As previously mentioned, the number of Hib cases has decreased dramatically in recent years and the rate of resistant streptococci has increased, making the data from these trials difficult to apply to other pathogens. In one small study, 29 of 56 children were randomized to receive dexamethasone for the management of pneumococcal meningitis.[65] Few audiologic and neurologic sequelae were observed in the dexamethasone-treated group compared with the placebo group, but the difference did not reach statistical significance.[65]

Other studies have demonstrated the critical importance of the timing of dexamethasone with respect to antimicrobial therapy. Significant differences in outcome have been observed when dexamethasone was given only before or at the time of administration of the first dose of parenteral antibiotic, as opposed to several hours after antibiotic administration.[5,64]

A meta-analysis by McIntyre and colleagues was designed to address important issues regarding the concomitant use of dexamethasone, including the value of dexamethasone for organisms other than Hib, the importance of the nature and timing of antibiotic therapy, the effect of dexamethasone on neurologic deficits other than hearing loss, and the frequency of adverse events.[5] Eleven randomized studies published between 1988 through 1996 were eligible for this analysis. One of the most significant findings of this analysis was that the administration of dexamethasone significantly reduced severe hearing loss in Hib meningitis. In pneumococcal meningitis, severe hearing loss was reduced in patients who received dexamethasone early (with or before parenteral antibiotics).[5] There was significant variation in hearing loss depending on the causative pathogen. In patients with meningococcal meningitis, only 1 child of 61 randomized to dexamethasone and none of the 50 controls had severe hearing loss. Although the efficacy of shorter treatment duration has not been extensively studied, similar outcomes were observed with 2 versus 4 days of therapy. Although not statistically significant, there was a trend toward less gastrointestinal (GI) bleeding in patients who were treated for only 2 days compared with patients who received 4 days of therapy (0.8% versus 3.0%, respectively).[5]

These studies, taken together, provide convincing evidence for the beneficial effects of adjunctive dexamethasone therapy. The risks associated with short-term steroid therapy are low and are far outweighed by the benefit of a reduction in neurologic complications. Therefore, children with bacterial meningitis should receive concomitant dexamethasone therapy.[2,4,60]

Thus, S.C. should receive dexamethasone therapy, 0.15 mg/kg per dose given IV Q 6 hr for 2 to 4 days. For S.C., who is 20 kg, this would be 3 mg Q 6 hr, with the first dexamethasone dose given 15 minutes before initiating ceftriaxone therapy.

The benefit of corticosteroid therapy in adults has recently been studied in a prospective, randomized double-blind multicenter trial.[62a] Three hundred one patients with acute bacterial meningitis were randomized to receive dexamethasone or placebo 15 to 20 minutes before or with the first dose of antibiotic every 6 hours for 4 days. Dexamethasone reduced the risk of unfavorable outcome, defined as a Glasgow Coma Scale score of 1 to 4 at 8 weeks (relative risk, 0.59; $P = 0.03$), and of death (relative risk, 0.48; $P = 0.04$). Among the patients with pneumococcal meningitis, 26% in the dexamethasone group and 52% in the placebo group had unfavorable outcomes (relative risk, 0.5; $P = 0.06$). While this was not statistically significant, patients with pneumococcal meningitis appeared to receive the most benefit from steroids. Neither GI bleeding nor other adverse effects were increased in the dexamethasone group.

In addition, an uncontrolled study demonstrated that patients infected with pneumococci benefited from dexamethasone therapy. In instances of overwhelming infection (as manifested by profoundly altered mental status) or when high bacterial inocula are present (as reflected by a positive CSF Gram's stain), dexamethasone therapy should be considered, particularly if Gram-positive cocci are seen on the Gram's stain.[2,43,62a,64] For such patients, the risk of neurologic complications is much greater than the potential for adverse drug effects.

Potential adverse effects associated with dexamethasone include GI bleeding, mental status changes (e.g., euphoria or encephalopathy), increases in blood glucose, and possibly elevations in blood pressure.[5,57–62] For S.C., the complete blood count (CBC), serum chemistries, and stool guaiac should be monitored daily while he is receiving dexamethasone. He also should be questioned about possible GI upset and assessed for changes in mental status (e.g., confusion, combativeness). Given the short duration of corticosteroid therapy, dexamethasone can be discontinued abruptly without tapering after 2 days.

Effect on Central Nervous System Penetration of Antibiotics

Another important issue to consider is whether dexamethasone, a potent anti-inflammatory agent, reduces the ability of some antimicrobials (e.g., the β-lactams) to penetrate across the blood–brain barrier into CSF. Because CSF penetration of the penicillins, cephalosporins, and other β-lactams is greatest when the meninges are inflamed, there is a hypothetical concern that concomitant dexamethasone may reduce CSF concentrations of these agents, resulting in reduced efficacy. Data to support or refute this hypothesis are limited. In animal models of pneumococcal meningitis, vancomycin penetration into the CSF was reduced in dexamethasone-treated animals compared with animals not treated with steroids.[66,67,67a] Unlike vancomycin, ceftriaxone penetration was not reduced in these animal models. However, decreased bactericidal activity was reported with cephalosporin- and penicillin-resistant *S. pneumoniae* isolates. Furthermore, only the combination of ceftriaxone and rifampin sterilized the CSF when dexamethasone was given in cases of highly resistant strains of *S. pneumoniae*.[67] In another cephalosporin-resistant pneumococcal meningitis animal model, dexamethasone did not decrease ceftriaxone levels in the CSF, but concomitant use of dexamethasone resulted in a higher number of failures due to decreased bacterial killing and bactericidal effect.[67b] Although LeBel and colleagues did not directly measure antibiotic concentrations in the CSF, they did not observe any significant differences in CSF bactericidal activity (a test in which CSF is serially diluted and tested for activity against the infecting pathogen) in steroid-treated versus placebo-treated children.[5] Furthermore, children given dexamethasone had similar, if not better, clinical responses (e.g., shorter duration of fever) than placebo controls,[5] and the rate of CSF sterilization did not differ.[5,60,62] Therefore, based on current evidence, vancomycin penetration into CSF does not appear to be reduced by dexamethasone administration in children, but decreased penetration of vancomycin is observed in adults.[64,66,67] In a rabbit meningitis model, the coadministration of dexamethasone and vancomycin resulted in 29% less penetration of vancomycin into the CSF. However, by increasing the daily dose of vancomycin in these rabbits, therapeutic CSF levels were achieved, suggesting that giving larger daily doses of vancomycin circumvents the steroid effect on CNS penetration.[68] Currently, it is unknown whether the decreased penetration of antibiotics secondary to dexamethasone administration is of clinical significance, especially in this era of penicillin- and cephalosporin-resistant pneumococcal isolates.[44,64] In adults receiving concomitant dexamethasone, experts suggest using the combination of ceftriaxone, vancomycin, and rifampin.[43,64]

Neisseria meningitidis Meningitis

Definitive Therapy

5. Twenty-four hours after admission, S.C.'s culture results from his blood and CSF samples are available. The CSF culture is growing *N. meningitidis,* also present in both of the two collected blood cultures. What modification in S.C.'s antimicrobial therapy is necessary at this time?

Once culture and sensitivity results become available, definitive therapy can be instituted, often with a single agent (Table 58-7).[4,6,31–33,53] As suspected, S.C.'s CSF culture is positive for *N. meningitidis.* Cefuroxime, a second-generation cephalosporin, also has activity against *N. meningitidis.* However, cefuroxime is less effective for meningitis than third-generation cephalosporins.[70,71] In a prospective, randomized

Table 58-7 Definitive Therapy for Bacterial Meningitis

Pathogen	Recommended Treatment	Alternative Agents
H. influenzae		
β-Lactamase-negative	Ampicillin	Cefotaxime or ceftriaxone
β-Lactamase-positive	Cefotaxime or ceftriaxone	Chloramphenicol
N. meningitidis	Penicillin G or ampicillin	Cefotaxime or ceftriaxone or chloramphenicol
S. pneumoniae	*Penicillin-sensitive[a]:* Penicillin G or ampicillin	Cefotaxime or ceftriaxone or chloramphenicol
	Intermediately penicillin-resistant[a]: Vancomycin + cefotaxime or ceftriaxone[e]	Cefotaxime or ceftriaxone and rifampin
	Highly penicillin-resistant[a]: Vancomycin + cefotaxime or ceftriaxone[d] ± rifampin	Cefotaxime or ceftriaxone and rifampin
S. agalactiae	Penicillin G or ampicillin + gentamicin	Cefotaxime or ceftriaxone and rifampin
L. monocytogenes	Ampicillin ± gentamicin	TMP-SMX
Enterobacteriaceae		
E. coli, Klebsiella species	Cefotaxime or ceftriaxone	Cefepime + gentamicin[b]
Enterobacter, Serratia species	TMP-SMX	Cefepime + gentamicin,[b] or ciprofloxacin,[c] or meropenem, cefepime[c]
P. aeruginosa	Ceftazidime + tobramycin[b]	Cefepime + tobramycin, or ciprofloxacin,[c] meropenem
S. aureus		
Penicillinase-producing	Nafcillin or oxacillin	Vancomycin[b]
Methicillin-resistant (MRSA)	Vancomycin[c] ± rifampin	TMP SMX[c] ± rifampin
S. epidermidis	Vancomycin[b] ± rifampin	TMP-SMX[c] ± rifampin

[a]Penicillin-sensitive strains defined as having MIC ≤0.1 μg/mL; intermediately resistant strains MIC >0.1–1.0 μg/mL; highly resistant strains MIC ≥2.0 μg/mL.
[b]Concomitant intrathecal therapy often required for optimal response.
[c]Limited experience or efficacy data for the agent against with this pathogen.
[d]Check cefotaxime or ceftriaxone if MIC ≤0.5; then susceptible in CSF isolates.
MIC, minimum inhibitory concentration; TMP SMX, trimethoprim-sulfamethoxazole.

trial involving 106 children with acute bacterial meningitis, 12% of the patients receiving cefuroxime had positive CSF cultures after 18 to 24 hours versus 2% of those who received ceftriaxone ($P = 0.11$), and 17% of cefuroxime-treated patients developed moderate to severe hearing loss compared with only 4% of those receiving ceftriaxone ($P = 0.05$).[70] Nearly identical findings to these also were noted in a retrospective analysis of four comparative trials of children treated with cefuroxime (159 patients) and ceftriaxone (174 patients) for bacterial meningitis.[71] The reason for the inferiority of cefuroxime relative to ceftriaxone most likely is related to reduced potency and the presence of an inoculum effect (described earlier).[45]

Because *N. meningitidis* is susceptible to penicillin and ampicillin currently, penicillin is the drug of choice. However, S.C.'s questionable history of amoxicillin rash makes the use of penicillin worrisome, and therapy previously begun with ceftriaxone should be continued.

Monitoring Therapy

6. **What subjective and objective data should be monitored to evaluate the efficacy and toxicity of treatment of patients with meningitis, and what specifically should be monitored in S.C.?**

The monitoring of patients with meningitis is similar in many respects to other infectious diseases. Clinical signs and symptoms attributable to the disease, such as fever, altered mental status, and stiff neck, need to be checked periodically throughout the day and monitored for resolution. S.C.'s temperature and mental status should be assessed at least four times a day. Accurate assessment of S.C.'s mental status can be difficult because of his young age. Thus, his baseline level of mental status should be evaluated (e.g., whether he is awake and alert, or lethargic and difficult to arouse). If awake and alert, S.C. should be observed for irritability, because this often is the only sign of altered mentation. Questions can be used to assess his orientation: Does he know where he is? Does he know his name? Can he recognize his mother or other family members? In general, signs of clinical improvement should be evident within 24 to 48 hours for most uncomplicated cases of acute bacterial meningitis,[5,6,37,70] and the corticosteroid therapy that S.C. is receiving may accelerate the clinical response.[5,61]

Laboratory tests should be monitored as well. A CBC with differential, serum electrolytes (e.g., Na, K, Cl, HCO_3), blood glucose, and renal function tests (e.g., BUN, SrCr) should be performed daily. Abnormal electrolyte results may require more frequent monitoring. Laboratory abnormalities such as leukocytosis and hyponatremia may take longer to normalize than clinical symptoms. If S.C. develops severe SIADH, as manifested by serum sodium values up to 120 mEq/L with altered mental status or seizures, fluid restriction and short-term (i.e., 6 to 12 hours) IV administration of 3% sodium chloride may be necessary.

CSF chemistries usually normalize after several days, although CSF protein may remain elevated for a week or more.[6,37] With effective therapy, the CSF culture usually is sterile after about 18 to 24 hours of therapy.[5,61,70] Delays in CSF sterilization are associated with a higher propensity for neurologic complications.[4,33] If S.C. responds to therapy in a straightforward manner, there is no need for him to undergo a repeat lumbar puncture. However, if the response is inadequate, as evidenced by persistent fever and/or deteriorating mental status, S.C. will require a repeat lumbar puncture to re-examine the CSF parameters.[6,37]

In addition to monitoring the therapeutic response, side effects of the antimicrobial regimen also need to be assessed frequently. Meningitis requires high-dose therapy, making the likelihood of adverse effects much greater. Currently, S.C. is being treated with ceftriaxone, a cephalosporin antibiotic. The adverse effects most often associated with ceftriaxone include hypersensitivity reactions, mild pain and phlebitis at the injection site, and GI complaints.[72] S.C. should be observed for the formation of a antibiotic-related skin rash or evidence of an accelerated allergic reaction (e.g., hives, wheezing). The IV catheter site should be observed daily for redness, tenderness, or pain upon palpation of the vein. S.C. should be watched closely for loose stools or diarrhea. Although diarrhea is a common side effect of most antimicrobials, this adverse effect is more likely to occur with ceftriaxone because approximately 40% to 50% of the dose is excreted unchanged into the bile. Mild diarrhea, which usually does not require discontinuation of therapy, occurs in 23% to 41% of children receiving ceftriaxone for meningitis therapy.[52,70] Less common but of concern is the potential for antibiotic-associated colitis.[72,73] If S.C. experiences diarrhea that is persistent, accompanied by fever and abdominal cramping, a stool sample should be tested for *Clostridium difficile* toxin. If positive, oral antibiotic therapy, preferably with metronidazole, should correct the problem (see Chapter 62, Infectious Diarrhea).

Ceftriaxone-Induced Biliary Pseudolithiasis

7. After 5 days of treatment, the nurse caring for S.C. notes that his appetite is markedly diminished, and he complains of an upset stomach. S.C. was afebrile and alert and oriented, but abdominal examination revealed "guarding," with pain localized in the right upper quadrant area. Laboratory data at this time are WBC count, 6,000 cells/mm³ (normal, 3,200 to 9,800); Hgb, 12.5 g/dL (normal, 14 to 19); Hct, 34% (normal, 39% to 49%); platelets, 120,000/mm³ (normal, 130,000 to 400,000); Na, 135 mEq/L; K, 3.6 mEq/L; Cl, 98 mEq/L; aspartate aminotransferase (AST), 35 U/L (normal, 0 to 35); alanine aminotransferase (ALT), 33 U/L (normal, 0 to 3.5); alkaline phosphatase, 110 MU/dL (normal, 30 to 120); total bilirubin, 1.2 mg/dL (normal, 0.1 to 1.0); and amylase 70 U/L. A stool guaiac is negative. What are possible causes of S.C.'s abdominal discomfort?

[SI units: WBC count, 6 * 10⁹ cells/L; Hgb, 125 g/L; Hct, 0.34; platelets, 120 * 10⁹/L; Na, 135 mmol/L; K, 3.6 mmol/L; Cl, 98 mmol/L; AST, 33 U/L; ALT, 33 U/L; alkaline phosphatase, 110 U/L; total bilirubin, 20.5 μmol/L; amylase, 70 U/L]

There are a number of possible etiologies for S.C.'s abdominal discomfort. His corticosteroid therapy may have caused acute GI bleeding. This is unlikely because the dexamethasone was discontinued 3 days ago and S.C.'s hemoglobin and hematocrit values are in the low-normal range. The negative stool guaiac result also argues strongly against a GI

bleed. Acute pancreatitis is unlikely given the normal amylase result. Viral or drug-induced hepatitis is another possibility but also is unlikely given his normal AST, ALT, and bilirubin results. An intra-abdominal infection also is possible, but this is improbable because he is afebrile and has a normal WBC count. Other causes such as acute cholecystitis or appendicitis require further diagnostic evaluation.

8. An abdominal ultrasound reveals sludge in the gallbladder. What is the significance of this finding in S.C., and how should this abnormality be managed?

The abnormality on S.C.'s abdominal ultrasound explains his right upper quadrant pain. S.C. has what appears to be a condition known as biliary pseudolithiasis (i.e., biliary "sludging"). Biliary sludging can occur in conditions of gallbladder hypomotility (e.g., recent surgery, burns, total parenteral nutrition) and in some instances can be drug induced. S.C. has been receiving ceftriaxone for treatment of his meningitis, and this drug can cause biliary pseudolithiasis.[74–77]

Antibiotic-associated biliary pseudolithiasis is seen almost exclusively with ceftriaxone.[72] The predominance of biliary excretion that occurs with ceftriaxone results in very high concentrations of the drug in gallbladder bile.[74] In selected circumstances, the biliary concentration of ceftriaxone may exceed solubility limits, resulting in formation of a fine, granular precipitate (i.e., sludge),[74] which differs in composition and ultrasound features from true gallstones.[70,75] The precipitate is composed of a ceftriaxone–calcium complex, the formation of which is dose dependent.[74,76] Given the high dosages required for meningitis therapy, it is not surprising that this adverse effect has occurred in S.C.[70,75] In the comparative randomized trial between ceftriaxone and cefuroxime cited previously, evidence of biliary pseudolithiasis on abdominal ultrasonography was observed in 16 of 35 (46%) patients who received ceftriaxone and in none of 35 patients receiving cefuroxime.[70] Pseudolithiasis usually appears 3 to 10 days following the start of therapy, and in the majority of instances it is clinically asymptomatic. Symptoms similar to acute cholecystitis are evident in some individuals and include nausea with or without vomiting and abdominal right upper quadrant pain. Although he has not vomited yet, S.C.'s symptoms fit this description. Approximately 10% to 20% of patients with evidence of biliary sludging on ultrasound are symptomatic.[75,77]

Prompt recognition of this adverse effect and discontinuation of ceftriaxone therapy are required to effectively manage biliary pseudolithiasis. Before this complication was recognized, a few patients underwent cholecystectomies, but this intervention is rarely necessary because the condition nearly always is reversible. Once S.C.'s ceftriaxone is discontinued, the condition should resolve gradually over a period of weeks to months; the clinical symptoms should disappear within a few days.[75,77] Cefotaxime can be substituted for ceftriaxone; cefotaxime is not associated with biliary complications, and the efficacy of these two agents is equivalent.[61,72] For S.C., the cefotaxime dosage would be 1,000 mg IV every 6 hours (see Table 58-6).

Chloramphenicol also could be considered. Although only bacteriostatic against most bacteria, it has bactericidal activity against the three common meningeal pathogens, *H. influenzae, S. pneumoniae,* and *N. meningitidis.*[6,16,33,78] Furthermore, chloramphenicol has excellent CSF penetration and frequently was used before the commercial availability of third-generation cephalosporins.[6,37,78] Aplastic anemia, an extremely rare but potentially fatal complication of therapy, has drastically limited the use of chloramphenicol.[78] More commonly, dose-related bone marrow suppression occurs, which can be minimized by maintaining peak serum concentrations of chloramphenicol <25 μg/mL.[78] The recommended dosage of chloramphenicol is 75 to 100 mg/kg per day, given IV in four divided doses.[53]

Duration of Therapy

9. What is the recommended duration of antimicrobial therapy for *N. meningitidis* meningitis, and for how long should S.C. be treated?

The optimal duration of therapy for meningitis is difficult to ascertain because few trials have been designed to address this issue.[79] Although general guidelines exist, the decision to discontinue therapy should be individualized based on the response to therapy, the presence of complicating factors (e.g., immunosuppression), and the specific causative pathogen. Table 58-8 lists the recommended treatment durations for uncomplicated cases of bacterial meningitis according to the specific pathogen.[6,53,55,79] Patients like S.C. with meningitis caused by *N. meningitidis* should be treated for 7 to 10 days.[53,79] Complicated cases such as those with delayed CSF sterilization require therapy for longer periods (up to 2 weeks or more).

S.C. had been responding well to the ceftriaxone therapy, and if he continues to respond well to the cefotaxime regimen outlined previously, there is no need for additional oral antibiotics upon discharge from the hospital. An oral second- or third-generation cephalosporin cannot be recommended in the treatment of meningitis because insufficient concentrations are achieved in the CSF. S.C. should be watched carefully for a possible relapse (e.g., the reappearance of signs and symptoms of meningitis), which would require readmission to the hospital for further evaluation and IV antibiotic therapy.

Prevention of N. meningitidis Meningitis

10. S.C. is ready to be discharged home. How can the potential spread of meningococcal disease be prevented in persons with whom S.C. has contact?

CHEMOPROPHYLAXIS OF CLOSE CONTACTS

Despite an excellent response to therapy, S.C. still may harbor *N. meningitidis* in his nasopharynx and could transmit this organism to individuals with whom he has close contact.[80]

Table 58-8	Duration of Therapy for Bacterial Meningitis
Etiology	*Duration of Therapy (0 days)*
H. influenzae	7–10
N. meningitidis	7–10
S. pneumoniae	10–14
Group B streptococci (*S. agalactiae*)	14–21
L. monocytogenes	14–21
Gram-negative bacilli	21

Therefore, chemoprophylaxis to reduce nasopharyngeal carriage of *N. meningitidis* is indicated for S.C. and his close contacts.[80,81] In this context, close contacts are defined as individuals who frequently sleep and eat in the same dwelling with an index case: a household member, day care center contacts, and any person directly exposed to the patient's oral secretions (e.g., boyfriend or girlfriend, mouth-to-mouth resuscitation or endotracheal intubation).[80,81] The potential for a close contact to become infected with *N. meningitidis* is 500 to 800 times greater than for the total population.[80] S.C.'s 7-year-old brother, who is at risk for invasive *N. meningitidis* disease, should receive chemoprophylaxis. Also, the children at the day care center or close contacts at the hospital who have been caring for S.C. may benefit from chemoprophylaxis. Because the risk of secondary disease is greatest within 2 to 5 days after exposure to the index case, chemoprophylaxis should be instituted as soon as possible and ideally within 24 hours.[80] Administering chemoprophylaxis 14 days or more after identification of the index case is probably of little value. The most frequently used regimen to reduce nasopharyngeal carriage of *N. meningitidis* for children >1 month is rifampin, given once daily in a dosage of 10 mg/kg per day for 2 days.[80,81] A suspension containing 10 mg/mL of rifampin (which requires extemporaneous compounding) is available; 20 mL will provide a 200-mg dose. The index patient should also receive prophylaxis if he or she was treated with penicillin or chloramphenicol as soon as he or she is able to tolerate oral medications. Because S.C. is receiving ceftriaxone, he does not need chemoprophylaxis. For adult close contacts, rifampin 600 mg twice a day for 2 days should be administered. Thus, S.C.'s brother, parents, and day care contacts should be treated with appropriate doses of rifampin as soon as he is diagnosed. Alternative chemoprophylactic regimens that have been shown to be effective for reducing nasopharyngeal carriage of *N. meningitidis* are ceftriaxone 250 mg or 125 mg intramuscularly in adults and children, respectively, and ciprofloxacin 500 mg orally as a single dose in adults. Because rifampin is not recommended for pregnant women, ceftriaxone would be a viable alternative.[80,81]

Prevention of Haemophilus influenzae Type b Meningitis
HIB VACCINATION RECOMMENDATIONS

11. S.C. and his brother were vaccinated for Hib. Are these vaccinations now routinely recommended?

Yes. S.C. appropriately received one of the Hib protein conjugate vaccines when he was 2 months of age.[84] Given the tremendous success that conjugated Hib vaccines have had on reducing the incidence of Hib meningitis in the United States, all children >2 months of age should receive the vaccination series with one of the three commercially available products.[84] HbOC (HibTITER) is a product that links polyribosylribitol phosphate (PRP), the antigen derived from Hib purified capsular polysaccharide, with a carrier protein (CRM_{197}) derived from a mutated variant of the diphtheria toxin protein, while PRP-OMP (PedvaxHIB) links PRP with the outer membrane complex protein of *N. meningitidis*.[80,84] The third product, PRP-T (ActHIB), is a PRP–tetanus toxoid conjugate. The linkage of PRP with a carrier protein is necessary to elicit an adequate immune response in children <15 months of age.[80,85] HbOC and PRP-OMP have been licensed since 1988 and 1989, respectively. In 1990, both products received FDA approval for use in infants 2 months of age or older. PRP-T was approved for use in infants 2 months of age or older by the FDA in early 1993. All three of these conjugate vaccines are equally effective.[24,25,84,85] Table 58-9 outlines the vaccination schedule for HbOC, PRP-OMP, and PRP-T as recommended by the Centers for Disease Control and Prevention Advisory Committee on Immunization Practices.[84] In general, the vaccines are well tolerated; fever, redness, and swelling at the injection site are the most common adverse effects and occur in <4% of patients.[25,80,85]

NEISSERIA MENINGITIDIS VACCINATION RECOMMENDATIONS

12. A 21-year-old college student who lives in a dormitory dies of *N. meningitidis* meningitis. Two additional cases are diagnosed in students living in the same dormitory. Should all individuals living in the dormitory be vaccinated? What are the current recommendations for the use of meningococcal vaccine?

N. meningitidis is responsible for causing both outbreaks (clusters of cases) as well as epidemics. Currently a meningococcal quadrivalent (Men A,C,Y,W-135) polysaccharide vaccine is available in the United States. Meningococci serogroups A, B, and C are responsible for causing >90% of cases. After vaccination, protective levels of antibody are usually achieved within 7 to 10 days. The vaccine has variable efficacy. Currently, there is no vaccine available for Men B.[80,81]

Although routine vaccination is not recommended for the general population, the Advisory Committee on Immunization Practices (ACIP) recommends meningococcal vaccination in certain high-risk groups: patients with underlying terminal complement deficiency or anatomic/functional asplenia, or persons traveling to endemic/epidemic areas.[80,81] In addition, vaccination is recommended in areas of outbreak or epidemic conditions.[80,81] In addition, college freshman should be educated about the benefits of vaccination, and vaccination should be provided or made easily available to those who wish to reduce their risk of disease.[83] College freshman living in a dormitory appear to have an increased risk of acquiring meningococci compared with persons of the same age not living in a dormitory.[83] However, vaccination of all freshmen who live in dormitories or residence halls is not recommended since it is unlikely to be cost effective for society as a whole. In the case mentioned in this question, however, it would be necessary to vaccinate all individuals living in the dormitory because it is considered an outbreak.[81,83]

Streptococcus pneumoniae Meningitis

Clinical Features, Predisposing Factors, and Diagnosis

13. A.L., a 58-year-old man with a long history of alcohol abuse, is admitted to the ED febrile and unresponsive. Over the past several days, A.L. has experienced intermittent episodes of fever, chills, SOB, and a worsening productive cough. A friend visiting A.L. called 911 when he could not arouse him. A.L.'s medical records indicate that he suffers from hypertension, adult-onset diabetes mellitus, peptic ulcer disease (PUD), and chronic obstructive airways disease (COAD). A splenectomy was performed 10 years ago after trauma to the abdomen. A.L. is divorced and lives alone in a low-income apartment. He has no known drug allergies. His records show him to be a smoker for >30 years. Current medications include hydrochlorothiazide 50 mg QOD, sustained-release theophylline (Theo-Dur) 300 mg PO TID, glipizide 5 mg PO BID, famotidine 20 mg PO HS, and ciprofloxacin 250 mg PO BID PRN for cough and increased sputum production.

On admission to the ED, A.L. had a temperature of 40°C, BP of 90/50 mm Hg, and pulse and respiratory rates of 115 beats/min and 25 breaths/min, respectively. His weight is 59 kg. A.L. was unresponsive but withdrew all extremities to painful stimuli. His pupils were equal and sluggishly reactive to light; papilledema and evidence of meningismus were present. Wheezes and crackles were heard throughout both lung fields, with dense consolidation noted in the left lower lobe. The remainder of his physical examination was noncontributory.

Stat laboratory tests revealed a WBC count of 18,000 cells/mm³ (normal, 3,200 to 9,800), with 80% PMNs, 15% bands, 3% lymphocytes, and 2% basophils; Hgb and Hct of 10.5 g/dL (normal, 14 to 18) and 34% (normal, 39 to 49%), respectively; and a platelet count of 250,000/mm³ (normal, 130,000 to 400,000). Serum chemistries were significant for K, 3.0 mEq/L (normal, 3.5 to 5.0); glucose, 250 mg/dL (normal, 70 to 110); AST and ALT, 190 mg/dL (normal, 0 to 35) and 140 mg/dL (normal, 0 to 3.5), respectively; BUN, 35 mg/dL (normal, 8 to 18); and SrCr, 2.4 mg/dL (normal, 0.6 to 1.2). The prothrombin time was high normal, and albumin was 3.1 mg/dL (normal, 4 to 6). A stat blood alcohol level of 100 mg/dL was reported, and a urine toxicology screen was negative. A.L.'s serum theophylline concentration was 18 mg/dL. Stool guaiac was positive.

A CT scan showed no evidence of mass lesions or cerebral hematoma. Lumbar puncture yielded CSF opening pressure, 200 mm Hg (normal, <20); protein, 120 mg/dL (normal, <50); glucose, 100 mg/dL (normal, 60% of plasma glucose); WBC count, 8,500 cells/mm³ (normal, <5 cells/mm³), 92% PMNs, 4% monohistiocytes, and 4% lymphocytes; and RBC count, 400/mm³. Gram-positive, lancet-shaped diplococci were visible on CSF Gram's stain. In addition, a sputum Gram's stain revealed numerous WBCs, few epithelial cells, and numerous Gram-positive cocci in pairs and in short chains. Blood, CSF, urine, and sputum cultures are pending.

What are the clinical and laboratory features of pneumococcal meningitis? What features of pneumococcal meningitis are present in A.L.?

Table 58-9 Recommended Vaccination Schedule for *Haemophilus influenzae* Protein Conjugated Vaccines

Vaccine (Trade Name)	Schedule				
	2 Months	4 Months	6 Months	12 Months	15 Months
HbOC (HibTITER)	Dose 1	Dose 2	Dose 3	—	Booster
PRP-T (ActHIB)	Dose 1	Dose 2	Dose 3	—	Booster
PRP-OMP (PedvaxHIB)	Dose 1	Dose 2	—	Booster	—

[SI units: WBC count, 18 * 10⁹ cells/L with 0.8 PMNs, 0.15 bands, 0.03 lymphocytes, and 0.02 basophils; Hgb, 105 g/L; platelets, 250 * 10⁹/L; K, 3.0 mmol/L; glucose, 13.9 mmol/L; BUN, 12.5 mmol/L urea; SrCr, 212 mmol/L; glucose, 5.5 mmol/L; WBC count, 8,500 * 10⁶ cells/L; RBC count, 400 * 10⁶/L]

A.L. presents to the ED with many signs and symptoms suggestive of pneumococcal meningitis. He is 56 years old, and *S. pneumoniae* is the most common bacterial etiology for meningitis in adults >30 years of age (see Table 58-1).[19,20] As is evidenced by A.L.'s presentation, invasive pneumococcal disease often is associated with significant morbidity, and mortality rates remain high.[20] Over the past several years, the incidence of *S. pneumoniae* meningitis in the United States has consistently ranged between 1.2 and 2.8 cases per 100,000 population per year.[19,20,24] Predisposing factors to invasive pneumococcal disease include advanced age, alcoholism, chronic pulmonary disease, and sickle cell disease.[6,37,80] In addition, individuals infected with the HIV, those with Hodgkin's disease, and patients who have undergone kidney, liver, or bone marrow transplantation also appear to be at higher risk.[6,80,86,87] Patients with CSF otorrhea or rhinorrhea induced by closed head trauma or neurosurgical procedures are more prone to develop pneumococcal meningitis as well.[20,80,87]

A.L. has many predisposing factors for pneumococcal meningitis. He has a low socioeconomic status, smokes, has a long history of alcohol abuse, has had a splenectomy, and suffers from diabetes and COAD. Underlying COAD is an important predisposing factor in that chronic colonization with pneumococci occurs in such patients. Intermittent use of ciprofloxacin by A.L. for acute exacerbations of COAD is unjustified. The poor activity of this antibiotic against *S. pneumoniae* is likely to select out this organism for infection. Furthermore, ciprofloxacin can increase serum theophylline concentrations by inhibiting its metabolism, another important reason why this agent is not a good therapeutic choice for productive cough in A.L.[88]

A diagnosis of pneumococcal meningitis in A.L. is supported by the high fever, stiff neck (meningismus), and altered mental status. He is unresponsive, which is a definite negative prognostic factor.[1,6] Results from CSF chemistries and microbiologic analysis are highly suggestive of pneumococcal meningitis. A.L. has an elevated opening CSF pressure and a markedly elevated CSF protein and WBC count with a predominance of neutrophils on differential examination. The normal CSF glucose level (100 g/dL) is misleading because A.L. is diabetic. The calculated ratio of CSF to serum glucose for A.L. is <50%, which is consistent with acute bacterial meningitis (see Table 58-3). The presence of Gram-positive, lancet-shaped diplococci in pairs on the CSF Gram's stain strongly supports the diagnosis of pneumococcal disease. The signs and symptoms of pneumococcal pneumonia (cough, SOB, increased sputum production, and pulmonary consolidation) as well as the sputum Gram's stain result also lend support to a diagnosis of invasive pneumococcal infection.

Empiric Therapy in Adults

14. What empiric therapy is appropriate for A.L. at this time?

Resistance among pneumococci to penicillin G has become an important concern worldwide and in the United States.[2,28,89] For this reason, susceptibility testing should be performed on all pneumococcal isolates obtained from sterile sites (e.g., blood, CSF).[2,89] For treatment of meningitis caused by strains intermediately resistant to penicillin, ceftriaxone and cefotaxime are the most useful agents because many of these isolates retain cephalosporin sensitivity.[2,8,90] Management of invasive pneumococcal infections in sites other than CSF (e.g., lungs, bloodstream) usually can be accomplished by increasing the dose of penicillin G to 20 to 24 million units/day. This approach is not possible with meningitis caused by intermediately resistant strains because further increases in the penicillin dose are likely to produce unacceptable neurotoxicity. Vancomycin and chloramphenicol are potential options, but relapses and clinical failures have been reported with both of these agents when given alone.[89,91,92] Many penicillin-resistant pneumococcal isolates also are resistant to chloramphenicol (defined as an MIC >4 µg/mL), and even against susceptible isolates, chloramphenicol may fail to elicit a bactericidal effect.[2,89,91,92] Third-generation cephalosporins cannot be relied on for treatment of meningitis caused by strains fully resistant to penicillin (MIC ≥2.0 µg/mL) because reduced cephalosporin sensitivity often occurs (MICs range from 2 to 8 µg/mL to both cefotaxime and ceftriaxone). *S. pneumoniae* strains in CSF with MICs >0.5 µg/mL to cefotaxime or ceftriaxone are considered resistant.[93] Reduced activity of ceftriaxone and cefotaxime against penicillin-resistant pneumococci affects the therapeutic ratio achieved in CSF and is the likely explanation for reports of clinical failure.[89,90] Optimal therapy for fully penicillin-resistant pneumococcal meningitis is unclear. Vancomycin alone in high dosage (3 to 4 g/day in adults) has been suggested.[2,89,91] The combination of vancomycin and ceftriaxone was superior to either agent given alone in a rabbit model of penicillin-resistant pneumococcal meningitis.[94] Ceftriaxone or vancomycin combined with rifampin also may be superior to either drug given alone.[89,91] Animal data suggest that the use of rifampin reduces early mortality in pneumococcal meningitis by reducing the release of proinflammatory bacterial cell components.[95] Thus, until more information is available, the combination of ceftriaxone or cefotaxime with vancomycin represents the most reasonable approach to empiric therapy for potential penicillin-resistant pneumococcal meningitis.

Until culture and susceptibility results are available, the recommended antibiotic in this situation is ceftriaxone 2 g given IV Q 12 hr and vancomycin 500 mg given IV Q 12 hr. A.L. weighs 59 kg, and because his renal function is not normal (SrCr, 2.4 mg/dL; creatinine clearance, 30 mL/min), a dosage adjustment was made. See Question 22 for vancomycin dosing in CNS infections.

Corticosteroid Therapy for Adult Meningitis

15. Should A.L. receive corticosteroid therapy in addition to his antibiotic therapy?

The issue of adjunctive corticosteroid therapy for A.L. needs to be addressed. As previously stated, the efficacy of dexamethasone in adults with meningitis has recently been studied.[62a] Clearly, A.L. presents with profoundly altered mental status, and his signs and symptoms are consistent with a fulminant course of disease. Given that he is unarousable, hypotensive, and tachycardic, A.L. likely will be admitted to the intensive care unit. Thus, his age, underlying medical problems, likely streptococcal meningitis, and deteriorating clinical status all point to a poor prognosis and argue for the use of adjunctive dexamethasone. On the other hand, A.L. is diabetic and has an elevated glucose concentration. He also suffers from PUD, which may be active given that he is anemic and has a positive stool guaiac result. High-dose dexamethasone therapy may cloud A.L.'s sensorium, making mental status assessment even more difficult. Although each of these issues is a concern, none appears to be so critical as to preclude the use of corticosteroids.[62a] Therefore, dexamethasone given in a dosage of 10 mg IV Q 6 hr could be instituted before starting ceftriaxone therapy and continued for up to 4 days, provided that the diagnosis of bacterial meningitis is confirmed. If corticosteroids are administered, the addition of rifampin to ceftriaxone is recommended.[43] To control blood glucose, a sliding-scale dosing schedule of regular insulin is recommended. A.L.'s PUD should be properly worked up and treated if necessary.

Treatment of Penicillin-Susceptible Pneumococcal Meningitis

16. Results from A.L.'s CSF, blood, and sputum cultures are available and are positive for *S. pneumoniae* at each site. Sensitivity testing in CSF revealed an MIC of 0.06 μg/mL to penicillin, 0.25 μg/mL to cefotaxime and ceftriaxone, 0.25 μg/mL to vancomycin, and 8 μg/mL to chloramphenicol. What therapy is indicated for A.L.?

Fortunately, A.L. has become infected with a strain of *S. pneumoniae* that is susceptible to penicillin G (see Table 58-5).[4,6,37] The dosage usually is 20 to 24 million units/day in adults with normal renal function (see Table 58-6). However, A.L. has renal impairment, which means he should receive a reduced penicillin dosage. One of the most useful methods for calculating the dose of penicillin G when renal function is compromised is the following equation[96]:

$$\text{Dose (in million units/day)} = \text{(Calculated creatinine clearance/7)} + 3.2$$

This equation should be used only when the calculated creatinine clearance is <40 mL/min.[96] For A.L., who has a calculated creatinine clearance of 30 mL/min (according to the method of Cockcroft and Gault), the daily dose would be approximately 8 million units, or 2 million units Q 6 hr. This revised regimen should provide penicillin serum concentrations similar to those achieved with high-dose therapy when kidney function is normal. Failure to adjust the dosage appropriately is equivalent to providing massive doses of penicillin, which may result in hyperkalemia (if the potassium-containing preparation is used), seizures, and encephalopathy.[96]

In patients unable to tolerate penicillin G, the best alternatives are ceftriaxone or cefotaxime (see Table 58-5).[4,6] First-generation cephalosporins (e.g., cefazolin) have good activity against pneumococci, but their limited CSF penetration makes these agents poor choices for therapy.[42,49] Conversely, the third-generation agent, ceftazidime, penetrates well into CSF, but its usefulness is limited by reduced activity against pneumococci in comparison to other third-generation agents.[48,49] Cefuroxime also has good pneumococcal activity but as previously mentioned is inferior to ceftriaxone and cefotaxime.[70] Vancomycin has more limited and variable CSF

penetration.[42,97] Therefore, vancomycin should be reserved for situations in which there is bacterial resistance or penicillin intolerance. TMP-SMX has excellent CSF penetration characteristics but is not active against many strains of *S. pneumoniae.* However, limited experience exists with this product for the treatment of pneumococcal meningitis.[42,98]

Prevention of Meningitis

17. Should A.L. have received pneumococcal vaccine? How effective is vaccination in preventing invasive pneumococcal disease?

Yes, he should have. The pneumococcal vaccine (Pneumovax 23, Pnu-Immune 23) provides protection against invasive pneumococcal disease.[80,81,87] The vaccine is composed of purified capsular polysaccharide antigens of 23 serotypes of *S. pneumoniae,* which are responsible for causing approximately 88% of the bacteremic pneumococcal disease in the United States.[80,87] Individuals like A.L. who are at high risk for pneumococcal infection should be given the vaccine. Persons with chronic cardiopulmonary diseases, diabetes, alcoholism, cirrhosis, CSF leaks, and asplenia, and those >65 years of age should be vaccinated with the pneumococcal vaccine.[87] Immunocompromised patients such as those with Hodgkin's disease, lymphoma, multiple myeloma, and chronic renal failure, patients who have undergone organ transplantation, and HIV-infected individuals also are at high risk for pneumococcal disease and should receive the vaccine.[87] Unfortunately, immunocompromised patients often fail to mount a sufficient immune response to the vaccine to fully protect them against infection.[80,87,99] Patients with asymptomatic HIV disease respond more favorably to the vaccine than those with advanced AIDS.[99] The antibody response in children <2 years of age also is poor or absent, and the vaccine is not recommended for these young children.[80]

Thus, given his underlying medical condition (splenectomy) and history of alcoholism, A.L. should receive the pneumococcal vaccine. A single dose is all that is required; subsequent doses may be necessary in ≥5 years.

Gram-Negative Bacillary Meningitis

18. R.R., a 40-year-old, 80-kg man, is admitted to the hospital for a cervical laminectomy with vertebral fusion. His surgical procedure was complicated by a dural tear. On the third postoperative day, drainage at his surgical excision site was noted, and R.R. was febrile to 38.2°C. A Gram's stain of the drainage revealed few Gram-positive cocci and moderate Gram-negative bacilli. Therapy with IV cefazolin 1 g Q 8 hr was begun. The following morning, R.R. was oriented to person, place, and time, but he was slightly obtunded and had a temperature of 40°C. Neck stiffness could not be assessed because of his recent surgery. A magnetic resonance imaging (MRI) scan of the head and neck was negative, and lumbar puncture yielded a CSF WBC count of 3,000 cells/mm³ (normal, <5 cells/mm³), with 95% PMNs; glucose of 20 mg/dL (normal, 60% of plasma glucose); and protein of 280 mg/dL (normal, <50). CSF Gram's stain showed numerous large Gram-negative rods. What important clinical and laboratory features of Gram-negative bacillary meningitis are manifested in R.R.?

[SI units: WBC count, 3 * 10⁹ cells/L; glucose, 1.11 mmol/L; protein, 2.8 g/L]

Epidemiology

R.R. has developed Gram-negative meningitis as a complication of his recent neurosurgical procedure. Although Gram-negative bacilli do not cause meningitis nearly as often as *H. influenzae, S. pneumoniae,* and *N. meningitidis,* they remain important pathogens both in the community and hospital setting.[1,19,20,30,33,55] During an 8-year period covering 1972 to 1979, 158 cases of Gram-negative bacillary meningitis were reported to the New York City Health Department, or approximately 20 cases per year for the population of 8 million.[30] Of 493 episodes of meningitis occurring over a 27-year period (1962 to 1988) at the Massachusetts General Hospital, enteric Gram-negative bacilli accounted for 33% of all nosocomial episodes and 3% of community-acquired cases.[1] Historically, mortality rates from Gram-negative bacillary meningitis have been extremely high, ranging from 40% to 70%. However, with the availability of newer antimicrobials such as third-generation cephalosporins, fatalities have declined to <40%.[19,30,33,55] Increasing resistance among certain Gram-negative bacilli, such as *Enterobacter* species and *P. aeruginosa,* presents a therapeutic dilemma in that mortality associated with these pathogens is high and therapeutic options are fewer.[31,32]

Predisposing Factors

Individuals at greatest risk for Gram-negative bacillary meningitis include neonates, the elderly, debilitated individuals, patients with open trauma to the head, and individuals like R.R. undergoing neurosurgical procedures.[19–21,30,55] Although meningitis is a rare complication of clean neurosurgical procedures (e.g., craniotomy, laminectomy), the consequences can be devastating when it does happen.[1,21,100]

Microbiology

E. coli and *K. pneumoniae* are the most common Gram-negative bacteria causing meningitis and represent about two thirds of all cases.[33,55,100] *E. coli* is the most common Gram-negative etiology of neonatal meningitis, whereas *K. pneumoniae* is isolated more often in the adult population.[22,33,55,100] The remaining one third of cases are divided evenly among *Proteus, Serratia, Enterobacter,* and *Salmonella* species, *P. aeruginosa,* and other less common bacilli.[33,55,100]

Clinical Features

In general, clinical laboratory features of Gram-negative bacillary meningitis are similar to other types of bacterial meningitis.[22,37,55,9100] Because of high virulence, Gram-negative bacillary meningitis often is a fulminant, rapidly progressive disease. An exception to this rule is meningitis after neurosurgery.[21] As is evidenced by R.R.'s clinical presentation, postneurosurgical Gram-negative bacillary meningitis can present in a more subtle fashion. In such patients, many of the symptoms of meningitis (e.g., altered mental status, stiff neck) are masked by underlying neurologic disease. Thus, a high index of suspicion is warranted in the postsurgical setting. In addition to Gram-negative bacilli, staphylococci also are associated with postneurosurgical meningitis.[21] The presence of what looks like staphylococci on R.R.'s wound drainage fluid is of concern, but the abundance of Gram-negative rods on his CSF Gram's stain supports the latter as being the most likely causative pathogen.

Treatment of Gram-Negative Bacillary Meningitis

19. What would be appropriate therapy for Gram-negative bacillary meningitis in R.R.?

Fewer choices are available for treatment of Gram-negative bacillary meningitis than for other meningitides. Ampicillin is active against only *E. coli, P. mirabilis,* and *Salmonella* species, but its low potency and a high likelihood of resistance severely limit its use.[33,55,100] Chloramphenicol has mediocre Gram-negative activity (except against *P. aeruginosa*) but is only bacteriostatic in activity against enteric bacilli.[33] Chloramphenicol treatment of Gram-negative bacillary meningitis historically has been associated with excessively high mortality.[30,33,55,100] Aminoglycosides are limited by their inability to achieve therapeutic CSF concentrations, as well as reduced activity in the acidic milieu of purulent CSF.[14,16,33,51] Intrathecal administration will produce therapeutic CSF concentrations, but repeated administration often is complicated by painful arachnoiditis. Even with this approach, mortality rates are high (>40%).[14,55] Unlike intrathecal administration, lumbar injections will not result in therapeutic CSF concentrations in the ventricle. Extended-spectrum penicillins (e.g., piperacillin) are active against most Gram-negative rods but require combination therapy with aminoglycosides for optimal results.[55] The third-generation cephalosporins represent by far the most useful group of agents for treating Gram-negative bacillary meningitis, given their high potency against many enteric Gram-negative bacilli and good CSF penetration. Experience with these agents spanning over a decade has resulted in the third-generation cephalosporins becoming the drugs of choice for Gram-negative bacillary meningitis.[4,33,101]

Empiric therapy for R.R. should include a third-generation cephalosporin, such as cefotaxime, ceftriaxone, or ceftazidime (see Table 58-5).[4,21,53] These three have excellent activity against *E. coli* and *K. pneumoniae* and are active against other enteric Gram-negative bacilli as well[33,101] (see Table 58-7). Resistance to third-generation cephalosporins among species of *Enterobacter, Citrobacter,* and *Serratia* is so problematic that these drugs cannot be relied on for the treatment of meningitis caused by these pathogens.[31–33,101,102] With this in mind, therapy of Gram-negative meningitis in situations in which resistance is more likely to be encountered (e.g., nosocomial or postneurosurgical meningitis) also may include an aminoglycoside based on susceptibility results. Of the third-generation cephalosporins currently available, the most experience has been accumulated with cefotaxime; success rates are >80% for treatment of Gram-negative bacillary meningitis caused by *E. coli* or *K. pneumoniae.*[33,101,103] Ceftriaxone has comparable efficacy to cefotaxime and is considered a good alternative.[33] Ceftizoxime penetrates CSF to about the same extent as cefotaxime and has virtually the same spectrum of activity, but published experience with this agent is limited.[33,104] Nonetheless, there is no compelling evidence to suggest that ceftizoxime is inferior to cefotaxime or ceftriaxone. Therefore, it represents another therapeutic option. Cefoperazone should not be considered for Gram-negative bacillary meningitis because its CSF penetration is erratic, and its potency compared with the other third-generation cephalosporins is inferior.[33,49]

For R.R., cefazolin should be discontinued, and treatment with cefotaxime (3 g IV Q 6 hr) should be instituted. The choice of cefotaxime for empiric therapy is appropriate while waiting for results from culture and sensitivity testing. Until these results are available, combination therapy with cefotaxime and an aminoglycoside (gentamicin) is not unreasonable. The dosage of IV gentamicin should be designed to achieve high peak serum concentrations (i.e., >6 μg/mL) while maintaining trough concentrations <2 μg/mL (see Table 58-6). If intrathecal administration is indicated based on culture and susceptibility data, a 5- to 10-mg intrathecal dose of gentamicin also may be administered daily until clinical improvement is noted.[13,14,55] Gentamicin is commercially available in a 2-mg/mL, preservative-free solution for intrathecal use. The most practical way to provide intrathecal gentamicin to R.R. is by performing a lumbar puncture each day and administering the drug by intralumbar injection. This also will allow daily sampling of CSF for cultures and chemistries. Although intraventricular administration of gentamicin is ideal, insertion of a ventricular reservoir (e.g., Ommaya reservoir) is not appropriate at this time because R.R. has just undergone major spinal surgery, and it is not clear yet whether prolonged therapy is required.

It is important to make the distinction between aminoglycoside therapy for Gram-negative bacillary meningitis in neonates versus adults. In adults, results from clinical trials support the use of combined IV and intrathecal therapy for reasons described previously.[33,55] However, in neonates, combined intraventricular and IV gentamicin produces higher mortality rates than IV gentamicin alone.[105] The reason for the poor clinical outcomes associated with direct instillation of gentamicin into ventricular fluid is unclear. Initially, the increased mortality was attributed to increased trauma related to repeated insertion of the intrathecal needle into the infant's fontanel. More recent evidence suggests that the direct intraventricular injection of aminoglycoside can cause an abrupt release of inflammatory cytokines (TNF and IL-1) from mononuclear cells that could have led to enhanced neurologic sequelae.[106] Whatever the reason, intraventricular and intrathecal therapy should not be given to neonates with Gram-negative bacillary meningitis (see Tables 58-5 and 58-6)[53] without due consideration of this increased risk.

Treatment of Enterobacter Meningitis

20. Culture results from R.R.'s wound drainage and CSF both are positive for *Enterobacter cloacae*. Sensitivity data reveal resistance to ceftriaxone, cefotaxime, ceftazidime, piperacillin, aztreonam, and chloramphenicol. Drugs to which the isolate is sensitive include imipenem, TMP-SMX, gentamicin, tobramycin, and ciprofloxacin. What alteration in antimicrobial therapy is most appropriate for R.R. at this time?

Treatment of meningitis caused by *Enterobacter* and related species (e.g., *Serratia, Citrobacter* species) presents a challenge in that resistance is encountered more commonly.[31,33,101] Furthermore, some isolates that are sensitive to third-generation cephalosporins can become resistant during therapy by virtue of possessing inducible, type I β-lactamases.[31] Thus, in contrast to Gram-negative bacillary meningitis caused by *E. coli* and *Klebsiella* species, alternative therapies are needed when treating meningitis caused by *Enterobacter, Serratia, Citrobacter,* and *Pseudomonas*

species. Based on the sensitivity profile of R.R.'s infecting strain, it is apparent that an extended-spectrum penicillin (e.g., piperacillin) would not be appropriate. Unfortunately, aztreonam, a monobactam antibiotic with good CSF penetration and Gram-negative activity comparable to ceftazidime, also is inactive against R.R.'s infecting strain.[107] The isolate is sensitive to imipenem, but the higher propensity for seizures compared with other β-lactams (including penicillin G) argues against its use in R.R.[108–110] Meropenem is not considered to be epileptogenic and is an alternative to imipenem for meningitis.[64,111] Clinical trials have evaluated the efficacy and safety of meropenem versus cefotaxime in the treatment of meningitis in children. Clinical outcomes were similar among the patients randomized to either group, and the incidence of seizures was similar in the treatment groups.[111,112] Ciprofloxacin, a fluoroquinolone antibiotic, offers the attractive features of excellent in vitro potency against Gram-negative bacilli (including *Enterobacter* and *Pseudomonas* species).[46,113] However, experience with ciprofloxacin in meningitis is limited, and achievable CSF levels are relatively low despite reasonable CSF penetration.[46] Furthermore, fluoroquinolones are associated with adverse CNS effects, including the potential to cause seizures.[114] Because there are limited clinical data on the use of meropenem and fluoroquinolones in adults, these agents should be reserved for the treatment of multiresistant isolates.[43,64] TMP-SMX has excellent activity against most Gram-negative bacteria, with the exception of *P. aeruginosa,* and penetrates into the CSF especially well.[43,50,98]

Thus, after consideration of the aforementioned options, TMP-SMX appears to be the best choice of therapy for R.R. Cefotaxime should be discontinued and therapy started with TMP-SMX 15 mg/kg per day (based on the trimethoprim component) given IV in three divided doses.[4,55,98] For R.R., this would be a dosage of 400 mg (trimethoprim component) Q 8 hr. Because of poor aqueous solubility, IV TMP-SMX must be prepared such that each 80 mg (5 mL) of TMP-SMX injectable solution is diluted with 75 to 125 mL of 5% dextrose in water. For R.R., 400 mg of TMP-SMX would be administered in approximately 500 mL of D_5W and each dose infused over 1 hour. Whether or not to discontinue gentamicin in R.R. at this time is less clear. Although there are no data demonstrating superiority of TMP-SMX combined with aminoglycosides over TMP-SMX alone, there is in vitro evidence of synergy, which may be of theoretical advantage.[115]

A review of antibiotic therapy for *Enterobacter* meningitis supports the contention that TMP-SMX is the most useful therapy currently available.[31] Although the study was uncontrolled and retrospective in design, infection was cured in all 7 patients receiving TMP-SMX, compared with 21 of 32 (65%) patients treated solely with third-generation cephalosporins. In all 11 instances of clinical failure, development of resistance during therapy was encountered.[31] In an earlier report describing TMP-SMX treatment of bacterial meningitis, including eight cases of Gram-negative bacillary meningitis caused by organisms known to be moderately susceptible to third-generation cephalosporins, clinical and bacteriologic cures were observed in all instances (two cases each of *E. cloacae, Serratia marcescens,* and *C. diversus;* one case each of *Proteus vulgaris* and *Morganella morganii*).[98] In contrast, TMP-SMX therapy failed to cure six cases of Gram-negative bacillary meningitis caused by *E. coli* (four cases) and *K.*

pneumoniae (two cases) despite documented sensitivity to the drug combination. Thus, TMP-SMX appears to be most useful for treatment of Gram-negative bacillary meningitis caused by organisms that are only moderately susceptible to third-generation agents, whereas cefotaxime and ceftriaxone remain the drugs of choice for meningitis caused by *E. coli* and *K. pneumoniae* (see Table 58-7).

Duration of Therapy

The optimal duration of therapy for Gram-negative bacillary meningitis has not been clearly established. Because of the high mortality and morbidity associated with these pathogens and the reduced susceptibility of enteric pathogens to antimicrobial agents, 21 days has been suggested (see Table 58-8).[43,53,55] Although R.R. does not appear to have a fulminant case of Gram-negative meningitis, a 21-day course of therapy is recommended with close follow-up.

Staphylococcus epidermidis Meningitis/Ventriculitis

Clinical Presentation of CSF Shunt Infections

21. T.A., a 21-year-old woman with a history of congenital hydrocephalus, is admitted to the neurosurgery unit for worsening mental status and fever. T.A. has a history of multiple revisions and placements of intraventricular shunts for control of hydrocephalus. Currently she has a ventriculoperitoneal (VP) shunt, which was placed 1 month ago and previously had been functioning normally. Over the past few days, T.A. has developed worsening obtundation, stiff neck, and a temperature of 39.5°C. A CT scan performed today reveals enlarged ventricles consistent with acute hydrocephalus.

T.A.'s medical history is noncontributory except for a seizure disorder for which she takes phenytoin 400 mg PO HS. She also takes Lo-Ovral for birth control. T.A. is allergic to sulfa drugs (severe skin rash). Her weight upon admission is 132 lb.

Laboratory analysis was significant for a WBC count of 14,000 cells/mm³ (normal, 3,200 to 9,800), with a differential of 85% PMNs and 10% lymphocytes; BUN and SrCr values were within the normal range at 19 mg/dL and 0.9 mg/dL, respectively.

A tap of T.A.'s shunt was performed, and the ventricular fluid was notable for total protein of 150 mg/dL (normal, <50), glucose of 40 mg/dL (normal, 60% of serum glucose), and a WBC count of 200 cells/mm³ (normal, <5 cells/mm³), with 85% PMNs and 10% lymphocytes. Gram's stain of the ventricular fluid showed numerous Gram-positive cocci in clusters. What are the subjective and objective findings of CSF shunt infections, and what manifestations of this type of infection are present in T.A.?

[SI units: WBC count, 14 * 10⁹ cells/L with 0.85 PMNs and 0.1 lymphocytes; BUN, 6.8 mmol/L urea; SrCr, 80 μmol/L; total protein, 1.0 g/L; glucose, 2.2 mmol/L; WBC count, 200 * 10⁶ cells/L with 0.85 PMNs and 0.1 lymphocytes]

T.A. appears to have meningitis with ventriculitis secondary to infection of her VP shunt. The most important way to manage hydrocephalus involves the use of devices that divert (shunt) CSF from the cerebral ventricles to other areas of the body such as the peritoneum (VP shunts) or atrium (VA shunts).[8,116,117] This approach alleviates increased CSF pressure and substantially reduces morbidity and mortality.[116,117] Unfortunately, infection of these devices is a common cause of shunt malfunction, as seen in T.A. The reported incidence of CSF shunt infections varies from 2% to 39% (usually between 10% and 11%) and depends on patient factors, surgical technique, and the type and duration of the procedure performed (i.e., shunt revision versus placement of a new device).[116,117] T.A., who has been hydrocephalic since birth and has a prior history of multiple shunt procedures, is at high risk for such an infection.

Clinical symptoms associated with infected CSF shunts vary widely from asymptomatic colonization to fulminant ventriculitis with meningitis.[116–118] Fever is common and in many instances is the only presenting symptom.[116] CSF findings also are slightly different in shunt infection compared with acute meningitis: the WBC count usually is not as elevated, the decrease in CSF glucose is less pronounced, and the protein value may be normal or slightly elevated.[116,117] CSF culture is positive in most patients not receiving concurrent antibiotics.[116,117] T.A.'s clinical presentation, CSF findings, and radiographic evidence of hydrocephalus are highly suggestive of a VP shunt infection. She is febrile and has altered mental status. The presence of a stiff neck strongly suggests meningeal involvement. Evaluation of T.A.'s ventricular fluid reveals a slightly elevated WBC count with a predominance of polymorphonuclear neutrophils, an elevated protein concentration, and a slightly lower than normal glucose concentration.

Skin microflora are the most common etiologies for CSF shunt infections.[116–119] Staphylococci account for 75% of all cases, with two thirds of these caused by coagulase-negative staphylococci (usually *S. epidermidis*) and one third by *S. aureus*.[118,119] Other less common pathogens include diphtheroids, enterococci, and *Propionibacterium acnes* (an anaerobic diphtheroid). Enteric Gram-negative bacilli are responsible for a small percentage of cases; these cases usually occur when the distal end of the shunt is inserted improperly into the peritoneal cavity.[118,119] The Gram-positive cocci in clusters on Gram's stain of T.A.'s CSF strongly suggest a staphylococcal shunt infection. Determining the coagulase status of the isolate will allow differentiation between *S. aureus* and *S. epidermidis*.

Treatment of CSF Shunt Infections

22. Culture and sensitivity tests of T.A.'s ventricular fluid are positive for *S. epidermidis*. The isolate is resistant to nafcillin but sensitive to vancomycin, rifampin, and TMP-SMX. How should T.A.'s CSF shunt infection be managed?

For T.A.'s CSF shunt infection to be optimally managed, a combined medical and surgical approach is required.[111,112,120] Antibiotic therapy directed against the causative organism, although essential, often is inadequate by itself. On average, antibiotic therapy by itself produces cure rates of <40%.[119] In contrast, antibiotic therapy plus surgical removal of the infected device produces clinical cure rates of >80%.[119] Because many patients cannot tolerate the complete removal of their shunt for long, externalization of the distal end of the shunt, or shunt removal and placement of an external drainage device, often is necessary during systemic antibiotic therapy. The presence of an externalized device permits sequential sampling of ventricular fluid and also provides a convenient way to administer antibiotic intraventricularly (see the following discussion).

GLYCOCALYX

Although *S. epidermidis* is not as virulent a pathogen as *S. aureus,* it is extremely difficult to eradicate this organism from prosthetic devices such as CSF shunts. This is because many strains of *S. epidermidis* produce a mucous film or slime layer known as glycocalyx, which allows the staphylococci to adhere tightly to the Silastic shunt material, protecting them against phagocytosis.[121,122] As expected, antibiotic failures are much more likely with slime-producing strains of *S. epidermidis.*

Vancomycin is the drug of choice for treatment of shunt infections caused by *S. epidermidis* and should be instituted immediately in T.A.[8,116,122] This is because a high percentage (>60%) of coagulase-negative staphylococci are resistant to methicillin (e.g., MRSE). Furthermore, methicillin-resistant staphylococci (both MRSA and MRSE) also are resistant to cephalosporins. T.A.'s isolate also is sensitive to TMP-SMX, as is the case with many strains of MRSE (and also MRSA).[8] However, it must be avoided because T.A. is allergic to this drug combination. Although many staphylococcal isolates (both *S. epidermidis* and *S. aureus*) are susceptible to rifampin, monotherapy with this drug is not recommended because of rapid emergence of resistance. Combination therapy with vancomycin and rifampin may be synergistic and sometimes is used.

VANCOMYCIN THERAPY

23. **What would be an appropriate dosage of vancomycin therapy in T.A.? What subjective or objective data should be monitored to evaluate the efficacy and toxicity of the treatment?**

Vancomycin therapy for T.A.'s CSF shunt infection requires the use of higher than usual doses, which is true for the treatment of other types of staphylococcal CNS infections as well.[8,53,123] For adults like T.A., vancomycin dosages of 20 to 30 mg/kg per day to a maximum of 2 g/day have been suggested. However, even higher dosages may be required in patients with fulminant disease (see Table 58-6).[8,53,91,123] For children with meningitis or infected shunts, the recommended dosage of vancomycin is 40 to 60 mg/kg per day, given IV in two to four divided doses (see Table 58-6).[8,53] Although specific recommendations are lacking, it is reasonable to target serum trough concentrations of vancomycin toward the higher end of the target range (i.e., approximately 15 to 20 μg/mL). With an every-12-hour dosing schedule, peak serum levels will approach or possibly exceed 40 μg/mL. It is unlikely, however, that peak serum concentrations of >60 μg/mL will be observed. Although the potential for toxicity may be greater, higher than usual vancomycin serum concentrations are warranted to ensure adequate penetration into the CSF.[91,123]

T.A., who weighs 132 lb, should be started on a vancomycin regimen of 1 g IV Q 12 hr (approximately 30 mg/kg per day) because her renal function is normal. Alternatively, the dose could be calculated using population estimates of vancomycin pharmacokinetic parameters to achieve a trough serum concentration of 15 μg/mL. In either case, trough serum concentrations should be obtained at steady state to assess whether the initial dosing regimen is adequate.

Anecdotal evidence suggests that very high dosages of vancomycin (≥3 g/day in adults with normal renal function) are associated with an increased risk of ototoxicity.[91,124] This observation is difficult to verify because hearing loss also is a potential sequela of meningitis. High-dose vancomycin therapy also has a greater likelihood of inducing the "red man syndrome."[125,126] This adverse effect, manifested by flushing and pruritus with or without hypotension, is related directly to the amount of drug infused over a given period of time.[125] It usually can be avoided or minimized by infusing vancomycin doses of 1,000 mg in ≥250 mL of solution (either D_5W or normal saline) over at least 1 hour. If red man syndrome is observed, slowing the infusion rate often ameliorates symptoms.[125] Pretreatment with antihistamines (diphenhydramine or hydroxyzine) may also minimize the reaction because the proposed mechanism partially involves histamine release.[126]

Another consideration for T.A. is the addition of rifampin to her vancomycin regimen. This is based on the excellent staphylococcal activity of rifampin, its good CSF penetration, and the potential for synergy between these two agents.[8,116] Whether rifampin plus vancomycin is superior to vancomycin alone has not been determined. For T.A., it is best to avoid rifampin because evidence supporting its efficacy is weak, and she currently is taking phenytoin and birth control pills. Rifampin is a potent inducer of hepatic microsomal enzymes, which can lower serum phenytoin concentrations (possibly resulting in seizure activity) and increase the possibility of an unplanned pregnancy (from reduced effectiveness of the birth control pill).

Intraventricular and Intravenous Dosing of Vancomycin

24. **Should T.A. receive intraventricular vancomycin? If so, what would be an appropriate dosage?**

T.A. has a long history of hydrocephalus and will require placement of an external drainage device after removal of her VP shunt. This makes intraventricular administration of vancomycin possible, and such treatment should be instituted promptly. The dosages used in the literature vary from 5 to 20 mg/day. Experts recommend 20 mg/day of intraventricular vancomycin; therefore, an intraventricular vancomycin dosage of 20 mg/day is recommended for T.A. Also, serial (daily) cultures of CSF are recommended to monitor her response to therapy. Some authors suggest adjusting intraventricular vancomycin doses to achieve trough CSF vancomycin concentrations of at least 5 μg/mL or CSF bactericidal activity of at least 1:8 against the infecting strain.[8,116] Until more information is available, monitoring serial CSF trough concentrations is more appropriate than CSF bactericidal titers, and serial trough levels should be obtained in T.A. To summarize, T.A. should receive combined IV and intraventricular vancomycin therapy as described previously. Therapy should be continued for at least 10 days after sterilization of her ventricular fluid is documented, at which time a new VP shunt can be placed.[116,116a,119]

In contrast to T.A.'s situation, vancomycin therapy for patients with staphylococcal meningitis not associated with a CSF shunt or indwelling ventricular catheter is more problematic. Because of this, therapy often is instituted with IV vancomycin alone.[91,123] Intrathecal vancomycin, although preferable, requires either daily lumbar puncture (for intralumbar therapy) or surgical placement of an intraventricular reservoir. If the response to therapy is inadequate within the first 24 to 48 hours, the addition of intrathecal vancomycin therapy (5 to 20 mg/day) is recommended.[91,123] However, in fulminant cases of staphylococcal meningitis, intrathecal vancomycin should be instituted as quickly as possible (i.e., with the first lumbar puncture) to optimize the response to therapy.

BRAIN ABSCESS

Epidemiology

Although not nearly as common as meningitis, abscesses of the brain parenchyma (brain abscess) remain an important type of CNS infection. The incidence of brain abscess has not varied since the preantibiotic era and is estimated to account for 1 in 10,000 hospital admissions.[127] On a busy neurosurgical service, 4 to 10 cases a year typically are seen.[127,128] For reasons that are not entirely clear, men are more likely to develop abscesses within the brain than women.[127,129] Brain abscess can occur at any age, but the median age is 30 to 40 years, with approximately 25% of cases occurring in children.[127,130,131]

Despite advances in antimicrobial therapy over the past several decades, mortality rates from brain abscess remained over 40% until just recently. Developments in imaging techniques such as CT and MRI scanning, which allow early recognition of abscesses and the ability to serially monitor the radiographic response to antimicrobial therapy, have had the most profound impact on reducing morbidity and mortality from brain abscess.[127,128,132] In a review of 102 cases of bacterial abscesses occurring over a 17-year period, mortality was 41% in the period before 1975 (pre-CT scan era), compared with 6% during 1975 to 1986, when CT scanning became routinely available.[128] With the combined medical and surgical approach currently recommended, mortality rates continue to average <10%.[127,128,132]

Predisposing Factors

Brain abscesses most commonly arise from a contiguous suppurative source of infection (e.g., sinusitis, otitis, mastoiditis, or dental infections).[127,129,133] In the United States, abscesses occurring as a complication of sinusitis are more common than abscesses arising from otitic or dental sources.[127] The formation of a single abscess cavity usually is found when infection develops from a contiguous source. In addition, the abscess nearly always is formed in close proximity to the primary focus of infection (Table 58-10).[127,133] For example, abscesses of sinusitic origin more commonly involve the frontal lobe, whereas otitic infections often lead to temporal lobe abscess formation.[133] Brain abscess also occurs as a consequence of metastatic spread of organisms from a primary site of infection (e.g., lung abscess, endocarditis, osteomyelitis, pelvic, and intra-abdominal infections).[124,126] In children, cyanotic congenital heart disease is a common predisposing factor for brain abscess.[130,131] Multiple abscesses suggest a metastatic source of infection.[127] As with meningitis, brain abscess occurs as an infrequent complication of head trauma or neurosurgery.[11,127,133] No identifiable source (cryptogenic abscess) is detected in as many as 30% of cases.[127,133]

Staging

Once an intracranial focus of infection is established, the evolution of brain abscess involves two distinct stages: cerebritis and capsule formation.[129,132] The cerebritis stage evolves gradually over the first 9 to 10 days of infection and is characterized by an area of marked inflammatory infiltrate that contains a necrotic center surrounded by an area of cerebral edema.[129,132] Capsule formation occurs about 10 to 14 days after the initiation of infection, and once formed, the capsule continues to thicken over a period of weeks.[129,132] The stage of abscess development has important implications for therapy. Although it is best to wait until the capsule is fully formed before attempting any type of surgical intervention, antimicrobial therapy alone may resolve the infection if discovered in the early cerebritis stage.[132]

Microbiology

The microbiology of brain abscess is distinctly different from that of meningitis. Streptococci are implicated in 60% to 70% of cases and include anaerobic as well as microaerophilic streptococci of the *S. milleri* group.[127,133,134] Other anaerobes,

Table 58-10	Predisposing Conditions, Microbiology, and Recommended Therapy for Bacterial Brain Abscess		
Predisposing Condition	*Usual Location of Abscess*	*Most Likely Organisms*	*Recommended Therapy*
Contiguous Site			
Otitic infection	Temporal lobe or cerebellum	Streptococci (anaerobic and aerobic), *B. fragilis*, Gram-negative bacilli	Penicillin G + metronidazole + cefotaxime or ceftriaxone
Sinusitis	Frontal lobe	Streptococci (predominantly), *Bacteroides* species, Gram-negative bacilli, *S. aureus*, *Haemophilus* species	Penicillin G + metronidazole + cefotaxime or ceftriaxone
Dental infection	Frontal lobe	*Fusobacteria* species, *Bacteroides* species, and streptococci	Penicillin G + metronidazole
Primary Infection			
Head trauma or neurosurgery	Related to site of wound	Gram-negative bacilli, staphylococci, streptococci, diphtheroids	Vancomycin + ceftazidime

particularly *Bacteroides* species (including *B. fragilis*) and *Prevotella* species, are found in up to 40% of cases, usually in mixed culture.[127,133] In recent years, staphylococci appear to be decreasing and enteric Gram-negative bacteria increasing as etiologic agents of bacterial brain abscess.[118] Although somewhat imprecise, there is a reasonable correlation between the various predisposing conditions and the microbiologic etiology of brain abscess (see Table 58-10).[127,128,131,133]

In the immunocompromised patient, a diverse group of microorganisms are capable of inducing abscesses within the brain. In patients with AIDS, *Toxoplasma gondii* is by far the most common infectious etiology of focal brain lesions.[135] Transplant patients and those receiving immunosuppressive therapy are susceptible to infection from *Nocardia* species.[136] In Mexico and other Central American countries, cysticercosis remains a common cause of intracerebral infection.[137]

Clinical and Radiologic Features

25. L.Y., a 40-year-old man, is brought to the ED by a friend. L.Y. complains of severe headache, fever, weakness in his left arm and leg, and increasing drowsiness. Over the past week, L.Y. has suffered from headaches, which have gradually worsened in intensity, and from intermittent episodes of fever. Despite getting plenty of sleep, L.Y. has been feeling increasingly drowsy over the past several days. When he noticed weakness in his left arm and difficulty concentrating this morning, he called a friend and asked to be taken in for evaluation.

L.Y. has a history of chronic sinusitis that has been treated with a variety of oral antibiotics. His last episode of sinusitis occurred about 1 month ago and was treated with a 10-day course of cephalexin. He denies any nausea or vomiting and has not experienced any seizures in the recent past. L.Y. was tested for HIV 6 months ago, and the result of his antibody test was negative. He takes no current medications, denies smoking and use of recreational drugs, and drinks alcohol only on social occasions a few times a month. L.Y. has no known drug allergies.

Physical examination reveals L.Y. to be in mild distress, with a temperature of 38.2°C. He is slightly lethargic and is oriented to person and place but not time (0 ×2). The strength in L.Y.'s left arm is 3/5; the strength in his left leg is 4/5. The remainder of his neurologic examination is grossly normal. L.Y. described moderate pain upon palpation of his frontal sinuses, and a purulent discharge is noted.

Laboratory evaluation shows a WBC count of 8,000 cells/mm³ (normal, 3,200 to 9,800), with 70% PMNs, 25% lymphocytes, and 5% monocytes; Hgb, Hct, platelets, and serum chemistries are within normal limits; and his BUN and SrCr are 16 mg/dL (normal, 8 to 18) and 1.2 mg/dL (normal, 0.6 to 1.2), respectively. L.Y.'s erythrocyte sedimentation rate (ESR) is 40 mm/hr (normal, 0 to 20).

A CT scan with contrast dye reveals a right frontal ring-enhancing lesion with a small amount of surrounding cerebral edema. L.Y. is admitted to the neurosurgery unit for further evaluation and treatment. What clinical signs and symptoms does L.Y. display that are suggestive of bacterial brain abscess? How can brain abscess be diagnosed in L.Y.?

[SI units: WBC count, 8 * 10⁹ cells/L with 0.7 PMNs, 0.25 lymphocytes, and 0.05 monocytes; Hgb, 145 g/L; Hct, 0.4; platelets, 120 * 10⁹/L; BUN, 5.7 mmol/L urea; SrCr, 106.1 μmol/L; ESR 40 mm/hr]

L.Y. has presented to the ED with many signs and symptoms suggestive of bacterial brain abscess. He is 40 years old and a man, both of which place him in a group with the highest likelihood of having a brain abscess. In contrast to the diffuse nature of meningitis, brain abscess presents as a focal neurologic process.[127,128] Notable in L.Y.'s presentation is left-sided (arm and leg) weakness. Symptoms of brain abscess range in severity from indolent to fulminant, and in most patients, the duration of symptoms at the time of presentation is ≤2 weeks.[127,128,130] Headache is the most common symptom of brain abscess, occurring in approximately 70% of cases. L.Y.'s clinical manifestations have become gradually worse over the past week, and his worsening headaches, increasing drowsiness, and difficulty in concentrating all are consistent with bacterial brain abscess.

L.Y. presents with the classic triad of fever, headache, and focal neurologic deficits. Although this triad should always be looked for, fewer than half of patients with confirmed bacterial brain abscess present in this manner.[127,128,131] The absence of fever does not rule out infection because fever is found in ≤50% of patients.[127,128] Focal neurologic deficits are present in approximately 50% of patients and vary in nature and severity in relation to the location and size of the abscess and surrounding cerebral edema.[127,128,131] Although L.Y. does not have a history of seizure activity, approximately one third of patients experience partial seizures that often become generalized.[127,131] Papilledema and nuchal rigidity occur in <25% of cases and often are not useful in confirming the diagnosis. Symptoms associated with a contiguous focus of infection should always be sought, and in some situations they may dominate the clinical picture.[127,128] L.Y. has a history of sinus infection, and the pain on palpation of his sinuses coupled with the purulent sinus drainage suggests active infection at this site.

As can be seen from L.Y.'s test results, laboratory evaluation usually is not very helpful when diagnosing brain abscess. L.Y. does not have a peripheral leukocytosis, but he does have an elevated ESR. A normal peripheral WBC count is not unusual in patients with intracranial suppuration. The ESR often is elevated in brain abscess, but this test is nonspecific and only indirectly supports the diagnosis.

L.Y. did not undergo a lumbar puncture because this procedure is contraindicated for diagnosing brain abscess.[40,127,128] The diagnostic yield from CSF is low because chemistries (e.g., protein, glucose, WBC) usually are normal and culture of the CSF in patients with brain abscess is unlikely to yield the causative pathogen. More important, performing a lumbar puncture in patients with space-occupying lesions of the brain may produce cerebral herniation as a consequence of the shifting pressure gradient induced within the cranial vault after insertion of the lumbar puncture needle.[40]

Of paramount importance is the abnormality detected on the CT scan of L.Y.'s brain. When dye is injected before the CT scan, brain abscesses will appear to "ring enhance." Furthermore, cerebral edema can be identified as a variable hypodense region immediately surrounding the abscess cavity. As stated earlier, CT and MRI scanning techniques have revolutionized the diagnosis and treatment of brain abscess.[127,128,132] The superiority of CT versus MRI is unclear. However, MRI is more sensitive in detecting cerebritis than CT, and MRI can be helpful in ruling out (or ruling in) an abscess when the CT scan is negative.[127,132] Assessment of the size and location of the lesion is possible with both techniques, which is invaluable in deciding which surgical intervention is indicated. In addition, serial radiographic studies can be used to evaluate antimicrobial response over time.[128,132] In general, a good correlation exists between the clinical and radiologic response to therapy of bacterial brain abscess.

Treatment

26. **How should L.Y.'s brain abscess be managed?**

Surgical Techniques

A combined medical and surgical approach is the best form of therapy for L.Y.'s brain abscess.[127,132] Response rates to antimicrobial therapy alone have been disappointing, and with a few exceptions surgical intervention is necessary to ensure optimal results. Medical therapy is indicated when multiple abscesses are present, when the abscess cavity is inaccessible surgically, for patients who are poor surgical candidates, and when the abscess is small (<4 cm).[127,132,138]

There are two types of surgical approaches for brain abscess: stereotactic needle aspiration and craniotomy for abscess excision.[132] Stereotactic aspiration of abscess contents can be performed under local anesthesia and produces lower morbidity and mortality than craniotomy.[19] Such an approach is highly effective, except when multiloculated abscesses are present.[132] With craniotomy, the abscess cavity can be excised completely, which often allows a shorter duration of antimicrobial therapy. Both techniques are effective, and the decision regarding which procedure is most appropriate must be individualized.

Antimicrobial Penetration Into Brain Abscess

Antimicrobial therapy is an essential component of brain abscess therapy.[133] Penetration of antibiotics into brain abscess fluid has not been studied as carefully as penetration into CSF, and as discussed earlier, the barrier involved is different (see Fig. 58-1).[15] Penicillins and cephalosporins penetrate adequately into abscess fluid, but certain agents, like penicillin G, may be susceptible to degradation by enzymes present within the abscess milieu.[127,133,139–141] Third-generation cephalosporins (e.g., cefotaxime, ceftriaxone, and ceftizoxime) are believed to penetrate sufficiently into the abscess and are good choices when Gram-negative bacteria are present.[127,141] Chloramphenicol penetrates very well into brain abscesses and has been used extensively in the past.[127,133,139] It has excellent anaerobic activity but also can be degraded (deacetylated) in purulent abscess fluid.[127] Metronidazole achieves abscess fluid concentrations equal to or in excess of serum levels and is bactericidal against strict anaerobes. The unique mechanism of action of metronidazole makes it particularly useful in the necrotic core of the cavity, where the oxidation-reduction potential is low and bacteria replicate slowly or are dormant. For these reasons, metronidazole has supplanted chloramphenicol for treatment of bacterial brain abscess.[127] Although data are limited, vancomycin and carbapenems appear to penetrate sufficiently into brain abscess fluid.[127,142] Although specific abscess-penetration data are unavailable, successful treatment of cerebral nocardiosis with TMP-SMX and CNS toxoplasmosis with clindamycin suggests that these com-

pounds also achieve adequate penetration into cerebral abscess cavities.[135,136]

Antibiotic Therapy

When antibiotic therapy should be instituted depends on the status of the patient and the stage of abscess development. For patients diagnosed during the cerebritis stage, before formation of a well-circumscribed capsule, surgery should be delayed and antimicrobial therapy begun in patients with significant symptoms.[127,132] If capsule formation already has taken place, it is better to delay initiation of antibiotics until after surgery to increase the microbiologic yield from tissue and fluid samples. If the disease is fulminant, antibiotics must be instituted promptly and surgical intervention performed as quickly as possible.[127,132]

L.Y.'s clinical presentation suggests an advanced brain abscess. The presence of ring enhancement on CT and the onset of symptoms over 2 weeks support this. Because he is not critically ill, antibiotic therapy should be delayed until surgery is performed. Specimens obtained from the surgical procedure should be sent for aerobic and anaerobic culture and a stat Gram's stain.

Initial antibiotic therapy for brain abscess needs to be sufficiently broad to cover the most likely pathogens (see Table 58-10).[127,129,131,133] In most cases, a combination of high-dose penicillin G and metronidazole is indicated. Penicillin will cover aerobic, anaerobic, and microaerophilic streptococci, whereas metronidazole will provide coverage for strict anaerobes, including *Bacteroides* and *Prevotella* species. If Gram-negative bacilli are suspected or documented, as in abscesses related to otitis, head trauma, or neurosurgery, a third-generation cephalosporin is indicated.[127] Staphylococcal abscesses should be treated with nafcillin or vancomycin.[127,129,143]

For L.Y., therapy with penicillin G 4 million units IV Q 4 hr and metronidazole 500 mg IV Q 8 hr should be started postoperatively (see Table 58-6). Because his abscess appears to originate from the sinus, the likelihood of Gram-negative infection is reduced. If there is evidence of Gram-negative bacteria on the Gram's stain of abscess fluid, therapy with cefotaxime 3 g IV Q 6 hr also should be included. Ceftriaxone 2 g IV Q 12 hr is a viable alternative to cefotaxime, particularly if the patient is going to be discharged to home on a prolonged course of therapy. Outpatient therapy is appropriate for CNS infections as long as patients are carefully selected and monitored, as described in a recent report.[144] Of interest, of the 24 patients treated on an outpatient basis, 46% received ceftriaxone 2 g IV once daily with a cure.[144] TMP-SMX is an alternative if the organism is resistant to cefotaxime. However, the large fluid volume required (particularly when 5% dextrose in water is used) for IV TMP-SMX administration may contribute to worsening cerebral edema.[124] Antimicrobial therapy for L.Y. should be revised once results from culture and sensitivity testing are available.

Adjunctive Corticosteroid Therapy

Adjunctive corticosteroid therapy for bacterial brain abscess is controversial.[127,132] Steroids may interfere with antibiotic penetration into abscesses and obscure the interpretation of serial CT scans when assessing response to therapy.[127,132] Therefore, steroids are indicated only if significant cerebral edema is present, particularly if it is accompanied by rapid neurologic deterioration.[127,132] L.Y. should not receive dexamethasone because his mental status is only mildly depressed and the cerebral edema seen on CT scan is not massive.

Adjunctive Anticonvulsant Therapy

L.Y. has shown no signs of seizure activity thus far and therefore does not require anticonvulsant therapy. However, anticonvulsants should be used in the acute setting when seizures are present.[127,132] Agents with activity against partial and complex partial seizures are preferred (e.g., phenytoin, carbamazepine). The long-term use of anticonvulsants depends on whether seizure activity persists. There is insufficient information regarding how long to continue anticonvulsants in such cases. Therefore, discontinuation of these agents must be individualized.

No formal guidelines are available regarding the optimal duration of therapy for bacterial brain abscess. Given the serious nature of the infection and the difficulty associated with antibiotic penetration, therapy with high-dose IV therapy should continue for at least 6 to 8 weeks.[127,132] The duration of therapy should be evaluated on a case-by-case basis. In an attempt to ensure complete eradication of infection, some experts recommend long-term (2 to 6 months) oral antibiotics after the IV course, provided agents with good oral absorption and activity against the offending pathogens are available.[127]

Monitoring Therapy

27. **How should L.Y. be monitored for therapeutic response and toxicity?**

Although L.Y. is on antibiotic therapy, weekly or biweekly CT scans should be obtained to evaluate abscess resolution. His clinical response to therapy also should be assessed daily. If therapy is effective, L.Y.'s mental status should improve gradually (e.g., he will become more alert and oriented) over a period of several days. L.Y.'s headaches and hemiparesis (weakness in his arm and leg) also should resolve eventually. However, it may take a week or longer to see a complete resolution of symptoms.[127,129] In general, radiologic improvement (i.e., reduction in abscess size) correlates reasonably well with clinical response, but not always.[127,129,132] Persistent symptoms or failure to detect a reduction in abscess size on CT scan or the appearance of new abscesses may indicate improper antimicrobial therapy or the need for more surgery.[127,132] Repeated surgical intervention with appropriate reculturing may be required in some instances to optimize therapy.

Adverse effects associated with the penicillin G therapy that L.Y. is receiving are similar to those of other β-lactam antibiotics. Seizures are a potential complication when high doses of penicillin are employed in the presence of a mass lesion in the brain.[6,96,110,145] L.Y. should be observed closely by those providing care and questioned regularly for any evidence of seizure activity. Metronidazole usually is well tolerated but may also cause neurotoxicity,[127,142,145,146] most commonly peripheral neuropathy.[146] L.Y. should be assessed for the presence of numbness or tingling in his hands or feet. Seizures, although uncommon, occasionally occur with metronidazole.[146] If L.Y. experiences peripheral neuropathy or seizures, a switch to chloramphenicol would be appropriate. Other adverse effects associated with metronidazole include mild nausea, brownish discoloration of the urine, and the potential for a disulfiram-like reaction with concomitant ethanol ingestion.[142] L.Y. should be counseled regarding the possibility of gastric upset and discoloration of the urine, and he should be strongly cautioned to avoid alcoholic beverages while receiving metronidazole. Given his young age, the absence of significant underlying diseases, and the relative early detection of his brain abscess, there is every reason to expect a good response to his treatment and, eventually, a complete resolution of his abscess.

REFERENCES

1. Durand ML et al. Acute bacterial meningitis in adults. N Engl J Med 1993;328:21.
2. Quagliarello VJ, Scheld WM. New perspectives on bacterial meningitis. Clin Infect Dis 1993;17:603.
3. Quagliarello VJ, Scheld WM. Bacterial meningitis: pathogenesis, pathophysiology, and progress. N Engl J Med 1992;327:864.
4. Scheld WM et al. Pathophysiology of bacterial meningitis: mechanism(s) of neuronal injury. J Infect Dis 2002;186(Suppl 2):S225.
5. McIntyre PB et al. Dexamethasone as adjunctive therapy in bacterial meningitis. A meta-analysis of randomized clinical trials since 1988. JAMA 1997;278:925.
6. Overturf GD. Pyogenic bacterial infections of the CNS. Neurol Clin 1986;4:69.
7. Silverberg AL, DiNubile MJ. Subdural empyema and cranial epidural abscess. Med Clin North Am 1985;69:361.
8. Morris A et al. Nosocomial bacterial meningitis, including central nervous system shunt infections. Infect Dis Clin North Am 1999;13:735.
9. Romanes GJ. Cunningham's Textbook of Anatomy, 12th ed. New York: Oxford University Press, 1981:28.
10. Bonadio WA. The cerebrospinal fluid: physiologic aspects and alterations associated with bacterial meningitis. Pediatr Infect Dis J 1992;11:423.
11. Bleck TP, Greenlee JE. Approach to the patient with central nervous system infections. In: Mandell GL et al, eds. Principles and Practice of Infectious Diseases, 5th ed. New York: Churchill Livingstone, 2000:950.
12. Gagnong WF. Review of Medical Physiology, 16th ed. Norwalk, CT: Appleton & Lange, 1993:551.
13. Allinson RR, Stach PE. Intrathecal drug therapy. Drug Intell Clin Pharm 1978;12:347.
14. Kaiser AB, McGee ZA. Aminoglycoside therapy of gram-negative bacillary meningitis. N Engl J Med 1975;293:1215.
15. Pardridge WM et al. Blood–brain barrier: interface between internal medicine and the brain. Ann Intern Med 1986;105:82.
16. Scheld WM. Drug delivery to the central nervous system: general principles and relevance to therapy for infections of the central nervous system. Rev Infect Dis 1989;11(Suppl 7):S1669.
17. Gripshover BM, Ellner JJ. Chronic meningitis. In: Mandell GL, eds. Principles and Practice of Infectious Diseases, 5th ed. New York: Churchill Livingstone, 2000:997.
18. Moris G et al. The challenge of drug-induced aseptic meningitis. Arch Intern Med 1999;159:1185.
19. Schlech WF III et al. Bacterial meningitis in the United States, 1978 through 1981. JAMA 1985;253:1749.
20. Wenger JD et al. Bacterial meningitis in the United States, 1986: report of a multistate surveillance study. JAMA 1990;162:1316.
21. Tenney JH. Bacterial infections of the central nervous system in neurosurgery. Neurol Clin 1986;4:91.
22. Unhanand M et al. Gram-negative enteric bacillary meningitis: a twenty-one-year experience. J Pediatr 1993;122:15.
23. Gellin BG, Broome CV. Listeriosis. JAMA 1989; 261:1313.
24. Adams WG et al. Decline of childhood Haemophilus influenzae type b (Hib) disease in the Hib vaccine era. JAMA 1993;269:221.
25. Progress toward elimination of Haemophilus influenzae type b invasive disease among infants and children, United States, 1998–2000. MMWR 2002; 51:234.
26. Schuchat A et al. Bacterial meningitis in the United States in 1995. N Engl J Med 1997;337:970.
27. Gold R. Epidemiology of bacterial meningitis. Infect Dis Clin North Am 1999;13:515.
28. Doern GV et al. Antimicrobial resistance among clinical isolates of Streptococcus pneumoniae in the Unite States during 1999–2000, including a comparison of resistance rates since 1994–1995. Antimicrob Agents Chemother 2001;45:1721.
29. Choi C. Bacterial meningitis. Clin Geriatr Med 1992;8:889.
30. Cherubin CE et al. Listeria and gram-negative bacillary meningitis in New York City, 1972–1979. Am J Med 1981;71:199.
31. Wolff MA et al. Antibiotic therapy for Enterobacter meningitis: a retrospective review of 13 episodes and review of the literature. Clin Infect Dis 1993;16:772.

32. Fong IW, Tomkins KB. Review of *Pseudomonas aeruginosa* meningitis with special emphasis on treatment with ceftazidime. Rev Infect Dis 1985; 7:604.

33. Cherubin CE et al. Treatment of gram-negative bacillary meningitis: role of the new cephalosporin antibiotics. Rev Infect Dis 1982;4(Suppl):S453.

34. Pomeroy SL et al. Seizures and other neurologic sequelae of bacterial meningitis in children. N Engl J Med 1990;323:1651.

35. Taylor HG et al. The sequelae of *Haemophilus influenzae* meningitis in school-age children. N Engl J Med 1990;323:1657.

36. Dodge PR et al. Prospective evaluation of hearing impairment as a sequelae of acute bacterial meningitis. N Engl J Med 1984;311:869.

37. Aronin SI et al. Community-acquired bacterial meningitis: risk stratification for adverse clinical outcomes and effect of antibiotic timing. Ann Intern Med 1998;129:862.

38. Keroack MA. The patient with suspected meningitis. Emerg Med Clin North Am 1987;5:807.

39. Verghese A, Gallemore G. Kerning's and Brudzinski's signs revisited. Rev Infect Dis 1987;9:1187.

40. Addy DP. When not to do a lumbar puncture. Arch Dis Child 1987;62:873.

41. Edberg SC. Conventional and molecular techniques for the laboratory diagnosis of infections of the central nervous system. Neurol Clin 1986;4:13.

42. Lutsar I et al. Antibiotic pharmacodynamics in cerebrospinal fluid. Clin Infect Dis 1998;27:1117.

43. Quagliarello VJ, Scheld WM. Treatment of bacterial meningitis. N Engl J Med 1997;336:708.

44. Andes DR et al. Pharmacokinetics and pharmacodynamics of antibiotics in meningitis. Infect Dis Clin North Am 1999;13:595.

45. Arditi M et al. Cefuroxime treatment failure and *Haemophilus influenzae* meningitis: case report and review of the literature. Pediatrics 1989;84:132.

46. Scheld WM. Quinolone therapy for infections of the central nervous system. Rev Infect Dis 1989;11(Suppl 5):S1194.

47. Scheld WM et al. Comparison of netilmicin with gentamicin in the therapy of experimental *Escherichia coli* meningitis. Antimicrob Agents Chemother 1978;13:899.

48. Norrby SR. Role of cephalosporins in the treatment of bacterial meningitis. Am J Med 1985;79(Suppl 2A):56.

49. Lutsar I, Friedland I. Pharmacokinetics and pharmacodynamics of cephalosporins in cerebrospinal fluid. Clin Pharmacokinet 2000;39:335.

50. Norrby SR. A review of the penetration of antibiotics into CSF and its clinical significance. Scand J Infect Dis Suppl 1978;14:296.

51. Bolan G, Barza M. Acute bacterial meningitis in children and adults. Med Clin North Am 1985;69:231.

52. Del Rio M et al. Ceftriaxone versus ampicillin and chloramphenicol for treatment of bacterial meningitis in children. Lancet 1983;1:1241.

53. Plotkin SA et al. Treatment of bacterial meningitis. Pediatrics 1988;81:904.

54. Saxon A et al. Immediate hypersensitivity reactions to beta-lactam antibiotics. Ann Intern Med 1987;107:204.

55. Rahal JJ, Simberkoff MS. Host defense and antimicrobial therapy in adult gram-negative bacillary meningitis. Ann Intern Med 1982;96:468.

56. Roche Laboratories. Rocephin Package insert. Nutley, NJ: Jan. 1994.

57. Fishman R. Steroids in the treatment of brain edema. N Engl J Med 1982;306:359.

58. deLemos RA, Haggerty RJ. Corticosteroids as an adjunct to treatment in bacterial meningitis. Pediatrics 1969;44:30.

59. Belsey MA et al. Dexamethasone in the treatment of acute bacterial meningitis: the effect of study design on the interpretation of results. Pediatrics 1969;44:503.

60. Syrogiannopoulos GA et al. Dexamethasone therapy for bacterial meningitis in children: 2- versus 4-day regimen. J Infect Dis 1994;169:853.

61. Odio CM et al. The beneficial effects of early dexamethasone administration in infants and children with bacterial meningitis. N Engl J Med 1991;324:1525.

62. Schaad UB et al. Dexamethasone therapy for bacterial meningitis in children. Lancet 1993;342:457.

62a. de Gans J et al. Dexamethasone in adults with bacterial meningitis. N Engl J Med 2002;347:1549.

63. Girgis NI et al. Dexamethasone treatment for bacterial meningitis in children and adults. Pediatr Infect Dis J 1989;8:848.

64. Saez-Lloren X et al. Antimicrobial and anti-inflammatory treatment of bacterial meningitis. Infect Dis Clin North Am 1999;13:619.

65. Kanra GY et al. Beneficial effects of dexamethasone in children with pneumococcal meningitis. Pediatric Infect Dis J 1995;14:490.

66. Cabellos C et al. Influence of dexamethasone on efficacy of ceftriaxone and vancomycin therapy in experimental meningitis. Antimicrob Agents Chemother 1995;39:2158.

67. Paris MM. Effect of dexamethasone on therapy of experimental penicillin and cephalosporin-resistant pneumococcal meningitis. Antimicrob Agents Chemother 1994;38:1320.

67a. Martinez-Lacasa J et al. Experimental study of the efficacy of vancomycin, rifampicin and dexamethasone in the therapy of pneumococcal meningitis. J Antimicrob Chemother 2002;49:507.

67b. Cabellos C et al. Evaluation of combined ceftriaxone and dexamethasone therapy in experimental cephalosporin-resistant pneumococcal meningitis. J Antimicrob Chemother 2000;45:315.

68. Ahmed et al. Pharmacodynamics of vancomycin for the treatment of experimental penicillin- and cephalosporin-resistant pneumococcal meningitis. Antimicrob Agents Chemother 1999;43:876.

69. Tuomanen E et al. Nonsteroidal anti-inflammatory agents in the therapy for experimental pneumococcal meningitis. J Infect Dis 1987;155:985.

70. Schaab UB et al. A comparison of ceftriaxone and cefuroxime for the treatment of bacterial meningitis in children. N Engl J Med 1990;322:141.

71. Lebel MH et al. Comparative efficacy of ceftriaxone and cefuroxime for treatment of bacterial meningitis. J Pediatr 1989;114:1049.

72. Neu HC. Third-generation cephalosporins: safety profiles after 10 years of clinical use. J Clin Pharmacol 1990;30:396.

73. Kelly CP et al. *Clostridium difficile* colitis. N Engl J Med 1994;330:257.

74. Shiffman ML et al. Pathogenesis of ceftriaxone-associated biliary sludge. Gastroenterology 1990;99:1772.

75. Schaad UB et al. Reversible ceftriaxone-associated biliary pseudolithiasis in children. Lancet 1988;2:1411.

76. Park HZ et al. Ceftriaxone-associated gallbladder sludge. Gastroenterology 1991;100:1665.

77. Heim-Duthoy KL et al. Apparent biliary pseudolithiasis during ceftriaxone therapy. Antimicrob Agents Chemother 1990;34:1146.

78. Feder HM et al. Chloramphenicol: a review of its use in clinical practice. Rev Infect Dis 1981;3:479.

79. Radetsky M. Duration of treatment in bacterial meningitis: a historical inquiry. Pediatr Infect Dis J 1990;9:2.

80. Peltola H. Prophylaxis of bacterial meningitis. Infect Dis Clin North Am 1999;13:685.

81. Recommendations of the Advisory Committee on Immunization Practices (ACIP): Prevention and control of meningococcal disease. MMWR 2000;49:1.

82. Cartwright KA. Early management of meningococcal disease. Infect Dis Clin North Am 1999;13:661.

83. Recommendations of the Advisory Committee on Immunization Practices (ACIP): Meningococcal disease and college students. MMWR 2000;49:11.

84. Immunization Practices Advisory Committee. *Haemophilus* b conjugate vaccines for prevention of *Hemophilus influenzae* type b disease among infants and children two months of age and older. MMWR 1991;40:1.

85. Ward JI et al. *Haemophilus influenzae* type b vaccines: lessons for the future. Pediatr 1988;81:886.

86. Redd SC et al. The role of human immunodeficiency virus infection in pneumococcal bacteremia in San Francisco residents. J Infect Dis 1990;162:1012.

87. Prevention of pneumococcal disease: Recommendations of the Advisory Committee on Immunization Practices (ACIP). MMWR 1997;46:1

88. Polk RE. Drug–drug interactions with ciprofloxacin and other fluoroquinolones. Am J Med 1989;87(Suppl 5A):76S.

89. Kaplan SL et al. Management of infections due to antibiotic-resistant *Streptococcus pneumoniae*. Clin Micro Rev 1998;11:628.

90. John CC. Treatment failure with use of a third-generation cephalosporin for penicillin-resistant pneumococcal meningitis: case report and review. Clin Infect Dis 1994;18:188.

91. Viladrich PF et al. Evaluation of vancomycin therapy for therapy of adult pneumococcal meningitis. Antimicrob Agents Chemother 1991;35:2467.

92. Friedland IR, Klugman KP. Failure of chloramphenicol therapy in penicillin-resistant pneumococcal meningitis. Lancet 1992;339:405.

93. NCCLS. Performance standards for antimicrobial susceptibility testing. Document M100-S5. 1995;15 NCCLS, Wayne, PA.

94. Friedland IR et al. Evaluation of antimicrobial regimens for treatment of experimental penicillin- and cephalosporin-resistant pneumococcal meningitis. Antimicrob Agents Chemother 1993;37:1630.

95. Nau R et al. Rifampin reduces early mortality in experimental *Streptococcus pneumoniae* meningitis. J Infect Dis 1999;179:1557.

96. Bryan SC, Stone WJ. "Comparably massive" penicillin G therapy in renal failure. Ann Intern Med 1975;82:189.

97. Farber BF, Moellering RC. Retrospective study of the toxicity of preparations of vancomycin from 1974 to 1981. Antimicrob Agents Chemother 1983;23:138.

98. Levitz RE, Quintiliani R. Trimethoprim-sulfamethoxazole for bacterial meningitis. Ann Intern Med 1984;100:881.

99. Rodriguez-Barradas MC et al. Antibody to capsular polysaccharides of *Streptococcus pneumoniae* after vaccination of human immunodeficiency virus-infected subjects with 23-valent pneumococcal vaccine. J Infect Dis 1992;165:553.

100. Berk SL, McCabe WR. Meningitis caused by gram-negative bacilli. Ann Intern Med 1980;93:253.

101. Corrado ML et al. Designing appropriate therapy in the treatment of gram-negative bacillary meningitis. JAMA 1982;248:71.

102. Tauber MG et al. Antibiotic therapy, endotoxin concentrations in cerebrospinal fluid, and brain edema in experimental *Escherichia coli* meningitis in rabbits. J Infect Dis 1987;156:456.

103. Cherubin CE, Eng RHK. Experience with the use of cefotaxime in the treatment of bacterial meningitis. Am J Med 1986;80:398.

104. Overturf GD et al. Treatment of bacterial meningitis with ceftizoxime. Antimicrob Agents Chemother 1984;25:258.

105. McCracken GH et al. Intraventricular gentamicin therapy in gram-negative bacillary meningitis in infancy. Lancet 1980;1:787.

106. Swartz MN. Intraventricular use of aminoglycosides in the treatment of gram-negative bacillary meningitis: conflicting views. J Infect Dis 1981;143:293.

107. Lentnek AL, Williams RR. Aztreonam in the treatment of gram-negative bacterial meningitis. Rev Infect Dis 1991;13(Suppl 7):S586.

108. Wong VK et al. Imipenem/cilastatin treatment of bacterial meningitis in children. Pediatr Infect Dis J 1991;10:122.

109. Calandra G et al. Factors predisposing to seizures in seriously ill infected patients receiving antibiotics: experience with imipenem/cilastatin. Am J Med 1988;84:911.

110. Eng RHK et al. Seizure propensity with imipenem. Arch Intern Med 1989;149:1881.

111. Klugman K et al. Randomized comparison of meropenem with cefotaxime for treatment of bacterial meningitis. Antimicrob Agents Chemother 1995;39:1140.

112. Odio CM et al. Prospective, randomized, investigator-blinded study of the efficacy and safety of meropenem vs. cefotaxime therapy in bacterial meningitis in children. Pediatric Infect Dis J 1999;18:581.

113. Wolff M et al. Penetration of ciprofloxacin into cerebrospinal fluid of patients with bacterial meningitis. Antimicrob Agents Chemother 1987;31:899.

114. Hooper DC, Wolfson JS. Fluoroquinolone antimicrobial agents. N Engl J Med 1991;324:384.117.

115. Parsley TL et al. Synergistic activity of trimethoprim and amikacin against gram-negative bacilli. Antimicrob Agents Chemother 1977;12:349.

116. Gardner P et al. Infections of central nervous system shunts. Med Clin North Am 1985;69:297.

116a. Bayston R. Epidemiology, diagnosis, treatment and prevention of cerebrospinal fluid shunt infections. Neurosurg Clin North Am 2001;36:703.

117. Yogev R Davis AT. Neurosurgical shunt infections. A review. Childs Brain 1980;6:74.

118. Schoenbaum SC et al. Infections of cerebrospinal fluid shunts: epidemiology, clinical manifestations, and therapy. J Infect Dis 1975;131:543.

119. Yogev R. Cerebrospinal fluid shunt infections: a personal view. Pediatr Infect Dis J 1985;4:113.

120. Walters BC et al. Cerebrospinal fluid shunt infection. J Neurosurg 1984;60:1014.

121. Younger JJ et al. Coagulase-negative staphylococci isolated from cerebrospinal fluid shunts: importance of slime production, species identification, and shunt removal to clinical outcome. J Infect Dis 1987;156:548.

122. Shapiro S et al. Origin of organisms infecting ventricular shunts. Neurosurgery 1988;22:868.

123. Gump DW. Vancomycin for treatment of bacterial meningitis. Rev Infect Dis 1981;3(Suppl):S289.

124. Brummett RE, Fox KE. Vancomycin- and erythromycin-induced hearing loss in humans. Antimicrob Agents Chemother 1989;33:791.

125. Polk RE et al. Vancomycin and the red-man syndrome: pharmacodynamics of histamine release. J Infect Dis 1988;157:502.

126. Sahai J et al. Influence of antihistamine pretreatment on vancomycin-induced red-man syndrome. J Infect Dis 1989;160:876.

127. Mathisen GE, Johnson JP. Brain abscess. Clin Infect Dis 1997;25:763.

128. Mampalam TJ, Rosenblum ML. Trends in the management of bacterial brain abscesses: a review of 102 cases over 17 years. Neurosurgery 1988;23:451.

129. Yoshikawa TT, Quinn W. The aching head. Intracranial suppuration due to head and neck infections. Infect Dis Clin North Am 1988;2:265.

130. Patrick, Kaplan SL. Current concepts in the pathogenesis and management of brain abscesses in children. Pediatr Clin North Am 1988;35:625.

131. Saez-Llorens X et al. Brain abscess in infants and children. Pediatr Infect Dis J 1989;8:449.

132. Rosenblum ML et al. Controversies in the management of brain abscesses. Clin Neurosurg 1986;33:603.

133. de Louvois J. The bacteriology and chemotherapy of brain abscess. J Antimicrob Chemother 1978;4:395.

134. Gossling J. Occurrence and pathogenicity of the *Streptococcus milleri* group. Rev Infect Dis 1988;10:257.

135. Luft BJ, Remington JS. Toxoplasmic encephalitis in AIDS. Clin Infect Dis 1992;15:211.

136. Simpson GL et al. Nocardial infections in the immunocompromised host: a detailed study in a defined population. Rev Infect Dis 1981;3:492.

137. Del Brutto OH et al. Therapy for neurocysticercosis: a reappraisal. Clin Infect Dis 1993;17:730.

138. Rosenblum ML et al. Nonoperative treatment of brain abscesses in selected high-risk patients. J Neurosurg 1980;52:217.

139. Black P et al. Penetration of brain abscess by systemically administered antibiotics. J Neurosurg 1973;38:705.

140. de Louvois J, Hurley R. Inactivation of penicillin by purulent exudates. Br Med J 1977;1:998.

141. Yamamoto M et al. Penetration of intravenous antibiotics into brain abscesses. Neurosurgery 1993;33:44.

142. Warner JF et al. Metronidazole therapy of anaerobic bacteremia, meningitis, and brain abscess. Arch Intern Med 1979;139:167.

143. Levy RM et al. Vancomycin penetration of a brain abscess: case report and review of the literature. Neurosurgery 1986;18:632.

144. Tice AD et al. Outpatient parenteral antimicrobial therapy for central nervous system infections. Clin Infect Dis 1999;29:1394.

145. Snavely SR, Hodges GR. The neurotoxicity of antibacterial agents. Ann Intern Med 1984;101:92.

146. Smilack JD et al. Tetracyclines, chloramphenicol, erythromycin, clindamycin, and metronidazole. Mayo Clin Proc 1991;66:1270.

CHAPTER 59

Endocarditis

Annie Wong-Beringer

INFECTIVE ENDOCARDITIS

Infective endocarditis (IE) is a microbial infection of the heart valves or other endocardial tissue and usually is associated with an underlying cardiac defect. In the past, IE was classified as either "acute bacterial endocarditis" or "subacute bacterial endocarditis" based on the clinical presentation and course of the untreated disease. However, this classification system is nonspecific and does not account for many nonbacterial causes of endocarditis, such as chlamydiae, rickettsiae, and fungi. Hence, the current system based on the causative organism is preferred because it provides information regarding the probable course of the disease, the likelihood of underlying heart disease, and the appropriate antimicrobial regimens.[1]

Pathogenesis[1,2]

The pathogenesis of endocarditis involves a complex series of events that ultimately results in the formation of an infected platelet–fibrin thrombus on the valve surface. This thrombus is called a *vegetation*.

The first step in the formation of the vegetation involves modification of the endocardial surface, which is normally nonthrombogenic. In patients with rheumatic heart disease, endocardial injury occurs as a result of immune complex deposition or hemodynamic disturbances. Valvular insufficiency caused by aortic stenosis or ventricular septal defects can produce regurgitant blood flow, high pressure gradients, or narrow orifices, resulting in turbulence and endocardial damage.

Once the endocardial surface of the valve is traumatized, small sterile thrombi consisting of platelets and fibrin are deposited, forming the lesion called *nonbacterial thrombotic endocarditis* (NBTE). NBTE occurs most commonly on the atrial surfaces of the mitral and tricuspid valves and on the ventricular surface of the aortic valve.

NBTE serves as a nidus for microbial colonization during periods of bacteremia. Table 59-1 lists procedures that cause bacteremia. Organisms such as *Streptococcus viridans,*

Table 59-1 Conditions and Procedures for Antibiotic Prophylaxis[a]

Cardiac Conditions

Prophylaxis Recommended

- Prosthetic cardiac valves, including bioprosthetic and homograft valves
- Previous bacterial endocarditis, even without heart disease
- Most congenital cardiac malformations
- Rheumatic and other acquired valvular dysfunction, even after valvular surgery
- Hypertrophic cardiomyopathy
- Mitral valve prolapse with valvular regurgitation and/or thickened leaflets

Prophylaxis Not Recommended

- Isolated secundum atrial septal defect
- Surgical repair without residua beyond 6 months of secundum atrial septal defect, ventricular septal defect, or patent ductus arteriosus
- Previous coronary artery bypass graft surgery
- Mitral valve prolapse without valvular regurgitation[b]
- Physiologic, functional, or innocent heart murmurs
- Previous Kawasaki disease without valvular dysfunction
- Previous rheumatic fever without valvular dysfunction
- Cardiac pacemakers and implanted defibrillators

Dental or Surgical Procedures

Prophylaxis Recommended

- Dental procedures known to induce gingival or mucosal bleeding, including professional cleaning
- Tonsillectomy and/or adenoidectomy
- Surgical operations that involve intestinal or respiratory mucosa
- Bronchoscopy with a rigid bronchoscope
- Sclerotherapy for esophageal varices
- Esophageal dilation
- Gallbladder surgery
- Cystoscopy
- Urethral dilation
- Urethral catheterization if urinary tract infection is present[c]
- Urinary tract surgery if urinary tract infection is present[c]
- Prostatic surgery
- Incision and drainage of infected tissue[c]
- Vaginal hysterectomy
- Vaginal delivery with infection[c]

Prophylaxis Not Recommended

- Dental procedures not likely to induce gingival bleeding, such as simple adjustment of orthodontic appliances or fillings above the gum line
- Injection of local intraoral anesthetic (except intraligamentary injections)
- Shedding of primary teeth
- Tympanostomy tube insertion
- Endotracheal intubation
- Bronchoscopy with a flexible bronchoscope, with or without biopsy
- Cardiac catheterization
- Endoscopy with or without gastrointestinal biopsy
- Cesarean section
- In the absence of infection for urethral catheterization, dilation and curettage, uncomplicated vaginal delivery, therapeutic abortion, sterilization procedures, or insertion or removal of intrauterine devices

[a]This table lists selected procedures and conditions but is not meant to be all-inclusive.
[b]Patients who have a mitral valve prolapse associated with thickening and/or redundancy of the valve leaflets may be at increased risk for bacterial endocarditis, particularly men ≥45 years of age.
[c]In addition to prophylactic regimen for genitourinary procedures, antibiotic therapy should be directed against the most likely bacterial pathogen.
[d]In patients who have prosthetic heart valves, a previous history of endocarditis, or surgically constructed systemic-pulmonary shunts or conduits, physicians may choose to administer prophylactic antibiotics even for low-risk procedures that involve the lower respiratory, genitourinary, or gastrointestinal tracts.
Reproduced with permission from Dajani AS et al. Prevention of bacterial endocarditis. Recommendations by the American Heart Association. JAMA 1997;277:1794. ©1997, American Medical Association.

Enterococcus species, *Staphylococcus aureus, Staphylococcus epidermidis, Pseudomonas aeruginosa,* and *Candida albicans* possess adherence factors that facilitate their colonization. In particular, platelet aggregation has been shown to be an important virulence factor in experimental streptococcal endocarditis; larger vegetations and multifocal embolic spread have been associated with strains that aggregate platelets.[3] Once the NBTE lesion becomes colonized by microorganisms, the surface is rapidly covered with a sheath of fibrin and platelets. This avascular encasement provides an environment protected from host defenses and is conducive to further bacterial replication and vegetation growth. Progression of the infection can be interrupted at any time by various host defense mechanisms, including blocking antibodies that interfere with bacterial adherence, serum bactericidal complement activity, hemodynamic forces that dislodge poorly adherent bacteria, and circulating prophylactic antibiotics.

The vegetation is thought to propagate by continuous reseeding of the thrombus by circulating organisms. As the vegetation enlarges, it takes on a laminar appearance caused by the alternating layers of bacteria and platelet–fibrin deposits. The bacterial colony count can be as high as 10^9 to 10^{10} bacteria per gram of valvular vegetation.

Endocarditis can result in life-threatening hemodynamic disturbances and embolic episodes. Without antimicrobial therapy and surgical intervention, IE is virtually 100% fatal.

Epidemiology

IE is among the leading causes of life-threatening infectious disease syndromes and accounts for approximately 15,000 to 20,000 new cases per year in the United States.[4l,4–7] The overall incidence appears to have risen over time, specifically among intravenous (IV) drug abusers and patients with prosthetic heart valves. The mean patient age reportedly has shifted from <30 years in the 1920s to about 55 years today. This increase in age is thought to be related to a decline in the incidence of acute rheumatic fever and rheumatic heart disease counterbalanced by degenerative valvular disease in an increasing elderly population. Specifically, the increasing longevity of the general population and advances in medical care have led to new predisposing factors resulting from increased exposure to more intense and invasive medical procedures. Men are affected more often than women (roughly 2:1), and the disease remains uncommon in children.

Predisposing Factors

Rheumatic heart disease was at one time the most common underlying cardiac defect associated with endocarditis; however, currently the predominant defect in documented cases of endocarditis is mitral valve prolapse and infection of prosthetic valves.[1,5-7] In addition, a growing population of IV drug abusers and a larger number of compromised hospitalized patients who are subjected to IV access procedures (e.g., IV catheterization, central venous catheterization for hyperalimentation, hemodialysis, and other shunt procedures) have resulted in a proportionate increase in the number of cases seen in these groups. As many as 30% of all cases seen at tertiary care hospitals in developed countries are nosocomially acquired; infected intravascular devices were the culprit in at least half the cases.[5] Other conditions associated with an increased incidence of IE include diabetes mellitus and HIV infection associated with IV drug abuse or long-term indwelling intravascular devices.[6,8] Congenital heart defects such as patent ductus arteriosus, ventricular septal defect, coarctation of the aorta, and tetralogy of Fallot are underlying causes in about 10% of cases. Degenerative cardiac lesions and idiopathic subaortic stenosis also have been associated with the development of endocarditis, but the actual contribution of these lesions is unknown. In addition, as many as one third of all patients have no recognizable underlying cardiac disease.

Bacteriology

Streptococci have been the predominant causative pathogens in IE, accounting for 60% to 80% of all cases historically.[1,5-7,9] However, when comparing epidemiologic studies in the aggregate over the past decades, staphylococci have assumed increased importance as a cause of IE. Specifically, S. viridans cases appear to have decreased by 35%, while S. aureus cases have increased by 50%. Among patients age >60 years with IE, streptococci account for 30% to 45% of cases; S. aureus accounts for 25% to 30% of cases, followed by Enterococcus species at 14% to 17%.[5] S. viridans group microorganisms (S. sanguis, S. bovis, S. mutans, and S. mitis) continue to be the most common streptococci isolated from patients with IE. Endocarditis in IV drug abusers often is due to S. aureus, whereas prosthetic valve endocarditis is more commonly caused by coagulase-negative staphylococci such as S. epidermidis. Gram-negative bacilli and fungi together account for <10% of all endocarditis cases and usually are associated with IV drug use, valvular prostheses, and hospital IV access procedures. Endocarditis caused by anaerobes and other organisms is rare. Polymicrobial infective endocarditis (caused by at least two organisms), while uncommon in the typical patient, is being recognized more frequently in IV drug abusers

and postoperative patients. *Candida* species, *S. aureus*, *P. aeruginosa*, *Serratia marcescens*, and non–group D streptococci are the organisms involved most frequently.

Site of Involvement

The site of heart valve involvement is determined by the underlying cardiac defect and the infecting organism.[1,2,4-6] The mitral valve is affected in >85% of cases caused by *S. viridans* when rheumatic heart disease is the underlying abnormality. The tricuspid valve is the common site of involvement in staphylococcal endocarditis associated with IV drug use. In addition, more than one heart valve may be affected simultaneously. Overall, the mitral valve is affected slightly more often than the aortic (55%), followed by the tricuspid (20%) and the pulmonic (1%) valves. However, recent studies have shown that aortic valve involvement is increasing in frequency and is associated with higher morbidity and mortality.

STREPTOCOCCUS VIRIDANS ENDOCARDITIS

Clinical Presentation

1. **A.G., a 57-year-old, 60-kg man with chief complaints of fatigue, a persistent low-grade fever, night sweats, arthralgias, and a 7-kg unintentional weight loss, is admitted to the hospital for evaluation. Visual inspection reveals a cachectic, ill-appearing man in no acute distress. Physical examination on admission is significant for a grade III/IV diastolic murmur with mitral regurgitation (insufficiency) that has increased from pre-existing murmur, a temperature of 100.5°F, petechial skin lesions, subungual splinter hemorrhages, and Janeway lesions on the soles of both feet. Nail clubbing, Roth spots, or Osler's nodes are not evident (see Figs. 59-1 to 59-5). The remainder of his physical examination is unremarkable. A.G.'s past medical history is significant for mitral valve prolapse and more recently a dental procedure involving the extraction of four wisdom teeth. The history of his present illness is noteworthy for the development of the aforementioned symptoms about 2 weeks after the dental procedure (about 2 months before admission). His only current medication is ibuprofen 600 mg QID.**

Relevant laboratory results include hemoglobin (Hgb), 11.4 g/dL; hematocrit (Hct), 34%; reticulocyte count, 0.5%; white blood cell (WBC) count, 85,000/mm³ with 65% polys and 1% bands; blood urea nitrogen (BUN), 21 mg/dL; and serum creatinine (SrCr), 1.8 mg/dL. A urinalysis (UA) reveals 2+ proteinuria and 10 to 20 red blood cells (RBCs) per high-power field (HPF). The erythrocyte sedimentation rate (ESR) on admission is elevated at 66 mm/hr and the rheumatoid factor (RF) is positive. Two-dimensional echocardiogram results were unrevealing.

To establish the diagnosis of IE, three blood cultures were obtained over 24 hours. All cultures obtained on day 1 are reported to be growing α-hemolytic streptococci. While confirmation and speciation of the organism is being performed, A.G. is started on penicillin G, 2 million units IV Q 4 hr (12 million U/day), and gentamicin, 120 mg (loading dose) followed by 60 mg Q 12 hr. Antimicrobial susceptibility results are pending. What clinical manifestations and laboratory abnormalities in A.G. are consistent with IE?

[SI units: Hgb, 114 g/L (normal, 140 to 180); Hct, 0.34 (normal, 0.39 to 0.49); reticulocyte count, 0.005 (normal, 0.001 to 0.024); WBC count, 85 × 10⁹/L with 0.65 polys and 0.01 bands (normal, 3.2 to 9.8 with 0.54 to 0.62 polys and 0.03 to 0.05 bands); BUN, 7.5 mmol/L of urea (normal, 2.9 to 8.9); and SrCr, 159 mmol/L (normal, 53 to 133)]

The clinical presentation of IE is highly variable and can involve almost any organ system.[1,4,5] A.G. appears pale and chronically ill and represents the typical patient with subacute disease (e.g., that caused by *S. viridans*). Nonspecific complaints consistent with endocarditis in A.G. include fatigue, weight loss, fever, night sweats, and arthralgias. Only fever is present in the majority (90%) of patients with endocarditis. The fever is characteristically low grade and remittent, with peaks in the afternoon and evening. The temperature rarely exceeds 103°F in subacute disease.[1,4,5] Fever may be absent or minimal in patients with congestive heart failure (CHF), chronic renal and liver failure, prior use of antimicrobial agents, or IE caused by less virulent organisms.[1,4,5] Musculoskeletal complaints such as arthralgias, myalgias, and back pain are common and may mimic rheumatic disease. Other symptoms can include lethargy, anorexia, malaise, nausea, and vomiting.[1] Because signs and symptoms are nonspecific and subtle, diagnosis often is difficult. In addition, the time from bacteremia to diagnosis often is prolonged because of the insidious progression of symptoms.[1,11] In particular, delayed diagnosis occurs more commonly in the elderly. Fever may be absent in 30% to 40% of patients >60 years of age while present in >90% of patients <40 years of age. Fewer of these patients have new or changed heart murmurs. The most common presenting complaints in the elderly with endocarditis are confusion, anorexia, fatigue, and weakness, which may be readily attributable to stroke, heart failure, or syncope.[10]

The temporal relationship between A.G.'s dental procedure and the onset of symptoms makes it the most obvious cause of bacteremia and subsequent endocarditis. Although it is assumed that prophylactic antibiotics were administered before the procedure, endocarditis can develop despite apparently adequate chemoprophylaxis.[12,13]

A.G. is noted to have an increase in his pre-existing diastolic murmur with mitral insufficiency, a finding consistent with endocarditis. Cardiac murmurs are present in >85% of patients with endocarditis. However, murmurs frequently are absent in patients with acute disease (e.g., staphylococcal endocarditis), right-sided disease (e.g., endocarditis in IV drug abusers), or mural infection.[1]

A.G. exhibits several peripheral manifestations of infective endocarditis, including conjunctival petechiae, Janeway lesions, and splinter hemorrhages. Overall, peripheral manifestations are found in 10% to 50% of cases, but none of these is pathognomonic for IE. These manifestations are usually a result of septic embolization of vegetations to distal sites or immune complex deposition. Mucocutaneous petechial lesions of the conjunctiva, mouth, or pharynx are present in 20% to 40% of patients, especially those with longstanding disease. These lesions generally are small, nontender, and hemorrhagic in appearance and occur as a result of vasculitis or peripheral embolization. Janeway lesions are painless, hemorrhagic, macular plaques most commonly found on the palms and soles (Fig. 59-1). Splinter hemorrhages are nonspecific findings that appear as red to brown linear streaks in the proximal portion of the fingers or toenails (Fig. 59-2). Other findings can include Roth spots (small, flame-shaped retinal hemorrhages with pale white centers found near the optic nerve) and Osler's nodes (purplish, nonhemorrhagic, painful nodules that develop on the subcutaneous pads of the fingers and toes or on palms and soles) (Fig. 59-3). Clubbing (broadening and

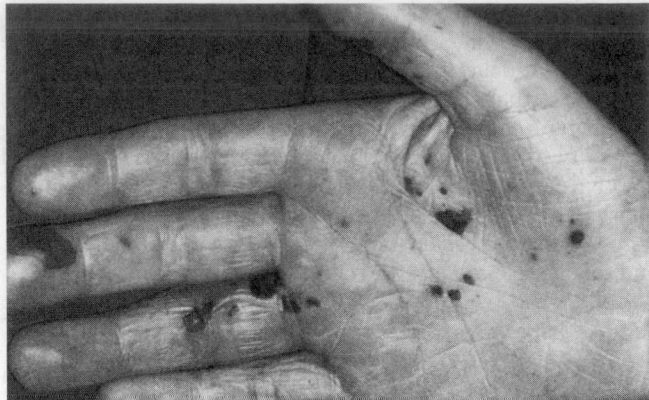

FIGURE 59-1. Janeway lesions. Extensive ecchymotic embolic lesions in a case of acute bacterial endocarditis.

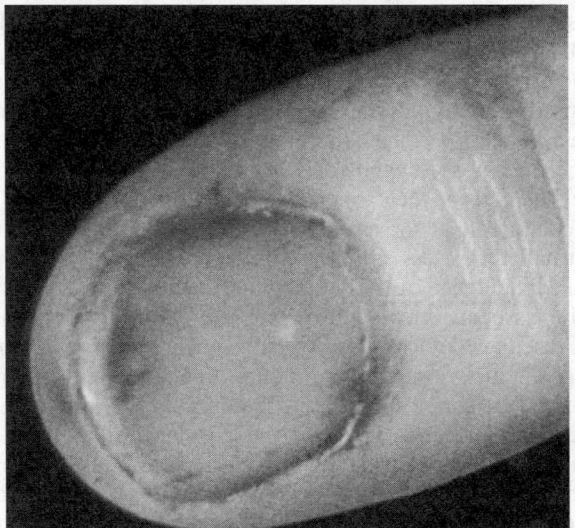

FIGURE 59-2. Splinter hemorrhages in the nailbed.

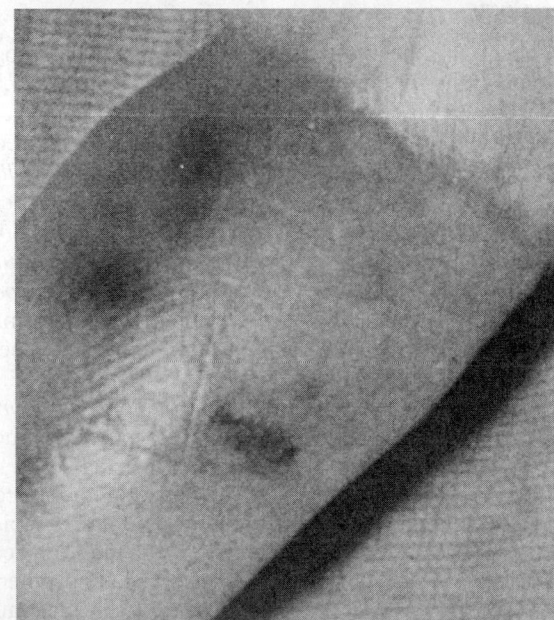

FIGURE 59-3. Osler's nodes on the tip of the index finger in a case of endocarditis caused by *S. aureus*.

thickening) of the nails also may be observed in patients with prolonged disease[1,11,14] (Fig. 59-4). Petechial skin lesions are also seen (Fig. 59-5).

Several laboratory findings are consistent with IE in A.G. A low Hgb and Hct with normal red cell indices suggest anemia of chronic disease. Of patients with subacute disease, 70% to 90% will have a normochromic, normocytic anemia as part of their initial presentation. Leukocytosis with a left shift, although not evident in A.G., commonly is seen in those with acute, fulminant disease such as staphylococcal endocarditis. The ESR nearly always is elevated in IE, but this finding is nonspecific and may be associated with several other disease entities. Rheumatoid factor (an IgM antiglobulin) and circulating immune complexes can be detected in most patients with longstanding disease, but both are nonspecific findings.[1]

Major embolic episodes and infarction involving the kidney, spleen, lung, and carotid artery develop as secondary complications in up to one third of cases.[1] A.G. exhibits some degree of renal damage, as evidenced by moderate hematuria and proteinuria. Erythrocyte and leukocyte cast formation also may be present. Alterations in A.G.'s renal function (increased BUN and creatinine) probably are a result of immune complex deposition (diffuse glomerulonephritis) or secondary to renal embolization (focal glomerulonephritis). Fortunately, renal impairment usually is reversible with the institution of effective antimicrobial therapy.[1,14]

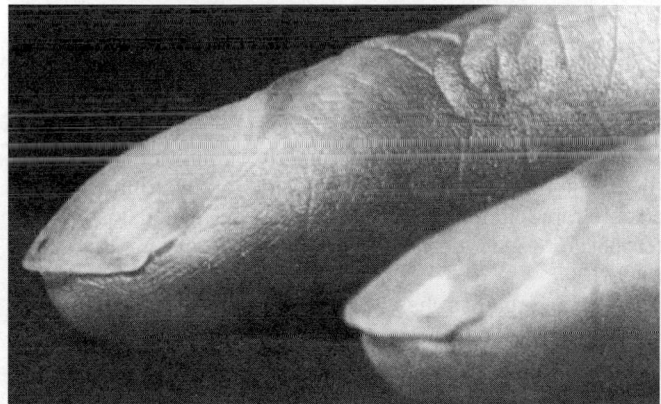

FIGURE 59-4. Clubbing of the fingers in longstanding subacute bacterial endocarditis.

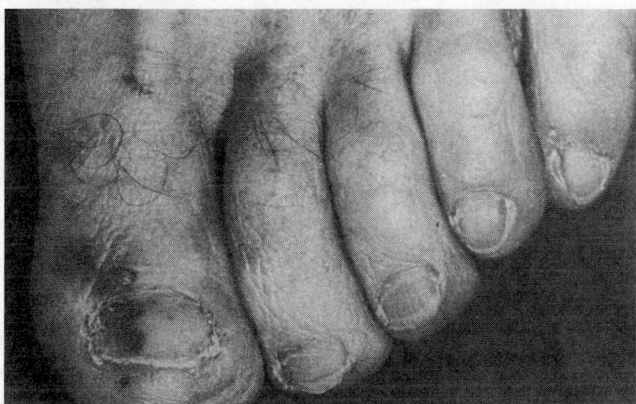

FIGURE 59-5. Petechial skin lesions in a case of acute staphylococcal endocarditis.

Cardiac complications occur most frequently. CHF is the most common cause of death in IE and is the most compelling indication for surgery. Infection-induced valvular damage is responsible for valvular insufficiency causing heart failure.[1,4,5,14] As many as two thirds of patients with endocarditis develop CHF. Infection of the aortic valve is more frequently associated with CHF than the mitral valve.[5] Other manifestations include paravalvular abscesses, pulmonary edema, and pericarditis.[5,14] Mitral valve injury caused by *S. viridans* generally is better tolerated hemodynamically than aortic valve injury caused by staphylococci. Although A.G. has no apparent signs of overt heart failure, he should be monitored closely for the development of hemodynamic instability.

Neurologic complications rank second to cardiac complications in frequency but may be the leading cause of death in patients with endocarditis. Stroke is the most common neurologic complication of IE.[14] A stroke syndrome in a patient with underlying valvular abnormalities should prompt the clinician to rule out IE. Other clinical manifestations include headache, mental status change, stroke or transient ischemic attack, seizures, brain abscess, or intracranial mycotic aneurysms.[1,5,14] Neurologic symptoms were noted in as many as 35% of patients in a recent study of *S. aureus* endocarditis in patients who were not drug addicts. A mortality rate of 74% was found for those with major neurologic manifestations compared with 56% in those without.[15]

Splenomegaly, although not part of A.G.'s findings, occurs in 20% to 60% of all cases and is more common in patients with a prolonged subacute presentation. In addition, metastatic abscesses can develop in virtually any organ secondary to systemic septic embolization. The most commonly involved metastatic foci are the spleen, kidney, liver, and iliac and mesenteric arteries.[5,14]

Diagnosis

2. How was the diagnosis of IE established in A.G.?

Blood Cultures
Although A.G.'s medical history (mitral valve prolapse, recent dental procedure) and clinical presentation are highly suggestive of IE, blood culture is the single most important diagnostic workup of a patient suspected to have IE.[1] Bacteremia secondary to endocarditis is continuous and low grade; >50% of the cultures have only 1 to 30 bacteria/mL. Despite the low concentration of organisms, bacteremia (when present) results in at least one of the first two blood cultures being positive in 95% of cases.[1,16] Administration of antibiotics within the previous 2 weeks may significantly decrease this yield.[17]

At least three sets of blood cultures collected by separate venipunctures should be obtained over the first 24 hours of presentation.[1] In a "stable" patient such as A.G. who has had the disease for several weeks or months, it is important to establish the exact microbiologic cause before initiating antimicrobial therapy. Patients who are acutely ill should have empiric therapy started as soon as the appropriate cultures are obtained to avoid further valvular damage or other complications.[1,5]

Echocardiography
Echocardiography is a valuable tool in establishing early diagnosis, identifying patients at high risk for complications,

and optimizing the timing and mode of surgical intervention by detecting and monitoring associated pathologic changes such as valvular abscess, as well as the presence and size of vegetations.[1,5,18–20] In an echocardiogram, high-frequency sound waves are applied, and the reflection by body tissues is processed by a transducer to create images. The transducer may be placed on the chest (transthoracic echocardiogram [TTE]) or in the esophagus (transesophageal echocardiogram [TEE]).[18] TEE is a rapid and noninvasive procedure with a 98% specificity for vegetations. However, sensitivity for vegetations may be <60% to 70% for adult patients with obesity, hyperinflated lungs due to emphysema, or a prosthetic valve. TEE is more costly and invasive but is significantly more sensitive in detecting vegetations while maintaining high specificity. All patients with suspected IE should have an echocardiogram on admission and repeated during their course as necessary.[5,18] Recent guidelines suggest that TTE should be used for patients with native valves who are good candidates for imaging, whereas TEE should be reserved for patients with prosthetic valves, patients with catheter-associated *S. aureus* bacteremia, and patients admitted with fever or bacteremia in the setting of IV drug use.[19–21]

In summary, IE should be suspected in any patient who has a documented fever and heart murmur. Prior cardiac disease, peripheral manifestations, splenomegaly, various laboratory abnormalities, and a positive echocardiogram strengthen the diagnosis, but microbiologic documentation is the most important factor in confirming IE. Disease entities with overlapping clinical presentation and laboratory abnormalities should be excluded using the appropriate tests.[1]

Standardized criteria (Duke criteria) for the clinical assessment of patients suspected of having IE were proposed by a group at Duke University in 1994[22] and are listed in Tables 59-2 and 59-3. These diagnostic criteria integrate clinical, laboratory, microbiologic, and echocardiographic data. Follow-up studies have found the Duke criteria to be highly sensitive, resulting in little underdiagnosis of IE.[1,5,23,24] A modified version has been proposed recently to overcome limitations such as misclassification of culture-negative endocarditis, the increasing role of TEE, the relative risk of IE with *S. aureus* bacteremia, and the overly broad categorization of "possible" causes.[25,26] However, the performance characteristics of the modified version have not been well studied.

A.G. possesses one major criterion (positive blood cultures) and three minor criteria (fever, predisposing heart condition, vascular and immunologic phenomena); therefore, he meets the diagnostic criteria for definite IE.[22]

Antimicrobial Therapy

General Principles

3. What would be a reasonable duration of antibiotic therapy for A.G.? When are serum bactericidal titers (SBTs) useful in managing bacterial endocarditis?

The avascular nature of the vegetation results in an environment that is devoid of normal host defenses (e.g., phagocytic cells and complement); this permits uninhibited growth of bacteria.[2] Therefore, to eradicate the causative organism, high doses of a parenterally administered, bactericidal antibiotic generally are administered for 4 to 6 weeks.[1,5,27] For some

---

Table 59-2 Proposed New Criteria for Diagnosis of Infective Endocarditis

Definite Infective Endocarditis

Pathologic Criteria

Microorganisms: Demonstrated by culture or histology in a vegetation, or in a vegetation that has embolized, or in an intracardiac abscess, or

Pathologic lesions: Vegetation or intracardiac abscess present, confirmed by histology showing active endocarditis

Clinical Criteria

Using specific definitions listed in Table 59-3; 2 major criteria *or* 1 major and 3 minor criteria *or* 5 minor criteria

Possible Infective Endocarditis

Findings consistent with infective endocarditis that fall short of "definite," but not "rejected"

Rejected

Firm alternative diagnosis for manifestations of endocarditis, *or*

Resolution of manifestations of endocarditis, with antibiotic therapy for ≤4 days, *or*

No pathologic evidence of infective endocarditis at surgery or autopsy, after antibiotic therapy for ≤4 days

Reprinted from Durack DT et al. New criteria for diagnosis of infective endocarditis: utilization of specific echocardiographic findings. Am J Med 1994;96:200, with permission from Excerpta Medica, Inc.

---

infections, it may be necessary to use two antibiotics to achieve synergistic activity against the organism.[28] For example, the addition of an aminoglycoside to penicillin results in a more rapid and complete bactericidal effect against the enterococci.[29] (See Question 16 for a detailed discussion of synergy.)

Once an organism has been identified, its in vitro susceptibility pattern is determined by the minimum inhibitory concentration (MIC) for various antibiotics. Standard Kirby-Bauer disk testing is inadequate in the setting of IE to aid in selection of antibiotics without the quantitative information provided by the MIC.[1] In addition, the minimum bactericidal concentration (MBC) may be useful in detecting tolerant strains, particularly in the setting of unexplained slow response or treatment failure. However, routine MBC determination is not recommended (see Question 15).[1] Treatment of endocarditis requires antibiotics with bactericidal activity; therefore, the serum concentration of the antibiotic must greatly exceed the MBC for the particular organism. For endocarditis caused by *S. viridans* acquired from the community, this usually is achieved without much problem because most isolates are sensitive to penicillin at an MIC of <0.125 µg/mL; corresponding MBCs are, at most, one or two tube dilutions higher.[30] However, the emergence of strains demonstrating resistance to penicillin and related β-lactams such as ceftriaxone is a significant problem, particularly among bloodstream isolates obtained from the nosocomial setting and neutropenic cancer patients.[30–33] The increasing prevalence of β-lactam–resistant clinical isolates highlights the im-

Table 59-3 Definitions of Terminology Used in the Proposed New Criteria

Major Criteria

Positive blood culture for infective endocarditis

- Typical microorganisms for infective endocarditis from two separate blood cultures

    1. Viridans streptococci,[a] *Streptococcus bovis,* HACEK group, *or*

    2. Community-acquired *Staphylococcus aureus* or enterococci, without a primary focus, *or*

- Persistently positive blood culture, defined as recovery of a microorganism consistent with infective endocarditis from:

    1. Blood cultures drawn ≥12 hr apart, *or*

    2. All of 3 or a majority of at least 4 separate blood cultures, with first and last drawn at least 1 hr apart

Evidence of endocarditis involvement

- Positive echocardiogram for infective endocarditis

    1. Oscillating intracardiac mass, on valve or supporting structures, or in the path of regurgitant jets, or on implanted material, without an alternative anatomic explanation, *or*

    2. Abscess, *or*

    3. New partial dehiscence of prosthetic valve, *or*

- New valvular regurgitation (increase or change in pre-existing murmur not sufficient)

Minor Criteria

- Predisposition: Predisposing heart condition or intravenous drug use

- Fever ≥38°C (100.4°F)

- *Vascular Phenomena:* Major arterial emboli, septic pulmonary infarcts, mycotic aneurysm, intracranial hemorrhage, conjunctival hemorrhages, Janeway lesions

- *Immunologic Phenomena:* Glomerulonephritis, Osler's nodes, Roth spots, rheumatoid factor

- *Microbiologic Evidence:* Positive blood culture but not meeting major criterion as noted previously,[b] or serologic evidence of active infection with organism consistent with infective endocarditis

- Echocardiogram: Consistent with infective endocarditis but not meeting major criterion as noted previously

[a]Including nutritional variants.
[b]Excluding single positive cultures for coagulase-negative staphylococci and organisms that do not cause endocarditis.
HACEK, *Haemophilus* species, *Actinobacillus actinomycetemcomitans, Cardiobacterium hominis, Eikenella* species, and *Kingella kingae.*
Reprinted from Durack DT et al. New criteria for diagnosis of infective endocarditis: utilization of specific echocardiographic findings. Am J Med 1994;96:200, with permission from Excerpta Medica, Inc.

portance of determining the MIC and continued close monitoring of the antibiotic susceptibility of *S. viridans.*

The SBT, commonly called a Schlichter test, is an in vitro modification of the MBC test. It measures the killing activity of the patient's serum (containing antibiotic) against the isolated organism.[34] To perform the test, a known inoculum of the patient's organism is added to serial dilutions of the patient's serum. The SBT is the highest dilution that kills 99% to 100% of the inoculum.

A great deal of controversy surrounds the value of the SBT in monitoring therapy for IE, the usefulness of peak versus trough SBT, and the appropriate SBT endpoint required for successful treatment of bacterial endocarditis.[1,34,35] The lack of agreement is due in part to the nonstandardized method for performing SBT, such as the inoculum size used and the timing of SBT samples, which leads to difficulty in test interpretation and correlation with clinical outcome.[1,34,35] In one large multicenter study using a standardized method, peak titers (dilutions) of ≥1:64 and trough titers of ≥1:32 were needed to predict bacteriologic cure in all patients.[35] On the other hand, the SBT was a poor predictor of failure, because many patients who were cured had much lower SBTs (e.g., <1:8). Until an accepted, standardized method is established, routine performance of SBT is not recommended. The SBT test may be useful in the following situations: (1) when endocarditis is caused by relatively resistant organisms (e.g., relatively penicillin-resistant *S. viridans,* MIC 0.1 to 0.5 μg/mL) when a synergistic combination of antibiotics might be beneficial; (2) when response to therapy has been suboptimal; and (3) when less well-established regimens are used for treatment.[1,34,35] Alternatively, in vitro synergy studies using the standard microtiter checkerboard tests or time-kill curves in broth may be performed to evaluate the synergistic potential of combination therapy in the above situations.[1]

4. **What antibiotic regimens are most useful for the treatment of *S. viridans* endocarditis?**

Patients with endocarditis caused by penicillin-sensitive strains of *S. viridans* and nonenterococcal group D streptococci (e.g., *S. bovis;* MIC <0.1 μg/mL) can be treated with any one of three regimens as outlined in the 1995 AHA treatment guidelines.[27] The suggested regimens (Table 59-4) are associated with cure rates of up to 98% and include: (1) high-dose parenteral penicillin for 4 weeks; (2) high-dose parenteral ceftriaxone for 4 weeks; and (3) 2 weeks of combined therapy with high-dose parenteral penicillin and an aminoglycoside.[27,36–42] In addition, results from recent trials indicate that combined therapy with once-daily dosing of ceftriaxone and an aminoglycoside for 2 weeks demonstrate comparable efficacy for selected patients.[45,46]

High-Dose Penicillin for 4 Weeks

The intravenous (IV) administration of 10 to 20 million units/day of penicillin G for 4 weeks resulted in a cure rate of 100% for 66 patients with nonenterococcal streptococcal endocarditis.[37] Another study using penicillin alone reported relapse in only 2 of 49 patients; however, both patients who relapsed received <4 weeks of therapy.[42] The large range of 12 to 18 million units/day of penicillin is recommended to allow flexibility in dosing based on the patient's renal function and disease severity.

Single Daily Ceftriaxone for 4 Weeks

Ceftriaxone has been shown to have excellent in vitro activity against viridans streptococcal strains isolated from patients with endocarditis. In one study, all 49 strains of viridans streptococci and 11 strains of *S. bovis* were inhibited at a concentration of <0.125 μg/mL of ceftriaxone; one strain of *S. sanguis* was inhibited at an MIC of 0.25 μg/mL.[44] Although no direct comparative trials have been performed evaluating

Table 59-4 Suggested Regimens for Therapy of Native Valve Endocarditis Caused by *Streptococcus viridans* and *Streptococcus bovis*

Antibiotic	Dose[a] and Route[b]	Duration
Penicillin-Susceptible (Minimum Inhibitory Concentration ≤0.1 µg/mL)		
Aqueous crystalline penicillin G[c]	*Adult:* 12–18 million units/24 hr IV either continuously or in 6 equally divided doses	4 wk
	Pediatric: 150,000–200,000 units/kg per 24 hr IV (max: 20 million units/ 24 hr) either continuously or in 6 equally divided doses	
Ceftriaxone sodium[c]	*Adult:* 2 g once daily IV or IM	4 wk
Aqueous crystalline penicillin G	*Adult:* 12–18 million units/24 hr IV either continuously or in six equally divided doses	2 wk
	Pediatric: 150,000–200,000 units/kg per 24 hr IV (max: 20 million units/ 24 hr) either continuously or in 6 equally divided doses	
	Adult: 1 mg/kg IM or IV (max: 80 mg) Q 8 hr	
With gentamicin sulfate[d]	*Pediatric:* 2–2.5 mg/kg IV (max: 80 mg) Q 8 hr	2 wk
Relatively Penicillin G Resistant (Minimum Inhibitory Concentration >0.1 µg/mL and <0.5 µg/mL)		
Aqueous crystalline penicillin G[e]	*Adult:* 18 million units/24 hr IV either continuously or in 6 equally divided doses	4 wk
	Pediatric: 200,000–300,000 units/kg per 24 hr IV (max: 20 million units/ 24 hr) either continuously or in 6 equally divided doses	
	Adult: 1 mg/kg IM or IV (max: 80 mg) Q 8 hr	
With gentamicin sulfate[d]	*Pediatric:* 2–2.5 mg/kg IV (max: 80 mg) Q 8 hr	2 wk
β-Lactam Allergic Patients		
Vancomycin hydrochloride[f]	*Adult:* 30 mg/kg per 24 hr IV in 2 equally divided doses (max: 2 g/24 hr unless serum concentrations are monitored)	4 wk
	Pediatric: 40 mg/kg per 24 hr IV in 2 or 4 equally divided doses (max: 2 g/24 hr unless serum concentrations are monitored)	

[a]Pediatric dosages are adapted from reference 36.
[b]Antibiotic doses for patients with impaired renal function should be modified appropriately. Vancomycin dosage should be reduced in patients with renal dysfunction; cephalosporin dosage may need to be reduced in patients with moderate to severe renal dysfunction.
[c]Preferred in most patients >65 years of age and in those with impairment of the eighth nerve or renal function.
[d]Dosing of gentamicin on a mg/kg basis produces higher serum concentrations in obese patients than in lean patients. Therefore, in obese patients, dosing should be based on ideal body weight. Other potentially nephrotoxic agents (e.g., nonsteroidal anti-inflammatory drugs) should be used cautiously in patients receiving gentamicin. A peak gentamicin serum concentration of 3 µg/mL and a trough concentration of <1 µg/mL are desirable.
[e]Cefazolin or other first-generation cephalosporins may be substituted for penicillin in patients whose penicillin hypersensitivity is not of the immediate type.
[f]Vancomycin dosage should be reduced in patients with impaired renal function. Vancomycin given on a mg/kg basis produces higher serum concentrations in obese patients than in lean patients. Therefore, in obese patients, dosing should be based on ideal body weight. Each dose of vancomycin should be infused over at least 1 hr to reduce the risk of the histamine-release red man syndrome. Peak serum concentrations of vancomycin should be obtained 1 hr after completion of the infusion and should be in the range of 30–45 µg/mL. Trough concentrations should be obtained within half an hour of the next dose and be in the range of 5–15 µg/mL.
Adapted from Wilson WR et al. Antibiotic treatment of adults with infective endocarditis due to streptococci, enterococci, staphylococci, and HACEK microorganisms. JAMA 1995;274:1706–1713. ©1995, American Medical Association.

ceftriaxone against high-dose penicillin for the treatment of streptococcal endocarditis, current data (based on open-label studies of ceftriaxone) indicate an efficacy rate comparable to that of high-dose penicillin when treatment is given for 4 weeks.[43,44] Of the 70 assessable patients who received ceftriaxone 2 g as a single daily dose for 4 weeks, all were cured, except for one patient who had a probable relapse 3 months after completion of therapy. All strains of viridans streptococci were inhibited by ceftriaxone at an MIC of ≤0.25 µg/mL in both studies. One study included only patients without cardiovascular risk factors or complications. Although the simplicity of single daily treatment with ceftriaxone is attractive for outpatient use, careful patient selection based on microbiologic, clinical, and host factors is critical to the success of treatment and the proper and timely management of potential complications. (See Question 32 for a detailed discussion of outpatient therapy.)

High-Dose Penicillin or Ceftriaxone Plus an Aminoglycoside for 2 Weeks

The combination of 2 weeks of streptomycin (or gentamicin) with 4 weeks of penicillin is synergistically bactericidal for most streptococci, including enterococci (see Question 16).[28,39] This in vitro synergy also has been correlated with a more rapid rate of eradication of *S. viridans* from cardiac vegetations in the rabbit model of endocarditis.[41] A shortened combination regimen consisting of high-dose penicillin G and streptomycin for 2 weeks is an effective alternative to the previously described regimens. The reported cure rate in 104 patients treated at the Mayo Clinics with this regimen was 99%.[38,39]

Although clinical experience with combination therapy has been primarily with penicillin and streptomycin, in vitro and animal data support the fact that streptomycin and gentamicin are reasonably interchangeable. Gentamicin is more widely used in clinical practice and serum concentrations are more readily available to monitor efficacy and toxicities. Experimental data suggest that a gentamicin dosing interval of once versus thrice daily does not affect the relative efficacy of penicillin plus gentamicin for treatment of viridans streptococcal endocarditis.[40]

Combination therapy with ceftriaxone and an aminoglycoside for 2 weeks was also evaluated recently in two studies.[45,46] In a noncomparative open-label study, a 2-week course of ceftriaxone 2 g plus netilmicin (3 mg/kg) (both given once daily) resulted in a clinical cure of 87% in 48 evaluable patients.[45] A second open-label study compared ceftriaxone 2 g alone versus the combination of ceftriaxone 2 g plus gentamicin (3 mg/kg), both given once daily, for the treatment of endocarditis caused by penicillin-susceptible streptococci.[46] Patients were randomized to either regimen; 26 monotherapy recipients and 25 combination therapy recipients were evaluable. Clinical cure was observed in 96% of the patients in both groups at completion of therapy and at 3-month follow-up. This study excluded patients with suspected or documented cardiac or extracardiac abscesses and those with prosthetic valve endocarditis. Although the aminoglycoside agent (netilmicin or gentamicin) was administered as a single daily dose in both studies, all of the patients had measurable serum trough levels. Therefore, the efficacy of "extended-interval dosing" of aminoglycoside (whereby trough levels are not detectable, allowing a drug-free interval) in short-course combination therapy will need to be confirmed in future studies.

Based on available data, the 2-week regimen of penicillin or ceftriaxone plus an aminoglycoside appears to be efficacious for uncomplicated cases of penicillin-susceptible *S. viridans* endocarditis. It is not currently recommended for patients with extracardiac complications or intracardiac abscesses. Patients infected with *Abiotrophia* species (formerly known as nutritionally variant viridans streptococci) or viridans streptococci that have a penicillin MIC >0.1 μg/mL, or patients who have prosthetic valve infections should not receive short-course therapy.[27]

Special Considerations

The risk of relapse may be higher in patients who have had symptoms for >3 months before the initiation of treatment.[1,27,47] These patients should be treated with 4 to 6 weeks of penicillin combined with an aminoglycoside for the first 2 weeks.[1,5,27,47]

Nutritionally deficient or variant streptococci (NVS) have been reclassified recently into a new genus, *Abiotrophia,* which includes *A. defectiva, A. adjacens* (renamed again as *Granulicatella adjacens*), and *A. elegans. Abiotrophia* species are slow-growing, fastidious organisms that are responsible for approximately 5% of IE cases. In the past, NVS has been the cause of most of the cases of endocarditis diagnosed as "culture-negative" initially due to its requirement for the addition of vitamin B_6 (pyridoxal HCl) to the culture media for laboratory growth. However, laboratory identification is no longer a significant problem with current culture media and laboratory techniques.[30]

NVS exhibits lower susceptibility to penicillin in vitro than other streptococci. Up to two thirds of NVS organisms have relatively high MICs to penicillin (0.2 to 2.0 μg/mL), and some show high-level resistance to penicillin (MIC >4

μg/mL).[30] In addition, tolerance to penicillin has been described in many strains.[30] An animal model of endocarditis indicates that a penicillin–aminoglycoside (streptomycin or gentamicin) combination is significantly better than penicillin alone in reducing bacterial counts of these organisms.[48] More importantly, endocarditis caused by NVS is associated with greater morbidity and mortality compared to IE caused by other streptococci. Higher mortality rate (14% versus 5%), more frequent complications of embolization (33% versus 11%) and CHF (33% versus 18%), and an increased rate of surgical intervention (33% versus 18%) were observed in a study comparing 49 patients with NVS endocarditis versus 130 patients infected with other oral streptococci.[30] High rates of bacteriologic failure and relapse may be expected in patients despite completion of the treatment course for strains highly susceptible to penicillin.[30] All patients infected with NVS or *Abiotrophia* should receive 4 to 6 weeks of penicillin (or ampicillin) in combination with gentamicin.[5,27] A 6-week course of combination therapy with penicillin and gentamicin is recommended for patients with symptoms >3 months in duration and those with prosthetic valve endocarditis caused by these strains.[5,27,30] Patients with endocarditis caused by relatively resistant viridans streptococci with penicillin MIC of >0.5 μg/mL or enterococci should receive a similar treatment regimen, as described above.[5,27]

Patients allergic to β-lactams should receive vancomycin 30 mg/kg per day divided into two doses for 4 to 6 weeks. In patients who have had minor reactions to penicillins (e.g., a delayed rash), a first-generation cephalosporin such as cefazolin (1 to 2 g Q 6 to 8 hr) may be cautiously substituted. Although the addition of an aminoglycoside to a cephalosporin or vancomycin enhances bactericidal activity in vitro, it is unknown whether the addition of an aminoglycoside confers any additional clinical benefit.[27]

Regimen Selection

5. What factors must be considered in selecting a regimen for A.G.? Which regimen should be used for A.G.?

For most cases of endocarditis caused by penicillin-sensitive *S. viridans* (in patients not allergic to penicillin), all three of the aforementioned regimens are equally acceptable; therefore, the choice should be based on their relative advantages and disadvantages. The 2-week regimen requires the shortest hospital stay, but it has the disadvantage of possible ototoxicity and nephrotoxicity secondary to aminoglycoside administration. Therefore, it may be prudent to consider the use of penicillin or ceftriaxone alone for 4 weeks in older persons (>65 years) and those with impaired renal or vestibular function. For those with uncomplicated *S. viridans* endocarditis who can manage the technical aspects of outpatient therapy, ceftriaxone monotherapy offers the convenience of single daily administration. The combined regimen consisting of penicillin (or ampicillin) and an aminoglycoside for 4 to 6 weeks can be used for patients infected with NVS or relatively penicillin-resistant strains, those with prosthetic valve infections, and those with longstanding disease (symptoms >3 months).[5,27,30,47]

Assuming the *S. viridans* isolated from A.G. is not resistant to penicillin and he has no other complicating factors, any of the suggested regimens would be appropriate. Because no compelling reason exists to use the 4-week regimens, the 2-week penicillin–aminoglycoside regimen is the most economical choice. Although A.G. has mild renal impairment, this is most likely secondary to the endocarditis and should improve once adequate antimicrobial therapy has been instituted. A.G. was begun on 12 million units/day of penicillin G, which would be reasonable for his age and mild renal impairment. If nephrotoxicity were a major concern in A.G., penicillin or ceftriaxone alone for 4 weeks would be reasonable. If gentamicin is used, A.G.'s dose should be adjusted appropriately and he should be evaluated frequently for signs of toxicity. Periodic peak and trough aminoglycoside concentrations should be monitored.

STAPHYLOCOCCUS EPIDERMIDIS: PROSTHETIC VALVE ENDOCARDITIS

Etiology

6. F.T., a 65-year-old man, presents with chief complaints of anorexia, fever, chills, and weight loss. His past medical history is significant for replacement of his mitral and aortic heart valves (both porcine) 1 year ago for aortic stenosis, mitral regurgitation, and mitral stenosis secondary to rheumatic heart disease. One month later he was readmitted with fever, a right pleural effusion, a pericardial friction rub, and pericarditis. The impression at that time was either postpericardiotomy or Dressler's syndrome. F.T. was sent home on anti-inflammatory agents but failed to improve. After continued complaints of anorexia, nausea, chills, and fever to 101°F, he returned to the hospital. On readmission his physical examination was noteworthy for a systolic ejection murmur at the left sternal border and 3+ pedal edema. Blood cultures were obtained and routine laboratory studies were performed. His history and clinical presentation were strongly suggestive of prosthetic valve endocarditis (PVE). What are the most likely agents responsible for PVE in F.T.?

PVE is a life-threatening infectious complication of artificial heart valve implantation that accounts for 7% to 25% of cases of IE in developed countries.[5,50] The prevalence of complications resulting in death has been as high as 20% to 40%.[51] The risk of PVE after surgery is approximately 1% at 12 months and 2% to 3% at 60 months.[5] PVE is categorized as early or late depending on the onset of clinical manifestations following cardiac surgery.[50,51] Early PVE occurs within 2 months following surgery and is thought to represent infection acquired during valve placement. It usually is caused by skin organisms that were implanted into the valve annulus (suture site where the valve is attached to cardiac muscle) at the time of surgery.[5,50,51] The most common organisms cultured from patients like F.T. with early PVE are coagulase-negative staphylococci (primarily *S. epidermidis* [>30%], most of which are resistant to methicillin), followed by *S. aureus* (20%), and Gram-negative bacilli (10% to 15%). Miscellaneous organisms such as diphtheroids and fungi account for the remainder.[50,51] On the other hand, streptococci are a more common cause of late PVE (>2 months after surgery).[50,51]

Nosocomial bacteremia and fungemia in a patient with prosthetic heart valves contribute to a significant risk for the development of PVE. One study noted that bacteremia due to staphylococci and Gram-negative bacilli resulted in 55% and 33% of subsequent PVE cases, respectively.[54] Another study observed the development of PVE in 25% (11/44) of patients following nosocomial candidemia.[55]

Prophylaxis

7. What measures can be taken to prevent early PVE?

The overall frequency of early PVE, despite antibiotic prophylaxis, is 1% to 4%.[53] Complications are severe and include valve dehiscence, acute heart failure, arrhythmias, and outflow obstruction. Although antibiotic prophylaxis before valve surgery (a "clean" procedure) has not been proven to reduce the frequency of early PVE, it is indicated nevertheless because the complications of infection are catastrophic. Animal data indicate that antibiotic prophylaxis reduces the infection rate.[53]

Cephalosporins

The antimicrobial regimen used most commonly for cardiac surgery prophylaxis consists of an antistaphylococcal cephalosporin, such as cefazolin, given in the operating room at the time of induction of anesthesia or within 60 minutes before the procedure. Drug administration should be timed to produce peak concentrations at the time when bacteremia may result from the procedure. Cephalosporins are frequently selected because they are active against most strains of *S. aureus*. Historically, they also were active against coagulase-negative staphylococci, but the current incidence of methicillin (and cephalosporin) resistance among coagulase-negative staphylococci is as high as 80% for nosocomial isolates.[51,52] Resistance is thought to be caused by an altered penicillin binding protein (PBP 2a); thus, cross-resistance to all other β-lactams is expected.[56]

When a first-generation cephalosporin cannot be used, vancomycin is the alternative prophylactic agent of choice. In a study comparing vancomycin (Vancocin), cefazolin (Ancef), and cefamandole (Mandol) for surgical prophylaxis in 321 patients undergoing cardiac or major vascular operations,[57] the overall surgical wound infection rates were 3.6%, 12.3%, and 11.5% ($P = 0.05$), respectively. Furthermore, no thoracic wound infections occurred in the vancomycin group; the rate was 7% ($P = 0.04$) in the cefazolin group and 4% in the cefamandole group. Given its demonstrated efficacy in the above study, vancomycin could be considered the prophylactic agent of choice for cardiovascular procedures including prosthetic valve replacement and implantation of prosthetic grafts if (1) the patient recently has received broad-spectrum antimicrobial therapy and is likely to be colonized with cephalosporin-resistant staphylococci or enterococci, or (2) the procedure is performed in a center experiencing outbreaks or a high endemic rate of surgical infection with methicillin-resistant staphylococci. Although the effectiveness of vancomycin prophylaxis appeared better than that of cefazolin, hypotension developed in eight patients treated with vancomycin, two patients treated with cefazolin ($P = 0.06$), and none treated with cefamandole. Five of the eight patients, however, were able to continue on vancomycin after slowing the rate of infusion to >1 hour or pretreating with diphenhydramine (Benadryl).

Vancomycin

8. What are the disadvantages of the routine use of vancomycin as a prophylactic agent?

Because the frequency of PVE is low, it would be nearly impossible to demonstrate a statistically significant decrease in its incidence following the use of vancomycin compared with conventional agents. Thus, the decision to use vancomycin rests on its superior in vitro activity for methicillin-resistant staphylococci. However, arguments against the use of vancomycin in this specific setting are compelling. First, the potential for vancomycin-related hypotension is of concern.[57] More importantly, recent emergence of vancomycin-resistant enterococci (VRE) heightens the need to limit vancomycin use, because the prior use of vancomycin, among other factors, has been associated with an increased risk of VRE infection or colonization. The increased incidence of VRE infection/ colonization has serious implications, including increased morbidity and mortality[58] and the transfer of resistant genes present in VRE to other Gram-positive organisms, such as *S. aureus.*[59]

In summary, the most appropriate prophylactic antibiotic for valve replacement surgery is patient and institution specific. The decision should be based on the patient's prior exposure to antibiotics and resultant colonization, in addition to the conditions at each institution, such as the infection rate, the types of organisms recovered, the number of procedures performed, and the feasibility of implementing effective infection control measures.

ADVERSE EFFECTS

9. What is the most common infusion-related adverse effect associated with vancomycin, and how can it be minimized?

The most common adverse effect associated with vancomycin administration is the so-called "red man" or "red neck" syndrome,[60,61] which most commonly causes erythema of the head and upper torso, pruritus, urticaria, and in some cases hypotension. It is mediated in part by histamine release, and the severity of the reaction is proportional to the quantity released (see Chapter 4, Anaphylaxis and Drug Allergies). The total dose of vancomycin administered and the rate of infusion are major determinants of the frequency and severity of this reaction. The reaction can be minimized by administering vancomycin over ≥ 1 hour. Cutaneous manifestations of the vancomycin-induced red man syndrome still can occur with a 1-hour infusion, but hypotension is uncommon.[57,60,61]

Several drugs used perioperatively and in anesthesia also cause histamine release; therefore, the possibility of additive toxicity with vancomycin cannot be dismissed. Most of the serious reactions caused by vancomycin have occurred in patients scheduled for surgery. Vancomycin-induced hypotension occurred in 7% of patients scheduled for cardiothoracic surgery, despite the 1-hour infusion time.[57]

ADMINISTRATION

10. When vancomycin is used to prevent PVE, when should it be administered relative to the time of surgery?

Vancomycin cannot be given in the operating room because it must be administered by infusion over 1 hour, and "on-call" administration may not provide sufficient time for the vancomycin infusion to achieve adequate serum and tissue levels. Therapeutic serum concentrations of vancomycin can be reliably maintained during surgery if the 15-mg/kg dose is infused over 1 hour just before initiation of anesthesia.[57]

Antibiotic-Impregnated Heart Valves

PVE following heart valve replacement surgery is rare, but early-onset infection is associated with a mortality rate of 23% to 41%.[51] Systemically administered antibiotic prophylaxis before surgery does not confer 100% protection. The infectious process typically begins at the sewing ring and extends to involve the adjacent area between the prosthesis and the annulus of the heart valve. Hence, investigators have evaluated the use of antibiotic-impregnated heart valve sewing rings for the prophylaxis and treatment of bacterial endocarditis. Various antibiotics including rifampin, gentamicin, and clindamycin have been studied with respect to their diffusion kinetics and duration of antimicrobial activity both in vitro and in animal experiments.[62–64] However, whether the combination of "local" and systemic antimicrobial prophylaxis enhances the prophylactic efficacy against PVE will require confirmation from clinical trials involving large number of patients.

Antimicrobial Therapy

11. What are the treatment options for F.T.?

As noted earlier, F.T. most likely is infected with coagulase-negative staphylococci. For those rare coagulase-negative staphylococci that remain sensitive to β-lactams (<20%), a penicillinase-resistant penicillin (nafcillin or oxacillin) is the drug of choice (Table 59-5).[83] For the treatment of PVE caused by methicillin-resistant, coagulase-negative staphylococci, vancomycin remains the cornerstone of therapy.[52] Most of the staphylococci remain sensitive to vancomycin at concentrations of <5 μg/mL; however, strains of staphylococci with intermediate susceptibility to vancomycin have emerged in the United States and elsewhere and are increasingly reported.[65,66]

The American Heart Association currently recommends the use of triple-drug combination therapy for the treatment of PVE caused by methicillin-resistant, coagulase-negative staphylococci based on experimental models of endocarditis and limited clinical data.[27] In a retrospective review of 75 episodes of PVE caused by methicillin-resistant *S. epidermidis* (MRSE),[67] 21 of 26 patients treated with vancomycin were cured compared with 10 of 20 patients treated with a β-lactam antibiotic ($P = 0.05$); however, the addition of either rifampin or an aminoglycoside to vancomycin appeared to produce superior results (18 of 20 cured) compared with vancomycin alone (3 of 6 cured, $P = 0.06$). A subsequent prospective multicenter study compared the efficacy of 6 weeks of vancomycin plus rifampin with and without gentamicin for the first 2 weeks for the treatment of PVE caused by MRSE.[51,52] The emergence of rifampin-resistant strains during therapy was reduced by the addition of gentamicin (6 of 15 versus 0 of 8, $P = 0.04$). Based on current data, a three-drug regimen (vancomycin, gentamicin, and rifampin) appears to be optimal for the medical treatment of PVE caused by MRSE, although toxicity would be expected to be greater. When isolates of MRSE are resistant to all available aminoglycosides, aminoglycoside treatment should be omitted. A fluoroquinolone active against the isolate may be considered as substitute for the aminoglycoside in the three-drug regimen. In addition, most patients who responded to medical treatment also required valve replacement surgery.[50,51]

Table 59-5 Treatment of Staphylococcal Endocarditis

Antibiotic	Dosage and Route[b]	Duration
Without Prosthetic Material[a]		
Methicillin-Susceptible Staphylococci		
NONPENICILLIN-ALLERGIC PATIENTS		
Nafcillin		
or	*Adult:* 2 g IV Q 4 hr	4–6 wk
	Pediatric: 150–200 mg/kg per 24 hr IV (max: 12 g/24 hr) in 4–6 equally divided doses	
	Adult: 2 g IV Q 4 hr	
Oxacillin	*Pediatric:* 150–200 mg/kg per 24 hr IV (max: 12 g/24 hr) in 4–6 equally divided doses	4–6 wk
With optional	*Adult:* 1 mg/kg IM or IV (max: 80 mg) Q 8 hr	3–5 days
addition of	*Pediatric:* 2–2.5 mg/kg IV (max: 80 mg) Q 8 hr	
gentamicin[b,c]		
PENICILLIN-ALLERGIC PATIENTS		
1. Cefazolin[d]	*Adult:* 2 g IV Q 8 hr	4–6 wk
	Pediatric: 80–100 mg/kg per 24 hr IV (max: 6 g/24 hr) in equally divided doses Q 8 hr	
With optional addition	*Adult:* See Nonpenicillin-allergic patient	
of Gentamicin[b]	*Pediatric:* See Nonpenicillin-allergic patient	
2. Vancomycin[b,e,f]	*Adult:* 30 mg/kg per 24 hr IV in 2 or 4 equally divided doses (max: 2 g/24 hr unless serum levels monitored)	4–6 wk
	Pediatric: 40 mg/kg per 24 hr IV in 2 or 4 equally divided doses (max: 2 g/24 hr unless serum levels monitored)	
Methicillin-Resistant Staphylococci		
Vancomycin[b,e,f]	*Adult:* 30 mg/kg per 24 hr IV in 2 or 4 equally divided doses (max: 2 g/24 hr unless serum levels monitored)	4–6 wk
	Pediatric: 40 mg/kg per 24 hr IV in 2 or 4 equally divided doses (max: 2 g/24 hr unless serum levels monitored)	
With Prosthetic Valve or Other Prosthetic Material[g]		
Methicillin-Resistant Staphylococci		
Vancomycin[b,e]	*Adult:* 30 mg/kg per 24 hr IV in 2 or 4 equally divided doses (max: 2 g/24 hr unless serum levels monitored)	≥6 wk
	Pediatric: 40 mg/kg per 24 hr IV in 2 or 4 equally divided doses (max: 2 g/24 hr unless serum levels monitored)	
With rifampin[h]	*Adult:* 300 mg PO Q 8 hr	≥6 wk
and	*Pediatric:* 20 mg/kg/24 hr PO (max: 900 mg/24 hr) in 2 equally divided doses	
With gentamicin[b,i,j]	*Adult:* 1 mg/kg IM or IV (max: 80 mg) Q 8 hr	2 wk
	Pediatric: 2–2.5 mg/kg per 24 hr IV (max: 80 mg) Q 8 hr	
Methicillin-Susceptible Staphylococci		
Nafcillin or oxacillin[k]	*Adult:* 2 g IV Q 4 hr	≥6 wk
	Pediatric: 150–200 mg/kg per 24 hr (max: 12 g/24 hr) in 4–6 equally divided doses	
With rifampin[h]	*Adult:* 300 mg PO Q 8 hr	≥6 wk
and	*Pediatric:* 20 mg/kg per 24 hr PO (max: 900 mg/24 hr) in 2 equally divided doses	
With gentamicin[b,i,j]	*Adult:* 1 mg/kg IM or IV (max: 80 mg) Q 8 hr	2 wk
	Pediatric: 2–2.5 mg/kg IV (max: 80 mg) Q 8 hr	

[a]Antibiotic doses should be modified appropriately for patients with impaired renal function. Shorter antibiotic courses have been effective in some drug addicts with right-sided endocarditis caused by *S. aureus*. See text for comments on the use of rifampin.
[b]Dosing of aminoglycosides and vancomycin on a mg/kg basis will give higher serum concentrations in obese than in lean patients.
[c]The benefit of additional aminoglycoside has not been established. The risk of toxic reactions because of these agents is increased in patients >65 years of age or those with renal or eighth nerve impairment.
[d]There is potential cross-allergenicity between penicillins and cephalosporins. Cephalosporins should be avoided in patients with immediate-type hypersensitivity to penicillin (see Chapter 4).
[e]Peak serum concentrations of vancomycin should be obtained 1 hour after infusion and should be in the range of 30–45 μg/mL for BID dosing and 20–30 μg/mL for QID dosing. Trough serum concentrations should be obtained within half an hour of the next dose and should be in the range of 5–15 μg/mL. Each vancomycin dose should be infused over 1 hour.
[f]See text for consideration of optional addition of gentamicin.
[g]Vancomycin and gentamicin doses must be modified appropriately in patients with renal failure.
[h]Rifampin is recommended for therapy of infections caused by coagulase-negative staphylococci. Its use in coagulase-positive staphylococcal infections is controversial. Rifampin increases the amount of warfarin sodium required for antithrombotic therapy.
[i]Serum concentration of gentamicin should be monitored and the dose should be adjusted to obtain a peak level of approximately 3 μg/mL.
[j]Use during initial 2 wk. See text on alternative aminoglycoside therapy for organisms resistant to gentamicin.
[k]First-generation cephalosporins or vancomycin should be used in penicillin-allergic patients. Cephalosporins should be avoided in patients with immediate-type hypersensitivity to penicillin and those infected with methicillin-resistant staphylococci.
Adapted from reference 36 and Wilson WR et al. Antibiotic treatment of adults with infective endocarditis due to streptococci, enterococci, staphylococci, and HACEK microorganisms. JAMA 1995;274:1706–1713. ©1995, American Medical Association.

While quinupristin/dalfopristin (Synercid) and linezolid (Zyvox) have activity against coagulase-negative staphylococci, clinical experience in the treatment of IE caused by these strains is lacking.

STAPHYLOCOCCUS AUREUS ENDOCARDITIS

Intravenous Drug Abuser Versus Nonabuser

12. T.J., a 36-year-old HIV-seropositive man with a long history of IV drug abuse, was admitted to the hospital 4 months after being released from the state prison. His chief complaints on admission were fever, night sweats, pleuritic chest pain, shortness of breath (SOB), dyspnea on exertion (DOE), and fatigue. Physical examination was remarkable for a temperature of 101.2°F, splenomegaly, and a pansystolic ejection murmur at the left sternal border, best heard during inspiration. The chest radiograph revealed diffuse nodular infiltrates. TTE was positive for a small vegetation on the tricuspid valve leaflet. Significant laboratory results included WBC count, 14,000/mm³ with 65% polys and 5% bands; CD4 cell count, 350/mm³; Hgb, 13.1 g/dL; Hct, 39%; and ESR 55 mm/hr (Westergren). IE was suspected. Blood cultures were obtained and all six samples were positive for coagulase-positive, Gram-positive cocci, later identified as methicillin-sensitive S. aureus (MSSA). How do the clinical presentation and prognosis of endocarditis in the IV drug abuser differ from in the nonabuser? What impact does HIV infection have on the risk and outcomes of endocarditis in the IV drug abuser?

[SI units: WBC, 14 × 10⁹/L with 0.65 polys and 0.05 bands (normal, 3.2 to 9.8 with 0.54 to 0.62 polys and 0.03 to 0.05 bands); Hgb, 131 g/L (normal, 140 to 180); Hct, 0.39 (normal, 0.39 to 0.49)]

The annual incidence of endocarditis among IV drug abusers is estimated at 1% to 5%; parenteral cocaine addicts have the highest risk.[68] The presentation, pathophysiology, and prognosis of endocarditis in those who acquire the disease secondary to IV drug abuse differ from those in nonabusers.[1,68,69] Although S. aureus is the pathogen in approximately 30% of all cases of native valve endocarditis, this organism is the most common cause of endocarditis (60% to 90%) in IV drug abusers.[68–70] S. aureus is part of the normal skin flora and is introduced when the illicit drug is injected. It is hypothesized that insoluble agents used to "cut" the drug damage the normal heart valve, preparing the surface for bacterial adherence and growth.

The following are differences between addicts and nonaddicts with S. aureus endocarditis: addicts were significantly younger, had fewer underlying diseases, had more right-sided (tricuspid) involvement (in contrast to the predominance of left-sided disease in the nonaddicts), were less likely to have heart failure or central nervous system (CNS) complications, exhibited fewer signs of peripheral involvement, and had a lower incidence of death.[69]

The prevalence of HIV seropositivity is 40% to 90% among IV drug abusers with IE.[68,70] One case-control study among an ongoing cohort of IV drug users suggested that HIV-related immunosuppression may be an independent risk factor for the development of endocarditis after controlling for confounding variables such as a history of endocarditis or sepsis before enrollment, injection duration, current injection frequency, and a recent history of abscess at injection sites.[72]

Notably, a significantly higher mortality rate was found in HIV-seropositive (CD4 cell counts <200/mm³) IV drug abusers with endocarditis compared with those who were seronegative in a retrospective study. However, the lack of antiretroviral therapy among HIV-seropositive patients in this study contributed to the observed differences in mortality.[73]

Antimicrobial Therapy

Methicillin-Sensitive Staphylococcus aureus

13. What are the therapeutic options for treating S. aureus endocarditis in T.J.?

The susceptibility of S. aureus to methicillin is the major determinant of which antibiotic is selected to treat T.J.'s endocarditis. T.J. is infected with MSSA. The therapy of choice for methicillin-sensitive strains is a penicillinase-resistant penicillin such as nafcillin or oxacillin[27] (see Table 59-5). Penicillin G rarely is appropriate because nearly all isolates of S. aureus produce penicillinase. Methicillin is no longer used because it is associated with a high incidence of interstitial nephritis.

Prospective, randomized, clinical trials have established that 4 to 6 weeks of therapy with high-dose (12 g/day) nafcillin is effective in most patients.[73,74] Recent clinical experience and in vitro studies indicate that vancomycin may be less efficacious than nafcillin as an antistaphylococcal agent.[27,81] Therefore, vancomycin should not be used to substitute for nafcillin merely for dosing convenience. IV drug addicts, for the reasons previously identified, have a higher response rate to appropriate therapy compared with nonaddicts, and 4 weeks of therapy is probably adequate. In one study, 31 addicts were successfully treated with 16 days of parenteral therapy followed by 26 days of oral dicloxacillin.[76]

Addicts with uncomplicated right-sided endocarditis caused by MSSA can be treated successfully with a 2-week course of combination therapy with a penicillinase-resistant penicillin and an aminoglycoside.[77–79] In one study, 47 of 50 patients (94%) were cured after treatment with the combination of IV nafcillin (1.5 g Q 4 hr) and tobramycin (1 mg/kg Q 8 hr) for a total of 2 weeks. Notably, two of three patients in this study who were treated with vancomycin relapsed, resulting in early termination of this arm of study. Thus, vancomycin should not be used to substitute for nafcillin in this regimen. In another study, 71 patients who completed the 2-week course of treatment with cloxacillin (2 g IV Q 4 hr) plus amikacin (7.5 mg/kg IV Q 12 hr) had a cure rate of 94%.[78] Of the four patients who failed, the treatment period had to be extended to achieve cure. In contrast to the prior study, a majority (72%) of patients had definite endocarditis with echocardiographic vegetations. Overall, none of the patients who responded promptly to treatment relapsed. In addition, the risk of nephrotoxicity secondary to 2 weeks of aminoglycoside therapy was minimal in this selected patient population. Alternatively, Ribera and associates demonstrated in a recent study that cloxacillin alone was as effective as combination therapy of cloxacillin plus gentamicin for the treatment of right-sided MSSA endocarditis; the treatment response exceeded 90% in the cloxacillin monotherapy arm.[80] Gentamicin administered at 1 mg/kg Q 8 hr for 7 days in the combination group did not improve treatment response.

Clinical studies thus far support the use of an abbreviated course of treatment in a defined group of IV drug abusers with right-sided endocarditis. These patients should have the following characteristics: (1) clinical and bacteriologic response within 96 hours of initiation of therapy; (2) no evidence of hemodynamic compromise, metastatic infection, or neurologic or systemic embolic complications either at the initiation or completion of 2 weeks of therapy; (3) no echographically demonstrable vegetations >2 cm³; (4) not infected with methicillin-resistant *S. aureus* (MRSA); and (5) not receiving antibiotics other than penicillinase-resistant penicillins such as first-generation cephalosporins and glycopeptides.[27,79] Recent evidence indicates that the addition of an aminoglycoside to the treatment regimen does not appear to improve overall response for patients who meet the above criteria for short-course therapy. Thus, emphasis should be shifted toward careful evaluation of all patients receiving this regimen for evidence of continuing infection or complications at the end of the 2-week treatment course before discontinuing therapy; extension of therapy with a β-lactam agent to at least 4 weeks' duration is prudent for those who demonstrate any evidence of active disease or complications. Finally, a 2-week treatment course should be avoided in patients with underlying HIV infection, such as T.J. While response to antibiotic therapy has been shown to be similar between asymptomatic HIV-seropositive and HIV-seronegative IV drug abusers, it is prudent to avoid short-course therapy in HIV-seropositive IV drug abusers until more definitive outcome data are available in this patient population, particularly those with CD4 cell counts <200/μL.[68]

ORAL REGIMEN

An oral treatment regimen consisting of ciprofloxacin (750 mg Q 12 hr) plus rifampin (300 mg Q 12 hr) has also been evaluated in addicts with uncomplicated right-sided endocarditis. In one small noncomparative study, 10 addicts were successfully treated with the combination of ciprofloxacin and rifampin for 4 weeks.[82] Ciprofloxacin was given IV (300 mg Q 12 hr) for the first 7 days, followed by oral administration (750 mg Q 12 hr) for the remaining 21 days of therapy. A more recent study prospectively compared the oral regimen with standard parenteral therapy for this subgroup.[83] Patients were randomized to receive 28 days of therapy with oral ciprofloxacin plus rifampin or oxacillin (2 g IV Q 4 hr) plus gentamicin (2 mg/kg IV Q 8 hr). Vancomycin (1 g IV Q 12 hr) was substituted for oxacillin in the penicillin-allergic patients. A total of 19 patients completed treatment with oral therapy compared with 25 patients with IV therapy. One of 19 patients in the oral group versus 3 of 25 in the IV group failed treatment; however, the difference in cure rates was not statistically significant. Cure was defined by negative blood cultures after 6 and 7 days posttreatment. Follow-up 1 month after treatment was available in only 30 patients; no failures were detected. Notably, approximately half of the study patients in either group had possible endocarditis, while only 21% versus 31% had definite infections. Given the small number of patients who completed treatment, therapeutic equivalency between the oral and parenteral regimens will need to be confirmed in larger trials. In addition, other issues that may complicate success with this oral regimen are the emerging quinolone resistance in *S. aureus* and the compliance and monitoring required of this regimen when administered in the outpatient setting. Nonetheless, it appears that a 4-week oral regimen with ciprofloxacin and rifampin may be a useful alternative treatment option in addicts with uncomplicated right-sided endocarditis.

PENICILLIN-ALLERGIC PATIENTS

Treatment of penicillin-allergic patients with *S. aureus* endocarditis is somewhat controversial. First-generation cephalosporins have been used with some success for the treatment of patients with mild penicillin allergy, but treatment failures with cefazolin are difficult to explain.[84] The stability of cefazolin when exposed to staphylococcal β-lactamase has been proposed as a mechanism for these failures.[85] Notably, staphylococci are capable of producing four penicillinase subtypes, to which the stability of cefazolin varies. These susceptibility differences are apparent upon MIC testing only if a larger-than-usual inoculum is used (i.e., >10⁶ organisms).[72] It is possible that treatment failures with cefazolin may be caused by a combination of the recalcitrant nature of the infection and the instability of cefazolin against a particular subtype of penicillinase produced by the staphylococcal strain, which is not readily detectable via routine MIC testing. Until further data are available, vancomycin should be used to treat patients with endocarditis caused by *S. aureus* who have immediate-type hypersensitivity to penicillin.

COMBINATION THERAPY

14. **Will the addition of another antibiotic enhance T.J.'s response to nafcillin?**

An enhanced response to combination therapy in the experimental animal model of MSSA endocarditis has prompted clinical trials to evaluate whether the addition of gentamicin to nafcillin confers any additional benefit. The combination of nafcillin and gentamicin resulted in more rapid clearing of organisms from the blood, but the response rates were similar to patients treated with nafcillin alone.[74,75] As expected, the group receiving gentamicin had a higher incidence of nephrotoxicity. Thus, for the routine management of endocarditis caused by MSSA, the addition of a second drug does not appear to offer additional benefit when a penicillinase penicillin is used. The addition of rifampin may be indicated in patients who remain bacteremic or who fail to improve clinically (usually nonaddicts).

Methicillin-Resistant Staphylococcus aureus: Vancomycin

15. **How would T.J.'s therapy differ if he were infected with MRSA?**

Although endocarditis caused by MRSA is relatively uncommon, it occurs in some communities of IV drug abusers with a much higher frequency. As a nosocomial pathogen, MRSA also can cause endocarditis in hospitalized patients.

Failure to correctly identify the organism's susceptibility may result in disastrous consequences. Detailed procedures for identifying these organisms have been published. Recent diagnostic methods based on the use of polymerase chain reaction to identify methicillin-resistant strains more rapidly have been described.[87] Methicillin resistance is heterotypic; in other words, only one in every 10⁶ organisms will be resistant.

The resistance mechanism is similar to that already discussed for *S. epidermidis* (see Question 7). As a result, MRSA should be considered resistant to all β-lactam antibiotics.[52]

TREATMENT OPTIONS

The treatment of choice for MRSA endocarditis is vancomycin; however, resistant strains of *S. aureus* have been identified following repeated and prolonged exposure to vancomycin therapy.[59,65] Vancomycin 30 mg/kg per day in two divided doses for a total of 4 to 6 weeks is recommended for adults with normal renal function. Ideal body weight should be used to dose vancomycin on a mg/kg basis in obese patients. Dosage adjustment for renal dysfunction is necessary. Serum vancomycin concentrations should be targeted for a trough level in the range of 5 to 20 μg/mL within 30 minutes of the next dose.[88] The prolonged distribution phase of vancomycin may affect the reproducibility of peak levels in general, so they are not practical to obtain. Dosage adjustment of vancomycin therapy based on measured trough levels is more reliable.

Although vancomycin is the drug of choice for MRSA endocarditis, response to treatment appears to be slower than with semisynthetic penicillins (e.g., nafcillin) for MSSA endocarditis.[95] The mean duration of bacteremia in patients with MSSA endocarditis has been reported to be 3.4 days for nafcillin alone and 2.9 days for the combination of nafcillin and gentamicin.[69,74] The median duration of bacteremia for MRSA endocarditis was 7 days for vancomycin alone and 9 days for vancomycin with rifampin.[95] Thus, the routine addition of rifampin to the treatment regimen for native valve endocarditis is not recommended.[27] While bacteremia with MRSA isolates responds more slowly to the antibiotics of choice than MSSA isolates, most patients respond to therapy without complications.

The addition of a second drug, such as an aminoglycoside or rifampin, for the routine management of endocarditis caused by MRSA is unnecessary,[89] and the coadministration of vancomycin with an aminoglycoside increases the potential for additive or synergistic nephrotoxicity (see Question 21).[90,91] Trimethoprim-sulfamethoxazole has been used successfully in a limited number of patients with right-sided native valve endocarditis caused by susceptible strains of *S. aureus* and may be an alternative to vancomycin.[92] However, a study of experimental staphylococcal endocarditis found trimethoprim-sulfamethoxazole to be inferior to cloxacillin, vancomycin, and teicoplanin.[93] Alternatively, minocycline has been shown to be a potential treatment alternative to vancomycin in experimental endocarditis caused by MRSA. Although both drugs are equally effective in decreasing the bacterial density of cardiac vegetations, the penetration of minocycline into vegetation was twice that of vancomycin.[94]

Animal models of IE show promise for the two newer agents with activity against MRSA, quinupristin/dalfopristin (Synercid) and linezolid (Zyvox). Clinical success has been reported in limited number of patients with MRSA endocarditis treated with quinupristin/dalfopristin.[99,100] A cure rate of 56% was reported for patients treated with quinupristin/dalfopristin for MRSA endocarditis in an international open trial that evaluated the drug in patients intolerant of or failed prior therapy.[100] On the other hand, linezolid was reported to achieve 50% clinical and microbiologic cure rates at 6-month follow-up in 32 patients with definite IE; MRSA was the causative agent in 7 of those patients. The most common adverse events reported in this group were gastrointestinal system effects and thrombocytopenia, each occurring in 15% of patients.[101] The degree of thrombocytopenia associated with linezolid has been shown to correlate with the extent of drug exposure, as measured by area under the concentration curve and duration of treatment.[102] Of note, treatment failure with linezolid for MRSA endocarditis due to persistent bacteremia has been described in two patients.[146] Thus, additional efficacy data are needed before quinupristin/dalfopristin and linezolid can be recommended for the treatment of IE due to MRSA.

ENTEROCOCCAL ENDOCARDITIS

Antimicrobial Therapy

Antibiotic Synergy

16. G.S., a 35-year-old woman, has been complaining of anorexia, weight loss, and fever for the past 2 months. Her past medical history is significant for an aortic aneurysm with insufficiency that resulted in an aortic valve replacement (porcine) 3 years before admission. Approximately 2 months before admission, G.S. had a cesarean section followed by a tubal ligation. She did not receive antibiotic prophylaxis for either procedure. Physical examination revealed a thin woman (5 foot 0 inches, 48 kg) in no acute distress with evidence of a systolic heart murmur, splinter hemorrhages, and petechiae on her soft palate. Her temperature was 100.2°F. Her WBC count was 14,000/mm³ with a slight left shift; all other laboratory results were within normal limits. She was not taking any medications and she has a documented allergy to penicillin (rash, urticaria, and wheezing). The working clinical diagnosis was probable bacterial endocarditis, which was confirmed when four sets of blood cultures grew Gram-positive cocci. Biochemical testing subsequently identified the organism as *Enterococcus faecalis*, highly resistant to streptomycin (MIC >2,000 μg/mL). Antibiotic therapy with gentamicin (50 mg IV Q 8 hr) and vancomycin (1,000 mg IV Q 12 hr) was begun. Why were two antibiotics prescribed for the treatment of enterococcal endocarditis in G.S.?

[SI unit: WBC, 14 × 10⁹/L]

Enterococci, unlike streptococci, are inhibited but not killed by penicillin or vancomycin alone.[29,103] The synergistic combination of penicillin (or ampicillin, piperacillin, or vancomycin) and an aminoglycoside is required to produce the desired bactericidal effect.[28,104] An antibiotic regimen is synergistic when a combination of antibiotics lowers the MIC to at least one fourth the MIC of either drug alone.[105] The mechanism of synergy against enterococci is caused by an increased cellular uptake of the aminoglycoside with agents that inhibit cell wall synthesis[106] (e.g., β-lactams and vancomycin). Because G.S. is allergic to penicillin, vancomycin was prescribed with an aminoglycoside. Relapse rates are unacceptably high if penicillin is used alone for the treatment of enterococcal endocarditis.[27,29] The addition of an aminoglycoside to penicillin therapy significantly increased the sterilization rate of vegetations in animal studies.[107,108] Numerous clinical studies have confirmed the in vitro synergy for penicillin in combination with streptomycin or gentamicin for enterococcal endocarditis.[109–111]

17. G.S. has enterococcal endocarditis caused by strains exhibiting high-level resistance to streptomycin. Why would (or would not) treatment with gentamicin achieve the desired synergy with vancomycin in G.S. with enterococcus highly resistant to streptomycin?

STREPTOMYCIN RESISTANCE

The combination of streptomycin and penicillin is synergistic for most enterococci that are sensitive to streptomycin (MIC <2,000 μg/mL).[29] However, as many as 55% of all enterococcal blood isolates are highly resistant to streptomycin (MIC >2,000 μg/mL), and the combination is not synergistic for isolates demonstrating this high-level resistance to streptomycin. In contrast, gentamicin in combination with penicillin, ampicillin, or vancomycin is synergistic for most blood isolates of enterococci, regardless of their susceptibility to streptomycin.[1,29,104] In addition, ototoxicity secondary to streptomycin therapy has been noted in nearly 30% of patients receiving the combination regimen for the treatment of enterococcal endocarditis. Unlike gentamicin-induced nephrotoxicity, streptomycin ototoxicity such as vestibular dysfunction is most often irreversible. Maintaining streptomycin peak serum concentrations below 30 μg/mL reduces the risk of ototoxicity, but laboratory assays for streptomycin levels are not readily available. For these reasons, gentamicin in combination with penicillin (or ampicillin) or vancomycin is recommended by most authorities for the treatment of aminoglycoside-susceptible and, in particular, streptomycin-resistant enterococcal endocarditis, as it was for G.S.[27] In cases of aminoglycoside-susceptible enterococcal isolates, either streptomycin or gentamicin in combination with an effective penicillin or vancomycin can be used successfully to treat endocarditis; however, other aminoglycosides cannot be used to substitute for gentamicin or streptomycin because of the uncertain correlation between in vitro synergy and in vivo efficacy.[27] Table 59-6 lists the suggested regimens for the treatment of enterococcal endocarditis.

GENTAMICIN RESISTANCE

Until fairly recently, enterococci exhibiting high-level resistance to gentamicin were uncommon. However, about 10% to 25% of the clinical isolates of *E. faecalis* and up to 50% of *E. faecium* are resistant to gentamicin.[112–114] It is anticipated that the prevalence of these isolates will continue to increase. In one medical center, high-level resistance to gentamicin was observed in 55% of enterococci found in patients.[113] In situations like these, all available aminoglycosides should be tested with penicillin (or ampicillin) for synergistic bactericidal activity. Without conclusive data, some groups favor long-term (8 to 12 weeks) therapy with high-dose penicillin (20 to 40 million units/day IV in divided doses) or ampicillin (2 to 3 g IV Q 4 hr) for treatment of these multiply resistant enterococci. Ampicillin plus the β-lactamase inhibitor sulbactam (Unasyn) would be substituted for β-lactamase–producing, high-level gentamicin-resistant enterococci. In light of the increasing prevalence of enterococci with high-level aminoglycoside resistance, the potential synergistic interaction between ampicillin/amoxicillin and a third-generation cephalosporin was explored recently in vitro and in experimental models of IE. A bactericidal synergistic effect was shown between amoxicillin and cefotaxime against 50 strains of *E. faecalis*. Amoxicillin MIC decreased from 0.25 to 1 μg/mL to 0.01 to 0.25 μg/mL for 48 of 50 strains tested.[115] A similar effect was demonstrated by others using the combination of amoxicillin and ceftriaxone.[116] Additionally, Brandt and colleagues demonstrated a synergistic bactericidal effect for amoxicillin in combination with imipenem against vancomycin-aminoglycoside–resistant *E. faecium* strains.[117] The authors speculated that saturation of different PBPs by different β-lactam agents may be the underlying mechanism for the synergy observed. Limited clinical data on 13 endocarditis cases caused by high-level aminoglycoside-resistant *E. faecalis* treated with the combination of high-dose ceftriaxone (4 g/day) and ampicillin appear to confirm the above synergistic interaction. All 16 evaluable patients were cured by 1 month of double β-lactam therapy with no evidence of relapse during a 3-month follow-up period. Of note, two patients experienced reversible neutropenia and were withdrawn from the study.[118] Double β-lactam therapy appears promising for infections caused by aminoglycoside-resistant *E. faecalis* strains as well as an aminoglycoside-sparing regimen for patients with renal insufficiency, but the above preliminary results need to be confirmed with a larger number of patients.

Gentamicin
DOSING

18. What is the optimal dosage of gentamicin for G.S.?

Because patients with enterococcal endocarditis require prolonged therapy with aminoglycosides, the optimal serum concentration should minimize toxicity without jeopardizing clinical cure. Early in vitro data indicated that the bactericidal activity of gentamicin against enterococci was not significantly different between concentrations of 5 μg/mL and 3 μg/L; however, the differences between 3 μg/mL and 1 μg/mL were significant.[119] In the rat model of endocarditis, the bacterial counts in vegetations at 5 and 10 days were compared between those treated with low-dose (1 mg/kg intramuscularly twice daily) and those treated with high-dose (5 mg/kg intramuscularly twice daily) gentamicin with penicillin.[120] Bacterial counts did not differ at 5 days, but at 10 days they were significantly lower in the rats receiving the high-dose regimen. In contrast, results in the rabbit model showed no difference in the amount of bacteria per gram of vegetation in high- and low-dose gentamicin treatment groups.[121] As for the influence of dosing interval of aminoglycosides on the efficacy of combination regimens in experimental enterococcal endocarditis, studies have demonstrated that multiple daily dosing is more effective in reducing bacterial titers in vegetations than single daily dosing,[122–124] in contrast to that shown with *S. viridans* endocarditis[40] (see Question 4). Thus, extended-interval dosing of aminoglycosides cannot be recommended for the treatment of enterococcal endocarditis at this time.

The only study comparing high-dose (>3 mg/kg per day) and low-dose (<3 mg/kg per day) gentamicin with penicillin in humans with enterococcal endocarditis evaluated 56 patients with enterococcal endocarditis seen over a 12-year period (36 with streptomycin-susceptible and 20 with streptomycin-resistant infections).[125] The relapse rate of patients infected with streptomycin-resistant organisms (n = 20) was not sig-

Table 59-6 Therapy for Endocarditis Caused by Enterococci (or *Streptococci viridans* with an MIC ≥0.5 μg/mL)^{a,b}

Antibiotic	Dose and Route	Duration
Nonpenicillin-Allergic Patient		
1. Aqueous crystalline penicillin G	*Adult:* 20–30 million units/24 hr IV given continuously or in 6 equally divided doses	4–6 wk
	Pediatric: 200,000–300,000 units/kg per 24 hr IV (max: 30 million units/24 hr) given continuously or in 6 equally divided doses	4–6 wk
With gentamicin^{c,d,e}	*Adult:* 1 mg/kg IM or IV (max: 80 mg) Q 8 hr	4–6 wk
or	*Pediatric:* 2–2.5 mg/kg IM or IV (max: 80 mg) Q 8 hr	4–6 wk
With streptomycin^{c,e,f}	*Adult:* 7.5 mg/kg IM (max: 500 mg) Q 12 hr	4–6 wk
	Pediatric: 15 mg/kg IM (max: 500 mg) Q 12 hr	4–6 wk
2. Ampicillin	*Adult:* 12 g/24 hr IV given continuously or in 6 equally divided doses	4–6 wk
	Pediatric: 300 mg/kg per 24 hr IV (max: 12 g/24 hr) in 4–6 equally divided doses	4–6 wk
With gentamicin^{c,d,e}	*Adult:* 1 mg/kg IM or IV (max: 80 mg) Q 8 hr	4–6 wk
or	*Pediatric:* 2–2.5 mg/kg IM or IV (max: 80 mg) Q 8 hr	4–6 wk
With streptomycin^{c,e,f}	*Adult:* 7.5 mg/kg IM (max: 500 mg) Q 12 hr	4–6 wk
	Pediatric: 15 mg/kg IM (max: 500 mg) Q 12 hr	4–6 wk
Penicillin-Allergic Patients^{g}		
Vancomycin^{h}	*Adult:* 30 mg/kg per 24 hr IV in 2 or 4 equally divided doses (max: 2 g/24 hr unless serum levels monitored)	4–6 wk
	Pediatric: 40 mg/kg per 24 hr IV in 2 or 4 equally divided doses (max: 2 g/24 hr unless serum levels monitored)	4–6 wk
With gentamicin^{c,d,e}	*Adult:* 1 mg/kg IM or IV (max: 80 mg) Q 8 hr	4–6 wk
or	*Pediatric:* 2–2.5 mg/kg IM or IV (max: 80 mg) Q 8 hr	4–6 wk
With streptomycin^{c,e,f}	*Adult:* 7.5 mg/kg IM or IV (max: 500 mg) Q 12 hr	4–6 wk
	Pediatric: 15 mg/kg IM (max: 500 mg) Q 12 hr	4–6 wk

^{a}Antibiotic doses should be modified appropriately in patients with impaired renal function.
^{b}Choice of aminoglycoside depends on the resistance level of the infecting strain. Enterococci should be tested for high-level resistance (streptomycin: MIC ≥2,000 μg/mL; gentamicin: MIC ≥500 μg/mL.)
^{c}Serum concentration of gentamicin should be monitored and dosage adjusted to obtain a peak level of approximately 3 μg/mL.
^{d}Dosing of aminoglycosides and vancomycin on a mg/kg basis gives higher serum concentrations in obese than in lean patients.
^{e}Serum concentrations of streptomycin should be monitored if possible and dose adjusted to obtain a peak level of approximately 20 μg/mL.
^{f}Desensitization should be considered; cephalosporins are not satisfactory alternatives.
^{g}Peak serum concentrations of vancomycin should be obtained 1 hour after infusion and should be in the range of 30–45 μg/mL for BID dosing and 20–30 μg/mL for QID dosing. Trough serum concentrations should be obtained within half an hour of the next dose and should be in the range of 5–15 μg/mL. Each dose should be infused over 1 hour.
Adapted from reference 36 and Wilson WR et al. Antibiotic treatment of adults with infective endocarditis due to streptococci, enterococci, staphylococci, and HACEK microorganisms. JAMA 1995;274:1706–1713. ©1995, American Medical Association.

nificantly different between the high- and low-dose treatment groups (n = 10 each). Furthermore, patients who received the higher doses of gentamicin experienced a greater prevalence of nephrotoxicity (10 of 10 versus 2 of 10, $P < 0.001$). Mean peak and trough concentrations of gentamicin in the patients who received the high doses were 5 μg/mL and 2.1 μg/mL, respectively; corresponding levels for patients receiving the low-dose regimen were 3.1 μg/mL and 1 μg/mL.

These data suggest that a gentamicin dosage of 3 mg/kg per day is adequate for most patients with uncomplicated enterococcal endocarditis. However, because of conflicting animal data and the lack of sufficient human data, dosing guidelines for the treatment of streptomycin-resistant strains have not been established. Until more definitive data are available, the dosing of aminoglycosides should be individualized.[27,125]

Based on available data, it would be reasonable to start G.S. on a gentamicin dosage of 1 mg/kg Q 8 hr (assuming his renal function is normal) and to maintain peak concentrations of 3 to 5 μg/mL and trough concentrations of <1 μg/mL.

IN COMBINATION WITH VANCOMYCIN

19. Why was vancomycin used in combination with gentamicin in G.S.? Is this combination effective against enterococci?

G.S. has a history of penicillin allergy. Most clinicians favor a combination of vancomycin and gentamicin for penicillin-allergic patients with enterococcal endocarditis, although vancomycin plus streptomycin is a suitable alternative.[27,29,125] The combination of vancomycin and gentamicin demonstrates bactericidal synergy for about 95% of enterococci strains. In contrast, the vancomycin and streptomycin combination demonstrates bactericidal synergy for about 65% of enterococci.[126] Because G.S. has PVE, she should receive approximately 30 mg/kg per day, or roughly 1.5 g/day (750 mg Q 12 hr), of vancomycin in combination with gentamicin (3 mg/kg per day). Serum levels of vancomycin and gentamicin should be monitored as previously discussed.

Duration of Therapy

20. How long should G.S. be treated?

Historically, enterococcal endocarditis has been treated with penicillin plus an aminoglycoside for 6 weeks; the overall cure rate with this regimen is about 85%.[27] Data indicate that 4 weeks of therapy is probably adequate for most patients with enterococcal endocarditis.[27,125,127] Nine of nine patients with uncomplicated enterococcal endocarditis treated for 4 weeks were cured, and none relapsed.[126] Other studies have reported similar results.[125]

However, patients with complicated courses should receive 6 weeks of therapy. These include patients infected with streptomycin-resistant organisms (such as G.S.), those who have had symptoms for >3 months before the initiation of antibiotics, and patients with PVE (such as G.S.).[17,125,127] Some clinicians recommend 6 weeks of therapy for all patients in whom the duration of illness cannot be firmly established; this accounts for many patients who present with subacute disease.

Increased Nephrotoxicity With Vancomycin Combination Therapy

21. Is the combination of vancomycin and an aminoglycoside more nephrotoxic than either drug alone?

The incidence of nephrotoxicity associated with vancomycin administration (alone) in humans is thought to be minimal or nonexistent.[128] In a three-arm study involving >200 patients,[91] nephrotoxicity was found in 5% of patients who received vancomycin alone, 22% of those receiving vancomycin with an aminoglycoside, and 11% of those receiving an aminoglycoside alone. The study was well designed in that an aminoglycoside control group was included for comparison on the incidence of nephrotoxicity. Patients in whom increases in the serum creatinine concentration may have been a result of clinical conditions and patients who received drugs known to alter renal function were excluded in the analysis of this study. Serial serum vancomycin and aminoglycoside concentrations as well as duration of therapy were reported and analyzed. The authors concluded that vancomycin trough concentrations >10 μg/mL and concurrent therapy with an aminoglycoside were risk factors associated with an increased incidence of nephrotoxicity. Based on the study data, it is difficult to ascertain the precise risk of nephrotoxicity relative to specific vancomycin trough concentrations >10 μg/mL. This issue needs to be studied further because a trough concentration in the range of 10 to 15 mg/L is advocated for the treatment of staphylococcal PVE.[27] A follow-up study by the same group supported the enhanced potential for nephrotoxicity when vancomycin is administered concurrently with an aminoglycoside.[129]

These studies suggest that an increased incidence of nephrotoxicity is likely when vancomycin and an aminoglycoside are given concomitantly. However, the relationship between the trough serum vancomycin concentration and the risk of nephrotoxicity in patients receiving combination therapy remains uncertain.

Glycopeptide Resistance

22. How do enterococci develop vancomycin resistance, and what are the therapeutic implications when managing a patient with glycopeptide-resistant enterococcal endocarditis?

The therapeutic challenges offered by a patient with endocarditis caused by enterococci exhibiting high-level resistance to aminoglycosides are compounded by the acquired resistance of enterococci to glycopeptide antibiotics such as vancomycin. VRE, particularly *E. faecium,* have emerged in the United States since 1987.[58,130] Because the use of prophylactic vancomycin has been increasing steadily since the mid-1980s, it should not be surprising to see increased resistance to this class of compounds. Between 1989 and 1993, the percentage of nosocomial enterococci reported as resistant to vancomycin in the United States rose more than 20-fold, from 0.3% to 7.9%.[130–132] Enterococcal isolates from intensive care units increased even more dramatically, from 0.4% to 13.6%, over the same time. More recent data from the Centers for Disease Control and Prevention's (CDC) National Nosocomial Infections Surveillance (NNIS) system indicated a 40% increase in VRE causing infections in intensive care units between 1999 and the prior 5-year period (1994 to 1998).[133] More importantly, epidemiologic studies conducted by the NNIS system as well as others have shown that VRE bacteremia is associated with significantly increased morbidity and mortality.[132,134]

While *E. faecalis* is responsible for 80% to 90% of infections caused by enterococci, *E. faecium* is more likely to exhibit resistance to glycopeptides compared with *E. faecalis;* more than 95% of VRE recovered in the United States are *E. faecium.*[131] Glycopeptide-resistant enterococci synthesize abnormal peptidoglycan precursors that lower the binding affinity of glycopeptides to peptidoglycans.[58,130] VRE can be broadly classified into three separate phenotypes (A, B, and C), based on three structurally different genes and gene products (e.g., altered ligases).[58] The majority (approximately 70%) of resistant enterococci are of the VanA phenotype, which are resistant to high levels of both vancomycin (MIC >256 μg/mL) and teicoplanin (MIC >16 μg/mL).[58,130] Expression of resistance is inducible, usually plasmid-mediated, and transferable to other organisms via conjugation. The VanB strains exhibit moderate vancomycin resistance (MIC 16 to 64 μg/mL) but remain susceptible to teicoplanin (MIC ≤2 μg/mL). Overall, the VanC isolates are the least resistant (vancomycin MIC 8 to 16 μg/mL; teicoplanin MIC ≤2 μg/mL) because of chromosomal-mediated constitutive expression (i.e., not inducible like VanA and VanB); however, VanC isolates usually are associated with the much less common *E. gallinarum* and *E. casseliflavus* infections.[58,130]

Several studies have implicated prior use of vancomycin as well as extended-spectrum cephalosporins and drugs with potent antianaerobic activity as risk factors for promoting infection and colonization with VRE.[58,130,131]

The emergence of VRE causing serious infections is indeed worrisome because few therapeutic alternatives exist for this organism due to the fact that synergistic combinations are required for bactericidal activity and a clinical cure. As might be anticipated with an organism that is still a relatively uncommon cause of serious infection, well-established guidelines for antimicrobial therapy are not available. To date, no articles have been published in which investigators have demonstrated successful treatment with any particular agent or combination of agents in a large series of patients infected with glycopeptide-resistant enterococci. As a result, practitioners must make decisions using the available data from in vitro synergy studies, experimental models of endocarditis, and scattered case reports. In addition, glycopeptide-resistant isolates often exhibit concomitant high-level resistance to aminoglycosides and/or high-level resistance to β-lactams (e.g., ampicillin, penicillin) secondary to either β-lactamase production or alteration in the target penicillin binding proteins.

Several antibiotic combinations appear promising in vitro and in preliminary animal models of endocarditis, but few data are currently available in humans. Those combinations include high-dose ampicillin (20 g/day) or ampicillin/sulbactam plus an aminoglycoside; vancomycin, penicillin or ceftriaxone and gentamicin; ampicillin and imipenem; ciprofloxacin and ampicillin; ciprofloxacin, rifampin, and gentamicin; teicoplanin and gentamicin[58] (teicoplanin is not available in the United States). New, promising agents under investigation include daptomycin, oritavancin, and tigecycline.

STREPTOGRAMIN AND OXAZOLIDINONE

Quinupristin/dalfopristin (Synercid) and linezolid (Zyvox) are two new agents with activity and proven efficacy against infections caused by VRE recently approved by the FDA in the United States. Quinupristin/dalfopristin (Synercid), available as a fixed 70:30 combination, is the first drug in the streptogramin class made available in the United States for human use. It belongs to the antibiotic family of macrolides/lincosamides/streptogramins. The agent received accelerated approval by the FDA in late 1999 specifically for the treatment of vancomycin-resistant E. faecium bacteremia. The combination is synergistic for glycopeptide-resistant enterococci with an MIC$_{90}$ of 2 μg/mL. The fixed product is generally bactericidal against susceptible streptococci and staphylococci (including methicillin-resistant strains), but it is bacteriostatic against E. faecium. Specifically, E. faecalis is not susceptible to the agent due to the presence of an efflux pump conferring resistance to dalfopristin. Emergence of resistance during therapy has been reported on rare occasions.[136] The recommended dosage is 7.5 mg/kg Q 8 to 12 hr (depending on the severity of infection).[135]

One report describes the largest clinical experience to date on the use of quinupristin/dalfopristin in the treatment of infections caused by multidrug-resistant E. faecium.[137] A total of 397 patients were enrolled in two prospective emergency-use studies. Treatment response varied by indication, with an overall success rate of 65%. Of the five clinically evaluable patients who were treated for endocarditis, only one (20%) responded. The low response rate observed with endocarditis is likely reflected by the need of bactericidal therapy for treatment success. An additional case of E. faecium endocarditis successfully treated by the combination of quinupristin/dalfopristin, doxycycline, and rifampin was reported by Matsumura and colleagues.[138] Arthralgias and/or myalgias were the most frequently reported events (10%) and also most frequently resulted in drug discontinuation.[137] A higher incidence of arthralgias/myalgias has been reported by others (up to 50%); those patients had significant comorbidities.[139] All cases were reversible upon cessation of therapy. Significant venous irritation occurred (46%) when the drug was administered via a peripheral vein. In addition, the dose should be diluted up to 500 to 750 mL, as long as the entire infusion can be given in 1 hour.[137,140] The drug is not compatible with saline solutions. Laboratory abnormalities most frequently observed

were increases in total and conjugated bilirubin in up to 34% of patients. As a result, liver function tests should be obtained once a week during therapy. Because quinupristin/dalfopristin is a potent inhibitor of the cytochrome P450 3A4 enzyme system, coadministration of drugs (e.g., cyclosporine, cisapride) metabolized by the same enzyme system should be avoided if possible, or done only with close monitoring of therapeutic levels.[135,140]

Linezolid (Zyvox) is the first drug in the oxazolidinone class to receive FDA approval for clinical use. Linezolid has bacteriostatic activity against enterococci, including vancomycin-resistant E. faecium and E. faecalis. It is also active against other Gram-positive cocci including S. pneumoniae and methicillin-resistant staphylococci.[135] Vancomycin-resistant E. faecium isolates resistant to linezolid have been encountered in the clinical setting.[141,142] Treatment experience with linezolid under the compassionate use protocol reported clinical and microbiologic cure rates of 50% at 6-month follow-up for patients with endocarditis. Vancomycin-resistant E. faecium was the causative organism for 19 of the 32 patients treated. Treatment response was not subgrouped by causative organisms in this report, which was presented in the form of a meeting abstract.[101] Adverse effects associated with linezolid are generally mild in nature and include nausea, headache, diarrhea, rash, and altered taste. Of greater concern is its potential to cause myelosuppression. Thrombocytopenia, leukopenia, anemia, and pancytopenia have all been reported. Up to 30% of patients treated have been reported to experience thrombocytopenia (platelet counts <100,000 platelets/mm^3).[135] In addition, linezolid is a weak monoamine oxidase inhibitor, which may potentiate the adrenergic effects of sympathomimetic agents (i.e., pseudoephedrine, phenylpropanolamine) and precipitate serotonergic syndrome when used concomitantly with selective serotonin reuptake inhibitors. Patients should be advised to avoid tyramine-containing foods (i.e., aged cheese, sausages, sauerkraut, wine) during therapy as well. Linezolid is available both orally and parenterally. Oral linezolid is completely bioavailable. A dosage of 600 mg BID is recommended for adults. Persistent MRSA bacteremia due to suboptimal serum concentrations of linezolid has been described,[143] suggesting a need to obtain serum drug concentrations in patients not responding appropriately to treatment.

CONTROL OF GLYCOPEPTIDE RESISTANCE

Considering the continuing rise in prevalence and therapeutic challenges associated with VRE, a control effort involving multiple disciplines is necessary to effect a decrease or prevent an increase in the number of patients colonized or infected by these organisms. The primary focus of control should be on limiting vancomycin use to those indications recommended by the CDC's Hospital Infection Control Practices Advisory Committee in 1994 and enforcing strict adherence to infection control practices to minimize cross-contamination of infected or colonized patients.[58,144]

Perhaps the biggest fear regarding VRE is that these enterococci may serve as a reservoir of resistance genes for other organisms, in particular staphylococci. Investigators have provided laboratory evidence that supports the potential for transfer of the VanA gene from enterococci to S. aureus, producing a vancomycin-resistant form.[130]

Selection pressure resulting from continued heavy use of vancomycin is evident in the recent emergence of vancomycin-intermediate *S. aureus* (VISA) and vancomycin-resistant *S. aureus* (VRSA). Cases of VISA have been reported in the United States and Japan.[65] While the mechanism of resistance for VISA is unique and does not appear to be mediated by the VanA gene, all patients had prior infections with MRSA and had received repeated and prolonged vancomycin therapy.[65] More alarming is the most recent recovery of a VRSA strain in a patient who had concurrent VRE infections.[145] This case represents the first demonstration of in vivo transfer of VanA gene from VRE to *S. aureus,* conferring high-level vancomycin resistance (MIC >1,012 μg/mL). The recent isolation of both VISA and VRSA underscores the importance of controlling the spread of vancomycin resistance through proper antibiotic stewardship and infection control practices.

FUNGAL ENDOCARDITIS CAUSED BY *CANDIDA ALBICANS*

Prognosis and Treatment

23. B.G., a 35-year-old male heroin addict, was admitted to the hospital with chief complaints of pleuritic chest pain and DOE. Physical examination revealed a cachectic man with a temperature of 104°F, a diastolic regurgitant heart murmur heard loudest during inspiration, splenomegaly, and pharyngeal petechiae. Funduscopic examination was noncontributory. On the chest radiograph, several pulmonary infiltrates with cavitation were evident. UA was significant for microscopic hematuria and RBC casts. An echocardiogram demonstrated vegetations on both the tricuspid and aortic heart valves. B.G. had evidence of moderate heart failure, although his hemodynamic status at that time was "stable." Six sets of blood cultures were drawn over 2 days and broad-spectrum empiric coverage consisting of vancomycin, gentamicin, and ceftazidime was initiated. Two days later, two of the cultures grew *C. albicans*, and a diagnosis of fungal endocarditis was established. What is B.G.'s prognosis, and how should his fungal endocarditis be managed?

Fungal endocarditis is a rare but life-threatening infection with a grave prognosis that is generally difficult to diagnose and even more difficult to treat.[1] Most cases are caused by *Candida* and *Aspergillus* species. Fungal endocarditis occurs primarily in IV drug abusers, patients with prosthetic heart valves, immunocompromised patients, those with IV catheters, or patients receiving broad-spectrum antibiotics.[147–150]

Management of fungal endocarditis generally requires early valve replacement and aggressive fungicidal therapy with a combination of high-dose amphotericin B (usually 1 mg/kg per day IV) and 5-flucytosine (5-FC; Ancobon) 150 mg/kg per day orally.[1,147–150] These antifungal agents should be prescribed for B.G. and his broad-spectrum antibiotic coverage with vancomycin, gentamicin, and ceftazidime should be discontinued.

B.G.'s clinical presentation and chest radiograph indicate that fragments of vegetation have already embolized to his lungs and possibly to other vital organs (e.g., spleen, kidneys). Because of the morbidity and mortality associated with major emboli and valvular insufficiency, B.G. should undergo surgery within 48 to 72 hours after antifungal therapy has been initiated. Delaying surgery beyond this time frame can increase B.G.'s risk of mortality.

The prognosis for B.G. is dismal even with proper medical and surgical treatment. In a recent series analyzing 270 cases of fungal IE occurring over a 30-year period, mortality for those who received combined medical and surgical management was 45%, compared to 64% for those who received antifungal therapy alone.[149] Despite initial response to treatment, the rate of relapse is high (30% to 40%), and relapse may occur up to 9 years following the initial episode of infection.[147–150] Most deaths in IV drug abusers with endocarditis are secondary to heart failure, a finding already evident in B.G.[1] In addition, replacement of a heart valve for fungal endocarditis in a heroin addict carries a significant risk of late morbidity and mortality.[149]

Combination Therapy With 5-Flucytosine and Amphotericin B

24. Why is it important to treat B.G.'s fungal endocarditis with the combination of 5-FC and amphotericin B? What is the optimal duration of therapy?

The importance of adding 5-FC (Ancobon) to amphotericin B (Fungizone) therapy has not been adequately studied; however, the poor prognosis associated with fungal endocarditis warrants the administration of 5-FC, despite its potential for causing bone marrow suppression and hepatotoxicity[149] (see Chapter 68, Prevention and Treatment of Infections in Neutropenic Cancer Patients, for a discussion of amphotericin B and 5-FC). The vegetations from his tricuspid or aortic heart valves already have broken off and caused pulmonary cavitation and possibly splenomegaly. His clinical presentation is consistent with a potentially fatal outcome; therefore, his blood isolates should be tested for in vitro susceptibility to amphotericin, to 5-FC, and to both of these drugs in combination. Fungi resistant to 5-FC alone may still be susceptible to the synergistic effect of the 5-FC–amphotericin B combination.[151] If the organism is resistant to 5-FC and in vitro synergy between these two antifungals is lacking, continued treatment with 5-FC is not indicated.

The optimal dose and duration of antifungal therapy for fungal endocarditis have not been determined by clinical studies; however, postoperative treatment with amphotericin B and 5-FC (if it has in vitro activity) for a minimum of 6 weeks (total dose, 1.5 to 3 g of amphotericin B) is recommended and is supported by the poor penetration of amphotericin B into heart valve tissue.[152] In patients with fungal PVE, some experts advocate secondary prophylaxis for a minimum of 2 years or lifelong suppressive treatment with an oral antifungal agent for nonsurgical candidates in light of the high rates of relapse.[1, 149–154]

Nephrotoxicity caused by amphotericin is often a serious dose-limiting factor to completion of therapy, particularly in patients who require a prolonged treatment course (see Chapter 66, Osteomyelitis and Septic Arthritis). Renal dysfunction secondary to the conventional formulation of amphotericin B may stabilize or improve with the switch to lipid-formulated amphotericin B products (i.e., Abelcet).[155] However, the efficacy of the new formulations in the treatment of endocarditis has been demonstrated only in anecdotal reports,[149,150,156] while the drug acquisition cost is substantially higher. Alternative antifungal agents may need to be considered in patients who experience significant renal toxicities.

Alternative Antifungals

25. If B.G. experiences significant toxicities because of prolonged combination treatment with amphotericin and 5-FC, what alternative antifungal agent(s) can be used to treat his fungal endocarditis?

Fluconazole (Diflucan) is a triazole compound active against *Candida* species, particularly *C. albicans* and *C. parapsilosis*. It also has a favorable toxicity profile compared with amphotericin and 5-FC.[157] Prolonged combination treatment with amphotericin and 5-FC often is limited by nephrotoxicity, bone marrow suppression, and/or hepatic damage. Limited experimental and clinical experience using fluconazole in the treatment of candidal endocarditis has been accumulating.

Fluconazole was effective in eradicating cardiac fungal vegetations caused by *C. albicans* and *C. parapsilosis* in a rabbit model.[158] Successful experience with fluconazole treatment of fungal endocarditis in humans has been described in only a few case reports.[159–164] Fluconazole-treated endocarditis patients were either intolerant of amphotericin or poor surgical candidates who required suppressive antifungal therapy after completion of a course of amphotericin therapy. Various *Candida* species (i.e., *C. albicans, C. parapsilosis,* and *C. tropicalis*) were treated with 200 to 600 mg of fluconazole daily over 45 days to 6 months or until death. Fluconazole therapy reduced or completely removed all cardiac vegetations and resolved clinical symptoms. However, because of the lack of adequate clinical experience, the use of fluconazole in treating fungal endocarditis cannot be advocated except in patients who require lifelong therapy because of the following situations: (1) the patient is a poor surgical candidate, (2) the patient has relapsed at least once since the initial infection episode, or (3) the patient has PVE.

Another potential alternative is caspofungin, which is a first-line agent in the echinocandin class.[198] Caspofungin was approved by the FDA for salvage therapy against invasive aspergillosis, esophageal candidiasis, and invasive candidiasis (primarily bloodstream infections and peritonitis). Caspofungin inhibits fungal cell wall synthesis by inhibiting β-1,3 glucan synthesis. It is fungicidal against most *Candida* species (including *C. albicans*), and its use is not associated with nephrotoxicity. Both characteristics make the drug an attractive treatment option for B.G. should toxicities develop after prolonged therapy with amphotericin B. However, no clinical experience exists currently to support the use of caspofungin in the treatment of endocarditis.

GRAM-NEGATIVE BACILLARY ENDOCARDITIS CAUSED BY *PSEUDOMONAS AERUGINOSA*

Prevalence

26. Fourteen months after completing his course of antifungal therapy, B.G. was readmitted to the hospital with a 48-hour history of fever, shaking chills, rigors, and night sweats. His vital signs at that time were blood pressure, 100/60 mm Hg; pulse, 120 beats/min; respirations, 24/min; and temperature, 103.7°F. A new-onset systolic murmur was noted on auscultation. Two-dimensional echocardiography revealed two small vegetations on the prosthetic valve. Empiric therapy consisting of amphotericin B, 5-FC, vancomycin, and gentamicin was initi-

ated. Three blood cultures drawn on the day of admission were positive for *P. aeruginosa* with the following antibiotic susceptibilities (MIC): gentamicin (8 μg/mL), tobramycin (2 μg/mL), piperacillin (64 μg/mL), and ceftazidime (2 μg/mL). A presumptive diagnosis of PVE caused by *P. aeruginosa* was made. Why was the finding of *Pseudomonas* expected in B.G.?

The prevalence of endocarditis caused by Gram-negative organisms has increased significantly in recent years, especially in IV drug abusers like B.G. and patients with prosthetic heart valves. Gram-negative organisms are responsible for about 15% to 20% of endocarditis cases in these populations.[165] Most Gram-negative endocarditis cases are caused by *Pseudomonas* species, *S. marcescens,* and *Enterobacter* species, although numerous other Gram-negative organisms have been known to cause endocarditis.[165–170] Geographic clustering of certain organisms causing endocarditis in narcotic addicts has been shown in the past, such as the association of *P. aeruginosa* with the Detroit area and *S. marcescens* with San Francisco.[171 174] These past epidemiologic findings are not necessarily true today. In narcotic addicts with Gram-negative endocarditis, the tricuspid, aortic, and mitral valves are involved in 50%, 45%, and 40% of cases, respectively.[165]

Antimicrobial Therapy

27. How should B.G.'s Gram-negative endocarditis be treated and monitored?

The regimen of amphotericin B, 5-FC, vancomycin, and gentamicin that was initiated empirically for B.G. pending the outcome of culture and sensitivity results should now be discontinued because *P. aeruginosa* has been cultured from B.G.'s blood. Proper antibiotic selection for the treatment of Gram-negative endocarditis should be based on antimicrobial susceptibility and synergy testing. A bactericidal combination of antibiotics usually is required to provide in vivo synergy and to prevent resistant subpopulations from emerging during therapy.[1,35] B.G., therefore, should be treated with ceftazidime (2 g IV Q 8 hr) with concurrent high-dose tobramycin (3 mg/kg IV Q 8 hr). The duration of therapy is not well defined, but most authorities recommend 4 to 6 weeks.[1,166,172] Despite the problems associated with using the SBT as a monitoring tool (see Question 3), therapy should be tailored to achieve a trough titer of at least 1:8.[28] Because B.G. should be receiving both ceftazidime and tobramycin on the same schedule (Q 8 hr), the trough titer should be drawn just before dose administration. Finally, the infected valve should be surgically excised for the reasons previously discussed.

Endocarditis caused by *P. aeruginosa* (as in B.G.) should be treated for at least 6 weeks with a combination of an aminoglycoside and an antipseudomonal penicillin (ticarcillin or piperacillin) or cephalosporin (ceftazidime).[1,172] The combination of an antipseudomonal penicillin and an aminoglycoside is synergistic in vitro and in the rabbit model of *P. aeruginosa* endocarditis,[175,176] and clinical experience has confirmed this finding in IV drug abusers. Combination therapy with high dosages of tobramycin or gentamicin (8 mg/kg per day) has been associated with a significantly higher cure rate and lower mortality rate compared with an older, "low-dose" regimen (2.5 to 5 mg/kg per day).[167,168,172] Aminoglycosides (tobramycin or gentamicin) should be dosed to produce peak and trough serum concentrations of 15 to 20 μg/mL and <2 μg/mL, respectively, to ensure maximum efficacy[1]; therefore, high-dose tobramycin should be selected for B.G.

For obvious reasons, peak and trough aminoglycoside concentrations should be routinely monitored in all patients receiving high-dose therapy for Gram-negative bacillary endocarditis. Of note, the use of extended-interval dosing of aminoglycoside has not been evaluated for the treatment of endocarditis caused by Gram-negative organisms; therefore, this dosing approach cannot be recommended at this time. The choice of aminoglycoside should be based on the in vitro activity of the organism (i.e., MIC), relative toxicity potential, and cost. In B.G.'s case, tobramycin should be selected over gentamicin because the isolated organism exhibited greater susceptibility to this aminoglycoside. Generally *P. aeruginosa* is more susceptible to tobramycin than to gentamicin. Thus, it is not at all surprising that the *P. aeruginosa* in B.G.'s blood cultures had a 2 μg/mL MIC for tobramycin compared with the 8 μg/mL MIC for gentamicin.

Data on the use of ceftazidime for the treatment of *P. aeruginosa* endocarditis are limited; however, it should be preferred over piperacillin in B.G. on the basis of its greater in vitro activity and good penetration into cardiac valvular tissue.[179]

Several compounds such as imipenem (Primaxin), aztreonam (Azactam), and ciprofloxacin (Cipro) have demonstrated excellent in vitro activity against many of the Gram-negative organisms causing endocarditis. However, clinical data regarding their use in the treatment of endocarditis are very limited.[180–183]

CULTURE-NEGATIVE ENDOCARDITIS

28. B.G.'s history, clinical presentation, and imaging studies are strongly suggestive of infective endocarditis. If his blood cultures had been negative after 48 hours of incubation, the working diagnosis would have been culture-negative endocarditis. What are the possible reasons for culture-negative endocarditis, and what measures should be taken to establish a microbiologic etiology?

The proportion of patients with culture-negative endocarditis has diminished considerably, presumably as a result of improved microbiologic culture techniques. Negative blood cultures are present in only 5% to 7% of patients who meet strict criteria for the diagnosis of IE and have not recently received antibiotics.[184]

The prior administration of antimicrobials is thought to account for most cases of culture-negative endocarditis.[185] B.G.'s blood cultures may remain negative for several days to weeks if he has taken antibiotics recently. The use of antibiotic absorbance resins or the addition of β-lactamases to the blood sample may remove or inactivate some antibiotics.[186,187]

Slow-growing and fastidious organisms such as Gram-negative bacilli in the *Haemophilus-Actinobacillus-Cardiobacterium-Eikenella-Kingella* group (HACEK), *Brucella, Coxiella,* chlamydiae, strict anaerobes, and fungi should be pursued in culture-negative patients. This usually is accomplished by the use of special culture media or by obtaining appropriate serologic acute and convalescent titers. Blood cultures should be saved for at least 3 weeks to detect slow-growing organisms.[185] The use of polymerase chain reaction to identify unculturable organisms in excised valvular speci-

mens or septic emboli has been helpful in some cases.[188] Of note, in the past NVS has been the cause of most of the cases of endocarditis diagnosed as "culture-negative" initially due to its requirement for the addition of vitamin B$_6$ (pyridoxal HCl) to the culture media for laboratory growth; however, laboratory identification is no longer a significant problem with current culture media and laboratory techniques.[30]

Empiric Therapy

29. Assume that the causative organism remains unidentified. Recommend an antimicrobial regimen for the empiric treatment of B.G.'s presumed culture-negative endocarditis.

In the hemodynamically stable patient, antibiotic therapy should be withheld until positive blood cultures are obtained.[1] Based on B.G.'s clinical presentation and echocardiographic findings, empiric antibiotics should be initiated as soon as necessary cultures have been collected. Because staphylococci and Gram-negative bacilli account for most organisms responsible for endocarditis in the narcotic addict with a prosthetic heart valve, B.G. should be started on a regimen consisting of an antistaphylococcal penicillin such as nafcillin, an aminoglycoside, and a third agent with Gram-negative coverage. Because B.G. may be experiencing a relapse caused by *C. albicans,* the addition of amphotericin B and flucytosine would be appropriate. If B.G. is from an area where methicillin-resistant staphylococci are prevalent, vancomycin should be substituted for nafcillin. A third-generation cephalosporin (ceftriaxone or ceftazidime) or piperacillin could be used depending on the Gram-negative pathogens common to the region and their anticipated susceptibilities. This regimen, which contains an aminoglycoside and piperacillin, also will provide coverage for enterococci.

The clinical status of B.G. and the positive echocardiogram indicate that early surgical valve excision and replacement are necessary.[189] Cultures obtained from excised valve may result in identification of the causative organism. His antimicrobial regimen may need to be altered if and when subsequent culture information becomes available. Other noninfective conditions, such as atrial myxoma, marasmic endocarditis, and rheumatic fever, may mimic culture-negative endocarditis and should be excluded from the differential diagnosis with the appropriate tests.[1]

PROPHYLACTIC THERAPY

Rationale and Recommendations

30. B.B., a 74-year-old man with poor dentition, is scheduled to have all of his remaining teeth extracted for subsequent fitting of dentures. His past medical history is significant for numerous infections of the oral cavity with abscess formation and mitral valve prolapse with valvular regurgitation. His only current medications are digoxin (Lanoxin) 0.125 mg/day and furosemide (Lasix) 40 mg Q am. What is the rationale for antibiotic prophylaxis?

Because infective endocarditis is associated with significant mortality and long-term morbidity, prevention in susceptible patients is of paramount importance.[1] Unfortunately, it is estimated that <10% of all cases are theoretically preventable.[13,53]

The incidence of endocarditis in patients undergoing procedures known to cause significant bacteremia, even without antibiotic prophylaxis, is low. In addition, endocarditis may develop following the administration of seemingly appropriate chemoprophylaxis. Therefore, it is not surprising that the efficacy of prophylaxis has never been established through placebo-controlled clinical trials. Approximately 6,000 patients would be necessary to demonstrate a statistical difference (if one exists) between untreated controls and a group receiving prophylaxis.[13,53]

Without conclusive clinical data from prospective trials, recommendations for antibiotic prophylaxis have been based largely on in vitro susceptibility data, evaluation of antibiotic regimens using animal models of endocarditis, and anecdotal experiences.[12,13,53,190,191]

Most authorities recommend antibiotic prophylaxis for patients at risk who are undergoing procedures associated with significant bacteremia. Table 59-1 lists the more common conditions and procedures for which antibiotic prophylaxis is currently recommended.

Prophylactic antibiotics are thought to provide protection by decreasing the number of organisms reaching the damaged heart valve from a primary source. Thus, antibiotics theoretically prevent bacterial multiplication on the valve and interfere with bacterial adherence to the cardiac lesion.[13,53]

The 1997 American Heart Association (AHA) recommendations for antibiotic prophylaxis before common medical procedures are outlined in Table 59-7.[13] Compared with pre-

---

Table 59-7   Endocarditis Prophylaxis Regimen for Patients Who Are at Risk

Drug	Dosage
Dental, Oral, or Upper Respiratory Tract Procedures[a]	
Standard Regimen	
Amoxicillin	*Adult:* 2.0 g
	Pediatric: 50 mg/kg PO 1 hr before procedure
Allergic to Penicillin	
Clindamycin	*Adult:* 600 mg
or	*Pediatric:* 20 mg/kg PO 1 hr before procedure
Cephalexin or cefadroxil[b]	*Adult:* 2.0 g
or	*Pediatric:* 50 mg/kg PO 1 hr before procedure
Azithromycin or	*Adult:* 500 mg
clarithromycin	*Pediatric:* 15 mg/kg PO 1 hr before procedure
Unable to Take Oral Medications	
Ampicillin (allergic to	*Adult:* 2.0 g IM/IV
penicillin)	*Pediatric:* 50 mg/kg IM/IV within 30 min before procedure
Clindamycin	*Adult:* 600 mg
or	*Pediatric:* 20 mg/kg IV within 30 min before procedure
Cefazolin[b]	*Adult:* 1.0 g
	Pediatric: 25 mg/kg IM/IV within 30 min before procedure
Genitourinary/Gastrointestinal (Excluding Esophageal) Procedures	
High-Risk Patients	
Ampicillin plus gentamicin	*Adult:* Ampicillin 2.0 g IM/IV plus gentamicin 1.5 mg/kg (max: 120 mg) within 30 min of starting the procedure; 6 hr later, ampicillin 1 g IM/IV or amoxicillin 1 g PO
Moderate-Risk Patients	
Amoxicillin or ampicillin	*Adult:* Amoxicillin 2.0 g PO 1 hr before procedure, or ampicillin 2.0 g IM/IV within 30 min of starting the procedure
Allergic to Ampicillin/Amoxicillin	
HIGH-RISK PATIENTS	
Vancomycin plus gentamicin	*Adult:* Vancomycin 1.0 g IV over 1–2 hr plus gentamicin 1.5 mg/kg IV/IM (max: 120 mg); complete injection/infusion within 30 min of starting the procedure
	Pediatric: Vancomycin 20 mg/kg IV over 1–2 hr plus gentamicin 1.5 mg/kg IV/IM; complete injection/infusion within 30 min of starting the procedure
MODERATE-RISK PATIENTS	
Vancomycin	*Adult:* Vancomycin 1.0 g IV
	Pediatric: 20 mg/kg IV over 1–2 hr; complete infusion within 30 min of starting the procedure

[a]Includes those with prosthetic heart valves and other high-risk patients.
[b]Cephalosporins should not be used in individuals with immediate-type hypersensitivity reaction (urticaria, angioedema, or anaphylaxis) to penicillins.
Reprinted from Dajani AS et al. Prevention of bacterial endocarditis. Recommendations by the American Heart Association. JAMA 1997;277:1794–1801. ©1997, American Medical Association.

vious (1990) guidelines,[192] the current recommendations are considerably less complicated and include the newer macrolides as treatment alternatives.

Dental and Upper Respiratory Tract Procedures

According to the 1997 AHA guidelines, antibiotic prophylaxis is recommended in susceptible persons (see Table 59-1) undergoing any dental procedure that is likely to cause bacteremia secondary to significant bleeding from hard and soft tissues.[13] Those procedures include periodontal surgery, scaling, and professional teeth cleaning. Simple adjustment of orthodontic appliances and spontaneous shedding of deciduous teeth do not require chemoprophylaxis. Endotracheal intubation also does not require prophylactic therapy.

Antimicrobial prophylaxis should be directed against the viridans group of streptococci because these organisms are the most common cause of endocarditis following dental procedures. Surgical procedures involving the upper respiratory tract (e.g., tonsillectomy/adenoidectomy, biopsy of respiratory mucosa, rigid bronchoscopy) may cause transient bacteremia with organisms that have similar antibiotic susceptibilities to those that occur after dental procedures; therefore, the same regimens are suggested. Amoxicillin is currently recommended for oral prophylaxis in susceptible persons undergoing dental or upper respiratory tract surgery. Oral clindamycin, clarithromycin, or azithromycin is recommended for patients with immediate-type hypersensitivity reaction to penicillins. Unlike past recommendations of the AHA, the current guidelines no longer recommend routine parenteral administration of prophylactic antibiotics in high-risk patients because of the logistical and financial barriers that have historically resulted in poor compliance with parenteral regimens.[209] In addition, other countries have accumulated considerable experience using oral regimens in patients with prosthetic heart valves without apparent failure. Patients who already are receiving continuous low-dose penicillin therapy for the secondary prevention of rheumatic fever should receive oral clindamycin, clarithromycin, or azithromycin to protect them against strains of *S. viridans* that have become relatively resistant to penicillin and amoxicillin.

Most cases of endocarditis that are caused by bacterial flora from the mouth do not follow dental procedures but rather are the result of poor oral hygiene. Therefore, it is important to advise patients with underlying cardiac abnormalities to maintain a high level of oral health. Furthermore, a recent large, population-based, case-control study involving 273 case/patients found that dental treatment did not increase the risk for IE among patients with known cardiac abnormalities.[212] Based on the study results, concerns for antimicrobial resistance, and cost, changes to restrict the use of antibiotic prophylaxis to the highest-risk patients before dental procedures may be expected with future guidelines issued by the AHA.

Gastrointestinal and Genitourinary Tract Procedures

The most common organisms responsible for bacteremia following gastrointestinal or genitourinary procedures are Gram-negative aerobes, *E. faecalis* (enterococcus), and anaerobes. Gram-negative organisms and anaerobes rarely cause endocarditis; therefore, in most cases requiring prophylaxis, therapy should be directed against enterococci.[13] Although the

use of ampicillin and an aminoglycoside (gentamicin) is still suggested to achieve synergy and bactericidal activity against enterococci in high-risk patients (e.g., those with a prosthetic heart valve, those who have had endocarditis previously, and those taking oral penicillin for rheumatic fever prophylaxis), "moderate-risk" patients may receive an oral 2-g dose of amoxicillin 1 hour before the procedure. This oral prophylactic regimen, without an aminoglycoside, for these procedures is different from past AHA and Medical Letter recommendations, presumably in an attempt to increase compliance and safety. "High-risk" patients who are allergic to penicillin should receive a combination of vancomycin and gentamicin.

Indications and Choice of Agent

31. Is prophylactic antibiotic therapy indicated for B.B.? If so, which antibiotic(s) should be used?

Based on the current recommendations, B.B. is a candidate for antibiotic prophylaxis. The mitral valve prolapse with valvular regurgitation places him in a higher risk category (as compared with other populations) for developing endocarditis. He also is scheduled to have all of his remaining teeth extracted, a procedure likely to result in bacteremia. According to Table 59-7, B.B. should receive a single 2-g oral dose of amoxicillin 1 hour before the procedure. Previous AHA guidelines recommended a higher dose (3 g) of amoxicillin to be administered before the procedure and followed by a second dose 6 hours after the procedure.[192] When the blood levels and tolerability of 2- and 3-g oral amoxicillin doses were compared in a crossover study involving 30 adult volunteers,[194] the 2-g doses resulted in adequate serum levels; concentrations 6 hours after dosing were well above the MICs for most oral streptococci. Furthermore, no adverse effects were noted with the 2-g dose versus a 10% incidence of gastrointestinal complaints with the 3-g dose.

HOME INTRAVENOUS ANTIBIOTIC THERAPY

32. T.M., a 48-year-old woman, developed *S. viridans* endocarditis following a dental procedure. Her past medical history is significant for rheumatic heart disease and chronic renal insufficiency (measured creatinine clearance, 50 mL/min). She is hemodynamically stable and has no evidence of vegetation on echocardiography. She is currently on day 7 of therapy with penicillin G, 2 million units IV Q 4 hr. The plan is to continue penicillin therapy for a total of 4 weeks. What are the considerations for using home IV therapy for the treatment of infective endocarditis? Is T.M. a candidate for home antibiotic therapy?

The successful use of home IV antibiotic therapy for the patient with endocarditis has been described, although the number of patients treated is relatively small compared with those treated for osteomyelitis.[195–197] The advantages of home therapy include economic benefits to the hospital for early discharge (the diagnosis-related-group [DRG] allocation for endocarditis is 18.4 days, which is shorter than the usual recommended duration of therapy) and the potential for greater acceptance by the patient.[5]

However, home treatment of endocarditis is not without risk.[197] Patients must be hemodynamically stable before discharge and free from the risk of sudden valve rupture. The drug abuser is obviously not a candidate for home treatment, nor is the patient receiving frequent doses of medication. The successful management of any infection amenable to home treatment requires careful patient evaluation for suitability and coordination of the health care provided by key personnel.

T.M. represents the typical patient with uncomplicated streptococcal endocarditis. If the sole reason for continued hospitalization is to administer IV antibiotics, she is a potential candidate for home therapy.

Ceftriaxone is an attractive option for outpatient therapy of uncomplicated endocarditis caused by penicillin-susceptible streptococci. The excellent in vitro activity of ceftriaxone and its long half-life of 6 to 9 hours allow once-a-day administration. The feasibility of intramuscular administration of ceftriaxone also obviates the need for IV access, thus avoiding any potential line-related complications when administered in the outpatient setting.

Clinical experience with the use of ceftriaxone in the treatment of patients with penicillin-susceptible streptococcal endocarditis was described in four open-label studies.[43–46] Two of the studies evaluated ceftriaxone monotherapy for 4 weeks; the other two evaluated combination therapy with ceftriaxone and an aminoglycoside for a 2-week duration. All infecting strains of streptococci in the first two studies were inhibited by ceftriaxone at an MIC of <0.25 μg/mL. In one study, ceftriaxone was given at a dosage of 2 g once daily for 4 weeks to most patients, with 15 receiving ceftriaxone for 2 weeks followed by amoxicillin 1 g four times daily for 2 weeks. Most of the patients received therapy predominantly as outpatients. All patients (n = 30) reported in this study responded favorably to treatment with ceftriaxone or ceftriaxone followed by amoxicillin.[43] Patients with cardiovascular risk factors such as heart failure, severe aortic insufficiency, or evidence of recurrent thromboembolic events were excluded from the study.

Only one probable relapse was noted at 3 months after therapy with presentation of febrile syndrome, elevated sedimentation rate, and negative bacterial blood culture. A more recent uncontrolled study extended the favorable results of the aforementioned study.[57] Treatment was completed in 55 of 59 patients. Patients were followed for 4 months to up to 5 years after the end of treatment with no clinical signs or laboratory evidence of relapse. Seventy-one percent of patients completed therapy without complications; however, 10 required valve replacement secondary to hemodynamic deterioration or recurrent emboli, while 4 required a change in therapy because of drug allergy. Adverse side effects were minor, but three patients had neutropenia that resolved after cessation of therapy.

Because of the lack of controlled trials comparing the efficacy of ceftriaxone against penicillin with or without an aminoglycoside in the treatment of penicillin-susceptible streptococcal endocarditis, ceftriaxone should be considered primarily in patients such as T.M. for whom home antibiotic therapy is a treatment option and who are hemodynamically stable with no evidence of vegetation.

The feasibility of home therapy depends on the following additional factors: (1) patient willingness; (2) adequate venous access; (3) psychosocial stability; (4) access to medical care if an emergency occurs; (5) ability to train T.M. (proper aseptic technique, catheter site care, antibiotic preparation, recognition of untoward effects of the antibiotic, and recognition of symptoms associated with worsening infection); and (6) insurance coverage for home IV therapy. These conditions can be accomplished only with the multidisciplinary involvement of the infectious disease physician, a social worker, a pharmacist, a specialty nurse, and the patient.[216] Home care, outpatient care, and other options will be used increasingly because health care reform mandates the decreased use of tertiary care facilities when possible.

REFERENCES

1. Bayer AS, Scheld WM. Endocarditis and intravascular infections. In: Mandell GL et al, eds. Principles and Practice of Infectious Diseases, 5th ed. New York: Churchill Livingstone, 2000:857.
2. Sullman PM et al. Pathogenesis of endocarditis. Am J Med 1985;78(6B):110.
3. Manning JE et al. An appraisal of the virulence factors associated with streptococcal endocarditis. J Med Microbiol 1994;40:110.
4. Bayer AS et al. Diagnosis and management of infective endocarditis and its complications. Circulation 1998;98:2936.
5. Mylonakis E, Calderwood SB. Infective endocarditis in adults. N Engl J Med 2001;345:18.
6. Cabell CH et al. Changing patient characteristics and the effect on mortality in endocarditis. Arch Intern Med 2002;162:90.
7. Strom BL et al. Dental and cardia risk factors for infective endocarditis. A population-based, case-control study. Ann Intern Med 1998;129:761.
8. Wilson LE et al. Prospective study of infective endocarditis among injection drug users. J Infect Dis 2002;185:1761.
9. Cabell CH, Abrutyn E. Progress toward a global understanding of infective endocarditis. Early lessons from the International Collboration on Endocarditis investigation. Infect Dis Clin North Am 2002;16:255.
10. Erbel R et al. Identification of high-risk subgroups in infective endocarditis and the role of echocardiography. Eur Heart J 1995;16:588.
11. Saccente M, Cobbs CG. Clinical approach to infective endocarditis. Cardiol Clin 1996;14:351.
12. Child JS. Risks for and prevention of infective endocarditis. Cardiol Clin 1996;14:327.
13. Dajani AS et al. Prevention of bacterial endocarditis. Recommendations by the American Heart Association. JAMA 1997;277:1794.
14. Sexton DJ, Spelman D. Current best practices and guidelines. Assessment and management of complications in infective endocarditis. Infect Dis Clin North Am 2002;16:507.
15. Roder BL et al. Neurological manifestations in Staphylococcus aureus endocarditis. A review of 260 bacteremic cases in non-drug addicts. Am J Med 1997;102:379.
16. Belli J, Waisbren BA. The number of blood cultures necessary to diagnose most cases of bacterial endocarditis. Am J Med Sci 1956;50:91.
17. Prazin GL et al. Blood culture positivity: suppression by outpatient antibiotic therapy in patients with bacterial endocarditis. Arch Intern Med 1982;142:263.
18. Sachdev M et al. Imaging techniques for diagnosis of infective endocarditis. Infect Dis Clin North Am 2002;16:319.
19. Heidenreich PA et al. Echocardiography in patients with suspected endocarditis: a cost-effective analysis. Am J Med 1999;107:198.
20. Cheitlin MD et al. ACC/AHA guidelines for the clinical application of echocardiography: executive summary: a report of the American College of Cardiology/American Heart Association Task Force on Practice Guidelines (Committee on Clinical Application of Echocardiography): developed in collaboration with the American Society of Echocardiography. J Am Coll Cardiol 1997;29:862.
21. Rosen AB et al. Cost-effectiveness of transesophageal echocardiography to determine the duration of therapy for intravascular catheter-associated Staphylococcus aureus bacteremia. Ann Intern Med 1999;130:810.
22. Durack DT et al. New criteria for diagnosis of infective endocarditis: utilization of specific echocardiographic findings. Am J Med 1994;96:200.
23. Dodds GA III et al. Negative predictive value of the Duke criteria for infective endocarditis. Am J Cardiol 1996;77:403.
24. Sekeres MA et al. An assessment of the usefulness of the Duke criteria for diagnosing active infective endocarditis. Clin Infect Dis 1997;24:1185.
25. Habib G et al. Value and limitations of the Duke criteria for the diagnosis of infective endocarditis. J Am Coll Cardiol 1999;33:2023.
26. Li JS et al. Proposed modificiations to the Duke criteria for the diagnosis of infective endocarditis. Clin Infect Dis 2000;30:63.
27. Wilson WR et al. Antibiotic treatment of adults with infective endocarditis due to streptococci, enterococci, staphylococci, and HACEK microorganisms. JAMA 1995;274:1706.

28. Le T, Bayer AS. Combination antibiotic therapy for bacterial endocarditis. Clin Infect Dis 2003;36:615.
29. Watanakunakorn C. Penicillin combined with gentamicin or streptomycin: synergism against enterococci. J Infect Dis 1971;124:581.
30. Johnson CC, Tunkel AR. Viridans streptococci and groups C and G streptococci. In: Mandell GL et al, eds. Principles and Practice of Infectious Diseases, 5th ed. New York: Churchill Livingstone, 2000:2167.
31. Alcaide F et al. In vitro activities of 22 B-lactam antibiotics against penicillin-resistant and penicillin-susceptible Viridans group streptococci isolated from blood. Antimicrob Agents Chemother 1995; 39:2243.
32. Carratala J et al. Bacteremia due to Viridans streptococci that are highly resistant to penicillin: Increase among neutropenic patients with cancer. Antimicrob Agents Chemother 1995;20:1169.
33. Doern GV et al. Emergence of high rates of antimicrobial resistance among viridans group streptococci in the United States. Antimicrob Agents Chemother 1996;40:891.
34. Wolfson JS, Swartz MN. Serum bactericidal activity as a monitor of antibiotic therapy. N Engl J Med 1985;312:968.
35. Weinstein MP et al. Multicenter collaborative evaluation of a standardized serum bactericidal test as a prognostic indicator in infective endocarditis. Am J Med 1985;78:262.
36. Bisno AL et al. Antimicrobial treatment of infective endocarditis due to viridans streptococci, enterococci and staphylococci. JAMA 1989;261:1471.
37. Karchmer AW et al. Single-antibiotic therapy for streptococcal endocarditis. JAMA 1979;241:1801.
38. Wilson WR et al. Short-term intramuscular therapy with procaine penicillin plus streptomycin for infective endocarditis due to viridans streptococci. Circulation 1978;57:1158.
39. Wilson WR et al. Short-term therapy for streptococcal infective endocarditis: combined intramuscular administration of penicillin and streptomycin. JAMA 1981;245:360.
40. Gavalda J et al. Effect of gentamicin dosing interval on therapy of viridans streptococcal experimental endocarditis with gentamicin plus penicillin. Antimicrob Agents Chemother 1995;39:2098.
41. Sande MA, Irvin RG. Penicillin-aminoglycoside synergy in experimental streptococcus viridans endocarditis. J Infect Dis 1974;129:572.
42. Malacoff RF et al. Streptococcal endocarditis (nonenterococcal, non-group A): single vs combination therapy. JAMA 1979;241:1807.
43. Stamboulian D et al. Antibiotic management of outpatients with endocarditis due to penicillin- susceptible streptococci. Rev Infect Dis 1991;13(Suppl 2):S160.
44. Francioli P et al. Treatment of streptococcal endocarditis with a single daily dose of ceftriaxone sodium for 4 weeks. JAMA 1992;267:264.
45. Francioli P et al. Treatment of streptococcal endocarditis with a single daily dose of ceftriaxone and netilmicin for 14 days: a prospective multicenter study. Clin Infect Dis 1995;21:1406.
46. Sexton DJ et al. Ceftriaxone once daily for four weeks compared with ceftriaxone plus gentamicin once daily for 2 weeks for treatment of endocarditis due to penicillin-susceptible streptococci. Endocarditis Treatment Consortium Group. Clin Infect Dis 1998;27:1470.
47. Hoen B. Special issues in the management of infective endocarditis caused by Gram-positive cocci. Infect Dis Clin North Am 2002;16:437.
48. Henry NK et al. Antimicrobial therapy of experimental endocarditis caused by nutritionally variant viridans group streptococci. Antimicrob Agents Chemother 1986;30:465.
49. Stein DS, Nelson KE. Endocarditis due to nutritionally deficient streptococci: Therapeutic dilemma. Rev Infect Dis 1987;9:908.
50. Karchmer AW, Longworth DL. Infections of intracardiac devices. Infect Dis Clin North Am 2002;16: 477.
51. Karchmer AW. Infections of prosthetic valves and intravascular devices. In: Mandell GL et al, eds.

52. Archer GL. Staphylococcus epidermidis and other coagulase-negative staphylococci. In: Mandell GL et al, eds. Principles and Practice of Infectious Diseases, 5th ed. New York: Churchill Livingstone, 2000:2092.
53. Durack DT. Prophylaxis of infective endocarditis. In: Mandell GL et al, eds. Principles and Practice of Infectious Diseases, 5th ed. New York: Churchill Livingstone, 2000:917.
54. Fang G et al. Prosthetic valve endocarditis resulting from nosocomial bacteremia: a prospective, multicenter study. Ann Intern Med 1993;119:560.
55. Nasser R et al. Incidence and risk of developing fungal prosthetic valve endocarditis after nosocomial candidemia. Am J Med 1997;103:25.
56. Hartman B, Tomasz A. Altered penicillin-binding proteins in methicillin-resistant strains of Staphylococcus aureus. Antimicrob Agents Chemother 1981;19:726.
57. Maki DG et al. Comparative study of cefazolin, cefamandole, and vancomycin for surgical prophylaxis in cardiac and vascular operations. J Thorac Cardiovasc Surg 1992;104:1423.
58. Murray BE. Vancomycin-resistant enterococcal infections. N Engl J Med. 2000;342:710.
59. Staphylococcus aureus resistant to vancomycin –United States, 2002. MMWR Morbid Mortal Wkly Rep 2002;51:565.
60. Polk RE et al. Vancomycin and the red man syndrome: pharmacodynamics of histamine release. J Infect Dis 1988;157:520.
61. Southorn PA et al. Adverse effects of vancomycin administered in the perioperative period. Mayo Clin Proc 1986;61:721.
62. Cimbollek M et al. Antibiotic-impregnated heart valve sewing rings for treatment and prophylaxis of bacterial endocarditis. Antimicrob Agents Chemother 1996;40:1432.
63. French BG et al. Rifampicin antibiotic impregnation of the St. Jude medical mechanical valve sewing ring: a weapon against endocarditis. J Thorac Cardiovasc Surg 1996;112:248.
64. Karck M et al. Pretreatment of prosthetic valve sewing ring with the antibiotic/fibrin sealant compound as a prophylactic tool against prosthetic valve endocarditis. Eur J Cardiovasc Thorac Surg 1990;4:142.
65. Fridkin S et al. Epidemiological and molecular characterization of infections caused by Staphylococcus aureus with reduced susceptibility to vancomycin, United States, 1997–2001. Clin Infect Dis 2003;36:429.
66. Schwalbe RS et al. Emergence of vancomycin resistance in coagulase-negative staphylococci. N Engl J Med 1987;316:927.
67. Karchmer AW et al. Staphylococcus epidermidis causing prosthetic valve endocarditis: microbiological and clinical observations as guides to therapy. Ann Intern Med 1983;98:447.
68. Miro JM et al. Infective endocarditis in intravenous drug abusers and HIV-1 infected patients. Infect Dis Clin North Am 2002;16:273.
69. Chambers HF et al. The National Collaborative Endocarditis Study Group. Staphylococcus aureus endocarditis: clinical manifestations in addicts and nonaddicts. Medicine (Baltimore) 1983;62:170.
70. Siddiq S et al. Endocarditis in an urban hospital. Arch Intern Med 1996;156:2454.
71. Mathew J et al. Clinical features, site of involvement, bacteriologic findings, and outcome of infective endocarditis in intravenous drug users. Arch Intern Med 1995;155:1641.
72. Manoff SB et al. Human immunodeficiency virus infection and infective endocarditis among injecting drug users. Epidemiology 1996;7:566.
73. Pulvirenti JJ et al. Infective endocarditis in injection drug users: importance of human immunodeficiency virus serostatus and degree of immunosuppression. Clin Infect Dis 1996;22:40.
74. Korzeniowski O, Sande MA. The National Collaborative Endocarditis Study Group: combination antimicrobial therapy for Staphylococcus aureus en-

docarditis in patients addicted to parenteral drugs and nonaddicts. Ann Intern Med 1982;97:496.
75. Abrams G et al. Single or combination therapy of staphylococcal endocarditis in intravenous drug abusers. Ann Intern Med 1979;90:789.
76. Parker RH, Fossieck BE. Intravenous followed by oral antimicrobial therapy for staphylococcal endocarditis. Ann Intern Med 1980;93:832.
77. Chambers HF et al. Right-sided endocarditis in intravenous drug abusers two-week combination therapy. Ann Intern Med 1988;104:619.
78. Torres-Tortosa M et al. Prospective evaluation of a two-week course of intravenous antibiotics in intravenous drug addicts with infective endocarditis. Eur J Clin Microbiol Infect Dis 1994;13:559.
79. DiNubile MJ. Short-course antibiotic therapy for right-sided endocarditis caused by Staphylococcus aureus in injection drug users. Ann Intern Med 1994;121:873.
80. Ribera E et al. Effectiveness of cloxacillin with or without gentamicin in short-term therapy for right-sided Staphylococcus aureus endocarditis: a randomized, controlled trial. Ann Intern Med 1996; 125:969.
81. Fortun J et al. Short-course therapy for right-sided endocarditis due to Staphylococcus aureus in drug abusers: cloxacillin versus glycopeptides in combination with gentamicin. Clin Infect Dis 2001; 33:120.
82. Dworkin RJ et al. Treatment of right-sided Staphylococcus aureus endocarditis in intravenous drug abusers with ciprofloxacin and rifampin. Lancet 1989;1071.
83. Heldman AW et al. Oral antibiotic treatment of right-sided staphylococcal endocarditis in injection drug users: prospective randomized comparison with parenteral therapy. Am J Med 1996;101:68.
84. Bryant RE, Alford RH. Unsuccessful treatment of staphylococcal endocarditis with cefazolin. JAMA 1978;239:1130.
85. Kernodle DS et al. Failure of cephalosporins to prevent staphylococcal surgical wound infections. JAMA 1990;263:961.
86. McDougal LK, Thornsberry CE. New recommendations for disc diffusion antimicrobial susceptibility tests for methicillin-resistant hetero-resistant staphylococci. J Clin Microbiol 1984;19:482.
87. Louie L et al. Evaluation of three rapid methods for detection of methicillin resistance in Staphylococcus aureus. J Clin Microbiol 2000;38:2170.
88. Karam CM et al. Outcome assessment of minimizing vancomycin monitoring and dosing adjustments. Pharmacotherapy 1999;19:257.
89. Perdikaris G et al. Vancomycin or vancomycin plus netilmicin for methicillin- and gentamicin-resistant Staphylococcus aureus aortic valve experimental endocarditis. Antimicrob Agents Chemother 1995;39:2289.
90. Faber BF, Moellering RC Jr. Retrospective study of the toxicity of preparations of vancomycin from 1974 to 1981. Antimicrob Agents Chemother 1983;23:138.
91. Rybak MJ et al. Nephrotoxicity of vancomycin, alone and with an aminoglycoside. J Antimicrob Chemother 1990;25:679.
92. Markowitz N, Quinn EL, Saravolatz LD. Trimethoprim-sulfamethoxazole compared with vancomycin for the treatment of Staphylococcus aureus infection. Ann Intern Med 1992;117:390.
93. DeGorgolas M et al. Treatment of experimental endocarditis due to methicillin-susceptible or methicillin-resistant Staphylococcus aureus with trimethoprim-sulfamethoxazole and antibiotics that inhibit cell wall synthesis. Antimicrob Agents Chemother 1995;39:953.
94. Nicholau DP et al. Minocycline versus vancomycin for treatment of experimental endocarditis caused by oxacillin-resistant Staphylococcus aureus. Antimicrob Agents Chemother 1994;38:1515.
95. Levine DP et al. Slow response to vancomycin or vancomycin plus rifampin in methicillin-resistant Staphylococcus aureus endocarditis. Ann Intern Med 1991;115:674.
96. Jacqueline C et al. Methicillin-resistant Staphylococcus aureus (MRSA) rabbit endocarditis experi-

mental model (REM): In vivo comparative activity between linezolid vs vancomycin. Abstract 671, 40th Interscience Conference on Antimicrobial Agents and Chemotherapy, September 17–20, 2000, Toronto.

97. Jacqueline C et al. Methicillin-resistant *Staphylococcus aureus* (MRSA) rabbit endocarditis model treated by linezolid or vancomycin: comparative in vivo efficacy of continuous infusion. Abstract B-786, 41st Interscience Conference on Antimicrobial Agents and Chemotherapy, December 16–19, 2001, Chicago.

98. Bozigar PS et al. Activity of quinupristin/dalfopristin compared to linezolid in the treatment of vancomycin-resistant *Enterococcus faecium* and methicillin-resistant *Staphylococcus aureus* in experimental model of endocarditis in rabbits. Abstract A-2093, 41st Interscience Conference on Antimicrobial Agents and Chemotherapy, December 16–19, 2001, Chicago.

99. Anwer S et al. Quinupristin/dalfopristin for treatment of MRSA endocarditis refractory to conventional therapy. Infect Dis Clin Pract 1998;7:414.

100. Drew RH et al. Treatment of methicillin-resistant *Staphylococcus aureus* infections with quinupristin-dalfopristin in patients intolerant of or failing prior therapy. J Antimicrob Chmeother 2000;46:775.

101. Dresser LD et al. Results of treating infective endocarditis with linezolid (LNZ). Abstract 2239, 40th Interscience Conference on Antimicrobial Agents and Chemotherapy, September 17–20, 2000, Toronto.

102. Forrest A et al. Pharmacostatistical modeling of hematologic effects of linezolid in seriously ill patients. Abstract 283, 40th Interscience Conference on Antimicrobial Agents and Chemotherapy, September 17–20, 2000, Toronto.

103. Wilkowske CJ et al. Antibiotic synergism: enhanced susceptibility of group D streptococci to certain antibiotic combinations. Antimicrob Agents Chemother 1970;10:195.

104. Drake TA, Sande MA. Studies of the chemotherapy of endocarditis: correlation of in vitro, animal model, and clinical studies. Rev Infect Dis 1983;5(Suppl 2):S345.

105. Eliopoulos GM, Moellering RC Jr. Antimicrobial combinations. In: Lorian V, ed. Antibiotics in Laboratory Medicine. Baltimore: Williams & Wilkins, 1996:330.

106. Moellering RC Jr, Weinberg AN. Studies on antibiotic synergisms against enterococci II: effect of various antibiotics on the uptake of C^{14}-labeled streptomycin by enterococci. J Clin Invest 1971;50:2580.

107. Moellering RC Jr et al. Synergy of penicillin and gentamicin against enterococci. J Infect Dis 1971;124(Suppl):S207.

108. Carrizosa J, Kaye D. Antibiotic synergism in enterococcal endocarditis. J Lab Clin Med 1976; 88:132.

109. Mandell GL et al. An analysis of 38 patients observed at New York Hospital–Cornell Medical Center. Arch Intern Med 1970;125:258.

110. Serra P et al. Synergistic treatment of enterococcal endocarditis. Arch Intern Med 1975;137:1562.

111. Koenig GM, Kaye D. Enterococcal endocarditis. Report of nineteen cases with long-term follow-up data. N Engl J Med 1961;264:257.

112. Eliopoulos GM. Aminoglycoside-resistant enterococcal endocarditis. Med Clin North Am 1993; 17:117.

113. Zervos MJ et al. Nosocomial infection by gentamicin-resistant *Streptococcus faecalis*: an epidemiological study. Ann Intern Med 1987;106:687.

114. Murray BE. The life and times of the enterococcus. Clin Microbiol Rev 1990;3:46.

115. Mainardi JL et al. Synergistic effect of amoxicillin and cefotaxime against *Enterococcus faecalis*. Antimicrob Agents Chemother 1995;39:1984.

116. Gavalda J et al. Efficacy of ampicillin plus ceftriaxone in treatment of experimental endocarditis due to *Enterococcus faecalis* strains highly resistant to aminoglycosides. Antimicrob Agents Chemother 1999;43:639.

117. Brandt CM et al. Effective treatment of multidrug-resistant enterococcal experimental endocarditis with combinations of cell wall-active agents. J Infect Dis 1996;173:909.

118. Gavalda J et al. Efficacy of ampicillin (A) plus ceftriaxone (Ctr) or cefotaxime (Cx) in treatment of endocarditis due to *Enterococcus faecalis* [abstract L1342]. In: Programs and Abstracts of the 41st Interscience Conference on Antimicrobial Agents and Chemotherapy (Chicago). Washington, DC: American Society for Microbiology, 2001:3.

119. Matsumoto JY et al. Synergy of penicillin and decreasing concentrations of aminoglycosides against enterococci from patients with infective endocarditis. Antimicrob Agents Chemother 1980;18:944.

120. Carrizosa J, Levison ME. Minimal concentrations of aminoglycosides that can synergize with penicillin in enterococcal endocarditis. Antimicrob Agents Chemother 1981;20:405.

121. Wright AJ et al. Influence of gentamicin dose size on the efficacies of combinations of gentamicin and penicillin in experimental streptomycin-resistant enterococcal endocarditis. Antimicrob Agents Chemother 1982;22:972.

122. Fantin B, Carbon C. Importance of the aminoglycoside dosing regimen in the penicillin-netilmicin combination for the treatment of *Enterococcus faecalis*-induced experimental endocarditis. Antimicrob Agents Chemother 1990;34:2387.

123. Marangos MN et al. Influence of gentamicin dosing interval on the efficacy of penicillin-containing regimens in experimental *Enterococcus faecalis* endocarditis. Antimicrob Agents Chemother 1997;39:519.

124. Tam VH et al. Once daily aminoglycosides in the treatment of Gram-positive endocarditis. Ann Pharmacother 1999;33:600.

125. Wilson WR et al. Treatment of streptomycin-susceptible and streptomycin-resistant enterococcal endocarditis. Ann Intern Med 1984;100:816.

126. Watanakunakorn C, Bakie C. Synergism of vancomycin-gentamicin and vancomycin–streptomycin against enterococci. Antimicrob Agents Chemother 1973;4:120.

127. Tompsett R, Berman W. Enterococcal endocarditis: duration and mode of treatment. Trans Am Clin Assoc 1977;89:49.

128. Wilhelm MP, Estes L. Vancomycin. Mayo Clin Proc 1999;74:928.

129. Rybak MJ et al. Prospective evaluation of the effect of an aminoglycoside dosing regimen on rates of observed nephrotoxicity and ototoxicity. Antimicrob Agents Chemother 1999;43:1549.

130. Murray BE. Diversity among multi-drug resistant enterococci. Emerging Infect Dis 1998;4:37.

131. Rice LB. Emergence of vancomycin-resistant enterococci. Emerg Infect Dis 2001;7:183.

132. Nosocomial enterococci resistant to vancomycin, United States, 1989–1993. MMWR Morbid Mortal Weekly Report 1993;42:597.

133. Fridkin S. ICU NNIS data 1999 vs 1994–98 on VRE.

134. Lodise TP et al. Clinical outcomes for patients with bacteremia caused by vancomycin-resistant enterococcus in a level 1 trauma center. Clin Infect Dis 2002;34:922.

135. Eliopoulos GM. Quinupristin-dalfopristin and linezolid: evidence and opinion. Clin Infect Dis 2003;36:473.

136. Dowzicky M et al. Characterization of isolates associated with emerging resistance to quinupristin/dalfopristin (Synercid) during the worldwide clinical program. Diagn Microbiol Infect Dis 2000;37:57.

137. Moellering RC et al. The efficacy and safety of quinupristin/dalfopristin for the treatment of infections caused by vancomycin-resistant *Enterococcus faecium*. Synercid Emergency-Use Study Group. J Antimicrob Chemother 1999;44:251.

138. Matsumura S, Simor AE. Treatment of endocarditis due to vancomycin-resistant *Enterococcus fae-*

cium with quinupristin/dalfopristin, doxycycline, and rifampin: a synergistic drug combination. Clin Infect Dis 1998;27:1554.

139. Olsen KM et al. Arthralgias and myalgias related to quinupristin-dalfopristin administration. Clin Infect Dis 2001;32:e83.

140. Fuller RE et al. Treatment of vancomycin-resistant enterococci, with a focus on quinupristin-dalfopristin. Pharmacotherapy 1996;16:584.

141. Gonzales RD et al. Infections due to vancomycin-resistant *Enterococcus faecium* resistant to linezolid. Lancet 2001;357:1179.

142. Herrero IA et al. Nosocomial spread of linezolid-resistant, vancomycin-resistant *Enterococcus faecium*. N Engl J Med 2002;346:867.

143. Sperber SJ et al. Persistent MRSA bacteremia in a patient with low linezolid levels. Clin Infect Dis 2003;36:675.

144. Centers for Disease Control and Prevention. Recommendations for preventing the spread of vancomycin resistance. Recommendations of the Hospital Infection Control Practices Advisory Committee (HICPAC). MMWR Morbid Mortal Wkly Rep 1995;44:1.

145. Tsiodras S et al. Linezolid resistance in a clinical isolate of *Staphylococcus aureus*. Lancet 2001;358:297.

146. Ruiz ME et al. Endocarditis caused by methicillin-resistant *Staphylococcus aureus*: treatment failure with linezolid. Clin Infect Dis 2003;35:1018.

147. Rubinstein E et al. Fungal endocarditis: analysis of 24 cases and review of the literature. Medicine 1975;54:331.

148. Melgar GR et al. Fungal prosthetic valve endocarditis in 16 patients. An 11-year experience in a tertiary care hospital. Medicine 1997;76:94.

149. Ellis ME et al. Fungal endocarditis: evidence in the world literature, 1965–1995. Clin Infect Dis 2001;32:50.

150. Pierrotti LC, Baddour LM. Fungal endocarditis, 1995–2000. Chest 2002;122:302.

151. Shadomy S et al. In vitro studies with combinations of 5-fluorocytosine and amphotericin B. Antimicrob Agents Chemother 1975;8:117.

152. Rubinstein E et al. Tissue penetration of amphotericin B in *Candida* endocarditis. Chest 1974;66:376.

153. Gilbert HM et al. Successful treatment of fungal prosthetic valve endocarditis: case report and review. Clin Infect Dis 1996;22:348.

154. Muehrcke DD et al. Surgical and long-term antifungal therapy for fungal prosthetic valve endocarditis. Ann Thorac Surg 1995;60:538.

155. Wong-Beringer A et al. Lipid formulations of amphotericin B: clinical efficacy and toxicities. Clin Infect Dis 1998;27:608.

156. Melamed R et al. Successful non-surgical treatment of *Candida tropicalis* endocarditis with liposomal amphotericin B (AmBisome). Scand J Infect Dis 2000;32:86.

157. Terrell CL. Antifungal agents. Part II. The Azoles. Mayo Clin Proc 1999;74:78.

158. Nguyen MH et al. *Candida* prosthetic valve endocarditis: Prospective study of six cases and review of the literature. Clin Infect Dis 1996;22:262.

159. Isalska BJ, Stanbridge TN. Fluconazole in the treatment of candidal prosthetic valve endocarditis. Br Med J 1988;297:178.

160. Martino P, Cassone A. Candidal endocarditis and treatment with fluconazole and granulocyte-macrophage colony-stimulating factor [letter]. Ann Intern Med 1990;112:966.

161. Roupie E et al. Fluconazole therapy of candidal native valve endocarditis [letter]. Eur J Clin Microbiol Infect Dis 1991;10:458.

162. Venditti M et al. Fluconazole treatment of catheter-related right-sided endocarditis caused by *Candida albicans* and associated with endophthalmitis and folliculitis. Clin Infect Dis 1992; 14:422.

163. Hernandez JA et al. Candidal mitral endocarditis and long-term treatment with fluconazole in a patient with human immunodeficiency virus infection [letter]. Clin Infect Dis 1992;15:1062.

164. Wells CJ et al. Treatment of native valve *Candida* endocarditis with fluconazole. J Infect 1995; 31:233.

165. Sande MA et al. Endocarditis in intravenous drug users. In: Kaye D, ed. Infective Endocarditis, 2nd ed. New York: Raven Press, 1992:345.

166. Watanakunakorn C. Antimicrobial therapy of endocarditis due to less common bacteria. In: Bisno AL, ed. Treatment of Infective Endocarditis. New York: Grune and Stratton, 1981:123.

167. Ellner JJ et al. Infective endocarditis caused by slow-growing, fastidious, gram-negative bacteria. Medicine 1979;58:145.

168. Cohen PS et al. Infective endocarditis caused by gram-negative bacteria: a review of the literature, 1945–1977. Prog Cardiovasc Dis 1980;22:205.

169. von Graevenitz A. Endocarditis due to nonfermentative gram-negative rods. An updated review. Eur Heart J 1987;8(Suppl J):331.

170. Tunkel AR et al. Enterobacter endocarditis. Scand J Infect Dis 1992;24:233.

171. Reiner NE. Regional pathogens in endocarditis. Ann Intern Med 1976;84:613.

172. Reyes MP, Lerner AM. Current problems in the treatment of infective endocarditis due to *Pseudomonas aeruginosa*. Rev Infect Dis 1983; 5:314.

173. Mills J, Crew D. *Serratia marcescens* endocarditis: a regional illness associated with intravenous drug abuse. Ann Intern Med 1976;84:29.

174. Cooper R, Mills J. *Serratia* endocarditis. A follow-up report. Arch Intern Med 1980;140:199.

175. Archer G, Fekety FR. Experimental endocarditis due to *Pseudomonas aeruginosa*. II. Therapy with carbenicillin and gentamicin. J Infect Dis 1977; 136:327.

176. Lerner SA et al. Effect of highly potent antipseudomonal B-lactam agents alone and in combination with aminoglycosides against *Pseudomonas aeruginosa*. Rev Infect Dis 1984;6(Suppl 3):S678.

177. Reyes MP et al. Treatment of patients with pseudomonas endocarditis with high-dose aminoglycoside and carbenicillin therapy. Medicine (Baltimore) 1978;57:57.

178. Komshian SV et al. Characteristics of left-sided endocarditis due to *Pseudomonas aeruginosa* in the Detroit Medical Center. Rev Infect Dis 1990;12:693.

179. Frank U. Penetration of ceftazidime into heart valves and subcutaneous and muscle tissue of patients undergoing open-heart surgery. Antimicrob Agents Chemother 1987;31:813.

180. Dickinson G et al. Efficacy of imipenem/cilastatin in endocarditis. Am J Med 1985;78(6A):117.

181. Scully BE, Neu HC. Use of aztreonam in the treatment of serious infection due to multiresistant gram-negative organisms, including *Pseudomonas aeruginosa*. Am J Med 1985;78:251.

182. Strunk RW et al. Comparison of ciprofloxacin with azlocillin plus tobramycin in the therapy of experimental *Pseudomonas aeruginosa* endocarditis. Antimicrob Agents Chemother 1985;28:428.

183. Brown NM et al. Ciprofloxacin treatment of bacterial endocarditis involving prosthetic material after cardiac surgery. Arch Dis Child 1997;76:68.

184. Brouqui P, Raoult D. Endocarditis due to rare and fastidious bacteria. Clin Microbiol Rev 2001; 14:177.

185. Hoen B et al. Infective endocarditis in patients with negative blood cultures: analysis of 88 cases from a one-year nationwide survey in France. Clin Infect Dis 1995;20:501.

186. Washington JA II. The role of the microbiology laboratory in the diagnosis and antimicrobial treatment of infective endocarditis. Mayo Clin Proc 1982;57:22.

187. Munro R et al. Is the antimicrobial removal device a cost-effective addition to conventional blood cultures? J Clin Pathol 1984;37:348.

188. Goldenberger D et al. Molecular diagnosis of bacterial endocarditis by broad-range PCR amplification and direct sequencing. J Clin Microbiol 1997;35:2733.

189. Alsip SG. Indications for cardiac surgery in patients with acute infective endocarditis. Am J Med 1985;78(6B):138.

190. Shulman ST et al. Prevention of bacterial endocarditis: a statement for health professionals by the Committee on Rheumatic Fever and Infective Endocarditis of the Council on Cardiovascular Disease in the Young. Circulation 1984;70:1123A.

191. Antibiotic prophylaxis of infective endocarditis recommendations from the endocarditis working party of the British Society for Antimicrobial Chemotherapy. Lancet 1990;335:88.

192. Dajani AS et al. Prevention of bacterial endocarditis. Recommendations by American Heart Association (AHA). JAMA 1990;264:2919.

193. Strom BL et al. Dental and cardiac risk factors for infective endocarditis. A population-based, case-control study. Ann Intern Med 1998;129:761.

194. Dajani AS et al. Oral amoxicillin as prophylaxis for endocarditis: what is the optimal dose? Clin Infect Dis 1994;18:157.

195. Nolet BR. Patient selection in outpatient parenteral antimicrobial therapy. Infect Dis Clin North Am 1998;12:835.

196. Huminer D et al. Home intravenous antibiotic therapy for patients with infective endocarditis. Eur J Clin Microbiol Infect Dis 1999;18:330.

197. Rehm SJ. Outpatient intravenous antibiotic therapy for endocarditis. Infect Dis Clin North Am 1998;12:879.

198. Wong-Beringer A, Kriengkauykiat J. Systemic antifungal therapy: new options, new challenges. Pharmacotherapy 2003;23:1441–1462.

CHAPTER 60

Respiratory Tract Infections

Steven P. Gelone, Judith O'Donnell

Infection of the respiratory tract continues to be the most common and important cause of short-term illness in the United States. It is typically the first infection to occur after birth, with pneumonia being the sixth leading cause of death and the number one infectious disease cause of death in the United States.[1,2] Respiratory tract infections occur more frequently than they are reported and often are thought of as inconveniences of life; however, they are responsible for more days of bed disability, restricted activity, and lost time from work and school than any other category of reported acute illness in America. Respiratory infections account for >40% of disability days secondary to acute illness,[2] and pneumonia and influenza are among the 10 leading causes of death in the overall population, with 80% to 90% of deaths occurring in the elderly (persons older than 65 years of age).[3,4] An estimated 2.2 million people worldwide die yearly because of acute respiratory infections.[5] In 1998, 91,871 people died in the United States as a direct result of pneumonia or influenza. The actual number is much larger, because this figure does not include individuals who died of pneumonia who had other diseases (e.g., HIV, tobacco- and alcohol-related diseases).[3]

The financial impact associated with respiratory infections in 1999 was $25.6 billion ($18.6 billion in direct costs and $7 billion in indirect costs).[1] These figures largely underestimate the financial impact of treating ambulatory respiratory infections. Statistics reported by the National Health Interview Sur-

vey estimate that 182 million episodes of respiratory infection occur for which no medical attention is sought.[2] Often, individuals with respiratory infections try home remedies or over-the-counter (OTC) medications for relief of their symptoms and only seek medical advice or treatment when these efforts fail. The estimated cost associated with the use of OTC medications in this population will contribute an additional $456 million annually to the treatment of respiratory infections.[1]

This chapter addresses the concepts relevant to the treatment and prevention of lower respiratory tract bacterial infections. Upper respiratory tract infections (see Chapter 96, Pediatric Infectious Diseases) and respiratory tract infections caused by viruses (with the exception of influenza) (see Chapter 72, Viral Infections) and fungi (see Chapter 71, Fungal Infections) are presented elsewhere in this book, as are the unique features of respiratory tract infections in immunocompromised hosts (see Chapter 68, Prevention and Treatment of Infections in Neutropenic Cancer Patients) and *Pneumocystis carinii* (see Chapter 70, Opportunistic Infection in HIV-Infected Patients).

Bronchial Infections
Acute Bronchitis

1. F.A., a 35-year-old woman, presents with a persistent cough following an acute respiratory viral infection that began 7 days ago. Although the nasal stuffiness and sore throat resolved 3 or 4 days ago, the cough has persisted and her sputum has become thick and mucoid; a burning, substernal pain is associated with each coughing episode. F.A. is currently afebrile. Coarse rales and rhonchi are heard on physical examination of her chest, and a tentative diagnosis of acute bronchitis is made. How should F.A. be assessed and managed?

Uncomplicated (acute) bronchitis (AB) is an isolated event characterized by inflammation of the tracheobronchial tree and clinically presents as cough of <2 to 3 weeks' duration with or without sputum production. Infectious causes of acute bronchitis are primarily viral and include influenza A and B, rhinovirus, coronavirus, parainfluenza virus 3, and respiratory syncytial virus. As a group, these agents are associated with 5% to 10% of all cases of acute uncomplicated bronchitis in adults. No evidence indicates that *S. pneumoniae, H. influenzae,* or *M. catarrhalis* produces AB in adults without underlying pulmonary disease.

As in F.A., cough—with or without sputum production—is the most prominent clinical feature of this disease. It usually begins early in the course of the syndrome and may persist after the acute infection is resolved. The initial dry, unproductive cough may progress to one with a productive mucoid sputum.

Most healthy adults with typical symptoms of bronchitis do not require diagnostic evaluation. The presence of a fever (≥38°C), heart rate ≥100 beats/min, respiratory rate ≥24 breaths/min, and signs of focal consolidation on chest examination such as rales, egophony, and fremitus are suggestive of the need for a more thorough diagnostic evaluation. Diagnostic studies to reveal a causative agent are not indicated.

The treatment of AB should be directed at symptom control. The use of antitussive agents to control cough, maintenance of adequate hydration, and the intermittent administration of antipyretics such as acetaminophen or ibuprofen should be employed. On the basis of the microbiology of AB, it is not surprising that randomized controlled clinical trials have failed to support a role for antibiotic therapy. Consistent with this, the U.S. Food and Drug Administration removed uncomplicated AB and secondary bacterial infections of AB as indications for randomized clinical trials in 1998. Since then, three meta-analyses have been published, all reporting no impact of antibiotic treatment on illness duration, activity limitation, or work loss, and all concluded that the routine use of antibiotics in adults with AB is not justified. Unfortunately, antibiotics are prescribed for acute bronchitis approximately 6 million times annually in the United States.[6,7] This practice has been documented to be a major source of antibiotic abuse. Encouragingly, data from the National Ambulatory Medical Care Survey (NAMCS) indicate that antibiotic prescriptions in adults with AB have decreased from 76% of cases in 1991–1992 to 59% of cases in 1998–1999 (*P* < 0.001).[8]

As described above, patients whose coughs are severe or prolonged (≥14 days) or present with the signs and symptoms enumerated above should be evaluated more thoroughly and may be candidates for antibiotic therapy.[9–11] In addition, the one common circumstance for which evidence supports antibiotic therapy in patients with uncomplicated AB is the suspicion of pertussis. Unfortunately, no clinical features allow clinicians to distinguish adults with persistent cough due to pertussis primarily because pertussis in adults with previous immunity does not lead to classic whooping cough seen in patients with primary infection. Therefore, treatment should be limited to adults with a high probability of exposure to pertussis, such as that associated with a documented outbreak. The use of antibiotics in this setting will decrease the shedding of the pathogen and the spread of disease.

Chronic Bronchitis
CLINICAL PRESENTATION

2. M.J., a 54-year-old man with a 40-year, 1-pack/day smoking history reports producing 2 cupfuls of whitish-clear, occasionally mucoid sputum per day over the past several years; he coughs up the largest volumes in the morning upon arising. M.J. has a raspy voice and a crackling cough, which often interrupts his talking. Two days ago, he noted that his sputum had increased in volume and had changed in appearance. A sputum sample, which was yellowish-green, tenacious, and purulent, was sent for culture; the Gram's stain showed few epithelial cells, moderate white cells, and a few Gram-positive cocci and Gram-negative rods with no predominant organisms. M.J. denies fever or chills and had no signs of pneumonia; a chest radiograph is negative for consolidation. M.J. has experienced similar episodes three or four times per year. What signs and symptoms in M.J.'s history are consistent with chronic bronchitis?

Chronic bronchitis (CB) is an inflammatory condition of the tracheobronchial tree in which chronic cough and excessive production of sputum are the prominent features. CB and emphysema are components of chronic obstructive pulmonary disease (COPD). In 1994, it was estimated that there were 14 million CB sufferers. Ninety percent of these patients sought treatment for acute exacerbations of CB, accounting for 10 million outpatient visits and 280,000 hospital admissions. Exacerbations may occur from any of the following: infection, smoking, air pollution, exposure to allergens, occupational exposure, or preclinical or subclinical asthma. The cost associated with the hospitalizations alone has been estimated to be $1.5 billion.[12] By definition, patients who cough up sputum daily or on most days over 3 or more consecutive months for >2 successive years presumptively have chronic bronchitis.[13] The diagnosis of CB is made only when other etiologies such as bronchiectasis, cardiac failure, and lung cancer have been excluded. M.J. meets these criteria.

Bronchitis is more common in men than women and more common after the age of 40 than earlier recognized.[14] A genetic basis has been noted with α_1-globulin deficiency, cystic fibrosis, immunoglobulin deficiencies, and primary ciliary dyskinesia. The most common cause of CB is smoking.[15] In M.J., cigarette smoking is an important factor associated with his disease. Smoking is an irritant to the respiratory airways and may stimulate the mucus-secreting goblet cells found in major and smaller bronchi. The increased amount of mucus is not readily cleared from smaller peripheral airways, creating airflow resistance; this accounts for the large volume of sputum cleared from larger airways. However, not all patients with CB have a history of smoking, and 6% to 10% of nonsmoking men will have persistent cough and sputum production.[14]

3. Has M.J.'s bronchitis worsened? What is the likelihood that M.J. has an infection?

Acute exacerbations of chronic bronchitis (AECB) are defined as a worsening of clinical symptoms with increased cough, sputum production, and dyspnea. Some patients report shortness of breath, fatigue, chest tightness, or an increasing cough with dyspnea as their only complaints. Some cases are accompanied by fever, and some patients have symptoms consistent with asthma. Hemoptysis may be seen during acute exacerbations as CB is the most common cause of hemoptysis in the developed world. As in M.J., the most reliable sign of worsening bronchitis is the patient's observation that his or her sputum has changed in amount, color, or consistency. These changes in sputum have been used as presumptive evidence of infection, but similar changes in sputum can be seen without documented infection.[15-17] As illustrated by M.J., patients may present without systemic symptoms of infection such as chills, fever, or leukocytosis.

MICROBIOLOGY

Although infections do not appear to promote the basic disease process or result in deterioration in pulmonary function, they are associated with the majority of exacerbations.[13] The organisms most commonly implicated are viral agents that often cause upper respiratory tract infections. Viruses including influenza A and B, parainfluenza virus 3, coronavirus, and rhinovirus, are associated with AECB in 7% to 64% of patients. Gump and colleagues found viral infections in 32% of patients during AECB compared with 1% of patients during remission periods.[17] The most commonly identified bacterial pathogens associated with acute exacerbations of CB are listed in Table 60-1.

Treatment of a bronchial infection must be directed at organisms found in the pulmonary tree rather than those commonly found in the oral cavity. The correct interpretation of a Gram's stain of a sputum sample depends on whether sputum or saliva has been sampled. Sputum, by definition, represents matter ejected from the lungs or bronchi and should contain, at most, a few white blood cells (WBCs) upon microscopic examination. Upon microscopic evaluation, a good sputum sample should have few epithelial cells. In contrast, saliva often contains large numbers of epithelial cells. The numbers of epithelial cells or WBCs in the sample is important because debilitated patients with pulmonary infection often have difficulty performing the physical maneuvers necessary to eject sputum from the lungs or bronchi. In the case of M.J., the Gram's stain would be interpreted as a good specimen (because of the low number of epithelial cells). The presence of moderate amounts of WBCs is consistent with infection, especially considering the recent change in the volume and appearance of M.J.'s sputum. However, using expectorated sputum cytology alone to assess the likelihood of an infection can be misleading as significant numbers of polymorphonuclear cells can be present throughout the course of CB with or without exacerbation.[18,19]

Many studies have shown that sputum in patients with CB culture grow potential respiratory pathogens when cultured during periods of exacerbations and remissions. Gump and colleagues demonstrated comparable recovery of *Streptococcus pneumoniae* and *Haemophilus influenzae* during periods of exacerbation and remission.[17] Patients with COAD and CB are more likely colonized with these organisms compared with healthy controls.[20] However, a quantitative increase in *S. pneumoniae* during an acute exacerbation is correlated with sputum purulence.[21] This association has not been shown for nontypeable *H. influenzae*.[22] For M.J., the finding of few Gram- positive and Gram-negative organisms with no predominant organism reflects normal oropharyngeal flora and likely colonization with *S. pneumoniae* and *Haemophilus* species. Consequently, this test result provides little additional information to guide antimicrobial therapy.

ANTIBIOTIC THERAPY

4. Should M.J. be given antibiotic therapy to treat his acute episode?

Mild to moderately ill patients without pneumonia, such as M.J., usually do not require antibiotics to treat exacerbations of CB.[23] History of occupational and environmental exposures should be conducted. If smoking is identified as the likely irritant (as in M.J), patients should be encouraged to participate in a comprehensive smoking cessation program. M.J. should be well hydrated and treated with scheduled postural drainage exercises to help mobilize the excessive mucus and improve his pulmonary function. In addition, the use of oral or aerosolized bronchodilators may be of some benefit during acute exacerbations. If his condition does not improve within 3 or 4 days, the initiation of antibiotic therapy should be considered.

Controversy exists regarding the use of antibiotics for AECB. The American Thoracic Society's guidelines regarding the management of exacerbations of chronic bronchitis state, "Although antibiotics have been used extensively for years to treat AECB, as well as for prophylaxis in stable bronchitis, their value for either purpose has not been established."[15,24] Of the many antibiotics used to treat AECB, only amoxicillin, the tetracyclines, trimethoprim- sulfamethoxazole (TMP-SMX), and chloramphenicol have been adequately studied.[25-33] Anthonisen and colleagues observed accelerated clinical recovery in patients treated with an antibiotic versus a placebo (68% versus 55%).[29] In addition, a modest but statistically significant improvement in peak expiratory flow rate (PEFR) also was observed. Saint and colleagues provided a meta-analysis of nine acceptable studies (of 214 reviewed) that addressed the need for antibiotic therapy for AECB.[34] Evaluated agents included tetracyclines, chloramphenicol, ampicillin, and TMP-SMX. These studies, conducted between 1957 and 1992, have shown an overall effect in favor of antibiotic therapy especially in those requiring hospitalization. More recently, newer macrolides (e.g., clarithromycin, azithromycin) and fluoroquinolones (including levofloxacin, gatifloxacin,

Table 60-1 Most Commonly Identified Bacterial Pathogens Associated With Acute Exacerbations of CB

Pathogen	Incidence
H. influenzae	24–26%
H. parainfluenzae	20%
S. pneumoniae	15%
M. catarrhalis	15%
K. pneumoniae	4%
S. marcescens	2%
P. aeruginosa	2%

and moxifloxacin) appear to be equally efficacious, but not superior to older therapies for this indication.[25-33] Table 60-2 serves as a useful guide in selecting antibiotics for AECB.

Independent of selection, predetermined outcome measures should be closely monitored. One of these measures is the infection-free interval (IFI) when persons with chronic bronchitis are not taking antibiotics. The IFI is hypothesized to relate to a decrease in colonization of the upper airways with bacteria, influence the cost of treatment of AECB, and aid in constraining antibiotic use in AECB.[37] The length of the infection-free period, as well as the change in the number of physician office visits and hospital admissions, with a particular antibiotic regimen is extremely important to identify in each patient. The longest infection-free period defines that antibiotic regimen as the regimen of choice for that specific patient for future exacerbations of their disease. Three comparative studies have been conducted with ciprofloxacin to evaluate the IFI as an outcome measure.[38,39] When compared with clarithromycin, the IFI for ciprofloxacin was 142 days versus 52 days ($P = 0.15$), compared to cefuroxime the IFI was 146 days versus 178 days ($P = 0.35$), and when compared to amoxicillin/clavulanate it was 163 days versus 178 days ($P = 0.81$). The infection-free period is a dynamic outcome measure that needs to be continually evaluated to determine the most appropriate therapy at any point in time in each patient.

ANTIBIOTIC PROPHYLAXIS

5. What strategies should be considered in the use of antibiotic prophylaxis if M.J. develops frequent exacerbations?

Prophylactic antibiotic therapy decreases the number of acute exacerbations of bronchitis in patients with frequent episodes.[14,40] In patients such as M.J. with infrequent exacerbations, prophylaxis does not appear to be beneficial and should be discouraged in this setting. Prophylaxis may be considered in patients with frequent, severe exacerbations, but used only during critical periods when patients are most susceptible. For example, daily doses of antibiotics 4 days a week during the winter months[41] or a 7-day course of antibiotics at the first sign of a "chest cold" have been suggested. As previously mentioned, amoxicillin, doxycycline, or TMP-SMX are preferred.[42,43] Caution should be exercised with the use of newer agents (e.g., antipneumococcal fluoroquinolones) because of a lack of additional benefit, including efficacy, cost effectiveness, adverse effects, and the development of bacterial resistance.

PNEUMONIA

Pneumonia is an inflammation of the lung parenchyma that is caused by infection. Considering that pneumonia is not a reportable disease and most community-acquired infections are treated on an outpatient basis, it is difficult to determine its true incidence morbidity. Approximately 4 million cases of community-acquired pneumonia (CAP) occur annually, with 25% requiring hospitalization.[44] Of those patients hospitalized for pneumonia, the average mortality rate is 10% to 12%.[45-47] Mortality depends on the type and number of underlying diseases, age of the patient, complications that occur during the hospitalization, and pathogen. Table 60-3 summarizes the mortality associated with various bacterial pneumonias. The aggregate cost of care in the United States has been estimated to be in excess of $4.4 billion annually.[45,47-50]

Normal Respiratory Tract Defenses

6. A.T., a 58-year-old man, is admitted to the hospital from home with fever, increased sputum production, tachypnea, and complaints of a knifelike chest pain that is made worse by coughing and breathing. Pertinent medical history includes a 12-year history of chronic bronchitis and chronic renal insufficiency. A.T. regularly produces 2 cups of sputum per day and continues to smoke 2.5 packs of cigarettes per day. He has been taking amoxicillin 250 mg BID prophylactically for the past 14 months.

Physical examination reveals an elderly man lying restlessly in bed, awake, and oriented to person but not place or time; temperature, 101.5°F (38.6°C), blood pressure (BP), 145/88 mm Hg; heart rate (HR), 105 beats/min; and respiratory rate (RR), 33 breaths/min. Chest examination reveals slight splinting on the right side with inspiration and fine crackling rales in the lower base of the right lung. Examination of the left lung is normal.

Significant laboratory results include the following: WBC count, 16,200 cells/mm³ (normal, 5,000 to 10,000 cells/mm³); differential polymorphonuclear neutrophils (PMNs), 82% (normal, 45% to 79%); bands, 9% (normal, 0% to 5%); lymphocytes, 8% (normal, 16% to 47%); hematocrit (Hct), 40% (normal, 37% to 47%); sodium, 141; potassium, 4.8; blood urea nitrogen, 32; creatinine, 3.8 mg/dL; glucose 148, mg/dL; arterial blood gases (ABGs), pH 7.46 (normal, 7.38 to 7.45), PO₂, 68 mm Hg (normal,

Table 60-2 Guide to Selecting Antibiotics for AECB[35]

Simple AECB	FEV₁ >35–50% of predicted	*H. influenzae*	Macrolide, doxycycline
	<4 AECB/year	*S. pneumoniae*	2nd/3rd generation cephalosporin
	No comorbidities	*M. catarrhalis*	Amoxicillin/clavulanate
	Low rate of penicillin resistance	Viruses	
Complicated AECB	FEV₁ <35–50% predicted	*H. influenzae*	Amoxicillin/clavulanate
	Increased age	*S. pneumoniae*	Fluoroquinolone
	≥4 AECB/year	*M. catarrhalis*	
	Comorbidities	Gram-negative bacilli	
	Increased risk of penicillin resistance		
Severe AECB	Recurrent antibiotic or steroid therapy	Gram-negative bacilli	Based on culture
	Bronchiectasis		

The relapse rates of selected antibiotics in the treatment of AECB has been reported to be 55% for amoxicillin, 22% for ciprofloxacin, 21% for macrolides, and 8% for amoxicillin/clavulanate.[36]

Table 60-3 Mortality Rates by Pathogen for Community-Acquired Pneumonia

Pathogen	Mortality Rate (%)
S. pneumoniae	12
H. influenzae	7.4
S. aureus	31.8
K. pneumoniae	35.7
P. aeruginosa	61
Legionella	14.7
C. pneumoniae	9.8
M. pneumoniae	1.4

80 to 100 mm Hg), PCO_2, 36 mm Hg (normal, 38 to 45 mm Hg), HCO_3, 24 mEq/L (normal, 22 to 26 mEq/L); and Gram's stain reveals <10 epithelial cells, 20 to 25 PMNs, and predominance of Gram-negative rods.

What are the normal respiratory defenses against infection?

[SI units: WBC count, 16.2×10^9/L (normal, 5 to 10); differential PMNs, 0.82 (normal, 0.45 to 0.79); bands, 0.09 (normal, 0 to 0.05); lymphocytes, 0.08 (normal, 0.16 to 0.47); Hct, 0.45 (normal, 0.37); PO_2, 9.06 kPa (normal, 10.66 to 13.33); PCO_2, 4.8 kPa (normal, 5.07 to 6)]

Preservation of normal respiratory tract function involves a complex system of local pulmonary lung defenses. Anatomic, functional, and mechanical barriers protect the tracheobronchial tree from inert particle and microbial invasion. In addition, an intricate system of cellular and humoral immune host defenses contribute to maintain the respiratory tract free of infection. Intrinsic defects in these normal defenses predispose the patient to respiratory infections.[51,52]

The hairs lining the nasal passages, ciliated epithelial cells on mucosal surfaces, production of mucus, salivary enzymes, and the mechanical process of swallowing minimize the passage of foreign material into the lower respiratory tract. Disease states, environmental factors, and age may alter the integrity and influence the function of these barriers.

Alteration in normal oropharyngeal flora by disease or antibiotics permit colonization of the oropharynx with more pathogenic bacteria. Colonization of the oropharynx in itself is not predictive of infection but predisposes the patient who may aspirate oropharyngeal secretions to infection.

Neurologic diseases and altered states of consciousness, which result in the loss of control of epiglottal and laryngeal function, predispose the patient to recurrent episodes of aspiration of upper respiratory tract secretions. Without an intact cough or gag reflex, the volume of upper respiratory secretions reaching the lower airways may exceed the local lung defenses, increasing the risk for infection. Patients at risk include any patient with altered consciousness secondary to disease or drugs (e.g., alcoholics, stroke victims, substance abusers, epileptics, surgical patients receiving general anesthesia, head injury patients, patients with any illness associated with obtundation).

A functioning mucociliary transport system, which traps and removes foreign material from the lower respiratory tract, is critical to the protection of the lungs. Diseases that alter mucus production and ciliary function severely compromise the body's ability to defend against infection.

Finally, defects in the cellular and humoral immune response compromise the host to invading pathogens.[53] These defenses include the pulmonary macrophages residing within the alveoli, polymorphonuclear leukocytes, and immunoglobulin and complement present in lung tissue. Deficiency of the latter substances is associated with an increase in the prevalence of infection with encapsulated organisms (i.e., S. pneumoniae, H. influenzae). These substances enhance the body's defense against bacterial invaders by functioning as opsonins to improve the efficiency of phagocytosis.

In the normal state, the lungs are repeatedly inoculated with microorganisms from the upper airway and inhaled aerosols, but pneumonia rarely occurs.[54] Defects in one or more of the aforementioned mechanisms expose the lung to an increased inoculum of microorganisms for a sufficient period, resulting in pneumonia.

Risk Factors

7. What factors present in A.T.'s case make him susceptible to pulmonary infection?

Most bacterial pneumonias probably result from the entry of pathogenic bacteria present in the mouth and upper respiratory tract into the lung. In the healthy state, the bacterial flora of the oropharynx consists of a mixture of aerobic bacteria (including *Streptococcus* species, *S. pneumoniae*) and anaerobic bacteria (including *Peptococcus* species, *Peptostreptococcus* species, *Fusobacterium* species, *Prevotella melaninogenica*, and various *Bacteroides* species such as *Bacteroides melaninogenicus* and *Bacteroides fragilis*).[55] Suppression of normal flora by broad-spectrum antibiotics (e.g., amoxicillin in A.T.) and the host's physiologic state can alter oropharyngeal flora.[56,57] These factors facilitate the colonization of the oropharynx with significant numbers of pathogenic Gram-negative aerobic bacteria and staphylococci. Gram-negative rods, including *Klebsiella* spp., are cultured from the sputum in 2% to 18% of healthy individuals, but the number of organisms is usually small.[58,59]

Gram-negative bacilli commonly occur in the oropharyngeal secretions of patients with moderate to severe acute and chronic illnesses who have had no exposure to broad-spectrum antibiotics.[60,61] Patients admitted to the hospital with acute illnesses are rapidly colonized with aerobic Gram-negative bacilli. Approximately 20% are colonized on the first hospital day, and this number increases with the duration of hospitalization and severity of illness.[57] Approximately 35% to 45% of hospitalized patients[57] and up to 100% of critically ill patients[59] will be colonized within 3 to 5 days of admission.

The elderly also have a higher prevalence of oropharyngeal colonization with Gram-negative rods. Colonization increases with the level of independence: for example, Gram-negative bacteria are recovered from the oropharyngeal cultures of 9% of the elderly living in apartments and 60% of elderly in acute hospital wards.[62] Altered pulmonary clearance resulting from a decrease in mucociliary transport, a decrease in cell-mediated immunity, altered immunoglobulin production and antibody response, and an increase in the severity of underlying diseases all contribute to increased colonization and pneumonia in the elderly.[53,63] Colonization of the upper respiratory tract with Gram-negative bacteria correlates with the development of infection as well.[57,59,60]

Colonization of the lower respiratory tract is well established in patients with chronic bronchitis such as A.T.[64] Whether a positive sputum culture represents a true pulmonary infection or simple colonization of the respiratory tract is difficult to determine. Additional data from the patient's history, physical examination, and laboratory tests are necessary to interpret the positive sputum culture.

Clinical Presentation

8. **What clinical signs, symptoms, and laboratory tests are consistent with pneumonia in A.T.?**

Nearly all patients with pneumonia have fever, cough (with or without sputum production), and a physical examination and chest radiograph revealing consolidation in one or more areas of the lung.[50] Tachypnea, fever, tachycardia, the chest examination, and chest radiograph findings represent an acute pulmonary process in this patient.

Although a number of tests are used to document pneumonia, a chest radiograph best distinguishes pneumonia from other disease states. Congestive heart failure, pulmonary embolism, and other diseases may mimic the signs and symptoms of pneumonia. In the majority of cases, a chest radiograph best differentiates between acute bronchitis, an infection that does not require antibiotics, and pneumonia, one that benefits from antimicrobial therapy. Consequently, a chest radiograph is recommended for all patients hospitalized for presumed pneumonia. The radiograph also may be useful in evaluating the severity of disease (multilobar versus single lobe involvement). Importantly, A.T. has not received a chest radiograph at this time; thus, a radiograph is recommended to confirm the diagnosis of pneumonia.

Attempts have been made to classify pneumonia as "typical" or "atypical." This categorization originated from the presumption that the presenting symptoms of pneumonia secondary to pathogens such as *S. pneumoniae, H. influenzae, Staphylococcus aureus,* and enteric Gram-negative bacteria ("typical") is different from that observed for Mycoplasma, Legionella, and Chlamydia ("atypical"). However, both the American Thoracic Society and the Infectious Diseases Society of America caution that this categorization is flawed. *S. pneumoniae* and viruses have been documented to cause a syndrome indistinguishable from that caused by *M. pneumoniae.* Consequently, reliance on the presence of specific symptoms in the etiology of pneumonia may be unreliable. The aforementioned difficulty with a pathogen-specific diagnosis commonly results in the empiric use of antibacterials in the treatment of pneumonia.

A.T. has many signs and symptoms of pneumonia. Fever, tachypnea, tachycardia, a productive cough, and a change in the amount or character of the sputum are common in patients with pneumonia. A.T. gives a history of pleuritic (knifelike) chest pain and examination of the chest shows splinting and an inspiratory lag on the right side during inspiration. All these signs are suggestive of a pneumonic process and usually are present on the affected side. Decreased breath sounds, dullness on chest percussion, and egophony (E to A changes) found during auscultation of the chest also are highly suggestive of consolidation. A.T. is also hypoxemic as evidenced by his PO_2 of 68 mm Hg. The chest radiograph is important in identifying and/or confirming a pulmonary infiltrate in patients with respiratory infections. A.T.'s WBC count is elevated with a left shift (predominance of PMNs and bands); this is consistent with bacterial infection.

Determination of Etiologic Agent

9. **How can the etiologic organism be determined?**

Adequately and appropriately collected sputum that is Gram stained and cultured remain the mainstays in identifying the etiologic organisms of acute pneumonias. Most often, sputum is collected by having the patient cough and expectorate lower respiratory tract secretions into a collection container; however, because the secretions must pass through the mouth, they may become contaminated with mouth flora. The sputum should be examined macroscopically and the color, consistency, amount, and odor should be recorded. Acceptable specimens should contain 25 PMNs/low-power field (LPF).[65] If there is a predominant organism on Gram's stain, empiric therapy can be directed toward the most likely organism. Patients with risk factors for pneumonia (e.g., elderly, hospitalized, chronically ill) often are colonized by multiple pathogens and a sputum culture is seldom helpful in identifying the specific causative organism.[66] In these cases, physical examination, chest radiograph, and changes in sputum production and quality continue to be the cornerstone for the diagnosis of pneumonia. In patients admitted to the hospital, blood cultures should be evaluated in making a diagnosis, as approximately 12% to 25% will have a positive blood culture with a respiratory pathogen. Empiric antibiotic therapy may be directed based on bacterial morphology or Gram's stain while awaiting the culture results to become available 24 to 48 hours later.

If a patient is unable to give an acceptable sputum specimen after three to four attempts, transtracheal aspiration, bronchoscopy, or open lung biopsy can be used to obtain sputum or tissue samples for laboratory analysis. However, these procedures are not without risk and should be used only when the etiology is crucial for diagnosis.

Table 60-4 Microbiology of Community-Acquired Pneumonia

Microbial Agent	Percentage
Bacteria	
S. pneumoniae	20–60
H. influenzae	3–10
S. aureus	3–5
Gram-negative bacilli	3–10
Atypical Agents	
Legionella species	2–8
M. pneumoniae	1–6
C. pneumoniae	4–6
Viral	2–15
No diagnosis	30–60

Microbiology

The major pathogens for CAP are summarized in Table 60-4.[50,53,67-70] These reports potentially are biased because most are based on studies of hospitalized patients and there is significant variation in the recovery of atypical pathogens, including viruses (influenza A and B), Legionella species, *C. pneumoniae,* and *M. pneumoniae*. Even with extensive diagnostic studies, the causative organism is identified in only 30% to 50% of cases. Several factors contribute to this low yield: (1) 20% to 30% of patients do not provide sputum samples, (2) 20% to 30% have received prior antimicrobial therapy, and (3) some pathogens can only be detected by using specialized techniques.

S. pneumoniae is the most common cause of pneumonia in all age groups, identified in 25% to 60% of all community-acquired bacterial pneumonias.[67] The sudden, rapid onset of dramatic rigor, pleuritic chest pain, a rust-colored sputum with Gram-positive diplococci, and leukocytosis are consistent with pneumococcal pneumonia.

H. influenzae is a significant pulmonary pathogen in infants and children. In recent years, *H. influenzae* also has been recognized as a significant pulmonary pathogen in adults. This trend may be related to the fact that the population is growing older and the number of patients with chronic lung diseases is increasing. The incidence of β-lactamase–producing *H. influenzae* has increased over the past several years, complicating antimicrobial selection.[71,72]

Gram-negative pneumonia in the community setting is increasing in incidence.[50,70] Most cases occur in patients who reside in nursing homes and long-term care facilities. In addition, alcoholic individuals are predisposed to Gram- negative pneumonia, often with *K. pneumoniae*.

The atypical pathogens of CAP are theoretically associated with an atypical clinical presentation, including subacute onset, nonproductive cough, extrapulmonary manifestations, and a chest radiograph that is characteristically worse than the patient's clinical appearance. However, a clear association between these organisms and an atypical presentation is debatable. Atypical pathogens account for 10% to 20% of all cases; however, frequency varies based on temporal and geographic epidemiologic patterns. Diagnostic tests for Legionella include culture, direct fluorescent antigen stain, or urinary antigen assays which are adequate for a presumptive diagnosis and empiric therapy.

Legionella pneumophila contributes significantly to the incidence of CAP.[70] Patients with altered immunologic function (e.g., elderly) and chronic diseases (e.g., COAD) are most susceptible to infection with this organism. Legionella is more common in middle-age and elderly adults and has the highest mortality rate of the atypical pathogens. Its presentation may be associated with significant GI complaints (nausea, vomiting) and electrolyte abnormalities. It is similar to serious pneumococcal pneumonia in that the clinical course of many patients is progressive despite administration of appropriate antibiotic therapy. The reported mortality rate is 15% to 25%, even with effective therapy.[47,73]

Mycoplasma (also called walking pneumonia) is more common in young adults.[50,74] Diagnostic tests are available (primarily an immunoglobulin [Ig] M enzyme immunoassay), but most laboratories do not provide these tests. Mycoplasma

carries virtually no mortality. *C. pneumoniae* reportedly accounts for 5% to 10% of all cases of CAP.[50,75] It has been associated with atherosclerotic disease; however, cause and effect continues to be debated. Diagnostic tests for this pathogen are not offered by most clinical laboratories.

Viral agents account for 2% to 15% of all cases of CAP.[50] Influenza A and B, adenovirus, and parainfluenza virus are most commonly reported in adults, whereas respiratory syncytial virus is most common in the pediatric population.

Epidemiologic factors may favor the presence of certain pathogens.[45] Patients with poor dental hygiene are likely to be infected with anaerobes, whereas HIV-coinfected individuals are more likely to be infected by *P. carinii*. A thorough travel and animal-contact history is important. Exposure to birds can be associated with *Chlamydia psittaci* (the cause of psittacosis), exposure to cattle or a parturient cat can be associated with *Coxiella burnetii* (the cause of Q fever), and travel to the southwestern United States can be associated with *Coccidioides immitis* infections. In addition, in the current age of bioterrorism, agents such as *Bacillus anthracis* (anthrax), *Francisella tularensis* (tularemia), and *Yersinia pestis* (plague) may need to be considered as potential causes of pneumonia.

Site of Care for Treatment of Community-Acquired Pneumonia

10. **How should A.T. be treated?**

Considering that hospitalization accounts for 89% to 96% of pneumonia costs, it is important to identify high-risk patients.[47] Risk factors for 30-day mortality have been derived by Fine and colleagues by using age, gender, laboratory data on admission, and comorbidities (Fig. 60-1).[44,44a] Patients in risk categories I and II have extremely low mortality rates associated with pneumonia and should be treated as outpatients. Patients in risk stratum III may require a brief hospitalization; those in categories IV and V should be hospitalized. These data do not include patients with HIV or other immunocompromised states. Furthermore, they do not take into account social issues such as home support and the likelihood of adherence with treatment requirements, all of which may necessitate hospitalization. Although not prospectively evaluated for this purpose, severity stratification also may identify candidates for oral antibiotics after initial parenteral therapy.

In the case of A.T., he is a 58-year old man (58 points), has a history of chronic renal insufficiency (10 points), a respiratory rate of ≥30 (20 points), and has an altered mental status (20 points). His score of 108 points places him in risk strata III, which carries a 30-day mortality risk of 8.2% to 9.3% (see Fig. 60-1). Based on his Pneumonia Severity Index (PSI) assessment and his clinical status, he should be admitted to the hospital.

INITIATION OF ANTIMICROBIAL TREATMENT

Initial antimicrobial therapy is largely empirical and should be guided by the results of the sputum Gram's stain, patient age, medical history, concomitant diseases, place of residence, clinical signs and symptoms, and allergy status. An approach to the patient with CAP is presented in Figure 60-2, and antibiotic regimens of choice are provided in Tables 60-5 through 60-7.[45] If no sputum is available for Gram's stain or

Step 1. Is the patient low risk (class I) based on history and physical examination and not a resident of a nursing home?
- Age 50 years or younger, and
- None of the coexisting conditions or physical examination findings listed in step 2

NO ☐→ Go to step 2

YES ☐→ Outpatient treatment is recommended

Step 2. Calculate risk score for classes II-V

Patient Characteristics	Points Assigned	Patient's Points
Demographic factors		
Age (in years)		
Males	Age	
Females	Age − 10	
Nursing home resident	+ 10	
Coexisting conditions		
Neoplastic disease	+ 30	
Liver disease	+ 20	
Congestive heart failure	+ 10	
Cerebrovascular disease	+ 10	
Renal disease	+ 10	
Initial physical examination findings		
Altered mental status	+ 20	
Respiratory rate ≥ 30/min	+ 20	
Systolic BP < 90 mmHg	+ 20	
Temperature < 35⁻ or ≥ 40° C	+ 15	
Pulse ≥ 125/min	+ 10	
Initial laboratory findings (score zero if not tested)		
ph < 7.35	+ 30	
BUN > 30 mg/dl	+ 20	
Sodium < 130 mEq/L	+ 20	
Glucose ≥ 250 mg/dl	+ 10	
Hematocrit < 30%	+ 10	
Po_2 < 60 mmHg or O_2 sat < 90%	+ 10	
Pleural effusion	+ 10	
Total score (sum of patient's points):		

30-Day Mortality Data by Risk Class

Total Score	Risk Class	Recommended Site of Treatment	Mortality Range Observed in Validation Cohorts. %
None (see step 1)	I	Outpatient	0.1
≤ 70	II	Outpatient	0.6
71–90	III	Outpatient	0.5–2.8
91–130	IV	Inpatient	8.2–9.3
> 130	V	Inpatient	27.0–29.2

FIGURE 60-1 **Application of the Pneumonia Patient Outcomes Research Team Severity Index to determine initial site of treatment.** Step 1 identifies patients in risk class 1 on the basis of age 50 years or younger and the absence of all comorbid conditions and vital sign abnormalities listed in step 2. For all patients who are not classified at risk class 1, the laboratory data listed in step 2 should be collected to calculate a pneumonia severity score. Risk class and recommended site of care based on the pneumonia severity score listed in the final table. Thirty-day mortality data are based on two independent cohorts of 40,326 patients. For additional information, see reference 96. BP, blood pressure; BUN, blood urea nitrogen. (Reproduced with permission from Metlay, Fine. Testing strategies in the initial management of patients with community-acquired pneumonia. Ann Intern Med 2003;138:109–118.)

the microbiological results do not identify a causative organism, antibiotics active against the most probable bacterial pathogens should be selected. (Tables 60-5 through 60-7). Of major concern is *S. pneumoniae,* which is the most commonly identifiable pathogen. Second are the atypical organisms, including *C. pneumonia, M. pneumoniae,* and *L. pneumophila.* Last, the likelihood of infection due to *H. influenzae* and *M. catarrhalis* needs to be addressed. Underlying conditions that predispose to specific pathogens, such as risks for aspiration,

alcohol abuse, smoking, and epidemiologic exposures, also should be considered in the empiric selection of therapy.

A summary and comparison of the IDSA, CDC, and ATS guidelines are provided in Table 60-7. For low-risk patients who may be treated safely in an ambulatory setting, the Infectious Diseases Society of America (IDSA) recommends doxycycline, a macrolide, or an antipneumococcal fluoroquinolone as preferred agents as these agents have activity against the most likely pathogens in this setting (*S. pneumo-*

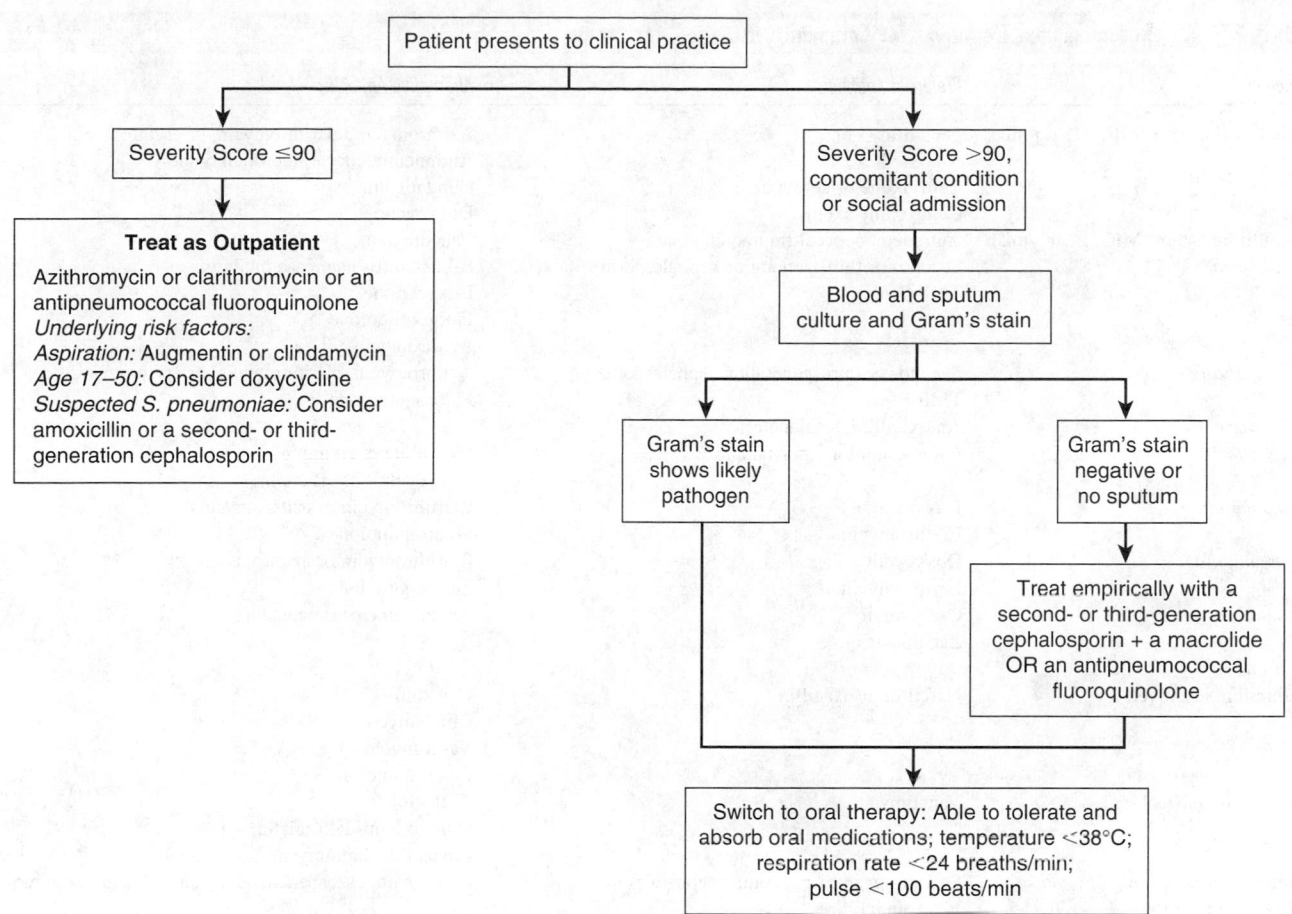

FIGURE 60-2 Approach to the patient with community-acquired pneumonia.

niae, M. pneumoniae, and *C. pneumoniae*).[3] In contrast, the Centers for Disease Control and Prevention (CDC) do not recognize the antipneumococcal fluoroquinolones as first line agents and prefer a macrolide, doxycycline, or an oral β-lactam with adequate antipneumococcal activity (cefuroxime axetil, amoxicillin, amoxicillin/clavulanic acid) in the outpatient treatment of CAP. The American Thoracic Society (ATS), in its newly published guidelines, separates CAP patients into two categories: 1) patients with risk factors for drug-resistant *S. pneumoniae* (DRSP), gram-negative infections and aspiration, or with cardiopulmonary disease and 2) patients without cardiopulmonary disease or without any of the aforementioned risk factors for infection. In patients without risk factors or cardiopulmonary disease, the ATS recognizes that fluoroquinolone use in this population may be unnecessary and recommends treatment with a macrolide or doxycycline. For more complex patients with risk factors or cardiopulmonary disease, oral therapy with a combination of an oral β-lactam (cefpodoxime, cefuroxime, amoxicillin, amoxicillin/clavulanic acid) and a macrolide *or* monotherapy with a fluoroquinolone may be utilized.

Summarizing the above recommendations: 1) in low risk patients, the use of a macrolide or doxycycline is accepted by all groups; 2) in moderate to high risk patients, the use of a combination of a cephalosporin and a macrolide is accepted by all groups; 3) the CDC recommendations are in favor of re-serving antipneumococcal fluoroquinolones; 4) the IDSA favors more broad use of the antipneumococcal fluoroquinolones; 5) the IDSA greater emphasizes an etiologic diagnosis; 6) the ATS places the most emphasis on atypical pathogens and the role of Gram-negative bacilli; 7) the ATS provides, arguably, the most complicated set of treatment recommendations; and 8) the ATS provides the best guidance on which patients should be admitted to an ICU.

For empiric treatment of the moderately ill hospitalized patient, the IDSA recommends an extended-spectrum cephalosporin (cefotaxime, ceftriaxone) plus a macrolide *or* monotherapy with an antipneumococcal fluoroquinolone. The recommendation to use combination therapy in the moderate to severely ill patient is a change from prior guidelines in which the addition of the macrolide had been optional. In part, this change is based on two recent retrospective studies demonstrating that the use of a macrolide plus a second- or third-generation nonantipseudomonal cephalosporin *or* an antipneumococcal fluoroquinolone alone in patients older than 65 years of age resulted in a decreased length of hospital stay and 30-day mortality.[76] Similarly, the CDC prefers a β-lactam (parenteral cefuroxime, cefotaxime, ceftriaxone, ampicillin/sulbactam) plus a macrolide as suitable treatment and reserves antipneumococcal fluoroquinolone use for select patient populations. The ATS supports the use of combination therapy with a macrolide and a β-lactam (cefotaxime, ceftri-

Table 60-5 Recommended Treatment for Community-Acquired Pneumonia

Pathogen	Preferred Antibiotic	Alternative Antibiotic
Penicillin-sensitive (MIC <1 μg/mL)	Penicillin G or V	Azithromycin, clarithromycin, or erythromycin
	Amoxicillin	Antipneumococcal fluoroquinolone
	Ceftriaxone or cefotaxime	Clindamycin
	Cefuroxime axetil	Doxycycline
Penicillin-resistant (MIC >2 mg/mL)	Antipneumococcal fluoroquinolone	Vancomycin
H. influenzae	Second- or third-generation cephalosporin	β-Lactam/β-lactamase inhibitor
	TMP-SMX	Doxycycline
		Fluoroquinolone
		Azithromycin
M. catarrhalis	Second- or third-generation cephalosporin	Azithromycin, clarithromycin, or erythromycin
	TMP-SMX	Fluoroquinolone
	Amoxicillin/clavulanate	
Legionella	Fluoroquinolone ± rifampin	Macrolide ± rifampin
		Doxycycline ± rifampin
M. pneumoniae	Doxycycline	Clarithromycin or azithromycin
	Erythromycin	Fluoroquinolone
C. pneumoniae	Doxycycline	Clarithromycin or azithromycin
	Erythromycin	Fluoroquinolone
Influenza A	Oseltamivir	Amantadine or rimantadine
	Zanamavir	
S. aureus		
Methicillin-sensitive	Nafcillin or oxacillin	Cefazolin
		Clindamycin
		Vancomycin
		Fluoroquinolone
Methicillin-resistant	Vancomycin	TMP-SMX
		Quinupristin-dalfopristin
		Linezolid, Daptomycin
Enterobacteriaceae (e.g., E. coli, Klebsiella, Proteus, Enterobacter)	Second- or third-generation cephalosporin Fluoroquinolone	Aztreonam, carbapenem, β-lactam/β-lactamase inhibitor
Anaerobes	Clindamycin	Carbapenem
	β-Lactam/β-lactamase inhibitor	
	Metronidazole + penicillin	
Pseudomonas aeruginosa	Aminoglycoside + antipseudomonal β-lactam (piperacillin, ceftazidime, cefepime, aztreonam, carbapenem)	Aminoglycoside + ciprofloxacin ciprofloxacin

axone, ampicillin/sulbactam) *or* fluoroquinolone monotherapy in patients with risk factors or cardiopulmonary disease. In the absence of risk factors, the ATS recommends azithromycin, β-lactam, or fluoroquinolone monotherapy. The ATS stresses the importance of providing empiric coverage for atypical organisms in all CAP patients. It is noteworthy that the recommendation to combine an antipneumococcal fluoroquinolone and a cephalosporin is based on the premise that DRSP, atypicals, and Gram-negative bacilli empirically should be covered in severely ill patients. In addition, the use of a β-lactam with a fluoroquinolone ensures adequate treatment of pneumonia potentially complicated by meningitis. To date, limited clinical evidence for this recommendation is available.[77]

For hospitalized patients admitted to the intensive care unit, both the IDSA and the ATS prefer combination therapy with an extended-spectrum cephalosporin (cefotaxime, ceftriaxone) plus either a macrolide or a fluoroquinolone. The goal is to provide optimal treatment for the two most common causes of severe pneumonia, *S. pneumoniae* and Legionella. Monotherapy with a fluoroquinolone is not recommended in the treatment of severely ill patients because data with seriously ill CAP patients are limited. The CDC continues to recommend combination therapy with a β-lactam (cefotaxime, ceftriaxone) and macrolide *or* fluoroquinolone monotherapy but recognizes efficacy of the latter has not been established in the critically ill. In addition, the CDC does not make reference to the β-lactam/fluoroquinolone combination.

A.T.'s treatment should be started empirically with antibiotics pending identification of the etiologic bacteria. The choice should be guided by the results of the sputum Gram's stain, patient age, medical history, concomitant diseases, place of residence, and clinical signs and symptoms. In A.T.'s case, the Gram's stain, which shows a predominance of one organism and many WBCs, should have the greatest influence on initial antimicrobial selection. Because A.T.'s Gram stain shows a predominance of Gram-negative bacilli, empiric therapy should be directed at *H. influenzae* and other Gram-negative bacilli. Based on A.T.'s age and history of previous amoxicillin prophylaxis, one can assume that the pathogen in question is not susceptible to amoxicillin. Consequently, an antibiotic regimen that is effective against ampicillin-resistant *H. influenzae* and other aerobic Gram-negative bacilli should generally be chosen. Second- or third-generation ceph-

Table 60-6 Usual Dosages of Agents Used to Treat Respiratory Tract Infections

Agent	Oral	Parenteral
Penicillins		
Penicillin V	500 mg QID	
Penicillin G		500,000–2 million units Q 4–6 hr
Ampicillin	500 mg QID	1–2 g Q 6 hr
Amoxicillin	500 mg TID	
Oxacillin/nafcillin	500 mg QID	1–3 g Q 6 hr
Ticarcillin		3–4 g Q 6 H
Piperacillin		3–4 g Q 6 hr
β-Lactamase Inhibitors		
Augmentin	500–875 mg BID	
Unasyn		1.5–3 g Q 6 hr
Timentin		3.1 g Q 4–6 hr
Zosyn		3.375–4.5 g Q 6–8 hr
Cephalosporins		
Cefazolin		1–2 g Q 8 hr
Cephalexin	500 mg QID	
Cefuroxime	500 mg BID	750–1,500 mg Q 8 hr
Cefaclor	500 mg TID	
Loracarbef	400 mg BID	
Cefotaxime		1–2 g Q 8 hr
Ceftriaxone		1 g Q 24 hr
Ceftazidime		1–2 g Q 8 hr
Cefpodoxime	400 mg BID	
Cefepime		1–2 g Q 12 hr
Carbapenems		
Imipenem		500 mg Q 6 hr
Meropenem		500–1,000 mg Q 8 hr
Macrolides		
Erythromycin	250–500 mg QID	1 g Q 6 hr
Clarithromycin	500 mg BID	
Azithromycin	500 mg QD	500 mg Q 24 hr
Fluoroquinolones		
Levofloxacin	500 mg QD	500 mg daily
Ciprofloxacin	500–750 mg BID	200–400 mg Q 12 hr
Gatifloxacin	400 mg QD	400 mg daily
Moxifloxacin	400 mg QD	400 mg daily
Aminoglycosides		
Gentamicin		1.7 mg/kg Q 8 hr or 5–7 mg/kg Q 24 hr
Tobramycin		1.7 mg/kg Q 8 hr or 5–7 mg/kg Q 24 hr
Amikacin		7.5 mg/kg Q 12 hr or 15–20 mg/kg Q 24 hr
Miscellaneous		
TMP-SMX	1 DS BID	10 mg/kg daily in 2–4 divided doses
Doxycycline	100 mg BID	100 mg Q 12 hr
Rifampin	300 mg BID	600 mg QD
Metronidazole	500 mg Q 12 hr	500 mg Q 8–12 hr
Vancomycin		1 g Q 12 hr

Table 60-7 Comparison of the IDSA, CDC, and ATS Guidelines for the Treatment of CAP

Patient Type	IDSA	CDC	ATS[b]
Low-risk, ambulatory care	Doxycycline, macrolide, or antipneumococcal FQ	Doxycycline, macrolide, oral β-lactam	*No risk factors:* macrolide or doxycycline *Risk factors:* β-lactam + macrolide or doxycycline; FQ monotherapy
Moderate risk, hospitalized	Cephalosporin + macrolide	Cephalosporin + macrolide	*No risk factors:* azithromycin monotherapy; β-lactam + doxycycline; FQ *Risk factors:* β-lactam + macrolide or doxycycline; FQ
High risk, ICU admission	Cephalosporin + macrolide Cephalosporin + FQ[a]	Cephalosporin + macrolide; FQ monotherapy[a]	*No Pseudomonas:* cephalosporin + macrolide *Pseudomonas:* anti-pseudomonal Cephalosporin + ciprofloxacin

[a]Limited controlled clinical data available to justify this recommendation.
[b]ATS risk factors include: 1) Cardiopulmonary disease: COPD or CHF; 2) risks for specific organisms: a) DRSP: age>65 years, β-lactam therapy within past 3 months, alcoholism, immunosuppressive illness or medications, exposure to a child in a day care center; b) enteric Gram-negatives: residence in a nursing home, underlying cardiopulmonary disease, multiple medical comorbidities, recent antibiotic therapy; c) *Pseudomonas aeruginosa:* structural lung diseases (bronchiectasis), corticosteroid therapy (> 10 mg prednisone equivalent per day), broad-spectrum antibiotic therapy for > 7 days in the past month, malnutrition.

alosporins, TMP-SMX, or fluoroquinolones are acceptable choices in this case. Ceftriaxone 1 g intravenously (IV) every 24 hours with or without the addition of a macrolide such as erythromycin or azithromycin *or* levofloxacin 250 mg IV daily would be reasonable selections for empiric treatment of A.T.'s pneumonia.

RESPONSE TO THERAPY

The response and outcome of patients with CAP depend largely on the microbial agent involved and the patient status at presentation. Poor prognostic factors include age older than 65 years; a coexisting disease such as diabetes, renal failure, heart failure, and COAD; clinical and laboratory findings as outlined in Figure 60-1; and recovery of *S. pneumoniae* or *Legionella*.[44,45,47]

Most patients with bacterial pneumonia improve clinically (decreased temperature and systemic toxicity) 24 to 48 hours after the initiation of effective antibiotic therapy. Chest radiograph resolution lags, taking 3 weeks in otherwise healthy, young adults and up to 12 weeks in elderly patients and those with complicated infections.[78,79] A subset of patients with bacterial pneumonia will do poorly. Factors associated with a poor outcome include involvement of multiple lobes of the lung, bacteremia, a history of alcoholism, age older than 60 years, and neutropenia. Despite the introduction of new anti-infectives, antibiotic therapy has not reduced the mortality rate in pneumococcal pneumonia with bacteremia, which remains at 20% to 30%.[47,80]

When the patient is clinically stable for 24 hours (temperature of <38°C; respiratory rate, <24 breaths/min; and pulse, <100 beats/min), conversion to the oral route can be considered. The patient must be able to take oral medications and have adequate gastrointestinal (GI) function to absorb the agent selected. Diarrhea is not a reason to avoid the oral route because it rarely causes significant reductions in absorption of medications.[45] Selecting an oral agent is simplified if culture and sensitivity data are available and if the parenteral agent is available in an oral formulation.

11. What is the impact of drug-resistant *S. pneumoniae* (DRSP) in the management of CAP?

Penicillin-Resistant S. pneumoniae

Pneumococcal antibacterial susceptibility has changed significantly over the past decade. Despite four decades of using penicillin, only modest rates of reduced susceptibility to penicillin were reported in the 1980s. The mechanism by which pneumococci become resistant to β-lactam antibiotics is through alteration in the binding proteins. This decrease in affinity results in variable increases in the MICs of different β-lactams. Strains with MICs of more than 0.1 μg/mL accounted for 3.8% of isolates in the 1980s; by 1994–1995, the rate was 24%, and by 1997 it was 43.8%.[81–83]

Although resistance rates are increasing, the clinical impact associated with DRSP is controversial. Much of the confusion over this issue is related to problems with designation of in vitro pneumococcal resistance to penicillin. The National Committee for Clinical Laboratory Standards (NCCLS)[84] currently designates pneumococcal isolates as susceptible if the MIC is ≤0.06 μg/mL, intermediate if the MIC value falls between 0.1 and 1.0 μg/mL, and resistant if

the MIC is ≥2.0 μg/mL. These current definitions are based on drug levels achieved in the CSF in cases of meningitis. However, much higher levels are attained in blood and lung. Although these categories appear to have clinical relevance for some agents used to treat otitis media and meningitis, they are inappropriate for guiding the treatment of pneumonia. Despite the report of treatment failures in otitis media and meningitis, studies of pneumococcal pneumonia indicate that pneumococcal resistance does not negatively affect treatment outcome. Available data show that mortality in CAP is only adversely affected by drug-resistant pneumococci when MIC ≥4 μg/mL. These data strongly suggest that ceftriaxone can be used for those isolates intermediately susceptible to penicillin.

The CDC suggests that susceptibility categories for *S. pneumoniae* when implicated as cause of pneumonia be redefined such that the susceptibility category will include all isolates with an MIC ≤1 μg/mL, the intermediate category would encompass isolates with an MIC of 2 μg/mL, and the resistant category would include isolates with an MIC ≥4 μg/mL.[19] The CDC has suggested that clinically relevant resistance to penicillin occurs when the MIC is ≥4 and is associated with increased mortality in patients with invasive disease.[85]

Penicillin resistance is also associated with resistance to other antimicrobial classes, including cephalosporins, macrolides, tetracyclines, and TMP-SMZ (Table 60-8). Antibiotics less affected by this broad-spectrum resistance include vancomycin, the fluoroquinolones, clindamycin, chloramphenicol, and rifampin.[77,81–83] Penicillin susceptibility should be tested for in all significant pneumococcal isolates.[86]

Macrolide-Resistant S. pneumoniae

Although high rates of in vitro macrolide resistance can coexist with penicillin resistance, there are few reports of macrolide failures in CAP due to drug-resistant pneumococci.[87] Pneumococcal resistance to macrolides is expressed as one of two phenotypes. The first, known as the M phenotype, is an efflux pump associated with the mefE gene that results in the efflux of all 14- and 15-membered macrolides from the cell.[88] M phenotype isolates typically have moderate

Table 60-8 Susceptibility of *Streptococcus pneumoniae* Based on Penicillin Susceptibility

Agent	% Susceptible to Indicated Agent		
	Pen-S	Pen-I	Pen-R
Cefuroxime axetil	99	76.3	0.7
Cefpodoxime proxetil	99.5	82.4	0.7
Cefepime	99.7	87.5	3.9
Cefotaxime	100	95.7	19.1
Erythromycin	96.6	81.7	50.7
Clarithromycin	94.9	63.5	38.9
Clindamycin	99.2	93.2	86.2
Tetracycline	96.1	86.7	63.2
TMP-SMX	89	72.4	23
Levofloxacin	97.4	96.9	97.1

Pen-S, penicillin sensitive; Pen-I, penicillin intermediate; Pen-R, penicillin resistant.

levels of macrolide resistance (MIC in the range of 1 to 32 μg/mL) and are almost always susceptible to clindamycin.[89] A second phenotype, called the MLSB phenotype, results from methylation of 23S ribosomal RNA and is encoded by the ermAM gene. Methylation results in blockade of the binding of macrolides, lincosamides, and group B streptogramin agents. The MLSB phenotype is associated with high level macrolide resistance (MIC >64 μg/mL) as well as resistance to clindamycin.

One investigation demonstrated the following: 1) macrolide use in the United States increased by 13% from 1993 to 1999 (17.7 million prescriptions versus 21.2 million prescriptions, respectively; the most dramatic increase was in children <5 years of age, a 320% increase over the same time frame); 2) macrolide resistance has doubled from 1995 to 1999 (10.6% in 1995 to 20.4% in 1999), mostly accounted for by increases in the M phenotype; and 3) the median MIC of the M phenotype increased from 4 μg/mL to ≥8 μg/mL, an MIC associated with treatment failures to clarithromycin and azithromycin.[90] The association between increasing macrolide use and the increasing prevalence of macrolide resistance, and more importantly the shift in the median MIC in M phenotype isolates, is disturbing. The impact of these results on future CAP guidelines remains to be determined. Clinicians need to be cognizant of the local patterns of *S. pneumoniae* susceptibility and should not assume that a macrolide-resistant, clindamycin susceptible isolate will respond to macrolide therapy.

Fluoroquinolones

12. What is the role of fluoroquinolones in treating CAP?

Historically, the fluoroquinolones have demonstrated excellent activity against aerobic Gram-negative bacilli and moderate activity against Gram-positive aerobes. In particular, older fluoroquinolones, such as ciprofloxacin and ofloxacin, have marginal activity against *S. pneumoniae*. Sporadic cases of breakthrough streptococcal infections have been reported in patients treated with older fluoroquinolones. Consequently, based on both in vitro data and clinical experience, the fluoroquinolones have not been recommended for the treatment of community-acquired respiratory tract infections. Beginning in 1996, several "new" antipneumococcal fluoroquinolones were approved by the Food and Drug Administration. These include levofloxacin (Levaquin), sparfloxacin (Zagam), trovafloxacin (Trovan), moxifloxacin (Avelox), and gatifloxacin (Tequin). All these compounds have excellent activity against pneumococcus while maintaining much of their Gram-negative aerobic activity.

Multiple trials have demonstrated these agents to be effective in treating CAP, including pneumococcal bacteremia and pneumonia due to penicillin-resistant strains.[91–93] Levofloxacin (given IV, orally, or both) was compared with ceftriaxone (which could be switched to oral cefuroxime axetil with or without erythromycin or doxycycline [at the investigator's discretion]).[91] Patients receiving levofloxacin had superior clinical and microbiologic response rates compared with those in the ceftriaxone treatment arm. Furthermore, the incidence of adverse effects was the same in both groups.

Based on the aforementioned results, reliable activity of fluoroquinolones against pathogens commonly associated with CAP (including penicillin-susceptible and penicillin-resistant pneumococci, *H. influenzae, M. catarrhalis,* and atypical organisms), and favorable dosing schedules and side effect profiles, many guidelines include the new antipneumococcal fluoroquinolones as potential options in the treatment of CAP.[45]

The major concern regarding the fluoroquinolones is that extensive use may result in increased resistance.[94,95] Although this argument may be raised regarding any antibiotic, the concern with the fluoroquinolones is that resistance with one agent somewhat affects all agents. Currently, pneumococcal resistance to the fluoroquinolones is low, but a report from Canada has demonstrated an association with increased fluoroquinolone use with resistance in *S. pneumoniae*.[96] In addition, the potential for development of resistance in other organisms (especially *Pseudomonas aeruginosa*) due the indiscriminate use of fluoroquinolones is a serious threat to this drug class.[97] The CDC working group on DRSP has issued a guideline outlining these concerns.[98] This group specifically states that fluoroquinolones should be used reserved for treatment of Gram-negative pathogens, for patients with β-lactam allergy, or for the treatment of penicillin-resistant pneumococcal pneumonia.

Antiviral Agents

13. What treatment options are available for influenza virus infection?

As outlined previously, viruses account for 2% to 15% of all cases of CAP. Influenza represents one organism that commonly may be associated with pneumonia. Influenza is an acute respiratory infection characterized by fever, headache, sore throat, myalgias, and a nonproductive cough. In some cases, it can progress to serious secondary complications such as bacterial and viral pneumonia. In addition to increased health care costs, loss of work days, and unnecessary antibiotics, influenza epidemics are responsible for a large number of deaths each year in the United States. Epidemics occur during the winter months nearly every year, with peak activity between late December and early March. The mainstay of protection against the disease has been the inactivated influenza vaccine. Antiviral agents are important adjuncts to the vaccine but do not serve as a substitute for preseason vaccination.

Both the influenza A and B viruses have two major surface glycoproteins that mediate immunity, hemagglutinin and neuraminidase. These two proteins play a critical role in viral replication. Hemagglutinin attaches virus to cells, whereas neuraminidase has several roles to facilitate the spread of the virus throughout the respiratory tract. The neuraminidase enzyme is responsible for releasing the virus from infected cells, preventing the formation of viral aggregates after the release, and potentially preventing viral inactivation. The active site of neuraminidase is almost identical in both influenza A and B.

Amantadine and rimantadine are compounds that indirectly interrupt the function of hemagglutinin by blocking the uncoating of the influenza A virus and preventing host penetration. When initiated within 48 hours of the onset of symptoms, both amantadine and rimantadine shorten the clinical course of the illness related to influenza A and enable patients to resume daily activities sooner. Until recently, these agents were the only antiviral agents available for the prevention and treatment of influenza A. However, their use has been limited by lack of activity against influenza B, emergence of resistance, and central nervous system effects, particularly with amantadine.

The neuraminidase inhibitors, zanamivir and oseltamivir, represent a new class of antivirals active against both influenza A and B.[99] They are sialic acid analogs that work by inhibiting the viral enzyme, neuraminidase. The function of neuraminidase is to cleave sialic acid residues on the cell surface, thereby promoting release of virus from infected cells. Blocking the activity of neuraminidase decreases the amount of virus released that can infect other cells. Resistance to the neuraminidase inhibitors can occur but seems to be less common and slower to develop than with the older antivirals amantadine and rimantadine. A comparison of these agents is provided in Table 60-9.

Zanamivir (Relenza) is indicated for the treatment of uncomplicated influenza illness in adults and children older than 12 years of age who have been symptomatic for no more than 48 hours.[100–102] Oseltamivir (Tamiflu) is approved for the treatment of uncomplicated influenza infection in adults 18 years or older who have been symptomatic for no more than 48 hours.[103,104] Studies have shown that when administered within 2 days of the onset of symptoms, both zanamivir and oseltamivir reduced the median duration of symptoms by approximately 1 day (6.5 to 5 days and 4.5 to 3 days, respectively). High-risk patients (i.e., the elderly, those with asthma), patients who had a febrile illness, and those treated within 30 hours of symptom onset showed the greatest improvement from zanamivir therapy (8 to 5.5 days). Neither neuraminidase inhibitor is approved for the prevention of influenza, but recent studies have demonstrated both to be approximately 60% to 80% effective when administered prophylactically. Likewise, there are no studies comparing the two neuraminidase inhibitors with each other or with amantadine or rimantadine.

Zanamivir is formulated as a dry powder for oral inhalation; its oral bioavailability is poor. The recommended dosage is two inhalations (5 mg each) twice daily for 5 days. Less than 20% of the inhaled dose is systemically absorbed; 70% to 90% of the inhaled drug deposits in the oropharynx. The half-life of systemically absorbed zanamivir is 3 to 5 hours and it is excreted unchanged in the urine. The manufacturer does not recommend a dosage adjustment in patients with renal insufficiency. The most common side effects encountered with zanamivir administration are nasal and throat irritation, headache, and bronchospasm.

Oseltamivir, available as a 75-mg oral capsule, is an ester prodrug that is hydrolyzed in the gut and liver to the active form, oseltamivir carboxylate. The recommended dosage is 75 mg twice daily for 5 days. Eighty percent of the drug is absorbed systemically, and the half-life (6 to 10 hours) of oseltamivir carboxylate is excreted in the urine by glomerular filtration. A dosage reduction to 75 mg daily is recommended in patients with a creatinine clearance <30 mL/min. The most common side effects experienced are nausea, vomiting, and headache. Food may improve GI tolerance.

Although there is limited clinical experience, no significant drug interactions have been reported with either agent. Neither zanamivir nor oseltamivir are substrates for cytochrome P450 metabolism and are not expected to alter the metabolism of other agents. The cost for 5-day therapy with zanamivir or oseltamivir is approximately $50.

The role of the neuraminidase inhibitors in the prevention and treatment of influenza is not clearly defined. It is widely accepted that influenza vaccination will continue to be the primary method of preventing influenza and its secondary complications. However, the neuraminidase inhibitors may be a reasonable alternative for those who cannot be vaccinated due to true egg allergy, those who are not likely to respond to the vaccination, or those who are at significantly high risk.

Effective treatment of influenza illness with any of the currently available antiviral agents is limited by the need for almost immediate diagnosis and intervention. When these agents are initiated within 2 days of the onset of symptoms, they can shorten the duration of the illness. This will require education of both the public and clinicians.[102,104] The role of the pharmacist may be in the early identification of patients who are potential candidates for antiviral therapy. Dialog with patients regarding symptoms and their duration will enable the pharmacist to make appropriate recommendations about the necessity of drug therapy and doctor visits. None of the four agents has been demonstrated to be effective in preventing serious influenza-related complications such as bacterial or viral pneumonia or exacerbation of underlying chronic conditions.

Table 60-9 Comparison of Current Antiviral Agents for Influenza

	Amantadine	Rimantadine	Oseltamivir	Zanamavir
Influenza activity	A	A	A and B	A and B
Route of administration	Oral	Oral	Oral	Oral inhalation
Treatment population	≥1 yr	≥14 yr	≥12 yr	≥18 yr
Prophylaxis population	≥1 yr	≥1 yr	No indication	No indication
Dosage	100 mg PO Q 12 hr	100 mg PO Q 12 hr	75 mg PO BID for 5 days	2 inhalations (5 mg each) PO BID for 5 days
Side effects	CNS, GI	CNS, GI (less than amantadine)	Nasal and throat discomfort, headache, bronchospasm	Nausea, vomiting, headache

CNS, central nervous system; GI, gastrointestinal.

Immunoprophylaxis

14. What agents are available for chemo/immunoprophylaxis against respiratory tract infections?

INFLUENZA VIRUS

In the United States, the primary option for reducing the effect of influenza is immunoprophylaxis with inactivated vaccine. Vaccinating persons at high risk for complications each year before seasonal increases in influenza virus circulation is the most effective means of reducing the effect of influenza. The inactivated influenza vaccines are standardized to contain the hemagglutinins of strains (usually two type A and one type B), representing the influenza viruses likely to circulate in the United States in the upcoming winter. The vaccines are made from highly purified, egg-grown viruses that have been made noninfectious. Because the vaccines are initially grown in embryonated hens' eggs, the final product might contain residual egg proteins. In addition, vaccine distributed in the United States might contain the preservative thimerosal, which contains mercury.

The effectiveness of influenza vaccination depends primarily on the age and immunocompetence of the recipient and the degree of similarity between viruses in the vaccine and in circulation. When strains are similar, vaccine prevents influenza illness in 70% to 90% of healthy adults aged younger than 65 years. Children as young as 6 months of age can develop protective levels of antibody after vaccination. Seroconversion rates have been reported to be 44% to ≥89% and increase with the age of the child. The effectiveness in preventing influenza-related illness in children between 1 to 15 years of age is 77% to 91%. In adults ≥65 years of age, the effectiveness of the vaccine has been reported to be 58%. Importantly, in this population it has been shown to prevent secondary complications and reduce the risk for influenza-related hospitalization and death.

Influenza vaccination is recommended for any person aged ≥6 months who are at increased risk for complications from influenza. These include persons ≥65 years of age; residents of nursing homes and other chronic care facilities; adults and children who have chronic pulmonary or cardiovascular system disorders, including asthma; adults and children who have required regular medical follow-up or hospitalization during the preceding year because of chronic metabolic conditions (including diabetes mellitus), renal dysfunction, hemoglobinopathies, or immunosuppression (including drug induced and HIV induced); children and adolescents (6 months to 18 years) who are receiving long-term aspirin therapy and therefore, might be at risk for experiencing Reye syndrome after influenza infection; and women who will be in the second or third trimester of pregnancy during influenza season.

Vaccination is also recommended in persons aged 50 to 64 years because this group has an increased prevalence of persons with high-risk conditions. In addition, age-based strategies are a more effective means of increasing vaccine coverage than patient-based methods, and 50 years is an age when other preventive services begin and when routine assessment of vaccination and other preventive services has been recommended. Finally, persons who are clinically or subclinically infected can transmit influenza virus to persons at high risk for complications. Thus, health care workers and household contacts of persons in groups at high risk should be vaccinated.

Influenza vaccination should ideally be administered in October through November. Those who are not vaccinated and fall into one of the groups listed above should still be offered vaccination throughout influenza season as long as vaccine supply is available. The most common adverse effects of vaccination include local reactions that are typically mild, fever, malaise, myalgia, headache, allergic reaction (in particular in those with an allergy to eggs), and thimerosal related reactions (usually local, delayed type hypersensitivity reactions).

Chemoprophylaxis

Chemoprophylactic drugs are not a substitute for vaccination, although they are critical adjuncts in the prevention and control of influenza. Both amantadine and rimantadine are indicated for the chemoprophylaxis of influenza A infection but not influenza B. Both drugs are approximately 70% to 90% effective in preventing illness from influenza A infection.[105-107] When used as prophylaxis, these antiviral agents can prevent illness while permitting subclinical infection and development of protective antibody against circulating influenza viruses. Therefore, certain persons who take these drugs will develop protective immune responses to circulating influenza viruses. Amantadine and rimantadine do not interfere with the antibody response to the vaccine.[106] Both drugs have been studied extensively among nursing home populations as a component of influenza outbreak-control programs, which can limit the spread of influenza within chronic care institutions.[106,108-111]

Among the neuraminidase inhibitor antivirals, zanamivir and oseltamivir, only oseltamivir has been approved for prophylaxis, but community studies of healthy adults indicate that both drugs are similarly effective in preventing febrile, laboratory-confirmed influenza illness (efficacy: zanamivir, 84%; oseltamivir, 82%).[112-114] Both antiviral agents have also been reported to prevent influenza illness among persons administered chemoprophylaxis after a household member was diagnosed with influenza.[115-117] Experience with prophylactic use of these agents in institutional settings or among patients with chronic medical conditions is limited in comparison with the adamantanes.[118-123] One 6-week study of oseltamivir prophylaxis among nursing home residents reported a 92% reduction in influenza illness.[118,124] Use of zanamivir has not been reported to impair the immunologic response to influenza vaccine.[115,125] Data are not available regarding the efficacy of any of the four antiviral agents in preventing influenza among severely immunocompromised persons.

CONTROL OF INFLUENZA OUTBREAKS IN INSTITUTIONS

Using antiviral drugs for treatment and prophylaxis of influenza is a key component of influenza outbreak control in institutions. In addition to antiviral medications, other outbreak-control measures include instituting droplet precautions and establishing cohorts of patients with confirmed or suspected influenza, re-offering influenza vaccinations to unvaccinated staff and patients, restricting staff movement between wards or buildings, and restricting contact between ill staff or visitors and patients.[126-128]

The majority of published reports concerning use of antiviral agents to control influenza outbreaks in institutions are based on studies of influenza A outbreaks among nursing home populations in which amantadine or rimantadine were used.[106,108–111,129] Less information is available concerning use of neuraminidase inhibitors in influenza A or B institutional outbreaks.[119,120,123,130,131] When confirmed or suspected outbreaks of influenza occur in institutions that house persons at high risk, chemoprophylaxis should be started as early as possible to reduce the spread of the virus. In these situations, having preapproved orders from physicians or plans to obtain orders for antiviral medications on short notice can substantially expedite administration of antiviral medications.

When outbreaks occur in institutions, chemoprophylaxis should be administered to all residents, regardless of whether they received influenza vaccinations during the previous fall, and should continue for a minimum of 2 weeks. If surveillance indicates that new cases continue to occur, chemoprophylaxis should be continued until approximately 1 week after the end of the outbreak. The dosage for each resident should be determined individually. Chemoprophylaxis also can be offered to unvaccinated staff who provide care to persons at high risk. Prophylaxis should be considered for all employees, regardless of their vaccination status, if the outbreak is caused by a variant strain of influenza that is not well-matched by the vaccine.

In addition to nursing homes, chemoprophylaxis also can be considered for controlling influenza outbreaks in other closed or semiclosed settings (e.g., dormitories or other settings where persons live in close proximity). For example, chemoprophylaxis with rimantadine has been used successfully to control an influenza A outbreak aboard a large cruise ship.[132]

To limit the potential transmission of drug-resistant virus during outbreaks in institutions, whether in chronic or acute-care settings or other closed settings, measures should be taken to reduce contact as much as possible between persons taking antiviral drugs for treatment and other persons, including those taking chemoprophylaxis

When determining the timing and duration for administering influenza antiviral medications for prophylaxis, factors related to cost, compliance, and potential side effects should be considered. To be maximally effective as prophylaxis, the drug must be taken each day for the duration of influenza activity in the community. However, to be most cost-effective, one study of amantadine or rimantadine prophylaxis reported that the drugs should be taken only during the period of peak influenza activity in a community.[129]

PERSONS AT HIGH RISK WHO ARE VACCINATED AFTER INFLUENZA ACTIVITY HAS BEGUN

Persons at high risk for complications of influenza still can be vaccinated after an outbreak of influenza has begun in a community. However, the development of antibodies in adults after vaccination takes approximately 2 weeks.[133,134] When influenza vaccine is administered while influenza viruses are circulating, chemoprophylaxis should be considered for persons at high risk during the time from vaccination until immunity has developed. Children aged younger than 9 years who receive influenza vaccine for the first time can require 6 weeks of prophylaxis (i.e., prophylaxis for 4 weeks after the first dose of vaccine and an additional 2 weeks of prophylaxis after the second dose).

PERSONS WHO PROVIDE CARE TO THOSE AT HIGH RISK

To reduce the spread of virus to persons at high risk during community or institutional outbreaks, chemoprophylaxis during peak influenza activity can be considered for unvaccinated persons who have frequent contact with persons at high risk. Persons with frequent contact include employees of hospitals, clinics, and chronic-care facilities; household members; visiting nurses; and volunteer workers. If an outbreak is caused by a variant strain of influenza that might not be controlled by the vaccine, chemoprophylaxis should be considered for all such persons, regardless of their vaccination status.

PERSONS WHO HAVE IMMUNE DEFICIENCIES

Chemoprophylaxis can be considered for persons at high risk who are expected to have an inadequate antibody response to influenza vaccine. This category includes persons infected with HIV, chiefly those with advanced HIV disease. No published data are available concerning possible efficacy of chemoprophylaxis among persons with HIV infection or interactions with other drugs used to manage HIV infection. Such patients should be monitored closely if chemoprophylaxis is administered.

OTHER PERSONS

Chemoprophylaxis throughout the influenza season or during peak influenza activity might be appropriate for persons at high risk who should not be vaccinated. Chemoprophylaxis can also be offered to persons who wish to avoid influenza illness. Health care providers and patients should make this decision on an individual basis.

Streptococcus pneumoniae

S. pneumoniae is the most common bacterial pathogen associated with respiratory tract infections. Severe infections can result from the dissemination of this organism to the bloodstream and the central nervous system. Pneumococcal infections cause an estimated 40,000 deaths annually in the United States. The currently available pneumococcal vaccine includes 23 purified capsular polysaccharide antigens from serotypes 1–5, 6B, 7F, 8, 9N, 9V, 10A, 11A, 12F, 14, 15B, 17F, 18C, 19A, 19F, 20, 22F, 23F, and 33F. After vaccination, an antigen specific antibody response develops within 2 to 3 weeks in ≥80% of healthy adults.[135] The levels of antibody to most antigens remains elevated for at least 5 years in healthy adults and decreases to prevaccination levels by 10 years.[136,137]

Pneumococcal vaccine has not been shown to be effective against nonbacteremic pneumococcal disease. Effectiveness against invasive disease is 56% to 81%.[138–141] Preliminary results of a cost-effectiveness analysis indicate that pneumococcal polysaccharide vaccine is cost-effective and potentially cost-saving among persons aged 65 years or older for prevention of bacteremia.[142]

The vaccine is both cost-effective and protective against invasive pneumococcal infection when administered to immunocompetent persons aged 2 years or older.[134] Therefore, all persons in the following categories should receive the 23-valent pneumococcal polysaccharide vaccine: patients aged 65 years or older, patients aged 2 to 64 years with chronic illness, patients aged 2 to 64 years with functional or anatomic asplenia, patients aged 2 to 64 years living in special environments or social settings, and immunocompromised patients. If vaccination status is unknown, patients in these categories should be administered pneumococcal vaccine. Children younger than 2 years of age can be administered a conjugated version of the pneumococcal vaccine. The effectiveness and indications are discussed in Chapter 96, Pediatric Infectious Diseases.

Pneumococcal polysaccharide vaccine generally is considered safe based on clinical experience since 1977, when the pneumococcal polysaccharide vaccine was licensed in the United States. Approximately half of patients who receive pneumococcal vaccine develop mild, local side effects (e.g., pain at the injection site, erythema, and swelling).[143,144] These reactions usually persist for less than 48 hours. Moderate systemic reactions (e.g., fever and myalgias) and more severe local reactions (e.g., local induration) are rare. Intradermal administration may cause severe local reactions and is inappropriate. Severe systemic adverse effects (e.g., anaphylactic reactions) rarely have been reported after administration of pneumococcal vaccine.

Routine revaccination of immunocompetent persons previously vaccinated with 23-valent polysaccharide vaccine is not recommended.[134] However, revaccination once is recommended for persons aged 2 years or older who are at highest risk for serious pneumococcal infection and those who are likely to have a rapid decline in pneumococcal antibody levels, provided that 5 years have elapsed since receipt of the first dose of pneumococcal vaccine. Revaccination 3 years after the previous dose may be considered for children at highest risk for severe pneumococcal infection who would be aged 10 years or younger at the time of revaccination. These children include those with functional or anatomic asplenia (e.g., sickle cell disease or splenectomy) and those with conditions associated with rapid antibody decline after initial vaccination (e.g., nephrotic syndrome, renal failure, or renal transplantation). Revaccination is contraindicated for persons who had a severe reaction (e.g., anaphylactic reaction or localized arthus-type reaction) to the initial dose.

Chemoprophylaxis

Oral penicillin V (125 mg, twice daily), when administered to infants and young children with sickle cell disease, has reduced the incidence of pneumococcal bacteremia by 84% compared with those receiving placebo.[145] Therefore, daily penicillin prophylaxis for children with sickle cell hemoglobinopathy is recommended before 4 months of age. Consensus on the age at which prophylaxis should be discontinued has not been achieved. However, children with sickle cell anemia who had received prophylactic penicillin for prolonged intervals (but without a prior severe pneumococcal infection or splenectomy) have discontinued penicillin therapy at 5 years of age with no increase in the incidence of pneumococcal bacteremia or meningitis.[116]

Oral penicillin G or V is recommended for prevention of pneumococcal disease in children with functional or anatomic asplenia.[117] Antimicrobial prophylaxis against pneumococcal infection may be particularly useful for asplenic children not likely to respond to the polysaccharide vaccine (e.g., those aged younger than 2 years or those receiving intensive

chemotherapy or cytoreduction therapy). However, the impact of this practice on the emergence of DRSP is not known.

The effectiveness of all vaccines depends on administration in those patients at highest risk. Data released from the National Health Interview Survey has shown that for influenza vaccine, persons aged 50 to 64 years were vaccinated 34% of the time, and those 65 years and older were vaccinated 65.6% of the time in 2002. For pneumococcal vaccine, those aged 65 years and older were vaccinated 55.7% of the time in 2002.[146] The role of pharmacists in identifying those patients who should be offered vaccination and potentially administering these vaccines may improve in increased rates of vaccination.

Aspiration Pneumonia
Predisposing Factors

15. R.G., a 38-year-old man, was brought to the ED after he was found unconscious, lying on his right side, near a pool of vomitus in a local municipal park. R.G. has a long history of binge drinking and has been admitted to the ED frequently for problems related to his alcoholism. Upon admission, R.G.'s vital signs were BP, 100/60 mm Hg; pulse, 110 beats/min; respirations, 32 breaths/min; and temperature, 38.0°C. A strong odor of alcohol and vomitus was noted. R.G.'s overall mental status is depressed; he has intermittent periods of disorientation and uncoordinated motor movements.

Crackling rales were heard in the middle and lower right lung fields; the left fields were clear. An ABG was drawn on room air, with the following results: pH, 7.46 (normal, 7.38 to 7.45); PO_2, 52 mm Hg (normal, 68 to 100 mm Hg); PCO_2, 35 mm Hg (normal, 38 to 45 mm Hg); and HCO_3, 24 mEq/L (normal, 22 to 26 mEq/L). Laboratory data include the following: WBC count, 12,000 cells/mm³ (normal, 5 to 10,000 cells/mm³); differential PMNs, 68% (normal, 45% to 79%); bands, 8% (normal, 0% to 5%); and lymphocytes, 24% (normal, 16% to 47%). During a period of consciousness, the physician obtained a sputum specimen from R.G. for Gram's stain and culture. A chest radiograph revealed density changes consistent with interstitial infiltrates in the dependent segments of the middle and lower right lung. A tentative diagnosis of aspiration pneumonitis is made. What factors predispose R.G. to aspiration pneumonitis? How can the aspirated material cause pneumonitis?

[SI units: PO_2, 6.93 kPa; PCO_2, 4.67 kPa; WBC count, 12 10⁹/L, with PMNs, 0.68; bands, 0.08; and lymphocytes, 0.24]

Several factors in R.G.'s history make him susceptible to aspiration. Alcohol intoxication has depressed his mental status as well as his cough and gag reflex, which may have led to aspiration of his vomitus. Table 60-10 lists conditions that predispose individuals to aspiration. Those conditions that cause or contribute to an altered state of consciousness are particularly important. The specific effect of the aspirated material on the lungs depends on the quantity and quality of the material aspirated. The latter can be categorized into three types: direct pulmonary toxin, particulate matter, and infected inoculum.[61,147]

Several toxic materials cause pneumonitis, the most common of which is gastric acid. When gastric acid enters the lungs, the sequence of events has been likened to a chemical burn. The aspirated secretions are neutralized rapidly over the first few minutes and this is accompanied by a shift of fluid

Table 60-10 Predisposing Conditions in Aspiration Pneumonia

Alterations of Consciousness
Alcoholism
Seizure disorders
General anesthesia
Cerebrovascular accident
Drug intoxication
Head injury
Severe illness with obtundation
Impaired Swallowing Mechanism
Neurologic disorders
Esophageal dysfunction
Nasogastric Feeding
Tracheotomy
Endotracheal Tube
Periodontal Disease

Reprinted with permission from Klein RS, Steigbigel NH. Seminars in Infectious Disease. New York: Thieme Medical Publishers, 1983;5.

into the involved area of the lung. An estimated 96% of patients will demonstrate signs of respiratory compromise within 1 hour of aspiration, and 100% within 2 hours. The two immediate consequences of aspiration of gastric acid are rapid, profound hypoxia and shock secondary to massive fluid shifts into lung tissue. In addition, atelectasis, hemorrhage, and pulmonary edema may occur.[61] Approximately 45% of healthy adults aspirate oropharyngeal secretions during deep sleep and 70% of patients with depressed consciousness aspirate pharyngeal secretions. Gastric juice has a pH ≤ 2.5 and contains few to no bacteria.[148,149] However, after the initial insult some patients will develop a secondary bacterial pneumonia.[150] The infection is due primarily to aspiration of oropharyngeal contents in a setting of diminished host defenses caused by the chemical pneumonitis.[151] Other toxic materials causing aspiration pneumonitis include hydrocarbons, mineral oil, bile, alcohol, and animal fats.[147]

A second category of aspirated material is fluid containing various amounts of bacteria. Oropharyngeal secretions are the most frequent source of this material. Bacterial pneumonia results when the normal host lung defenses have been damaged or altered and when the bacteria inoculum exceeds the body's ability to contain and eliminate it. Infection due to aspirated bacteria may result in a pneumonia with little or no tissue destruction, necrotizing pneumonia, lung abscess, or empyema.

A third category of aspirated material consists of particulate matter. When relatively large particles are aspirated, sudden aphonia, cyanosis, and respiratory distress occur; the patient can progress rapidly toward death. Smaller particles reaching the lower airways cause local irritation with bronchospasm and infection if they are not removed. Many of these cases occur in young children following the ingestion of coins, peanuts, teeth, vegetables, or other small particles. Rapid removal of these particles usually results in the rapid reversal of symptoms without significant sequelae.

Clinical Course

16. What is the expected clinical course of aspiration pneumonia in R.G.?

The clinical course of a patient such as R.G. who has aspirated gastric contents and/or oropharyngeal secretions is variable; three courses have been identified. Shock will occur in 20% to 30% of patients with documented aspiration[148,152]; respiratory function continues to deteriorate in many of these patients, and approximately 25% die. Mortality rates may be higher in severely ill patients.[153] Early clinical signs and symptoms of gastric aspiration include fever, tachypnea, rales, cough, cyanosis, wheezing, apnea, and shock. A second group of patients will resolve the pneumonitis completely over a few days to weeks without complication. A third group will develop bacterial pneumonia following an initial period of improvement.

Treatment

17. How should R.G. be treated?

R.G.'s initial treatment should primarily consist of supportive measures. Attention should be directed toward respiratory support and correction of his fluid and electrolyte status. In addition, any particulate matter present in the airways should be removed.

Pulmonary edema secondary to massive fluid shifts into the lung can contribute to a decrease in the intravascular volume. If this occurs, aggressive supportive therapy with ventilation, oxygen supplementation, and fluid replacement is indicated.

The use of corticosteroids to reduce inflammation in the setting of aspiration pneumonia is not warranted. There are no well-designed studies, and data supporting their use are anecdotal. In one published report, the use of steroids in the treatment of aspiration in humans was suggested to be harmful.[154] Although no difference was found in mortality, the incidence of Gram-negative pneumonia was more frequent in those patients receiving steroids. Therefore, if steroids are used in patients with aspiration pneumonia, their potential risks must be weighed against their unproven benefit. Because bacteria play little or no role in the initial events following aspiration, antibiotic therapy should be withheld until bacterial involvement is established.

Prophylactic antibiotics are not beneficial in this setting and may contribute to a change in the oropharyngeal flora that may, in turn, predispose the patient to pneumonia secondary to resistant bacterial organisms. On the other hand, if the patient has been hospitalized for >3 days at the time of aspiration, empiric antimicrobial therapy may be justified, particularly if the patient is elderly, debilitated, or is believed to be deteriorating clinically.

Clinical Presentation

18. R.G.'s pulmonary symptoms improved during the next 3 days, but now he has a temperature of 38.5°C with an increase in sputum production. How should he be assessed?

Patients such as R.G. with mild aspiration pneumonia usually resolve their respiratory difficulties within a few days following the insult. If an infection occurs, there is occasionally a short period of clinical improvement before signs and symptoms present. Criteria used to identify bacterial pneumonia following aspiration include (1) a new fever or a significant rise in temperature from the patient's baseline, (2) a new or extending pulmonary infiltrate after the initial 36- to 48-hour period, (3) an increase in WBCs or a change in the differential WBC count, (4) a change in sputum characteristics with purulence, and (5) the presence of pathogenic bacteria in a transtracheal aspirate.

Microbiology

19. What bacterial organisms are likely to be responsible for R.G.'s infectious pneumonia?

In the setting of aspiration pneumonitis, the bacterial pathogen is difficult to predict because large numbers of potential bacterial pathogens are present in sputum.

Most cases of aspiration pneumonia are caused by a wide spectrum of Gram-positive and Gram-negative anaerobic and aerobic bacteria representing the complex microbial flora of the oropharynx and upper GI tract. In approximately 50% of cases, aerobic bacteria have been recovered, and in 60% to 90% of cases, anaerobes have been recovered.[57,155] Tables 60-11 and 60-12 list the most common bacteria recovered from patients with aspiration pneumonia. A large percentage of community-acquired aspiration pneumonias are caused by anaerobes alone, followed by mixed or polymicrobial etiologies. In contrast, a larger percentage of hospital-acquired aspiration pneumonias are caused by aerobic bacteria; they also

Table 60-11 Bacteriology of Aspiration Pneumonia

Community-Acquired Pneumonia
Streptococcus pneumoniae
Peptococcus sp.
Peptostreptococcus sp.
Microaerophilic streptococci
Fusobacterium sp.
Bacteroides melaninogenicus
Bacteroides sp.
Streptococcus sp.
Special Patients (Alcoholics, Diabetics [±Nursing Home Residents])
Staphylococcus aureus
Klebsiella pneumoniae
Escherichia coli
Anaerobes included above
Hospital-Acquired Pneumonia
Pseudomonas aeruginosa
S. aureus
S. pneumoniae
Anaerobes included above
Escherichia coli
Enterobacter cloacae
Serratia marcescens
Other Gram-negative bacilli

Table 60-12 Etiology of Aspiration-Associated Lung Infections

	No. of Patients	Anaerobes Only	Aerobes Only	Mixed
Community-acquired	54	32 (59%)	5 (10%)	17 (31%)
Hospital-acquired	47	8 (18%)	17 (36%)	22 (47%)

Adapted from references 63 and 156.

are usually polymicrobial in nature. The aerobic bacteria recovered from patients with hospital-acquired aspiration pneumonia include S. aureus, various Enterobacteriaceae, and P. aeruginosa. Understanding the differences in the bacterial etiology in these two settings facilitates the selection of antimicrobial therapy. The bacterial etiology of aspiration pneumonia in children is similar to that of adults.[74,157]

When a patient develops aspiration pneumonia in the community setting, mouth anaerobes and Gram-positive aerobic bacteria such as group A streptococcus, and S. pneumoniae, are the most common pathogens. However, some patients with community-acquired aspiration pneumonia are more likely to be infected with S. aureus or Gram-negative pathogens because of oropharyngeal colonization. These individuals include alcoholics (as in the case of R.G.), elderly patients housed in long-term care nursing facilities,[63] patients receiving enteral feedings,[158] and patients treated chronically with antacids and/or H_2 receptor antagonists such as famotidine or ranitidine. In the latter individuals, Gram-negative flora are recovered from the stomach because they are better able to survive in a more alkaline pH.[148,159,160] In addition, the oropharynx of these individuals frequently is colonized with the same bacteria found in the gastric flora.[161] In patients in which this occurred, 60% developed Gram-negative pneumonia. Information suggests that the use of sucralfate reduces bacterial colonization of the stomach of critically ill patients while maintaining adequate stress ulcer prophylaxis. The initial experience with this substitution has reduced the frequency of nosocomial pneumonia.[162,163]

Treatment

ANTIMICROBIAL THERAPY

20. How should antibiotics be used in aspiration pneumonia? How should R.G. be treated?

Antibiotic therapy should be selected on the basis of several criteria: the clinical setting in which the aspiration occurred, knowledge of the patient's medical history, the Gram's stain of a reliably obtained sputum, and aerobic and anaerobic culture results of lower respiratory tract secretions. Table 60-13 lists common antibiotics and dosages used to treat aspiration pneumonia.

As noted previously, anaerobes are often the sole or dominant bacteria involved in patients with community-acquired aspiration pneumonia. Preferred therapy for aspiration pneumonia is clindamycin. The selection of a cephalosporin should be based on its ability to effectively inhibit anaerobes inhabiting the oropharynx (e.g., Peptostreptococcus, Peptococcus). Metronidazole also has been used to treat anaerobic pleuropulmonary infections,[164,165] but the results have been mixed due, in part, to the severity of infections treated (e.g., lung abscess). Metronidazole effectively inhibits Gram-negative obligate anaerobic bacteria, such as B. fragilis and other Prevotella species, but fails to effectively inhibit facultative anaerobic bacteria, such as Peptococcus species and Peptostreptococcus species.[156] Other agents that can be used IV include a β-lactamase–inhibitor combination or the combination of metronidazole plus penicillin.

Treatment of aspiration pneumonia in the elderly, in patients from extended-care facilities, in patients with extensive medical histories, and in alcoholics (as in the case of R.G.)

Table 60-13   Suggested Antimicrobial Dosages for Treatment of Aspiration Pneumonia[a]

Drug	Adult		Pediatric[b]	
	Dose	Interval (hr)	Total Daily Dose (mg/kg/24 hr)	Interval (hr)
Penicillins				
Ampicillin	1–2 g	Q 4–6	100–200	Q 4–6
Mezlocillin	2–3 g	Q 4–6	200–300	Q 4–6
Nafcillin	1–2 g	Q 4–6	100–200	Q 4–6
Penicillin (procaine) (IM)	0.6–1.2 million units	Q 12	50,000 units	Q 12
Penicillin G (for anaerobic infection)	1–2 million units	Q 4–6	50,000–100,000 units	Q 4–6
Piperacillin	2–5 g	Q 4–8	200–300	Q 4–6
Ticarcillin	2–3 g	Q 4–6	200–300	Q 4–6
Other Antibacterials				
Aztreonam	1–2 g	Q 8–12	50–100	Q 6–8
Chloramphenicol	250–500 mg	Q 6–8	50–100	Q 6–8
Ciprofloxacin	400 mg	Q 12		
Clindamycin	600–900 mg	Q 6–8	25–40	Q 6–8
Doxycycline	100 mg	Q 12		
Erythromycin	250–500 mg	Q 6	40	Q 6
Imipenem	0.5–1 g	Q 6–8	60	Q 6
Metronidazole	500 mg	Q 8	25–60	Q 8–12
TMP-SMX[c]	10 mg/kg	Q 12	10 mg	Q 12
Vancomycin	500–1,000 mg	Q 6–12	40	Q 6–12
Cephalosporins				
Cefamandole	1–2 g	Q 4–6		
Cefazolin	1–2 g	Q 8	50–100	Q 8
Cefoperazone	1–2 g	Q 8–12	50–100	Q 8–12
Cefotaxime	1–2 g	Q 6–8	50–100	Q 6–8
Cefotetan	1–2 g	Q 8–12		
Cefoxitin	1–2 g	Q 4–6	50–100	Q 4–6
Ceftazidime	1–2 g	Q 8–12	50–100	Q 8–12
Ceftizoxime	1–2 g	Q 8–12	50–100	Q 8–12
Ceftriaxone	1–2 g	Q 12–24	50–75	Q 12–24
Cefuroxime	0.75–1.5 g	Q 6–8	50–100	Q 6–8
Aminoglycosides				
Amikacin	5–7.5 mg/kg	Q 8–12	15–30	Q 8–12
Gentamicin	1.7 mg/kg	Q 8	6–7.5	Q 8
Tobramycin	1.7 mg/kg	Q 8	6–7.5	Q 8

[a]Intravenous doses administered over 30 to 60 minutes; in patients with normal clearance.
[b]Infants and children older than 1 month.
[c]TMP-SMX, trimethoprim-sulfamethoxazole. TMP-SMX dosed at 10 mg/kg of TMP.

should include agents with activity against Gram-negative rods. Appropriate therapy choices might be a β-lactamase–inhibitor combination or a fluoroquinolone plus clindamycin.

Due to colonization with more resistant organisms, aspiration pneumonia in the hospital setting should be treated with a regimen active against both Gram-negative pathogens and anaerobes. *P. aeruginosa* should be considered as a possible pathogen in high risk units (e.g., intensive care unit) or in those patients at high risk (i.e., neutropenic patients or moderate to severe thermal injury patients). Effective regimens include a β-lactamase–inhibitor combination (piperacillin/tazobactam [Zosyn] and ticarcillin/ clavulanate [Timentin]), ciprofloxacin, aztreonam or an antipseudomonal cephalosporin plus clindamycin or metronidazole, or a carbapenem. An empiric regimen should be modified when the results of the sputum culture are known. The addition of vancomycin to cover methicillin-resistant *S. aureus* (MRSA) should be guided by local epidemiologic data, sputum Gram's stain, and culture and sensitivity results. In patients with effusion or an

empyema, drainage of the collection will likely be required to achieve a clinical cure.

Parenteral antibiotics should be continued until the patient has responded clinically to the therapy as outlined previously (see Fig. 60-1). Oral antibiotic therapy should be continued for 2 to 4 weeks, depending on the patient. In patients with lung abscesses, particularly with inadequate drainage, 6 weeks or more may be needed. Oral combination options in treating aspiration pneumonia include amoxicillin/clavulanate or clindamycin or metronidazole plus a fluoroquinolone.

Hospital-Acquired Pneumonia
Risk Factors

21. A.A., a 68-year-old man, is admitted to the hospital from an extended-care nursing facility because of an acute change in mental status, fever, dyspnea with respiratory difficulty, cough, and sputum production. His medical history is notable for insulin-dependent diabetes mellitus since the age of 10, a right-sided cerebrovascular accident that left him with residual weakness, and a recent *Escherichia coli* urinary tract infection that was treated with oral TMP-SMX DS for 10 days. Because of poor nutrition, A.A. has been receiving nutritional supplements through a flexible nasogastric feeding tube for the past 2 months.

Physical examination reveals a restless, elderly man with the following vital signs: BP, 147/87 mm Hg; pulse, 110 beats/min; respirations, 28 breaths/min; and temperature, 39°C. His head is without obvious trauma and his neck is supple. Crackling rales with diminished breath sounds are noted in the middle and upper right lung fields. The chest radiograph shows a pulmonary infiltrate involving the right middle and upper lobes of the right lung with lobar consolidation. Because A.A. is relatively uncooperative and cannot give a good sputum specimen, a specimen of lower respiratory tract secretions was collected by transtracheal aspiration. This specimen was sent to the laboratory for Gram's stain and culture.

The Gram's stain showed Gram-negative rods with 4% neutrophils. ABGs included a PaO_2 of 34 mm Hg on room air (normal, 80 to 100 mm Hg); his current PaO_2 is 52 mm Hg, and 80 to 100 mm Hg with 4 L/min of supplemental oxygen. Other laboratory values include the following: Hct, 39% (normal, 37% to 47%); WBC count, 16,000 cells/mm³ (normal, 5 to 10,000 cells/mm³); PMNs, 88% (normal, 45% to 79%); bands, 10% (normal, 0% to 5%); lymphocytes, 2% (normal, 16% to 47%); blood urea nitrogen (BUN), 12 mg/dL (normal, 7 to 20 mg/dL); and creatinine, 1.0 mg/dL (normal, 0.8 to 1.2 mg/dL).

Medications on admission include oral famotidine 20 mg QD. A tentative diagnosis of a hospital-acquired Gram-negative pneumonia is made. A.A. is intubated and placed on a ventilator. In addition, intravenous fluids are started to maintain a urine output of 50 mL/hr. What are the risk factors for pneumonia in A.A.?

[SI units: PaO_2, 4.53 and 6.93 kPa, respectively; Hct, 0.39; WBC count, 16 × 10⁹/L; PMNs, 0.88; bands, 0.1; lymphocytes, 0.02; BUN, 4.28 mmol/L of urea (normal, 2.5 to 7.14); creatinine 88.4 μmol/L (normal, 70.72 to 106.08)]

Although A.A. is just now being admitted to the hospital, his diagnosis should be considered hospital-acquired pneumonia (HAP) because he resides in a nursing home. Patients residing in nursing homes have an increased incidence of nosocomial pneumonias and oropharyngeal colonization with Gram-negative bacteria. In addition, poor infection control practices contribute to the cross-contamination of patients with pathogenic bacteria.[166] Nursing homes generally have flora similar to a hospital and this is reflected by his Gram's stain, which is consistent with a Gram-negative pneumonia. Other risk factors associated with developing hospital-acquired pneumonia are listed in Table 60-14. The most significant risk factor is intubation, which increases the risk by 7- to 21-fold.

An important contributing factor in the cause of a pneumonia is colonization of the oropharynx. Several factors may contribute to the colonization of A.A.'s oropharynx with Gram-negative bacteria.[167] He is disabled because of a cerebrovascular accident, which has left him with right-sided weakness; this chronic condition also may predispose him to changes in oropharyngeal flora. A.A. is prone to aspiration of these secretions because the residual effects of the stroke and nasogastric tube used for nutritional support have decreased his airway protection. Finally, an altered immune response in diabetics and the elderly can further contribute to the establishment of a respiratory infection in A.A. (see Table 60-15). The use of drugs that inhibit the production of gastric acid, such as famotidine, increases the possibility of oropharyngeal colonization.[160,161] Finally, the use of broad-spectrum antibiotics may inhibit the growth of many normal flora, which allows Gram-negative bacteria and other multiple-resistant bacteria to colonize the oropharynx.[168–170]

Treatment

22. **How does the bacteriology of HAP differ from CAP?**

The major difference in the bacteriology between CAP and HAP is a shift to Gram-negative pathogens in HAP. Gram-negative bacilli commonly colonize oropharyngeal secretions of patients with moderate to severe acute and chronic illnesses without exposure to broad-spectrum antibiotics.[60,61] Patients admitted to the hospital with acute illnesses are rapidly colonized with Gram-negative organisms. Approximately 20% are colonized on the first hospital day, and this number increases with the duration of hospitalization and severity of illness.[57] Approximately 35% to 45% of hospitalized patients[57] and up to 100% of critically ill patients[59] will be colonized within 3 to 5 days of admission.

Table 60-16 lists the most common bacteria associated with hospital-acquired or nosocomial pneumonia. Virtually all reports indicate that Gram-negative bacteria account for 50% to 70% of all cases.[171–176] The most common bacterium within this category is *P. aeruginosa*. In patients who are ventilator dependent, *Acinetobacter* species often is reported as the most common Gram-negative pathogen. *S. aureus,* which accounts for 10% to 20% of all cases hospital-acquired pneumonia, is the most commonly identified Gram-positive organism. Other organisms with special risk factors include Le-

Table 60-14 Risks for Nosocomial Pneumonia

Intubation or tracheostomy
Age older than 70 years
Chronic lung disease
Poor nutrition status
Depressed consciousness
Thoracic or abdominal surgery
Immunosuppressive therapy

Table 60-15 Conditions Associated With Gram-Negative Colonization

Prolonged hospitalization
Alcoholism
Antibiotic exposure
Diabetes
Advanced age
Coma
Pulmonary disease
Intubation
Azotemia
Major surgery
Neutropenia

Table 60-16   Microbiology of Nosocomial Pneumonia

Pathogen	% of Cases
Gram-negative Bacilli	50–70
Pseudomonas aeruginosa	
Acinetobacter species	
Enterobacter species	
Staphylococcus aureus	15–30
Anaerobic bacteria	10–30
Haemophilus influenzae	10–20
Streptococcus pneumoniae	10–20
Legionella	4
Viral	10–20
Cytomegalovirus	
Influenza	
Respiratory syncytial virus	
Fungi	
Aspergillus	<1%

Table 60-17   Treatment for Nosocomial Pneumonia

Mild, Early Onset (<5 Days of Hospitalization), Low Risk
Cephalosporins: cefuroxime, cefotaxime, ceftriaxone
β-Lactamase–inhibitor combination: ampicillin-sulbactam, ticarcillin-
    clavulanate, piperacillin-tazobactam
Penicillin allergy: antipneumococcal fluoroquinolone or clindamycin
    plus azithromycin
Severe, Late Onset (>5 Days of Hospitalization), High Risk
Aminoglycoside or ciprofloxacin plus one of the following:
1. Antipseudomonal b-lactam: ceftazidime, cefepime, piperacillin
2. β-Lactamase–inhibitor combination: ticarcillin-clavulanate,
    piperacillin-tazobactam
3. Imipenem or meropenem
4. Aztreonam
The addition of vancomycin should be based on Gram's stain results
Severe Pneumonia Defined as Follows:
Respiratory failure
Need for mechanical ventilation or requires >35% O_2 to maintain Pao_2
    >90%
Rapid progression on chest radiograph to show multiple lobe involve-
    ment or cavitation
Evidence of severe sepsis
    Hypotension (systolic <90 mm Hg or diastolic <60 mm Hg)
    Vasopressors required for > 4 hr
    Oliguria with urinary output < 20 mL/hr
    Acute renal failure requiring dialysis

gionella, which is associated with high-dose corticosteroid use and outbreaks secondary to water supplies and cooling systems,[73,177] and Aspergillus, which is associated with neutropenia or organ transplantation.[178]

SELECTING ANTIBIOTIC THERAPY

23.   How should antibiotic therapy be started in A.A.?

Knowledge of the potential pathogens and the local institution's bacteria–antibiotic sensitivities permits the rational selection of an initial empiric regimen. The American Thoracic Society has published guidelines for the treatment of HAP.[176] The likelihood of an infection with a potential pathogen is based on the onset of HAP (early, <5 days into hospitalization versus late, >5 days), severity of the condition, and underlying risk factors. These guidelines are outlined in Table 60-17.[176] In general, patients with early-onset disease who are not severely ill and have no risk factors can be treated with a single agent, including non-antipseudomonal second- or third-generation cephalosporins, β-lactam–inhibitor combinations, or an antipneumococcal fluoroquinolone. Empiric therapy in those with late-onset or severe disease should include a combination of antibiotics active against *Pseudomonas*. This regimen usually includes an antipseudomonal cephalosporin, such as ceftazidime or cefepime, plus either an aminoglycoside or ciprofloxacin/levofloxacin. The addition of vancomycin should be considered if the Gram's stain shows many Gram-positive cocci in clusters. Risk factors for modifying therapy and recommendations are provided in Table 60-17.[176]

Considering the high mortality associated with HAP,[179,180] aggressive broad-spectrum empiric antibiotic therapy should be initiated and then modified when the results of sputum culture are known. The choice of empiric antibiotic therapy should be guided by the results of the Gram's stain and an analysis of the patient's risk factors for oropharyngeal colonization or altered pulmonary host factors. When these are present, as in the case of A.A., coverage for infection due to Gram-negative bacteria is indicated.

If culture results are negative or inconclusive (because of known specimen contamination with mouth flora) the patient's response to the initial antibiotic therapy should be used to evaluate modification of the antibiotic regimen. If the patient responds to the initial therapy, those antibiotics should be continued. If the patient is not responding to the initial antibiotic therapy, one should consider whether (1) the pathogen is not covered in the initial choice of antibiotic therapy, (2) the dose of antibiotic is insufficient, and (3) any other factors are responsible for the failure to respond to therapy. Such factors include poor pulmonary clearance of necrotic tissue and cellular debris, lung abscesses, and severely altered host defenses with a rapidly fatal underlying disease.

Of note, if one of the following organisms is isolated (*Serratia, Pseudomonas,* indole positive *Proteus, Citrobacter,* or *Enterobacter* species), in vitro reports indicating susceptibility should be questioned, as these organisms often possess an inducible β-lactamase gene (also referred to as a type I β-lactamase enzyme).[181] In vitro testing may show these organisms to be susceptible to third-generation cephalosporins and extended-spectrum penicillins; however, they are likely to fail in the clinical setting. As a possible scenario, after initiation with one of these agents, the patient initially will respond; however, after approximately 1 week, the patient's condition will begin to worsen. Because treatment with the β-lactam agent induces the expression of the type I enzyme, a subsequent specimen sent after approximately 1 week is likely to show an organism that is resistant to the third-generation cephalosporins and extended-spectrum penicillins.[181] Although cefepime is more likely to be active against these isolates, a large inoculum of organisms (e.g., that present in pneumonia) can result in β-lactamase degradation of the cephalosporin.[182] Considering this phenomenon will not be identified using in vitro testing, cefepime should be used cautiously in these patients.[99] The preferred therapy in these patients include TMP-SMX, a fluoroquinolone, or a carbapenem.[181] In addition, in some centers *Acinetobacter* species have become resistant to many commonly used antibacterial agents. Treatment of this sometimes multiply-resistant pathogen requires the use of very high doses of ampicillin-sulbactam (up to 24 g per day) or colistin.[182a,b]

In summary, A.A. could be started empirically with cefepime. In addition, gentamicin or ciprofloxacin could be added for synergy for possible *Pseudomonas* infection. When culture results are known, the antibiotic regimen can be modified and individualized for the patient. Therapy is generally continued for 2 weeks. A.A.'s clinical response should be monitored to determine whether the selected antibiotics are effective in treating this infection. These parameters include a decrease in temperature and heart rate, as well as a decrease in the WBC count with resolution of the left shift. Mental status and sensorium are good monitoring parameters in older individuals.

BROAD-SPECTRUM β-LACTAMS

24. **Can the broad-spectrum β-lactam antibiotics, such as cefepime (Maxipime), be used as monotherapy in the treatment of A.A.'s pneumonia?**

In the past, the aminoglycosides were considered the antibiotics of choice in the treatment of nosocomial Gram-negative infections. However, the availability of a large number of relatively nontoxic antibiotics with broad-spectrum antibacterial coverage has minimized the role of aminoglycosides as the agents of choice for these infections. Many of the newer antibiotics have been studied in the treatment of hospital-acquired pneumonias and are effective. Monotherapy with newer β-lactam antibiotics or high-dose ciprofloxacin is a useful alternative choice to the aminoglycosides in the treatment of patients with Gram-negative pneumonia. However, when choosing empiric therapy for a suspected or documented pneumonia caused by *Pseudomonas,* combination therapy probably is preferred.[176] The potential advantages of combination antibiotic therapy include a broad antibacterial coverage, improved bactericidal activity because of synergy between the agents, and suppression of resistance that may develop to one of the antibiotics. In particular, patients with bacteremic pseudomonal pneumonia treated with combination therapy have a lower mortality rate compared with those treated with monotherapy.[183] However, more recent studies do not confirm additional benefit with combination therapy over monotherapy in the treatment of pseudomonal infection.[183a]

AMINOGLYCOSIDES

25. **What pharmacokinetic and pharmacodynamic characteristics must be considered in the dosing of aminoglycosides in patients with hospital-acquired pneumonia?**

Individualization of aminoglycoside dosing is required in patients receiving these drugs.[184–186] The efficacy and toxicity of aminoglycosides correlates with aminoglycoside plasma concentrations and therapeutic outcome in patients with Gram-negative pneumonia.[187] Patients in whom 1-hour postinfusion peak plasma concentrations exceeded 7 μg/mL

had successful outcomes more often than those with lower plasma concentrations. These results suggest that all patients with pneumonia should be dosed individually and monitored using aminoglycoside plasma concentrations.

The aminoglycosides are concentration-dependent killing antibiotics. Their rate and extent of killing organisms is maximized by increasing the peak serum concentration to >10 times the MIC of the pathogenic organism. In addition to maximizing the killing properties of this class of agents, in vitro evidence has demonstrated that this concentration goal also minimizes the development of resistance. The use of once-daily dosing strategies to minimize nephrotoxicity of the aminoglycosides has been studied extensively. Single doses of gentamicin and tobramycin (5 to 7 mg/kg per day) and of amikacin (15 to 20 mg/kg per day) have been reported to be as effective as standard dosing of these agents in controlled clinical trials. However, none of the trials has enrolled a sufficient number of patients required to demonstrate a difference. There are several advantages of single-dose aminoglycoside therapy: (1) it is no more or less nephrotoxic, (2) clinicians are ensured that every patient will achieve a therapeutic peak serum level on the first dose, (3) it is the only safe and effective way to achieve serum peak levels of 10 to 20 times the MIC for difficult-to-treat organisms such as *P. aeruginosa,* and (4) it is a more efficient dosing regimen (less doses and administration times per day; fewer serum level measurements are required).

Despite the use of individualized aminoglycoside dosing, morbidity and mortality rates due to Gram-negative pneumonia remain high. This is because the success of antibiotic therapy depends on the ability of the antibiotic to reach the site of infection and remain biologically active.[188] Concentrations of the aminoglycosides in bronchial secretions range from 1 to 5 μg/mL (approximately 30% to 40% of serum concentrations) 2 to 4 hours after parenteral administration.[189] These concentrations may be insufficient to inhibit the growth of many Gram-negative bacteria in this setting, especially *Pseudomonas*. Whether once-daily dosing will allow for this phenomenon to be overcome remains to be determined.

In addition, the bioactivity of the aminoglycosides is influenced by the local tissue pH. In contrast to the penicillins and cephalosporins, whose activities are little affected over a pH range of 6.0 to 8.0, a 2- to 16-fold increase in the MIC of most Gram-negative bacteria occurs when the pH is decreased from 7.4 to 6.8.[190] Therefore, more antibiotic would have to be present in an acidic environment to inhibit the bacteria. The pH of endobronchial fluid in patients with normal lung physiology and pneumonia averages 6.6. Therefore, to achieve bronchial secretion aminoglycoside concentrations exceeding the MICs of most Gram-negative bacteria, much larger doses will be required.

Inactivation of the aminoglycosides at the site of infection also has been demonstrated. The aminoglycosides bind to purulent exudates and cellular debris, which inactivates their antimicrobial effects.[191–193] In summary, the aminoglycosides penetrate poorly into bronchial secretions and are less active at the site of infection because of local pH effects and binding to cellular debris. Thus, higher dosages must be used, which may in turn place patients at higher risk for ototoxicity and nephrotoxicity.

BRONCHIAL PENETRATION OF ANTIBIOTICS

26. What factors govern the penetration of antibiotics into bronchial secretions? Is penetration into bronchial secretions critical to the effectiveness of an antibiotic used in the treatment of pneumonia?

An important factor to consider in the selection of an antibiotic used to treat pneumonia is its ability to reach the site of infection (i.e., the lung tissue or bronchopulmonary secretions). Antibiotic concentrations in bronchial secretions do not necessarily reflect the lung tissue concentrations but do represent the ability of the antibiotic to cross the bronchoalveolar barrier.[189]

Many anatomic, physicochemical, and host factors influence drug penetration into respiratory tissue and secretions.[189] Active transport mechanisms for drugs have not been identified in respiratory tissues; therefore, passive diffusion is responsible for the transfer of antibiotics into respiratory tissue. The degree of diffusion is determined by the ability of the antibiotic to reach high free concentrations in the serum. The transfer of an antibiotic into tissue may be slower than its elimination from the serum. Furthermore, elimination of the antibiotic from the tissue site occurs more slowly than from the serum; thus, serum concentrations may not reflect antimicrobial concentrations in lung tissue. The results of studies investigating the penetration of antibiotics into bronchial secretions should be interpreted cautiously because most of these studies have analyzed the amount of antibiotic present in samples of expectorated sputum or saliva, which may significantly underestimate the amount of antibiotic present in respiratory secretions. The use of fiberoptic bronchoscopy with a protected sampling device has been helpful in the study of antibiotic penetration into respiratory secretions, but this procedure is impractical in the routine management of patients with pneumonia.

LOCALLY ADMINISTERED ANTIBIOTICS: PROPHYLAXIS

27. Can locally administered antibiotics be used to prevent Gram-negative pneumonias?

The morbidity and mortality rates from hospital-acquired Gram-negative pneumonia have not been reduced despite aggressive treatment with high-dose parenteral antibiotics. Lack of improved outcomes may be the result of poor antibiotic penetration into the bronchial secretions and the local conditions at the site of infection. Consequently, several investigators have studied the efficacy of endotracheal instillation or aerosolization of antibiotics to prevent Gram-negative pneumonias in patients at risk for oropharyngeal colonization.[194–198] Most patients treated have been seriously ill individuals who were admitted to the intensive care unit unconscious and with tracheotomy to provide long-term ventilatory support. Endotracheal instillation and aerosolization of antibiotics significantly reduced oropharyngeal colonization with Gram-negative pathogens as well as the incidence of pneumonia. However, other investigators have observed the emergence of colonization with antibiotic-resistant Gram-negative organisms and pneumonia caused by these pathogens.[196–198] In summary, endotracheally instilled and aerosolized antibiotics can be used to prevent or reduce oropharyngeal colonization in high-risk patients when used for short periods with close microbiologic monitoring. Routine and long-term use cannot be recommended because of a lack of well-controlled clinical trials and the possible emergence of resistance.[199,200]

AEROSOLIZED ANTIBIOTICS

28. Can aerosolized antibiotics be used to treat patients with Gram-negative pneumonias?

The efficacy of locally administered antibiotics to treat bronchopneumonia has been studied to a limited extent.[199] Klastersky and others compared the effects of endotracheally instilled gentamicin with intramuscular gentamicin in patients with pneumonia.[201] A favorable outcome occurred in all seven patients receiving endotracheally instilled gentamicin versus only two of eight patients receiving intramuscular gentamicin.

In a second study, these investigators compared the effects of endotracheally instilled sisomicin with placebo in a similar patient population.[202] All patients received systemic antibiotics consisting of parenteral sisomicin and carbenicillin. A more favorable outcome occurred in those patients receiving endotracheally instilled sisomicin versus those receiving a placebo (78% and 45%, respectively). In patients in whom the infecting organism was sensitive to both carbenicillin and sisomicin, a more favorable response occurred in those patients receiving endotracheal sisomicin versus placebo (79% and 54%, respectively). When the infecting organism was sensitive to sisomicin only, a favorable outcome occurred in 79% versus 28%, respectively. The development of resistant organisms was not a problem in either case.

In a third study, these same investigators compared the effects of parenteral mezlocillin and endotracheally administered sisomicin with and without parenteral sisomicin to determine the benefit of concomitant parenteral aminoglycoside.[203] The clinical outcome in both groups was similar; however, resistant bacteria were isolated from the sputum of the groups that were administered endotracheal sisomicin. These findings strongly support the recommendation that this form of therapy only be used in those patients unresponsive to maximal doses of parenteral therapy.

Administration

29. How is local antibiotic therapy administered?

Local antibiotic therapy may be administered by direct endotracheal instillation or aerosolization. The antibiotic usually is diluted with normal saline before administration. In the case of direct instillation, gentamicin/tobramycin (40 to 80 mg) or amikacin (500 mg) is diluted in 5 to 10 mL of normal saline and instilled directly into the trachea through a catheter or through an endotracheal tube. The patient is then rotated from side to side to promote distribution. Delivery of the antibiotic into the oropharynx by aerosolization is accomplished by use of an atomizer or nebulizers to deliver the antibiotic to the lungs. The aerosolized route is preferred and the dosage is 300 to 600 mg every 8 hours for gentamicin and tobramycin diluted in a smaller volume (1 to 3 mL).[199,200]

Bronchial and Serum Concentrations

30. What concentration of aminoglycoside can be achieved in bronchial secretions by this route of administration, and is any of the antibiotic absorbed?

The concentration of the aminoglycoside in bronchial secretions after parenteral administration (IV or intramuscularly) is low and usually <2 μg/mL.[189] When the aminoglycosides are delivered by either endotracheal instillation or aerosolization, bronchial fluid antibiotic concentrations are substantially higher.[204–207] Bronchial fluid concentrations are significantly higher when the aminoglycosides are given by endotracheal instillation than by aerosol. These values usually exceed 200 μg/mL and remain elevated for the dosing interval[206]; when aerosolization is used, bronchial fluid concentrations usually exceed 20 μg/mL.[205,206]

Absorption of the aminoglycosides from the lung differs with the method of local administration used. Various doses of aminoglycosides have been administered, which makes quantification of the amount of the drug absorbed difficult. When 80 mg of gentamicin is administered by endotracheal instillation, serum concentrations >2.5 μg/mL are achieved, suggesting that a substantial amount of the administered drug is absorbed.[196,204,205] Approximately 10% to 15% of the dose administered by endotracheal instillation is excreted into the urine.[208] When similar doses of antibiotic are administered by aerosolization, serum concentrations are low or undetectable; approximately 2% to 5% of the dose is excreted into the urine. For this reason, aerosolization is the preferred route of administration. As with parenteral aminoglycoside administration, patients with renal dysfunction should be monitored carefully for drug accumulation.

Adverse Effects

31. What adverse effects are associated with local antibiotic administration?

As noted previously, the emergence of antibiotic-resistant bacteria is of major concern because these may be responsible for subsequent bacterial infections. This phenomenon is more frequently associated with prophylactic aerosolized antibiotics.

Endotracheal instillation or aerosolization of antibiotics may cause cough, bronchial irritation, and in some individuals, bronchospasm. These effects most often have been associated with polymyxin-B and have resulted in episodes of acute respiratory failure.[209,210] Polymyxin can stimulate the release of histamine, which is believed to be responsible for these adverse effects; it also can decrease ventilatory function.[209] The aminoglycosides have been relatively well tolerated, although minor alterations in ventilatory function have been reported.[211]

Studies evaluating the incidence of aminoglycoside nephrotoxicity and ototoxicity associated with local antibiotic administration are unavailable; however, the incidence should be low. Patients with renal dysfunction may accumulate this drug, and serum concentrations of the aminoglycoside should be monitored.

32. What preventive measures are effective for hospital-acquired or nosocomial pneumonia?

The substantial risk of pneumonia in the intensive care unit has prompted aggressive methods to prevent this disease.[212,213] The most important recommendations include the use of the semi-upright position to reduce the risk of aspiration[214] and infection control (including hand washing) to prevent the spread of pathogens from one patient to the next. As mentioned previously in the discussion of aspiration pneumonia, the use of sucralfate in lieu of H_2-antagonists to prevent GI ulcers should be advocated, because this practice has shown to reduce the frequency of nosocomial pneumonia.[188] The use of antibiotic rotation (6 months of ceftazidime then 6 months of ciprofloxacin) has been shown by Kollef and colleagues to reduce the number of ventilator-associated pneumonia cases and decrease the incidence of resistant Gram-negative bacterial infections.[215] Although these results are encouraging, more data are required before this practice becomes commonplace. The use of "selective decontamination" to decrease the bacterial burden in the GI tract is not advocated. This practice has been extensively studied in $>4,000$ patients and has been shown to reduce the frequency of pneumonia in the intensive care unit, but it has had no impact on mortality.[216,217] This fact, coupled with the costs of the antibiotic regimens and the potential for the emergence of resistance, makes it difficult to recommend this approach. Finally, as described previously, the use of inhaled or aerosolized antibiotic therapy should be discouraged.[199,200]

Pneumonia in Cystic Fibrosis
Special Treatment Considerations

33. K.P., an 18-year-old man with cystic fibrosis (CF), has been well until 3 days ago when he noted "chest tightness" and a progressive deterioration of pulmonary function requiring supplemental oxygen. Other symptoms include an increased cough with sputum production, decreased appetite, and weight loss.

On physical examination, K.P. is a cachectic young male in moderate respiratory distress. Vital signs include the following: BP, 110/60 mm Hg; pulse, 120 beats/min; respirations, 35 breaths/min; and temperature, 38.5°C. Examination of the chest reveals an increased chest diameter with diffuse bilateral rales; there are no wheezes. K.P.'s height is 64 inches, weight is 42 kg, and serum creatinine (SrCr) is 1.0 mg/dL. Are there special considerations in the treatment of pneumonia in patients with CF?

[SI unit: SrCr, 88.4 μmol/L]

CF is a genetically linked disease affecting exocrine gland secretions throughout the body (See Chapter 98, Cystic Fibrosis.).[218] Progressive pulmonary disease is the major determinant of the morbidity and mortality of patients with this illness. The presence of airway mucus plugging is likely to contribute to the development of significant respiratory dysfunction and the establishment of infection; recurrent respiratory infections play a major role in the pathogenesis of the chronic pulmonary disease seen in these patients. Symptoms associated with an infectious exacerbation include an increased frequency and duration of cough or increased shortness of breath, increased sputum production, change in the appearance of sputum, decreased exercise tolerance, decreased appetite, and a feeling of increased chest congestion.

MICROBIOLOGY

Early in the disease, *S. aureus* is an important pathogen; but later, colonization and infection with *P. aeruginosa* frequently develops. Multiple bacterial isolates with differing antimicrobial sensitivity patterns often are found.[219] In addition, infection due to *Burkholderia cepacia* is emerging as a significant problem in patients with CF.[220,221] The role of *B. cepacia* as a pathogen in CF patients is difficult to determine because many patients recover from acute infections despite the use of antimicrobials with little activity against this organism. Most strains demonstrate variable sensitivity patterns to many of the presently used antibiotics. Therefore, antibiotic therapy should be based on known in vitro sensitivity testing.

Vigorous chest percussion with postural drainage and systemic antibiotics have been the mainstay of therapy in the treatment of pulmonary infections in patients with CF. It is unclear whether combination antibiotic therapy is required to treat these patients, but it frequently is used to treat Gram-negative pulmonary infections in CF patients. Combination therapy usually consists of an aminoglycoside or ciprofloxacin and an antipseudomonal β-lactam (piperacillin, ceftazidime, cefepime, aztreonam, imipenem, or meropenem). Therapy generally is continued for 14 to 21 days.

DOSING CONSIDERATIONS

Altered drug elimination in CF patients has been reported for several different types of drugs.[222–225] Jusko and colleagues studied the pharmacokinetics of dicloxacillin in patients with CF and reported that the total body clearance and renal clearance of this drug were increased.[222] In another study, when specific techniques to assess the glomerular infiltration rate were used, tobramycin renal clearance was not increased out of proportion to the glomerular filtration rate. These results suggest that alterations in the nonrenal clearance are responsible for the increased clearance of the aminoglycosides. The underlying reasons for these changes are unclear. In addition, changes in the pharmacokinetics of antibiotics are neither consistent nor predictable. Patients with CF may require higher dosages to achieve therapeutic plasma concentrations of some antibiotics.[200,226] Therefore, dosages must be carefully individualized and serum levels (in the case of the aminoglycosides) should be monitored.

LOCAL ANTIBIOTIC ADMINISTRATION

34. **Because such high doses or parenteral aminoglycosides are required in CF patients, can aerosolized aminoglycosides be used instead?**

Aerosolized antibiotics have been advocated for CF patients with acute pulmonary infections,[227–230] because several factors limit the use of intravenous administration. Because most antibiotics penetrate variably into lung tissue, they usually are administered in maximal doses to facilitate passive diffusion, which also increases the risk of systemic toxicity. In contrast, inhaled antibiotics deliver large concentrations of antibiotics to the site of infection while producing negligible serum concentrations, which should reduce the risk of systemic toxicity.

However, several potential problems are associated with aerosolized antibiotics. Prolonged administration selects out resistant organisms in the bronchial airways, and this may have deleterious consequences because of the recurrent nature of pulmonary infections in CF patients. To be effective, the antibiotic must be delivered to the alveoli. This requires particles <2 μm wide, but most commercially available nebulizers generate particles between 2.5 and 4.5 μm wide,[231] which are deposited primarily in the oropharynx and smaller airways. Also, studies using radioisotope-labeled aerosolized particles have shown that there is a heterogeneous pattern of deposition in CF patients,[232] which may limit the therapeutic effectiveness of this delivery route. Bronchospasm has occurred in patients given aerosolized gentamicin, which also may limit the delivery of antibiotic to the site of infection. Although nephrotoxicity and ototoxicity have not been associated with the administration of aerosolized aminoglycosides, long-term studies have not been performed.

To date, there are few well-controlled studies evaluating the effectiveness of aerosolized antibiotics in CF patients. Stephens and colleagues administered aerosolized tobramycin along with parenteral antibiotics and reported that the clinical outcomes of those receiving the combination of parenteral and aerosolized antibiotics did not differ from those receiving parenteral antibiotics alone.[228] Steinkamp and colleagues evaluated the clinical effectiveness of long-term, prophylactic tobramycin aerosol therapy in 14 CF patients.[230] The best clinical outcomes occurred in individuals who were defined as moderately ill and had mild lung disease. Drug toxicity and the emergence of resistant organisms were minimal in the study population. Although aerosolized antibiotics have reportedly slowed the rate of pulmonary function decline in uncontrolled trials,[233] these positive results are difficult to differentiate from the natural course of CF, which is characterized by significant variability in the rate of lung function deterioration. Ramsey and colleagues conducted a placebo-controlled, parallel-design, cross-over study of 71 patients with stable pulmonary status and *P. aeruginosa* detected in their sputum.[234] Tobramycin 600 mg three times daily or placebo was delivered for 28 days by ultrasonic nebulizer. The dose was based on previous studies showing that sputum tobramycin concentrations >10 times the MIC for *P. aeruginosa* or a minimum sputum concentration of 400 μg/mL were required to ensure bacterial killing. The results showed a small but significant improvement in pulmonary function in favor of the tobramycin group. They also showed a 100-fold reduction in the density of *P. aeruginosa* in sputum, a modest reduction in PMN count, a reduction in pulmonary exacerbations, and a lower rate of systemic antibiotic use. More recently, Ramsey and colleagues conducted two double-blind, placebo-controlled trials of intermittent inhaled tobramycin in patients with CF. These studies used a new formulation of tobramycin for inhalation that is preservative free and less likely to induce local adverse reactions. Patients treated with tobramycin had a statistically significant increase in FEV_1, a decrease in the density of *P. aeruginosa,* and a decrease in hospitalization relative to the placebo group. An increase in the percentage of resistant *P. aeruginosa* was noted in the tobramycin-treated patients, but it did not reach statistical significance.[235]

In summary, aerosolized antibiotics provide tangible clinical benefits in this patient population. The development of resistance subsequent to aerosolized therapy is concerning, but the clinical significance of these findings are unknown. This route can be used as an adjunct to parenteral therapy in patients with severe, acute exacerbations of pulmonary infections that are unresponsive to maximal parenteral doses.[226,234–236]

The optimal dose of aerosolized antibiotics is unknown. The regimens found to be most effective include gentamicin or tobramycin, 300 to 600 mg three times daily, administered via a jet nebulizer.[226,235]

REFERENCES

1. Dixon RE. Economic costs of respiratory tract infections in the United States. Am J Med 1985; 78(Suppl 6B):45.
2. U.S. Department of Commerce, Bureau of the Census. Statistical Abstract of the United States. 113th Ed. Washington, DC: U.S. Government Printing Office, 1993.
3. Centers for Disease Control and Prevention. Trends in morbidity and mortality: pneumonia, influenza, and acute respiratory conditions, January 2001. www.cdc.gov/nchs/about/major/nhis/released200306.htm
4. Lui KJ, Kendal AP. Impact of influenza epidemics on mortality in the United States from October 1972 to May 1985. Am J Public Health 1987;77:712.
5. Chretien J et al. Acute respiratory infections in children: burden during the first five years of life. N Engl J Med 1984;310:982.
6. Gonzales R et al. What will it take to stop physicians from prescribing antibiotics in acute bronchitis. Lancet 1995;345:665.
7. Gonzales R et al. Antibiotic prescribing for adults with colds, upper respiratory tract infections and bronchitis by ambulatory care physicians. JAMA 1997;278:901.
8. Steinman MA et al. Changing antibiotic use in community-based outpatient practice, 1991-1997. Ann Intern Med 2003;138:523.
9. Franks P et al. The treatment of acute bronchitis with trimethoprim and sulfamethoxazole. J Fam Pract 1984;19:185.
10. Verheij TJM et al. Effects of doxycycline in patients with acute cough and purulent sputum: a double-blind placebo-controlled study. Br J Gen Pract 1994;44:400.
11. Orr PH et al. Randomized placebo-controlled trials for acute bronchitis: a critical review of the literature. J Fam Pract 1993;36:507.
12. Niederman MS et al. Treatment cost of acute exacerbations of chronic bronchitis. Clin Ther 1999;21:576.
13. Sethi S. Infectious etiology of acute exacerbations of chronic bronchitis. Chest 2000;117:380S.
14. Reynolds HY. Chronic bronchitis and acute infectious exacerbations. In: Mandell GL et al., eds. Principles and Practice of Infectious Diseases. 3rd Ed. New York: John Wiley and Sons, 1990.
15. American Thoracic Society. Standards for the diagnosis and care of patients with chronic obstructive pulmonary disease (COPD) and asthma. Am Rev Respir Dis 1987;136:225.
16. Burrows B et al. The course and prognosis of different forms of chronic airways obstruction in a sample from the general population. N Engl J Med 1987;317:1309.
17. Gump DW et al. Role of infection in chronic bronchitis. Am Rev Respir Dis 1976;113:465.
18. Chodosh S. Treatment of acute exacerbations of chronic bronchitis: state of the art. Am J Med 1991;91(Suppl 6A):87S.
19. Chodosh S. Examination of sputum cells. N Engl J Med 1970;282:854.
20. Bartlett J. Diagnostic accuracy of transtracheal aspiration bacteriologic studies. Am Rev Respir Dis 1977;115:777.
21. Gump DW et al. Role of infection in chronic bronchitis. Am Rev Respir Dis 1976;113:465.
22. Pollard JA et al. Incidence of *Moraxella catarrhalis* in the sputa of patients with chronic lung disease. Drugs 1986:31(Suppl 3):103.
23. Nicotra MB et al. Antibiotic therapy of acute exacerbations of chronic bronchitis: a controlled study using tetracycline. Ann Intern Med 1982;97:18.
24. Celli BR et al. ATS statement: standards for the diagnosis and care of patients with chronic obstructive pulmonary disease. Am J Respir Crit Care Med 1995;152(Suppl 2):S77.
25. Anzueto A et al. Etiology, susceptibility, and treatment of acute bacterial exacerbations of complicated chronic bronchitis in the primary care setting: ciprofloxacin 750 mg BID versus clarithromycin 500 mg BID. Curr Ther 1998;20:1.

26. Ball P et al. Acute exacerbations of chronic bronchitis: an international comparison. Chest 1998; 113(Suppl 3):1995.
27. Chodosh S et al. Efficacy and safety of a 10 day course of 400 mg or 600 mg of grepafloxacin once daily for treatment of acute bacterial exacerbations of chronic bronchitis: comparison with a 10 day course of 500 mg of ciprofloxacin twice daily. Antimicrob Agents Chemother 1998;42:114.
28. Rodnick JE et al. The use of antibiotics in acute bronchitis and acute exacerbations of chronic bronchitis. West J Med 1988;149:347.
29. Anthonisen NR et al. Antibiotic therapy in exacerbations of chronic obstructive pulmonary diseases. Ann Intern Med 1987;106:196.
30. Elmes PC et al. Prophylactic use of oxytetracycline for exacerbations of chronic bronchitis. BMJ 1957;2:1272.
31. Nicotra MB et al. Antibiotic therapy of acute exacerbations of chronic bronchitis. Ann Intern Med 1982;97:18.
32. Petersen ES et al. A controlled study of the effect of treatment on chronic bronchitis: an evaluation using pulmonary function tests. Acta Med Scand 1967; 182:293.
33. Jorgensen AF et al. Amoxicillin in treatment of acute uncomplicated exacerbations of chronic bronchitis: a double-blind, placebo-controlled multicentre study in general practice. Scand J Prev Health Care 1992;10:7.
34. Saint S et al. Antibiotics in chronic obstructive pulmonary disease exacerbations: a meta-analysis. JAMA 1995;273:957.
35. Flaherty KR et al. The spectrum of acute bronchitis: using baseline factors to guide empirical therapy. Postgrad Med 2001;109:39.
36. Adams SG et al. Antibiotics are associated with lower relapse rates in outpatients with acute exacerbations of COPD. Chest 2000;117:1345.
37. Anzueto A et al. The infection-free interval: its use in evaluating antimicrobial treatment of acute exacerbation of chronic bronchitis. Clin Infect Dis 1999; 28:1344.
38. Chodosh S et al. Randomized, double-blind study of ciprofloxacin and cefuroxime axetil for treatment of acute bacterial exacerbations of chronic bronchitis: The Bronchitis Study Group. Clin Infect Dis 1999;27:727.
39. Read RC. Infection in acute exacerbations of chronic bronchitis: a clinical perspective. Respir Med 1999;93:252.
40. Black P et al. Prophylactic antibiotic treatment for CB. Cochrane Database of Systematic Reviews 2003;1:DD004105.
41. Recommendations of the Immunization Practices Advisory Committee (ACIP). Pneumococcal polysaccharide vaccine. MMWR 1989;38:64.
42. Johnston RN et al. Five year chemoprophylaxis for chronic bronchitis. BMJ 1969;4:265.
43. Pridie RB et al. A trial of continuous winter chemotherapy in chronic bronchitis. Lancet 1960; 2:723.
44. Fine MJ et al. A prediction rule to identify low risk patients with community-acquired pneumonia. N Engl J Med 1997;336:243.
45a. Metlay SP, Fine MJ. Testing strategies in the initial management of patients with community-acquired pneumonia. Ann Intern Med 2003;138: 109–118.
45. Bartlett JG et al. Practice guidelines for the management of community-acquired pneumonia in adults. Clin Infect Dis 2000;31:347.
46. Garibaldi RA. Epidemiology of community-acquired respiratory tract infections in adults: incidence, etiology, and impact. Am J Med 1985;78:32S.
47. Fine MJ et al. Prognosis and outcomes of patients with community-acquired pneumonia. JAMA 1996;275:134.
48. Centers for Disease Control and Prevention. Pneumonia and influenza death rates—United States, 1979–1994. MMWR 1995;44:535.

49. Niederman MS et al. The cost of treating community-acquired pneumonia. Clin Ther 1998;20:820.
50. Bartlett JG et al. Community-acquired pneumonia. N Engl J Med 1995;333:1618.
51. Pennington JE. Respiratory tract infections: intrinsic risk factors. Am J Med 1984;76(Suppl 5A):34.
52. Skerett SJ. Host defenses against respiratory infections. Med Clin North Am 1994;78:941.
53. Mundy LM et al. Community-acquired pneumonia: impact of immune status. Am J Respir Crit Care Med 1995;152:1309.
54. Toews GB. Pulmonary clearance of infectious agents. In: Pennington JE, ed. Respiratory Infections: Diagnosis and Management. New York: Raven Press, 1983.
55. Lorber B, Swenson R. Bacteriology of aspiration pneumonia: a prospective study of community- and hospital-acquired cases. Ann Intern Med 1974; 81:329.
56. Petersdorf RG et al. A study of antibiotic prophylaxis in unconscious patients. N Engl J Med 1957;257:1001.
57. Tillotson JR, Finland M. Bacterial colonization and clinical super-infection of the respiratory tract complicating antibiotic treatment of pneumonia. J Infect Dis 1969;119:597.
58. Rosenthal S, Tager IB. Prevalence of Gram-negative rods in the normal pharyngeal flora. Ann Intern Med 1975;83:355.
59. Johanson WG et al. Changing pharyngeal bacterial flora of hospitalized patients. N Engl J Med 1969;28:1137.
60. Johanson WG et al. Nosocomial respiratory infections with Gram-negative bacilli: the significance of colonization of the respiratory tract. Ann Intern Med 1972;77:701.
61. Klein RS, Steigbigel NH. Aspiration pneumonia. Semin Infect Dis 1983;5:274.
62. Valenti WM et al. Factors predisposing to oropharyngeal colonization with Gram-negative bacilli in the aged. N Engl J Med 1978;298:1108.
63. Verghese A, Berk SL. Bacterial pneumonia in the elderly. Medicine (Baltimore) 1983;62:271.
64. Haas H et al. Bacterial flora of the respiratory tract in chronic bronchitis: comparison of transtracheal, fiberbronchoscopic, and oropharyngeal sampling methods. Am Rev Respir Dis 1977;116:41.
65. Murray PR, Washington JA. Microscopic and bacteriologic analysis of expectorated sputum. Mayo Clin Proc 1975;50:339.
66. Dal Nogare AR. Nosocomial pneumonia in the medical and surgical patient. Med Clin North Am 1994;78:1081.
67. Marrie TJ et al. Community-acquired pneumonia requiring hospitalization: a 5-year prospective study. Rev Infect Dis 1989;11:586.
68. Fekety FR Jr et al. Bacteria, viruses, and mycoplasmas in acute pneumonia in adults. Am Rev Respir Dis 1971;104:499.
69. Farr BM et al. Predicting death in patients hospitalized with community-acquired pneumonia. Ann Intern Med 1991;115:428.
70. Fang GD et al. New and emerging etiologies for community-acquired pneumonia with implications for therapy: a prospective multi-center study of 359 cases. Medicine 1990;69:307.
71. Thornsberry C et al. Surveillance of antimicrobial resistance in *Streptococcus pneumoniae, Haemophilus influenzae* and *Moraxella catarrhalis* in the United States in 1996–1997 respiratory season. Diagn Microbiol Infect Dis 1997;29:249.
72. Thornsberry C et al. International surveillance of resistance among respiratory tract pathogens in the United States, 1997–1998. 38th Interscience Conference on Antimicrobial Agents and Chemotherapy, San Diego, September 24, 1998. Abstract E-22.
73. Edelstein PH. Legionnaires' disease. Clin Infect Dis 1993;16:741.
74. Brook I. Percutaneous transtracheal aspiration in the diagnosis and treatment of aspiration pneumonia in children. J Pediatr 1980;96:1000.

75. Grayston JT et al. A new *Chlamydia psittaci* strain, TWAR, isolated in acute respiratory tract infections. N Engl J Med 1986;315:161.

76. Gleason PP et al. Associations between initial antimicrobial therapy and medical outcomes for hospitalized elderly patients with pneumonia. Arch Intern Med 1999;159:2562.

77. Krumpe PE et al. Intravenous and oral mono- or combination-therapy in the treatment of severe infections: ciprofloxacin versus standard antibiotic therapy. Ciprofloxacin Study Group. J Antimicrob Chemother 1999;43(Suppl A):117.

78. Mittl RL Jr et al. Radiographic resolution of community-acquired pneumonia. Am J Respir Crit Care Med 1994;149:630.

79. Jay SJ et al. The radiographic resolution of *Streptococcus pneumoniae* pneumonia. N Engl J Med 1975;293:798.

80. Austrian R et al. Pneumococcal bacteremia with special reference to bacteremic pneumococcal pneumonia. Ann Intern Med 1964;60:759.

81. Thornsberry C et al. Surveillance of antimicrobial resistance in *Streptococcus pneumoniae, Haemophilus influenzae,* and *Moraxella catarrhalis* in the United States in 1996–1997 respiratory season. The Laboratory Investigator Group. Diagn Microbiol Infect Dis 1997;29(4):249.

82. Doern GV. Antimicrobial use and the emergence of antimicrobial resistance with *Streptococcus pneumoniae* in the United States. Clin Infect Dis 2001; 33(Suppl 3):S187.

83. Doern GV et al. Antimicrobial resistance among clinical isolates of *Streptococcus pneumoniae* in the United States during 1999–2000, including a comparison of resistance rates since 1994–1995. Antimicrob Agents Chemother 2001;45(6):1721.

84. Mufson MA. Penicillin-resistant *Streptococcus pneumoniae* increasingly threatens the patient and challenges the physician. Clin Infect Dis 1998; 27(4):771.

85. Pallares R et al. Resistance to penicillin and cephalosporin and mortality from severe pneumococcal pneumonia in Barcelona, Spain. N Engl J Med 1995;333:474.

86. Whitney CG et al. Increasing prevalence of multidrug resistant *Streptococcus pneumoniae* in the United States. N Engl J Med 2003;343:1917.

87. Yu VL et al. An international prospective study of pneumococcal bacteremia: correlation with in vitro resistance, antibiotics administered, and clinical outcome. Clin Infect Dis 2003;37:230.

88. Lonks JR et al. Failure of macrolide antibiotic treatment in patients with bacteremia due to erythromycin-resistant *Streptococcus pneumoniae.* Clin Infect Dis 2002;35:556.

89. Sutcliffe J et al. *Streptococcus pneumoniae* and *Streptococcus pyogenes* resistant to macrolides but sensitive to clindamycin: a common resistance pattern mediated by an efflux system. Antimicrob Agents Chemother 1996;40:1817.

90. Johnston NJ et al. Prevalence and characterization of the mechanisms of macrolide, lincosamide, and streptogramin resistance in isolates of **Streptococcus pneumoniae.** Antimicrob Agents Chemother 1998;42:2425.

91. File T et al. A multicenter, randomized study comparing the efficacy and safety of intravenous and/or oral levofloxacin versus ceftriaxone and/or cefuroxime axetil in the treatment of adults with community-acquired pneumonia. Antimicrob Agents Chemother 1997;41:1965.

92. Ortqvist A et al. Oral empiric treatment of community-acquired pneumonia: a multi-center, double blind, randomized study comparing sparfloxacin with roxithromycin: the Scandinavian Sparfloxacin Study Group. Chest 1996;110(6):1499.

93. Dowell ME et al. A randomized, double-blind, multicenter comparative study of gatifloxacin 400 mg IV and PO versus ceftriaxone ±erythromycin in treatment of community-acquired pneumonia requiring hospitalization. 39th Interscience Conference on Antimicrobial Agents and Chemotherapy, San Francisco, September 26, 1999. Abstract 2241.

94. Hooper DC. Expanding uses of fluoroquinolones: opportunities and challenges. Ann Intern Med 1998;129:908.

95. Applebaum PC et al. Role of the newer fluoroquinolones against penicillin-resistant *Streptococcus pneumoniae.* Infect Dis Clin Pract 1999;8:374.

96. Chen DK et al. Decreased susceptibility of *Streptococcus pneumoniae* to fluoroquinolones in Canada: Canadian Bacterial Surveillance Network. N Engl J Med 1999;34:233.

97. Low DE et al. Strategies for stemming the tide of antimicrobial resistance. JAMA 1998;273:394.

98. Heffelfinger JD et al. Management of community-acquired pneumonia in the era of pneumococcal resistance: a report from the Drug-Resistant Streptococcus Pneumoniae Therapeutic Working Group. Arch Intern Med 2000;160(10):1399.

99. Acar J. Rapid emergence of resistance to cefepime during treatment [Letter]. Clin Infect Dis 1998; 26(6):1484.

100. Monto AS et al. Zanamivir in the prevention of influenza among healthy adults. JAMA 1999;282:31.

101. Hayden FG et al. Efficacy and safety of the neuraminidase inhibitor zanamivir in the treatment of influenza virus infections. N Engl J Med 1997; 337:874.

102. Hayden FG et al. Use of the selective neuraminidase inhibitor oseltamivir to prevent influenza. N Engl J Med 1999;341:1336.

103. Treanor JJ et al. Efficacy and of the oral neuraminidase inhibitor oseltamivir in treating acute influenza. JAMA 2000;283:1016.

104. Winquist AG et al. Neuraminidase inhibitors for treatment of influenza A and B infections. MMWR 1999;48(RR-14):1.

105. Demicheli V et al. Prevention and early treatment of influenza in healthy adults. Vaccine 2000;18:957.

106. Uyeki TM et al. Large summertime influenza A outbreak among tourists in Alaska and the Yukon Territory, 2003. volume 36:1095–1102 Clin Infect Dis (in press).

107. Gross PA et al. Time to earliest peak serum antibody response to influenza vaccine in the elderly. Clin Diagn Lab Immunol 1997;4:491.

108. Brokstad KA et al. Parenteral influenza vaccination induces a rapid systemic and local immune response. J Infect Dis 1995;171:198.

109. Tominack RL, Hayden FG. Rimantadine hydrochloride and amantadine hydrochloride use in influenza A virus infections. Infect Dis Clin North Am 1987;1:459.

110. Nicholson KG. Use of antivirals in influenza in the elderly: prophylaxis and therapy. Gerontology 1996;42:280.

111. Wintermeyer SM, Nahata MC. Rimantadine: a clinical perspective. Ann Pharmacother 1995;29:299.

112. Gravenstein S et al. Zanamivir: a review of clinical safety in individuals at high risk of developing influenza-related complications. Drug Saf 2001;24:1113.

113. Bowles SK et al. Use of oseltamivir during influenza outbreaks in Ontario nursing homes, 1999–2000. J Am Geriatr Soc 2002;50:608.

114. Guay DR. Amantadine and rimantadine prophylaxis of influenza A in nursing homes: a tolerability perspective. Drugs Aging 1994;5:8.

115. Peters PH Jr et al. Long-term use of oseltamivir for the prophylaxis of influenza in a vaccinated frail older population. J Am Geriatr Soc 2001;49:1025.

116. Faletta JM et al. Discontinuing penicillin prophylaxis in children with sickle cell anemia. J Pediatr 1995;127:685.

117. American Academy of Pediatrics. 1994 Red book: report of the Committee on Infectious Diseases. Elk Grove Village, IL: American Academy of Pediatrics, 1994:371.

118. Patriarca PA et al. Safety of prolonged administration of rimantadine hydrochloride in the prophylaxis of influenza A virus infections in nursing homes. Antimicrob Agents Chemother 1984;26:101.

119. Arden NH et al. Roles of vaccination and amantadine prophylaxis in controlling an outbreak of influenza A (H3N2) in a nursing home. Arch Intern Med 1988;148:865.

120. Monto AS et al. Zanamivir in the prevention of influenza among healthy adults: a randomized controlled trial. JAMA 1999;282:31.

121. Hayden FG et al. Use of the selective oral neuraminidase inhibitor oseltamivir to prevent influenza. N Engl J Med 1999;341:1336.

122. Monto AS et al. Zanamivir prophylaxis: an effective strategy for the prevention of influenza types A and B within households. J Infect Dis 2002;186:1582.

123. Schilling M et al. Efficacy of zanamivir for chemoprophylaxis of nursing home influenza outbreaks. Vaccine 1998;16:1771.

124. Lee C et al. Zanamivir use during transmission of amantadine-resistant influenza A in a nursing home. Infect Control Hosp Epidemiol 2000;21:700.

125. Parker R et al. Experience with oseltamivir in the control of a nursing home influenza B outbreak. Can Commun Dis Rep 2001;27:37

126. Webster A et al. Coadministration of orally inhaled zanamivir with inactivated trivalent influenza vaccine does not adversely affect the production of antihaemagglutinin antibodies in the serum of healthy volunteers. Clin Pharmacokinet 1999;36(Suppl 1):51.

127. Patriarca PA et al. Prevention and control of type A influenza infections in nursing homes: benefits and costs of four approaches using vaccination and amantadine. Ann Intern Med 1987;107:732.

128. Gomolin IH et al. Control of influenza outbreaks in the nursing home: guidelines for diagnosis and management. J Am Geriatr Soc 1995;43:71.

129. Garner JS. Guideline for isolation precautions in hospitals: Hospital Infection Control Practices Advisory Committee. Infect Control Hosp Epidemiol 1996;17:53.

130. Paradise JL et al. Otitis media in 2253 Pittsburgh-area infants: prevalence and risk factors during the first two years of life. Pediatrics 1997;99:318.

131. Bradley SF. Prevention of influenza in long-term-care facilities. Long-Term-Care Committee of the Society for Healthcare Epidemiology of America. Infect Control Hosp Epidemiol 1999;20:629.

132. Shijubo N et al. Experience with oseltamivir in the control of nursing home influenza A outbreak. Intern Med 2002;41:366.

133. Centers for Disease Control and Prevention. Prevention and control of influenza: recommendations of the Advisory Committee on Immunization Practices. MMWR 2003;52(RR-08):1.

134. Centers for Disease Control and Prevention. Prevention of pneumococcal disease: recommendations from the Committee on Immunization Practices (ACIP). MMWR 1997;46(RR-08):1.

135. Musher DM et al. Pneumococcal polysaccharide vaccine in young adults and older bronchitics: determination of IgG responses by ELISA and the effect of adsorption of serum with non-type-specific cell wall polysaccharide. J Infect Dis 1990;161:728.

136. Mufson MA et al. G. Long-term persistence of antibody following immunization with pneumococcal polysaccharide vaccine. Proc Soc Exp Biol Med 1983;173:270.

137. Mufson MA et al. Pneumococcal antibody levels one decade after immunization of healthy adults. Am J Med Sci 1987;293:279.

138. Shapiro ED, Clemens JD. A controlled evaluation of the protective efficacy of pneumococcal vaccine for patients at high risk of serious pneumococcal infections. Ann Intern Med 1984;101:325.

139. Sims RV et al. The clinical effectiveness of pneumococcal vaccine in the elderly. Ann Intern Med 1988;108:653.

140. Shapiro ED et al. The protective efficacy of polyvalent pneumococcal polysaccharide vaccine. N Engl J Med 1991;325:1453.

141. Farr BM et al. Preventing pneumococcal bacteremia in patients at risk: results of a matched case-control study. Arch Intern Med 1995;155:2336.

142. Lin JD et al. The cost effectiveness of pneumococcal vaccination [Abstract]. Abstracts of the American Public Health Association 124th Annual Meeting and Exposition, New York, NY, November 17–21,1996, p. 328.
143. Centers for Disease Control and Prevention. Recommendations of the Immunization Practices Advisory Committee: pneumococcal polysaccharide vaccine. MMWR 1989;38:64.
144. Fedson DS, Musher DM. Pneumococcal vaccine. In: Plotkin SA, Mortimer EA Jr, eds. Vaccines. 2nd Ed. Philadelphia: WB Saunders, 1994:517.
145. Garner CV, Pier GB. Immunologic considerations for the development of conjugate vaccines. In: Cruse JM, Lewis RE, eds. Conjugate Vaccines. Basel, Switzerland: Karger, 1989;11.
146. Centers for Disease Control and Prevention. National Health Interview Survey. http://www.cdc.gov/nip/coverage/default.htm#NHIS, accessed, June 18, 2003.
147. Bartlett JG, Gorbach SL. The triple threat of aspiration pneumonia. Chest 1975;68:560.
148. Gianella RA et al. Gastric acid barrier to ingested microorganisms in man: studies in vivo and in vitro. Gut 1972;13:251.
149. Drasar BS et al. Studies on the intestinal flora: I. The bacterial flora of the gastrointestinal tract in health and achlorhydric persons. Gastroenterology 1969;56:71.
150. Bynum LJ, Pierce AK. Pulmonary aspiration of gastric contents. Am Rev Respir Dis 1976;114:1129.
151. Huxley EJ et al. Pharyngeal aspiration in normal adults and patients with depressed consciousness. Am J Med 1978;64:564.
152. LeFrock JL et al. Aspiration pneumonia: a ten-year review. Am Surg 1979;45:305.
153. Landay MJ et al. Pulmonary manifestations of acute aspiration of gastric contents. Am J Roentgenol 1978;131:587.
154. Wolfe JE et al. Effects of corticosteroids in the treatment of patients with gastric aspiration. Am J Med 1977;63:719.
155. Bartlett JG et al. The bacteriology of aspiration pneumonia. Am J Med 1974;56:202.
156. Ingham HR et al. The activity of metronidazole against facultatively anaerobic bacteria. J Antimicrob Chemother 1980;6:343.
157. Brook I, Finegold SM. Bacteriology of aspiration pneumonia in children. Pediatrics 1980;65:1115.
158. Pingleton SD et al. Enteral nutrition in patients receiving mechanical ventilation: multiple sources of tracheal colonization include the stomach. Am J Med 1986;80:827.
159. Drasar BS et al. Studies of the intestinal flora. Gastroenterology 1969;56:71.
160. Muscroft TJ et al. The microflora of the postoperative stomach. Br J Surg 1981;68:560.
161. DuMoulin GC et al. Aspiration of gastric bacteria in antacid-treated patients: a frequent cause of postoperative colonization of the airway. Lancet 1982;1:242.
162. Tryba M. Risk of acute stress bleeding and nosocomial pneumonia in ventilated intensive care unit patients: sucralfate versus antacids. Am J Med 1987;83(Suppl 3B):117.
163. Driks MR et al. Nosocomial pneumonia in intubated patients given sucralfate as compared with antacids of histamine type 2 blockers. N Engl J Med 1987;317:1376.
164. Sanders CV et al. Metronidazole in the treatment of anaerobic infections. Am Rev Respir Dis 1979;120:337.
165. Perlino CA. Metronidazole vs clindamycin treatment of anaerobic pulmonary infection. Arch Intern Med 1981;141:1424.
166. Garibaldi RA et al. Infections among patients in nursing homes: policies, prevalence, and problems. N Engl J Med 1981;305:731.
167. Johanson WG et al. Changing pharyngeal bacterial flora of hospitalized patients: emerging Gram-negative bacilli. N Engl J Med 1969;281:1137.

168. Mackowiak PA et al. Pharyngeal colonization by Gram-negative bacilli in aspiration-prone persons. Arch Intern Med 1978;138:1224.
169. Johanson WG et al. Association of respiratory tract colonization with adherence of Gram-negative bacilli to epithelial cells. J Infect Dis 1979;139:667.
170. Johanson WG et al. Bacterial adherence to epithelial cells in bacillary colonization of the respiratory tract. Am Rev Respir Dis 1980;121:55.
171. Rouby JJ et al. Nosocomial bronchopneumonia in the critically ill: histologic and bacteriologic aspects. Am Rev Respir Dis 1992;146:1059.
172. Bartlett JG et al. Bacteriology of hospital-acquired pneumonia. Arch Intern Med 1986;146:868.
173. Prod'hom G et al. Nosocomial pneumonia in mechanically ventilated patients receiving antacid, ranitidine, or sucralfate as prophylaxis for stress ulcer: a randomized controlled trial. Ann Intern Med 1994;120:653.
174. Rello J et al. Impact of previous antimicrobial therapy on etiology and outcome of ventilator-associated pneumonia. Chest 1993;104:1230.
175. Fridkin SK et al. Magnitude and prevention of nosocomial prevention infections in the intensive care unit. Infect Dis Clin North Am 1997;11:479.
176. American Thoracic Society. Hospital-acquired pneumonia in adults: diagnosis, assessment of severity, initial antimicrobial therapy, and preventative strategies. A consensus statement. Am Rev Respir Crit Care Med 1995;153:1711.
177. Stout JE et al. Ubiquitousness of *Legionella pneumophila* in water supply of a hospital with endemic Legionnaires' diseases. N Engl J Med 1982;306:466.
178. Rhame FS. Prevention of nosocomial aspergillosis. J Hosp Infect 1991;18:466.
179. Celis RT et al. Nosocomial pneumonia: a multivariant analysis of risk and prognosis. Chest 1988;93:318.
180. Fagon JY et al. Nosocomial pneumonia in ventilated patients: a cohort study evaluating attributable mortality and hospital stay. Am J Med 1993;94:281.
181. Chow JW et al. Enterobacter bacteremia—clinical features and emergence of antibiotic resistance during therapy. Ann Intern Med 1991;115:585.
182. Medeiros AA. Relapsing infection due to Enterobacter species: lessons of heterogeneity [Editorial; Comment]. Clin Infect Dis 1997;25(2):341.
182a. Smolyakov R et al. Nosocomial multi-drug resistant Acinetobacter baumannii bloodstream infection: risk factors and outcome with ampicillin-sulbactam treatment. J Hosp Infect 2003;54:32–38.
182b. Garnacho-Montero J, et al. Treatment of multi-drug-resistant Acinetobacter baumannii ventilator-associated pneumonia (VAP) with intravenous colistin: A comparison with imipenem-susceptible VAP. Clin Infect Dis 2003;36:1111–1118.
183. Hilf M et al. Antibiotic therapy for *Pseudomonas aeruginosa* bacteremia: outcome correlations in a prospective study of 200 patients. Am J Med 1989;87:540.
183a. Klibanov OM, Raasch RH, Rublein JC. Single versus combined therapy for gram-negative infections. Ann Pharmacother 2004;38:332–337.
184. Barza M et al. Predictability of blood levels of gentamicin in man. J Infect Dis 1975;132:165.
185. Zaske DE et al. Wide interpatient variations in gentamicin dose requirements for geriatric patients. JAMA 1982;248:3122.
186. Flint LM et al. Serum level monitoring of aminoglycoside antibiotics. Arch Surg 1985;120:99.
187. Moore RD et al. Association of aminoglycoside plasma levels with therapeutic outcome in Gram-negative pneumonia. Am J Med 1984; 77:657.
188. Moore RD et al. Association of aminoglycoside levels with therapeutic outcome in Gram-negative pneumonia. Am J Med 1984;77:657.
189. Bergogne-Berezin E. Pharmacokinetics of antibiotics in respiratory secretion. In: Pennington JE, ed. Respiratory Infections: Diagnosis and Management. New York: Raven Press, 1983.

190. Bodem CR et al. Endobronchial pH: relevance of aminoglycoside activity in Gram-negative bacillary pneumonia. Am Rev Respir Dis 1983;127:39.
191. Vaudaux P. Peripheral inactivation of gentamicin. J Antimicrob Chemother 1981;8(Suppl A):17.
192. Levy J et al. Bioactivity of gentamicin in purulent sputum from patients with cystic fibrosis or bronchiectasis: comparison with activity in serum. J Infect Dis 1983;148:1069.
193. Mendelman PM et al. Aminoglycoside penetration, inactivation, and efficacy in cystic fibrosis sputum. Am Rev Respir Dis 1985;132:761.
194. Greenfield S et al. Prevention of Gram-negative bacillary pneumonia using aerosol polymyxin as prophylaxis: I. Effect on the colonization pattern of the upper respiratory tract of seriously ill patients. J Clin Invest 1973;52:2935.
195. Klick JM et al. Prevention of Gram-negative bacillary pneumonia using polymyxin aerosol as prophylaxis: II. Effect on the incidence of pneumonia in seriously ill patients. J Clin Invest 1975;55:514.
196. Klastersky J et al. Endotracheally-administered gentamicin for the prevention of infections of the respiratory tract in patients with tracheostomy: a double-blind study. Chest 1974;65:650.
197. Feeley TW et al. Aerosol polymyxin and pneumonia in seriously ill patients. N Engl J Med 1975;293:471.
198. Klastersky J et al. Endotracheal antibiotics for the prevention of tracheobronchial infections in tracheotomized unconscious patients. Chest 1975;68:302.
199. Wood GC et al. Aerosolized antimicrobial therapy in acutely ill patients. Pharmacotherapy 2000;20:166.
200. Ramsey BW et al. Management of pulmonary disease in patients with cystic fibrosis. N Engl J Med 1996:335:179.
201. Klastersky J et al. Endotracheal gentamicin in bronchial infections in patients with tracheostomy. Chest 1972;61:117.
202. Klastersky J et al. Endotracheally administered antibiotics for Gram-negative bronchopneumonia. Chest 1979;75:586.
203. Sculier JP et al. Effectiveness of mezlocillin and endotracheally-administered sisomicin with or without parenteral sisomicin in the treatment of Gram-negative bronchopneumonia. J Antimicrob Chemother 1982;9:63.
204. Lake KB et al. Combined topical pulmonary and systemic gentamicin: the question of safety. Chest 1975;68:62.
205. Baran D et al. Concentration of gentamicin in bronchial secretions of children with cystic fibrosis or tracheostomy. Int J Clin Pharmacol 1975;12:336.
206. Odio W et al. Concentrations of gentamicin in bronchial secretions after intramuscular and endotracheal administration. J Clin Pharmacol 1975;15:518.
207. Stillwell PC et al. Endotracheal tobramycin in Gram-negative pneumonitis. Drug Intell Clin Pharm 1988;22:577.
208. Klastersky J, Thys JP. Local antibiotic therapy for bronchopneumonia. In: Pennington JE, ed. Respiratory Infections: Diagnosis and Management. New York: Raven Press, 1983.
209. Dickie KJ, de Groot WJ. Ventilatory effects of aerosolized kanamycin and polymyxin. Chest 1974;63:694.
210. Wilson FE. Acute respiratory failure secondary to polymyxin-B inhalation. Chest 1981;79:237.
211. Dally MB et al. Cystic fibrosis: ventilatory effects of aerosol gentamicin. Thorax 1978;33:54.
212. Craven DE et al. Preventing nosocomial pneumonia: state of the art and perspectives for the 1990s. Am J Med 1991;91:44S.
213. Kollef MH. The prevention of ventilator associated pneumonias. N Engl J Med 1999;340:627.
214. Torres A et al. Pulmonary aspiration of gastric contents in patients receiving mechanical ventilation: the effect of body position. Ann Intern Med 1992;116:540.

215. Kollef MH et al. Scheduled change of antibiotic classes: a strategy to decrease the incidence of ventilator associated pneumonia. Am Rev Respir Crit Care Med 1997;154(4 Pt 1):1040.

216. Gastinne H et al. A controlled trial in intensive care units of selective decontamination of the digestive tract with nonabsorbable antibiotics. N Engl J Med 1992;326:594.

217. Selective Decontamination of the Digestive Tract Trialists' Collaborative Group. Meta-analysis of randomized controlled trials of selective decontamination of the digestive tract. BMJ 1993; 307:525.

218. Wood RE et al. Cystic fibrosis. Am Rev Respir Dis 1976;113:833.

219. Thomassen MJ et al. Multiple isolates of *Pseudomonas aeruginosa* with differing antimicrobial susceptibility patterns from patients with cystic fibrosis. J Infect Dis 1979;140:873.

220. Isles A et al. *Pseudomonas cepacia* infection in cystic fibrosis: an emerging problem. J Pediatr 1984;104:206.

221. Tablan OC et al. *Pseudomonas cepacia* colonization in patients with cystic fibrosis: risk factors and clinical outcome. J Pediatr 1985;107:382.

222. Jusko WJ et al. Enhanced renal excretion of dicloxacillin in patients with cystic fibrosis. Pediatrics 1975;56:1038.

223. Ziemniak JA et al. The bioavailability of pharmacokinetics of cimetidine and its metabolites in juvenile cystic fibrosis patients: age-related differences as compared to adults. Eur J Clin Pharmacol 1984;26:183.

224. Isles A et al. Theophylline disposition in cystic fibrosis. Am Rev Respir Dis 1983;127:417.

225. Levy J et al. Disposition of tobramycin in patients with cystic fibrosis: a prospective controlled study. J Pediatr 1984;105:117.

226. Beringer PM. New approaches to optimizing antimicrobial therapy in patients with cystic fibrosis. Curr Opin Pulmon Med 1999;5:371.

227. Hodson ME et al. Aerosol carbenicillin and gentamicin treatment of *Pseudomonas aeruginosa* infection in patients with cystic fibrosis. Lancet 1981;2:1137.

228. Stephens D et al. Efficacy of inhaled tobramycin in the treatment of pulmonary exacerbations in children with cystic fibrosis. Pediatr Infect Dis 1983;2:209.

229. Cooper DM et al. Comparison of intravenous and inhalation antibiotic therapy in acute pulmonary deterioration in cystic fibrosis. Am Rev Respir Dis 1985;131:A242.

230. Steinkamp G et al. Long-term tobramycin aerosol therapy in cystic fibrosis. Pediatr Pulmonol 1989;6:91.

231. Swift DL. Aerosols and humidity therapy: generation and respiratory deposition of therapeutic aerosols. Am Rev Respir Dis 1980;122(Suppl):71.

232. Alderson PO et al. Pulmonary disposition of aerosols in children with cystic fibrosis. J Pediatr 1974;84:479.

233. MacLusky I et al. Inhaled antibiotics in cystic fibrosis: is there a therapeutic effect? J Pediatr 1986;108:861.

234. Ramsey BW et al. Efficacy of aerosolized tobramycin in patients with cystic fibrosis. N Engl J Med 1993;328:1740.

235. Ramsey BW et al. Intermittent administration of inhaled tobramycin in patients with cystic fibrosis. N Engl J Med 1999;340:23.

236. Meehan TP et al. Quality of care, process, and outcomes in elderly patients with pneumonia. JAMA 1997;278:2080.

Tuberculosis

Michael B. Kays

History

Tuberculosis (TB) is an ancient disease, and evidence of TB dates as far back as prehistoric times, with evidence being found in pre-Columbian and early Egyptian remains. However, it did not become a problem until the 17th and 18th centuries, when crowded living conditions of the industrial revolution contributed to its epidemic numbers in Europe and the United States. Early physicians referred to it as *phthisis* (from the Greek term for wasting) because its presentation consisted of weight loss, cough, fevers, and hemoptysis. Although its characteristics were well known, an etiologic agent was not clearly defined until 1882, when Koch isolated and cultured *Mycobacterium tuberculosis* and demonstrated its infectious nature. With this knowledge, early treatment in the mid-1800s to the early 1900s consisted of removing patients with TB from the community and placing them in a sanatorium for bed rest and fresh air. With the advent of radiographic film, pulmonary cavitary lesions were found to be pivotal in the evolution of the disease. Therapy then included procedures such as pneumoperitoneum, thoracoplasty, and plombage to reduce the size of the cavitary lesion. Some of these therapies continue to be used for severe and refractory cases. The modern era of medical therapy for TB did not begin until 1944, with the discovery of streptomycin and para-aminosalicylic acid shortly thereafter. The addition of isoniazid (INH) in 1952 and rifampin in the late 1960s greatly increased the hopes for eventual elimination of TB in the United States.[1]

Incidence/Epidemiology

Although the incidence of TB in the United States has declined dramatically since 1900, TB continues to be one of the deadliest diseases in the world. Globally, there were an estimated 8.3 million new TB cases and 1.8 million deaths from the disease in 2000.[2] Most of the new TB cases were in adults aged 15 to 49 years, and the total number of new cases increased at a rate of 1.8% per year between 1997 and 2000.[2] The vast majority of TB cases occurred in developing countries, where inadequate resources hinder proper treatment of the disease and where HIV infection may be common. Assuming lifelong TB infection, approximately 30% of the world population (1.8 billion people) were infected with *M. tuberculosis* in 2000.[2]

In the United States, the TB case rate declined from 53.0 per 100,000 population in 1953, when the CDC began conducting TB surveillance, to 9.1 cases per 100,000 population in 1988.[3] However, there was a resurgence of TB in the United States from the late 1980s to the early 1990s, in large part due to the HIV/AIDS epidemic and the emergence of multidrug-resistant TB (MDR-TB). At its peak in 1992, 26,673 TB cases (10.5 per 100,000 population) were reported.[3] As a result of this resurgence, an advisory committee was established by the Department of Health and Human Services to provide recommendations for the elimination of TB in the United States. The committee urged the establishment of a national goal of TB elimination (<1 case per million of population) by the year 2010. The plan incorporated identification of populations more susceptible to TB infection, the use of biotechnology in diagnosis and treatment, and computer telecommunication to track cases.[4] These recommendations, along with the basics of infection control, prompt initiation of treatment, and ensuring completion of TB therapy, have been successful in reducing the TB case rate in the United States. The number of TB cases reached its recent low in 2001, with 15,989 cases (5.6 per 100,000 population) being reported, a 40% decrease from 1992.[3]

In 2001, the number of TB cases was greatest in adults aged 25 to 44 years (5,630 cases) and in the Black, non-Hispanic ethnic group (4,796 cases).[3] However, the TB case rates per 100,000 population were greatest for adults aged ≥65 years (9.1) and in the Asian/Pacific Islander ethnic group (32.7). In 2001, TB cases were reported in 3.3% of residents in correctional facilities, 6.1% of homeless persons, 2.8% of residents in long-term care facilities, 2.3% of injection drug users, 7.2% of non-injection drug users, and 15.2% of persons with excess alcohol use.[3] In 1992, 72% of reported TB cases were among U.S.-born persons, while 27% were among foreign-born persons.[3] However, there was an equal distribution (50%) in the number of TB cases among these two groups in 2001, and the TB case rate per 100,000 population was more than eight times higher in foreign-born persons (26.6) compared to U.S.-born persons (3.1).[3] In 1991, 4 states reported that ≥50% of their total TB cases were among foreign-born persons, compared to 23 states in 2001.[3] Of these 23 states, the total number of TB cases among foreign-born persons was ≥70% in California, Massachusetts, Minnesota, Washington, Hawaii, New Hampshire, and Vermont.[3] The top five countries of origin for TB cases among foreign-born persons were Mexico, the Philippines, Vietnam, India, and China.[3] MDR-TB, defined as resistance to both INH and rifampin, declined from 2.5% of total TB cases in 1993 to 1.0% in 2001. However, the proportion of MDR-TB cases reported in foreign-born persons increased from 31% (150 of 482 cases) in 1993 to 73% (101 of 138 cases) in 2001.[3] Although the reporting of HIV status is incomplete, available data in 2001 show that 24% of TB cases in adults aged 25 to 44 years in the United States were HIV positive.[3] Continued commitment to TB control and treatment programs is essential to the goal of TB elimination.

Etiology

TB is caused by *M. tuberculosis*, an aerobic, non–spore-forming bacillus that resists decolorization by acid alcohol after staining with basic fuchsin. For this reason, the organism is often referred to as an acid-fast bacillus (AFB). It is also different from other organisms in that it replicates slowly: once every 24 hours instead of every 20 to 40 minutes, as with some other organisms. *M. tuberculosis* thrives in environments where the oxygen tension is relatively high, such as the apices of the lung, the renal parenchyma, and the growing ends of bones.[1]

Transmission

Tubercle bacilli are transmitted through the air by aerosolized droplet nuclei that are produced when a person with pulmonary or laryngeal TB coughs, sneezes, speaks, or sings. Droplet nuclei may also be produced by other methods, such as aerosol treatments, sputum induction, bronchoscopy, endotracheal intubation, suctioning, or autopsy, and through manipulation of lesions or processing of secretions in the hospital or laboratory.[5] These droplet nuclei, which contain one to three *M. tuberculosis* organisms, are small enough (1 to 5 μm) to remain airborne for long periods of time and to reach the alveoli within the lungs when inhaled. Tubercle bacilli are not transmitted on inanimate objects such as dishes, clothing, or bedding, and organisms deposited on skin or intact mucosa do not invade tissue.

Several factors influence the likelihood of transmission of *M. tuberculosis,* including the number of organisms expelled into the air, the concentration of organisms in the air (determined by the volume of the space and its ventilation), the length of time an exposed person breathes the contaminated air, and presumably the immune status of the exposed individual.[5] Family household contacts, especially children, and persons working or living in an enclosed environment (e.g., hospitals, nursing homes, prisons) with an infected person are at a significantly increased risk for becoming infected. Individuals with impaired cell-mediated immunity, such as HIV-infected persons or transplant patients, are thought to be more likely to become infected with *M. tuberculosis* after exposure than persons with normal immune function.[5]

Several techniques are effective in limiting airborne transmission of *M. tuberculosis* by reducing the number of droplet nuclei in a given airspace. Adequate room ventilation with fresh air is very important, especially in the health care setting, where a rate of six or more room-air exchanges per hour is desirable.[5,6] Ultraviolet irradiation of air in the upper part of the room can also reduce the number of viable airborne tubercle bacilli. If masks are to be used on coughing patients with infectious TB, they should be fabricated to filter droplet nuclei and molded to fit tightly around the patient's nose and mouth.[5] However, the most important means of reducing transmission of *M. tuberculosis* is by treating the infected patient with effective antituberculosis therapy.

Pathogenesis

Latent Infection Versus Active Disease

LATENT INFECTION

A clear distinction should be made between latent infection and active disease (TB). Latent infection occurs when the tubercle bacilli are inhaled into the body. After inhalation, the droplet nuclei containing *M. tuberculosis* settle into the bronchioles and alveoli of the lungs. Development of infection in the lung is dependent on both the virulence of the organism and the inherent microbicidal ability of the alveolar macrophages.[7,8] In the nonimmune (susceptible) host, the bacilli initially multiply unopposed by normal host defense mechanisms. The organisms are then taken into alveolar macrophages by phagocytosis and may remain viable, multiplying within the cells for extended periods of time. After 14 to 21 days of replication, the tubercle bacilli spread via the lymphatic system to the hilar lymph nodes and through the bloodstream to many other organs of the body. Fortunately, certain organs and tissues in the body, such as the bone marrow, liver, and spleen, are resistant to subsequent multiplication of these bacilli. Organs with high blood flow and PaO_2, such as the upper lung zones, kidneys, bones, and brain, are particularly favorable for growth of the organisms. The organisms replicate for 2 to 12 weeks until they reach 10^3 to 10^4 in number, then a specific T lymphocyte-mediated immune response develops, which can be detected by a reaction to the tuberculin skin test, and prevents further replication.[5]

In persons with intact cell-mediated immunity, activated T lymphocytes and macrophages form granulomas that limit multiplication and spread of the bacilli by walling off the infection from the surrounding environment.[5] The organisms tend to localize in the center of the granuloma, which is frequently necrotic. Although small numbers of tubercle bacilli may remain viable within the granuloma, proliferation of *M. tuberculosis* is halted when cell-mediated immunity develops. At this point, the majority of persons with pulmonary TB infections are clinically asymptomatic and there is no radiographic evidence of the infection.[8] In some patients, there may be a healed, calcified lesion on the chest radiograph, but bacteriologic studies are negative.[1,9] A positive tuberculin skin test is usually the only indication that the person has been infected with *M. tuberculosis*. Individuals with latent TB infection are not infectious and thus cannot transmit the organism.[5]

ACTIVE DISEASE (TB)

Approximately 10% of individuals who acquire TB infection and do not receive therapy for the latent infection will develop active TB disease. The risk of developing active disease is highest in the first 2 years after infection, when half of the cases occur.[5] Physical or emotional stress can destroy the balance between the immune system and the infection, leading to active disease. The ability of the host to respond to the organism may also be reduced by certain diseases such as diabetes mellitus, silicosis, and diseases associated with immunosuppression (e.g., HIV infection, corticosteroids, and immunosuppressive agents). The likelihood of developing active TB disease is greater in persons with these diseases.[5,10] HIV-infected persons, especially those with low $CD4^+$ T-cell counts, develop active TB disease rapidly after becoming infected with *M. tuberculosis;* up to 50% of these individuals may develop active disease in the first 2 years after infection.[11] In addition, persons with untreated latent TB infection who acquire HIV infection will develop active TB disease at a rate of approximately 5% to 10% per year.[12,13] Other factors that may contribute to the development of active disease include gastrectomy, intestinal bypass surgery, alcohol abuse, chronic renal failure, hematologic disease, reticuloendothelial disease, and intravenous (IV) drug use. The elderly, adolescents, and children <2 years of age may also be at an increased risk of developing active disease.[5,9]

DIAGNOSIS

Signs and Symptoms

Subjective Findings

1. M.W., a 36-year-old woman, is admitted to the hospital with a 2-month history of cough, which has recently become productive. She is also experiencing fatigue and night sweats and has lost 10 lb. Other medical problems include diabetes mellitus, which is controlled with 10 units of NPH insulin daily, and poor nutritional status secondary to frequent dieting. M.W. works as a volunteer in a nursing home several days a week. Recently, it was discovered that two patients she had been caring for had undiagnosed active TB.

Physical examination was normal, but M.W.'s chest radiograph revealed bibasilar infiltrates. A tuberculin purified protein derivative (PPD) skin test, sputum collections for cultures and susceptibility testing, and a sputum AFB smear were ordered as part of M.W.'s diagnostic workup. Initial laboratory tests were within normal limits.

The result of her tuberculin PPD skin test, read at 48 hours, was a palpable induration of 14 mm. Her sputum smear was positive for AFB, and additional sputum cultures for *M. tuberculosis* were ordered to confirm the diagnosis of active TB disease. What subjective and objective findings does M.W. have that are consistent with TB?

M.W.'s history of cough (which gradually became productive), bibasilar infiltrates, fatigue, and night sweats are classic symptoms of TB.[4,5] The cough may be nonproductive early in the course of the illness, but with subsequent inflammation and tissue necrosis, sputum is usually produced and is key to most diagnostic studies. The sputum may contain blood (hemoptysis) in patients with advanced cavitary disease, which is particularly worrisome because cavitary lesions harbor large numbers of organisms and the pulmonary location allows for airborne transmission.[1,9] Anorexia from TB, along with frequent dieting, may have resulted in M.W.'s weight loss. Other symptoms of TB may include fever, pleuritic pain secondary to inflammation of lung parenchyma adjacent to the pleural space, and general malaise. Dyspnea is unusual unless there is extensive disease.[5]

Objective Findings

M.W. has a chest radiograph consistent with a lower respiratory tract infection. In pulmonary TB, nodular infiltrates are usually found in the apical or posterior segments of the upper lobes, but markings may be found in any segment. M.W. also has a positive sputum smear for AFB, a positive PPD skin test (14 mm), and diabetes mellitus, which is a risk factor for TB. Although her laboratory test results were within normal limits, peripheral blood leukocytosis and anemia are the most common hematologic manifestations of TB.[5] The increase in white blood cell count is usually slight, and an increase in peripheral blood monocytes and eosinophils may be observed on the differential.

Potential Misdiagnoses

Many patients with active pulmonary TB have no acute symptoms, and cases are often found following routine chest radiographs for other illnesses. Because many of the symptoms of TB also occur in persons with pre-existing pulmonary disease or pneumonia, they may be overlooked and not attributed to TB.

A lack of clinical symptoms may also contribute to misdiagnosis of TB. A report from a private urban hospital showed that over a 1-year span, almost 50% of the cases of active TB were misdiagnosed because classic symptoms were absent.[14] More than one third of the patients with active TB had no sweats, chills, or malaise, and <50% were febrile. Cough was evident in 80% of these patients, and only 25% had hemoptysis. Although dullness over the apices of the lungs and posttussive rales are expected in TB, less than one third of these patients had any abnormal pulmonary signs on physical examination. Similarly, TB was not suspected in 42% of patients with active disease in a community hospital.[15] The lack of specific clinical symptoms underscores the importance of skin testing, sputum smears for AFB, and chest radiographs as diagnostic tools in individuals suspected of having TB.

Tuberculin PPD Skin Test

2. What is the tuberculin PPD skin test? How should the results be interpreted in M.W.?

The tuberculin PPD skin test (Mantoux method) is a limited diagnostic tool used for the detection of infection with *M. tuberculosis,* and it is not necessary for the diagnosis of active TB disease.[16] When an infection with *M. tuberculosis* occurs, a delayed hypersensitivity reaction to the tubercle bacilli or to its components usually develops in the host. This reaction develops within 2 to 12 weeks after initial infection.[5,17] The abbreviation "PPD" refers to the purified protein derivative of *M. tuberculosis,* which is prepared from a culture of tubercle bacilli. The solutions are available as 1, 5, or 250 tuberculin units (TU) per 0.1 mL, although the 5-TU preparation (formerly referred to as intermediate-strength PPD) is the most commonly used in the United States. The 250-TU/0.1 mL PPD has limited usefulness in the diagnosis of TB infection and is not recommended by the Centers for Disease Control and Prevention (CDC) because the preparation is not standardized, making accurate interpretation difficult. It has, however, occasionally been used to assess the immunologic status of the patient.[9]

The skin test is performed by injecting 0.1 mL of solution containing 5-TU PPD intradermally into the volar or dorsal surface of the forearm.[5,16] The injection is made using a one-quarter to one-half inch, 27-gauge needle and a tuberculin syringe. The solution should be injected just beneath the surface of the skin with the needle bevel upward or downward, being sure to avoid subcutaneous tissue.[5,18] A discrete, pale elevation of the skin (a wheal) 6 to 10 mm in diameter should be produced when the injection is performed correctly. If the first injection was administered improperly, another test dose can be given at once, selecting a site several centimeters away from the original injection site.[5] If the patient has previously been infected with *M. tuberculosis,* sensitized T cells are recruited to the skin site, where they release cytokines.[19] These cytokines induce an induration (raised area) through local vasodilatation, edema, fibrin deposition, and recruitment of other inflammatory cells to the area.[5,16,20] Typically, the reaction to tuberculin begins 5 to 6 hours after injection, with maximal induration observed at 48 to 72 hours. Therefore, the test should be read between 48 and 72 hours after injection because tests read after 72 hours tend to underestimate the actual size of the induration.[5] For standardization, the diameter of the induration should be measured transversely to the long axis of the forearm and recorded in millimeters.[5,18] The diameter of the induration should be measured, not the erythematous zone surrounding the induration.

An induration ≥5 mm in diameter read 48 to 72 hours after injection is considered to be a positive reaction in persons with a recent history of close contact with someone with active TB, persons with fibrotic changes on the chest radiograph consistent with old TB, organ transplant patients, and other immunosuppressed patients (receiving the equivalent of >15 mg per day of prednisone for >1 month), or HIV-positive persons.[5,16,21,22] M.W.'s reaction to the PPD is positive (14 mm), and she has no history of a previously positive PPD skin test. The skin test may remain positive throughout M.W.'s life.[9]

An induration size of 10 mm is used as the cut point for positivity in persons with clinical conditions that put them at increased risk for TB, such as diabetes mellitus, silicosis, chronic renal failure, leukemia, lymphoma, gastrectomy, jejunoileal bypass, and weight loss of >10% of ideal body weight.[5] In addition, an induration ≥10 mm is considered to be positive in recent immigrants (<5 years) from countries with a high prevalence of TB, injection drug users, residents and employees of high-risk congregate settings (e.g., prisons, nursing homes, homeless shelters), mycobacteriology laboratory personnel, children <4 years of age, or infants, children, and adolescents exposed to adults in high-risk categories.[5] For individuals with no risk factors for TB, an induration ≥15 mm is required for a positive reaction.

False-positive tuberculin skin tests may be caused by infections secondary to other mycobacterial species that cross-react with the *M. tuberculosis* antigen, including vaccination with a bacillus of Calmette-Guerin (BCG) vaccine. These cross-reacting mycobacteria are common in many areas of the United States, especially in the Southeast.[16] False-positive readings with some PPD preparations have also been reported, possibly because of impurities in the solutions.[16,23] Only experienced persons should read the Mantoux PPD skin tests, because the risk of error in performance and interpretation is high. In a study of 1,036 persons who each received two injections of 5-TU PPD from the same vial (one in each arm), 14.5% had an induration >10 mm in one arm and an induration <10 mm in the other arm. This was thought to be caused by variability in the reading of the tests.[24]

M.W.'s positive reaction to 5-TU PPD alone does not imply active TB disease; it merely signifies that she has previously been infected with *M. tuberculosis.* However, because she also has symptoms consistent with active TB disease and a positive sputum smear for AFB, a preliminary diagnosis of active TB disease can be made.

3. Because M.W.'s Mantoux PPD skin test is positive, does this confirm her diagnosis of active TB?

No. To confirm the diagnosis of active TB disease, *M. tuberculosis* must be detected and isolated from sputum, gastric aspirate, spinal fluid, urine, or tissue biopsy, depending on the site of infection.[5] As was done in M.W., the detection of AFB in stained smears examined microscopically is the first bacteriologic evidence of the presence of mycobacteria in a clinical specimen. It is the easiest and fastest procedure and can provide the clinician with a preliminary confirmation of the diagnosis. Sputum samples for AFB stain and culture are best obtained early in the morning on at least 3 separate days.[25] Smears may be prepared directly from clinical specimens or from concentrated preparations.[5] This is done by placing the specimen on a glass slide under a microscope with a Ziehl-Neelsen or fluorochrome stain (not a Gram's stain). However, studies have shown that 5,000 to 10,000 bacilli per milliliter of specimen must be present to allow AFB to be detected in stained smears.[5,26] Therefore, a negative AFB smear does not rule out active TB disease, and patients with active TB and negative AFB smears may play an important role in the ongoing transmission of *M. tuberculosis.*

Additional limitations of the AFB smear are its inability to differentiate among mycobacterial species and between viable and nonviable organisms. In many areas of the United States, *Mycobacterium avium* complex organisms are being isolated more frequently from the sputum of patients in whom a diagnosis of TB is highly probable, such as the elderly and patients with HIV infection.[27] This has resulted in a marked decrease in the specificity and positive predictive value of the sputum smear, in some cases to as low as 50%.[28] During the past 10 to 15 years, nucleic acid amplification (NAA) techniques have been developed that enhance and expedite the direct identification of *M. tuberculosis* in clinical specimens. These technologies allow the amplification of specific target sequences of nucleic acids in *M. tuberculosis* that can be detected by a nucleic acid probe within hours. In the research laboratory, a positive result can be obtained from specimens containing as few as 10 bacilli, but the sensitivity is somewhat less in the clinical laboratory.[5] The AMPLIFIED *Mycobacterium .tuberculosis* Direct Test (MTD, GenProbe) and Amplicor *Mycobacterium tuberculosis* Test (Roche) are NAA assays available for commercial use in the United States.[27] The AMPLIFIED MTD test is approved by the U.S. Food and Drug Administration (FDA) for use in both smear-positive and smear-negative specimens; the Amplicor test is approved only for smear-positive specimens. These tests will accurately diagnose nearly every case of sputum smear-positive pulmonary TB (sensitivity 95%, specificity 98%); the tests will also diagnose approximately half of the smear-negative, culture-positive pulmonary TB cases, and the specificity remains approximately 95%.[5,27] As a result, the CDC currently recommends that AFB smear and NAA be performed on the first sputum smear collected.[29] If the AFB smear and NAA are both positive, TB is diagnosed with near certainty. If the AFB smear is negative and the NAA is positive, additional sputum samples should be obtained, and if positive, the patient can be presumed to have TB. If the AFB smear is positive and the NAA is negative, the patient can be presumed to have nontuberculous mycobacteria. If both the AFB smear and the NAA are negative, additional samples should be tested by NAA. If negative, the patient can be presumed not to have infectious TB.[27,29]

Some patients may have a negative AFB smear, but a sufficient number of organisms may be present to produce a positive culture. Only 10 to 100 organisms are needed for a positive culture.[5,30] As a result of the limitations of the AFB smear, a positive culture for *M. tuberculosis* is necessary to definitively diagnose TB. In addition, the culture is of paramount importance, since it is the only widely available technology that allows drug susceptibility testing.[27] *M. tuberculosis* organisms grow slowly, so depending on the type of media and detection system, it may take several weeks for the cultures to become positive.[1,5] Broth-based culture systems such as BACTEC, MGIT, MB/BacT, Septi-Check, and ESP, when combined with DNA probes, can produce positive results in 2 weeks or less for sputum smear-positive specimens and within 3 weeks for smear-negative specimens.[27]

4. **Should M.W. be tested for HIV infection?**

Yes, it should be considered, because TB may be the first manifestation of HIV infection.[1,31] Approximately 37% of HIV-infected patients develop active TB disease within 5 months compared with 5% of exposed persons with intact immune defenses.[11,32] A complete discussion of TB and HIV infection can be found in Questions 24 to 28 and Chapter 69, Pharmacotherapy of Human Immunodeficiency Virus Infection.

5. **Would a negative tuberculin skin test have eliminated the possibility of infection with *M. tuberculosis* in M.W.?**

No, a negative response to 5-TU PPD in M.W. would not necessarily have excluded infection with *M. tuberculosis.* The PPD skin test has a reported false-negative rate of 25% during the initial evaluation of persons with active TB.[5] This high false-negative rate appears to be due to poor nutrition and general health, overwhelming acute illness, or immunosuppression. False-negative results usually occur in persons who have had no prior infection with *M. tuberculosis,* who have only recently been infected, or who are anergic. Factors that may result in a false-negative tuberculin skin test are shown in Table 61-1.

Anergy (decreased ability to respond to antigens) may be caused by severe debility, old age, immaturity in newborns, high fever, sarcoidosis, corticosteroids, immunosuppressive drugs, hematologic disease, HIV infections, overwhelming

Table 61-1   Factors Associated With False-Negative Tuberculin Skin Tests

Factors related to the person being tested
  Bacterial, viral, or fungal infections
  Live virus vaccinations (measles, mumps, polio, varicella)
  Chronic renal failure
  Severe protein depletion
  Diseases affecting lymphoid organs (Hodgkin's disease, lymphoma, chronic leukemia)
  Corticosteroids, immunosuppressive agents
  Age (newborns, elderly)
Factors related to the method of administration
  Subcutaneous injection
  Injecting too little antigen
Factors related to the tuberculin used
  Improper storage (exposure to light and heat)
  Improper dilution
  Contamination
Factors related to reading the test and recording the results
  Inexperienced reader
  Error in recording

Adapted from reference 5.

TB, recent viral infection, live-virus vaccinations, and malnutrition.[5] If anergy is suspected, control skin tests (*Candida, mumps,* and/or *trichophyton*) should also be placed in the contralateral arm. If the control test results are positive and the PPD test result is negative, infection with *M. tuberculosis* is less likely. The CDC changed its recommendations regarding anergy skin testing in HIV-infected patients with a negative PPD. They cited problems with standardization and reproducibility, a low risk for TB associated with a diagnosis of anergy, and the lack of apparent benefit of therapy for latent TB infection in anergic HIV-infected patients. Therefore, the use of anergy testing in conjunction with PPD is no longer routinely recommended in this population.[33]

Booster Phenomenon (PPD Skin Test)

6. S.N., a 50-year-old hospital employee receiving his initial tuberculin skin test (PPD-Mantoux), had a 7-mm induration. Because of his age and previous hospital employment, it was decided to retest him 1 week later to rule out any "booster" effect. The result of the repeated skin test was 12 mm. He denied any known exposure to persons with active TB. What is the significance of this reaction? Should S.N. be placed on INH therapy for latent TB infection?

Some persons experience a significant increase in the size of a tuberculin skin test reaction that may not be caused by *M. tuberculosis* infection.[5,34] This reaction, known as the "booster" phenomenon, is not fully understood but may be caused by the tuberculin skin test itself when tests are performed every 1 to 2 years. It may also be caused by infection with other mycobacteria, remote TB, or prior BCG vaccination. When caused by a previous skin test, it can occur as soon as 1 week after the previous test. The incidence of this reaction appears to increase with age.[35] Therefore, S.N.'s reaction may not represent infection with *M. tuberculosis*.

Because serial tuberculin testing is recommended for hospital employees, it becomes important to distinguish a possible booster reaction from a recent infection with *M. tuberculosis*. Some hospitals advocate the use of two-step skin testing in new employees.[36] Persons who exhibit an increase in the size of the induration from <10 mm to >10 mm, as in the case of S.N., may be mistaken for a recent converter and given INH to treat a latent infection unnecessarily. To determine whether a reaction is caused by "boosting" rather than an infection, a second identical skin test should be administered 7 to 21 days after the first. The results of this test should be read in 48 to 72 hours. If the repeat test is positive (>10 mm), the reaction should be classified as a booster reaction and the subject should not be treated with INH. If the repeat test is <10 mm but changes to positive (with a 6-mm increase) after 1 year, the person should be classified as a recent converter and managed accordingly (see Question 15). One report suggested using a 15-mm induration as the appropriate baseline in hospital employees tested annually.[37]

The increase in reaction size in S.N. is most likely caused by the booster phenomenon. Because he is >35 years old, he would not be an ideal candidate for INH therapy. S.N. should be given a repeat skin test next year and evaluated as previously described. He should not receive a two-step test in the future because this is done only on initial evaluation of an employee.

BCG Vaccine

7. C.T., a 25-year-old female refugee from Cambodia, was given a routine physical examination upon entering this country. As part of this examination, she received a tuberculin skin test with 5-TU PPD. The test result was positive with an induration of 12 mm. She denied previous treatment for TB, but she remembered receiving a TB vaccine (BCG) several years ago. What is BCG vaccine? Does this positive skin test indicate infection with *M. tuberculosis*?

BCG is a live vaccine derived from an attenuated strain of *M. bovis,* and it is used in many foreign countries with a high prevalence of TB to prevent the disease in persons who are tuberculin negative (no immunity to TB infection). Many different BCG vaccines are available worldwide, and they differ with respect to immunogenicity, efficacy, and reactogenicity. Additional factors, such as the genetic variability in the subjects vaccinated, the nature of the mycobacteria endemic in different parts of the world, and the use of different doses and different immunization schedules, may contribute to the varied degrees of protection afforded by the vaccine.[38] The protective effect derived from BCG vaccines in case-control studies has ranged from 0% to 80%.[39] Two meta-analyses concerning the efficacy of BCG vaccination for preventing TB attempted to calculate estimates of the protective efficacy of the vaccines. The results of the first meta-analysis indicated an 86% protective effect against meningeal and miliary TB in children in 10 randomized clinical trials and a 75% protective effect in eight case-control studies.[40] In the second meta-analysis, the overall protective effect of BCG vaccines was 51% in 14 clinical studies and 50% in 12 case-control studies.[41] Vaccine efficacy rates were higher in studies where persons were vaccinated during childhood compared to persons vaccinated at older ages.[41] Unfortunately, neither study was able to determine the vaccine's efficacy for preventing pulmonary TB in adolescents and adults.

Prior vaccination with BCG usually results in a positive tuberculin skin test, but skin test reactivity does not correlate with protection against TB.[5,39] There is no reliable method of distinguishing tuberculin reactions caused by BCG vaccination from those caused by natural mycobacterial infections.[5,39] Therefore, it is prudent to consider "positive" reactions to 5-TU of PPD in BCG-vaccinated persons as indicating infection with *M. tuberculosis,* especially among persons from countries with a high prevalence of TB.[5] As a result, C.T. should be treated as though she has a positive tuberculin skin test (see Question 15). Because she is from an area of the world with a high drug-resistance rate, the possibility of infection with organisms that are resistant to INH should also be considered (see Question 22).

Adverse reactions to the BCG vaccine vary according to the type, dose, and age of the vaccine. Osteitis, prolonged ulceration at the vaccination site, lupoid reactions, regional suppurative lymphadenitis, disseminated BCG infection, and death have all been reported.[39]

BCG vaccine is not recommended for use in the routine prophylaxis of TB in the United States. The risk of exposure to TB in this country is relatively low, and other methods of control (e.g., treatment of high-risk groups) are usually adequate. BCG vaccination should be considered for infants or children who are tuberculin negative and are continually exposed to a highly infectious, untreated patient with active TB, or children continually exposed to a patient with infectious pulmonary TB caused by *M. tuberculosis* strains resistant to INH and rifampin.[39,42] BCG vaccination of health care workers should be considered in settings where many patients are infected with MDR-TB, transmission of MDR-TB strains to health care workers and subsequent infection are likely, and comprehensive infection control precautions have been unsuccessful.[39] BCG vaccination is not recommended during pregnancy or for HIV-infected children or adults in the United States.[39]

TREATMENT OF ACTIVE DISEASE

Initial Therapy

Regimens

8. **M.W.'s HIV test was negative. How should treatment be initiated in M.W., pending the results of the sputum culture and susceptibility testing? Can she transmit infection during treatment?**

The overall goals for the treatment of TB are to cure the individual patient and to minimize the transmission of *M. tuberculosis* to other persons. The primary goals of antituberculosis chemotherapy are to kill the tubercle bacilli rapidly, prevent the emergence of drug resistance, and eliminate persistent bacilli from the host's tissues to prevent relapse.[43] To accomplish these goals, treatment must be tailored to and supervision must be based on each patient's clinical and social circumstances (patient-centered care). Effective treatment of TB requires a substantial period (minimum 6 months) of intensive drug therapy with at least two bactericidal drugs that are active against the organism. The initial phase of treatment is crucial for preventing the emergence of resistance and for the ultimate outcome of TB therapy.

Four basic regimens are recommended for the treatment of adults with TB caused by organisms that are known or presumed to be drug susceptible (Table 61-2).[43] Since M.W. has not been treated previously for TB, she should be started on INH, rifampin, pyrazinamide, and ethambutol. Previous guidelines recommended the addition of ethambutol (or streptomycin) only if the local prevalence of INH-resistant *M. tuberculosis* was ≥4%.[25,42,44] In the United States, however, 7.1% of *M. tuberculosis* isolates recovered from patients with no previous history of TB in 2001 were resistant to INH.[3] Because of the relatively high likelihood of TB caused by INH-resistant organisms, four drugs are necessary in the initial 8-week treatment phase. The initial four-drug regimen may be administered daily throughout the 8-week period (regimen 1), daily for the first 2 weeks and then twice weekly for 6 weeks (regimen 2), or three times weekly throughout (regimen 3).[43] On the basis of clinical experience, administration of drugs for 5 days per week is considered to be equivalent to 7-day-a-week administration, and either may be considered "daily." However, 5-day-a-week administration should always be given by directly observed therapy (DOT).[43] Drug dosages for these recommended regimens are listed in Table 61-3. In addition, two fixed-dose combination preparations are available in the United States: Rifamate contains INH 150 mg and rifampin 300 mg per capsule, and Rifater contains INH 50 mg,

rifampin 120 mg, and pyrazinamide 300 mg per tablet. These formulations are a means of minimizing inadvertent monotherapy, especially when DOT is not possible, and they may decrease the risk of acquired drug resistance while reducing the number of capsules or tablets that must be ingested each day.[43]

Ethambutol can be discontinued as soon as the results from susceptibility testing demonstrate that the isolate is susceptible to INH and rifampin. However, these results may not be available for 6 to 8 weeks after treatment is started. The incidence of streptomycin resistance has increased globally; therefore, streptomycin is no longer considered interchangeable with ethambutol unless the organism is known to be susceptible to the drug or the patient is from an area where streptomycin resistance is unlikely.[43]

M.W., who is diabetic and has a poor nutritional status, should also be given pyridoxine 25 mg/day because she may be at greater risk for the development of INH-induced peripheral neuropathy (see Question 17).

The high risk of transmission of *M. tuberculosis* to other patients and health care workers mandates that hospitalized persons with suspected or confirmed infectious TB be placed in respiratory isolation until they are determined not to have TB, they are discharged from the hospital, or they are confirmed to be noninfectious.[25] Based on M.W.'s subjective and objective findings, she should be placed in respiratory isolation without hesitation. M.W.'s symptoms of TB should improve within the first 4 weeks. She would be considered to be noninfectious when she is receiving effective drug therapy, is improving clinically, and has had negative results for three consecutive sputum AFB smears collected on different days.[25] Patients who have responded clinically may be discharged to home despite positive smears if their household contacts have already been exposed and these contacts are not at increased risk of TB (e.g., infants, HIV-positive and immunosuppressed persons). In addition, patients discharged to home with positive smears must agree not to have contact with other susceptible persons.[25]

Contact Investigation

9. **If M.W. is a risk to the community, does anyone need to know?**

Yes. Each case of active TB must be reported to the local and/or state public health departments.[5,25] This not only ensures proper therapy by monitoring adherence to therapy, but it also ensures that contact and source case investigations will be performed. Caseworkers will attempt to evaluate all people who have been in close contact to M.W. so they may be evaluated for latent TB infection or active disease as well. Reporting of cases also permits record-keeping and surveillance to determine if public health efforts are achieving their goal of preventing the spread of TB.[25]

Continuation Therapy

Regimens

10. **Six weeks later, M.W.'s sputum culture** positive for *M. tuberculosis*. Drug susceptibility tests ism was susceptible to both INH and r men should be used for continued t should treatment be continued?

Table 61-2 Treatment Regimens for Pulmonary Tuberculosis Caused by Drug-Susceptible Organisms

Regimen	Drugs	Initial Phase Interval and Doses (minimal duration)	Regimen	Drugs	Continuation Phase Interval and Doses[c] (minimal duration)	# Total Doses (minimal duration)	Rating[a] (Evidence)[b] HIV−	Rating[a] (Evidence)[b] HIV+
1	INH RIF PZA EMB	7 days/wk for 56 doses (8 wk) or 5 days/wk for 40 doses (8 wk)[d]	1a	INH/RIF	7 days/wk for 126 doses (18 wk) or 5 days/wk for 90 doses (18 wk)[d]	182–130 (26 wk)	A (I)	A (II)
			1b	INH/RIF	Twice weekly for 36 doses (18 wk)	92–76 (26 wk)	A (I)	A (II)[e]
			1c[f]	INH/RPT	Once weekly for 18 doses (18 wk)	74–58 (26 wk)	B (I)	E (I)
2	INH RIF PZA EMB	7 days/wk for 14 doses (2 wk) then twice weekly for 12 doses (6 wk) or 5 days/wk for 10 doses (2 wk)[d] then twice weekly for 12 doses (6 wk)	2a	INF/RIF	Twice weekly for 36 doses (18 wk)	62–58 (26 wk)	A (II)	B (II)[e]
			2b[f]	INH/RPT	Once weekly for 18 doses (18 wk)	44–40 (26 wk)	B (I)	E (I)
3	INH RIF PZA EMB	3 times weekly for 24 doses (8 wk)	3a	INH/RIF	3 times weekly for 54 doses (18 wk)	78 (26 wk)	B (I)	B (II)
4	INH RIF EMB	7 days/wk for 56 doses (8 wk) or 5 days/wk for 40 doses (8 wk)[d]	4a	INH/RIF	7 days/wk for 217 doses (31 wk) OR 5 days/wk for 155 doses (31 wk)[d]	273–195 (39 wk)	C (I)	C (I)
			4b	INH/RIF	Twice weekly for 62 doses (31 wk)	118–102 (39 wk)	C (II)	C (II)

[a]Definitions of evidence ratings: A, preferred; B, acceptable alternative; C, offer when A and B cannot be given; E, should never be given.

[b]Definitions of evidence ratings: I, randomized clinical trial; II, data from clinical trials that were not randomized or were conducted in other populations; III, expert opinion.

[c]Patients with cavitation on initial chest radiograph and positive cultures at completion of 2 months of therapy should receive a 7-month continuation phase (31 weeks; either 217 doses [daily] or 62 doses [twice weekly]).

[d]Five-day-a-week administration is always given by directly observed therapy (DOT). Rating for 5 day/week regimens is A (III).

[e]Not recommended for HIV-infected patients with CD41 cell counts <100 cells/mL.

[f]Options 1c and 2b should be used only in HIV-negative patients who have negative sputum smears at the time of completion of 2 months of therapy and who do not have cavitation on the initial chest radiograph.

EMB, ethambutol; INH, isoniazid; PZA, pyrazinamide; RIF, rifampin; RPT, rifapentine.

Reprinted from reference 43.

Table 61-3 Drugs Used in the Treatment of Tuberculosis in Adults and Children

Drug	Dosing (maximum dose)	Primary Side Effects	Dose Adjustment in Renal Impairment	Comments
First-Line Agents				
Isoniazid	*Adult:* 5 mg/kg (300 mg) daily; 15 mg/kg (900 mg) once, twice, or thrice weekly *Pediatric:* 10–15 mg/kg (300 mg) daily; 20–30 mg/kg (900 mg) twice weekly	Increased aminotransferases (asymptomatic), clinical hepatitis, peripheral neuropathy, CNS effects, lupus-like syndrome, hypersensitivity reactions	No	Peripheral neuropathy preventable with pyridoxine 10–25 mg; increased serum level of phenytoin. Hepatitis more common in older patients and alcoholics.
Rifampin	*Adult:* 10 mg/kg (600 mg) once daily, twice weekly, or thrice weekly *Pediatric:* 10–20 mg/kg (600 mg) once daily or twice weekly	Pruritus, rash, hepatotoxicity, GI (nausea, anorexia, abdominal pain), flu-like syndrome, thrombocytopenia, renal failure	No	Orange-red discoloration of body secretions (sweat, saliva, tears, urine). Drug interactions due to induction of hepatic microsomal enzymes (warfarin, antiretroviral agents, corticosteroids, diazepam, lorazepam, triazolam, quinidine, oral contraceptives, methadone, sulfonylureas).
Rifabutin	*Adult:* 5 mg/kg (300 mg) once daily, twice weekly, or thrice weekly *Pediatric:* unknown	Neutropenia, uveitis, GI symptoms, polyarthralgias, hepatotoxicity, rash	No	Orange-red discoloration of body secretions (sweat, saliva, tears, urine). Weaker inducer of hepatic microsomal enzymes than rifampin.
Rifapentine	*Adult:* 10 mg/kg (600 mg) once weekly during continuation phase *Pediatric:* not approved	Similar to rifampin	Unknown	Drug interactions due to induction of hepatic microsomal enzymes (see rifampin)
Pyrazinamide	*Adult:* 20–25 mg/kg (2 g) daily; 40–55 kg: 2 g twice weekly or 1.5 g thrice weekly; 56–75 kg: 3 g twice weekly or 2.5 g thrice weekly; 76–90 kg: 4 g twice weekly or 3 g thrice weekly *Pediatric:* 15–30 mg/kg (2 g) daily; 50 mg/kg twice weekly (2 g)	Hepatotoxicity, nausea, anorexia, polyarthralgias, rash, hyperuricemia, dermatitis	Yes	Monitor aminotransferases monthly.
Ethambutol	*Adult:* 15–20 mg/kg (1.6 g) daily; 40–55 kg: 2 g twice weekly or 1.2 g thrice weekly; 56–75 kg: 2.8 g twice weekly or 2 g thrice weekly; 76–90 kg: 4 g twice weekly or 2.4 g thrice weekly	Optic neuritis, skin rash, drug fever	Yes	Routine vision tests recommended; 50% excreted unchanged in urine

Continued

Table 61-3   Drugs Used in the Treatment of Tuberculosis in Adults and Children—cont'd

Drug	Dosing (maximum dose)	Primary Side Effects	Dose Adjustment in Renal Impairment	Comments
Second-Line Agents				
Cycloserine	*Pediatric:* 15–20 mg/kg (1 g) daily; 50 mg/kg (2.5 g) twice weekly	CNS toxicity (psychosis, seizures), headache, tremor, fever, skin rashes	Yes	May exacerbate seizure disorders or mental illness. Some toxicity preventable by pyridoxine (100–200 mg/day). Monitor serum concentrations (peak 20–35 µg/mL desirable).
Ethionamide	*Adult:* 10–15 mg/kg per day (1 g), usually 500–750 mg/day in 2 divided doses *Pediatric:* 10–15 mg/kg per day (1 g)	GI effects (metallic taste, nausea, vomiting, anorexia, abdominal pain), hepatotoxicity, neurotoxicity, endocrine effects (alopecia, gynecomastia, impotence, hypothyroidism), difficulty in diabetes management	Yes	Must be given with meals and antacids. Monitor aminotransferases and thyroid-stimulating hormone monthly.
Streptomycin	*Adult:* 15–20 mg/kg per day (1 g), usually 500–750 mg/day in 1 daily dose or 2 divided doses *Pediatric:* 15–20 mg/kg per day (1 g)	Vestibular and/or auditory dysfunction of eighth cranial nerve, renal dysfunction, skin rashes, neuromuscular blockade	Yes	Audiometric and neurologic examinations recommended; 60–80% excreted unchanged in urine. Monitor renal function.
Amikacin	*Adult:* 15 mg/kg per day (1 g); >60 years, 10 mg/kg per day (750 mg) *Pediatric:* 20–40 mg/kg per day (1 g)	Ototoxicity, nephrotoxicity	Yes	Less vestibular toxicity than streptomycin. Monitoring similar to streptomycin.
Capreomycin	*Adult:* 15 mg/kg per day (1 g); >60 years, 10 mg/kg per day (750 mg) *Pediatric:* 15–30 mg/kg per day (1 g)	Nephrotoxicity, ototoxicity	Yes	Monitoring similar to streptomycin
Para-aminosalicylic acid (PAS)	*Adult:* 15 mg/kg per day (1 g); >60 years, 10 mg/kg per day (750 mg) *Pediatric:* 15–30 mg/kg per day (1 g) as single dose or twice-weekly dose	GI intolerance, hepatotoxicity, malabsorption syndrome, hypothyroidism	Yes	Monitor liver enzymes and thyroid function.
Levofloxacin	*Adult:* 8–12 g/day in 2 or 3 doses *Pediatric:* 200–300 mg/kg per day in 2 to 4 divided doses	Nausea, diarrhea, headache, dizziness	Yes	Do not give with divalent and/or trivalent cations (aluminum, magnesium, iron, etc.).
Moxifloxacin	*Adult:* 500 to 1,000 mg/day	Nausea, diarrhea, headache, dizziness	No	See levofloxacin
Gatifloxacin	*Adult:* 400 mg/day *Adult:* 400 mg/day	Nausea, diarrhea, headache, headache	Yes	See levofloxacin

CNS, central nervous system; GI, gastrointestinal.
Adapted from reference 43.

Successful treatment of uncomplicated TB can now be completed in 6 months (26 weeks) if INH, rifampin, pyrazinamide, and ethambutol are used for the first 2 months (8 weeks) and if patient adherence to the regimen and the organism's susceptibility can be ensured.[43] Therefore, after 8 weeks of DOT with INH, rifampin, pyrazinamide, and ethambutol, M.W.'s regimen may be reduced to INH and rifampin daily (5 days or 7 days per week) or two or three times per week under continued DOT for an additional 18 weeks (see Table 61-2). Since M.W. is HIV negative and her chest radiograph did not reveal cavitary lesions, she may also be a candidate for weekly administration of INH and rifapentine, as long as her sputum AFB smear is negative after completing the initial 8 weeks of therapy.[43]

One study of 160 patients with both pulmonary and extrapulmonary TB demonstrated the effectiveness of a primarily twice-weekly treatment regimen. It consisted of INH 300 mg, rifampin 600 mg, pyrazinamide 1.5 to 2.5 g, and streptomycin 750 to 1,000 mg intramuscularly daily for 2 weeks, followed by the same drugs twice weekly at higher doses (except rifampin) for an additional 6 weeks. The regimen was then reduced to INH and rifampin twice weekly for the remaining 16 weeks (4 months). All doses were administered by DOT. Three months after beginning therapy, 75% of all patients studied had negative sputum cultures, and all patients were culture negative at 20 weeks. There was a 1.6% relapse rate (two patients), and only minor adverse effects were reported. Another important feature of this regimen is that it is highly cost effective. Among the 6- and 9-month regimens, it is the second lowest in cost, primarily because of the least number of patient–health care worker encounters (62 directly observed doses).[45]

If pyrazinamide cannot be included in the initial regimen, therapy should be initiated with INH, rifampin, and ethambutol for the first 8 weeks. Therapy should be continued with INH and rifampin for 31 weeks given either daily or twice weekly.[43] If drugs other than INH and rifampin are used in the initial phase, treatment must be continued for 18 to 24 months.[42]

Twice-weekly administration of INH (900 mg) and rifampin (600 mg) is recommended for M.W. because this approach requires fewer doses and should result in substantial cost savings.[43,45] In addition, the relapse rate for the twice- and thrice-weekly INH–rifampin continuation regimens is significantly lower than the once-weekly regimen of INH and rifapentine 600 mg.[46,47] Five characteristics were identified to be independently associated with increased relapse risk in the INH–rifapentine group: having a positive sputum culture at 2 months; having cavitation on chest radiograph; being underweight; having bilateral pulmonary involvement; and being a non-Hispanic white person.[47] A potential explanation for these results is the high protein binding of rifapentine (97%); therefore, a study was conducted to evaluate the safety and tolerability of rifapentine 600 mg, 900 mg, and 1,200 mg once weekly (with INH 15 mg/kg) in 150 HIV-negative patients.[48] There was a trend toward more adverse events possibly related to study therapy in the 1,200-mg treatment arm ($P = 0.051$), but the 900-mg dose appeared to be safe and well tolerated.[48] However, relapse rates for the higher-dose rifapentine regimens are not available at this time.

Treatment with INH and rifampin should be continued for a minimum total duration of 26 weeks. Recent recommendations suggest that a full course of therapy is determined more accurately by the total number of doses taken, not solely by the duration of therapy.[43] Thus, 26 weeks is the minimum duration of treatment and accurately indicates the amount of time the drugs are given only if there are no interruptions in drug administration.[43] Pyridoxine 10 to 25 mg/day should be continued throughout the treatment period. If M.W. is symptomatic or her smear or culture is positive after 3 months of therapy, she should be re-evaluated for possible nonadherence with therapy or infection with drug-resistant tubercle bacilli. These are the two most common reasons for treatment failure. Evaluation should include a second culture and a second susceptibility test, consideration of DOT (if not already instituted), and consultation with experts in the treatment of TB.[25]

Directly Observed Therapy

11. What is DOT, and why is it important that M.W. be placed on it?

DOT involves a health care provider or another responsible person observing as the patient ingests and swallows the TB medications. DOT is the preferred core management strategy for all patients with TB.[25,43] The purpose of DOT is to ensure adherence to TB therapy. DOT not only ensures completion of therapy, but it also reduces the risk of developing drug resistance. By improving these two factors, it also reduces the risk to the community. DOT can be used with daily or two- or three-times-per-week regimens. It may be used in the office or clinic setting or at the patient's home, school, workplace, or other mutually agreed-upon place.[42,43] Often, enablers or incentives, such as food or transportation, are used to improve adherence to DOT. A comprehensive review of DOT-related articles by a consensus panel of public health experts found that the completion rate of TB therapy exceeds 90% when DOT, as recommended by the CDC, is used along with enablers.[49] Although DOT is recommended for all patients, many public health departments do not provide it for cost reasons. However, a study reporting the cost–benefit analysis of DOT versus self-administered therapy found that although the initial cost of DOT was greater, when the costs of relapse and failure were included in the model, DOT was significantly less expensive, with differences up to $3,999 versus $12,167.[50] When drug resistance develops because DOT was not used, the cost of salvage therapy goes up to $180,000 per patient.[51] It is therefore widely accepted that TB patients should receive DOT.[50–52]

Despite this, some clinicians believe DOT is not worth the added expense or may alienate the patient receiving it. One unblinded, randomized trial of 216 patients with drug-susceptible TB found that TB therapy completion rates were equivalent in two groups who either received DOT or administered their own medications. This study demonstrates the need for additional, prospective research on the topic.[53]

Multiple Drug Therapy

12. Why is multiple drug therapy indicated for the treatment of active TB disease? What is the role of each drug in the treatment of TB?

The key to treating active TB disease is multiple drug therapy for a sufficient period of time; this is necessary to kill the organisms and to prevent development of resistant strains of *M. tuberculosis*. Most cavitary lesions contain 10^{9-12} organisms, and the frequency of mutations that confer resistance to a single drug is approximately 10^{-6} for INH and streptomycin, 10^{-8} for rifampin, and 10^{-5} for ethambutol.[43] Because of the large numbers of organisms involved, there is a very high likelihood that patients with active TB disease will harbor organisms with random mutations that confer drug resistance to a given drug. If a single drug is given, it would reduce the number of drug-susceptible organisms but leave the drug-resistant organisms to replicate. By employing multiple drug therapy, the likelihood of encountering organisms with mutations to multiple drugs is reduced. For example, the frequency of concurrent mutations to INH and rifampin would be 10^{-14} (10^{-6} for INH and 10^{-8} for rifampin), making simultaneous resistance to both drugs unlikely in an untreated patient.[43] Therefore, monotherapy has no place in the treatment of active TB disease.[1,43,51]

Multiple drug therapy also serves to sterilize the sputum and lesions as quickly as possible. The drugs available for the treatment of TB vary in their ability to accomplish this task.[43] Drugs effective against tubercle bacilli can be divided into first-line and second-line agents (see Table 61-3). The foundation of treatment should be with first-line agents such as INH, rifampin, pyrazinamide, and ethambutol. INH has been shown to possess the most potent ability to kill rapidly multiplying *M. tuberculosis* during the initial phase of therapy (early bactericidal activity), followed by ethambutol, rifampin, and streptomycin.[54-56] Drugs that have potent early bactericidal activity more rapidly decrease the infectiousness of the patient and reduce the likelihood of developing resistance within the bacillary population.[43] Pyrazinamide has weak early bactericidal activity during the first 2 weeks of therapy and is less effective at preventing emergence of drug resistance than INH, rifampin, and ethambutol.[43,54,57] Therefore, pyrazinamide should not be combined with only one other agent when treating active TB disease. Rifampin also has activity against intracellular organisms that are usually dormant but undergo periods of active growth. This ability to penetrate and destroy the persistent intracellular organisms makes rifampin extremely valuable in short-course chemotherapy regimens.[58]

Pyrazinamide is most effective against tubercle bacilli in the acidic environment within the macrophage or areas of tissue necrosis. Pyrazinamide is most effective in sterilizing lesions when used in the first 2 months of treatment, but it does not offer substantial sterilizing activity after 2 months. Pyrazinamide is an essential component of the short-course regimens and must be prescribed for regimens as short as 6 months to be effective.[42,43]

Ethambutol is bacteriostatic at low doses and bactericidal at higher doses. It is moderately effective against the fast-growing bacilli. It has little sterilizing activity and is primarily used to prevent the emergence of drug-resistant organisms.[42]

Streptomycin is bactericidal against the rapidly multiplying extracellular organisms and is effective when given daily for 2 months followed by two- or three-times-weekly administration thereafter.[59] In the past, streptomycin was administered by intramuscular (IM) injection, but these IM injections were painful. Therefore, although it is not labeled for IV use,

streptomycin may be given in 50 to 100 mL 5% dextrose in water or normal saline and infused over 30 to 60 minutes.[60] Also, like all aminoglycosides, streptomycin can cause ototoxicity and nephrotoxicity.[42,43,60]

The other drugs used in the treatment of TB (capreomycin, amikacin, cycloserine, ethionamide, para-aminosalicylic acid, fluoroquinolones) are usually reserved for cases involving drug-resistant organisms, treatment failure, drug toxicity, or patient intolerance to the other agents. Their use is discussed in Question 23.

Monitoring Drug Therapy

Subjective Findings

13. What subjective and objective findings should be followed to ensure therapeutic efficacy and minimize drug toxicity? Should M.W. be followed closely after completion of her treatment regimen?

M.W. should be asked about the occurrence of adverse reactions secondary to the INH and rifampin (see Table 61-3). Specifically, she should be asked about gastrointestinal (GI) complaints of anorexia, nausea, vomiting, or abdominal pain, which may be an indication of possible hepatitis. Because she has diabetes and is at greater risk for the development of peripheral neuropathy, she should be questioned about numbness and tingling in her extremities. INH-induced peripheral neuropathy, however, should not be a problem in M.W. because she is also taking pyridoxine, which should prevent this adverse effect. M.W. also should be examined for and questioned about petechiae or bruises, since thrombocytopenia is occasionally seen with intermittent rifampin therapy. This effect purportedly occurs more frequently with intermittent rifampin therapy, but it is rare at the currently recommended intermittent rifampin dosage of 10 mg/kg per day (approximately 600 mg).[42]

In a study comparing 6-month versus 9-month antituberculosis therapies of mostly INH and rifampin in 1,451 patients, the incidence of side effects was similar between the two groups. Adverse effects occurred in 7.7% of patients in the 6-month arm compared with 6.4% in the 9-month arm, a difference that was not statistically significant (95% confidence interval, 0.0% to 4.6%).[61] Hepatic disturbances occurred in 1.6% of patients in the 6-month regimen, a nonsignificant difference from patients in the 9-month regimens (1.2%). Hematologic disturbances were rare at 0.2% and 0.0% in the 6-month and 9-month groups, respectively. Other reported effects, GI problems, rash, and arthralgias, were minor and infrequent in both regimens.[61]

Objective Findings

A pretreatment complete blood count, platelet count, blood urea nitrogen (BUN), hepatic enzymes (serum aminotransferases), bilirubin, and serum uric acid should be evaluated. Baseline visual examination should also be performed for patients receiving ethambutol. These tests are performed to detect any abnormality that may complicate or necessitate modification of the prescribed regimen. They should be repeated if the patient experiences any evidence of drug toxicity or has abnormalities at baseline.[42,43]

M.W. is >35 years of age and may be at increased risk for development of drug-induced hepatotoxicity. INH can cause asymptomatic increases in serum transaminases as well as clinical hepatitis.[43] Pyrazinamide has also been associated with hepatotoxicity, but the incidence is less common at dosages of 25 mg/kg per day. Transient asymptomatic hyperbilirubinemia may occur in patients receiving rifampin, and clinical hepatitis that typically has a cholestatic pattern may also occur.[43] Therefore, the patient should be instructed about possible signs and symptoms of hepatotoxicity, primarily nausea, vomiting, abdominal pain, anorexia, and jaundice. Monthly serum liver function tests (LFTs) are no longer recommended because they may be costly and lead to unnecessary alarm secondary to transient, asymptomatic elevations associated with therapy. The CDC now recommends that medical personnel ask the patient about symptoms once monthly.[42]

Sputum cultures and smears for AFB should be ordered every 2 to 4 weeks initially and then monthly after the sputum cultures become negative. With appropriate therapy, sputum cultures should become negative in >85% of patients after 2 months. At this point, the patient will usually need only one more sputum smear and culture at the completion of therapy. Radiologic examination (chest radiography) is not as important as sputum examination, but it may be useful at the completion of therapy to serve as a comparison for any future films.

Patients who are culture positive at 2 months need to be carefully re-examined. Drug susceptibility testing should be performed to rule out acquired drug resistance, and special attention should be given to drug adherence (i.e., DOT should be used). If drug resistance is identified, the regimen should be modified on an individual basis (see MDR-TB, Question 23). Sputum cultures should also be obtained monthly until negative cultures are achieved.[42]

Routine follow-up usually is not required after the successful completion of chemotherapy with INH and rifampin. However, it may be prudent to re-examine the patient 6 months after completion of therapy or at the first sign of any symptoms suggestive of active TB. This is especially important in patients who were slow to respond to therapy or who have significant radiologic findings at the completion of therapy. These recommendations are only for patients with organisms fully susceptible to the medications being used.[42]

Patients who are culture negative but have radiographic abnormalities consistent with TB should have an induced sputum or bronchoscopy performed to establish a microbiologic diagnosis. They will then likely have to be monitored radiographically. Patients with extrapulmonary TB should be evaluated according to the site of involvement.[42,43]

Treatment Failure

14. If M.W. does not respond to her current therapy, should one more drug be added to her regimen?

No. Unfortunately, adding a single drug to a failing regimen is the most common and devastating mistake in TB therapy today. This is essentially the same as monotherapy, because one can assume that the organisms are resistant to the medications currently being used. Resistance to the new drug will eventually develop, further reducing the patient's chance of cure. At least two, and preferably three, new drugs to which susceptibility can be inferred should be added to lessen the probability of further acquired drug resistance. Empiric retreatment regimens may include a fluoroquinolone, an in-

jectable agent like streptomycin, amikacin, or capreomycin, and an additional oral agent such as para-aminosalicylic acid, cycloserine, or ethionamide.[43] New susceptibilities should be obtained and treatment adjusted accordingly.[1,43,51,62]

TREATMENT OF LATENT TB INFECTION

15. M.W.'s 38-year-old husband, S.W., is skin tested with 5-TU strength PPD to determine whether he is infected with *M. tuberculosis*. He has a 10-mm reaction to the skin test, which is classified as "positive." He does not have any clinical symptoms or radiographic findings suggestive of active TB at this time. Is he at risk of developing active disease? What are the current recommendations for drug therapy for persons with latent TB infection? Should S.W. be treated?

Because S.W. is a household contact of a person with active TB disease and has a positive PPD skin test, he is at great risk of becoming infected and developing active disease (Table 61-4). During the first year after infection of the source

Table 61-4   High-Priority Candidates for Treatment of Latent Tuberculosis Infection

Treatment should be recommended for the following persons with a positive tuberculin skin test, regardless of age:

1. Persons with known or suspected HIV infection[a]

2. Close contacts of persons with infectious TB[a]

3. Recent tuberculin skin test converters (≥10-mm increase within a 2-year period for those <35 years of age; >15 mm increase for those ≥35 years of age)

4. Persons with medical conditions that have been reported to increase the risk of TB (e.g., diabetes, prolonged corticosteroid therapy, immunosuppressive therapy, some IV hematologic and reticuloendothelial disease, injection drug use, end-stage renal disease, and clinical situations associated with rapid weight loss)

Treatment should be recommended for the following persons in high-incidence groups with a positive tuberculin test who are <35 years of age and do not have additional risk factors:

1. Foreign-born persons from high-prevalence countries (e.g., Mexico, Philippines, Vietnam, India, Latin America, Asia, and Africa)

2. Medically underserved low-income populations, including high-risk racial or ethnic minority populations, especially Black non-Hispanic, Hispanic, and American Indian/Alaska Native, and Asian/Pacific Islander

3. Residents of facilities for long-term care (e.g., correctional institutions, nursing homes, and mental institutions)

Infected persons <35 years of age with no additional risk factors for TB with a positive test (>15 mm) may also be considered for treatment based on individual assessment of risk and benefits.

---

[a]Persons in these categories may be given treatment in the absence of a positive tuberculin test in some circumstances.
HIV, human immunodeficiency virus; TB, tuberculosis.
Reprinted with permission from reference 21.

case, a household contact's risk of developing active disease is 2% to 4%; persons with a positive skin test are at the greatest risk.[42]

Treatment of latent TB infection (formerly known as preventive therapy) prevents active TB disease in persons who have positive tuberculin skin tests and persons who are at risk for reactivation of active TB; therefore, it is strongly recommended.[25,63–65] Treatment decreases the population of tubercle bacilli and reduces future morbidity from TB in the groups at high risk for developing active disease.[66,67] In clinical studies, INH has been shown to prevent TB in up to 93% of persons who receive the drug, depending on the duration of therapy and patient adherence to the prescribed regimen.[65] Although debate regarding the issue continues, the benefits of treating latent TB infection are generally believed to outweigh the risks of INH-induced hepatitis because every TB-infected person is at risk for developing active disease throughout his or her lifetime.[42,68]

S.W. is infected with *M. tuberculosis,* but he does not currently have active TB disease. In 2000, the CDC recommended four regimens for the treatment of latent TB infection.[65] Daily INH for 9 months was the preferred regimen. Studies in HIV-negative persons indicated that 12 months of INH was more effective than 6 months, but subgroup analysis of several studies suggested that the maximal benefit on INH is likely achieved by 9 months. Daily INH for 6 months and twice-weekly INH for 6 or 9 months are also recommended treatment options for latent TB infection.[65] Because of concerns about INH toxicity and poor adherence due to the relatively long duration of therapy, shorter rifampin-based regimens were also recommended. Rifampin and pyrazinamide, daily for 2 months or twice weekly for 2 to 3 months, and daily rifampin monotherapy for 4 months were recommended alternatives to INH therapy.[65] However, in April 2001, severe and fatal hepatitis was reported in two patients receiving rifampin and pyrazinamide for latent TB infection.[69] Both patients developed anorexia and malaise, and LFTs revealed an alanine aminotransferase (ALT) and an aspartate aminotransferase (AST) greater than 20 times the upper limit of normal. The total bilirubin peaked at 17.8 mg/dL and 27.5 mg/dL in the first and the second patient, respectively.[69] In August 2001, the CDC reported an additional 21 cases of liver injury associated with the 2-month rifampin–pyrazinamide regimen.[70] Of these 21 cases, 16 patients recovered and 5 patients died of liver failure. The onset of liver injury occurred during the second month of the 2-month course in all five patients who died.

To reduce the risk of liver injury associated with rifampin–pyrazinamide therapy, the American Thoracic Society and the CDC, with the endorsement of the Infectious Diseases Society of America, have published revised recommendations for the treatment of latent TB infection.[70] For persons not infected with HIV, daily INH therapy for 9 months remains the preferred regimen, and 4 months of daily rifampin is an acceptable alternative. Two months of daily rifampin and pyrazinamide may be useful when completion of longer treatment courses is unlikely and when the patient can be closely monitored. The 2-month rifampin–pyrazinamide regimen should be used with caution, especially in patients taking medications associated with liver injury or those with alcoholism. No more than a 2-week supply of INH and pyrazinamide should be dispensed at a time to facilitate periodic clinical assessments of the patient. Serum aminotransferases and bilirubin should be measured at baseline and at 2, 4, and 6 weeks of treatment in patients receiving the rifampin–pyrazinamide regimen.[70]

S.W. should be placed on INH 300 mg/day, given as a single daily dose, for at least 6 months and preferably up to 9 months.[65,70] Even though he has a higher chance of developing liver damage (2.3%) because of his age, he also has a high risk of developing active TB. In this case, the benefits of treatment outweigh the possible risks of hepatitis. S.W. should be educated and questioned frequently about the clinical symptoms of hepatitis, such as GI complaints. Pretreatment serum aminotransferases and bilirubin should be assessed to rule out pre-existing liver disease. The need for monthly or routine monitoring of these values is controversial.

ADVERSE DRUG EFFECTS

Isoniazid

Hepatitis

16. After 2 months of INH therapy, S.W. was found to have an aspartate aminotransferase (AST) of 130 U/L (normal, 7 to 40). Discuss the presentation, prognosis, and mechanism of INH-induced hepatitis. What are the risk factors for developing hepatitis? Should INH be discontinued to prevent further liver damage?

[SI unit: AST, 130 U/L]

Approximately 10% to 20% of INH recipients develop elevated serum aminotransferase levels.[43] However, most patients with mild, subclinical hepatic damage do not progress to overt hepatitis and recover completely even while continuing INH therapy. In contrast, continuation of INH in patients with clinical symptoms may result in severe hepatocellular toxicity, which is associated with a higher fatality rate than seen in patients whose INH was discontinued immediately.[43] However, the risk of death from TB is estimated to be 11 times higher than the risk of death from INH hepatitis.[71]

INH-induced hepatitis is clinically, biochemically, and histologically indistinguishable from viral hepatitis. Viral hepatitis, however, primarily affects young adults, while INH hepatitis occurs more frequently in older patients.[72] The development of INH hepatitis has been linked to several factors, including acetylator phenotype, age, daily alcohol consumption, and concurrent rifampin use. Additionally, women may be at a higher risk of death, especially during the postpartum period.[71]

The mechanisms responsible for INH hepatotoxicity remain unclear. Previously, it was thought that rapid acetylators had a greater risk for INH hepatitis than slow acetylators. Rapid acetylators of INH form monoacetylhydrazine, a compound that can cause liver damage, more rapidly than slow acetylators.[73] However, rapid acetylators also would eliminate this compound at a faster rate, and this should equalize the risk of toxicity between slow and fast acetylators.[74] One study demonstrated a different incidence of hepatitis between Asian males and females. Because both groups were fast acetylators, this study suggests that hepatitis is probably caused by factors other than acetylator phenotype.[75] Thus, it appears that acetylator status alone does not explain the development of INH hepatitis.

Some evidence supports the theory that INH-induced hepatitis is a hypersensitivity reaction; however, many patients can tolerate INH on rechallenge, discounting this theory.[76,77]

Age and concurrent daily alcohol ingestion are probably more significant factors to consider in the development of INH hepatitis.[42] Progressive liver damage is rare in persons <20 years of age. It occurs in approximately 0.3% of persons ages 20 to 34 years, 1.2% of those ages 35 to 49 years, and 2.3% of persons >50 years of age.[42] One prospective cohort study demonstrated a low incidence of INH hepatitis. Of 11,141 patients receiving INH alone for the treatment of latent TB infection, only 11 (0.1% of those starting and 0.15% of those completing therapy) developed clinical hepatitis.[78] Previous studies suggested a higher incidence of clinical hepatitis in patients receiving INH alone, and a meta-analysis of six studies estimated the rate to be 0.6%.[43] These findings confirm that further study of INH hepatitis is warranted.

As mentioned earlier, whether biochemical monitoring of liver function is of value in the detection of liver toxicity secondary to INH is controversial. The American Thoracic Society and the CDC do not recommend routine monitoring of LFTs unless symptoms suggest hepatitis.[42] However, of 1,000 patients receiving INH, 47 of 64 patients with extremely high AST levels were asymptomatic.[79] Similar findings occurred in 5 of 83 health care workers receiving INH therapy for latent TB infection. As a result, some clinicians maintain that monthly serum LFTs should be performed.[80] Subclinical hepatic injury occurs early in treatment and is reversible during the first 3 months if detected early with routine LFTs.[79]

High-risk patients should be followed with routine monitoring of LFTs. This includes those who consume alcohol daily, persons >35 years of age, those taking other hepatotoxic drugs, those with pre-existing liver disease, IV drug abusers, Black and Hispanic women, and all postpartum women. INH should be discontinued if the AST level exceeds three to five times the upper limit of the normal value.[42]

Because S.W.'s AST is three times the upper range of the normal value and he is >35 years old, INH should be discontinued temporarily until the AST returns to normal. At that time, INH should be resumed and the LFTs should be rechecked. If the AST increases again, the drug should be discontinued and S.W. should be followed frequently for development of active TB. In addition to laboratory monitoring, S.W. should be reminded of the importance of reporting any GI signs and symptoms that might suggest hepatitis. Of all patients with INH hepatitis, 55% experience GI signs and symptoms such as nausea, anorexia, vomiting, and abdominal discomfort. Some patients (35%) complain of a viral-like illness, and others are asymptomatic until the onset of jaundice (10%). Other patients have had hepatomegaly (33%), hyperbilirubinemia (25%), and prolonged prothrombin times (35%).[81]

17. C.M., a 50-kg, 35-year-old woman, is being treated for active TB disease with INH 1,200 mg and rifampin 600 mg twice weekly. Is 1,200 mg of INH twice weekly an appropriate dose for a 50-kg patient? What INH side effects, other than hepatotoxicity, should be anticipated?

The usual twice-weekly INH dose is 15 mg/kg, with a maximum dose of 900 mg; therefore, C.M. should be receiving no more than 900 mg rather than 1,200 mg of INH. Al-

though high doses or serum concentrations are not usually directly related to hepatitis, elevated serum INH concentrations are associated with increased central nervous system (CNS) effects, ranging from somnolence to psychosis and seizure. GI complaints are also higher at doses >20 mg/kg.

Peripheral Neuropathy

Although uncommon at the recommended daily and intermittent doses, INH may cause a peripheral neuropathy by interfering with pyridoxine (vitamin B_6) metabolism.[43,65] As many as 20% of patients experience this problem when the INH dosage exceeds 6 mg/kg per day. Clinically, the patient usually experiences numbness or tingling in the feet or hands. In patients with medical conditions where neuropathy is common, such as diabetes, alcoholism, HIV infection, malnutrition, and renal failure, supplemental pyridoxine 25 mg/day should be given with INH.[43,65] Women who are pregnant or breast-feeding and persons with seizure disorders should also receive supplemental pyridoxine with INH.[65]

Allergic Reactions

Allergic reactions consisting of arthralgias, skin rash, fever, and swelling of the tongue have also occurred. INH has been associated with arthritic symptoms and systemic lupus erythematosus; approximately 20% of patients receiving INH develop antinuclear antibodies.[43]

Other Reactions

Other reactions that may occur with INH are dry mouth, epigastric distress, CNS stimulation and depression, psychoses, hemolytic anemia, pyridoxine-responsive anemia, and agranulocytosis.[76]

Drug Interactions

In addition to the previously mentioned adverse reactions, INH is a relatively potent inhibitor of several cytochrome P450 isoenzymes (CYP2C9, CYP2C19, CYP2E1) but has minimal effects on CYP3A.[43] INH inhibits the hepatic metabolism of phenytoin and carbamazepine, resulting in increased plasma concentrations of these drugs. Patients receiving either of these two drugs with INH should be observed for signs of phenytoin or carbamazepine toxicity, such as nystagmus, ataxia, headache, nausea, or drowsiness. Plasma phenytoin and carbamazepine concentrations should be monitored periodically so that the doses can be adjusted if necessary. Carbamazepine also may induce INH hepatitis by inducing its metabolism to toxic metabolites.[82] In addition, INH inhibits the metabolism of diazepam and triazolam. Rifampin has the opposite effect on hepatic metabolism and to a stronger degree; INH–rifampin combination therapy induces the metabolism of diazepam, phenytoin, and other agents metabolized by the cytochrome P450 system.[83]

Rifampin

Flu-like Syndrome

18. One month after beginning her twice-weekly DOT regimen, C.M. developed symptoms of myalgias, malaise, and anorexia. Laboratory data were normal except for a slightly decreased platelet count. Could C.M.'s symptoms be related to her drug therapy? What adverse reactions other than hepatotoxicity should be anticipated in a patient receiving rifampin?

A flu-like syndrome has been reported in about 1% of patients receiving intermittent rifampin administration. This syndrome is rarely seen with usual dosages of 600 mg twice weekly, but the incidence increases with twice-weekly doses of >900 mg. The incidence also increases if the dosage interval is increased to 1 week or longer.[84,85] Unless the symptoms are severe, discontinuation of the drug is unnecessary. Because C.M. is receiving rifampin 900 mg twice weekly, her dose should be reduced to 600 mg and administered daily until the symptoms subside. The temporary administration of a nonsteroidal anti-inflammatory drug has been used to alleviate the flu-like symptoms. Twice-weekly therapy may then be resumed as long as the dose of rifampin does not exceed 600 mg.

Hepatotoxicity

Rifampin may also cause hepatotoxicity, but in <1% of patients taking the drug. Therefore, the risk of drug-induced hepatotoxicity is greater for INH than for rifampin. Although elevated liver enzymes are seen on occasion, rifampin is more likely to produce cholestasis, as manifested by increases in alkaline phosphatase and bilirubin levels. Elevations of all LFTs may be seen transiently during the first month of rifampin therapy but are usually benign.[43]

Thrombocytopenia

The platelet count should be monitored closely because thrombocytopenia is also more frequently associated with intermittent or interrupted rifampin administration. It is thought that this reaction may be caused by IgG and IgM antibodies to rifampin. With rifampin, these antibodies may fix complement onto the platelets, resulting in platelet destruction. It is thought that a sufficient quantity of antibodies builds up when treatment is intermittent or interrupted. When thrombocytopenia occurs with rifampin, its use is contraindicated from then on because the problem will likely recur.[86,87]

Miscellaneous Reactions

In addition to the side effects associated with high-dose, intermittent therapy, 3% to 4% of patients taking normal doses of rifampin may experience adverse reactions.[86] The most common of these are nausea, vomiting, fever, and rash. Other reactions to rifampin include the hepatorenal syndrome (hemolysis, leukopenia, anemia, and arthralgias) as part of a suspected drug-induced lupus syndrome.[43,88] The development of these latter reactions requires discontinuation of the drug.

Acute Renal Failure

Acute renal failure has also occurred rarely with rifampin.[43] This hypersensitivity reaction may occur with both intermittent and daily administration and may last as long as 12 months.[84] Rifampin should be discontinued and other drugs such as pyrazinamide and ethambutol should be given in reduced doses. However, both rifampin and INH may be given in normal dosages to patients with pre-existing renal failure.[89,90]

Another important problem associated with rifampin is caused by its chemical makeup. It is an orange-red crystalline powder that is distributed widely in body fluids. As a result, it may discolor saliva, tears, urine, and sweat.[43] Patients using rifampin should be warned of this effect and cautioned not to use soft contact lenses because of possible discoloration. This effect may also be used to monitor adherence to rifampin therapy.

Drug Interactions

Rifampin is a potent inducer of cytochrome P450 isoenzymes, especially CYP3A4.[43] The rifamycins differ in their ability to induce cytochrome P450 isoenzymes: rifampin is the most potent, rifapentine is intermediate, and rifabutin is the least potent enzyme inducer.[43] Rifampin increases the metabolism of protease inhibitors, nonnucleoside reverse transcriptase inhibitors, macrolide antibiotics, azole antifungal agents, corticosteroids, oral contraceptives, warfarin, cyclosporine, tacrolimus, theophylline, phenytoin, quinidine, diazepam, propranolol, metoprolol, sulfonylureas, verapamil, nifedipine, diltiazem, enalapril, and simvastatin.[43,83] While the patient is receiving rifampin, it may be necessary to monitor serum concentrations of the aforementioned drugs, where appropriate, or increase their dosages. Also, women who are taking rifampin and oral contraceptives should use an alternative birth control method. When treating any patient with rifampin, the health care professional should carefully evaluate all concomitant medications for the possibility of drug–drug interactions.

INH–Rifampin

Hepatotoxicity

19. Does the combination of INH and rifampin cause hepatotoxicity more frequently than either drug alone?

The use of these two agents together has been controversial. Some evidence initially suggested that the use of INH and rifampin together might lead to a greater incidence of hepatotoxicity in some patients. Many believed this might be caused by rifampin inducing the metabolism of INH to either monoacetylhydrazine or products of hydrolysis, both of which may lead to hepatotoxins. In an attempt to answer this question, Steele and coworkers performed a meta-analysis looking at the incidence of hepatitis in all studies between 1966 and 1989 using regimens that contained INH without rifampin, rifampin without INH, and regimens containing both drugs. They found that the incidence of clinical hepatitis was greater in regimens containing both INH and rifampin (2.7%) versus regimens of INH alone (1.6%), but this effect was additive, not synergistic, and therefore expected.[77] The use of the two drugs together, therefore, is not contraindicated. However, caution should be used in high-risk groups such as the elderly, alcoholics, those taking additional hepatotoxic agents, and those with pre-existing liver disease.[91]

Ethambutol

Optic Neuritis

20. S.E., a 65-year-old woman, was placed on INH 300 mg/day, rifampin 600 mg/day, pyrazinamide 900 mg/day, and ethambutol 1,200 mg/day for initial treatment of active TB. Two months after the initiation of therapy, she began to complain of blurred vision. A routine eye examination and visual field tests resulted in a diagnosis of optic neuritis. There was no evidence of glaucoma, cataracts, or retinal damage. Laboratory tests were within normal limits except for an elevated serum uric acid (9.7 mg/dL; normal, 2 to 8 mg/dL) and a slightly elevated serum creatinine (SCr) (1.4 mg/dL; normal, 0.6 to 1.3 mg/dL). No symptoms of joint pain were associated with the elevated serum uric acid, and there was no past history of gout. Her calculated creatinine clearance (Cl_{Cr}) based on her weight of 60 kg was 50 mL/min. Could the visual problem and increased uric acid levels be related to her medications?

[SI units: uric acid, 576.96 μmol/L; SCr, 123.76 μmol/L; Cl_{Cr}, 0.83 mL/sec]

S.E.'s decrease in visual acuity is compatible with ethambutol-induced optic neuritis. This condition is characterized by central scotomas, loss of green color vision, or less commonly a peripheral vision defect. The intensity of these ocular effects is related to the duration of continued therapy after decreased visual acuity is first noted. The optic neuritis is related to the dose and duration of therapy. Optic neuritis is rare at doses of 15 mg/kg but has occurred.[92–94] The incidence is estimated to be 6% for doses of 25 mg/kg and 15% for doses >35 mg/kg. Recovery, which may take many months, is usually but not always complete when the drug is discontinued.

The optic neuritis manifested in S.E. is probably caused by the use of a higher ethambutol dose (20 mg/kg) with mildly impaired renal function (estimated Cl_{Cr} 50 mL/min). Because ethambutol adds no additional benefit to the INH–rifampin regimen after the first 2 months unless drug-resistant organisms are suspected, it can be discontinued. Because ethambutol is excreted by the kidney (50% to 80%), the dosage interval for ethambutol should have been increased based on the decline in creatinine clearance. If the Cl_{Cr} is 10 to 50 mL/min, the interval should be increased from 24 to 36 hours; if the Cl_{Cr} is <10 mL/min, it should be increased to 48 hours.[89] S.E.'s visual acuity should be monitored closely through periodic eye examinations, and she should be instructed to contact her physician immediately if she experiences any further visual changes.

S.E.'s elevated serum uric acid also may be attributed to her ethambutol as well as a decline in her renal function, but it is more likely caused by pyrazinamide, which decreases the tubular secretion of urate.[61] Asymptomatic hyperuricemia secondary to drugs usually does not require treatment.

SPECIAL TREATMENT CONSIDERATIONS
The Elderly
Incidence

21. G.H., a 75-year-old man recently confined to a nursing home, becomes disoriented, refuses to eat, and has a productive cough. Physical examination reveals a thin man who is having slight difficulty breathing. Laboratory findings are essentially normal with the exception of a slightly elevated BUN of 25 mg/dL (normal, 10 to 20 mg/dL) and SCr of 1.3 mg/dL (normal, 0.6 to 1.3 mg/dL). A chest radiograph reveals infiltrates in the right lower lobe; he has a history of congestive heart failure, which is well controlled. Blood, urine, and sputum samples are sent for culture and susceptibility testing; the initial Gram's stain is negative. Because the nursing home has recently had two cases of active TB, a PPD skin test and sputum smear for AFB are ordered as well. The PPD skin test induration is 16 mm, and the sputum smear is positive for AFB. G.H.'s admission skin test was negative. Discuss the presentation of TB in the elderly and the appropriate treatment of active disease in G.H. Is the incidence of drug side effects greater in the elderly? Should other patients in close contact with G.H. receive INH therapy?

[SI units: BUN, 8.93 mmol/L of urea (normal, 3.57 to 7.14); SCr, 114.92 μmol/L (normal, 53.04 to 88.4)]

The incidence of new TB infections has increased in the geriatric population living in nursing homes. The case rate of 39.2 per 100,000 is greater than that of elderly patients living at home (18.7 per 100,000).[95,96] Although active TB disease in the elderly has been attributed to a decrease in the immune system followed by reactivation of an earlier infection, active disease is a common, endemic infection in nursing homes in patients with no previous immunity (negative skin test) to *M. tuberculosis*.[97–99] The incidence of positive skin tests increases after patients have been in the nursing home >1 month. Therefore, all patients entering a nursing home should be tested with 5-TU PPD. If the initial test is negative and a source case is present in the nursing home (as illustrated by this case), this test should be repeated in 1 month. The rate of tuberculin skin test conversion (from negative to positive) in this population is approximately 5%. If these recent converters are not treated with INH, approximately 8% of women and 12% of men will progress from infection to active disease within 2 years.[100]

Diagnosis

The diagnosis of active TB in elderly patients may be extremely difficult because the classic symptoms of TB (cough, fever, night sweats, weight loss) are often absent, and elderly patients may describe their symptoms poorly. The chest radiograph and PPD skin test may be the only clues indicating a TB infection.[98,101] Frequently, the chest radiograph is atypical, resembling pneumonia or worsening heart failure. Chest radiographs in the elderly are less likely to have upper lobe infiltration but more commonly have extensive infiltration of both lungs.[102] If the patient's clinical diagnosis is caused by granuloma breakdown (reactivation), the chest radiograph often shows apical infiltrates or nodules. However, if the disease is progressing from an initial infection, as in the case of G.H., lower lobe infiltrates may be present.[100] TB in this population may present clinically with changes in activities of daily living, chronic fatigue, cognitive impairment, anorexia, or unexplained low-grade fever. Nonspecific signs and symptoms that range in severity from subacute to chronic and that persist for a period of weeks to months must alert clinicians to the possibility of unrecognized TB.[103] Sputum examination for *M. tuberculosis* and AFB smear and culture should be performed in all patients, including the elderly.

Treatment of Active Disease in the Elderly

The principles of TB treatment are the same for the elderly as for any other age group. Because G.H. has clinical symptoms of a respiratory infection, positive sputum smears for AFB, and a positive skin test, he should be treated with a four-drug regimen for active TB disease. The vast majority of TB cases in elderly patients are caused by drug-susceptible strains of *M. tuberculosis;* however, notable exceptions would be older patients who are from a country or region where the prevalence of drug-resistant strains is high, persons who have been inadequately treated in the past, or persons who acquired the infection from a recent contact known to be infected with drug-resistant *M. tuberculosis*.[103] His drug regimen could include INH 300 mg, rifampin 600 mg, pyrazinamide 20 to 25 mg/kg, and ethambutol 15 to 20 mg/kg daily for 8 weeks followed by INH and rifampin daily or two or three times a week for 16 weeks (DOT). He could also receive INH, rifampin, pyrazinamide, and ethambutol daily for 2 weeks, followed by twice a week for 6 weeks, then INH and rifampin twice a week for 16 weeks.[103] Some clinicians prefer treating the elderly with 9-month regimens of INH and rifampin. He should also receive pyridoxine 10 to 50 mg with each dose.[42]

Adverse Drug Effects

Although there have been reports of higher incidences of hepatitis in elderly patients receiving INH, INH and rifampin are generally well tolerated in this age group, with major side effects of hematologic or hepatic abnormalities occurring in 3% to 4% of patients.[104] Therefore, serum aminotransferases should be assessed at baseline, and G.H. should be observed monthly for clinical signs of hepatitis. Serum aminotransferases can also be monitored monthly, although this remains controversial because transient, asymptomatic rises do occur among the elderly.[100,104]

Although uncommon at 600 mg, rifampin given twice weekly may cause a higher incidence of flu-like symptoms. Because potential drug interactions with INH and rifampin are possible, any medication added to the patient's regimen should be carefully evaluated. Ethambutol may cause optic neuritis, even at the lower doses, in conjunction with an age-related decline in renal function. G.H. has an increased serum creatinine and should have his vision monitored carefully.

Treatment of Latent Infection in the Elderly

Treatment of elderly patients with positive skin tests but no active TB disease with INH 300 mg daily for 6 to 9 months is essential if a source case is present in the nursing home. A 15-mm cutoff for skin test positivity is used for persons >35 years, so that the benefits of using INH therapy clearly outweigh the risks (see Table 61-4).[96] Stead and colleagues reported only 1 case of active disease in patients receiving therapy for latent TB infection compared with 69 cases in untreated patients. In patients with recently converted skin tests, 1 patient in the group receiving INH therapy developed active disease compared with 45 who received no treatment.[98]

Multidrug-Resistant Organisms

Definition/Etiology

22. **M.S., an ill-appearing 22-year-old Asian man, is admitted to the hospital with signs and symptoms of pneumonia. He is coughing and his chest radiograph indicates bilateral infiltrates. He is placed in respiratory isolation pending the results of sputum testing for *M. tuberculosis*. He states that he was diagnosed with TB 3 months ago and started on a regimen of INH, rifampin, pyrazinamide, and ethambutol. He stopped taking his medication after 1 month, and he is HIV negative. What is the likelihood of acquired drug resistance?**

Drug-resistant *M. tuberculosis* became increasingly prevalent in the United States in the late 1980s to early 1990s, although this has improved in recent years.[3,21,105–107] In 2001, the incidence of INH resistance in the United States was 7.1%, and the incidence of resistance to both INH and rifampin (multidrug resistance) was 1.0%.[3] Resistance in *M. tuberculosis* is either primary or acquired. Primary drug resistance oc-

curs when a patient harbors a resistant strain before any drugs have been administered. Acquired drug resistance occurs when resistant subpopulations are selected by inappropriate therapy.[51] The World Health Organization (WHO) conducted a global survey of drug resistance in *M. tuberculosis* and showed that resistance to at least one antituberculosis drug occurs in a median of 9.9% of strains in patients never having received treatment ("primary") and in 36.0% of strains in patients who received treatment for at least 1 month ("acquired"). Based on these results, acquired drug resistance is a larger problem.[107]

Acquired drug resistance may be the result of treatment errors, such as addition of a single drug to a failing regimen, inadequate primary regimen, failure to recognize resistance, and, most importantly, nonadherence to the prescribed regimen. Sporadic ingestion, inadequate dosages, or malabsorption of medications can cause susceptible *M. tuberculosis* strains to become resistant to multiple drugs within a few months.[47,108,109] These resistant organisms can then be transmitted to persons who have never received treatment, leading to primary resistance in these patients.

Patterns and prevalence of drug resistance vary throughout the world, with areas such as Russia, Asia, the Dominican Republic, and Argentina showing the highest rates of MDR-TB.[107] As mentioned earlier, the incidence of MDR-TB in the United States has declined. Nonetheless, it is important to note the populations at risk: HIV-infected persons and those in group or institutional settings such as hospitals, prisons, nursing homes, and homeless shelters.[110]

M.S. is Asian and therefore may have primary resistance from his country of origin, making a detailed exposure history essential. M.S. is also an example of the problem of treatment failure caused by nonadherence and the acquisition of drug-resistant organisms.

Treatment

23. **How should M.S. be treated, and can he be cured?**

M.S.'s current regimen should be re-evaluated, drug susceptibility testing should be done, and he should be referred to a specialist or consultation from a specialized treatment center.[43] Current drug susceptibility testing in most institutions takes several weeks; this can be decreased to 3 weeks with the use of the BACTEC system. Definitive randomized or controlled clinical studies have not been performed in patients with organisms resistant to multiple drugs. When initiating or revising therapy, clinicians should always attempt to use at least three previously unused drugs to which there is in vitro susceptibility, and one of these agents should be injectable.[43] A new regimen should contain at least four drugs, possibly more, depending on the severity of the disease and the resistance pattern. If resistance to INH and rifampin is suspected, M.S. should be started on a regimen of pyrazinamide, ethambutol, a fluoroquinolone (levofloxacin, ciprofloxacin, moxifloxacin, or gatifloxacin), and an injectable agent (streptomycin, amikacin, capreomycin), pending the results of susceptibility testing (Table 61-5).[43] Treatment should be continued for 18 to 24 months.[43,111]

The fluoroquinolone antibiotics (ciprofloxacin, levofloxacin, moxifloxacin, and gatifloxacin) are active against mycobacteria, including *M. tuberculosis*, and they penetrate

Table 61-5 Potential Regimens for Patients With Tuberculosis with Various Patterns of Drug Resistance

Resistance	Suggested Regimen	Duration of Therapy	Comments
Isoniazid and rifampin (± streptomycin)	Pyrazinamide, ethambutol, fluoroquinolone, amikacin[a]	18–24 months	Consider surgery.
Isoniazid, streptomycin, and pyrazinamide	Rifampin, pyrazinamide, ethambutol, amikacin[a]	6–9 months	Anticipate 100% response and <5% relapse rate.
Isoniazid and ethambutol (± streptomycin)	Rifampin, pyrazinamide, fluoroquinolone, amikacin[a]	6–12 months	Efficacy should be comparable to above regimen.
Isoniazid, rifampin, and ethambutol (± streptomycin)	Pyrazinamide, fluoroquinolone, amikacin,[a] plus 2 additional agents[b]	20 months after conversion	Consider surgery.
Isoniazid, rifampin, and pyrazinamide (± streptomycin)	Ethambutol, fluoroquinolone, amikacin,[a] plus 2 additional agents[b]	24 months after conversion	Consider surgery.
Isoniazid, rifampin, pyrazinamide, and ethambutol (± streptomycin)	Fluoroquinolone, amikacin,[a] plus 3 additional agents[b]	24 months after conversion	Surgery, if possible

[a]If TB is resistant to amikacin and streptomycin, capreomycin is a good alternative. Injectable agents usually are continued for 4–6 months if toxicity does not intervene. All the injectable drugs are given daily (or twice or thrice weekly) and may be administered intravenously or intramuscularly.
[b]Potential agents from which to choose: ethionamide, cycloserine, or para-aminosalicylic acid. Others that are potentially useful but of unproven utility include clofazimine and amoxicillin-clavulanate. Clarithromycin, azithromycin, and rifabutin are unlikely to be active.
Reprinted with permission from Iseman MD. Drug therapy: treatment of multidrug-resistant tuberculosis. N Engl J Med 1993;329:784–791. ©1993 Massachusetts Medical Society. All rights reserved.

rapidly into mammalian cells. These two features are critical in treating intracellular pathogens such as *M. tuberculosis*. Also, in vitro studies do not show any cross-resistance between fluoroquinolones and other antimycobacterial drugs.[112–114] Ciprofloxacin and ofloxacin have been used long term for the treatment of mycobacterial infections and were well tolerated, with few serious adverse effects.[114] Levofloxacin is also frequently used for MDR-TB instead of ofloxacin because of its reduced toxicity and higher concentrations in relation to minimum inhibitory concentrations (MICs).[114,115] Other medications used for MDR-TB include para-aminosalicylic acid, cycloserine, ethionamide, and capreomycin. These are all associated with numerous side effects and should not be prescribed without the guidance of an expert in the treatment of MDR-TB (see Table 61-3).

Outcome

While previously untreated drug-susceptible TB is curable in 98% to 99% of cases, the cure rate of MDR-TB is not as promising. Goble and colleagues showed that in 171 patients taking an average of 5.7 drugs over 51 months for treatment of MDR-TB, the overall response rate was only 56%. Outcomes are slightly improved with surgical resection.[108]

HIV
TREATMENT OF LATENT INFECTION WITH MDR-TB

24. L.W., the 26-year-old roommate of M.S., was recently found to be HIV positive. Currently, he does not have symptoms of active TB. His PPD skin test is 6 mm. What is the possibility that M.S. has infected L.W. with drug-resistant *M. tuberculosis*? How should he be managed?

The risk is high that L.W. is infected with drug-resistant *M. tuberculosis*. HIV-infected persons are much more likely to become infected than immunocompetent persons. His risk is estimated to be 113 times that of a person with no known risk factors.[106]

Because L.W. is at high risk of infection with multidrug-resistant organisms, he should be started on two drugs for treatment of latent TB infection.[65,106] He could be started on pyrazinamide 20 to 25 mg/kg per day and ethambutol 15 to 20 mg/kg per day for 12 months. Another possible regimen would be pyrazinamide and a fluoroquinolone (levofloxacin, ofloxacin, or ciprofloxacin), although this regimen has been poorly tolerated.[42,116] The specific regimen for L.W. should also take into consideration the drug susceptibility results of his roommate, M.S.

25. Because he is HIV positive, what is L.W.'s prognosis?

One initial study of HIV-infected patients with MDR-TB showed immediate progression to active TB disease after infection and a median survival of only 2.1 months.[117] However, a more recent study showed improved results, with the median survival time being 6.8 months in similar patients.[118] Nonetheless, the mortality of HIV-positive patients remains significantly higher than HIV-negative patients. If L.W. develops MDR-TB and had AIDS, his risk of death would increase to 72% to 89%, even with aggressive multidrug treatment.

26. F.R., a 32-year-old man diagnosed with AIDS 6 months ago, is experiencing mild pleuritic chest pain with a productive cough. He also has experienced weight loss, fatigue, and night sweats over the past 2 weeks. A chest radiograph reveals bilateral infiltrates. Sputum samples are ordered for AFB smear and culture, and a PPD skin test is placed. The AFB smear is positive, and the induration from the PPD is 6 mm. His CD4+ T cell count is 150/mm³. He is currently receiving zidovudine, lamivudine, and indinavir for his HIV disease with no complaints. How does TB present and what is its frequency in a patient with AIDS? How effective is skin testing in the diagnosis of latent TB infection? How should F.R. be treated?

HIV infects CD4+ T cells, leading to a decrease in cell-mediated immunity. This absence of immunity allows the rapid development of active TB disease in a person who is infected with *M. tuberculosis*.[11,31,44,119–121] The lungs are most frequently affected (74% to 79% of cases); however, extra-pulmonary disease also occurs much more frequently in patients with HIV infection than in patients without HIV infection (45% to 72% versus 17.5%).[119,121] Patients with AIDS have a much greater chance of extrapulmonary disease than asymptomatic HIV-infected persons. Infection with *M. tuberculosis* may be difficult to distinguish from other HIV-related pulmonary opportunistic infections (e.g., *Pneumocystis carinii, M. avium* complex). TB often precedes other opportunistic pulmonary infections and should be ruled out in any patient with HIV infection.[119] Several studies have identified predictors of poor survival in HIV-infected patients, such as low CD4+ cell counts, MDR-TB, no DOT, and a history of IV drug abuse.[122] New therapies, such as the fluoroquinolones and immunomodulating agents, may improve the outcome in these patients, but more clinical research is needed to assess their value.[123]

PPD and Treatment of Active Disease

A PPD skin test should be applied to HIV-infected patients, although only about 30% to 50% of patients with AIDS and TB will respond to a PPD skin test with an induration >10 mm. Therefore, an induration of >5 mm is considered to be a positive reaction in this population (see Table 61-4).[42,65,124] F.R.'s reaction to PPD (6 mm) should be considered positive. Based on his symptoms and positive AFB smear, he should be started on multiple drug therapy for treatment of active TB disease. Recommendations for the treatment of TB in HIV-infected adults are the same as those for HIV-uninfected persons, with a few important exceptions (see Table 61-2).[43] These exceptions include the potential for drug–drug interactions between rifamycins and antiretroviral agents, and the potential for the development of acquired rifamycin resistance with highly intermittent therapy.[43,125,126] However, antiretroviral therapy should not be withheld simply because the patient is being treated for TB, and a rifamycin should not be excluded for the treatment regimen for fear of interactions with certain antiretroviral agents.[43] Exclusion of a rifamycin will likely delay sputum conversion, prolong the duration of therapy, and possibly result in a poor outcome.

As noted earlier, rifampin is a potent inducer of cytochrome P450 isoenzymes (especially 3A4), rifapentine is intermediate in potency, and rifabutin is the least potent inducer.[43] Rifabutin is highly active against *M. tuberculosis*, so it has been recommended in place of rifampin for the treatment of active TB in HIV-infected patients receiving protease inhibitors or nonnucleoside reverse transcriptase inhibitors.[43] Data from clinical trials also suggest that rifabutin- and rifampin-based regimens are equally efficacious.[43] However, protease inhibitors and nonnucleoside reverse transcriptase

inhibitors may either induce or inhibit cytochrome P450 isoenzymes, depending on the specific drug. As a result, these drugs may alter the serum concentrations of rifabutin.[43,126] Since F.R. is receiving indinavir, a cytochrome P450 3A4 inhibitor, the dose of rifabutin must be decreased to reduce the likelihood of clinical toxicity associated with increased concentrations of rifabutin (leukopenia, uveitis, arthralgias, skin discoloration).[126] Therefore, he should be started on rifabutin 150 mg, INH 300 mg, pyrazinamide 20 to 25 mg/kg, and ethambutol 15 to 20 mg/kg daily for the first 8 weeks of therapy. The CDC has also updated its guidelines for the use of rifampin for treatment of TB in HIV-infected patients receiving protease inhibitors and nonnucleoside reverse transcriptase inhibitors.[125] Based on these guidelines, rifampin can be used in the following patients: (1) a patient whose antiretroviral regimen includes the nonnucleoside reverse transcriptase inhibitor efavirenz and two nucleoside reverse transcriptase inhibitors; (2) a patient whose antiretroviral regimen includes the protease inhibitor ritonavir and one or more reverse transcriptase inhibitors; or (3) a patient whose antiretroviral regimen includes the combination of two protease inhibitors (ritonavir and saquinavir hard-gel or soft-gel capsules).[125]

After this initial period, if no drug resistance is evident on susceptibility testing, F.R. can be treated with INH and rifabutin daily or two or three times a week for a minimum of 26 weeks. Since he is receiving indinavir, the rifabutin dose for intermittent therapy should be 300 mg.[126] Although not applicable to F.R. because his CD4+ T cell count is 150 cells/mL, twice-weekly continuation therapy with INH and rifampin or INH and rifabutin is not recommended for HIV-infected patients with CD4+ cell counts <100 cells/mL due to an increased frequency of acquired rifamycin resistance.[43,126,127] In addition, the once-weekly continuation regimen of INH and rifapentine is contraindicated in HIV-infected patients because of a high rate of relapse with organisms that have acquired resistance to the rifamycins.[43]

Because the margin of error is probably less in HIV-infected patients, special care to ensure adherence is required. In other words, DOT is highly recommended in this population. Furthermore, if the patient is slow to respond, prolonged therapy (>6 months) should also be considered. In addition to the antituberculosis medications, pyridoxine should be given to prevent peripheral neuropathy.

DRUG INTERACTIONS

27. Are there any interactions between TB and antiretroviral agents to consider in F.R.'s therapy?

There are many. Since 1995, the FDA has approved several products in the protease inhibitor class of antiretroviral drugs: ritonavir (Norvir), saquinavir hard-gel capsule (Invirase), saquinavir soft-gel capsule (Fortovase), indinavir (Crixivan), nelfinavir (Viracept), amprenavir (Agenerase), and lopinavir plus ritonavir (Kaletra). These products are the most potent antiretroviral agents available to treat HIV-infected patients, but they have many drug–drug interactions that are important to consider. First, all of the protease inhibitors are cytochrome P450 3A4 inhibitors, and ritonavir is the most potent inhibitor in the class. As a result, drugs affected by this interaction, such as rifabutin, will have elevated concentrations. In addition to their effect on other drugs, the protease inhibitors are affected by other drugs that affect the cytochrome P450 system, such as rifampin, which is a potent inducer of the cytochrome P450 system. The protease inhibitor concentrations are reduced by 35% to 80% with concomitant rifampin administration. This reduction is somewhat less with rifabutin. A summary of these effects can be found in Table 61-6.[128–130]

At present, three nonnucleoside reverse transcriptase inhibitors are available in the United States: nevirapine (Viramune), delavirdine (Rescriptor), and efavirenz (Sustiva). These agents are metabolized by cytochrome P450, but they affect other drugs metabolized by cytochrome P450 3A4 to varying degrees. Nevirapine is an inducer of CYP 3A4 isoenzymes, delavirdine is an inhibitor of CYP 3A4 isoenzymes, and efavirenz is a mixed inducer/inhibitor. Therefore, their interactions cannot be summarized as a class. Table 61-7 lists the effects of coadministration of rifamycins and nonnucleoside reverse transcriptase inhibitors on the metabolism of each other. The nucleoside reverse transcriptase inhibitors, such as zidovudine and lamivudine, are not metabolized by the cytochrome P450 system, making drug interactions unlikely.[130]

MALABSORPTION

As mentioned earlier, inadequate therapy of TB is one of the main reasons for treatment failure and development of acquired drug resistance. This can occur in many ways, such as nonadherence to therapy or malabsorption of the medications. Researchers have found considerable evidence for malabsorption of antituberculosis medications in HIV-infected patients. In one study, 19 of 20 serum rifampin concentrations were found to be subtherapeutic. This phenomenon is particularly common with rifampin and ethambutol. It can also contribute to the slow response often seen in HIV-infected patients with TB.[109,131–133] Therefore, serum concentrations of rifampin (or rifabutin) and ethambutol should be monitored in F.R.[109,131–133]

Therapy of Latent Infection in HIV

28. Why should N.M., an HIV-infected person with a positive PPD skin test and no clinical symptoms, receive treatment for his latent TB infection?

The risk that N.M. will develop active TB disease is substantial. Pape and colleagues conducted a randomized, placebo-controlled trial of INH therapy in HIV-infected patients and found that patients receiving placebo were six times more likely to develop active TB than those receiving INH. The patients receiving INH were also less likely to progress to AIDS.[134] INH 300 mg daily for 9 months is, therefore, recommended for N.M.[65] Some clinicians suggest that these patients receive INH for life because eventual failure of the immune system will allow infection to progress to active

---

Table 61-6 Effects of Coadministration of Rifamycins (Rifabutin, Rifampin) and Protease Inhibitors on the Systemic Exposure of Each Drug

PI	Rifabutin		Rifampin	
	Effect of Rifabutin on PI	Effect of PI on Rifabutin	Effect of Rifampin on PI	Effect of PI on Rifampin
Saquinavir	45% decrease	NR	80% decrease	NR
Ritonavir	NR	293% increase	35% decrease	Unchanged[a]
Indinavir	34% decrease	173% increase	92% decrease	NR
Nelfinavir	32% decrease	200% increase	82% decrease	NR
Amprenavir	14% decrease	200% increase	81% decrease	NR

[a]Data from only two subjects.
Data in this table are expressed as a percentage change in the area under the concentration-time curve of the concomitant treatment relative to that of treatment with the drug alone. These are average changes, but the effect of these interactions in individual patients may be substantially different. Rifampin is a potent inducer of CYP3A but is not itself a CYP3A substrate. For example, concomitant delavirdine, a CYP3A inhibitor, does not change serum concentrations of rifampin. Therefore, although few data are currently available, it is likely that PIs will not substantially increase the serum concentrations of rifampin, and the same is true of rifapentine. No data exist regarding the magnitude of these bidirectional interactions when the rifamycin is administered twice or thrice weekly.
NR, not reported; PI, protease inhibitor.
Reprinted with permission from Burman WJ et al. Therapeutic implications of drug interactions in the treatment of human immunodeficiency virus-related tuberculosis. Clin Infect Dis 1999;28:419–430. ©1999 by the Infectious Diseases Society of America. All rights reserved.

Table 61-7 Effects of Coadministration of Rifamycins (Rifabutin, Rifampin) and Currently Approved Nonnucleoside Reverse Transcriptase Inhibitors

NNRTI	Rifabutin		Rifampin	
	Effect of Rifabutin on NNRTI	Effect of NNRTI on Rifabutin (Predicted)[a]	Effect of Rifampin on NNRTI	Effect of NNRTI on Rifampin (Predicted)[a]
Nevirapine	16% decrease	NR (decrease)	37% decrease	NR (unchanged)
Delavirdine	80% decrease	342% increase	96% decrease	Unchanged
Efavirenz	Unchanged	38% decrease	13% decrease	Unchanged

[a]Predicted using existing knowledge regarding metabolic pathways for the two drugs.
Data are given as effect on the area under the serum concentration-time curve of each drug.
NNRTI, nonnucleoside reverse transcriptase inhibitor; NR, not reported.
Reprinted with permission from Burman et al. Therapeutic implications of drug interactions in the treatment of human immunodeficiency virus-related tuberculosis. Clin Infect Dis 1999;28:419–430. ©1999 by the Infectious Diseases Society of America. All rights reserved.

disease.[119] Therapy for MDR-TB was addressed in Question 24. Therapy should also be considered in nonanergic, HIV-infected, PPD-negative patients who have been in recent contact with an infectious TB patient. The effectiveness of INH therapy in anergic, HIV-infected patients has not been established.[33]

Pregnancy

29. E.F., a 25-year-old woman who is being treated with INH 15 mg/kg and rifampin 600 mg twice a week for uncomplicated pulmonary TB, thinks she might be pregnant. Her obstetrician is concerned about the possible teratogenic effects of INH and rifampin and urges her to have a therapeutic abortion. What are the risks of TB and its treatment to the mother and the fetus? Are these drugs teratogenic? Should a therapeutic abortion be recommended?

Risks/Teratogenicity

Although there are always concerns regarding the use of any medication during pregnancy, it is now recognized that untreated TB represents a far greater risk to a pregnant woman and her fetus than treatment.[42,135,136] INH, rifampin, ethambutol, and streptomycin have all been reported to be teratogenic in animals, but no direct correlation with human malformation has been reported. Animal data may suggest a teratogenic potential, but because of genetic and environmental differences, these data cannot always be extrapolated to humans.[137] A comprehensive review of the literature by Snider and colleagues revealed that INH, rifampin, and ethambutol are all relatively safe to use in normal dosages during pregnancy.[136] Treatment can be started with these three drugs and should be continued for 9 months.[43]

Pyrazinamide has been used safely in pregnancy in other countries, but its teratogenic potential has not been adequately studied for the FDA to recommend its use.[42,43] It should, therefore, be reserved for cases of suspected drug resistance. All pregnant women receiving INH also should receive pyridoxine 25 mg/day because of the possibility of CNS toxicity. Rifampin has been used in only a small number of pregnant patients. The incidence of limb malformations was slightly increased but was not statistically different from the control population; several infants also were reported to have hypoprothrombinemia or an increased tendency to hemorrhage.

Streptomycin should not be used during pregnancy except as a last alternative because it has been associated with mild to severe ototoxicity in the infant. This ototoxicity can occur throughout the gestational period and is not confined to the first trimester. With the exception of streptomycin ototoxicity, the occurrence of birth defects in women being treated for TB with the above agents is no greater than that of healthy pregnant women[136,137–140] (Table 61-8). Therefore, administration of antituberculosis drugs is not an indication for termination of pregnancy.[43]

Lactation

When the baby is born, E.F. may breast-feed while continuing her medication. Drug concentrations are small and neither cause toxicity nor provide a sufficient concentration for the treatment or prevention of TB in the nursing infant.[42,43,136]

Pediatrics

30. A.M., a 3-year-old African-American boy, is suspected of having TB. His father has been receiving treatment for TB for the past 2 months. A.M. has a productive cough, fever, and general malaise. His sputum is positive for AFB, and his PPD skin test is positive (10 mm). What is the incidence of TB in children? How should A.M. be treated?

The incidence of TB in children <15 years of age declined from 1,718 cases (3.0 per 100,000 population) in 1993 to 931 cases (1.5 per 100,000 population) in 2001.[3] Because of the high risk of disseminated TB in infants and children, treatment should be started as soon as the diagnosis of TB is suspected. In general, the regimens recommended for adults are also the regimens of choice for infants, children, and adolescents, with the exception that ethambutol is not used routinely in children.[43] Although it is no more toxic, ethambutol is often avoided because it is difficult to assess visual acuity in children. A.M. should be started on INH 10 to 15 mg/kg per day, rifampin 10 to 20 mg/kg per day, and pyrazinamide 15 to 30 mg/kg per day.[42,43] Many experts prefer to treat children with three drugs (rather than four) in the initial phase because the bacillary population is usually low and it may be difficult for an infant or child to ingest four drugs. If resistance is suspected, ethambutol 15 to 20 mg/kg per day or streptomycin 20 to 40 mg/kg per day should be added to the regimen until susceptibility of the organism to INH, rifampin, and pyrazinamide is known.

Table 61-8 Pregnancy Outcomes Among Women Receiving Antituberculosis Therapy and in a Normal Population

Drug	Spontaneous Abortion	Stillbirth	Premature Birth	Malformed Infant
Isoniazid	0.34	0.61	1.88	1.09
Ethambutol	0.16	0.78	4.08	2.19
Rifampin	1.67	2.15	0.48	3.35
Streptomycin	0.97	0.0	0.0	16.91
Normal populations	6.8[a]	2.2[b]	7.1[b]	1.4–6.0[c] 2.3–13.8[b]

Rates are expressed as percentages of all conceptions that were not electively aborted.
[a]Based on fetal deaths at 12–20 weeks' gestation.[138]
[b]Based on Collaborative Perinatal Study data for whites.[139]
[c]Based on reports in 16 series of malformations noted at birth.[140]
Reprinted with permission. Snider DE et al. Treatment of tuberculosis during pregnancy. Am Rev Respir Dis 1980:122;65.

If resistance is not suspected in A.M. and this is confirmed by susceptibility testing, he should receive the INH, rifampin, and pyrazinamide daily for 8 weeks. He can then continue to take the INH and rifampin daily or two or three times a week (DOT) for an additional 4 months. The dosage for INH and rifampin in a two-or-three-times-weekly regimen would be 20 to 30 mg/kg per dose and 10 to 20 mg/kg per dose, respectively (see Table 61-3).

A.M. should be examined routinely for signs and symptoms of hepatitis. Although antituberculosis medications are generally well tolerated in children, LFTs two to three times normal are common. These elevations are often benign and transient; however, the incidence of hepatitis in children taking INH with rifampin has been reported to be four to six times greater than that in children receiving INH alone. Most of the hepatitis cases occurred within the first 3 months of therapy; hepatitis generally was associated with higher-than-recommended doses of INH or rifampin.[77,135,141]

Extrapulmonary Tuberculosis and Tuberculous Meningitis

31. R.U., a 64-year-old man, is brought to the emergency room following a 4-day period during which he became progressively disoriented, febrile to 40.5°C, and obtunded. He also had severe headaches during this time. Physical examination revealed some nuchal rigidity and a positive Brudzinski's sign (neck resistant to flexion). An initial diagnosis of possible meningitis was made, and a lumbar puncture was ordered. The cerebrospinal fluid (CSF) appeared turbid, and laboratory analysis revealed an elevated protein concentration of 200 mg/dL, a decreased glucose concentration of 30 mg/dL, and a white blood cell (WBC) count of 500/mm³ (85% lymphocytes). A Gram's stain of the spinal fluid and a sputum smear for AFB were negative; other laboratory tests were within normal limits. A diagnosis of tuberculous meningitis was presumed. Discuss the presentation and prognosis of tuberculous meningitis. How should R.U. be treated?

[SI units: WBC count, 500 × 10⁹/L (0.85 lymphocytes)]

Tuberculous meningitis is only one of the extrapulmonary complications of infection with *M. tuberculosis*. Successful treatment of extrapulmonary TB may usually be accomplished in 6 to 9 months with an acceptable relapse rate,[42,43,142] but some forms, such as bone/joint TB, miliary TB, or tuberculous meningitis in children and infants, may require 12 months of therapy.[42] Because specimens for culture and susceptibility testing may be difficult or impossible to obtain from a site, response to treatment must be based on clinical and radiographic improvement.

Tuberculous meningitis in older persons usually is caused by hematogenous dissemination of the tubercle bacilli from a primary site, usually the lungs. In its early stages, tuberculous meningitis often is confused with aseptic meningitis because the Gram's stain is negative. The most common signs and symptoms of tuberculous meningitis are headache, fever, restlessness, irritability, nausea, and vomiting. A positive Brudzinski's sign and neck stiffness may be present. As illustrated by R.U., the CSF is usually turbid, with increased protein and decreased glucose concentrations. There is an increase in the CSF WBC count with a predominance of lymphocytes. Culture of the CSF for *M. tuberculosis* may not be helpful since rates of positivity for clinically diagnosed cases range from 25% to 70%.[143]

Early recognition and treatment are essential for a favorable outcome. In a study by Kennedy and colleagues, four of five patients whose treatment was delayed for 7 or more days died.[144] Treatment usually must be based on a suspected diagnosis of tuberculous meningitis and must be started before culture and susceptibility test results are received. Multiple drug therapy should be used because irreversible brain damage or death may occur as soon as 2 weeks after the onset of infection, not the onset of clinical symptoms.[143]

Treatment

Treatment should be initiated in R.U. with daily administration of INH 300 mg, rifampin 600 mg, pyrazinamide 20 to 25 mg/kg, and ethambutol 15 to 20 mg/kg for the first 2 months.[43] After this initial phase of treatment, R.U. should receive daily INH and rifampin treatment for an additional 7 to 10 months, although the optimal duration of therapy is unknown.[43] In addition, because R.U. is older, pyridoxine 10 to 50 mg/day should be given to prevent peripheral neuropathy due to INH. Rifampin may impart a red to orange color to the spinal fluid.

INH readily penetrates into the CSF, with CSF concentrations reaching up to 100% of those in the serum. Rifampin is often included in tuberculous meningitis regimens and may be associated with reduced morbidity and mortality; however, even with inflammation, its CSF concentrations are only 6% to 30% of those found in the serum. Ethambutol should be used in the highest dosage to achieve bactericidal concentrations in the CSF because its CSF concentrations are only 10% to 54% of those in the serum. Streptomycin penetrates into the CSF poorly even with inflamed meninges.[145,146] Table 61-9 lists the most commonly used drugs and their CSF concentrations.

Table 61-9 Cerebrospinal Fluid Concentrations in Tuberculosis Meningitis

Drug	Dose	C_{max} (mg/dL)	MIC (mg/dL)	T_{max} (hr)	% Serum Concentration
Isoniazid	1.8–3.1 mg/kg	1.77–4.10	0.05–0.20	3.25–4.25	100
Rifampin	600 mg	0.24–2.40	0.5	3–6	6–30
Ethambutol	15–35 mg/kg	0.30–4.21	1–2		10–54
Pyrazinamide	3 g	50	20	5	100

C_{max}, maximum CSF concentration with inflamed meninges; MIC, minimum inhibitory concentration; T_{max}, time to achieve maximum CSF concentration.
Adapted with permission from reference 143.

CORTICOSTEROIDS

The adjunctive use of corticosteroids in the treatment of tuberculous meningitis has been controversial. A comprehensive literature review by Dooley and colleagues indicated that corticosteroids in moderate to severe tuberculous meningitis might reduce sequelae and prolong survival. CSF parameters may be improved, including reduction of intracranial pressure. Dexamethasone dosages of 8 to 12 mg/day (or prednisone equivalent) for 6 to 8 weeks are recommended. The dosage can then be tapered slowly after symptoms subside.[147] Because R.U. is obtunded, he may be considered to have a moderate case, and corticosteroids may therefore be indicated for him at this time.

Solid Organ Transplant Patients

32. **M.S., age 66, had a history of TB as a child. He recently underwent a renal transplant. Will he develop TB, and if so, what pharmacologic concerns should be addressed?**

The risk of developing TB is 36- to 74-fold greater among solid organ transplant recipients than in the general population. The overall mortality rate in this population is 29%. The increased risk of developing TB is largely caused by the immunosuppressive therapy given to prevent transplant rejection. Although some patients may acquire the TB nosocomially, most will develop it as reactivation of dormant TB. More than half of the patients will develop pulmonary disease. However, many will also develop disseminated or extrapulmonary disease, which is difficult to diagnose and therefore may cause a delay in diagnosis.[148] Patients should be treated with a standard TB regimen.[42,43] Attention should be paid to potential interactions with rifampin, which may increase the metabolism of cyclosporine, tacrolimus, and other medications. In addition, transplant recipients, in particular liver transplant recipients, may be at an increased risk of developing INH hepatitis. It is recommended that all transplant patients receive a tuberculin skin test and that chemoprophylaxis be offered to all high-risk patients.[148]

Acknowledgement

The author would like to acknowledge Shaun Berning for her contribution as author of this chapter in the 7th edition.

REFERENCES

1. Peloquin CA, Berning SE. Infection caused by *Mycobacterium tuberculosis*. Ann Pharmacother 1994;28:72.
2. Corbett EL, Watt CJ, Walker N, et al. The growing burden of tuberculosis. Global trends and interactions with the HIV epidemic. Arch Intern Med 2003;163:1009.
3. Centers for Disease Control and Prevention. Reported tuberculosis in the United States, 2001. Atlanta: U.S. Department of Health and Human Services, CDC, September 2002.
4. Centers for Disease Control and Prevention. A strategic plan for the elimination of tuberculosis in the United States. MMWR Morbid Mortal Wkly Rep 1989;38(Suppl S-3).
5. American Thoracic Society/Centers for Disease Control and Prevention. Diagnostic standards and classification of tuberculosis in adults and children. Am J Respir Crit Care Med 2000;161:1376.
6. Centers for Disease Control and Prevention. Guidelines for preventing the transmission of *Mycobacterium tuberculosis* in health-care facilities. MMWR 1994;43(RR-13).
7. Edwards D, Kirkpatrick CH. The immunology of mycobacterial diseases. Am Rev Respir Dis 1986;134:1062.
8. Dannenberg AM. Immune mechanisms in the pathogenesis of pulmonary tuberculosis. Rev Infect Dis 1989;11:S369.
9. American Thoracic Society/Centers for Disease Control. Diagnostic standards and classification of tuberculosis. Am Rev Respir Dis 1990;142:725.
10. Barnes PF et al. Tuberculosis in patients with human immunodeficiency virus infection. N Engl J Med 1991;324:1644.
11. Daley CL et al. An outbreak of tuberculosis with accelerated progression among persons infected with the human immunodeficiency virus. N Engl J Med 1992;326:231.
12. Selwyn PD et al. A prospective study of the risk of tuberculosis among intravenous drug users with human immunodeficiency virus infection. N Engl J Med 1989;320:545.
13. Markowitz N et al. Tuberculin and anergy testing in HIV-seropositive and HIV-seronegative persons. Ann Intern Med 1993;119:185.
14. MacGregor RR. A year's experience with tuberculosis in a private urban teaching hospital in the post-sanatorium era. Am J Med 1975;58:221.
15. Counsel SR et al. Unsuspected pulmonary tuberculosis in a community teaching hospital. Arch Intern Med 1989;149:1274.
16. Seibert AF, Bass JB. Tuberculin skin testing: guidelines for the 1990's. J Respir Dis 1990;11:225.
17. Daniel T et al. Improving methods for detecting infected persons at risk of developing disease. Am Rev Respir Dis 1986;134:409.
18. Howard A et al. Bevel-down superior to bevel-up in intradermal skin testing. Ann Allergy Asthma Immunol 1977;78:594.
19. Tsicopoulos A et al. Preferential messenger RNA expression of Th1-type cells (IFN-gamma+, IL-2+) in classical delayed-type (tuberculin) hypersensitivity reactions in human skin. J Immunol 1992;148:2058.
20. Colvin RB et al. Delayed-type hypersensitivity skin reactions in congenital afibrinogenemia: lack of fibrin deposition and induration. J Clin Invest 1979;63:1302.
21. Snider DE. Recognition and elimination of tuberculosis. Adv Intern Med 1993;38:169.
22. Centers for Disease Control and Prevention. Screening for tuberculosis and tuberculosis infection in high-risk populations and the use of preventive therapy for tuberculosis in the United States. Recommendations of the Advisory Council for the elimination of tuberculosis. MMWR 1990;39(No. RR-8):1.
23. Lanphear BP et al. A high false-positive rate of tuberculosis associated with Aplisol: an investigation among health care workers. J Infect Dis 1994;169:703.
24. Chaparas SD. Tuberculin test: variability with the Mantoux procedure. Am Rev Respir Dis 1985;132:175.
25. Horsburgh CR et al. Practice guidelines for the treatment of tuberculosis. Clin Infect Dis 2000;31:633.
26. Hobby GL et al. Enumeration of tubercle bacilli in sputum of patients with pulmonary tuberculosis. Antimicrob Agents Chemother 1973;4:94.
27. Schluger NW. Changing approaches to the diagnosis of tuberculosis. Am J Respir Crit Care Med 2001;164:2020.
28. Wright PW et al. Sensitivity of fluorochrome microscopy for detection of *Mycobacterium tuberculosis* versus nontuberculous mycobacteria. J Clin Microbiol 1998;36:1046.
29. Centers for Disease Control and Prevention. Nucleic acid amplification tests for tuberculosis. MMWR Morbid Mortal Wkly Rep 2000;49:593.
30. Yeager HJ et al. Quantitative studies of mycobacterial populations in sputum and saliva. Am Rev Respir Dis 1967;95:998.
31. Centers for Disease Control. Tuberculosis and human immunodeficiency virus infections: Recommendations of the Advisory Committee for the elimination of tuberculosis. MMWR Morbid Mortal Wkly Rep 1989;38:236.
32. Dooley SW et al. Nosocomial transmission of tuberculosis in a hospital unit for HIV-infected patients. JAMA 1991;267:2632.
33. Centers for Disease Control and Prevention. Anergy skin testing and preventive therapy for HIV-infected persons: revised recommendations. MMWR Morbid Mortal Wkly Rep 1997;46(RR-15):1.
34. Comstock GW et al. Tuberculin conversions: true or false. Am Rev Respir Dis 1978;118:215.
35. Thompson JN et al. The booster phenomenon in serial tuberculin testing. Am Rev Respir Dis 1979;119:587.
36. Snider DE et al. Tuberculin skin testing of hospital employees: infection, "boosting," and two-step testing. Am J Infect Control 1984;12:305.
37. Bass JB et al. Choosing an appropriate cutting point for conversion in annual tuberculin skin testing. Am Rev Respir Dis 1985;132:379.
38. Bretscher PA. A strategy to improve the efficacy of vaccination against tuberculosis and leprosy. Immunol Today 1992;13:342.
39. Centers for Disease Control and Prevention. The role of BCG vaccine in the prevention and control of tuberculosis in the United States. MMWR Morbid Mortal Wkly Rep 1996;45 (RR-4):1.
40. Rodrigues LC et al. Protective effect of BCG against tuberculous meningitis and miliary tuberculosis: a meta-analysis. Int J Epidemiol 1993;22:1154.
41. Colditz GA et al. Efficacy of BCG vaccine in the prevention of tuberculosis: meta-analysis of the published literature. JAMA 1994;271:698.
42. American Thoracic Society. Treatment of tuberculosis and tuberculosis infection in adults and children. Am J Respir Crit Care Med 1994;149:1359.
43. American Thoracic Society/Centers for Disease Control and Prevention/Infectious Diseases Society of America. Treatment of tuberculosis. Am J Respir Crit Care Med 2003;167:603.

44. Centers for Disease Control. Initial therapy for tuberculosis in the era of multidrug-resistance: Recommendations of the Advisory Counsel for the elimination of tuberculosis. MMWR Morbid Mortal Wkly Rep 1993;42(No. RR-7):1.

45. Cohn DL et al. A 62-dose, 6-month therapy for pulmonary and extrapulmonary tuberculosis: a twice-weekly, directly observed and cost-effective regimen. Ann Intern Med 1990;112:407.

46. Tam CM et al. Rifapentine and isoniazid in the continuation phase of treating pulmonary tuberculosis. Am J Respir Crit Care Med 1998;157:1726.

47. Benator D et al. Rifapentine and isoniazid once a week versus rifampicin and isoniazid twice a week for treatment of drug-susceptible pulmonary tuberculosis in HIV-negative patients: a randomised clinical trial. Lancet 2002;360(9332):528.

48. Bock NN et al. A prospective, randomized, double-blind study of the tolerability of rifapentine 600, 900, and 1,200 mg plus isoniazid in the continuation phase of tuberculosis treatment. Am J Respir Crit Care Med 2002;165:1526.

49. Chaulk CP, Kazandijan VA. Directly observed therapy for treatment completion of pulmonary tuberculosis. JAMA 1998;279:943.

50. Burman WJ et al. A cost-effectiveness analysis of directly observed therapy vs. self-administered therapy for treatment of tuberculosis. Chest 1997;112:6370.

51. Mahmoudi A et al. Pitfalls in the care of patients with tuberculosis. JAMA 1993;270:65.

52. Iseman MD et al. Directly observed treatment of tuberculosis: we can't afford not to try it. N Engl J Med 1993;328:576.

53. Swarenstein M et al. Randomised controlled trial of self-supervised and directly observed treatment of tuberculosis. Lancet 1998;352:1340.

54. Jindani A et al. The early bactericidal activity of drugs in patients with pulmonary tuberculosis. Am Rev Respir Dis 1980;121:939.

55. Chan SL et al. The early bactericidal activity of rifabutin measured by sputum viable counts in Hong Kong patients with pulmonary tuberculosis. Tuber Lung Dis 1992;73:33.

56. Sirgel FA et al. The early bactericidal activity of rifabutin in patients with pulmonary tuberculosis measured by sputum viable counts: a new method of drug assessment. J Antimicrob Chemother 1993;32:867.

57. Botha FJH et al. The early bactericidal activity of ethambutol, pyrazinamide, and the fixed combination of isoniazid, rifampicin, and pyrazinamide (Rifater) in patients with pulmonary tuberculosis. S Afr Med J 1996;86:155.

58. Dickinson JM et al. Experimental models to explain the high sterilizing activity of rifampin in the chemotherapy of tuberculosis. Am Rev Respir Dis 1981;123:376.

59. Stradling P et al. Twice-weekly streptomycin plus isoniazid for tuberculosis. Am Rev Respir Dis 1981;123:367.

60. Peloquin CA, Berning SE. Comment: intravenous streptomycin [letter]. Ann Pharmacother 1993;27:1546.

61. Combs DL et al. USPHS tuberculosis short-course chemotherapy trial 21: effectiveness, toxicity, and acceptability: the report of final results. Ann Intern Med 1990;112:397.

62. Heifets LB, Lindholm-Levy PJ. Bacteriostatic and bactericidal activity of ciprofloxacin and ofloxacin against Mycobacterium tuberculosis and Mycobacterium avium complex. Tubercle 1987;68:267.

63. Centers for Disease Control and Prevention. Screening for tuberculosis and tuberculosis infection in high-risk populations: recommendations of Advisory Council for the Elimination of Tuberculosis. MMWR Morb Mortal Wkly Rep 1995;44(RR-11):19.

64. Centers for Disease Control and Prevention. Prevention and treatment of tuberculosis among patients infected with human immunodeficiency virus: principles of therapy and revised recommendation. MMWR Morb Mortal Wkly Rep 1998;47(RR-20):1.

65. Centers for Disease Control and Prevention. Targeted tuberculin testing and treatment of latent tuberculosis infection. MMWR Morb Mortal Wkly Rep 2000;49(RR-6):1.

66. Falk A et al. Prophylaxis with isoniazid in inactive tuberculosis. Chest 1978;77:44.

67. Ferebee SH. Controlled chemoprophylaxis trials in tuberculosis: a general review. Adv Tuberc Res 1970;17:28.

68. Taylor WC et al. Should young adults with a positive tuberculin test take isoniazid? Ann Intern Med 1981;94:808.

69. Centers for Disease Control and Prevention. Fatal and severe hepatitis associated with rifampin and pyrazinamide for the treatment of latent tuberculosis infection, New York and Georgia, 2000. MMWR Morb Mortal Wkly Rep 2001;50:289.

70. Centers for Disease Control and Prevention. Update: Fatal and severe liver injuries associated with rifampin and pyrazinamide for latent tuberculosis infection, and revisions in American Thoracic Society/CDC recommendations, United States, 2001. MMWR Morb Mortal Wkly Rep 2001;50:733.

71. Snider DE. Isoniazid-associated hepatitis deaths: a review of available information [letter]. Am Rev Respir Dis 1992;146:1643.

72. Comstock GW et al. The competing risks of tuberculosis and hepatitis for adult tuberculin reactors. Am Rev Respir Dis 1975;11:573.

73. Ellard GA. Variations between individuals and populations in the acetylation of isoniazid and its significance for the treatment of pulmonary tuberculosis. Clin Pharmacol Ther 1976;19:610.

74. Ellard GA et al. The hepatic toxicity of isoniazid among rapid and slow acetylators of the drug. Am Rev Respir Dis 1978;118:628.

75. Kopanoff DE et al. Isoniazid-related hepatitis. Am Rev Respir Dis 1976;117:991.

76. Girling DJ. Adverse effects of antituberculosis drugs. Drugs 1982;23:56.

77. Steele MA et al. Toxic hepatitis with isoniazid and rifampin. Chest 1991;99:465.

78. Nolan CM et al. Hepatotoxicity associated with isoniazid preventive therapy: a 7-year survey from a public health tuberculosis clinic. JAMA 1999;281:1014.

79. Black M. Isoniazid and the liver. Am Rev Respir Dis 1974;110:1.

80. Stuart RL et al. Isoniazid toxicity in health care workers. Clin Infect Dis 1999;28:895.

81. Maddrey WC et al. Isoniazid hepatitis. Ann Intern Med 1973;79:1.

82. Wright JM et al. Isoniazid-induced carbamazepine toxicity and vice versa: a double drug interaction. N Engl J Med 1982;307:1325.

83. Strayhorn VA et al. Update on rifampin drug interactions, III. Arch Intern Med 1997;157:2453.

84. Sanders WE. Rifampin. Ann Intern Med 1976;85:82.

85. Zierski M et al. Side-effects of drug regimens used in short-course chemotherapy for pulmonary tuberculosis: a controlled clinical study. Tubercle 1980;61:41.

86. Girling DJ. Adverse reactions to rifampicin in antituberculosis regimens. J Antimicrob Chemother 1977;3:115.

87. Lee CH et al. Thrombocytopenia, a rare but potentially serious side effect of initial daily and interrupted use of rifampicin. Chest 1989;96:202.

88. Berning SE, Iseman MD. Rifamycin-induced lupus syndrome. Lancet 1997;319:1521.

89. Bennett WM et al. Drug therapy in renal failure: dosing guidelines for adults. Ann Intern Med 1980;93(Pt 1).62.

90. Andrew OT et al. Tuberculosis in patients with end-stage renal disease. Am J Med 1980;68:59.

91. Cross FS et al. Rifampin-isoniazid therapy of alcoholic and nonalcoholic tuberculosis patients in a U.S. Public Health Service cooperative therapy trial. Am Rev Respir Dis 1980;122:349.

92. Citron KM. Ocular toxicity from ethambutol. Thorax 1986;41:737.

93. Schlid HS, Fox BC. Rapid-onset reversible ocular toxicity from ethambutol therapy. Am J Med 1991;90:404.

94. Alvarez KL, Krop LC. Ethambutol-induced ocular toxicity revisited [letter]. Ann Pharmacother 1993;27:102.

95. Centers for Disease Control and Prevention. Tuberculosis morbidity, United States, 1992. MMWR Morbid Mortal Wkly Rep 1993;42:696.

96. Centers for Disease Control and Prevention. Prevention and control of tuberculosis in facilities providing long-term care to the elderly. Recommendation of the Advisory Committee for elimination of tuberculosis. MMWR Morbid Mortal Wkly Rep 1990; 39(No. RR-10):7.

97. Dutt AK, Stead WW. Tuberculosis. Clin Geriatr Med 1992;8:761.

98. Stead WW et al. Tuberculosis as an endemic and nosocomial infection among elderly in nursing homes. N Engl J Med 1985;312:1483.

99. Rajagopalan S, Yoshikawa TT. Tuberculosis in long-term-care facilities. Infect Control Hosp Epidemiol 2000;21:611.

100. Nagami P et al. Management of tuberculosis in elderly person. Compr Ther 1984;10:57.

101. Rudd AJ. Tuberculosis and the aged. J Am Geriatr Soc 1985;33:566.

102. Chan CH et al. The effect of age on the presentation of patients with tuberculosis. Tuberc Lung Dis 1995;76:290.

103. Rajagopalan S. Tuberculosis and aging: a global health problem. Clin Infect Dis 2001;33:1034.

104. van den Brande P et al. Aging and hepatotoxicity of isoniazid and rifampin in pulmonary tuberculosis. Am J Respir Crit Care Med 1995;152:1705.

105. Snider DE et al. Drug-resistant tuberculosis. Am Rev Respir Dis 1991;144:732.

106. Centers for Disease Control and Prevention. Management of persons exposed to multidrug-resistant tuberculosis. MMWR Morbid Mortal Wkly Rep 1992;41(RR-11):61.

107. Cohn DL et al. Drug-resistant tuberculosis: review of the worldwide situation and the WHO/IUATLD global surveillance project. Clin Infect Dis 1997;24(Suppl 1):S121.

108. Goble M et al. Treatment of 171 patients with pulmonary tuberculosis resistant to INH and rifampin. N Engl J Med 1993;328:527.

109. Berning SE et al. Malabsorption of antituberculosis medications by a patient with AIDS. N Engl J Med 1992;327:1817.

110. Centers for Disease Control and Prevention. National action plan to combat multidrug-resistant tuberculosis. MMWR Morbid Mortal Wkly Rep 1992;41(RR-11):5.

111. Iseman MD. Drug therapy: treatment of multidrug-resistant tuberculosis. N Engl J Med 1993;329:784.

112. Leysen DC et al. Mycobacterial and the new quinolones. Antimicrob Agents Chemother 1989;33:1.

113. Baohong J et al. In vitro and in vivo activities of levofloxacin against Mycobacterium tuberculosis. Antimicrob Agents Chemother 1995;39:1341.

114. Berning SE et al. Long-term safety of ofloxacin and ciprofloxacin in the treatment of mycobacterial infections. Am J Respir Crit Care Med 1995;151:2006.

115. Peloquin CA et al. Levofloxacin for drug-resistant Mycobacterium tuberculosis. Ann Pharmacother 1998;32:268.

116. Horn DL et al. Limited tolerance of ofloxacin and pyrazinamide prophylaxis against tuberculosis. Lancet 1994;343:171.

117. Fischl MA et al. Clinical presentation and outcome of patients with HIV infection and tuberculosis caused by multiple drug resistant bacilli. Ann Intern Med 1992;117:184.

118. Park MM et al. Outcome of MDR-TB patients, 1983–1993: prolonged survival with appropriate therapy. Am J Respir Crit Care Med 1996;153:317.

119. Mehta JB, Morris F. Impact of HIV infection on mycobacterial disease. Am Fam Physician 1992;45:2203.

120. Snider DE. Recognition and elimination of tuberculosis. Adv Intern Med 1993;38:169.

121. Girling DJ et al. Extrapulmonary tuberculosis. Br Med Bull 1988;44:738.

122. Daley CL. Current issues in the pathogenesis and management of HIV-related tuberculosis. AIDS Clin Rev 1997;98:289.

123. Schluger NW. Issues in the treatment of active tuberculosis in human immunodeficiency virus-infected patients. Clin Infect Dis 1999;28:130.

124. Centers for Disease Control and Prevention. Clinical update: impact of HIV protease inhibitors on the treatment of HIV-infected tuberculosis patients with rifampin. MMWR Morbid Mortal Wkly Rep 1996;45:921.

125. Centers for Disease Control and Prevention. Updated guidelines for the use of rifabutin and rifampin for the treatment and prevention of tuberculosis among HIV-infected patients taking protease inhibitors or nonnucleoside reverse transcriptase inhibitors. MMWR Morbid Mortal Wkly Rep 2000;49:185.

126. Burman WJ, Jones BE. Treatment of HIV-related tuberculosis in the era of effective antiretroviral therapy. Am J Respir Crit Care Med 2001; 164:7.

127. Centers for Disease Control and Prevention. Notice to readers: Acquired rifamycin resistance in persons with advanced HIV disease being treated for active tuberculosis with intermittent rifamycin-based regimens. MMWR Morbid Mortal Wkly Rep 2002;51:214.

128. Piscitelli SC et al. Drug interactions in patients infected with human immunodeficiency virus. Clin Infect Dis 1996;23:685.

129. Antoniskis D et al. Combined toxicity of zidovudine and antituberculosis chemotherapy. Am Rev Respir Dis 1992;145:430.

130. Burman WJ et al. Therapeutic implications of drug interactions in the treatment of human immunodeficiency virus-related tuberculosis. Clin Infect Dis 1999;28:419.

131. Peloquin CA et al. Malabsorption of antimycobacterial medications. N Engl J Med 1993; 329:1122.

132. Peloquin CA et al. Low antituberculosis drug concentrations in patients with AIDS. Ann Pharmacother 1996;30:919.

133. Peloquin CA. Using therapeutic drug monitoring to dose the antimycobacterial drugs. Clin Chest Med 1997;18:79.

134. Pape JW et al. Effect of isoniazid prophylaxis on incidence of active tuberculosis and progression of HIV infection. Lancet 1993;342(8866):268.

135. Starke JR, Correa AG. Management of mycobacterial infection and disease in children. Pediatr Infect Dis J 1995;14:455.

136. Snider DE et al. Treatment of tuberculosis during pregnancy. Am Rev Respir Dis 1980;122:76.

137. Vallejo JG et al. Tuberculosis and pregnancy. Clin Chest Med 1992;13:693

138. Werner EE et al. The Chidren of Kauai. Honolulu: University of Hawaii Press, 1971.

139. Niswander KR, Gordon M. Women and Their Pregnancies. Washington, DC: USGPO, 1972:40.

140. Haskasalo JK. Cumulative detection rates of congenital malformation in a 10-year study. Acta Pathol Microbiol Scand (A) 1973;242 (Suppl):12.

141. Centers for Disease Control and Prevention. Adverse drug reactions among children treated for tuberculosis. MMWR Morbid Mortal Wkly Rep 1980;29:589.

142. Dutt AK. Treatment of extrapulmonary tuberculosis. Semin Respir Infect 1989;4:225.

143. Garg RK. Tuberculosis of the central nervous system. Postgrad Med J 1999;75:133.

144. Kennedy DH et al. Tuberculous meningitis. JAMA 1979;241:264.

145. Davidson PT, Le HQ. Drug treatment of tuberculosis, 1992. Drugs 1992;43.651.

146. Holdiness MR. Cerebrospinal fluid pharmacokinetics of the antituberculosis drugs. Clin Pharmacokinet 1985;10:532.

147. Dooley DP et al. Adjunctive corticosteroid therapy for tuberculosis: a critical reappraisal of the literature. Clin Infect Dis 1997;25:872.

148. Singh N, Paterson DL. Mycobacterium tuberculosis infection in solid-organ transplant recipients: impact and implications for management. Clin Infect Dis 1998;27:1266.

CHAPTER 62

Infectious Diarrhea

Gail S. Itokazu, David T. Bearden, Larry H. Danziger

Worldwide, infectious diarrhea continues to be a significant cause of morbidity and mortality.[1-3] Infectious diarrheas are caused by the ingestion of food or water contaminated with pathogenic microorganisms or their toxins. The spectrum of infection caused by these enteropathogens includes asymptomatic carriage to a life-threatening diarrheal illness requiring urgent medical attention. The ingestion of pathogenic microorganisms may also cause clinical syndromes that manifest primarily as a systemic illness, such as infection caused by hepatitis A, brucellosis, and listeriosis; or with neurologic manifestations such as paresthesias following the ingestion of mushrooms and ciguatoxin.[1] This chapter focuses on the di-

agnosis and management of common microbial causes of acute infectious diarrhea.

DEFINITIONS

Diarrhea is often defined as three or more episodes of loose stool or any loose stool with blood during a 24-hour period.[2] Acute diarrhea is defined as diarrhea of <2 weeks' duration, while diarrhea lasting >14 days is defined as persistent diarrhea and diarrhea lasting >30 days is defined as chronic diarrhea. The severity of diarrhea may be classified as mild if it does not limit activity, moderate if it forces a change in activities, or severe if it does not allow continuation of usual activities.[4]

Infectious diarrheas are classified as either noninflammatory or inflammatory diarrheas, and such a classification is used to guide the overall treatment plan. Noninflammatory diarrhea is generally a less severe illness, presenting as watery stools without blood, fecal white blood cells (WBCs), or occult blood; patients are afebrile and without significant abdominal pain.[2] Noninflammatory diarrheas are typically caused by rotaviruses, Norwalk-like viruses, *Staphylococcus aureus*, *Bacillus cereus*, *Clostridium perfringens*, *Cryptosporidium parvum*, and *Giardia lamblia*.[3] Inflammatory diarrhea is generally a more severe illness, presenting as bloody diarrhea with large numbers of fecal leukocytes; patients are febrile and complain of severe abdominal pain.[3] Inflammatory diarrheas are generally caused by invasive pathogens, including *Campylobacter jejuni*, *Shigella* species, nontyphoidal *Salmonella*, *Clostridium difficile*, Shiga toxin–producing *Escherichia coli*, and *Entamoeba histolytica*.[3] However, the distinction between noninflammatory and inflammatory diarrhea is not always clear-cut: some enteropathogens cause illnesses that may be characteristic of either noninflammatory or inflammatory diarrhea.

PREVALENCE

In the 1990s, >3 million deaths worldwide were attributed to infectious diarrhea, with most deaths occurring in developing countries.[2] The morbidity and mortality from diarrheal illnesses are largely attributed to dehydration,[3] and the populations at highest risk for this complication are the very young, the elderly, and the immunocompromised.[3,4] In developing countries infectious diarrhea is commonly attributed to inadequate sewage and water treatment systems, resulting in the rapid spread of enteropathogens to food and water supplies. In developed countries persons at risk for infectious diarrhea include international travelers and individuals in institutional settings such as day care centers, hospitals, and extended care facilities, where maintenance of good hygiene is often difficult. The increased reliance on foreign food supplies is a means by which exposure to food-borne pathogens from other parts of the world may occur.[2] Finally, worldwide, the increasing numbers of immunocompromised hosts, including HIV-infected persons and organ transplant recipients, represent a population who are more susceptible to intestinal infections.[4]

ETIOLOGY

Microbial causes of infectious diarrhea include bacteria, viruses, protozoa, or fungi (Table 62-1). In the United States, the most commonly confirmed microbial causes of infectious diarrhea in children requiring hospitalization are viruses (19.3%), followed by bacteria (5.1%) and parasites (0.7%). Approximately 75% of hospitalizations for diarrheal illnesses in this population are of unknown origin.[15]

PATHOGENESIS

Bacterial Virulence Factors

Enteropathogens possess a number of virulence factors, including toxins, adhesions, and invasive properties, that contribute to the organism's pathogenicity.[2] Enterotoxins target

the small bowel, leading to net movement of fluid into the gut lumen and resulting in voluminous quantities of watery stools and potentially life-threatening dehydration. Watery diarrhea may also be caused by an alteration in the absorptive function of the villus tip, as seen with rotaviruses and Norwalk-like viruses.[5] Cytotoxins target the colon, causing direct mucosal damage leading to fever and bloody diarrhea.

The invasive properties of bacteria such as those identified in *Shigella* species and invasive strains of *E. coli* allow these bacteria to invade and destroy epithelial cells, causing bloody/mucoid stools.[5] Some enteropathogens induce a vigorous host response (e.g., release of proinflammatory cytokines from intestinal epithelial cells) that can lead to diarrhea.[5] Adhesins allow enteropathogens to attach to and colonize the gastrointestinal (GI) mucosa, facilitating invasion, dissemination, toxin delivery, or host cell lysis.[6]

Only a small number of organisms are needed to cause symptomatic illness, further contributing to the pathogenicity of enteropathogens. For *Shigella* and some parasitic cysts, only 10 to 100 organisms are necessary to cause illness, a number far less than the usual 10^5 to 10^8 organisms required for other enteropathogens.[5]

Host Defenses

The human GI tract possesses numerous defense mechanisms to protect against enteric infection. For example, because many bacteria cannot survive in an acidic environment, the normal gastric acidity of the stomach prevents viable pathogens from passing from the stomach into the small intestine. Intestinal peristalsis moves bacteria and their toxins along and out of the GI tract. GI mucus and mucosal tissue integrity provide physical barriers against infection. Intestinal immunity, including the local production of antibody, contributes to the host's ability to resist enteric infection. Finally, the normal bacterial flora compete for space and nutrients with potentially pathogenic organisms, or produce substances that may be inhibitory to enteropathogens.[5]

Predisposing Factors

Predisposing factors to GI infection include travel history, compromised immune status, outbreaks of food-borne or water-borne illnesses, personal hygiene, and use of pharmacologic agents. For example, a diarrheal illness in the setting of recent travel to a developing country suggests travelers' diarrhea caused by the pathogens endemic to that area. HIV-infected patients are prone to infectious diarrhea caused by *Salmonella*, *Cryptosporidium*, and numerous other enteropathogens.[4] Outbreaks of diarrheal illnesses should raise suspicions of illness caused by *S. aureus*, *B. cereus*, *C. perfringens*, *Shigella*, *Salmonella*, *Campylobacter*, or noncholera *Vibrio*.[4] In the day care setting, agents spread by the fecal–oral route such as *Shigella*, *G. lamblia*, and *Cryptosporidium* should be considered.[4] Diarrhea in the setting of hospitalization or recent exposure to antibiotics increases the likelihood of *C. difficile* colitis.[2] Drugs that increase stomach pH (H_2-receptor antagonists, proton pump inhibitors, or antacids) increase the risk of infection with *Salmonella* because these bacteria do not survive well in the normally acidic stomach. (Table 62-2).

Table 62-1 Predisposing Factors, Symptoms, and Therapy of Gastrointestinal Infections

Pathogen	Predisposing Factors	Symptoms	Diagnostic Evaluations	Drug of Choice[a]	Alternative[a]
Salmonella (nontyphoidal)	Ingestion of contaminated poultry, raw milk, custards, and cream fillings; foreign travel	Nausea, vomiting, diarrhea, cramps, fever, tenesmus Incubation: 8–48 hr	Fecal leukocytes, stool culture	Fluoroquinolone, third-generation cephalosporins[b]	Ampicillin, amoxicillin, TMP-SMX, chloramphenicol, azithromycin
Salmonella (typhoid fever)	Ingestion of contaminated food, foreign travel. Minimum infective dose: 10–100 organisms.	Fever, dysentery, cramps, tenesmus Incubation: 12–24 hr	Fecal leukocytes	Fluoroquinolone, third-generation cephalosporins	Chloramphenicol, TMP-SMX, ampicillin, amoxicillin
Shigella	Ingestion of contaminated food, foreign travel. Minimum infective dose: 10–100 organisms.	Fever, dysentery, cramps, tenesmus Incubation: 12–24 hr	Fecal leukocytes	Fluoroquinolone[b]	Azithromycin, TMP-SMX, ampicillin, ceftriaxone[b]
Campylobacter	Day care centers, contaminated eggs, raw milk, foreign travel	Mild to severe diarrhea; fever, systemic malaise Incubation: 24–72 hr	Fecal leukocytes, stool culture	Erythromycin, azithromycin, fluoroquinolone[b]	Tetracycline, aminoglycosides, third-generation cephalosporins, chloramphenicol
Clostridium difficile	Antibiotics, antineoplastics	Mild to severe diarrhea, cramps	C. difficile toxin, C. difficile culture, colonoscopy	Metronidazole[b]	Vancomycin[b]
Staphylococcal food poisoning	Contaminated meat, milk, exposed foods	Nausea, diarrhea onset <4 hr, resolves in 24–48 hr Incubation: 2–4 hr	Stool cultures	Supportive therapy only	
Travelers' diarrhea (Escherichia coli)	Contaminated food (vegetables and cheese), water, foreign travel	Nausea, vomiting mild to severe diarrhea, cramps Incubation: 16–48 hr	Stool culture	See Table 62-3	
Shiga toxin–producing Escherichia coli (E. coli O157:H7)	Beef, raw milk, water	Diarrhea, headache bloody stools Incubation: 48–96 hr	Stool cultures on MacConkey's sorbitol	Supportive therapy only	
Cryptosporidiosis	Immunosuppression, day care centers, contaminated water, animal handlers	Mild to severe diarrhea (chronic or self-limited); large fluid volume	Stool screening for oocytes, PCR, ELISA	See Chapter 70, Opportunistic Infections in HIV-Infected Patients	
Viral gastroenteritis	Community-wide outbreaks, contaminated food	Nausea, diarrhea (self-limited), cramps Incubation: 16–48 hr	Special viral studies	Supportive therapy only	

[a]See text for doses and duration of therapy. See text for details.
[b]Not all cases require antibiotic therapy. See text for details.
ELISA, enzyme-linked immunosorbent assay; HAART, highly active antiretroviral therapy; PCR, polymerase chain reaction; TMP-SMX, trimethoprim-sulfamethoxazole.
From reference 14.

Table 62-2 Pharmacologic Agents That May Promote Gastrointestinal Infection

Drug	Mechanism
Antacids, H₂-receptor antagonists, proton pump inhibitors	Increased gastric pH; viable pathogens passed to lower gut
Antibiotics	Eradication of normal (anaerobic) flora
Antidiarrheals	Decreased gut motility; bacterial growth
Immunosuppressives	Inhibition of gut immune defenses

CLINICAL PRESENTATION

The patient's symptoms and their onset, severity, and duration help in determining the cause of a GI infection. Watery diarrhea associated with nausea and vomiting occurring within hours of exposure to a contaminated food source suggests the ingestion of preformed toxins such as those produced by *S. aureus* or *B. cereus*.[4] In contrast, abdominal cramps and diarrhea within 8 to 16 hours (longer incubation period) after consumption of contaminated meats and gravies suggests infection with *C. perfringens*.[1] Bloody diarrhea and fever should raise suspicion of infection with invasive pathogens such as *Salmonella, Shigella,* and *Campylobacter*. Voluminous watery diarrhea without fever should raise suspicion of infection with noninvasive pathogens including enterotoxigenic *E. coli* and *Vibrio cholerae*.[6] Some invasive organisms, however (e.g., *Campylobacter, Aeromonas, Shigella, Vibrio parahaemolyticus*), may initially cause watery diarrhea, followed by bloody diarrhea.[2] In the United States, Shiga toxin–producing *E. coli* (STEC) is the most common cause of bloody diarrhea and should be suspected, especially if fever is absent.[7] Persistent diarrhea in travelers is associated with parasites such as *G. lamblia, Cryptosporidium,* or *Isospora belli* and bacteria such as enteropathogenic *E. coli,* enterotoxigenic *E. coli,* STEC, *Shigella, C. jejuni,* and *Aeromonas*.[8]

Complications related to infectious diarrhea include dehydration and electrolyte losses. Severe vomiting following staphylococcal food poisoning, or gastroenteritis caused by rotaviruses or Norwalk viruses may lead to metabolic alkalosis. Other complications include toxic megacolon and intestinal perforation following *Shigella,* STEC, and *C. difficile* infection; hemolytic uremic syndrome following STEC and *Shigella* infection; reactive arthritis following *Shigella, Salmonella,* and *Campylobacter* infection; and metastatic infection following *Salmonella* infection.[6]

MANAGEMENT OF PATIENTS WITH INFECTIOUS DIARRHEA

Infectious diarrhea is generally a self-limiting infection, and most patients never seek medical attention. In many cases, replacement of fluid and electrolytes is all that is required.[4] Medical evaluation is warranted for patients with profuse watery diarrhea with dehydration, dysentery, temperature ≥101.3°F, six or more unformed stools within a 24-hour period, or illness of >48 hours' duration. Others requiring medical evaluation of a diarrheal illness include patients >50 years of age with severe abdominal pain, patients ≥70 years of age, and immunocompromised patients (e.g., AIDS, organ transplant recipient, or cancer chemotherapy patient).[4]

The evaluation of any diarrheal illness should also consider the possibility of a noninfectious cause for the illness, such as medications, inflammatory bowel disease, radiation colitis, or malabsorption syndromes.[9]

Initial management of diarrheal illnesses focuses on the need for rehydration and correction of electrolyte disturbances. Patients are then evaluated to determine the need for further medical evaluation, including the benefit of antimotility and antisecretory drugs and antimicrobials. Most patients with noninflammatory diarrhea require only supportive therapy, while some patients with inflammatory diarrhea may benefit from antimicrobial therapy.[2]

Rehydration Therapy

Replacement of fluids is based on the degree of dehydration. Manifestations of mild to moderate volume depletion include decreased skin turgor, dry skin, dry axillae, dry mucous membranes,[10] thirst,[11] and dizziness due to postural hypotension.[10] More severe volume depletion is characterized by cold clammy extremities, agitation and confusion due to decreased cerebral blood flow, hypotension, tachycardia, cyanosis, and low urine output (usually <15 mL/hr).[10–12] When assessing the severity of volume depletion, the clinician should also consider the contribution of drugs capable of altering the physiologic responses to dehydration (e.g., β-blockers, sympatholytics) or underlying diseases, including autonomic neuropathy, that may lead to postural hypotension.[10]

Depending on the degree of volume depletion and ongoing losses, fluids and electrolytes may be replaced intravenously (IV) or orally. Otherwise healthy individuals with acute diarrhea who are not dehydrated can replace fluid losses with sport drinks, diluted fruit juices, and other flavored soft drinks; sodium losses can be replaced with salted crackers, broths, and soups.[4] Special attention should be given to fluid therapy in elderly and immunosuppressed patients. For these patients, oral replacement solutions containing 45 to 75 mEq/L of sodium (Pedialyte or Rehydralyte solutions) are recommended in the United States.[4] In developing countries, the oral replacement solution recommended by the World Health Organization (water, glucose 20 g/L, sodium 90 mEq/L, potassium 20 mEq/L, chloride 35 mEq/L, and citrate 30 mEq/L) is an essential component in the management of diarrheal illnesses.[12] This oral replacement solution is effective because sodium absorption is accelerated in the presence of glucose.[12] Once dehydration is corrected, high-sodium formulas should be diluted to prevent hypernatremia or edema.

For patients who are severely dehydrated and unable to drink on their own or those with intestinal ileus, fluids and electrolytes should be administered IV.[11] Readily available IV solutions include Ringer's lactate[11] and normal saline to which potassium and bicarbonate may be added as necessary to replace electrolytes.[13]

Laboratory Tests

Stool assays testing positive for leukocytes (≥3 leukocytes per high-power microscopic field in four or more fields),[3] markers of fecal leukocytes (lactoferrin), or occult blood suggest inflammatory diarrhea caused by invasive pathogens [3,4,14] Pathogens commonly cultured in these patients include *Shigella, Salmonella, Campylobacter, Aeromonas, Yersinia,* noncholera *Vibrio,* and *C. difficile.*[4] However, the absence of leukocytes in a stool specimen does not rule out inflammatory diarrhea.[14] The mean sensitivity of fecal leukocytes for the prototypical inflammatory diarrhea disease agent *Shigella* averages 73% (range, 49% to 100%).[14] The absence of fecal WBCs suggests a noninflammatory diarrhea.

A definitive diagnosis of infectious diarrhea is often made by culture of the pathogen or isolation of the toxin (e.g., *C. difficile*) from a stool sample. Careful selection of patients in whom stool cultures are performed should maximize the cost-effectiveness of performing this test.[14] Stool cultures are recommended in patients with one of the following: severe diarrhea; oral temperature ≥101.3°F; bloody stools; or stools containing leukocytes, lactoferrin, or occult blood. Cultures are also recommended in patients with persistent diarrhea who have not been given empiric antimicrobials.[4] Some enteropathogens are also identified from cultures of extraintestinal sites such as the blood, bone marrow, and other metastatic sites of infection. The diagnosis of parasitic causes of infectious diarrhea is made by microscopic examination of the stool specimen for ova and parasites. More sensitive tests to diagnose parasitic infections include direct immunofluorescence staining (DFA) to detect *G. lamblia* and *Cryptosporidium,* and enzyme immunoassay (EIA) to detect *G. lamblia* and *Cryptosporidium* antigen.[14]

Drug Therapy

Bismuth Subsalicylate

Experimentally, bismuth subsalicylate (Pepto-Bismol) has both antisecretory and antibacterial properties.[15] It is effective for the prevention and treatment of travelers' diarrhea and may be considered an alternative to antibiotics. Adverse effects of bismuth subsalicylate include constipation, black tongue, and darkened stools.[16] Salicylate toxicity may be a significant problem for patients with renal dysfunction or bleeding disorders, elderly patients, or patients taking aspirin products.

Loperamide and Diphenoxylate/Atropine

The antimotility agents loperamide and diphenoxylate/atropine provide symptomatic relief by slowing intestinal transit time, facilitating the absorption of intestinal contents.[4] Advantages of loperamide over diphenoxylate/atropine include its availability as an over-the-counter preparation, and a lower risk for side effects because it does not cross the blood–brain barrier.[17] Diphenoxylate/atropine may cause drowsiness, dizziness, dry mouth, and urinary retention. Antimotility drugs are not recommended in patients with febrile dysentery because of the potential to prolong the illness.[4,17] However, loperamide has been used without adverse consequences in adults who have dysentery primarily caused by *Shigella* but are not critically ill.[18] Antimotility drugs are not recommended in children because of the potential for harmful effects, including ileus.[17]

Probiotics

Probiotics are live microbial mixtures (bacteria and yeasts) administered to restore the normal intestinal flora, thereby reduc-

ing intestinal colonization with pathogenic organisms.[19] In addition, probiotics may produce pathogen-inhibiting substances, inhibit pathogen adhesion to the GI tract, inhibit the action of microbial toxins, and stimulate immune defense mechanisms.[17,20] Interest in probiotics stems in part from their potential to decrease the use of antibiotics. Disadvantages of probiotics include a lack of well-controlled trials supporting their efficacy, lack of quality controls on the manufacturing of these agents, and risk of systemic infection, particularly in the immunocompromised host.[20] There is some evidence supporting the use of probiotics for rotavirus diarrhea in children[17,20] and as an adjunct for the treatment of recurrent *C. difficile* colitis.[20]

Miscellaneous Agents

Adsorbents include pectins and activated clays (attapulgite).[17] Overall, adsorbents confer little if any benefit in adults with acute diarrheal illnesses.[17] Attapulgite absorbs water and makes stools more formed.[4] Experimentally, activated clay will adsorb toxins, bacteria, and rotavirus and strengthen the mucosal barrier.[17] Octreotide has been used as a last resort in AIDS-associated diarrhea.[4]

Antimicrobials

Since most cases of infectious diarrhea are self-limiting, routine use of antibiotics is not necessary.[2,9] For selected cases of infectious diarrhea, antimicrobials decrease the duration of illness, decrease the severity of illness, prevent invasive infection, and prevent person-to-person transmission of pathogens.[9] In general, antimicrobials are recommended for patients with severe illness, patients with conditions that compromise normal enteric defenses, or immunocompromised patients. Antibiotics are also necessary to treat extraintestinal complications of enteric infection, such as bacteremia and osteomyelitis. Empiric antimicrobial therapy without additional laboratory testing may be considered in the following settings: (1) suspected bacterial diarrhea based on clinical presentation (i.e., fever and stools positive for fecal leukocytes, lactoferrin, or occult blood); (2) persistent diarrhea for >2 weeks and if *Giardia* is suspected; and (3) travelers' diarrhea.[4]

Trimethoprim-sulfamethoxazole (TMP-SMX), the aminopenicillins, tetracyclines, and nalidixic acid have been used extensively for the treatment of enteric infections because of their ease of administration, relative safety, and low cost. However, the emergence of enteric pathogens resistant to one or all of these agents is limiting their usefulness in both domestically and internationally acquired infectious diarrhea.[9] Depending on the microbial etiology of diarrhea, alternatives to these agents include the fluoroquinolones, third-generation cephalosporins (e.g., ceftriaxone, cefotaxime, cefixime), and azithromycin.[21] More recently, a number of enteropathogens, including *Salmonella* species and *Campylobacter* species, are demonstrating less susceptibility to fluoroquinolones.[9] Increasing fluoroquinolone resistance is in part related to the widespread use of these antibiotics in agriculture and veterinary medicine.[9] Although fluoroquinolones are not approved for use in children because lesions on cartilage tissue have been reported in juvenile animals,[21] clinical trials using fluoroquinolones in children have been performed because of the emergence of multidrug-resistant enteropathogens in some geographic areas, and no problems have been reported related to these antibiotics.[22,23]

Prevention

Measures to prevent the spread of enteropathogens include good personal hygiene and proper handling, cooking, and storage of foods. Persons traveling to areas that have suboptimal sewage and water systems should follow the rule, "boil it, cook it, peel it, or forget it." In addition, vaccines to prevent typhoid fever are available.

TREATMENT OVERVIEW

1. B.K., a 78-year-old man, presented to his physician with a GI illness of 1 day's duration. His illness began with vomiting and was followed by abdominal pain, nausea, and nonbloody, watery diarrhea. He denies any fever. He has been drinking undiluted apple juice which in retrospect seemed to worsen his diarrhea. B.K.'s history is significant for dining with several friends at a seafood restaurant 2 nights ago. They all shared an appetizer of raw oysters, and he has since learned that the friends he dined with are experiencing a similar illness. B.K. has no significant medical history; he has not recently been hospitalized, he has not been in contact with small children, he has not traveled abroad, and he has not taken antibiotics. On physical examination B.K. is alert and oriented; his examination is significant for decreased skin turgor, dry mucous membranes, and dry axillae. What is your general approach to the management of this patient's diarrheal illness?

The most common complication of any diarrheal illness is dehydration; if severe, dehydration can lead to hypovolemia, shock, and death. Thus, replacement of fluid and electrolyte losses is the cornerstone of therapy. Once these issues have been addressed, patients are assessed for the need for further medical evaluation and specific drug therapy.

2. What specific plan for rehydration would you recommend for B.K.? Would evaluation of a stool sample for the presence of WBCs or blood provide useful information to assist in the management of his illness?

B.K.'s clinical presentation is that of a nontoxic-appearing elderly man with signs and symptoms of mild to moderate volume depletion (decreased skin turgor, dry mucous membranes, dry axillae). First, he should stop drinking the undiluted apple juice, which compared to oral replacement solutions has a high osmolarity that contributes to increased stool output.[12] Instead, an oral rehydration solution containing 45 to 90 mEq/L of sodium can be used to manage his fluid and electrolyte losses.[4]

Further medical evaluation to determine if B.K.'s illness is likely to be an inflammatory or noninflammatory diarrhea will assist in assessing the role of drug therapy. Patients with inflammatory diarrhea may benefit from specific antibiotic therapy, while those with noninflammatory diarrhea are generally managed with supportive fluids and electrolytes. A stool specimen should be sent to the laboratory to look for WBCs or blood.

VIRAL GASTROENTERITIS

Clinical Presentation

3. B.K.'s stool is negative for WBCs and blood. In the meantime, because of B.K.'s history of dining with friends who have a similar illness, the physician calls the Board of Health to ask about the possibility of other similar illnesses. The physician is told of an ongoing investigation of a likely outbreak of Norwalk-like virus gastroenteritis associated with food served at the restaurant where B.K and his friends had dinner. Why are B.K.'s clinical presentation and epidemiologic history consistent with gastroenteritis caused by Norwalk-like viruses?

Viruses are estimated to cause 30% to 40% of cases of infectious diarrhea in the United States.[24] Of the common viral causes of gastroenteritis, B.K.'s history suggests Norwalk-like viruses as the likely pathogens. Norwalk-like viruses are responsible for major outbreaks of food-borne viral illnesses in both adults and children.[25] These viruses are spread by the fecal–oral route through the consumption of contaminated water or foods (e.g., inadequately cooked clams and oysters harvested from contaminated waters), by person-to-person contact, or by exposure to recreational waters.[25] Outbreaks of gastroenteritis caused by Norwalk-like viruses have occurred in restaurants, schools, and day care centers.[25] Illness typically begins within 12 to 48 hours after exposure to the virus and generally lasts 1 to 3 days.[25] GI illness is generally mild. Signs and symptoms include nausea, vomiting, diarrhea, abdominal cramps, myalgias, headache, and chills.[25] Fever occurs in one third to one half of cases. Prevention of illness is aimed at proper food handling practices.[25]

Rotaviruses and astroviruses cause infectious diarrhea primarily in children. Rotaviruses are responsible for 30% to 60% of all cases of severe watery diarrhea in children.[24] After an incubation period of 1 to 3 days, patients present with fever, vomiting, nonbloody and watery diarrhea that in normal hosts lasts 5 to 7 days.[24] Since rotavirus is spread by the fecal–oral route, preventive measures include proper hand washing and disposal of contaminated items.

The morbidity and mortality of viral gastroenteritides are primarily due to fluid and electrolyte losses. Thus, supportive measures to correct these deficits and replace ongoing losses is the mainstay of treatment for viral gastroenteritis.[24] However, probiotics have been found to decrease the duration of diarrhea caused by the rotavirus.[167] In young children hospitalized with acute diarrhea primarily caused by rotavirus; a randomized, double-blind placebo-controlled trial demonstrated that a mixture of lactobacillus strains administered early (<60 hours) in the course of illness decreased the duration of the diarrheal illness from 130 hours to 80 hours ($P = 0.003$). The lactobacillus strains used in this study were selected for their potential probiotic characteristics.[167]

VIBRIO SPECIES

Vibrio species are curved gram-negative rods whose natural habitat is environmental waters. Toxigenic *V. cholerae* 01 and 0139 cause epidemic cholera in humans,[26] while the non-*cholerae Vibrio* species such as *V. parahaemolyticus* cause gastroenteritis and extraintestinal infections.[27]

Vibrio Cholerae

Clinical Presentation

4. M.M., a 50-year-old, previously healthy man, is brought to the emergency department (ED) by his family because of severe watery diarrhea, vomiting, and altered mental status. At the onset of diarrhea approximately 24 hours ago, he began drinking oral rehydrating solution left over from his recent trip to Latin America. Over the past several hours he has not been able to drink on his own, and his family noted "white flecks" in his stools. M.M.'s history is significant for return from Latin America 1 day ago; there he visited relatives, several of whom were recovering from mild cases of cholera. In the ED, M.M.'s temperature is 40°C, his blood pressure is 70/40 mm Hg, and heart rate is 130 beats/min. His weight is 61 kg, which is 8 kg below his normal weight. Physical examination reveals a critically ill man with sunken eyes, poor skin turgor, dry mucous membranes, and dry axillae. The physician's assessment is severe dehydration, most likely secondary to *V. cholerae*. What should be the first step in the management of this patient with severe dehydration?

M.M. shows signs of severe dehydration, as manifested by his altered mental status, sunken eyes, poor skin turgor, dry mucous membranes, dry axillae, low blood pressure, and increased heart rate. His loss of >10% of his normal body weight is also indicative of severe dehydration.[11] Potential complications of M.M.'s diarrheal illness include acidosis as a result of bicarbonate losses through stool along with lactic acidosis from shock, and renal failure due to hypovolemia.[11]

Fluid and electrolyte replacement is the mainstay of treatment for patients with cholera. The watery stools of patients with cholera stools have high concentrations of sodium, potassium, and bicarbonate.[11] In the United States, Ringer's lactate solution is the only readily available IV solution with the electrolyte composition required to treat cholera.[11] Vigorous IV hydration to restore his intravascular volume should be instituted. Monitoring of blood pressure and normalization of heart rate are mandatory. Once M.M. is able to drink, oral rehydration can be instituted even while rehydration with IV fluids is ongoing.[11] For the management of cholera, the use of oral replacement solutions containing <75 mEq/L of sodium is inappropriate because of the large amounts of sodium lost through cholera stools.[11]

5. Why is M.M.'s clinical presentation and epidemiologic history consistent with a severe diarrheal illness caused by toxin-producing *V. cholerae*?

The incubation period of *V. cholerae* is typically 1 to 3 days and ranges from a few hours to 5 days.[11] The spectrum of illness caused by *V. cholerae* includes asymptomatic carriage (most persons), mild to moderate watery diarrhea, and life-threatening dehydration.[3,11] M.M. is one of the few (2% to 5%) persons with severe dehydration that could lead to hypovolemic shock and death within hours. The watery and colorless stools with "white flecks" of mucus are referred to as rice-water stools. Patients may lose up to 1 L of fluid per hour during the first 24 hours and may lose up to 10% of their body weight.[11] The watery diarrhea is due to the cholera toxin, which promotes the secretion of fluids and electrolytes by the small intestine.[3] Hypoglycemia may occur in severe cholera, especially in children.[11]

V. cholerae 01 is transmitted by the fecal–oral route and spread via contaminated water and foods such as improperly preserved fish, raw oysters, and undercooked shellfish such as crabs.[11] In the United States, *V. cholerae* has been virtually eliminated because of modern sewage and water treatment systems. Nevertheless, as in M.M., cases of cholera are still seen in travelers, especially travelers to parts of Latin American, Africa, or Asia where cholera is epidemic, or travelers

who bring contaminated seafood back to the United States. Domestic cases of cholera arise from the consumption of contaminated, undercooked seafood from the Gulf Coast.[26]

Treatment

6. Would M.M. benefit from the administration of antibiotics?

Antibiotics are beneficial in patients with cholera because they shorten the extent and duration of diarrhea.[28] In adults, recommended antibiotic regimens include doxycycline 300 mg as a single dose, tetracycline 500 mg four times daily for 3 days, ciprofloxacin 250 mg orally daily for 3 days, ciprofloxacin 1,000 mg orally as a single dose, or erythromycin 250 mg orally four times daily for 3 days.[11,28] TMP-SMX or erythromycin can be used when tetracyclines are contraindicated,[28] although TMP-SMX is not effective for *V. cholerae* 0139.[28] Fluoroquinolone-resistant *V. cholerae 01* has been reported from India.[29]

Vibrio parahaemolyticus

Clinical Presentation

7. C.T., a 45-year-old man, presents to his family physician with a 1-day history of nonbloody, watery diarrhea. His history is significant for return 2 days ago from the coastal areas of Florida. The evening before leaving Florida, he and his wife dined at seafood restaurant; they ate the same meal, except that C.T. also ate an appetizer of raw oysters. His wife is not ill. He has no significant medical history. His physical examination reveals no signs or symptoms of dehydration. Why is C.T.'s clinical presentation and epidemiologic history consistent with non-*cholerae Vibrio* gastroenteritis?

In the United States, *V. parahaemolyticus* is commonly isolated in waters along the Gulf Coast and Florida. In a survey of *V. parahaemolyticus* infection in the United States, 59% were cases of gastroenteritis, 34% were cases of wound infection, and 5% were cases of septicemia.[27] *V. parahaemolyticus* gastroenteritis is caused by the consumption of undercooked fish or shellfish harvested from contaminated waters. Following a median incubation period of 17 hours (range, 4 to 90 hours),[30] clinical manifestations of gastroenteritis include diarrhea, abdominal cramps, nausea, vomiting, and fever. Bloody diarrhea occurs in 9% to 29% of cases.[27,30] In Japan, *V. parahaemolyticus* is a frequent cause of watery diarrhea because of the consumption of raw fish and shellfish.[3]

Treatment

8. Should a course of antibiotics be prescribed for C.T.?

In healthy adults, *V. parahaemolyticus* gastroenteritis is usually a mild, self-limiting illness lasting a median of 2.4 to 6 days.[31] Antibiotics have not been shown to shorten the course of uncomplicated infection[31] but may be helpful for patients with severe diarrhea.[27] Antibiotics are used to treat wound infections and septicemia.[27] When indicated, ceftazidime with doxycycline, or doxycycline with ciprofloxacin or an aminoglycoside is recommended.[30] Individuals with liver disease or alcoholism are at risk for severe *Vibrio* infections, including septicemia.[27] Persons should avoid eating raw or undercooked shellfish and exposing wounds to seawater, especially during the warmer months, when water temperatures are especially favorable for the multiplication of *Vibrio*.[30]

STAPHYLOCOCCUS AUREUS, BACILLUS CEREUS, AND CLOSTRIDIUM PERFRINGENS

Clinical Presentation

S. aureus, B. cereus, and *C. perfringens* are important causes of toxin-mediated food-borne illnesses. GI symptoms typically begin within 24 hours of ingestion of contaminated foods, which is in contrast to the longer incubation periods for illnesses caused by *Salmonella, Shigella,* and *Campylobacter. B. cereus* causes two different intestinal syndromes: short-incubation disease (emetic syndrome) and long-incubation disease (diarrheal syndrome).[24]

9. T.N., a 30-year-old woman, presents to her family physician with an acute onset of nausea and vomiting. Her history is significant for attending a Chinese buffet 3 hours ago with friends who are experiencing a similar illness. The buffet included a variety of beef, fish, and chicken dishes, fried rice, and desserts, including cream-filled pastries. T.N. is alert and oriented, and her physical examination is normal. Why are T.N.'s clinical presentation and epidemiologic history consistent with food poisoning caused by *S. aureus* or short-incubation disease *B. cereus*? Should empiric antibiotics be prescribed?

The rapid onset of T.N.'s GI symptoms after eating suggests a food-borne illness caused by the ingestion of preformed toxins. Food-borne illnesses are often grouped by their usual incubation period: <6 hours, 8 to 16 hours, and >16 hours. The rapid onset (within 6 hours) of nausea and vomiting after the ingestion of contaminated foods suggests that the illness is caused by preformed toxins produced by *S. aureus* or short-incubation disease *B. cereus* (emetic syndrome). Diarrhea and abdominal cramps may also occur. Although cooking kills the toxin-producing bacteria, it does not destroy toxin that has already been produced. Foods implicated in staphylococcal food poisoning include salads, cream-filled pastries, and meats;[24] foods implicated in *B. cereus* food poisoning include fried rice, dried foods, and dairy products. [24]

In contrast, the features of T.N.'s illness are not consistent with signs and symptoms of toxin-mediated illness caused by *C. perfringens* or long-incubation disease *B. cereus* (diarrheal syndrome). These bacteria are associated with the onset of diarrhea and abdominal cramps within 8 to 16 hours after the ingestion of contaminated foods, and vomiting is not a prominent symptom in these illnesses. *C. perfringens* or long-incubation disease *B. cereus* produces heat-labile toxins that are produced in vivo after ingestion of contaminated foods, thus explaining the longer incubation period compared to illness caused by the ingestion of performed toxins. Foods implicated in *C. perfringens* food poisoning include improperly stored beef, fish, poultry dishes, pasta salads, and dairy products; foods implicated in long-incubation *B. cereus* food poisoning include meats, vanilla sauce, cream-filled baked goods, and salads.[24]

Illnesses caused by these toxin-producing bacteria usually resolve within 24 hours. Antibiotic therapy is not indicated.[24]

DYSENTERY

Dysentery is a severe manifestation of inflammatory diarrhea characterized by bloody/mucoid stools, abdominal cramps, and tenesmus (painful straining when passing stools). *Shigella dysenteriae* type 1 is the most common cause of dysentery; other causes include *Salmonella, Campylobacter,* enteroinvasive *E. coli,* and *E. histolytica* (see Chapter 74, Parasitic Infections, for the treatment of *E. histolytica* infection).[5] In developing countries, shigellosis is common in children; in the United States and Europe, foreign travelers, institutionalized persons, and homosexual men are most often infected.[9]

Shigellosis

Clinical Presentation

10. M.T., a 60-year-old, ill-appearing man, was admitted to the hospital for bloody diarrhea and fever. Two days prior to admission he developed fever, abdominal cramps, and six or seven nonbloody, watery stools per day. His diarrhea has since worsened to 10 to 12 small-volume stools with blood and mucus, and he describes painful straining while passing his stools. His history is significant for return 3 days ago from a trip to Bangladesh. On the day of his departure, he participated in a local celebration where he had close contact with the local villagers and failed to adhere to the good hygiene measures he had practiced during his vacation. M.T. lives alone in Florida. He has no significant medical history, has no known drug allergies, and takes no medications. On admission his temperature is 101°F. Physical examination reveals an acutely ill man with abdominal tenderness and signs and symptoms of mild dehydration. Why are his clinical presentation and epidemiologic history consistent with the dysentery syndrome, most likely due to *Shigella* species? What potential complications may occur in patients with dysentery?

Symptoms of the *Shigella* dysentery syndrome begin within 24 to 48 hours following ingestion of these bacteria.[24] Early clinical findings of the dysentery syndrome include fever, abdominal cramps, and voluminous watery diarrhea.[6] Three to 5 days after the onset of illness, patients experience a decrease in fever and have GI symptoms suggesting involvement of the large bowel, including small-volume and bloody/mucoid stool, fecal urgency, and tenesmus.[6] Complications of bacillary dysentery include the hemolytic uremic syndrome (HUS) and toxic megacolon.[32] Bacteremia is uncommon because *Shigella* only rarely penetrate the intestinal mucosa.

M.T.'s epidemiologic history and onset of symptoms are consistent with his return 3 days ago from Bangladesh, where shigellosis is not uncommon. Since transmission of *Shigella* is usually via person-to-person contact, it is likely that M.T. acquired his infection during the celebration with local villagers. Of the four *Shigella* species, dysentery occurs most frequently with *S. dysenteriae* type 1, followed by *S. flexneri. S. sonnei* and *S. boydii* generally cause a self-limited, watery diarrhea.

Treatment

11. Should antimotility agents be started in patients with dysentery?

Antimotility agents are not recommended in patients with high fever and bloody diarrhea because they may worsen the illness. [4,18] However, in adults with bacillary dysentery primarily caused by *Shigella* species who are not critically ill, the combination of ciprofloxacin and loperamide did not prolong fever or extend the excretion of enteric bacterial pathogens. [18] Rather, the combination decreased the number of unformed stools and shortened the duration of diarrhea.

12. **Would M.T. benefit from antibiotics to treat his dysentery, presumed to be caused by *Shigella* species? If so, what choices are available?**

Antimicrobial therapy for *Shigella* bacillary dysentery is beneficial because treatment decreases the duration and severity of illness and shortens the period of fecal excretion of *Shigella,* thereby reducing the period of infectivity to others. [32]

Since the early 1940s, when sulfonamides were the drugs of choice for the treatment of bacillary dysentery, [33] antibiotic therapy for shigellosis has evolved as these bacteria developed resistance to the preferred drugs from each era. [9] Currently, worldwide resistance of *Shigella* species to sulfonamides, tetracycline, ampicillin, and TMP-SMX makes these agents unsuitable for empiric therapy, but they may have a role after the results of susceptibility testing are available. [9]

In the 1990s fluoroquinolones emerged as the drugs of choice for the treatment of shigellosis. [9] Norfloxacin 400 mg twice daily for 5 days [34] and ciprofloxacin 500 mg twice daily for 3 to 5 days [18,35] were as effective as the comparator regimens. For patients with mild to moderate disease, a single dose of ciprofloxacin 1 g [36] or norfloxacin 800 mg [37] is effective. However, limitations of single-dose therapy should be considered. In patients with *S. dysenteriae* type 1 infection, a single dose of ciprofloxacin is less effective than 5 days of ciprofloxacin, [36] which may be related to the reduced antimicrobial sensitivity of this particular *Shigella* species. Likewise, a single dose of norfloxacin (and 5 days of TMP-SMX) is less effective in patients with more severe illness. [37] Finally, in the setting of empiric therapy, coinfection with other enteropathogens capable of causing dysentery (e.g., *Campylobacter*) and for which the efficacy of a single dose of an antibiotic is not available needs to be considered. [38]

More recently, the role of fluoroquinolones for the treatment of shigellosis is being threatened with the emergence of *S. dysenteriae* type 1 with decreased susceptibility to fluoroquinolones. [9,39] Alternatives to fluoroquinolones include ceftriaxone [21,40] and azithromycin. [21,41] In adults with bloody/mucoid stools, clinical success was similar for patients treated with oral azithromycin (500 mg on day 1, then 250 mg daily for 4 days) or oral ciprofloxacin (500 mg Q 12 hr for 5 days) (89% versus 82%, respectively; $P > 0.2$). [41] For the subset of patients infected with *S. dysenteriae* type 1, the failure rates for ciprofloxacin and azithromycin were 29% and 17%, respectively. [41] Interestingly, differences in treatment responses may be observed between adults and children. [42]

If susceptible, TMP-SMX (160/800 mg twice daily for 3 to 5 days), [37,43] ampicillin (but not amoxicillin) [44] 500 mg Q 6 hr for 5 days, [35,45] a fluoroquinolone [21] (ciprofloxacin, levofloxacin, ofloxacin, or norfloxacin) for 3 to 5 days, [9] or ceftriaxone [21] can be used. Nalidixic acid is recommended for children. [43]

13. **What specific empiric antimicrobial regimen would be appropriate to treat M.T.'s presumed case of shigellosis?**

In the United States the most common *Shigella* species identified is *S. sonnei* (55% to 60%), followed by *S. flexneri*. [46,47] Susceptibility data from *Shigella* isolates collected throughout the United States during 1985 and 1986 indicated that 32% were resistant to ampicillin, 7% were resistant to TMP-SMX, and 0.4% were resistant to nalidixic acid. [46] Isolates from patients with a history of foreign travel were more likely to be resistant to TMP-SMX (20%) compared with isolates from patients with no history of foreign travel (4%). More recently, higher resistance rates were reported for *Shigella* species from Oregon, where 63% were ampicillin resistant and 59% were TMP-SMX resistant. [47] The origin of these resistant isolates may have been migrant workers traveling to Latin American and Mexico, where multidrug-resistant *Shigella* is widespread. Until definitive culture and susceptibility results are available, empiric therapy can be started with a fluoroquinolone or ceftriaxone. [21] Shigellosis is treated with 3 to 5 days of antibiotics; in patients with mild to moderate illness, a single dose of a fluoroquinolone may be adequate.

Person-to-Person Transmission

14. **F.F., a 30-year-old woman, presents to her physician with watery diarrhea of 3 days' duration. Over the past few days she has been caring for her 2-year-old son, who is recovering from a similar illness. During the past week, several children at the day care center her son attends have been diagnosed with shigellosis. On examination, F.F. is afebrile and her physical examination is completely normal. She judges her diarrhea to be about the same and possibly better compared to the previous day. Is F.F.'s belief that she has the same infection as her son justified?**

F.F.'s belief that she has the same infection as her son is justified because person-to-person transmission of *Shigella* is the most common means of spreading this infection. [6] Since only small numbers (as few as 200 viable cells) of bacteria may cause infection in healthy hosts, [43] it is likely that during the care of her son, she inadvertently became infected herself. Good hygiene is important to limit person-to-person transmission of *Shigella*. [43]

15. **Should F.F. receive a course of antibiotics to treat her diarrheal illness, which is likely to be caused by *Shigella* species?**

Left untreated, shigellosis is usually a self-limiting illness lasting approximately 7 days. [43] For this reason, and because *Shigella* species readily develop resistance following exposure to antimicrobials, some experts recommend that antibiotic therapy be prescribed only for patients with severe shigellosis. [33] On the other hand, because effective antibiotic therapy shortens the period of fecal excretion of these bacteria, thereby reducing the risk for person-to-person transmission, others recommend antibiotic therapy for all infected persons. [4,9,43]

SALMONELLA

Salmonellae are facultative anaerobic Gram-negative rods that are widely found in nature, including the GI tracts of domesticated and wild mammals, reptiles, and birds. [48] *Salmonella* infections are classified into the following syndromes:

gastroenteritis, bacteremia with or without GI involvement, localized infection, enteric fever, and chronic carrier state.[48] Nontyphoidal Salmonellae (e.g., *S. typhimurium, S. enteritidis*) are important causes of reportable food-borne disease,[49] whereas typhoidal Salmonellae (*S. typhi, S. paratyphi*) cause typhoid fever.[49]

Nontyphoidal Salmonellosis

Uncomplicated Gastroenteritis in the Immunocompetent Host
CLINICAL PRESENTATION

16. B.B., a 35-year-old, previously healthy man, presents to the ED with a 1-day history of abdominal pain, nausea, and vomiting, that was followed by nonbloody, loose stools of moderate volume. One day before the onset of his symptoms, he attended a turkey dinner at the local community center. He was subsequently notified by the Board of Health of an outbreak of *Salmonella* gastroenteritis from food served at the gathering. On physical examination, B.B. does not appear toxic and is afebrile. His physical examination is normal. Why are B.B.'s clinical presentation and history consistent with *Salmonella* gastroenteritis?

B.B. displays some of the typical clinical manifestations of *Salmonella* gastroenteritis, which include diarrhea, nausea, vomiting, abdominal cramps, headache, chills, and myalgias. Although loose stools without blood of moderate volume are a common finding, fulminant bloody diarrhea may also occur. Fever is present in about 50% of patients. The onset of B.B.'s symptoms is also consistent with *Salmonella* gastroenteritis, which usually begins 8 to 48 hours after ingestion of contaminated food or water.[24]

In the United States, more than 95% of *Salmonella* infections are food-borne. Salmonellae are transmitted to humans by the ingestion of contaminated water or foods such as poultry (chickens, turkeys, ducks), poultry products (eggs), and dairy products.[49] The most common *Salmonella* serotypes identified in the United States are *S. typhimurium* and *S. enteritidis*.[49]

TREATMENT

17. Should B.B. receive a course of antibiotics for uncomplicated nontyphoidal *Salmonella* gastroenteritis?

For otherwise healthy individuals like B.B. with uncomplicated nontyphoidal *Salmonella* gastroenteritis, antibiotics are not routinely recommended. In these individuals, *Salmonella* gastroenteritis is typically a self-limiting illness lasting 2 to 5 days. When antibiotics are used, they demonstrate only a modest reduction (<1 to 3 days) in the duration of illness[49] or provide no clinical benefit.[49,50] However, in one study, patients who were most severely ill benefited the most from antibiotic therapy.[51] Additional arguments against the routine use of antibiotics in patients with uncomplicated *Salmonella* gastroenteritis include higher relapse rates,[44,52] the promotion of widespread resistance to antibacterials,[51] adverse drug effects,[50] and, though controversial,[49] prolongation of the fecal excretion of pathogens.[51,52] During an outbreak of *Salmonella* gastroenteritis, ciprofloxacin was an effective adjunct to measures to contain the spread of infection;[53] while during another outbreak, ciprofloxacin failed to eradicate convalescent fecal excretion.[52]

Given B.B.'s mild illness (i.e., not toxic-appearing, no fever, and no blood in stools) and absence of a significant medical history, B.B. does not have risk factors (see Question 18) associated with the development of complications from *Salmonella* gastroenteritis. Otherwise-healthy patients such as B.B. with mild to moderate *Salmonella* gastroenteritis will likely have an uncomplicated, self-limiting illness requiring only supportive therapy, including replacement of fluids and electrolytes.[48]

Nontyphoidal Salmonella Gastroenteritis in Patients at Risk for Invasive Salmonella Infection
PREEMPTIVE THERAPY AGAINST INVASIVE INFECTION

18. W.M., a 75-year-old man, attended the same dinner as B.B. and presents to his physician with an illness similar to B.B.'s. W.M.'s past medical history is significant for a renal transplant 1 year ago. Would antimicrobial therapy be beneficial for W.M.?

Overall, <5% of patients with *Salmonella* gastroenteritis become bacteremic.[48] However, for some patients who have risk factors that compromise their body's ability to contain infections, *Salmonella* gastroenteritis may be complicated with bacteremia and other extraintestinal infections. Patients at risk for bacteremia include infants <3 months of age, patients >65 years of age, patients with HIV infection and AIDS, uremia, or malignancy, and patients who have undergone renal transplantation.[4] Patients at risk for localized infection include those with prosthetic joints.[24] Decreased stomach acidity as a result of age, gastric surgery, or drug therapy allows Salmonellae to advance to the small intestine, thereby increasing the risk for *Salmonella* infection.[48] Because of W.M.'s renal transplant and age, he is at risk for invasive *Salmonella* infection and therefore should receive preemptive antibiotics for his gastroenteritis.[49]

19. What antimicrobial options are available for the treatment of nontyphoidal *Salmonella* gastroenteritis in patients like W.M. with risk factors for invasive infection? What empiric antibiotic would be appropriate for W.M.?

If susceptible, antimicrobials used for nontyphoidal *Salmonella* gastroenteritis include ampicillin, amoxicillin, TMP-SMX, third-generation cephalosporins (cefotaxime or ceftriaxone), and fluoroquinolones.[21,24,48] However, in the setting of empiric therapy when susceptibilities are unknown, a third-generation cephalosporin (e.g., cefotaxime or ceftriaxone) or a fluoroquinolone[21] would be recommended[49] because of the worldwide emergence of multidrug-resistant *Salmonella,* including *S. typhimurium* definitive phage type 104 (DT104). These multidrug-resistant *Salmonella* are resistant to ampicillin, chloramphenicol, TMP-SMX, streptomycin, and tetracycline. Of recent concern is the emergence of *Salmonella* with reduced susceptibility to fluoroquinolones (MIC >0.25 µg/mL).[49] Infections caused by *Salmonella* with reduced susceptibility to fluoroquinolones may not respond to therapy with these antibiotics.[54] Resistance to nalidixic acid is a sensitive and specific means of screening for Salmonellae with reduced susceptibility to fluoroquinolones.[49] Ceftriaxone-resistant nontyphoidal *Salmonella* have also been identified.[49] For preemptive therapy against invasive *Salmonella* infection, antibiotics are administered for 48 to 72 hours or until the patient is afebrile.[24]

Treatment of Invasive Nontyphoidal Salmonella

20. Four hours later, B.T., a 70-year-old man who attended the same turkey dinner as B.B. and W.M., presents to the ED with complaints of severe abdominal pain, bloody diarrhea, new-onset right hip pain, and a temperature of 102°F. His medical history is significant for leukemia and a right hip prosthesis. Would B.T. benefit from antibiotic therapy?

B.T. is presenting with signs and symptoms of *Salmonella* gastroenteritis (abdominal pain, bloody diarrhea), bacteremia (high fever), and localized infection (right hip pain) likely involving his prosthetic hip. B.T.'s past medical history for leukemia places him in the high-risk group for invasive *Salmonella* infection. *Salmonella* bacteremia without other infectious complications can usually be treated with 10 to 14 days of therapy. A longer duration of treatment and surgery may be required for metastatic infections, including osteomyelitis and endovascular infection.[49] For B.T., empiric antimicrobial therapy may include selected third-generation cephalosporins (cefotaxime or ceftriaxone) or a fluoroquinolone.[21]

Enteric Fever

Enteric fever is an acute systemic illness most commonly caused by *S. typhi,* though other Salmonellae (*S. paratyphi*) may cause this illness. When enteric fever is caused by *S. typhi* it is referred to as typhoid fever, and when caused by other Salmonellae it is referred to as paratyphoid fever.

Clinical Presentation

21. B.C., a 49-year-old obese woman, is admitted to the hospital with fever, abdominal pain, headache, anorexia, and constipation for the past week. One day before admission, she noted a new red rash on her chest. Her recent travel history includes return from the Indian subcontinent 10 days ago, where she visited her family, including a 7-year-old nephew who was recovering from typhoid fever. B.C.'s medical history is significant for gallstones. She lives with her husband, who did not accompany her on this trip.

On admission, B.C. is a moderately ill woman who is alert and oriented; her temperature is 39°C and her heart rate is 60 beats/min. Physical examination is significant for a maculopapular rash on her chest, splenomegaly, and hepatomegaly. Her peripheral WBC is $3.0 \times 10^6/mm^3$. Two sets of blood cultures are sent to the microbiology laboratory. Why are her clinical and laboratory findings and history consistent with the diagnosis of enteric fever, likely secondary to *S. typhi*?

B.C. displays the classic signs and symptoms of enteric fever, including fever, headache, abdominal pain, splenomegaly, and rash. The faint salmon-colored maculopapular rash on her trunk is referred to as rose spots.[48] Bradycardia is considered a common finding in enteric fever but is not consistently observed. Manifestations of severe typhoid fever (which B.C. does not display) include delirium, obtundation, stupor, coma, and shock.[23] B.C.'s low WBC count is also consistent with the diagnosis of typhoid fever. Complications of typhoid fever include intestinal hemorrhage and perforation, encephalopathy, and pneumonia.[23] Relapse of infection occurs in 5% to 10% of patients, usually within 2 to 3 weeks after resolution of fever.[23]

The incubation period of B.C.'s illness is consistent with the usual 7 to 14 days for typhoid fever. During the incubation period, Salmonellae multiply within macrophages and monocytes, and systemic manifestations of typhoid fever appear when bacteria are released into the bloodstream. B.C.'s travel history also supports the diagnosis of typhoid fever. In the United States, 81% of typhoid fever cases are attributed to international travel during the previous 6 weeks; 57% of these are from travel to the Indian subcontinent.[55] It is likely that B.C acquired her infection through the ingestion of contaminated food or water while visiting her family.

Treatment

22. Would B.C. benefit from a course of antimicrobials to treat her presumed case of typhoid fever? If so, what options are available?

Antimicrobials are indicated for the treatment of typhoid fever because they shorten the duration[48] and severity of illness, decrease the incidence of complications, and decrease mortality to an average of <1%.[23] Until the late 1980s, the standard treatment for typhoid fever was 10 to 14 days of chloramphenicol, TMP-SMX, or ampicillin. The advent of the parenteral third-generation cephalosporins cefotaxime and ceftriaxone and fluoroquinolones led to studies demonstrating that shorter courses of these newer agents are as effective as the standard drugs used to treat typhoid fever. In adults or children with typhoid fever caused by *S. typhi* or *S. paratyphi* that are susceptible to ampicillin, chloramphenicol, and TMP-SMX, 3 to 7 days of ceftriaxone (3 to 4 g/day) is as effective as 2 weeks of chloramphenicol.[56] Clinical cure for either regimen is ≥91%.[56] Of the parenteral third-generation cephalosporins, ceftriaxone has been most studied and is preferred because of lower relapse rates[57] and more rapid defervescence.[58] A short course of a fluoroquinolone is more rapidly effective and is associated with lower rates of stool carriage than the standard first-line agents chloramphenicol and TMP-SMX; cure rates are ≥96%. Thus, for fully susceptible isolates, recommended antibiotic regimens include 5 to 7 days of a fluoroquinolone or 10 to 14 days of TMP-SMX, ampicillin, or chloramphenicol.[23]

During the late 1980s and early 1990s, the emergence of multidrug resistant *S. typhi* that are simultaneously resistant to chloramphenicol, ampicillin, and TMP-SMX caused outbreaks of typhoid fever in India, Pakistan, Bangladesh, Vietnam, the Middle East, and Africa.[23] With the emergence of multidrug-resistant *S. typhi,* fluoroquinolones became the preferred treatment for enteric fever in both adults and children. In adults with enteric fever, 63% of whom were infected with multidrug-resistant *S. typhi,* a 5-day course of oral ofloxacin (200 mg Q 12 hr for 5 days) was superior to a 5-day course of ceftriaxone (3 g/day).[59] Ceftriaxone failures were successfully treated with ofloxacin.[59] In children with uncomplicated typhoid fever, a 2- to 3-day course of ofloxacin (7.5 mg/kg twice daily) achieved cure rates of ≥89%. In this study, 86% of isolates were multidrug resistant (i.e., resistant to chloramphenicol, TMP-SMX, ampicillin, and tetracycline), and all were susceptible to ofloxacin.[60] In children with typhoid fever, oral azithromycin (10 mg/kg per day, maximum 500 mg/day) was as effective as ceftriaxone (75 mg/kg per day, maximum 2.5 g/day), with clinical response rates of 91% and 97%, respectively.[61] Likewise, in adults oral azithromycin (1 g on day 1, then 500 mg daily on days 2 to 6) was as effective as oral ciprofloxacin 500 mg twice daily for 7 days (100% cure rate for both treatment groups).[62] In this study, approximately one third of patients were infected with multidrug-resistant *Salmonella*. [62] Thus, treatment options for multidrug-resistant *S. typhi* include a fluoroquinolone, ceftriaxone, or azithromycin.[23]

More recently, the efficacy of fluoroquinolones for the treatment of enteric fever has been questioned. Clinical failure rates of patients with enteric fever following treatment with fluoroquinolones increased from 9% in 1997 to 35% in 1999.[63] Following 12 to 14 days of ciprofloxacin for the treatment of typhoid fever, the overall condition of 32 patients did not improve, and all cases were successfully treated with ceftriaxone.[64] In this report, the ciprofloxacin MICs of *S. typhi* isolates ranged from 0.0625 to 0.5 μg/mL, and ceftriaxone MICs were <0.0625 μg/mL. Finally, a retrospective review revealed that compared to typhoid fever caused by nalidixic acid–susceptible isolates, infection with nalidixic acid–resistant *S. typhi* (which is a marker for isolates with decreased fluoroquinolone susceptibility) was less responsive to short courses of ofloxacin, with treatment failure rates of <5% versus 50%, respectively. Thus, short courses of ofloxacin (i.e., <5 days) are not recommend for the treatment of infections caused by nalidixic acid–resistant *S. typhi*.[65]

Fully fluoroquinolone-resistant isolates have been detected in India, and rarely isolates with high-level resistance to ceftriaxone.[23] Optimal treatment for fluoroquinolone-resistant isolates has not been determined. Azithromycin, ceftriaxone, or maximum recommended doses of fluoroquinolones for 10 to 14 days can be used. [23] The efficacy of combinations of these antibiotics is being evaluated. [23]

Finally, the re-emergence of chloramphenicol-susceptible *S. typhi* may mean that chloramphenicol may once again be effective.[23]

23. **What empiric antibiotic regimen should be initiated for B.C.'s typhoid fever?**

Uncomplicated cases of typhoid fever may be treated with oral antibiotics, while severe cases are treated with parenteral therapy.[23] In the United States, a study on the susceptibilities of 350 *S. typhi* isolates collected during 1996 and 1997 reported that all isolates were susceptible to ceftriaxone and ciprofloxacin, and 7% were resistant to nalidixic acid.[55] Thus, until susceptibility data are known, a fluoroquinolone or ceftriaxone can be used to treat B.C.'s presumptive typhoid fever.[21,23,55]

Adjunctive Treatment

24. **Besides the administration of antibiotics, are there adjunctive therapies from which B.C. could benefit?**

For cases of severe typhoid fever (with altered mental status or shock), mortality is decreased to 10% when chloramphenicol is combined with dexamethasone (3 mg/kg IV followed by 1 mg/kg Q 6 hr IV for eight doses) compared to chloramphenicol alone (56% mortality).[66] However, the benefit of steroids when the more potent fluoroquinolones are used is unknown.[67]

Chronic Typhoid Carriers

Clinical Presentation

25. **Fourteen months after being discharged from the hospital, B.C.'s stool is still positive for *S. typhi*. During this time, her husband has had two episodes of typhoid fever. Why is B.C.'s clinical syndrome consistent with the chronic carrier state?**

Although most patients excrete viable *S. typhi* in their stools for 3 to 4 weeks following recovery from their illness, 1% to 4% excrete *Salmonella* from stool or urine for >1 year after infection and are referred to as chronic carriers. B.C.'s risk factor for becoming a chronic carrier is her history of biliary tract disease (gallstones), which allows the sequestration of organisms in her diseased biliary tract.[48] Although chronic carriage of *S. typhi* is not a problem for B.C., she serves as a reservoir for disseminating infection to others.

Treatment

26. **What therapeutic options are available to cure B.C.'s chronic carrier state?**

Treatment options for chronic *S. typhi* carriers like B.C. include a prolonged course of antibiotics, cholecystectomy, or suppressive antimicrobial therapy.[23] Fifty percent to 90% of chronic carriers may be cured following prolonged courses of antibiotics,[68–71] but some studies have demonstrated less efficacy when anatomic abnormalities (e.g., cholelithiasis) are present.[72] Relapse is usually detected within the first several months after completing antimicrobial therapy,[73] but it may occur as long as 24 months after completing therapy.[72] Antimicrobial regimens that have been effective include amoxicillin 2 g three times daily for 28 days,[70] ampicillin 1 g four times daily for 90 days,[69] ampicillin 1.5 g four times daily plus probenecid for 6 weeks,[68] TMP-SMX 160/800 mg twice a day for 3 months,[71] ciprofloxacin 500 to 750 mg twice a day for 3 to 4 weeks,[73–75] or norfloxacin 400 mg twice daily for 4 weeks.[76] Follow-up in these studies ranged from 10 to 12 months after completion of therapy.

Prevention

27. **B.C.'s sister is planning a trip to the Indian subcontinent and is concerned about developing typhoid fever. What can she do to reduce her risk for developing typhoid fever?**

In the United States, the parenteral vaccine can be administered to persons ≥2 years of age and is 51% to 77% effective in preventing typhoid fever. Limitations of the parenteral vaccine include adverse effects such as local pain and swelling, fever, headache, and malaise.[23] The Ty21a oral vaccine produces protective efficacy ranging from 42% to 96%,[23] is well tolerated, and can be administered to persons ≥6 years of age. A new *S. typhi* Vi conjugate vaccine under investigation provides >91.5% efficacy in children 2 to 5 years of age.[23] B.C.'s sister should consult her physician regarding the need for typhoid vaccination. However, because the vaccine may not be fully protective, good hygiene still is necessary to minimize her risk for acquiring typhoid fever.

ESCHERICHIA COLI O157:H7

Epidemiology

28. P.J., a 3-year-old girl, is brought to the ED because of "stomach pains" and nonbloody diarrhea that has progressed to bloody diarrhea over the past 48 hours. Five days before the onset of diarrhea, the family celebrated the Fourth of July at a fast-food restaurant; P.J.'s parents ate fish sandwiches, while P.J. ate a hamburger. P.J.'s mother noted that unlike previous hamburgers eaten at the restaurant, this hamburger was not thoroughly cooked because the juices from the hamburger were still pinkish. P.J. has no significant medical history. During the week, she attends a day care center.

On physical examination P.J. is afebrile, with signs of mild to moderate dehydration. A stool sample is negative for fecal leukocytes. The physician assesses her illness as bloody diarrhea, possibly caused by STEC. The plan is to admit P.J. to the hospital for hydration, observation, and further workup. What clinical and laboratory findings and epidemiologic history are consistent with the diagnosis of STEC as the cause of P.J.'s illness?

E. coli O157:H7 is a strain of *E. coli* that produces Shiga toxins as one of its mechanisms of causing GI illness. A second virulence factor of STEC strains is their ability to attach to and damage the intestinal mucosa.[77] These *E. coli* bacteria cause a spectrum of infection, including asymptomatic carriage, mild and nonbloody diarrhea, bloody diarrhea (hemorrhagic colitis), HUS, and thrombotic thrombocytopenia purpura.[78]

E. coli O157:H7 should be suspected in the setting of abdominal cramps with nonbloody diarrhea that progresses to bloody diarrhea over 1 to 2 days.[77] Unlike bloody diarrhea associated with *Shigella* species or *Campylobacter* species, fever is often absent or of low grade because this pathogen is not invasive.[107] However, patients with severe illness are more likely to have fever.[79]

STEC is most commonly spread by consumption of undercooked beef products that are contaminated with *E. coli* O157:H7, although other modes of acquiring this infection have been reported (see Question 32). The incubation period for this infection is usually 3 to 4 days, which is consistent with P.J.'s recent history of eating undercooked hamburger. In most instances, the illness resolves in 5 to 7 days.[77] Fecal leukocytes may or may not be found in stool samples.[80]

Laboratory Diagnosis

29. How can the diagnosis of *E. coli* O157:H7 infection be confirmed?

In the United States, *E. coli* O157:H7 is the most common STEC serotype identified as causing this infection.[80] Unlike other *E. coli,* O157:H7 does not rapidly ferment sorbitol, thus allowing the use of special culture media (Sorbitol-MacConkey) to help in the identification of this organism.[78] Because of sorbitol-fermenting organisms and non-O157 STEC, further testing for Shiga toxins or the genes encoding them is increasingly performed.[77,78,80]

Hemolytic Uremic Syndrome

30. Forty-eight hours after admission to the hospital, P.J. is pale and has developed several "bruises" on her extremities. The nurse recorded only a minimal output of darkened urine during the past 24 hours. New laboratory tests reveal blood urea nitrogen (BUN), 150 mg/dL (normal, 5 to 25); serum creatinine (SrCr), 6 mg/dL (normal, 0.3 to 0.7); serum potassium (K), 6.8 mEq/L (normal, 3.5 to 5.5); WBC count, 20,000 ×10⁹/L (normal, 5,000 to 15,000); hemoglobin (Hgb), 5 g/dL (normal, 11 to 13); platelets, 50,000 cells/mm³ (normal, 150,000 to 350,000); and urinalysis is positive for blood and protein. The stool specimen sent on admission is positive for *E. coli* O157:H7. What complication of *E. coli* O157:H7 infection does P.J. now display?

[SI units: BUN, 53.55 mmol/L of urea (normal, 1.79 to 8.93); SrCr, 530.4 μmol/L (normal, 26.52 to 62.88); K, 6.8 mmol/L (normal, 3.5 to 5.5); WBC count, 20 ×10⁹/L (normal, 5 to 15); Hgb, 50 g/L (normal, 110 to 130); platelets, 50 ×10⁹/L (normal, 150 to 350)]

The new clinical and laboratory findings support the diagnosis of HUS, a well-known complication of STEC infection. HUS is characterized by the triad of thrombocytopenia, microangiopathic hemolytic anemia, and acute renal failure with oliguria.[81] On physical examination, P.J.'s "bruises" on her extremities are consistent with thrombocytopenia, which is confirmed by the low platelet count. Her pale appearance is consistent with anemia and is confirmed by the low Hgb; the dark urine is due to the color imparted from bilirubin because of red cell lysis (hemolytic anemia). Finally, P.J.'s decreased urine output and increased serum creatinine and BUN concentrations are consistent with renal failure.

P.J. has several risk factors for HUS: her age (i.e., children aged <5 to 15 years, median age 4 to 8 years),[79,81,82] fever,[79,82] increased peripheral WBC count,[79,83] and the season of the year (i.e., summer).[81] Although not present in this case, another possible risk factor for developing HUS is treatment with antimotility or antidiarrheal agents,[84] although this has not been universally confirmed.[79,83] In addition to young age, age >65 years appears to be a risk factor for HUS.[79] The progression of *E. coli* O157:H7 gastroenteritis to HUS typically becomes apparent about 1 week after the onset of diarrhea.[79,81,82] Three percent to 7% of children[85] may develop HUS, with a mortality rate ranging from 3% to 5%. In adults, *E. coli* O157:H7 infection progresses to HUS in as many as 27% of patients, with a higher rate in patients >65 years old.[79] HUS-related mortality has reached 42% in patients >15 years old[79]; elderly nursing home patients have a mortality rate of up to 88%.[86]

Treatment

31. Would P.J. benefit from drug therapy, including antimicrobial, antimotility, or antidiarrheal agents?

Other than supportive measures to manage the complications associated with illness caused by *E. coli* O157:H7, there is no specific drug therapy for this infection.[77] In retrospective and prospective[87] studies, antibiotics have not influenced the severity of illness,[88] the duration of diarrhea, or the duration of other GI symptoms.[87] When TMP-SMX was started a mean of 7 days after the onset of diarrhea, the duration of *E. coli* O157:H7 excretion was not altered.[87]

The effect of antibiotic administration on the risk of *E. coli* O157:H7 complications (e.g., HUS) remains controversial. A prospective cohort study of 71 children with diarrhea caused by *E. coli* O157:H7 found that antibiotic treatment increased the risk of progression to HUS.[83] Previous publications have supported these findings,[85,87,88] whereas others have reported that antibiotics do not increase the risk of progression to HUS.[84,79] A meta-analysis of these and other studies revealed no association between antibiotic administration and development of HUS.[89] Antibiotic selection, timing of administration, STEC strain, and patient selection are variable in the selected studies and complicate the analysis. Thus, the role of antibiotics in the management of *E. coli* O157:H7 infection remains controversial. Currently, clinicians do not recommend antibiotic treatment for STEC. Clinicians must carefully weigh empiric antibiotic treatment prior to organism identification.

Antimotility drugs are not recommended for patients with *E. coli* O157:H7 infection because they have been variably associated with an increased risk of progression to HUS,[84,85] although other studies have failed to find an association.[79,83] Although the explanation for the increased risk is unknown, the reduction of bowel motility may decrease the clearance of organisms from the GI tract, thereby increasing the absorption of toxins. Administration of antimotility drugs within the first 3 days of illness has been associated with a longer duration of bloody diarrhea.[90]

Prevention

32. **P.J.'s family members want to know what they could have done to prevent this infection. Upon discharge from the hospital, is it safe for P.J. to return to her day care center?**

STEC is often spread to humans by consumption of contaminated beef products that are not thoroughly cooked.[78] Because thorough cooking kills this organism, meat should be well cooked (i.e., juices from meat should be clear, not pink). In addition, this infection can be acquired by consuming other contaminated foods, including water, unpasteurized milk, apple cider, lettuce, and sprouts.[77,78]

Finally, because contact with infected persons commonly results in transmission of this infection to others,[85,86,88] P.J. should have two consecutive stool cultures that are negative for *E. coli* O157:H7 before returning to day care.[91]

CAMPYLOBACTER JEJUNI

Worldwide, *C. jejuni* is one of the most common causes of gastroenteritis.[92] In the United States, *C. jejuni* accounts for >99% of *Campylobacter* species isolated[92]; other species include *C. fetus* and *C. coli*. Whereas infection with *C. jejuni* is more commonly associated with GI symptoms, patients with *C. fetus* infection are more likely to present with a systemic illness.[93]

Clinical Presentation

33. **M.U., a 20-year-old, previously healthy woman, presents to the Student Health Center at her college in Minnesota with a history of malaise, fever, diarrhea, abdominal pain, and bloody diarrhea for the past 24 hours. One day ago she dined at a restaurant where she ate a chicken sandwich that she recalls not finishing because the meat was not thoroughly cooked. For the past 2 months, she has been attending college. She has no significant medical history and no recent travel history. On physical examination, M.U. is not acutely ill. The physician tells her that over the past week, several students with GI symptoms similar to hers have been diagnosed with *C. jejuni* enteritis, and all had recently eaten at the same restaurant. Why are M.U.'s epidemiologic history and clinical presentation consistent with *Campylobacter* enteritis?**

Symptoms of *Campylobacter* enteritis are first noticed 24 to 72 hours following exposure to contaminated foods. Clinical manifestations of enteritis include diarrhea and fever (90%), abdominal cramps, and either loose and watery or bloody stools.[92] M.U. does not exhibit signs or symptoms of complications from her presumed *Campylobacter* infection, including bacteremia (<1% of cases, and most commonly in immunosuppressed persons, the very young, or the elderly), meningitis, cholecystitis, pancreatitis, peritonitis, GI hemorrhage, and reactive arthritis. Guillain-Barré syndrome is an important but uncommon (<1 case per 1,000 cases of *C. jejuni* infection) postinfectious complication of *C. jejuni* enteritis.[92]

Campylobacter is often found in animals such as chicken, cattle, dogs, and cats. In industrialized nations, the most important means of acquiring *Campylobacter* infection is from the consumption and handling of chicken.[92] Human infection occurs after ingestion of improperly cooked foods, unpasteurized foods, and contaminated water, or contact with pets (e.g., birds and cats). Person-to-person transmission is not a major mode of spreading *Campylobacter* infection. Prevention of *Campylobacter* infection involves careful food preparation and cooking practices.[92]

Treatment

34. **Would M.U. benefit from antimicrobial therapy for her *Campylobacter* enteritis?**

Since *C. jejuni* enteritis is typically an acute, self-limited illness that resolves within 1 week,[92] antibiotic therapy is usually not necessary.[93] Antibiotics are recommended for the treatment of *Campylobacter* enteritis in patients with symptoms lasting >1 week, high fevers, or bloody stools; pregnant women, and immunocompromised hosts.[92,94] Based on M.U.'s clinical presentation (fever with bloody stools), antimicrobial therapy is warranted.

When administered early in the course of the illness (i.e., before determining the cause of the diarrhea), antimicrobial therapy will shorten the duration and the severity of illness and the duration of fecal excretion of pathogens.[51,94,95] On the other hand, when initiated late (i.e., after determining the cause of the diarrhea), antibiotics do not alter the clinical course of *Campylobacter* gastroenteritis.[166]

35. **What empiric antimicrobial therapy could be initiated to treat M.U.'s presumed case of *C. jejuni* enteritis?**

Until recently, fluoroquinolones were considered the drugs of choice for *Campylobacter* infection.[92] However, in some European countries the rate of fluoroquinolone-resistant *Campylobacter* is as high as 50% to 55%[97]; in Thailand and Spain it is 72% to 84%; and in the United Kingdom it is 18%.[92] In the United States, of the *Campylobacter* species causing human illness in Minnesota, fluoroquinolone resistance increased from 1.3% in 1992 to 10.2% in 1998, while resistance to erythromycin remained low at 2%. Worldwide, the emergence of fluoroquinolone-resistant *Campylobacter* is in part attributed to the widespread use of fluoroquinolones in food animals (e.g., poultry) and in veterinary medicine.[92,96] For patients who are very ill, gentamicin, imipenem, cefotaxime, or chloramphenicol can be used.[93] *Campylobacter* species are inherently resistant to vancomycin, rifampin, and trimethoprim.[92]

Currently, the drug of choice for *C. jejuni* infection is erythromycin for 5 days[21,92] (500 mg orally twice daily for adults and 40 mg/kg per day in two divided doses for children).[93] Clarithromycin and azithromycin[97] are also effective but more expensive.[92] In travelers with *Campylobacter* enteritis, azithromycin is as effective as ciprofloxacin in shortening the duration of illness, although there is a trend toward a shorter duration of illness in patients treated with azithromycin versus ciprofloxacin (39.6 hours versus 51.5 hours, respectively). The slower clinical response in the patients treated with ciprofloxacin may be related to the finding that 50% of *Campylobacter* isolates were resistant to ciprofloxacin, while all isolates were susceptible to azithromycin.[97] For M.U., empiric therapy with erythromycin can be started.

TRAVELERS' DIARRHEA

Etiology and Clinical Presentation

36. **E.J. and B.R. are healthy 23-year-old women spending their Christmas vacation traveling through the interior of Mexico. Prior to leaving on vacation, they discussed with their physician ways to avoid acquiring travelers' diarrhea. The physician instructed them about when they could consider the self-administration of medications, should they develop diarrhea, and provided samples of medications for them to take on their trip. Contrary to their physician's recommendations, the day they arrived in Mexico they both began eating fresh fruits and vegetables from local vendors and drinking unbottled water. On the third day of their vacation, B.R. noted some mild abdominal cramps and during the past 24 hours passed three or four unformed stools without blood. In contrast, E.J. is feeling feverish and passed six or seven loose bloody stools. Neither woman feels dizzy or thirsty, and both are drinking normally. Why are the illnesses of B.R. and E.J. consistent with the diagnosis of travelers' diarrhea, and what risk factors do they have for acquiring this infection?**

Travelers' diarrhea is defined as three or more loose, unformed stools per day plus at least one symptom of enteric infection (e.g., abdominal cramps, nausea, vomiting, fever, dysentery, fecal urgency, tenesmus, or the passage of bloody/mucoid stools).[98] Cramps, bloody stools, and fever and/or vomiting occur in 60%, 15%, and 10% of patients, respectively.[99] Clinical manifestations of travelers' diarrhea typically begin within 24 to 48 hours after consuming fecally contaminated foods. Forty percent of travelers who develop diarrhea have a mild, self-limiting illness of 1 to 2 days' duration.[98]

These travelers' major risk factors for acquiring travelers' diarrhea are their destination (a developing country with poor sanitation facilities) and the consumption of food items that are often contaminated with enteropathogens (fresh fruits and vegetables from local vendors and unbottled water).[126] Infectious agents are the major cause of travelers' diarrhea; bacteria represent 80% of the cases in which a pathogen is identified.[98] Bacterial pathogens include enterotoxigenic *E. coli,*

enteroaggregative *E. coli, Shigella* species, *C. jejuni, Salmonella* species, and *Aeromonas* species.[100] Enterotoxigenic *E. coli* is a common enteropathogen in travelers to Latin America and Africa. *Campylobacter* is an important cause of infectious diarrhea in the coastal areas of Mexico and Southeast Asia during the winter or dry seasons. *E. histolytica, G. lamblia,* and enteroviruses are generally less important causes of travelers diarrhea.[100] As many as 20% to 50% of cases of diarrhea lack a specific pathogen.[100]

General Management

37. **What general approach should B.R. and E.J. take to manage their illnesses?**

The general approach to the management of travelers' diarrhea includes maintaining adequate hydration, avoiding continued ingestion of contaminated foods, and, depending on the severity of symptoms, determining the need for drug therapy and/or medical evaluation. Neither traveler shows signs and symptoms of dehydration, including thirst, dizziness, and altered mental status; and both are drinking normally. They should continue to drink fluids including tea, broth, carbonated beverages, and fruit juices. Electrolytes can be replaced by eating salted crackers or similar sources of sodium chloride.[16] In travelers able to drink fluids ad libitum, a modified World Health Organization oral rehydration solution was found to offer no benefit over the administration of loperamide alone.[101]

Travelers need to avoid consumption of foods at high risk for contamination with enteropathogens, including unbottled water, ice cubes, raw milk, unpeeled fruits and vegetables, uncooked foods, and raw seafood from unreliable restaurants and street vendors.[16] Instead, they should eat well-cooked foods that are served steaming hot and should drink boiled or commercially bottled beverages.[16]

38. **What drug therapies could B.R. and E.J. consider using to reduce the duration and severity of travelers' diarrhea?**

Bismuth Preparations and Loperamide
Bismuth preparations and loperamide can be used to relieve abdominal cramps and frequent stools.[17]

Antibiotics
Many antimicrobial agents have been shown to shorten the duration and severity of illness. However, because of the increasing antimicrobial resistance of enteropathogens that cause travelers' diarrhea, currently only fluoroquinolones and to a lesser extent TMP-SMX can be recommended for the empiric treatment of travelers' diarrhea.[98] Compared to placebo, fluoroquinolones[102–105] and TMP-SMX[102] decreased the average duration of illness from 50 to 93 hours to 20 to 34 hours.[98] Most[18,104,106,107] but not all studies[108] demonstrated even faster (<24 hours) relief of symptoms when antibiotics were combined with loperamide.[104,106] Tetracyclines are of limited value because of the high frequency of enteropathogens that are resistant to this class of antibiotics.[38,98,108] TMP-SMX can be used in children, although resistance is rising, and if *Campylobacter* is a likely pathogen, erythromycin should be added.[98]

The selection of drug therapy for travelers' diarrhea is in part based on the individual's severity of illness. Patients with mild illness (e.g., one or two stools per 24 hours with mild or absent symptoms) may opt to forego specific drug therapy or elect to use loperamide or bismuth preparations.[98] For patients with mild to moderate illness (e.g., more than two stools per 24 hours without distressing symptoms), loperamide or bismuth preparations with or without a single dose of a fluoroquinolone can be used. If distressing symptoms are present, loperamide plus a fluoroquinolone is recommended; symptoms should be reassessed after 24 hours and the antibiotic discontinued if diarrhea has stopped. For travelers with severe illness (e.g., fever or bloody stools, more than six stools per 24 hours), 1 to 3 days of a fluoroquinolone is recommended,[98] and antimotility drugs should be avoided.

39. Based on the severity of their illnesses, what specific drug therapy could B.R and E.J. consider taking?

B.R.'s presentation is that of a mild to moderate illness with some distressing symptoms. For her, either a bismuth preparation, or loperamide plus a single dose of a fluoroquinolone may be used (Table 62-3). Loperamide is more effective than bismuth subsalicylate in decreasing the number of unformed stools[15]; it also is more convenient to administer than the liquid bismuth subsalicylate. Concurrent administration of bismuth preparations and a fluoroquinolone should be avoided because of the chelation of fluoroquinolones by bivalent cations,[98] resulting in reduced bioavailability of fluoroquinolones.[109]

In contrast, E.J. has a more severe illness characterized by bloody stools and fever; medical evaluation may be warranted. Antimotility drugs should be avoided because of their potential to worsen her illness. A fluoroquinolone, taken either as a single dose or a 3-day course, should be started[4,98] (see Table 62-3).

Prophylaxis

40. Upon hearing of the travels of B.R. and E.J., classmates J.G. and T.M. begin planning their summer vacation through the interior of Mexico. They want to prevent any diarrheal illness that could interfere with their travel plans. Except for migraines, for which T.M. takes 1 to 2 g/day of aspirin, neither student has a significant past medical history. Besides avoiding the consumption of potentially contaminated food and drink, what drug

therapies can be used to minimize the likelihood of developing travelers' diarrhea?

Specific drug therapies effective in preventing travelers' diarrhea include bismuth subsalicylate or selected antibiotics. The use of prophylactic drugs should not exceed 3 weeks (see Table 62-3).

Bismuth Subsalicylate
Bismuth subsalicylate, two tablets (524 mg/dose) four times daily for a maximum of 3 weeks,[110] has a protective efficacy of 65%.[100]

Antibiotics
Although some antibiotics provide up to 80% to 100% protection against travelers' diarrhea, they should be reserved for situations in which the risk of acquiring travelers' diarrhea outweighs the risks associated with antibiotic prophylaxis, including adverse drug reactions, increased bacterial resistance, and expense. Antibiotic prophylaxis can be considered for travelers in whom the inconvenience of even a short diarrheal illness is unacceptable. Prophylactic antimicrobials can also be considered in travelers in whom a bout of diarrhea would not be well tolerated (e.g., patients with decreased gastric acidity or underlying diseases such as inflammatory bowel disease, AIDS, or diabetes mellitus requiring insulin).[100] The protective efficacy for TMP-SMX ranges from 79% to 94%; for fluoroquinolones it is 80% to 100%.[100]

41. What specific drug therapies would be reasonable for T.M. and J.G. to take as prophylaxis against travelers' diarrhea?

The fluoroquinolones provide a higher protective efficacy against travelers' diarrhea than bismuth preparations. In addition, for T.M. bismuth subsalicylate would not be a good choice because her concurrent use of aspirin increases her risk for salicylate toxicity.

The fluoroquinolones (e.g., ciprofloxacin, levofloxacin, norfloxacin, ofloxacin) are effective for the prophylaxis of travelers' diarrhea.[100] Trials comparing either placebo with norfloxacin 400 mg once a day or ciprofloxacin 500 mg once a day for 7 to 15 days reported significantly fewer diarrheal illnesses with antimicrobial therapy: 26% to 64% versus 2% to 7%.[111–113] Fluoroquinolones may cause photosensitivity reactions. Phototoxic reactions are lower (<2.4%) for some flu-

---

Table 62-3 Prophylaxis and Therapy of Travelers' Diarrhea in Adults

Drug	Prophylaxis[a]	Treatment[a]
Bismuth Subsalicylate	2 tablets chewed with meals and HS (8 tablets/day)	1 oz Q 30 min for a total dose of 8 oz/day
Loperamide		4-mg load, followed by 2 mg after each loose stool (max, 16 mg/day)
TMP-SMX	160–800 mg/day	320–1,600 mg once, or 160–800 mg BID for 3 days
Norfloxacin	400 mg/day	400 mg BID for 3 days
Ciprofloxacin	500 mg/day	500 mg BID for 3 days
Ofloxacin	300 mg/day	300 mg BID for 3 days
Levofloxacin	500 mg/day	500 mg QD for 3 days

[a]Many cases of travelers' diarrhea require neither prophylaxis nor therapy.
TMP-SMX, trimethoprim-sulfamethoxazole.
Adapted from references 17, 98, and 100.

oroquinolones (ciprofloxacin, ofloxacin, norfloxacin, and enoxacin) compared with other agents in this class (10% to 15% for lomefloxacin, fleroxacin).[114,122,124]

CLOSTRIDIUM DIFFICILE–ASSOCIATED DIARRHEA
Mild to Moderate Infection
Clinical Presentation and Diagnosis

42. B.W., a 35-year-old woman, is admitted to a 10-bed medical ward for the treatment of *Streptococcus pneumoniae* meningitis. Upon arrival, she is started on ceftriaxone (Rocephin) 2 g IV Q 12 hr and improves over the next few days. On day 7 of antibiotic therapy, she complained of feeling warm with cramping abdominal pain and diarrhea. She began passing mucoid, greenish, foul-smelling watery stools, and had a temperature of 101°F. Microscopic examination of a stool sample was positive for fecal leukocytes. The physician's assessment of B.W.'s clinical and laboratory findings is antibiotic-associated diarrhea (AAD), most likely caused by *C. difficile*. What is the most likely mechanism for this patient's AAD?

AAD is a common complication of antimicrobial therapy.[115] The mechanisms by which antibiotics cause diarrhea include allergic and toxic effects on intestinal mucosa, alteration of GI motility (e.g., erythromycin), and alteration of normal intestinal flora. Changes in the normal bowel flora may lead to changes in carbohydrate or bile acid metabolism by intestinal bacteria or to overgrowth of pathogenic bacteria, either of which may be followed by diarrhea.[116] Bacteria known to be associated with AAD include *C. perfringens, S. aureus, Klebsiella oxytoca, Candida* species, and *C. difficile*.[116] *C. difficile* infection is most clinically relevant and is the focus of this section.

C. difficile is a spore-forming, Gram positive anaerobic bacillus capable of causing a wide spectrum of syndromes, including asymptomatic carriage, diarrhea of varying severity, colitis with or without formation of pseudomembranes, toxic megacolon, colonic perforation, and death.[115]

The pathogenesis of *C. difficile* infection involves disruption of the normal colonic flora, most commonly by antibiotics; however, antineoplastic drugs[117] and tacrolimus[118] have been implicated as well (Table 62-4). Alteration of the colonic

microflora is followed by overgrowth of toxin-producing strains of *C. difficile*.[116] These toxins are responsible for causing colonic inflammation and the clinical manifestations of this infection.[115,118]

43. Why is B.W.'s history and presentation consistent with AAD caused by *C. difficile*?

B.W.'s major risk factor for acquiring *C. difficile*-associated diarrhea (CDAD) is the fact that she received an antibiotic within the last 2 weeks. *C. difficile* is a common cause of nosocomial diarrhea. The clinical and laboratory findings consistent with CDAD include mucoid, greenish, foul-smelling watery stools and crampy abdominal pain. Patients usually present with low-grade fevers, but temperature may be >104°F.[115] Peripheral leukocytosis is common, with CDAD a common cause of WBC >30,000 cells/mm³.[120,121] Fecal leukocytes are variably present in CDAD and are not clinically useful for diagnosis.[123]

Other clinical manifestations associated with CDAD include hypovolemia, dehydration, hypoalbuminemia, electrolyte abnormalities, shock, and a reactive arthritis.[115] The onset of symptoms of CDAD varies widely from a few days after the start of antibiotic therapy to 8 weeks after the agent is discontinued.[115] Other risk factors for acquiring CDAD are admission to a hospital in which *C. difficile* is endemic or in which there is an ongoing outbreak of *C. difficile* infection.

44. How can the diagnosis of CDAD be confirmed?

Several tests are available to make the diagnosis of *C. difficile* infection. The rapid tests latex agglutination and EIA are commonly used in clinical laboratories. The latex agglutination test detects antigens to *C. difficile*; EIA detects toxins A and/or B produced by *C. difficile*.[115] Limitations of the latex agglutination test are that it also detects antigens to other intestinal bacteria, and it does not differentiate toxin-producing strains from non–toxin-producing strains.[115] Of the *C. difficile* strains isolated from various populations, 5% to 25% do not produce toxins (nontoxigenic) and do not cause colitis or diarrhea.[119]

Cytotoxin tissue culture assay for toxin B (considered the gold standard) or culture for *C. difficile* can also be used to diagnose this infection. Compared with the rapid tests, they are more labor intensive and have a longer turnaround time. In addition, like the latex agglutination test, culture for *C. difficile* does not distinguish between toxigenic and nontoxigenic strains.[119]

Colonoscopy with biopsy is used to make the diagnosis of *C. difficile* colitis rapidly. The characteristic colonic changes are raised, yellowish nodules or plaque-like pseudomembranes, often with skip areas of normal mucosa.[115] Because the characteristic pseudomembranes may be scattered throughout the colon, the diagnosis of pseudomembranous colitis may be missed with colonoscopy.

45. How can B.W.'s CDAD be differentiated from enigmatic AAD?

Only 10% to 20% of cases of AAD are positive for toxigenic *C. difficile;* the remaining cases have an unknown etiology and are referred to as simple, benign, or "nuisance" diarrhea.[115,120] The clinical presentation of benign diarrhea is

Table 62-4	Medications Implicated in *Clostridium difficile*–Associated Diarrhea
Commonly Implicated	**Rarely Implicated**
Cephalosporins	Aminoglycosides
Clindamycin	Fluoroquinolones
Ampicillin	Rifampin
Less Commonly Implicated	Tetracycline
	Chloramphenicol
Erythromycin	Vancomycin
Clarithromycin	Metronidazole
Azithromycin	Antineoplastic agents
Other penicillins	
Trimethoprim-sulfamethoxazole	

From references 115 and 119.

similar to many cases of CDAD in that it is a self-limited illness that resolves with nonspecific supportive measures and discontinuation of antibiotics.[115] Despite these similarities, these clinical entities can be differentiated from one another by several objective measures. In benign diarrhea, *C. difficile* or its toxins and leukocytes are not identified in stool samples, and intestinal lesions are not found on colonoscopy.[115] Other clinical features that suggest CDAD rather than enigmatic diarrhea are constitutional symptoms, no antibiotic dose relationship to the illness, and hospital-wide epidemics of diarrhea.[120]

Treatment

46. B.W.'s stool sample is positive for *C. difficile* toxin. What is the general plan for managing B.W.'s CDAD?

After replacement of fluids and electrolytes, there are three options to manage B.W.'s diarrhea. The first is to discontinue the offending drug (if possible), which in B.W.'s case is probably the antibiotic ceftriaxone. In approximately 25% of cases, discontinuation of the offending agent with concomitant fluid and electrolyte replacement leads to resolution of symptoms within 48 to 72 hours.[125] Thus, patients with mild diarrhea may not require any treatment other than discontinuation of the offending agent.[115,119]

Because B.W. is being treated for bacterial meningitis, a life-threatening infection, discontinuing antibiotics is not an option. A second option is to change her antimicrobial therapy to an agent less likely to cause CDAD. B.W. is taking a cephalosporin, which, like ampicillin, amoxicillin, and clindamycin, is frequently implicated as a cause of *C. difficile* diarrhea (see Table 62-4). In contrast, antibiotics such as TMP-SMX, fluoroquinolones, and aminoglycosides are less commonly associated with *C. difficile* infection.[115,119] Unfortunately, none of these antimicrobials is a suitable alternative for treating *S. pneumoniae* meningitis.

The third and most reasonable option for B.W. is to receive therapy directed against *C. difficile* while continuing to take ceftriaxone for the treatment of her bacterial meningitis.

METRONIDAZOLE AND VANCOMYCIN

47. What antibiotics could be prescribed to treat B.W.'s CDAD?

The oral agents most commonly used to treat CDAD are metronidazole and vancomycin. In a randomized trial that enrolled patients with CDAD and colitis, there was no significant difference in the efficacy of these drugs after 10 days of treatment.[125] Overall, >95% of patients treated for a first episode of CDAD with oral metronidazole or vancomycin are

expected to respond to therapy.[125,126] Recent reports have shown increases in *C. difficile* resistance to metronidazole and vancomycin, but the clinical significance in treatment selection is unknown.[127] Antibiotic sensitivities are therefore not routinely performed on *C. difficile*.

Metronidazole is well absorbed after oral administration and is excreted through the biliary tract before reaching the colon. Common adverse reactions include nausea, vomiting, diarrhea, dizziness, confusion, and an unpleasant metallic taste.[115] A disulfiram-like reaction may occur when alcohol or alcohol-containing medications are taken concurrently with metronidazole.[128] Because metronidazole is a carcinogen and in some animal species a mutagen, it should be used in pregnancy only if clearly needed. Similarly, metronidazole's safety in children has not been proven, and many prefer not to use it in this population if other options exist.[115]

Oral vancomycin produces fecal concentrations that are several hundred times the concentration needed to inhibit toxin-producing strains of *C. difficile*.[126] A 7- to 10-day course of oral vancomycin (125 to 500 mg orally four times daily) is recommended for the treatment of CDAD, with all dosing regimens equally effective.[115,126,129,130] Because of equal efficacy and high concentrations in the colon with all doses, 125 mg is the most commonly prescribed dose. Although oral vancomycin is not well absorbed, measurable serum concentrations have been found in patients with both normal and compromised renal function.[131,132]

Oral vancomycin is recommended when patients (1) fail to respond to metronidazole; (2) are infected with *C. difficile* resistant to metronidazole; (3) cannot tolerate metronidazole (e.g., allergy, or concurrent use of ethanol-containing products); (4) are pregnant or <10 years of age; (5) are critically ill because of *C. difficile* infection; or (6) have evidence of diarrhea caused by *S. aureus*.[115]

48. What antibiotic regimen would you recommend for treatment of B.W.'s CDAD?

When antibiotic therapy is required for patients who are not critically ill as a result of their *C. difficile* infection, metronidazole (250 to 500 mg orally four times daily or 500 to 750 mg orally three times daily) for 7 to 10 days is recommended as first-line treatment.[115,133] Oral metronidazole and oral vancomycin are equally efficacious,[125] but vancomycin use should be limited to prevent emergence of vancomycin-resistant organisms.[133] In addition, oral vancomycin is significantly more expensive than a course of oral metronidazole. Some of this cost differential can be offset by using the IV vancomycin preparation to prepare an oral solution (Table 62-5).

Table 62-5 Costs of Oral Drug Therapy for *Clostridium difficile*–Associated Diarrhea

Drug	Regimen	Cost[a]
Metronidazole tablets (generic)	500 mg TID × 10 days	$21.86/10 days
Vancomycin capsules (Vancocin)	125 mg QID × 10 days	$257.28/10 days
Vancomycin solution (Vancocin)	125 mg QID × 10 days	$185.40/10 days
Vancomycin solution[b] (generic)	125 mg QID × 10 days	$109.70/10 days

[a]AWP Red Book 2002.
[b]Prepared from intravenous formulation.

Once therapy directed against *C. difficile* is initiated, diarrhea or cramping should subside within 2 to 4 days. If B.W.'s symptoms do not improve, vancomycin can be tried.[120]

49. **Following resolution of B.W.'s CDAD, is it necessary to send a follow-up stool sample to determine whether it is negative for *C. difficile* toxin?**

After resolution of diarrhea, obtaining a follow-up stool sample to determine whether it is negative for *C. difficile* toxin is not recommended as part of routine practice because most patients with positive tests will not develop a recurrence of their diarrhea.[115] In addition, approximately 5% of normal adults carry small numbers of *C. difficile* in their feces, whereas colonization rates are much higher (30% to 50%) in hospitalized patients and newborns.[115,119]

BACITRACIN

50. **What other oral therapies have been used to treat CDAD?**

In a randomized, double-blind trial, oral bacitracin (80,000 to 25,000 units/day) was as effective as oral vancomycin (500 to 2,000 mg/day) in resolving symptoms of CDAD. However, although the difference was not statistically significant, there was a trend toward a slower clinical response with bacitracin. Compared with vancomycin, the clinical response to bacitracin is slower and less certain, possibly because of resistance to bacitracin.[115] The recurrence rate is similar for both antibiotics.[134,135]

EXCHANGE RESINS

Anion-binding resins (e.g., cholestyramine, colestipol) are not as reliable or as rapidly effective as oral metronidazole or vancomycin.[115] If prescribed, they are recommended only for mild CDAD.[115,136] The rationale for using exchange resins for CDAD is their ability to bind to toxin B produced by *C. difficile*[136]; however, resins have a limited binding capacity for toxins that is probably inadequate for severe cases.[115] Other limitations of exchange resins include their inability to eradicate the pathogenic organisms responsible for toxin production and their ability to bind to vancomycin, which may reduce the efficacy of the antibiotic.[115] Severe constipation is a side effect of exchange resins.[115]

PROBIOTICS

Probiotic microorganisms are introduced into the normal flora to counteract disturbances and reduce the colonization with pathogenic species.[19] Although orally administered *Lactobacillus* species and the yeast *Saccharomyces boulardii* have been used to treat CDAD, no data support the use of probiotics alone to treat CDAD. However, adjunctive use has been suggested in prevention of CDAD and in recurrences (see Question 58). Reports of isolated adverse effects, including rare fungemia, with ingestion of viable *S. boulardii* have been reported.[137]

ANTIDIARRHEALS

51. **What is the role of antidiarrheal agents in patients with CDAD?**

Opiates and other antiperistaltic agents should be avoided in patients with CDAD. Although these types of drugs may relieve diarrheal symptoms, they may also delay toxin removal from the GI tract. Patients with antibiotic-associated pseudomembranous colitis have deteriorated during therapy with antimotility medications.[138]

Transmission

52. **H.T., a 76-year-old man with multiple medical conditions, is admitted to the same 10-bed ward as B.W. His medical history is significant for a stroke that has left him bedridden in a nursing home. His only medications are those used to manage his hypertension. On day 4 of his hospitalization, H.T. complained of severe abdominal pain and watery, loose stools with blood. Physical examination revealed a toxic-appearing man with a temperature of 38.5°C. A stool specimen is positive for *C. difficile* toxin, and colonoscopy reveals pseudomembranes and colitis. A surgical consultant recommends an emergent colectomy because of impending bowel perforation secondary to the *C. difficile* infection. What are H.T.'s risk factors for acquiring *C. difficile*–associated pseudomembranous colitis during his hospitalization?**

H.T.'s risk factors for acquiring *C. difficile* infection include his advanced age, bedridden status,[139] underlying diseases,[140] and admission to the hospital. *C. difficile* infection is spread when hospital personnel or equipment contaminated with *C. difficile* spores come into contact with susceptible patients.[119] Physical proximity to an infected patient has been associated with an increased risk of CDAD.[141] Therefore, measures to prevent the spread of *C. difficile* infection include proper handwashing before and after contact with infected patients, and the use of gloves and enteric isolation precautions when in contact with infected patients with diarrhea. Contaminated equipment should be properly disinfected.[115]

Although *C. difficile* is often thought of as a nosocomial pathogen, it is being increasingly isolated in outpatient settings.[142,143] A European study found that up to 28% of all cases occurred without previous hospitalization.[142]

53. **Over the next few days, all 10 patients on the ward with B.W. and H.T. are found to have *C. difficile* toxin in their stools. Five patients have diarrhea and the other five are asymptomatic. What is the role of antibiotic therapy directed at *C. difficile* in controlling this outbreak?**

Neither oral metronidazole nor vancomycin is reliably effective in eradicating the carrier state (i.e., asymptomatic, fecal excretion), and neither is recommended for use in this situation.[144] The lack of efficacy of these drugs is probably related to the fact that unlike the vegetative forms of *C. difficile*, the spores of *C. difficile* are resistant to the action of antibiotics.[115] Furthermore, compared with placebo, vancomycin administration is associated with a significantly higher rate of *C. difficile* carriage 2 months after treatment.[144] Restricting the use of clindamycin can be an effective component in efforts to control nosocomial epidemics of CDAD.[139]

54. **What effect will the current CDAD outbreak have on the outcomes of the infected patients and on health care costs?**

In a prospective study, hospitalized patients who developed CDAD had a 3.6-day increase in length of stay.[145] This increase was accompanied by a doubling of hospital costs. While 3-month mortality rates were higher in CDAD patients (48% versus 22%), no significant differences were observed when adjustments were made for severity of underlying illness. The current outbreak is likely to increase hospital costs and increase individual lengths of stay.

Severe *C. difficile* Infection

Oral Treatment

55. What treatment is recommended for patients like H.T. who are critically ill from a *C. difficile* infection? What criteria are used to characterize patients as "critically ill"?

Of patients with antibiotic-associated pseudomembranous colitis who require surgical intervention (colectomy), up to 57% die.[146] Although the precise definition of "critically ill" is not clear, it has included patients with pseudomembrane formation, fever >40°C, marked abdominal tenderness, and marked leukocytosis.[133] H.T. meets these criteria for being critically ill.

Nonoral Treatment

56. Three days after oral vancomycin is initiated, H.T. develops an ileus and cannot take anything by mouth. What therapeutic options are available to treat H.T.'s pseudomembranous colitis?

Adequate antibiotic levels in the colon are necessary to treat *C. difficile*–associated pseudomembranous colitis. If the oral route is not feasible (e.g., patients with an ileus or bowel obstruction), the clinician must choose an agent that is either secreted or excreted into the GI tract in its active form. IV vancomycin is not the most desirable agent in this situation because it is not secreted into the GI tract. In contrast, metronidazole is eliminated by both renal and hepatic routes; bactericidal concentrations are achieved in both serum and bile.[147]

The literature contains few reports of successful attempts to treat CDAD or pseudomembranous colitis with IV metronidazole (500 mg Q 6 to 8 hr).[148–150] Likewise, unsuccessful attempts to treat CDAD with IV metronidazole have been reported.[150,151] When oral therapy is not feasible in patients with CDAD, some experts recommend IV metronidazole 500 to 750 mg three or four times daily with concurrent use of enteral vancomycin.[115] The clinical response of *C. difficile* infection to IV vancomycin in a patient who did not survive was difficult to ascertain.[126]

In adults, enteral vancomycin 500 mg four times daily can be given through an ileostomy or colostomy (if present). Several reports of successful outcomes using intercolonic vancomycin (as an adjunct to oral or IV antibiotics) in patients with CDAD have been documented. Rectal doses of vancomycin have varied from 500 mg Q 4 to 8 hr to 1,000 mg/L Q 8 hr.[152] Because patients with CDAD are at risk for colonic perforation, enteral vancomycin should be administered cautiously.

Relapse

57. One week after discharge from the hospital, B.W. once again developed abdominal pain and diarrhea. Her clinic physician assumed these symptoms could not be related to a relapse of her CDAD because she had responded so well to metronidazole. What is the likelihood that CDAD has recurred?

Regardless of the antibiotic regimen prescribed for CDAD, symptomatic relapse occurs in 5% to 30% of patients who respond to their initial treatment regimen.[115,119] Relapses occur 2 weeks to 2 months (median of 7 days) after treatment has been discontinued.[153]

In most instances, relapses are caused by germination of dormant spores that are intrinsically resistant to antibiotics. However, reinfection with *C. difficile* from external sources may account for up to half of all second episodes.[154] In rare instances, either vancomycin[155] or metronidazole may have caused CDAD.[156]

Risk factors for recurrent CDAD include increasing age, low quality-of-health score,[153] use of additional antibiotics, spring onset, and multiple prior episodes of *C. difficile* infection.[157] Twenty-four percent of patients experiencing their first episode of CDAD experience a relapse, and 65% of patients with a prior history of CDAD relapse.[158]

58. How should patients such as B.W. who relapse after therapy for CDAD be treated?

The majority of infections resulting from relapse are not related to bacterial resistance and respond to retreatment with the same antibiotic used for initial treatment of the *C. difficile* infection.[119] Thus, an appropriate approach for B.W. is to administer another 7- to 10-day course of oral metronidazole.

For patients with multiple recurrences of CDAD, the optimal management plan is unresolved.[115] Different approaches have been tried, including (1) high-dose vancomycin (2,000 mg/day)[159]; (2) a 4- to 6-week course with vancomycin, after which the dose is tapered over a 1- to 2-month period[159,160]; (2) exchange resins[136,161]; (3) "pulse" dosing every 2 to 3 days[159]; or (4) a combination of vancomycin and rifampin (600 mg orally twice daily).[162] Tapered and pulse therapy with vancomycin were shown to be most effective in a clinical trial comparing multiple strategies.[159] When combined with standard antibiotic therapy, a clinical trial with the probiotic *S. boulardii* for cases of relapsing CDAD noted a 65% response rate verses a 36% response rate for combination therapy with placebo.[158] The relapse rate was reduced to 17% when *S. boulardii* was combined with high-dose vancomycin.[163]

CRYPTOSPORIDIUM PARVUM

Clinical Presentation

59. C.K., a 35-year-old, previously healthy man, presents to his family physician with complaints of 15 days of watery diarrhea and a 5-lb weight loss. He heard an announcement by the Board of Health of a community-wide outbreak of cryptosporidiosis from contaminated water supplies and is concerned that he has this illness. Why are C.K.'s clinical presentation and epidemiologic history consistent with cryptosporidiosis? Should antimicrobials be prescribed to treat cryptosporidiosis in otherwise healthy persons like C.K.?

C.K. presents with persistent diarrhea, defined as diarrhea lasting >14 days. Common microbial causes of persistent watery diarrhea include parasites such as *C. parvum*, *Isospora belli*, *Microsporidia*, and *G. lamblia*. *C. parvum* causes a watery diarrheal illness (cryptosporidiosis) in both normal and immunocompromised patients. The spectrum of infection ranges from asymptomatic carriage to a persistent noninflammatory diarrhea.[164] In immunocompetent patients like C.K., cryptosporidiosis is generally a self-limiting illness lasting approximately 2 weeks.[164] Other manifestations of cryptosporidiosis include nausea, vomiting, abdominal cramps, weight loss, and fever.[164] In contrast, in immunocompromised patients cryptosporidiosis may be a debilitating chronic diarrhea associated with malabsorption and significant weight loss (see Chapter 70, Opportunistic Infections in HIV-Infected Patients).

The most important mode of acquiring cryptosporidial infection is via water contaminated with cryptosporidium oocysts.[164] In a 1993 outbreak, a contaminated water supply was responsible for 370,000 cases of cryptosporidiosis in Milwaukee, Wisconsin.[164] Other means of spreading this infection include animal contact (cattle and sheep), person-to-person contact (e.g., health care workers, day care personnel), and exposure to recreational waters.[164]

Treatment

No antimicrobial agent is known to eradicate *C. parvum*, though some agents suppress infection.[164] In general, asymptomatic patients and immunocompetent hosts require no specific therapy other than replacement of fluids and electrolytes.[164] Nitazoxanide is approved for the treatment of diarrhea caused by *C. parvum* in children 1 to 11 years old.[165] In HIV-negative patients, half of whom were children, compared to patients who received placebo, cure rates were significantly higher following a 3-day course of nitazoxanide. In HIV-positive children, nitazoxanide was no more effective than placebo.

REFERENCES

1. Tauxe RV et al. Food-borne disease. In: Mandell GL et al, eds. Principles and Practice of Infectious Diseases, 5th ed. Philadelphia: Churchill Livingstone, 2000:1150.
2. Ilnyckyj A. Clinical evaluation and management of acute infectious diarrhea in adults. Gastroenterol Clin North Am 2001;30:599.
3. Turgeon DK et al. Laboratory approaches to infectious diarrhea. Gastroenterol Clin North Am 2001;30:693.
4. DuPont HL et al. Guidelines on acute infectious diarrhea in adults. Am J Gastroenterol 1997;92:1962.
5. Guerrant RL et al. Principles and syndromes of enteric infection. In: Mandell GL et al, eds. Principles and Practice of Infectious Diseases, 5th ed. Philadelphia: Churchill Livingstone, 2000:1076.
6. Gorbach SL. Infectious diarrhea and bacterial food poisoning. In: Sleisenger MH, Fortran JS, eds. Gastrointestinal Diseases, 5th ed. Philadelphia: WB Saunders, 1993:1128.
7. Talan D, et al. Etiology of bloody diarrhea among patients presenting to United States emergency departments: prevalence of *Escherichia coli* O157:H7 and other enteropathogens. Clin Infect Dis 2001;32:573.
8. DuPont HL et al. Persistent diarrhea in travelers. Clin Infect Dis 1996;22:124.
9. Oldfield EC et al. The role of antibiotics in the treatment of infectious diarrhea. Gastroenterol Clin North Am 2001;30:817.
10. Hypovolemic states. In: Rose BD, et al, eds. Clinical Physiology of Acid–Base and Electrolyte Disorders, 5th ed. New York: McGraw-Hill, 2001:415.
11. Swerdlow DL et al. Cholera in the Americas. Guidelines for the clinician. JAMA 1992;267:1495.
12. Duggan C et al. The management of acute diarrhea in children: oral rehydration, maintenance, and nutritional therapy. Centers for Disease Control and Prevention. MMWR Recomm Rep 1992;41(RR-16):1.
13. Powell DW. Approach to the patient with diarrhea. In: Goldman L et al, eds. Cecil Textbook of Medicine, 21st ed. Philadelphia: W.B. Saunders, 2000:702.
14. Hines J et al. Effective use of the clinical microbiology laboratory for diagnosing diarrheal diseases. Clin Infect Dis 1996;23:1292.
15. Jin S et al. Trends in hospitalizations for diarrhea in united states children from 1979 through 1992: estimates of the morbidity associated with rotavirus. JAMA 1996;15:397.
16. Johnson PC et al. Comparison of loperamide with bismuth subsalicylate for the treatment of acute travelers' diarrhea. JAMA 1986;255:757.
17. Wolfe MS. Protection of travelers. Clin Infect Dis 1997;25:177.
18. Murphy GS et al. Ciprofloxacin and loperamide in the treatment of bacillary dysentery. Ann Intern Med 1993;118:582.

19. Sullivan A, Nord CE. Probiotics in human infections. J Antimicrob Chemother 2002;50:625.
20. Elmer GW. Probiotics: "living drugs." Am J Health-Syst Pharm 2001;58:1101.
21. The choice of antimicrobial drugs. Med Lett Drugs Ther 2001;43:69.
22. Ha V et al. Two or three days of ofloxacin treatment for uncomplicated multidrug-resistant typhoid fever in children. Antimicrob Agents Chemother 1996;40:958.
23. Parry CM et al. Typhoid fever. N Engl J Med 2002;347:1770.
24. Graman PS et al. Gastrointestinal and intraabdominal infections. In Reese RE, Betts RF, eds. A Practical Approach to Infectious Diseases, 5th ed. Philadelphia: Lippincott Williams & Wilkins, 2003:403.
25. Bresee J S et al. Foodborne viral gastroenteritis: challenges and opportunities. Clin Infect Dis 2002;35:748.
26. Steinberg EB et al. Cholera in the United States, 1995–2000; trends at the end of the twentieth century. J Infect Dis 2001;184:799.
27. Daniels NA et al. *Vibrio parahaemolyticus* infections in the United States, 1973–1998. J Infect Dis 2000;181:1661.
28. Seas C et al. Practical guidelines for the treatment of cholera. Drugs 1996;51:966.
29. Garg P et al. Emergence of fluoroquinolone-resistant strains of *Vibrio cholerae* O1 biotype El Tor among hospitalized patients with cholera in Calcutta, India. Antimicrob Agents Chemother 2001;45.1605.
30. Daniels NA et al. Emergence of a new *Vibrio parahaemolyticus* serotype in raw oysters: A prevention quandary. JAMA 2000;284:1541.
31. Potasman I et al. Infectious outbreaks associated with bivalve shellfish consumption: a worldwide perspective. Clin Infect Dis 2002;35:921.
32. Salam MA et al. Antimicrobial therapy for shigellosis. Clin Infect Dis 1991;13(Suppl 4).
33. Weissman JP et al. Changing needs in the antimicrobial therapy of shigellosis. J Infect Dis 1973; 127:611.
34. Rogerie F et al. Comparison of norfloxacin and nalidixic acid for treatment of dysentery caused by *Shigella dysenteriae type 1* in adults. Antimicrob Agents Chemother 1986;29:883.
35. Bennish ML et al. Therapy for shigellosis, II: Randomized, double-blind comparison of ciprofloxacin and ampicillin. Infect Dis 1990;162:711.
36. Bennish ML et al. Treatment of shigellosis, III. Comparison of one- or two-dose ciprofloxacin with standard 5-day therapy. Ann Intern Med 1992; 117:727.
37. Gotuzzo E et al. Comparison of single-dose treatment with norfloxacin and standard 5-day treatment with trimethoprim-sulfamethoxazole for acute shigellosis in adults. Antimicrob Agents Chemother 1989;33:1101.

38. Petruccelli BP et al. Treatment of travelers' diarrhea with ciprofloxacin and loperamide. J Infect Dis 1992;165:557.
39. Sarkar K et al. *Shigella dysenteriae type 1* with reduced susceptibility to fluoroquinolones. Lancet 2003;361(9359):785.
40. Varsano I et al. Comparative efficacy of ceftriaxone and ampicillin for treatment of severe shigellosis in children. J Pediatr 1991;118:627.
41. Khan WA et al. Treatment of shigellosis, V. Comparison of azithromycin and ciprofloxacin. Ann Intern Med 1997;126:697.
42. Salam MA et al. Treatment of shigellosis, IV. Cefixime is ineffective in shigellosis in adults. Ann Intern Med 1995;123:505.
43. DuPont HL. Shigella species (bacillary dysentery). In: Mandell GL et al, eds. Principles and Practice of Infectious Diseases, 5th ed. Philadelphia: Churchill Livingstone, 2000:2363.
44. Nelson JD, Haltalin KS. Amoxicillin less effective than ampicillin against *Shigella* in vitro and in vivo: relationship of efficacy to activity in serum. J Infect Dis 1974;129(Suppl):S222.
45. Gilman RH et al. Randomized trial of high and low dose ampicillin therapy for treatment of severe dysentery due to *Shigella dysenteriae type I*. Antimicrob Agents Chemother 1980;17:402.
46. Tauxe RV et al. Antimicrobial resistance of *Shigella* isolates in the USA: the importance of international travelers. J Infect Dis 1990;162:1107.
47. Replogle ML et al. Emergence of antimicrobial-resistant shigellosis in Oregon. Clin Infect Dis 2000;30:515.
48. Miller SI et al. *Salmonella* (including *Salmonella typhi*). In: Mandell et al, eds. Principles and Practice of Infectious Diseases, 5th ed. Philadelphia: Churchill Livingstone, 2000:2344.
49. Hohmann EL. Nontyphoidal salmonellosis. Clin Infect Dis 2001;32:263.
50. Nelson JD et al. Treatment of *Salmonella* gastroenteritis with ampicillin, amoxicillin, or placebo. Pediatrics 1980;65:1125.
51. Wistrom J et al. Empiric treatment of acute diarrheal disease with norfloxacin. A randomized, placebo-controlled study. Ann Intern Med 1992; 117:202.
52. Neill MA et al. Failure of ciprofloxacin to eradicate convalescent fecal excretion after acute salmonellosis: experience during an outbreak in health care workers. Ann Intern Med 1991;114:195.
53. Ahmad F et al. Use of ciprofloxacin to control a *Salmonella* outbreak in a long-stay psychiatric hospital. J Hosp Infect 1991;17:171.
54. Aarestrup FM et al. Is it time to change fluoroquinolone breakpoints for *Salmonella* spp.? Antimicrob Agents Chemother 2003;47:827.
55. Ackers ML et al. Laboratory-based surveillance of *Salmonella serotype typhi* infections in the United States: antimicrobial resistance on the rise. JAMA 2000;283:2668.

56. Islam A et al. Randomized treatment of patients with typhoid fever by using ceftriaxone or chloramphenicol. J Infect Dis 1988;158:742.

57. Shehla H et al. Multidrug resistant typhoid fever in 58 children. Scand J Infect Dis 1992;24:175.

58. Gupta A. Multidrug-resistant typhoid fever in children: epidemiology and therapeutic approach. Pediatr Infect Dis J 1994;13:134.

59. Smith M et al. Comparison of ofloxacin and ceftriaxone for short-course treatment of enteric fever. Antimicrob Agents Chemother 1994;38:1716.

60. Ha V et al. Two or three days of ofloxacin treatment for uncomplicated multidrug-resistant typhoid fever in children. Antimicrob Agents Chemother 1996;40:958.

61. Frenck RW et al. Azithromycin versus ceftriaxone for the treatment of typhoid fever in children. Clin Infect Dis 2000;31:1134.

62. Girgis NI et al. Azithromycin versus ciprofloxacin for treatment of uncomplicated typhoid fever in a randomized trial in Egypt that included patients with multidrug resistance. Antimicrob Agents Chemother 1999;43:1441.

63. John M. Decreasing clinical response of quinolones in the treatment of enteric fever. Indian J Med Sci 2001;55:189.

64. Dutta P et al. Ceftriaxone therapy in ciprofloxacin treatment failure typhoid fever in children. Indian J Med Res 2001;113:210.

65. Wain J et al. Quinolone-resistant Salmonella typhi in Vietnam: molecular basis of resistance and clinical response to treatment. Clin Infect Dis 1997; 25:1404.

66. Hoffman SL et al. Reduction of mortality in chloramphenicol-treated severe typhoid fever by high-dose dexamethasone. N Engl J Med 1984; 310:82.

67. Parry CM et al. Typhoid fever [correspondence]. N Engl J Med 2003; 348:1182.

68. Kaye D et al. Treatment of chronic enteric carriers of Salmonella typhi with ampicillin. Ann NY Acad Sci 1967;145:429.

69. Phillips WE. Treatment of chronic typhoid carriers with ampicillin. JAMA 1971;217:913.

70. Nolan CM et al. Treatment of typhoid carriers with amoxicillin. JAMA 1978; 239:2352.

71. Pichler H et al. Treatment of chronic carriers of Salmonella typhi and Salmonella paratyphi with trimethoprim-sulfamethoxazole. J Infect Dis 1973; 128(Suppl):S743.

72. Kaye D et al. Treatment of chronic enteric carriers of Salmonella typhosa with ampicillin. Ann NY Acad Sci 1967;145:429.

73. Ferreccio C et al. Efficacy of ciprofloxacin in the treatment of chronic typhoid carriers. J Infect Dis 1988;157:1235.

74. Diridl G et al. Treatment of chronic Salmonella carriers with ciprofloxacin [letter]. Eur J Clin Microbiol 1986;5:260.

75. Sammalkorpi K et al. Treatment of chronic Salmonella carriers with ciprofloxacin [letter]. Lancet 1987;2:164.

76. Gotuzzo E et al. Use of norfloxacin to treat chronic typhoid carriers. J Infect Dis 1988;157:1221.

77. Mead PS, Griffin PM. Escherichia coli O157:H7. Lancet 1998;352:1207.

78. Karch H, et al. Epidemiology and diagnosis of Shiga toxin-producing Escherichia coli infections. Diagn Microbiol Infect Dis 1999;34:229.

79. Dundas S et al. The central Scotland Escherichia coli O157:H7 outbreak: risk factors for the hemolytic uremic syndrome and death among hospitalized patients. Clin Infect Dis. 2001;33:923.

80. Klein EJ et al. Shiga toxin-producing Escherichia coli in children with diarrhea: a prospective point-of-care study. J Pediatr 2002;141:172.

81. Banatvala N et al. The United States National Prospective Hemolytic Uremic Syndrome Study: microbiologic, serologic, clinical, and epidemiologic findings. J Infect Dis 2001;183:1063.

82. Ikeda K et al. Predictors for the development of haemolytic uraemic syndrome with Escherichia

coli O157:H7 infections: with focus on the day of illness. Epidemiol Infect 2000;124:343.

83. Wong CS et al. The risk of the hemolytic-uremic syndrome after antibiotic treatment of Escherichia coli O157:H7 infections. N Engl J Med 2000; 342:1930.

84. Cimolai N et al. Risk factors for the progression of Escherichia coli O157:H7 enteritis to hemolytic-uremic syndrome. J Pediatr 1990;116:589.

85. Slutsker L et al. A nationwide case-control study of Escherichia coli O157:H7 infection in the United States. J Infect Dis 1998;177:962.

86. Carter AO et al. A severe outbreak of Escherichia coli O157:H7-associated hemorrhagic colitis in a nursing home. N Engl J Med 1987;317:1496.

87. Proulx F et al. Randomized, controlled trial of antibiotic therapy for Escherichia coli O157:H7 enteritis. J Pediatr 1992;121:299.

88. Pavia AT et al. Hemolytic-uremic syndrome during an outbreak of Escherichia coli O157:H7 infections in institutions from mentally retarded persons: clinical and epidemiologic observations. J Pediatr 1990;116:544.

89. Safdar N et al. Risk of hemolytic uremic syndrome after antibiotic treatment of Escherichia coli O157:H7 enteritis: a meta-analysis. JAMA 2002;288:996.

90. Bell BP et al. Prediction of hemolytic uremic syndrome in children during a large outbreak of Escherichia coli O157:H7 infections. Pediatrics 1997;100:127.

91. Belongia EA et al. Transmission of Escherichia coli O157:H7 infection in Minnesota child day-care facilities. JAMA 1993;269:883.

92. Allos BM. Campylobacter jejuni infections: update on emerging issues and trends. Clin Infect Dis 2001;32:1201.

93. Blaser MJ. Campylobacter and related species. In: Mandell GL et al, eds. Principles and Practice of Infectious Diseases, 5th ed. Philadelphia: Churchill Livingstone, 2000:2276.

94. Salazar-Lindo E et al. Early treatment with erythromycin of Campylobacter jejuni-associated dysentery in children. J Pediatr 1986;109:355.

95. Goodman LJ et al. Empiric antimicrobial therapy of domestically acquired acute diarrhea in urban adults. Arch Intern Med 1990;150:541.

96. Smith DE et al. Quinolone-resistant Campylobacter jejuni infection in Minnesota, 1992–1998. N Engl J Med 1999;340:1525.

97. Kuschner RA et al. Use of azithromycin for the treatment of Campylobacter enteritis in travelers to Thailand, an area where ciprofloxacin resistance is prevalent. Clin Infect Dis 1995;21:536.

98. Adachi JA et al. Empirical antimicrobial therapy for traveler's diarrhea. Clin Infect Dis 2000; 31:1079.

99. Ericsson CD et al. Travelers' diarrhea: approaches to prevention and treatment. Clin Infect Dis 1993;16:616.

100. Rendi-Wagner P et al. Drug prophylaxis for travelers' diarrhea. Clin Infect Dis 2002;34:628.

101. Caeiro JP et al. Oral rehydration therapy plus loperamide versus loperamide alone in the treatment of traveler's diarrhea. Clin Infect Dis 1999; 28:1286.

102. Ericsson CD et al. Ciprofloxacin or trimethoprim/sulfamethoxazole as initial therapy for travelers' diarrhea. Ann Intern Med 1987;106:216.

103. DuPont HL et al. Five versus three days of ofloxacin therapy for travelers' diarrhea: a placebo controlled study. Antimicrob Agents Chemother 1992;36:87.

104. Ericsson CD et al. Treatment of travelers' diarrhea with sulfamethoxazole and trimethoprim and loperamide. JAMA 1990;263:257.

105. Salam I et al. Randomised trial of single-dose ciprofloxacin for travellers' diarrhoea. Lancet 1994;344(8936):1537.

106. Ericsson CD et al. Single dose ofloxacin plus loperamide compared with single dose or three days

of ofloxacin in the treatment of traveler's diarrhea. J Travel Med 1997;4:3.

107. Ericsson CD et al. Optimal dosing of trimethoprim-sulfamethoxazole when used with loperamide to treat travelers' diarrhea. Antimicrob Agents Chemother 1992;36:2821.

108. Taylor DN et al. Treatment of travelers' diarrhea: ciprofloxacin plus loperamide compared with ciprofloxacin alone. Ann Intern Med 1991;114:731.

109. Radandt JM et al. Interactions of fluoroquinolones with other drugs: mechanisms, variability, clinical significance, and management. Clin Infect Dis 1992;14:272.

110. DuPont HL et al. Prevention of travelers' diarrhea by the tablet formulation of bismuth subsalicylate. JAMA 1987;257:1347.

111. Scott DA et al. Norfloxacin for the prophylaxis of travelers' diarrhea in U.S. military personnel. Am J Trop Med Hyg 1990;42:160.

112. Johnson PC et al. Lack of emergence of resistant fecal flora during successful prophylaxis of travelers' diarrhea with norfloxacin. Antimicrob Agents Chemother 1986;30:671.

113. Rademaker CMA et al. Results of a double-blind placebo-controlled study using ciprofloxacin for prevention of travelers' diarrhea. Eur J Clin Microbiol Infect Dis 1989;8:690.

114. Ferguson J et al. Phototoxicity in quinolones: comparison of ciprofloxacin and grepafloxacin. J Antimicrob Chemother 1997;40(Suppl)A:93.

115. Fekety R. Guidelines for the diagnosis and treatment of Clostridium difficile-associated diarrhea and colitis. Am J Gastroenterol 1997;92:739.

116. Hogenauer C et al. Mechanisms and management of antibiotic-associated diarrhea. Clin Infect Dis 1998;27:702.

117. Husain A et al. Gastrointestinal toxicity and Clostridium difficile diarrhea in patients treated with paclitaxel-containing chemotherapy regimens. Gynecol Oncol 1998;71:104.

118. Sharma AK et al. Clostridium difficile diarrhea after use of tacrolimus following renal transplantation. Clin Infect Dis 1998;27:1540.

119. Johnson S et al. Clostridium difficile-associated diarrhea. Clin Infect Dis 1998;26:1027.

120. Bartlett JG. Antibiotic-associated diarrhea. Clin Infect Dis 1992;15:573.

121. Wanahita A et al. Conditions associated with leukocytosis in a tertiary care hospital, with particular attention to the role of infection caused by Clostridium difficile. Clin Infect Dis 2002;34: 1585.

122. Martin SJ et al. Levofloxacin and sparfloxacin: new quinolone antibiotics. Ann Pharmacother 1998;32:320.

123. Savola KL et al. Fecal leukocyte stain has diagnostic value for outpatients but not inpatients. J Clin Microbiol 2001;39:266.

124. Scheife RT et al. Photosensitizing potential of ofloxacin. Int J Dermatol 1993;32:413.

125. Teasly DG et al. Prospective randomized study of metronidazole versus vancomycin for clostridium-associated diarrhea and colitis. Lancet 1983; 2:1043.

126. Tedesco F et al. Oral vancomycin for antibiotic-associated pseudomembranous colitis. Lancet 1978; 2:226.

127. Pelaez T et al. Reassessment of Clostridium difficile susceptibility to metronidazole and vancomycin. Antimicrob Agents Chemother 2002;46: 1647.

128. Edwards DL et al. Disulfiram-like reaction associated with intravenous trimethoprim-sulfamethoxazole and metronidazole. Clin Pharm 1986;5:999.

129. Fekety R et al. Treatment of antibiotic-associated Clostridium difficile colitis with oral vancomycin: comparison of two-dosage regimens. Am J Med 1989;86:15.

130. Keighley MRD et al. Randomized controlled trial of vancomycin for pseudomembranous colitis and post-operative diarrhea. Br Med J 1978;2:1667.

131. Dudley NM et al. Absorption of vancomycin. Ann Intern Med 1984;101:144.
132. Spizter PG, Eliopoulous GM. Systemic absorption of vancomycin in a patient with pseudomembranous colitis. Ann Intern Med 1984;100:523.
133. Reinke CM et al. ASHP therapeutic position statement on the preferential use of metronidazole for the treatment of Clostridium difficile-associated disease. Am J Health-Syst Pharm 1998;55:1407.
134. Dudley MN et al. Oral bacitracin versus vancomycin therapy for Clostridium difficile-induced diarrhea. Arch Intern Med 1986;146:1101.
135. Young GP et al. Antibiotic-associated colitis due to Clostridium difficile: double-blind comparison of vancomycin with bacitracin. Gastroenterology 1985;89:1038.
136. Ariano RE et al. The role of anion-exchange resins in the treatment of antibiotic-associated pseudomembranous colitis. Can Med Assoc J 1990;142:1049.
137. Pletincx M et al. Fungemia with Saccharomyces boulardii in a 1-year-old girl with protracted diarrhea. J Pediatr Gastroenterol Nutr 1995;21:113.
138. Novak E et al. Unfavorable effect of atropine–diphenoxylate therapy in the therapy of lincomycin diarrhea. JAMA 1976;235:1451.
139. Climo MW et al. Hospital-wide restriction of clindamycin: effect on the incidence of Clostridium difficile-associated diarrhea and cost. Ann Intern Med 1998;128:989.
140. Kyne L et al. Underlying disease severity as a major risk factor for nosocomial Clostridium difficile diarrhea. Infect Control Hosp Epidemiol 2002;23:653.
141. Chang VT, Nelson K. The role of physical proximity in nosocomial diarrhea. Clin Infect Dis 2000;31:717.
142. Karlstrom O et al. A prospective nationwide study of Clostridium difficile-associated diarrhea in Sweden. Clin Infect Dis 1998;26:141.

143. Beaugerie L et al. Antibiotic-associated diarrhoea and Clostridium difficile in the community. Aliment Pharmacol Ther 2003;17:905.
144. Johnson SJ et al. Treatment of asymptomatic Clostridium difficile carriers (fecal excretors) with vancomycin or metronidazole. Ann Intern Med 1992;117:297.
145. Kyne L et al. Health care costs and mortality associated with nosocomial diarrhea due to Clostridium difficile. Clin Infect Dis 2002;34:346.
146. Dallal RM et al. Fulminant Clostridium difficile: an underappreciated and increasing cause of death and complications. Ann Surg 2002;235:363.
147. Lamp KC et al. Pharmacokinetics and pharmacodynamics of the nitroimidazole antimicrobials. Clin Pharmacokinet 1999;36:353.
148. Bolton RP et al. Faecal metronidazole concentrations during oral and intravenous therapy for antibiotic-associated colitis due to Clostridium difficile. Gut 1986;27:1169.
149. Kleinfeld DI et al. Parenteral therapy for antibiotic-associated pseudomembranous colitis [letter]. J Infect Dis 1988;157:389.
150. Friedenberg F et al. Intravenous metronidazole for the treatment of Clostridium difficile colitis. Dis Colon Rectum 2001;44:1176.
151. Guzman R et al. Failure of parenteral metronidazole in the treatment of pseudomembranous colitis [letter]. J Infect Dis 1988;158:1146.
152. Apisarnthanarak A et al. Adjunctive intracolonic vancomycin for severe Clostridium difficile colitis: case series and review of the literature. Clin Infect Dis 2002;35:690.
153. McFarland LV et al. Recurrent Clostridium difficile disease: epidemiology and clinical characteristics. Infect Cont Hosp Epidemiol 1999;20:43.
154. Barbut F et al. Epidemiology of recurrences or reinfections of Clostridium difficile-associated diarrhea. J Clin Microbiol 2000;38.2386.
155. Hecht J, Olinger E. Clostridium difficile colitis secondary to intravenous vancomycin. Dig Dis Sci 1989;34:148.

156. Saginur R et al. Colitis associated with metronidazole therapy. J Infect Dis 1980;141:772.
157. Fekety R et al. Recurrent Clostridium difficile diarrhea: Characteristics of and risk factors for patients enrolled in a prospective, randomized, double-blinded trial. Clin Infect Dis 1997;24:324.
158. McFarland LV et al. A randomized placebo-controlled trial of Saccharomyces boulardii in combination with standard antibiotics for Clostridium difficile disease. JAMA 1994;271:1913.
159. McFarland LV et al. Breaking the cycle: treatment strategies for 163 cases of recurrent Clostridium difficile disease. Am J Gastroenterol 2002;97:1769.
160. Tedesco F et al. Approach to patients with multiple relapses of antibiotic-associated pseudomembranous colitis. Am J Gastroenterol 1985;80:867.
161. Pruksananonda P et al. Multiple relapses of Clostridium difficile-associated diarrhea responding to an extended course of cholestyramine. Pediatr Infect Dis J 1989;8:175.
162. Buggy BP et al. Therapy of relapsing Clostridium difficile-associated diarrhea and colitis with the combination of vancomycin and rifampin. Clin Gastroenterol 1987;9:155.
163. Surawicz CM et al. The search for a better treatment for recurrent Clostridium difficile disease: use of high-dose vancomycin combined with Saccharomyces boulardii. Clin Infect Dis 2000;31:1012.
164. Chen XM et al. Cryptosporidiosis. N Engl J Med 2002;346:1723.
165. Med Lett Drugs Ther 2003;45:29.
166. Anders BJ et al. Double-blind placebo-controlled study of erythromycin for treatment of Campylobacter enteritis. Lancet 1982;1:131.
167. Rosenfeldt V et al. Effect of probiotic lactobacillus strains in young children hospitalized with acute diarrhea. Pediatr Infect Dis J 2002;21:411.

CHAPTER 63

Intra-Abdominal Infections

Jill S. Burkiewicz, Carrie A. Quigley

Despite the introduction of newer, more potent antimicrobial agents and improvements in diagnostic and surgical techniques, the treatment of intra-abdominal infections remains a therapeutic challenge. Improvements in radiographic techniques that allow better localization of abscesses and early drainage, improved nutritional management, and the selection of appropriate antimicrobial agents all contribute to a decrease in mortality from intra-abdominal infections.

Intra-abdominal infections are those contained within the peritoneal cavity, which extends from the undersurface of the diaphragm to the floor of the pelvis or the retroperitoneal space. Intra-abdominal infections may present as localized infections, a diffuse inflammation throughout the peritoneum, or infections in visceral organs such as the liver, biliary tract, spleen, pancreas, or female pelvic organs. Abscesses may form in any of the potential spaces within the abdomen, between bowel loops, or in the solid organs. If localization of the infection site is delayed, multiple organ failure, which is associated with a high mortality, is likely to occur.

Antimicrobial therapy should be selected on the basis of the microbiology of the infecting pathogens, in vitro susceptibility data, an understanding of the pharmacokinetic and pharmacodynamic properties of the antimicrobial agents, the results of well-designed clinical trials, and cost.[1]

INFECTIONS OF THE BILIARY TRACT

Cholangitis and Cholecystitis

Cholangitis is inflammation of the biliary ductal system. Acute cholangitis can develop from an infectious, chemical, ischemic, or idiopathic process. Historically, the most common cause of biliary obstruction resulting in cholangitis has been cholelithiasis obstructing the common bile duct.[2] Other principal etiologies of obstruction include strictures formed after surgery or endoscopy, parasitic infections, and neoplasm of either the biliary system (cholangiocarcinoma) or the head of the pancreas (adenocarcinoma). Under normal conditions, bile is a sterile fluid. However, bacterial colonization of the biliary tract by enteric bacteria can occur in patients with biliary pathology, especially patients with gallstone disease.[2] Colonization of the biliary tree, or bactibilia, is associated with obstruction to the outflow of bile.[3] In acute infectious cholangitis, the progression of obstruction leads to biliary stasis and proliferation of bacteria within the biliary tree. Once infection occurs, increased pressure and edema result in increased permeability of the surrounding tissues, promoting systemic spread of bacteria and resulting in sepsis.[2,3]

Cholecystitis (inflammation of the gallbladder) is associated with obstruction of the cystic duct, which normally drains the contents of the gallbladder into the common bile duct. The pathogenesis of infection is similar in cholangitis and cholecystitis: biliary stasis results in bacterial proliferation and subsequent infection.

Clinical Presentation and Diagnosis

1. L.K., a 59-year-old woman, presents to the hospital with a 2-day history of abdominal pain and tenderness, localized to the right upper quadrant, fever to 38.9°C, and rigors. She complains of nausea, with three episodes of emesis occurring in the past 24 hours. L.K. appears jaundiced and reports dark-colored urine. Her laboratory values are white blood cell (WBC) count, $15 \times 10^3/mm^3$ (normal, 3.2 to 9.8), with a shift to the left; serum creatinine (SCr), 1.9 mg/dL (normal, 0.6 to 1.2); total bilirubin, 4 mg/dL (normal, 0.1 to 1); and alkaline phosphatase, 220 U/L (normal, 30 to 120). What evidence of cholangitis exists in L.K.? How does cholecystitis differ from cholangitis?

[SI units: WBC count, 15×10^9/L (normal, 3.2 to 9.8); SCr, 167.96 μmol/L (normal, 50 to 110); total bilirubin, 68.4 μmol/L (normal, 2 to 18)]

Acute cholangitis presents with varying degrees of severity. The clinical presentation ranges from mild discomfort that resolves with conservative management to overwhelming sepsis. Charcot's triad—fever, jaundice, and abdominal pain—is the classical description of cholangitis.[4] The clinical signs and symptoms of cholangitis, as exemplified by L.K., include high fevers (>38.5°C), chills, jaundice, and abdominal pain. Abdominal pain localized to the right upper quadrant is often the presenting symptom and is accompanied by nausea and vomiting. In severe cases of cholangitis, bacteremia may occur, leading to septic shock.

As illustrated by L.K., laboratory evidence of cholangitis reveals leukocytosis with a predominance of immature neutrophils (shift to the left). Other abnormal laboratory values may include elevated bilirubin (usually in the range of 2 to 4 mg/dL), alkaline phosphatase, liver transferases, and amylase levels. L.K. has a total bilirubin of 4 mg/dL and an alkaline phosphatase of 220 U/L.

Clinical and laboratory findings of acute cholecystitis are similar to those of acute cholangitis. Both diseases are associated with leukocytosis, fever, acute right upper quadrant pain and tenderness, nausea and vomiting, and elevations in liver transferases, total bilirubin, alkaline phosphatase, and amylase levels. The differences between the diseases are subtle, but patients with cholecystitis generally present with milder fevers (38 to 38.5°C), prominent rebound tenderness, guarding during physical examination, minimal elevations in bilirubin, alkaline phosphatase, and amylase, and less commonly mild jaundice (bilirubin <60 mmol/L).[5] Radiologic diagnosis includes ultrasonography, which reveals distention of the gallbladder, often with stones. Conversely, patients with cholangitis generally have an increase in the diameter of the common bile duct, but there is no increase in gallbladder size. If the ultrasound is inconclusive, biliary scintigraphy may be performed.[5]

Bacteriology

2. Which organisms are likely to be associated with infection in L.K.? Are blood cultures helpful in identifying the pathogen(s)?

The most prevalent biliary tract pathogens include *Escherichia coli*, *Klebsiella* species, *Enterococcus*, *Enterobacter cloacae*, and anaerobes, including *Bacteroides* species and *Clostridium* species.[2] Anaerobes are detected in >15% of patients and commonly are involved in polymicrobic infections.[2] Other possible pathogens include *Streptococcus viridans* and *Staphylococcus aureus*. *Pseudomonas aeruginosa* may be introduced after endoscopy or surgery.[3] Bacteriologic findings are similar in infectious cholecystitis.[2] However, anaerobes are uncommon pathogens. (Table 63-1).

Obstruction of the common bile duct results in increased ductal pressure that forces bacteria through the hepatic sinusoids and into the systemic circulation.[2] As a result, blood cultures obtained from a patient with signs of systemic infection, such as rigors and hypotension, are often positive. The organisms isolated in bacteremia are similar to those found in the biliary tract. However, *Enterococcus* and anaerobes are rarely isolated from the blood of a bacteremic patient.

A three-step approach is suggested in the treatment of acute biliary tract infections[2,4,5]: (1) drainage of the biliary tree by surgery or interventional radiology; (2) appropriate antibacterial therapy; and (3) supportive measures.

Treatment of both cholecystitis and cholangitis requires drainage of obstructed biliary fluid.[6] In patients with cholangitis, endoscopic retrograde cholangiopancreatography (ERCP) is used to relieve biliary ductal system blockage by removing the obstructive stone or stricture in the common bile duct. Alternatively, percutaneous transhepatic cholangiopancreatography (PTCA) can be used to drain bile by passing a catheter through the intrahepatic duct. Cholecystitis requires removal of the gallbladder (cholecystectomy) or drainage (cholecystostomy) in older, more debilitated patients.[6] Endoscopic or surgical treatment of the obstruction often is necessary to avoid recurrences.[6] The timing of surgery in patients with uncomplicated cholecystitis remains controversial.[5]

Table 63-1 Common Pathogens in Intra-Abdominal Infection

Disease	Pathogens	Comments
Primary peritonitis	*E. coli, K. pneumoniae, S. pneumoniae*, group A streptococci, occasional anaerobes	Predominately in spontaneous bacterial peritonitis in cirrhotics. Anaerobes less likely than aerobes.
Secondary peritonitis	*E. coli, B. fragilis*, other aerobic gram-negative rods and anaerobes, enterococci	Generally polymicrobial with both aerobic and anaerobic pathogens. Enterococci are associated with chronic surgical infection, particularly in patients receiving broad-spectrum antimicrobials such as cephalosporins.
Chronic ambulatory peritoneal dialysis	*S. epidermidis, S. aureus*, diphtheroids, gram-negative rods	
Cholecystitis, cholangitis	*E. coli, K. pneumoniae* anaerobes, other gram-negative rods	Necessity for antimicrobials that achieve high biliary concentrations is unknown.

Antimicrobial Therapy

3. Based on the expected pathogens, what empiric antimicrobial therapy should be suggested for L.K.?

Treatment of cholangitis must be started empirically and should be directed at the most likely pathogens: *E. coli* and *Klebsiella* species. The need to empirically cover anaerobes is less certain. However, anaerobic coverage is generally recommended, particularly in patients in serious clinical condition, such as the elderly and those with previous bile duct–bowel anastamosis.[2] Enterococci are less commonly encountered pathogens; empiric coverage is not necessary unless the patient is clinically septic. Historically, combination therapy with an aminoglycoside or second- or third-generation cephalosporin, plus metronidazole or clindamycin, has been used empirically to treat cholangitis. However, aminoglycosides have been associated with renal and cochlear toxicity and require close monitoring of drug levels and renal function. Furthermore, the risk of renal toxicity has been suggested to be greater in patients with obstructive jaundice.[7] As a result, less toxic antibacterials (e.g., extended-spectrum penicillins, third- and fourth-generation cephalosporins, carbapenems) have been studied in the treatment of biliary tract infections. Successful monotherapy with cefoperazone, cefepime, piperacillin, and imipenem has been reported.[1,8] Combinations of extended-spectrum penicillins with β-lactamase inhibitors are also an option. As a result, empiric therapy has shifted to monotherapy with a single agent or β-lactamase inhibitor combination.

The efficacy of fluoroquinolones in the treatment of acute biliary tract infections also has been documented.[9,10] Fluoroquinolones offer coverage of Enterobacteriaceae without the risk of nephrotoxicity but generally have poor activity against anaerobes. It may be necessary to add anaerobic coverage by combining fluoroquinolones that have poor anaerobic activity (e.g., ciprofloxacin, levofloxacin) with clindamycin or metronidazole. Some fluoroquinolones, such as moxifloxacin and garenoxacin, have anaerobic activity and are being investigated as monotherapy for biliary tract infections.[11]

Aminoglycoside therapy should be avoided in L.K. because her age, elevated SCr, and hyperbilirubinemia place her at higher risk for the development of aminoglycoside-induced nephrotoxicity. Alternatively, a less toxic, broad-spectrum agent that adequately covers common biliary tract pathogens should be considered. L.K. should be treated with intravenous (IV) ampicillin/sulbactam 1.5 g Q 6 hr.

BILIARY CONCENTRATIONS

4. The physician caring for L.K. prefers to use an antibiotic that concentrates in the bile. What is the benefit of using an antibiotic that is excreted into bile?

Common bile duct obstruction is a factor that affects and may prevent the entry of antibiotics into the bile, but the need for high biliary concentrations of antibiotics in the treatment of cholangitis is unclear.[12] Table 63-2 summarizes the concentrations of several antibiotics in bile relative to serum.[7,13,14] Nagar and colleagues reviewed the biliary excretion of several antibiotics and concluded that a number of antibiotics with excellent in vitro susceptibility are poorly excreted into bile

but are still clinically effective.[14] Because all patients with biliary tract infections require endoscopy or surgery to relieve obstruction, the biliary excretion of antibiotics may not have an effect on outcome. Highly excreted versus moderately excreted antibiotics have been studied.[12] The investigators concluded that serum levels were more important than biliary levels in reducing the septic complications of biliary tract surgery. These authors concluded that biliary excretion of any antibiotic is minimal in the presence of obstruction.[12]

The treatment of L.K.'s biliary tract infection must include biliary drainage. Ampicillin/sulbactam should be continued for a duration of 7 to 10 days.

PRIMARY PERITONITIS

Peritonitis is an inflammation of the peritoneal lining that occurs in response to chemical irritation or bacterial invasion; this chapter addresses infectious peritonitis only. The etiology of peritonitis is important because it can determine the treatment approach. Most often, peritonitis is secondary to contamination of the peritoneum by gastrointestinal (GI) bacteria that have been released by inflammation, perforation, or trauma; this is called *secondary peritonitis*. Some clinicians use the term *tertiary* or *persistent* peritonitis to describe intra-abdominal infection associated with a higher morbidity and mortality.[15] Less often, patients develop primary or "spontaneous" bacterial peritonitis that has no apparent connection with an intra-abdominal event (e.g., appendicitis). In this form of peritonitis, there is no obvious intra-abdominal source of bacterial contamination.

Primary peritonitis often is associated with alcoholic cirrhosis and occurs in up to 25% of patients with chronic liver disease and ascites. However, it also is associated with other postnecrotic liver diseases (including hepatitis, cryptogenic cirrhosis, cardiac cirrhosis, and biliary cirrhosis), nephrosis, and peritoneal dialysis.[15,16] In adults, the presence of peritoneal fluid appears to be an essential factor for the development of spontaneous bacterial peritonitis (SBP); end-stage liver disease need not be present.[4] Thus, SBP also has been reported in patients with nephrotic syndrome, malignancies, congestive heart failure, and severe viral hepatitis.[15]

Table 63-2 Concentration in Bile Relative to Serum[14]

Bile Less Than Serum	Bile Equal to Serum	Bile Greater Than Serum
Penicillin G	Ampicillin	Nafcillin
Phenoxypenicillins	Cefazolin	Cefamandole
Amoxicillin	Cefotaxime	Cefoxitin
Cefuroxime	Gentamicin	Cephradine
Ceftazidime	Amikacin	Cefoperazone
Ceftizoxime	Sulfamethoxazole	Cefotetan
Vancomycin		Ciprofloxacin
		Erythromycin
		Clindamycin
		Doxycycline
		Metronidazole
		Rifampin

Adapted from references 12 and 13.

Spontaneous Bacterial Peritonitis

Signs and Symptoms

SBP is generally characterized by fever, chills, vomiting, abdominal pain, signs of peritoneal irritation, and impending shock and hepatic coma. In contrast to secondary peritonitis, which is generally an acute event, this process can develop over days to weeks. Bowel sounds become hypoactive, and rebound tenderness appears as the abdominal pain becomes progressively more severe.[15] However, these signs are not invariably present, and asymptomatic bacterial ascites sometimes occurs.[4] Cloudy ascitic fluid with an elevated leukocyte count ($>250/mm^3$) is indicative of peritoneal infection.[17]

Primary Peritonitis in Cirrhotics

Pathogenesis

5. R.S., a 47-year-old man with Laennec's (alcohol-related) cirrhosis and massive abdominal ascites, presents with a 4-day history of fever to 38.4°C, decreasing mental status, decreased urine output, and abdominal pain. Ascitic fluid obtained by paracentesis was cloudy. Cell count, differential, and culture of the ascitic fluid are pending. Laboratory values are WBC count, $12.2 \times 10^3/mm^3$ (normal, 3.2 to 9.8), and total bilirubin, 4.4 mg/dL (normal, 0.1 to 1). What organisms are likely to be cultured from R.S.'s ascitic fluid?

[SI units: WBC count, $12.2 \times 10^9/L$ (normal, 3.2 to 9.8); total bilirubin, 75.2 μmol/L (normal, 2 to 18)]

Enteric bacteria, most commonly *E. coli* or *K. pneumoniae,* are recovered in approximately 60% to 70% of patients with SBP, and nonenteric organisms, usually *S. pneumoniae* or other streptococci, are recovered in 25% of patients[15,16] (see Table 63-1). Staphylococci, anaerobes, and microaerophilic organisms are rarely reported. Anaerobes, when present, are almost invariably seen in the setting of a polymicrobial infection.[15] Bacteremia occurs in up to 75% of patients with peritonitis due to aerobes, but it is rarely present in patients with anaerobic peritonitis.[15]

Although the pathogenesis of SBP is unclear, several mechanisms have been suggested. In cirrhotics such as R.S., hematogenous spread is the most likely route of infection.[15] In advanced cirrhosis, the majority of portal blood flow may bypass the liver, permitting circulating bacteria to bypass the hepatic reticuloendothelial filtering system, a major site for their removal from the blood.[15]

Changes in the intestinal mucosa also may serve as a source of bacteremia.[15] Congestion of the splanchnic veins and lymphatics secondary to portal hypertension may result in inflammation and edema of the bowel wall and increased intestinal permeability. Under certain circumstances, bacteria are known also to cross the intact intestinal wall.[17,18] Bacterial translocation from the GI tract to mesenteric lymph nodes is implicated in the pathogenesis of SBP. Another local defense mechanism of the peritoneum is its capacity to exude opsonins, polymorphonuclear leukocytes (PMNs), and macrophages into the peritoneal cavity, where phagocytosis and destruction of bacteria can take place. However, in cirrhotic patients, this host defense mechanism is compromised because macrophages phagocytize bacteria poorly in the presence of ascites.[4,17]

In children, SBP occurs primarily in girls, and almost exclusively in children <10 years of age. Although pre-existing cirrhosis may be present, peritonitis generally occurs after necrotic liver disease, nephrotic syndrome, or urinary tract infections, and the infecting organisms are almost invariably *S. pneumoniae* or β-hemolytic streptococci. In the preantibiotic era, primary peritonitis accounted for about 10% of all pediatric abdominal emergencies. It now accounts for $<1\%$ to 2% of cases, perhaps because of the widespread use of antimicrobials for minor upper respiratory tract illness.[15] The spread of *S. pneumoniae* from the vagina may explain the higher frequency of SBP in the female pediatric population. The possibility of transfallopian spread also is suggested by the development of primary peritonitis in women using intrauterine devices (IUDs) and by perihepatitis caused by organisms infecting the female genitalia: gonococci and chlamydia (Fitz-Hugh-Curtis syndrome).[15]

Antimicrobial Therapy

6. What antimicrobial therapy should be considered for R.S. pending ascitic fluid culture results? How long should therapy be continued, and how should the response to therapy be monitored?

EMPIRIC

A Gram's stain of spun ascitic fluid may be helpful in selecting empiric antimicrobial therapy. Although a positive Gram's stain is diagnostic, 40% of patients with signs and symptoms of SBP have negative cultures.[17] Empiric therapy generally is aimed at likely pathogens, primarily *E. coli* and other Gram-negative enteric bacteria. Historically, ampicillin or a first-generation cephalosporin plus an aminoglycoside was used as empiric therapy.[15] While this regimen covers the expected pathogens, patients with SBP are particularly sensitive to the nephrotoxic effects of aminoglycosides.[18] Single-agent therapy with a third-generation cephalosporin or fluoroquinolone is also efficacious and avoids the risk of nephrotoxicity associated with aminoglycoside use.[18–20] β-Lactam/β-lactamase inhibitor combinations provide coverage of expected pathogens, and there are some data to support their use.[21] Single-agent empiric therapy is used until culture and sensitivity data are available.

THERAPEUTIC ENDPOINTS

In a prospective study, a PMN count of <250 cells/mm^3 in ascitic fluid was determined to be a suitable endpoint for termination of antibiotic therapy.[22] Patients who received "conventional" therapy in which the therapeutic endpoint was determined empirically received antibiotic courses that were significantly longer than those whose duration was determined by the PMN count. Mortality correlated with the severity of underlying liver disease rather than the duration of antibiotic therapy.

Antibiotic therapy is generally continued for at least 5 days.[18] Evidence shows that the PMN count in ascitic fluid generally decreases to $<250/mm^3$ in approximately 5 days,[22] and this is a reasonable therapeutic endpoint. In a clinical trial, a 5-day course of cefotaxime was as effective as a 10-day course.[23] The efficacy of a short duration of therapy has been confirmed in later trials.[24] Early recognition of SBP and prompt antibiotic therapy have reduced single-event mortality to 20% to 40%.[17] However, the long-term prognosis for these patients remains poor as a result of underlying liver disease.

R.S. should receive empiric therapy with an antimicrobial agent effective against *E. coli, S. pneumoniae,* and other common Gram-negative enteric pathogens such as *Klebsiella* species (e.g., IV cefotaxime 1 g Q 8 hr). Antimicrobial therapy should be tailored to the specific bacteria when culture and sensitivity results are available and should be continued for at least 5 days.

Prognosis

A poor short-term outcome of SBP is associated with increasing hepatic encephalopathy, renal insufficiency, hyperbilirubinemia, and hypoalbuminemia. A temperature $>38°C$ indicates a relatively intact host defense mechanism and is associated with increased survival. Although they occur less often, enteric bacteremias are associated with a significantly higher mortality than infections caused by nonenteric pathogens. Gram-negative infections are associated with a significantly higher mortality than infections caused by Gram-positive organisms.[4]

Prophylaxis

7. **After treatment is completed, should prophylactic antimicrobial therapy be initiated in R.S.?**

Recurrence rates for primary peritonitis are high, ranging from 43% at 6 months to 74% at 2 years.[25] Thus, prophylactic antimicrobial therapy with broad-spectrum agents has been advocated to reduce recurrence rates.[18] However, the risks and benefits must be carefully evaluated.

Long-term selective decontamination aimed at eliminating aerobic Gram-negative bacilli is effective and safe in preventing recurrent SBP in cirrhotic patients. Prospective, placebo-controlled, randomized studies in cirrhotic subjects with ascites have evaluated the efficacy of oral norfloxacin,[26] ciprofloxacin,[27] and trimethoprim-sulfamethoxazole (TMP-SMX).[16] Relative to placebo, each of these agents decreased the recurrence rate of SBP: 12% versus 35% for norfloxacin 400 mg/day; 3.6% versus 22% for ciprofloxacin 750 mg weekly; and 3% versus 27% for double-strength TMP-SMX five times weekly (Monday through Friday). None of these prophylactic regimens reduced mortality.

Concerns have been raised regarding the rapid emergence of bacterial resistance in cirrhotic patients receiving norfloxacin prophylaxis. In one study to determine the influence of prophylactic norfloxacin (400 mg/day) on fecal flora, fluoroquinolone-resistant isolates developed during treatment.[28] A second study documented the emergent problem of fluoroquinolone-resistant SBP in patients on long-term norfloxacin prophylaxis. Notably, the rate of TMP-SMX–resistant Gram-negative bacilli was also very high in patients receiving long-term norfloxacin, ruling out TMP-SMX as a viable alternative to norfloxacin.[29] Therefore, prophylactic antibiotics for selective decontamination should be used with caution.[17,18]

Cost analyses have determined the economic benefit of long-term antimicrobial prophylaxis for SBP in cirrhotics.[30] In a review of the literature, existing studies were stratified into three categories: antibiotic prophylaxis in all, antibiotic prophylaxis in none, or antibiotic prophylaxis in high-risk patients. High risk was defined as cirrhotic patients with high serum bilirubin (>2.5 mg/dL) and low ascitic fluid protein (<1 g/dL). Long-term antibiotic prophylaxis was particularly cost-effective when restricted to the group of patients at high risk for SBP. Notably, the highest cost per patient per day was associated with the group receiving no prophylaxis.

Prophylactic antibiotics are generally recommended in two situations: (1) secondary prophylaxis in patients with cirrhosis and ascites with a prior history of SBP and (2) primary prophylaxis in patients with cirrhosis who are admitted for acute upper GI hemorrhage.[17,18,31] Future studies may determine if primary prophylaxis reduces morbidity and mortality in patients with cirrhosis and ascites with no prior history of SBP, but currently use is not recommended in this population.

R.S. has cirrhosis, a previous episode of SBP, and a high total bilirubin; thus, he is at high risk for recurrence. Prophylactic antimicrobial therapy should be considered and may be a cost-effective measure. Any of the aforementioned prophylactic regimens would be appropriate for R.S. A specific choice for prophylactic therapy for R.S. would depend on institutional resistance patterns.

Penetration of Antimicrobial Agents Into the Peritoneum

8. **The physician asks if the agents chosen for treatment and prophylaxis of peritonitis in R.S. will penetrate the peritoneum. What properties determine the penetration of antibiotics into the peritoneum?**

The penetration of antimicrobial agents into tissues or abscess cavities depends on the serum-to-tissue fluid concentration gradient; the binding of the antimicrobial to serum and tissue proteins; the diffusibility of the drug, based on its molecular size and pKa; and lipid solubility.[32] In general, the β-lactam antimicrobials have been shown to achieve peritoneal tissue fluid concentrations that exceed typical minimum inhibitory concentrations (MICs) for most commonly encountered facultative Gram-negative and anaerobic bacteria.[32,33]

Continuous Ambulatory Peritoneal Dialysis–Associated Peritonitis

9. **S.K., a 23-year-old woman with diabetes mellitus and end-stage renal disease, has undergone continuous ambulatory peritoneal dialysis (CAPD) daily for the past year. She presents with abdominal pain and a cloudy dialysate fluid. S.K. maintains a residual urine volume of 150 mL per day. Against which bacteria should empiric antimicrobial therapy be directed? How should antimicrobial agents be administered?**

PATHOGENESIS

Approximately 80% of patients undergoing CAPD develop peritonitis during the first year of dialysis, and recurrent infection occurs in 20% to 30% of patients. Infections are caused primarily by Gram-positive bacteria (60% to 70% of cases), with coagulase-negative staphylococci responsible for approximately 40% of all infections (see Table 63-1). Gram-negative bacteria are isolated in approximately 25% of cases; anaerobes, fungi, and mycobacteria constitute the remainder of the commonly observed pathogens. The source of most Gram-positive infections is the patient's own skin flora.[34] The source and portal of entry of other bacteria are unclear, although transmural migration of bacteria has been suggested, and continuous spread from the skin along the peritoneal dialysis cuff to the peritoneum has been demonstrated. Patients may present with abdominal pain and tenderness, but fever is not a consistent finding. Often the only clue to the presence of infection is a cloudy dialysate, although bacteria may be seen on examination of a centrifuged specimen. Fortunately, most patients do not have positive blood cultures.[15]

ANTIMICROBIAL THERAPY

The optimal antimicrobial regimen and appropriate dose, route, and duration of therapy for the treatment of CAPD-associated peritonitis are unclear because of a paucity of randomized, controlled trials. In general, empiric antibiotic therapy should be directed against both Gram-positive and facultative Gram-negative enteric bacteria until cultures of peritoneal fluid are available. After IV administration, most antimicrobial agents reach therapeutic concentrations within the peritoneal cavity. Intraperitoneal administration of antibiotics also can be employed because this produces high concentrations of antibiotics at the site of infection. Most agents readily cross the peritoneal membrane, with 50% to 80% of the intraperitoneal dose reaching the systemic circulation. Approximately 70% to 80% of patients can be treated on an outpatient basis with IV and/or intraperitoneal instillation of antimicrobials. Oral treatment of peritonitis in CAPD with fluoroquinolones may be emerging as an option, but further studies of oral versus intraperitoneal agents are needed.[35]

Revised treatment recommendations for CAPD-associated peritonitis provide a systematic approach for antimicrobial management, antibiotic selection, dosing guidelines, duration of therapy, and prophylaxis.[36] Empiric coverage of Gram-positive and Gram-negative organisms with a first-generation cephalosporin (e.g., cefazolin) in combination with ceftazidime is recommended. Because of emerging resistance, vancomycin is no longer recommended as empiric therapy. Since residual renal function is an independent predictor of survival, the routine use of nephrotoxic aminoglycosides should be avoided in patients who are not anuric and who have a residual urine volume of >100 mL per day. In anuric patients, cefazolin plus an aminoglycoside is an appropriate empiric regimen.

Culture and sensitivity results should guide changes to empiric therapy. If enterococci alone are isolated, the cephalosporins should be discontinued. Guidelines recommend the administration of ampicillin, with addition of an aminoglycoside based on sensitivity.[36] However, considering the high rate of ampicillin-resistant enterococci, many clinicians recommend vancomycin for enterococci until sensitivity results are available. If *S. aureus* alone is isolated, appropriate therapy depends on sensitivity to methicillin. When methicillin-sensitive *S. aureus* (MSSA) is isolated, ceftazidime should be discontinued and the first-generation cephalosporin continued. Both antibiotics may be discontinued, and guidelines rec-

ommend that vancomycin or clindamycin should be initiated with rifampin (600 mg/day orally) if methicillin-resistant *S. aureus* (MRSA) is isolated. However, many clinicians would consider vancomycin monotherapy appropriate at this time. Clindamycin or vancomycin alone is recommended when methicillin-resistant *S. epidermidis* (MRSE) is isolated. In <20% of cases, cultures are negative. If there is no evidence of a Gram-negative infection and the patient is improving after 5 days of empiric coverage, a first-generation cephalosporin alone should be continued.

When a single ceftazidime-sensitive Gram-negative organism is cultured (e.g., *E. coli, Klebsiella,* or *Proteus*), the first-generation cephalosporin should be stopped.[36] When Gram-negative organisms are cultured, therapy should be adjusted based on local sensitivity patterns. Ceftazidime may be continued, but many clinicians prefer to switch to a non-antipseudomonal agent active against the Gram-negative organism cultured, such as ceftriaxone. Anaerobic coverage with metronidazole in combination with ceftazidime, or a β-lactamase inhibitor combination, is considered if an anaerobic Gram-negative organism is cultured. For infections caused by *P. aeruginosa,* double coverage is recommended. Ceftazidime is continued and a second agent with activity against the isolated organism is added, such as ciprofloxacin, aztreonam, or an aminoglycoside. Table 63-3 lists antimicrobial dosing guidelines for the treatment of peritonitis associated with CAPD.[36] Separate consensus guidelines are now available with recommendations regarding the treatment of peritonitis in children receiving peritoneal dialysis.[37]

The use of ceftazidime in these guidelines has been met with some concern over the potential emergence of ceftazidime-resistant Enterobacteriaceae.[38] These guidelines do not represent the only way to treat peritoneal dialysis patients with peritonitis. Local bacterial flora and resistance patterns should be considered.

Since S.K. is not anuric, her empiric treatment regimen should not include an aminoglycoside. S.K. should receive ceftazidime plus cefazolin given intraperitoneally. The clinician should follow culture and sensitivity results to adjust therapy based on guidelines, local sensitivity patterns, and therapeutic response.

FUNGAL PERITONITIS

10. **Two years later, S.K. again presents with abdominal pain and cloudy dialysate fluid.** *Candida albicans* **is cultured from the dialysate fluid. No other organisms are present. How should S.K. be treated?**

Fungal peritonitis is a rare complication of CAPD, accounting for only 3% of all episodes.[39] In patients undergoing CAPD, *Candida* can attach to the peritoneal catheter; thus, even prolonged antimicrobial therapy with amphotericin B, parenteral and locally instilled, may not eradicate the infection. There are other problems. Penetration of amphotericin B into the peritoneal fluid is minimal because it is extensively bound to serum protein, and intraperitoneal instillation of amphotericin B often is irritating to the mucosa. Antifungal therapy appears merely to suppress the infection, and removal of the catheter may be required to eradicate the infection.[15,39] Fluconazole is active against *C. albicans* but has no activity against certain types of non-albicans *Candida,* such as *C. glabrata.*

Table 63-3   Antibiotic Dosing Recommendations for CAPD (Only) Patients With and Without Residual Renal Function[a]

Drug	CAPD Intermittent Dosing (once/day)		CAPD Continuous Dosing (per liter exchange)	
	Anuric	Nonanuric	Anuric	Nonanuric
Aminoglycosides				
Amikacin	2 mg/kg	Increase anuric doses by 25%	MD 24 mg	Increase all MD by 25%
Gentamicin	0.6 mg/kg		MD 8 mg	
Tobramycin	0.6 mg/kg		MD 8 mg	
Cephalosporins				All LD same as anuric
Cefazolin	15 mg/kg	20 mg/kg	LD 500 mg, MD 125 mg	MD increase by 25%
Cephalothin	15 mg/kg	ND	LD 500 mg, MD 125 mg	MD, ND
Cephalexin	500 mg PO, QID	ND	As intermittent	MD, ND
Cefuroxime	400 mg PO/IV, QD	ND	LD 200 mg, MD 100–200 mg	MD, ND
Ceftazidime	1,000–1,500 mg	ND	LD 250 mg, MD 125 mg	MD, ND
Ceftizoxime	1,000 mg	ND	LD 250 mg, MD 125 mg	MD, ND
Penicillins				All LD same as anuric
Piperacillin	4,000 mg IV, BID	ND	LD 4 g IV, MD 250 mg	MD, ND
Ampicillin	250–500 mg PO, BID	ND	MD 125 or 250–500 mg PO, BID	MD, ND
Dicloxacillin	250–500 mg PO, QID	ND	250–500 mg PO, QID	MD, ND
Oxacillin	ND	ND	MD 125 mg	MD, ND
Nafcillin	ND	No change	MD 125 mg	MD, no change
Amoxicillin	ND	ND	LD 250–500 mg, MD 50 mg	MD, ND
Penicillin G	ND	ND	LD 50,000 U, MD 25,000 U	MD, ND
Quinolones				
Ciprofloxacin	500 mg PO, BID	ND	LD 50 mg, MD 25 mg	ND
Ofloxacin	400 mg PO, then 200 mg PO, QD	ND	As intermittent	ND
Others				
Vancomycin	15–30 mg/kg q.5–7 d	Increase anuric doses by 25%	MD 30–50 mg/L	Increase MD by 25%
Aztreonam	ND	ND	LD 1000 mg, MD 250 mg	ND
Clindamycin	ND	ND	LD 300 mg, MD 150 mg	ND
Metronidazole	250 mg PO, BID	ND	As intermittent	ND
Rifampin	300 mg PO, BID	ND	As intermittent	ND
Antifungals				All LD same as anuric
Amphotericin	NA	NA	MD 1.5 mg	NA
Fluconazole	200 mg QD	ND	As intermittent	ND
Itraconazole	100 mg Q 12 hr	ND	100 mg Q 12 hr	100 mg Q 12 hr
Combinations				All LD same as anuric
Ampicillin/sulbactam	2 g Q 12 hr	100 mg Q 12 hr	LD 1000 mg, MD 100 mg	ND
Trimeth/ sulfamethoxazole	320/1,600 mg PO, Q 1–2 days	ND	LD 320/1600 mg PO, MD 80/400 mg PO	ND

CAPD patients with residual renal function may require increased doses or more frequent dosing, especially when using intermittent regimens. For penicillins: "No change" is for those predominantly hepatically metabolized, or hepatically metabolized and renally excreted; "ND" means no data, but these are predominantly renally excreted, therefore probably an increase in dose by 25% is warranted; "NA" = not applicable, that is, drug is extensively metabolized and therefore there should be no difference in dosing between anuric and nonanuric patients. Anuric = <100 mL urine/24 hours; nonanuric = >100 mL/24 hours. These data for CAPD only.

[a]The route of administration is IP unless otherwise specified. The pharmacokinetic data and proposed dosage regimens presented here are based on published literature reviewed through January 2000, or established clinical practice. There is no evidence that mixing different antibiotics in dialysis fluid (except for aminoglycosides and penicillins) is deleterious to the drugs or patients. Do not use the same syringe to mix antibiotics.

BID, twice per day; IP, intraperitoneally; IV, intravenous; LD, loading dose; MD, maintenance dose; NA, not applicable; ND, no data; PO, oral; QID, four times per day; QD, once per day.

Reprinted with permission from: Keane WF, et al. Adult peritoneal dialysis-related peritonitis treatment recommendations: 2000 update. Perit Dial Int. 2000;20:400.

S.K.'s treatment should include temporary catheter removal and administration of antifungal agents. Antifungal therapy with amphotericin B (IV and/or intraperitoneal) or fluconazole (oral, 200 mg/day) should be continued for 10 to 14 days.[39,40]

SECONDARY PERITONITIS

Pathogenesis and Epidemiology

Secondary peritonitis usually occurs after contamination of the peritoneal cavity or its surrounding structures by intestinal contents.[15,41] Intra-abdominal infections most often occur after perforation of the GI tract (e.g., appendicitis, diverticulitis, perforated ulcer, abdominal trauma, bowel neoplasm). The most common type of intra-abdominal infection is generalized peritonitis after penetrating or blunt abdominal trauma.

Localization of intra-abdominal infections without eradication of bacteria results in intraperitoneal or visceral abscesses. Intraperitoneal abscesses occur most often in the right lower quadrant in association with appendicitis or a perforated peptic ulcer. Visceral abscesses generally are found in the pancreas but occasionally occur in the liver, spleen, or kidney.[4]

Normal Gastrointestinal Flora

Because intra-abdominal infections result from perforation of the intestinal tract, the normal flora of the perforated segment of the intestinal tract determine the initial bacterial inoculum (Fig. 63-1). The stomach of fasting individuals contains very few bacteria (i.e., <100 colony-forming units [CFU]/mL) because of the combined effects of gastric motility and the bactericidal activity of normal gastric fluid, which has a pH of 1 to 2.[13] The bacterial population of the stomach can be altered by drugs or diseases that increase gastric pH or decrease gastric motility. Thus, patients with bleeding or obstructing duodenal ulcers, gastric ulcers, or gastric carcinomas have an increased number of oral anaerobes and facultative Gram-negative bacteria colonizing the stomach.

The upper small intestine (duodenum and jejunum) usually contains relatively few bacteria and harbors mainly oral flora. The lower small intestine serves as a transitional zone between the sparsely populated stomach and the abundant mi-

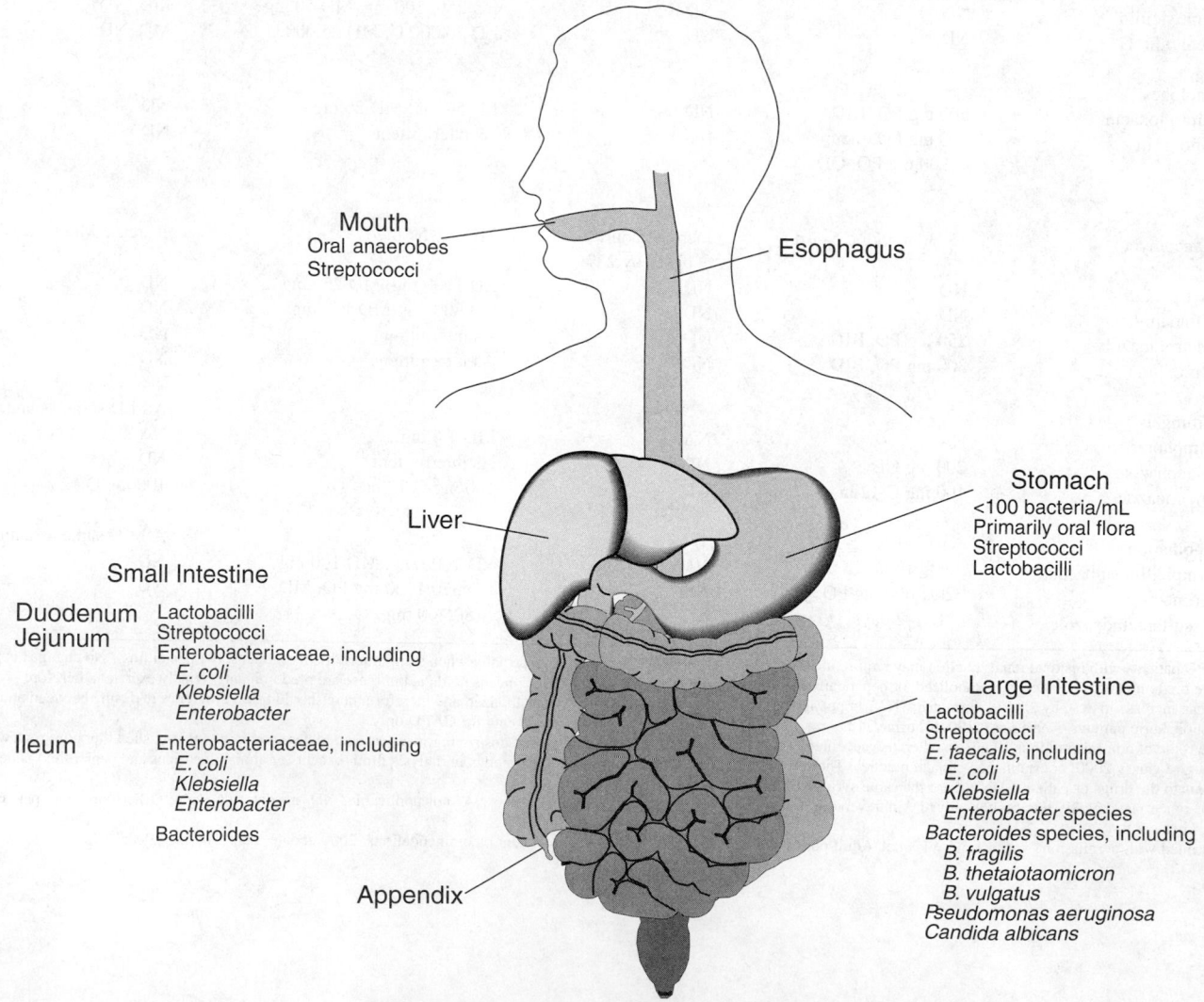

FIGURE 63-1 Microflora of the gastrointestinal tract.

crobial flora of the colon.[4] The biliary tree is generally sterile, although colonization with aerobic Gram-negative bacilli (particularly *E. coli* and *Klebsiella*) is more likely in patients with biliary tract stones, jaundice, or morbid obesity and in patients >60 years of age.[2] In the ileum, facultative Gram-negative and Gram-positive species as well as obligate anaerobes are encountered. As the distal ileum is approached, the quantity and variety of bacteria increase. Substantial numbers of anaerobic bacteria are present, including *Bacteroides* species as well as *E. coli* and enterococci.[1,4,15]

In the large bowel, anaerobic bacteria, particularly *Bacteroides* species, predominate. In the distal colon, bacterial counts average 10^{11} CFU/mL of feces, with anaerobes outnumbering other organisms by a ratio of 1,000:1.[4] Although large numbers of *Clostridia,* anaerobic cocci, and non–spore-forming anaerobic rods are present, the most prevalent anaerobes are *Bacteroides* species. Among the facultative aerobes, *E. coli* is the most frequently isolated species.[1,4,15] The majority of fecal weight consists of viable bacteria.[4] Given these differences in regional microflora populations, it is not surprising that trauma to the colon (which contains large numbers of bacteria) carries a much higher risk of intra-abdominal infection than trauma to the stomach or jejunum.[42]

Diagnosis

11. T.R., a 49-year-old man, presents with severe abdominal pain and nausea. Endoscopy reveals a perforated duodenal ulcer. Vital signs include temperature of 101°F and tachycardia (pulse, 110 beats/min). Bowel sounds are absent. Laboratory values are WBC count, $17 \times 10^3/\text{mm}^3$ (normal, 3.2 to 9.8), and blood urea nitrogen (BUN), 30 mg/dL (normal, 8 to 18). What signs and symptoms of an intra-abdominal infection does T.R. display? What bacteria should be considered as potential pathogens if T.R. has an intra-abdominal infection?

[SI units: WBC count, $17 \times 10^9/\text{L}$ (normal, 3.2 to 9.8); BUN, 11 mmol/L (normal, 3 to 6.5)]

Signs and Symptoms of Infection

Making the diagnosis of a localized intra-abdominal infection may be difficult, despite the presence of signs and symptoms typical of severe infection. The patient may experience pain and voluntary guarding of the abdomen, with shallow, rapid respirations. Generalized abdominal pain usually is followed by a rigid, "board-like" tensing of the abdominal muscles.[4] Inflammation around the intestines and peritoneal cavity results in local paralysis and reflex rigidity of the abdominal wall muscles and the diaphragm, causing rapid and shallow respirations.[4] Bowel sounds may be faint or absent with concomitant abdominal distention, nausea, and vomiting. Fever usually is present with tachycardia and decreased urine output secondary to fluid loss into the peritoneum. These signs usually are accompanied by an elevated WBC count of 17,000 to 25,000/mm³ with a predominance of neutrophils (left shift). The hematocrit (Hct) and BUN may be elevated as a result of dehydration. Initially, patients are usually alkalotic as a result of vomiting and hyperventilation, but in the later stages of peritonitis, acidosis usually occurs. Untreated peritonitis results in generalized sepsis and hypovolemic shock.[4]

A Gram's stain should be performed immediately on infected material to identify potential pathogens. The presence of pleomorphic Gram-negative bacilli, a strong odor, or tissue gas is strongly suggestive of infection with anaerobes, particularly *B. fragilis.* Cultures using appropriate media for the isolation of both facultative and anaerobic bacteria should be performed before antimicrobial therapy is initiated. Plain abdominal x-rays or sonography may help to localize sites of intra-abdominal abscesses.

12. Given these findings, what are the most likely pathogens for T.R.'s intra-abdominal infection?

Infecting Pathogens

The microbiology of intra-abdominal infection was first documented >60 years ago when anaerobic and facultative Gram-negative bacteria were identified in patients with appendicitis.[43] Studies consistently document a mixed culture of aerobes and anaerobes.[15] The presence of anaerobic bacteria in the culture is indicative of a polymicrobial infection.[15]

The most commonly isolated facultative bacterium is *E. coli,* which is found in approximately 60% of cultures. A variety of other Gram-negative bacteria also are isolated, including *Klebsiella* species, *Proteus* species, *Enterobacter* species, and *P. aeruginosa* (Table 63-4).[44-46] Highly antibiotic-resistant strains of *P. aeruginosa, Enterobacter* species, and enterococci often are isolated from patients who develop intra-abdominal infections while hospitalized.[15] *B. fragilis* is the most important anaerobe recovered from intra-abdominal sites because of its particular virulence factors. It is the most frequently isolated anaerobe following perforation of the colon.[15] Anaerobic cocci (peptostreptococci) and facultative Gram-positive cocci, such as enterococci, are also isolated.[44-46] Although rarely isolated in pure culture from intra-abdominal infections, *B. fragilis* and *E. coli* are the most commonly isolated pathogens found in blood culture samples after bacteremia from intra-abdominal infection.[4]

In summary, T.R. is likely to have an intra-abdominal infection caused by mixed flora, containing both aerobic and anaerobic bacteria. His current clinical status, highlighted by an elevated temperature, is probably secondary to the presence of facultative Gram-negative bacteria such as *E. coli, Proteus, Klebsiella,* or *Enterobacter. P. aeruginosa, Candida* species, or other resistant bacteria are less likely to be present

Table 63-4   Bacteriology of Intra-Abdominal Infections[44-46]

Bacteria	% of Patients
Facultative and Aerobic	
Escherichia coli	24–81
Proteus sp.	3–6
Klebsiella or *Enterobacter* sp.	6–19
Streptococci (including enterococci)	11–42
Staphylococci	2–9
Pseudomonas aeruginosa	2–16
Anaerobes	
Bacteroides fragilis	31–43
Other *Bacteroides* sp.	9–41
Peptostreptococci	6
Clostridium sp.	3–18
Fusobacterium sp.	<2.5

unless T.R. has recently undergone prolonged hospitalization or received broad-spectrum antimicrobial agents.

13. If T.R. were left untreated, what would be the typical course of an intra-abdominal infection? What roles do the facultative (e.g., coliform) and anaerobic bacteria play in the infection?

Studies suggest that synergy between anaerobic and facultative bacteria is important in abscess formation, and that coliform bacteria are responsible for early mortality in intra-abdominal infections, whereas anaerobic bacteria are primarily responsible for the late complication of intra-abdominal abscess formation.[47] Although many *Bacteroides* species possess capsules or capsule-like material located on the surface, only the capsular polysaccharide of *B. fragilis* appears capable of potentiating abscesses.[48]

Several possible mechanisms have been proposed to explain the increased virulence of the combination of facultative and anaerobic bacteria:

1. Production of enzymes by one bacterium may permit tissue invasion by the other bacteria.[47]
2. Critical growth factors or nutrients produced by one organism may permit survival of another pathogen at the site of infection.
3. Aerobic bacteria may lower local oxygen concentrations and the oxidation-reduction potential, producing the appropriate environment for the replication of anaerobic species.
4. One organism may protect another from natural host defenses. For example, *B. fragilis* reduces opsonization of *E. coli* by leukocytes.[47]

Antimicrobial Therapy

Empiric Therapy

14. How should T.R. be managed? Based on clinical studies, what empiric antimicrobial therapy is appropriate for T.R. at this time?

Therapy for intra-abdominal infection should include surgical intervention and drainage, antimicrobial therapy directed at facultative Gram-negative bacteria and obligate anaerobes, fluid therapy, and support of vital functions. Surgical debridement and drainage in conjunction with appropriate antimicrobial therapy have been shown to decrease the morbidity and mortality associated with this disease.[15,49] Therapy with an agent with activity against *P. aeruginosa* is desirable if the infectious process develops while the patient is hospitalized or has received broad-spectrum antimicrobials. This is not necessary in T.R.

In general, when an intra-abdominal infection is present, antimicrobial agents should be started immediately after appropriate specimens (e.g., blood, peritoneal fluid, abscess drainage) are obtained for culture and sensitivity and before any surgical procedures are performed.[1] The appropriate dosage and parenteral route should be used to ensure adequate systemic and tissue concentrations, especially in patients in whom shock or poor perfusion of the muscles or GI tract precludes the use of oral or intramuscular (IM) routes of administration. Therefore, antimicrobial therapy is generally empiric, based on the expected pathogens at the site of infection. Table 63-5 outlines dosing recommendations for antibiotics commonly used in the treatment of intra-abdominal infections.

The antimicrobial regimen should provide coverage against facultative and anaerobic Gram-negative bacilli such as *E. coli* and *B. fragilis,* respectively, because they are the most common intra-abdominal pathogens.

Clindamycin combined with gentamicin is historically the standard antimicrobial therapy against which other treatment regimens for intra-abdominal infections should be compared.[15] Although the standard regimen is clearly efficacious, the potential for nephrotoxicity secondary to aminoglycosides and clindamycin-associated enterocolitis have led investigators to search for alternative therapies. Multiple regimens have been found to be efficacious for the treatment of intra-abdominal infections in randomized, controlled clinical trials.[8,44,45,50–55] Many of these regimens were taken into consideration in the Surgical Infection Society Guidelines. For mild to moderate community-acquired intra-abdominal infections, monotherapy with cefotetan or cefoxitin, β-lactam/β-lactamase inhibitors, or carbapenems is recommended.[56] For severe infections, monotherapy with imipenem/cilastatin[56] or combination therapy with clindamycin or metronidazole with a third- or fourth-generation cephalosporin, ciprofloxacin, aztreonam, or an aminoglycoside is recommended.[56]

Meropenem and imipenem/cilastatin, because of their broad spectrum of activity, should be reserved as last-line agents in the treatment of more resistant Gram-negative organisms. These antimicrobials should be used only in patients suspected of having multiple resistant pathogens.

Piperacillin/tazobactam, ticarcillin/clavulanic acid, and ampicillin/sulbactam are the β-lactam/β-lactamase inhibitors that may be used in the treatment of intra-abdominal infections. However, ampicillin/sulbactam should not be used in severe infections due to its inferior activity against nosocomial Gram-negative organisms. Clinical efficacy, cost, and the impact on the cost of care should all be considered when choosing a regimen.

T.R. should receive antimicrobial therapy with activity against facultative Gram-negative bacteria and anaerobes, including *B. fragilis.* IV cefotetan 1 g Q 12 hr would be an appropriate treatment for T.R.'s mild to moderate infection.

Duration of Antimicrobial Therapy

15. For how long should T.R. receive antimicrobial therapy?

Recommendations for the duration of therapy for intra-abdominal infection vary from 5 to 7 days and depend primarily on the patient's clinical response to therapy.[56] In general, antimicrobial therapy should be continued until the patient's temperature, WBC count, and differential are within normal limits. T.R.'s antimicrobial therapy should be continued for 5 to 7 days or until his temperature and WBC count fall to within normal limits.

Monotherapy

16. K.B. is a 52-year-old, 86-kg, nonobese man with colon carcinoma. One day after undergoing surgical resection of the colon, he develops a fever of 102°F, shaking chills, and abdomi-

Table 63-5   Treatment of Intra-Abdominal Infection

Regimen	Dosage
Combination Therapy[a]	
1) Metronidazole (or clindamycin)	500 (600) mg IV Q 8 hr
plus	
Aminoglycoside	5 mg/kg/day IV Q 24 hr
or	(normal renal function)
2) Metronidazole (or clindamycin)	500 (600) mg IV Q 8 hr
plus	
Aztreonam	1 g Q 8 hr
or	
3) Metronidazole (or clindamycin)	500 (600) mg IV Q 8 hr
plus	
2nd- or 3rd-generation cephalosporin	(see below)
Monotherapy	
Cefotaxime (Claforan)[a,b,c]	1 g Q 6–8 hr
Cefotetan (Cefotan)[a,b]	1–2 g Q 12 hr
Cefoxitin (Mefoxin)[a,b]	1–2 g Q 6 hr
Ceftizoxime (Cefizox)[a,b]	1 g Q 8 hr
Ceftriaxone (Rocephin)[a,b,c]	1 g Q 24 hr
Ertapenem (Invanz)	1 g Q 24 hr
Piperacillin (Pipracil)[d]	4 g Q 6 hr
Imipenem-cilastatin (Primaxin)[a,e]	0.5 g Q 6 hr
Meropenem (Merem)	1 g Q 8 hr
Ticarcillin-clavulanic acid (Timentin)[a,f]	3.1 g Q 6–8 hr
Ampicillin-sulbactam (Unasyn)[f]	3 g Q 6 hr
Piperacillin-tazobactam (Zosyn)[f]	3.375 g Q 6–8 hr

[a]Ampicillin or vancomycin may need to be added if enterococci are suspected. Use vancomycin in penicillin-allergic patients. This combination covers *B. fragilis, E. coli,* and enterococci.
[b]Cephalosporins have excellent activity against *E. coli,* moderate to good coverage of *B. fragilis,* and no activity against enterococci.
[c]Cefotaxime and ceftriaxone have limited anaerobic activity; thus, the addition of agents such as metronidazole may be necessary.
[d]The ureidopenicillins have moderate aerobic and anaerobic activity and excellent enterococcal activity. However, these agents should be reserved for suspected or documented pseudomonal infection.
[e]Imipenem has excellent activity versus *B. fragilis;* however, its activity against multidrug-resistant Gram-negative bacilli such as *Pseudomonas aeruginosa* and *Enterobacter cloacae,* suggests that its use be restricted to the treatment of infection secondary to these organisms.
[f]Ampicillin/sulbactam, piperacillin/tazobactam, and ticarcillin/clavulanic acid have excellent activity versus *B. fragilis,* approaching that of metronidazole. Ticarcillin/clavulanic acid, however, has limited enterococcal activity, whereas ampicillin/sulbactam has excellent activity against this organism but only moderate aerobic gram-negative activity. Piperacillin/tazobactam is active against both enterococcus and most Gram-negative aerobes.

nal pain. **Laboratory values are WBC count, 16.2 ×10³/mm³ (normal, 3.2 to 9.8), and creatinine, 1.3 mg/dL (normal, 0.6 to 1.2). What empiric therapy would be appropriate for K.B.?**

[SI units: WBC count, 16.2 ×10⁹/L (normal, 3.2 to 9.8); creatinine, 115 μmol/L (normal, 50 to 110)]

A number of potent, broad-spectrum antimicrobials have been evaluated as single agents for the treatment of intra-abdominal infections.[8,44,45,50–55] Second- and third-generation cephalosporins, imipenem/cilastatin, meropenem, piperacillin/tazobactam, and ampicillin/sulbactam have all been compared with combination drug regimens containing aminoglycosides. In a comparative phase III trial of ertapenem versus piperacillin/tazobactam, the two agents were shown to be similar in efficacy and safety. Results from this study suggest that ertapenem may be another suitable option for the treatment of mixed aerobic and anaerobic intra-abdominal infections.[57] Moxifloxacin and garenoxacin also have anaerobic coverage and are being investigated as monotherapy for this indication. Since monotherapy has been shown to be efficacious in numerous trials, combination therapy is now rarely used.

K.B. is a high-risk patient because he has been exposed to a heavy bacterial inoculum resulting from colonic perforation. K.B. should be started on piperacillin/tazobactam 3.375 g IV Q 6 hr. Therapy should be continued until the results of blood and peritoneal fluid cultures are available.

Enterococcal Infection

17. **K.B.'s peritoneal fluid cultures reveal a mixed infection with *E. coli, B. fragilis, C. albicans,* and *Enterococcus*. Blood cultures are negative. Should he receive additional antimicrobial therapy active against *Enterococcus*?**

Although *Enterococcus* is commonly cultured in patients with secondary peritonitis, its pathogenicity has been questioned and there is ambivalence regarding the necessity for antimicrobial coverage for this organism. *Enterococcus* can cause serious infections (e.g., endocarditis, urinary tract infections), although it often has been considered relatively nonvirulent in the setting of polymicrobial infections such as intra-abdominal abscess.

An important issue is whether empiric treatment should have included antibiotics directed specifically against *Enterococcus*. Some investigators believe that enterococci are commensal organisms that need not be treated in most clinical settings. They point to clinical studies in which antibiotic regimens lacking in vitro activity against enterococci have been successful. The pathogenicity of enterococci lies in its ability to enhance the formation of abscesses.[15]

In general, enterococcal coverage is warranted only if *Enterococcus* is present in blood cultures, is the sole organism on culture, or is the predominant organism on Gram's stain.[15] Because K.B.'s blood cultures are negative and ascitic culture has demonstrated mixed pathogens, enterococcal coverage is not necessary. K.B. should be treated with an antimicrobial regimen that has activity against Gram-negative coliforms and anaerobes.

Antifungal Therapy: Treatment of Candida

18. Should K.B.'s antimicrobial therapy include an agent with antifungal activity?

The need to treat *Candida* species as a solitary isolate or as part of a polymicrobial infection is controversial. Certainly, *Candida* has the potential to cause peritonitis, intraperitoneal abscesses, and subsequent candidemia. Parenteral administration of amphotericin B is the standard for fungal peritonitis.[15] However, concern over the toxicity of amphotericin is warranted, and the risk/benefit ratio must be assessed carefully for each patient. To date, there are no clinical trials assessing the efficacy and safety of lipid-based amphotericin B or caspofungin in the treatment of intra-abdominal fungal infections. The use of antifungal agents such as fluconazole may offer decreased toxicity in these patients. However, the potential risk of the development of resistance must be addressed in clinical trials.

Therapy with an IV antifungal agent is not warranted at this time unless positive blood cultures for *Candida* are isolated or K.B. fails to respond to appropriate antimicrobial therapy.

Antimicrobial Irrigations

19. K.B.'s physician wishes to irrigate the peritoneum with aminoglycosides to achieve high local concentrations. Is irrigation with antimicrobial agents rational or effective in the treatment of intra-abdominal infections?

Some clinicians are reluctant to irrigate the peritoneal cavity for fear of spreading local infection, further damaging the mesothelium, diluting opsonins, or suspending bacteria in a fluid medium, where they are less amenable to phagocytosis. However, most animal studies demonstrate that gravity and the movement of the diaphragm during respiration spread bacteria throughout the peritoneal cavity even in the absence of irrigation. In addition, free circulation of fluids within the peritoneal cavity facilitates lymphatic clearance of microorganisms and toxins.[58]

Although data are limited, systemic antibiotic therapy and antibiotic irrigations appear to be equally efficacious for both the prevention and treatment of postoperative infections.[59,60]

However, the clinician must recognize the potential for systemic toxicity resulting from systemic absorption of antimicrobial agents from the peritoneal cavity. Most antimicrobials are readily absorbed from mucosal surfaces, especially when they are inflamed. When large volumes of irrigating solution containing antibiotics are used (especially in combination with IV doses), systemic drug concentrations can markedly exceed the therapeutic range. Neuromuscular blockade, renal failure, and ototoxicity have been reported after absorption of aminoglycosides from mucosal surfaces. Although a greater margin of safety exists for many of the penicillins and cephalosporins, the potential for toxicity is still of concern.[61]

There are few data to support the superiority of antibiotic-containing irrigating solutions over systemic therapy. Given the potential for systemic toxicity secondary to absorption of antimicrobial agents from the peritoneum, the paucity of controlled trials documenting the efficacy of this method of administration, and the proven efficacy of systemic therapy, it seems prudent to use systemic therapy alone for the treatment of intra-abdominal infections. If irrigation of contaminated tissue is desired, antibiotic-free dialysate should be used.[61]

Anaerobic Bacteria

20. The surgical resident continues K.B. on piperacillin/tazobactam for the treatment of his intra-abdominal infection. Should culture and sensitivity results be used to monitor for anaerobic activity?

With the introduction of broad-spectrum antimicrobial agents with in vitro activity against *B. fragilis* and a significant problem of increasing resistance, the choice of a specific antianaerobic agent has become more complex. Multiple mechanisms of resistance are encountered, and resistance rates differ among various geographic areas of the United States. Although *Bacteroides* resistance to metronidazole is rare,[15,62] resistance to clindamycin is increasing.[15] Isolates resistant to β-lactams are common in some centers, but the resistance rates may be decreasing.[62] In general, the carbapenems and the β-lactamase inhibitor combinations continue to be active against *Bacteroides*. However, resistant strains have been isolated. It is important to be aware of institution-specific resistance patterns.

The Working Group on Anaerobic Susceptibility Testing of the National Committee for Clinical Laboratory Standards (NCCLS) has suggested that susceptibility testing should be performed in four settings:

1. To determine patterns of susceptibility of anaerobes to new antimicrobial agents
2. To periodically monitor susceptibility patterns on a geographic basis
3. To periodically monitor susceptibility patterns in local institutions
4. To assist occasionally in the management of individual patients[63]

Because most anaerobes are cultured in the setting of mixed flora, isolation of individual components of a complex mixture can be time consuming. In addition, most anaerobes are very slow growing, and it may take days to weeks for a definitive culture and sensitivity report. If specimens are not collected and transported in optimal media or in a timely manner, inaccurate or misleading results may be reported. The methods for susceptibility testing of anaerobic bacteria are not well standardized, and many hospital laboratories do not have the funds or expertise to perform extensive culture and sensitivity testing.[64] In fact, Dougherty maintains that routine cultures may be unnecessary because few routine cultures affect the choice of antibiotic regimen, and empiric therapy usually determines outcome.[65] Therefore, empiric therapy must be aimed at the most likely pathogens, and the clinician must be aware of the usual sensitivity patterns at the institution. Routine susceptibility testing for patient-specific cases is not recommended because of the prolonged length of time to achieve results.

Intra-Abdominal Abscess

21. W.D. is a 40-year-old man who has undergone abdominal surgery. Two weeks postoperatively, he develops abdominal pain and purulent material begins to drain from his abdominal wound. An intra-abdominal abscess is visualized by plain films. How did this abscess develop? What considerations should be taken into account in the selection of appropriate antimicrobial agents?

Abscesses are collections of necrotic tissue, bacteria, and WBCs that form over a period of days to years. They generally result from chronic inflammation and the body's attempt to localize organisms and toxic substances by formation of an avascular fibrous wall. This isolates bacteria and the liquid core from opsonins and antimicrobial agents.

Microbiology
Although pathogens encountered in abscesses are similar to other intra-abdominal infections, abscesses pose a therapeutic challenge because they typically contain large bacterial inocula that are likely to include small subpopulations of resistant bacteria.[49] Furthermore, the rate of penetration of antibiotics into abscesses is hindered by the low surface-to-volume ratio and the presence of a fibrous capsule.

Although surgical debridement and drainage of W.D.'s abscess is crucial, adjunctive therapy with antimicrobial agents is warranted. The optimal antimicrobial agent must rapidly penetrate into the abscess in adequate concentrations and possess the antimicrobial spectrum that provides optimal activity in the treatment of intra-abdominal abscesses.[15,49] W.D. should be placed on an antimicrobial regimen that covers Gram-negative bacteria and anaerobes, such as imipenem/cilastatin.

INFECTIONS AFTER ABDOMINAL TRAUMA

Risk factors for infection after penetrating abdominal trauma include the number, type, and location of injuries; the presence of hypotension; large transfusion requirements; prolonged operation; advanced age; and the mechanism of injury.[66]

Most investigators stress the importance of instituting antimicrobial therapy as close to the time of trauma as possible. Fullen and colleagues[67] demonstrated a significant reduction in the incidence of postoperative infections when antibiotics were administered before laparotomy for surgical repair of trauma, compared with patients whose antibiotics were initiated during or after surgery.

Antimicrobial Therapy
Penetrating Trauma

22. J.K., a 23-year-old man, is admitted to the emergency department within 1 hour after sustaining a gunshot wound to the stomach, colon, and right thigh. He is to undergo emergency laparotomy. What antimicrobial therapy is appropriate at this time?

As with other types of intra-abdominal infections, the use of antibiotics active against both aerobic and anaerobic pathogens has become the cornerstone of therapy for peritoneal contamination after penetrating abdominal trauma.

Anti-infective therapy has been studied in patients who have sustained penetrating trauma to the abdomen (usually from knife or gunshot wounds). Generally, second- and third-generation cephalosporins that may be less toxic and less costly are compared with clindamycin plus gentamicin. In several comparative trials, single-drug therapy with cefoxitin was as effective as the combination of clindamycin or metronidazole plus an aminoglycoside.[68,69] However, in evaluating these studies, it is important to note that the majority of patients did not sustain injuries to the colon, where the risk of infection is highest. In studies that did include patients with perforations of the colon and rectum or colonic perforation alone, cephalothin and clindamycin in combination with an aminoglycoside were equally efficacious. Therefore, mono therapy with the cephalosporins has become the typical treatment regimen, while aminoglycosides are not frequently used for reasons previously discussed.

J.K. should be started on an antimicrobial regimen with activity against enteric aerobes and facultative anaerobes such as IV cefoxitin 1 g Q 6 hr.

23. How long should antibiotic therapy be administered to J.K.?

Consensus guidelines regarding the duration of therapy were recently published by the Eastern Association for the Surgery of Trauma (EAST) Practice Management Group. These investigators reviewed all literature from 1976 to 1997 regarding the duration of antimicrobial use following penetrating abdominal trauma. They concluded that antimicrobial use should not exceed 24 hours in patients with a hollow viscus injury. Those without this type of injury should receive a one-time preoperative dose of an antimicrobial agent with aerobic and anaerobic coverage.[66] The efficacy of regimens using shortened courses of antibiotic administration has also been studied.[70–72]

The shortest duration of therapy that has been shown to be effective has been 12 hours. Several investigators have demonstrated that a short course (<48 hours) of antimicrobial therapy is as efficacious as 5- to 7-day courses of therapy if antimicrobial therapy is promptly instituted.[73,74] Several other trials have had low infection rates using a 24-hour regimen, suggesting there is no additional benefit in providing a longer duration of treatment.[70–72,75]

Because antimicrobial therapy carries a risk of adverse reactions and the development of resistance and may be costly, short-term therapy seems warranted if it can be instituted soon after the injury.[66] If the initial dose of antibiotic is administered >3 to 4 hours after injury, therapy should be continued for 3 to 7 days because the incidence of infection in this circumstance is high.

Antimicrobial therapy was instituted soon after J.K. sustained the colonic injury; therefore, a short course of antimicrobial therapy is appropriate. The combination regimen should be continued for 24 hours.

Appendectomy

24. **K.S. is a 13-year-old girl with a 2-day history of periumbilical pain migrating to the right lower quadrant, abdominal distention, fever of 102°F, diarrhea, and decreased bowel sounds. Her WBC count is 16.1 ×10³/mm³ (normal, 3.2 to 9.8). A presumptive diagnosis of acute appendicitis is made. What antimicrobial therapy is indicated, and for how long should it be continued?**

[SI unit: WBC count, 16. 1 ×10⁹/L (normal, 3.2 to 9.8)]

Clinical manifestations commonly encountered with acute appendicitis include right lower quadrant abdominal pain, rebound tenderness, and low-grade fever complicated by nausea, vomiting, and anorexia.[4]

A variety of antimicrobial agents are effective in the treatment of peritoneal contamination associated with acute appendicitis.[76–80] Unfortunately, the majority of studies involved patients without gangrenous or perforated appendices, which are associated with the highest risk of infection. In several well-designed, randomized, placebo-controlled trials, the combination of clindamycin or metronidazole plus an aminoglycoside has been compared with imipenem, β-lactams (e.g., cefoxitin), and β-lactamase inhibitor combinations (e.g., ampicillin plus sulbactam). These single agents were found to be as efficacious as combination therapy.[24,77,79] Patients with gangrenous or perforated appendices who were afebrile for 48 hours were treated with regimens that ranged in duration from a single dose[80] to 3 or more days.[78]

Overall, the studies justify the use of single-agent therapy with a β-lactam or β-lactamase inhibitor combination that possesses antimicrobial activity directed at both Gram-negative aerobes and anaerobes. The appropriate duration of therapy is not as clear. In patients with uncomplicated appendicitis, single-dose therapy is probably sufficient, but patients with gangrenous or perforated appendicitis should be treated for 3 or more days.

K.S. should receive a preoperative dose of any of the aforementioned β-lactam antimicrobials with activity against facultative Gram-negative and anaerobic bacteria (e.g., one dose of IV cefotetan 1 g). Cost, availability, potential side effects, and ease of administration can be used to guide selection of a specific agent. If a gangrenous or perforated appendix is found during surgery, antimicrobial therapy should be continued for a minimum of 3 days or until K.S. has been afebrile for 48 hours (e.g., IV cefotetan 1 g Q 12 hr).

REFERENCES

1. Bohnen JM. Antibiotic therapy for abdominal infection. World J Surg 1998;22:152.
2. Westphal JF, Brogard JM. Biliary tract infections: a guide to drug treatment. Drugs 1999;57:81.
3. Carpenter HA. Bacterial and parasitic cholangitis. Mayo Clin Proc 1998;73:473.
4. Levison ME, Bush LM. Peritonitis and other intraabdominal infections. In: Mandell GL et al. eds. Mandell, Douglas, and Bennett's Principles and Practice of Infectious Diseases. Philadelphia: Churchill Livingstone, 2000:821.
5. Indar AA, Beckingham IJ. Acute cholecystitis. Br Med J 2002;325:639.
6. Podnos YD et al. Intra-abdominal sepsis in elderly persons. Clin Infect Dis 2002;35:62.
7. Gumaste VV. Antibiotics and cholangitis. Gastroenterology 1995;109:323.
8. Solomkin JS et al. Results of a multicenter trial comparing imipenem/cilastatin to tobramycin/clindamycin for intra-abdominal infections. Ann Surg 1990;212:581.
9. Sung JJ et al. Intravenous ciprofloxacin as treatment for patients with acute suppurative cholangitis: a randomized, controlled clinical trial. J Antimicrob Chemother 1995;35:855.
10. Karachalios GN et al. Treatment of acute biliary tract infections with ofloxacin: a randomized, controlled clinical trial. Int J Clin Pharmacol Ther 1996;34:555.
11. Goldstein EJ. Intra-abdominal anaerobic infections: bacteriology and therapeutic potential of newer antimicrobial carbapenem, fluoroquinolone, and desfluoroquinolone therapeutic agents. Clin Infect Dis 2002;35:S106.
12. Keighley MR et al. Antibiotics in biliary disease: the relative importance of antibiotic concentrations in the bile and serum. Gut 1976;17:495.
13. Sinanan MN. Acute cholangitis. Infect Dis Clin North Am 1992;6:571.
14. Nagar H, Berger SA. The excretion of antibiotics by the biliary tract. Surg Gynecol Obstet 1984; 158:601.
15. Johnson CC et al. Peritonitis: update on pathophysiology, clinical manifestations, and management. Clin Infect Dis 1997;24:1035.
16. Singh N et al. Trimethoprim-sulfamethoxazole for the prevention of spontaneous bacterial peritonitis in cirrhosis: a randomized trial. Ann Intern Med 1995;122:595.
17. Mowat C, Stanley AJ. Review article: spontaneous bacterial peritonitis—diagnosis, treatment and prevention. Aliment Pharmacol Ther 2001;15:1851.
18. Garcia-Tsao G. Current management of the complications of cirrhosis and portal hypertension: variceal hemorrhage, ascites, and spontaneous bacterial peritonitis. Gastroenterology 2001;120:726.
19. Navasa M et al. Randomized, comparative study of oral ofloxacin versus intravenous cefotaxime in spontaneous bacterial peritonitis. Gastroenterology 1996;111:1011.
20. Terg R et al. Oral ciprofloxacin after a short course of intravenous ciprofloxacin in the treatment of spontaneous bacterial peritonitis: results of a multicenter, randomized study. J Hepatol 2000;33:564.
21. Ricart E et al. Amoxicillin-clavulanic acid versus cefotaxime in the therapy of bacterial infections in cirrhotic patients. J Hepatol 2000;32:596.
22. Fong TL et al. Polymorphonuclear cell count response and duration of antibiotic therapy in spontaneous bacterial peritonitis. Hepatology 1989;9:423.
23. Runyon BA et al. Short-course versus long-course antibiotic treatment of spontaneous bacterial peritonitis. A randomized controlled study of 100 patients. Gastroenterology 1991;100:1737.
24. Franca A et al. Five days of ceftriaxone to treat spontaneous bacterial peritonitis in cirrhotic patients. J Gastroenterol 2002;37:119.
25. Such J, Runyon BA. Spontaneous bacterial peritonitis. Clin Infect Dis 1998;27:669.
26. Gines P et al. Norfloxacin prevents spontaneous bacterial peritonitis recurrence in cirrhosis: results of a double-blind, placebo-controlled trial. Hepatology 1990;12:716.
27. Rolachon A et al. Ciprofloxacin and long-term prevention of spontaneous bacterial peritonitis: results of a prospective controlled trial. Hepatology 1995;22:1171.
28. Dupeyron C et al. Rapid emergence of quinolone resistance in cirrhotic patients treated with norfloxacin to prevent spontaneous bacterial peritonitis. Antimicrob Agents Chemother 1994;38:340.
29. Fernandez J et al. Bacterial infections in cirrhosis: epidemiological changes with invasive procedures and norfloxacin prophylaxis. Hepatology 2002; 35:140.
30. Das A. A cost analysis of long-term antibiotic prophylaxis for spontaneous bacterial peritonitis in cirrhosis. Am J Gastroenterol 1998;93:1895.
31. Williams CN. Prophylaxis for spontaneous bacterial peritonitis. Can J Gastroenterol 1999;13:549.
32. Gerding DN, Hall WH. The penetration of antibiotics into peritoneal fluid. Bull NY Acad Med 1975;51:1016.
33. Wittman DH, Schassan HH. Penetration of eight beta-lactam antibiotics into the peritoneal fluid. A pharmacokinetic investigation. Arch Surg 1983;118:205.
34. Vargemezis V, Thodis E. Prevention and management of peritonitis and exit-site infection in patients on continuous ambulatory peritoneal dialysis. Nephrol Dial Transplant 2001;16(Suppl 6):106.
35. Passadakis P, Oreopoulos D. The case for oral treatment of peritonitis in continuous ambulatory peritoneal dialysis. Adv Perit Dial 2001;17:180.
36. Keane WF et al. Adult peritoneal dialysis-related peritonitis treatment recommendations: 2000 update. Perit Dial Int 2000;20:396.
37. Warady BA et al. Consensus guidelines for the treatment of peritonitis in pediatric patients receiving peritoneal dialysis. Perit Dial Int 2000;20:610.
38. Korzets Z, Lang R. On the recent recommendations of the Ad Hoc Advisory Committee on Peritonitis Management—or should ceftazidime be used as initial empiric therapy? Perit Dial Int 2001;21:319.
39. Goldie SJ et al. Fungal peritonitis in a large chronic peritoneal dialysis population: a report of 55 episodes. Am J Kidney Dis 1996;28:86.

40. Piraino B. Peritonitis as a complication of peritoneal dialysis. J Am Soc Nephrol 1998;9:1956.
41. Elsakr R et al. Antimicrobial treatment of intra-abdominal infections. Dig Dis 1998;16:47.
42. Tyburski JG et al. Infectious complications following duodenal and/or pancreatic trauma. Am Surg 2001;67:227.
43. Altemeier WA. The bacterial flora of acute appendicitis with peritonitis. Ann Surg 1938;107:517.
44. Ohlin B et al. Piperacillin/tazobactam compared with cefuroxime/metronidazole in the treatment of intra-abdominal infections. Eur J Surg 1999; 165:875.
45. Dupont H et al. Monotherapy with a broad-spectrum beta-lactam is as effective as its combination with an aminoglycoside in treatment of severe generalized peritonitis: a multicenter randomized controlled trial. The Severe Generalized Peritonitis Study Group. Antimicrob Agents Chemother 2000;44:2028.
46. Christou NV et al. Management of intra-abdominal infections. The case for intraoperative cultures and comprehensive broad-spectrum antibiotic coverage. The Canadian Intra-abdominal Infection Study Group. Arch Surg 1996;131:1193.
47. Onderdonk AB et al. Microbial synergy in experimental intra-abdominal abscess. Infect Immun 1976;13:22.
48. Onderdonk AB et al. The capsular polysaccharide of *Bacteroides fragilis* as a virulence factor: comparison of the pathogenic potential of encapsulated and unencapsulated strains. J Infect Dis 1977;136:82.
49. Sirinek KR. Diagnosis and treatment of intra-abdominal abscesses. Surg Infect (Larchmt) 2000; 1:31.
50. Cohn SM et al. Comparison of intravenous/oral ciprofloxacin plus metronidazole versus piperacillin/tazobactam in the treatment of complicated intraabdominal infections. Ann Surg 2000;232:254.
51. Study Group of Intraabdominal Infections. A randomized controlled trial of ampicillin plus sulbactam vs. gentamicin plus clindamycin in the treatment of intraabdominal infections: a preliminary report. Rev Infect Dis 1986;8(Suppl 5):S583.
52. Intra-abdominal Infection Study Group. Results of the North American trial of piperacillin/tazobactam compared with clindamycin and gentamicin in the treatment of severe intra-abdominal infections. Eur J Surg Suppl 1994:61.
53. Brismar B et al. Piperacillin-tazobactam versus imipenem-cilastatin for treatment of intra-abdomi-

54. Barie PS et al. A randomized, double-blind clinical trial comparing cefepime plus metronidazole with imipenem-cilastatin in the treatment of complicated intra-abdominal infections. Cefepime Intra-abdominal Infection Study Group. Arch Surg 1997; 132:1294.
55. Wilson SE. Results of a randomized, multicenter trial of meropenem versus clindamycin/tobramycin for the treatment of intra-abdominal infections. Clin Infect Dis 1997;24(Suppl 2):S197.
56. Mazuski JE et al. The Surgical Infection Society Guidelines on Antimicrobial Therapy for Intra-Abdominal Infections: An Executive Summary. Surg Infect (Larchmt) 2002;3:161.
57. Solomkin JS et al. Ertapenem versus piperacillin/tazobactam in the treatment of complicated intraabdominal infections: results of a double-blind, randomized comparative phase III trial. Ann Surg 2003;237:235.
58. Hau T et al. Irrigation of the peritoneal cavity and local antibiotics in the treatment of peritonitis. Surg Gynecol Obstet 1983;156:25.
59. Noon GP et al. Clinical evaluation of peritoneal irrigation with antibiotic solution. Surgery 1967; 62:73.
60. Burnett WE ea. The treatment of peritonitis using peritoneal lavage. Ann Surg 1967;145:675.
61. Carver P. Postoperative use of antibiotic irrigations. Clin Pharm 1987;6:352.
62. Snydman DR et al. Multicenter study of in vitro susceptibility of the *Bacteroides fragilis* group, 1995 to 1996, with comparison of resistance trends from 1990 to 1996. Antimicrob Agents Chemother 1999;43:2417.
63. Brown WJ. National Committee for Clinical Laboratory Standards agar dilution susceptibility testing of anaerobic gram-negative bacteria. Antimicrob Agents Chemother 1988;32:385.
64. Thornsberry C. Antimicrobial susceptibility testing of anaerobic bacteria: review and update on the role of the National Committee for Clinical Laboratory Standards. Rev Infect Dis 1990;12(Suppl 2):S218.
65. Dougherty SH. Antimicrobial culture and susceptibility testing has little value for routine management of secondary bacterial peritonitis. Clin Infect Dis 1997;23(Suppl 2):S258.
66. Luchette FA et al. Practice management guidelines for prophylactic antibiotic use in penetrating abdominal trauma: the EAST Practice Management Guidelines Work Group. J Trauma 2000;48:508.

67. Fullen WD et al. Prophylactic antibiotics in penetrating wounds of the abdomen. J Trauma 1972; 12:282.
68. Tally FP et al. Randomized prospective study comparing moxalactam and cefoxitin with or without tobramycin for the treatment of serious surgical infections. Antimicrob Agents Chemother 1986; 29:244.
69. Nichols RL et al. Risk of infection after penetrating abdominal trauma. N Engl J Med 1984;311:1065.
70. Bozorgzadeh A et al. The duration of antibiotic administration in penetrating abdominal trauma. Am J Surg 1999;177:125.
71. Demetriades D et al. Short-course antibiotic prophylaxis in penetrating abdominal injuries: ceftriaxone versus cefoxitin. Injury 1991;22:20.
72. Fabian TC et al. Duration of antibiotic therapy for penetrating abdominal trauma: a prospective trial. Surgery 1992;112:788.
73. O'Donnell V et al. Evaluation of carbenicillin and a comparison of clindamycin and gentamicin combined therapy in penetrating abdominal trauma. Surg Gynecol Obstet 1978;147:525.
74. Oreskovich MR et al. Duration of preventive antibiotic administration for penetrating abdominal trauma. Arch Surg 1982;117:200.
75. Delgado G, Jr. et al. Characteristics of prophylactic antibiotic strategies after penetrating abdominal trauma at a level I urban trauma center: a comparison with the EAST guidelines. J Trauma 2002; 53:673.
76. Berne TV et al. Surgically treated gangrenous or perforated appendicitis. A comparison of aztreonam and clindamycin versus gentamicin and clindamycin. Ann Surg 1987;205:133.
77. Lau WY et al. Randomized, prospective, and double-blind trial of new beta-lactams in the treatment of appendicitis. Antimicrob Agents Chemother 1985;28:639.
78. Heseltine PN et al. Imipenem therapy for perforated and gangrenous appendicitis. Surg Gynecol Obstet 1986;162:43.
79. Lau WY et al. Cefoxitin versus gentamicin and metronidazole in prevention of post-appendicectomy sepsis: a randomized, prospective trial. J Antimicrob Chemother 1986;18:613.
80. Foster MC et al. A randomized comparative study of sulbactam plus ampicillin vs. metronidazole plus cefotaxime in the management of acute appendicitis in children. Rev Infect Dis 1986;8(Suppl 5):S634.

CHAPTER 64

Urinary Tract Infections

Douglas N. Fish

INTRODUCTION

This chapter begins with a brief review of urinary tract infections (UTIs) but focuses on the management of patients with UTIs. For a more detailed discussion of the etiology, pathophysiology, and diagnosis of UTIs, the reader is referred to some excellent texts and review articles.[1–9] Additionally, a glossary of associated terms is supplied at the end of this chapter.

Epidemiology

UTIs occur frequently in both community and hospital environments and are the most common bacterial infections in humans.[1] UTIs encompass a spectrum of clinical entities ranging in severity from asymptomatic infection to acute pyelonephritis with sepsis.[1,6] Approximately 7 million cases of acute cystitis and 250,000 cases of acute pyelonephritis occur annually in the United States.[4] The direct costs associated with the diagnosis and treatment of UTIs have been estimated at $1.6 billion annually in the United States.[8] After 1 year of age and until about age 50, UTI is predominantly a disease of females. From ages 5 through 14, the incidence of bacteriuria is 1.2% among girls and 0.03% among boys. One percent to 3% of women between the ages of 15 and 24 have bacteriuria; the incidence increases 1% to 2% for each ensuing decade of life until approximately 10% of women are bacteriuric after age 70.[1,7] Approximately 25% to 40% of women in the general population will experience a urinary tract infection during their lifetime.[4] Women have more UTIs than men probably because of anatomic and physiologic differences. The female urethra is relatively short and allows bacteria easy access to the bladder. In contrast, males are partly protected because the urethra is longer and antimicrobial substances are secreted by the prostate.[1,7]

The incidence of urinary tract infections in neonates is about 1% and is most frequent among males, many of whom prove to have congenital structural abnormalities.[10] The mortality rate among newborns with UTIs was earlier reported to be as high as 10%[10]; more recently this rate has decreased because of an increased awareness of the high frequency of UTI in children, improved diagnostic techniques, and more effective management.[11]

UTIs again become a problem for males after the age of 50, when prostatic obstruction, urethral instrumentation, and surgery influence the infection rate. Infection in younger males is rare and requires careful evaluation for urinary tract pathology.[12,13]

In general, 10% to 20% of the elderly living at home have bacteriuria. This increases to 20% to 50% in extended care facilities and 30% in hospitals.[14,15] The frequency of infection also tends to rise with increasing age for those 65 years or older. Most of the UTIs in these patients are asymptomatic but are still important because they often result in symptomatic infection.[14,15] Whether bacteriuria in old age is associated with decreased survival is controversial.[16,17] However, the presence of asymptomatic bacteriuria and decreased functional ability of institutionalized persons are associated.[18] The reasons for higher UTI rates in elderly persons include the high prevalence of prostatic hypertrophy in males, incomplete bladder emptying caused by underlying diseases or medications, dementia, and urinary and fecal incontinence.[7,14,15]

Etiology

Community-Acquired Infections

Most UTIs are caused by Gram-negative aerobic bacilli from the intestinal tract (Table 64-1). *Escherichia coli* cause 75% to 90% of community-acquired, uncomplicated UTIs.[1,19] Coagulase-negative staphylococci (i.e., *Staphylococcus saprophyticus*) account for an additional 5% to 20% of UTIs in younger women.[1,2,4] Other Enterobacteriaceae (*Proteus mirabilis, Klebsiella*) and *Enterococcus faecalis* also are common pathogens.[1,2,19] Uncomplicated infections are nearly always caused by only a single organism.

Hospital-Acquired Infections

E. coli is still a common pathogen in hospital-acquired or other complicated UTIs but is responsible for only 15% to 20% of these infections. Other Gram-negative organisms such as *Pseudomonas aeruginosa, Proteus, Enterobacter, Serratia,* and *Acinetobacter* cause significantly more infections (up to 25%) than in community-acquired infections.[4,20,21] *Enterococcus* is also a common pathogen in hospital-acquired infections and causes approximately 25% of infections.[20,21] UTIs caused by *Staphylococcus aureus* are usually the result of hematogenous spread, although this pathogen may also be associated with urinary catheterization.[1,22,23] Finally, *Candida albicans* is a common pathogen in hospital-acquired infections and may be involved in 20% to 30% of cases.[20,21] In contrast to uncomplicated infections that are usually monomicrobial, hospital-acquired UTIs associated with structural abnormalities or indwelling urinary catheters are often caused by multiple organisms.[1,20,22,23]

Pathogenesis

The most common pathway for the spread of bacteria to the urinary tract is the ascending route. A UTI usually begins with heavy and persistent colonization of the vaginal vestibule with intestinal bacteria, especially in women with recurrent UTIs. Once introital (i.e., vaginal vestibule and urethral mucosa) colonization has occurred, colonization of the urethra leads to retrograde infection of the bladder.[3,24]

The bladder has additional defense mechanisms that prevent spread of the infection after urethral colonization occurs. Urination washes bacteria out of the bladder and is effective if urine can flow freely and the bladder is emptied completely. Elements in the urine, including organic acids (which contribute to a low pH) and urea (which contributes to a high osmolality), are antibacterial. The bladder mucosa also has antibacterial properties.[1,2] Lastly, several substances including IgA and glycoproteins (e.g., Tamm-Horsfall protein) are actively secreted into the urine and act to prevent adherence of bacteria to uroendothelial cells.[3]

Focal renal involvement may result from the spread of bacteria via the ureters and may be facilitated by vesicoureteral reflux or decreased ureteral peristalsis. Reflux can be produced by cystitis alone or by anatomic defects. Ureteral peristalsis is decreased by pregnancy, ureteral obstruction, or Gram-negative bacterial endotoxins.[1,3]

Predisposing Factors

Extremes of age, female gender, sexual activity, use of contraception, pregnancy, instrumentation, urinary tract obstruction, neurologic dysfunction, renal disease, previous antimicrobial use, and expression of A, B, and H blood group oligosaccharides on the surface of epithelial cells are among the many predisposing factors for the development of UTIs.[3–5,25,26]

The overall likelihood of developing a UTI is approximately 30 times higher in women than in men.[2] The incidence of bacteriuria in pregnant women is 4% to 10%, which is at least twice that of similarly aged nonpregnant women.[1,27] The inci-

Table 64-1	Urinary Tract Infections
Organisms Commonly Found	**Antibacterial of Choice**
Uncomplicated UTI	
Escherichia coli	TMP-SMX[c]
Proteus mirabilis	TMP-SMX[c]
Klebsiella pneumoniae	TMP-SMX[c]
Enterococcus faecalis	Amoxicillin
Staphylococcus saprophyticus	First-generation cephalosporin or TMP-SMX
Complicated UTI[a,b]	
Escherichia coli	First-, second-, or third-generation cephalosporin; TMP-SMX[c]
Proteus mirabilis	First-, second-, or third-generation cephalosporin
Klebsiella pneumoniae	First-generation cephalosporin; fluoroquinolone
Enterococcus faecalis	Ampicillin or vancomycin ± aminoglycoside
Pseudomonas aeruginosa	Antipseudomonal penicillin ± aminoglycoside; ceftazidime; cefepime; fluoroquinolone; carbapenem
Enterobacter	Fluoroquinolone; TMP-SMX; carbapenem
Indole-positive *Proteus*	Third-generation cephalosporin; fluoroquinolone
Serratia	Third-generation cephalosporin; fluoroquinolone
Acinetobacter	Carbapenem; TMP-SMX
Staphylococcus aureus	Penicillinase-resistant penicillin; vancomycin

[a]Oral therapy when appropriate.
[b]Drug selection based on culture and susceptibility testing when possible.
[c]Caution in communities with increased resistance (>10–20%). Fluoroquinolone, nitrofurantoin, cephalosporins should be used in areas with increased TMP-SMX resistance.
TMP-SMX, trimethoprim-sulfamethoxazole; UTI, urinary tract infection.

dence of acute symptomatic pyelonephritis in pregnant women with untreated bacteriuria also is high. Many factors probably contribute to the increased susceptibility of the pregnant female to infection; these include hormonal changes, anatomic changes, progressive urinary stasis, and glucose in the urine.[27]

Instrumentation of the urinary tract (i.e., urethral and ureteral catheterization) is an important predisposing factor for hospital-acquired UTIs in particular. As many as 67% of nosocomial UTIs are preceded by urinary tract instrumentation.[23] Other urologic procedures, such as cystoscopy, transurethral surgery, prostate biopsy, and upper urinary tract endoscopy, are much less likely to result in infection unless there is pre-existing bacteriuria or other contaminated sites (e.g., prostate, renal stones).

Any obstruction to the free flow of urine (e.g., urethral stenosis, stones, tumor) or mechanical difficulty in evacuating the bladder (e.g., prostatic hypertrophy, urethral stricture) predisposes patients to UTIs. Furthermore, infections associated with urethral or renal pelvic obstruction can lead to rapid destruction of the kidney and sepsis.[1]

Renal disease increases the susceptibility of the kidney to infection.[1] The incidence of UTI among renal transplant recipients has been reported to range from 35% to 80%.[28]

Patients with spinal cord injuries, stroke, atherosclerosis, or diabetes may have neurologic dysfunction that can cause UTIs. The neurologic dysfunction may cause urinary retention, which may lead to catheterization. Furthermore, prolonged immobilization facilitates hypercalciuria and stone formation in some of these patients.[1,3,4]

Previous antimicrobial use has been shown to increase the relative risk for UTI in women by approximately threefold to sixfold.[5] This increased infection risk applies to prior antimicrobial use (within the previous 15 to 28 days) for treatment of UTIs as well as non-urinary tract infections. The proposed mechanism for increased risk is alteration of normal flora of the urogenital tract and predisposition to colonization with pathogenic bacterial strains.[5]

Diabetes mellitus has often been associated with an increased risk for UTIs because of glucose in the urine, which both promotes bacterial growth and impairs leukocyte function. Diabetes is also often associated with anatomic and immunologic abnormalities of the urinary tract that increase risk of infection, often because of increased need for urinary tract instrumentation.[29,30] Several studies have documented a twofold to threefold increase in UTIs in diabetic women compared with nondiabetic women.[31,32] It has recently been suggested that patients with diabetes who have no neurologic complications resulting in bladder dysfunction and who have not undergone instrumentation are not at increased risk compared with nondiabetic patients.[3] However, with autonomic neuropathy affecting the bladder (i.e., cystopathy) or following instrumentation, UTIs in diabetic patients are both more frequent and more severe.[3,31] Increased rates of complications such as pyelonephritis have been documented in such diabetic patients.[29,30]

Studies also have supported an association between sexual intercourse and UTIs.[26,33] Frequent sexual intercourse is an established UTI risk factor among otherwise healthy women.[3,26] Specific contraceptive practices, particularly the use of spermicides, have also been associated with increased risk for UTI. The use of a diaphragm, cervical cap, or condom in combination with spermicidal jelly has been shown to increase the risk of UTI compared with the use of the barrier method alone.[26,34,35] Although the greatest risk has been associated with the spermicide nonoxynol-9, the use of other types of spermicidal jellies has also been associated with a significantly higher risk for UTI.[36] Oral contraceptive use has also now been associated with increased risk of UTI.[26] The exact mechanisms of infection related to sexual intercourse, contraceptives, and associated factors are still unclear but appear to be related to alterations in vaginal flora that allow for bacterial overgrowth and subsequent infection.[37,38]

Clinical Presentation

Symptoms commonly associated with lower UTIs (e.g., cystitis) include burning on urination (dysuria), frequent urination, suprapubic pain, blood in the urine (hematuria), and back pain. Patients with upper tract infection (e.g., acute pyelonephritis) also may present with loin pain, costovertebral angle (CVA) tenderness, fever, chills, nausea, and vomiting.[1,6]

These signs and symptoms correlate poorly with either the presence or the extent of the infection. Symptoms common to lower UTIs often are the only positive findings in upper UTIs (i.e., subclinical pyelonephritis).[1,6] The probability of true infection in women who present with one or more symptoms of UTI is only about 50%.[39] However, the presence of certain factors enhance the probability of true infection in these patients (history of previous UTI, dysuria, back pain, pyuria, hematuria, and bacteriuria); other symptoms significantly decrease the probability of true infection (absence of dysuria or back pain, history of vaginal discharge or irritation).[39] It has also been determined that the combination of dysuria and frequency in the absence of vaginal discharge or irritation increases the probability of true infection to greater than 90%.[39] Fever, chills, flank pain, nausea and vomiting, or CVA tenderness are also highly suggestive of acute pyelonephritis rather than cystitis.[4,6] Many elderly patients with UTI are asymptomatic without pyuria. Additionally, because many patients have frequency and dysuria, it is difficult to distinguish between noninfectious and infectious causes based on symptoms.[1] Nonspecific symptoms such as failure to thrive and fever may be the only manifestations of UTI in neonates and children younger than 2 years of age.[1]

Laboratory Diagnosis

The urinalysis (UA) is a series of laboratory tests commonly performed in patients suspected of having a UTI. A technician first performs a macroscopic analysis by describing the color of the urine; measuring its specific gravity; and estimating the pH and glucose, protein, ketone, blood, and bilirubin contents using a rapid "dipstick" method. Then the urine sediment, obtained by centrifugation, is examined under a microscope for the presence and quantity of leukocytes, erythrocytes, epithelial cells, crystals, casts, and bacteria.

Microscopic examination of the urine sediment in patients with documented UTIs reveals many bacteria (usually >20 per high-power field [HPF]). A Gram's stain of the uncentrifuged ("unspun") urine will show at least one organism per immersion oil field and usually correlates with a positive urine culture. Pyuria (i.e., ≥8 white blood cells [WBCs] per mm^3 of unspun urine or 2 to 5 WBCs/HPF of centrifuged urine) frequently is seen in patients with UTIs. WBC casts in the urine strongly suggest acute pyelonephritis.[1]

A rapid diagnostic "dipstick" test for the detection of bacteriuria, the nitrite test, detects nitrite formation from the reduction of nitrates by bacteria. This test is both widely available and easily performed; however, at least 10^5 bacteria per milliliter are necessary to form enough nitrite for the reaction to occur. Although a positive nitrite reading is useful, false-negative results do occur. The leukocyte esterase test detects the esterase activity of leukocytes in the urine. A positive test correlates well with significant pyuria[40]; however, both false-negative and false-positive findings can occur with the leukocyte esterase panel.

The major criterion used for the diagnosis of a UTI is the urine culture. Proper interpretation of these cultures depends on appropriate urine collection techniques. Urinating into a sterile collection cup using the midstream clean-catch technique is the most practical method of urine collection. This method of urine specimen collection is especially useful for males but is less useful in female patients because contamination is extremely difficult to avoid.[1] The external urethral area must first be thoroughly cleaned and rinsed, then the urine specimen collected after initiation of the urine stream (hence "midstream").

Suprapubic bladder aspiration, although unpleasant from a patient's point of view, generally is not painful and is quite reliable. It is not practical for routine office or clinic practice, but may be especially useful when voided urine samples repeatedly yield questionable results or when patients have voiding problems. Because contamination is negligible, any number of bacteria found by this method reflects infection.[1]

Urinary catheterization for a urine culture sample yields fairly reliable results if performed carefully. Infections may result from the procedure itself because organisms may be introduced into the bladder at the time of catheterization.

Urine must be plated on culture media within 20 minutes of collection to avoid erroneously high colony counts from bacterial growth in urine at room temperature. Otherwise, it should be refrigerated promptly until it can be cultured. Colony counts also can be affected by the concentration of bladder urine; bacterial counts are higher in first-voided morning urines compared with those obtained from the same patient later in the day.

Urine cultures in the bacteriology laboratory usually are evaluated by the pour-plate or streak-plate method. Greater than 10^5 colonies of bacteria per milliliter cultured from a midstream urine specimen confirms a UTI. A single, carefully collected urine specimen provides 80% reliability, and two consecutive cultures of the same organism are virtually diagnostic.[1,2]

It is important to understand that the classic definition of UTI as $\geq 10^5$ bacteria per milliliter is fairly insensitive in accurately diagnosing patients with UTI. Approximately 30% to 50% of actual cases of acute cystitis have $< 10^5$ bacteria per milliliter.[4,41] Particularly in a symptomatic patient, using a definition of $\geq 10^2$ bacteria per milliliter is much more sensitive and avoids failure to diagnose the infection in many patients.[4]

Diagnosis of UTI in men also requires different interpretation of laboratory data. Contamination of urinary specimens is much less likely to occur in men compared with women, and numbers of bacterial colonies in specimens are therefore much lower. Greater than 10^3 bacteria per milliliter is thus highly suggestive of UTI in men.[12,13,42]

Diagnosis of UTI in children is particularly difficult because of the difficulties and high contamination rates associated with commonly used methods such as the clean-catch technique. Suprapubic aspiration is the most accurate urine collection method in children, followed by urinary bladder catheterization.[9] Although clean-catch and bag methods (i.e., collecting urine into a bag placed around the urogenital area) are most prone to contamination and inaccurate results, they are also the most preferred methods for parents and healthcare personnel because they are simple and noninvasive. The choice of diagnostic tests for children will therefore be based on the experience, skill, and preferences of those involved with the child, and no one technique will be ideal in every setting.[9]

Simplified culture methods such as the filter-paper method (e.g., Testuria-R), dip-slide method (e.g., Uricult), and pad-culture method (Microstix) are as reliable as the traditional laboratory methods for bacterial identification and quantification. The filter-paper method is relatively inexpensive, but it does not differentiate between Gram-positive and Gram-negative organisms. The dip-slide and pad-culture methods are accurate, differentiate between Gram-positive and Gram-negative organisms, and are similar in cost. The dip-slide method has the added advantages of ease in storage and a nitrite indicator pad.

LOWER URINARY TRACT INFECTION
Initiation of Therapy

1. V.Q., a 20-year-old woman (married, no children) with no previous history of UTI, complains of burning on urination, frequent urination of a small amount, and bladder pain. She has no fever or CVA tenderness. A clean-catch midstream urine sample shows Gram-negative rods on Gram's stain. A culture and sensitivity (C&S) test is ordered, and the results of a STAT UA are as follows: appearance, straw-colored (normal, straw); specific gravity, 1.015 (normal, 1.001 to 1.035); pH, 8.0 (normal, 4.5 to 7.5); and protein, glucose, ketones, bilirubin, and blood are all negative (normal, all negative); WBCs, 10 to 15 cells/mm³ (normal, 0 to 2 cells/mm³); RBCs, 0 to 1 cells/mm³ (normal, 0 to 2 cells/mm³); bacteria: many (normal, 0 to rare); epithelial cells, 3 to 5 cells/mm³ (normal, 0 to few cells/mm³). Based on these findings, V.Q. is presumed to have a lower UTI. What should be the goals of therapy and treatment plan at this time?

Drug treatment of a lower UTI often is started before C&S results are known because the most probable infecting organism and its sensitivity to antibiotics can be predicted. Approximately 75% to 90% of community-acquired infections are caused by Enterobacteriaceae (especially *E. coli*). Although these organisms may be sensitive to ampicillin, amoxicillin, and the sulfonamides such as trimethoprim-sulfamethoxazole (TMP-SMX), resistance to these agents is common. Ampicillin resistance has been reported in as many as 25% to 70% of community-acquired isolates; resistance nationwide is currently about 35% to 40%.[1,4,19,43] Trimethoprim-sulfamethoxazole has been a traditional agent of choice for many years; however, recent data indicate that TMP-SMX resistance has significantly increased in recent years and may be as high as 16% to 20% among community-acquired *E. coli* isolates.[19,43,44] Another relatively common organism is *S. saprophyticus*. Most strains are susceptible to sulfonamides, TMP-SMX, penicillins, and cephalosporins. Alternative medications and doses can be found in Table 64-2.

Table 64-2   Commonly Used Oral Antimicrobial Agents for Acute Urinary Tract Infections[1,2,4,45–49]

Drug	Usual Dose Adult	Pediatric	Pregnancy[a]	Breast Milk[a]	Comments[b]
Amoxicillin	250 mg Q 8 hr or 3 g single dose	20–40 mg/kg/day in 3 doses	Crosses placenta (cord) = 30% (maternal)[c]	Small amount present	Watch for resistant organisms
Amoxicillin + potassium clavulanate	500 + 125 mg Q 12 hr	20 mg/kg/day (amoxicillin content) in 3 doses	Unknown	Unknown	
Ampicillin	250–500 mg Q 6 hr	50–100 mg/kg/day in 4 doses	Crosses placenta	Variable amount (*milk*) = 1–30% (serum)[c]	Watch for resistant organisms. Should be taken on an empty stomach
Cefadroxil	0.5–1 g Q 12 hr	15–30 mg/kg/day in 4 doses	Crosses placenta	Enters breast milk (*milk*) = 20% (serum)[c]	Alternate choices for patients allergic to penicillins, although cross-hypersensitivity can occur. May be associated with high failure rates
Cephalexin	250–500 mg Q 6 hr	15–30 mg/kg/day in 4 doses	Crosses placenta		
Cephradine	250–500 mg Q 6 hr	15–30 mg/kg/day in 4 doses	Crosses placenta (cord) = 10% (maternal)[c]		
Norfloxacin[d]	400 mg Q 12 hr	Avoid	Arthropathy in immature animals	Unknown	Useful for Pseudomonal infection. *Avoid antacids and ditrivalent cations and sucralfate. May cause dizziness*
Ciprofloxacin[d]	250–500 mg Q 12 hr	Avoid	Arthropathy in immature animals	Unknown	Alternate choices for patients allergic to beta-lactams
Gatifloxacin	200 mg Q 24 hr	Avoid	Arthropathy in immature animals	Unknown	First-line agents for prostatitis
Levofloxacin	250 mg Q 24 hr	Avoid	Arthropathy in immature animals	(milk) = 100% (serum)[c]	
Nitrofurantoin	50–100 mg Q 6 hr	5–7 mg/kg/day in 4 doses	Hemolytic anemia in newborn	Variable amounts; not detectable to 30%; may cause hemolysis in G6PD-deficient baby	Alternate choice. *To be taken with food or milk. May cause brown or rust-yellow discoloration of urine.* See Questions 47–49
Doxycycline Tetracycline	100 mg Q 12 hr 250–500 mg Q 6 hr	Avoid Avoid	Congenital limb abnormalities; cataracts; tooth discoloration and dysplasia; inhibition of bone growth in fetus; hepatic toxicity and azotemia with IV use in pregnant patients with renal dysfunction or with overdosage	(milk) = 30–40% (serum)[c] Risk may be less because of binding to milk calcium, but best to avoid (milk) = 20–140% (serum)[c]	Effective for urethritis. Avoid in children <8 yr. Alters bowel flora to favor resistant organisms. *To be taken 1 hr before or 2 hr after meals (doxycycline may be taken with food or milk). Avoid simultaneous ingestion of dairy products, antacids, laxatives, iron products. May cause photosensitivity*
Sulfisoxazole	0.5–1 g Q 6 hr	50–100 mg/kg/day in 4 doses	Crosses placenta; hemolysis in newborn with G6PD deficiency; displacement of bilirubin may lead to hyperbilirubinemia and kernicterus; teratogenic in some animal studies	Enters breast milk; displacement of bilirubin may lead to neonatal jaundice; may cause hemolysis in G6PD deficient baby	Alters bowel flora to favor resistant organisms. *To be taken on an empty stomach with a full glass of water. Photosensitivity may occur*
Sulfamethoxazole (SMX)	1 g Q 12 hr	60 mg/kg/day in 2 doses			
Trimethoprim (TMP)	100 mg Q 12 hr		Crosses placenta (cord) = 60%; (maternal) folate antagonism; teratogenic in rats	(*milk*) >1 (serum)[c]	Alternate choice
TMP-SMX	160 + 800 mg Q 12 hr or 0.48 + 2.4 g single dose	10 mg/kg/day (TMP component in 2 doses)	Crosses placenta (cord) = 60%; (maternal) folate antagonism; teratogenic in rats	(*milk*) >1 (serum)[c]	*To be taken on an empty stomach with a full glass of water. Photosensitivity may occur.* Monitor HIV-infected patients closely for development of adverse hematologic reactions First-line agent for prostatitis

[a]Also see Chapter 47, Teratogenicity and Drugs in Breast Milk.
[b]Includes unique patient consultation information in italics.
[c]Denotes drug concentration.
[d]May increase theophylline concentrations when given concurrently. Carefully monitor theophylline serum concentrations during quinolone use.

The goals of therapy in the treatment of acute cystitis are to effectively eradicate the infection and prevent associated complications, while at the same time minimizing adverse effects and costs associated with drug therapy. To accomplish these goals, selection of a specific antimicrobial agent should be made after consideration of the following factors: (1) pathogens likely to be causing the infection, (2) resistance rates to various antimicrobials within the specific geographic area, (3) desired duration of therapy, (4) clinical efficacy and toxicity profiles of various agents, and (5) costs of specific agents. Because resistance rates among various pathogens vary considerably among geographic areas, clinicians involved in the management of patients with UTIs must be familiar with resistance rates prevalent within the specific area within which they practice.[19]

Duration of Therapy

2. What treatment duration options are available for V.Q.?

Outpatients with acute, uncomplicated UTIs can be treated successfully with a 7- to 14-day course of oral medications, a 3-day course of therapy, or by single-dose therapy.[1,4] A urine C&S may be obtained before antibacterial therapy and repeated 2 to 3 weeks after the completion of therapy,[1,2,4] although this practice is seldom necessary in young adult females with a lower urinary tract infection.[1,4]

The duration of therapy for UTIs has been shortened considerably. The traditional 7- to 14-day course of antibiotic therapy now is considered excessive for most patients with uncomplicated infections.[4,49] A 3-day antibiotic treatment regimen is just as effective as a 10-day regimen in eradicating urinary tract organisms, although this is somewhat antibiotic class-specific.[4,49–55] TMP-SMX, amoxicillin-clavulanic acid (Augmentin), and the fluoroquinolones are recommended as the preferred agents for 3-day treatment regimens.[4,49–55] Other β-lactams and nitrofurantoin are more appropriately reserved for longer treatment courses of 7 to 14 days.[4,48,51] Longer treatment courses are also used in cases of treatment failure following regimens of shorter duration. Because of the relatively high incidence of E. coli resistance to ampicillin and amoxicillin, some experts do not recommend these agents for initial, empiric use.[2,4,48] Although TMP-SMX is still recommended as the preferred agent for acute, uncomplicated UTIs, this agent also may not be a suitable choice for empiric therapy in certain geographic areas because of increasing resistance. Use of trimethoprim or TMP-SMX has been discouraged in geographic areas where the incidence of E. coli resistance exceeds 15% to 20%.[44,49,56,57] The fluoroquinolones have become favored agents in many geographic areas with high rates of resistance to ampicillin, TMP-SMX, and trimethoprim because of excellent activity against common urinary pathogens and the ability to use short 3-day courses of therapy. The choice of a specific agent should be based on geographic sensitivities as well as any patient allergies and the relative cost of the agents under consideration.

Even a single dose of an antibiotic may be effective. Bacteria disappear from the urine within hours after antibacterial therapy has been initiated.[49] This, coupled with the urinary bladder's ability to defend itself through micturition, acidification, and inherent antibacterial activity, gives theoretic support to the clinical evidence that a large single dose of an antibiotic can eradicate a UTI.

Single-Dose Therapy

3. Would a 3-day course of therapy or single-dose therapy be preferred for V.Q.?

A single antibiotic dose is reasonably effective in treating acute, lower UTIs in young, adult females.[4,7,49,55,58] Commonly used regimens are TMP-SMX (two or three double-strength tablets), trimethoprim 400 mg, amoxicillin-clavulanate 500 mg, amoxicillin 3 g, ampicillin 3.5 g, nitrofurantoin 200 mg, ciprofloxacin 500 mg, and norfloxacin 400 mg.[1,48] Again, choice of a specific agent should be based on local sensitivity patterns, patient allergies, and relative drug costs. Female patients with history or clinical presentation suggestive of complicated infection (e.g., systemic manifestations of infection, renal disease, anatomic abnormalities of the urinary tract, diabetes mellitus, pregnancy), a history of antibiotic resistance, or a history of relapse after single-dose therapy should not receive single-dose regimens. Single-dose therapy is also not appropriate for males with UTIs. Because V.Q. does not have any of these contraindications, she could potentially receive single-dose therapy with an appropriate agent.

The advantages of single-dose treatment of UTIs include improved compliance, cost savings, proven efficacy in a defined population of patients (i.e., young women with acute, uncomplicated lower UTIs), minimal side effects, and a potentially decreased incidence of bacterial resistance associated with antibiotic overuse. Furthermore, failure to eradicate the organism with a single dose of an antibiotic may help identify patients who have subclinical pyelonephritis and require more intensive evaluation of their urinary tract.

There also are some concerns about single-dose therapy.[4,7,48,49] First, sample sizes in most of the comparative studies to date have been relatively small. Consequently, it is difficult to determine whether differences in effectiveness or in incidence of side effects between single-dose and multiple-dose therapy are clinically significant. Meta-analysis of studies comparing single-dose with multiple-dose TMP-SMX therapy has demonstrated that single-dose therapy is significantly less effective in eradicating bacteriuria than regimens of either ≥5 days (83% versus 93%, respectively, $P < 0.001$) or ≥7 days in duration (87% versus 94%, respectively; $P = 0.014$).[49] Although side effects with the longer courses of therapy were more common (11% to 13% with single-dose versus 19% to 28% with longer regimens), they were mild and well tolerated.[49] While fewer studies have directly compared single-dose versus 3-day therapies, numerous studies have shown that 3-day courses are as effective as courses of longer duration.[49] A 3-day course of therapy is therefore currently recommended for uncomplicated cystitis.

A second area of concern relates to recurrences in patients treated with single-dose therapy. Recurrent infections may represent either a relapse caused by incomplete eradication of more deep-seated kidney infection or a true reinfection in a high-risk patient. If it is assumed that patients who receive single-dose therapy are selected properly, then reinfection is a more likely explanation. However, it has also has been suggested that relapse following single-dose therapy actually suggests subclinical upper urinary tract infection.[4] In either case, single-dose therapies have been associated with higher rates of recurrence compared to therapies of longer duration.[49]

Finally, the safety of single-dose therapy in patients with subclinical pyelonephritis needs further evaluation, and these regimens are not currently recommended in this setting. Based on the preceding information, a 3-day antibiotic course is reasonable in V.Q. and is the preferred initial treatment regimen in other patients with acute, uncomplicated lower tract infection as well.[4]

When using short-course (i.e., 1- or 3-day) regimens, it is important to counsel the patient that the clinical signs and symptoms of infection may often not be completely resolved for 2 to 3 days following initiation of therapy. Therefore, symptoms that persist after beginning therapy (or actually completing therapy, in the case of single-dose regimens) are not necessarily indicative of treatment failure.

Trimethoprim-Sulfamethoxazole

4. TMP-SMX, 1 double-strength tablet BID for 3 days is prescribed for V.Q. Is this appropriate therapy?

Yes. TMP-SMX (co-trimoxazole, Bactrim, Septra) has been shown to be effective for single- and multiple-dose therapy for uncomplicated cystitis.[49] Gram-positive and Gram-negative organisms, with the notable exceptions of *P. aeruginosa, Enterococcus,* and anaerobes, generally are susceptible to TMP-SMX.[59] Although TMP-SMX may appear active against enterococci in vitro, clinical efficacy against this pathogen is variable and does not always correlate well with in vitro susceptibilities. The efficacy of this drug combination largely depends on the sensitivity of the organism to trimethoprim, although *Neisseria gonorrhoeae* is relatively more susceptible to the sulfonamide component. Individually, trimethoprim and sulfamethoxazole are bacteriostatic, but in combination they are bactericidal against most urinary pathogens.[59] Furthermore, this combination is almost uniformly successful in the treatment of uncomplicated UTIs, even against organisms that originally were resistant to either agent alone. Although rates of trimethoprim resistance have increased over the past several years,[19,44] resistance rates remain relatively low in many geographic areas and trimethoprim alone would be effective in managing many simple UTIs.

The ratio of trimethoprim to sulfamethoxazole in the available tablet products is 1:5 (e.g., 80 mg trimethoprim/400 mg sulfamethoxazole). This combination has been chosen to achieve peak serum concentrations of the two drugs that approximate a 1:20 ratio. This ratio is optimal for synergistic activity against most microorganisms, although the drugs remain synergistic and bactericidal in ratios ranging from 1:5 to 1:40 in vitro.[59] Urinary concentrations of trimethoprim and sulfamethoxazole far exceed the minimum inhibitory concentrations (MICs) for most susceptible urinary pathogens, accounting for the combination's effectiveness in the management of UTIs. Therefore, good in vitro activity, excellent clinical success, relatively low resistance rates among common pathogens in many geographic areas, and low cost make TMP-SMX a reasonable choice in V.Q. Many consider TMP-SMX the initial agent of choice in the treatment of acute, un-

complicated lower UTI in geographic areas where the incidence of TMP-SMX resistance among *E. coli* is <20%.[4,49]

Interpretation of Culture and Sensitivity

5. C&S studies in V.Q. show a few *Klebsiella* and >10⁵ bacteria per milliliter of *P. mirabilis,* which are sensitive to ampicillin, cephalosporins, trimethoprim, TMP-SMX, and gentamicin. The *Proteus* is intermediately sensitive to sulfonamides, carbenicillin, and nalidixic acid and is resistant to tetracycline. Based on V.Q.'s clinical presentation and recent culture reports, did she have a true UTI?

Yes. Most women with either lower or upper urinary tract infection have >100,000 bacterial colonies per milliliter of urine. As previously mentioned, a major revision in the diagnostic criteria for symptomatic UTI has been the abandonment of the absolute requirement for growth of at least 10^5 bacterial colonies per milliliter of urine. In one group of patients, the criterion of ≥ 100 bacteria per milliliter provided excellent sensitivity and specificity for the purpose of correctly diagnosing and treating women with symptomatic infection.[41] This same criterion should also be applied to lower UTIs when *S. saprophyticus* is isolated because UTIs caused by this pathogen often are associated with low urine bacterial colony counts, suboptimal growth on commonly used media, and negative findings on nitrite screening.

Mixed flora (≥ 2 organisms) is rare except in severely debilitated persons and other complicated infections. Thus, mixed flora in the setting of uncomplicated infection frequently suggests contamination, and a repeat specimen should be obtained.

6. What is the correlation between sensitivity of the organism to a particular drug and treatment outcome in acute cystitis?

Bacterial susceptibility to different antimicrobial drugs usually is tested by placing discs impregnated with antibacterial agents on an agar surface that has been seeded with the infecting organism. Bacterial sensitivity or susceptibility is indicated by a zone of inhibited growth around the disc containing the drug. Most discs are impregnated with a quantity of drug that correlates with achievable serum concentrations. However, drugs useful in the treatment of UTIs are excreted primarily by the kidney, and urine concentrations of these drugs may be 20 to 100 times greater than serum concentrations. Therefore, an organism that is only intermediately sensitive, or even "resistant" to the concentration of antibacterial drug in the testing disc might be sensitive to the high concentration of drug present in the urine.

Although in vitro susceptibility testing is not always predictive of whether patients will adequately respond to therapy, recent studies clearly show that patients infected with a resistant pathogen are at increased risk of treatment failure.[54,57,58,60–63] Several studies reported clinical response to infection in only 35% to 61% of patients with organisms resistant to TMP-SMX compared to 86% to 92% of patients infected with susceptible organisms.[54,57,60,61] Another study found that patients infected with TMP-SMX-resistant pathogens were 17 times more likely to experience therapy failure compared to those patients with susceptible strains.[62] Although 50% to 60% of patients with resistant organisms may experience failure of TMP-SMX therapy, antimicrobial therapy is usually chosen empirically without the benefit of C&S testing results. Appropriateness of antibiotic therapy is thus usually judged according to subsequent clinical response. If the infecting organism is sensitive, the urine will usually be sterile in 24 to 48 hours. If a urine specimen collected 48 hours after initiation of therapy is not sterile and the patient has been taking the medication properly, the antibiotic may be inappropriate or the focus of infection may be deeper (e.g., pyelonephritis, abscess, obstruction). If the urine specimen in the patient is sterile and the patient is symptomatically better, the appropriate antimicrobial is being used (regardless of sensitivity studies), and the full course of therapy should be completed.

7. **Was it necessary to order a pretreatment urine C&S for V.Q.?**

Some investigators question the value of pretreatment urine cultures.[4] Women with a lower UTI usually have pyuria on urinalysis and respond rapidly to antimicrobial treatment. Pyuria appears to be a better predictor of treatable infection than the colony count obtained on urine culture. Furthermore, the urine culture accounts for a large portion of the cost of managing a patient with a urinary tract infection. Consequently, in patients with uncomplicated, acute, lower UTI, it is more cost-effective to order a urinalysis and, if pyuria is present, to forego a urine culture. Instead, the patient should be empirically treated with a conventional 3- to 7-day course of antibiotic therapy. If she remains symptomatic 48 hours later, a C&S test can be ordered.

Fluoroquinolone Therapy

8. **I.B., a 48-year-old woman, presents with a community-acquired UTI. She has experienced a rash with TMP-SMX and has a Type I hypersensitivity reaction to penicillins. What is the role of fluoroquinolones in the treatment of I.B.'s community-acquired UTI?**

Several fluoroquinolones are indicated for the treatment of uncomplicated and/or complicated UTI; these include norfloxacin, ciprofloxacin, levofloxacin, and gatifloxacin. The fluoroquinolones are usually administered orally in the treatment of UTI and have excellent in vitro activity against most Gram-negative organisms, including *P. aeruginosa*.[64] They are also active in vitro against many Gram-positive organisms including *S. saprophyticus*.[64] Although resistance to the fluoroquinolones may be more common in complicated infections, resistance to these agents among organisms causing acute uncomplicated UTI is usually less than 1% to 2%.[19] The activity of many fluoroquinolones in vitro is antagonized by urine (acidic pH, divalent cations); however, this is unlikely to be clinically significant because urine concentrations are several hundredfold greater than serum levels.[64]

Although the fluoroquinolones are as effective as TMP-SMX in the treatment of uncomplicated UTIs, they are not recommended as first-line therapy because they are more expensive and provide no additional treatment benefits.[4,7,49,64] There also are concerns regarding the overuse of fluoroquinolones and the promotion of drug resistance among community-acquired pathogens. However, these agents are appro-

priate alternatives for patients with allergies to first-line agents or for patients infected with organisms resistant to multiple antibiotics, such as *P. aeruginosa*. Fluoroquinolones are also now recommended as first-line agents in geographic areas with >20% resistance of *E. coli* to TMP-SMX.[49] Finally, the fluoroquinolones have been effective in treating patients with structural or functional abnormalities of the urinary tract and other types of complicated infections.[64,65]

A fluoroquinolone is appropriate for I.B. because it will be effective and because she has experienced previous adverse reactions to penicillins and sulfas. The fluoroquinolones are considered similar in efficacy in this setting[65,66]; choice of a specific agent should be based on comparative costs and compliance considerations. The duration of fluoroquinolone therapy in I.B. would be 3 days.

Drug Interactions

9. **I.B. also is taking Maalox for a duodenal ulcer. What is the likelihood that this antacid will affect the action of the fluoroquinolones?**

It is imperative that the clinician questions I.B. regarding other medications (both prescription and nonprescription) that she may be taking. Products containing divalent and trivalent cations (Mg^{2+}, Ca^{2+}, Zn^{2+}, Al^{2+}, Fe^{2+}) invariably cause significantly decreased fluoroquinolone absorption (20% to 70% decrease in area under the concentration curve [AUC]), and this may result in therapeutic failures.[67] Although this interaction can be avoided by taking the antacids or other products at least 2 hours before or 4 to 6 hours after the fluoroquinolone dose, this is complicated and inconvenient for the patient.[68] Patients simply should avoid these products while taking fluoroquinolones. Interactions of the fluoroquinolones with H_2-receptor antagonists and proton pump inhibitors are usually not clinically significant, and these agents can be used for patients with gastrointestinal (GI) ulcers.[67,68]

Some older fluoroquinolones also interfere with theophylline metabolism, especially enoxacin (60% to 240% increase in AUC) and ciprofloxacin (20% to 90% increase in AUC).[67] Norfloxacin increases the theophylline AUC by approximately 15%.[69] Therefore, theophylline levels should be monitored closely in patients receiving these quinolones and theophylline together. Levofloxacin and gatifloxacin do not significantly alter methylxanthine metabolism.[67,70,71] Whereas ciprofloxacin interferes with the metabolism of caffeine, other newer agents do not.[67,70,71] Although the clinical significance of the interaction between caffeine and most fluoroquinolones is minimal, patients should be monitored carefully for signs and symptoms of caffeine toxicity. This is especially important for patients ingesting large quantities of caffeine and in older patients.

There have been isolated reports of a clinical interaction between certain quinolones (such as ciprofloxacin) and warfarin. Although there seems to be no truly relevant pharmacokinetic or pharmacodynamic interactions, patients receiving both warfarin and quinolone therapy should nevertheless be carefully monitored for changes in their anticoagulation.[67,72] There also have been isolated cases of increased toxicity with coadministration of quinolones and nonsteroidal anti-inflammatory drugs (NSAIDs), phenytoin, and cyclosporine; whether these interactions truly exist is unknown.[67,72]

HOSPITAL-ACQUIRED ACUTE URINARY TRACT INFECTION

10. P.M., an alert, 70-year-old woman with chest pain, was hospitalized to rule out acute myocardial infarction. This is her third hospitalization for chest pain in the past 6 months. A urinary catheter was temporarily placed as part of her routine medical care. Two days after admission, she complained of burning on urination and bladder pain. TMP-SMX double strength, 1 tablet BID was ordered after microscopic examination of the urine indicated a UTI. Why was this empiric therapy appropriate?

Hospital-acquired (or nosocomial) UTIs occur in about one-half million patients per year and most are associated with the use of indwelling bladder catheters. Approximately 10% to 30% of catheterized patients develop infection.[23] Complications of catheter-associated UTI are significant. Nosocomial UTIs are the source of up to 15% of all nosocomial bloodstream infections, occurring in about 4% of all catheterized patients[73]; the associated mortality rate is approximately 15%.[23] Nosocomial UTIs also prolong hospitalization by an average of 2.5 days and cost an additional $600 to $700.[20,23,73] Prevention is the best way to manage nosocomial UTIs, but in hospitalized patients who develop UTI symptoms, antibiotic treatment usually is initiated.

The sensitivity of hospital-acquired pathogenic bacteria to antimicrobial agents differs from community-acquired bacteria, and these susceptibilities frequently vary from one hospital to another. Therefore, the microbiology department of a particular hospital should be consulted to determine current trends in the antibiotic susceptibility of bacteria acquired in that setting. In general, *E. coli* is still the predominant urinary tract pathogen. However, an increased proportion of infections is caused by other Gram-negative bacteria such as *Proteus* and *Pseudomonas*, as well as Gram-positive pathogens such as *Staphylococcus* and *Enterococcus* and yeast (e.g., *Candida*).[20,21,23]

Repeated courses of antibiotic therapy, anatomic defects of the urinary tract, old age, increased hospital length of stay, and repeated hospital admissions are associated with a higher incidence of infection with antibiotic-resistant organisms.[23,74,75] *Pseudomonas, Proteus, Providencia, Morganella, Klebsiella, Enterobacter, Citrobacter,* and *Serratia* are particularly difficult to eradicate because they usually are less susceptible to commonly used antimicrobial agents.

P.M. is elderly, hospitalized, and has been repeatedly exposed to potentially resistant organisms during her previous hospitalizations. Because prompt treatment is deemed necessary, oral TMP-SMX is a reasonable first choice since *E. coli* still is the most likely causative agent, and P.M. is only mildly ill with signs and symptoms of lower UTI. However, oral fluoroquinolones are more commonly used in this setting because of the high potential for infection with resistant pathogens.[75] Cultures of P.M.'s urine should be performed and, once C&S test results are known, therapy promptly changed according to susceptibility reports. To achieve the most cost-effective therapy, oral agents should be administered to all patients capable of taking medications by mouth unless the isolated pathogens are resistant to oral medications or underlying GI dysfunction makes adequate absorption of oral antibiotics questionable.

11. If P.M. had additional symptoms of fever, chills, flank pain, and vomiting, how would her treatment differ?

In seriously ill patients with possible sepsis, broad-spectrum parenteral antibiotics with activity against *Pseudomonas aeruginosa* usually are preferred as initial therapy (Table 64-3). Several agents are suitable choices, including antipseudomonal cephalosporins (e.g., ceftazidime, cefepime), extended-spectrum penicillins (e.g., piperacillin/tazobactam, ticarcillin-clavulanate), carbapenems (imipenem-cilastatin, meropenem), intravenous fluoroquinolones (ciprofloxacin), and aztreonam. These antibiotics appear to be at least as effective as the aminoglycosides and lack the ototoxic and nephrotoxic potential. On the other hand, these newer agents are more costly and may be associated with the emergence of resistant organisms and superinfection with organisms such as *Enterococcus* and *Candida*.

In general, antipseudomonal β-lactam antibiotics remain the drugs of choice for nosocomial urologic sepsis. The combination of a β-lactam and an aminoglycoside may be advantageous in neutropenic patients. Once the susceptibility pattern of the infecting organism is known, therapy should be altered to single-agent therapy whenever possible to decrease the risks of drug toxicity and to decrease drug costs.

ACUTE PYELONEPHRITIS
Signs and Symptoms

12. L.B., a 45-year-old woman with diabetes, comes to the emergency department (ED) complaining of frequent urination, fever, shaking chills, and flank pain. She takes 20 units of NPH insulin SC every morning. Positive physical findings include a temperature of 103°F, a pulse of 110 beats/min, blood pressure (BP) of 90/60 mm Hg, and CVA tenderness. A Gram's stain of L.B.'s urine reveals Gram-negative rods, and a STAT UA demonstrates glucosuria, macroscopic hematuria, 20 to 25 WBCs/mm[3], numerous bacteria, and WBC casts. She also has a blood sugar level of 400 mg/dL (normal, 70 to 105 mg/dL). L.B. is admitted to the hospital with a diagnosis of acute bacterial pyelonephritis, and routine laboratory tests including a blood chemistry profile, complete blood count (CBC) with differential, and specimens of urine and blood for C&S are ordered. L.B. is started on IV normal saline, 1 g of ampicillin IV Q 6 hr, and a sliding-scale schedule of regular insulin based on Q 6 hr blood sugars. Which signs and symptoms in L.B. are consistent with a kidney infection?

[SI units: blood sugar, 22.20 mmol/L (normal, 3.88 to 5.82)]

It is not always possible to differentiate clinically between upper and lower urinary tract infections. Symptoms common in lower UTIs often are the only positive findings in upper UTIs (i.e., subclinical pyelonephritis).[1,4,6,76,77] However, L.B. does manifest signs and symptoms of systemic infection consistent with acute bacterial pyelonephritis, including tachycardia, hypotension, fever, shaking chills, flank pain, CVA tenderness, hematuria, and WBC casts. In addition, her diabetes may predispose her to renal infections, possibly because diabetic patients have altered antibacterial defense mechanisms.[6,76,77]

Table 64-3 Parenteral Antimicrobial Agents Commonly Used in the Treatment of Urinary Tract Infections

Class	Drug	Average Adult Daily Dose		Usual Dosage Interval[a]	Comments
		UTI	Sepsis		
Penicillins	Ampicillin	2–4 g	8 g	Q 4–6 hr	Use should be based on local susceptibility patterns
	Ampicillin/sulbactam	6 g	12 g	Q 6 hr	
Extended-spectrum penicillin	Ticarcillin/clavulanate	9–12 g	18 g	Q 4–6 hr	
	Piperacillin	12 g	18 g	Q 4–6 hr	
	Piperacillin/tazobactam	9 g	18 g	Q 4–6 hr	
First-generation cephalosporins	Cefazolin	1.5–3 g	6 g	Q 8–12 hr	More effective than second- or third-generation cephalosporins against Gram-positive organisms
Second-generation cephalosporins	Cefoxitin	3–4 g	8 g	Q 4–8 hr	Intermediate between first- and third-generation cephalosporins against Gram-negative organisms
	Cefuroxime	2.25 g	4.5 g	Q 8 hr	
	Cefotetan	1–4 g	6 g	Q 12 hr	
Third-generation cephalosporins	Cefotaxime	3–4 g	8 g	Q 6–8 hr	Better coverage than first- and second-generation cephalosporins against Gram-negative organisms. Ceftazidime and cefepime are most effective against *Pseudomonas*. All generations of cephalosporins are ineffective against *Enterococcus faecalis* and methicillin-resistant Staphylococci
	Ceftizoxime	2–3 g	8 g	Q 8–12 hr	
	Ceftriaxone	1 g	2 g	Q 12–24 hr	
	Ceftazidime	1.5–3 g	6 g	Q 8–12 hr	
Fourth-generation cephalosporins	Cefepime	1–2 g	4 g	Q 12 hr	
Carbapenems	Imipenem/cilastatin	1 g	2 g	Q 6 hr	The most broad-spectrum coverage of any antibiotics listed. Resistance may develop especially with *Pseudomonas*. Toxic in some pregnant animals
	Meropenem	1.5–3 g	3 g	Q 8 hr	
	Ertapenem	0.5–1 g	1 g	Q 24 hr	
Monobactam	Aztreonam	1–2 g	6–8 g	Q 8–12 hr	Active against Gram-negative aerobic pathogens, including *Pseudomonas sp.*
Aminoglycosides	Gentamicin	3 mg/kg	5 mg/kg	Q 8 hr	Potent against Gram-negative bacteria including *Pseudomonas*. Associated with possible eighth nerve toxicity in the fetus. Amikacin should be reserved for multiresistant bacteria
	Tobramycin	3 mg/kg	5 mg/kg	Q 8 hr	
	Amikacin	7.5 mg/kg	15 mg/kg	Q 12 hr	
Quinolones	Ciprofloxacin	400–800 mg	800 mg	Q 12 hr	Use for resistant organisms. Change to oral therapy when indicated
	Ofloxacin	400–800 mg	800 mg	Q 12 hr	
	Levofloxacin	250–500 mg	500 mg	Q 24 hr	
	Gatifloxacin	200–400 mg	400 mg	Q 24 hr	

[a]Assuming normal renal function.

Treatment
Triage for Hospitalization

13. Why was L.B. hospitalized?

Most patients with clinical pyelonephritis have relatively mild infection and can potentially be managed as outpatients. In such cases, the need for hospitalization often is determined by the patient's social situation and ability to maintain an adequate fluid intake and tolerate oral medications.[6,7,76] Patients like L.B. with evidence of bacteremia (e.g., fever, shaking chills) or sepsis (e.g., hypotension) should be hospitalized and treated with parenteral antibiotics.[6,7,76] It also is prudent to hospitalize L.B. because her acute pyelonephritis may predispose her to diabetic ketoacidosis.

Although it is customary to obtain blood cultures in patients with moderate-to-severe pyelonephritis, a recent study found that blood cultures were of low yield in the setting of acute uncomplicated pyelonephritis, rarely provided any additional information not already obtained from the urine culture, and were not helpful in the clinical management of pa-

tients.[78] However, blood cultures may be positive in up to 25% of patients with severe or complicated pyelonephritis and are still recommended for patients such as L.B.[6,76]

Antimicrobial Choice

14. Was ampicillin appropriate treatment for L.B.?

Ampicillin is not an appropriate choice for L.B. because diabetic patients (and patients treated with corticosteroids) are prone to colonization with unusual or more resistant organisms. Like lower tract UTIs, pyelonephritis is often classified as uncomplicated or complicated. L.B.'s infection would be classified as a complicated infection because of her underlying diabetes.[6,76] *E. coli* remains the predominant pathogen in complicated pyelonephritis, but other Gram-negative organisms (e.g., *Klebsiella, Proteus, Pseudomonas*) are found relatively more frequently.[6] Because L.B. is acutely ill and has Gram-negative organisms in her urine, she should be treated with an antibiotic that has a better spectrum of activity against Gram-negative organisms. Broad-spectrum antibiotics appropriate for initial therapy would include parenteral third-generation cephalosporins (e.g., ceftriaxone), intravenous fluoroquinolones (e.g., ciprofloxacin, levofloxacin), aztreonam, and piperacillin/tazobactam; aminoglycosides are also sometimes recommended as monotherapy.[6,7,79,80] It is not always necessary to initially treat patients with antipseudomonal therapy; thus, agents such as ceftriaxone with relatively less activity against *Pseudomonas* are often appropriate as initial therapy in patients such as L.B. Because most hospital laboratories can report C&S results within 48 hours, these antibiotics can be replaced with more specific ones if appropriate.

Serum Versus Urine Concentrations

15. Is it necessary to achieve bactericidal concentrations of antimicrobials in the serum, or are high urinary concentrations adequate for L.B.? How long should she be treated? How should therapeutic success be determined?

When the renal parenchyma is infected (e.g., pyelonephritis as opposed to uncomplicated cystitis), adequate tissue concentrations of antimicrobial agents are needed. Therefore, antibiotics that achieve bactericidal concentrations in serum and kidney tissues should be selected. Patients requiring hospitalization should be treated with parenteral antibiotics until fluids can be taken orally and the patient is symptomatically improved and afebrile for 24 to 48 hours. This should be followed with a course of oral antibiotics for a total duration of antimicrobial therapy of 14 to 21 days; less severe infections not requiring hospitalization are usually treated with courses of 7 to 14 days in duration. Although it is customary to observe the patient in the hospital for 24 hours after switching from parenteral to oral antibiotics before discharge, this is probably of limited benefit.[81] Specimens for C&S should be obtained on the second day of therapy (to rule out treatment failure), 2 to 3 weeks after the completion of therapy, and again at 3 months.[1,6]

For patients who have relapsed after 14 days, re-treatment for 6 weeks usually is curative. There have been reports of successful therapy with 5 days of treatment[78]; however, longer courses are recommended.[7,76,80]

Oral Therapy

16. When would you recommend oral therapy for the initial treatment of acute pyelonephritis?

Patients with mild, acute pyelonephritis (no nausea, vomiting, or signs of sepsis) can be managed with oral antibiotics such as TMP-SMX for 14 days.[6,76,80,82] This regimen is as effective as 6 weeks of TMP-SMX and significantly better than 6 weeks of ampicillin. The fluoroquinolones may be useful for patients infected with resistant organisms because of their excellent in vitro activity against Gram-negative organisms and high kidney tissue concentrations (2-fold to 10-fold greater than serum).[64] Agents such as amoxicillin-clavulanate, cefixime, or cefuroxime also can be used in this setting.

SYMPTOMATIC ABACTERIURIA
Clinical Presentation

17. R.D., a 22-year-old woman, complains of urinary frequency and painful urination, which have developed over the past 4 to 5 days. UA reveals 10 to 15 WBCs/mm³ (normal, 0 to 2 WBCs/mm³), but no bacteria are seen on a Gram's stain of the urine. Phenazopyridine 200 mg TID is prescribed. What is a reasonable assessment of R.D.'s clinical presentation?

Acute urethral syndrome is defined as symptoms consistent with lower UTI but with no organisms evident on Gram's stain or culture. The lack of detectable pathogens may mean that the urine specimen is sterile or that the concentration of the organism in the urine sample is small. Patients with these findings still may have a UTI even though the voided urine is sterile or contains $<10^5$ microorganisms per milliliter.[83,84] The causative organisms and the pathogenesis of infection in these cases are the same as for lower UTIs. Other organisms that may cause urethritis in this setting are *Chlamydia trachomatis, N. gonorrhoeae,* and *Trichomonas vaginalis.*[83,84]

Most cases of urinary tract infection with low bacterial counts are associated with bacteriuria or *C. trachomatis* and also demonstrate pyuria (>8 WBCs/mm³).[83,84] Conversely, pathogens are seldom present in patients with the acute urethral syndrome when pyuria is absent. Because R.D. is symptomatic, has 10 to 15 WBCs/mm³ in her urine, and no bacteria on Gram's stain, infection with *C. trachomatis* or some other more atypical pathogen is likely.

Antibiotic Treatment

18. Should R.D. be treated with antibiotics?

Yes. A double-blind, placebo-controlled study evaluated the use of doxycycline 100 mg twice daily in patients with UTI and low bacterial counts.[85] Clinical cure of bacteriuria and pyuria was significantly greater in the doxycycline-treated group, but doxycycline did not alter symptoms in patients without pyuria. Because *E. coli,* other Gram-negative bacteria, and *C. trachomatis* are the usual causes of acute urethral syndrome, an antibiotic like doxycycline with activity against *Chlamydia* is reasonable initial treatment for patients like R.D. presenting with urinary tract symptoms (without bacteriuria) if pyuria also is present. All tetracyclines and sulfonamides, with or without trimethoprim, also are likely to be effective in such patients, but doxycycline has been best studied to date. Of the fluoroquinolones, newer agents such as levofloxacin and gatifloxacin offer promise as alternatives to doxycycline but have not been well studied in this setting.[84] Azithromycin as a single dose also has a major role in treating chlamydial infections (see Chapter 65, Sexually Transmitted Diseases).

Prolonged therapy of 2 to 4 weeks in duration and treatment of sexual partners may be required to prevent reinfection through intercourse. Prolonged therapy is appropriate if the patient has a history consistent with *Chlamydia* urethritis; a sexual partner with recent urethritis; a recent new sexual partner; a gradual, rather than abrupt, onset of symptoms that has occurred over a period of days (as in R.D.); and no hematuria.[83] However, patients without such a history can be managed with a short course of antibiotics like any other patient with a lower UTI.

Phenazopyridine

19. Was phenazopyridine appropriate for R.D.?

Phenazopyridine, a urinary tract analgesic, often is prescribed alone or along with an antibacterial agent for the symptomatic relief of dysuria. Although 200 mg three times a day may relieve dysuria, it is ineffective in the actual eradication of true UTIs. Phenazopyridine plus an antibiotic is not any better than an antibiotic alone; therefore, the drug is not likely to be of significant value in R.D. and should seldom be prescribed for such patients.

Although most patients have resolution of symptoms within 24 to 48 hours after beginning therapy, some patients with severe dysuria or delayed response to antibiotic therapy may benefit symptomatically from a short trial (1 to 2 days) of phenazopyridine.[4] The need for and duration of analgesic therapy must be individualized.

Side Effects

20. What side effects have been associated with phenazopyridine?

Phenazopyridine is an azo dye and may discolor the urine to an orange-red, orange-brown, or red color that can stain clothes. Other adverse effects of phenazopyridine occur following an acute overdose or as a result of accumulation in older patients or in patients with decreased renal function who take the drug chronically. In vivo, about 50% of phenazopyridine is metabolized to aniline, which can cause methemoglobinemia and hemolytic anemia. The hemolytic anemia associated with phenazopyridine occurs primarily in patients with glucose-6-phosphate dehydrogenase (G6PD) deficiency.[86] Cases of reversible acute renal failure and allergic hepatitis have also been rarely reported following brief exposure to phenazopyridine.[86]

ASYMPTOMATIC BACTERIURIA
Antibiotic Treatment

21. A.K., an asymptomatic 6-year-old girl, is found to have significant bacteriuria on routine screening. Should she be treated with an antimicrobial agent?

The management of patients with asymptomatic bacteriuria depends on the clinical setting in which it is found. Asymptomatic bacteriuria occurs in a heterogeneous group of patients with different prognoses and risks. Some patients will have significant bacteriuria ($>10^5$ bacteria per milliliter of urine) without pyuria. Others may have pyuria without significant bacteriuria. The patients in this latter group probably have self-limiting infections and do not require treatment if they are asymptomatic. However, because asymptomatic patients with significant bacteriuria and pyuria may develop overt pyelonephritis, therapy is probably warranted if significant bacteriuria is confirmed on successive cultures.[1]

Although the management of asymptomatic bacteriuria is inconsistent, the potential for long-term complications from UTIs must be considered. Patients who appear to benefit most from antibiotic treatment are those with complicating factors. These include urinary tract structural abnormalities, immunosuppressive therapy, and procedures requiring urinary tract instrumentation or manipulation.[2] Short-course regimens (i.e., single-dose or 3-day) are usually recommended when treatment is desired.[2] The treatment of asymptomatic bacteriuria in women with diabetes has recently been shown not to reduce complications and is not currently recommended.[87]

UTIs in infants and preschool children (predominantly girls) occasionally are associated with renal tissue damage.[88] Asymptomatic bacteriuria of childhood also is important because it may be a manifestation of an anatomic or mechanical defect in the urinary tract. Therefore, it should be evaluated fully. However, because most cases of renal scarring as a result of bacteriuria occur within the first 5 years of life, it is controversial whether treatment should be limited to infants and preschool children or whether all children should be treated regardless of age.[11] Screening for bacteriuria in children and treating those with positive cultures, regardless of their clinical presentation, seems reasonable and is frequently recommended.[11,88] Treatment of A.K., although still controversial, seems prudent because renal damage resulting from asymptomatic bacteriuria generally occurs during childhood. Should the decision be made to treat, principles of therapy are similar to those for symptomatic infections.

Pregnant Patients and the Elderly

22. The decision to treat the asymptomatic bacteriuria of A.K. was based primarily on the increased probability of renal damage during childhood. What other population groups should be treated for asymptomatic bacteriuria?

Without urinary tract obstruction, UTIs in adults rarely lead to progressive renal damage.[2,4] Therefore, asymptomatic bacteriuria does not require treatment in adult patients who have no evidence of mechanical obstruction or renal insufficiency. However, aggressive antimicrobial therapy is appropriate during pregnancy because as many as 40% of pregnant women with asymptomatic bacteriuria later develop symptomatic UTIs, particularly pyelonephritis. In addition, studies have confirmed associations between acute pyelonephritis during pregnancy with increased rates of preterm labor, premature delivery, and lower birth-weight infants.[26] The treatment of asymptomatic bacteriuria in pregnancy is therefore justified to decrease the risk of associated complications.

Treatment can be based on in vitro susceptibility testing or by selecting the least expensive, least toxic agent. Tetracyclines should be avoided because they may stain and weaken the forming dentition of the unborn child. Sulfonamides should be avoided in late pregnancy because they can contribute to kernicterus in the neonate. Fluoroquinolones should be avoided during pregnancy because of the risk of arthropathies (see Question 38).

Bacteriuria in the elderly is common.[14,15] However, although bacteriuria in this population often leads to symptomatic infection, clinical studies have consistently documented no beneficial outcomes in treated patients compared with nontreated patients.[14] Consequently, therapy is not recommended for the asymptomatic older patient because the expense, side effects, and potential complications of drug therapy appear to outweigh the benefits.[14] Patients experiencing symptomatic infections should be treated as usual.

RECURRENT URINARY TRACT INFECTIONS
Relapse Versus Reinfection

23. T.W., a 28-year-old woman with a history of recurrent infections, recently was treated for an *E. coli* UTI with TMP-SMX for 10 days. A repeat UA was scheduled, but she canceled her appointment because she "felt fine." Eight weeks later, she returned to the clinic with signs and symptoms of another UTI. The only other medication she has taken is an oral contraceptive. Why would C&S testing of a urine sample be especially useful at this time?

Recurrent infections develop in approximately 20% to 30% of women with acute cystitis.[2,4] Repeat C&S data should help determine whether this infection represents a relapse or a reinfection. *Relapse* refers to a recurrence of bacteriuria caused by the same microorganism that was present before the initiation of therapy. Most relapses occur within 1 to 2 weeks after the completion of therapy and are caused by persistence of the organism in the urinary tract. Relapses often are associated with an inadequately treated upper UTI, structural abnormalities of the urinary tract, or chronic bacterial prostatitis.[1]

Reinfection implies recurrence of bacteriuria with a different organism than was present before therapy. Reinfections may occur at any time during or after the completion of treatment, but most appear several weeks to several months later. Approximately 80% of recurrences are due to reinfection.[1] Reinfections generally are due to introital colonization with Enterobacteriaceae from the lower intestinal tract[1]; of these, *E. coli* is the most common. Certain *E. coli* strains have been shown to adhere to vaginal epithelial cells and, in women with recurrent UTI, adherence of these organisms to epithelial cells is increased.[24,89] That T.W. was symptom free for 8 weeks suggests that this is a reinfection.

Oral Contraceptives as a Risk Factor

24. Is there an association between T.W.'s use of oral contraceptives and her risk of contracting a UTI?

Information regarding the association between oral contraceptive use and UTIs is controversial. The two most recent studies to examine this association disagree in their conclusions. A well-designed prospective study examined 796 women and found the incidence of UTI to be exactly the same between oral contraceptive users and nonusers.[35] However, a subsequent case-control study in 229 women with recurrent UTI and 253 control subjects found that oral contraceptive users were at significantly higher risk for recurrent infection.[26] The association between oral contraceptive use and risk of UTI remains unclear.

The association between diaphragm use and urinary tract infection is much stronger. Diaphragm users are approximately three times more likely to develop a UTI than women using other contraceptive methods, especially when the diaphragm is used in conjunction with spermicidal jelly.[26,35] Possible explanations include urethral obstruction by the diaphragm together with increased vaginal colonization by coliform organisms caused by the spermicide. Use of a spermicide-coated condom also has been shown to increase the risk of UTI.[26,90]

Treatment for Reinfection

25. Pending the C&S results, what therapy should be instituted in T.W.?

T.W. has a history of recurrent infections and now probably has a reinfection. Because reinfection is not caused by failure of previous therapy, TMP-SMX may be a reasonable choice once again. The probability that a resistant organism will be responsible for the infection increases when the interval between infectious episodes is short. If several months elapse between each episode of antimicrobial therapy, normal fecal bacterial flora become re-established and the risk of infection with resistant pathogens is reduced.

The alteration of fecal flora caused by the sulfonamides and tetracyclines makes these drugs poor choices for repeated use in cases of frequent reinfection, especially when C&S results are unknown. The development of bacterial resistance also may limit the usefulness of these agents for chronic antimicrobial therapy.[19,43]

26. If T.W. developed an adverse reaction to TMP-SMX, what are some other therapeutic alternatives?

Nitrofurantoin is effective against 80% to 90% of *E. coli* strains. It does not significantly alter the fecal or introital flora, and the development of resistance in previously sensitive strains does not often occur.[19,43,91] Therefore, it generally is a useful agent for the treatment of recurrent *E. coli, S. saprophyticus,* and *Enterococcus* infections. On the other hand, *Proteus, Enterobacter,* and *Klebsiella* tend to be somewhat resistant to this drug (susceptibility <60%).[19]

Nitrofurantoin is absorbed orally. Food substantially decreases the rate of absorption, but increases the total bioavailability of nitrofurantoin from both the macrocrystalline capsules and the microcrystalline tablets by about 40%. This effect lengthens the duration of therapeutic urine concentrations by about 2 hours.[92] Nitrofurantoin barely reaches detectable levels in the plasma because it is eliminated rapidly (half-life, 20 minutes) into the urine and bile; urine levels are 50 to 250 mg/L.[92] Thus nitrofurantoin is used only for UTIs. While the Kirby-Bauer disc sensitivity test measures the sensitivity of an organism to the expected serum levels of most antibiotics, in the case of nitrofurantoin the test measures sensitivity to urinary levels.

The fluoroquinolones also are useful in this setting. However, their widespread use should not be encouraged in light of their high cost and selection of resistant organisms.[48] Cephalexin and trimethoprim also have been recommended as alternative agents in this setting.[2]

Evaluation Procedures (Localization)

27. Greater than 10⁵ bacteria per milliliter of *P. mirabilis*, sensitive to ampicillin and TMP-SMX, are cultured in T.W.'s urine. One week after completing her second course of TMP-SMX therapy, signs and symptoms of a UTI again appear. How should T.W. be assessed at this time?

One should first attempt to rule out common causes for relapse. Inadequate therapy resulting from patient noncompliance with the prescribed treatment, inappropriate antibiotic selection, or bacterial resistance to the prescribed agent should be considered if significant bacteriuria persists despite treatment. Next, one must consider renal infections (e.g., subclinical pyelonephritis), which cause the most relapsing UTIs.[1,2] Finally, if these common causes are not present, radiologic tests to rule out surgically correctable structural abnormalities of the urinary tract should be performed (e.g., intravenous pyelogram). Infected kidney stones and unilateral atrophic kidneys are common but correctable abnormalities in females.

Radiologic tests are indicated when UTIs start to recur in children, in men younger than 50 years of age, and in patients with UTIs associated with bacteremia, ureteral colic, or passage of stones. These populations are most likely to have surgically correctable lesions. In contrast, these procedures rarely are necessary in adult women and elderly men until the common causes of relapse in these populations have been eliminated.[4,22,93] Chronic bacterial prostatitis, a frequent cause of recurrent infections in males, need not be considered in this case.

Treatment of Relapse
Trimethoprim-Sulfamethoxazole

28. Pending C&S results, TMP-SMX is again prescribed. Is this still a reasonable medication for T.W. at this time?

Because the *P. mirabilis* cultured during the last recurrence was still susceptible to TMP-SMX, this agent would again be a reasonable choice until C & S results are obtained. Alternatively, use of a different agent (e.g., fluoroquinolone) could be considered because the relapse occurred within 1 week of completing the previous treatment and resistance may have developed.[4]

29. How long should this therapy be continued?

The duration of therapy for relapsing infections usually is 14 days. In patients who relapse after a second 2-week course of therapy, treatment for 6 weeks should be instituted.[1,2,93] If relapse occurs after a 6-week course, some experts recommend longer courses of 6 months to 1 year.[1,2] These prolonged courses should be reserved for children, adults who have continuous symptoms, or adults who are at high risk for developing progressive renal damage. Asymptomatic adults without evidence of obstruction should not receive these longer courses. T.W. should be treated for at least 2 weeks and perhaps as long as 6 weeks.

Trimethoprim

30. T.W. was previously treated with TMP-SMX and experienced nausea and vomiting after taking the medication. Why would trimethoprim alone be an appropriate substitute?

Trimethoprim alone and in combination with sulfamethoxazole is active in vitro against many of the Enterobacteriaceae associated with UTIs and is an effective alternative to TMP-SMX in the management of both chronic and acute UTIs.[1,2,4,93] It would be especially appropriate for T.W. because GI intolerance to TMP-SMX is most commonly attributed to the sulfamethoxazole component, and trimethoprim is associated with a lower incidence of side effects. There is some concern for the potential development of resistant organisms, but

studies using trimethoprim alone have failed to demonstrate a significant increase in bacterial resistance.[94] Trimethoprim is used for the treatment of acute, uncomplicated UTIs in a dosage of 200 mg/day.

Chronic Prophylaxis

31. T.W. was treated successfully with trimethoprim for 6 weeks. Is prophylactic antimicrobial therapy indicated? If so, how long should it be continued?

Chronic UTIs may be managed by treating each recurrent infection with an appropriate antibacterial. A single dose or longer course may be used. More commonly, chronic UTIs are managed by administering chronic, low-dose prophylactic therapy. The frequency of urinary infections probably is the main determinant of whether chronic suppressive therapy should be used, because data suggest that repeated treatment of recurrent infections eventually will result in a decreased incidence of subsequent infections.[1,95] Long-term prophylactic therapy clearly reduces the frequency of symptomatic infections in nearly all patients.[14]

From a cost-effectiveness standpoint, women having more than one episode of cystitis per year may benefit from antimicrobial prophylaxis.[93,94] For women with three or more episodes of cystitis per year, prophylaxis clearly is more cost-effective than treating individual infections. Therefore, chronic antimicrobial prophylaxis should be considered in any patient with two or more episodes of UTI per year.[93,95]

The duration of prophylactic therapy also is determined by the frequency of infection. Women with three or more UTIs in the 12 months before a 6-month course of antimicrobial prophylaxis have a significantly higher recurrence rate (75%) in the 6 months following prophylaxis than women who had only two infections in the 12 months before prophylaxis (26% recurrence rate).[96] Therefore, prophylaxis should be continued for 6 months in patients with less than three UTIs per year and for at least 12 months in patients with three or more UTIs per year.

Before chronic antimicrobial suppressive therapy is initiated, active infections must be completely eradicated with a full course of appropriate antibiotic therapy. The low doses of antimicrobials used for chronic prophylaxis suppress bacterial growth but do not eliminate active infection. Furthermore, surgically correctable anatomic abnormalities that predispose the patient to recurrent infections (e.g., obstruction, stones) should be ruled out. Patients with urologic abnormalities respond poorly to prophylactic therapy.[93,94] Age also should be considered when contemplating chronic antimicrobial therapy. An asymptomatic, elderly patient taking many other medications is usually not an ideal candidate for chronic prophylactic treatment because of problems of noncompliance, cost, and potential drug interactions or toxicities.[93,94] However, younger patients are good candidates for long-term suppressive therapy.[93,95]

Because T.W., a 28-year-old woman, has had at least three UTIs in the past few months, has undergone extensive evaluation, and has just been successfully treated with a standard course of trimethoprim, a 12-month course of antimicrobial prophylaxis would seem reasonable. She also should be evaluated at regular intervals for recurrent UTIs and for the development of resistant organisms.[1,2,94,95]

32. What drugs can be used for long-term suppressive therapy?

Although numerous drugs are used for prophylaxis, TMP-SMX may be the drug of choice for chronic antimicrobial therapy due to extensive experience, proven efficacy, infrequent toxicities, and low cost.[93,95] TMP-SMX also has the effect of decreasing vaginal colonization with uropathogens.[95] TMP-SMX one-half tablet daily is commonly prescribed for chronic UTI prophylaxis; thrice-weekly TMP-SMX is also an effective, well-tolerated and convenient prophylactic regimen.[93,95]

Successful prophylaxis, however, is significantly decreased in patients with urologic abnormalities or renal dysfunction. Also, infections that are not eradicated by a short-term therapeutic trial of TMP-SMX are not likely to respond to a long-term regimen.[94] Finally, enterococci may colonize introitally in patients taking chronic TMP-SMX.[96]

Fluoroquinolones are effective for chronic suppressive therapy but should be used only when antimicrobial resistance exists among cultured organisms or if the patient is intolerant to other recommended drugs. Cephalosporins also have been recommended as being appropriate for long-term prophylactic therapy, but are perhaps best reserved for patients intolerant to or failing prophylaxis with other agents.[93–95]

When selecting a drug for chronic antimicrobial therapy, one must consider efficacy, the likelihood that resistant organisms will develop, long-term toxicity, convenience, and cost to the patient. The most commonly used agents are listed in Table 64-4.

Based on the available information, it appears that T.W. could be switched to TMP-SMX. Although she has a history of GI distress because of this drug, this may not be a problem with the lower doses used for prophylaxis. If it is, trimethoprim alone, nitrofurantoin, or a fluoroquinolone also should be effective.

SPECIAL CASES
Prostatitis

Prostatitis is a common but poorly understood entity. Many clinicians group all prostatic diseases into one category but, in fact, the types and causes of prostatitis are many. The most prevalent forms include acute and chronic bacterial prostatitis, chronic calculus prostatitis, nonbacterial prostatitis, and prostatodynia.[12,13,97]

Acute Bacterial Prostatitis

Acute bacterial prostatitis is characterized by the sudden onset of chills and fever; perineal and low back pain; urinary urgency and frequency; nocturia, dysuria, and generalized malaise; and prostration. Patients also may complain of myalgias, arthralgias, and symptoms of bladder outlet obstruction. Rectal examination usually discloses an exquisitely tender, swollen prostate that is firm and warm to the touch. The pathogens generally can be identified by culture of the voided urine and usually are similar to those causing UTIs in women (see Table 64-1). In patients with acute bacterial prostatitis, prostatic massage should be avoided because of patient discomfort and the risk of bacteremia.[12,13]

Chronic Bacterial Prostatitis

Chronic bacterial prostatitis is one of the most common causes of recurrent UTIs in men. Except in males with spinal cord injuries, infectious stones, or obstructive abnormalities of the urinary tract, recurrent infections are almost always relapses caused by persistence of bacteria in the prostate. Normally, males secrete a prostatic antibacterial factor; however, this substance is absent in men with chronic prostatitis.[97] Simple UTIs will often eventually involve the prostate gland, where bacteria are difficult to eradicate.

The clinical manifestations of chronic bacterial prostatitis are highly variable and, in many patients, are asymptomatic. The disease usually is suspected when a male treated for UTI relapses, and the diagnosis is confirmed by examination of expressed prostatic secretions.[12,97] To ensure accurate localization (i.e., to distinguish prostatic from urethral bacteria), segmented urine samples are taken. The first 10 mL of voided urine represents the urethral sample, the midstream urine collected represents the bladder sample, and the first 10 mL voided immediately after prostatic massage represents the prostate sample. When the bladder sample is sterile or nearly so, bacterial prostatitis is diagnosed if the bacterial count in the prostate sample is at least one logarithm greater than that in the urethral sample. The bacterial pathogens responsible for chronic prostatitis often are similar to those of acute prostatitis and UTIs in general (see Table 64-1).[12,13,97]

Table 64-4	**Antimicrobial Agents Commonly Used for Chronic Prophylaxis Against Recurrent UTIs**[1,2,4,93-96]	
Agent	*Adult Dose*	*Comments*[a]
Nitrofurantoin	50–100 mg nightly	Contraindicated under 1 month of age. *To be taken with food or milk. May cause brown or rust-yellow discoloration of urine*
Trimethoprim	100 mg nightly	Not recommended in children <12 yr
Trimethoprim 80 mg + Sulfamethoxazole 400 mg	0.5–1 tab nightly or 3 × per week	Not recommended for use in infants <2 months. *To be taken on an empty stomach with a full glass of water. Photosensitivity may occur*
Norfloxacin	200 mg/day	Avoid antacids; monitor theophylline levels
Cephalexin	125–250 mg/day	
Cefaclor	250 mg/day	
Cephradine	250 mg/day	
Sulfamethoxazole	500 mg/day	

[a]Includes unique patient consultation information in italics.

Treatment

33. **D.G., a 60-year-old man, experienced his first UTI at age 40, with symptoms of frequency, dysuria, nocturia, perineal pain, chills, and fever, but no flank pain. Acute prostatitis was diagnosed. *E. coli* was cultured from the urine, and treatment with a sulfonamide was successful. After 12 asymptomatic years, acute prostatitis caused by *E. coli* recurred and again responded to sulfonamide therapy. Two more *E. coli* infections that responded to sulfonamide therapy occurred over the next 8 years. Why were sulfonamides appropriate treatment for D.G.'s acute episodes of bacterial prostatitis?**

Most antibacterial drugs appropriate for UTIs, including sulfonamides, can be used to treat acute bacterial prostatitis because the diffuse, intense inflammation of the prostate gland allows many drugs to readily penetrate into the prostatic fluid and tissues. Antimicrobial therapy should be continued for at least 1 month to prevent the development of chronic prostatitis.[12,13,97]

In addition to antibiotics, other supportive measures may provide symptomatic relief to patients with acute bacterial prostatitis. These measures include liberal hydration, NSAIDs for pain relief, sitz baths, and stool softeners.[98]

In retrospect, sulfonamides were appropriate for D.G. because they effectively treated his infections.

34. **Taking into account the pathophysiology of prostatitis, what would be a reasonable choice of therapy for D.G. should he have future recurrences of prostatitis?**

Because inflammation is minimal in patients with chronic prostatitis, most antibiotics that are acidic do not readily cross the prostatic epithelium into the alkaline prostatic fluid. Theoretically, the high alkalinity of prostatic fluids should impair the diffusion of trimethoprim and enhance the diffusion of the tetracyclines, certain sulfonamides, and the macrolide antibiotics, such as erythromycin. Nevertheless, TMP-SMX historically has the best documented cure rates in the treatment of acute and chronic bacterial prostatitis. Long-term therapy of chronic bacterial prostatitis with TMP-SMX for 4 to 16 weeks is associated with a cure rate of 32% to 71%, which significantly exceeds the cure rate associated with short-term therapy of 2 weeks or less.[12,13,98]

The fluoroquinolones have become well-accepted alternatives to TMP-SMX and are even considered by many to be the agents of choice for the management of prostatitis.[98] A number of studies have documented bacteriologic cure in 80% to 90% of patients treated with norfloxacin, ciprofloxacin, or levofloxacin for 4 to 12 weeks, rates comparable to or substantially higher than those achieved with agents such as TMP-SMX.[12,13,98] The fluoroquinolones have assumed an important role in the treatment of prostatitis due to their bactericidal activity against common pathogens and excellent penetration into prostatic tissues and fluid. The fluoroquinolones are often used as initial empiric therapy of prostatitis and are also excellent alternatives to other agents in patients who are unresponsive or intolerant to conventional therapy, or in those infected with resistant organisms.[12,13,98] Fluoroquinolones also have been used for chronic suppressive therapy (one-half normal doses) in patients who relapse after conventional treatment.[1]

D.G. should be treated with TMP-SMX for a minimum of 6 weeks; some authorities recommend a 2- to 3-month total

course of therapy.[98] If an adequate trial of TMP-SMX is unsuccessful, fluoroquinolone therapy can be used. Alternatively, a fluoroquinolone could be used as initial therapy.

If D.G. continues to develop recurrent infections following a trial of fluoroquinolone therapy, chronic low-dose treatment with TMP-SMX, fluoroquinolones, or nitrofurantoin can alleviate the symptoms of episodic bladder infection associated with chronic bacterial prostatitis. Infections eventually recur with greater frequency in most of these patients, although some become asymptomatic, even with chronic bacteriuria. Chronic, low-dose antibacterial therapy sterilizes the bladder, alleviates symptoms, confines bacteria to the prostate, and prevents infection of and damage to the rest of the urinary tract. Chronic bacterial prostatitis is one of the few indications for continuous antibiotic therapy.

Urinary Tract Infection and Sexual Intercourse

35. **On routine screening, asymptomatic bacteriuria is noted in W.W., a 30-year-old pregnant woman in her first trimester. Five years ago, during her first pregnancy, she developed acute bacterial pyelonephritis, which required hospitalization and treatment with parenteral antibiotics. Since that time, she has had recurrent UTIs, apparently related to sexual intercourse. These subsided when she began taking a single dose of nitrofurantoin after coitus, but she discontinued the practice before this pregnancy because she was afraid of the potential effects of this drug on the fetus. What is the association between sexual intercourse and the occurrence of UTIs?**

Studies strongly support an association between sexual intercourse and symptomatic UTIs.[1,2,26,35,93] One recent study demonstrated a direct relationship between the number of days with intercourse within the previous week and the risk of developing a UTI.[35] The relative risk of infection in women with 1, 4, and 7 days of intercourse within the previous week was 1.4, 3.5, and 9.0, respectively, compared with women who were sexually inactive within the previous week. Another study found that the risk of UTI was doubled in women having intercourse more than 4 times per month compared to those women who did not.[26] Studies also indicate that introital colonization by fecal bacteria has a definite role in recurrent infections related to intercourse. The migration of these colonizing bacteria into the bladder appears to be facilitated during intercourse, but the exact mechanism remains unclear.[1,2,35,93] Because UTIs are uncommon in males, transmission of an infection from the male is unlikely. Occasionally, bacteria harbored under the foreskin of an uncircumcised male may be transmitted to his partner through intercourse.[3]

36. **Was it rational to manage these infections with a single dose of an antibiotic after intercourse?**

Postcoital antibiotic prophylaxis often is recommended when recurrent UTIs are thought to result from sexual intercourse. Theoretically, a single dose of an antimicrobial agent produces bactericidal activity in the urine before bacteria have a chance to multiply, and the infection is averted. Patients should be instructed to empty their bladder just after intercourse and before taking the medication to minimize the number of bacteria present in the bladder and to eliminate unnecessary dilution of the drug in the urine. Because most drugs effective for UTIs are rapidly excreted by the kidney and reach high urinary concentrations, this regimen appears reasonable and does lower the incidence of postcoital infections. However, it has the same drawbacks as does any other type of antibiotic prophylaxis, and is not recommended in patients with structural abnormalities of the urinary tract or decreased renal function. It also is important to treat symptomatic infection before beginning prophylaxis.

Depending on the frequency of intercourse, postcoital prophylaxis may result in less antibiotic use compared with continuous prophylaxis. TMP-SMX probably is the drug of choice; however, other agents such as nitrofurantoin, fluoroquinolones, and cephalexin may be used.[99]

Urinary Tract Infection and Pregnancy

37. **Because W.W.'s UTI is asymptomatic at this time, should treatment be withheld because of her pregnancy?**

Treatment should not be withheld because acute symptomatic pyelonephritis may develop in pregnant women with untreated bacteriuria. In addition, there is evidence that maternal UTIs during pregnancy are associated with increased rates of preterm labor, premature delivery, and lower birthweight infants.[26] Although a cause-and-effect relationship has not been definitely established, current recommendations are in favor of treating maternal UTIs during pregnancy.

Screening pregnant women is appropriate because bacteriuria is so common. The high frequency of bacteriuria early in pregnancy and its rarity late in pregnancy suggests that screening should be done early in pregnancy, particularly during the 16th gestational week.[100] Treatment with an appropriate antimicrobial agent is then recommended for all pregnant patients with significant bacteriuria.[100]

Teratogenicity

38. **Which antimicrobial agents are contraindicated in W.W.?**

The use of antibiotics in pregnancy has been reviewed thoroughly elsewhere.[45,46,101] As indicated in Table 64-2, tetracyclines are contraindicated in pregnant women and in nursing mothers because they can cause permanent yellow, grayish-brown, or brown discoloration of the teeth in the fetus or nursing infant. In addition, tetracyclines have been associated with the development of fatty liver and nephropathy in the pregnant female. Thus, tetracyclines should always be avoided in pregnant and nursing mothers.

Sulfonamides and sulfonamide combinations (e.g., TMP-SMX) can cause kernicterus in neonates if given to mothers during the third trimester of pregnancy or to lactating women. The sulfonamides displace unconjugated bilirubin from plasma albumin, thereby allowing bilirubin to enter the brain; this induces encephalopathy in the newborn. The risk of kernicterus with TMP-SMX may be lower than that previously seen with older drugs (e.g., sulfasoxazole) that were more highly protein-bound and administered in high doses of up to several grams per day. However, TMP-SMX should still be considered to be relatively contraindicated during the third trimester and alternative agents used whenever possible. Sulfonamides in breast milk can cause hemolytic anemia in infants with G6PD deficiency.

Teratogenicity attributed to TMP-SMX has not been reported to date, although the total number of women who have taken this drug during the first trimester (when the fetus is most susceptible to teratogenic effects) is too small to make any conclusion about its safety. Fetal malformations have been associated with other folic acid antagonists, so it may be best to avoid the use of TMP-SMX and trimethoprim during pregnancy or nursing.

Nitrofurantoin is often recommended during pregnancy because teratogenic effects have not been observed clinically. However, in vitro investigations suggest a slight mutagenic potential. Nitrofurantoin also could cause hemolytic anemia in a G6PD-deficient nursing infant; however, only small amounts have been detected in breast milk.[45,46,101] The fluoroquinolones are contraindicated in pregnancy because of the arthropathy observed in immature animals.[67]

The penicillins, cephalosporins, and aminoglycosides appear to be relatively safe for use during pregnancy, although caution with the aminoglycosides is warranted because of possible eighth nerve toxicity in the fetus. These drugs, along with the others listed in Tables 64-2 and 64-3, cross the placental barrier; thus, the risk of toxicity or teratogenicity to the fetus always must be considered before deciding to treat a pregnant patient with a UTI.

In this case, a cephalosporin or sulfisoxazole could be safely prescribed for treatment of W.W.'s UTI. Ampicillin or amoxicillin would also be reasonable choices if W.W. resided in a geographic area where rates of resistance to these agents were known to be low. W.W. was correct in discontinuing her nitrofurantoin before pregnancy because the risk to the fetus, though small, tends to offset the advantage of antimicrobial prophylaxis. However, W.W. must receive proper follow-up care (also see Chapter 47, Teratogenicity and Drugs in Breast Milk).

39. **How long should W.W. be treated?**

Few studies have compared single-dose and 3-day therapy to conventional therapy for 7 days in pregnant patients. However, initial trials demonstrated that cure rates of single-dose therapy were lower than 7- to 10-day therapy.[26] Although more recent trials have shown that single-dose therapy effectively eradicates bacteriuria in pregnancy, these studies were conducted in a small number of patients. Therefore, it is recommended that pregnant patients receive either a 3-day regimen or a 7- to 10-day regimen rather than single-dose therapy.[26]

Irrespective of the duration of therapy, appropriate follow-up of patients is crucial. Clinicians must document elimination of pathogens 1 to 2 weeks after therapy and follow the patient monthly for the remainder of gestation. If bacteriuria recurs, therapy should be given for relapse or reinfection and the patient evaluated radiologically for structural abnormalities.[1,26]

Urinary Catheters

Catheter-associated UTIs are the most common type of hospital-acquired infection and may occur in up to 30% of catheterized patients.[23] Catheterization and other forms of urologic instrumentation are involved in 65% to 75% of all hospital-acquired UTIs, and catheter-associated UTI accounts for up to 30% of all nosocomial infections. These UTIs also are a major cause of nosocomial Gram-negative bacteremia.

Catheter infection may occur by bacterial entry from several routes. The urethral meatus and the distal third of the urethra normally are colonized by bacteria; therefore, initial catheter insertion can introduce bacteria into the bladder. Bacteria contaminating catheter junctions and the urine collection bag can migrate through the catheter lumen to the bladder, initiating infection.[23] The extraluminal space in the urethra also has been considered a potential route of contamination. The risk of infection is directly related to catheter insertion technique, care of the catheter, duration of catheterization, and the susceptibility of the patient. A diagnostic or single, short-term catheterization is associated with a much lower risk of infection than indwelling, long-term catheterization. Despite careful technique, the risk of contaminating a sterile bladder with urethral bacteria is always present. The incidence of infection following a single catheterization is 1% in healthy young women and 20% in debilitated patients. Each reinsertion of the catheter introduces a risk of infection.[23]

Infections have been reduced dramatically by the closed, sterile drainage system, the most common type of catheter currently in use. With this system, the drainage tube leads from the catheter directly to a closed plastic collection bag. The overall incidence of infection from the closed system with careful insertion and maintenance is about 20%; the risk increases to 50% after 14 days of catheterization. If the system is disconnected or contaminated accidentally, the infection rate is similar to that of an open system.[23]

Condom catheters appear to be associated with a lower incidence of bacteriuria than indwelling urethral catheters. These catheters avoid problems associated with insertion of a tube directly into the urinary tract; nevertheless, urine within the catheters may have high concentrations of organisms so that colonization of the urethra and subsequent cystitis may develop.[23]

To prevent bacterial contamination of the bladder when the catheter is inserted, the periurethral area should be cleansed carefully with soap and water followed by some type of antiseptic solution. An iodophor solution often is recommended. Once the catheter is in place, proper maintenance of the closed system is imperative to minimize the incidence of infections. Thus, caregivers must be trained in the techniques of obtaining urine samples from closed systems. Application of antibacterial substances to the collection bag and to the catheter-urethral interface or the use of silver-coated catheters do not decrease the incidence of bacteriuria.[23,102]

40. J.W., an 18-year-old man, was hospitalized following a diving accident that resulted in a spinal cord injury with paralysis. Included among several initial interventions was insertion of an indwelling catheter with a closed drainage system because of bladder incontinence. Two weeks after admission to the hospital, J.W. has an asymptomatic UTI. How should this be treated?

A systemic antibiotic selected specifically for the infecting organism will result in a sterile urine. However, reinfection, often by a resistant organism, occurs in one-third to one-half of these cases if closed drainage catheterization is continued during therapy.[1,23] For this reason, it generally is recommended that systemic antimicrobial therapy be initiated after or just before catheter removal.[1,23] Because long-term catheterization is necessary in many patients and because bacteriuria is an inevitable consequence of long-term catheteriza-

tion, it is often recommended that asymptomatic patients (like J.W.) be left untreated to avoid the complications of recolonization and potential bacteremia with highly resistant organisms.[1,23] However, therapy must be started if fever, flank pain, or other symptoms indicative of UTI develop.[1,23] The strictest adherence to good catheter care is the primary concern in the chronically catheterized patient. Recatheterization with a new, sterile unit is necessary whenever catheter contamination is suspected.

41. Is systemic antimicrobial prophylaxis useful for J.W.?

The benefits of systemic antibiotics in preventing catheter-induced UTIs are not clear. Studies using closed drainage systems with diligent catheter care indicate that systemic antibiotics decrease the daily and overall incidence of infection in patients with sterile urines before catheterization.[103] The preventive effect of the antimicrobial agents is greatest for short-term catheterizations or during the first 4 to 7 days of long-term catheterization.[103] Thereafter, the rate of infection increases. Although the overall infection rate remains lower than that of untreated patients, the emergence of resistant organisms is significant. Therefore, in deciding to use systemic antimicrobials, one must consider the patient's underlying diseases or risk factors, probable duration of catheterization, and the potential complications of drug toxicity or resistant organisms that may result from the chronic use of antimicrobial agents. Because long-term catheterization is anticipated for J.W., antimicrobial prophylaxis for J.W. is not recommended.

42. C.A., a 60-year-old woman admitted for coronary bypass, is catheterized for urinary incontinence. Two days after removal of the catheter, she still has asymptomatic bacteriuria. How should she be treated?

Catheter-acquired bacteriuria that persists 48 hours after catheter removal should be treated with either a single large dose or a 3-day regimen of TMP-SMX, even if the patient is asymptomatic.[104] Older women (>65 years) probably should be treated with a 10-day course; however, the optimal duration in this age group is unknown. Whether these treatment regimens can be used in males requires further study.

Renal Failure

43. K.M., a 55-year-old man with a history of hypertension and chronic renal failure, develops a UTI. His creatinine clearance (Cl_{Cr}), determined from a recent 24-hour urine collection, is 20 mL/min. What antimicrobial agent should be prescribed?

[SI unit: SrCr, 0.33 mL/sec]

The major problem in selecting an antimicrobial agent to treat a UTI in a patient with renal failure is how to achieve adequate urine concentrations of the drug without causing systemic toxicity. The ideal drug would be (1) inherently nontoxic, even at high serum concentrations, making dosage adjustments unnecessary; (2) excreted unchanged in the urine (i.e., not metabolized); and (3) eliminated by renal tubular secretion rather than glomerular filtration. Because renal tubular secretion remains active in all but the most severe cases of renal failure, antibiotics eliminated by this mechanism would reach adequate urinary levels. Unfortunately, no such ideal drug exists.

Nitrofurantoin, doxycycline, and many of the sulfonamides are substantially metabolized by the liver and generally produce low urine levels in uremic patients. The aminoglycosides are eliminated almost exclusively by the kidneys, but uremic patients are at high risk of drug-induced toxicities and alternative agents are usually recommended. The penicillins, the cephalosporins, and trimethoprim are partially metabolized by the liver but are also eliminated by the kidney to a significant extent. These agents are suitable for use in renal failure according to the criteria described above. Certain fluoroquinolones, specifically ciprofloxacin, levofloxacin, and gatifloxacin, are highly excreted in the urine through a combination of filtration and tubular secretion and reach extremely high urinary concentrations. These agents are also considered safe and effective in the treatment of UTI in patients with renal failure.

ADVERSE DRUG REACTIONS AND DRUG INTERACTIONS
Sulfonamides
Hemolytic Anemia

44. G.R., a 45-year-old black man with an 8-year history of congestive heart failure, was admitted to the hospital with increasing shortness of breath. His hematocrit (Hct) was stable at around 42% (normal in males, 40% to 49%) and his total serum bilirubin was 0.8 mg/dL (normal, 0.2 to 1.1 mg/dL). Sixteen days after admission, an *E. coli* UTI was diagnosed and G.R. was treated with TMP-SMX 160 mg/800 mg twice daily. Four days after beginning TMP-SMX, the Hct suddenly dropped to 25% and the hemoglobin (Hgb) to 8.4 g/dL (normal in males, 14 to 18 g/dL). There were no signs of bleeding, but his sclerae became icteric. After seven days of TMP-SMX therapy the Hct was still 25%, but the reticulocyte count had risen to 6.6% (normal, 0.5% to 1.5%) and the total serum bilirubin was 3.0 mg/dL. The TMP-SMX was discontinued, and over a period of 2 weeks the Hct steadily rose to 40%. What mechanism might explain G.R.'s sulfonamide-induced hemolytic anemia? Is his presentation typical? Are there any other drugs used to treat UTIs that can cause a similar reaction?

[SI units: Hct, 0.39 to 0.43, 0.25, and 0.40, respectively (normal, 0.40 to 0.49); bilirubin, 13.7 and 51.3 μmol/L, respectively (normal, 3.4 to 18.8); Hgb, 84 g/L (normal, 140 to 180 g/L); reticulocyte count, 0.066 (normal, 0.005 to 0.015)]

Hemolytic anemia is associated with sulfonamide administration and can be mediated by several mechanisms including abnormally high blood levels, acquired hypersensitivity as reflected by the development of a positive Coombs' test, genetically determined abnormalities of red blood cell metabolism (e.g., G6PD deficiency), or an "unstable" hemoglobin in red blood cells (e.g., Hgb Zurich, Hgb Towns, Hgb H).[105,106]

In this case, hemolytic anemia caused by G6PD deficiency could be confirmed by measuring red blood cell levels of this enzyme. (See Chapter 87, Drug-Induced Blood Disorders, for a discussion of G6PD deficiency.) Although the defect appears to be most common and severe in Mediterranean males, one variant affects as many as 11% of American black males.[106]

Acute hemolytic anemia induced by sulfonamides in G6PD-deficient patients does not appear to be a dose-related phenomenon. It usually is abrupt in onset and occurs within the first week of therapy. Typical symptoms inclu... fever, vertigo, jaundice, hepatosplenomegaly, and o... ally, hypotension. Hematocrit and hemoglobin values ma... precipitously and may be reduced to 30% to 50% of the no... mal values, as illustrated by G.R.; leukocytosis and reticulocytosis are common; and acute renal failure may result from the hypotension and hemoglobinuria. A mild hemolytic episode is characterized by reticulocytosis without a significant fall in hemoglobin or hematocrit.[121] Nitrofurantoin has also been reported to induce G6PD-deficiency hemolysis.[106]

Clinical illness, as well as drug administration, may precipitate hemolysis in patients with G6PD deficiency. Patients with chronic bacterial infections of the urinary or upper respiratory tract who receive chronic or repetitive courses of certain drugs are particularly predisposed to hemolysis.[106]

Patients with enzyme deficiencies, especially those enzymes associated with the pentose-phosphate shunt (as is G6PD), can develop hemolytic reactions when taking drugs commonly used to treat UTIs. Future use of sulfonamides or nitrofurantoin should be avoided in G.R.

Rash and Drug Fever

45. J.P., a 63-year-old diabetic woman taking glipizide 10 mg/day, developed an acute UTI for which TMP-SMX 160 mg/800 mg twice daily for 10 days was prescribed. Seven days later she presented to the ED with a pruritic maculopapular rash and fever. Are the rash and fever in J.P. typical of that caused by the sulfonamides?

Yes. Rash is one of the more common side effects associated with sulfonamide use and occurs in approximately 1% to 2% of patients treated with TMP-SMX. Various hypersensitivity skin and mucous membrane reactions have been reported including morbilliform, scarlatinal, urticarial, erysipeloid, pemphigoid, purpuric, and petechial rashes. Erythema nodosum, exfoliative dermatitis, photosensitivity reactions, and the Stevens-Johnson syndrome also are associated with sulfonamides. Skin eruptions usually appear after 1 week of treatment, although more rapid onset may occur in a sensitized person.[59] The hypersensitivity reactions that occurred in J.P. signify that an alternate drug should be used to treat future UTIs.

Trimethoprim-Sulfamethoxazole
Trimethoprim-Sulfamethoxazole Folate Deficiency

46. D.M., a 50-year-old epileptic woman, has been taking prophylactic TMP-SMX nightly for 3 months for chronic recurrent UTI. She also takes phenytoin 300 mg/day, which effectively controls her seizures, and diazepam 2 mg TID. She smokes 1 pack of cigarettes/day and drinks 1 pint of gin/day. Routine CBC after a clinic visit shows a Hgb of 9 g/dL (normal in females, 13.5 to 16.7 g/dL), a Hct of 30% (normal in females, 40% to 49%), a mean corpuscular volume (MCV) of 105 mm³ (normal, 80 to 100 mm³), and a mean corpuscular hemoglobin concentration (MCHC) of 32% (normal, 32% to 36%). Could TMP-SMX account for D.M.'s megaloblastic anemia?

[SI units: Hgb, 90 g/L (normal, 135 to 167); Hct, 0.30 (normal, 0.40 to 0.49); MCV, 105 fL (normal, 80 to 100); MCHC, 0.32 (normal, 0.32 to 0.36)]

On rare occasions, megaloblastic anemia secondary to folate deficiency has been associated with the use of TMP-SMX.[59] Sulfonamides inhibit folic acid synthesis in bacterial

lo not affect the human cell to a sig-
when given in high doses. It is espe-
nts with known or questionably defi-
ch as pregnant women, older persons,
tion or malnutrition, alcoholics, pa-
ulsants, or those with chronic hemol-
disease). Concomitant administration
e these effects without interfering with
antimicrobial activity.[?] It is doubtful that significant folate
deficiency would occur following short-term TMP-SMX therapy or in patients without the above risk factors.

In D.M., both phenytoin and alcohol undoubtedly contributed to folate deficiency anemia. Whether or not TMP-
SMX was a significant factor may be questioned, but an alternate antibacterial may be preferable in a patient already at risk
for folate deficiency.

Nitrofurantoin
Gastrointestinal Disturbance

47. J.R., a 45-year-old, 110-pound woman, is given nitrofurantoin 100 mg QID for 14 days for an acute UTI. She complains
of nausea and GI upset after the ingestion of each dose of nitrofurantoin. How can this effect be minimized?

Nausea is a fairly common complication of nitrofurantoin
therapy, and the patient's compliance with the prescribed regimen may be severely affected by this common side effect. It
is not fully known whether the mechanism by which nitrofurantoin produces nausea is central or local, but a central component may be present because nausea occurs after parenteral
administration. The following approaches can be used to decrease nitrofurantoin-induced nausea:

- *Take Each Dose With Food.* All manufacturers of nitrofurantoin recommend that the drug be taken with food or
  milk. If the nausea is a locally mediated effect, the food
  may serve as a buffer; if the nausea is centrally mediated,
  then food may slow the rate of absorption and lower the
  peak serum concentration of the drug. Interestingly, however, food may also increase the bioavailability of nitrofurantoin. Slowing of absorption is particularly beneficial in
  decreasing the incidence of nausea and vomiting associated
  with the microcrystalline product.[107]
- *Change to a Macrocrystalline Product.* Use of the macrocrystalline preparation results in significantly fewer adverse
  effects without affecting clinical cure rates. The larger particle size of the macrocrystalline preparation results in a
  slower rate of dissolution and absorption and lower serum
  levels. This may decrease the nausea and vomiting associated with the microcrystalline product.[107] A disadvantage of
  the macrocrystalline form is the cost, which may be 2 to 10
  times that of the microcrystalline form, depending on the
  product source.
- *Lower the Dose.* Nausea and vomiting appear to be dose-
  related and occur more frequently in small persons.[107]
  The minimum effective dose of nitrofurantoin generally is
  stated to be 5 mg/kg per day and the average dose is usually
  7 mg/kg per day. At daily doses greater than 7 mg/kg,
  the incidence of nausea appears to increase significantly, so
  the dose in this 110-pound (50 kg) patient could be decreased.

Pneumonitis

48. J.R. tolerated the macrocrystalline form taken with meals
and continued her regimen. However, 10 days later she presented with dyspnea, tachypnea, coughing, and wheezing. Examination revealed a temperature of 38.4°C, pulse of 115
beats/min, and soft inspiratory and expiratory rhonchi with a
few bibasilar rales. Nitrofurantoin was stopped, and inhaled β2-
agonists and steroids were administered. Symptoms gradually
disappeared after a few days; however, rechallenge with a single
50-mg dose of nitrofurantoin caused a recurrence of the respiratory distress. What is the nature of the apparent nitrofurantoin-
induced respiratory reaction that occurred in J.R.?

Several hundred cases of nitrofurantoin-induced pulmonary reactions have been reported.[108] Acute, subacute, and
chronic reactions have been described. The acute form, illustrated by J.R., often manifests within several days of initiating
the drug with a sudden flu-like syndrome consisting of fever,
dyspnea, and cough. The subacute form tends to occur after at
least a month of exposure; symptoms include fever and dyspnea. The chronic form tends to be more insidious with
milder dyspnea and low-grade fever. In all forms, rales are
commonly heard and pulmonary infiltrates can be demonstrated on chest radiograph. Although eosinophilia frequently
occurs with the acute form, it may be absent with the subacute
and chronic forms. Antinuclear antibodies are elevated in the
latter two forms. Discontinuation of nitrofurantoin results in
complete symptomatic recovery after several weeks; however,
permanent fibrotic changes may persist with the chronic pulmonary reaction. Although steroids are frequently administered when the adverse reaction is diagnosed, their efficacy
has not been demonstrated. Rechallenge with oral nitrofurantoin results in rapid reappearance of pulmonary symptoms in
those who have suffered an acute reaction.[108]

Neurotoxicity

49. G.T., a 55-year-old woman, has been taking nitrofurantoin
100 mg QID for an acute UTI. Pertinent history includes hypertension and moderate renal failure. Medications include lisinopril, hydrochlorothiazide, and allopurinol. On the tenth day of
therapy, she complains that both her hands and feet feel numb
and weak. Physical examination shows significant sensory loss to
the hands and feet as well as no ankle reflexes, although knee
and arm reflexes are present. What are the characteristics of the
neuropathy that is associated with nitrofurantoin therapy?

Peripheral neuropathy usually is characterized by symmetric dysesthesia and paresthesia in the distal extremities, which
progresses in a central and ascending fashion. It usually occurs within the first 60 days of treatment, although neuropathy can be recognized up to 6 weeks after discontinuation of
therapy in 16% of patients. Symptom severity is unrelated to
the total nitrofurantoin dose. Although generally reversible,
more severe cases may require up to several months to completely resolve; a small number of patients may develop permanent neuropathy. Renal failure is a risk factor for toxicity,
but neuropathy has been reported in patients with normal renal function as well.[92,107]

Nitrofurantoin excretion is impaired in renal failure; however, serum levels do not rise proportionately, suggesting that
the drug might be sequestered in an extravascular space. It has

been postulated that neurotoxicity is due to accumulation of nitrofurantoin in neural tissue, or that toxic metabolites are involved.[92,107] In view of the inability to achieve adequate urinary concentrations of nitrofurantoin even in mild renal failure, G.T. should not be given this drug.

GLOSSARY

Acute pyelonephritis: Inflammation of the kidney, with flank pain and tenderness, bacteriuria (often bacteremia), pyuria, and fever.

Bacteriuria: Bacteria cultured from urine when it is obtained by either suprapubic aspiration, catheterization, or from a freshly voided specimen. Asymptomatic bacteriuria exists if colony counts exceed 10^5 per milliliter in a patient without UTI symptoms. Clinically significant bacteriuria probably exists if colony counts are $\geq 10^2$ per milliliter in patients with UTI symptoms.

Chronic pyelonephritis: A chronic, inflammatory condition of the kidney with associated calyceal dilation and overlying cortical scarring. A nonspecific pathologic appearance of the kidney seen with many disease entities, only one of which is bacterial infection of the kidney.

Complicated urinary tract infection: Infections associated with conditions that increase the risk for acquiring infection, the potential for serious outcomes, or the risk for therapy failure. Such conditions are often associated with abnormalities that may interfere with normal urine flow or the voiding mechanism. Infections in men, children, and pregnant women are considered complicated. Other examples of complicated infections include those associated with structural and neurologic abnormalities of the urinary tract, metabolic/hormonal abnormalities, impaired host responses, and those caused by unusual pathogens (e.g., yeasts, *Mycoplasma*).

Cystitis: An inflammation of the bladder and urethra with dysuria, frequency, urgency, pyuria, clinically significant bacteriuria, and suprapubic tenderness on examination.

Prostatitis: An inflammatory condition affecting the prostate. It may be acute or chronic. Frequently, specific bacterial organisms cannot be detected.

Pyuria: White blood cells in the urine. A WBC count of $\geq 8/mm^3$ of uncentrifuged urine or 2 to 5 per HPF in centrifuged urine sediment is consistent with a UTI.

Subclinical pyelonephritis:

A kidney infection, but with lower UTI signs and symptoms only. Uncomplicated urinary tract infection:

Infections occurring in otherwise healthy persons, usually women, who have none of the underlying risk factors known to increase the risk for treatment complications or failure (see complicated UTIs).

Urethritis: An inflammation of the urethra with dysuria. The etiologic organisms most commonly implicated are *Neisseria gonorrhoeae, Ureaplasma urealyticum, Chlamydia trachomatis,* and herpes simplex virus.

Urinary tract infection: Microorganisms (bacteria, fungi, viruses) in the urinary tract, including the bladder, prostate, kidneys, and collecting duct. Although fungi and viruses are occasional etiologic agents, UTIs are predominantly caused by bacteria.

Vaginitis: Inflammation of the vagina with dysuria, vaginal discharge, and vaginal odor. Common etiologic agents include *Candida albicans, Gardnerella vaginalis,* and trichomonads.

REFERENCES

1. Sobel JD et al. Urinary tract infections. In: Mandell GL et al., eds. Principles and Practice of Infectious Diseases. 5th Ed. New York: Churchill Livingstone, 2000:773.
2. Bacheller CD et al. Urinary tract infections. Med Clin North Am 1997;81:719.
3. Sobel JD. Pathogenesis of urinary tract infections: role of host defenses. Infect Dis Clin North Am 1997;11:531.
4. Hooton TM et al. Diagnosis and treatment of uncomplicated urinary tract infection. Infect Dis Clin North Am 1997;11:551.
5. Smith HS et al. Antecedent antimicrobial use increases the risk of uncomplicated cystitis in young women. Clin Infect Dis 1997;25:63.
6. Bergeron MG. Treatment of pyelonephritis in adults. Med Clin North Am 1995;79:619.
7. Krieger J. Urinary tract infections: what's new? J Urol 2002;168:2351.
8. Foxman B et al. Urinary tract infection: self-reported incidence and associated costs. Ann Epidemiol 2000;10:509.
9. Craig JC. Urinary tract infection: new perspectives on a common disease. Curr Opin Infect Dis 2001;14:309.
10. Jodal U. The natural history of bacteriuria in childhood. Infect Dis Clin North Am 1987;1:713.
11. Hansson S et al. The natural history of bacteriuria in childhood. Infect Dis Clin North Am 1997;11:499.
12. Lipsky BA. Prostatitis and urinary tract infection in men: what's new; what's true? Am J Med 1999;106:327.
13. Lummus WE et al. Prostatitis. Emerg Med Clin North Am 2001;19:691.
14. Nicolle LE. Asymptomatic bacteriuria in the elderly. Infect Dis Clin North Am 1997;11:647.
15. Nicolle LE. Urinary tract infection in long-term-care facility residents. Clin Infect Dis 2000;31:757.
16. Heinamaki P et al. Mortality in relation to urinary characteristics in the very aged. Gerontology 1986;32:167.
17. Matsumoto T. Urinary tract infections in the elderly. Curr Urol Rep 2001;2:330.
18. Abrutyn E et al. Does asymptomatic bacteriuria predict mortality and does antimicrobial treatment reduce mortality in elderly ambulatory women? Ann Intern Med 1994;120:827.
19. Gupta K et al. Antimicrobial resistance among uropathogens that cause community-acquired urinary tract infections in women: a nationwide analysis. Clin Infect Dis 2001;33:89.
20. Tambyah PA et al. The direct costs of nosocomial catheter-associated urinary tract infection in the era of managed care. Infect Control Hosp Epidemiol 2002;23:27.
21. Laupland KB et al. Incidence and risk factors for acquiring nosocomial urinary tract infection in the critically ill. J Crit Care 2002;17:50.
22. Ronald AR et al. Complicated urinary tract infections. Infect Dis Clin North Am 1997;11:583.
23. Warren JW. Catheter-associated urinary tract infections. Infect Dis Clin North Am 1997;11:609.
24. Schoolnik GK. How Escherichia coli infect the urinary tract. N Engl J Med 1989;320:804.
25. Shleinfeld J et al. Association of Lewis blood group phenotype with recurrent tract infections in women. N Engl J Med 1989;307:773.
26. Scholes D et al. Risk factors for recurrent urinary tract infection in young women. J Infect Dis 2000;182:1177.
27. Patterson TF et al. Detection, significance, and therapy of bacteriuria in pregnancy. Infect Dis Clin North Am 1997;11:593.
28. Tolkoff-Rubin NE et al. Urinary tract infection in the immunocompromised host. Infect Dis Clin North Am 1997;11:707.
29. Stapleton A. Urinary tract infections in patients with diabetes. Am J Med 2002;113(Suppl 1A):80S.
30. Meiland R et al. Management of bacterial urinary tract infections in adult patients with diabetes mellitus. Drugs 2002;62:1859.
31. Patterson JE et al. Bacterial urinary tract infections in diabetics. Infect Dis Clin North Am 1997;11:735.
32. Boyko EJ et al. Diabetes and the risk of acute urinary tract infection among postmenopausal women. Diabetes Care 2002;25:1778.
33. Foxman B et al. First time urinary tract infection and sexual behavior. Epidemiology 1995;6:162.
34. Hooton TM et al. Effects of recent sexual activity and use of a diaphragm on the vaginal microflora. Clin Infect Dis 1994;19:274.
35. Hooton TM et al. A prospective study of risk factors for symptomatic urinary tract infection in young women. N Engl J Med 1996;335:468.
36. Handley MA et al. Incidence of acute urinary tract infection in young women and use of male condoms with and without nonoxynol-9 spermicides. Epidemiology 2002;13:431.
37. Eschenbach DA et al. Effects of vaginal intercourse with and without a condom on vaginal flora and vaginal epithelium. J Infect Dis 2001;183:913.

38. Gupta K et al. Effects of contraceptive method on the vaginal microbial flora: a prospective evaluation. J Infect Dis 2000;181:595.

39. Bent S et al. Does this woman have an acute uncomplicated urinary tract infection? JAMA 2002; 287:2701.

40. Jou WW et al. Utility of dipstick urinalysis as a guide to management of adults with suspected infection or hematuria. South Med J 1998;91:266.

41. Kunin CM et al. A reassessment of the importance of "low-count" bacteriuria in young women with acute urinary symptoms. Ann Intern Med 1993; 119:454.

42. Dimitrakov J et al. Recent developments in diagnosis and therapy of the prostatitis syndromes. Curr Opin Urol 2001;11:87.

43. Mazzulli T. Resistance trends in urinary tract pathogens and impact on management. J Urol 2002;168(Suppl):1720.

44. Gupta K et al. Increasing prevalence of antimicrobial resistance among uropathogens causing acute uncomplicated cystitis in women. JAMA 1999; 281:736.

45. Chow AW et al. Pharmacokinetics and safety of antimicrobial agents during pregnancy. Rev Infect Dis 1985;7:287.

46. Dashe JS et al. Antibiotic use in pregnancy. Obstet Gynecol Clin North Am 1997;24:617.

47. Briggs GG et al. Drugs in Pregnancy and Lactation. 5th Ed. Baltimore: Williams & Wilkins, 1998.

48. Nicolle LE. Urinary tract infection: traditional pharmacological therapies. Dis Mon 2003;49:111.

49. Warren JW et al. Guidelines for antimicrobial treatment of uncomplicated acute bacterial cystitis and acute pyelonephritis in women. Clin Infect Dis 1999;29:745.

50. Travani A et al. Short-course ciprofloxacin treatment of acute uncomplicated urinary tract infection in women: the minimum effective dose. The Urinary Tract Infection Study Group. Arch Intern Med 1995;155:485.

51. Raz R et al. 3-day course of ofloxacin versus cephalexin in the treatment of urinary tract infections in postmenopausal women. Antimicrob Agents Chemother 1996;40:2200.

52. Iravani A et al. A trial comparing low-dose, short-course ciprofloxacin and standard 7 day therapy with co-trimoxazole or nitrofurantoin in the treatment of uncomplicated urinary tract infection. J Antimicrob Chemother 1999;43(Suppl):67.

53. Krcmery S et al. Ciprofloxacin once versus twice daily in the treatment of complicated urinary tract infections. German Ciprofloxacin UTI Study Group. Int J Antimicrob Agents 1999;11:133.

54. McCarty JM et al. A randomized trial of short-course ciprofloxacin, ofloxacin, or trimethoprim/sulfamethoxazole for the treatment of acute urinary tract infection in women. Ciprofloxacin Urinary Tract Infection Group. Am J Med 1999;106:292.

55. Richard GA et al. Single-dose fluoroquinolone therapy of acute uncomplicated urinary tract infection in women: results from a randomized, double-blind, multicenter trial comparing single-dose to 3-day fluoroquinolone regimens. Urology 2002;59:334.

56. Le TP et al. Empirical therapy for uncomplicated urinary tract infections in an era of increasing antimicrobial resistance: a decision and cost analysis. Clin Infect Dis 2001;33:615.

57. Raz R et al. Empiric use of trimethoprim-sulfamethoxazole (TMP-SMX) in the treatment of women with uncomplicated urinary tract infections, in a geographical area with a high prevalence of TMP-SMX-resistant uropathogens. Clin Infect Dis 2002;34:1165.

58. Masterton RG et al. High-dosage co-amoxiclav in a single dose versus 7 days of co-trimoxazole as treatment of uncomplicated lower urinary tract infection in women. J Antimicrob Chemother 1995; 35:129.

59. Masters PA et al. Trimethoprim-sulfamethoxazole revisited. Arch Intern Med 2003;163:402.

60. Talan DA et al. Comparison of ciprofloxacin (7 days) and trimethoprim-sulfamethoxazole (14 days) for acute uncomplicated pyelonephritis in women: a randomized trial. JAMA 2000;283:1583.

61. Noskin GA et al. Disappearance of the uncomplicated urinary tract infection: the impact of emerging resistance. Clin Drug Invest 2001;21(Suppl):13.

62. Brown PD et al. Prevalence and predictors of trimethoprim-sulfamethoxazole resistance among uropathogenic *Escherichia coli* isolates in Michigan. Clin Infect Dis 2002;34:1061.

63. Gupta K et al. Outcomes associated with trimethoprim/sulfamethoxazole (TMP/SMX) therapy in TMP/SMX resistant community-acquired UTI. Int J Antimicrob Agent. 2002;19:554.

64. Hooper DC. Quinolones. In: Mandell GL et al., eds. Principles and Practice of Infectious Diseases. 5th Ed. New York: Churchill Livingstone, 2000:404.

65. Richard GA et al. Levofloxacin versus ciprofloxacin versus lomefloxacin in acute pyelonephritis. Urology 1998;52:51.

66. Pisani E et al. Lomefloxacin versus ciprofloxacin in the treatment of complicated urinary tract infections: a multicenter study. J Chemother 1996;8:210.

67. Fish DN. Fluoroquinolone adverse effects and drug interactions. Pharmacotherapy 2001;21(Suppl 2):253S.

68. Nix DE et al. Effects of aluminum and magnesium antacids and ranitidine on the absorption of ciprofloxacin. Clin Pharmacol Ther 1989;46:700.

69. Ho G et al. Evaluation of the effect of norfloxacin on the pharmacokinetics of theophylline. Clin Pharmacol Ther 1988;44:35.

70. Martin SJ et al. Levofloxacin and sparfloxacin: new quinolone antibiotics. Ann Pharmacother 1998; 32:320.

71. Fish DN et al. The clinical pharmacokinetics of levofloxacin. Clin Pharmacokinet 1997;32:101.

72. Davis R et al. Ciprofloxacin: an updated review of its pharmacology, therapeutic efficacy and tolerability. Drugs 1996;51:1019.

73. Saint S. Clinical and economic consequences of nosocomial catheter-associated bacteriuria. Am J Infect Control 2000;28:68.

74. Nguyen-Van-Tam SE et al. Risk factors for hospital-acquired urinary tract infection in a large English teaching hospital: a case-control study. Infection. 1999;27:192.

75. Wagenlehner FM et al. Spectrum and antibiotic resistance or uropathogens from hospitalized patients with urinary tract infections: 1994-2000. Int J Antimicrob Agents 2002;19:557.

76. Miller O et al. Urinary tract infection and pyelonephritis. Emerg Med Clin North Am 2001;19:655.

77. Wing DA. Pyelonephritis. Clin Obstet Gynecol 1998;41:515.

78. McMurray BR et al. Usefulness of blood cultures in pyelonephritis. Am J Emerg Med 1997;15:137.

79. Bailey RR et al. Prospective, randomized, controlled study comparing two dosage regimens of gentamicin/oral ciprofloxacin switch therapy for acute pyelonephritis. Clin Nephrol 1996;46:183.

80. Roberts JA. Management of pyelonephritis and upper urinary tract infections. Urol Clin North Am 1999;26:753.

81. Caceres VM et al. The clinical utility of a day of hospital observation after switching from intravenous to oral antibiotic therapy in the treatment of pyelonephritis. J Fam Pract 1994;39:337.

82. Stamm WE et al. Acute renal infection in women: treatment with trimethoprim-sulfamethoxazole or ampicillin for two- or six-weeks: a randomized trial. Ann Intern Med 1987;106:341.

83. Stamm WE et al. Causes of acute urethral syndrome in women. N Engl J Med 1980;303:409.

84. Hamilton-Miller JM. The urethral syndrome and its management. J Antimicrob Chemother 1994; 33(Suppl A):63.

85. Stamm WE et al. Treatment of acute urethral syndrome. N Engl J Med 1981;304:956.

86. Phenazopyridine Hydrochloride. In: American Hospital Formulary Service. American Society of Hospital Pharmacists. Bethesda, MD, 2003:3419.

87. Harding GK et al. Antimicrobial treatment in diabetic women with asymptomatic bacteriuria. N Engl J Med 2002;347:1576.

88. Sherbotie JR et al. Management of urinary tract infections in children. Med Clin North Am 1991; 75:327.

89. Svanborg C et al. Bacterial virulence in urinary tract infection. Infect Dis Clin North Am 1997; 11:513.

90. Fihn SD et al. Use of spermicide-coated condoms and other risk factors for urinary tract infection caused by Staphylococcus saprophyticus. Arch Intern Med 1998;158:281.

91. McOsker CC et al. Nitrofurantoin: mechanism of action and implications for resistance development in common uropathogens. J Antimicrob Chemother 1994;33(Suppl A):23.

92. Hooper DC. Urinary tract agents: nitrofurantoin and methenamine. In: Mardell GL et al., eds. Principles and Practice of Infectious Diseases. 5th Ed. New York: Churchill Livingstone, 2000:376.

93. Stapleton A et al. Prevention of urinary tract infection. Infect Dis Clin North Am 1997;11:719.

94. Nicolle LE et al. Recurrent urinary tract infection in adult women: diagnosis and treatment. Infect Dis Clin North Am 1987;1:793.

95. Hooton TM. Recurrent urinary tract infection in women. Int J Antimicrob Agents 2001;17:259.

96. Stamm WE et al. Antimicrobial prophylaxis of recurrent urinary tract infections: a double-blind, placebo-controlled trial. Ann Intern Med 1980; 92:770.

97. Roberts RO et al. A review of clinical and pathological prostatitis syndromes. Urology 1997; 49:809.

98. Pewitt EB et al. Urinary tract infection in urology, including acute and chronic prostatitis. Infect Dis Clin North Am 1997;11:623.

99. Stapleton A et al. Post-coital antimicrobial prophylaxis for recurrent urinary tract infection. JAMA 1990;264:703.

100. Andriole VT et al. Epidemiology, natural history, and management of urinary tract infections in pregnancy. Med Clin North Am 1991;75:359.

101. Christensen B. Which antibiotics are appropriate for treating bacteriuria in pregnancy? J Antimicrob Chemother 2000;46(Suppl 1):29.

102. Riley D et al. A large randomized clinical trial of a silver-impregnated urinary catheter: lack of efficacy and staphylococcal superinfection. Am J Med 1995;98:349.

103. Mountokalakis T et al. Short-term versus prolonged systemic antibiotic prophylaxis in patients treated with indwelling catheters. J Urol 1985; 134:506.

104. Harding GKM et al. How long should catheter-acquired urinary tract infection in women be treated? Ann Intern Med 1991;144:713.

105. Zinner SH et al. Sulfonamides and Trimethoprim. In: Mardell GL et al., eds. Principles and Practice of Infectious Diseases. 5th Ed. New York: Churchill Livingstone, 2000:394.

106. Beutler E. Glucose-6-phosphate dehydrogenase deficiency. N Engl J Med 1991;324:169.

107. Guay DR. An update on the role of nitrofurans in the management of urinary tract infections. Drugs 2001;61:353.

108. Ben-Noun L. Drug-induced respiratory disorders: incidence, prevention and management. Drug Saf 2000;23:143.

Sexually Transmitted Diseases

Jeffery A. Goad

Although descriptions of sexually transmitted diseases (STDs) can be discerned in the earliest written records, only recently have the common STDs been differentiated from each other; unique STD syndromes continue to be described today. For example, of the common STDs, bacterial vaginosis was not described clearly as a syndrome (initially called *Haemophilus vaginalis* vaginitis) until the 1950s; herpes simplex virus (HSV) type 2 (the cause of genital herpes) was not differentiated from HSV type 1 until the 1960s; the spectrum of genital chlamydial infections was not well worked out until the 1970s; and the newest sexually transmitted pathogen, HIV, was not recognized until the 1980s. Since 1980, eight new sexually transmitted pathogens have been identified. They include the human papillomaviruses (HPV), human T-lymphotropic virus

(HTLV-I and II), *Mycoplasma genitalium, Mobiluncus* species, HIV-1 and 2, and the human herpes virus type 8 (now associated with Kaposi's sarcoma).[1] As the medical aspects of STDs have become better understood, social attitudes toward the diagnosis and therapy for STDs have become more enlightened.

This chapter reviews both the older and the more recently defined STDs. However, of special note are the observations of an overall decrease in the prevalence of gonorrhea in the United States and Europe, although higher rates are being reported in minority and adolescent groups. In addition, a sharp increase in *Chlamydia trachomatis,* as well as viral STDs (HSV, human papillomavirus, and HIV), has been noted in the 1990s. AIDS is discussed in Chapter 69, Pharmacotherapy of Human Immunodeficiency.

GONORRHEA

Gonorrhea is caused by *Neisseria gonorrhoeae,* a Gram-negative diplococcus. In 130 AD, Galen coined the term gonorrhea (Greek for "flow of seed") for the syndrome associated with this infection because he believed the urethral exudate was semen.

Although the role of the gonococcus in causing urethral discharge in men has been known for >100 years, the manifestations of gonorrhea in women have not been studied as well until recently. In the 1930s, sulfonamides became the first form of effective antimicrobial therapy for gonorrhea, but then penicillins and tetracyclines became the mainstay of therapy. Newer antimicrobials are required now in many areas of the world, including the United States, because high levels of resistance to these two antimicrobial classes have developed.

In the United States, the incidence of gonorrhea rose steadily (15% per year) from the early 1960s through 1975, fell 74% between 1975 and 1997, and, since 1998, has been fairly stable but still higher than the Centers for Disease Control and Prevention's (CDC's) goal of less than 100 cases per 100,000 people (Fig. 65-1).[2] Despite the growing fear of AIDS and other viral STDs and aging of the baby boom generation, the incidence of gonorrhea in heterosexuals rose sharply in 1985 for the first time in a decade. Since 1985 it has declined, but this has been largely limited to whites and Asians. The rate among African Americans was about 27 times greater than the rate in non-Hispanic whites in 2001. The highest incidence of gonorrhea is in men aged 20 to 24 years and in females aged 15 to 19 years.[3] Additional demographic risk factors for gonorrhea include low socioeconomic status, urban residence, unmarried marital status, illicit drug use, prostitution, and a history of gonorrhea.[4,5] The risk of gonorrhea was much higher in homosexual men than in heterosexual men in the past, but the incidence of gonorrhea dropped rapidly in homosexual men during the 1980s AIDS epidemic in large part because of a reduction in sexual risk behaviors. Since 1988, the rate of gonococcal isolates from homosexual men has increased from 4% to a high of 17% in 2001, which suggests a reversal in sexual risk behaviors.[3,6]

Uncomplicated Gonorrhea
Transmission

1. J.C., a 23-year-old male naval officer recently stationed in the Philippines, complains of dysuria, meatal pain, and a profuse yellow urethral discharge for 2 days. He admits to extramarital sex with a prostitute over the past week. He is accompanied by his pregnant wife, B.C., who is asymptomatic. J.C. engages in vaginal sex but there is no history of oral or anal sex with either partner.

Assuming the prostitute has gonorrhea, what is the likelihood that J.C. and B.C. have been infected?

After one or two episodes of vaginal intercourse with an infected prostitute, a man has approximately a 50% risk of acquiring a urethral infection; the risk increases with repeated exposures and high prevalence among commercial sex workers.[7] The prevalence of infection in women, such as B.C., who are secondary sex contacts of infected men has been reported to be as high as 80% to 90%.[8] Therefore, the likelihood that J.C. and B.C. are infected is high. Because J.C. had sex with a prostitute, both J.C. and B.C. should be tested for HIV infection.

Signs and Symptoms: Males

2. What signs and symptoms in J.C. are consistent with the diagnosis of gonorrhea? Describe J.C.'s anticipated clinical course if he is untreated.

In males, gonorrhea usually becomes clinically apparent 1 to 7 days after contact with an infected source. A purulent discharge associated with dysuria is the first sign of infection and both are exhibited by J.C. The discharge, which is presumably caused by chemotactic factors such as C5a that are released when antigonococcal antibody binds complement, may become more profuse and blood-tinged as the infection progresses. Some strains of gonorrhea have a propensity to cause asymptomatic or minimally symptomatic infection and show negative Gram's stain, probably owing to different auxotypes.[9]

Patients with asymptomatic or minimally symptomatic disease may serve as reservoirs for the infection, evading treat-

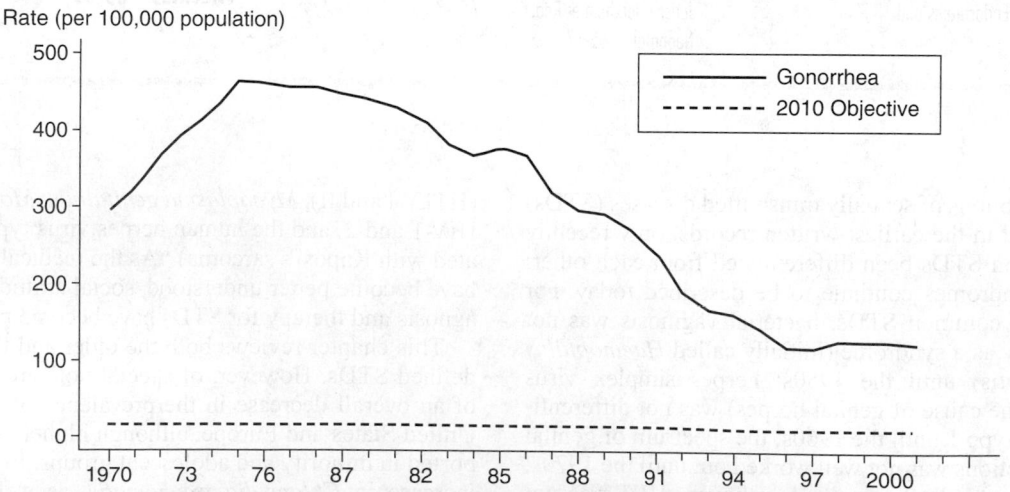

FIGURE 65-1 Gonorrhea—Reported Rates: United States, 1970–2001 and the Healthy People 2010 objective. Centers for Disease Control and Prevention, Gonococcal Isolate Surveillance Project (GISP) Annual Report - 2001.[2] Note: Healthy People 2010 (HP2010) objective for gonorrhea is 19.0 cases per 100,000 population.

ment for prolonged periods of time.[10] At one time, only females were thought to have asymptomatic gonorrhea, but now it is known that men may be asymptomatic carriers as well.[11]

In the preantimicrobial era, gonococci occasionally spread to the epididymis, causing unilateral epididymitis; the prevalence was 5% or more in patients in some studies. Now epididymitis occurs in <1% of men with gonorrhea. Urethral stricture after repeated attacks and sterility after epididymitis are rare complications of gonococcal infection because antibiotics are so effective.

Diagnosis: Males

3. **Intracellular Gram-negative diplococci were seen on the Gram's stain of J.C.'s urethral exudate. Is any further diagnostic testing required?**

Demonstration of intracellular Gram-negative diplococci in the Gram-stained exudate confirms the diagnosis. Until recently, some experts recommended that cultures be reserved for individuals with negative Gram's stain of urethral exudate. However, today cultures are recommended for all patients to permit isolation and testing of the bacteria for antibiotic susceptibility. Cultures usually are performed on Thayer-Martin medium, an enriched chocolate agar to which vancomycin, colistimethate, and nystatin have been added. Cultures from the throat should be obtained if J.C. was exposed by cunnilingus to the prostitute. In J.C.'s case, a urethral culture is indicated.

Signs and Symptoms: Females

4. **B.C., J.C.'s wife, is asymptomatic. What symptoms would be consistent with gonorrhea in B.C.? Will the symptoms differ because she is pregnant? What is the natural course of gonorrhea in women if left untreated?**

Because the endocervical canal is the primary site of urogenital gonococcal infection in women, the most common symptom is vaginal discharge as a result of mucopurulent cervicitis. Many women with gonorrhea have abnormalities of the cervix, including purulent or mucopurulent endocervical discharge, erythema, friability, and edema of the zone of ectopy.[8] The incubation period for urogenital gonorrhea in women is variable.[12] Pelvic inflammatory disease results in

10% to 20% of women with acute gonococcal infection and can lead to infertility and chronic pelvic pain.[8] The assessment of signs and symptoms in women with gonorrhea often is confounded by nonspecific signs and symptoms and a high prevalence of coexisting infection, especially with *C. trachomatis* or *Trichomonas vaginalis.*

Although lower genital tract symptoms in women may disappear, they remain carriers of *N. gonorrhoeae* and should be treated. Complications of urogenital gonorrhea in pregnancy include spontaneous abortion, premature rupture of the fetal membranes, premature delivery, and acute chorioamnionitis.[13,14] Other complications include gonococcal arthritis (see Question 16) conjunctivitis, and ophthalmia neonatorum in the newborn.[15] For these reasons, it is critical that B.C. be worked up thoroughly for gonorrhea.

Diagnosis: Females

5. **How should gonorrhea be ruled out in B.C.?**

B.C. should undergo an endocervical culture, which is positive in 80% of women with gonorrhea and is still considered the "gold standard."[16] This test should be a part of every pelvic examination of sexually active women. Nucleic acid amplification tests, such as polymerase chain reaction (PCR), may yield sensitivities and specificities in the 90% to 100% range, but results must be confirmed with endocervical culture in low-prevalence communities (i.e., <4%).[17] In B.C., anal cultures also could be performed because the rectum can serve as a reservoir for gonococci.

Treatment

6. **Compare the various drug regimens used for uncomplicated gonorrhea.**

Many antimicrobial regimens effectively treat uncomplicated gonorrhea; the recommendations of the CDC are summarized in Table 65-1. Single-dose treatment strategies with a β-lactam or quinolone in combination with doxycycline or azithromycin, to eradicate coexisting chlamydial infections that can't be ruled out, is the preferred regimen.[18] The CDC's 2001 Sexually Transmitted Disease Surveillance Program reported on national trends in antimicrobial prescribing for initial therapy of uncomplicated gonorrhea (Fig. 65-2). Accord-

---

Table 65-1 CDC Recommendations for Treatment of Uncomplicated Gonorrhea

Presentation	Drugs of Choice (% Cured)	Dosage	Alternatives for Allergic Patients (% Cured)
Urethritis, cervicitis[a], rectal	Ceftriaxone (99.1)	125 mg IM once	Spectinomycin 2 g IM once (98.2), ciprofloxacin 500 mg PO once (99.8), ofloxacin 400 mg PO once (98.4)
	Cefixime (97.1)[b]	400 mg PO once	Azithromycin 2 g PO once[c]
	Ciprofloxacin	500 mg PO once	
	Ofloxacin	400 mg PO once	
	Levofloxacin	250 mg PO once	
Pharyngeal	Ceftriaxone	125 mg IM once	Spectinomycin (52)[d]
	Ciprofloxacin	500 mg PO once	Ofloxacin 400 mg PO once

[a]Because a high percentage of patients with gonorrhea have coexisting *Chlamydia trachomatis* infections, many clinicians recommend treating all patients with gonorrhea with a 7-day course of doxycycline, as recommended for treatment of chlamydia.
[b]In July of 2002, Wyeth discontinued cefixime (Suprax); no other company makes or sells cefixime.
[c]This expensive alternative is active against uncomplicated gonococcal infections and *C. trachomatis,* but causes significant gastrointestinal upset.
[d]Reserved only for patients who cannot tolerate cephalosporins or quinolones. A follow-up pharyngeal culture is recommended 3 to 5 days after treatment with spectinomycin to test for cure.

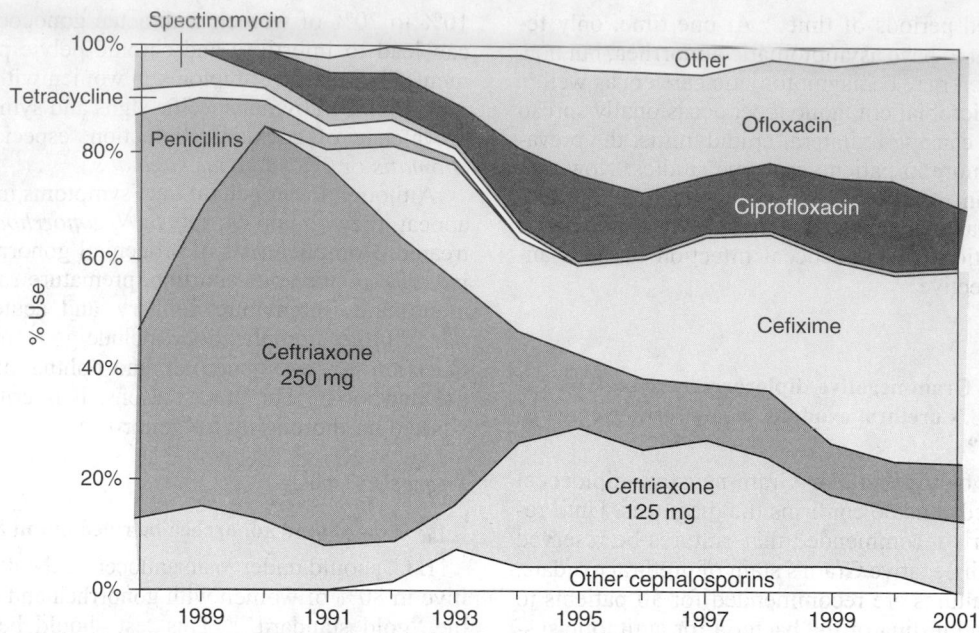

FIGURE 65-2 2001 CDC Gonococcal Isolate Surveillance Project (initial therapy of uncomplicated gonorrhea)[2]

ing to this surveillance program, ceftriaxone followed by cefixime were the most commonly prescribed agents. Cefixime, however, was discontinued by the manufacturer, and no other U.S. company currently makes it.[19] Cefixime went off patent in 2002. In California and Hawaii, the rate of quinolone resistance combined with the unavailability of cefixime make ceftriaxone the drug of choice.[20]

The 1985 CDC recommendations removed tetracycline as a therapy of choice because of the emergence of tetracycline-resistant *N. gonorrhoeae*. The 1987 guidelines removed aqueous procaine penicillin G as a treatment choice because of its unacceptable toxicity (pain upon injection, procaine reactions) and relatively high resistance rates. Amoxicillin combined with probenecid also no longer is recommended be-

cause of relatively high resistance rates. The 1998 CDC guidelines recommended ceftriaxone (Rocephin) as a single, small-volume injection in the deltoid or cefixime (Suprax) as a single oral dose as therapy for gonorrhea because of the ever-growing problem of plasmid and chromosomally mediated resistance.[21] The 2002 CDC guidelines reaffirm the same treatment strategy.

Many strains of *N. gonorrhoeae* exhibit plasmid-mediated resistance to penicillin and tetracycline (penicillinase-producing *N. gonorrhoeae* [PPNG] and/or tetracycline-resistant *N. gonorrhoeae* [TRNG]) (Fig. 65-3). In addition, significant levels of chromosomally mediated resistance to penicillin, tetracycline, and cefoxitin have been reported.[2] In 2001, all isolates in the Gonococcal Isolate Surveillance Project (GISP) were suscepti-

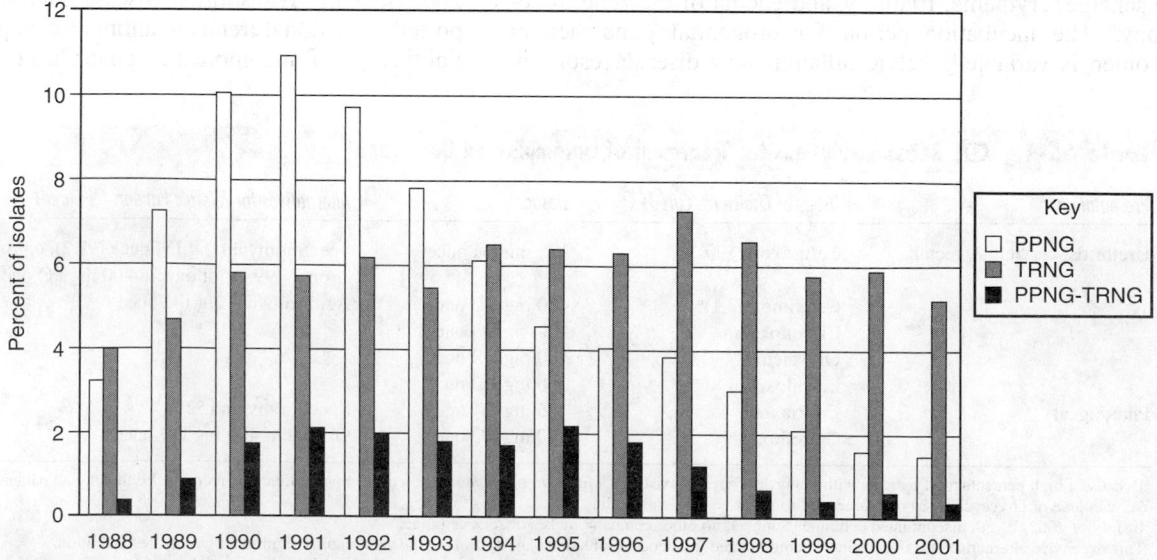

FIGURE 65-3 Gonococcal Isolate Surveillance Project (GISP)—trends in plasmid-mediated resistance to penicillin and tetracycline, 1988–2001.[2]

ble to ceftriaxone. Because a high percentage of patients with gonorrhea also have coexisting *C. trachomatis* infections, a concurrent 7-day course of doxycycline or single dose azithromycin is recommended (see Question 28). Acceptable alternative regimens are listed in Table 65-1. The final decision regarding the most appropriate therapy is patient specific.

CEFTRIAXONE

Ceftriaxone is a third-generation cephalosporin that is highly effective against penicillin-susceptible and penicillin-resistant strains of gonococci. It is given as a single, small-volume intramuscular (IM) injection (e.g., 125 mg diluted with normal saline or 1% lidocaine solution). Ceftriaxone also eradicates anal and pharyngeal gonorrhea. Pregnant women can be treated safely with ceftriaxone or cefixime (FDA pregnancy category B). Other cephalosporins (notably ceftizoxime, cefuroxime, cefpodoxime) have been found to be as effective, although coverage for pharyngeal infections has not been studied as well. Cefixime appears to be effective against pharyngeal infection, but few patients with pharyngeal gonococcal infection have been studied.

Quinolones are preferable to cephalosporins in patients with true penicillin allergy. Ceftriaxone and spectinomycin are ineffective against *C. trachomatis* and in the prevention of postgonococcal urethritis, whereas ofloxacin and levofloxacin for 7 days have similar efficacy to doxycycline.[18] Spectinomycin, quinolones, and ampicillin plus probenecid are inactive against incubating syphilis.

SPECTINOMYCIN

Spectinomycin (Trobicin) is not a first-line drug for the treatment of gonorrhea. There has not been a published case of *N. gonorrhoeae* resistant to spectinomycin since 1994.[2] Spectinomycin should be reserved for the treatment of patients who have failed treatment with ceftriaxone or who are allergic to penicillin. It is not effective in the treatment of pharyngeal gonorrhea, incubating syphilis, or *C. trachomatis*.[22] Spectinomycin currently is recommended for pregnant, penicillin-allergic patients (Table 65-1).

QUINOLONES

The quinolones are effective therapy for gonorrhea. A single oral dose of ciprofloxacin, ofloxacin, or levofloxacin achieves over a 98% cure against susceptible strains of *N. gonorrhoeae*.[18] The quinolones have variable activity against *C. trachomatis* but lack activity against *Treponema pallidum*.

7. How should J.C.'s urethritis be treated? B.C. has a history of periorbital edema and urticaria secondary to penicillin. Because she is totally asymptomatic and the results of her cultures are pending, should she be treated empirically? If so, what drug(s) would you recommend?

Because J.C. has gonococcal infection limited to the urethra (uncomplicated), a number of treatment regimens are possible, as outlined in Question 6. Ceftriaxone or cefixime is the preferred treatment. With the current unavailability of cefixime, alternative oral agents may need to be considered if ceftriaxone is not appropriate. Quinolones should be avoided because J.C.'s gonorrheal infection was likely obtained in the Philippines, where quinolone resistance occurs in over half of all isolates.[23] Although not mentioned as alternative agents in

the 2002 CDC guidelines, cefpodoxime (200 mg PO) and cefuroxime (1 g PO) are active in vitro against PPNG, CMRNG, and TRNG; have limited clinical evidence to support their use; and are FDA approved to treat uncomplicated *N. gonorrhoea*.[24-26] Because no single-dose therapy for gonorrhea and chlamydia is highly effective, additional concurrent therapy needs to be administered. Doxycycline or azithromycin are two effective therapies that he could be given to adequately cover the potential of a chlamydia coinfection. Single-dose azithromycin 2 g orally has been used to treat concurrent gonorrhea and chlamydia, but it is expensive, poorly tolerated because of increased gastrointestinal (GI) side effects, and less effective than standard combination therapy.[27]

SEXUAL PARTNERS

B.C. also should be treated even though she appears asymptomatic. All partners who have had sexual exposure to patients with gonorrhea within 60 days should be treated. If the patient has not been sexually active for 60 days, the most recent sexual partner should be treated. This is especially true when the partner is pregnant because gonorrhea during pregnancy is associated with chorioamnionitis and prematurity, as well as with neonatal infection. Pregnant women can be treated safely with cephalosporins, but because B.C. is allergic to penicillin, spectinomycin plus azithromycin is the treatment of choice. Doxycycline and quinolones should be avoided during pregnancy.

FOLLOW-UP

8. How does one determine whether the drug therapy of gonorrhea has been effective in J.C. and B.C.?

If recommended therapies are used for treatment of uncomplicated gonorrhea (see Table 65-1), a test of cure is not necessary for either B.C. or J.C. since cure rates are close to 100%.[8,18] However, a follow-up culture is recommended only when spectinomycin is used to treat pharyngeal gonorrhea and disseminated disease.[18] If symptoms persist in J.C., who was treated with ceftriaxone, cultures should be done to rule out other causes of urethritis.

ANTIBIOTIC-RESISTANT *NEISSERIA GONORRHOEAE*

9. J.C. states that he was treated with penicillin in the past for a gonococcal infection. Why are penicillins not prescribed routinely today?

Failure of penicillin to eradicate the gonococcus can be the result of plasmid (e.g. PPNG) or chromosomally mediated resistant *N. gonorrhoeae* (CMRNG) antibiotic resistance. PPNG contain plasmids, which determine the production of β-lactamase, an enzyme that hydrolyzes the β-lactam ring of penicillin G or ampicillin. Chromosomally mediated resistance does not involve β-lactamase production and often is associated with increased resistance to other β-lactams. The clinical significance of CMRNG is questionable because high serum levels of approved antibiotics can be achieved above the MIC (minimum inhibitory concentration), such that treatment failure is unlikely. However, to date, CMRNG remain largely susceptible to ceftriaxone. High-level tetracycline resistance is defined by gonococci that carry plasmid-encoded resistance to 16 μg/mL or more of tetracycline. These strains

Table 65-2 Antimicrobial Regimens Recommended by the CDC for Treatment of Acute Pelvic Inflammatory Disease

Treatment Setting, Drugs, Schedule	Advantage	Disadvantage	Clinical Considerations
Inpatient			
Regimen A Cefotetan 2 g IV Q 12 hr or cefoxitin 2 g IV Q 6 hr plus doxycycline 100 mg IV or PO[a] Q 12 hr) Continue doxycycline (100 mg PO BID) after discharge to complete 10–14 days of therapy	Optimal coverage of *N. gonorrhoeae* (including resistant strains) and *C. trachomatis*	Possible suboptimal anaerobic coverage	Penicillin-allergic patients also may be allergic to cephalosporins; doxycycline use in pregnant patients may cause reversible inhibition of skeletal growth in the fetus and discoloration of teeth in young children
Regimen B Clindamycin 900 mg IV Q8 hr plus gentamicin or tobramycin (1.5–2 mg/kg IV Q 8 hr)[b] Continue clindamycin 450 mg PO QID or doxycycline 100 mg PO BID after discharge to complete 14 days of therapy	Optimal coverage of anaerobes and Gram-negative enteric rods	Possible suboptimal coverage of *N. gonorrhoeae* and *C. trachomatis*	Patients with decreased renal function may not be good candidates for aminoglycoside treatment or may need a dosage adjustment
Alternative regimen Ofloxacin 400 mg IV every 12 hours or levofloxacin 500 mg IV once daily with or without metronidazole 500 mg IV every 8 hours or ampicillins/sulbactam 3 g IV every 6 hours plus doxycycline 100 mg PO or IV every 12 hours.	Optimal coverage of *N. gonorrhoeae* and *C. trachomatis*	Inadequate coverage of anaerobes necessitates use of metronidazole or ampicillin/sulbactam	Not appropriate in pregnancy or in young children
Outpatient			
Regimen A Ofloxacin 400 mg PO BID or levofloxacin 500 mg PO once daily with or without metronidazole 500 mg PO BID or clindamycin 450 mg PO QID for total of 14 days	Adequate coverage against *N. gonorrhoeae* and *C. trachomatis*	Lack of anaerobic coverage necessitates use of metronidazale	Levofloxacin has comparable efficacy to ofloxacin, but needs to be administered only once daily
Regimen B Ceftriaxone 250 mg IM in a single dose or cefoxitin 2 g IM in a single dose and probenecid, 1 g orally administered concurrently in a single dose or other parenteral third-generation cephalosporin (e.g., ceftizoxime or cefotaxime) plus doxycycline 100 mg PO BID for 14 days with or without metronidazole 500 mg PO BID for 14 days	Good to excellent coverage of *N. gonorrhoeae* and optimal coverage of *C. trachomatis*	Possible suboptimal anaerobic coverage necessitating the addition of metronidazole	Optimal cefphalosporin is unclear; more complicated regimen requiring combination of parenteral and oral therapies

[a]Because of the pain involved with doxycycline infusions and the comparable PO/IV bioavailability, IV therapy should be replaced with PO as soon as possible.
[b]Single daily dose aminoglycosides may be substituted.
Adapted from reference 18.

are known as TRNG. Although not of major concern in the United States, development of resistance to alternative therapies is a continuing concern.

The first cases of PPNG infection were reported in the United States in 1976.[28] PPNG are especially prevalent in Southeast Asia, the Far East, and West Africa where the prevalence often exceeds 50%. In the United States, the percent of PPNG strains reached a peak of about 11% in 1991; since then, cases have steadily declined to just under 2% in 2001, according to the CDC's Gonococcal Isolate Surveillance Project[2] (Fig. 65-3). Strains of TRNG were first identified in 1985, but fortunately most TRNG isolates still are sensitive to β-lactam antibiotics. The use of tetracycline was officially abandoned by the CDC in 1985 and penicillin in 1987. In the late 1990s, we have seen a plateau in the number of TRNG and PPNG plus TRNG cases at about 5% and 1%, respectively.

Because about 21% of gonococcal isolates are resistant to tetracycline and/or penicillin within the United States, it is still not acceptable to use these agents in the initial management of uncomplicated genital gonorrhea. Clinicians should get a travel history to identify patients who have traveled recently or whose sexual contacts have traveled recently to areas where multiple drug resistance is endemic. In endemic or hyperendemic areas (areas where PPNG accounts for 3% or greater of all gonococcal isolates), ceftriaxone IM or cefixime orally are the drugs of choice. Antibiotic susceptibility testing is recommended for all isolates associated with children, apparent treatment failure, and patients with complicated gonococcal disease.

Quinolone-resistant *N. gonorrhoeae* (QRNG) was first reported in 1990 and is reported to be 0.2% of isolates in the continental United States.[2,18] As early as 1992, Cleveland,

Ohio,[29] and in 1995, Seattle, Washington,[30] reported outbreaks of QRNG. In the 2001 GISP report, Hawaii QRNG made up 14.3% of isolates, whereas in California the rate approached 7%.[2] In other geographic regions, strains exhibiting resistance to ciprofloxacin are as high as 63% in the Philippines, 48.8% in Hong Kong, with slightly lower rates occurring in the rest of Asia.[31,32] For this reason, quinolones are not recommended for gonorrhea acquired in Hawaii, California, or Asia.[20] Resistance to fluoroquinolones is associated with mutations of GyrA and is commonly identified in strains that produce β-lactamase and strains exhibiting chromosomally mediated resistance to penicillin and tetracycline.[33] *N. gonorrhoeae* strains may exhibit decreased susceptibility or complete resistance to quinolones. Ciprofloxacin-resistant strains may not respond to therapy with recommended doses of fluoroquinolones, and the clinical importance of strains with decreased susceptibility is unknown.[34] The CDC recommends that as long as QRNG isolates remain <1%, fluoroquinolone regimens may be used with confidence.[20]

If J.C. had been treated initially with ceftriaxone, he probably would have been free of gonococcal infection within 3 days. Patients whose test-of-cure culture yields strains of PPNG should be treated with single doses of ceftriaxone 125 mg IM or spectinomycin 2 g IM. To date, ceftriaxone fully resistant strains of *N. gonorrhoeae* have not been reported. Because J.C. most likely acquired *N. gonorrhoeae* in the Philippines, QRNG should be considered when selecting an appropriate antibiotic.

Anorectal and Pharyngeal Gonorrhea
Epidemiology

10. M.B. is a 24-year-old, sexually active, homosexual man with a 2-month history of perianal itching, painful defecation, constipation, a bloody mucoid rectal discharge, and a sore throat. Sigmoidoscopy revealed rectal mucosal inflammation but no apparent ulcers or fissures. Stool examination for parasites was negative and a Venereal Disease Research Laboratory (VDRL) test was nonreactive. Both rectal and pharyngeal cultures revealed *N. gonorrhoeae*. How does gonorrhea in homosexual men compare with gonorrhea in heterosexual men?

The most prevalent bacterial STD among the homosexual male population is gonorrhea.[35] Rectal infection occurs rarely in strictly heterosexual men, whereas in the male homosexual population, anorectal (25%) and pharyngeal (10% to 25%) gonococcal infections occur more often.[8,36] Because pharyngeal[36,37] and anorectal gonococcal infections are often asymptomatic, there may be a large reservoir of carriers in the homosexual male population that may only be detected with more sensitive DNA amplification techniques.[38] By comparison, very few urethral gonococcal infections are asymptomatic. In addition, recent data indicate that pharyngeal infections may be an important source of urethral gonorrhea in homosexual men spread by fellatio.[36]

Signs and Symptoms

11. Are M.B.'s signs and symptoms consistent with gonorrhea?

Rectal gonorrhea produces the syndrome of proctitis with anorectal pain, mucopurulent anorectal discharge, constipa-

tion, tenesmus, and anorectal bleeding. The differential diagnosis of proctitis in the homosexual male includes rectal infection with *N. gonorrhoeae*, *C. trachomatis*, HSV, and syphilis. Proctitis, limited to the distal rectum, should be differentiated from proctocolitis often caused by *Shigella* species, *Campylobacter* species, or *Entamoeba histolytica* in homosexual men. Rectal symptoms should not be attributed to trauma until specific infections are excluded. The evidence of rectal infection in homosexual men declined because of changing sexual practices in the AIDS era, but may be on the rise again.[39]

Treatment

12. How should M.B.'s diagnosis be managed?

The treatment of choice for patients such as M.B. with anorectal and/or pharyngeal gonorrhea is ceftriaxone 125 mg IM as a single dose (see Table 65-1). Azithromycin or doxycycline should be given to those with rectal gonorrhea to treat possible coexisting rectal chlamydial infection. Patients such as M.B. with either anorectal or pharyngeal gonorrhea should be advised to avoid further unprotected sexual activity and should be counseled and tested for infection with HIV.

13. What are alternative regimens for patients with isolated anal or pharyngeal gonorrhea?

Women with anorectal gonorrhea alone should be treated with ceftriaxone. Alternative regimens for isolated anorectal infection include spectinomycin or a quinolone. Patients with anorectal gonorrhea who are allergic to penicillin should be treated with 2 g of spectinomycin hydrochloride IM, which is nearly 100% effective for anorectal gonorrhea. However, it is only 43% effective against pharyngeal gonococcal infection.[40,41] In patients who are truly allergic to penicillin, ciprofloxacin 500 mg, gatifloxacin 400mg, or ofloxacin 400mg orally one time are all nearly 100% effective for pharyngeal or anorectal gonorrhea.[42] Although manufacturers do not recommend quinolones in patients less than 18 years and in pregnancy, the CDC recommends that children weighing more than 45 kg may be treated with an appropriate adult regimen, including a quinolone.[18] If spectinomycin is used, a pharyngeal culture should be obtained 3 to 5 days after treatment to ensure erradication.[8]

Prevention

14. What measures have been used to prevent the sexual transmission of infection?

Condoms, when used properly, appear to provide a high degree of protection against the acquisition and/or transmission of STDs.[43] Previous studies indicated that the use of the spermicide nonoxynol-9 had activity against gonorrhea and chlamydia, whereas more recent studies show no effect.[44–46] In light of recent evidence that suggests nonoxynol-9 might actually increase the chance of acquiring HIV, the CDC recommends that it should not be used for the prevention of HIV infection.[47] Thus, widespread use of this agent for the purpose of decreasing the risk of STDs cannot be recommended at this time. Topical antibacterial agents, urinating, washing, or douching after intercourse are of little value in preventing the transmission of STDs.[48]

The prophylactic administration of antibiotics immediately before or soon after sexual intercourse reduces the risk of infection,[49] but can result in selection and transmission of antibiotic-resistant strains of *N. gonorrhoeae*. Routine antibiotic prophylaxis after all casual sexual encounters is not cost-effective and could cause more disease than is prevented. Development of an effective vaccine and public health measures, such as education, are the best hopes for preventing gonorrhea.

PELVIC INFLAMMATORY DISEASE

The term pelvic inflammatory disease (PID) commonly has been used for a variety of acute and chronic conditions caused by ascending, surgical, or trauma-related infections in the female genital tract. This term does not denote the primary infection site (the fallopian tubes) nor the causative microorganisms. PID also has been used to connote an infection that occurs acutely when either vaginal or cervical microorganisms traverse the sterile endometrium and ascend to the fallopian tubes. Acute salpingitis also may be used to describe an acute infection of the fallopian tubes. Therefore, the terms PID and salpingitis will be used interchangeably in the following discussion to denote an acute infection involving the fallopian tubes.

PID affects 1 million women annually in the United States.[53] Approximately 85% of all cases of acute PID occur by sexual transmission in women of reproductive age, another 15% occur after procedures that require instrumentation, including intrauterine device insertion, abortion, or dilation and curettage.[50,51] Acute PID develops in an estimated 1 in 8 sexually active 15-year-old women, but only 1 in 80 women 24 years of age.[52] Other risk markers and factors include use of an IUD,[54] douching,[55,56] bacterial vaginosis[57,58], and smoking.[59] Two-thirds of PID cases resulting in infertility are asymptomatic, while up to a third are incorrectly diagnosed due to low specificity of diagnostic techniques. In the United States, infertility occurs in about 12.1% of women after the first episode of PID and is probably responsible for the upswing in ectopic pregnancy in the early 1980s.[60,61] The estimated cost of direct medical expenditures for PID and its sequalae was estimated to be $1.88 billion in 1998 with most of this cost associated with treatment of acute PID.[62]

Etiology

The etiology of PID is often polymicrobial, but most cases are caused by *C. trachomatis* followed by *N. gonorrhoeae*.[63–66] Other organisms associated with PID include *Mycoplasma hominis*[67] and *Ureaplasma urealyticum,* but a causative role is questionable.[60] Facultative enteric Gram-negative bacilli and a variety of anaerobic bacteria have also been isolated from the upper genital tract of 25% to 50% of women with acute PID.[50]

Signs and Symptoms

The onset of symptoms of abdominal pain attributable to PID caused by either gonococci or chlamydia often occurs soon after the menstrual period. The onset of chlamydial PID is slower than that of gonococcal disease, the duration of pain is longer, and the clinical manifestations are milder.[60,68] Symptoms of vaginal discharge, menorrhagia, and dysuria commonly are associated with PID. Signs include uterine and adnexal tenderness and a mucopurulent endocervical exudate. Clinical diagnosis has a sensitivity for PID of about 65% to 85%, whereas laparoscopy is about 100% specific, thus making the combination of laparoscopy and clinical impression the gold standard.[69,70] Unfortunately, laparoscopy is often not readily available for acute cases nor is it diagnostic for endometritis; thus, clinical impression is still heavily relied on. A key to reducing the incidence of PID may be through active screening of *Chlamydia* in young sexually active women.[71,72]

Clinical Sequelae

An abscess may form in the pelvic or abdominal cavity and in one or both fallopian tubes. Chronic abdominal pain develops in 18% of women with PID and may be the result of pelvic adhesions surrounding the tubes and ovaries.[51] After a single episode of PID, tubal occlusion and fibrosis secondary to fallopian tube inflammation (salpingitis) result in 12% infertility, 25% infertility after two episodes, and 50% infertility after three or more episodes.[60] Other sequalae include ectopic pregnancy (9%)and chronic pelvic pain (18%).[73] The risk of ectopic pregnancy is increased approximately eightfold after one or more episodes of PID.[51]

Diagnosis and Treatment

15. B.O., a 19-year-old, sexually active woman, complains of mild dysuria, a purulent vaginal discharge, fever, and moderately severe, bilateral, lower abdominal pain of 3 days' duration. Examination confirms uterine and adnexal tenderness, a purulent cervical exudate, and a temperature of 39°C. Laboratory examinations show a nonreactive VDRL and negative urinalysis. A pregnancy test performed at this time was negative. The peripheral white blood cell (WBC) count was mildly elevated (11,000/mm³) with 70% polymorphonuclear leukocytes. Does B.O. have PID? How should she be treated?

[SI unit: WBC count, 11×10^9/L]

Although fever and leukocytosis are often absent in mild or subacute PID, these findings in a woman with adnexal tenderness and cervical exudate increase the likelihood of acute PID. Treatment of PID varies with the severity of the infection and is based on the assumption that the precise bacteriologic cause often is unknown (Table 65-2). An estimated 75% of PID is treated orally.[74] The 2002 CDC recommendations[18] for outpatient therapy include ofloxacin 400 mg twice daily or levofloxacin 500 mg daily with or without metronidazole 500 mg twice daily for 14 days. Ofloxacin and levofloxacin lack anaerobic coverage, often necessitating the addition of metronidazole, which also has the advantage of covering bacterial vaginosis, a common contributor to PID.[75] Metronidazole is widely used by clinicians even though its application is theoretical as the role of anaerobes in PID is not well understood.

Alternatively, the CDC recommends a single dose of IM ceftriaxone or IM cefoxitin plus probenecid, followed by doxycycline with or without metronidazole for 14 days. Tetracyclines no longer are used for treatment of PID as monotherapy because they lack optimal activity against Gram-negative

Table 65-3   Treatment of Disseminated Gonococcal Infection[a]

No Penicillin Allergy

Parenteral

Ceftriaxone 1 g IV or IM Q 24 hr or cefotaxime 1 g IV Q 8 hr or ceftizoxime 1 g IV Q 8 hr and doxycycline 100 mg PO BID[b] or erythromycin base 500 mg PO QID[b] (if pregnant)

Oral

Cefixime 400 mg PO BID or ciprofloxacin 500 mg PO BID or ofloxacin 400 mg PO BID

Penicillin Allergy

Parenteral

Ciprofloxacin 500 mg IV Q 12 hr or ofloxacin 400 mg IV Q 12 hr or spectinomycin 2 g IM Q 12 hr and doxycycline 100 mg PO BID[b] or erythromycin base 500 mg PO QID[b] (if pregnant)

Oral

Ciprofloxacin 500 mg PO BID or ofloxacin 400 mg PO BID

[a]Duration of treatment is 7 days.
[b]For possible concomitant chlamydial infection, treat for 7 days.

aerobic and anaerobic organisms and against some strains of *N. gonorrhoeae.* However, a tetracycline or an alternative drug active against *C. trachomatis* should always be included.

Patients such as B.O. with moderate to severe PID should be hospitalized and treated empirically with parenteral antibiotics after a cervical discharge has been obtained for Gram's stain and culture. Intravenous (IV) cefotetan or cefoxitin plus doxycycline for 14 days are the CDC's first-line drugs of choice. Parenteral therapy should be given for at least 24 hours beyond the first signs of improvement and IV doxycycline converted to oral doxycycline as soon as the patient can tolerate it.[18] Substantial clinical improvement is usually seen within 3 days and patients receiving outpatient therapy for PID should be reevaluated within 3 days. Oral doxycycline should be continued to complete 14 days of therapy. Clindamycin plus gentamicin can be used alternatively in penicillin-allergic and pregnant females.[18] Because B.O. is sexually active, any sexual partners within the previous 60 days, (or if >60 days, then the most recent sexual partner) should be empirically treated because of the risk of gonococcal or chlamydial urethritis as well as to reduce the risk of reinfection.[18]

COMPLICATED GONORRHEA
Disseminated Gonococcal Infection
Signs and Symptoms

16. S.P., a 28-year-old, sexually active woman, was seen for stiffness and pain of the right wrist and left ankle and fever (38°C). On physical examination, the knee and wrist joints were found to be hot, red, and swollen; papules and pustular lesions were observed on S.P.'s legs and forearms. A latex fixation test for rheumatoid factor was negative. A tap of the right knee yielded an effusion with a WBC count of 34,000/ mm³ (80% polymorphonuclear [PMN] leukocytes). Cultures of the skin lesions were negative, but *N. gonorrhoeae* was isolated from the throat,

cervix, blood, and synovial fluid. A chest radiograph, echocardiogram, and electrocardiogram all were normal, and no murmur could be appreciated. Assess S.P.'s clinical presentation.

[SI unit: WBC count, 34 × 10⁹/L]

S.P.'s signs, symptoms, and laboratory findings are consistent with gonococcal bacteremia, which today occurs in <1% of women and men with gonorrhea. The most common manifestation of gonococcemia is the gonococcal arthritis-dermatitis syndrome or disseminated gonococcal infection exhibited by S.P. Symptoms include fever, occasional chills, a mild tenosynovitis of the small joints, and skin lesions; the latter primarily involving the distal extremities are petechial, papular, pustular, and hemorrhagic in appearance.[76,77]

Diagnosis of disseminated gonococcal infection (DGI) is made by Gram's stain and culture. However, blood cultures are positive in only 33% of DGI cases, even when patients are cultured early in the course of the infection.[78] The low positive yield from blood cultures may be due to the low inoculum and/or intermittent bacteremic period. Routine culture of the urethra, cervix, pharynx, and rectum should be performed in any patient suspected of having DGI.

Treatment

17. How should S.P. be managed? How quickly will she respond to therapy?

Patients like S.P. with gonococcal arthritis and bacteremia should be hospitalized for treatment with ceftriaxone 1 g IM or IV daily until clinical improvement, such as decreased fever and pain, is sustained for 24 to 48 hours, at which time therapy may be switched to an appropriate oral agent (see Table 65-3).[18,79] Such agents include cefixime 400 mg orally twice daily or ciprofloxacin 500 mg orally twice daily for a total of 7 days. Levofloxacin may be preferable owing to the convenience of once-daily administration. Because patients with gonococcal arthritis caused by PPNG are encountered, therapy should be initiated with ceftriaxone. An alternative therapy for the patient who is allergic to penicillin is a quinolone or spectinomycin 2 g IM every 12 hours.[18]

Symptoms and signs of tenosynovitis should be improved markedly within 48 hours. Septic gonococcal arthritis with purulent synovial fluid may require repeated aspiration and will resolve more slowly.

Treatment of Gonococcal Endocarditis and Meningitis

18. How should gonococcal endocarditis and meningitis be treated?

Gonococcal endocarditis and meningitis, occurring in only 1% to 3% of DGIs, require high-dose IV therapy such as ceftriaxone (1 to 2 g IV every 12 hours) for 10 days or more in the case of meningitis and for 3 to 4 weeks in the case of endocarditis.[8,18]

Neonatal Disseminated Gonococcal Infection: Treatment

19. How should neonatal DGI and meningitis be managed?

Neonatal DGI and meningitis should be treated with ceftriaxone (25 to 50 mg/kg IV every 24 hours) for at least 10 to 14 days.

CHLAMYDIA TRACHOMATIS

C. trachomatis was first isolated from patients with lymphogranuloma venereum (LGV). However, chlamydial genital infections were not studied extensively until improved procedures for culture isolation and serology were developed and applied during the 1960s and 1970s.[80] Despite the use of reliable nonculture diagnostic tests since the 1980s, young sexually active women are not routinely screened annually.[81]

In U.S. family planning clinics, the chlamydial test positivity, a proxy for prevalence, is 5.6% in 15- to 24-year-old women and probably much lower for men, although men are infrequently screened.[82] High rates of asymptomatic infection are observed among both men and women leading to serious sequelae if not treated.

C. trachomatis, an intracellular obligate parasite, is a difficult organism to demonstrate in clinical specimens because this requires cell culture techniques that routinely are not available to the practitioner. Because few practitioners have access to facilities for isolation of *C. trachomatis,* most chlamydial infections are diagnosed and treated based on clinical impression and nonculture techniques. Nonculture diagnostic tests, including nucleic acid amplification tests (NAATs) and non-NAATs such as direct immunofluorescence assay (DFA) and enzyme immunoassay (EIA) are generally sensitive methods for detecting *C. trachomatis*. Ligase chain reaction (LCR) and PCR are two NAATs with wide commercial availability, are relatively simple to use, can be performed using urine or genital swab specimens, and are more sensitive than non-NAATs.[16] Caution should be exercised if interpreting these nonculture tests <3 weeks after treatment because false positives may occur as the result of the continued excretion of dead organisms (a test of cure is not necessary unless symptoms persist or reinfection is suspected).

The variety of clinical syndromes that are now known to be caused by *C. trachomatis* are cervicitis, urethritis, bartholinitis, endometritis, salpingititis, and perihepatitis in women, and urethritis, epididymitis, prostatitis, proctitis, and Reiter's syndrome in men.[83] It is interesting to note that the spectrum of chlamydial infections closely resembles those caused by the gonococcus, which is why many patients presenting with these syndromes are treated with drugs effective against both organisms (Table 65-4).

C. trachomatis is sensitive to the tetracyclines, erythromycin, azithromycin, and ofloxacin, but is unresponsive to the penicillins, cephalosporins, aminoglycosides, clarithromycin, most fluoroquinolones (except ofloxacin and some newer generation quinolones), and metronidazole.[84,85]

Nongonococcal Urethritis
Etiology

20. T.K., a 26-year-old, sexually active man, complains of mild dysuria and a mucoidlike urethral discharge that started about 15 days after his last intercourse. He had no fever, lymphadenopathy, penile lesions, or hematuria. A Gram's stain smear of an anterior urethral specimen showed 20 PMNs per oil immersion (1,000) field and no intracellular Gram-negative diplococci. What pathogens are associated with nongonococcal urethritis (NGU)?

In the United States, NGU is the most common STD in men.[83,86] Depending on the diagnostic technique and study design, causative organisms identified include *C. trachomatis* in 35% to 50%,[83] *Ureaplasma urealyticum* in 9% to 42%,[87] *Mycoplasma genitalium* in 15% to 25%,[88] *Trichomonas vaginalis* in 5% to 15%[89] and up to 20% had no identifiable cause.[87] The variety of pathogens and disparity among identification techniques require sound clinical judgment and an algorithmic laboratory testing approach to correctly identify and treat the cause.

Signs and Symptoms

21. Describe the clinical presentation of a person with NGU. Is T.K.'s presentation consistent with NGU? How does one differentiate between NGU and gonococcal urethritis?

T.K.'s presentation is typical. Compared with gonococcal urethritis, nongonococcal urethritis typically produces less se-

---

Table 65-4 Clinical Parallels Between Genital Infections Caused by *N. gonorrhoeae* and *C. trachomatis*

Site of Infection	Resulting Clinical Syndrome	
	N. gonorrhoeae	*C. trachomatis*
Men		
Urethra	Urethritis	Nongonococcal urethritis, post-gonococcal urethritis
Epididymis	Epididymitis	Epididymitis
Rectum	Proctitis	Proctitis
Conjunctiva	Conjunctivitis	Conjunctivitis
Systemic	Disseminated gonococcal infection	Reiter's syndrome
Women		
Urethra	Acute urethral syndrome	Acute urethral syndrome
Bartholin's gland	Bartholinitis	Bartholinitis
Cervix	Cervicitis	Cervicitis
Fallopian tube	Salpingitis	Salpingitis
Conjunctiva	Conjunctivitis	Conjunctivitis
Systemic	Disseminated gonococcal infection	Arthritis-dermatitis (Reiter's syndrome)

Reprinted with permission from Schachter J. Chlamydial infections. N Engl J Med 1978;298:428, 490, 540.

vere and less frequent dysuria and less penile discharge. Chlamydial urethral infection is completely asymptomatic more often than gonococcal urethral infection. The incubation period for gonococcal urethritis is 2 to 7 days, whereas the incubation period for NGU is typically 2 to 3 weeks.

Nonetheless, NGU and gonococcal urethritis cannot be reliably differentiated solely on the basis of symptoms and signs. If there is objective evidence of a urethral discharge (expressed by milking the urethra), Gram's stain with >5 WBCs per oil immersion field in the urethral secretion, positive leukocyte esterase test demonstrating ≥10 WBCs per high-power field, the diagnosis of NGU is made by excluding the presence of *N. gonorrhoeae* by Gram's stain and/or culture.

Treatment

22. **How should T.K. be treated?**

Azithromycin 1 g orally (single dose) should be administered in the clinic to increase compliance.[18] Doxycycline can be given in a dose of 100 mg two times a day for 7 days. Doxycycline and azithromycin are considered equally effective against NGU.[90–92] Doxycycline is less expensive and has been used more extensively than azithromycin. Erythromycin, in a dosage equivalent to 500 mg of base or stearate (800 mg ethylsuccinate) orally every 6 hours for 7 days, is an alternative CDC-approved regimen. Ofloxacin 300 mg twice daily or levofloxacin 500 mg once daily for 7 days is a third alternative, but it offers no significant advantages over the previously mentioned agents, may not treat *U. urealyticum* adequately, and is significantly more expensive.[93] Ciprofloxacin should be avoided as treatment failures have been reported.[94] Patient counseling should emphasize the need to use a condom or abstain from sexual intercourse at least until the prescribed course of therapy has been completed (or 7 days after single-dose therapy) by the patient and his sexual partner(s).[83] There is some indication that the proportion of NGU caused by *C. trachomatis* might be declining, potentially being replaced by an increased proportion of *U. urealyticum,* which is variably cured at 2 weeks by azithromycin (73%) and doxycycline (65%).[90]

RECURRENT INFECTION

23. **T.K. was treated with doxycycline 100 mg BID for 7 days. He remained asymptomatic for 14 days after completion of his therapy, when he again noticed similar symptoms of dysuria and a mucoidlike urethral discharge. How should T.K.'s recurrent infection be treated?**

The major problem encountered in the treatment of NGU is the high rate of recurrent infections. Approximately 15% to 30% of patients experience recurrent urethritis within 6 weeks after completing a course of tetracycline,[95] and up to 50% of patients with nonchlamydial NGU suffer relapse after 2 months.[87] The rate of recurrence is highest in patients with idiopathic urethritis; that is, those not infected with *C. trachomatis* or *U. urealyticum.* Recurrence suggests re-exposure to an untreated partner, whereas persistent urethritis (without improvement during therapy) suggests the presence of tetracycline-resistant *U. urealyticum,* infection with *T. vaginalis* or HSV, urethral stricture, or chronic prostatitis.[96] NGU that persists or recurs should be re-treated with the initial agent[18] if the patient was not compliant or the sexual partner was not treated. For patients with persistent symptoms who were compliant with the initial regimen and were not re-exposed, the CDC recommends using metronidazole 2 g orally in a single dose plus 7 days of erythromycin.[18]

Men with acute epididymitis often have chlamydial or gonococcal infection, particularly if they are younger than 35 years of age or have a urethral discharge. Older men with epididymitis more often are infected with *Escherichia coli* or other urinary pathogens. If testicular tenderness is present with urethritis, and the clinical impression is consistent with epididymitis caused by chlamydia or gonorrhea, some experts recommend ceftriaxone 250 mg IM single dose plus doxycycline 100 mg orally twice for 10 days. For a nonsexually transmitted etiology of epididymitis, ofloxacin 300 mg orally BID or levofloxacin 500 mg orally once daily for 10 days may be used.[18]

Sexual Partners

24. **A.C., T.K.'s girlfriend, comes into the clinic 3 weeks after T.K.'s last visit. She is worried that she may have a similar infection, although she has no signs or symptoms. What clinical manifestations of chlamydial infections are seen in women? Should A.C. be treated for suspected chlamydial infection?**

In the absence of cultures for chlamydia, empirical treatment of women who are sexual partners of men with NGU is recommended. Routine partner referral for presumptive therapy is not indicated for nonchlamydial NGU.[87] Many partners are asymptomatic, but from 30% to 70% are culture positive if tested. A.C. should be examined carefully for mucopurulent cervicitis and salpingitis. Although many women with chlamydial infection of the cervix are asymptomatic, at least one-third have evidence of mucopurulent discharge and hypertrophic ectopy.[97] Gram's stain of appropriately collected mucopurulent endocervical discharge from these patients shows many PMNs and an absence of gonococci.

Regardless of findings, treatment should be initiated with the same doxycycline regimen used for nongonococcal urethritis. If A.C. is pregnant, tetracyclines and fluoroquinolones should be avoided. Amoxicillin 500 mg three times daily for 7 days, azithromycin (1 g single dose) or erythromycin (500 mg four times daily for 7 days) should be prescribed. The estolate form of erythromycin should be avoided in pregnancy because of the increased risk of hepatotoxicity. Azithromycin appears to be safe and effective during pregnancy.[98,99] High rates of gastrointestinal complaints limit the use of erythromycin and if amoxicillin is used, a test of cure should be recommended owing to its low efficacy.[83] Coinfection with chlamydia is common in heterosexual men and women with gonorrhea. Therefore, drug regimens effective against both organisms are recommended in patients with gonorrhea to prevent postgonococcal chlamydial morbidity (epididymitis, mucopurulent cervicitis, salpingitis) and to reduce the genital reservoir of *C. trachomatis.*

Lymphogranuloma Venereum
Etiology and Signs and Symptoms

25. **S.F., a 32-year-old male student who recently arrived from Uganda, presents to the STD clinic with a chief complaint of pain and swelling in the groin. He reports the appearance of a small**

ulcer on his penis about 2 weeks ago, which resolved rapidly. Upon examination, he has a bubo (inflammatory swelling of one or more lymph nodes in the groin) with surrounding erythema on his right side. S.F. also has a fever (39°C). Laboratory findings are remarkable for a mild leukocytosis (WBC count, 12,000 cells/mm³). What organisms are responsible for LGV? Describe its clinical course. What subjective and objective manifestations in S.F. are consistent with LGV?

[SI unit: WBC count, 12,000 × 10⁹/L]

Lymphogranuloma venereum is rare in the United States, occurring mainly in Africa, India, Southeastern Asia, South America, and the Caribbean.[100] The cause of LGV is usually *C. trachomatis* serovars L1, L2, or L3, which is different from those serovars responsible for chlamydia urethritis. Three stages of LGV infection are recognized in heterosexual men.[101] During stage I, a small genital papule or vesicle appears from 3 to 30 days after exposure. The patient usually is asymptomatic, and the ulcer heals rapidly, leaving no scar. This primary lesion is consistent with the penile ulcer reported by S.F. Many patients with LGV recall no primary lesion.

Stage II is characterized by acute painful lymphadenitis with bubo formation (the inguinal syndrome); it often is accompanied by pain and fever, as illustrated by S.F. Without treatment, the buboes may rupture, forming numerous sinus tracts that drain chronically. Adenopathy above and below the inguinal ligament results in the "groove sign," which is considered pathognomonic for LGV in 10% to 20% of cases.[102] Healing occurs slowly, and most patients suffer no serious sequelae. Patients in this stage also may present with an anogenitorectal syndrome, which is accompanied by proctocolitis and hyperplasia of intestinal and perirectal lymphatic tissue. Late or tertiary manifestations include perirectal abscesses, rectovaginal fistulas (in women), rectal strictures, and genital elephantiasis.[101] Appropriate treatment of stage II LGV usually prevents these late complications.

An acute anorectal syndrome of LGV occurs in homosexual men who acquire the infection through rectal receptive intercourse. In these cases, a primary anal ulcer may be noted with associated inguinal adenopathy (anal lymphatics drain to inguinal nodes). Subsequently, acute hemorrhagic proctocolitis occurs with tenesmus, rectal pain, constipation, and a mucopurulent, bloody rectal discharge. Rectal biopsy may show granulomatous colitis, mimicking Crohn's disease. Perirectal pelvic adenopathy also occurs.

Treatment

26. How should S.F. be treated?

Current CDC recommendations for LGV include treatment with oral doxycycline (100 mg every 12 hours) or erythromycin (500 mg base every 6 hours) for 21 days.[18] Surgical intervention may be needed for later forms of the disease. Azithromycin once weekly for 3 weeks may be effective, but clinical data on its use are lacking.[18]

SYPHILIS
Epidemiology

Syphilis is caused by a Gram-negative spirochete, *Treponema pallidum*. The rates of primary and secondary syphilis in the United States probably increased in the late 1980s related to crack cocaine use, but from 1990 to 2000, rates have decreased to those reported in 1941, representing more than an 86% decrease since 1990.[103,104] In 2001, however, rates increased 2.1%, the first increase since 1990, although exclusively in males, and primarily in men who have sex with men.[105] Another concern is that syphilis appears to facilitate transmission of HIV, and recent outbreaks of syphilis have been associated with HIV-positive men who have sex with men.[105,106] In the late 1980s, the incidence of syphilis increased in the heterosexual population and declined in homosexual males. Coincident with the increase in heterosexuals, rates of congenital syphilis and women with syphilis rose sharply in 1990 (Fig. 65-4). Part of the increased reporting of congenital syphilis was due to a change in the case definition

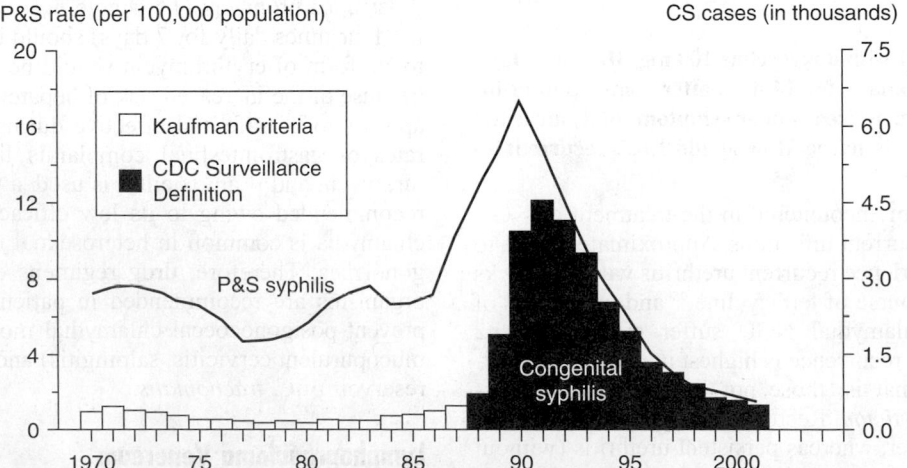

FIGURE 65-4 Congenital syphilis—reported cases for infants younger than 1 year of age and rates of primary and secondary syphilis among women: United States, 1970–2001. Note that the surveillance case definition for congenital syphilis changed in 1988. (From Division of STD Prevention. Sexually Transmitted Disease Surveillance, 2001. U.S. Department of Health and Human Services, Public Health Service. Atlanta: Centers for Disease Control and Prevention, February 2003.)

from the Kaufman criteria to the CDC Surveillance definition. From 2000 to 2001, congenital syphilis dropped by nearly 21%.[105] The Healthy People (HP) 2010 goal (0.2 cases per 100,000 people) is significantly lower than the HP 2000 goal (4 cases per 100,000). Although we met the HP 2000 goal, we still have far to go in the next decade to surpass the HP 2010 goal (Fig. 65-5).

The clinical manifestations of syphilis have not changed appreciably since their first description. However, early diagnosis, treatment, and greater physician/patient awareness of the disease have reduced the incidence of its severe forms. Penicillin continues to be the mainstay of therapy. Vaccine development, although premature, hopefully will advance as more is learned about the biology of *T. pallidum*.

Clinical Stages

27. D.M., a 27-year-old homosexual man, presents to the STD clinic with complaints of malaise, headache, and fever of 4 days' duration. He also reveals that he had a sore on his penis about 8 weeks ago, but it resolved. Upon examination, he is afebrile and has a widespread maculopapular skin rash that also involves the soles of his feet; general lymphadenopathy also is appreciated. Medical history is unremarkable except for one episode of gonorrhea 2 years ago that was treated with procaine penicillin. Laboratory findings include a normal peripheral WBC count, a negative serology for HIV antigen, and a positive rapid plasma reagin (RPR) test and fluorescent treponemal antibody absorption (FTA-Abs) test. Describe the clinical course of syphilis. Are D.M.'s symptoms consistent with this infection?

Primary Stage

The average incubation period for syphilis is 3 weeks and ranges from 10 to 90 days.[107] During this incubation period, *T. pallidum* can be demonstrated in the lymph and blood. The primary chancre develops at the site of inoculation as a painless papule that becomes ulcerated and indurated. The ulcer is nontender and filled with spirochetes. The chancre usually involves the penis in the heterosexual male; the penis or anus in the homosexual male; and the vulva, perineum, or cervix in the female. Occasionally, the lip or tongue is involved. Regional lymph nodes are enlarged, firm, and nontender. Unfortunately, the typical chancre described earlier often is missed, particularly in women or homosexual men.[108] Without treatment, the primary chancre resolves spontaneously, usually in 2 to 6 weeks. The differential diagnosis of genital ulcers also includes chancroid and genital herpes. Like chancroid, genital herpes produces painful, superficial, nonindurated ulcers with tender inguinal adenopathy. However, unlike chancroid, lesions of genital herpes characteristically proceed through a vesicular state and often are associated with urethritis, cervicitis, and constitutional symptoms, such as fever and chills. Syphilis can be differentiated from herpes by a nonpainful versus painful lesion, a papular versus vesicular appearance, and single versus multiple lesions. Chancroid is more difficult to tell apart from syphilis, although chancroid tends to have a more tender lesion, jagged border, and striking inguinal lymphadenopathy.[109]

Secondary Stage

Approximately 6 weeks after a chancre first appears, the untreated patient begins to manifest signs and symptoms of the secondary stage of syphilis. This is illustrated by D.M.

Skin lesions of secondary syphilis may erupt in a variety of patterns and are usually widespread in distribution. A macular syphilid often is the earliest manifestation in this stage. The lesion is round or oval, occurs primarily on the trunk, and is rose or pink in color. As lesions mature, they become papular or nodular with scaling (the so called papulosquamous rash). The differential diagnosis of diffuse papulosquamous rashes includes psoriasis, pityriasis rosea, and lichen planus. In syphilis, the palms and soles are characteristically involved, and oral lesions (mucous patches) may occur. Generalized lymphadenopathy usually is present, and patching alopecia may be seen. The most infectious lesion of secondary syphilis

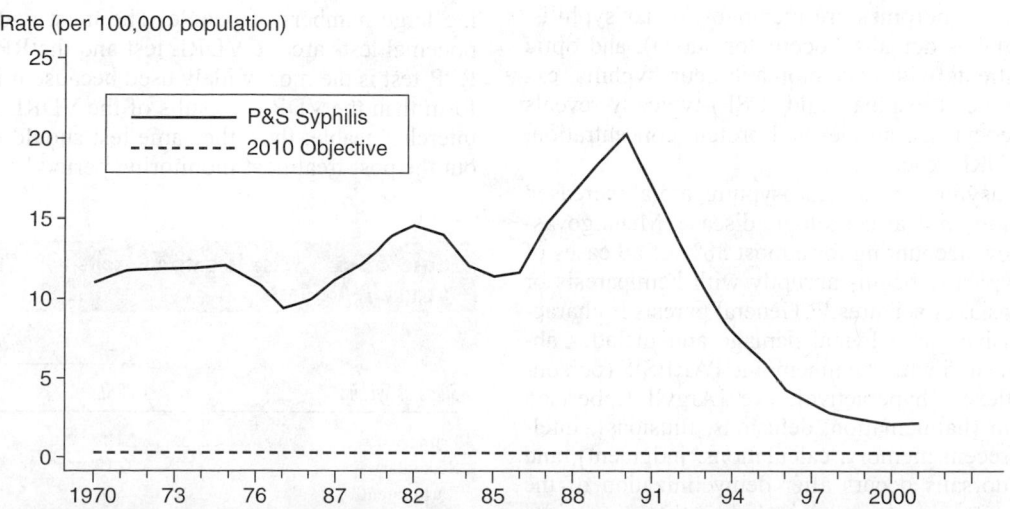

FIGURE 65-5 Primary and secondary syphilis—reported rates: United States, 1970–2001 and the Healthy People 2010 objective (0.2 cases per 100,000). (From Division of STD Prevention. Sexually Transmitted Disease Surveillance, 2001. U.S. Department of Health and Human Services, Public Health Service. Atlanta: Centers for Disease Control and Prevention, February 2003.)

is condyloma latum. Condylomata lata are characteristically wet, indurated lesions occurring primarily in the perineum or around the anus as a result of direct spread from the primary lesion.[109]

Laboratory studies sometimes reveal anemia, leukocytosis, or an increased erythrocyte sedimentation rate. Other manifestations of secondary syphilis include mild hepatitis, aseptic meningitis, uveitis, neuropathies, and glomerulonephritis.[110]

Latent Stage

By definition, untreated, asymptomatic persons with serologic evidence for syphilis have latent syphilis. The latent stage is divided into two phases: the early latent (<1 year's duration) and late latent (>1 year's duration). In the Oslo study of patients with untreated syphilis, 25% experienced secondary relapses, usually within the first year.[111] Patients who relapse to the secondary stage are infectious; those in the late latent stage are not infectious and are immune to reinfection with *T. pallidum*.

Tertiary Stage

Morbidity and mortality of syphilis in adults are due primarily to a variety of late manifestations involving the skin, bones, central nervous system (CNS), and cardiovascular system. Infectious granulomas (gummas), the characteristic lesions of tertiary syphilis, now are observed infrequently. Most gummas respond quickly to specific therapy, although if critical organs are involved (heart, brain, liver), they can be fatal.[112]

The most common manifestations of syphilitic cardiovascular disease are aortic insufficiency and aortitis, with aneurysm of the ascending aorta.

Neurosyphilis may be classified as asymptomatic early or late, meningeal, parenchymatous, or gummatous. Although neurosyphilis has been a rare complication for more than 40 years because of the widespread of use of penicillin, syphilitic meningitis, an early form of neurosyphilis, may be increasing in HIV-positive patients.[113,114] Late neurosyphilis may be asymptomatic or accompanied by a variety of manifestations; the most common syndromes are meningovascular syphilis, general paresis, tabes dorsalis (locomotor ataxia), and optic atrophy.[113] In patients with asymptomatic neurosyphilis, examination of the cerebrospinal fluid (CSF) typically reveals mononuclear pleocytosis, an elevated protein concentration, and a positive VDRL reaction.

Patients with asymptomatic neurosyphilis are at increased risk for developing clinical neurologic disease. Meningovascular syphilis, now accounting for almost 38% of all cases of neurosyphilis, typically begins abruptly with hemiparesis or hemiplegia, aphasia, or seizures.[115] General paresis is characterized by extensive parenchymal damage and includes abnormalities associated with the mnemonic PARESIS (personality, affect, reflexes [hyperactive], eye [Argyll Robertson pupil], sensorium [hallucination, delusions, illusions], intellect [decreased recent memory, calculations, judgment], and speech). Tabes dorsalis occurs after demyelinization of the spinal cord. Symptoms observed include an ataxic, wide-based gait and foot slap; paresthesias; bladder irregularities; impotence; areflexia; and loss of position, deep pain, and temperature sensation. The Argyll Robertson pupil, seen in both paresis and tabes dorsalis, is a small, irregular pupil that reacts to accommodation but not to light.

Laboratory Tests

28. Evaluate D.M.'s laboratory findings.

Dark-Field Examination

Exudate expressed from the chancre or from condyloma latum is examined with a dark-field microscope. The diagnosis of syphilis is made if spirochetes with characteristic corkscrew morphology and mobility are present. Dark-field examination is the most specific and sensitive method, but only when the microscopist is experienced in the diagnosis of syphilis.[116] Three dark-field examinations on consecutive days should be performed before considering the test negative in suspected primary syphilis.

Serologic Tests

Serologic tests become reactive during the primary stage, but as shown in Table 65-5, they may be negative at the time of presentation with primary syphilis. When the history or examination suggest primary syphilis, a VDRL should be sent to the laboratory, or an RPR test should be performed in the clinic (see discussion on nontreponemal tests, following). If initial serology and dark-field examinations are negative, the serology should be repeated in 1 to 4 weeks to exclude primary syphilis. If the dark-field examination is positive, an RPR may still be ordered to establish a baseline for follow-up after treatment.

Serologic tests are essentially always positive during secondary syphilis.[109] Two types of tests are used for the serodiagnosis of syphilis: nontreponemal tests, which measure serum concentrations of reagin (antibody to cardiolipin), and treponemal tests, which detect the presence of antibodies specific for *T. pallidum*.

NONTREPONEMAL TESTS

Nontreponemal tests are not specific for *T. pallidum* but can be quantified. They are inexpensive and useful for screening large numbers of people. The most widely used nontreponemal tests are the VDRL test and the RPR Card test. The RPR test is the most widely used because it is simpler to perform than the VDRL. Results of the VDRL and RPR are not interchangeable; thus, the same test should be used throughout the post-treatment monitoring period.[117]

Table 65-5 False-Negative Results with VDRL and FTA-Abs Tests

Stage of Syphilis	Percentage	
	VDRL	FTA-Abs
Primary	24%	14%
Secondary	<0.1%	<0.1%
Early latent	5%	1%
Late latent	28%	5%

FTA-Abs, fluorescent treponemal antibody absorption; VDRL, Venereal Disease Research Laboratory.

The result reported in the quantitative VDRL test is the most dilute serum concentration with a positive reaction. This test may be used to follow the decline in VDRL titer after effective therapy (see Question 31). In some individuals, a sero-fast reaction occurs in which nontreponemal antibodies may remain at a low titer for a long time and even their entire lives. When false-positive tests occur (Table 65-6), the titer usually is low (e.g., VDRL or RPR titer ≤1:8).[118] In secondary syphilis, sensitivity of the RPR and VDRL approach 100% owing to the high antibody concentrations.[119]

TREPONEMAL TESTS

Specific treponemal tests are most useful to confirm a positive nontreponemal test. The FTA-Abs test is the most commonly used treponemal test. Because the FTA-Abs test requires fluorescence microscopy, it is relatively difficult and expensive to perform and not appropriate for screening.

The *Treponema pallidum* immobilization (TPI) test, the microhemagglutination (MHA-TP) test, and the hemagglutination test for syphilis (HATTS) are three other treponemal tests. The TPI test is used rarely because of its cost and complexity. The MHA-TP and HATTS tests are both easier to perform and less expensive than the FTA-Abs test, but they are less sensitive in primary syphilis. Treponemal tests should not be used to assess treatment response because antibody titers correlate poorly with disease progression. A newer test is the *T. pallidum* latex agglutination (TPLA) test, which, in one study, was 100% sensitive and specific for nearly all stages of syphilis and took only 10 minutes to complete.[117,120] This test, however, is not in widespread use.

Treatment

29. How should D.M. be treated?

Penicillin G is the drug of choice for the treatment for all stages of syphilis (Table 65-7).[18] Every effort should be made to rule out penicillin allergy before choosing other antimicrobials that have been studied much less extensively than penicillin in the treatment of syphilis. Because *T. pallidum* has not developed antimicrobial resistance, treatment regimens for syphilis have changed relatively little over the years.

Table 65-6   Causes of False-Positive VDRL and FTA-Abs Tests

VDRL	FTA-Abs
Technical error	Technical error
Other spirochetal diseases (yaws, bejel, pinta)	Genital herpes
	Heroin addiction
Lupus erythematosus	Leprosy
Hashimoto's thyroiditis	Mononucleosis
Malaria	Collagen vascular disease
Mononucleosis	Pregnancy
Pregnancy	
Immunizations	
IV narcotic abuse	

FTA-Abs, fluorescent treponemal antibody absorption; IV, intravenous; VDRL, Venereal Disease Research Laboratory.

Table 65-7   Treatment Guidelines for Syphilis

Stage	Recommended	Alternative
Early (primary, secondary, or latent <1 year)[a]	Benzathine penicillin G 2.4 MU single dose IM (1.2 MU in each hip)	Doxycycline 100 mg orally BID or 200 mg orally QD × 2 wk or Tetracycline 500 mg orally QID × 2 wk or Ceftriaxone 1 g IM/IV QD × 8–10 days or Ceftriaxone 500 mg IM QD × 2 wk Azithromycin 2 g × 1 dose or azithromycin 500 mg QD × 2 wk
Late (>1 year's duration, unknown duration, late-latent)	Lumbar puncture: CSF normal: Benzathine penicillin G 2.4 MU/wk IM × 3 wk CSF abnormal: Treat as neurosyphilis	Lumbar puncture: CSF normal: Doxycycline 100 mg PO BID × 28 days or Tetracycline 500 mg PO QID × 28 days CSF abnormal: Treat as neurosyphilis
Neurosyphilis[b] (asymptomatic or symptomatic)	Aqueous penicillin G 18–24 MU IV per day × 10–14 days[c]	Aqueous procaine penicillin G 2.4 MU IM QD *plus* probenecid 500 mg QID, both for 10–14 days
Congenital	Aqueous penicillin G 100,000–150,000 units/kg/day, administered as 50,000 units/kg/dose IV Q 12 hr during the first 7 days of life, and Q 8 hr thereafter for a total of 10 days[d] or Procaine penicillin G 50,000 units/kg/dose IM a day in a single dose for 10 days	Only if CSF normal: benzathine penicillin G 50,000 units/kg IM in a single dose
Syphilis in pregnancy	According to stage	According to stage

[a]Some experts recommend repeating this regimen after 7 days for HIV-infected patients.
[b]Benzathine penicillin G does not achieve treponemicidal levels in the cerebrospinal fluid and has given inferior results for treatment of neurosyphilis. Because of the shorter duration of therapy compared with latent syphilis treatment, some experts recommend giving benzathine penicillin G, 2.4 MU IM weekly for 3 weeks after the completion of these neurosyphilis regimens.
[c]Administered as 3 to 4 MU IV every 4 hours or continuous infusion.
[d]All infants born to women treated during pregnancy with erythromycin must be treated with penicillin at birth.
Adapted from references 18 and 43.

As shown in Table 65-7, recommended therapy for primary, secondary, or latent syphilis (with negative findings in the CSF) of <1 year's duration is a single, intramuscular 2.4 MU dose of benzathine penicillin G. If penicillin is contraindicated, tetracycline (500 mg PO QID) or doxycycline (100 mg PO BID or 200 mg PO QD) for 2 weeks are the main alternatives.[18] If the patient is allergic to penicillin, not pregnant, and is contraindicated or cannot tolerate tetracycline or doxycycline, a 14-day regimen of azithromycin (500 mg PO QD) or ceftriaxone (500 mg IM QD) may be used (see Table 65-7).[121] The CDC lists an alternative regimen of azithromycin 2 g in one dose or ceftriaxone 1 g IM or IV for 8 to 10 days.[18] The use of erythromycin as an alternative is no longer recommended by the CDC because of its low efficacy. The optimal dose, duration, and efficacy of these alternative regimens are not well defined, necessitating close follow-up of patients. If compliance and follow-up cannot be ensured, the patient should be skin tested for hypersensitivity to penicillin. If the patient is truly allergic, he or she should be desensitized with oral penicillin in incrementally greater doses over a 4-hour period after which a full course of penicillin may be given.[18,122] Latent syphilis (>1 year's duration) and cardiovascular syphilis are treated with intramuscular benzathine penicillin G weekly (2.4 MU) for a total of 3 weeks. The alternative regimen is doxycycline (100 mg PO BID) or tetracycline (500 mg PO QID) for 28 days with close serologic and clinical follow-up. CSF examination is recommended if nonpenicillin therapy is being considered.

Neurosyphilis

30. Would D.M.'s treatment differ if his CSF had tested positive for syphilis?

Neurosyphilis can present at any stage of syphilis. When conventional IM doses of benzathine penicillin G are administered, no measurable levels of penicillin are obtained in the CSF, but that doesn't mean it is not in the CNS tissue itself.[121] It was recognized many years ago that treatment failures, as well as late clinical progression to neurosyphilis, can occur after treatment with the recommended IM regimen.[123,124] After one dose, benzathene penicillin reaches peak plasma concentration slower (13 to 24 hours) but with more prolonged treponemicidal plasma concentrations (7 to 10 days) than procaine penicillin (1 to 4 hours to peak; 12- to 24-hour treponemicidal plasma concentrations).[121] However, the CDC guidelines recommend treatment of neurosyphilis with aqueous penicillin G, 3 to 4 MU IV every 4 hours, or 18 to 24 MU per day continuous infusion, for 10 to 14 days.[18] Alternatively, neurosyphilis can be treated with procaine penicillin (2.4 MU IM per day) plus probenecid (500 mg orally every 6 hours) for 10 to 14 days. Some experts add benzathine penicillin G (2.4 MU IM once a week for 3 weeks) after the completion of aqueous penicillin G or procaine penicillin in the hope of providing persistent treponemicidal blood/tissue/CSF levels; the duration of therapy is the same as that for late syphilis stage. Penicillin-allergic patients should be skin tested to confirm allergy. If an allergy is confirmed, the patient should be desensitized and treated with an appropriate penicillin regimen. The World Health Organization also recommends in penicillin-allergic nonpregnant patients 30 days of doxycycline 200 mg orally twice daily or tetracycline 500 mg orally four times daily.[125]

Follow-Up

31. D.M. was treated with a single IM dose of benzathine penicillin (2.4 MU). How should his response to therapy be monitored?

Physical examination and a quantitative VDRL or RPR test for primary and secondary syphilis should be repeated at least 6 and 12 months after therapy.[18] Retreatment should be considered when the RPR or VDRL titer does not decline by fourfold in 6 months. Patients who also are infected with HIV should have serologic testing every 3 months for 1 year and then a follow-up at 2 years.[109] Patients with latent syphilis should be retested 6, 12, and 24 months after treatment. Close nontreponemal serologic test monitoring is necessary if antibiotics other than penicillin are used; CSF examination should be performed in these patients at their last follow-up visit. Patients with neurosyphilis should be monitored serologically every 6 months; CSF examinations should be repeated at 6-month intervals until normal. If still abnormal at 2 years, re-treatment should be considered. Return of lesions, a fourfold increase in titer, or a titer of 1:8 that does not fall at least fourfold within 12 months indicates the need for retreatment because of relapse or reinfection. Suspected treatment failures, especially if there is an abnormal CSF, should be treated as described for neurosyphilis. However, false-positive serologic results should be ruled out (see Table 65-6).

In 2 years, most patients with early syphilis become seronegative. However, if the disease is treated during the late stages, complete seroreversal may not occur. Patients treated with oral doxycycline or erythromycin are less likely to become seronegative.[126] Therapy is considered adequate in patients who never become seronegative if the titer decreases fourfold. Although the disease process may be halted in patients with tertiary syphilis, existing damage to the cardiovascular system or nervous system cannot be reversed.

Pregnancy

32. N.W., a 27-year-old woman in the 19th week of gestation, has a positive VDRL and FTA-Abs. How should N.W. be managed? How would management be altered in the face of penicillin allergy?

Although pregnancy has been a reported cause of false-positive nontreponemal tests,[110] the presence of both a positive treponemal test and a nontreponemal test virtually excludes a false-positive reaction.[116] The next step is to determine whether N.W. already has been treated adequately. If she has previously received adequate treatment and follow-up and shows no evidence of persistence or recurrence of syphilis, then she requires no further therapy. Pregnancy has no known effect on the clinical course of syphilis.[127] However, her infant should be observed carefully. If N.W. has not been treated previously for syphilis, then she should be treated with penicillin in the same doses recommended for nonpregnant women; some experts recommend a second dose 1 week later of 2.4 MU of benzathine penicillin.[18]

The goal of therapy should be to treat the mother with syphilis as soon as possible. Syphilis transmission can occur transplacentally as early as 9 to 10 weeks' gestation and by direct contact with lesions in the birth canal.[127,128] If the mother is left untreated, up to 50% of fetuses born to mothers with primary or secondary syphilis may be aborted, stillborn, or born with congenital syphilis (see Question 34).[129,130]

There is no completely satisfactory alternative for the pregnant woman allergic to penicillin. Tetracycline, as well as doxycycline, should be avoided during pregnancy, especially during the second or third trimester, because of tetracycline's known effects on the fetus (tooth staining and inhibition of bone growth).[131]

Erythromycin has been used to treat pregnant patients with syphilis. However, the mean transplacental transfer rate (ratio of the concentration between fetal and maternal blood levels) of erythromycin is only 3%.[132] This may explain why some patients treated with erythromycin aborted or gave birth to stillborn infants. Therefore, erythromycin is no longer recommended as therapy for syphilis in the pregnant patient.[18] A woman with a history of allergy to penicillin should be skin tested; if allergy is confirmed, she should be desensitized and treated with penicillin.[18] It is possible that newer cephalosporins and azithromycin may ultimately prove to be more acceptable alternatives to penicillin G in the pregnant woman with syphilis who is allergic to penicillin, but data are insufficient at this time to recommend their use. Sadly, even with adequate detection and treatment, some fetal infection may still occur.[133] However, more recent evidence suggests that adequate treatment with the appropriate penicillin dose can prevent up to 98% of fetal infection.[134]

During pregnancy, the patient should be followed up with monthly quantitative VDRL titers to evaluate the effectiveness of therapy; thereafter, she should be followed up as any other syphilitic patient.

Jarisch-Herxheimer Reaction

33. N.W. was treated with an IM injection of 2.4 MU of benzathine penicillin G. Six hours later, she complained of diffuse myalgias, chills, headache, and an exacerbation of her rash. She was tachypneic, but normotensive. What has happened? How should N.W. be managed?

N.W. has developed the Jarisch-Herxheimer reaction (JHR), a benign, self-limited complication of antitreponemal antibiotic therapy that develops in a high proportion of patients within a few hours after treatment of secondary syphilis and less often after primary. The cause of JHR is not well understood, but is probably related to release of cytokines.[135] Clinical manifestations include fever, chills, myalgias, headache, tachycardia, and hypotension. The pathogenesis of the syndrome is uncertain, but the reaction is not an allergic reaction to penicillin. It typically begins 1 to 2 hours after antibiotic administration and normally subsides spontaneously even while antibiotics are continued.[136] Notably, JHR can occur after administration of many antimicrobials and is not exclusive to penicillins, nor is it exclusive to syphilis treatment, occurring in other spirochetal diseases such as Lyme disease and relapsing fever.[137] Usually self-limiting in nonpregnant patients, the primary risk of this reaction in pregnant women is miscarriage, premature labor, or fetal distress.[138] Pregnant women should seek medical attention if contractions or a change in fetal movements are noted. Close monitoring of the JHR should be observed for patients with ophthalmic or neurologic syphilis. For these patients, prednisolone 10 to 20 mg three times a day for 3 days given 24 hours before syphilis

treatment may prevent fever, but will not control local inflammation.[121] More recently, tumor necrosis factor alpha was used to prevent JHR with some success in a similar spirochete disease.[139] Although there is no proven effective preventive therapy, some experts still recommend antipyretics, hydration, and patient education[30]; antibiotic therapy should not be discontinued.

Neonatal

34. How should N.W.'s baby be treated if a diagnosis of congenital syphilis is confirmed?

Infants born to mothers treated for syphilis during pregnancy should be carefully examined at birth, at 1 month, every 2 to 3 months for 15 months, and then every 6 months until the VDRL is negative or stable at a low titer. Newborn serology is difficult to interpret because of transplacental transfer of nontreponemal and treponemal IgG to the infant. Treatment decisions then are largely based on evidence of syphilis in the mother, adequacy of maternal treatment, comparison of maternal and neonate nontreponemal serology, and/or presence of clinical or laboratory evidence of syphilis in the neonate. Aqueous penicillin G 50,000 units/kg per dose IV every 12 hours should be used during the first 7 days of life and every 8 hours thereafter for a total of 10 days.[18] Procaine penicillin G 50,000 U/kg per dose IM once a day for at least 10 days is an alternative regimen. If more than 1 day of therapy is missed, the CDC recommends restarting the entire course. In addition, infants should be treated at birth, even if they are asymptomatic, when maternal treatment is unknown or inadequate, or when infant follow-up cannot be guaranteed. In most cases, a CSF examination should be performed before treatment is begun to rule out neurosyphilis. Although benzathine penicillin (50,000 U/kg IM) as a single dose is recommended by some clinicians to treat infants who may not be followed up, data on the efficacy of this treatment are lacking and any abnormalities in the infant examination (i.e., abnormal or uninterpretable CSF, long-bone radiographs, CBC, and platelets) should preclude its use.

CHANCROID

Chancroid or soft chancre is a painful genital ulcer disease that often is associated with tender inguinal adenopathy. It is caused by *Haemophilus ducreyi,* a Gram-negative bacillus.

Chancroid is endemic in developing countries and some areas of the United States, but its incidence in the United States has steadily declined from nearly 5,000 cases in 1987 to 38 cases in 2001.[3] Chancroid and other genital ulcers have been implicated in the transmission of HIV. In the United States, up to 18% of people with genital ulcers were also HIV seropositive.[140]

Signs and Symptoms

35. E.J., a 31-year-old uncircumcised man, presents to the STD clinic with complaints of tender lesions on the penis and inguinal regions. He noticed the penile lesions on the external surface of the prepuce (foreskin) 2 days before his visit. The lesions were sharply demarcated but were not indurated; the base of the penile ulcer was covered by a yellow-gray purulent exudate.

Right inguinal adenitis was present and extremely painful on palpation. A dark-field examination of the purulent exudate was negative. Gram's stain revealed a mixture of Gram-positive and Gram-negative flora. E.J. claims to have no drug allergies. What is the natural course of chancroid? Does E.J. have signs or symptoms consistent with chancroid? What diagnostic procedures are necessary?

Uncircumcised males may have an increased risk of chancroid infection and may not respond to therapy as well as circumcised males.[141] The chancroid ulcer appears 3 to 10 days after exposure and begins as a tender red papule that becomes pustular and ulcerates within 2 days. As illustrated by E.J., the ulcer may be covered by a grayish or yellow exudate. Multiple ulcers and tender inguinal lymph nodes, which may become fluctuant, are seen in about 50% of cases.[142] Aspiration of fluctuant nodes may be necessary to prevent rupture. Gram's stain can be misleading because of the polymicrobic nature of the ulcer and culture and because isolation of *H. ducreyi* is difficult, requiring specialized specimen collection and growth media.[18,143]

Treatment

36. **How should E.J.'s chancroid be treated?**

Most strains of *H. ducreyi* produce a TEM-type β-lactamase, and many strains are resistant to the antimicrobials that traditionally were used to treat chancroid, such as sulfonamides and tetracycline.[144,145] The drugs of choice today are azithromycin (1 g orally), ceftriaxone (250 mg IM once), ciprofloxacin (500 mg orally twice daily for 3 days), or erythromycin (500 mg orally three times a day for 7 days).[18] Ciprofloxacin is contraindicated in pregnant and lactating women and children 17 years of age or younger. Because E.J. has no history of penicillin hypersensitivity, azithromycin or ceftriaxone as a single dose is the preferred treatment. Single-dose therapy may not be as effective if the patient is coinfected with HIV and uncircumsized.[18,141]

BACTERIAL VAGINOSIS

Bacterial vaginosis (BV) (formerly called nonspecific vaginitis, leukorrhea, *Gardnerella vaginalis,* or *Haemophilus vaginalis*) is associated with an increased, malodorous vaginal discharge. The normal vaginal lactobacillus flora is overgrown by *Mobiluncus* species, *Bacteroides* species, *Peptococcus* species, *M. hominis,* and increased numbers of *Gardnerella.*

The prevalence of BV varies widely due to differing diagnostic criteria, demographics, and lack of a national reporting system, but it probably represents the most common cause of vaginal disharge.[146] Many sexually active women are infected with *G. vaginalis* at any one time; yet less than 50% are symptomatic or have signs of abnormal vaginal discharge.[147] The evidence for definitive risk factors in BV is inconclusive. Intrauterine devices,[148] lack of lactobacilli,[149] and douching[150] have been associated with BV, whereas smoking, abnormal Pap smears, and timing in relation to menstrual cycle have not.[149,150] There is conflicting information on the role of heterosexual transmission since some nonsexually active postpubertal women had BV,[149] whereas longitudinal cohort studies showed increased incidence of BV after single and multiple

sexual experiences.[151,152] A study in sexually active lesbians showed strong evidence for sexual transmission.[153] Occasionally, *G. vaginalis* is found to colonize the urethras of men, but treatment of male sexual partners does not prevent the recurrence of BV in women.[18]

Signs, Symptoms, and Diagnosis

37. **S.D. is a 19-year-old, sexually active girl with a 1-week history of a moderate vaginal discharge that has a "fishy" odor, most notable after coitus. She has no complaints of vaginal pruritus or burning. On examination, the discharge appears gray, homogeneous, and notably malodorous. A wet mount of the vaginal secretion revealed few leukocytes and numerous "clue cells." The vaginal pH was 4.8, and a characteristic fishy odor was noted when the discharge was mixed with 10% KOH. Does S.D. have signs and symptoms consistent with BV? What diagnostic tests are required?**

S.D.'s symptoms and signs are typical of BV. The clinical diagnosis can be confirmed by a vaginal Gram's stain that shows overgrowth of the vagina with *G. vaginalis* and other organisms noted earlier.

A small drop of 10% KOH mixed with vaginal secretion will yield a transient "fishy" odor because of the increased production of biogenic diamines (positive amine test). A wet preparation of the specimen will reveal "clue cells" (exfoliated vaginal epithelial cells with adherent coccobacillary pathogens), pH >4.5, and the characteristic KOH "whiff" test.[154] If there are many white cells, other infections (e.g., *T. vaginalis*) should be suspected. Self-diagnosis is correct only about 3% to 4% of the time because most women attribute symptoms to poor hygiene.[155]

Treatment

38. **How should S.D. be treated?**

Oral metronidazole 500 mg twice a day for 7 days is the most effective treatment of BV. Initially, up to 95% of women respond to this regimen, while only 82% still report cure after 4 weeks, indicating the need for follow-up if symptoms persist or reappear.[146,156] Although the FDA approved Flagyl ER (750 mg once daily for 7 days), the CDC reports that adequate trials to evaluate its comparable efficacy to twice-daily metronidazole have not been done. Ampicillin no longer is considered an alternative treatment because approximately 50% of women develop recurrent symptoms within 6 weeks.[146,157] Clindamycin cream 2%, one full applicator (5 g) intravaginally at bedtime for 7 days or metronidazole 0.75% gel, one full applicator (5 g) intravaginally, once daily for 5 days are CDC-approved topical recommendations.[18,158] Patients should be told that clindamycin is oil based and may weaken latex condoms or diaphragms. Alternatively, the CDC recommends metronidazole 2 g orally in a single dose, clindamycin 300 mg orally two times a day for 7 days, or clindamycin ovules 100 g intravaginally once daily at bedtime for 3 days. Because of the limited published experience with oral clindamycin regimens, some experts recommend combining the single-dose metronidazole with the 7-day clindamycin regimen.[159]

In the absence of signs of BV, isolation of flora from the vagina is not an indication for treatment. To date, there is insufficient evidence that treatment of sexual partners is beneficial. BV has been associated with pregnancy complications such as preterm labor and premature delivery. If the decision is made to treat BV during pregnancy, the CDC-recommended therapy is metronidazole 250 mg orally three times daily for 7 days. Recent teratogenic data suggest that metronidazole may not be harmful to the fetus, but clindamycin cream should not be used because an increase in preterm delivery was noted.[18,160]

TRICHOMONIASIS
Signs and Symptoms

39. N.J. is a 32-year-old woman with a recent history of profuse vaginal discharge with vaginal irritation. A wet-mount examination of vaginal secretions revealed numerous trichomonads. Examination confirms the presence of an increased, yellow vaginal discharge. What subjective and objective clinical data support a diagnosis of trichomoniasis?

Trichomoniasis is an STD caused by the protozoan *T. vaginalis*. The prevalence in women ranges from 5% to 10% and up to 60% in commercial sex workers.[161] Trichomoniasis in women is asymptomatic about 20% to 50% of the time.[162] In men, *T. vaginalis* presumably infects the urethra, although the site of infection (urethra versus prostate) is uncertain. Men with *T. vaginalis* infection usually are asymptomatic. Classic symptoms of trichomoniasis in women include yellowish-green frothy discharge, pruritus, dysuria, and the "strawberry" cervix (cervical microhemorrhages). The latter is typically seen in only 2%[163] to 25% of cases, whereas a vaginal pH higher than 5 or 6 occurs in almost all cases.[164] The Pap smear was reported to have a 48.4% error in diagnosis when used alone.[163] Direct microscopic observation of trichomoniasis using a wet mount suffers from low sensitivity, but is up to 99% specific.[165] Broth culture is considered to be the gold standard for identification of trichomoniasis, but it requires up to a 7-day incubation period and the culture system is not widely available.[163] The best approach to diagnosis requires clinical and laboratory confirmation.

Treatment
Metronidazole

40. How should N.J.'s trichomoniasis be treated?

The only drugs effective for the treatment of *T. vaginalis* are the nitroimidazoles. In the United States, metronidazole is the only available nitroimidazole. The preferred dose for men or women is a single 2-g dose of metronidazole; sexual partners should be treated simultaneously. If the 2-g dose is not tolerated or the patient does not become asymptomatic, use 500 mg orally twice daily for 7 days. If this is ineffective, the dose can be increased to 2 g orally daily for 3 to 5 days.[18] If the latter dosage regimen is used, the patient should be monitored closely for signs of peripheral neuropathy. Cure rates are reported to be 90% to 95%, especially when sexual partners are concomitantly treated.[18,166] Assuming that a patient has not been reinfected, approximately 5% of *T. vaginalis* isolates from initial treatment failures may be resistant to metronidazole, necessitating dosage increases to overcome low ferrodoxin levels or a change to another drug, such as furazolidone

or paromomycin cream.[167,168] At this time, however, use of alternative agents to metronidazole requires further clinical evaluation before they can be recommended. If patients are allergic to metronidazole, they can be desensitized and then treated.[169]

ADVERSE EFFECTS

41. N.J. was treated with metronidazole 500 mg twice a day for 7 days. On the fourth day of therapy while attending a party, N.J. developed a severe headache, followed by nausea, sweating, and dizziness. Could N.J.'s symptoms be caused by metronidazole?

Minor side effects associated with metronidazole therapy include nausea, vomiting (especially with single-dose therapy), headache, skin rashes, and alcohol intolerance. The alcohol intolerance may be due to a metronidazole-induced inhibition of aldehyde dehydrogenase, which results in the build-up of high serum acetaldehyde levels, although this mechanism is questionable.[170] Severe "Antabuse reactions" are uncommon, but according to the manufacturer, patients still should be warned about the possibility of nausea, vomiting, flushing, and respiratory distress after ethanol ingestion, although reliable evidence is lacking.[171]

Pregnancy

42. S.G., a 31-year-old woman, is in her first trimester of pregnancy and has a history of recurrent trichomoniasis. She now complains of a frothy, yellow vaginal discharge. The preliminary diagnosis of trichomoniasis is confirmed by a wet-mount examination of vaginal secretions that revealed numerous trichomonads. S.G. has read much of the lay press on metronidazole and is concerned about her own safety as well as that of her fetus. Can metronidazole be used for S.G.?

Metronidazole is mutagenic in facultative bacteria and contains a nitro-reductase enzyme. Long-term, high-dose metronidazole in laboratory mice is associated with the development of pulmonary and hepatic tumors. Midline facial defects have been documented in humans, but two recent literature reviews indicate that metronidazole is not a teratogen.[172,173] However, caution should still be exercised if metronidazole must be administered within the first trimester.

TREATMENT

43. How should S.G. be treated?

During pregnancy, trichomoniasis is associated with premature rupture of the membranes, preterm delivery, and low birth weight; thus, all symptomatic women should be treated with 2 g metronidazole orally in a single dose.[18] In asymptomatic women, however, studies do not support the use of treatment with metronidazole to reduce preterm delivery.[174] Since metronidazole is discouraged during the first trimester, clotrimazole cream 100 mg intravaginally at bedtime for 7 days has been studied, but it is not as effective as oral metronidazole.[175]

GENITAL HERPES

The word *herpes* is of Greek origin and means "to creep." HSV is a DNA-containing virus that consists of two antigenic distinct serotypes: HSV-1 and HSV-2. HSV-1 is the primary cause of herpes labialis (cold sores), herpes keratitis, and herpetic encephalitis. Genital herpes and neonatal herpes primarily are the result of HSV-2 infections. However, up to 30% of all reported cases of primary genital herpes are due to HSV-1 infections acquired through oral sex.[176,177]

Etiology

Most infants are exposed to HSV-1 early in life with over half being positive for HSV-1 antibodies before 18 years and more than 90% of the population positive by 70 years of age.[178] The infection often is asymptomatic and generally is acquired through primary infection of the respiratory tract. The initial, primary disease is a gingivostomatitis characterized by vesicles in the oral cavity and occasionally an elevated temperature; life-threatening encephalitis or keratitis may appear during this interval. Usually after primary exposure, HSV-1 enters cells of the trigeminal ganglion, where it may remain latent for the lifetime of the host.[179]

Initial HSV-2 infections usually follow puberty and coincide with the onset of sexual activity, although transfer to a neonate from an infected mother can occur. After primary infection, the virus enters a state of latency in the sacral dorsal root ganglia in many infected individuals; a high percentage of infected persons may never manifest the disease clinically.[179,180]

In both HSV-1 and HSV-2 infections, the latent virus can reactivate. Recurrent disease may occur even when circulating antibody and sensitized lymphocytes are present. Clinically, the lesions periodically erupt usually at the same location, and the interval between episodes varies widely between individuals.

Epidemiology

Although herpes was recognized several thousand years ago, genital herpes was not described formally until the 18th century. The seroprevalence of genital herpes has increased dramatically in the United States—from 16.4% in the late 1970s to 21.9% in the early 1990s, making it the most common STD with over 45 million people infected in the United States.[181] In 2001, U.S. physicians saw more than 150,000 new patients presenting with herpes simplex.[3]

The prevalence of antibody to genital herpes is greater among women (25.6%) than men (17.6%) and among blacks (45.9%) than whites (17.6%).[181] Demographic characteristics obtained at the University of Washington indicate that the mean number of lifetime sexual partners before acquisition of the disease was 8.8 in women compared with 32.8 in men, with the overall chance of acquiring HSV-2 of 5 per 1,000 sex contacts.[182] The mean time from the last sexual exposure to the onset of disease was 5.8 days.[180]

Signs and Symptoms

44. B.J., a 28-year-old, sexually active man, complains of painful penile lesions and tender inguinal adenopathy. The lesions are vesicular and limited to the scrotum, glands, and shaft of the penis. The onset of the lesions was preceded by a 1-week period of fever, malaise, headache, and itching. Viral culture of the lesions was positive for HSV infection. Describe the typical course and clinical presentation of herpes genitalis in men and women. What subjective and objective clinical data in B.J. are compatible with herpes genitalis?

Most initial episodes of genital herpes, especially in the male, are symptomatic. As illustrated by B.J., the symptoms usually start about 1 week after the initial exposure with prodromal signs of tingling, itching, paresthesia, and/or genital burning.[183] The prodromal stage, which can last from a few hours to several days, is followed by the appearance of numerous vesicles. The vesicles eventually erupt, resulting in painful genital ulcers. The pain and edema associated with genital herpetic lesions, especially if they are infected secondarily, can be severe enough to result in dysuria and urinary retention. Bilaterally distributed lesions of the external genitalia are characteristic. The lesions usually are limited to the glands, corona prepuce, and shaft of the penis in the man and to the vulva and vagina in the woman. However, lesions can occur on the buttocks, thighs, and urethra.[180] In addition, women with primary and nonprimary genital HSV-2 infections have concomitant HSV cervicitis at rates of 90% and 70%, respectively.[184,185] Rectal and perianal HSV-2 infections increasingly are being recognized. HSV proctitis usually is seen in homosexual men and heterosexual men who engage in anorectal intercourse. Symptoms include anorectal pain and discharge, tenesmus, and constipation.

Prior infection with HSV-1 appears to ameliorate the severity of the first episode of genital herpes, but does not appear to affect the rate of recurrece.[186] In primary infections, the local symptoms of pain, itching, and urethral or vaginal discharge last from 11 to 14 days, with a complete disappearance of lesions in 3 to 6 weeks.[180,187] The clinical course of primary herpes is presented in Figure 65-6. Of importance, however, is that only one-third of patients seropositive for HSV-2 recall signs or symptoms of herpes, indicating the importance of subclinical and asymptomatic disease.[188]

Recurrence

45. Is B.J.'s infection likely to recur?

Most patients experience a recurrence of their initial infection. The rate of recurrent infections varies among individual patients. In one study, 38% experienced at least 6 episodes, and 20% had more than 10 recurrences.[186] Natural infection with HSV-2 induces type-specific immunity against exogenous reinfection, but does not affect recurrences.[189] The severity of the primary episode as well as the host's immune response to the disease appear to influence the subsequent recurrence rate.[190] Recurrent infections usually appear at or near the site of the initial infection, and prodromal symptoms are reported by about 50% of persons with recurrent infection. Men appear to have slightly more frequent recurrences. In contrast to primary infections, there are fewer lesions and they are often unilateral.[180] Constitutional symptoms such as lymphadenopathy, fever, and malaise generally are milder. Recurrent infections are shorter in duration (average, 1 week); local symptoms such as pain and itching last 4 to 5 days and the lesions themselves last 7 to 10 days.[180] By about 5 years after the initial infection, recurrence rates tend to decrease.[191] Genital infections with HSV-1, however, recur infrequently and decrease by 50% between 1 and 2 years after infection.[192]

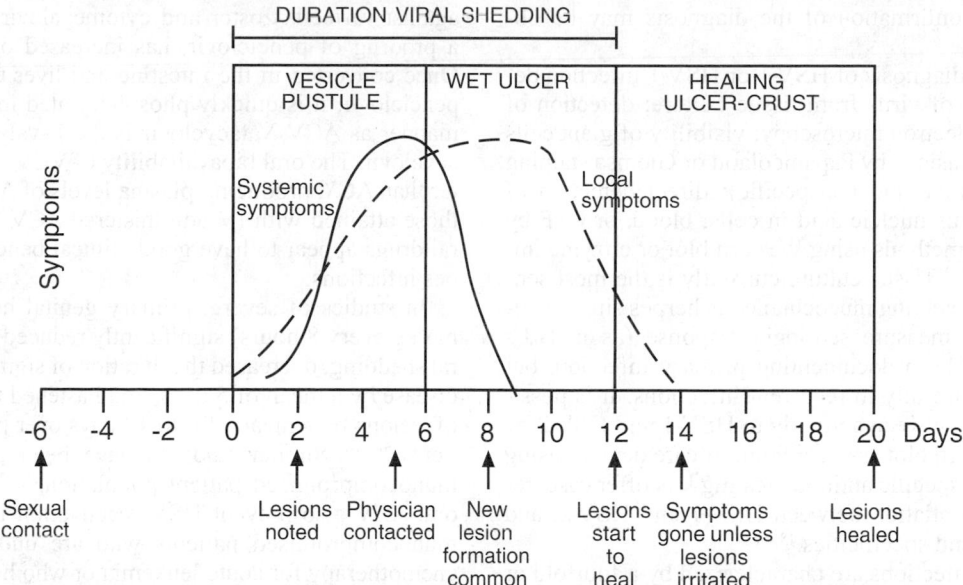

DURATION VIRAL SHEDDING

FIGURE 65-6 The clinical time course of primary genital herpes infections. (Reprinted with permission from reference 180.)

Transmission

46. **B.J. states that this is the first time he has had such lesions and that he has had only one sexual partner for the last 14 months. His sexually active female partner has no history of herpes genitalis or any other STD. The couple is very curious as to how B.J. acquired his infection. How is HSV transmitted?**

Transmission of HSV occurs by direct contact with active lesions or from a symptomatic or asymptomatic person shedding virus at a peripheral site, mucosal surface, or secretion.[193] Genital HSV-2 infections usually are acquired through sexual (vaginal or anorectal) intercourse, whereas genital HSV-1 infections are acquired via oral-genital sexual practices. Because HSV is inactivated readily by drying and exposure to room temperature, aerosol and fomite spread are unusual means of transmission.[194] Condoms may act as an effective barrier to viral transmission, although this method does not offer complete protection for men.[195,196]

A patient with genital herpes is contagious only when he or she is shedding the virus. The patient begins to shed virus during the prodromal phase, which may be several hours to days before the actual lesions first appear. Subclinical or asymptomatic viral shedding is an important means of sexual transmission from a public health standpoint.[197,198] Lesions are most contagious during the ulcerative phase. The median duration of viral shedding as defined from onset to the last positive culture is about 12 days.[180] The mean time from the onset of vesicles to the appearance of the crust stage (approximately 10.5 days) correlates well with the duration of viral shedding. However, there is considerable overlap between the duration of viral shedding and the duration of crusting. Therefore, patients should be advised to refrain from sexual activity until the lesions have completely healed. Women appear to require a longer total lesion healing time than men, 19.5 and 16.5 days, respectively.[180] The mean duration of viral shedding from the cervix is 11.4 days.

A genital herpes infection may be acquired from an individual who has never had symptomatic genital lesions. States of asymptomatic or subclinical viral shedding occur in the majority of women with recurrent genital herpes as a result of reactivation of latent infection. These recurrent infections can have a primary disease presentation, causing the patient to blame the most proximate sexual partner when in actuality, the exposure could have occurred in the distant past.[199] Serologic and virologic typing can be used to determine whether this is a true primary infection. Using sensitive detection techniques such as polymerase chain reaction (PCR), women with recurrent HSV infections demonstrated viral shedding up to 28% of the time, but the relation between a PCR-positive HSV test and true communicability has yet to be determined.[200] A recent study of men and women seropositive for HSV-2, but with no previous history of symptomatic genital herpes, demonstrated viral shedding in the genital tract at a rate similar to those who reported symptomatic infection.[201] For asymptomatic viral shedding treatment is not indicated. Seropositive HSV patients also should be counseled to practice safer sex, using male or female condoms, at all times, not just during symptomatic episodes.

Diagnostic Tests

47. **An HSV antibody test (Western blot) of B.J.'s serum taken on day 1 of the illness was negative. However, 20 days later, the HSV-2 antibody was positive. Viral cultures of B.J.'s genital lesions grew HSV-2. A genital Pap smear and serologic antibody detection tests were negative in B.J.'s asymptomatic sexual partner. How are these laboratory tests to be interpreted?**

The accuracy with which herpes genitalis can be diagnosed without the aid of laboratory tests generally is quite good, especially if the infection is recurrent in nature. However, because of the potentially severe psychological and physiologic ramifications of such a diagnosis, either virologic and/or serologic confirmation of the diagnosis may be obtained.

The laboratory diagnosis of HSV-1 or HSV-1 infection depends on isolation of virus from tissue culture; detection of viral particles by electron microscopy; visibility of giant cells or intranuclear inclusions by Papanicolaou or Giemsa staining (which are insensitive and nonspecific); direct detection of herpes simplex virus nucleic acid in cells, blood, or CSF by PCR; or serologic methods using Western blot or enzyme immunoassay (EIA).[183] Tissue culture currently is the most sensitive method for detecting mucocutaneous herpes simplex infection. Tests that measure serologic response (as in B.J.'s partner) are valuable in documenting primary infection, but they are not very usefully in recurrent infections. It is possible to differentiate between antibody to HSV-1 and HSV-2 by means of the Western blot assay.[202] Point of care devices using HSV-1 and HSV-2 specific antibody testing kits offer ease, reduced time, differentiation between HSV-1 and HSV-2, and high sensitivities and specificities.[18,203]

Primary HSV infections are characterized by a fourfold or greater rise in the HSV antibody titer as seen in B.J.'s case. Fewer than 10% of patients with recurrent episodes of disease experience a serologic rise in antibody titer between acute and convalescent sera.[190]

B.J.'s partner's results need to be interpreted cautiously. The negative Pap smear is not completely diagnostic. A nonreactive serology (absence of HSV antibodies) implies the absence of a primary infection, although false-negative reactions have occurred. Absence of antibody to HSV-2 by Western blot would be good evidence against asymptomatic carriage.

Treatment

48. How should B.J.'s lesions be managed? Because the likelihood of recurrence of genital herpes is high, what treatment and prevention measures are recommended currently?

The great anxiety commonly associated with the diagnosis of genital herpes is because there is presently no cure available for the condition. Therapies ranging from antiviral agents and photoinactivation to investigational vaccines have been tried. Currently, only acyclovir (ACV), famciclovir (FCV), and valacyclovir (VCV) are used to treat and prevent genital herpes outbreaks.

The ideal anti-HSV agent should (1) prevent infection, (2) shorten the clinical course, (3) prevent the development of latency, (4) prevent recurrence in patients with established latency, (5) decrease transmission of disease, and (6) eradicate established latent infection.[180] To date, no agent has been successful in achieving all of these goals.

All three agents, ACV, FCV, and VCV, are effective for the short-term treatment of some HSV infections. In general, ACV has been in clinical use longer than FCV or VCV and thus has more data to support its role in the treatment and suppression of mucocutaneous and visceral HSV infections. Acyclovir, a nucleoside analog, is a substrate for HSV-specific thymidine kinase. Through a series of phosphorylation steps, ACV is transformed to ACV-triphosphate, a competitive inhibitor of viral DNA polymerase. Acyclovir has potent in vitro activity against both HSV-1 and HSV-2 and is least active

against varicella-zoster and cytomegalovirus.[204] Famciclovir, a prodrug of penciclovir, has increased oral bioavailability. Once converted in the intestine and liver to the active form, penciclovir, it is quickly phosphorylated in HSV in a similar manner as ACV. Valacyclovir is the L-valyl ester prodrug of acyclovir. The oral bioavailability of VCV is significantly better than ACV, producing plasma levels of ACV comparable to those attained with IV administered ACV.[205] All three antiviral drugs appear to have good clinical benefit for genital herpes infections.

In studies of severe, primary genital herpes, IV ACV (5 mg/kg every 8 hours) significantly reduced the duration of viral shedding, decreased the duration of signs and symptoms of disease by a mean of 5 days, and hastened the time to healing of lesions by a mean of 6 to 12 days over placebo-treated patients.[206,207] Similar findings have been shown in the immunocompromised patient population.[208–210] Intravenous and oral ACV also prevent HSV reactivation in seropositive immunocompromised patients who are undergoing induction chemotherapy for acute leukemia or who have just undergone transplantation.[211,212] For patients with HIV, doses of 400 mg orally three times daily or 200 mg five times daily have been used for recurrent episodes.[18] Currently, IV therapy is recommended only for patients with severe genital or disseminated infections who cannot take oral medication.

Topical therapy with ACV ointment (5% in polyethylene glycol) has minimal effect on the duration of viral shedding, symptoms, and lesion healing in first-episode primary genital herpes and has no effect on the recurrence rate.[213] Currently, topical ACV is not recommended for primary genital herpes. Penciclovir 1% cream is applied every 2 hours while awake and has been shown to be effective for treatment of herpes simplex labialis,[214] but insufficient data exist to recommend its use for genital herpes infections.

The introduction of oral products such as ACV, FCV, and VCV (Table 65-8) have replaced the use of topical ACV, and they are indicated for B.J. Like IV therapy, the oral antivirals speed the healing and resolution of symptoms of first and recurrent episodes of genital HSV-2 infections.[215] Treatment of primary infection after the first week of infection does not appear to change the natural history of recurrent outbreaks; thus, patients should be educated about risk of sexual transmission and prompt recognition of signs and symptoms and the early use of antivirals.[216] The frequency of recurrence decreases with time in most patients. Recurrent episodes of genital HSV-2 infection can be treated with any of the three available oral antivirals (see Table 65-8). Rather than having to go into clinic, patients with recurrent infection should have a supply of their antiviral drug with them to allow early initiation of therapy, which may abort or reduce symptoms by 1 to 2 days.[217,218]

Daily suppressive therapy with ACV, FCV, or VCV reduces the frequency of recurrent episodes up to 70% among patients with frequent (more than six episodes per year) genital herpes.[18, 219–221] Recurrent outbreaks diminish over time; thus, after each year of continuous suppressive therapy, an effort should be made to discontinue therapy (especially with FCV and VCV where long-term suppressive data are not available).[18] The use of suppressive therapy does not completely eliminate viral transmission. However, a recent randomized controlled clinical trial of serodiscordant HSV-2–positive

Table 65-8   Antiviral Chemotherapy of Genital HSV-2 Infections

	Acyclovir	Valacyclovir	Famciclovir	Duration	Comments
First clinical episode	400 mg PO TID or 200 mg PO 5 × per day	1 g PO BID	250 mg PO TID	7–10 days	May extend treatment duration if healing is incomplete
Episodic recurrent infection	400 mg PO TID or 200 mg PO 5 × per day or 800 mg PO BID	500 mg PO BID or 1 g QD	125 mg PO BID	5 days	Most effective if initiated within the first 24 hr of onset of lesions or during the prodrome
Daily suppressive therapy	400 mg PO BID[a]	500 mg PO QD[b] or 1 g PO QD	250 mg PO BID	Daily	Reduces the frequency of genital herpes recurrences by ≥75% among patients who have frequent recurrences (i.e., ≥6 recurrences per year); use should be re-evaluated at 1 yr
Severe disseminated	5–10 mg/kg IV Q 8 hr	Not indicated	Not indicated	Variable	Hospitalize and treat until clinical resolution of symptoms. Follow-up IV therapy with PO acyclovir to complete 10 days
HIV-infected: Episodic	400 mg PO TID or 200 mg 5 × per day	1 g PO BID[c]	500 mg PO BID	5–10 days	Treat until clinical resolution of lesions
HIV-infected: Suppressive	400–800 mg PO BID-TID	500 mg PO BID[d]	500 mg PO BID		

Note: Regimen recommendations derived from 2002 CDC Recommendations.[18]
[a]Safety and efficacy up to 6 years have been documented with the use of acyclovir.
[b]Valacyclovir 500 mg QD appears less effective in patients with more than10 episodes per year. Thus, 1 g QD should be used in these patients.
[c]Dosages up to 8 g/day have been used, but an association with a syndrome resembling either hemolytic uremic syndrome or thrombotic thrombocytopenic purpura was observed.
[d]Effective in decreasing both the rate of recurrences and the rate of subclinical shedding among HIV-infected patients.

couples demonstrated a statistically significant decrease in the rate of transmission to uninfected partners when infected partners took 500 mg per day of VCV.[222] This 8-month study was restricted to heterosexual partners with less than 10 recurrences per year. The CDC recommends various dosing regimens for VCV, but the 500 mg once daily dose appears to be less effective than the 1-g once-daily dose in patients with frequent recurrent episodes (i.e., >10 episodes per year).[18] Immunocompromised patients may require higher doses or more frequent intervals for suppression.[223] An increased frequency of resistant strains has been reported in immunocompromised hosts who have used long-term therapy.[224] All ACV-resistant strains are also resistant to VCV, and most are resistant to FCV as well. Foscarnet 40 mg/kg IV every 8 hours until clinical resolution may be used for severe ACV-resistant genital HSV infections.[18] Cidofovir 1% gel (not commercially available in the United States, but may be compounded by pharmacists) applied once daily for 5 days may be an alternative to IV foscarnet, but more studies are needed.[18,225]

B.J. is not yet a candidate for daily suppressive ACV therapy. A summary of the indications for ACV, FCV, and VCV is outlined in Table 65-8.

ADVERSE EFFECTS

49. **What adverse effects secondary to ACV, FCV, or VCV should be anticipated?**

Overall, all forms of ACV, including VCV, and FCV seem to be relatively free of frequent adverse reactions largely because of the drugs' affinity for viral thymidine kinase over cellular kinase.

Hematuria and an increase in blood urea nitrogen and serum creatinine may occur, primarily in patients with underlying renal disease or those receiving concomitant nephrotoxic agents. Transient elevations in serum creatinine are associated more frequently with IV than with oral administration. In addition, severe local reactions are possible with IV administration. In immunocompromised patients, VCV at a dosage of 8 g/day was associated with symptoms resembling a hemolytic uremic syndrome or thrombotic thrombocytopenic purpura, but in normal therapeutic doses, this has not occurred according to the manufacturer. When given intravenously in high doses or when significant dehydration exists, ACV has been shown to crystallize in the renal collecting tubules of animals leading to renal insufficiency.[226] Acyclovir should not be rapidly infused or administered at concentrations greater than 10 mg/mL. If oral ACV or VCV is administered to produce plasma levels equivalent to IV doses, similar changes in renal function may be observed. Dose adjustment is necessary for all three antiviral agents in patients with decreased renal function.

Although neurotoxicity is a rare side effect, case reports of coma and delirium have been reported in patients with renal failure and renally adjusted ACV dosages.[227,228]

Intravenous ACV occasionally has been associated with cutaneous irritation and phlebitis, reversible leukopenia,[209] and transient elevations of liver transaminases.[229] Oral ACV did not produce any clinical or laboratory side effects that were significantly different from placebo in clinical trials.[230–232]Patients receiving oral ACV, VCV, or FCV may complain of nausea, dizziness, diarrhea, and headaches.

Topical ACV usually is well tolerated. Local reactions, including transient pain, burning, or rash, have been reported with the 5% ACV ointment, although discontinuation of therapy often was not necessary. Adverse reactions related to penciclovir cream in one study were similar to placebo,[214] but some sources report up to a 50% incidence of mild erythema.[233]

Patient Education and Counseling

50. What are the roles for education and counseling in patients with genital herpes? Are other forms of local or symptomatic care useful?

Most genital herpes infections are benign, and lesions heal spontaneously unless the patient is immunocompromised or the lesions have become infected secondarily. The patient should be instructed to keep the involved areas clean and dry. To prevent autoinoculation, the patient should be told not to touch the lesions and to wash his hands immediately afterward if he comes in contact inadvertently. Local anesthetics provide relief from the pain of genital lesions, but they should be avoided if possible because they counteract efforts to keep the lesions dry. Local corticosteroid therapy is contraindicated because it may predispose the patient to secondary bacterial infections.

Patient counseling is an important facet in the therapy of genital herpes and should include the source contact and any future partner. Health care practitioners should attempt to relieve patients' feelings of guilt and anxiety; discussion of long-term consequences should take place after the acute symptoms of the infection have resolved.

For individuals with frequent recurrences, efforts should be made to identify and avoid stimulatory factors such as sunlight, trauma, or emotional stress. The limitations of therapy and the decreased severity and frequency of recurrences with time should be explained to the patient. The periods of infectivity and the need to avoid sexual activity during these times also should be emphasized, although subclinical or asymptomatic shedding does occur, indicating the need for continuous barrier protection. Women with herpes genitalis should be scheduled for a routine Pap smear every year and should be instructed to discuss the problem with their physicians if they become pregnant.

Currently, there is no completely effective way to prevent the transmission of HSV-2 infection. Barrier forms of contraception, in particular condoms, may reduce the transmission of HSV, but this may be limited only to male-to-female transmission owing to the large area that herpes lesions may occupy on the female.[195] Nonoxynol-9, a spermicide that has in vitro anti-HSV activity, is ineffective in the treatment of established genital HSV infection and may actually increase the risk of transmission of HSV by causing genital ulceration.[234]

Complications

51. M.F. is a 23-year-old, sexually active female student with a history of frequent and severe recurrences of genital herpes since her initial infection 3 years ago. M.F. has tried numerous therapies including topical ether, photoinactivation, and BCG vaccines. None of these therapies has provided M.F. with any relief of her symptoms, nor have they decreased the frequency of her recurrences. M.F. has read much in the lay press about herpes and is concerned about the possible complications of the disease, especially cervical cancer. What are the potential complications of herpes genitalis?

Previous research suggested that HSV-2 might be an oncogenic agent responsible for carcinoma of the cervix. The theoretical association between HSV-2 and carcinoma of the cervix was most likely biased by cross-sectionally designed studies, misclassification, confounding with HPV, now known to cause cervical cancer, and lack of power. Lehtinen and colleagues[235] conducted the largest longitudinal nested case-control study using nearly 20 years of seroepidemiologic and epidemiologic data combined with a meta-analysis to conclude that it is very unlikely that HSV-2 is associated with the development of invasive cervical carcinoma.

Pregnancy

52. A.P., a 26-year-old woman in her 32nd week of gestation, was hospitalized with complaints of painful genital lesions, headache, fever, increased vaginal discharge, and dysuria of 1 week's duration. Multiple ulcerative lesions consistent with genital herpes were present on the cervix, vulva, labia minora, and thighs. How should A.P. be treated?

Neonatal herpes is a devastating systemic infection of the newborn, associated with high morbidity and mortality. In 1994, assuming an average incidence of 265 cases of neonatal HSV per year, the estimated annual cost to the health care system was $10.5 million.[1] HSV-2 usually is transmitted to the newborn during passage through an infected birth canal, although ascending infections in newborns delivered by cesarean section 6 hours after the membranes have ruptured have been known to occur.[236] The risk of transmission to the newborn is greatest in mothers who acquire an initial infection late in the third trimester and lower in mothers with recurrent infection or those who acquire herpes in the first trimester.[18] A primary episode of clinically apparent HSV-2 will result in neonatal HSV-2 50% of the time; 33% of the time in asymptomatic primary infection; 4% if lesions are due to recurrent infection; and 0.04% in nonprimary asymptomatic infection.[237]

Herpes genitalis infections in pregnant women occur more frequently than in nonpregnant women, with 3% to 4% of all pregnant women having a known history of recurrent HSV-2 infection.[238] Unfortunately, a large proportion of those infections occurring during pregnancy are limited to the cervix and are totally asymptomatic, often eluding diagnosis.

Pregnant patients with a history of recurrent genital herpes should be examined carefully when they present in labor for evidence of active disease. Surveillance cultures should be performed from the cervix and vulva even if lesions are absent. The safety of systemic ACV and VCV in pregnant women has not been established in controlled trials and therefore is not clearly indicated for A.P. Some small studies suggest ACV administered for several weeks before delivery may decrease recurrent outbreaks and lessen the need for herpes-related cesarian section,[239] whereas a larger randomized clinical trial did not show a benefit on reducing the need for a caesarian section with primary infection.[240] The manufacturer of Zovirax (ACV) maintains an extensive database of fetal complications related to ACV use. To date, there does not appear to be clear evidence that ACV causes birth defects.[241] Nevertheless, firm conclusions recommending the use of ACV in pregnancy cannot be made at this time. The decision to treat HSV with ACV during pregnancy should depend on the clinical severity of infection. Fetal exposure data to FCV or VCV is too limited to recommend their use at this time. If the mother has an active herpes genitalis infection at the time of delivery (either active genital lesions or asymptomatic HSV-2 cervicitis), the baby should be delivered by cesarean section within 4 hours after the membranes have ruptured to prevent exposure of the neonate to the virus.[180] However, if no genital lesions are present at the time of delivery, vaginal delivery can be recommended.[18,242]

GENITAL WARTS

53. S.L., a 19-year-old woman, presents to the women's health clinic for her annual pelvic examination. One week later, her Pap smear is read as showing koilocytosis. A colposcopy is subsequently performed, revealing changes consistent with cervical flat warts. What is the cause of S.L.'s infection? How should she be managed?

Human papillomaviruses (HPV), primarily types 6 and 11, now are recognized as the cause of genital warts, or condylomata acuminata. Other types, including 16 and 18, are strongly associated with cervical cancer.[243] These cause Pap smear changes, including koilocytosis and cervical dysplasia. In women, visible warts occur on the labia, the introitus, and the vagina. Subclinical lesions also commonly occur on these sites and on the cervix as in S.L.'s case. They are visible only by colposcopy after applying acetic acid.

The goal of HPV therapy is the removal of symptomatic warts. Several therapeutic options are available and include patient-administered treatments such as podofilox 0.5% solution or gel and imiquimod 5% cream and provider administered products such as topical treatments (podophyllin 10% to 25%, trichloroacetic acid 80% to 90%, and cryotherapy), surgery (laser or scalpel), and intralesional interferon.[18] None of these treatments has been shown to eradicate HPV infection or alter the natural history of HPV.

Podophyllin, compounded as a 10% or 25% solution in tincture of benzoin, is applied by the health care provider to visible warts. After application, it is washed off 3 to 4 hours later and then reapplied once or twice a week until the warts have disappeared. Podofilox 0.5% solution or gel, the active component of podophyllin resin, may be applied by the patient with a cotton swab, or podofilox gel with a finger, to visible genital warts twice a day for 3 days, followed by 4 days of no therapy. A total of four cycles, 0.5 mL/day, or application of an area >10 cm² should not be exceeded. Podofilox solution is not suitable for use with perianal warts, whereas the gel is more practical for this region. Podophyllin is potentially neurotoxic if absorbed in large amounts. Podofilox has the advantage over podophyllin resin in that it has a longer shelf life, does not need to be washed off, and has less systemic toxicity.[244] Therefore, it should be applied in limited doses and should also be avoided in pregnancy. The rate of wart recurrence after podophyllin therapy is extremely high, probably 50%. With high cost of clinic care and the high recurrence rate, home treatment of HPV with podofilox solution may be more cost effective and equally efficacious.[245]

Imiquimod induces cytokines and activates the cell-mediated immune system. In initial trials, complete clearance of warts was seen in 37% to 50% of immunocompetent patients, but up to 20% had recurrence of the warts.[246] A 5% cream may be applied with a finger at bedtime three times per week up to 16 weeks. It is usually left on for 6 to 10 hours before it is washed off with soap and water. Imiquimod may take as long as 8 weeks before warts are cleared. Mild to moderate local irritation occurs in more than half of the patients who use it, especially when used daily instead of three times weekly.[246]

Cryotherapy by application of liquid nitrogen can be more effective than podophyllin, but requires special equipment and highly trained personnel to avoid over- or undertreating warts. Pain and skin blistering after treatment is not unusual. Cryotherapy is associated with little systemic toxicity and is useful against oral, anal, urethral, and vaginal warts.

Trichloroacetic acid (80% to 90%) is used topically in the treatment of some genital warts, but its efficacy is uncertain. To date, interferons are not recommended because of expense, frequent occurrence of toxicity when given systemically, and limited efficacy for intralesional administration. Cases refractory to topical drug therapy should be considered for surgical treatment.

VACCINES

Prevention and control of sexually transmitted diseases have largely revolved around education and antimicrobials. Immunization, however, holds the promise of protecting large numbers of people before they are at risk for STDs as well as targeting those who already have the infection. Hepatitis B is an example of an STD with a highly effective vaccine that is now mandatory for school-aged children. A candidate STD vaccine furthest along in development is the HPV vaccine.

An HPV-16 virus–like protein (VLP) vaccine is in phase III studies, and the results of a large preliminary study are encouraging. Koutsky and colleagues[247] showed in a double-blind randomized trial of HPV-16 VLP vaccine that nearly 100% of women vaccine recipients were protected against acquiring HPV-16, the serotype associated with cervical cancer. Although development of cervical cancer was not an endpoint, the established relation between HPV and cervical cancer suggests that this vaccine may also prevent cancer. The vaccine contains no actual papillomavirus and thus has no risk of giving HPV to the vaccine recipient. Duration of immunity and optimal vaccination strategy must still be determined. The vaccine will most likely be combined with targeted screening as this strategy appears to be the most cost effective.[248] A therapeutic vaccine for HPV is in much earlier testing stages than the preventive vaccine. The ideal HPV therapeutic vaccine would decrease the progression of HPV infection and cervical cancer. The current HPV-16 VLP vaccine would most likely not be appropriate because the late proteins are not expressed reliably in the basal epithelial cells that generate condylomata.[249]

REFERENCES

1. Institute of Medicine: Committee on Prevention and Control of Sexually Transmitted Diseases: The hidden epidemic: confronting sexually transmitted diseases. Washington, D.C.: National Academy Press, 1997. (Eng T, Butler W, eds.)

2. U.S. Department of Health and Human Services. Sexually Transmitted Disease Surveillance 2001 Supplement: Gonococcal Isolate Surveillance Project (GISP) Annual Report 2001. 2002; pg. 28 [Last accessed October (available at http://www.cdc.gov/std/GISP2001/)]

3. U.S. Department of Health and Human Services.Sexually Transmitted Disease Surveillance, 2001. 2002; pg. [Last accessed September(available at http://www.cdc.gov/std/stats/2001PDF/Survtext2001.pdf)]

4. Handsfield IIH et al. Localized outbreak of penicillinase-producing Neisseria gonorrhoeae. Paradigm for introduction and spread of gonorrhea in a community. JAMA 1989;261(16):2357.

5. Mertz KJ et al. Gonorrhea in male adolescents and young adults in Newark, New Jersey: implications of risk factors and patient preferences for prevention strategies. Sex Transm Dis 2000;27(4):201.

6. CDC. Resurgent bacterial sexually transmitted disease among men who have sex with men—King County, Washington, 1997-1999. MMWR Morb Mortal Wkly Rep 1999;48(35):773.

7. Holmes KK et al. An estimate of the risk of men acquiring gonorrhea by sexual contact with infected females. Am J Epidemiol 1970;91(2):170.

8. Hook EW et al. Gonococcal infections in the adult. In: Holmes KK, ed. Sexually Transmitted Diseases, 3rd Ed. New York: McGraw-Hill Health Professions Division, 1999;451.

9. Whittington WL et al. Unique gonococcal phenotype associated with asymptomatic infection in men and with erroneous diagnosis of nongonococcal urethritis. J Infect Dis 2000;181(3):1044.

10. Turner CF et al. Untreated gonococcal and chlamydial infection in a probability sample of adults.[comment]. JAMA. 2002;287(6):726.

11. Mehta SD et al. Unsuspected gonorrhea and chlamydia in patients of an urban adult emergency department: a critical population for STD control intervention. Sex Transm Dis 2001;28(1):33.

12. Emmert DH et al. Sexually transmitted diseases in women. Gonorrhea and syphilis. Postgrad Med 2000;107(2):181, 189, 193.

13. CDC: Control of Neisseria gonorrhoeae infection in the United States: report of an external consultants' meeting convened by the division of STD prevention, National Center for HIV, STD, and TB Prevention, Centers for Disease Control and Prevention (CDC), October 2001. Atlanta, GA.:19.

14. Watts DH et al. Sexually transmitted diseases, including HIV infection in pregnancy. In: Holmes KK, ed. Sexually Transmitted Diseases, 3rd Ed. New York: McGraw-Hill Health Professions Division, 1999;1089.

15. Brocklehurst P. Update on the treatment of sexually transmitted infections in pregnancy—2. Int J STD AIDS 1999;10(10):636; quiz 642.

16. Johnson RE et al. Screening tests to detect Chlamydia trachomatis and Neisseria gonorrhoeae infections—2002. MMWR Recomm Rep 2002;51(RR-15):1.

17. Diemert DJ et al. Confirmation by 16S rRNA PCR of the COBAS AMPLICOR CT/NG test for diagnosis of Neisseria gonorrhoeae infection in a low-prevalence population. J Clin Microbiol 2002; 40(11):4056.

18. CDC. Sexually transmitted diseases treatment guidelines 2002. Centers for Disease Control and Prevention. MMWR Recomm Rep 2002;51(RR-6):1.

19. CDC. Discontinuation of cefixime tablets—United States. MMWR Morb Mortal Wkly Rep 2002; 51(46):1052.

20. CDC. Increases in fluoroquinolone-resistant Neisseria gonorrhoeae—Hawaii and California, 2001. MMWR Morb Mortal Wkly Rep 2002;51(46): 1041.

21. CDC. 1998 guidelines for treatment of sexually transmitted diseases. Centers for Disease Control and Prevention. MMWR Recomm Rep 1998; 47(RR-1):1.

22. McCormack WM. Treatment of gonorrhea. Ann Intern Med 1979;90(5):845.

23. Aplasca De Los Reyes MR et al. A randomized trial of ciprofloxacin versus cefixime for treatment of gonorrhea after rapid emergence of gonococcal ciprofloxacin resistance in the Philippines. Clin Infect Dis 2001;32(9):1313.

24. Thorpe EM et al. Comparison of single-dose cefuroxime axetil with ciprofloxacin in treatment of uncomplicated gonorrhea caused by penicillinase-producing and non-penicillinase-producing Neisseria gonorrhoeae strains. Antimicrob Agents Chemother 1996;40(12):2775.

25. Thompson EM et al. Oral cephalosporins: newer agents and their place in therapy. Am Family Phys 1994;50(2):401.

26. Tapsall JW et al. The sensitivity of 173 Sydney isolates of Neisseria gonorrhoeae to cefpodoxime and other antibiotics used to treat gonorrhea. Pathology 1995;27(1):64.

27. Handsfield HH et al. Multicenter trial of single-dose azithromycin vs. ceftriaxone in the treatment of uncomplicated gonorrhea. Azithromycin Gonorrhea Study Group. Sex Transm Dis 1994;21(2):107.

28. Siegel MS et al. Penicillinase-producing Neisseria gonorrhoeae: results of surveillance in the United States. J Infect Dis 1978;137(2):170.

29. CDC. Decreased susceptibility of Neisseria gonorrhoeae to fluoroquinolones—Ohio and Hawaii, 1992–1994. MMWR Morb Mortal Wkly Rep 1994; 43(18):325.

30. CDC. Fluoroquinolone resistance in Neisseria gonorrhoeae—Colorado and Washington, 1995. MMWR Morb Mortal Wkly Rep 1995;44(41):761.

31. World Health Organization. Antimicrobial resistance in Neisseria gonorrhoeae. 2001;pg. 65 [Last accessed at http://www.who.int/emc/amrpdfs/Antimicrobial_resistance_in_Neisseria_gonorrhoeae.pdf)]

32. Kam KM et al. Ofloxacin susceptibilities of 5,667 Neisseria gonorrhoeae strains isolated in Hong Kong. Antimicrob Agents Chemother 1993; 37(9):2007.

33. Knapp JS et al. Molecular epidemiology, in 1994, of Neisseria gonorrhoeae in Manila and Cebu City, Republic of the Philippines. Sex Transm Dis 1997;24(1):2.

34. Fox KK et al. Antimicrobial resistance in Neisseria gonorrhoeae in the United States, 1988–1994: the emergence of decreased susceptibility to the fluoroquinolones. J Infect Dis 1997;175(6):1396.

35. Tracking the hidden epidemics:trends in STDs in the United States, 2000:36. [Last accessed 2000 (available at http://www.cdc.gov/nchstp/dstd/Stats_Trends/Trends2000.pdf)]

36. Lafferty WE et al. Sexually transmitted diseases in men who have sex with men. Acquisition of gonorrhea and nongonococcal urethritis by fellatio and implications for STD/HIV prevention. Sex Transm Dis 1997;24(5):272.

37. Jebakumar SP et al. Value of screening for oropharyngeal Chlamydia trachomatis infection. J Clin Pathol 1995;48(7):658.

38. Page-Shafer K et al. Increased sensitivity of DNA amplification testing for the detection of pharyngeal gonorrhea in men who have sex with men. Clin Infect Dis 2002;34(2):173.

39. Handsfield HH et al. Trends in sexually transmitted diseases in homosexually active men in King County, Washington, 1980-1990. Sex Transm Dis 1990;17(4):211.

40. Hutt DM et al. Epidemiology and treatment of oropharyngeal gonorrhea. Ann Intern Med 1986; 104(5):655.

41. Judson FN et al. Comparative study of ceftriaxone and spectinomycin for treatment of pharyngeal and anorectal gonorrhea. JAMA 1985;253(10):417.

42. Stoner BP et al. Single-dose gatifloxacin compared with ofloxacin for the treatment of uncomplicated gonorrhea: a randomized, double-blind, multicenter trial. Sex Transm Dis 2001;28(3):136.

43. Feldblum PJ et al. The effectiveness of barrier methods of contraception in preventing the spread of HIV. AIDS 1995;9 Suppl A:S85.

44. Roddy RE et al. Effect of nonoxynol-9 gel on urogenital gonorrhea and chlamydial infection: a randomized controlled trial. JAMA 2002;287(9):1117.

45. Louv WC et al. A clinical trial of nonoxynol-9 for preventing gonococcal and chlamydial infections. J Infect Dis 1988;158(3):518.

46. Cook RL et al. Do spermicides containing nonoxynol-9 prevent sexually transmitted infections? A meta-analysis. Sex Transm Dis 1998; 25(3):144.

47. CDC. Nonoxynol-9 spermicide contraception use—United States, 1999. MMWR Morb Mortal Wkly Rep 2002;51(18):389.

48. Barrett-Connor E. The prophylaxis of gonorrhea. Am J Med Sci 1975;269(1):4.

49. Harrison WO et al. A trial of minocycline given after exposure to prevent gonorrhea. N Engl J Med 1979;300(19):1074.

50. CDC. Pelvic inflammatory disease: guidelines for prevention and management. MMWR Recomm Rep 1991;40(RR-5):1.

51. Westrom L. Incidence, prevalence, and trends of acute pelvic inflammatory disease and its consequences in industrialized countries. Am J Obstet Gynecol 1980;138(7 Pt 2):880.

52. WHO. Pelvic inflammatory disease in nongonococcal urethritis and other slected sexually transmitted diseases of public health importnace. WHO Techn Rep Ser 1981;660:89.

53. Wiesenfeld HC et al. Lower genital tract infection and endometritis: insight into subclinical pelvic inflammatory disease. Obstet Gynecol 2002; 100(3):456.

54. Kessel E. Pelvic inflammatory disease with intrauterine device use: a reassessment. Fertil Steril 1989;51(1):1.

55. Wolner-Hanssen P et al. Association between vaginal douching and acute pelvic inflammatory disease. JAMA 1990;263(14):1936.

56. Ness RB et al. Douching and endometritis: results from the PID evaluation and clinical health (PEACH) study. Sex Transm Dis 2001;28(4):240.

57. Larsson PG et al. Incidence of pelvic inflammatory disease after first-trimester legal abortion in women with bacterial vaginosis after treatment with metronidazole: a double-blind, randomized study. Am J Obstet Gynecol 1992;166(1 Pt 1):100.

58. Peipert JF et al. Bacterial vaginosis as a risk factor for upper genital tract infection. Am J Obstet Gynecol 1997;177(5):1184.

59. Marchbanks PA et al. Cigarette smoking as a risk factor for pelvic inflammatory disease. Am J Obstet Gynecol 1990;162(3):639.

60. Westrom L et al. Pelvic inflammatory disease. In: Holmes KK, ed. Sexually Transmitted Diseases, 3rd Ed. New York: McGraw-Hill Health Professions Division, 1999;783.

61. Ory HW. Ectopic pregnancy and intrauterine contraceptive devices: new perspectives. The Women's Health Study. Obstet Gynecol 1981;57(2):137.

62. Rein DB et al. Direct medical cost of pelvic inflammatory disease and its sequelae: decreasing, but still substantial. Obstet Gynecol 2000;95(3):397.

63. Stacey CM et al. A longitudinal study of pelvic inflammatory disease. Br J Obstet Gynaecol 1992; 99(12):994.

64. Bevan CD et al. Clinical, laparoscopic and microbiological findings in acute salpingitis: report on a United Kingdom cohort. Br J Obstet Gynaecol 1995;102(5):407.

65. Mardh PA et al. Chlamydia trachomatis infection in patients with acute salpingitis. N Engl J Med 1977;296(24):1377.

66. Eschenbach DA et al. Polymicrobial etiology of acute pelvic inflammatory disease. N Engl J Med 1975;293(4):166.

67. Cassell GH et al. Mycoplasmas as agents of human disease. N Engl J Med 1981;304(2):80.

68. Svensson L et al. Differences in some clinical and laboratory parameters in acute salpingitis related to culture and serologic findings. Am J Obstet Gynecol 1980;138(7 Pt 2):1017.

69. Kahn JG et al. Diagnosing pelvic inflammatory disease. A comprehensive analysis and considerations for developing a new model. JAMA 1991;266(18):2594.

70. Gaitan H et al. Accuracy of five different diagnostic techniques in mild-to-moderate pelvic inflammatory disease. Infect Dis Obstet Gynecol 2002;10(4):171.

71. Scholes D et al. Prevention of pelvic inflammatory disease by screening for cervical chlamydial infection. N Engl J Med 1996;334(21):1362.

72. Addiss DG et al. Decreased prevalence of *Chlamydia trachomatis* infection associated with a selective screening program in family planning clinics in Wisconsin. Sex Transm Dis 1993;20(1):28.

73. Westrom L et al. Pelvic inflammatory disease and fertility. A cohort study of 1,844 women with laparoscopically verified disease and 657 control women with normal laparoscopic results. Sex Transm Dis 1992;19(4):185.

74. Washington AE et al. Cost of and payment source for pelvic inflammatory disease. Trends and projections, 1983 through 2000. JAMA 1991;266(18):2565.

75. Walker CK et al. Anaerobes in pelvic inflammatory disease: implications for the Centers for Disease Control and Prevention's guidelines for treatment of sexually transmitted diseases. Clin Infect Dis 1999;28 Suppl 1:S29.

76. Bayer AS. Gonococcal arthritis syndromes: an update on diagnosis and management. Postgrad Med 1980;67(3):200, 207.

77. Mehrany K et al. Disseminated gonococcemia. Int J Dermatol 2003;42(3):208.

78. Ross JD. Systemic gonococcal infection. Genitourin Med 1996;72(6):404.

79. Wise CM et al. Gonococcal arthritis in an era of increasing penicillin resistance. Presentations and outcomes in 41 recent cases (1985-1991). Arch Intern Med 1994;154(23):2690.

80. Schachter J. Biology of *Chlamydia trachomatis*. In: Holmes KK, ed. Sexually Transmitted Diseases, 3rd Ed. New York: McGraw-Hill Health Professions Division, 1999;391.

81. CDC. *Chlamydia trachomatis* genital infections—United States, 1995. MMWR Morb Mortal Wkly Rep 1997;46(9):193.

82. U.S. Department of Health and Human Services. Sexually Transmitted Disease Surveillance 2001 Supplement: *Chlamydia* Prevalence Monitoring Project Annual Report 2001:14. [Last accessed October 2002(available at http://www.cdc.gov/std/chlamydia2001/CT2001text.pdf)]

83. Stamm WE: *Chlamydia trachomatis* infections of the adult. In: Holmes KK, ed. Sexually Transmitted Diseases, 3rd ed. New York: McGraw-Hill Health Professions Division, 1999:407.

84. Ridgway GL. Treatment of chlamydial genital infection. J Antimicrob Chemother 1997;40(3):311.

85. Rice RJ et al. Susceptibilities of *Chlamydia trachomatis* isolates causing uncomplicated female genital tract infections and pelvic inflammatory disease. Antimicrob Agents Chemother 1995;39(3):760.

86. Hughes G et al. New cases seen at genitourinary medicine clinics: England 1997. Commun Dis Rep CDR Suppl 1998;8(7):S1.

87. Burstein GR et al. Nongonococcal urethritis—a new paradigm. Clin Infect Dis 1999;28 Suppl 1:S66.

88. Horner P et al. Role of *Mycoplasma genitalium* and *Ureaplasma urealyticum* in acute and chronic nongonococcal urethritis. Clin Infect Dis 2001;32(7):995.

89. Krieger JN. Trichomoniasis in men: old issues and new data. Sex Transm Dis 1995;22(2):83.

90. Stamm WE et al. Azithromycin for empirical treatment of the nongonococcal urethritis syndrome in men. A randomized double-blind study. JAMA 1995;274(7):545.

91. Steingrimsson O et al. Single dose azithromycin treatment of gonorrhea and infections caused by *C. trachomatis* and *U. urealyticum* in men. Sex Transm Dis 1994;21(1):43.

92. Martin DH et al. A controlled trial of a single dose of azithromycin for the treatment of chlamydial urethritis and cervicitis. The Azithromycin for Chlamydial Infections Study Group. N Engl J Med 1992;327(13):921.

93. Tartaglione TA et al. The role of fluoroquinolones in sexually transmitted diseases. Pharmacotherapy 1993;13(3):189.

94. Hooton TM et al. Ciprofloxacin compared with doxycycline for nongonococcal urethritis. Ineffectiveness against *Chlamydia trachomatis* due to relapsing infection. JAMA 1990;264(11):1418.

95. Handsfield HH et al. Differences in the therapeutic response of chlamydia-positive and chlamydia-negative forms of nongonococcal urethritis. J Am Vener Dis Assoc 1976;2(3):5.

96. Stimson JB et al. Tetracycline-resistant Ureaplasma urealyticum: a cause of persistent nongonococcal urethritis. Ann Intern Med 1981;94(2):192.

97. Tait IA et al. Chlamydial infection of the cervix in contacts of men with nongonococcal urethritis. Br J Vener Dis 1980;56(1):37.

98. Wehbeh HA et al. Single-dose azithromycin for Chlamydia in pregnant women. J Reprod Med 1998;43(6):509.

99. Adair CD et al. *Chlamydia* in pregnancy: a randomized trial of azithromycin and erythromycin. Obstet Gynecol 1998;91(2):165.

100. Perine PL et al. *Lymphogranuloma venereum*. In: Holmes KK, ed. Sexually Transmitted Diseases, 3rd Ed. New York: McGraw-Hill Health Professions Division, 1999:23.

101. Mabey D et al. Lymphogranuloma venereum. Sex Transm Infect 2002;78(2):90.

102. Schachter J et al. Lymphogranuloma venereum. Br Med Bull 1983;39(2):151.

103. CDC. Primary and secondary syphilis—United States, 1998. MMWR Morb Mortal Wkly Rep 1999;48(39):873.

104. CDC. Primary and secondary syphilis—United States, 2000-2001. MMWR Morb Mortal Wkly Rep 2002;51(43):971.

105. U.S. Department of Health and Human Services. Sexually Transmitted Disease Surveillance 2001 Supplement: Syphilis Surveillance Report. February 2003:14. [Last accessed at http://www.cdc.gov/std/Syphilis2001/default.htm)]

106. CDC. Outbreak of syphilis among men who have sex with men—Southern California, 2000. MMWR Morb Mortal Wkly Rep 2001;50(7):117.

107. Sparling P: Natural history of syphilis. In: Holmes KK, ed. Sexually Transmitted Diseases, 3rd Ed. New York: McGraw-Hill Health Professions Division, 1999:473.

108. Chapel TA. The variability of syphilitic chancres. Sex Transm Dis 1978;5(2):68.

109. Musher D: Early syphilis. In: Holmes KK, ed. Sexually Transmitted Diseases, 3rd Ed. New York: McGraw-Hill Health Professions Division, 1999:479.

110. Birnbaum NR et al. Resolving the common clinical dilemmas of syphilis. Am Fam Physician 1999;59(8):2233, 2245.

111. Gjestland T. The Oslo study of untreated syphilis: an epidemiologic investigation of the natural course of syphilitic infection based on a restudy of the Boeck-Bruusgaard material. Acta Derm Venereol 1955;35(Suppl 34):I.

112. Garnett GP et al. The natural history of syphilis. Implications for the transmission dynamics and control of infection. Sex Transm Dis 1997;24(4):185.

113. Swartz M et al. Late syphilis. In: Holmes KK, ed. Sexually Transmitted Diseases, 3rd Ed. New York:

McGraw-Hill Health Professions Division, 1999;487.

114. Flood JM et al. Neurosyphilis during the AIDS epidemic, San Francisco, 1985–1992. J Infect Dis 1998;177(4):931.

115. Pezzini A et al. Meningovascular syphilis: a vascular syndrome with typical features? Cerebrovasc Dis 2001;11(4):352.

116. Larsen SA et al. Laboratory diagnosis and interpretation of tests for syphilis. Clin Microbiol Rev 1995;8(1):1.

117. Clyne B et al. Syphilis testing. J Emerg Med 2000;18(3):361.

118. Farnes SW et al. Serologic tests for syphilis. Postgrad Med 1990;87(3):37, 45.

119. Hook EW, 3rd et al. Acquired syphilis in adults. N Engl J Med 1992;326(16):1060.

120. Matsumoto M et al. Latex agglutination test for detecting antibodies to Treponema pallidum. Clin Chem 1993;39(8):1700.

121. Pao D et al. Management issues in syphilis. Drugs 2002;62(10):1447.

122. Wendel GD, Jr. et al. Penicillin allergy and desensitization in serious infections during pregnancy. N Engl J Med 1985;312(19):1229.

123. Hooshmand H et al. Neurosyphilis. A study of 241 patients. JAMA 1972;219(6):726.

124. Berry CD et al. Neurologic relapse after benzathine penicillin therapy for secondary syphilis in a patient with HIV infection. N Engl J Med 1987;316(25):1587.

125. WHO: Guidelines for the Management of Sexually Transmitted Infections. Vol 2003. Geneva: WHO Department of HIV/AIDS, 2001:1.

126. Felman YM et al. Syphilis serology today. Arch Dermatol 1980;116(1):84.

127. Genc M et al. Syphilis in pregnancy. Sex Transm Infect 2000;76(2):73-9.

128. Nathan L et al. In utero infection with *Treponema pallidum* in early pregnancy. Prenat Diagn 1997;17(2):119.

129. Fiumara N. The incidence of prenatal syphilis at the Boston City Hospital. N Engl J Med 1952;247:48.

130. Larkin JA et al. Recognizing and treating syphilis in pregnancy. Medscape Womens Health 1998;3(1):5.

131. Niebyl JR. Teratology and Drugs in Pregnancy. In: Danforth DN, Scott JR, eds. Danforth's Obstetrics and Gynecology, 8th Ed. Philadelphia: Lippincott Williams & Wilkins, 1999 [Online: accessed August 1, 2003].

132. Heikkinen T et al. The transplacental transfer of the macrolide antibiotics erythromycin, roxithromycin and azithromycin. Bjog 2000;107(6):770.

133. Mascola L et al. Congenital syphilis. Why is it still occurring? JAMA 1984;252(13):1719.

134. Alexander JM et al. Efficacy of treatment for syphilis in pregnancy. Obstet Gynecol 1999;93(1):5.

135. Radolf JD et al. *Treponema pallidum* and *Borrelia burgdorferi* lipoproteins and synthetic lipopeptides activate monocytes/macrophages. J Immunol 1995;154(6):2866.

136. Silberstein P et al. A case of neurosyphilis with a florid Jarisch-Herxheimer reaction. J Clin Neurosci 2002;9(6):689.

137. Negussie Y et al. Detection of plasma tumor necrosis factor, interleukins 6, and 8 during the Jarisch-Herxheimer reaction of relapsing fever. J Exp Med 1992;175(5):1207.

138. Klein VR et al. The Jarisch-Herxheimer reaction complicating syphilotherapy in pregnancy. Obstet Gynecol 1990;75(3 Pt 1):375.

139. Fekade D et al. Prevention of Jarisch-Herxheimer reactions by treatment with antibodies against tumor necrosis factor alpha. N Engl J Med 1996;335(5):311.

140. Mertz KJ et al. Etiology of genital ulcers and prevalence of human immunodeficiency virus coinfection in 10 US cities. The Genital Ulcer

Disease Surveillance Group. J Infect Dis 1998; 178(6):1795.

141. Schmid GP. Treatment of chancroid, 1997. Clin Infect Dis 1999;28 Suppl 1:S14.

142. Hammond GW et al. Epidemiologic, clinical, laboratory, and therapeutic features of an urban outbreak of chancroid in North America. Rev Infect Dis 1980;2(6):867.

143. Allan RR et al. Chancroid and *Haemophilus ducreyi*. In: Holmes KK, ed. Sexually Transmitted Diseases, 3rd Ed. New York: McGraw-Hill Health Professions Division, 1999:515.

144. Knapp JS et al. In vitro susceptibilities of isolates of Haemophilus ducreyi from Thailand and the United States to currently recommended and newer agents for treatment of chancroid. Antimicrob Agents Chemother 1993;37(7):1552.

145. National guideline for the management of chancroid. Clinical Effectiveness Group (Association of Genitourinary Medicine and the Medical Society for the Study of Venereal Diseases). Sex Transm Infect 1999;75(Suppl 1):S43.

146. Hillier SL et al. Bacterial vaginosis. In: Holmes KK, ed. Sexually Transmitted Diseases, 3rd Ed. New York: McGraw-Hill Health Professions Division, 1999:563.

147. West RR et al. Prevalence of *Gardnerella vaginalis:* an estimate. Br Med J (Clin Res Ed) 1988;296(6630):1163.

148. Avonts D et al. Incidence of uncomplicated genital infections in women using oral contraception or an intrauterine device: a prospective study. Sex Transm Dis 1990;17(1):23.

149. Amsel R et al. Nonspecific vaginitis. Diagnostic criteria and microbial and epidemiologic associations. Am J Med 1983;74(1):14.

150. Holst E et al. Bacterial vaginosis: microbiological and clinical findings. Eur J Clin Microbiol 1987;6(5):5361.

151. Barbone F et al. A follow-up study of methods of contraception, sexual activity, and rates of trichomoniasis, candidiasis, and bacterial vaginosis. Am J Obstet Gynecol 1990;163(2):510-4.

152. Hawes SE et al. Hydrogen peroxide-producing lactobacilli and acquisition of vaginal infections. J Infect Dis 1996;174(5):1058.

153. Berger BJ et al. Bacterial vaginosis in lesbians: a sexually transmitted disease. Clin Infect Dis 1995;21(6):1402.

154. Hay P et al. Evaluation of a novel diagnostic test for bacterial vaginosis: 'the electronic nose'. Int J STD AIDS 2003;14(2):114.

155. Ferris DG et al. Women's use of over-the-counter antifungal medications for gynecologic symptoms. J Fam Pract 1996;42(6):595.

156. Lugo-Miro VI et al. Comparison of different metronidazole therapeutic regimens for bacterial vaginosis. A meta-analysis. JAMA 1992; 268(1):92.

157. Spiegel CA et al. Anaerobic bacteria in nonspecific vaginitis. N Engl J Med 1980;303(11):601.

158. Livengood CH, 3rd et al. Comparison of once-daily and twice-daily dosing of 0.75% metronidazole gel in the treatment of bacterial vaginosis. Sex Transm Dis 1999;26(3):137.

159. Joesoef MR et al. Bacterial vaginosis: review of treatment options and potential clinical indications for therapy. Clin Infect Dis 1999;28 Suppl 1:S57.

160. Joesoef MR et al. Intravaginal clindamycin treatment for bacterial vaginosis: effects on preterm delivery and low birth weight. Am J Obstet Gynecol 1995;173(5):1527.

161. Krieger JN et al. *Trichomonas vaginalis* and trichomoniasis. In: Holmes KK, ed. Sexually Transmitted Diseases, 3rd Ed. New York: McGraw-Hill Health Professions Division, 1999;587.

162. Pabst KM et al. Disease prevalence among women attending a sexually transmitted disease clinic varies with reason for visit. Sex Transm Dis 1992; 19(2):88.

163. Petrin D et al. Clinical and microbiological aspects of *Trichomonas vaginalis*. Clin Microbiol Rev 1998;11(2):300.

164. Haefner HK. Current evaluation and management of vulvovaginitis. Clin Obstet Gynecol 1999; 42(2):184.

165. Egan ME et al. Diagnosis of vaginitis. Am Fam Physician 2000;62(5):1095.

166. Heine P et al. *Trichomonas vaginalis:* a reemerging pathogen. Clin Obstet Gynecol 1993;36(1):137.

167. Narcisi E et al. In vitro effect of tinidazole and furazolidone on metronidazole-resistant *Trichomonas vaginalis*. Antimicrob Agents Chemother 1996;40(5):1121.

168. Nyirjesy P et al. Difficult-to-treat trichomoniasis: results with paromomycin cream. Clin Infect Dis 1998;26(4):986.

169. Pearlman MD et al. An incremental dosing protocol for women with severe vaginal trichomoniasis and adverse reaction to metronidazole. Am J Obstet Gynecol 1996;174(3):934.

170. Visapaa JP et al. Lack of disulfiram-like reaction with metronidazole and ethanol. Ann Pharmacother 2002;36(6):971.

171. Williams CS et al. Do ethanol and metronidazole interact to produce a disulfiram-like reaction? Ann Pharmacother 2000;34(2):255.

172. Burtin P et al. Safety of metronidazole in pregnancy: a meta-analysis. Am J Obstet Gynecol 1995;172(2 Pt 1):525.

173. Friedman GD. Cancer after metronidazole. N Engl J Med 1980;302(9):519.

174. Gulmezoglu AM. Interventions for trichomoniasis in pregnancy. Cochrane Database Syst Rev 2002(3):CD000220.

175. duBouchet L et al. Multicenter comparison of clotrimazole vaginal tablets, oral metronidazole, and vaginal suppositories containing sulfanilamide, aminacrine hydrochloride, and allantoin in the treatment of symptomatic trichomoniasis. Sex Transm Dis 1997;24(3):156.

176. Wald A et al. A randomized, double-blind, comparative trial comparing high- and standard-dose oral acyclovir for first-episode genital herpes infections. Antimicrob Agents Chemother 1994; 38(2):174.

177. Langenberg AG et al. A prospective study of new infections with herpes simplex virus type 1 and type 2. Chiron HSV Vaccine Study Group. N Engl J Med 1999;341(19):1432.

178. Smith JS et al. Age-specific prevalence of infection with herpes simplex virus types 2 and 1: a global review. J Infect Dis 2002;186 Suppl 1:S3.

179. Whitley RJ et al. Immunologic approach to herpes simplex virus. Viral Immunol 2001;14(2):111.

180. Corey L. Genital herpes. In: Holmes KK, ed. Sexually Transmitted Diseases, 3rd Ed. New York: McGraw-Hill Health Professions Division, 1999;285.

181. Fleming DT et al. Herpes simplex virus type 2 in the United States, 1976 to 1994. N Engl J Med 1997;337(16):1105.

182. Corey L. Challenges in genital herpes simplex virus management. J Infect Dis 2002;186 Suppl 1:S29.

183. Hirsch M. Herpes simplex virus. In: Mandell GL, Douglas RG, Bennett JE, eds. Principles and Practice of Infectious Diseases, 4th ed. New York: Churchill Livingstone, 1995:1336.

184. Barton IG et al. Association of HSV-1 with cervical infection. Lancet 1981;2(8255):1108.

185. Corey L et al. Genital herpes simplex virus infections: clinical manifestations, course, and complications. Ann Intern Med 1983;98(6):958.

186. Benedetti J et al. Recurrence rates in genital herpes after symptomatic first-episode infection. Ann Intern Med 1994;121(11):847.

187. Davis LG et al. Genital herpes simplex virus infection: clinical course and attempted therapy. Am J Hosp Pharm 1981;38(6):825.

188. Koutsky LA et al. Underdiagnosis of genital herpes by current clinical and viral-isolation procedures. N Engl J Med 1992;326(23):1533.

189. Koelle DM et al. Antigen-specific T cells localize to the uterine cervix in women with genital herpes simplex virus type 2 infection. J Infect Dis 2000; 182(3):662.

190. Reeves WC et al. Risk of recurrence after first episodes of genital herpes. Relation to HSV type and antibody response. N Engl J Med 1981; 305(6):315.

191. Benedetti JK et al. Clinical reactivation of genital herpes simplex virus infection decreases in frequency over time. Ann Intern Med 1999; 131(1):14.

192. Engelberg R et al. Natural history of genital herpes simplex virus type 1 infection. Sex Transm Dis 2003;30(2):174.

193. Wald A et al. Virologic characteristics of subclinical and symptomatic genital herpes infections. N Engl J Med 1995;333(12):770.

194. Langenberg A et al. Development of clinically recognizable genital lesions among women previously identified as having "asymptomatic" herpes simplex virus type 2 infection. Ann Intern Med 1989;110(11):882.

195. Wald A et al. Effect of condoms on reducing the transmission of herpes simplex virus type 2 from men to women. JAMA 2001;285(24):3100.

196. Dobbins JG et al. Herpes in the time of AIDS: a comparison of the epidemiology of HIV-1 and HSV-2 in young men in northern Thailand. Sex Transm Dis 1999;26(2):67.

197. Rooney JF et al. Acquisition of genital herpes from an asymptomatic sexual partner. N Engl J Med 1986;314(24):1561.

198. Mertz GJ et al. Risk factors for the sexual transmission of genital herpes. Ann Intern Med 1992;116(3):197.

199. Diamond C et al. Clinical course of patients with serologic evidence of recurrent genital herpes presenting with signs and symptoms of first episode disease. Sex Transm Dis 1999;26(4):221.

200. Wald A. Herpes. Transmission and viral shedding. Dermatol Clin 1998;16(4):795, xiv.

201. Wald A et al. Reactivation of genital herpes simplex virus type 2 infection in asymptomatic seropositive persons. N Engl J Med 2000; 342(12):844.

202. Ashley RL et al. Comparison of Western blot (immunoblot) and glycoprotein G-specific immunodot enzyme assay for detecting antibodies to herpes simplex virus types 1 and 2 in human sera. J Clin Microbiol 1988;26(4):662.

203. Ashley-Morrow R et al. Time course of seroconversion by HerpeSelect ELISA after acquisition of genital herpes simplex virus type 1 (HSV-1) or HSV-2. Sex Transm Dis 2003;30(4):310.

204. Balfour HH, Jr. Antiviral drugs. N Engl J Med 1999;340(16):1255.

205. Jacobson MA et al. Phase I trial of valaciclovir, the L-valyl ester of acyclovir, in patients with advanced human immunodeficiency virus disease. Antimicrob Agents Chemother 1994;38(7):1534.

206. Leung DT et al. Current recommendations for the treatment of genital herpes. Drugs 2000;60(6): 1329.

207. Peacock JE, Jr. et al. Intravenous acyclovir therapy of first episodes of genital herpes: a multicenter double-blind, placebo-controlled trial. Am J Med 1988;85(3):301.

208. Ioannidis JP et al. Clinical efficacy of high-dose acyclovir in patients with human immunodeficiency virus infection: a meta-analysis of randomized individual patient data. J Infect Dis 1998;178(2):349.

209. Straus SE et al. Acyclovir for chronic mucocutaneous herpes simplex virus infection in immunosuppressed patients. Ann Intern Med 1982;96(3): 270.

210. Shepp DH et al. Oral acyclovir therapy for mucocutaneous herpes simplex virus infections in immunocompromised marrow transplant recipients. Ann Intern Med 1985;102(6):783.

211. Wade JC et al. Oral acyclovir for prevention of herpes simplex virus reactivation after marrow transplantation. Ann Intern Med 1984;100(6):823.

212. Saral R et al. Acyclovir prophylaxis of herpes-simplex-virus infections. N Engl J Med 1981; 305(2):63.

213. Corey L et al. Double-blind controlled trial of topical acyclovir in genital herpes simplex virus infections. Am J Med 1982;73(1A):326.

214. Spruance SL et al. Penciclovir cream for the treatment of herpes simplex labialis. A randomized, multicenter, double-blind, placebo-controlled trial. Topical Penciclovir Collaborative Study Group. JAMA 1997;277(17):1374.

215. Au E et al. Antivirals in the prevention of genital herpes. Herpes 2002;9(3):74.

216. Nadelman CM et al. Herpes simplex virus infections. New treatment approaches make early diagnosis even more important. Postgrad Med 2000;107(3):189, 199.

217. Drake S et al. Improving the care of patients with genital herpes. BMJ 2000;321(7261):619.

218. Strand A et al. Aborted genital herpes simplex virus lesions: findings from a randomised controlled trial with valaciclovir. Sex Transm Infect 2002;78(6):435.

219. Patel R et al. Valaciclovir for the suppression of recurrent genital HSV infection: a placebo controlled study of once daily therapy. International Valaciclovir HSV Study Group. Genitourin Med 1997;73(2):105.

220. Diaz-Mitoma F et al. Oral famciclovir for the suppression of recurrent genital herpes: a randomized controlled trial. Collaborative Famciclovir Genital Herpes Research Group. JAMA 1998;280(10):887.

221. Gold D et al. Acyclovir prophylaxis for herpes simplex virus infection. Antimicrob Agents Chemother 1987;31(3):361.

222. Corey L et al. Once Daily Valacyclovir Reduces Transmission of Genital Herpes (LB-3). ICAAC, San Diego, CA, 2002.

223. Conant MA et al. Valaciclovir versus aciclovir for herpes simplex virus infection in HIV-infected individuals: two randomized trials. Int J STD AIDS 2002;13(1):12.

224. Chatis PA et al. Resistance of herpesviruses to antiviral drugs. Antimicrob Agents Chemother 1992;36(8):1589.

225. Lalezari J et al. A randomized, double-blind, placebo controlled trial of cidofovir gel for the treatment of acyclovir-unresponsive mucocutaneous herpes simplex virus infection in patients with AIDS. J Infect Dis 1997;176(4):892.

226. Perazella MA. Crystal-induced acute renal failure. Am J Med 1999;106(4):459.

227. Revankar SG et al. Delirium associated with acyclovir treatment in a patient with renal failure. Clin Infect Dis 1995;21(2):435.

228. Kitching AR et al. Neurotoxicity associated with acyclovir in end stage renal failure. N Z Med J 1997;110(1043):167.

229. Corey L et al. Intravenous acyclovir for the treatment of primary genital herpes. Ann Intern Med 1983;98(6):914.

230. Mertz GJ et al. Double-blind placebo-controlled trial of oral acyclovir in first-episode genital herpes simplex virus infection. JAMA 1984;252(9):1147.

231. Bryson YJ et al. Treatment of first episodes of genital herpes simplex virus infection with oral acyclovir. A randomized double-blind controlled trial in normal subjects. N Engl J Med 1983;308(16):916.

232. Reichman RC et al. Treatment of recurrent genital herpes simplex infections with oral acyclovir. A controlled trial. JAMA 1984;251(16):2103.

233. Penciclovir. Gold Standard Media: Clinical Pharmacology, 2003.

234. Wilkinson D et al. Nonoxynol-9 for preventing vaginal acquisition of sexually transmitted infections by women from men. Cochrane Database of Systematic Reviews. 2002(4): CD003939.

235. Lehtinen M et al. Herpes simplex virus and risk of cervical cancer: a longitudinal, nested case-control study in the Nordic countries. Am J Epidemiol 2002;156(8):687.

236. Kibrick S. Herpes simplex infection at term. What to do with mother, newborn, and nursery personnel. JAMA 1980;243(2):157.

237. Scott LL. Prevention of perinatal herpes: prophylactic antiviral therapy? Clin Obstet Gynecol 1999;42(1):134,quiz 174.

238. Prober CG et al. Use of routine viral cultures at delivery to identify neonates exposed to herpes simplex virus. N Engl J Med 1988;318(14):887.

239. Tyring SK et al. Valacyclovir for herpes simplex virus infection: long-term safety and sustained efficacy after 20 years' experience with acyclovir. J Infect Dis. 2002;186(Suppl 1):S40.

240. Watts DH et al. A double-blind, randomized, placebo-controlled trial of acyclovir in late pregnancy for the reduction of herpes simplex virus shedding and cesarean delivery. Am J Obstet Gynecol 2003;188(3):836.

241. Reiff-Eldridge R et al. Monitoring pregnancy outcomes after prenatal drug exposure through prospective pregnancy registries: a pharmaceutical company commitment. Am J Obstet Gynecol 2000;182(1 Pt 1):159.

242. Prober CG et al. Low risk of herpes simplex virus infections in neonates exposed to the virus at the time of vaginal delivery to mothers with recurrent genital herpes simplex virus infections. N Engl J Med 1987;316(5):240.

243. Schiffman MH. Recent progress in defining the epidemiology of human papillomavirus infection and cervical neoplasia. J Natl Cancer Inst 1992;84(6):394.

244. Longstaff E et al. Condyloma eradication: self-therapy with 0.15-0.5% podophyllotoxin versus 20-25% podophyllin preparations—an integrated safety assessment. Regul Toxicol Pharmacol 2001;33(2):117.

245. Lacey CJ et al. Randomised controlled trial and economic evaluation of podophyllotoxin solution, podophyllotoxin cream, and podophyllin in the treatment of genital warts. Sex Transm Infect 2003;79(4):270.

246. Perry CM et al. Topical imiquimod: a review of its use in genital warts. Drugs 1999;58(2):375.

247. Koutsky LA et al. A controlled trial of a human papillomavirus type 16 vaccine. N Engl J Med 2002;347(21):1645.

248. Kulasingam SL et al. Potential health and economic impact of adding a human papillomavirus vaccine to screening programs. JAMA 2003;290(6):781.

249. Kahn JA et al. Human papillomavirus vaccines. Pediatr Infect Dis J 2003;22(5):443.

CHAPTER 66

Osteomyelitis and Septic Arthritis

Ralph H. Raasch

Osteomyelitis is an inflammation of the bone marrow and surrounding bone caused by an infecting organism. It can occur in any bone of the body and often leads to serious morbidity, even with early diagnosis and treatment. Despite the continued refinement of diagnostic procedures (e.g., radionuclide imaging, magnetic resonance imaging), advances in antimicrobial therapy, and the use of prophylactic antibiotics before orthopedic procedures, osteomyelitis continues to be a serious problem from both a diagnostic and therapeutic standpoint.

Previously, osteomyelitis was more common in children and the elderly, and the causative microorganisms were usually Gram-positive cocci such as streptococci and staphylococci. Although *Staphylococcus aureus* remains the most common causative organism, the prevalence of infection caused by Gram-negative and anaerobic bacilli is increasing, and it can affect all age groups.[1]

Bone can be infected by three routes: hematogenous spread of bacteria from a distant infection site, direct infection of bone from an adjacent or contiguous source of infection, and infection of bone due to vascular insufficiency. Table 66-1 summarizes important characteristics of these types of osteomyelitis.[1] Patients with recurrent osteomyelitis are considered to have chronic osteomyelitis.

BONE ANATOMY AND PHYSIOLOGY

Understanding the pathophysiology of osteomyelitis requires a basic understanding of bone anatomy and physiology. Figure 66-1 is a graphic representation of a long bone of the body. The bone is divided into three sections: the epiphysis, located at the end of the bone; the metaphysis; and the diaphysis. The epiphysis and metaphysis are separated by the epiphyseal growth plate. This is the rapidly growing area of the bone, and a large number of blood vessels supply this area. Surrounding most of the bone is a fibrous and cellular envelope. The external portion of this envelope is called the periosteum, and the internal portion is referred to as the endosteum.

The blood vessels that supply bone tissue are located predominantly in the bone's epiphysis and metaphysis. The nutrient arteries enter the bone at the metaphyseal side of the epiphyseal growth plate and lead to capillaries that form sharp loops within the growth plate. These capillaries lead to large sinusoidal veins that eventually exit the metaphysis of the bone through a nutrient vein. Within the sinusoidal veins, blood flow is slowed considerably, and infection can begin if bacteria settle in this area.

Variations exist in the vasculature of bone in different age groups, leading to different forms of osteomyelitis. In neonates and adults, vascular communications are present between the epiphysis and metaphysis, which may allow infection to spread from the metaphysis to the epiphysis and the adjacent joint. However, during childhood, this area often is protected from infection because the epiphyseal plate separates the vascular supply for these two regions.

HEMATOGENOUS OSTEOMYELITIS

Hematogenous osteomyelitis classically has been a disease of children, although the number of cases reported in adults is increasing. Osteomyelitis in children tends to be acute and hematogenous and is often responsive to antibiotic therapy

Table 66-1 Features of Osteomyelitis

Feature	Hematogenous	Adjacent Site of Infection	Vascular Insufficiency
Usual age of onset (yr)	1–20; 50	50	50
Sites of infection	Long bones, vertebrae	Femur, tibia, skull, mandible	Feet
Risk factors	Bacteremia	Surgery, trauma, cellulitis; joint prosthesis	Diabetes, peripheral vascular disease
Common bacteria	*Staphylococcus aureus*, Gram-negative bacilli; usually one organism	*S. aureus*, Gram-negative bacilli; anaerobic organisms; often mixed infection	*S. aureus*, coagulase-negative staphylococci, Gram-negative and anaerobic organisms; usually mixed infection
Clinical findings			
Initial episode	Fever, chills, local tenderness, swelling; limitation of motion	Fever, warmth, swelling; unstable joint	Pain, swelling, drainage, ulcer formation
Recurrent episode	Drainage	Drainage, sinus tract	As above

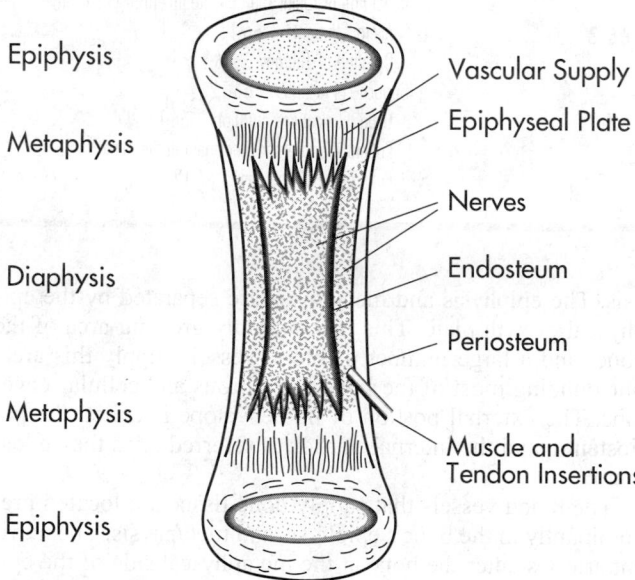

Epiphysis

Metaphysis

Diaphysis

Metaphysis

Epiphysis

Vascular Supply

Epiphyseal Plate

Nerves

Endosteum

Periosteum

Muscle and Tendon Insertions

FIGURE 66-1 Long bone anatomy. (Adapted from Triffitt JT. Organic matrix of bone tissue. In: Urist MR, ed. Fundamental and Clinical Bone Physiology. Philadelphia: JB Lippincott, 1980:46.)

alone. In comparison, osteomyelitis in adults tends to be subacute or chronic and commonly results from trauma, prosthetic devices, or other insult. As a result, surgical débridement often is needed in addition to antibiotics when managing osteomyelitis in adults.

Infection in children develops primarily in the metaphysis of the rapidly growing long bones of the body, probably because the slow blood flow in these areas allows bacteria to settle and multiply. The acute infectious process (e.g., edema, inflammation, small vessel thrombosis) causes a rise in pressure within the bone that compromises blood flow and eventually leads to necrosis. Released cytokines alter bone integrity by promoting osteoclast activity. Eventually, the elevated pressure and necrosis may cause devitalized bone to fragment from healthy bone (sequestra). With continued spread of the infection into outer layers of the bone and soft tissue, abscess and draining sinus tracts form.[1,2]

In children, hematogenous infection most commonly occurs in the long bones, as a single focus in the femur and tibia.[1] In adults, the vertebrae are more commonly involved, and infection usually occurs in the fifth and sixth decades of life.[3] In neonates, hematogenous osteomyelitis is an especially serious disease that often involves multiple bones, especially the long bones. Rapid spread across the epiphyseal plate can involve the adjacent joint, making immediate, aggressive treatment crucial.[4]

The most common organism causing hematogenous osteomyelitis in children is *S. aureus*. This is due partly to the proclivity of this bacterial species to settle and adhere to bone and cartilage. In adults, S. *aureus* is also the most common causative pathogen. However, Gram-negative bacilli (*Escherichia coli, Klebsiella, Proteus, Salmonella,* and *Pseudomonas*) are responsible for an increasing number of cases of osteomyelitis. Intravenous (IV) drug abuse often leads to infection with *Pseudomonas aeruginosa,* whereas *Salmonella* species is a common cause in patients with hemoglobinopathies such as sickle cell anemia.[1,2]

The clinical features of hematogenous osteomyelitis vary depending on the patient's age and the site of infection. In children, infection usually is characterized by an abrupt onset of high fever and chills, localized pain, tenderness, and swelling. Unfortunately, systemic symptoms often are absent in neonates, delaying the diagnosis. Therefore, a diagnosis must be made on the basis of localized symptoms such as edema and restricted limb movement. Systemic symptoms are also less common in adults. Patients with vertebral osteomyelitis may present with the insidious onset of localized back pain and tenderness.[1,3]

ACUTE OSTEOMYELITIS

Usual Clinical Presentation

1. **C.D., an 11-year-old boy, was sent home early from school yesterday because of fever and leg pain. His right leg began to hurt above the knee about 4 days ago, and he began to limp last night. C.D. and his parents deny any trauma to the area. He has never been sick before except for two episodes of acute otitis me-**

dia when he was 2 years old. In the pediatrician's office today, maximal tenderness is noted over his right distal femur without right knee joint effusion. There are no visible signs of swelling, warmth or trauma. His white blood cell (WBC) count is 9,500 cells/mm³ (normal, 5,000 to 10,000), with a normal WBC differential. A plain radiograph of the leg is normal, but the erythrocyte sedimentation rate (ESR) is 55 mm/hr (normal, 0 to 15). Two blood cultures are obtained, and C.D. is sent home with directions for bed rest and use of acetaminophen as needed for fever. However, 2 days later, he is admitted to the hospital because of severe pain and tenderness in his right leg and a fever of 39.2°C. Two blood cultures are positive for *S. aureus*, and the C-reactive protein (CRP) is 10 mg/dL (normal, <2.0). Plain radiographs are again normal, but a bone scan is positive for inflammation in the right distal femur. What findings in C.D. are consistent with hematogenous osteomyelitis?

[SI units: WBC, 9,500 ×10⁹/L (normal, 5,000 to 10,000); ESR, 55 mm/hr (normal, 0 to 15); CRP, 10 mg/dL (normal, <2.0)]

C.D. displays most of the usual signs and symptoms of acute hematogenous osteomyelitis in children. He is a previously healthy child who developed acute localized pain and tenderness of the right distal femur, abrupt onset of high fever, and an elevated ESR. The plain radiograph of C.D.'s leg was normal on two occasions before hospitalization; however, plain radiographs of bone are usually normal during the first 2 weeks of infection. Bone scans usually are able to detect bone changes earlier in the course of disease, and C.D.'s bone scan upon hospitalization detected inflammation in the right proximal tibia.² Although C.D. did not have a bone biopsy sent for culture, his clinical picture, a positive bone scan, and blood cultures positive for *S. aureus* establish the diagnosis of osteomyelitis.²,⁵ As in many cases of osteomyelitis, the specific event that caused bacteremia in C.D. and allowed bacterial dissemination to bone is unknown.

Several laboratory tests should be obtained in every child suspected of having osteomyelitis. Although these tests are not specific for the diagnosis of osteomyelitis, they help confirm the clinical diagnosis. A complete blood count (CBC) and an ESR are routinely obtained. The serum CRP, when elevated, is a measure of systemic inflammation.

An increased WBC count is consistent with osteomyelitis, but significant leukocytosis is absent in many children with osteomyelitis at the initial examination. Thus, C.D.'s high-normal WBC count of 9,500/mm³ is not unusual. In adults, leukocytosis does occur, but it is more commonly associated with an acute infection than with recurrent disease. When leukocytosis is present, the WBC count rarely exceeds 15,000/mm³.²

Although the ESR and the CRP are relatively nonspecific, most patients with osteomyelitis have ESR values >20 mm/hr and a CRP >2.0 mg/dL.² Therefore, the increased ESR and CRP in C.D. are consistent with osteomyelitis. Destructive changes of bone can be seen in plain radiographs, although these do not appear for at least 2 weeks after the onset of symptoms.² Bone scans can detect inflammation of bone more quickly than plain radiographs. Hence, a normal plain film does not rule out acute osteomyelitis if obtained within the first 2 weeks of infection. The bone scan in C.D. was extremely helpful because it detected acute osteomyelitis before the appearance of osteomyelitis on plain film.

Predisposing factors for hematogenous osteomyelitis include any risk factors that promote bacteremia (e.g., indwelling catheters in the neonate, hemodialysis shunts, central venous catheters used for chemotherapy or parenteral nutrition). A distant focus in the gastrointestinal or urinary tract can lead to bacteremia and predispose a patient to the development of osteomyelitis. IV drug abuse leading to bacteremia can be a predisposing factor for osteomyelitis in young adults. None of these factors seem to have predisposed C.D. to the development of osteomyelitis. In children like C.D. who have no history of fractures or penetrating injury, the most common cause for acute hematogenous osteomyelitis is *S. aureus*.¹,²,⁶

Patient Workup

2. What additional patient and diagnostic information should be obtained before C.D. receives his first dose of antibiotics?

Before C.D. receives a course of antibiotic therapy, he should be assessed for drug allergies, especially penicillin allergy. Patient interviews, discussions with his parents, and a comprehensive review of his medical record are necessary, especially if a history of allergy is reported. Details of an allergic reaction, including symptoms, onset of the reaction, probable causative agent, treatment, and exposure to related compounds, should be sought.

Cultures of blood and bone aspirate material are the best ways to identify the specific bacterial etiology for osteomyelitis and are often part of the initial workup. However, cultures taken after antibiotics are started often are negative, thereby necessitating the use of empiric broad-spectrum antibiotic therapy for several weeks. As a result, the cost of therapy and the risk of toxicity increase.

In C.D.'s case, the positive blood culture and bone scan established the diagnosis of osteomyelitis without the need to do a bone culture. However, if C.D.'s blood cultures had been negative, a bone aspirate for culture to identify the pathogen would be recommended.¹,² Once material has been obtained for culture, initial empiric therapy should be started as soon as possible.

Treatment

Empiric Antibiotic Therapy

3. C.D. has no history of drug allergies and has received amoxicillin in the past for episodes of acute otitis media without incident. What antibiotic treatment should be started? What is the relevance of bone concentrations or protein binding of antibiotics in the selection of therapy for osteomyelitis?

For initial antimicrobial treatment of hematogenous osteomyelitis, the agent chosen should be administered IV at high dosages to achieve adequate levels in the infected bone. It is important to initiate treatment as soon as possible to improve the chances for complete eradication of infection and to avoid the need for surgery. Thus, empiric antibiotic therapy often is instituted before culture and sensitivity results are known.

Based on the epidemiology of C.D.'s infection and the results of the blood culture, he should be treated for *S. aureus* osteomyelitis. The initial treatment should be with an IV penicillinase-resistant penicillin (e.g., oxacillin or nafcillin) or with cefazolin. Because C.D. acquired his infection outside of the hospital, the possibility that oxacillin-resistant *S. aureus* (ORSA) is responsible for his infection is low. ORSA is resistant to all β-lactam antibiotics. Although *S. aureus* is the most common cause of osteomyelitis, efforts to culture the responsible pathogen should be undertaken to determine whether the empiric treatment is appropriate or if an adjustment in the regimen is indicated. If ORSA is cultured, vancomycin should be used. Because of much more limited experience in treating ORSA osteomyelitis, clindamycin or linezolid should be used only in vancomycin-intolerant patients. Other organisms that may cause osteomyelitis include *Staphylococcus epidermidis, Streptococcus pyogenes, Streptococcus pneumoniae, Haemophilus influenzae,* and *P. aeruginosa.* In the neonate with osteomyelitis, *S. aureus* and *Streptococcus* species are commonly responsible.[1] Because C.D.'s blood culture grew *S. aureus* and he is not allergic to penicillin, he is placed on IV oxacillin therapy at 150 mg/kg per day Q 6 hr. His prior exposure to amoxicillin is irrelevant except to establish the absence of a penicillin allergy.

Under circumstances of negative cultures or while blood or bone cultures are pending, the age of the child with acute osteomyelitis is important in the selection of appropriate empiric antibiotics. Table 66-2 summarizes recommended drugs and dosages in children with acute osteomyelitis.[1,6,7]

Antibiotic Bone Penetration and Protein Binding

The importance of selecting an antibiotic that penetrates into bone when treating osteomyelitis is unclear. Data are available on the bone-penetrating qualities of many antibiotics. In general, bone tissue concentrations for the antibiotics are several times greater than the minimum inhibitory concentration (MIC) values for the infecting pathogens being treated with these agents. However, the relationship between bone concentrations and outcome of therapy is not established.[1,2,8,9]

Theoretically, how extensively an antibiotic is protein bound may influence the drug's clinical efficacy because it is believed that the free drug, rather than the protein-bound drug, diffuses from plasma into tissue. However, studies evaluating the penetration of highly protein-bound drugs, such as cefazolin (90% protein bound), suggest the contrary. High levels of cefazolin are achieved within bone after a single 1-g IV dose, exceeding levels achieved with cephalothin, a drug with only 20% protein binding. In addition, cefazolin and ceftriaxone, two highly protein-bound drugs, usually are effective in treating osteomyelitis, provided high dosages are given and the responsible pathogen is susceptible. In summary, antibiotic bone concentrations and protein binding of antibiotics (when appropriate dosages are used) are not significant factors in the selection of appropriate therapy for osteomyelitis.[1,9]

Duration of Therapy

4. The *S. aureus* grown from C.D.'s blood culture is resistant to penicillin but sensitive to oxacillin and cefazolin. Is oxacillin the best antibiotic choice for C. D., or would other antibiotics, given less frequently, also be adequate therapy?

Continuing to treat C.D. with oxacillin (or nafcillin) every 6 hours follows treatment recommendations for staphylococcal osteomyelitis. Antistaphylococcal penicillins achieve high levels in bone and usually provide effective therapy as long as the treatment regimen is followed with frequent doses for an adequate duration of treatment. Changing C.D. to cefazolin would allow slightly less frequent dosing (every 8 hours), a potential advantage for home treatment. The use of vancomycin should be discouraged in C.D.'s case because cultures grew an oxacillin-sensitive organism, and overuse of vancomycin predisposes to selection of resistant strains.[10] While the logistics of outpatient therapy in C.D. are being investigated, he should remain on oxacillin while in the hospital.

5. Both of C.D.'s parents work, and their work schedules would prevent them from leaving their jobs to transport C.D. to

Table 66-2 Empiric Antibiotics for Acute Osteomyelitis in Children

Host	Likely Etiologies	Antibiotics	Dosage (mg/kg/day)	Dosage (doses/day)
Neonate	Staphylococcus aureus Group B streptococci Gram-negative bacilli	Nafcillin + cefotaxime *or* Nafcillin + gentamicin	100 150 100 5–7.5	4 3 4 3
<3 yr	S. aureus Haemophilus influenzae type b	Cefuroxime *or* Ceftriaxone *or* Nafcillin + cefotaxime	150 50 150 100	4 2 4 4
≥3 yr	S. aureus	Nafcillin *or* Oxacillin *or* Cefazolin *or* Clindamycin	150 150 100 30–40	4 4 3 3
After puncture wound through shoe Child with sickle cell disease	P. aeruginosa Salmonella sp. S. aureus	Ceftazidime Nafcillin + cefotaxime	150 150 100	3 4 4

an outpatient antibiotic treatment center. Is C.D. a candidate for outpatient IV antibiotic therapy at home, or could oral antibiotic treatment be considered at this time? Must C.D. remain in the hospital to receive his oxacillin?

Initially, all patients should receive IV antibiotics because early, aggressive therapy offers the best chance to cure the infection. The technology to treat C.D. as an outpatient with IV oxacillin is available[11,12]; thus, he does not necessarily need to stay in the hospital to complete his therapy. A peripheral central catheter (PICC) can be inserted to begin treatment.[1,2,12,13] Continuous infusion pumps (i.e., CAD pumps) are small, comfortable to wear, and programmable so that a set dose can be delivered at designated intervals. The pump has to be changed (drug cassette replaced) only every 24 hours. Once-a-day IV therapy can also be considered with ceftriaxone or ertapenem. However, these drugs would not be preferred because of their unnecessary broad spectrum and likely higher MICs against *S. aureus* in comparison to oxacillin or nafcillin. Whether C.D. should go home on IV antibiotics should be decided in concert with his parents. If they do not have the resources or are unwilling to oversee IV treatment at home, C.D. should remain hospitalized to assess the first week of treatment. In any case, expecting an 11-year-old boy like C.D. to complete several weeks of IV therapy at home is overly optimistic. Furthermore, catheter complications such as dislodgment, infection, or occlusion are a concern. As discussed in Question 6, C.D. may be able to complete most of his course of treatment with oral antibiotics. However, oral antibiotics should not be given to C.D. until the effectiveness of the first week of IV therapy can be assessed. The total duration of IV and oral therapy for C.D. should be 4 weeks.[1,2,6,13]

Use of Oral Antibiotics and Serum Bactericidal Titers

6. After 1 week of IV oxacillin, C.D. is afebrile and the pain and tenderness in his right leg are significantly reduced. The ESR is 40 mm/hr, and CRP is 2.0 mg/dL. The plan is to switch C.D. to oral antibiotics to complete a 4-week course of treatment at home. What is an appropriate dosing regimen, and how often should he return to the clinic for evaluation?

[SI units: ESR, 40 mm/hr; CRP, 2.0 mg/dL]

Because IV therapy for several weeks is inconvenient and expensive even at home, patients like C.D. who have responded to IV antibiotics can be switched to oral therapy. Again, this decision must be made in concert with C.D.'s parents, who must understand the vital importance of frequent antibiotic doses in these circumstances.

To monitor oral antibiotic therapy, investigators have used serum bactericidal titers (SBTs) to assess serum antimicrobial levels because assays of β-lactam antibiotics generally are unavailable. The SBT is the highest dilution of C.D.'s serum that exerts a bactericidal effect in vitro against the *S. aureus* cultured from his blood. In other words, the SBT is the highest serum dilution at which no growth of organism is seen (lack of turbidity in the serum) in the test tube. Peak and trough SBTs can be ascertained depending on whether the serum sample was obtained immediately after an antibiotic dose (peak SBT), or immediately before a dose (trough SBT).[14]

In early reports of oral therapy for staphylococcal osteomyelitis, children were treated with IV antibiotics until fever and local signs of infection (swelling, erythema, tender-

ness) resolved. The duration of IV therapy was usually 14 days. Oral therapy then was instituted in doses necessary to achieve a trough SBT of at least 1:2. Initial recommendations were that the peak SBT should be >1:16, but subsequent evaluation indicated that peak SBTs were not predictive of cure in acute osteomyelitis. To achieve a trough SBT of >1:2, dicloxacillin or cephalexin was given in oral doses of at least 100 mg/kg per day. Probenecid given before these antibiotics increased the trough SBT in some patients.[14,15] Subsequent investigators have questioned the necessity of measuring SBTs. They advocate treating patients for 4 to 5 days with IV antibiotics, then switching to high-dose oral therapy to complete 3 to 4 weeks of treatment. The antibiotics and dosages used are dicloxacillin (100 mg/kg per day), cephradine (150 mg/kg per day), cephalexin (100 mg/kg per day), and clindamycin (40 mg/kg per day). Patients are switched to oral drugs (e.g., dicloxacillin, cephradine, cephalexin, or clindamycin) after fever and pain have subsided and the CRP is <2.0 mg/dL.[16,17] SBTs are not monitored. In 50 patients treated this way, there were no relapses of infection for 1 year of follow-up.[16] Nevertheless, clinicians may continue to monitor trough SBTs to assess compliance and dose adequacy when the patient is switched from IV to oral therapy, especially in children.

Thus, C.D. is a candidate for oral therapy, assuming his parents agree to supervise treatment once he leaves the hospital. C.D. has responded promptly to the IV therapy: his fever, leg pain, and tenderness have resolved, the ESR is reduced, and the CRP is normal. The CRP changes more quickly in response to adequate antimicrobial therapy than does the ESR.[18] However, oral therapy will work only if C.D. is compliant. Therefore, assurances must be in place to guarantee that all doses will be taken. C.D.'s parents have made arrangements with his sixth-grade teacher to help him take his oral antibiotic during the day.

C.D. can complete his 4-week course of antibiotics with oral dosing of cephalexin capsules or suspension, which seems to taste better (and hence is usually better tolerated) than dicloxacillin suspension. Dosages should begin at 25 mg/kg Q 6 hr and then be increased as needed to achieve a trough SBT of at least 1:2. There is no evidence that a given dosage increase (or decrease) causes a proportional change in SBT. Close follow-up of C.D. (weekly) is required under these circumstances to monitor compliance and clinical response to therapy. SBTs should be monitored weekly and parenteral therapy should be reinitiated promptly if C.D.'s compliance is not perfect, the goal SBTs are not achieved, or symptoms (or increased ESR or CRP) recur.[6,13] Initial oral therapy with a quinolone is not appropriate for C.D. because resistance by staphylococci has emerged to ciprofloxacin and because quinolone use is contraindicated in children.

Duration of Follow-Up for Recurrent Infection

7. C.D. has completed 4 weeks of treatment for his acute staphylococcal osteomyelitis. Clinical evidence shows that the osteomyelitis is completely resolved, and the ESR and CRP are normal. For how long should C.D. be followed for possible recurrence of his infection?

Relapses of osteomyelitis can occur years after the initial acute episode.[1,2] In C.D.'s case of uncomplicated acute osteomyelitis, he should be evaluated for recurrence at least every 3 months for at least 2 years.

SECONDARY OSTEOMYELITIS

Osteomyelitis Secondary to a Contiguous Source Infection

8. T.S., a 45-year-old man, suffered a closed fracture of his left distal fibula 2 weeks ago in a tractor accident. His fracture was set by open reduction and on the day of surgery he was started on cefazolin, which was continued for 24 hours. The postoperative course was unremarkable until 2 days ago, when he developed pain and swelling in his left calf. Evaluation for deep venous thrombosis was negative. On presentation, his left calf is tender, warm, swollen, and erythematous, and he is afebrile. Other physical findings are within normal limits. Laboratory data, including WBC count, ESR, serum creatinine, and blood urea nitrogen (BUN), are normal. However, plain bone films and bone scan are consistent with left fibula inflammation, due either to bone healing or infection. What findings in T.S. are characteristic of secondary osteomyelitis?

Few of the systemic signs and symptoms usually associated with acute osteomyelitis are seen in secondary osteomyelitis. The objective findings usually present in hematogenous disease, such as fever, leukocytosis, and an elevated ESR, are absent. The most common subjective complaint in acute contiguous osteomyelitis is pain in the area of infection, which often is accompanied by localized tenderness, swelling, and erythema. Because several weeks may pass before the patient becomes symptomatic, radiographic studies at the time of diagnosis may reveal abnormalities consistent with bone deterioration.[1,2]

T.S.'s case illustrates the usual findings in secondary osteomyelitis. Probable infection has arisen in his left calf at a site adjacent to the surgical repair of a fracture of his left distal fibula. T.S.'s localized symptoms, along with the absence of fever and leukocytosis, are characteristic of secondary osteomyelitis.

Clinical Presentation

T.S.'s case is consistent with osteomyelitis secondary to a contiguous focus of infection. In these cases, bone becomes infected from an exogenous source, or infection can occur through spread of an infection from adjacent tissue to bone. Any orthopedic procedure may result in infection, but as illustrated by T.S., 80% of surgically related osteomyelitis cases follow open reductions of fractures.[1] The bones most commonly involved are the hip, tibia, femur, and fibula.

Other associated situations are caused by contiguous spread of an infection. These include any penetrating injury, such as a gunshot wound or a nail puncture, or soft tissue infections such as pressure sores or those involving the fingers and toes.

Unlike hematogenous osteomyelitis, which occurs mostly in children, acute contiguous infection occurs more often in adults >50. This is explained by the higher incidence of precipitating factors within this age group, such as hip fractures, orthopedic procedures, oral cancers, sternotomy incisions for cardiac surgery, and craniotomies.[1,2]

Common Pathogens

Whereas hematogenous osteomyelitis usually involves a single pathogen, coinfection with several organisms is common in contiguous-spread osteomyelitis. Thus, although *S. aureus* is the most common pathogen, it is often part of a mixed infection. Other organisms responsible for infection include *Pseudomonas, Proteus, Streptococcus,* and *Klebsiella* species, *E. coli,* and *S. epidermidis.* Most cases of osteomyelitis involving the mandible, pelvis, and small bones (e.g., those of the hands and feet) are caused by Gram-negative organisms. *Pseudomonas* often is isolated from infections after puncture wounds of the foot.[1,7]

Anaerobes also are associated with contiguous-spread osteomyelitis. The anaerobic organisms most commonly isolated are *Bacteroides* species and anaerobic cocci. Possible predisposing factors include previous fractures or injuries resulting from human bites. Adjacent soft tissue infections also may lead to anaerobic infections of bone, as in the case of sacral osteomyelitis secondary to severe decubitus ulcers. Periodontal infections and paranasal sinusitis have been known to cause anaerobic osteomyelitis involving the cranium and jaw.[19]

To establish the pathogenic organisms, T.S. should undergo surgical re-evaluation and biopsy of involved bone at the probable site of infection.[1,2,9] The bone films and bone scan will help localize the possible infectious process to direct the surgical biopsy.

Initial Treatment

9. T.S. returns to the operating room for surgical exploration, and bone tissue is obtained for culture. He has no drug allergies. The initial postoperative antibiotic order is for oxacillin, 2 g Q 6 hr. Is this adequate antibiotic treatment for C.P.?

T.S. has undergone surgery to obtain bone material for culture because cultures of adjacent wound or sinus tract material are not predictive of the bacteria actually infecting the bone.[20] Because the infecting organisms in T.S. could have been acquired by trauma from his accident or in the hospital during or after his surgery, antibiotic coverage for *S. aureus* and Gram-negative bacilli is necessary. T.S. already has been started on oxacillin, but the dosage should be maximized to 2 g Q 4 hr. Nafcillin could be substituted for oxacillin; however, a third-generation cephalosporin (cefotaxime, ceftriaxone, or ceftazidime) or a quinolone (ciprofloxacin) should be added for Gram-negative coverage. Ciprofloxacin (400 mg Q 12 hr) or ceftazidime (2 g Q 8 hr) is preferred in cases involving *P. aeruginosa*. If a high rate of ORSA (>25% of isolates) is found locally, then vancomycin (1 g Q 12 hr) should be substituted for oxacillin or nafcillin. Despite concerns that tissue penetration of vancomycin is inferior to that of β-lactams, it usually is adequate for effective treatment.[21] Third-generation cephalosporins or quinolones should not be relied on to treat serious staphylococcal infection; therefore, combined therapy with antistaphylococcal penicillins or vancomycin is necessary.[1,9] Oxacillin and vancomycin have activity against Gram-positive anaerobes but not against an important Gram-negative anaerobe, *Bacteroides fragilis*. If *B. fragilis* is cultured from bone, additional therapy with clindamycin or metronidazole is indicated. While cultures are pending for C.P., his antibiotic regimen is changed to oxacillin 2 g IV Q 4 hr and ciprofloxacin 400 mg IV Q 12 hr.

OSTEOMYELITIS CAUSED BY *PSEUDOMONAS*

10. The bone biopsy from T.S. grows *P. aeruginosa*, which is sensitive to piperacillin, ceftazidime, imipenem, gentamicin, tobramycin, and ciprofloxacin. His leg pain is no worse than it was 2 days ago, and he remains afebrile. How should T.S. now be treated? Is he a candidate for oral therapy?

Traditional aggressive therapy for T.S. would include gentamicin or tobramycin plus a second agent active against *Pseudomonas,* such as piperacillin, ceftazidime, or ciprofloxacin. More recently, anti-*Pseudomonal* therapy with a β-lactam plus ciprofloxacin combination has been used with increasing frequency to avoid the complications of aminoglycosides. Thus, oxacillin should be discontinued. There is reasonable experience treating *Pseudomonas* osteomyelitis with ceftazidime, 2 g Q 8 hr, with gentamicin added, to complete a 4-week course of therapy.[1,9] T.S. should receive this combination as initial therapy. However, the therapeutic gentamicin serum levels needed to treat osteomyelitis are not well established. Thus, the therapeutic aminoglycoside levels defined previously are probably not relevant to current therapy with two active agents. To facilitate antibiotic therapy at home, T.S. is a candidate for once-daily dosing of gentamicin.[1] Because his renal function is normal, a single daily dose of 4 to 7 mg/kg can be administered. Although there are only a few reports of extended-dose aminoglycoside use in osteomyelitis, for other Gram-negative infections there is considerable evidence that once-a-day therapy is as effective as multiple daily doses and possibly less toxic.[22–24] At home, T.S. should have serum creatinine and trough gentamicin concentrations measured weekly. Desired trough levels are <1 μg/mL.

In an effort to avoid aminoglycoside toxicity, some investigators have administered cephalosporins or ciprofloxacin alone for 4 to 6 weeks to treat osteomyelitis caused by *Pseudomonas.* However, these studies are inadequate because they involved small case series without control groups or their follow-up time was too short (6 months).[25–27] Furthermore, studies do not yet support the use of oral quinolones (ciprofloxacin) alone in these cases.[28] To provide the best chance of cure, T.S. should receive ceftazidime and gentamicin for the entire 4-week course of therapy. The relative effectiveness of ceftazidime plus ciprofloxacin is unknown. T.S.'s antibiotic therapy can be reasonably accomplished at home. If gentamicin nephrotoxicity occurs or if he develops an allergic reaction to ceftazidime, oral ciprofloxacin (750 mg orally Q 12 hr) can be used to complete the full 4-week course of therapy. He should be followed closely thereafter for at least 2 years to detect recurrent infection.

OSTEOMYELITIS ASSOCIATED WITH VASCULAR INSUFFICIENCY

11. H.L., a 63-year-old man, presents to the diabetes clinic with an ulcer on the superior surface of his left foot. This lesion began as a red spot about 3 months ago but is now an ulcer approximately 3 cm wide ×2 cm deep. He has not paid much attention to it because it is not very painful. The ulcer is not foul smelling. H.L. has had type 2 diabetes mellitus for 20 years and is currently treated with regular and NPH insulin injections twice daily. Otherwise, he has no other complaints, but notes that his foot sore began after he started using a new pair of work boots about 4 months ago. Laboratory data obtained earlier today show a normal WBC count and differential, normal electrolytes, BUN, and creatinine. However, his fasting blood glucose is 240 mg/dL (normal, 65 to 110), and the ESR is 65 mm/hr (normal, 0 to 15). What findings in H.L. are consistent with secondary osteomyelitis?

[SI units: fasting plasma glucose, 13.3 mmol/L (normal, 3.6 to 6.1); ESR, 65 mm/hr (normal, 0 to 15)]

H.L. suffers from chronic lower extremity vascular insufficiency as a result of type 2 diabetes. Patients like H.L. with impaired blood flow usually develop osteomyelitis in the toes or small bones of the feet. Often infection first presents as cellulitis, as in H.L.'s case, which commonly progresses to deep ulcers. Finally, the infection spreads to the underlying bone. In many cases of osteomyelitis associated with vascular insufficiency, multiple pathogens can be cultured from surgical specimens or the wound. The most commonly isolated pathogens are *S. aureus;* however, Gram-negative and anaerobic bacteria also are often recovered.

Similar to contiguous-spread osteomyelitis, systemic signs of infection such as fever and leukocytosis are often absent in patients who develop bone infection secondary to vascular insufficiency. Local symptoms such as pain, swelling, and erythema usually dominate the picture.[1,2,29]

H.L. may have a bone infection that underlies a chronic, cutaneous ulcer on the surface of his left foot. Because of likely diabetic neuropathy, the skin lesion may not be very painful, and poor blood supply to the site likely contributed to the development of a chronic infection and possibly secondary osteomyelitis. Clinically, osteomyelitis is suggested by his elevated ESR and fasting glucose (consistent with infection). In addition, diabetic foot ulcers that are >2 cm wide and >2 cm deep are often predictive for underlying osteomyelitis.[29]

Antibiotic Selection

12. H.L.'s wound is débrided, and material obtained from a deep wound swab is sent to the microbiology laboratory for cultures. He is hospitalized to receive wound care and to begin antibiotics. He has no drug allergies, and he is started on cefazolin (1 g IV Q 8 hr) and ciprofloxacin (750 mg PO Q 12 hr). Is this appropriate initial therapy?

The antibiotic treatment selected for H.L. should be active against both Gram-positive and Gram-negative aerobic bacteria. Because anaerobic, Gram-negative bacteria are cultured from bone in diabetes patients with osteomyelitis <15% of the time, empiric anaerobic coverage may not be necessary at this stage of treatment. An antistaphylococcal agent (cefazolin, oxacillin, or vancomycin) plus a third-generation cephalosporin (cefotaxime, ceftazidime) or a quinolone (ciprofloxacin, ofloxacin) for Gram-negative coverage is the regimen most often used empirically. If anaerobic bacteria are believed to be clinically involved (e.g., foul-smelling wound), clindamycin or metronidazole (Flagyl) should be added to the regimen, or ampicillin/sulbactam (Unasyn) could be used as the antistaphylococcal agent. Hence, the initial regimen of cefazolin and ciprofloxacin for H.L. is rational. At least 2 weeks of IV treatment with cefazolin is preferred. After 2 weeks of IV cefazolin, he can be switched to oral cephalexin (500 mg orally Q 6 hr) or amoxicillin/clavulanic acid (Augmentin, 850 mg orally Q 12 hr) if his ulcer is healing. The overall duration of combination therapy is 6 weeks.

H.L. should also be made aware that osteomyelitis associated with diabetic foot ulcers is difficult to treat because poor circulation may impair antibiotic delivery to the site of infection. Despite surgical débridement of the infection followed by appropriate treatment with long-term IV antibiotic therapy, cure rates are low. Even minor amputations (one or two toes) are unsuccessful in eradicating infection. Unfortunately, radical surgical approaches such as transmetatarsal, below-the-knee, or above-the-knee amputations often are necessary to cure these infections.[1,2,29,30]

CHRONIC OSTEOMYELITIS

Clinical Presentation

13. A.D., a 28-year-old man, sustained a fracture of the left humerus after a fall 4 years ago. Two years ago, a draining sinus tract developed after bone grafting was performed for malunion of the fracture. A.D. has continued to notice slight drainage from the sinus tract since the bone graft. He has taken various oral antibiotics intermittently, including cephalexin and ciprofloxacin, which he stopped taking 6 months ago. One month ago, he noted increased sinus drainage, pain, swelling, and erythema of his left upper arm. Ciprofloxacin was restarted, and a swab culture of the sinus drainage grew *S. epidermidis, Corynebacterium* species, *Peptostreptococcus micros,* and *Bacteroides* species. A.D.'s ciprofloxacin was stopped after 2 weeks, and 7 days later, surgical débridement of bone and tissue was performed because of increased drainage and poor appearance of the wound. Gentamicin-impregnated polymethylmethacrylate (PMMA) beads were placed in the tissue adjacent to the débrided bone during surgery. Bone cultures grew *Proteus mirabilis, P. micros,* and *B. fragilis.* The *Proteus* was resistant to ampicillin, cefazolin, and ticarcillin but sensitive to cefotaxime, ceftriaxone, imipenem, gentamicin, and ciprofloxacin. Antibiotic sensitivities for the *Bacteroides* were not done. What aspects of A.D.'s case are characteristic of chronic osteomyelitis?

Inadequate treatment of an acute episode of osteomyelitis can lead to formation of necrotic, infected bone and recurrent symptoms consistent with chronic disease. Persistent symptoms or signs lasting ≥10 days correlate with chronic osteomyelitis and the development of necrotic bone.[1] Draining sinus tracts often develop from the bone to the skin in cases of chronic osteomyelitis.

A.D. developed a chronic bone infection after the injury. The persistence of sinus tract drainage in his left upper arm indicates an indolent infection of bone that was periodically suppressed, but not treated, by his courses of oral antibiotics. Cultures of sinus drainage now grow multiple organisms, and components of the topical normal bacterial flora were found. These cultures usually do not correlate with the organisms actually causing bone infection.[20] A.D.'s long course of bone involvement with drainage and local symptoms, and lack of any remarkable systemic symptoms, is classic for chronic osteomyelitis.

Surgery and Oral Antibiotics

14. Oral ciprofloxacin, 750 mg BID, was restarted 1 month ago when A.D.'s left arm became more painful and drainage increased. Was his poor response to therapy unexpected? How should he have been managed?

A.D.'s poor response should have been expected for three reasons. Antibiotic therapy was started before surgical débridement of avascular tissue; he was given an antibiotic that is ineffective against two of the cultured organisms, *B. fragilis* and *Peptostreptococcus;* and the oral route of antibiotic administration probably did not produce sufficiently high tissue levels.

Surgery plays an important role in the treatment of chronic osteomyelitis. Bone necrosis will progress if decompression and drainage of the infected area is not carried out as soon as possible. Furthermore, without initial surgical removal of necrotic bone and other poorly vascularized, infected material, even IV antibiotics are likely to fail. Additional surgical procedures include microvascular techniques that allow transplantation of a muscle flap to areas of infected bone.[31]

After surgery, it is important to achieve high levels of antibiotics that have been selected based on culture results from specimens obtained by deep aspiration or bone biopsy. Antibiotics should not be selected based on culture results from sinus tract drainage, as was done in A.D.'s case, because these cultures do not correlate with the actual etiologic organisms. The use of oral rather than parenteral antibiotics immediately after surgery has been explored.[26] The results for ofloxacin and ciprofloxacin were somewhat positive, but the relapse rates for *S. aureus* and *P. aeruginosa* infections were 20% to 30%. Thus, the IV route remains the standard initially. Although the optimal duration of therapy for chronic osteomyelitis is not well studied,[1,2,9] parenteral therapy is generally recommended for 6 to 8 weeks, followed by 3 to 12 months of oral antibiotic therapy, depending on the healing rate.[2,9]

Finally, A.D. should continue to be evaluated by an orthopedic surgeon because he may require further surgical treatment to eradicate chronically infected bone.

Intravenous Antibiotics

15. What would be reasonable antibiotic therapy for A.D.?

On the basis of the bone culture and sensitivity results, A.D. needs high-dose therapy directed at *P. mirabilis* and *B. fragilis.* For purposes of convenience and possible future home therapy, ceftriaxone (2 g IV Q 24 hr) should be started for coverage of *Proteus.* The anaerobic activity of ceftriaxone is inadequate for infections caused by *Bacteroides.* Therefore, metronidazole (500 mg IV Q 8 hr) also should be started. Clindamycin could be used as an alternative to metronidazole for anaerobic coverage plus activity against *Staphylococcus* species. However, metronidazole should be considered because its oral bioavailability is excellent, an important consideration when A.D. is converted to oral antibiotics. The newer carbapenem ertapenem (Invanz) is useful in these circumstances because it will cover the *Proteus* (since the organism is susceptible to imipenem) and anaerobes (*Bacteroides*) and can be given once daily (1 g IV Q 24 hr).

After 6 to 8 weeks of parenteral therapy (which can be completed at home), A.D. can be converted to oral therapy with high-dose ciprofloxacin (750 mg twice a day) and metronidazole (500 mg three times a day). Treatment with oral antibiotics should continue for at least 6 to 8 weeks, but it can be continued for several additional months based on resolution of the sinus tract drainage, pain, and tenderness in A.D.'s arm. If the sinus tract does not heal or if A.D.'s arm remains painful, surgical exploration and bone cultures must be repeated.

Local Antibiotics

16. What are the rationale for and effectiveness of local antibiotic administration (the PMMA beads) inserted during A.D.'s orthopedic surgery?

To deliver high concentrations of antibiotics to poorly vascularized sites of bone infection, various materials containing antibiotics have been placed at the infection site during surgery.[32] Plaster pellets, fibrin, collagen, hydroxyapatite, and PMMA impregnated with antibiotic, usually an aminoglycoside or vancomycin, have been used. The dosage form is designed to slowly release antibiotics from the material.[33] The most commonly reported experience with local antibiotic delivery has been with antibiotic-impregnated PMMA cement or beads inserted during joint arthroplasty. Unfortunately, recurrent infection rates have been comparable in patients treated with local antibiotic insertion and those treated with systemic antibiotics.[34] Thus, there is no evidence that the PMMA beads will improve A.D.'s outcome when added to systemic therapy. Local delivery of antibiotics should never replace systemic antibiotics in the treatment of chronic osteomyelitis.[9]

OSTEOMYELITIS ASSOCIATED WITH PROSTHETIC MATERIAL

Usual Clinical Presentation

17. J.G., a 63-year-old man, underwent bilateral hip replacements 5 years ago for chronic osteoarthritis. He is seen today in the orthopedic clinic because his left hip pain has worsened and he has been unable to bear weight for 3 months. His hip is painful and warm, but his temperature is 37.5°C. Aspiration of fluid from the hip reveals a total nucleated cell count of 55,000/mm³ with 94% neutrophils. Gram's stain of this fluid shows 4+ polymorphonuclear leukocytes (PMNs) and 1+ Gram-positive cocci. His peripheral WBC count is 8,800 cells/mm³. He is started on antibiotic therapy with vancomycin and cefotaxime pending culture results, and he is scheduled for operative evaluation and possible removal of his prosthetic joint. Does J.G. have a prosthetic joint infection?

[SI unit: WBC, 8,800 ×10⁹ cells/L]

Joint replacement surgery has become a common orthopedic procedure for patients with significant joint destruction as a result of rheumatoid arthritis (RA) and other disabling diseases. Prosthetic knee, shoulder, elbow, or hip devices made of metallic alloys are cemented to adjacent bone to reestablish joint function. Infection of these foreign bodies can occur because of hematogenous dissemination of bacteria or by contiguous spread from a topical wound. *Staphylococcus* species are most commonly involved in prosthetic joint infections, followed by *Streptococcus* species, Gram-negative bacilli, and anaerobes. Bacteria infect bone adjacent to the joint prosthesis, including the bone–cement interface, which results in a loosened and less functional prosthesis.[35]

Chronic pain, swelling, erythema, and tenderness over a prosthetic joint are typical findings associated with prosthetic joint infection. J.G. has a relatively lengthy duration of symptoms associated with his left hip, which also could be caused by joint loosening, but the cell count and differential from the joint aspirate suggest joint infection. Also, the predominance of neutrophils in his joint fluid and Gram-positive cocci on Gram's stain are consistent with an infected prosthesis. As is often the case, he has no obvious source of infection on his skin or other site from which bacteria could disseminate. Occasionally, sources of infection with hematogenous dissemination to the prosthetic joint are identified, such as dental infections, cellulitis, or urinary tract infections. Given the Gram's stain result, J.G. should be covered for *Staphylococcus* and *Streptococcus* species with vancomycin, pending the results of cultures and sensitivities. *Staphylococcus* species, including coagulase-negative species such as *S. epidermidis,* are the most commonly isolated bacteria responsible for prosthetic infection. These coagulase-negative *Staphylococci* are especially adherent to prosthetic material, and although coagulase-negative *Staphylococci* are usually considered a contaminant in culture, when a prothesis is in place, it should be considered a likely pathogen. Coagulase-negative *Staphylococci* are often resistant to oxacillin but are susceptible to vancomycin. Because Gram-negative bacteria also can infect these joints, it is reasonable to add Gram-negative coverage to J.G.'s regimen until the results of joint fluid cultures are available.

Surgery

18. Does J.G. need surgery and antibiotics to cure his infection?

Yes. Surgery to remove J.G.'s hip prosthesis and chronic antibiotics for 6 weeks are the current recommendations for optimal eradication of prosthetic joint infection.[1,35,36] A two-stage orthopedic procedure is involved: removal of the infected prosthesis, placement of an antibiotic-filled spacer or block, joint immobilization, and antibiotics for 6 weeks. If the joint space remains culture negative, a new joint prosthesis is reinserted. Because avascular bone cement and prosthetic material can become seeded with bacteria, complete removal of this material is necessary to have the greatest chance of curing the infection. Six weeks of systemic antibiotic therapy in combination with orthopedic surgery results in restoration of joint function in 85% to 95% of cases. High rates of treatment failure (approximately 70%) occur if the joint prosthesis is not removed and chronic suppressive antibiotics are not given.[37,38]

Antibiotics

19. Because the pelvic portion of J.G.'s hip prosthesis is so firmly attached to bone, the surgeon decides not to remove this portion of the prosthesis because doing so would require a pelvic fracture. Instead, his hip is débrided and the acetabular lining material is replaced. Purulent material is sent for culture. The removed lining material and three swabs of the left hip prosthesis grow oxacillin-susceptible *S. aureus*. How should J.G. be treated?

To prevent recurrence of his infection, J.G. will need to take antibiotics indefinitely, perhaps for the rest of his life if his original prosthesis remains in place. However, lifelong therapy is impractical, expensive, and likely to provoke adverse effects. J.G. should be treated initially with oxacillin (2 g IV Q 4 hr) for at least 2 weeks, although the optimal duration of this initial parenteral therapy is unknown. Thereafter, he should be managed with oral antibiotics. Limited success has been reported with the use of ciprofloxacin plus rifampin, both given orally, in patients with prosthetic joint infections caused by *Staphylococcus* species in which the implant was not removed. In 18 patients with a short duration of symptoms (<21 days), ciprofloxacin (750 mg orally twice daily) and rifampin (450 mg orally twice daily) were given for 3 months. Twelve patients who completed the protocol had no evidence of infection at 24 months of follow-up.[39] J.G.'s symptoms have lasted 3 months, suggesting that his infection may not respond to therapy as well as that reported. Nevertheless, a prolonged course of ciprofloxacin and rifampin could be tried for at least 3 months.[39] Another option for oral therapy is linezolid (Zyvox). However, there are limited data on the use of linezolid for prosthetic joint infection, and chronic use is associated with thrombocytopenia. If linezolid is used for >2 weeks, J.G.'s platelet count should be followed weekly.[40]

SEPTIC ARTHRITIS

20. S.F. is a 48-year-old man with hemophilia A and chronic bilateral knee hemarthroses. He has been HIV seropositive for 8 years; his last CD4 count 2 months ago was 280 cells/mm³ (normal, >800). One week ago, he underwent uncomplicated bilateral knee arthroplasty. Cefazolin prophylaxis was administered before surgery and for 24 hours postoperatively. Soon after surgery, he noted intermittent chills and sweats accompanied by documented fevers. Two blood cultures drawn 3 days postoperatively were negative, and he was started on ampicillin/sulbactam (Unasyn) and gentamicin. However, two more blood cultures drawn 3 days later are positive for *P. aeruginosa*, sensitive to ceftazidime, piperacillin, imipenem, ciprofloxacin, and gentamicin. The surgical sites are unremarkable. His antiretroviral medications are zidovudine and lamivudine (Combivir) and efavirenz (Sustiva). What is a rational antibiotic therapy plan for S.F.?

Antibiotic treatment for S.F. should be designed to treat his *Pseudomonas* bacteremia and also to eradicate and then suppress *Pseudomonas* that may have seeded his prosthetic joints. As long as he is without symptoms related to his knees (pain, swelling, redness, tenderness), it will be impossible to tell whether the joint has become infected without removing the prosthesis. The conservative approach is to treat S.F. with combined antipseudomonal antibiotics—ceftazidime (2 g IV Q 8 hr) and once-daily gentamicin for 6 weeks—followed by chronic suppressive therapy with oral ciprofloxacin for the rest of his life.[35] There is no evidence that adjunctive rifampin improves outcomes in Gram-negative infections. Also, rifampin would interact significantly with S.F.'s antiretroviral therapy, particularly efavirenz.[41]

Nongonococcal Arthritis

21. A.W., a 44-year-old man, is referred to a rheumatology clinic for right knee swelling. Four days ago, his right knee became painful and swollen and he became unable to flex the joint. He also noted a temperature of 100.5° to 102.0°F for at least 5 days. A joint effusion is present on physical examination and is aspirated for cell count, Gram's stain, and culture. His medical history is unremarkable except for an episode of hives after receiving cephalexin for an episode of cellulitis 6 months ago. A.W.'s WBC count is 12,000 cells/mm³, and his ESR is 40 mm/hr. The synovial fluid from his right knee contains 80,000 WBCs/mm³ with 90% neutrophils, and the Gram's stain shows Gram-positive cocci. Culture results are pending. His temperature is 38.5°C. What findings in A.W. are consistent with septic arthritis?

[SI units: WBC count, 12,000 and 80,000 ×10⁹ cells/L, respectively; neutrophils, 0.90; ESR, 40 mm/hr]

Septic arthritis or infectious arthritis usually is acquired hematogenously. The highly vascular synovium of the joint allows easy passage of bacteria from blood into the synovial space. Bacteremia, secondary to *Neisseria gonorrhoeae* or *S. aureus* in particular, often is associated with the development of joint infections. Septic arthritis also can develop secondary to the spread of osteomyelitis into the joint. This is especially a problem in children <1 year of age who still have capillaries perforating the epiphyseal growth plate.

Several factors predispose patients to the development of infectious arthritis. Trauma can directly inoculate the synovium or allow infecting organisms to penetrate the synovium more easily. Patients with certain systemic disorders, such as diabetes mellitus, rheumatoid arthritis, osteoarthritis, chronic granulomatous disease, cancer, or chronic liver disease, are more susceptible to the development of infection. Endocrine factors can predispose pregnant or menstruating women to the development of gonococcal arthritis. In the menstruating patient, this can be partially explained by the increased endocervical shedding of *N. gonorrhoeae*.[42,43]

Usual Clinical Presentation

A.W. has had an acute onset of monoarticular joint pain and swelling, with reduced range of motion and fever. These findings are classic for septic, nongonococcal arthritis. The tap of his joint effusion with a predominance of neutrophils in the joint fluid confirms the diagnosis. In these circumstances, A.W.'s knee has been infected hematogenously from a distant, usually unrecognized, source of infection. The knee is involved most commonly, and *S. aureus* is the usual causative organism. However, if A.W. had a urinary tract infection as well, Gram-negative bacilli would more commonly be responsible for joint infection. Occasionally, a predisposing factor is present in the involved joint, such as pre-existing arthritis (i.e., RA) or trauma.[42,43]

A single joint is involved in 90% of bacterial or suppurative arthritis cases. As in A.W.'s case, the joint most commonly involved is the knee. Other potential sites of infectious arthritis in adults include the hip, shoulder, sternoclavicular, and sacroiliac joints; the ankle and elbow are common sites of infection in children. The wrist and interphalangeal joints of the hand also may be involved, but in these cases, the infectious pathogens are most often *N. gonorrhoeae* and *Mycobacterium tuberculosis*.[42] The most common systemic indication of infectious arthritis is fever. Localized symptoms include pain, decreased mobility of the involved joint, and swelling.

As illustrated by A.W., 90% of patients also have joint effusion on physical examination. When evaluating a patient who may have a joint infection, any purulent joint effusion should be considered septic until a thorough workup proves otherwise. On the other hand, noninfectious conditions may be present, such as single joint involvement with synovial effusions (e.g., acute RA, gout, chondrocalcinosis).[42]

Aspirated joint fluid should be cultured because isolation of bacteria is the only definitive diagnostic test for bacterial arthritis. A.W.'s joint fluid picture also is typical. The leukocyte count in the synovial fluid usually is significantly elevated, with counts ranging from 50,000 to 200,000 cells/mm³. Leukocyte counts of <20,000 rarely are seen during infection, except in early cases of bacterial arthritis or in patients with disseminated gonococcal infection (DGI). Synovial fluid from an infected joint also may have a decreased glucose concentration, but this is seen in only about 50% of cases.[42]

Another laboratory finding in A.W. that is consistent with infectious arthritis is the elevated ESR. Although this value is higher in the case of bacterial infection, viral or fungal arthritis also may be associated with this finding. Increased WBC counts in serum are common in younger patients but rare in adults. Anemia also may be associated with infection, especially in patients with chronic involvement or in cases where predisposing factors such as RA are present.[43]

When attempting to determine the most likely pathogen, the patient's age must be taken into consideration. In adults (e.g., A.W.) and in children >2 years of age, *S. aureus* is the most common cause of bacterial arthritis. However, in adults <30, *N. gonorrhoeae* is more likely to be the etiologic agent. Bacterial arthritis in children <2 years of age may also be a result of *H. influenzae* type b, although *H. influenzae* vaccination has decreased the incidence of infection caused by this bacteria.[44] *Streptococci,* such as group A β-hemolytic *Streptococci,* can cause infection in children and adults. Other organisms such as group B *Streptococci,* anaerobic *Streptococci,* and gram-negative bacteria can cause infection. Gram-negative bacilli are responsible for approximately 15% of cases and often infect multiple joints. Infections with these organisms usually are associated with predisposing factors such as RA, osteoarthritis, or heroin use. The organism most commonly isolated from patients with bacterial arthritis who have a history of IV drug abuse is *P. aeruginosa.*[42,43]

Initial Antimicrobial Therapy: Treatment in β-Lactam–Allergic Patients

22. A.W. describes his reaction to cephalexin as intense pruritic skin lesions over his trunk and upper extremities that appeared acutely (several hours) after he had received several doses. He did not experience wheezing or shortness of breath, and his reaction was treated symptomatically with diphenhydramine and discontinuation of the cephalexin. He had received several types of oral antibiotics before this episode of pruritus without difficulty but has not taken antibiotics since then. How should A.W. be treated?

Treatment of nongonococcal arthritis includes drainage of purulent joint fluid (by needle aspiration or surgery) and appropriate antibiotic therapy. Because *S. aureus* is most likely involved, initial empiric therapy with a penicillinase-resistant penicillin, a cephalosporin, or vancomycin should be initi-

ated. However, A.W.'s reaction to cephalexin is worrisome because readministration of a penicillin or cephalosporin could cause allergic symptoms. Fortunately, an alternative, effective non–β-lactam treatment is available. Because A.W.'s septic arthritis is probably caused by *S. aureus* and, perhaps, streptococci, vancomycin (1 g IV Q 12 hr), which covers both organisms, should be started as soon as possible. In patients who are not allergic to penicillin, oxacillin and nafcillin (2 g IV Q 4 hr) are recommended for OSSA infections. β-Lactams and vancomycin penetrate joint effusions adequately for Gram-positive infections.[45] If A.W. acquired his infection in the hospital, vancomycin also would be initially indicated because of the possibility that ORSA is involved. In a nonallergic patient, therapy then can be changed on the basis of sensitivity testing to oxacillin if the organism is susceptible.

Duration of Therapy

23. How long should A.W. be treated? How should the efficacy of treatment be monitored?

Although few studies have been carried out to determine the optimal duration of therapy for bacterial arthritis, the current recommendation is 2 to 3 weeks; some investigators recommend that treatment be extended to 4 weeks for infectious arthritis caused by *S. aureus* or Gram-negative bacilli.[42,43,45]

A.W. should be treated for at least 3 weeks.[15,43] His response to therapy should be monitored clinically (resolution of symptoms, fever, and falling ESR) as well as by periodic evaluation of joint fluid. Frequent aspirations of joint fluid, initially on a daily basis, should be done, with evaluation of cell count and fluid culture. Effective therapy results in a diminishing WBC count in the joint fluid and negative cultures, usually within 3 to 4 days of treatment. A poorer outcome (permanent joint dysfunction) can result if joint fluid cultures are still positive after 6 days of treatment for Gram-positive infection. If fluid cultures are persistently positive, more aggressive surgical management is necessary to preserve joint function.[42,46]

Most joint fluid cultures become negative after 7 days of treatment with IV antibiotics. Joint inflammation and other symptoms also should improve by this time. However, the duration of articular symptoms before antibiotic therapy is begun correlates with the subsequent time required to sterilize the synovial fluid. Therefore, delay in initiating antibiotic treatment may necessitate a longer course of therapy.

As in hematogenous osteomyelitis, oral antibiotics have been used in septic arthritis to complete a course of treatment if the initial response to IV therapy is adequate. Oral therapy should not be considered until the patient is afebrile, joint fluid cultures are negative, the ESR is normal, and there is decreased joint pain and increased joint mobility.[43] There are case series with generally positive results, but adequately controlled, randomized clinical trials comparing IV and oral therapy are not available.[15] Because of A.W.'s allergy to cephalexin, the choice of adequate oral therapy to complete at least 3 weeks of treatment is difficult. Because of the continuing emergence of resistance among Gram-positive organisms to ciprofloxacin, use of this agent is not recommended. Oral clindamycin could be used, but published experience in adults is minimal and there would be concern about the possible development of antibiotic-associated colitis. Use of linezolid (Zyvox) in septic arthritis is also not extensively reported in the literature. If the *S. aureus* isolated from A.W. is sensitive to trimethoprim-sulfamethoxazole, this agent may be an alternative to clindamycin for oral treatment. However, published experience with this mode of treatment also is lacking. A.W. should be advised that parenteral treatment with vancomycin, which can be accomplished at home, would be the most effective mode of treatment. Finally, injections of antibiotics into the joint space are of no value. Most antibiotics readily penetrate the joint space and enter the synovial fluid.[42,43,45]

Gonococcal Arthritis

24. **A.S., age 19, presents to the walk-in clinic with right knee and right shoulder pain, nausea, and vomiting. Upon physical examination, her right knee is swollen and she has decreased range of motion of her right shoulder. Several erythematous, papular skin lesions are noted on both hands. She also has a vaginal discharge. Her temperature is 38.2°C, and her WBC count is 15,000 cells/mm³. She gives a history of having two recent sexual partners. Cultures of blood, joint fluid, and vaginal discharge are obtained; joint fluid Gram's stain shows heavy PMNs, but no organisms are seen. Why is A.S. considered to have gonococcal arthritis?**

[SI unit: WBC, 15,000 ×10⁹ cells/L]

Usual Clinical Presentation

Polyarticular arthritis in a young, sexually active adult, as is the case with A.S., is caused most commonly by *N. gonorrhoeae*. Arthritis in multiple joints is one of the most common features of DGI. Unlike nongonococcal arthritis, which is almost exclusively monoarticular, gonococcal arthritis involves multiple joints in approximately 50% of cases. Clinically, patients present initially with a migratory polyarthralgia and later with fever, dermatitis, and tenosynovitis. Skin lesions are an important clue to the diagnosis of disseminated gonococcal disease and often begin as tiny erythematous papules and develop into larger vesicles. Other symptoms, such as purulent and swollen joints, are present in only 30% to 40% of patients. As in hematogenously acquired nongonococcal arthritis, the synovial fluid leukocyte count usually is elevated, but to a lesser degree. Unfortunately, *N. gonorrhoeae* is recovered in <50% of purulent joint effusions; however, blood cultures often are positive for this organism and coupled with the patient's clinical presentation can be used to make a definitive diagnosis.[42,47]

A.S. has systemic signs of infection, skin lesions, and multiple joint involvement, which are classic for DGI. Her history of recent sexual activity and the presence of a vaginal discharge are consistent with gonococcal infection, although evidence of mucosal infection with *N. gonorrhoeae* is not necessary for disseminated infection to occur.[42,47]

Patient Workup and Treatment in the Clinic

25. **What additional workup should be done in A.S.? Can she be treated immediately in the clinic?**

A.S. should be evaluated for other sexually transmitted diseases, specifically syphilis and HIV infection. Serologic testing for syphilis (rapid plasma reagent [RPR] or venereal disease research laboratory [VDRL] testing) and for antibody to HIV should be obtained. In addition, A.S. should have a pregnancy test because some of the antibiotics that may be used in A.S. are contraindicated during pregnancy, including doxycycline and ciprofloxacin.

Because of possible penicillinase production by *N. gonorrhoeae,* recommended therapy is with ceftriaxone (1 g intramuscularly or IV Q 24 hr) initially. A.S. should receive her first dose of ceftriaxone in the clinic today. Parenteral treatment should continue for 1 to 2 days after improvement begins; at that point, oral therapy (levofloxacin 500 mg once daily or ciprofloxacin 500 mg twice a day) can be started. Quinolone-resistant *N. gonorrhoeae* are currently prevalent in California and Hawaii, so the use of ciprofloxacin or levofloxacin as treatment in these locations is not recommended. Effective therapy should be continued with ceftriaxone. The duration of antibiotic treatment is 7 days.[48]

A.S.'s sexual partners should also be evaluated and treated for relevant sexually transmitted diseases.

Full Course of Therapy

26. **Results of RPR and pregnancy testing in A.S. are negative. How should she complete her course of therapy?**

DGI should be treated for 7 days. A.S. also should begin treatment with azithromycin (1 g orally once) or doxycycline (100 mg orally twice a day for 7 days) for the possibility of concomitant chlamydial infection. A.S. can complete her course of treatment for DGI orally, although parenteral therapy is recommended until signs and symptoms resolve. This usually takes 2 to 4 days.[47] She will have to return to the clinic for daily ceftriaxone administration unless other arrangements for parenteral therapy can be made. Current recommendations from the Centers for Disease Control and Prevention are that oral treatment should be with either ciprofloxacin 500 mg orally twice daily or levofloxacin 500 mg orally daily (except in California and Hawaii). Improvement in symptoms usually occurs within 48 hours.[47,48] Treatment guidelines for DGI are included in the gonorrhea section of Chapter 65, Sexually Transmitted Diseases.

REFERENCES

1. Lew DP, Waldwogel FA. Osteomyelitis. N Engl J Med 1997;336:999.
2. Mader JT, Calhoun J. Osteomyelitis. In: Mandell GL et al, eds. Principles and Practice of Infectious Diseases, 5th ed. New York: Churchill Livingstone, 2000:1175.
3. Tay BK et al. Spinal infections. J Am Acad Orthop Surg. 2002;10:188.

4. Jackson MA et al. Pyogenic arthritis associated with adjacent osteomyelitis: identification of the sequela-prone child. Pediatr Infect Dis J 1992;11:9.
5. Mandel S et al. *Staphylococcus aureus* bone and joint infection. J Infect 2002;44:143.
6. Gutierrez KM. Osteomyelitis. In: Long SS et al, eds. Principles and Practice of Pediatric Infectious Diseases, 2nd ed. New York: Churchill Livingstone, 2003:467.

7. Laughlin TJ et al. Soft tissue and bone infections from puncture wounds in children. West J Med 1997;166:126.
8. Fitzgerald RH Jr et al. Pathophysiology of osteomyelitis and pharmacokinetics of antimicrobial agents in normal and osteomyelitic bone. In: Esterhai JL Jr et al, eds. Musculoskeletal Infection. Park Ridge: American Academy of Orthopaedic Surgeons, 1990:387.

9. Haas DW, McAndrew MP. Bacterial osteomyelitis in adults: evolving considerations in diagnosis and treatment. Am J Med 1996;101:550.

10. Hospital Infection Control Practices Advisory Committee. Recommendations for preventing the spread of vancomycin resistance. Am J Infect Control 1995;23: 87.

11. Gilbert DN et al. Outpatient parenteral antimicrobial-drug therapy. N Engl J Med 1997;337:829.

12. Osman DR, Berbari EF. Outpatient intravenous antimicrobial therapy for the practicing orthopaedic surgeon. Clin Orthop Rel Res 2002;403:80.

13. Sonnen GM, Henry NK. Pediatric bone and joint infections. Diagnosis and antimicrobial management. Pediatr Clin North Am 1996;43:933.

14. Weinstein MP et al. Multicenter collaborative evaluation of a standardized serum bactericidal test as a predictor of therapeutic efficacy in acute and chronic osteomyelitis. Am J Med 1987;83:218.

15. Syrogiannopoulos GA, Nelson JD. Duration of antimicrobial therapy for acute suppurative osteoarticular infections. Lancet 1988;1:37.

16. Peltola H et al. Simplified treatment of acute staphylococcal osteomyelitis of childhood. Pediatrics 1997;99:846.

17. Karwowska A et al. Epidemiology and outcome of osteomyelitis in the era of sequential intravenous-oral therapy. Pediatr Infect Dis J 1998;17:1021.

18. Roine I et al. Serial serum C-reactive protein to monitor recovery from acute hematogenous osteomyelitis in children. Pediatr Infect Dis J 1995;14:40.

19. Brook I, Frazier EH. Anaerobic osteomyelitis and arthritis in a military hospital: a 10-year experience. Am J Med 1993;94: 21.

20. Perry CR et al. Accuracy of cultures of material from swabbing of the superficial aspect of the wound and needle biopsy in the preoperative assessment of osteomyelitis. J Bone Joint Surg [Am] 1991;73:745.

21. Graziani AL et al. Vancomycin concentrations in infected and non-infected human bone. Antimicrob Agents Chemother 1988;32:1320.

22. Nicolau DP et al. Experience with a once-daily aminoglycoside program administered to 2,184 adult patients. Antimicrob Agents Chemother 1995;39:650.

23. Ali MZ, Goetz MB. A meta-analysis of the relative efficacy and toxicity of single daily dosing versus multiple daily dosing of aminoglycosides. Clin Infect Dis 1997;24:769.

24. Bailey TC et al. A meta-analysis of extended-interval dosing versus multiple daily dosing of aminoglycosides. Clin Infect Dis 1997;24:786.

25. Sheftel TG, Mader JT. Randomized evaluation of ceftazidime or ticarcillin and tobramycin for the treatment of osteomyelitis caused by gram-negative bacilli. Antimicrob Agents Chemother 1986;29:112.

26. Gentry LO, Rodriguez GG. Oral ciprofloxacin compared with parenteral antibiotics in the treatment of osteomyelitis. Antimicrob Agents Chemother 1990;34:40.

27. Stengel D et al. Systematic review and meta-analysis of antibiotic therapy for bone and joint infections. Lancet Infect Dis 2001;1:175.

28. Lew DP, Waldwogel FA. Quinolones and osteomyelitis: state-of-the-art. Drugs 1995;49(Suppl 2):100.

29. Lipsky BA. Osteomyelitis of the foot in diabetic patients. Clin Infect Dis 1997;25:1318.

30. Lipsky BA, Berendt AR. Principles and practice of antibiotic therapy of diabetic foot infections. Diab Metab Res Rev 2000;16(Suppl 1):S42.

31. Eckardt JJ et al. An aggressive surgical approach to the management of chronic osteomyelitis. Clin Orthop 1994;298:229.

32. Kanellakopoulou K, Giamarellos-Bourboulis EJ. Carrier systems for the local delivery of antibiotics in bone infections. Drugs 2000;59:1223.

33. Humphrey JS et al. Pharmacokinetics of a degradable drug delivery system in bone. Clin Orthop Rel Res 1998;349:218.

34. Nelson CL et al. A comparison of gentamicin-impregnated polymethylmethacrylate bead implantation to conventional parenteral antibiotic therapy in infected total hip and knee arthroplasty. Clin Orthop Rel Res 1993;295:96.

35. Brause BD. Infections with prostheses in bones and joints. In: Mandell GL et al, eds. Principles and Practice of Infectious Diseases, 5th ed. New York: Churchill Livingstone, 2000:1196.

36. Gillespie WJ. Prevention and management of infection after total joint replacement. Clin Infect Dis 1997;25:1310.

37. Tsukayama DT et al. Infection after total hip arthroplasty. J Bone Joint Surg [Am] 1996;78:512.

38. Brandt CM et al. *Staphylococcus aureus* prosthetic joint infection treated with prosthesis removal and delayed reimplantation arthroplasty. Mayo Clin Proc 1999;74:553.

39. Zimmerli W et al. Role of rifampin for treatment of orthopedic implant-related staphylococcal infections. JAMA 1998;279:1537.

40. Bassetti M et al. Linezolid treatment of prosthetic hip infections due to methicillin-resistant *Staphylococcus aureus* (MRSA). J Infect 2001;43:148.

41. Finch CK et al. Rifampin and rifabutin drug interactions: an update. Arch Intern Med 2002;162:985.

42. Smith JW, Hasan MS. Infectious arthritis. In: Mandell GL et al, eds. Principles and Practice of Infectious Diseases, 5th ed. New York: Churchill Livingstone, 2000:1175.

43. Shirtliff ME, Mader JT. Acute septic arthritis. Clin Microbiol Rev 2002;15:524.

44. Bowerman SG et al. Decline in bone and joint infections attributable to *Haemophilus influenzae* type b. Clin Orthop Rel Res 1997;341:128.

45. Hamed KA et al. Pharmacokinetic optimisation of the treatment of septic arthritis. Clin Pharmacokinet 1996;31:156.

46. Goldenberg DL. Septic arthritis. Lancet 1998;351:197.

47. Cucurull E, Espinoza LR. Gonococcal arthritis. Rheum Dis Clin North Am 1998;24:305.

48. Centers for Disease Control and Prevention 2002 sexually transmitted diseases treatment guidelines. MMWR 2002;51:38.

CHAPTER 67

Traumatic Skin and Soft Tissue Infections

James P. McCormack, Glen Brown

Skin and soft tissue infections refer to infections involving any or all layers of the skin (epidermis, dermis), subcutaneous fat, fascia, or muscle. Many terms or classifications are used to describe various skin and soft tissue infections, and these often are based on the site of infection and causative organism(s). However, these terms or classifications add little to the understanding and treatment of these infections. In fact, confusion in terminology may be detrimental if treatment is delayed until a causative organism is identified.[1]

Although mild skin and soft tissue infections often are self-limiting, moderate to severe infections can progress to complicated infections such as septic arthritis, osteomyelitis, or systemic infections (bacteremia) if not treated appropriately. Soft tissue infections in diabetic patients can lead to gangrene and loss of limb, whereas necrotizing soft tissue infections, even with appropriate treatment, are fatal in 30% to 50% of patients.[2]

This chapter focuses on skin and soft tissue infections that are primarily the result of a break in the skin following an abrasion, skin puncture, ulceration, surgical wound, intentional or unintentional insertion of a foreign body, or blunt soft tissue contusion. Superficial skin infections such as impetigo, infections that originate within the hair follicle (e.g., folliculitis, furuncles, carbuncles) or sweat pores, styes, acne, diaper rash, and skin infestations are not discussed.

The treatment of traumatic skin and soft tissue infections often is empiric and based on the severity and site of infection, the patient's underlying immunocompetence, and the triggering event (e.g., abrasion, bite, insertion of a foreign object) because attempts to isolate the causative organism often are futile.[3,4] The organisms that should be considered when empirically treating patients with a traumatic skin or soft tissue infection are outlined in Table 67-1.

CELLULITIS

Definition and Causative Organisms

1. T.E., age 25, presents to her family doctor with a 2- to 3-day history of worsening pain, redness, and swelling on her left leg following an abrasion that occurred sliding into second base during a softball tournament. The area is warm to the touch with a defined erythematous border. Over the past 24 to 36 hours, the leg has become increasingly painful and "tight." Mild lymphadenopathy is present, and T.E. has a temperature of 38.2°C. The presumptive diagnosis is a moderate cellulitis, and cloxacillin (Tegopen, Cloxapen) is prescribed. Why is cloxacillin appropriate empiric treatment for T.E.?

Cellulitis (an acute inflammation of the skin and subcutaneous fat) is characterized by local tenderness, pain, swelling, warmth, and erythema with or without a definite entry point. Cellulitis is usually secondary to trauma or an underlying skin lesion that allows bacterial penetration into the skin and underlying tissues. Local treatment (i.e., cleaning/irrigation of the site with soap and water) is all that is required for mild cellulitis in patients with no evidence of a systemic infection. In T.E., however, her elevated temperature, increasing pain, and lymphadenopathy suggest a more serious infection. Antibiotics, in addition to local wound care, should be prescribed for T.E. Cellulitis most often is caused by group A β-hemolytic streptococci (*Streptococcus pyogenes*) and, less often, *Staphylococcus aureus* (see Table 67-1).[3,4] However, wound cultures often are negative and fail to identify the causative organism.[3,4] Other organisms (*Escherichia coli, Pseudomonas aeruginosa, Klebsiella pneumoniae*) also can cause cellulitis but should be suspected only in immunocompromised patients or in patients

Table 67-1   **Potential Organisms Causing Skin and Soft Tissue Infections**

	Gram-Positive		Gram-Negative			Anaerobes		
	Staphy-lococcal	Strepto-coccal	E. coli, Klebsiella, Proteus	Pasteurella multocida	Eikenella corrodens	Oral Anaerobes	Clostridium Species	Bacteroides fragilis
Cellulitis	X	X						
Diabetic soft tissue	X	X	X					X
Necrotizing infections	X	X	X			X	X	X
Erysipelas		X						
Animal bites	X	X	X	X		X		
Human bites	X	X	X		X	X		

X, organisms that should be covered empirically with appropriate antibiotic therapy.

who fail to respond to antibiotics that have activity limited to Gram-positive organisms.

Empiric Antibiotic Therapy for Moderate Cellulitis

Oral cloxacillin (Tegopen, Cloxapen) is appropriate empiric therapy for cellulitis in an otherwise healthy individual such as T.E. Cloxacillin has good activity against staphylococcal and streptococcal organisms and is better tolerated than erythromycin (E-Mycin) or clindamycin (Cleocin). Dicloxacillin (Dynapen), another antistaphylococcal penicillin, produces slightly higher total serum concentrations than cloxacillin but is more highly protein bound, resulting in slightly lower free-serum concentrations.[5] Flucloxacillin (Floxapen; not available in the United States) provides similar total serum concentrations to dicloxacillin (Dynapen) but is less protein bound and produces higher free concentrations than either cloxacillin or dicloxacillin.[5] These small differences in pharmacokinetics do not affect clinical outcome, and the choice between these agents should be based on cost. If the cellulitis is well demarcated and there are no pockets of pus or evidence of vein thrombosis, penicillin (V-Cillin K, Pen-Vee K) alone can be appropriate because the causative organism is likely to be streptococcal. Many other available antibiotics that have activity against staphylococcal and streptococcal organisms have been evaluated for effectiveness in skin and soft tissue infections. In a recent surveillance study in the United States, all 405 isolates of *S. pyogenes* isolated from skin and soft tissue infections were sensitive to penicillin. *S. pyogenes* was also 100% susceptible to ceftriaxone, vancomycin, levofloxacin, and moxifloxacin; 6% of the organisms were resistant to azithromycin.[6] While many antibiotics are effective for the treatment of cellulitis, none is more effective than cloxacillin or dicloxacillin. Cephalexin (Keflex) is probably as effective and as well tolerated as cloxacillin or dicloxacillin and is comparable in cost. Cephalexin has been shown to be just as effective as more expensive agents (ofloxacin).[7] The Gram-negative activity of cephalexin (not seen with cloxacillin or dicloxacillin) is not required for most cases of cellulitis in otherwise healthy patients. In many emergency departments (EDs), a single dose of a long-acting parenterally administered cephalosporin (e.g., ceftriaxone), followed by oral therapy with one of the above agents, is often the preferred treatment regimen. This regimen is not more effective than oral therapy alone, and ceftriaxone (Rocephin) signifi-cantly adds to the cost of treatment. A single dose of ceftriaxone is as expensive as (if not more so) a 10-day course of appropriate oral therapy.

In this case, antibiotic treatment is required, and T.E. should receive the least expensive of cloxacillin, dicloxacillin, or cephalexin. Although some of the newer macrolides and quinolones are effective in treating cellulitis, they do not provide any therapeutic advantage over older and less expensive agents.

In addition to systemic therapy, T.E. should be instructed to keep the area clean with soap and water (if an open wound is present) and to protect the area.

Treatment for the Penicillin-Allergic Patient

2. What agents could be chosen if T.E. were allergic to penicillin?

Oral erythromycin (E-mycin) or clindamycin (Cleocin) could be chosen in patients with a documented history of penicillin or cephalosporin allergy. Erythromycin causes nausea, vomiting, diarrhea, and cramps in 30% to 40% of patients, but this can be decreased by taking it with food. Clindamycin causes diarrhea in 20% of patients and can cause serious toxicity secondary to pseudomembranous colitis. Erythromycin is much less expensive than clindamycin, and unless a patient has documented gastrointestinal (GI) intolerance to erythromycin, it is preferred over clindamycin. In addition, trimethoprim-sulfamethoxazole (Bactrim, Septra) has very good activity against Gram-positive organisms, and although it has not been significantly evaluated or compared against other antibiotics for soft tissue infections, it would be a useful inexpensive alternative in a patient with an allergy to penicillin.

Dosages of Antibiotics

3. What dose should be prescribed for T.E.?

The recommended dosages in the literature for cloxacillin (Tegopen, Cloxapen) and dicloxacillin (Dynapen) are 250 to 500 mg orally Q 6 hr and 125 to 250 mg orally Q 6 hr, respectively. Although lower dosages of dicloxacillin can be used, cloxacillin and dicloxacillin produce relatively similar free serum concentrations and should be prescribed at similar dosages. The dosage for mild to moderate infections should be 250 mg orally Q 6 hr; for moderate to severe infections, it should be 500 mg orally Q 6 hr. Dosages up to 1,000 mg orally Q 6 hr have been used, but GI intolerance (usually diarrhea) may occur. These dosages also apply to cephalexin and erythromycin. The dosage for Pen-V is 250 to 500 mg orally Q 6 hr; for oral clindamycin, the dosage is 150 to 450 mg orally Q 6 hr. Because cloxacillin is the drug chosen for T.E., a dosage of 250 mg orally Q 6 hr should be sufficient. However, if she were more severely ill, the higher dosage of 500 mg orally Q 6 hr could be chosen.

Treatment Duration

4. **For how long should T.E. be treated?**

The usual duration of therapy for cellulitis is 10 days, or 4 to 5 days after the patient has become afebrile and has improved clinically. T.E. should be counseled to expect a response within 1 to 2 days after therapy begins (although erythema may persist longer). In addition, she should be instructed to return for re-evaluation if the condition does not improve or worsens over the next few days.

Evaluation of Therapy

5. **What further diagnostic evaluation should be undertaken for T.E.?**

In otherwise healthy individuals, identification of the causative organism in cases of cellulitis is unnecessary. Needle aspiration, fine-needle aspiration biopsy, and punch biopsy have isolated the causative organism in only about 15% to 25% of patients.[3,4] Appropriate empiric treatment is effective in most patients, and an attempt to isolate the organism does not contribute to the success of treatment and adds significantly to the cost of care. Although organisms often are not cultured, attempts to identify the organism are recommended if initial treatment fails and when treating immunocompromised patients, patients with potential joint or tendon damage, and patients with life-threatening infections requiring hospitalization. In these cases, a swab of the primary wound and a needle aspiration or punch biopsy of the leading edge of the cellulitis should be obtained for Gram's stain and culture before initiating antimicrobial therapy. Blood for cultures should be drawn in addition to wound cultures in these patients. Anaerobic cultures need to be drawn only when the wound contains necrotic tissue, the wound is foul smelling, or crepitus is present. Even if wound and blood cultures are obtained, many infections will be culture negative (74%).[3] Culture information, in conjunction with clinical course, can be used to modify subsequent treatment. Because T.E. has only a moderate cellulitis, cultures are not required and therapy can be given empirically.

Role of Topical Antibiotics

6. **What role do topical antibiotics play in treating T.E.'s cellulitis?**

The value of topical antibiotics in treating skin infections is questionable. Most topical antibiotics have not been evaluated in appropriately designed trials. Although mupirocin produced positive bacteriologic results over placebo in treating some types of wound infections,[8,9] most of the studies showed no important clinical differences.[9] Mupirocin has been compared favorably to erythromycin and cloxacillin in the treatment of patients with impetigo, minor wound infections, and mild cellulitis; however, most cases of mild cellulitis will improve with only local wound care (e.g., cleansing or irrigation of the area). In patients with moderate to severe infections, mupirocin or any topical antibiotics (neomycin, bacitracin, polymyxin B) should not be used to replace or augment systemic antibiotics. Topical antibiotics likely do little but add to the cost of therapy, and they occasionally cause a contact dermatitis.[9] Therefore, T.E. should not be treated with topical antibiotics because her moderate cellulitis should be managed adequately by her systemic antimicrobial therapy.

Empiric Antibiotic Therapy for Moderate to Severe Cellulitis

7. **J.M., age 34, presents to the ED with a 3- to 4-day history of increasing pain around his left hip, secondary to an injury he received falling on the sidewalk. In addition, he has a fever and feels weak, lethargic, and nauseated. Examination reveals a swollen, warm, and extremely tender hip. J.M. has a temperature of 39.8°C and appears quite ill. A diagnosis of moderate to severe cellulitis is made, and J.M. is hospitalized because of the severity of the infection. J.M. has no other underlying medical problems. What empiric antibiotic regimen would be reasonable for J.M.?**

In moderate to severely ill patients, when hospitalization is required, antibiotics should be administered parenterally. The parenteral agent of choice is nafcillin (Nafcil, cloxacillin in Canada). Some clinicians add penicillin G (2 million units Q 6 hr) to nafcillin to ensure coverage against streptococcal organisms because the minimum inhibitory concentrations for penicillin against streptococci are lower than those with nafcillin. However, this "double coverage" is unnecessary if high-dose nafcillin (2 g intravenously [IV] Q 6 hr) is used. Cefazolin (2 g IV Q 8 hr) would be an appropriate alternative if it is less expensive than nafcillin. Second- and third-generation cephalosporins (cefuroxime [Zinacef], cefoxitin [Mefoxin], ceftriaxone [Rocephin], cefotaxime [Claforan]) and some quinolones may be as effective as nafcillin but provide no clinical advantages and are more expensive. Linezolid is also effective for the treatment of complicated skin and soft tissue infections, but it is no more effective than cloxacillin.[10]

Therefore, J.M. should receive either nafcillin or cefazolin, whichever is less expensive. Once J.M. has become afebrile and has clinically improved for 2 days, the parenteral antibiotic should be discontinued and appropriate oral therapy (cloxacillin) initiated to complete at least a 10-day course (2 weeks if the patient responds slowly).

Penicillin Allergy

8. **Two days after starting therapy, J.M. develops a maculopapular skin rash. What alternative therapy should be chosen?**

Regardless of when during the course of therapy a drug rash occurs (early or late), the precipitant drug should be discontinued because there is a chance, although small, that the reaction could worsen. In patients who develop a penicillin allergy and who still require parenteral therapy, clindamycin, erythromycin, vancomycin (Vancocin), or linezolid (Zyvoxam) could be chosen. Because all of these agents are equally effective, the decision of which drug to use in J.M. should be based on cost and dosing convenience (clindamycin 600 mg IV Q 8 hr, erythromycin 500 mg IV Q 6 hr, vancomycin 1,000 mg IV Q 12 hr, and linezolid 600 mg IV Q 12 hr). The administration of IV erythromycin is inconvenient because of its significant local irritative properties, and vancomycin, clindamycin, or linezolid is preferred for J.M. The choice between these agents should be based on cost.

Culture and Sensitivity Results

9. After 48 hours of therapy, culture and sensitivity results are available. What changes, if any, should be made in J.M.'s treatment?

If cultures show only streptococcal organisms, in a patient who is not allergic to penicillin, therapy should be switched to penicillin G because it is effective, well tolerated, and less expensive than nafcillin (Nafcil). If cultures show staphylococcal species (*S. aureus*) that are sensitive to methicillin, the initial empiric therapy should be continued. If the organisms are resistant to methicillin, therapy should be switched to vancomycin 15 mg/kg IV Q 12 hr or linezolid 600 mg IV Q 12 hr. The choice between these two agents should be based on oral bioavailability, side effect profile, and cost. Because J.M. has developed a presumed penicillin allergy, he should continue with his existing therapy of either clindamycin or vancomycin.

Switching to Oral Therapy

10. After 72 hours of therapy, J.M. has improved considerably and has been afebrile for 24 hours. Can he be switched to oral therapy?

Once J.M. has been afebrile for at least 24 hours and is virtually asymptomatic, other than some continuing tenderness around the site of the infection, oral therapy can replace IV therapy, assuming J.M. can tolerate oral medications. Although clinicians often switch to an oral version of the drug that was given parenterally, this may not always provide the patient with the most convenient and cost-effective therapy. Clinicians should select the oral agent on the basis of culture results, convenience, and cost.

Intravenous Drug Abuser

11. M.C., age 22, presents to the ED with a 3- to 4-day history of pain in her left forearm. On examination, she has a swollen and erythematous area of approximately 8 × 12 cm in the antecubital fossa of the left arm. The area is warm and tender to the touch. M.C. has a temperature of 39.2°C. She admits to injecting heroin daily; track marks are present on both arms. She states that she uses "filtered tap water" as a diluent for her narcotics and that her arm "has only been hurting for the last 3 days." There are no signs of lymphangitis or thrombophlebitis. What tests are needed to confirm the diagnosis?

M.C. has all the cardinal signs of cellulitis (i.e., induration, edema, erythema, and tenderness to touch). Given her history of an injury (injection), her presentation is compatible with cellulitis. No additional tests are required unless, on clinical examination, there is a suspicion of additional injury beyond the injection site or of a deeper infection (e.g., osteomyelitis). Obtaining a specimen from the infection site (by aspiration) to identify the organism(s) is unnecessary unless the patient has a concurrent condition that could impair her immunologic response.[4] The sensitivity of needle aspiration at the edge of the wound or at the site of greatest inflammation in identifying the infecting organism is only about 10%.[2] Therefore, aspiration of the wound is not warranted. The sensitivity of needle aspiration increases to 25% in patients with underlying immunologic dysfunction (e.g., diabetes, malignancy, poor peripheral circulation) and may be beneficial in identifying the infecting organism(s) in these patients.[4] Because M.C. gives no history of any disease that could impair her host defenses, needle aspiration is unnecessary. For patients such as M.C. with signs and symptoms (e.g., fever) where the injury is a significant risk for bacteremia and potentially for endocarditis, blood cultures are warranted. Blood cultures should be drawn before antibiotics are started to assess the presence of bacteria. If the blood cultures return positive, further assessment for potential endocarditis is warranted.

Causative Organisms

12. Are the suspected organisms in this patient population similar to those found in other patients with cellulitis?

A wide range of organisms can cause cellulitis in an IV drug abuser because of the potential for direct inoculation of any organism with the drug of abuse. Despite the efforts of an IV drug abuser to make as sterile an IV product as possible, the IV drug abuser commonly is injecting a contaminated solution. Although almost any organism can be found, the infecting bacteria causing cellulitis in an IV drug abuser are similar to those found in normal hosts. β-Hemolytic group A streptococci and staphylococci, particularly *S. aureus,* are the most common infecting organisms.[11,12] *Staphylococcus epidermidis* and Gram-negative organisms, including *P. aeruginosa,* are rarely the causative organisms unless the drug abuser has taken oral cephalexin concurrent with his or her injections, which is common in IV drug abusers.[11] In areas with a high prevalence of methicillin-resistant *S. aureus,* a similar resistance pattern may be seen in IV drug abusers with cellulitis.[13] Some investigators report a high incidence of anaerobic bacteria in cellulitis of IV drug abusers and hypothesize that these result from the transfer of oral flora.[14]

Empiric Antibiotic Therapy

Antibiotic therapy directed at eradicating all possible infecting organisms is not required. Because streptococci and staphylococci account for >94% of all infecting organisms in IV drug abusers with soft tissue infections,[11] therapy need cover only the sensitivity patterns of these organisms in the treatment area. Cloxacillin, dicloxacillin, or nafcillin is appropriate therapy (see Question 1). Oral therapy is appropriate for mild cases of cellulitis. Infections that involve a large area or that are associated with lymphangitis should be treated with parenteral antibiotics. Likewise, infections involving the hand should be treated parenterally.[15] If methicillin-resistant *S. aureus* is prevalent in the treatment area, antibiotic coverage should address this sensitivity pattern. Because there is no evidence to suggest that M.C. comes from an area where methicillin-resistant *S. aureus* is prevalent and because she has not taken cephalexin prophylactically, treatment with cloxacillin, dicloxacillin, or nafcillin is appropriate. If treatment does not result in some resolution of inflammation within 48 hours, antimicrobial coverage should be expanded to cover Gram-negative organisms. The anaerobic organisms found in IV drug abusers with cellulitis usually respond to treatment with penicillins or cephalosporins.[14]

For patients not responding to initial therapy and for patients with signs or symptoms of a systemic response (e.g., rigors, hypotension), parenteral nafcillin 2 g IV Q 6 hr, with gentamicin (Garamycin) 2 mg/kg Q 8 hr or 6 mg/kg IV Q 24 hr (assuming normal renal function), is appropriate empiric therapy. The combination of nafcillin with gentamicin provides coverage against the other common organisms causing cellulitis (i.e., *S. aureus, E. coli,* and *K. pneumoniae*). Although some clinicians suggest that a third-generation cephalosporin or a quinolone be chosen over an aminoglycoside because of concerns about toxicity, an aminoglycoside is effective, safe, and inexpensive when used for a short period (5 to 7 days).[16] However, in patients with poor renal function (estimated creatinine clearance <60 mL/min or 1 mL/sec), the aminoglycoside should be replaced with either ciprofloxacin (Cipro) 500 mg orally Q 12 hr (400 mg IV Q 12 hr if parenteral therapy is required) for moderate infections, or 750 mg orally Q 12 hr (400 mg IV Q 12 hr if parenteral therapy is required) for severe infections, or another quinolone such as gatifloxacin or levofloxacin, or a third-generation cephalosporin such as cefotaxime (Claforan) 1 g IV Q 8 hr (2 g IV Q 8 hr if severe) or ceftriaxone (Rocephin) 1 g IV Q 24 hr (2 g IV Q 24 hr if severe), whichever is the least expensive. The degree of dosage reduction or interval extension would be based on the degree of renal impairment.

Treatment of cellulitis in an IV drug abuser should include rest, immobilization and elevation of the infected arm, antibiotics, and surgical drainage or débridement as required. If any sign of pus collection in the wound is noted, the wound must be surgically explored and drained. If no area of pus collection can be seen or palpated, immobilization and elevation, combined with systemic antibiotic therapy, is appropriate treatment. The wound should be assessed daily for local tenderness, pain, erythema, swelling, ulceration, necrosis, and wound drainage until it shows signs of resolution to ensure that subsequent surgical treatment is not required.[15]

SOFT TISSUE INFECTIONS IN DIABETIC PATIENTS

Skin and soft tissue infections are common in patients with diabetes mellitus. Approximately 25% of diabetic patients report a history of skin and soft tissue infections,[17] and 5% to 15% of diabetic patients may undergo limb amputation.[18] In addition to the cost associated with treating skin and soft tissue infections, functional disability can occur, which can significantly decrease the quality of life.

Predisposing Factors

Diabetic patients are at particular risk for foot problems, primarily because of the neuropathies and peripheral vascular diseases associated with longstanding diabetes. The decreased pain sensation allows the patient to continue to bear weight in the presence of skin damage, thereby promoting the formation of an ulcer. In addition, minor trauma (e.g., cuts, foreign body insertion) may go unnoticed and, when left untreated, can become infected and extensive. Although these infections are common, preventive measures can reduce the frequency of amputations.[18]

Causative Organisms

13. **P.U., a 67-year-old man with diabetes, presents to his general practitioner for a routine checkup and has no specific complaints. P.U. has a 15-year history of poorly controlled type 2 diabetes and a 3-year history of recurrent foot ulcers. On examination, the physician sees that one ulcer on the underside of the foot, which had previously healed over, is open and inflamed; purulent fluid can be expressed from the wound. P.U. reports no pain around the area and was unaware that the ulcer had worsened. His temperature is normal, and he shows no other signs of a systemic infection. Does P.U. have an active infection, and is antibiotic therapy required?**

All open wounds, in diabetic and nondiabetic patients, will become colonized with bacteria, but only infected wounds should be treated with antibiotic therapy.[19] It often is difficult to determine whether an open wound is infected, but signs and symptoms such as purulent drainage, erythema, pain, and swelling around the area are suggestive of infection. Based on his symptoms, P.U. should be considered to have an infection that requires treatment.

Empiric Antibiotic Therapy

14. What treatment should P.U. receive?

Mild infections can be treated empirically like other soft tissue infections[19] because these are commonly caused by aerobic Gram-positive cocci. A penicillinase-resistant penicillin (e.g., cloxacillin, nafcillin) will be effective in most cases. However, a culture of either the drainage or the infected site should be obtained to help guide future treatment. Other potentially useful oral agents for mild infections include cephalexin or cotrimoxazole. The choice between these agents should be based on allergy status and cost. If anaerobes are suspected, metronidazole or clindamycin should be added to the regimen. In addition, for all diabetic patients with soft tissue infections, osteomyelitis must be ruled out. In patients with significant vascular compromise, crepitus, or gangrene, a radiograph should be taken to identify any bone involvement.

In moderate to severe infections, antibiotic coverage should be expanded because multiple organisms may be responsible for the infection. An average of two to six organisms are cultured from foot ulcers in patients with diabetes. The following organisms (in no particular order) are found in >20% of wounds in patients with diabetes: *S. aureus, S. epidermidis, Enterococcus faecalis,* other streptococci, *Proteus* species, *E. coli, Klebsiella* species, *Peptococcus* species, *Peptostreptococcus* species, and *Bacteroides* species.[19] These infections are often polymicrobial, but treatment can be effective even if not all cultured pathogens are covered.[19] To determine the pathogens most accurately, a specimen of infected tissue should be obtained that is not directly communicating with an ulcer. If this is not possible, cultures of purulent exudate or curettage should be obtained, versus superficial swab, to determine the true pathogens in the wound.[20] Although antibiotics are important, drainage and surgical débridement to remove all the infected or necrotic tissue are essential and are considered by some to be the mainstay of treatment.[19]

Cultures of the affected areas may not be that useful unless bone involvement is suspected. Although anaerobic organisms often are difficult to culture, anaerobic organisms must be considered if an abscess or devitalized, necrotic, foul-smelling tissue is present or the wound is a result of abdominal surgery. Empiric coverage for *E. faecalis* is required only for severe (necrotizing) infections Even if enterococci are found in the wound, enterococcal coverage probably is needed only if it is the predominant organism.

There are no "best" regimens for the treatment of diabetic soft tissue infections. Clindamycin 600 mg IV Q 8 hr with ciprofloxacin 400 mg or a third-generation cephalosporin is a very effective combination that will provide coverage against most potential pathogens (Gram-positive, Gram-negative, and anaerobes), with the exception of *E. faecalis.* However, clindamycin can cause *Clostridium difficile* associate diarrhea, and the parenteral formulation is expensive. Aminoglycosides are associated with serious toxicity if used for an extended period and should probably be avoided in diabetic patients with pre-existing renal impairment. A β-lactam/β-lactamase inhibitor combination such as piperacillin and tazobactam (Tazocin), or ticarcillin/clavulanic acid or ampicillin/sulbactam provides similar coverage but also adds coverage against enterococci and could be chosen over other combinations if it is less expensive.

Other single-agent therapies could include the use of a carbapenem (imipenem or meropenem), but the increased cost of these agents should limit use to patients unresponsive to other therapies.

In many cases, diabetic foot infections are difficult to treat, but aggressive treatment can prevent extension of the infection, development of osteomyelitis, and on occasion loss of limb. Treatment should be continued for 3 to 4 days after all signs of infection are absent. Oral therapy should be considered once the infection has begun to improve. Because P.U. is an elderly diabetic patient and does not appear to be severely ill, the least expensive of a ciprofloxacin/clindamycin or piperacillin/tazobactam, cefoxitin, cefotetan, ceftizoxime, or cefmetazole should be chosen as empiric therapy. In addition, ampicillin and sulbactam (Unasyn) or ticarcillin and clavulanate (Timentin) could be chosen if it is less expensive than the aforementioned agents or if local sensitivity patterns suggest that organisms typically found in these types of infections are routinely resistant to the other less expensive agents. The broad spectrum of carbapenems (e.g., imipenem, meropenem) may appear desirable, but frequent use contributes to isolation in individual patients and patient populations of more resistant pathogens, such as *Stenotrophomonas.* Their use should be limited when possible.

Postamputation Antibiotic Treatment

15. Unfortunately, despite aggressive antibiotic therapy and débridement, P.U.'s infection spreads and an amputation is required. How long should antibiotics be prescribed following surgery in P.U.?

The best option for uncontrollable, life-threatening infections often is amputation to remove the infected area. Once the infected area has been removed, antibiotic therapy is no longer required. However, if it was impossible to remove all of the infected tissue, treatment should be continued as just described.

Prevention

16. What could have been done to prevent this complication in P.U.?

Many of the foot problems associated with diabetes can be prevented with proper foot care (Table 67-2),[18] and these preventive measures must be stressed. Diabetic patients with neuropathies or those who are elderly should take care of their feet regularly (every 1 to 2 days).

NECROTIZING SOFT TISSUE INFECTIONS
Definitions, Terminology, and Causative Organisms

Skin and soft tissue infections are described as *necrotizing* when the inflammation is rapidly progressing and necrosis of the skin or underlying tissue is present. The following clinical signs are associated with necrotizing infections, but not with simple cellulitis: edema beyond the area of erythema, skin blisters or bullae, localized pallor or discoloration, gas in the subcutaneous tissues (crepitus), and the absence of lymphangitis and lymphadenitis. Necrotizing soft tissue infections may progress rapidly to cause additional local effects (i.e., necrosis and loss of skin sensation) and severe systemic effects (e.g., hypotension, shock).

Group A β-hemolytic streptococci, *Pseudomonas,* other Gram-negative organisms, *Clostridium perfringens,* peptostreptococci, *B. fragilis,* and *Vibrio* species can cause necrotizing infections.[1]

Necrotizing cellulitis involves the skin and subcutaneous tissues. Necrotizing fasciitis involves both superficial and deep fascia, and necrotizing infections involving the muscle are termed *myonecrosis.* These terms can be used to describe all three of these processes. Gas gangrene is myonecrosis caused by a *Clostridium* subspecies, most commonly *C. perfringens* (70%).[1] Gas in a wound is not necessarily indicative of gas gangrene caused by *C. perfringens.* Gram-negative organisms (e.g., *E. coli, Proteus, Klebsiella*), or anaerobic streptococci can produce gas in a wound. Air also could have been introduced at the time of the injury. Gas gangrene is charac-

Table 67-2	**Foot Care for the Diabetic Patient**

- Inspect feet daily for cuts, blisters, or scratches. Pay particular attention to the area between the toes and use a mirror to examine the bottom of the foot.
- Wash feet daily in tepid water and dry thoroughly.
- Apply lotion to feet to prevent calluses and cracking.
- Ensure that shoes fit properly (not too tight or too loose), and inspect them daily.
- Trim nails regularly, making sure to cut straight across the nail.
- Do not use chemical agents to remove corns or calluses.

terized by acute onset of worsening pain that is usually out of proportion to the degree of injury.

Clostridial myonecrosis (true gas gangrene), streptococcal gangrene (caused by group A β-hemolytic streptococci), and synergistic bacterial gangrene (caused by anaerobic and aerobic bacteria, usually Gram-negative) are other terms used to describe necrotizing skin and soft tissue infections. Fournier's gangrene (a type of synergistic bacterial gangrene of the scrotum), nonclostridial crepitant gangrene (nonclostridial gas gangrene), and necrotizing fasciitis (all necrotizing soft tissue infections other than clostridial myonecrosis, or sometimes just streptococcal gangrene) are other commonly used terms.[1]

Empiric Antibiotic Therapy

17. M.T., a 45-year-old alcoholic man who lives on the streets of the city, presents to the ED with a broken nose and facial lacerations, which he received after a fight outside one of the local taverns. On examination, in addition to the facial wounds, an area of severe inflammation, erythema, and necrosis is found on his left calf. The area is very painful, crepitation is felt over the area, and a purulent discharge is present. M.T. states this is secondary to a knife wound he suffered approximately 1 week ago. What treatment should be provided?

In addition to setting the broken nose and suturing the facial lacerations, the clinician should evaluate the infection on M.T.'s calf. A Gram's stain and culture of the purulent discharge should be evaluated before initiating antimicrobial therapy. Because crepitus is present, the area should be incised and a specimen of the infected tissue should be obtained for Gram's staining and culture.[1]

The primary treatment for necrotizing soft tissue infections involves extensive débridement of the area to remove all necrotic tissue and drain the area. Thus, a surgical consultation will be required for M.T. In addition, IV antibiotics are required. In this case, gas in the tissues could be caused by many organisms, and empiric antibiotic therapy should be broad spectrum and should include coverage against Gram-positive organisms, the Enterobacteriaceae, and *B. fragilis*. Clindamycin and penicillin plus gentamicin is appropriate empiric therapy for M.T. If aminoglycosides were contraindicated, cefoxitin, ceftizoxime, cefotetan, or cefmetazole would likely suffice in the mild to moderately ill patient. Penicillin G (3 million units Q 4 hr) should be added to this regimen to provide additional coverage against *C. perfringens*. If the Gram's stain of the discharge shows only Gram-positive rods (which would likely be clostridial subspecies), the therapy could be streamlined to high-dose penicillin.

Recently, a number of cases of "flesh-eating disease" have been reported in the press. Flesh-eating disease is usually a necrotizing fasciitis caused by virulent strains of group A streptococci. High-dose penicillin G (3 million units Q 4 hr) plus clindamycin (900 mg IV Q 8 hr) are the drugs of choice for this condition.[21,22] There are few, if any, clinical trials to guide antibiotic selection. This combination is recommended because certain penicillin-binding proteins may not be expressed by streptococci during certain phases, which may be the reason for the occasional failure of penicillin to treat these infections. Although there are only experimental model data, clindamycin is more effective in fulminant streptococcal in-

fections, potentially because it inhibits protein synthesis. Clindamycin may have adjunctive activities that contribute to reduced morbidity from Gram-positive pathogens. In vitro evidence suggests that clindamycin suppresses toxin production by *S. aureus* isolates.[22]

Adjunctive therapy for streptococcal necrotizing skin infections could include IV immunoglobulin G (IVIG) 2 g/kg as a single dose or 0.4 mg/kg daily for 2 days.[23–25] IVIG is thought to work by binding to the superantigens released by the streptococcal bacteria that are involved in the systemic effects of the infection. The optimal dosage and duration of IVIG therapy are unknown, as is the response to the variability between commercial lots of IVIG products.

Therapy for necrotizing fasciitis should be altered based on the patient's clinical response and culture results.

ERYSIPELAS

Signs, Symptoms, and Causative Organisms

18. D.D., a 70-year-old man, presents to the ED with a red, swollen face. He describes the area as "a swollen red spot" that has appeared over the past 2 days. He also describes feeling unwell for the previous 3 days and having a fever. On examination, D.D. has a bright red, shiny, edematous lesion on his right cheek that is 0.4 cm wide. It is a continuous lesion with a clearly demarcated border. What signs and symptoms support the diagnosis of erysipelas in D.D.?

Erysipelas is a superficial skin infection caused by streptococci, predominantly group A, although groups C or G and group B in children also may cause the infection.[26] Erysipelas is diagnosed based on characteristics of the skin lesion and concurrent systemic symptoms.[26] Patients with erysipelas have associated systemic symptoms of high fever, chills, frequent history of rigors, and general malaise. This constellation of systemic symptoms differentiates erysipelas from other local skin disorders. The lesion is a continuous, indurated, edematous area, and the most common site of infection is the face. Early in the course, the lesion is bright red, but it may turn to brown as the lesion ages or grows. The lesion spreads peripherally with no islands of unaffected tissue. The initial lesion results from a small break in the skin that becomes infected, although signs of the initial wound often are not evident. The streptococci may originate from a prodromal respiratory infection, although culture of the respiratory tract at the time of the lesion eruption will rarely produce positive cultures.

D.D. has the classic signs and symptoms of erysipelas: a well-demarcated, edematous, red lesion with associated systemic signs. No further diagnostic tests are required because aspiration of the lesion or a superficial swab is not useful in detecting the offending organism.

Empiric Antibiotic Therapy

19. What antibiotic therapy should be initiated for D.D.?

Erysipelas will respond promptly to antibiotics with activity against group A streptococci.[26] Oral penicillin V 250 to 300 mg (depending on available dosage form) Q 6 hr or parenteral penicillin G (1 million units IV Q 6 hr) should reduce the systemic symptoms (e.g., fever, malaise) within 24 to 48 hours.[26] It will take several more days for the skin lesion to resolve. If D.D. does not feel better within 72 hours after initiation of antibiotics, he should be instructed to return for reassessment. If D.D. has an allergy to penicillins, a macrolide such as erythromycin is also effective. Antibiotic therapy should be continued for 10 days even if signs and symptoms resolve quickly to avoid a relapse, which could lead to chronic infection or scarring.

ACUTE TRAUMATIC WOUNDS

20. J.K., a 25-year-old construction worker, presents to the ED with a deep cut on his left forearm suffered when he accidentally put his hand through a plate glass window. Fourteen stitches are required to close the wound. Is oral antibiotic therapy required for J.K.?

Although almost all traumatic wounds are contaminated with bacteria,[27] routine oral antibiotic therapy is not indicated unless there is evidence of an infection. Contaminated wounds do become infected more often than noncontaminated wounds, but prophylactic antibiotic therapy does not appear to decrease the chance of infection.[27] For all traumatic wounds, aggressive wound care (e.g., irrigation, removal of foreign objects) is required. A meta-analysis of randomized trials of prophylactic antibiotics in patients presenting to an ED for nonbite wounds suggested that there is no evidence that oral antibiotics protect against infection.[28] A course of antibiotic therapy should be given only to immunocompromised patients (e.g., those with diabetes mellitus, peripheral vascular disease, HIV/AIDS, chronic corticosteroid use, leukopenia). Other potential candidates for antibiotic therapy include wounds with pus, contamination by feces, and delays in cleansing (>3 hours) of the wound.[29] Antibiotic therapy would be similar to that given for cellulitis (see Question 1). Patients with risk factors for the development of infective endocarditis (i.e., mitral valve prolapse with regurgitation, an indwelling nonnative cardiac valve, a previous history of endocarditis, a history of congenital heart malformations, surgically constructed systemic-pulmonary shunts, and cardiomyopathy) should receive prophylactic amoxicillin (Amoxil) 3 g orally followed by 1.5 g in 6 hours or erythromycin 1,000 mg orally followed by 500 mg orally in 6 hours if the patient is penicillin allergic.[30] Because J.K. has no risk factors, all that is required is removal of any glass fragments, irrigation, and suturing of the area.

21. K.M., a 7-year-old boy, presents 30 minutes after falling and scraping his elbow on the pavement. The father requests an antibiotic ointment for the wound. You look at his elbow and notice a 1-inch square mildly abraded area. What treatment would you recommend?

All minor injuries such as scratches, cuts, and abrasions should be thoroughly cleaned with soap and water. The evidence on the use of a topical antibiotic as a preventive measure is contradictory. Placebo was compared with povidone ointment and a topical antibiotic combination (cetrimide/bacitracin/polymyxin) in children with minor dermatologic injuries.[31] The incidence of clinical infection was significantly different in placebo (12.5%) versus the topical antibiotic group (1.6%). There was no difference in the incidence of clinical infection between povidone and the topical antibiotic group. In addition, there was no significant difference between any of the preparations in the incidence of microbiologic infections. A randomized, double-blind, prospective trial comparing white petrolatum with bacitracin ointment in wound care following dermatologic surgery showed no difference between the groups in the incidence of wound infection.[32] Some patients can develop skin sensitivities to topical antibiotics. K.M.'s wound should be thoroughly washed and inspected, but a topical antibiotic ointment would not be required.

ANIMAL BITE WOUNDS

Evaluation of Dog and Cat Bites

22. P.J., a 14-year-old boy, presents to the ED 3 hours after being bitten on the leg by a neighbor's dog. He has a laceration, 14 cm long, on his medial calf. Four distinct puncture marks, suggestive of teeth marks, also are present on the calf. There is no suggestion of bone injury. P.J. was healthy before the attack and has no chronic illness. Should P.J. receive any treatment other than suturing of his laceration?

Any wound caused by an animal that results in the skin being cut or punctured should be examined to ensure no underlying tissue damage has occurred. This is especially true in patients with bites of the hand or around other joints. The wound should be washed with clean water as soon as possible after the bite.[33] Irrigation of the wound, including puncture sites, should be extensive to reduce the risk of infection. Obtaining specimens for cultures is not required and wound irrigation should begin as soon as possible.[33]

P.J.'s wound should be evaluated for deep tissue injury, devascularization of any tissue, and bone injury.[33] Loose suturing or closure with adhesive strips is appropriate for lacerations following irrigation.[33] Although the safety of closure of bite wounds has been debated, a good therapeutic response has been obtained following the closure of wounds.[34] P.J. should be instructed to keep his leg elevated and immobilized until signs of any infection have resolved.[35]

The need for antibiotics is controversial and guided by wound characteristics. The patient should receive a course of antibiotics[36] if the wound involves the hand or is near joints,[33] involves deep punctures or is difficult to irrigate, if the patient is immunocompromised (e.g., diabetes, splenectomy), or if the wound is not well perfused. Antibiotics are not required for dog bites in which no deep tissue injury is present and the wound can be well irrigated, particularly if the wound is on the lower extremities in healthy adults or children.[37]

Prophylaxis for rabies is required only if the animal is from an area with endemic rabies or if the bite was the result of an unprovoked attack by a wild animal.[33,35,38] Contact the local health board to determine the recent rabies risk in the area. If P.J. has not received a tetanus toxoid booster within the past 5 years, a booster should be administered. If P.J. has never been immunized for tetanus, tetanus immune globulin should be administered in addition to the tetanus toxoid (see Question 26).[38]

Causative Organisms and Empiric Antibiotic Therapy

23. Because P.J. has several punctures that are difficult to irrigate, he is a candidate for antibiotic therapy. Which antibiotic(s) should he receive?

The selection of the appropriate antibiotic is based on the most likely pathogens from the specific animal bite. Animals have different oral flora, which alters the potential pathogens associated with bites. The most common pathogens in dog bites are β-hemolytic streptococci, *S. aureus, Pasteurella multocida,* anaerobic bacteria (particularly *Bacteroides* species), and *Fusobacterium* species.[38] Although *P. multocida* often is considered the primary pathogen of dog bites, it occurs in only 25% of infections; therefore, antibiotic coverage also must address the other common pathogens.[38] A combination of penicillin V 500,000 IU orally Q 6 hr with a penicillinase-resistant drug such as dicloxacillin or cloxacillin 500 mg orally Q 6 hr will provide coverage for the predominant organisms in dog bites. The more expensive alternative of amoxicillin-clavulanate (Augmentin) has not been demonstrated to be superior to the combination of cloxacillin and penicillin V.[39] If the patient is allergic to penicillin, tetracycline or doxycycline provides adequate coverage. Doxycycline is preferred over tetracycline because it is more convenient to administer (twice daily for doxycycline versus four times a day for tetracycline), can be used in patients with decreased renal function, may be taken with food, and is only a little more expensive (in the generic form) than tetracycline.

If the penicillin-allergic patient cannot take a tetracycline, a fluoroquinolone, such as levofloxacin 500 mg PO daily, could be used. In all cases, patients should be instructed to watch for a positive response; if the wound does not improve or worsens within 48 hours, the patient will need to be re-evaluated.

Antibiotic treatment should not extend beyond 5 days unless signs of an infection remain.[33] Appropriate therapy for P.J. would be penicillin V and a penicillinase-resistant penicillin (e.g., dicloxacillin or cloxacillin) orally.

For cat bites, the role of *P. multocida* appears more significant because this organism can be found in the oral flora of up to 75% of cats. Although antibiotic treatment is not required for some dog bites, reports of a >50% incidence of infection after cat bites[35] suggest that all patients with cat bites should receive antibiotics. Because *P. multocida* often is resistant to penicillinase-resistant penicillins and first-generation cephalosporins, use of these agents in cat bites should be avoided. Either the combination of penicillin plus a penicillinase-resistant penicillin or amoxicillin-clavulanate is appropriate for cat bites, and the choice between these regimens should be based on cost.

If the patient presents with an established infection, parenteral therapy is warranted if the infection is over a joint, has lymphatic spread, or involves the hand or head. If the patient has not responded to oral therapy, parenteral second-generation cephalosporins such as cefoxitin 1 g IV Q 6 hr, cefotetan 1 g IV Q 12 hr, or ceftizoxime or cefmetazole 1 g IV Q 8 hr have activity against *P. multocida,* streptococci, staphylococci, and anaerobes.[35] The value of parenteral administration of clindamycin or erythromycin is limited by poor activity against *P. multocida.*[3,35] The poor activity of quinolones against anaerobes has limited their use, despite good activity against *P. multocida.*[40] Parenteral therapy should be continued until resolution of the wound is evident, and therapy should then be continued with oral antibiotics. Treatment should continue for at least 7 days or until all clinical signs of the infection have resolved.

HUMAN BITE WOUNDS

Evaluation of Human Bites

24. **E.D., a 40-year-old man, presents with a sore arm 24 hours after receiving a bite to his left forearm by his neighbor in a "discussion over property boundaries." E.D. was previously healthy and has no chronic diseases. A 6 ×8-cm area of his left forearm is swollen and erythematous and includes several distinct puncture marks consistent with a human bite. No joint deformity or bone abnormality is detected on clinical examination. How should E.D. be treated?**

Treating a human bite is similar to any other laceration and includes cleansing, irrigating, exploring, débriding, draining, excising, and suturing as required.[38,41] All human bites should be cleansed as soon as possible, and any lacerations or punctures irrigated copiously. Surgical exploration with débridement, drainage, or excision should be undertaken if deeper tissues may have been injured or if pus collection could have occurred. Exploration for damage to subcutaneous nerves, tendons, joints, or vascularity is particularly important in bites to the hand, especially the knuckles, because subsequent infections could seriously affect hand function. Because E.D. presents 24 hours after the injury, thorough exploration and irrigation of all lacerations or punctures is required. If there is evidence of pus accumulation in his wound, the area should be explored and drained. E.D. also should receive systemic antibiotic therapy to eradicate potential infecting organisms. Tetanus toxoid booster should be administered if E.D. has not received a booster in the past 10 years.

Empiric Antibiotic Therapy and Causative Organisms

25. Which antibiotic should be prescribed for E.D.?

If E.D. had been seen within 12 hours of the injury, the wound could likely have been treated adequately with simple irrigation. This is especially true if the human bite does not involve the hand.[37] If the hand has been bitten or the patient is immunocompromised, a course of antibiotics using oral agents is appropriate.

If the wound is severe (i.e., involves subcutaneous tissues, a joint, or a large area) or if the patient is unlikely to be compliant with oral antibiotics, parenteral administration of antibiotics is required.[33] The most common pathogens in human bites are β-hemolytic streptococci, *S. aureus, Eikenella corrodens,* and *Corynebacterium* subspecies.[38] Anaerobic bacteria, including *Bacteroides* subspecies, also are commonly involved.[38] Treatment with a combination of penicillin G and a penicillinase-resistant penicillin is appropriate.[38] Therapy with a penicillinase-resistant penicillin or a first-generation cephalosporin alone is not appropriate because *E. corrodens* commonly is resistant to these antibiotics.[35,40] If the anaerobic flora of the patient's community is often resistant to penicillin, alternative anaerobic coverage with amoxicillin-clavulanate may be required.[38] If parenteral therapy is required, a second-generation cephalosporin with antianaerobic activity (e.g., cefoxitin, cefotetan, ceftizoxime) is appropriate.[38] Cefuroxime should not be used as single-agent therapy because it lacks activity against anaerobes and *E. corrodens.*[40] Third-generation cephalosporins and quinolones have good activity against

E. corrodens, but they cannot be recommended because of their inferior activity against anaerobic organisms.[35] Fluoroquinolones, such as levofloxacin or moxifloxacin, have good activity against the organisms of bite infections, with the exception of poor activity against *Fusobacterium* species.[42] Azithromycin is the macrolide with the best activity against bite organisms.[43]

TETANUS PROPHYLAXIS

26. G.T., a 48-year-old woman, presents to the ED 1 hour after receiving a 2-cm laceration to her foot from stepping on a nail while walking around her neighborhood. Examination of the wound found it to be clean, with no subcutaneous extension. The wound was closed with superficial sutures, and no antibiotics, systemic or topical, were prescribed. Should G.T. receive tetanus prophylaxis?

Tetanus is a preventable disease through primary prophylaxis and appropriate wound management. Every child should receive primary prophylaxis of three separate doses of tetanus toxoid. This provides adequate coverage for at least 10 years.[44] Tetanus can develop in patients who have not been immunized or who have not received a booster dose within the past 10 years. If G.T. has received her primary tetanus immunization and had a booster dose within the previous 10 years, no additional tetanus prophylaxis is required for her wound (Table 67-3). If her primary immunization status is unknown or >10 years has elapsed since her last dose, a single 0.5-mL subcutaneous tetanus toxoid dose should be administered. If primary immunization is unknown or incomplete, G.T. should receive the initial 0.5-mL dose immediately and should be scheduled to complete the primary immunization over the next 2 months. For adults, the combination product of tetanus and diphtheria toxoid is the recommended treatment because this will enhance protection against diphtheria.

If G.T. had presented with a dirty wound (contaminated with dirt, feces, soil, or saliva) or if the wound had resulted from a burn, frostbite, missile (bullet), crush, or avulsion, she should receive passive tetanus immunization with tetanus immune globulin in addition to the tetanus toxoid described above. A single 250-U intramuscular dose of tetanus immune globulin will provide passive immunization in addition to the active immunization produced from exposure to the tetanus toxoid (see Table 67-3).

Table 67-3 Tetanus Prophylaxis in Routine Wound Management: Adults[41]

History of Adsorbed Tetanus Toxoid	Clean, Minor Wounds		All Other Wounds[a]	
	Td[b]	TIG	Td[b]	TIG
Unknown or <3 doses	Yes	No	Yes	Yes
≥3 doses	No[c]	No	Yes[d]	No

[a]Including, but not limited to, wounds contaminated with dirt, feces, soil, and saliva, puncture wounds, avulsions, and wounds resulting from missiles, crushing, burns, frostbite.
[b]For children <7 years old, diphtheria-tetanus-pertussis (DTP) is preferred to tetanus toxoid alone. For persons ≥7 years, Td is preferred to tetanus toxoid alone.
[c]Yes, if >10 years since last dose.
[d]Yes, if >5 years since last dose. (More frequent boosters are not needed and can accentuate the side effects.)
Td, tetanus and diphtheria toxoid; TIG, tetanus immune globulin.

REFERENCES

1. Lewis RT. Necrotizing soft tissue infections. Infect Dis Clin North Am 1992;6:693.
2. Sachs MK. Cutaneous cellulitis. Arch Dermatol 1991;127:493.
3. Hook EW et al. Microbiologic evaluation of cutaneous cellulitis in adults. Arch Intern Med 1986; 146:295.
4. Sachs MK. The optimum use of needle aspiration in the bacteriologic diagnosis of cellulitis in adults. Arch Intern Med 1990;150:1907.
5. Sutherland R et al. Flucloxacillin, a new isoxazolyl penicillin, compared with oxacillin, cloxacillin, and dicloxacillin. Br Med J 1970;4:455.
6. Critchley IA et al. Antimicrobial susceptibilities of *Streptococcus pyogenes* isolated from respiratory and skin and soft tissue infections. Diagnostic Microbiol Infect Dis 2002;42:129.
7. Powers RD. Soft tissue infections in the emergency department: the case for the use of simple antibiotics. South Med J 1991;84:1313.
8. Stevens DL et al. Randomised comparison of linezolid (PNU-100766) versus oxacillin-dicloxacillin for treatment of complicated skin and soft tissue infections. Antimicrob Agents Chemotherapy 2000; 44:3408.
9. Ward A, Campoli-Richards DM. Mupirocin: a review of its antibacterial activity, pharmacokinetic properties and therapeutic use. Drugs 1986;32:425.
10. Hirschmann JV. Topical antibiotics in dermatology. Arch Dermatol 1988;124:1691.
11. Beaufoy A. Infections in intravenous drug users: a two-year review. Can J Infect Control 1993;8:7.
12. Orangio GR et al. Soft tissue infections in parenteral drug abusers. Ann Surg 1984;199:97. 15

13. Sheagren JN. Treatment of skin and skin infections in the patient at risk. Am J Med 1984;76(5B):180.
14. Bergstein JM et al. Soft tissue abscesses associated with parenteral drug abuse: presentation, microbiology, and treatment. Am Surg 1995;61:1105.
15. Hausman MR, Lisser SP. Hand infections. Orthop Clin North Am 1992;23:171.
16. McCormack JP, Jewesson PJ. A critical reevaluation of the therapeutic range of the aminoglycosides. Clin Infect Dis 1992;14:320.
17. LeFrock JL, Joseph WS. Lower extremity infections in diabetics. Infect Surg 1986;5:135.
18. Most RS, Sinnock P. The epidemiology of lower extremity infections in diabetic individuals. Diabetes Care 1983;6:87.
19. Cunha BA. Antibiotic selection for diabetic foot infections: a review. J Ankle Foot Surg 2000;39:253.
20. Committee of Antimicrobial Agents. Management of diabetic foot infections: a position paper. Can J Infect Dis 1996;7:361.
21. Bisno AL, Stevens DL. Streptococcal infections of skin and soft tissues. N Engl J Med 1996;334:240.
22. Seal DV. Necrotizing fasciitis. Curr Opin Infect Dis 2001;14:127.
23. Perez CM et al. Adjunctive treatment of streptococcal toxic shock syndrome using intravenous immunoglobulin: case report and review. Am J Med 1997;102:111.
24. Kaul R et al. Intravenous immunoglobulin therapy for streptococcal toxic shock syndrome: a comparative observational study. Clin Infect Dis. 1999; 28:800.
25. Cawley MJ et al. Intravenous immunoglobulin as adjunctive treatment for streptococcal toxic shock

syndrome associated with necrotizing fasciitis: case report and review. Pharmacotherapy 1999;19:1094.
26. Eriksson B et al. Erysipelas: clinical and bacteriologic spectrum and serological aspects. Clin Infect Dis 1996;23:1091.
27. Langford JH et al. Topical antimicrobial therapy in minor wounds. Ann Pharmacother 1997;31:559.
28. Rodgers KG. The rational use of antimicrobial agents in simple wounds. Emerg Med Clin North Am 1992;10:753.
29. Cummings P, Del Beccaro MA. Antibiotics to prevent infection of simple wounds: a meta-analysis of randomised studies. Am J Emerg Med 1995;13:396.
30. Eron LJ. Targeting lurking pathogens in acute traumatic and chronic wounds. J Emerg Med 1999; 17:189.
31. Dajani AS et al. Prevention of bacterial endocarditis: recommendations by the American Heart Association. JAMA 1990;264:2919.
32. Smack DP et al. Infection and allergy incidence in ambulatory surgery patients using white petrolatum vs bacitracin ointment. JAMA 1996;276:972.
33. Anderson CR. Animal bites. Guidelines to current management. Postgrad Med J 1992;92:134.
34. Medeiros I, Saconato H. Antibiotic prophylaxis for mammalian bites. Cochrane Database of Systematic reviews. 2002; issue 4
35. Goldstein EJ. Bite wounds and infection. Clin Infect Dis 1992;14:633.
36. Dire DJ. Emergency management of dog and cat bite wounds. Emerg Med Clin North Am 1992; 10:719.
37. Higgins MAG et al. Managing animal bite wounds. J Wound Care 1997;6:377.

38. Griego RD et al. Dog, cat, and human bites: a review. J Am Acad Dermatol 1995;33:1019.

39. Smith PF et al. Treating mammalian bite wounds. J Clin Pharm Ther 2000;25:85.

40. Goldstein EJ, Citron DM. Comparative susceptibilities of 173 aerobic and anaerobic bite wound isolates to sparfloxacin, temafloxacin, clarithromycin, and older agents. Antimicrob Agents Chemother 1993;37:1150.

41. Bunzli WF et al. Current management of human bites. Pharmacotherapy 1998;18:227.

42. Goldstein EJC et al. Comparative in vitro activities of azithromycin, Bay y3118, levofloxacin, sparfloxacin, and 11 other oral antimicrobial agents against 194 aerobic and anaerobic bite wound isolates. Antimicrob Agent Chemother 1995;39:1097.

43. Goldstein EJC et al. Activities of HMR3004, and HMR3647 compared to those of erythromycin, azithromycin, clarithromycin, roxithromycin and eight other antimicrobial agents against unusual aerobic and anaerobic human and animal bite pathogens isolated from skin and soft tissue infections in humans. Antimicrob Agent Chemother 1998;42:1127.

44. Advisory Committee on Immunization Practices, CDC. Diphtheria, tetanus, and pertussis: guidelines for vaccine use and other preventative measures. MMWR 1991;40:(RR10).

CHAPTER 68

Prevention and Treatment of Infections in Neutropenic Cancer Patients

Richard H. Drew

Many patients with malignancy have had their lives prolonged through therapeutic advances in chemotherapy, immunotherapy, and bone marrow transplantation. Despite such advances, infectious complications continue to be a major cause of morbidity and mortality in these patients, often replacing the primary disease as the leading cause of death.[1] While newer broad-spectrum antimicrobial agents and chemotherapeutic agents have altered the frequency and types of infectious complications in patients with both solid and hematologic malignancies, the management of infections in immunocompromised hosts remains a major challenge to health care professionals.

This chapter focuses on the prevention, diagnosis, and management of infectious complications in patients with neutropenia secondary to cancer chemotherapy. The following topics are addressed: principles of prophylactic antimicro-

bials, empiric antibiotic selection in the febrile patient, modification and duration of therapy, monotherapy versus combination regimens, empiric antifungal and antiviral use, and the use of myeloid colony-stimulating factors.

RISK FACTORS FOR INFECTION

Patients are rendered "immunocompromised" when there is a significant disruption or deficiency of one of the host defenses as a result of the underlying disease or chemotherapy. These risk factors include neutropenia, iatrogenic damage to skin and mucosal barriers, and impairment in both humoral (antibody and complement) and cell-mediated immune defenses. Bacteria, fungi, viruses, and protozoa may infect various sites, depending on the specific immunodeficiency (Table 68-1).

Neutropenia

Granulocytes, or granular leukocytes, represent an important defense against bacterial and fungal infections. *Neutropenia* (a reduction in the number of circulating granulocytes or

Acknowledgment: The author would like to acknowledge Dr. Hiliary D. Mandler, the author of this chapter in the previous edition. Some of her work remains in this edition.

Table 68-1   Most Common Pathogens Causing Infections in Neutropenic Cancer Patients

Immunologic Defect	Underlying Condition(s)	Pathogen(s)			
		Bacteria	Fungi	Parasites	Viruses
Neutropenia	Cancer chemotherapy, acute leukemia	S. aureus, coagulase-negative staphylococci, enterococci, E. coli, K. pneumoniae, P. aeruginosa	Candida spp, Aspergillus spp, Fusarium		
T-helper lympho-cyte (cell-mediated immunity)	Immunosuppressive therapy, Hodgkin's disease, transplanta-tion	Listeria monocytogenes, Nocardia asteroides, Legionella, Salmonella, mycobacteria	Cryptococcus, Aspergillus, Candida, H. capsulatum, Mucoraceae	Pneumocystis carinii, Toxoplasma gondii	Herpes simplex, varicella-zoster, cytomegalovirus
Gamma-globulin (humoral immunity)	Splenectomy, chronic lymphocytic leukemia, hypogam-maglobulinemia, bone marrow trans-plantation	S. pneumoniae, H. influen-zae, N. meningitidis		P. carinii, Babesia spp.	
Damage to physical barriers	Surgical procedures	S. aureus; coagulase-negative staphylococci, S. pyogenes; Enterobac-teriaceae; P. aeruginosa, Bacteroides spp.	Candida spp.		
	Indwelling catheters, venipuncture	S. aureus, coagulase-negative staphylococci, Corynebacterium	Candida spp.		
	Chemotherapy, en-doscopy, radiation	S. aureus, coagulase-negative staphylococci, streptococci, Enterobac-teriaceae, P. aeruginosa, Bacteroides	Candida spp.		Herpes simplex
Microbial colonization	Chemotherapy, antibi-otics, hospitalization	S. aureus, coagulase-negative staphylococci, Enterobacteriaceae, P. aeruginosa, Legionella	Candida spp., Aspergillus		
Transplantation	Bone marrow		Candida spp.	Toxoplasma gondii, P. carinii	Cytomegalovirus, hepatitis B and C, Epstein-Barr virus

Modified from Armstrong D. History of opportunistic infection in the immunocompromised host. Clin Infect Dis 1993;17(Suppl 2):S318.

neutrophils) predisposes the host to infections. The terms *granulocytopenia* and *neutropenia* often are used interchangeably. The degree of neutropenia is expressed in terms of the absolute neutrophil count (ANC) or the total number of granulocytes (polymorphonuclear leukocytes and band forms) present in the circulating pool of white blood cells (WBCs).

The quantitative relationship between neutropenia and outcome of infections was established more than 30 years ago.[2] It was discovered that the risk of infection in the neutropenic patient is proportional to both the severity and duration of neutropenia. In general, the risk of infection is low when the ANC exceeds 1,000 cells/mm³, with the frequency and severity of infection inversely proportional to the ANC.[2] As the ANC drops below 500 cells/mm³, the risk of infection rapidly increases. The risk of developing bacteremia is further increased as the ANC drops below 100 cells/mm³.[2] Conversely, recovery of the ANC is the most important factor determining the outcome of infectious complications in neutropenia.

Febrile patients with short durations of neutropenia (<1 week) or in whom neutropenia is not severe (<100 cells/mm³) generally respond promptly to empiric antibiotics and rarely develop serious infections.[2] In contrast, patients rendered neutropenic for >1 week (e.g., those receiving more intensive chemotherapy regimens) and/or are severely neutropenic are more vulnerable to serious infection.[2]

Damage to Physical Barriers

The intact skin and mucosal surfaces of the body constitute the host's primary physical defense against microbial invasion. The integrity of this physical barrier may be disrupted by tumor, treatment (e.g., surgery, irradiation), or various medical procedures (e.g., insertion of intravenous [IV] or urinary catheters, venipuncture, measurement of rectal temperature).[3] Device-related infections, including those associated with central IV catheters, are commonly caused by migration of skin flora (e.g., coagulase-negative staphylococci) through the cutaneous insertion site.[3] Infections secondary to damaged mucosal lining of the gastrointestinal (GI) tract usually are caused by the enteric bacteria as well as fungi such as *Candida* spp.[3]

Alterations in the Immune System

Patients with immunoglobulin deficiencies (e.g., hypogammaglobulinemia, chronic lymphocytic leukemia, or splenectomy) are at increased risk for infections with encapsulated bacteria that must undergo antibody opsonization for efficient phagocytosis. Such bacteria include *Neisseria meningitidis, Haemophilus influenzae,* and *Streptococcus pneumoniae.*[1,3] Hodgkin's disease, organ transplantation, and HIV disease can disrupt the cellular immune system, increasing the risk for infections with obligate and facultative intracellular organisms such as mycobacteria, *Listeria, Toxoplasma,* viruses, and fungi.[1,3]

Some chemotherapeutic regimens have profound effects on both cellular and humoral defenses. Corticosteroids exert their immunosuppressive effects on the cellular immune system, particularly at the T-lymphocyte and macrophage level. Therefore, patients receiving corticosteroids have increased susceptibility to infections with viral, bacterial, protozoal, and fungal infections.[4] Infectious complications secondary to glucocorticoid use appear to be dose dependent. The risk of infection increases with daily doses >10 mg or cumulative doses >700 mg of prednisone or its equivalent.[4] Thus, patients receiving corticosteroids in either high doses or for prolonged periods are at increased risk for a wide spectrum of infections caused by bacteria, fungi, and other opportunistic pathogens.[4]

Colonization

Microbial colonization can be a prerequisite to infection in neutropenic patients. *Colonization* may be defined as the recovery of an organism from any particular site (e.g., stool, nasopharynx) without clinical signs of infection. Most infections in neutropenic patients are caused by the host's endogenous microflora or hospital-acquired pathogens that have colonized the alimentary tract, upper respiratory tract, and/or skin.[5]

Bone Marrow Transplantation

Transplantation of bone marrow predisposes patients to the development of opportunistic infections secondary to both intensive immunosuppressive therapy and transmission.[6,7] These infections may be acquired from blood products or may represent reactivation of latent host infection.[6,7] The types of infections are detailed in other chapters (see Chapter 35, Solid Organ Transplantation, and Chapter 92, Hematopoietic Cell Transplantation.)

MOST COMMON PATHOGENS

1. B.C., a 41-year-old woman, was admitted to the cancer center for placement of a central IV catheter for administration of chemotherapy to treat acute nonlymphocytic leukemia in relapse. She was diagnosed 2 years ago and was treated with cytarabine plus daunorubicin, which resulted in a complete remission for 33 months. This admission, she will be treated with high-dose cytarabine plus mitoxantrone for reinduction. What are the most likely pathogens to cause infection in patients like B.C. during periods of chemotherapy-induced neutropenia?

Bacteria are the primary pathogens associated with infection in febrile neutropenic patients (see Table 68-1).[8] Bacteremia is most often caused by aerobic Gram-negative bacilli (especially *Pseudomonas aeruginosa, Escherichia coli,* and *Klebsiella pneumoniae*) or aerobic Gram-positive cocci (i.e., coagulase-negative staphylococci, *Staphylococcus aureus,* enterococci, and streptococcal species).[9,10] Over the past decade, the proportion of Gram-negative infections has decreased with a proportional increase in Gram-positive infections.[9–12] Gram-positive bacteria now account for 60% to 70% of microbiologically documented infections in neutropenic cancer patients.[12] This is thought to be due (in part) to the frequent use of indwelling intravascular catheters, use of more intensive chemotherapy regimens, and the widespread use of broad-spectrum antibiotics for prophylactic and therapeutic use. All of these factors can contribute to the development of infection in patients like B.C.

Methicillin-resistant *S. aureus* (MRSA) and *Staphylococcus epidermidis,* streptococci (including *S. pneumoniae* and viridans streptococci), and *Corynebacterium* species have become important pathogens in some cancer centers.[9–12] Moreover, enterococcal infections are increasing in frequency because of routine use of broad-spectrum antibiotics.[13] Meningitis caused by the intracellular organism *Listeria monocytogenes* is observed in patients with defective cellular immunity caused by disease or prolonged corticosteroid use. In general, anaerobic bacteria are an infrequent cause of infection in granulocytopenic patients with hematologic malignancies.[14] However, they may occur more frequently in patients with GI malignancies.[14]

Invasive fungal infections are a major cause of morbidity and mortality among neutropenic cancer patients and patients undergoing bone marrow transplantation.[15] Patients with prolonged neutropenia (>7 days) are at high risk of developing systemic fungal infections. In one report, approximately 50% of patients who die during prolonged periods of neutropenia had evidence of deep-seated mycoses at autopsy.[16]

Viral infections are generally a reactivation of latent infection. These may include herpes simplex virus and varicella-zoster virus.[9] Other viruses, such as cytomegalovirus, can be acquired during hematopoietic stem cell transplantation.[7]

PROPHYLAXIS AGAINST INFECTION

Infection Control

Exogenous contamination can be prevented by strict protective isolation of patients in specially designed rooms that maintain a sterile environment. These laminar airflow rooms are ventilated with air that is passed through a high-efficiency particulate air (HEPA) filter, which removes >99% of all particles larger than 3 microns. Total protective isolation is accomplished by strict isolation in conjunction with the administration of sterile food and water, local skin care, and intensive microbial surveillance.[7] However, this regimen is burdensome to the patient and health care personnel, difficult to accomplish and maintain, and expensive. Thus, it continues to be used in only a few treatment centers.

Antimicrobial Prophylaxis

2. **What is the role of oral antimicrobial prophylaxis during the neutropenic period?**

Studies have demonstrated that the early administration of oral antibiotics (both antibacterials and antifungals) during the afebrile, neutropenic period in select "high-risk" patients can result in a reduction in the number of febrile episodes and subsequent risk of infection.[17] The goals of such prophylactic antibiotic regimens have been aimed at reducing potentially pathogenic endogenous microflora or preventing the acquisition of new microorganisms in the neutropenic patient.[17] Potential benefits must outweigh the risks of antibiotic-related adverse effects, the development of resistance, and the potential for superinfection. Therefore, prophylaxis is generally considered only in patients with neutropenia expected to be severe (<100 cells/mm³) or prolonged (<7 days).[9]

Nonabsorbable Antibacterials

The alimentary tract is recognized as an important reservoir of potential pathogens. Therefore, gut decontamination with and without total protective isolation has been investigated. The rationale behind the use of selective decontamination regimens is based on animal studies that demonstrated that selective elimination of aerobic GI flora, while maintaining anaerobic flora, prevented colonization with potentially pathogenic aerobic Gram-negative bacteria. Early studies focused on the use of nonabsorbable antimicrobials such as gentamicin, polymyxin B, and colistin to eradicate selected bowel flora. These agents, when administered orally, undergo minimal systemic absorption, thereby potentially reducing intestinal colonization while reducing the potential for systemic toxicity.

Oral, nonabsorbable antibacterial regimens have not shown consistent efficacy in preventing infection in the neutropenic cancer patient.[17] A major problem with these regimens has been poor patient compliance and tolerance, often because of their unpleasant taste. Lack of compliance in one study was associated with an increased frequency of infection caused by Gram-negative bacilli in neutropenic patients.[18] Of additional concern is the development of aminoglycoside resistance from the nonabsorbable aminoglycoside-containing regimens. Finally, colistin use has recently been identified as a risk factor for staphylococcal infections.[11] Therefore, nonabsorbable antibacterial agents have been supplanted by oral, absorbable antibiotics.[9,17]

Trimethoprim-Sulfamethoxazole

Several studies have demonstrated the benefit of trimethoprim-sulfamethoxazole (TMP-SMX) in reducing bacterial infections when compared to placebo in febrile neutropenic patients.[19–21] Its benefit in reducing mortality, however, is less clear. In contrast, its role in preventing *Pneumocystis carinii* pneumonia has been established in many immunocompromised patient populations, independent of the presence of neutropenia.[7,9,20] The potential benefits of TMP-SMX prophylaxis must be carefully balanced against the potential for drug-induced bone marrow suppression, hypersensitivity reactions, the emergence of resistant organisms (such as *E. coli*), and the development of superinfections. Patients at high risk for developing *P. carinii* pneumonia (i.e., patients with acute lymphocytic leukemia receiving intensive chemotherapy, AIDS, allogeneic bone marrow transplantation) should be strongly considered for TMP-SMX prophylaxis.[9] In the absence of these risk factors, routine use of TMP-SMX prophylaxis for neutropenia is not currently recommended.[9]

Fluoroquinolones

Data regarding the use of fluoroquinolones (e.g., ciprofloxacin, norfloxacin, and ofloxacin) for preventing infection in neutropenic cancer patients have been summarized.[22–24] Comparative studies of ofloxacin[25] or ciprofloxacin[26] versus TMP-SMX suggest that these agents are equal or superior to TMP-SMX in preventing infectious episodes due to Gram-negative pathogens in neutropenic patients. Of concern, however, is the increasing frequency of Gram-positive infections observed in patients receiving fluoroquinolone prophylaxis,[27,28] combined with the emergence of resistant Gram-negative bacilli (especially *E. coli*)[29] caused by the widespread use of these agents. In addition, fluoroquinolone prophylaxis does not appear to reduce mortality in this patient population.[24] Attempts to use rifampin in combination with ciprofloxacin[30] and ofloxacin[22] to enhance the Gram-positive spectrum have not been successful.[30] Because the benefits of fluoroquinolone prophylaxis may be offset by the emergence of resistant organisms, routine prophylactic use in neutropenic patients should be avoided.[9]

Antifungals

3. **What is the role of antifungal prophylaxis in neutropenic patients?**

As previously stated, patients with prolonged neutropenia (>7 days) are at high risk of developing systemic fungal infections. Because of the increased frequency with which such infections are encountered, difficulties in establishing a diagnosis, and poor response rates in patients with serious invasive infection who are immunocompromised, effective prophylactic strategies are necessary in select high-risk patients.

NONABSORBABLE ANTIFUNGALS

Various nonabsorbable antifungal agents have been studied for use in fungal prophylaxis in neutropenic patients. Topical agents, such as oral nystatin,[18,31] clotrimazole,[32] and oral amphotericin B[33] have been studied. Of these agents, only oral amphotericin B and clotrimazole have been successful in reducing the frequency of oropharyngeal candidiasis. None of the antifungals have a role as primary prophylaxis of invasive fungal infections.[9]

SYSTEMIC ANTIFUNGALS

The use of systemic antifungals for empiric or prophylactic therapy has been extensively studied. Early trials with the imidazoles miconazole and ketoconazole met with limited success. The toxicities associated with these agents and the availability of newer, less toxic azole antifungals currently limit their clinical utility in this setting.

In addition to its in vitro activity against many *Candida* spp (such as *C. albicans*), itraconazole is active in vitro against *Aspergillus* species. Randomized, placebo-controlled trials[34,35] as well as comparisons with amphotericin B[36] have demonstrated its efficacy in reducing systemic *Candida* infections in this patient population. A previous limitation to itraconazole's potential efficacy was the availability of a tablet formulation whose bioavailability following oral administration was significantly dependent on gastric acidity. An oral solution with improved bioavailability and an IV formulation have been introduced.

Studies have demonstrated that fluconazole prophylaxis has decreased the frequency of both superficial (e.g., oropharyngeal candidiasis) and systemic fungal infections in bone marrow transplant patients[37,38] but not in patients with leukemia.[39,40] When fluconazole 400 mg/day was compared with placebo for fungal prophylaxis in bone marrow transplant recipients, it significantly reduced the incidence of invasive candidiasis and delayed the initiation of empiric amphotericin B from day 17 to day 21.[30] In contrast, in a study of patients with acute leukemia undergoing chemotherapy, fluconazole prophylaxis was not associated with a reduction in invasive fungal infections or need for empiric amphotericin B.[40] Despite its potential role, concern over its lack of reliable in vitro activity against molds limits its expanded use in high-risk patients. An increased frequency of isolation of non-albicans *Candida* (such as *C. krusei, C. glabrata,* and *C. parapsilosis*) has also been noted in some institutions.[41] Finally, fluconazole may not have a significant impact in reducing mortality in these patients.[42] Therefore, routine use of fluconazole should be reserved for higher-risk patients with neutropenia (e.g., patients undergoing allogeneic hematopoietic stem cell transplantation until engraftment).[7]

Fluconazole is available as both oral and IV formulations, and its oral bioavailability is not significantly influenced by changes in gastric acidity. Like itraconazole, the IV formulation enables fluconazole to be administered to critically ill patients or patients who have difficulty swallowing. However, unlike itraconazole, it is not contraindicated in patients with significant renal impairment. Despite such potential advantages, fluconazole's efficacy in preventing invasive fungal infections was inferior to that of itraconazole in a randomized, comparative trial performed in 140 patients receiving allogeneic hematopoietic stem cell transplants.[43] In this trial, proven invasive fungal infections occurred in 6 of 71 (9%) itraconazole recipients and 17 of 61 (25%) fluconazole-treated patients. While overall mortality was not different,

fewer fungal deaths were reported in the itraconazole-treated patients (9% versus 18%), but this difference was not statistically different ($P = 0.13$).

The prophylactic role of IV amphotericin B has also been investigated.[42,44] In one such evaluation, amphotericin B 0.5 mg/kg given three times weekly was compared with fluconazole 400 mg/day in 90 patients with acute leukemia.[44] Although efficacy against fungal infections was similar in both groups, more side effects were observed with the amphotericin B regimen. There are limited published data on the efficacy of lipid-based formulations of amphotericin B (e.g., amphotericin B lipid complex and liposomal amphotericin B) for prophylaxis. One recent study compared liposomal amphotericin B versus a combination with fluconazole and itraconazole.[45] No significant differences were detected in terms of efficacy, but toxicity was noted more frequently in the patients receiving liposomal amphotericin B. Lipid-based amphotericin B preparations are generally reserved for patients with underlying renal dysfunction. The efficacies of the echinocandin caspofungin and the new azole voriconazole have not yet been established for prophylaxis.

Patients receiving cytotoxic chemotherapy for solid tumors have lower rates of invasive fungal infections compared with patients with hematologic malignancies and those receiving allogeneic bone marrow transplantation. This is primarily because of the differences in the duration of neutropenia. In patients receiving cytotoxic chemotherapy for solid tumors, antifungal prophylaxis may not be beneficial and may actually increase the potential for superinfection with resistant fungi. Such patients should be managed with empiric antifungal therapy should they develop persistent fever and neutropenia.

Antivirals

The use of antiviral prophylaxis varies with patient population. High-risk patients (e.g., those receiving allogeneic bone marrow transplants, those with acute leukemia undergoing induction or reinduction therapy, or those with a past history of infection during neutropenia) who are seropositive for *Herpes simplex* virus may require acyclovir prophylaxis during periods of neutropenia.[7,9] Bone marrow transplant patients seropositive for varicella-zoster virus should also be considered for acyclovir prophylaxis.[7,9] In addition, bone marrow transplant recipients at increased risk of cytomegalovirus infection (such as CMV-seropositive patients and CMV-seronegative recipients with a CMV-seropositive donor) should be considered for either ganciclovir prophylaxis or pre-emptive therapy if early evidence of infection is observed.[7,9]

In summary, the routine need for prophylaxis with oral antimicrobials (antibiotics and/or antifungals) remains controversial. Use of these agents may not reduce the need for empiric, systemic antimicrobials. Also, the impact of these agents on the selection of multiresistant bacteria (i.e., vancomycin-resistant enterococci, quinolone-resistant streptococci and *E. coli*) and fungi (azole-resistant *Candida* species) remains a major therapeutic dilemma. Caution must be exercised with the widespread use of antifungal prophylaxis, because prolonged use can potentially select out resistant molds and yeast.

INFECTIONS IN NEUTROPENIC CANCER PATIENTS

Clinical Signs and Symptoms

4. Seven days after completing chemotherapy, B.C. developed a fever of 102°F (orally). Vital signs are blood pressure (BP), 109/70 mm Hg; pulse, 102 beats/min; and respirations, 25 breaths/min. Physical examination demonstrates a clear oropharynx without exudates or plaques. Chest and cardiac examination are normal. The exit site for the Hickman catheter is clean and nontender without signs of erythema or induration. The perineum and rectum are nontender, and no masses are noted.

Laboratory data are hematocrit (Hct), 20% (normal, 33% to 43%); hemoglobin (Hgb), 7 g/dL (normal, 14 to 18); WBC count, 1,400 cells/mm³ (normal, 3,200 to 9,800) with 3% polymorphonuclear leukocytes (PMNs) (normal, 54 to 62), 1% band forms (normal, 3 to 5), 70% lymphocytes (normal, 25 to 33), and 22% monocytes (normal, 3 to 7); platelet count, 17,000 cells/L (normal, 130,000 to 400,000); blood glucose, 160 mg/dL (normal, 70 to 110); serum creatinine (SrCr), 1.1 mg/dL (normal, 0.6 to 1.2); blood urea nitrogen (BUN), 24 mg/dL (normal, 8 to 18).

What are the signs and symptoms of infection in B.C.? What are the most common sites and sources of infection in patients like B.C.?

[SI units: Hct, 0.2 (normal, 0.33 to 0.43); Hgb, 70 g/L (normal, 140 to 180); WBC count, 1.4 × 10⁹/L (normal, 3.2 to 9.8) with 0.03 PMNs (normal, 0.54 to 0.62), 0.01 band forms (normal, 0.03 to 0.05), 0.7 lymphocytes (normal, 0.25 to 0.33), and 0.22 monocytes (normal, 0.03 to 0.07); platelets, 17 × 10⁹/L (normal, 130 to 400); glucose, 8.88 mmol/L (normal, 3.89 to 6.11); SrCr, 97.24 mmol/L (normal, 53.04 to 106.08); BUN, 8.57 mmol/L urea (normal, 2.86 to 6.43)]

B.C. has an ANC of 48 cells/mm³ (1,400 WBC/mm³ × [0.03 PMN + 0.01 bands]) and is therefore at high risk for infection. Fever in neutropenic patients is defined as a single oral temperature of ≥38.3°C (101°F) or a temperature of >38.0°C (100.4°F) for >1 hr.[9,46] As her case illustrates, fever is the earliest (and often the only) sign of infection in neutropenic patients.[9,47,48]

Although the lung is the most common site of serious infection in neutropenic cancer patients, fever and a dry cough are often the only presenting signs of pneumonia.[49] The impaired inflammatory response in these patients often makes sputum production scant, and sputum Gram stains often contain few polymorphonuclear cells. Radiologic evidence of a pulmonary infection can be minimal or absent, and the chest examination is frequently nondiagnostic. Pneumonia has a high mortality rate in neutropenic patients, especially if it occurs in conjunction with bacteremia.[9] In the presence of shock, a mortality rate of approximately 80% has been observed in these patients.[50]

Invasive procedures such as venipuncture, central IV catheter placement (e.g., Hickman catheter), and skin biopsies are associated with cellulitis and systemic infections. However, detecting skin and soft tissue infections is also difficult because the typical signs and symptoms of infection (e.g., pain, heat, erythema, swelling) are often absent.[49] This phenomenon exists due to the lack of adequate numbers of granulocytes, as well as the suppression or absence of other components of the inflammatory response.[2] Colonization of these lesions may result in local infection and the potential for systemic dissemination of bacteria and fungi. Bacteremia occurs primarily from entry of bacteria through the skin or through unrecognized ulcerations in the GI and perirectal areas.[9]

Confirmation of Infection

5. How can an infection be confirmed in patients such as B.C.?

Because of the frequent lack of physical signs and symptoms of infection, the clinician must obtain an accurate history and conduct a careful physical examination at the first sign of fever.[49,51] A detailed search for subtle signs and symptoms of inflammation at the most common sites, such as the oropharynx, bone marrow aspiration sites, lung, periodontium, skin, vascular catheter access sites, nail beds, and perineum (including the anus), is necessary. Before antibiotics are initiated, specimens of the blood, urine, and other suspected sites of infection should be obtained for culture. Any indwelling urinary or IV catheter should be considered as a potential focus of infection and, if possible, should be removed and cultured.[9] Other diagnostic tests such as chest radiographs should be obtained if signs and symptoms point to the respiratory tract as a potential infection site.[9] Finally, a complete blood count and assessment of organ function (such as liver and kidney function) may assist in drug dosing and monitoring for treatment-related toxicities.[9]

An infectious cause for fever can be documented either clinically or microbiologically in up to 60% of neutropenic cancer patients.[8] Forty percent of these febrile episodes have a documented microbiologic origin; the remaining 20% are attributed to infection based on clinical findings alone.[8] Although molecular diagnostic technology may allow the detection of certain infections in the future, these techniques are not used routinely in clinical practice today.[52]

Impact of Colonization

6. Routine surveillance cultures of swabs taken from B.C.'s axillae, nasopharynx, and rectum grew *C. jeikeium* (axillae), *S. aureus* (axillae and nasopharynx), and *Enterococcus faecium* (rectum). What is the significance of these culture results? Should routine, serial surveillance cultures be performed in patients such as B.C.?

Several factors influence the colonization and subsequent infection by microorganisms in cancer patients such as B.C. Organisms isolated from infected patients can be found in endogenous flora or acquired during hospitalization.[5] The sources of and factors contributing to colonization are numerous and include staff-to-staff and patient-to-patient transmission (e.g., lack of frequent and adequate hand hygiene), direct transmission from the environment (e.g., inadequately disinfected bathtubs, sinks, toilet bowls), foods (e.g., raw fruits and vegetables), inhalation from contaminated fomites (e.g., respirators, ventilating systems), and IV access devices.[53]

In addition to immunosuppression, the underlying malignancy and chemotherapy diminish the cancer patient's resistance to colonization and infection. For example, chemotherapy induces changes in the microbial binding receptors on epithelial cells in the oropharynx. This allows Gram-negative bacilli to adhere to these surfaces, changing the composition of the oropharyngeal flora from a mixture of Gram-positive aerobes and anaerobes to Gram-negative aerobic bacteria.[54] Colonization with resistant organisms is enhanced by prior antibiotic administration, which may suppress the growth of normal anaerobic flora in the GI tract. This anaerobic suppression may promote the overgrowth of resistant microorganisms.[54] For example, *P. aeruginosa* and *K. pneumoniae* are not commonly found in the stools of normal healthy adults, but they are recovered from the stools of hospitalized cancer patients.

Organisms that colonize cancer patients differ in their invasiveness and propensity to cause infection.[5,55] Colonization with *P. aeruginosa* is more likely to result in infection than is colonization with less virulent organisms such as *E. coli* or *S. epidermidis.*[56] However, if the host is profoundly impaired, organisms generally considered to be less virulent may become pathogenic.

The acquisition of and subsequent colonization by potentially pathogenic microbes may be detected by serial "surveillance" cultures of specimens obtained from various body sites such as the nasopharynx, axilla, urine, and rectum. Such surveillance cultures can provide information about the dynamic changes in microflora during hospitalization that may be useful for infection control purposes. However, little clinically useful information is gained when infection is absent.[57] Therefore, surveillance cultures are generally restricted to select patients for infection control purposes. In such cases, culture of the anterior nares (for MRSA) or rectal samples (for vancomycin-resistant enterococci or multidrug-resistant Gram-negative bacilli) may be performed.

In summary, B.C.'s surveillance culture results indicate that she is colonized with several potential pathogens associated with infection in the immunocompromised host, but these results are probably not useful in selecting empiric antibiotics for her fever.

EMPIRIC ANTIBIOTIC THERAPY

Rationale

7. Should B.C. be started on antibiotic therapy immediately? Is this rational in view of the fact that neither the source of her fever nor the pathogen has been established?

All febrile patients with either an ANC of <500 cells/mm³ or 500 to 1,000 cells/mm³ and predicted to be <500 cells/mm³ should be considered to have a potentially life-threatening infection.[9] In addition, afebrile neutropenic patients with signs or symptoms of infection should also receive antibiotic therapy. Once blood cultures and cultures from suspected sources of infection are obtained, these patients should be promptly started on broad-spectrum antibacterials.[9] Early studies in the 1950s and 1960s documented the poor prognosis of neutropenic patients whose Gram-negative infections were untreated during the first 24 to 48 hours following the onset of fever. Crude mortality rates secondary to *P. aeruginosa* bacteremia approached 91%.[56] This finding was confirmed in the 1970s when it was demonstrated that withholding antibiotics until a pathogen was isolated resulted in an unacceptably high mortality rate in neutropenic patients. Prompt use of empiric, broad-spectrum antibiotics over the past two decades has contributed to reductions in infectious

mortality rates to <30%, depending on the causative organism.[58] These observations emphasize the need for timely institution of empiric antibiotic therapy to prevent early morbidity and mortality.

Optimal Antibacterial Spectrum

8. What pathogen- and patient-specific factors should be considered when initiating empiric therapy for B.C.?

Empiric antibiotic regimens should provide broad-spectrum coverage against the potential Gram-negative bacilli most commonly isolated from neutropenic cancer patients: *E. coli, K. pneumoniae, P. aeruginosa,* staphylococcal and streptococcal species.[9] Because the mortality from untreated bacteremia caused by *P. aeruginosa* was high in early studies,[56] empiric regimens have traditionally included antimicrobials with antipseudomonal activity. Despite advances in the development in antibacterials since the 1960s, the empiric management of febrile neutropenic patients continues to be complicated by the changing spectrum of bacterial pathogens and their antimicrobial susceptibilities.

Selecting an initial empiric regimen for a given patient should take into account likely pathogens, their frequency of isolation, and institutional susceptibility patterns. Patient-related considerations should include allergies, concomitant treatments (e.g., prior or concomitant nephrotoxins), and organ dysfunction (e.g., renal or hepatic) that may limit antibiotic selection. Attempts should be made to identify low-risk patients for whom oral antimicrobial therapy may be an option.[9] Finally, dosing schedules, acquisition costs, and the potential for significant toxicities should be considered.

In addition to broad-spectrum activity, antibacterial regimens should have potent bactericidal activity against the infecting pathogen. The rationale for bactericidal therapy is that when defense mechanisms are impaired (e.g., in neutropenia), antibiotic agents that kill rather than inhibit bacterial growth would be optimal. However, no comparative trials of bacteriostatic versus bactericidal antibiotics have been conducted in humans. Rather, the need for bactericidal activity has been based on studies relating the bactericidal activity of patients' serum during antibiotic therapy to their clinical response.[59]

In summary, many organisms, including those recovered from surveillance cultures, may be pathogens in B.C. Those associated with a high mortality rate during the first 48 hours should be empirically treated pending culture and sensitivity results. Therefore, an empiric regimen with optimal activity against commonly isolated Gram-negative bacilli (including *P. aeruginosa*) should be promptly administered to B.C.

Initial Empiric Antibiotic Regimens

9. What would be a reasonable initial empiric antibiotic regimen for B.C.?

Practice guidelines prepared by the NCCN[60] and the Infectious Diseases Society of America[9] identify antimicrobial options for the treatment of fever in the neutropenic cancer patient. The ideal antibiotic regimen for empiric management in this setting remains controversial. Various antibiotics, alone and in combination, have been studied extensively.[9] Monotherapy regimens commonly include a third-generation cephalosporin (e.g., ceftazidime), a fourth-generation cephalosporin (e.g., cefepime), or a carbapenem (e.g., imipenem-cilastatin or meropenem). The combination regimens most frequently recommended (excluding those containing vancomycin) are an aminoglycoside (e.g., gentamicin, tobramycin, or amikacin) plus an antipseudomonal ureidopenicillin with or without a β-lactamase inhibitor (e.g., piperacillin, piperacillin-tazobactam), an aminoglycoside with an antipseudomonal cephalosporin (e.g., ceftazidime, cefepime), or an aminoglycoside in combination with a carbapenem (e.g., imipenem-cilastatin or meropenem). [9,60] Although recommended by some sources, [60] combination β-lactam antibiotics are less frequently used. Comparisons of efficacy rates between studies are complicated by differences in the definitions of neutropenia, the incidence of documented infections, criteria used to assess clinical response, and statistical methodology. [46] Guidelines have been proposed recently to establish standards for evaluating antimicrobial therapy in this population. [46] Despite such limitations, no striking differences regarding efficacy have been observed between these empiric approaches. [9]

Oral Antibiotics

Carefully selected ("low-risk") adult febrile neutropenic patients may be candidates for oral antibiotic therapy, either as initial therapy or as follow-up to IV antibiotics ("sequential therapy"). [9,61,62] Such an option is generally restricted to younger patients (<60 years) with ANC ≥100 cells/mm³ with short durations of neutropenia (<7 days) and whose cancer is in partial or complete remission. Patients must be without microbiologic or clinical evidence of infection (other than fever), they must be clinically stable, and they must be closely observed. Recently, an international collaborative study established and validated a risk scoring system in adults that incorporated these principles to identify low-risk patients for whom oral therapy may be an option. [63]

Trials have confirmed the value of oral ciprofloxacin in combination with amoxicillin-clavulanate in low-risk adult patients with febrile neutropenia. Freifeld and others compared oral ciprofloxacin (30 mg/kg per day in three divided doses) combined with amoxicillin-clavulanate (40 mg/kg per day in three divided doses) to IV ceftazidime. [64] Treatment was equally successful in both groups, but the ceftazidime group required significantly more modifications in the initial regimen compared with the oral group. Conversely, more patients receiving ciprofloxacin with amoxicillin-clavulanate were unable to tolerate the oral regimen. Similarly, Kern and colleagues evaluated the efficacy of oral ciprofloxacin (750 mg twice daily) in combination with amoxicillin-clavulanate (625 mg three times daily) versus IV ceftazidime and amikacin. [65] As with the previous trial, the oral regimen was found to be as effective as IV antibiotics. Clindamycin may be used in place of amoxicillin-clavulanate if the patient is allergic to β-lactam antibiotics. [9] Cefixime has been used effectively as an alternative regimen in low-risk pediatric patients initially receiving IV therapy, [66] but there is not adequate experience with cefixime as an initial therapy. [9]

Intravenous Monotherapy

10. Can any of the more potent, extended-spectrum β-lactams be used as monotherapy in febrile neutropenic patients?

CEPHALOSPORINS

The antipseudomonal third-generation cephalosporin ceftazidime and the fourth-generation agent cefepime have been extensively studied as monotherapy for empiric therapy in febrile neutropenic patients. In general, these agents are safe and have potent broad-spectrum activity in vitro against many Gram-negative and some Gram-positive pathogens.

Numerous comparative clinical studies in both adults and children have been performed to evaluate the efficacy of ceftazidime as initial empiric monotherapy in febrile neutropenic cancer patients. [67–81] Overall, ceftazidime was as effective as the standard regimen in patients with documented infections and unexplained fever. In some of these trials, the efficacy of ceftazidime in patients with documented staphylococcal infections was suboptimal. Select clinical trials have empirically added antistaphylococcal coverage with a glycopeptide (e.g., vancomycin) and have shown improved outcomes in these patients. [82,83] In addition, pathogens (particularly Gram-negative pathogens) that produce either type 1 β-lactamase or extended-spectrum β-lactamases (such as *K. pneumoniae*) are not likely to respond to ceftazidime monotherapy. [84,85] These may be seen more frequently in patients with prolonged hospitalization or those who have received prior antimicrobial therapy. [84] Therefore, local in vitro susceptibilities of common Gram-negative pathogens should be examined prior to the routine use of ceftazidime as monotherapy.

Cefepime is a fourth-generation cephalosporin with a U.S. Food and Drug Administration (FDA)–approved indication for monotherapy for empiric management of infection in patients with febrile neutropenia. The potential advantage of this agent over third-generation cephalosporins is its low affinity for major chromosomally mediated β-lactamases. [86,87] Compared with ceftazidime, cefepime has more potent activity in vitro against select Gram-positive bacteria (methicillin-susceptible *Staphylococcus* species, viridans streptococci, and *S. pneumoniae*). [87] Randomized, comparative studies have evaluated the role of cefepime as monotherapy in both adults and children with febrile neutropenia. [68,69,71,73,74,88–95] The improved Gram-positive activity (relative to ceftazidime) may decrease the empiric need for vancomycin in some patients. However, this advantage is less likely in institutions with a high rate of MRSA, as cefepime and other cephalosporins are inactive against this pathogen.

CARBAPENEMS

The carbapenems are a unique class of antibiotics with broad-spectrum activity against numerous Gram-positive and Gram-negative bacteria, including anaerobes. Imipenem (in combination with the dehydropeptidase inhibitor cilastatin) and meropenem are two currently available agents in this class. Both imipenem-cilastatin[77,79,81,88,96–105] and meropenem[70,72,76,78,104,106–110] have been studied as monotherapy for febrile, neutropenic patients. The third member of this class available in the United States, ertapenem, possesses microbiologic activity similar to that of the other carbapenems, although it lacks in vitro activity against *Acinetobacter* species and *Pseudomonas,* including *P. aeruginosa.* [111] Considering this lack of activity, ertapenem would not be appropriate as empiric therapy for febrile neutropenic patients and has not been evaluated in this setting.

Clinical outcomes with imipenem-cilastatin monotherapy have been comparable with those of the β-lactam plus aminoglycoside combinations[81,96,100,103] as well as combination of two β-lactams.[98] Although proven to be effective, imipenem-cilastatin has generally been associated with a higher incidence of nausea and vomiting compared with ceftazidime or meropenem.[79,112] The GI side effects generally are dose-related (3 to 4 g/day) and associated with the rate of IV administration.[99] Therefore, dosages of 2 g/day (divided Q 6 hr) are generally given to patients with normal renal function.[113]

Meropenem has a broad spectrum of activity (similar to that of imipenem-cilastatin) but is generally associated with fewer GI side effects. Meropenem monotherapy for febrile neutropenia has been evaluated in both adults and children,[70,72,76,78,104,106–110] and the results have supported the value of meropenem as empiric monotherapy for use in febrile neutropenic patients.

In summary, several studies have demonstrated that monotherapy with cefepime, ceftazidime, or a carbapenem (imipenem-cilastatin or meropenem) is appropriate as initial empiric antibiotic therapy in febrile neutropenic patients. There are no convincing data to support one choice over the others as empiric monotherapy. However, routine carbapenem use may be associated with increased drug acquisition cost (relative to cephalosporins) and increased potential for development of carbapenem resistance. Therefore, many institutions have elected to reserve the carbapenems for patients who have either failed to respond to prior empiric therapy or who have a history of infections with pathogens resistant to third- and fourth-generation cephalosporins.

Regardless of the empiric regimen selected, patients must be closely monitored for nonresponse, emergence of secondary infections, adverse effects, and the development of drug-resistant organisms.

ALTERNATIVE INTRAVENOUS MONOTHERAPY REGIMENS

Monobactams, fluoroquinolones, and β-lactam/β-lactamase inhibitor combinations have shown efficacy in the management of febrile neutropenic patients. Monobactams and fluoroquinolones have been particularly useful as empiric alternatives in patients with β-lactam allergies.

Monobactams. Aztreonam, the only monobactam currently available in the United States, demonstrates in vitro activity only against Gram-negative aerobic bacilli.[114] While its in vitro potency against Gram-negative bacteria is comparable to that of ceftazidime, aztreonam lacks activity against Gram-positive bacteria or anaerobes.[114] Considering the lack of Gram-positive activity, aztreonam should not be used as monotherapy in this patient population. Empiric use with aztreonam has been evaluated in combination with either a β-lactam (piperacillin)[115] or vancomycin.[116]

Fluoroquinolones. Select fluoroquinolones offer a new approach to the empiric management of febrile neutropenic patients. Most agents in this class are rapidly bactericidal against many Gram-negative bacilli. However, they demonstrate variable potency in vitro against certain Gram-positive bacteria, such as *S. pneumoniae, S. aureus,* and *E. faecalis.* Of the currently available fluoroquinolones, ciprofloxacin is generally considered the most active in vitro against *P. aerugi-*

nosa. However, recent surveys have demonstrated only 60% to 70% of *P. aeruginosa* isolates are susceptible to ciprofloxacin.[117,118]

Ciprofloxacin has been studied as both monotherapy[119–123] and as part of combination regimens[124–127] as initial empiric therapy in febrile neutropenic patients. However, monotherapy with ciprofloxacin has met with mixed success. An EORTC trial comparing ciprofloxacin 400 to 600 mg/day versus piperacillin plus amikacin was terminated prematurely because of significantly poorer response rates in the patients treated with ciprofloxacin (65%) compared with the combination group (91%) ($P < 0.002$).[122] This finding may be due in part to the suboptimal ciprofloxacin dosage used as well as the impact of fluoroquinolone prophylaxis on the institution's nosocomial flora. An additional study demonstrated more favorable results with ciprofloxacin monotherapy.[123] However, the consensus is that the fluoroquinolones should not be used as monotherapy.[9]

β-Lactam/β-Lactamase Inhibitor Combinations

Randomized trials have compared piperacillin-tazobactam monotherapy to various antibiotics.[89,102,128–131] Although the results look promising, experience with this agent as monotherapy is limited relative to the carbapenems and antipseudomonal cephalosporins, and it cannot be routinely recommended.[9]

In summary, the diversity of organisms causing infection in neutropenic cancer patients makes it difficult to recommend one single regimen for empiric use in all institutions. Because institutional differences in prevailing pathogens exist, antibiotic selection should be based on the experience and susceptibility patterns in each institution.[132] Patient-related factors also play a role, depending on the presumed site of infection as well as patient allergies. Published studies provide useful information on drug selection but may not be applicable to all institutions.

Antimicrobial Combinations
RATIONALE FOR USE

Prior to the introduction of third- and fourth-generation cephalosporins and carbapenems, the empiric use of antibacterial combinations in febrile neutropenic cancer patients was favored because these regimens offered broad-spectrum activity against bacteria commonly infecting cancer patients. In addition, these combinations offered the potential, in select circumstances, to provide an additive or synergistic effect. Finally, they offered the potential to minimize the development of bacterial resistance. However, infections in neutropenic patients have shifted from Gram-negative to Gram-positive pathogens, against which traditional combination regimens (selected primarily for their activity against Gram-negative pathogens) have limited efficacy. Despite this concern, many clinicians continue to favor antibiotic combinations.

Synergy. Antibiotic *synergy* is defined as an interaction between antimicrobial agents in which the effect produced by the combination is greater than the sum of their individual activity. Various in vitro methods may be used to test for synergistic activity between antibacterials, and these methods may result in differing conclusions between similar combinations.

Studies published more than two decades ago reported that the outcome in neutropenic cancer patients with documented

Gram-negative bacteremia was significantly improved with the use of antibacterial combinations with the potential for demonstrating synergy in vitro when compared with nonsynergistic combinations.[133,134] De Jongh and associates reported their observations in a small number of patients with profound persistent neutropenia (<100 cells/mm³).[134] In 18 patients whose regimen demonstrated in vitro synergism or partial synergism against the infecting pathogen, 8 showed clinical improvement. In contrast, none of the 13 patients receiving nonsynergistic antibiotic regimens responded. This difference was statistically significant ($P < 0.005$). While these results are of interest, this study was performed using older, less potent Gram-negative agents. It is unknown whether synergistic combinations of newer antimicrobials, such as quinolones with carbapenems or pipcracillin, would result in similar findings.

Prevention of Resistant Strains. Another argument in favor of antibiotic combination use is that these combinations may prevent or delay the emergence of resistance during therapy. While resistant bacterial strains have emerged during therapy with monotherapy, it is not clear whether combination therapy will prevent the emergence of resistance during therapy.

11. B.L., a 13-year-old boy, presented with a 3-week history of "always being tired" and a persistent sore throat. Initial evaluation revealed anemia, thrombocytopenia, and a WBC count of 130,000 cells/L (normal, 3,200 to 9,800 cells/mm³) with a predominance of immature lymphoblasts. Further evaluation demonstrated that B.L. had "high-risk" acute lymphocytic leukemia. Remission induction treatment was initiated with teniposide plus cytarabine followed by prednisone, vincristine, and L-asparaginase. Seven days after induction chemotherapy, B.L. developed a fever (102°F) and chills. The ANC was 48 cells/mm³. SrCr and BUN were 1.0 mg/dL (normal, 0.6 to 1.2 mg/dL) and 15 mg/dL (normal, 8 to 18 mg/dL), respectively. The physician wants to empirically start B.L. on ceftazidime plus gentamicin combination regimen. What is the role of this combination in the empiric management of febrile neutropenia? Are there any differences in efficacy between these combinations?

[SI units: SrCr, 88.4 mmol/L (normal, 53.04 to 106.08); BUN, 5.36 mmol/L urea (2.86 to 6.43)]

Aminoglycoside Plus β-Lactam Combinations. Until the 1980s, most febrile neutropenic patients were treated with two-drug combination regimens that contained an aminoglycoside (gentamicin, tobramycin, or amikacin) plus a β-lactam antibiotic, such as an antipseudomonal penicillin or a third-generation cephalosporin. This combination is one of the most established empiric treatment regimens for the management of febrile neutropenia.[9]

Numerous studies have been conducted to evaluate the efficacy of combination therapy of an aminoglycoside with an antipseudomonal cephalosporin. Both ceftazidime[67,81,85,106–108,131,135–146] and cefepime[138,139,147,148] have been evaluated as part of a combination regimen. Cephalosporins without antipseudomonal activity (e.g., ceftriaxone) have also been investigated in combination with aminoglycosides, although this regimen is not routinely recommended.[149]

The duration of combination therapy consisting of an aminoglycoside plus a cephalosporin has also been evaluated.

A study conducted by the EORTC evaluated the effectiveness of full-course versus short-course amikacin plus ceftazidime in neutropenic patients with Gram-negative bacteremia.[150] A better outcome was demonstrated with full-course amikacin plus ceftazidime than with a short course (3 days) of amikacin plus a full course of ceftazidime. These data confirm the superiority of combined therapy of ceftazidime plus a full course of an aminoglycoside in profoundly neutropenic patients with Gram-negative bacteremia.

Carbapenem antibiotics are more frequently evaluated as monotherapy in this patient population. Therefore, relative to the numerous trials examining the role of combination therapy with cephalosporins, there are limited studies examining the combination of an aminoglycoside with either impenem-cilastatin[101,142] or meropenem[106] in this patient population. However, in one such evaluation, the combination of imipenem-cilastatin plus amikacin was found to be superior to imipenem-cilastatin monotherapy.[151]

Aminoglycosides have generally been considered the backbone of combination regimens because of their potential for bactericidal action against various bacteria. However, the addition of an aminoglycoside is associated with increased costs for therapeutic monitoring.[152,153] The benefit of an aminoglycoside for empiric therapy has not been consistently demonstrated.[152,153] In addition, there is an increased potential for the development of nephrotoxicity and ototoxicity.[153] This concern is especially relevant in patients receiving concomitant nephrotoxins such as cisplatin and cyclosporine. Despite these issues, B.L. may benefit from the empiric institution of an aminoglycoside/β-lactam combination because he is profoundly neutropenic (ANC <50 cells/mm³). Serum concentrations of the aminoglycosides should be monitored as needed to achieve optimal outcomes while reducing the risks of toxicity.

12. Seven days into therapy, despite rehydration, B.L.'s SrCr and BUN rose to 2.0 g/dL and 45 mg/dL, respectively. Because B.L. has developed nephrotoxicity (thought to be secondary to the aminoglycoside), what other combination regimens (excluding those containing aminoglycosides) could be used? Are these regimens as effective as aminoglycoside-containing regimens?

[SI units: SrCr, 176.8 mmol/L; BUN, 16.07 mmol/L urea]

Double β-Lactam Combinations. Although numerous β-lactam combinations (usually consisting of either moxalactam or a cephalosporin plus an antipseudomonal penicillin) have been studied, overall response rates have not been significantly different from those of patients treated with aminoglycoside/β-lactam regimens. However, experience is limited with double β-lactam combinations in patients with neutropenia or patients with documented infections caused by *P. aeruginosa,* and the available results are somewhat disturbing. Winston and associates observed a lower response in patients with profound, persistent neutropenia who were treated with moxalactam plus piperacillin (48%) compared with those treated with moxalactam plus amikacin (77%).[154] Because the number of patients studied was small, these differences approached but did not achieve statistical significance ($P < 0.08$). A poorer response in patients with infection caused by *P. aeruginosa* was observed. One of five patients treated with moxalactam plus piperacillin versus seven of nine patients treated with moxalactam plus amikacin responded ($P < 0.06$). Two patients with bacteremia caused by *P. aeruginosa* initially susceptible to the double β-lactam regimen relapsed with isolates resistant to multiple β-lactam antibiotics. These results are compatible with the selection of bacteria producing high amounts of the chromosomally mediated β-lactamase, which is capable of inactivating third-generation cephalosporins as well as other less stable β-lactams.

Other Combinations. As previously stated, ciprofloxacin has been studied in combination with other antibacterials (either an aminoglycoside or a β-lactam) as initial empiric therapy for treatment of suspected infection in febrile neutropenic patients.[124–127] These studies, however, were associated with increased Gram-positive infections in ciprofloxacin-treated patients. In addition, the in vitro activity of ciprofloxacin against *P. aeruginosa* has declined significantly (to <70% in many institutions).[117,118] Therefore, if used as part of combination therapy, ciprofloxacin should be combined with an antimicrobial with favorable in vitro activity against this pathogen.

In summary, given the limited experience with these regimens in patients with profound persistent neutropenia or infections caused by *P. aeruginosa*, empiric therapy with double β-lactam regimens should not routinely be used as primary therapy. They can be considered, however, in cases where combination therapy is indicated, but the addition of an aminoglycoside may be contraindicated.

Empiric Vancomycin

13. B.L. is begun on a three-drug regimen of ceftazidime, tobramycin, and vancomycin. What is the rationale for adding vancomycin to the regimen?

As previously discussed, the number of infections due to Gram-positive pathogens is increasing. Because cephalosporins lack activity against methicillin-resistant staphylococci, vancomycin is often added to empiric regimens. A growing proportion of *S. aureus* infections are methicillin resistant (as many as 50% in some institutions).[155] However, excessive use of vancomycin has been associated with the rise in vancomycin resistance among Gram-positive organisms, such as the vancomycin-resistant enterococci (VRE).[155] Finally, newly emergent resistance in *S. aureus* has been seen in the form of vancomycin intermediately resistant *S. aureus* (VISA) and, most recently, case reports of *S. aureus* fully resistant to vancomycin (VRSA).[155]

Clinical studies evaluating the need for vancomycin as initial empiric therapy have reached different conclusions, primarily due to differences in the measured endpoints.[156] For example, febrile neutropenic patients with cancer had more rapid resolution of fever, fewer days of bacteremia, and a lower frequency of treatment failure when vancomycin was added to an initial regimen of an antipseudomonal penicillin plus an aminoglycoside.[157,158] Similarly, the addition of vancomycin to ceftazidime showed improved results compared with ceftazidime alone or with a three-drug combination.[159] However, other studies have concluded that mortality was not increased when vancomycin therapy was delayed.[160–162] The mortality from staphylococcal infections is generally considered to be low (<4%) during the first 48 hours after the onset of fever.[156] In contrast, the mortality associated with viridans streptococcal infections may be higher among patients who are not initially treated with vancomycin.[163] Some strains of viridans streptococci are either resistant or tolerant to penicillin, but antibacterials such as piperacillin, cefepime (not ceftazidime), and carbapenems demonstrate excellent activity in vitro against these strains.[163,164]

There has been considerable debate over whether vancomycin should be included in the initial empiric regimen for febrile neutropenic patients. Many clinicians believe that this decision should be based on both patient and institution factors.[9] At institutions where these fulminant Gram-positive infections are rare, vancomycin should not be routinely used unless culture results indicate the need. However, for institutions frequently isolating invasive Gram-positive bacterial pathogens (e.g., those caused by viridans streptococci), vancomycin should probably be included in the initial empiric regimen. Other patients in whom empiric vancomycin should be considered in the initial regimen include the following:

- Patients with clinically suspected, serious catheter-related infections[9,165]
- Patients receiving intensive chemotherapy (e.g., high-dose cytarabine) that produces substantial mucosal damage and subsequent risk for penicillin-resistant streptococcal infections (i.e., viridans streptococci)[9,165,166]
- Patients receiving prior fluoroquinolone prophylaxis[167]
- Patients with a previous history of colonization with β-lactam–resistant pneumococci or methicillin-resistant *S. aureus*
- Patients with blood cultures positive for Gram-positive bacteria prior to identification and susceptibility testing
- Patients with hypotension or other evidence of cardiovascular compromise.[9,165,166]

Vancomycin has been studied in combination with various antibiotics, including imipenem-cilastatin, meropenem, ceftazidime, cefepime, and various aminoglycosides. The addition of vancomycin to an aminoglycoside-containing regimen should be done with caution, since data support an increased risk of aminoglycoside-induced nephrotoxicity in patients receiving these agents concomitantly with vancomycin.[168] Vancomycin should be discontinued after 3 to 5 days if a Gram-positive infection is not identified.[9]

Newer options exist for the treatment of invasive Gram-positive infections. Linezolid is an oxazolidinone that can be administered IV or orally.[155] It is associated with thrombocytopenia and secondary neutropenia, especially when given for prolonged periods. Considering the reduced marrow reserve in cancer chemotherapy patients, these adverse events are of particular concern. Quinupristin-dalfopristin is available for IV administration only, and concerns regarding potential drug interactions and patient tolerability may limit its use.[155] Further studies are needed with both agents before they could be routinely recommended as an alternative to vancomycin in this patient population.

In the case of B.L., empiric use of vancomycin is not warranted based on the previous discussion, and it should be discontinued unless cultures indicate the need for this antibiotic.

ANTIBIOTIC DOSING, ADMINISTRATION, AND MONITORING CONSIDERATIONS

Intermittent Versus Continuous Infusion of Intravenous Antibiotics

14. Should B.L.'s antibiotics be given intermittently (i.e., divided doses) or as a continuous infusion?

β-lactam antibiotics exhibit time-dependent (i.e., concentration-independent) pharmacodynamic activity.[169] Studies with these agents in both animal and in vitro models of infection suggest that prolonged exposure of bacteria to drug concentrations above the minimum inhibitory concentration (MIC) of the organism for a significant period of time may be linked to improved bacterial killing and survival.[169] Based on these observations and the poor prognosis of neutropenic cancer patients with bacteremia, recent noncomparative, open-label trials were conducted to evaluate the role of continuous infusions of β-lactams (i.e., ceftazidime) in the empiric treatment of suspected infection in cancer patients.[170–172] These noncomparative trials showed that continuous-infusion ceftazidime was a treatment option and should be evaluated in larger, comparative trials.

In contrast to β-lactam antibiotics, aminoglycosides exhibit concentration-dependent (time-independent) pharmacodynamic activity in both animal and in vitro models of infection.[169] Despite such properties, improved response with continuous rather than intermittent infusion of the aminoglycoside has been reported.[173] Such reports are difficult to evaluate, since many of the patients were entered into the studies after "failing" to respond to previous antibiotic regimens. Patients often differed significantly in their immune status (e.g., differences in incidence of neutropenia between study groups, uncontrolled use of granulocyte transfusions), and the total daily dose of the aminoglycoside was often greater in the continuous infusion group. In the only randomized, prospective study conducted to date, no significant difference in efficacy was observed between the two modes of administration.[173] The most convincing argument against the continuous infusion of aminoglycosides relates to the incidence of toxicity. Studies in established animal models of aminoglycoside-induced nephrotoxicity showed that the uptake of aminoglycosides into renal cortical tissue increased and glomerular function decreased more when the drug was infused continuously rather than given as single or divided doses.[174]

In conclusion, the maintenance of β-lactam antibiotic concentrations above the MIC of the suspected pathogen (as might be provided by continuous infusion) appears rational. However, data demonstrating improved effects with newer, more potent agents in cancer patients are unavailable. Considering the potential for toxicity with this route of administration, B.L. should not receive tobramycin by continuous infusion. Although consideration could be given to administering ceftazidime by continuous infusion, this method of administration would require an IV line dedicated for continuous drug administration. This technique may limit B.L.'s ability to receive intermittent tobramycin infusions unless additional IV ports or lines are available for use. Lastly, there are no data showing that this method is superior to intermittent administration.

Consolidated ("Once-Daily") Aminoglycoside Dosing

15. What is the role of consolidated ("once-daily") aminoglycoside dosing in febrile neutropenic patients such as B.L.?

Because of the concentration-dependent pharmacodynamic properties of aminoglycosides and the convenience of administration, studies have been conducted to describe both the pharmacokinetic properties and efficacy of consolidated dosing of aminoglycosides in animals and in neutropenic patients. Pharmacokinetic studies with amikacin[175,176] and gentamicin[177,178] have not revealed pharmacokinetic differences when compared with other populations. Several clinical studies have included consolidated aminoglycoside dosing for amikacin,[106,135,137,139,148,179,180] gentamicin,[147,181–183] and tobramycin.[140] However, most of the studies in this population were not designed to evaluate differences between consolidated aminoglycoside dosing compared to similar regimens using intermittent dosing.[9,184] In general, the various studies suggest that consolidated dosing is as effective and possibly less nephrotoxic than traditional dosing. Therefore, consolidated dosing of aminoglycosides appears reasonable in neutropenic patients.[184]

Outpatient Administration

Continued administration of antimicrobials in the outpatient setting has been suggested in a subset of low-risk patients.[63,179,185–187] The criteria used to eligibility for outpatient therapy are generally similar to those established and previously discussed for oral therapy. Therefore, outpatient administration of parenteral antibiotics can be considered in a subset of low-risk patients with close medical follow-up. Studies are underway to describe the economic and quality-of-life issues that may be associated with this strategy to quantify the benefits and limitations.

Antibiotic-Related Hematologic Abnormalities

16. B.L. is changed to a combination of piperacillin plus cefoperazone. Seven days later, persistent epistaxis is noted. Relevant laboratory values were Hgb, 13.1 g/dL; Hct, 38%; WBC count, 1,100 cells/mm³ (30% polys, 60% lymphocytes); prothrombin time, 20 seconds (control, 12); platelet count, 280,000 cells/mL; no fibrin split products. What are the possible drug-induced causes of B.L.'s hematologic problems?

[SI units: Hgb, 131 g/L; Hct, 0.38; WBC count, 1.1×10^9/L with 0.3 polys, 0.6 lymphocytes]

Coagulopathy caused by hypoprothrombinemia or platelet dysfunction has been infrequently associated with the use of moxalactam, cefoperazone, cefotetan, cefmetazole, and cefamandole.[188] Two mechanisms for the hypoprothrombinemia have been proposed. One hypothesis is that the significant biliary excretion of some compounds suppresses intestinal bacteria (e.g., *B. fragilis*) that produce vitamin K, a necessary cofactor in the synthesis of four clotting factors.[188] The methylthiotetrazole (MTT) moiety located at the three-position of the cephem or oxa-cephem nucleus of some β-lactams has been proposed as the cause of hypoprothrombinemia.[188] The prevalence of coagulopathy, however, may be greater in high-risk patients regardless of the antibiotic(s) administered.[188,189] Patients at high risk for coagulopathy disorders include older patients, malnourished patients, surgical patients, patients with renal disease, and patients with hematologic malignancy, such as B.L.[188,189] Coagulopathy may be minimized in these patients by administering vitamin K prophylactically to avoid the consequences of vitamin K deficiency.

In summary, B.L.'s antibiotic regimen (piperacillin plus cefoperazone) is a possible cause of his hematologic problems. The additive effects of these two drugs could have predisposed B.L. to bleeding episodes. Because of this risk, cefoperazone would be seldom used in this patient population. The hypoprothrombinemia induced by cefoperazone is best treated with administration of vitamin K. Fresh-frozen plasma can be given to patients who exhibit severe hemorrhage. Alternative antibiotics that do not contain a methylthiotetrazole group (i.e., cefepime, ceftazidime) and have less potent antiplatelet effects should be substituted if antibiotic therapy is to continue, and vitamin K 10 mg should be administered weekly during antibiotic therapy. Coagulopathy from other than drug-induced causes also needs to be evaluated.

HOST FACTORS INFLUENCING RESPONSE TO THERAPY

17. What factors may have influenced B.L.'s clinical response to antimicrobial therapy?

The most important prognostic determinants of a favorable outcome in patients with neutropenia and Gram-negative bacteremia are the recovery of the granulocyte count and the selection of agents with appropriate antimicrobial activity against the pathogen.[9] Patients with profound, persistent neutropenia (<100 cells/mm³ that does not rise during therapy or an initial ANC of 100 to 500 cells/mm³ that declines during therapy) tend to respond to antibiotics less favorably than patients whose bone marrow recovers.[9] The initial granulocyte count appears to be less important than the trend toward granulocyte recovery in influencing the patient's overall response to therapy. The site of infection also influences outcome. Septic shock and pneumonia are associated with high mortality in bacteremic neutropenic patients.[9,51]

MODIFYING INITIAL EMPIRIC ANTIBIOTIC THERAPY
Afebrile Within 3 to 5 Days

18. M.H., a 24-year-old woman with a recent diagnosis of ovarian cancer, developed neutropenia (ANC <150 cells/mm³) following chemotherapy. Five days after becoming neutropenic, she developed a fever of 101°F and was begun on an empiric antibiotic regimen of ceftazidime 2 g IV Q 8 hr. Although she remained febrile, her initial cultures remained negative at 48 hours. Should M.H. be continued on the same regimen, or should modifications be made? How do the culture results influence this decision? How long should empiric therapy be continued?

Following initiation of empiric antibiotics, a minimum of 3 days (72 hours) of empiric treatment are generally required to determine initial efficacy in the absence of worsening of clinical status. Further treatment is based on whether the fever has resolved, whether the patient's condition has improved or deteriorated, and whether an etiologic pathogen has been identified.[9] Adjustments to empiric antibiotic therapy should be made prior to 3 days if pneumonia or bacteremia is documented or if the patient's condition deteriorates.

No Etiology Identified

Premature withdrawal of antibiotics may predispose these patients to recrudescence of bacterial infection and increase the risk of infection-related morbidity and mortality. In a clinical study, 142 cancer patients with unexplained fever who became afebrile following empiric antibiotics were randomized to continue or discontinue antibiotic therapy after 7 days.[190] The patients whose neutropenia resolved had no infectious sequelae regardless of whether antibiotics were continued or discontinued. For persistently neutropenic patients randomized to continue or discontinue antibiotic therapy until their ANC was >500 cells/mm³, the percentages of patients remaining febrile without infections complications were 94% and 41%, respectively.

In general, if the fever resolves following initiation of empiric antibacterials but no identifiable etiology is identified, empiric therapy should be continued for a minimum of 7 days.[9] Patients for whom no infection is identified after 3 days of treatment, who are afebrile for 48 hours or more, and who have an ANC of at least 500 cells/mm³ for 2 consecutive days can be considered for treatment discontinuation. Although it is most desirable that the patient's ANC be at least 500 cells/mm³, discontinuing antibacterials after 14 days can be considered for patients with prolonged neutropenia in the absence of infection, with no disruption in mucous membranes and integument, and in whom no invasive procedures or ablative chemotherapy is planned. Patients at higher risk of infectious complications (ANC <500 cells/mm³ at day 7 with initially severe neutropenia [ANC <100 cells/mm³] or mucositis or who are clinically unstable) should continue antibacterial treatment.[9]

M.H.'s slow response to empiric ceftazidime suggests that this regimen may be suboptimal. However, it is prudent to wait at least 72 hours to make that assessment in the absence of clinical worsening. If at 72 hours M.H. becomes afebrile and remains so for 5 to 7 days, it would be reasonable to discontinue ceftazidime after 7 days as long as she appears clinically well and has no apparent evidence of infection. Although it is desirable for M.H.'s ANC to be >500 cells/mm³ before treatment is stopped, therapy may be discontinued before this time as long as she is closely monitored for recurrent fever and/or evidence of new infection.

Etiology Identified

19. On day 3, M.H.'s temperature is normal (97.6°C). However, two sets of blood cultures drawn 3 days ago have grown S. aureus resistant to methicillin and susceptible to vancomycin. Her ANC is 170 cells/mm³. How should therapy be modified in M.H.? For how long should antibiotics be continued?

Pizzo and colleagues treated 78 neutropenic cancer patients with documented Gram-positive bacteremias with a single drug (e.g., oxacillin, nafcillin) or a broad-spectrum combination regimen that provided Gram-positive coverage (carbenicillin plus cephalothin plus gentamicin).[191] Of the 15 patients treated with pathogen-directed therapy who remained neutropenic for >7 days, 7 developed a secondary infection. In contrast, none of the 24 patients who continued to receive the broad-spectrum combination regimen developed any secondary infections.

For patients such as M.H. for whom an infectious cause of fever is identified but who are afebrile at 3 to 5 days, additional antimicrobials or antibiotic dosage adjustments (based on antimicrobial susceptibility tests and antibiotic serum concentrations) may be required.[9] Despite such modifications, broad-spectrum antibacterial coverage should be maintained in patients who remain persistently neutropenic.[9] If M.H.'s neutropenia resolves, broad-spectrum antimicrobials may be discontinued and narrow-spectrum therapy directed against the infecting pathogen should be continued for an appropriate duration. However, because M.H. remains neutropenic, the ceftazidime should be continued for a minimum of 7 days or until her ANC is >500 cells/mm³. Vancomycin should be added to treat the staphylococcal bacteremia and should be continued for an appropriate treatment course of 10 to 14 days (assuming an uncomplicated infection).

Persistent Fever During the First 3 to 5 Days

No Etiology Identified

20. S.B. is a 55-year-old woman with chronic myelogenous leukemia (CML). She was admitted to the hospital with a 4-day history of fevers and night sweats. On admission, her temperature was 102.3°F and her WBC count was 100,000 cells/mm³ with an ANC of 500 cells/mm³. Blood and urine cultures were obtained, and ceftazidime plus tobramycin was empirically started. Over the next 3 days, S.B. remained persistently febrile and neutropenic. All cultures remained negative. How should she be treated?

One of the most challenging and controversial aspects of empiric antibacterial therapy in the neutropenic host is the management of patients without a microbiologically documented infection who remain persistently febrile on broad-spectrum antibacterial therapy. A persistent fever may be due to tumor lysis, an infection caused by resistant bacteria, slow response to appropriate therapy, drug-related fever, superinfection, infections caused by nonbacterial pathogens (e.g., fungi, viruses), inadequate serum or tissue levels of antibiotics, or an avascular infection (e.g., abscess). By days 3 to 5 following the initiation of empiric antibiotics, S.B. should be reassessed in an attempt to identify any one or more of these causes.[9] A meticulous physical examination and a thorough review of all culture results should be done. If indicated, additional cultures, diagnostic imaging of suspected areas of infection, and serum drug concentrations should be obtained.

Based on the results and reassessment, options for management are to continue the current empiric regimen, change antimicrobials, or add empiric antifungal therapy with or without changes to antibacterial therapy[9] (Table 68-2). Each of these treatment options will be discussed separately.

Recent guidelines published by the Infectious Diseases Society of America (IDSA) suggest that even if fever persists after 5 days, the initial empiric regimen can be continued without modification as long as the patient remains stable and does not clinically deteriorate.[9] This treatment decision arm works best in patients with neutropenia expected to resolve within the subsequent 5 days.[9] Additional consideration should be given to discontinuing vancomycin (if applicable) in the ab-

sence of evidence for a Gram-positive infection. Treatments are generally continued for a minimum of 4 to 5 days after the resolution of neutropenia.[9] The need for further antibiotics can then be reassessed. Patients for whom neutropenia does not resolve generally receive at least 2 weeks of therapy, at which time treatment needs can be reassessed.[9]

Modify Initial Antibiotics

21. S.B., on day 4, continues to feel "lousy" and has started to complain of abdominal pains. What is the significance of this complaint? Should her antibiotic regimen be modified again?

In neutropenic patients with evidence of disease progression, the initial empiric regimen is generally modified (see Table 68-2). Such evidence may include catheter site drainage, abdominal pain, or pulmonary infiltrates. In such cases (or in the event of drug-related toxicities), consideration should be given to adding antibiotics or changing to a different antibiotic regimen. Because S.B. has developed new abdominal pains suggestive of enterocolitis, her antibiotic regimen should be modified. Although cefepime provides excellent coverage against the common Gram-negative pathogens, it has limited activity against select Gram-positive pathogens (such as MRSA or VRE) and anaerobes. A change from cefepime to imipenem-cilastatin or another broad-spectrum regimen with both aerobic and anaerobic activity should be considered.

Antifungal Therapy

22. S.B.'s antibiotic regimen was changed to imipenem-cilastatin plus tobramycin. Despite the change, she continues to have a low-grade fever and does not feel better. What is S.B.'s risk for developing a systemic fungal infection? What is the significance of fungal infections in neutropenic cancer patients?

The incidence of invasive fungal infections in febrile neutropenic patients varies between studies due to differences in definitions, methods of detection, specific patient populations studied, and the prior use of antifungal prophylaxis.[192] In one retrospective review, the incidence of documented invasive fungal infections in patients with leukemia was 27% (32 of 119).[16] However, the diagnosis of invasive fungal infection was established before death in only nine of the patients. In general, patients with hematologic malignancies have a higher incidence of fungal infections than those with solid tumors.[192] Early diagnosis and prompt treatment of such systemic fungal diseases are critical to patient survival.[192] Therefore, patients with protracted fever and granulocytopenia for ≥5 days despite the administration of broad-spectrum antibiotics should be considered for empiric antifungal therapy.

Most fungal infections in neutropenic cancer patients are caused by *Candida* and *Aspergillus* species.[193–195] Other less common but important pathogenic fungi are those associated with zygomycosis (e.g., *Mucor, Rhizopus* species) and other emerging pathogens (non-albicans *Candida, Trichosporon beigelii, Malassezia* species, *Cryptococcus neoformans,* and *Fusarium* species).[193–195]

It is difficult to compare clinical trials evaluating empiric antibiotic therapy in neutropenic cancer patients due to clinical trial design elements such as inclusion of low-risk pa-

Table 68-2   Modifications Following Initial Empiric Antibacterials in Patients With Neutropenia and Fever

Clinical Condition	Suspected Pathogen(s) and Type of Modification(s)
Afebrile within 3–5 days of treatment	
No etiology identified	Low risk: change to ciprofloxacin + amoxicillin-clavulanate (adults) or cefixime (children).
	High risk: continue antibiotic therapy.
Etiology identified	Adjust antibiotics to most appropriate therapy based on infection.
Persistent fever (3–5 days) without clinical or microbiologic evidence of infection	No evidence of progressive infection: continue antibiotics.
	Consider empiric antifungal therapy, especially if resolution of neutropenia is not imminent (e.g., amphotericin B).
	If initial regimen did not include vancomycin: re-evaluate risk factors for Gram-positive infection, consider adding vancomycin.
Positive Gram stain from	Gram-positive: add vancomycin, pending further identification (especially in blood culture institutions with high rate of methicillin-resistant *S. aureus*)
	Gram-negative: if monotherapy, consider adding aminoglycoside to carbapenem or β-lactam therapy.
Head, Eyes, Ears, Nose, Throat	
Necrotizing ulceration/gingivitis	If initial regimen did not include carbapenem or β-lactam/β-lactamase inhibitor (i.e., piperacillin-tazobactam), consider adding clindamycin or metronidazole or switch to carbapenem (imipenem-cilastatin or meropenem).
	Consider adding antifungal therapy.
Vesicular lesions	Add antiviral therapy for *Herpes simplex* virus: (e.g., acyclovir).
Oral mucositis	Evidence of candidiasis: add oral clotrimazole, nystatin, or fluconazole.
Sinus tenderness	Suspicion of *Aspergillus* or mucormycosis: add amphotericin B or voriconazole.
	Reassess antistaphylococcal activity of empiric regimen; consider vancomycin.
Gastrointestinal Tract	
Esophagitis	*Candida* and/or *Herpes simplex:* Add antifungal agent; if no response, add acyclovir. Assess CMV risk and (if high) consider ganciclovir or foscarnet.
Acute abdominal pain/perianal	If initial regimen did not include carbapenem or β-lactam/β-lactamase intenderness hibitor (i.e., piperacillin-tazobactam), consider adding clindamycin or metronidazole or switch to imipenem-cilastatin or meropenem
	Consider enterococcal coverage.
	Consider antifungal coverage.
Respiratory Tract	
Interstitial pneumonitis	*Pneumocystis carinii:* Institute trial of TMP-SMX or pentamidine.
	Legionella: Add macrolide.
	CMV: Add ganciclovir if high risk.
Focal lesion on chest radiograph	If evidence of fungal infection, add voriconazole or amphotericin B (1.0–1.5 mg/kg per day) (if *Aspergillus* spp suspected).
	Consider growth factors (G-CSF, GM-CSF).
	Consider antibiotic coverage for pathogen causing atypical pneumonia.
Central venous catheter tunnel infection	Remove catheter. Consider adding empiric vancomycin therapy. Adjust based on culture and susceptibility results.

CMV, cytomegalovirus; TMP-SMX, trimethoprim-sulfamethoxazole.
Based on: National Comprehensive Cancer Network's Fever and Neutropenia Guidelines, 2003, and Hughes WT et al. 2002 guidelines for the use of antimicrobial agents in neutropenic patients with cancer. Clin Infect Dis 2002;34:730.

tients, lack of blinding, changes in concomitant antibacterials obscuring antifungal therapy endpoints, prior antifungal prophylaxis, use of composite endpoints of safety and efficacy, and different endpoint criteria.[192] While select studies have also demonstrated that empiric antifungal therapy can decrease fungal-related deaths, overall mortality has not been affected.[196,197] This is the case particularly for patients with invasive disease and persistent neutropenia.

EMPIRIC AMPHOTERICIN B THERAPY

23. Why should amphotericin B therapy be considered in S.B.?

Historically, amphotericin B deoxycholate is most commonly used in this setting because of its reliable activity in vitro against most *Candida* and *Aspergillus* species.[198,199] Pizzo and associates demonstrated the impact of empiric amphotericin B deoxycholate in persistently febrile neutropenic patients.[200] After 7 days of empiric broad-spectrum antibiotics, 50 patients with unexplained fever, prolonged granulocytopenia, and evidence of GI colonization with *Candida* species were randomized to one of three groups. Patients in group 1 continued to receive broad-spectrum antibiotics, those in group 2 had their antibiotics discontinued, and those in group 3 had amphotericin B added empirically to their antibiotic regimen. Infectious complications (e.g., bacterial or fungal infection, shock) developed in 9 of 16 patients (56%) in group 2 within 3 days of stopping antibiotics. Of the 16 patients in group 1 who continued to receive antibiotics until neutropenia resolved, an infectious complication developed in 6 (38%), 5 of which were caused by fungal infections. In the 18 patients randomized to receive amphotericin B, only 2 patients developed infectious complications. One of these infections in the latter group was caused by an amphotericin B–resistant organism (*P. boydii*).

Amphotericin B is still considered by many to be the empiric antifungal drug of choice in this patient population.[198] Recent comparative trials have evaluated the role of lipid-based formulations of amphotericin B in the treatment of suspected or documented infections in this population.[201–209] Liposomal amphotericin B,[201–203,205] amphotericin B lipid complex,[203] and amphotericin B colloidal dispersion[204] have demonstrated reductions in nephrotoxicity compared to amphotericin B deoxycholate. In addition, liposomal amphotericin B offers the potential for reducing infusion-related side effects.[202] However, efficacy appears comparable between the preparations, and the lipid formulations are substantially more expensive based on acquisition costs. Therefore, their use is generally restricted to patients with underlying renal dysfunction or those with significant risk factors for amphotericin B-induced nephrotoxicity. Although there are limited data to suggest that the continuous infusion of amphotericin B deoxycholate may also reduce nephrotoxicity,[210] efficacy regarding this method of administration has not been established and cannot be recommended at this time.

When initiated as empiric therapy, amphotericin B is generally continued (in the absence of a documented fungal infection) in a clinically stable patient until the resolution of neutropenia. Clinically stable patients without evidence of fungal infection but with persistent neutropenia often receive a 2-week course of therapy. Patients with documented (invasive) fungal infections are treated with variable durations of treatment, depending on the fungal diagnosis.

ALTERNATIVES TO AMPHOTERICIN B

In centers where mold infections with *Aspergillus* and drug-resistant *Candida* species (e.g., *C. krusei* and some strains of *C. glabrata*) are uncommon, fluconazole may be an acceptable empiric alternative to amphotericin B.[211,212] Patients with suspected aspergillosis or for whom fluconazole was used as prophylaxis should be excluded. Itraconazole may also prove to be an alternative in these patients, and it has reduced toxicity relative to amphotericin B.[213] Caspofungin, an injectable echinocandin, has demonstrated in vitro activity against *Candida* species and *Aspergillus* species but has had limited published experience as empiric therapy in this population.[214] Finally, voriconazole (a new azole antifungal agent with increased activity against *Aspergillus* and non-albicans

Candida relative to fluconazole) has also been tested in this population.[205] This trial concluded that voriconazole should be considered as an alternative to amphotericin B preparations for empiric therapy in this population. However, voriconazole has not yet received FDA approval for this indication.

Antiviral Therapy

Empiric use of antiviral agents in the febrile neutropenic patient are not indicated without evidence of viral disease.[9] In contrast, clinical evidence of herpes simplex or varicella-zoster virus involving the skin or mucous membranes should be treated with antivirals (e.g., acyclovir, valacyclovir, famciclovir).[9] With the exception of patients undergoing bone marrow transplantation,[215] cytomegalovirus is an uncommon source of infection in the febrile neutropenic patient.

ANTIMICROBIAL ADJUVANTS

24. S.B. became afebrile 2 days after amphotericin B was initiated, yet she remained neutropenic with an ANC of 480 cells/mm³. An induction chemotherapy regimen consisting of idarubicin plus cytarabine was initiated for her CML. Because the chemotherapy will further reduce her ANC 7 to 10 days after treatment, is there any way to facilitate marrow recovery and reduce the duration of neutropenia in S.B.?

As previously discussed, the duration of neutropenia is the most important factor affecting outcome in neutropenic cancer patients. Because of this, there has been considerable interest in enhancing the immune system in these patients.

Granulocyte Transfusions

One of the earliest approaches used to boost the patient's defense against infections was the transfusion of WBCs. In the 1970s, granulocyte transfusions were used adjunctively in patients with persistent neutropenia and documented infections who, despite appropriate antibiotics, failed to respond after 24 to 48 hours. This approach had limited value because of the difficulties in obtaining adequate cells for transfusion, as well as the problems with alloimmunization and risk of infection transmission. In addition, the questionable efficacy of WBC transfusions has decreased the use of this strategy.[216] Therefore, granulocyte transfusions are not indicated routinely in this population.

Myeloid Colony-Stimulating Factors

The introduction of hematopoietic colony-stimulating factors (CSFs) such as G-CSF (filgrastim) or GM-CSF (sargramostim) in clinical practice has raised the hopes of improving survival in cancer patients.[217] CSFs act on various stages of cell proliferation and differentiation in the bone marrow (see Chapter 89, Adverse Effects of Chemotherapy). Studies in cancer patients receiving myelosuppressive or myeloablative chemotherapy have demonstrated that concurrent use of the CSFs can reduce the duration of neutropenia.[217] Rash, bone pain, headache, fever, and myalgias have been reported as side effects with both G-CSF and GM-CSF.[217] Bone pain is usually mild to moderate and often responds to nonopiate analgesics (acetaminophen or ibuprofen). The pain usually resolves upon discontinuation. A flu-like syndrome consisting of fever, chills, rigors, headache, and GI symptoms has been reported in many patients receiving GM-CSF.[217] The selection of one CSF agent over another is often based on practitioner preference rather than clinical data.

Because these agents have not demonstrated a consistent and significant effect on other infection-related parameters (e.g., duration of fever, use of antibiotics, or costs of treatment),[217] both the American Society of Clinical Oncology[218] and the Infectious Diseases Society of America[9] recommend against the routine use of CSFs for febrile neutropenic patients. The exception would be patients with clinical instability (hypotension or multiorgan system failure secondary to sepsis) or infections (pneumonia, severe cellulitis, sinusitis, invasive fungal infection) that are expected to worsen, and in whom there is an expected prolonged delay in recovery from neutropenia.

G-CSF administration, although likely to reduce the duration of her chemotherapy-induced neutropenia, is not indicated in S.B., who is otherwise stable.

REFERENCES

1. Zinner SH. New pathogens in neutropenic patients with cancer: an update for the new millennium. Int J Antimicrob Agents 2000;16:97.
2. Bodey G. Quantitative relationships between circulating leukocytes and infection in patients with acute leukemia. Ann Intern Med 1966;64:328.
3. Viscoli C, Castagnola E. Treatment of febrile neutropenia: what is new? Curr Opinion Infect Dis 2002;15:377.
4. Stuck AE et al. Risk of infectious complications in patients taking glucocorticosteroids. Rev Infect Dis 1989;11:954.
5. Schimpff SC et al. Origin of infection in acute nonlymphocytic leukemia. Significance of hospital acquisition of potential pathogens. Ann Intern Med 1972;77:707.
6. De Bock R, Middelheim AZ. Febrile neutropenia in allogeneic transplantation. Int J Antimicrob Agents 2000;16:177.
7. Dykewicz CA, Centers for Disease Control and Prevention, Infectious Diseases Society of America, and American Society of Blood and Marrow Transplantation. Summary of the Guidelines for Preventing Opportunistic Infections Among Hematopoietic Stem Cell Transplant Recipients. Clin Infect Dis 2001;33:139.
8. Barton TD, Schuster MG. The cause of fever following resolution of neutropenia in patients with acute leukemia. Clin Infect Dis 1996;22:1064.
9. Hughes WT et al. 2002 guidelines for the use of antimicrobial agents in neutropenic patients with cancer. Clin Infect Dis 2002;34:730.
10. Coullioud D et al. Prospective multicentric study of the etiology of 1051 bacteremic episodes in 782 cancer patients. CEMIC (French-Belgian Study Club of Infectious Diseases in Cancer). Suppor Care Cancer 1993;1:34.
11. Cordonnier C et al. Epidemiology and risk factors for gram-positive coccal infections in neutropenia: toward a more targeted antibiotic strategy. Clin Infect Dis 2003;36:149.
12. Zinner SH. Changing epidemiology of infections in patients with neutropenia and cancer: emphasis on Gram-positive and resistant bacteria. Clin Infect Dis 1999;29:490.
13. Murray BE. Vancomycin-resistant enterococci. Am J Med 1997;102:284.
14. Mathur P et al. A study of bacteremia in febrile neutropenic patients at a tertiary-care hospital with special reference to anaerobes. Med Oncol 2002;19:267.
15. De Pauw BE. Treatment of documented and suspected neutropenia-associated invasive fungal infections. J Chemother 2001;13(Spec No 1):181.
16. DeGregorio MW et al. Fungal infections in patients with acute leukemia. Am J Med 1982;73:543.
17. Cruciani M. Antibacterial prophylaxis. Int J Antimicrob Agents 2000;16:123.
18. Schimpff SC et al. Infection prevention in acute nonlymphocytic leukemia. Laminar air flow room reverse isolation with oral, nonabsorbable antibiotic prophylaxis. Ann Intern Med 1975;82:351.
19. EORTC International Antimicrobial Therapy Project Group. Trimethoprim-sulfamethoxazole in the prevention of infection in neutropenic patients. J Infect Dis 1984;150:372.
20. Hughes WT et al. Successful intermittent chemoprophylaxis for *Pneumocystis carinii* pneumonitis. N Engl J Med 1987;316:1627.
21. Wade JC et al. A comparison of trimethoprim-sulfamethoxazole plus nystatin with gentamicin plus nystatin in the prevention of infections in acute leukemia. N Engl J Med 1981;304:1057.
22. Bow EJ et al. Quinolone-based antibacterial chemoprophylaxis in neutropenic patients: effect of augmented Gram-positive activity on infectious morbidity. National Cancer Institute of Canada Clinical Trials Group. Ann Intern Med 1996;125:183.
23. Cruciani M et al. Prophylaxis with fluoroquinolones for bacterial infections in neutropenic patients: a meta-analysis. Clin Infect Dis 1996;23:795.
24. Engels EA et al. Efficacy of quinolone prophylaxis in neutropenic cancer patients: a meta-analysis. J Clin Oncol 1998;16:1179.
25. Kern W, Kurrle E. Ofloxacin versus trimethoprim-sulfamethoxazole for prevention of infection in patients with acute leukemia and granulocytopenia. Infection 1991;19:73.
26. Lew MA et al. Ciprofloxacin versus trimethoprim/sulfamethoxazole for prophylaxis of bacterial infections in bone marrow transplant recipients: a randomized, controlled trial. J Clin Oncol 1995;13:239.
27. Horvathova Z et al. Bacteremia due to methicillin-resistant staphylococci occurs more frequently in neutropenic patients who received antimicrobial prophylaxis and is associated with higher mortality in comparison to methicillin-sensitive bacteriemia. Int J Antimicrob Agents 1998;10:55.
28. Oppenheim BA et al. Outbreak of coagulase negative staphylococcus highly resistant to ciprofloxacin in a leukaemia unit. Br Med J 1989;299:294.
29. Carratala J et al. Emergence of quinolone-resistant *Escherichia coli* bacteremia in neutropenic patients with cancer who have received prophylactic norfloxacin. Clin Infect Dis 1995;20:557.
30. Gomez-Martin C et al. Rifampin does not improve the efficacy of quinolone antibacterial prophylaxis in neutropenic cancer patients: results of a randomized clinical trial. J Clin Oncol 2000;18:2126.
31. Young GA et al. A double-blind comparison of fluconazole and nystatin in the prevention of candidiasis in patients with leukaemia. Antifungal Prophylaxis Study Group. Eur J Cancer 1999;35:1208.
32. Owens NJ et al. Prophylaxis of oral candidiasis with clotrimazole troches. Arch Intern Med 1984;144:290.
33. Akiyama H et al. Fluconazole versus oral amphotericin B in preventing fungal infection in chemotherapy-induced neutropenic patients with haematological malignancies. Mycoses 1993;36:373.
34. Nucci M et al. A double-blind, randomized, placebo-controlled trial of itraconazole capsules as antifungal prophylaxis for neutropenic patients. Clin Infect Dis 2000;30:300.
35. Menichetti F et al. Itraconazole oral solution as prophylaxis for fungal infections in neutropenic patients with hematologic malignancies: a randomized, placebo-controlled, double-blind, multicenter trial. GIMEMA Infection Program. Gruppo Italiano Malattie Ematologiche dell' Adulto. Clin Infect Dis 1999;28:250.
36. Harousseau JL et al. Itraconazole oral solution for primary prophylaxis of fungal infections in patients with hematological malignancy and profound neutropenia: a randomized, double-blind, double-placebo, multicenter trial comparing itraconazole and amphotericin B. Antimicrob Agents Chemother 2000;44:1887.
37. Chandrasekar PH, Gatny CM. Effect of fluconazole prophylaxis on fever and use of amphotericin in neutropenic cancer patients. Bone Marrow Transplantation Team. Chemotherapy 1994;40:136.
38. Goodman JL et al. A controlled trial of fluconazole to prevent fungal infections in patients undergoing bone marrow transplantation. N Engl J Med 1992;326:845.
39. Ellis ME et al. Controlled study of fluconazole in the prevention of fungal infections in neutropenic patients with haematological malignancies and bone marrow transplant recipients. Eur J Clin Microbiol Infect Dis 1994;13:3.
40. Winston DJ et al. Fluconazole prophylaxis of fungal infections in patients with acute leukemia. Results of a randomized placebo-controlled, double-blind, multicenter trial. Ann Intern Med 1993;118:495.
41. Safdar A et al. Hematogenous infections due to *Candida parapsilosis*: changing trends in fungemic patients at a comprehensive cancer center during the last four decades. Eur J Clin Microbiol Infect Dis 2002;44:11.
42. Gotzsche PC, Johansen HK. Routine versus selective antifungal administration for control of fungal infections in patients with cancer. Cochrane Database of Systematic Reviews 2002;CD000026.
43. Winston DJM. Intravenous and oral itraconazole versus intravenous and oral fluconazole for long-term antifungal prophylaxis in allogeneic hematopoietic stem-cell transplant recipients: A multicenter, randomized trial. Ann Intern Med 2003;138:705.
44. Bodey GP et al. Antifungal prophylaxis during remission induction therapy for acute leukemia fluconazole versus intravenous amphotericin B. Cancer 1994;73:2099.
45. Mattiuzzi GN et al. Liposomal amphotericin B versus the combination of fluconazole and itraconazole as prophylaxis for invasive fungal infections during induction chemotherapy for patients with acute myelogenous leukemia and myelodysplastic syndrome. Cancer 2003;97:450.
46. Feld R et al. Methodology for clinical trials involving patients with cancer who have febrile neutropenia: updated guidelines of the Immunocompromised Host Society/Multinational Association for Supportive Care in Cancer, with emphasis on outpatient studies. Clin Infect Dis 2002;35:1463.
47. Gurwith MJ et al. Granulocytopenia in hospitalized patients: I. Prognostic factors and etiology of fever. Am J Med 1978;64:121.

48. Gill FA et al. The relationship of fever, granulocytopenia and antimicrobial therapy to bacteremia in cancer patients. Cancer 1977;39:1704.

49. Bodey GP. Unusual presentations of infection in neutropenic patients. Int J Antimicrob Agents 2000;16:93.

50. Malik I et al. Clinical characteristics and therapeutic outcome of patients with febrile neutropenia who present in shock: need for better strategies. J Infect 2001;42:120.

51. Dompeling EC et al. Evolution of the clinical manifestations of infection during the course of febrile neutropenia in patients with malignancy. Infection 1998;26:349.

52. Bille J. Laboratory diagnosis of infections in febrile neutropenic or immunocompromised patients. Int J Antimicrob Agents 2000;16:87.

53. Newman KA, Schimpff SC. Hospital hotel services as risk factors for infection among immunocompromised patients. Rev Infect Dis 1987;9:206.

54. Fainstein V et al. Patterns of oropharyngeal and fecal flora in patients with acute leukemia. J Infect Dis 1981;144:10.

55. Kurrle E et al. Risk factors for infections of the oropharynx and the respiratory tract in patients with acute leukemia. J Infect Dis 1981;144:128.

56. Schimpff SC et al. Significance of *Pseudomonas aeruginosa* in the patient with leukemia or lymphoma. J Infect Dis 1974;130(Suppl):S24.

57. de Jong PJ et al. The value of surveillance cultures in neutropenic patients receiving selective intestinal decontamination. Scand J Infect Dis 1993;25:107.

58. Hathorn JW, Lyke K. Empirical treatment of febrile neutropenia: evolution of current therapeutic approaches. Clin Infect Dis 1997;24(Suppl 2):S256.

59. Schimpff SC et al. Three antibiotic regimens in the treatment of infection in febrile granulocytopenic patients with cancer. The EORTC International Antimicrobial Therapy Project Group. J Infect Dis 1978;137:14.

60. NCCN practice guidelines for fever and neutropenia. National Comprehensive Cancer Network. Oncology (Huntington) 1999;13:197.

61. Castagnola E et al. Clinical and laboratory features predicting a favorable outcome and allowing early discharge in cancer patients with low-risk febrile neutropenia: a literature review. J Hematother Stem Cell Res 2000;9:645.

62. Koh A, Pizzo PA. Empirical oral antibiotic therapy for low-risk febrile cancer patients with neutropenia. Cancer Invest 2002;20:420.

63. Klastersky J et al. The Multinational Association for Supportive Care in Cancer risk index: A multinational scoring system for identifying low-risk febrile neutropenic cancer patients. J Clin Oncol 2000;18:3038.

64. Freifeld A et al. A double-blind comparison of empirical oral and intravenous antibiotic therapy for low-risk febrile patients with neutropenia during cancer chemotherapy. N Engl J Med 1999; 341:305.

65. Kern WV et al. Oral versus intravenous empirical antimicrobial therapy for fever in patients with granulocytopenia who are receiving cancer chemotherapy. International Antimicrobial Therapy Cooperative Group of the European Organization for Research and Treatment of Cancer. N Engl J Med 1999;341:312.

66. Paganini HR et al. Oral administration of cefixime to lower risk febrile neutropenic children with cancer. Cancer 2000;88:2848.

67. Jacobs RF et al. Ceftazidime versus ceftazidime plus tobramycin in febrile neutropenic children. Infection 1993;21:223.

68. Mustafa MM et al. Comparative study of cefepime versus ceftazidime in the empiric treatment of pediatric cancer patients with fever and neutropenia. Pediatr Infect Dis J 2001;20:362.

69. Chuang YY et al. Cefepime versus ceftazidime as empiric monotherapy for fever and neutropenia in children with cancer. Pediatr Infect Dis J 2002; 21:203.

70. Fleischhack G et al. Meropenem versus ceftazidime as empirical monotherapy in febrile neutropenia of paediatric patients with cancer. J Antimicrob Chemother 2001;47:841.

71. Kebudi R et al. Randomized comparison of cefepime versus ceftazidime monotherapy for fever and neutropenia in children with solid tumors. Med Pediatr Oncol 2001;36:434.

72. Feld R et al. Meropenem versus ceftazidime in the treatment of cancer patients with febrile neutropenia: a randomized, double-blind trial. J Clin Oncol 2000;18:3690.

73. Chandrasekar PH, Arnow PM. Cefepime versus ceftazidime as empiric therapy for fever in neutropenic patients with cancer. Ann Pharmacother 2000;34:989.

74. Wang FD et al. A comparative study of cefepime versus ceftazidime as empiric therapy of febrile episodes in neutropenic patients. Chemotherapy 1999;45:370.

75. Antabli BA et al. Empiric antimicrobial therapy of febrile neutropenic patients undergoing haematopoietic stem cell transplantation. Int J Antimicrob Agents 1999;13:127.

76. Lindblad R et al. Empiric monotherapy for febrile neutropenia: a randomized study comparing meropenem with ceftazidime. Scand J Infect Dis 1998;30:237.

77. Aparicio J et al. Randomized comparison of ceftazidime and imipenem as initial monotherapy for febrile episodes in neutropenic cancer patients. Eur J Cancer 1996;32A:1739.

78. Equivalent efficacies of meropenem and ceftazidime as empirical monotherapy of febrile neutropenic patients. The Meropenem Study Group of Leuven, London and Nijmegen. J Antimicrobial Chemother 1995;36:185.

79. Freifeld AG et al. Monotherapy for fever and neutropenia in cancer patients: a randomized comparison of ceftazidime versus imipenem. J Clin Oncol 1995;13:165.

80. De Pauw BE et al. Ceftazidime compared with piperacillin and tobramycin for the empiric treatment of fever in neutropenic patients with cancer. A multicenter randomized trial. The Intercontinental Antimicrobial Study Group. Ann Intern Med 1994;120:834.

81. Miller JA et al. Efficacy and tolerability of imipenem-cilastatin versus ceftazidime plus tobramycin as empiric therapy of presumed bacterial infection in neutropenic cancer patients. Clin Ther 1993;15:486.

82. Vancomycin added to empirical combination antibiotic therapy for fever in granulocytopenic cancer patients. European Organization for Research and Treatment of Cancer (EORTC) International Antimicrobial Therapy Cooperative Group and the National Cancer Institute of Canada-Clinical Trials Group. J Infect Dis 1991;163:951.

83. Rubin M et al. Gram-positive infections and the use of vancomycin in 550 episodes of fever and neutropenia. Ann Intern Med 1988;108:30.

84. Ariffin H et al. Ceftazidime-resistant *Klebsiella pneumoniae* bloodstream infection in children with febrile neutropenia. Int J Infect Dis 2000;4:21.

85. Fanci R et al. Management of fever in neutropenic patients with acute leukemia: current role of ceftazidime plus amikacin as empiric therapy. J Chemother 2000;12:232.

86. Cunha BA, Gill MV. Cefepime. Med Clin North Am 1995;79:721.

87. Kennedy HF et al. Antimicrobial susceptibility of blood culture isolates of viridans streptococci: relationship to a change in empirical antibiotic therapy in febrile neutropenia. J Antimicrob Chemother 2001;47:693.

88. Biron P et al. Cefepime versus imipenem-cilastatin as empirical monotherapy in 400 febrile patients with short duration neutropenia. CEMIC (Study Group of Infectious Diseases in Cancer). J Antimicrob Chemother 1998;42:511.

89. Bohme A et al. Piperacillin/tazobactam versus cefepime as initial empirical antimicrobial therapy in febrile neutropenic patients: a prospective randomized pilot study. Eur J Med Res 1998;3:324.

90. Borbolla JR et al. Comparison of cefepime versus ceftriaxone-amikacin as empirical regimens for the treatment of febrile neutropenia in acute leukemia patients. Chemotherapy 2001;47:381.

91. Engervall P et al. Cefepime as empirical monotherapy in febrile patients with hematological malignancies and neutropenia: a randomized, single-center phase II trial. J Chemother 1999; 11:278.

92. Jandula BM et al. Treatment of febrile neutropenia with cefepime monotherapy. Chemotherapy 2001;47:226.

93. Montalar JS. Cefepime monotherapy as an empirical initial treatment of patients with febrile neutropenia. Med Oncol 2002;19:161.

94. Tamura K et al. Cefepime or carbapenem treatment for febrile neutropenia as a single agent is as effective as a combination of 4th-generation cephalosporin plus aminoglycosides: comparative study. Am J Hematol 2002;71:248.

95. Yamamura D et al. Open randomized study of cefepime versus piperacillin-gentamicin for treatment of febrile neutropenic cancer patients. Antimicrob Agents Chemother 1997;41:1704.

96. Au E et al. Randomised study comparing imipenem/cilastatin to ceftriaxone plus gentamicin in cancer chemotherapy-induced neutropenic fever. Ann Acad Med Singapore 1994;23:819.

97. Bodey G et al. Imipenem or cefoperazone-sulbactam combined with vancomycin for therapy of presumed or proven infection in neutropenic cancer patients. Eur J Clin Microbiol Infect Dis 1996;15:625.

98. Bohme A et al. A randomized study of imipenem compared to cefotaxime plus piperacillin as initial therapy of infections in granulocytopenic patients. Infection 1995;23:349.

99. Bohme A et al. Prospective randomized study to compare imipenem 1.5 grams per day vs. 3.0 grams per day in infections of granulocytopenic patients. J Infect 1998;36:35.

100. Erjavec Z et al. Comparison of imipenem versus cefuroxime plus tobramycin as empirical therapy for febrile granulocytopenic patients and efficacy of vancomycin and aztreonam in case of failure. Scand J Infect Dis 1994;26:585.

101. Kojima A et al. A randomized prospective study of imipenem-cilastatin with or without amikacin as an empirical antibiotic treatment for febrile neutropenic patients. Am J Clin Oncol 1994;17:400.

102. Marra F et al. Piperacillin/tazobactam versus imipenem: a double-blind, randomized formulary feasibility study at a major teaching hospital. Eur J Clin Microbiol Infect Dis 1998;31:355.

103. Ozyilkan O et al. Imipenem-cilastatin versus sulbactam-cefoperazone plus amikacin in the initial treatment of febrile neutropenic cancer patients. Korean J Intern Med 1999;14:15.

104. Shah PM et al. Empirical monotherapy with meropenem versus imipenem/cilastatin for febrile episodes in neutropenic patients. Infection 1996;24:480.

105. Rolston KV et al. A comparison of imipenem to ceftazidime with or without amikacin as empiric therapy in febrile neutropenic patients. Arch Intern Med 1992;152:283.

106. Akova M et al. Comparison of meropenem with amikacin plus ceftazidime in the empirical treatment of febrile neutropenia: a prospective randomised multicentre trial in patients without previous prophylactic antibiotics. Meropenem Study Group of Turkey. Int J Antimicrob Agents 1999; 13:15.

107. Behre G et al. Meropenem monotherapy versus combination therapy with ceftazidime and amikacin for empirical treatment of febrile neutropenic patients. Ann Hematol 1998;76:73.

108. Cometta A et al. Monotherapy with meropenem versus combination therapy with ceftazidime plus amikacin as empiric therapy for fever in granulocytopenic patients with cancer. The International Antimicrobial Therapy Cooperative Group of the European Organization for Research and Treatment of Cancer and the Gruppo Italiano Malattie

Ematologiche Maligne dell' Adulto Infection Program. Antimicrob Agents Chemother 1996;40:1108.

109. Duzova A et al. Monotherapy with meropenem versus combination therapy with piperacillin plus amikacin as empiric therapy for neutropenic fever in children with lymphoma and solid tumors. Turk J Pediatr 2001;43:105.

110. Vandercam B et al. Meropenem versus ceftazidime as empirical monotherapy for febrile neutropenic cancer patients. Ann Hematol 2000;79:152.

111. Cunha BA. Ertapenem. A review of its microbiologic, pharmacokinetic and clinical aspects. Drugs Today 2002;38:195.

112. Raad II et al. How should imipenem-cilastatin be used in the treatment of fever and infection in neutropenic cancer patients? Cancer 1998;82:2449.

113. Cometta A, Glauser MP. Empiric antibiotic monotherapy with carbapenems in febrile neutropenia: a review. J Chemother 1996;8:375.

114. Asbel LE, Levison ME. Cephalosporins, carbapenems, and monobactams. Infect Dis Clin North Am 2000;14:435.

115. Fishman A et al. Aztreonam plus piperacillin: empiric treatment of neutropenic fever in gynecology-oncology patients receiving cisplatin-based chemotherapy. Eur J Gynaecol Oncol 1998;19:126.

116. Raad II et al. A comparison of aztreonam plus vancomycin and imipenem plus vancomycin as initial therapy for febrile neutropenic cancer patients. Cancer 1996;77:1386.

117. Johnson DM et al. Potency and antimicrobial spectrum update for piperacillin/tazobactam (2000): emphasis on its activity against resistant organism populations and generally untested species causing community-acquired respiratory tract infections. Eur J Clin Microbiol Infect Dis 2002;43:49.

118. Livermore DM. Multiple mechanisms of antimicrobial resistance in *Pseudomonas aeruginosa:* our worst nightmare? Clin Infect Dis 2002;34:634.

119. Giamarellou H et al. Monotherapy with intravenous followed by oral high dose ciprofloxacin versus combination therapy with ceftazidime plus amikacin as initial empiric therapy for granulocytopenic patients with fever. Antimicrob Agents Chemother 2000;44:3264.

120. Marra CA et al. A new ciprofloxacin stepdown program in the treatment of high-risk febrile neutropenia: a clinical and economic analysis. Pharmacotherapy 2000;20:931.

121. Petrilli AS et al. Oral ciprofloxacin vs. intravenous ceftriaxone administered in an outpatient setting for fever and neutropenia in low-risk pediatric oncology patients: randomized prospective trial. Med Pediatr Oncol 2000;34:87.

122. Meunier F et al. Prospective randomized evaluation of ciprofloxacin versus piperacillin plus amikacin for empiric antibiotic therapy of febrile granulocytopenic cancer patients with lymphomas and solid tumors. The European Organization for Research on Treatment of Cancer International Antimicrobial Therapy Cooperative Group. Antimicrob Agents Chemother 1991;35:873.

123. Johnson PR et al. A randomized trial of high-dose ciprofloxacin versus azlocillin and netilmicin in the empirical therapy of febrile neutropenic patients. J Antimicrob Chemother 1992;30:203.

124. Griggs JJ et al. Ciprofloxacin plus piperacillin is an equally effective regimen for empiric therapy in febrile neutropenic patients compared with standard therapy. Am J Hematol 1998;58:293.

125. Peacock JE et al. Ciprofloxacin plus piperacillin compared with tobramycin plus piperacillin as empirical therapy in febrile neutropenic patients. A randomized, double-blind trial. Ann Intern Med 2002;137:77.

126. Flaherty JP et al. Multicenter, randomized trial of ciprofloxacin plus azlocillin versus ceftazidime plus amikacin for empiric treatment of febrile neutropenic patients. Am J Med 1989;87:278S.

127. Chan CC et al. Randomized trial comparing ciprofloxacin plus netilmicin versus piperacillin plus netilmicin for empiric treatment of fever in neutropenic patients. Antimicrob Agents Chemother 1989;33:87.

128. Bauduer F et al. A randomized prospective multicentre trial of cefpirome versus piperacillin-tazobactam in febrile neutropenia. Leuk Lymphoma 2001;42:379.

129. Del Favero A et al. A multicenter, double-blind, placebo-controlled trial comparing piperacillin-tazobactam with and without amikacin as empiric therapy for febrile neutropenia. Clin Infect Dis 2001;33:1295.

130. Hazel DL et al. Piperacillin-tazobactam as empiric monotherapy in febrile neutropenic patients with haematological malignancies. J Chemother 1997;9:267.

131. Hess U et al. Monotherapy with piperacillin/tazobactam versus combination therapy with ceftazidime plus amikacin as an empiric therapy for fever in neutropenic cancer patients. Support Care Cancer 1998;6:402.

132. Ramphal R. Is monotherapy for febrile neutropenia still a viable alternative? Clin Infect Dis 1999;29:508.

133. Klastersky J et al. Significance of antimicrobial synergism for the outcome of Gram negative sepsis. Am J Medl Sci 1977;273:157.

134. De Jongh CA et al. Antibiotic synergism and response in Gram-negative bacteremia in granulocytopenic cancer patients. Am J Med 1986;80:96.

135. Ariffin H et al. Single-daily ceftriaxone plus amikacin versus thrice-daily ceftazidime plus amikacin as empirical treatment of febrile neutropenia in children with cancer. J Pediatr Child Health 2001;37:38.

136. Bosi A et al. An open evaluation of triple antibiotic therapy including vancomycin for febrile bone marrow transplant recipients with severe neutropenia. J Chemother 1999;11:287.

137. Charnas R et al. Once daily ceftriaxone plus amikacin vs. three times daily ceftazidime plus amikacin for treatment of febrile neutropenic children with cancer. Writing Committee for the International Collaboration on Antimicrobial Treatment of Febrile Neutropenia in Children. Pediatr Infect Dis J 1997;16:346.

138. Cordonnier C et al. Cefepime/amikacin versus ceftazidime/amikacin as empirical therapy for febrile episodes in neutropenic patients: a comparative study. The French Cefepime Study Group. Clin Infect Dis 1997;24:41.

139. Erman M et al. Comparison of cefepime and ceftazidime in combination with amikacin in the empirical treatment of high-risk patients with febrile neutropenia: a prospective, randomized, multicenter study. Scand J Infect Dis 2001;33:827.

140. Gibson J et al. A randomised dosage study of ceftazidime with single daily tobramycin for the empirical management of febrile neutropenia in patients with hematological diseases. Int J Hematol 1994;60:119.

141. Hoffken G et al. An open, randomized, multicentre study comparing the use of low-dose ceftazidime or cefotaxime, both in combination with netilmicin, in febrile neutropenic patients. German Multicentre Study Group. J Antimicrob Chemother 1999;44:367.

142. Laszlo D et al. Randomized trial comparing netilmicin plus imipenem-cilastatin versus netilmicin plus ceftazidime as empiric therapy for febrile neutropenic bone marrow transplant recipients. J Chemother 1997;9:95.

143. Marie JP et al. Piperacillin/tazobactam plus tobramycin versus ceftazidime plus tobramycin as empiric therapy for fever in severely neutropenic patients. Support Care Cancer 1999;7:89.

144. Nucci M, Biasoli I, Braggio S et al. Ceftazidime plus amikacin plus teicoplanin or vancomycin in the empirical antibiotic therapy in febrile neutropenic cancer patients. Oncol Reports 1998;5:1205.

145. Pizzo PA et al. A randomized trial comparing ceftazidime alone with combination antibiotic therapy in cancer patients with fever and neutropenia. N Engl J Med 1986;315:552.

146. Rossini F et al. Amikacin and ceftazidime as empirical antibiotic therapy in severely neutropenic patients: analysis of prognostic factors. Support Care Cancer 1994;2:259.

147. Cornely OA et al. A randomized monocentric trial in febrile neutropenic patients: ceftriaxone and gentamicin vs cefepime and gentamicin. Ann Hematol 2002;81:37.

148. Sanz MA et al. Cefepime plus amikacin versus piperacillin-tazobactam plus amikacin for initial antibiotic therapy in haematology patients with febrile neutropenia: results of an open, randomized, multicentre trial. J Antimicrob Chemother 2002;50:79.

149. Furno P et al. Ceftriaxone versus beta-lactams with antipseudomonal activity for empirical, combined antibiotic therapy in febrile neutropenia: a meta-analysis. Support Care Cancer 2000;8:293.

150. Ceftazidime combined with a short or long course of amikacin for empirical therapy of gram-negative bacteremia in cancer patients with granulocytopenia. The EORTC International Antimicrobial Therapy Cooperative Group. N Engl J Med 1987;317:1692.

151. Kojima A et al. A randomized prospective study of imipenem-cilastatin with or without amikacin as an empirical antibiotic treatment for febrile neutropenic patients. Am J Clin Oncol 1994;17:400.

152. Furno P et al. Monotherapy or aminoglycoside-containing combinations for empirical antibiotic treatment of febrile neutropenic patients: a meta-analysis. Lancet Infect Dis 2002;2:231.

153. Paul M et al. Beta-lactam versus beta-lactam-aminoglycoside combination therapy in cancer patients with neutropaenia. Cochrane Database of Systematic Reviews 2002;CD003038.

154. Winston DJ et al. Moxalactam plus piperacillin versus moxalactam plus amikacin in febrile granulocytopenic patients. Am J Med 1984;77:442.

155. Eliopoulos GM. Quinupristin-dalfopristin and linezolid: evidence and opinion. Clin Infect Dis 2003;36:473.

156. Feld R. Vancomycin as part of initial empirical antibiotic therapy for febrile neutropenia in patients with cancer: pros and cons. Clin Infect Dis 1999;29:503.

157. Shenep JL et al. Vancomycin, ticarcillin, and amikacin compared with ticarcillin-clavulanate and amikacin in the empirical treatment of febrile, neutropenic children with cancer. N Engl J Med 1988;319:1053.

158. Karp JE et al. Empiric use of vancomycin during prolonged treatment-induced granulocytopenia. Randomized, double-blind, placebo-controlled clinical trial in patients with acute leukemia. Am J Med 1986;81:237.

159. Kramer BS et al. Randomized comparison between two ceftazidime-containing regimens and cephalothin-gentamicin-carbenicillin in febrile granulocytopenic cancer patients. Antimicrob Agents Chemother 1986;30:64.

160. Dompeling EC et al. Early identification of neutropenic patients at risk of Gram-positive bacteraemia and the impact of empirical administration of vancomycin. Eur J Cancer 1996;32A:1332.

161. Koya R et al. Analysis of the value of empiric vancomycin administration in febrile neutropenia occurring after autologous peripheral blood stem cell transplants. Bone Marrow Transplant 1998;21:923.

162. Granowetter L et al. Ceftazidime with or without vancomycin vs. cephalothin, carbenicillin and gentamicin as the initial therapy of the febrile neutropenic pediatric cancer patient. Pediatr Infect Dis J 1988;7:165.

163. Shenep JL. Viridans-group streptococcal infections in immunocompromised hosts. Int J Antimicrob Agents 2000;14:129.

164. Kennedy HF et al. Antimicrobial susceptibility of blood culture isolates of viridans streptococci: relationship to a change in empirical antibiotic therapy in febrile neutropenia. J Antimicrob Chemother 2001;47:693.

165. Adcock KG et al. Evaluation of empiric vancomycin therapy in children with fever and neutropenia. Pharmacotherapy 1999;19:1315.

166. Blijlevens NM et al. Empirical therapy of febrile neutropenic patients with mucositis: challenge of risk-based therapy. ClinMicrobiol Infect 2001; 7(Suppl 4):47.

167. Razonable RR et al. Bacteremia due to viridans group streptococci with diminished susceptibility to levofloxacin among neutropenic patients receiving levofloxacin prophylaxis. Clin Infect Dis 2002;34:1469.

168. Rybak MJ et al. Prospective evaluation of the effect of an aminoglycoside dosing regimen on rates of observed nephrotoxicity and ototoxicity. Antimicrob Agents Chemother 1999;43:1549.

169. Craig WA. Does the dose matter?. Clin Infect Dis 2001;33(Suppl 3):S233.

170. Dalle JH et al. Continuous infusion of ceftazidime in the empiric treatment of febrile neutropenic children with cancer. J Pediatr Hematol Oncol 2002;24:714.

171. Egerer G et al. Efficacy of continuous infusion of ceftazidime for patients with neutropenic fever after high-dose chemotherapy and peripheral blood stem cell transplantation. Int J Antimicrob Agents 2000;15:119.

172. Marshall E et al. Low-dose continuous-infusion ceftazidime monotherapy in low-risk febrile neutropenic patients. Support Care Cancer 2000; 8:198.

173. Bodey GP et al. The role of schedule of antibiotic therapy on the neutropenic patient. Infection 1980;Suppl 1:75.

174. Powell SH et al. Once-daily vs. continuous aminoglycoside dosing: efficacy and toxicity in animal and clinical studies of gentamicin, netilmicin, and tobramycin. J Infect Dis 1983; 147:918.

175. Krivoy N et al. Pharmacokinetic analysis of amikacin twice and single daily dosage in immunocompromised pediatric patients. Infection 1998;26:396.

176. Tod M et al. Population pharmacokinetic study of amikacin administered once or twice daily to febrile, severely neutropenic adults. Antimicrob Agents Chemother 1998;42:849.

177. MacGowan AP et al. The pharmacokinetics of once daily gentamicin in neutropenic adults with haematological malignancy. J Antimicrob Chemother 1994;34:809.

178. Peterson AK, Duffull SB. Population analysis of once-daily dosing of gentamicin in patients with neutropenia. Austr NZ J Med 1998;28:311.

179. Paganini HG. Outpatient, sequential, parenteral-oral antibiotic therapy for lower risk febrile neutropenia in children with malignant disease. Cancer 2003;97:1775.

180. Suwangool P et al. Empirical antibiotic therapy in febrile neutropenic patients with single-daily dose amikacin plus ceftriaxone. J Med Assoc Thailand 1993;76:314.

181. Bakri FE et al. Once-daily versus multiple-daily gentamicin in empirical antibiotic therapy of febrile neutropenia following intensive chemotherapy. J Antimicrob Chemother 2000;45:383.

182. Tomlinson RJ et al. Once daily ceftriaxone and gentamicin for the treatment of febrile neutropenia. Arch Dis Child 1999;80:125.

183. Warkentin D et al. Toxicity of single daily dose gentamicin in stem cell transplantation. Bone Marrow Transplant 1999;24:57.

184. Aiken SK, Wetzstein GA. Once-daily aminoglycosides in patients with neutropenic fever. Cancer Control 2002;9:426.

185. Davis DD, Raebel MA. Ambulatory management of chemotherapy-induced fever and neutropenia in adult cancer patients. Ann Pharmacother 1998;32:1317.

186. Kern WV. Risk assessment and risk-based therapeutic strategies in febrile neutropenia. Curr Opinion Infect Dis 2001;14:415.

187. Rolston KV et al. Early empiric antibiotic therapy for febrile neutropenia patients at low risk [review]. Infect Dis Clin North Am 1996;10:223.

188. Shevchuk YM, Conly JM. Antibiotic-associated hypoprothrombinemia: a review of prospective studies, 1966–1988. Rev Infect Dis 1990;12:1109.

189. Grasela TH, Jr et al. Prospective surveillance of antibiotic-associated coagulopathy in 970 patients. Pharmacotherapy 1989;9:158.

190. Pizzo PA et al. Duration of empiric antibiotic therapy in granulocytopenic patients with cancer. Am J Med 1979;67:194.

191. Pizzo PA et al. Treatment of gram-positive septicemia in cancer patients. Cancer 1980;45:206.

192. Bennett JEP. Forum report: issues in clinical trials of empirical antifungal therapy in treating febrile neutropenic patients. Clin Infect Dis 2003; 36:S117.

193. Hagen EA et al. High rate of invasive fungal infections following nonmyeloablative allogeneic transplantation. Clin Infect Dis 2003;36:9.

194. Martino R, Subira M. Invasive fungal infections in hematology: new trends. Ann Hematol 2002; 81:233.

195. Ninin E et al. Longitudinal study of bacterial, viral, and fungal infections in adult recipients of bone marrow transplants. Clin Infect Dis 2001;33:41.

196. Gotzsche PC, Johansen HK. Meta-analysis of prophylactic or empirical antifungal treatment versus placebo or no treatment in patients with cancer complicated by neutropenia. Br Med J 1997; 314:1238.

197. Guiot HF et al. Risk factors for fungal infection in patients with malignant hematologic disorders: implications for empirical therapy and prophylaxis. Clin Infect Dis 1994;18:525.

198. Gotzsche PC, Johansen HK. Routine versus selective antifungal administration for control of fungal infections in patients with cancer. Cochrane Database of Systematic Reviews 2000;CD000026.

199. Bennett JEP. Forum report: issues in clinical trials of empirical antifungal therapy in treating febrile neutropenic patients. Clin Infect Dis 2003;36:S117.

200. Pizzo PA et al. Empiric antibiotic and antifungal therapy for cancer patients with prolonged fever and granulocytopenia. Am J Med 1982;72:101.

201. Prentice HG et al. A randomized comparison of liposomal versus conventional amphotericin B for the treatment of pyrexia of unknown origin in neutropenic patients. Br J Haematol 1997;98:711.

202. Walsh TJ et al. Liposomal amphotericin B for empirical therapy in patients with persistent fever and neutropenia. National Institute of Allergy and Infectious Diseases Mycoses Study Group. N Engl J Med 1999;340:764.

203. Wingard JR et al. A randomized, double-blind comparative trial evaluating the safety of liposomal amphotericin B versus amphotericin B lipid complex in the empirical treatment of febrile neutropenia. L Amph/ABLC Collaborative Study Group. Clin Infect Dis 2000;31:1155.

204. White MH et al. Randomized, double-blind clinical trial of amphotericin B colloidal dispersion vs. amphotericin B in the empirical treatment of fever and neutropenia. Clin Infect Dis 1998;27:296.

205. Walsh TJ et al. Voriconazole compared with liposomal amphotericin B for empirical antifungal therapy in patients with neutropenia and persistent fever. N Engl J Med 2002;346:225.

206. Blau IW, Fauser AA. Review of comparative studies between conventional and liposomal amphotericin B (Ambisome) in neutropenic patients with fever of unknown origin and patients with systemic mycosis. Mycoses 2000;43:325.

207. Dupont B. Overview of the lipid formulations of amphotericin B. J Antimicrob Chemother 2002;19(Suppl 1):31.

208. Frothingham R. Lipid formulations of amphotericin B for empirical treatment of fever and neutropenia. Clin Infect Dis 2002;35:896.

209. Johansen HK, Gotzsche PC. Amphotericin B lipid soluble formulations vs amphotericin B in cancer patients with neutropenia. Cochrane Database of Systematic Reviews 2000;CD000969.

210. Eriksson U et al. Comparison of effects of amphotericin B deoxycholate infused over 4 or 24 hours: randomised controlled trial. Br Med J 2001;322:579.

211. Malik IA et al. A randomized comparison of fluconazole with amphotericin B as empiric anti-fungal agents in cancer patients with prolonged fever and neutropenia. Am J Med 1998;105:478.

212. Winston DJ et al. A multicenter, randomized trial of fluconazole versus amphotericin B for empiric antifungal therapy of febrile neutropenic patients with cancer. Am J Med 2000;108:282.

213. Boogaerts M et al. Intravenous and oral itraconazole versus intravenous amphotericin B deoxycholate as empirical antifungal therapy for persistent fever in neutropenic patients with cancer who are receiving broad-spectrum antibacterial therapy. A randomized, controlled trial. Ann Intern Med 2001;135:412.

214. Groll AH, Walsh TJ. Caspofungin: pharmacology, safety and therapeutic potential in superficial and invasive fungal infections. Expert Opin Invest Drugs 2001;10:1545.

215. Fassas AB et al. Cytomegalovirus infection and non-neutropenic fever after autologous stem cell transplantation: high rates of reactivation in patients with multiple myeloma and lymphoma. Br J Haematol 2001;112:237.

216. Illerhaus G et al. Treatment and prophylaxis of severe infections in neutropenic patients by granulocyte transfusions. Ann Hematol 2002;81:273.

217. Dale DC. Colony-stimulating factors for the management of neutropenia in cancer patients. Drugs 2002;62(Suppl 1):1.

218. Ozer H et al. 2000 update of recommendations for the use of hematopoietic colony-stimulating factors: evidence-based, clinical practice guidelines. American Society of Clinical Oncology Growth Factors Expert Panel. J Clin Oncol 2000;18:3558.

Pharmacotherapy of Human Immunodeficiency Virus Infection

Andrew D. Luber

INTRODUCTION

New advances in the management of human immunodeficiency virus (HIV) infection have resulted in a renewed sense of optimism and hope among patients and clinicians. Research into the areas of viral pathogenesis and kinetics has made a direct impact on the clinical management of HIV-infected patients and has led to the development of new and more potent antiretroviral agents, regimens, and classes of antiretroviral therapy. These highly active antiretroviral therapies (HAART) have dramatically altered the natural progression of infection and significantly improved the quality of life for many HIV-infected patients. As a result, there has been a pronounced decline in the reported number of new AIDS related opportunistic infections and deaths.[1,2] For many, the use of HAART-containing regimens has shifted the outlook of HIV infection from a fatal to a potentially manageable disease.

Despite these remarkable advances, clinicians working in the area of HIV remain cautious. Although many will benefit from these new and more potent regimens, data have shown that up to 50% of patients will fail therapy,[3] and approximately 40% will have to change regimens within the first year because of drug-related adverse events.[4] Many concerns, including the development of resistance, long term toxicities/adverse events, patient compliance, the management of HAART failures, and methods to control and prevent the rampant spread of HIV throughout Third World countries remain.

This chapter focuses on the antiretroviral management of HIV infection. Although many therapeutic options exist, a thorough understanding of viral pathogenesis and its implications on clinical practice is essential for clinicians managing HIV-infected patients. By understanding the principles of therapy as they relate to viral pathogenesis, clinicians will be able to rapidly assimilate new data as they become available. Consensus panel recommendations have been published that can be used as a framework for clinical decision making.[5–7] Given the complexity of therapy, this chapter focuses only on management of adult HIV infection; the reader is referred to the various Consensus Panel Guidelines on treatment of perinatal transmission, pediatric HIV, and postexposure prophylaxis for both occupational and nonoccupational HIV exposures (located at www.hivatis.org).

EPIDEMIOLOGY

Despite a dramatic decline in the number of AIDS-related opportunistic infections and deaths in industrialized countries,[1,2] infection with HIV remains a leading killer throughout many regions of the world. Unfortunately, access to newer, more potent antiretroviral regimens and monitoring techniques are often limited by economics and politics. Infected patients residing in countries with a strong economic standing have access (North America, Western Europe, Australia, and New Zealand), whereas others must make do with scarce resources (Africa, South and Southeast Asia, the Pacific, Latin America, and the Caribbean). This is extremely alarming given that roughly 90% of all infected patients worldwide reside in developing regions of the world.[8]

As of December 2002, worldwide estimates of persons living with HIV and AIDS have been calculated to be a staggering 42 million people: 38.6 million among adults (19.2 million women) and 3.2 million among children less than 15 years of age. In 2002, 5 million people were newly infected and 3 million people died of HIV. Dramatic increases in newly HIV-infected patients occurred in Eastern Asia/Pacific, Eastern Europe/Central Asia and the Caribbean with increases of 29%, 21%, and 16%, respectively, in 2002 as compared with 2001. Estimates are that roughly 45 million new infections will occur between 2002 and 2012, with roughly 40% occurring in Asia and the Pacific if intervention strategies are not immediately implemented. Intervention strategies to educate and protect young people have been highly effective in Ethiopia, South Africa, Uganda, and Zambia with some regions showing a 33% decline in new infections among young women between 1995 and 2001.[8] Intervention and treatment strategies are often difficult to implement in Third World countries because of social, political, financial and resource limitations.

In the United States, deaths from HIV in men and woman ages 25 to 44 years remain a leading cause of mortality. An estimated 900,000 people in the United States are HIV infected, with 25% of patients unaware that they are HIV-positive.[4,9,10] HIV infection has increased among certain ethnic populations with young, disadvantaged people being at greatest risk. In the year 2000, 54% of all new HIV infections in the United States occurred among African Americans despite the fact that they make up only 13% of the entire US population.[8] In addition, 64% of newly infected females in 2001 were African American, and most were infected either through injection drug use or having sexual intercourse with men who have sex with men. Among men aged 25 to 44 AIDS remains the leading cause of death for African-American men and is the third leading cause of death among Hispanic men.

Transmission through sexual intercourse remains a predominant route of infection with large increases in the incidence among heterosexual men and women. For example, in the United Kingdom, 50% of all new infections in 2001 were obtained through heterosexual transmission compared with 33% in 1998.[8] Patients older than 50 years of age also represent another rapidly expanding group. Lack of concern regarding risks of pregnancy, widespread use of Viagra, and limited knowledge of HIV/AIDS have contributed to this rise in new infections among this age group.

Among homosexual men, the rates of newly infected patients have stopped declining and have leveled off and slightly increased. It appears that high-risk sexual behavior among gay men is increasing; in San Francisco, self-reported sexual behavior has shown increased rates of unprotected anal sex, even among couples in which one partner was HIV infected and the other was not.[8] Of particular concern to health officials has been the increased incidence of outbreaks of syphilis and methicillin-resistant *Staphylococcus* skin infections among gay communities, which could serve as a marker for future infections with HIV.[11]

PATHOPHYSIOLOGY

HIV infection can be acquired through unprotected sexual intercourse (both anal and vaginal), injectable drug use, receipt of tainted blood products, and mother-to-infant transmission (both perinatal infection and via contaminated breast milk).[5] Infection can also be acquired from occupational exposures among healthcare workers after needle sticks from HIV-infected patients. Rarely, HIV infection has been documented after oral sex.[12-15]

Unprotected sexual intercourse has accounted for roughly 75% to 85% of all documented HIV infections to date.[8] Transmission between sexual partners depends on a number of factors, including the HIV viral subtype, stage of infection in the index partner, genetic susceptibility to infection of the potential host and potentially the fitness, or pathogenicity of the infecting viral strain. Infectivity via male-to-male receptive anal intercourse represents the greatest sexual risk factor followed by male-to-female and female-to-male transmission, respectively.[16]

HIV attacks and binds to specific cells of the immune system including monocytes, macrophages and T-cell lymphocytes (also known as CD4 cells, helper T cells, T cells).[17-20] These cells display specific receptor proteins known as CD4 receptors to which HIV binds. Once bound to the CD4 receptor, coreceptor proteins are required for fusion (CCR-5, CXCR-4).[21,22] CXCR-4 is predominantly found on T lymphocytes and among viral strains that are syncytium inducing, whereas CCR-5 is found on both monocytes and T lymphocytes and among viral strains that are non-syncytium inducing.[22,23] The CD4–coreceptor complex causes conformational changes to key HIV proteins (gp41 and gp120) allowing for a more close association between the virus and host cell.[24,25] HIV fuses with the cell releasing its contents, including the virus' genetic material (RNA) and specific enzymes necessary for replication, into the host cell's cytoplasm (Fig. 69-1). The single-stranded viral RNA is transcribed via reverse transcriptase into a double-stranded proviral DNA that is subsequently incorporated into the host cell's genetic material via the integrase enzyme. HIV then uses the infected cell's machinery to translate, transcribe, and produce immature viral particles that bud and break from the infected cell. For these immature virions to become infectious, the protease enzyme must cleave large precursor polypeptides into functional proteins.[26,27] Once complete, the mature virion is free to infect new host cells and subsequently produce more infectious virus. Over time, HIV-infected host cells are destroyed either (1) by a direct cytolytic effect of the virus (e.g., formation of syncytium induction, cellular dysfunction), (2) by the identification and elimination of the infected cell by the host's immune response (e.g., via cytotoxic T-cell lymphocytes), or (3) by the cell's natural life cycle coming to completion.[20] In addition, HIV infection inhibits the production of new CD4 cells.[28]

Upon infection, HIV invades, uses, and eventually destroys key cells of the immune system, specifically the CD4 lymphocyte. The CD4 cell is responsible for a number of functions; however, its main role is to regulate the host's cell-mediated immunity. Most of these cells, and consequently most infectious HIV virions (~99%), reside inside lymph nodes and other tissues found throughout the body.[19,29-31]

Once infected, an initial burst of viremia with subsequent viral "seeding" of various tissues (e.g., lymph nodes) and cells (CD4, macrophages and monocytes) occurs.[29,32] Initially, the immune system reacts by producing antibodies against HIV; however, given the rapid production of new HIV particles and the development of various new viral strains as a result of in-

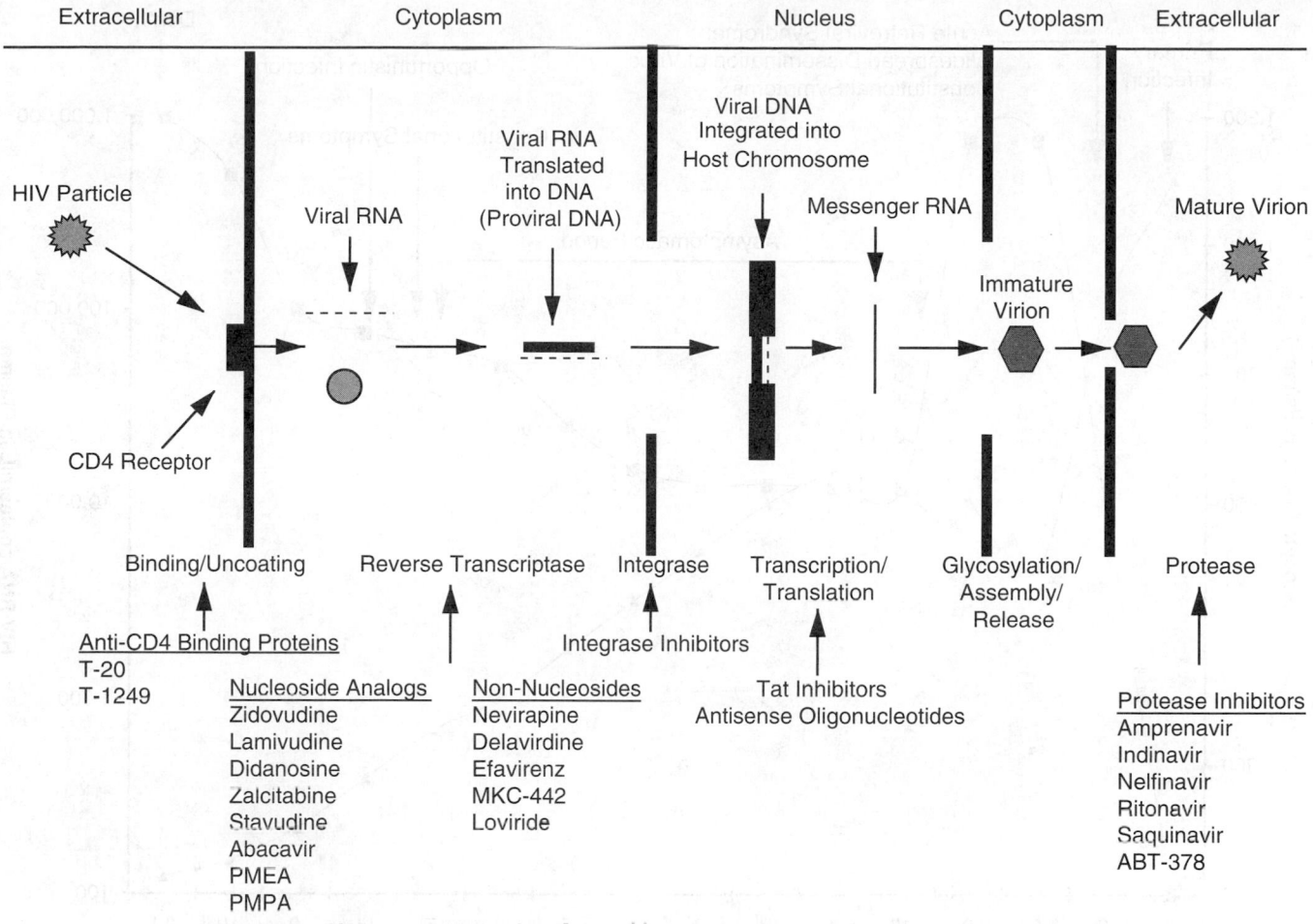

FIGURE 69-1 Schematic representation of HIV-1 life cycle showing sites of activity for the various anti retroviral agents. (Adapted and updated from Reference 258.)

efficient viral replication, the antibody response is always one step behind the virus.[33] After this burst of viremia, a transient depletion of CD4 cells occurs (Fig. 69-2). Initially, patients may complain of nonspecific symptoms such as fever, lymphadenopathy, rash, fatigue, and night sweats.[34,35] This phase of infection is known as the *acute retroviral syndrome*. In most cases, patients are unaware that they are infected. Within 6 months, the host's immune response is able to control the infection to a point where the number of virus particles produced per day equals the number of particles destroyed per day. This steady-state viral load is often referred to as the patient's viral "set point." The higher the set point, the greater risk for disease progression. The larger the viral population in a host, the greater the chance for more widespread viral infection with destruction of immune cells and lymphoid tissue. Why some patients establish higher or lower viral set points is currently under investigation, but this may be a consequence of differences in immune responses, viral subtypes, viral fitness or a combination of these factors. This new understanding of viral pathogenesis theoretically allows clinicians a window of opportunity to alter the natural course of disease. If patients with acute infection can be identified, potent antiretroviral regimens to reduce the set point can be initiated and potentially lower the overall risk for disease progression.

Once the initial burst of viremia has been controlled and the viral set point established, infection with HIV results in a constant battle between the virus and immune system. Mathematical models have calculated the daily production of HIV at 10 billion particles per day.[19,36–38] To keep the infection in check, the body must produce an equally sufficient immune response. Over time, HIV depletes the body of T cells and places the host at an increased risk for opportunistic infections (Fig. 69-3). Direct measurements of HIV concentrations in plasma (viral load) can predict disease progression (see below).[39–41] Higher viral load measurements represent an inability of the host to control infection and a greater risk for infection and destruction of other tissues and cells. Long-term, "nonprogressors" (e.g., patients with asymptomatic HIV infection for >10 years; 5% of all HIV-infected patients) consistently have lower baseline viral load values than patients with rapidly progressive disease (e.g., within 5 years of infection; 20% of all HIV-infected patients).[42,43] In addition, recent data have shown that patients infected with viral strains that are compromised in their ability to replicate (known as viral fitness) results in newly infected patients with higher CD4 cell counts on establishment of their set points.[44] The clinical implications of this are currently unknown; however, given that HAART may compromise viral fitness, transmission of HIV from patients

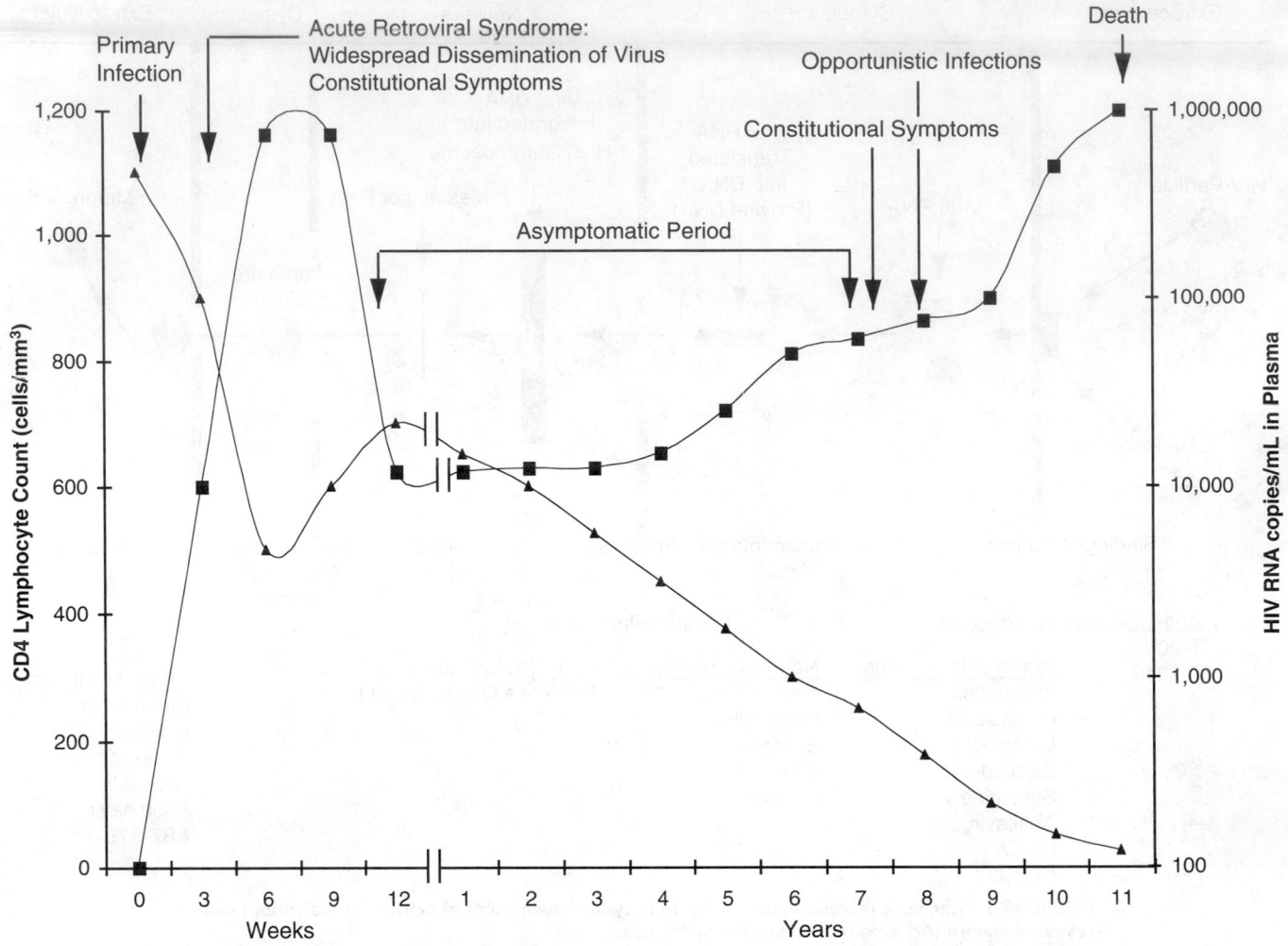

FIGURE 69-2 Sample disease course for an untreated HIV-infected individual showing relationship among immunologic, virologic, and clinical outcomes over time. Constitutional symptoms include fever, night sweats, and weight loss. ■ Viral load values; ▲ CD4 T lymphocytes. (Adapted from References 25 and 29.)

receiving HAART may result in lower viral set points and higher CD4 cell counts on newly HIV-infected patients compared with patients infected with "fit" viruses.

Without intervention, the natural progression of HIV infection results in depletion of 50 to 100 T cells per year.[29,45] The severity of immune dysfunction, as evidenced by T-cell loss, is highly predictive of the potential for developing specific types of opportunistic infections. For example, *Pneumocystis carinii* pneumonia rarely occurs when T-cell counts are >200 cells/mm³, whereas retinitis from *Cytomegalovirus* infection infrequently occurs in patients with CD4 counts >75 cells/mm³. The diagnosis of AIDS is made when a significant amount of immune deterioration has occurred, either by direct depletion of CD4 cells or because of the development of new opportunistic infection (Tables 69-1 and 69-2).[29,46] It is important to recognize that not every patient with HIV has a diagnosis of AIDS. On average, without appropriate interventions, death occurs within 10 to 15 years after infection.[29,46]

The interplay between viral load and CD4 cell counts has been compared with that of a train heading toward a particular destination. The T-cell count is the location of the train, the viral load is the speed of the train, and the destination is immune system deterioration and eventual death. In addition, vi-

ral fitness may represent the size of the engine; a fit virus has a powerful engine whereas an unfit virus does not. Speeding trains (e.g., high viral load measurements) have more powerful engines (viral fitness) and are farther along on their course (e.g., lower T-cell values) and therefore closer to their destinations (e.g., immune deterioration and death) than are slower trains. In a situation analogous to pulling the break lever of the train, new, potent, antiretroviral regimens decrease viral load and subsequently slow disease progression. These new regimens have been shown to dramatically alter the course of infection and have resulted in fewer opportunistic infections and deaths (see below).[10,47]

PHARMACOTHERAPY

Pharmacotherapy of HIV has been directed at inhibiting key areas of the HIV life cycle (see Fig. 69-1; Table 69-3). A great deal of research has been focused on agents that target inhibition of the reverse transcriptase enzyme. Reverse transcriptase inhibitors, such as zidovudine, didanosine, zalcitabine, lamivudine, abacavir, tenofovir and stavudine, inhibit this enzyme by incorporating false nucleic acids into the newly produced proviral DNA.[48] This results in a DNA strand that can-

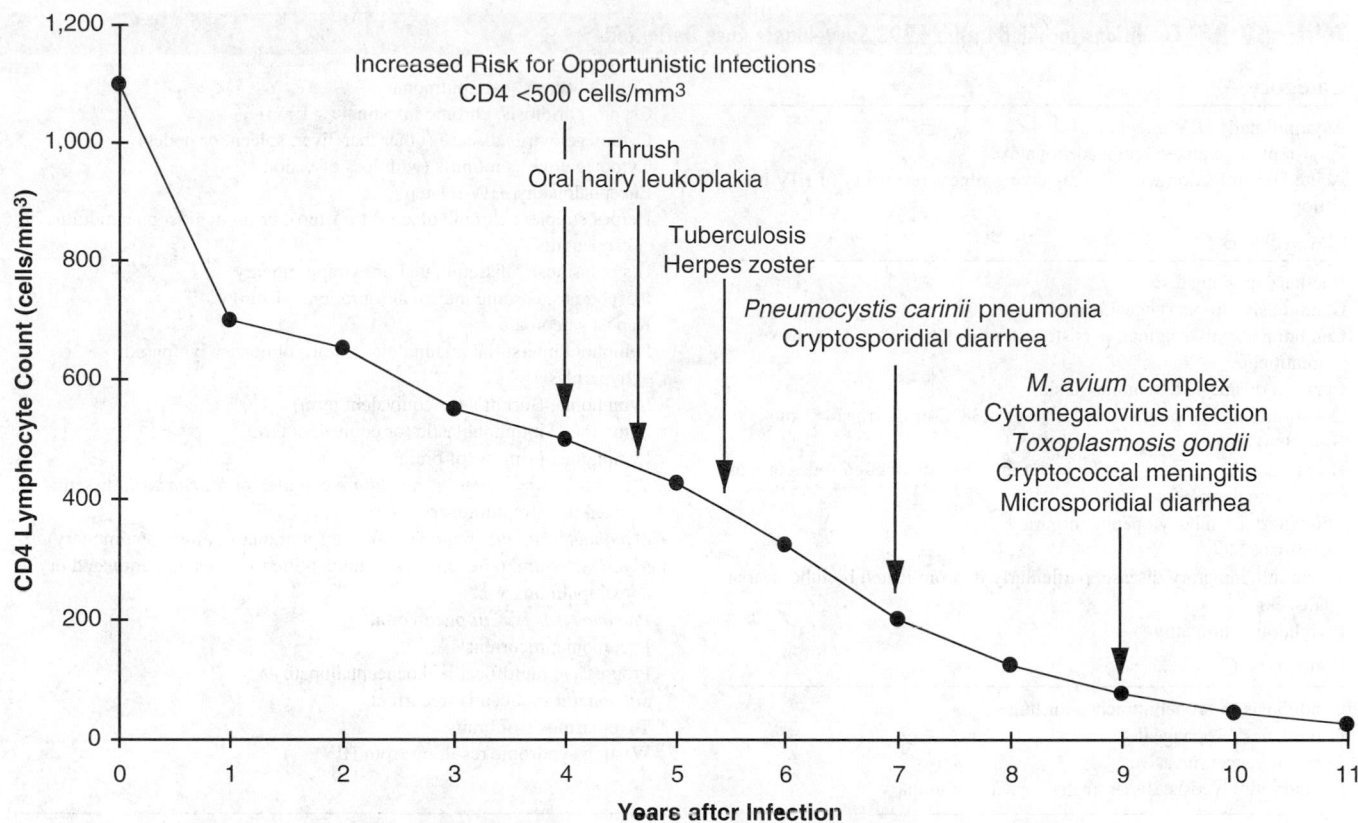

FIGURE 69-3 Relative risk for development of opportunistic infections based on CD4 lymphocyte counts over time.

Table 69-1   1993 Revised Classification System for HIV Infection and the Expanded CDC Surveillance Case Definition for AIDS in Adults and Adolescents[a]

	Clinical Categories		
CD4 + T-Cell Categories	(A) Asymptomatic, Acute (Primary) HIV	(B) Symptomatic, Not (A) or (C) Conditions	(C) AIDS-Indicator Conditions
1. >500/mm³	A1	B1	C1
2. 200–499/mm³	A2	B2	C2
3. <200/mm³ (AIDS indicator T-cell count)	A3	B3	C3

[a]The modifications to the prior 1986 Surveillance Case Definition, which have been included in the 1993 revision, include the use of CD4 cell count (<200 cells/mm³) or CD4 cell percent (<14%) and the additional AIDS-indicating conditions of pulmonary tuberculosis, recurrent pneumonia, and invasive cervical cancer (see Table 69-2).

not continue elongation. Non-nucleoside reverse transcriptase inhibitors (NNRTIs), such as delavirdine, nevirapine, and efavirenz, inhibit reverse transcriptase by directly binding to the enzyme itself.[49] Agents that target the protease enzyme (saquinavir, amprenavir, nelfinavir, indinavir, lopinavir, atazanavir, ritonavir, tipranavir) inhibit activity by directly binding to the catalytic site; this results in the production of immature, noninfectious virions.[50,51] Unlike reverse transcriptase translation, which occurs relatively early in the course of the HIV life cycle, protease enzyme activity occurs late in virion development. As a result, inactivation of the protease enzyme inhibits viral replication in any infected cell regardless of the current stage of HIV replication within that cell. In contrast, reverse transcriptase inhibitors can protect newly infected cells only before formation and insertion of proviral DNA into the host cell's genetic material. Subsequently, these agents provide no benefit for those infected cells that are ac-

tively producing new strains of virus. Fusion inhibitors such as T-20 work by preventing HIV and CD4 cells from being pulled closer together after binding to CD4 and CCR5 or CXCR-4 coreceptors. Through direct attachment to a double coil–coil complex at the gp41–gp120–CD4 receptor area, T-20 prevents fusion from occurring.[25] Other areas under investigation include development of agents that prevent binding of HIV to the CD4 receptor (attachment inhibitors), coreceptor blockers (e.g., via CCR5 and CXCR-4 blockade), neutralizing antibodies against CD4 and coreceptors, inhibition of the integrase enzyme, and altered translation and transcription of proviral DNA (e.g., Tat inhibitors, antisense oligonucleotide).

With the development of newer, more potent antiretroviral regimens, researchers have speculated about the possibility of eradicating HIV from an infected patient. This would require complete inhibition of viral replication in all cell lines and body stores where HIV resides (Fig. 69-4).[19] One problem

Table 69-2   Conditions Included in the 1993 Surveillance Case Definition

Category A

Asymptomatic HIV infection

Persistent generalized lymphadenopathy

Acute HIV infection with accompanying illness or history of HIV infection

Category B

Bacillary angiomatosis

Candidiasis, oropharyngeal (thrush)

Candidiasis, vulvovaginal; persistent, frequent, or poorly responsive to treatment

Cervical dysplasia/carcinoma in situ

Constitutional symptoms, such as fever >38°C or diarrhea >1 mo

Hairy leukoplakia

Herpes zoster (shingles), involving at least two distinct episodes or more than one dermatome

Idiopathic thrombocytopenia purpura

Listeriosis

Pelvic inflammatory disease, particularly if complicated by tubo-ovarian abscess

Peripheral neuropathy

Category C

Candidiasis of bronchi, trachea, or lungs

Candidiasis, esophageal

Cervical cancer, invasive

Coccidioidomycosis, disseminated or extrapulmonary

Cryptococcosis, extrapulmonary

Cryptosporidiosis, chronic intestinal (>1 mo)

Cytomegalovirus disease (other than liver, spleen, or nodes)

Cytomegalovirus retinitis (with loss of vision)

Encephalopathy, HIV-related

Herpes simplex: chronic ulcer(s) (>1 mo); or bronchitis, pneumonitis, or esophagitis

Histoplasmosis, disseminated or extrapulmonary

Isosporiasis, chronic intestinal (duration >1 mo)

Kaposi sarcoma

Lymphoid interstitial pneumonia and/or pulmonary lymphoid hyperplasia[a]

Lymphoma, Burkitt's (or equivalent term)

Lymphoma, immunoblastic (or equivalent term)

Lymphoma, primary, of brain

Mycobacterium avium-intracellulare complex or *M. kansasii,* disseminated or extrapulmonary

Mycobacterium tuberculosis, any site (pulmonary[b] or extrapulmonary)

Mycobacterium, other species or unidentified species, disseminated or extrapulmonary

Pneumocystis carinii pneumonia

Pneumonia, recurrent[b]

Progressive multifocal leukoencephalopathy

Salmonella septicemia, recurrent

Toxoplasmosis of brain

Wasting syndrome resulting from HIV

[a]Children <13 yr old.
[b]Added in the 1993 expansions of the AIDS surveillance case definition for adolescents and adults.

Table 69-3   Characteristics of Antiretroviral Agents for the Treatment of Adult HIV Infection[5,9,231–233]

Drug	Dose	Pharmacokinetic Parameters	Administration Considerations
Nucleoside Reverse Transcriptase Inhibitors			
Zidovudine (AZT; ZDV) **Retrovir** *Preparations* Syrup: 10 mg/mL Capsule: 100 mg Tablet: 300 mg Injection: 10 mg/mL	200 mg TID or 300 mg BID or with 3TC as Combivir, 1 tablet BID; or with 3TC and abacavir as Trizivir 1 tablet BID; 600 mg QD under investigation	*Oral bioavailability:* 60% *Serum $t_{1/2}$:* 1.1 hr *Intracellular $t_{1/2}$:* 3 hr *Elimination:* hepatic glucuronidation; renal excretion of glucuronide metabolite	Can be administered without regard to meals (manufacturer recommends administration 30 min before or 1 hr after a meal)
Didanosine (ddI) **Videx** *Preparations* Pediatric powder for oral solution (when reconstituted as solution containing antacid): 10 mg/mL Chewable tablets with buffers: 25, 50, 100, 150 mg	Non-EC formulation: >60 kg: 200 mg BID <60 kg: 125 mg BID; 300–400 mg QD EC tablets: >60 kg: 400 mg QD <60 kg: 250 mg QD	*Oral bioavailability:* 30–40% with tablet; 30% with powder *Serum $t_{1/2}$:* 1.6 hr *Intracellular $t_{1/2}$:* 25–40 hr *Elimination:* renal excretion ~50%	Food decreases absorption (↓55%); administer ddI on empty stomach (1 hr before or 2 hr after meal) When administering chewable tablets, at least 2 tablets per dose should be administered to ensure adequate buffering capacity
Buffered powder for oral solution: 100, 167, 250 mg Enteric-coated tablets: 125, 200, 250, 400 mg			Antacid buffer in tablets/powder may cause significant drug interactions with various medications; separate administration by at least 2 hr

Table 69-3   Characteristics of Antiretroviral Agents for the Treatment of Adult HIV Infection[5,9,231–233]—cont'd

Drug	Dose	Pharmacokinetic Parameters	Administration Considerations
Nucleoside Reverse Transcriptase Inhibitors—cont'd			
Zalcitabine (ddC) **Hivid** *Preparations* Syrup: 0.1 mg/mL (investigational) Tablets: 0.375 and 0.75 mg	0.75 mg TID	*Oral bioavailability:* 85% *Serum $t_{1/2}$:* 1.2 hr *Intracellular $t_{1/2}$:* 3 hr *Elimination:* renal excretion ~70%	Administer on empty stomach
Stavudine (d4T) **Zerit** *Preparations* Solution: 1 mg/mL Capsules: 15, 20, 30, 40 mg Sustained release: 37.5, 50, 75, 100 mg	>60 kg : 40 mg BID <60 kg: 30 mg BID Sustained release: >60 kg–100 mg QD; <60 kg–75 mg QD	*Oral bioavailability:* 86% *Serum $t_{1/2}$:* 1.0 hr *Intracellular $t_{1/2}$:* 3.5 hr *Elimination:* renal excretion ~50%	Can be administered without regard to meals
Lamivudine (3TC) **Epivir** *Preparations* Solution: 10 mg/mL Tablets: 150 mg	150 mg PO BID or with ZDV as Combivir, 1 tablet BID or with zidovudine and abacavir as Trizivir 1 tablet BID 300 mg QD <50 kg: 2 mg/kg BID	*Oral bioavailability:* 86% *Serum $t_{1/2}$:* 3–6 hr *Intracellular $t_{1/2}$:* 12 hr *Elimination:* 70% unchanged in urine	Can be administered without regard to meals
Emtricitabine (FTC) **Emtriva** *Preparations* Capsules: 200 mg	200 mg QD for patients with calculated creatinine clearance (CrCl) >50 mL/min Dose needs to be adjusted for renal dysfunction: CrCl 30–49 mL/min: 200 mg Q 48 hr CrCl 15–29 mL/min: 200 mg Q 72 hr CrCl <15 mL/min: 200 mg Q 96 hr	*Oral bioavailability:* 93% *Serum $t_{1/2}$:* 10 hr *Intracellular $t_{1/2}$:* 39 hr *Elimination:* 86% recovered in urine	Can be administered without regard to meals
Tenofovir (Viread) *Preparations* Tablets: 300 mg	300 mg QD for patients with creatinine clearance >60 mL/min; should not be used for patients with creatinine clearance <60 mL/min	*Oral bioavailability:* 25% fasting; 39% with high-fat meal *Serum $t_{1/2}$:* 17 hr *Intracellular $t_{1/2}$:* 10–50 hr *Elimination:* primarily by glomerular filtration and active tubular secretion	Should be taken with food
Abacavir **Ziagen** *Preparations* Tablets: 300 mg Oral solution: 20 mg/mL	300 mg Q 12 hr, or with zidovudine and lamivudine as Trizivir 1 tablet BID 600 mg QD under investigation	*Oral bioavailability:* 83% *Serum $t_{1/2}$:* 1.5 hr *Intracellular $t_{1/2}$:* 3.3 hr *Elimination:* hepatic metabolism (non–cytP450; alcohol dehydrogenase and glucuronyltransferase) with renal elimination of metabolites (82%)	Can be administered without regard to meals Alcohol raises abacavir levels by 41%
Hydroxyurea **Hydrea** *Preparations* Capsules: 500 mg	500 mg BID	*Oral bioavailability:* 79% *Serum $t_{1/2}$:* 3.5–4.5 hr *Intracellular $t_{1/2}$:* Unknown *Elimination:* hepatic metabolism with renal elimination	Administer on empty stomach For those unable to swallow capsules, empty capsules into a glass of water and drink immediately
Non-Nucleoside Reverse Transcriptase Inhibitors[a]			
Nevirapine **Viramune** *Preparations* Suspension: 10 mg/mL (investigational) Tablets: 200 mg	200 mg PO QD × 14 days, then 200 mg PO BID (400 mg PO QD under investigation)	*Oral bioavailability:* >90% *Serum $t_{1/2}$:* 25–30 hr *Intracellular $t_{1/2}$:* Unknown *Elimination:* metabolized by cytP450 (3A4 inducer) with 80% glucuronide metabolite being eliminated in urine	Can be administered without regard to meals
Delavirdine **Rescriptor** *Preparations* Tablets: 100 and 200 mg	400 mg TID (four 100-mg tabs in ≥3 oz water to produce slurry); 600 mg BID under investigation	*Oral bioavailability:* 85% *Serum $t_{1/2}$:* 5.8 hr *Intracellular $t_{1/2}$:* Unknown *Elimination:* metabolized by cytP450 (3A4 inhibitor) with 51% being eliminated in urine as metabolites	Can be administered without regard to meals

continued

Table 69-3   Characteristics of Antiretroviral Agents for the Treatment of Adult HIV Infection[5,9,231–233]—cont'd

Drug	Dose	Pharmacokinetic Parameters	Administration Considerations
Non-Nucleoside Reverse Transcriptase Inhibitors—cont'd			
Efavirenz **Sustiva** *Preparations* Capsules: 50, 100, 200, 600 mg	600 mg QHS	*Oral bioavailability*: 60–70% *Serum $t_{1/2}$*: 40–55 hr *Intracellular $t_{1/2}$*: Unknown *Elimination*: hepatically metabolized (3A4 mixed inhibitor/inducer)	Avoid taking with high-fat meals, levels ↑50% (increased risk for CNS toxicity)
Protease Inhibitors			
Indinavir **Crixivan** *Preparations* Capsule: 200, 333, and 400 mg	800 mg Q 8 hr (BID dosing ineffective when sole protease inhibitor) Indinavir/ritonavir—800/200 BID; 800/100 BID; 400/400 mg BID; 1,200/100 400 mg QD under investigation	*Oral bioavailability*: 65% *Serum $t_{1/2}$*: 1.5–2 hr *Intracellular $t_{1/2}$*: Unknown *Elimination*: hepatically metabolized via cytP450 3A4 (inhibitor)	Must be taken on empty stomach (1 hr before or 2 hr after a meal); may take with skim milk or low-fat meal. Adequate hydration necessary (at least 1.5 liters of liquid per 24 hr) to minimize risk of nephrolithiasis
Ritonavir **Norvir** *Preparations* Oral solution: 80 mg/mL Capsules: 100 mg	600 mg Q 12 hr (day 1–2: 300 mg BID; day 3–5: 400 mg BID; day 6–13: 500 mg BID; day 14: 600 mg BID)	*Oral bioavailability*: Unknown *Serum $t_{1/2}$*: 3–5 hr *Intracellular $t_{1/2}$*: Unknown *Elimination*: extensive hepatic metabolism via cytP450 3A4 > 2D6 (potent 3A4 inhibitor)	Take with food if possible to improve tolerability Dose should be titrated upward to minimize gastrointestinal adverse events Refrigerate capsules
Nelfinavir **Viracept** *Preparations* Powder for oral suspension: 50 mg per 1 level scoop (200 mg per 1 level teaspoon) Tablets: 250 and 625 mg	750 mg TID or 1,250 mg BID	*Oral bioavailability*: 20–80% *Serum $t_{1/2}$*: 3.5–5 hr *Intracellular $t_{1/2}$*: Unknown *Elimination*: hepatic metabolism via cytP450 3A4	Administer with meal or light snack (levels increased 2–3 fold)
Saquinavir **Fortovase** (soft gel capsules) **Invirase** (hard gel capsules) *Preparations* Soft gel capsules: 200 mg Hard gel capsule: 200 mg	1,200 mg TID (soft gel capsule) Hard gel cap should be used only in combination with ritonavir Saquinavir/ritonavir—400/400 BID, 1,000/100 BID; 1,600/100 QD under investigation Hard gel capsules should be administered with ritonavir given that the bioavailability of hard gel capsules is equivalent to soft gel capsules with significantly less gastrointestinal side effects Saquinavir/atazanavir 1,600/400 QD under investigation	*Oral bioavailability*: 4% hard gel capsule; soft gel capsule not determined *Serum $t_{1/2}$*: 1–2 hr *Intracellular $t_{1/2}$*: Unknown *Elimination*: hepatic metabolism via cytP450 3A4 (inhibitor)	Take with full meal (levels increase 6-fold) Soft gel capsules should be refrigerated or can be stored at room temperature for up to 3 months
Amprenavir **Agenerase** *Preparations* Capsules: 50, 150 mg Solution: 15 mg/mL	1,200 mg PO BID Amprenavir/ritonavir—1,200/200 QD (FDA-approved); 600/100–200 BID; 750–900/100–200 BID under investigation	*Oral bioavailability*: Not determined *Serum $t_{1/2}$*: 7.1–10.6 hr *Intracellular $t_{1/2}$*: Unknown *Elimination*: hepatic metabolism via cytP450 3A4 (inhibitor)	Can be taken without regard to meals but should not be taken with high-fat meals
Lopinavir/ritonavir **Kaletra** *Preparations* Capsules: 133.3 mg lopinavir + 33.3 mg ritonavir per capsule Solution: 80 mg lopinavir + 20 mg ritonavir per mL	3 capsules BID (4 capsules BID with efavirenz or nevirapine) 6 capsules QD under investigation	*Oral bioavailability*: Not determined *Serum $t_{1/2}$*: 5–6 hr *Intracellular $t_{1/2}$*: Unknown *Elimination*: hepatic metabolism via cytP450 3A4 (inhibitor)	Take with food (increases area under the curve by 48%)
Atazanavir **Reyataz** *Preparations* Tablets: 200 and 300 mg	400 mg QD Atazanavir/ritonavir—300/100 QD under investigation Atazanavir/saquinavir—400/1,600 QD under investigation	*Oral bioavailability*: 60–70% *Serum $t_{1/2}$*: 6–7 hr *Intracellular $t_{1/2}$*: Unknown *Elimination*: hepatic metabolism via cytP450 3A4 (modest inhibitor)	None

Table 69-3   **Characteristics of Antiretroviral Agents for the Treatment of Adult HIV Infection[5,9,231–233]—cont'd**

Drug	Dose	Pharmacokinetic Parameters	Administration Considerations
Entry Inhibitors			
Fuzeon (Enfurvitide, T-20)	90 mg SC BID in upper arm, thigh, or abdomen	*Oral bioavailability:* Not applicable *Serum $t_{1/2}$:* 3.8 hr *Intracellular $t_{1/2}$:* Not applicable *Elimination:* nonrenal, nonhepatic	Reconstitute with 1.1 mL of sterile water for injection; gently tap vial for 10 sec and then roll gently between hands to avoid foaming and ensure all drug is off vial walls After reconstitution, use immediately or refrigerate for 24 hr. Refrigerated T-20 should be brought to room temperature before injection.

[a]In clinical trials, the non-nucleoside reverse transcriptase inhibitor (NNRTI) was discontinued because of rash in 7% of patients taking nevirapine, 4.3% of patients taking delavirdine, and 1.7 % of patients taking efavirenz. Rare cases of Stevens-Johnson have been reported with all three NNRTIs.

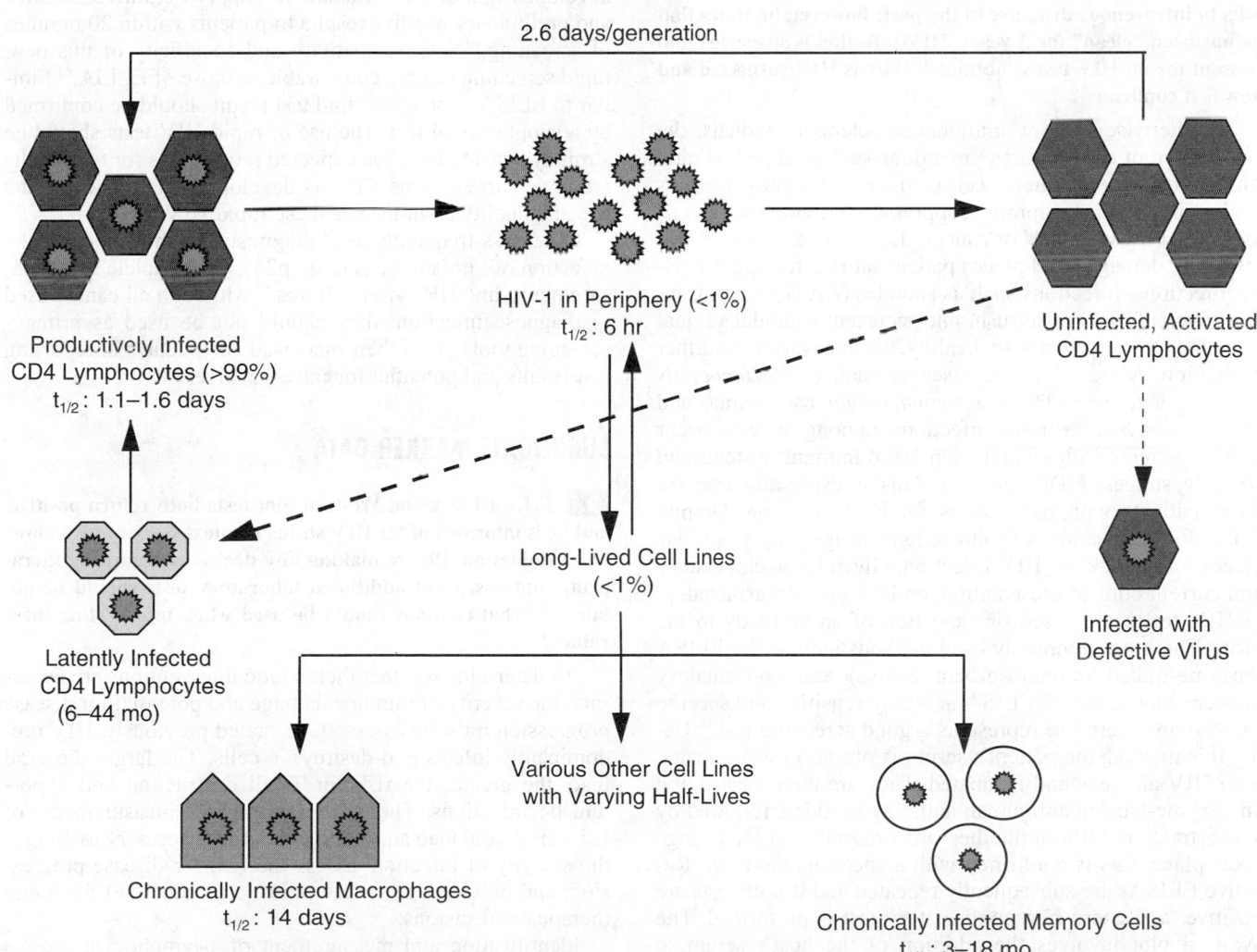

FIGURE 69-4 Schematic summary of HIV-1 infection dynamics within various cell lines of the immune system. Solid lines represent major route of progression, dashed lines represent minor route of progression. (Adapted and updated from Reference 19).

that exists is that some cell lines have shorter half-lives than others (e.g., peripheral T cells, ~1 to 2 days versus macrophages 14 days).[52,53] In addition, long-lived infected T cells with half-lives lasting more than 6 to 44 months have been identified.[54,55] This would require complete HIV suppression for 60 years or more to eradicate infection![54–56] Another complicating factor is the potential for HIV to reside in sites that are unaffected by antiretroviral agents and thereby serve as sanctuaries for smoldering HIV infection (e.g., central nervous system [CNS], testes). Once therapy is discontinued, these sites could theoretically release unaffected virions, which could then repopulate the host. As a result of this situation, research has been shifted toward immune-based therapies that can identify and destroy HIV-infected cells.

DIAGNOSIS

1. E.J. is a 27-year-old man who presents to your clinic with new complaints of fevers, night sweats, weight loss, and a white exudate in his mouth. He states that these symptoms have been present for the past 4 to 6 weeks. On physical examination, it is concluded that E.J. has thrush due to *Candida albicans*. E.J. admits to intravenous drug use in the past; however, he states that he has been "clean" for 3 years. HIV infection is suspected and consent for an HIV test is obtained. Why is HIV suspected and how is it confirmed?

In otherwise healthy, immunocompetent individuals, the appearance of opportunistic infections such as thrush is rare. This is because an intact cell-mediated immunity protects against infection. In immunosuppressed individuals, such as those infected with HIV or cancer, the immune system is significantly damaged and places patients at risk for opportunistic infections. Infections such as shingles (*Herpes zoster*), active tuberculosis, oral thrush, and recurrent candidal vaginal infections in an otherwise healthy person warrants further evaluation. More advanced diseases such as *Pneumocystis carinii* pneumonia, *Mycobacterium avium* bacteremia, and *Cytomegalovirus* retinitis infections, among others, occur only in patients with severely depressed immune systems and strongly suggest HIV infection. This is especially true for those patients with risk factors for HIV infection. Despite E.J.'s discontinuation of intravenous drugs, his prior use places him at risk for HIV infection. Given his social history and current clinical presentation, an HIV test is warranted.

HIV testing is based on detection of an antibody to the virus. The most commonly used methods include the ELISA (enzyme-linked immunosorbent assays) and confirmatory Western blot tests.[57–59] ELISA is highly sensitive and specific (>99%) and therefore represents a good screening test.[59] Using this method, the patient's serum is placed in wells coated with HIV antigens and incubated. They are then washed and an enzyme-labeled antihuman antibody is added, followed by a substrate. If HIV antibodies are present, a color change takes place; this is confirmed with a spectrophotometer. Reactive ELISAs are subsequently repeated and if both tests are positive, a Western blot confirmatory test is performed. The Western blot involves the addition of the host's serum to known HIV antigens that have been separated by gel electrophoresis. After washing and incubation, antihuman immune globulins linked to an enzyme or radioactive probe are

added. The spectrum of band patterns on the gel is then interpreted and compared to controls for HIV diagnosis.

Although these tests when used together are highly specific and sensitive, there are situations where both false-negatives and false-positives can occur.[60] The most troublesome is the situation in which a patient is truly infected but both ELISA and Western blot results are negative. Once infected, it may take up to 1 to 2 months for a person to develop antibodies to HIV.[61] Because both these tests rely on antibody detection, this "window" period of acute infection could result in a false-negative test for HIV. If this is suspected, clinicians may wish to order a HIV PCR or bDNA test (viral load measurement; see below); measurements greater than 2,000 copies/mL are present only among patients who are HIV infected. In all situations, a confirmatory Western blot test should be performed to rule out false-positives and mislabeled samples.

Results of the ELISA test take up to 1 to 2 weeks, and this delay means that patients must contact their providers for test results. According to the Centers for Disease Control and Prevention (CDC), in the year 2000 approximately one-third of individuals who tested positive for HIV didn't return to the clinic to learn their results.[10] Newer test methods have been developed that allow clinicians to supply definitive negative and preliminary positive results to patients within 20 minutes of screening.[10,62] The sensitivity and specificity of this new, rapid screening test are comparable to those of ELISA.[62] Similar to ELISA, a positive rapid test result should be confirmed by a supplemental test. The use of rapid HIV tests should be strongly considered when expected return rates for test results are low. Currently, the CDC is developing guidelines on the use and quality assurance of these rapid HIV tests.

Other less frequently used diagnostic methods include the detection of viral antigens (e.g., p24), viral nucleic acid measurements, and HIV viral cultures.[59] Although all can be used to diagnose infection, they should not be used as primary screening tools given their increased cost, delays in reporting test results and potential for false-positives.[60,63]

SURROGATE MARKER DATA

2. E.J.'s ELISA and Western blot tests both return positive, and he is informed of his HIV status the next week at his follow-up examination. Before making any decisions regarding therapeutic options, what additional laboratory tests should be obtained? What cautions should be used when interpreting these values?

To determine whether therapeutic interventions are necessary, the severity of immune damage and potential for disease progression must be assessed. As stated previously, HIV predominantly infects and destroys T cells. The larger the viral load, the greater the risk for T-cell destruction and opportunistic infections. Therefore, quantitative measurements of E.J.'s HIV viral load and T-cell counts are necessary to "stage" the severity of infection, assess the risk for disease progression, and provide a reference point (e.g., baseline) for future therapeutic decisions.

Identification and measurement of T-lymphocyte subsets (e.g., CD4; CD8) are based on flow cytometry readings of fluorescent-labeled monoclonal antibodies.[5,46] These values can display wide variability on repeated laboratory evaluations, even in clinically stable patients. Samples from a patient can display up to 30% intra- and interlaboratory, as well as intrapatient variability.[5] In at least one study, enough interlaboratory variability existed to potentially result in conflicting treatment recommendations in 58% of patients (e.g., initiating therapy when T-cell counts fell below 500 cells/mm³).[64] Consequently, it is important to realize that assessment of T-cell measurements should always be interpreted as trends and not as individual values.

The measurement of HIV viral load can be performed by one of two methods: reverse transcriptase–polymerase chain reaction (RT-PCR) or branched-chain DNA (bDNA) assay.[65,66] Measurements using RT-PCR are obtained when viral RNA is amplified and counted. In contrast, bDNA amplifies and enumerates the signal from target probes attached to the viral RNA. Both methods report HIV RNA in plasma as the number of copies per milliliter, with results being roughly equivalent when newer versions of bDNA assays are used.[5] It should be recognized that plasma viral RNA values measure the amount of free virus in the periphery and not the lymph nodes. Because viral concentrations are substantially greater in the lymph node, plasma measurements of HIV indirectly reflect spill over from replication in that compartment.[67,68]

Similar to CD4 counts, viral load measurements (copies/mL) can vary by as much as threefold (0.5 log) in either direction.[5] When obtaining a patient's baseline value, a number of issues must be considered. On initial infection with HIV, a burst of viremia occurs until the host's immune responses are able to control the infection. Subsequently, viral load measurements obtained during the first 6 months of infection may not accurately reflect a true baseline value.[5] In addition, factors that activate the immune system, such as the development of a new opportunistic infection or immunizations,[69] can result in transient elevations of viral load measurements. In these situations, levels obtained within 4 weeks of the event may not accurately reflect the baseline viral load measurement.[5] Therefore, to make an accurate assessment, it is recommended that at least two separate viral load measurements, which are obtained within 1 to 2 weeks of each other, be performed before making decisions regarding therapeutic options.[6] As with T-cell values, viral load measurements should be evaluated as trends between levels and not as individual values.

E.J. should have a baseline T-cell count and viral load measurement obtained. It is recommended that the viral load test be repeated within 1 to 2 weeks to confirm the value. A complete blood count, electrolyte panel, and renal and liver function tests should also be performed. These laboratory values help in selecting therapeutic options (see below) and establish baseline values in the event that problems are encountered in the future.

ANTIRETROVIRAL THERAPY

3. E.J.'s T-cell count and viral load measurement (two separate levels obtained within the past 2 weeks) return at 225 cells/mm³ and 145,000 copies/mL (by RT-PCR assay). Should antiretroviral therapy be initiated?

The decision to initiate antiretroviral therapy should consider the potential benefits of therapy to the potential risk of therapy, including both short-term and long-term side effects

and potential for the development of drug resistance (and cross-resistance; see below). Antiretroviral therapy should be offered to any patient who is symptomatic, regardless of T-cell count and viral load measurements. "Symptomatic" refers to any new opportunistic infection or increases in constitutional symptoms (e.g., fevers, night sweats, unexplained weight loss). These events suggest a faltering immune system that necessitates therapy. In patients who are asymptomatic, assessment of the patient's surrogate marker data (T-cell count, viral load measurements), concurrent medical conditions, medication adherence history, if any, and motivation to initiate therapy are necessary. In addition, given increasing transmission rates of drug-resistant HIV to newly infected patients that could limit treatment responses, a drug resistance test should be considered before initiating therapy.

Knowledge of both the T-cell count and the baseline viral load values is necessary to "stage" the severity of infection. In otherwise healthy, immunocompetent persons, T-cell measurements are >1,200 cells/mm³. In patients who have been chronically infected with HIV, significant T-cell destruction occurs. When T-cell counts fall below 500 cells/mm³, patients are at increased risk for opportunistic infections (see Fig. 69-3). The optimal time to initiate antiretroviral therapy among asymptomatic HIV-infected patients is unknown. Data from both clinical trials and observational cohort studies have shown a clear benefit for antiretroviral therapy when CD4 cell counts are less than 200 cells/mm³. In contrast, the benefits of therapy among asymptomatic patients with CD4 cell counts over 200 cells/mm³ is currently unknown and must be carefully weighed against the potential for both short- and long-term toxicities and other considerations. In the MACS cohort study of untreated HIV-infected patients, the 3-year risk of progression to AIDS was 38.5% for patients with CD4 cell counts between 201 and 350 cells/mm³ and 14.3% among patients with CD4 cell counts greater than 350. Among treated patients, one large collaborative analysis showed improved prognosis among patients who initiate therapy above 200 cells/mm³.[70] Another large cohort study showed clinical benefit when therapy was initiated when the CD4 cell count was greater than 350 cells/mm³. However, 40% experienced adverse drug events requiring discontinuation of therapy within the first year, and 20% were no longer on treatment after 2 years.[4] Consequently, many clinicians use the 350 cells/mm³ value as a time to consider initiating discussions with the patient about the pros and cons of starting antiretoviral therapy. The viral load value at baseline also needs to be considered. As can be seen from Figure 69-5 and Table 69-4 from the MACS cohort study, the higher the baseline viral load measurement, the greater the risk for more rapid disease progression. Note that this trend was found across all CD4 cell counts. Among asymptomatic patients with baseline viral load measurements greater than 55,000 copies/mL (RT-PCR), therapy may be necessary depending on the CD4 cell count. If the CD4 cell count is less than 350 cells/mm³, therapy should be considered; if the CD4 cell count is greater than 350 cells/mm³, clinicians may elect to initiate therapy or follow-up patients more carefully over time and initiate therapy if there is a greater than expected decline in CD4 cell counts (e.g., >30% decline).

As a result of these data, the Department of Health and Human Services published guidelines on when to consider

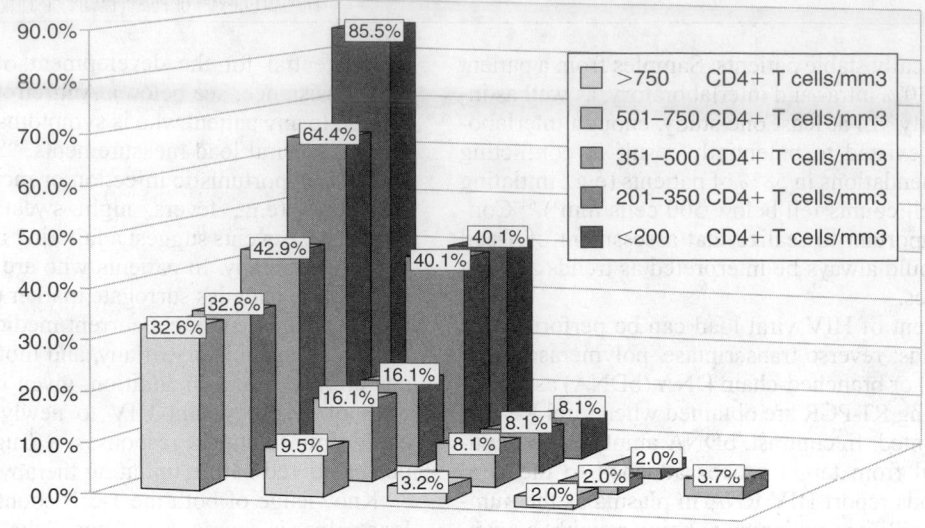

MACS bDNA:	>30K	10K–30K	3K–10K	501K–3K	<500
RT-PCR:	>55K	20K–55K	7K–20K	1.5K–7K	<1500

FIGURE 69-5 Relation between CD4 cell count strata and baseline viral load measurements and risk for developing AIDS within 3 years. (From Reference 5.)

Table 69-4 Risk of Progression to AIDS-Defining Illness in a Cohort of Homosexual Men Predicted by Baseline CD4+ T-Cell Count and Viral Load[a]

CD4 ≤ 200 Plasma Viral Load (copies/mL)[b]			% AIDS (AIDS-defining complication)[c]		
bDNA	RT-PCR	n	3 years	6 years	9 years
≤500	≤1,500	0[e]	–	–	–
501–3,000	1,501–7,000	3[e]	–	–	–
3,001–10,000	7,001–20,000	7	14.3	28.6	64.3
10,001–30,000	20,001–55,000	20	50.0	75.0	90.0
>30,000	>55,000	70	85.5	97.9	100.0

CD4 201–350[d] Plasma Viral Load (copies/mL)			% AIDS (AIDS-defining complication)		
bDNA	RT-PCR	n	3 years	6 years	9 years
≤500	≤1,500	3[e]	–	–	–
501–3,000	1,501–7,000	27	0	20.0	32.2
3,001–10,000	7,001–20,000	44	6.9	44.4	66.2
10,001–30,000	20,001–55,000	53	36.4	72.2	84.5
>30,000	>55,000	104	64.4	89.3	92.9

CD4 > 350 Plasma Viral Load (copies/mL)			% AIDS (AIDS-defining complication)		
bDNA	RT-PCR	n	3 years	6 years	9 years
≤500	≤1,500	119	1.7	5.5	12.7
501–3,000	1,501–7,000	227	2.2	16.4	30.0
3,001–10,000	7,001–20,000	342	6.8	30.1	53.5
10,001–30,000	20,001–55,000	323	14.8	51.2	73.5
>30,000	>55,000	262	39.6	71.8	85.0

[a]Data from the Multi-Center AIDS Cohort Study (MACS) adapted from reference 3 by Alvaro Muñoz, Ph.D. (personal communication).

[b]MACS numbers reflect plasma HIV RNA values obtained by version 2.0 bDNA testing. RT-PCR values are consistently 2–2.5 fold higher than first generation bDNA values, as indicated. It should be noted that the current generation bDNA assay (3.0) gives similar HIV-1 RNA values as RT-PCR except at the lower end of the linear range (<1,500 copies/mL).

[c]In this study AIDS was defined according to the 1987 CDC definition and does not include asymptomatic individuals with CD4+ T cells <200 mm³.

[d]A recent evaluation of data from the MACS cohort of 231 individuals with CD4+ T cell counts >200 and <350 cells/mm³ demonstrated that of 40 (17%) individuals with plasma HIV RNA <10,000 copies/mL, none progressed to AIDS by 3 years (Alvaro Muñoz, personal communication). Of those individuals with plasma viremia of 10,000–20,000 copies/mL, 4% and 11% progressed to AIDS at 2 and 3 years, respectively. Plasma HIV RNA was calculated as RT-PCR values from measured bDNA values.

[e]Too few subjects were in the category to provide a reliable estimate of AIDS risk.

bDNA, branched-chain DNA; RT-PCR, reverse transcriptase–polymerase chain reaction.

antiretroviral therapy in HIV-infected persons[5] (Table 69-5). These guidelines provide general principles for when to initiate therapy in an antiretroviral-naive patient; however, they are not absolute. The decision to initiate therapy should not be taken lightly nor should it be based solely on surrogate marker data. Antiretroviral regimens may improve the quality and duration of a patient's life, but they are not without significant risks and problems. Once therapy is initiated, antiretroviral therapy is a lifetime commitment! For some patients, this may be a difficult realization because it marks a significant point in their lives when they go from an otherwise healthy to a potentially sick HIV-infected patient. In addition, the fear of adverse events and toxicities and potential alterations to lifestyles may provide barriers to the initiation of appropriate therapeutic interventions. These guidelines, therefore, should be used as a springboard for discussions with the patient regarding the risks and benefits of therapy. It is critical for practitioners to talk openly with patients about their fears and concerns and make an assessment about their motivation to initiate therapy and ability to take a complex regimen. The patient should always make the final decision after careful discussions with the practitioner.

E.J. has a number of significant risk factors for disease progression. He is clinically symptomatic with oral thrush and nonspecific constitutional symptoms (e.g., fevers, night sweats, and weight loss). Second, his surrogate maker data place him at risk for greater disease progression (T-cell count <350 cells/mm³ and viral load >55,000 copies/mL). Finally, his risk for disease progression, as evidenced by his T-cell count and viral load measurement, is high. Using Table 69-4, his chance for an AIDS-defining event over the next 3, 6 and 9 years are roughly 64%, 89% and 93%, respectively. Based on these data, E.J. should be advised to start antiretroviral therapy.

4. After careful discussions, E.J. agrees to initiate therapy. What should be the goals of therapy? What other factors/information needs to be considered in order to select an appropriate regimen?

Before developing a patient specific regimen, it is important to recognize the benefits and limitations of therapy and identify obtainable and realistic goals.

Goals of Therapy
Goal 1: Preserve and Strengthen the Immune System
The single most important goal of therapy should be to preserve and strengthen the host's immune system and thereby prevent opportunistic infections. Using a potent regimen, that is, one that significantly suppresses HIV replication, is crucial to obtaining this goal. The ability to measure viral loads has shown that maximal viral suppression often results in significant increases in T-cell counts and improved clinical outcomes.[71-74] Based on our understanding of viral pathogenesis, this is not surprising. Lower amounts of replicating virus results in decreased risk for T-cell infection and destruction and, subsequently, a more intact immune response. Therefore, therapy should suppress viral replication as much as possible, preferably to nondetectable levels in the plasma, for as long as possible.[5,6]

There are a number of caveats to this goal. First, it should be recognized that this might not be easily obtainable in all patients. For example, a patient with an initial viral burden of 1,000,000 copies/mL is different from another patient with an initial viral burden of only 10,000 copies/mL. In the latter patient, viral suppression to nondetectable levels may be a realistic goal, whereas in the former patient it may require a much more potent regimen that may result in increased risk for adverse drug events. In situations in which viral suppression to

---

Table 69-5   Indications for the Initiation of Antiretroviral Therapy in the Chronically HIV-1–Infected Patient

The optimal time to initiate therapy in asymptomatic individuals with >200 CD4+ cells is not known. This table provides general guidance rather than absolute recommendations for an individual patient. All decisions to initiate therapy should be based on prognosis as determined by the CD4+ T-cell count and level of plasma HIV RNA, the potential benefits and risks of therapy shown in Table 69-4, and the willingness of the patient to accept therapy.

Clinical Category	CD4+ T-Cell Count	Plasma HIV RNA	Recommendation
Symptomatic (AIDS, severe symptoms)	Any value	Any value	Treat
Asymptomatic, AIDS	CD4+ T cells <200/mm³	Any value	Treat
Asymptomatic	CD4+ T cells >200/mm³ but <350/mm³	Any value	Treatment should generally be offered, though controversy exists.[a]
Asymptomatic	CD4+ T cells >350/mm³	>55,000 (by bDNA or RT-PCR)[b]	Some experts would recommend initiating therapy, recognizing that the 3-year risk of developing AIDS in untreated patients is >30% and some would defer therapy and monitor CD4+ T-cell counts more frequently.
Asymptomatic	CD4+ T cells >350/mm³	<55,000 (by bDNA or RT-PCR)[b]	Many experts would defer therapy and observe, recognizing that the 3-year risk of developing AIDS in untreated patients is <15%.

[a]Clinical benefit has been demonstrated in controlled trials only for patients with CD4+ T cells <200/mm³. However, most experts would offer therapy at a CD4+ T-cell threshold <350/mm³. A recent evaluation of data from the MACS cohort of 231 individuals with CD4+ T-cell counts >200 and <350 cells/mm³ demonstrated that of 40 (17%) individuals with plasma HIV RNA <10,000 copies/mL, none progressed to AIDS by 3 years (Alvaro Muñoz, personal communication). Of those individuals with plasma viremia of 10,000–20,000 copies/mL, 4% and 11% progressed to AIDS at 2 and 3 years respectively. Plasma HIV RNA was calculated as RT-PCR values from measured bDNA values.
[b]Although there was a 2–2.5 fold difference between RT-PCR and the first bDNA assay (version 2.0), with the current bDNA assay (version 3.0), values obtained by bDNA and RT-PCR are similar except at the lower end of the linear range (<1,500 copies/mL).

nondetectable levels is not obtainable, the goal of therapy should be to suppress viral replication to as low as possible for as long as possible. Second, as stated previously, most HIV infection resides in the lymph node and not the plasma. Lymph node biopsies have shown that viral suppression in the plasma indirectly reflects viral replication in these compartments as well.[75,76] Although viral replication may be suppressed to low or nondetectable levels, it does not represent eradication of HIV from an infected patient. Studies have documented HIV infection in reservoir tissues despite persistently undetectable viral load values in the plasma.[76–79]

Goal 2: Prevent the Development of Resistance and Preserve Future Treatment Options

An additional benefit derived from using potent antiretroviral regimens is the ability to suppress the development of resistant virus. In any given viral population the potential exists for a spontaneous mutation to occur, which results in a resistant isolate. The larger the population, the greater the risk. HIV replication is a highly error-prone process, especially the reverse transcriptase enzyme. Given the high rate of viral replication, the potential exists for the daily production of thousands of replication-competent viral mutants to each and every site on the HIV genome (about 10,000 nucleotides in length).[7,38] Under selective pressures from inadequate antiretroviral therapies, isolates with reduced susceptibility to the given regimen eventually flourish and repopulate the host. This is of particular concern given the potential for cross-resistance between antiretroviral agents (see following discussion of resistance). Therefore, the use of a potent regimen that fully suppresses or significantly lowers the viral population reduces the potential for mutations and the development of cross-resistance.

Even though there are currently 16 FDA approved antiretroviral agents to use in combination therapies, many of these agents display similar resistance profiles.[7] As a result, it is possible to develop resistance to one or more agents in a given regimen, which could cause the loss of activity to other agents with similar resistance profiles despite the fact that the patient has not received therapy with that agent (i.e., cross-resistance). If viral replication occurs while the patient is on therapy along with sufficient selective pressure on the virus from the given regimen, drug resistance may occur. Whether drug resistance develops is a consequence of the genetic barrier associated with the individual agents. Some agents have low genetic barriers; that is, only one or two critical changes in the virus are necessary for resistance to occur. An example of a class of agents with a low genetic barrier is the nonnucleoside reverse transcriptase inhibitors (NNRTIs). One critical point mutation in the viral genome is required for loss of activity among this class of agents.[7] In contrast, the protease inhibitors (PIs) have a wide genetic barrier in that it takes multiple viral changes to incur significant loss of activity.[7,81,82] It should be recognized, however, that just because an agent has a low genetic barrier does not mean it is virologically inferior or less potent. Potent HAART regimens containing NNRTIs have been shown to be highly effective and provide durable treatment responses.[92,93,99] It is also important to realize that the potency of the regimen as a whole is critical to determining whether or not drug resistance develops. If viral replication is suppressed, the development of

resistance will be minimal. However, if viral replication does occur, the greater the replication, the greater the risk for development of resistance.[5,6] In situations in which viral replication does occur, having an agent(s) in the antiretroviral regimen with a low genetic barrier may be risky and could result in the loss of activity of the individual agent and/or the development of cross-resistance to other agents. As a result, it is critical to select an antiretroviral regimen that is potent enough to suppress viral replication and allows the patient to adhere to therapy (either through ease of dosing and/or minimization of adverse drug events that may limit adherence to therapy).

Given the increased rate of transmission of resistant viruses to newly HIV-infected patients,[82–85] many clinicians are obtaining resistance test before initiation of therapy to help in the selection of appropriate agents in the antiretroviral regimen.[7] If a regimen is initiated that contains an agent(s) to which the virus has already developed resistance, the potency of the entire regimen may be insufficient to allow for complete viral suppression and further antiretroviral resistance may develop.

Goal 3: Select a Regimen That the Patient Will Take

Maximal viral suppression should not be obtained at the expense of a patient's overall health and safety. Adherence to an antiretroviral regimen can be a complex and difficult task.[4,86–89] The patient's ability to adhere to therapy may be the difference between a regimen that fails and one that results in a clinical benefit. Many regimens require strict adherence to therapy to ensure maximal viral suppression. In addition, unpleasant adverse events may make tolerating these regimens difficult. Data from studies evaluating the incidence of noncompliance among HIV-infected individuals have shown that at least 10% of patients on PIs miss a dose each day and that at least 20% miss a dose every 2 days.[88] Although the exact amount of adherence needed to maintain viral suppression is unknown, brief "drug holidays" (3 days or more) have resulted in viral breakthrough.[90] The four most common reasons for skipping antiretroviral doses among HIV-infected patients were simple forgetfulness, a change in daily routine, being too busy with other things, and being away from home.[90,91] Therefore, factors that have been associated with poor adherence include (1) the number of medications—the greater the number, the greater the likelihood of poor compliance; (2) the complexity of the regimen—special meal requirements, escalating/de-escalating doses, number of times per day that pills must be taken; (3) special storage requirements; (4) interference of medication with lifestyle and daily activities; and (5) poor communication with primary care providers and other healthcare professionals.[90,91] Incorporating these factors into the selection of a patient-specific regimen may improve adherence and subsequently, the chance for an improved clinical outcome.

In hopes of improving patient adherence, many investigators, clinicians, and pharmaceutical companies have been working on developing simpler regimens and dosing schedules for antiretroviral therapies for HIV. Interventions include (1) combining drugs to optimize drug–drug interactions (boosting of PI levels by drugs that inhibit hepatic metabolism); (2) using fixed-dosing formulation products (e.g., lopinavir/ritonavir in one dosing form, the combination of zidovudine, epivir, and abacavir into 1 tablet); (3) removing drug–food requirements where possible; (4) developing agents with longer half-lives; and (5) treatment strategies that use less frequent dosing schedules (e.g., once or twice daily regimens).

Goal 4: Minimize Both Short- and Long-Term Adverse Drug Events

Treatment with HAART has been shown to be highly effective in suppressing HIV replication and improving survival among HIV-infected patients. Although great strides have been made in improving the dosing and tolerability to these agents, both short- and long-term adverse events could minimize drug adherence and subsequent response to therapy.

Changes in body composition (known as lipodystrophy), increases in lipids and triglyccrides, bone and joint fractures, increased risks for cardiac disease, and the development of lactic acidosis have both patients and clinicians concerned.[92] In addition, both acute and long-term adverse events can be fatal if not properly identified and managed.

Clinical trials have shown that up to 40% of patients discontinue their initial HAART regimen in the first year because of adverse drug events.[4] It is therefore critical to select a patient-specific HAART regimen that minimizes the risk for adverse drug events where possible (Fig. 69-6). Many agents can be used to treat HIV infection, but many potential

Clinical symptom	NRTIs						NNRTIs		Protease Inhibitors					
	ABC	AZT	ddC	ddI	d4T	3TC	EFV	NVP	APV	IDV	LPV	NFV	RTV	SQV
Abdominal pain														
Alterations of taste														
CNS symptoms							■							
Diarrhea			■				■	■	■		■	■	■	■
Drug rash	■						■	■						
Fat accumulation							?	?						
Fat loss					■		?	?						
Fatigue														
Fever	■							■						
Headaches														
Hypersensitivity syndrome	■													
Kidney stones										■				
Myalgia														
Nausea													■	
Pancreatitis				■										
Paraesthesias														
Polyneuropathy			■		■									
Sleep disturbances							■							
Stomatitis														
Vertigo							■							
Vomiting														
Laboratory tests														
Amylase↑														
Bilirubin↑														
Cholesterol↑											■		■	
Creatinine↑														
Cytopenias		■												
Glucose↑														
GOT/GPT↑								■						
Lactate↑					■									
Macrocytosis														
Triglycerides↑														

FIGURE 69-6 Known and expected adverse drug events for various FDA-approved antiretroviral agents used for treatment of HIV. See text for drug abbreviations. (From Reference 242.)

regimens will be eliminated from the long list of possibilities by patients' medical/social histories, familial risk factors, and drug–drug interactions. Therefore, a thorough assessment of the patient's medical history, social habits, and prior and current medication histories are essential. In addition, many patients are well educated about their disease and may have preferences regarding therapeutic options. Including the patient in all aspects of the decision-making process may help to limit the number of viable options and make the selection of an appropriate regimen easier.

5. Upon questioning, E.J. states that he has had two bouts of alcohol-induced pancreatitis in the past. The last episode was approximately 1 year ago. He admits to occasional binge drinking even though he knows it's not good for him. E.J. has no known drug allergies and is currently taking only temazepam periodically to help him sleep. He is employed as a construction worker and during the day hours is extremely busy. His complete blood count, electrolyte, and liver and renal panel all return within normal limits. E.J. has no particular preference for a specific regimen and appears highly motivated to take control of his disease. What factors should be considered when selecting an appropriate antiretroviral regimen?

The selection of a patient-specific regimen can be a complex decision. Many potential combinations can be used, but a number of general principles should be followed:

General Rules of Therapy

1. Initiate therapy when the potential clinical benefits outweigh the potential risks. As discussed previously, the initiation of HAART should take into consideration the potential benefits of initiating therapy compared with the potential short- and long-term risks. Many of the current HAART regimens have been shown to reduce viral replication to below nondetectable levels in most of patients studied and have resulted in durable treatment responses.[5,6,81,92,93] Reasons for these improved response rates compared with older HAART regimens include the simplification of the regimens (e.g., less pills per day, less frequent dosing per day, use of fixed-dose combination products), improvement in overall potency of the regimens as a whole, and minimization of short-term side effects. Consequently, if the correct patient-specific HAART regimen is selected as initial therapy, the patient should be able to adhere to therapy and gain both a virologic and clinical benefit from the regimen.

2. Select the type of antiretroviral regimen. The use of HAART is preferred as initial therapy. Monotherapy with any agent should be avoided because clinical trials have shown these regimens to be inferior to combination therapies.[5,6,71,95–99] In addition, the use of dual nucleoside-only–containing regimens should be avoided because initial viral suppression may not be sustained.[5,6,71,95–99] In general, clinicians prefer two types of initial HAART strategies—NNRTI- or PI-based. Clinical trials have shown NNRTI-based strategies to be superior to single PI-based HAART and have produced long-term durable treatment responses.[94,100,259,260] Although not investigated in head-to-head trials with NNRTIs, boosted PI-based HAART (e.g., lopinavir/ritonavir) have been shown to re-

sult in similar overall viral response rates and durable treatment responses.[81] Recent data have shown equivalent virologic response rates between nevirapine and efavirenz; thus, the choice of agent is based on potential adverse events and drug–drug interactions (see text that follows).[100] The use of triple-nucleoside–only based regimens (e.g., zidovudine, lamivudine, and abacavir) has also been investigated.[101–103] This strategy minimizes patient exposure to multiple classes of antiretroviral agents, thereby preserving future treatment options and potentially minimizing both short- and long-term side effects. Conflicting clinical trial data using this strategy exist with two large trials, one showing benefit and another showing inferiority when compared with NNRTI-based HAART.[101–103] In general, the response rates using zidovudine, lamivudine, and abacavir are decreased when the viral load is elevated, probably as a consequence of limited potency of the regimen. As a result, clinicians may elect to reserve this strategy for patients with lower viral loads (e.g., <100,000 copies/mL) and for patients in whom adherence may be an issue (zidovudine, lamivudine, and abacavir comes in a fixed-dose formulation). For patients with very high viral loads, a more potent regimen may be necessary to fully suppress viral replication. Strategies that use four or more antiretroviral agents have been investigated with good results (e.g., triple nucleosides and lopinavir/ritonavir or an NNRTI).[104] Given concerns about adverse events, some clinicians elect to use these more potent regimens until viral control is obtained for a period of time (e.g., 6 to 12 months) and then de-intensify the regimen to standard three-drug HAART.[105] Each interventional strategy comes with potential benefits and risks that should be considered before selection of a given regimen (Table 69-6).

3. Avoid regimens with overlapping toxicities. In general, the concomitant use of the D's (ddI, ddC, and d4T) should be avoided because there is concern over an increased risk for pancreatitis and neuropathies. An exception to this rule is the concomitant use of ddI and d4T. Clinical trials have shown this combination to be effective[106–108] and could offer an alternative to patients who are unwilling to or unable to take zidovudine-containing regimens. The use of ddI and d4T in combination with hydroxyurea has fallen out of favor because of increased adverse events (especially among patients with advanced disease).

4. AZT and d4T should not be used together because both in vitro and in vivo studies have shown these agents to be antagonistic.[5,6,109–112]

5. If PI-based HAART is desired, consider using a dual PI-boosted regimen. The use of combination PIs in a given regimen is based on a number of considerations including increased tolerability, maximal viral suppression, and a beneficial drug–drug interaction. Various combinations of boosted PIs have been evaluated in combination with ritonavir and include saquinavir, lopinavir, indinavir, amprenavir, tipranavir, and atazanavir. Ritonavir, a potent inhibitor of cytochrome p450 metabolism, interacts significantly with a number of agents, including other PIs.[51] This hepatic inhibition can be exploited to decrease the metabolism or increase the absorption of the other PIs (e.g., saquinavir levels are increased >20-fold when administered with ritonavir[113]). The end result is a regimen

Table 69-6   Advantages and Disadvantages of Class-Sparing Regimens

Regimen	Possible Advantages	Possible Disadvantages	Drug Interaction Complications	Impact on Future Options
PI-based HAART regimen (NNRTI-sparing)	• Clinical, virologic, and immunologic efficacy well documented • Continued benefits sometimes seen despite viral breakthrough • Resistance requires multiple mutations • Targets HIV at two steps of viral replication (RT and PI)	• May be difficult to use and adhere to • Long-term side effects may include lipodystrophy[a], hyperlipidemia, and insulin resistance	• Mild to severe inhibition of cytochrome P450 pathway; ritonavir is most potent inhibitor, but this effect can be exploited to boost levels of other PIs	• Preserves NNRTIs for use in treatment failure • Resistance primes for cross-resistance with other PIs
NNRTI-based HAART regimen (PI-sparing)	• Sparing of PI-related side effects • Generally easier to use and adhere to compared with PIs	• Comparability to PI-containing regimens with regard to clinical endpoints unknown • Resistance conferred by a single or few mutations	• Fewer drug-drug interactions compared with PIs	• Preserves PIs for later use • Resistance usually leads to cross-resistance across entire NNRTI class
Triple NRTI regimen (NNRTI- and PI-sparing)	• Generally easier to use and adhere to compared with PIs • Sparing of PI and NNRTI side effects • Resistance to 1 NRTI does not confer cross-resistance to entire class	• Comparability to PI-containing regimens with regard to clinical endpoints unknown • Long-term virologic efficacy with high baseline plasma viral load (i.e., >100,000 copies/mL) may be suboptimal	• Generally manageable drug interaction problems	• Preserves both PI and NNRTI classes for later use • Limited cross-resistance within the NRTI class

[a]Some side effects being attributed to protease inhibitor therapy, such as lipodystrophy, have not been proven to be strictly associated with the use of protease inhibitor-containing regimens. Lipodystrophy has also been described uncommonly in patients on NRTIs alone and in patients on no antiretroviral therapy.
HAART, highly active antiretroviral therapies; NRTI, nucleoside reverse transcriptase inhibitor; NNRTI, non-nucleoside reverse transcriptase inhibitors; PI, protease inhibitor.

with more potent viral suppression than a HAART regimen using either agent alone. In addition, this combination allows for more convenient twice-daily dosing, often lowers the total daily pill burden, and removes the need for drug–food requirements. Given that ritonavir can cause significant gastrointestinal side effects in some patients at increased doses and that only small amounts of ritonavir are needed to inhibit metabolism, low doses of the agent are sufficient (e.g., 100 to 200 mg). In addition, because the levels of the affected PI are significantly elevated, increased adverse events can be seen and may require dosage adjustments (see Therapeutic Drug Monitoring). It should also be remembered that ritonavir interacts with a number of medications and depending on the severity of the interaction may require dosage adjustments of other agents or the inability to use ritonavir in the given regimen.[5,6]

6. What initial antiretroviral regimen should E.J. receive?

When selecting a patient-specific regimen, the following steps should be followed:

Step 1: Determine Which HAART-Based Regimen Will Be Used
After careful review of the pros and cons of each interventional strategy listed in Table 69-6, it is important to assess the patient's motivation and ability to take a potent HAART regimen to minimize medication nonadherence, potential treatment failures, and drug resistance. If concern exists regarding

nonadherence, therapy should probably not be started until the patient is ready and motivated. NNRTI-based HAART should be avoided in nonadherent patients given the low genetic barrier of these agents. A familial history or current medical condition consisting of coronary artery disease, hyperlipidemia, or diabetes mellitus, may result in avoiding the PIs if possible.[92] In addition, recent data suggest that there may be different effects of the nucleoside analogs on body habitus changes and lipid alterations, which may result in the preferential selection of some agents over others.[93,114] As discussed above, elevated viral load measurements may require additional potency from four or more antiretroviral agents in the HAART regimen and viral load measurements less than 100,000 copies/mL may benefit from single class nucleoside-based therapy.

After discussions with E.J., it appears that he is highly motivated to take control of his disease and is willing to initiate therapy. In addition, given E.J.'s high viral load and risk for disease progression, the use of a highly potent regimen appears necessary to ensure complete viral suppression. Subsequently, the use of a HAART-containing regimen is appropriate. Given his current surrogate marker measurements, single-class triple nucleoside therapy may not be appropriate. In addition, given E.J.'s current viral load measurement of 145,000 copies/mL, standard HAART with either PIs or NNRTIs should be sufficient. Potential treatment options are listed in Table 69-7.

Table 69-7 Recommended Antiretroviral Agents for Initial Treatment of Established HIV Infection

This table provides a guide to the use of available treatment regimens for individuals with no prior or limited experience on HIV therapy. In accordance with the established goals of HIV therapy, priority is given to regimens in which clinical trials data suggest the following: sustained suppression of HIV plasma RNA (particularly in patients with high baseline viral load), sustained increase in CD4+ T-cell count (in most cases over 48 weeks), and favorable clinical outcome (i.e., delayed progression to AIDS and death). Particular emphasis is given to regimens that have been compared directly with other regimens that perform sufficiently well with regard to these parameters to be included in the "Strongly Recommended" category. Additional consideration is given to the regimen's pill burden, dosing frequency, food requirements, convenience, toxicity, and drug interaction profile compared with other regimens.

It is important to note that all antiretroviral agents, including those in the "Strongly Recommended" category, have potentially serious toxic and adverse events associated with their use.

Antiretroviral drug regimens comprise one choice each from columns A and B. Drugs are listed in alphabetical, not priority, order.

	Column A	Column B
Strongly recommended	Efavirenz	Didanosine + lamivudine
	Indinavir	Stavudine + didanosine[e]
	Nelfinavir	Stavudine + lamivudine
	Ritonavir + indinavir[a,b]	Zidovudine + didanosine
	Ritonavir + lopinavir[a,c]	Zidovudine + lamivudine
	Ritonavir + saquinavir[a] (SGC[d] or HGC[d])	
Recommended as alternatives	Abacavir	Zidovudine + zalcitabine
	Amprenavir	
	Delavirdine	
	Nelfinavir + saquinavir-SGC	
	Nevirapine	
	Ritonavir	
	Saquinavir-SGC	
No recommendation: Insufficient data[f]	Hydroxyurea in combination with antiretroviral drugs	
	Ritonavir + amprenavir[a]	
	Ritonavir + nelfinavir[a]	
	Tenofovir[i]	
Not recommended: Should not be offered	All monotherapies, whether from column A or B[g]	
	Saquinavir-HGC[h]	
		Stavudine + zidovudine
		Zalcitabine + didanosine
		Zalcitabine + lamivudine
		Zalcitabine + stavudine

[a]See text for more information on optimizing protease inhibitor exposure with ritonavir.
[b]Based on expert opinion.
[c]Co-formulated as Kaletra.
[d]Saquinavir-SGC, soft-gel capsule (Fortovase); saquinavir-HGC, hard-gel capsule (Invirase).
[e]Pregnant women may be at increased risk for lactic acidosis and liver damage when treated with the combination of stavudine and didanosine. This combination should be used in pregnant women only when the potential benefit clearly outweighs the potential risk.
[f]This category includes drugs or combinations for which information is too limited to allow a recommendation for or against use.
[g]Zidovudine monotherapy may be considered for prophylactic use in pregnant women with low viral load and high CD4+ T-cell counts to prevent perinatal transmission.
[h]Use of saquinavir-HGC (Invirase) is not recommended, except in combination with ritonavir.
[i]Data from clinical trials are limited to use in salvage. Data from trials of tenofovir as initial therapy may be available in the near future.

Step 2: Selection of Agents in the Regimen (Tables 69-8 and 69-9; Fig. 69-6)

EXCLUSION OF ABSOLUTE CONTRAINDICATIONS AND DRUG INTERACTIONS

The next step requires the selection of agents for the regimen. In many situations, absolute contraindications and significant drug–drug interactions limit potential agents for use in the regimen. As can be seen from Table 69-8, both ddI and ddC are absolute contraindications given a history of alcohol abuse and pancreatitis. Both agents can cause pancreatitis with the greatest risk seen among patients with a medical history similar to E.J.'s. The remaining reverse transcriptase inhibitors, including zidovudine (AZT), lamivudine (3TC), stavudine (d4T), tenofovir (TDF), and abacavir, are all potential options. Any agent in the NNRTI or PI class can be administered safely with temazepam.

Step 3: Quality-of-Life Considerations

When selecting a regimen, assessment of quality-of-life issues, potential adverse drug events, and patient requests should be given as much consideration as drug–drug interactions and absolute contraindications. In some situations, these issues could be the difference between a regimen that is effective and one that is not. Considering E.J.'s lifestyle and work requirements, it is best to select a regimen that will minimally interfere with his daily activities. In E.J.'s situation, middle-of-the-day dosing could present a problem given his busy work schedule. Subsequently, the selection of a regimen with once- or twice-daily dosing would be optimal (see Table 69-3). All combinations of the remaining nucleosides can be given once or twice daily and therefore represent viable options (see Table 69-3). As stated above, any of these agents can be used in combination except AZT and d4T. Examples of

Table 69-8   Absolute Contraindications for Antiretroviral Agents Used for Treatment of HIV Infection[a]

Agent	Drug–Drug Interactions	Prior Medical History	Significant Social History
Nucleoside Reverse Transcriptase Inhibitors			
Zidovudine (AZT; ZDV)	IV induction with ganciclovir (AZT should be held or dose ↓ to 100 mg Q 8 hr); high dose probenecid (e.g., for cidofovir administration—hold AZT dose for day of cidofovir infusion); d4T, ribavirin	Use with caution in patients with risk factors for liver disease given concern over development of lactic acidosis and severe hepatomegaly with steatosis	None
Didanosine (ddI)	IV pentamidine; ddC	History of pancreatitis or neuropathies (use with caution); use with caution in patients with risk factors for liver disease given concern over lactic acidosis and severe hepatomegaly with steatosis. Fatal lactic acidosis has been reported in pregnant women who received a combination of d4T and ddI—use in pregnancy only when benefits outweigh potential risks	Currently drinking alcohol or history of alcohol abuse
Zalcitabine (ddC)	IV pentamidine, ddI; d4T	History of pancreatitis or neuropathies (use with caution); use with caution in patients with risk factors for liver disease given concern over lactic acidosis and severe hepatomegaly with steatosis	Currently drinking alcohol or history of alcohol abuse
Stavudine (d4T)	ddC, AZT	History of peripheral neuropathies (use with caution); use with caution in patients with risk factors for liver disease given concern over lactic acidosis and severe hepatomegaly with steatosis. Fatal lactic acidosis has been reported in pregnant women who received a combination of d4T and ddI—use in pregnancy only when benefits outweigh potential risks	None
Lamivudine (3TC)	None	Use with caution in patients with risk factors for liver disease given concern over lactic acidosis and severe hepatomegaly with steatosis	None
Abacavir	Unknown	Previous hypersensitivity syndrome characterized by fevers, abdominal pain, malaise, and rash; should not be restarted because fatalities have been reported; use with caution in patients with risk factors for liver disease given concern over lactic acidosis and severe hepatomegaly with steatosis	Unknown
Tenofovir	Cidofovir, adefovir; use with caution when coadministered with nephrotoxic agents	Calculated creatinine clearance <60 mL/min or serum creatinine >1.5 mg/dL; use with caution in patients with risk factors for liver disease given concern over lactic acidosis and severe hepatomegaly with steatosis	None
Non-Nucleoside Reverse Transcriptase Inhibitors			
Nevirapine	Rifampin	Previous severe rash, fever to nevirapine; use with caution in patients with hepatic disease	Unknown
Efavirenz	Astemizole, terfenadine, cisapride, midazolam, triazolam, ergot alkaloids	Previous severe rash, fever to efavirenz; should not be used in pregnant women given increased teratogenicity potential	Unknown
Delavirdine	Terfenadine, astemizole, midazolam, cisapride, rifabutin, rifampin, triazolam, ergot derivatives, phenytoin, carbamazapine, phenobarbital, pimozide, simvastatin, lovastatin, ergot alkaloids	Previous severe rash, fever to delavirdine	Unknown
Protease Inhibitors			
Indinavir	Rifampin, terfenadine, astemizole, cisapride, triazolam, midazolam, ergot alkaloids, simvastatin, lovastatin, St. John's wort	None	Use with caution in patients with history of nephrolithiasis (especially patients who are unable to maintain adequate hydration)

Table 69-8   Absolute Contraindications for Antiretroviral Agents Used for Treatment of HIV Infection[a]—cont'd

Agent	Drug–Drug Interactions	Prior Medical History	Significant Social History
Protease Inhibitors—cont'd			
Saquinavir	Rifampin, rifabutin, terfenadine, astemizole, cisapride, triazolam, midazolam, ergot alkaloids, simvastatin, lovastatin, St. John's wort, garlic	None	None
Nelfinavir	Rifampin, terfenadine, astemizole, cisapride, triazolam, midazolam, ergot alkaloids, simvastatin, lovastatin	None	None
Ritonavir	disulfiram, metronidazole, amioderone, astemizole, bepridil, bupropion, cisapride, clozapine, encainide, flecainide, midazolam, quinidine, terfenadine, pimozide, triazolam, ergot alkaloids, simvastatin, lovastatin, St. John's wort Given the increased risk for adverse drug–drug interactions, any new medication should be evaluated for potential interactions when administered with ritonavir	None	Currently drinking alcohol: risk for disulfiram-like reaction
Amprenavir	Astemizole, terfenadine, rifampin, midazolam, triazolam, bepridil, ergot alkaloids, cisapride, simvastatin, lovastatin, St. John's wort	None	None
Kaletra (lopinavir/ritonavir)	See ritonavir drug interaction list	None	None
Atazanavir	Not fully clarified at time of writing; however, atazanavir is a mild cyp3A4 inhibitor, therefore potential drug–drug interactions Use caution when atazanavir is used with rifampin and drugs with narrow therapeutic indexes that are metabolized by cyp3A4 Drugs that increase gastric pH decrease atazanavir bioavailability (H_2 blockers, proton pump inhibitors)	None	None

[a]Avoid use of any agent in patients with history of previous hypersensitivity reactions to the given agent.

potential regimens include zidovudine, epivir and efavirenz or nevirapine; tenofovir, epivir, and efavirenz or nevirapine; stavudine, epivir, and efavirenz or nevirapine; or all of the above options replacing efavirenz or nevirapine with lopinavir/ritonavir.

7. E.J. is starting zidovudine, lamivudine, and efavirenz. How should therapy be monitored? Are any additional laboratory tests necessary?

Short-Term Assessments

Three important criteria determine whether an antiretroviral regimen is effective: clinical assessment, surrogate marker responses, and regimen tolerability.[5,6] In patients who are clinically symptomatic (e.g., increase in constitutional symptoms such as fatigue, night sweats, and weight loss; new opportunistic infections), the initiation of an appropriate antiretroviral regimen often results in resolution of symptoms, increases in strength and energy, and improvements in overall general health. In some patients, however, the effect may not be as prominent. A careful assessment of clinical symptoms should therefore be regularly performed at all follow-up appointments.

In all patients, regardless of clinical status, assessment of repeat viral load and T-cell counts are necessary. Once therapy is initiated, it often takes up to 3 to 4 months for maximal viral suppression to occur.[5,6] This delay is a result of viral suppression within different compartments of the body. The tis-

Table 69-9   Drug Interactions Involving Protease Inhibitors and Non-Nucleoside Reverse Transcriptase Inhibitors: Effect of Drug on Levels (AUCs)/Dose

Drug Affected	Ritonavir	Saquinavir[a]	Nelfinavir	Amprenavir	Lopinavir/Ritonavir
Indinavir (IDV)	Levels: IDV ↑ 2–5× Dose: IDV 400 mg BID + RTV 400 mg BID, or IDV 800 mg BID + RTV 100 or 200 mg BID	Levels: IDV no effect SQV ↑ 4–7×[b] Dose: Insufficient data	Levels: IDV ↑ 50% NFV ↑ 80% Dose: Limited data for IDV 1,200 mg BID + NFV 1,250 mg BID	Levels: APV AUC ↑ 33% Dose: No change	Levels: IDV AUC and C_{min} increased Dose: IDV 600 mg BID
Ritonavir (RTV)	•	Levels: RTV no effect SQV ↑ 20×[c] Dose: Invirase or fortovase 400 mg BID + RTV 400 mg BID	Levels: RTV no effect NFV ↑ 1.5× Dose: RTV 400 mg BID + NFV 500–750 mg BID	Levels: APV AUC ↑ 2.5-fold Dose: Limited data for APV 600–1,200 mg BID + RTV 100–200 mg BID	Lopinavir is co-formulated with ritonavir as Kaletra
Saquinavir (SQV)	•	•	Levels: SQV ↑ 3–5× NFV ↑ 20%[b] Dose: Standard NFV fortovase 800 mg TID or 1,200 mg BID	Levels: APV AUC ↓ 32% Dose: Insufficient data	Levels: SQV[b] AUC and C_{min} increased Dose: SQV 800 mg BID, LPV/r standard
Nelfinavir (NFV)	•	•	•	Levels: APV AUC ↑ 1.5-fold Dose: Insufficient data	No data
Amprenavir (APV)	•	•	•	•	Levels: APV AUC and C_{min} increased Dose: APV 600–750 mg BID, LPV/r standard

Drug Affected	Nevirapine	Delavirdine	Efavirenz
Indinavir (IDV)	Levels: IDV ↓ 28% NVP no effect Dose: IDV 1,000 mg/Q 8 hr NVP standard	Levels: IDV ↑ >40% DLV no effect Dose: IDV 600 mg Q 8 hr DLV: standard	Levels: IDV ↓ 31% Dose: IDV 1,000 mg Q 8 hr EFV standard
Ritonavir (RTV)	Levels: RTV ↓ 11% NVP no effect Dose: Standard	Levels: RTV ↑ 70% DLV: no effect Dose: DLV: standard RTV: no data	Levels: RTV ↑ 18% EFV ↑ 21% Dose: RTV 600 mg bid (500 mg BID for intolerance) EFV standard
Saquinavir (SQV)	Levels: SQV ↓ 25% NVP no effect Dose: No data	Levels: SQV ↑ 5×[c] DLV no effect Dose: Fortovase 800 mg TID DLV standard (monitor transaminase levels)	Levels: SQV ↓ 62%[c] EFV ↓ 12% Co-administration not recommended
Nelfinavir (NFV)	Levels: NFV ↑ 10% NVP no effect Dose: Standard	Levels: NFV ↑ 2× DLV ↓ 50% Dose: No data (monitor for neutropenic complications)	Levels: NFV ↑ 20% Dose: Standard
Amprenavir (APV)	No data	No data	Levels: APV AUC ↓ 36% Dose: APV 1,200 mg TID as single PI, or 1,200 mg BID + RTV 200 mg BID EFV standard
Lopinavir/Ritonavir (LPV/RTV)	Levels: LPV Cmin ↓ 55% Dose: Consider LPV/r 533/133 mg BID in PI-experienced patients NVP standard	Levels: LPV levels expected to increase Dose: Insufficient data	Levels: LPV AUC ↓ 40% EFV: no change Dose: Consider LPV/r 533/133 mg BID in PI-experienced patients EFV: standard
Nevirapine (NVP)	•	No data	Levels: NVP: No effect EFV: AUC ↓ 22%
Delavirdine (DLV)	No data	•	No data

[a]Several drug interaction studies have been completed with saquinavir given as Invirase or Fortovase. Results from studies conducted with Invirase may not be applicable to Fortovase.
[b]Conducted with Fortovase
[c]Conducted with Invirase

sues and cells with the longest viral half-lives account for most of the observed delay. If therapy were assessed solely at the 3- to 4-month time point and the regimen were subtherapeutic, the potential would exist for the development of a resistant isolate and/or increased viral seeding of other tissues and cells within the body. Therefore, a repeat "midpoint" viral load value should be obtained within 4 to 8 weeks of initiation of therapy.[5,6] This midpoint value allows clinicians to assess the magnitude of response and ensures declining viral load measurements. Therapy with an effective regimen will result in at least a threefold (0.5 log) and tenfold decrease (1.0 log) in viral load counts by weeks 4 and 8, respectively.[5,6,66] The viral load should continue to decline over the next 12 to 16 weeks, and in most patients it will become undetectable.[5,6]

Long-term response to therapy correlates with the magnitude of viral suppression upon initiation of a regimen. The greater the suppression, the greater the durability of response to that regimen.[115,116] The speed and magnitude of suppression, however, can be affected by a number of factors including clinical status of the patient (e.g., more advanced disease—low T-cell counts, high viral load value), adherence to therapy, and overall potency of the regimen.[5,6] When the virologic response is less than optimal (either at the midpoint or the 3- to 4-month measurement), evaluation of compliance should be assessed, repeat viral load measurements performed, drug levels of key antiretroviral agents evaluated for subtherapeutic values and/or a change in therapy considered (e.g., intensifying therapy with additional agents).

In response to declining viral replication, T-cell destruction decreases and subsequently CD4 counts increase. The magnitude of this rebound can vary significantly, with some patients experiencing large increases and others experiencing little or no change. Given that T-cell changes do not occur rapidly, once therapy is initiated, repeat T-cell counts should be obtained at the 3- to 4-month follow-up visit.[5,6]

Finally, failure either by surrogate marker data or clinical symptomatology can occur when inadequate serum concentrations of antiretrovirals are obtained. This can occur for many reasons; however, the most common is failure to adhere to the prescribed regimen. It is important to determine whether the regimen was too complex for the patient or an adverse event occurred. In both situations, selection of an alternative, more appropriate regimen should be used. Drug exposures can also be affected by the addition of new drugs or herbal products. Both garlic and St. John's wort have been shown to lower the levels of a number of nonboosted PIs; many other agents have not been investigated.[117,118] In addition, certain medications require specific food–drug requirements to ensure optimal exposure (see Table 69-3). Therefore careful evaluation of new drugs, herbs, and dosing habits should be performed at each follow-up visit. If after discussions with the patient, the clinician does not identify adverse events, adherence issues, and new drug–drug, drug–herb, or drug–food interactions as potential causes of failure, then changing to another viable regimen should be considered or malabsorption or increased metabolism be assessed by serum drug concentrations.

8. E.J.'s viral load values at 4 and 14 weeks after initiation of therapy are 7,000 copies/mL and nondetectable, respectively. His T-cell counts have increased from 225 to 525 cells/mm³. In addition, E.J. states that his night sweats and fevers have disappeared, he "feels great" and that he has had no drug-related problems. Is the therapy effective? How should therapy be monitored?

E.J.'s response to the zidovudine, lamivudine, and efavirenz appears to be effective on many different levels. Clinically, he states his symptoms have subsided and his overall health is much improved. Virologically his midpoint and follow-up viral load measurements have responded appropriately and are now below the level of assay detection. Lastly, his T-cell counts have increased by 300 cells/mm³. In addition, E.J. has experienced no drug-related adverse events. Given the response to date, no changes are required and the current regimen should be continued.

Long-Term Assessments

Once the prescribed regimen has been stabilized, the overall long-term goals of therapy should be to maintain maximal viral suppression, sustain clinical and immunologic improvements, and maintain continued drug tolerability. Periodic assessments of viral load measurements and T-cell counts should be performed every 3 to 4 and 3 to 6 months, respectively.[5,6] These surrogate marker data allow clinicians to monitor viral activity, immunologic status, and trends between time periods. In addition, these laboratory values help clinicians determine whether therapy should be continued (see the following). Clinical assessment of the patient, and tolerability to the prescribed regimen, should also be performed at the 3- to 6-month follow-up visits. These visits should involve discussions regarding regimen tolerability, clinical signs and symptoms of disease progression (e.g., new opportunistic infections), new signs and symptoms of constitutional symptoms, and patient concerns. These visits also allow clinicians to fine tune or change the regimen when necessary.

Treatment Failure

9. E.J. has remained on AZT, 3TC, and efavirenz for over 2 years. To date, his T-cell counts have remained stable at 550 cells/mm³, and his viral load measurements have remained below the level of assay detection. He presents with new complaints of fevers and malaise. E.J. reports that he has been compliant with therapy and has not started any new medications. Repeat laboratory tests now show E.J.'s viral load is 3,000 copies/mL and his T-cell count is 375 cells/mm³ (both repeated and validated). Should E.J.'s regimen be changed?

Up to 50% of patient on HAART eventually fail therapy.[3,4] Reasons for failure are not fully known; however, risk factors include a history of low T-cell counts, high viral loads, and extensive use of antiretroviral agents.[3,4] Assessment of regimen failure should be based on data similar to that used when therapy is initiated: (1) clinical symptoms, (2) surrogate marker data, and (3) regimen tolerability and compliance.[5–7,10]

In many patients, the first sign of failure is a change in clinical signs and symptoms. These changes can be subtle (e.g., increase in constitutional symptoms, new onset of oral thrush) or more severe (e.g., new opportunistic infections). These situations suggest a failing regimen and necessitate a change in therapy.

Assessment of efficacy should also involve evaluation of surrogate marker data (e.g., T cells and viral load). In many situations, changes to these markers occur before any noticeable clinical signs and symptoms or opportunistic infections. Therefore, careful evaluation of surrogate marker data may allow clinicians an opportunity to intervene before any significant immune destruction occurs. Virologic failure, defined as new or continued viral replication despite appropriate antiretroviral therapy, suggests a failing regimen. For example, patients with repeated detection of virus in plasma after initial suppression to undetectable levels should be evaluated as potential treatment failures. In patients in whom viral suppression to nondetectable levels was not achieved, a significant increase in viral replication (defined as a threefold increase or greater) should also be viewed as a treatment failure.[5,6,66]

When assessing viral load measurements it is important to remember that these values can increase as a result of vaccinations or other concurrent infections (see Question 2). Therefore, a thorough medical history should be performed to rule out other causes for increasing viral load measurements. In addition, it is important to remember that laboratory values should be interpreted as trends over time and not as individual measurements. A repeat viral load should be performed and evaluated within 4 weeks of the initial viral load increase. In some cases, transient viral "blips" occur (increases in viral load measurements just above the level of assay detection, e.g., 200 to 500 copies/mL), which again become nondetectable at the next follow-up visit.[119,120] Although these transient blips may not directly reflect treatment failure, they may represent the potential for future viral breakthrough either because of patient nonadherence or insufficient antiretroviral potency. Careful follow-up of these patients is therefore required, and/or intensification with another agent may be necessary.

In response to increasing viral replication, T-cell destruction occurs. A significant decrease in CD4 cells is defined as a decrease of >30% from baseline.[5,6,66] Persistently declining T-cell counts, with or without increasing viral load measurements, represent a treatment failure and strongly suggest a change in therapy should be made.

Other potential causes for failure include nonadherence and drug–drug interactions. When a patient has not taken the prescribed regimen as directed (including not adhering to drug–food requirements), discussions regarding tolerability, number of doses missed, duration of nonadherence, and lifestyle changes should take place. The decision to reinitiate a prescribed regimen should take into account the future likelihood of adherence and the potential development of resistant strains. In those patients with a history of long-standing nonadherence, the success of reinitiating the prescribed regimen may be limited. Unfortunately, the precise effect of the duration and extent of nonadherence on the development of resistance has not been fully evaluated. However, for the virus to mutate, enough drug pressure must be placed on the virus; this requires at least 50% patient adherence to ensure adequate drug exposures.[121]

Significant drug–drug, drug–food, and drug–herb interactions could also contribute to therapeutic failure. Interactions between a new medication or herbal product could decrease the bioavailability or increase the metabolism of the HIV medications leading to low serum concentrations.[117,118] In addition, many medications require certain drug–food requirements to allow maximal drug absorption and concentrations. A careful review of all new medications and their potential for clinically significant drug interactions should be evaluated at all visits (see Table 69-9).

Currently, E.J. has a number of signs and symptoms that suggest a failing regimen. First, he is experiencing new symptoms of fevers and malaise not attributable to any other cause. Second, his viral load value has become detectable at 3,000 copies/mL without evidence of concurrent infections or vaccinations in the past 4 weeks. Lastly, his T-cell counts have declined from 550 cells/mm^3 to 375 cells/mm^3. In addition, it appears that E.J. has been adhering to his therapy and has not started any new medications that could affect the efficacy of his current regimen. A change in therapy is therefore necessary.

10. What potential antiretroviral regimen(s) can be considered for E.J. ?

In addition to the general rules of therapy described in Question 5, a number of other issues should be considered when selecting an alternative regimen for a patient failing therapy.

General Rules for Changing Therapies[5,6]

1. If possible, the new regimen should contain all new antiretroviral agents to which the patient is naive. If this is not possible, the new regimen should contain at least two new agents that are not currently contained in the failing regimen. The potential for cross-resistance between antiretroviral drugs should be considered when choosing new regimens, and therefore resistance testing may provide useful information in certain situations (see Question 12).

2. Given that antiretroviral drug resistance is more likely to occur with increased and prolonged viral replication in the presence of antiretroviral agents, changes to therapy should occur close to the time of treatment failure.

3. As in the treatment of tuberculosis, one new drug should never be added to a failing regimen to prevent the development of resistance. An exception to this rule is if the initial response to therapy among newly infected patients has not reached the desired virologic goal (e.g., nondetectable viral load measurements). In this situation, some clinicians opt to intensify therapy with an additional agent provided that the viral load measurement were trending downward and not leveled off or increased between visits (suggesting potential for the development of resistance). In addition, it is probably best to use agents with wide genetic barriers (e.g., abacavir or tenofovir) to intensify therapy and minimize the risk of losing valuable agents with small genetic barriers (e.g., NNRTIs) if the potency of the regimen as a whole is insufficient.

4. If possible, never re-initiate a regimen that the patient has failed in the past; an isolate resistant to the failed regimen could continue to reside within various compartments of the body. If a regimen to which the patient had previously failed were restarted, unimpeded viral replication of the resistant strain would occur, repopulate the host, and eventually result in treatment failure. In some situations (e.g., patients with advanced disease, limited treatment options and prior exposure to most antiretroviral agents), it may be necessary to re-initiate agents or regimens in combination

with additional agents with the goal of suppressing viral replication.

5. When treatment failure is a direct result of drug toxicity, the offending agent should be replaced with an alternative drug from a similar class provided that the potential for cross-resistance is minimal.

6. If an agent in a given regimen must be discontinued or held, it is recommended that all agents in the regimen be stopped and restarted simultaneously to prevent the development of resistance.

It should be recognized that many alternative regimens are based on theoretical benefits or limited data. In addition, many potential options could be limited in some patients based on prior antiretroviral use, toxicity, or past intolerances. Therefore, the clinician should carefully discuss these issues with the patient before changing therapy.

Because E.J. is failing to respond to his current regimen, a new antiretroviral regimen must be chosen. As previously discussed, combined use of ddI and ddC should be avoided because the risk for pancreatitis may be increased. The new regimen should also take into consideration quality-of-life issues. In E.J.'s situation, middle-of-the-day dosing could present a problem, and therefore, twice-daily dosing would represent an optimal dosing schedule. Using the rules above, quality-of-life considerations, and the remaining antiretroviral agents, many regimens could be used. For example, the combination of tenofovir (TDF) plus abacavir (ABC) and lopinavir/ritonavir meets all of the above criteria and therefore represents a viable option.

Considerations in Antiretroviral-Experienced Patients

11. H.G. is a 46-year-old, HIV-positive man with an extensive history of treatment with a variety of antiretroviral agents. He took AZT monotherapy in the late 1980s and early 1990s. When 3TC became available, he took the combination of AZT and 3TC until he failed therapy about 5 years ago. At that time, he began experiencing AZT-induced myopathies. Since that time, H.G. has been "on and off" various regimens without sustained clinical benefit. He is currently taking d4T, ddI, ritonavir, and saquinavir with a CD4 count and viral load measurement of 55 cells/mm³ and 48,000 copies/mL (by RT-PCR assay), respectively. These laboratory values have been stable for the last 9 months. How do patients with extensive antiretroviral histories differ from antiretroviral-naive patients? Are there any special considerations when selecting therapeutic regimens for patients such as H.G.?

Patients who have been infected for 10 or more years may have been treated with many different regimens, both experimental and FDA approved. As a result, many potential regimens have already been exhausted and therefore may not represent viable therapeutic options. From a clinician's perspective, the ideal scenario is to evaluate a newly infected patient who does not have a history of extensive antiretroviral therapy. In many cases, however, this is not possible. Although many patients with antiretroviral drug histories can be appropriately managed with therapies that successfully inhibit viral replication, data from clinical trials and clinical experience suggest that many of these patients will exhibit a decreased response to therapy (e.g., less viral load suppression).[71,95,122] In

addition, the durability of viral suppression often is not sustained.[5,6] This may reflect the development of resistant viral isolates that display cross-resistance to various antiretroviral agents.

Patients who have taken several antiretroviral regimens often present other unique situations for clinicians that require the clinician to consider the following factors when selecting or changing drug therapy:

1. *Regimen tolerability*[123–125]: Patients with advanced HIV disease display decreased tolerability to many medications, including antiretroviral agents. Although this is not fully understood, it is probably a result of HIV-induced immune alterations and cytokine dysregulations. Subsequently, clinicians evaluating patients with advanced disease should be alert for possible drug-induced adverse events.

2. *Drug interactions:* Many patients with advanced disease take numerous medications for primary or secondary prophylaxis of various opportunistic infections, as well as other medications. Subsequently, the risk for a drug–drug interaction is increased. Therefore, any addition of a new medication, either prescription or over-the-counter, should be carefully evaluated for potential interactions with the patient's current antiretroviral regimen (see Tables 69-8 and 69-9). In addition, any change to the current antiretroviral regimen should also be checked against the patient's current medication list.

3. *Altered bioavailability:* HIV-infected patients with advanced disease may have unreliable absorption of many medications. Reasons for this finding include episodes of severe diarrhea, anorexia, weight loss, wasting and gastric achlorhydria. As a result, the bioavailability of some agents, especially certain PIs that require specific dietary requirements, may be affected (see Table 69-3). Any changes in dietary habits or bowel function should be carefully assessed as to the potential impact on the patient's antiretroviral regimen.

4. *Antiretroviral drug histories:* The most useful information to guide the choice of alternative regimens is a detailed drug history. Among patients with extensive prior antiretroviral use, it is critical to identify previously failed regimens and determine the precise cause of the failures. In an experienced patient who has taken many different regimens over a lifetime, the number of remaining viable agents and regimens may be limited. Therefore, it is important to determine whether prior regimens truly failed or whether drug discontinuation was the result of some other cause (such as regimen intolerability or an inadequate trial period). In addition, detailed knowledge of regimen intolerabilities and which agent(s) caused the adverse event will help in the selection of an appropriate regimen. In some situations, the offending agent may be reinitiated if the adverse event was minimal or can be appropriately managed.

RESISTANCE, VIRAL GENOTYPING, PHENOTYPING, AND VIRAL FITNESS

12. Will viral genotyping and phenotyping assist in selecting an appropriate therapeutic regimen for H.G.? What are these tests? What are their limitations and when should they be used?

What is viral fitness, and does it have a role in clinical decision-making?

Viral genotyping and phenotyping are tests that assess viral resistance patterns to antiretroviral agents. Genotyping evaluates mutations in the virus' genetic material, whereas phenotyping assesses the ability of the virus to grow in the presence of increasing concentrations of antiretroviral agents. There are three potential causes for the development of resistance:

1. Initial infection with a resistant isolate from a source patient[82–85]
2. Natural selection of a resistant isolate as a consequence of inefficient, error-prone viral replication[38,126,127]
3. Generation of resistant isolates via selective pressures from antiretroviral therapies that do not fully suppress viral replication[7,128–137]

Mutations are generated when naturally occurring amino acids in the HIV genome are replaced with alternative amino acids. For example, resistance to lamivudine (3TC) occurs when the amino acid methionine (M) is replaced by valine (V) at the 184th amino acid in the protein chain.[7,138] This mutation is subsequently referred to as an M184V mutation. These amino acid substitutions subsequently can change the proteins that are produced and may alter the shape, size or charge of the viral enzyme's substrate or primer.[139–141] Subsequently, binding to the active site by antiretroviral agents is decreased, their affinity for natural substrates is increased, or there is increased removal of the antiretroviral agent from the enzyme by the virus (known as pyrophosphorylation).[142] Whether a mutation results in a clinically resistant, less viable, or indifferent isolate depends on which amino acid(s) is replaced. In addition, certain mutations or combination of mutations have been shown to produce viral isolates that display increased sensitivity to various antiretroviral agents (known as hypersusceptibility). Alterations to certain key amino acids could potentially result in cross-resistance between various antiretrovirals.[7]

Two key enzymes have been extensively studied with regard to their potential for development of resistance: reverse transcriptase (RT) and protease. Replication via the RT enzyme is a highly error-prone process. Given that the HIV genome is roughly 10,000 nucleotides in length and that mutations via the RT enzyme occur roughly once in every 10,000 nucleotides copied, it has been estimated that a mutation occurs with every viral replication. With up to 10 billion particles of virus being produced per day, the potential exists for 1,000 to 10,000 mutations occurring at each site in the HIV genome every day.[38] The protease enzyme is composed of two identical monomers that combine to form a symmetrical pocket catalytic site. Key mutations inside this pocket that result in the development of resistance have been identified.[143–145] Because the protease enzyme is composed of proteins formed from amino acids, mutations outside the catalytic site could also cause conformational changes to the enzyme that results in the development of resistance. The interactions between mutations both inside and outside the catalytic site could result in a synergistic, hypersusceptible, antagonistic, or indifferent viral response to the various PIs. These interactions are currently under investigation. Key mutations to the antiretroviral agents are identified in Figure 69-7 and are updated periodically by expert panels of clinicians.

Over time, countless viral subpopulations known as "quasi-species" develop. It is important to recognize that in any given host at any given time many different quasi species can exist. In addition, within any compartment of the body (e.g., CNS versus gut versus testes) there also can exist many different quasi species. Because these mutant strains represent only a small number of isolates in the total viral population, they must have some replicative disadvantage when compared with the "wild-type" virus.[128,129] Under selective pressures from antiretroviral therapies, however, the potential exists for these mutant isolates to replicate. For example, if wild-type viral replication is inhibited by an antiretroviral regimen and if any one viral strain of the quasi-species is more fit for growth in the presence of that regimen, then the viral mutant will have a competitive advantage and could overtake the wild-type virus in the general population.[146] It should be recognized that for resistance to develop, viral replication must occur. When viral replication is completely inhibited, the development of resistant isolates is uncommon.

Genotypic analysis involves sequencing the viral isolates genetic material via polymerase chain reaction (PCR) amplification. Mutations associated with resistance to a given agent are identified by analysis of key sequences of the RT or protease enzymes. These tests can be rapidly processed; however, they are limited in that only one sequence can be detected at a time and whether or not the single sequence that is being analyzed is a key mutation is unknown. In addition, these tests detect mutations only if they are present in more than 25% of all HIV isolates in the body. Because pressures from antiretroviral therapies select resistant isolates, these tests may not provide information regarding rare, yet potentially clinically significant isolates.[5] Phenotypic analysis involves growing virus in the presence of various concentrations of drug and then determining viral susceptibilities (e.g., inhibitory concentrations [IC_{50}]). Phenotyping is limited because it evaluates only one viral isolate at a time and subsequently could fail to identify other clinically relevant isolates. In addition, the amount of drug required to inhibit viral growth within a test tube may not represent concentrations required in a given patient or within various compartments of the body.[5] Evaluations of an individual patient's drug concentrations to their respect viral isolates IC_{50} values have shown promising results.[147–149] This relationship, known as an inhibitory quotient (IQ), is currently under investigation (see Therapeutic Drug Monitoring).

Simply knowing the mutation patterns of a given viral isolate may or may not be clinically relevant. Although the development of certain key mutations during antiretroviral therapies have been directly correlated with clinical failure, it should be recognized that many of these isolates were derived via selective pressures from monotherapy regimens.[131–136] The clinical relevance of mutations that occur when combination therapy is used is under investigation. Key mutations derived from clinical trials represent the most useful resistance test data.

Genotyping and phenotyping have the potential to provide useful information to clinicians who manage HIV-infected patients. Evidence to date suggests that these tests are effective

---

Guide to Antiretroviral Resistance Mutations

These tables give an overview of mutations associated with resistance to antiretrovirals. Although the interaction between mutations is complex and cannot be fully represented in a concise table format, these tables may still aid in the interpretation of genotypic analysis results. The tables list mutations seen frequently and/or considered significant. Results of genotypic testing always indicate mutations in the majority virus population only (>20%). Mutations caused by previous antiretrovirals may be present only in minority virus populations and may thus not be detected, but will reemerge if the drug(s) in question is resumed. Any mutations reported on previous genotypic testing of a given patient should be taken into account when deciding on future treatment.

How to read these tables:

Bold underlined: Major mutation commonly associated with high level resistance
Bold: Common mutation that can be associated with resistance
Italicized: Not always associated with resistance; possible polymorphism

Nucleosides and Nucleotides

	41/50	65	67	69	69*	70	74	75	115	151	178	184	210	215	219	333	Notes
AZT	**41**		67		**69***	**70**				**151**			210	**215**	219	**333**	184 restores AZT sensitivity in presence of 41 + 215.
3TC					**69***					**151**		**184**				**333**	333 resistant to AZT + 3TC
ddI		65			**69***		**74**			**151**		*184*					
ddC		65		69	**69***		74			**151**		184					Incomplete data
d4T	50				**69***			75		**151**	178						Multiple AZT mutations also □ d4T resistance
ABC		65			**69***		74		**115**	**151**		184					Multiple mutations required
ADV		**65**			**69***					**151**							184 increases ADV sensitivity

69* = 69SSS insertion, which leads to cross-resistance for the class and is difficult to identify in genotypic testing.
151 = leads to cross-resistance to NRTI class when present along with ≥3 mutations.

Non-Nucleoside Reverse Transcriptase Inhibitors (NNRTIs)

	100	103	106	108	179	181	188	190	225	236	Notes
DLV		**103**				**181**				236	NNRTI resistance occurs quickly if viral suppression is incomplete. K103N and Y181C are the most common mutations and lead to cross-resistance. Y181C alone may not lead to EFV resistance.
EFV	100	**103**		108	179	**181**	188		225		
NVP	100	**103**	106	108		**181**	188	190			

Protease Inhibitors

	10	20	24	30	32	33	36	46	47	48	50	54	63	71	73	77	82	84	88	90	Notes
APV	10						*36*	*46*	*47*		**50**	54	63	71			**82**	84			Primary mutation: I50 V
IDV	10	20	24		32		*36*	**46**		*48*		54	63	71	73		**82**	84		90	Requires ≥3 mutations
NFV	10			**30**			*36*	*46*		*48*				71		**77**		84	88	90	Primary mutation: D30N
RTV	10	20			32	33	*36*	*46*				54	63	71			**82**	84		90	Multiple mutations required
SQV	10	20	24	30			*36*	*46*		**48**		**54**	63	71	73		**82**	84		**90**	Primary mutations: G48V & L90M

Reprinted with permission from Medscape, Inc, 1999. Website: http://hiv.medscape.com/updates/quickguide

FIGURE 69-7 Patterns of genotypic resistance for the various classes of antiretroviral agents. The potential for cross-resistance exists when more than one agent shows similar mutation patterns. For example, the potential for cross-resistance between indinavir, ritonavir, and saquinavir, but not nelfinavir, exists when a V82 mutation is present. In contrast, a D30 mutation appears to be specific for nelfinavir alone. It should be recognized that in vitro mutations do not necessarily correlate with in vivo resistance. (From Reference 7.)

at predicting which agents will not work, but they are less useful in predicting those that will work.[5,7,150] For example, if testing identifies resistance to an agent, it is highly unlikely this agent will be effective. However, if testing identifies an agent as susceptible, it does not necessarily predict that this agent will be effective. Clinical trials evaluating the use of genotyping and phenotyping for selection of alternative antiretroviral regimens have been promising.[5,6,151,154–157] Given that each test uses only one viral isolate for analysis, it is possible to obtain different resistance patterns when using both genotyping and phenotypic testing. For example, certain key genotypic mutations produce predictable loss of activity on phenotypic analysis (e.g., the need for increasing concentration of drug). If one test is performed on one sample of blood and the other test performed on a different sample of blood, discordant results could be obtained if different isolates are analyzed (especially among patients with extensive treatment histories and numerous viral quasi-species). As with all clinical decisions made

for HIV-infected patients, careful assessment of the results in combination with the treatment history are essential for proper clinical decision making.

In early treatment failures (e.g., first- or second-regimen failures), expert clinicians can often predict which resistance mutations are likely to be present and consequently resistance testing may be unnecessary. In extensive treatment failures, the use of a genotype or phenotype may be limited in that many viral quasi-species exist and changes to therapy are made based on that viral isolates resistance pattern. Consequently, once the predominant species is eliminated by the current regimen, the next quasi-species will grow and become the predominant species. These tests most likely benefit clinicians in the middle areas, where knowledge of the potential mutation patterns is difficult to predict and there still exist treatment options or new drugs to use.[81] When using a new antiretroviral agent in situations of extensive viral resistance, using one or both of these tests may allow for selection of a regimen that is potent enough for full viral suppression without the loss of activity of the new agent(s).

Only viral isolates that have a competitive advantage can survive in antiretroviral therapy. This occurs as a result of a change in the virus's genetic make-up that results in different protein formation and subsequently a different viral enzyme. For the virus to change from its preferred form (completely sensitive virus, known as wild-type), these genetic changes often impair viral ability to grow (known as fitness).[43,44,152,153] Viral fitness is measured during phenotypic evaluation in that the virus must be amplified and counted. During amplification, the replicative capacity (RC) of the virus can be measured and compared with a reference wild-type, sensitive virus. A wild-type viral isolate has an RC between 70% and 120%; isolates with values less than 70% are considered to be less fit than wild-type virus. In general, the more genotypic changes that occur to a viral isolate, the more compromised the virus and the lower the fitness. However, in some situations the interplay between mutations may result in a viral isolate that is relatively fit. The decrease in fitness needed to make a significant impact on virologic response is unknown. In addition, is it the change in fitness from baseline (e.g., from 120% to 40%) or the absolute % fitness that's critical? Recent data have shown that unfit viruses may allow for preserved immune function despite persistent viral replication.[153] This may be important for patients with limited treatment options in that they may be able to stay on a HAART regimen that produces an unfit virus but does not cause significant T-cell depletion. In these situations, it may be best to keep patients on their current therapy despite measurable viral load measurements (provided their CD4 cell counts are stable) until newer treatment options become available.

Given H.G.'s extensive antiretroviral drug history and his current failure to a highly aggressive regimen, a genotypic or phenotypic analysis may provide some insights into potential therapeutic options. In addition, because his CD4 and viral load measurement are stable, an RC may provide useful information.

SPECIAL CIRCUMSTANCES
Immune System Reconstitution

13. Results from H.G.'s genotype analysis suggest that a regimen containing tenofovir, 3TC, lopinavir/ritonavir, and nevirapine may be useful. After thorough discussions with H.G., and careful evaluation of potential drug–drug interactions, this regimen is initiated. Within 2 weeks, H.G.'s T-cell counts increased from 55 to 127 cells/mm³; however, he now complains of progressive visual loss in his right eye. Physical examination shows macular edema and retinal inflammation consistent with *Cytomegalovirus* infection. Is this a treatment failure? Should H.G.'s antiretroviral regimen be discontinued or changed?

If H.G.'s therapy were evaluated based solely on the rules of therapy (see Questions 7, 8, and 9), this situation would represent a treatment failure. This case, however, is an example of immune reconstitution with disease reactivation after the initiation of potent antiretroviral therapies.[159–162] In patients with advanced HIV disease (e.g., CD4 <100 cells/mm³), significant immune dysfunction occurs, which results in an inability to mount an appropriate response to subclinical infections. As a result, these infections replicate unimpeded and often remain undetected by the host (quiescent disease). When potent antiretroviral therapies are initiated, immune function is often restored leading to symptoms that can be used to identify and eliminate smoldering infections. During the first 12 weeks of therapy, this increased immune response primarily results from redistribution of memory cells.[163–166,240–242] Because of this phenomenon, inflammation at the site of infection often occurs.

The immune reconstitution syndrome can present in any organ system where quiescent disease exists (e.g., CNS, eyes, lymph nodes). Most cases have occurred within 1 to 4 weeks after the initiation of potent antiretroviral therapies. Of particular interest, these cases often occur despite significant increases in T-cell counts to levels well above those generally associated with the respective opportunistic infections.

Although most reports of immune system reconstitution and inflammatory responses have involved infections, one report describes the recurrence of hypersensitivity reactions to trimethoprim-sulfamethoxazole (TMP-SMX).[167] All patients had undergone desensitization protocols or dose reductions and were taking TMP-SMX for *Pneumocystis carinii* pneumonia prophylaxis (n = 4). On initiation of HAART, patients experienced fever (4/4), maculopapular rash (2/4), and leukocytosis (4/4). The fevers did not resolve until TMP-SMX was discontinued. As a result, clinicians should be aware of the possibility of recurrence of hypersensitivity reactions after the initiation of HAART therapies.

In this case, H.G. presents with signs and symptoms of immune reactivation–associated cytomegalovirus (CMV) retinitis including (1) recent initiation of a potent antiretroviral regimen, which increased T-cell counts from 55 to 127 cells/mm³; (2) new onset of visual complaints; and (3) inflammation consistent with CMV retinitis on physical examination. Because the new opportunistic infection is a result of immune reconstitution and not clinical failure, the regimen does not need to be discontinued or changed. Appropriate treatment for CMV, however, should be implemented.

Discordant Surrogate Markers

14. H.G. was successfully treated for CMV retinitis and the regimen of tenofovir, 3TC, lopinavir/ritonavir, and nevirapine was continued. Over the following 6 months, H.G.'s T-cell counts increased to 325 cells/mm³ and his viral load value declined to 5,000 copies/mL (using bDNA assay). At the last two clinic visits H.G.'s viral load (copies/mL) and CD4 counts (cells/mm³) were 2,000/275 and <500/225, respectively. H.G. reports no new clinical complaints or adverse drug events. In addition, H.G. states that he has been compliant with therapy. Are changes to therapy necessary?

In most cases, declines in viral load measurements result in increases in CD4 cell counts and increasing viral load measurements result in declining CD4 cell counts. Given that HIV replication results in T-cell destruction, these observations are not surprising. In roughly 20% of cases, however, T cells decline along with viral load decline or T cells increase along with viral load increases.[5,168,169] These situations are referred to as discordant surrogate marker data and present unique considerations for clinicians.

Although no consensus recommendations exist for treatment options, an understanding of HIV pathophysiology provides rationale for clinical decision making. If the end result of HIV replication is T-cell destruction, then therapeutic decisions should always be based on trends in CD4 cell counts. In the current situation despite declining viral load measurements H.G.'s T-cell counts continue to trend downward and many clinicians would opt to change therapy. When T-cells counts increase despite increasing viral load measurements, decisions regarding therapeutic options are not as well defined. Reasons for this disparity are unclear; however, they may represent a window of time before HIV-induced T-cell destruction. Although these patients may continue to observe a clinical benefit from the current antiretroviral regimen for a period of time, data suggest that long-term stability of the CD4 count is unlikely.[170] Because this may be an early warning sign of impending CD4 cell destruction, many clinicians would change antiretroviral therapies. Other clinicians, however, might opt to follow up patients carefully and change therapies at the first sign of T-cell declines or new clinical signs and symptoms. In these situations, other potential causes of viral load increases (e.g., recent infection, vaccination) should be carefully evaluated to prevent inappropriately changing nonfailing regimens.

Therapeutic Drug Monitoring

15. **P.P. is a 30-year-old HIV-positive man who has failed prior antiretroviral regimens. Based on phenotypic resistance testing, it appears that a regimen including amprenavir boosted by ritonavir may be able to overcome the viral isolate's resistance pattern. Will plasma measurements of P.P.'s antiretroviral drug levels be useful? What measurement should be used, which agent(s) should be measured, and how should the samples be collected?**

Pharmacokinetic evaluations of various antiretrovirals, including the NNRTIs and PIs, have shown wide interpatient variability in drug exposures among cohorts of patients taking the same dose of drug under the same conditions.[50,171,172] In real world conditions, many other factors help to significantly increase this interpatient variability (e.g., missed doses, various antiretroviral regimens used, inappropriate drug–food requirements, drug–drug or drug–herb interactions).[261] Reasons for varying drug levels are currently unknown but may reflect a genetic predisposition to metabolism or absorption. Although most patients fall around the median value, interpatient variability results in some patients having low- or high-drug exposures.[50] For many of these agents, a drug exposure–viral suppression relation exists (e.g., the higher the exposure, the greater the viral suppression).[50,171–175] In addition, excessive drug exposures often lead to increased risks for adverse drug events.[172] Consequently, many clinicians and researchers have expressed an interest in evaluating antiretroviral drug exposures via therapeutic drug monitoring (TDM) for patients infected with HIV in hopes of improving clinical outcomes or minimizing adverse drug events.

Many questions remain as to which sample or series of samples is most appropriate for evaluating antiretroviral drug exposure. Currently, it is not known whether HIV viral suppression is concentration dependent (i.e., whether higher drug concentrations provide greater viral inhibition) or whether it is related to total drug exposure (i.e., area under the curve [AUC]). Given that sampling AUC in clinical practice is not practical and given that viral breakthrough may be more likely to occur when drug exposure is at its lowest point, many clinicians and investigators using TDM choose to sample the trough value (the level immediately before the next dose). It should be recognized, however, that the trough value is not always the minimum concentration during a dosing interval or a 24-hour time period (i.e., the C_{min}). For a drug like nelfinavir which displays diurnal variations in plasma concentrations and delayed oral absorption, the C_{min} actually occurs 2 hours after the evening dose and not immediately before the morning dose.[176,177] In contrast, the NNRTIs have long plasma half-lives, which result in relatively constant blood levels, thereby allowing for convenient sampling of these agents any time after the dose.[179,180] This is especially important for efavirenz, which is usually taken in the evening.

If the trough value is used, careful coordination of patient and physician (or appropriate office staff) is necessary to obtain the sample at the appropriate time. In many situations, this can be difficult. Consequently, investigators have evaluated the use of population pharmacokinetic data to sample the level at any time after the last dose and back-calculate the expected trough value. This method of random sampling will be available to clinicians commercially in the near future.

Many factors can affect the trough values of various antiretroviral agents. For agents with relatively short plasma half-lives, such as the PIs, the level may reflect only the last two or three doses taken by the patient. Thus, assessment of patient medication adherence during the previous few days is necessary. In contrast, it is possible that patients may not have been completely adherent to therapy between clinic visits, but were compliant in the days immediately before sampling the level; this could result in the drug level appearing to be therapeutic in a patient with incomplete viral suppression. This pattern of behavior, known as "white coat syndrome," could lead to inappropriate clinical decision making and must be considered before any changes to therapy.

In addition, levels can be affected by whether or not the patient took their medication with the appropriate food restrictions or requirements. Because drug–drug and/or drug–herb interactions could raise or lower the trough levels, all concomitant medications—including over-the-counter medications, vitamins, and minerals—must be carefully evaluated.

Another factor that can affect interpretation of drug levels over time is intrapatient variability. Although not fully evaluated, it appears that under pharmacokinetic conditions (e.g., study conditions in which dosing, concomitant food administration, drug–drug interactions, and adherence all are controlled) the day-to-day variability of drug levels over time is minimal.[178,181,182] In real-world situations, however, where patients take their medications under conditions that vary from day to day, the levels could be highly variable at clinic visits over time.

Lastly, it should be recognized that there are no standardized laboratory methods for evaluating plasma levels of antiretroviral medications used to treat HIV, resulting in wide interlaboratory variability.[183,184] In addition, there may be *intra*laboratory variability from day to day as a result of operator error. Thus, clinicians should remain alert for levels that seem inappropriate for the given clinical situation and have them re-evaluated before any clinical decision making.

In general, TDM levels costs between $65 and $80 per drug level (plus shipping charges). It takes approximately 7 days for the results to be reported back to the clinician; this may be faster or slower depending on the specific laboratory. TDM may or may not be covered by insurance providers, depending on the third party payor. Currently, TDM is commercially available for the PIs and NNRTIs. The plasma or serum levels of NRTIs provide little useful clinical information because the intracellular triphosphate moiety is the active component of these agents. Recently, researchers have begun to evaluate the intracellular triphosphate concentrations of the NRTIs in various cell lines, including peripheral blood mononuclear cells (PBMC). Many clinicians have expressed interest in evaluating the intracellular triphosphate levels of various NRTIs in clinical practice. It should be recognized, however, that PBMCs need to be processed in a very precise manner immediately after extraction from the patient and cannot merely be frozen and evaluated at a later date. In addition, very few laboratories in the world are able to perform these complex assays; those that can are providing these tests predominantly for research purposes only.

The interpretation of the level itself will vary according on the clinical situation. Among treatment-naive patients with wild-type viral isolates, the key assessment is whether the level is above or below the mean or median population value. If it is below the desired level, the clinician should consider giving more drug or using a pharmacokinetic boosting technique. If it is above the desired level and the patient is experiencing drug toxicity, a dose reduction should be considered. Clinical trials evaluating TDM among antiretroviral-naive patients initiating PI-based HAART have shown improved clinical responses compared with those with standard of care without TDM.[185–187]

Among patients with antiretroviral resistance, the interpretation of the level is much more complex and may require the additional assessment of phenotypic resistance data. Clinical data have shown correlations between individual patient drug levels of PIs and their phenotypic resistance profile (known as the inhibitory quotient [IQ])[146,188]; however, interpretation of these data has been made complicated because various pharmaceutical companies have used varying methods to calculate the IQ.[189] There are two critical issues: 100% human serum cannot be used to measure in vitro phenotypic resistance; and TDM laboratories normally report plasma drug levels as total drug levels (i.e., protein-bound plus unbound drug) and not as the "free" unbound active drug. As a result, the clinician must use a protein correction factor to adjust for one or both of these factors, thus calculating the total drug concentration required to inhibit the individual patient's viral isolate. One method is to use population pharmacokinetic data for PI protein binding in conjunction with current phenotypic data performed without protein.[190] It should be recognized that this method may not be accurate for highly protein-bound drugs such as ritonavir, lopinavir, nelfinavir, and saquinavir. Another method is to use the patient's drug level and phenotypic resistance data to calculate a "virtual phenotypic IC_{50} value" (patient IQ) and then compare this with reference population drug levels and resistance data (reference IQ). This normalized IQ (NIQ = patient IQ/reference IQ) will be reported back to clinicians as a ratio value; when the number is <1, the NIQ suggests the patient's exposure is suboptimal and may require dosage adjustment. Limited data are available to validate the NIQ with clinical outcome[191]; however, data will constantly be adjusted and validate the NIQ as data from clinical practice are received. To date, prospective, randomized clinical trials evaluating dose adjustments based on the IQ are lacking and currently underway.

When evaluating data from TDM and phenotypic resistance testing there are many questions to which conclusive answers are not currently available:

1. Is the IC_{50} value the most appropriate inhibitory concentration to aim for when performing TDM, or should the IC_{95} value be used?
2. How high above the IC_{50} or IC_{95} values must the drug levels be to obtain maximal viral suppression, and can this level be achieved without causing drug toxicity?
3. Is the target level above the IC_{50} or IC_{95} value similar in patients with different clinical scenarios (e.g., those with extensive resistance, high viral loads, and low CD4+ cell counts compared with those with limited resistance, low viral loads, and high CD4+ cell counts)?
4. What is the impact of viral quasi-species when evaluating a target inhibitory concentration for TDM (especially among patient with extensive viral resistance)?
5. Is the activity of the entire antiretroviral regimen, and not just the pharmacokinetic parameters of one or more agents, sufficient to suppress viral replication?
6. What is the role, if any, of the intracellular pharmacokinetics of these agents?

In the current case, knowledge of P.P.'s amprenavir trough level and the IC_{50} value from the phenotype may help to ensure optimal drug exposure and thereby potentially improve his chances of getting an optimal antiviral response.

Metabolic Complications of Antiretroviral Therapies

16. J.F. is a 37-year-old HIV-positive man who has been taking d4T, ddI, ritonavir, and saquinavir for the past 4 years. Since starting this regimen, J.F.'s T-cell counts have increased from 65 to 475 cells/mm³, and his viral load has declined from 70,000 to <500 copies/mL (using RT-PCR). J.F. is concerned because he has noticed that his arms and legs have gotten quite thin and the veins in his calves are now very pronounced. In addition, his cheeks have "disappeared," and he can't seem to get the extra weight off around his belly. Otherwise, he "feels fine." On physical examination, you notice an abnormal accumulation of fat on his posterior neck and upper back. Laboratory tests reveal increased total cholesterol at 8.2 mmol/L (normal, <5.17 mmol/L), triglycerides at 3.8 mmol/L (normal, <2.82 mmol/L), and a fasting blood glucose of 230 mg/dL (normal, <115mg/dL) with no evidence of ketones or sugar on urine analysis. Before starting this regimen, all laboratory values were within normal limits. J.F. admits to smoking two packs of cigarettes per day, occasional alcohol consumption, poor dietary habits including eating fast foods, and rarely exercising. Are the changes in laboratory values and body shape a result of his current antiretroviral regimen? Is J.F. at increased risk for cardiovascular disease since starting HAART? What interventions, if any, may help?

The discovery and widespread use of HAART in clinical practice have resulted in significant antiviral, clinical, and survival benefit among HIV-infected individuals. Although these agents represent a significant advance in the management of HIV infection, data are limited with regard to their long-term safety and adverse event profiles. Reports of metabolic complications, including abnormal distribution of body fat, lipid abnormalities (e.g., hypercholesteremia, hypertriglyceridemia, increases in LDL and decreases in HDL), and new-onset diabetes have concerned both patients and providers.[91,193–200] With patients living longer as a direct consequence of these highly active antiretroviral regimens, concerns regarding premature vascular complications may be warranted. Case reports have documented coronary artery disease, myocardial infarctions, and vascular complications among relatively young HIV-infected patients taking HAART-containing regimens.[201–204] Large observational studies have suggested an increased risk for cardiovascular disease among patients taking HAART. However, it should be recognized that the overall incidence of clinical events was very low, even among patients taking antiretroviral therapy.[205–208] Despite extensive research, the precise cause of these abnormalities is unknown. One theory is that a sequence of the HIV-1 protease enzyme contains similar homologies with a number of human proteins (e.g., low density lipoprotein-receptor-related protein, cytoplasmic retinoic-acid binding protein).[193] The effect on these proteins by PIs could inhibit adipocyte growth or promote adipocyte lysis,[209] leading to alterations in serum lipid concentrations, visceral fat accumulation, and impaired insulin signaling. Another hypothesis is that PIs interfere with retinoid signaling within adipocytes (excessive levels of certain retinoids can resemble the lipodystrophy syndrome).[210] Given that nucleoside analogs appear to inhibit mitochondrial DNA polymerase-γ, they have been implicated for causing lipoatrophy.[211] Although data suggest HAART increases the risk for lipodystrophy, similar reports have been published identifying patients with these complications before receiving HAART.[196,198] As a result, these abnormalities may be a consequence of HIV infection itself or pre-existing metabolic disorders that may become exacerbated by HAART.

In June of 1997, the Food and Drug Administration reported the first cases of PI-induced hyperglycemia.[194] A total of 83 patients were identified in which new-onset hyperglycemia or worsening of pre-existing diabetes occurred. Thirty-three percent of patients required hospitalization, and six patients experienced life-threatening hyperglycemia (five of whom experienced ketoacidosis). The mean duration of PI therapy before any symptoms was 76 days and occurred among all available PI agents (nelfinavir, indinavir, saquinavir, ritonavir).

Up to 40% of patients on PI-based HAART experience impaired glucose intolerance due to significant insulin resistance.[212] Patients with risk factors, including type 2 diabetes mellitus and receiving PI-based HAART therapy are at an increased risk.[91] PI-based regimens should be avoided, if possible, in these patients. Fasting glucose levels are recommended before and during therapy (e.g., every 3 to 6 months) with PI-based HAART.[91] In many cases, the hyperglycemia will respond to diet and exercise modifications; however, if pharmacologic interventions are necessary, insulin "sensitizers" (troglitazone, metformin) may be effective.[91,213] For more pronounced hyperglycemia, oral sulfonyureas or insulin may be appropriate, although oral agents may not work as well in HIV-infected patients compared with non–HIV-infected patients.[91] Whether a specific PI agent alters glucose metabolism to a greater extent than another is unknown; however, anecdotal reports of patients changing agents with subsequent clinical response have been reported.[196] Although the discontinuation of PI therapy may help to control the hyperglycemia, the potential benefit of sustained viral suppression with HAART-containing regimens outweigh the potential risks for complications in those patients in whom hyperglycemia can be controlled.

Elevations in serum levels of triglycerides, total cholesterol, LDL, along with mild decreases in HDL, have also been reported after the initiation of HAART.[91,214,215] The precise cause of these hyperlipidemias is unknown but may be a result of impaired clearance and increased synthesis of triglyceride-rich lipoproteins.[196] In some instances, these abnormalities have been identified as early as 2 weeks after the initiation of therapy.[91] Although all PIs have been implicated, these laboratory abnormalities appear to occur more frequently in regimens containing ritonavir and are limited among patients receiving saquinavir or atazanavir.[193,216–218,265] The NNRTIs can also cause lipid alterations, although it appears to be at a lower incidence than the PIs.[99,218] In addition, both efavirenz and nevirapine have been shown to increase HDL concentrations among patients receiving HAART.[99,218] Recent data have also suggested different effects of the nucleoside analog on lipid alterations. Two prospective clinical trials have shown greater increases in triglycerides and total cholesterol levels among patients receiving stavudine-based HAART compared with zidovudine or tenofovir-based regimens.[92,113]

The management of HAART-associated hyperlipidemias should involve dietary modifications and regular physical exercise with pharmacologic interventions reserved for those patients at risk for complications (e.g., severely elevated triglyceride levels with increased risk for pancreatitis, familial or history of coronary artery disease). When drug therapy is warranted, hydroxymethylglutaryl coacetyl-A reductase inhibitors (HMG-CoA) may be used for hypercholesterolemia and fibric acid derivatives for hypertriglyceridemia.[91,213] Both HMG-CoA reductase inhibitors and PIs are metabolized by the hepatic cytochrome p450 enzyme systems potentially resulting in a significant drug–drug interaction (e.g., decreased clearance of the HMG-CoA reductase inhibitor resulting in an increased risk for rhabdomyolysis, myositis, and transaminase elevations). Pharmacokinetic studies have shown significant increases in simvastatin levels, modest increases in atorvastatin levels, and significant decreases in pravastatin levels when concomitantly administered with ritonavir.[219] Consequently, simvastatin should not be used among patients receiving ritonavir-based HAART, whereas atorvastatin can be used with caution. Among patients who experience increases in lipids or triglycerides and who are virologically controlled, it may be possible to switch out the PI for another agent that has a lower propensity for raising these laboratory values (e.g., nucleoside analogs, lower incidence PI, such as atazanavir or an NNRTI).[220–225] It should be recognized that a detailed history of prior resistance must be known before switching therapies so as to prevent virologic failure.[226] If an agent was substituted and there was underlying resistance to that agent, virologyic failure could occur given that the potency of the new regimen would then be compromised. Clinical trials investigating switching abacavir for PIs have shown promising results while maintaining continued virologic control.[224,227] Variable results have been shown when switching an NNRTI for a PI, and recent data have shown beneficial changes in lipids when atazanavir was switched for nelfinavir among patients experiencing hyperlipidemia.[217,221,222] Current studies are evaluating the role of tenofovir as a switch agent for both PIs and stavudine-containing HAART. The goals of therapy for HIV-infected patients are the same for non–HIV-infected patients and follow the National Heart Association guidelines.[91]

Alterations in body composition, both fat loss (arms, legs, face, buttocks) and fat accumulation (dorsocervical fatty deposits, e.g., buffalo humps, increased abdominal girth) are commonly observed among patients taking HAART. Incidence of this adverse event ranges from 5% to 64% and varies according to differing case definitions.[193,213] Compared with non–HIV-infected controls, fat loss appears to be the most predominant clinical finding.[228] Although not fully defined, it appears that baseline body mass index; duration of exposure to antiretroviral agents; CD4 nadir at time of initiation of HAART and CD4 response to therapy; increasing age, gender, and duration of HIV infection all are risk factors for this complication.[193,211,229] In general, the nucleoside analogs are believed to be responsible for lipoatrophy,[91,193] and the PIs are believed to be responsible for the lipo-accumulation.[91,211] It should be recognized that because these agents are often given in combinations that contain both classes of agents, it is difficult to precisely identify which class of agents is responsible for which adverse event.

The precise causes of this syndrome are unknown but for the nucleoside analogs it is believed that these agents inhibit mitochondrial DNA polymerase-γ.[211] Because some nucleoside analogs inhibit DNA polymerase-γ to a greater extent than others (e.g., stavudine) and have been implicated in causing lipoatrophy to a greater extent, switch studies involving the substitution of one agent for another have been investigated.[224,225,227] Although the substitution of stavudine with zidovudine or abacavir has shown statistically significant increases in arms, legs, and trunk using objective radiographic tests (e.g., dual-energy x-ray absorptiometry, computed tomography scans), these initial improvements are so modest that they may not be clinically significant.[230–232] Longer follow-up is needed to see whether these improvements continue and whether lipoatrophy is reversible. The use of recombinant human growth hormone, an agent with lipolytic effects, has been shown to decrease the size of buffalo humps and abdominal girth[223]; however, once this agent is discontinued, the growth often returns. Given that lipodystrophy may be a result of impaired insulin signaling, investigations have tried using insulin sensitizers such as metformin and rosiglitazone with limited success.[233,234] Surgical excision or liposuction may be effective; however, recurrences have been reported.[236,237] In addition, caution should be exercised when using surgical interventions for abdominal girth because of concerns about intestinal perforation and intraperitoneal bleeding. For facial wasting, injection of fat or synthetic polymers into the recessed areas of the cheeks has shown good results but requires frequent readministration, is costly, and lacks long-term safety data.[238–240]

Other long-term complications that should be recognized are nucleoside-associated lactic acidosis, osteonecrosis, and osteopenia.[91,213] Lactic acidosis has been predominantly associated with stavudine use (but can occur among all nucleoside analogs) and has been managed by discontinuing therapy until lactate levels return to normal and then reinitiating therapy with a non-stavudine or non-nucleoside analog–containing HAART regimen, if possible.[241]

Currently, J.F. has elevated serum levels of cholesterol, lipids, and fasting blood sugars. In addition, he has the classic clinical presentation of body habitus changes with thinning of his arms, legs, and face, as well as accumulation of central fat and a modest buffalo hump on his neck. Although the current antiretroviral regimen has been effective in lowering J.F.'s viral load and increasing his T-cell counts, interventions are necessary to prevent long-term complications such as premature heart disease and other vascular complications. Initially, nonpharmacologic interventions such as diet, exercise, and life-style modifications (e.g., smoking cessation) should be tried. In addition, given the increased reported incidence of these adverse events with ritonavir- and stavudine-containing regimens, modification of J.F.'s current antiretroviral regimen may be reasonable and should be based on treatment history, resistance profiles, and drug intolerances. If these interventions fail, sulfonylurea agents, gemfibrozil, atorvastatin, metformin, or troglitazone should be considered.

Limited interventions are currently available for treatment of the buffalo hump. J.F. could consider surgery or recombinant human growth hormone; however, he should be advised that the hump might return. In addition, if the facial lipoatrophy is of significant concern, J.F. should consult a dermatologist who specializes in HIV associated facial reconstruction.

Structured Treatment Interruptions and Target-Controlled Interventions

17. T.D. is a 32-year-old HIV-infected man who initiated antiretroviral therapy with stavudine, lamivudine, and lopinavir/ritonavir 2 years ago when he was first diagnosed with HIV at a routine physical exam. At that time his CD4 cell count was 125 cells/mm^3 and his viral load was 85,000 copies/mL. T.D. has done well with his current regimen; he has been without any adverse drug events, and his CD4 cell counts and viral load measurements have been stable at 575 cells/mm^3 and nondetectable ($<$50 copies/mL), respectively. T.D. is concerned about long-term adverse events from HAART and asks you if he can stop therapy or at least minimize his exposure to these agents. Can therapy be discontinued once it is stable, and, if so, how should it be monitored? Are there any interventions that can be implemented so as to minimize drug exposures and potentially long-term adverse events?

Although HAART-based therapies have been shown to improve survival and minimize the risk for development of opportunistic infections, these agents are not benign and do have significant adverse events associated with their use.[242] In addition, given the improved survival rates from HAART, new and more complex long-term adverse events are now just being recognized. In the past, the goal of antiretroviral therapy was to prolong survival; now, with the use of HAART, the management of HIV has shifted to a chronic health mainte- nance disease. Consequently, any intervention that can de- crease the risk for long-term adverse events or minimize drug exposures over time may represent a key strategy for manag- ing infection with HIV, provided that the intervention does not cause immunologic harm to the patient. Unfortunately, for many patients merely decreasing the doses of the current agents is not an option because it may allow for exposures of subtherapeutic concentrations of drug that could allow for vi- ral breakthrough and the development of resistance.

Two strategies have been investigated: structured treatment interruptions (STI) and CD4/viral load–guided discontinua- tions of therapy. It should be recognized that limited data ex- ist for both strategies; long-term follow-up and large random- ized, prospective controlled clinical trials are lacking. In addition, the impact of these interventions on minimizing long-term adverse events is also lacking.[243]

STI interventions involve starting and stopping HAART at controlled time points in hopes of minimizing drug exposure, maintaining immunologic control, and minimizing drug resis- tance. Various dosing schedules have been used (e.g., 7 days on, 7 days off; 3 months on, 2 months off) with mixed re- sults.[244–251] The difficulty in this strategy is adhering to the dosing schedule, especially for interventions that are not eas- ily remembered. In addition, short-term adverse drug events may occur when therapy is re-initiated, including the acute retroviral syndrome.[252–254]

It appears that antiviral resistance may occur using STI in- terventions; caution should be exercised when using regimens that contain agents with low genetic barriers and/or long half- lives.[255,256] For example, if the regimen of zidovudine, lamivu- dine and efavirenz was to be cycled on and off using an STI strategy, and all agents were discontinued at the same time, zi- dovudine and lamivudine drug exposures would be eliminated from the plasma in a few days. In contrast, given the long half-life of efavirenz, efavirenz drug levels may remain in the plasma for days after zidovudine and lamivudine are no longer there. This monotherapy may allow for the selection of mutant viruses that develop resistance to efavirenz (and cross- resistance to the other NNRTIs). Although there is excitement about the potential of using STIs in the community, this inter- vention strategy is controversial and should only be used among patients who are highly motivated and in whom close follow-up can be ensured.

Target-controlled therapy involves a strategy in which pa- tients have their therapy discontinued and re-initiated only when certain target values are reached (e.g., CD4 cell counts).[247,248] This intervention is of particular interest for pa- tients who either initiated therapy in the past when their CD4 cell counts were above 350 cells/mm³ or for patients whose immune systems have improved to values above 350 cells/mm³ for extended periods of time. Clinical trial data us- ing target values of CD4 cells counts falling below 350 cells/mm³ or a decline of 25% to 30% from baseline have shown promising results.[247,248] Some trials also have included target viral load measurements of greater than 50,000 to 100,000 copies/mL.[247,248] In general, patients in these trials have been well controlled on HAART, are clinically stable, and have been virologically controlled on their regimen for extended periods of time before the initiation of target control intervention. This strategy may not be appropriate for patients

who experienced severe immune damage before initiation of HAART for concerns over rapid decline in immune function once therapy has been discontinued (e.g., CD4 cell counts <100 cells/mm³ or patients who experienced an opportunistic infection as their AIDS diagnosis). It should also be recog- nized that this strategy should be used only for patients in whom careful follow-up can be assured.

Given that T.D. has experienced a good response to therapy (e.g., CD4 cell counts and viral load measurements) and his CD4 cell counts have been above 350 cells/mm³, he may be a good candidate for target-controlled intervention. In addition, given the increased risk for potential facial lipoatrophy with stavudine, it may be reasonable to switch zidovudine, didano- sine, or tenofovir for stavudine when therapy needs to be re- initiated.

KEEPING CURRENT

The management of HIV infection is a constantly evolving process. This, combined with the wealth of data that have been presented at meetings and in journals, has made staying informed about current issues and new developments a daunt- ing task. As a result, many clinicians, even those actively car- ing for HIV-infected patients, remain cautious and often con- fused as to which therapeutic options to use.

New technologies for the dissemination of medical infor- mation have been constantly evolving. The internet has al- lowed clinicians from various regions of the world to ex- change ideas, teach new concepts, and obtain access to limited resources. In addition, many research centers, patient advocacy groups, and academic institutions have posted sites on the internet that have resulted in access to large amounts of high-quality medical information. Unfortunately, this new technology has also allowed for the dissemination of incom- plete, misleading, or inaccurate information. In essence, the worldwide web is an unpoliced medium in which any person or group can publish without restriction. Therefore, clinicians must remain cautious and carefully evaluate the information obtained from various websites.

When evaluating the quality of a website, clinicians should look for a few basic standards[257]:

1. *Author qualifications.* Is the author qualified to write the article or perform the research? Is his or her affiliation or relevant credentials provided?
2. *Attribution.* Are references provided to confirm state- ments? Are all relevant copyrighted information noted?
3. *Currency.* When was the content posted? Is the website updated regularly?
4. *Disclosure.* Who owns the website? Is there a conflict of interest between what is being posted and any commercial interest?

Any internet site that fails to meet these basic competen- cies should be viewed with caution. In general, the most ac- curate and informative websites for HIV-specific information come from academic institutions, government organizations, medical societies, and patient advocacy groups. Table 69-10 is a list of high-quality websites that provide timely and accurate information. A periodic evaluation of these sites often pro- vides enough information to stay up-to-date on current issues and controversies.

Table 69-10   HIV Internet Resources

Government Sites

Adult AIDS Clinical Trials Resources: http://www.actis.org/
American Foundation for AIDS Research: http://www.amfar.org
Centers for Disease Control and Prevention.:http://www.cdc.gov
Centers for Disease Control Prevention Information Network:
   http://www.cdcnac.org/
Community Provider AIDS Training Center: http://itsa.ucsf.edu/
   warmline/
Consensus Panel Guidelines On-line: http://www.hivatis.org/trtgdlns.html
CDC National AIDS Clearinghouse: http://www.cdcnac.org
Government HIV Mutation Charts: http://hiv-web.lanl.gov
Henry J. Kaiser Foundation: http://www.kff.org/archive/aidshiv.html
HIV/AIDS Treatment Information Network: http://www.hivatis.org
International AIDS Vaccine Initiative: http://www.iavi.org/
Morbitity and Mortality Weekly: http://www2.cdc.gov/mmwr/
MMWR AIDS resource:
   http://www.cdc.gov/nchstp/hiv_aids/pubs/mmwr.htm
National Institute of Allergy and Infectious Diseases:
   http://www.niaid.nih.gov
National Prevention Information Network: http://www.cdcnpin.org
Pediatric HIV Resource Page: http://www.pedhivaids.org/
Post Exposure Prevention WebSite: http://epi-center.ucsf.edu/PEP/
   pepnet.html
United Nations AIDS WebSite: http://www.unaids.org/

University Sites

Harvard AIDS Institute: http://www.hsph.harvard.edu/hai.html
Johns Hopkins AIDS Service: http://www.hopkins-aids.edu
University of California, HIV/AIDS Program: http://hivinsite.ucsf.edu

AIDS Treatment/Advocacy Groups

AIDS Treatment Project United Kingdom: http://www.atp.org.uk/
Bulletin of Experimental Treatment for AIDS (BETA):
   http://www.sfaf.org/beta
Project Inform: http://www.projinf.org
San Francisco AIDS Foundation: http://www.sfaf.org/index.html
Treatment Action Group: http://www.aidsnyc.org/tag

Other Relevant Sites

The AIDS Map: http://www.aidsmap.com
AIDS Education Global Information System: http://www.aegis.com
Clinical Care Options: http://www.clinicalcareoptions.com
HIV Drug Interactions: http://www.hiv-druginteractions.org
HIV and Hepatitis.com: http://hivandhepatitis.com
HIV Pharmacology: http://www.hivpharmacology.com/
HIV Resistance Web: http://www.hivresistanceweb.com/
   Immunenet: http://www.aids.org
Medscape: http://www.medscape.com
Physician's Research Network: http://www.prn.org
The Body for Clinicians: http://www.thebodypro.com
Retroviral Conference: http://www.retroconference.org

CONCLUSIONS

Despite significant advances made in the management of HIV-infected persons, a cure still appears well out of reach. Health care providers are in a unique position to assist both clinicians and patients in the general management of HIV infection. A basic understanding of drug–drug interactions, absolute contraindications, and adverse event profiles for antiretroviral agents can go a long way toward substantially improving patient compliance, minimizing adverse events, and improving clinical outcomes. Although the pharmacologic management of HIV is rapidly evolving, a basic understanding of viral pathogenesis and its implications on the clinical management of infected patients will provide a framework that can be used to evaluate new information as it becomes available.

REFERENCES

1. CDC. HIV/AIDS Surveillance report. 2001:13(2).
2. Palella FJ et al. Declining morbidity and mortality among patients with advanced Human Immunodeficiency virus infection. N Engl J Med 1998; 338:853.
3. Fatkenheuer G et al. Virological treatment failure of protease inhibitor therapy in an unselected cohort of HIV-infected patients. J AIDS 1997;11:F113.
4. D'Arminio MA et al. Insights into the reasons for discontinuation of the first highly active antiretroviral therapy (HAART) regimen in a cohort of antiretroviral naïve patients. I.CO.N.A. study group. Italian cohort of antiretroviral-naïve patients. AIDS 2000;14:499.
5. CDC. Guidelines for the use of antiretroviral agents in HIV-Infected adults and adolescents February 4, 2002; HIV AIDS Treatment Information Service: Online resource: www.hivatis.org/trtgdlns.html.
6. Yeni P et al. Antiretroviral therapy for HIV infection in 2002: updated recommendations of the International AIDS Society—USA Panel. JAMA 2002;288:222.
7. D'Aquila RT et al. Drug resistance mutations in HIV-1. Topics HIV Med 2002;10:11.
8. World Health Organization/UNAIDS. AIDS epidemic update. December 2002. Available at http://www.unaids.org. Accessed May 2003.
9. Fleming P, Byers RH, Sweeney PA, Daniels D, Karon JM, Janssen RS. HIV prevalence in the United States, 2000. [Abstract]. In: Program and abstracts of the 9th Conference on Retroviruses and Opportunistic Infections, Seattle, Washington, February 24–28, 2002. Alexandria, Virginia: Foundation for Retrovirology and Human Health.
10. CDC. Advancing HIV Prevention: New Strategies for a Changing Epidemic—United States, 2003.
11. CDC. Primary and secondary syphilis among men who have sex with men—New York City, 2001. MMWR 2002;51:853.
12. Lifson AR et al. HIV seroconversion in two homosexual men after receptive oral intercourse with ejaculation: implications for counseling concerning safe sexual practices. Am J Public Health 1990; 80:1509.
13. Rozenbaum W et al. HIV transmission by oral sex. Lancet 1988;1:1395.
14. Lance HC et al. HIV seroconversion and oral intercourse. Am J Public Health1991;81:658.
15. Page-Shafer K et al. Risk of HIV infection attributable to oral sex among MSM and in the MSM population: the HIV Oral Transmission (HOT) Study. Abstract TuPeC4872. Presented at the 14th International AIDS Conference. July 2002. Barcelona, Spain.
16. Royce RA et al. Sexual transmission of HIV. N Engl J Med 1997;15:1072.
17. Fauci AS. The human immunodeficiency virus: infectivity and mechanisms of pathogenesis. Science 1988;239:617.
18. Fahey JL et al. Quantitative changes in T helper or T suppressor/cytotoxic lymphocyte subsets that distinguish acquired immune deficiency syndrome from other immune disorders. Am J Med 1984;76:95.
19. Perelson AS et al. HIV-1 dynamics in vivo: virion clearance rate, infected cell life-span, and viral generation time. Science 1996;271:1582.

20. Pantaleo G et al. The immunopathogenesis of human immunodeficiency virus infection. N Engl J Med 1993;328:327.

21. Deng HK et al. Identification of a major co-receptor for primary isolates of HIV-1. Nature 1996;381:661.

22. Dragic T et al. HIV-1 entry into CD4+ cells is mediated by the chemokine receptor CC-CKR-5. Nature 1996;381:667.

23. Berson JF et al. A seven transmembrane domain receptor involved in fusion and entry of T-cell trophic human immunodeficiency virus type 1 strains. J Virol 1996;70:6288.

24. Levy J. Infection by human immunodeficiency virus—CD4 is not enough. N Engl J Med 1996;335:280.

25. Wild C et al. A synthetic peptide from HIV-1 gp41 is a potent inhibitor of virus-mediated cell-cell fusion. AIDS Res Hum Retroviruses 1993;9:1051.

26. Kohl NE et al. Active human immunodeficiency virus protease is required for viral infectivity. Proc Natl Acad Sci 1988;85:4686.

27. Bugelski PJ et al. HIV protease inhibitors: effects on viral maturation and physiologic function in macrophages. J Leukoc Biol 1994;56:374.

28. Hellerstein M et al. Directly measured kinetics of circulating T lymphocytes in normal and HIV-1 infected humans. Nature Med 1999;5:83.

29. Fauci AS. Immunopathogenic mechanisms of HIV infection. Ann Intern Med 1996;124:654.

30. Fox CH et al. Lymphoid germinal centers are reservoirs of human immunodeficiency virus type 1 RNA. J Infect Dis 1991;164:1051.

31. Pantaleo G et al. HIV infection is active and progressive in lymphoid tissue during the clinically latent stage of disease. Nature 1993;362:355.

32. Daar ES et al. Transient high levels of viremia in patients with primary human immunodeficiency virus type 1 infection. N Engl J Med 1991;324:954.

33. Richman DD et al. Rapid evolution of the neutralizing antibody response to HIV type 1 infection. Proc Natl Acad Sci U S A 2003;100(7):4144.

34. Schacker T et al. Clinical and epidemiologic features of primary HIV infection. Ann Intern Med 1996;125:257.

35. Tindall B, Cooper DA. Primary HIV infection: host responses and intervention strategies. AIDS 1991;5:1.

36. Ho DD et al. Rapid turnover of plasma virions and CD4 lymphocytes in HIV-1 infection. Nature 1995;373:123.

37. Wei X et al. Viral dynamics in human immunodeficiency virus type 1 infection. Nature 1995;373:117.

38. Coffin JM. HIV population dynamics in vivo: implications for genetic variation, pathogenesis, and therapy. Science 1995;267:483.

39. Mellors JW et al. Prognosis in HIV-1 infection predicted by the quantity of virus in plasma. Science 1996;272:1167.

40. O'Brien WA et al. Changes in plasma HIV-1 RNA and CD4 lymphocyte counts and the risk of progression to AIDS. N Engl J Med 1996;334:426.

41. Mellors JW et al. Plasma viral load and CD4+ lymphocytes as prognostic markers of HIV-1 infection. Ann Intern Med 1997;126(12):946.

42. Pantaleo G et al. Studies in subjects with long-term nonprogressive human immunodeficiency virus infection. N Engl J Med 1995;332:209.

43. O'Brien TR et al. Serum HIV-1 RNA levels and time to development of AIDS in the multicenter hemophilia cohort study. JAMA 1996;276:105.

44. Leigh Brown AJ et al. Transmission fitness of drug-resistant human immunodeficiency virus and the prevalence of resistance in the antiretroviral-treated population. J Infect Dis 2003;187(4):683.

45. Moss AR, Bacchetti P. Natural history of HIV infection. AIDS 1989;3:55.

46. Stein DS et al. CD4 lymphocyte cell enumeration for prediction of clinical course of human immunodeficiency virus disease: a review. J Infect Dis 1992;165:352.

47. Sepkowitz KA. Effect of HAART on natural history of AIDS-related opportunistic disorders. Lancet 1998;351:228.

48. Yarchoan R, Broder S. Development of antiretroviral therapy for the acquired immunodeficiency syndrome and related disorder: a progress report. N Engl J Med 1987;316:557.

49. Merluzzi VJ et al. Inhibition of HIV-1 replication by a nonnucleoside reverse transcriptase inhibitor. Science 1990;250:1411.

50. Deeks SG et al. HIV-1 protease inhibitors: a review for clinicians. JAMA 1997;277:145.

51. Acosta E et al. Pharmacodynamics of human immunodeficiency virus type 1 protease inhibitors. Clin Infect Dis 2000;30(Suppl 2):S151.

52. Siliciano R. Latent reservoirs of HIV. (Absract S-36). Presented at the 37th International Conference on Antimicrobial Agents and Chemotherapy (ICAAC). Toronto, Ontario, Canada. September 28-October 1, 1997.

53. Perelson AS et al. Decay characteristic of HIV-1 infected compartments during combination therapy. Nature 1997;387:188.

54. Finzi D et al. Latent infection of CD4+ T cells provides a mechanism for lifelong persistence of HIV-1, even in patients on effective combination therapy. Nature Med 1999;5:512.

55. Zhang L et al. Quantifying residual HIV-1 replication in patients receiving combination antiretroviral therapy. N Engl J Med 1999;340:1605.

56. Pomerantz RJ. Residual HIV-1 disease in the era of highly active antiretroviral therapy. N Engl J Med 1999;340:1672.

57. Steckelberg JM, Cockerill FR. Serologic testing for human immunodeficiency virus antibodies. Mayo Clin Proc 1988;63:373.

58. Proffitt MR, Lieberman-Yen B. Laboratory diagnosis of human immunodeficiency virus infection. Infect Dis Clin North Am 1993;7:203.

59. Diagnostic tests for HIV. Med Lett 1997;39:81.

60. Cordes RJ, Ryan ME. Pitfalls in HIV testing: application and limitations of current tests. Postgrad Med 1995;98:177.

61. Gaines H et al. Antibody response in primary human immunodeficiency virus infection. Lancet 1987;1249.

62. Malia K et al. Alternative Serologic and Nucleic Acid Supplemental Test Evaluation for the Diagnosis of Human Immunodeficiency Virus Type-1 Infection. Abstract 662. Presented at the 10th Conference on Retroviruses and Opportunistic Infections. February 2003. Boston, MA.

63. Rich J et al. Misdiagnosis of HIV infection by HIV-1 plasma viral load testing: a case series. Ann Intern Med 1999;130:37.

64. Sax PE et al. Potential clinical implications of interlaboratory variability of CD4 T-lymphocyte counts in patients infected with human immunodeficiency virus. Clin Infect Dis 1995;21:1121.

65. Clementi M et al. Clinical use of quantitative molecular methods in studying human immunodeficiency virus type 1 infection. Clin Microbiol Rev 1996;9:135.

66. Saag MS et al. HIV viral load markers in clinical practice. Nature Med 1996;2:625.

67. Lafeuillade A et al. Human immunodeficiency virus type 1 kinetics in lymph nodes compared with plasma. J Infect Dis 1996;174:404.

68. Harris M et al. Correlation of virus load in plasma and lymph node tissue in human immunodeficiency virus infection. J Infect Dis 1997;176:1388.

69. Brichacek B et al. Increased plasma human immunodeficiency virus type 1 burden following antigenic challenge with pneumococcal vaccine. J Infect Dis 1996;174:1191.

70. Egger M et al. Art Cohort Collaboration. Progression of HIV-1 infected drug-naïve patients starting potent antiretroviral therapy: multicohort analysis of 12,040 patients. Abstract LB-18. Presented at the 41st Interscience Conference on Antimicrobial Agents and Chemotherapy. September 2001. Chicago IL.

71. Hammer SM et al. A controlled trial of two nucleoside analogues plus indinavir in persons with human immunodeficiency virus infection and CD4 cell counts of 200 per cubic millimeter or less. N Engl J Med 1997;337:725.

72. Cameron DW et al. Randomised placebo-controlled trial of ritonavir in advanced HIV-1 disease. Lancet 1998;351:543.

73. Clendeninn NJ et al. Study 511: analysis of long-term virologic data from the nelfinavir (NFV) 511 protocol using 3 HIV-RNA assays. (Abstract 372) Presented at the 5th Conference on Retroviruses and Opportunistic Infections. Chicago, IL. February 1-5, 1998.

74. Marschner IC et al. Use of changes in plasma levels of human immunodeficiency virus type 1 RNA to assess the clinical benefit of antiretroviral therapy. J Infect Dis 1998;177:40.

75. Cohen OJ et al. Decreased human immunodeficiency virus type 1 plasma viremia during antiretroviral therapy reflects downregulation of viral replication in lymphoid tissue. Proc Natl Acad Sci 1995;92:6017.

76. Wong JK et al. Recovery of replication-competent HIV despite prolonged suppression of plasma viremia. Science 1997;278:1291.

77. Finzi D et al. Identification of a reservoir for HIV-1 in patients on highly active antiretroviral therapy. Science 1997;278:1295.

78. Chun T et al. Presence of an inducible HIV-1 latent reservoir during highly active antiretroviral therapy. Proc Natl Acad Sci 1997;94:13193.

79. Lafeuillade A et al. Residual human immunodeficiency virus type 1 RNA in lymphoid tissue of patients with sustained plasma RNA of <200 copies/ml. J Infect Dis 1998;177:235.

80. Havlir DV et al. Drug susceptibility in HIV infection after viral rebound in patients receiving indinavir-containing regimens. JAMA 2000;283:229.

81. King M et al. Impact of baseline CD4 cell count and viral load on durability of virologic response through 96 weeks of lopinavir/ritonavir and nelfinavir in a phase III clinical trial. Abstract 470. Presented at the 9th Conference on Retroviruses and Opportunistic Infections. February 2002. Seattle, WA.

82. Hecht FM et al. Sexual transmission of an HIV-1 variant resistant to multiple reverse-transcriptase and protease inhibitors. N Engl J Med 1998;339:307.

83. Yerly S et al. Transmission of antiretroviral-drug-resistant HIV-1 variants. Lancet 1999;354:729.

84. Boden D et al. HIV-1 drug resistance in newly infected individuals. JAMA 1999;282:1135.

85. Little SJ et al. Reduced antiretroviral drug susceptibility among patients with primary HIV infection. JAMA 1999;282:1142.

86. Chesney MA. Factors affecting adherence to antiretroviral therapy. Clin Infect Dis 2000;30(Suppl 2):S171.

87. Max B et al. Management of the adverse effects of antiretroviral therapy and medication adherence. Clin Infect Dis 2000;30(Suppl 2):S96.

88. Vanhove GF et al. Patient compliance and drug failure in protease inhibitor monotherapy. JAMA 1996;276:1955.

89. Mehta S et al. Potential factors affecting adherence with HIV therapy J AIDS. 1997;11:1665.

90. Chesney MA. Compliance: how physicians can help. HIVInsite.ucsf.edu-University of California, San Francisco; San Francisco General Hospital electronic website. 1/21/98.

91. Stone VE. Strategies for optimizing adherence to highly active antiretroviral therapy: lessons from research and clinical practice. Clin Infect Dis 2001; 33:865.

92. Schambelan M et al. Management of metabolic complications associated with antiretroviral therapy for HIV-1 infection: recommendations of an international AIDS society—USA Panel. J AIDS 2002; 31:257.

93. Staszewski S et al. Efficacy and safety of tenofovir DF (TDF) versus stavudine (d4T) when used in combination with lamivudine and efavirenz in antiretroviral naïve patients: 96-week preliminary interim results. Abstract 564b. Presented at the 10th Conference on Retroviruses and Opportunistic Infections. February 2003. Boston, MA.

94. Staszewski S et al. Efavirenz plus zidovudine and lamivudine, efavirenz plus indinavir and indinavir

plus zidovudine and lamivudine in the treatment of HIV-1 infections in adults (48 weeks). N Engl J Med 1999;341:1865.

95. Gulick RM et al. Treatment with indinavir, zidovudine, and lamivudine in adults with human immunodeficiency virus infection and prior antiretroviral therapy. N Engl J Med 1997;337:734.

96. Delta Coordinating Committee. Delta: a randomised double-blind controlled trial comparing combinations of zidovudine plus didanosine or zalcitabine with zidovudine alone in HIV-infected individuals. Lancet 1996;348:283.

97. Hammer SM et al. A trial comparing nucleoside monotherapy with combination therapy in HIV-infected adults with CD4 cell counts from 200-500 per cubic millimeter. N Engl J Med 1996;335:1081.

98. Collier AC et al. Combination therapy with zidovudine and didanosine compared to zidovudine alone in HIV-1 infection. Ann Intern Med 1993;119:786.

99. Katlama C et al. Safety and efficacy of lamidudine-zidovudine combination therapy in antiretroviral-naive patients: a randomized controlled comparison with zidovudine monotherapy. JAMA 1996;276:118.

100. van Leth F et al. Results of the 2NN Study: A Randomized Comparative Trial of First-line Antiretroviral Therapy with Regimens Containing Either Nevirapine Alone, Efavirenz Alone or Both Drugs Combined, Together with Stavudine and Lamivudine. Abstract 176. Presented at the 10th Conference on Retroviruses and Opportunistic Infections. February 2003. Boston, MA.

101. Staszewski S et al. Abacavir-lamivudine-zidovudine in antiretroviral naïve HIV-infected adults. JAMA 2001;285:1155.

102. Matheron M et al. Metabolic and clinical evaluation of lipodystrophy syndrome in HIV-1-infected adults receiving initial HAART with or without a protease inhibitor: 48 week data. Abstract 670. Presented at the 8th Conference on Retroviruses and Opportunistic Infections. February 2001. Chicago, IL.

103. Department of Health and Human Services. No tice to physicians: Important interim results from a Phase III, randomized, double-blind comparison of three protease inhibitor-sparing regimens for the initial treatment of HIV infection (AACTG Protocol A5095). Letter to physicians. March 10, 2003.

104. Parenti D et al. The compact quad, Combivir/abacavir/efavirenz (COM/ABC/EFV) preliminary 48-wk results (COL30336). In: abstracts of the 39th IDSA Meeting, Orlando, FL, October 25-28, 2001, Poster No. 697

105. De Truchis P et al. An open-label study to evaluate safety and efficacy of switch to Trizivir (TZV) maintenance treatment after first line quadruple induction therapy: (AZLF3002-Suburbs). In: Posters of the 8th European Conference on Clinical Aspects and Treatment of HIV Infection. Athens, Greece, October 28–31, 2001. Poster # 76.

106. Pedneault L et al. Stavudine (d4T), didanosine (ddI) and nelfinavir combination therapy in HIV-1 infected subjects: antiviral effect and safety (Abstract 241). Presented at the 4th Conference on Retroviruses and Opportunistic Infections. Washington DC. January 22–26, 1997.

107. Raffi F et al. A pilot trial of antiviral activity and safety of didanosine-stavudine combination therapy in HIV-infected subjects: the Quintet trial. (Abstract I-123) Presented at the 37th International Conference on Antimicrobial Agents and Chemotherapy (ICAAC). Toronto, Ontario. September 28–October 1, 1997.

108. Reynes J et al. Stadi pilot study: Once daily administration of didanosine (ddI) in combination with stavudine (d4T) in antiretroviral naive patients. (Abstract I-128a) Presented at the 37th International Conference on Antimicrobial Agents and Chemotherapy (ICAAC). Toronto, Ontario. September 28-October 1, 1997.

109. Merrill DP et al. Lamivudine or stavudine in two- and three-drug combinations against human immunodeficiency virus type 1 replication in vitro. J Infect Dis 1996;173:355.

110. Hoggard P et al. Intracellular metabolism of zidovudine and stavudine in combination. [Letter.] J Infect Dis 1996;174:671.

111. Havlir DV et al. Combination zidovudine (ADV) and stavudine (d4T) therapy versus other nucleosides: Report of two randomized trials (ACTG 290 and 298). (Abstract 2). Presented at the 5th Conference on Retroviruses and Opportunistic Infections. Chicago, IL. February 1–5, 1998.

112. Sommadossi JP et al. Impairment of stavudine (d4T) phosphorylation in patients receiving a combination of zidovudine (ZDV) and d4T (ACTG 290). (Abstract 3). Presented at the 5th Conference on Retroviruses and Opportunistic Infections. Chicago, IL. February 1–5, 1998.

113. Hsu A et al. Assessment of single- and multiple-dose interactions between ritonavir and saquinavir (Abstract LB.B. 6041) Presented at the 11th International Conference on AIDS. July 1996. Vancouver, British Columbia.

114. Kumar P, Rodriguez-French A, Thompson M et al. Prospective study of hyperlipidemia in ART-naive subjects taking Combivir/abacavir (COM/ABC), COM/nelfinavir (NFV), or stavudine (d4T)/lamivudine (3TC)/NFV (ESS40002). Program and abstracts of the 9th Conference on Retroviruses and Opportunistic Infections; February 24-28, 2002; Seattle, Washington. Abstract 33.

115. Kempf D et al. The duration of viral suppression during protease inhibitor therapy for HIV-1 infection is predicted by plasma HIV-1 RNA at the nadir. AIDS 1998;12:F9.

116. Montaner J et al. Full suppression of viral replication to below 20 copies/ml is needed to achieve a durable antiviral response. (Abstract 105). Presented at the 6th European Conference on Clinical Aspect and Treatment of HIV-Infection. October 13, 1997. Hamburg, Germany.

117. Piscitelli SC The effect of garlic supplementation on the pharmacokinetics of saquinavir. Clin Infect Dis 2002,34.234.

118. Piscitelli SC et al. Indinavir concentrations and St John's wort. Lancet 2000,12.547.

119. Havlir D et al. Are Episodes of Transient Viremia ("Blips" in HIV RNA) Predictive of Virologic Failure in Heavily Treatment-Experienced Patients? Abstract 93. Presented at the 9th Conference on Retroviruses and Opportunistic Infections. February 2002. Seattle WA.

120. Di Mascio M et al. Viral Blip Dynamics during HAART. Abstract 94. Presented at the 9th Conference on Retroviruses and Opportunistic Infections. February 2002. Seattle, WA.

121. Bangsberg DR et al. Adherence to protease inhibitors, HIV-1 viral load, and development of drug resistance in an indigent population. AIDS 2000;14:357.

122. Montaner JS et al. A randomized, double-blind trial comparing combinations of nevirapine, didanosine, and zidovudine for HIV-infected patients: the INCAS trial. JAMA 1998;279:930.

123. Bayard PJ et al. Drug hypersensitivity reactions and human immunodeficiency virus disease. J AIDS 1992;5:1237.

124. Coopman SA et al. Cutaneous disease and drug reactions in HIV infection. N Engl J Med 1993;328:1670.

125. Carr A et al. Allergic manifestations of human immunodeficiency virus (HIV) infection. J Clin Immunol 1991;11:55.

126. Najera I et al. pol gene quasispecies of human immunodeficiency virus: mutations associated with drug resistance in virus from patients undergoing no drug therapy. J Virol 1995;69:23.

127. Mohri H et al. Quantitation of zidovudine-resistant human immunodeficiency virus type 1 in the blood of treated and untreated patients. Proc Natl Acad Sci 1993;90:25.

128. Moyle GJ. Current knowledge of HIV-1 reverse transcriptase mutations selected during nucleoside

analogue therapy: the potential to use resistance data to guide clinical decisions. J Antimicrob Chemother 1997;40:765.

129. Moyle GJ. Use of viral resistance patterns to antiretroviral drugs in optimising selection of drug combinations and sequences. Drugs 1998;52:168.

130. Mayers D. Rational approaches to resistance: nucleoside analogues. AIDS 1996;10(Suppl 1):S9.

131. Larder BA et al. HIV with reduced sensitivity to zidovudine (AZT) isolated during prolonged therapy. Science 1989;243:1731.

132. Kozal MJ et al. Didanosine resistance in HIV-infected patients switched from zidovudine to didanosine monotherapy. Ann Intern Med 1994;121:263.

133. Schmit J et al. Resistance-related mutations in the HIV-1 protease gene of patients treated for 1 year with the protease inhibitor ritonavir (ABT-538). AIDS1996;10:995.

134. Richman DD et al. Nevirapine resistance mutations of human immunodeficiency virus type 1 selected during therapy. J Virol.1994;68:1660.

135. Kellam P et al. Zidovudine treatment results in the selection of human immunodeficiency virus type 1 variants whose genotypes confer increasing levels of drug resistance. J Gen Virol 1994;75:341.

136. D'Aquila RT et al. Zidovudine resistance and HIV-1 disease progression during antiretroviral therapy. Ann Intern Med 1995;122:401.

137. Frost S, McLean AR. Quasispecies dynamics and the emergence of drug resistance during zidovudine therapy of HIV infection. AIDS 1994;8:323.

138. Schinazi RF et al. Characterization of human immunodeficiency viruses resistant to oxathiolane-cytosine nucleosides. Antimicrob Agents Chemother 1993;37:875.

139. Erickson JW, Burt SK. Structural mechanisms of HIV drug resistance. Annu Rev Pharmacol Toxicol 1996;36:545.

140. Arts EJ, Wainberg MA. Mechanisms of nucleoside analog antiviral activity and resistance during human immunodeficiency virus reverse transcription. Antimicrob Agents Chemother 1996;40:527.

141. Caliendo AM et al. Effects of zidovudine-selected human immunodeficiency type 1 reverse transcriptase amino acid substitutions on processive DNA synthesis and viral replication. J Virol 1996;2146.

142. Mellors J. New Insights into Mechanisms of HIV-1 Resistance to Reverse Transcriptase Inhibitors. Abstract L6. Presented at the 9th Conference on Retroviruses and Opportunistic Infections. February 2002. Seattle, WA.

143. Condra JH et al. In vivo emergence of HIV-1 variants resistant to multiple protease inhibitors. Nature 1995;374:569.

144. Erickson JW, Burt SK. Structural mechanisms of HIV drug resistance. Annu Rev Pharmacol Toxicol 1996;36:545.

145. Roberts NA. Drug-resistance patterns of saquinavir and other HIV proteinase inhibitors. AIDS 1995;9(Suppl 2):S27.

146. Condra JH, Emini EA. Preventing HIV-1 drug resistance. Science Med 1997;4:2.

147. Hsu A et al. The Ctrough inhibitory quotient predicts virologic response to ABT-378/ritonavir (ABT-378/r) therapy in treatment-experienced patients. AIDS 2000;14(Suppl 4):S12.

148. Kempf D et al. Response to ritonavir (RTV) intensification in indinavir (indinavir) recipients is highly correlated with virtual inhibitory quotient. Program and abstracts of the 8th Conference on Retroviruses and Opportunistic Infections; February 4-8, 2001; Chicago, Illinois. Abstract 523.

149. Piscitelli SC et al. The relative inhibitory quotient (RIQ): a method for predicting response to protease inhibitors. Program and abstracts of the 8th European Congress on Clinical Aspects and Treatment of HIV Infection; October 28-31, 2001; Athens, Greece. Abstract 164.

150. Stephenson J. HIV drug resistance testing shows promise. JAMA 1999;281:309.

151. Durant J et al. Drug-resistance genotyping in HIV-1 therapy: the VIRADAPT randomised controlled trial. Lancet 1999;353:2195.

152. Baxter JD et al. A pilot study of the short-term effects of antiretroviral management based on plasma genotypic antiretroviral resistance testing (GART) in patients failing antiretroviral therapy. Abstract LB8. Presented at the 6th Conference on Retroviruses and Opportunistic Infections. February 1999. Chicago, IL.

153. Deeks SG et al. Continued Reverse Transcriptase Inhibitor Therapy is Sufficient to Maintain Short-Term Partial Suppression of Multi-drug Resistant Viremia. Abstract 640. Presented at the 10th Conference on Retroviruses and Opportunistic Infections. February 2003. Boston, MA.

154. Markowitz M. Resistance, fitness, and potency. Mapping the paths to virological failure. JAMA 2000;283:250.

155. Katzenstein DA et al. Phenotypic susceptibility and virological outcome in nucleoside-experienced patients receiving three or four antiretroviral drugs. AIDS 2003;17(6):821.

156. Haubrich RH et al. The clinical relevance of non-nucleoside reverse transcriptase inhibitor hypersusceptibility: a prospective cohort analysis. AIDS 2002;16(15):F33.

157. Call SA et al. Phenotypic drug susceptibility testing predicts long-term virologic suppression better than treatment history in patients with human immunodeficiency virus infection. J Infect Dis 2001;183(3):401.

158. Cohen C et al. Phenotypic resistance testing significantly improves response to therapy: a randomized trial (VIRA3001). Abstract 237. Presented at the 7th Conference on Retroviruses and Opportunistic Infections. February 2000. San Francisco, CA.

159. Race EM et al. Focal mycobacterial lymphadenitis following initiation of protease-inhibitor therapy in patients with advanced HIV 1 disease. Lancet 1998;351:252.

160. Freeman WR et al. Ophthalmologic manifestations of immune recovery in AIDS patients on HAART therapy. (Abstract 757) Presented at the 5th Conference on Retrovirus and Opportunistic Infections. February 1-5, 1998. Chicago, IL.

161. Jacobson MA et al. Failure of highly active antiretroviral therapy (HAART) to prevent CMV retinitis despite marked CD4 count increase. (Abstract 353) Presented at the 4th Conference on Retrovirus and Opportunistic Infections. January 22–26, 1997. Washington, DC.

162. Gilquin J et al. Acute CMV infection in AIDS patients receiving combination therapy including protease inhibitors. (Abstract 354) Presented at the 4th Conference on Retrovirus and Opportunistic Infections. January 22-26, 1997. Washington, DC.

163. Michelet C et al. Viral ocular involvement after initiation of antiprotease inhibitor therapy. (Abstract 315) Presented at the 4th Conference on Retrovirus and Opportunistic Infections. January 22-26, 1997. Washington, DC.

164. Parker NG et al. Biphasic kinetics of peripheral blood T cells after triple combination therapy in HIV-1 infection: a composite of redistribution and proliferation. Nature Med 1998;4:208.

165. Roederer M. Getting to the HAART of T cell dynamics. Nature Med 1998;4:145.

166. Gray CM et al. Changes in CD4+ and CD8+ T cell subsets in response to highly active antiretroviral therapy in HIV type-1 infected patients with prior protease inhibitor experience. AIDS Res Hum Retroviruses 1998;14:561.

167. Lederman MM et al. Immunologic responses associated with 12 weeks of combination antiretroviral therapy consisting of zidovudine, lamivudine, and ritonavir: results of AIDS Clinical Trials Group Protocol 315. J Infect Dis. 1998;178:70.

168. Race E et al. Recurrence of trimethoprim-sulfamethoxazole TMP/SMX hypersensitivity following initiation of protease inhibitor (PRI) in patients with advanced HIV-1. (Abstract 535) Presented at the 4th Conference on Retrovirus and Opportunistic Infections. January 22-26, 1997. Washington, DC.

169. Rabound JM et al. Variation in plasma RNA levels, CD4 cell counts, and p24 antigen levels in clinically stable men with human immunodeficiency virus infection. J Infect Dis 1996;174:191.

170. Piketty C et al. Discrepant responses to triple combination antiretroviral therapy in advanced HIV disease. AIDS 1998;12:745.

171. Tenoriio A et al. Immunologic course of antiretroviral treated HIV-infected patients with a plateau response to therapy. . (Abstract 168). Presented at the 6th Conference on Retroviruses and Opportunistic Infections. January 31- February 4, 1999. Chicago, IL.

172. Acosta EP et al. Position paper on therapeutic drug monitoring of antiretroviral agents. AIDS Res Hum Retroviruses 2002;18:825.

173. Back et al. Therapeutic drug monitoring in HIV infection: current status and future directions. AIDS 2002;16(Suppl 1):S5.

174. Murphy RL et al. Antiviral effect and pharmacokinetic interaction between nevirapine and indinavir in persons infected with human immunodeficiency virus type 1. J Infect Dis 1999;179:1116.

175. Schapiro JM et al. The effect of high-dose saquinavir on viral load and T-cell counts in HIV-infected patients. Ann Intern Med 1996; 124:1039.

176. Acosta EP et al. Indinavir concentrations and antiviral effect. Pharmacotherapy 1999;19:708.

177. Baede-van Dijk P et al. Analysis of variation in plasma concentrations of nelfinavir and its active metabolite M8 in HIV-positive patients. AIDS 2001;15:991.

178. Burger DM et al. Treatment failure on nelfinavir-containing triple therapy can largely be explained by low nelfinavir plasma concentrations. AIDS 2000;14(Suppl 4):P258.

179. Marzolini C et al. Efavirenz plasma levels can predict treatment failure and central nervous system side effects in HIV-1 infected patients. AIDS 2001;15:71.

180. Veldkampa AI et al. High exposure to nevirapine in plasma is associated with an improved virological response in HIV-1 infected individuals. AIDS 2001;15:1089.

181. Joshi AS et al. Population pharmacokinetics of efavirenz in phase II studies and relationship with efficacy. Program and abstracts of the 40th Interscience Conference on Antimicrobial Agents and Chemotherapy; September 17-20, 2000; Toronto, Ontario, Canada. Abstract 1201.

182. Luber AD et al. Serum drug levels of amprenavir display limited inter- and intra-patient variability. AIDS 2000;14(Suppl 4):S28.

183. Acosta E et al. Pharmacodynamics of human immunodeficiency virus type 1 protease inhibitors. Clin Infect Dis 2000;30(Suppl 2):S151.

184. Aarnoutse R et al. An international interlaboratory quality control (QC) program for therapeutic drug monitoring (TDM) in HIV infection. Program and abstracts of the 8th Conference on Retroviruses and Opportunistic Infections. February 5-8, 2001. Chicago, Illinois. Abstract 734.

185. Luber AD, Merry C. Standard methods to measure HIV drug concentrations. Lancet 2001;358:930.

186. Burger DM et al. Therapeutic drug monitoring of indinavir in treatment-naïve patients improves therapeutic outcome after 1 year: results from Athena. Program and abstracts of the 2nd International Workshop on Clinical Pharmacology of HIV Therapy; April 2-4, 2001; Noordwijk, The Netherlands. Abstract 6.2a.

187. Burger DM et al. Therapeutic drug monitoring of nelfinavir 1250mg bid in treatment-naïve patients improves therapeutic outcome after 1 year: results from Athena. Program and abstracts of the 2nd International Workshop on Clinical Pharmacology of HIV Therapy; April 2-4, 2001; Noordwijk, The Netherlands. Abstract 6.2b.

188. Fletcher CV et al. Viral dynamics of concentration-targeted vs standard dose therapy with zidovudine (ZDV), lamivudine (3TC), and indinavir (IDV). (Abstract 322). Present at the 39th Interscience Conference on Antimicrobial Agents and Chemotherapy (ICAAC). San Francisco, CA. 1999.

189. Kempf D al. Response to ritonavir (RTV) intensification in indinavir (indinavir) recipients is highly correlated with virtual inhibitory quotient. Program and abstracts of the 8th Conference on Retroviruses and Opportunistic Infections; February 4-8, 2001;Chicago, Illinois. Abstract 523.

190. Becker S et al. Pharmacokinetic parameters of protease inhibitors and the Cmin/IC50 ratio: call for consensus. J Acquir Immune Defic Syndr 2001;27:210.

191. Luber AD, Hardy WD. Therapeutic drug monitoring: step by step. HIV/AIDS Annual Update 2001; iMedOptions, LLC; Milford, MA. Available online at http://hiv.medscape.com/update2001.

192. Piscitelli SC et al. The relative inhibitory quotient (RIQ): a method for predicting response to protease inhibitors. Program and abstracts of the 8th European Congress on Clinical Aspects and Treatment of HIV Infection; October 28-31, 2001; Athens, Greece. Abstract 164.

193. Dube MP, Sattler FR. Metabolic complications of antiretroviral therapies. AIDS Clin Care 1998; 10(6):41.

194. Carr A et al. A syndrome of peripheral lipodystrophy, hyperlipidaemia and insulin resistance in patients receiving HIV protease inhibitors. AIDS 1998;12:F51.

195. Lumpkin MM. FDA public health advisory: reports of diabetes and hyperglycemia in patients receiving protease inhibitors for the treatment of human immunodeficiency virus (HIV). June 11, 1997.

196. Eastone JA. New-onset diabetes mellitus associated with use of protease inhibitors. (Letter). Ann Intern Med 1997;11:948.

197. Dube MP et al. Protease inhibitor-associated hyperglycemia. Lancet 1997;350:713.

198. Miller KD et al. Visceral abdominal-fat accumulation associated with use of indinavir. Lancet 1998;351:871.

199. Lo JC et al. "Buffalo hump" in men with HIV-1 infection. Lancet 1998;867.

200. Viraben R, Aquilina C. Indinavir-associated lipodystrophy. AIDS 1998;12:F37.

201. Miller KD et al. Visceral abdominal fact accumulation associated with the use of indinavir. Lancet 1998;351:871.

202. Henry K et al. Severe premature coronary artery disease with protease inhibitors. Lancet 1998;351:1328.

203. Behrens G et al. Vascular complications associated with use of HIV protease inhibitors. (Letter). Lancet 1998;351:1958.

204. Gallet B et al. Vascular complications associated with use of HIV protease inhibitors. (Letter). Lancet 1998;351:1958.

205. Vittecog D et al. Vascular complications associated with use of HIV protease inhibitors. (Letter). Lancet 1998;351:1959.

206. Friis-Møller N et al. Exposure to HAART Is Associated with an Increased Risk of Myocardial Infarction: The D:A:D Study. Abstract 130. Presented at the 10th Conference on Retroviruses and Opportunistic Infections. February 2003. Boston, MA.

207. Moore RD et al. Increasing Incidence of Cardiovascular Disease in HIV-infected Persons in Care. Abstract 132. Presented at the 10th Conference on Retroviruses and Opportunistic Infections. February 2003. Boston, MA.

208. Klein D et al. Hospitalizations for Coronary Heart Disease and Myocardial Infarction Among Men with HIV-1 Infection: Additional Follow-up. Abstract 747. Presented at the 10th Conference on Retroviruses and Opportunistic Infections. February 2003. Boston, MA.

209. Bozzette S et al. Cardiovascular and cerebrovascular events in patients treated for human immunodeficiency virus infection. N Engl J Med 2003;348:602.

210. Lenhard JM et al. HIV protease inhibitors block adipogenesis and increase lipolysis in vitro. (Ab-

stract 666). Presented at the 6th Conference on Retroviruses and Opportunistic Infections. January 31–February 4, 1999. Chicago, IL.

211. Lenhard JM et al. Indinavir enhances retinoic acid signaling: nelfinavir, saquinavir, and ritonavir inhibit effects in vitro. (Abstract 667). Presented at the 6th Conference on Retroviruses and Opportunistic Infections. January 31–February 4, 1999. Chicago, IL.

212. Brinkman K et al. Mitochondrial toxicity induced by nucleoside-analogue reverse-transcriptase inhibitors is a key factor in the pathogenesis of antiretroviral therapy related lipodystrophy. Lancet 1999;354:1112.

213. Hadigan C et al. Metabolic abnormalities and cardiovascular disease risk factors in adults with HIV and lipodystrophy. Clin Infect Dis 2001;32:130.

214. Currier J. Management of metabolic complications of therapy. AIDS 2002;16:S171.

215. Distler O et al. Hyperlipidemia and inhibitors of HIV protease. Curr Opin Clin Nutr Metab Care 2001;4:99.

216. Mooser V, Carr A. Antiretroviral therapy associated hyperlipidemia in HIV disease. Curr Opin Lipidol 2001;3:313.

217. Schooley R. Treatment complications. (Session 627). Presented at the 12th World AIDS Conference. July 2, 1998. Geneva, Switzerland.

218. Sanne I et al. Results of a phase 2 clinical trial at 48 weeks (AI424-007): a dose-ranging, safety, and efficacy comparative trial of atazanavir at three doses in combination with didanosine and stavudine in antiretroviral-naive subjects. J Acquir Immune Defic Syndr 2003;32:18.

219. Squires K et al. Atazanavir (ATV) QD and Efavirenz (EFV) QD with fixed-dose ZDV + 3TC: comparison of antiviral efficacy and safety through Wk 24 (AI424). ICSSC Abstract 11-10761

220. Fichtenbaum CJ et al. Pharmacokinetic interactions between protease inhibitors and statins in HIV seronegative volunteers: ACTG study A5047. AIDS 2002;16:569.

221. Murphy R et al. Long-term efficacy and safety of atazanavir (ATV) with stavudine (d4T) and lamivudine (3TC) in patients previously treated with nelfinavir (NFV) or ATV: 108-week results of BMS study 008/044. Program and abstracts of the 10th Conference on Retroviruses and Opportunistic Infections; February 10-14, 2003; Boston, Massachusetts. Abstract 555.

222. Negredo F et al. Virological, immunological, and clinical impact of switching from protease inhibitors to nevirapine or to efavirenz in patients with human immunodeficiency virus infection and long-lasting viral suppression. Clin Infect Dis 2002;34:504.

223. Martinez E et al. Impact of switching from human immunodeficiency virus type 1 protease inhibitors to efavirenz in successfully treated adults with lipodystrophy. Clin Infect Dis 2000;31:1266.

224. Carr A et al. HIV protease inhibitor substitution in patients with lipodystrophy: a randomized, controlled, open-label, multicenter study. AIDS 2001;15:1811.

225. Clumeck N et al. Simplification with abacavir-based triple nucleoside therapy versus continued protease inhibitor-based highly active antiretorviral therapy in HIV-1-infected patients with undetectable plasma HIV-1 RNA. AIDS 2001;15:1517.

226. Saag MS et al. Switching antiretroviral drugs for treatment of metabolic complications in HIV-1 infection: summary of selected trials. Topics HIV Med 2002;10:47.

227. Opravil M et al. Simplified maintenance therapy with abacavir + lamivudine+zidovudine in patients with long-term suppression of HIV-1 RNA. In: Abstracts of the 39th Interscience Conference on Antimicrobial Agents and Chemotherapy. San Francisco, CA, September 26-29, 1999. Poster 120.

228. Keiser P et al. Simplification of protease inhibitor (PI) based highly active antiretroviral regimens

with abacavir (ABC) improves hyperlipidemia and maintains viral suppression in HIV-1 infected adults (ESS40003). Abstract WePeC6267. Presented at the XIV International AIDS Conference. 2002. Barcelona, Spain.

229. Grunfeld C. Basic science and metabolic disturbances. Presented at the XIV International AIDS Conference. July 2002. Barcelona, Spain.

230. Lichtenstein KA et al. Clinical assessment of HIV-associated lipodystrophy in an ambulatory population. AIDS 2001;15:1389.

231. Carr A et al. Abacavir substitution for nucleoside analogues in patients with HIV lipoatrophy: a randomized trial. JAMA 2002;288:207.

232. John M et al. A randomized, controlled, open-label study of revision of antiretroviral regimens containing stavudine and or a protease inhibitor to zidovudine/lamivudine/abacavir to prevent or reverse lipoatrophy. Abstract 700-T. Presented at the 9th Conference on Retroviruses and Opportunistic Infections. February 2002. Seattle, WA.

233. McComsey G et al. Improvements in lipodystrophy are observed after 24 weeks when stavudine is replaced by either abacavir or zidovudine. Abstract 701-T. Presented at the 9th Conference on Retroviruses and Opportunistic Infections. February 2002. Seattle, WA.

234. Kotler D et al. Growth hormone (Serostim®) effectively reduces visceral adipose tissue (VAT) and non-HDL cholesterol. Abstract LbOr18. Presented at the XIV International AIDS Conference. 2002. Barcelona, Spain.

235. Martinez E et al. A randomized, double-blind, placebo-controlled, comparative study on the effects of metformin or gemfibrozil in lipodystrophic HIV-1-infected patients receiving protease inhibitors. Antivir Ther 2001;6:21.

236. Sutinen J et al. Rosiglitazone in the treatment of HAART associated lipodystrophy (HAL): a randomized, double-blind, placebo-controlled study. Abstract LB13. Presented at the 9th Conference on Retroviruses and Opportunistic Infections. February 2002. Seattle, WA.

237. Gervasoni C et al. Long-term Efficacy of Buffalo Hump Surgical Treatment in Patients Continuing Antiretroviral Therapy. Abstract 723. Presented at the 10th Conference on Retroviruses and Opportunistic Infections. February 2003. Boston, MA.

238. Piliero P et al. Ultrasound-assisted Liposuction of HIV-related Buffalo Humps. Abstract 724. Presented at the 10th Conference on Retroviruses and Opportunistic Infections. February 2003. Boston, MA.

239. Vanantin MA et al. Polylactic Acid Implants (New-Fill) in the Correction of Facial Lipoatrophy in HIV-Infected Patients (VEGA Study): Results at 72 Weeks. Abstract 719. Presented at the 10th Conference on Retroviruses and Opportunistic Infections. February 2003. Boston, MA.

240. Lafaurie M et al. Treatment of Facial Lipoatrophy with Injections of Polyactic Acid in HIV-infected Patients. Abstract 720. Presented at the 10th Conference on Retroviruses and Opportunistic Infections. February 2003. Boston, MA.

241. Guaraldi G et al. Autologous Fat Transfer for Treating Facial Wasting in HIV Body Fat Redistribution Syndrome. Abstract 722. Presented at the 10th Conference on Retroviruses and Opportunistic Infections. February 2003. Boston, MA.

242. Lonergan JT et al. Incidence and outcome of hyperlactatemia associated with clinical manifestations in HIV-infected adults receiving NRTI-containing regimens. Abstract 624. Presented at the 8th Conference on Retroviruses and Opportunistic Infections. February 2001. Chicago, IL.

243. Flepp M et al. Modern anti-HIV therapy. Swiss Med Wkly 2001;131:207.

244. Hatano H et al. Metabolic and anthropometric consequences of interruption of highly active antiretroviral therapy. AIDS 2000;14:1935.

245. Deeks SG et al. Continued Reverse Transcriptase Inhibitor Therapy is Sufficient to Maintain Short-

Term Partial Suppression of Multi-Drug Resistant Viremia. Abstract 640. Presented at the 10th Conference on Retroviruses and Opportunistic Infections. February 2003. Boston, MA.

246. Katlama C et al. Long-term Benefit of Treatment Interruption in Salvage. Therapy (GIGHAART ANRS 097). Abstract 68. Presented at the 10th Conference on Retroviruses and Opportunistic Infections. February 2003. Boston, MA.

247. Lawrence J et al. CPCRA 064: A Randomized Trial Examining Structured Treatment Interruption for Patients Failing Therapy with Multi-drug Resistant HIV. Abstract 67. Presented at the 10th Conference on Retroviruses and Opportunistic Infections. February 2003. Boston, MA.

248. Ananworanich J, HIV-NAT 001.4: A Prospective Randomized Trial of Structured Treatment Interruption in Patients with Chronic HIV Infection. Abstract 64. Presented at the 10th Conference on Retroviruses and Opportunistic Infections. February 2003. Boston, MA.

249. Ruiz L et al. A Multi-center, Randomized Controlled Clinical Trial of Continuous vs Intermittent HAART Guided by CD4+ T-cell Counts and Plasma HIV-1 RNA Levels. Abstract 65. Presented at the 10th Conference on Retroviruses and Opportunistic Infections. February 2003. Boston, MA.

250. Dybul M. Treatment interruptions in chronic HIV infection. Presented at the XIV International AIDS Conference. July 2002. Barcelona, Spain.

251. Dybul M et al. Short-cycle structured intermittent treatment of chronic HIV infection with highly active antiretroviral therapy. AIDS 2000;14:1935.

252. Deeks S, Hirschel B. Supervised interruptions of antiretroviral therapy. AIDS 2002;16(Suppl 4):S157.

253. Kilby JM et al. Recurrence of the acute HIV syndrome after interruption of antiretroviral therapy in a patient with chronic HIV-1 infection: a case report. Ann Intern Med 2000;133:435.

254. Colven R et al. Retroviral rebound syndrome after cessation of suppressive antiretroviral therapy in three patients with chronic HIV infection. Ann Intern Med 2000;133:430.

255. Daar ES et al. Acute HIV syndrome after discontinuation of antiretroviral therapy in a patient treated before seroconversion. Ann Intern Med 1998;128:827.

256. Jackson JB et al. Identification of the K103N resistance mutation in Ugandan women receiving nevirapine to prevent HIV-1 vertical transmission. AIDS 2000;14:F111.

257. Deeks SG. International perspectives on antiretroviral resistance. Nonnucleoside reverse transcriptase inhibitor resistance. J Acquir Immune Defic Syndr 2001;26(Suppl 1):S25.

258. Silberg WM et al. Asssessing, controlling, and assuring the quality of medical information on the internet: caveat lector et viewor—let the reader and viewer beware. JAMA 1997;277:1244.

259. Hirsch MS, D'Aquila RT. Therapy for human immunodeficiency virus infection. N Engl J Med 1993;328:1686.

260. Arribas JR et al. High effectiveness of efavirenz-based HAART in HIV-1 infected patients with less than 100 CD4 cells/mL and opportunistic diseases. The EfaVIP-1 study. Abstract TuPeB4444. Presented at the 14th International AIDS Conference. July 2002. Barcelona Spain.

261. Robbins G et al. Antiretroviral strategies in naive HIV+ subjects: comparisons of sequential 3-drug regimens (ACTG 384). Program and abstracts of the XIV International AIDS Conference; July 7-12, 2002; Barcelona, Spain. [Abstract LbOr20A].

262. Gibbons SE et al. The Liverpool Therapeutic Drug Monitoring Service—a summary of the service and examples of use in clinical practice. AIDS 2000;14(Suppl 4):S89.

CHAPTER 70

Opportunistic Infections in HIV-Infected Patients

Angela D.M. Kashuba, Marjorie D. Robinson

AIDS is characterized by the gradual erosion of immune competence and the development of opportunistic infections (OIs) and malignancies. OIs account for approximately 90% of the mortality and morbidity associated with AIDS. In 1997, the Centers for Disease Control and Prevention (CDC) estimated that approximately 60,000 AIDS-related opportunistic illnesses had occurred in the United States during 1996.[1] This report represents the first calendar year in which the overall incidence of AIDS-associated OIs did not increase in the United States; the 1996 figure represented a decline of 6% compared with 1995. This trend has continued and may be attributed to the early use of combination antiretroviral therapy, which delays the progression from HIV infection to AIDS and death.[1,2] Patients with HIV infection are susceptible to an array of diseases, but most OIs are caused by a few common pathogens, including *Pneumocystis carinii,* cytomegalovirus (CMV), fungi, and mycobacteria. Persons with AIDS also are susceptible to neoplastic diseases (lymphoma and Kaposi's sarcoma) and other conditions such as wasting syndrome.[2,3]

The 1993 revised classification system for HIV infection and expanded surveillance case definition for AIDS included stratification for the CD4+ lymphocyte count, as well as subgrouping by clinical categories (see Table 70-1). These AIDS-defining OIs or malignancies may also occur in asymptomatic HIV-infected patients (Table 70-1).[3]

Table 70-1   Conditions Included in the 1993 Surveillance Case Definition

Category A	Category C (continued)
Asymptomatic HIV infection	Cryptosporidiosis, chronic intestinal (>1 month)
Persistent generalized lymphadenopathy	Cytomegalovirus disease (other than liver, spleen, or nodes)
Acute HIV infection with accompanying illness or history of HIV infection	Cytomegalovirus retinitis (with loss of vision)
	Encephalopathy, HIV-related
Category B	Herpes simplex: chronic ulcer(s) (>1 month); or bronchitis, pneumonitis, or esophagitis
Bacillary angiomatosis	Histoplasmosis, disseminated or extrapulmonary
Candidiasis, oropharyngeal (thrush)	Isosporiasis, chronic intestinal (>1 month's duration)
Candidiasis, vulvovaginal; persistent, frequent, or poorly responsive to treatment	Kaposi's sarcoma
Cervical dysplasia/carcinoma in situ	Lymphoid interstitial pneumonia and/or pulmonary lymphoid hyperplasia[a]
Constitutional symptoms, such as fever >38°C or diarrhea >1 month	Lymphoma, Burkitt's (or equivalent term)
Hairy leukoplakia	Lymphoma, immunoblastic (or equivalent term)
Herpes zoster (shingles), involving at least two distinct episodes or more than one dermatome	Lymphoma, primary, of brain
Idiopathic thrombocytopenia purpura	*Mycobacterium avium-intracellulare* complex or *M. kansasii,* disseminated or extrapulmonary
Listeriosis	*Mycobacterium tuberculosis,* any site (pulmonary[b] or extrapulmonary)
Pelvic inflammatory disease, particularly if complicated by tubo-ovarian abscess	Mycobacterium, other species or unidentified species, disseminated or extrapulmonary
Peripheral neuropathy	*Pneumocystis carinii* pneumonia
	Pneumonia, recurrent[b]
Category C	Progressive multifocal leukoencephalopathy
	Salmonella septicemia, recurrent
Candidiasis of bronchi, trachea, or lungs	Toxoplasmosis of brain
Candidiasis, esophageal	Wasting syndrome due to HIV
Cervical cancer, invasive	
Coccidioidomycosis, disseminated or extrapulmonary	
Cryptococcosis, extrapulmonary	

[a]Children younger than 13 years old.
[b]Added in the 1993 expansions of the AIDS surveillance case definition for adolescents and adults.

The Natural History of Opportunistic Infections

The Decline of the CD4+ Lymphocyte

Within the immune system, the CD4+ lymphocyte functions as a "helper cell" that modulates the actions of the other key cellular components of the immune system. The eventual loss of CD4+ lymphocytes is the underlying pathophysiologic problem that leads to AIDS. (See Chapter 69, Pharmacotherapy of Human Immunodeficiency Virus Infection, and comprehensive immunology texts for a more detailed explanation of immune function and inflammation associated with HIV infection).[4,5] The infected CD4+ lymphocyte can function normally for a period of time but eventually becomes dysfunctional, as manifested by an abnormal response to soluble mitogens.[6,7] It is this cellular functional deficit, compounded by the eventual decline in the absolute number of CD4+ lymphocytes, that leads to OIs, malignancies, and neurologic dysfunctions. The CD4+ count declines gradually over several years in the untreated HIV-infected person. The average rate of decline of CD4+ lymphocyte cells (CD4 slope) is approximately 40 to 80 cells/mm³ per year in the absence of antiretroviral therapy. An accelerated decline in the CD4+ count occurs at 1.5 to 2 years, just before an AIDS-defining diagnosis.[8,9] Without therapy, the course of infection averages approximately 10 years from the time of initial infection to an

AIDS-defining diagnosis. There is individual variation in the decline of the CD4+ count. Some patients have a rapid decline after the acute retroviral presentation, whereas approximately 5% to 15% have a CD4+ count of ≥500 for >8 years; these patients are considered chronic nonprogressors.[10]

The CD4+ count dictates the need for OI prophylaxis, affects the differential diagnosis of the OI, and is an independent indicator of prognosis. For these reasons, the CD4+ count has become a primary surrogate marker of immune suppression and antiretroviral activity.[11] HIV-1 RNA is the other clinical surrogate marker most predictive of survival and antiretroviral activity.

OIs range from relatively minor events (e.g., oral candidiasis or oral hairy leukoplakia) to sight-threatening episodes of CMV retinitis, or life-threatening *P. carinii* pneumonia (PCP). The risk for specific OIs varies with the degree of immunosuppression.[12–14] Asymptomatic patients with moderate immunosuppression (CD4+ counts 200 to 500) may become infected with herpes viruses or *Candida* species. Massive destruction of the immune system occurs when the CD4+ count is <200, which increases the risk for opportunistic pathogens (e.g., PCP), opportunistic tumors, wasting, and neurologic complications. With a CD4+ count of 50 to 100, invasive candidiasis, cerebral toxoplasmosis, cryptococcosis, and various protozoal infections are observed. When the

CD4+ falls below 50, the patient is in an advanced immuno-suppressed state, which is associated with non-Hodgkin's lymphoma, CMV, and disseminated *Mycobacterium avium* complex (MAC) (Fig. 70-1). Without treatment, the median survival associated with a CD4+ count <200 is 3.1 years, and the time to an AIDS-defining infection ranges from 18 to 24 months. The median survival after an AIDS-defining complication is 1.3 years.[8,11,12,14]

The Effect of Opportunistic Infections on Viral Load and Survival

Acute OIs upregulate HIV replication, resulting in higher HIV-1 RNA concentrations in the plasma and lymphoid tissues of HIV-infected patients.[15–19] This enhanced replication is presumably caused by antigen-mediated activation of HIV-1 replication in latently infected cells. To assess the impact of OIs on survival, data from a cohort of 2,081 HIV-infected patients followed (in the pre-protease inhibitor era) for a mean of 30 months were analyzed.[21] CD4+ counts and incidence of opportunistic disease were used as independent variables. These investigators found that PCP, CMV, MAC, esophageal candidiasis, Kaposi's sarcoma, non-Hodgkin's lymphoma, progressive multifocal leukoencephalopathy (PML), dementia, wasting syndrome, toxoplasmosis, and cryptosporidiosis were independently associated with death.[21] Additionally, data from a prospective longitudinal study of HIV infection in homosexual men initiated in 1984 (Multicenter AIDS Cohort Study [MACS]) demonstrated that plasma HIV-1 RNA concentrations strongly predict the rate of decline of the absolute CD4+ count as well as clinical progression to AIDS and death.[16a]

Impact of Antiretroviral Agents on the Natural History of Opportunistic Infections

Reduction in the Incidence of Opportunistic Infections and Death

The introduction of protease inhibitors, combination therapy, prophylaxis therapy, and improved medical care has reduced the incidence of OIs and death resulting from AIDS in HIV-positive patients. Highly active antiretroviral therapy (HAART) usually consists of two nucleoside reverse transcriptase inhibitors, in addition to one or more protease inhibitors or one nonnucleoside reverse transcriptase inhibitor. HAART generally refers to an antiretroviral regimen that can be expected to reduce the viral load in antiretroviral-naïve patients to <50 copies/mL. A panel of experts convened by the Department of Health and Human Services (DHHS) and the Henry J. Kaiser Family Foundation recommended HAART as the standard of care for all HIV-infected patients.[21] These potent antiretroviral agents and effective management of OIs have led to an improved quality of life and prolonged duration of survival among HIV-infected patients in the United States.[22–25] A significant decrease in the incidence of OIs and death was first reported in February 1996, when preliminary data from a pivotal study became available. The data demonstrated that the addition of ritonavir to an existing reverse transcriptase regimen in severely immunocompromised patients decreased the incidence of OIs and death.[26] Several studies[26–30] since have shown a decrease in the incidence of OIs in AIDS patients receiving HAART therapy. One such study, a retrospective cohort design of patients in an HIV outpatient clinic observed from Dec. 1, 1994, through Jan. 1, 1998, demonstrated a significant decline in OIs in 1996 and 1997. The most common conditions with reported reduced incidence included Kaposi's sarcoma, HIV wasting, and infections such as PCP, MAC, and CMV.[27]

Since the introduction of the protease inhibitors, the CDC has reported a deceleration in the rate of AIDS diagnosis.[29] This finding was observed in homosexual men and in intravenous (IV) drug users but was not observed in heterosexual exposure groups. Notably, a decrease in incidence of OIs was not observed in HIV-positive, non-Hispanic Blacks and Hispanics. The decline in AIDS-associated mortality is probably the result of improved medical care, increased use of HAART therapy, and effective prophylaxis. Unfortunately, the number of deaths caused by AIDS has increased among women and heterosexual transmission groups.

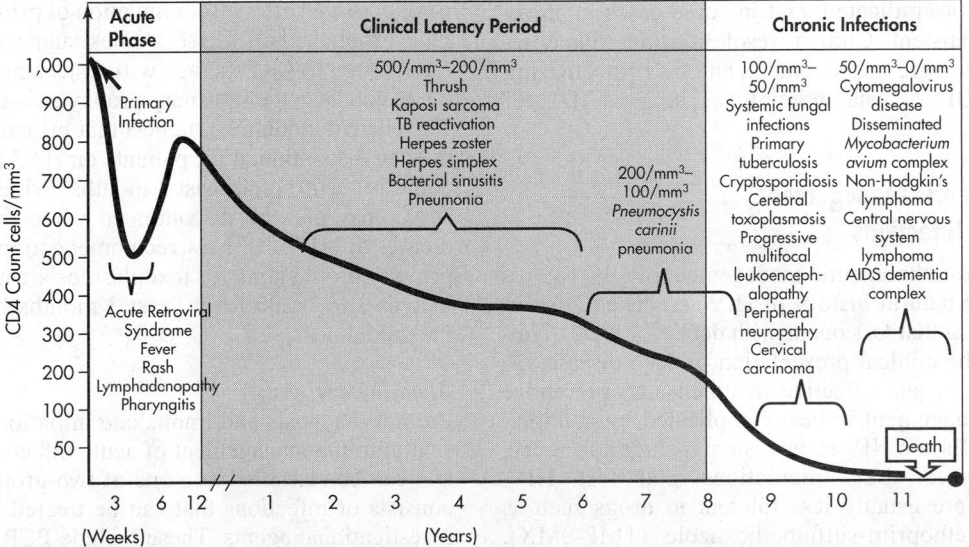

FIGURE 70-1 Natural history of CD4+ cell count in the average HIV patient without antiretroviral therapy from the time of HIV transmissions to death. (Illustration by Mary Van, Pharm.D.)

Changes in the Natural History of Opportunistic Infections

OIs and cancers result from longstanding immunosuppression from HIV infection.[12–14] Several studies have reported a change in the natural history of certain OIs following the initiation of antiretroviral agents.[31,32] Before HAART, approximately 40% of all AIDS patients developed CMV retinitis, with the most cases occurring at CD4$^+$ counts of <100. Currently, a decrease in the incidence of CMV retinitis and a decline in the rate of retinitis progression have been noted.[32,33]

Ironically, HAART therapy also has been associated with a worsening or an unmasking of occult OIs in patients with advanced AIDS. When antiretroviral therapy strengthens the immune system, inflammatory symptoms in response to infection are more clinically pronounced.[31,34] A subclinical MAC infection syndrome, characterized by severe fever, leukocytosis, and lymphadenitis, was observed in five patients after initiating HAART.[31] CMV retinitis occurred in five patients previously treated with HAART despite a marked improvement in CD4$^+$ counts (195 cell/mm^3) before diagnosis.[33] Elevated liver function tests (LFTs) and hepatitis C viremia have been documented after the initiation of HAART.[34]

The initiation of HAART typically results in an increase in CD4$^+$ lymphocytes and a decrease in HIV-1 RNA to undetectable levels. It is unclear whether the CD4$^+$ lymphocytes associated with HAART therapy are as functional as the cells previously lost over the course of the HIV infection. It is also unknown whether this increase in total CD4$^+$ lymphocytes reflects an increase in memory subtypes, and whether these subtypes mediate a subclinical inflammatory response.[35]

Improvement or Resolution of Opportunistic Infections

With the initiation of HAART, reports of improvement or resolution of some OIs have recently been published.[36–40] These OIs include Kaposi's sarcoma,[36] PML,[37] CMV,[32,33] microsporidiosis, cryptosporidiosis,[38] and molluscum contagiosum,[39] a viral infection caused by a member of the Poxviridae family. Furthermore, there are reports of restored immunity and clinical improvement in patients with chronic hepatitis B infection (not classified as a CDC-defined AIDS indicator condition) upon the initiation of HAART.[40] These infections were not eradicated, and in some cases improvement was only transient. Clinical resolution most likely results from immunologic improvement, and the protective immunity against OI is sustained only as long as HAART remains effective.

Pharmacotherapeutic Management of Opportunistic Infections

Successful pharmacotherapeutic management of OIs requires understanding the natural history of HIV-associated OIs, including recognizing that OIs occur with declining CD4$^+$ lymphocyte counts, the clinical presentation of each disease, diagnostic techniques, and effective treatment and preventive strategies.[41,42] Management issues, complicated by multiple-drug therapy for OIs and HIV suppression, include adherence, toxicities, resistance, drug interactions, and cost. HIV-infected patients are usually less tolerant to drugs such as flucytosine, trimethoprim-sulfamethoxazole (TMP-SMX), and pyrimethamine. Therapeutic options are often limited; therefore, more efficacious agents (e.g., for the treatment of cryptosporidia and microsporidia) and less toxic agents (e.g., than pyrimethamine and sulfadiazine) need to be developed.[43]

In 1995, the United States Public Health Service (USPHS) and the Infectious Diseases Society of America (IDSA) issued guidelines for the prevention of OIs in HIV-infected patients; these were revised in 1997,[47] 1999,[48] and 2002.[49] Nineteen OIs, or groups of OIs, are addressed, and recommendations are included for preventing exposure to opportunistic pathogens, preventing first episodes of disease by chemoprophylaxis or vaccination (primary prophylaxis), and preventing disease recurrence (secondary prophylaxis).

Primary Prophylaxis

Primary prophylaxis is defined as therapy that is initiated before the appearance of an OI in high-risk asymptomatic persons. It is used to prevent the initial occurrence of an infection. Primary prevention of OIs is important, considering the inevitable immune depletion associated with chronic HIV infection.[42–45] PCP and MAC prophylaxis have significantly prolonged survival and delayed the onset of illness (see sections about PCP and MAC prophylaxis).[44,45]

The guidelines strongly recommend primary prophylaxis against PCP, toxoplasmosis, *Mycobacterium tuberculosis*, MAC, and varicella-zoster virus (VZV). Vaccinations to prevent *Streptococcus pneumoniae*, hepatitis B virus, hepatitis A virus, and influenza virus infection generally are recommended for all HIV-infected patients. Primary prophylaxis for fungal infections (*Cryptococcus neoformans* and *Histoplasma capsulatum*), CMV, and bacterial infections are not routinely recommended for most patients, except in unusual circumstances (Table 70-2).

DISCONTINUATION OF PRIMARY PROPHYLAXIS THERAPY

HAART has diminished the incidence of several OIs.[31,32,36,39] Therefore, it may be possible to discontinue prophylactic OI therapy when CD4$^+$ counts rise above the threshold associated with risk for infection. These data have been particularly encouraging in patients who had PCP prophylaxis discontinued with an increase in CD4$^+$ counts.[49,53–55] In one observational PCP prophylaxis study, no episodes of PCP were observed after discontinuation of primary and secondary PCP prophylaxis.[53] These studies suggest that patients who respond to HAART therapy with a sustained increase in CD4$^+$ count can have their primary prophylaxis safely discontinued. The current guidelines suggest that primary PCP prophylaxis may be discontinued for patients on HAART when the CD4$^+$ count is >200 for at least 3 months. Primary prophylaxis for MAC may also be discontinued when the CD4$^+$ count increases to >100.[49,56] New recommendations for discontinuing primary prophylaxis for toxoplasmosis when the CD4$^+$ count increases to >200 for at least 3 months have been added to the guidelines.

Acute Therapy

Prompt diagnosis and immediate initiation of therapy are essential to the management of acute infections. Most common OIs can be classified into one of two groups. The first group consists of infections that can be treated by conventional or investigational agents. These include PCP, tuberculosis (TB), cryptococcosis, and histoplasmosis. Treatment may result in either effective or moderately effective resolution. These in-

Table 70-2   Primary Prophylaxis of OIs in HIV-Infected Adults and Adolescents

| Pathogen | Indication | Preventive Regimens | | |
		First Choice	Alternatives	D/C Prophylaxis
Strongly Recommended as Standard of Care				
Pneumocystis carinii	CD4$^+$ count <200 or oropharyngeal candidiasis	Trimethoprimsulfamethoxazole (TMP-SMX), 1 DS PO QD or TMP-SMX 1 SS PO QD	TMP/SMX 1 DS PO TIW; dapsone 50 mg BID or 100 mg/day; dapsone 50 mg QD plus pyrimethamine 50 mg QW plus leucovorin, 25 mg PO QW; dapsone, 200 mg PO plus pyrimethamine 75 mg PO plus leucovorin, 25 mg PO QW; aerosolized pentamadine, 300 mg QM via Respirgard II nebulizer, atovaquone, 1,500 mg PO QD; TMP/SMX 1 DS 3 times/week	Patients on HAART with sustained ↑ in CD4 >200 cells for ≥3 months may discontinue PCP prophylaxis. Reintroduce if CD4$^+$ <200.
Mycobacterium tuberculosis Isoniazid sensitive	Tuberculin skin test (TST) reaction ≥5 mm or prior positive result without treatment or contact with case of active tuberculosis regardless of TST result	Isoniazid 300 mg PO plus pyridoxine 50 mg PO QD × 9 months or isoniazid 900 mg PO plus pyridoxine, 100 mg PO BIW × 9 months	Rifampin 600 mg PO QD × 4 months or rifabutin 300 mg PO QD × 4 months: PZA 15–20 mg/kg PO QD × 2 months + rifampin 600 mg PO QD × 2 months or rifabutin 300 mg PO QD × 2 months	
Isoniazid resistant	Same; high probability of exposure to multidrug resistance tuberculosis	Rifampin 600 mg PO QD or rifabutin 300 mg PO QD × 4 months	Pyrazinamide 20 mg/kg PO QD × 2 months; plus either rifampin 600 mg PO QD × 2 months or rifabutin 300 mg PO QD × 2 months	
Multidrug resistant (INH and RIF)	Same; high probability of exposure to isoniazid-resistant tuberculosis	Choice of drugs requires consultation with public health authorities	None	
Toxoplasma gondii	IgG antibody to *Toxoplasma* and CD4$^+$ count <100	TMP-SMX, 1 DS PO QD	TMP-SMZ, 1 SS PO QD: dapsone, 50 mg PO QD plus pyrimethamine, 50 mg PO QW plus leucovorin, 25 mg PO QW; dapsone 200 mg PO QW + pyrimethymine 75 mg PO QW + leucovorin 25 mg PO QW: atovaquone, 1,500 mg PO QD with or without pyrimethamine 25 mg PO QD plus leucovorin, 10 mg PO QD	Patients on HAART with sustained ↑ in CD4 >200 for ≥3 months. Restart if CD4 <200.

Continued

Table 70-2   Primary Prophylaxis of OIs in HIV-Infected Adults and Adolescents—cont'd

| Pathogen | Indication | Preventive Regimens | | | D/C Prophylaxis |
		First Choice	Alternatives		
Mycobacterium avium complex	CD4$^+$ count <50	Azithromycin, 1,200 mg PO QW or clarithromycin 500 mg PO BID	Rifabutin, 300 mg PO QD; azithromycin, 1,200 mg PO QW plus rifabutin, 300 mg PO QD		Patient on HAART with sustained ↑ in CD4 >100 for ≥3 months may discontinue MAC prophylaxis. Restart if CD4 <50–100.
Varicella-zoster virus (VZV)	Significant exposure to chickenpox or shingles for patients who have no history of either condition or, if available, negative antibody to VZV	Varicella zoster immune globulin (VZIG) 5 vials (1.25 mL each) IM administered ≤96 hr after exposure, ideally within 48 hr	—		—

Usually Recommended

Pathogen	Indication	First Choice	Alternatives		D/C Prophylaxis
Streptococcus pneumoniae	CD4$^+$ >1200	23 valent polysaccharide Pneumococcal vaccine 0.5 mL IM	None		
Hepatitis B virus	All susceptible (anti-HBc-negative) patients	Hepatitis B vaccine 3 doses	None		
Influenza virus	All patients (annually before influenza season)	Inactivated trivalent influenza virus vaccine 0.5 mL/IM/yr	Rimantadine, 100 mg PO BID, or amantadine, 100 mg PO BID (influenza A only)		
Hepatitis A virus	All susceptible (anti-HAV-negative) patients, or patients with chronic liver disease (including hep B or C)	Hepatitis A vaccine; two doses	None		

Not Recommended For Most Patients; Indicated For Use Only in Unusual Circumstances

Pathogen	Indication	First Choice	Alternatives		D/C Prophylaxis
Bacteria	Neutropenia	Granulocyte colony-stimulating factor (G-CSF) 5–10 μg/kg SC QD × 2–4 wk or granulocyte macrophage colony-stimulating factor (GM-CSF) 250 μg/m² SC × 2–4 wk	None		
Cryptococcus neoformans	CD4$^+$ count <50	Fluconazole 100–200 mg PO QD	Itraconazole, 200 mg PO QD		
Histoplasma capsulatum	CD4$^+$ count <100, endemic geographic areas	Itraconazole 200 mg PO QD	None		
Cytomegalovirus (CMV)	CD4$^+$ count <50 and CMV antibody positive	Oral ganciclovir 1 g PO TID	None		

Adapted from USPHS/IDSA Guidelines. MMWR Morbid Mortal Wkly Rep June 14, 2002;51(RR-8):1–52.

fections may recur if chronic suppressive or secondary prophylaxis is discontinued without an accompanying elevation in the CD4+ count and viral load suppression. The second group includes pathogens for which no therapeutic regimen is currently effective (Table 70-3). These include cryptosporidiosis, microsporidiosis, and PML.[41]

Secondary Prophylaxis or Chronic Suppressive Therapy

Secondary prophylaxis is used to prevent recurrence of an OI once the patient has developed signs and symptoms of active infection. In some cases, secondary prophylaxis regimens can be discontinued after patients achieve a certain CD4+ level. The USPHS and IDSA strongly recommend secondary prophylaxis for PCP, toxoplasmosis (reduced dosage), MAC, CMV, *Salmonella* species, and infections caused by endemic fungi and *C. neoformans*.[49]

DISCONTINUATION OF SECONDARY PROPHYLAXIS OR CHRONIC SUPPRESSIVE THERAPY

In 1999, the USPHS/IDSA guidelines first reported that stopping primary or secondary prophylaxis for certain pathogens was safe if HAART led to an increase in the CD4+ count to above specified threshold levels. The 2002 USPHS/IDSA guidelines incorporated more data to support these initial recommendations and expanded recommendations to other pathogens. Criteria for discontinuing chemoprophylaxis are based on specific clinical studies and vary by duration of CD4+ count increase and duration of treatment of the initial episode of disease (in the case of secondary prophylaxis).

Multiple case series have reported that maintenance therapy for CMV can be discontinued safely in patients whose have maintained a CD4+ count of >100 to 150 for >6 months on HAART.[31,32,50–52,57,58] Whereas CMV retinitis typically reactivated <6 to 8 weeks after stopping CMV therapy in the pre-HAART era, these patients have remained disease free for >30 to 95 weeks. Plasma HIV RNA levels varied among these patients, demonstrating that the CD4+ count is the primary determinant of immune recovery to CMV. The decision to stop CMV prophylaxis should be made in consultation with an ophthalmologist and will be influenced by factors such as the magnitude and duration of CD4+ increases and viral load suppression, anatomic location of retinal lesions, and vision in the contralateral eye. Regular ophthalmic examination is critical.[31,32,49,57–59]

Secondary PCP prophylaxis may be discontinued among patients whose CD4+ counts have increased to >200 for >3 months while on HAART. Secondary prophylaxis for disseminated MAC may be discontinued among patients who have completed 12 months of MAC therapy, have no signs or symptoms of MAC, and have had a CD4+ count of >100 for >6 months in response to HAART. Similarly, secondary prophylaxis for toxoplasmosis may be discontinued in patients who have completed initial therapy, have no signs or symptoms of infection, and have had CD4+ counts of >200 for >6 months. Using the same criteria, patients with cryptococcosis can discontinue secondary prophylaxis if they have had CD4+ counts of >100 to 200 for >6 months.

Although there are considerable data concerning the discontinuation of primary and secondary prophylaxis, there are no data regarding restarting prophylaxis if the CD4+ count decreases again to levels at which the patient is likely to again be at risk for OIs. For primary prophylaxis, it is unknown whether the same threshold at which prophylaxis can be stopped should be used or whether the threshold below which initial prophylaxis is recommended should be used. For prophylaxis against PCP, current guidelines use a CD4+ count of 200 as the threshold for restarting both primary and secondary prophylaxis.

PNEUMOCYSTIS CARINII PNEUMONIA

As an indication of the relative obscurity of this organism, no comprehensive text on PCP was available until 1983.[60] Recently, this organism has been reclassified from a protozoan to a fungus on the basis of ribosomal RNA sequence comparisons.[61] The morphologic resemblance of *P. carinii* to a protozoan has led to its life cycle being described as a cyst form, with up to eight sporozoites per cyst. The trophozoite or extracystic form has different staining characteristics (i.e., it does not stain with toluidine-blue O or Grocott-Gomori stains) compared with the cyst or sporozoites.

Clinical Presentation

1. J.R. is a 38-year-old, HIV-seropositive man who was diagnosed 5 years ago when he had an outbreak of herpes zoster. He refused antiretroviral therapy and was determined to treat himself using natural teas and herbs. J.R. developed a mild, nonproductive cough that has persisted for the last 4 weeks. He has also had a low-grade fever but denies any chills or pleuritic chest pain. His chest radiograph demonstrates a diffuse, symmetric, interstitial infiltrate. Arterial Pao2 is 80 mm Hg (normal, 80 to 105). His last CD4+ count approximately 3 months ago was 180

Table 70-3 Acute Management of Opportunistic Infections

Group I[a]		Group II
A	*B*	
Infections effectively treated	Moderate chance of effective treatment	No currently effective therapeutic regimen
• *Pneumocystis carinii* pneumonia	• Cytomegalovirus	• Cryptosporidiosis
• Tuberculosis	• *Mycobacterium avium* complex	• Microsporidiosis
• Cryptococcosis		• Progressive multifocal
• Histoplasmosis		leukoencephalopathy

[a]A and B may recur if secondary prophylaxis is discontinued.
Adapted from reference 40.

cells/mm³ (normal, approximately 1,000 cells/mm³) and his viral load was 60,000 copies/mL. He refused primary PCP prophylaxis. Following hypertonic saline nebulization for sputum induction and subsequent bronchoalveolar lavage, examination of the specimens with the modified Giemsa stain revealed both intracystic bodies and extracystic trophozoites. How is the clinical presentation of J.R. consistent with PCP?

The clinical features of PCP in AIDS patients differ from non-AIDS patients in that a more subtle onset, with mild fever, a cough, tachypnea, and dyspnea, is typically seen in HIV- infected patients.[62] J.R.'s low-grade fever and mild, nonproductive cough of 4 weeks' duration are consistent with this description of PCP. His history of HIV infection and the finding of trophozoites on Giemsa stain further support a diagnosis of PCP. The characteristic diffuse interstitial pulmonary infiltrates on J.R.'s chest radiograph are consistent with PCP. Limited data exist with regard to the latent state of *P. carinii* after infection of the host. Some investigators hypothesize that most persons are asymptomatic unless the immune system of the host becomes impaired. Others believe that the infection is caused by reinfection as opposed to reactivation.[63]

Antimicrobial Selection

2. A diagnosis of PCP is made and J.R. agrees to be treated. What patient factors are important to consider when selecting an antimicrobial? What would be a reasonable drug for J.R., and how might his course of PCP be monitored?

The treatment of acute PCP is determined by the degree of clinical severity on presentation. The arterial oxygen status on presentation is an important indicator of overall outcome. In one study, surviving patients had a mean P_{O_2} of 70 mm Hg, whereas the mean P_{O_2} of the nonsurvivors was 55 mm Hg.[64] Key factors to consider when initiating therapy for PCP include the arterial blood gas findings, whether it is an initial or repeat episode of PCP, the need for parenteral therapy, and a prior history of adverse drug reactions or hypersensitivity. Concomitant therapy must also be considered.

Patients with PCP often can be classified as having mild, moderate, or severe disease, based on their oxygenation. Patients with mild PCP often have a room air alveolar-arterial (A-a) oxygen gradient of <35, patients with moderate disease have a gradient of 36 to 45, and patients with severe cases have a gradient >45. With the advent of corticosteroid use for moderate to severe cases of PCP (discussed later), it is useful to calculate the (A-a) gradient. The A-a gradient (normal range, 5 to 15 mm Hg) can be calculated as $P_{IO_2} - 1.25\ P_{CO_2} - P_{O_2}$, where P_{IO_2} is the partial pressure of oxygen (150 mm Hg in room air), and P_{CO_2} and P_{O_2} are arterial levels of CO_2 and O_2, respectively, expressed in millimeters of mercury (mm Hg).[65]

Several other clinical tests have been used to identify and monitor PCP. The lactate dehydrogenase (LDH) concentration in serum or bronchoalveolar lavage fluid has been used to diagnose and monitor therapy and to predict outcome during PCP. However, many patients have overlapping diseases, preventing LDH from being used alone. Chest radiographs also are variable. The most common picture is one of bilateral diffuse interstitial pneumonitis, but atypical patterns, such as pleural effusion, cavities, pneumatoceles, and nodules, may

occur as well. A normal chest radiograph is associated with a better clinical outcome.

The natural course of PCP among untreated HIV-infected patients is progressive dyspnea and hypoxemia. The increased experience with treatment of PCP in AIDS patients (compared with non–HIV-infected patients) indicates that a longer duration of therapy is needed.[60] Despite the greater appreciation of PCP in AIDS patients, some patients may not respond to therapy; many experience worsening hypoxemia during the first 3 to 5 days after treatment is started. This period of clinical worsening is least tolerated by those patients with moderate to severe PCP (P_{O_2} <70 mm Hg). In the sicker patients, this period may lead to respiratory failure and the need for intubation with continued critical care. Although many would associate the need for intensive care unit admission as a poor prognostic factor, many patients do well despite the need for mechanical ventilation and IV antibiotics. In light of the now-appreciated role of corticosteroids, patients with PCP and respiratory failure may be viewed as manageable if treated aggressively (Table 70-4).

Trimethoprim-Sulfamethoxazole

The decision to hospitalize a patient is based on the severity of his or her illness. Patients who present with mild PCP with reasonable oxygenation and without evidence of clinical deterioration can be managed as outpatients. Patients with reasonably good gas exchange (i.e., P_{O_2} >70 mm Hg), but with signs of clinical deterioration, most often are admitted to the hospital and given oxygen by nasal cannula and are usually started on IV TMP-SMX (15 to 20 mg/kg daily TMP, 75 to 100 mg/kg daily SMX) for 21 days. The dosing of IV TMP-SMX must be modified in patients with renal dysfunction. Trimethoprim reversibly inhibits dihydrofolate reductase, and sulfamethoxazole competes with para-aminobenzoic acid (PABA) in the production of dihydrofolate, synergistically blocking thymidine biosynthesis. TMP-SMX is always the first choice for the treatment of PCP unless the patient has a history of life-threatening intolerance. In the treatment of PCP, TMP-SMX is either as effective as, or superior to, all alternative agents. A good response may be expected in >70% of patients receiving TMP-SMX.

TMP-SMX is often prescribed because of its availability as an oral formulation. Tablets are >90% bioavailable. The usual dose is 15 mg/kg (dosed by the TMP component) Q 8 hr for 21 days. Since one double-strength tablet of TMP-SMX contains 160 mg TMP plus 800 mg SMX, a standard regimen is two double-strength tablets three times per day (or Q 8 hr). Taking two double-strength tablets Q 6 hr (eight double-strength tablets per day) does not improve efficacy and causes increased toxicity (gastrointestinal [GI] intolerance, nausea, vomiting, anorexia, and abdominal pain).

Although the TMP-SMX regimen is very efficacious, 25% to 50% of patients may be intolerant. Adverse effects include an erythematous, maculopapular, morbilliform rash and, less commonly, severe urticaria, exfoliative dermatitis, and Stevens-Johnson syndrome. GI intolerance (nausea, vomiting, abdominal pain) is common. Hematologic side effects may include leukopenia, anemia, and/or thrombocytopenia. Neurologic toxicities and hepatitis also may occur. The role of excessive doses, plasma concentration monitoring, and metabolic capability (i.e., rapid or slow acetylation of SMX)

Table 70-4 Treatment of *Pneumocystis carinii* Pneumonia

Regimen	Dose	Route	Adverse Effects/Comments
Approved			
TMP-SMX	5 mg/kg TMP + 25 mg/kg SMX Q 6–8 hr × 21 days (2 DS tablets Q 8 hr)	IV, PO	Hypersensitivity, rash, fever, neutropenia ↑ LFTs, nephrotoxicity (15 mg/kg/day preferred to 20 mg/kg/day because of reduced toxicity)
Pentamidine isethionate	4 mg/kg IV daily over 60–90 min × 21 days	IV	Pancreatitis, hypotension, hypoglycemia, hyperglycemia, nephrotoxicity
Trimetrexate + leucovorin	45 mg/m² IV/day × 21 days 20 mg/m² PO or IV Q 6 hr × 24 days	IV PO/IV	Hematologic, GI, CNS, rash
Atovaquone[a]	750 mg BID with meals × 21 days (suspension)	PO	Headache, nausea, diarrhea, rash, fever, ↑ LFTs
Trimethoprim[a] + dapsone	15 mg/kg/day	PO	Pruritus, GI intolerance, bone marrow suppression
	100 mg/day × 21 days	PO	Methemoglobinemia, hemolytic anemia (contraindicated in G6PD deficiency)
Clindamycin + primaquine	600 mg IV Q 8 hr or 300–450 mg PO Q 6 hr	PO or IV	Rash, diarrhea
	15–30 mg (base) daily × 21 days	PO	Methemoglobinemia, hemolytic anemia (contraindicated in G6PD deficiency)
Prednisone	Within 72 hr of anti-*Pneumocystis* therapy 40 mg Q 12 hr × 5 days, then 40 mg QD × 5 days then 20 mg/day × 11 days	PO	Initiation in patients with moderately severe or severe disease Po₂ <70 mm Hg or A-a gradient >35 mm Hg
Investigational			
Difluoromethylornithine (DFMO, eflornithine)	400 mg/kg daily by continuous infusion or in four divided doses × 41–21 days, followed by 4-6 wk oral therapy	IV	Myelosuppression, GI toxicity

Used only in mild to moderate PCP.

CNS, central nervous system; DS, double strength; GI, gastrointestinal; G6PD, glucose-6 phosphate dehydrogenase; IV, intravenous; PCP, *Pneumocystis carinii* pneumonia; PO, oral; LFTs, liver function tests; TMP-SMX, trimethoprim-sulfamethoxazole.

in the development of hypersensitivity reactions remains unclear and is under investigation.[66,67] Most patients who develop a mild hypersensitivity (skin rash) reaction can be managed with antipruritics or antihistamines without discontinuation of TMP-SMX. In some patients with mild hypersensitivity reactions the agent can be restarted after the rash has resolved, using gradual dosage escalation or rapid oral desensitization to reduce adverse effects (Table 70-5).[68] Patients with severe adverse reactions should be switched to another agent rather than being rechallenged with this drug.

Because J.R. appears to have a mild to moderate case of PCP (Po₂, 80 mm Hg), has not previously experienced an episode of PCP, and has no history of adverse effects to TMP-SMX, an outpatient course of TMP-SMX would be reasonable.

Alternatives to TMP-SMX

3. J.R. experienced exfoliative dermatitis on day 7 of TMP-SMX treatment. What other drugs could be prescribed to treat his PCP?

Because J.R. presents with a significant adverse effect to TMP-SMX, it should be discontinued and he should not be rechallenged or desensitized. Instead, he should be treated with an alternative regimen (see Table 70-2).[70]

IV pentamidine isethionate can be used to treat acute PCP. The mechanism of action against the organism is unknown but may be related to interference with oxidative phosphorylation, inhibition of nucleic acid biosynthesis, or interference with dihydrofolate reductase. Pentamidine generally is more toxic than TMP-SMX.[70,72] In a 5-year review of 106 courses of IV pentamidine, 76 (72%) had adverse reactions (nephrotoxicity, dysglycemia, hepatotoxicity, hyperkalemia, and hyperamylasemia). Drug discontinuation occurred in 31 (18%) of the severe cases. Nephrotoxicity and hypoglycemia were the most common causes of drug discontinuation. Nephrotoxicity occurred in 25% to 50% of the patients and was associated with dehydration and concurrent use of nephrotoxic drugs. Hypoglycemia was noted in 5% to 10% of patients after 5 to 7 days of treatment, or several days after discontinuation of treatment. Hyperglycemia is a consequence of de-

Table 70-5 TMP-SMX Desensitization Schedule

Time

Hours: Rapid TMP-SMX Desensitization Schedule[a]

0	0.004/0.02 mg	1:100,000 (5 mL)
1	0.04/0.2 mg	1:1,000 (5 mL)
2	0.4/2.0 mg	1:100 (5 mL)
3	4/20 mg	1:10 (5 mL)
4	40/200 mg	5 mL
5	160/800 mg	Tablet

Days: Eight Day TMP-SMX Desensitization Schedule (QID)[b,c]

1	1:1,000,000
2	1:100,000
3	1:10,000
4	1:1,000
5	1:100
6	1:10
7	1:1
8	Standard suspension—1 mL
≥9	1 DS tablet/day

[a]Serial 10-fold dilutions were given hourly over a 4-hour period.
[b]TMP-SMX given four times daily for 7 days in doses of 1 mL, 2 mL, 4 mL, and 8 mL in accordance with dilution schedule.
[c]40 mg/TMP, 200 mg SMX/5 mL.
Adapted from references 67 and 68.

creased β-cells and results in diabetes mellitus in 2% to 9% of patients. Other less common adverse effects and toxicities include thrombocytopenia, orthostatic hypotension, ventricular tachycardia, leukopenia, nausea, vomiting, abdominal pain, and anorexia.[72]

Patients receiving IV pentamidine should be monitored closely, and serum concentrations of glucose, potassium, blood urea nitrogen (BUN), and creatinine should be obtained daily or Q other day during treatment. Other tests for periodic monitoring include a complete blood count (CBC), LFTs, amylase, lipase, and calcium.[72] Renal toxicity often responds to a reduction in the dosage of pentamidine to 3 mg/kg per day or 4 mg/kg Q 48 hr (creatinine clearance <10 mL/min); however, the drug should be discontinued in patients who develop signs and symptoms of pancreatitis. Risk factors for pentamidine-induced pancreatitis include prior episodes of pancreatitis and concurrent therapy with other drugs known to cause pancreatitis. The prior use of didanosine or stavudine may be a risk factor for pancreatitis during pentamidine therapy.[73]

The daily pentamidine dose of 4 mg/kg is based on clinical tolerance rather than target plasma concentrations. The exact mechanisms for elimination of pentamidine are not well understood. The drug is not excreted by renal mechanisms, and no metabolites have been identified.[71] The half-life of pentamidine is prolonged with multiple dosing and may increase up to 12 days after the last dose.[71] Nebulized pentamidine should not be considered as an alternative to IV pentamidine.

Trimetrexate (Neutrexin), a lipid-soluble derivative of methotrexate, is a highly potent inhibitor of dihydrofolate reductase. It was first studied as salvage therapy in patients failing to respond to available drugs. The ability of trimetrexate to enhance survival in these often-fatal situations gave hope to the future of this treatment. However, results of subsequent studies have not been as promising. Nonetheless, trimetrexate has been approved for patients with moderately severe and severe cases of PCP who are intolerant or unresponsive to TMP-SMX.[75] Most clinicians reserve trimetrexate for hospitalized patients intolerant of both TMP-SMX and IV pentamidine. Serious complications associated with trimetrexate administration include bone marrow suppression, oral or GI ulcerations, renal dysfunction, and hepatotoxicity. Patients receiving trimetrexate should be monitored for myelosuppression with daily CBCs and platelet counts. They should also be given leucovorin (80 mg/m² daily) to counteract trimetrexate-associated leukopenias. Leucovorin should be continued for 3 to 5 days after completion of trimetrexate therapy (45 mg/m² IV once daily over 60 to 90 minutes for 21 days).[75] Comparative studies with TMP-SMX demonstrate faster resolution of the A-a oxygen gradient and overall superiority of TMP-SMX.[75,76]

Atovaquone (Mepron) suspension, 750 mg twice a day, is available for treatment of mild to moderate PCP.[76–81] Atovaquone interrupts protozoan pyrimidine synthesis and demonstrates activity against *P. carinii* and *Toxoplasma gondii* in animal models. Thus, this compound may benefit patients with more than one OI. Atovaquone is approved by the U.S. Food and Drug Administration (FDA) for the treatment of mild to moderate PCP in patients intolerant of TMP-SMX. Atovaquone is also an alternative for primary and secondary prophylaxis for both PCP and toxoplasmosis.[49] Atovaquone is well tolerated compared with other PCP therapies. Adverse effects include rash, fever, increased LFTs, and emesis. A comparative study with oral TMP-SMX in patients with mild to moderate PCP demonstrated fewer side effects with atovaquone but greater efficacy with TMP-SMX.[80] When compared with IV pentamidine in the treatment of mild to moderate PCP, atovaquone and pentamidine were equally efficacious, but significantly more toxicities occurred with pentamidine.[81] Most atovaquone studies were performed using the moderately absorbed oral tablets; reformulation of this drug as a suspension has improved bioavailability by at least 30%. Concomitant administration of fatty foods with atovaquone doubles the absorption.

An oral regimen of dapsone plus trimethoprim is another alternative to TMP-SMX. Dapsone-trimethoprim can be used to treat mild to moderate PCP in patients intolerant of TMP-SMX. Dapsone is a sulfone antimicrobial that is used for leprosy. Although monotherapy (200 mg daily) with dapsone is ineffective for the treatment (not prophylaxis) of PCP, the addition of TMP (20 mg/kg daily) to dapsone (100 mg/day) is an effective alternative regimen.[76,82] In a small comparative trial of TMP-dapsone versus TMP-SMX, response rates of 93% and 90% were observed, respectively.[85] When dapsone is coadministered with TMP, the resulting plasma concentrations for both drugs are higher than when either drug is taken alone. In combination with TMP, a pyrimidine, synergistic inhibition of folic acid synthesis occurs.[83] Dapsone-TMP should not be used in sulfonamide-allergic patients with a history of type I hypersensitivity reaction, toxic epidermal necrolysis, or Stevens-Johnson syndrome. Dapsone is associated with hematologic toxicities, including hemolytic anemia, methemoglobinemia, neutropenia, and thrombocytopenia. Patients with glucose-6-phosphate dehydrogenase (G6PD) deficiency cannot detoxify hydrogen peroxide[84] and are at an increased risk for hematologic toxicity from dapsone.

Clindamycin-primaquine has activity in animal models against *P. carinii*. A few trials with small sample sizes have reported success rates of 70% to 100% with clindamycin (600 mg IV Q 6 hr or 600 mg orally three times a day) given in conjunction with 30 mg/day of primaquine base. Although skin rashes are common with this combination, they often subside with continued therapy. Some patients experience toxicities (fever, rash, granulocytopenia, and methemoglobinemia) requiring discontinuation.[76,84,86] As with dapsone, before starting primaquine, patients should be screened for G6PD deficiency. Patients who test positive for G6PD deficiency are at risk for developing hemolytic anemia.[84]

A double-blind efficacy and toxicity study of 181 patients with mild to moderate PCP compared three oral drug regimens: TMP-SMX versus dapsone-TMP versus clindamycin-primaquine. The doses of TMP-SMX and dapsone-TMP were weight based, and the dosage of clindamycin-primaquine was 600 mg clindamycin three times daily and primaquine 30 mg daily. All patients with moderately severe PCP (A-a oxygen gradient >45) were treated with prednisone (40 mg twice daily for 5 days, then once daily for 3 weeks). The three groups differed in toxicities. Rash was the most frequent dose-limiting toxicity: TMP-SMX, 19%; dapsone-TMP, 10%; clindamycin-primaquine, 21% ($P = 0.2$). Hematologic toxicities were observed more frequently in the clindamycin-primaquine arm. Elevated LFTs (five times above baseline) were more frequent in the TMP-SMX arm ($P = 0.003$). The clindamycin-primaquine group demonstrated better quality of life scores at day 7, but by day 21 these differences became less significant.[87] TMP-SMX, dapsone-TMP, and clindamycin-primaquine demonstrated equal efficacy in patients with mild to moderate PCP.

J.R. should be hospitalized to better manage his severe adverse reaction and to complete his treatment of PCP. Because of his severe reaction to TMP-SMX, dapsone-TMP will not be administered because dapsone is a sulfone with a high risk of cross-reaction in patients who present with severe sulfa allergies. IV pentamidine is an option for J.R., but it is associated with an extensive adverse effect profile and should be reserved for patients with a more severe PCP presentation. Trimetrexate is used as a parenteral alternative to treat severe PCP in patients who are intolerant of or not responsive to TMP-SMX and IV pentamidine. Although it may be better tolerated, it is not as potent as TMP-SMX or IV pentamidine. Atovaquone is a reasonable option for patients with mild PCP who are intolerant to TMP-SMX and have no evidence of GI dysfunction, but it is not as effective as TMP-SMX or IV pentamidine. Clindamycin-primaquine is as efficacious as TMP-SMX for the treatment of mild to moderate PCP and can be administered orally. Consequently, it is the drug of choice in this patient.

The decision was made to start J.R. on oral clindamycin-primaquine for his mild to moderate PCP. J.R. tested negative for G6PD deficiency and was treated with clindamycin- primaquine for 14 days, completing a 21-day course of PCP therapy (see Table 70-3).

Initiation of Corticosteroids

4. Should J.R. receive corticosteroid therapy with PCP treatment? When should corticosteroids be initiated, and what would be a reasonable regimen for patients with PCP?

Corticosteroids have an important role in the management of patients with acute PCP who are clinically ill and have a low Po_2 <70 mm Hg or (A-a) oxygen gradient >35.[88–91] Many patients who are started on PCP therapy have an acute period of clinical deterioration, which may be associated with an acute inflammatory reaction to the rapid killing of *Pneumocystis* organisms. Particularly among patients with moderate to severe PCP ([A-a] oxygen gradient >35 mm Hg or Po_2 <70 mm Hg on room air), the use of prednisone during the first 72 hours of treatment may prevent fatal acute deterioration.[93] Preliminary data suggest that corticosteroids may also have some benefit in patients exhibiting acute respiratory failure after 72 hours of conventional PCP therapy.[94] The recommended dosing of prednisone is 40 mg given orally twice daily for 5 days, then 40 mg/day for 5 days, and then 20 mg/day for 11 days, for a total of 21 days. Patients requiring IV corticosteroids may receive methylprednisolone at 75% of the prednisone dose. The impact of this therapy on further immunosuppression has not been clearly defined. The major concern is activation of latent infections (such as TB) or exacerbation of an active undiagnosed condition (especially fungal infections). However, the beneficial role of corticosteroids as adjunctive therapy outweighs the relative risk of short-term steroid use in this population.[92] More common side effects of short-term corticosteroids include ulcerative esophagitis, increased appetite, weight gain, sodium and fluid retention, headache, and elevated LFTs. While corticosteroids are being given, it may be prudent for patients with a history of candidiasis to receive suppressive fluconazole therapy; those with a positive TB skin test should receive suppressive TB therapy. Corticosteroids should be used with caution in the presence of uncontrolled diabetes, active GI bleeding, and uncontrolled hypertension.

Considering his mild hypoxemia (Po_2 >70 mm Hg), J.R. is not a candidate for corticosteroid therapy.

Prophylaxis

5. J.R. was hospitalized and responded well to treatment. He now is a candidate for secondary prophylaxis. What secondary prophylaxis would be a good choice for J.R. when he is discharged from the hospital?

The early recognized efficacy of TMP-SMX prophylaxis[44] led to the eventual widespread application of prophylaxis and the development of guidelines for PCP prophylaxis (see Tables 70-2 and 70-6).[49,95,96] A clear relationship between the CD4+ count and the occurrence of PCP led researchers to conclude that most of the initial episodes of PCP could be prevented or delayed by instituting primary prophylaxis. Studies that examined HIV-infected patients who were not receiving antiretroviral agents or antimicrobial prophylaxis observed a PCP prevalence of 8.4%, 18.4%, and 33.3% at 6, 12, and 36 months, respectively, in patients with a CD4+ count of <200.[97] These data have formed the basis on which patients receive PCP prophylaxis. In addition to patients with CD4+ counts of <200, other patients at risk for PCP include those with a CD4+ count of <14%, a history of an AIDS-defining illness, a history of oropharyngeal candidiasis, and possibly those with CD4+ counts of 200 to 250.[49] J.R. refused primary prophylaxis and developed PCP. Since the expected relapse

Table 70-6 Antibiotic Regimens for Prophylaxis of *Pneumocystis carinii* Pneumonia

Regimen	Dose	Route
Approved		
TMP-SMX	160 mg TMP + 800 mg SMX daily, BID or 3 × wk (1 DS/day, 1 SS/day or 1 DS 3 × wk)	PO
Dapsone	50 mg BID or 100 mg QD	PO
Dapsone plus	50 mg/day	PO
pyrimethamine plus	50 mg/wk	PO
leucovorin	25 mg/wk	
Dapsone plus	200 mg/wk	
pyrimethamine plus	75 mg/wk	
leucovorin	25 mg/wk	
Aerosolized pentamadine isethionate	300 mg every month	Via Respirgard II nebulizer
Atovaquone	1,500 mg QD	PO
Investigational		
Pentamidine isethionate	2 wk induction (5 doses), then 60 mg 2 × wk	By Fisoneb nebulizer
Pentamidine isethionate	4 mg/kg 4 × wk	IV/IM
Atovaquone suspension	750 mg/day	PO
Pyrimethamine plus[a] sulfadoxine	25 mg/day	PO
Clindamycin plus primaquine	500 mg 1–2 × wk or 3 × month	
plus dapsone	150 mg QID	PO
Trimetrexate plus leucovorin	15 mg primaquine base daily	
	50 mg daily	
	Less than treatment doses	IV

[a]Fansidar is rarely used because of severe hypersensitivity reaction.
DS, double strength; IM, intramuscularly; IV, intravenously; PO, orally; SS, single strength.

rate without prophylaxis among patients (before the use of protease inhibitors) has been documented to be 66% at 12 months' follow-up, secondary prophylaxis is necessary for J.R. to prevent recurrence.

The same agents and dosing schedules are recommended for primary (before an acute event) and secondary (after an acute event) prophylaxis of PCP.[49,100–102] TMP-SMX, one double-strength tablet daily, is the most efficacious prophylactic regimen; a single-strength tablet daily is less toxic and nearly as efficacious.[105] Anti-*Pneumocystis* prophylaxis (TMP-SMX or dapsone) increases survival by 9 to 12 months, improves quality of life, and decreases hospitalization.[26,29,43,49] Patients with a history of non–life-threatening rash or fever due to TMP-SMX, such as J.R., may benefit from rechallenge with the original (or half) dose, or a dose-escalation technique (desensitization regimen). Desensitization is preferred over switching to an alternative agent and appears to be more successful than the direct rechallenge method.[98,99] Desensitization involves initiating very low doses of TMP-SMX and gradually increasing to the maximum dose over days to weeks (see Table 70-5).

The alternative agents used for prophylaxis include dapsone alone, dapsone plus pyrimethamine (with leucovorin), atovaquone suspension, and aerosolized pentamidine administered by the Respirgard II nebulizer (see Tables 70-2 and 70-6). TMP-SMX confers additional protection against toxoplasmosis and certain bacterial infections. Regimens containing dapsone plus pyrimethamine or atovaquone with or without pyrimethamine also protect against toxoplasmosis.[49,70,100–102] Investigational prophylaxis agents with unproven efficacy include

oral clindamycin-primaquine, intermittently administered IV pentamidine, oral pyrimethamine-sulfadiazine, IV trimetrexate, and aerosolized pentamidine administered by other nebulizing devices.[49] TMP-SMX is more efficacious than dapsone or aerosolized pentamidine in the prevention of PCP.[100]

Extrapulmonary (e.g., lymph nodes, spleen, liver, bone marrow, adrenal gland, GI tract) *P. carinii* has been noted in patients receiving inhaled pentamidine prophylaxis,[103,104] a finding rarely observed with IV administration. In addition, aerosolized pentamidine alters the usual chest radiograph findings associated with PCP, complicating the diagnosis of this disease. Upper lobe infiltrates, cystic lesions, pneumothoraces, cavitary lesions with nodular infiltrates, and pleural effusions have been associated with aerosolized pentamidine prophylaxis. Pentamidine prophylaxis is more expensive than TMP-SMX or dapsone but less expensive than atovaquone suspension.

The current guidelines for primary prophylaxis indicate that it may be possible to discontinue prophylactic antimicrobial therapy when CD4$^+$ counts rise above the threshold associated with risk for infection (i.e., <200 for PCP).[49–53,106] Reports from three observational studies, one randomized trial, and a combined analysis of eight prospectively followed European cohorts support discontinuing secondary PCP prophylaxis in patients whose CD4$^+$ counts have increased to >200 for at least 3 months.[107–112] The most recent guidelines recommend that prophylaxis be reintroduced if the CD4$^+$ count decreases to <200, or if PCP recurs at a CD4$^+$ count of >200.

J.R. responded well to his PCP treatment with clindamycin-primaquine in the hospital. However, because this regimen is unproven for secondary prophylaxis, it cannot be recommended. Considering his intolerance to TMP-SMX, the best selections would be dapsone (with or without pyrimethamine) or atovaquone suspension.

Children

The prophylaxis of PCP in children needs further clinical research. The CD4$^+$ threshold of 200 is unreliable in infants because they have higher normal values for lymphocyte counts. The current guidelines recommend administering primary PCP prophylaxis to (1) HIV-infected or HIV-indeterminate children born to HIV-infected mothers aged 1 to 12 months (prophylaxis should be discontinued for children subsequently determined not to be infected with HIV); (2) HIV-infected children ages 1 to 5 years with a CD4$^+$ count <500 or CD4$^+$ percentage <15%; and (3) HIV-infected children ages 6 to 12 years old with a CD4$^+$ count <200 or CD4$^+$ percentage <15%. The recommended regimen is oral TMP-SMX (150/750 mg/m^2 per day) twice daily three times a week on consecutive days. Acceptable alternative dosing strategies include a single oral dose given three times a week on consecutive days, or two divided doses daily, or two divided doses three times per week on alternate days. HIV-infected children with a history of PCP should be administered lifelong secondary prophylaxis to prevent recurrence, since the safety of discontinuing secondary prophylaxis among HIV-infected children has not been studied extensively.[49]

Pregnancy

Primary and secondary PCP prophylaxis is recommended for all HIV-infected women who are pregnant. TMP-SMX is the recommended agent, and dapsone is an alternative. Because of the theoretical risk of teratogenicity from drug exposure during the first trimester, withholding prophylaxis until the second trimester may be considered. As an alternative during this time, aerosolized pentamidine is not systemically absorbed and may be administered during the first trimester.[49]

TOXOPLASMA ENCEPHALITIS

Clinical Presentation

6 W.O. is a 40-year-old man discovered to be HIV positive during admission to a detoxification program for alcohol and heroin dependency. W.O. presented to the AIDS clinic with esophageal candidiasis, a CD4$^+$ count of 60 cells/mm^3 (normal, approximately 1,000 cells/mm^3), a viral load of 150,000 copies/mL, and a *Toxoplasma* immunoglobulin G (IgG) titer of 1:256. W.O. was started on HAART therapy. He remained well until 2 years later, when he presented to the emergency department (ED) reporting two seizures in the past 24 hours. His medications at that time included daily indinavir, stavudine, didanosine, and inhaled pentamidine 300 mg monthly. His temperature was 100.1°F, and he was observed to have difficulty walking. His CD4$^+$ count is 90 cells/mm^3 (previously 230 cells/mm^3), viral load is 70,000 copies/mL (previously 4,000), and white blood cell (WBC) count is 4,200 cells/L (normal, 3,800 to 9,800). A magnetic resonance image (MRI) of the head reveals several ring-shaped lesions in the brain stem. *Toxoplasma* encephalitis is presumptively diagnosed. Should W.O. be isolated from other patients and health care workers to prevent the spread of this organism?

Toxoplasma gondii is a parasitic protozoan that can infect people and is spread by environmental factors, such as the consumption of raw or undercooked meats and contact with cats. Immunocompetent persons infected with *T. gondii* may develop mild symptoms resembling infectious mononucleosis. However, these symptoms are generally transient and associated with minimal problems (except in pregnant women). Recrudescent disease from *T. gondii* is problematic in patients with a suppressed cellular immune system, including those infected with HIV. Any HIV-positive patient infected with *T. gondii* is at risk for developing clinical disease, particularly at CD4$^+$ counts <100, as illustrated by W.O.[113,114] W.O. presents with encephalitis (an inflammation of the brain or brain stem), the most frequent manifestation of *T. gondii* in HIV-positive patients.

All HIV-infected patients should be tested for IgG antibody to *T. gondii* following HIV diagnosis to detect latent infection. In the United States, as many as 70% of healthy adults are seropositive to *Toxoplasma*. The prevalence of *Toxoplasma* encephalitis among HIV-positive patients varies depending on the geographic region. In the United States, only 3% to 10% of AIDS patients actually develop encephalitis. In countries such as France, El Salvador, and Tahiti, where uncooked meat commonly is ingested, seropositivity is >90% by the fourth decade of life. *Toxoplasma* encephalitis may develop in as many as 25% to 50% of AIDS patients in these countries.[113]

The two major routes of transmission of *Toxoplasma* to humans are oral and congenital. W.O. need not be isolated from other patients and health care workers. HIV-infected patients should be advised not to eat raw and undercooked meat (internal temperature of meat should be at least 165 to 170°F), especially patients who are IgG negative for *T. gondii*. Patients should wash their hands after touching uncooked meats and soil, and fruits and vegetables must be washed before eating. HIV-infected patients should avoid stray cats, keep their cats inside, and change the litter box daily. If no one else is available to change the litter box, patients should wash their hands thoroughly afterwards.[49]

Diagnosis

7 Is there sufficient clinical evidence to establish a presumptive diagnosis of *Toxoplasma* encephalitis in W.O.?

The diagnosis of *Toxoplasma* encephalitis usually is presumptive because demonstration of cysts or trophozoites in brain tissue is required for a definitive diagnosis. The clinical signs and symptoms of *Toxoplasma* encephalitis can be either focal (indicating a specific region of the brain that is infected or inflamed) or generalized (indicating diffuse inflammation of the brain). *Toxoplasma* encephalitis usually occurs in patients with CD4$^+$ counts of <100. Serum titers of antibodies against *T. gondii* typically reflect past infection with the organism and unfortunately do not help delineate whether acute infection is present. Without prophylaxis, 45% of seropositive HIV-infected patients will develop encephalitis as a reactivation of a latent infection. Most patients with encephalitis have single or multiple lesions demonstrated on computed tomography scan or MRI of the head. Brain biopsy is reserved for patients with symptoms of encephalitis who are seronegative and for those who do not respond to presumptive antitoxoplasmosis therapy.[113–115] Because of the nonspecific diagnosis of *Toxoplasma* encephalitis, a high index of suspicion for other causes of encephalitis (e.g., central nervous system [CNS] lymphoma or TB) should be maintained throughout the treatment period for presumed *Toxoplasma* encephalitis.[116] W.O. has overwhelming clinical evidence suggestive of *Toxoplasma* encephalitis. He is HIV positive, with a CD4$^+$ count of <100, and he has a positive *Toxoplasma* titer of 1:256 IgG and a ring-shaped lesion in the brain stem on MRI. The development of this infection, in addition to the decline in CD4$^+$ T cells and the increase in plasma HIV RNA concentrations, may signal antiretroviral failure. W.O.'s current antiretroviral therapy should be reassessed, including his adherence to the regimen.

Prophylaxis

8. **Should W.O. have been receiving prophylactic therapy for *T. gondii*?**

Similar to many other OIs associated with HIV, therapy for toxoplasmosis can be categorized into primary prophylaxis, treatment of acute disease, and secondary prophylaxis. Primary prophylaxis is currently recommended in HIV-infected patients with CD4$^+$ counts of <100 who are also IgG positive for *T. gondii* (see Table 70-2). Many of the agents used to prevent PCP have activity against *T. gondii* and afford protection: TMP-SMX, dapsone-pyrimethamine, and atovaquone with or without pyrimethamine are effective as primary prophylaxis for *T. gondii*.[49,117–120] The increased use of PCP prophylaxis with these agents has significantly decreased the incidence of *Toxoplasma* encephalitis.[2,29] The double-strength TMP-SMX tablet daily dose is recommended as first-line prophylaxis. Current data do not support the use of macrolides or aerosolized pentamidine for *Toxoplasma* prophylaxis. Similarly, data are conflicting regarding the efficacy of pyrimethamine as monotherapy for primary prophylaxis.[121,122]

Primary prophylaxis may be discontinued in patients who have responded to HAART with an increase in the CD4$^+$ counts to >200 for >3 months. Multiple observational studies[123–125] and two randomized trials[126,127] have reported minimal risk in discontinuing *Toxoplasma* encephalitis prophylaxis in these patients. In these studies, median follow-up ranged from 7 to 22 months. Primary prophylaxis should be reinstituted when CD4$^+$ counts drop below 200.

W.O. is currently receiving inhaled pentamidine for PCP prophylaxis. Because of the localized delivery of inhaled pentamidine, this agent has no anti-toxoplasmosis activity, so W.O. was at risk for the development of *Toxoplasma* encephalitis. Considering his CD4$^+$ count and IgG seropositivity, he should have received primary prophylaxis for *T. gondii*.

Treatment

Acute Therapy

9. **How should W.O.'s presumptive *Toxoplasma* encephalitis be treated?**

Approximately 80% of patients with acute *Toxoplasma* encephalitis can be treated successfully with a combination of sulfadiazine 4 g/day in three or four daily divided doses and pyrimethamine as a single 200-mg loading dose, followed by 50 mg/day as a single daily dose plus leucovorin 10 to 25 mg orally Q day.[113,114] Induction therapy should be continued for 6 weeks after resolution of symptoms (a treatment course of approximately 8 weeks) followed by maintenance therapy (secondary prophylaxis). Sulfadiazine toxicity may limit the completion of a full course of therapy in as many as 40% of patients.[129] However, successful desensitization has been documented.[130] W.O.'s clinical and radiologic response should be monitored closely and other diagnoses considered if there is no improvement.

Alternative therapy includes pyrimethamine plus leucovorin with clindamycin 600 to 900 mg IV Q 6 to 8 hr or 300 to 450 mg orally Q 6 hr for at least 6 weeks. One controlled trial compared the efficacy and tolerability of pyrimethamine plus sulfadiazine versus pyrimethamine plus clindamycin. Although both regimens were effective, pyrimethamine-sulfadiazine was found to be superior to pyrimethamine-clindamycin. The risk of progression of *Toxoplasma* encephalitis was higher for patients who received pyrimethamine-clindamycin therapy. Furthermore, the rate of relapse was twice as high in the pyrimethamine-clindamycin group. The rate of side effects was similar with both regimens; however, pyrimethamine-clindamycin led to fewer discontinuations than pyrimethamine-sulfadiazine (11% versus 30%, respectively).[131]

10. **W.O. is treated with sulfadiazine-pyrimethamine. What are the limitations to the use of the sulfadiazine component for the treatment of *Toxoplasma* encephalitis?**

As with other sulfonamides in HIV patients, rashes commonly occur with sulfadiazine therapy.[129] Similar to TMP-SMX, various desensitization regimens have been recommended[68,130]; however, it may be simpler to use alternative regimens.

Renal function should be monitored throughout therapy.[132–136] Elevated serum creatinine levels, hematuria, or decreased urine output may occur secondary to sulfadiazine-induced crystalluria. The water solubility of sulfadiazine is less than that of other sulfonamides; therefore, hydration (2 to 3 L daily) is needed to prevent crystalline nephropathy, and aggressive hydration and alkalinization can be used in cases of crystal formation. Although few manufacturers market sulfadiazine, this drug is available from the CDC and from Eon Labs Manufacturing, Inc.[137,138]

11. **What toxicities are associated with the pyrimethamine component?**

Pyrimethamine can suppress bone marrow function; thus, concomitant therapy with other medications that suppress marrow function (e.g., zidovudine [AZT] or ganciclovir) may not be tolerated. Leucovorin (10 to 25 mg/day) is always given in conjunction with pyrimethamine to maintain bone marrow function, although it may not always be successful. Folic acid (not folinic acid) should be avoided because it can be used for growth by protozoal organisms, potentially antagonizing pyrimethamine-sulfadiazine activity.[139–141] Vitamin preparations containing large quantities of folic acid should be discontinued during therapy for *T. gondii*.

W.O. is not taking any medications that would make him particularly susceptible to the myelosuppressive effects of pyrimethamine and he is not neutropenic. Consequently, he should be given sulfadiazine and pyrimethamine.

Suppressive Therapy (Secondary Prophylaxis)

12. **Once W.O. has completed acute therapy for his** *Toxoplasma* **encephalitis, should he receive suppressive therapy?**

Most antiprotozoal agents do not eradicate the cyst form of *T. gondii*. Therefore, patients should be administered lifelong suppressive therapy unless immune reconstitution occurs as a consequence of HAART. The combination of pyrimethamine plus sulfadiazine plus leucovorin is very effective. Pyrimethamine (25 to 75 mg/day) plus sulfadiazine (500 to 1,000 mg orally four times daily) plus leucovorin is significantly more efficacious than taking this combination twice weekly.[142] A commonly used regimen for patients who cannot tolerate sulfa drugs is pyrimethamine plus clindamycin.[131] However, only the combination of pyrimethamine plus sulfadiazine provides protection against PCP as well. Additionally, one retrospective chart review of 35 patients receiving maintenance therapy for *Toxoplasma* encephalitis suggested that sulfadiazine-pyrimethamine was more effective than clindamycin-pyrimethamine or pyrimethamine alone.[143] Low-dose, intermittent pyrimethamine monotherapy has been associated with an unacceptably high rate of mortality.[144]

Patients receiving secondary prophylaxis are at low risk for recurrence of *Toxoplasma* encephalitis when they have completed initial therapy for *Toxoplasma* encephalitis, remain asymptomatic, and have a sustained increase in their CD4+ count to >200 after HAART therapy for >6 months. Clinicians may obtain an MRI of the brain as part of the evaluation to determine whether to discontinue therapy. Secondary prophylaxis should be reintroduced if the CD4+ count decreases to <200.

Children aged >12 months who qualify for PCP prophylaxis and who are receiving an agent other than TMP-SMX or atovaquone should have serologic testing for *Toxoplasma* antibody. Severely immunosuppressed children who are not receiving TMP-SMX or atovaquone who are found to be seropositive for *Toxoplasma* should receive prophylaxis for both PCP and toxoplasmosis (i.e., dapsone plus pyrimethamine). Children with a history of toxoplasmosis should be given lifelong prophylaxis to prevent recurrence. The safety of discontinuing primary or secondary prophylaxis among HIV-infected children receiving HAART has not been studied extensively.

In pregnancy, TMP-SMX can be administered for prophylaxis against *Toxoplasma* encephalitis as described for PCP. Because of the possible risk associated with pyrimethamine treatment and the low incidence of *Toxoplasma* endocarditis during pregnancy, chemoprophylaxis with pyrimethamine-containing regimens can reasonably be deferred until after pregnancy. In rare cases, HIV-infected pregnant women who have serologic evidence of toxoplasmic infection have transmitted *Toxoplasma* to the fetus in utero. However, there are no specific guidelines for continuing secondary prophylaxis during pregnancy. Pregnant HIV-infected women who have active toxoplasmosis or evidence of a primary toxoplasmic infection should be evaluated and managed in consultation with appropriate specialists. Infants born to women who have serologic evidence of infections with HIV and *Toxoplasma* should be evaluated for congenital toxoplasmosis.

W.O. will be continued on sulfadiazine-pyrimethamine for suppressive therapy for his *Toxoplasma* encephalitis since his CD4+ count has decreased to <100. W.O. is currently receiving aerosolized pentamidine for PCP prophylaxis, but since sulfadiazine-pyrimethamine is also protective against PCP, the aerosolized pentamidine can be discontinued. Clindamycin-pyrimethamine is an inferior option because it does not protect against PCP.[49,131]

Alternative Therapies

13. **What treatment options exist for patients who cannot tolerate sulfadiazine and do not wish to undergo desensitization?**

Clindamycin can be substituted for sulfadiazine in the acute treatment of toxoplasmosis (900 to 1,200 mg IV Q 6 hr or 300 to 450 mg orally Q 6 hr) plus pyrimethamine and leucovorin at standard doses.[145–149] Monotherapy with atovaquone,[150–154] trimetrexate, and the tetracyclines, doxycycline and minocycline, has been successful.[114–155]

Combination therapy with pyrimethamine and folinic acid plus azithromycin (1.2 to 1.5 g/day), clarithromycin (1 g twice a day), or atovaquone (750 mg orally four times per day) was relatively successful in noncomparative trials with limited numbers of patients.[114,154,156]

CYTOMEGALOVIRUS RETINITIS

Diagnosis

14. **P.Z., a 39-year-old man with AIDS, complains of floating spots, light flashes, and difficulty reading road signs when he drives. His most recent BUN was 17 mg/dL (normal, 8 to 25) and serum creatinine (SrCr) was 0.8 mg/dL (normal, 0.5 to 1.7). His CD4+ count was 40 cells/mm³ (normal, approximately 1,000), and his viral load was 80,000 copies/mL 3 months ago. His current weight is 63 kg. P.Z.'s medications include nelfinavir, stavudine, lamivudine (3TC), dapsone (PCP prophylaxis), and azithromycin (MAC prophylaxis). He has a history of hematologic intolerance to AZT and TMP-SMX. His WBC count is 1,200 cells/L (normal, 3,800 to 9,800) with 63% polymorphonuclear neutrophil leukocytes. P.Z. is known to have a positive CMV IgG antibody titer. Funduscopic examination reveals alternating areas of hemorrhage and scar tissue (a "cottage cheese and ketchup" appearance) in the proximity of the retina in his left eye. What is the likely cause of P.Z.'s visual problems?**

[SI units: BUN, 6.07 mmol/L (normal, 2.9 to 8.9); SrCr, 70.72 µmol/L (normal, 44 to 150); WBC count, 1.2 ×10⁹/L (normal, 3.8 to 9.8) with 0.63 polymorphonuclear neutrophil leukocytes]

P.Z. appears to have an inflammation of the retina (retinitis), most likely because of CMV. Many HIV patients have been previously infected with CMV, and reactivation typically occurs when CD4+ counts are <50. Before HAART, the prevalence of CMV disease in HIV patients with a CD4+ count of <50 was 20% to 40%, and the incidence varied between 15 and 20 per 100 patient-years. Since the introduction of HAART, more than a fivefold decrease in the incidence of CMV disease has been reported by several authors. The current incidence of CMV disease in HIV patients is approximately 3 to 5 per 100 patient-years in the United States.[157] More than 90% of homosexual men are antibody positive. Although CMV can cause colitis, pneumonitis, and hepatitis, retinitis is the most common manifestation of active infection. CMV retinitis in HIV patients accounts for 75% to 85% of CMV end-organ disease. A panel of physicians with clinical and virologic expertise was convened by the International AIDS Society to review the available data and develop recommendations for treatment and diagnosis of CMV disease.[42] Diagnosis is usually presumptive because biopsy is difficult given the inaccessibility of the retina. Serology is indicative of previous CMV infection but not active disease. Cultures (serum, urine, and/or saliva) may be useful for monitoring therapy, considering that patients frequently have disseminated CMV disease. Patients with positive cultures for CMV, while receiving therapy, may be at a higher risk for relapse.[158] Typically, the diagnosis of CMV retinitis is based on observations made during a dilated retinal examination and indirect ophthalmoscopy, as was done for P.Z. Lesions appear as fluffy, white, retinal patches with retinal hemorrhage.

Once CMV retinitis is diagnosed, the patient should be thoroughly examined for extraocular CMV disease. P.Z. will require regular ophthalmologic examinations, along with retinal photographs, for life. As with HIV therapy, CMV-DNA quantification in plasma or blood cells by quantitative branched-chain DNA (b-DNA) or polymerase chain reaction (PCR) may have a role in evaluating treatment efficacy and predicting symptomatic development of CMV disease.[159–161]

Drug Therapy

15. **What are the treatment options for CMV retinitis, and which one would be preferred for P.Z.?**

Several treatment options exist for CMV retinitis: IV ganciclovir, foscarnet, or cidofovir for induction and maintenance therapy. Alternatives include combined IV ganciclovir plus foscarnet, intraocular ganciclovir implants, or intraocular injections of ganciclovir, foscarnet, cidofovir, or fomivirsen sodium (Vitravene).[42,162–164] The efficacy of combined parenteral ganciclovir and foscarnet is similar to monotherapy, but it is more toxic. This latter therapy should be reserved for patients with refractory disease (Table 70-7).[165]

Intraocular implants and intraocular injections of ganciclovir have similar efficacy in the treatment of CMV retinitis, but their benefit is localized and they may lead to an increased risk of contralateral retinitis and extraocular CMV disease. Concomitant systemic anti-CMV therapy is therefore recommended (e.g., oral or IV ganciclovir). The choice of agents typically depends on drug efficacy, toxicity, stage of disease, and quality-of-life issues.

Ganciclovir

Ganciclovir is an acyclic nucleoside with CMV activity superior to acyclovir.[167,168] Similar to other nucleosides, ganciclovir must be taken into cells and phosphorylated before it can compete with endogenous nucleotides for binding to viral DNA polymerase.[169] Ganciclovir is poorly absorbed orally (bioavailability, approximately 5% to 9%) and its disposition is biexponential following IV administration (terminal half-life, approximately 2.5 hours). The total body clearance is highly dependent on glomerular filtration and tubular secretion.[170]

The induction dose of ganciclovir is 5 mg/kg per dose Q 12 hr IV for 14 to 21 days. It is approximately 80% effective in delaying the progression of CMV retinitis.[42,171–173] The dose-limiting toxicity is bone marrow suppression, with neutropenia occurring in approximately 50% of patients. Thrombocytopenia is also observed. Absolute neutrophil counts (ANCs) and platelets should be monitored weekly during ganciclovir therapy. If the ANC falls to $<1,000$ cells/mm^3 or the platelet count to $<50,000/$ mm^3, the monitoring frequency should be increased to twice weekly.[42,174] Ganciclovir is available in two other dosage forms, oral capsules and an intraocular implant (see Table 70-7).[42,49] Dosage adjustments must be made in patients with renal dysfunction (Table 70-8).

Patients who develop ganciclovir-induced bone marrow suppression can be given granulocyte colony-stimulating factor (G-CSF). Both G-CSF (filgrastim) and granulocyte-macrophage colony-stimulating factor (GM-CSF [sargramostim])[175,176] have been used successfully. Although neither of these agents is FDA approved for this indication, use of the colony-stimulating factors may result in sight-saving or life-prolonging therapy. Because GM-CSF may stimulate HIV replication in macrophage cell lines,[177,178] patients should receive concomitant antiretroviral therapy.

Valgancyclovir

Valganciclovir is an oral monovalyl ester prodrug that is rapidly hydrolyzed to ganciclovir. The absolute bioavailability of ganciclovir from valganciclovir is 60%, and a dose of 900 mg results in ganciclovir blood concentrations similar to those obtained with a dose of 5 mg/kg of IV ganciclovir. The effects of oral valganciclovir to those of IV ganciclovir as induction therapy for newly diagnosed CMV retinitis were recently compared in patients with AIDS.[179] Seventy-seven percent of patients in the IV ganciclovir group and 72% of patients in the valganciclovir group had a satisfactory response to induction therapy. The median times to progression of retinitis were 125 days in the IV ganciclovir group and 160 days in the oral valganciclovir group. The mean values for the area under the curve for the ganciclovir dosage interval were similar at both induction doses and maintenance doses. The frequency and severity of adverse events were similar in the two groups. Based on these data, oral valganciclovir is as effective as IV ganciclovir for induction treatment and is convenient and effective for the long-term management of CMV retinitis in patients with AIDS.

Cidofovir

Cidofovir is a nucleotide analog that is phosphorylated intracellularly to an active diphosphate metabolite. It is the most potent of all the available anti-CMV compounds and is active against herpes simplex virus (HSV) and VZV, including the acyclovir-resistant isolates. Cidofovir does not require viral activation. Because nucleotide analogs do not require virally encoded kinases for their activity, they remain a treatment option for patients who have failed to respond to ganciclovir. Cidofovir is poorly absorbed orally (bioavailability, $<5\%$) and has an intracellular half-life of 17 to 65 hours, resulting in once-weekly induction and every-other-week maintenance therapy. This feature substantially enhances the quality of life relative to foscarnet or ganciclovir, which must be administered much more frequently.

Eighty percent of this poorly soluble agent is excreted unchanged in the urine via filtration and tubular secretion. Cid-

Table 70-7 Treatment of CMV Retinitis[a]

	IV Ganciclovir	IV Foscarnet	Combination IV Ganciclovir and IV Foscarnet Sodium	IV Then Oral Ganciclovir	Intraocular Ganciclovir Implant	IV Cidofovir
Dosing regimens	Induction: 5 mg/kg Q 12 hr for 14–21 days; Maintenance: 5 mg/kg QD; Refractory disease: Induction: 7.5 mg/kg Q 12 hr for 14–21 days; Maintenance: 10 mg/kg QD (Note: dosage should be adjusted for creatinine clearance <70 mL/min, see Table 70-8.)	Induction: 90 mg/kg Q 12 hr for 14–21 days; Maintenance: 90–120 mg/kg QD; 750–1,000 mL of 0.9% saline or D5W solution with each dose	Prior ganciclovir: Induction: both IV foscarnet 90 mg/kg Q 12 hr and IV ganciclovir 5 mg/kg QD for 14–21 days; Maintenance: both IV foscarnet 90–120 mg/kg and IV ganciclovir 5 mg/kg QD; Prior foscarnet sodium: Induction: both IV ganciclovir 5 mg/kg Q 12 hr and IV foscarnet 90–120 mg/kg QD; Reinduction: IV ganciclovir 5 mg/kg and IV foscarnet 90 mg/kg Q 12 hr for 14–21 days	Induction: same as IV ganciclovir; Maintenance: 3,000–6,000 mg/day in 3 divided doses with food	Surgical: intraocular implantation of ganciclovir (4.5 mg) implant releasing 1 µg/hr (duration 6–8 months; then replacement required every 5–8 months)	Induction: 5 mg/kg every wk for 2 wk; Maintenance: 5 mg/kg every 2 wk (Note: dose reduction to 3 mg/kg for ↑ serum creatinine by 0.3–0.4 mg/dL above baseline, all doses given with probenecid and IV fluid)
Select adverse effects	Neutropenia, thrombocytopenia; catheter sepsis	Nephrotoxicity; electrolyte abnormalities; anemia; catheter sepsis; nausea/irritability; genital ulceration	Same as IV ganciclovir and IV foscarnet	Neutropenia/diarrhea/nausea	Surgical complications: transient blurred vision; infection; hemorrhage	Nephrotoxicity; neutropenia; probenecid adverse effects (rash, fever, nausea, fatigue; uveitis; alopecia; hypotonia
Important drug interactions	↑ Neutropenia; with zidovudine, cancer chemotherapy ↑ Didanosine levels	↑ Nephrotoxicity with other nephrotoxic drugs (e.g., amphotericin B, aminoglycosides, IV pentamidine)	Same as IV ganciclovir and IV foscarnet	Same as IV ganciclovir		↑ Nephrotoxicity with other nephrotoxic drugs (e.g., amphotericin B, aminoglycosides, IV pentamidine, NSAIDs) Probenecid: ↑ Level of most proximal tubular-excreted drugs
Adjunctive therapy	G-CSF/GM-CSF effective for neutropenia	IV or oral hydration essential; potassium, calcium/magnesium supplements, antiemetics may be required	Same as both IV ganciclovir and IV foscarnet	Same as IV ganciclovir	Systemic anti-CMV therapy recommended (oral ganciclovir, 4,500 mg/day)	Probenecid and IV hydration essential; antiemetics, antihistamine, acetaminophen premedication commonly used for probenecid toxicity
Advantages	Systemic therapy; anti-HSV activity	Systemic therapy; anti-HSV (acyclovir-resistant) activity; anti-HIV activity	Increased efficacy compared with either IV ganciclovir or IV foscarnet alone; improved response for relapsed disease	Systemic therapy; oral administration; fewer catheter/sepsis complications	Longest time to retinitis progression in treated eye; no IV dosing or catheter required	Systemic therapy; no indwelling catheter required; infrequent dosing

Table 70-7 Treatment of CMV Retinitis[a]

	IV Ganciclovir	IV Foscarnet	Combination IV Ganciclovir and IV Foscarnet Sodium	IV Then Oral Ganciclovir	Intraocular Ganciclovir Implant	IV Cidofovir
Disadvantage	Hematologic toxicity; requires daily infusions; indwelling catheter	Nephrotoxicity; requires daily infusions/indwelling catheter; supplemental hydration required; prolonged infusion time; requires infusion pump or controlled rate infusion device	Same as IV ganciclovir and IV foscarnet; prolonged daily infusion time and impact on quality of life	Faster time to retinitis progression; high pill count; poor oral bioavailability (6%)	↑ Fellow eye and extraocular disease; requires surgery; postintraocular surgical complications	Requires probenecid and IV hydration; probenecid toxicity; nephrotoxicity (may be prolonged)
Monitoring requirement	Induction therapy: (a) CBC with WBC differential, platelet count weekly; (b) serum creatinine weekly Maintenance therapy: (a) CBC with WBC differential, platelet count weekly; (b) Serum creatinine every 2–4 wk	Induction therapy: (a) serum creatinine twice weekly; (b) serum Ca^{++}, albumin Mg^{--}, phosphates, and K$^+$ twice weekly; (c) hemoglobin and hematocrit weekly Maintenance therapy: (a) serum creatinine weekly; (b) serum Ca^{++}, albumin Mg^{--}, phosphates, and K$^+$ weekly; (c) hemoglobin and hematocrit every 2–4 wk	Same as both IV ganciclovir and IV foscarnet	Induction therapy: IV ganciclovir Maintenance therapy: oral ganciclovir (a) CBC with WBC differential, platelet count every 2 wk; (b) serum creatinine every 2–4 wk	No specific laboratory monitoring required for implant; if oral ganciclovir therapy is added, follow monitoring guidelines as outlined	Within 48 hr before each induction and maintenance: (a) serum creatinine quantitation proteinuria; (b) WBC with differential cell count; monitor intraocular pressure and slit-lamp examination at least monthly
Precautions and contraindications	Moderate to severe thrombocytopenia (platelet counts <25 × 10^9/L)	Concomitant use with other nephrotoxic drugs (e.g., amphotericin B, aminoglycosides, or IV pentamadine) or in patients with preexisting moderate to severe renal insufficiency (serum Creatine >168 µmol/L or creatinine clearance <50 mL/min)	Same as both IV ganciclovir and IV foscarnet	Use with caution in patients with immediately sight-threatening (zone 1) retinitis	External ocular or nasolacrimal infection; patients with ↑ risk of postoperative intraocular infection	Same as IV foscarnet except baseline parameters are baseline serum creatinine level (>1.5 mg/dL) or creatinine clearance (<55 mL/min), or 2+ proteinuria (after IV fluid) Discontinue therapy for 3+ proteinuria, if serum creatinine level increases by 0.5 mg/dL above baseline, or intraocular pressure decreases by 50% of baseline value

[a]Fomivirsen intravitreal injection:
Induction therapy: 330 µg (0.05 mL) every other week for 2 doses (day 1 and day 15).
Maintenance dose: 330 µg (0.05 mL) once every 4 weeks (monthly).
Primary adverse effects: uveitis (ocular inflammation); increased intraocular pressure.
Adapted from Consensus Statement: International AIDS Society–USA The Treatment of Cytomegalovirus diseases. *Arch Intern Med* 1998;158:957, and product information.

Table 70-8 Dosage Adjustment for Cytomegalovirus Medications

Drug	Normal Dosage	CrCl (mL/min/1.73 m²)	Adjusted Dosage
Cidofovir	Induction dose: 5 mg/kg IV QW × 2 Maintenance dose: 5 mg/kg IV QOWK	Increase in serum creatinine of 0.3–0.4 above baseline Increase in serum creatinine of 0.5 above baseline or 3+ proteinuria Cidofovir is contraindicated in patients with preexisting renal failure: 1. SrCr concentrations >1.5 mg/dL 2. Calculated CrCl of <55 mL/min 3. Urine protein ≥100 mg/dL (>2+ proteinuria)	3 mg/kg Discontinue cidofovir

Foscarnet

Normal Dosage:
Induction dose:
IV Q 8 hr to 90 mg/kg IV Q 12 hr
Maintenance dose:
90–120 mg/kg IV QD

CrCl (mL/min/kg):	Induction Dose		Maintenance Dose	
	Low Dose	High Dose	Low Dose	High Dose
>1.4	60 mg/kg Q 8 hr	90 mg/kg Q 12 hr	90 mg/kg Q 24 hr	120 mg/kg Q 24 hr
1.0–1.4	45 mg/kg Q 8 hr	70 mg/kg Q 12 hr	70 mg/kg Q 24 hr	90 mg/kg Q 24 hr
0.8–1.0	50 mg/kg Q 12 hr	50 mg/kg Q 12 hr	50 mg/kg Q 24 hr	65 mg/kg Q 24 hr
0.6–0.8	40 mg/kg Q 12 hr	80 mg/kg Q 24 hr	80 mg/kg Q 48 hr	105 mg/kg Q 48 hr
0.5–0.6	60 mg/kg Q 24 hr	60 mg/kg Q 24 hr	60 mg/kg Q 48 hr	80 mg/kg Q 48 hr
0.4–0.5	50 mg/kg Q 24 hr	50 mg/kg Q 24 hr	50 mg/kg Q 48 hr	65 mg/kg Q 48 hr
<0.4	Not recommended		Not recommended	

Ganciclovir

Normal Dosage:
Oral (maintenance only):
1,000 mg PO TID

CrCl (mL/min):	Maintenance dose:
≥70	1,000 mg TID
50–69	1,500 mg QD or 500 mg TID
25–49	1,000 mg QD or 500 mg BID
10–24	500 mg QD
<10	500 mg TIW after dialysis

IV:
Induction dose: 5 mg/kg Q 12 hr
Maintenance dose: 5 mg/kg QD or 6 mg/kg QD × 5 days/wk

CrCl (mL/min):	Induction dose:	Maintenance dose:
>70	5 mg/kg Q 12 hr	5 mg/kg Q 24 hr
50–69	2.5 mg/kg Q 12 hr	2.5 mg/kg Q 24 hr
25–49	2.5 mg/kg Q 24 hr	1.25 mg/kg Q 24 hr
10–24	1.25 mg/kg Q 24 hr	0.625 mg/kg Q 24 hr
<10	1.25 mg/kg 3× Q wk following hemodialysis	0.625 mg/kg 3× Q wk following hemodialysis

Modified from reference 47 and product information.

ofovir is nephrotoxic; however, administration of probenecid (2 g administered 3 hours before the start of infusion and two 1-g doses administered at 2 and 8 hours after infusion) blocks tubular secretion and reduces nephrotoxicity. Prehydration with 1 L of normal saline is required 1 hour before each dose and, if tolerated, repeated concomitantly with or after the cidofovir infusion. Because nephrotoxicity is the most significant dose-limiting toxicity, other nephrotoxic agents should be discontinued (e.g., nonsteroidal anti-inflammatory drugs [NSAIDs], aminoglycosides), and renal function should be carefully monitored throughout therapy (BUN, SrCr, proteinuria) (see Table 70-7). Dosage adjustments must accompany deterioration in renal function (see Table 70-8).

The CBC should be checked at baseline because neutropenia has been reported in approximately 20% of patients in clinical trials. Hypotony (reduction in intraocular pressure) and uveitis (inflammation of the uveal tract of the eye) have also been reported. Thus, monthly intraocular pressure checks and slit-lamp examinations of the retina are necessary.[42,179,180]

The role of cidofovir remains unclear. It offers the advantage of weekly and biweekly dosing, but its toxicity greatly limits its utility. Cidofovir appears to be as efficacious as foscarnet and ganciclovir in the treatment of CMV retinitis, but no comparative studies have been performed. Finally, the efficacy of cidofovir in the treatment of extraocular CMV (e.g., GI disease, pneumonitis, encephalitis) remains to be established.[42,179,180]

Foscarnet

Foscarnet is a pyrophosphate analog that acts by selectively inhibiting viral DNA polymerases and reverse transcriptase. At doses currently recommended for induction therapy (60 mg/kg Q 8 hr or 90 mg/kg IV Q 12 hr), peak plasma foscarnet concentrations are attained that should inhibit CMV in vitro (see Table 70-7).[181] The dose-limiting toxicity of foscarnet is nephrotoxicity, probably because its poor solubility results in crystallization in nephrons.[174,182]

In one prospective randomized trial, patients receiving foscarnet for CMV retinitis survived approximately 4 months longer than those receiving ganciclovir.[183] However, foscarnet-treated patients with reduced creatinine clearance (<1.2 mL/min per kilogram) had a poor survival rate. Whether the improvement was because of the anti-HIV activity of foscarnet or the ability of foscarnet-treated patients to continue receiving AZT (which was not the case with ganciclovir) is unknown and remains controversial.[184,185]

Because P.Z. has a low ANC, the bone marrow–suppressive effects of ganciclovir are of concern. Adjunctive therapy with G-CSF is an option. Because he has good renal function (SrCr of 0.8 mg/dL), foscarnet or cidofovir probably would be preferred.

NEPHROTOXICITY

16. **P.Z. will receive foscarnet, 90 mg/kg IV over 2 hours Q 12 hr. How can the risk of nephrotoxicity be minimized?**

During foscarnet therapy, adequate hydration is important to prevent nephrotoxicity. To establish diuresis, 750 to 1,000 mL of normal saline or 5% dextrose should be administered before the first infusion of foscarnet. With subsequent infusions, 500 to 1,000 mL should be administered, depending on the foscarnet dose. Careful dosage titration based on P.Z.'s estimated creatinine clearance may also minimize nephrotoxicity (see Table 70-8). The serum creatinine clearance should be measured at least twice weekly and the dosage recalculated if the creatinine clearance changes. CMV infection itself may also cause an acute increase in the serum creatinine due to acute interstitial nephritis. Drugs with nephrotoxic potential, such as amphotericin B or aminoglycosides, should be avoided if possible.[182,183]

ADVERSE EFFECTS

17. **What toxicities other than nephrotoxicity have been associated with foscarnet therapy?**

Hypocalcemia can occur because foscarnet, a pyrophosphate analog, can bind to unbound calcium. Electrolyte complications can be minimized by avoiding high foscarnet plasma concentrations. Therefore, foscarnet should be infused slowly over 1 to 2 hours.[187] Unbound serum calcium and phosphate levels should be monitored twice weekly during induction therapy and weekly during maintenance therapy, ideally when foscarnet is at its highest concentration. Fatal hypocalcemia occurred in an AIDS patient receiving both foscarnet and parenteral pentamidine; thus, coadministration of these drugs should be avoided.[185]

Penile ulceration from foscarnet has been problematic, especially in uncircumcised men. Characterized as a fixed-drug eruption, careful attention to genital hygiene may minimize the potential for penile ulceration. Other adverse events associated with foscarnet include seizures, hypomagnesemia, anemia, nausea, fever, and rash. Twice-weekly albumin, magnesium, and potassium levels are required during induction therapy and then weekly during maintenance therapy. In general, patients tolerate foscarnet more poorly than ganciclovir.[186]

DOSAGE ADJUSTMENTS

18. **After 12 days of foscarnet therapy, P.Z.'s SrCr has increased from 0.8 mg/dL to 1.2 mg/dL despite the coadministration of 2 L of normal saline daily. What dosage adjustments should be made for the remainder of the foscarnet treatment?**

[SI units: SrCr, 70.72 and 106.08 µmol/L, respectively]

Ganciclovir, foscarnet, and cidofovir are highly dependent on renal elimination, and dosages (or dosing intervals) should be adjusted for even a modest reduction in renal function (see Table 70-8). For example, the creatinine clearance threshold for dosage reduction of ganciclovir is 70 mL/1.73 m² per minute; for dosage reduction of foscarnet, it is 1.6 mL/min per kilogram. In contrast, the renal threshold for acyclovir and many other drugs is a creatinine clearance of <50 mL/min. Therefore, careful monitoring of renal function is important throughout CMV therapy. P.Z.'s estimated creatinine clearance is 1.2 mL/min per kilogram; therefore, his foscarnet induction dosage should be adjusted to 70 mg/kg IV Q 12 hr (see Table 70-8).[42,184]

Ganciclovir–Foscarnet Combination

In a prospective randomized controlled trial of patients with persistent or relapsed retinitis, ganciclovir and foscarnet monotherapy were compared with combination low-dose therapy.[165] Mortality and adverse effects were similar in all three groups. However, combination therapy was associated with significantly delayed time to retinitis progression (median 1.3 and 2 months with foscarnet and ganciclovir monotherapy, respectively, versus 4.3 months in the combination arm). However, the overall prolonged daily infusion time (up to 4 hours/day) and adverse effects detracted from quality of life.[165] Consequently, combination therapy should be reserved for more refractory cases of CMV retinitis[189,190] (see Relapse and Refractory Retinitis).

Suppression Therapy

19. **P.Z. completes 21 days of foscarnet induction therapy. How can his CMV retinitis be suppressed in the future?**

The currently available antiviral agents used to treat CMV disease are not curative. Following induction therapy, chronic maintenance therapy is indicated for the remainder of P.Z.'s life, unless immune reconstitution occurs as a result of HAART. Regimens that have been shown to be effective in randomized controlled clinical trials include parenteral or oral ganciclovir, parenteral foscarnet, combined parenteral ganciclovir and foscarnet, parenteral cidofovir, and (for retinitis only) ganciclovir administration via intraocular implant or repetitive intravitreous injections of fomivirsen. Oral valganciclovir is approved for both acute induction and maintenance therapy, but the published clinical data are limited. The current guidelines do not include this as a preferred option for maintenance, but this may change in the near future. In uncontrolled case series, repeated intravitreous injections of ganciclovir, foscarnet, and cidofovir have been shown to be effective for prophylaxis of CMV retinitis. However, since this therapy is effective only locally and does not protect the contralateral eye or other organ systems, it is usually combined with oral ganciclovir.

Foscarnet 90 mg/kg Q 12 hr as IV induction for 14 to 21 days is usually followed by IV foscarnet 90 to 120 mg/kg per day as a single daily maintenance dose. The maintenance dose of 120 mg/kg per day is more efficacious but may be more toxic than the lower maintenance dose.[188,191] Ganciclovir IV induction (5 mg/kg per dose Q 12 hr) may be followed by IV ganciclovir maintenance (5 mg/kg per day five to seven times per week). Ganciclovir IV induction may also be followed by oral ganciclovir 3,000 to 6,000 mg daily in three divided doses administered with food. Cidofovir, with induction doses of 5 mg/kg IV each week for 2 weeks followed by a maintenance dose of 5 mg/kg IV every 2 weeks, offers a more convenient dosing schedule and negates the need for an indwelling IV catheter (see Table 70-7).

Current guidelines suggest that discontinuation of prophylaxis may be considered in patients with CMV retinitis who are taking HAART with a sustained (>6 months) increase in the $CD4^+$ count to >100 to 150. These patients must have remained disease free for >30 weeks. The decision to discontinue suppression should be based on the magnitude and duration of the $CD4^+$ increase and viral load suppression, the anatomic location of the retinal lesions, and the degree of vision loss. An ophthalmology consultation is recommended.[49] All patients who have had anti-CMV maintenance therapy discontinued should continue to undergo regular ophthalmo-logic monitoring for early detection of CMV relapse as well as for immune reconstitution uveitis.

Relapse or Refractory CMV Retinitis

20. **After 5 months of maintenance therapy with foscarnet, a routine funduscopic examination reveals retinal CMV disease progression. How should P.Z.'s retinitis be managed at this time?**

Most patients with CMV disease eventually relapse.[42,191] For the first relapse, repeating induction therapy followed by maintenance therapy with the same drug is beneficial in most patients. Because P.Z. has tolerated foscarnet therapy thus far, he should receive another course of induction therapy. After reinduction, P.Z. should receive a higher maintenance dosage (120 g/kg daily).[49]

It is important to distinguish between relapse and refractory disease. Relapse, as in the case of P.Z., is defined as recurrence of clinically apparent viral activity and is usually caused by a decline in immune function, insufficient delivery of drug into the eye, or resistant CMV strains. Relapse can be effectively managed by repeat induction therapy of the same drug.[42] If the relapse is due to a resistant virus, the patient may benefit from a change in therapy. Ganciclovir-resistant CMV strains occur by two mechanisms. DNA polymerase mutation at the UL54 gene is observed in approximately 20% of ganciclovir-resistant strains. This mutation usually confers resistance to cidofovir and, to a lesser extent, foscarnet.[42,192,193] Most ganciclovir-resistant CMV strains have UL97 mutations. UL97 mutations are incapable of monophosphorylating ganciclovir. Cidofovir and foscarnet are appropriate alternatives to treat strains with UL97 mutations. Patients who receive extensive ganciclovir treatment (>6 to 9 months) may present with highly ganciclovir-resistant strains containing UL54 and UL97 mutations.[194] Cidofovir may be considered in most patients who relapse while receiving ganciclovir or foscarnet. Although ganciclovir- and foscarnet-resistant strains of CMV have been reported, their precise role in the clinical failure of these regimens is not known.[194] Because of the different mechanisms of action of ganciclovir and foscarnet, strains resistant to one drug may retain sensitivity to the other.[192,195] Resistant or relapsing CMV retinitis may be treated by administration of local ocular therapy via intravitreal injection of ganciclovir, foscarnet, or fomivirsen. Fomivirsen is a phosphorothioate oligonucleotide that inhibits the replication of the human CMV through an antisense mechanism. Fomivirsen has potent activity against CMV, including strains resistant to ganciclovir, foscarnet, and cidofovir. Fomivirsen demonstrates a 30-fold greater local activity than ganciclovir.[196–198] Ganciclovir intraocular implants are also a potential option (see Local Therapy of CMV).

Refractory CMV retinitis is defined by disease progression because of ineffective therapy. This phenomenon is observed in two clinical situations: when the disease persists with minimal or no response during induction therapy, and when long-term control is inadequate with maintenance therapy. Refractory CMV disease has been defined in clinical trials as two relapses occurring within 10 weeks despite repeat induction and maintenance therapy. Treatment options for refractory CMV retinitis include reinduction with ganciclovir at higher dosages (7.5 mg/kg per dose Q 12 hr, followed by maintenance doses of 10 mg/kg per day) or reinduction using combination therapy (IV ganciclovir plus foscarnet).[42] Refractory CMV retinitis can be treated with local ocular therapy via intravitreal injection of ganciclovir, foscarnet, or fomivirsen as well as intraocular implants.[196–198]

Local Treatment

Intravitreal Injections

21. **What is the role of intravitreal injections in CMV retinitis?**

Intravitreal administration of ganciclovir or foscarnet through a small-gauge needle is a method of selectively delivering the drug to the site of infection.[42,199–201] Ganciclovir and foscarnet doses of 0.2 to 2 mg and 1.2 to 2 mg, respectively, are administered two or three times per week for active disease, followed by weekly maintenance injections. Intravitreal fomivirsen induction—330 µg (0.05 mL) once a week for 2 doses (day 1 and day 15) followed by maintenance doses once every 4 weeks—also has been used.[198] Potential complications of intravitreal injections include bacterial endophthalmitis, vitreous hemorrhage, and retinal detachment. Ocular inflammation, with iritis and vitreitis, is the most frequently observed adverse experience with fomivirsen (25%); this complication usually responds to topical corticosteroids.[198] Intravitreous therapy is relatively uncommon because intraocular implants are available. Importantly, in contrast to systemic therapy, local instillation of a drug is associated with a higher risk of CMV disease developing in the contralateral eye as well as extraocular sites (see Table 70-7).

Intraocular Ganciclovir Implants

22. **Is P.Z. a candidate for ganciclovir intraocular implants?**

The intraocular implant is a surgically implantable delivery device (Vitrasert implant) capable of delivering ganciclovir into the vitreous humor at a constant rate of approximately 1 µg/hr over a period of 5 to 8 months.[162,202–204] The implant delivers a much higher concentration into the vitreous cavity than can be achieved with systemic therapy. Implants may be an acceptable initial choice for newly diagnosed patients or patients with imminent sight-threatening disease. Surgical complications, such as retinal detachments, infections, and hemorrhage, can occur during or after the procedure. To reduce the risk of contralateral retinitis or extraocular CMV disease, patients receiving the intraocular implant should also be given oral ganciclovir (1,000 mg three times a day) (see Table 70-7).[205]

P.Z. should be reinduced with foscarnet therapy and maintained on a higher foscarnet dose. Neither alternating regimens nor intravitreal administration of antiviral agents is appropriate at present.

Oral Ganciclovir

23. **What is the role of oral ganciclovir in the treatment of CMV retinitis? Would P.Z. be a candidate for oral ganciclovir (Cytovene) therapy?**

Oral ganciclovir is available in the United States for the suppressive treatment of CMV retinitis in AIDS patients. When taken with food, oral ganciclovir at a dosage of 1,000 mg three times a day provides daily drug exposure (e.g., area under the curve [AUC]) that is approximately 75% that of IV doses (5 mg/kg). Peak concentrations associated with oral dosing are substantially lower, but trough levels are higher than with IV dosing. The bioavailability of oral ganciclovir is increased by 22% when administered with food. Therefore, patients should be counseled to take all doses with food to maximize their drug exposure.[206] Although oral ganciclovir is a viable alternative to IV ganciclovir as maintenance therapy, the time to relapse may be sooner.[206] As with the IV formulations, neutropenia or anemia occurs in 40% to 60% of patients; however, the risk appears to be less with oral administration.

An esterified ganciclovir, valganciclovir, has recently become available. This agent yields an AUC approximately equivalent to that associated with the IV administration of ganciclovir. The maintenance dosage is two 450-mg tablets of valganciclovir once daily. Valganciclovir is currently not in the guidelines as a preferred agent for prophylaxis, but it may be in the near future.

The expense of oral versus parenteral ganciclovir is controversial. Cost comparisons must take into consideration catheter-associated costs as well as the additional cost of catheter-associated complications, such as sepsis. Furthermore, quality-of-life issues may weigh in favor of oral ganciclovir. Oral ganciclovir appears to suppress CMV disease effectively and is a maintenance therapy option for patients with stable, non–sight-threatening disease. The limited bioavailability decreases its efficacy; however, larger dosages (e.g., 4,500 or 6,000 mg daily) appear more efficacious.[42,205–207] Considering his previous history of neutropenia, P.Z. should not receive oral ganciclovir. Furthermore, oral ganciclovir is less effective as maintenance therapy in sight-threatening cases of retinitis, which exists in P.Z.

24. **What is the role of oral ganciclovir for initial CMV prevention?**

The role of oral ganciclovir for primary prophylaxis of CMV retinitis has been evaluated in two studies.[208,209] Oral ganciclovir decreased the 1-year incidence of disease by approximately 50% in one study[208] but did not demonstrate appreciable efficacy in the second investigation.[209] These two studies had important differences in study design that likely explain the disparate results. One cost-effectiveness study estimated that oral ganciclovir prophylaxis would cost >$1.7 million per year of anticipated life expectancy.[210] These issues, in addition to ganciclovir-induced adverse effects such as neutropenia and anemia, the lack of proven survival benefit, and the risk for ganciclovir-resistant CMV are concerns that should be addressed when deciding whether to institute prophylaxis in individual patients. Prophylaxis with oral ganciclovir is not currently "strongly recommended as standard of care" by the guidelines, but rather is "usually recommended" for patients who are seropositive and have a CD4+ count of <50 (see Table 70-2).[42,49]

Acyclovir offers no protection against CMV, and valacyclovir is not recommended because of an unexplained higher mortality trend in patients given the drug for CMV disease prevention.[49] Therefore, oral ganciclovir is the oral systemic agent currently used. The exact role of oral ganciclovir in the prevention and management of CMV retinitis remains unclear.

CRYPTOCOCCAL MENINGITIS

Clinical Presentation and Prognosis

25. A.S., age 28, is infected with HIV. She weighs 48 kg. Her boyfriend was an IV drug user who died of AIDS 2 years ago. She presents with a fever (103°F) and a 2-week history of "splitting headaches." Laboratory test results include hemoglobin (Hgb), 11.2 g/dL (normal, 12.1 to 15.3 for females); WBC count, 4,100 cells/mm³ (normal, 3,800 to 9,800); platelets, 73,000/L (normal, 150,000 to 450,000); SrCr, 0.9 mg/dL (normal, 0.5 to 1.7); glucose, 94 mg/dL (normal, 65 to 115); and CD4⁺ count, 92 cells/mm³. She is highly nonadherent and has not been to the clinic in more than a year, at which time she was prescribed indinavir, AZT, and 3TC. Physical examination reveals no nuchal rigidity. With the exception of moderate lethargy, her neurologic examination is unremarkable. Her chest radiograph and three sets of blood cultures for bacteria and fungi are negative. A computed tomography (CT) scan is nondiagnostic. Lumbar puncture reveals the following cerebrospinal fluid (CSF) findings: glucose, 45 mg/dL (normal, 40 to 80); protein, 90 mg/dL (normal, 15 to 45); WBC count, 10 cells/mm³ (normal, <5); and a cryptococcal antigen titer of 1:2,048. The intracranial pressure (ICP) is 240 mm H_2O (normal, 80 to 220). How is A.S.'s clinical presentation typical of a patient with AIDS and cryptococcal meningitis? What is her likely prognosis?

[SI units: Hgb, 112 g/L (normal, 121 to 153); WBC count, 4.1 ×10⁹/L (normal, 3.8 to 9.8); platelets, 73 ×10⁹/L (normal, 150 to 450); SrCr, 79.56 µmol/L (normal, 44 to 150); peripheral glucose, 5.2 mmol/L (normal, 3.6 to 6.3); CSF glucose, 2.5 mmol/L (normal, 60% to 70% of peripheral glucose); CSF protein, 0.9 g/L]

In the pre-HAART era, cryptococcosis developed in approximately 6% to 10% of AIDS patients in the United States, with meningitis being the most common clinical presentation.[211] In the era of HAART and azole prophylaxis, a significant decline in the incidence of cryptococcosis has been observed.[29,211] After HIV encephalopathy and toxoplasmosis, cryptococcosis is the most common CNS infection associated with AIDS.[211] The initial portal of entry is the lungs, where the organism is normally contained by an intact immune system. Cryptococcal disease typically develops in patients with profound defects in cell-mediated immunity (i.e., CD4⁺ counts <100). Unlike bacterial meningitis, cryptococcal CNS infection has a much more insidious onset; the most common symptoms are fever and headache. Less frequent signs and symptoms include nausea and vomiting, meningismus, photophobia, and altered mental status. Focal neurologic deficits and seizures are observed in <10% of patients. CSF glucose is decreased, whereas CSF proteins are usually elevated. CSF cryptococcal antigen titer and CSF culture are frequently positive. These findings, along with the clinical presentation, form the basis for the diagnosis. The overall outcome is poor, with a mean survival of 5 months. Relapse within 6 months occurs in 50% of patients who do not receive suppressive therapy. Altered mental status at baseline, CSF WBC count of <20 cells/mm³, high CSF cryptococcal antigen titer (>1:1,000), and an elevated initial CSF opening pressure of >200 mm H_2O have all been associated with a poor prognosis.[211]

A.S.'s CD4⁺ count is 92. She has a temperature of 103°F and has experienced "splitting headaches" for about a week. Her clinical presentation is typical of an AIDS patient with cryptococcal meningitis. The CSF WBC count of 10 cells/mm³, high cryptococcal antigen titer, and ICP >200 mm H_2O, suggest a poorer prognosis.[212]

Treatment

Amphotericin B

26. How should A.S.'s acute cryptococcal meningitis be managed?

The current treatment recommended for cryptococcal meningitis is amphotericin B, 0.7 mg/kg per day IV, plus flucytosine (100 mg/kg per day) given orally in four divided doses as induction therapy. Once the patient is stable (e.g., afebrile, with resolution of symptoms), then consolidation therapy with oral fluconazole 400 mg daily for 10 weeks can be initiated. Following consolidation therapy, daily suppressive therapy with fluconazole 200 mg should be continued indefinitely unless immune reconstitution occurs with HAART.[212]

Although the aforementioned regimen is highly effective, the ability to rapidly reduce A.S.'s ICP will also significantly improve her clinical course. Removal of 10 to 20 mL of spinal fluid by repeat lumbar puncture is recommended for patients with an ICP >200 mm H_2O (A.S.'s ICP is 240 mm H_2O). Additional interventions to consider to reduce A.S.'s elevated ICP include administration of acetazolamide (a carbonic anhydrase inhibitor that decreases CSF production) and the insertion of an intraventricular shunt.[211,212]

27. What is the evidence for adding flucytosine to amphotericin B in the acute treatment of A.S.? What are the disadvantages of this combination?

Amphotericin B binds to sterols in the fungal cell membrane, resulting in leakage of cytoplasmic contents.[213] Flucytosine is an antimetabolite type of antifungal drug that is activated by deamination within the fungal cells to 5-fluorouracil. It inhibits fungal protein synthesis by replacing uracil with 5-flurouracil in fungal RNA, and it also inhibits thymidylate synthetase via 5-fluorodeoxy-uridine monophosphate, interfering with fungal DNA synthesis. Although in vitro data have demonstrated synergy between amphotericin B and flucytosine, the addition of the latter agent remains controversial, particularly in AIDS patients, because of the potential for bone marrow toxicity.[211,214] Flucytosine, a purine analog, is approximately 10% converted to 5-fluorouracil, an antimetabolite.

A classic prospective study conducted in HIV-negative patients favored the use of the combination.[215] The protocol randomized patients to receive either amphotericin B monotherapy (0.4 mg/kg per day IV for 6 weeks followed by 0.8 mg/kg per day IV every other day for 4 weeks) or amphotericin B plus flucytosine (150 mg/kg per day orally divided Q 6 hr) for 6 weeks. Fewer failures or relapses, more rapid CSF sterilization, and less nephrotoxicity occurred in the combination group, while overall mortality was no different. However, approximately one fourth of the patients in the combination arm developed leukopenia, thrombocytopenia, or both.

The addition of flucytosine to the therapeutic regimen in HIV-positive patients warrants careful monitoring. In a retrospective review of 89 AIDS patients with cryptococcal meningitis confirmed by CSF culture, no survival difference was noted between those who received amphotericin B monotherapy and those who were treated with the combination.[216] Flucytosine-induced bone marrow suppression, possibly exacerbated by amphotericin B–induced renal dysfunction, resulted in discontinuation of flucytosine in more than half of the patients. Neutropenia, thrombocytopenia, and diarrhea are more common with sustained blood levels >100 mg/dL. However, not all patients with high blood concentrations experienced adverse effects, suggesting variable patient responses. If flucytosine is chosen as adjunctive therapy, renal function and CBCs should be monitored closely. Whether prospective evaluation of flucytosine blood levels to maintain peak levels <100 mg/ dL reduces the incidence of toxicity remains unknown. A.S. is at increased risk of granulocytopenia because of her HIV disease and her concomitant myelotoxic AZT therapy.

The comparative trial forming the basis for the current recommendations for treatment of acute cryptococcal meningitis in HIV-positive patients evaluated a higher dose of IV amphotericin B (0.7 mg/kg per day) with or without flucytosine given at a lower dose (25 mg/kg per dose orally Q 6 hr) for 2 weeks. The study evaluated 381 patients with an acute first episode of cryptococcal meningitis. The second part of this trial re-randomized stable or improved patients to either a fluconazole or itraconazole treatment arm for an additional 8 weeks as consolidation therapy. Sixty percent and 51% of patients receiving amphotericin B plus flucytosine, and amphotericin B alone, respectively, had sterile CSF cultures at 2 weeks of therapy. No significant differences were noted between groups in the percentage of patients who were culture negative at 2 weeks. Importantly, the addition of flucytosine to amphotericin B was not associated with a significant increase in drug toxicities at 2 weeks. Fluconazole and itraconazole were similar in efficacy. However, multivariate analysis revealed two factors that were independently associated with a higher rate of CSF sterilization: the addition of flucytosine and the randomization to fluconazole. Consequently, amphotericin with flucytosine is the preferred initial regimen.

INTRATHECAL OR INTRAVENTRICULAR AMPHOTERICIN B

28. Should A.S. also receive intrathecal or intraventricular amphotericin B?

Although amphotericin B does not penetrate readily into CSF, IV therapy for cryptococcal meningitis is adequate in most patients. One small retrospective review of 13 patients with a first episode of cryptococcal meningitis and underlying malignancy favored insertion of an Ommaya reservoir (a device inserted into the ventricle of the brain to enable the repeated injection of drugs into the CSF).[217] However, the number of subjects was small, and complications from using the Ommaya reservoir occurred in 30% of these patients (e.g., chemical ventriculitis, bacterial superinfection, headache, fever, and tinnitus). Considering the lack of clear efficacy and documented complications associated with the direct instillation of amphotericin into CSF, this method of administration should be avoided.

Fluconazole

29. Could A.S. be treated with fluconazole instead of amphotericin B for acute cryptococcal meningitis?

Fluconazole, one of the triazole antifungal agents, inhibits a fungal cytochrome P450 enzyme necessary for the conversion of lanosterol to ergosterol. Without ergosterol, the fungal cell membrane becomes defective and loses its selective permeability properties.[221] Unlike ketoconazole or itraconazole, fluconazole is well absorbed orally even in the presence of an elevated gastric pH. Fluconazole has excellent CNS penetration and a good safety profile,[221] but its role as initial therapy for the treatment of acute cryptococcal meningitis remains controversial. In a prospective, randomized, multicenter trial, the National Institute of Allergy and Infectious Diseases (NIAID) Mycoses Study Group and the AIDS Clinical Trial Group (ACTG) compared amphotericin B with 200 mg/day of oral fluconazole (following a 400-mg loading dose) for 10 weeks in 194 patients.[222] The dose of amphotericin B (mean dose, 0.4 to 0.5 mg/kg daily) and the possible addition of flucytosine were left to the discretion of the individual investigators. Although the overall mortality was similar (14% for amphotericin B versus 18% for fluconazole), more fluconazole-treated patients died during the first 2 weeks of treatment (15% versus 8%; $P = 0.25$). Furthermore, the median time to the first negative CSF culture in the successfully treated patients was shorter in the amphotericin B group compared with fluconazole (16 days versus 30 days). In a small, prospective, randomized trial of 20 male patients with AIDS, oral fluconazole (400 mg daily) for 10 weeks was compared with IV amphotericin B (0.7 mg/kg daily for 1 week, followed by the same dose thrice weekly for 9 weeks) combined with flucytosine (150 mg/kg daily).[223] There were four deaths in the fluconazole group and none in the amphotericin B group ($P = 0.27$). Eight of the 14 patients in the fluconazole group failed to respond to treatment, whereas none of the amphotericin B patients failed to respond. The mean duration of positive CSF cultures was 41 days in the fluconazole group and 16 days in the amphotericin B group ($P = 0.02$). These results, taken together, have led most clinicians to choose amphotericin, with or without fluconazole, as initial treatment for severe cryptococcal meningitis. Although increased doses of fluconazole have been proposed, it is unknown whether these will result in improved outcomes. Considering the severity of her meningitis, A.S. should be treated acutely with amphotericin and not fluconazole.

Itraconazole

30. What is the role of itraconazole (Sporanox) in the treatment of cryptococcal meningitis?

Although CSF penetration of itraconazole is poor, it has been efficacious in an animal model of cryptococcal meningitis.[224] In a small, uncontrolled trial, all symptoms resolved and cultures were negative in 10 of 14 AIDS patients with cryptococcal meningitis. The median survival of these patients exceeded 10.5 months. In another small, controlled trial, 42% (5 of 12) of itraconazole-treated patients (200 mg orally twice daily) responded completely, compared with 100% (10 of 10) of patients who received amphotericin B (0.3 mg/kg daily IV) plus flucytosine (150 mg/kg daily) for 6 weeks ($P = 0.009$).[225] The lack of efficacy may be the result of erratic absorption of itraconazole capsules and poor penetration into the CSF. The suspension and IV formulations of itraconazole offer better bioavailability and thus may result in improved outcomes. In both studies, itraconazole generally was well tolerated, but its role as initial therapy for acute cryptococcal meningitis remains to be clarified.

In a comparative study of amphotericin B plus flucytosine versus amphotericin B alone for 2 weeks, patients were randomized to receive either fluconazole or itraconazole for an additional 8 weeks of consolidation therapy. Itraconazole produced a lower rate of CSF sterilization than fluconazole. The researchers concluded that itraconazole could be used in consolidation therapy of cryptococcal meningitis only for patients who could not tolerate fluconazole.[212] Itraconazole appears to have a limited role in the treatment of cryptococcal meningitis in HIV-positive patients.

Duration of Therapy

31. **For how long should treatment continue for A.S.'s cryptococcal meningitis?**

Once A.S. completes 2 weeks of acute induction therapy with amphotericin B and flucytosine, she should be switched, if stable, to oral fluconazole 400 mg daily for consolidation therapy. However, itraconazole could be used if A.S. is intolerant to fluconazole. Consolidation should be continued for an additional 8 to 10 weeks, followed by lifelong suppressive therapy with fluconazole 200 mg daily[212] (see Maintenance Therapy).

Maintenance Therapy

32. **Should A.S. receive maintenance therapy following successful treatment?**

After induction and consolidation treatment of cryptococcal meningitis, A.S. and all AIDS patients should receive maintenance therapy indefinitely, unless immune reconstitution occurs as a result of HAART.[49, 211, 212] A higher relapse rate and a shorter life expectancy have been observed in patients who did not receive chronic secondary prophylaxis.[216] Fluconazole (200 mg once daily) has emerged as the suppressive treatment of choice. In a randomized, placebo-controlled trial of 61 AIDS patients, four recurrent cases of meningitis developed in the placebo group and none in the fluconazole group ($P = 0.03$).[226] One multicenter, comparative trial randomized patients to receive either weekly amphotericin B 1 mg/kg daily IV or 200 mg/day of fluconazole orally.[227] Of 189 patients enrolled, 18% of the patients in the amphotericin B group relapsed, compared with 2% in the fluconazole group. Serious toxicities were more frequent in the amphotericin B group. Although data are limited, four of five patients maintained on itraconazole (200 to 400 mg/day) for 3 to 12 months had a threefold to sixfold decline in CSF cryptococcal antigen titers. The fifth patient refused repeat lumbar punctures (see previous section on itraconazole). Thus, itraconazole should be used only as an alternative to fluconazole.[212,228]

According to the OI guidelines, adult and adolescent patients are at low risk for recurrence of cryptococcosis when they have completed a course of initial therapy, remain asymptomatic, and have a sustained increase (e.g., >6 months) in their CD4$^+$ counts to >100 to 200 after HAART. This has been evaluated in limited numbers of patients. Nonetheless, discontinuing chronic maintenance therapy among such patients is reasonable. Recurrences may happen,

and certain specialists may perform a lumbar puncture to determine if the CSF is culture negative before stopping therapy. Maintenance therapy should be reinitiated if the CD4$^+$ count decreases to 100 to 200.

Primary Prophylaxis

33. **What is the role of primary prophylaxis in cryptococcal meningitis?**

Primary prophylaxis against cryptococcal disease in HIV-infected patients has been studied in a few clinical trials.[229,230] In one open-label study, fluconazole (100 mg/day) was administered to all patients (329 HIV-infected patients) with CD4$^+$ counts <68. These results were compared with 337 historical controls from the pre-HAART era.[229] Sixteen cases of cryptococcal meningitis occurred in the historical controls (4.8%) compared with only one case in the fluconazole group (0.3%). In a prospective, randomized ACTG study, fluconazole 200 mg/day was compared with clotrimazole troches (10 mg five times a day) for the prevention of fungal infections in 428 patients with advanced HIV disease. After a median follow-up of 35 months, 32 cases of invasive fungal infection were confirmed. Of these, the majority (17 of 32) were cryptococcosis: 2 cases in the fluconazole group and 15 cases in the clotrimazole group. The greatest benefit derived from fluconazole was observed in patient with CD4$^+$ counts of <50.[230] However, no effect on survival was noted.

The risk for fluconazole resistance has been a concern with primary prophylaxis because fluconazole resistance has been reported in HIV-infected patients receiving long-term therapy.[231] In addition to the potential for resistance, other concerns include the lack of survival benefits associated with prophylaxis, the possibility of drug interactions, and cost. In light of these concerns, the CDC currently does not recommend primary prophylaxis for this disease (see Table 70-2).[49] Fluconazole in a daily dose of 100 to 200 mg is reasonable for patients with a CD4$^+$ count of <50.

Investigational Therapies

34. **What other acute therapies are under investigation for cryptococcal meningitis?**

The combination of fluconazole plus flucytosine appears to be superior to fluconazole alone. High-dose fluconazole alone (800 to 1,600 mg/day for up to 6 months) was compared with high-dose fluconazole and flucytosine (150 mg/kg daily for 4 weeks) in 36 AIDS patients.[232] Nine of 12 (75%) patients in the combination group survived and became CSF culture negative, whereas only 7 of 24 (29%) patients on fluconazole monotherapy had similar outcomes. In a dose-escalation trial of high-dose fluconazole with or without flucytosine, a significant increase in efficacy was observed as fluconazole doses were increased. Potentially, combination fluconazole and flucytosine are useful because of the excellent oral bioavailability of both agents, which is particularly important in developing countries. A randomized trial of 58 AIDS patients with cryptococcal meningitis compared fluconazole and flucytosine with fluconazole monotherapy. Thirty patients received fluconazole 200 mg once daily for 2 months and flucytosine 150 mg/kg daily for the first 2 weeks versus 28 patients who received only fluconazole 200 mg once daily for 2 months. Those who were surviving after 2 months received fluconazole maintenance therapy at a dose of 200 mg three times a week for 4 months. Combination therapy significantly increased the survival rate compared with monotherapy. No serious adverse effects were observed in either group. Fluconazole and short-term flucytosine may be a cost-effective and safe regimen in developing countries.[233]

MYCOBACTERIUM TUBERCULOSIS

Clinical Presentation

35. C.J., a 45-year-old male prison inmate with AIDS, presents with fever, cough, and occasional night sweats. A tuberculin purified protein derivative (PPD) skin test is negative, but C.J. is assumed to be anergic based on his response to other skin test antigens. Two acid-fast bacilli (AFB) sputum smears are also negative. Chest radiograph reveals hilar adenopathy with a questionable right middle lobe localized infiltrate. No cavitary lesions are seen. Why is infection with *M. tuberculosis* a strong possibility in C.J.? His antiretroviral medications include saquinavir/ritonavir, stavudine, and 3TC. Three months ago his CD4$^+$ count was 320 cells/mm^3 (normal, approximately 1,000 cells/mm^3) and his viral load was 5,200 copies/mL.

One third of the global population is infected with *M. tuberculosis,* with 7 to 8 million new cases every year. Mortality is 2 to 3 million people annually, making TB the most common infectious cause of death worldwide.[234] The incidence of TB in the United States from 1985 to 1992 increased by 20%, approximately 40,000 more cases than expected.[235–237] Factors associated with this resurgence include the HIV epidemic, urban homelessness, drug abuse, and the dismantling of public health TB control resources. At that time, HIV disease was believed to be a major factor contributing to the emergence of multidrug-resistant TB. The recognized link between HIV and TB, along with an increase in clinical and public health resources, has subsequently resulted in a decline in the incidence of TB in the United States.[236] Nevertheless, TB is the leading cause of death in HIV-infected persons worldwide, and pulmonary TB is an AIDS-defining illness. Furthermore, *M. tuberculosis* strains resistant to isoniazid and rifampin, with or without resistance to other agents, have become a major public health concern.[235,238–240] Multidrug-resistant *M. tuberculosis* (MDRTB) is defined by resistance to both isoniazid and rifampin. In 1991 in New York City, 33% of *M. tuberculosis* cases were resistant to at least one drug and 19% were resistant to both isoniazid and rifampin.[241] These drug-resistant strains have been identified primarily in large urban areas (e.g., New York and Miami), in coastal or border communities, and in institutional settings.[237,238] Nine outbreaks of MDRTB in hospital and prison settings in New York and Florida in 1990 were investigated by the CDC. A high prevalence of HIV infection (range, 20% to 100%), a high mortality rate (72% to 89%), and a short median duration of survival (range, 4 to 16 weeks) were common to these outbreaks. Multidrug-resistant strains have been transmitted to health care workers and prison staff.[237]

A Community Programs for Clinical Research on AIDS (CPCRA) survey evaluating MDRTB in eight metropolitan regions in the United States observed drug-resistant isolates among 37% of all HIV-positive patients versus 18% of HIV-

negative patients in New York City. In areas outside of New York City, resistance rates were approximately 15% in both groups.[242]

C.J. presents with fever, cough, night sweats, and a right middle lobe infiltrate with hilar adenopathy, consistent with TB. Furthermore, his HIV status in combination with his incarceration increases the probability of *M. tuberculosis* infection, including multidrug-resistant isolates. C.J. will be started with the standard four-drug regimen: isoniazid, rifampin (or rifabutin), pyrazinamide, and ethambutol.[243] (See Chapter 61, Tuberculosis, for a more comprehensive approach to TB treatment.)

36. Sputum cultures from C.J. document *M. tuberculosis* resistant to both isoniazid and rifampin. Why are the negative tuberculin skin test, negative sputum smears for AFB, and lack of cavitary lesions in C.J. still consistent with *M. tuberculosis* infection?

The clinical presentation of TB is often different in patients with HIV infection. As many as one half to two thirds of AIDS patients presenting with TB have evidence of extrapulmonary sites of infection.[234] These extrapulmonary sites include lymph nodes, bone marrow, spleen, liver, CSF, and blood. *M. tuberculosis* was rarely cultured from blood before the AIDS era; however, bacteremia is well documented today.[243] HIV-infected patients with TB infection are also at risk for developing tuberculous meningitis.[245] The chest radiograph in HIV-infected patients may reveal hilar or mediastinal adenopathy or localized infiltrates in the middle or lower lung fields.

In HIV-infected patients, it is unusual to see typical apical infiltrates or cavitations. Furthermore, concomitant PCP may confuse interpretation of chest radiographs. In addition, AFB smears of sputum are negative in approximately 40% of HIV-infected patients despite a positive culture, as in this patient.[246] Finally, anergy is extremely common in HIV disease. Only 10% to 40% of HIV-infected patients with TB have a positive tuberculin skin test. Anergy testing is not generally recommended because of lack of standardization of anergy test reagents, poor reproducibility, and a failure to show efficacy of prophylaxis in anergic patients.[49,247] Thus, definitive diagnosis of TB rests on positive cultures from sputum or other tissue and body fluid specimens.

Treatment

37. How should C.J. be treated?

C.J.'s organism is resistant to both isoniazid and rifampin (by definition, MDRTB). These two agents should be discontinued, and at least two more drugs should be added to his regimen. The organism must be known to be susceptible to at least three agents in the regimen.[238,243] Treatment additions for C.J. may include an aminoglycoside (e.g., streptomycin, kanamycin, amikacin), capreomycin, and a fluoroquinolone (e.g., ofloxacin, ciprofloxacin, levofloxacin).[238,243] C.J.'s physician decided to treat him with pyrazinamide, 20 mg/kg orally daily (maximum dose, 2 g), ethambutol 15 mg/kg orally daily (maximum dose, 2.5 g), amikacin 15 mg/kg daily IV or intramuscularly, and levofloxacin 500 mg orally or IV daily.

The optimal duration of treatment for MDRTB has not been established. The National Jewish Center for Immunology and Respiratory Medicine treats MDRTB for 24 months after sputum cultures become negative. Parenteral medication is continued for 4 to 6 months if toxicity remains manageable (e.g., amikacin ototoxicity, nephrotoxicity).[235,237,240] Intermittent therapy (administered two or three times per week) is allowable as long as it is directly observed.[238] All patients infected with organisms resistant to either isoniazid or rifampin should have their ingestion of antitubercular medications directly observed. Although directly observed drug regimens are labor intensive, they are overall cost effective.[238]

Whenever isoniazid- or rifampin-resistant organisms are isolated, a medical expert should be consulted. Because many patients suffer from adverse events related to their antituberculosis regimens (particularly GI effects), the National Jewish Center recommends that initial therapy begin in the hospital to monitor toxicity.[238] To minimize side effects, this center also initiates therapy with small doses of each agent followed by gradual escalation to the target dose over 3 to 10 days.

In patients with organisms resistant only to isoniazid, suggested regimens include rifampin or rifabutin, pyrazinamide, and ethambutol daily for 14 days then twice weekly for 6 to 9 months, or for 4 months after sputum conversion. If the organism is resistant only to rifampin, suggested regimens include isoniazid, pyrazinamide, and ethambutol plus streptomycin daily for 8 weeks, then isoniazid, pyrazinamide, and streptomycin two or three times per week for 30 weeks. An alternative to this regimen for rifampin resistance includes isoniazid, pyrazinamide, and ethambutol plus streptomycin daily for 2 weeks, then the same regimen two or three times a week for 6 weeks, followed by isoniazid, pyrazinamide, and streptomycin two or three times a week for 30 weeks.

If the organism is sensitive to both isoniazid and rifampin, then the preferred regimen consists of isoniazid, rifampin, pyrazinamide, and ethambutol or streptomycin for 2 months. The third and fourth drugs (pyrazinamide and ethambutol or streptomycin) may be discontinued after 2 months. The dosing regimens for HIV-infected patients and for non–HIV-infected patients are the same. Treatment should continue for 9 months for both non–HIV-infected and HIV-infected patients. If HIV-positive patients demonstrate a slow or suboptimal response, therapy should be prolonged on an individual basis.[235,240] All HIV-infected patients receiving isoniazid are at risk for peripheral neuropathy and should receive pyridoxine (Table 70-9).[49,237,238]

38. **How should C.J.'s response to therapy be monitored?**

C.J.'s response to therapy should be monitored by drug efficacy and toxicity. Efficacy may be assessed by the resolution of symptoms. Symptoms usually improve within 4 weeks, and sputum cultures become negative within 3 months. C.J. should be monitored for a decrease in the frequency of his fevers and night sweats, as well as improvement in his cough. Sputum smear and culture should be monitored at least monthly until a negative culture is documented. Chest radiography may be the last parameter to improve.[238,240,243] In some patients, recurrence of symptoms may be caused by nontuberculous complications associated with HIV. This paradoxical reaction is associated with the initiation of antiretroviral

Table 70-9 **Tuberculosis Treatment Recommendations for Patients Coinfected with HIV and Tuberculosis**

Induction	Maintenance	Comments
Rifampin-Based Therapy (no Concurrent Use of PIs or NNRTIs)		
INH/RIF/PZA/EMB (or SM) daily × 2 months	INH/RIF daily or 2–3×/wk × 18 wk	RIF-containing regimens used with caution with protease inhibitors and NNRTIs.
INH/RIF/PZA/EMB (or SM) daily × 2 wk, then 2–3 per wk × 6 wk	INH/RIF 2–3×/wk × 18 wk	HIV status should be assessed at 3-month intervals to determine need for antiretroviral therapy.
INH/RIF/PZA/EMB (or SM) 3×/wk × 8 wk	INH/RIF/PZA/EMB (or SM) 3×/wk × 4 months	
Rifabutin-Based Therapy (Concurrent Use of PIs or NNRTIs)		
INH/RFB/PZA/EMB daily × 8 wk	INH/RFB daily or 2×/wk × 18 wk	Monitor for RFB toxicity—arthralgias, uveitis, leukopenia.
INH/RFB/PZA/EMB daily × 2 wk, then 2×wk × 6 wk • Nucleoside analogs and nucleotides: not contraindicated/ no dosage changes recommended	INH/RFB 2×/wk × 18 wk	Dose modifications of RFB and PIs/NNRTIs when given concurrently (see Table 70-10).
Streptomycin-Based Therapy (Concurrent Use of PIs or NNRTIs)		
INH/SM/PZA/EMB daily × 8 wk	INH/SM/PZA 2-3×/wk × 30 wk	SM is contraindicated in pregnant women.
INH/SM/PZA/EMB daily × 2 wk, then 2–3 ×/wk × 6 wk	INH/SM/PZA 2-3×/wk × 30 wk	If SM cannot be continued for 9 months, add EMB and treatment should be extended to 12 months.

APV, amprenavir; EFV, efavirenz; EMB, ethambutol; IDV, indinavir; INH, isoniazid; NNRTI, nonnucleoside reverse transcriptase inhibitor; NFV, nelfinavir; PI, protease inhibitor; PZA, pyrazinamide; RFB, rifabutin; RIF, rifampin; SM, streptomycin.
Adapted from MMWR 2002:51(RR-8):1–52, and references 47, 68.

therapy[248] and is the consequence of immune reconstitution. Recovery of delayed hypersensitivity occurs with increases in CD4$^+$ counts, resulting in increased reactions to mycobacterial antigens. Continuation of antimycobacterial and antiviral treatment is recommended, and a short course of prednisone may be considered for severe symptoms.[248]

The second monitoring parameter is drug toxicity. Recommended baseline tests include LFTs, serum creatinine, CBC, and platelet count. Baseline uric acid is required for patients receiving pyrazinamide. Patients receiving ethambutol require baseline visual acuity and red-green color perception assessment. Reassessment should be performed at least once monthly. Laboratory monitoring usually is not recommended unless symptoms suggest toxicity. Isoniazid and, secondarily, rifampin and pyrazinamide are the agents most associated with hepatotoxicity (also see Chapter 61). C.J. is not receiving isoniazid or rifampin but is receiving pyrazinamide. Therefore, if transaminase levels increase to greater than five times the upper limits of normal, pyrazinamide should be discontinued and an alternative agent given. When his LFTs return to their normal limits, pyrazinamide can be reintroduced.[243]

Prophylaxis

HIV-Infected Persons: Multidrug-Resistant Tuberculosis

39. **An HIV-infected nurse inadvertently entered C.J.'s room without taking adequate precautions and suctioned respiratory secretions. Four weeks later, her tuberculin skin test converted to positive. What prophylactic regimen should be initiated for this nurse?**

There is no known prophylactic regimen with proven efficacy against MDRTB,[49,238] but several regimens have been recommended: pyrazinamide (25 to 30 mg/kg daily) combined with ethambutol (15 to 25 mg/kg daily); pyrazinamide with ofloxacin (400 mg twice daily); and pyrazinamide combined with ciprofloxacin (750 mg twice daily).[238,249] Other fluoroquinolones, such as levofloxacin, are associated with good in vitro activity and may prove beneficial. Considering that C.J. is HIV infected, multidrug prophylaxis should continue for 12 months.[49,249] The choice of drugs must be based on susceptibility tests and consultation with public health authorities (see Table 70-2).[49]

HIV-Infected Persons: Drug-Susceptible Tuberculosis

40. **K.D., a 26-year-old HIV-infected man, comes in for a routine clinic visit. It is discovered that he is a household contact of a person known to have active, untreated, drug-susceptible TB. His CD4$^+$ count is 350 cells/mm³. A tuberculin skin test (5 tuberculin units of PPD) and two other skin test antigens are administered, and he is instructed to return to the clinic in 48 hours. His PPD has been negative in the past, and he has demonstrated delayed hypersensitivity responsiveness. How should the results of K.D.'s skin tests be interpreted, and should he receive prophylaxis considering his known exposure to TB?**

The CDC and the American Thoracic Society currently recommend 9 months of isoniazid prophylaxis (300 mg orally daily) plus pyridoxine (50 mg orally daily) for all HIV-infected persons who have at least a 5-mm induration reaction to PPD and no evidence of active TB (negative chest radiograph and no clinical symptoms), unless otherwise contraindicated and regardless of bacille Calmette-Guérin (BCG) vaccination status. The administration of BCG vaccine to HIV-infected persons is contraindicated because of the potential to cause disseminated disease.[49] A >5-mm reaction in HIV-infected persons contrasts to a ≥10-mm cutoff for HIV-negative persons.[49,243] Few isoniazid prophylaxis failures have been reported, although this finding has not been systematically studied. Additional preferred regimens in instances of questionable compliance include isoniazid 900 mg twice weekly plus pyridoxine 50 mg twice weekly for 9 months, both administered under direct observed therapy (DOT). A short-course preferred regimen includes rifampin (600 mg/day) plus pyrazinamide (20 mg/kg daily) for 2 months (see Table 70-2).[49,250]

An inverse relationship exists between anergy and a CD4$^+$ count of <500.[251] If K.D. proves to be anergic, he should still be given isoniazid prophylaxis, considering his exposure history.[49] All HIV-infected persons, irrespective of age, PPD results, or prior course of chemoprophylaxis, should be given chemoprophylaxis if they are in close contact with persons who have active TB. Prophylaxis also should be considered for anergic, HIV-infected persons who are members of groups known to have a prevalence of TB infection of ≥10%. In the United States, these groups include IV drug users, prison inmates, residents of homeless shelters, and persons born in Latin American, Asian, or African countries with high rates of TB. The efficacy of primary prophylaxis in this group has been demonstrated.[49,240,243] Before any prophylactic regimen is begun, active TB needs to be ruled out. K.D. should undergo chest radiography and clinical evaluation to rule out active disease. HIV-infected patients who are anergic or have a negative reaction when tested do not require prophylaxis if they are not close contacts of TB-infected patients.[49,240,243] The CDC no longer recommends routine anergy testing, because several studies have demonstrated inconsistent results.[49,252]

HIV-Infected Persons: Protease Inhibitors or Nonnucleoside Reverse Transcriptase Inhibitors

41. **F.C., a 36-year-old HIV-infected woman, diagnosed 6 months ago, was found to have active TB (pulmonary infiltrates on chest radiographs, sputum AFB stain and culture positive, culture pansensitive). She is taking indinavir, 3TC, AZT, and fluconazole, and CD4$^+$ count is 300 cells/mm³. What factors must be considered when selecting TB therapy for F.C.?**

The use of protease inhibitors in the treatment of HIV patients coinfected with TB increases the potential for drug interactions with rifamycin derivatives (rifampin, rifabutin). Because the rifamycins are potent inducers of the hepatic cytochrome P450 system (e.g., CYP3A4), they can induce metabolism of the protease inhibitors, resulting in subtherapeutic levels. Conversely, the protease inhibitors elevate rifamycin serum levels by inhibiting their metabolism and increasing toxicities, such as uveitis (inflammation of the uveal tract of the eye) (also see Chapter 61).

According to recent guidelines,[244] rifampin should not be coadministered with amprenavir, indinavir, lopinavir/ritonavir, nelfinavir, saquinavir, atazanavir, and delavirdine. Rifampin can be used with ritonavir, ritonavir plus saquinavir, efavirenz, and possibly nevirapine. Rifabutin may be used in place of rifampin but should not be used with the hard-gel formulation of saquinavir (Invirase) or delavirdine. The data are limited on the interaction between rifabutin and soft-gel saquinavir (Fortovase). Rifabutin should be given at 50% of the usual dose (i.e., reduce from 300 mg to 150 mg/day) with indinavir, nelfinavir, or amprenavir. Rifabutin should be used at 25% of the usual dose (i.e., 150 mg every other day or three times a week), with ritonavir, ritonavir plus saquinavir, lopinavir/ritonavir, or atazanavir. When rifabutin is administered with indinavir as a single protease inhibitor, the dosage of indinavir should be increased from 800 mg/8 hr to 1,000 mg/8 hours. Rifabutin should be given with efavirenz at dosages of 450 to 600 mg/day. There are no data on using rifabutin in the HAART setting of efavirenz plus a protease inhibitor. In this situation, rifabutin dosing may need to be decreased. Rifabutin can be used in full doses with nevirapine.

The CDC has recommended three treatment options for patients receiving protease inhibitors and nonnucleoside reverse transcriptase inhibitors. If the patient has not yet been started on a protease inhibitor or NNRTI, it may be best to delay therapy and start antituberculosis medication immediately. If the patient is receiving a protease inhibitor or NNRTI, some physicians may decide to discontinue this treatment for the duration of the antituberculosis medication. If the decision is made to continue or initiate protease inhibitor or NNRTI therapy, an antituberculosis regimen must be selected that modifies the doses of rifampin or rifabutin (see Table 70-9).[243,253]

There are currently five options for concomitant TB and antiretroviral therapy; the first three are CDC-recommended options. These are initiating therapy with regimens that do not contain a protease inhibitor or an NNRTI (e.g., abacavir, 3TC, AZT), using a concomitant protease inhibitor or NNRTI with streptomycin-based therapy with no use of rifamycins, and initiating rifabutin-based therapy with dose adjustments of the concomitant protease inhibitor or NNRTI (see Table 70-9).[244] The other two options are not recommended by the CDC. They are using isoniazid, ethambutol, and pyrazinamide for 18 to 24 months[254] with concomitant protease inhibitor or NNRTI therapy, and using efavirenz 800 mg/day (plus two NRTIs) plus rifampin 600 mg/day or 600 mg twice weekly.[69]

Discontinuing the protease inhibitor in F.C. is not an option considering the rapid viral replication and the risk of developing resistant isolates, especially considering that she recently was started on protease inhibitor therapy and is clinically responsive. New data indicate that rifampin can be used for the treatment of active TB in three situations: (1) in a patient whose antiretroviral regimen includes the NNRTI efavirenz and two NRTIs; (2) in a patient whose antiretroviral regimen includes the protease inhibitor ritonavir and one or more NRTIs; and (3) in a patient whose antiretroviral regimen includes the combination of two protease inhibitors (ritonavir and either saquinavir hard-gel capsule [HGC] or saquinavir soft-gel capsule [SGC]). In addition, the updated guidelines recommend substantially reducing the dosage of rifabutin (150 mg two or three times per week) when it is administered to patients taking ritonavir (with or without saquinavir HGC or saquinavir SGC) and increasing the dose of rifabutin (either 450 mg or 600 mg daily or 600 mg two or three times per week) when rifabutin is used concurrently with efavirenz.

Half the usual rifabutin dose, 150 mg daily or 300 mg twice weekly, is recommended when coadministered with indinavir, nelfinavir, or amprenavir (see Table 70-9 and Chapter 61).

Considering that F.C. is receiving indinavir, she will be treated with a rifabutin-based regimen. She will receive isoniazid, rifabutin, pyrazinamide, and ethambutol daily for 8 weeks followed by isoniazid and rifabutin daily or twice weekly for 18 weeks. An alternative regimen could be isoniazid, rifabutin, pyrazinamide, and ethambutol daily for 2 weeks, then two times weekly for 6 weeks, followed by isoniazid and rifabutin, twice weekly for 18 weeks. Considering the indinavir-associated reduction in metabolism, rifabutin should be administered 150 mg daily or 300 mg twice weekly (see Table 70-9).

Drug Interactions

42. **What additional non–antiretroviral-related drug interactions are of concern to patients like F.C. who are taking antituberculosis medications?**

Rifampin induces hepatic microsomal enzymes and therefore increases the metabolism of many drugs frequently prescribed for HIV-positive patients. For example, serum concentrations of fluconazole and ketoconazole are decreased by 25% and 80%, respectively,[255,256] and dapsone concentrations are lowered by as much as 90% with concomitant administration of rifampin. Rifampin may induce acute withdrawal when given with methadone. The activity of oral contraceptives and warfarin anticoagulants also may be reduced. Rifampin also lowers serum concentrations of theophylline, anticonvulsants, corticosteroids, sulfonylureas, and digoxin.

F.C. is receiving rifabutin rather than rifampin. Rifabutin also induces hepatic microsomal enzymes, but the effect is less pronounced. Rifabutin reduces the activity of several agents, including warfarin, barbiturates, benzodiazepines, β-adrenergic blockers, chloramphenicol, clofibrate, corticosteroids, cyclosporine, diazepam, digitalis, doxycycline, haloperidol, oral hypoglycemics, ketoconazole, phenytoin, theophylline, quinidine, and verapamil. A significant reduction in activity is observed with oral contraceptives, dapsone, and methadone (Tables 70-10 and 70-11).

Cytochrome P450 system inhibitors, such as certain macrolides, quinolones, and antifungal azoles, prolong the half-life of rifabutin. The macrolides erythromycin and clarithromycin result in a fourfold increase in rifabutin.[49,237] F.C. is concomitantly taking fluconazole; thus, rifabutin serum levels might increase when given with fluconazole, leading to possible uveitis.[236] However, F.C. is currently taking half the usual dose of rifabutin, minimizing the risk for rifabutin-induced uveitis.

Table 70-10   Recommendations for Coadministering Rifampin and Rifabutin With Nonnucleoside Reverse Transcriptase Inhibitors and Protease Inhibitors

Antiretroviral	Use in Combination With Rifabutin	Use in Combination With Rifampin	Comments
Saquinavir Hard-gel capsules (HGC)	Possibly[a], if regimen also includes ritonavir	Possibly, if regimen also includes ritonavir	Coadministration of saquinavir SGC with usual-dose rifabutin (300 mg QD or 2–3 times/week) is a possibility. However, pharmacokinetic data and clinical experience are limited.
Soft-gel capsules (SGC)	Probably[b]	Possibly, if antiretroviral regimen also includes ritonavir	The combination of saquinavir SGC or saquinavir HGC and ritonavir, coadministered with 1) usual-dose rifampin (600 mg QD or 2–3 times/week), or 2) reduced-dose rifabutin (150 mg 2-3 times/week) is a possibility. However, the pharmacokinetic data and clinical experience are limited. Coadministration of saquinavir HGC or saquinavir SGC with rifampin (in the absence of ritonavir) is not recommended because rifampin markedly decreases concentrations of saquinavir.
Ritonavir	Probably	Probably	If the combination of ritonavir and rifabutin is used, then a substantially reduced-dose rifabutin regimen (150 mg 2–3 times/week) is recommended. Coadministration of ritonavir with usual-dose rifampin (600 mg QD or 2–3 times/week) is possible; pharmacokinetic data and clinical experience are limited.
Indinavir	Yes	No	There is limited, but favorable, clinical experience with coadministration of indinavir[c] with a reduced daily dose of rifabutin (150 mg) or with the usual dose of rifabutin (300 mg 2–3 times/week) Coadministration of indinavir with rifampin is not recommended because rifampin markedly decreases concentrations of indinavir.
Nelfinavir	Yes	No	There is limited, but favorable, clinical experience with coadministration of nelfinavir[d] with a reduced daily dose of rifabutin (150 mg) or with the usual dose of rifabutin (300 mg 2–3 times/week). Coadministration of nelfinavir with rifampin is not recommended because rifampin markedly decreases concentrations of nelfinavir.
Amprenavir	Yes	No	Coadministration of amprenavir with a reduced daily dose of rifabutin (150 mg) or with the usual dose of rifabutin (300 mg 2–3 times/week) is a possibility, but there is no published clinical experience. Coadministration of amprenavir with rifampin is not recommended because rifampin markedly decreases concentrations of amprenavir.
Atazanavir	Yes	No	Coadministration of atazanavir with a reduced dose of rifabutin (150 mg every other day, or three times per week) is a possibility, but there is no published clinical experience. Coadministration of atazanavir with rifampin is not recommended because rifampin markedly decreases concentrations of atazanavir
Lopinavir/ ritonavir	Yes	No	Coadministration of lopinavir/ritonavir with a reduced dose of rifabutin (150 mg every other day, or three times per week) is a possibility, but there is no published clinical experience. Coadministration of lopinavir/ritonavir with rifampin is not recommended because rifampin markedly decreases concentrations of atazanavir
Nevirapine	Yes	Possibly	Coadministration of nevirapine with usual-dose rifabutin (300 mg QD or 2–3 times/week) is possible based on pharmacokinetic study data. However, there is no published clinical experience for this combination. Data are insufficient to assess whether dose adjustments are necessary when rifampin is coadministered with nevirapine. Therefore, rifampin and nevirapine should be used only in combination if clearly indicated and with careful monitoring.

Table 70-10 **Recommendations for Coadministering Rifampin and Rifabutin With Nonnucleoside Reverse Transcriptase Inhibitors and Protease Inhibitors—cont'd**

Antiretroviral	Use in Combination With Rifabutin	Use in Combination With Rifampin	Comments
Delavirdine	No	No	Contraindicated because of the marked decrease in concentrations of delavirdine when administered with either rifabutin or rifampin.
Efavirenz	Probably	Probably[e]	

[a]Despite limited data and clinical experience, the use of this combination is potentially successful.
[b]Based on available data and clinical experience, the successful use of this combination is likely.
[c]Usual recommended dose is 800 mg q 8 hr. Some experts recommend increasing the indinavir dose to 1,000 mg q 8 hr if indinavir is used in combination with rifabutin.
[d]Usual recommended dose is 750 mg TID or 1,250 mg BID. Some experts recommend increasing the nelfinavir dose to 1,000 mg if used TID and in combination with rifabutin.
[e]Usual recommended dose is 600 mg QD. Some experts recommend increasing the efavirenz dose to 800 mg QD if efavirenz is used in combination with rifampin.
Adopted from MMWR 2000; 49:23.

Table 70-11 **Drug Interactions With TB and MAC Medications**

Affected Drug	Interacting Drug(s)	Mechanism	Recommendation
Atovaquone	Rifampin	Induction of metabolism—↓ drug levels	Concentrations might not be therapeutic; avoid combination or ↑ atovaquone dose
Clarithromycin	Ritonavir, indinavir	Inhibition of metabolism—↑ drug levels by 77% (w/ritonavir) and 53% with indinavir	No adjustments needed in normal renal function; adjust if CrCl is <30 mL/min
Clarithromycin	Nevirapine	Induction of metabolism—↓ in clarithromycin AUC by 35%, ↑ in AUC of 14-OH clarithromycin by 27%	Effect on *Mycobacterium avium* prophylaxis might be decreased; monitor closely
Clarithromycin	Rifabutin, rifampin	Induction of hepatic metabolism—clarithromycin concentration ↓ 50% (w/rifabutin) to 120% (w/rifampin)	Clinical significance of ↓ clarithromycin levels unknown
Ketoconazole, rifampin	Isoniazid	↓ serum concentration of ketoconazole ↑ hepatotoxicity	Possible antifungal treatment resistance May consider discontinuing one or both agents if >5× baseline
Quinolones	Didanosine, antacids, iron products, calcium products, sucralfate	Chelation that results in marked ↓ in quinolone drug levels	Administer interacting drug at least 2 hours after quinolone
Rifabutin	Fluconazole	Inhibition of metabolism—significant ↑ in rifabutin drug levels	Monitor for rifabutin, toxicity such as uveitis, nausea, neutropenia
Antifungals, dapsone, methadone, theophylline, oral contraceptives, phenytoin, digoxin, warfarin (all drugs metabolized via CYP450)	Rifampin	Induction of metabolism-significant decrease in drug levels	Monitor drug levels (theophylline, phenytoin, digoxin) Monitor prothrombin time with warfarin Use alternative birth control
Theophylline, warfarin, digoxin	Ciprofloxacin	Inhibition of metabolism— ↑ theophylline levels, ↑ digoxin levels, ↑ anticoagulant effects	Monitor theophylline and digoxin levels and prothrombin time

CYP450, cytochrome P450 enzyme system; NNRTIs, nonnucleoside reverse transcriptase inhibitors; PIs, protease inhibitors.
Modified from MMWR 1999;48(RR-10).

MYCOBACTERIUM AVIUM COMPLEX INFECTION

Clinical Presentation

43. M.E., an HIV-infected 38-year-old woman with a history of IV drug use, presents with fevers, drenching night sweats, a poor appetite, and a 20-lb weight loss (>15% of baseline) over the past 4 months. M.E. has refused all antiretroviral therapy for the past year because of drug intolerance. She has a past medical history of recurrent herpes zoster, PCP, and cryptococcal meningitis. Her current medications include one TMP-SMX double-strength tablet once daily and an occasional acyclovir dose when she feels the herpes zoster "is beginning to start"; she refuses MAC prophylaxis therapy. Physical examination reveals a cachectic woman with mild hepatosplenomegaly. Pertinent laboratory test results include hematocrit (Hct), 23% (normal, 36% to 44.6%); WBC count, 3,500 cells/L (normal, 3,800 to 9,800) with 68% neutrophils, 2% bands, 22% lymphocytes, and 8% monocytes; absolute CD4$^+$ count, 25 cells/mm^3; viral load, 200,000 copies/mL; aspartate transferase (AST), 135 IU/L (normal, 0 to 35); alanine aminotransferase (ALT), 95 IU/L (normal, 0 to 35); and alkaline phosphatase, 186 IU/L (normal, 30 to 120). Skin testing reveals anergy. The chest radiograph is unremarkable. Based on these findings, a presumptive diagnosis of MAC infection is made. Why is M.E.'s clinical presentation consistent with MAC infection?

[SI units: Hct, 0.23; WBC count, 3.5 ×10^9/L with 0.68 neutrophils, 0.02 bands, 0.22 lymphocytes, 0.08 monocytes; AST, 135 U/L (normal, 0 to 35); ALT, 95 U/L (normal, 0 to 35); alkaline phosphatase, 186 U/L (normal, 30 to 120)]

Disseminated MAC infection is common in end-stage AIDS patients. On autopsy, MAC organisms are observed in the lungs, spleen, colon, adrenals, kidneys, brain, and skin.[258,259] MAC reduces survival; increased mortality is observed in AIDS patients with disseminated MAC, compared to AIDS patients without disseminated MAC.[258] The predominant organism in HIV-positive patients is *M. avium* (97% of typeable isolates) followed by *Mycobacterium intracellulare* (3%).[260] The risk of developing disseminated MAC infection is strongly associated with a CD4$^+$ count of <100; the highest risk is in patients with a CD4$^+$ count <50.[14,258] Age, sex, and race do not influence the risk of disseminated MAC infection.[49,258] The overall prognosis is poor, with a mean survival of 3 to 7 months. Poor prognostic indicators include prior OI, severe anemia, AZT dose interruption, and low total lymphocyte count.[261]

M. avium is a ubiquitous organism found in food, water, soil, and house dust. The most likely portal of entry is either the GI or respiratory tract. Sputum and stool samples frequently are colonized with MAC, although the significance of this finding remains controversial. Common presenting symptoms associated with MAC infection include fever, night sweats, anorexia, malaise, profound weight loss (>10% body weight), anemia, lymphadenopathy, and diarrhea.[262] M.E.'s fevers, drenching night sweats, poor appetite, 20-lb weight loss, and mild hepatosplenomegaly are consistent with MAC infection. In particular, her CD4$^+$ count of 25 puts her at risk for this OI.

Treatment

Initiation

44. Why is it appropriate to initiate M.E.'s drug therapy before blood culture results have documented the presence of MAC?

Disseminated MAC is best diagnosed by peripheral blood cultures. The finding of AFB on a blood smear is diagnostic, but the results are variable.[262,263] Conventional culture methods using solid media may have a turnaround time of as long as 8 weeks; however, newer radiometric broth systems signaling the release of C^{14}-labeled CO$_2$ from mycobacteria may detect bacterial growth in 7 to 10 days.[262,263] Identification of the organism (*M. tuberculosis* versus atypical mycobacteria) by conventional biochemical methods may take weeks to months. Newer techniques using DNA probes make diagnosis possible within several hours.[263] Quantitative blood cultures have been useful to monitor the effects of drug therapy but may not be practical on a routine clinical basis. Radiometric broth methods also may provide in vitro drug susceptibility in another 7 to 10 days. Even with the availability of all of the newer laboratory tests, results generally are not available for 2 to 3 weeks. In view of this lag time, it is in the patient's best interest to initiate empiric therapy as quickly as possible. Although MAC is typically isolated from blood, the organism can also be demonstrated via acid-fast smears of lymph node, liver, or bone marrow biopsies. Because these organs are rich in monocytes, the target cells for MAC infection, the organism load may be high (up to 10^{10} CFU/mL). Granuloma formation or inflammation may be absent because of profound suppression of cell-mediated immunity in end-stage AIDS patients.[263,264]

45. What is the relevance of M.E.'s discontinued antiretroviral therapy to her development of MAC infection?

The incidence of disseminated MAC in AIDS patients residing in the United States before HAART was 30% to 40%. Treatment with protease inhibitors and the widespread use of primary MAC prophylaxis since mid-1996 substantially lowered the incidence of disseminated MAC infection.[264–266] HIV also is known to infect monocytes and macrophages. In in vitro macrophage culture studies, the intracellular growth rate of *M. avium* was greatly enhanced in HIV-infected cells.[267] Conversely, if macrophages taken from HIV-infected patients were infected with *M. avium,* latent HIV virus began to replicate in some of these cultures.[267] Consequently, the two organisms may act synergistically, leading to a hastened deterioration of the host.[262] Because M.E. has discontinued antiretroviral therapy, the resultant increase in viral load has contributed to her development of MAC.

Drug Susceptibility as a Basis for Treatment

46. Should M.E.'s therapy be based on in vitro drug susceptibility results?

Correlation between in vitro drug susceptibility results and clinical efficacy has not been clearly established for MAC. Numerous reasons may account for this finding. First, results are method dependent; MAC isolates are more sensitive to antibiotics if broth is used rather than agar.[263,268] Second, current in vitro methods are cell free, which does not take into account the intracellular nature of MAC infection. Thus, drugs that have excellent intracellular penetration may be useful clinically, even if in vitro minimum inhibitory concentration (MIC) data suggest otherwise. Conversely, drugs that have favorable MIC data may be ineffective clinically if they do not reach the intracellular environment.[267,268] An in vitro drug susceptibility testing system that incorporates murine macrophages is under development[267,268] and eventually may be a better predictor of clinical outcome. Clinical laboratories in the United States widely use the radiometric broth macrodilution utilizing Bactec Technology.[268,269]

Drug susceptibility studies also may not correlate with clinical efficacy because in vitro results for individually tested drugs may show resistance, but combination therapy may be additive or synergistic.[270] Finally, some antimycobacterial agents exhibit large differences between the MIC and maximum bactericidal concentration (MBC). This finding may reflect the difficulty in eradicating this organism, particularly in a severely immunocompromised host. Despite these limitations, many clinicians still use in vitro drug susceptibility data as a guide to therapy. Only recently have large-scale, randomized, comparison clinical trials been undertaken using these results. In summary, in vitro tests for susceptibility, while used, may not predict clinical efficacy.

Drug Therapy

47. **What drug regimens could be selected to treat M.E.?**

The CDC currently recommends a two- or three-drug MAC regimen, and at least one of these drugs must be a macrolide. Clarithromycin (500 mg orally twice daily) is the preferred agent; azithromycin is an alternative. Ethambutol (15 to 25 mg/kg orally daily) is recommended as the second agent. Several drugs can be used as the third agent, including rifabutin (300 mg daily), ciprofloxacin (500 to 750 mg daily), and amikacin (15 mg/kg daily). The choice of the third agent depends on the severity of the illness, drug interactions, hepatic and renal function, patient tolerability, patient compliance, and cost. Amikacin (15 mg/kg daily) has been used in acute MAC therapy, but it is toxic and does not appear to have a role in long-term therapy. Long-term therapy may be discontinued in patients who have completed a course of >12 months of treatment for MAC, remain asymptomatic, and have a sustained increase (e.g., >6 months) in their CD4+ count to >100 after HAART.[49]

In the late 1980s, it was controversial whether patients with disseminated MAC infection should be treated at all. The results of early, uncontrolled trials were disappointing, with poor microbiologic response rates, little improvement in clinical symptoms, and a high incidence of adverse drug reactions. More recent clinical trials have been associated with improvement or eradication of MAC bacteremia and improvement in clinical symptoms. These improved results probably can be attributed to earlier diagnosis, longer follow-up, more potent antiretroviral therapy, and newer anti-MAC agents that penetrate intracellular spaces more effectively.[270]

The macrolides have potent antimycobacterial activity. Several studies have shown clarithromycin to be efficacious against MAC.[271,272] In a small placebo-controlled trial, seven of eight patients who received 2 g daily of clarithromycin monotherapy eradicated *M. avium* from their blood cultures after 4 weeks. In contrast, all five placebo patients showed increases in CFU/mL. In an uncontrolled, monotherapy trial of azithromycin (500 mg daily), patients showed a mean decrease from 2,028 CFU/mL to 136 CFU/mL. Fevers and night sweats resolved in most patients.[273] However, bacteriologic relapse occurred after treatment was discontinued and in 10 patients who elected to continue azithromycin therapy (250 mg daily), suggesting the emergence of resistance. In another investigation, all isolates initially were susceptible to clarithromycin, but after 12 weeks of monotherapy (1 to 4 g daily), in vitro resistance developed in 16 of 72 (22%) patients.[275]

Since monotherapy can lead to breakthrough bacteremia and resistance, MAC infections should be treated with a combination of at least two agents, including a macrolide plus ethambutol. Although clarithromycin and azithromycin have excellent activity against MAC, clarithromycin is preferred because the emergence of resistance is more likely with azithromycin.[271-273] Both macrolides demonstrate excellent intracellular penetration and have prolonged half-lives.[276-278] GI toxicity (e.g., nausea, vomiting, diarrhea, abdominal pain, and anorexia) is the most frequent adverse effect with either agent.[272,273] These effects may be dose related. Data show that patients receiving 4 g daily of clarithromycin are more likely to have their therapy discontinued because of GI upset than patients receiving lower doses.[279] The dosage of clarithromycin is 500 mg orally twice daily, and the dosage of azithromycin is 500 mg daily.

Ethambutol (15 to 25 mg/kg daily orally) is preferred as the second agent.[274] In a monotherapy study, 800 mg of ethambutol was more effective than either clofazimine or rifampin.[279] One or more of the following drugs can be added to the macrolide/ethambutol combination: rifabutin, rifampin, ciprofloxacin, and clofazimine, with or without amikacin. Isoniazid and pyrazinamide are not effective for the treatment of MAC.[267,269,252]

Although four-drug regimens have been used, one study observed that a three-drug macrolide regimen (clarithromycin, ethambutol, rifabutin) was more effective than a four-drug regimen (ciprofloxacin, clofazimine, ethambutol, rifampin).[280] Benefits of the macrolide regimen included more rapid clearing of MAC bacteremia and a longer duration of survival. Rifabutin, at 600 mg daily, induced uveitis in approximately one third of patients. Subsequently, the rifabutin dosage was lowered to 300 mg daily, and the incidence of uveitis decreased to 5.6%. Although clearance of bacteremia was superior at the higher rifabutin dose, no differences in survival were observed. Several recent studies have demonstrated no bacteriologic or clinical benefit with the addition of clofazimine. Clarithromycin and ethambutol, with and without clofazimine, were investigated for the treatment of MAC bacteremia. Survival was found to be significantly decreased in the clofazimine arm; 61% of the patients died versus 38% in the two-drug arm. Based on this analysis, the FDA no longer recommends the addition of clofazimine to clarithromycin and ethambutol.[281]

M.E. will be placed on a regimen containing clarithromycin 500 mg twice daily and ethambutol 15 mg/kg daily. The choice to use two drugs rather than three is based on M.E.'s poor adherence profile. Other considerations for the addition of a third-line agent include the severity of the illness, potential drug interactions, tolerability, hepatic and renal function, and cost. M.E. must be counseled regarding the slow response to treatment. If she improves, therapy should be continued and HAART therapy should be reinstituted.

MONITORING THERAPY

48. How should M.E. be monitored?

The primary goals of MAC therapy are to eradicate or reduce the number of *M. avium* organisms, decrease symptoms, enhance quality of life, and prolong survival. M.E. should be monitored for symptomatic relief (temperature spikes and frequency of night sweats), as well as a microbiologic response (CFU/mL). Clinical improvement may not be observed for 2 to 4 weeks, whereas eradication of bacteremia frequently takes longer (4 to 12 weeks). If no improvement in clinical manifestations is observed in 4 to 8 weeks, a mycobacterial blood culture should be repeated along with susceptibility testing. If resistance is observed or suspected, two new drugs should be added based on susceptibility testing plus or minus the macrolide. If the organism is found to be susceptible to macrolides, therapy should be continued and adherence, absorption, tolerance, and drug interactions should be considered.[282,283] If the problem is determined to be drug absorption, IV agents can be considered. M.E. also should be followed for development of toxicities related to drug therapy. Furthermore, because many drugs used to treat MAC infections are associated with drug interactions, this issue must be considered each time a new drug is prescribed. In some cases, drug doses will need to be modified or alternative drugs selected to prevent adverse events or therapeutic failures (see Table 70-10).[284]

Prophylaxis

49. What drug(s) should be used to provide primary prophylaxis against MAC infection?

The current official guidelines recommend oral therapy with clarithromycin (500 mg twice daily) or azithromycin 1,200 mg every week for persons with a CD4+ count <50. Although the combination of azithromycin and rifabutin is more effective than azithromycin alone, the increased cost, adverse events, potential for drug interactions, and absence of a survival benefit preclude this regimen from being routinely recommended. If neither clarithromycin nor azithromycin is tolerated, rifabutin 300 mg daily may be used[49] (Tables 70-2 and 70-12).

Before the use of macrolides, rifabutin was the agent of choice for primary prophylaxis. However, no survival benefit has been demonstrated with the use of this agent, and the drug is associated with high cost, complex drug interactions, and an increased risk for uveitis.[49,284]

Six hundred eighty-two patients with AIDS, CD4+ counts <100, and negative MAC blood cultures were randomized to receive clarithromycin (500 mg orally twice daily) or placebo.[45] The clarithromycin arm had a 69% reduction in MAC bacteremia and fewer (16% versus 6%) cases of MAC infection. Significantly more patients in the clarithromycin arm survived during the 10-month follow-up (68% versus 59%), with an accompanying longer median duration of survival. This trial was the first prospective MAC prophylaxis study demonstrating a survival benefit and a reduced risk of disseminated MAC infection.[45]

In a randomized, double-blind placebo-controlled trial, 182 MAC-negative patients with AIDS and CD4+ counts <100 (median 44) were treated with azithromycin 1,200 mg every week or placebo.[285] Azithromycin reduced MAC bacteremia by 57% and infection (23.3% versus 8.2%). Survival benefit

Table 70-12 Drugs Commonly Used in the Treatment of *Mycobacterium avium* Complex Infection[a]

Agents	Dose	Toxicities
Initial Therapy Agents		
Clarithromycin	500 mg PO BID[b]	Nausea, vomiting, diarrhea, abdominal pain, serum transferase elevations, bitter taste
Azithromycin	500 mg PO daily	Nausea, vomiting, diarrhea, abdominal pain, serum transferase elevations
Ethambutol	15-25 mg/kg/day PO	Optic neuritis,[c] nausea and vomiting
Rifabutin[d]	300 mg/day PO	Nausea, vomiting, diarrhea, serum transferase elevations, hepatitis, neutropenia, thrombocytopenia, rash, orange discoloration of body fluids, uveitis
		↑ clearance of other drugs due to hepatic microsomal enzyme induction[e]
Secondary Agents		
Ciprofloxacin	500-750 mg PO BID	Nausea, vomiting, diarrhea, abdominal pain, headache, rare insomnia, hallucinations, seizures
Amikacin	10-15 mg/kg/day IV or IM	Nephrotoxicity, ototoxicity

[a]Macrolide + ethambutol +/− one or more of the drugs listed above.
[b]Clarithromycin dose >500 mg BID is associated with an increased mortality.
[c]Visual testing should be done monthly in patients receiving >15 mg/kg/day.
[d]Rifabutin dose 300-600 mg/day; but should not exceed 300 mg/day if given with clarithromycin or fluconazole.
[e]Common drug interactions include protease inhibitors (see Table 70-10).

was not evaluated. GI disturbance was observed more commonly in the azithromycin arm.[285]

Azithromycin 1,200 mg every week, rifabutin 300 mg daily, and a combination of both drugs in the same doses were compared in patients with AIDS and CD4$^+$ counts <100. The incidence of MAC bacteremia was 13.9% in the azithromycin monotherapy arm, 23.3% in the rifabutin monotherapy arm, and 8.3% in the azithromycin–rifabutin combination arm. Time to death was not significantly different among the treatments; however, the combination arm had an increased incidence of adverse drug effects. Although combination therapy was superior to azithromycin alone, its use is considered second-line because of the increased cost, toxicity, and lack of survival benefit.[286]

In a similar trial, patients with AIDS and CD4$^+$ counts <100 were randomized to receive clarithromycin 500 mg twice daily, rifabutin 450 mg daily, or both.[287] In the midst of the trial, the rifabutin dosage was reduced to 300 mg daily because of a drug interaction with clarithromycin that resulted in rifabutin-induced uveitis. MAC bacteremia occurred in 9% of patients in the clarithromycin monotherapy arm, 15% of patients in the rifabutin monotherapy arm, and 7% of patients receiving the combination. Time to death was not significantly different among the arms, but the combination was more toxic.

The decision to use clarithromycin or azithromycin (both first-line recommendations for primary prophylaxis) is based on patient compliance and the potential for drug interactions. Azithromycin (1,200 mg once weekly) may be preferable in a patient who has difficulty with compliance. In contrast to clarithromycin, azithromycin does not affect the cytochrome P450 enzyme system and is therefore less likely to interact with other drugs. M.E. would have benefited from MAC prophylaxis when her CD4$^+$ count decreased to <50.

Patients whose CD4$^+$ count increases from 100 for >3 months may discontinue primary prophylaxis (see Table 70-2).[49] However, prophylaxis should be reintroduced if the CD4$^+$ count decreases to <50 to 100.

ENTERIC INFECTIONS

50. A.B. is a 38-year-old woman with a 4-year history of HIV infection and a CD4$^+$ count of 160 (normal, approximately 1,000). She reports two or three watery, unformed bowel movements per day for approximately 6 weeks, with accompanying abdominal pain. She has refused antiretroviral therapy and is currently taking only one TMP-SMX double-strength tablet each day. What GI pathogens should be considered in the differential diagnosis in HIV-infected patients who develop diarrhea?

GI complications are common in HIV patients (e.g., enteric infections, gastric achlorhydria, pancreatitis, cholangitis, hepatitis, proctitis, Kaposi's sarcoma, lymphoma, carcinoma, and HIV enteropathy). Enteric infections can be caused by fungal, viral, bacterial, or protozoan pathogens. In general, clinical manifestations caused by GI infections appear with a decline in the CD4$^+$ count. Similar to A.B., most patients present with a change in bowel habits, predominantly diarrhea.[288] When evaluating infectious diarrhea, several factors should be considered. The diarrhea first must be categorized as acute or chronic. Acute diarrhea is defined as "greater than or equal

to three loose or watery stools for >10 days with fever, blood in the stool, and/or weight loss."[69] In acute diarrhea in patients with AIDS, all potential etiologies should be evaluated, including medication, dietary, or psychosomatic causes. Acute diarrhea is usually associated with bacterial causes, such as *Salmonella, Shigella, Campylobacter jejuni,* or *Clostridium difficile.*

Chronic diarrhea is defined as "greater than two to three loose or watery stools per day for >30 days."[69] Chronic infectious diarrhea also can be caused by protozoans, such as *Microsporidia, Isospora, Cyclospora, Cryptosporidia, Entamoeba histolytica,* and *Giardia.* Chronic diarrhea may also have a viral etiology (e.g., HSV or CMV). Bacteria can also be associated with chronic diarrhea, primarily *Salmonella, Shigella, C. jejuni, C. difficile,* and MAC (Table 70-13).

Fungal Infections

In acute infectious diarrhea, fungal infections are rare; they tend to be isolated to the oropharynx and esophagus and are predominantly caused by *Candida* species, primarily *C. albicans.* Other fungal infections in AIDS patients do not commonly involve the GI tract. However, patients with disseminated histoplasmosis may develop diarrhea (see Table 70-12).

Viral Infections

Viruses that infect the GI tract of AIDS patients are unlike those associated with diarrhea in non–HIV-infected patients (e.g., rotaviruses, enteric adenoviruses, Norwalk agent, coronavirus, and coxsackieviruses). More common among HIV patients are CMV and herpes simplex infections. Disseminated CMV infection is common in HIV-infected patients with advanced disease, and although retinitis is the most common CMV infection (see Questions 14 to 25), up to 2% of patients have GI involvement.[291] CMV usually involves the colon, and the common presentation is diarrhea. Tissue biopsy is preferred for a definitive diagnosis. CMV infection of the pancreas, liver, gallbladder, and biliary tree also has been described.[292] The IV agents used to treat CMV retinitis may also be used to treat CMV disease in the GI tract. In contrast to the treatment of CMV retinitis, therapy for colitis lasts 3 to 6 weeks. Data support the use of ganciclovir over foscarnet for CMV colitis, whereas the efficacy of cidofovir is unknown. Regular ophthalmologic screening for CMV retinitis is recommended for all patients with CMV GI tract disease.[42]

The other common cause of viral GI disease is herpes simplex. The clinical presentation is similar to that of disseminated CMV, but the site of infection and biopsy findings differentiate the viruses. HSV type 1 primarily is associated with ulcerated esophageal lesions. In contrast, HSV type 2 is often the cause of proctitis. Although not usually associated with diarrhea, proctitis may result in bloody mucous stools. HSV also can cause large, painful perianal lesions. Herpes simplex GI lesions usually are treated with acyclovir; if herpes-resistant virus is suspected, foscarnet is used (see Table 70-12).[69]

Bacterial Infections

Bacteria such as *Salmonella, Shigella,* and *Campylobacter* cause lower GI disease in HIV patients, but these organisms are generally more virulent in HIV-negative patients. The

Table 70-13 Enteric Infections Associated with Infectious Diarrhea

Enteric Infections	Treatment
Fungal	
Candida albicans[a]	Fluconazole 100–400 mg PO QD; or ketoconazole 200–400 mg PO QD or amphotericin B 0.3–0.5 mg/kg IV; efficacy of fluconazole is 85%
Histoplasmosis	Itraconazole 300 mg PO TID × 3 days, then 200 mg PO BID (liquid formulation has better absorption, limited data available on IV)
	Alternative: amphotericin B 0.8-1.5 mg/kg IV
Viral	
Cytomegalovirus	Ganciclovir 5 mg/kg IV BID × 2–3 wk or foscarnet 40–60 mg/kg Q 8 hr × 2–3 wk (efficacy of antiretroviral treatment is 75%)
Herpes simplex virus[a]	Acyclovir 200–800 mg PO 5×/day or 5 mg/kg IV Q 8 hr × 2–3 wk
Bacterial	
Salmonella spp.	Ciprofloxacin 500–750 mg PO BID × 14 days or TMP-SMX 1–2 DS PO BID × 14 days or ampicillin 2 g PO/day or 6 g/day IV × 14 days or third-generation cephalosporin or chloramphenicol; treatment may be extended to ≥4 wk
Shigella spp.	Ciprofloxacin 500 mg PO BID × 3 days or TMP-SMX 1 DS PO BID × 3 days; antiperistaltic agents (Lomotil or loperamide) are contraindicated
Campylobacter jejuni	Ciprofloxacin 500 mg PO BID × 3–5 days or erythromycin 500 mg PO QID × 5 days
Clostridium difficile	Metronidazole 250–500 mg PO QID × 10-14 days or vancomycin 125 mg PO QID × 10–14 days; antiperistaltic agents (Lomotil or loperamide) are contraindicated
Protozoa	
Isospora	TMP-SMX 1 DS BID; alternative: pyrimethamine 75 mg with folinic acid 10 mg
Cyclospora	TMP-SMX 1 DS BID
Microsporidia	Albendazole 400-800 mg PO BID × 3>wk; efficacy is established for *Septata intestinalis, E. bieneusi:* best results are with highly active antiretroviral therapy
	Alternative: metronidazole, atovaquone, and thalidomide
Cryptosporidia	No effective treatment; paromomycin, nitazoxanide, octreotide, azithromycin (marginal benefits and no cure)

[a]Primarily esophagitis.
Adapted from references 288 and 289.

frequency of acute infectious diarrhea caused by *Salmonella* for patients with AIDS is 5% to 15%. *Salmonella* bacteremia is considered an AIDS-defining diagnosis. The clinical features include fever and watery stools, with variable fecal WBCs. Diagnosis is made based on stool and blood cultures. In contrast to immunocompetent persons, antibiotics are recommended for treatment of *Salmonella* in HIV-infected patients; ciprofloxacin (750 mg twice daily for 2 weeks) is the preferred regimen. Alternative regimens include ampicillin (8 to 12 g IV daily for 1 to 4 weeks), amoxicillin (500 mg orally three times daily to complete a 2- to 4-week course), TMP-SMX (5 to 10 mg/kg daily IV or orally for 2 to 4 weeks), or a third-generation cephalosporin. Eradication of *Salmonella* has been demonstrated only with ciprofloxacin. Bacteremia may be more frequent compared with non–HIV-infected patients and may recur despite antibiotic therapy. For recurrent therapy, ciprofloxacin (500 mg orally twice daily) is preferred for several months. TMP-SMX (5 to 10 mg/kg TMP component daily IV or orally) may be considered as an alternative. Lifelong treatment may be required (see Table 70-13).[293,294]

The frequency of *Shigella* is 1% to 3% in acute infectious diarrhea in AIDS patients; *S. sonnei* accounts for approximately 70% of the reported U.S. cases. *S. flexneri* is also reported in young homosexual men. Person-to-person spread is the main route of transmission. *Shigella* causes dysentery, fever, and abdominal cramps, which precede voluminous watery stools. Bloody mucoid stools with fecal urgency may also develop. Fecal WBCs are common, and diagnosis is made by stool culture. Mild to severe cases of *Shigella* bacteremia have been reported, lasting an average of 7 days if untreated. Because this is a self-limiting illness and resistance is common, treatment is recommended only in severely ill patients. Antibiotic therapy should be selected based on susceptibility patterns. Ciprofloxacin (500 mg orally twice daily) or TMP-SMX (1 double-strength tablet orally twice daily for 3 days) both are effective regimens. Antiperistaltic agents are contraindicated. As with *Salmonella, Shigella* infections are associated with an increased frequency of bacteremia in HIV-infected patients, which may require prolonged therapy (see Table 70-13).[294,295]

C. jejuni accounts for 4% to 8% of cases of acute infectious diarrhea in AIDS patients. *Campylobacter* enteritis is associated with a prodrome of fever, headaches, myalgia, and malaise 12 to 24 hours before diarrhea and abdominal pain. Diarrhea varies from loose bowel movements to voluminous watery and grossly bloody stools. Fecal leukocytes are variable, and the diagnosis is made by stool culture. *Campylobacter* enteritis is self-limiting, lasting only several days; however, some HIV-infected persons have symptoms lasting

>1 week and may relapse if left untreated. Antibiotics are recommended for patients with high fevers, bloody stools, more than eight stools per day, and symptoms for >1 week without improvement. Erythromycin (500 mg orally four times daily for 5 days) and ciprofloxacin (500 mg orally twice daily for 3 to 5 days) are the preferred agents. Quinolone-resistant isolates have been documented. Alternatives to erythromycin or ciprofloxacin include tetracycline, clindamycin, and ampicillin (see Table 70-12).[294,296]

HIV patients should take preventive measures against potential enteric pathogens. Close attention to hand hygiene is recommended, as is not handling or eating raw or uncooked poultry, fruits, vegetables, and nonpasteurized dairy products. Fortunately, the widespread use of TMP-SMX for PCP prophylaxis has reduced the frequency of these bacterial infections. Disseminated MAC disease, *M. tuberculosis, Helicobacter pylori,* and *C. difficile* also can cause diarrhea in HIV-infected patients.[49,288]

Protozoal Infections

As a group, protozoal infections are the most common cause of diarrhea among HIV-infected patients. Opportunistic protozoans such as *Cryptosporidium, Isospora belli,* and *Microsporidia* are well-known GI pathogens. Other nonopportunistic protozoans such as *Giardia lamblia, Entameba histolytica,* and *Cyclospora cayetanensis* also cause disease.[288]

Cryptosporidium, a coccidioidin protozoan with a life cycle that occurs entirely within a single host, can be transmitted from animals to humans by fecal water contamination or person-to-person fecal–oral spread.[297] HIV-infected patients should be advised to wash their hands after contact with fecal material (e.g., changing diapers), exposure to pets, gardening, or contact with soil, and they should avoid oral–anal sexual practices. HIV-infected patients also should avoid drinking water from lakes and swallowing water during recreational activities. Outbreaks of cryptosporidiosis have been linked to municipal water supplies.[298] HIV-infected patients should avoid eating raw oysters because the oocysts can survive in oysters for >2 months.[49] In patients with AIDS, the frequency of chronic infectious diarrhea due to cryptosporidiosis is 10% to 30%.[66] In contrast to the explosive onset that occurs in non-HIV patients, acute cryptosporidiosis in AIDS patients is more insidious and progresses in severity as the degree of immunosuppression increases. Intestinal cryptosporidiosis may be complicated by concurrent biliary involvement, leading to jaundice and hepatosplenomegaly. Although the diagnosis of cryptosporidiosis formerly depended on intestinal tissue biopsy, newer techniques such as staining oocysts in stool (modified acid-fast methods) and fluorescent antibody assays have been developed.[299] No known prophylaxis exists; however, one MAC prophylaxis study suggested that clarithromycin and rifabutin also may prevent cryptosporidiosis.[300] After >10 years, the treatment of cryptosporidiosis remains investigational and studies have progressed slowly. Supportive care that includes fluid and electrolytes, parenteral hyperalimentation, and antidiarrheal agents often is necessary.

The long-acting somatostatin analog octreotide acetate (50 to 500 μg three times daily subcutaneously or IV at 1 μg/hr) also has been used with limited benefit in some patients. However, it is expensive and the parenteral administration is inconvenient for many patients.[299] Trials of α-difluoromethylornithine (DFMO) and oral spiramycin have yielded inconsistent results. Other drugs such as IV spiramycin, letrazuril, hyperimmune bovine colostrum, transfer factor (a dialyzable leukocyte extract obtained from cow lymph nodes), and IGX-CP (an oral formulation of chicken egg yolks immunized with *Cryptosporidium* antigen) are under investigation, but preliminary results are not encouraging.[299]

Paromomycin (500 to 750 mg orally four times per day with food for 21 days, then 500 mg orally twice daily) is a poorly absorbed aminoglycoside antibiotic commonly used to treat HIV-infected patients with cryptosporidiosis.[289] Paromomycin, 1 g twice daily plus azithromycin 600 mg daily for 4 weeks followed by paromomycin alone, 1 g twice daily for 8 weeks, was associated with improvement of symptoms and a significant reduction in oocyst excretion. Azithromycin, an azalide antibiotic, when used alone, is ineffective.[301]

Nitazoxanide (NTZ) is an antimicrobial compound with activity against protozoans, helminths, and bacterial organisms. This drug has recently been approved for use; the usual dosage is 500 mg orally twice daily for 3 days.[69,299,302] Data have demonstrated a 30% favorable response rate in HIV-negative but not HIV-positive subjects. Higher doses or longer durations of therapy may be needed in HIV-infected patients.

Several reports suggest that treatment with HAART results in improved immune function and subsequent resolution of cryptosporidiosis.[38,303]

I. belli, a coccidioidin protozoan, has a life cycle similar to that of *Cryptosporidium.* The frequency of *I. belli* is 1% to 3% in chronic infectious diarrhea in patients with AIDS. *Isospora* is rarely identified as a cause of diarrhea (<1%) in the United States and Europe, in contrast to Africa, Haiti, and Latin America.[304] Clinically, these patients develop diarrhea, steatorrhea, cramping, and weight loss. In AIDS patients, as well as infants or children without AIDS, this disease may become a protracted illness.[299,304] Similar to *Cryptosporidium,* the diagnosis of isosporiasis is made with acid-fast stains. *Isospora* oocysts are larger and morphologically distinct. Importantly, and in contrast to cryptosporidiosis, isosporiasis can be treated with TMP-SMX (160 mg daily and 800 mg daily, respectively). Chronic suppressive therapy often is needed and can be accomplished with lower doses of TMP-SMX or pyrimethamine-sulfadoxine (see Table 70-12).

Microsporidium (a ubiquitous, obligate intracellular protozoan parasite) characterizes the four genera (out of hundreds) of *Microsporidia* known to cause human disease; it is responsible for 15% to 30% of chronic infectious diarrhea in AIDS patients. Among AIDS patients, the cornea, liver, peritoneum, and small intestine have been reported to be infected with *Microsporidium.*[290] The primary species associated with AIDS patients are *Enterocytozoon bieneusi* or *Septata intestinalis.* These can be identified in intestinal biopsy specimens using electron microscopy and hematoxylin-and-eosin–stained paraffin-embedded sections. Albendazole (400 to 800 mg orally twice daily for >3 weeks) has been found to be efficacious in the treatment of *S. intestinalis.* Some patients have been successfully treated with metronidazole, atovaquone, and thalidomide (see Table 70-12).[290,305,306] Several reports suggest that infection resolves with HAART therapy.[38,49]

GI manifestations of HIV infection become increasingly common in the advanced stages of HIV infection. A.B.

presents with chronic infectious diarrhea (two or three watery stools for >30 days). Review of her current medications (to rule out a medication source for diarrhea) revealed only low-dose TMP-SMX. CMV, MAC, *Microsporidia, Isospora,* and *Cyclospora* are common in patients with a CD4+ count <100. Stool analyses, including ova and parasites, AFB smears, bacterial culture, *C. difficile* toxin assay, and *Microsporidia* assay, were ordered. A fecal WBC examination was also ordered. The AFB smear of stool showed *Cryptosporidia* oocysts. A.B. was empirically treated with paromomycin, 500 mg orally four times a day with food for 21 days, then 500 mg orally twice daily with food for chronic suppressive therapy. Baseline auditory and renal function assessment should be done before initiation of therapy to monitor for ototoxicity and nephrotoxicity. A.B. should be treated symptomatically with nutritional supplements and antidiarrheal agents (Lomotil or loperamide). HAART therapy with immune recovery may reverse the progression of her enteritis and should be recommended.

ESOPHAGEAL DISEASE

51. **P.J. is a 45-year-old, HIV-positive man who was started on AZT, 3TC, and saquinavir when he was diagnosed 1 year ago. P.J. is a heroin user and has not been seen in the clinic since his initial presentation. He appears today complaining of difficult, painful swallowing and diffuse pain. Upon examination, localized white plaques are observed in the oral cavity. His CD4+ count is 280 (normal, approximately 1,000). What is the most likely cause of this patient's dysphagia and odynophagia?**

Esophagitis in HIV-positive patients generally is caused by *Candida* (50% to 75% of cases), CMV (10% to 20%), HSV (2% to 5%), and aphthous ulcers (10% to 20%).[69] Symptoms include dysphagia, odynophagia, and thrush (with *Candida* infections). Oral ulcers are common with HSV, rare with *Candida,* and uncommon with CMV or aphthous ulcers. Pain is usually diffuse in *Candida* infections and more focused with HSV, CMV, and aphthous ulcers. Fever is primarily associated with CMV.

Up to 75% of AIDS patients develop oral candidiasis, a consequence of a failing immune system and fungal colonization of the oropharynx. Patients with localized white plaques in the oral cavity likely have oral candidiasis (thrush) and should be started on antifungal therapy. Initially, patients may be treated with local antifungal therapy (e.g., "swish and swallow" nystatin suspension 3 million units four or five times daily or clotrimazole troches four or five times daily). If no response is noted or symptoms of esophageal involvement develop (e.g., dysphagia or odynophagia), these patients should be treated with a systemic agent; the azoles are preferred. Many patients with thrush without esophagitis do not respond to topical treatment and also require systemic azole therapy.

Esophagitis due to *C. albicans* increases in frequency as HIV progresses. Not all patients with thrush develop esophagitis; however, patients who experience esophageal symptoms generally will have esophagitis. Diagnosis is made using endoscopy and microbiology. Multiple white or gray plaques are observed endoscopically; they may be discrete or appear as continuous exudates.[307] Esophageal candidiasis must be treated as a systemic infection; local antifungal

agents should never be used. Therapy should be initiated with oral fluconazole (Diflucan) 200 mg orally, then 100 mg orally daily for 2 to 3 weeks (up to 400 mg daily). Fluconazole is the preferred azole because of fewer toxicities, fewer drug–food interactions, and a reduced potential for drug–drug interactions. Alternative oral therapies include itraconazole (Sporanox) oral solution or ketoconazole (Nizoral). If azole-resistant candidiasis or severe disease is diagnosed, parenteral amphotericin B (0.3 to 0.5 mg/kg daily IV with or without flucytosine 100 mg/kg daily) should be used.[308]

CMV esophagitis should be considered in patients who do not respond to a 1-week course of an antifungal. CMV esophagitis is confirmed via endoscopic biopsy demonstrating erythema and single or multiple discrete erosive lesions, usually located distally.[42,292] Acute treatment consists of ganciclovir 5 mg/kg IV per dose twice daily or foscarnet 40 to 60 mg/kg IV per dose Q 8 hr for 2 to 3 weeks. Maintenance therapy, if used, is usually half the dose used for induction treatment. Patients with CMV esophagitis have a poor prognosis.

Diagnosis of esophageal disease caused by HSV is by endoscopy, which reveals erythema and erosions. These small shallow ulcers usually coalesce. HSV can be successfully treated with acyclovir. Aphthous ulcers are similar in appearance and location to CMV, and negative results for *Candida,* HSV, and CMV are suggestive of aphthous ulcers. Acute treatment involves prednisone 40 mg daily for 7 to 10 days, tapered to 10 mg/week. Thalidomide, 200 mg daily, is a promising regimen; one trial demonstrated a 53% response compared with 7% in the placebo group.[309]

A presumptive diagnosis of *Candida* esophagitis can be made for P.J. because he presents with oral pharyngeal candidiasis, dysphagia, and odynophagia. P.J. should be empirically treated with fluconazole, 200 mg daily for 14 to 21 days. If he is unresponsive to fluconazole, endoscopy with biopsy and culture should be performed to confirm the diagnosis. If candidiasis is confirmed, P.J. should be checked for medication adherence and potential drug interactions. If the patient is adherent and does not have malabsorption, parenteral amphotericin B should be considered. Anecdotally, fluconazole doses have been increased in some patients with refractory candidiasis, with successful clinical outcomes. This may be an option prior to amphotericin therapy.[310] Relapse is common in patients who do not receive secondary prophylaxis. Chronic suppressive therapy (fluconazole 100 to 200 mg daily) should be considered in all patients responsive to fluconazole therapy who have frequent or severe recurrent esophagitis. However, this practice has been documented to increase the probability of azole resistance.[49,311]

HIV WASTING SYNDROME

52. **J.R. is a 38-year-old woman who has been followed in the HIV clinic for 8 years. She has been treated with antiretroviral therapy for 5 years from the time she developed PCP. She has chronic oral candidiasis managed with intermittent fluconazole. Her last CD4+ count was 90 (normal, approximately 1,000). Over the last two visits, J.R.'s weight has declined from a baseline weight of 140 lb to 115 lb. She reports two or three loose stools per day, intermittent fevers, loss of appetite, and a generalized weakness for at least 5 weeks. What is the potential cause of J.R.'s weight loss, and how should it be managed?**

Rapid disease progression is associated with significant weight loss in HIV-infected patients. Wasting syndrome can be defined as "the unintentional weight loss of >10% of baseline body weight plus chronic diarrhea (more than two loose stools a day for >30 days) or chronic weakness with unexplainable fever that is intermittent or constant for >30 days."[312]

The pathophysiology of HIV wasting syndrome is not clearly understood, but it is characterized by depletion of both adipose and lean body tissue. Because weight loss may also signal an opportunistic infection (e.g., enteric infection, PCP, or MAC), these etiologies must be ruled out.[2] Wasting syndrome may be multifactorial, resulting from decreased nutritional intake or absorption, accelerated nutrient metabolism, stress, or a combination of these factors.[312,314] J.R. meets the criteria for wasting with an unintentional 18% weight loss accompanied by chronic diarrhea and weakness.

Three appetite stimulants are routinely used to treat HIV-related wasting (Table 70-14). Megestrol acetate is an oral synthetic progestin related to progesterone. This drug is widely used for the treatment of hormone-responsive malignancies, but it is also approved for HIV-infected patients who have lost at least 10% of their ideal body weight. Megestrol 400 to 800 mg daily has been associated with weight gains of up to 10 kg.[315,316] However, a significant portion of the observed weight gain appears to be fat mass rather than lean tissue. Hypergonadism, diabetes, and adrenal insufficiency are the most serious side effects. Other side effects include impotence, diarrhea, reduced testosterone levels, hyperglycemia, and alopecia.

Dronabinol (delta-9-tetrahydrocannabinol), the psychoactive component of marijuana, 2.5 mg twice daily has been approved for AIDS-related weight loss. The dronabinol significantly increases appetite,[317] increases body weight (primarily fat), and improves mood. Besides stimulating appetite, dronabinol also has antiemetic effects, which are useful in patients with nausea and vomiting associated with the wasting syndrome. Euphoria, dizziness, confusion, and somnolence occur in 18% of dronabinol-treated patients. A reduction in the dose of dronabinol to 2.5 mg 1 hour before supper or bedtime may reduce adverse events. Because of its potential for misuse, dronabinol should be used with caution in patients with a history of substance abuse. Patients should be counseled to avoid driving, operating machinery, or other potentially hazardous activity until it is established that they can safely perform these activities. Alcohol or other CNS depressants may result in additive CNS depression.

Cyproheptadine is an antihistamine reported to stimulate appetite in HIV-infected patients. The use of cyproheptadine 12 mg daily has been associated with minimal weight gain as a result of an increase in daily caloric intake. This drug, although used for the treatment of anorexia, is not approved by the FDA for HIV wasting (see Table 70-14).

Anabolic steroids and testosterone have been shown to increase muscle mass and strength in people with HIV wasting syndrome. Products include oxandrolone (Oxandrin), nan-

Table 70-14 HIV Wasting Regimens

Agent	Dose	Side Effects	Comments
Approved			
Megestrol acetate[a]	400–800 mg daily	Impotence, GI disturbances and endocrine effects	Dose must be tapered before discontinuation
Dronabinol[a]	2.5 mg twice daily (before lunch and dinner)	Euphoria, dizziness, confusion, sedation	Use with caution in patients with a history of drug abuse
Somatropin (rhGH)[b]	0.1 mg/kg/day SC (6 mg/day)	Edema, arthralgias, myalgias, paresthesias, diarrhea	Long-term effect unknown / Expensive agent
Unlabeled Use			
Oxandrolone[b]	5–20 mg/day	Elevated LFTs	FDA orphan drug
Oxymetholone[b]	25–50 mg/day	Irritability and aggression	Monitor glucose tolerance
Testosterone[b]	200–400 mg IM Q 2 wk	Irritability, aggression, gynecomastia, acne	Endogenous testosterone levels must be <400 ng/dL for all anabolic steroid administration
→ Cypionate or enanthate	4 or 6 mg/day		
→ Testoderm scrotal patch	5 mg/day		
→ TTS patch	5 mg/day		
→ Androderm			
Nandrolone[b] decanoate	100–200 mg IM Q 2 wk	Elevated hemoglobin and hematocrit, dysmenorrhea	Anabolic steroid
Thalidomide	300–400 mg/day	Teratogenicity, somnolence, rash, peripheral neuropathy	FDA orphan drug / Enhanced sedation with other CNS depressants
Cyproheptadine[a]	12–20 mg/day	Sedation	Antihistamine

[a]Appetite stimulants: weight gain predominantly fat, not lean body mass.
[b]Significant increases in lean body mass.
CNS, central nervous system; GI, gastrointestinal; IM, intramuscularly; LFTs, liver function tests; SC, subcutaneously.

drolone (Deca-Durabolin), oxymetholone (Anadrol-50), and testosterone.[318,319] Oxandrolone at a dosage of 15 mg daily significantly increases body weight but does not improve body strength. The usual dosage for males is 10 to 20 mg twice daily; for females the range is 5 to 20 mg daily. This drug has a low androgenic effect, so it is particularly useful in women. Most weight gain is lean body mass. Minimal hepatotoxicity has been associated with this agent.[318] Oxandrolone can be administered orally, which may improve adherence.[318,320]

Nandrolone (Deca-Durabolin) increases body weight, muscle mass, and strength. Nandrolone has a high anabolic effect and a low androgenic effect. The dosage of nandrolone for males is 100 to 200 mg intramuscularly every 1 to 2 weeks and for females 25 mg intramuscularly per week or 50 mg intramuscularly every 2 weeks.[320,321]

Oxymetholone is not recommended for use in women because of its high androgenic potential. Hepatic toxicity is common, so LFTs must be carefully monitored. Doses of 50 mg twice daily are used in HIV-infected male patients.[320] In an open-label study, oxymetholone produced a mean weight gain of 5.7 kg with improvement in the Karnofsky score in HIV-infected patients with wasting syndrome.[322] It has high androgenic and some anabolic effects, so it may be better suited for HIV-infected men.

A decrease in testosterone correlates with a decrease in lean body mass in AIDS patients.[319] Testosterone administration produces a significant increase in lean body mass (mean of 1.2 kg) in HIV-positive patients without wasting syndrome. It is available as long-acting intramuscular injections (enanthate and cypionate), short-acting intramuscular injections (propionate), and a transdermal system (2.5 mg/24 hours; 4 mg/24 hours; 5 mg/24 hours; 6 mg/24 hours). The transdermal systems differ in release rate, surface area, and total testosterone content. Testosterone should be used in patients with low endogenous testosterone levels (<400 ng/dL in men). Testosterone has been associated with improved mood, libido, and energy in clinical trials. It is also associated with acne, gynecomastia, alopecia, and testicular atrophy. Testosterone has been shown to be less effective than oxandrolone or nandrolone for weight gain.[323,324] In clinical practice, testosterone is sometimes combined with megestrol acetate or nandrolone, but this combination has not been studied.

Growth hormones (which directly influence nitrogen balance and muscle protein synthesis) have been used in the treatment of HIV wasting syndrome. These include recombinant human insulin–like growth factor-1 (rhIGF-1) and somatropin (Serostim), a recombinant human growth hormone (rhGH). Disturbances in growth hormone–insulin- like growth factor-1 axis have been described in HIV-positive subjects. In one placebo-controlled trial, 10 mg daily of rhIGF-1 subcutaneously failed to significantly increase weight or lean body mass.[325] Subcutaneous injections of somatropin (0.1 mg/kg daily) have been associated with increases in lean body mass and functional performance.[326] Adverse events include edema, arthralgia, diabetes, acute pancreatitis, and carpal tunnel syndrome. The questionable long-term benefits and the tremendous expense of growth hormone diminish its appeal (see Table 70-14).[321]

Several cytokine modulators are used in the treatment of HIV wasting. These include pentoxifylline (Trental), thalidomide, ketotifen, and omega-3 fatty acids (fish oil). Altered metabolism of cytokines, tumor necrosis factor (TNF), interleukin-1 (IL-1), or interferon-α may play a role in the wasting syndrome. As an example, an elevation in serum TNF-α has been noted in HIV patients with advanced disease. Thalidomide and pentoxifylline, which decrease TNF-α, have been used in patients with HIV wasting syndrome Thalidomide has been associated with significant weight gain.[320,327] However, thalidomide is associated with numerous adverse effects, including somnolence, rash, teratogenicity, and peripheral neuropathy (additive with other drugs known to cause peripheral neuropathy). It may also be associated with an elevation in HIV-RNA levels; however, more recent studies are needed for confirmation. Pentoxifylline, a drug used to prevent intermittent claudication, has also been evaluated as treatment for the HIV wasting syndrome. Unfortunately, since pentoxifylline has failed to stimulate the appetite or increase weight gain, it does not have a role in the treatment of HIV wasting.[320]

Exercise has been considered as a possible intervention for HIV wasting. The preliminary results of one study demonstrated an increase in lean body mass and strength after patients underwent an 8-week course of progressive resistance training.[328]

J.R. must be assessed for possible OIs and treated accordingly. Once the diarrhea has resolved, medications to reverse HIV wasting may be started. The patient's lack of appetite should be addressed first with the use of megestrol acetate (400 mg/day oral suspension). In addition, the patient should be started on oxandrolone (10 mg/day orally). A pregnancy test should be performed because most anabolic agents should not be administered to pregnant women. Because of their high androgenic effects, oxymetholone and testosterone should be avoided in J.R.

HIV-ASSOCIATED MALIGNANCIES

53. **Despite an extensive microbiologic workup, no organism was identified, and other causes for J.R.'s change in bowel habits were evaluated. What neoplastic conditions could be contributing to J.R.'s GI status?**

In addition to the OIs described under enteric infections, GI malignancy is common in patients with HIV. As the CD4$^+$ count declines, patients may develop Kaposi's sarcoma (see following section), lymphoma, and invasive cervical cancer. The reason for the increased occurrence of malignancy is unknown, but it may be related to impaired immune function. In addition, effective antiretroviral therapy and prophylactic anti-infective therapy have extended the life span of patients with AIDS, increasing the likelihood that malignancies will be detected.[329,330] J.R. has been on HAART therapy and prophylactic anti-infective therapy for many years; thus, she may be at risk for malignancy.

Kaposi's Sarcoma

Kaposi's sarcoma (KS) previously was well described in non–HIV-infected patients, and its course was fairly uneventful. Consequently, limited studies of innovative chemotherapy regimens were conducted in the past. In contrast, KS in HIV-infected patients is more invasive and is associated with increased morbidity and mortality.[330] Although KS occurs predominantly in homosexual men, the incidence of KS has increased in IV drug users, recipients of blood products, women, and children. The risk of developing KS is 20,000 times greater for HIV-infected patients than for non–HIV-infected persons. The incidence of KS as a presenting AIDS illness has significantly declined since the early 1990s, and this may be indirectly due to HAART.[331] An infectious etiology has been suggested in recent studies. DNA sequencing in KS tissue has detected a herpes virus. A new human herpes virus 8 (HHV-8) has been observed in biopsies of classic KS, African KS, and HIV-positive KS. This finding suggests that HHV-8 is either a causative agent or a recurrent passenger virus (i.e., an "innocent bystander").[332,333]

Other studies have suggested that the pathogenesis of KS in HIV patients is related to the existence of cells with the potential to become KS lesions. Cytokines released from activated immune cells potentially stimulate the proliferation of KS precursor cells at a time when the immune function for such cells is becoming progressively impaired. Furthermore, some cells may produce a growth factor for KS cells (e.g., angiogenic factors), and the expression of the tat gene by HIV may produce growth factors that induce vascular KS-like tumors.[329,334–336]

KS presents with three types of lesions: flat, raised, or nodular. The lesions occur primarily on the skin, oral mucosa, GI tract, and lungs. KS lesions may be asymptomatic or painful; intestinal or pulmonary lesions may be associated with significant clinical symptoms such as dyspnea or diarrhea. Cutaneous disease involves initially small, flat lesions that progress to reddish or purple nodules.[336] They are generally asymptomatic and follow a pattern of cutaneous lymphatic drainage. Progression of KS leads to lesions in the oral cavity in approximately one third of cases.[333] KS has a multifactorial presentation without a primary lesion; therefore, staging according to a standard tumor-node-metastasis (TNM) classification is not appropriate. A staging system proposed in 1989 by the ACTG Oncology Committee divides patients into good- or poor-risk groups based on tumor characteristics, the patient's immunity (measured by CD4+ count), and the severity of systemic HIV-associated illness.[334,335] Whether staging and the choice or response to therapy are correlated is unclear.

The growth of KS is stimulated by inflammatory cytokines, which are increased in acute OIs and active HIV replication. Successful management of KS includes optimal antiretroviral therapy, prophylactic therapy, and effective treatment of OIs. Mild disease is not treated; therefore, management of KS can be divided into local therapy and systemic therapy.[335] Local therapy involves the use of topical liquid nitrogen cryotherapy, intralesional injections of vinblastine 0.01 to 0.02 mg/lesion every 2 weeks for 3 doses, and low-dose radiation therapy (e.g., 400 rads every week for 6 weeks). Local therapy is used in slowly progressive KS without life-threatening organ involvement. Systemic therapy involves the use of interferon-α, 18 to 36 million IU daily intramuscularly or subcutaneously for 10 to 12 weeks, followed by 18 million units per day with additional chemotherapeutic agents. These include paclitaxel (Taxol) 100 to 135 mg/m² IV every 2 to 3 weeks; doxorubicin (Adriamycin), bleomycin, plus either vincristine or vinblastine (ABV) or bleomycin plus vincristine; liposomal daunorubicin (DaunoXome) 40 to 60 mg/m² IV

every 2 weeks; or liposomal doxorubicin (Doxil) 10 to 20 mg/m².[335]

The use of interferon-α for KS in patients with AIDS has been well studied alone and in combination with antiretroviral therapy.[337,338] Early studies demonstrated that AIDS patients receiving high doses of interferon developed neutropenia and neurologic toxicity, and that nonresponders had high circulating levels of endogenous interferon.[337–340] Later, in vitro data indicated that interferon-α was synergistic with zidovudine against HIV. As a result, interferon therapy was investigated in combination with zidovudine.[338,339] Unfortunately, increasing doses of both interferon-α and zidovudine caused neutropenia, hepatitis, and neurologic toxicity. However, patients who could tolerate the combination had partial or complete remissions and had increased CD4+ counts. The hematologic toxicity caused by this combination has prompted researchers to evaluate the concurrent use of colony-stimulating factors such as G-CSF and GM-CSF. Preliminary results indicate that colony-stimulating factors can attenuate the hematologic toxicity.[340] Although interferon may be helpful for certain patients with KS, many cannot tolerate this agent. For this reason, drugs that inhibit the effects of angiogenic factors are under study. Patients with progressive disease, widespread skin involvement (>25 lesions), extensive cutaneous KS unresponsive to local treatment, and/or visceral organ involvement (especially lung KS) require chemotherapeutic agents. Newer products such as liposomal anthracyclines demonstrate comparable clinical efficacy with reduced toxicities.[341] Experimental therapies include foscarnet, ganciclovir, and cidofovir because of their in vitro activity against HHV-8.[342] Intralesional β-human chorionic gonadotropin injections also have produced favorable responses.[343]

Non-Hodgkin's Lymphoma

Non-Hodgkin's lymphoma (NHL) is more common in people infected with HIV, particularly those with low CD4+ counts (median, 100 cells/mm³).[344] Unlike KS, NHL occurs in all risk groups of HIV-infected patients and does not predominantly occur in homosexual men.[346] High-grade NHLs account for approximately 3% of initial AIDS-defining illnesses in adults and adolescents.[345] The reason for the increased incidence is unknown; however, similar to KS, cytokine dysregulation may play a role.[329]

HIV patients often have disseminated disease at the time of diagnosis. In fact, many patients with systemic NHL have extranodal disease (87% to 95%). Patients also may present with GI involvement at sites such as the oral cavity, esophagus, small bowel, large bowel, appendix, and anorectum. Involvement of the subcutaneous and soft tissue, epidural space, myocardium, and pericardium has been reported. Patients with CNS lymphomas often present with altered mental status, which may be mistaken for cerebral toxoplasmosis or HIV dementia. Only brain biopsy definitively diagnoses CNS NHL. Poor prognostic risk factors for patients with NHL include a CD4+ count of <100, bone marrow involvement, Karnofsky performance status <70, stage IV disease, and a history of a prior AIDS-defining illness. Patients having none of the aforementioned prognostic risk factors have a threefold greater survival rate compared with patients with one or more of these risk factors.[345,347]

The treatment of NHL is determined by organ involvement. Patients with evidence of CNS lymphoma often require local radiation or intrathecal chemotherapy. Several systemic chemotherapy regimens have been evaluated,[348] including cyclophosphamide with doxorubicin, vincristine, and prednisone (CHOP); cyclophosphamide with methyl GAG, bleomycin, prednisone, doxorubicin, and vincristine (NHL-7); cyclophosphamide combined with vincristine, intrathecal methotrexate, doxorubicin, and prednisone (L-17); and methotrexate, bleomycin, doxorubicin, cyclophosphamide, and dexamethasone (m-BACOD). Of these regimens, low-dose m-BACOD and low-dose CHOP are considered to be the standard therapies for NHL.[349]

Patients with NHL tend to have more advanced HIV disease accompanied by reduced bone marrow reserves. As a result, patients with poor prognostic factors do not tolerate full doses of chemotherapy and often develop leukopenia. These patients benefit from low-dose treatment. Patients with good prognostic risk factors may benefit from full-dose chemotherapy along with a colony-stimulating factor (e.g., G-CSF, GM-CSF) and may still be able to remain on antiretroviral therapy.[347,350]

Because J.R. presents with pathogen-negative, persistent, large-volume chronic diarrhea, KS and NHL must be ruled out. J.R. has shown no visible skin lesions or oral lesions of KS, and endoscopy revealed a small GI tumor. Tissue biopsy ruled out KS and confirmed NHL, which was found to be stage II. The bone marrow aspirate was also positive for NHL. The prognostic risk factors for J.R. include a CD4+ count <100 and a past history of an AIDS-defining illness (PCP). Consequently, low-dose m-BACOD was initiated with GM-CSF as needed. J.R. will be monitored for resolution of diarrhea as well as toxicities (e.g., hematologic). Her HAART therapy also should be re-evaluated.

Cervical Intraepithelial Neoplasia

54. L.P., a 38-year-old woman, was heterosexually infected with HIV. She also has a history of human papillomavirus (HPV) infection successfully treated with imiquimod cream 5%. During a routine HIV clinic visit, a "cheesy" vaginal discharge is noted. L.P. states that her vagina has been itching. Physical examination is unremarkable with the exception of her vaginal discharge. A potassium hydroxide stain of vaginal secretions is positive for hyphae, indicating a yeast infection. CBC values include Hgb, 13.3 g/dL (normal, 12.1 to 15.3); WBC count, 5,500 cells/L (normal, 3,800 to 9,800); and platelets, 95,000/mm³ (normal, 150,000 to 450,000). Notably, for the first time, L.P.'s CD4+ count has declined to 435 cells/mm³ (normal, approximately 1,000). She has received no prior antiretroviral therapy. Is L.P.'s gynecologic presentation typical of a woman with early HIV disease?

[SI units: Hgb, 130 g/L (normal, 121 to 153); WBC count, 5.5 ×10⁹/L (normal, 3.8 to 9.8); platelets, 95 ×10⁹/L (normal, 150 to 450)]

Four gynecologic disorders occur more frequently, with greater severity, and with less responsiveness in HIV-infected women[351–353]: HPV, associated cervical intraepithelial neoplasia, *Candida* vaginitis, and pelvic inflammatory disease (PID). All are considered CDC HIV-associated conditions.[3,354] Cervical neoplasia is a CDC AIDS-defining illness.[3] Consequently, L.P.'s presentation with vaginitis is typical. Her vaginal yeast infection should be treated with an antifungal agent

such as fluconazole (100 mg/day orally) for at least 7 days. She should be followed closely to ensure that her infection resolves, since HIV-positive patients may not respond to the standard duration of therapy.

55. L.P. returns to the clinic in a week and her vaginal infection has cleared. A routine Pap smear is performed on this visit, demonstrating cellular changes consistent with a low-grade squamous intraepithelial lesion. What therapeutic intervention should follow this abnormal Pap smear?

Women at increased risk of precancerous cervical cytology include those with HIV infection or HPV infection and cigarette smokers.[355–357] HPV infections, types 16, 18, and 33, are more prevalent among HIV-positive women than HIV-negative women and have been causally implicated in the development of preinvasive and invasive cervical neoplasms.[358] Furthermore, the greater the degree of immunosuppression (CD4+ count <200), the higher the risk for cervical intraepithelial neoplasia.[359] Rapidly progressive cervical malignancy and death have been reported in HIV-infected women.[355,360,361]

All HIV-infected women should have Pap smears every 6 months in the first year of diagnosis.[49] In HIV-infected women, approximately 15% of low-grade squamous intraepithelial lesions progress to high-grade lesions, including moderate to severe dysplasia or carcinoma in situ.[362,363] Because the risk of progression may be greater in HIV-infected women, many gynecologists recommend colposcopic examination (microscopic inspection of the entire cervical area) with directed biopsy.

If a biopsy confirms precancerous cellular changes, as in L.P., a surgical procedure is indicated to destroy or remove the dysplastic tissue.[363] Options include laser therapy, electrosurgery (LEEP), and cryotherapy. Postsurgical complications may include prolonged bleeding or infertility because of cervical stenosis.[365,366] After surgery, L.P. should have follow-up Pap smears every 3 months for at least 1 year.[363,364] The risk of recurrence is much higher in HIV-infected women.[358]

Pharmacologic Intervention

56. What pharmacologic intervention has proven to be successful in the treatment of cervical intraepithelial neoplasia? Is L.P. a candidate for this therapy?

Interferon has been suggested for the treatment of cervical intraepithelial neoplasia.[367] Many uncontrolled studies have been performed, but the number of women who have been evaluated is insufficient to recommend use of this agent. The best results were observed in one small study with systemic administration, but most patients experienced adverse effects.[367] In an additional trial, 15 women were treated with interferon-β, 2 million IUs intramuscularly daily for 10 days, and their outcomes were compared with 15 women treated with saline.[368] After >6 months, 14 of 15 (93%) of the treated women had a complete response compared with 6 of 15 (40%) of the controls. In a placebo-controlled trial using the same dosage regimen,[369] women with earlier-stage cervical intraepithelial neoplasia disease responded, but women with more advanced disease responded poorly. A flu-like syndrome characterized by fever, chills, headache, malaise, arthralgia, and myalgia was the most common adverse effect, although these symptoms were better tolerated with continued treatment.[367]

Topical interferon-α is associated with a lower incidence of adverse effects, but this route of administration appears less efficacious.[368,369] Intralesional interferon injections have been tried, but they are inferior to the systemic route, and expert personnel are required for administration.[370,371] In one trial, women with grade II cervical intraepithelial neoplasia were randomized to receive intramuscular β-interferon, intralesional β-interferon, a combination of both, or conventional therapy. Combination therapy demonstrated the best response with respect to lesion progression.[368] L.P. should not be treated with either local or systemic interferon-β Systemic therapy appears somewhat more effective in small-scale trials, but it is not well tolerated. The exact role of interferons in the treatment of cervical intraepithelial neoplasia, particularly in HIV-infected women, remains uncertain.

Acknowledgments

We would like to acknowledge Gene D. Morse, PharmD.; Alice M. O'Donnell, PharmD.; and Mark J. Shelton, PharmD., for their contributions to this chapter in previous editions.

REFERENCES

1. Centers for Disease Control and Prevention. Update: trends in AIDS incidences, United States, 1996. MMWR Morbid Mortal Wkly Rep 1997;46:861.
2. Centers for Disease Control and Prevention. Surveillance for AIDS-defining opportunistic illnesses, 1992–1997. MMWR Morbid Mortal Wkly Rep 1999;48(SS-2).
3. Centers for Disease Control and Prevention. 1993 revised classification system for HIV infection and expanded surveillance case definition for AIDS among adolescents and adults. MMWR Morbid Mortal Wkly Rep 1992;41(RR–17):1.
4. Cohen O et al. The immunology of human immunodeficiency virus infection. In: Mandell GL et al., eds. Principles and Practice of Infectious Diseases. New York: Churchill Livingstone, 2000:1374.
5. Paul WE. Fundamental Immunology. New York: Lippincott Williams & Wilkins, 1998.
6. Lane HC et al. Qualitative analysis of immune function in patients with the acquired immunodeficiency syndrome. N Engl J Med 1985;313:79.
7. Clerici M et al. Detection of three distinct patterns of T helper cell dysfunction in asymptomatic, human immunodeficiency virus-seropositive patients independent of CD4+ cell numbers and clinical settings. J Clin Invest 1989;84:1892.
8. Pantaleo G et al. The immunopathogenesis of human immunodeficiency virus infection. N Engl J Med 1993;328:327.
9. Niu MT et al. Primary human immunodeficiency virus type 1 infection: review of pathogenesis and early treatment intervention in humans and animal retrovirus infections. J Infect Dis 1993;168:1490.
10. Munoz A et al. Long-term survivors with HIV-1 infection: incubation period and longitudinal patterns of CD4+ lymphocytes. J Acquir Immune Defic Syndr Hum Retrovirol 1995;8:496.
11. Fauci AS et al. Immunopathogenic mechanisms of HIV infection. Ann Intern Med 1996;124:654.
12. Crowe SM et al. Predictive value of CD4+ lymphocyte numbers for the development of opportunistic infections and malignancies in HIV-infected persons. J Acquir Immun Defic Syndr Hum Retrovirol 1991;4:770.
13. Holmberg SD et al. The spectrum of medical conditions and symptoms before acquired immunodeficiency syndrome in homosexual and bisexual men infected with the human immunodeficiency virus. Am J Epidemiol 1996;141:395.
14. Moore RD et al. Natural history of opportunistic disease in an HIV-infected urban clinical cohort. Ann Intern Med 1996;124:633.
15. Welles SL et al. Prognostic value of plasma human immunodeficiency virus type 1 (HIV-1) RNA levels in patients with advanced HIV-1 disease and with little or no prior zidovudine therapy. J Infect Dis 1996;174:696.
16. Coombs SL. Association of plasma human immunodeficiency virus type 1 RNA level with risk of clinical progression in patients with advanced infection. J Infect Dis 1996;174:704.
16a. Mellors JW et al. Plasma viral load and CD4+ lymphocyte as prognostic markers of HIV-1 infection. Ann Intern Med 1997;126:946.

17. Donovan RM et al. Changes in virus load markers during AIDS-associated opportunistic diseases in human immunodeficiency virus-infected persons. J Infect Dis 1996;174:401.
18. Galetto-Lacour A et al. Prognostic value of viremia in patients with long-standing human immunodeficiency virus infection. J Infect Dis 1996;173:1388.
19. Chaisson RE et al. Impact of opportunistic disease on survival in patients with HIV infection. AIDS 1998;12:29.
20. Guidelines for the use of antiretroviral agents in HIV-infected adults and adolescents. The Department of Health and Human Services and The Henry J. Kaiser Family Foundation. AIDS Treatment Information Service (ATIS). Available at: http://www.aidsinfo.nih.gov/guidelines/ . Accessed March 1, 2003.
21. Sepkowitz KA. The effect of HAART on the natural history of AIDS-related opportunistic conditions. Lancet 1998;351:228.
22. Mourton Y et al. Impact of protease inhibitors on AIDS-defining events and hospitalizations in 10 French AIDS reference centres. AIDS 1997;11:101.
23. Mars ME et al. Protease inhibitors lead to a change of infectious diseases unit activity [Abstract]. In: Programs and Abstracts of the 4th Conference on Retroviruses and Opportunistic Infections. Washington, DC: IDSA Foundation for Retrovirology and Human Health, 1997.
24. Cameron B et al. Prolongation of life and prevention of AIDS in advanced HIV immunodeficiency with ritonavir [Abstract]. In: Programs and Abstracts of the 3rd Conference on Retroviruses and Opportunistic Infections. Washington, DC: January–February, 1996.
25. Micheals S et al. Difference in the incidence rates of opportunistic infections before and after the availability of protease inhibitors [Abstract]. In: Programs and Abstracts of the 5th Conference on Retroviruses and Opportunistic Infections. Chicago: 1998.
26. Palella F et al. Reducing morbidity and mortality among patients with advanced human immunodeficiency virus infection. N Engl J Med 1998;338:853.
27. Hammer SM et al. A controlled trial of two nucleoside analogues plus indinavir in persons with human immunodeficiency virus infection and CD4+ cell counts of 200 per cubic millimeter or less. N Engl J Med 1997;337:725.
28. Centers for Disease Control and Prevention. Update: trends in AIDS incidences, death and prevalence, United States, 1996. MMWR Morbid Mortal Wkly Rep 1997;46:165.
29. Race EM et al. Focal mycobacterial lymphadenitis following initiation of protease inhibitor therapy in patients with advanced HIV-1 disease. Lancet 1998;351:252.
30. Whitcup SM et al. Therapeutic effect of combination antiretroviral therapy on cytomegalovirus retinitis. JAMA 1997;277:1519.
31. Tural C et al. Lack of reactivation of cytomegalovirus retinitis after stopping maintenance therapy in HIV+ patients. J Infect Dis 1998;177:1080.
32. Jacobson MA et al. Cytomegalovirus retinitis after initiation of highly active antiretroviral therapy. Lancet 1997;349:1443.

33. Rutschmann OT et al. Impact of treatment with HIV protease inhibitors on hepatitis C viremia in patients co-infected with HIV. J Infect Dis 1998;177:783.
34. Autran B et al. Positive effects of combined antiviral therapy on the CD4+ T cell homeostasis and function in advanced HIV disease. Science 1997;227:112.
35. Murphy M et al. Regression of AIDS-related Kaposi's sarcoma following treatment with an HIV-1 protease inhibitor. AIDS 1997;11:26.
36. Elloitt B et al. 2–5 year remission of AIDS-associated progressive multifocal leukoencephalopathy with combined antiretroviral therapy. Lancet 1997;349:850.
37. Carr A et al. Treatment of HIV-1 associated microsporidiosis and cryptosporidiosis with combination antiretroviral therapy. Lancet 1998;351:256.
38. Hicks CB et al. Resolution of intractable molluscum contagiosum in a human immunodeficiency virus infected patient after institution of antiretroviral therapy with ritonavir. Clin Infect Dis 1997;24:1023.
39. Carr A, Cooper DA. Restoration of immunity to chronic hepatitis B infection in HIV-infected patients on protease inhibitor. Lancet 1997;349:996.
40. Masur H. Management of opportunistic infections associated with human immunodeficiency virus infection. In: Mandell GL et al., eds. Principles and Practice of Infectious Diseases, 5th ed. New York: Churchill Livingstone, 2000:1500.
41. Whitley RJ et al. Consensus statement. Guidelines for the treatment of cytomegalovirus diseases in patients with AIDS in the era of potent antiretroviral therapy. Arch Intern Med 1998;158:957.
42. Sepkowitz KA. Effect of prophylaxis on the clinical manifestations of AIDS-related opportunistic infections. Clin Infect Dis 1998;26:806.
43. Fischl MA et al. Safety and efficacy of sulfamethoxazole and trimethoprim chemoprophylaxis for Pneumocystis carinii pneumonia in AIDS. JAMA 1988;259:1185.
44. Pierce MD et al. A randomized trial of clarithromycin as prophylaxis against disseminated Mycobacterium avium complex infection in patients with advanced acquired immunodeficiency syndrome. N Engl J Med 1996;335:384.
45. Kaplan JE et al. Prevention of opportunistic infections in persons infected with human immunodeficiency virus. Clin Infect Dis 1995;21(Suppl 1):S1.
46. Centers for Disease Control and Prevention. 1997 USPHS/IDSA guidelines for the prevention of opportunistic infections in persons infected with human immunodeficiency virus. MMWR Morbid Mortal Wkly Rep 1997;46:1.
47. Centers for Disease Control and Prevention. 1999 USPHS/IDSA guidelines for the prevention of opportunistic infections in persons infected with human immunodeficiency virus. MMWR Morbid Mortal Wkly Rep 1999;48(RR-10):1.
48. Centers for Disease Control and Prevention. 2002 USPHS/IDSA guidelines for the prevention of opportunistic infections in persons infected with human immunodeficiency virus. MMWR Morbid Mortal Wkly Rep 2002;51:1.

49. MacDonald JC et al. Lack of reactivation of cytomegalovirus (CMV) retinitis after stopping CMV maintenance therapy in AIDS patients with sustained elevations in CD4 T cells in response to highly active antiretroviral therapy. J Infect Dis 1998;177:1182.

50. Jabs DA et al. Discontinuing anticytomegalovirus therapy in patients with immune reconstitution after combination antiretroviral therapy. Am J Ophthalmol 1998;126:817.

51. Jouan M et al. Discontinuation of maintenance therapy for cytomegalovirus retinitis in HIV-infected patients receiving highly active antiretroviral therapy. RESTIMOP Study Team. AIDS 2001;15:23.

52. Schneider MME et al. Discontinuation of Pneumocystis carinii pneumonia (PCP) prophylaxis in HIV-1 infected patients treated with highly active antiretroviral therapy. Lancet 1999;353:201.

53. Furrer H et al. Discontinuation of primary prophylaxis against PCP in HIV-1 infected adults treated with combination ARVT. Swiss HIV cohort study. N Engl J Med 1999;340:1301.

54. Weverling GJ et al. Discontinuation of Pneumocystis carinii pneumonia prophylaxis after start of highly active antiretroviral therapy in HIV-1 infection. EUROSIDA study group. Lancet 1999;353:1293.

55. Dworkin MS et al. Risk for preventable opportunistic infections in persons with AIDS after antiretroviral therapy increases CD4+ T lymphocyte counts above prophylaxis thresholds. J Infect Dis. 2000; 182:611.

56. Reed JB et al. Regression of cytomegalovirus retinitis associated with protease inhibitors treatment in patients with AIDS. Am J Ophthalmol 1997; 124:199.

57. Vrabec TR et al. Discontinuation of maintenance therapy in patients with quiescent cytomegalovirus retinitis and elevated CD4+ counts. Ophthamology 1998;105:1259.

58. Torriani FJ et al. Lack of progression after discontinuation of maintenance therapy (MT) for cytomegalovirus retinitis (CMVR) in AIDS patients responding to highly antiretroviral therapy (HAART). J Infect Dis 1998;177:1182.

59. Young LS. Pneumocystis carinii pneumonia. In: Walzer PD, ed. Pneumocystis carinii Pneumonia (rev. ed.). New York: Marcel Dekker, 1993.

60. Edman JC et al. Ribosomal RNA sequence shows Pneumocystis carinii to be a member of fungi. Nature 1988;334:519.

61. Masur H. Pneumocystosis. In: Dolin R et al., eds. AIDS Therapy. Philadelphia: Churchill Livingstone, 1999:299.

62. Beard C, Navin T. Molecular epidemiology of Pneumocystis carinii pneumonia. Emerg Infect Dis 1996;2:147.

63. Montgomery AB. Pneumocystis carinii pneumonia in patients with the acquired immunodeficiency syndrome. Pathophysiology and therapy. AIDS Clin Rev 1991;127.

64. Rose PD. Clinical Physiology of Acid–Base and Electrolyte Disorders, 3rd ed. NewYork: McGraw-Hill, 1989.

65. Sattler FR, Jelliffe RW. Pharmacokinetic and pharmacodynamic considerations for drug dosing in the treatment of Pneumocystis carinii pneumonia. In: Walzer PD, ed. Pneumocystis carinii Pneumonia. New York: Marcel Dekker, Inc., 1993:467.

66. Lee BL et al. Altered patterns of drug metabolism in patients with acquired immunodeficiency syndrome. Clin Pharmacol Ther 1993;53:529.

67. Gluckstein D, Ruskin J. Rapid oral desensitization to trimethoprim-sulfamethoxazole (TMP-SMX): use in prophylaxis for Pneumocystis carinii pneumonia in patients with AIDS who were previously intolerant to TMP-SMX. Clin Infect Dis 1995;20:849.

68. Bartlett JG. 1999 Medical Management of HIV Infection. Baltimore: Port City Press, 1999.

69. Warren E et al. Advances in the treatment and prophylaxis of Pneumocystis carinii pneumonia. Pharmacotherapy 1997;17:900.

70. Conte JE Dr et al. Intravenous or inhaled pentamidine for treating Pneumocystis carinii pneumonia in AIDS. A randomized trial. Ann Intern Med 1990;113:203.

71. O'Brien J et al. A 5-year retrospective review of adverse drug reactions and their risk factors in human immunodeficiency virus-infected patients who were receiving intravenous pentamidine therapy for Pneumocystis carinii. Clin Infect Dis 1997;24:854.

72. Foisey M et al. Pancreatitis during intravenous pentamidine therapy in an AIDS patient with prior exposure to didanosine. Ann Pharmacother 1994; 28:1025.

73. Comtois R et al. Higher pentamidine levels in AIDS patients with hypoglycemia and azotemia during treatment of Pneumocystis carinii pneumonia. Am Rev Respir Dis 1992;146:740.

74. Sattler FR et al. Trimetrexate with leucovorin verus trimethoprim-sulfamethoxazole for moderate to severe episodes of Pneumocystis carinii pneumonia in patients with AIDS: a prospective, controlled multicenter investigation of the AIDS Clinical Trials Group Protocol 029/031. J Infect Dis 1994; 170:165.

75. Fishman JA. Treatment of infection due to Pneumocystis carinii. Antimicrob Agents Chemo 1998; 42:1309.

76. Dohn MN et al. Open-label efficacy and safety trial of 42 days of 566C80 for Pneumocystis carinii pneumonia in AIDS patients. J Protozool 1991; 38:220S.

77. Falloon J et al. A preliminary evaluation of 566C80 for the treatment of Pneumocystis pneumonia in patients with the acquired immunodeficiency syndrome. N Engl J Med 1991;325:1534.

78. Gutteridge WE. 566C80, an antimalarial hydroxynaphthoquinone with broad spectrum: experimental activity against opportunistic parasitic infections of AIDS patients. J Protozool 1991;38:141S.

79. Hughes W et al. Comparison of atovaquone (566C80) with trimethoprim-sulfamethoxazole to treat Pneumocystis carinii pneumonia in patients with AIDS. N Engl J Med 1993;328:1521.

80. Dohn MN et al. and the Atovaquone Study Group. Oral atovaquone compared with intravenous pentamidine for Pneumocystis carinii pneumonia in patients with AIDS. Ann Intern Med 1994;121:174.

81. Safrin S et al. Dapsone as a single agent is suboptimal therapy for Pneumocystis carinii pneumonia. J Acquir Immune Defic Syndr 1991;4:244.

82. Lee BL et al. Dapsone, trimethoprim, and sulfamethoxazole plasma levels during treatment of Pneumocystis pneumonia in patients with the acquired immunodeficiency syndrome (AIDS). Ann Intern Med 1989;110:606.

83. Sin DD, Shafran SD. Dapsone and primaquine induced methemoglobinemia in HIV-infected individuals. J Acquir Immune Defic Syndr Hum Retrovirol 1996;12:477.

84. Medina I et al. Oral therapy for Pneumocystis carinii pneumonia in the acquired immunodeficiency syndrome. A controlled trial of trimethoprim-sulfamethoxazole versus trimethoprim-dapsone. N Engl J Med 1990;323:776.

85. Noskin GA et al. Salvage therapy with clindamycin/primaquine for Pneumocystis carinii pneumonia. Clin Infect Dis 1992;14:183.

86. Safrin S et al. Comparison of three regimens for the treatment of mild to moderate Pneumocystis carinii pneumonia in patients with AIDS. Ann Intern Med 1996;124:792.

87. Bozzette SA et al. A controlled trial of early adjunctive treatment with corticosteroids for Pneumocystis carinii pneumonia in the acquired immun-odeficiency syndrome. California Collaborative Treatment Group. N Engl J Med 1990; 323:1451.

88. Nielsen TL et al. Adjunctive corticosteroid therapy for Pneumocystis carinii pneumonia in AIDS: a randomized European multicenter open label study. J Acquir Immune Defic Syndr Hum Retrovirol 1992;5:726.

89. Gagnon S et al. Corticosteroids as adjunctive therapy for severe Pneumocystis carinii pneumonia in the acquired immunodeficiency syndrome. A double-blind, placebo-controlled trial. N Engl J Med 1990;323:1444.

90. Montaner JS et al. Corticosteroids prevent early deterioration in patients with moderately severe Pneumocystis carinii pneumonia and the acquired immunodeficiency syndrome (AIDS). J Acquir Immune Defic Syndr Hum Retrovirol 1990;113:14.

91. Bozzette SA, Morston SC. Reconsidering the use of adjunctive corticosteroids in Pneumocystis pneumonia? J Acquire Immune Defic Syndr Hum Retrovirol 1995;8:345.

92. Sistek CJ et al. Adjuvant corticosteroid therapy for Pneumocystis carinii pneumonia in AIDS patients. Ann Pharmacother 1992;26:1127.

93. LaRocco A Jr et al. Corticosteroids for Pneumocystis carinii pneumonia with acute respiratory failure. Experience with rescue therapy. Chest 1992;102:892.

94. Kovacs JA et al. Prophylaxis for Pneumocystis carinii pneumonia in patients infected with human immunodeficiency virus. Clin Infect Dis 1992;14: 1005.

95. Loannidis JP et al. A meta-analysis of the relative efficacy and toxicity of Pneumocystis carinii prophylaxis regimens. Arch Intern Med 1996; 156:177.

96. Phair J et al. The risk of Pneumocystis carinii pneumonia among men infected with human immunodeficiency virus type 1. N Engl J Med 1990; 322:161.

97. Para MF et al. for the ACTG 268 Study Team. ACTG 286 Trial: gradual initiation of trimethoprim/sulfamethoxazole (T/S) as primary prophylaxis for Pneumocystis carinii pneumonia (PCP). In: Abstracts of the 4th Conference on Retroviruses and Opportunistic Infections, Washington, DC, 1997. Abstract No. 2.

98. Leoung GS et al. Trimethoprim-sulfamethoxazole (TMP-SMZ) dose escalation versus direct rechallenge for Pneumocystis carinii pneumonia prophylaxis in human immunodeficiency virus-infected patients with previous adverse reaction to TMP-SMZ. J Infect Dis 2001;184:992.

99. Bozzette S et al. A randomized trial of three anti-Pneumocystis agents in patients with advanced human immunodeficiency virus infection. N Engl J Med 1995;332:693.

100. Opravil M et al. Once-weekly administration of dapsone/pyrimethamine versus aerosolized pentamidine as combined prophylaxis for Pneumocystis pneumonia and toxoplasmic encephalitis in human immunodeficiency virus-infected patients. Clin Infect Dis 1995;20:531.

101. El-Sadr W et al. Atovaquone compared with dapsone for the prevention of Pneumocystis carinii pneumonia in patients with HIV infection who cannot tolerate trimethoprim, sulfonamides, or both. N Engl J Med 1998;339:1889.

102. Telzak EE, Armstrong D. Extrapulmonary infection and other unusual manifestations of Pneumocystis carinii. In: Walzer PD, ed. Pneumocystis carinii Pneumonia. New York: Marcel Dekker, Inc., 1993:361.

103. Noskin GA et al. Extrapulmonary infection with Pneumocystis carinii in patients receiving aerosolized pentamidine. Rev Infect Dis 1991;13:525.

104. Selik MA et al. Trends in infectious diseases and cancers among persons dying of HIV infection in the United States from 1987 to 1992. Ann Intern Med 1995;123:933.

105. Lopez Bernaldo de Quiros JC et al; Grupo de Estudio del SIDA 04/98. A randomized trial of the discontinuation of primary and secondary prophylaxis against Pneumocystis carinii pneumonia after highly active antiretroviral therapy in patients with HIV infection. Grupo de Estudio del SIDA 04/98. N Engl J Med 2001;344:159.

106. Dworkin M et al. Risk for preventable opportunistic infections in persons with AIDS after antiretroviral therapy increases CD4+ T lymphocyte counts above prophylaxis thresholds. J Infect Dis 2000;182:611.

107. Lopez Bernaldo de Quiros JC et al. for the Grupo de Estudio del SIDA 04/98. Randomized trial of the discontinuation of primary and secondary prophylaxis against Pneumocystis carinii pneumonia after highly active antiretroviral therapy in patients with HIV infection. N Engl J Med 2001;344:159.

108. Kirk O et al. Can chemoprophylaxis against opportunistic infections be discontinued after an increase in CD4 cells induced by highly active antiretroviral therapy? AIDS 1999;13:1647.

109. Soriano V et al. Discontinuation of secondary prophylaxis for opportunistic infections in HIV-infected patients receiving highly active antiretroviral therapy. AIDS 2000;14:383.

110. Ledergerber B et al. Discontinuation of secondary prophylaxis against *Pneumocystis carinii* pneumonia in patients with HIV infection who have a response to antiretroviral therapy. Eight European study groups. N Engl J Med 2001;344:168.

111. Montoya JG, Remington JS. *Toxoplasma gondii.* In: Mandell GL et al., eds. Principles and Practice of Infectious Diseases, 5th ed. New York: Churchill Livingstone, 2000:2858.

112. Murray HW. Toxoplasmosis. In: Dolin R et al., eds. AIDS Therapy. Philadelphia: Churchill Livingstone, 1999:307.

113. Matthews C et al. Early biopsy versus empiric treatment with delayed biopsy of non-responders in suspected HIV-associated cerebral toxoplasmosis: a decision analysis. AIDS 1995;9:1243.

114. Harrison PB et al. Focal brain lesions on computed tomography in patients with acquired immune deficiency syndrome. Can Assoc Radiol J 1990;41:83.

115. Girard PM et al. Dapsone-pyrimethamine compared with aerosolized pentamidine as primary prophylaxis against *Pneumocystis carinii* pneumonia and toxoplasmosis in HIV infection. The PRIO Study Group. N Engl J Med 1993; 328:1514.

116. Hardy WD et al. A controlled trial of trimethoprim-sulfamethoxazole or aerosolized pentamidine for secondary prophylaxis of *Pneumocystis carinii* pneumonia in patients with the acquired immunodeficiency syndrome. AIDS Clinical Trials Group Protocol 021. N Engl J Med 1992;327:1842.

117. Carr A et al. Low-dose trimethoprim-sulfamethoxazole prophylaxis for toxoplasmic encephalitis in patients with AIDS. Ann Intern Med 1992;117:106.

118. Podzamczer D et al. Intermittent trimethoprim-sulfamethoxazole compared with dapsone-pyrimethamine for the simultaneous primary prophylaxis of *Pneumocystis* pneumonia and toxoplasmosis in patients infected with HIV. Ann Intern Med 1995;122:755.

119. Leport C et al. Pyrimethamine for primary prophylaxis of *Toxoplasma* encephalitis in patients with HIV infection: a double-blind, randomized trial. J Infect Dis 1996;173:91.

120. Jacobson M et al. Primary prophylaxis with pyrimethamine for *Toxoplasma* encephalitis in patients with advanced HIV disease. Results of a randomized trial. J Infect Dis 1994;169:384.

121. Dworkin M et al. Risk for preventable opportunistic infections in persons with AIDS after antiretroviral therapy increases CD4+ T lymphocyte counts above prophylaxis thresholds. J Infect Dis 2000;182:611.

122. Kirk O et al. Can chemoprophylaxis against opportunistic infections be discontinued after an increase in CD4 cells induced by highly active antiretroviral therapy? AIDS 1999;13:1647.

123. Furrer H et al. Stopping primary prophylaxis in HIV-1-infected patients at high risk of toxoplasma encephalitis. Swiss HIV Cohort Study. Lancet 2000;355:2217–8.

124. Mussini C, Pezzotti P, Govoni A, et al. Discontinuation of primary prophylaxis for *Pneumocystis carinii* pneumonia and toxoplasmic encephalitis in human immunodeficiency virus type I-infected patients: the changes in opportunistic prophylaxis study. J Infect Dis 2000;181:1635.

125. Miro JM et al. Discontinuation of primary and secondary *Toxoplasma gondii* prophylaxis is safe in HIV-1 infected patients after immunological recovery with HAART: final results of the GESIDA 04/98 Study [Abstract L16]. Presented at the 39th Interscience Conference on Antimicrobial Agents and Chemotherapy, San Francisco, 2000.

126. de la Hoz Caballer B et al. Management of sulfadiazine allergy in patients with acquired immunodeficiency syndrome. J Allergy Clin Immunol 1991;88:137.

127. Tenant-Flowers M et al. Sulfadiazine desensitization in patients with AIDS and cerebral toxoplasmosis. AIDS 1991;5:311.

128. Katlama C et al. Pyrimethamine-clindamycin versus pyrimethamine-sulfadiazine as acute and long- term therapy for toxoplasmic encephalitis in patients with AIDS. Clin Infect Dis 1996;22:268.

129. Molina JM et al. Sulfadiazine-induced crystalluria in AIDS patients with *Toxoplasma* encephalitis. AIDS 1991;5:587.

130. Oster S et al. Resolution of acute renal failure in toxoplasmic encephalitis despite continuance of sulfadiazine. Rev Infect Dis 1990;12:618.

131. Christin S et al. Acute renal failure due to sulfadiazine in patients with AIDS. Nephron 1990; 55:233.

132. Ventura MG et al. Sulfadiazine revisited. J Infect Dis 1989;160:556.

133. Simon DI et al. Sulfadiazine crystalluria revisited. The treatment of *Toxoplasma* encephalitis in patients with acquired immunodeficiency syndrome. Arch Intern Med 1990;150:2379.

134. Remington J. Availability of sulfadiazine, United States. JAMA 1993;269:461.

135. EON Labs Manufacturers, Inc. Laurelton, NY. Available at: http://www.EONLABS.COM.

136. Holliman RE. Folate supplements and the treatment of cerebral toxoplasmosis. Scand J Infect Dis 1989;21:475.

137. Frenkel JK et al. Relative reversal by vitamins (p-aminobenzoic, folic, and folinic acids) of the effects of sulfadiazine and pyrimethamine on *Toxoplasma,* mouse and man. Antibiot Chemother 1957;VII:630.

138. Eyles DE et al. The effect of metabolites on the antitoxoplasmic action of pyrimethamine and sulfadiazine. Am J Trop Med 1960;9:277.

139. Podzamczer D et al. Twice weekly maintenance therapy with sulfadiazine-pyrimethamine to prevent recurrent toxoplasmosis encephalitis in patients with AIDS. Spanish Toxoplasmosis Study Group. Ann Intern Med 1995;123:175.

140. Leport C et al. Long-term follow-up of patients with AIDS on maintenance therapy for toxoplasmosis. Eur J Clin Microbiol Infect Dis 1991; 10:191.

141. Bhatti N et al. Low-dose alternate-day pyrimethamine for maintenance therapy in cerebral toxoplasmosis complicating AIDS. J Infect Dis 1990;21:119.

142. Ruf B et al. Role of clindamycin in the treatment of acute toxoplasmosis of the central nervous system. Eur J Clin Microbiol Infect Dis 1991;10:183.

143. Rolston KV. Treatment of acute toxoplasmosis with oral clindamycin. Eur J Clin Microbiol Infect Dis 1991;10:181.

144. Dannemann BR et al. Treatment of acute toxoplasmosis with intravenous clindamycin. The California Collaborative Treatment Group. Eur J Clin Microbiol Infect Dis 1991;10:193.

145. Katlama C. Evaluation of the efficacy and safety of clindamycin plus pyrimethamine for induction and maintenance therapy of toxoplasmic encephalitis in AIDS. Eur J Clin Microbiol Infect Dis 1991;10:189.

146. Foppa CU et al. A retrospective study of primary and maintenance therapy of toxoplasmic encephalitis with oral clindamycin and pyrimethamine. Eur J Clin Microbiol Infect Dis 1991;10:187.

147. Araujo FG et al. In vitro and in vivo activities of the hydroxynaphthoquinone 566C80 against the cyst form of *Toxoplasma gondii.* Antimicrob Agents Chemother 1991;36:326.

148. Araujo FG et al. Remarkable in vitro and in vivo activities of the hydroxynaphthoquinone 566C80 against tachyzoites and tissue cysts of *Toxoplasma gondii.* Antimicrob Agents Chemother 1991; 35:293.

149. Gianotti N et al. Efficacy and safety of atovaquone (556C80) in the treatment of cerebral toxoplasmosis (CT) and *Pneumocystis carinii* pneumonia (PCP) in

150. White A et al. Comparison to natural history data of survival of toxoplasmic encephalitis patients treated with atovaquone. Paper presented at the IXth International Conference on AIDS in affiliation with the IVth STD World Congress, Berlin, 1993.

151. Torres RA et al. Atovaquone for salvage treatment and suppression of toxoplasmic encephalitis in patients with AIDS. Clin Infect Dis 1997;24:422.

152. Chang HR et al. In vitro and in vivo effects of doxycycline on *Toxoplasma gondii.* Antimicrob Agents Chemother 1990;34:775.

153. Alder J et al. Treatment of experimental *Toxoplasma gondii* infection by clarithromycin-based combination therapies. J Acquir Defic Syndr Hum Retrovirol 1994;7:1141.

154. Salmon-Ceron D. Cytomegalovirus infection. HIV Medicine 2001;2:255.

155. Jennens ID et al. Cytomegalovirus cultures during maintenance DHPG therapy for cytomegalovirus (CMV) retinitis in acquired immunodeficiency syndrome (AIDS). J Med Virol 1990;30:42.

156. Shinkai M et al. Utility of urine and leukocyte cultures and plasma DNA polymerase chain reaction for identification of AIDS patients at risk for developing human cytomegalovirus disease. J Infec Dis 1997;175:302.

157. Dodt KK et al. Development of cytomegalovirus (CMV) disease may be predicted in HIV-infected patients by CMV polymerase chain reaction and the antigenemia test. AIDS 1997;11:F21.

158. Bowen EF et al. Cytomegalovirus (CMV) viremia detected by polymerase chain reaction identifies a group of HIV-positive patients at high risk of CMV disease. AIDS 1997,11:889.

159. Jacobson MA. Treatment of cytomegalovirus retinitis in patients with the acquired immunodeficiency syndrome. N Engl J Med 1997;337:105.

160. Masur H et al. Advances in the management of AIDS-related cytomegalovirus retinitis. Ann Intern Med 1996;125:126.

161. Parenteral cidofovir for cytomegalovirus retinitis in patients with AIDS: the HPMPC Peripheral Cytomegalovirus Retinitis Trial. A randomized, controlled trial. Studies of Ocular Complications of AIDS Research Group in collaboration with the AIDS Clinical Trials Group. Ann Intern Med 1997;126:264.

162. Combination foscarnet and ganciclovir therapy vs monotherapy for the treatment of relapsed cytomegalovirus retinitis in patients with AIDS. The Cytomegalovirus Retreatment Trial. The Studies of Ocular Complications of AIDS Research Group in collaboration with the AIDS Clinical Trials Group. Arch Ophthalmol 1996;114:23.

163. Musch DC et al. Treatment of cytomegalovirus retinitis with a sustained-release ganciclovir implant. The Ganciclovir Implant Study Group. N Engl J Med 1997;337:83.

164. Mar E et al. Effect of 9-(1,3-dihydroxy-2-propoxymethyl)guanine on human cytomegalovirus replication in vitro. Antimicrob Agents Chemother 1983;24:518.

165. Smee DF et al. Anti-herpesvirus activity of the acyclic nucleoside 9-(1,3-dihydroxy-2-propoxymethyl)guanine. Antimicrob Agents Chemother 1983;23:676.

166. Biron KK et al. A human cytomegalovirus mutant resistant to the nucleoside analog 9-([2-hydroxy-1-(hydroxymethyl)ethoxy]methyl)guanine (BW B759U) induces reduced levels of BW B759U triphosphate. Proc Natl Acad Sci USA 1986;83: 8769.

167. Fletcher CV et al. Evaluation of ganciclovir for cytomegalovirus disease. DICP 1989;23:5.

168. Crumpacker CS. Ganciclovir. N Engl J Med 1996; 335:721.

169. Peters BS et al. Cytomegalovirus infection in AIDS. Patterns of disease, response to therapy and trends in survival. J Infect Dis 1991;23:129.

170. Weisenthal RW et al. Long-term outpatient treatment of CMV retinitis with ganciclovir in AIDS patients. Br J Ophthalmol 1989;73:996.

171. SOCA. Morbidity and toxic effects associated with ganciclovir or foscarnet therapy in a randomized cytomegalovirus retinitis trial. Arch Intern Med 1995;155:65.

172. Jacobson MA et al. Ganciclovir with recombinant methionyl human granulocyte colony-stimulating factor for treatment of cytomegalovirus disease in AIDS patients. AIDS 1992;6:515.

173. Hardy WD. Combined ganciclovir and recombinant human granulocyte-macrophage colony-stimulating factor in the treatment of cytomegalovirus retinitis in AIDS patients. J Acquir Immun Defic Syndr Hum Retrovirol 1991;4:S22.

174. Koyanagi Y et al. Cytokines alter production of HIV-1 from primary mononuclear phagocytes. Science 1988;241:1673.

175. Perno CF et al. Effects of bone marrow stimulatory cytokines on human immunodeficiency virus replication and the antiviral activity of dideoxynucleosides in cultures of monocyte/macrophages. Blood 1992;80:995.

176. Martin DF et al. A controlled trial of valganciclovir as induction therapy for cytomegalovirus retinitis. N Engl J Med 2002;346:1119.

177. Cundy KC et al. Clinical pharmacokinetics of cidofovir in human immunodeficiency virus-infected patients. Antimicrob Agents Chem 1995;39:1247.

178. Lalezari JP et al. Intravenous cidofovir for peripheral cytomegalovirus retinitis in patients with AIDS. Ann Intern Med 1997;126:257.

179. Aweeka F et al. Pharmacokinetics of intermittently administered intravenous foscarnet in the treatment of acquired immunodeficiency syndrome patients with serious cytomegalovirus retinitis. Antimicrob Agents Chemother 1989;33:742.

180. Deray G et al. Foscarnet nephrotoxicity: mechanism, incidence and prevention. Am J Nephrol 1989;9:316.

181. SOCA. Mortality in patients with the acquired immunodeficiency syndrome treated with either foscarnet or ganciclovir for cytomegalovirus retinitis. Studies of Ocular Complications of AIDS Research Group, in collaboration with the AIDS Clinical Trials Group. N Engl J Med 1992;326:213.

182. Jacobson MA et al. Foscarnet treatment of cytomegalovirus retinitis in patients with the acquired immunodeficiency syndrome. Antimicrob Agents Chemother 1989;33:736.

183. Youle MS et al. Severe hypocalcaemia in AIDS patients treated with foscarnet and pentamidine. Lancet 1988;1:1455.

184. Jayaweera DT. Minimising the dosage-limiting toxicities of foscarnet induction therapy. Drug Safety 1997;16:258.

185. Jacobson MA et al. Foscarnet therapy for ganciclovir-resistant cytomegalovirus retinitis in patients with AIDS. J Infect Dis 1991;163:1348.

186. Holland GN et al. Dose-related difference in progression rates of cytomegalovirus retinopathy during foscarnet maintenance therapy. Am J Ophthalmol 1995;199:576.

187. Foscarnet-ganciclovir cytomegalovirus retinitis trial 4. Visual outcomes. Studies of Ocular Complications of AIDS Research Group in collaboration with the AIDS Clinical Trials Group. Ophthalmology 1994;101:1250.

188. Jacobson MA et al. Randomized phase I trial of two different combination foscarnet and ganciclovir chronic maintenance therapy regimens for AIDS patients with cytomegalovirus retinitis: AIDS Clinical Trials Group protocol 151. J Infect Dis 1994;170:189.

189. Jacobson MA et al. A dose-ranging study of daily maintenance intravenous foscarnet therapy for cytomegalovirus retinitis in AIDS. J Infect Dis 1993; 168:444.

190. Jabs DA et al. Cytomegalovirus retinitis and viral resistance: ganciclovir resistance. J Infect Dis 1998;177:770.

191. Chou S et al. Frequency of UL97 phosphotransferase mutations related to ganciclovir resistance in clinical cytomegalovirus isolates. J Infect Dis 1995;172:239.

192. Smith IL et al. High-level resistance of cytomegalovirus to ganciclovir is associated with alterations in both UL97 and DNA polymerase genes. J Infect Dis 1997;176:69.

193. Fausto B et al. Single amino acid changes in the DNA polymerase confer foscarnet resistance and slow-growth phenotype, while mutations in the UL97-encoded phosphotransferase confer ganciclovir resistance in three double-resistant human cytomegalovirus strains recovered from patients with AIDS. J Virol 1996;70:1390.

194. Azad RF. Antiviral activity of a phosphorothioate oligonucleotide complementary to human cytomegalovirus RNA when used in combination with antiviral nucleoside analogs. Antiviral Res 1995;28:101.

195. Kuppermann BD. Therapeutic options for resistant cytomegalovirus retinitis. J Acquir Immun Defic Syndr Hum Retroviral 1997;14:S13.

196. Perry CM, Balfour JA. Fomivirsen. Drugs 1999; 57:375.

197. Cochereau-Massin I et al. Efficacy and tolerance of intravitreal ganciclovir in cytomegalovirus retinitis in acquired immune deficiency syndrome. Ophthalmology 1991;98:1348.

198. Cantrill HL et al. Treatment of cytomegalovirus retinitis with intravitreal ganciclovir. Long-term results. Ophthalmology 1989;96:367.

199. Young SH et al. High dose intravitreal ganciclovir in the treatment of cytomegalovirus retinitis. Med J Aust 1992;157:370.

200. Martin DF. Treatment of cytomegalovirus retinitis with an intraocular sustained-release ganciclovir implant: a randomized controlled clinical trial. Arch Ophthalmol 1994;112:1531.

201. Marx JL et al. Use of the ganciclovir implant in the treatment of recurrent cytomegalovirus retinitis. Arch Ophthalmol 1996;114:815.

202. Musch DC et al. Treatment of cytomegalovirus retinitis with a sustained-release ganciclovir implant. N Engl J Med 1997;337:83.

203. Drew WL et al. Oral ganciclovir as maintenance treatment for cytomegalovirus retinitis in patients with AIDS. N Engl J Med 1995;333:615.

204. Syntex. Cytovene package insert. Palo Alto, CA: 1996.

205. Anderson RD et al. Ganciclovir absolute bioavailability and steady-state pharmacokinetics after oral administration of two 3000 mg/d dosing regimens in human immunodeficiency virus- and cytomegalovirus-seropositive patients. Clin Ther 1995;17:425.

206. Spector SA et al. Oral ganciclovir for the prevention of cytomegalovirus disease in persons with AIDS. N Engl J Med 1996;334:1491.

207. Brosgart CL et al. A randomized, placebo-controlled trial of the safety and efficacy of oral ganciclovir for prophylaxis of cytomegalovirus disease in HIV-infected individuals. Terry Beirn Community Programs for Clinical Research on AIDS. AIDS 1998;12:269.

208. Rose DN, Sacks HS. Cost-effectiveness of cytomegalovirus (CMV) disease prevention in patients with AIDS: oral ganciclovir and CMV polymerase chain reaction testing. AIDS 1997;11:883.

209. Powderly WG. AIDS commentary: cryptococcal meningitis and AIDS. Clin Infect Dis 1993; 17:837.

210. Van der Horst CM et al. Treatment of cryptococcal meningitis associated with the acquired immunodeficiency syndrome. N Engl J Med 1997;337:15.

211. Goodman L, Gilman A, eds. The Pharmacological Basis of Therapeutics. New York: Macmillan, 1995:1236.

212. Shadomy S et al. In vitro studies with combination 5-fluorocytosine and amphotericin B. Antimicrob Agents Chemother 1975;8:117.

213. Bennett JE et al. A comparison of amphotericin B alone and combined with flucytosine in the treatment of cryptococcal meningitis. N Engl J Med 1979;301:126.

214. Chuck SL et al. Infections with cryptococcal meningitis and AIDS. N Engl J Med 1989; 321:794.

215. Polsky B et al. Intraventricular therapy of cryptococcal meningitis via a subcutaneous reservoir. Am J Med 1986;81:24.

216. Wong-Beringer et al. Lipid formulations of amphotericin B: clinical efficacy and toxicities. Clin Infect Dis 1998;27:603.

217. Walsh TJ et al. Liposomal amphotericin B for empirical therapy in patients with persistent fever and neutropenia. N Engl J Med 1999;340:764.

218. Sharkey PK et al. Amphotericin B lipid complex compared with amphotericin B in the treatment of cryptococcal meningitis in patients with AIDS. Clin Infect Dis 1996;22:315.

219. Grant SM et al. Fluconazole: a review of its pharmacodynamic and pharmacokinetic properties, and therapeutic potential in superficial and systemic mycoses. Drugs 1990;39:877.

220. Saag MS et al. Comparison of amphotericin B with fluconazole in the treatment of acute AIDS-associated cryptococcal meningitis. The NIAID Mycoses Study Group and the AIDS Clinical Trials Group. N Engl J Med 1992;326:83.

221. Larson RA et al. Fluconazole compared with amphotericin B plus flucytosine for cryptococcal meningitis in AIDS. Ann Intern Med 1990; 113:183.

222. Perfect JR et al. Penetration of imidazoles and triazoles into cerebrospinal fluid of rabbits. J Antimicrob Chemother 1985;16:81.

223. deGans J et al. Itraconazole compared with amphotericin B plus flucytosine in AIDS patients with cryptococcal meningitis. AIDS 1992;6:185.

224. Bozzette SA et al. A controlled trial of maintenance therapy with fluconazole after treatment of cryptococcal meningitis in the acquired immunodeficiency syndrome. N Engl J Med 1991;324:580.

225. Powderly WG et al. A controlled trial of fluconazole or amphotericin B to prevent relapse of cryptococcal meningitis in patients with the acquired immunodeficiency syndrome. The NIAID AIDS Clinical Trials Group and Mycoses Study Group. N Engl J Med 1992;326:793.

226. deGans J et al. Itraconazole as maintenance treatment for cryptococcal meningitis in the acquired immune deficiency syndrome. Br Med J 1988; 296:339.

227. Nightingale SD et al. Primary prophylaxis with fluconazole against systemic fungal infections in HIV-positive patients. AIDS 1992;6:191.

228. Powderly et al. A randomized trial comparing fluconazole with clotrimazole troches for the prevention of fungal infections in patients with advanced human immunodeficiency virus infection. N Engl J Med 1995;332:700.

229. Darouiche RO. Oropharyngeal and esophageal candidiasis in immunocompromised patients: treatment issues. Clin Infect Dis 1998;26:259.

230. Milefchik E et al. High dose fluconazole with and without flucytosine for AIDS-associated cryptococcal meningitis. Paper presented at the IX International Conference on AIDS, Berlin, 1993.

231. Mayanja-Kizza H et al. Combination therapy with fluconazole and flucytosine for cryptococcal meningitis in Ugandan patients with AIDS. Clin Infect Dis 1998;26:1362.

232. Chambers HF. Tuberculosis in the HIV-infected patient. In: Sande MA, Volberding PA, eds. The Medical Management of AIDS. Philadelphia: WB Saunders, 1999:353.

233. American Thoracic Society. Treatment of tuberculosis infection in adults and children. Clin Infect Dis 1995;21:9.

234. Centers for Disease Control and Prevention. Tuberculosis morbidity, United States, 1996. MMWR Morbid Mortal Wkly Rep 1997:46:695.

235. Centers for Disease Control and Prevention. Initial therapy for tuberculosis in the era of multidrug resistance: recommendations of the advisory council for the elimination of tuberculosis. MMWR Morbid Mortal Wkly Rep 1993;42(RR-7):1.

236. Iseman MD. Treatment of multidrug-resistant tuberculosis. N Engl J Med 1993;329:784.

237. Goble M et al. Treatment of 171 patients with pulmonary tuberculosis resistant to isoniazid and rifampin. N Engl J Med 1993;328:527.

238. American Thoracic Society. Treatment of tuberculosis and tuberculosis infection in adults and children. Am J Respir Crit Care Med 1994;149:1359.

239. Frieden TR et al. The emergence of drug-resistant tuberculosis in New York City. N Engl J Med 1993;328:521.

240. Gordin FM et al. The impact of human immunodeficiency virus infection of drug-resistant tuberculosis. Am J Respir Crit Care Med 1996;154:1478.

241. Centers for Disease Control and Prevention. Prevention and treatment of tuberculosis among patients infected with human immunodeficiency virus: principles of therapy and revised recommendations. MMWR Morbid Mortal Wkly Rep 1998;47(RR-20):1.

242. CDC. Updated guidelines for the use of rifabutin or rifampin for the treatment and prevention of tuberculosis among HIV-infected patients taking protease inhibitors or nonnucleoside reverse transcriptase inhibitors. MMWR 2000;49:185.

243. Berenguer J et al. Tuberculous meningitis in patients infected with the human immunodeficiency virus. N Engl J Med 1992;326:668.

244. Smith RL et al. Factors affecting the yield of acid-fast sputum smears in patients with HIV and tuberculosis. Chest 1994;106:684.

245. Centers for Disease Control and Prevention. Anergy skin testing and preventive therapy for HIV-infected persons: revised recommendations. MMWR Morbid Mortal Wkly Rep 1997;46(RR-15):1.

246. Narita M et al. Paradoxical worsening of tuberculosis following antiretroviral therapy in patients with AIDS. Am J Respir Crit Care Med 1998;158:157.

247. Villarino ME et al. Management of persons exposed to multidrug-resistant tuberculosis. MMWR Morbid Mortal Wkly Rep 1992;41(RR-11):1.

248. Gordon F et al. A randomized trial of 2 months of rifampin and pyrazinamide versus 12 months of isoniazid for the prevention of tuberculosis in HIV-positive, PPD positive patients. In Program and Abstracts: 5th Conference on Retroviruses and Opportunistic Infections. Chicago, 1998. Abstract LB5.

249. Brix D et al. Correlation of in vivo cellular immunity with CD4+ number and disease progression in HIV seropositive patients. Paper presented to the 5th International Conference on AIDS, Montreal, 1989.

250. Chin DP et al. Clinical utility of a commercial test based on the polymerase chain reaction for detecting Mycobacterium tuberculosis in respiratory specimens. Am J Respir Crit Care Med 1995;151:1872.

251. Centers for Disease Control and Prevention. Clinical update: impact of HIV protease inhibitors on the treatment of HIV-infected tuberculosis patients with rifampin. MMWR Morbid Mortal Wkly Rep 1996;45:921.

252. Havlin D, Barnes P. Tuberculosis in patients with human immunodeficiency virus infection. N Engl J Med 1999;340:367.

253. Englehard D et al. Interaction of ketoconazole with rifampin and isoniazid. N Engl J Med 1984;311:1681.

254. Lazar JD et al. Drug interactions with fluconazole. Rev Infect Dis 1990;12:327.

255. Piscitelli SC et al. Drug interactions in patients with human immunodeficiency virus. Clin Infect Dis 1996;23:685.

256. Chaisson RE et al. Incidence and natural history of Mycobacterium avium-complex infections in patients with advanced human immunodeficiency virus disease treated with zidovudine. Am Rev Respir Dis 1992;146:285.

257. Von Reyn CF et al. The international epidemiology of disseminated Mycobacterium avium complex infection in AIDS. AIDS 1996;10:1025.

258. Yakrus MA et al. Geographic distribution, frequency and specimen source of Mycobacterium avium complex serotypes isolated from patients with acquired immunodeficiency syndrome. J Clin Microbiol 1990;28:926.

259. Sathe SS et al. Severe anemia is an important negative predictor for survival with disseminated Mycobacterium avium-intracellulare in acquired immunodeficiency syndrome. Am Rev Respir Dis 1990;142:1306.

260. Benson CA. Disease due to the Mycobacterium avium complex in patients with AIDS: epidemiology and clinical syndrome. Clin Infect Dis 1994;18:S218.

261. Woods GL. Disease due to the Mycobacterium avium complex in patients infected with human immunodeficiency virus: diagnosis and susceptibility testing. Clin Infect Dis 1994;18(Suppl 3):S227.

262. Currier JS et al. Preliminary ACTG 320 OI data analysis (presentation). 23rd AIDS Clinical Trials Group Meeting, Washington, DC, 1997.

263. Baril L et al. Impact of highly active antiretroviral therapy on onset of Mycobacterium avium complex infection and cytomegalovirus disease in patients with AIDS. AIDS 2000;14:2593.

264. Hoffner SE et al. Control of disease progress in Mycobacterium avium-infected AIDS patients. Res Microbiol 1992;143:391.

265. Yajko DM. In vitro activity of antimicrobial agents against the Mycobacterium avium complex inside macrophages from HIV-1-infected individuals: the link to clinical response to treatment? Res Microbiol 1992;143:411.

266. Inderlied CB. Microbiology and minimum inhibitory concentration testing for Mycobacterium avium prophylaxis. Am J Med 1997;102:2.

267. Heifets L et al. Radiometric broth macrodilution method for determination of minimal complex isolates: proposed guidelines. Denver: National Jewish Center for Immunology and Respiratory Medicine, 1993.

268. Ellner JJ et al. Mycobacterium avium infection and AIDS: a therapeutic dilemma in rapid evolution. J Infect Dis 1991;163:1326.

269. Heifets LB et al. Clarithromycin minimal inhibitory and bactericidal concentrations against Mycobacterium avium. Am Rev Respir Dis 1992;145:856.

270. Heifets LB et al. Individualized therapy versus standard regimens in the treatment of Mycobacterium avium infections. Am Rev Respir Dis 1991;144:1.

271. Young LS et al. Azithromycin for treatment of Mycobacterium avium-intracellulare complex infection in patients with AIDS. Lancet 1991;338:1107.

272. Chaisson RE et al. Clarithromycin therapy for bacteremic Mycobacterium avium complex disease. A randomized, double-blind, dose-ranging study in patients with AIDS. AIDS Clinical Trials Group Protocol 157 Study Team. Ann Intern Med 1994;15;121(12):905.

273. Ishiguro M et al. Penetration of macrolides into human polymorphonuclear leukocytes. J Antimicrob Chemother 1989;24:719.

274. Mor N et al. Accumulation of clarithromycin in macrophages infected with Mycobacterium avium. Pharmacotherapy 1994;14:100.

275. Girard AE et al. Pharmacokinetic and in vivo studies with azithromycin (CP-62,993), a new macrolide with an extended half-life and excellent tissue distribution. Antimicrob Agents Chemother 1987;31:1948.

276. Barradel LB et al. Clarithromycin: a review of its pharmacological properties and therapeutic use in Mycobacterium avium-intracellulare complex infections in patients with acquired immune deficiency syndrome. Drugs 1993;46:289.

277. Kemper CA et al. The individual microbiologic effect of three antimycobacterial agents, clofazimine, ethambutol, and rifampin, on Mycobacterium avium complex bacteremia in patients with AIDS. J Infect Dis 1994;170:157.

278. Shafran SD et al. A comparison of two regimens for the treatment of MAC bacteremia in AIDS: rifabutin, ethambutol and clarithromycin versus rifampin, ethambutol, clofazimine and ciprofloxacin. N Engl J Med 1996;335:377.

279. Chaisson RE et al. Clarithromycin ethambutol with or without clofazimine for the treatment of bacteremic Mycobacterium avium complex disease in patients with HIV infection. AIDS 1997;11:311.

280. Masur H et al. Recommendations on prophylaxis and therapy for disseminated Mycobacterium avium complex for adults and adolescents infected with human immunodeficiency virus. MMWR Morbid Mortal Wkly Rep 1993;42:14.

281. Dube MP et al. Successful short-term suppression of clarithromycin-resistant Mycobacterium avium complex bacteremia in AIDS. California Collaborative Treatment Group. Clin Infect Dis. 1999;28:136.

282. Flexner C. HIV-Protease inhibitors. New Engl J Med 1998;338:1281.

283. Oldfield EC 3rd et al. Once weekly azithromycin therapy for prevention of Mycobacterium avium complex infection in patients with AIDS: a randomized, double-blind, placebo-controlled multicenter trial. Clin Infect Dis 1998;26:611.

284. Havlir DV et al. Prophylaxis against disseminated Mycobacterium avium complex with weekly azithromycin, daily rifabutin or both. California Collaborative Treatment Group. N Engl J Med 1996;335:392.

285. Benson CA et al. Clarithromycin or rifabutin alone or in combination for primary prophylaxis of Mycobacterium avium complex disease in patients with AIDS: a randomized, double-blind, placebo-controlled trial. The AIDS Clinical Trials Group 196/Terry Beirn Community Programs for Clinical Research on AIDS 009 Protocol Team. J Infect Dis 2000;181:1289.

286. Kotler DP. The gastrointestinal and hepatobiliary systems of HIV infection. In: Wormser GP, ed. AIDS and Other Manifestations of HIV Infection. New York: Lippincott-Raven, 1998:505.

287. Flanigan TP et al. Prospective trial of paromomycin for cryptosporidiosis in AIDS. Am J Med 1996;100:370.

288. Weiss LM. Microsporidiosis. In: Dolin R et al., eds. AIDS Therapy. Philadelphia: Churchill Livingstone, 1999:336.

289. Jacobson MA et al. Retinal and gastrointestinal disease due to cytomegalovirus in patients with the acquired immune deficiency syndrome: prevalence, natural history, and response to ganciclovir therapy. Quob J Med 1988;67:473.

290. Wu GD et al. A comparison of routine light microscopy, immunohistochemistry, and in situ hybridization for the detection of cytomegalovirus in gastrointestinal biopsies. Am J Gastroenterol 1989;84:1517.

291. Profeta S et al. Salmonella infections in patients with acquired immunodeficiency syndrome. Arch Intern Med 1985;145:670.

292. Rompalo A, Quinn TC. Enteric bacterial diseases. In: Dolin R et al., eds. AIDS Therapy. Philadelphia: Churchill Livingstone, 1999:350.

293. Blaser MJ et al. Recurrent shigellosis complicating human immunodeficiency virus infection: failure of preexisting antibodies to confer protection. Am J Med 1989;86:105.

294. Bernard E et al. Diarrhea and Campylobacter infections in patients infected with the human immunodeficiency virus. J Infect Dis 1989;159:143.

295. Juranels DD. Cryptosporidiosis: sources of infection and guidelines for prevention. Clin Infect Dis 1995;21(Suppl 1):S57.

296. Vakil NB et al. Biliary cryptosporidiosis in HIV-infected people after the waterborne outbreak of cryptosporidiosis in Milwaukee. N Engl J Med 1996;34;19.

297. Flanigan, TP. Cryptosporidium, Isospora, and Cyclospora infections. In: Dolin R et al., eds. AIDS Therapy. Philadelphia: Churchill Livingstone, 1999:328.

298. Holmberg SD et al. Possible effectiveness of clarithromycin and rifabutin for cryptosporidiosis chemoprophylaxis in HIV Disease. JAMA 1998;279:384.

299. Smith NH et al. Combination drug therapy for cryptosporidiosis in AIDS. J Infect Dis 1998;178;900.

300. Amadi B et al. Effect of nitazoxanide on morbidity and mortality in Zambian children with cryptosporidiosis: a randomized, controlled trial. Lancet 2002;360:1375.

301. Grube H et al. Resolution of AIDS associated cryptosporidiosis after treatment with indinavir. Am J Gastroenterol 1997;92:726.

302. Goodgame RW. Understanding intestinal spore-forming protozoa: *Cryptosporidia, Microsporidia, Isospora,* and *Cyclospora.* Ann Intern Med 1996;124:429.

303. Anwar-Bruni DM et al. Atovaquone is effective treatment for the symptoms of gastrointestinal microsporidiosis in HIV-1 infected patients. AIDS 1996;10:619.

304. Sharpstone D et al. The treatment of microsporidial diarrhoea with thalidomide. AIDS 1996;9:659.

305. Blackstone MO. Endoscopic Interpretation. New York: Raven Press, 1984:19.

306. Reef SE et al. Opportunistic *Candida* infections in patients infected with human immunodeficiency virus: prevention issues and priorities. Clin Infect Dis 1995;21(Suppl 1):S99.

307. Jacobson JM et al. Thalidomide for the treatment of oral aphthous ulcers in patients with human immunodeficiency virus infection. New Institute of Allergy and Infection Disease AIDS Clinical Trials Group. N Engl J Med 1997;336:1489.

308. Duswald KH et al. High-dose therapy with fluconazole ≥800 mg/day. Mycoses 1997;40:267.

309. Maenza JR et al. Risk factors for fluconazole-resistant candidiasis in human immunodeficiency virus-infected patients. J Infect Dis 1996;173:219.

310. Revision of the Centers for Disease Control and Prevention surveillance case definition for acquired immunodeficiency syndrome. MMWR Morbid Mortal Wkly Rep 1987;36(Suppl 1):3S.

311. Talal AH, Dieterich DT. Gastrointestinal and hepatic manifestation of AIDS. In: Sande MA, Volberding P, eds. The Medical Management of AIDS. Philadelphia: WB Saunders, 1999;195.

312. Beisel WR. Malnutrition as a consequence of stress. In: Suskind RM, ed. Malnutrition and the Immune Response. New York: Raven Press, 1997.

313. Von Roenn JH et al. Megestrol acetate in patients with AIDS-related cachexia. Ann Intern Med 1994;121:393.

314. Oster MH et al. Megestrol acetate in patients with AIDS and cachexia. Ann Intern Med 1994;121:400.

315. Goster R et al. Dronabinol effects on weight in patients with HIV infection. AIDS 1992;6:127.

316. Berger JR et al. Oxandrolone in AIDS-wasting myopathy. AIDS 1996;10:1657.

317. Engelson ES et al. Effects of testosterone upon body composition. Acquir Immun Defic Syndr Hum Retrovirol 1996;11:510.

318. Balog DL et al. HIV wasting syndrome: treatment update. Ann Pharmacother 1998;32:446.

319. Grinspoon SK et al. An etiology and pathogenesis of hormonal and metabolic disorders in HIV infection. Baillieres Clin Endocrinol Metab 1994;4:735.

320. Hengge UR et al. Oxymetholone promotes weight gain in patients with advanced human immunodeficiency virus (HIV-1) infection. Br J Nutrition 1996;75:129.

321. Miller K et al. Transdermal testosterone administration in women with acquired immunodeficiency syndrome wasting: a pilot study. J Clin Endocrinol Metab 1998;83:2717.

322. Grinspoon S et al. Effects of androgen administration in men with the AIDS wasting syndrome. A randomized, double-blind, placebo-controlled trial. Ann Intern Med 1998;128:18.

323. Waters D et al. Recombinant human growth hormone, insulin-like growth factor, and combination therapy in AIDS-associated wasting: a randomized, double-blind, placebo-controlled trial. Ann Intern Med 1996;125:865.

324. Schambelan M et al. Recombinant human growth hormone in patients with HIV-associated wasting. A randomized, placebo-controlled trial. Serostim Study Group. Ann Intern Med 1996;125:873.

325. Minor JR, Piscitelli SC. Thalidomide in diseases associated with human immunodeficiency virus infection. Am J Health-Syst Pharm 1996;53:429.

326. Roubenoff R et al. Feasibility of increasing lean body mass in HIV-infected adults using progressive resistance training. Nutrition 1997;13:271.

327. Pluda JM et al. Parameters affecting the development of non-Hodgkin's lymphoma in patients with severe human immunodeficiency virus infection receiving antiretroviral therapy. J Clin Oncol 1993;11:1099.

328. Kaplan LD, Northfelt DW. Malignancies associated with AIDS. In: Sandle MA, Volberding PA, eds. The Medical Management of AIDS. Philadelphia: WB Saunders, 1999;467.

329. Jacobson LP et al. Impact of potent antiretroviral therapy on the incidence of Kaposi's sarcoma and non-Hodgkin's lymphomas among HIV-1-infected individuals. Multicenter AIDS Cohort Study. J Acquir Immun Defic Syndr Hum Retrovirol 1999;21(Suppl 1):S34.

330. Chang Y et al. Identification of herpesvirus-like DNA sequences in KS tissue from HIV-1 infected men. Science 1994;266:1565.

331. Huang YQ et al. Human herpes virus-like nucleic acid in various forms of Kaposi sarcoma. Lancet 1995;345.759.

332. Krown SE et al. Kaposi's sarcoma in the acquired immune deficiency syndrome: a proposal for uniform evaluation, response and staging criteria. J Clin Oncol 1989;7:1201.

333. Krown S. Kaposi sarcoma. In: Dolin R et al., eds. AIDS Therapy. New York: Churchill Livingstone, 1999:580.

334. Gao SJ et al. Seroconversion to antibodies against Kaposi's sarcoma-associated herpes-virus-related latent nuclear antigens before development of Kaposi's sarcoma. N Engl J Med 1996;335:233.

335. Lane HC. The role of alpha-interferon in patients with human immunodeficiency virus infection. Semin Oncol 1991;18(Suppl 7):46.

336. Kovacs JA et al. Combined zidovudine and interferon-alpha therapy in patients with Kaposi sarcoma and the acquired immunodeficiency syndrome (AIDS). Ann Intern Med 1989;111:280.

337. Fischl MA. Antiretroviral therapy in combination with interferon for AIDS-related Kaposi's sarcoma. Am J Med 1991;90:2S.

338. Krown SE et al. Interferon-alpha, zidovudine, and granulocyte-macrophage colony-stimulating factor: a phase I AIDS Clinical Trials Group study in patients with Kaposi's sarcoma associated with AIDS. J Clin Oncol 1992;10:1344.

339. Uthyakumar S et al. Randomized cross-over comparison of liposomal daunorubicin versus observation for early Kaposi's sarcoma. AIDS 1996;10:515.

340. Kedes DH et al. Sensitivity of Kaposi's sarcoma-associated herpesvirus replication to antiviral drugs. Implications for potential therapy. J Clin Invest 1997;99:2082.

341. Gill PS et al. The effects of preparations of human chorionic gonadotropin on AIDS-related Kaposi's sarcoma. N Engl J Med 1997;336:1115.

342. Moore RD et al. Non-Hodgkin's lymphoma in patients with advanced HIV infection treated with zidovudine. JAMA 1991;265:2208.

343. Pluda JM et al. Development of non-Hodgkin lymphoma in a cohort of patients with severe human immunodeficiency virus (HIV) infection on long-term antiretroviral therapy. Ann Intern Med 1990;113:276.

344. Armenian HK et al. Risk factors for non-Hodgkin's lymphoma in acquired immunodeficiency syndrome. Am J Epidemiol 1996;143:374.

345. Krown S. Non-Hodgkin lymphoma. In: Dolin R et al., eds. AIDS Therapy. New York: Churchill Livingstone, 1999:592.

346. Tirelli U et al. Prospective study with combined low-dose chemotherapy and zidovudine in 37 patients with poor-prognosis AIDS-related non-Hodgkin's lymphoma. French-Italian Cooperative Study Group. Ann Oncol 1992;3:843.

347. Kaplan LD et al. Low-dose chemotherapy with standard-dose m-BACOD chemotherapy for non-Hodgkin's lymphoma associated with human immunodeficiency virus infection. National Institute of Allergy and Infectious Diseases AIDS Clinical Trials Group. N Engl J Med 1997;336:1641.

348. Pluda JM et al. Hematologic effects of AIDS therapies. Hematol Oncol Clin North Am 1991;5:229.

349. Centers for Disease Control and Prevention. AIDS in women, United States. MMWR Morbid Mortal Wkly Rep 47:845,1990.

350. Feingold AR et al. Cervical cytological abnormalities and papillomavirus in women infected with human immunodeficiency virus. J Acquir Immun Defic Syndr Hum Retrovirol 1990;3:896.

351. Irwin KL et al. Pelvic inflammatory disease in human immunodeficiency virus-infected women. Obstet Gynecol 1994;83:480.

352. Watts DH et al. Comparison of gynecologic history and laboratory results in HIV-positive women with CD4+ lymphocyte counts between 200 and 500 cells/microl and below 100 cells/microl. J Acquir Immune Defic Syndr Hum Retrovirol 1999;20:455.

353. Maiman M et al. Human immunodeficiency virus infection and cervical neoplasia. Gynecol Oncol 1990;38:377.

354. Schiffman MH. Recent progress in defining the epidemiology of human papillomavirus infection and cervical neoplasia. J Natl Cancer Inst 1992;84:394.

355. Winkelstein W Jr. Smoking and cervical cancer—current status: a review. Am J Epidemiol 1990;131:945.

356. Newman MD, Wofsy CB. Women and HIV disease. In: Sande MA, Volberding PA, eds. The Medical Management of AIDS. Philadelphia: WB Saunders, 1999;537.

357. Vermund SH et al. High risk of human papillomavirus infection and cervical squamous intraepithelial lesions among women with symptomatic human immunodeficiency virus infection. Am J Obstet Gynecol 1991;165:392.

358. Rellihan MA et al. Rapidly progressing cervical cancer in a patient with human immunodeficiency virus infection. Gynecol Oncol 1990;36:435.

359. Monfardini S et al. Unusual malignant tumors in 49 patients with HIV infection. AIDS 1989;3:449.

360. Nasiell K et al. Behavior of mild cervical dysplasia during long-term follow up. Obstet Gynecol 1986;67:665.

361. Cervical cytology: evaluation and management of abnormalities. ACOG Technical Bulletin #183. Int J Gynaecol Obstet 1993;43:212.

362. Kurman RJ et al. Interim guidelines for management of abnormal cervical cytology. JAMA 1994;271:1866.

363. Ferenczy A et al. Loop electrosurgical excision procedure for squamous intraepithelial lesions of the cervix: advantages and potential pitfalls. Obstet Gynecol 1996;87:332.

364. Wetchler SJ. Treatment of cervical intraepithelial neoplasia with the CO_2 laser: laser versus cryotherapy. A review of effectiveness and cost. Obstet Gynecol Surv 1984;39:469.

365. Bornstein J et al. Treatment of cervical intraepithelial neoplasia and invasive squamous cell carcinoma by interferon. Obstet Gynecol Surv 1993;48:251.

366. Rotola A et al. Beta-interferon treatment of cervical intraepithelial neoplasia: a multicenter clinical trial. Intervirol 1995;38:325.

367. Costa S et al. Intramuscular alpha-interferon treatment of human papillomavirus lesions in the lower female genital tract. Cervix LFGT 1988;6:203.

368. Byrne MA et al. The effect of interferon on human papillomaviruses associated with cervical intraepithelial neoplasia. Br J Obstet Gynecol 1986;93:1136.

369. Ylikoski M et al. Topical treatment with human leukocyte interferon of HPV 16 infections associated with cervical and vaginal intraepithelial neoplasias. Gynecol Oncol 1990;36:353.

370. Puligheddu P et al. Activity of interferon-alpha in condylomata with dysplastic lesion of the uterine cervix. Eur J Gynecol Oncol 1988;9:161.

371. Frost L et al. No effect of intralesional injection of interferon on moderate cervical intraepithelial neoplasia. Br J Obstet Gynecol 1990;97:626.

CHAPTER 71

Fungal Infections

John D. Cleary, Stanley W. Chapman, Margaret Pearson

Mycotic (fungal) infections, once observed only occasionally, are now the fourth most commonly encountered nosocomial infection. This increase can, in part, be attributed to the growing numbers of immunocompromised hosts as a result of organ transplants, cancer chemotherapy, and the AIDS epidemic. Practitioners must be abreast of current concepts in medical mycology that affect the treatment and monitoring of patients with fungal infections. This chapter reviews the mycology, diagnosis, antimycotics, and therapeutics for common mycotic infections. For a more in-depth presentation of the basic biology of fungi, as well as the epidemiology, pathogenesis, immunology, diagnosis, and monitoring of mycotic infections, see Kwon-Chung and Bennett's *Medical Mycology.*[1] In addition, other chapters in this book address specific areas of antifungal therapy and should be reviewed by the reader. These topics include the treatment of fungal meningitis (see Chapter 58, Central Nervous System Infections); endocarditis (see Chapter 59, Endocarditis); intra-abdominal and hepatosplenic infections (see Chapter 63, Intra-Abdominal Infections); bone and joint infections (see Chapter 66, Osteomyelitis and Septic Arthritis and Chapter 67, Traumatic Skin and Soft Tissue Infections); and infections in immunocompromised patients with and without HIV infections (see Chapter 68, Prevention and Treatment of Infections in Neutropenic Cancer Patients and Chapter 70, Opportunistic Infections in HIV-Infected Patients). The treatment of uncommon fungal infections (e.g., paracoccidioidomycosis, alternariosis or fusariosis, mucormycosis, and pseudallescheriasis) is not presented.

MYCOLOGY
Morphology

The pathogenic fungi that infect humans are nonmotile eucaryotes that reproduce by sporulation and exist in two forms: filamentous molds and unicellular yeasts. These forms are not mutually exclusive and, depending on the growth conditions, a fungus may exist in one or even both of these forms (Table 71-1). The dimorphic fungi (e.g., *Histoplasma capsulatum and Blastomyces dermatitidis*) grow as a mold in nature (27°C) but quickly convert to the parasitic yeast form after infecting the host (37°C). This mycelium-to-yeast conversion is an important factor in the pathogenesis of disease caused by these organisms. Other pathogenic fungi, such as *Aspergillus* species, grow only as a mold form, whereas *Cryptococcus neoformans* usually grows as a yeast form. *Candida* species grow with a modified form of budding whereby newly budded cells remain attached to the parent cells and form pseudohyphae. Fungi are aerobic and are easily grown on routine culture media similar to that used to grow bacteria. Most fungi

Table 71-1 Organism Classification

Hyphae (Molds)
  Hyalohyphomycoses
    Aspergillus species, *Pseudallescheria boydii*
    Dermatophytes: *Epidermophyton floccosum, Trichophyton* species,
      Microsporum species
  Phaeohyphomycoses
    Alternaria species, *Anthopsis deltoidea, Bipolaris hawaiiensis,*
      Cladosporium species, *Curvularia geniculata, Exophiala*
      species, *Fonsecaea pedrosoi, Phialophora* species, *Fusarium*
      species
  Zygomycetes
    Absidia corymbifera, Mucor indicus, Rhizomucor pusillus
Dimorphic Fungi
    Blastomyces species, *Coccidioides* species, *Paracoccidioides*
      species, *Histoplasma* species, *Sporothrix* species
Yeasts
    Candida species, *Cryptococcus neoformans*

Table 71-2 Clinical Classification of Mycoses

Classification	Site Infected	Example
Superficial	Outermost skin and hair	Malasseziasis (Tinea versicolor)
Cutaneous	Deep epidermis and nails	Dermatophytosis
Subcutaneous	Dermis and subcutaneous tissue	Sporotrichosis
Systemic	Disease of ≥1 internal organ	
Opportunistic		Candidiasis
		Cryptococcosis
		Aspergillosis
		Mucormycosis
Nonopportunistic		Histoplasmosis
		Blastomycosis
		Coccidioidomycosis

grow best at 25 to 35°C. Fungi that cause only cutaneous and subcutaneous disease grow poorly at temperatures >37°C. This temperature-selective growth explains, at least in part, why these organisms rarely disseminate from a primary focus in the skin or subcutaneous tissues.

Classification

Fungal infections are best classified by the area of the body infected (Table 71-2). Superficial mycoses involve only the outermost keratinized layers of the skin (stratum corneum) and hair. The cutaneous mycoses extend deeper into the epidermis and may also infect the nails. The subcutaneous mycoses infect the dermis and subcutaneous tissues: entry into these sites is by inoculation or implantation of dirt or vegetative matter. The systemic mycoses cause disease of the internal organs of the body. Standard definitions that are useful in daily patient care for invasive fungal infections have been developed for epidemiologic and clinical trials. The guidelines are referenced under each infection. The respiratory tract is the most common primary portal of entry into the patient, and infection in the lungs may be symptomatic or asymptomatic. Systemic infection with *Candida* usually results from a primary focus in the gastrointestinal (GI) tract or skin. In each case, the organism may spread hematogenously from the primary focus throughout the body, resulting in disseminated disease. The opportunistic mycoses occur primarily in the immunocompromised host and require more aggressive treatment. The list of fungi that cause opportunistic infection is rapidly expanding, especially with the AIDS epidemic.[2] The nonopportunistic fungi (primary pathogens) usually cause disease in the immunologically normal host. However, some primary pathogens result in unique clinical syndromes when infection occurs in the immunocompromised host, such as histoplasmosis in AIDS.[1]

Pathogenesis of Infection
Endogenous
Fungal infection may be acquired from both exogenous and endogenous sources. The only fungi known to be normal flora (commensals) in humans are *Pityrosporum obiculare*, which causes the noninflammatory superficial condition of tinea versicolor, and *Candida* species. Infections with these yeast organisms primarily develop from the patient's own normal flora (endogenous infection). These endogenous fungal infections of the skin or mucous membranes occur when host resistance is lowered and the organism proliferates in high numbers. Excess heat and humidity, oral contraceptive use, pregnancy, diabetes, malnutrition, and immunosuppression facilitate endogenous local infection by both *Pityrosporum* and *Candida*. Systemic candidal infections occur in the immunocompromised host when the organism colonizing the patient's skin or GI tract is disseminated hematogenously throughout the body.

Exogenous
Exogenous infections occur when the fungus is acquired from an environmental source. In the case of dermatophytes (ringworm fungi), the organism may be acquired from dirt, animals, or another infected individual. The subcutaneous mycoses result from direct inoculation of infected material, often a thorn or other vegetable matter, through the skin. Infections of the skin and subcutaneous tissues by *Aspergillus* and the agents causing mucormycosis (e.g., *Rhizopus, Absidia, Mucor*) have resulted from contaminated wound dressings and cast materials.[3] Exogenous fungi colonized or carried on the hands of health care workers can infect patients; therefore, these health care workers, especially in intensive care units, must wash their hands to prevent cross-infection between patients.[4] Other than candidal infections, the systemic mycoses are primarily the result of inhalation of dust contaminated by the infectious spores, with a primary focus of infection in the lungs. If local or systemic host defenses are unable to control the primary infection, the organism may be spread hematogenously to other organs. Some of the systemic mycoses have defined geographic (endemic) areas in which the fungus is more commonly encountered in the environment. For example, histoplasmosis and blastomycosis occur most often in the regions of the Mississippi and Ohio River valleys, whereas coccidioidomycosis is endemic to the southwestern United States and the Central Valley of California.

Host Defenses

Host defenses against fungal infection involve both nonimmune (also known as nonspecific or natural resistance) and immune (also known as specific or acquired resistance) mechanisms. Nonimmune resistance plays a primary role in preventing colonization and invasion of a susceptible tissue. The normal bacterial flora of the skin and mucous membranes prevent colonization (colonization resistance) by more pathogenic bacteria and fungi. Patients treated with broad-spectrum antibiotics are at greater risk for colonization and infection by fungi because of the alteration in their bacterial flora. The barrier function of the intact skin and mucous membranes is also an important defense against fungal infection. Skin defects, whether the result of intravenous (IV) catheters, burns, surgery, or trauma, predispose individuals to local invasion and fungemia, especially with *Candida* species. When these physical barriers are breached, the polymorphonuclear leukocyte (neutrophil) is the cell involved earliest in host defense against fungi. The antifungal activity of neutrophils involves phagocytosis and intracellular killing but also may include extracellular killing by secreted lysosomal enzymes. Neutropenia is the most common neutrophil defect predisposing to fungal infection, but functional defects of neutrophils, such as those occurring in patients with chronic granulomatous disease of childhood and myeloperoxidase deficiency, have also been associated with an increased frequency of fungal infections, especially with *Candida* and *Aspergillus.*

Antibody and complement may have some role in resistance to certain fungal infections, but they are not the primary effectors of acquired resistance. Cellular immunity, mediated by antigen-specific T lymphocytes, cytokines, and activated macrophages, is the primary acquired (immune) host defense against fungi. Patients with defective cellular immunity (e.g., immunosuppressed organ transplant recipients, patients with lymphomas and AIDS, and those treated with corticosteroids or cytotoxic agents) are at greatest risk for fungal infection. The immunodeficiency noted in these patients is also the primary reason for the poor therapeutic outcome despite appropriate antifungal therapy. An additional factor associated with an increased risk for fungal infection is the use of total parenteral nutrition.[1]

ANTIMYCOTICS
Mechanisms of Action

Table 71-3 lists the FDA-approved topical and systemic antimycotics for the treatment of fungal infections. Griseofulvin and potassium iodide have limited clinical utility and are not used to treat systemic fungal infections. Griseofulvin inhibits growth by inhibiting fungal cell mitosis caused by polymerization of cell microtubules, thereby disrupting mitotic spindle formation. It has activity only against the dermatophyte fungi. The antifungal mechanism of potassium iodide is unclear. It is effective only in the treatment of lymphocutaneous sporotrichosis.

The eight antifungal drugs used for systemic disease fall into five structural classes that act by four mutually exclusive mechanisms. *Amphotericin B and nystatin,* polyene macrolides, act principally by binding to ergosterol in the fungal cell membrane, effectively creating pores in the cell membrane and leading to depolarization of the membrane and cell leakage.[5] Although liposomal nystatin is in clinical trials, it is unlikely to be marketed in the United States. Amphotericin B binds with greater affinity to ergosterol than to cholesterol.[6] This phenomenon is believed to be mediated through both hydrophilic hydrogen bonding and hydrophobic, nonspecific van der Waals forces. Investigations using P^{31} nuclear magnetic resonance spectroscopy to study the interactions of polyene macrolides with sterols documented that the presence of the double bond in the side chain of ergosterol (not present in cholesterol) accounts for the greater affinity of amphotericin B for ergosterol.[5] Unfortunately, amphotericin B also binds to

Table 71-3 Antifungal Agents Approved for Use

Agent (Brand Name)	Formulation
Systemic Agents	
Amphotericin B (Abelcet, AmBisome, Amphotec)	IV
Caspofungin (Cancidas)	IV
Fluconazole (Diflucan)	IV, tablet, oral suspension
Fluorocytosine [Flucytosine] (Ancobon)	Capsule
Griseofulvin (generic)	Tablet, oral suspension
Itraconazole (Sporanox)	IV, capsule, oral solution
Ketoconazole (Nizoral)	Tablet
Miconazole (Monistat)	IV
Potassium iodide	Solution
Terbinafine (Lamisil)	Tablet
Voriconazole (Vfend)	IV, tablet
Topicals, Class I	
Amphotericin B	Cream, lotion, ointment, oral suspension[a]
Butenafine (Mentax)	Cream
Butoconazole (Femstat)	Ointment
Ciclopirox (Loprox)	Cream, lotion
Clioquinol (Vioform)	Cream, ointment
Clotrimazole	Cream, lotion, lozenge, pessary, solution, tablet
Econazole (Spectazole)	Cream
Haloprogin (Halotex)	Cream, solution
Ketoconazole (Nizoral)	Cream shampoo
Miconazole	Aerosol, cream, lotion, pessary, spray, suppository, vaginal tablet
Naftifine (Naftin)	Cream, gel
Nystatin	Cream, lozenge, ointment, powder, suspension, tablet
Oxiconazole (Oxistat)	Cream, lotion
Povidone iodine	Douche, gel, suppository
Sodium thiosulfate (Exoderm)	Lotion
Sulconazole (Exelderm)	Cream, solution
Terbinafine (Lamisil)	Cream
Terconazole (Terazol 7)	Cream, suppository
Tioconazole (Vagistat)	Ointment
Tolnaftate (generic)	Cream, gel, powder, solution, spray
Triacetin (Fungoid)	Cream, solution, spray
Undecylenic acid	Cream, foam, ointment, powder, soap

[a]No longer available in United States
Classification identified in Federal Register[201]

sterols of mammalian cells (i.e., cholesterol), a fact that is believed to account for most of the toxic effects of amphotericin B. Alteration in the lipid content of the pathogens membrane may play a role in the development of resistance,[7] although this alone is apparently not sufficient to affect that development.[8] However, the lethal antifungal effects of amphotericin B are the result of not only cell leakage resulting from ergosterol binding, but also immune stimulation and oxygen-dependent killing.[6,9]

5-Flucytosine (5-FC), a fluorinated cytosine analog, is believed to act principally by inhibiting nucleic acid synthesis. It is actively transported into susceptible cells by the enzyme cytosine permease, where it is metabolically transformed by deamination to the toxic metabolite 5-fluorouracil. Fluorouracil, when converted to 5-fluorouridine triphosphate, functions as an antimetabolite. It is incorporated into fungal RNA, where it is substituted for uracil and thereby disrupts protein synthesis.[10,11] 5-Fluorouracil may also be converted to fluorodeoxyuridine monophosphate, which inhibits thymidylate synthase and thus disrupts DNA synthesis.[11,12]

The azole *antifungals* and the *allylamines* (naftifine and terbinafine) appear to act by the same principal mechanism: inhibition of sterol biosynthesis by interference with either cytochrome P450–dependent lanosterol C14-demethylase (azoles) or squalene epoxidase (allylamines), critical enzymes in the biosynthesis of ergosterol.[13–16] The superior affinity of the triazoles (fluconazole, itraconazole, voriconazole) for fungal versus mammalian enzyme, as compared to the imidazoles (ketoconazole, miconazole), generally is believed to account for their reduced toxicity and improved efficacy.[15] The consequence of sterol biosynthesis inhibition is a faulty cell membrane with altered permeability. In general, the allylamines and older azoles are viewed as fungistatic in their action. The newer triazoles (voriconazole, posaconazole, and ravuconazole) demonstrate fungicidal activity against some fungal species.[17–19] The clinical relevance of *in vitro* fungicidal versus fungistatic action is the subject of considerable debate. Nevertheless, it seems logical that fungicidal action, if it can also be achieved *in vivo,* might be preferable in immunosuppressed hosts.

Lipopeptides are potent antifungal agents and include the structural class of *echinocandins* (anidulafungin, micafungin, and caspofungin). All share a common mechanism: they act by interfering with 1,3-β-D-glucan, preventing synthesis of essential cell wall polysaccharides that protect the cell from osmotic and structural stresses. The result is inhibition of fungal cell wall biosynthesis. Targeting the cell wall (as opposed to the cell membrane, which is the target of polyene, azole and allylamine) has been an important step in selective inhibition of fungal versus mammalian cells; the fungal cell wall does not share target-associated toxicity with the mammalian cell wall.[20]

Antifungal Spectrum and Susceptibility Testing

The evaluation of *in vitro* antifungal activity has long challenged investigators. Results are influenced substantially by many factors, including selection of culture medium, pH, inoculum size, incubation period, and other factors. Historically, attempts to use *in vitro* assay results to evaluate the susceptibility of clinical isolates to antifungal agents, to monitor therapeutic progress, and to compare the efficacy of antifungal drugs have led to frustration. More recently, novel techniques for susceptibility testing, evolution of antifungal pharmacodynamics, and knowledge of mechanisms of antifungal resistance which allow for identification of resistant isolates for validation of *in vitro* measurement systems have advanced methods for and interpretation of antifungal susceptibility testing.[21]

In 1997, the National Committee for Clinical Laboratory Standards (NCCLS) recommended a standardized method for determining *in vitro* antifungal susceptibilities for yeasts.[22] This method stipulates test medium, inoculum size and preparation, incubation time and temperature, end-point reading and quality control limits for amphotericin B, flucytosine, fluconazole, ketoconazole, and itraconazole. Minimum inhibitory concentration (MIC) values for use in clinical interpretation are specified for fluconazole, itraconazole, and flucytosine against *Candida* species after 48 hours of incubation. For fluconazole and itraconazole, a newly described breakpoint, susceptible-dose dependent (S-DD), was developed based on data supporting a trend toward better response with higher drug levels for isolates with higher MICs.[23] The S-DD range includes MICs of 16 and 32 µg/mL and >0.125 through < 0.5 µg/mL for fluconazole and itraconazole, respectively. *Candida* isolates with MICs less than these ranges are considered susceptible, and isolates with greater MICs are considered resistant. Owing to rapid development of resistance and limited data on correlation of MIC with outcome for flucytosine monotherapy, proposed interpretive breakpoints for this agent are based on a combination of historical data and results from animal studies. *Candida* isolates with a flucytosine MIC ≤4 µg/mL are considered susceptible, isolates with MIC >16 µg/mL are considered resistant, and isolates with MICs between these values are considered intermediate. Limitations of the M27-A methodology have precluded development of amphotericin B interpretive breakpoints nor have interpretive criteria been proposed for ketoconazole MICs. An E-Test (AB Biodisk; Piscataway, NJ) is commercially available. Difficulties in end-point determination using this method are from the result of frequent, nonuniform growth of the fungus on the agar medium; yet when properly performed, correlation between the E-Test and M27-A methods has been satisfactory for the azole antifungal agents against most *Candida.*[24,25] Other techniques under development for antifungal susceptibility testing for yeasts include disk-based testing, flow cytometry, and direct measurement of alterations in ergosterol synthesis.[21]

Recently the NCCLS also approved a standardized method for determining *in vitro* antifungal susceptibilities for certain spore-producing molds, namely *Aspergillus* spp., *Fusarium* spp., *Rhizopus* spp., *Pseudallescheria boydii,* and *Sporothrix schenckii.* To date, *in vitro* correlations with *in vivo* outcomes have not been established.[26] An E-Test to evaluate mold susceptibilities to the systemic antimycotics is also being studied. Results appear dependent on the antifungal agent investigated, incubation time, and fungal species being tested.[27] Despite these recent advances, the determination of *in vitro* susceptibilities or resistance in clinical practice is of limited utility and not readily available.

Susceptibility testing for clinical isolates is not routinely recommended; however, published data on the susceptibility of the identified species of yeast or mold should guide the clinician's therapeutic choice. Clinical isolates from patients failing high-dose therapy (i.e., refractory oral pharyngeal candidiasis) or unusual pathogenic yeasts in AIDS patients can be sent for testing.[21] Testing should be performed in a laboratory whose staff is trained in mycoses. Despite these limitations, certain generalities should be emphasized. First, amphotericin B, the echinocandins and pneumocandins have broad *in vitro* activity and clinical efficacy against the yeasts and filamentous molds. Of note, echinocandins and pneumocandins have intrinsically less activity against *Candida parapsilosis*, *Candida guilliermondii*, and *Cryptococcus neoformans*. The azole antifungals generally have clinically significant activity against only the yeasts and most dimorphic fungi. Additionally, itraconazole, voriconazole, posaconazole, and ravuconazole have excellent *in vitro* activity against Aspergillus species, with clinical efficacy demonstrated for itraconazole and voriconazole. Clinical data on treatment of aspergillosis using posaconazole or ravuconazole are forthcoming.

New Frontiers for Antifungal Therapy

Various investigative efforts have been directed toward both enhancing efficacy and reducing the toxicity of older antifungal drugs, including biochemical modifications of the agent, improved delivery systems, and combination therapy. The most significant strides have occurred with release of a new lipopeptide, improved delivery of amphotericin B by formulating it with a lipid, and the incorporation of itraconazole or voriconazole into a water-soluble sugar, cyclodextrin. Other novel delivery systems under investigation for antifungal compounds include cochleate lipid cylinders, nanoparticles or nanospheres, and coating of small hydrophobic lysosomes by hydrophilic polymers. Combination therapy has the potential advantage of targeting multiple sites for additive or synergistic antifungal activity and may prove to be an important advance in the management of fungal disease.

Even more challenging are the attempts to discover or design new prototype antifungal compounds. Substantial hurdles exist because both mammalian cells and fungal cells are eukaryotes and share many similar biochemical processes, unlike bacterial cells, which are prokaryotes. Traditionally, the drug discovery process depended on the ability to detect compounds (either natural products or synthetic compounds) that selectively inhibit or destroy fungal cells. This process is accomplished by either or both of two approaches: (1) the evaluation of existing compounds (natural or synthetic) for potentially useful antifungal activity and (2) the design and synthesis of new compounds that selectively block fungal targets. The former approach relies on a supply of compounds with structural diversity and a reliable biologic assay to detect antifungal activity. The latter depends on knowledge of the basic biology of the pathogen that can be exploited in drug design and synthesis. Recent advances in genomic sequencing of *C. albicans*, *C. glabrata*, *A. fumigatus*, and *C. neoformans* have allowed for use of this information within the search for new targets. Other less conventional drug discovery approaches include targeting known traditional virulence factors (e.g., adhesions, secreted enzymes). This approach is based on the principle that killing of the microbe need not occur in order for an anti-infective agent to be efficacious in reduction of disease.

Lead compounds that appear promising for antimycotic therapy include nikkomycins, sordarins, and lytic peptides. Nikkomycins inhibit chitin synthase. Chitin synthase catalyzes the polymerization of B-(1,4) linkages of *N*-acetyl glucosamine, which is critical to yeast cell membrane stabilization. Phase I and II clinical trials have been completed in the therapy of phaeohyphomycosis. Sordarins interfere with elongation factor-2, which is essential for protein synthesis, whereas lytic peptides bind to cell membrane sterols, thereby reducing cell membrane stability. Sordarins and lytic peptides are still in early development.

SUPERFICIAL AND CUTANEOUS MYCOSES
Tinea Pedis: Treatment

1. C.W., a 28-year-old male construction worker, is evaluated for a chronic case of "athlete's foot." He wears boots all day at work and notes intense itching of both feet throughout the day. He has been using tolnaftate powder (Tinactin) for 1 week with no real therapeutic benefit. On examination, the web spaces between all the toes are white, macerated, and cracked. A few vesicles are also present over the dorsum of the foot at the base of the toes. Scrapings of the lesions examined as a potassium hydroxide preparation reveal branching, filamentous hyphae compatible with a dermatophyte infection. The diagnosis of "athlete's foot" is made. What therapeutic options are available for C.W.?

Selection of antifungal therapy should be based on the extent and type of infection. Superficial or cutaneous infections should initially be approached topically. Any follicular, nail, or widespread (>20% of body surface area [BSA]) infection should be treated systemically under medical supervision owing to poor penetration of topical applications. Topical antifungals have been reviewed as a class by the FDA advisory review panel on over-the-counter (OTC) antimicrobial drug products and on an individual basis as newer products have been released. To receive a class 1 recommendation, each agent (or combination) must have been tested in well-designed clinical trials that show the drug microbiologically and clinically effective against dermatophytosis or candidiasis with insignificant toxicity (irritation). Class I agents are listed in Table 71-3. Class II agents (camphor, candicidin, coal tar, menthol, phenolates, resorcinol, tannic acid, thymol, tolindate) are considered to have higher risk-benefit ratios associated with their pharmacotherapy. Class III agents (benzoic acid, borates, caprylic acid, oxyquinolines, iodines, propionic acid, salicylates, triacetin, gentian violet) lack adequate scientific data to determine efficacy. Topical therapy with any class I agent applied twice daily to the affected area for 2 to 6 weeks should be adequate. Therapy should be titrated to response.

Because C.W. could continue tolnaftate powder for 2 to 6 weeks or switch to an antifungal cream or lotion (e.g., miconazole), these products should be applied to the web spaces between all the affected toes twice daily. C.W. should also be careful to use nonocclusive footwear (e.g., cotton rather than synthetic fiber socks, and leather rather than vinyl boots). Application of an absorbent or antifungal powder to his footwear would also be helpful (see Chapter 38, Dermatotherapy).

Tinea Unguium (Onychomycosis): Treatment

2. If C.W. also suffered from an infection of the toenail (onychomycosis), what additional therapy could be offered to him?

Onychomycosis is typically caused by either a dermatophyte, a hyphal fungi, or *Candida*. Nail scrapings and culture should be performed to help plan initial therapy. Once culture results are known, therapy can be initiated with either terbinafine 250 mg/day or itraconazole 200 mg/day for 6 (fingernail) to 12 (toenail) weeks. However, in some cases successful therapy of tinea unguium can require 3 to 6 months for fingernails and 6 to 12 months for toenails. Therapy should be considered successful when several millimeters of healthy nail have emerged from the nailfold to the margin of infected nail, or when a 25% reduction in size of the infected site has been achieved.

For dermatophyte nail or paronychial infections, griseofulvin therapy could be used if an azole or allylamine is contraindicated. Griseofulvin (microsized or ultramicrosized) administered orally at 10 mg/kg per day and titrated to response should be effective.[28] Owing to the large doses given for prolonged periods, C.W. should be monitored closely at each prescription refill for signs and symptoms of adverse reactions. Terbinafine or itraconazole most commonly causes symptoms of headache, rash, and GI distress. Griseofulvin is more toxic, often causing hypersensitivity (urticaria, angioedema, type II hypersensitivity reactions), photosensitivity dermatitis, GI distress, and neurologic complications (headache, paresthesias, altered sensorium).[28]

Antimycotic pulse therapy is a novel approach to the treatment of onychomycosis. An FDA-approved alternative to daily therapy can now include a course of itraconazole 200 mg twice daily for 1 week in 2 consecutive months for fingernail infections. Double-blind, placebo-controlled trials revealed that this regimen was associated with a 77% clinical response and 73% mycologic response.[29] Overall responses and toxicity to therapy were more desirable with pulse regimens then with traditional regimens. Comparative studies demonstrate promising results for itraconazole pulse therapy for toenail infections[30] and fluconazole pulse therapy administered as a 150- to 450-mg dose once weekly for up to 12 months for mild disease.[31–32] Relapse rates after pulse (intermittent) terbinafine for 4 months have been frequent and longer courses of therapy are under study to enhance long-term efficacy.[33] Longer courses of therapy are being evaluated.

Removal of the nail as the sole therapy is not recommended because of the high relapse rate without concomitant systemic therapy. Likewise, IV antifungals are not indicated.

3. Describe the role of corticosteroids, antibacterials, or other additives to the antimycotic regimen in C.W.

Many patients with superficial, cutaneous, or nail infections will suffer additional morbidity associated with local inflammation and secondary bacterial infections. Inflammation is caused primarily by a type IV hypersensitivity reaction. Topical corticosteroids in conjunction with antifungals will often relieve itching and erythema secondary to inflammation. Bacterial (Proteus or Pseudomonas species) superinfection can also occur in these inflamed or macerated areas and may require concomitant topical antibacterial therapy. Pharmaceutical manufacturers of OTC preparations often combine a drying agent or astringent (e.g., alcohol, starch, talc, camphor) to their preparations to increase desquamation of the stratum corneum. Hyperhidrosis also can be relieved by these pharmaceutical additions. However, such combination treatments should not be used routinely because they increase the risk of toxicity and have not been proven to increase efficacy. If required for symptomatic relief, they should be used only for the initial days of treatment.

The affected web spaces between C.W.'s toes are macerated and cracked and vesicles are present at the base of his toes. A topical corticosteroid cream will probably facilitate the healing process and make him more comfortable during the first few days of antifungal therapy. The selection of topical corticosteroid formulations is presented in Chapter 38, Dermatotherapy.

SUBCUTANEOUS MYCOSES
Sporotrichosis
Treatment Options

4. O.M., a 62-year-old man, has had a painless, slowly enlarging ulcer on his left hand for the past 4 months. He is an avid gardener but can identify no antecedent local trauma. The primary lesion began as a red papule that slowly enlarged and then ulcerated. At the same time the ulcer developed, O.M. also noted painless, red nodules that spread proximally up his arm. He denies any chills, fever, weight loss, or cough. The ulcer has slowly enlarged despite daily application of a povidone-iodine ointment and 2 weeks of cephalexin treatment. On physical examination, O.M. is afebrile. A 1.5-cm^2 ulcer is present on the dorsum of the left hand. Extending proximally from the ulcer is a palpable cord and multiple nontender, erythematous nodules distributed linearly up the forearm, elbow, arm, and axilla. A culture of this ulcer obtained 4 weeks ago is now growing *Sporothrix schenckii*. What is the recommended therapy for O.M.?

Sporothrix schenckii is the dimorphic fungi found in the soil and on many plants. Infection is usually secondary to inoculation into the skin from a thorn or sharp plant matter. *S. schenckii* infection most commonly causes lymphocutaneous disease (Fig. 71-1) as illustrated by this case. Rarely, extracutaneous disease may occur and usually involves the lungs, bones, or joints.

Heat Treatment
In the 1930s and 1940s, local heat was applied to very mild plaque or lymphocutaneous disease.[34] Germination rates of this dimorphic fungus actually can be decreased by increased temperature, and heat therapy 1 hour/day for 3 months is effective in 90% of patients with plaques (very mild disease).[35,36] Heat treatment could be particularly useful in pregnant patients when pharmacotherapy may be contraindicated.

Itraconazole
Itraconazole is more active *in vitro* against *S. schenckii* than other imidazoles or saturated solution of potassium iodide (SSKI) and has dramatically improved the therapy of sporotrichosis. SSKI is seldom used for therapy secondary to treatment limiting toxicity. Cure rates for sporotrichosis cutaneous

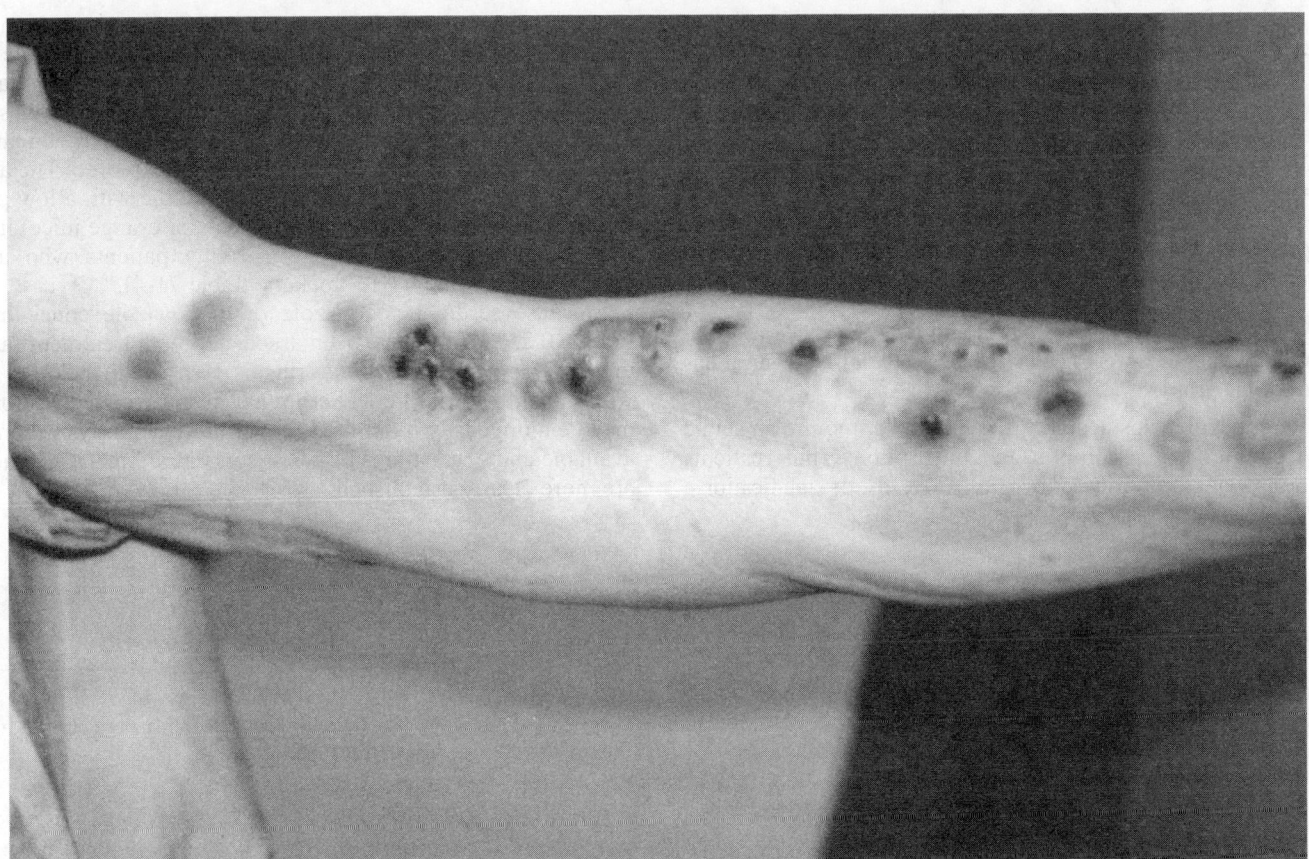

FIGURE 71-1 Lymphocutaneous sporotrichosis.

and lymphocutaneous disease are >90% with itraconazole 100 to 200 mg/day for 3 to 6 months. For extracutaneous disease, higher dosages of itraconazole (200 mg twice daily) for 1 to 2 years achieve response rates of 81%, but relapse frequently occurs (27%) after therapy is stopped.[35–38] The toxicity and safety profile for itraconazole also appears favorable in these patients. Patients with extracutaneous disease who are unable to tolerate the higher itraconazole dosages or whose disease continues to progress should be treated with amphotericin B. An amphotericin A total dose of 2.0 to 2.5 g is most often recommended. Although voriconazole, posaconazole and ravuconazole demonstrate amphotericin B *in vitro* activity against *S. schenckii,* (albeit less than itraconazole), their role in the treatment of sporotrichosis has not been defined.[18,39] Neither ketoconazole or fluconazole is effective in the treatment of sporotrichosis.[36]

Terbinafine

Terbinafine has good *in vitro* activity against *S. schenckii.* Clinical data, although not abundant, also suggest *in vivo* efficacy.[40] An unpublished clinical trial comparing 250 mg or 500 mg BID for 3 months for lymphocutaneous disease revealed responses equivalent to itraconazole. Adverse reactions common in this population included GI distress (dysgeusia, dyspepsia, diarrhea), skin rash, and weight gain. Greater clinical experience and peer review of the aforementioned trial will further define the role of terbinafine in the treatment of sporotrichosis.

Therefore, in the case of O.M., she has lymphocutaneous disease; itraconazole 100 mg/day for a minimum of 3 months is the treatment of choice. If significant improvement is not observed in the first 6 weeks, the itraconazole dosage should be increased to 200 mg/day and continued for 6 months or until both the ulcer and lymphangitis have resolved. Most patients will respond to this dosage, but an occasional patient may require dosages of 300 or 400 mg/day.

Itraconazole Dosing

5. **What instructions should O.M. receive for taking his itraconazole dose?**

The peak serum concentrations of itraconazole capsules are ninefold higher when the drug is taken with food (i.e., 0.18 μg/mL with food and 0.02 μg/mL in fasting subjects).[41] The influence of food on absorption appears to be somewhat dependent on the nature of the food. High-carbohydrate meals decrease the absorption of itraconazole, and high-lipid content meals appear to increase itraconazole absorption.[42,43] Patients who have difficulty eating (e.g., AIDS patients, cancer patients receiving antineoplastic therapy) may not absorb enough from the capsule to achieve therapeutic plasma concentrations following a typical oral dose.[44] Although itraconazole manifests nonlinear serum pharmacokinetics (i.e., administering the total dose in two divided doses is associated with higher peak serum concentrations than a single larger dose), no clinical benefit of splitting the dose has been demonstrated. Therefore, O.M. could be instructed to take his itraconazole capsule with his highest fat content meal of the day or itraconazole solution could be substituted to improve absorption.

Itraconazole oral solution is a cyclodextrin formulation that has 55% bioavailability in a fed patient; this increases in a fasting patient. Furthermore, bioavailability of this formulation is not affected by level of gastric acidity. Average serum concentration in a cohort of patients with advanced HIV infection was 2,719 ng/mL following a 28-day twice daily dosing regimen.[45] O.M. should take his itraconazole solution on an empty stomach twice a day if this formulation is selected.

6. **How would instructions for taking itraconazole capsules be modified if O.M. were achlorhydric as a result of medications or AIDS gastropathy?**

Itraconazole capsules, like ketoconazole, require an acidic environment for dissolution and absorption. Thus, patients who are achlorhydric, either as a result of medications, surgery, or underlying disease (e.g., AIDS gastropathy), may not absorb itraconazole adequately.[44,46] Use of ketoconazole in achlorhydric patients has historically required concomitant administration of 4 mL, 0.2 N hydrochloric acid aqueous solution.[47] Etching of tooth enamel by the acid concerned many clinicians, and other alternatives have been explored. The administration of ketoconazole and itraconazole with a low pH liquid (e.g., 8 to 16 fluid ounces of a cola or orange juice) improves absorption in 65.2% of healthy patients who are achlorhydric or taking H_2-blockers (Table 71-4).[48,49]

Because serum ketoconazole or itraconazole concentrations <0.25 μg/mL have been associated with treatment failures, therapeutic drug monitoring is justified in patients in whom therapy is failing.[50] Serum antimycotic concentrations may be more easily monitored in the future as assays become available and correlations between concentration and efficacy are more clearly established.

Table 71-4 Significant Drug Interactions[51-60, 153, 154]

Interacting Agent(s)	Antifungal	Class[a]	Onset	Manifestation
ACE inhibitors	KI	2	D	Hyperkalemia
Acetazolamide	AmphoB		R	Development of severe hyperchloremic acidosis which may be due to additive or synergistic renal effects
Anticholinergics	KTZ	2	R	Antifungal should not be administered concomitantly because of a ↓ in antifungal absorption
Anticonvulsants				
Carbamazepine, phenytoin, mephenytoin	MIC, KTZ, FCZ, ITZ, VOR, CAS	2	D	A significant ↑ in phenytoin serum concentrations appears possible with concomitant FCZ therapy. ITZ serum concentrations have been reduced and therapeutic failures have occurred. Data extrapolated for KTZ and MIC. Carbamazepine and phenytoin are likely to significantly ↓ VOR and CAS concentrations through CYP450 induction
Antituberculars				
Isoniazid	KTZ	2	D	Combination can lead to a significant ↓ in serum antifungal concentrations, potentially leading to treatment failure
Rifabutin	VOR	1	R	↓ VOR C_{max} and AUC with concomitant ↑ rufabutin kinetic parameters
Rifampin	KTZ, FCZ, ITZ, VOR	2	D	Combination can lead to a significant ↓ in serum antifungal concentrations, potentially leading to treatment failure
Chemotherapeutic Agents				
Doxorubicin, carmustine, cyclophosphamide, fluorouracil	AmphoB	2	D	Enhanced pharmacologic effect of chemotherapeutic agent, secondary to ↑ cellular uptake
Corticosteroids	KTZ, ITZ, CAS	2	D	A twofold ↑ in serum methylprednisolone observed with concomitant KTZ. A similar reaction with prednisone has been observed. ↑ systemic effects of inhaled budesonide after ITZ. Dexamethasone may hepatically induce metabolism of ITZ. Dexamethasone may hepatically induce metabolism of CAS, thus ↓ serum concentrations of CAS
Didanosine	KTZ, ITZ	2	R	Acid neutralizing agents in didanosine will prevent ITZ absorption. KTZ extrapolated
Digoxin	AmphoB	2	D	AmphoB-induced hypokalemia can lead to ↑ digoxin toxicity
Fluoxetine	ITZ	3	D	Norfluoxetine inhibits CYP3A4 allowing for possible ↑ ITZ concentrations
Gastrointestinals				
Antacids	KTZ, FCZ, ITZ	2	R	Poor dissolution of dosage form, therefore ↓ azole availability. Specifically, KTZ and ITZ should be administered 2 hr postantacid dose. Be sure to note drugs like didanosine also contain buffers like antacids
H_2-blockers[b]	KTZ, FCZ, ITZ	2	R	Antifungal should not be administered with H_2-blocker because of ↓ in antifungal absorption
Sucralfate	KTZ	2	R	A 20% ↓ in KTZ absorption
Omeprazole	KTZ, VOR	2	R	↑ omeprazole concentration via CYP2C19 inhibition by VOR. Data theoretical for KTZ; agents should not be administered together

Table 71-4   Significant Drug Interactions[51-60, 153, 154]—cont'd

Immunologic agents				
Cyclosporine	KTZ, ITZ, FCZ, AmphoB	2	D	A significant ↑ in serum cyclosporine concentration can result in ↑ toxicity
	CAS			Enhanced nephrotoxicity
				Elevations in transaminases may result in hepatic toxicity; CAS AUC ↑ by 35%
Sirolimus	VOR	1	R	↑ C$_{max}$ and AUC of sirolimus
Tacrolimus	VOR, CAS	1	R	↑ tacrolimus C$_{max}$ and AUC necessitating tacrolimus dose reduction
	CAS	2	R	
Leukocyte transfusion	AmphoB	1	R	Severe pulmonary leukostasis is observed with potential for respiratory failure
Lithium	KI	2	D	Hypothyroidism
NSAIDs	AmphoB	2	R	Combination has additive/synergistic nephrotoxicity
Oral contraceptives	FCZ, griseofulvin	1	D	↓ oral contraceptive efficacy
Pentamidine	AmphoB	2	D	Combination has additive/synergistic nephrotoxicity
Potassium-sparing diuretics	KI	2	D	Hyperkalemia. Spironolactone reduced potassium requirements, preventing hypokalemia in neutropenic patients receiving AmphoB
Quinidine	KTZ, VOR	2	D	↑ quinidine serum concentrations have been observed
Sedative Hypnotics				
Benzodiazepines, ethanol, barbiturates	ITZ, KTZ, VOR, Griseofulvin	3	D	A 20% ↓ in chlordiazepoxide clearance has been demonstrated with KTZ. Long-acting barbiturates are likely to significantly decrease plasma VOR concentrations. An ↑ in griseofulvin clearance also has been observed with concomitant barbiturate or ethanol consumption
Sulfonylureas	MIC, KTZ, FCZ, ITZ, VOR	2	D	Antifungal therapy significantly ↑ sulfonylurea concentrations
Theobromines	FCZ, KTZ	2	R	Antifungal therapy can inhibit theophylline absorption
Warfarin	MIC, KTZ, FCZ, ITZ, VOR	1	D	Poorly documented mechanism. Antifungals hypothesized to ↓ warfarin protein binding and hydroxylation by liver. ↑ the risk of bleeding. Prolongation of prothrombin time with VOR

[a]Classification: 1, major; 2, moderate; 3, minor.
[b]Clinically significant interaction that the authors recommend the reader should focus upon.
ACE, angiotensin-converting enzyme; AmphoB, amphotericin B; D, delayed; FCZ, fluconazole; ITZ, itraconazole; KI, potassium iodide; KTZ, ketoconazole; MIC, miconazole; VOR, voriconazole; NSAIDs, nonsteroidal anti-inflammatory drugs; R, rapid.

Other significant drug interactions with the azole antifungals revolve around their ability to inhibit the cytochrome (CYP) P450 enzyme system. CYP3A4 is the major isoenzyme inhibited by ketoconazole and itraconazole and one of the major isoenzymes inhibited by voriconazole. In addition to the interactions documented in Table 71-4,[51-60] there are numerous other agents that are substrates to cytochrome P450 3A4 but for which there are no clinical studies evaluating an interaction. As azole antifungals could increase serum concentrations and therefore increase activity of these substrates, caution should be exercised during concomitant use. Alternatively, agents that either induce or inhibit the CYP450 system may decrease or increase, respectively, antifungal drug concentrations. Voriconazole has the propensity to inhibit CYP2C19 and CYP2C9.

SYSTEMIC MYCOSES
Candida Infection

7. L.K., a 21-year-old, 5'8", 170-lb, otherwise healthy man, was admitted to the hospital 16 days ago following a gunshot wound to the abdomen. He has undergone three exploratory laparotomies with repair and resection of damaged small intestine. He was placed on total parenteral nutrition to allow his bowel to rest and Solu-Medrol for stress on admission day 6. Three days ago, he developed a fever of 39.1°C and chills; his blood pressure (BP) of 100/70 mm Hg had dropped >30 mm Hg (systolic). Vancomycin and meropenem were promptly begun after obtaining cultures. Despite 3 days of antibiotics he remains febrile. His physical examination reveals a Hickman catheter in the right subclavian that is functioning normally; no inflammatory changes are evident at the exit site. A single erythematous nodule about 0.5 cm wide is noted near the left wrist. The funduscopic examination of both eyes is normal. A chest radiograph is also normal. The white blood cell (WBC) count is currently 10,950 cells/mm³. What subjective and objective data in this case are sufficiently suspicious of a possible *Candida* infection to warrant further diagnostic evaluations in L.K.?

Epidemiology

Although L.K. might be infected with bacterial pathogens that are not susceptible to vancomycin and meropenem, the possibility of a candidal infection should be considered. In epidemiologic studies, *Candida* species are the most common nosocomial fungal pathogens. *Candida* species were responsible for 72.2% of mycoses in hospitalized cases, and *Candida albicans* accounted for 55% of these cases in the Centers for Disease Control, National Nosocomial Infections Surveillance System. Attributable mortality associated with disseminated candidiasis from all species is 38%. These statistics may well be an underestimate of the true occurrence because systemic candidiasis is difficult to diagnose. For example, autopsies in neutropenic patients with hematologic malignancies indicate that diagnosis of systemic candidal infection is made in 30% to 50% of patients at postmortem.[61-63] Therefore, the morbidity for systemic candidiasis may be even higher because of the limited number of autopsies actually performed and our limited ability to diagnose systemic disease.

Characteristics

The diagnosis and monitoring of therapeutic outcomes for systemic candidal infection are difficult because the characteristics of systemic candidal infection are subtle. Salient clinical features include constitutional symptoms (e.g., fever, chills, hypotension) and evidence of end-organ dissemination such as nodular skin lesions that are usually erythematous, endophthalmitis, liver abscess, and spleen abscess. In addition, only about 50% of patients or fewer will have a single positive *Candida* blood culture.

Risk Factors

Risk factors for candidemia include central venous catheters, broad-spectrum antibiotic use, extensive surgical procedures, *Candida* colonization, total parenteral nutrition, neutropenia or neutrophil dysfunction, and immunosuppression (e.g., premature infants, burn patients, AIDS patients).[62-64]

L.K. has chills and a temperature of 39.1°C and is hypotensive. He is probably immunosuppressed as a result of multiple surgeries and corticosteroids. His Hickman catheter could serve as a possible portal of entry for an infectious agent, and his broad-spectrum antibiotic therapy with vancomycin and meropenem would be expected to be adequate for most of the likely bacterial pathogens. Because L.K. still has manifestations of an infection despite 3 days of antibiotics, additional diagnostic studies appear warranted.

Diagnostic Tests

8. **What diagnostic tests could be ordered for L.K. to evaluate a possible fungal infection?**

The diagnosis of fungal infection may be made with varying levels of certainty. Sometimes, the diagnosis is absolutely certain, such as when a pathogenic fungus from a clinical specimen is isolated and identified. This is referred to as a definitive or microbiologically confirmed diagnosis. At other times, the physician can determine only that there is a high probability of infection. This is designated as a presumptive diagnosis. To illustrate, a patient with a chest radiograph showing nodular lesions and a high complement fixation antibody against *H. capsulatum* would have a presumptive diagnosis of histoplasmosis. This may be as certain a diagnosis as is possible without performing a more invasive procedure to obtain lung tissue. In this event, a trial of drug therapy may be undertaken on the presumptive diagnosis alone. A diverse spectrum of tests is available for clinicians to diagnose and monitor therapeutic responses.

DIRECT EXAMINATION

Direct examination of the specimen is often useful in diagnosing fungal infection. Traditionally, the specimen is treated with 10% KOH to digest the cells and debris, resulting in clear visualization of the hyphae or yeast. Treatment of cerebrospinal fluid (CSF) specimens with KOH is not necessary because this fluid is naturally clear. India ink can be added to CSF to increase contrast and outline the organisms. Calcofluor white, a fluorescent fabric brightener that binds to fungi and fluoresces brilliantly when viewed under the ultraviolet microscope, also can be used to assist in recognition of fungal elements.

Histologic examination of biopsy specimens is an important tool for diagnosing and monitoring the presence of fungal infection, but identification of the precise species of fungus involved may be difficult. This is because only the tissue phase can be observed, and the fungal organisms in the specimen may be few. Because recognizing a fungus in hematoxylin- or eosin-stained sections may be difficult, a number of special stains have been developed.[64] Periodic acid–Schiff staining capitalizes on the presence of linked sugar groups in the fungal cell wall. Material with these sugar groups is stained intensely magenta, thus increasing the contrast and making visualization of the fungal form easier. Likewise, several silver precipitation stains, such as Gomori methenamine silver (sometimes also called Grocott's method), have been developed. These rely on the presence of a charge on the surface of the fungus to reduce oxidized silver to metallic silver. This process coats the fungus with a black layer, again outlining the form.[65] The pathologist then examines the slide and determines whether the fungus is growing as a yeast or a mold. Sometimes this is all that can be determined. The size of the organism, manner of budding, and the presence or absence of septae can all help narrow the possibilities. The mucicarmine stain imparts a deep red color to complex polysaccharides, such as mucin. It will also stain the thick capsule of *C. neoformans*. Because no other yeast has a positive mucicarmine stain, the definitive diagnosis of cryptococcosis can be made.[64]

Monoclonal antibodies against many fungi are now available. Immunohistochemical procedures using these sera on biopsy specimens will enable the pathologist to detect the presence of a fungus, and determine its identity.[66-68] Reagents for in situ oligonucleotide probe hybridization to detect fungi in tissue are being developed and will also be extremely helpful.[69]

CULTURE

The most definitive method for diagnosing or monitoring a fungal infection is with culture. Sputum, bronchial lavage specimens, transbronchial biopsies, fine-needle aspirates, biopsy tissue specimens, CSF, bone marrow, urine, or blood specimens should be inoculated onto several different types of fungal media, some of which contain antibiotics to inhibit bacterial overgrowth. Swab specimens have a very low yield, especially for hyphal fungi and should be avoided in follow-up cultures. Yeast may grow rapidly and be isolated within 24 to 48 hours, but many fungi grow slowly and 4 to 6 weeks of incubation may be necessary to isolate and identify the organism. When the fungus has grown, it may be identified by a variety of methods. Yeasts are usually recognized by their patterns of metabolic activity on a variety of substrates, whereas mycelial organisms may produce characteristic spores and fruiting bodies that are used for identification. Occasionally, a mycelial organism will be slow in producing recognizable spores, and immunologic testing for a characteristic isoantigen may be used for identification.

ANTIGEN DETECTION

Fungi synthesize polysaccharides that cannot be broken down by human enzymatic systems. These polysaccharides may accumulate within the body and be excreted in the urine. These fungal antigens can be detected by using antibodies that specifically recognize a particular species of fungus, thereby providing a diagnosis. The most commonly used antigen detection test is a latex agglutination test for cryptococcal antigen. This assay can be performed on serum or CSF. Antigenemia is present in 80% to 100% of patients with culture-proven cryptococcal meningitis. This test can also be used to monitor patient response to therapy by determining the end-point dilution for the positive reaction and following this end-point over time as the patient is treated. If treatment is successful, the titer will decline.[70,71]

Tests (quantitative PCR, ELISA, latex agglutination) for other fungal antigens are not as well established. Latex particle agglutination tests to detect candidal antigens are available, but their utility has not been clearly demonstrated. Several studies have reported only 25% to 87% sensitivities of the commercially available tests for candidal antigens, with specificities of 43% to 100%.[72-74] Still under development are procedures for detecting the substance D-arabinitol in urine and serum. D-arabinitol is synthesized by *Candida*, whereas human beings synthesize and excrete L-arabinitol. Tests to detect the D-stereoisomer, using either gas chromatography or a rapid enzymatic assay show promise for detecting invasive disease.[75-77] Assays for detecting *H. capsulatum* antigen in serum and urine have been reported.[78] Antigen can be detected in the blood of 50% and the urine of 80% to 90% of patients with systemic histoplasmosis. However, patients with blastomycosis and paracoccidioidomycosis may also have positive cross-reactions. The ELISA for detection of *Aspergillus* galactomannan (GXM) antigen in serum was approved in May 2003. Owing to the reported false-positive and false-negative rates, it is unclear if this assay will improve therapeutic decision making for patients at risk for this infection.

ANTIBODY DETECTION

Detection of antibody can be useful for some fungal diseases but not for others. Serologic diagnosis of systemic candidiasis is complicated because most people have anti-*Candida* antibodies. A rising titer is not specific for infection and may indicate only colonization. Furthermore, dissemination of *Candida* is most likely in people who are immunocompromised and therefore may not respond by producing antibody.[79] On the other hand, seropositivity can be demonstrated in >90% of patients with symptomatic histoplasmosis.[80] The most important serologic tests use the complement fixation, immunodiffusion, and enzyme immunoassay (EIA) techniques. Appropriate evolution of serologic results requires an understanding of the sensitivity, specificity, and predictive value of each methodology. In general, serologic tests allow only a presumptive diagnosis of mycotic infections.

SKIN TESTING

Antigens to be used for skin tests for delayed hypersensitivity have been developed for the dimorphic fungi. However, these are most useful as epidemiologic tools to define the geographic foci of infection. A large percentage of people living in the areas endemic for these organisms will have had asymptomatic, self-limited infection with these agents, making the skin tests less useful in diagnosing clinical illness. Furthermore, patients with severe disease with any of the dimorphic fungi may develop a state of immunologic anergy in which all skin tests are negative. In general, skin testing can help only to narrow the diagnostic probabilities and cannot be used to monitor therapy or diagnose infection.

Although any of the aforementioned tests could be ordered for L.K., a direct examination of his blood and urine specimens along with an assessment of signs/symptoms of disseminated candidiasis are reasonable first steps in his evaluation. A blood and urine specimen from L.K. should also be cultured on different fungal media. Because a candidal infection is suspected, the culture could isolate *Candida* within 24 to 48 hours. Cultures and histopathologic examination of a biopsy specimen of skin lesions are often helpful not only in confirming a diagnosis of disseminated candidal infection, but also in monitoring response to therapy. The other fungal tests previously described need not be ordered immediately and should await the results from direct examination and culture.

Necessity of Treatment

9. The clinical laboratory reports that a single blood culture obtained from 2 days ago is growing *Candida* species. In addition, a secondary finding of many budding yeast in the urine was reported on urinalysis (UA). Why is therapy necessary in L.K. with only a single positive blood culture?

In the past, most experts withheld antifungal therapy unless a patient had sustained candidemia or had evidence of end-organ disease. However, more recent studies of candidemia noted an 85.6% mortality rate in the untreated patients compared to a 41.8% mortality rate in patients who were treated early. Isolation of *Candida* from the bloodstream of patients is now viewed seriously, and therapy should be initiated immediately. Delays in therapy of up to 1 week can increase mortality rates by 23%.[81] Removal of risk factors may improve the clinical outcome of candidemia, and removal of central venous catheters is believed to improve morbidity and mortality.[82,83] However, removal of centrally inserted catheters may make pharmacotherapy difficult, and L.K.'s other risk factors (e.g., broad-spectrum antibiotics) are perhaps of even greater importance.

Treatment Options

10. What therapeutic options are available to treat candidemia? Which option would be best for L.K.?

Therapeutic options are individualized and based on the competence of a patient's host defenses. In immunocompetent patients, amphotericin B, caspofungin, or fluconazole decrease morbidity and mortality associated with this disease.[84,85] Caspofungin 70 mg loading dose then 50 mg/day parenterally was demonstrated as effective as amphotericin B in neutropenic and non-neutropenic patients; however, amphotericin B cleared the bloodstream fastest.[84] In the largest well-controlled comparative trial, 206 non-neutropenic patients were randomized to amphotericin B 0.5 to 0.6 mg/kg per day or fluconazole 400 mg/day for 14 days. Mortality was <9% in both groups with no significant difference in successful outcomes (amphotericin B, 80%; fluconazole, 72%). However, less toxicity was noted in the fluconazole group.[85] Therefore, fluconazole 400 mg/day is probably equally as effective as amphotericin B for non-neutropenic patients infected with susceptible *Candida*. In another large clinical trial, higher dosages of fluconazole (12 mg/kg/day) alone or in combination with amphotericin B for a minimum of 3 days, followed by step-down therapy to fluconazole, was performed to evaluate the effect of combination therapy on improving clinical efficacy. Outcomes were not different from previously reported success rates. Yet, the fluconazole treatment group experienced higher APACHE II scores, making evaluation of the comparison difficult.[86] In contrast, another clinical trial the combination of amphotericin B and flucytosine appears more effective than single-agent therapy.[87,88] Treatment of candidemia in neutropenic patients is reviewed in Question 29 and in Chapter 70, Opportunistic Infections in HIV-Infected Patients.

L.K. should be treated with amphotericin B, with the total dose based on clinical response and resolution of positive cultures (see Question 12). The efficacy of this therapy should be monitored by assessing the previously identified patient-specific signs and symptoms of candidemia. Combination therapy should be tried in patients who are not responding clinically along with a complete examination for focal sites of infection (septic thrombi or intra-abdominal abscess).

11. This fungal species has now been identified as *C. non-albicans*. How does this affect the therapeutic options for L.K.?

Historically, isolation of a non-albicans *Candida* from any patient's blood has been a matter of concern because of increasing *in vitro* susceptibilities, clinical resistance observed in animal models, and uncontrolled case reports. Intrinsic resistance (*C. lusitaniae* to amphotericin B, *C. parapsilosis* to caspofungin, and *C. kruseii* to fluconazole) or acquired resistance (*C. tropicalis* or *Torulopsis [Candida] glabrata* against fluconazole) has been reported.[87–89] Acquired *in vitro* fluconazole drug resistance is probably associated with altered fungal cell membrane permeability, antifungal efflux pumps, and/or changes in the cytochrome P450 enzyme. In uncontrolled, observational studies, fluconazole resistance *in vitro* is up to 9%.[87–89] However, a large, multicenter study of 232 non-neutropenic patients was unable to demonstrate a relationship between a yeast's minimum inhibitory concentration and patient outcome.[89] Our inability to demonstrate a relationship is probably a result of our poor understanding or inadequate management of risk factors for infection. For example, the removal of a colonized IV catheter is probably a more important predictor of outcome than minimum inhibitory concentration of the isolated yeast. Also, the therapeutic environment is changing with higher doses, new formulations of older agents, and new agents used in therapeutic regimens.

Therefore, the true rate of acquired clinical resistance to azoles and ultimate failure is unknown. We recommend vigilant monitoring and aggressive therapy of infections caused by *non-albicans Candida*. In patients in whom susceptibilities are available, fluconazole should be avoided when the minimum inhibitory concentrations are >16 µg/mL. An antifungal should be avoided if the organism has intrinsic resistance.

Amphotericin
DOSING

12. How should amphotericin B desoxycholate be dosed and administered to L.K.?

The amphotericin B desoxycholate dose and duration of therapy should be individualized based on the severity of infection and immunocompetence of the patient. Candidemic (or other mycotic infections discussed in this chapter) patients who are clinically stable and have no evidence of deep-seated infection should be initiated on amphotericin B 0.3 mg/kg per day for at least 14 days. Patients who are unstable or have deep-seated (organ involvement) infections should be treated with 0.5 to 0.6 mg/kg per day for at least 14 days. Patients who develop concomitant septic shock should receive a minimum daily amphotericin B dose of 1.0 mg/kg. In some centers, this daily dose is administered in a twice-daily, divided-dose schedule and/or flucytosine (100 to 150 mg/kg per day) is added to the initial few days of treatment. Once the patient is stable, therapy should be changed to one of the applicable regimens discussed previously.

The dose of amphotericin B should be based on lean body mass. However, owing to the difficulty in measuring, many clinicians use ideal body weight (IBW). Tissues that contain large numbers of macrophages sequester significant amounts of amphotericin B (liver, 17.5% to 40.3%; spleen, 0.7% to 15.6%; kidney, 0.6% to 4.1%; lung, 0.4% to 13%), but it does not distribute well into adipose tissue (<1.0%).[90,91] Because L.K. is 5 feet, 8 inches tall and not obese, his lean body weight should be about 70 kg (LBW = 50 kg + 2.3 + height in inches >5 ft). Therefore, amphotericin B 35 mg/day (0.5 mg/kg) should be initiated because L.K. is not clinically stable and is likely to need the higher-dose regimen. Half the full dose should be given on the first day of therapy and the full dose given on subsequent days. In more seriously ill patients, the full dose of amphotericin B can be initiated immediately. Although the optimal dosing regimen to initiate amphotericin B is not well established, most clinicians gradually titrate the dose upward to minimize infusion-related reactions. Test dosing with 1 mg before the first dose is not currently used in this titration because of the immeasurably low incidence of anaphylactoid reactions.

Peak amphotericin B serum concentrations achieved after parenteral administration are a function of dose, frequency of dosing, and rate of infusion. When the amphotericin B total dose is <50 mg, the serum concentration is directly proportional to the dose; doses >50 mg show a plateau in serum concentrations. After administration, amphotericin B undergoes biphasic elimination: peak serum concentrations drop rapidly (initial $t_{1/2}$, 24 to 48 hours), but low concentrations (0.5 to 1.0 µg/mL) are detectable for up to 2 weeks (terminal $t_{1/2} = \sim 15$ days).[92] The long terminal-elimination half-life has been used as a justification for the common practice of every-other-day amphotericin B dosing, in which twice the daily dose is given every other day. Every-other-day regimens have not been carefully evaluated but are rationalized based on the potential for reduced nephrotoxicity. Administration of 0.5 mg/kg per day or 1.0 mg/kg every other day results in trough amphotericin B concentrations with sufficient postdose antifungal effects that inhibit the common pathogenic fungi.[93] Once L.K.'s clinical status has improved, the potential for renal toxicity could outweigh the concerns of potential reduced efficacy, and implementation of amphotericin B every-other-day therapy should be considered.

PREMEDICATION

Premedication to prevent amphotericin B infusion–related reactions and a test dose of amphotericin B are not needed for L.K. Most practices of premedicating and administering test doses are performed out of ritual rather than predicated on scientific study, and acute allergic reactions are extremely rare.[94] Until clinical trials clarify the risk-to-benefit ratio of premedications, concomitant therapy should be restricted to acetaminophen for fever or headache and heparin to prevent thrombophlebitis when possible.

INFUSION REACTIONS

13. L.K. has no complaints except for fevers and shaking chills that occur during his 6- to 8-hour amphotericin B infusion for the past 3 days. He has been receiving acetaminophen 650 mg 30 minutes before amphotericin B infusion, but he has refused today's amphotericin B dose. What measures can be taken to minimize these infusion-related reactions?

Adverse reactions are common with amphotericin B administration and are best classified as acute infusion-related, dose-related, or idiosyncratic reactions. Infusion-related reactions include an acute symptom complex of fever, chills, nau-

sea, vomiting, headache, hypotension, and thrombophlebitis. Dose-related reactions also may be acute (e.g., cardiac arrhythmias) or chronic (e.g., renal dysfunction with secondary electrolyte imbalances and anemia).

Many infusion-related reactions appear to be mediated by amphotericin B–induced cytokine (interleukin-1β, tumor necrosis factor, prostaglandin E_2) expression by mononuclear cells.[95,96] Hydrocortisone is extremely effective in suppressing cytokine expression[95] and also blunts the fever and chills associated with amphotericin B administration.[97] However, hydrocortisone does not reduce the frequency of chronic dose-related toxicity such as renal insufficiency, and corticosteroid-induced immunosuppression could decrease amphotericin B fungicidal activity.[98] Nonsteroidal anti-inflammatory drugs (NSAIDs) also prevent fever, most likely by the suppression of prostaglandin E_2 expression.[99] However, NSAIDs cannot be recommended for routine use because of their potential for additive nephrotoxicity when used with amphotericin B.

The mild to moderate elevations in temperature and the other infusion-related symptoms usually subside when the infusion is completed, and tolerance to these effects develops over 3 to 5 days. L.K. initially should be counseled that these reactions will abate over the next few days without intervention. If assessment of the reactions suggests the need for more aggressive premedication, a short course of hydrocortisone should be initiated as outlined in Table 71-5. A dose of

---

Table 71-5 Amphotericin B Desoxycholate Infusion Protocol

A. Administration

Dilute amphotericin in D_5W; the final concentration should not exceed 0.1 mg/mL. Initial dosing (0.25 mg/kg based on ideal body mass) should not exceed 30 mg. Infuse the dose over 0.75–4 hr immediately after a meal. Record temperature, pulse rate, and blood pressure every 30 min for 4 hr. If patient develops significant chills, fever, respiratory distress, or hypotension, administer adjunctive medication before the next infusion. If initial dose is tolerated, advance to maximum dose by the 3rd–5th day. Consult an infectious diseases clinician for any questions concerning maximum daily dose, total dose, and duration of therapy.

B. Adjunctive Medications

1. Heparin 1,000 units may diminish thrombophlebitis for peripheral lines. Observe the contraindications to the use of heparin (e.g., thrombocytopenia, ↑ risk of hemorrhage, concomitant anticoagulation).
2. Administration of 250 mL of normal saline before amphotericin B may help ↓ renal dysfunction.
3. Acetaminophen administered 30 min before amphotericin B infusion may ameliorate the fever.
4. Hydrocortisone 0.7 mg/kg (Solu-Cortef) can be added to the amphotericin infusion. Hydrocortisone is given to ↓ infusion-related reactions. It should be used only for significant fever (>2.0°F elevation from baseline) and chills during infusions and should be discontinued as soon as possible (3–5 days). It is not necessary to add hydrocortisone if the patient is receiving supraphysiologic doses of adrenal corticosteroids.
5. Meperidine hydrochloride 25–50 mg may be used parenterally in adults to ameliorate chills.

C. Laboratory

1. At least twice weekly for first 4 weeks, then weekly: Hct, reticulocyte count, magnesium, potassium, BUN, creatinine, bicarbonate, and UA. The GFR may fall 40% before stabilizing in these patients. Discontinue for 2–5 days if renal function continues to deteriorate and reinstate after improvement. Hct often falls 22–35% of the initial level.
2. Monitor closely for hypokalemia and hypomagnesemia. Supplementation with a nonchloride potassium is preferable for metabolic (renal tubular) acidosis associated with hypokalemia.

D. Caveats

1. Electrolytes. Addition of an electrolyte to an amphotericin solution causes the colloid to aggregate and probably results in suboptimal therapeutic effect. This includes IV piggyback medications containing electrolytes or preservatives.
2. Filtering. The colloidal solution is partially retained by 0.22-micron pore membrane filter: do not use filters if possible.
3. The infusion bottle need not be light-shielded.

E. Patients Needing Closer Monitoring

1. Addisonian patients tolerate infusion poorly. Treatment with corticosteroids improves patient tolerance.
2. Patients should receive neither granulocyte transfusion nor indium scanning.
3. Patients with anuria or previous cardiac history may have an ↑ risk of arrhythmias, and slower infusions are recommended.

BUN, blood urea nitrogen; GFR, glomerular filtration rate; Hct, hematocrit; IV, intravenous; UA, urinalysis.

meperidine 25 to 50 mg by rapid IV infusion reduces amphotericin B–induced rigors and can be repeated every 15 minutes as required while monitoring for signs and symptoms of opiate toxicity. Administration of an average meperidine dose of 45 mg has been found to resolve chills three times faster than placebo.[100] The mechanism of this pharmacologic effect is currently under investigation.

Faster amphotericin B infusion rates (<4 to 6 hours) are associated with the earlier onset of infusion-related reactions but not with more severe infusion reactions.[101,102] Many patients prefer rapid infusions (1 to 2 hours) because the infusion-related reactions abate quickly upon completion of the amphotericin B infusion. Electrocardiographic evaluations of 1-hour infusions indicate that this rate of amphotericin infusion is safe at currently recommended doses in patients without renal or heart disease. However, rapid infusions are not safe in all patients because cardiac arrhythmias[103,104] appear to be dose and infusion rate related.[105] If infused too rapidly, high serum concentrations of amphotericin B can precipitate severe cardiac adverse events. Arrhythmias have been reported most often in patients who are anuric or have previous cardiac disease.[106] Continuous infusion is not recommended based on the pharmacodynamics of this agents and the concentration dependence of activity.

NEPHROTOXICITY

14. On day 4 of therapy with amphotericin B, L.K.'s serum creatinine (SrCr) and blood urea nitrogen (BUN) are 2.3 mg/dL and 42 mg/dL, respectively. How could amphotericin B exacerbate L.K.'s renal dysfunction and how could it be prevented from worsening?

[SI units: SrCr, 203.32 μmol/L; BUN, 14.99 mmol/L]

Renal dysfunction is the adverse event that most often limits treatment with amphotericin B. The renal toxicity results from amphotericin B–mediated damage to renal tubules, which results in electrolyte wasting and disrupts the tubuloglomerular feedback mechanism. The clinical manifestations of amphotericin B–induced renal damage include azotemia, renal tubular acidosis, hypokalemia, and hypomagnesemia.[94] Generally, amphotericin B–related renal toxicity is reversible within 2 weeks after therapy has been discontinued. Administration of normal saline (250 mL) immediately before amphotericin B administration can decrease amphotericin B–induced nephrotoxicity[107] and should be initiated before L.K.'s next dose. However, amphotericin B should not be admixed with normal saline because sodium causes amphotericin B to precipitate into an inactive particulate in IV admixture formulations.[108] The cumulative dose of amphotericin deoxycholate should be kept below 3 g; other nephrotoxins should be avoided (especially diuretics; see Table 71-4); and patients with already compromised renal function should be closely monitored.[108] Hypokalemia and hypomagnesemia also should be monitored closely, and replacement therapy should be initiated as soon as significant declines in potassium or magnesium are detected. These measures to prevent further renal deterioration should be implemented and the amphotericin B therapy continued cautiously in this patient with systemic candidiasis. Anemia, associated with decreased renal production of erythropoietin, should resolve after amphotericin B is discontinued and need not be treated.[109]

15. L.K. has developed significant renal dysfunction resulting from acute tubular necrosis. How should his dose of systemic antifungal drugs be altered?

Renal elimination of the antimycotics varies tremendously. For systemically administered amphotericin B, only 5% to 10% of unchanged drug is eliminated in urine and bile during the first 24 hours,[94] and there is no evidence it is metabolized to a significant extent. Therefore, no substantial dosage adjustment is required for patients with chronic renal or hepatic failure. Although many clinicians will withhold amphotericin B doses if acute renal dysfunction develops during therapy, concerns of drug-induced nephrotoxicity in L.K. must be balanced against the high likelihood of mortality in untreated patients with deep-seated infections.[50,61–63] Alternative systemic antifungal therapy (i.e., azoles) that is less nephrotoxic can also be considered.

Ketoconazole and itraconazole undergo first-pass metabolism and have a biphasic dose-dependent elimination.[41,42] These agents are extensively metabolized and excreted in the bile; small amounts of unchanged drug are excreted in the urine. Therefore, there is no need to adjust dosages in patients with renal dysfunction or in patients undergoing dialysis.[110] Fluconazole and voriconazole, unlike ketoconazole and itraconazole, are not extensively metabolized. More than 90% of a fluconazole dose is excreted in urine, of which about 80% is measured as unchanged drug and about 20% as metabolites.[111] Because fluconazole is excreted primarily unchanged in the urine, dosages should be adjusted in patients with renal insufficiency (Table 71-6).[94,110–117] Fluconazole or voriconazole may be reasonable alternatives in L.K., but the dosage must be adjusted for renal function based on published nomograms.[117]

16. What is the role of an amphotericin B formulated with a lipid?

Lipid formulations of amphotericin B have been approved by the FDA for patients who are unable to tolerate generic amphotericin B (Table 71-7). In addition, the admixture of amphotericin B in 10% or 20% lipid emulsion has been used for treating systemic mycotic infections. The lipid carriers differ tremendously for each of the amphotericin formulations. The liposomal formulation is a spherical carrier that contains amphotericin both on the inside and outside of the vesicle. Imagine the lipid complex as a snowflake shape, and the colloidal dispersion shaped like a Frisbee with amphotericin bound to the structure. The differences in structure appear to have no effect on therapeutic outcome but confer different protection against amphotericin adverse effects.[118] Amphotericin B admixture with a lipid emulsion cannot be recommended until a stable formulation can be established.[119]

Limited data are available to assist in the management of this case. A single large controlled trial has evaluated amphotericin B lipid complex for the treatment of disseminated candidiases. Amphotericin B 0.6 to 1.0 mg/kg per day for 14 days was slightly, but not significantly, superior to the lipid complex formulation at 5 mg/kg per day for mycologic efficacy (68% versus 63%) or survival. However, renal dysfunction defined as a doubling in serum creatinine was 47% with amphotericin B and 28% with this lipid formulation. Because of the significant cost, lipid formulations of amphotericin B should be reserved for patients who suffer severe adverse

Table 71-6 Pharmacokinetic Properties of Systemically Active Antifungals[41–45, 94, 110–117, 166, 167, 203–211]

Characteristic	Imidazoles			Triazoles				Other		
	MCZ[a]	KCZ[a]	ICZ[a]	FCZ[a]	VCZ[a]	PCZ[a]	RCZ[a]	CFG	5FC	TBF
Absorption										
Relative bioavailability	<10	75[b]	99.8 (40)[b]	(85–92)[b]	96[d]	≈100	ND	NA	75–90[b]	70%
C_{max} (µg/mL)	1.90	3.29	0.63	1.4	2.3–4.7[d]	0.366	0.76	12.09, .94	70–80	1.34–1.7
T_{max} (hr)	1.0	2.6	4.0	1.0–4.0	1.2	8.7	ND	1	<2	1.5
AUC^c (µg/hr/mL)	ND	12.9 (13.6)	1.9 (0.7)	42	9.31–13.22[d]	4.4	13.84–119.12	97.63–100.5	ND	4.74–10.48
Distribution										
Protein binding (%)	91–93	99	99.8	11	58	ND	ND	97	2–4	>99
CSF/serum conc. (%)	<10	<10	<10	60	≈50	ND	ND	ND	60	<10
Excretion										
Beta $t_{1/2}$ (hr)	2.1	8.1[d]	17[d]	23–45	6	35	157	9–10	2.5–6.0	36
Active drug in urine (%)	1	2	<10	60–80	5	<14	ND	2	0	80

[a]Above parameters are estimated from the administration of currently recommended doses. Miconazole [MCZ] 7.4–14.2 mg/kg/day (500–1,000 mg) parenterally, ketoconazole [KCZ] 2.8 mg/kg/day orally (200 mg), itraconazole [ICZ] 1.4–2.8 mg/kg/day orally (100–200 mg), fluconazole [FCZ] 0.7–1.4 mg/kg/day orally, voriconazole [VCZ] 400(200) mg Q 12 hr orally on day 1 (2–10) and 6 (3) mg/kg Q 12 hr hours parenterally on day 1 (2–10), posaconazole [PCZ] 200 mg/day orally, ravuconazole [RCZ] 400 mg/day orally, caspofungin [CFG] 70 (50) mg parenterally on day 1 (2–14), flucytosine [5FC] 150 mg/kg/day parenterally, and terbinafine [TBF] 250 mg/day orally.
[b]With meals (fasting), absorption altered by gastric acidity.
[c]Dose and/or infusion dependent.
[d]Absorption decreased when administered with high fat meal; C_{max} and AUC reduced by 34% and 24%, respectively.
AUC, area under the concentration-time curve; C_{max}, maximum concentration; CSF, cerebrospinal fluid; ND, no data; T_{max}, time of maximum concentration; $t_{1/2}$, half-life.

Table 71-7 Amphotericin B Formulations

Category	Amphotericin B (Fungizone®)	Amphotericin B Lipid Complex (ABLC©; Abelcet)	Amphotericin B Colloidal Dispersion (Amphotec®)	Liposomal Amphotericin B (AmBisome®)		Amphotericin B in Lipid Emulsion (ABLE)
FDA-approved indication	Life-threatening fungal infections; Visceral leishmaniasis	Refractory/ intolerant to AmB	Invasive Aspergillosis in patients refractory/ intolerant to AmB	Empirical therapy in neutropenic FUO; Refractory/intolerant to AmB; Visceral leishmaniasis		NA
Formulation						
Sterol	None	None	Cholesterol sulfate	Cholesterol sulfate (3)[a]		Safflower and Soybean Oils
Phospholipid	None	DMPC and DMPG(7:3)[a]	None	EPC & DSPG(10:4)[a]		10–20 g/100 mL; EPC >2.21 g/100 mL; Glycerin >258 g/100 mL
Amphotericin B (Mole %)	34	33	50	10		Variable
Particle size (nm)	<10	1,600–11,000	122(±48)	80–120		333–500
Manufacturer	Generic	Enzon	Intermune	Fujisawa Pharmaceuticals		Not applicable
Stability	1 week at 2–8°C or 24 hr at 27°C	15 hr at 2–8°C or 6 hr at 27°C	24 hr at 2–8°C	24 hr at 2–8°C		Unstable
Dosage and rate	0.3–1.0 mg/kg/day over 1–6 hr	5.0 mg/kg/day at 2.5 mg/kg/hr	3–4 mg/kg/day over 2 hr	3.0–5.0 mg/kg/d over 2 hr		Investigational: 1.0 mg/kg/day over 1–8 hrs
Lethal dose 50%	3.3 mg/kg	10–25 mg/kg	68 mg/kg	175 mg/kg		Unknown
Pharmacokinetic Parameters						
Dose	0.5 mg/kg	5.0 mg/kg × 7 days	5.0 mg/kg × 7 days	2.5 mg/kg × 7 days	5 mg/kg × 7 days	0.8 mg/kg/day × 13 days
Serum Concentrations						
Peak	1.2 µg/mL	1.7 µg/mL	3.1 µg/mL	31.4 µg/mL	83.0 µg/mL	2.13 µg/mL
Trough	0.5 µg/mL	0.7 µg/mL		4.0 µg/mL		0.42 µg/mL
Half-life	91.1 hrs	173.4 hrs	28.5 hrs	6.3 hrs	6.8 hrs	7.75 hrs
Volume of Distribution	5.0 L/kg	131.0 L/kg	4.3 L/kg	0.16 L/kg	0.10 L/kg	0.45 L/kg
Clearance	38.0 mL/hr/kg	436.0 mL/hr/kg	0.117 mL/hr/kg	22.0 mL/hr/kg	11.0 mL/hr/kg	37.0 m/hr/kg
Area Under the Curve	14 µg/mL × hr	17 µg/mL × hr	43.0 µg/mL × hr	197 µg/mL × hr	555 µg/mL × hr	26.37 µg/mL × hr

[a]Molar ratio of each component, respectively.
AMB, amphotericin B; DSPG, distearolyphosphatidyglycerol; DMPC, dimyristoyl phosphatidycholine; DMPG, dimyristoyl phosphatidyglycerol; EPC, egg phosphatidylcholine; FUO, fever of unknown origin; NA, not applicable.

reactions to, or are failing, generic amphotericin B. Indications for the lipid formulations are further reviewed in the discussion of Aspergillosis and Cryptococcosis.

Antimycotic Prophylaxis

17. What measures could have been undertaken to prevent invasive fungal infections in L.K.?

Selective GI decontamination or systemic antimycotic pharmacotherapy can be used in high-risk, immunocompromised, or surgical patients to prevent the development of fungal infections and could have been used for L.K. In critically ill surgical patients, the risk of invasive infection may be reduced by greater than 50% with systemic fluconazole prophylaxis. However, there is no change in patient survival.[120]

Selective GI decontamination in high-risk patients would ideally include the use of a nonabsorbable antifungal such as amphotericin B or nystatin. Oral amphotericin B decreases systemic candidal infections threefold to fivefold in high-risk patients.[121,122] Yet, the problems of questionable antifungal stool concentrations,[123,124] decreasing azole cost, and poor compliance have led to preferential azole (clotrimazole, miconazole, ketoconazole) use. However, systemic antifungals could increase adverse effects and potential drug interactions because of systemic absorption. The tradeoff can be improved patient compliance in regimens using an azole.[125] Azoles are more effective in preventing oral pharyngeal candidiasis (OPC) than placebo.[126,127] However, only small studies[125,128,129] with inadequate sample sizes have compared the clinical efficacy of azoles to polyene antifungals (e.g., amphotericin B) for prevention of either oropharyngeal or systemic candidiasis. Reduced rates for oropharyngeal and systemic candidiasis have been noted in noncomparative studies using fluconazole[122,130] and itraconazole.[131] Rates of superficial and systemic fungal infections are similar in patients treated with amphotericin B or fluconazole prophylaxis.[121,122,130]

Selective GI decontamination with 4 to 12 million units/day of oral nystatin or 400 mg/day of amphotericin oral suspension to ensure adequate fecal concentrations is one approach over systemic azoles.[124] Once prophylaxis is begun, it should be continued until L.K. develops a systemic infection or until immunosuppression ends. If L.K. is discharged from the hospital and treated as an outpatient, a systemic azole (imidazole or triazole) administered once daily is preferable to a polyene to improve adherence. However, allow us to reemphasize, systemic therapy increases the risk of resistance, adverse effects, drug interactions (see Table 71-4), and sometimes cost (Table 71-8).

Candiduria
Treatment

18. M.Y., a 24-year-old man, has been hospitalized in the surgical intensive care unit with multiple trauma injuries resulting from a motor vehicle accident. Shortly after admission, he underwent an exploratory laparotomy for a ruptured spleen and lacerated liver. He subsequently suffered respiratory and renal failure. M.Y. is currently intubated and on mechanical ventilation. Since admission, he has been nutritionally supported with central hyperalimentation and has been receiving broad-spectrum antibiotics (gentamicin, ampicillin, and metronidazole). A Foley catheter is in place. Two recent UAs show budding yeast and cultures were positive for >100,000 colony-forming units of *C. albicans*. M.Y. is currently afebrile, his funduscopic examination is normal, and no macronodular skin lesions are present. The WBC count is 8,900 cells/mm³, and three sets of blood cultures drawn over the past 2 days are negative. How should M.Y.'s candiduria be treated?

[SI unit: 8.9×10^9/L]

Eradication of fungi in the urine (specifically *C. albicans*) should begin with removal of the indwelling urinary catheter and alleviation of risk factors for fungal disease. If catheter removal does not clear the urine within 48 hours, pharmacotherapy should be considered. If M.Y. is scheduled for a genitourinary procedure, he should receive systemic therapy because the rate of candidemia after surgery is high (10.8%). In addition, any patient at high risk for dissemination into the blood should be treated (e.g., patients with diabetes, genitourinary abnormalities, renal insufficiency, or immunosuppression).[132]

Bladder irrigation with amphotericin B has been commonly used and concentrations of 150 μg/mL effectively kill 5×10^6 *C. albicans* in the urine within 2 hours.[133] However, clinical studies evaluating the efficacy of continuous amphotericin B 150 μg/mL irrigations or intermittent irrigations (15 to 30 mg/100 mL) retained for 1 hour × 3 to 7 days are limited and often have had serious design flaws. In two comparative studies, bladder irrigation for 5 days with amphotericin B 50 μg/mL appeared to be superior to fluconazole 100 mg/day as measured by microbiologic cure rates. However, 2

Table 71-8 Antimycotic Prophylaxis Regimens and Costs

Agent	Dose/Day	Formulation	Recommended Regimen	Cost ($)/day[a]
Selective GI Decontamination				
Amphotericin B	400 mg	Oral suspension[b]	Swish and swallow QID	4.00[b]
Nystatin	4–12 million units	Oral suspension	Swish and Swallow QID	16.60–40.80
Systemic				
Clotrimazole	30–80 mg	Trouche	TID–QID	11.43–40.64
Ketoconazole	200–400 mg	Oral	QD	2.78–5.56
Itraconazole	200–400 mg	Oral	QD	15.56–31.11
Fluconazole	50–400 mg	Oral	QD	5.15–26.48

[a]From 2002 Red Book AWP Price.
[b]Made from parenteral formulation, no longer commercially available.

to 4 weeks after infection, cure rates were equal but mortality rates were higher in the amphotericin B–treated groups. Amphotericin B failures may have been associated with dissemination of yeast from the urinary tract.[134,135] Systemic antifungal therapy with flucytosine 100 to 150 mg/kg/day × 7 days[136] and azoles (fluconazole 0.6 to 1.4 mg/kg/day × 7 days)[137–139] also has been used in noncomparative or nonrandomized studies.

Caution must be used when selecting pharmacotherapy for M.Y. because it is difficult to differentiate among cystitis, urethritis, or systemic infection in the presence of funguria. Similarly, it is difficult to differentiate colonization from infection because canduric patients are usually asymptomatic. Funguria cannot be used to determine the location or severity of invasion. Signs and symptoms of systemic disease should be monitored diligently until a diagnosis of colonization, cystitis, or urethritis is confirmed and the risk of dissemination is excluded. Therefore, M.Y.'s Foley catheter should be replaced with a condom catheter and further treatment should await a definitive diagnosis or persistence of candiduria beyond 48 hours.

Blastomycosis
Etiology

19. C.P., a 17-year-old girl, is admitted to the hospital with a chronic pneumonia that has not responded to antibiotics. Three months ago, she developed a chronic cough that eventually became productive of purulent sputum, which was occasionally streaked with blood. Two months ago, she developed "boils" on her lower extremities and back, which drained spontaneously. She was hospitalized at another hospital but failed to respond to amoxicillin and erythromycin. C.P. denies fever, chills, or night sweats but has lost 11 pounds. Her temperature is 38.2°C. There is a 2-cm² subcutaneous, fluctuant, tender mass over the right mandible and a second fluctuant mass about 4 cm wide on the lower back. There are also several 0.5- to 1-cm² ulcers with heaped-up, hyperkeratotic margins on the lower extremities (Fig. 71-2). Rales are heard at the right lung base. C.P.'s leukocyte count is slightly elevated at 13,500 cells/mm³. A chest radiograph shows a masslike infiltrate in the right midlung field (Fig. 71-3). A wet preparation of ulcer scrapings and material aspirated from a subcutaneous abscess reveal numerous broad-based, budding yeast forms with refractile cell walls and multiple nuclei typical of *B. dermatitidis.*

Cultures of sputum, skin scrapings, and abscess material eventually confirmed the diagnosis. What was the likely portal of entry for C.P.'s disseminated blastomycosis? Why should it be treated?

[SI unit: WBC count, 13.5 × 10⁹/L]

Typical of the other endemic mycoses, the primary portal of entry for *B. dermatitidis* is the lungs. A pulmonary origin for C.P.'s infection is also supported by her history of cough with purulent, blood-streaked sputum, evident about a month before cutaneous lesions appeared on her legs and back. An acute pulmonary infection is most often asymptomatic and when symptomatic usually requires only observation. Chronic pulmonary or extrapulmonary blastomycosis will develop in an unknown number of these patients. C.P.'s rales at the base of her right lung and persistent pneumonia that is unrespon-

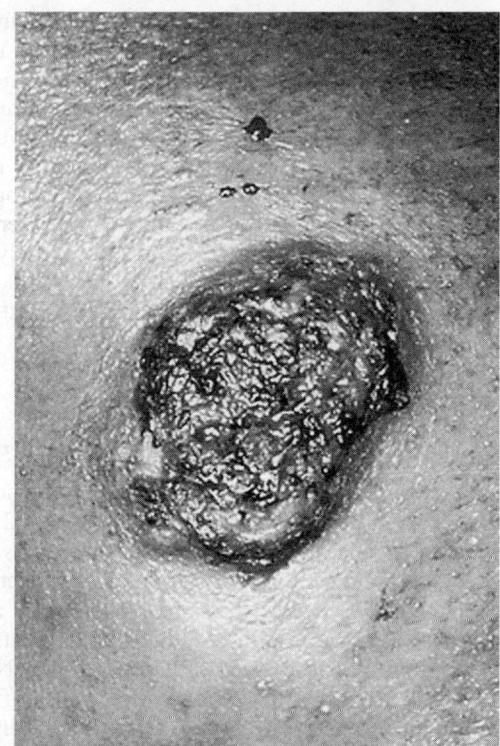

FIGURE 71-2 Disseminated *Blastomyces dermatitidis* skin ulcers.

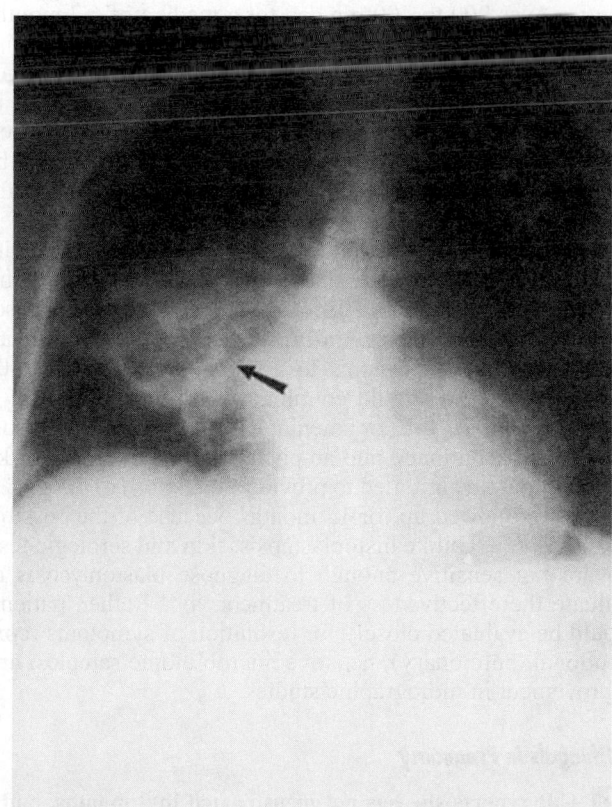

FIGURE 71-3 Chest radiograph of pulmonary *Blastomyces dermatitidis.*

sive to antibiotics indicate that she has a chronic pulmonary infection and will require therapy. Chronic pulmonary disease often presents with radiographic studies that can be mistaken for tuberculosis or lung cancer; the masslike infiltrate in her right lung on chest radiograph also is consistent with chronic pulmonary disease. Extrapulmonary infections may involve the skin (verrucous or ulcerative lesions), bone, genitourinary system (prostatitis, epididymo-orchitis), or CNS (meningitis or brain abscess). If untreated, these chronic pulmonary or extrapulmonary infections will be fatal in at least 21% of patients.[140] Because C.P. presents with pulmonary and cutaneous evidence of blastomycosis, she should be treated.

Treatment

20. What specific therapy should be initiated for C.P.?

Until recently, amphotericin B was considered the treatment of choice for blastomycosis and total doses of >2 g were associated with 97% cure rates and low relapse rates. However, toxicity was observed in 70% of patients.[140] Ketoconazole and itraconazole currently are advocated as safe and effective alternatives to amphotericin B in patients with non–life-threatening, non-CNS infections. The NIAID-Mycoses Study Group confirmed the effectiveness of azoles for the treatment of chronic pulmonary and extrapulmonary disease caused by the endemic mycoses, blastomycosis, and histoplasmosis. In uncontrolled evaluations of chronic pulmonary and extrapulmonary infections (excluding life-threatening or CNS), ketoconazole at dosages of 400 to 800 mg/day resulted in cure rates of about 89%, failure rates of about 6%, and relapse rates of about 5%.[141] In similar studies, itraconazole capsules 200 to 400 mg/day for a median of 6.2 months resulted in cure rates of 88% to 95%.[142] Fluconazole was ineffective at dosages <400 mg/day. However, higher dosages (400 to 800 mg/day) are as effective as ketoconazole in non–life-threatening disease.[143] Although these trials are neither comparative nor controlled, itraconazole appears to be less toxic than ketoconazole and to have the best benefit (efficacy) to risk (toxicity) ratio.

C.P. has mild to moderate disease and can be treated with an initial itraconazole dosage of 200 mg/day. If no clinical improvement is seen within 2 weeks or if the disease progresses despite therapy, the dosage of itraconazole can be titrated upward in 100-mg increments to a maximum dosage of 400 mg/day. Treatment should continue for at least 6 months. If C.P. develops severe or meningeal disease, itraconazole should be discontinued and amphotericin B 0.3 to 0.5 mg/kg per day should be initiated to provide a total dose of 1.5 g. C.P. should be followed up for 12 months because of the possible risk of relapse. Unlike histoplasmosis, skin and serologic testing are not sensitive enough to diagnose blastomycosis or evaluate the effectiveness of treatment.[141,144] Rather, patients should be evaluated closely for resolution of symptoms (constitutional, pulmonary), negative microbiologic samples, and improvement in radiographic studies.

Antifungals in Pregnancy

21. C.P. reports she has not menstruated in 3 months, and a urine pregnancy test is positive. How does this information change the therapeutic options for her?

The data on the safety of antimycotics for treating patients who are pregnant or lactating are limited but comprehensively reviewed according to FDA categories of the teratogenic risks of drugs (see Chapter 47, Teratogenicity and Drugs in Breast Milk).[145,146] The systemic azoles are categorized risk factor C.[147] However, we believe they are contraindicated in pregnant or lactating women who are breast-feeding because of their potential teratogenicity and endocrine toxicity in the fetus or newborn. Like the azoles, griseofulvin and flucytosine have been classified as risk factor C. This suggests that there are animal studies, but no human studies, demonstrating significant adverse effects (embryotoxicity and teratogenicity). These agents should not be used in C.P. because the risk clearly outweighs the therapeutic benefit. There are few or no data on the secretion of these agents in breast milk. Therefore, breast-feeding should be discouraged in women receiving these antifungal agents.

Amphotericin B and terbinafine are classified as risk factor B. Therapeutic agents in this category have no fetal risk based on animal studies, or when risk has been found in animals, controlled human studies have not confirmed the results. To our knowledge, there have been no reports of the use of terbinafine in pregnancy. Therefore, we are concerned by this arbitrary designation and recommend avoiding terbinafine in pregnancy until published data support a B classification. Furthermore, considerable clinical experience with amphotericin B in pregnant women has documented successful treatment of systemic mycoses with no excess toxicity to either the mother or fetus. Thus, amphotericin B formulations have been the mainstay of antifungal therapy in pregnancy.

Histoplasmosis
Treatment

22. J.N., a 47-year-old man with severe rheumatoid arthritis, has been maintained on daily prednisone for the past 6 years; his current dosage is 20 mg/day. For the past 4 weeks, he has experienced daily fevers to 38.4°C, drenching night sweats, anorexia, and an 8.2-kg weight loss. His prednisone dosage was increased to 40 mg/day with little clinical effect. On admission to the hospital, J.N. appears chronically ill and has many of the stigmata of chronic steroid therapy. His temperature is 37.8°C with an associated rapid heart rate of 105 beats/min. A shallow mouth ulcer is present on the hard pallet. The liver is enlarged to a total span of 18 cm, and the spleen is palpable 3 cm below the left costal margin. Stool is positive for occult blood. A chest radiograph shows bilateral interstitial infiltrates (Fig. 71-4A). He is pancytopenic, with a hematocrit (Hct) of 29% (normal, 39% to 45%), a WBC count of 3,500 cells/mm³ (normal, 4,000–11,000 cells/mm³), and platelet count of 78,000 cells/mm³ (normal, 130 to 400,000 cells/mm³). The bilirubin is normal but the aminotransferases are elevated to about 1.5 times normal, and serum lactate dehydrogenase is 10 times over normal. A UA reveals 8 to 10 WBCs/high-power field. The SrCr is 1.9 mg/dL, and BUN is 42 mg/dL. A bone marrow aspirate and biopsy of the mouth ulcer reveals multiple, small intracellular yeast forms compatible with *H. capsulatum* in macrophages and polymorphonuclear leukocytes (Fig. 71-4B). Cultures of blood and urine, bone marrow aspirate, and mouth ulcer biopsy grew *H. capsulatum*. What should be the primary antifungal therapy in this case of systemic *H. capsulatum*? What clinical parameters should be monitored to assess the efficacy and toxicity of J.N.'s therapy?

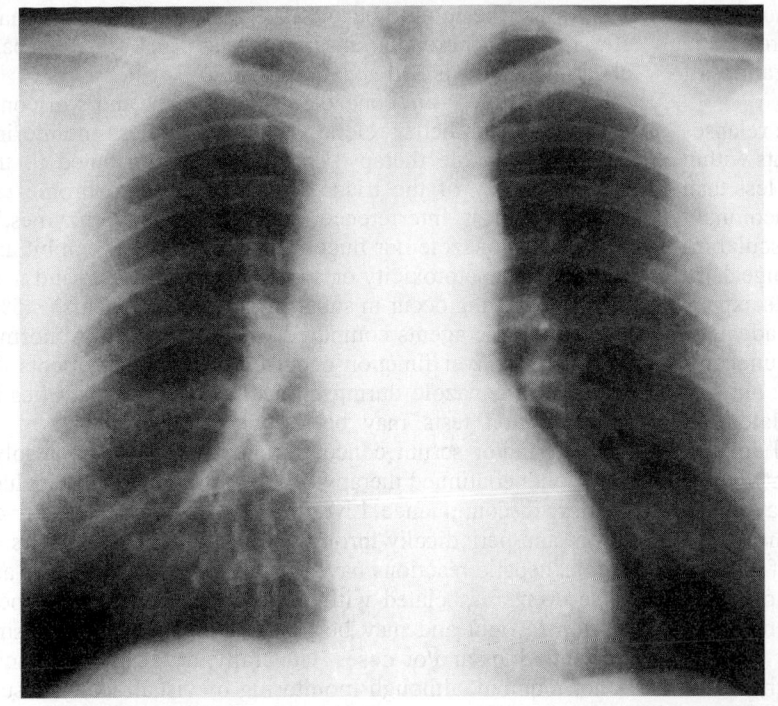
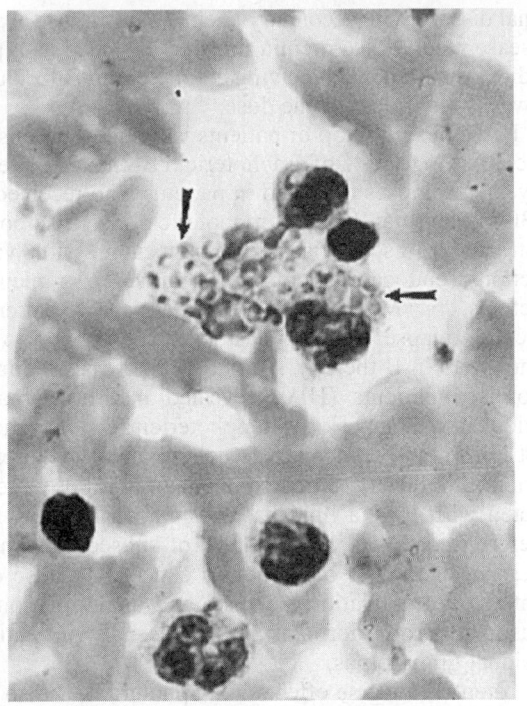

FIGURE 71-4 Histoplasmosis infection. A. Chest radiograph showing bilateral interstitial infiltrate. **B.** Gram's stain of peripheral blood showing leukocytes with intracellular organisms.

[SI units: Hct, 0.29; WBC count, 3.5 × 10⁹/L; SrCr, 167.96 μmol/L; BUN, 14.99 mmol/L urea]

The treatment benefits of antifungal therapy in systemic histoplasmosis have not been well investigated. However, the treatment options for histoplasmosis are outlined in Table 71-9.[148] Accordingly, J.N. should be treated with amphotericin B 0.3 to 0.5 mg/kg per day or itraconazole 2.8 mg/kg per day, and his course of therapy should be monitored for both efficacy and toxicity. Amphotericin B was selected for this case.

Blood and urine cultures, pancytopenia (except anemia in amphotericin B treated patients), constitutional symptoms, serum lactate dehydrogenase (LDH,) and hepatosplenomegaly are excellent measures for evaluating outcome to antifungal therapy of J.N.'s histoplasmosis. Anemia and chest radiographs are poor measures of treatment response. Chest radiographs often reflect calcified granulomas in chronic disease with scarring, which rarely resolve even with extensive therapy. Therefore, evaluation of deterioration on radiograph but not of improvement is possible. In addition, amphotericin B–induced

Table 71-9 Treatment of Histoplasmosis

Disease	Primary	Secondary
Acute Pulmonary	Resolves spontaneously	Not applicable
Prolonged symptomatology (>2 wk)	ITZ 50–100 mg/day (3–6 mo)[a]	AmphoB 0.3–0.5 mg/kg/day[a]
Immunocompromised[c]	AmphoB lipid formulation[c]	AmphoB 0.3–0.5 mg/kg/day
Respiratory distress	AmphoB 0.5–1.0 mg/kg/day	ITZ 1.5–2.8 mg/kg/day (≥6 mo)[a]
(Pao₂ <70 mm Hg)	(TD 250–500 mg) ± corticosteroids	ITZ (has not been investigated in life-threatening situations)
Chronic Pulmonary		
Active	ITZ 1.5–2.8 mg/kg/day (≈9 mo)[a,b]	AmphoB 0.5 mg/kg/day[b]
Inactive		Or KTZ 400 mg/day (≈6 mo)
Histoplasmoma	No treatment	Not applicable
Mediastinal fibrosis	Surgery[d]	Not applicable
Systemic Disease	AmphoB (total dose recommended: 35 mg/kg) or ITZ 2.8 mg/kg/day[a]	Fluconazole 400–800 mg/d[e]

[a]Treatment should be continued until the patient is symptom free and culture negative for 3 months. The recommendations for duration of therapy or total doses should be used only as guides for initial therapy.
[b]Indicated only for serious symptoms (i.e., hemoptysis).
[c]Lipid formulations of amphotericin B are preferable to generic amphotericin B in HIV-infected patients.[150]
[d]ITZ 200 mg QD or BID for 6–18 months for most patients.
[e]Fluconazole should only be used in patients who cannot take ITZ.
AmphoB, amphotericin B deoxycholate; ITZ, itraconazole; KTZ, ketoconazole.

renal disease with secondary anemia can confuse evaluation of disease resolution. Anemia must be excluded as a prognostic indicator in patients receiving amphotericin B for durations of 3 weeks regardless of the dose.[109]

Diligent follow-up of patients is required because relapses occur in 5% to 15% of amphotericin B–treated patients within 3 years. Relapses occurred in patients who received less than a 30 mg/kg total dose of amphotericin B, or had concomitant untreated Addison's disease, immunosuppression, vascular infections (endocarditis, grafts, aneurysms), or meningeal infections.[148,149] More than 90% of HIV-positive patients experience a relapse of histoplasmosis subsequent to adequate amphotericin B therapy. A double blind trial in immunocompromised patients (HIV) revealed that liposomal amphotericin B was superior to amphotericin B deoxycholate. It is not known how itraconazole compares to liposomal amphotericin B in the HIV infected population. If this patient was infected with HIV, a lipid based amphotericin may have been preferred.[150] Even the initiation of subsequent immunosuppressive therapy is of particular concern because of the potential for reactivation (relapse) and dissemination of histoplasmosis from dormant foci, especially in patients with residual granulomas.

Potential adverse effects to amphotericin B also should be monitored in J.N. (e.g., infusion-related reactions, nephrotoxicity, anemia, hypokalemia, neurotoxicity, thrombophlebitis). In addition, J.N.'s adrenal status should be monitored closely because of his long-term corticosteroid therapy and his histoplasmosis. Patients who are addisonian secondary to histoplasmosis infections appear to experience more episodes of amphotericin B–induced acute hypotension.

Azole Adverse Effects

23. After treatment with a total amphotericin B dose of 750 mg, clinical improvement of J.N.'s histoplasmosis is subjectively and objectively documented. The clinician selected ketoconazole 400 mg/day as an oral substitute for his amphotericin B regimen due to the patient's economic circumstances. Six weeks later, J.N. complains of impotence and wonders whether this could be caused by his medication. What is the likelihood that ketoconazole is the cause of J.N.'s impotence?

Ketoconazole has been associated with more adverse reactions and greater potential for drug interactions compared with miconazole, itraconazole, and fluconazole. Fortunately, the most common side effects of ketoconazole are nausea and vomiting. GI distress appears to be dose-related because a substantially smaller percentage of patients experience these effects when receiving ketoconazole dosages of 400 mg/day compared with dosages of 800 mg/day.[149] Endocrine and hepatic toxicities are the most significant adverse effects of ketoconazole requiring monitoring. Dose-splitting from daily to twice daily may decrease the nausea and vomiting. Dose-related endocrinologic toxicities (hypoadrenalism, oligospermia, and diminished libido in males) have been observed during ketoconazole therapy secondary to inhibition of mammalian sterol synthesis,[15,151] and usually resolve with drug discontinuation. Therefore, J.N.'s complaints of impotence might well be attributed to his ketoconazole. Liver enzymes

should also be monitored because there is an approximate 10% risk of elevation in transaminases and an occasional case of serious hepatitis and hepatic failure.[15,151]

The triazoles—itraconazole, fluconazole, and voriconazole—are much better tolerated and require less monitoring than ketoconazole therapy. This has been attributed to the greater affinity of the triazoles for fungal cytochrome enzymes and less interference with mammalian enzymes.[152] Neither itraconazole nor fluconazole (6 mg/kg/d) exhibit any substantial hepatotoxicity or antiandrogenic effects, and nausea and vomiting occur in substantially fewer patients (<5%) receiving these agents compared with imidazoles. Abnormal elevations in liver function occurred in 2.7% of patients receiving voriconazole during clinical trials. Abnormalities in liver function tests may be associated with higher azole dosages and/or serum concentrations, but generally resolve either with continued therapy or dosage modification, including drug discontinuance. Liver function should be determined before and periodically throughout azole therapy as cases of serious hepatic reactions have been reported.[152] A unique adverse events associated with voriconazole is enhanced perception to light and may be associated with higher plasma concentrations and/or doses. Generally, drug discontinuance is not required, although monitoring of visual acuity, visual field, and color perception is advised if therapy lasts longer than 28 days. Preliminary data with ravuconazole suggest an adverse effects profile similar to fluconazole. Diarrhea, asthenia, flatulence, and eye pain have been reported with posaconazole therapy.[153,154] Based on these data, J.N. should be given a trial of itraconazole.

Azole Drug Interactions

24. J.N. chose to continue his ketoconazole therapy. He now returns with Cushnoid signs and symptoms. What potential drug/disease state interaction could be implicated as a cause of this serious problem in J.N.?

Drug interactions with systemic azoles and polyenes can lead to mild inconveniences or life-threatening events (see Table 71-4 and Question 9). The interaction between azoles and glucocorticoids is not as serious as the interaction reporting Q-T prolongation and ventricular arrhythmias with nonsedating H_1-selective antihistamines.[155] However, the interaction with corticosteroids can be multifaceted and is therapeutically challenging. It has been suggested that using corticosteroids can lead to a broad spectrum of responses, including decreased immune activation and inhibition of phagocytosis while in contrast finding no change in organism growth and animal survival.[98] Although it is clinically possible that corticosteroids could affect outcome, no clinical trial has addressed this important question. Drug interaction trials have measured an increase in corticosteroid serum concentrations leading to recommendations to decrease the steroid dose by 50% when ketoconazole is used concomitantly. The interaction has been suggested between glucocorticoids and other azoles.[156] In addition, dexamethasone has been demonstrated to increase the clearance of caspofungin. Recommendations for caspofungin dosage adjustments are being developed by the manufacturer.

Coccidioidomycosis
Serologic Tests

25. F.W., a 32-year-old Filipino woman and a lifelong resident of the Central Valley in California, is admitted to the hospital with a third recurrence of coccidioidal meningitis. Approximately 4 years ago, she was treated with a total amphotericin B dose of 2.2 g, which resulted in a good clinical response. Nine months later, she relapsed and received a second course of amphotericin B to a total of 1.6 g. She did well over the next 18 months and was able to return to work as a secretary. However, over the past 4 months, F.W. has noted chronic headaches, has been unable to concentrate at work, and is reported by family members to have a very labile personality. A CT scan of the brain reveals mild hydrocephalus. An opening pressure of 19 mm Hg (normal, 10 mm Hg) was documented at lumbar puncture. Analysis of the CSF showed 110 WBCs/mm³ (normal, 0 WBCs/mm³); glucose, 18 mg/dL (normal, 60% of serum glucose); and protein, 190 mg/dL (normal, <50 mg/dL). Complement fixation antibodies were positive in the CSF at a titer of 1:32. How should serologic tests for coccidioidomycosis be interpreted?

The most important serologic tests for fungal infections use complement fixation (CF), immunodiffusion, and EIA techniques. Tests for complement fixing antibodies (i.e., CF) to the dimorphic fungi (see Table 71-1) are well established and various antigens have been used. Coccidioidin is the mycelial phase antigen for *Coccidioides immitis*. Of patients with coccidioidomycosis, 61% will have coccidioidin CF titers of at least 1:32 and 41% will have titers of 1:64. Rising titers are a bad prognostic sign, and falling titers indicate clinical improvement. Therefore, F.W.'s CSF CF titer of 1:32 is consistent with active coccidioidomycosis. Immunodiffusion testing for coccidioidomycosis using coccidioidin reveals that seropositive results appear 1 to 3 weeks after onset of primary infection in 75% of patients and this positivity usually disappears within 4 months if the infection resolves.[157] IgG- and IgM-specific EIA using a combination of antigens for *C. immitis* have been developed. These tests offer sensitivities of >92% and specificities of 98% for serum and CSF. EIA reactivity appears earlier than CF reactivity.[158,159]

Antifungal Central Nervous System Penetration

26. What is a pharmacokinetic explanation for the treatment failure of F.W.? How might this problem be overcome?

F.W. has received prolonged parenteral amphotericin B administration and the CSF still contains fungal organisms. Treatment failures in this case may be due, in part, to the limited penetration of amphotericin B into the CSF.[94] Because amphotericin B is highly bound to lipid (90% to 95%), CSF concentrations achieved are only 2% to 4% of the serum concentration[94,152]; peritoneal, synovial, and pleural fluid concentrations are slightly <50% of the serum concentrations. Augmentation of systemic antifungal administration with intraventricular or intrathecal administration may improve the outcome for antifungals with poor penetration into the CSF.[160–165] Intrathecal amphotericin B doses in adults normally range from 0.25 to 0.5 mg diluted in 5 mL of 5% glucose.[161,162] A few studies suggest that doses >0.7 mg improve

the cure rate and decrease relapse.[165] Cisternal or intraventricular administration is recommended as the routes of choice because of flow characteristics of CSF from the ventricles to the spinal cord.[160,165,166] When lumbar administration is necessary, amphotericin B is administered in a hypertonic solution of 10% glucose and the patient is placed in a Trendelenburg position in an attempt to improve distribution of the drug to the basilar meninges and ventricles and reduce local toxicity. Voriconazole, caspofungin, and the lipid amphotericin formulations have not been evaluated.[166,167]

Flucytosine and the systemic azoles might be alternatives to amphotericin B (see Table 71-5). Flucytosine is not significantly bound to protein and penetrates the CSF, vitreous, and peritoneal fluids; its volume of distribution approximates that of total body water.[168] Flucytosine concentration in the CSF is 74% of the serum concentration, resulting in its extensive use in treatment of CNS mycoses. Unfortunately, flucytosine has no activity in coccidioidomycosis and, therefore, cannot be used in F.W.

The volume of distribution of fluconazole approaches that of total body water,[169,170] and concentrations of fluconazole in CSF are approximately 60% of simultaneous serum concentrations. Ketoconazole has only about 1% of the dose present as free drug because it is highly bound to plasma proteins (>80%) and to erythrocytes (15%). Therefore, ketoconazole penetrates poorly into the CSF except with dosages of 1,200 mg/day. Itraconazole is similar to ketoconazole in that it is >99% protein bound. However, itraconazole concentrates intracellularly in host alveolar macrophages and that may account for its efficacy against fungal CNS infection despite its inability to penetrate into the CSF.[171] Data on terbinafine penetration are currently unavailable. Therefore, fluconazole might be an alternative to CNS instillation of amphotericin B based only on pharmacokinetic considerations.

Preliminary studies with fluconazole, investigated at dosages of 400 mg/day, are promising for control of disease in patients with coccidioidomycosis meningitis. However, relapse rates are high once fluconazole therapy is stopped.[172] Early reports with itraconazole appear promising.[172,173] Ketoconazole, which must be given at very high doses and results in significant toxicity, should be used only if other therapies are contraindicated.[152,174,175]

Intrathecal Amphotericin

27. What adverse events might be observed with the intrathecal administration of an antifungal in F.W.?

Cisternal antifungal administration has been associated with headaches, nausea, vomiting, cranial nerve paresis, and cisternal hemorrhage caused by needle trauma.[160, 176–178] An Ommaya reservoir often is used to facilitate intraventricular administration of amphotericin B. Common complications of these devices include shunt occlusion, bacterial colonization or bacterial meningitis, parkinsonian symptoms, and seizures.[160,176–179] Lumbar administration has been used because it is simpler, but it often must be discontinued because of chemical arachnoiditis, headache, transient radiculitis, paresthesia, nerve pulses, difficulty voiding, impaired vision, vertigo, and tinnitus.[179] Acute toxic delirium, demyelinating peripheral neuropathy, and spinal cord injury have also been reported.[180–182] Regardless of the substantial and serious adverse effects, intrathecal administration may be effective in treating patients with meningitis who have severe disease or who are pharmacologic nonresponders.

Aspergillosis
Empiric Therapy (Neutropenic Host)

28. **M.Z., an otherwise healthy 29-year-old man, presented for allogeneic bone marrow transplantation (BMT) 12 days ago. He has had no serious complications associated with his chloroquine-induced aplastic anemia during his 7-month wait for BMT. On BMT days −5 to −2, induction therapy was initiated with cyclophosphamide (50 mg/kg) and total body irradiation, and then bone marrow from his HLA-compatible brother was infused on day 0. The onset of neutropenia was noted on day 3 and the WBC count was 50 cells/mm³. M.Z. has complained of only stomatitis and diarrhea before day 5. On that morning, he was complaining of fever, chest pain, and headache. On physical examination, his temperature is 37°C. Empiric anti-infectives were added but by day 8 he was not clinically improving. What therapeutic options should be considered for this patient?**

Empiric antifungal therapy in a neutropenic host should be initiated when a patient is febrile for >96 hours on appropriate anti-infectives. Routine empiric therapy for a patient without evidence of deep-seated fungal infection historically has been amphotericin B 0.3 to 0.6 mg/kg per day or fluconazole 200 to 400 mg/day until the absolute neutrophil count is >500 cells/mm³.[183] Therapy results in resolution of signs and symptoms in up to 64% of patients. However, there have been recent efforts to improve the delivery system for amphotericin B to reduce its toxicity. These have included formulating it as a lipid complex, a liposome, colloidal dispersion, or admixing amphotericin B with a lipid emulsion (see Table 71-7). A motivation for developing these formulations was the observation that serum triglycerides and cholesterol decrease adverse drug reactions and may improve efficacy.[118,184,185]

Because mold infections are of concern in this neutropenic patient population, drug therapy that is highly active against these organisms should be considered. A large, well-controlled, double-blind comparison of amphotericin B 0.6 mg/kg per day versus liposomal amphotericin B 3.0 mg/kg per day can guide us in this case. Patients who were febrile >96 hours and neutropenic (<500 cells/mm³) experienced equal survival and clinical success of approximately 50% for both agents. However, there were significantly fewer fungal infections that emerged on liposomal amphotericin B. Liposomal amphotericin B–treated patients also experienced significantly lower rates of adverse reactions (approximately twofold).[184] Therefore, a lipid formulation provides greater protection against emergent fungal infections during neutropenic fevers. This is probably because of the ability to deliver larger amphotericin B doses.

29. **What is the role of lipid formulations of amphotericin B in other disease states?**

The advantage of the lipid formulations is clear in the treatment of diseases such as aspergillosis, which require long-term therapy that can result in patient intolerance to generic amphotericin B.[118] Multiple uncontrolled or retrospective trials have observed that all four lipid formulations of amphotericin B appear to be less nephrotoxic and may be more effective than amphotericin B desoxycholate. A single large randomized, double-blind trial and a historical controlled trial support these observations.[185,186]

There are also a few well-controlled prospective comparative trials to guide our decision-making process for fungal infections that require a shorter course of therapy. In addition to the data presented for candidemia (Question 16), liposomal and lipid complex amphotericin B have been evaluated for treatment of cryptococcal meningitis and histoplasmosis in HIV-infected patients.[150,187,188] Each lipid agent appears safer and more effective than amphotericin B desoxycholate. However, secondary to the high acquisition cost and relatively low rates of toxicity with short course therapy, generic amphotericin B should be selected over the lipid formulation unless a patient is clearly intolerant, requires extended therapy, or experiences a treatment failure.

Of particular interest are the ongoing studies and case reports in which Intralipid 10% to 20% combined with amphotericin B (1 to 2 mg/mL) is administered at a dosage of 1 mg/kg/day. This practice cannot be recommended until a prospective, randomized, control trial documents efficacy and reduced toxicity of these lipid emulsion—amphotericin B formulations as compared with amphotericin B alone. Our current concerns are the inability to formulate a pharmaceutically stable product,[189] difficulty assessing whether inline filtering is required, and the delivery of excessive calories.[190]

Treatment of Aspergillosis

30. **Chest auscultation on day 8 reveals right-sided rales with a friction rub. Chest radiograph shows a nodular infiltrate in the right middle lobe. Fiberoptic bronchoscopy identified eroded bronchioles with necrotic tissue, and methenamine silver nitrate stain of a biopsy sample revealed fragmented, closely septated hyphal bodies branched at 45° angles. The samples were sent to microbiology for cultures. All previous blood and sputum cultures have been negative, except that *Aspergillus niger* growing from sputum before admission was classified as a "contaminant." The diagnosis at this time is probable aspergillosis. What treatment steps should be taken?**

Drug therapy should be approached by first determining whether the infection is likely to be invasive or noninvasive disease (Fig. 71-5). Most patients inhale *Aspergillus* species and never become symptomatic or develop only mild hypersensitivity pneumonitis. Invasive infections are more likely to occur in immunocompromised patients, especially those with prolonged neutropenia associated with bone marrow transplantation. A classic observation reported by radiology is a "halo" sign or a "crescent" sign identified on CT, highly suggestive of this infection. Additionally, an ELISA for a surface protein, galactomannan, has been reported to have high sensitivity in the diagnosis of invasive disease. However, the clinical utility of this assay is still under investigation. Administration of piperacillin or piperacillin-tazobactam has been associated with false positive galactomannan.[191] The subjective and objective data in this case clearly represent invasive symptomatic disease and there is a need for aggressive treatment.

Aspergillosis is a model for invasive mold infections that have a propensity to invade blood vessels and tissue. Antimycotic pharmacotherapy should be initiated rapidly and aggressively (Table 71-10) in conjunction with removal or reversal of immunosuppression if possible. Definite or probable inva-

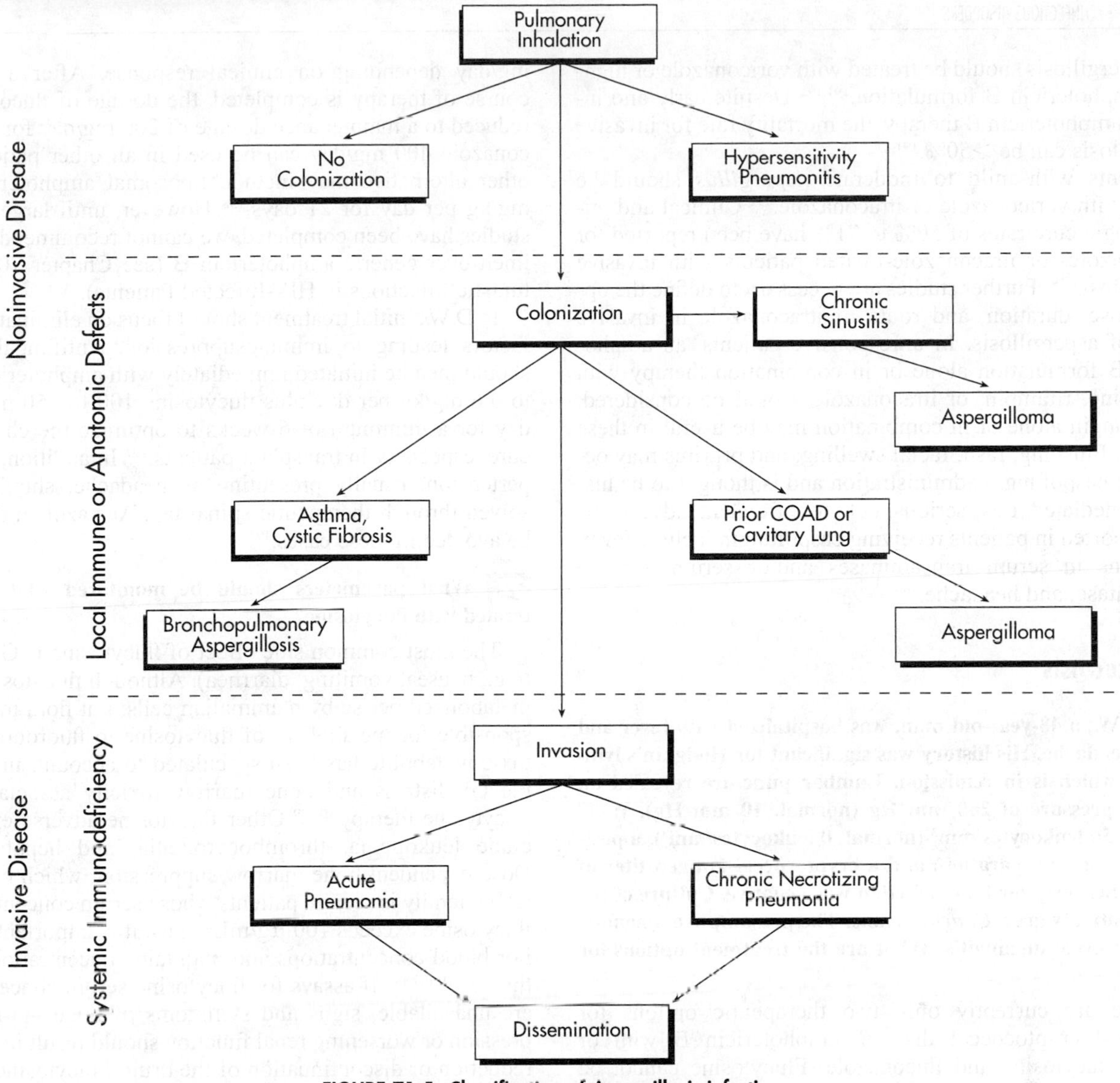

FIGURE 71-5 Classification of Aspergillosis infections.

The figure shows a flowchart starting from "Pulmonary Inhalation" branching into:
- Noninvasive Disease: No Colonization, Hypersensitivity Pneumonitis
- Local Immune or Anatomic Defects: Colonization → Chronic Sinusitis → Aspergilloma; Asthma, Cystic Fibrosis → Bronchopulmonary Aspergillosis; Prior COAD or Cavitary Lung → Aspergilloma
- Invasive Disease / Systemic Immunodeficiency: Invasion → Acute Pneumonia, Chronic Necrotizing Pneumonia → Dissemination

Table 71-10   Therapeutic Options for Treatment of Aspergillosis

Disease	Primary	Secondary
Hyalohyphomycetes		
Aspergillosis		
Allergic bronchopulmonary	Prednisone 1 mg/kg/day followed by 0.5 mg/kg/day or QOD × 3–6 mo; no antifungal therapy	ITZ 200 mg BID × 4 months[a]
Aspergilloma	Observation	Surgery[b]
Systemic (invasive)		
Serious	Voriconazole 6 mg/kg/day LD, 4 mg/kg/day divided twice daily	Amphotericin B lipid Formulation,[d] or AmphoB 1.0–1.5 mg/kg/day[c]
Mild/moderate	Voriconazole 6 mg/kg/day LD, 4 mg/kg/day divided twice daily	Amphotericin B Lipid Formulation,[d] or AmphoB 0.5–0.6 mg/kg/day[c] or ITZ 200 mg TID loading dose × 3 days then 200 mg BID with meals (6-mo minimum)

[a]Treatment should be continued until the patient is symptom free and culture negative for 3 months. Noted durations or total doses should be used only as a compass to help guide therapy.
[b]Indicated only for serious symptoms (e.g., hemoptysis).
[c]Lipid formulations of amphotericin B should be utilized preferentially in these patients.
[d]Liposomal amphotericin B at doses up to 15 mg/kg/d appears safe in Phase I/II trials.[202]
AmphoB, amphotericin B; ITZ, itraconazole.

LIVERPOOL
JOHN MOORES UNIVERSITY
AVRIL ROBARTS LRC
TEL. 0151 231 4022

sive aspergillosis should be treated with voriconazole or high-dose amphotericin B formulation.[191,192] Despite early and intensive amphotericin B therapy, the mortality rate for invasive aspergillosis can be >50%.[191]

Patients with mild to moderate *Aspergillus* should be treated with voriconazole or itraconazole.[192] Clinical and microbiologic cure rates of 50% to 71% have been reported for voriconazole- or itraconazole-treated patients with invasive aspergillosis.[191] Further studies are necessary to define the optimal dose, duration, and route of itraconazole in invasive forms of aspergillosis. In unresponsive patients, an amphotericin B formulation alone or in combination therapy with flucytosine, rifampin, or itraconazole should be considered. Caspofungin alone or in combination may be useful in these patients. Flushing, rash, facial swelling, and pruritus may occur with caspofungin administration and is thought to be histamine mediated. Less serious, but more frequent, adverse effects reported in patients receiving caspofungin include fever, elevations in serum transaminases and/or serum alkaline phosphatase, and headache.[166]

Cryptococcosis

31. **D.W., a 48-year-old man, was hospitalized with fever and severe headache. His history was significant for Hodgkin's lymphoma, which is in remission. Lumbar puncture revealed an opening pressure of 280 mm Hg (normal, 10 mm Hg), WBC count of 50 leukocytes/mm³ (normal, 0 leukocytes/mm³), a positive India ink preparation, and a cryptococcal antigen titer of 1:4,096. Serology for HIV infection was negative. Culture of the CSF eventually grew *C. neoformans*. The presumptive diagnosis is cryptococcal meningitis. What are the treatment options for D.W.?**

There are currently only two therapeutic options for meningeal cryptococcal disease: amphotericin B with or without flucytosine and fluconazole. Flucytosine cannot be used alone for therapy or prophylaxis because of the rapid development of resistance. Patients, whether infected with HIV or not, have improved treatment outcomes when the combination of amphotericin B and flucytosine is used.[193,194] Furthermore, when flucytosine (100 to 150 mg/kg/day divided into four daily doses) is used in combination therapy, the dose of amphotericin B may be reduced to 0.3 to 0.6 mg/kg/day, which decreases the frequency of dose-related amphotericin B toxicity. In patients who cannot be treated with flucytosine, the dosage of amphotericin B must be increased to >0.6 mg/kg/day.

Fluconazole is an alternative to amphotericin B in HIV-infected patients with cryptococcal meningitis. However, one must be mindful of the following caveats: sterilization of the CSF occurs more rapidly and mortality is lower during the first 2 weeks of therapy in patients treated with amphotericin B as compared to fluconazole.[195,196] Early mortality was especially high in fluconazole-treated patients who presented with altered mental status.[193,195,197] Thus, initial therapy of cryptococcal meningitis in patients with mental status changes should be initiated with amphotericin B for at least 2 weeks or until the patient has stabilized clinically. At this point, fluconazole may be substituted at an initial dosage of 400 mg/day. The dosage may be titrated upward to a dosage of 800

mg/day depending on clinical response. After a 10-week course of therapy is completed, the dosage of fluconazole is reduced to a maintenance dosage of 200 mg/day for life. Fluconazole 400 mg/day can be used in all other patients. Another alternative may include liposomal amphotericin B 4 mg/kg per day for 21 days.[188] However, until larger clinical studies have been completed, we cannot recommend this regimen over generic amphotericin B (see Chapter 70, Opportunistic Infections in HIV-Infected Patients).

In D.W., initial treatment should focus on elimination of all factors leading to immunosuppression. Antifungal therapy should then be initiated immediately with amphotericin B 0.3 to 0.6 mg/kg per day plus flucytosine 100 to 150 mg/kg per day for a minimum of 6 weeks to optimize the chance of a cure, especially in transplant patients.[197] In addition, CSF hypertension, usually presenting as headache, should be resolved through therapeutic spinal tap. Acetazolamide should be avoided in these cases.[198]

32. **What parameters should be monitored while D.W. is treated with flucytosine?**

The most common side effect of flucytosine is GI distress (e.g., nausea, vomiting, diarrhea). Although flucytosine is not metabolized per se by mammalian cells, gut flora may be responsible for metabolism of flucytosine to fluorouracil. This toxic metabolite has been speculated to account, in part, for the GI distress and bone marrow toxicity associated with flucytosine therapy.[10,199] Other flucytosine adverse effects include leukopenia, thrombocytopenia, and hepatotoxicity. Dose-dependent bone marrow suppression, which can be fatal, generally is seen in patients whose serum concentration of flucytosine exceeds 100 μg/mL. Thus, it is important to monitor blood concentrations and maintain concentrations below this level.[197,199] If assays for flucytosine serum concentrations are unavailable, signs and symptoms of bone marrow suppression or worsening renal function should result in a dosage reduction or discontinuation of the drug. Flucytosine is eliminated by glomerular filtration, with 80% to 95% of the dose excreted unchanged in the urine. Renal excretion of flucytosine is directly related to creatinine clearance, and dosages should be adjusted based on creatinine clearance to prevent accumulation to toxic concentrations in patients with renal impairment.[110,167] Patients with creatinine clearances of 10 to 40 mL/min should have the dosage of flucytosine reduced by 50% (usual dose, 37.5 mg/kg Q 12 hr). For patients with creatinine clearance <10 mL/min, dosing should be initiated at 37.5 mg/kg/day with frequent monitoring of flucytosine serum concentrations. Dosage adjustment and close monitoring also are required for patients receiving hemodialysis and it is recommended that the dose be given postdialysis.

33. **When is combination antifungal therapy indicated?**

In vitro results of antifungal combinations against many common mycotic pathogens have been variable. Combination antifungals have been found to be synergistic, additive, antagonistic, or to have no effect. These *in vitro* evaluations involved the concurrent administration of amphotericin B formulations with flucytosine, rifampin, echinocandins, or azoles. The azoles have been concurrently administered with flucytosine, rifampin, sulfamethoxazole, echinocandins, and nikkomycins. These incomplete and inconsistent findings have been attributed to variable incubation times, variable concentrations of antifungal agents, and the sequence of antifungal addition.[200] As a result, clinical decisions about combination therapy should be based on patient-specific *in vivo* evaluations. Because of the limited clinical data, combination antifungal therapy should be initiated cautiously. Except for the treatment of cryptococcal meningitis, combination therapy should be reserved for cases of treatment failure with no other established pharmacologic options for therapy or mold infections with high mortality rates.

REFERENCES

1. Kwon-Chung KJ, Bennett JE, eds. Medical Mycology. Malvern, PA: Lea & Febiger, 1992.
2. Rinaldi MG. Systemic fungal infections: diagnosis and treatment II—emerging opportunists. Infect Dis Clin North Am 1989;3:65.
3. Khardori N et al. Cutaneous Rhizopus and Aspergillus infections in five patients with cancer. Arch Dermatol 1989;125:952.
4. Wingard JR. Importance of Candida species other than *C. albicans* as pathogens in oncology patients. Clin Infect Dis 1995;20:115.
5. Brajtburg J et al. Amphotericin B: current understanding of mechanisms of action. Antimicrob Agents Chemother 1990;34:183.
6. Gruda I et al. Application of different spectra in the UV-visible region to study the formation of amphotericin B complexes. Biochem Biophys Acta 1980;602:260.
7. Hitchcock CA et al. The lipid composition and permeability to azole of an azole-and polyene-resistant mutant of *Candida albicans*. J Med Vet Mycol 1987;25:29.
8. Pierce AM et al. Lipid composition and polyene antibiotic resistance of *Candida albicans*. Can J Biochem 1978;56:135.
9. Brajtburg J et al. Stimulatory, permeabilizing, and toxic effects of amphotericin B on L cells. Antimicrob Agents Chemother 1984;26:892.
10. Diasio RB et al. Mode of action of 5-fluorocytosine. Biochem Pharmacol 1978;27:703.
11. Chouini-Lalanne N et al. Study of the metabolism of flucytosine in Aspergillus species by ^{19}F nuclear magnetic resonance spectroscopy. Antimicrob Agents Chemother 1989;33:1939.
12. Polak A, Scholer HJ. Mode of action of 5-fluorocytosine and mechanisms of resistance. Chemotherapy 1975;21:113.
13. van den Bossche H et al. Hypothesis on the molecular basis of the antifungal activation of N-substituted imidazoles and triazoles. Biochem Soc Trans 1983;11:665.
14. van den Bossche H. Biochemical targets for antifungal azole derivatives: hypothesis of the mode of action. In: McGinnis M, ed. Current Topics in Medical Mycology. New York: Springer-Verlag, 1985:313.
15. Bodey GP. Azole antifungal agents. Clin Infect Dis 1992;14(Suppl 1):S161.
16. Petranyi G et al. Allylamine derivative: new class of synthetic antifungal agents inhibiting fungal squalene epoxidase. Science 1984;244:1239.
17. Barchiesi F et al. *In vitro* activity of posaconazole against clinical isolates of dermatophytes. J Clin Microbiol 2001;39:4208.
18. Fung-Tome JC et al. *In vitro* activity of a new oral triazole, BMS-207147 (ER-30346). Antimicrob Agents Chemother 1998;42:313.
19. Manavathu EK et al. Organism-dependent fungicidal activities of azoles. Antimicrob Agents Chemother 1998;42:3018.
20. Walsh TJ et al. New targets and delivery systems for antifungal therapy. Med Mycol 2000;38(Suppl 1):335.
21. Rex JH et al. Antifungal susceptibility testing: practical aspects and current challenges. Clin Microbiol Rev 2001;14:643.
22. National Committee for Clinical Laboratory Standards. Reference method for broth dilution antifungal susceptibility testing of yeasts. Approved standard NCCLS document M27-A. National Committee for Clinical Laboratory Standards, Wayne, PA, 1997.
23. Rex JH et al. Development of interpretive breakpoints for antifungal susceptibility testing: conceptual framework and analysis of *in vitro-in vivo* correlation data for fluconazole, itraconazole, and *Candida* infections. Clin Infect Dis 1997;24:235.
24. Martin-Mazuelos E et al. A comparative evaluation of E test and broth microdilution methods for fluconazole and itraconazole susceptibility testing of *Candida* spp. J Antimicrob Chemother 1999;43:477.
25. Morace G et al. Multicenter comparative evaluation of six commercial systems and the National Committee for Clinical Laboratory Standards M27-1. Broth microdilution method for fluconazole susceptibility testing of *Candida* species. J Clin Microbiol 2002;40:2953.
26. National Committee for Clinical Laboratory Standards. Reference method for broth dilution antifungal susceptibility testing of yeasts. Approved standard NCCLS document M38-P. National Committee for Clinical Laboratory Standards, Wayne, PA, 2001.
27. Espinel-Ingroff A et al. E-test method for testing susceptibilities of *Aspergillus* spp. to the new triazoles voriconazole and posaconazole and to established antifungal agents: comparison with NCCLS broth microdilution method. J Clin Microbiol 2002;40:2101.
28. Schering-Plough Healthcare Products. Fulvicin package insert. Liberty Corner, NJ: January 1994.
29. Odom RB et al. A multicenter, placebo-controlled, double-blind study of intermittent therapy with itraconazole for the treatment of onychomycosis of the fingernail. J Am Acad Dermatol 1997;36:231.
30. Havu V et al. A double-blind, randomized study comparing itraconazole pulse therapy with continuous dosing for the treatment of toenail onychomycosis. Br J Dermatol 1997;36:230.
31. Scher RK et al. Once-weekly fluconazole (150, 300, or 450 mg) in the treatment of distal subungual onychomycosis of the toenail. J Am Acad Dermatol 1998;38:S77.
32. Ling MR et al. Once-weekly fluconazole (450 mg) for 4, 6, or 9 months of treatment for distal subungual onychomycosis of the toenail. J Am Acad Dermatol 1998;38:S95.
33. Gupta AK. Single-blinded, randomized, prospective study of sequential itraconazole and terbinafine pulse compared with terbinafine pulse for the treatment of toenail onychomycosis. J Am Acad Dermatol 2001;44:485.
34. Vanderveen EE et al. Sporotrichosis in pregnancy. Cutis 1982;30:761.
35. Kan VL, Bennett J. Efficacies of four antifungal agents in experimental murine sporotrichosis. Antimicrob Agents Chemother 1988;32:1619.
36. Bennett JE. *Sporothrix schenckii*. In: Mandell GL et al., eds. Principles and Practice of Infectious Diseases. 3rd Ed. New York: Churchill Livingstone, 1990:1972.
37. Restrepo A et al. Itraconazole therapy in lymphangitic and cutaneous sporotrichosis. Arch Dermatol 1986;122:413.
38. Breeling JL, Weinstein L. Pulmonary sporotrichosis treated with itraconazole. Chest 1993;103(1):313.
39. McGinnis MR et al. Sporothrix schenckii sensitivity to voriconazole, itraconazole, and amphotericin B. Med Mycol 2001;39:369.
40. Pappas PG et al. Treatment of lymphocutaneous sporotrichosis with terbinafine: results of randomized double-blind trial. Paper presented to 39th Annual Infectious Diseases Society of America Meeting, San Francisco. 2001:648.
41. Wishart JM. The influence of food on the pharmacokinetics of itraconazole in patients with superficial fungal infection. J Am Acad Dermatol 1987;220.
42. Barone JA et al. Food interaction and steady state pharmacokinetics of itraconazole capsules in healthy male volunteers. Antimicrob Agents Chemother 1993;37:778.
43. Lelawongs P et al. Effect of food and gastric acidity on absorption of orally administered ketoconazole. Clin Pharm 1988;7:228.
44. Smith D et al. The pharmacokinetics of oral itraconazole in AIDS patients. J Pharm Pharmacol 1992;44:618.
45. Zhao Q et al. Pharmacokinetics of intravenous itraconazole followed by itraconazole oral solution in patients with human immunodeficiency virus infection. J Clin Pharmacol 2001;41:1319.
46. Janssen Pharmaceuticals. Sporonox Oral Suspension package insert. Piscataway, NJ: January 1998.
47. Janssen Pharmaceuticals. Nizoral package insert. Piscataway, NJ: January 1998.
48. Chin TWF et al. Effects of Coca-Cola on the oral absorption of ketoconazole in the presence of achlorhydria. Paper presented to 33rd Interscience Conference on Antimicrobial Agents and Chemotherapy, New Orleans, October 17, 1993.
49. Lange D et al. Effect of a cola beverage on the bioavailability of itraconazole in the presence of H2 blockers. J Clin Pharmacol 1997;37(6):535.
50. Meunier-Carpentier F et al. Fungemia in the immunocompromised host: changing patterns, antigenemia, high mortality. Am J Med 1981;71:363.
51. Tatro DS, ed. Drug Interaction Facts. St. Louis: Facts and Comparisons, 1998.
52. Feron B et al. Interaction of sucralfate with antibiotics used for selective decontamination of the gastrointestinal tract. Am J Hosp Pharm 1993;50:2550.
53. Hoechst Marion Roussel. Allegra package insert. Kansas City, MO. January 1998.
54. Present CA. Amphotericin B induction of sensitivity to Adriamycin, BCNU plus cyclophosphamide in human neoplasia. Ann Intern Med 1977;86:47.
55. Kivisto KT et al. Plasma buspirone concentrations are greatly increased by erythromycin and itraconazole. Clin Pharmacol Ther 1997;62:348.
56. Cleary JD. Unpublished data, 2002.
57. Antoniskis D, Larsen RA. Acute, rapidly progressive renal failure with simultaneous use of amphotericin B and pentamidine. Antimicrob Agents Chemother 1990;34:470.
58. McNalty RM et al. Transient increase in plasma quinidine concentrations during ketoconazole-quinidine therapy. Clin Pharm 1989;8:222.
59. Wright DG et al. Lethal pulmonary reactions associated with the combination use of amphotericin B and leukocyte transfusions. N Engl J Med 1981;304:1185.
60. Dutcher JP et al. Granulocyte transfusion therapy and amphotericin B adverse reactions? Am J Hematol 1989;31:102.
61. Rex JH et al. Practice guidelines for the treatment of candidiasis. Clin Infect Dis 2000;30:662.
62. Pfaller MA et al. Trends in antifungal susceptibility of *Candida* spp. isolated from pediatric and adult patients with bloodstream infections: SENTRY Antimicrobial Surveillance Program, 1997 to 2000. J Clin Microbiol 2002;40:852.
63. Pfaller M, Wenzel R. Impact of the changing epidemiology of fungal infections in the 1990s. Eur J Clin Microbiol Infect Dis 1992;11:287.
64. Woods GL, Gutierrez Y. Diagnostic Pathology of Infectious Diseases. Philadelphia: Lea & Febiger, 1993.

65. Arrington JB. Bacteria, fungi, and other microorganisms. In: Prophet EB et al., eds. Laboratory methods in histotechnology. Armed Forces Institute of Pathology. Washington, DC; American Registry of Pathology: Washington DC, 1992:203.

66. Jensen HE et al. The use of immunohistochemistry to improve sensitivity and specificity in the diagnosis of systemic mycoses in patients with hematologic malignancies. J Pathol 1997;181:100.

67. Jansen HE et al. Diagnosis of systemic mycoses by specific immunohistochemical tests. APMIS 1996;104:241.

68. Diaz Ponce H. et al. Indirect immunofluorescent assay (IFA) in buffy coat as a rapid diagnostic test for invasive candidiasis. Arch Med Res 1995; 26(SpecNo):S41.

69. Lischewski A et al. Detection and identification of Candida species in experimentally infected tissue and human blood by rRNA-specific fluorescent in-situ hybridization. J Clin Microbiol 1997;35:2943.

70. Coovadia YJ, Solwa Z. Sensitivity and specificity of a latex agglutination test for detection of cryptococcal antigen in meningitis. S Afr Med J 1987; 71:510.

71. Loshi G et al. Coagglutination (CoA) test for the rapid diagnosis of cryptococcal meningitis. J Med Microbiol 1989;29:189.

72. Herent P et al. Retrospective evaluation of two latex agglutination tests for detection of circulating antigens during invasive candidiasis. J Clin Microbiol 1992;30:2158.

73. Phillips P et al. Nonvalue of antigen detection immunoassays for diagnosis of candidemia. J Clin Microbiol 1990;28:2320.

74. Mitsutake K et al. Enolase antigen, mannan antigen, Cand-Tec antigen, and beta-glucan in patients with candidemia. J Clin Microbiol 1996;34:1918.

75. Lehtonen L et al. Diagnosis of disseminated candidiasis by measurement of urine D-arabinitol/L-arabinitol ratio. J Clin Microbiol 1996;34:2175.

76. Walsh TJ et al. Diagnosis and therapeutic monitoring of invasive candidiasis by rapid enzymatic detection of serum D-arabinitol. Am J Med 1995; 99:164.

77. Christensson B et al. Diagnosis of invasive candidiasis in neutropenic children with cancer by determination of D-arabinitol/L-arabinitol ratios in urine. J Clin Microbiol 1997;35:636.

78. Wheat LJ et al. Diagnosis of disseminated histoplasmosis by detection of H. capsulatum antigen in serum and urine specimens. N Engl J Med 1986;314:83.

79. Crislip MA, Edwards JE. Candidiasis, in systemic fungal infections: diagnosis and treatment II. Infect Dis Clin North Am 1989;2:103.

80. Wheat LJ. Histoplasmosis in systemic fungal infections: diagnosis and treatment I. Infect Dis Clin North Am 1988;2:841.

81. Wey SB et al. Risk factors for hospital-acquired candidemia: a matched case-control study. Arch Intern Med 1989;149(10):2349.

82. Walsh TH, Rex JH. All catheter-related candidemia is not the same: assessment of the balance between risks and benefit of removal of vascular catheters. Clin Infect Dis 2002;34:600.

83. Nucci M, Anaisse E. Should vascular catheters be removed from all patients with candidemia? An evidence-based review. Clin Infect Dis 2002;34:601.

84. Mora-Duarte J et al. Comparison of caspofungin and amphotericin B for invasive candidiasis. N Engl J Med 2002;347:2020.

85. Rex JH et al. A randomized trial comparing fluconazole with amphotericin B for the treatment of candidemia in patients without neutropenia. N Engl J Med 1994;331:1325.

86. Rex JH et al. A randomized and blinded multicenter trial of high-dose fluconazole plus placebo vs. fluconazole plus amphotericin B as therapy of candidemia and its consequences in non-neutropenic patients. Clin Infect Dis 2003;36(10):1221.

87. Abele-Horn M. A randomized study comparing fluconazole with amphotericin B/5-flucytosine for the treatment of systemic Candida infections in intensive care patients. Infection 1996;2496:426.

88. Wingard JR. Infections due to resistant Candida species in patients with cancer who are receiving chromotherapy. Clin Infect Dis 1994; 19(Suppl.1):S49.

89. Rex JH et al. Antifungal susceptibility testing of isolates from a randomized, multicenter trial of fluconazole versus amphotericin B as treatment of nonneutropenic patients with candidemia. Antimicrob Agents Chemother 1995;39:40.

90. Christiansen KJ et al. Distribution and activity of amphotericin in humans. J Infect Dis 1985;152:1037.

91. Collette N et al. Tissue concentrations and bioactivity of amphotericin B in cancer patients treated with amphotericin B-deoxycholate. Antimicrob Agents Chemother 1989;33:362.

92. Daneshmend TK, Warnock DW. Clinical pharmacokinetics of systemic antifungal drugs. Clin Pharmacokinet 1983;8:17.

93. Ernst EJ et al. Postantifungal effects of echinocandin, azole, and polyene antifungal agents against Candida albicans and Cryptococcus neoformans. Antimicrob Agents Chemother. 2000;44(4):1108.

94. Gallis HA et al. Amphotericin B: 30 years of clinical experience. Rev Infect Dis 1990;12:308.

95. Cleary JD et al. Inhibition of interleukin 1 release from endotoxin- or amphotericin B- stimulated monocytes. Antimicrob Agents Chemother 1992; 36:977.

96. Cleary JD, Chapman SW. Pharmacologic modulation of prostaglandin E$_2$ (PGE$_2$) production by bacterial endotoxin (LPS) or amphotericin B (AB) stimulated mononuclear cells (MNCs). Paper presented to 31st Annual Interscience Conference on Antimicrobial Agents and Chemotherapy Meeting, Chicago, September 19, 1991.

97. Tynes BS et al. Reducing amphotericin B reactions. Am Rev Respir Dis 1963;87:264.

98. Hoeprich PD. Clinical use of amphotericin B and derivative: lore, mystique, and fact. Clin Infect Dis 1992;14:S114.

99. Gigliotti F et al. Induction of prostaglandin synthesis as the mechanism responsible for the chills and fever produced by infusing amphotericin B. J Infect Dis 1987;156:784.

100. Burks LC et al. Meperidine for the treatment of shaking chills and fever. Arch Intern Med 1980;140:483.

101. Cleary JD et al. Effect of infusion rate on amphotericin B-associated febrile reactions. Drug Intell Clin Pharm 1988;22:769.

102. Oldfield EC III et al. Randomized, double-blind trial of 1-versus 4-hour amphotericin B infusion durations. Antimicrob Agents Chemother 1990; 34:1402.

103. Butler WT et al. Electrocardiographic and electrolyte abnormalities caused by amphotericin B in dog and man. Proc Soc Exp Biol Med 1964; 116:857.

104. Cleary JD et al. Amphotericin B overdose in pediatric patients with associated cardiac arrest. Ann Pharmacother 1993;27:715.

105. Fields BT et al. Effect of rapid intravenous infusion of serum concentrations of amphotericin B. Appl Microbiol 1971;22:615.

106. Bowler WA et al. Risk of ventricular dysrhythmias during 1-hour infusions of amphotericin B in patients with preserved renal function. Antimicrob Agents Chemother 1992;36(11):2542.

107. Branch RA. Prevention of amphotericin B–induced renal impairment: a review on the use of sodium supplementation. Arch Intern Med 1988; 148:2389.

108. Fisher MA et al. Risk factors for amphotericin B-associated nephrotoxicity. Am J Med 1989; 87:547.

109. Lin AC et al. Amphotericin B blunts erythropoietin response to anemia. J Infect Dis 1990; 161:348.

110. Bennett WM et al. Drug prescribing in renal failure: Dosing guidelines for adults. Am J Kidney Dis 1983;3:155.

111. Grant SM, Clissold SP. Fluconazole: a review of its pharmacodynamic and pharmacokinetic properties and therapeutic potential in superficial and systemic mycoses. Drugs 1990;39:877.

112. Daneshmend TK, Warnock DW. Clinical pharmacokinetics of systemic antifungal drugs. Clin Pharmacokinet 1983;8:17.

113. Daneshmend TK, Warnock DW. Clinical pharmacokinetics of ketoconazole. Clin Pharmacokinet 1988;14:13.

114. VanCauteren H et al. Itraconazole pharmacologic studies in animals and humans. Rev Infect Dis 1987;9(Suppl 1):S43.

115. Hardin TC et al. Pharmacokinetics of itraconazole following oral administration to normal volunteers. Antimicrob Agents Chemother 1988;32:1310.

116. Novartis Pharmaceuticals. Lamisil package insert. Summit, NJ: January 1998.

117. Graybill JR. New antifungal agents. Eur J Clin Microbiol Infect Dis 1989;8:402.

118. Wong-Beringer A et al. Lipid formulations of amphotericin B: clinical efficacy and toxicities. Clin Infect Dis 1998;27:603.

119. Cleary JD. Amphotericin B formulated in a lipid emulsion. Ann Pharmacother 1996;30:409.

120. Pelz RK et al. Double-blind placebo-controlled trial of fluconazole to prevent candidal infections in critically ill surgical patients. Ann Surg 2001;233:542.

121. Viscoli C et al. Fluconazole versus amphotericin B as empirical antifungal therapy of unexplained fever in granulocytopenic cancer patients: a pragmatic, multicentre, prospective and randomised clinical trial. Eur J Cancer 1996;32A(5):814.

122. Ezdinli EZ et al. Oral amphotericin for Candidiases in patients with hematologic neoplasms. J Am Med Assoc 1979;242:258.

123. Degregorio MW et al. Candida infections in patients with acute leukemia: ineffectiveness of nystatin prophylaxis and relationship between oropharyngeal and systemic candidiasis. Cancer 1982;50:2780.

124. Hofstra W et al. Concentrations of nystatin in feces after oral administration of various doses of nystatin. Infection 1979;7:166.

125. Shepp DH et al. Comparative trial of ketoconazole and nystatin for prevention of fungal infection in neutropenic patients treated in a protective environment. J Infect Dis 1985;152:1257.

126. Cuttner J et al. Clotrimazole treatment for prevention of oral candidiasis in patients with acute leukemia undergoing chemotherapy. Am J Med 1986; 81:771.

127. Yeo E et al. Prophylaxis of oropharyngeal candidiasis with clotrimazole. J Clin Oncol 1985; 3:1668.

128. Owens NJ et al. Prophylaxis of oral candidiasis with clotrimazole trochees. Arch Intern Med 1984;290.

129. Slotman GJ, Burchard KW. Ketoconazole prevents Candida sepsis in critically ill surgical patients. Arch Surg 1987;122:147.

130. Samonia G et al. Prophylaxis of oropharyngeal candidiasis with fluconazole. Rev Infect Dis 1990;12:5369.

131. Tricot G et al. Ketoconazole vs itraconazole for antifungal prophylaxis in patients with severe granulocytopenia: preliminary results of two non-randomized studies. Rev Infect Dis 1987;9:S94.

132. Ang BSP et al. Candidemia from a urinary tract source: microbiological aspects and clinical significance. Clin Infect Dis 1993;17:662.

133. Fong IW et al. Fungicidal effect of amphotericin B in urine: in vitro study to assess feasibility of bladder washout for localization of site of candiduria. Antimicrob Agents Chemother 1991; 35(9):1856.

134. Vergis EN et al. A randomized controlled trial of oral fluconazole and local amphotericin B for treatment of Candida funguria in hospitalized patients. Paper presented to Infectious Diseases Society Meeting. San Francisco, September 14, 1997.

135. Jacobs LG et al. Oral fluconazole compared with bladder irrigation with amphotericin B for treat-

ment of fungal urinary tract infections in elderly patients. Clin Infect Dis 1996;22:30.

136. Fujihior S et al. Flucytosine in the treatment of urinary fungal infections: clinical efficacy and background factors. Jpn J Antibiot 1991;44:14.

137. Graybill JR et al. Ketoconazole therapy for fungal urinary tract infections. J Urol 1983;29:68.

138. Symoens J et al. An evaluation of two years of clinical experience with ketoconazole. Rev Infect Dis 1980;2:674.

139. Ikemoto H. A clinical study of fluconazole for the treatment of deep mycoses. Diag Microbiol Infect Dis 1989;12(Suppl 4):239S.

140. Parker JD et al. A decade of experience with blastomycosis and its treatment with amphotericin B. Am Rev Respir Dis 1969;99:895.

141. National Institute of Allergy and Infectious Diseases Mycoses Study Group. Treatment of blastomycosis and histoplasmosis with ketoconazole: results of a prospective, randomized clinical trial. Ann Intern Med 1985;103:861.

142. Bradsher RW. Blastomycosis in systemic fungal infections: diagnosis and treatment I. Infect Dis Clin North Am 1988;2:877.

143. Pappas PG. Treatment of blastomycosis with higher doses of fluconazole. Clin Infect Dis 1997;25:200.

144. Chapman SW. *Blastomyces dermatitidis*. In: Mandell GL et al, eds. Principles and Practice of Infectious Diseases. New York: Churchill Livingstone, 1990;1999.

145. Fed Reg 1980;44:37434.

146. King CT et al. Antifungal therapy during pregnancy. Clin Infect Dis 1998;27:115.

147. Pursley TJ. Fluconazole- induced congenital anomalies in three infants. Clin Infect Dis 1996;22:336.

148. Wheat LJ. Histoplasmosis in systemic fungal infections: diagnosis and treatment I. Infect Dis Clin North Am 1988;2:841.

149. Sutliff WD et al. Histoplasmosis cooperative study. Am Rev Respir Dis 1964;89:641.

150. Johnson PC et al. Safety and efficacy of liposomal amphotericin B compared with conventional amphotericin B for induction therapy of histoplasmosis in patients with AIDS. Ann Intern Med 2002; 137:105.

151. Pont A et al. Ketoconazole blocks adrenal steroid synthesis. Ann Intern Med 1982;97:370.

152. Lyman CA, Walsh TJ. Systemically administered antifungal agents. Drugs 1992;44:9.

153. Beale M et al. Randomized, double-blind study of the safety and antifungal activity of ravuconazole relative to fluconazole in esophageal candidiasis. Paper presented to 42nd Interscience Conference on Antimicrobial Agents Chemotherapy, San Diego, September 27, 2002.

154. Hachem RY et al. An open, non-comparative multicenter study to evaluate efficacy and safety of posaconazole (SCH 56592) in the treatment of invasive fungal infections refractory to or intolerant to standard therapy. Paper presented to 42nd Interscience Conference on Antimicrobial Agents Chemotherapy, San Diego, September 27, 2002.

155. Honig PK et al. Terfenadine-ketoconazole interactions: pharmacokinetic and electrocardiographic consequences. JAMA 1993;269:1513.

156. Glynn AM et al. Effects of ketoconazole on methylprednisolone pharmacokinetics and cortisol secretion. Clin Pharmacol Ther 1986;39:654.

157. Stevens DA. *Coccidioides immitis*. In: Mandell GL et al., eds. Principles and Practice of Infectious Diseases. New York: Churchill Livingstone, 1990:1989.

158. Peter JB. Use and Interpretation of Tests in Medical Microbiology. 3rd Ed. Santa Monica, CA: Specialty Laboratories, 1992.

159. Galgiani JN et al. New serologic tests for early detection of coccidioidomycosis. J Infect Dis 1991;163:671.

160. Ratcheson RA, Ommaya AK. Experience with the subcutaneous cerebrospinal fluid reservoir: a preliminary report of 60 cases. N Engl J Med 1968;279:1.

161. Salaki JS. Fungal and yeast infections of the central nervous system: a clinical review. Medicine 1984;63:108.

162. Oldfield EC et al. Prediction of relapse after treatment of coccidioidomycosis. Clin Infect Dis 1997;25(5):1205.

163. Shehab ZM et al. Imidazole therapy of coccidioidal meningitis in children. Pediatr Infect Dis J 1988;7:40.

164. Galgiani JN et al. Fluconazole therapy for coccidioidal meningitis. Ann Intern Med 1993;119:28.

165. Labadie EL, Hamilton RH. Survival improvement in Coccidioidal meningitis by high dose intrathecal amphotericin B. Arch Intern Med 1986; 146:2013.

166. Caspofungin package insert Merck Pharmaceuticals. Caspofungin package insert. Bluebell, PA: January 2003.

167. Pfizer Pharmaceuticals. Vfend package insert. Groton, CT: January 2003.

168. Vermes A et al. Flucytosine: a review of its pharmacology, clinical indications, pharmacokinetics, toxicity and drug interactions. J Antimicrob Chemother. 2000;46(2):171.

169. Brammer KW, Tarbit MH. A review of the pharmacokinetics of fluconazole (UK-49,858) in laboratory animals and man. In: Fromtling RA ed. Recent Trends in the Discovery, Development and Evaluation of Antifungal Agents. Barcelona: JR Prous Science Publishers, 1987:141.

170. Brammer KW et al. Pharmacokinetics and tissue penetration of fluconazole in humans. Rev Infect Dis 1990;12(Suppl 3):S318.

171. Phillips P et al. Tolerance to and efficacy of itraconazole in treatment of systemic mycoses: preliminary results. Rev Infect Dis 1987; 9(Suppl1):S87.

172. Knoper SR, Galgiani JN. Coccidioidomycosis. Infect Dis Clin North Am 1988;2:861.

173. Armstrong D. Problems in management of opportunistic fungal diseases. Rev Infect Dis 1989; 11:1591.

174. Galgiani JN et al. Ketoconazole therapy of progressive coccidioidomycoses: comparison of 400 and 800 mg doses and observations at higher doses. Am J Med 1988;84:603.

175. Craven PC et al. High-dose ketoconazole for treatment of fungal infections of the central nervous system. Ann Intern Med 1983;98:160.

176. Witorsch P et al. Intraventricular administration of amphotericin B. J Am Med Assoc 1965;194:109.

177. Sung JP et al. Intravenous and intrathecal miconazole therapy for systemic mycoses. West J Med 1977;126:5.

178. Harrison HR et al. Amphotericin B and imidazole therapy for coccidioidal meningitis in children. Pediatr Infect Dis 1983;2:216.

179. Fisher JF, Dewald J. Parkinsonism associated with intraventricular amphotericin B. J Antimicrob Chemother 1983;12:97.

180. Winn RE et al. Acute toxic delirium: neurotoxicity of intrathecal administration of amphotericin B. Arch Intern Med 1979;139:706.

181. Haber RW, Joseph MJ. Neurologic manifestations after amphotericin B therapy. Br Med J 1962;1:230.

182. Carnevale NT et al. Amphotericin-induced myelopathy. Arch Int Med 1980;140:1189.

183. Anaissie EJ et al. Management of invasive candidal infections: results of a prospective, randomized, multicenter study of fluconazole versus amphotericin B and review of the literature. Clin Infect Dis 1996;23(5):964.

184. Patterson TF. New agents for treatment of invasive aspergillosis. Clin Infect Dis 2002;35:367.

185. Bowden R et al. A double-blind, randomized, controlled trial of amphotericin B colloidal dispersion versus amphotericin B for treatment of invasive aspergillosis in immunocompromised patients. Clin Infect Dis 2002;35:359.

186. White MH et al. Amphotericin B colloidal dispersion vs. amphotericin B as therapy for invasive aspergillosis. Clin Infect Dis 1997;24:635.

187. Leenders ACAP. Liposomal amphotericin B (AmBisome) compared with amphotericin B both fol-

lowed by oral fluconazole in the treatment of AIDS-associated cryptococcal meningitis. AIDS 1997;11:1463.

188. Sharkey PK et al. Amphotericin B lipid complex compared with amphotericin B in the treatment of cryptococcal meningitis in patients with AIDS. Clin Infect Dis 1996;22:329.

189. Cleary JD, Ziska DS. Lipid-associated amphotericin B. Florida J Hosp Pharm 1994;14:19.

190. Sacks GS et al. Nutritional impact of lipid-associated amphotericin B formulations. Ann Pharmacotherapy 1997;31:121.

191. Stevens DA et al. Practice guidelines for diseases caused by *Aspergillus*. Infectious Diseases Society of America. Clin Infect Dis 2000;30:696.

192. Herbrecht R et al. Voriconazole versus amphotericin B for primary therapy of invasive aspergillosis. N Engl J Med 2002;347:408.

193. Larsen RA et al. Fluconazole compared with amphotericin B plus flucytosine for cryptococcal meningitis in AIDS: a randomized trial. Ann Intern Med 1990;113:183.

194. Bennett JE et al. A comparison of amphotericin B alone and combined with flucytosine in the treatment of cryptococcal meningitis. N Engl J Med 1979;301:126.

195. Saag MS et al. Comparison of amphotericin B with fluconazole in the treatment of acute AIDS associated cryptococcal meningitis. N Engl J Med 1992; 326:83.

196. Dismukes WE et al. Treatment of cryptococcal meningitis with combination amphotericin B and flucytosine for 4 as compared with 6 weeks. N Engl J Med 1987;317:334.

197. Hibberd PL, Rubin RH. Clinical aspects of fungal infection in organ transplant recipients. Clin Infect Dis 1994;19:S33.

198. Newton PN et al. A randomized, double-blind, placebo-controlled trial of acetazolamide for the treatment of elevated intracranial pressure in cryptococcal meningitis. Clin Infect Dis 2002;35:769.

199. Kauffman CA, Framd PT. Bone marrow toxicity associated with 5-fluorocytosine therapy. Antimicrob Agents Chemother 1977;11:244.

200. Craven PC, Graybill JR. Combination of oral flucytosine and ketoconazole as therapy for experimental cryptococcal meningitis. J Infect Dis 1984;149:584.

201. Fed Reg 1982;47:12480.

202. Walsh TJ et al. Safety, tolerance, and pharmacokinetics of high-dose liposomal amphotericin B (AmBisome) in patients infected with Aspergillus species and other filamentous fungi: Maximum tolerated dose study. Antimicrob Agents Chemother 2001;45:3487.

203. Stone JA et al. Single- and multiple-dose pharmacokinetics of caspofungin in healthy men. Antimicrob Agents Chemother 2002;46:739.

204. Hajdu R et al. Preliminary animal pharmacokinetics of the parenteral antifungal agent MK-0991 (L-743,872). Antimicrob Agents Chemother 1997;41:2339.

205. Patterson BE et al. UK-109,496, a novel, widespectrum triazole derivative for the treatment of fungal infections: disposition in man. In: Program and Abstracts of the 35th Interscience Conference on Antimicrob Agents Chemother, San Francisco, CA. September 18, 1995. Abstract F79, p.126. American Society for Microbiology, Washington, DC.

206. Schwartz S et al. Successful treatment of cerebral aspergillosis with a novel triazole (voriconazole) in a patient with acute leukaemia. Br J Haematol 1997;97:663.

207. Courtney R et al. Effect of food and antacid on the pharmacokinetics of posaconazole in healthy volunteers. Paper presented to 42nd Interscience Conference on Antimicrobial Agents Chemotherapy. San Diego, September 27, 2002.

208. Courtney R et al. Effect of cimetidine of the pharmacokinetics of posaconazole in healthy volunteers Paper presented to 42nd Interscience Conference on Antimicrobial Agents Chemotherapy. San Diego, September 27, 2002.

209. Ezzet F et al. The pharmacokinetics of posaconazole in neutropenic oncology patients. Paper presented to 42nd Interscience Conference on Antimicrobial Agents Chemotherapy. San Diego, September 27, 2002.

210. Krieter P et al. Pharmacokinetics and excretion of 14C-posaconazole following oral administration in healthy male subjects. Paper presented to 42nd Interscience Conference on Antimicrobial Agents Chemotherapy. San Diego, September 27, 2002.

211. Grasela DM et al. Ravuconazole: multiple ascending oral dose study in healthy subjects. Paper presented to 42nd Interscience Conference on Antimicrobial Agents Chemotherapy. San Diego, September 27, 2002.

CHAPTER 72

Viral Infections

Milap C. Nahata, Neeta Bahal O'Mara, Sandra Benavides

Viral infections are common causes of human disease. An estimated 60% of illnesses in developed countries result from viruses, compared with only 15% from bacteria. These may include the common cold, chickenpox, measles, mumps, influenza, bronchitis, gastroenteritis, hepatitis, poliomyelitis, rabies, and numerous diseases caused by the herpesvirus. Most of the U.S. population is affected each year by at least one upper respiratory tract infection, such as the common cold or influenza.[1] Although most of these patients have a self-limiting illness, certain viral infections, such as influenza, can cause significant mortality, particularly in the elderly. For example, in the worldwide influenza epidemic of 1918 and 1919, 500 million people became infected and 20 million died.[1] Influenza vaccines can reduce the impact of this illness in susceptible populations, but there are no vaccines against many other potentially severe viral infections, including herpes encephalitis, neonatal herpes, and emerging viral infections, such as West Nile Virus. Therefore, the need for safe and effective antiviral agents is obvious.

Substantial progress has been made in antiviral chemotherapy as a result of advances in molecular virology and genetic engineering. Antiviral agents can be designed to inhibit functions specific to viruses; this maximizes their therapeutic benefits while minimizing adverse effects to the host cell.

Current technology also permits rapid diagnosis of viral diseases. It is now possible to make a specific diagnosis of several viral illnesses within hours to a few days; previously, specific diagnosis took days to months. This has made it possible to select an appropriate antiviral drug early for the treatment of acute viral infection.

The primary objective of this chapter is to describe the etiology, pathogenesis, and treatment of common viral infections. Specific case presentations illustrate the optimal use of antiviral drugs in patients with viral infections.

HERPES SIMPLEX VIRUS INFECTIONS

Herpesvirus is an extremely important pathogen in humans. It causes many illnesses, including herpes encephalitis and neonatal herpes, which are associated with significant mortality and sequelae, and genital herpes, which causes substantial pain and emotional suffering. Fortunately, antiviral drugs can decrease the morbidity, mortality, and duration of symptoms in most cases.[2]

Herpes Encephalitis

Herpes simplex virus (HSV) encephalitis is the most common sporadic viral infection of the central nervous system (CNS). The estimated incidence is approximately 2.3 cases per million population per year, although this may be an underestimate because of the difficulty in diagnosing this disease. It can occur at any age and is characterized by the acute onset of fever, headache, decreased consciousness, and seizures. Any child with fever and altered behavior should be evaluated carefully. This is a devastating infection: without treatment, mortality approaches 70%, and only 2.5% of patients recover enough to lead normal lives.[2]

HSV-1 is the etiologic agent in most patients with herpes encephalitis, but HSV-2 is more common in newborns. The infection may be localized to the brain or involve cutaneous and mucous membranes. Although any area of the brain can be involved, the orbital region of the frontal lobes and portions of the temporal lobes are affected most often.

Herpes encephalitis often is difficult to diagnose and is always a very serious disease. A computed tomography (CT) scan usually is indicated to rule out other conditions, including a brain abscess or other space-occupying lesions that may produce similar symptoms. The CT or radionucleotide scans may be unremarkable early in the course of the disease.

Cerebrospinal fluid (CSF) examination usually reveals pleocytosis (predominately lymphocytes) with 50 to 2,000 white blood cells (WBCs)/mm³. Polymorphonuclear leukocytosis and red blood cells (RBCs) also may be seen. Many patients have an elevated protein level in the CSF (median, 80 mg/dL). The presence of antibody to HSV-1 is useful in making the diagnosis.

The electroencephalogram (EEG) is the most sensitive but least specific test. There usually are CT or brain scan abnormalities, but these may take a day or two longer to appear. The EEG, CT, and brain scan findings compatible with HSV encephalitis can be mimicked by other conditions, and a brain biopsy is required to clearly establish the diagnosis. Rapid diagnosis of herpes encephalitis by a polymerase chain reaction assay of HSV DNA in the CSF is available at certain medical centers. This is a highly sensitive, specific, and rapid method for the diagnosis of herpes encephalitis.[3]

Clinical Presentation

1. **R.F., a 7-year-old boy weighing 20 kg, was seen in the emergency department (ED) after a seizure. Over the previous 3 days, R.F. had decreased appetite, headache, and fever (101° to 102°F) and was lethargic and disoriented. His leukocyte count was 13,000/mm³ with a shift to the left. Ceftriaxone (50 mg/kg given intravenously [IV] Q 12 hr) and dexamethasone (0.15 mg/kg IV Q 6 hr) were initiated for presumed bacterial meningitis. Phenobarbital (5 mg/kg IV Q 24 hr) was given for seizure control. The CSF was normal, and no bacteria could be identified. Over the next 2 days, R.F. became increasingly less responsive and lapsed into a coma. A CT scan of the brain revealed decreased density in a localized area of the left temporal lobe. Because of a high suspicion of herpes encephalitis, a brain biopsy was performed. Acyclovir 10 mg/kg IV Q 8 hr was started immediately after the procedure. HSV-1 was isolated from the biopsy specimen 24 hours later. What findings in R.F. are consistent with the diagnosis of herpes encephalitis? Why was a brain biopsy performed?**

[SI unit: leukocytes, 13 × 10⁹]

Fever, headache, lethargy, and disorientation are common features of herpes encephalitis. As illustrated by R.F., the CSF examination can be normal in some patients. The CT scan showing decreased density in the left temporal lobe is suggestive of herpes encephalitis. Finally, a negative CSF culture

also suggests the absence of a bacterial infection. However, these findings cannot establish the diagnosis of herpes encephalitis.

Brain biopsy is the most definitive diagnostic procedure for herpes encephalitis. Biopsy is particularly important because other treatable conditions, including cryptococcosis and aspergillosis, can be missed by other diagnostic procedures. The morbidity (bleeding) caused by brain biopsy is low (1%) in medical centers with extensive experience.

Treatment: Acyclovir

2. **As expected, a specific pathogen (HSV-1) was isolated from the biopsy specimen in R.F. What is the treatment of choice for R.F.'s herpes encephalitis?**

Two studies comparing acyclovir and vidarabine have demonstrated that IV acyclovir (10 mg/kg Q 8 hr for 10 days) is the treatment of choice in patients with herpes encephalitis.[4,5] The mortality was 19% to 28% in the acyclovir-treated group and 50% to 54% in the vidarabine-treated group. Of great importance was the fact that nearly half of the acyclovir-treated patients returned to normal life, compared with only 13% to 15% of those treated with vidarabine.[6] In addition, acyclovir is less toxic than vidarabine. Currently, vidarabine is not marketed in the United States.

Acyclovir-resistant herpes is not an important consideration in the management of herpes encephalitis in most patients, but it can be important in AIDS or other immunocompromised patients who receive multiple repeated courses of acyclovir (see Chapter 70, Opportunistic Infections in HIV-Infected Patients). Foscarnet has been successfully used in immunocompromised patients with acyclovir-resistant HSV.[7,8]

Acyclovir is the treatment of choice for R.F. because it has been shown to decrease morbidity in patients with herpes encephalitis.

ACYCLOVIR PHARMACOKINETICS

3. **Why is the acyclovir dosage regimen appropriate based on the serum concentrations required for the inhibition of viral replication? How should the effect of acyclovir be monitored in R.F.?**

In adults receiving single IV doses of acyclovir 2.5 to 5 mg/kg, a peak plasma concentration of 3.4 to 6.8 μg/mL has been reported.[9,10] The mean peak and trough plasma concentrations were 9.9 and 0.7 μg/mL, respectively, after multiple doses of 5 mg/kg every 8 hours.[11] At larger IV doses of 10 to 15 mg/kg, the peak plasma concentrations of acyclovir have ranged from 10 to 30 μg/mL[12] (Tables 72-1 and 72-2).

Limited data are available on acyclovir pharmacokinetics in children, particularly premature infants. Acyclovir pharmacokinetics for children >1 year of age are similar to those of adults[13] (see Table 72-1). In neonates receiving acyclovir 5 to 15 mg/kg IV Q 8 hr, the peak and trough serum concentrations have ranged from 3.1 to 38 μg/mL and 0.23 to 30 μg/mL, respectively.[14,15] Acyclovir distributes into all tissues, with the highest concentrations occurring in the kidney (10 times the plasma concentration) and the lowest concentrations in the CSF (25% to 70% of plasma concentration).[12] For R.F., the regimen is appropriate (Table 72-3). Although the phar-

Table 72-1 Pharmacokinetic Properties of Antiviral Drugs

Drug	Dose Used in Study	Peak Serum Concentrations (μg/mL)	% Recovered Unchanged in Urine	Elimination Half-Life (hr)
Acyclovir[12,20,21,139,140]	5 mg/kg IV	9.8	52–82	1.8–3.1
Amantadine[81]	100–300 mg/day	0.2–0.6	52–88	15–20
Famciclovir[141,142]	500 mg PO	3.3–4[a]	60–73[a]	2.3–3.0[a]
Oseltamivir[b, 143]	100 mg × 1	0.2–5	5	6.7–8.2
Ribavirin[102]	0.82 mg/kg × 20 hr	1–3	—	6.5–11
Rimantadine[c, 144]	100–200 mg/day	0.11–0.42	8	24–37
Valacyclovir[145, 146]	1,000 mg PO	5.7–6.7[d]	46–80[d]	2.5–3.3[d]
Zanamivir[147, 148]	10 mg IN BID	0.054–0.097	5	2.5–5.1

[a]Pharmacokinetic properties of active metabolite, penciclovir.
[b]Serum concentration 10-fold lower and nasal wash concentration 1,000-fold higher after administration of aerosolized rimantadine, 20 μg/L of air than oral rimantadine, 200 mg.
[c]Tracheal concentration 1 μg/mL; cerebrospinal fluid concentration about 60% of plasma concentration.
[d]Pharmacokinetic properties of active metabolite, acyclovir.

Table 72-2 Clinical Pharmacokinetics of Antiviral Drugs

Drug	Type of Patient	Total Clearance	Volume of Distribution	Elimination Half-Life (hr)	Comments
Acyclovir[10,13,15,20]	Adults	307 mL/min/1.73 m²	59 L/1.73 m²	2.5–3.0	Use 100% of recommended dose but extend dosage interval to 12 and 24 hr if Cl_{Cr} ranges from 25–50 and 10–25 mL/min/1.73 m², respectively; use 50% of recommended dose Q 24 hr if Cl_{Cr} ranges from 0–10 mL/min/1.73 m².
	Neonates	98–122 mL/min/1.73 m²	24–30 L/1.73 m²	3.2–4.1	
Amantadine[102]	Adults	2.5–10.5 L/hr	1.5–6.1 L/kg	22.6–37.7	Adjust doses in renal failure: 20 mg on day 1 and then 100 mg/day if Cl_{Cr} 30–50; 200 mg on day 1 and then 100 mg QOD if Cl_{Cr} 15–29; 200 mg Q 7 days if Cl_{Cr} <15 mL/min/1.73 m₂.
Famciclovir[141,142,149]	Adults	0.37–0.48 L/hr/kg	1.5 L/kg	2.2–3.0	Use 100% of recommended dose but extend dosage interval to 12 and 24 hr if Cl_{Cr} ranges from 40–59 and 20–39 mL/min, respectively; use 250 mg Q 48 hr if Cl_{Cr} <20 mL/min.
Oseltamivir[79,143]	Adults	18.8 L/hr (renal clearance)	NA	6.7–8.2	Use 75 mg/day in patients if Cl_{Cr} 10–30 mL/min. The effect of hepatic impairment has not been determined.
	Pediatrics (1–12 yr)	0.63 L/h/kg	NA	7.8	Dosage recommendations are based on body weight and age. Use 30 mg BID if patient is 15 kg and 1–3 yr, 45 mg if patient is 15–23 kg and 4–7 yr, 60 mg if patient is 23–40 kg and 8–12 yr and normal adult dose if >40 kg and >13 years.
	Adolescents	0.32 L/h/kg	NA	8.1 hr	

Continued

Table 72-2 Clinical Pharmacokinetics of Antiviral Drugs—cont'd

Drug	Type of Patient	Total Clearance	Volume of Distribution	Elimination Half-Life (hr)	Comments
Rimantadine[150,151]	Adults	20–48 L/hr	25 L/kg	29–37	Because it undergoes extensive metabolism, dose may have to be adjusted in patients with severe liver disease. Dose adjustments may also be necessary in elderly and in those with severe renal failure (Cl_{Cr} <10 mL/min). Manufacturer recommends 50% reduction in such cases.
Valacyclovir	See acyclovir				
Zanamivir[80]	Adults	2.5–10.9 L/hr	15.9 L	2.5–5.1	4–17% of inhaled dose systemically absorbed. Although only limited studies with renal or hepatic impairment, dosing adjustment likely unnecessary.
Valganciclovir	See ganciclovir				

Table 72-3 FDA-Indicated Drugs for Various Viral Infections

Disease	Drug	Dosage (Age Group)	Route	Duration
Herpes encephalitis	Acyclovir (Zovirax)[a]	*Adults:* 10 mg/kg Q 8 hr *6 mo–12 yr:* 500 mg/m² Q 8 hr	IV	10 days
Neonatal herpes	Acyclovir (Zovirax)	10–20 mg/kg Q 8 hr	IV	14–21 days
Mucocutaneous herpes (immunocompromised patients)	Acyclovir (Zovirax)	*Adults:* 5 mg/kg Q 8 hr	IV	7 days
Varicella-zoster (immunocompromised patients)	Acyclovir (Zovirax)[a]	*Adults:* 10 mg/kg Q 8 h *Children:* 500 mg/m² Q 8 hr	IV IV	7 days
Herpes zoster (normal host)	Acyclovir (Zovirax) or famciclovir (Famvir) valacyclovir (Valtrex)	800 mg 5×/day 500 mg TID 1,000 mg TID	PO PO PO	7–10 days 7 days 7 days
Varicella (chickenpox)	Acyclovir (Zovirax)	*Adults and children >2 yr:* 20 mg/kg (≤800 mg) QID	PO	5 days
Herpes keratitis	Trifluridine 1% ophthalmic solution (Viroptic)	1 drop Q 2 hr; then 1 drop Q 4 hr	Topical	Until corneal ulcer reepithelialized, 7 days
Cytomegalovirus retinitis (immunocompromised patients)	Ganciclovir (Cytovene)	5 mg/kg Q 12 hr; then 5 mg/kg/day or 6 mg/kg, 5 days a week	IV	14–21 days for induction; maintenance
	Cidofovir (Vistide)	5 mg/kg Q week ×2, then Q 2 weeks	IV	Maintenance
	Foscarnet (Foscavir)	90 mg/kg Q 12 hr, then 90 mg/kg Q day	IV	Induction ×2 weeks; maintenance
	Valganciclovir (Valcyte)	900 mg BID, 900 mg QD	PO	Induction ×21 days; maintenance
Influenza A	Amantadine (Symmetrel)	*Adults and children >9 yr:* 100 mg BID *Children 19 yr:* 4.4–8.8 mg/kg/day but <150 mg/day	PO	10 days (treatment), 14–21 days (protection with vaccine), 90 days (protection without vaccine)

Table 72-3   FDA-Indicated Drugs for Various Viral Infections—cont'd

Disease	Drug	Dosage (Age Group)	Route	Duration
	Rimantadine (Flumadine)	*Adults and children ≥10 yr:* 100 mg BID *Children 1–10 yr:* 5 mg/kg/day (<150 mg/day)	PO	7 days (treatment) up to 6 wk for prophylaxis (not approved for treatment in children)
Influenza A and B	Oseltamivir (Tamiflu)	*Adults:* 75 mg BID *Adults:* 75 mg QD	PO PO	5 days (treatment) Up to 6 weeks for prophylaxis
	Zanamivir	*Adults and children >12 yr:* 10 mg (2 inhalations) BID	Inhalation	5 days treatment
Respiratory syncytial virus	Ribavirin (Virazole)	6 g in 300 mL over 12–18 hr/day	Inhalation	3–7 days

*a*Foscarnet 40 mg/kg IV Q 8 hr is recommended for acyclovir-resistant herpes simplex virus or varicella-zoster virus.

macokinetics in children >1 year are similar to those in adults, higher dosages are needed in view of its relatively poor distribution into CSF.

In clinical trials of acyclovir, HSV-1 clinical isolates have a mean ID_{50} of 0.46 μg/mL.[21] However, antiviral susceptibility testing can be affected by many variables, including the amount of inoculum and the testing method used. The results of antiviral susceptibility tests are usually reported as ID_{50} (the serum concentration necessary to produce 50% inhibition of the viral cytopathic effect) ID_{90} may correlate better than ID_{50} with clinical outcome, but the results are unpredictable.[17] Consequently, the clinical status of patients is monitored for efficacy of acyclovir. Most patients begin to improve within 48 hours after starting treatment.

ADVERSE EFFECTS

4. What type of adverse effects can occur as a result of IV acyclovir therapy in R.F.? How should these be monitored, and how can they be minimized?

Acyclovir is a relatively safe drug, but renal toxicity associated with IV acyclovir should be considered (Table 72-4). Blood urea nitrogen (BUN) and serum creatinine (SrCr) levels can increase in approximately 5% to 10% of patients. These changes appear to be reversible. Acyclovir is relatively insoluble: maximum urine solubility at 37°C is 1.3 mg/mL. Therefore, a transient crystal nephropathy may occur at high acyclovir concentrations.[18]

Other common adverse effects include gastrointestinal (GI) complaints such as nausea and vomiting and neurologic disturbances including lethargy, tremors, confusion, hallucinations, and seizures.[18,19] Neurotoxicity appears to be more common in patients with impaired renal function and tends to be reversible. Transient elevation of liver enzymes may occur. Finally, IV acyclovir can cause phlebitis and pain at the injection site.[18] This can be minimized by administering acyclovir at a concentration of about 5 mg/mL (maximum, 7 mg/mL).[19]

Renal function tests, including BUN, SrCr, and urine output, should be monitored closely. To minimize the risk of acyclovir nephrotoxicity, R.F. should be well hydrated and each acyclovir dose should be infused over 1 hour. In addition, the IV infusion site should be inspected for inflammation and pain, and R.F. should be asked about pain at the infusion site.

CONVERSION TO ORAL THERAPY

5. After 7 days of IV acyclovir, R.F. is alert, responsive, actively moving about, and eating a normal diet. The intern suggests switching him to oral acyclovir and discontinuing IV therapy. Why is this not appropriate?

Oral therapy is inappropriate for R.F. Based on studies in adults, the absorption of acyclovir after oral administration is variable, slow, and incomplete. The bioavailability of acyclovir is low (F = 0.15 to 0.30) and decreases with increasing doses.[20] The mean peak plasma concentration, occurring at 1.5 to 2 hours, has ranged from only 0.15 to 1.3 μg/mL after multiple acyclovir doses of 200 to 600 mg Q 4 hr.[20,21] Thus, the concentrations of acyclovir in the CSF may be inadequate for R.F. Therapy with IV acyclovir should be continued to complete a 10-day course (see Table 72-3).

Neonatal Herpes

Most neonates acquire herpes from the infected genital secretions of the mother at delivery. The incidence ranges from 1 in 3,000 to 5,000 deliveries per year in the United States. The infection can present in one of three forms: localized to the skin, eye, and mouth (45%); encephalitis (35%); or disseminated disease (25%). The effects of neonatal herpes can be devastating, and severe handicaps persist in many afflicted children.[22] The mortality has ranged from 15% in those with CNS involvement to 50% in those with disseminated disease.[23] Neonatal HSV-1 infections also may be acquired after birth through contact with family members with symptomatic or asymptomatic oral-labial HSV-1 infection or from nosocomial

Table 72-4 FDA-Indicated Drugs for Various Viral Infections

Adverse Effects of Approved Antiviral Drugs

Drug	Adverse Effects
Acyclovir	Local irritation and phlebitis (9%); increased SrCr and BUN (5–10%); nausea and vomiting (7%); itching and rash (2%); increased liver transaminases (1–2%); CNS toxicity (1%)
Amantadine	Nausea, dizziness (light-headedness), and insomnia (5–10%); depression, anxiety, irritability, hallucination, confusion, dry mouth; constipation, ataxia, headache, peripheral edema, and orthostatic hypotension (1–5%)
Cidofovir	Nephrotoxicity (59%); nausea, vomiting, fever, asthenia, neutropenia (24%), rash, headache, diarrhea, alopecia, anemia, abdominal pain
Famciclovir	Headache (6–9%); nausea (4–5%); diarrhea (1–2%)
Foscarnet	Renal dysfunction (14%); fever, nausea, anemia, diarrhea, seizure, headache, vomiting, bone marrow suppression (10%)
Ganciclovir	Decreased Hgb, Hct, WBC count, and platelet count; fever, diarrhea, anorexia, vomiting, neuropathy, nausea, rash; retinal detachment (11%)
Oseltamivir	Nausea, vomiting (9–10%); vertigo (1%)
Ribavirin	Worsening of respiratory status, bacterial pneumonia, pneumothorax, apnea, ventilator dependence; cardiac arrest, hypotension; rash and conjunctivitis
Rimantadine	CNS (insomnia, dizziness, headache, nervousness, fatigue) and GI (nausea, vomiting, anorexia, dry mouth abdominal pain) (1–3%)
Trifluridine	Burning or stinging upon instillation (4.6%); palpebral edema (2.8%); keratopathy, hypersensitivity reaction, stromal edema, hyperemia, increased intraocular pressure
Valacyclovir	Headache (13–17%); nausea (10–16%); vomiting (1–7%); diarrhea (1–5%)
Valgancyclovir	Decreased Hgb, Hct, WBC count, and platelet count; diarrhea, nausea, vomiting, abdominal pain, fever, headache, insomnia, peripheral neuropathy, retinal detachment
Zanamivir	Bronchospasm, decline in respiratory function, especially if underlying respiratory disease; nasal/throat irritation; headache (2%); cough (2%)

BUN, blood urea nitrogen; CNS, central nervous system; GI, gastrointestinal; Hgb, hemoglobin; Hct, hematocrit; ScCr, serum creatinine; WBC, white blood cell.

transmission. When the virus is transmitted from the mother, clinical evidence of infection in the neonate usually is present 5 to 17 days after birth. Although skin vesicles are the hallmark of infection, at least one third to one half of neonates never have skin lesions.[24] In 70% of patients, the disease may progress from isolated skin lesions to involve other organs, including the lungs, liver, spleen, CNS, and eyes.

Diagnosis of this infection can be made by direct fluorescent antibody examination of epithelial cells from the infant or the mother. Examination of the base of a vesicular lesion may show giant cells and intranuclear inclusions, which are characteristic of HSV infections. Serologic test results also are helpful in making a specific diagnosis of neonatal herpes.

Risk Factors

6. S.P., an 18-year-old woman, was admitted to labor and delivery with premature rupture of the membranes. Four hours later, S.P. vaginally delivered a 2.5-kg baby boy, R.P., who had an estimated gestational age of 33 weeks. Twenty-four hours after delivery, S.P. reported the onset of vesicles in the genital area; she had a history of previous episodes of genital herpes. The last infection was during her first trimester of pregnancy. Is R.P. at risk of developing herpes infection?

R.P. is at risk of acquiring herpes infection because the mother had genital herpes during the first trimester and because he was delivered vaginally rather than by cesarean section. The risk of a newborn acquiring the disease from an infected mother with primary disease is about 35%; that from a mother with reactivation is 3%.

Treatment: Acyclovir

7. Ten days after birth, R.P. developed poor feeding patterns, irritability, and respiratory distress. Three days later, skin lesions appeared. How should R.P. be treated?

R.P. is manifesting signs of HSV infection and should be treated with antiviral therapy (see Table 72-3). The drug of choice for neonatal herpes simplex virus infections is acyclovir.[24–26] Vidarabine was the first antiviral agent used in the treatment of neonatal HSV. Because of the drastic reduction in morbidity, it became the standard of therapy to which other antiviral agents were compared. In clinical trials comparing vidarabine with acyclovir, acyclovir was shown to be as effective as vidarabine in infants with skin, eye, mouth (SEM) involvement, encephalitis, and disseminated HSV infection.[27] Although both agents were equally effective, acyclovir was safer and easier to administer, making it the standard of care for neonatal HSV.

Administration

8. What dosage of acyclovir should R.P. receive?

An IV dosage of 30 mg/kg given in three divided doses has been shown to be effective in the treatment of neonatal herpes.[27] The use of 45 to 60 mg/kg may have additional benefits in decreasing morbidity and mortality, but a higher frequency of hematologic abnormalities has been seen with the 60-mg/kg dose.[28] The minimum duration of therapy should be 14 days, although longer courses (up to 21 days) may be indicated in infants with CNS involvement or disseminated disease.[29]

The role of prolonged oral suppressive therapy in newborns with SEM involvement has been investigated. Acyclovir, given orally at 300 mg/m² per dose three times daily, resulted in a reduction in the recurrences of lesions. Half of these patients developed neutropenia. One patient had lesions resistant to acyclovir.[30] Because the long-term benefits cannot be fully attributed to the use of suppressive acyclovir, suppressive therapy for patients with SEM involvement is not recommended.[31]

Oral-Facial Herpes

Both primary and recurrent oral-facial HSV-1 infections can be asymptomatic. Gingivostomatitis and pharyngitis are the most common clinical manifestations of a first episode of HSV-1 infection, and recurrent herpes labialis is most commonly caused by reactivated HSV infection. Clinical features include fever, malaise, myalgias, inability to eat, and irritability. Immunocompromised patients with oral-facial herpes have severe pain, extensive lesions, and prolonged viral shedding; thus, they are candidates for antiviral therapy.

Herpes labialis (cold sores) is the most common oral-facial HSV infection. Clinical features include pain or paresthesia and erythematous or papular lesions followed by vesiculation and swelling. These lesions usually crust and heal in the next few days. Viral cultures often are positive within 2 to 3 days. Rapid diagnosis can be made by visualizing viral particles in vesicular fluid with electron microscopy or fluorescent antibody staining of cells from vesicles.

Indications for Antiviral Treatment

9. M.K., a 26-year-old man, developed pain and erythematous skin lesions on his face and around his mouth over a 2-day period after contact with a person with active lesions. Over the next 2 days, significant swelling was noted. M.K. has no previous history of cold sores or any other illnesses. Should he be treated with antiviral drugs?

Most patients with herpes labialis have a self-limiting benign course. Antiviral drugs (e.g., acyclovir) are indicated only when the patient has a primary infection, an underlying illness, or a compromised immune system that may lead to prolonged illness or dissemination.

Although ice, ether, lysine, silver nitrate, and smallpox vaccine have been used to treat cold sores, no data support their efficacy. Aspirin and acetaminophen sometimes are suggested for symptomatic relief.

10. P.L., a 16-year-old boy diagnosed with acute lymphocytic leukemia 8 months ago, now is admitted for a bone marrow transplant. Admission laboratory tests reveal that he has antibodies against HSV-1 and that 4 months ago, during a course of chemotherapy, he developed an oral-facial herpes infection. What is the significance of these findings for P.L., who is about to undergo a bone marrow transplant?

Immunosuppressed patients have more frequent and severe mucocutaneous HSV infections. Therefore, IV acyclovir

should be considered to suppress the reactivation of oral-facial HSV infections.[32,33] Oral therapy with famciclovir is approved for use in HIV-infected patients,[34] but efficacy in other immunocompromised patients is not yet established.

Acyclovir
TREATMENT

11. P.L. did not receive antiviral therapy. Two weeks later, he developed oral-mucosal and skin lesions on his face, which were painful and associated with malaise. HSV was identified from the lesion by an immunofluorescence technique. What is the treatment of choice for P.L.?

Acyclovir is administered IV at 5 mg/kg Q 8 hr for 7 days[18] or until the lesions are healed, followed by oral acyclovir 200 mg three times daily for about 6 months. In patients with marrow transplants and culture-proven recurrent mucocutaneous herpes simplex, oral acyclovir (400 mg five times daily for 10 days) is significantly more effective than placebo in reducing pain, virus shedding, new lesion formation, and lesion healing time.[35] Furthermore, oral acyclovir is as effective as or more effective than IV acyclovir in bone marrow recipients or topical acyclovir in immunosuppressed patients.[36] Studies have shown that oral valacyclovir has similar pharmacokinetic parameters as IV acyclovir and may be used as an alternative to IV therapy.[37] The immunocompromised patients in these studies included those receiving corticosteroids, those with leukemia, and recipients of renal allografts.[35, 37]

12. N.B., a 43-year-old woman, experiences 8 to 10 cold sores a year. These typically are preceded by "colds" or sun exposure. She requests a prescription for acyclovir to "prevent" cold sores when she feels one coming on. What is the role of acyclovir in immunocompetent patients with recurrent herpes labialis?

Acyclovir (Zovirax) 5% cream and ointment, docosanol (Abreva) 10% cream, and penciclovir (Denavir) 1% cream are approved by the U.S. Food and Drug Administration (FDA) for the treatment of recurrent herpes labialis in immunocompetent patients. Clinical trials showed that each agent resulted in decreased healing time and decreased pain associated with herpes lesions.[38-44] Penciclovir also decreases viral shedding. Some data have indicated that penciclovir cream may be more effective than acyclovir cream and ointment.[41,42] An advantage of docosanol over the other agents is that it is available without a prescription. These agents must be applied within 1 hour of the first sign or symptom of a cold sore and then Q 2 hr for 4 days while awake.

Oral antiviral medications can decrease the duration of pain and healing time in immunocompetent patients. Oral acyclovir 400 mg five times daily for 5 days started within 1 hour of the development of a cold sore was more effective than placebo in reducing mean duration of pain and healing time in immunocompetent patients with a history of one to five episodes of herpes labialis per year.[45] Valacyclovir, penciclovir, and famciclovir showed similar clinical efficacy. Frequency of dosing and cost should be considered when choosing a particular agent.

Daily suppressive therapy may be recommended in patients with six or more recurrences per year. In immunocompetent patients with six or more episodes of herpes labialis, oral acyclovir 400 mg twice daily for 4 months was more effective than placebo in decreasing the number of recurrences in patients with herpes labialis.[46] Valacyclovir and acyclovir are equally efficacious in decreasing the number of recurrences in patients on daily suppressive therapy.

N.B. may be treated with either a topical or an oral antiviral. She should be instructed to start treatment as soon as the first sign or symptom of the cold sore appears.

RESISTANCE

13. **How should an acyclovir-resistant HSV infection be treated?**

The incidence of acyclovir-resistant herpes is higher in immunocompromised patients compared with immunocompetent patients. Current estimates of HSV resistance in the immunocompromised population are about 5%; some populations, such as bone marrow transplant patients, have a resistance rate approaching 30%.[47,48] IV foscarnet 40 mg/kg Q 8 hr was found to be more effective and less toxic than IV vidarabine 15 mg/kg per day in patients with AIDS and mucocutaneous herpetic lesions unresponsive to IV acyclovir.[49] More concerning, however, are the reports of foscarnet-resistant HSV, particularly in the bone marrow transplant population.[50,51] Cidofovir has been used with moderate success in such cases.[50]

Herpes Keratitis

Drug of Choice

14. **Z.F., a 20-year-old man, complains of acute pain, blurred vision, swelling of the conjunctival tissue around the cornea (chemosis), and vesicles on the eyelids. The conjunctivitis and characteristic dendritic lesions of the cornea are consistent with the diagnosis of herpes keratitis. What is the antiviral drug of choice?**

HSV infections of the eye are the most common causes of corneal blindness in the United States. HSV-1 is the common pathogen in adults and children beyond the neonatal period. Z.F. should be treated with a topical antiviral drug because drug therapy has been shown to enhance healing.[52] Three drugs have been approved to treat this condition: trifluridine, idoxuridine, and vidarabine.

Trifluridine is at least as effective as vidarabine[52] and is superior to idoxuridine. Trifluridine is the drug of choice because it is thought to be more effective than vidarabine when amoeboid ulcers are present, and idoxuridine is associated with more local adverse effects than vidarabine. Daily suppressive therapy with acyclovir 400 mg given twice daily decreased the recurrence rate of HSV keratitis from 32% in the placebo group to 19% in the treatment group, and the patients who benefited most from suppressive therapy were those with the most recurrences.[53]

VARICELLA-ZOSTER INFECTIONS

Chickenpox

Chickenpox used to be a common childhood infection, but the incidence has decreased by up to 84% in states with moderate rates of use of the varicella-zoster virus (VZV) vaccine since 1995.[54] This vaccine is now considered a routine childhood vaccine by the American Academy of Pediatrics (see Chapter 95, Immunizations.) Before the vaccine was available, approximately 3.5 million cases occurred per year in the United States: 60% of cases occurred in children 5 to 9 years of age and 80% occurred in those <10 years of age. Although it is a benign disease in most patients, complications and mortality (7 per 10,000 cases) can occur in patients <5 and >20 years of age, and in immunocompromised patients.

This is a highly contagious disease. Children are considered infectious from 2 days before the onset of rash until all vesicles have crusted (usually 4 to 6 days after the onset of rash). After household exposure, >90% of susceptible individuals become infected. Thus, the history can assist in making a diagnosis. A smear of cells scraped from the lesions will show multinucleated giant cells. Viruses also can be identified in vesicular lesions by electron microscopy, or antigen can be detected by countercurrent immunoelectrophoresis. Chickenpox is a primary varicella-zoster infection, whereas herpes zoster (shingles) is caused by reactivation of VZV.

Clinical Presentation

15. **A.V., a 10-year-old boy, was admitted to the hospital for evaluation and treatment of possible recurrent chickenpox with progressive lesions. According to his mother and his physician, he had a mild case of chickenpox at age 4 years. At admission, A.V. had a 10-day history of progressive vesicular and pustular lesions that began on his neck and spread to his back, trunk, extremities, and face. Although he had been febrile (up to 40.5°C orally) over the past 3 days, his temperature on admission was 37°C. A.V. had episodes of vomiting during the 4 days before admission. On admission, he was alert, cooperative, and well oriented but had overt ataxia with abnormal cerebellar signs. Lesions consistent with VZV infection were extensive and confluent over the face, neck, chest, and back. Stages of lesions varied from tiny thin-walled vesicles with an erythematous base to umbilicated vesicles. Few crusted lesions were present. Blood analysis revealed a BUN of 9 mg/dL, SrCr of 0.2 mg/dL, and slightly elevated serum transaminase levels (AST 65 IU/L [normal, 0 to 34] and ALT 122 IU/L [normal, 0 to 34]). Because of the possibility of cerebellar involvement with VZV infection and possible underlying immunodeficiency, therapy with acyclovir 550 mg IV Q 8 hr (1,500 mg/m² per day) was instituted. Oral diphenhydramine also was prescribed for itching, but A.V. required only two doses on the first hospital day.**

New lesions were noted on the second day of acyclovir therapy, but by the third day, no new lesions appeared and previous lesions were healing. The ataxia improved daily. He was discharged on day 7 with no further complaints of nausea and vomiting. Follow-up serologic evaluation demonstrated a fourfold rise in the optical density for the VZV enzyme-linked immunosorbent assay (ELISA) from day 20 to day 60 after the onset of infection. These results suggested primary VZV infection. Why is the use of acyclovir in A.V. appropriate?

[SI units: BUN, 3.213 mmol/L; SrCr, 15.25 μmol/L; AST, 1.084 μkat/L; ALT, 2.034 μkat/L]

Antiviral Treatment

Neonates, adults, immunocompromised hosts, patients with progressive varicella, and those with extracutaneous complications can benefit from acyclovir therapy. In clinical trials, acyclovir has been shown to be effective in preventing dissemination of VZV infection, accelerating cutaneous healing, and decreasing fever and pain.[55,56] A.V. had a prolonged progressive course of varicella and demonstrated an extracutaneous manifestation of varicella infection (e.g., ataxia with abnormal cerebellar signs). Because of the concern of possible cerebellar involvement, the use of IV acyclovir was appropriate in A.V.

16. **C.J., an 8-year-old boy, developed a case of chickenpox and was kept home from school. Four days later, his 15-year-old brother, K.J., began to exhibit similar symptoms. What is the role of acyclovir in immunocompetent patients with chickenpox? Should C.J. or K.J. be treated with acyclovir?**

Three studies in children (2 to 18 years of age) have shown that oral acyclovir 20 mg/kg (when initiated within 24 hours of disease onset) four times daily for 5 days was more effective than placebo in accelerating healing and decreasing the formation of new lesions, fever, and itching. However, acyclovir produced only modest benefits (usually healing 1 day sooner than placebo) and was not effective in reducing the complications of varicella.[57] Thus, acyclovir is not indicated for C.J.

Adolescents and adults are more likely to develop complications (e.g., pneumonia, encephalitis) than children. Acyclovir 800 mg orally four times daily for 5 days in adolescents and 800 mg orally five times daily for 5 days in adults (initiated within 24 hours of disease onset) was more effective than placebo in decreasing the number of lesions, time for healing, fever, and itching. The effect of acyclovir on severe complications could not be assessed.[23,58,59] Thus, acyclovir therapy should be considered in those at increased risk of severe chickenpox—for example, those like K.J. who are >14 years of age or those with chronic respiratory or skin disease.[60] No data are available to show if famciclovir and valacyclovir are as effective as acyclovir.

Supportive Treatment

17. **What is the role of supportive treatment in A.V. and C.J.?**

Cool baths and application of calamine or other topical antipruritic agents may decrease itching. In severe cases, a systemic antipruritic/antihistamine preparation may be useful because some degree of sedation may be desired. In A.V. and C.J., aspirin should not be used because Reye's syndrome has been associated with the use of salicylates in chickenpox or flu-like illness (see Chapter 93, Pediatric Considerations).

Shingles (Herpes Zoster)

Herpes zoster infections are caused by the reactivation of dormant VZV in the sensory neurons. Reactivation is thought to occur because of waning immunity. The incidence of herpes zoster is higher in immunocompromised patients (e.g., those with HIV or cancer or those receiving immunosuppressive medications), and the incidence of zoster increases with age. It tends to be more severe in the elderly.

Acute herpes zoster infection is characterized by pain, which is described as deep aching or burning. It may be accompanied by excessive sensitivity to touch. Many patients develop a rash that presents initially as erythematous patches and progresses to vesicles that crust in 7 to 10 days. By 1 month, the rash is usually gone, but scarring can occur.

Postherpetic neuralgia (PHN) is pain that continues >1 month after the onset of the rash. It is estimated that 10% to 70% of patients experience PHN. PHN is the most common complication of acute herpes zoster and its prevention is important because PHN pain is difficult to treat.

The goal of pharmacotherapy in acute herpes zoster is to inhibit viral replication to reduce pain and duration of rash. Ultimately, it is hoped that by inhibiting the virus, nerve damage can be prevented and the incidence and severity of PHN can be decreased. Unfortunately, no therapy can prevent all cases of PHN.

Antiviral Therapy in Immunocompetent Patients

18. **E.O. is a 72-year-old, previously healthy man who complains of a burning pain under his left arm for the last 2 days. The pain radiates across his chest. The pain is worse when the area is touched. This morning, he noticed a rash that starts under his arm and continues to his midline. Pertinent laboratory findings include BUN of 15 mg/dL (normal, 8 to 18) and SrCr of 2.0 mg/dL (normal, 0.6 to 1.2). A diagnosis of herpes zoster is made. What therapy should be initiated?**

[SI units: BUN, 5.4 mmol/L; SrCr 177 μmol/L]

Acyclovir is the standard antiviral agent against which new therapies are compared. In immunocompetent patients, oral acyclovir 800 mg five times daily for 7 to 10 days is beneficial in reducing acute pain during the first 28 days. Acyclovir therapy should be initiated within 72 hours of the onset of the rash. The effects of acyclovir in reducing PHN and chronic pain are unclear. Although a number of trials showed no benefit in reducing PHN, a meta-analysis of four trials of acyclovir treatment in herpes zoster showed a 42% reduction in the incidence of PHN at 6 months.[61]

Famciclovir (Famvir) is approved for the treatment of acute herpes zoster infection. Famciclovir is rapidly absorbed and converted to the active drug penciclovir in the intestine. The bioavailability of famciclovir is higher than acyclovir, resulting in higher concentrations of active drug in the infected cells. In addition, the half-life of famciclovir is considerably longer compared with acyclovir, allowing less frequent administration. In a large clinical trial comparing famciclovir with acyclovir, famciclovir 500 mg three times daily was as effective as acyclovir 800 mg five times a day in reducing the duration of acute pain and healing of the rash.[62] In another study comparing famciclovir with placebo, famciclovir did not decrease the incidence of PHN but reduced the duration of PHN versus placebo.[63]

A limitation of acyclovir is its poor oral bioavailability (15% to 30%). In an attempt to overcome this, valacyclovir (Valtrex), a prodrug of acyclovir, was developed. Valacyclovir is rapidly and extensively absorbed and converted to acyclovir in the body after oral administration. In clinical trials, valacyclovir 1 g three times daily was equally effective as acyclovir 800 mg five times a day in terms of rash progression and time to rash healing, and valacyclovir was more effective than acyclovir in relieving zoster-associated pain.[64]

E.O. should be started on acyclovir, famciclovir, or valacyclovir for the treatment of his herpes zoster. Famciclovir or valacyclovir may be preferred because compliance with a three-times-daily regimen will likely be better than with acyclovir, which must be administered five times a day. Therapy should be initiated as soon as possible because most of the clinical trials began therapy within 72 hours of the rash onset. Although therapy may not prevent PHN, it may have an effect on the duration of pain. Because all of these agents are renally eliminated, the dosage should be adjusted based on E.O.'s creatinine clearance (see Table 72-2).

19. **Should E.O. receive a corticosteroid to treat or prevent the pain associated with herpes zoster?**

The use of corticosteroids such as prednisone or prednisolone remains controversial.[65] A number of studies have examined the effect of steroids on pain during acute neuralgia and on the development of PHN. Early studies indicated benefit for both acute pain and PHN, but these studies were small and uncontrolled, lacked statistical analysis, and used various corticosteroid regimens. Recent studies suggest possible relief of the acute pain but no decrease in PHN.[66–69] Adverse effects of the corticosteroids and the theoretical possibility of dissemination of herpes zoster resulting from their use should be considered when deciding whether to initiate therapy. Based on recent studies demonstrating lack of benefit in preventing PHN, the theoretical concerns of herpes zoster dissemination, and the beneficial effects of antiviral agents such as acyclovir, famciclovir, and valacyclovir for acute pain, corticosteroids should not be used in E.O.

20. **Two months after the onset of the rash, E.O. continues to complain of pain. A diagnosis of PHN is made. What FDA-approved treatments for PHN should be prescribed for E.O.?**

Although many different agents have been studied, the only FDA-approved treatment for PHN is topical capsaicin. Capsaicin depletes substance P, a mediator that transmits pain from the periphery to the CNS. The largest double-blind, placebo-controlled trial of capsaicin evaluated 143 patients with PHN for at least 6 months. After 6 weeks of treatment with capsaicin 0.075% cream, pain scores were reduced in 21% and 6% of the capsaicin and placebo groups, respectively. Following the double-blind phase of the study, a subset of patients continued to use capsaicin cream for up to 2 years, and most patients experienced prolonged pain relief.[70]

Capsaicin cream is an option for E.O. Capsaicin should be applied three or four times per day. A common adverse effect is a burning sensation after application, which is intolerable in up to one third of patients. The burning sensation usually lessens with continued use. E.O. should be counseled about this adverse effect.

Antiviral Therapy in Immunocompromised Patients

21. **R.F. is a 68-year-old woman seen in the ED with a chief complaint of vesicles on her face associated with severe pain. She has a history of polymyalgia rheumatica and possible temporal arteritis causing headaches that generally are responsive to steroids. She had been having increasing headaches on the right side of her forehead 5 days before admission. Two days before admission, her family physician increased the dosage of prednisone from 30 mg/day to 60 mg/day. Vesicles developed on her face 1 day before admission. She was admitted for pain control and diagnosed with herpes zoster infection. Six hours after admission, R.F. began having visual hallucinations, hearing noises, and talking to herself. A lumbar puncture was performed with**

the following results: 3 WBCs (2 lymphocytes and 1 monocyte); 3 RBCs; protein, 84 mg/dL; and glucose, 86 mg/dL. Herpes zoster was isolated from the CSF. IV acyclovir was started at a dosage of 10 mg/kg Q 8 hr. Why is antiviral therapy indicated in R.F.? Should her prednisone be continued or discontinued?

Antiviral therapy is indicated for R.F. Acyclovir may halt the progression of acute herpes zoster infection in immunocompromised hosts such as R.F., who has been taking large doses of corticosteroids.[71]

In a placebo-controlled trial, IV acyclovir 500 mg/m^2 Q 8 hr for 7 days, halted the progression of herpes zoster in immunocompromised patients. In patients with cutaneous dissemination of disease, there was a more rapid clearance of the herpes zoster virus from vesicles. Pain relief occurred faster in patients who received acyclovir and fewer acyclovir-treated patients reported PHN, but the differences were not statistically significant.[71] There are no data available regarding the use of famciclovir or valacyclovir in severe herpes zoster infection in an immunocompromised host.

Systemic corticosteroids are of unproven usefulness and may slow the healing of lesions. Therefore, if possible, R.F.'s prednisone should be slowly tapered.

ACYCLOVIR TOXICITY

22. **On the fourth day of acyclovir therapy, R.F. developed severe nausea and vomited three times. The laboratory data showed a BUN of 45 mg/dL and SrCr of 3.2 mg/dL (baseline BUN 10 mg/dL and SrCr 1.0 mg/dL). Why must R.F.'s acyclovir dosage be altered?**

[SI units: BUN, 16.07 and 3.57 mmol/L, respectively; SrCr, 282.88 and 88.40 μmol/L, respectively]

Nausea and vomiting have been reported with acyclovir therapy in patients with herpes zoster infections.[18] Similarly, elevations of SrCr and BUN can occur in association with acyclovir therapy. This may be secondary to acyclovir crystallization in the renal tubules, particularly when fluid intake is inadequate (see Table 72-4). Because R.F.'s creatinine clearance is between 10 and 25 mL/min per 1.73 m^2, the acyclovir dosage interval should be extended to 24 hours. Every effort should be made to maintain adequate hydration for the duration of acyclovir therapy. (See Table 72-2 and Chapter 2, Interpretation of Clinical Laboratory Tests, for creatinine clearance calculation.)

INFLUENZA

Influenza is an acute infection caused by the virus of the Orthomyxoviridae family. Epidemics of influenza usually are caused by the type A virus; type B virus generally is associated with sporadic infection. Infection is transmitted by the inhalation of virus-containing droplets ejected from the respiratory tract of a person with influenza. It can be spread by direct contact, large droplets, or articles recently contaminated by nasopharyngeal secretions. The incubation period is typically 2 days (range, 1 to 4 days).

Influenza A viruses are classified into subtypes of hemagglutinin (H) and neuraminidase (N) surface antigens. Three subtypes of hemagglutinin (H_1, H_2, H_3) and two subtypes of neuraminidase (N_1, N_2) have caused influenza in humans. Infection with a virus of one subtype may confer little or no protection against viruses of other subtypes. In addition, significant antigenic variation (antigenic drift) within a subtype may occur over time. Thus, infection or vaccination with one strain may not protect against a distantly related strain of the same subtype. This is why major epidemics of influenza continue to occur and influenza vaccines are reformulated each year with current viral strains to maximize immunity.

Persons at highest risk for influenza infection (Table 72-5) should receive the influenza vaccine each year. Each year's vaccine contains three virus strains (generally two type A and one type B) that are likely to circulate in the community for the upcoming season. The efficacy depends on the similarity of the components of the vaccine to the circulating viruses that year and the immunocompetence of the host. If there is a good match with the circulating viruses, the vaccine can prevent illness in approximately 70% to 90% of healthy adults and children. It appears to be effective in preventing hospitalization and pneumonia in 70% of elderly persons living in the community and in 50% to 60% of elderly persons residing in nursing homes. However, the efficacy of the vaccine in preventing illness is often only 30% to 40% among the frail elderly. Despite the lower efficacy, the illness is less severe and the risk of complications is reduced in vaccinated individuals.

Individuals who can transmit influenza to persons at high risk include physicians, nurses, and other personnel in both hospital and ambulatory settings; employees of nursing homes and chronic care facilities; providers of home care services; and household members, including children.

Persons at high risk and those who may transmit the virus to those at high risk should be vaccinated annually. Table 72-6 describes the types of vaccines, dosage, number of doses, and route of administration for four age groups. The optimal time for vaccine administration is between mid-October and mid-November, because influenza activity peaks between late December and early March in the United States. Vaccinating an individual too early in the season could result in waning antibody concentrations before the influenza season is over.

Because the influenza vaccine is an inactivated vaccine and contains no infectious viruses, it cannot cause influenza. The most common adverse effect is soreness at the administration site lasting for up to 2 days.[72] Fever, malaise, myalgia, and other systemic reactions occur infrequently; these may develop within 6 to 12 hours after the vaccine is given and persist for 1 to 3 days.[72,73] Immediate hypersensitivity to egg protein (hives, angioedema, allergic asthma, or systemic anaphylaxis) occurs rarely. Persons with anaphylactic hypersensitivity and those with acute febrile illness should not be given the vaccine. However, minor illnesses with or without fever are not contraindications for the influenza vaccine, particularly in children with a mild upper respiratory tract infection or allergic rhinitis. When the vaccine is contraindicated, an antiviral drug (amantadine, rimantadine, or oseltamivir) should be used for prophylaxis.[74]

Clinically, it is impossible to differentiate between influenza A and B. Definitive diagnosis can be made by the isolating the virus from throat washings or sputum and a significant increase in antibody titers during the convalescent period.

Clinical Presentation

23. K.B., a 40-year-old woman, comes into the pharmacy and says she has "the flu." She recently started a new job and is afraid she will lose her job if she misses too many days from work. What questions would you ask her to differentiate the common cold from an influenza infection?

It can be difficult to differentiate the common cold from an influenza infection. Influenza infections typically occur from December through March in the United States. Patients with influenza generally experience more systemic symptoms,

Table 72-5 Persons Who Should Receive the Influenza Vaccine[74]

- All healthy children ages 6–35 months
- All persons ≥65 yr
- Nursing home or chronic care facility residents
- Children and adults with chronic pulmonary or cardiovascular disease
- Children and adults who have required medical follow-up because of chronic metabolic diseases (e.g., diabetes mellitus), renal dysfunction, hemoglobinopathies, or immunosuppression (due to medications or diseases such as HIV)
- Children (6 mo–18 yr) receiving long-term aspirin therapy
- Women who will be in the second or third trimester of pregnancy during influenza season
- Health care workers who come in contact with high-risk individuals
- Household members of person in high-risk groups

Table 72-6 Influenza Vaccines[74]

Age	Type of Vaccine[a]	Dosage	Number of Doses	Route[b]
6–35 mo	Split virus only[c]	0.25 mL	1 or 2[d]	IM
3–8 yr	Split virus only[c]	0.5 mL	1 or 2[d]	IM
9–13 yr	Split virus only[c]	0.5 mL	1	IM
>13 yr, including adults	Whole or split virus	0.5 mL	1	IM

[a]2002-2003 available vaccines contain 15 µg of A/Moscow/10/99(H3N2)-like, A/New Caledonia/20/99(H1N1)-like, B/Hong Kong/330/2001-like antigens. The products are Fluzone whole- or split-virus vaccine; Fluvirin purified surface antigen vaccine; Fluogen split vaccine; and Flushield split vaccine.
[b]The recommended site is the deltoid muscle for adults and older children and the anterolateral aspect of the thigh in infants and young children.
[c]Only split-virus vaccines should be used in children because they cause fewer febrile reactions; adverse effects of whole-virus and split-virus vaccines are similar in adults.
[d]Two doses given at least 1 month apart for children <9 years who are receiving the vaccine for the first time.
IM, intramuscular.

such as fever >102°F, headache, myalgia, and cough. Rhinorrhea, nasal congestion, and sneezing are more pronounced in patients with the common cold. Sore throat can occur with both a cold and the flu. Bacterial sore throat (e.g., strep throat) is differentiated from a viral sore throat in that a viral sore throat usually has a slower onset and the throat pain is less severe. Lymph nodes are only slightly enlarged and not tender in a viral sore throat, whereas with a bacterial sore throat, lymph nodes are large and tender.[75]

K.B. should be questioned about her symptoms and exposure to other sick people to help differentiate an influenza infection from the common cold.

Treatment

24. K.B. describes symptoms consistent with an influenza infection for the past 24 hours. What treatment options exist for the treatment of influenza? Why is she a candidate for a neuraminidase inhibitor agent such as zanamivir or oseltamivir?

Two agents for the treatment of influenza A and B in adults were approved in 1999. Zanamivir (Relenza) and oseltamivir (Tamiflu) work by selectively inhibiting the enzyme neuraminidase, an enzyme necessary for viral replication and spread. When administered within 2 days of onset of illness, zanamivir and oseltamivir reduce influenza symptoms by approximately 1 day.[76–78] Oseltamivir is indicated for patients 1 year of age and older; zanamivir is indicated for patients 7 years of age and older.[82]

Zanamivir is available as an oral powder for inhalation. For the treatment of influenza infection, 10 mg (two inhalations) twice a day for 5 days should be used. Patients should inhale two doses separated by at least 2 hours on the first day and then two doses separated by 12 hours on days 2 through 5.[80] Bronchospasm after use can occur, and if bronchodilators are also prescribed, the bronchodilator should be used before zanamivir.[80] Proper use of the delivery system (Rotadisk Diskhaler) is important, and patients should be instructed on proper use, with a demonstration of delivery technique, by the pharmacist.

Oseltamivir is pharmacologically related to zanamivir but has significantly better oral bioavailability, allowing oral dosing. The dosage of oseltamivir for the treatment of influenza is 75 mg twice a day for 5 days.[79] As with zanamivir, treatment with oseltamivir must be started within 2 days of the onset of symptoms. Common side effects include nausea, vomiting, and headache.[79]

Amantadine and rimantadine are efficacious in the treatment of infections caused by influenza A viruses. These agents prevent penetration of the host cell by influenza A viruses and prevent assembly of the virus during the replication cycle of the virus.[81] Amantadine and rimantadine have been shown to decrease the duration of illness due to influenza A by 1 day. Amantadine is approved for patients ≥1 year of age. Rimantadine is not approved for the treatment of influenza in children.[82]

Amantadine and rimantadine are administered as 100 mg twice daily in the treatment of influenza A. Patients should begin treatment within 48 hours of symptom onset. Treatment is continued for 24 to 48 hours after the symptoms have resolved or for a maximum of 3 to 5 days to prevent the development of resistant viruses.[74] Five percent to 10% of otherwise healthy adults taking amantadine have reported

insomnia, nausea, and dizziness. CNS adverse effects (depression, anxiety, irritability, hallucinations, dream abnormalities, and nervousness) occur in 1% to 5% of patients receiving amantadine therapy. Rimantadine has similar adverse effects, but the incidence of these adverse effects is lower. Amantadine is excreted unchanged by the kidney, so renal clearance of amantadine is reduced in the elderly and in patients with renal dysfunction. A reduction in dosage is recommended in patients with creatinine clearance <50 mL/min per 1.73 m². Elderly patients and those with impaired renal function should be monitored closely for adverse effects and the dosage should be decreased if adverse effects occur. In patients >65 years of age or those unable to tolerate the CNS toxicity, a daily dose of 100 mg is indicated.

To date, no data exist comparing the efficacy between amantadine and rimantadine with the neuraminidase inhibitors. Advantages of the neuraminidase inhibitors include the efficacy against influenza B or resistant influenza A. Because the causative agent is unknown and symptoms have been present for <2 days, K.B. may benefit from an neuraminidase inhibitor. Oral oseltamivir is easier to administer than inhaled zanamivir. Although oseltamivir will not cure influenza, it may reduce the severity and duration of symptoms by about 1 day. Because K.B. is concerned about missing too much time from work, she should be treated with a 5-day course of oseltamivir.

25. J.T., a 74-year-old man, is brought to the ED from a nursing home with chief complaints of fever (103°F), shaking chills, cough, headache, malaise, anorexia, and photophobia. He has been ill for the past 48 hours but suddenly became worse this evening. On physical examination, he appeared flushed, his skin was hot and moist, and he was working hard to breathe. Vital signs were blood pressure, 150/90 mm Hg; pulse, 108 beats/min; respiratory rate, 22 breaths/min; temperature, 103°F. Rales were audible on auscultation of both lungs. A chest roentgenogram showed bilateral infiltrates but no consolidation. Blood gas studies showed significant hypoxia, with a PaO_2 of 50 mm Hg and a $PaCO_2$ of 50 mm Hg. J.T.'s medical history was significant for chronic bronchitis and a stroke 16 months ago.

Blood, sputum, and urine cultures were obtained, and J.T. was started on antibiotics (gentamicin 140 mg loading dose, then 90 mg Q 12 hr IV piggyback and clindamycin 900 mg Q 8 hr IV piggyback). Gram's stain of the sputum sample showed many WBCs but no bacteria. He was started on oxygen therapy at 4 L/min via nasal cannula.

Twenty-four hours later, his respiratory symptoms worsened and arterial blood gases deteriorated slightly (PaO_2, 40 mm Hg; $PaCO_2$, 55 mm Hg). J.T. was intubated and a sputum sample was obtained and sent to the virology lab. Three days later, influenza A virus was isolated from the sputum. Blood, urine, and sputum cultures were all negative for bacterial pathogens.

Why is this presentation consistent with influenza infection? Is antiviral treatment indicated in J.T.?

[SI units: PaO_2, 6.665 and 5.332 kPa, respectively; $PaCO_2$, 6.665 and 7.332 kPa, respectively]

Although symptoms of influenza may vary depending on age, most patients with influenza A have an abrupt onset of fever, chills, cough, and headache. In elderly patients like J.T. and those with underlying diseases, the course of influenza can worsen quickly, and patients are more likely to require hospitalization.

Antiviral therapy in J.T. is inappropriate. None of the antiviral agents has been studied in patients presenting with symptoms after 48 hours of onset. In addition, the antiviral agents have shown efficacy only in uncomplicated influenza.[74]

Prevention

26. Over the next 3 weeks, two other nursing home patients develop influenza A infections. What measures should be taken to prevent a further outbreak of influenza among other residents?

Influenza Vaccines

The nursing home residents and staff should receive influenza vaccine plus chemoprophylaxis with amantadine, rimantadine, oseltamivir, or zanamivir. The Centers for Disease Control and Prevention (CDC) recommends immunization of all high-risk groups[74] (see Table 72-5). The top-priority groups include all healthy children from ages 6 to 35 months; adults and children with chronic cardiovascular or pulmonary disease severe enough to warrant regular medical care during the preceding year; residents of nursing homes and other chronic care facilities; and physicians, nurses, and other personnel who have extensive contact with high-risk patients. Second in priority are otherwise healthy adults >65 years of age and children with chronic metabolic diseases severe enough to warrant regular follow-up during the preceding year. However, the efficacy of influenza vaccine is incomplete (70%).[74] Therefore, the CDC recommends the use of amantadine, rimantadine, or oseltamivir in high-risk individuals who may not develop an adequate antibody response (e.g., patients with HIV infection) to supplement the protection by vaccine.[84]

Amantadine and Rimantadine

Prophylactic amantadine and rimantadine therapy are approximately 63% and 72% effective, respectively, in preventing further cases of influenza A.[83] The recommended dosage of amantadine and rimantadine is 200 mg/day (100 mg twice daily) to prevent influenza A infections. Treatment should begin as soon as possible and continued for 14 days if given with vaccine because the development of antibodies may take up to 2 weeks after vaccination and throughout influenza season if the vaccine is not given.

Oseltamivir

Analysis of clinical trials of oseltamivir in the prevention of influenza showed a decreased incidence of laboratory-confirmed influenza: 4.8% in the placebo group and 1.2% in the treatment group.[85] The incidence of influenza in a skilled nursing facility was 4.4% in the placebo group and 0.4% in the oseltamivir group. In addition, oseltamivir lowered the rate of infection in patients exposed to influenza at home from 12% to 1%. Zanamivir also showed decreases in subsequent cases among individuals exposed to influenza in the home setting, although zanamivir is currently not indicated for prophylaxis of influenza.[86,87]

Because oseltamivir has activity against influenza B, it may be a better option in the prevention of outbreaks in institutional settings, although comparative studies between neuraminidase inhibitors and amantadine or rimantadine have not been published.

Emergence of Resistance

27. What can be done to minimize emergence of resistance and transmission of influenza A virus to close contacts and family members?

Although amantadine and rimantadine are effective in the prevention and treatment of influenza A, resistant strains have been isolated from treated patients as well as close contacts.[88] Amantadine-resistant strains are cross-resistant with rimantadine and vice versa. Antiviral-resistant strains have been reported as early as 2 days after starting antiviral treatment.[89] Typically, resistant strains are not more virulent or transmissible than susceptible strains, but the clinical significance of this resistance is unknown.[90,91]

The emergence of resistance may be minimized by limiting treatment to those who are likely to have severe disease or who might develop complications, and limiting the duration of treatment. However, the close contacts to be protected can receive prophylaxis with amantadine or rimantadine. Strains resistant to both zanamivir and oseltamivir have developed after treatment with these agents.[92–94] The clinical implication of resistant strains to these antiviral agents is unknown.

RESPIRATORY SYNCYTIAL VIRUS INFECTIONS

Respiratory syncytial virus (RSV) is an important pathogen causing bronchiolitis and bronchopneumonia. RSV infection commonly affects infants <2 years of age, with more than one half of the infants becoming infected in the first 2 years of life. Of these infants, approximately 1% to 2% will require hospitalization.[95] Children with underlying congenital heart disease or lung disease may be at increased risk of mortality due to RSV.[96] Patients with RSV infection before 3 years of age appear to be at an increased risk of wheezing and asthma during childhood.[97–99]

RSV infections usually occur in the winter. The chest radiograph and blood gases often are abnormal, and the virus can be isolated in the nasopharyngeal secretions. Virus isolation, serologic tests during illness, and increased antibody titers during convalescence can establish the diagnosis.

Clinical Presentation and Ribavirin Therapy

28. J.R., a 6-month-old infant who is lethargic, tachypneic, and cyanotic, is brought to the ED. J.R.'s medical history is significant for congenital HIV. He has a fever (102°F), and his breathing is labored; wheezing is audible on expiration. The chest roentgenograms show a flattened diaphragm and hyperinflated lung parenchyma. Because of hypoxemia and hypercarbia, J.R. is placed on ambient oxygen to maintain the alveolar oxygen pressure at >60 mm Hg. RSV is present in the respiratory secretions. What type of therapy is indicated for J.R., who has underlying immunodeficiency?

The goal of therapy is to decrease airway resistance in a patient like J.R.[100] Treatment of RSV is highly individualized, depending on the presenting signs and symptoms. Oxygen is first-line therapy. Decreases in airway resistance may be achieved with the use of bronchodilators or corticosteroids. Bronchodilators have led to minimal clinical improvement. The use of corticosteroids in the treatment of RSV is controversial. Although individual studies differ on the clinical benefits of oral corticosteroids, a meta-analysis found that oral corticosteroids may decrease the length of stay, duration of symptoms, and clinical scores in patients with mild to moderate disease.[101] The use of either bronchodilators or corticosteroids must be individualized based on the patient's clinical presentation.[100]

Ribavirin (1-β-D-ribofuranosyl-1,2,4-triazole-3-carboxamide; Virazole), an antiviral agent that possesses unique inhibitory activity against a large number of both DNA and RNA viruses, is indicated for the treatment of infections caused by RSV. The virus is inhibited at serum concentrations of 16 μg/mL.[102] Early studies with ribavirin showed significant clinical improvement compared to placebo in both healthy children and those with underlying disease.[103] These studies reported clinical recovery and improvement in arterial oxygenation. Subsequent studies found ribavirin to be ineffective in patients with a variety of risk factors.[104,105] Consequently, the routine use in previously healthy infants and children has not been clearly established. Current recommendations for the use of ribavirin are children with underlying congenital heart disease or immunosuppressive disorders, or patients with severe or worsening RSV infection.[106] Whether ribavirin decreases the long-term sequelae and severity of illness in high-risk groups (including premature infants, patients with bronchopulmonary dysplasia, congenital heart disease, cystic fibrosis, and immunodeficiency) has not been determined. Because J.R. has an underlying immunodeficiency, ribavirin should be started.

RSV immune globulin (RSV-IGIV, Respigam) is an IV product made from the blood of donors with high titers of RSV-neutralizing antibodies. The use of RSV-IGIV has been evaluated in children at high risk for severe infections and in previously healthy children. Although administration of RSV-IGIV was safe, studies have shown no efficacy with the use of immune globulins in the treatment of RSV.[107,108] Thus, they are not recommended for use in the treatment of RSV.[109]

Administration of Ribavirin

29. **How is ribavirin administered, and what precautions should be taken during drug administration in J.R.?**

Ribavirin is administered as an aerosol through a collision generator that generates particles small enough (1 to 2 μm wide) to reach the lower respiratory tract. This ensures that high concentrations of ribavirin penetrate the respiratory secretions at the site of viral replication while minimizing systemic absorption. The concentration of the ribavirin solution in the reservoir is 20 mg/mL (6 g in 300 mL of sterile water). The dose is administered over 12 to 18 hours, although in nonventilated patients, 2 g over 2 hours three times daily (using a 60-mg/mL solution) has been successfully used.[105] Ribavirin therapy is continued for 3 to 7 days.[102]

Ribavirin is approved for use in patients requiring mechanical ventilation. However, ribavirin is hygroscopic, and aerosol particles can deposit in the tubing and around the expiratory valve of a ventilator. The precipitated drug can obstruct the expiratory valve and alter the peak end-expiratory pressure.[110] Ribavirin has been safely used in such patients,[111,112] but close monitoring of respiratory therapy is advised to prevent this problem. In addition to the inspection of tubing, modifications of standard ventilatory circuits have been suggested.

Adverse Effects

30. **What are the important adverse effects of ribavirin?**

The most common adverse effects of ribavirin are rash, initial mild bronchospasm upon drug initiation, and reversible skin irritation.[113] Although long-term follow-up data are limited, a study evaluating the effects of ribavirin in patients 1 year after administration showed a reduction in the incidence and severity of reactive airway disease and also in hospitalizations related to respiratory illness. Further long-term evaluation is still necessary.[114]

Ribavirin is contraindicated in women who are or may become pregnant during exposure to the drug. Although there are no human data, ribavirin has been found to be teratogenic and/or embryolethal in nearly all animal species in which it has been tested. Teratogenesis was evident after a single oral dose of 2.5 mg/kg in the hamster and after daily oral doses of 10 mg/kg in the rat. Malformation of the skull, palate, eye, jaw, skeleton, and GI tract were noted in animals. Ribavirin has reduced the survival of fetuses and offspring of animals tested. It is lethal to the rabbit embryo in daily oral doses as small as 1 mg/kg. There are no studies that address teratogenicity in humans, but female hospital personnel who are pregnant or may be pregnant should avoid exposure to this drug.[102]

It is important to consider the environmental effects of ribavirin on the personnel involved with its administration. One study found no detectable plasma or urine concentrations of ribavirin in 19 nurses,[115] whereas another reported its presence in the RBCs of a nurse caring for a patient who received ribavirin via oxygen tent.[116] The ribavirin concentration in the air was highest when it was administered via oxygen tent, followed by mist mask, and was lowest after administration via endotracheal tubes of mechanically ventilated patients.[116] This has led to several recommendations: (1) ribavirin aerosol should be administered solely via endotracheal tube of mechanically ventilated patients in a closed filtered system[95]; (2) children receiving ribavirin should be placed in a containment chamber equipped with a high-efficiency particulate air filter exhaust in an isolation room with negative air pressure[102]; (3) disposable full-body coverings and either a powered air-purifying respirator or disposable particulate respirator should be made available to all health care personnel[102]; (4) men and women planning to have children should not care for patients receiving ribavirin via oxygen tents.[116] ICN Pharmaceuticals markets an aerosol delivery system for oxygen and ribavirin that decreases the liberation of ribavirin into the environment.[102]

31. **S.N. is a 7-month-old boy born prematurely at 31 weeks' gestation. He has bronchopulmonary dysplasia (BPD) and uses oxygen at home. RSV season will begin next month. What treatments to prevent RSV infection are available? Why is S.N. a candidate for such treatment?**

Two products are available for the prevention of RSV infections. RSV-IGIV may be used to prevent or decrease the severity of lower respiratory tract infections caused by RSV in children <24 months old with BPD or a history of premature birth before 35 weeks' gestation. Infants who were born prematurely and who have underlying pulmonary disease (e.g., BPD), cardiovascular disease, or immunodeficiency states are at higher risk for death because of RSV than other infants.

In a large study of infants with BPD and/or prematurity, monthly infusions of RSV-IGIV during RSV season (starting in mid-November and continuing for three to five monthly doses) decreased the number of RSV lower respiratory tract infections, hospital admissions, duration of hospitalizations, and days in the intensive care unit.[118] Other studies have demonstrated similar results.[119]

Palivizumab (Synagis), a humanized monoclonal antibody made from recombinant DNA, is active against RSV and is indicated for children at high risk of RSV respiratory tract infections (e.g., infants with BPD or a history of premature birth <35 weeks' gestation). The efficacy of palivizumab was demonstrated in a randomized, double-blind, placebo-controlled trial involving 1,502 children who had a history of prematurity or BPD.[120] Children received monthly intramuscular injections of placebo or palivizumab for 5 months during RSV season. Palivizumab-treated children had a reduction in RSV hospitalizations and intensive care admissions and had shorter hospitalizations for RSV disease. Palivizumab is preferred over RSV-IGIV for most high-risk infants because it is easier to administer (intramuscularly versus IV), does not interfere with the response of live vaccines such as measles-mumps-rubella or varicella vaccine, and is not likely to transmit blood-borne diseases because it is synthesized in a laboratory rather than derived from human blood.[121]

Based on S.N.'s age, history of prematurity, and history of BPD, he is a candidate for palivizumab therapy.[109,121]

Dosage and Administration

32. How are the doses of RSV-IGIV and palivizumab calculated, and how should they be given?

RSV-IGIV 750 mg/kg is given as an IV infusion. The dose of palivizumab is 15 mg/kg given intramuscularly. For both products, the first dose is given before the start of RSV season, and then monthly doses are given throughout RSV season. In the Northern Hemisphere, RSV season is typically November through April.

Because adverse reactions to RSV-IGIV may be related to the infusion rate, infusion titration is important. During the initial 15 minutes, RSV-IGIV should be infused at 1.5 mL/kg per hour (using a 50-mg/mL solution). The infusion rate can then be increased to 3 mL/kg per hour for the next 15 minutes and, if tolerated, the rate can be increased to a maximum of 6 mL/kg per minute.

HANTAVIRUS INFECTIONS

Rodents are the primary reservoir hosts of Hantavirus, and the deer mouse (*Peromyscus maniculatus*) is the main reservoir in the United States. These viruses apparently do not cause illness in the reservoir hosts, but infection in humans occurs when infected saliva, urine, and feces are inhaled as aerosols produced by the animal. Most patients recall exposure to rodents or rodent feces within 6 weeks of the onset of illness.[122] Person-to-person transmission has not been documented.

Four serotypes of hantavirus have been identified. The case definition used by the CDC includes clinical evidence of (1) febrile illness characterized by unexplained adult respiratory distress syndrome (ARDS) or acute bilateral pulmonary interstitial infiltrates; (2) an autopsy finding of noncardiogenic pulmonary edema resulting from an unexplained respiratory illness (laboratory evidence consists of a positive serology [i.e., presence of hantavirus-specific immunoglobulin M or rising titers of immunoglobulin G]); (3) positive immunohistochemistry for hantavirus antigen in a tissue specimen; or (4) positive polymerase chain reaction for hantavirus RNA in a tissue specimen.[123]

Hantavirus infection can cause three different clinical diseases: hemorrhagic fever with renal syndrome, nephropathia epidemica, and hantavirus pulmonary syndrome (HPS). Hemorrhagic fever with renal syndrome and nephropathia epidemica occur outside of the United States, whereas HPS occurs only in the Western Hemisphere, including North America.[124] As of May 2003, there have been 336 cases of HPS in the United States, with 38% of the cases resulting in death.[125] Most have occurred in the Southwestern United States during spring and summer.

Clinical Presentation

33. K.C., a previously healthy 55-year-old woman, presented with an abrupt onset of fever, cough, myalgia, and shortness of breath. K.C. lives in western Texas and has not traveled out of state during the past 6 months. Diagnostic evaluation, including a complete blood count with differential and blood and sputum cultures, was negative. On day 3, K.C. remained febrile and had vomiting, hypotension, hypoxemia, and bilateral diffuse infiltrates on the chest radiograph.

Abnormal laboratory findings included a leukocyte count of 22,000/mm³ with a shift to the left, platelet of 70,000/mm³, and albumin concentration of 2 g/dL. K.C. suddenly developed ARDS. The hantavirus immunoglobulin M ELISA titer, performed from K.C.'s serum specimen at the CDC, was elevated. What signs and symptoms are consistent with hantavirus infection?

The clinical features of patients with HPS include fever, myalgia, headache, and cough. Abdominal pain, nausea, and/or vomiting also may be present. The physical examination has been unreliable. Laboratory abnormalities may include leukocytosis, thrombocytopenia, and hypoalbuminemia. The chest radiograph may be normal initially and can progress rapidly to bilateral infiltrates and ARDS. Other viral pneumonias do not typically progress to ARDS as rapidly as hantavirus infections. Because of the nonspecific signs and symptoms, some patients may be misdiagnosed as having influenza.

Treatment

34. How should K.C. be treated?

Supportive treatment is important. Oxygen therapy and mechanical ventilation may be necessary. Hypotension can be treated with vasopressor agents and judicious use of IV crystalloids to prevent worsening of pulmonary edema. Universal precautions and respiratory isolation should be instituted.[124]

There is no FDA-approved drug to treat hantavirus infections. Based on one study in 242 patients, IV ribavirin was more effective than placebo in reducing the mortality and the morbidity (oliguria and hemorrhage) in patients in China. Ribavirin was given IV as a loading dose of 33 mg/kg followed by 16 mg/kg Q 6 hr for 4 days, and 8 mg/kg Q 8 hr for the next 3 days. Each dose was infused over 30 minutes. Reversible anemia was the main adverse effect of ribavirin.[126]

In an open-label trial conducted by the CDC, IV ribavirin was made available to patients with suspected HPS. Of the 64 patients definitively diagnosed with HPS, the mortality rate was 47% in patients who received ribavirin compared with 50% to those who did not. Upon review of the results of the open-label trial, a panel of experts concluded that the trial was inconclusive and a placebo-controlled trial was needed.[127]

K.C. should receive supportive treatment, including vasopressors, fluids, oxygen, and mechanical ventilation, if necessary. K.C. is a candidate for inclusion in the CDC's placebo-controlled IV ribavirin trial.

WEST NILE VIRUS

West Nile Virus (WNV) was first identified in the United States in 1999 in New York City. Since that time, the virus has had rapid geographic expansion and has infected individuals in all but four states in the continental United States.[128] Although WNV normally occurs in tropical climates, the increase in international travel and changes in weather patterns have led to its spread.

WNV is a member of the Flaviviridae family. Culicine mosquitoes (including *Culex pipiens, C. restuans,* and *C. quinquefasciatus*) are the vectors, and they infect both birds and humans. Infection with the virus involves direct inoculation by the infecting mosquito. WNV can infect a number of vertebrates, including horses. Transmission requires a mosquito bite, and transmission from person to person or bird to bird is not known to occur. Birds are reservoir hosts. Because of the seasonal variations in the life cycle of the mosquito, cases are most commonly seen during the summer and early fall.

Diagnosis is usually made by high clinical suspicion and laboratory tests. WNV can cause a wide range of illness, from an asymptomatic disease to West Nile fever to encephalitis. Mortality is low except in those with encephalitis. Mortality rates in the elderly, particularly those >70 years of age, can be nine times higher than in the general population.[129] The CDC classification of WNV encephalitis consists of the following: (1) febrile illness with neurologic symptoms plus isolation of the WNV antigen or genomic sequence from a tissue, blood, CSF, or other body fluids; (2) WNV IgM antibody in a CSF sample; (3) a fourfold rise in the antibody titer to WNV; and (4) demonstration of an IgM and IgG to WNV in a single serum sample.

Clinical Presentation

35. A.G. is an 84-year-old woman. She is very active and runs for the yearly flower festival in the community. She was brought to the ED by her granddaughter, who found her at home, confused and complaining of a headache, fatigue, and increasing muscle weakness. She is found to have a temperature of 103°F. Her Mini-Mental Status Exam score was 21 of 30. She has decreasing muscle strength and an erythematous, macular, papular rash on her arms and legs. The complete blood count and electrolytes were normal, with the exception of slightly decreased sodium. The CSF had increased white blood cells, increased protein and normal glucose, and positive IgM antibody to WNV. A CT scan showed no abnormalities. What signs and symptoms are indicative of WNV encephalitis?

Acute signs and symptoms of WNV include sudden onset of fever, anorexia, weakness, nausea, vomiting, eye pain, headache, altered mental status, and stiff neck. A rash may be present on the arms, legs, neck, and trunk. The rash is typically erythematous, macular, and papular with or without morbilliform eruption. Laboratory parameters may show normal or elevated WBC counts. Low serum sodium concentrations may be seen in patients with encephalitis. CSF usually shows pleocytosis, with mostly an elevation of lymphocytes, elevated protein levels, and normal glucose levels. Magnetic resonance imaging (MRI) shows some enhancement of the leptomeninges or the periventricular areas in approximately one third of patients, but no other abnormalities or evidence of acute disease are present on either CT or MRI examination.

With disease progression, further muscle weakness and hyporeflexia may be seen. Patients may progress to a diffuse, flaccid paralysis similar to Guillain-Barré syndrome. Ataxia, extrapyramidal signs, cranial nerve abnormalities, myelitis, optic neuritis, and seizures may be seen.

Treatment

36. What treatment options are available to A.G.?

Currently, treatment of WNV infection is supportive. Patients with febrile infection usually have a self-limiting course. In more severe cases, patients with muscle weakness and signs of encephalitis will require admission to an intensive care unit, and many will need mechanical ventilation. The available antiviral medications do not have any activity against WNV in vivo, although ribavirin inhibits replication in vitro.[130] Combination therapy of high-dose ribavirin and interferon-α-2b has been used in patients with severe disease with minimal success. Although doses have not been established, the doses required to inhibit the virus are 2 million units of interferon and 2,400 mg of ribavirin daily.[131] Further studies are necessary to determine the effectiveness of these agents and the appropriate dose and duration of therapy.

SEVERE ACUTE RESPIRATORY DISTRESS SYNDROME

Severe acute respiratory distress syndrome (SARS) was first identified in China in early 2003. Since that time the viral syndrome has been reported in several countries in East Asia, North America (particularly Canada), and Europe. As of May 2003, nearly 7,000 cases have been reported, with a case fatality rate of about 4% to 7%.[132] Many of the cases reported in Asia and Canada have been traced to a single index case, with outbreaks clustered in apartments, hotels, or health care facilities. There is some evidence to suggest that increased age (>60 years) may be associated with an increased mortality risk.[133]

The disease is thought to be spread by airborne microdroplets. Geography and a history of recent travel to affected areas are thought to be very important to an individual's likelihood of contracting the disease. In a sample of 100 suspected patients in the United States, 94% traveled within the 10 days before illness onset to an area listed in SARS case definitions.[134] While travel to an affected area is a risk factor for acquisition of SARS, it is not known whether domestic or international flights represent a risk factor.

Because the etiology of the SARS epidemic remains to be definitively identified, diagnosis is usually made on the basis of clinical criteria as outlined by the CDC. In the absence of a definitive etiology, the diagnosis of SARS is based upon criteria that make a case either suspect or probable. Patients who are considered suspected cases have the following features:[135] documented temperature >100.4°F, one or more respiratory symptoms, close contact within 10 days of onset of symptoms with person being investigated for or suspected of having SARS, or travel to an area with documented transmissions as defined by the World Health Organization (WHO).[136] A patient who is considered a probable case is one with radiographic evidence of pneumonia or respiratory distress syndrome or autopsy findings consistent with respiratory distress syndrome without an etiology.

Efforts to identify the syndrome have led to the isolation of a novel coronavirus from patients who met the case definition of SARS. Inoculations of a Vero E6 cell line with throat swab specimens from patients with the diagnosis of SARS showed cytopathologic features. Electron microscopy indicated morphologic features consistent with coronavirus. The uniqueness of the potential coronavirus was also established by polymerase chain reaction techniques. In addition, immunohistochemical testing revealed reactivity with group I corona family polyclonal antibodies.[137]

Clinical Presentation

37. N.Z. is a 48-year-old Asian female who recently returned from a 2-week business trip to Taiwan. Two days after her return, she complained of fatigue, myalgia, chills, and headache. On the third day, she awoke feeling feverish and diaphoretic. She measured her temperature as 101°F. She complained of a sore throat with cough and shortness of breath as she climbed stairs. She visited her local physician, who noted rales during chest auscultation. As there was concern for SARS, the patient was admitted and placed under quarantine in a local hospital. A chest radiograph revealed bilateral interstitial infiltrates. A routine pneumonia workup was performed with pulse oximetry, blood cultures, and sputum Gram's stain and culture. Blood was also collected for antibody analysis. Complete blood count and clinical chemistries were analyzed, and the tests were remarkable only for lymphopenia. What signs and symptoms in N.Z. suggest that this is a case of SARS?

A typical incubation period for SARS is 2 to 7 days. The subsequent clinical course has been characterized by rapid onset of high fever, myalgia, chills, rigor, and sore throat followed by shortness of breath, nonproductive cough, and radiographic evidence of pneumonia.[138] While the majority of cases of infection are self-limited, this may be followed by hypoxemia, which may progress to the need for intubation and mechanical ventilation. Typically, patients do not manifest neurologic or GI symptoms.

For patients suspected of having SARS in the United States, initial diagnostic testing should include a chest radiograph, pulse oximetry, blood cultures, and sputum Gram's stain and culture (to include testing for influenza A, influenza B, and RSV). It is also important to save additional specimens for later testing. The clinical study that can retrospectively indicate that someone has been infected with SARS is the detection of the SARS coronavirus antibody, which is obtained from convalescent serum at >21 days.

Treatment

38. What treatment options are available to N.Z.?

Currently, treatment for SARS is empiric as SARS signs and symptoms are nonspecific and not readily distinguishable from those associated with a wide variety of other potential pathogens, including bacteria, viruses, and atypical bacteria (including intracellular pathogens). Antibiotics whose spectrum of activity includes bacteria associated with atypical pneumonia (e.g., macrolides) may be given, depending on the severity of the presentation.[138] Ribavirin has also been widely used empirically in Canada.[139] Although doses varied from hospital to hospital, most patients received a loading dose of 2 g IV, followed by 1 g IV Q 6 hr for 4 days, then 500 mg Q 8 hr for 3 days. Recent in vitro data, however, have confirmed the lack of activity of ribavirin against this coronavirus. In addition, oseltamivir has been used empirically in the treatment of SARS. The majority of U.S. patients suspected of having SARS recovered or were clinically stabilized without targeted antiviral therapy.[134]

THE COMMON COLD

The most common viral infection is the common cold. In the United States, approximately 62 million cases of the common cold occur annually.[153] An estimated 20 million and 22 million days of absence from work and school, respectively, occur. The frequency of the occurrence of a cold is greater in younger children and decreases with increasing age. Although the common cold is self-limiting, otitis media in occurs in approximately 20% of children following infection.[154]

Many viruses have been isolated from patients with respiratory infections, but rhinovirus is the most common viral pathogen.[155] Rhinovirus accounts for approximately 34% of all respiratory illnesses. Over 100 different serotypes of rhinovirus exist, and the prevalence of each varies with time and geography. Other pathogens include coronavirus, parainfluenza, RSV, adenovirus, and enterovirus. Because of the number of pathogens known to cause the common cold, development of an effective vaccine remains difficult.

Treatment for the common cold is directed at pharmacologic treatment of symptoms. Nonsteroidal anti-inflammatory drugs, oral or intranasal decongestants, antihistamines, and antitussives may be used. Currently there are no specific antiviral treatments for the common cold.

Prevention

39. J.C. comes into the pharmacy asking for an herbal product that will help him prevent colds this upcoming cold season. He states that last year he had three colds and his neighbor had none. His neighbor had mentioned an herbal product he had been taking. J.C. cannot remember the name of the product but wonders if there are any products that may be helpful.

Zinc

Zinc, a dietary supplement, has been studied in both the prevention and treatment of the common cold. The proposed mechanism of action is that the rhinovirus 3C protease is inhibited by zinc, and the inhibition of this enzyme prevents viral replication. In vitro, zinc has been shown to have antiviral activity. Several trials conducted in the past several decades have produced conflicting results on the benefits of zinc in decreasing symptom severity or duration. A meta-analysis found no clear evidence to support the use of zinc lozenges in the treatment or prevention of the common cold. Patients who took zinc lozenges for the common cold complained of mouth irritation, unpleasant taste, feeling sick, and diarrhea. Zinc is not recommended for treatment or prophylaxis of the common cold.[156]

Echinacea

Echinacea is an herbal product extracted from the *Echinacea* plant, which belongs to the Compositae family. Echinacea is thought to stimulate the immune system, specifically phagocytosis. Clinical trials using Echinacea have shown positive results in decreasing the incidence of infection when compared to placebo, but the results remain inconclusive. No benefits were shown in decreasing the severity and duration of the common cold when compared to placebo. In trials evaluating the effectiveness of Echinacea in the treatment of the common cold, two of eight trials found a decrease in the severity and duration of symptoms. Because the current data are inconclusive, the use of Echinacea in the prevention or treatment of the common cold is not recommended.[157]

REFERENCES

1. Reid AH et al. The 1918 Spanish influenza: integrating history and biology. Microbes Infect 2001; 3:81.
2. Whitley RJ et al. Herpes simplex virus. Clin Infect Dis 1998;26:541.
3. Aurelius E et al. Rapid diagnosis of herpes simplex encephalitis by nested polymerase chain reaction assay of cerebrospinal fluid. Lancet 1991;337:189.
4. Skoldenberg B et al. Acyclovir versus vidarabine in herpes simplex encephalitis. Lancet 1984;2:707.
5. Whitley RJ et al. Vidarabine versus acyclovir therapy in herpes simplex encephalitis. N Engl J Med 1986;314:144.
6. Skoldenberg B. Herpes simplex encephalitis. Scand J Infect Dis Suppl 1996;100:8.
7. Naik HR et al. Foscarnet therapy for acyclovir-resistant herpes simplex virus 1 infection in allogeneic bone marrow transplant recipients. Clin Infect Dis 1995;21:1514.
8. Safrin S et al. A controlled trial comparing foscarnet with vidarabine for acyclovir-resistant mucocutaneous herpes simplex in the acquired immunodeficiency syndrome. N Engl J Med 1991;325:551.
9. Whitley RJ et al. Pharmacokinetics of acyclovir in humans following intravenous administration. Am J Med 1982;73(1A):165.
10. de Miranda P et al. Acyclovir kinetics after intravenous infusion. Clin Pharmacol Ther 1979; 26:718.
11. Fiddian AP, Brigden D. Acyclovir: an update of the clinical applications of this antiherpes agent. Antiviral Res 1984;4:99.
12. Laskin OL et al. Pharmacokinetics and tolerance of acyclovir, a new antiherpes virus agent, in humans. Antimicrob Agents Chemother 1982;21:393.
13. Blum MR et al. Overview of acyclovir pharmacokinetic disposition in adults and children. Am J Med 1982;73(1A):186.
14. Yeager AS. Use of acyclovir in premature and term neonates. Am J Med 1982;73(1A):205.
15. Hintz M et al. Neonatal acyclovir pharmacokinetics in patients with herpes virus infection. Am J Med 1982;73(1A):210.
16. Collins P et al. Sensitivity of herpes, virus isolates from acyclovir clinical trials. Am J Med 1982;73(1A):380.
17. Swierkosz EM, Biron KK. Antimicrobial agents and susceptibility testing. In: Murray PR et al, eds. Manual of Clinical Microbiology, 6th ed. Washington, DC: ASM Press, 1995:1417.
18. GlaxoWellcome. Zovirax (acyclovir). Product Information. Research Triangle Park, 2001.
19. Wagstaff AJ et al. Aciclovir. A reappraisal of its antiviral activity, pharmacokinetic properties and therapeutic efficacy. Drugs 1994;47:153.
20. Laskin OL. Acyclovir: pharmacology and clinical experience. Arch Intern Med 1984;144:1241.

21. Bryson YJ et al. Treatment of first episodes of genital herpes simplex virus infection with oral acyclovir. N Engl J Med 1983;308:916.
22. Forsgren M, Malm G. Herpes simplex virus and pregnancy. Scand J Infect Dis Suppl 1996; 100:14.
23. Feder HM Jr. Treatment of adult chickenpox with oral acyclovir. Arch Intern Med 1990;150:2061.
24. Kohl S. The diagnosis and treatment of neonatal herpes simplex virus infection. Pediatr Ann 2002; 31:726.
25. Kimberlin DW. Advances in the treatment of neonatal herpes simplex infections. Rev Med Virol 2001;11:157.
26. Whitley RL. Neonatal herpes simplex virus infections. J Med Vir 1993;Suppl 1:13.
27. Whitley R et al. A controlled trial comparing vidarabine with acyclovir in neonatal herpes simplex virus infection. N Engl J Med 1991;324:444.
28. Kimerlin DW et al. Safety and efficacy of high-dose intravenous acyclovir in the management of neonatal herpes simplex virus infections. Pediatrics 2001;108:230.
29. American Academy of Pediatrics. Herpes simplex. In: Peter G, ed. 1997 Red Book: Report of the Committee on Infectious Diseases, 24th ed. Elk Grove Village, IL: American Academy of Pediatrics, 1997:266.
30. Kimberlin DW et al. Administration of oral acyclovir suppressive therapy after neonatal herpes simplex virus disease limited to the skin, eyes and mouth: results of a Phase I/II trial. Pediatr Infect Dis J 1996;15:247.
31. Gutierrez K, Arvin AM. Long term antiviral suppression after treatment for neonatal herpes infection. Pediatr Infect Dis J 2003;22:371.
32. Saral R et al. Acyclovir prophylaxis of herpes simplex virus infections: a randomized, double-blind, controlled trial in bone marrow transplant recipients. N Engl J Med 1981;305:63.
33. Gluckman E et al. Prophylaxis of herpes infections after bone marrow transplantation by oral acyclovir. Lancet 1983;2:706.
34. Schacker T et al. Famciclovir for the suppression of symptomatic and asymptomatic herpes simplex virus reactivation in HIV-infected persons. Ann Intern Med 1998;128:21.
35. Shepp DH et al. Oral acyclovir therapy for mucocutaneous herpes simplex virus infections in immunocompromised marrow transplant patients. Ann Intern Med 1985;102:783.
36. Whitley RJ et al. Infections caused by herpes simplex virus in the immunocompromised host: natural history and topical acyclovir therapy. J Infect Dis 1984;150:323.
37. Hoglund M et al. Comparable aciclovir exposures produced by oral valaciclovir and intravenous aciclovir in immunocompromised cancer patients. J Antimicrob Chemother 2001;47:855.
38. Spruance SL et al. Acyclovir cream for treatment of herpes simplex labialis: results of two randomized, double-blind, vehicle-controlled, multicenter clinical trials. Animicrob Agents Chemother 2002; 46:2238.
39. Raborn GW et al. Effective treatment of herpes simplex labialis with penciclovir cream: combined results of two trials. J Am Dent Assoc 2002;133:303.
40. Sacks SL et al. Clinical efficacy of topical docosanol 10% cream for herpes simplex labialis: a multicenter, randomized, placebo-controlled trial. J Am Acad Dermatol 2001;45:222.
41. Lin L et al. Topical application of penciclovir cream for the treatment of herpes simplex facialis/labialis: a randomized, double-blind, multicentre, aciclovir-controlled trial. J Dermatol Treat 2002;13:67.
42. Femiano F et al. Recurrent herpes labialis: efficacy of topical therapy with penciclovir compared with acyclovir (aciclovir). Oral Diseases 2001;7:31.
43. Spruance SL et al. Penciclovir cream for the treatment of herpes simplex labialis. JAMA 1997; 277:1374.
44. Raborn GW et al. Penciclovir cream for recurrent herpes simplex labialis: an effective new treatment. Interscience Conference Antimicro Agents Chemother 1996;36:178.
45. Spruance SL et al. Treatment of recurrent herpes simplex labialis with oral acyclovir. J Infect Dis 1990;161:185.
46. Rooney JF et al. Oral acyclovir to suppress frequently recurrent herpes labialis: a double-blind, placebo-controlled trial. Ann Intern Med 1993; 118:268.
47. Rabella N et al. Antiviral susceptibility of herpes simplex viruses and its clinical correlates: a single center's experience. Clin Infec Dis 2002;34:1055.
48. Morfin F et al. Herpes simplex virus resistance to antiviral drugs. J Clin Virol 2003;26:29.
49. Safrin S et al. A controlled trial comparing foscarnet with vidarabine for acyclovir resistant mucocutaneous herpes simplex in the acquired immunodeficiency syndrome. N Engl J Med 1991;325:551.
50. Bryant P et al. Successful treatment of foscarnet-resistant herpes simplex stomatitis with intravenous cidofovir in a child. Pediatr Infect Dis J 2001; 20:1083.
51. Chen Y et al. Resistant herpes simplex virus type 1 infection: an emerging concern after allogenic stem cell transplantation. Clin Infect Dis 2000;31:927.
52. Wilhelmus K. Interventions for herpes simplex virus epithelial keratitis. Cochrane Database Syst Rev 2001;1.
53. Herpetic Eye Disease Study Group. Oral acyclovir for herpes simplex virus eye disease. Arch Ophthalmol 2000;118:1030.

54. Seward JF et al. Varicella disease after introduction of varicella vaccine in the United States, 1995–2000. JAMA 2002;287:606.

55. Carcao MD et al. Sequential use of intravenous and oral acyclovir therapy of varicella in immunocompromised children. Pediatr Infect Dis J 1998; 17:626.

56. Masaoka T et al. Varicella-zoster virus infection in immunocompromised patients. J Med Vir 1993; Suppl 1:82.

57. Klassen TP et al. Acyclovir for treating otherwise healthy children and adolescents. Cochrane Database Sys Rev 2003;(1).

58. Whitley RJ. Therapeutic approaches to varicella-zoster virus infections. J Infect Dis 1992;166(Suppl 1):S51.

59. Wallace MR et al. Treatment of adult varicella with oral acyclovir: a randomized placebo-controlled trial. Ann Intern Med 1992;117:358.

60. Committee on Infectious Diseases. The use of acyclovir in otherwise healthy children with varicella. Pediatrics 1993;91:674.

61. Crooks RT et al. Zoster-associated chronic pain: an overview of clinical trials with acyclovir. Scand J Infect Dis Suppl 1991;80:62.

62. deGreef H. Famciclovir, a new oral antiherpes drug; results of the first controlled clinical study demonstrating its efficacy and safety in the treatment of uncomplicated herpes zoster in immunocompetent patients. Int J Antimicrob Agents 1995;4:241.

63. Tyring S et al. Famciclovir for the treatment of acute herpes zoster: effects on acute disease and postherpetic neuralgia: a randomized, double-blind placebo-controlled trial. Ann Intern Med 1995; 123:89.

64. Beutner KR et al. Valacyclovir compared to acyclovir for improved therapy of herpes zoster in immunocompetent adults. Antimicrob Agents Chemother 1995;39:1546.

65. Ernst ME et al. Oral corticosteroids for herpes zoster pain. Ann Pharmacother 1998;32:1099.

66. Santee JA. Corticosteroids for herpes zoster: what do they accomplish? Am J Clin Dermatol 2002; 3:517.

67. Wood MJ et al. A randomized trial of acyclovir for seven days or twenty-one days with and without prednisolone for treatment of acute herpes zoster. N Engl J Med 1994;330:896.

68. Whitley RJ et al. Acyclovir with and without prednisone for the treatment of herpes zoster. Ann Intern Med 1996;125:376.

69. Whitley RJ et al. Acyclovir plus steroids for herpes zoster [letter]. Ann Intern Med 1997;126:832.

70. Watson CP et al. A randomized vehicle-controlled trial of topical capsaicin in the treatment of postherpetic neuralgia. Clin Ther 1993;15:510.

71. Balfour HH Jr et al. Acyclovir halts progression of herpes zoster in immunocompromised patients. N Engl J Med 1983;308:1448.

72. Margolis KL et al. Frequency of adverse reactions after influenza vaccination. Am J Med 1990;88:27.

73. Nichol KL et al. Side effects associated with influenza vaccination in healthy working adults. Arch Intern Med 1996;156:1546.

74. Prevention and control of influenza: recommendations of the Advisory Committee on Immunization Practices (ACIP). MMWR 2003;52(No. RR-8):1.

75. Covington TR, ed. Handbook of Nonprescription Drugs, 13th ed. Washington, DC: American Pharmaceutical Association, 2002.

76. Hayden FG et al. Use of oral neuraminidase inhibitor oseltamivir in experimental influenza. Randomized controlled trials for prevention and treatment. JAMA 1999;282:1240.

77. The Management of Influenza on the Southern Hemisphere trial (MIST) study group. Randomized trial of efficacy and safety of inhaled zanamivir in treatment of influenza A and B virus infections. Lancet 1998;352:1877.

78. Jefferson T et al. Neuraminidase inhibitors for preventing and treating influenza in healthy adults. Cochrane Database Syst Rev 2003;1.

79. Roche Laboratories. Oseltamivir. Product information. Nutley, NJ, 2000.

80. Glaxo Wellcome Inc. Zanamivir. Product information. Research Triangle, NC, 2001.

81. Endo Pharmaceuticals Inc. Symmetrel. Product information. Wilmington, DE, 2000.

82. Uyeki TM. Influenza diagnosis and treatment in children: a review of studies on clinically useful tests and antiviral treatment for influenza. Pediatr Infect Dis J 2003;22:164.

83. Jefferson TO et al. Amantadine and rimantadine for preventing and treating influenza A in adults. Cochrane Database Syst Rev 2003;1.

84. Miotti PG et al. The influence of HIV infection on antibody responses to a two-dose regimen of influenza vaccine. JAMA 1989;262:779.

85. Hayden FG et al. Use of selective oral neuraminidase inhibitor oseltamivir to prevent influenza. N Engl J Med 1999;341:1336.

86. Hayden FG et al. Inhaled zanamivir for the prevention of influenza in families. N Engl J Med 2000;18:1282.

87. Monto AS et al. Zanamivir in the prevention of influenza in healthy adults: a randomized controlled trial. JAMA 1999;282:31.

88. Englund JA et al. Common emergence of amantadine- and rimantadine-resistant influenza A viruses in symptomatic immunocompromised adults. Clin Infect Dis 1998;26:1418.

89. Hayden FG et al. Recovery of drug-resistant influenza A virus during therapeutic use of rimantadine. Antimicrob Agents Chemother 1991; 35:1741.

90. Monto AS, Arden NH. Implications of viral resistance to amantadine in control of influenza A. Clin Infect Dis 1992;15:362.

91. Hayden FG et al. Recovery of drug-resistant influenza A virus during therapeutic use of rimantadine. Antimicrob Agents Chemother 1991; 35:1741.

92. Barnett JM et al. Zanamivir susceptibility monitoring and characterization of influenza virus clinical isolates obtained during phase II clinical efficacy studies. Antimicrob Agents Chemother 2000;44:78.

93. Gubareva LV et al. Selection of influenza virus mutants in experimentally infected volunteers treated with oseltamivir. J Infect Dis 2001; 183:523.

94. Jackson HC et al. Management of influenza: use of new antivirals and resistance in perspective. Clin Drug Invest 2000;20:447.

95. Lugo RA, Nahata MC. Pathogenesis and treatment of bronchiolitis. Clin Pharm 1993;12:95.

96. Shay DK et al. Bronchiolitis-associated mortality and estimates of respiratory syncytial virus-associated deaths among US children 1979–1997. J Infect Dis 2001; 183:16.

97. Stein RT et al. Respiratory syncytial virus in early life and risk of wheeze and allergy by age 13 years. Lancet 1999;354:541.

98. Nafstad P et al. Early respiratory infections and childhood asthma. Pediatrics 2000;106:e38.

99. Peter JM et al. Links between respiratory syncytial virus bronchiolitis and childhood asthma: clinical and research approaches. Pediatr Infect Dis J 2003;22:S58.

100. Panitch HB. Respiratory syncytial virus bronchiolitis: supportive care and therapies designed to overcome airway obstruction. Pediatr Infect Dis J 2003;22;S83.

101. Kellner JD et al. Efficacy of bronchodilator therapy in bronchiolitis: a meta-analysis. Arch Pediatr Adolesc Med 1996;150:1166.

102. ICN Pharmaceuticals. Product information. Virzole (ribavirin for inhalation solution). Costa Mesa, CA: ICN Pharmaceuticals, May 1996.

103. American Academy of Pediatrics, Committee on Infectious Diseases. Use of ribavirin in the treatment of respiratory syncytial virus infection. Pediatrics 1993;92:501.

104. Wheeler JG et al. Historical cohort evaluation of ribavirin efficacy in respiratory syncytial virus infection. Pediatr Infect Dis J 1993;12:209.

105. Englund JA et al. High-dose, short-duration ribavirin aerosol therapy compared with standard ribavirin therapy in children with suspected respiratory syncytial virus infection. J Pediatr 1994; 125:635.

106. American Academy of Pediatrics, Committee on Infectious Diseases. Reassessment of the indications for ribavirin therapy in respiratory syncytial virus infections. Pediatrics 1996;97:137.

107. Rodriguez WJ et al. Respiratory syncytial virus (RSV) immune globulin intravenous therapy for RSV lower respiratory tract infection in infants and young children at high risk for severe RSV infections. Pediatrics 19997;99:454.

108. Rodriguez WJ et al. Respiratory syncytial virus immune globulin treatment of RSV lower respiratory tract infection in previously healthy children. Pediatrics 1997;100:937.

109. American Academy of Pediatrics, Committee on Infectious Diseases, Committee on Fetus and Newborn. Respiratory syncytial virus immune globulin intravenous: Indications for use. Pediatrics 1997;99:645.

110. Hall CB. Ribavirin and respiratory syncytial virus. Am J Dis Child 1986;140:331.

111. Smith DW et al. A controlled trial of aerosolized ribavirin in infants receiving mechanical ventilation for severe respiratory syncytial virus infection. N Engl J Med 1991;325:24.

112. Meert KL et al. Aerosolized ribavirin in mechanically ventilated children with respiratory syncytial virus lower respiratory tract disease: a prospective, double-blind, randomized trial. Crit Care Med 1994;22:566.

113. Janai HK et al. Ribavirin: adverse drug reactions, 1986 to 1988. Pediatr Infect Dis J 1990;9:209.

114. Edell D et al. Early ribavirin treatment of bronchiolitis. Effect on long-term respiratory morbidity. Chest 2002;122:935.

115. Rodriguez WJ et al. Environmental exposure of primary care personnel to ribavirin aerosol when supervising treatment of infants with respiratory syncytial virus infections. Antimicrob Agents Chemother 1987;31:1143.

116. Harrison R et al. Assessing exposure of healthcare personnel to aerosols of ribavirin, California MMWR 1988;37:560.

117. Fackler JC et al. Precautions in the use of ribavirin at the Children's Hospital. N Engl J Med 1990; 322:634.

118. Groothius JR et al. Prophylactic administration of respiratory syncytial virus immune globulin to high-risk infants and young children. N Engl J Med 1993;329:1524.

119. PREVENT Study Group. Reduction of RSV hospitalization among premature infants and children with bronchopulmonary dysplasia using respiratory syncytial virus immune globulin prophylaxis. Pediatrics 1997;99:93.

120. The IMpact-RSV Study Group. Palivizumab, a humanized respiratory syncytial virus monoclonal antibody, reduces hospitalizations from respiratory syncytial virus infection in high-risk infants. Pediatrics 1998;102:531.

121. Committee on Infectious Diseases. Prevention of respiratory syncytial virus infections: Indications for the use of palivizumab and update on the use of RSV-IVIG. Pediatrics 1998;102:1211.

122. Khan AS et al. Hantavirus pulmonary syndrome: the first 100 cases. J Infect Dis 1996;173:1297.

123. Centers for Disease Control. Update: hantavirus pulmonary syndrome, United States, 1993. MMWR 1993;42:816.

124. Mertz GJ et al. Hantavirus infection. Disease-a-Month 1998;44:89.

125. Centers for Disease Control and Prevention. Case Information: Hantavirus pulmonary syndrome case count and descriptive statistics as of May 7, 2003. Available at http://www.cdc.gov/ncidod/diseases/hanta/hps/noframes/caseinfo.htm. Accessed May 28, 2003.

126. Huggins JW et al. Prospective, double-blind, concurrent, placebo-controlled clinical trial of intravenous ribavirin therapy of hemorrhagic fever with renal syndrome. J Infect Dis 1991;164:119.

127. Mertz G et al. Hantavirus infections in the United States: diagnosis and treatment. Adv Exp Med Biol 1996;394:153.

128. Centers for Disease Control and Prevention. Epidemic/epizootic West Nile Virus in the United States: revised guidelines for surveillance, prevention, and control. April 2001.

129. Nash D et al. The outbreak of West Nile Virus infection in the New York City area in 1999. N Engl J Med 2001;344:1807.

130. Petersen LR et al. West Nile Virus: a primer for the clinician. Ann Intern Med 2002;137:173.

131. Anderson JF, Rahal JJ. Efficacy of interferon alpha-2b and ribavirin against West Nile Virus in vitro. Emerg Infect Dis 2002;8:107.

132. CDC. Severe acute respiratory syndrome, Singapore, 2003. MMWR 2003;52:411.

133. Donnelly C et al. Epidemiological determinants of spread of causal agent of severe acute respiratory syndrome in Hong Kong. Lancet, published online May 7, 2003.

134. CDC. Update: Outbreak of severe acute respiratory syndrome, worldwide, 2003. MMWR 2003; 52:269.

135. CDC SARS website "case definition," updated April 20, 2003, at http://www.cdc.gov/ncidod/sars/casedefinition. Accessed April 26, 2003.

136. CDC. Outbreak of severe acute respiratory syndrome, worldwide, 2003. MMWR 2003;52:226.

137. Ksiazek TG et al. A novel coronavirus associated with severe acute respiratory syndrome. N Engl J Med 2003;348:1953.

138. CDC. Update: Outbreak of severe acute respiratory syndrome, worldwide, 2003. MMWR 2003; 52:255.

139. Booth CM et al. Clinical features and short-term outcomes of 144 patients with SARS in the greater Toronto area. JAMA 2003;289 (in press, JAMA-Express available online at http://jama.ama-assn.org/cgi/reprint/289.21.JOC30885v1.pdf).

140. Van Dyke RB et al. Pharmacokinetics of orally-administered acyclovir in patients with herpes progenitalis. Am J Med 1982;73(1A):172.

141. Straus SE et al. Acyclovir for chronic mucocutaneous herpes simplex virus infection in immunosuppressed patients. Ann Intern Med 1982; 96:270.

142. Pue MA et al. Linear pharmacokinetics of penciclovir following administration of single oral doses of famciclovir 125, 250, 500 and 750 mg to healthy volunteers. J Antimicrob Chemother 1994;33:119.

143. Smith Kline Beecham Pharmaceuticals. Famciclovir. Product information. Philadelphia, 1997.

144. Bardsley-Elliot A, Noble S. Oseltamivir. Drugs 1999;58:851.

145. Wills RJ et al. Rimantadine pharmacokinetics after single and multiple doses. Antimicrob Agents Chemother 1987;31:826.

146. Soul-Lawton J et al. Absolute bioavailability and metabolic disposition of valacyclovir, the L-valyl ester of acyclovir, following oral administration to humans. Antimicrob Agents Chemother 1995; 39:2759.

147. Glaxo Wellcome Inc. Valacyclovir hydrochloride. Product Information. Research Triangle, NC, 1997.

148. Cass LMR et al. Pharmacokinetics of zanamivir after intravenous, oral, inhaled, or intranasal administration to healthy volunteers. Clin Pharmacokinet 1999;36(Suppl 1):1.

149. Dunn CJ, Goa KL. Zanamivir. A review of its use in influenza. Drugs 1999;58:761.

150. Filer CW et al. Metabolic and pharmacokinetic studies following oral administration of 14C-famciclovir to healthy subjects. Xenobiotica 1994; 24:357.

151. Wills RJ et al. Pharmacokinetics of rimantadine hydrochloride in patients with chronic liver disease. Clin Pharmacol Ther 1987;31:826.

152. Hayden FG et al. Comparative single-dose pharmacokinetics of amantadine hydrochloride and rimantadine hydrochloride in young and elderly adults. Antimicrob Agents Chemother 1985; 28:216.

153. Centers for Disease Control and Prevention. Vital and health statistics. Current estimates from the National Health Interview survey, 1996. October 1999.

154. Heikkinen T et al. The common cold. Lancet; 361:51.

155. Monto AS. Epidemiology of viral respiratory infections. Am J Med 2002;112:4S.

156. Marshall I. Zinc for the common cold. Cochrane Database Syst Rev 2003;1.

157. Melchart D et al. Echinacea for preventing and treating the common cold. Cochrane Database Syst Rev 2003;1.

Viral Hepatitis

Curtis D. Holt

Table 73-1   Hepatitis Nomenclature

Hepatitis Type	Antigen	Corresponding Antibody	Comments
A	Hepatitis A virus (HAV)	Hepatitis A antibody (anti-HAV)	RNA virus; present in stool and serum early in course of hepatitis A
B	Hepatitis B surface antigen (HBsAg)	Hepatitis B surface antibody (anti-HBs)	DNA virus; found in serum in >90% of patients with acute hepatitis B, anti-HBs appears following infection and confers immunity
	Hepatitis B core antigen (HBcAg)	Hepatitis B core antibody (anti-HBc)	Anti-HBc detected in serum during and after acute infection
	Hepatitis B envelope antigen (HBeAg)	HB envelope antibody (anti-HBe)	HBeAg correlates with infectivity; suggestive of active viral replication
C	Hepatitis C antigen (HCAg)	Hepatitis C antibody (anti-HCV)	RNA virus; previously known as post-transfusion NANB hepatitis
D	Hepatitis D antigen (HDAg)	Hepatitis D antibody (anti-HDV)	Defective RNA virus; requires presence of HBsAg
E	Hepatitis E antigen (HEAg)	Hepatitis E antibody (anti-HEV)	RNA virus present in stool; cause of enteric NANB hepatitis
G	Hepatitis G antigen (HGAg)	Not available	RNA-like virus; named GBV-A, GBV-B, and GBV-C; thought to be of tamarin origin

NANB, non-A, non-B hepatitis.

Table 73-2   Comparison of the Etiologic Forms of Hepatitis A, B, C, D, E, and G

	HAV	HBV	HCV	HDV	HEV	HGV
Virus	HAV	HBV	HCV	HDV	HEV	HGV
Genome	RNA	DNA	RNA	RNA	RNA	RNA
Family	Picornavirus	Hepadnavirus	Flavivirus	Satellite	Calicivirus	Flavivirus
Size (nm)	27	42	30–60	40	32	Unknown
Incubation (days) [mean]	15–50 [30]	45–180 [80]	15–160	21–140 [35]	15–65 [42]	14–35 [na]
Transmission						
Oral	Yes	Rare	Rare	No	Yes, common	Unknown
Percutaneous	Rare	Common	Common	Common	Unknown	Yes
Sexual	No	Common	Common	Common	No	Rare
Perinatal	No	Common	Rare	Common	Rare	Yes, rare
Onset	Sudden	Insidious	Insidious	Insidious	Sudden	Yes, rare
Clinical illness	70-80% adults 5% children	10–15%	5–10%	10%	70–80% adults	Unknown
Icteric presentation						
Children	<10%	30%	25%	Unknown	Unknown	Unknown
Adults	30%	5–20%	5–10%	25%	Common	Unknown
Peak ALT (U/L)	800–1,000	1,000–1,500	300–800	1,000–1,500	800–1,000	Unknown
Incidence of acute liver failure (%)	<1	<1	<1	2–7.5	<1; higher in pregnant women	Unknown
Serum diagnosis						
Acute infection	Anti-HAV IgM	HBsAg Anti-HBc IgM	HCV-RNA (anti-HCV)	Anti-HDV IgM	Anti-HEV IgG (seroconversion)	HGV RNA
Chronic infection		HBsAg Anti-HBc IgG	Anti-HCV (ELISA) RIBA	Anti-HDV IgG	NA	HGV RNA
Viral markers	HAV RNA	HBV-DNA DNA polymerase	HCV-RNA	HDV-RNA	Viruslike particles	HGV RNA
Immunity	Anti-HAV IgG	Anti-HBs	NA	NA	Anti-HEV IgG	Unknown
Case-fatality rate	0.1–2.7% 0.15–1.7%	1–3%	1–2%	<1% coinfect	0.5–4% 1.5–21% pregnant women	Unknown
Complete recovery	>97%	85–97%	50%	90%	99%	Unknown
Incidence of chronic infection	0%	2–7% >90% neonates	50%	80% superinfect ≤5% coinfection	0%	Unknown
Carrier state	No	Yes	Yes	Yes	No	Unknown
Risk of hepatocellular carcinoma	No	Yes	Yes	Yes	No	No
Drug treatment	None	Interferon, lamivudine Adefovir	Interferon, ribavirin + interferon pegylated Interferon pegylated Interferon + ribavirin	Interferon	None	Unknown

NA, not applicable.

Table 73-3   Etiologies of Chronic Hepatitis

Viral Infections	Isoniazid
Hepatitis viruses (B, C, D)	Sulfonamides
Cytomegalovirus (CMV)	Propylthiouracil
Epstein-Barr virus (EBV)	*Metabolic Disorders*
Rubella virus	Wilson's disease
Drug-Induced	α_1-Antitrypsin deficiency
Methyldopa	*Autoimmune Hepatitis*
Nitrofurantoin	

One of the first references to epidemic jaundice was ascribed to the philosopher Hippocrates. Over the centuries several epidemics, usually associated with poor hygiene, were observed, especially during wartime. The possibility of a viral etiology was considered as recently as the turn of the 20th century. Since the 1970s, five distinctly separate hepatitis viruses have been identified with liver disease as their major clinical manifestation, all of which have been characterized and cloned. A sixth virus also has been identified but has yet to be implicated in liver disease. Five of these viruses are RNA viruses, and one is a DNA virus. The mode of transmission differs, as do the natural history and outcomes. Individual viral types can be distinguished by serologic assays and, in some instances, by genotyping. Although significant progress in the area of disease prevention has occurred, advances in treatment have been limited because of the large amount of virus produced and rapid mutation. People with chronic hepatitis C produce approximately 1 trillion virus particles daily, compared with 100 billion particles daily for those infected with chronic hepatitis B and 10 billion particles daily for those with HIV infection. This chapter reviews the virology, epidemiology, pathogenesis, clinical manifestations, diagnosis, natural history, prevention, and treatment strategies for viral hepatitis.

CAUSATIVE AGENTS AND CHARACTERISTICS

Viral hepatitis is a major cause of morbidity and mortality in the United States.[1,2] At least six distinct agents are responsible for viral hepatitis.[3] These hepatotrophic viruses are identified by the letters A through G as follows: (1) type A hepatitis caused by hepatitis A virus (HAV), (2) type B hepatitis caused by hepatitis B virus (HBV), (3) type C hepatitis caused by hepatitis C virus (HCV), (4) delta hepatitis caused by the HBV-associated hepatitis D virus (HDV), (5) type E hepatitis caused by the hepatitis E virus (HEV), and (6) type G hepatitis, caused by the hepatitis G virus (HGV) (Table 73-1). Hepatitis A through E viruses primarily affect the liver and have the potential to cause inflammation and hepatocellular necrosis, whereas the clinical manifestations of HGV are unknown.[4,5] These viruses differ in their immunologic characteristics and epidemiologic patterns (Table 73-2). Fecal-oral transmission is the primary mode of infection for HAV and HEV, whereas percutaneous transmission is characteristic of HBV, HCV, and HDV.[6-10] HGV also appears to be transmitted percutaneously, primarily through volunteer blood donors.[11,12] Several other viruses primarily affect nonhepatic organ systems and may secondarily induce a hepatitis-like syndrome. These include the Epstein-Barr virus (infectious mononucleosis); cytomegalovirus; herpes simplex viruses; varicella-zoster virus; and rubella, rubeola, and mumps viruses (Table 73-2).

Definitions of Acute and Chronic Hepatitis

Viral hepatitis may present as either an acute or chronic illness. Acute hepatitis is defined as an illness with a discrete date of onset with jaundice or increased serum aminotransferase concentrations >2.5 times the upper limit of normal.[13,14] Acute viral hepatitis infection is a systemic process and lasts as long, but not exceeding, 6 months.

Chronic hepatitis is an inflammatory condition of the liver that involves ongoing hepatocellular necrosis for 6 months or more beyond the onset of acute illness.[15,16] The etiologies of chronic hepatitis are shown in Table 73-3. The most common cause of chronic hepatitis is chronic viral hepatitis, caused by HBV or HCV.[17-19] Drug-induced and autoimmune chronic hepatitis occur less frequently, while metabolic disorders and HDV chronic hepatitis are relatively rare.[20-24] Neither HAV nor HEV infections cause chronic hepatitis. The long-term effects of HGV continue to be investigated.[25]

Serologic Evaluation in Presumed Chronic Hepatitis

The diagnostic evaluation of a patient with presumed chronic hepatitis should include hepatitis serologies. Appropriate tests include hepatitis B surface antigen (HBsAg) and hepatitis C antibody (anti-HCV). If HBsAg is present, further testing for hepatitis B envelope antigen (HBeAg) and HBV-DNA is indicated to document the presence of active viral replication and assess the viral load. Testing for hepatitis D antibody (anti-HDV) also should be performed in patients with hepatitis B to evaluate the possibility of coexisting delta hepatitis. If the hepatitis serology is negative, rare but treatable causes of chronic active hepatitis should be excluded. These include alcoholic liver disease, Wilson's disease, α-antitrypsin deficiency, and drug-induced chronic active hepatitis. Drugs associated with reversible chronic active hepatitis syndrome include methyldopa,[26] nitrofurantoin,[27] isoniazid,[28] and rarely, sulfonamides[29] and propylthiouracil.[30]

Following exclusion of these conditions, the patient should be evaluated for the presence of circulating immunologic markers associated with the autoimmune (idiopathic) form of chronic hepatitis. These tests include anti–smooth muscle antibody, antimitochondrial antibody, antinuclear antibody titers, and increased serum immunoglobulins.

HEPATITIS A VIRUS
Virology and Epidemiology

Hepatitis A virus (HAV) is a 27-nm-diameter single-stranded RNA virus that is classified as a picornavirus (see Table 73-2).[31] HAV appears to replicate within the liver; however, enterocytes may also support viral replication.[31] Four distinct human HAV genotypes contain 11 structural and nonstructural proteins co-translationally and post-translationally cleaved by a viral protease.[31,32] HAV has a single serotype that remains detectable in intact virions.[31,32]

HAV has a worldwide distribution.[6,33-35] The prevalence of infection is related to the quality of the water supply, level of sanitation, and age.[35,36] However, incidence data are unreliable because the disease is frequently mild and often unrecognized, resulting in underreporting.[33–36] The primary mode of transmission is person-to-person via the fecal-oral route.[33–36] HAV is passed into the stool in high titer. Considering that the virus resists degradation by environmental conditions, gastric acid, and digestive enzymes in the upper gastrointestinal (GI) tract, it is readily spread within a population.[37] Fecally contaminated water or food also is a significant mode of transmission.[33,34,37] Children are considered an important reservoir of infection for others.[38,39]

In the United States, the reported incidence of HAV is 10.8 cases per 100,000, and it is usually associated with outbreaks in lower socioeconomic groups or common-source outbreaks (e.g., day-care centers).[34,36,37,39] Rates in males are greater than those in females by about 20%.[34,37] Children aged 5 to 14 years and Native Americans have the highest incidence of HAV.[34,36] Additionally, cyclic outbreaks of HAV have been reported among users of injecting and non-injecting drugs and in men who have sex with men.[38] Considering the widespread presence of hepatitis A antibody (anti-HAV), the virus has a high attack rate, with 70% to 90% of those exposed ultimately becoming infected.[33,34]

The most common risk factors for acquiring HAV include close contact with a person positive for HAV (26%), employment or attendance at a day-care center (14%), injection drug use (11%), recent travel (4%), and association with a suspected food- or water-borne outbreak (3%).[6,33,34,36,38,40] Up to 42% of reported HAV infections have no known source for infection.[34] Exceedingly rare causes of HAV include transfusion of blood or blood products collected from donors during the viremic phase of their infection and from contact with experimentally infected nonhuman primates.[9,34,36,41] Percutaneous transmission is rare because there is no asymptomatic carrier state for HAV, and the incubation period is brief.[1,35,39,40,42] Occupations at risk for HAV include sewage workers, hospital cleaning personnel, day-care staff, and pediatric nurses.[36,39,41] Furthermore, HAV is the most common preventable (e.g., vaccination) infection in travelers visiting locations with poor hygienic conditions.[39,43]

Pathogenesis

Theoretically, HAV infection results in both a cytopathic and immunologic hepatocyte injury; however, the exact mechanism of injury is unknown.[37,43,44] Viral replication occurs within the liver, based on immunohistochemical analysis in primates. The presence of IgM in sinusoidal cells and hepatitis A viral antigen (HAVAg) in Kupffer cells likely results in the histologic manifestations and functional impairment observed in HAV disease.[39,45] In addition, circulating T lymphocytes have been isolated from the liver of patients with acute HAV infection.[39,46]

Nonspecific mechanisms of hepatocyte injury may involve natural killer (NK) cells and lymphokine-activated killer (LAK) cells, which are believed to precede the initiation of damage caused by cytotoxic T lymphocytes (CTLs).[39,47] Subsequent hepatocyte death results in viral elimination and eventual resolution of the clinical illness.

Natural History

HAV is typically a benign, self-limited infection, with recovery within 2 months of disease onset. Two atypical courses of acute HAV infection have also been described: prolonged cholestasis and relapsing hepatitis.[39,40] In patients with prolonged cholestasis, the duration of jaundice exceeds 12 weeks and is associated with pruritus, fatigue, loose stools, and weight loss. Aminotransferase concentrations during this period are less than 500 IU/L. Spontaneous recovery often occurs, yet corticosteroids have been administered to facilitate resolution of the cholestatic phase. Relapsing or polyphasic HAV occurs in 6% to 12% of both adult and pediatric patients and can be characterized by an initial phase of acute infection followed by remission (duration of 4 to 15 weeks), with subsequent relapse. Aminotransferase concentrations often normalize during the time of remission but increase to more than 1,000 IU/L with relapse. Also HAV RNA is detectable in the serum, and HAV is usually recovered from the stool during relapse. The pathogenesis of relapsing hepatitis has not been elucidated. Fulminant hepatitis A is rare, occurring in 0.014% to 3.0% of the population infected with HAV, but it is often fatal.[39,40,49] Patients older than age 40 or younger than age 11 are more susceptible to HAV-induced fulminant hepatic failure. Chronic HAV does not exist. Typically, the course of HAV includes an incubation phase, an acute hepatitis phase, and a convalescent phase.

Clinical Manifestations

1. **E.T., a 34-year-old medical sales representative, presents to the emergency department (ED) with acute onset of jaundice and "dark urine." He was in good health until 2 weeks ago, when he noted feeling fatigued and weak, which he attributed to his demanding work schedule. He also recalled having a mild headache, loss of appetite, muscle pain, diarrhea, and low-grade fevers from 99 to 101°F. He attributed these symptoms to the flu and took acetaminophen with plenty of fluids. His symptoms persisted until yesterday, when they seemed to resolve unexplainably. He then noted his urine was cola-colored. This morning he noted jaundice of his eyes and skin and sought medical attention.**

E.T.'s medical history includes a recent respiratory tract infection, treated successfully with cefuroxime axetil. His social history is significant for frequenting the local oyster bar, where he regularly ingests raw oysters. He denies smoking and recent travel outside the United States, but admits to occasional alcohol consumption. E.T. has no history of sexual exposure, needle use, or transfusions. His current medications include diazepam 5 mg PO HS PRN for "muscle spasms," but he has not taken diazepam for "several months." He also has a seizure disorder sustained after a motorcycle accident 2 years before admission, for which he takes phenytoin 400 mg PO HS.

Physical examination is significant for a well-developed, well-nourished man in no acute distress. He is alert and oriented, with a temperature of 99°F. His sclerae and skin are icteric, and his abdomen is positive for a tender, enlarged liver and right upper quadrant (RUQ) pain. Laboratory tests reveal the following values: hemoglobin (Hgb), 16 g/dL (normal, 12.3 to 16.3 g/dL); hematocrit (Hct), 44% (normal, 37.4% to 47.0%); white blood cell (WBC) count, 5,500 cells/mm³ (normal, 3.28 to 9.29 × 10³); aspartate transaminase (AST), 120 U/L (normal, 5 to 40 U/L); alanine aminotransferase (ALT), 240 U/L (normal, 5 to 40 U/L); alkaline phosphatase, 86 U/L (normal, 21 to 91 U/L); total biliru-

bin, 3.2 mg/dL (normal, 0.2 to 1.0 mg/dL); direct bilirubin, 1.5 mg/dL (normal, 0 to 0.2 mg/dL); and phenytoin concentration, 12 mg/L (normal, 10 to 20 mg/L). The albumin, prothrombin time (PT), blood glucose, and electrolytes all are within normal limits. E.T. is negative for anti-HCV, HBeAg, HBsAg, and hepatitis B core antibody (anti-HBc), but is positive for IgM anti-HAV. What clinical features and serologic markers are consistent with viral hepatitis in E.T.?

[SI units: Hgb, 160 g/L (normal, 123 to 163); Hct, 0.44% (normal, 0.374 to 0.47%); WBC count, 5,500 × 10⁹ cells/L (normal, 3280 to 9290 × 10⁹); AST, 120 U/L (normal, 5 to 40); ALT, 240 U/L (normal, 5 to 40); alkaline phosphatase, 86 U/L (normal, 21 to 91); total bilirubin, 54.72 μmol/L (normal, 3.42 to 17.1); direct bilirubin, 25.65 μmol/L (normal, 0 to 4)]

The incubation period for HAV is 15 to 45 days (average, 30) following inoculation (see Table 73-2). The host is usually asymptomatic during this stage of the infection; thus, E.T. is beyond the inoculation phase of the disease. Because HAV titers are highest in the acute-phase fecal samples, and the period of infectivity is between 14 and 21 days before the onset of jaundice to 7 or 8 days following jaundice, he should be considered infectious at this time. In HAV infections, acute-phase serum and saliva are less infectious than fecal samples, whereas urine and semen samples are not infectious. Family members and persons recently in immediate contact with E.T. should be notified to limit the possibility of disease transmission.

The symptoms of acute viral hepatitis caused by HAV, HBV, HCV, HDV, and HEV are similar. However, the onset of symptoms in HAV infection are less insidious than those seen with HBV and HCV infection.[37–39] Generally, symptoms of HAV are present a week or more before the onset of jaundice. E.T. has signs and symptoms of acute HAV infection, including the nonspecific prodromal symptoms of fatigue, weakness, anorexia, nausea, and vomiting. Abdominal pain and hepatomegaly are common. Less common symptoms include fever, headache, arthralgias, myalgias, and diarrhea. Within 1 to 2 weeks of the onset of prodromal symptoms, patients may enter an icteric phase with symptoms, including clay-colored stools, dark urine, scleral icterus, and frank jaundice. The dark urine is due to bilirubin, generally occurring shortly before the onset of jaundice. E.T. should be questioned about the presence of pale stools (light gray or yellow), which usually is observed during the icteric phase. His scleral icterus is strongly suggestive of viral hepatitis. Icteric infections usually occur in adults, and are 3.5 times more common than the nonicteric presentation that are seen in children.[50]

The results of E.T.'s liver function tests (LFTs) (e.g., elevations in AST, ALT, and bilirubin) also are consistent with viral hepatitis. Serum transaminase concentrations increase during the prodromal phase (usually ALT > AST) of HAV infection, peaking before the onset of jaundice. These concentrations are often >500 IU/L, and decline at an initial rate of 75% per week, followed by a slower rate of decline thereafter. Serum bilirubin peaks following aminotransferase activity and rarely exceed 10 mg/dL. Bilirubin levels decline more slowly than aminotransferases and generally normalize within 3 months.

Extrahepatic Manifestations

2. Are there any additional complications that E.T. could develop from his acute HAV infection?

With the appearance of jaundice, prodromal pruritus and extrahepatic manifestations can occur, usually in patients with a more protracted illness. Thus E.T. should be monitored for additional manifestations of HAV infection, including immune complex–associated rash, leukocytoclastic vasculitis, glomerulonephritis, cryoglobulinemia (less than with HCV), and arthritis. Rare extrahepatic manifestations include epidermal necrolysis, fatal myocarditis, renal failure in the presence of hepatic failure (hepatorenal syndrome), optic neuritis, and polyneuritis.[39,51–53] Hematologic abnormalities, although infrequently reported, include thrombocytopenia, aplastic anemia, and red cell aplasia.[39,51]

Diagnosis and Serology

Several diagnostic methods are available for detecting HAVAg (antigen) and anti-HAV (antibody). HAV can be detected in stool specimens 1 to 2 weeks preceding clinical illness. Viral RNA can be detected in body fluids and serum using the polymerase chain reaction (PCR), an expensive method usually reserved for research purposes. Because most patients present when the virus is no longer in stool, serum antibody can be detected by radioimmunoassay (RIA) or enzyme-linked immunosorbent assay (ELISA). Two classes of anti-HAV antibodies are detectable: IgM and IgG (Fig. 73-1). Detection of IgM to HAV in a patient who presents with clinical characteristics of hepatitis or in an asymptomatic patient with elevated transaminases is consistent with acute HAV infection. HAV IgG appears following IgM and is indicative of previous exposure and immunity to HAV, whereas a rising IgG is consistent with recent exposure.[37,39,54] Anti-HAV IgM is commonly present throughout the disease course (16 to 40 weeks), usually peaking early and declining to undetectable levels 3 to 4 months after the initial infection.[39,55] One quarter of patients infected with HAV have IgM present for up to 6 months, and occasionally longer. HAV IgG appears early in the convalescent phase and is detectable for decades after the acute infection resolves, with a slowly declining titer.[39,56] Both ELISA and RIA methods of antibody detection are sensitive, specific, and reliable to diagnose acute HAV infection. E.T. has a positive IgM anti-HAV, consistent with acute HAV infection. E.T. has a negative IgM anti-HBc test, ruling out acute HBV infection.[39,57]

Treatment

General Measures

HAV infection is usually a self-limited disease that does not require specific therapy. Many treatments have been recommended for acute viral hepatitis, but none significantly alter the course of the disease. The patient with acute viral hepatitis may be treated as an outpatient if symptoms are mild to moderate and regular medical evaluation occurs. Patients infected with hepatitis A usually do not require hospitalization, unless they develop complications of hepatic insufficiency, such as encephalopathy or hemorrhage secondary to hypoprothrombinemia. Patients should continue their normal activities as much as possible while avoiding physical exhaustion. Intravenous (IV) fluid and electrolyte replacement is necessary in some patients with severe nausea and vomiting. Patients should abstain from alcohol during the acute phase of the disease. Following resolution of symptoms and serum

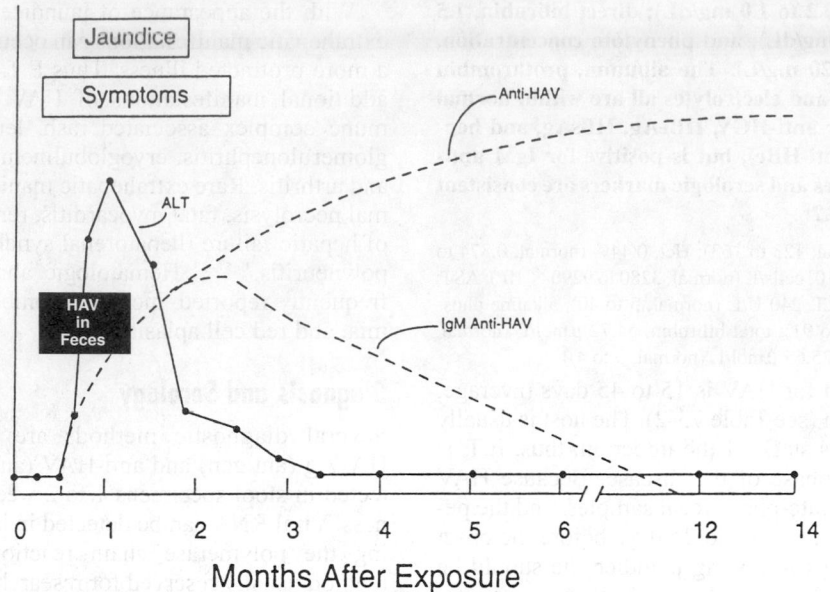

FIGURE 73-1 Typical course of hepatitis A. ALT, alanine aminotransferase, anti-HAV, antibody to HAV, HAV, hepatitis A virus. (Reproduced with permission from reference 54.)

biochemical abnormalities, moderate alcohol intake no longer is contraindicated.

Pharmacologic Treatment

Supportive measures are the only treatment required in most HAV infection cases. In patients with severe cholestasis, a short course of prednisolone (30 mg/day with a rapid taper) may minimize the severity of symptoms such as pruritus and malaise and reduce the serum bilirubin concentration. Prolonged courses of corticosteroids are not recommended. Similar to any etiology, any patient with fulminant hepatic failure should be evaluated for liver transplantation.

Adjustment of Medication Doses

3. Should E.T.'s medications be adjusted during the acute phase of hepatitis A infection?

Dosage adjustments for hepatically eliminated drugs in the setting of liver disease are difficult to predict. This is because hepatic metabolism is complex, involving numerous oxidative and conjugative pathways that are variably affected in hepatic disease. In renal disease, creatinine serves as an endogenous marker to predict the clearance of renally eliminated drugs. Unfortunately, in hepatic disease, there are no reliable endogenous markers to predict drug hepatic clearance. Laboratory tests that approximate the synthetic function of the liver (albumin, PT) and biliary clearance (bilirubin) are used to estimate the degree of hepatic impairment, but these tests are not dependable in predicting alterations in pharmacokinetic parameters for hepatically metabolized drugs.

Because of the difficulty in predicting hepatic drug clearance, unnecessary and potentially hepatotoxic medications are best avoided during the acute phase of the illness. When drug therapy is indicated with agents that undergo hepatic elimination, it is prudent to use the lowest doses possible to achieve the desired therapeutic effect. Data from small pharmacokinetic studies in patients with acute viral hepatitis are shown in Table 73-4.[58–76]

E.T. should be advised to discontinue diazepam (Valium) because this medication undergoes extensive hepatic biotransformation and limited data suggest this agent accumulates in the setting of acute viral hepatitis.[63] If E.T. should re-

Table 73-4 Half-Life Data for Various Agents in Acute Viral Hepatitis Compared With Normal Controls

Drug	$t_{1/2}$ (hr)	
	Normal Controls	Acute Viral Hepatitis
Acetaminophen[58]	2.1	3.2
Aspirin[58]	0.4	No change[a]
Carbamazepine[59]	12	Increased
Chlordiazepoxide[60]	11.1	91
Chloramphenicol[61]	4.6	11.6
Clofibrate[62]	17.5	No change
Diazepam[63]	37.2	74.5
Lidocaine[64]	3.7	6.4
Lorazepam[65]	21.7	No change
Meperidine[66]	3.4	7
Nitrendipine[67]	2.2	No change
Norfloxacin[68]	4.3	No change
Oxazepam[69]	5.1	No change
Phenobarbital[70]	86	No change
Phenytoin[71]	13.2	No change
Quinine[72]	10	17
Rifampin[73]	2.5	6.5
Theophylline[74]	7.7	19.2
Tolbutamide[75]	5.9	4.0
Warfarin[76]	25	No change

[a]No change indicates that the difference between patients with acute viral hepatitis and normal controls is not statistically significant.
$t_{1/2}$, half-life.

quire drug therapy for muscle spasms, he should either decrease the diazepam dose or consider using an alternative agent (e.g., lorazepam) that does not accumulate in acute viral hepatitis.[65] Patients with acute viral hepatitis do not require phenytoin dosage adjustments.[71] Because E.T.'s plasma phenytoin concentration is within the desired therapeutic range, no dosage adjustment is needed at this time.

Prevention of Hepatitis A

Prevention of hepatitis A infection can be achieved through immunoprophylactic measures. Immunoprophylaxis may be passive, active, or a combination of both. In passive immunization, temporary protective antibody in the form of immunoglobulin is administered. In active immunization, a vaccine is administered to induce the formation of protective antibody. Prophylaxis can be administered before exposure (pre-exposure prophylaxis) or after exposure has occurred (postexposure prophylaxis).

Pre-Exposure Prophylaxis

4. **M.D., a 22-year-old student, is preparing for a 2-week vacation to Thailand. He plans to travel 3 months from now and wonders if he should receive prophylaxis for HAV.**

IMMUNOGLOBULIN

Before hepatitis A vaccine was available, the sole therapy for pre-exposure prophylaxis of hepatitis A infection was immunoglobulin. Immunoglobulin is an injectable solution containing a full complement of antibodies normally present in human serum. Current preparations are manufactured by cold ethanol fractionation of pooled plasma collected from at least 1,000 human donors, providing protective levels of anti-HAV. Although passive immunization with immunoglobulin alone is highly effective in preventing hepatitis A virus infection,[77] the duration of protection is short. When used for pre-exposure prophylaxis, a dose of 0.02 mL/kg of immunoglobulin administered intramuscularly (IM) confers protection for less than 3 months, and an IM dose of 0.06 mL/kg confers protection for greater than or equal to 5 months.[38,39,77] Patients with continued exposure to hepatitis A require IM administration of immunoglobulin 0.06 mL/kg every 5 months for adequate protection.[38,78]

VACCINE

Active immunization with hepatitis A vaccine has largely supplanted the use of immunoglobulin for pre-exposure prophylaxis of infection caused by HAV. Formulations of inactivated hepatitis A vaccine available in the United States include Havrix (SmithKline Beecham) and Vaqta (Merck). Both vaccines are formalin-inactivated preparations of attenuated HAV strains. The manufacturers use differing units to express antigen content of their respective vaccines. Havrix dosages are expressed in ELISA units (EL.U.), and Vaqta dosages are expressed as units (U) of hepatitis A antigen

Dosing Regimen

Havrix is available in two formulations that differ according to age: for persons 2 to 18 years of age, 720 EL.U. (0.5 mL) per dose in a two-dose schedule; and for persons older than 18 years of age, 1,440 EL.U. (1.0 mL) per dose in a two dose schedule (Table 73-5).[38,39] This vaccine is usually injected IM into the deltoid muscle using a needle length appropriate for the person's age and size, with a booster dose administered 6 to 12 months later. Of note, the pediatric Havrix formulation (three-dose schedule) is no longer available. In comparison, Vaqta is available in two formulations, and the formulations differ according to the person's age: for persons 2 to 17 years of age, 25 U (0.5 mL) in a two-dose schedule; for persons older than 17 years of age, 50 U (1.0 mL) per dose in a two-dose schedule (Table 73-5).[38,39] Likewise, this vaccine is usually injected IM into the deltoid muscle with a booster dose administered 6 to 18 months later for persons 2 to 17 years of age and 6 to 12 months later for persons older than 17 years of age.[38]

The levels of anti-HAV necessary to prevent infection have not been definitively established. The manufacturer-specified protective levels for Havrix and Vaqta are >20 mIU/mL and >10 mIU/mL, respectively. The immune response to each preparation has been rapid and complete, with >94% of patients achieving protective antibody levels 1 month after vaccination.[38,78] Following administration of a second dose, 100% of vaccine recipients achieve protective antibody titers.[38,79] Additionally, both vaccines are extensively immunogenic in children and adolescents with 97% to 100% of persons aged 2 to 18 years achieving protective antibody levels 1 month after receiving the first dose; 100% achieve protective levels 1 month following the second dose.[38]

Efficacy, Safety, and Duration of Response

The efficacy of the hepatitis A vaccine is well-established with protective efficacy of 94% to 100%.[80-82] The vaccine is well tolerated with soreness at the injection site, headache, myalgia, and malaise as the most commonly reported adverse effects. A recent postmarketing surveillance study of >6 million doses of vaccine revealed <0.01% of patients reporting adverse events.[83]

The duration of protection has not been studied extensively; however, the little data that exist suggest persistence of protective antibody titers for periods of 6 years with Havrix and 5 to 6 years with Vaqta.[38] Estimates of antibody persistence derived from pharmacokinetic models of antibody decline indicate that protective concentrations of antibody could be present for >20 years.[38,84,85] The U.S. Advisory Committee on Immunization Practices (ACIP) does not have a recommendation regarding the need for booster doses at this time.

Table 73-5	Recommended Doses of Hepatitis A Vaccines	
Age at Vaccination	Dose (Volume)[a]	Schedule (Months)[b]
Havrix		
Children 2–18 yr	720 EL.U. (0.5 mL)	0, 6–12
Adults >18 yr	1,440 EL.U. (1.0 mL)	0, 6–12
Vaqta		
Children 2–17 yr	25 U (0.5 mL)	0, 6–18
Adults >17 yr	50 U (1.0 mL)	0, 6

[a]Enzyme-linked immunosorbent assay (ELISA) units.
[b]Zero months represents timing of the initial dose; subsequent numbers represent months after the initial dose.
From reference 78.

Indications

The ACIP recommends administering hepatitis A vaccination for several high-risk groups including: travelers to countries with high endemicity of infection (South and Central America, Africa, South and Southeast Asia, Caribbean, and the Middle East), travelers to countries with intermediate endemicity of infection (Eastern and Southern Europe and the former Soviet Union), children living in communities with high rates of hepatitis A infection and periodic hepatitis A outbreaks (Alaskan Native villages, American Indian reservations), men who have sex with men, intravenous drug users, researchers or persons who have occupational risk for hepatitis A (health-care workers), persons with clotting factor disorders, and persons with chronic liver disease who are at increased risk for fulminant hepatitis A.[38]

Children living in areas in which the incidence of HAV is at least twice the national average should be routinely vaccinated.[38] These children include those who live in states (Arizona, Alaska, Oregon, New Mexico, Utah, Washington, Oklahoma, South Dakota, Idaho, Nevada, and California), counties, or communities in which the average annual rate of HAV during 1987–1997 was ≥20 cases per 100,000 population. Children who live in states (Missouri, Texas, Colorado, Arkansas, Montana, and Wyoming), counties, or communities in which the annual rate of HAV during 1987–1997 was ≥10 cases per 100,000 population but <20 cases per 100,000 population should also be considered for vaccination.[79]

Because M.D. will not travel for another 3 months, he should receive either Havrix 1,440 EL.U. or Vaqta 50 units as soon as possible and no later than 1 month before travel. This initial injection will provide adequate protection from HAV infection during his travel, and he can receive the booster injection upon his return, at least 6 months after the first injection.

Postexposure Prophylaxis

5. L.W., a 26-year-old man, recently was diagnosed with HAV infection. He attends college and works part-time as a retail clerk. He lives with his wife and infant daughter. Which of L.W.'s contacts require postexposure prophylaxis for HAV?

The ACIP recommends using immunoglobulin for postexposure prophylaxis of hepatitis A disease. The recommended dose is 0.02 mL/kg, administered IM as soon as possible but no later than 2 weeks after exposure. Contacts who have received a dose of hepatitis A vaccine at least 1 month before exposure do not need immunoglobulin, because protective antibody titers are achieved in >95% of patients 1 month after vaccination.[38,78]

Administration of immunoglobulin within 2 weeks of exposure to HAV is 80% to 90% effective in preventing acute HAV infection.[38,86] In most cases, when given early, immunoglobulin prevents both clinical and subclinical HAV illness.[87] Protection following immunoglobulin administration is immediate and complete; however, long-lasting immunity to HAV does not develop.

Immunoglobulin is recommended for close personal contacts (household and sexual) of persons with acute hepatitis A infection. L.W.'s wife and infant daughter should receive prophylactic administration of immunoglobulin. Vaccination is not required at this time. Prophylaxis is not recommended for casual contacts at work or school.

Other situations in which immunoglobulin administration may be indicated include hepatitis A infection in day-care centers and in settings with infected persons who prepare and serve food. Immunoglobulin is recommended for all staff and children in day-care settings when a case of hepatitis A virus infection is diagnosed among employees or attendees.[38,78] When a food handler is diagnosed with hepatitis A, immunoglobulin is recommended for other food handlers at the same location. Given the improbability of disease transmission to persons consuming food prepared or served by workers infected with hepatitis A, the routine administration of immunoglobulin in this setting is not recommended.[38,78]

Unvaccinated patients with continued exposure to hepatitis A require intramuscular administration of immunoglobulin 0.06 mL/kg every 5 months for adequate protection.[38] When immunoglobulin is required for infants or pregnant women, preparations that do not contain thimerosal should be used.[38] Additionally, immune globulin does not appear to impede the immune response to inactivated vaccines or to oral poliovirus vaccine or yellow fever vaccine.[88] However, immune globulin may interfere with the response to live attenuated vaccines such as measles, mumps, rubella (MMR) vaccine and varicella vaccine when administered as either individual or combination vaccines.[88] Therefore, MMR and varicella vaccine should be delayed for at least 3 months following administration of immune globulin for HAV prophylaxis. Immune globulin should not be given within 2 weeks after the administration of MMR or varicella vaccine. Finally, if immune globulin is administered within 2 weeks of MMR, the person requires revaccination, but not sooner than 3 months after the immune globulin administration for MMR.[88] Serologic tests for varicella vaccination should be performed 3 months after immune globulin administration to determine if revaccination is required.

HEPATITIS B VIRUS
Virology

Hepatitis B virus (HBV) is a partially double-stranded DNA virus that is a member of the Hepadnaviridae family of viruses (see Table 73-2).[19,89–92] Unlike HAV, which has only one serotype and causes a self-limited infection, HBV is antigenically complex, contains four major serotypes (adw, ayw, adr, and ayr), and results in an acute illness with or without a chronic disease state. Intact HBV virions are 42 nm wide and contain four open reading frames (S, P, C, and X) that encode four major proteins (surface, polymerase, core, and X protein, respectively) associated with viral replication.[19,89–94] On the surface, coating HBV, is an antigen called the hepatitis B surface antigen (HBsAg), which is the virus's major envelope protein. This antigen is found in patients with acute or chronic HBV infection and chronic carriers. Two additional proteins, L and M, are also present in the viral envelope. The function of the L protein appears to be viral binding to the hepatocyte surface, whereas the function of the M protein is unknown. Inside the surface envelope of the intact hepatitis B virion is a 27-nm structure called the internal nucleocapsid core, which consists of several copies of the viral core protein or hepatitis B core antigen (HBcAg) surrounding the viral DNA and the virally encoded polymerase. The hepatitis Be antigen (HBeAg) is a secreted product of the nucleocapsid core of

HBV, and its presence is also indicative of viral replication.[89–94] In addition to intact virions, several subviral particles (S proteins) are produced that are not infectious; however, they are severely immunogenic and promote the formation of neutralizing antibodies.[89–94] These particles were used to develop the first HBV vaccines.

Our understanding of HBV replication is based on experiments performed in animals; thus, extrapolation of these results to human disease must be made with caution.[92,94,95] The life cycle of HBV can be summarized as follows: (1) viral binding and entry; (2) viral uncoating in the cytoplasm through direct membrane fusion; (3) synthesis of complete double-stranded DNA in the nucleus, catalyzed by HBV viral DNA polymerase; (4) synthesis of RNA that forms the template for DNA synthesis by host RNA polymerase; (5) translation of viral transcripts in the cytoplasm, which yields the viral envelop, core, precore, and X proteins, as well as the viral DNA polymerase; (6) encapsidation/packaging of RNA in the cytoplasm with production of viral cores; (7) RNA synthesis of minus strand DNA by reverse transcriptase (RT); and (8) envelopment of viral cores with excretion of infective virions, or transport of viral core back into the nucleus (Fig. 73-2). The final step of replication facilitates horizontal spread of infection throughout the liver.

A basic understanding of the HBV life cycle has provided unique opportunities for drug development. Of special importance, the HBV polymerase functions as both a reverse transcriptase (RT) for synthesis of the negative DNA strand from genomic RNA and as an endogenous DNA polymerase. Because the HBV polymerase is remotely related to the RT enzymes of retroviruses (e.g., HIV), it is apparent that some inhibitors of HIV polymerase/RT might have activity against the HBV polymerase. Thus, reverse transcriptase inhibitors such as lamivudine and adefovir have been evaluated for treating and preventing HBV.

Epidemiology

Approximately 5% of the world's population is infected with HBV.[1,8,17,91,96] More than 1.25 million cases occur in the United States, many of which occur in immigrants from endemic areas and Alaskan natives (6.4%).[1,8,89,91,96] However, the incidence of acute HBV has been on the decline in the United States.[1,8,89,91,96] Over the past decade, HBV has been reduced from a rate of 438,000 infections per year in the late 1980s to an estimated 185,000 cases in 1997. This reduction has occurred in all age, racial/ethnic, and high-risk groups. The most significant reduction is in children and health care workers, groups with the highest rate of vaccination. The reduced incidence of HBV infection may be attributed to changes in behavior, which has led to decreased transmission of infection. High-risk groups in the United States for acquiring HBV infection include certain ethnic groups (Alaskan natives, Pacific Islanders), first-generation immigrants from regions of high endemicity (southeast Asia), injection drug users, gay men, African Americans (compared with white Americans), and males (more than females).[1,91,96–98] The most prominent risk factors associated with acute HBV include heterosexual contact (42%), men having sex with men (15%), and injection drug use (21%).[91,96–98] HBV vaccination opportunities include clinics for sexually transmitted disease (and contacts) and in prisons and holding centers for incarceration.

The epidemiology of chronic HBV infection is less well known than that of acute disease. Within the United States, it is estimated that 0.2% of the population is HBsAg positive.[91,96–98] African Americans are more likely to be HBsAg positive than whites, with the highest reported rates among Asian Americans, especially those from China and Southeast Asia. In population-based surveys, HBV is responsible for 1% to 14% of chronic liver disease with chronic infection more likely to develop in infants compared with adults.[8]

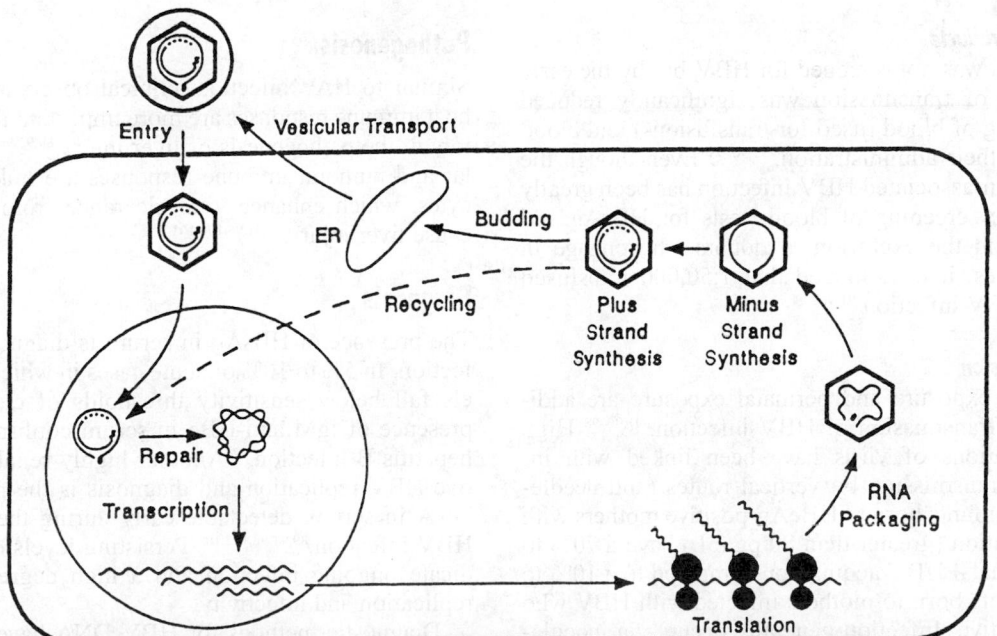

FIGURE 73-2 Life cycle of hepatitis B virus. (Reproduced with permission from Ganem D. Hepadnaviridae: the viruses and their replication. In: Fields BN. Ed. Fundamental Virology. 3rd Ed. Philadelphia: Lippincott-Raven, 1996:1199.)

Transmission

HBV is a parenterally transmitted virus acquired via sexual contact, contaminated blood or blood products, or perinatal exposure. These modes of transmission of HBV are summarized in the following sections.

Sexual Transmission

Sexual activity is the most significant mode of HBV transmission in areas of the world, including North America, where the prevalence of infection is low.[91,96–99] Heterosexual intercourse accounts for the majority of United States infections (26%). In heterosexuals, factors associated with an enhanced risk of HBV infection include duration of sexual activity, number of sexual partners, and history of sexually transmitted diseases. Sexual partners of injection drug users, prostitutes, and clients of prostitutes are at a very high risk for infection. Sexual partners of infected individuals are at high risk for infection, even in the absence of high-risk behavior. Studies of household and sexual contacts have reported that 0% to 3% of the spouses or sexual partners and 4% to 9% of the children are HBsAg positive. Since the majority of patients with chronic HBV infection are unaware of their infection and are "silent carriers," sexual transmission is likely to be a significant mode of worldwide transmission. The use of condoms appears to reduce the risk of sexual transmission.[91,96–98]

From 1980 to 1985, a very high rate of HBV infection was observed in homosexual men, accounting for 20% of all reported cases of infection.[91,96–98] Multiple sexual partners, anal-receptive intercourse, and duration of sexual activity were the most common factors associated with HBV acquisition in this population. Current rates of HBV infection in this population have fallen and are estimated to be about 8%, possibly as a result of modifications of sexual behavior in response to HIV. Similar to heterosexuals, the use of condoms in this population may also reduce the risk of sexual transmission.

Blood and Blood Products

Previously, blood was not screened for HBV, but by the early 1970s, this risk of transmission was significantly reduced through screening of blood (used for transfusions) and blood products before their administration.[91,96–98] Even though the risk of transfusion-associated HBV infection has been greatly reduced with the screening of blood (tests for HBsAg and anti-HB core) and the exclusion of donors who engage in high-risk activities, it is estimated that 1:50,000 transfused units transmit HBV infection.[91,96–98]

Perinatal Transmission

Early childhood exposure and perinatal exposure are additional modes of transmission of HBV infection.[91,96–98] High serum concentrations of virus have been linked with increased risk of transmission by vertical routes (and needle-stick exposure). Infants born to HBeAg-positive mothers with high viral replication (greater than 80 pg/mL) have a 70% to 90% risk of perinatal HBV acquisition compared to a 10% to 40% risk in infants born to mothers infected with HBV who are HBeAg-negative. Infection generally occurs via inoculation of the infant at the time of birth or soon thereafter and even with active and passive immunization, 10% to 15% of babies may acquire HBV infection at birth.

In developing countries with high prevalence rates and in regions of the United States with high endemicity, children born to HBsAg-positive mothers with HBV are at risk for acquiring HBV infection in the perinatal period, with infection rates reported to be between 7% and 13%.[91,96–98] In addition, children of HBsAg-positive mothers who are not infected at birth remain at very high risk of early childhood infection, with 60% of those born to HBsAg-positive mothers becoming infected by the age of 5 years. Unfortunately, the mechanism of the later infection, which is neither perinatal nor sexual, is not known. Furthermore, even though HBsAg is detectable in breast milk, breast-feeding is not believed to be a primary mode of HBV transmission.

Injection Drug Use

Recreational drug use in the United States and Europe is an important mode of HBV transmission, accounting for approximately 23% of all patients.[91,96–98] The risk of HBV infection increases with duration of recreational drug use; thus, serologic markers of ongoing or prior HBV infection are usually present after 5 years of drug use.

Other Modes of Transmission

Other risk factors for transmission of HBV include working in a health care setting, transfusion and dialysis, acupuncture, tattooing, travel abroad, and living in institutions.[91,96–98] Sporadic cases of HBV transmission have been attributed to nonpercutaneous transmission by way of small breaks in the skin, biting, or mucous membranes. Although HBsAg is found in saliva, tears, sweat, semen, vaginal secretions, breast milk, cerebrospinal fluid, ascites, pleural fluid, synovial fluid, gastric juice, urine, and, rarely, feces of HBsAg-positive persons, only semen, saliva, and serum actually contain infectious HBV in experimental transmission studies. Thus, kissing is not considered to be a significant means of HBV transmission, but biting could be.

Pathogenesis

Similar to HAV infection, clinical observations suggest that host immune responses are more important than virologic factors in the pathogenesis of liver injury.[89,91,96,100,101] Host cellular and humoral immune responses are linked to T lymphocytes, which enhance viral clearance from hepatocytes and cause liver injury.[89,91,96,100,101]

Diagnosis

The presence of HBsAg in serum is diagnostic for HBV infection. In 5% to 10% of acute cases in which the HBsAg levels fall below sensitivity thresholds of current assays, the presence of IgM anti-HBc in serum confirms a recent acute hepatitis B infection.[57] Another highly reliable marker of active HBV replication and diagnosis is the presence of HBV DNA in serum, detectable early during the course of acute HBV infection.[89,91,96,102,103] Persisting levels of HBV DNA indicate ongoing infection and a high degree of active viral replication and infectivity.

Diagnostic methods for HBV DNA have expanded in recent years.[89,91,96,104,105] Tests detecting HBV DNA can be classified as: 1) dependent on hybridization of labeled probe to the DNA with quantification (Genostics assay; branched DNA

[bDNA]) and 2) PCR-based assays in which viral DNA is amplified with detection through gel electrophoresis. Genostics and bDNA are moderately sensitive in detecting DNA in HBsAg-negative and HBeAg-positive patients and they have high specificity. Values obtained by these assays are not interchangeable and are used primarily as research tools.

Serology

Serologic patterns of HBV infection are depicted in Table 73-6. Within the first several weeks after exposure, HBsAg appears in the blood and is present for several weeks before serum concentrations of aminotransferases increase and symptoms become apparent (Fig. 73-3A).[55,89,91,96,106,107] Clinical illness usually follows HBV exposure by 1 to 3 months. HBsAg can be detected in serum until the clinical illness resolves. The antibody to HBsAg (anti-HBs) often appears after a short "window" period during which neither HBsAg nor anti-HBs are detectable. Anti-HBs persists for years after HBV infection, conferring immunity to reinfection (Fig. 73-3A).

HBeAg is detectable early during the acute phase of the disease and persists in chronic hepatitis B infection. HBeAg is a marker of active HBV replication, and its presence correlates with circulating HBV particles. The presence of both HBeAg and HBsAg indicates a high level of viral replication and infectivity. Hepatitis B envelope antibody (anti-HBe) becomes detectable as HBeAg levels decline in acute or chronic hepatitis B. The appearance of anti-HBe suggests resolution of HBV infection.

Hepatitis B core antigen does not circulate freely in the bloodstream and is not measured. Anti-HBc, the antibody directed against HBcAg, is usually detected 1 to 2 weeks after the appearance of HBsAg and just before the onset of clinical symptoms, and persists for life. The detection of IgM anti-HBc is the most sensitive diagnostic test for acute HBV infection. During the recovery phase of infection, the predominant form of anti-HBc is in the IgG class. The presence of this antibody suggests prior or ongoing infection with HBV. Patients immunized against HBV do not develop anti-HBc; therefore, the presence of this antibody differentiates successful vaccination from actual HBV infection.

Natural History

Of those patients with acute HBV infection, only 1% develop fulminant hepatic failure (FHF).[47,89,91,108] These patients generally have coagulopathy, encephalopathy, and cerebral edema.[47,108] The cause of fulminant infection is a heightened immune response to the virus, provided that HDV or HCV coinfections are ruled out. Patients with acute liver failure often have early clearance of HBsAg, which may complicate the diagnosis, but a positive IgM antibody to HBcAg generally confirms the diagnosis.

Up to 12% (average 5%) of immunocompetent patients acutely infected with HBV remain chronically infected (historically defined as detectable HBsAg in serum for 6 months or longer) (Fig. 73-3B).[89,96,108,109] In these patients, HBsAg generally remains detectable indefinitely and anti-HBs fails to appear.

The risk of chronicity following neonatal-acquired infection is high (>90%), possibly because neonates have immature immune systems. Fifty percent of infected neonates have evidence of active viral replication. Furthermore, patients who have a reduced ability to clear viral infections—including those receiving chronic hemodialysis, immunosuppression following transplantation, chemotherapy, or patients with HIV infection—may have a greater risk for developing chronic HBV infection.[89,110] The outcomes of these patients are mainly determined by the presence or absence of viral replication and by the severity of liver damage.[110,111] Approximately 50% of all chronic carriers have ongoing viral replication, especially with elevated aminotransferases, and 15% to 20% of these develop cirrhosis within 5 years.[89,96,110,111] Spontaneous loss of HBeAg (7% to 20% per year) has been reported, possibly a result of the use of antiviral therapy, whereas loss of HBsAg occurs less frequently (1% to 2% per year). In general, chronic carriers remain infected throughout their entire life.[55,106,107] In one study, the 5-year survival rate was 97% in patients with early histologic changes, including chronic persistent hepatitis (in which inflammation is limited to the portal areas), compared with 86% in patients with chronic active hepatitis (in which liver cell necrosis and inflammation are present in the hepatic parenchyma) and 55% in patients with documented cirrhosis.[112] Asymptomatic HBV carriers tend to have mild disease manifestations with few complications, even with a long period of follow-up. Finally, the risk of hepatocellular carcinoma (HCC) is increased up to 300-fold in chronic carriers with active viral replication (HBeAg-positive).[113,114]

Clinical Manifestations

6. W.H. is a 35-year-old man who developed nausea, vomiting, anorexia, scleral icterus, and jaundice within the past month. Within the past week he became increasingly lethargic, confused, disoriented, and lapsed into a coma. He is admitted to the ED, intubated, and transferred to the intensive care unit.

W.H.'s social history is significant for IV drug use for the past 10 years and alcohol abuse (none for the previous 5 years). Physical findings include an older-than-age-appearing, hypertensive (blood pressure, 158/99 mm Hg), bradycardic (heart rate, 58

Table 73-6	Common Serologic Patterns of Hepatitis B Virus Infection				
HbsAg	HbeAg	Anti-HBs	Anti-Hbe	Anti-HBc	Interpretation
+	+	−	−	±	Incubation period
+	+	−	−	+ (IgM)	Acute HBV infection (typical case); chronic HBV carrier with high infectivity
−	−	+	±	+ (IgG)	Recovery from HBV infection
+	±	−	±	+ (IgG)	Chronic HBV carrier; chronic hepatitis B
−	−	+	−	−	Successful immunization with HBV vaccine

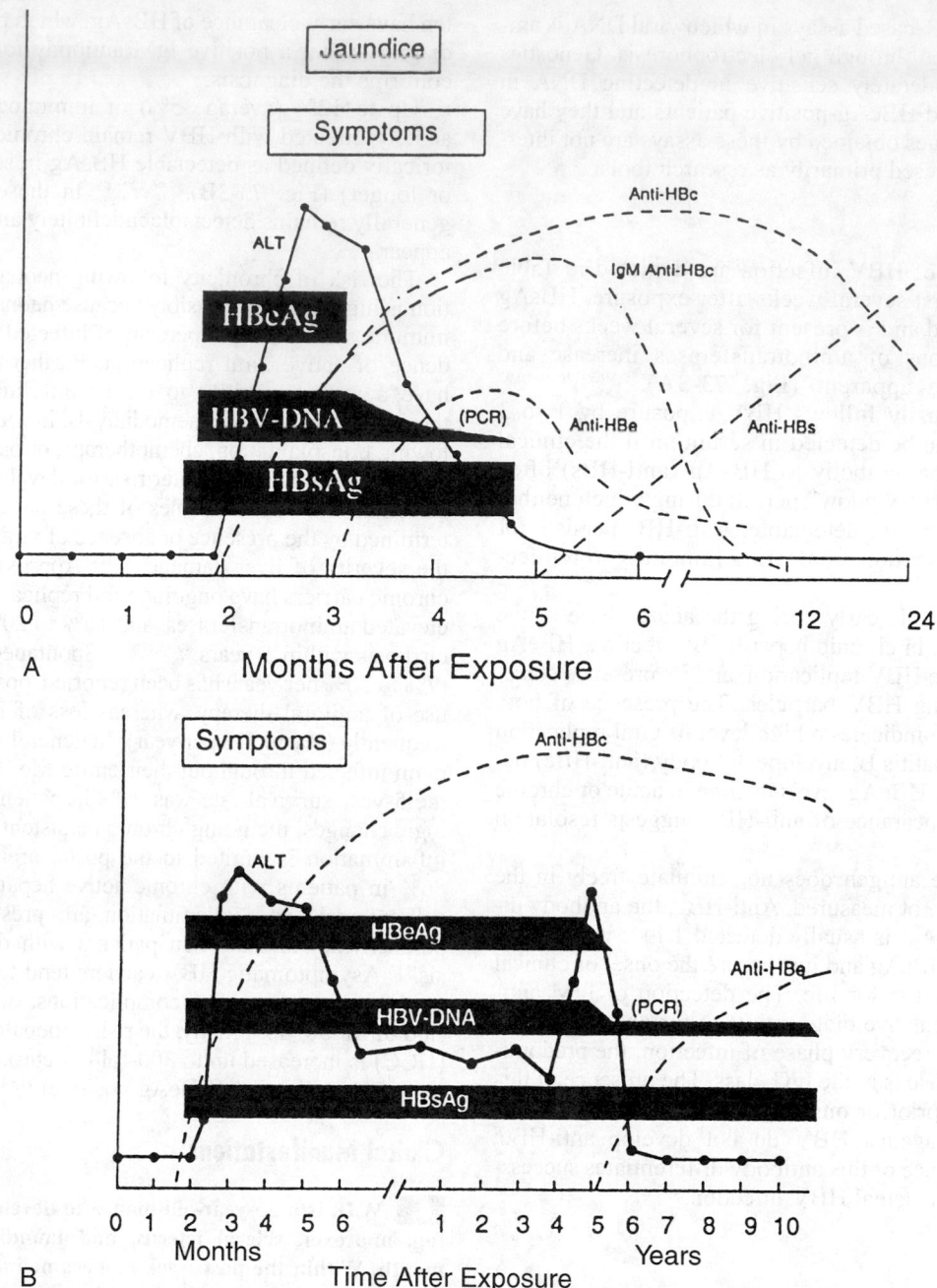

FIGURE 73-3 A. Sequence of events after acute hepatitis B virus infection with resolution. ALT, alanine aminotransferase; anti-HBc, hepatitis B core antibody; anti-Hbe, hepatitis B envelope antibody; anti-HBs, hepatitis B surface antibody; HbeAg, hepatitis B e antigen; HbsAg, hepatitis B surface antigen; HBV DNA; hepatitis B virus DNA; IgM anti-HBc, IgM antibody to hepatitis B core virus; PCR, polymerase chain reaction. (Reprinted with permission from reference 54.) **B. Sequence of events after acute hepatitis B virus infection converts to chronicity.** ALT, alanine aminotransferase; anti-HBc, hepatitis b core antibody; anti-Hbe, hepatitis B envelope antibody; HbeAg; hepatitis B e antigen; HbsAg, hepatitis B surface antigen; HBV DNA, hepatitis B virus DNA; PCR, polymerase chain reaction; (Reprinted with permission from reference 54.)

beats/min) man in respiratory distress (respiratory rate, 26 breaths/min) with severe jaundice, scleral icterus, and decreased hepatic dullness to percussion (reduced hepatic mass). He shows sluggish pupillary response and increasing muscle tone; neurologic examination reveals him to be stuporous and nonarousable.

The laboratory evaluation shows the following results: Hct, 42%; Hgb, 14 g/dL; platelets, 85,000/mm³ (normal, 150,000 to 300,000/mm³); PT, 25.8 sec (control, 12 sec), international normalized ratio, 3.8; AST, 555 U/L (normal, 5 to 40 U/L); ALT, 495 U/L (normal, 5 to 40 U/L); alkaline phosphatase, 101 U/mL (normal, 21 to 91 U/mL); and total bilirubin, 8.4 mg/dL (normal, 0.1 to 1.2 mg/dL). Hepatitis serologic tests are positive for HBsAg, HBeAg, IgM anti-HBc, and HBV DNA. IgM anti-HAV, IgM anti-HDV, and anti-HCV are negative. STAT blood gases reveal a metabolic acidosis with a compensatory respiratory alkalosis. W.H.'s serum creatinine is 1.8 mg/dL (normal, 0.5 to 1.2 mg/dL) with a recent reduction in urine output.

What clinical findings does W.H. have that support the diagnosis of acute hepatitis and acute liver failure?

[SI units: Hct, 0.42; Hgb, 140 g/L; AST, 555 U/L (normal, 5 to 40); ALT, 495 U/L (normal, 5 to 40); alkaline phosphatase, 101 U/L (normal, 21 to 91); total bilirubin, 143.6 μmol/L (normal, 1.7 to 20.5)]

The clinical features of acute HBV infection are similar to those described for HAV infection. W.H.'s initial symptoms included a recent history of nausea, vomiting, anorexia, scleral icterus, and jaundice. These are consistent with diagnosis of acute hepatitis B. His serologies, notably a positive IgM anti-HBc and HBV DNA, also support this diagnosis.

Acute Liver Failure

The most significant complication of acute HBV infection is acute liver failure (ALF), defined as the onset of hepatic encephalopathy within 8 weeks of the onset of symptoms (Table 73-7).[49,91,96,108] W.H. has several symptoms consistent with acute liver failure. These include recent onset of hepatic encephalopathy, lethargy, confusion, coma, coagulopathy, hemodynamic instability, declining liver function, and acidosis. Patients with ALF often have cerebral edema (80% mortality rate), a complication of a disrupted blood-brain barrier that allows protein-rich fluid to cross into the extracellular spaces of the brain tissue leading to edema and increased intracranial pressure (ICP) (vasogenic model). Toxins also can induce cerebral damage, edema, and subsequent increases in ICP in patients with an intact blood-brain barrier (cytotoxic model) (Table 73-7). Clinical symptoms (sluggish pupillary response and increasing muscle tone) develop when the ICP exceeds 30 mm Hg.[49,91,96,108,115–117] Cerebral edema in the confinement of the cranial vault raises the ICP, which may reduce intracerebral perfusion. The edema can result in cerebral ischemia if the cerebral-perfusion pressure (CPP) (systemic blood pressure minus ICP) is not maintained above 40 mm Hg.

W.H. has symptoms of cerebral edema and may benefit from 100 to 200 mL of a 20% solution of mannitol (0.3 to 0.4 g/kg) administered by rapid IV infusion to induce an osmotic diuresis with a subsequent decrease in ICP. The dose may be repeated at least once after several hours.[49,91,96,116,117] Because

W.H. also has a blood pressure of 158/99 mm Hg, has a heart rate of 58 beats/min, and is at risk for intracranial hemorrhage, an ICP monitoring device should be placed.[49,108,118,119] Although placement of this device is invasive, and bleeding is a potential complication, ICP monitoring devices provide important prognostic information. Patients with a CPP >40 mm Hg that is refractory to mannitol therapy are not candidates for liver transplantation.

W.H. also has a coagulopathy typical of ALF. Decreased levels of clotting factors II, V, VII, IX, and X normally synthesized by the liver account for his prolonged PT and elevated INR.[49,108,120] In addition, consumption of clotting factors by low-grade disseminated intravascular coagulation (DIC) is common in ALF. W.H. is also thrombocytopenic and at risk for GI ulceration.[49,108,116] A platelet transfusion should be considered if his counts drop to <50,000/mm³. Since he is not actively bleeding, fresh frozen plasma is not indicated at this time.[49,108,121]

W.H. also should be monitored for cardiovascular and renal abnormalities as a result of his ALF.[49,108,116] These resemble those associated with cirrhosis and septic shock in certain respects, but differ in others. Although W.H. is hypertensive, most patients with ALF are hypotensive and hypovolemic and present with interstitial edema due to low levels of oncotic proteins. Functional renal failure, also known as hepatorenal syndrome (HRS) or acute tubular necrosis (ATN), occurs in 43% to 55% of patients with ALF.[49,108] In HRS, renal blood flow is reduced, renin and aldosterone levels are increased, and levels of atrial natriuretic factor are unchanged.[122,123]

As seen in W.H., patients may develop acid-base disturbances, including a respiratory alkalosis as a result of CNS-mediated hyperventilation or a lactic acid–induced metabolic acidosis.[49,108] Hyponatremia, hypokalemia, hypocalcemia, hypomagnesemia, hypoglycemia, and pancreatitis are additional findings associated with ALF. Thus, sodium, potassium, calcium, magnesium, blood glucose, and amylase should be monitored closely in W.H.[49,108] Finally, pulmonary complications (hypoxemia, aspiration, adult respiratory distress syndrome [ARDS], and pulmonary edema) or sepsis (bacterial, fungal) occur in patients with ALF.[49,108,116]

Prognosis

7. **What is W.H.'s prognosis?**

Although the incidence of ALF is ≤1%, the prognosis for these patients is poor once encephalopathy has developed.[49,108,116,124] Survival depends on the etiology and degree of hepatic destruction, the ability of the remaining liver cells to regenerate, and the management of complications that may develop during the course of illness. Survival rates often depend on the etiology of ALF. In one series, patients with non-A, non-B hepatitis and halothane or drug hepatotoxicity had worse survival rates (20% and 12.5% survival, respectively) compared with those with hepatitis A, hepatitis B, or acetaminophen overdose (66.7%, 38.9%, and 52.9% survival, respectively).[124] Age younger than 14 years, worsening grade of encephalopathy, reduced liver size, and significantly abnormal LFT values (e.g., serum bilirubin, aminotransferases, alkaline phosphatase, PT, and serum albumin) also are poor prognostic indicators in patients with ALF (Table 73-8).[49,124] Because W.H. has evidence of encephalopathy, cerebral

Table 73-7   Principal Causes of Acute Liver Failure

Cause	Agents Responsible
Viral hepatitis	Hepatitis A, B, C, D, E virus
Toxins	Carbon tetrachloride
	Amanita phalloides
	Phosphorus
Vascular events	Ischemia
	Veno-occlusive disease
	Heatstroke
	Malignant infiltration
Miscellaneous	Wilson's disease
	Acute fatty-liver of pregnancy
	Reye's syndrome
Drug-related injury	Acetaminophen
	Idiosyncratic

Table 73-8 Criteria for Predicting Death and the Need for Liver Transplantation in Patients With Acute Liver Failure

Cause of Acute Liver Failure	Criteria
Acetaminophen poisoning	pH. <7.3 (irrespective of grade of encephalopathy)
	OR
	PT >100 sec *AND*
	Serum creatinine >3.4 mg/dL (300 μmol/L) in patients with grade III or grade IV encephalopathy
All other causes	PT >100 sec
	OR
	Any 3 of the following variables (irrespective of grade of encephalopathy):
	Age <10 yr or >40 yr; liver failure caused by non-A, non-B hepatitis, halothane-induced hepatitis, or idiosyncratic drug reactions; duration of jaundice before encephalopathy >7 days; PT >50 sec; serum bilirubin >17.5 mg/dL (300 μmol/L)

PT, prothrombin time.
From reference 124.

edema, and abnormal LFTs, he has a poor prognosis (Table 73-8).

Treatment

8. Outline an appropriate treatment plan for W.H.'s ALF.

The primary therapy in ALF is supportive care for the comatose patient. Systemic therapies with heparin, prostaglandins, or insulin and glucagon have shown limited efficacy.[49,108] Blood or plasma exchange, hemodialysis, or other methods implemented to detoxify the blood or improve the coma grade do not result in long-term benefits if liver mass is not reconstituted as well.[125,126] Thiopental may be useful in lowering ICP, but corticosteroids and prolonged hyperventilation are of no value.[49,108] W.H. could benefit from prophylactic H_2 blockers because they have been shown to reduce the incidence of upper GI hemorrhage.[49,108,127] Blood products (packed red blood cells, fresh frozen plasma, or platelets) should be given as needed if W.H. develops active bleeding, and pulmonary artery monitoring should be implemented to guide management of intravascular volume and gas exchange. W.H. should be closely monitored for additional complications, especially cardiac abnormalities (arrhythmias), hemodynamic changes, renal failure, acidosis, pulmonary complications, and sepsis.

In cases in which prognostic information indicates <20% chance of survival without transplantation, liver transplantation is indicated (see Table 73-8). In patients with acetaminophen poisoning resulting in ALF, a pH <7.3, a pT >100 seconds) and a serum creatinine (>3.4 mg/dL) with grade III or IV encephalopathy usually require transplantation.[124,128] Other causes of ALF, a PT >100 seconds, or any three of the following variables (irrespective of grade of encephalopathy)—age younger than 10 years or older than 40 years; liver failure caused by non-A, non-B hepatitis, halothane-induced hepatitis, or idiosyncratic drug reactions; duration of jaundice before encephalopathy >7 days; PT >50 seconds; or serum bilirubin >17.5 mg/dL—indicate a need for transplanta-

tion.[124,128] Several strategies to prevent death have been used before liver transplantation with some success. These include hepatic assist devices (e.g., bioartificial liver), auxiliary partial heterotopic transplants, and partial liver graft from living related donors.[49,108]

Extrahepatic Manifestations

9. What are the extrahepatic manifestations of acute or chronic HBV infection?

Extrahepatic manifestations such as arthralgias, rash, angioneurotic edema, and polyarteritis nodosa have been reported in patients with acute or chronic HBV infection.[89,96] Chronic and, to a lesser extent, acute HBV infection have been associated with immune complex–associated membranoproliferative glomerulonephritis. Neurologic complications of HBV infection include Guillain-Barré syndrome and a polyneuropathy. Pericarditis and pancreatitis are infrequent complications of HBV infection. Additional complications of chronic HBV infection include portal hypertension with variceal and esophageal bleeding, encephalopathy, ascites, spontaneous bacterial peritonitis, and hepatorenal syndrome. Although hepatocellular carcinoma (HCC) is not considered extrahepatic, many patients with HBV may develop HCC.[89,96,114]

Coinfection with other viruses has been reported in patients with HBV infection. For example, markers of prior or active HBV infection are present in more than 80% of patients with AIDS, with approximately 10% of these cases seropositive for HBsAg.[129] HIV has also been reported to coexist in up to 13% of patients with chronic HBV infection.[130] Compared with patients with HBV infection alone, HBV/HIV coinfected patients have significantly higher levels of viral replication, lower ALT levels, and less severe histologic disease. HBV infection does not reduce survival in HIV-positive patients; however, as these patients live longer, hepatic decompensation and manifestations of HBV may occur.

Prevention of Hepatitis B

Comprehensive strategies should be implemented to prevent and maintain protection against HBV infection and should be widely available to eliminate transmission that occurs during infancy and childhood as well as during adolescence and adulthood. Thus, alterations in sexual behavior, screening of high-risk patients and blood products, developing needle exchange programs, and cultural outreach and education may impact HBV transmission. The goals of preventive therapy should be to identify persons who require immunoprophylaxis for the prevention of infection and provide long-term protection through vaccination to decrease the risk of chronic HBV infection and its subsequent complications, as well as minimizing adverse effects and cost of therapy.

Pre-Exposure Prophylaxis

10. P.G., a 55-year-old nursing student, is going to start her clinical rotations. She has no history of hepatitis and has not yet been immunized. She is 5′2″ and weighs 80 kg. What prophylactic regimen should P.G. receive to prevent hepatitis secondary to HBV?

The available vaccines are manufactured using recombinant DNA technology. Both Recombivax HB (10 mg HBsAg/mL) and Engerix-B (20 mg HBsAg/mL) are yeast-derived HBV vaccines that induce an immunologic response similar to the plasma-derived vaccine (non longer used). Because P.G. will come in contact with potentially infectious bodily secretions during her rotations, she should be immunized against hepatitis B with either Recombivax HB or Engerix-B.

DOSING REGIMEN

The recommended doses of available hepatitis B vaccines are shown in Table 73-9.[131–133] The preferred vaccination schedule uses a three-dose regimen. The first dose is followed 1 month later by a second dose, and the third dose is administered 6 months after the initial dose. The first two doses function as priming doses, inducing anti-HBs in >85% of normal persons. The third dose serves as a booster dose, significantly increasing the anti-HBs titer and conferring optimal protection. The third dose can be administered up to 12 months after the initial dose with comparable efficacy. A four-dose series has been approved for high-risk patients in whom rapid protection is desired. If this schedule is followed, the fourth dose at 12 months is necessary to ensure protective antibody titers.

The recommended doses for the yeast-derived recombinant hepatitis B vaccines were based on dose-response studies that determined the optimal dose necessary to achieve protective antibody titers. Dose-response studies with Recombivax HB in healthy adults using 1.25, 2.5, 5, 10, and 20 μg of HBsAg all elicited an immune response. Those patients receiving the 10- or 20-μg dose developed substantially higher antibody titers than those receiving lower doses. No significant difference was observed between the 10- and 20-μg dose; thus, the 10-μg dose was selected as the standard adult dose of Recombivax HB. Similar analyses were performed to determine the 5-μg adolescent and pediatric dosage.[134] Dose-response trials with Engerix-B demonstrated an optimal immune response at higher dosages. The reason for the differing doses necessary to elicit an adequate immune response is unknown. Some have speculated that differences in the manufacturing process (yeast culture, purification methods) may influence the immunogenicity of the final product. For this reason, hepatitis B vaccines produced by different manufacturers may not be equally immunogenic on a microgram-for-microgram basis.[135] Relative potency comparisons are not clinically important because comparative trials using Recombivax HB and Engerix-B in the recommended dosages have demonstrated equivalent immunogenicity and tolerability. P.G. can be immunized with either product, provided she receives the manufacturer's recommended dosage with each injection.

Hepatitis B vaccine should be administered as an IM injection in the deltoid muscle of adults and children or in the anterolateral thigh muscle of neonates and infants. The immunogenicity of hepatitis B vaccine is significantly lower when injections are given in the buttocks, probably because the greater amount of fat tissue in the buttocks inhibits interfacing of vaccine and antigen-recognition leukocytes. The results of a small vaccination series suggest that healthy adults who do not respond to HBV injection to the buttocks have a significantly higher response when vaccinated in the arm.[136] P.G. should be immunized with either Recombivax HB (10 μg) or Engerix-B (20 μg) administered as a 1-mL IM injection in the deltoid muscle.

EFFICACY

Recombinant yeast derived vaccines (e.g., Recombivax HB, Engerix-B) produce similar results.[137] While a measurable immune response is readily achieved with the current HBV vaccine, a quantitative titer of circulating anti-HBs necessary to prevent infection has not been clearly substantiated. A protective antibody response has been defined as anti-HBs levels ≥10 mIU/mL.[133] This threshold was derived from early HBV vaccine trials in homosexual men, where vaccine recipients with serum antibody levels ≥10 sample ratio units (SRU) were protected from HBV infection.[138–140,141] A serum antibody level of 10 SRU is roughly equivalent to 10 mIU/mL when the international standard is used.[142] For this reason, an anti-HBs level of ≥10 mIU/mL is considered a protective antibody titer and is the standard used by the U.S. ACIP. Although HBV infections have occurred in vaccine recipients with a detectable immune response, almost all infections have been asymptomatic, identified only through the presence of anti-HBc. These infections have been limited largely to patients with no response or a poor response to vaccination.[140,143]

NONRESPONDERS

11. P.G. has completed her three-dose vaccination series with Engerix-B. Routine hepatitis serology testing, performed before volunteering for a drug study, reveals that P.G. is anti-HBs negative. Why did P.G. not respond to the hepatitis B vaccine, and how should she be managed?

Two important determinants of vaccine efficacy appear to be the age at vaccination and underlying immune function. In healthy recipients, the immune response to vaccination decreases with advancing age. In one study, 99% of patients age 0 to 19 years, 93% of those age 20 to 49 years, and 73% of those older than 50 years of age achieved protective anti-HBs levels (≥10 SRU) after three doses of the hepatitis B vaccine.[144]

Table 73-9 Recommended Doses of Currently Licensed Hepatitis B Vaccines[a]

Group	Recombivax HB		Engerix-B	
	Dose (μg)	(mL)	Dose (μg)	(mL)
Birth to 10 years old	—	—	10	(0.5)
Birth to 19 years old	5	(0.5)	—	—
Children and adolescents 11–19 years	—	—	10	(0.5)
Adolescents 11–15 years[b]	10	(1.0)	—	—
Adults ≥20 years of age	10	(1.0)	20	(1.0)
Dialysis patients and other immunocompromised hosts	40	(1.0)	40[c]	(2.0)

[a]One dose administered 3 times—at time 0, 1 month, and 6 months.
[b]One dose administered—at time 0 and 4–6 months.
[c]Two 1.0 mL doses administered at 1 site, in a 4-dose schedule at 0, 1, 2, and 6 months.
From references 131–133.

Immunocompromised patients, including those receiving hemodialysis,[145] those infected with HIV,[146] or children receiving cytotoxic chemotherapy,[147] respond poorly to the HBV vaccine. Patients who smoke [148–150] or are obese[148,149] also have a reduced response. P.G. has two risk factors for a poor response to the hepatitis B vaccine: she is older than 50 years of age and she is moderately obese (ideal body weight for her height is 50 kg).

Vaccine recipients who respond poorly to hepatitis B vaccine have been classified either as hyporesponders who can probably be protected by additional doses of vaccine or as true nonresponders. Patients with inadequate initial response to the HBV vaccine series should be revaccinated. Of hyporesponders (anti-HBs levels <10 mIU/mL), 50% to 90% develop a protective level following a single booster injection [151–153] or after repeating the entire three-dose series.[147,156] Sixty percent of patients not responding to a primary vaccination series with Engerix B produced an immune response after a three-dose series with HBVax II (Recombivax), suggesting a repeat course with the alternative HBV vaccine may be a reasonable approach in some patients.[154] Revaccination of nonresponders (no detectable anti-HBs) is less successful, and protective levels, if achieved, are not sustained.[155] True nonresponders to HBV vaccination are rare in the immunocompetent population, and these persons may have a genetic predisposition toward nonresponsiveness.[156] P.G. should be revaccinated with a booster dose of hepatitis B vaccine. Her anti-HBs levels can be rechecked 1 month after the injection. If she still has not responded, it is reasonable to administer an additional two injections to complete a second vaccination series.

INTERCHANGEABILITY OF HBV VACCINES

12. T.M., a 32-year-old laboratory technician, received the first two doses of hepatitis B vaccine with Recombivax HB. He has relocated recently and is due for the third injection. The employee health service at his new job uses only Engerix-B for hepatitis B vaccination. Can hepatitis B vaccines produced by different manufacturers be used interchangeably?

While it is recommended that patients receive the complete vaccination series with the same product, data suggest this is not absolutely necessary to induce a protective antibody titer. In a study to determine whether a hepatitis B vaccination series initiated with Recombivax HB could be completed with Engerix-B, healthy adults received 10 µg of Recombivax HB at baseline and 1 month. At 6 months, the subjects were randomized to receive either Engerix-B 20 µg or Recombivax HB 10 µg. One month after the third dose, 100% of those who had received Engerix-B and 92% of those who had received Recombivax HB had protective anti-HBs levels.[157]

Chan and colleagues studied the booster response to either recombinant hepatitis B vaccine or plasma-derived vaccine in children who had been vaccinated originally with the plasma-derived product (Heptavax-B). Children were randomized to either 5 µg of the plasma-derived vaccine or 20 µg of Engerix-B. One month after the booster injection, all vaccine recipients had significant elevations in their anti-HBs titers, suggesting recombinant hepatitis B vaccines elicit an adequate booster response in persons who originally received the plasma-derived vaccine.[158] According to the ACIP, the immune response from one or two doses of a vaccine produced by one manufacturer, when followed by subsequent doses from a different manufacturer, is comparable with that resulting from a full course of vaccination with a single vaccine.[133]

T.M. may complete the hepatitis B vaccine series with Engerix-B provided he receives the recommended dosage of 20 µg administered as a 1-mL intramuscular injection to the deltoid region. This dose will significantly increase his circulating anti-HBs titer, thus conferring optimal protection from HBV infection.

DURATION OF RESPONSE

13. Does T.M. require a booster injection for sustained protection from HBV infection?

The duration of vaccine-induced immunity has been evaluated in many long-term studies.[141,159–166] The duration of detectable anti-HBs appears proportional to the peak antibody response achieved after vaccination, and protective anti-HBs levels were sustained in 68% to 85% of patients receiving the plasma-derived HBV vaccine in studies with follow-up ranging from 6 to 12 years.[159–163] Importantly, the protective efficacy of the HBV vaccine in these trials was high, even in patients with anti-HBs levels <10 mIU/mL. HBsAg was only rarely detected and most HBV events consisted of asymptomatic seroconversion to anti-HBc. These studies suggest that successful HBV vaccination is associated with long-lasting protection without the need for additional booster doses for up to 12 years.

The mechanism of sustained protection from HBV, despite low or nondetectable anti-HBs levels, is thought to be related to the phenomenon of immunologic memory in previously sensitized B lymphocytes. This amnestic response, in combination with the long incubation period of HBV, may allow the synthesis of protective antibodies quickly enough to block infection in patients rechallenged with HBV.[167]

In summary, there is no need for routine administration of HBV vaccine booster doses to immunocompetent persons following successful vaccination. Immunocompromised patients may require a persistent minimum level of protective antibody, and the ACIP does recommend annual antibody testing for patients receiving chronic hemodialysis with administration of a booster dose when antibody levels are <10 mIU/mL.[133] Based on available evidence, T.M. does not require a scheduled booster dose of hepatitis B vaccine.

INDICATIONS

14. Why is it appropriate for T.M. to be vaccinated with hepatitis B vaccine, and who should be vaccinated with this vaccine?

The ACIP has recommended pre-exposure hepatitis B vaccination for the following high-risk groups: health care workers with exposure to blood, staff of institutions for the developmentally disabled, hemodialysis patients, recipients of blood products, household and sexual contacts of HBV carriers, international travelers to HBV-endemic areas, injecting drug users, sexually active homosexual men, bisexual men, and inmates of long-term correctional facilities.[133] Because T.M. is a hospital laboratory technician, he is at high risk for exposure to hepatitis B and should be vaccinated.

UNIVERSAL HEPATITIS B VACCINATION

In addition to the previously listed high-risk groups, all infants should receive hepatitis B vaccination. This recommendation is based on data suggesting the practice of vaccinating only high-risk persons had little impact on decreasing the incidence of HBV disease. Populations at risk for HBV disease (injecting drug users, persons with multiple sexual partners) generally are not vaccinated before they begin engaging in high-risk behaviors. In addition, many persons who become infected have no identifiable risk factors for infection and thus would not be recognized as candidates for vaccination. A program designed to immunize children before they initiate high-risk behaviors is likely to have a greater impact in reducing the incidence of HBV infection. As a means to achieve this goal, the hepatitis B vaccine now is incorporated into the existing pediatric vaccination schedule. The first dose is administered during the newborn period (preferably before the infant is discharged from the hospital) but no later than 2 months of age.[133] The recommended vaccination schedule is shown in Table 73-10.

15. R.M. is a mother of two children aged 11 years and 2 months. Her infant daughter just received a second dose of hepatitis B vaccine as part of her routine well-baby care. R.M. wonders if her son, who did not receive the hepatitis B vaccine during his normal childhood immunizations, should receive the vaccine now.

The Centers for Disease Control and Prevention (CDC) has recently addressed the issue of immunizing children and adolescents born before 1991 who are potentially at risk for hepatitis B infection. The current recommendations suggest that adolescents who have not received three doses of hepatitis B vaccine should initiate or complete the series at ages 11 to 15 years. A schedule of 0, 1 to 2, and 4 to 6 months is recommended.[168] It is anticipated that universal vaccination of all infants and previously unvaccinated adolescents aged 11 to 12 years, in addition to ongoing immunization of high-risk persons, will reduce the incidence of acute hepatitis B infection, hepatitis B–associated chronic liver disease, and HCC. R.M. should receive either Recombivax HB 5 μg or Engerix-B 10 μg as an intramuscular injection in the deltoid with repeat doses 1 to 2 months and 4 to 6 months from the initial injection.

ADVERSE EFFECTS

HBV vaccination generally has been well-tolerated. The most common side effect is pain at the injection site, observed in 10% to 20% of patients. Transient febrile reactions occur in <5% of recipients, and other reactions, including nausea, rash, headache, myalgias, and arthralgias, are observed in <1% of recipients.

Postexposure Prophylaxis
PERCUTANEOUS EXPOSURE

16. K.N., a 26-year-old medical student, presents to the ED after accidentally sticking herself with a contaminated needle while drawing blood from an HBsAg-positive patient. K.N. was not vaccinated previously and had no known prior episodes of hepatitis or liver disease. Her tetanus status is current. She weighs 56 kg. How should K.N. be managed for percutaneous exposure to hepatitis B?

Following exposure to HBV, prophylactic treatment with hepatitis B vaccination and possibly passive immunization with hepatitis B immunoglobulin (HBIG) should be considered. The ACIP recommendations for postexposure immunoprophylaxis following hepatitis B exposure are shown in Table 73-11.

K.N.'s percutaneous exposure warrants active immunization with HBV and passive immunization with HBIG. The source of K.N.'s exposure is HBsAg-positive, and K.N. had not been vaccinated previously with the hepatitis B vaccine. She should receive a single dose of HBIG 0.06 mL/kg (3.4 mL) as an intramuscular injection in either the gluteal or deltoid region as soon as possible after exposure, preferably within 24 hours. HBIG is prepared from plasma of persons preselected for high titer anti-HBs. The anti-HBs of HBIG in the United States is 1:100,000 as determined by radioimmunoassay. HBIG is superior to immunoglobulin in the prevention of hepatitis B infection following percutaneous exposure.[169] K.N. also should receive active immunization with intramuscular hepatitis B vaccine (at a separate site) simultaneously with HBIG. The second and third doses should be given 1 month and 6 months later. Passively acquired antibodies against hepatitis B virus from HBIG or immunoglobulin

Table 73-10 Recommended Schedules of Hepatitis B Vaccination for Infants Born to HBsAg (−) Mothers

Hepatitis B Vaccine	Age of Infant
Option 1	
Dose 1	Birth (before hospital discharge)
Dose 2	1–2 months[a]
Dose 3	6–18 months[a]
Option 2	
Dose 1	1–2 months[a]
Dose 2	4 months[a]
Dose 3	6–18 months[a]

[a]Hepatitis B vaccine can be administered simultaneously with diphtheria-tetanus-pertussis, *Haemophilus influenza* type b conjugate, measles-mumps-rubella, and oral polio vaccines.
From reference 133.

Table 73-11 Guide to Postexposure Immunoprophylaxis for Exposure to Hepatitis B Virus

Type of Exposure	Immunoprophylaxis
Perinatal	Vaccination + HBIG
Sexual	Vaccination + HBIG
Household contact	
Chronic carrier	Vaccination
Acute case	None unless known exposure
Acute case, known exposure	HBIG ± vaccination
Infant (<12 months) acute case in primary caregiver	HBIG + vaccination
Inadvertent (percutaneous/permucosal)	Vaccination ± HBIG

[a]HBIG, hepatitis B immunoglobulin.
From references 133 and 171.

will not interfere with active immunization via hepatitis B vaccine.[170]

If the HBsAg status of the donor source of a percutaneous exposure is unknown, recommendations for prophylaxis of HBV infection depend on whether the donor source is at high risk or at low risk for being HBsAg-positive. High-risk donor sources include homosexual men, IV drug abusers, patients undergoing hemodialysis, residents of mental institutions, immigrants from endemic areas, and household contacts of HBV carriers. Additional ACIP recommendations for hepatitis B prophylaxis following percutaneous exposure are shown in Table 73-12.

SEXUAL EXPOSURE

17. **What are the current recommendations for a person who has had sexual contact with an HBsAg-positive person?**

Sexual transmission of hepatitis B is an important cause of HBV infection, accounting for approximately 30% to 60% of all new cases annually.[171] Passive immunization with a single 5-mL dose of hepatitis B immunoglobulin (HBIG) was found highly effective in preventing hepatitis B infection following sexual exposure when compared with a control globulin (with no anti-HBs activity).[172] The CDC recommends that susceptible persons exposed to HBV through sexual contact with a person who has acute or chronic HBV infection should receive postexposure prophylaxis with 0.06 mL/kg of HBIG as a single IM dose within 14 days of the last exposure. Patients also should receive the standard three-dose immunization series with hepatitis B vaccine beginning at the time of HBIG administration.[171]

PERINATAL EXPOSURE

18. **S.L., a 3.2-kg boy, was just born to an HBsAg-positive mother. Is S.L. at risk for acquiring HBV infection, and how should he be managed?**

In many Asian and developing countries, perinatal (vertical) transmission accounts for most hepatitis B infections. Infants born to HBV-infected mothers have a >85% risk of acquiring HBV during the perinatal period.[173] Of those who become infected, 80% to 90% become chronic HBsAg carriers.[174-176] Although fulminant cases have been reported, most hepatitis infections in neonates are asymptomatic. Despite the usually innocuous initial disease, significant adverse consequences are associated with chronic HBsAg carriage in neonates. Chronic hepatitis B infection is associated with chronic liver disease and has been clearly implicated as a major risk factor in the development of primary HCC.[177,178]

Mothers who are chronic carriers of hepatitis B, although not acutely infected, pose the risk of transmitting the hepatitis B virus to their infants. The risk is related to the presence of HBsAg and HBeAg (suggesting a high degree of viral replication and infectivity). The likelihood that S.L. will develop HBV infection is high. S.L. requires immediate therapy with HBIG (to provide immediate high titers of circulating anti-HBs) and simultaneous vaccination with hepatitis B vaccine (to induce long-lasting protective immunity). Screening pregnant women for the presence of HBeAg and administration of hepatitis B immunoglobulin and hepatitis B vaccine is 85% to 98% effective in preventing HBV infection and the chronic carrier state.[173,174,176,179,180] This compares with a 71% efficacy rate for administration of hepatitis B immunoglobulin alone. Simultaneous administration of HBIG and hepatitis B vaccine does not adversely affect the production of anti-HBs in neonates.[174,176]

Infants born to mothers who are HBsAg positive should receive simultaneous IM injections of the appropriate doses of hepatitis B vaccine (see Table 73-9) and HBIG (0.5 mL) within 12 hours of birth. The injections should be administered at separate sites. S.L. should receive HBIG (0.5 mL) as soon as possible after birth, administered as an intramuscular

---

Table 73-12   **Recommendations for Hepatitis B Prophylaxis Following Percutaneous Exposure[133]**

Exposed Person	Treatment When Source Is Found to Be		
	HBsAg-Positive	HBsAg-Negative	Unknown or Not Tested
Unvaccinated	Administer HBIG × 1[a] and initiate hepatitis B vaccine	Initiate hepatitis B vaccine[b]	Initiate hepatitis B vaccine[b]
Previously vaccinated			
Known responder	Test exposed person for anti-HBs[c] 1. If inadequate, hepatitis B vaccine booster dose 2. If adequate, no treatment	No treatment	No treatment
Known responder	HBIG × 1[a] as soon as possible, repeat in 1 month *OR* HBIG × 1[a] plus 1 dose of hepatitis B vaccine	No treatment	If known high-risk source, may treat as if source were HBsAg positive
Response unknown	Test exposed person for anti-HBs[c] 1. If inadequate, HBIG × 1[a] plus hepatitis B vaccine booster dose 2. If adequate, no treatment	No treatment	Test exposed person for anti-HBs[c] 1. If inadequate, hepatitis B vaccine booster dose 2. If adequate, no treatment

[a]HBIG dose 0.06 mL/kg IM.
[b]For dosing information see Table 73-9.
[c]Adequate anti-HBs is ≥10 mIU.

injection. He also should receive 0.5 mL of either Recombivax HB (5 μg) or Engcrix-B (10 μg) as an intramuscular injection at a separate site.

19. **What would the management plan be if the HBsAg status of S.L.'s mother was unknown?**

The ACIP has developed recommendations for the prevention of perinatal HBV infection. This includes the routine testing of all pregnant women for HBsAg during an early prenatal visit. HBsAg testing should be repeated late in the pregnancy for women who are HBsAg-negative but who are at high risk of HBV infection or who have had clinically apparent hepatitis. Women admitted for delivery who have not had prenatal HBsAg testing should have blood drawn for testing. While test results are pending, the infant should receive hepatitis B vaccine within 12 hours of birth (see Table 73-9). If the mother is found later to be HBsAg-positive, her infant should receive HBIG as soon as possible within 7 days of birth. The second and third doses of vaccine should be administered at 1 and 6 months, respectively. If the mother is found to be HbsAg-negative, her infant should continue to receive hepatitis B vaccine as part of the routine vaccination series.[133]

COMBINATION VACCINE

Recently the Food and Drug Administration (FDA) licensed a combined HAV and HBV vaccine (Twinrix, GlaxoSmithKline Biologicals, Rixensart, Belgium) for use in persons aged ≥18 years.[38,181] Twinrix is composed of the same antigenic components used in Havrix and Engerix-B. Each dose of Twinrix contains at least 720 EL.U. of inactivated HAV and 20 μg or recombinant hepatitis B surface antigen (IIDsAg). Trace amounts of thimerosal (<1 μg) is also present from the manufacturing process.

Primary immunization consists of three doses, given on a 0-, 1-, and 6- month schedule, the same that is used for single antigen hepatitis B vaccine.[38,181] Any person 18 years of age or older having an indication for both hepatitis A and hepatitis B vaccine can be given Twinrix, including patients with chronic liver disease, users of illicit injectable drugs, men who have sex with men, and persons with clotting factor disorders who receive therapeutic blood products.[38,181] For international travel, hepatitis A vaccine is recommended; hepatitis B vaccine is recommended for travelers to areas of high or intermediate hepatitis B endemicity who plan to stay for longer than 6 months and have frequent close contact with the local population.[38,181]

Data from 11 clinical trials in adult patients aged 17 to 70 years indicated, at 1 month after completion of the three-dose series, that seroconversion for anti-HAV (titer ≥20 mIU/mL) was elicited in 99.9% of vaccinees, and protective antibodies against HBsAg (anti-HBs ≥10 mIU/mL) were elicited in 98.5% of vaccinees.[38,181] Thus, the efficacy of Twinrix likely is comparable with existing single antigen hepatitis vaccines. The persistence of anti-HAV and anti-HBs following administration is similar to that following single antigen hepatitis A and B vaccine administration at 4 years follow-up. Observed adverse effects were generally similar in type and frequency to those reported following vaccination with monovalent hepatitis A and B vaccines and no serious vaccine-related adverse events were observed in clinical trials.[38,181]

Clinical Features and Treatment of Chronic Hepatitis B

20. **C.R., a 28-year-old man, presents to the ED with jaundice, complaints of incapacitating fatigue, and vague intermittent abdominal pain for the past month. C.R. was diagnosed with hepatitis B 2 years before admission. His social history includes IV drug abuse (none for 2 years) and alcohol abuse (none for 2 years). Several weeks ago, C.R. noted darkening of his urine and yellowing of his eyes.**

Physical examination reveals a thin man in no apparent distress. He is afebrile, and blood pressure, heart rate, and respiratory rate are within normal limits. Moderate scleral icterus is noted. The abdomen is soft and nondistended. The liver is enlarged, nontender, and smooth with an edge palpable 5 cm below the costal margin and a span of 15 cm. The spleen is palpable. The cardiac, pulmonary, neurologic, and extremity examinations all are within normal limits.

C.R.'s laboratory evaluation is significant for Hct, 44%; Hgb, 15 g/dL; WBC count, 8.8 cells/mm³; platelets, 225,000/mm³ (normal, 150,000 to 300,000/mm³); PT, 15.4 sec (control, 12 sec), international normalized ratio, 1.8; AST, 326 U/L (normal, 5 to 40 U/L); ALT, 382 U/L (normal, 5 to 40 U/L); alkaline phosphatase, 142 U/mL (normal, 21 to 91 U/L); total bilirubin, 4.2 mg/dL (normal, 0.1 to 1.2 mg/dL); and albumin, 2.8 g/dL (normal, 3.5 to 4.5 g/dL). Hepatitis serologic tests are positive for HBsAg, HBeAg, and anti-HBc and negative for IgM anti-HBc, IgM anti-HAV, and anti-HCV. HBV DNA is reported as <200 pg/mL. A liver biopsy reveals periportal inflammation as well as piecemeal and bridging necrosis. What clinical findings does C.R. have that support the diagnosis of chronic hepatitis B infection?

[SI units: Hct, 0.44; Hgb, 150 g/L; WBC count, 8.8 × 10⁹ cells/L; AST, 326 U/L (normal, 5 to 40); ALT, 382 U/L (normal, 5 to 40); alkaline phosphatase, 142 U/L (normal, 21 to 91); total bilirubin, 71.8 μmol/L (normal, 1.7 to 20.5); albumin, 28 g/L (normal, 35 to 45)]

The chronic occurrence of jaundice and hepatosplenomegaly with significantly elevated AST and ALT in a young patient such as C.R. is suggestive of chronic hepatitis. Although alcoholic hepatitis secondary to long-term alcohol abuse is consistent with these clinical features, his serologic tests are positive for HBV. Hepatitis serology with positive HBsAg and HBeAg suggest ongoing viral replication and a high degree of infectivity.

Serum concentrations of aminotransferases can range from slightly abnormal to greatly elevated, with ALT concentrations generally greater than AST. Serum bilirubin concentrations >3.0 mg/dL are common, serum concentration of alkaline phosphatase usually is increased, and the PT may be prolonged. Patients such as C.R. with a prolonged PT and low serum albumin concentration generally have a more severe form of chronic hepatitis.

Liver biopsy is important for the diagnosis, treatment, and prognosis of patients with chronic hepatitis. C.R.'s liver biopsy reveals the classic triad of periportal inflammation as well as piecemeal and bridging necrosis. The liver biopsy and hepatitis serologic test results are consistent with a diagnosis of chronic hepatitis B infection.

Treatment of chronic HBV infection requires knowledge of the natural history of the untreated disease and the potential benefits of intervention. Currently only α-interferon, lamivudine, and adefovir are approved by the U.S. Food and

Drug Administration (FDA) for treating chronic HBV infection.

21. Does C.R. require treatment for chronic hepatitis secondary to hepatitis B?

The decision to treat C.R. depends on the severity of symptoms, the serum biochemistries, and the liver biopsy results. Symptom-free patients with moderate elevations in aminotransferases and liver biopsies demonstrating mild chronic HBV infection probably should not be treated. These patients should be monitored every 3 to 6 months with routine serum biochemistries and by liver biopsy at yearly intervals.

C.R. has evidence of severe chronic HBV infection. He is symptomatic with jaundice, severe fatigue, and abdominal pain, and the results of his LFTs suggest his disease is advanced (decreased albumin, elevated PT). Therefore, he should be treated to reduce the replication of HBV, resolve the hepatocellular damage, and prevent long-term adverse hepatic sequelae.

Goals of Therapy

22. What are the goals of therapy for chronic hepatitis secondary to HBV?

Progression of chronic hepatitis to cirrhosis is thought to be related to continued replication of the hepatitis B virus. Loss of active viral replication usually is associated with a decrease in infectivity, a reduction in inflammatory cells within the liver, and a fall of serum aminotransferase activities into the normal range. The disappearance of detectable HBeAg and HBV DNA is considered an indicator of loss of active viral replication.

The goal of therapy in chronic HBV infection is eradication of viral carriage, which will resolve ongoing hepatocellular damage and development of cirrhosis and HCC. Clinical trials for chronic HBV infection have used the following markers as endpoints for successful therapy: seroconversion from HBeAg-positive to HBeAg-negative (with appearance of anti-HBe), reductions in serum aminotransferase activity, elimination of circulating HBV DNA, and improvement in liver histology. The elimination of HBsAg (termination of HBV carrier state) has been difficult to achieve in clinical trials.

Drug Therapy

23. Would initiating therapy during the acute phase of the HBV infection have benefited C.R.?

Pharmacologic interventions in the management of acute hepatitis B have been disappointing. Early studies demonstrated a transient decrease in serum aminotransferase activity and bilirubin concentration associated with corticosteroids. However, more recent studies have resulted in a higher incidence of relapse[182,183] and mortality[184–186] in patients receiving corticosteroids. Other therapies, including hepatitis B immunoglobulin (HBIG)[187] and α-interferon,[188] have been ineffective in managing acute viral hepatitis secondary to HBV. Nucleoside and nucleotide reverse transcriptase inhibitors reduce HBV DNA levels in patients with chronic disease[89,90,92,189–198]; however, their use in acute HBV infection requires further investigation.[189–191] Thus, administration of antivirals during the acute phase of HBV infection is not recommended in C.R.

INTERFERONS

24. What drug therapy should C.R. receive to treat chronic HBV-associated infection?

Previously, the most effective agents for treating chronic hepatitis B have been interferons,[199,200] which appear to activate their target cells by binding to specific cell surface receptors to induce synthesis of effector proteins.[201,202] These intracellular proteins induce the antiviral, antiproliferative, and immunomodulatory actions of the interferons. Gene expression, upregulation of NK cells, cytotoxic T cells, and macrophages are induced by interferons.[201,202] Their antiviral activity possibly arises from their ability to abate viral entry into the host cells and modulate several steps of the viral replication cycle (e.g., viral uncoating, inhibition of mRNA, and protein synthesis).

Three classes of interferons (α, β, and γ) are secreted endogenously by different cells in response to foreign stimuli (Table 73-13). α-Interferon is produced by peripheral monocytes, macrophages, and B lymphocytes in response to viral infection. β-Interferon is produced by fibroblasts and epithelial cells in response to viral infection. γ-Interferon is pro-

---

Table 73-13 Comparison of Interferons Used to Treat Viral Hepatitis

Agent[a]	Trade	Source	Indication	Dose/Route	Comments
α-Interferons					
Interferon α-2a	Roferon-A	Recombinant	HCV	3 MU TIW IM/SC × 12 months	Most commonly used interferon for HCV
Interferon α-2b	Intron-A	Recombinant	NANB/HCV	3 MU TIW IM/SC × 6 months	Previous standard of care for HCV
Interferon α-n1	NA	Lymphoblastoid	Not FDA approved for HCV	3 MU TIW IM/SC × 12 months	Originally thought to have higher relapse rate versus recombinant α-interferons (6 months); response rate with 12 months of therapy
Interferon α-con-1	Infergen	Recombinant	HCV	9 μg TIW SC × 6 months	Has greater in vitro effects versus other interferons; proposed enhanced efficacy against HCV type 1 genotype

[a]Interferons may decrease hepatic cytochrome P450 metabolism of drugs.
NA, not applicable; NANB, non-A, non-B hepatitis; TIW, three times weekly.

Table 73-14   Clinical Trials Using Interferon to Treat Chronic HBV

Author	Interferon	Dosage	Duration (Months)	N	HbeAg Clearance (%)	HBV DNA Clearance (%)
Hoofnagle	Alfa-2b	10 million U TIW	4	31	32	32
Brook	Alfa-2b	5–10 million U/m² TIW	6	37	41	32
Saracco	Lymphoblastoid	5 million U/m² TIW	6	33	21	79
Perillo	Alfa-2b	5 million U/day	4	41	37	nm
Lak	Alfa-2b	10 million U TIW	4	79	15	nm
Wong	Alfa-2b	10 million U/m² TIW	3	50	24	nm
Brunetto	Alfa-2a	9 million U TIW then 3 million U TIW	4 then 2	30	anti-HBe (+)	67
Hadziyannis	Alfa-2b	3 million U TIW	4	25	anti-HBe (+)	78
Pastore	Lymphoblastoid	5 million U/m² TIW	6	10	anti-HBe (+)	85
Pattovich	Lymphoblastoid	5 million U/m² TIW	6	60	anti-HBe (+)	27

Anti-HBe, hepatitis B envelope antibody; nm, not measured; TIW, three times weekly.
From references 200, 203–209.

duced by T lymphocytes and differs from both α- and β-interferons in that it possesses more immunoregulatory than antiviral effects.

Three varieties of α-interferon are commercially available: recombinant interferon alfa-2a (Roferon-A, Hoffmann-LaRoche), recombinant interferon alfa-2b (Intron A, Schering Corp.), and consensus interferon (Infergen, Amgen). Consensus interferon (primarily studied for HCV infection) was developed by scanning subtypes of α-interferon and assigning the most frequently observed amino acid at each position to form a consensus molecule (see Table 73-13). The DNA coding sequence was then synthesized and cloned in a recombinant system. Interferon alfa-2a (Roferon-A) and interferon alfa-2b (Intron-A) differ by a single amino acid substitution. The clinical significance of these differences is unknown. Although several of these agents have been used to treat chronic hepatitis B infection, most clinical data are with interferon alfa-2b (Intron-A), which remains the only FDA-approved interferon (INF) for the treatment of chronic HBV infection (Table 73-14).

In addition, interferon α-2a and interferon α-2b have been chemically conjugated to polyethylene glycol (PEG) forms to make "pegylated" interferons. These "pegylated" interferons are used for treatment of HCV infection (see section on Hepatitis C). These agents are known to have increased serum half-life resulting in a prolonged antiviral effect, as well as less immunogenicity. Their efficacy in HBV infection is under clinical investigation.

Efficacy

α-Interferon is moderately effective in treating chronic hepatitis B.[203–208] Patients receiving α-interferon may experience a virologic response based on clearance of HBeAg (27%; range, 15% to 41%) or HBV DNA (47%; range, 32% to 79%) compared with 9% of untreated controls. Normalization of ALT values is observed in 47% of α-interferon–treated patients versus 13% in untreated controls. Clearance of HBsAg occurs in only 10% to 15% of patients after completion of therapy.[203,204–208] In one long-term follow-up study of patients responding to α-interferon, delayed clearance of HBsAg was observed in 65% of patients 3 years after completion of therapy.[209] Relapse after successful therapy is rare. In another

prospective study, 103 patients with chronic hepatitis B treated with 2 to 5 million units of α-interferon for 4 to 6 months compared with untreated patients demonstrated greater HBeAg and HBsAg clearance rates (56% versus 28% and 11.6% versus 0%, respectively; $P < 0.001$) at 5 years.[210] All patients with loss of HBeAg also lost HBV DNA and had newly detectable anti-HBeAg antibodies. A trend toward greater survival and fewer clinical complications was also seen in the treatment group. For these reasons, a trial with INF is reasonable for C.R. However, no long-term follow-up data are available to demonstrate reductions in cirrhosis or hepatocellular cancer in patients receiving α-interferon therapy.

Predictors of Response

25. Is C.R. likely to respond to α-interferon therapy?

Certain patient variables can predict the response to therapy with α-interferon (Table 73-15). The most reliable predictor of a positive response to α-interferon appears to be the pretreatment level of HBV DNA.[89,91,92] Patients with HBV DNA levels <200 pg/mL are more likely to respond to therapy than those with higher levels.[89,91,204] In addition, data suggest that HBeAg seroconversion with INF treatment is associated with improved survival and reduced complications. Other predictors of a positive response include a short duration of disease, negative HIV status, high pretreatment aminotransferase levels, and active liver disease demonstrated by liver biopsy.[89,91,92,209,,211,212]

Table 73-15   Factors Predictive of a Sustained Response to Interferon-Alfa in Patients With Chronic Hepatitis

Chronic hepatitis B
Short duration of disease
High serum, aminotransferase concentrations[a]
Active liver disease with fibrosis[a]
Low HBV DNA concentrations
Wild-type (HBcAg positive) virus
Absence of immunosuppression

[a]One of the most commonly associated factors with a high degree of response to therapy.

C.R. is a reasonable candidate for α-interferon therapy. His liver biopsy is consistent with chronic disease, he has high pretreatment aminotransferase levels, his HBV DNA is <200 pg/mL, and his duration of chronic hepatitis is short. Before initiating α-interferon, serologic testing for HIV should be performed to assist in the evaluation of C.R.'s response to therapy (Fig. 73-4).

Adverse Effects

26. **What adverse effects to α-interferon should be monitored in C.R.?**

Adverse effects associated with α-interferon therapy are common (Table 73-16). These have been categorized as early side effects that rarely limit the use of INF, and late side effects that may necessitate dose reduction or discontinuation of therapy altogether.[200,213,214] The early side effects of α-interferon therapy generally appear hours after administration and resemble an influenza-like syndrome with fever, chills, anorexia, nausea, myalgias, fatigue, and headache. Virtually all patients receiving α-interferon experience these toxicities, and they tend to resolve after repeated exposure to the drug. Administration of α-interferon at bedtime may decrease the severity of

Table 73-16	Serious Adverse Events Reported With Interferon-α Therapy
Central Nervous System	**Cardiovascular**
Psychosis	Cardiac arrhythmias
Depression/suicide	Sudden death
Delirium/confusion	Dilated cardiomyopathy
Extrapyramidal ataxia	Hypotension
Paresthesia	**Other**
Seizures	Retinopathy
Relapse in substance abuse	Hearing loss
Hematologic	Pulmonary interstitial fibrosis
Granulocytopenia	Acute renal failure
Thrombocytopenia	Hyperthyroidism
Anemia	Hypothyroidism
Dermatologic	Systemic lupus erythematosus
Psoriasis	
Erythema multiforme	
Gastrointestinal	
Autoimmune hepatitis	
Primary biliary cirrhosis	
Hepatic decompensation	

From references 200, 213, 214, and 215.

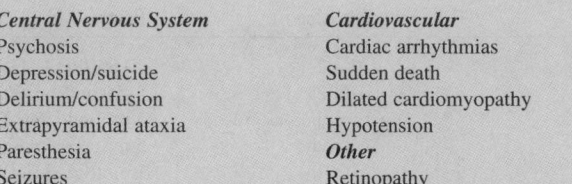

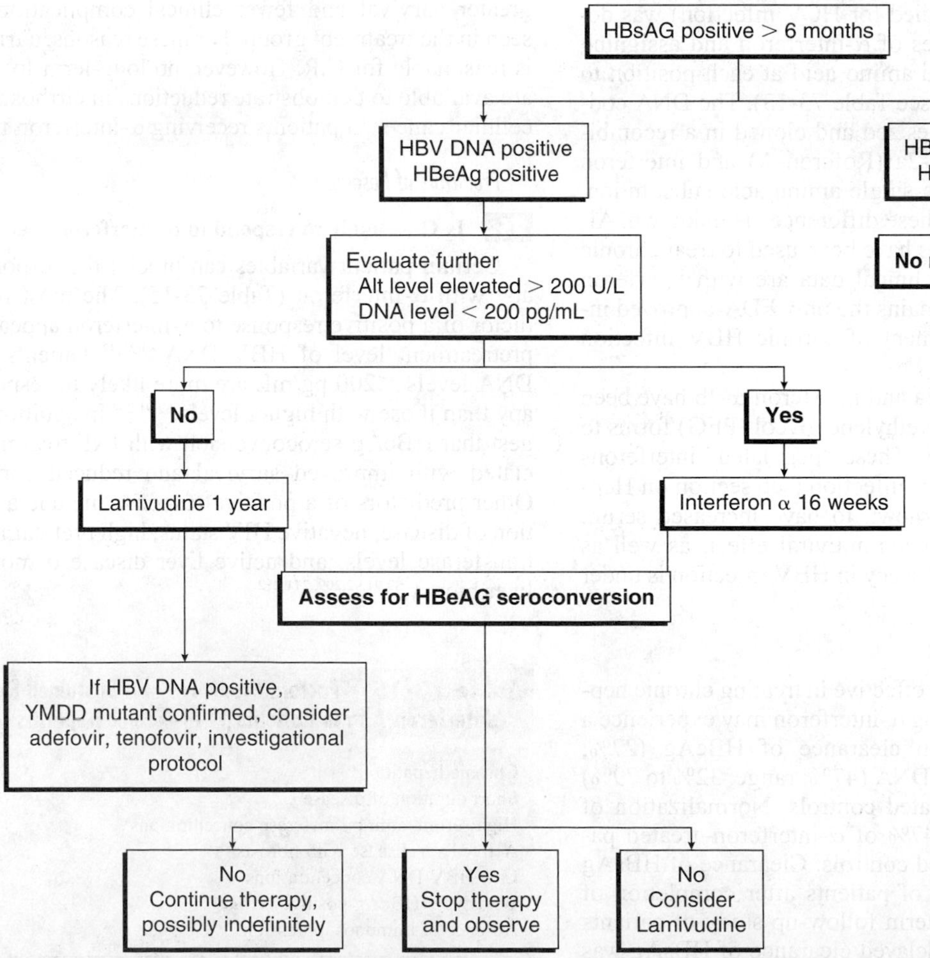

FIGURE 73-4 Hepatitis B Virus Treatment Algorithm. (Adapted from reference 92.)

early side effects. Acetaminophen can be used to treat early side effects of α-interferon therapy, but should be limited to 2 g/day to minimize the risk of hepatotoxicity. The late side effects usually are observed after 2 weeks of therapy and are more serious. These toxicities limit the use of α-interferon and include worsening of the influenza-like syndrome, alopecia, bone marrow suppression, bacterial infections, thyroid dysfunction (both hypothyroidism and hyperthyroidism), and psychiatric disturbances (depression, anxiety, delirium). C.R. should be questioned at each clinic visit about new or worsening symptoms as well as any changes in mood or the ability to perform daily tasks of living. Additional monitoring parameters include a complete blood count (CBC) with differential and platelet count after weeks 1 and 2 of therapy and monthly thereafter during treatment.

Dosing

27. **What dose of α-interferon should C.R. receive?**

Interferon doses of 2.5 to 10 million units can be administered subcutaneously (SC) daily or three times weekly for 1 to 12 months. The manufacturer of INF alfa-2b recommends 30 to 35 million U/week, administered subcutaneously or intramuscularly as 5 million U/day or 10 million units three times weekly for 16 weeks. Some authorities believe thrice-weekly administration of α-interferon is associated with more severe flulike symptoms and headache when compared with daily administration. In contrast, severe bone marrow suppression tends to occur less often with thrice-weekly administration.[214,215] Treatment questions that still need to be adequately assessed are the optimal schedule of INF administration (daily versus every other day versus three times weekly) and the benefit of combining INF with other antiviral agents (see below) for the treatment of HBV infection. However, because C.R. has normal WBC and platelet counts, he should initially receive INF alfa-2b as a 5-million-unit subcutaneous injection daily for 16 weeks. The subcutaneous route of administration is preferred in C.R. to decrease the possibility of hematoma formation because his PT is prolonged. If conventional doses of INF lead to liver failure, development of sepsis, or bleeding, low-dose therapy may be of benefit based on results from a trial in patients with decompensated cirrhosis.[216]

The dose should be decreased by 50% if granulocyte or platelet counts decline to <750/mm³ and 50,000/mm³, respectively.[217] Profound thrombocytopenia (<30,000/mm³) or neutropenia (<500/mm³); serious changes in mood or behavior; and intractable nausea, vomiting, or fatigue warrant the immediate discontinuation of α-interferon.

NUCLEOSIDE ANALOGS

28. **If C.R. does not respond to α-interferon, what additional antiviral therapies are available?**

Although INF has been important in the treatment of chronic HBV infection, patients included in most clinical trials represented a highly select group of chronic HBV carriers. Specifically, patients with decompensated liver disease were excluded because they often have leukopenia and thrombocytopenia as a result of hypersplenism, which limits the dose of INF that can be administered. The FDA has approved lamivu-

dine (Epivir-HBV) for use in patients with compensated liver disease who had evidence of active viral replication and liver inflammation caused by chronic hepatitis B infection. Nucleoside analogs represent an alternative approach to treatment.[89,91,92,189–198]Lamivudine, the (−) enantiomer of 3′–thiacytidine is an oral 2′, 3′–dideoxynucleoside that inhibits DNA synthesis by terminating the nascent proviral DNA chain and interferes with the reverse transcriptase activity of HBV.[218,219]

Lamivudine has gained FDA approval for the treatment of HIV infection, and pilot trials in humans demonstrated that dosages of 5 to 600 mg/day of the drug were well tolerated and reduced serum levels of HBV DNA.[89,91,92,219] Doses of ≤20 mg resulted in incomplete suppression of HBV DNA, whereas doses of ≥100 mg led to virtually complete suppression. Increase in viral replication following cessation of therapy, however, was significant. Subsequently, lamivudine was studied in a randomized, double-blind trial in 32 patients with chronic, replicative HBV, including 17 nonresponders to INF.[195] Patients received 25, 100, or 300 mg of oral lamivudine daily for 12 weeks with a follow-up period of an additional 24 weeks. Results demonstrated that the drug was well tolerated, and levels of HBV DNA became undetectable in 70%, 100%, and 100% of patients who received the 25-, 100-, or 300-mg doses, respectively. HBV DNA reappeared following cessation of therapy in most patients; however, six patients (19%), including five INF-nonresponders, had sustained suppression of HBV DNA along with normalization of ALT levels. Three-year trials have had similar results, with improvement in inflammation scores in the treated group and clearance of HBV DNA in the majority of patients by the end of treatment.[220]

In a larger trial, Chinese patients with chronic hepatitis B were randomly assigned to receive 25 mg of lamivudine (N = 142), 100 mg of lamivudine (N = 143), or placebo (N = 73) once a day for 12 months.[196] Results at 12 months demonstrated that lamivudine was associated with substantial histologic improvement in 56% of patients receiving the 100-mg dose of lamivudine, 49% of patients receiving 25 mg of lamivudine, and 25% of those receiving placebo. In addition, the percent reduction of HBV DNA and aminotransferase levels was significant with the 100-mg group (98% and 72%, respectively) compared with the 25-mg (93% and 65%, respectively) or placebo groups (23% and 64%, respectively).

In one randomized, placebo-controlled trial patients received 100 mg lamivudine or placebo as initial therapy for chronic hepatitis B for 52 weeks.[221] Patients receiving lamivudine were more likely to have a histologic response, loss of HBeAg in serum, sustained suppression of HBV DNA to undetectable levels, and reduced incidence of hepatic fibrosis. Additional findings were that lamivudine recipients were more likely to experience HBeAg seroconversion (loss of HBeAg), undetectable levels of serum HBV DNA, and the appearance of antibodies against HBeAg. HBeAg responses were maintained in most patients for 16 weeks following discontinuation of therapy. Additional trials are necessary to determine whether administration of lamivudine will improve the rates of serologic and virologic responses, and whether it should be considered as first-line therapy over INF. However, lamivudine appears to benefit patients similar to C.R.

Adverse Effects

29. What adverse effects to lamivudine should be monitored in C.R.?

Lamivudine has been well tolerated in patients receiving the drug for chronic HBV infection. The most commonly reported adverse effects have been headache, fatigue, nausea, and abdominal discomfort. Less common adverse effects include laboratory abnormalities such as transient asymptomatic elevation in amylase, lipase, and creatinine kinase levels.[89,91,92,96,194-196,219]

30. What is the risk of development of resistance in CR?

Lamivudine Resistance

Considering the high rate of viral turnover and the error prone nature of the polymerase (particularly the reverse transcriptase), acquisition of resistance mutations would be predicted. The most common mutation leading to lamivudine resistance is a specific point mutation in the highly conserved methionine motif of the HBV polymerase.[89,91,92,96,114,224] In this mutation, the methionine residue is changed to a valine or isoleucine. These genotypic mutations in the YMDD locus associated with a reduced sensitivity to lamivudine occur following long-term therapy (e.g., 52 weeks). This motif is thought to be representative of the active site of the enzyme, similar to that associated with HIV reverse transcriptase, leading to lamivudine resistance.[89,91,92,96,194-196,219,222,223] YMDD mutants appear to cause an acute increase in aminotransferase concentrations without affecting histologic responses. Lamivudine-resistant HBV mutants generally are detectable after 6 months or more of continuous therapy. Integrated data from four studies show a 24% (range, 16% to 32%) incidence at 1 year, increasing to 47% to 56% at 2 years of therapy and 69% to 75% at 3 years of therapy.[89,91,92,96,114,224]

In these patients median HBV-DNA was rapidly reduced and remained low or undetectable throughout the follow-up period. The authors concluded that the drug was well tolerated and that seroconversion might be associated with a reduced rate of HCC, liver failure, and death.

NEW DRUG THERAPIES
Adefovir

31. If C.R. does not respond to α-interferon or lamivudine, what new drug therapies are available?

Adefovir dipivoxil (Hepsera, Gilead) was approved by the FDA in September 2002 for the treatment of chronic hepatitis B in adults with evidence of active viral replication and either evidence of persistent elevations in serum aminotransferases (ALT or AST) or histologically active disease.[225] Adefovir dipivoxil is the oral prodrug of an acyclic nucleotide monophosphate analogue, 9-(2-phosphonylmethoxyethyl)-adenine (PMEA). The active drug is a selective inhibitor of numerous species of viral nucleic acid polymerases and reverse transcriptases. It has broad-spectrum antiviral activity against retroviruses, hepadnaviruses, and herpesviruses. Orally administered adefovir dipivoxil exhibits an inhibitory effect on both the HIV and HBV reverse transcriptases. Importantly, it appears that adefovir is capable of inhibiting the enzymatic activity of both wild type and YMDD mutant variants of both of these viruses.

Recently, two trials reported the results of adefovir for the treatment of patients who were HBeAg negative[226] and HBeAg positive.[227] The first of these trials, patients with chronic hepatitis B who were negative for hepatitis B e antigen (HBeAg) were randomly assigned to receive either 10 mg of adefovir dipivoxil (N = 123) or placebo (N = 61) once daily for 48 weeks.[226] The primary end-point in this trial was histologic improvement. At week 48, 64% of patients who had baseline liver biopsy specimens available in the adefovir dipivoxil group had improvement in histologic liver abnormalities (77 of 121), as compared with 33% of patients in the placebo group (19 of 57). Additionally, serum hepatitis B virus (HBV) DNA levels were reduced to less than 400 copies per milliliter in 61 of 123 patients (51%) receiving adefovir and in 0 of 61 patients (0%) receiving placebo. The median decrease in log-transformed HBV DNA levels was also greater with adefovir-treated patients compared with patients taking placebo (3.91 versus 1.35 log copies per milliliter; $P < 0.001$). Biochemical markers (alanine aminotransferase levels) had normalized at week 48 in 84 of 116 (72%) of patients receiving adefovir compared with 17 of 59 (29%) of those receiving placebo. No HBV polymerase mutations associated with resistance to adefovir were identified within the study period. Adefovir resulted in significant histologic, virologic, and biochemical improvement, with an adverse event profile similar to that of placebo. Emergence of adefovir-resistant HBV polymerase mutations was not observed; however, long-term follow-up is required to validate these findings.

In the second clinical trial adefovir was given to hepatitis B e antigen-positive patients with chronic hepatitis B.[227] Patients were randomly assigned to receive 10 mg or 30 mg of adefovir dipivoxil or placebo daily for 48 weeks. The primary end-point was histologic improvement in the 10-mg group as compared with the placebo group. After 48 weeks of treatment, significantly more patients who received 10 mg or 30 mg of daily adefovir had histologic improvement (53% and 59%, respectively) versus 25% in placebo patients. In addition, a significant reduction in serum HBV DNA levels, undetectable levels (less than 400 copies per milliliter) of serum HBV DNA, normalization of alanine aminotransferase levels, and HBeAg seroconversion were associated with adefovir. Adefovir-associated resistance mutations were identified in the HBV DNA polymerase gene within the study period. The safety profile of the 10-mg dose of adefovir dipivoxil was similar to that of placebo. However, more adverse events and renal laboratory abnormalities were observed in the group receiving 30 mg/day of adefovir. In summary, adefovir dipivoxil led to histologic liver improvement, reduced serum HBV DNA and alanine aminotransferase levels, and increased rates of HBeAg seroconversion without adefovir-associated resistance. Again, long-term follow-up is required to validate these findings. Thus C.R. could receive adefovir 10 mg/day orally if he does not respond to interferon or lamivudine.

Investigational Agents

The safety and efficacy of other antiviral agents for the treatment of chronic HBV infection, including entecavir (BMS-200475),[91,92,228] tenofovir (PMPA),[91,92,228] fluorocytidine (Fd4C),[229] clevudine [L-FMAU (1-(2-fluoro-5-methyl-β-L-arabinofuranosyl-uracil)],[91,231] emtricitabine [Coviracil (2R,5S)-5-fluoro-1-[2-(hydroxymethyl)-1,3-oxathiolan-5-

yl]cytosine],[91,228,230,232] DAPD (1-β-D-2,6-diaminopurine dioxolane),[231] epavudine (L-dT, NV-02B),[233,234] and epcitabine (L-dC, NV-02C),[233,234] are under investigation. Although several drugs have failed to treat HBV effectively,[234–239] agents such as DAPD, clevudine, and tenofovir may prove effective against HBV isolates that are resistant to lamivudine.[240–242] Novel agents such as glycosidase inhibitors, hammerhead ribozymes (short RNA molecules that possess endoribonuclease activity capable of degrading target RNA), and antisense phosphodiester oligodeoxynucleotides (short fragments of DNA that are complimentary to HBV-RNA which result in inhibition of RNA translation) are also under investigation.[243] Pending the results of these trials and the arrival of HBV protease inhibitors and cytokine therapies, combination antiviral therapy as demonstrated in HIV patients, may enhance response rates, reduce the progression of liver disease, and ultimately enhance survival in patients with chronic HBV infection.[244,245]

Therapeutic Vaccines

Theradigm-HBV (Cytel, San Diego, CA) is a therapeutic vaccine consisting of the viral protein HBcAg peptide, a T-helper peptide (tetanus toxoid peptide) that enhances immunogenicity, and two palmitic acid molecules (Table 73-17). The vaccine appears to be well tolerated, has dose-dependent response rates, and appears to work by inducing HBV-specific MHC class I-restricted CTLs. Phase I and II studies in patients with chronic HBV are in progress.[246] Another therapeutic vaccine undergoing clinical investigation for chronic HBV is HBV/MF59.[247] This vaccine combines the HBV "Pre S2 and S" antigens with an MF59 adjuvant (enhances immune responses).

Liver Transplantation

32. As C.R. continues to decompensate from his chronic HBV infection, what nonpharmacologic interventions are available?

One-year survival rates for patients with cholestatic or alcoholic liver disease are >90% in most transplant centers.[110] Historical data for liver transplants in patients with chronic HBV infection are associated with 1-year survival of 50% compared with non–HBV-infected recipients. In one report, 51 HBsAg-positive patients who received a liver transplant for postnecrotic cirrhosis were compared with 38 patients transplanted with evidence of HBV immunity (HBsAg-negative and anti–HBs-positive).[110] Early post-transplant mortality was similar between the groups but delayed mortality was greater in the HBsAg-positive arm (63 versus 80%, respectively, in patients who survived at least 60 days, or 45.1% and 63.2%, respectively, overall). Recurrent HBV infection was the primary cause of death in HBsAg-positive patients.[110] Patients with active viral replication preceding transplantation as indicated by HBeAg or HBV DNA positivity are less likely to have graft or overall survival compared with those without active viral replication.[248] Reinfection of the allograft takes place in up to 100% of liver recipients, but morbidity is higher in HBeAg-positive patients. HBV DNA levels may be a better predictor of outcome than HBeAg positivity.[248] For this reason, pretransplant HBV DNA status has become the preferred predictor of outcome following transplantation. Because of poor outcomes, several centers have excluded HBsAg-positive patients (in the presence of viral replication) from undergoing liver transplantation. However, this policy is not universally accepted, and with appropriate post-transplant

Table 73-17 Therapeutic Options for the Treatment of Hepatitis B

Drug	Status of Development	Comments
Antivirals		
Adenosine arabinoside (Ara-A)		Neurotoxic
Adenosine arabinoside 5′-monophosphate (Ara-AMP)		
Acyclovir		Limited efficacy
Ganciclovir		Limited efficacy; poor bioavailability
Val-ganciclovir	Phase III trials under way	Enhanced bioavailability
Famciclovir	Phase III trial under way	Limited efficacy; adequate safety profile; converted to penciclovir
Lamivudine	Phase III trial completed	Significant efficacy; good safety profile; escape mutants possible with long-term therapy
Immunomodulators		
INF alfa-2a, INF alfa-2b INF-β, INF-γ	FDA approved	Moderate efficacy and poor tolerability; limited efficacy data in decompensated cirrhosis
Corticosteroids		Significant toxicity; may enhance HBV replication
Thymosin	Phase III trial completed	Minimal efficacy; well tolerated
Levamisole		Limited efficacy as monotherapy; significant toxicity with INF
IL-2		Limited efficacy; significant toxicity
Ribavirin		Limited efficacy; significant toxicity
Therapeutic vaccines	Phase II trial under way	Data unavailable
Other Agents		
IL-12		
Entecavir, emtricitabine, FD4C, L-FMAU, DAPD, AT-61	Phase I/II trials under way	Good efficacy in vitro
HBV protease inhibitors	Awaiting phase I trials	
Pegylated interferons	Awaiting phase I trials	

IL, interleukin; INF, interferon.

prophylactic strategies, patients who are nonresponders to drug therapy can undergo successful liver transplantation.

33. **What are the current recommendations for prevention of recurrent hepatitis B infection following liver transplantation?**

The most efficacious approach to preventing HBV recurrence following transplantation has been with high-dose IV hepatitis B immunoglobulin (HBIG) in the anhepatic and postoperative periods.[248,249] Samuel and colleagues reported that 110 HBsAg-positive patients treated with daily IV HBIG in the early postoperative period to maintain their serum anti-HBs levels ≥100 IU/L had an overall survival (84%) that approached that observed in other patients transplanted without HBV infection.[248] These data have been confirmed in a large retrospective analysis of patients (N = 334) undergoing transplantation for HBV infection in Europe. Furthermore, the European trial demonstrated that patients receiving long-term HBIG administration (>6-months' duration) compared with patients receiving short-term HBIG (<6-months' duration) had a lower risk for recurrent HBV infection (35% versus 75%) and longer 3-year actuarial survival (78% versus 48%).[248]

HBIG DOSAGE, ADMINISTRATION, AND ADVERSE EFFECTS

Several liver transplant centers routinely administer immunoprophylaxis with IV HBIG 10,000 IU (10 vials, 50 mL in 250 mL of saline) in the anhepatic (recipient liver excised) phase, then 10,000 IU (50 mL infused over 4 to 6 hours) for the next 6 days postoperatively. HBIG (10,000 IU) is administered on a monthly basis for life, or is discontinued if HBsAg becomes positive, indicating treatment failure. This regimen achieves trough anti-HBs titers of approximately 500 IU/L and up to 2,000 IU/L; however, the link of specific titers and protection from recurrence is controversial at this time. Because the HBIG preparation that is routinely given to liver transplant patients intravenously in the postoperative setting is formulated for intramuscular administration and contains thimerosal, patients should be closely monitored (once a month) for thimerosal toxicity, including neurotoxicity (tremor), cardiac abnormalities (arrhythmias), acidosis, and GI disturbances (nausea, abdominal pain). Patients may also experience a serum sickness–like syndrome (fever, myalgias) that is reversible after discontinuation of HBIG therapy. An IV preparation of HBIG is now undergoing phase III trials in patients undergoing liver transplantation for chronic HBV infection.

Long-term concerns associated with HBIG administration include the potential for HBV reinfection from extrahepatic sites despite adequate anti-HBs titers, emerging mutant viruses that no longer bind to the immunoglobulin, and the prohibitive high cost of therapy (>$60,000/year).[249,250] Current data suggest that pharmacokinetic modeling and use of maintenance therapy with intramuscular administration of HBIG (e.g., 2.5 to 10 mL every 2 to 3 weeks) may achieve similar outcomes and reduce the cost associated with IV administration of the intramuscular preparation.[251,252]

34. **What is the role of oral antiviral agents in liver transplant recipients with HBV?**

As previously described, the availability of nucleoside analogs such as lamivudine and adefovir are impacting the management of patients with HBV infection, and they also may have a role in patients who undergo transplants for chronic HBV infection.[89,91,219,253–257] Lamivudine monotherapy is effective in converting HBV-DNA–positive patients to negative status before and after liver transplantation. However, emerging mutations at the YMDD locus in transplant and nontransplant recipients also have been observed, rendering lamivudine ineffective.[89,91,219,258,259] Nucleoside analogs are still considered investigational at this time for HBV prophylaxis following transplantation because they have not been FDA approved for this indication in the United States. Future considerations for preventing recurrent HBV infection following transplantation include combining nucleoside analogs, HBIG, or both; however, optimal management strategies continue to be determined. Currently, patients transplanted for chronic HBV infection should be managed as part of an investigational protocol.

HEPATITIS D VIRUS
Virology and Epidemiology

Hepatitis D virus (HDV) is a small, single-stranded RNA animal virus (36 nm) that is similar to defective RNA plant viruses (see Table 73-2).[260–262] It was discovered in the late 1970s, found in the nuclei of infected hepatocytes, and present in some but not all HBV-infected patients. HDV appears to replicate exclusively in the liver via extensive base-pairing that results in the formation of an unbranched rodlike genome. Although replication of the virus can occur within hepatocytes in the absence of HBV, the latter is required for coating the HDV virions and allowing for their cellular spread. The HDV genome is replicated by an RNA intermediate (antigenome) that depends on the host's RNA-dependent RNA polymerase. During replication, the genomic (positive strand) HDV RNA becomes the template for successive rounds of minus-strand synthesis. The multimeric minus strand then serves as a template for positive strand synthesis. Subsequently, autocleavage and ligation form circular genomes that are produced from this multimeric precursor.

Fifteen million persons are infected with HDV, with the highest incidence reported in Italy, Eastern Europe, the Amazon Basin, Colombia, Venezuela, Western Asia, and the South Pacific.[1,261–263] In the United States, an estimated 7,500 HDV cases occur annually.[1,262,263] The prevalence of HDV is greatest among persons with percutaneous exposure (e.g., injection drug users) and hemophiliacs (20% to 53% and 48% to 80%, respectively) and may be affected by additional factors such as age of infection.[1,262] The modes of transmission of HDV are similar to those reported for HBV infection. Thus, HDV clearly represents a potential infectious hazard to patients susceptible to HBV and those who are chronic HBV carriers.[262,264] Because infection by HDV requires the presence of active HBV, preventing HBV infection will prevent HDV infection in a susceptible patient.[1,261,262,263]

Pathogenesis

Limited data suggest that HDVAg (antigen) and HDV RNA may possess direct cytotoxic effects on hepatocytes, whereas other findings implicate the immune response in pathogenesis.[261,262,265] Furthermore, several autoantibodies associated with chronic HDV infection may play a role in propagating liver disease and could partially explain the differences in disease severity observed in patients with HDV plus HBV compared with those with HBV alone.

Diagnosis and Serology

ELISA and RIA tests for total and IgM anti-HDV are available commercially, whereas detection methods for HDV RNA are available only on a research basis to distinguish ongoing from previous HDV infection.[262,266] Measurement of anti-HDV is generally not useful for early diagnosis because detectable antibody levels are usually achieved late in the clinical course of the infection (Fig. 73-5A). Anti-HDV IgM is detectable before anti-HDV IgG in acute HDV coinfection and is diagnostic for acute HDV infection. Anti-HDV IgM levels are not sustained in self-limiting HDV infection but may persist in patients with chronic HDV infection. Also, anti-HDV IgM does not distinguish coinfection (HBV and HDV acquired simultaneously) from superinfection (HDV acquired in chronic HBV carrier) (Fig. 73-5B).

Differentiation between coinfection and superinfection is made by the presence or absence of anti-HBc IgM. In acute coinfection, serum anti-HDV IgM and HDV RNA appear together with anti-HBc IgM, whereas in patients with superinfection, HDV markers are present in the absence of anti-HBc IgM. The presence and titer level of anti-HDV, in the case of persistent infection, also correlate with the severity of disease. Titers of anti-HDV IgG of greater than 1:1,000 indicate ongoing viral replication.

HDVAg is present in the serum in the late incubation period of acute infection and lasts into the symptomatic phase in

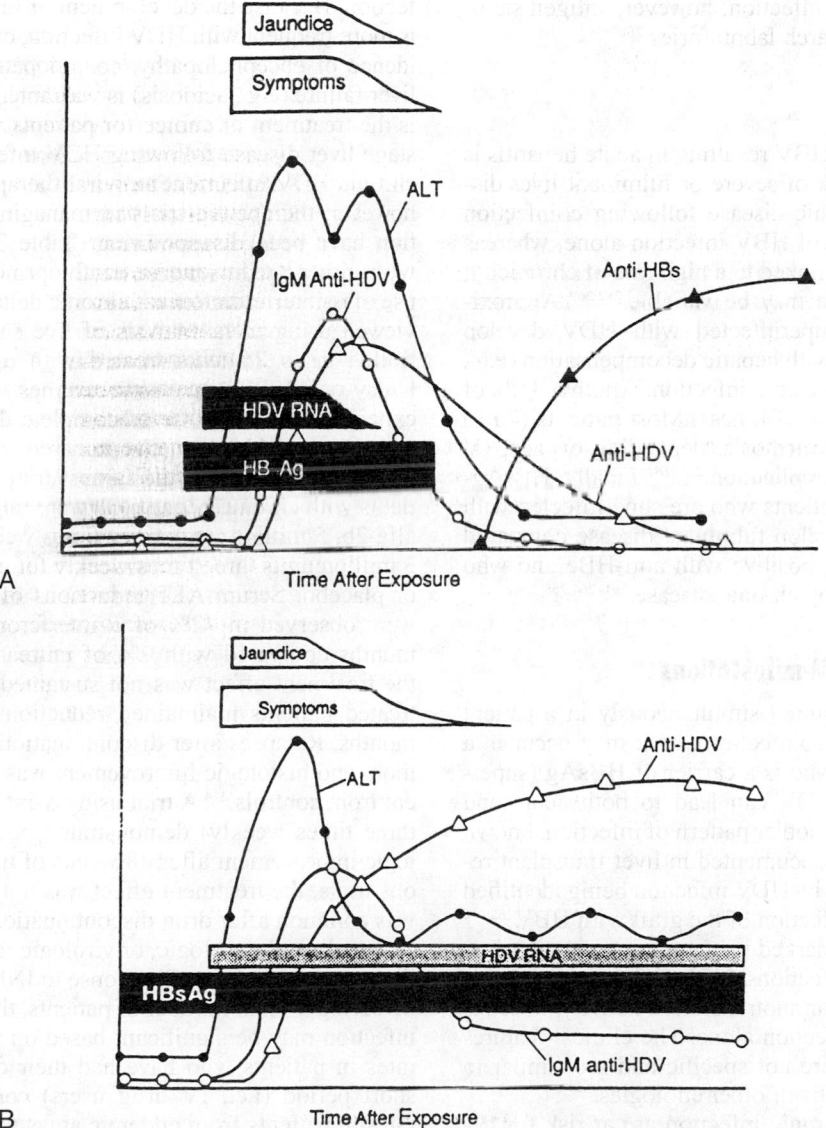

FIGURE 73-5 A. Typical course of acute icteric HBV with HDV coinfection. ALT, alanine aminotransferase; anti-HBs, hepatitis B surface antibody; anti-HDV, antibody to delta hepatitis virus; HbsAg, hepatitis B surface antigen; HDV RNA, delta hepatitis RNA; IgM anti-HDV, IgM antibody to delta hepatitis virus.
B. Typical course of acute icteric HBV with HDV superinfection. ALT, alanine aminotransferase; anti-HBs, hepatitis B surface antibody; anti-HDV, antibody to delta hepatitis virus; HbsAg, hepatitis B surface antigen; HDV RNA, delta hepatitis RNA; IgM anti-HDV, IgM antibody to delta hepatitis virus.

up to 20% of patients. Because this antigen is transient, repeat testing may be required to detect its presence. The clinical utility of HDVAg detection by ELISA and RIA is limited by the necessity of precise timing of a sample and by its availability only as a research test. In addition, during persistent infection, HDVAg may not be detectable because it is complexed with anti-HDV.

HDV RNA is an early marker of infection in patients with both acute and chronic HDV infection.[262,266,267] HDV RNA is detectable in 90% of patients during the symptomatic phase of HDV infection. HDV RNA levels are nondetectable following symptomatic resolution but remain elevated in chronic infection. A significant correlation exists among HDV RNA detection by hybridization assay, positive results for IgM anti-HDV in serum, and positive immunohistochemistry for HDVAg in liver biopsies. Detection of HDVAg by immunohistochemical analysis of liver tissue is the best diagnostic method for persistent HDV infection; however, antigen staining is only available in research laboratories.[266]

Natural History

Coinfection with HDV and HBV resulting in acute hepatitis is correlated with a higher risk of severe or fulminant liver disease.[262,268] The rate of chronic disease following coinfection with HDV is similar to that of HBV infection alone, whereas superinfection with HDV is linked to a high rate of chronicity; however, the clinical course may be variable.[262,269] Approximately 15% of patients superinfected with HDV develop rapidly progressive disease with hepatic decompensation (e.g., cirrhosis) within 12 months of the infection. Another 15% of patients have a benign course of illness. Most patients (70%) have a slow progression to cirrhosis, depending on age, IV drug use, and level of viral replication.[261–264] Finally, HBsAg-positive, HBeAg-positive patients who are superinfected with HDV are more likely to develop fulminant disease compared with those who are HBsAg-positive with anti-HBe and who are superinfected and develop chronic disease.[261–264,268]

Clinical and Extrahepatic Manifestations

Delta infection may be acquired simultaneously in a patient with acute HBV infection (coinfection), or it may occur in a patient with chronic HBV who is a carrier of HBsAg (superinfection). Infection with HDV can lead to both acute and chronic forms of hepatitis. Another pattern of infection, known as latent HDV infection, is documented in liver transplant recipients and is characterized by HDV infection being identified in the liver graft before reinfection of the graft with HBV.[262,270] Acute HDV coinfection is marked by symptoms seen in other acute hepatotrophic viral infections. HDV infection also has a unique biphasic increase in aminotransferase activity, which is rarely observed in HBV infection alone. The clinical features of chronic HDV infection are not specific and are similar to those seen in chronic hepatitis of other etiologies.

Patients who develop chronic infection are at risk for developing cirrhosis and hepatic decompensation. In contrast to patients with chronic HBV infection, there is a negative association between HDV and HCC.[262,263,264,271] Potential reasons for this could be that the delta agent has direct tumor protective effects; delta markers in HCC patients disappear because the time between infection and cancer detection is longer than in patients with HCC from other causes, or HDV predisposes to early mortality before HCC can develop.[262,271]

Prevention

HDV replication is dependent on HBV replication; therefore, successful immunization with HBV vaccine also prevents HDV infection.[261,262,264] Unfortunately, no immunoprophylactic therapies are available for patients with chronic HBV infection who are also at risk for superinfection with HDV. Prevention of HDV superinfection is based on behavioral modification, such as the use of condoms to prevent sexual transmission and needle exchange programs to minimize transmission by IV drug use.

Treatment

Supportive care is the general strategy used to treat HDV infection. Because the development of fulminant hepatic failure is more frequent with HDV infection, close monitoring for evidence of encephalopathy, coagulopathy, and other signs of liver failure (e.g., acidosis) is warranted. Liver transplantation is the treatment of choice for patients with fulminant or end-stage liver disease following HDV infection. In patients with chronic HDV infection, antiviral therapy has been attempted; however, therapeutic trials in managing chronic HDV infection have been disappointing (Table 73-18).[262,269] Treatment with either prednisone or azathioprine is ineffective.[272] The use of α-interferon to treat chronic delta hepatitis has been reviewed using meta-analysis of five small, randomized, controlled trials. Patients treated with α-interferon (5 million U/day or 9 million units three times weekly) for 12 months experienced a 30% rate of complete disease remission (normalization of ALT values) compared with 1% observed in untreated controls.[273] In the largest trial published to date, patients with chronic hepatitis D were randomized to either INF alfa-2b, 5 million units three times weekly for 4 months then 3 million units three times weekly for an additional 8 months, or placebo. Serum ALT reductions of >50% from baseline were observed in 42% of α-interferon–treated patients at 4 months compared with 7% of untreated controls. However, the treatment effect was not sustained because only 26% of treated patients maintained reductions in ALT levels at 12 months. Relapses after discontinuation of therapy were common, and histologic improvement was not statistically different from controls.[274] A trial using α-interferon (9 million units three times weekly) demonstrated both virologic and histologic improvement after 48 weeks of therapy. As in the previous trials, the treatment effect was not sustained, and relapse was common after drug discontinuation.[275]

No clinical, serologic, or virologic factors consistently predict response or lack of response to INF. In uncontrolled trials involving a small number of patients, the duration of the HDV infection may be significant based on the improved response rates in patients who have had their disease for a relatively short period (i.e., IV drug users) compared with response rates in patients from endemic areas whose infections are acquired early in life. However, because of the nature of these reports, verification of this association is needed.

Clearly, more efficacious therapies for HDV are needed. Suramin and ribavirin possess anti-HDV efficacy in animal models; however, clinical reports suggest that toxicity and lack of response, respectively, may limit the use of these

Table 73-18   Efficacy of Interferon in Chronic HDV

					Response (%)	
Author	N	Interferon	Dosage	Duration (Months)	Primary	Sustained
Rosina/Rizzetto	12	Alfa-2b	5 million U TIW	3	33	8
	12	None			17	0
Rosina	31	Alfa-2b	5 million U TIW then 3 million U TIW	4 then 8	45	25
	30	None			27	0
Farci	14	Alfa-2a	9 million U TIW	12	71	36
	14	Alfa-2a	3 million U TIW	12	29	0
	13	None			8	0
Gaudin	11	Alfa-2b	5 million U TIW then 3 million U TIW	4 then 8	66	9
	11	None			36	18
Puoti	21	Alfa-2b	10 million U TIW and 6 million U TIW	6 and 6	14	9

TIW, three times weekly.
From references 200, 274, and 275.

agents.[276] Results from a pilot trial that evaluated the efficacy of 100 mg of oral lamivudine in five patients with HDV (all were positive for HBsAg, antibody to HDV, and HDV RNA) for 12 months demonstrated that serum levels of HBV DNA were reduced in all five patients. However, all patients remained HBsAg-and HDV-RNA positive, and serum ALT and liver histology did not improve.[277] Nucleoside analogs such as lamivudine and transribozyme and antisense probes require further evaluation in controlled clinical trials.[278]

Additionally, in patients with chronic HDV infection who received 100 mg of oral lamivudine for 24 weeks followed by a combination of high-dose interferon (9 MU TIW) and 100 mg of oral lamivudine for 16 weeks, biochemical and histologic were not significantly improved compared with baseline characteristics.[279]

In patients with decompensated cirrhosis caused by HDV, liver transplantation is the most appropriate intervention because INF may precipitate hepatic decompensation.[248,250,275] The presence and amount of HBV DNA before transplantation is the most significant outcome marker, often predicting the post-transplant reinfection rate. Patients who receive a liver transplant for chronic HDV infection have a lower incidence of post-transplant HBV infection than do those with HBV infection alone (67% versus 32%, respectively).[248] This is thought to be related to an inhibitory effect of HDV on HBV replication. Furthermore, 3-year survival is higher for patients with HDV cirrhosis than for patients undergoing transplantation for HBV cirrhosis alone (88% versus 44%, respectively) and is similar to patients undergoing liver transplantation for other indications.[248]

HEPATITIS C VIRUS
Virology

Before the development of methods to identify hepatitis C virus (HCV), most post-transfusion hepatitis cases were designated as non-A, non-B (NANB) hepatitis. HCV is recognized now as the most common cause of chronic NANB transfusion-associated hepatitis.[280–283] HCV is a single-stranded, 50-nm RNA virus related to the flaviviruses, a family that includes the yellow fever virus and two animal viruses, bovine viral diarrhea virus, and classic swine fever virus (see Table 73-2).[280,284,285]

The genome of HCV contains a single outer reading frame (ORF) capable of encoding a large viral protein precursor that, when cleaved, results in a series of structural (nucleocapsid core and the envelops 1 and 2) and nonstructural (NS2, NS3, NS4a, NS4b, NS5a, and NS5b) proteins. [284,286,287]The aminoterminal region of NS3 encodes a viral serine protease that cleaves viral peptides, whereas the carboxyl end functions as a helicase, which is essential in unwinding of viral RNA during replication. The NS5b protein functions as an RNA-dependent RNA polymerase; the function of the NS5a protein is unknown, but it may play a role in regulating replication. Furthermore, the positive strand RNA of HCV functions as a template for synthesis of negative strand RNA, as a template for translation of viral proteins, and as genomic RNA to be packaged into new virions. Unlike HBV, HCV has no DNA intermediate and therefore cannot integrate into the host genome. [284,286,287]

The replication process of HCV is poorly understood because there is no in vitro or in vivo study model system. Available data suggest that viral binding and uptake into the hepatocytes occur through membrane fusion and receptor-mediated endocytosis[284,286,287] (see Table 73-2). In primates, HCV RNA is detectable within 3 days of infection, persisting in serum during peak ALT elevation. Detection appears to be associated with the appearance of viral antigens in hepatocytes, the major site of HCV replication. The importance of extrahepatic sites for replication (e.g., mononuclear cells) has not been determined. Kinetic studies in HCV-infected patients have depicted a high viral turnover that may partially explain the rapid emergence of viral diversity in patients with chronic HCV infection and the persistence of the infection, through immune escape, following acute exposure. Mechanisms pertaining to viral packaging and release from the hepatocytes are poorly understood.

Epidemiology

The worldwide seroprevalence based on antibody to HCV (anti-HCV) is approximately 1%. Geographic variations exist, from 0.4% to 1.1% in North America to 9.6% to 13.6% in North Africa.[280,285,288] The prevalence of anti-HCV in the United States has been estimated to be 1.8%, corresponding to an estimated 3.9 million persons infected nationwide. Of these, 2.7 million persons are chronically infected (based on positive HCV RNA), with approximately 230,000 new infections per year.[280,285,288] HCV is the etiologic agent in more than 85% of cases associated with post-transfusional NANB hepatitis.[280,282,283] Following HCV antibody screening of blood donors in the early 1990s, transfusion-related reports of HCV have been dramatically reduced, and non–transfusion-related cases have emerged (e.g., injection drug users).[280,285,289] Sporadic infection with HCV (infection without an identifiable risk factor) accounts for up to 40% of reported HCV infections.[280,282,285] HCV is transmitted through percutaneous (e.g., blood transfusion, needlestick inoculation, high-risk behavior) [280,282,285] and nonpercutaneous (e.g., sexual contact, perinatal exposure) routes. [280,282,285,290,291] The latter appears to occur to a lesser extent than with HBV.

HCV infection occurs among persons of all ages, but the highest incidence is among persons aged 20 to 39 years with a male predominance. African Americans and whites have similar incidence rates of acute disease, whereas persons of Hispanic ethnicity have higher rates. In the general population, the highest prevalence rates of chronic HCV infection are found among persons aged 30 to 49 years and among males. [280,282,285] Unlike the racial/ethnic pattern of acute disease, African Americans have a substantially higher prevalence of chronic HCV infection than do whites.

In the United States, the predominant HCV genotype is type 1, with subtypes 1a and 1b accounting for 70% of cases. [280,282,285] Knowledge of the genotype or serotype (genotype-specific antibodies) of HCV is helpful in making recommendations and counseling regarding therapy. Patients with genotypes 2 and 3 are almost three times more likely to respond to therapy with interferon α or the combination of interferon α and ribavirin. Furthermore, when using combination therapy, the recommended duration of treatment depends on the genotype. For these reasons, testing for HCV genotype is often clinically helpful. Once the genotype is identified, it need not be tested again; genotypes do not change during the course of infection. However, since HCV has a high mutation rate during replication, several so-called quasispecies, a heterogeneous population of HCV isolates that are closely related, may exist in an infected individual.[280,286,287] The number of quasispecies increases over the course of infection which allows HCV to escape the host's immune system, leading to persistent infection.

Percutaneous Transmission

Before the routine use of blood screening, the incidence of acute HCV infection among transfusion recipients in the 1970s was approximately 5% to 10%.[292] Subsequently, blood donor screening using a first-generation anti-HCV test reduced the risk of transfusion-related hepatitis to 0.6% per patient and 0.03% per unit transfused.[280,289] Following the use of more sensitive second- and third-generation assays for anti-HCV, the risk and incidence of transfusion-related hepatitis approaches that reported in hospitalized patients who have not received a transfusion.

The incidence of HCV infection is 48% to 90% among injection drug users, and the risk of acquiring the infection in these persons is as high as 90%.[280,283,293] Of injection drug users with acute NANB hepatitis, 75% are anti-HCV positive, and unlike transfusion-related hepatitis, the incidence of HCV infection associated with injection drug use has not de-

clined.[280,283,293] Additional risk factors for HCV infection include the presence of HBV or HIV infections.[280,283,293] Other populations at risk for acquiring HCV include patients receiving chronic hemodialysis (up to 45%)[280,283,293] and health care workers (0% to 4% seroconversion following needlestick).[280,283,293,294]

Nonpercutaneous and Sporadic Transmission

Nonpercutaneous transmission includes transmission between sexual partners and from mother to child. This route of transmission is less efficient compared with the percutaneous route, and is supported by data assessing sexual transmission of HCV. Sexual partners of index patients with anti-HCV have an incidence of HCV infection ranging from 0% to 27%, whereas low-risk (anti-HCV negative) index subjects without liver disease or high-risk behavior (injection drug use or promiscuity) have an incidence of anti-HCV of 0% to 7%.[280,283] In contrast, sexual partners of subjects with liver disease and/or high-risk behavior have an incidence of anti-HCV ranging between 11% and 27%.[280,290] Also, the sexual partners of homosexual men and promiscuous heterosexuals with HCV have shown an increase in anti-HCV positivity.

Compared with the high incidence of perinatal transmission of HBV from mothers to infants, perinatal transmission of HCV infection is relatively low; however, high titers of circulating HCV in the mother may enhance the risk of infection in the infant.[280] Additional concerns and areas for investigation related to mother-to-infant transmission of HCV include the timing of transmission (in utero, time of birth), the relative risk associated with breast-feeding, and the natural history of perinatally acquired infection.

In sporadic HCV infection, up to 40% of patients acquire HCV infection without a known or identifiable risk factor.[280] This type of HCV infection may be related to a prevalent nonpercutaneous or percutaneous route that has yet to be identified.

Pathogenesis

The pathogenesis of liver damage as a result of HCV infection most likely results from both direct and indirect, immune-mediated response instigated by the virus. Direct cellular injury may be caused by the accumulation of intact virus or viral proteins.[287,295] The direct mechanism of injury is supported by the observation that patients with high concentrations of HCV RNA (quantified through branched chain DNA assay) have greater lobular inflammatory activity compared with those with minimal inflammation. Whether specific genotypes (i.e., 1, 1b, 2) are correlated with severe disease continues to be assessed. European data suggest that type 1 genotype is associated with higher viral replication, and infection with the type 1b genotype is associated with more progressive liver disease.[287,296] One reason why HCV genotype 1 may be more difficult to treat than genotypes 2 or 3 is that genotype one has a longer half-life (2.9 hours) than that of genotypes 2 or 3 (2.0 hours).[280,297] Viral half-life can be defined as the time for the original amount of virus to be decreased by half, or in this case, die. Other data do not support these findings and have shown that patients with type 2 genotypes have more severe liver disease.[298] Duration of infection is another factor that may be related to disease severity because the expression of genotypes may change over time making the correlation between genotype and severity of disease problematic.

Immune-mediated mechanisms for hepatic injury have been based on the presence of CD8+ and CD4+ lymphocytes in portal, periportal, and lobular areas in patients with HCV infection.[287,295] Hepatic CD8+ lymphocytes are activated through an alternative antigen-independent pathway that stimulates CTLs, which initiate hepatocellular injury. Helper/inducer T cells (CD4+) have also been implicated in the pathogenesis of chronic HCV infection; however, other data suggest that CD4+ cells may play a protective role against hepatocellular injury. Autoimmune mechanisms of hepatocellular injury (e.g., anti–liver-kidney microsomal antibodies) may play a minor role in the pathogenesis of liver injury.[287,295]

Diagnosis
Serologic Tests
A test for antibodies to HCV is the initial screening test for suspected HCV infection.[280,285,299,300,301] There are two types of antibody tests: the enzyme immunoassay (EIA) and the recombinant immunoblot assay (RIBA). These serologic assays were developed using recombinant antigens derived from cloned HCV transcripts to substantiate a diagnosis of HCV.

Predictive values of a positive third generation EIA test are about 99% (in immunocompetent patients), which obviates the need for a confirmatory RIBA test in the diagnosis of patients with clinical liver disease.[280,285,299,300,301] A negative EIA test is adequate to exclude a diagnosis of chronic HCV infection in non-immunocompromised individuals.[280,285,300,301] Occasionally, patients undergoing hemodialysis and those with immune deficiencies may have false-negative EIAs. On the other hand, false-positive results can occur in healthy persons without any identifiable risk factors and normal aminotransferases, and in patients with autoimmune disorders.[280,285,299,300–302] In these groups, the results should be confirmed using an assay for HCV RNA to diagnose chronic HCV infection. Anti-HCV antibodies usually are detected in serum late during the course of acute hepatitis C. However, in many cases, seroconversion may take up to a year or longer following exposure to HCV. Anti-HCV is detectable in serum for a variable length of time after acute infection, but it is not protective and its presence does not differentiate between acute, chronic, or resolved infection. The clinical symptoms, changes in HCV RNA, and serologic changes in acute and chronic HCV infection are shown in Figure 73-6A and B.

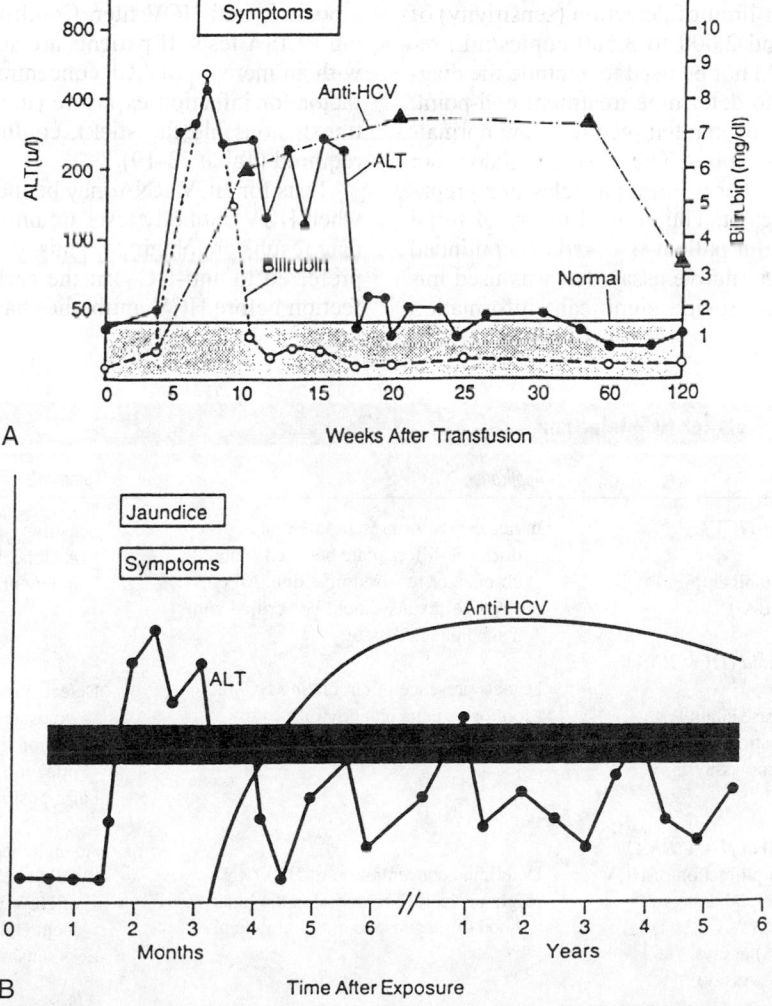

FIGURE 73-6 A. Typical course of acute hepatitis C virus. ALT, alanine aminotransferase; anti-HCV, hepatitis C antibody; **B. Typical course of chronic hepatitis C virus.** ALT, alanine aminotransferase; anti-HCV, hepatitis C antibody.

Qualitative HCV RNA Assays

Acute or chronic HCV infection in a patients with EIA positivity should be confirmed by a qualitative HCV RNA (PCR) assay with a lower limit of detection of 50 IU/mL or less (approximately 100 viral gene/mL). [280,285,300,301,302] Qualitative tests detect HCV as early as 1 to 2 weeks after exposure and detect the presence of circulating HCV RNA (viral copies/mL). Results are reported as either "positive" or "negative" and are used to monitor patients receiving antiviral therapy. A single positive qualitative assay for HCV RNA confirms active replication but does not exclude viremia and may only detect a transient decline in viral load below the level of detection of the assay. [280,285,300-302] A follow-up qualitative HCV RNA needs to be obtained to confirm the lack of active HCV replication. [280,285,300-302]

Quantitative HCV RNA Assays

In comparison, quantitative tests are less sensitive than qualitative tests and are used to determine the concentration of HCV RNA with assays such as semiquantitative PCR-based Amplicor assay (qPCR) or branched DNA (bDNA) signal amplification. [280,285,300-302] The lower limit of detection with the second generation bDNA and Amplicor assays are 250,000 viral equivalents/mL and 200 viral copies/mL, respectively. The newest qualitative HCV viral load test and third-generation bDNA test have a lower limit of detection (sensitivity) of 50 copies per millimeter and 2,000 to 3,500 copies/mL, respectively. These tests should not be used to exclude the diagnosis of HCV infection or to determine treatment end-point. An HCV RNA standard has been attempted to allow normalization of reported viral titers in IUs. The reported IU does not correlate with the actual number of viral particles in a preparation and variability does exist. The clinical utility of serial HCV viral concentrations in a patient is based on continued use of the same specific quantitative assay that was used initially. [280,285,300-302] These tests provide significant information with respect to response to treatment in patients receiving antiviral therapy.

Biochemical Markers

Testing for serum ALT concentrations are not sensitive markers for assessing disease activity and at best have a weak correlation with the histopathologic findings on a liver biopsy. [280,285,300-302] Nevertheless, serial determination of ALT over time appears to be a better indicator of liver injury than is a single ALT test.

Biopsy

Liver biopsy can determine the extent of liver injury due to HCV. [280,285,300-302] Although some histologic findings are characteristic of HCV infection, such as portal lymphoid aggregates, steatosis, and bile duct injury, these alone are not sufficiently specific to establish a diagnosis of hepatitis C. There are currently no reliable, readily available tests for detection of HCV antigens in the liver.

Selection of Tests

All patients with elevated liver aminotransferases without an obvious source, especially those with known risk factors, should be tested for HCV. A diagnosis of acute hepatitis C can be initiated in a patient with symptoms of acute hepatitis and a positive anti-HCV titer. Confirmation is established by using ELISA tests. If patients are anti-HCV positive by ELISA with an increase in ALT concentration and have a known risk factor for infection exposure (intravenous drug abuse, blood transfusions, needle stick), confirmatory assays may not be required (Table 73-19).

Tests for HCV RNA may be indicated for diagnosing HCV when HCV antibody tests are unreliable and when indeterminate results are obtained. Thus, direct testing of HCV RNA is preferred to anti-HCV in the early stages of acute HCV infection before HCV antibodies have been produced, when an-

---

Table 73-19 Diagnostic Tests for HCV Infection

Test/Type	Application	Comments
Hepatitis C Virus Antibody (Anti-HCV) EIA (enzyme immunoassay) Supplemental assay (i.e., recombinant immunoblot strip assay [RIBA])	Indicates past or present infection, but does not differentiate between acute, chronic, or resolved infection. All positive EIA results should be verified with a supplemental assay	Sensitivity >97% EIA alone has low positive predictive value in low prevalence populations
Hepatitis C Virus Ribonucleic Acid (HCV RNA) Qualitative tests[a] Reverse transcriptase polymerase chain reaction (RT-PCR) amplification of HCV RNA by in-house or commercial assays (e.g., Amplicor HCV)	Detects presence of circulating HCV RNA Monitor patients on antiviral therapy	Detects virus as early as 1–2 weeks after exposure Detection of HCV RNA during course of infection might be intermittent False-positive/negative results might occur
Hepatitis C Virus Ribonucleic Acid (HCV RNA) Quantitative tests[a] RT-PCR amplification of HCV RNA by in-house or commercial assays (e.g., Amplicor HCV Monitor) Branched chain DNAb (bDNA) assays (e.g., Quantiplex HCV RNA Assay)	Determine concentration of HCV RNA Might be useful for assessing the likelihood of response to antiviral therapy	A single negative RT-PCR is not conclusive Should not be used to exclude the diagnosis of HCV infection or to determine treatment endpoint Less sensitive than qualitative RT-PCR

[a]Currently not U.S. Food and Drug Administration approved; lack standardization.

tibody tests are unreliable (e.g., immunocompromised patients), when intermediate results are reported (e.g. RIBA 2 in blood donors), in differentiation between active and past infection, and in the evaluation of patients with chronic liver disease in whom antibody tests are intermediate.

Natural History
Nonimmunocompromised Patients
Once established, infection with HCV persists in most patients.[280,284,285,303] Because disease progression is often asymptomatic, patients are typically diagnosed when they receive routine biochemical testing during a physical examination or before blood donation, for example. Because NANB hepatitis (e.g., hepatitis C) was established in 1974, comprehensive data pertaining to the natural history of the disease are limited. However, it is known that HCV infection leads to progressive liver disease. Following an asymptomatic period, histologic or clinical cirrhosis can be identified in 8% to 42% of patients as early as 15 months following the infection.[280,284,285,303] Ten percent of patients may also have decompensated liver disease as evidenced by splenomegaly, ascites, coagulopathy, and esophageal varices. In nonimmunocompromised patients, the time between acute infection and manifestations of chronic liver disease is usually 20 to 30 years with rare instances of terminal disease occurring within 3 to 5 years following acute infection. Patients with chronic HCV infection are also at increased risk for HCC.[280,284,285,303]

Patients receiving dialysis have a greater incidence of HCV infection compared with the general population (6% to 22%) because they receive multiple blood transfusions.[304] Kidney transplant recipients also have a high incidence of HCV infection (6% to 28%), which may be acquired through dialysis before transplant or from the allograft or blood products following transplantation.[305] Following kidney transplantation, elevation in aminotransferases is more common in anti–HCV-positive compared with anti–HCV-negative patients (48% and 14%, respectively) and cirrhosis has been reported with the former.[306,307] While HCV infection is associated with liver failure, differences in overall patient and graft survival between HCV-positive and HCV-negative patients do not appear to be significant. Long-term studies are needed to confirm these findings.

Immunocompromised Patients
Chronic HCV infection is the most common indication for orthotopic liver transplantation (OLT) in the United States with up to 40% of patients receiving a transplant for the disease.[308–311] Recurrence rates of HCV following transplantation are 100%, possibly because of viremia at the time of transplant.[308–311] In addition, de novo acquisition of HCV from the donor liver or from blood products may occur. One-year follow-up studies indicate that 50% of patients with viremia following transplant (HCV RNA) have normal biopsies with no histologic evidence of HCV infection, 40% have mild chronic hepatitis, and 10% have progressive liver damage with chronic active hepatitis and bridging fibrosis or cirrhosis.[308,309] Histologic evidence of disease may also be present even when aminotransferase levels are normal. Reports suggest that high viral loads, as measured by quantitative HCV RNA, have been correlated with early acute hepatitis in the allograft and that

genotype 1b may predispose OLT recipients to more severe histologic disease compared with patients transplanted with other genotypes.[308–310] Controlled trials are needed to further evaluate the relationship between genotype, viral load, amount of immunosuppression, and immunomodulating coinfections (e.g., CMV) and the course of post-transplant HCV infection.

HIV Coinfection
The incidence of HCV infection in HIV-infected patients is variable with up to 100% infection reported in HIV-positive injection drug users.[308] In other populations, such as homosexual men, the incidence is marginally greater than that reported in the general population. Some studies suggest that HCV patients who are coinfected with HIV may also have more severe hepatic injury and a worse outcome than those infected with HCV alone, while other reports contradict these findings.[308,312–314] These conflicting reports may be affected by several factors, including the duration of HCV infection before HIV infection, the route of HCV infection, the genotype associated with infection, and patient selection.

HBV Coinfection
As mentioned above, both HBV and HCV are transmitted parenterally and coinfection is not uncommon, particularly in intravenous drug users and in countries with a high prevalence of HBV infection.[90,280] Coinfection with chronic HBV and HCV results in more severe liver disease than infection with either virus alone, including increased risk of liver cancer and fulminant hepatitis.[90,280,315,316]

Clinical and Extrahepatic Manifestations
Most patients with acute HCV infection are asymptomatic.[280,285,303,317] In contrast, patients with chronic HCV infection generally complain of fatigue. Nonspecific symptoms are similar to those seen in with HBV infection and include nausea, anorexia, abdominal discomfort, and depression. Once patients develop cirrhosis and portal hypertension, they may experience intractable ascites, spontaneous bacterial peritonitis, GI or esophageal bleeding, poor synthetic function (hypoalbuminemia or prolonged PT), or encephalopathy.[280,285,303,317] Jaundice occasionally occurs in acute HCV infection but is usually present in chronic infection as a result of decompensated liver disease.

Significant extrahepatic manifestations may also develop as a result of HCV infection.[280,285,303,318] They include membranoproliferative glomerulonephritis, mixed cryoglobulinemia, porphyria cutanea tarda, leukocytoclastic vasculitis, focal lymphocytic sialadenitis, corneal ulcers, idiopathic pulmonary fibrosis, and rheumatoid arthritis.

Prevention of Hepatitis C
Pre-Exposure Prophylaxis
No vaccines are effective against HCV, and current measures to prevent hepatitis C infection have largely focused on identifying high-risk uninfected persons and counseling them on risk-reducing strategies to prevent infection.

The CDC and NIH have recently published recommendations that address these issues.[280,283] Suggested primary preventive measures are that in health care settings, adherence to universal (standard) precautions for the protection of medical personnel and patients be implemented and that HCV-positive individuals should refrain from donating blood, organs, tissues, or semen. In some situations, the use of organs and tissues from HCV-positive individuals may be considered. For example, in emergency situations the use of a donor organ in which the HCV status is either positive or unknown may be considered in a HCV-negative recipient after full disclosure and informed consent. Strategies should be developed to identify prospective blood donors with any prior history of injection drug use. Such individuals must be deferred from donating blood.

Furthermore, safer sexual practices, including the use of latex condoms, should be strongly encouraged in persons with multiple sexual partners. In monogamous long-term relationships, transmission is rare.[280,283] Although HCV-positive individuals and their partners should be informed of the potential for transmission, there are insufficient data to recommend changes in current sexual practice in persons with a steady partner. It is recommended that sexual partners of infected patients should be tested for antibody to HCV.

In households with an HCV-positive member, sharing razors and toothbrushes should be avoided.[280,283] Covering open wounds is recommended. Injection needles should be carefully disposed of using universal precaution techniques. It is not necessary to avoid close contact with family members or to avoid sharing meals or utensils. There is no evidence to justify exclusion of HCV-positive children or adults from participation in social, educational, and employment activities.

Additionally, pregnancy is not contraindicated in HCV-infected individuals. Perinatal transmission from mother to baby occurs in less than 6% of instances.[280,283] There is no evidence that breast-feeding transmits HCV from mother to baby; therefore, it is considered safe. Babies born to HCV-positive mothers should be tested for anti-HCV at 1 year.

Finally, needle exchange and other safer injection drug use programs may be beneficial in reducing parenterally transmitted diseases.[280,283] Expansion of such programs should be considered in an effort to reduce the rate of transmission of hepatitis C. It is important that clear and evidenced-based information be provided to both patients and physicians regarding the natural history, means of prevention, management, and therapy of hepatitis C.

Postexposure Prophylaxis

Immunoglobulin is no longer recommended for postexposure prophylaxis of hepatitis C infection because it is not effective.[280,283,319]

Treatment of Acute Hepatitis C

35. R.D. is a 37-year-old, 95-kg professional athlete with multiple arm tattoos and a remote history of IV drug use. In 1993, an unscheduled physical examination was performed on R.D. because of the severe fatigue he experienced following inscription of a tattoo. Laboratory tests at that time revealed the following results: ALT, 350 U/L (normal, 5 to 40 U/L); serum anti-HCV positive (RIBA-2); and an HCV RNA level of 800,000 viral equivalents/mL (bDNA). What were the clinical and serologic features of HCV in R.D. (at that time), and what drug therapy could have been used to treat his acute hepatitis C?

R.D. clearly had a clinical picture consistent with acute IICV infection, including symptoms of fatigue, elevated ALT, and positive anti-HCV RIBA-2 assay and HCV RNA levels. α-Interferon has been studied in patients with acute HCV in an effort to reduce the severity and rate of progression of chronic infection. Limited data suggest that patients with acute HCV infection receiving α-interferon had a lower rate of chronic infection (36% to 61%) compared with patients who did not receive therapy (80% to 100%).[320,321] However, these studies have included relatively few patients and used varying dosages and durations (6 months to 1 year). One recent report in Germany evaluated 44 patients with acute hepatitis C.[322] Patients received 5 million units of interferon alfa-2b subcutaneously daily for 4 weeks and then three times per week for another 20 weeks. Serum HCV RNA concentrations were measured before and during therapy and 20 weeks after the end of therapy. At the end of therapy, 43 of 44 patients had undetectable concentrations of HCV RNA in serum and normal serum alanine aminotransferase concentrations. Therapy was well tolerated in all but one patient, who stopped therapy after 12 weeks because of side effects. Thus, if early identification is possible, interferon therapy in the acute phase of the disease appears to be rational. Thus, R.D. could have been started on α-interferon to minimize his risk for developing chronic HCV infection.

Treatment of Chronic Hepatitis C

36. Initially, R.D.'s hepatologist did not initiate INF therapy. R.D. now presents to the clinic confused (encephalopathic), with mild ascites, and scleral icterus. Significant laboratory findings are as follows: total bilirubin, 4.2 ng/mL (normal, 0.2 to 1.0 ng/mL); direct bilirubin, 2.2 ng/mL (normal, 0 to 0.2 ng/mL); ALT, 350 U/L (normal, 5 to 40 U/L); and AST, 330 U/L (normal, 5 to 40 U/L). What pharmacologic agents are effective in the management of patients with chronic hepatitis C?

R.D. appears to have an atypical accelerated progression of hepatitis C infection based on the current status of his disease. Chronic hepatitis develops in approximately 80% of patients with acute hepatitis C infection. Of patients chronically infected with HCV, approximately 8% to 42% develop histologic or clinical cirrhosis and disability from end-stage liver disease.[280,283,285,303] Up to 10% of cases are associated with decompensated disease with splenomegaly, ascites, coagulopathy, and esophageal varices as early as 15 months after the episode of acute HCV infection. The lack of specific immunoprophylaxis and significant morbidity and mortality associated with chronic HCV infection highlight the need for effective antiviral therapy. Previously, symptomatic patients with chronic hepatitis C infection without decompensated liver disease could be managed with α-interferon[323-338] (Table 73-20) or INF plus ribavirin[339-341] (Table 73-21) based on controlled studies confirming effectiveness. Furthermore, patients without evidence of fibrosis or significant inflammatory activity are at extremely low risk for the development of cirrhosis or serious hepatic complications, therefore they can usually defer therapy. Conversely, patients with advanced cirrhosis are poor candidates for current interferon-based treatment regimens because of the increased treatment associated morbidity seen in these patients and the possible precipitation of decompensation or frank hepatic failure.

Table 73-20   Efficacy of Interferon in Chronic Hepatitis C

Author	Interferon	Dosage	Duration (Months)	Response (%) Primary	Sustained	Relapse
Davis[323]	Alfa-2b	1 or 3 million U TIW	6	45	22	50
Di Bisceglie[324]	Alfa-2b	2 million U TIW	6	48	10	80
Saracco[325]	Alfa-2b	1 or 3 million U TIW	6	46	20	60
Weiland[326]	Alfa-2b	3 million U TIW	9	58	20	64
Gomez-Rubio[327]	Alfa-2b	5 million U TIW then 1.5 million U TIW	2 then 16	40	25	33
Marcellin[328]	Alfa-2b	1 or 3 million U TIW	6	42	14	44
Saez-Royuela[329]	Alfa-2c	7.5 million U TIW then 5 million U TIW then 2.5 million U TIW	3 then 3 then 6	50	30	33
Causse[330]	Alfa-2b	1 or 3 million U TIW	6	43	17	70
Reichen[331]	Alfa-2b	3 million U TIW	13	28	14	NA
Poynard[332]	Alfa-2b	3 million U TIW	18	45	22	50
		3 million U TIW then 1 million U TIW	18	27	9.9	63
		3 million U TIW then none	18	30	8.1	79
Diodati[333]	Alfa-2a	6, 3, 1 million U TIW (taper)	12	47	27	40
Negro[334]	Alfa-2a	6 million U TIW	9	46	17	47
		6 million U TIW	3 + 3 (6 months apart)	45	10	60
Chemello[335]	Alfa-2a	6 million U TIW	12	72	49	36
		3 million U TIW	12	55	31	40
		6 million U TIW	6	74	28	62
Rumi[337]	Alfa-nl	6 then 3 million U TIW	12	24	17	NA
	Alfa-2a			26	16	NA
Tong[348]	CIFN	3 or 9 µg	12	52 and 55	7 and 20	NA
	Alfa-2b	15 µg (3 million U)	12	54	19.6	NA

NA, not available; TIW, three times weekly.

Table 73-21   Treatment Response to Interferon Plus Placebo Versus Interferon Plus Ribavirin

	Interferon Plus Placebo (3MU TIW, 24 weeks)	Interferon Plus Placebo (3MU TIW, 48 weeks)	Interferon Plus Ribavirin (3MU TIW, 24 weeks)	Interferon Plus Ribavirin (3MU TIW, 24 weeks)
End of therapy response (%)	29	24	33	50
Overall sustained virologic response (%)	6	13	31	38
Sustained Virologic Response (%)				
Genotype 1	2	7	16	28
Genotype non-1	16	29	69	66

Based on references 200, 339, and 340.

GOALS OF THERAPY

The goals of therapy for treating HCV infection are: 1) eradicate the virus; 2) decrease morbidity and mortality; 3) normalize biochemical markers; 4) improve clinical symptoms; 5) prevent spread of the disease; 6) prevent progression to cirrhosis and hepatocellular carcinoma; and 7) prevent the development of end-stage liver disease and its manifestations. These goals may be in part achieved through pharmacologic therapy.

Interferon

ASSESSMENT OF INTERFERON RESPONSE/EFFICACY

Several tests are used to assess therapy in HCV infection. These include biochemical markers such as ALT (less reliable), histologic markers (improvement in HAI), clinical progression and mortality, and viral load (HCV RNA). Patterns of response with respect to viral load can be summarized as follows: 1) nonresponder: no reduction in HCV RNA during treatment; 2) partial responder: reduced HCV RNA during treatment, increased HCV RNA following treatment period; 3) relapser: HCV RNA undetectable during treatment followed by high HCV RNA at the end of therapy; and 4) sustained responder: nondetectable HCV RNA throughout the treatment period and beyond the end of therapy (Fig. 73-7).

In one of the largest trials published to date, patients with chronic hepatitis C were randomly assigned to 3 million units or 1 million units of interferon α-2b three times weekly for 24 weeks or placebo.[323] Response to therapy was assessed by serial measurements of ALT values and liver biopsy results before and after treatment. Of 58 patients treated with 3 million units of α-interferon, approximately one-third had normalized ALT values compared with 16% of patients treated with 1 million units of α-interferon and less than 5% of untreated controls. Improvement in liver histology was noted in patients receiving α-interferon. The responses to α-interferon were rapid (in general within 12 weeks). Unfortunately, end of treatment response was only poor following discontinuation of α-interferon.

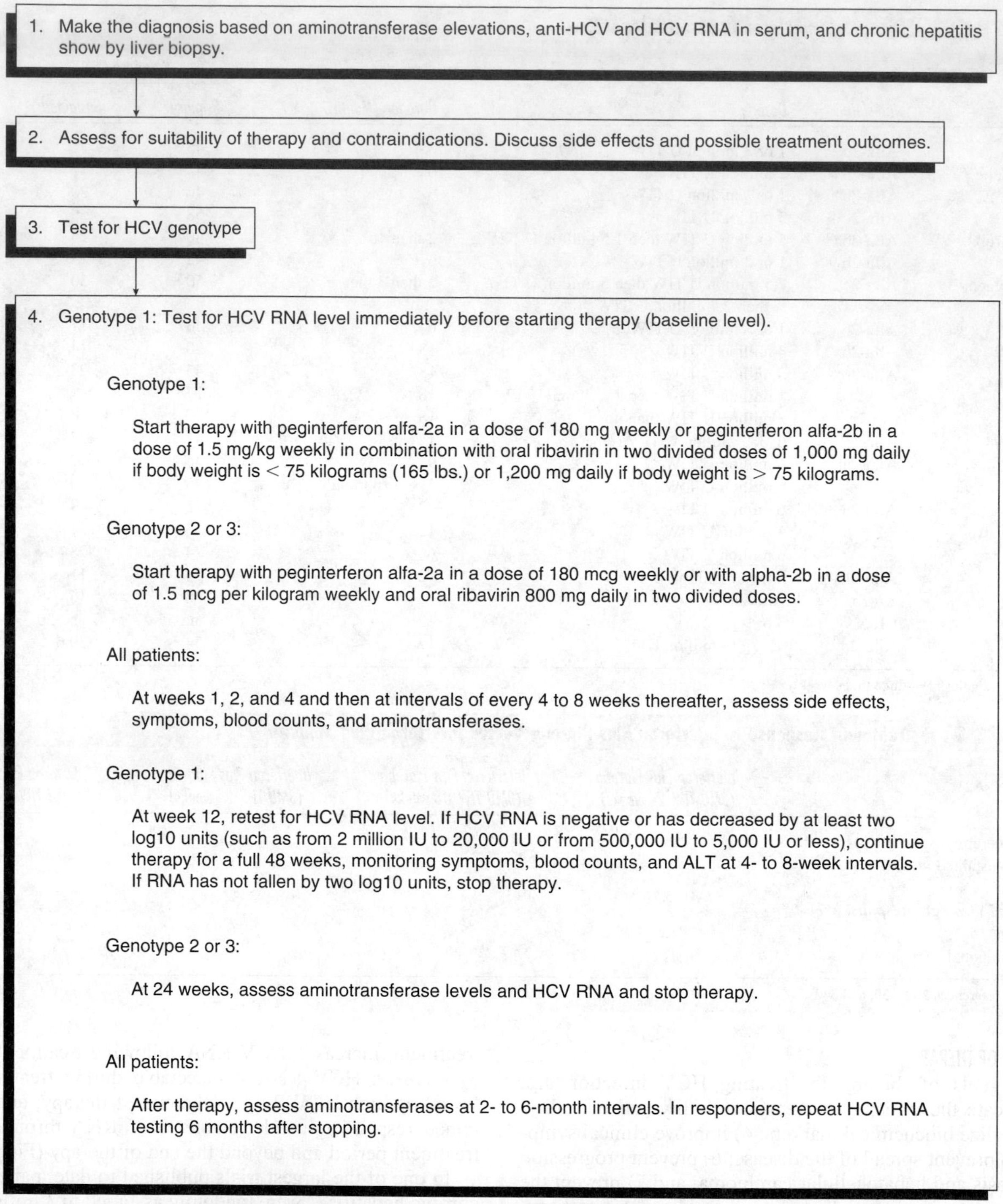

1. Make the diagnosis based on aminotransferase elevations, anti-HCV and HCV RNA in serum, and chronic hepatitis show by liver biopsy.

2. Assess for suitability of therapy and contraindications. Discuss side effects and possible treatment outcomes.

3. Test for HCV genotype

4. Genotype 1: Test for HCV RNA level immediately before starting therapy (baseline level).

Genotype 1:

Start therapy with peginterferon alfa-2a in a dose of 180 mg weekly or peginterferon alfa-2b in a dose of 1.5 mg/kg weekly in combination with oral ribavirin in two divided doses of 1,000 mg daily if body weight is < 75 kilograms (165 lbs.) or 1,200 mg daily if body weight is > 75 kilograms.

Genotype 2 or 3:

Start therapy with peginterferon alfa-2a in a dose of 180 mcg weekly or with alpha-2b in a dose of 1.5 mcg per kilogram weekly and oral ribavirin 800 mg daily in two divided doses.

All patients:

At weeks 1, 2, and 4 and then at intervals of every 4 to 8 weeks thereafter, assess side effects, symptoms, blood counts, and aminotransferases.

Genotype 1:

At week 12, retest for HCV RNA level. If HCV RNA is negative or has decreased by at least two log10 units (such as from 2 million IU to 20,000 IU or from 500,000 IU to 5,000 IU or less), continue therapy for a full 48 weeks, monitoring symptoms, blood counts, and ALT at 4- to 8-week intervals. If RNA has not fallen by two log10 units, stop therapy.

Genotype 2 or 3:

At 24 weeks, assess aminotransferase levels and HCV RNA and stop therapy.

All patients:

After therapy, assess aminotransferases at 2- to 6-month intervals. In responders, repeat HCV RNA testing 6 months after stopping.

FIGURE 73-7 Algorithm for treatment of hepatitis C. (Based on reference 280.)

Because of the suboptimal response of interferon in early clinical trials, several strategies were attempted to enhance efficacy.[323–338] Explored strategies included longer courses of therapy, higher doses of interferon, and utilization of different formulations of interferon.[342–351] Also, patients developed anemia, thrombocytopenia, neutropenia, and neurologic adverse effects with the prolonged regimens or higher dosing schedules. Ultimately, there did not appear to be a significant difference in efficacy or tolerability between different forms of interferon (e.g., interferon α, consensus interferon).[342–350]

37. Are there additional INF formulations that R.D. could receive that may be more efficacious than α-interferon monotherapy for treating chronic HCV infection?

Additional Treatment Strategies
RIBAVIRIN PLUS INTERFERON
In 1998, reports were published on the results of blinded, placebo-controlled trials of hepatitis C–infected patients with combination therapy utilizing interferon and ribavirin for

treatment naïve patients[339–341] (See Table 73-21) and in patients with relapsing HCV.[342] In a double-blind, U.S. multicenter trial, patients with chronic HCV infection were randomly assigned to receive recombinant INF alfa-2b plus placebo for 24 weeks or 48 weeks, or the combination of INF alfa-2b and ribavirin for 24 weeks or 48 weeks.[339] INF alfa-2b was administered subcutaneously at a dosage of 3 million units three times per week, and oral ribavirin (or matched placebo) was given in daily divided doses of 400 mg (AM) and 600 mg (PM) in patients <75 kg or 600 mg twice daily in patients >75 kg. Efficacy was determined based on sustained virologic response (absence of HCV RNA 24 weeks after treatment was discontinued), biochemical response (reduction in serum aminotransferases), and histologic response (hepatic inflammation and fibrosis based on biopsy).

Greater sustained virologic response took place in patients receiving combination therapy with ribavirin for either 24 weeks (70 of 228 patients; 31%) or 48 weeks (87 of 228 patients; 38%) than in patients who received INF alone for 24 weeks (13 of 231 patients; 6%) or 48 weeks (29 of 255 patients; 13%). The rate of sustained biochemical response similarly was greater among patients who received INF and ribavirin for 24 or 48 weeks than among those who received INF alone. Histologic improvement was observed most often in patients receiving the combination regimen for either 24 weeks (57%) or 48 weeks (61%) compared with INF alone for either 24 weeks (44%) or 48 weeks (41%). Dose-limiting adverse effects were most commonly associated with combination therapy. Eight percent of ribavirin patients required dosage reduction for hemoglobin concentrations <10 g/dL. Hemoglobin concentrations remained depressed, yet stable, with the dosage reduction throughout the rest of the trial period and returned to baseline within 4 to 8 weeks after treatment was stopped at 24 or 48 weeks. Dyspnea, pharyngitis, pruritus, rash, nausea, insomnia, and anorexia were also more common with combination therapy than with INF alone. However, the most common reason for discontinuation of therapy was depression, which ranged from 2% to 9% in all groups. Despite the favorable outcomes with combination therapy, no difference in overall survival was described between the treatment groups.

Similarly, another placebo-controlled, multicenter, randomized trial was performed in 832 patients with compensated chronic HCV infection.[340] Patients were assigned to one of three regimens: 3 million units interferon alfa-2b three times per week plus oral ribavirin (400 mg followed by 600 mg daily if <75 kg or 600 mg twice daily if >75 kg) for 48 weeks; 3 million units interferon alfa-2b three times per week plus oral ribavirin (400 mg followed by 600 mg daily if <75 kg or 600 mg twice daily if >75 kg) for 24 weeks; or 3 million units interferon alfa-2b three times per week plus placebo for 48 weeks. The primary study end-point was loss of detectable HCV RNA (serum HCV RNA <100 copies/mL) at week 24 after treatment. A sustained virologic response was observed in 119 (43%) of the 277 patients treated for 48 weeks with the combination regimen, 97 (35%) of the 277 patients treated for 24 weeks with the combination regimen, and 53 (19%) of the 278 patients treated for 48 weeks with INF alone.

Discontinuation of therapy for adverse events was more frequent with combination therapy (19%) and monotherapy (13%) given for 48 weeks than combination therapy given for 24 weeks (8%).

PREDICTORS OF TREATMENT OUTCOME

These studies have resulted in identification of several independent factors predicting sustained virologic response to combination therapy.[280,351,352] The most significant of which is HCV genotype. Generally, genotype 1-infected patients have poor response to interferon/ribavirin irrespective of viral load and require 48 weeks of therapy. However, patients with HCV other than genotype 1 with viral load less than 2 million copies/mL have higher response rates and require only 24 weeks of therapy. Additional host factors have recently been identified and may help predict response to and duration of therapy, allowing combination therapy to be tailored more effectively.[280,351,352] In addition to HCV genotype non-1, other factors that predict a good response to interferon/ribavirin include age younger than 40 years, female gender, and little to no portal fibrosis on biopsy.[280,351,352] In addition, African American patients with chronic HCV infection have lower response rates than whites to interferon monotherapy and are predominantly infected with genotype 1.[280,351,352]

Based on previous studies, R.D. could have benefited from the combination of ribavirin plus INF. However, there are new interferon-based therapies that are considered to be the standard of care for patients with chronic HCV infection.

Current Treatment Strategies

38. What new interferon-based drug therapy could provide R.D. with therapeutic advantages over interferon alone or interferon plus ribavirin?

Although the advent of combination interferon/ribavirin therapy has led to significant improved clearance of serum HCV RNA and improved both biochemical and histologic evidence of chronic hepatitis, there are still numerous patients with chronic infection who are not adequately treated.[280,339–341,351,352] Thus, research in the last few years has examined methodologies for enhancing the effectiveness of interferon-based treatments. The most promising of these explorations has been the development of pegylated interferons.[280,353–356] These compounds are formed through the attachment of polyethylene glycol (PEG) to an interferon molecule, thus changing the pharmacokinetic and pharmacodynamic properties of the drug (Table 73-22).[280,353–356] Of importance, the PEG moiety significantly increases the half-life of interferon, resulting in sustained serum concentrations and permitting once weekly dosing.[280,353–356] The current "standard of care" is pegylated interferon plus ribavirin for the majority of patients with chronic hepatitis C infection. However, there remain subgroups of patients in whom standard interferon plus ribavirin combination or pegylated monotherapy may be preferable. Treatment groups are discussed below.

PEGYLATED INTERFERONS

There are currently two forms of pegylated interferons that are FDA approved for treatment of HCV infection. The linear 12 kDa pegylated interferon, peginterferon α2b (Pegintron; Schering-Plough Corporation), was the first to be FDA approved.[280,353,357,358] The 40kDa pegylated interferon, peginterferon alfa 2a (Pegsys;Hoffman La Roche), has also recently received FDA approval (Table 73-23).[280,353,359–361]

Table 73-22   Contraindications to α-Interferon Plus Ribavirin

Interferon	Ribavirin
Absolute neutrophil <1.5	Unstable cardiac disease
Platelets <75,000/mm³	Severe COPD, asthma
Severe depression	Renal dysfunction
Psychiatric instability	Serum creatinine >1.5 mg/dL
Active substance abuse	Creatinine clearance <50 mL/min
Uncontrolled autoimmune disorders	Anemia
Thyroid	Hgb <13 g/dL in males
Diabetes	Hgb <12 g/dL in females
Rheumatoid arthritis	Hemoglobinopathies
Elevated anti-nuclear antibodies	Thalassemias, sickle cell anemia

Note: Pregnancy risk:
   a) Contraindicated in women who are pregnant or by men whose female partners are pregnant
   b) Negative pregnancy test should be obtained before therapy
   c) Women of childbearing potential and men capable of inducing pregnancy must use two reliable forms of birth control during treatment; contraception should be continued for 6 months following discontinuation of treatment

Efficacy

In a recent dose-finding study, peginterferon α2b (12 kDa) was compared to interferon α-2b for the initial treatment of compensated chronic hepatitis C.[357] Patients received either interferon α-2b 3 MIU three-times-weekly (TIW) or peginterferon α2b 0.5 μg/kg, 1.0 μg/kg, or 1.5 μg/kg once-weekly (QW). Subjects were treated for 48 weeks and then followed for an additional 24 weeks. All three peginterferon α2b doses significantly improved virologic response rates (loss of detectable serum HCV RNA) compared with interferon α-2b. Unlike the end-of-treatment virologic response, the sustained virologic response rate was not dose-related above 1.0 μg/kg peginterferon α2b because of a higher relapse rate among patients treated with 1.5 μg/kg peginterferon α2b, particularly among patients infected with genotype 1. All three peginterferon α2b doses decreased liver inflammation to a greater extent than did interferon α2b, particularly in subjects with sustained responses. Adverse events and changes in laboratory values were mild or moderate.

In another trial using the 40 kDa pegylated interferon dosage form, peginterferon alfa-2a was compared with interferon alfa-2a in the initial treatment of patients with chronic hepatitis C.[359] Five hundred thirty-one patients with chronic hepatitis C were randomized to receive either 180 μg of peginterferon alfa-2a subcutaneously once per week for 48 weeks or 6 million units of interferon alfa-2a subcutaneously three times per week for 12 weeks, followed by 3 million units three times per week for 36 weeks. Patients were assessed at week 72 for a sustained virologic response that was defined as an undetectable level of hepatitis C virus RNA (<100 copies per milliliter). Peginterferon alfa-2a was associated with a higher rate of virologic response than was interferon alfa-2a at week 48 (69% versus 28%) and at week 72 (39% versus 19%). Sustained normalization of serum alanine aminotransferase concentrations at week 72 was also more common in the peginterferon group than in the interferon group (45% versus 25%). The two groups were similar with respect to the reported adverse events. Authors concluded that in these patients, a regimen of peginterferon alfa-2a given once weekly is more effective than a regimen of interferon alfa-2a given TIW.

These trials demonstrate that monotherapy with pegylated interferons is superior to conventional interferon alone. Current trials have evaluated the role of combination pegylated interferon plus ribavirin for the treatment of chronic hepatitis C infection.[358,361]

Manns and colleagues compared the combination of peginterferon α2b (1.5 μg/kg per week) plus ribavirin 800 mg/day to peginterferon α2b (1.5 μg/kg per week with a reduction to 0.5 μg/kg per week after 4 weeks) plus ribavirin 1,000 to 1,200 mg/day and to interferon α-2b plus ribavirin.[358] No difference in the sustained response was observed between the lower dose of peginterferon α2b (12 kD) plus ribavirin and standard interferon α-2b plus ribavirin. The difference in the overall treatment response between peginterferon α2b (12 kD) (1.5 μg/kg) plus ribavirin and interferon α-2b plus ribavirin was 6% adjusted for viral genotype and presence of cirrhosis at baseline. As with other interferon-based therapies, patients with genotype 1 infection, regardless of their pretreatment viral load, had a lower response to peginterferon α2b (12 kD) plus ribavirin compared with patients infected with other viral genotypes. The superior efficacy of peginterferon plus ribavirin over standard interferon plus ribavirin was only seen in patients with genotype 1 infection. One-third of patients with both genotype 1 infection and a high viral load (>2,000,000 copies/mL, >800,000 IU/mL) responded to therapy in both groups. Similarly, the efficacy of peginterferon plus ribavirin was the same as that observed with standard interferon plus ribavirin in patients with bridging fibrosis and/or cirrhosis.

Table 73-23   Comparative Pharmacokinetics of Pegylated Interferons

Parameter	Interferon alfa	Peginterferon alfa 2b (12 kD)	Peginterferon alfa 2a (40 kD)
Absorption	Rapid	Rapid	Sustained
Distribution	Wide	Wide	Blood, organs
Clearance	—	10-fold reduction (hepatic/renal)	100-fold reduction (hepatic)
Elimination half-life (hr)	3–5	30–50	50–80
Weight-based dosing	No	Yes	No
Increased concentration with multiple dosing	No	Yes	Yes
Protected from degradation	No	Probable	Yes

Other researchers have compared the efficacy and safety of peginterferon α-2a plus ribavirin, interferon α-2b plus ribavirin, and peginterferon α-2a alone in the initial treatment of chronic hepatitis C.[361] In this trial, patients were randomly assigned to three treatment groups who received at least one dose of study medication consisting of 180 µg of peginterferon α-2a once weekly plus ribavirin 1,000 or 1,200 mg/day (depending on body weight), weekly peginterferon α-2a plus daily placebo or 3 million units of interferon α-2b TIW plus daily ribavirin for 48 weeks. A significantly greater proportion of patients receiving peginterferon α-2a plus ribavirin had a sustained virologic response (defined as the absence of detectable HCV RNA 24 weeks after cessation of therapy) compared with patients who received interferon α-2b plus ribavirin (56% versus 44%; $P < 0.001$) or peginterferon α-2a alone (56% versus 29%; $P < 0.001$). The proportions of patients with HCV genotype 1 who had sustained virologic responses were 46%, 36%, and 21%, respectively, for the three regimens. Among patients with HCV genotype 1 and high baseline levels of HCV RNA, the proportions of those with sustained virologic responses were 41%, 33%, and 13%, respectively. The overall safety profiles of the three treatment regimens were similar. Based on these results, it appears that peginterferon α-2a plus ribavirin is superior to interferon alfa-2b plus ribavirin or peginterferon alfa-2a alone in the treatment of chronic hepatitis C.

Predictors of Treatment Outcome for Pegylated Interferons

Independent variables associated with a favorable response to peginterferon plus ribavirin include genotype non-1, low pretreatment HCV RNA level, light body weight, young age, and the absence of bridging fibrosis/cirrhosis.[280,358,361] The most appropriate dose of ribavirin administered in combination with peginterferon alfa-2b is controversial.[280,283] The FDA-approved ribavirin dose of 800 mg is lower than that approved for standard interferon alfa-2b. The FDA-approved dose was selected because of concerns regarding additive toxicities associated with peginterferon and ribavirin. Additional data from trials of peginterferon alfa-2a have suggested that the 800 mg dose is sufficient for treatment of non-genotype 1 infection, but that higher doses (1,000 mg/1,200 mg based on a 75 kg weight) are necessary for effective treatment of genotype 1.

Adverse Effects/Monitoring

39. **What adverse effects might be expected if pegylated interferon plus ribavirin are used in D.R., and what are appropriate monitoring parameters?**

In the clinical trials with pegylated interferon and ribavirin, adverse effects resulted in discontinuation of treatment in approximately 10% to 14% of patients.[357–363] Adverse events were similar between those patients receiving peginterferon plus ribavirin and those receiving interferon plus ribavirin, except for a higher frequency of injection site reactions and a higher frequency of neutropenia in the peginterferon plus ribavirin group. Side effects in both groups included influenza-like symptoms, hematologic abnormalities, and neuropsychiatric symptoms.[357–363] The education of patients, their family members, and caregivers about side effects and their prospective management is an integral aspect of treatment.

Regular monitoring of neuropsychiatric side effects, cytopenias, and adherence to HCV therapy is mandatory (see Table 21-24). Psychological conditions, particularly depression, are common among persons with hepatitis C and are frequent side effects of interferon.[354–363] Patients' mental health should be assessed before initiation of antiviral therapy and monitored regularly during therapy. Antidepressants, such as selective serotonin re-uptake inhibitors, may be useful in the management of depression associated with antiviral therapy.[354–363]

In certain patients with persistent cytopenias despite dose reductions, treatment with hematopoietic growth factors (i.e., erythropoietin, granulocyte colony stimulating factor) may be useful to reduce symptoms and maintain adherence to antiviral therapy.[354–363] However, this therapy is costly and the optimal dosage is not yet clear. Additionally, it is not known if the use of hematopoietic growth factors will enhance the likelihood of sustained virologic response (SVR). Thus, the potential benefits of these agents need confirmation in prospectively designed trials before they can be recommended.

Of special importance, severe hemolysis from ribavirin may occur in patients with renal insufficiency.[354–363] In these patients, the ribavirin dose should either be reduced or discontinued. Finally, lactic acidosis may be a rare complication of combination therapy in patients undergoing therapy for HIV and HCV. Thus D.R. should be monitored closely to minimize the risk of severe adverse effects in initiated pegylated interferon plus ribavirin therapy.

Choosing Interferon Formulations

Pegylated interferons offer the convenience of once weekly versus three times weekly dosing, but pegylated interferons are associated with a greater incidence of cytopenias and injection site reactions compared with standard interferon. Moreover, there are subsets of patients in which treatment response with standard interferon alfa-2b plus ribavirin is the same with as pegylated interferons plus ribavirin. These include patients with non genotype-1 infection and patients with compensated cirrhosis.[280,285] When deciding whether to treat a patient with pegylated interferons or standard interferon in combination with ribavirin, the patient and provider should weigh the risks and benefits of the two treatment regimens (see Fig. 73-7). For example, in the patient with compensated cirrhosis, particularly if he or she has leukopenia before therapy, standard interferon might be the preferred treatment because of a short half-life and reduced likelihood of dose reductions for cytopenias.

Interferon or Pegylated Interferon Monotherapy

For patients with contraindications to the use of ribavirin, such as those with unstable cardiac disease, anemia, renal insufficiency, or those who might conceive while receiving treatment or within 6 months of completing therapy, interferon monotherapy or pegylated interferons should be considered.[280,285] Pegylated interferons have been shown to be superior to standard interferon α in the treatment of hepatitis C, and pegylated interferons are the treatment of choice in select patients.[280,285]

As a result of recent trials, combination therapy is the treatment of choice for naïve patients, that is patients who have received neither interferon nor ribavirin therapy and who are able to tolerate ribavirin. Pegylated interferons plus ribavirin offer the convenience of once-weekly dosing, but with only a slight increase in efficacy and an increase in adverse events compared with standard interferon α plus ribavirin.[280,285] The FDA-approved dose of ribavirin is 800 mg, but higher doses (1,000/1,200 mg based on a 75 kg weight) may be improve efficacy in patients with genotype 1 infection. A ribavirin dose of 800 mg appears adequate for treatment of genotype non-1 infection. While the results using pegylated interferons plus ribavirin are encouraging, the benefits of treatment on important clinical outcomes such as prevention of complications of advanced liver disease and the prevention of hepatocellular carcinoma remain to be demonstrated. Finally, there are no clinical trials that demonstrate the superiority of one type of pegylated interferon compared to the other (e.g., pegylated interferon α-2a versus pegylated interferon α-2b).

Treatment Options for Relapse of Chronic Hepatitis C

40. What is the role for combination therapy in patients who have relapse of chronic HCV infection?

As noted previously, HCV relapse rates (based on HCV RNA reappearance) often occur following discontinuation of INF therapy despite longer courses of treatment. Based on previous trials, the combination of ribavirin plus INF may reduce HCV relapse. Results from these trials were recently confirmed in 345 patients with chronic active HCV who relapsed following INF.[342,362] One hundred seventy-three patients were randomly assigned to receive either standard dose interferon alfa-2b with ribavirin (400 mg [AM] and 600 mg [PM] in patients <75 kg or 600 mg twice daily in patients >75 kg) for 6 months or INF and placebo.[342] The primary endpoints of the study were the disappearance of HCV RNA from the serum and histologic improvement at the end of the 24-week follow-up period. Upon the completion of treatment, serum levels of HCV RNA were undetectable in 141 of 173 patients who received combination therapy compared with INF alone (82% versus 47%; $P < 0.001$). Serum HCV RNA continued to be undetectable in 84 patients (49%) in the combination group and in only 8 patients (5%) in the INF alone group ($P < 0.001$) at 6 months. Patients who achieved a virologic response also had sustained normalization of serum ALT concentrations and histologic improvement. Of note, patients with the greatest response were those with low viral load and genotypes 2 or 3. As in previous trials, patients receiving combined therapy had a significant reduction in their hemoglobin concentrations, but otherwise had a safety profile similar to that of INF alone. These results appear to be as good or better than those in patients receiving higher doses and longer courses of INF. Thus, patients with chronic HCV infection without decompensated liver disease who relapse, may benefit from combination therapy.

Adjunctive Therapies

41. In addition to INF alone, or the combination of INF plus ribavirin, or pegylated interferons, are there any other therapeutic options available for R.D.?

INF responders have lower serum iron, iron saturation, and hepatic iron levels (which is believed to up regulate cellular immune responses) than do INF nonresponders.[363] In pilot trials, iron reduction by phlebotomy has been correlated with an improvement in aminotransferase levels in patients with chronic HCV infection and iron overload. These limited data suggest an enhanced response to INF may be achieved through iron reduction by phlebotomy.

Other approaches to treating chronic HCV infection include INF in combination with ursodeoxycholic acid.[364] This combination produced a more sustained biochemical response than did treatment with INF alone, but there was no sustained, histologic improvement, or survival benefit. Preliminary results of INF in combination with thymosin suggest an additive effect, but further controlled trials are required to validate these findings.[365] Also, granulocyte colony-stimulating factor (G-CSF) combined with INF has been suggested to enhance HCV clearance compared with INF alone.[366] Agents such as amantadine,[367] nonsteroidal anti-inflammatory drugs,[368] pentoxifylline,[369] vitamin E,[370] omega-3 fatty acid supplements,[371] and herbal remedies such as glycyrrhizin (licorice root),[372] silymarin (milk thistle),[373] and sho-saiko-to (TJ-9)[374] are unproven for the routine management of HCV. These agents are thought to have anti-inflammatory or antifibrotic effects on the liver, which may lead to normalization of biochemical markers (i.e., ALT). Data from patients receiving IL-10 (Tenovil), which inhibits the Th1 T-cell subset, suggest that formation of liver scar tissue may be reduced.[375] In vitro studies with novel agents such as VX-497 (Vertex Pharmaceuticals), which inhibits inosine monophosphate dehydrogenase, have shown antiviral activity based on the proposed mechanism of action of ribavirin, and may reduce lymphocyte migration and proliferation involved in the immune system response to HCV infection.

Other experimental targets for anti-HCV drugs include the HCV NS3 protease and helicase enzymes (i.e., HCV protease and helicase inhibitors), which are thought to be essential enzymes in HCV replication.[376–378] Ribozymes (LY466700, Heptazyme) that can be synthesized to selectively inhibit disease-causing proteins by interfering with RNA synthesis are also awaiting clinical investigation.[376–378] Finally, an experimental vaccine has also been studied in chimpanzees; however, no efficacy or safety data are available with this agent in humans.[379] R.D. should not be initiated on these agents at this time.

Summary of HCV in Nonimmunocompromised Patients

Overall, many factors have been identified that are associated with an increased or decreased likelihood of response to INF therapy in patients infected with HCV. Analyses have generally shown that a decreased pretreatment HCV RNA titer is associated with more favorable response, that genotypes other than type 1b exhibit higher sustained response rates compared with genotype 1b, and that responders have less fibrosis and less inflammatory changes than nonresponders. Furthermore, most trials conducted using INF(s) or combinations thereof exclude patients with decompensated liver disease (cirrhosis), patients with HCC, patients with cryoglobulinemia or associated membranoproliferative glomerulonephritis, and children infected with HCV. Additional experience is needed in these areas to definitively assess therapy for HCV infection.

Treating Hepatitis C Following Liver Transplantation

42. While discussing treatment options for HCV infection, R.D. experiences a sudden loss of consciousness. He is admitted to the intensive care unit where he will be emergently evaluated for a liver transplant. What are the therapeutic options for preventing or treating HCV-infected patients following liver transplantation?

Uncontrolled trials have reported the efficacy of α-interferon in treating hepatitis C following transplantation.[380–382] In one report, 11 patients were treated with α-interferon (3 million units three times weekly for 6 months).[380] After therapy was stopped, only one patient had normal liver enzyme levels and INF was not correlated with precipitating allograft rejection. In a similar trial, 4 of 18 patients (22%) had a sustained biochemical response (normal aminotransferase levels) at the end of treatment and in 6-month follow-up.[382] HCV RNA levels were reduced in both responders and nonresponders, but returned to pretreatment levels after discontinuation of INF. Sustained effects were not observed, nor were improvements in histology. Only one patient had an INF-associated, biopsy-proven delayed rejection episode. In contrast to these reports, others have identified INF therapy with precipitating rejection, possibly because of its ability to up-regulate the expression of human leukocyte antigen (HLA) class I and II antigens.[383]

Similar to the nontransplant population, the combination of INF and ribavirin or ribavirin alone has also been assessed in liver transplant recipients for treating recurrent HCV infection following transplantation.[384,385,386] Data from pilot and randomized, noncomparative trials suggest that combination therapy is effective but poorly tolerated.[384] Furthermore, transplant recipients appear to have a high incidence of hemolysis, thrombocytopenia, and mental status changes with combination therapy. Transplant recipients should also be closely monitored for rejection during and following cessation of INF plus ribavirin therapy. Finally, the use of pegylated interferons alone or in combination with ribavirin has also been considered following liver transplantation.[384] However, any combination therapy could be considered (based on response criteria for interferon as listed above) in the following areas in liver transplant patients transplanted for HCV: 1) as prophylaxis for HCV immediately following liver transplantation (first transplant); 2) as prophylaxis for HCV immediately following liver transplantation (second transplant for recurrent HCV); 3) in patients with HCV recurrence without decompensation with worsening symptoms; and 4) in patients with recurrent HCV with decompensation. These areas are clearly controversial and warrant clinical investigation.

HEPATITIS E VIRUS
Virology, Epidemiology, Transmission, and Pathogenesis

Hepatitis E virus (HEV) is an icosahedral, nonenveloped virus of the Caliciviridae family between 32 and 34 nm wide that was initially identified by immune electromicroscopy in the stool samples of infected persons (see Table 73-2).[387,388] The HEV genome is a single-stranded polyadenylated RNA and unlike HAV, has an RNA genome that encodes for nonstructural proteins through overlapping open reading frames (ORFs). Several ORFs encode for nonstructural proteins, structural proteins, or proteins of undetermined function. The HEV polyprotein has several sequences, including an RNA-dependent RNA-polymerase, and RNA helicase, and a virally encoded cysteine protease.

HEV occurs in endemic areas such as Africa, Southeast and Central Asia, Mexico, and Central and South America as both epidemic and sporadic infections.[387,389] Sporadic infections also occur in nonendemic areas and are usually associated with travel into areas of endemicity. The attack rate (the percentage of exposed patients who become infected) of HEV is low compared with HAV (1% versus 10%, respectively). In endemic areas, outbreaks usually occur between 5 and 10 years apart and are often associated with times of heavy rainfall, after floods or monsoons, or following the recession of flood waters.[387,389,390] The overall case fatality rate for the general endemic population is 0.5% to 4%, whereas for reasons unknown, pregnant women have a much greater case fatality rate of 20%.[387,391] In particular, the fetal complication rate is increased, especially if the infection occurs in the third trimester of pregnancy.[387,392] The frequency of death in utero and immediately following birth is also greater than seen with acute hepatitis of other etiologies.[387,392]

Transmission of HEV is via the fecal-oral route, and the most common source of transmission is ingestion of fecally contaminated water.[387,389,391] Poor climactic conditions in conjunction with inadequate personal hygiene and sanitation have led to epidemics of HEV infection. Secondary attacks usually are much lower than that observed with HAV ranging from 0.7% to 2.2% versus 50% to 75%, respectively.[387,389,391] The mechanism for this difference could be related to the instability of HEV to its environment, differences in the quantity of virus needed to propagate infection, or a greater frequency of subclinical disease.

Interference with the production of cellular macromolecules, alteration of cellular membranes, and alteration of lysosomal permeability are some of the proposed mechanisms of hepatic injury.[393,394] In addition, immune-mediated mechanisms are believed to be responsible for lysis of virally infected hepatocytes by direct lymphocyte cytotoxicity or antibody-mediated cytotoxicity.

Diagnosis

Initial assays for detection of anti-HEV used electromicroscopy to detect HEVAg on the surface of HEV particles in stool and serum and immunohistochemistry to detect the antigen in liver tissue.[387,389,391] Fluorescent antibody-blocking assay is currently used to detect anti-HEV reacting to HEVAg in serum, and although highly specific, this assay lacks sensitivity (50%) in acute HEV infection.[387,389] Additional cloning and sequencing of HEV has led to the development of Western blot assays and ELISAs that detect anti-HEV by using recombinant expressed proteins from the structural region of the virus. Reverse transcriptase polymerase chain reaction (RT-PCR) has also been used to confirm the diagnosis of HEV by detecting HEV RNA from serum, liver, or stool.[387,389,393] Clinically, HEV is a diagnosis of exclusion.

Clinical Manifestations, Serology, and Natural History

The incubation period following exposure is listed in Table 73-1. Two phase of illness have been described, including a prodromal and preicteric phase as described for HAV infection. Peak serum aminotransferase levels reflect the onset of the icteric phase and generally return to baseline by 6 weeks.[387,394] Stool is often positive for HEV RNA at the onset of the icteric phase and persists for an additional 10 days beyond this period. Viral shedding may also occur for up to 52 days after the onset of icterus. Detection in the serum occurs during the preicteric phase, before detection of virus in the stool, and becomes undetectable following the peak in aminotransferase activity. Because HEV RNA is not detectable in the serum during symptoms, diagnostic tests using HEV RNA have limited utility and a correlation between PCR detection and infectivity has not been observed. Serologically, HEV IgM becomes detectable before the peak rise in ALT, whereas antibody titers peak with peak ALT levels and subsequently decline. In most patients HEV IgM is present for 5 to 6 months following the onset of illness. HEV IgG appears after HEV IgM and remains detectable for up to 14 years after acute infection; however, the duration of protective immunity has not been fully elucidated.[387,395]

In nonfatal cases, acute HEV hepatitis is followed by complete recovery without any chronic complications. There appears to be protection from reinfection; however, the duration of protection is variable. Fulminant hepatitis has also been associated with HEV infection and has a high association with pregnancy.[387,389,390,392] Maternal mortality was reported to be 1.5% for HEV infection occurring in the first trimester of pregnancy, 8.5% for those in the second trimester, and 21% for those infected in the third trimester.

Prevention and Treatment

No immunoprophylactic measures exist for HEV disease, and effective prevention strategies are dependent on improved sanitation in endemic areas. Travelers going to endemic areas should be educated on drinking water, eating ice, or eating uncooked shellfish or uncooked and peeled fruits and vegetables. Drinking water should be boiled to inactivate HEV. No vaccines or postexposure prophylaxis are available to prevent HEV infection; however, vaccines to induce an active immune response are under development.

HEPATITIS G VIRUS
Virology

In 1995 the genomes of two previously unidentified RNA viruses were cloned from experimentally inoculated tamarins.[396–398] The original inoculate was obtained from a surgeon (initials G.B.) with non-A, non-B (NANB) hepatitis who was thought to have HCV. The viruses were subsequently named GB virus A (GBV-A) and GB virus B (GBV-B).[396–398] However, another unknown RNA virus related to GBV-A and GBV-B was discovered (using representational difference analysis) and was designated GB virus C (GBV-C).[396–398] Similar methods were also implemented in the discovery of one more previously unknown virus, designated TT virus (TTV), obtained from a patient with the initials T. T. In 1996, another independent research group isolated a novel RNA virus (designated HGV) that was associated with hepatitis.[396–398] Sequencing studies comparing GBV-C and HGV have shown these isolates to be 2 genotypes of the same virus. Apparently, only humans and higher primates can be infected by human GBV-C/HGV.[396–398]

GBV-C/HGV is a single-stranded enveloped RNA virus that consists of 9,100 to 9,400 nucleotides (Table 73-2).[396–398] GBV-C/HGV belongs to the Flaviviridae viruses, and temporarily to the hepacivirus genus together with HCV since the genomic organization of this virus resembles HCV. The biological functions of many GBV-C/HGV proteins have not been entirely defined, although the capsid region of this virus is defective and core proteins are not encoded, unlike with HCV. Recently, an envelope region that encodes a surface glycoprotein as well as protease, helicase regions have been identified.[396–398] Additional phylogenetic analysis has depicted four genotypes: genotype 1 (GBV-C; originated from West Africa), genotype 2 (TTV; originated from the United States), and genotype 3 and 4 (originated from Asia).

Epidemiology

GBV-C/HGV is spread worldwide and infection has been observed in healthy persons and in intravenous drug users, men who have sex with men, patients receiving multiple transfusions, and patients with fulminant hepatic failure.[396,397,399] Viremia has been reported to be between 1% and 4% among healthy populations in Europe and North America and even higher rates (10% to 33%) have been documented in residents of South America and Africa.[396–398] The prevalence of resolved GBV-C/HGV infections (using envelope antibodies) appears to be more common than the occurrence of viremic infections. Rates of resolved infections described in blood donors are 3% to 15% in Europe, 3% to 8% in North America, 20% in Africa and South America, and 3% to 6% in Asia.[396–398]

Transmission

Transmission of GBV-C/HGV has been primarily associated with blood transfusions and infections have been observed in the presence of other hepatitis viruses (e.g., HBV, HCV).[396–398] Additional modes of transmission include injection drug use, hemodialysis, sexual contact, and vertical/perinatal transmission.[396] Also, GBV-C/HGV RNA has been isolated in saliva, suggesting that close social contact may be a possible mode of transmission.[396–398]

Pathogenesis and Diagnosis

The pathogenesis and serologic presentation of GBV-C/HGV are poorly described. The natural course of GBV-C/HGV infection appears to vary from an acute self-limited episode to a chronic infection that may persist from years to decades.[396–398,400] GBV-C/HGV may cause mild acute hepatitis, but despite persistent infection, it does not appear to cause clinically significant chronic hepatitis.[396] Diagnosis is usually established through detection of the virus by RT-PCR methodology (HGV RNA).[396,401] Additionally, first generation EIA tests have been utilized to detect specific antibodies to the envelope glycoprotein to diagnose previous infection; however, the specificity and sensitivity of these tests have not been fully elucidated. Reliable serologic assays are needed.

Clinical Manifestations and Treatment

Clinical and extrahepatic manifestations of GBV-C/HGV are unknown, but the virus has been found to be in serum for many years in patients with several types of liver diseases.[396–402,403] However, no causal relationship has been established between GBV-C/HGV and acute, fulminant, and chronic non B–C-D hepatitis.[396,397,398,402,403] The role of the GBV-C/HGV in human hepatitis remains unclear. Published studies provide further evidence that GBV-C/HGV may not be a significant cause of acute or chronic liver disease.[396] One report demonstrated that 15% of children with chronic hepatitis C or hepatitis B are infected with GBV-C/HGV; however, GBV-C/HGV coinfection does not appear to cause more severe liver disease. In another report, serum HCV RNA concentrations, liver histology and response to treatment with interferon-α did not differ between patients with and without GBV-C/HGV coinfection. Loss of serum HGV RNA did not correlate with a biochemical response whereas loss of serum HCV RNA did. These results show that GBV-C/HGV coinfection frequently occurs in individuals infected with HCV and that GBV-C/HGV does not influence the severity of liver disease or response to treatment with interferon-α in patients with chronic hepatitis C. Because the significance of GBV-C/HGV is unclear, screening of blood donors for this virus is not presently justified. Currently there are no agents used to treat or prevent GBV-C/HGV infection.[396]

SUMMARY

Viral hepatitis continues to be a significant worldwide infectious disease. To date, prevention strategies through universal vaccination are the most efficient methods for minimizing the incidence of HAV, HBV and HDV. Patient education with respect to the common ways of spreading these infections may also result in behavioral modifications that reduce the overall incidence of infection. However, once HBV and HCV progress to chronic infection, more efficacious and better tolerated antiviral therapies are needed to treat these infections. Similarly, therapeutic modalities that reduce the progression of these diseases are necessary to prevent end-stage liver disease and development of additional complications (encephalopathy, intractable ascites, coagulation disorders, and HCC). As a better understanding of viral replication is established, as well as appropriate models for study, new agents may become available in the near future. Furthermore, more diagnostic tools are needed to better identify new hepatitis viruses and monitor response to drug therapies. The economic impact and quality of life of these patients remains to be fully elucidated.

REFERENCES

1. Alter MJ et al. The epidemiology of viral hepatitis in the United States. Gastroenterol Clin North Am 1994;23:437.
2. Hadler SC. Vaccines to prevent hepatitis B and hepatitis A infections. Infect Dis Clin North Am 1990; 4:29.
3. Wilkinson SP et al. Clinical course of chronic lobular hepatitis: report of five cases. Q J Med 1978; 60:421.
4. Ishak KG. Light microscopic morphology of viral hepatitis. Am J Clin Pathol 1976;65:787.
5. Berenguer M et al. Hepatitis G virus infection in patients with hepatitis C virus infection undergoing liver transplantation. Gastroenterology 1996;111: 1569.
6. Melnick J. Proper and classification of hepatitis A virus. Vaccine 1992;10 (Supp l).S24.
7. Purcelli RH. Enterically transmitted non-A, non-B hepatitis. In: Popper H, Shaffner F, eds. Progress in Liver Diseases. New York: Grune and Stratton, 1990;9:371.
8. Margolis H et al. Hepatitis B: evolving epidemiology and implications for control. Semin Liver Dis 1991;11:84.
9. Kiyasu PK et al. Diagnosis and treatment of the major hepatotrophic viruses. Am J Med Sci 1993; 306:248.
10. Bonino F et al. Delta agent (type D) hepatitis. Semin Liver Dis 1986;6:28.
11. Linnen J et al. Molecular cloning and disease association of hepatitis G virus: a transfusion-transmission agent. Science 1996;271:505.
12. Matsuko K et al. Infection with hepatitis GB virus C in patients on maintenance hemodialysis. N Engl J Med 1996;334:1485.
13. Wrobleski F et al. Serum glutamic oxaloacetate transaminase activity as an index of liver cell injury: a preliminary report. Ann Intern Med 1995; 43:360.
14. Losowsky, MS. The clinical course of viral hepatitis. Clin Gastroenterol 1980;91:3.
15. Davis S. Chronic hepatitis. In: Kaplowitz N, ed. Liver and Biliary Diseases. 2nd Ed. Baltimore, MD: Williams & Wilkins, 1996;327.

16. Wright R. Type B hepatitis: progression to chronic hepatitis. Clin Gastroenterol 1980;9:97.
17. Maddrey WC. Chronic hepatitis. Dis Mon 1993; 39:53.
18. Dienstag JL. Non-A, non-B hepatitis: recognition, epidemiology, and clinical features. Gastroenterology 1983;85:439.
19. Lau JYN et al. Molecular virology and pathogenesis of hepatitis B. Lancet 1993;342:1335.
20. Maddrey WC et al. Drug-induced chronic liver disease. Gastroenterology 1977;72:1348.
21. Dossing M et al. Drug-induced hepatic disorders. Drug Saf 1993;9:441.
22. Brewer GJ et al. Wilson's disease. Medicine 1992; 71:139.
23. Hoofnagle JH et al. Therapy of chronic delta hepatitis: overview. Prog Clin Biol Res 1993;382:337.
24. Czaja AJ. Natural history of chronic active hepatitis. In: Czaja AJ, Dickerson ER, eds. Chronic Active Hepatitis: The Mayo Clinic Experience. New York: Marcel Dekker, 1986:9.
25. Mphahlele MJ et al. HGV: the identification, biology, and prevalence of an orphan virus. Liver 1998; 18:14395.
26. Maddrey WC et al. Severe hepatitis from methyldopa. Gastroenterology 1975;68:351.
27. Black M et al. Nitrofurantoin-induced chronic active hepatitis. Ann Intern Med 1980;92:62.
28. Maddrey WC et al. Isoniazid hepatitis. Ann Intern Med 1973;79:1.
29. Tonder M et al. Sulfonamide-induced chronic liver disease. Scand J Gastroenterol 1974;9:93.
30. Weiss M et al. Propylthiouracil-induced hepatic damage. Arch Intern Med 1980;140:1184.
31. Lemon S et al. Genetic, antigenic, and biological difference between strains of hepatitis A virus. Vaccine 1992;10(Suppl 1):S40.
32. Schultheiss T et al. Proteinase 3C of hepatitis A virus (HAV) cleaves the HAV polyprotein P2-P3 at all sites including VP1/2A and 2A/2B. Virology 1994;198:275.
33. Shapiro C et al. Worldwide epidemiology of hepatitis A infection. J Hepatol 1993;18(Suppl 2):S11.

34. Shapiro C et al. Epidemiology of hepatitis A: seroepidemiology and risk groups in the USA. Vaccine 1992;10 (Suppl 1):S59.
35. Melnick J. History and epidemiology of hepatitis A virus. J Infect Dis 1995;171(Suppl 1):S2.
36. Hoffman F et al. Hepatitis A as an occupational hazard. Vaccine 1992,10(Suppl 1).382.
37. Gust ID et al. Hepatitis A. Prog Liver Dis 1990; 306:248.
38. Centers for Disease Control. Prevention of hepatitis A through active or passive immunization: recommendations of the Advisory Committee on Immunization Practices (ACIP). MMWR 1999;48:RR12:1.
39. Cuthbert JA. Hepatitis A: old and new. Clin Micro Rev 2001;14:38.
40. Gingrich GA et al. Serological investigation of an outbreak of hepatitis A in rural day care center. Am J Public Health 1983;73:1190.
41. Shapiro CN. Transmission of hepatitis viruses. Ann Intern Med 1994;120:82.
42. Sheretz RJ et al. Transmission of hepatitis A by transfusion of blood products. Arch Intern Med 1994;144:1579.
43. Steffen R et al. Epidemiology and prevention of hepatitis A in travelers. JAMA 1994;272:885.
44. Margolis H et al. Identification of virus components in circulating immune complexes isolated during hepatitis A virus infection. Hepatology 1990;11:31.
45. Scoit R et al. Hepatitis A: a kupffer cell disease? J Clin Pathol 1986;39:1160.
46. Vallbracht A et al. Liver-derived cytotoxic T cells in hepatitis A virus infection. J Infect Dis 1989; 160:209.
47. Baba H et al. Cytolytic activity of natural killer cells and lymphokine activated killer cells against hepatitis A infected fibroblasts. J Clin Lab Immunol 1993;40:47.
48. Akriviadis et al. Fulminant hepatitis A in intravenous drug users with chronic liver disease. Ann Intern Med 1989;110:838.
49. Lee WM. Acute liver failure. N Engl J Med 1993; 329:1862.
50. Romero R et al. Viral hepatitis in children. Semin Liver Dis 1994;14:289.

51. Schiff E. Atypical clinical manifestations of hepatitis A. Vaccine 1992;10(Supp 1):S18.
52. Cook D et al. Relapsing hepatitis A infections with immunological sequelae. Can J Gastroenterol 1989;3:145.
53. Scoit R et al. Cholestatic features in hepatitis A. J Hepatol 1986;3:172.
54. Hoofnagle JH et al. Serologic diagnosis of acute and chronic hepatitis. Semin Liver Dis 1991;11:73.
55. Glikson M et al. Relapsing hepatitis A: a review of 14 cases and literature survey. Medicine 1992; 71:14.
56. Lemon SM. Type A viral hepatitis: new developments in an old disease. N Engl J Med 1985; 313:1059.
57. Kryger P et al. Acute type B hepatitis among HBsAg negative patients detected by anti-HBc IgM. Hepatology 1982;2:50.
58. Jorup-Ronstrom C et al. Reduction of paracetamol and aspirin metabolism during viral hepatitis. Clin Pharmacokinet 1986;11:250.
59. Puente M et al. Increase in serum carbamazepine concentrations after acute viral hepatitis. Ann Pharmacother 1998;32:1369.
60. Roberts RK et al. Effect of age and parenchymal liver disease on the disposition and elimination of chlordiazepoxide (Librium). Gastroenterology 1978;75:479.
61. Narang APS et al. Pharmacokinetic study of chloramphenicol in patients with liver disease. Eur J Clin Pharmacol 1981;20:479.
62. Gugler R et al. Clofibrate disposition in renal failure and acute and chronic liver disease. Eur J Clin Pharmacol 1979;15:341.
63. Klotz U et al. The effects of age and liver disease on the disposition and elimination of diazepam in adult man. J Clin Invest 1975;55:347.
64. Williams RL et al. Influence of viral hepatitis on the disposition of two compounds with high hepatic clearance: lidocaine and indocyanine green. Clin Pharmacol Ther 1976;20:290.
65. Kraus JW et al. Effects of aging and liver disease on disposition of lorazepam. Clin Pharmacol Ther 1978;24:411.
66. McHorse TS et al. Effect of acute viral hepatitis in man on the disposition and elimination of meperidine. Gastroenterology 1975;68:775.
67. Dylewicz P et al. Bioavailability and elimination of nitrendipine in liver disease. Eur J Clin Pharmacol 1987;32:563.
68. Eandi M et al. Pharmacokinetics of norfloxacin in healthy volunteers and patients with renal and hepatic damage. Eur J Clin Microbiol 1983;2:253.
69. Shull HJ et al. Normal disposition of oxazepam in acute viral hepatitis and cirrhosis. Ann Intern Med 1976;84:420.
70. Alvin J et al. The effect of liver disease in man on the disposition of phenobarbital. J Pharmacol Exp Ther 1975;192:224.
71. Blaschke TF et al. Influence of acute viral hepatitis on phenytoin kinetics and protein binding. Clin Pharmacol Ther 1975;17:685.
72. Karbwang J et al. The pharmacokinetics of quinine in patients with hepatitis. Br J Clin Pharmacol 1993;35:444.
73. Holdiness MR. Clinical pharmacokinetics of the antitubercular drugs. Clin Pharmacokinet 1984; 9:511.
74. Staib AH et al. Pharmacokinetics and metabolism of theophylline and patients with liver disease. Int J Clin Pharmacol Ther Toxicol 1980;18:500.
75. Williams RL et al. Influence of acute viral hepatitis on disposition and plasma binding of tolbutamide. Clin Pharmacol Ther 1977;21:301.
76. Williams RL et al. Influence of acute viral hepatitis on disposition and pharmacologic effect of warfarin. Clin Pharmacol Ther 1976;20:90.
77. Winokur PL, Stapleton JT. Immunoglobulin prophylaxis for hepatitis A. Clin Infect Dis 1992; 14:580.
78. Centers for Disease Control. Prevention of hepatitis A through active or passive immunization: recommendations of the Advisory Committee on Immu-

nization Practices (ACIP). MMWR 1996;45 (RR-15):1.
79. Westblom TU et al. Safety and immunogenicity of an inactivated hepatitis A vaccine: effect of dose and vaccination schedule. J Infect Dis 1994; 169:996.
80. Werzberger A et al. A controlled trial of formalin inactivated hepatitis A vaccine in healthy children. N Engl J Med 1992;327:453.
81. Innis BL et al. Protection against hepatitis A by an inactivated vaccine. JAMA 1994;271:1328.
82. Riedemann S et al. Placebo-controlled efficacy study of hepatitis A vaccine in Valdivia, Chile. Vaccine 1992;10(Supp 1):S152.
83. Niu MT et al. Two-year review of hepatitis A vaccine safety: data from the Vaccine Adverse Event Reporting System (VAERS). Clin Infect Dis 1998;26:1475.
84. Totos G et al. Hepatitis A vaccine: persistence of antibodies 5 years after the first vaccination. Vaccine 1997;15:1252.
85. Van Damme P et al. Inactivated hepatitis A vaccine; reactogenicity, immunogenicity, and long-term antibody persistence. J Med Virol 1994; 44:446.
86. Landrigan PJ et al. The protective efficacy of immune serum globulin in hepatitis A: a statistical approach. JAMA 1973;223:74.
87. Krugman S. Effect of human immune serum globulin on infectivity of hepatitis A virus. J Infect Dis 1976;134:70.
88. Centers for Disease Control. Prevention of hepatitis A through active or passive immunization: recommendations of the Advisory Committee on Immunization Practices (ACIP). MMWR 2002; 51(RR-2):1.
89. Lee WM. Hepatitis B virus infection. N Engl J Med 1997;337:1733.
90. Lok A et al. Management of hepatitis B: 2000—summary of a workshop. Gastroenterology 2001; 120:1828.
91. Lok A et al. Chronic hepatitis B. Hepatology 2001;34:1225.
92. Malik AH et al. Chronic hepatitis B virus infection: treatment strategies for the new millennium. Ann Intern Med 2000;132:723.
93. Locarnini S et al. The hepatitis B virus and common mutants. Semin Liver Dis 2003;23:5.
94. Kann M et al. Recent studies on replication of the hepatitis B virus. J Hepatol 1995;22(Suppl 1):9.
95. Ganem D. Hepadnaviridae: the viruses and their replication. In: Fields BN, ed. Fundamental Virology. 3rd Ed. Philadelphia: Lippincott-Raven, 1996:1199.
96. Befeler A et al. Hepatitis B. Infect Dis Clin North Am 2000;14:617.
97. McMahon B et al. A comprehensive programme to reduce the incidence of hepatitis B infection and its sequelae in Alaskan natives. Lancet 1987;2:1134.
98. Alter M. Epidemiology and prevention of hepatitis B. Semin Liver Dis 2003;23:39.
99. Perillo RP. Hepatitis B: transmission and natural history. Gut 1993;S43.
100. Rehermann B. Immune responses in hepatitis B virus infection. Semin Liver Dis 2003;23:21.
101. Guidotti, LG. Intracellular inactivation of the hepatitis B virus by cytotoxic T lymphocytes. Immunity 1996;4:25.
102. Zaaijer H et al. Comparison of methods for detection of hepatitis B virus DNA. J Clin Microbiol 1994;32:2088.
103. Ke-Qin H et al. Molecular diagnostic techniques for viral hepatitis. Gastroenterology Clin North Am 1994;23:479.
104. Koff RS. Hepatitis B today: clinical and diagnostic overview. Pediatr Infect Dis 1993;12:428.
105. Schmilovitz-Weiss H et al. Viral markers in the treatment of hepatitis B and C. Gut 1993;S26.
106. Kumar S et al. Serologic diagnosis of viral hepatitis. Postgrad Med 1992;92:55.
107. Sjogren MH. Serologic diagnosis of viral hepatitis. Gastroenter Clin North Am 1994;23:45.

108. Shakil AO et al. Fulminant hepatic failure. Surg Clin North Am 1999;79:77.
109. Hyams KC. Risks of chronicity following acute hepatitis B virus infection. Clin Infect Dis 1995; 20:992.
110. Wright TL et al. Hepatitis B virus. In Richman DD et al., eds. Clinical Virology. New York: Churchill Livingstone, 1996:663.
111. Fattovich G et al. Natural history and prognostic factors for chronic hepatitis B. Gut 1991;32:294.
112. Weissberg J et al. Survival in chronic hepatitis B: an analysis of 379 patients. Ann Intern Med 1984;101:613.
113. Beasley R. Hepatitis B: the major etiology of hepatocellular carcinoma. Cancer 1988;61:1942.
114. Fattovich G. Natural history and prognosis of hepatitis B. Semin Liv Dis 2003;23:47.
115. Lee WM. Acute liver failure Am J Med 1994; 96(Suppl 1A):3S.
116. Hoofnagle JH et al. Fulminant hepatic failure: summary of a workshop. Hepatology 1995;21:240.
117. Aldersley MA et al. Hepatic disorders. Drugs 1995;49:83.
118. Lidofsky SD et al. Intracranial pressure monitoring and liver transplantation for fulminant hepatic failure. Hepatology 1992;16:1.
119. Larsen FS et al. Brain edema in liver failure: basic physiologic principles and management. Liver Transpl 2002;8:983.
120. Gazzard BG et al. Early changes in coagulation following a paracetamol overdose and a controlled trial of fresh frozen plasma therapy. Gut 1975;16:617.
121. Pereria LMMB et al. Coagulation factor V and VIII/V ratio as predictors to outcome in paracetamol induced fulminant hepatic failure: relation to other prognostic indicators. Gut 1992;33:98.
122. Guarner F et al. Renal function in fulminant hepatic failure: hemodynamics and renal prostaglandins. Gut 1987;28:1643.
123. Roberts LR et al. Ascites and hepatorenal syndrome: pathophysiology and management. Mayo Clin Proc 1996;71:874.
124. O'Grady JG et al. Early indicators of prognosis in fulminant hepatic failure. Gastroenterology 1989;97:4439.
125. Berger RL et al. Exchange transfusion in the treatment of fulminating hepatitis. N Engl J Med 1966;274:497.
126. Denis J et al. Treatment of encephalopathy during fulminant hepatic failure by hemodialysis with high permeability membrane. Gut 1978;19:787.
127. MacDougall BR et al. H2 receptor antagonist in the prevention of acute upper gastrointestinal hemorrhage in fulminant hepatic failure: a controlled trial. Gastroenterology 1978;74:464.
128. Pauwels A et al. Emergency liver transplantation for acute liver failure: evaluation of London and Clichy criteria. J Hepatol 1993;17:124.
129. Scharschmidt B et al. Hepatitis B in patients with HIV infection: relationship to AIDS and patient survival. Ann Intern Med 1992;117:837.
130. Thio CL. Hepatitis B in the human immunodeficiency virus-infected patient: epidemiology, natural history, and treatment. Semin Liver Dis 2003; 23:125.
131. Merck and Company. Recombivax HB package insert. West Point, PA: August 1998.
132. SmithKline Beecham Pharmaceuticals. Engerix-B package insert. Philadelphia, PA: July 1998.
133. Centers for Disease Control. Recommendations of the immunization practices advisory committee (ACIP). Hepatitis B virus: a comprehensive strategy for eliminating transmission in the United States through universal childhood vaccination. MMWR 1991;40;(RR-13):1.
134. West DJ. Clinical experience with hepatitis B vaccines. Am J Infect Control 1989;17:172.
135. Ellis RW et al. Plasma-derived and yeast-derived hepatitis B vaccines. Am J Infect Control 1989; 17:181.
136. Ukena T et al. Site of injection and response to hepatitis B vaccine [letter]. N Engl J Med 1985; 313:579.

137. Dentico P et al. Long-term immunogenicity safety and efficacy of a recombinant hepatitis B vaccine in healthy adults. Eur J Epidemiol 1992;8:650.

138. Szmuness W et al. Hepatitis B vaccine: demonstration of efficacy in a controlled clinical trial in a high-risk population in the United States. N Engl J Med 1980;303:833.

139. Francis DP et al. The prevention of hepatitis B with vaccine: report of the CDC multi-center efficacy trial among homosexual men. Ann Intern Med 1982;97:362.

140. Szmuness W et al. A controlled clinical trial of the efficacy of the hepatitis B vaccine (Heptavax B): a final report. Hepatology 1981;1:377.

141. Hadler SC et al. Long-term immunogenicity and efficacy of hepatitis B vaccine in homosexual men. N Engl J Med 1986;315:209.

142. Hollinger FB et al. Response to hepatitis B vaccine in a young adult population. In: Szmuness W et al., eds. Viral Hepatitis: 1981 International Symposium. Philadelphia: Franklin Institute Press, 1982:451.

143. Coutinho RA et al. Efficacy of a heat inactivated hepatitis B vaccine in male homosexuals: outcome of a placebo controlled double blind trial. Br Med J 1983;286:1305.

144. Wainwright RB et al. Duration of immunogenicity and efficacy of hepatitis B vaccine in a Yupik Eskimo population. JAMA 1989;261:2362.

145. Stevens CE et al. Hepatitis B vaccine in patients receiving hemodialysis: immunogenicity and efficacy. N Engl J Med 1984;311:496.

146. Collier AC et al. Antibody to human immunodeficiency virus (HIV) and suboptimal response to hepatitis B vaccination. Ann Intern Med 1988;109:101.

147. Hovi L et al. Impaired response to hepatitis B vaccine in children receiving anticancer chemotherapy. Pediatr Infect Dis J 1995;14:931.

148. Wood RC et al. Risk factors for lack of detectable antibody following hepatitis B vaccination of Minnesota health care workers. JAMA 1993;270:2935.

149. Roome AJ et al. Hepatitis B vaccine responsiveness in Connecticut public safety personnel. JAMA 1993;270:2931.

150. Winter AP et al. Influence of smoking on immunological responses to hepatitis B vaccine. Vaccine 1994;12:771.

151. Jilg W et al. Immune response to hepatitis B revaccination. J Med Virol 1988;24:377.

152. Goldwater PN. Randomized, comparative trial of 20 μg vs 40 μg Engerix B vaccine in hepatitis B vaccine non-responders. Vaccine 1997;15:353.

153. Clemens R et al. Booster immunization of low- and non-responders after a standard three dose hepatitis B vaccine schedule-results of a post marketing surveillance. Vaccine 1997;15:349.

154. Boxall E, Dennis M. HBVax II in non-responders to Engerix B. Vaccine 1998;16:877.

155. Weissman JY et al. Lack of response to recombinant hepatitis B vaccine in nonresponders to the plasma vaccine. JAMA 1988;260:1734.

156. Alper CE et al. Genetic prediction of non-responsiveness to hepatitis B vaccination. N Engl J Med 1989;321:708.

157. Bush LM et al. Evaluation of initiating a hepatitis B vaccination schedule with one vaccine and completing it with another. Vaccine 1991;9:807.

158. Chan CY et al. Booster response to recombinant yeast-derived hepatitis B vaccine in vaccinees whose anti-HBs response were initially elicited by a plasma-derived vaccine. Vaccine 1991;9:765.

159. Tabor E et al. Nine-year follow-up study of a plasma-derived hepatitis B vaccine in a rural African setting. J Med Virol 1993;40:204.

160. Milne A et al. Hepatitis B vaccination in children: five year booster study. NZ Med J 1992;105:336.

161. Coursaget P et al. Twelve-year follow-up study of hepatitis B immunization of Senegalese infants. J Hepatol 1994;21:250.

162. Wainwright RB et al. Protection provided by hepatitis B vaccine in a Yupik Eskimo population: results of a 10-year study. J Infect Dis 1997;175:674.

163. Trivello R et al. Persistence of anti-HBs antibodies in health care personnel vaccinated with plasma-derived hepatitis B vaccine and response to recombinant DNA HB booster vaccine. Vaccine 1995;13:139.

164. Resti M et al. Ten-year follow-up study of neonatal hepatitis B immunization: are booster injections indicated? Vaccine 1997;15:1338.

165. Yuen MF et al. Twelve-year follow-up of a prospective randomized trial of hepatitis B recombinant DNA yeast vaccine versus plasma-derived vaccine without booster doses in children. Hepatology 1999;29:924.

166. Huang LM et al. Long term response to hepatitis B vaccination and response to booster in children born to mothers with hepatitis Be antigen. Hepatology 1999;29:954.

167. West DJ, Calandra GB. Vaccine induced immunologic memory for hepatitis B surface antigen: implications for policy on booster vaccination. Vaccine 1996;14:1019.

168. Centers for Disease Control and Prevention. Immunization of adolescents. MMWR 1996;45 (RR-13):1.

169. Szmuness W et al. Passive-active immunization against hepatitis B: immunogenicity studies in adult Americans. Lancet 1981;1:575.

170. Centers for Disease Control and Prevention. 1998 Guidelines for treatment of sexually transmitted diseases. MMWR 1998;47(RR-1):1.

171. Seeff LB et al. Type B hepatitis after needle-stick exposure: prevention with hepatitis B immune globulin. Ann Intern Med 1978;88:285.

172. Redeker AG et al. Hepatitis B immune globulin as a prophylactic measure for spouses exposed to acute type B hepatitis. N Engl J Med 1975;293:1055.

173. Xu ZY et al. Prevention of perinatal acquisition of hepatitis B virus carriage using vaccine: preliminary report of a randomized, double-blind placebo-controlled and comparative trial. Pediatrics 1985;76:713.

174. Beasley RP et al. Prevention of perinatally transmitted hepatitis B virus infections with hepatitis B immune globulin and hepatitis B vaccine. Lancet 1983;2:1099.

175. Beasley RP et al. Efficacy of hepatitis B immune globulin for prevention of perinatal transmission of the hepatitis B virus carrier state: final report of a randomized double-blind, placebo controlled trial. Hepatology 1983;3:135.

176. Wong VCW et al. Prevention of the HBsAg carrier state in newborn infants of mothers who are chronic carriers of HBsAg and HBcAg by administration of hepatitis B vaccine and hepatitis B immunoglobulin: double-blind randomized placebo-controlled study. Lancet 1984;1:921.

177. Beasley RP et al. Hepatocellular carcinoma and hepatitis B virus: a prospective study of 22,707 men in Taiwan. Lancet 1981;2:1129.

178. Beasley RP. Hepatitis B virus as the etiologic agent in hepatocellular carcinoma: epidemiologic considerations. Hepatology 1982;2(Suppl):21.

179. Stevens CE et al. Yeast-recombinant hepatitis B vaccine: efficacy with hepatitis B immune globulin in prevention of perinatal hepatitis B virus transmission. JAMA 1987;257:2612.

180. Stevens CE et al. Perinatal hepatitis B virus transmission in the United States: prevention by passive-active immunization. JAMA 1985;253:1740.

181. Centers for Disease Control and Prevention. FDA approval for a combined hepatitis A and B vaccine. MMWR 2001;50;37:806.

182. Evans AS et al. Adrenal hormone therapy in viral hepatitis: II. The effect of cortisone in the acute disease. Ann Intern Med 1953;38:1134.

183. Blum AL et al. A fortuitously controlled study of steroid therapy in acute viral hepatitis. Am J Med 1969;47:82.

184. Ware AJ et al. A controlled trial of steroid therapy in massive hepatic necrosis. Am J Gastroenterol 1974;62:130.

185. Gregory PB et al. Steroid therapy in severe viral hepatitis: a double blind, randomized trial of methyl-prednisolone versus placebo. N Engl J Med 1976;294:681.

186. European Association for the Study of the Liver (EASL). Randomized trial of steroid therapy in acute liver failure. Gut 1979;20:620.

187. Acute Hepatic Failure Study Group. Failure of specific immunotherapy in fulminant type B hepatitis. Ann Intern Med 1977;86:272.

188. Sanchez-Tapias JM et al. Recombinant α2-interferon therapy in fulminant viral hepatitis. J Hepatol 1987;5:205.

189. Hoofnagle JH. Therapy of viral hepatitis. Digestion 1998;59:563.

190. Hoofnagle JH et al. New therapies for chronic hepatitis B. J Viral Hepatitis 1997;4(Suppl 1):41.

191. Schlam SW et al. New nucleoside analogues for chronic hepatitis B. J Hepatol 1995;22(Suppl 1):52.

192. Clerq E. Perspectives for the treatment of hepatitis B virus infections. Int J Antimicrob Agents 1999;81.

193. Van Thiel DH et al. Lamivudine treatment of advanced and decompensated liver disease due to hepatitis B. Hepatogastroenterology 1997;44:808.

194. Nevens F et al. Lamivudine therapy for chronic hepatitis B: a six month randomized dose ranging study. Gastroenterology 1997;113:1258.

195. Dienstag JL et al. A preliminary trial of lamivudine for chronic hepatitis B infection. N Engl J Med 1995;25:1657.

196. Ching-lung L et al. A one year trial of lamivudine for chronic hepatitis B. N Engl J Med 1998;2:61.

197. Heathcote J. Treatment of HBe Ag-positive chronic hepatitis B. Semin Liver Dis 2003;23:69.

198. Hadziyannis SJ. Treatment of HBeAg-negative chronic hepatitis B. Semin Liver Dis 2003;23:81.

199. Malaguanrnera M et al. Interferon, cortisone, and antivirals in the treatment of chronic viral hepatitis. Pharmacotherapy 1997;17:998.

200. Saracco G et al. A practical guide to the use of interferons in the management of hepatitis virus infections. Drugs 1997;53:74.

201. Cirelli R et al. Interferons: an overview of their pharmacology. Clin Immunother 1996;5(Suppl 1):22.

202. Farber JM et al. Interferon-γ in the management of infectious diseases. Ann Intern Med 1995;123:216.

203. Hoofnagle JH et al. Randomized, controlled trial of recombinant human α-interferon in patients with chronic hepatitis B. Gastroenterology 1988;95:1318.

204. Perrillo RP et al. Prednisone withdrawal followed by recombinant alpha interferon in the treatment of chronic type B hepatitis: a randomized, controlled trial. Ann Intern Med 1988;109:95.

205. Perrillo RP et al. A randomized, controlled trial of interferon alfa-2b alone and after prednisone withdrawal for the treatment of chronic hepatitis B. N Engl J Med 1990;323:295.

206. Perez V et al. A controlled trial of high dose interferon, alone and after prednisone withdrawal, in the treatment of chronic hepatitis B: long term follow up. Gut 1993;33(Suppl):S91.

207. Korenman J et al. Long-term remission of chronic hepatitis B after alpha-interferon therapy. Ann Intern Med 1991;114:629.

208. Niederau C et al. Long-term follow-up of the HBeAg-positive patients treated with interferon alfa for chronic hepatitis B. N Engl J Med 1996;334:1422.

209. Brook MG et al. Which patients with chronic hepatitis B virus infection will respond to α-interferon therapy? A statistical analysis of predictive factors. Hepatology 1989;10:761.

210. Perrillo RP et al. Therapy for hepatitis B virus infection. Gastroenterol Clin North Am 1994;23:581.

211. Wong DKH et al. Effect of alpha interferon treatment in patients with hepatitis B e antigen-positive chronic hepatitis B: a meta-analysis. Ann Intern Med 1993;119:312.

212. Renault PF, Hoofnagle JH. Side effects of alpha interferon. Semin Liver Dis 1989;9:273.

213. Woo MH et al. Interferon alfa in the treatment of chronic viral hepatitis B and C. Ann Pharmacother 1997;31:330.

214. Perrillo RP. The management of chronic hepatitis B. Am J Med 1994;96(Suppl. 1A):34S.

215. Perrillo RP et al. Low-dose, titratable interferon alfa in decompensated liver disease caused by chronic infection with hepatitis B virus. Gastroenterology 1995;109:908.

216. Schering Corporation. Intron-A package insert. Kenilworth, NJ: May 1992.

217. Schalm SW et al. Contrasting features and responses to treatment of severe chronic active liver disease with and without hepatitis Bs antigen. Gut 1976;17:781.

218. Doong SL et al. Inhibition of the replication of hepatitis B virus in vitro by 2', 3'-dideoxy-3'-thiacytidine and related analogues. Proc Natl Acad Sci USA 1991;88:8495.

219. Jarvis B et al. Lamivudine: a review of its therapeutic potential in chronic hepatitis B. Drugs 1999;58:101.

220. Dienstag JL et al. Histological outcome during long-term lamivudine therapy. Gastroenterology 2003;124:105.

221. Dienstag JL et al. Lamivudine as initial treatment for chronic hepatitis B in the United States. N Engl J Med 1999;341:1256.

222. Honkoop P et al. Lamivudine resistance in immunocompetent chronic hepatitis B: incidence and patterns. J Hepatol 1997;26:1393.

223. Chang TT et al. Enhanced HbeAg seroconversion rates in chinese patients on lamivudine [abstract]. Hepatology 1999;30(Suppl 2):420A.

224. Lai CL et al. Prevalence and clinical correlates of YMDD variants during lamivudine therapy for patients with hepatitis B. Clin Infect Dis 2003; 36:687.

225. FDA Consum 2002;36:4.

226. Hadziyannis SJ et al. Adefovir dipivoxil for the treatment of hepatitis Be antigen-negative chronic hepatitis B. N Engl J Med 2003;348:800.

227. Marcellin P et al. Adefovir dipivoxil for the treatment of hepatitis Be antigen-positive chronic hepatitis B. N Engl J Med 2003;348:808.

228. Sommadossi J-P. Anti-hepatitis B specific L-nucleosides [abstract]. Antiviral Ther 1999;4 (Suppl 4):8.

229. Colancio JM et al. The identification and development of antiviral agents for the treatment of chronic hepatitis B infection. Prog Drug Res 1998;50:259.

230. Delaney W, et al. Evolving therapies for the treatment of chronic hepatitis B infection. Expert Opin Investig Drugs 2002;11:169.

231. Chin R et al. Two novel antiviral agents, DAPD and L-FMAU, which are active against wild type and lamivudine resistant HBV [abstract]. Hepatology 1999;30(Suppl 2):421A.

232. Gish RG et al. Emtricitabine (FTC): activity against hepatitis B virus in a phase I/II study [abstract]. Poster 83 presentation at the 39th ICAAC, September 26–29, 1999 San Francisco, California.

233. Cretton-Scott E et al. Pharmacokinetics of beta-L-thymidine and beta-L-2'-deoxycytidine in woodchucks and monkeys [abstract]. Antiviral Ther 1999;4(Suppl 4):8.

234. Bassendine MF et al. Adenine arabinoside therapy in HBsAg positive chronic liver disease: a controlled study. Gastroenterology 1981;80:1016.

235. Hoofnagle JH et al. Randomized controlled trial of adenine arabinoside monophosphate for chronic type B hepatitis. Gastroenterology 1984; 86:150.

236. Perrillo RP et al. Comparative efficacy of adenine arabinoside 5' monophosphate and prednisone withdrawal followed by adenine arabinoside 5' monophosphate in the treatment of chronic active hepatitis type B. Gastroenterology 1985;88: 780.

237. Hultgren C et al. The antiviral compound ribavirin modulates the T helper (Th) 1/Th 2 subset balance

238. Ruiz-Moreno M et al. Levamisole and interferon in children with chronic hepatitis B. Hepatology 1993;18:264.

239. Hernandez B et al. Cellular kinases involved in the phosphorylation of beta-L-thymidine and beta-L-2'-deoxycytidine, two specific anti-hepatitis B virus agents [abstract]. Antiviral Ther 1999; 4(Suppl 4):49.

240. Le Guerhier F et al. 2'3'-Dideoxy-2'3'dideoxyhydro-beta-L-fluorocytidine (beta-L-FD4C) exhibits a more potent antiviral effect than lamivudine in chronically WHV infected woodchucks [abstract]. Hepatology 1999;30(Suppl 2):421A.

241. Ying C et al. Inhibition of the replication of the DNA polymerase M550V variant of hepatitis B virus by adefovir, tenofovir, L-FMAU, DAPD, penciclovir and lobucavir [abstract]. Antiviral Ther 1999;4(Suppl 4):27.

242. Onbo-Nita SK et al. Screening of new antivirals for wild-type hepatitis B virus and three lamivudine-resistant mutants [abstract]. Antiviral Ther 1999;4(Suppl 4):33.

243. Von Weizsacker F et al. Gene therapy for chronic viral hepatitis: ribozymes, antisense oligonucleotides, and dominant negative mutants. Hepatology 1997;26:251.

244. Yalcin K et al. Comparison of 12 month courses of interferon α-2b-lamivudine combination therapy and interferon α-2b monotherapy among patients with untreated chronic hepatitis B. Clin Infect Dis 2003;36:1516.

245. Barbaro G et al. Long-term efficacy of interferon α-2b and lamivudine in combination compared to lamivudine monotherapy in patients with chronic hepatitis B. J Hepatol 2001;35:406.

246. Livingston BD et al. The hepatitis B virus-specific CTL responses induced in humans by lipopeptide vaccination are comparable to those elicited by acute viral infection. J Immunol 1997;159:1383.

247. Wright T et al. Phase I study of a potent adjuvant hepatitis B vaccine (HBV/MF59) for therapy of chronic hepatitis B [abstract]. Hepatology 1999;30(Suppl 2):421A

248. Samuel D et al. Liver transplantation in European patients with the hepatitis B surface antigen. N Engl J Med 1993;329:1842.

249. Terrault NA et al. Prophylaxis in liver transplant recipients using a fixed dosing schedule of hepatitis B immunoglobulin. Hepatology 1996;24:1327.

250. Waters J et al. Loss of the common 'a' determinant of hepatitis B surface antigen by a vaccine induced escape mutant. J Clin Invest 1992;90:2543.

251. McGory RW et al. Improved outcome of orthotopic liver transplantation for chronic hepatitis B cirrhosis with aggressive passive immunization. Transplantation 1996;9:1358.

252. Burbach GJ et al. Intravenous or intramuscular anti-HBs immunoglobulin for the prevention of hepatitis B reinfection after orthotopic liver transplantation. Transplantation 1997;63:478.

253. Poterucha JJ. Liver transplantation and hepatitis B. Ann Intern Med 1997;126:805.

254. Perrillo RP. Treatment of post-transplantation hepatitis B. Liver Transpl Surg 1997;3(Suppl 1):S8.

255. Brumage LK et al. Treatment for recurrent viral hepatitis after liver transplantation. J Hepatol 1997;26:440.

256. Bain JA et al. Efficacy of lamivudine in chronic hepatitis B patients with acute viral replication and decompensated cirrhosis undergoing liver transplantation. Transplantation 1996;10:1456.

257. Grellier L et al. Lamivudine prophylaxis against reinfection in liver transplantation for hepatitis B cirrhosis. Lancet 1996;348:1212.

258. Ling R et al. Selection of mutations in the hepatitis B virus polymerase during therapy of transplant recipients with lamivudine. Hepatology 1996;24:711.

259. Bartholomew MM et al. Hepatitis-B-virus resistance to lamivudine given for recurrent infection after orthotopic liver transplantation. Lancet 1997;349:20.

in hepatitis B and C virus-specific immune responses. J Gen Virol 1998;79:2381.

260. Wang KS et al. Structure, sequence, and expression of the hepatitis delta viral genome. Nature 1986;323:508.

261. Bean R. Latest discoveries on the infection and coinfection with hepatitis D virus. Am Clin Lab 2002;21:25.

262. Taylor JM. Hepatitis delta virus. Intervirology 1999;42:173.

263. Rizzetto M et al. Hepatitis delta virus disease. Prog Liver Dis 1986;8:417.

264. Hoofnagle JH. Type D (delta) hepatitis JAMA 1989;261:1321.

265. Lai M. The molecular biology of hepatitis delta virus. Ann Rev Biochem 1995;64:259.

266. Negro F et al. Diagnosis of hepatitis delta virus infection. J Hepatol 1995;22 (Suppl 1):136.

267. Smedile A et al. The clinical significance of hepatitis D RNA in serum as detected by a hybridization-based assay. Hepatology 1996;6:1297.

268. Govindarajun S et al. Fulminant B viral hepatitis: role of the delta agent. Gastroenterology 1984; 86:1417.

269. Rosino F et al. Interferon for HDV infection. Antiviral Res 1994;24:165.

270. Ottobrelli A et al. Patterns of delta hepatitis reinfection and disease following liver transplantation. Gastroenterology 1991;101:1649.

271. Raimondo G et al. Delta infection in hepatocellular carcinoma positive for hepatitis B surface antigen. Ann Intern Med 1984;101:343.

272. Rosina F et al. A randomized controlled trial of a 12-month course of recombinant human interferon-α in chronic delta (type D) hepatitis: a multicenter Italian study. Hepatology 1991;13:1052.

273. Farci P et al. Treatment of chronic hepatitis D with interferon alfa-2a. N Engl J Med 1994;330:88.

274. Rizzetto M et al. Chronic hepatitis in carriers of hepatitis B surface antigen, with intrahepatic expression of the delta antigen. Ann Intern Med 1983; 98:437.

275. Hadziyannis SJ. Use of α-interferon in the treatment of chronic delta hepatitis. J Hepatol 1991;13:S21.

276. Rasshofer R et al. Interference of antiviral substances with replication of hepatitis delta virus RNA in primary woodchuck hepatocytes. In Gerin J et al., eds. The Delta Hepatitis Virus. New York: Wiley Liss, 1992:223.

277. Lau DT et al. Lamivudine for chronic delta hepatitis. Hepatology 1999;30:546.

278. Madejon A et al. In vitro inhibition of the hepatitis delta virus replication mediated by interferon and trans-ribozyme or antisense probes. J Hepatol 1998;29:385.

279. Wolters LM et al. Lamivudine-high dose interferon combination therapy for chronic hepatitis B patients co-infected with the hepatitis D virus. J Viral Hepatitis 2000;7:428.

280. Seef LB et al. Appendix: The National Institutes of Health Consensus Development Conference Management of hepatitis C 2002. Clin Liver Dis 2003;7:261.

281. Stevens CE et al. Epidemiology of hepatitis C virus: a preliminary study in volunteer blood donors. JAMA 1990;263:49.

282. Alter MJ et al. Risk factors for acute non-A, non-B hepatitis in the United States and association with hepatitis C virus infection. JAMA 1990;264: 2231.

283. Centers for Disease Control and Prevention. Recommendations for prevention and control of hepatitis C virus (HCV) infection and HCV-related chronic disease. MMWR 1998;47(RR-19):1.

284. Cuthbert JA. Hepatitis C: progress and problems. Clin Micro Rev 1994;7:505.

285 Flamm SL. Chronic hepatitis C infection. JAMA 2003;289:2413.

286. Bartenschlager R. Replication of hepatitis C virus. Baillieres Clin Gastroenterol 2000;14:241.

287. Kohara M. Hepatitis C virus replication and pathogenesis. J Derm Sci 2000;22:161.

288. Alter MJ et al. The prevalence of hepatitis C virus infection in the United States. N Engl J Med 1999;341:556.

289. Donahue JG et al. The declining risk of post-transfusion hepatitis C virus infection. N Engl J Med 1992;327:369.

290. Akahane Y et al. Hepatitis C virus infection in spouses of patients with type C chronic liver disease. Ann Intern Med 1994;120:748.

291. Ohto H et al. Transmission of hepatitis C virus from mothers to infants. N Engl J Med 1994;330:744.

292. Aach RD, Kahn RA. Post-transfusion hepatitis: current perspectives. Ann Intern Med 1980;92:539.

293. Alter MJ. Epidemiology of community-acquired hepatitis C. In: Hollinger FB et al., eds. Viral Hepatitis and Liver Disease. Baltimore: Williams &Wilkins, 1991:410.

294. Kiyosawa K et al. Hepatitis C in hospital employees with needlestick injuries. Ann Intern Med 1991;115:367.

295. Gonzales-Peralta R et al. Pathogenesis of hepatocellular damage in chronic hepatitis C virus infection. Gastrointest Dis 1995;6:28.

296. Pol S et al. The changing relative prevalence of hepatitis C virus genotypes: evidence in hemodialyzed patients and kidney recipients. Gastroenterology 1995;108:581.

297. Neumann AU et al. Differences in hepatitis C virus (HCV) dynamics between HCV of genotype 1 and genotype 2 [abstract]. Hepatology 1999;30(Suppl 2):191A.

298. Mahaney K et al. Genotypic analysis of hepatitis C virus in American patients. Hepatology 1994;20:1405.

299. De Medina M et al. Hepatitis C: diagnostic assays. Semin Liver Dis 1995;15:33.

300. Centers for Disease Control and Prevention. Guidelines for laboratory testing and result reporting of antibody to hepatitis C virus. MMWR 2003;52(RR-3):1.

301. Wilber J et al. Serological and virological diagnostic tests for hepatitis C virus infection. Semin Gastro Dis 1995;6:13.

302. Gretch DR et al. Assessment of hepatitis C viremia using molecular amplification technologies: correlation and clinical implications. Ann Intern Med 1995;123:321.

303. Seef LB. Natural history of hepatitis C. Hepatology 1997;26(Suppl 1):21S

304. Chan T et al. Prevalence of hepatitis C virus infection in hemodialysis patients: a longitudinal study comparing the results of RNA and antibody assays. Hepatology 1993;17:5.

305. Chan T et al. Prospective study of hepatitis C virus infection among renal transplant recipients. Gastroenterology 1993;104:862.

306. Klauser R et al. Hepatitis C antibody in renal transplant recipients. Transplant Proc 1992;24:286.

307. Gane E. Management of chronic viral hepatitis before and after renal transplantation. Transplantation 2002;74:427.

308. Garcia G et al. Hepatitis C virus infection in the immunocompromised patient. Semin Gastro Dis 1995;6:35.

309. Ghobrial RM et al. A 10-year experience of liver transplantation for hepatitis C: analysis of factors determining outcome in over 500 patients. Ann Surg 2001;234:384.

310. Charlton M. Hepatitis C infection in liver transplantation. Am J Transplant 2001;1:197.

311. Gane EJ et al. Long-term outcome of hepatitis C infection after liver transplantation. N Engl J Med 1996;334:815.

312. Eyster ME et al. Natural history of hepatitis C virus infection in multitransfused hemophiliacs: effect of coinfection with human immunodeficiency virus: the multicenter hemophilia cohort study. J AIDS 1993;6:602.

313. Sulkowski MS et al. Hepatitis C virus infection as an opportunistic disease in persons infected with human immunodeficiency virus. Clin Infect Dis 2000;30:S77.

314. Sulkowski MS et al. Hepatitis C in the HIV-infected person. Ann Intern Med 2003;138:197.

315. Liaw YF. Hepatitis C superinfection in patients with chronic hepatitis B virus infection. J Gastroenterol 2002;37(Suppl 13):65.

316. El-Serag HB. Hepatocellular carcinoma and hepatitis C in the United States. Hepatology 2002;36(5 Suppl 1):S74.

317. Hoofnagle JH. Hepatitis C: the clinical spectrum of disease. Hepatology 1997;26(Suppl 1):15S.

318. Koof RS et al. Extrahepatic manifestations of hepatitis C. Semin Gastro Dis 1995;15:101.

319. Centers for Disease Control and Prevention. Recommendations for follow-up of health-care workers after occupational exposure to hepatitis C virus. MMWR 1997;46:603.

320. Viladomiu L et al. Interferon alfa in acute post-transfusion hepatitis C: a randomized controlled trial. Hepatology 1992;15:767.

321. Lampertico P et al. A multicenter randomized controlled trial of recombinant interferon alfa 2b in patients with acute transfusion-related hepatitis C. Hepatology 1994;19:19.

322. Jaeckel E et al. Treatment of acute hepatitis C with interferon alfa-2b. N Engl J Med 2001;245:1452.

323. Davis GL et al. Treatment of chronic hepatitis with recombinant interferon alfa: a multicenter randomized, controlled trial. N Engl J Med 1991;321:1501.

324. Di Bisceglie AM et al. Recombinant interferon alfa therapy for chronic hepatitis C: a randomized, double-blind, placebo-controlled trial. N Engl J Med 1989;321:1506.

325. Saracco G et al. A randomized controlled trial of interferon alfa-2b as therapy for chronic nonA nonB hepatitis. J Hepatol 1990;11:S43.

326. Weiland O et al. Therapy of chronic post-transfusion nonA nonB hepatitis with interferon alfa-2b: Swedish experience. J Hepatol 1990;11(Suppl 1):S57.

327. Gomez-Rubio M et al. Prolonged treatment (18 months) of chronic hepatitis C with recombinant alfa-interferon in comparison with a control group. J Hepatol 1990;11:S63.

328. Marcellin P et al. Recombinant human alfa-interferon in patients with chronic nonA nonB hepatitis C: a multicenter randomized controlled trial from France. Hepatology 1991;13:393.

329. Saez-Royuela F et al. High dose of recombinant alfa-interferon or gamma-interferon for chronic hepatitis C: a randomized controlled trial. Hepatology 1991;13:327.

330. Causse X et al. Comparison of 1 or 3 MU of interferon-alfa 2b and placebo in patients with chronic nonAnonB hepatitis. Gastroenterology 1991;101:497.

331. Reichen J et al. Fixed versus titrated interferon-alfa 2B in chronic hepatitis C: a randomized controlled multicenter trial. The Swiss Association for the study of the liver. J Hepatol 1996;25:275.

332. Poynard T et al. A comparison of three interferon alfa-2b regimens for the long-term treatment of chronic nonA, nonB hepatitis. N Engl J Med 1995;332:1457.

333. Diodati G et al. Treatment of chronic hepatitis C with recombinant interferon alfa-2a: results of a randomized controlled clinical trial. Hepatology 1994;19:1.

334. Negro F et al. Continuous versus intermittent therapy for chronic hepatitis C with recombinant interferon alfa-2a. Gastroenterology 1994;107:479.

335. Chemello L et al. Randomized trial comparing three different regimens of alpha-2a interferon in chronic hepatitis C. Hepatology 1995;22:700.

336. Imai Y et al. Recombinant interferon-α-2a for treatment of chronic hepatitis C: results of a multicenter randomized controlled dose study. Liver 1997;17:88.

337. Rumi et al. A prospective randomized comparing lymphoblastoid interferon to recombinant interferon alfa 2a as therapy for chronic hepatitis C. Hepatology 1996;24:1366.

338. Farrell GC et al. Lymphoblastoid interferon alfa-n1 improves the long-term response to a 6-month course of treatment in chronic hepatitis C compared with recombinant interferon alfa-2b: results of an international randomized controlled trial. Hepatology 1998;27:1121.

339. McHutchison JG et al. Interferon alfa-2b alone or in combination with ribavirin as initial treatment for chronic hepatitis C. N Engl J Med 1998; 339:1485.

340. Reichard O et al. Randomised, double-blind, placebo-controlled trial of interferon α-2b with and without ribavirin for chronic hepatitis C. Lancet 1998;351:83.

341. Poynard T et al. Randomised trial of interferon α2b plus ribavirin for 48 weeks or for 24 weeks versus interferon α2b plus placebo for 48 weeks for treatment of chronic infection with hepatitis C virus. Lancet 1998;352:1426.

342. Davis GL et al. Interferon alfa-2b alone or in combination with ribavirin for the treatment of relapse of chronic hepatitis C. N Engl J Med 1998; 339:1493.

343. Iino S et al. Treatment of chronic hepatitis C with high-dose interferon α-2b: a multicenter study. Dig Dis Sci 1993;38:612.

344. Reichard O et al. High sustained response rate and clearance of viremia after treatment with interferon α2b for 60 weeks. Hepatology 1994;19:280.

345. Picciotto A et al. Interferon therapy in chronic hepatitis C: evaluation of a low dose maintenance schedule in responder patients. J Hepatol 1993; 17:359.

346. Lee WM. Therapy of hepatitis C: interferon alfa-2a trials. Hepatology 1997;26(Suppl 1):89S.

347. Farrell GC. Therapy of hepatitis C: interferon alfa-n1 trials. Hepatology 1997;26(Suppl 1):96S.

348. Keefe. Therapy of hepatitis C: consensus interferon trials. Hepatology 1997;26(Suppl 1):101S.

349. Tong MJ et al. Treatment of chronic hepatitis C with consensus interferon: a multicenter, randomized, controlled trial. Hepatology 1997;26:747.

350. Calleri G et al. Natural beta interferon in acute type-C hepatitis patients: a randomized controlled trial. Ital J Gastroenterology Hepatology 1998; 30:181.

351. McHutchison JG et al. Predicting response to initial therapy with interferon plus ribavirin in chronic hepatitis C using serum HCV RNA results during therapy. J Viral Hepatitis 2001;8:414.

352. McHutchison JG. Hepatitis C advances in antiviral therapy: what is accepted treatment now. J Gastroenterol Hepatol 2002;17:431.

353. McHutchison JG. Current therapy for hepatitis C: pegylated interferon and ribavirin. Clin Liver Dis 2002;7:149.

354. Baker DE. Pegylated Interferons. Rev Gastro Disord 2001;2:87

355. Luxon BA et al. Pegylated interferons for the treatment of chronic hepatitis C infection. Clin Ther 2002;24:1363.

356. Perry CM. Peginterferon alfa2a (40kD): a review of its use in the management of chronic hepatitis C. Drugs 2001;61:2263.

357. Linsay KL et al. A randomized, double-blind trial comparing pegylated interferon alfa-2b to interferon alfa-2b as initial treatment for chronic hepatitis C. Hepatology 2001;34:395.

358. Manns MP et al. Peginterferon alfa-2b plus ribavirin compared with interferon alfa-2b plus ribavirin for initial treatment of chronic hepatitis C: a randomised trial. Lancet 2001;358:958.

359. Zeuzem S et al. Peginterferon alfa-2a in patients with chronic hepatitis C. N Engl J Med 2000; 343:1666.

360. Heathcote EJ et al. Peginterferon alfa-2a in patients with chronic hepatitis C and cirrhosis. N Engl J Med 2000;343:1673.

361. Fried MW et al. Peginterferon alfa-2a plus ribavirin for chronic hepatitis C virus infection. New Engl J Med 2002;347:975.

362. Saracco G et al. A randomized 4-arm multicenter study of interferon alfa-2b plus ribavirin in the treatment of patients with chronic hepatitis C relapsing after interferon monotherapy. Hepatology 2002;36:959.

363. Arber N et al. Elevated serum iron predicts response to interferon treatment in patients with chronic HCV infection. Dig Dis Sci 1995; 40:2431.

364. Shinichi K et al. Efficacy of combination therapy of interferon-α with ursodeoxycholic acid in chronic hepatitis C: a randomized controlled trial. J Gastroenterol 1997;32:56.

365. Sherman KE et al. Combination therapy with thymosin alpha 1 and interferon for the treatment of chronic hepatitis C infection: a randomized, placebo-controlled double-blind trial. Hepatology 1998;27:1128.

366. Van Thiel DH et al. A preliminary experience with GM-CSF plus interferon in patients with HBV and HCV resistant to interferon therapy. J Viral Hepatitis 1997;4(Suppl 1):101.

367. Smith JP. Treatment of chronic hepatitis C with amantadine-hydrochloride [abstract]. Gastroenterology 1996;110:A1330.

368. Andreone P et al. Interferon alpha increases prostaglandin E2 production by cultured liver biopsy in patients with chronic viral hepatitis: can non-steroidal anti-inflammatory drugs improve the response to interferon? J Hepatol 1993; 19:228.

369. Lebovics E et al. Pentoxifylline enhances response of chronic hepatitis C to interferon α-2b: a double-blind randomized controlled trial [abstract]. Hepatology 1996;24:402A.

370. Parola M et al. Vitamin E dietary supplementation protects against carbon tetrachloride-induced chronic liver damage and cirrhosis. Hepatology 1992;16:1014.

371. Gross JB et al. Vitamin E or omega-3 fatty acid concentrate (Omacor) as suppressive treatment for patients with chronic hepatitis [abstract]. Hepatology 1999;30(Suppl 2):191A.

372. Van Rossim TGJ et al. Review article: glycyrrhizin as a potential treatment for chronic hepatitis C. Aliment Pharmacol Ther 1998;12:199.

373. Pares A et al. Effects of silymarin in alcoholic patients with cirrhosis of the liver: results of a controlled, double-blind, randomized and multicenter trial. J Hepatol 1998;28:615.

374. Kayano K et al. Inhibitory effects of the herbal medicine Sho-saiko-to (TJ-9) on cell proliferation and pro-collagen gene expression in cultured rat hepatic stellate cells. J Hepatol 1998;29:642.

375. Nelson DR et al. A pilot study of recombinant human interleukin 10 (Tenovil) in patients with chronic hepatitis C who failed interferon-based therapy [abstract]. Hepatology 1999;30(Suppl 2):189A.

376. Davis GL et al. Future options for the management of hepatitis C. Semin Liver Dis 1999; 19(Suppl 1):103.

377. McHutchison JG et al. Future therapy of hepatitis C. Hepatology 2002;36:S245.

378. Bisceglie AM. Hepatitis C-virology and future antiviral targets. Am J Med 1999;107:45S.

379. Delpha E et al. Therapeutic vaccination of chronically infected chimpanzees with the hepatitis C virus E1 protein [abstract]. Antiviral Ther 1999;4(Suppl 4):12.

380. Wright H et al. Preliminary experience with α-2b-interferon therapy in viral hepatitis in allograft recipients. Transplantation 1992;53:121.

381. Wright T et al. Interferon-alpha therapy for hepatitis C virus infection after liver transplantation. Hepatology 1994;20:773.

382. Sheiner PA et al. The efficacy of prophylactic interferon alfa-2b in preventing recurrent hepatitis C after liver transplantation. Hepatology 1998;28:831.

383. Feray C et al. An open trial of interferon alfa recombinant for hepatitis C after liver transplantation. Hepatology 1995;22:1084.

384. Bizollon T et al. Pilot study of the combination of interferon alfa and ribavirin as therapy of recurrent hepatitis C after liver transplantation. Hepatology 1997;26:500.

385. Gane E et al. A randomized study comparing ribavirin and interferon alfa monotherapy for hepatitis C recurrence after liver transplantation. Hepatology 1998;27:1403.

386. Gane E. Pre- and post-transplant treatment of hepatitis C. J Gastroenterol Hepatol 2000; 15 (Suppl:E):187.

387. Mast EE, Krawczynski K. Hepatitis E: an overview. Annu Rev Med 1996;47:257.

388. Bradley DW. Hepatitis E virus: a brief review of the biology, molecular virology, and immunology of a novel virus. J Hepatol 1995;22(Suppl 1):140.

389. Purdy MA et al. Hepatitis E. Gastroenterol Clin North Am 1994;23:537.

390. Khuroo M et al. Spectrum of hepatitis E virus infection in India. J Med Virol 1990;43:281.

391. Mast E et al. Hepatitis E: an overview. Annu Rev Med 1996;47:257.

392. Tsega E et al. Acute sporadic viral hepatitis in Ethiopia: causes, risk factors, and effects on pregnancy. Clin Infect Dis 1992;14:961.

393. Longer C et al. Experimental hepatitis E: pathogenesis in cynomolgus macaques (Macaca fascicularis). J Infect Dis 1992;168:602.

394. Chauhan A et al. Hepatitis E virus transmission to a volunteer. Lancet 1993;1:149.

395. Khuroo M et al. Hepatitis E and long term antibody status. Lancet 1993;2:1355.

396. Tucker TJ, Smuts HE. Review of the epidemiology, molecular characterization and tropism of the hepatitis G virus/GBV-C. Clinica Laborio 2001;47:239.

397. Halasz R et al. GB virus C/hepatitis G virus. Scand J Infect Dis 2001;33:572.

398. Tucker TJ et al. GBV/HGV genotypes: proposed nomenclature for genotypes 1-5. J Med Virol 2000;62:82.

399. Frey SE et al. Evidence for probable sexual transmission of the hepatitis G virus. Clin Infect Dis 2002;34:1033.

400. Lazdina U et al. Humoral and cellular immune response to the GBV virus C/hepatitis G virus envelope 2 protein. J Med Virol 2000;62:334.

401. Schlueter V et al. Reverse transcription PCR detection of hepatitis G virus. J Clin Microbiol 1996;34:2660.

402. Matsumura MM et al. Hepatitis G virus coinfection influences the liver histology of patients with chronic hepatitis C. Liver 2000;20:397.

403. Kapoor RK et al. Clinical implications of hepatitis G virus (HGV) infection in patients of acute viral hepatitis and fulminant hepatic failure. Int J Med Res 2000;112:121.

Parasitic Infections

J.V. Anandan

MALARIA

Distribution and Mortality

Malaria is considered the world's most important parasitic disease, responsible for an estimated 300 to 500 million cases and annual deaths in excess of 2 million.[1-3] Approximately 7 million U.S. travelers visit malaria-endemic areas each year. The distribution of the four *Plasmodium* species of malaria varies worldwide, with *Plasmodium falciparum,* which has the highest mortality, primarily acquired in sub-Saharan Africa, Haiti, the Dominican Republic, the Amazon region in South America, and parts of Asia and Oceania.

Life Cycle

Malarial infection is transmitted by the female mosquito of the genus *Anopheles,* which injects the asexual forms or sporozoites into the human host during a blood meal. After a lapse of about 9 to 16 days and an asexual multiplication stage in the liver called exoerythrocytic schizogony, daughter cells, or merozoites, are released into the blood to infect red blood cells (RBCs). The merozoites develop into the characteristic ring or trophozoite forms in RBCs and then go through another asexual reproductive stage called erythrocytic schizogony to produce more merozoites. When the infected red blood cells rupture, the merozoites invade new blood cells and repeat the erythrocyte cycle. In 1 or 2 weeks, a subpopulation of merozoites differentiates into the sexual forms, resulting in male and female gametocytes. If the gametocytes in the host blood are ingested by a female *Anopheles* mosquito during a blood meal, fertilization and an asexual division in the mosquito midgut will propagate the infective sporozoites to complete the cycle.

The characteristic malarial paroxysms of chills and fever in patients usually coincide with the periodic release of merozoites and other pyrogens in the blood. In *P. falciparum* infections, this periodicity may not always be apparent (Fig. 74-1). However, intervals of 48 hours between paroxysms are reported for *Plasmodium vivax, Plasmodium ovale,* and *P. falciparum* (tertian periodicity), and 72 hours for *Plasmodium malariae* (quartan periodicity). Unlike infections caused by *P. falciparum* and *P. malariae,* infections with *P. vivax* and *P. ovale* have a latent form of the exoerythrocytic phase that can persist in the host liver for months to years. This latent form can produce relapses of erythrocytic infection.

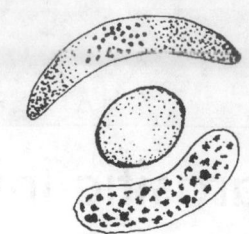

FIGURE 74-1 *P. falciparum* gametocytes.

Epidemiology

Although malaria is epidemic to the tropics, approximately 1,402 cases were diagnosed in the United States in 2000.[4] Of the 825 U.S. civilians who acquired malaria while abroad, 190 (23%) reported that they had been on a chemoprophylaxis regimen recommended by the Centers for Disease Control and Prevention (CDC). Malaria transmission in the United States has occurred from the blood of immigrants and travelers, local transmission, military personnel, and rarely through blood transfusions.[2,5–8] In terms of the species of *Plasmodium* identified in the United States, 43.6% represented *P. falciparum,* and >75% of these infections were acquired in Africa.[4] Transfusion malaria often is the result of *P. malariae,* which can persist in the blood without symptoms for extended periods.[9] Malaria also can be transmitted congenitally and through contaminated needles.[8]

Drug Resistance

Chloroquine-resistant *P. falciparum* (CRPF) is widespread and present in all malaria-endemic areas of the world except Mexico, the Caribbean, Central America (north of the Panama Canal), Haiti, the Dominican Republic, and parts of the Middle East.[10–12] However, *P. falciparum* malaria, resistant to chloroquine and mefloquine, has been isolated to Thailand, Cambodia, and Myanmar (Burma). Chloroquine-resistant *P. vivax* is an emerging problem in Papua New Guinea, Irian Jaya (Indonesia), Myanmar, and Columbia.[10–14] Most fatal cases of imported malaria in the United States are the result of travelers' failure to comply with appropriate chemosuppressive regimens, delays in seeking treatment, misdiagnosis by physicians or laboratories, and inappropriate antimalarial regimens.[2,10] Prophylactic drug regimens for individuals traveling to endemic areas are problematic (see Question 5).[10–16]

Acute Malaria

Signs and Symptoms

1. **A.R., a 26-year-old male student, presents to the emergency department (ED) with complaints of malaise, myalgia, headache, and fever of 4 days' duration. The native of Kenya, West Africa, recently visited his parents and returned to the United States 3 weeks ago. Two days before admission, he had an abrupt onset of coldness and chills, followed 1 hour later by a high fever, headache, nausea, and vomiting. The episode of chills and fever lasted about 24 hours, after which he became asymptomatic. On the afternoon of admission, he again had a bout of chills that preceded a fever of 40°C.**

Physical examination reveals a slender Black male who is acutely ill and complaining of severe abdominal pain. Abdominal examination reveals a soft, tender spleen that is slightly enlarged. Blood pressure (BP) is 110/70 mm Hg; pulse, 120 beats/min, respiration rate, 32 breaths/min, and temperature, 40°C. Laboratory findings include hemoglobin (Hgb), 11 g/dL (normal, 12 to 16); hematocrit (Hct), 34% (normal, 36% to 47%); white blood cell (WBC) count, 3,300 cells/mm³ (normal, 4,000 to 11,000) with 76% neutrophils (normal, 45% to 65%), 23% lymphocytes (normal, 15% to 35%), and 1% monocytes (normal, 1% to 6%); platelets 83 × 10³/mm³ (normal, 150 to 450); and bilirubin 1.0 mg/dL (normal, 0.1 to 1). Urinalysis reveals trace amounts of albumin and the presence of urobilinogen. Thick and thin films of A.R.'s blood are prepared. A Giemsa stain of the thin film demonstrates *P. falciparum* gametocytes. Why is the presentation of A.R. consistent with *P. falciparum* malaria?

[SI units: Hgb, 110 g/L (normal, 120 to 160); Hct, 0.34 (0.36 to 0.47); WBC count, 3.3 × 10⁹/L (normal, 4 to 11) with 0.76 neutrophils (normal, 0.45 to 0.65), 0.23 lymphocytes (normal, 0.15 to 0.35), 0.01 monocytes (normal, 0.01 to 0.06); platelets, 83 × 10⁹/L (normal, 150 to 450); bilirubin, 18 μmol/L (normal, 2 to 18)]

A.R. recently visited Kenya, West Africa, where *P. falciparum* is endemic.[8,17,18] *P. vivax* malaria accounts for about 60% of all cases of malaria reported in the United States. However, the prevalence of *P. falciparum* malaria has been increasing and accounts for about 43% of all malarial cases.[4] The incubation period for *P. falciparum* is 8 to 12 days, and infected persons usually experience prodromal symptoms (primarily headache, muscle aches and pains, malaise, nausea, and vomiting) the second week after exposure.[8,17] This time frame is consistent with A.R.'s onset of symptoms. However, the incubation period and the onset of primary symptoms for *P. falciparum* malaria can be delayed for months.[17,19] History of travel to an endemic area, the typical paroxysmal episode of chills and fever, thrombocytopenia and jaundice, and the identification of *P. falciparum* gametocytes in A.R.'s blood confirm the diagnosis of malaria.

Treatment

2. **How should the *P. falciparum* malaria in A.R. be treated? How would A.R.'s treatment differ from that used for other *Plasmodium* species?**

P. falciparum malaria is the most severe form of malaria and has the highest mortality rate.[8,17,19–25] The fever spikes, unlike those associated with *P. vivax* and *P. ovale* malaria, normally are very high (40° to 41°C), and complications (including confusion, vomiting, diarrhea, severe abdominal pain, hypoglycemia, renal failure, and encephalopathy) are common.[17–22]

QUINIDINE AND QUININE

A.R. is very ill and may be unable to tolerate oral medications because of nausea and vomiting. He should be admitted to an acute care unit and started on intravenous (IV) quinidine gluconate.[8,10,17,26,27] For doses of IV quinidine, see Table 74-1. If >48 hours of parenteral therapy is required, the dosage of quinidine should be reduced by one third to one half.[19]

Because IV quinidine is not routinely used in cardiology care, it may not be available in all hospitals. Because of the serious nature of *P. falciparum* malaria, small stocks of the drug should be kept on hand, or a procedure needs to be established in the hospital to acquire IV quinidine on short notice from an alternative source.[26] Oral quinine and clindamycin may be used until IV quinidine is available.[8,26]

Table 74-1   Drug Therapy of Parasitic Infection[2,12,19,26,31,37,39,40,43,64,74,81,106,132,139]

Drug of Choice	Dosage	Adverse Effects
Amebiasis (Including Cyst Passers)		
Asymptomatic		
Iodoquinol	*Adults:* 650 mg PO TID × 20 days	Rash, acne, thyroid enlargement
or	*Children:* 30–40 mg/kg per day PO TID × 20 days	
Diloxanide furoate	*Adults:* 500 mg PO TID × 10 days	Flatulence, abdominal pain
or	*Children:* 20 mg/kg per day PO TID × 10 days	
Paromomycin	*Adults:* 25–35 mg/kg/day PO TID × 7 days	Nausea, vomiting
	Children: Same as adults	
Mild to Moderate Gastrointestinal Disease		
Metronidazole	*Adults:* 750 mg PO TID × 10 days	Nausea, headache, metallic taste, disulfiram reac-
followed by	*Children:* 35–50 mg/kg per day PO TID × 10 days	tion with alcohol, paresthesia
Iodoquinol	*Adults:* 650 mg PO TID × 20 days	Rash, acne, thyroid enlargement
	Children: 30–40 mg/kg per day PO TID × 20 days	
Severe Gastrointestinal Disease		
Metronidazole	*Adults:* 750 mg PO TID × 10 days	Nausea, headache, metallic taste, disulfiram reac-
followed by	*Children:* 35–50 mg/kg per day PO TID × 10 days	tion with alcohol, paresthesia
Iodoquinol	*Adults:* 650 mg PO TID × 20 days	Rash, acne, thyroid enlargement
	Children: 30–40 mg/kg per day PO TID × 20 days	
Alternatives		
Dehydroemetine	*Adults:* 1–1.5 mg/kg per day IM × 5 days (max, 90 mg/day)	Arrhythmias, hypotension; ECG: P-R, Q-T, QRS
followed by	*Children:* Same as adults	prolongation, S-T depression
Iodoquinol	*Adults:* 650 mg PO TID × 20 days	Rash, acne, thyroid enlargement
	Children: 35–40 mg/kg per day PO TID × 20 days	
Amebic Liver Abscess		
Metronidazole	*Adults:* 750 mg PO TID × 10 days	Nausea, headache, metallic taste, disulfiram reac-
followed by	*Children:* 35–50 mg/kg per day PO TID × 10 days	tion with alcohol, paresthesia
Iodoquinol	*Adults:* 650 mg PO TID × 20 days	Rash, acne, thyroid enlargement
or	*Children:* 30–40 mg/kg per day PO TID × 20 days	
Alternatives		
Dehydroemetine	*Adults:* 1–1.5 mg/kg per day IM × 5 days (max, 90 mg/day)	Arrhythmias, hypotension; ECG: P-R, Q-T, QRS
followed by	*Children:* Same as adult	prolongation, S-T depression
Diloxanide furoate	*Adults:* 500 mg PO TID × 10 days	
or	*Children:* 20 mg/kg per day PO TID × 10 days	
Paromomycin	*Adults:* 25–30 mg/kg per day PO TID × 7 days	Nausea, vomiting
	Children: Same as adults	
Ascariasis (Roundworm)		
Albendazole	*Adults/Pediatric:* 400 mg once	Nausea and headache
or		
Mebendazole	*Adults and children:* 100 mg BID PO × 3 days	Diarrhea, abdominal pain
Enterobiasis (Pinworm)		
Pyrantel pamoate	*Adults and children:* 11 mg/kg PO once (max, 1 g), repeat in 2 wk	
or		
Albendazole	*Adult/Pediatric:* 400 mg once; Repeat in 2 weeks	
Filariasis		
Diethylcarbamazine	*Adults:* Day 1, 50 mg PO; day 2, 50 mg TID; day 3, 100 mg TID; days 4–14, 6 mg/kg per day in 3 doses	Severe allergic/febrile reactions, gastrointestinal disturbance, rarely encephalopathy
	Children: Day 1, 25–50 mg; day 2, 25–50 mg TID; day 3, 50–100 mg TID; days 4–14, 6 mg/kg per day in 3 doses	

continued

Table 74-1   Drug Therapy of Parasitic Infection[2,12,19,26,31,37,39,40,43,64,74,81,106,132,139] **—cont'd**

Drug of Choice	Dosage	Adverse Effects
Flukes (Trematodes)[a]		
Praziquantel	*Adults and children:* 75 mg/kg per day in 3 doses × 1 day (exceptions: *C. sinensis* and *P. westermani,* × 2 days)	Malaise, headache, dizziness, sedation, fever, eosinophilia
Giardiasis		
Metronidazole *or*	*Adults:* 250 mg PO TID with meals × 5 days *Children:* 15 mg/kg per day PO TID × 5 days	Nausea, headache, metallic taste, disulfiram reaction with alcohol, paresthesia
Quinacrine[b]	*Adult:* 100 mg PO TID × 5 days *Pediatric:* 2 mg/kg TID × 5 days (Maximum 300 mg/day)	Gastrointestinal yellow staining of skin and psychosis

Nitazoxanide[c]	*Pediatric:* 12–47 months
	  100 mg (5 ml) Q 12 hr × 3 days
	  4–11 yr
	  200 mg (10 ml) Q 12 hr × 3 days
		Abdominal pain, diarrhea, vomiting and headache

Hookworm		
Mebendazole	*Adults and children:* 100 mg PO BID × 3 days	Diarrhea, abdominal pain
Lice		
1% Permethrin (NIX)	Topical administration	Occasional allergic reaction, mild stinging, erythema
Leishmaniasis		
Sodium stibogluconate	*Adult:* 20 mg SB/kg IV or IM × 20–28 days *Pediatric:* Same as adult	Gastrointestinal, malaise, headache arthralgias, myalgias, anemia, neutropenia, thrombocytopenia; ECG abnormalities (St- and T-wave changes)
or Liposomal Amphotericin B	*Adult:* 3 mg/kg/day (days 1–5) And 3 mg/kg/days 4 & 21 *Pediatric:* Same as adult	Hypotension, chills, headache, anemia, thrombocytopenia, fever, and ↑ serum creatinine
Malaria		
All Plasmodia Except Chloroquine-Resistant		
PARENTERAL THERAPY		
Quinidine gluconate	*Adults:* Loading dose 10 mg/kg of salt (6.2 mg base) diluted in 250 mL normal saline and infused IV over 2 hr, followed by a continuous IV infusion of 0.02 mg/kg/min (0.012 mg base) for 72 hr; switch to oral quinine 650 mg Q 8 hr as soon as possible Pediatric: Same as adult	ECG: Q-T and QRS prolongation; hypotension, syncope, arrhythmias; cinchonism
ORAL THERAPY		
Chloroquine Phosphate	*Adult:* 1 g (600 mg base), then 500 mg 6 hr later, then 500 mg at 24 and 48 hours later. *Pediatric:* 10 mg base (max. 600 mg base) then 5 mg base/kg 6 hr later, then 5 mg/base at 24 and 48 hr	Gastrointestinal, headache, pruritus, malaise, and cinchonism
Chemoprophylasis		
Chloroquine phosphate	*Adult:* 500 mg (base) once weekly (beginning 1–2 wks before departure and continuing through stay and up to 4 wks after returning) *Pediatric:* 5 mg/kg base once weekly Up to adult dose (300 mg base)	Dose-related: vertigo, nausea, dizziness, lightheadedness, headache, visual disturbances, toxic psychosis and seizures
Chloroquine Resistant Therapy (CRF)		
Mefloquine *or*	*Adult:* 750 mg followed by 500 mg 12 hr later *Pediatric:* 15 mg/kg followed 8–12 hr later by 10 mg/kg	Nausea, vomiting, abdominal pain, arthralgias, chills, dizziness, tinnitus and A-V block

Atovaquone/ proguanil	*Adult:* 2 tablets BID × 3 days
	Pediatric: 11–20 kg: 1 adult tablet/day × 3 days
	  21–30 kg: 2 adult tablets/day × 3 days
	  31–40 kg: 3 adult tablets/day × 3 days
	  >40 kg: 2 adult tablets BID × 3 days	

Table 74-1 **Drug Therapy of Parasitic Infection**[2,12,19,26,31,37,39,40,43,64,74,81,106,132,139]—cont'd

Drug of Choice	Dosage	Adverse Effects
Chemoprophylaxis-CRF		

Mefloquine	*Adult:* 250 mg once weekly
	  Beginning 1–2 weeks before departure, continuing through stay and
	  for 1–4 wk after return
	Pediatric: <15 kg: 5 mg/kg once weekly
	  15–19 kg: 1/4 tablet once weekly
	  20–30 kg: 1/2 tablet once weekly
	  31–45 kg: 3/4 tablet once weekly	

or Doxycycline	>45 kg: 1 tablet once weekly *Adult:* 100 mg daily beginning 1–2 days before departure continuing during stay and 1 wk after return	Nausea, diarrhea and monilial rash
Quinine sulfate	*Adults:* 650 PO TID × 3 days	Cinchonism
plus Pyrimethamine- sulfadoxine (Fansidar)	*Children:* 25 mg/kg per day PO TID × 3 days *Adults:* 3 tablets at once (withhold until febrile episode) *Children:* 1/2–2 tablets (depends on age)[c]	Gastrointestinal, erythema multiforme, Stevens-Johnson syndrome, toxic epidermal necrolysis
or Mefloquine	*Adults:* 1,250 mg once *Children:* 25 mg/kg once (>45 kg)	Dose-related: vertigo, nausea, dizziness, lightheadedness, headache, visual disturbances, toxic psychosis seizures
Prevention of Relapses (*P. vivax* and *P. ovale*)		
Primaquine phosphate	*Adults:* 26.3 mg/day (15 mg base) × 14 days; this follows chloroquine or mefloquine regimen	Abdominal cramps, nausea, hemolytic anemia in G6PD
Scabies		
5% Permethrin (Elimite cream)	Topical administration	Rash, edema, erythema
Alternatives		
Ivermectin Lindane (Kwell)	*Adult:* 200 mg/kg PO; repeat in 2 wks Apply topically once.	Nausea, diarrhea, dizziness vertigo and pruritus Not recommended in pregnant women, infants, and patients with massively excoriated skin Local skin irritation
Crotamiton 10% (Eurax)	Topically	
Tapeworm[d]		
Praziquantel	*Adults and children:* 5–10 mg/kg PO × 1 dose	Malaise, headache, dizziness, sedation, eosinophilia, fever
Hydatid Cysts[e]		
Albendazole	*Adults:* 400 mg BID × 8–30 days, repeat if necessary *Children:* 15 mg/kg/day × 28 days, repeat if necessary (surgical resection may precede drug therapy)	Diarrhea, abdominal pain, rarely hepatotoxicity, leukopenia
Trichomoniasis		
Metronidazole	*Adults:* 2 g PO × 1 day or 250 mg PO TID × 7 days *Children:* 15 mg/kg per day PO TID × 7 days	Nausea, headache, metallic taste, disulfiram reaction with alcohol, paresthesia

[a]*Schistosoma haematobium, S. mansoni, S. japonicum, Clonorichis sinensi, Paragonimus westermani.*
[b]Quinacrine is available in the United States: Panorama Compounding Pharmacy, Van Nuys, CA 91406
[c]Same dose is recommended in children with *Cryptosporium parvum*
[d]*Diphyllobothrium latum* (fish), *Taenia solium* (pork), and *Dipylidium caninum* (dog), except for *Hymenolepis nana* where the dose is 25 mg/kg × 1 dose.
[e]*Echinococcus granulosus, Echinococcus multilocularis.* For neurocysticercosis: 400 mg BID × 8–30 days
BID, twice daily; ECG, electrocardiograph; G6PD, glucose-6-phosphate dehydrogenase; IM, intramuscularly; PO, orally; TID, three times daily.

While receiving the IV quinidine, A.R.'s electrocardiogram and BP should be monitored closely.[8,10,19] Supportive care, including fluid and electrolyte management, dialysis, blood transfusion, and mechanically assisted ventilation, are important adjunctive therapies in seriously ill patients. The serum concentration of quinidine should be determined once daily during the continuous infusion. Quinidine levels should remain between 6.1 and 18.5 μmol/dL. The quinidine infusion should be slowed or stopped if the QRS complex exceeds 25% of baseline, if hypotension is unresponsive to fluid challenge, or if the quinidine serum concentration is >18.5 μmol/dL.[17] When A.R. can be switched to oral therapy, he should receive oral quinine sulfate 650 mg Q 8 hr to complete 3 days of therapy.[17,19,26] The quinine is administered for 7 days if *P. falciparum* is acquired in Thailand.[19,26]

MANAGING CHLOROQUINE-RESISTANT *PLASMODIUM FALCIPARUM*

If A.R. does not respond to the quinidine or quinine regimen within 48 to 72 hours (i.e., failure to reduce parasitemia to <1% and continued fever over this period), other adjunctive therapies must be considered.[19,26] One of the recommended drug treatments for CRPF infection is three tablets of the combination of 25 mg pyrimethamine and 500 mg sulfadoxine (Fansidar) as a single dose on the third day of the quinine regimen; quinine would be discontinued on the third day. Other alternatives added to quinine therapy include doxycycline 100 mg twice daily for 7 days (doxycycline should overlap the quinine for 2 to 3 days before the latter is discontinued) or clindamycin 900 mg three times a day for 5 days.[26] If the patient cannot tolerate oral doxycycline, IV doxycycline 100 mg Q 12 hr can be substituted.[17] An alternative in a patient who can tolerate oral therapy and in whom it is not contraindicated (i.e., history of seizures, or endemic area where *P. falciparum* is not resistant to the agent) is mefloquine 750 mg initially, followed by 500 mg 12 hours later.[26] Recently, the combination of atovaquone 250 mg and proguanil 100 mg (Malarone) has been approved, and this can be administered to A.R. The dose of Malarone is two tablets twice daily for 3 days.[12,26] Although exchange transfusion as been suggested as an adjunct therapy for serious *P. falciparum* malaria, the role of this intervention remains questionable.[22]

MANAGING OTHER *PLASMODIA* SPECIES

A patient infected with one of the other species of *Plasmodia* (*P. vivax, P. ovale,* or *P. malariae*) should receive oral chloroquine phosphate (Aralen). The initial dose is 1 g (600 mg base) followed by 500 mg (300 mg base) 6 hours later; subsequently, 500 mg (300 mg base) is administered daily for 2 days.[26] For patients who cannot tolerate the oral doses of chloroquine, parenteral doses of quinidine can be administered (see Question 2 for doses).[26] Patients with *P. ovale* and *P. vivax* also should be given primaquine to prevent relapses from the latent exoerythrocytic stages in the liver. The adult dosage of primaquine is 26.3 mg/day (15 mg base) for 14 days or 79 mg (45 mg base) weekly for 8 weeks; this should follow the chloroquine regimen.

Chemoprophylaxis and Pregnancy

3. R.P., a male medical resident from Colombia, is planning to visit his seriously ill mother. His wife, J.P., who is 16 weeks pregnant, and their 4-year-old daughter will accompany him. What prophylactic medications for malaria should be administered to each member of the family?

All travelers to endemic areas should receive chemoprophylaxis for malaria. In Latin America, including Colombia, all four types of malaria are present.[26] R.P. and his family may have to take prophylactic therapy for all malarial species, including a regimen that will protect them against CRPF infections. To verify whether a country is included in the CRPF list or to obtain other relevant information on malaria prophylaxis, R.P. should call the CDC, which provides a touch tone–activated, computer-assisted service (404-332-4555).[26,28] Pregnant women are at greater risk for malaria infection and its complications (especially severe hemolytic anemia and splenomegaly) and should be advised not to travel to areas endemic for malaria, if possible.[4,12,29] Current publications that provide updated information on parasitic diseases and immunization requirements include *Medical Letter, Morbidity and Mortality Weekly Reports, Health Information for International Travel,* and various Internet sites.[12,17,26,28,29]

CHLOROQUINE AND PRIMAQUINE PHOSPHATE

Chloroquine phosphate is an effective chemoprophylactic agent against all species of *Plasmodia* except drug-resistant *P. falciparum*. The adult dosage of chloroquine phosphate is 500 mg (300 mg base) once weekly beginning 1 week before departure and continuing for 4 weeks after last exposure. The pediatric dosage of chloroquine is 5 mg/kg base (8.3 mg chloroquine phosphate) once weekly beginning 1 week before departure and continuing for 4 weeks after exposure. A suspension of chloroquine in chocolate syrup can be prepared for children (5 mg/mL). Chloroquine prophylaxis is safe during pregnancy, and the benefits outweigh the risk of malaria and the drug's possible side effects.[8,10,12,26,30–37]

By taking the chloroquine 1 week before travel, the patient can achieve adequate antimalarial chloroquine levels in the blood by the second week. Potential side effects also can be detected early. A weekly dose of 0.5 g of chloroquine phosphate produces average plasma concentrations of chloroquine between 0.47 to 0.78 μmol/L. Most strains of *P. vivax* and *P. falciparum* are susceptible to plasma levels between 0.046 and 0.093 μmol/L, respectively.[38,39] Mefloquine (Lariam) 250 mg (salt) once weekly beginning 1 week before departure and continuing for 4 weeks after leaving a malarious area is an alternative regimen to chloroquine.[26,40] However, mefloquine is not recommended during pregnancy or in children weighing <5 kg because the safety of this agent has not been established in these populations.[26] Recently *P. vivax* was reported to be resistant to chloroquine in Columbia, and despite the lack of data on mefloquine in pregnancy (J.P. is in the second trimester), J.P. may have to be given this agent.[4,35,41] Chloroquine suppresses the asexual erythrocytic forms of the malaria parasite and has no action against the exoerythrocytic phase of *P. vivax* and *P. ovale*.[40,41] However, primaquine phosphate prevents relapses of *P. vivax* and *P. ovale* by inhibiting the exoerythrocytic stage; it also has a significant gametocytocidal effect against all species.[8,10,26] To prevent an attack after departure from an area where *P. vivax* and *P. ovale* are present, the clinician should also prescribe primaquine phosphate 26.3 mg/day (15 mg base) for 14 days to coincide with the last 2 weeks of the chloroquine regimen. Primaquine should not be administered to pregnant patients.[26] The major toxicity of concern, aside from the teratogenic risk, is hemolytic anemia in patients with RBC glucose-6-phosphate dehydrogenase (G6PD) deficiency.[12,35,42,43]

PROPHYLAXIS FOR CHLOROQUINE-RESISTANT *PLASMODIUM FALCIPARUM*

Prophylaxis for CRPF also can be achieved by taking mefloquine in the doses indicated above instead of using the chloroquine regimen.[26] An alternative to mefloquine is doxycycline 100 mg/day beginning 1 day before travel and continuing for the duration of the stay and for 4 weeks after leaving the malarial area. Travelers such as R.P. should be advised to take measures to reduce contact with infected mosquitoes by wearing long-sleeved shirts and trousers, applying insect repellent containing 31% to 35% N,N-diethyl-metatoluamide (DEET) (e.g., HourGuard-12, Amway Corp., NY; Deet Plus, Sawyer Products), sleeping in a screened room, or using netting impregnated with permethrin.[17,44] An alternative to the mefloquine chemoprophylaxis regimen in CRPF areas is the combination of atovaquone 250 mg and proguanil 100 mg (Malarone) administered once daily taken 1 to 2 days before departure and continued for 1 week after return.[2,26] The pediatric dosage (Malarone Pediatric) contains 62.5 mg of atovaquone and 25 mg of proguanil.[25,26] Instead of doxycycline, R.P. could take Malarone as chemoprophylaxis. The advantage of Malarone is that it can also be used as treatment. The recommended therapeutic dose of Malarone for CRPF is two tablets twice daily for 3 days.[26] In a recent study conducted in nonimmune volunteers, azithromycin (Zithromax) 250 mg daily was suggested as an alternative regimen for malaria prophylaxis.[45] Both prophylaxis and treatment of CRPF pose special problems in pregnancy. Pyrimethamine has teratogenic effects and sulfonamides are contraindicated in early pregnancy; however, chloroquine, quinine, and quinidine have been suggested as safe treatments during pregnancy.[17,26,32,37] Although not associated with abortions, low birthweight, neurologic retardation, or congenital malformations, mefloquine is associated with an increased risk of stillbirth.[46]

R.P. and J.P. should reconsider their decision to travel together because of the risks of malarial infection during pregnancy. In view of the recent report of *P. vivax* resistance to chloroquine in Columbia, the family members should consider using mefloquine.[41] The risks and benefits of mefloquine in pregnancy (J.P. is in her second trimester) should be communicated to the family.[35] Physical barriers (e.g., clothes, mosquito nets), insect repellent, and a short stay in the endemic area also should be helpful.[2,44]

Malaria Vaccine

4. Why couldn't J.P. be vaccinated as an alternative to prophylaxis with 8-aminoquinolines such as chloroquine?

Currently, no vaccination is available. As a result of successful in vitro *P. falciparum* cultivation and advances in genetic engineering and monoclonal antibody research, some progress has been made, but this vaccine is probably a few years away.[42,47–51] The malaria plasmodium undergoes many transformations during its development, and each stage expresses a different plasmodial genome that generates a large number of antigens. The development of a malaria vaccine relies on the identification and characterization of these antigens and the subsequent production of monoclonal antibodies.[49]

At present, three types of vaccines against *P. falciparum* are under study: a merozoite vaccine that would induce immunity against the erythrocytic forms of plasmodia in the blood, a sporozoite vaccine that would protect against the exoerythrocytic or liver phase, and a gamete vaccine ("transmission blocking") that would prevent transmission of malaria in epidemic areas.[49] When a vaccine for malaria is available, it is expected to provide an immune response for at least 1 year. The safety of these vaccines to the fetus and mother during pregnancy will need evaluation. Trials in animal models and in limited human populations have provided evidence of protection, but the efficacy of these vaccines has been low and the duration of protection rather brief.[49]

Multidrug-Resistant Plasmodium falciparum Malaria

5. T.S., a permanent U.S. resident of Cambodian origin, is planning to travel to the Thai-Kampuchean refugee camp. What antimalarial agents should he use for chemoprophylaxis?

T.S. is traveling to the Thai-Burma border, where *P. falciparum* malaria is epidemic. Chemoprophylaxis against malaria in this region of southeast Asia has become progressively difficult because of the appearance of *P. falciparum* strains resistant to chloroquine, pyrimethamine-sulfadoxine, quinine, and even mefloquine.[12 16,17,26,52 58]

T.S. will have to take chemoprophylaxis against both *P. vivax* and multidrug-resistant *P. falciparum*. Mefloquine (Lariam) 250 mg once weekly starting 1 week before travel and continuing weekly for the duration of the stay and for 4 weeks after leaving Thailand is recommended.[26] Upon return from his visit, primaquine phosphate should be added to T.S.'s regimen to prevent an attack of *P. vivax*, because mefloquine has no effect on the exoerythrocytic phase of *P. vivax* (see Question 3 for doses of primaquine).[26] Another alternative drug for prophylaxis against *P. falciparum* malaria for T.S. would be doxycycline 100 mg taken once daily beginning 1 to 2 days before departure and continuing for 4 weeks after he returns from Thailand.[2,26]

A new drug, ginghaosu, has been undergoing field trials and may prove to be useful for resistant *P. falciparum*. Ginghaosu, a plant extract (artemisinin compounds), has been used for many centuries in China for fever and malaria.[13,19,26,43,57–59] Artemisinin and its derivatives are considered moderately to significantly neurotoxic. The antimalarial agent halofantrine (Halfan) may be another alternative to mefloquine, but this agent has been associated with fatal arrhythmias.[26] Clinical trials of fosmidomycin, tefenoquine, and other new antimalarial agents are ongoing.[15,59–61]

Side Effects of Antimalarials

6. A.K., a 36-year-old Malaysian man, is seen in the ED with a 2-day history of fever, chills, and bouts of diarrhea following his return from West Malaysia, where he was visiting his parents for 3 weeks. A.K. had not taken any prophylaxis for malaria. A blood smear stained with Giemsa solution demonstrated *P. vivax*, and A.K. was given chloroquine 1 g (600 mg base) initially, to be followed by 500 mg (300 mg base) 6 hours later and 500 mg at 24 and 48 hours. Upon completion of the chloroquine regimen, A.K. was instructed to take primaquine 26.5 mg/day (15 mg base) for 14 days. However, A.K. was seen again in the ED a day later with complaints of abdominal pain, severe headache, vomiting, and a "bitter taste" in the mouth. What subjective evidence does A.K. exhibit that is compatible with the toxicity of antimalarials?

The major side effects of chloroquine (e.g., nausea, abdominal pain, pruritus, vertigo, headache, and visual disturbances)[8,39,43] usually are associated with large doses such as those needed for A.K.'s therapy. The gastrointestinal (GI) complaints and severe headache experienced by A.K. are consistent with chloroquine therapy, and the bitter taste he described is experienced by all patients who are given chloroquine or other 8-aminoquinoline preparations. Because A.K. also will be taking primaquine after the course of chloroquine, he should be told that he probably will experience some GI upset with this drug as well. Abdominal cramps associated with primaquine may be relieved by antacids or by taking the drug after meals. The severe nausea and vomiting may have dehydrated A.K., and he should be encouraged to replenish his fluids. Table 74-1 lists the adverse effects of antimalarials.

Glucose-6-Phosphate Dehydrogenase Deficiency

7. Why is A.K. at risk for primaquine sensitivity?

Primaquine sensitivity, or G6PD deficiency, is an inherited error of metabolism transmitted by a gene of partial dominance located on the X chromosome. Patients with this enzyme deficiency are sensitive to the 8-aminoquinolines, sulfonamides, para-aminosalicylates, nitrofurantoin, sulfone, aspirin, quinine, quinidine, nalidixic acid, and methylene blue.[39,62,63] G6PD in RBCs preserves glutathione in the reduced form (see Fig. 87-2 in Chapter 87, Drug-Induced Blood Disorders) by regenerating nicotinamide adenine dinucleotide phosphate (NADPH). Reduced glutathione protects RBC membranes from increased oxidant stress. Patients with low levels of glutathione and impaired regeneration of NADPH, as seen with G6PD deficiency, are susceptible to the oxidizing effect of drugs.[39,62,63] Hemolysis reportedly occurs on the third day of drug ingestion and usually is manifested as abdominal discomfort, anemia, and hemoglobinuria.[39]

The incidence of G6PD deficiency in the Southeast Asian refugee population is approximately 5.2%.[62] Because A.K. is a native of Malaysia and may have G6PD deficiency, he may be at risk of hemolysis if primaquine is ingested. Therefore, he should be screened for G6PD deficiency before being treated with this drug.

Although a number of simple and satisfactory screening tests for G6PD deficiency are available, the fluorescent spot test is the simplest, most reliable, and most sensitive. The spot test is based on the addition of a reagent containing NADPH to a hemolysate of the patient's RBCs. After an incubation period, the mixture is spotted on filter paper and examined under long-wave ultralight. Fluorescence of the mixture on the filter paper will indicate the presence of NADPH generated by G6PD. In patients who have G6PD deficiency, it will fluoresce only weakly, or no fluorescence will be detected. There are large variants among those with the mutant gene, and if A.K. has a variant with relatively mild episodic clinical manifestations (variant A, with 10% to 60% residual enzyme activity),

he may be treated with primaquine at 45 mg/week for 8 weeks.[8,43]

AMEBIASIS

Prevalence and Mortality

Amebiasis, caused by the small protozoan parasite *Entamoeba histolytica* (Fig. 74-2), results in amebic dysentery and hepatic abscess.[64–68] Approximately 10% of the world's population (predominately in Latin America, Africa, and Asia) is infected, and about 100,000 die annually from this infection.[64,65] In the United States, amebiasis is considered endemic in homosexual men because 20% to 30% of this population are infected with *E. histolytica* or *Entamoeba dispar* (see Fig. 74-2).[64,68] Most of these individuals are infected with *E. dispar,* an antigenically different strain from the pathogenic *E. histolytica* that does not seem to cause symptomatic invasive disease.[64] Amebiasis can be asymptomatic, or it can present as colitis or dysentery. Extraintestinal lesions, primarily abscesses in the liver, also can be characteristic.[64–74]

Life Cycle

The amebic parasite or trophozoite lives in the lumen of the colon and the colonic mucosa (Fig. 74-3). Trophozoites do not survive outside the host body and, if ingested, will be destroyed by gastric juice. In contrast, the encysted trophozoites can survive drying and freezing: they are killed only by temperatures in excess of 55°C or by hyperchlorination of water.[64,68] Infection occurs by ingestion of cysts present in contaminated water or food. Once ingested by the host, each cyst dissolves in the alkaline media of the small intestine and undergoes asexual division to produce eight trophozoites.[64,68]

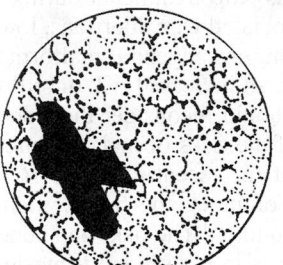

FIGURE 74-2 *E. histolytica.*

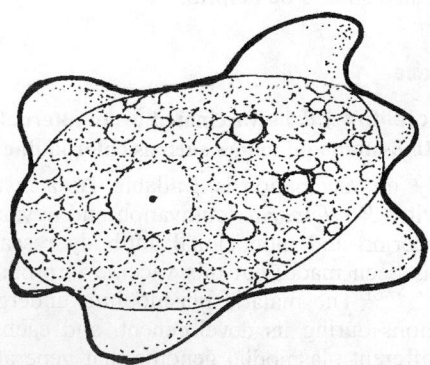

FIGURE 74-3 *E. histolytica* trophozoite.

The trophozoites, which represent the invasive form of *E. histolytica,* then move to the large bowel, invade the mucosal crypts, and produce ulcerations.[64,68] Ulcerations of the bowel wall may result in amebic dysentery, inflammatory lesions in the bowel (amebomas), amebic appendicitis, and perforation of the colon or intestine.[64,68] The amebae also can enter into the portal vein, which transports them to the liver, where they can initiate multiple abscesses.[64,68,70] Cases of genital and cutaneous amebiasis are rare but have been reported.[67,72,73]

Amebic Dysentery

Diagnosis

8. **M.B., a 35-year-old homosexual man, presented to the ED with a 10-day history of abdominal pain and multiple, loose watery stools with occasional streaks of blood. Upon physical examination, he is a thin man with abdominal distress. His vital signs are temperature, 38°C; pulse, 88 beats/min; and BP 120/80 mm Hg. He has no skin lesions, jaundice, or lymphadenopathy. The examination is remarkable for slight abdominal distention with some right lower quadrant tenderness. Rectal examination reveals some tenderness and brown liquid stool positive for occult blood. Proctosigmoidoscopy demonstrates colonic mucosa that is diffusely edematous and friable. A biopsy specimen could not be obtained because M.B. was uncooperative and combative. Initial laboratory findings are Hgb, 13.4 g/dL; Hct, 40%; leukocyte count, 13,800 cells/mm³ with 68% neutrophils, 14% bands, 5% lymphocytes, and 13% monocytes; albumin, 3.1 g/dL (normal, 3.5 to 5). A liver scan and liver function tests are normal.**

On ultrasound examination, a tender mass palpable in the lower right quadrant proves to be a 3-cm collection of fluid consistent with an abdominal abscess. During an exploratory operation, the clinician drains 100 mL of a brownish-yellow material. Smears of the drained material are positive for *F. histolytica* trophozoites, and culture of the material is negative for bacteria. Fresh stool tested for *E. histolytica* by TechLab's *E. histolytica* II antigen detection test (Blacksburg, VA) is positive.

How was amebic colitis differentiated from ulcerative colitis in M.B.? What is the significance of obtaining serology in M.B.?

[SI units: Hgb, 130.4 g/L; Hct, 0.40; leukocyte count, 13.8 × 10⁹/L with 0.68 neutrophils, 0.14 bands, 0.05 lymphocytes, and 0.13 monocytes; albumin, 31 g/L (normal, 35 to 50)]

M.B.'s abdominal symptoms, elevated temperature, right lower quadrant tenderness, and occult blood in the stool examination, together with the proctosigmoidoscopic findings, strongly suggest either a bacterial or a protozoan infection.[64,65,68] Stool examination confirms that M.B. has amebiasis; the presence of *E. histolytica* in the abdominal abscess and bloody stools confirms the diagnosis of amebic colitis. Serum antibody tests are useful especially when the parasite is absent from the stool or abscess material and are considered highly sensitive (>90%).[71,75] The TechLab *E. histolytica* II antigen detection test, which detects specific antibody to the amebae in stool, is helpful in nonendemic areas for the differential diagnosis between ulcerative colitis and amebic colitis.[71,75] Although in M.B. a positive finding of *E. histolytica* in the smear from the abdominal abscess is diagnostic, TechLab's *E. histolytica* II test will document the presence of *E. histolytica.*[71] However, the test may not differentiate between

acute and chronic disease in an area of high endemicity.[64,65] The TechLab test is specific for *E. histolytica* and does not cross-react with the nonpathogenic *E. dispar.*[71] When appropriate stool samples are not available in these cases, endoscopic or colonoscopic specimens may be critical for diagnosis, and positive serology will confirm the diagnosis of acute amebiasis.[64,68] In invasive amebiasis, serum antibodies are found in 90% of individuals by day 7 of illness.[68] A positive antibody test of the stool with the TechLab antigen detection test identifies a majority of patients with invasive amebic colitis; the absence of serum antibodies to *E. histolytica* after 7 days of symptoms is evidence against a diagnosis of invasive amebiasis.[64,68,71] M.B.'s positive antibody test for *E. histolytica* in the stool and identification of *E. histolytica* in the abdominal abscess confirm the diagnosis of amebiasis.

Drugs

9. **What are the major drugs that can be used to treat M.B.? What regimen might be preferred?**

The two classes of drugs that can be used to treat M.B.'s amebiasis are the luminal-acting drugs, which act only in the bowel lumen, and the tissue amebicides, which have activity in the bowel wall, liver, and other extraintestinal tissues.[26,43,64,74] Luminal-acting drugs achieve high concentrations in the bowel, but only minimal systemic absorption takes place. These drugs include diiodohydroxyquin or iodoquinol (Yodoxin), diloxanide furoate (Furamide), and paromomycin (Humatin). Tetracycline should be considered a secondary bowel amebicide because it is not active against liver amebae.[43,64] Tetracycline modifies the enteric bowel flora and reduces amebic colonization, and it is usually combined with another luminal-acting agent when used for intestinal amebiasis.[43]

M.B. needs to be treated with a tissue amebicide in combination with a luminal agent because he has positive serology, which indicates tissue invasion by *E. histolytica.* Tissue amebicides are well absorbed and attain adequate systemic levels to treat extraintestinal amebiasis.[26,43,64,68] Because the concentrations of the tissue drugs in the bowel may be insufficient to eradicate *E. histolytica,* they must be combined with a luminal-acting agent to treat both serious intestinal amebiasis and extraintestinal amebic lesions.[26,43] The tissue amebicides include metronidazole (Flagyl), chloroquine phosphate (Aralen), emetine, and dehydroemetine. Chloroquine is effective only as a liver amebicide.[43] Dehydroemetine can be obtained from the CDC.[43] Diloxanide can be obtained from Panorama Compounding Pharmacy, Van Nuys, California (800-247-9767).[26]

M.B.'s acute amebic dysentery should be treated with a combination of metronidazole and a luminal agent, such as iodoquinol or diloxanide furoate. If M.B. is too ill to tolerate the oral tablets, a loading dose of 15 mg/kg of metronidazole can be administered IV over 1 hour followed by a maintenance dose of 500 mg Q 6 hr.[68] A single oral dose of 2.4 g of metronidazole for 2 to 3 days is equally effective[64] (for doses of other agents, see Table 74-1).

M.B. needs to be monitored and his stool should be examined over the ensuing 3 months. A colonoscopy could document the cure. The relapse rate of amebic colitis is around 10%.[70]

AMEBIC CYST PASSER

10. P.C., a 47-year-old man whose stool was found to be positive for *E. histolytica* cysts on routine examination, was completely asymptomatic. Would you treat P.C.? What are other drug regimens for amebiasis?

P.C. is an asymptomatic cyst passer and the infection may be chronic. Invasive amebiasis and extraintestinal disease are potential threats to P.C., and he is a source of infection to others.[64,68] For these reasons, he should be treated with a full course of a luminal amebicide (diloxanide or iodoquinol).[64,65,68] To verify the eradication of the infection, P.C.'s stool should be examined monthly for 3 months. (For other treatment regimens for amebiasis, see Table 74-1 or reference 26.)

11. If P.C. is not treated, what complications might be encountered?

Failure to treat P.C. may lead to significant medical problems. Amebic liver abscess is one of the most common complications of amebiasis, with the right lobe of the liver being involved in 90% of all cases.[64,68,70,75–77] Patients usually present with fever, tenderness over an enlarged liver, leukocytosis, an elevated sedimentation rate, and anemia.[68,70,78] Liver scans (using radioactive isotopes with either technetium-99 or gallium), magnetic resonance imaging (MRI), ultrasonography, and serology (enzyme immunoassay or TechLab) usually confirm the presence of an abscess.[64,68,70,75,76] Liver abscesses can extend to the lungs through fistulas and can cause empyemas and lung abscesses.[66,70] Amebic peritonitis also may result from liver abscesses.[64,68] Other complications include amebic pericarditis, brain abscess, amebic strictures secondary to dysentery, and cutaneous amebiasis.[64–68,70,75] Management of these complications includes exploratory surgery to drain the abscesses, needle aspiration directed by radiologic monitoring, appropriate cultures of aspirate fluid, and drug therapy with metronidazole combined with a luminal agent such as iodoquinol.[43,64,68,70,78,79] Most patients respond within 3 days with decreased pain, anorexia, and fever.[70] Lesions may take 4 to 10 months to resolve; healing can be monitored through periodic radiologic studies.[70,75]

TREATMENT DURING PREGNANCY

12. C.R., a 24-year-old woman, presented with a 5-day history of watery stools, bloody mucus, and fever after returning from Thailand. She initially was treated with ampicillin, to which she did not respond. She is 22 weeks pregnant, and her medical history includes rheumatic fever at age 5 and heart murmurs. Her temperature is 38.2°C and her abdomen is soft but nontender; she complains of severe cramps. Fresh stool is positive for occult blood, and the wet mount demonstrates trophozoites with ingested RBCs. A trichrome stain shows *E. histolytica* trophozoites. Bacterial culture is negative for pathogenic bacteria. An abdominal computed tomography (CT) scan is negative for abdominal or liver amebiasis, and an antiamebic antibody test is negative. A diagnosis of intestinal amebiasis is made. How would you treat C.R.? If C.R. subsequently develops amebic colitis, how would you treat her, and what are some toxicities of concern with the selected regimens?

C.R. needs to receive a luminal amebicide to treat her intestinal amebiasis. However, because she is 22 weeks preg-nant and has an underlying cardiovascular problem, the therapeutic options are limited. Metronidazole, iodoquinol, and emetine are not preferred regimens for C.R. because of their potential adverse effects to mother or fetus. A drug that has minimal systemic effects would be optimal so as not to jeopardize her fetus. Paromomycin, a nonabsorbable aminoglycoside, is effective and has been used in pregnant patients.[74] C.R. should receive paromomycin 25 to 35 mg/kg per day in three divided doses for 7 days.[26,68] The most common side effect of paromomycin is GI upset, manifested as increased frequency of stools.[43,74] At the end of the course of therapy, C.R.'s stools should be tested to verify a cure. A serology for serum amebic antibodies also should be evaluated. If her serology is positive, a full course of metronidazole followed by a luminal agent, either iodoquinol or diloxanide furoate, must be considered.[26,64] Because C.R. would be in the third trimester of pregnancy during this period, her fetus would be less susceptible to the teratogenic effects of the drugs if she develops amebic colitis or hepatic amebiasis.

Used concomitantly with a luminal amebicide, metronidazole remains the drug of choice for all patients with severe amebic colitis, hepatic abscess, and extraintestinal amebiasis.[43,68,70,74] The most common side effects include nausea, diarrhea, furry tongue, and glossitis.[43,74] Metronidazole causes disulfiram-like effects if alcohol is consumed concomitantly.[43] Of major concern are the reports of carcinogenicity in rodents and mutagenic activity of metronidazole in bacteria.[74] The clinical significance of carcinogenicity in the human population has not been fully assessed because a cause-and-effect relationship between use of the drug and malignancy has not been documented adequately.[43,74] Although metronidazole is considered safe in C.R., who now is in her third trimester, it should be avoided if possible during the first trimester of pregnancy.[43,74]

If amebic colitis or hepatic amebiasis develops, C.R. needs to receive either iodoquinol or diloxanide furoate to follow her metronidazole regimen. If iodoquinol is selected, the side effects associated with usual dosages include nausea and vomiting, abdominal discomfort, diarrhea, headache, and occasionally enlargement of the thyroid gland.[43,68,74]

If diloxanide furoate is selected instead of iodoquinol, this agent is essentially free of side effects with the exception of some minor GI symptoms such as flatulence (belching and abdominal distention) and stomach cramps.[43,74] This may be preferable to iodoquinol for C.R.

C.R. should not receive either emetine or dehydroemetine because of her history of rheumatic disease and heart murmurs; these two drugs can cause serious cardiovascular toxicity, such as arrhythmias, hypotension, and precordial pain.[43,64] Emetine and dehydroemetine were previously used for severe amebic dysentery and hepatic abscess but are rarely indicated today because of their unacceptable side effects.

GIARDIASIS

Prevalence and Transmission

Giardiasis, manifested as nausea, abdominal cramping, and diarrhea, is caused by the protozoan *Giardia lamblia*.[80–83] The disease is endemic in large areas of the world, especially where sanitation and sanitary habits are poor.[81] Although the prevalence is low in most developed countries, a number of outbreaks of giardiasis have been reported in Russia, Eastern Europe, and the United States.[80-83] *G. lamblia* is the most commonly reported pathogen in infectious diarrhea among Americans.[84] Water-borne outbreaks of giardiasis occur more often than food-borne outbreaks.[84-86] Giardia seems more prevalent in children, older debilitated individuals, those with dysgammaglobulinemias (specifically those with a deficiency of IgA), and the homosexual population.[80-83,87]

Life Cycle

G. lamblia exists in two forms: the trophozoite and the cyst (Fig. 74-4). The cyst is excreted in the stool, and if it is ingested in contaminated water or food, it will excyst in the stomach to produce trophozoites.[80-83] The trophozoites migrate to the small intestine and produce the GI symptoms characteristic of giardiasis. Symptoms appear 5 to 15 days after ingestion of the cyst.[83]

Diagnosis

Signs and Symptoms

13. J.T., a 23-year-old female student, has just returned from Mexico after spending a month there with a local church group. Two days before returning to the United States, J.T. had a bout of diarrhea with "offensive yellow stools." She now complains of nausea, abdominal discomfort, and occasional foul-smelling diarrhea alternating with constipation. J.T. indicates that she has lost about 10 lb over the previous 2 weeks. Three stool samples are examined for ova and parasites, and a stool culture is ordered. Two of the three stool samples are positive for *G. lamblia* cysts, and the culture is negative for bacterial pathogens. Why is this a typical presentation of giardiasis?

The symptoms of giardiasis are variable. Some patients present with profuse watery stools, abdominal distention, and cramping for several weeks; others complain only of mild abdominal discomfort, flatulence, and occasional loose stools.[81-83] J.T.'s symptoms are typical and consistent with the description of giardiasis. Symptoms usually begin about 2 weeks after transmission of the infection and include anorexia, nausea, and diarrhea with bulky, foul-smelling stools.[80-83] The acute phase of giardiasis can be followed by a period of chronic intermittent diarrhea alternating with constipation.[82,83] During this period, anorexia and malabsorption

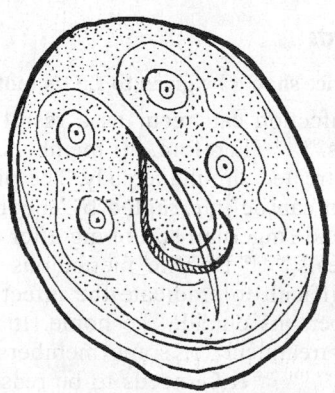

FIGURE 74-4 *G. lamblia* cyst.

will cause weight loss. Malabsorption from severe or chronic giardiasis can result in steatorrhea and deficiencies in vitamins A and B_{12}.[82,88,89] *G. lamblia* cysts usually are found in the stool, although there may be periods when cysts are difficult to detect because of a low count.[81-83] The onset of symptoms, foul-smelling stools, and weight loss are consistent with symptomatic giardiasis in J.T.

14. If the stool examination had been negative for *G. lamblia*, what alternative steps would have been necessary to make a diagnosis in J.T.?

Bacterial infection caused by *Salmonella, Shigella,* or *Campylobacter* was ruled out by a negative stool culture in J.T.[80,82] The next step would be to use the Entero-Test in an attempt to obtain a diagnosis of giardiasis.[81] The Entero-Test consists of a gelatinous capsule attached to a string. The patient swallows the capsule and the other end of the string is secured to the face with tape. After 4 to 6 hours, the string is pulled up and the bile-stained end is examined under a microscope. The Entero-Test sample obtained from the duodenum will demonstrate the trophozoite rather than the cyst and reportedly has a better yield than a stool examination.[82]

Several other tests to detect *Giardia* antigen in the stool have become commercially available.[81,82] These tests have a sensitivity of 85% to 98% and a specificity of 90% to 100%.[82,90,91] However, stool samples are still important to document *G. lamblia*.[90] An immunofluorescence assay using monoclonal antibody against *Giardia* cysts is available (Meridian Diagnostics, Cincinnati). Some clinicians may prefer to use these newer tests rather than the Entero-Test. However, if the Entero-Test is negative, most clinicians would initiate a therapeutic trial rather than subject a patient to other invasive diagnostic procedures.[81,82] As a last resort, endoscopy with duodenal fluid sampling and biopsy may be performed.[82,92-94]

TREATMENT

15. How should J.T. be treated?

Metronidazole is the drug of choice for giardiasis in J.T.[26] Metronidazole 250 mg three times daily for 7 days is as effective as quinacrine in the treatment of giardiasis.[26,43,81,82] Although metronidazole was reported to be mutagenic in bacteria and carcinogenic at high dosages in animals, there is no evidence that it represents a risk in humans at this time.[81,82]

Quinacrine (Atabrine) administered 100 mg three times daily for 5 days, with cure rates of 90% to 95%, was once considered the drug of choice for giardiasis but is no longer commercially available; it may be obtained from Panorama Compounding Pharmacy (see Question 9).[26,81,82]

Furazolidone (Furoxone) is an alternative to metronidazole and is available in the United States as a tablet and suspension for the treatment of giardiasis.[26,41,80-82] Furazolidone has cure rates of 80% to 90%, and the adult dosage is 100 mg four times daily for 7 days.[82]

Furazolidone, which is available as a suspension, is preferred by some clinicians for children. However, metronidazole should be considered the drug of choice for giardiasis in both adults and children.

Tinidazole (Fasigyn), an analog of metronidazole, is not available in the United States but is also highly effective for giardiasis.[26,83] Other alternatives are paromomycin (25 to 35 mg/kg per day in three divided doses for 7 days), albendazole (400 mg daily for 5 days), and an investigational agent, nitazoxanide (100 to 500 mg twice daily for 3 to 7 days).[88,95–97]

Following therapy, diarrhea usually subsides within 1 to 2 days and completely resolves in about 10 days.[80–83] Cyst excretion is disrupted 2 days after initiation of therapy.[81–83] Complete normalization of intestinal functions, especially recovery from malabsorption, may require 4 to 8 weeks.[82] If J.T. does not respond to one course of therapy, she may need a second course of metronidazole.[81–83]

ENTEROBIASIS

Prevalence

Enterobiasis is an intestinal infection caused by the pinworm *Enterobius vermicularis* (Fig. 74-5). Pinworm is the most common helminthic infection in the United States and has an estimated annual incidence of 42 million.[98–100] A study of elementary school children documented a 15% to 20% prevalence rate of pinworm infection.[101] Enterobiasis is a cosmopolitan disease that usually affects all members of a family when one member is infected. Therefore, all household residents must be treated simultaneously. Institutionalized patients and preschool children in day care centers may be at greater risk for acquiring enterobiasis.[98–104]

Life Cycle

Infection is initiated with the ingestion of pinworm eggs, which reach the mouth on soiled hands or contaminated food and drink. After ingestion, the eggs hatch in the intestine, releasing the larvae, which attach to the jejunum or upper ileum.[103] After copulation, the female worm migrates to the lower bowel and produces eggs. Under the stimulus of air or change in temperature, the female releases eggs in the perianal skin.[103] Cutaneous irritation in the perianal region produced by migrating females and the presence of eggs can cause severe pruritus.[98,103]

Signs and Symptoms

16. L.C., a 6-year-old boy, is brought in by his mother, K.C., to see the family physician. K.C. states that L.C. was sent home from school because of inattention and disruptive behavior. L.C. has been very irritable and complained of abdominal discomfort and perianal pain on two occasions the previous week. A cellophane tape swab placed over the perianal skin demonstrates the translucent eggs of *E. vermicularis*. Explain the symptoms observed in L.C. What pathologic changes are associated with enterobiasis?

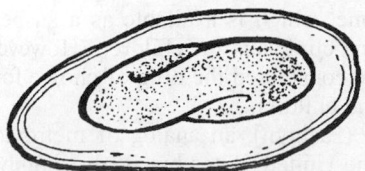

FIGURE 74-5 *E. vermicularis* ovum.

Pinworm infection may be asymptomatic, but the most common symptom is intense pruritus ani caused by the presence of the sticky pinworm eggs in the perianal skin. Pruritus can cause constant scratching and may result in dermatitis and secondary bacterial infections.[98,103,104] A heavy load of worms can cause anorexia, restlessness, and insomnia, resulting in behavioral changes, as illustrated in L.C.[98,104]

Generally, pinworms do not cause any serious intestinal pathology.[98,104] Rarely, *E. vermicularis* ectopic lesions can be caused by a gravid worm that has migrated from the perianal region into the vagina, uterus, or fallopian tubes. The adult worm may travel through the fallopian tubes to the peritoneal cavity.[100,102] The association between cystitis in young females and enterobiasis presumably results when the female worm enters the urethra and makes its way into the bladder carrying enteric bacteria.[104]

Treatment

Pyrantel Pamoate, Mebendazole, and Albendazole

17. How should L.C. be treated?

Three different preparations are available to treat pinworm infection in L.C.: pyrantel pamoate (Antiminth), mebendazole (Vermox), and albendazole (Albenza).[26,103,104–106] Either pyrantel pamoate or mebendazole can be considered for this patient. L.C. should receive a single dose of 11 mg/kg (maximum, 1 g) of pyrantel pamoate followed by a second dose in 2 weeks.[26,103,106] Some patients experience mild GI upset, headache, and fever from this therapy.[26,106] Pyrantel pamoate acts as a depolarizing neuromuscular blocking agent releasing acetylcholine, which inhibits cholinesterase, thereby leading to paralysis of the worm and expulsion from the host's intestinal tract.[99]

Mebendazole is as effective as pyrantel for enterobiasis, with a cure rate of 90% to 100%.[103,106] Mebendazole, a broad-spectrum antihelmintic agent that also is given as a single dose (100 mg), is repeated in 2 weeks.[26] Because mebendazole is poorly absorbed, few systemic side effects are associated with its use, except abdominal pain or diarrhea.[103,106] Albendazole, another broad-spectrum antihelmintic, is administered as 400 mg once and repeated in 2 weeks.[26] Both albendazole and mebendazole inhibit microtubule function and deplete glycogen stores in worms, leading to their death.[99,106]

Household Contacts

18. What advice should be given to L.C.'s mother?

Pinworm infection can recur as a result of reinfection within families.[99,104] Therefore, all members of L.C.'s family need to be treated simultaneously. The pinworm's cycle of transmission can be interrupted by encouraging careful handwashing and fingernail scrubbing after using the toilet and before meals.[99,104] Despite meticulous precautions, it still may be difficult to eradicate the infection because of contact with persons outside the home. It may be necessary to repeat treatment for some members of the family at a later date.[98,101,104] K.C. needs to be reassured that pinworm infection in the home does not represent substandard hygiene.[104]

CESTODIASIS

Description

Cestodiasis (tapeworm infection) is caused by members of the phylum Platyhelminths (flat worms), which include, among others, *Taenia solium* (pork tapeworm), *Taenia saginata* (beef tapeworm), *Diphyllobothrium latum* (broad fish tapeworm), and *Hymenolepis nana* (dwarf tapeworm).[107–111]

The tapeworm's body is made up of an anterior attachment organ called a scolex, accompanied by a chain of segments or proglottids called a strobila. The strobila grows throughout the life of the tapeworm, with the extension taking place just posterior to the scolex.[107,108] At the end of the strobila, mature or gravid segments contain eggs enclosed in the uterus, which, because of its characteristic shape and size, may be used for identifying tapeworm species.[107,108]

Tapeworms remain attached to the mucosal wall of the upper jejunum by the scolex, which contains two to four muscular cup-shaped suckers. The parasite lacks an alimentary canal and obtains nutrients directly from the host's intestine. A protrusible structure called a rostellum is located in the center of the scolex and may contain hooks in some species.[107–111] The scolex, proglottids, and eggs are very specific for each species and are used for definitive diagnosis.[110]

Tapeworms cause disease in humans in either the adult or larval stage.[109] The symptoms in the host primarily are GI when the adult form is present. Larvae or cysticerci become encysted in various visceral organs, causing a disease called cysticercosis.[108,109,112–119]

Life Cycle

Pork tapeworm (*T. solium*) and beef tapeworm (*T. saginata*) infections are caused by ingestion of poorly cooked meat. The larva or cysticercus is released from the contaminated meat by bile salts and matures in the host jejunum in about 2 months.[108,110] The pork tapeworm has been reported to reach a length of 10 to 20 feet, and adult beef tapeworms can measure up to 30 feet. Gravid proglottids, which contain the eggs, are passed in the host's feces and are the source of infection in animals. When ingested by animals, the embryos are released from the eggs; these migrate through the lymphatics and blood, developing into cysticerci (encysted larvae) in various muscles.[108,110]

Cysticercosis, the systemic infection caused by the larval stage of *T. solium,* is usually acquired by ingestion of the eggs in contaminated food or by autoinfection.[108] The eggs of *T. solium,* when ingested by the host, are digested by gastric juices and develop into the larvae (oncospheres), which penetrate the small bowel and migrate through the bloodstream throughout the body to produce human cysticercosis. Clinical manifestations range over a broad spectrum of symptoms and include both neurogenic and psychiatric: increased intracranial pressure, chronic severe headache, intellectual deterioration, decreased visual acuity, and focal and generalized seizures.[108,109,114–118]

Epidemiology

The pork tapeworm occurs worldwide and is prevalent in Mexico, Latin America, Slavic countries, Africa, Southeast Asia, India, and China.[108,109,111] The beef tapeworm is cosmopolitan but is found predominantly in Ethiopia, Europe, Japan, the Philippines, Latin America, and the Middle East.[110] Both occur in the United States, although the prevalence is low.[108,111]

D. latum (broad fish tapeworm) inhabits the ileum in the human host, and infection is acquired by ingesting raw or inadequately cooked freshwater fish.[110,111,119] *D. latum* also infects other fish-eating animals, including the fox, mink, bear, walrus, and seal. These animals can serve as reservoirs.[108]

Broad tapeworm disease, or diphyllobothriasis, is common in Finland, Scandinavia, Russia, the lake regions of North Italy, Switzerland, and France.[110] In North America, the highest incidence of infection has been reported in Alaska and Canada.[108,110]

H. nana (dwarf tapeworm) is cosmopolitan in distribution, with a high incidence in children in the tropics and subtropics.[110] It is the most common human tapeworm in the United States, particularly in the southeastern section. The infection is passed primarily from person to person by contaminated hands or fomites.

Taenia saginata and *Taenia solium*

Signs and Symptoms

19. B.R., a 10-year-old boy from Mexico, has moved to the United States with his parents. The school nurse saw him on several occasions when he complained of vague abdominal discomfort and pain. Upon questioning, B.R. reports seeing "white noodle-like" objects in his stools. B.R. is seen in the clinic. A cellophane impression of the perianal region and three stool samples over several days demonstrate infection with *T. saginata* (Fig. 74-6). IgE level and eosinophil count are within normal limits. Explain the presenting symptoms in B.R.

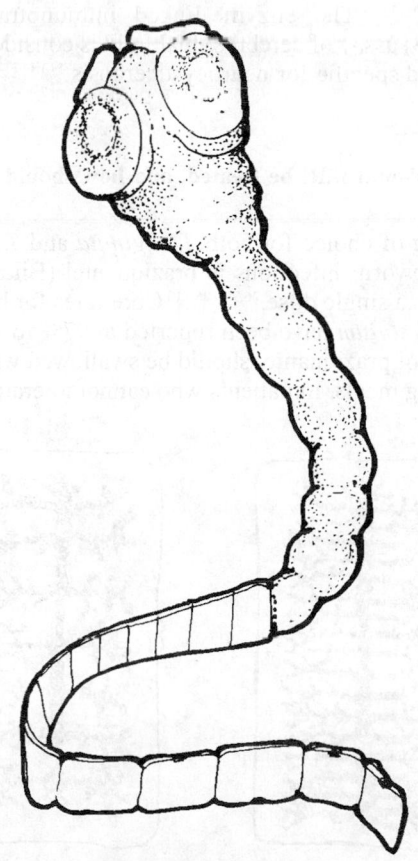

FIGURE 74-6 *T. saginata.*

Patients with tapeworm infections (either *T. saginata,* as in B.R., or *T. solium*) present with symptoms ranging from mild epigastric or abdominal pain to a burning sensation, general weakness, weight loss, headache, constipation, and diarrhea.[110,111] Complications from *T. saginata* include appendicitis, obstruction of pancreatic ducts, and intestinal obstruction.[108,110,111] Because the adult worm is weakly immunogenic, some patients present with moderate eosinophilia and elevated IgE levels.[111] However, B.R. did not. He reported worm segments ("white noodle-like" objects) in the stool. This is commonly the way diagnosis is made. Segments are sometimes found in underclothing. An alternative diagnostic method is to use anal swabs (the "Scotch tape" method) as used for pinworm ova.[111]

Diagnosis

20. How can *T. saginata* infection be differentiated from *T. solium* in B.R.?

The eggs of *T. saginata* and *T. solium* are identical and, when found in the stool, will not aid in diagnosis. The presence of gravid proglottids (Fig. 74-7) or a scolex in the stool is necessary to determine the species.[108,110]

Placing gravid proglottids from B.R.'s stool between two slides and injecting India ink into the central uterine system will demonstrate the characteristic anatomic differences.[108,111]

An intact scolex recovered from B.R.'s stool after treatment also will confirm the species. The scolex of *T. saginata* has no hooklets ("unarmed"), whereas that of *T. solium* contains a double row of hooklets ("armed").[108] With *T. solium,* the diagnosis of neurocysticercosis is made based on history, symptoms, and identification of neurologic lesions by CT scanning and MRI.[108–111] The enzyme-linked immunotransfer blot (CDC-ETIB) assay of cerebrospinal fluid is considered highly sensitive and specific for neurocysticercosis.[113,117]

Treatment

21. How should B.R. be treated, and how should therapy be evaluated?

The drug of choice for both *T. saginata* and *T. solium* intestinal tapeworm infections is praziquantel (Biltricide) 5 to 10 mg/kg as a single dose.[26,99,106,110] Cure rates for both *T. saginata* and *T. solium* have been reported at 97% to 100%.[106,110] The tablets of praziquantel should be swallowed whole with a liquid during meals. In patients who cannot tolerate the single dose because of severe nausea and vomiting, praziquantel may be administered in divided doses; the interval between doses should be 4 to 6 hours.[120] Praziquantel kills the adult worm but does not kill the eggs. The intact or disintegrating segments appear in the stool over a week.[110] Stool specimens should be re-examined to confirm that there is no regrowth of *T. solium* (5 weeks after treatment) and *T. saginata* (3 months after treatment).[110]

Eggs may be released when gravid segments of *T. solium* disintegrate after treatment, and the release of embryos from the eggs can cause cysticercosis. To minimize this possibility, the clinician should give a purgative (magnesium sulfate 15 to 30 g) 2 hours after administration of praziquantel when *T. solium* infection is suspected.[106] B.R. should be told that segments of the tapeworm will be passed for several days after treatment.

Diphyllobothrium latum and Hymenolepsis nana

22. Could B.R. have *D. latum* or *H. nana* infection? How are these treated?

Infection with *D. latum* is highly unlikely in B.R. because diphyllobothriasis is almost exclusively found among raw fish–eating populations of the Baltic countries, Alaska, and Canada,[108,111] and B.R. is from Mexico. In addition, neither the characteristic operculate eggs (Fig. 74-8) nor the distinctive almond-shaped scolex of *D. latum* were found during stool examination.

H. nana (dwarf tapeworm) infection is worldwide and is a possibility in B.R. It is unusual to find proglottids of *H. nana* because they usually disintegrate before passage.[111] Instead, identification is made by the presence of the characteristic eggs (Fig. 74-9).

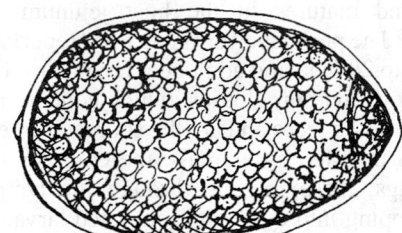

FIGURE 74-8 *D. latus* ovum.

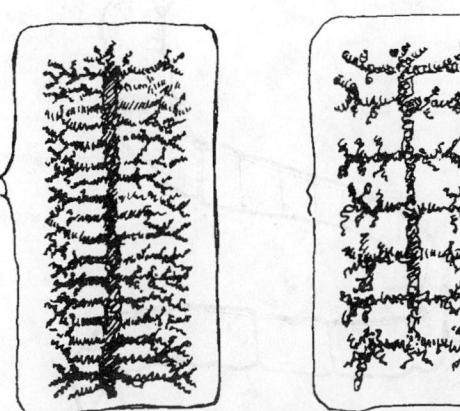

FIGURE 74-7 *T. solium* and *T. saginata* gravid segments.

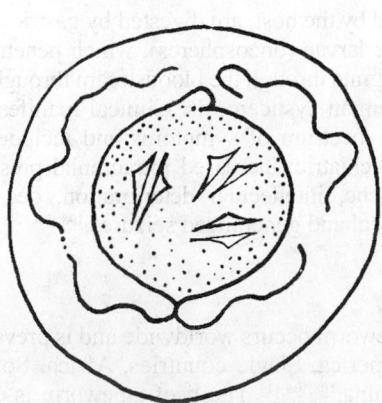

FIGURE 74-9 *H. nana* ovum.

Treatment of *D. latum* is identical to that of *T. saginata* except that a purgative is not necessary after therapy. *H. nana* infections are treated with praziquantel 25 mg/kg as a single dose.[26]

Cysticercosis and Other Complications

23. If B.R. were infected with *T. solium* rather than *T. saginata* and subsequently developed neurocysticercosis, how should this be treated?

Neurocysticercosis, the deposition of the larval cysts (fluid-filled bladder containing the invaginated scolex) of *T. solium* in the cerebral parenchyma, meninges, spinal cord, and the ventricular system, is considered the most common parasitic disease of the central nervous system.[109,113–118] However, there is continuing debate regarding the efficacy of anthelminthic therapy and the optimal dosages of these agents for neurocysticercosis.[109,113,115,121–128] If B.R. had subarachnoid or intraventricular cysticercosis, these would normally be treated with surgery. However, because of the risk of neurosurgical procedures, others have suggested anthelminthic therapy.[125] If it were parenchymal disease (cerebral cysticercosis) and multiple cysts, B.R. would receive medical treatment.[109,112] Hydrocephalus (blockage of the foramen of Monroe or sylvian aqueduct), if present, and elevated intracranial pressure are relieved by a ventriculoperitoneal shunt or temporary ventriculostomy.[109] B.R. may need only symptomatic therapy (e.g., anticonvulsants) if he presented with seizures and the CT scan showed granuloma or calcified cysts.[109,126] Seizures, which occur in 70% to 90% of these cases, are the most common manifestation of neurocysticercosis. For seizures, B.R. would be started on an anticonvulsant with either phenytoin (doses to attain serum levels of 10 to 20 µg/mL) or carbamazepine (doses to attain serum levels of 5 to 12 µg/mL) before any surgical or medical therapy. Phenobarbital is the preferred anticonvulsant in children.[126] If B.R. had parenchymal neurocysticercosis, corticosteroids, which are used empirically to ameliorate B.R.'s inflammatory reaction to dying parasites, would be initiated 1 to 2 days before anthelminthic therapy and continued for 4 to 7 days after completion of therapy. However, administration of corticosteroids may not prevent adverse effects in B.R.[109] Dexamethasone 4 to 16 mg/day (or an equivalent dose of prednisone) is the suggested dose for corticosteroid.[26,109,112] Albendazole 400 mg for 8 to 30 days is the preferred agent and may be more cost-effective than praziquantel.[128] However, praziquantel 50 to 100 mg/kg/day in three divided doses for 30 days has also been recommended for parenchymal neurocysticercosis.[26,122,124] The comparative eradication rates for parenchymal brain cysticercosis for albendazole and praziquantel are 80% to 85% and 60% to 70%, respectively.[125] Praziquantel 75 mg/kg/day in three divided doses Q 2 hr as a single-day dosage treatment has also been suggested in a recent paper.[125] Because dexamethasone may lower the levels of praziquantel, cimetidine 800 mg/day may be administered concurrently with it.[124] A brain CT scan and an electroencephalogram obtained 1 to 3 months after the end of treatment can be used in B.R. to monitor the resolution or reduction in the size of cysts and seizure activity.[109,114,121]

24. If B.R. had *D. latum* instead of *T. saginata*, what would be some subjective and objective findings?

If B.R. had been infected with *D. latum* instead of *T. saginata,* he may complain of being tired and possibly sleepy, which may be manifestations of anemia. *D. latum* can cause a megaloblastic anemia because the tapeworm competes with the host for dietary vitamin B_{12}.[110] Although 40% of patients with *D. latum* infection have reduced levels of vitamin B_{12}, <2% actually develop anemia from this deficiency.[110] Decreased levels of other nutritional elements have included ascorbic acid, folic acid, and riboflavin.[111] In those who do develop deficiency in vitamin B_{12} from *D. latum* infection, manifestations may include glossitis, tachycardia, and neurologic symptoms such as weakness, paresthesia, and motor coordination disturbances.[108,110,111]

Praziquantel: Side Effects

25. What are the common side effects of praziquantel that B.R. should be informed about?

Praziquantel, which is used for *T. saginata* infections, is associated with headache, dizziness, drowsiness, nausea, abdominal pain, myalgia, and urticaria.[99,106,120] The side effects usually appear about 2 hours after administration and dissipate within 48 hours. The tablets of praziquantel should never be chewed but should be swallowed whole with fluids, preferably during meals. Chewing the tablets can induce retching and vomiting because of the bitter taste.[106]

PEDICULOSIS

Prevalence

Pediculosis (lice infections) may be caused by head lice (*Pediculus humanus capitis*) (Fig. 74-10), body lice (*P. humanus*), or crab lice (*Phthirus pubis*). Lice infections may be present in all socioeconomic groups but are seen more often among the poor because of crowded living conditions and infrequent washing.[129–131]

Life Cycle

Head and body lice have similar life cycles, but their habitat preferences distinguish the two varieties.[129] The adult fertilized female lays eggs, which remain glued to hair or seams of clothing (Fig. 74-11). The oval-shaped eggs (nits) hatch in 7 to 10 days and produce nymphs, which go through a number of molts to evolve into mature adults.[129] Both larvae and adults feed on the host's blood. The lice penetrate the host skin

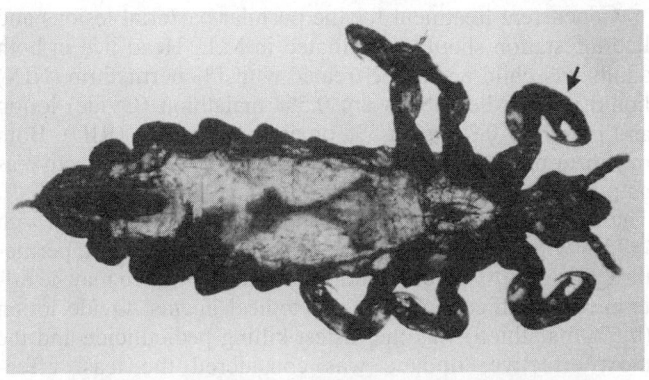

FIGURE 74-10 *Pediculus humanus capitis* (head lice).

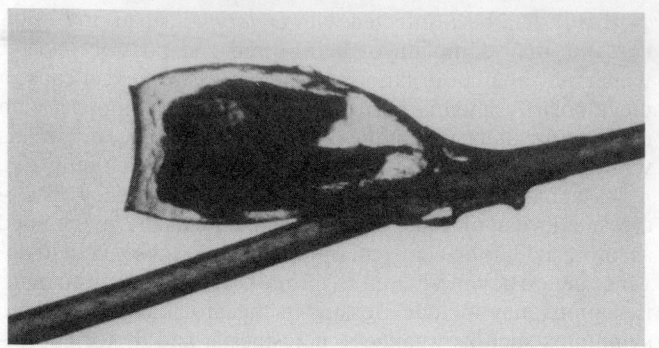

FIGURE 74-11 Nit or egg of lice on hair shaft.

by use of stylets within their head and attach themselves by a circlet of teeth on their proboscis.[129] Crab lice usually are found in pubic hair, although these organisms may also be found on eyebrows, eyelashes, and axillary hairs.[129,130]

Epidemiology

The highest incidence of head lice is seen among schoolchildren.[129] The incidence of all types of lice infestation in the United States has been estimated to be 6 to 12 million cases.[131] Head and body lice are transferred between hosts by personal and clothing contact, whereas crab lice are transmitted by sexual contact.[132]

Signs and Symptoms

26. **M.L., a 54-year-old homeless man, lives in a city shelter and is brought to the clinic by his welfare worker. M.L. has excoriations and numerous pustular lesions all over his body. The welfare worker states that M.L. has "lice all over his body." Why are the symptoms in M.L. consistent with lice infection?**

The most common complaint of patients with head and body lice is pruritus of the scalp, ears, neck, and other body parts. However, with severe infestations, as seen in M.L., intractable itching and scratching can result in folliculitis, hemorrhagic macules or papules, postinflammatory skin thickening, and pigmentation.[129,131,132] In contrast, schoolchildren who are exposed frequently to head lice may have only minor pruritus affecting the scalp, ears, and neck.[129,131]

Treatment

27. **How should M.L. be treated for lice infection of the head, body, and genital areas?**

Concurrent treatment for the pustular bacterial lesions and lice infestation should be initiated in M.L. Head lice in both adults and children can be treated with 1% permethrin (NIX) liquid rinse. Alternatives are 0.5% malathion (Ovide) lotion and pyrethrin 0.3% plus 3% piperonyl butoxide (RID). Both pyrethrin preparations and malathion 0.5% are as effective as gamma benzene hexachloride or lindane 1% (Kwell).[26,131–137] The eradication rate for lindane is 65% to 85%, compared with >95% with the new synthetic derivative of pyrethrin, permethrin (NIX).[132–135] Recent studies indicate that there may be differences in efficacy among the topical agents. Ovide lotion (0.5% malathion) was the fastest-killing pediculicide and the most effective; lindane was considered the least effec-

tive.[132,133,137] There is a growing concern that lice are becoming resistant to the pyrethrin products in the United States.[132–137]

PYRETHRIN, LINDANE, AND MALATHION

Pyrethrin, which contains extracts of chrysanthemum flowers, acts by blocking the transmission of nerve impulses in lice and kills them in a few minutes.[131] Approximately 30 to 50 mL of the pyrethrin lotion should be massaged into M.L.'s scalp, left for about 10 minutes, then rinsed out. The treatment should be followed by a plain shampoo. Nits can be removed from the hair by applying a solution containing equal parts of water and vinegar and using a sturdy fine-tooth comb to remove the nits.[129,131] Some investigators are not impressed with "combing" as an effective method to remove nits.[135] The whole course of treatment should be repeated within 7 to 10 days to eradicate the organisms hatched after initial therapy.[129,131] Patients who have a history of ragweed allergy occasionally react to pyrethrin preparations.[134] If M.L. has an allergy to pyrethrin, malathion lotion 0.5% may be an alternative. Malathion should be left on for 12 to 24 hours.

For the body and pubic lice in M.L., a pyrethrin combination lotion should be applied. It may be necessary to leave the lotion on for 4 to 6 hours to eradicate crab lice.[129] The applications should be followed by a warm bath. The treatment should be repeated in 7 to 10 days. The pruritus in M.L. can be symptomatically treated with an antihistamine and a low-potency topical steroid.[129]

Alternative treatment for head lice for patients in whom the infestations are not eradicated with either permethrin 1% or lindane are 5% permethrin cream (Elimite) applied to the scalp overnight, or petrolatum (approximately 40 g) applied to the scalp and left overnight with a shower cap.[129] After the application of the petrolatum, a shampoo should be used for 7 to 10 days to remove the residue. Children 2 years or younger should not be treated for lice, and only manual removal should be attempted.[131]

PETROLATUM

To remove pubic lice from M.L.'s eyelids or eyelashes, plain petrolatum ointment can be used.[129,132] Petrolatum is applied to the eyelashes and lid margins with cotton swabs three or four times daily. This regimen will either suffocate the lice or physically remove them.[129,132]

DECONTAMINATION MEASURES

Treatment for pediculosis should include thorough decontamination to avoid reinfection. All personal articles of clothing, including bedding, should be washed (preferably in the hot cycle of the washer, or in hot water). Hairbrushes, combs, and other plastic articles can be decontaminated by soaking in rubbing alcohol or pediculicide.[129,131] In institutions and schools where lice infestations are a problem, outer clothing (coats, hats, scarves) of individuals should be isolated in separate plastic bags at the beginning of the day. This measure will reduce reinfection significantly.

Toxicity

28. **What are the toxicities of the common pediculicides?**

Lindane can cause neurologic symptoms, including tremors, ataxia, insomnia, and seizures in patients who are exposed to it over extended periods.[131,132,134] It also is reported to cause aplastic anemia.[132] However, when it is applied for 10 minutes to treat head or body lice, it is considered safe and effective in both adults and children.[132] In clinical studies of >3,500 patients, the only adverse effects reported with permethrin were local irritative symptoms (2.1% to 5.9%).[138] Malathion, an organophosphate cholinesterase inhibitor, is degraded rapidly by hepatic enzymes in humans and occasionally can cause some local irritation.[131,139] These agents are not contraindicated during pregnancy and may be used for treatment.[26,138]

SCABIES

Prevalence

Scabies is caused by *Sarcoptes scabiei* var. *hominis*.[139–141] The female mite burrows into the skin of the host and lays eggs, which hatch into larvae after 72 to 84 hours. After a number of molts, the adult mites mate and the male dies. The female gravid mite continues to burrow into new areas of skin, primarily in web spaces between the fingers, wrists, elbows, periumbilical skin, and buttocks.[141] The hallmark of scabies is intense itching with erythematous papules and excoriations. In infants, scabies may be vesicular or bullous; secondary pyoderma is not uncommon. Transmission is by intimate contact, and institutional epidemics have been reported.[140–142]

Treatment

29. T.R., a 4-year-old girl, has a pruritic rash with excoriations in the interdigital areas of both hands. Her mother states that T.R.'s 7-year-old brother, G.R., has a similar rash affecting his hands, groin, and feet. The lesions are scraped and microscopic examination reveals mites and ova of *S. scabiei*. How should T.R. and G.R. be treated? What special instructions and precautions should accompany therapy?

LINDANE, PERMETHRIN, AND CROTAMITON

The agents available for treatment of scabies include lindane 1% (Kwell), crotamiton 10% (Eurax), and permethrin 5% cream (Elimite).[26,142–146] The agent that has been used most extensively is lindane, but its safety remains a point of contention.[132,145,146] When lindane is left on the skin too long (especially excoriated skin), percutaneous absorption can cause neurotoxicity.[132] Crotamiton 10% is presumably safe for infants and pregnant women, but definitive data do not exist. A single application of permethrin 5% cream is more effective than crotamiton or lindane.[143–146] However, it has been suggested that ivermectin (Stromectol) (200 μg/kg every 2 weeks for three doses) may be added to the topical therapy if there is no response to permethrin alone. Although ivermectin is not FDA-label approved for scabies, there have been a significant number of studies using this agent both topically and systemically for scabies.[132,147,148] Studies indicate that two doses of ivermectin of 400 μg/kg separated by a week can be used for scabies epidemics, and the cure rate has been around 100% with this regimen.[132]

T.R. and G.R. should have their nails trimmed to minimize further excoriation. They then should be bathed using a soft washcloth to remove loose crusts. Thereafter, permethrin cream should be massaged into the skin from the head (including the scalp) to the soles of the feet.[139,142] The cream should be left on for 8 to 14 hours before they are bathed again. If crotamiton is selected, it should be applied to the entire body (including the scalp) and left on for 24 hours after the initial bath. A second 24-hour application is recommended before the children are bathed again. When lindane is used, it is applied to the entire body (avoiding the eyes and mucous membranes) and left on the body for approximately 8 hours.[139] After 6 to 8 hours, a cool bath should be taken. Pruritus from scabies may be treated symptomatically with an oral antihistamine such as hydroxyzine (Vistaril) or diphenhydramine (Benadryl), or with a low-potency topical steroid.

Clothes and linens belonging to T.R. and G.R. should be freshly laundered, and they should be re-examined after a week. If there is evidence of active infestation (positive microscopic findings), a second treatment course may be initiated in these patients. They should be informed that pruritus may persist for >10 days. Pruritus usually results from retained parts of the mites.

REFERENCES

1. Dorsey G et al. Difficulties in the prevention, diagnosis, and treatment of imported malaria. Arch Intern Med 2000;160:2505.
2. Dardick K. Educating travelers about malaria: dealing with resistance and patient noncompliance. Cleveland Clin J Med 2002;69:469.
3. Jerrard DA et al. Malaria: a rising incidence in the United States. J Emerg Med 2002;23:23.
4. Malarial Surveillance, United States, 2000. MMWR 2002;51:(SS5):9.
5. Center for Disease Control and Prevention. Malaria in an immigrant and travelers, Georgia, Vermont, and Tennessee, 1996. MMWR 1997;46:536.
6. Local transmission of *Plasmodium vivax* malaria, Virginia, 2002.MMWR 2002;51:922.
7. Wallace M et al. Malaria among United States troops in Somalia. Am J Med 1996;100:49.
8. Strickland GT, Taylor TE. Infections of the blood and reticuloendothelial system: malaria. In: Strickland GT, ed. Hunter's Tropical Medicine and Emerging Infectious Diseases. Philadelphia: WB Saunders, 2000:614.

9. Vinetz JM et al. *Plasmodium malariae* infection in asymptomatic 74-year-old Greek woman with splenomegaly. N Engl J Med 1998;338:367.
10. Krogstad DJ. Plasmodium species (malaria). In: Mandell GL et al, eds. Principles and Practice of Infectious Diseases. New York: Churchill Livingstone, 2000:2817.
11. Kain KC et al. Malaria deaths in visitors to Canada and in Canadian travelers. A case series. CMAJ 2001;164:654.
12. Kain KC et al. Malaria chemoprophylaxis in the age of drug resistance. I. Currently recommended drug regimens. Clin Infect Dis 2001;33:226.
13. Nosten F et al. Effects of artesunate-mefloquine combination on the incidence of *Plasmodium falciparum* malaria and mefloquine resistance in Western Thailand: A prospective study. Lancet 2000; 356:297.
14. Centers for Disease Control and Prevention. Malaria deaths following inappropriate malaria chemoprophylaxis, United States, 2001. MMWR 2001;50:597.

15. Blum PG, Stephens D. Severe falciparum malaria in five soldiers from East Timor: A case series and literature review. Anaesthesia Intensive Care 2001; 29:426.
16. Shanks GD et al. Malaria chemoprophylaxis in the age of drug resistance. II. Drugs that may be available in the future. Clin Infect Dis 2001;33:381.
17. Murphy GS, Oldfield EC III. Falciparum malaria. Infect Dis Clin North Am 1996;10:747.
18. Wellems TE, Plowe CV. Chloroquine-resistant malaria. J Infect Dis 2001;184:770.
19. White NJ. The treatment of malaria. N Engl J Med 1996;335:800.
20. Murphy SC, Breman JG. Gaps in the childhood malaria burden in Africa: cerebral malaria, neurological sequelae, anemia, respiratory distress, hypoglycemia, and complication of pregnancy. Am J Trop Med Hyg 2001;64:57.
21. Breman JG. The ears of the hippopotamus: manifestations, determinants, and estimates of the malaria burden. Am J Trop Med Hyg 2001;64:28.

22. Riddle MS et al. Exchange transfusion as an adjunct therapy in severe *Plasmodium falciparum* malaria: a meta-analysis. Clin Infect Dis 2002; 34:1192.

23. Newton CRJC, Warrell DA. Neurological manifestations of falciparum malaria. Ann Neurol 1998; 43:695.

24. Taylor WRJ, White NJ. Malaria and the lung. Clin Chest Med 2002;23:457.

25. Sehdev PS. Atovaquone/proguanil for *Plasmodium falciparum* malaria. Pediatr Infect Dis J 2002; 21:787.

26. Drugs for parasitic infections. Med Lett Drugs Ther April 2002:1-12. (Available online at www.medletter.com).

27. Centers for Disease Control and Prevention. Availability and use of parenteral quinidine gluconate for severe or complicated malaria. MMWR 2000; 49:1138.

28. Angus BJ. Malaria on the World Wide Web. Clin Infect Dis 2001;33:651.

29. Croft A. Malaria: prevention of malaria for travellers. JAMA 1997;278:1767.

30. Na Bangchang K et al. Mefloquine pharmacokinetics in pregnant women with active falciparum malaria. Trans R Soc Trop Med Hyg 1994;88:321.

31. Phillips-Howard P, Wood D. The safety of antimalarial drugs in pregnancy. Drug Safety 1996; 14:131.

32. Massele AY et al. Chloroquine blood concentrations and malaria prophylaxis in Tanzanian women during the second and third trimester of pregnancy. Eur J Clin Pharmacol 1997;52:299.

33. Steketee RW et al. The burden of malaria in pregnancy in endemic areas. Am J Trop Med Hyg 2001;64:28.

34. Steketee RW et al. Malaria parasite infection during pregnancy and at delivery in mother, placenta, and newborn: efficacy of chloroquine and chloroquine and mefloquine in rural Malawi. Am J Trop Med Hyg 1996;55:24.

35. Samuel BU, Barry M. The pregnant traveler. Infect Dis Clin North Am 1998;12:325.

36. Schultz LJ et al. Evaluation of maternal practices, efficacy, and cost-effectiveness of alternative antimalarial regimens for use in pregnancy: chloroquine and sulfadoxine-pyrimethamine. Am J Trop Med Hyg 1996;55:87.

37. Alecrim WD et al. *Plasmodium falciparum* infection in the pregnant patient. Infect Dis Clin North Am 2000;14:83.

38. White NJ. Antimalarial pharmacokinetics and treatment regimens. Br J Clin Pharmacol 1992;34:1.

39. Tracy JW, Webster LT Jr. Drugs used in the chemotherapy of protozoal infections. Malaria. In: Gilman AG et al, eds. The Pharmacological Basis of Therapeutics. New York: McGraw-Hill, 2001; 1069.

40. Advice to travelers. Med Lett Drugs 2002;44:33.

41. Soto J et al. *Plasmodium vivax* clinically resistant to chloroquine in Columbia. Am J Trop Med Hyg 2001;65:90.

42. Newton P, White N. Malaria: New developments in treatment and prevention. Annu Rev Med 1999; 50:179.

43. Rosenthal PJ, Goldsmith RS. Antiprotozoal drugs. In: Katzung BG, ed. Basic and Clinical Pharmacology. Norwalk, CT: Appleton & Lange, 2001;882.

44. Fradin MS. Mosquitoes and mosquito repellents: a clinician's guide. Ann Intern Med 1998;128:931.

45. Andersen SL et al. Successful double-blinded, randomized, placebo-controlled field trial of azithromycin and doxycycline as prophylaxis for malaria in Western Kenya. Clin Infect Dis 1998;26:146.

46. Nosten F et al. The effects of mefloquine treatment in pregnancy. Clin Infect Dis 1999;28:808.

47. Whitty CJM et al. Malaria. Br Med J 2002; 325:1221.

48. Hoffman SL. Plasmodium, human and anopheles genomics and malaria. Nature 2002;415:702.

49. Richie TL, Saul A. Progress and challenges for malaria vaccines. Nature 2002;415:694.

50. Alloueche A et al. Protective efficacy of the RTSS/AS02 *Plasmodium falciparum* malaria vaccine is strain specific. Am J Trop Med Hyg 2003; 68:97.

51. Carvalho LJ et al. Malaria vaccine: candidate antigens, mechanisms, constraints and prospects. Scand J Immunol 2002;56:327.

52. Schwobel B et al. Therapeutic efficacy of chloroquine plus sulfhadoxime/pyrimethamine compared with monotherapy with either chloroquine or sulfhadoxime/pyrimethamine in uncomplicated *Plasmodium falciparum* malaria in Loas. Trop Med Int Health 2003;8:19.

53. Hogh B et al. Atovaquone/proguanil versus chloroquine/proguanil for malaria prophylaxis in non-immune travelers: results from a randomized, double-blind study. Lancet 2000;356:1888.

54. Taylor WR et al. Chloroquine/doxycycline combination versus chloroquine, and doxycycline alone for the treatment of *Plasmodium falciparum* and *Plasmodium vivax* malaria in Northeastern Irian Jaya, Indonesia. Am J Trop Med Hyg 2001;64:223.

55. Fischer PR, Bialek R. Prevention of malaria in children. Clin Infect Dis 2002;34:493.

56. Looareesuwan S et al. Malarone (atovaquone and proguanil): A review of its clinical development for treatment of malaria. Malarone Clinical Trials Group. Am J Trop Med Hyg 1999;60:533.

57. Brockman A et al. *Plasmodium falciparum* Antimalarial drug susceptibility of the northwestern border of Thailand during five years of extensive use of artesunate-mefloquine. Trans R Soc Trop Med Hyg 2000;94:537.

58. McGready R et al. Artemisinin antimalarials and pregnancy: a prospective treatment study of 539 episodes of multidrug-resistant *Plasmodium falciparum*. Clin Infect Dis 2001;33:2009.

59. Meshnick SR. Artemisinin: mechanisms of action, resistance and toxicity. Int J Parasitol 2002; 32:1655.

60. Lell B et al. Fosmidomycin, a novel chemotherapeutic agent for malaria. Antimicrob Agents Chemother 2003;47:735.

61. Lell B et al. Malaria chemoprophylaxis with tefenoquine: a randomized study. Lancet 2000;355:2041.

62. Quak SH et al. Glucose-6-phosphate dehydrogenase deficiency in Singapore. Ann Acad Med Singapore 1996;25:45.

63. Hundsdoerfer P et al. Chronic haemolytic anemia and glucose-6-phosphate dehydrogenase deficiency. Case report and review of the literature. Acta Haematol 2002;108:102.

64. Ravdin JI, Petri WA. *Entamoeba histolytica* (Amebiasis). In: Mandell GL et al, eds. Principles and Practice of Infectious Diseases. New York: Churchill Livingstone, 2000:2798.

65. Haque R et al. Amebiasis. N Engl J Med 2003;348:1565.

66. Shamsuzzaman SM, Hashiguchi Y. Thoracic amebiasis. Clin Chest Med 2002;23:479.

67. Parshad S et al. Primary cutaneous amoebiasis: case report with review of the literature. Int J Dermatol 2002;41:676.

68. Jackson TFGH, Gathiram V. Intestinal and genital infections. Amebiasis. In: Strickland GT, ed. Hunter's Tropical Medicine and Emerging Infectious Diseases. Philadelphia: WB Saunders, 2000;577.

69. Stanley SL Jr. Protective immunity to amebiasis: new insights and new challenges. J Infect Dis 2001;184:504.

70. Hughes MA, Petri WA. Amebic liver abscess. Infect Dis Clin North Am 2000;14:565.

71. Haque R et al. Diagnosis of amebic liver abscess and intestinal infection with the TechLab *Entamoeba histolytica* II antigen detection and antibody tests. J Clin Microbiol 2000;38:3235.

72. Citronberg RJ, Semel D. Severe vaginal infection with *Entamoeba histolytica* in a woman who recently returned from Mexico: case report and review. Clin Infect Dis 1995;20:700.

73. Hejase MJ et al. Amebiasis of the penis. Urology 1996;48:151.

74. Tracy JW, Webster LT Jr. Drugs used in the chemotherapy of protozoal infections (continued). Ameblasis, giardiasis, trichomoniasis, trypanosomiasis, leishmaniasis and other protozoal infections. In: Gilman AG et al, eds. The Pharmacological Basis of Therapeutics. New York: McGraw-Hill, 2001:1097.

75. Petri WA Jr, Singh U. Diagnosis and management of amebiasis. Clin Infect Dis 1999;29:1117.

76. Kimura KL et al. Amebiasis: Modern diagnostic imaging with pathological and clinical correlation. Semin Roentgenol 1997;32:250.

77. Hira PR et al. Invasive amebiasis: Challenges in diagnosis in non-endemic country (Kuwait). Am J Trop Med Hyg 2001;65:341.

78. Reed SL. Amebiasis and infection with free-living amebas. In: Braunwald E et al., eds. Harrison's Principle of Internal Medicine. New York: McGraw-Hill, 2001:1199.

79. Cushing AH et al. Metronidazole concentrations in a hepatic abscess. Pediatr Infect Dis 1985; 4:697.

80. Wright SG. Giardiasis. In: Strickland GT, ed. Hunter's Tropical Medicine and Emerging Infectious Diseases. Philadelphia: WB Saunders, 2000:589.

81. Hill DR. *Giardia lamblia*. In: Mandell GL et al., eds. Principle and Practice of Infections Diseases. New York: Churchill Livingstone, 2000:2888.

82. Gardner TB, Hill DR. Treatment of giardiasis. Clin Microbiol Rev 2001;14:114

83. Ortega YR, Adam RD. Giardia. Overview and update. Clin Infect Dis 1997;25:545.

84. Furness BW, Beach MJ, Roberts JM. Giardiasis surveillance, United States, 1992–1997. MMWR 2000;49:1.

85. Hopkins RS et al. Water-borne disease in Florida: continuing threats require vigilance. J Florida Med Assoc 1997;84:441.

86. Mintz ED et al. Foodborne giardiasis in a corporate office setting. J Infect Dis 1993;167:250.

87. Olivares JL et al. Vitamin B12 and folic acid in children with intestinal parasitic infection. J Am Coll Nutrition 2002;21:109.

88. Ortiz JJ et al. Randomized clinical study of nitazoxanide compared to metronidazole in the treatment of symptomatic giardiasis in children from Northern Peru. Alimentary Pharmacol Therap 2001;15:1409.

89. Farthing MJG. The molecular pathogenesis of giardiasis. J Pediat Gastroenterol Nutrition 1997; 24:79.

90. Hanson KL, Cartwright CP. Use of an enzyme immunoassay does not eliminate the need to analyze multiple stool specimens for sensitive detection of *Giardia lamblia*. J Clin Microbiol 2001;39:474.

91. Soliman MM et al. Comparison of serum antibody response to *Giardia lamblia* of symptomatic and asymptomatic patients. Am J Trop Med Hyg 1998;58:232.

92. Oberhuber G, Stolte M. Symptoms in patients with giardiasis undergoing upper gastrointestinal endoscopy. Endoscopy 1997;29:716.

93. Oberhuber G et al. Giardiasis: a histologic analysis of 527 cases. Scan J Gastroenterol 1997;32:48.

94. Aronson NE et al. Biliary giardiasis in a patient with human immunodeficiency virus. J Clin Gastroenterol 2001;33:167.

95. Nashte OCA et al. Treatment of patients with refractory giardiasis. Clin Infect Dis 2001;33:22.

96. Abboud P et al. Successful treatment of metronidazole-and albendazole-resistant giardiasis with nitrazoxanide in a patient with acquired immunodeficiency syndrome. Clin Infect Dis 2001; 31:1792.

97. Rossignol JF et al. Treatment of diarrhea caused by *Giardia intestinalis* and *Entamoeba histolytica* or *E. dispar*: a randomized, double-blind, placebo-controlled study by nitazoxanide. J Infect Dis 2001;184:381.

98. Mahmoud AAF. Intestinal nematodes (roundworms). In: Mandell GL et al., eds. Principles and

Practice of Infectious Diseases. New York, Churchill Livingstone, 2000:2938.

99. Tracy JW, Webster LT Jr. Drugs used in the chemotherapy of helminthiasis. In: Gilman AG et al., eds. The Pharmacological Basis of Therapeutics. New York: McGraw-Hill, 2000:1121.

100. Tandan T et al. Pelvic inflammatory disease associated with *Enterobius vermicularis.* Arch Dis Child 2002;86:439.

101. Wagner ED, Eby W. Pinworm prevalence in California elementary school children, and diagnostic methods. Am J Trop Med Hyg 1983;32:998.

102. Wu ML et al. *Enterobius vermicularis.* Arch Path Lab Med 2003;124:647.

103. Grencis RK, Cooper ES. Enterobius, trichuris, capillaria, and hookworm including *Ancylostoma caninum.* Gastroenterol Clin North Am 1996; 25:579.

104. Bundy DA, Cooper E. Nematodes limited to the intestinal tract (*Enterobius vermicularis, Trichuris trichiura,* and *Capillaria philippinensis*): Enterobiasis. In: Strickland GT et al., eds. Hunter's Tropical Medicine and Emerging Infectious Diseases. Philadelphia: WB Saunders, 2000:719.

105. Savioli L et al. Use of drugs during pregnancy. Am J Obstet Gynecol 2003;118:5.

106. Goldsmith RS. Clinical Pharmacology of antihelminthic drugs. In: Katzung BG, ed. Basic and Clinical Pharmacology. Norwalk, CT: Appleton & Lange, 2001:903.

107. White AC Jr., Weller PF. Cestodes. In: Braunwald E et al., eds. Harrison's Principles of Internal Medicine. New York: McGraw-Hill, 2001:1248.

108. Markell EK et al. Medical Parasitology. Philadelphia: WB Saunders, 1999.

109. Garcia HH, Del Brutto OH. *Taenia solium* cysticercosis. Infect Dis Clin North Am 2000;14:97.

110. Schantz PM. Tapeworms (cestodiasis). Gastroenterol Clin North Am 1996;25:637.

111. Schantz PM et al. Tapeworm infections. In: Strickland GT, ed. Hunter's Tropical Medicine and Emerging Infectious Diseases. Philadelphia: WB Saunders, 2000:854.

112. Proano J et al. Medical treatment for neurocysticercosis characterized by giant subarachnoid cysts. N Engl J Med 2001;345:879.

113. Del Brutto OH et al. Proposed diagnostic criteria for neurocysticercosis. Neurology 2001;57:177.

114. Garcia HH et al. Current consensus guidelines for treatment of neurocysticercosis. Clin Microbiology Rev 2002;15:747.

115. Evans CAW et al. Larval cestode cysticercosis. In: Strickland GT, ed. Hunter's Tropical Medicine and Emerging Infectious Diseases. Philadelphia: WB Saunders, 2000:862.

116. Sotelo J. Neurocysticercosis: Eradication of cysticercosis is an attainable goal. Br Med J 2003; 326:51.

117. Garcia HH et al. Circulating parasite antigen in patients with hydrocephalus secondary to neurocysticercosis. Am J Trop Med Hyg 2002;66:427.

118. Gilman RH et al. and the Cysticercosis Working Group in Peru. Prevalence of taeniasis among neurocysticercosis patients is related to severity of cerebral infection. Neurology 2000;55:1062.

119. Schantz PM. Dangers of eating raw fish. N Engl J Med 1989;320:1143.

120. Antihelminths. In: Kastrup EK et al, eds. St. Louis: Drug Facts and Comparisons, 2003:1474.

121. Garcia HH et al. Albendazole therapy for neurocysticercosis: a prospective, double-blind trial comparing 7 versus 14 days of treatment. Neurology 1997;48:1421.

122. Rajshekar V. Incidence and significance of adverse effects of albendazole therapy in patients with a persistent solitary cysticercus granuloma. Acta Neurol Scand 1998;98:121.

123. Del Brutto OG et al. Single-day praziquantel versus 1-week albendazole for neurocysticercosis. Neurology 1999;52:1081.

124. Yee T et al. High-dose praziquantel with cimetidine for refractory neurocysticercosis: a case report with clinical and MRI follow-up. West J Med 1999;170:112.

125. Sotelo J, Jung H. Pharmacokinetic optimization of the treatment of neurocysticercosis. Clin Pharmacokinet 1998;34:503.

126. Carpio A, Hauser WA. Prognosis for seizures recurrence in patients with newly diagnosed neurocysticercosis. Neurology 2002;59:1730.

127. Del Brutto OH. Albendazole therapy for subarachnoid cysticerci: clinical and neuroimaging analysis of 17 patients. J Neurol Neurosurg Psychiatry 1997;62:659.

128. Venkatesan P. Albendazole. J Antimicrob Chemother 1998;41:145.

129. Mathieu ME, Wilson BB. Lice (pediculosis). In: Mandell GL et al, eds. Principles and Practice of Infectious Diseases. New York: Churchill Livingstone, 2000:2972.

130. Elston DM. What's eating you? Cutis 1999; 63:259.

131. Mazurek CM, Lee NP. How to manage head lice. West J Med 2000;172:342.

132. Wendel K, Rompalo A. Scabies and pediculosis: An update of treatment regimens and general review. Clin Infect Dis 2002;35(Suppl 2):S146.

133. Meniking TL et al. Comparative efficacy of treatments for *Pediculosis capitis* infestations. Update 2000. Arch Dermatol 2001;137:287.

134. Roberts RJ. Head lice. N Engl J Med 2002; 346:1645.

135. Meinking TL et al. An observer-blinded study of 1% permethrin crème rinse with and without adjunctive combing in patients with head lice. J Pediatr 2002;141:665.

136. Bartels CL et al. Head lice resistance: Itching that just won't stop. Ann Pharmacother 2001;35:109.

137. Meinking TL et al. Comparative In vitro pediculicidal efficacy of treatments in a resistant head lice population in the United States. Arch Dermatol 2002;138:220.

138. Andrews EB et al. Postmarketing surveillance study of permethrin cream rinse. Am J Public Health 1992;82:857.

139. Scabicides/pediculicides. In: Kastrup EK et al., eds. St. Louis: Drug Facts & Comparisons, 2003:1699.

140. Mathieu ME, Wilson BB. Scabies. In: Mandell GL et al., eds. Principles and Practice of Infectious Diseases. New York: Churchill Livingstone, 2000:2974.

141. Paller AS. Scabies in infants and small children. Semin Dermatol 1993;12:3.

142. Haag ML et al. Attack of scabies: what to do when an attack occurs. Geriatrics 1993;48:45.

143. Quarterman MJ, Leshher JL Jr. Neonatal scabies treated with permethrin 5% cream. Pediatr Dermatol 1994;11:264.

144. Centers for Disease Control and Prevention. Sexually transmitted diseases treatment guidelines 2002. MMWR 2002;51(RR-6):67.

145. Franz TJ et al. Comparative percutaneous absorption of lindane and permethrin. Arch Dermatol 1996;132:901.

146. Elgart ML. A risk-benefit assessment of agents used in the treatment of scabies. Drug Safety 1996;14:386.

147. Currie B et al. Ivermectin for scabies. Lancet 1997;350:1551.

148. Usha V, Gopalakrishnan Nair TV. A comparative study of oral ivermectin and topical permethrin cream for the treatment of scabies. J Am Acad Dermatol 2000;42:236.

Tick-Borne Diseases

Tom E. Christian

OVERVIEW

Ticks belong to the class Arachnida, which includes scorpions, spiders, and mites. As a vector of human illness worldwide, ticks are second in importance only to mosquitoes. Ticks transmit more infectious agents than any other arthropod. Disease may be spread by ticks either by transmission of microorganisms or by injection of tick toxin into a host. Bacterial, rickettsial, protozoal, and viral disease pathogens can be transmitted from ticks to humans[1] (Table 75-1).

Tick Genus

Only two of the three families of ticks are of medical significance to humans: the soft-bodied ticks, *Argasidae,* and the hard-bodied ticks, *Ixodidae.*[1] Three of the 13 genera of *Ixodidae* transmit disease in the United States: *Dermacentor, Ixodes,* and *Amblyomma.* Among the five genera of *Argasidae,* only *Ornithodoros* are known to transmit pathogens to humans in the United States. Most hard ticks have a 2-year life

cycle, comprising the larval, nymphal, and adult stages. They require one blood meal during each stage before they can progress to the next stage, and they usually remain attached to the host for hours or days. In contrast, soft ticks may have multiple nymphal stages, and both nymphal and adult forms can feast on blood more than once, usually for only 30 minutes. However, *Argasidae* can survive many years without blood sustenance and are long-lived.[1] Humans are the inadvertent hosts for the life cycle of almost all ticks and tick-borne diseases.

LYME DISEASE

Lyme disease, or more accurately Lyme borreliosis, is a multisystem spirochetal disease transmitted by a tick bite.[1-10] Although the responsible spirochete, *Borrelia burgdorferi,* was not identified until 1982,[1] late manifestations of a dermatitis produced by a *Borrelia* species were described in Europe more than a century ago.[10]

Table 75-1   Tick-Borne Diseases

Disease	Causative Agent	Tick Vector	Host	Region
Lyme	*Borrelia burgdorferi*	*Ixodes*	Wild rodents	Worldwide
Relapsing fever (endemic)	*Borrelia* species	*Ornithodoros*	Wild rodents	Worldwide
Southern tick-associated rash illness	*Borrelia lonestari*	*Amblyomma*	?	South-central U.S.
Tularemia	*Francisella tularensis*	*Dermacentor* *Amblyomma*	Rabbits	North America
Rocky Mountain spotted fever	*Rickettsia rickettsii*	*Dermacentor*	Wild rodents, ticks	Western Hemisphere
Boutonneuse fever	*Rickettsia conorii*	*Ixodes*	Wild rodents, dogs	Africa, India, Mediterranean
North Asian tick typhus	*Rickettsia sibirica*	*Ixodes*	Wild rodents	Mongolia, Siberia
Queensland tick typhus	*Rickettsia australis*	*Ixodes*	Wild rodents, marsupials	Australia
Q fever	*Coxiella burnetii*	*Dermacentor* *Amblyomma*	Sheep, goats, cattle, ticks, cats	Worldwide
Babesiosis	*Babesia* species	*Ixodes*	Mice, voles	Europe, North America
Ehrlichiosis				
Human monocytic erlichiosis	*Ehrlichia chaffeensis*	*Amblyomma* *Dermacentor*	Deer, mice, dogs	United States, Mexico, Europe, Africa, Middle East
Human granulocytic erlichiosis	*Anaplasma phagocytophilia* *Ehrlichia ewingii*	*Ixodes pacificus* *Ixodes* *Dermacentor* *Amblyomma*	Deer, mice, rodents	United States, Europe U.S.
Colorado tick fever	*Coltivirus* species	*Dermacentor*	Ticks	North America
Tick-borne encephalitis	*Flavivirus*	*Ixodes*	Rodents	Eurasia
Tick paralysis	Neurotoxin	*Dermacentor*	N/A	North America, Europe, Australia, South Africa

Spirochete Identification and Pathology

There are three genomic subgroups of *B. burgdorferi* worldwide that probably account for the clinical variations observed in the disease. The North American strains identified to date belong to the *B. burgdorferi sensu stricto* group. Although all three groups have been found in Europe, most isolates are *Borrelia garinii* or *Borrelia afzelii*. An example of a disease variation is the condition of acrodermatitis chronica atrophicans (Table 75-2), a skin lesion associated only with *B. afzelii* infection.

Lyme disease is a multisystem condition, affecting the skin, eyes, joints, and cardiovascular system, as well as the central and peripheral nervous systems. The gastrointestinal (GI) and reticuloendothelial systems are involved less often. The ailment is named for the villages of Lyme and Old Lyme, Connecticut, where arthritic complications of this disease were first recognized. Lyme disease accounts for 96% of cases of vector-borne illness in the United States, with >15,000 cases reported annually.[3,6] Worldwide, it is probably the most commonly reported human disease borne by ticks.[11]

Tick Vector

Spirochetal Behavior

The tick acquires the *B. burgdorferi* spirochete from feeding on an infected host. The spirochete remains dormant in the tick's midgut until the tick feeds again, at which time the spirochete acquires a mammalian plasminogen, allowing it to penetrate the midgut wall and invade the salivary glands and other tissues of the tick. The spirochete then passes through the salivary ducts of the tick and is injected through the skin of the new host with the tick bite. Therefore, few spirochetes are transmitted from the tick to its host during the first 24 to 36 hours of attachment. However, an infected nymphal tick invariably transfers spirochetes when attached to its host for >72 hours.[12]

Tick Identification

Nymphal and larval ticks are small, <3 mm—the size of a freckle or poppy seed. Therefore, the tick often goes unnoticed, and fewer than half of patients with Lyme disease recall having been bitten by a tick. The tick feeds on small, medium, or large mammals; lizards; or birds during its larval and nymphal (immature) stages. Adult ticks parasitize only medium or large mammals; they do not feed on small mammals, birds, or lizards.[1] Humans are inadvertent hosts of any stage of the tick.[1] Although the tick can feed on many different animals, each tick species has preferred hosts. For example, the immature *Ixodes scapularis* prefers to be hosted by the white-footed mouse, whereas the mature tick prefers white-tailed deer. Collectively, these tick species, *I. scapularis* (formerly *dammini*), *I. ricinus, I. persulcatus*, and *I. pacificus*, have been referred to as the *Ixodes ricinus* complex.[11] In the Northeastern and Midwestern United States, *I. scapularis* is the primary vector, whereas *I. pacificus* is the primary vector in the Western United States. In Europe, *I. ricinus* is the vec-

Table 75-2 Lyme Borreliosis Stages

Early Localized Infection: Usually Days After Tick Bite

Erythema migrans skin rash
Myalgia, arthralgia, headache, stiff neck, fatigue, lethargy
Viral-like syndrome, fever, chills

Early Disseminated Disease: Days to Months After Bite

Musculoskeletal: Fibromyalgia, Arthralgia

Migratory arthritis
Large or small joint swelling, especially the temporomandibular joint
Painful, unilateral hand/finger swelling (Europe)

Heart (5% of Untreated Patients in U.S.)

Cardiomyopathy, congestive heart failure, myocarditis or pericarditis
Conduction defects, varying degrees of atrioventricular or bundle branch
   block, but permanent pacing not indicated
Arrhythmias

Nervous System (Neuroborreliosis)

Cranial nerve (Bell's) palsy
Meningitis, lymphocytic
Radiculoneuritis, myelitis
Sensory or motor peripheral neuropathy
Ataxia
Encephalomyelitis

Eye

Iritis, conjunctivitis, choroiditis, uveitis, optic neuritis, retinal vasculitis,
   panophthalmitis, optic disk edema, keratitis

Lymph

Generalized or localized lymphadenopathy

Skin

Multiple secondary erythema migrans lesions in 50% with primary erythema migrans; lymphocytoma (lymphadenosis benigna cutis) rare in
   the United States, but 1% in Europe

Liver

Hepatitis, recurrent; abnormal liver function tests

Lung

Acute respiratory distress syndrome

Kidney

Microscopic hematuria or proteinuria

Testicle

Orchitis

Late Disease: Months to Years After Bite

Musculoskeletal (62% in U.S., less common in Europe)

Persistent (10% of untreated in U.S.) or intermittent arthritis of ≥1 large
   joints, especially the knee

Skin (10% in Europe, rare in the U.S.)

Acrodermatitis chronica atrophicans (unique to Lyme borreliosis)

Fibromyalgia

Late Neurologic

Peripheral neuropathy, subacute encephalopathy (memory impairment,
   sleep disturbance, dementia) and in Europe, progressive encephalomyelitis

---

tor, whereas *I. persulcatus* is the primary vector in Asia.[4] The discovery of *B. burgdorferi*–like organisms from *I. ovatus* in Japan and *Haemaphysalis longicornis* in China, both of which parasitize domestic animals and humans, demonstrates greater diversity of endemic vectors and cycles in Asia. Therefore, the geographic distribution of Lyme disease matches the geographic range of the specific *Ixodes* species that harbor Lyme *Borrelia*.

Host Identification

Host type and the host's ability to harbor and transmit the spirochete to the tick (i.e., reservoir competency) are important considerations in understanding the epidemiology and prevalence of Lyme disease. The reservoir-competent white-footed mouse and the reservoir-incompetent (i.e., incapable of harboring and transmitting the spirochete) white-tailed deer are the preferred hosts for the immature and adult forms of *I. scapularis* in the Northeastern United States, respectively.[1,4] Subadult *I. pacificus* organisms preferentially feed on Western fence lizards, which are reservoir incompetent. Deer are not important hosts for mature *I. pacificus* organisms.[4] Similarly, in the Southern United States, immature *I. scapularis* ticks feed primarily on lizards. However, the cotton mouse and cot-

ton rat appear to be the predominant reservoir hosts for the spirochete in the South.[12] In Europe, various reservoir-competent mice and vole species are reported hosts for *I. ricinus*.[1] In addition, Norway rats are reservoir competent and may contribute to the risk of disease to visitors of urban parks in London, Prague, Baltimore, or Bridgeport, Connecticut.

How is Lyme borreliosis transmitted to humans in the Western United States if the preferred hosts are not reservoir competent? It is suggested that the dusky-footed wood rat and kangaroo rat, which can support *B. burgdorferi*, are the hosts of the spirochete for the few immature *I. pacificus*, which incidentally feed on the rats. Thus, an estimated 1% to 3% of *I. pacificus* organisms are infected with spirochetes, contrasting with infection rates for *I. scapularis* in the Northeastern United States of 20% to 50%.[4] In Europe, *I. ricinus* infection rates vary from 4% to 40%. In addition, bird parasitism by ticks enables the ticks to be carried long distances, even intercontinentally, during spring and fall migrations. Birds can bring ticks into new areas and also serve as maintenance hosts.[1]

Thus, the complex interplay of spirochete, host, and vector in a particular area influences the risk of Lyme disease after a tick bite. Borrelia also have been detected in soft-bodied ticks, mosquitoes, and horse and deer flies, and erythema migrans has developed after deer fly bites.[12] Lyme borreliosis is not transmitted directly between people.[7]

Stages and Laboratory Testing of Lyme Borreliosis

The clinical features of Lyme borreliosis were historically divided into three stages: early localized (stage 1), early disseminated (stage 2), and chronic, persistent, or late disease (stage 3) (see Table 75-2). Many believe that "chronic" Lyme borreliosis is an unproven entity,[13,14] although others disagree.[15] The stages may overlap, and not all stages appear sequentially. Patients may not have symptoms of any of the disease stages and may suffer no sequelae. Although Lyme disease may be debilitating, it is not life threatening.

The most specific marker of Lyme borreliosis is a characteristic skin rash termed erythema migrans. This solitary skin lesion occurs in 80% to 90% of patients with the disease.[5,6] No other physical finding of Lyme borreliosis is diagnostic. Except for direct isolation and culture of *B. burgdorferi* from body sites, no laboratory gold standard currently exists. Laboratory diagnosis of Lyme borreliosis is problematic because sufficiently sensitive and specific tests are lacking; deficiencies in laboratory standardization confound the issue. Therefore, the diagnosis of Lyme borreliosis is based on the presence of clinical findings, combined with a thorough history.[16,17] Positive results of blood tests for an antibody response to the spirochete only support a diagnosis of Lyme borreliosis. The IgM antibody response develops 4 weeks after infection, peaks at 6 to 8 weeks, and declines to the normal range after 4 to 6 months. In some patients, IgM levels may remain high or reappear. The IgG antibody response begins 6 to 8 weeks after disease onset, peaks at 4 to 6 months, and may remain elevated indefinitely.[18] In the absence of erythema migrans, serologic tests for antibody response often are used to help confirm the diagnosis of Lyme borreliosis. However, overusing serologic testing and relying too much on the results of serologic tests have resulted in excessive and inaccurate diagnoses of Lyme borreliosis.[9] Overdiagnosis of Lyme borreliosis also occurs due to its resemblance to other diseases.[4]

Treatment

The stage of Lyme borreliosis disease and the extent of infection should govern the treatment strategy of this disease.[14] However, the optimal drug, dosage, and duration of therapy for Lyme borreliosis are not firmly established. Treatment failures occur with all regimens, and despite treatment for early erythema migrans, 5% to 10% of patients are treated unsuccessfully. Poor patient compliance, use of ineffective antibiotic regimens, intra-articular corticosteroid injections before or during antibiotic treatment for arthritic complications, and ongoing immune responses imitating active infection can affect the success rate of therapy. *B. burgdorferi* can invade fibroblasts (abundant in the skin), lymphocytes, and other cells and can elude destruction by potent antibiotics such as ceftriaxone.[15,20] However, to effect a cure, it is not necessary to continue antibiotic treatment until all symptoms have resolved.[6] There is a growing tendency to use longer treatment periods of months or even years, especially in the United States. However, few scientific investigations support such prolonged

treatment regimens.[21,22] One study has shown favorable outcomes in 80% to 90% of patients with chronic Lyme disease using a 3- to 6-month regimen of tetracycline therapy.[23] Controlled trials of long- versus short-term treatment strategies are still needed (Table 75-3). Finally, it is important to distinguish fibromyalgia and chronic fatigue from active Lyme borreliosis because the symptoms of fibromyalgia do not respond to antibiotic therapy. This is true whether or not Lyme borreliosis originally triggered the fibromyalgia.[6,15] Fibromyalgia responds well to other therapies. Lyme encephalomyelitis may be confused with multiple sclerosis, yet it is conjectural whether Lyme may indirectly initiate an episode of it.[24]

1. J.S., age 38, visits his local physician with symptoms of low-grade fever and muscle aches 3 days after deer hunting in Washington state. After hunting for approximately 6 hours, he noticed a small tick on his thigh and immediately destroyed it. A small, itchy spot that he felt at the site of the tick bite is no longer symptomatic. The temporal relationship of the tick bite with his symptoms of fever and myalgias prompts his physician to collect blood samples for Lyme borreliosis antibody testing. Antibiotic therapy also is initiated. Why is the blood test not likely to be of value? Why is empiric antibiotic therapy not appropriate for J.S.?

The antibody response to *B. burgdorferi* is not detectable for the first 4 weeks after a tick bite.[6] Therefore, the blood tests for antibodies to *B. burgdorferi* are unlikely to be positive, as J.S.'s tick bite occurred only 3 days ago.

The risk of developing Lyme borreliosis can be affected by the rate of transmission of the spirochete from infected ticks to humans; the length of time before the tick is removed during its bite; the prevalence of spirochete infestation of ticks in an area, which varies with the tick species; and the reservoir competency of host animals in the region.

Although transmission rates of Lyme borreliosis from an infected tick bite are estimated at approximately 10%, the risk is reduced dramatically if the tick is removed within 24 hours of attachment, as in J.S.'s case. The small, itchy spot experienced by J.S. probably represented a hypersensitivity reaction to the bite.

Empiric antibiotic treatment for J.S. would be warranted if he were hunting in an area highly endemic for Lyme borreliosis. Specifically, if the probability of *B. burgdorferi* infection after a tick bite is ≥3.6%, then empiric prophylactic therapy is indicated. If the probability of infection is 1% to 3.5%, then immediate treatment may be preferred to waiting for signs and symptoms of Lyme borreliosis to develop. However, empiric therapy is not warranted if the probability of infection is <1%. The product of the prevalence of spirochete-infected ticks and the spirochete-to-human transfer rate is used to calculate the probability of infection after a tick bite.

The prevalence of *B. burgdorferi* infection of *I. pacificus* ticks in the Western United States is 1% to 3%. If an assumed transmission rate from spirochete to human after a tick bite is set at 10%, the product of 0.1% to 0.3% produces a probability of infection of <1% for J.S. The duration of the tick bite is the most important factor in transmission rates.[4] Because J.S. was hunting in Washington state, which is not endemic for Lyme borreliosis, and because he removed the tick within 6 hours of when it became attached to his thigh, empiric antibiotic therapy for J.S. is not warranted in the absence of symp-

Table 75-3   Treatment Recommendations for Lyme Borreliosis

Erythema Migrans, Early, Uncomplicated

Adults: Doxycycline (Vibramycin) 100 mg PO BID × 14–21 days
or
Amoxicillin (Polymox) 500 mg PO TID × 14–21 days
or
Cefuroxime axetil (Ceftin) 500 mg PO BID × 14–21 days
Children (<8 yr): Amoxicillin 50 mg/kg per day PO in 3 divided doses
    (max, 500 mg/dose) × 14–21 days or cefuroxime 30 mg/kg per day PO
    in 2 divided doses (max, 500 mg/dose) × 14–21 days
Children (≥8 yr): May use doxycycline 1–2 mg/kg PO in 2 divided doses
    (max, 100 mg/dose) × 14–21 days

Erythema Migrans With Signs of Dissemination

Cardiac Disease: third-degree heart block

Adults: Ceftriaxone (Rocephin) 2 g IV QD × 14–21 days
or
Cefotaxime (Claforan) 2 g IV TID × 14–21 days
or
Penicillin G (Pfizerpen) 3–4 MU IV Q 4 hr × 14–21 days
or
For first- or second-degree heart block: doxycycline or amoxicillin in doses
    as noted above × 14–21 days
Children: Ceftriaxone IV 75–100 mg/kg/day divided
    BID × 14–21 days

Cardiac Disease: third-degree heart block—cont'd
or
Cefotaxime IV 150–200 mg/kg per day divided TID ×14–21 days
or
Penicillin G IV 50,000–100,000 U/kg Q 4 hr × `4–21 days

Neurologic or Ocular Disease

Cranial nerve palsy as an isolated early finding: at dosages as noted above
    for early erythema migrans × 14–21 days
Meningitis, radiculitis, or encephalitis: IV drugs at dosages as noted above
    for third-degree heart block × 14–28 days
or
Doxycycline 100 mg IV BID × 14–28 days

Late Disease

Lymphocytoma or Acrodermatitis

Oral regimens for 28 days

Arthritis without neurologic disease

Adults: Doxycycline 200 mg/day PO × 28 days
or
Amoxicillin 500 mg PO QID × 28 days
Children: Amoxicillin 50 mg/kg divided TID × 28 days

Note: Tetracyclines are relatively contraindicated for pregnant or breast-feeding women.
BID, twice a day; IV, intravenously; PO, orally; QD, per day; TID, three times a day.

toms of acute Lyme disease.[12,25] Routine prophylactic treatment of a tick bite is not recommended by most clinicians.[14,20] Single-dose doxycycline prophylaxis within 3 days after a tick bite has been shown to reduce the incidence of Lyme borreliosis.[26] However, the appropriateness of this practice outside of centers with clinicians who are experienced in the identification of engorged nymphal *I. scapularis* ticks is in question.[27]

ERYTHEMA MIGRANS
Signs, Symptoms, and Disease Course

2. **K.T., a 34-year-old woman, presents with right knee pain and multiple, large, discrete skin rashes that she has had for the past 10 days. Three months ago, in July, she visited friends in Massachusetts and spent much of her time engaged in outdoor activities (e.g., hiking, biking, swimming). Two months ago, her husband noticed a circular area of intense redness, approximately 9 cm wide, in her left armpit. The rash grew considerably larger over the next 2 weeks and had a red outer border. K.T. attributed the expansion of the rash to scratching the mildly itchy area. The rash gradually disappeared. In late August, K.T. experienced fatigue, nausea, and headache for a week and thought it was "summer flu." In early September, she experienced right knee pain; ibuprofen produced some relief. Upon examination, she was afebrile and had mild soft tissue swelling of the right knee. Her white blood cell (WBC) count was normal. Electrocardiogram (ECG) was normal. Serum samples contained anti-**body titers to *B. burgdorferi* of 1:60 and 1:400 for IgM and IgG, respectively. A Venereal Disease Research Laboratory (VDRL) test for syphilis and a pregnancy test were negative.**

K.T. is started on a 4-week course of oral doxycycline 100 mg twice daily. What characteristics of K.T.'s skin rash are consistent with the erythema migrans of Lyme borreliosis?

The erythema migrans of Lyme borreliosis usually develops within 30 days (median, 7 days) of a (usually asymptomatic) tick bite at the site of inoculation of the spirochete.[5,11] The rash begins as an erythematous (red) macule or papule typically in the groin, gluteal fold, axilla, torso, popliteal fossa, or thigh.[28] In children, erythema migrans is often found on the head at the hairline, neck, arms, or legs.[28,29] It expands outwardly at 2 to 3 cm per day to a diameter of 5 to 70 cm (mean, 16 cm), occasionally with some central clearing.[28] The classic annular or ringlike patch may have complex concentric inner erythematous circles, resembling a bull's eye or target, especially in European cases.[28] Most (63%) cases of erythema migrans in the United States lack central clearing.[25] The rash may be warm to the touch and is usually painless, but some patients have mild burning or itching.[5,29] In contrast, hypersensitivity reactions to insect bites, which are commonly intensely pruritic, occur within 24 hours.[11] Up to 50% of patients with erythema migrans have multiple secondary lesions that most likely represent blood-borne spread of the spirochete to other skin sites rather than multiple tick bites.[11] If untreated, erythema migrans generally fades within several weeks; if treated, it usually resolves in several days.

Low-grade fever and other nonspecific symptoms, such as fatigue, malaise, lethargy, headache, stiff neck, myalgia, arthralgia, and regional or generalized lymphadenopathy, may accompany erythema migrans. In the United States, 80% to 90% of patients with Lyme borreliosis display erythema migrans.[5,6] Some may not have the other early symptoms of the disease. Some clinicians prefer abandoning the term "flu-like illness" in favor of "viral-like syndrome" to describe the nonspecific symptoms of early Lyme disease because cough, rhinitis, sinusitis, and GI symptoms do not usually occur.[15]

There are pitfalls in the diagnosis of erythema migrans. Erythema migrans rashes often are confused with other conditions, resulting in underdiagnosis of Lyme borreliosis, include vesicular rashes, urticarial rashes, atypical rashes, fleeting rashes, and multiple rashes with initial negative serology. Lesions commonly misdiagnosed as erythema migrans include streptococcal cellulitis, urticaria, dermal hypersensitivity reaction, *Rhus* contact dermatitis, granuloma annulare, arthropod hypersensitivity reactions, tinea corporis, and serum sickness rashes.[28,30]

K.T.'s skin rash was large (>9 cm) and red and had a red outer border. It gradually faded over a few weeks. These characteristics are consistent with a diagnosis of erythema migrans.

Serologic Testing

3. What might have been the rationale for the laboratory tests that were undertaken in K.T., and what would be reasonable interpretations of laboratory tests in patients with Lyme disease?

An antibody titer measured by enzyme-linked immunosorbent assay (ELISA) is considered positive for IgM when it is ≥1:100 and positive for IgG when it is ≥1:130. K.T.'s results (IgM of 1:60 and IgG of 1:400) support a diagnosis of Lyme borreliosis because the IgM can naturally fall by this time, yet IgG levels may remain elevated indefinitely. Syphilis and other known biologic causes (periodontal spirochetes) of false-positive serologic testing should be excluded. An ECG might have shown atrioventricular (AV) nodal block because Lyme carditis can occur within days or as long as 9 months after the onset of erythema migrans in 5% of untreated U.S. patients.[6] Rheumatoid factor or antinuclear antibody tests usually are negative in Lyme borreliosis. These tests help differentiate rheumatoid arthritis or systemic lupus erythematosus from Lyme borreliosis. The WBC count is normal or mildly elevated in Lyme borreliosis. K.T. had a normal WBC and ECG. Pregnancy was ruled out before initiating a tetracycline. Most interesting in K.T. is the presence of secondary erythema migrans lesions, which develop in up to 50% of untreated patients in the United States and represent disseminated infection.[25] Lyme borreliosis as the etiology of arthritis should always be ruled out before corticosteroids are injected into a joint because intra-articular corticosteroids administered before antibiotic therapy in Lyme borreliosis arthritis predispose the patient to treatment failure.[31] Steroid injections were appropriately not used in K.T. but could provide temporary symptomatic relief after the completion of antibiotic therapy.

The presence of erythema migrans as an early indicator of Lyme borreliosis gives physicians the best opportunity for early diagnosis and treatment, which can prevent the sequelae of disseminated disease.

LYME BORRELIOSIS TREATMENT
Antibiotics

4. Why was doxycycline (Vibramycin) chosen to treat K.T.?

The optimal therapy for Lyme borreliosis has not been firmly established, and treatment failures have occurred with all regimens studied to date. Treatment failure may be considered if minor symptoms of continued infection such as fatigue, headache, or arthralgias persist for several weeks after initial treatment or if progression to neurologic disease ensues.

B. burgdorferi is susceptible to macrolides, amoxicillin, tetracyclines, and some second- and third-generation cephalosporins, based on in vitro data. It is only moderately sensitive to penicillin G (Pfizerpen) and is resistant to rifampin (Rimactane), co-trimoxazole (Bactrim), aminoglycosides, chloramphenicol (Chloromycetin), and the fluoroquinolones.

Penicillin, tetracycline, and erythromycin historically were the drugs of choice for the treatment of Lyme borreliosis because they are given orally, are relatively inexpensive, and appeared to have good in vitro activity. Unfortunately, disappointing in vivo results were found with all these agents except penicillin. Perhaps tetracycline and erythromycin were underdosed, given in too short a duration, or intrinsically have larger time-to-kill ratios than penicillin. In Europe, in particular, penicillin still is used with continued success. Amoxicillin (Polymox) has better absorption and a longer serum half-life than penicillin V (Veetids) and continues to be effective in treating Lyme disease.

Compared with the third-generation cephalosporins, the second-generation drug cefuroxime axetil (Ceftin) is available in an oral dosage form and has good in vitro activity as well as in vivo performance. It is more expensive than oral amoxicillin or tetracyclines. Of the third-generation cephalosporins, ceftriaxone (Rocephin) has the strongest in vitro activity. The long half-life of ceftriaxone allows the convenience of once-daily dosing in an outpatient program. However, ceftriaxone is expensive and has a higher incidence of diarrhea than other β-lactams, probably because of partial biliary excretion. Risk factors for the development of ceftriaxone-induced biliary disease include age <18 years, daily ceftriaxone dose >40 mg/kg, female gender, and administration of prior courses of the drug.[32] Cefotaxime (Claforan) is an alternative to ceftriaxone that is comparable in cost but must be dosed more frequently.

The macrolides clarithromycin (Biaxin) and azithromycin (Zithromax) have excellent in vitro activity, rivaling that of ceftriaxone. However, like erythromycin, treatment failures are documented for azithromycin. A comparison study of azithromycin and amoxicillin in the treatment of erythema migrans found that azithromycin had lower response rates and higher treatment failure and relapse rates than amoxicillin.[33] Azithromycin has better tissue penetration than ceftriaxone and has been used for treatment failures of the latter, but a potential disadvantage of azithromycin is its limited ability to cross the blood–brain barrier, which may be important in preventing central nervous system (CNS) infection by the spirochete. Clarithromycin warrants further investigation because it showed promise in one study of 41 patients with early Lyme borreliosis.[34] It achieves and maintains bactericidal concentrations both intracellularly and extracellularly, unlike β-lactams or azithromycin.[34] The combination of a macrolide with lysosomotropic agents, especially hydroxychloroquine, anecdotally has been suggested to be associated with increased efficacy.[15]

Doxycycline is well absorbed orally and is less expensive than third-generation cephalosporins that must be administered parenterally. A cost-comparison study of oral doxycycline with IV ceftriaxone for early Lyme or Lyme arthritis concluded that ceftriaxone treatment is no more effective than doxycycline and is substantially more expensive.[35] Doxycycline has a long serum half-life of 18 to 22 hours. In addition, doxycycline is lipid soluble compared with the water-soluble β-lactams, accumulates intracellularly, and penetrates into the cerebrospinal fluid (CSF) at concentrations of at least 10% of serum levels even in the absence of meningeal inflammation. Doxycycline can complex with divalent or trivalent cations in the gut, and absorption may be decreased as a result. Compared with other tetracyclines, doxycycline has the least affinity for divalent calcium cations, and oral absorption is reduced by only 20% if given with milk. The major side effect of doxycycline is phototoxicity, which is of concern because Lyme borreliosis usually occurs during sunny times of the year. A less recognized side effect is the risk of doxycycline-induced esophageal ulceration. Patients should be instructed not to take doxycycline or other tetracyclines for 1 to 2 hours before going to bed or lying down and to take the medication while standing up with at least 100 mL of clear fluid, especially the capsule form.[36] Despite less in vitro activity compared with some β-lactam antibiotics, *B. burgdorferi* is sufficiently susceptible to doxycycline, and clinical experience with doxycycline has been favorable.[14] Minocycline (Minocin) has been used by some clinicians.[15,37]

In conclusion, doxycycline was a suitable choice for K.T., and the 4-week duration of therapy matches the recommendation for adult arthritis treatment outlined in Table 75-3.

Treatment-Resistant Lyme Arthritis

5. K.T. continues to have knee inflammation for 1 year despite treatment and now is considered to have treatment-resistant Lyme arthritis. Why should antibiotic therapy be repeated (or not repeated) for K.T.'s arthritis?

Treatment-resistant Lyme arthritis, which develops in approximately 10% of U.S. Lyme arthritis patients has been associated with an increased frequency of the class II major histocompatibility complex allele, HLA-DRB1*0401 human leukocyte antigen, and an immune response to OspA.[38,39] Patients with these markers may be predestined for the development of chronic arthritis despite antibiotic therapy.[38,39] The HLA-DRB1*0401 allele is associated with lack of response to antibiotic therapy and autoimmunity.[38,39] Destructive changes in the involved joint may occur, with the synovium showing vascular proliferation, villous hypertrophy, and a lymphoplasma cellular infiltrate similar to other inflammatory arthritides. In these patients, persistent arthritis is not the result of the persistence of active infection by the spirochete in a protected site.

Such patients often respond well to synovectomy, again suggesting that the presence of synovitis may not be the result of persistence of the infection.

If K.T. is HLA-DRB1*0401 positive and has antibody reactivity to the outer surface protein OspA of *B. burgdorferi*, she will likely be resistant to treatment. Repeat antibiotics are ineffective in this case. Remittive agents such as hydroxychloroquine or methotrexate may be helpful. Synovectomy may be offered.

Neuroborreliosis

6. E.C., a 54-year-old man, presents with symptoms of late Lyme encephalopathy, including memory deficits, somnolence, and irritability. CSF analyses confirm the diagnosis. Should E.C. be treated with antibiotics? If so, for how long?

Neurologic complications of Lyme borreliosis are the major morbidity of the disease.[11] Lyme encephalopathy is the most common late-stage neurologic syndrome in the United States.[11] Although the acute neurologic manifestations of Lyme borreliosis can remit spontaneously, IV antibiotic therapy hastens the resolution of symptoms and prevents the more chronic sequelae (e.g., mild cognitive dysfunction or low-grade peripheral neuropathies) of persistent CNS infection. The development of these other syndromes in E.C. may be evidence of irreversible neurologic damage. Therefore, the approach to diagnosis and treatment should be aggressive. Lumbar puncture should be performed if there is strong clinical suspicion of neurologic disease. IV antibiotic therapy is indicated according to most clinicians (see Table 75-3),[14] although others believe that there is no evidence that IV ceftriaxone is superior to tetracyclines or macrolide/hydroxychloroquine combinations in this setting.[15] As for other stages of Lyme borreliosis, the optimal duration of therapy is not firmly established. Most authorities recommend a minimum of 2 to 4 weeks.[14] Other candidates for intensive IV regimens of antibiotic therapy include patients with third-degree AV block or acute Lyme meningitis or radiculopathy.[14]

All patients with Lyme borreliosis should be treated with antibiotics because most cases can be managed effectively with appropriately chosen antibiotics. Recommendations are based on the stage of disease and the extent of the infection.[14] In conclusion, E.C. should be treated aggressively with a parenteral third-generation cephalosporin such as ceftriaxone 2 g IV daily for 2 to 4 weeks.

LABORATORY TESTING OF LYME BORRELIOSIS

7. P.S., a 35-year-old asymptomatic man with a history of a tick bite from a nonendemic Lyme borreliosis area, just tested positive on ELISA. He was tested because he expressed a fear of Lyme borreliosis. Why is this positive result alone sufficient (or insufficient) to begin treatment for Lyme borreliosis? What other tests could be considered to help confirm the diagnosis?

The *B. burgdorferi* spirochete is long and narrow, with flagella. A flagellar 41-kD protein is similar to flagellar proteins on other spirochetes, and cross-reactivity can occur. The outer surface proteins (Osp) include two of the major elicitors of antibody response in late Lyme disease, termed OspA and OspB. The OspA antigen was used for vaccine development.

Problems of standardization, sensitivity, and specificity have caused significant interlaboratory and intralaboratory variations in test results in the serodiagnosis of Lyme borreliosis.[16,17] Serologic testing for an antibody response to the spirochete is incapable of distinguishing between active infection and prior exposure. However, demonstration of local CSF antibody production and comparison with serum concentrations is highly useful in the diagnosis of neuroborreliosis, especially in European cases.[10] Despite these problems, detection of the antibody response to *B. burgdorferi* is the most commonly used laboratory procedure for the diagnosis of Lyme borreliosis.

Immunofluorescent assay (IFA) detection of antibody response was the first tool used in the diagnosis of Lyme borreliosis. However, this test is labor intensive and interpretation of the results is subjective; it has been replaced by ELISA analysis. Even with ELISA, however, 5% to 7% of test results may be false positives. The Western blot (immunoblotting) test has been shown to increase the specificity of ELISA results, but it is also insensitive in early Lyme borreliosis.[5] However, this two-step approach using a flagella-based ELISA has increased the sensitivity and specificity of antibody testing.[40] Western blotting supplements ELISA testing but does not confirm it, as they are not independent tests.[41]

The polymerase chain reaction (PCR) test can detect as few as 1 to 10 chromosomal genomes of *B. burgdorferi* by gene amplification. Unfortunately, it is so sophisticated and sensitive that it is subject to false-positive results by the accidental contamination of a sample with small quantities of the target DNA. PCR testing requires meticulous laboratory standards and quality assurance.[40] It cannot differentiate between actively infecting spirochetes and dead ones because it searches only for DNA.[8] In patients with acute Lyme borreliosis, spirochetes or spirochetal DNA circulates in the blood only intermittently or at such low levels that PCR serologic testing is unlikely to prove generally useful. New subunit serologic assays that are quicker and perhaps more sensitive and specific are commercially available. Whether these will replace the current recommendation of a sensitive ELISA followed by Western blot for serologic testing remains to be seen.[11,42]

Direct cultivation of *B. burgdorferi* from the patient's tissue or fluid or PCR detection is the irrefutable diagnostic procedure for Lyme borreliosis.[42] Direct biopsy of erythema migrans lesions or techniques of cutaneous lavage of the margin of the lesions sometimes are successful.[42] Isolation of the organism from the blood is difficult and generally not likely to be useful in the diagnosis of patients without erythema migrans.

In summary, P.S. should not be treated for active Lyme borreliosis based solely on one positive ELISA test. Although the Western blot might help to establish a diagnosis, only a careful history and physical examination in combination with the serologic testing will accurately diagnose Lyme borreliosis. The erythema migrans rash is key to early diagnosis.

Lyme Prevention

8. **P.S. is alarmed that his family members may contract Lyme borreliosis. How do you advise him?**

Most vector-borne diseases are prevented through vector control. This has proven difficult for tick-borne diseases be-cause of a lack of efficacy or environmental concerns. Methods tried include habitat destruction by fire, chemical spraying, eradication of host deer, or protection of mice from tick infestation.

The prevention of Lyme borreliosis has been limited thus far to personal protection efforts. Tick repellents may be applied to the skin or clothing. N,N-diethyl-m-toluamide (DEET) skin repellents (Repel Sportsmen) combined with a permethrin (Permanone) clothing repellent offer the best overall protection.[4,6]

DEET has been tested against *Ixodid* ticks for repellence and found to be more effective than dibutyl phthalate, dimethyl phthalate, pyrethrum, and two combination products. Although DEET was considered safe historically, studies suggest that up to 50% of an applied dose may be absorbed through the skin and distributed to fat, liver, and muscle tissue. Half of it is excreted as metabolites in the urine over 5 days. However, because DEET is lipid soluble, it can accumulate in fatty tissue and the brain.

Adverse DEET effects reported in adults include tingling, dryness, and some desquamation around the nasal area after repeated application of a 50% DEET solution to the face and arms. Two days after discontinuation of the solution, these side effects usually resolve. More severe adverse reactions in adults include acute hypersensitivity reactions with permanent scarring as a result of hemorrhagic blistering as well as anaphylaxis and an episode of acute manic psychosis. An adult case of cardiovascular toxicity consisting of hypotension and bradycardia has been reported.

In children, on the other hand, serious reactions have been reported, including hypersensitivity, toxic encephalopathy, other CNS toxicities, and a death. These are rare events, though, and if the products are used according to their labeling, the risk is low.[5] Prolonged or excessive application is not recommended. The use of a 100% DEET repellent is unnecessary and should be avoided in small children. In theory, the final concentration of DEET on the skin after application of any percentage DEET-containing product can increase due to evaporation of the solvent vehicle. It may be prudent to use the lowest effective concentration of DEET-containing repellents, such as those containing 20% to 30%. Guidelines for minimizing DEET toxicity include applying it sparingly, avoiding inhalation or introduction into the eyes, washing repellent-treated skin when coming inside, avoiding use on children's hands (which are prone to have contact with the eyes or mouth), and applying it only to intact skin or clothing.

Physical barriers to ticks, such as wearing protective garments, long pants, and long-sleeved shirts, tucking shirts into pants and pants into boots, and wearing closed-toed shoes, should help to prevent infection. Ticks can be easier to spot on light-colored clothing. Checking the body for ticks regularly is recommended; any that are found should be promptly removed. Avoiding tick habitats minimizes the potential for infection. Vaccinations for Lyme borreliosis for humans have been withdrawn from the market.

ENDEMIC RELAPSING FEVER

Physicians in ancient Greece recognized relapsing fever as a distinct disease entity,[43] but the agent of the disease was not identified until the late 19th century. Relapsing fever exists in two forms: epidemic and endemic. The bacterial spirochete *Borrelia recurrentis,* the agent responsible for epidemic relapsing fever, is transmitted between humans by the human body louse. Epidemic relapsing fever prevails in crowded conditions and occurs in the Middle East, Africa, and Asia; it has not been reported in the United States in recent years.[43-46] Mortality rates of up to 40% have been reported in some epidemics. Endemic relapsing fever is caused by a variety of *Borrelia* species, occurs worldwide, and is spread by ticks.

Spirochete Identification

In Europe and Africa, the identified responsible spirochetes are *Borrelia hispanica, Borrelia duttoni,* and *Borrelia crocidurae;* in North America, the species are *Borrelia hermsii, Borrelia turicatae,* and *Borrelia parkeri.*[43,44] Other *Borrelia* species may produce Lyme-like diseases or relapsing fevers worldwide. For example, *Borrelia lonestari* has tentatively been identified as the etiologic agent of Southern tick-associated rash illness (STARI) in the south-central United States.[47] The terms "tick-borne" relapsing fever and "endemic" or "sporadic" relapsing fever are considered interchangeable. In contrast to epidemic relapsing fever, death from tick-borne relapsing fever is rare, and most patients recover.[43]

As the name implies, this disease is characterized by intermittent bouts of fever of variable duration. The *Borrelia* have the genetic ability to alter their outer surface proteins extensively. This capacity of the spirochetes to vary their surface antigens, thus eluding host defenses, is the presumed explanation for the recurrent nature of relapsing fever.[43,44]

Tick Vector

Tick Identification

The predominant tick vector for relapsing fever is of the genus *Ornithodoros,* a soft-bodied tick. These ticks feed on wild rodents or domestic animals and, incidentally, on humans. In Europe, *O. erraticus* is one *Ornithodoros* species that transmits *Borrelia.* In North America, three tick species carry the agents of endemic relapsing fever with apparent strict specificity. In fact, the names of the responsible *Borrelia* species have been adopted from the three tick species that transmit them: *O. hermsii, O. parkeri,* and *O. turicata.* Although the ticks themselves may serve as reservoir hosts, the *Borrelia* usually circulate between wild rodents and ticks. The basis for this rather strict association of one spirochete species with one tick species is unknown but may involve species-specific interactions between the *Borrelia* and the tick's salivary glands. For example, although *B. hermsii* is able to escape a tick's midgut and establish infection in all three species of North American ticks, salivary transmission of the spirochete to a new host occurs only in *O. hermsii.*[48] On the other hand, the assumption that relapsing fever-causing *Borrelia* are associated only with soft-shelled ticks is challenged by the isolation of *B. miyamotoi* from *I. persulcatus,* the hard-bodied vector tick for Lyme disease in Japan.[42] Similar to Lyme borreliosis, greater worldwide variations of endemic cycles and vectors for tick-borne relapsing fever may exist than in North America.

Tick Geography

In North America, relapsing fever is an uncommon disease largely confined to the geographic distribution of the tick species that harbor the *Borrelia.* These ticks are usually found in the remote natural settings of the mountains and semiarid plains of the far west and Mexico. In the United States, most cases of relapsing fever are caused by *B. hermsii.* It can develop when people visit tick- or rodent-infested cabins or summer homes.[48] *O. hermsii* inhabits forested mountain areas, usually at high altitudes, and has been pinpointed as the common source of relapsing fever outbreaks from human exposure in mountain cabins. However, this tick has created disease at lower altitudes, even at sea level. *O. turicata* and rarely *O. parkeri* transmit their respective *Borrelia* in the semiarid plains, the former creating outbreaks in people visiting caves, especially limestone ones in central Texas.[44]

Spirochetal Behavior

Ticks acquire spirochetes from blood feeding on small wild rodents. If high levels of *Borrelia* are present in the animal's blood, large numbers of spirochetes will be ingested by the tick and reside in the tick's midgut. During the next few days, the spirochetes invade the midgut wall, traverse the hemolymph system, and within a few weeks infect the salivary glands as well as other tick tissues and organs. They endure through tick molting and by now are practically absent in the midgut. Females may develop infected ovaries and transmit *Borrelia* to offspring in some *Ornithodoros* species, but this is rare in *O. hermsii.*[44,48] Having infected the tick's salivary glands, the spirochetes are poised to invade the next host that the tick feeds upon.

Tick Behavior

In contrast to the hard-bodied ticks, these ticks feed rapidly, often detaching after 30 to 90 minutes.[44] They feed at night while people are sleeping, and their bite is usually painless. Therefore, most people are unaware that they have been bitten.[48]

Disease Characterization

The hallmark of endemic relapsing fever is an abrupt onset of high fever (often >39°C) after an incubation period of 4 to 18 days.[44,45] The patient may develop shaking chills, severe headache, tachycardia, abdominal pain, myalgias, arthralgias, nausea, vomiting, and malaise. The fever usually breaks in 3 to 6 days in untreated patients. After a variable afebrile period of 3 to 36 days, (usually 7 days), cyclical periods of fever and constitutional symptoms reappear. Each febrile attack progressively diminishes in severity. Three to five relapses typically occur in untreated patients. A transient skin rash lasting 1 to 2 days appears in 6% to 28% of patients, typically when the primary fever has broken. The rash may be localized or generalized and consists of petechiae, macules, papules, or erythema migrans. In 5% to 10% of cases, neurologic involvement is evident as peripheral neuropathy, altered sensorium, or pupillary abnormalities.[43]

Routine laboratory testing is of little value. However, moderate anemia is common as well as an increased erythrocyte sedimentation rate. Leukocyte counts may be normal or elevated, and thrombocytopenia is regularly encountered but is considered nonspecific.[44,45]

The diagnosis of relapsing fever is made by direct observation of the spirochete on a peripheral blood smear. The observation of the smear is enhanced with Wright's or Giemsa staining. Further enhancement may be obtained by staining fixed smears with acridine orange. Antibody serology tests, although available, are not standardized. Skin biopsy of the rash demonstrating the spirochete is unreliable. Direct culture of the spirochete from the blood into a special culture medium is the most specific diagnostic tool, but it is a slow technique confined to research laboratories.

Treatment

Successful treatment regimens usually include a 7- to 10-day course of antibiotics. Tetracyclines are preferred (500 mg orally four times a day) or doxycycline (100 mg orally two times a day). Erythromycin is also effective at dosages of 500 mg orally four times a day. Hospitalization and administration of IV antibiotics may be required in severely ill patients.

9. O.T. is a 52-year-old man who visits his family practitioner with a sudden onset of high fever, severe headache, malaise, nausea, vomiting, and abdominal pain. He returned a week ago, at the end of July, from a stay in a rustic cabin on the north rim of the Grand Canyon. The clinician orders a manual complete blood count (CBC) and chemistry panel and asks the laboratory to observe a blood smear with Giemsa stain. What clues does the physician have to suspect endemic relapsing fever as the diagnosis?

The disease occurs more often in males, and the nonspecific constitutional symptoms exhibited by O.T. match the customary features of the ailment. The history is more revealing. The patient visited a location and setting where prior outbreaks of relapsing fever have been documented. In addition, cases of endemic relapsing fever peak in the summer months.

10. After confirming the presence of *Borrelia* in the blood smear, the physician prescribes a 10-day course of tetracycline. Two hours after the first dose, O.T.'s wife calls the physician's office with concerns that the disease is worsening. O.T. is experiencing an increased temperature, is feeling faint and chilled, and has a rapid pulse and respiration rate. A skin lesion appears. What is most likely happening? Is this a drug reaction?

Up to 54% of patients with relapsing fever experience a reaction to the first dose of antibiotic, called a Jarisch-Herxheimer reaction (see Chapter 65, Sexually Transmitted Diseases).[44,45] It is more common and severe (and may be fatal) in louse-borne relapsing fever than in tick-borne, and it may also occur in other spirochetal diseases such as syphilis or Lyme. The dramatic reaction consists of a rise in temperature, chills, myalgias, tachycardia, hypotension, increased respiratory rate, vasodilation, and occasionally exacerbation of skin lesions.

Treatment of the reaction consists of supportive care. Severe reactions may require hospitalization for monitoring of vital signs and management of hypovolemia. Although this is a reaction to the administration of an antibiotic drug, it is not an allergic response, and the antibiotic should be continued.

Southern Tick-Associated Rash Illness (STARI)

11. M.G., a 46-year-old man living in southern Missouri, recently developed a rash resembling erythema migrans after a Lone Star tick bite. Since this tick is not known as a vector for Lyme borreliosis, what could be the cause?

Amblyomma americanum (the Lone Star tick) is found through the southeast and south-central United States and along the Atlantic coast as far north as Maine. This tick aggressively bites humans in the Southern states, as opposed to *I. scapularis* ticks. Spirochetes detected by microscopy and DNA analysis, but not yet cultivated in vitro, have been found in 1% to 3% of Lone Star ticks and are named *Borrelia lonestari*.[47] It is believed to be the agent of STARI and is more closely related to the relapsing fever group of *Borrelia* than to Lyme *Borrelia* based upon DNA sequencing. A skin rash almost indistinguishable from erythema migrans is the major finding. Whether antibiotic treatment is required for STARI is being determined.

OTHER BACTERIAL DISEASES: TULAREMIA AND EHRLICHIOSIS

Tularemia

Etiology and Epidemiology

In 1911, McCoy investigated a plague-like disease in wild ground squirrels harvested in Tulare County, California, and discovered tularemia's cause.[49] The bacteria is a small, nonmotile, aerobic, nonencapsulated, Gram-negative coccobacillus now named *Francisella tularensis* in honor of Francis for his fieldwork and contributions to tularemia research.[49] Two tularemia strains, the more virulent biovar A and the less virulent biovar B, are recognized based on biologic differences. Type A tularemia, found exclusively in North America, is fatal in up to 5% of cases.[49,50] The important reservoir hosts for the bacteria are hares, rabbits, and ticks. Before 1950, most human cases of the disease developed from direct contact with infected animals, usually hares or rabbits, and tularemia cases that occur in the fall or winter are usually associated with hunting season exposure. However, tick bite transmission now accounts for more than half of tularemia cases west of the Mississippi River in the United States. Other modes of transmission include ingestion of or contact with infected meat, water, or soil; inhalation of aerosolized bacteria; or bites from infected animals, mosquitoes, or deer flies.[49] Direct person-to-person spread of the disease is rare.

Tularemia is found in North America, Europe, Russia, Japan, and the Middle East. Most U.S. cases occur in the South and Midwest, primarily in Arkansas, Missouri, Oklahoma, and Kansas.[51] The North American tick vectors are *Dermacentor variabilis* (dog tick), *Amblyomma americanum* (lone star tick), and *Dermacentor andersoni* (wood tick). Tick-borne tularemia occurs most often in the spring and summer, matching the likelihood of exposure. Reported cases of tularemia in the United States have steadily declined since 1950 from a case report high of 2,291 in 1939 to current levels of <200 per year since 1967.

Clinical Presentation

The clinical manifestations of tularemia are related to the mode of transmission. Classically, six types of tularemia presentation are identified: ulceroglandular, glandular, typhoidal, oculoglandular, oropharyngeal, and pneumonic.[49] The last three forms are presumably not tick-borne, reflecting the potential avenues of transmission of the microorganism.

Ulceroglandular is the most common form of tularemia, accounting for 75% to 80% of cases.[49] It is characterized by an ulcer that forms at the site of the tick bite, usually on the lower extremities, perineum, buttocks, or trunk. The lesion starts as a firm, erythematous papule that ulcerates and heals over several weeks. It is accompanied by regional, painful lymphadenopathy, usually inguinal or femoral. Glandular tularemia is defined by painful, swollen lymph nodes without an accompanying skin lesion. Ten percent of tularemia cases are termed typhoidal and are characterized by fever, chills, headache, debilitation, abdominal pain, and prostration. Fever and chills are common with all forms of tularemia.

After exposure to the bacteria and an incubation period of 3 to 6 days, patients become ill with a sudden onset of fever, chills, headache, cough, arthralgias, myalgias, fatigue, and malaise. The severity of symptoms is quite variable, ranging from a mild, limited disease (probably type B tularemia) to rare cases of septic shock (probably type A tularemia). Common complications are mild hepatitis, secondary pneumonia, and pharyngitis. With antibiotic treatment of uncomplicated tularemia, mortality rates are 1% to 3%. Increased morbidity and mortality are seen in the typhoidal forms.

Diagnosis

Laboratory diagnosis of tularemia is limited to the demonstration of an antibody response to the bacteria. Routine laboratory testing is of little help in establishing the diagnosis. Because an antibody response to the illness requires 10 to 14 days for detection, treatment is usually empiric. The diagnosis is based on clinical suspicion from the epidemiologic history and the presence of compatible findings. The customary serologic test demonstrates *F. tularensis* antibody agglutination. Although a single agglutination test with a titer of 1:160 or more in a suspected case is highly suggestive of a tularemia diagnosis, a fourfold or greater rise in titers between the acute and convalescent stages is diagnostic.[49]

Treatment

In adults, streptomycin 7.5 to 10 mg/kg intramuscularly (IM) or IV Q 12 hr for 7 to 14 days is the treatment of choice.[49] Pediatric dosing is 20 to 40 mg/kg IM divided twice daily for 7 to 14 days.

12. Streptomycin is considered the drug of choice for tularemia but is often unavailable commercially or is available only on an individual case basis. What other antibiotics are alternatives? What are their drawbacks?

Some clinicians believe that gentamicin is the best alternative aminoglycoside for the treatment of nonmeningitic tularemia.[49] Its advantages compared with streptomycin include lower minimal inhibitory concentrations (MICs), less vestibular toxicity, and wider commercial availability. Considered comparable in efficacy to streptomycin treatment, gentamicin therapy has been associated with increased treatment failure and relapse.[52] However, some of the case reports and studies of gentamicin may have involved inadequate durations of therapy, treatment delays, or sicker patients. Tobramycin (Nebcin) has been associated with lower cure rates and higher failure rates than gentamicin or streptomycin, despite having MIC activity similar to gentamicin. Again, this might reflect study difficulties rather than a drug deficiency.

Initial cure rates and response to tetracycline are equivalent to those for gentamicin, but therapy with tetracycline has resulted in twice as many relapses. Perhaps bactericidal agents are required for successful tularemia treatment.[52]

Reported cure rates for chloramphenicol therapy of tularemia are significantly lower than those for streptomycin. Chloramphenicol is considered bacteriostatic like tetracycline. Chloramphenicol does penetrate into the CSF, with or without inflamed meninges, better than aminoglycosides or tetracyclines. Therefore, when tularemic meningitis is suspected, chloramphenicol plus streptomycin should be considerd.[49]

Newer cephalosporins such as ceftriaxone (Rocephin) and ceftazidime (Fortaz) possess favorable MIC data for *F. tularensis;* but inadequate clinical responses were obtained with ceftriaxone therapy in reported studies.[52] A successful 14-day course of imipenem-cilastatin (Primaxin) in one tularemia case has been reported, but more studies are needed before its use can be routinely recommended.[52] Of the fluoroquinolones studied, ciprofloxacin (Cipro) has the optimal minimum bacteriocidal concentration (MBC) in vitro data. Promising results for ciprofloxacin treatment have been documented.[49,53] However, because pneumonia is a common complication of tularemia, concern exists about the potential for overwhelming streptococcal meningitis or sepsis during ciprofloxacin therapy.[52] Fluoroquinolones should not be used in children.

Unfortunately, in many of the reported studies of antimicrobial therapy for tularemia, short courses of treatment (≤ 7 days) were used. To prevent tularemia from worsening or relapse, longer regimens (14 days) should be used.[52] Jarisch-Herxheimer reactions can occur with antibiotic treatment of tularemia.[52] Antibiotic prophylaxis for people exposed to those with tularemia is not recommended, but prophylactic antibiotics might be employed for suspected bioterrorism attacks of tularemia. There are no tularemia vaccines available in the United States.[49]

Ehrlichiosis

Ehrlichial Species Identification

Two tick-borne ehrlichial human diseases have emerged in recent years: human monocytic ehrlichiosis (HME), caused almost exclusively by *Ehrlichia chaffeensis,* and human granulocytic ehrlichiosis (HGE), caused by *Anaplasma phagocytophilia, Ehrlichia equi,* and *Ehrlichia ewingii.*[54–56] Previously, ehrlichial diseases were primarily of veterinary interest because infections were usually found in domesticated animals, including sheep, cattle, dogs, and horses. A human mononucleosis-like disease first described in Japan in 1954 is caused by *Ehrlichia sennetsu,* a rickettsial-like bacteria having a fish fluke vector. The disease is termed Sennetsu fever and is now indigenous to Japan and Southeast Asia.[56,57] Ehrlichial species, named in honor of the German microbiologist Paul Ehrlich, are now known to be obligate, intracellular, pleomorphic, Gram-negative coccobacilli that parasitize white blood cells.

In 1987, the first reported case of human ehrlichial infection in the United States was found in a soldier at Fort Chaffee, Arkansas. It was initially misinterpreted as being the same agent that infects dogs, *Ehrlichia canis.* Subsequent studies revealed that it was a unique species, *E. chaffeensis.* More than 750 cases of HME have now been reported in many states, Europe, and Africa.[55] One human case of asymptomatic HME by *E. canis* has been detailed.[55] Retrospective analysis revealed that 10% to 20% of unconfirmed, presumptive diagnoses of Rocky Mountain spotted fever (RMSF) were actually HME. The number of HME cases is greater than RMSF in several states today.[59]

The neutrophilic form of ehrlichiosis was first described in 1994. The responsible agents are closely related or identical to the veterinary pathogens *Ehrlichia equi* and *Ehrlichia phagocytophilia* that infect horses and sheep, respectively.[54,55] HGE agents are now recognized as identified above. Since HGE's discovery, >450 cases have been diagnosed, especially in Minnesota, Wisconsin, Northern California, and more recently the Northeastern United States, Arkansas, and Florida.[55]

Tick Vectors and Disease Hosts

The primary tick vector of HME is *A. americanum,* the lone star tick, and its geographic distribution matches that of most cases of HME, occurring in the south central and southeastern Unites States.[55] *E. chaffeensis* also has been recovered in *Dermacentor variabilis, Ixodes pacificus,* and *Amblyomma cajennense.*[55,57] Cases of HME that have been diagnosed in the northeastern United States are probably caused by *A. americanum.* HME cases in Europe, Africa, Washington, Utah, and Wyoming suggest other vectors. The most likely reservoirs for *E. chaffeensis* are white-tailed deer, small rodents, and dogs. Dogs experimentally infected with *E. chaffeensis* have ehrlichemia for 26 days, but direct transmission to humans has not been demonstrated. HME begins with the introduction of *E. chaffeensis* into the skin of a host from the bite of an infected tick. The bacteria spread throughout the body hematogenously. They become established within the cells of monocytic macrophages in the spleen, lymph nodes, liver, bone marrow, lung, and kidney. Characteristic, microscopically visible intracellular inclusion bodies called morulae (for their mulberry-like appearance) develop. Each morula is actually a membrane-bound bacterial colony that grows and divides within the monocyte's cytoplasm.[57] Cellular necrosis in heavily infected cells occurs, and it is believed that cell rupture and the subsequent release of bacteria allows infection of more monocytes, repeating the cycle.

Tick vectors that harbor the HGE agent include *I. scapularis* and *I. pacificus,* which are also Lyme borreliosis transmitters. In Europe, *Ixodes ricinus* is the vector. The main reservoir for *A. phagocytophilia* is the white-footed mouse. Other bacterial hosts include white-tailed deer, cotton mice, wood rats, and coyotes. Cats, horses, and dogs may become infected but are not natural hosts.[55] The events after introduction into a patient's skin of the HGE agent by tick bite are unknown. Rather than directly attacking mature granulocytes, it is suspected that the bacteria infects a myeloid precursor in the bone marrow and survives or multiplies throughout granulocytic cellular maturation.

About 75% or more of patients with ehrlichiosis report a tick bite or tick exposure within 3 weeks of illness onset.[57,58] Tick removal from the body is less likely to be effective for disease prevention than it is in Lyme borreliosis due to the rapid transmission of HGE during the nymphal tick bite.[60] Tick exposure is defined by geography and season. Simply being in an area where ticks can be found, particularly during spring and summer, constitutes exposure.

Clinical and Laboratory Findings

Human ehrlichiosis usually presents as a nonspecific, febrile, flu-like illness resembling RMSF. It begins 7 to 10 days after a tick bite.[55,61] Patients may be entirely asymptomatic, but there have been occasional fatalities from the complications of renal failure, respiratory failure, shock, or encephalopathy. HME and HGE share similar clinical features.[59] Both display fever as the major symptom in nearly 100% of cases.[59,61] The other common symptoms of malaise, myalgia, headaches, and rigors are found in virtually all cases of HGE but somewhat less in HME.[57] Other less common symptoms for both diseases include diaphoresis, nausea, vomiting, cough, diarrhea, abdominal pain, arthralgia, pharyngitis, rash, and confusion.

As with many other tick-borne diseases, serologic findings of antibody response to ehrlichiosis assist only by retrospectively confirming the diagnosis. Currently, indirect IFA serology is the gold standard for both HGE and HME.[55] However, the following signs often are noted: hypertransaminasemia, leukopenia (often with a shift to the left), thrombocytopenia, and anemia.[57,59] These may provide clues that increase the suspicion for HME or HGE. A peripheral blood smear showing neutrophilic morulae is diagnostic for HGE, but negative results do not rule out the diagnosis.[61] In HME, peripheral blood smears are rarely diagnostic. HME morulae are more likely to be identified in macrophages with biopsy or postmortem specimens of the liver, spleen, or bone marrow anecdotally. In summary, a peripheral blood smear examination for morulae should probably be undertaken because this method is the quickest and easiest for making a provisional diagnosis.

13. **Because the clinical findings of HME and HGE are similar, how can they be differentiated?**

The nonspecific manifestations and laboratory findings of HME and HGE are considered indistinguishable.[62] Although considered an uncommon finding, skin rash is consistent with ehrlichiosis, but rash is much less common than the 80% incidence seen in RMSF. Ehrlichial skin rashes are usually maculopapular but may be variable. In HME, skin rashes are present in only 6% of patients at disease onset, 25% during the first week, and 36% to 40% overall.[55,59] In HGE, skin rashes occur in only 10% or fewer of patients: in one study, only 1 of 41 patients (2%) with confirmed HGE had a rash.[61] Therefore, if a skin rash is present, HME is much more likely than HGE[59] (Table 75-4).

HME and HGE can be differentiated by serologic evaluation or PCR. Treatment should never be delayed pending the results of testing because the mortality rate is 2% to 3% for HME and 0.5% to 1% for HGE.[55] Delays in diagnosis and treatment are related to a substantial proportion of deaths from the disease.[57]

Ehrlichiosis as Opportunist/Immunosuppressor

Opportunistic cases of ehrlichiosis have appeared in AIDS patients, and death from overwhelming HME infection has occurred in other immunocompromised patients. Animal models of *A. phagocytophilia* infection have shown impaired defense responses such as defects in granulocyte emigration and phagocytosis, suppressed CD4 and CD8 counts, and impaired lymphoproliferation of isolated lymphocytes.[62] HGE fatalities have been associated with concomitant candidiasis, cryptococcal pneumonia, severe herpesvirus infection, and invasive pulmonary aspergillosis. Theoretically, opportunistic infections may be secondary to ehrlichial-mediated impairment of the immune response.[62]

Table 75-4   Tick-Borne Disease Findings

	LB	RF	Tularemia	HME	HGE	RMSF	Babesiosis	CTF
Rash	+++	+	+	++	+	+++		+/-
Fever	++	++++	+-+++	++++	++++	++++	++	+
Rigors	-	+++	+-+++	+++	++++	+++	++	-
Headache	++	++++	+-+++	+++	++++	++++	+	+
Myalgia	++	+	+-+++	+++	++++	++++	++	+++
Anemia		++		++	++	+++	+++	+
Nausea/vomiting	+	+++		++	++	+++	+	+
Cough	+	++	+	+	++		+	
Confused	+	+		+	++	++		+
Malaise	++++	++	+-+++	++++	++++	++++	++	
Arthralgias	+++	++	+	++	+		+	
LFTs	+	++	++	++++	++++	++	+	+
Increased WBCs	+	+	+/-			+/-		-
Decreased WBCs	-		-	++	+++	+/-		++
ESR		++	-				+	+
Decreased platelet count		+++		+++	++++	++	++	+

Caution: Routine laboratory testing is of little value in diagnosing or differentiating tick-borne diseases.

+, ≤25% association; -, not usually associated; CTF, Colorado tick fever; ESR, erythrocyte sedimentation rate; HGE, human granulocytic ehrlichiosis; HME, human monocytic ehrlichiosis; LB, Lyme borreliosis; LFTs, liver function tests; RF; relapsing fever; RMSF, Rocky Mountain spotted fever; WBCs, white blood cell counts.

Treatment and Prevention

Tetracycline 500 mg orally four times a day or doxycycline (Vibramycin) 100 mg orally or IV twice daily for 14 days is the drug of choice for both HME and HGE.[55,57] In children <8 years old, doxycycline is given at a dosage of 3 to 4 mg/kg per day divided into two daily doses. For those >8 years old but weighing <45 kg, 3 mg/kg of doxycycline Q 12 hr is used; adult doses are used for children weighing >45 kg. (See RMSF for a discussion of the pediatric use of doxycycline.) If tetracyclines are absolutely contraindicated, rifampin 600 mg orally once daily for 7 to 10 days is an alternative.[63] Chloramphenicol (Chloromycetin) appears ineffective in vitro and should not be used.[55] Fluoroquinolones may prove to be effective. Ineffective antibiotics for ehrlichiosis include gentamicin (Garamycin), ceftriaxone (Rocephin), co-trimoxazole (Bactrim), erythromycin (E-Mycin), metronidazole (Flagyl), clindamycin (Cleocin), sulfonamides, and penicillin.

Prevention of ehrlichial disease is preferable to treatment. Tick avoidance and detection strategies, as outlined for Lyme borreliosis, are recommended.[59] There is no evidence supporting the routine administration of prophylactic antibiotics for ehrlichial disease prevention in patients with known tick bites.[59] Ehrlichial vaccines may be developed.[55]

14. G.K., a 78-year-old man living outside Duluth, Minnesota, presents with an influenza-like illness in late May. He has a 2-day history of fever, shaking chills, headache, myalgias, nausea, and anorexia. On examination, his temperature is 39.4°C, but other physical findings are unremarkable. No skin rashes are found. During questioning, he stated he had multiple tick bites about 3 weeks ago while he was fur trapping. The physician suspects ehrlichiosis and prescribes doxycycline 100 mg PO twice daily for 2 weeks. Blood is drawn for serology, CBC with differential, chemistry profile, C-reactive protein, and a Wright's stain microscopic examination. Immediately available abnormal results include neutrophilic morulae on microscopy, a WBC count of $2.5 \times 10^9/L$ (normal, 4.0 to 10.7), a platelet count of $80 \times 10^9/L$ (normal, 150 to 450), C-reactive protein of 136 mg/L (normal, 4 to 8), aspartate aminotransferase (AST) of 150 U/L (normal, 16 to 40), and lactate dehydrogenase of 700 U/L (normal, 80 to 175). Serology is still pending. Two days later, G.K. defervesced and was feeling better. How does this case fulfill a diagnosis of HGE?

First of all, G.K.'s history is significant for HGE. He was in the right place, the upper Midwest United States, and was outdoors during the right season; most patients are diagnosed with HGE in May through August.[61] The usual incubation period from tick bite to illness onset ranges from 1 to 60 days.[61]

G.K.'s symptoms are also important. Nearly 100% of patients with HGE have a fever of ≥37.6°C. Other symptoms in G.K. consistent with HGE are rigors (shaking chills), headache, myalgias, nausea, and anorexia.[61] Matching laboratory findings include neutrophilic morulae, found in 62% of patients.[61] The observed leukopenia and thrombocytopenia strongly support the diagnosis. Evidence of mild to moderate hepatic injury, as seen by the elevated liver enzyme results, and the elevated C-reactive protein also are helpful in HGE diagnosis.[61] Finally, the good response to doxycycline, with fever resolution in 2 days, is customary with tetracycline treatment of HGE.[57]

THE RICKETTSIA: ROCKY MOUNTAIN SPOTTED FEVER

Rocky Mountain Spotted Fever

RMSF is the most prevalent and virulent rickettsial disease in the United States. As early as 1872, it is believed that RMSF infected White settlers of the Northwest, and it may have been prevalent in Native Americans of the region before that. Most cases occurred in women of the Shoshone tribe because, according to Indian legend, men sought to avoid the "evil spirits" of certain foothills and valleys and sent only women into the areas known to be dangerous. RMSF was first described in residents of the Bitterroot, Snake, and Boise River valleys of Montana and Idaho in the late 1800s. Howard Ricketts discovered the causative agent, *Rickettsia rickettsii*, in 1906. The parasite is small (0.3 by 1.5 μm), pleomorphic, Gram negative and is an obligate intracellular coccobacillus that can survive only briefly outside of a host.[64,65]

Epidemiology

Today, RMSF is reported in every U.S. state except Vermont and Hawaii; Canada; Mexico; Central America, including Costa Rica and Panama; and South America, including Brazil and Colombia.[64,66] It has not been documented outside of the Western Hemisphere. The term "Rocky Mountain spotted fever" is actually a misnomer today. It became a reportable disease by the CDC in 1920. Since then, the disease has shifted eastward from the Rocky Mountain states, and the greatest incidence of RMSF now occurs in North Carolina, Oklahoma, Virginia, Maryland, Georgia, Missouri, Arkansas, South Carolina, and Tennessee.[64] Most RMSF infections arise from tick exposure in rural or suburban locations, yet rare outbreaks in urban environments have occurred.

RMSF incidence rates for all age groups are 1.5 per million population per year. The prevalence is highest in children ages 5 to 9 years, with a peak of 3.2 per million.[67] Another peak prevalence is seen in men >60 years old.[67] Other risk factors are male gender, residence in wooded areas, and exposure to dogs that may bring ticks into households and yards.

Tick Vectors and Hosts

In the east, south, and west coasts of the United States, tick vectors for RMSF have been identified as the dog tick, *Dermacentor variabilis*. In the Rocky Mountains states, the wood tick, *Dermacentor andersoni*, is the vector. In Mexico, it is *Rhipicephalus sanguineus* and *Amblyomma cajennense*, with the latter also being responsible in Central and South America.

The *Dermacentor* tick feeds on humans only during its adult stage.[64] Larval *Dermacentor* ticks may be infected while feeding on small mammals that develop sufficient rickettsemia for transmission, such as chipmunks, ground squirrels, cotton rats, snowshoe hares, and meadow voles. Dogs are not reservoirs for *R. rickettsia* but may introduce infected ticks into households. Adult ticks transmit the rickettsia transovarially to their progeny with high efficiency and establish newly infected tick lines. However, if the rickettsia burden is large in the adult tick, it may cause tick death, thereby reducing infected tick lines. Therefore, there must be non-tick reservoirs, as mentioned previously, to develop newly infected tick generational lines; otherwise, RMSF would slowly disappear. In summary, ticks are both vectors and hosts for *R. rickettsia*.

Disease Course, Symptoms, and Fatalities

R. rickettsia is usually transmitted to humans from an infected tick bite.[64,66] The organism can also gain access to humans via broken skin if an infected tick is being crushed with bare fingers, and such crushing may generate infectious aerosols that may be inhaled. Conjunctival contact with infected tick tissues or feces provides another route for rickettsial entry.

After introduction of the organisms into the body, the rickettsia spread hematogenously with a predilection for the vascular endothelium, especially in capillaries. During an incubation period of 2 to 14 days, induced phagocytosis allows rickettsial entry into endothelial cells, where they replicate by binary fission in the cytoplasm and nuclei of infected cells. This induces a generalized vasculitis leading to activation of clotting factors, capillary leakage, and microinfarctions in various organs.[66] In severe infections, hypotension and intravascular coagulation may coexist and culminate in cell, tissue, or organ destruction.

Dehydration is an early sign of RMSF, followed by increased vascular permeability, edema, decreased plasma volume, hypoproteinemia, reduced serum oncotic pressure, and prerenal azotemia.[64] RMSF is a multisystem disease, but a particular organ may be the major focus of the disease. If the brain or lungs are severely infected, death may ensue. An increased severity of illness is associated with edema, particularly in children, and hypoalbuminemia.[64] Hypotension is present in 17% of patients and hyponatremia in 56%. Extensive infection of the pulmonary microvascular endothelium may cause noncardiogenic pulmonary edema. The principal cardiac manifestation of RMSF is arrhythmias, which are noted in 7% to 16% of patients. CNS involvement or RMSF encephalitis is usually first noticed as confusion or lethargy and is apparent in 26% to 28% of cases.[64] Delirium or stupor, ataxia, coma, or seizures may also occur.[67] Multiple other neurologic signs of RMSF infection may be present, and an RMSF-associated first case of Guillain-Barré syndrome has been reported.[66] A common finding in RMSF is myalgia (72% to 83%) or tenderness, which are manifestations of skeletal muscle necrosis. Striking creatinine kinase elevations have been described.[64] Thrombocytopenia resulting from consumption of platelets during intravascular coagulation processes occurs in 35% to 52% of patients. However, true disseminated intravascular coagulation with attendant hypofibrinogenemia is exceptional even in severe or fatal cases.[62] Blood loss or hemolysis in some may cause anemia, which is seen in 30% of patients and reflects blood vessel damage.[62] Fatalities usually occur 8 to 15 days after illness onset if no treatment is given or if treatment is delayed.

"Fulminant" RMSF is best defined as a disease with a rapidly fatal course with death occurring in ≤5 days. This form of disease is characterized by an early onset of neurologic signs and late or absent skin rash; it is highly associated with glucose-6-phosphate dehydrogenase deficiency in Black males.[64] RMSF surveillance studies determined a case-to-fatality ratio of 3.3% to 4%, and the risk factors identified were older age, delay in treatment or no treatment, and treatment with chloramphenicol compared to tetracycline.[67,68] There is not a significant difference in case-fatality ratios for Black compared to White individuals.[68] Data were insufficient to fully assess the confounder of illness severity with antibiotic choice. In the preantibiotic era, RMSF mortality rates were as high as 30%, but they have fallen to as low as 1.1%, in 1996, presumably due to the increased use of tetracyclines for treatment.[68]

The classically defined triad of RMSF symptoms at initial presentation comprises fever, rash, and history of tick exposure, but this is found in only a minority of cases.[66,67,69,70] The RMSF skin rash typically begins as pink, 1- to 5-mm blanchable macules that later become papules. It begins on the ankles, wrists, and forearms and soon thereafter involves the palms or soles. It then spreads to the arms, thighs, and trunk and typically evolves into a petechial exanthem. The utility of these findings in the differential diagnosis is limited because rash may be absent, transient, or late; may never become petechial; or may have an unusual distribution.

Diagnosis

As for most tick-borne diseases, confirmatory serologic analysis is only retrospective in nature, and antirickettsial treatment should begin immediately to prevent morbidity and mortality. Immunohistologic demonstration of *R. rickettsii* in biopsy specimens of rash lesions is the only approach that can yield diagnostic results in a timely manner, but this approach is applicable only to those presenting with a skin rash.[64]

The best serologic test for RMSF is the IFA test, but antibodies typically appear only after 10 to 14 days.[66] More striking laboratory abnormalities of RMSF disease include a normal leukocyte count with a shift to the left, hyponatremia, thrombocytopenia, elevated serum transaminases or creatinine kinase, and CSF pleocytosis. Unfortunately, these findings are observed late in the disease course and are not helpful in early disease recognition.[64]

Clinical findings and history are key to early diagnosis and successful treatment. In a febrile, tick-exposed person with a rash, RMSF should be considered.[64] RMSF should be strongly considered in febrile children, adolescents, or men >60 years of age, especially if they reside in or have traveled to the southern Atlantic or south-central United States from May through September. A delay in treatment for RMSF beyond 5 days of symptom onset increases the mortality rates from 6% to 22%.[69,71]

Treatment

In vitro, the MIC for *R. rickettsia* is 0.5 μg/mL for chloramphenicol, 0.25 μg/mL for tetracycline, and 0.06 μg/mL for doxycycline.[67] The recommended treatment is doxycycline 100 mg orally or IV two times a day for at least 7 days and for 2 days after the temperature is normal.[70] Chloramphenicol is reserved for use in pregnancy.[66] The erythromycins, penicillins, sulfonamides, aminoglycosides, and cephalosporins are not effective. Although fluoroquinolones have shown activity in other spotted fever rickettsial diseases, there are no reports of their use in human RMSF disease and they cannot be recommended at this time.[70]

15. **Can tetracyclines be given safely to young children with RMSF?**

In 1994, the American Academy of Pediatrics (AAP) Committee on Infectious Diseases revised the RMSF treatment options for young children after considering chloramphenicol's potential toxicity and the dental staining concerns for tetracyclines. The AAP now acknowledges tetracyclines as acceptable treatment in children of any age with RMSF. Doxycycline should be the tetracycline agent of choice in pediatric RMSF because it is dosed less frequently than other tetracyclines, which may improve compliance, and does not bind calcium as strongly as other tetracyclines. Therefore, it is less likely than tetracycline to stain developing teeth. Others investigating tetracycline tooth staining have determined that

five or fewer courses of oral tetracycline in children resulted in tooth darkening undetectable to an untrained eye. These results favor doxycycline as the treatment of choice in children with RMSF. The dosage is 4.4 mg/kg orally divided into two doses on day 1 followed by 2.2 mg/kg per day orally each day for 7 to 10 days or 2 to 3 days after the fever abates and clinical improvement occurs.[70]

Prevention

In addition to the same guidelines for prevention of Lyme borreliosis, keeping pets free of ticks should reduce exposure. Ticks must not be crushed in a way that might introduce rickettsia into cutaneous lesions, mucous membranes, or the conjunctiva.[64] No RMSF vaccine is available.[64] Antirickettsial antibiotic prophylaxis after a tick bite is not warranted.[64]

THE PROTOZOA: BABESIOSIS

Babesiosis

History

In Biblical times, an illness infecting Pharaoh Ramses II's cattle was referred to as the plague or "divine murrain" (hemoglobinuria) (Exodus 9:3). This may be the first reported epidemic of babesiosis.[72–74] Investigating the deaths of 30,000 to 50,000 head of Romanian cattle with febrile hemoglobinuria in 1888, Babes described an intraerythrocytic organism that was thought to be bacterial, and it was named *Haematococcus bovis*.[72,73,75,76] While investigating a hemolytic cattle fever in Texas in 1893, Smith and Kilborne established that the causative organism was a protozoan and introduced the concept of arthropod-borne transmission of this disease.[72,73,75,76] The first human case of babesiosis was definitively identified in a 33-year-old Yugoslavian cattle farmer in 1957. His febrile hemoglobinuria and intraerythrocytic organisms were attributed to the bovine pathogen *Babesia divergens*.[72,73,75,76] He had undergone a previous splenectomy and died of the disease. Inquiry after his death revealed that his cattle were infected with a bovine babesial species. Also identified were the possible tick vectors *Ixodes ricinus* and *Dermacentor sylvarum*.[73] To date, rare and often fatal human cases of babesiosis in Europe have been caused by *B. divergens, B. bovis,* and in one case *B. microti*.[72] European cases present with a fulminant, febrile illness 1 to 3 weeks after a tick bite. In 84% of cases, the patients have been asplenic. Coma and death has occurred in >50% of cases. Usual findings are hemoglobinuria, hemolysis, jaundice, chills, sweats, myalgia, pulmonary edema, and renal insufficiency.[72,73]

The first human babesiosis case in a person with an intact spleen was reported in 1969 in a patient from Nantucket Island, Massachussetts.[72] Since then, "Nantucket fever" has been found to be caused by the babesial rodent agent *B. microti*.[72,73,77] In contrast to most European cases and those reported in California, human babesiosis in endemic areas of the Great Lakes regions and the northeastern United States commonly occurs in normosplenic patients.[72–77] The presenting complaints are usually nonspecific and consist of malaise, fatigue, low-grade fever or shaking chills, headache, generalized musculoskeletal complaints, emotional lability, nausea, emesis, and weight loss. Fatal cases have been found in distinct areas of Wisconsin, Missouri, Rhode Island, and

California. Severe, nonfatal cases have occurred in Minnesota, Washington state, and California.[77] Additional cases have been reported in New York, Connecticut, Maryland, Virginia, Georgia, as well as in Mexico.[72] Members of *Babesia* and *Theileria* genuses are called piroplasms due to their pear-shaped appearance of dividing parasites within erythrocytes.[73] A different type of *Babesia*-like piroplasm has emerged in the western United States: designated WA-1, it was originally isolated in a resident of Washington state.[75] In Missouri a pathogen called MO-1 has caused a human case of babesiosis.[75,76] These implicated organisms are genetically and antigenically related to *B. gibsoni,* which causes severe hemolytic anemia in dogs. Phylogenetically they are related to members of the *Theileria* species, which cause morbidity and mortality in African and Eurasian cattle, even to the exclusion of some *Babesia* members.[77] The implications of this finding may include the possible existence of a lymphocytic exoerythrocytic stage of parasite development and attendant features of chronicity, immune suppression, and perhaps lymphoproliferation.[75,77]

Babesia, Ticks, and Hosts

There are 99 species of *Babesia,* and they have a wide geographic range.[75] They are probably the most common mammalian intraerythrocytic parasites, and they are not as host specific as once thought.[72] They are transmitted by *Ixodes, Boophilus, Dermacentor, Haemaphysalis,* and *Rhipicephalus* ticks. *B. microti* is transmitted in the northeastern United States by *I. scapularis,* the deer tick of Lyme borreliosis, and in the United Kingdom by *I. trianguliceps.*[72] In Europe, bovine babesiosis is transmitted by *I. ricinus.* In the western United States, *I. pacificus* is the probable vector. High infection rates of *B. microti* in field mice (*Microtus pennsylvanicus*) and white-footed mice (*Peromyces leucopus*) have been found on Nantucket Island in Massachusetts during investigations of transmission cycles. The white-footed mouse is the most common host for *I. scapularis* here, accounting for 90% of such animal hosts. Other reservoirs for *B. microti* are chipmunks, meadow voles, shrews, and rats.[75] *Babesia* also are transmitted from the larval to nymphal stage of the tick (that is, transstadial transmission occurs).[72,75]

Symptoms and Diagnosis

16. **H.W., age 64, spent July on Martha's Vineyard. A week later, he felt fatigued and lost his appetite. He presents in the middle of August with complaints of fever, headache, drenching sweats, aches and pains, and occasional dark-colored urine. He does not recall a tick bite. On physical examination, he has splenomegaly, hepatomegaly, but no palpable lymphadenopathy. Laboratory tests show a normochromic, normocytic anemia, decreased hemoglobin, hemoglobinuria, thrombocytopenia, and increased liver enzymes; otherwise, the chemistry panel is normal. His temperature is 40°C. Examination of a Giemsa-stained blood smear reveals the presence of unpigmented ring-shaped intraerythrocytic parasites, some forming tetrads that resemble a Maltese cross in appearance. No schizonts or gametocytes are present. The physician institutes a clindamycin and quinine regimen. What was the clue to the diagnosis of babesiosis?**

The babesiosis diagnosis was confirmed by the direct observation of the parasite inside the red blood cells. Although this is a commonly used tool, it is subject to false-negative results because the rate of parasitemia, ranging from 5% to 85%, is typically low.[72] Although both *P. falciparum,* the cause of malaria, and *B. microti* have ring forms, a few features rule out malaria in H.W. There is an absence of the brownish pigment deposits (hemozoin) commonly seen in malaria. The Maltese cross tetrads of merozoites, although rarely seen, are characteristic of *B. microti,* whose larger ring forms may have a pale area compared with *P. falciparum.*[76]

Because blood smear inspection is not often successful in diagnosing babesiosis, some advocate the use of serology, particularly the IgM indirect IFA procedure and/or PCR.[73,78] PCR may be especially useful for monitoring the disease course and response to therapy in an individual patient. It also could delineate the complete clinical spectrum of the disease and determine its geographic distribution.[73]

Most patients with *B. microti* babesiosis are asymptomatic.[72] This form of babesiosis may be viewed as a distinct occult, asymptomatic disease with few known sequelae. This has been demonstrated from seropositivity surveillance studies. One study showed that babesial infection is as prevalent in children as in adults, but the disease appears to be more severe in adults >50 years old.[75] A number of transfusion-acquired infections have been documented, indicating the existence of the asymptomatic form of babesiosis, which may become a hazard to blood supplies.[73] A second form of babesiosis is a potentially life-threatening hemolytic one that occurs in people predisposed to severe infection because of advanced age, immune suppression, or prior splenectomy.[73]

In the northeastern United States, infections commonly occur in patients with spleens, as in H.W. Clinically apparent cases are most common in 50- to 60-year-old patients, most of whom do not recall a tick bite. Most symptoms of babesiosis are due to hemolysis or the systemic inflammatory responses to parasitemia.[76] The usual incubation period is 1 to 6 weeks after the tick bite. Nonspecific symptoms that are gradual in onset appear first, as in H.W.'s case, followed several days later by the other symptoms H.W. displayed. A hallmark of the disease is hemolytic anemia of varying severity. The other physical examination and laboratory findings in H.W. are consistent with *B. microti* infection.[72,73] A high index of suspicion for babesiosis should be maintained in any patient with an unexplained febrile illness who lives in or has traveled to a region where the infection is endemic during June and July, as in H.W.'s case, particularly if there is a history of tick bite.[72]

Treatment

17. **Why were clindamycin and quinine chosen to treat H.W.? What other drugs have been used?**

The discovery of a human babesiosis treatment regimen that combines clindamycin (Cleocin) and quinine was a fortuitous one.[73,77] An 8-week-old infant with presumed transfusion-acquired malaria was initially treated with chloroquine. Because of a lack of response, treatment was switched to quinine plus clindamycin, and the patient defervesced.[76] A correct diagnosis of babesiosis was made early and subsequently confirmed serologically. Although this treatment combination is used, occasional failures have occurred. Dosing recommendations for adults are clindamycin 600 mg orally three times a day plus quinine 650 mg orally three times a day for 7 to 10 days; children should receive clindamycin 20 to 40 mg/kg per day orally divided into three doses plus quinine 25 mg/kg per day orally divided into three doses.[72,75,76]

Atovaquone (Mepron), the hydroxynaphthoquinone derivative used for *Toxoplasmosis gondii* infections in AIDS patients, has been used with substantial success in patients with *B. microti* infection refractory to conventional therapy. Combination therapy with azithromycin and atovaquone may cure this disease.[79] This regimen can now be considered the treatment of choice for adults since it is as effective as the clindamycin with quinine combination yet has fewer side effects. The dosing is atovaquone 750 mg orally Q 12 hr plus azithromycin 500 to 600 mg orally on day 1 and 250 to 600 mg on subsequent days for 7 to 10 days.[75,80] This treatment has yet to be tested in children.[75,76] Exchange blood transfusions with the aforementioned therapy may be life-saving for patients with severe babesiosis.[75] Rapidly increasing parasitemia leading to massive intravascular hemolysis and renal failure mandates immediate treatment for this form of the disease.[72]

Babesiosis prevention is the same as for other tick-borne diseases. Splenectomized patients should avoid areas where babesiosis is endemic. Although developed for use in cattle, vaccines are not available for humans.[75]

THE VIRUSES: COLORADO TICK FEVER AND TICK-BORNE ENCEPHALITIS

Colorado Tick Fever

Disease History

"Mountain fever" has been described since the first immigrants arrived in the Rocky Mountains. It was renamed Colorado tick fever (CTF) once a clinical picture of the disease was established.[81]

Virus Identification

CTF is caused by a double-stranded RNA virus formerly classified as an orbivirus, an intraerythrocytic virus. Now at least 22 strains of CTF virus are known and taxonomically reside in the family Reoviridae, genus *Coltivirus* (group A).[82] The virus is an arbovirus because it replicates inside ticks.[81] The primary nidus of infection is thought to be CTF invasion of hematopoietic cell lines, accounting for the pathology.[82] Infection of erythrocytes in particular has been detected.[82]

Ticks and Host Reservoirs

CTF is a viral illness transmitted by the bite of an infected tick.[81–83] Although at least eight tick species have been found to be infected with the virus, *Dermacentor andersoni* is the primary vector that transmits the illness to humans.[82] *D. andersoni* feeds on numerous mammals, but ground squirrels, porcupines, and chipmunks are the primary reservoirs for CTF virus.[82,83] Transovarial transmission of CTF virus in the tick has been documented.[81]

Prevalence

CTF is contracted in forested mountain areas at higher elevations of the Rocky Mountain regions in the United States and Canada, especially on the south-facing brush slopes and dry rocky surfaces of mountains east of the Continental Divide.[82] Neutralizing CTF antibodies are found in up to 15% of peren-

nial campers.[81] In Colorado, the number of CTF cases is 20 times that for RMSF, but the incidence has dramatically declined there since the 1980s.[81,82] CTF may be acquired in Utah, Wyoming, Montana, Idaho, South Dakota, California, Oregon, Washington, Nevada, New Mexico, Alberta, and British Columbia.[83] Approximately 200 to 300 cases are reported annually in the United States.[82] April and May are the peak months for CTF.[82]

Symptoms

18. T.M., a previously healthy 28-year-old native of Atlanta, Georgia, returns from a 1-week late spring camping trip in the eastern Colorado Rocky Mountains. Four days later, he experiences fever, chilliness, aching back and leg muscles, and headache. He recalls no tick bites and has no skin rashes. Suspecting RMSF, his physician prescribes doxycycline. T.M.'s symptoms and fever initially resolve, but 2 days later his symptoms return. Physical examination at this time reveals a temperature of 39°C. Routine laboratory tests are normal, although leukopenia is observed with a WBC count of 2.4×10^9/L. Why do T.M.'s symptoms suggest a diagnosis of CTF?

CTF symptoms usually start 3 to 6 days after a tick bite, although about half of patients do not remember getting a tick bite.[81,83] The most common initial symptoms are fever of rapid onset, headache, and chills without true rigors, and myalgias.[81,83] Rash is uncommon.[83] A biphasic or "saddle-back" pattern of fever and other symptoms occurs in 50% of CTF patients.[81–83] Initial symptoms last about 2 days, followed by an afebrile period of around 2 days; then the fever recurs, sometimes higher than the first bout, lasting up to 3 days.[81] Rarely, a third bout of fever occurs.[81] CTF infection is usually self-limiting and sequelae are rare, although fatigue and malaise may last for months.[83] Three-week periods of convalescence are reported in 70% of patients >30 years of age, compared with <1 week in 60% of the patients <20 years of age. However, children experience complications more frequently than adults.[82] A prolonged convalescence does not imply persistent viremia, although viremia may be prolonged for 3 to 4 months.[81,82]

Laboratory Findings

Moderate to significant leukopenia is the most important finding in CTF. Leukocyte counts are usually normal on the first day but decrease to 2 to 3×10^9/L by the fifth or sixth day.[81] However, in one third of confirmed CTF cases, the leukocyte counts remained about 4.5×10^9/L. Counts return to normal within a week of fever abatement in most cases.[81] Occasionally, mildly elevated levels of creatinine phosphokinase and aspartate aminotransferase are reported.[81]

Diagnosis and Treatment

The CTF diagnosis is made either serologically with IFA staining of erythrocytes, complement fixation, or immunoperoxidase staining or by culture of the virus after introduction into suckling mice.[81–83] Reverse transcriptase and plaque reduction neutralization of serum sample or postinfection IgM capture assays may be diagnostic.[82] Treatment is limited to supportive care.[82] A few deaths have been reported, all with hemorrhagic signs.[81] Lifelong immunity is generally conferred by CTF infection.

Tick-Borne Encephalitis

Tick-borne encephalitis (TBE) was described first by the Austrian physician Shneider in 1931.[84] The Soviet scientist Zilber proved that the disease is caused by a virus that can be spread to humans by a tick bite in 1937. Today TBE is divided into two subtypes, Eastern and Western, and is endemic to Central and Eastern Europe, Russia, and the Far East, with some overlap in geographic locale.[84] The highest incidence of TBE is in Latvia, the Urals, and western Siberia.

The etiologic agent is an RNA virus of the family Flaviviridae and in the genus *Flavivirus*. Although 8 to 14 species of ticks have been found to be infected with TBE virus, the Western subtype is transmitted to humans by *I. ricinus* and the Eastern subtype by *I. persulcatus*.[84,85] Occasional TBE cases have followed the consumption of infected unpasteurized milk directly without a tick vector.[84] The virus reservoirs are small rodents. Ticks are vectors, and humans are accidental hosts of the virus.[84] Ticks can become infected for life by the virus at larval, nymphal, or adult stages and can transmit it transovarially and transstadially.[84]

As the disease name implies, the ultimate outcome of the infectious process is manifested as CNS involvement with symptoms of aseptic meningitis, meningoencephalitis, and meningoencephalomyelitis. TBE begins as a febrile headache with a biphasic course for the Western subtype and straightforward progression from febrile headache to CNS manifestations for the Eastern subtype. Treatment is supportive. Human TBE vaccines are available in some countries.[84,86]

THE TOXINS: TICK PARALYSIS

Tick Paralysis

19. A.M., a 3-year-old girl residing in Spokane, Washington, complains of weakness in both legs. The next day, she begins experiencing flaccid paralysis in both legs and the lower trunk, although she is alert and oriented. Her mother discovers a tick attached to A.M.'s scalp under her hair and removes it. A.M. is back to full health in 2 days. What happened?

Tick paralysis (tick toxicosis) occurs worldwide in humans and many animals and was first described by the explorer Hovell in Australia in 1824.[87,88] Although 43 tick species worldwide can produce tick paralysis in animals and humans, it is predominantly caused in humans by *Dermacentor andersoni* in North America. The other ticks implicated are *D. variabilis, A. americanum, A. maculatum, I. scapularis,* and *I. pacificus*.[88] In Australia, *I. holocyclus* is the culprit.

Most human cases occur during the spring and summer in Australia and the United States. In the United States, it is most common in the Pacific Northwest and Rocky Mountain states.[87,88] Female ticks are predominantly responsible.[87] In children girls are more commonly affected, but in adults more males are affected.[87]

The presumed cause of the disease is the secretion of a neurotoxin present in the saliva of a tick, which must usually be attached for 2 to 7 days before symptoms develop.[87] The toxin affects motor neurons and decreases acetylcholine release.[87,89] Paresthesias and symmetric weakness in the lower extremities with motor difficulties progress to an ascending flaccid paralysis in several hours or days.[85] Cerebral senso-

rium is usually spared, and the blood and CSF are normal.[88] Ataxia also may be seen early and may progress to respiratory paralysis with death in 10% to 12% of cases.[87,88]

In North America, tick removal commonly results in complete recovery within hours to days. In Australia, the disease is more acute and paralysis may continue to progress for 2 days after tick removal. Recovery from the disease in Australia may take several weeks. Treatment is supportive. Antitoxin derived from dogs is the treatment of choice in animals but not humans due to the risk of serum sickness or acute reactions.[87]

MIXED INFECTIONS

20. Because the tick vectors and mammalian hosts are the same for babesiosis, HGE, and Lyme borreliosis in the northeastern United States, all three diseases could, theoretically, be transmitted to a human from one tick bite. Is there evidence of human coinfection with more than one tick-borne disease?

Human coinfection by the agents of Lyme borreliosis, babesiosis, and ehrlichiosis is common, especially in endemic areas.[90,91] Some believe that coinfection may alter the natural course for each disease, while others have found only an increase in clinical manifestations, especially flu-like symptoms in concurrent Lyme borreliosis with babesiosis or HGE.[90,91]

Dual infection may affect the choice of initial antibiotic therapy. For example, although amoxicillin is widely used to treat early Lyme borreliosis, it is not effective for HGE.[92] However, doxycycline is useful in both of these diseases. Thus, some cases of Lyme borreliosis that were believed to be treatment failures may actually have been confounded by coinfection. Serologic surveillance has shown that approximately 10% of Lyme disease patients in southern New England are coinfected with babesiosis.[92] Patients with concurrent Lyme borreliosis and babesiosis have more symptoms and a longer duration of illness compared to patients with single infections.[90–92] When moderate to severe Lyme borreliosis is diagnosed, the possibility of concomitant babesial or ehrlichial diseases should be considered in regions where both diseases have been reported.[92] Neutropenia and thrombocytopenia are associated with HGE, anemia and thrombocytopenia are associated with babesiosis, and neither is routinely found in Lyme borreliosis. For Lyme borreliosis patients who experience a prolonged flu-like illness that fails to respond to appropriate antiborrelial therapy, clinicians should consider testing for babesiosis and HGE.[91]

SUMMARY

Most of the research into tick-borne human disease demonstrates a close historical relationship of endemic tick–deer–rodent cycles for various microorganisms. These cycles are almost exclusively identified as having occurred at the geologic sites of the terminal moraines of Ice Age glaciers. Given the recent explosion of deer populations in the United States and Europe, the increase in tick-borne human diseases may reflect the reduction of natural deer predators and/or the continued expansion of human populations from urban to rural environments, where increasing numbers of deer and ticks are located. Therefore, it is likely that we will continue to encounter increasing cases of tick-borne human disease of known or unknown origin.

REFERENCES

1. Parola P, Raoult D. Ticks and tickborne bacterial diseases in humans: an emerging infectious threat. Clin Infect Dis 2001;32:897.
2. Anderson JF. The natural history of ticks. Med Clin North Am 2002;86:205.
3. Wilson ME. Prevention of tick-borne diseases. Med Clin North Am 2002;86:219.
4. Steere AC. Lyme disease: a growing threat to urban populations. Proc Natl Acad Sci USA 1994;91:2378.
5. Shapiro ED, Gerber MA. Lyme disease: fact versus fiction. Pediatr Annals 2002;31:170.
6. Steere AC. Lyme disease. N Engl J Med 2001; 345:115.
7. Baumgarten JM et al. Lyme disease, Part 1: Epidemiology and etiology. Cutis 2002;69:349.
8. Montiel NJ et al. Lyme disease, Part II: Clinical features and treatment. Cutis 2002;69:443.
9. Reid MC et al. The consequences of overdiagnosis and overtreatment of Lyme disease: an observational study. Ann Intern Med 1998;128:354.
10. Pfister HW et al. Lyme borreliosis: basic science and clinical aspects. Lancet 1994;343:1013.
11. Coyle PK, Schutzer SE. Neurologic aspects of lyme disease. Med Clin North Am 2002:86:261.
12. Sood SK et al. Duration of tick attachment as a predictor of the risk of Lyme disease in an area in which Lyme disease is endemic. J Infect Dis 1997; 175:996.
13. Sigal LH. Misconceptions about Lyme disease: confusions hiding behind ill-chosen terminology. Ann Intern Med 2002;136:413.
14. Wormser GP et al. Practice guidelines for the treatment of Lyme disease. Clin Infect Dis 2000;31:1.
15. Donta ST. Tick-borne diseases. Med Clin North Am 2002;86:341.
16. Marques AR. Lyme disease: an update. Curr Allergy Asthma Rep 2001;1:541.
17. Magnarelli LA. Current status of laboratory diagnosis for Lyme disease. Am J Med 1995;98(Suppl 4A):4A.
18. Kalish RA et al. Persistence of immunoglobulin M or immunoglobulin G antibody responses to Borrelia brugdorferi 10 to 20 years after active Lyme disease. Clin Infect Dis 2001;33:780.
19. Dorward DW et al. Invasion and cytopathic killing of human lymphocytes by spirochetes causing Lyme disease. Clin Infect Dis 1997;25(Suppl 1):S2.
20. Anon. Treatment of Lyme disease. Med Lett Drugs Ther 1997;39:47.
21. Wormser GP et al. Duration of treatment for Lyme borreliosis: time for a critical reappraisal. Wien Klin Wochenschr 2002;114:613.
22. Klempner MS et al. Two controlled trials of antibiotic treatment in patients with persistent symptoms and a history of Lyme disease. N Engl J Med 2001; 345:85.
23. Donta ST. Tetracycline therapy for chronic Lyme disease. Clin Infect Dis 1997;25(Suppl 1):S52.
24. Halperin JJ et al. Practice parameters for the diagnosis of patients with nervous system Lyme borreliosis (Lyme disease). Neurology 1996;46:619.
25. Nadelman RB, Wormser GP. Erythema migrans and early Lyme disease. Am J Med 1995;98(Suppl 4A):4A.
26. Nadelman RB et al. Prophylaxis with single-dose doxycycline for the prevention of Lyme disease after an Ixodes scapularis tick bite. N Engl J Med 2001;345:79.
27. Nadelman RB, Wormser GP. Letter. N Engl J Med 2001;345:1349.
28. Edlow JA. Erythema migrans. Med Clin North Am 2002;86:239.
29. Gerber MA et al. Lyme disease in children in southeastern Connecticut. N Engl J Med 1996;335:1270.
30. Feder HM, Whitaker DL. Misdiagnosis of erythema migrans. Am J Med 1995;99:412.
31. Rahn DE, Malawista SE. Lyme disease: recommendations for diagnosis and treatment. Ann Intern Med 1991;114:472.
32. Ettestad PJ et al. Biliary complications in the treatment of unsubstantiated Lyme disease. J Infect Dis 1995;171:356.

33. Luft BJ et al. Azithromycin compared with amoxicillin in the treatment of erythema migrans. Ann Intern Med 1996;124:785.
34. Dattwyler RJ et al. Clarithromycin in treatment of early Lyme disease: a pilot study. Anitimicrobial Agents Chemother 1996;468.
35. Eckman MH et al. Cost effectiveness of oral as compared with intravenous antibiotic therapy for patients with early Lyme disease. N Engl J Med 1997;337:357.
36. Foster JA, Sylvia LM. Doxycycline-induced esophogeal ulceration. Ann Pharmacother 1994;28: 1185.
37. Muellegger RR et al. No detection of Borrelia burgdorferi-specific DNA in erythema migrans lesions after minocycline treatment. Arch Dermatol 1995;131:678.
38. Guerrau-de-Arellano M, Huber BT. Development of autoimmunity in Lyme arthritis. Curr Opin Rheumatol 2002;14:388.
39. Massarotti EM. Lyme arthritis. Med Clin North Am 2002;86:297.
40. Johnson BJ et al. Serodiagnosis of Lyme disease: accuracy of a two-step approach using a flagella-based ELISA and immunoblotting. J Infect Dis 1996;174:346.
41. Wormser GP et al. A limitation of 2-stage serological testing for Lyme disease: enzyme immunoassay and immunoblot assay are not independent tests. Clin Infect Dis 2000;30:545.
42. Bunikis J, Barbour AG. Laboratory testing for suspected Lyme disease. Med Clin North Am 2002; 86:311.
43. Diego D, Barbour AG. Neuroborreliosis during relapsing fever: review of the clinical manifestations, pathology, and treatment of infections in human and experimental animals. Clin Infect Dis 1998;26:151.
44. Dworkin MS et al. Tick-borne relapsing fever in North America. Med Clin North Am 2002;86:417.
45. Dworkin MS et al. Tick-borne relapsing fever in the northwestern United States and southwestern Canada. Clin Infect Dis 1998;26:122.
46. Parotam RH. Borreliosis in the Arabian Gulf states: report of a case from Kuwait. Clin Infect Dis 1996;22:1114.
47. Storch GA. New developments in tick-borne infections. Pediatr Ann 2002;31:200.
48. Schwan TG. Ticks and Borrelia: model systems for investigating pathogen-arthropod interactions. Infect Agents Dis 1996;5:167.
49. Choi E. Tularemia and Q fever. Med Clin North Am 2002;86:393.
50. Bryant KA. Tularemia: lymphadenitis with a twist. Pediatr Ann 2002;31:187.
51. Tularemia, United States, 1900–2000. MMWR 2002;51:182.
52. Enderlin G et al. Streptomycin and alternative agents for the treatment of tularemia: review of the literature. Clin Infect Dis 1994;19:42.
53. Perez-Castrillon JL et al. Tularemia epidemic in northwestern Spain: clinical description and therapeutic response. Clin Infect Dis 2001; 33:573.
54. Zaidi SA, Singer C. Gastrointestinal and hepatic manifestations of tickborne diseases in the United States. Clin Infect Dis 2002;34:1206.
55. Olano JP, Walker DH. Human erhlichioses. Med Clin North Am 2002;86:375.
56. Buller RS et al. Ehrlichia ewingii, a newly recognized agent of human ehrlichiosis. N Engl J Med 1999;341:148.
57. Weinstein RS. Human ehrlichiosis. Am Fam Phys 1996;54:1971.
58. Jacobs RF. Human monocytic ehrlichiosis: similar to Rocky Mountain spotted fever but different. Pediatr Ann 2002;31:180.
59. Smith RP, Tobin EH. Case studies in emerging infections II: bacterial infections. Hosp Physician 1997;2:2.
60. des Vinges F et al. Effect of tick removal on transmission of Borrelia burgdorferi and Ehrlichia phagocytophilia by Ixodes scapularis nymphs. J Infect Dis 2001;183:773.

61. Bakken JS, Dumler JS. Human granulocytic ehrlichiosis. Clin Infect Dis 2000;31:554.
62. Dumler JS. Is human granulocytic ehrlichiosis a new Lyme disease? Review and comparison of clinical, laboratory, epidemiological and some biological features. Clin Infect Dis 1997;25(Suppl 1):S43.
63. Buitrago MI et al. Human granulocytic ehrlichiosis during pregnancy treated successfully with rifampin. Clin Infect Dis 1998;27:213.
64. Walker DH. Rocky Mountain spotted fever: a seasonal alert. Clin Infect Dis 1995;20:1111.
65. Brady WJ et al. Dermatological emergencies. Am J Emerg Med 1994;12:217.
66. Sexton DJ, Kaye KS. Rocky Mountain spotted fever. Med Clin North Am 2002;86:351.
67. Dalton MJ et al. National surveillance for Rocky Mountain spotted fever, 1981–1992: epidemiologic summary and evaluation of risk factors for fatal outcome. Am J Trop Med 1995;52:405
68. Holman RC et al. Analysis of risk factors for fatal Rocky Mountain spotted fever: evidence for superiority of tetracyclines for therapy. J Infect Dis 2001;184:1437.
69. Thorner AR et al. Rocky Mountain spotted fever. Clin Infect Dis 1998;27:1353.
70. Donovan BJ et al. Treatment of tick-borne diseases. Ann Pharmacother 2002;36:1590.
71. Kirkland KB et al. Therapeutic delay and mortality in cases of Rocky Mountain spotted fever. Clin Infect Dis 1995;20:1118.
72. Boustani MR, Gelfand JA. Babesiosis. Clin Infect Dis 1996;22:611.
73. Pruthi RK et al. Human babesiosis. Mayo Clin Proc 1995;70:853.
74. Shulman ST. Ticks! Pediatr Ann 2002;31:154.
75. Krause PJ. Babesiosis. Med Clin North Am 2002; 86:361.
76. Lantos PM, Krause PJ. Babesiosis: similar to malaria but different. Pediatr Ann 2002;31:192.
77. Persing DH, Conrad PA. Babesiosis: new insights from phylogenetic analysis. Infect Agents Dis 1995;4:182.
78. Krause PJ et al. Efficacy of immunoglobulin m serodiagnostic test for rapid diagnosis of acute babesiosis. J Clin Micr 1996;34:2014.
79. Krause PJ et al. Persistent parasitemia after acute babesiosis. N Engl J Med 1998;339:160.
80. Krause PJ et al. Atovaquone and azithromycin for the treatment of babesiosis. N Engl J Med 2000;343:1454.
81. Sanford JP. Arbovirus infections. In: Isselbacher KJ et al, eds. Harrison's Principles of Internal Medicine. New York: McGraw-Hill, 1994;840.
82. Klasco R. Colorado tick fever. Med Clin North Am 2002;86:435.
83. Midoneck SR et al. Colorado tick fever in a resident of New York City. Arch Fam Med 1994;3:731.
84. Dumpis U et al. Tick-borne encephalitis. Clin Infect Dis 1999;28:882.
85. Lotric-Furlan S et al. Is an isolated initial phase of a tick-borne encephalitis a common event? [letter]. Clin Infect Dis 2000;30:987.
86. Bratu S, Lutwick LI. Active immunization against human tick-borne diseases. Expert Opin Biol Ther 2002;2:187.
87. Greenstein P. Tick paralysis. Med Clin North Am 2002;86:441.
88. Dworkin MS et al. Tick paralysis: 33 human cases in Washington state, 1946–1996. Clin Infect Dis 1999;29:1435.
89. Centers for Disease Control and Prevention. Tick paralysis, Washington. MMWR 1996;45:325.
90. Thompson C et al. Coinfecting deer-associated zoonoses: Lyme disease babesiosis, and ehrlichiosis. Clin Infect Dis 2001;33:676.
91. Krause PJ et al. Disease-specific diagnosis of coinfecting tickborne zoonoses: babesiosis, human granulocytic ehrlichiosis and Lyme disease. Clin Infect Dis 2002;34:1184.
92. Nadelman RB et al. Simultaneous human granulocytic ehrlichiosis and Lyme borreliosis. N Engl J Med 1997;337:27.

LIVERPOOL JOHN MOORES UNIVERSITY
LEARNING & INFORMATION SERVICES

Anxiety Disorders

Sara Grimsley Augustin

Continued

LIVERPOOL JOHN MOORES UNIVERSITY
LEARNING & INFORMATION SERVICES

OVERVIEW

Anxiety can be described as an uncomfortable feeling of vague fear or apprehension accompanied by characteristic physical sensations. It is a normal and often beneficial response to situations that humans perceive as threatening, frightful, or otherwise disturbing. Anxiety serves the therapeutic purpose of alerting us to take appropriate measures for dealing with such stressful circumstances. Thus, unlike other mental disorders such as schizophrenia or depression, anxiety can be both a normal emotion and a psychiatric illness.[1] Anxiety involves two basic components: mental features (e.g., worry, fear, difficulty concentrating) and physical symptoms (e.g., racing heart, shortness of breath, trembling, pacing).

Sometimes, the anxiety experienced by a person is excessive for the situation (in intensity or duration) or very distressing, to the point that it interferes with daily functioning. When the harmful effects of anxiety outweigh the beneficial, this constitutes pathologic anxiety or anxiety disorders. Pathologic anxiety can be differentiated according to whether it occurs (1) as a primary anxiety disorder, (2) as a secondary anxiety disorder due to medical causes or substances, (3) in response to acute stress (e.g., loss of a loved one, marital or family problems), or (4) as a symptom associated with other psychiatric disorders. This differentiation can be difficult but is important in guiding optimal treatment.

Classification and Diagnosis of Anxiety Disorders

The characterization and classification of pathologic anxiety have changed substantially during the past few decades. In the 1960s, a major emphasis in psychiatric nosology focused on separating anxiety states and their treatment from depression and its treatment. At that time, all pathologic anxiety conditions were included in one group referred to as "anxiety neurosis." Differentiation of specific anxiety disorders began in 1980, with the publication of the third edition of the *Diagnostic and Statistical Manual of Mental Disorders (DSM-III)*. Since then, much research has been conducted to greatly expand our knowledge about the various anxiety disorders. The fourth edition of the *Diagnostic and Statistical Manual of Mental Disorders (DSM-IV)* classifies primary anxiety disorders into six types: generalized anxiety disorder (GAD), panic disorder, phobic disorders (including social anxiety disorder), obsessive-compulsive disorder (OCD), post-traumatic stress disorder (PTSD), and acute stress disorder.[1] The additional category of "Anxiety Disorder Not Otherwise Specified" is used for cases not meeting the diagnostic criteria for any of these six types or for cases in which it cannot be determined whether the anxiety disorder is primary or secondary. Each disorder involves an unhealthy level of anxiety, but the characteristic type and severity of symptoms, as well as courses of

illness, vary from one disorder to another. Efficacy of drug and nondrug treatments also varies between disorders, indicating underlying biologic differences. The DSM-IV secondary anxiety disorders include "anxiety disorder due to a general medical condition" and "substance-induced anxiety disorder."[1]

Neurobiology of Anxiety

A neurocircuit arising from the output pathways of the central nucleus of the amygdala is thought to mediate fear and anxiety responses in humans.[2] Dysregulated or exaggerated output through various amygdala-related circuits may be a common element underlying the different anxiety disorders, but the specific type of dysfunction probably differs among the various disorders. Several neurotransmitter systems have been linked to the neurobiology of anxiety: the inhibitory amino acid, γ-aminobutyric acid (GABA); the monoamine neurotransmitters, serotonin and norepinephrine; the excitatory amino acid, glutamate; and the neuropeptides, cholecystokinin (CCK), corticotrophin-releasing factor (CRF), neuropeptide Y (NPY), and substance P.[2,3] Much of the evidence for these biologic processes has come from research on drugs that are used either to treat anxiety or to induce anxiety. Discovery of the anxiolytic effects of benzodiazepines in the early 1960s marked the beginning of this era of research. However, the anxiety-reducing properties of alcohol and barbiturates were recognized long before that time.

GABA and Benzodiazepines

GABA is synthesized from the amino acid precursor glutamate, and its primary role is to serve as an inhibitory regulator for other neurotransmitter systems such as norepinephrine, serotonin, and dopamine. Benzodiazepines work by facilitating GABA. Three subtypes of GABA receptors have been identified: GABA-A, GABA-B, and GABA-C. GABA-A receptors are involved in anxiety-related effects.[4] Each GABA-A receptor is composed of a combination of various subunits, of which at least 18 different types have been identified (α1 to α6, β1 to β3, γ1 to γ3, δ, ρ1 to ρ3, ε, and θ).[4,5] Various combinations of these subunits make up GABA-A receptors in different brain areas and determine specific pharmacologic effects. Benzodiazepines work at receptors containing α1, α2, α3, or α5 subunits in combination with γ2 and any of the β subunits. Individual differences in sensitivity to benzodiazepines may be related in part to genetic polymorphisms in specific GABA-A receptor subunits.[6,7] The functional roles of GABA-B and GABA-C receptors are not well understood, but the muscle relaxant agent baclofen is an agonist at GABA-B receptors. Preliminary evidence suggests that decreased functioning of GABA-B receptors may be associated with addic-

LIVERPOOL JOHN MOORES UNIVERSITY
LEARNING & INFORMATION SERVICES

tive disease processes.[8] GABA receptors containing ρ subunits are referred to as GABA-C receptors.

The GABA-A receptor is a ligand-gated structure that possesses binding sites for benzodiazepines, barbiturates, the convulsant drug picrotoxin, and ethanol.[6] This oligomeric transmembrane glycoprotein is arranged around a chloride ion channel, as depicted in Figure 76-1. Binding of GABA to the GABA-A receptor promotes the direct opening of the chloride ion channel, causing an influx of chloride ions into the neuron. This inward shift of ions hyperpolarizes and stabilizes the membrane, resulting in a net inhibitory effect on neuronal firing. Benzodiazepines are allosteric modulators of the GABA-A receptor, and their binding to this receptor potentiates the chloride conduction which occurs when GABA works alone. Benzodiazepines depend on the presence of GABA for their activity and have little effect on chloride ion permeability in its absence. Other allosteric modulators of the GABA-A receptor include barbiturates, anesthetics, ethanol, and neuroactive steroids.[6] This correlation explains the cross-tolerance observed among the benzodiazepines, barbiturates, and ethanol.

In addition to centrally located GABA-A receptors, benzodiazepines also bind to peripheral benzodiazepines receptors (PBRs).[9] These PBRs are located in various peripheral tissues (adrenal glands, kidneys, lungs, ovaries, testes) as well as nonneuronal brain tissue. Although the clinical effects of benzodiazepines are not mediated through PBRs, their identification has been useful as a proposed measure of central GABA-A receptors. Studies of platelet and lymphocyte PBRs have found abnormally decreased PBR densities in all primary anxiety disorders except OCD, and these abnormalities can be reversed by chronic benzodiazepine therapy.[9] The neuropeptide known as "diazepam binding inhibitor" (DBI) is thought to be an anxiogenic endogenous ligand for PBRs, and overproduction of DBI may be involved in the pathogenesis of anxiety.[6]

The spectrum of activity of various benzodiazepine receptor ligands is depicted in Table 76-1. Endogenous modulators of GABA-A receptors include naturally occurring benzodiazepine-like compounds, β-carboline esters, and the neurosteroids, allopregnanolone and pregnanolone.[6] Certain β-carbolines are GABA-A receptor inverse agonists and produce effects opposite to those of the benzodiazepines by decreasing GABA-mediated chloride conduction. The clinical consequences of this action include anxiogenic, proconvulsant, and activating effects. In contrast to inverse agonists,

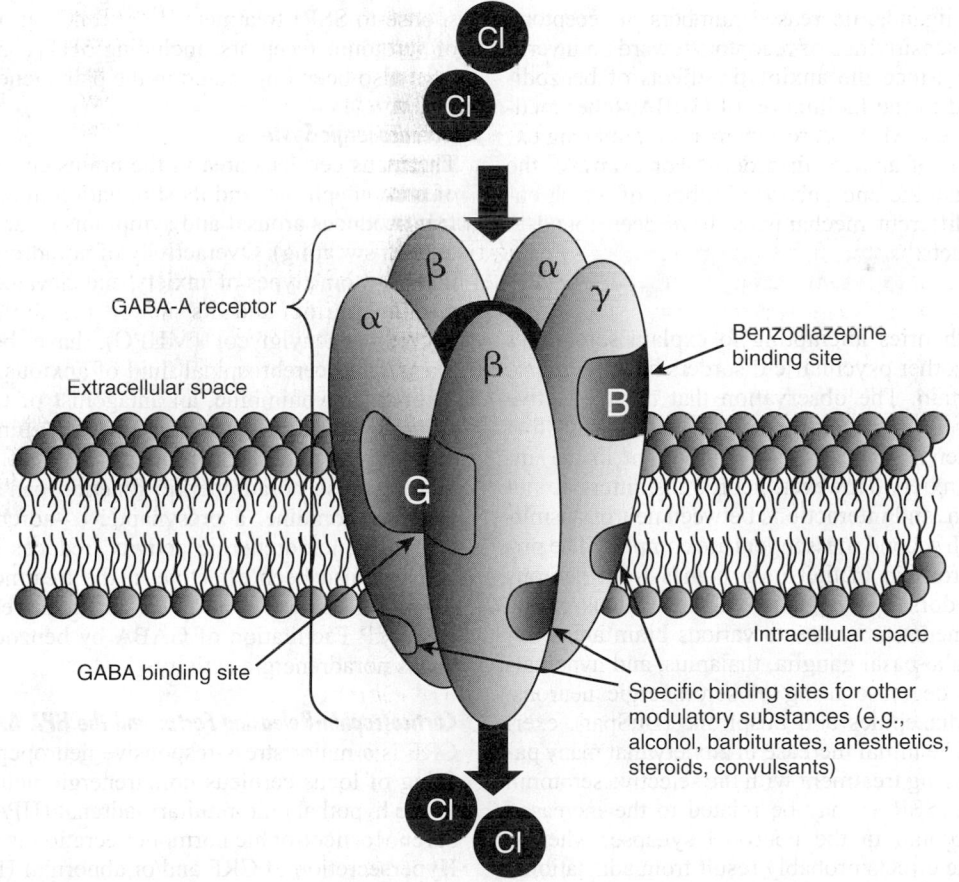

FIGURE 76-1 The GABA-A receptor complex. The GABA-A receptor is composed of five subunits arranged cylindrically around a chloride ion channel. Various arrangements of α, β, and γ subunits may combine to form the GABA-A receptor. δ, ε, π, and ρ subunits also have been identified, but their pharmacologic properties have not been fully characterized. The chloride ion channel is closed in the resting state. Binding of GABA alone partially opens the channel, allowing moderate chloride ion influx. Concurrent binding of both GABA and a benzodiazepine causes full opening of the channel with high influx of chloride ions, stabilization of the cell membrane, and decreased neuronal firing.

Table 76-1   Spectrum of Activity of GABA-A Receptor Ligands

	GABA-A Receptor Ligand Class				
	Agonist	*Partial Agonist*	*Antagonist*	*Partial Inverse Agonist*	*Full Inverse Agonist*
Example	Diazepam	Abecarnil	Flumazenil	B-CCE	DBI
Change in GABA-mediated chloride ion conduction	↑↑	↑	None	↓	↓↓
Clinical effects	Anxiolytic Sedative/hypnotic Anticonvulsant Muscle relaxant	Anxiolytic Sedative/hypnotic Anticonvulsant Muscle relaxant	None[a]	Anxiogenic Proconvulsant Activating	Anxiogenic Proconvulsant Activating

[a]Unless administered in the presence of another benzodiazepine receptor ligand, then will result in reversal of the pharmacologic effects of that agent.
B-CCE, ethyl-β-carboline-3-carboxylate; DBI, diazepam binding inhibitor; GABA, gamma-aminobutyric acid.

which bind to the receptor and exert an opposite effect, the GABA-A receptor antagonist flumazenil competitively occupies the receptor and blocks (or reverses) binding of other ligands without affecting GABA-mediated chloride conduction. Flumazenil has been a useful tool in researching possible abnormalities of GABA receptor function underlying various anxiety disorders. Currently, proposed theories related to this system include abnormally low levels of GABA or other endogenous receptor ligands, decreased numbers of receptors, and changes in the sensitivities of receptors toward an inverse agonist direction.[6,3] Since the anxiolytic effects of benzodiazepines are related to the facilitation of GABA, other medications that enhance GABA neurotransmission are being explored for treatment of anxiety disorders.[9] For example, the anticonvulsants tiagabine and gabapentin, both of which enhance GABA by different mechanisms, have been found to have anxiolytic effects.[10]

Serotonin Systems

Although several theories attempting to explain serotonin's role in anxiety and other psychiatric disorders have been proposed, none is certain. The observation that most effective anxiolytics affect serotonin neurotransmission indicates that this neurotransmitter is somehow very important in the underlying cause of anxiety. However, neurotransmitters do not function in isolation, and interactions between neurotransmitter systems and with second messengers are complex. The primary source of serotonin in the brain comes from neurons originating in the dorsal and median raphe nucleus of the brainstem.[2] These neurons innervate various brain areas, including the amygdala, basal ganglia, thalamus, and hypothalamus. Agents that decrease firing of serotonergic neurons, such as the benzodiazepines and buspirone (BuSpar), exert anxiolytic effects. The initial increase in anxiety that many patients experience during treatment with the selective serotonin reuptake inhibitors (SSRIs) may be related to the increased availability of serotonin in the neuronal synapse, whereas their later anxiolytic effects probably result from adaptational changes, including up- or down-regulation of different types of serotonin receptors, and inhibitory effects on noradrenergic transmission and CRF release.[2,11] Treatment with SSRIs is also associated with significant increases in GABA concentrations in certain brain regions as measured by proton magnetic resonance spectroscopy.[12]

A popular hypothesis is that anxiety represents a state of relative serotonin excess in certain brain areas. However, not all neurobiologic studies support this theory and some suggest an opposite effect.[2,3] A functional polymorphism in the human serotonin transporter promoter (5HTT) gene has been identified, which is associated with anxiety-related personality traits. This suggests a genetic vulnerability to anxiety related to the serotonin system.[13] This gene may also influence response to SSRI treatment.[14] Dysfunction of various subtypes of serotonin receptors, including $5HT_{1A}$, $5HT_{2A}$, and $5HT_{2C}$, have also been implicated in the pathogenesis of anxiety.[3]

Noradrenergic Systems

The locus ceruleus area in the brainstem is the major source of norepinephrine, and its stimulation in response to stress or fear produces arousal and symptoms of anxiety (tachycardia, tremor, sweating). Overactivity of noradrenergic neurons may underlie some types of anxiety, and elevated concentrations of norepinephrine and its major metabolite, 3-methoxy-4-hydroxy phenylglycol (MHPG), have been found in the plasma and cerebrospinal fluid of anxious patients.[15] Administration of yohimbine, an antagonist of the presynaptic α_2-adrenergic autoreceptor, increases norepinephrine release in the locus ceruleus and produces anxiety in humans. Drugs that decrease noradrenergic function can possess anxiolytic effects. Clonidine, a presynaptic α_2-adrenergic agonist that decreases noradrenergic activity, reduces anxiety symptoms and has also been effective in the treatment of alcohol and opiate withdrawal syndromes characterized by symptoms of anxiety.[15] Facilitation of GABA by benzodiazepines also reduces noradrenergic activity.

Corticotrophin-Releasing Factor and the HPA Axis

CRF is a major stress-responsive neuropeptide that increases firing of locus ceruleus noradrenergic neurons.[2,16] Activation of the hypothalamic-pituitary-adrenal (HPA) axis by pituitary adrenocorticotrophic hormone secretion is controlled by CRF. Hypersecretion of CRF and/or abnormal HPA axis regulation are hypothesized to underlie some states of abnormal anxiety, most notably PTSD.[17] In animal studies, early life stress causes an increase in CRF function and is associated with lifelong impairments in the regulation of fear and anxiety responses.[3] CRF antagonists are being explored as potential anxiolytic medications.[10]

Cholecystokinin System

Cholecystokinin (CCK) is an abundant neuropeptide in the central nervous system (CNS) with widely distributed receptors. The CCK system appears to play a major role in normal anxiety responses, and abnormalities in this system have been associated with some anxiety disorders.[3] Exogenous administration of CCK-B (brain), which is an agonist at CCK-4 receptors, induces anxiety in animals and humans. This effect can be blocked by pretreatment with a CCK receptor antagonist. CCK-B has complex interactions with other neurotransmitter systems, and appears to increase noradrenergic firing in the locus ceruleus.[3] It also interacts with the serotonin and GABA systems and has modulatory effects on HPA axis stress activation. Current research is targeting development of new anxiolytic compounds that work through the CCK system.

Epidemiology and Clinical Significance of Anxiety Disorders

As a group, the anxiety disorders are the most common of psychiatric illnesses. Epidemiologic surveys indicate that one in four Americans suffer from an anxiety disorder at some time in their life and that 17% are affected in any given year.[18,19] Most anxiety disorders are more common in women than in men.[19]

In 1990, the economic burden of anxiety disorders on society was estimated to be between $42 and $46.6 billion, including both direct and indirect costs.[20] Direct treatment costs primarily involve outpatient visits because hospitalization for treatment of anxiety disorders is not usually necessary. Medication expenses make up only about 2% of the total economic burden. Indirect costs of anxiety disorders can be substantial, especially in the workplace. Lost productivity and absenteeism due to anxiety is estimated to cost employers $4.1 billion annually, or approximately $256 per suffering worker in 1990.[20] Unemployment, dependence on public assistance programs, and alcohol and other substance abuse also contribute to the societal burden of anxiety disorders.

Today, most anxiety disorders are highly treatable with medications, cognitive or behavioral therapies, or combinations thereof. However, fewer than one-third of those who suffer seek help, and many who do are not properly diagnosed.[19,20] Most medical care for anxiety disorders is rendered in nonpsychiatric settings. Patients commonly present to primary care providers complaining of physical symptoms that cannot be medically explained, while the anxiety continues unrecognized. A large portion of primary care patients with medically unexplained symptoms, especially those who are high utilizers of health care services, actually have undetected anxiety or depressive disorders.[21] Screening tools have been developed to help identify anxiety and other psychiatric disorders in primary care patients in an attempt to improve their recognition and treatment. These include the Primary Care Evaluation of Mental Disorders (PRIME-MD), the Symptom Driven Diagnostic Screen-Primary Care (SDDS-PC), and the Well-Being Life Chart (WBLC).

Because anxiety is a feeling with which everyone is familiar, there is a tendency to trivialize the impact it can have on a sufferer's functioning and quality of life. An increased understanding about pathologic anxiety is needed in society in general and health care professionals in particular so that people seek and receive the treatment they need. Widespread public educational campaigns have been initiated to help increase awareness about anxiety disorders and their potential treatments. Practitioners must be knowledgeable about the clinical characteristics and treatment options for various disorders and must be able to share this information with patients and other health care professionals. A list of consumer and professional resources for information about anxiety disorders and treatment can be found at the end of the chapter in Table 76-15. Patients need to make the best use of their anxiolytic medications, which can result in decreased disability associated with the illness and improved quality of life.

Clinical Assessment and Differential Diagnosis of Anxiety

1. J.K., a 66-year-old man, complains to his physician of having trouble sleeping, feeling nervous, and worrying constantly. J.K.'s wife passed away 1 year ago, and he recently retired from his job as an accountant. Since then, he has become very involved in his hobbies of gardening and writing short stories but claims that he often cannot concentrate well enough to write. J.K. has mild chronic obstructive pulmonary disease (COPD) and suffered a myocardial infarction (MI) 2 years ago. His currently prescribed medications include lisinopril (Zestril), furosemide (Lasix), atorvastatin (Lipitor), niacin, and sucralfate. He also takes over-the-counter (OTC) diphenhydramine and pseudoephedrine for allergies, naproxen for back pain, and docusate sodium PRN for constipation. J.K. states that he drinks several cups of coffee each morning, and drinks one or two glasses of beer several nights a week to help him calm down when he has had a stressful day. He denies any history of psychiatric illness but states that he has always been a "high-strung" individual. What factors should be considered in the clinical assessment and differential diagnosis of J.K.'s symptoms of anxiety?

A diagnostic decision tree such as that in Figure 76-2 can be used to assist the clinician in differentiating among various causes of anxiety and between the different anxiety disorders. According to DSM-IV criteria for primary anxiety disorders, the symptoms are not secondary to any medical (drug or disease) causes. As illustrated in Table 76-2, the potential "organic" or secondary sources for anxiety symptoms are numerous.

Secondary Causes of Anxiety
ANXIETY SECONDARY TO MEDICAL CONDITIONS

A diagnosis *of anxiety disorder due to a general medical condition* is warranted when symptoms are believed to be the direct physiologic consequence of a medical condition.[1] In patients such as J.K. who have a number of medical conditions, all of these illnesses must be considered as possible underlying precipitants of anxiety. A complete physical and laboratory workup, with a thorough medical and psychiatric history, also are needed to exclude other, possibly reversible, causes before a primary anxiety disorder diagnosis is considered. In most cases of new-onset anxiety in elderly persons, symptoms can be attributed to some medical or substance-related cause.

Hypoglycemia, hyperthyroidism, electrolyte abnormalities, and angina pectoris are notably associated with anxiety

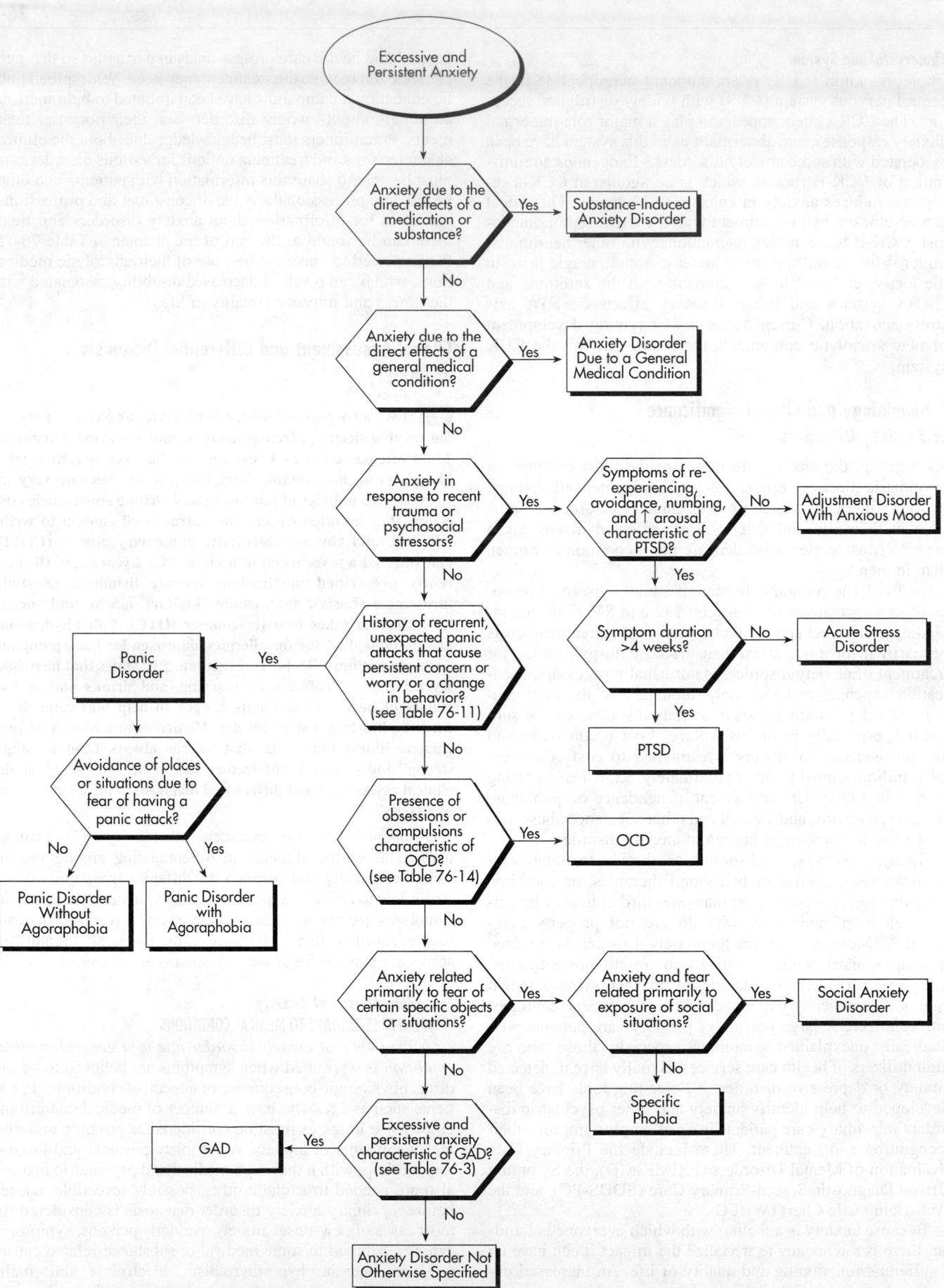

FIGURE 76-2 Diagnostic decision tree for anxiety disorders. GAD, generalized anxiety disorder; OCD, obsessive-compulsive disorder; PTSD, post-traumatic stress disorder.

Table 76-2   Secondary Causes of Anxiety

Medical Illnesses

Endocrine and metabolic disorders: hyperthyroidism, hypoglycemia, Addison's disease, Cushing's disease, pheochromocytoma, PMS, electrolyte abnormalities, acute intermittent porphyria, anemia

Neurologic: seizure disorders, multiple sclerosis, chronic pain syndromes, traumatic brain injury, CNS neoplasm, migraines, myasthenia gravis, Parkinson's disease, vertigo, essential tremor

Cardiovascular: mitral valve prolapse, CHF, arrhythmias, post-MI, hyperdynamic β-adrenergic state, hypertension, angina pectoris, postcerebral infarction

GI: PUD, Crohn's disease, ulcerative colitis, irritable bowel syndrome

Respiratory: COPD, asthma, pneumonia, pulmonary edema, respirator dependence, pulmonary embolus

Others: HIV infection, systemic lupus erythematosus

Psychiatric

Depression, mania, schizophrenia, adjustment disorder, personality disorders, delirium, dementia, eating disorders

Drugs

CNS stimulants: amphetamines, caffeine, cocaine, diethylpropion, ephedrine, MDMA (Ecstasy), methylphenidate, nicotine (and withdrawal), PCP, phenylephrine, pseudoephedrine

CNS depressant withdrawal: barbiturates, benzodiazepines, ethanol, opiates

Psychotropics: antipsychotics (akathisia), bupropion, buspirone, SSRIs, TCAs, venlafaxine

Cardiovascular: captopril, enalapril, digoxin, disopyramide, hydralazine, propafenone, procainamide, reserpine

Others: albuterol, aminophylline, baclofen, bromocriptine, cycloserine, dapsone, dronabinol, efavirenz, fluoroquinolones, interferon alfa, isoniazid, isoproterenol, levodopa, lidocaine, mefloquine, metoclopramide, monosodium glutamate, nicotinic acid, NSAIDs, pergolide, quinacrine, sibutramine, statins, steroids, triptans, theophylline, thyroid hormone, vinblastine, yohimbine

CHF, congestive heart failure; CNS, central nervous system; COPD, chronic obstructive pulmonary disease; GI, gastrointestinal; MI, myocardial infarction; NSAIDs, nonsteroidal anti-inflammatory drugs; PCP, phencyclidine; PMS, premenstrual syndrome, PUD, peptic ulcer disease; SSRIs, selective serotonin reuptake inhibitors; TCAs, tricyclic antidepressants.

symptoms.[22] Persons with chronic medical conditions such as COPD, Parkinson's disease, cardiomyopathy, post-MI, Graves' disease, and primary biliary cirrhosis have prevalences of anxiety that are markedly increased compared with healthy controls.[22] Medical illness in general, and especially in older patients such as J.K., is associated with higher rates of both anxiety and depression compared with the general population.[22] In some cases, the anxiety is physically induced by the medical condition, but reactional anxiety also may occur in response to being faced with a medical illness, especially a serious illness. In either case, the presence of anxiety may complicate the medical picture and have a negative impact on the course of illness. Successful management of the medical condition often relieves anxiety in such cases, but short-term use of anxiolytic medications or nondrug therapies (biofeedback, psychotherapy) also can be very helpful.

SUBSTANCE-RELATED ANXIETY

When evaluating for possible causes of anxiety, it also is important to consider all medications a person is taking, including OTC drugs such as cough and cold preparations.[23] A diagnosis of *substance-induced anxiety disorder* is warranted when anxiety symptoms occur in relation to substance intoxication or withdrawal or when medication use causes the symptoms. Among the medications that J.K. is taking, pseudoephedrine might be contributing to his anxiety. Other medications that can cause anxiety are listed in Table 76-2. Psychoactive substance abuse, withdrawal from CNS depressants (e.g., alcohol, barbiturates, benzodiazepines), excessive caffeine intake, and nicotine withdrawal may go unrecognized as underlying precipitants of anxiety. In some cases, a person

may begin use of substances such as alcohol in an attempt to self-medicate for anxiety and may continue a cycle of dependency during which withdrawal efforts can worsen the anxiety.[14] J.K.'s current pattern of alcohol use, though not excessive at present, may represent an early stage of this cycle if his anxiety continues.

ANXIETY ASSOCIATED WITH OTHER PSYCHIATRIC ILLNESSES

Although anxiety is the hallmark characteristic of anxiety disorders, it is not unique to this diagnostic category. Virtually any psychiatric illness may present with anxiety symptoms. Schizophrenia, bipolar disorder (both depressive and manic phases), eating disorders, dysthymia, and major depression are notably associated with anxiety, and diagnostic differentiation can sometimes be difficult.[1] For example, J.K.'s symptoms of having trouble sleeping, having difficulty concentrating, and worrying too much may be core target symptoms of either anxiety or depression, or possibly both. If anxiety symptoms occur only in relation to another psychiatric disorder, then a separate anxiety disorder diagnosis is precluded. Anxiety in these cases may be alleviated with successful treatment of the primary psychiatric disorder. However, benzodiazepine or other anxiolytics are often used as adjunctive therapy.

Individuals with other psychiatric disorders can also have a primary anxiety disorder. In fact, comorbidity with anxiety disorders is the rule rather than the exception.[18] Depression, in particular, is notably associated with anxiety disorders, and there are marked degrees of comorbidity between the two.[25] Concurrent anxiety and depression are associated with greater disability, poorer treatment outcomes, and higher suicide rates than either noncomorbid illness.[26]

PERSONAL AND ENVIRONMENTAL STRESSORS

Other factors that should be considered in J.K. are the recent changes in his life (retiring, losing his spouse). Stressful or traumatic life events may be anxiety provoking for anyone. Anxiety in response to life stressors may be severe and functionally detrimental, but could be considered appropriate for the circumstances. Usually, this type of anxiety is self-limiting and brief, subsiding over days to weeks as the person adapts to the new situation. However, some people may have serious difficulty adjusting, with prolonged, excessive, or debilitating symptoms that progress to a primary and sometimes chronic disorder. If the person has no history of an anxiety disorder and the symptoms last only a few months, a diagnosis of *adjustment disorder with anxious mood* may be appropriate. If the symptoms are severe enough and continue for a prolonged period, a primary anxiety disorder may be present. The initial onset of a chronic anxiety disorder often occurs during a stressful time period. Short-term or intermittent therapy with anxiolytic medication or counseling can be extremely beneficial in helping persons cope during times of acute stress. In contrast, management of primary anxiety disorders usually requires more extended treatment.

In summary, the factors in J.K.'s case that warrant further investigation before a primary anxiety disorder diagnosis can be made include his medical illnesses (COPD, post-MI), his use of pseudoephedrine and caffeine, possible depression, and his adjustment to the recent changes in his life. These factors need to be addressed, and treated or corrected if possible, before a diagnosis of an anxiety disorder can be made and an appropriate treatment plan defined.

GENERALIZED ANXIETY DISORDER
Epidemiology and Clinical Course

GAD is one of the most common anxiety disorders, with a lifetime prevalence of 3.9% to 6.6%.[1,19] The onset of GAD is usually gradual and may be associated with increased life stressors. Although the mean age of onset for GAD is 21 years, the high-risk period for onset ranges from the early teens to the mid-fifties.[19] GAD appears to be twice as common in females than males, and affected women often experience premenstrual exacerbation of symptoms.[27] The typical course of GAD is often described as being chronic but recurrent, but much is unknown about the long-term course of illness. Without treatment, it appears that less than half of GAD cases undergo remission. Degrees of impairment in role functioning and quality of life are comparable to that in major depression.[26]

Most people with GAD also have at least one other psychiatric disorder, most commonly depression or another anxiety disorder. At least two-thirds of GAD patients have another psychiatric illness, and >90% experience psychiatric comorbidity at some time in their life.[18,26] Common comorbid disorders include panic disorder, social anxiety disorder, simple phobia, OCD, and major depression.[26,28] GAD commonly precedes the development of these other disorders, and coexistence of GAD with these other conditions, particularly major depression, is associated with marked disability, high utilization of health care resources, and relatively poor treatment outcomes.[19,26] Alcohol abuse and dependence also are common in GAD patients and frequently result from attempts at self-medication of anxiety symptoms.[29] The observation that GAD rarely occurs in isolation has prompted debate about whether it is actually a primary anxiety disorder or merely a prodromal or residual phase of another disorder. A 5-year longitudinal study found significant diagnostic stability in GAD, supporting its existence as a distinct anxiety disorder.[30]

Diagnostic Criteria

The DSM-IV criteria for GAD are presented in Table 76-3. GAD is characterized by unrealistic or excessive anxiety and worry about life issues for a duration of 6 months or longer.[1] The patient usually has great difficulty in controlling the worry, which is accompanied by at least three of the associated symptoms listed in Table 76-3. Although some types of physical symptoms are similar between GAD and other anxiety disorders, the course of the symptoms varies between disorders. If the anxiety is related solely to another anxiety disorder (e.g., obsession with germs, fear of being in social situations), a diagnosis of GAD is not warranted.

In children with GAD (also called overanxious disorder of childhood), the duration requirement for symptoms is only 1 month.[1] Excessive worries in this younger population typically involve performance in school or sports, punctuality, perfectionism, and the possibility of catastrophic events. Children with GAD commonly seek excessive reassurance and approval from others.

Etiology and Pathophysiology

Genetic factors play a modest, but significant, role in the etiology of GAD. The genes involved in the hereditary development of GAD are thought to be the same as those in major depression, with environmental factors determining which disorder is expressed in an individual.[3,31] Biologic studies in

---

Table 76-3 Diagnostic Criteria for GAD

A. Unrealistic or excessive anxiety and worry about life circumstances for a period of at least 6 months, during which the person has been bothered more days than not by these concerns

B. The person has difficulty controlling anxiety and worry

C. The anxiety and worry are associated with at least three of the following symptoms:
  1. Restlessness or feeling keyed up or on edge
  2. Easy fatigue
  3. Difficulty concentrating or mind going blank
  4. Irritability
  5. Muscle tension
  6. Sleep disturbances

D. If another psychiatric disorder is present, the focus of the anxiety and worry is unrelated to it

E. The anxiety, worry, or physical symptoms cause significant distress or impairment in social, occupational, or some other important aspect of functioning

F. The disturbance is not due to the direct effects of a substance, medication, or general medical condition and does not occur only during the course of a mood disorder, a psychotic disorder, or a pervasive developmental disorder

Adapted from Reference 1.
GAD, generalized anxiety disorder.

GAD have found abnormalities in the noradrenergic, serotonergic, and CCK systems, as well as in GABA-A receptor function.[3] Several studies report decreased α_2-adrenergic receptors in GAD patients, and this is thought to represent down-regulation of receptors in response to high catecholamine levels. Abnormally low levels of lymphocyte peripheral benzodiazepine receptors (PBRs) have been reported by several investigators. GAD patients also have been found to have enhanced anxiety response to CCK-4 administration compared with normal controls, suggesting an increased sensitivity of the CCK system in GAD.

Treatment of Generalized Anxiety Disorder

Nonpharmacologic Treatments

Management of GAD can involve both nonpharmacologic and pharmacologic therapies. Nondrug treatments such as supportive psychotherapy, dynamic psychotherapy, cognitive therapy, relaxation training, and meditation exercises often are helpful in relieving anxiety and improving coping skills.[32] Cognitive therapy is aimed at identifying negative thought patterns that may provoke or worsen anxiety and changing them to be more positive. Combined cognitive-behavioral therapy (CBT) has been associated with significant reductions in anxiety that are maintained over 6 to 12 months, as well as decreased psychiatric comorbidity in GAD.[32] Controlled comparisons of cognitive therapies and benzodiazepine treatment have reported comparable efficacies in GAD.[32] Although psychosocial treatments are commonly recommended as first-line therapy for GAD and other anxiety disorders, they are vastly underused.[33] Reasons for this include cost and time requirements as well as a limited availability of trained therapists. The decline in use of psychosocial therapies for anxiety disorders over the past decade also correlates with the explosion in medication options for treating anxiety disorders.

Benzodiazepines

Benzodiazepines are the most widely prescribed anxiolytic agents today, and their efficacy in treating GAD and many other anxiety disorders is well established.[29,34,35] The benzodiazepines offer distinct clinical advantages over older agents such as barbiturates, meprobamate, paraldehyde, and alcohol. These advantages include more specific anxiolytic effects, lower fatality rates from acute toxicity and overdose (when taken alone), better side effect profiles, lower potential for abuse, and less dangerous interactions with other drugs. Currently, use of these older nonbenzodiazepine agents as anxiolytics is generally considered inappropriate because of the many advantages of benzodiazepines and other newer agents.

MECHANISM OF ACTION

In humans, benzodiazepines have four distinct effects: anxiolytic, anticonvulsant, muscle relaxant, and sedative-hypnotic. These agents are used to treat a wide variety of medical and psychiatric conditions, including muscle spasms, seizures, anxiety disorders, acute agitation, and insomnia.[34] Certain benzodiazepines are commonly used to decrease anxiety and apprehension and induce sedation before surgery and other medical procedures.

As described in the Neurobiology of Anxiety section, the mechanism of action of benzodiazepines involves potentiation of GABA by binding to sites on the central GABA-A receptor. There are four types of GABA-A receptors that are benzodiazepine sensitive; these are distinguished by the type of α subunit they contain (α_1, α_2, α_3, or α_5).[4,6] Benzodiazepine binding sites on α_1-GABA-A and α_2-GABA-A receptors were formerly called BZ-1 and BZ-2 receptors, respectively, but there is a trend away from use of the latter terminology. GABA-A receptors possessing α_4 or α_6 subunits are not sensitive to benzodiazepines. Receptors with a α_1 subunit are widely distributed throughout most brain areas and are the most abundant type. Benzodiazepine interaction at these α_1-GABA-A receptors produces sedative and amnestic effects, whereas anxiolytic effects are associated with binding to the α_2-GABA-A receptor.[4,5] This latter type of GABA-A receptor is localized mainly in the limbic system, cerebral cortex, and striatum. GABA-A receptors with α_3 subunits are linked with noradrenergic, serotonergic, and cholinergic neurons.

Currently available benzodiazepine anxiolytics do not have selective activity at any of the four GABA-A receptor subtypes. Research is aimed at developing benzodiazepine compounds with specific affinity for the α_2-GABA-A receptor, which would produce anxiolytic effects without sedative and amnestic effects.[10] Agents that are partial agonists at α_2-GABA-A receptors are also being studied as potential benzodiazepine anxiolytics; these would be associated with minimal tolerance, dependence, and withdrawal.[10] Zolpidem (Ambien) and zaleplon (Sonata) are examples of selective α_1-GABA-A receptor agonists that have been introduced as selective hypnotic agents.

CLINICAL COMPARISON OF BENZODIAZEPINES

Approximately 35 benzodiazepine compounds are marketed worldwide, and even though numbers of benzodiazepine prescriptions are declining, they remain the most frequently prescribed psychotropic medications in the world. Of the 13 benzodiazepines commercially available in the United States, 7 are marketed as antianxiety agents, and 6 as oral sedative-hypnotics. These indications reflect the manufacturers' labeling decisions, because the anxiolytics can be effective sedatives and vice versa. The benzodiazepine halazepam (Paxipam), which was not widely used, was discontinued in 2001.

Midazolam (Versed), a short-acting, water-soluble benzodiazepine, is indicated only for induction of sedation before surgery or for short diagnostic or endoscopic procedures. It was previously marketed only in parenteral formulation, but an oral syrup form is now available. Clonazepam (Klonopin) was originally approved only as an anticonvulsant, but is now also indicated for the treatment of panic disorder. Clonazepam and most of the other benzodiazepines also have many unlabeled uses, including treatment of anxiety and agitation associated with various medical or psychiatric illnesses, GAD, and other anxiety disorders, irritable bowel syndrome, premenstrual syndrome, chemotherapy-induced nausea and vomiting, catatonia, tetanus, involuntary movement disorders (restless legs syndrome, periodic limb movements of sleep, akathisia, tardive dyskinesia, essential tremor), and spasticity associated with various neurologic disorders (cerebral palsy, paraplegia).[34] Table 76-4 compares the clinical profiles of marketed oral benzodiazepines.

Table 76-4   Clinical Comparison of Benzodiazepine Agents

Drug (Trade Name, Generic)	FDA-Approved Indications	Usual Dosage Range ≤65 Years of Age	Maximum Recommended Dosage ≥65 Years of Age	Approximate Dosage Equivalencies	Year Introduced
Chlordiazepoxide (Librium, Limbitrol,[a] Librax,[b] generic)	Anxiety, preoperative anxiety, acute alcohol withdrawal	15–100 mg/day	40 mg/day	50	1960
Diazepam (Valium, generic)	Anxiety, muscle relaxant, acute alcohol withdrawal, preoperative anxiety, anticonvulsant	4–40 mg/day	20 mg/day	10	1963
Oxazepam (Serax, generic)	Anxiety, alcohol withdrawal	30–120 mg/day	60 mg/day	30	1965
Flurazepam (Dalmane, generic)	Sedative-hypnotic	15–30 mg HS	15 mg HS	30	1970
Clorazepate (Tranxene, Tranxene-SD, generic)	Anxiety, alcohol withdrawal, anticonvulsant	15–60 mg/day	30 mg/day	15	1972
Clonazepam (Klonopin, Klonopin wafer, generic)	Anticonvulsant, panic disorder	0.5–12.0 mg/day	3 mg/day	0.5	1975
Lorazepam (Ativan, generic)	Anxiety, anxiety associated with depression	2–6 mg/day	3 mg/day	1.5–2.0	1977
Alprazolam (Xanax, Xanax XR, generic)	Anxiety, anxiety associated with depression, panic disorder	0.5–6.0 mg/day (up to 10 mg/day for panic disorder)	2 mg/day	1.0	1981
Temazepam (Restoril, generic)	Sedative-hypnotic	15–30 mg HS	15 mg HS	30	1981
Triazolam (Halcion, generic)	Sedative-hypnotic	0.125–0.25 mg HS	0.125 mg HS	0.25	1983
Quazepam (Doral)	Sedative-hypnotic	7.5–15 mg HS	7.5 mg HS	15	1990
Estazolam (Prosom, generic)	Sedative-hypnotic	1–2 mg HS	1 mg HS	2.0	1991

[a]Combination product containing amitriptyline.
[b]Combination product containing clidinium bromide (classified as a gastrointestinal antispasmodic agent).

Buspirone

Buspirone (BuSpar) was marketed in the United States in 1986 as the first of a nonbenzodiazepine class of anxiolytics, the azapirones. This class differs pharmacologically and clinically from the benzodiazepines and also contains several other investigational anxiolytics such as gepirone and ipsapirone.[29,36] Buspirone does not interact with GABA receptors and works as a partial agonist of the serotonin type 1A (5-hydroxytryptamine [5HT1A]) receptor (i.e., it binds to the receptor but exerts less of an effect than a full agonist).[37] This partial agonist activity results in reduced serotonin neurotransmission. In addition, buspirone enhances dopaminergic neurotransmission by blocking presynaptic dopamine receptor-2 autoreceptors and also facilitates noradrenergic activity.[36] Buspirone has been found to be superior to placebo and comparably effective to the benzodiazepines in some, but not all, studies in the treatment of GAD.[29,38–40] Buspirone and other azapirones lack general CNS depressant effects and are relatively free of the potential for abuse and dependence. In addition to their anxiolytic activity, azapirones may be useful in the treatment of depression as well as a wide variety of other psychiatric and neurologic disorders.[36,41] Buspirone is preferred over benzodiazepines in patients with a history of substance abuse or dependence, and those who are elderly or medically ill, but probably offers no clinical advantages over antidepressant agents for GAD in most patients.

Antidepressant Agents

Antidepressants have now surpassed benzodiazepines as the recommended first-line treatment for most anxiety disorder patients, even though benzodiazepines are probably still the most widely prescribed anxiolytics.[42] One important clinical difference between these two medication classes is that the anxiolytic effects of benzodiazepines occur almost immediately, whereas the effects of antidepressants occur gradually over several weeks. For this reason, it is common practice for short-term benzodiazepine therapy to be prescribed in combination with an antidepressant during initial treatment of many anxiety disorders.

The first indication that antidepressants might be effective in the treatment of anxiety disorders appeared in the late 1970s, when certain tricyclic antidepressants (TCAs) and monoamine oxidase (MAO) inhibitors were found to be useful in treating panic disorder. The TCA clomipramine (Anafranil) emerged as an effective treatment for OCD soon thereafter, and as shown in Table 76-5, SSRIs have since gained first-line status for treating all five primary anxiety disorders.[43] The distinction between anxiolytics and antidepressants is continually narrowing.

Early controlled studies found trazodone, doxepin, imipramine, and amitriptyline to be comparably effective or even superior to benzodiazepines in treating GAD.[29] Although the benzodiazepines work quicker and TCA treatment is often associated with initial increases in anxiety (especially with higher dosages), continued TCA therapy is usually effective if the side effects can be tolerated. However, the discovery of the TCAs' anxiolytic potential came too late for these agents to ever be widely used for treating anxiety disorders because attention soon turned to the much safer and better tolerated SSRIs.

Paroxetine (Paxil) is the best-studied SSRI in GAD, and was FDA approved for this indication in 2001. Paroxetine is superior to placebo and as effective as the TCAs in treating GAD, but it is much better tolerated.[45,46] Results from a large fixed-dose study suggest that a paroxetine dosage of 20 mg/day is effective for most GAD patients, although some may need 30 to 40 mg/day for optimal benefits.[47] As with TCAs, some patients experience an initial increase in anxiety during SSRI treatment, so that lower-than-normal SSRI starting doses should be used in GAD patients. A low paroxetine

Table 76-5 **Summary of Comparative Medication Treatment Options for Anxiety Disorders**

Disorder	First-Line Treatments[a]	Second-Line Treatments	Possible Alternatives
Generalized anxiety disorder	Venlafaxine XR Buspirone Benzodiazepines Paroxetine Escitalopram	Nefazodone Sertraline Citalopram	Tricyclic antidepressants[b] Fluoxetine Mirtazapine Hydroxyzine
Panic disorder	Paroxetine Sertraline Fluoxetine Alprazolam Clonazepam	Fluvoxamine Citalopram Clomipramine Lorazepam Escitalopram	Venlafaxine Nefazodone Mirtazapine Imipramine Valproic acid Diazepam
Social anxiety disorder	Paroxetine Sertraline Venlafaxine XR	Fluvoxamine Citalopram Clonazepam Alprazolam Escitalopram	Phenelzine[b] Nefazodone Bupropion Buspirone[c] Topiramate Gabapentin
Post-traumatic stress disorder	Sertraline Paroxetine	Fluoxetine Fluvoxamine Venlafaxine Nefazodone Citalopram	Amitriptyline[b] Imipramine[b] Phenelzine[b] Mirtazapine Trazodone[c] Carbamazepine Valproic acid Lamotrigine Topiramate Atypical antipsychotics[c]
Obsessive-compulsive disorder	Paroxetine Fluoxetine Sertraline Fluvoxamine	Clomipramine[b] Venlafaxine Citalopram Escitalopram	Clonazepam[c] Antipsychotic agents[c] Buspirone[c] Pindolol[c] Nefazodone Lithium[c]

[a]FDA-approved indications.
[b]Documented efficacy but not recommended for first-line treatment because of undesirable clinical properties (side effects, potential toxicity, drug interactions).
[c]Adjunctive therapy only.

starting dose of 10 mg/day is recommended for the first week in GAD patients to minimize initial side effects. Compared with benzodiazepines, paroxetine's anxiolytic effects are slower in onset but reportedly superior to benzodiazepines after 8 weeks of treatment.[46] Paroxetine maintenance therapy significantly decreases the risk of GAD relapse at 6 months.[48] The most common side effects of paroxetine in GAD patients are sedation, nausea, dry mouth, constipation, asthenia, headache, and sexual dysfunction. With long-term therapy, weight gain may be problematic.

The combination serotonin/norepinephrine reuptake inhibitor, venlafaxine (Effexor XR formulation), was the first antidepressant to be approved by the U.S. Food and Drug Administration (FDA) for the treatment of GAD. Several large controlled studies have shown venlafaxine XR to be effective in reducing anxiety associated with depression as well as in the treatment of pure GAD.[38,49–51] The recommended venlafaxine starting dose is 37.5 mg/day, and the effective dosage range for GAD is 75 to 225 mg/day.[51] Many patients respond to doses of 75 to 150 mg/day, although some may require up

to 225 mg/day. The side effect profile of venlafaxine is similar to the SSRIs, with nausea being the most common complaint. Nausea is dose related and usually subsides after 1 to 2 weeks of continued therapy. Other common side effects of venlafaxine include dizziness, asthenia, dry mouth, sweating, and either sedation or insomnia. Significant increases in blood pressure are not usually seen within the dosage range used for GAD (75 to 225 mg/day), but can occur with higher venlafaxine doses. Long-term studies report that GAD response to venlafaxine is maintained during 6 months of continued treatment.[50]

SSRIs other than paroxetine also can be beneficial in treating GAD. Escitalopram (Lexapro) received FDA-approval for GAD in late 2003, and preliminary reports suggest efficacy for citalopram (Celexa).[43,52] Sertraline (Zoloft), fluvoxamine (Luvox, generic), and fluoxetine (Prozac) are reportedly effective in alleviating anxiety symptoms in patients with depression.[29,53,54] Fluoxetine may be more likely than other SSRIs to cause anxiety as an initial side effect.[43] Fluoxetine use in depressed patients with prominent anxiety or psychomotor agitation has been associated with poor response in some studies, although others report it to be comparably effective and as well tolerated as other SSRIs in this population.[54,55]

Nefazodone (Serzone) and mirtazapine (Remeron) are two other non-SSRI antidepressants that appear promising in the treatment of GAD, but controlled studies are lacking.[29] Depression trials indicate that these two agents have significant anxiolytic effects.[56,57] They are associated with especially low incidences of causing anxiety as a side effect, which is attributed to their serotonin receptor type-2 blocking activity. (See Chapter 79, Mood Disorders I: Major Depressive Disorders, for more information regarding the clinical use of various antidepressant agents.)

Although decreases in anxiety symptoms during antidepressant treatment may appear within the first 2 weeks, response is gradual and generally continues over 8 to 12 weeks or longer. Therefore, optimal trials of antidepressants in GAD should allow at least 8 weeks of adequate doses before a lack of response is determined. Continued improvements may occur over 4 to 6 months in some GAD patients treated with antidepressants.[48,50]

Overall, advantages of antidepressants over benzodiazepines in treating GAD include their superior efficacy for cognitive symptoms such as excessive worry and their better coverage for common comorbid disorders such as depression and other anxiety disorders. Antidepressants also lack potential for abuse and dependence, although nearly all antidepressants can cause a withdrawal syndrome upon abrupt discontinuation. Advantages for benzodiazepines over antidepressants include rapid onset of anxiolytic effects, better efficacy for physical anxiety symptoms, appropriateness for as-needed use, lower medication costs for generic forms, and better overall tolerability in some patients. Compared with antidepressants and benzodiazepines, buspirone is effective in treating cognitive anxiety symptoms and is not associated with abuse or dependence; however, it has a delayed onset of anxiolytic effects and is not appropriate for as-needed use.

β-Blockers

β-Adrenergic receptor blocking agents such as propranolol (Inderal) are very effective in reducing certain physical symptoms of anxiety (tremor, flushing, tachycardia) that result from activation of the sympathetic nervous system.[58] These agents are especially effective in preventing performance anxiety or "stage fright" by suppressing peripheral autonomic activity but they do not modify cognitive symptoms of anxiety. β-Blockers are not as effective as benzodiazepines in the treatment of anxiety disorders and are not recommended as a primary treatment option for GAD.

Antihistamines

H₁-receptor blocking agents such as hydroxyzine (Vistaril) and diphenhydramine (Benadryl) have been used for years in the treatment of anxiety and insomnia. Because of their potent sedative effects, these antihistamines generally are used on an as-needed basis for insomnia or for their calming effects in a variety of patient types. Although these drugs are considered benign and diphenhydramine is available over the counter, they do possess significant anticholinergic effects, which can produce problems such as confusion, cognitive impairment, nausea, and constipation. Elderly patients, especially those who are medically ill or have dementia, are particularly vulnerable to these side effects, and diphenhydramine is considered inappropriate for use in the elderly.[59] There is no evidence for the efficacy of diphenhydramine in the treatment of primary anxiety disorders.

Several studies have reported hydroxyzine to be beneficial in treating GAD. A large placebo-controlled study in nonelderly patients demonstrated superiority of hydroxyzine (50 mg/day given in three divided doses) over placebo.[60] Hydroxyzine was as effective as benzodiazepine therapy over 3 months of treatment, although it did not work as quickly. No anticholinergic, cognitive impairment, or weight gain adverse effects were reported in hydroxyzine-treated patients and it was very well tolerated. Minimal sedation was reported with the relatively low daily hydroxyzine dose used in this study. Abrupt discontinuation of hydroxyzine after 3 months was not associated with significant withdrawal symptoms. Hydroxyzine is an inexpensive drug and may be a treatment option for GAD in some patients, but controlled comparisons with antidepressant agents are needed to better define its current role in therapy. It is not a good choice of therapy for elderly persons or GAD patients with comorbid depression or other anxiety disorders.

Clinical Presentation and Assessment of GAD

2. N.K., a 25-year-old woman, has been employed as a bank clerk for the past 5 years. She had an excellent work record until 6 months ago, when excessive absences and a tendency to become easily upset at customers and co-workers became noticeable. Upon clinical assessment, N.K. complains of being tired, irritable, and tense, with frequent stomach upset and diarrhea. She has no history of mental illness; however, she admits to being stressed and worrying too much about "just little things," which she cannot seem to control no matter how hard she tries. N.K. denies experiencing episodic "attacks" of severe anxiety (which might be indicative of panic disorder), or of having obsessive-compulsive thoughts or behaviors.

N.K.'s physical examination is unremarkable, and she has no history of mental illness in her family, although her mother was a "nervous person." N.K. denies any past or present use of any illicit substances or alcohol. Her mental status examination reveals the following: *Appearance and behavior:* N.K. is neatly groomed and dressed and speaks coherently, but she constantly fidgets and taps her right foot. She states that she often has difficulty falling asleep but generally remains asleep throughout the night. *Mood:* N.K. is anxious and worried about the clinician's evaluation and admits to occasionally feeling depressed because of her anxiety. *Sensorium:* N.K. is oriented to person, place, and time. *Thoughts:* N.K. denies any auditory or visual hallucinations.

N.K. states that at times she has difficulty speaking, is unable to relax, and startles easily. She realizes that work has been difficult for her lately, and her supervisor has told her that her job is in immediate jeopardy unless she improves her performance. N.K. states that she just wants to be able to perform her job well, relax, and enjoy life. Her insight and judgment are good, and she is motivated to obtain treatment. N.K. denies any suicidal ideation. The physician's provisional diagnosis is GAD (DSM-IV criteria). What clinical features of GAD are present in N.K., and how can her symptoms be assessed objectively?

N.K. exhibits the following target symptoms associated with GAD: excessive worry that is difficult to control, irritability, tension and inability to relax, fatigue, and sleep disturbances. Other typical symptoms of anxiety present in N.K. include gastrointestinal (GI) problems (upset stomach and diarrhea), being startled easily, difficulty speaking, and fidgeting. These target symptoms are not necessarily diagnostic of any particular disorder, but other factors in association with these symptoms are consistent with GAD. The absence of physical or other psychiatric illnesses, as well as use of any illicit substances or alcohol, excludes possible secondary causes of anxiety. The 6-month duration of symptoms is consistent with a diagnosis of GAD, and N.K. is at a common age for onset of GAD. More important, the symptoms are causing significant occupational impairment for N.K. and interfering with her quality of life; therefore, a diagnosis of GAD is appropriate in N.K.

The Hamilton Anxiety Rating Scale (HAM-A) is a useful assessment tool to evaluate clinical anxiety and it is the standard instrument used in GAD clinical trials. A HAM-A score of >18 is generally correlated with significant anxiety and a score of ≤7 to 10 is associated with remission.[61] The HAM-A can be used to assess baseline anxiety symptoms in patients such as N.K. and to monitor response throughout treatment. The Sheehan Disability Scale is a patient-rated instrument, which is commonly used to assess functional impairment due to GAD and other anxiety disorders. A score of ≤1 reflects mild disability.[61]

Indications for and Goals of Treatment

3. Based on the information presented in N.K.'s case, how can it be determined whether treatment is indicated? What are the goals of treatment?

N.K. meets the diagnostic criteria for GAD and is suffering significant disability from her anxiety disorder. She also has insight into her illness and desires treatment to be able to improve her job performance and quality of life. Appropriate treatment of GAD can help achieve these goals and therefore is indicated for patients such as N.K. Desired outcomes of treatment include reductions in N.K.'s cognitive (worrying, irritability) and somatic (GI symptoms, fatigue, insomnia) symptoms of anxiety, improved performance at work, and an increased ability to relax and "enjoy life."

Selection of Treatment

4. What factors should be considered in the process of selecting the most appropriate treatment option for N.K.?

Treatment options for GAD may include both pharmacologic and nondrug therapies. Psychosocial treatments such as CBT can be effective in treating GAD, but use of these therapies alone is generally reserved for patients with mild to moderate symptoms, those in whom anxiety is mainly related to stressful life events, or when immediate symptom relief is not necessary. In N.K.'s case, prompt treatment is needed because she feels that her job is in immediate jeopardy owing to impairments associated with her anxiety. Therefore, pharmacotherapy in combination with psychological therapy, if available, is indicated in N.K.

Among potential drug therapies, the benzodiazepines, buspirone, paroxetine, and venlafaxine are all considered first-line treatments for GAD.[29] A primary consideration when choosing among these options is whether any comorbid psychiatric conditions are present. For example, venlafaxine and paroxetine are good initial choices for patients with concurrent depression, which is common in GAD patients. They are also preferred over benzodiazepines in patients with past or present alcohol or substance abuse. Paroxetine may be the best choice if another anxiety disorder is present, since it is FDA approved for all five primary anxiety disorders. Other medical or psychiatric disorders may also be present, which can guide selection toward a treatment that may be dually effective.

Another important consideration when selecting treatment for GAD is how fast therapeutic effects are needed. Benzodiazepines reduce anxiety very quickly, within a few hours, whereas the antidepressants and buspirone have delayed onsets of anxiolytic effects. Medication cost is another potential factor, and generic benzodiazepines are by far the least expensive anxiolytic medications.

In N.K.'s case, a benzodiazepine may be a good initial choice because of the need for quick symptom relief relating to her problems at work. N.K. is young and healthy with no past or present history of substance or alcohol use that might make benzodiazepines unsuitable for her. GAD is often chronic, and antidepressants or buspirone are usually preferred over benzodiazepines for long-term treatment. Therefore, one of these agents would also be appropriate to use in this case. Combination benzodiazepines-SSRI therapy during initial treatment of anxiety disorders is well tolerated and may result in synergistic anxiolytic effects and quicker response.[62,63]

Benzodiazepine Treatment
Factors Influencing Benzodiazepine Selection

5. The physician decides to treat N.K.'s GAD with venlafaxine XR and also wants to prescribe a benzodiazepine for quick control of her anxiety during the first several weeks until the onset of venlafaxine's anxiolytic effects appear. What factors are important in the selection of a particular benzodiazepine agent for N.K.?

Of the available benzodiazepines, none has demonstrated clear superior efficacy in the treatment of anxiety. However, certain agents have been used much more extensively than others. Although diazepam (Valium, generic) is the most frequently prescribed benzodiazepine in the world, alprazolam (Xanax, generic) is the most commonly used in the United States and accounts for approximately one-third of all benzodiazepine prescriptions.[42] Lorazepam (Ativan, generic) is the next most popular, followed by clonazepam (Klonopin, generic) and then diazepam. Alprazolam and clonazepam are the only benzodiazepines that are FDA approved for the treatment of panic disorder, although other benzodiazepines also can be effective.

Because the overall anxiolytic efficacies of benzodiazepines are similar, other factors must be considered when selecting one agent over another. The one major area of clinically significant differences between benzodiazepines is their pharmacokinetic properties. These are generally the main factors considered in drug selection (Table 76-6).

PHARMACOKINETICS AND METABOLISM

Benzodiazepines can be differentiated pharmacokinetically according to their elimination half-lives and their metabolism to active or inactive compounds (Fig. 76-3; see Table 76-6). Diazepam and chlordiazepoxide (Librium) have half-lives between 10 and 40 hours but are metabolized by hepatic oxidative pathways to the active metabolite desmethyldiazepam (DMDZ), which has a half-life of at least 100 hours.[64] Demethylation of diazepam to DMDZ is mediated by several cytochrome P450 (CYP) isozymes, including CYP

2C19, CYP 3A4, and to a lesser extent, CYP 2B6. CYP 2C19 appears to be the predominate pathway with usual therapeutic diazepam doses, but CYP 3A4 becomes more important with high doses, in overdose cases, and in CYP 2C19 poor metabolizers.[65] The other major active diazepam metabolite, temazepam, is formed through CYP 3A4–mediated hydroxylation.

As shown in Figure 76-3, the prodrugs quazepam (Doral) and clorazepate (Tranxene) also are metabolized to DMDZ.[64] Because of the exceedingly long half-life of this active metabolite, chronic dosing of any benzodiazepines that are converted to DMDZ can lead to drug accumulation and prolonged clinical effects. This can be especially detrimental in

Table 76-6 Pharmacokinetic Comparison of Benzodiazepine Agents

Drug	Elimination Half-Life (hr)[a]	Active Metabolites	Protein Binding	Pathway of Metabolism	Rate of Onset After Oral Administration
Chlordiazepoxide	>100	Desmethyldiazepam	96%	Oxidation	Intermediate
Diazepam	>100	Desmethyldiazepam	98%	Oxidation (CYP 3A4, CYP 2C19)	Very fast
Oxazepam	5–14	None	87%	Conjugation	Slow
Flurazepam	>100	Desalkylflurazepam, hydroxyethylflurazepam	97%	Oxidation	Fast
Clorazepate	>100	Desmethyldiazepam	98%	Oxidation	Fast
Lorazepam	10–20	None	85–90%	Conjugation	Intermediate
Alprazolam	12–15	Insignificant	80%	Oxidation (CYP 3A4)	Fast
Temazepam	10–20	Insignificant	98%	Conjugation	Intermediate
Triazolam	1.5–5	Insignificant	90%	Oxidation (CYP 3A4)	Intermediate
Quazepam	47–100	2-oxoquazepam, desalkyloxoquazepam	>95%	Oxidation	Fast
Estazolam	24	Insignificant	93%	Oxidation	Intermediate
Clonazepam	20–50	Insignificant	85%	Oxidation, reduction (CYP 3A4)	Intermediate
Midazolam	1–4	None	97%	Oxidation (CYP 3A4)	NA

[a]Parent drug + active metabolite.
NA, not applicable.

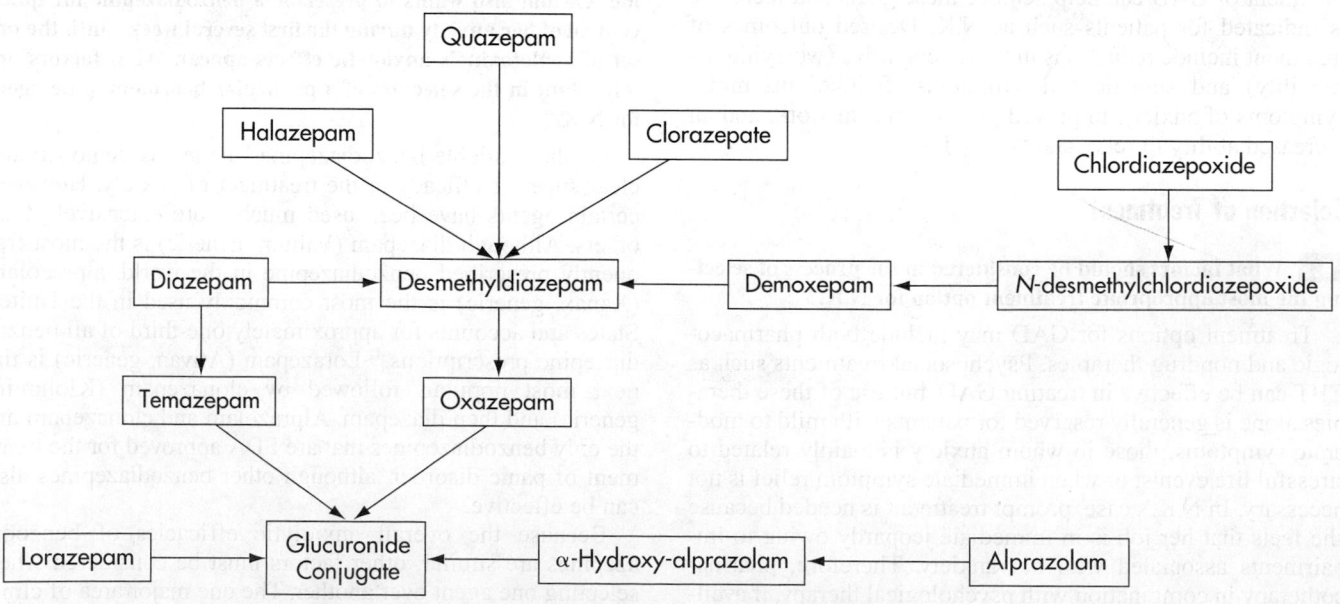

FIGURE 76-3 Metabolic pathways of benzodiazepines.

the elderly, those with liver disease, or persons taking other drugs that interfere with benzodiazepine metabolism. Although their long durations of action make once-daily dosing possible, small, divided daily doses often are used clinically to minimize side effects.

Clonazepam undergoes various routes of hepatic metabolism, including oxidative hydroxylation, reduction, and acetylation.[64] At least five metabolites have been identified, but their pharmacologic activity is uncertain. One main metabolite, 7-amino clonazepam, is known to be inactive. The specific enzymes responsible for clonazepam metabolism have not been confirmed, but there is evidence that it is a substrate for CYP 3A4.[66] The elimination half-life of clonazepam ranges from 20 to 50 hours, making once-daily dosing feasible. A new formulation of orally disintegrating clonazepam tablets (Klonopin wafer) has been introduced and is indicated for the treatment of panic disorder. This product dissolves quickly on the tongue and is promoted as being especially convenient because it can be taken without water.

Alprazolam (Xanax) and lorazepam (Ativan) have intermediate half-lives of 10 to 20 hours, and oxazepam (Serax) has a short to intermediate half-life of 5 to 14 hours. Alprazolam is a triazolobenzodiazepine that is metabolized by CYP 3A4 to an active metabolite, α-hydroxy alprazolam, which has a short half-life of approximately 2 hours and is considered clinically insignificant. Alprazolam, lorazepam, and oxazepam usually need to be taken on a TID to QID dosing schedule for sustained clinical effects, but an extended-release (XR) preparation of alprazolam that allows QD or BID dosing has become available. Alprazolam XR may be associated with less CNS side effects than the immediate-release form because peak alprazolam blood levels are lower.[67] Lorazepam, temazepam (Restoril), and oxazepam undergo phase II metabolism by glucuronidation and are believed to be substrates for the uridine diphosphate-glucuronosyltransferase (UGT) 2B7 isozyme.[68] These agents are free of active metabolites and are unlikely to accumulate with chronic administration, so are preferred over long-acting agents in patients with liver disease and in the elderly. Unlike phase I oxidative metabolism, phase II glucuronidation processes do not appear to decline with age.[68] However, the clearance of oxazepam has been found to be significantly decreased in the "old-old" (older than 80).[69]

Benzodiazepines are readily absorbed within 2 to 3 hours after oral administration.[64] They are widely distributed in the body and accumulate preferentially in lipid-rich areas such as the CNS and fat tissue. Lipid solubility varies between the agents, resulting in differences in rates of absorption and speed of onset, as well as duration of clinical effects (see Table 76-6). Diazepam and clorazepate have the highest lipid solubilities and the quickest onsets of action, which can be desirable when rapid anxiolysis is needed; however, both can produce an unpleasant "drugged" or "high" feeling in some patients. Highly lipophilic benzodiazepines are also more quickly redistributed out of the brain, which decreases their actual duration of action. For example, even though diazepam has a very long half-life, its clinical effects last for a shorter period than lorazepam, which has a relatively short half-life.

Diazepam, lorazepam, chlordiazepoxide, and midazolam also are available for parenteral (intravenous [IV] and intramuscular [IM]) administration.[64] These routes are usually reserved for treatment of severe agitation or seizures or for induction of preoperative sedation and anxiolysis. IM diazepam should be injected into the deltoid muscle, because administration into other sites can result in erratic and unpredictable absorption.[70] IM chlordiazepoxide is absorbed slowly, resulting in lower peak plasma levels compared with oral or IV administration, which limits its usefulness.[70] IM injection of both chlordiazepoxide and diazepam can be very painful. Lorazepam is the preferred agent when parenteral dosing is needed for quick control of anxiety or agitation because it is rapidly and completely absorbed after IM injection and peak levels occur in approximately 1 hour.[70] The absorption of sublingual lorazepam, alprazolam, and triazolam (Halcion) is comparable to or slightly faster than oral absorption. A special formulation of diazepam for rectal administration (Diastat) is indicated for the treatment of acute repetitive seizures, and midazolam has been successfully administered by buccal and intranasal routes to terminate seizures.[64] When benzodiazepines are used in the treatment of GAD and other anxiety disorders, oral administration is the standard route.

Benzodiazepines can also be classified according to potency, and "high potency" anxiolytic benzodiazepines include alprazolam, lorazepam, and clonazepam. These high-potency agents appear to cause less CNS side effects than equivalent doses of low-potency agents and are preferred by many clinicians for this reason. Cost is another important factor in benzodiazepine selection. Brand-name benzodiazepines can be relatively expensive, but all are available in less costly generic versions except the newer XR (alprazolam) and wafer (clonazepam) formulations. Potential drug interactions should also be considered in the selection of an agent, because they can alter pharmacokinetics and clinical effects (see Question 10).

Because N.K. is young and healthy and is not taking any other medications, treatment with a benzodiazepine should not be accompanied by any pharmacokinetic impairments. Nevertheless, most clinicians still prefer to use shorter-acting high-potency agents such as lorazepam or alprazolam for patients such as N.K. Appropriate starting doses would be lorazepam 0.5 to 1 mg three times daily or alprazolam 0.25 to 0.5 mg three times daily. Dosages can be increased every 3 to 4 days, if needed, within the dosage ranges indicated in Table 76-4. N.K. should notice a decrease in her anxiety symptoms within the first few days of treatment. Prescription of a generic formulation is recommended to reduce treatment costs.

Adverse Effects and Patient Counseling

6. Lorazepam 0.5 mg TID is prescribed for N.K in addition to the venlafaxine XR. What side effects may occur with benzodiazepine treatment and how should N.K. be counseled regarding benzodiazepine therapy?

Overall, benzodiazepines are very safe and well-tolerated medications. Unlike most other psychotropic classes, drug discontinuation due to side effects is extremely rare. Sedation and feelings of tiredness are the most common side effects of the benzodiazepines, but sedation also can be beneficial in alleviating the insomnia that often accompanies anxiety. Tolerance usually develops to the sedative effects of benzodiazepines within 1 to 2 weeks of continued treatment, which is a major reason why benzodiazepine sedative-hypnotics are recommended for only short-term use.[34,71] Fortunately, tolerance does not appear to develop to the anxiolytic or muscle relaxant effects of benzodiazepines.[34]

In addition to sedation, patients taking benzodiazepines may report cognitive impairment such as difficulty concentrating or memory problems.[72] Benzodiazepines can cause anterograde amnesia (decreased memory for new information after taking the drug), which is dose related and reversible upon medication discontinuation. Tolerance does often develop to the cognitive adverse effects, but they can also persist throughout therapy in some patients.[73] High-potency benzodiazepines may be more likely to cause memory impairment than low-potency agents.[34] Use of alcohol during benzodiazepine therapy greatly increases the risks for memory problems and sedation, as well as for other more dangerous effects. Elderly individuals are more sensitive to the sedative, cognitive, and psychomotor effects of the benzodiazepines, and tolerance to these effects may occur more slowly than in the nonelderly.[69,74] Long-term use even of low benzodiazepine doses in the elderly has been reported to significantly increase the risk of cognitive decline.[75]

The effects of benzodiazepines on memory and cognition are not always negative. For example, amnesia is considered a beneficial result of presurgical benzodiazepine administration. Severe anxiety itself can interfere with concentration and cognitive functioning, and these may be improved by successful anxiolytic treatment. In addition, low-dose lorazepam has been found to actually facilitate retrieval of previously learned information, suggesting it may improve long-term memory function.[76]

Other psychomotor effects such as problems with balance and coordination and delayed reaction time also can occur during benzodiazepine treatment.[72] These effects are also dose related, but usually subside within a few weeks of continued treatment. Interestingly, initial psychomotor impairment with low doses of shorter-acting agents (lorazepam and alprazolam) has been followed by improvements in psychomotor performance (over baseline) during chronic treatment.[77] However, it is important that patients starting on benzodiazepine therapy be cautioned about possible adverse psychomotor effects. Benzodiazepine use before driving has been associated with a 1.5-to 6.5-fold increased risk of being in a vehicle accident, especially in elderly individuals.[78,79] Residual daytime effects after taking a long-acting benzodiazepine the previous night may even pose a hazard while driving the next day.

The link between benzodiazepine use and falls is well documented and may result from a combination of balance impairment, sedation, and muscle relaxant effects.[69,80] A number of studies have shown that use of benzodiazepines in the elderly is related to falls and hip fractures, especially during the first 2 weeks of their use.[80,81] Rapid dosage escalation and use of doses that are too high (of either long-acting or short-acting agents) have been identified as major risk factors, but even use of low doses of short-acting agents greatly increases the fall risk in the elderly.[80,81] This potential hazard of benzodiazepines is critically significant because hip fractures are a leading cause of loss of functional independence and nursing home placement in older people. Although tolerance can develop to the psychomotor effects of benzodiazepines, elderly or other vulnerable individuals may experience persistent impairment. Benzodiazepines are probably best avoided in the ambulatory older population.

Paradoxical disinhibition, with increased anxiety, irritability, and agitation, can occur infrequently with benzodiazepines.[82,83] Such effects have been mainly observed in elderly or developmentally disabled patients. Other unusual behaviors, such as increased anger, hostility, and violence, have been attributed to benzodiazepine use in a small number of cases.[82] Most of these reports were anecdotal and involved patients with pre-existing psychiatric disorders such as bipolar disorder, schizophrenia, or personality disorders. It is difficult to confirm that benzodiazepines caused these paradoxical reactions because such disorders are commonly associated with behavioral problems, and benzodiazepines are often used in their treatment. Nevertheless, media attention has focused on cases that have reportedly led to aggressive or self-destructive acts, which has resulted in the removal of triazolam from some foreign markets.[82] These effects may reflect an expression of underlying anger or psychopathology, which is facilitated by reduction in anxiety rather than a direct effect of the benzodiazepines. In the case of triazolam, adverse behavioral effects have been linked to excessive doses and inappropriately long durations of use.[82] Overall, there is no convincing evidence that benzodiazepines actually cause violent or suicidal behaviors, but there is some evidence to the contrary.[82–84]

Benzodiazepines also have been associated with clinical depression, although evidence supporting a causal relationship is very limited.[25,34] This belief may result from confusion regarding statements that benzodiazepines are CNS depressants. In fact, some benzodiazepines, most notably alprazolam, have been reported to have antidepressant effects.[34] In addition, use of benzodiazepines during the initial weeks of antidepressant therapy can improve and possibly hasten antidepressant response in depression.[25,85]

Respiratory depression is another potential adverse effect of benzodiazepines, but it is usually clinically relevant only in patients with severe respiratory disease, in overdose situations (see Question 12), or when combined with alcohol or substances that depress breathing. It is recommended that benzodiazepines be avoided in patients with sleep apnea. Respiratory complications are encountered most often with IV administration. IV midazolam has been associated with a number of deaths due to cardiorespiratory arrest during its use for conscious sedation, most often in patients premedicated with narcotics or in those with chronic obstructive airways disease. Severe respiratory depression also has occurred with the concurrent use of benzodiazepines and loxapine (Loxitane) or clozapine (Clozaril).

In summary, N.K. should be told that she may experience sedation and difficulties in thinking, concentration, or memory during the first week or so of therapy, but these side effects should resolve once her body gets used to the drug. She should be extremely careful while driving or performing other tasks that require psychomotor skills, especially during the first week. It also is imperative that N.K. be counseled against the use of alcohol while she is taking benzodiazepines.

Benzodiazepine Abuse and Dependence

7. Two weeks later, N.K. contacts her clinician to discuss a medication concern. She reports that the medication has been extremely effective in relieving her anxiety, and she is currently taking venlafaxine XR, 150 mg Q AM, and lorazepam, 0.5 mg TID, as directed by her physician. However, her mother has told her that she will become addicted to lorazepam, and she wonders if she should stop taking it because of this concern. What potential for abuse and dependence is associated with benzodiazepines? How should N.K. be counseled regarding "becoming addicted" to lorazepam?

Concerns related to abuse and dependence are probably the major drawback to the clinical use of benzodiazepines. These agents are classified as schedule IV controlled substances, reflecting a relatively limited abuse and dependence liability. There may be differences within the class regarding abuse potential. Diazepam, alprazolam, and lorazepam are reported to be more likely to be abused than are oxazepam and chlordiazepoxide.[35] This difference in abuse potential is commonly attributed to the quicker onset of effects for drugs such as diazepam, which may be associated with a subjective euphoric sensation. The XR alprazolam formulation is reported to have a lower abuse potential than immediate-release alprazolam because of its slower onset of effects and lower maximum plasma concentrations.[67]

Abuse is related to drug use outside the therapeutic setting and is characterized by recreational use, continued use despite negative consequences, dose escalation, and loss of control over use. Patients without a history of substance abuse who take benzodiazepines for therapeutic purposes are unlikely to escalate doses or use them in ways characteristic of abuse.[86] Misuse and abuse of benzodiazepines is limited primarily to those with a current or past history of abusing other substances, including alcohol.[86] A consensus among experts is that benzodiazepines are drugs of abuse, but only in drug abusers. Despite this fact, concern over abuse issues has led to negative attitudes and considerable controversy about benzodiazepine use among both health professionals and patients. Clinicians can play an important role in resolving some of the misunderstandings that surround benzodiazepine use and abuse. One important aspect is the differentiation between addiction, physical dependence, and benzodiazepine discontinuation syndromes.

BENZODIAZEPINE WITHDRAWAL SYMPTOMS

Although the term *addiction* historically has been used loosely to describe a variety of drug abuse patterns, a currently accepted definition refers to a behavioral pattern of drug abuse, characterized by overwhelming involvement with the use of a drug, the securing of its supply, and a high tendency to relapse after discontinuation.[35,86] The inclusion of drug abuse in this definition implies drug use outside the therapeutic setting or in an unacceptable or unsafe manner. Physical dependence refers to the need to continue using a drug to relieve or avoid physical withdrawal symptoms and may or may not be associated with abuse.

Three types of benzodiazepine discontinuation syndromes have been described: relapse, rebound, and withdrawal.[86,87] *Relapse* indicates a recurrence of the original anxiety symptoms that follow discontinuation of treatment and may be expected in those with chronic anxiety disorders. The time frame for onset of relapse may vary from weeks to months after drug discontinuation and may be misinterpreted as symptoms of withdrawal. The *rebound* syndrome also is similar to the original anxiety, but symptoms are more intense. It usually occurs within hours to days after the drug is discontinued and lasts for only a few days, after which symptoms may lessen to that of relapse (the original anxiety).

The benzodiazepine *withdrawal* syndrome implies some degree of physical dependence, and its onset, duration, and severity can vary according to dose, duration of treatment, speed of withdrawal, and elimination half-life of the agent used.[86,87] Withdrawal symptoms that follow discontinuation of agents with short half-lives usually appear within 1 to 2 days and may be more short-lived, but more intense, than after discontinuation of long-acting benzodiazepines. Withdrawal symptoms usually appear 4 to 7 days after discontinuation of long-acting agents and may last several weeks. Symptoms of benzodiazepine withdrawal, which are listed in Table 76-7, are generally mild when the drug is tapered gradually during discontinuation.[87]

Increased risk of withdrawal and severity of symptoms is associated with a quicker rate of discontinuation, larger daily doses, long-term (>3 to 4 months) treatment, and high-potency agents (alprazolam, lorazepam, clonazepam).[87] Patient-specific variables that have been linked to increased withdrawal severity include a diagnosis of GAD or panic disorder (these patients seem to be more sensitive to the somatic symptoms of withdrawal), higher levels of anxiety before drug discontinuation, a history of alcohol or other substance abuse, and presence of a personality disorder.[35,86] Rarely, serious symptoms such as seizures or psychosis may occur during benzodiazepine withdrawal. Risk factors for seizures include head injury, alcohol dependence, electroencephalogram abnormalities, and use of other drugs that lower the seizure threshold.

MINIMIZATION OF ABUSE AND DEPENDENCE AND PATIENT COUNSELING

Clinically, the potential problems with benzodiazepine abuse and dependence can be avoided or minimized in several ways. First is the identification of patients who are susceptible to abuse and are using nonbenzodiazepine treatments in such cases. Patients with past or present alcoholism or other substance abuse are considered at highest risk for benzodiazepine abuse.[86] Second, patients should be counseled about the likely duration of benzodiazepine use, the possibility of withdrawal symptoms, and the importance of gradual drug tapering when therapy is to be discontinued. The distinction between "addiction" and appropriate therapeutic use, which may be accompanied by some degree of physical dependence, also should be explained. Discussion about these issues should occur at the onset of therapy, so that patients understand the importance of not abruptly discontinuing benzodiazepine therapy on their own.

Table 76-7 Symptoms of Benzodiazepine Withdrawal

Common	Less Common	Rare
Anxiety	Nausea	Confusion
Insomnia	Depression	Delirium
Irritability	Ataxia	Psychosis
Muscle aches/weakness	Hyperreflexia	Seizures
Tremor	Blurred vision	Catatonia
Loss of appetite	Fatigue	

N.K. should be advised that as long as the medication is helping her anxiety and she is taking it according to her physician's instructions, her use of lorazepam does not constitute addiction. However, her body may become accustomed to the drug, so if she stops taking it abruptly, she could experience increased anxiety and other withdrawal symptoms. When lorazepam is to be discontinued, the dose will be decreased gradually over a sufficient period to minimize withdrawal symptoms.

Duration of Treatment

8. **Two weeks later at her clinic appointment, N.K. is still doing well and has shown further improvements in her GAD symptoms. She has been taking the prescribed lorazepam and venlafaxine doses for 1 month, and her venlafaxine has been increased to the current dose of 150 mg/day during this time. How long should medication therapy continue?**

GAD is a chronic disorder that can fluctuate in severity and often requires long-term treatment. Relapse after discontinuation of benzodiazepine monotherapy is reported to occur in 50% to 80% of GAD patients; however, some of these cases may actually involve benzodiazepine withdrawal.[87] These relapse rates also do not take into account the concurrent use of other medications which may prevent relapse, such as venlafaxine. Although long-term use of benzodiazepines is generally safe and effective, it is desirable to limit treatment to the shortest duration necessary because of the physical dependence potential.[29,35] When benzodiazepines are used for acute anxiolytic effects during initiation of antidepressant treatment for GAD, they are commonly limited to short-term (2 to 6 weeks) therapy. N.K. has shown good response after 1 month of combined lorazepam and venlafaxine XR therapy. Since the anxiolytic effects of venlafaxine usually occur between 2 and 4 weeks of therapy and she is taking a therapeutic venlafaxine dose, it is appropriate to start discontinuing lorazepam at this time. N.K. is unlikely to experience significant withdrawal symptoms after only 1 month of treatment, but the dose should still be gradually decreased over several weeks, according to tolerability of the taper.[87]

There is no consensus about the optimal duration of drug therapy for GAD. However, recent recommendations suggest that effective medication treatment be continued for at least 6 to 12 months after response.[29] Continuation treatment with antidepressants such as venlafaxine and paroxetine significantly reduces the risk of GAD relapse over 6 months.[48,50] Therefore, venlafaxine XR therapy should be continued for another 5 to 11 months in N.K.'s case. After that time period, gradual venlafaxine discontinuation may be considered. Chronic GAD can be accompanied by substantial distress and disability, and reinstitution of treatment is warranted if relapse occurs. The need for continued treatment should be reassessed regularly during long-term GAD therapy.

Management of Benzodiazepine Withdrawal

9. **G.S., a 43-year-old man, has been taking diazepam 40 mg/day for 6 months for its muscle relaxant effects after sustaining a dislocated shoulder and other injuries in a car accident. Four days ago, G.S. was unable to refill his prescription for financial reasons. A brief mental status examination reveals mild confusion and irritability. Physically, G.S. is trembling and complains of overall body aching and an upset stomach. His medical history indicates no current medical problems or psychiatric illnesses, and G.S. denies the use of tobacco, alcohol, or other drugs of abuse. How should G.S. be treated?**

Because G.S. has not taken his prescribed diazepam for 4 days, it is likely that he is experiencing a withdrawal syndrome from long-term benzodiazepine use. His mental and physical symptoms are consistent with benzodiazepine withdrawal. Diazepam 10 to 20 mg orally should be administered and repeated within 1 to 2 hours if needed. Resumption of his previous diazepam dosage of 40 mg/day should effectively treat his withdrawal symptoms. Because his acute injury occurred 6 months ago, it may be desirable to begin discontinuation of the benzodiazepine.

Various time periods and dosage-reduction schedules for benzodiazepine discontinuation have been proposed. Even when managing withdrawal from low-dose benzodiazepine use, doses should be reduced slowly over 4 to 16 weeks.[87] The rate of the drug taper should always be monitored closely and individualized to the patient, but a general recommendation is a 10% to 25% decrease in the dosage every 1 to 2 weeks. The first half of the benzodiazepine taper (down to 50% of the original dose) is generally easier and can proceed more quickly than the last half of the taper, which usually requires a much longer time period.[87] In G.S.'s case, the discontinuation period may take several months.

In general, the same benzodiazepine the patient has been taking should be used to manage withdrawal. However, because withdrawal symptoms are more severe during discontinuation of short-acting compared with long-acting benzodiazepines, substitution of a long-acting agent at an equivalent dosage, which is then tapered, can decrease the severity of withdrawal symptoms from short-acting agents.[87] In difficult cases, adjunctive medications have been used to ease tolerability of the gradual withdrawal. Carbamazepine (Tegretol) has been effective in attenuating the symptoms of withdrawal from benzodiazepines as well as alcohol. Propranolol decreases some physical withdrawal symptoms (tremor, tachycardia), but does not affect the associated anxiety or decrease the seizure risk. There are conflicting, but mostly negative, reports about the usefulness of trazodone and valproate (Depakene, Depakote) in treating benzodiazepine withdrawal symptoms. Other drugs that have been studied, but found not to be beneficial, include clonidine, buspirone, and ondansetron.[87,88] CBTs, combined with gradual drug taper, also have been effective in facilitating successful benzodiazepine discontinuation.

Benzodiazepine Drug Interactions

10. **R.G., a 24-year-old female college student, has been taking alprazolam 1 mg TID for treatment of GAD for almost a year. She states that alprazolam has been very helpful for her GAD but complains to her physician that she is feeling especially stressed lately because she is trying to keep up with extremely difficult schoolwork while making arrangements for her upcoming wedding. She has no medical illnesses but states that she also feels depressed. R.G. recently started taking an oral contraceptive (Ortho-Novum 1/35), smokes two packs of cigarettes per day, and drinks up to six cups of coffee per day. Nefazodone**

(Serzone), 100 mg BID, is prescribed for treatment of her depression. **What potential drug interactions with alprazolam are present in this case?**

Reported drug interactions with benzodiazepines are summarized in Table 76-8 and can be divided into two primary types: pharmacodynamic and pharmacokinetic. The most significant pharmacodynamic drug interactions involve other CNS depressants such as alcohol or barbiturates. These combinations can lead to additive CNS and respiratory depressant effects that can be deadly. Important pharmacokinetic drug interactions mainly involve agents that either inhibit or induce benzodiazepine metabolism.[89] Because the benzodiazepines have a relatively wide margin of safety, elevated plasma levels and/or prolonged elimination half-lives are unlikely to cause any serious toxicity. However, they can lead to increased sedative and psychomotor effects, which may be clinically significant in certain cases. Conversely, increased benzodiazepine metabolism by hepatic enzyme inducers may result in medication ineffectiveness. As indicated in Table 76-8, most pharmacokinetic drug interactions with benzodiazepines involve CYP 3A4–or CYP 2C19–mediated mechanisms.

In R.G.'s case, the most important drug interaction is between alprazolam and the newly prescribed antidepressant nefazodone. Nefazodone, a potent CYP 3A4 inhibitor, can cause a twofold increase in plasma alprazolam levels.[90] Therefore, the dosage of alprazolam should be reduced by half, over

Table 76-8   Drug Interactions With Benzodiazepines

Interacting Drug(s)	Effect on Object Drug	Clinical Significance/Comments
Hepatic enzyme inducers: carbamazepine, phenobarbital, phenytoin, and rifampin	Decreased Cps and clinical effects of benzodiazepines	Triazolam and midazolam may be ineffective in patients taking rifampin.[226] Carbamazepine greatly decreases the Cps and clinical effects of midazolam, alprazolam, and clonazepam, possibly rendering them ineffective.[227,228]
Hepatic CYP 3A4 inhibitors: ketoconazole, itraconazole, nefazodone, fluvoxamine, fluoxetine, erythromycin, clarithromycin, cimetidine, oral contraceptives, diltiazem, nelfinavir, indinivir, ritonavir, saquinavir, verapamil	Significantly increased Cps of benzodiazepines that undergo oxidative metabolism (alprazolam, triazolam, diazepam, chlordiazepoxide, clonazepam)	Benzodiazepine dosage reductions may be required because of increased clinical effects such as sedation and psychomotor impairment; effects are greatest on alprazolam, triazolam, and midazolam.[229] Ketoconazole and itraconazole should be avoided in patients taking alprazolam or triazolam.[231] Benzodiazepine dosage reductions are recommended when nefazodone, fluoxetine, or fluvoxamine are added to alprazolam, diazepam, or triazolam.[90, 229]
Ritonavir	Initial inhibition of alprazolam and triazolam metabolism, followed by later induction of metabolism	Reduced benzodiazepine dosage is needed initially if ritonavir is added to therapy; a dosage increase may be required later.[232]
Grapefruit juice	Increased Cps of diazepam, alprazolam, and triazolam	Increased benzodiazepine clinical effects (sedation, psychomotor impairment) are possible.[229,233]
Omeprazole	Increased diazepam Cp and prolonged half-life	Increased benzodiazepine clinical effects (sedation, psychomotor impairment) are possible.[89]
Antacids, ranitidine	Decreased rate of benzodiazepine absorption	Possible delayed onset of benzodiazepine clinical effects; separation of administration times is recommended.
Valproic acid, probenecid	Significantly decreased clearance of lorazepam	Lorazepam dosage reductions may be required.[235]
Estrogen-containing oral contraceptives	Decreased Cps of benzodiazepines that undergo glucuronidation (lorazepam, oxazepam, temazepam) and increased Cps of benzodiazepines that undergo oxidative CYP 3A4 metabolism (alprazolam)	Decreased or increased clinical effects of benzodiazepines are possible.[68,89,27]
Central nervous system depressants (alcohol, barbiturates, and opioids)	Increased central nervous system depressant effects of benzodiazepines (sedation, psychomotor impairment)	Avoid use of alcohol with benzodiazepines; exercise caution with use of other depressants.
Alprazolam	Increased digoxin Cp	Digoxin toxicity is possible; monitoring of digoxin level and possible digoxin dosage reduction are recommended.[236]
Benzodiazepines	Respiratory depression and adverse cardiovascular effects reported on addition of benzodiazepines in several patients taking clozapine	Caution with benzodiazepine use in patients taking clozapine.
Benzodiazepines	Possible decreased efficacy of levodopa in Parkinson's disease	Drug interaction is not well established; monitor for possible effect.
Benzodiazepines	Increased or decreased efficacy of neuromuscular blocking agents	Drug interaction is not well established; monitor for possible effect.

Cps, plasma concentration; CYP, cytochrome P450.

several days according to tolerability, when nefazodone is started. Several other antidepressants also can interfere with the metabolism of various benzodiazepines, which is an important issue because these drug combinations are very frequently prescribed.[89]

Estrogen-containing oral contraceptives also can inhibit the CYP 3A4 metabolism of benzodiazepines such as alprazolam, potentially resulting in increased side effects.[27] Thus, a reduction in the benzodiazepine dosage may be needed when oral contraceptives are added to benzodiazepine therapy. In R.G.'s case, her alprazolam dosage is already being decreased because of the nefazodone. The clearance of benzodiazepines that undergo glucuronidation (lorazepam, oxazepam, and temazepam) can be accelerated by oral contraceptives, but this interaction is thought to be clinically insignificant.[27,68]

Cigarette smoking increases the clearance of some benzodiazepines (clorazepate, lorazepam, oxazepam), but has no effect on others (diazepam, midazolam, chlordiazepoxide).[91] Overall, the effect of smoking is unpredictable and is most likely to be important in patients who either stop or start smoking while taking a benzodiazepine. These patients may experience increased or decreased clinical effects, respectively. R.G. should be urged to quit smoking for the sake of her general health as well as to prevent substantial risks for serious cardiovascular events that occurs in smokers taking oral contraceptives. If R.G. does quit, careful monitoring will be needed to determine whether any alprazolam dosage reduction is necessary.

R.G. also should be encouraged to decrease her coffee consumption because caffeine can increase anxiety and possibly decrease the effectiveness of alprazolam. Caffeine has been found to decrease diazepam concentrations by approximately 22%, but studies with other benzodiazepines are lacking.[89] Caffeine has been successfully used to counteract benzodiazepine-related sedation and cognitive impairment.

Benzodiazepine Use in Pregnancy and Lactation

11. At her clinic visit 8 months later, R.G is doing very well. She has graduated from college, is happily married, and states that she and her husband have decided to start a family. R.G. stopped taking the nefazodone shortly after it was started because of the side effects and has successfully quit smoking. She also has discontinued her oral contraceptive and plans to become pregnant soon. R.G. continues to take alprazolam 0.5 mg BID to TID, and wonders whether she should also stop taking this drug before she becomes pregnant. What is the teratogenic potential of alprazolam? What alternative treatments are available for the management of R.G.'s anxiety?

Early reports implicated diazepam in causing several birth deformities, including cleft lip and/or cleft palate and limb and digit malformations, but later studies failed to support this association.[92] The most recent evidence suggests that benzodiazepine use during the first trimester increases the risk for oral clefts by approximately 2.4-fold, but the absolute risk is <1%. Alprazolam and lorazepam have not been found to have teratogenic effects, but it is always advisable to avoid drug use during pregnancy when possible, especially in the first trimester.[92] In patients such as R.G., the benzodiazepine should be tapered and discontinued before she becomes pregnant. Nondrug treatments for her GAD such as relaxation

therapy, meditation, and biofeedback or cognitive therapy may be helpful. It also appears that many of the stressors in her life have resolved. If necessary, single or repeated small doses of benzodiazepines during the second and third trimesters are unlikely to have important adverse effects on the baby. Alprazolam and lorazepam are the preferred agents to use.[92] Chronic or large doses, especially of long-acting agents, should be avoided because they may accumulate in the fetus because of its limited metabolic capacity. Perinatal sequelae reported in newborns whose mothers took benzodiazepines during pregnancy include withdrawal symptoms, sedation, muscle weakness, hypotonia, apnea, poor feeding, and impaired temperature regulation.[92] There is also some concern about possible long-term neurobehavioral effects from prenatal benzodiazepine exposure, but the evidence to support this is questionable.[92]

Pregnancies sometimes are unplanned, and the clinical situation of unexpected pregnancy in a woman maintained on benzodiazepines also can arise. The general course of action in such cases is often to discontinue all medications immediately. However, it is unwise to abruptly stop benzodiazepine treatment in someone who has been receiving chronic therapy because the resultant withdrawal syndromes can be detrimental to both mother and child. Benzodiazepine dosages should be tapered as quickly as possible to the lowest dosage necessary and discontinued if possible. Most benzodiazepine anxiolytics are classified as pregnancy category D, indicating that there is some evidence of fetal risk but that the benefits of the medication may outweigh these risks in certain patients.[92] The postpartum period is a time of heightened risk for recurrence of anxiety disorders, and new mothers should be monitored carefully for signs of relapse.[94] Untreated maternal anxiety can adversely affect development of the infant by leading to behavioral inhibition, which is a risk factor for development of psychiatric illness later in life.[93] Benzodiazepines are excreted readily in breast milk, and it is generally recommended that they be avoided by nursing mothers.[95] (Also see Chapter 47, Teratogenicity and Drugs in Breast Milk.)

Benzodiazepine Overdose and Use of Flumazenil

12. S.P. is a 17-year-old young man who is brought to the hospital by his mother. S.P. is almost unconscious, and his breathing is slow and shallow. His mother states that he took a whole bottle of diazepam (5 mg, #30) sometime during the previous night. S.P.'s medical history is significant for a severe head injury sustained from a car accident 8 months ago. He currently takes carbamazepine (Tegretol) 200 mg TID for seizure prophylaxis. S.P.'s mother believes that diazepam is the only drug that he ingested because no other medications are missing. What signs and symptoms are consistent with benzodiazepine overdose? Why is it inappropriate to administer the benzodiazepine antagonist flumazenil in this case?

Benzodiazepine overdose is characterized by respiratory and CNS depression, both of which are evident in this case (S.P. is almost unconscious, with slow and shallow breathing). Overdose with benzodiazepines (as the sole ingested agent) is rarely life-threatening, and full recovery is the usual outcome.[96] Flumazenil is a benzodiazepine receptor antagonist that is effective in reversing the sedation associated with benzodiazepine intoxication. Its effects on respiratory depression are inconsistent, but improved breathing may occur secondarily to increased consciousness.[96]

The primary clinical use of flumazenil is in reversing benzodiazepine-induced conscious sedation (primarily midazolam) in patients who have been sedated for minor surgical or diagnostic procedures. Its use for this purpose is generally safe and effective and facilitates patient recovery and discharge by decreasing the postprocedural monitoring period.[97] Flumazenil also is approved for treating benzodiazepine overdose, but this use is controversial because of potentially serious complications and questions about its cost-effectiveness.[97] Flumazenil administration does not appear to decrease mortality or length of hospital stay in cases of benzodiazepine overdose; therefore, its use for this purpose has become limited.[97]

There are several reports of flumazenil-induced seizures or cardiac arrhythmias, including a few fatal cases, with its use in comatose patients who had ingested multiple drugs.[96] These overdoses often included TCAs and carbamazepine, which are quite dangerous. The anticonvulsant effects of benzodiazepines apparently protect against TCA-induced seizures, and the rapid reversal of their effects with flumazenil removes this protection. Flumazenil is contraindicated in cases of overdose involving TCAs or carbamazepine or overdoses of other agents that decrease the seizure threshold. Toxicology screening and an electrocardiogram (ECG) should be performed in uncertain cases before flumazenil is administered. Physical symptoms suggestive of TCA overdose include dry mucous membranes, mydriasis, and motor twitching or rigidity. Flumazenil should also be avoided in patients with increased intracranial pressure or a known history of seizures or head injury, in those who have been receiving chronic benzodiazepine therapy, and in patients with a history of recent illicit drug abuse (cocaine, heroin) because it can precipitate seizures in these situations. Administration of flumazenil should occur only in settings prepared for seizure management.

Flumazenil reverses benzodiazepine-induced sedation or coma within 1 to 2 minutes after IV administration. The most common side effects include agitation, dizziness, nausea, general discomfort, tearfulness, anxiety, and a sensation of coldness.[96] Its use in patients with panic disorder can induce panic attacks. Rapid or excessive infusion has been associated with tachycardia and hypertension. The elimination half-life of flumazenil is 41 to 79 minutes, and resedation may occur after 1 to 2 hours when its effects wear off, especially when large doses of long-acting benzodiazepines are involved. Repeated flumazenil doses or an IV infusion may be indicated in these cases. Full recovery should be verified (3 to 4 hours of stable alertness) before patients are discharged after flumazenil administration, and they should be advised to avoid driving or performing other potentially hazardous activities for 24 hours. Flumazenil undergoes extensive hepatic metabolism to inactive metabolites.[96] Dosage reductions are recommended in patients with liver dysfunction, but flumazenil pharmacokinetics are not altered significantly by gender, age, or renal impairment.

Flumazenil administration is not appropriate in S.P.'s case because of his history of head injury and seizures. Instead, management should involve general supportive measures and mechanical ventilation, if indicated. It is probably too late for use of activated charcoal or gastric lavage in this case because the ingestion occurred the previous night. These interventions often can be beneficial in managing benzodiazepine overdose, although gastric lavage may provide no extra benefit over administration of activated charcoal alone. A psychiatric evaluation also is indicated in this case to identify and address the reasons for S.P.'s overdose.

Physiologic Variables Influencing Benzodiazepines

13. B.G., a 68-year-old man, is brought to the emergency department (ED) by his wife after being involved as the driver in a minor car accident. He has no physical injuries except for several small abrasions caused by the car airbag deployment. However, B.G. appears drowsy, is mildly confused, and has an unsteady gait. A toxicology screen reveals no alcohol or other substances, except for the diazepam that his doctor prescribed several months ago. B.G.'s wife states that he has been taking 1 tablet (5 mg) two or three times daily and that it has been remarkably effective in improving his mood and anxiety. B.G., who is 5'8" tall and weighs 250 lb, is a recovering alcoholic with moderate liver disease caused by years of heavy drinking. He has been successful in maintaining his sobriety for almost 2 years now. Besides the diazepam, the only other medications that B.G. takes are occasional OTC omeprazole (Prilosec) and cimetidine (Tagamet) for heartburn. It is determined that B.G. is suffering from adverse effects of diazepam, probably caused by drug accumulation. What factors could be influencing diazepam's disposition in this patient?

Benzodiazepine pharmacokinetics can be affected by various physiologic factors, including age, gender, obesity, hepatic and renal disease, and ethnicity (Table 76-9). Several of these factors are present in this case and may have contributed to the accumulation of diazepam with resulting adverse consequences. This case also illustrates the potential dangers of psychomotor impairment due to benzodiazepines.

The first factor is B.G.'s age. It is well known that older people have longer half-lives of most benzodiazepines, sometimes two to three times longer than nonelderly individuals. This effect is most often attributed to an age-related decrease in the ability to metabolize drugs by oxidative hepatic pathways.[69] Reductions in both CYP 3A4 and CYP 2C19 activity have been reported to occur with aging. The glucuronidation metabolic pathways are minimally affected with age so no such effect is seen with lorazepam or oxazepam.[68,69] Although some studies indicate reduced clearance of various benzodiazepines in the elderly (especially males), others have found comparable rates of benzodiazepine clearance between young and elderly groups. Other factors that may contribute to the longer benzodiazepine half-lives in the elderly include decreased hepatic blood flow and increased volumes of distribution of lipid-soluble compounds (due to decreased muscle mass and increased fat), the latter of which can increase a drug's half-life in the absence of any clearance changes.[69] As described in Question 6, a prolonged elimination half-life may lead to drug accumulation, and older patients are already more sensitive to the sedative and psychomotor effects of benzodiazepines.[69] For these reasons, the recommended benzodiazepine dosages for patients older than 65 are generally one-third to one-half of those used in healthy adults (see Table 76-4). In addition, long-acting benzodiazepines (flurazepam,

Table 76-9   Physiologic Factors Influencing Benzodiazepine Pharmacokinetics

Factor	Physiologic and Pharmacokinetic Effects	Clinical Significance/Comments
Aging	Increased elimination half-life due to increased Vd of all benzodiazepines[69,237]	Lower benzodiazepine dosages, and possibly less frequent dosing intervals, recommended in the elderly
	Decreased clearance of benzodiazepines that undergo oxidative hepatic metabolism (see Table 76-6)[69,238]	Benzodiazepines that undergo glucuronidation (lorazepam, oxazepam) preferred in the elderly
	Decreased plasma proteins may lead to increased free fraction of highly protein bound benzodiazepines (see Table 76-6)[69]	Possible increased clinical effects
	Decreased gastric acidity may lead to increased rate of benzodiazepine absorption[69]	Possible faster onset of clinical effects
Gender	Age-related decrease in hepatic oxidative metabolism of benzodiazepines more pronounced in males	Elderly males may require especially low benzodiazepine dosages
	Increased CYP 3A4 and CYP 2C19 activity in premenopausal women may result in higher clearance of drugs that undergo oxidative metabolism[27]	Possible decreased plasma benzodiazepine concentrations and shorter duration of clinical effects of oxidatively metabolized agents in premenopausal women
	Decreased glucuronidation in women may result in slower clearance of benzodiazepines metabolized by conjugation[27]	Women may have longer elimination half-lives of lorazepam and temazepam and may require less frequent dosing
	Increased Vd in women due to lower lean body mass and higher adipose tissue[27]	Possible longer elimination half-lives in women, especially the elderly, and greater drug accumulation
	Lower plasma protein binding in women[27]	Clinical significance unknown
Obesity	Increased benzodiazepine elimination half-lives due to increased Vd[69]	Increased chance of drug accumulation in obese patients; dosage reductions may be indicated
Liver disease	Decreased clearance and increased elimination half-lives of long-acting benzodiazepines and alprazolam in cirrhosis and hepatitis; no changes with oxazepam or triazolam[68]	Avoid long-acting benzodiazepines, or use significantly lower doses to avoid drug accumulation
	Increased elimination half-life of lorazepam in cirrhosis but not acute hepatitis	Decreased lorazepam dose or increased dosing interval recommended in cirrhosis
Kidney disease	Decreased plasma protein binding may lead to increased free fraction of highly protein bound benzodiazepines (see Table 76-6)[99]	Dosage reductions may be necessary
Ethnicity	Decreased oxidative metabolism (via CYP 2C19) of diazepam and alprazolam in Asians[100]	Asians may require lower doses of diazepam, alprazolam, and possibly other benzodiazepines

CYP, cytochrome P450; Vd, volume of distribution.

chlordiazepoxide, and diazepam) meet the Beers' criteria for medications that are considered inappropriate to use in community-dwelling elderly patients.[59] These include agents that have unnecessarily poor safety risks and/or poor efficacy. Because of increasing recognition that short-acting benzodiazepines pose risks similar to those of the long-acting agents, it is advisable to limit use of any benzodiazepines in ambulatory elderly patients.

Gender also may influence benzodiazepine clearance.[27,98] Studies examining gender effects have yielded mixed results, probably because of wide interindividual differences. In elderly patients, some investigators have found lower clearances of clorazepate, diazepam, and alprazolam in men compared with those in women.[98] Women have been reported to have higher CYP 3A4 and CYP 2C19 activities, which may partially explain these findings. The increased CYP 3A4 activity in women disappears after menopause, which may lead to a need for lower benzodiazepine dosages during the postmenopausal period. In contrast to oxidation, women have slower glucuronidation metabolic processes than men, resulting in lower clearance of agents such as temazepam and oxazepam.[27,68]

Obesity and liver impairment are other physiologic factors that apply to B.G.'s case. Obesity increases the volume of distribution of benzodiazepines and increases the extent of accumulation of long-acting agents, which may necessitate dosage reductions.[69] Significant changes in the elimination half-lives

of lorazepam and oxazepam are not observed in obese patients. As expected, liver dysfunction can reduce the benzodiazepine elimination rates and prolong their half-lives, resulting in recommendations for decreased dosage requirements. The elimination half-lives of diazepam and lorazepam usually return to normal on recovery from acute viral hepatitis. The pharmacokinetics of oxazepam or triazolam are unaffected by liver disease.

Decreased protein binding is the most prominent change in benzodiazepine pharmacokinetics observed in patients with renal insufficiency, and increased free fractions of highly protein-bound benzodiazepines may lead to increased clinical effects.[105] However, no significant changes in clearance or volume of distribution have been noted. Impairment of lorazepam elimination was reported in two patients with renal dysfunction, but the elimination half-life of benzodiazepines undergoing glucuronidation is generally not significantly altered in renal disease.[99] Regarding ethnicity, up to 20% of Asians are CYP 2C19 poor metabolizers, and slower metabolism with decreased clearance of a variety of CYP 2C19 substrates, including diazepam, have been reported in Asian subjects.[100] In CYP 2C19 poor metabolizers, diazepam metabolism depends mainly on CYP 3A4.

In summary, the physiologic factors that can alter benzodiazepine disposition in B.G. are his age, obesity, male gender, and liver disease. Accumulation of diazepam due to these combined effects probably led to his mental status changes. In addition to these factors, cimetidine and omeprazole can both significantly impair the metabolism of diazepam, resulting in decreased clearance and increased side effects (see Table 76-8).[89]

If continued benzodiazepine therapy is deemed necessary for B.G., lorazepam or oxazepam would be the best agents to use because they would be least affected by aging, obesity, liver disease, or drug interactions. Benzodiazepine dosage equivalencies, which are based on relative potencies, can be used to determine an equivalent dose for the selected agent (see Table 76-4). However, these equivalencies are only general guidelines and dosing conversions should take patient variables and usual dosage ranges into consideration. For example, B.G. had been taking 10 to 15 mg/day of diazepam, so the calculated equivalent lorazepam dosage is 2 to 3 mg/day. Because of his age, a somewhat lower initial dose of 0.5 to 1.0 mg twice a day would be indicated, accompanied by careful monitoring for adverse effects or withdrawal symptoms. However, switching to a nonbenzodiazepine agent would probably be a better treatment option for B.G.

Buspirone Therapy

14. Several days after recovery from his diazepam intoxication, B.G. expresses a desire to discontinue benzodiazepine use. He is being criticized by his fellow Alcoholics Anonymous program members for taking a drug associated with dependency. The decision is made to switch B.G. from diazepam to buspirone. How does the clinical profile of buspirone compare with that of the benzodiazepines? What factors in B.G.'s case make buspirone a good choice?

Clinical Comparison With Benzodiazepines

Buspirone was the first agent marketed as an anxiolytic that lacks CNS depressant effects. In contrast to the benzodiazepines, it produces no significant sedation, cognitive or psychomotor impairment, or respiratory depression, and it lacks muscle relaxant and anticonvulsant effects.[37] Buspirone has minimal reinforcing properties or potential for abuse, and it is not classified as a controlled substance. It does not produce physical dependence or withdrawal syndromes on discontinuation, even after long-term therapy.[37,39] It also does not interact with alcohol or other CNS depressants and is relatively safe in overdose situations.[37] Buspirone would appear to be an ideal anxiolytic drug. However, there are mixed findings regarding its overall efficacy in GAD, which limits its clinical usefulness.

Buspirone is as effective as benzodiazepines such as alprazolam, oxazepam, lorazepam, diazepam, and clorazepate in the treatment of GAD.[39,40] Its superiority over placebo has been reported in many, but not all, trials. In a controlled comparison with venlafaxine XR, buspirone was no more effective than placebo in treating GAD.[38] Like antidepressants, buspirone is more effective than benzodiazepines in treating the cognitive symptoms of anxiety. However, its anxiolytic effects have a more gradual onset than the benzodiazepines, which have a rapid onset. Initial effects are observed within the first 7 to 10 days, but 3 to 4 weeks may be needed for optimal results. Buspirone must be taken on an ongoing basis if it is to be effective and should not be taken intermittently or "as needed."

Buspirone Adverse Effects

Buspirone's most common side effects include nausea, dizziness, headache, and initial nervousness.[40] Some patients may experience mild drowsiness or fatigue on initiation of therapy. There have been isolated cases of hypomania, mania, abnormal movements, oral dyskinesias, extrapyramidal symptoms, generalized myoclonus, and psychosis. Overall, the adverse effect profile is very favorable, making buspirone a better-tolerated drug than benzodiazepines in some patients. Buspirone's low sedation potential and lack of cognitive and respiratory depressant effects make it useful in older patients. It also is safe, effective, and well tolerated in elderly anxious patients who have a variety of chronic medical conditions. Buspirone does not adversely affect sexual functioning and has improved sexual functioning in some GAD patients.[36]

Antidepressant Effects and Other Potential Uses for Buspirone

In addition to its anxiolytic efficacy, a plethora of other uses for buspirone have been described. Numerous studies report its antidepressant efficacy, both in depression associated with GAD and in primary major depression.[36] It has been successfully used to augment response to standard antidepressants in treatment-resistant depression, although not all reports are positive.[36] Effective antidepressant dosages of buspirone generally are higher (40 to 60 mg/day) than those required for anxiolytic effects alone (15 to 30 mg/day). Buspirone also controls agitation and aggression in patients with a variety of disorders, including dementia, mental retardation, traumatic brain injury, attention deficit hyperactivity disorder, and autism.[36] It may be effective in the treatment of premenstrual dysphoric disorder, social anxiety disorder, PTSD, schizophrenia, nicotine dependence, sleep apnea, migraine and chronic tension headaches, tardive dyskinesia, cerebellar ataxia, and Huntington's disease.[36] It also is useful for certain SSRI-associated side effects such as bruxism and sexual dysfunction.[36] Interestingly, buspirone has been associated with increases in T-cell counts in patients with HIV infection.[101]

In summary, the factors that make buspirone a good choice of anxiolytic therapy in B.G. include its lack of potential for abuse, dependence, or interaction with alcohol; its lack of cognitive, psychomotor, or sedative effects; and its overall good safety profile in elderly individuals. Buspirone also has been reported to reduce alcohol consumption and craving, so this may provide additional benefit because B.G. is a recovering alcoholic.[36]

Switching From Benzodiazepine to Buspirone Therapy

15. How should patients be switched from benzodiazepine to buspirone therapy?

Because buspirone has no CNS depressant effects and is not cross-tolerant with the benzodiazepines, it is not effective in preventing or treating benzodiazepine withdrawal. Thus, when patients are being converted from benzodiazepine to buspirone therapy, the benzodiazepine must still be discontinued gradually. Because it takes several weeks for full therapeutic effects of buspirone to occur, it can be initiated before the benzodiazepine taper begins. This may indirectly ease benzodiazepine withdrawal by providing extra anxiolytic coverage during the benzodiazepine taper period.[102]

It was previously believed that patients who had been treated with benzodiazepines in the past did not respond as well to buspirone as benzodiazepine-naive patients. It is now evident that buspirone can work well in this population as long as the benzodiazepine is tapered slowly enough to prevent withdrawal.[29,102] B.G. has been taking diazepam for several months and needs to be withdrawn gradually over a period of at least several weeks, based on how he tolerates the taper. B.G. can be started on buspirone at this time. The usual recommended starting dosage of buspirone is 15 mg/day given in two to three divided doses, but a lower dosage (10 mg/day) is indicated in B.G. because of his liver disease (see Buspirone Pharmacokinetics). Twice-daily dosing is preferred to facilitate compliance and is comparable in efficacy and tolerability to three-times-daily dosing.[103] The daily dosage is usually increased in 5-mg/day increments every 3 to 4 days. Optimal anxiolytic doses generally range from 20 to 30 mg/day, with 60 mg/day being the manufacturer's recommended maximum. There are no specific guidelines for adjusting dosages in patients with liver impairment; therefore, dosage titrations in B.G. should be made slowly, according to his response and side effects. "Dividose" 15-mg tablets are available; these tablets are scored and notched, so they may be broken into 5-, 7.5-, or 10-mg pieces. A 30-mg "Dividose" tablet is also available, as well as generic buspirone products.

Buspirone Patient Counseling

16. **What patient counseling information should be provided to B.G. regarding buspirone therapy?**

Patients starting buspirone therapy should be advised that it is important to take the drug regularly and that it may take 1 to 2 weeks before they notice beneficial results. Otherwise, they may believe that the medication is ineffective. This is particularly pertinent in patients who have previously taken benzodiazepines and are accustomed to their rapid anxiolytic effects. B.G. should also be counseled on the most common side effects of buspirone, such as nausea, dizziness, headache, and nervousness. Education about how buspirone's profile differs from that of the benzodiazepines in terms of potential for physical dependence also is beneficial for patients who have taken benzodiazepines in the past.

Buspirone Pharmacokinetics and Drug Interactions

Buspirone is completely absorbed, but it undergoes extensive first-pass metabolism, which reduces its absolute bioavailability to approximately 5%.[37] Administration with food may significantly increase bioavailability by decreasing the first-pass effect. Buspirone has an active metabolite, 1-pyrimidinylpiperazine (1-PP), which is present in much higher concentrations than buspirone at therapeutic doses. 1-PP acts on the noradrenergic system rather than serotonin and functions as an α_2-adrenergic antagonist. Some of the side effects of buspirone, such as nervousness, are attributed to this active metabolite.[35,37] The contribution of 1-PP to buspirone's anxiolytic effects is uncertain. The mean elimination half-life of buspirone is short, approximately 2 to 3 hours, but 1-PP is longer acting. An extended-release buspirone formulation with once-daily dosing is under investigation.[104] This product has threefold greater bioavailability than regular buspirone and is associated with much lower levels of the undesirable 1-PP metabolite.

The clearance of buspirone is significantly reduced in patients with kidney or liver disease, but there is little change in side effects or tolerability.[37] Nevertheless, it is recommended that lower buspirone dosages be used in patients with compromised renal or hepatic function and that it be avoided in cases of severe impairment. Buspirone pharmacokinetics are not significantly affected by age or gender, so no dosage adjustments are needed in the elderly.[37]

Important drug interactions with buspirone are summarized in Table 76-10.[37] Buspirone is metabolized by CYP 3A4 and coadministration of CYP 3A4 inhibitors, including grapefruit juice, can result in enormous increases in buspirone levels. In many cases, the half-life of buspirone remained unchanged, suggesting that these interactions are mainly due to inhibition of CYP 3A4–mediated first-pass metabolism in the gut. Because of buspirone's extremely wide margin of safety and tolerability, even very large increases in its plasma levels may be clinically insignificant. However, severe parkinsonian symptoms have been attributed to increased buspirone levels during ritonavir coadministration.[105] In contrast to CYP 3A4 inhibitors, some hepatic enzyme inducers can render buspirone ineffective. Regarding pharmacodynamic drug interactions, buspirone should be avoided in combination with MAO inhibitors, like any other serotonergic drug. Buspirone does not have synergistic CNS depressant effects with agents such as alcohol.

PANIC DISORDER
Diagnostic Criteria

The DSM-IV criteria for panic disorder are presented in Table 76-11.[1] The hallmark characteristic of panic disorder is the occurrence of sudden and distinct panic attacks, which are

Table 76-10	Buspirone Drug Interactions	
Interacting Drug(s)	*Clinical Significance/Comments*
CYP 3A4 inhibitors: nefazodone, fluoxetine, fluvoxamine, erythromycin, itraconazole, ketoconazole, diltiazem, verapamil, grapefruit juice, and ritonavir	Significant increases in buspirone Cp have been reported with these agents, but adverse clinical effects not always apparent. Buspirone dosage reductions are recommended when coadministered with erythromycin, fluvoxamine, nefazodone, fluoxetine, or itraconazole.
Rifampin	Highly significant decreases in buspirone Cp; avoid concurrent use.
Haloperidol	Buspirone may increase haloperidol Cp, but one study found no interaction.
Monoamine oxidase inhibitors	Possible serotonin syndrome; avoid concurrent use.

Cp, plasma concentration; CYP, cytochrome P450.

Table 76-11 **Diagnostic Criteria for Panic Disorder**

A. The presence of at least two unexpected panic attacks, characterized by at least four of the following symptoms, which develop abruptly and reach a peak within 10 min:
   1. Palpitations, pounding heart, or accelerated heart rate
   2. Sweating
   3. Trembling or shaking
   4. Sensations of shortness of breath or smothering
   5. Feeling of choking
   6. Chest pain or discomfort
   7. Nausea or abdominal distress
   8. Feeling dizzy, unsteady, light-headed, or faint
   9. Derealization or depersonalization
   10. Fear of losing control or going crazy
   11. Fear of dying
   12. Numbness or tingling sensations
   13. Chills or hot flushes

B. At least one of the attacks has been followed by at least one of the following symptoms for a duration of at least 1 month:
   1. Persistent concern about having another attack
   2. Worry about the implications or consequences of the attack
   3. A significant change in behavior because of the attack

C. The symptoms are not due to the direct effects of a medication, substance, or general medical condition

D. The panic attacks are not better accounted for by another psychiatric or anxiety disorder (e.g., phobias, OCD)

E. May occur with or without agoraphobia (see text)

OCD, obsessive-compulsive disorder.
Adapted from Reference 1.

marked by a tremendous wave of symptoms and feelings listed in Table 76-11. At least four of these symptoms are required for a full panic attack, and the term "limited symptom attack" refers to those involving less than four symptoms. Three types of panic attacks have been defined with regard to the context in which they occur: unexpected or uncued panic attacks (the attack is not associated with a situational trigger); situationally bound panic attacks (the attacks invariably occur on exposure to a situational trigger); and situationally predisposed panic attacks (the attacks are more likely to, but do not invariably, occur upon exposure to a situational trigger).[1]

The DSM-IV criteria for panic disorder require the occurrence of at least two unexpected or uncued panic attacks that are followed by persistent worry or concern about having another panic attack or a significant change in behavior related to the attacks. Although panic attacks are the hallmark symptom of panic disorder, their occurrence does not always indicate panic disorder.[1] Depressive disorders and other anxiety disorders can also be associated with occasional panic attacks. Situationally bound panic attacks are more characteristic of specific phobias or social anxiety disorder than panic disorder, and situationally predisposed panic attacks may occur in either panic or phobic disorders. Nocturnal panic attacks, which awaken a person from sleep, are almost always indicative of panic disorder. Because panic attacks occur unpredictably, they often lead to generalized anxiety or constant fear of sudden attacks. Two subtypes of panic disorder have been identified: without agoraphobia or with agoraphobia.[1] *Agoraphobia* refers to a fear of being in situations from which escape might be difficult or embarrassing in the event of a panic attack. Mild to moderate agoraphobia involves selective avoidance of certain places or situations such as shopping malls, theaters, grocery stores, elevators, and driving alone. Some people may be unable to go anywhere unless accompanied by a companion. In severe cases of agoraphobia, the sufferer may become completely housebound.

Epidemiology and Clinical Course

Approximately 7% to 10% of the general population experiences a single isolated panic attack at some time in their life. Approximately 3% to 4% of persons experience recurrent panic attacks that don't fulfill the diagnostic criteria for panic disorder; however, these persons still can be significantly affected. Full-fledged panic disorder is estimated to affect 1% to 2% of Americans at some time in their life.[19] Women are affected two to three times more often than men and are more likely to develop agoraphobia.[27] The onset of panic disorder usually occurs in the late teens to mid-thirties, and it is rarely seen in the elderly.[19] Most persons report onset of the disorder at some particularly stressful time in their life; in women, this often includes the prenatal and postpartum periods.[27,94]

Panic disorder is accompanied by marked degrees of psychiatric comorbidity; 50% to 60% of patients suffer a major depressive episode at some point. Other common comorbid conditions include social anxiety disorder, GAD, OCD, PTSD, personality disorders, alcohol abuse, and bipolar disorder.[1,106] Patients with comorbid disorders have more severe symptoms, show slower and poorer response to treatments, are less likely to experience full remission, and have a greatly elevated suicide risk (particularly when depression or substance abuse are present) than those with panic disorder alone.[106-108] Panic disorder causes significant functional disability in areas of work, family relationships, and overall quality of life.[19]

Panic disorder is associated with very high rates of health care service utilization.[108] Because of the physical manifestations of panic attacks, repeated ED visits and costly diagnostic tests (including laboratory tests, ECGs, coronary angiograms, echocardiograms, electroencephalograms, GI endoscopic studies, and pulmonary function tests) are common.[109] About 25% to 32% of patients making ED visits related to chest pain actually have panic disorder. The poor recognition of panic disorder in primary care settings further increases use of medical services, because patients are determined to uncover the hidden medical reason for their terrifying symptoms. Panic disorder is the underlying cause of symptoms in an estimated 10% to 30% of patients referred to specialty vestibular, respiratory, or neurology clinics, and up to 60% of those referred for cardiology consultation.[1] The vast majority of panic disorder patients do not complain of feeling anxious and report only physical symptoms, such as chest pain, GI problems, headache, dizziness, and shortness of breath, which contributes to misdiagnosis.[109] It is not uncommon for patients to have been in the health care system for ≥10 years before they are correctly diagnosed.

The long-term course of panic disorder is highly variable.[1] Some patients experience episodic periods of remission and relapse, whereas others suffer almost continuously. Follow-up studies conducted several years after treatment reveal that approximately one-third of patients are still well and in remission; 40% to 50% of patients are improved but experience persistent symptoms, and another 20% to 30% are unchanged or worse.[1,110]

Etiology and Pathophysiology

There is substantial evidence that panic disorder is biologically based. A neuroanatomic model for panic disorder has been proposed in which the anxiety and fear response to threatening stimuli are mediated through the amygdala.[3,8] Various projections from the amygdala, including the hypothalamus and the locus ceruleus, trigger autonomic and neuroendocrine responses that result in anxiety and panic attacks. Patients with panic disorder have a heightened anxiety sensitivity (fear of anxiety-related sensations), and a wide variety of substances and situations are capable of triggering the neural fear network that activates the anxiety and panic response.[8] Acute panic attacks are thought to be caused by dysregulated firing in the locus ceruleus as described previously (see Neurobiology of Anxiety), and hyperresponsiveness of the norepinephrine system may be an underlying cause for panic disorder.[11,15]

Experimental provocation of panic attacks is an important component of panic disorder research. Administration of certain substances induce panic attacks almost consistently in persons with panic disorder, but not in normal healthy subjects.[3,8] These substances include caffeine, noradrenalin, sodium lactate, hypertonic sodium chloride, concentrated carbon dioxide (CO_2), yohimbine, flumazenil, and CCK-B agonists. Administration of effective medication treatments for panic disorder blocks the effects of these panic-inducing substances. Challenge studies such as these provide evidence for possible abnormalities in GABA-A receptor, noradrenergic, serotonergic, and CCK functioning that underlie panic disorders. Decreased GABA-A benzodiazepine binding sites, abnormal regulation of neuroactive steroids that modulate GABA-A receptors, hyperactivation of the HPA axis, and CCK-B receptor gene polymorphism are among the findings.[111,112] People with panic disorder have also been found to have lower brain GABA levels than healthy controls.[113]

Hypersensitivity to 35% CO_2 inhalation, as evidenced by precipitation of panic attacks, robustly distinguishes panic disorder patients from normal controls as well as those with other anxiety disorders such as OCD and GAD.[8] This association is specific enough that CO_2 hypersensitivity is considered a biologic trait marker, at least for a subset of panic disorder patients. This sensitivity appears to be genetically influenced, because relatives of people with panic disorder who do not have panic disorder themselves also have increased panicogenic reactions to CO_2 challenge.[114] Effective treatment of panic disorder with medication significantly decreases the sensitivity to CO_2 inhalation.[115] Brain imaging studies also have demonstrated abnormal patterns of cerebral glucose metabolism in certain brain areas in patients with panic disorder.[8]

Panic disorder definitely runs in families; first-degree relatives of people with panic disorder have an 8 to 21 times greater risk of developing panic disorder than relatives of unaffected people.[1,31] Genetic and environmental influences both contribute to this familial pattern. The inherited component is thought to involve heightened anxiety sensitivity, which confers increased vulnerability for developing panic disorder. Heightened anxiety sensitivity in panic disorder has been associated with "catastrophic cognitions," in which harmless normal physical sensations are misinterpreted as being dangerous and cause for fear.[110] These negative cognitive patterns are often unconscious and may be integral in potentiating recurrent panic attacks in a biologically predisposed individual.

Developmental experiences also may be important in the etiology of panic disorder. Several studies have shown that distressing childhood events such as separation from parents and abuse are associated with markedly increased risks of developing panic disorder later in life.[8] Behavioral inhibition during childhood, characterized by excessive fear and avoidance of novel stimuli, is also extremely common in panic disorder patients. Obviously, no one biologic abnormality can explain panic disorder, and further research is needed to define the complex interplay of the various pathophysiologic, genetic, and cognitive findings in this illness.

Treatment of Panic Disorder

Approximately 70% to 90% of panic disorder patients can experience substantial relief with currently available treatments, which include both pharmacologic therapies and CBTs.[106,110] Medications are most beneficial for reducing panic attacks initially, and their effects on phobic avoidance generally occur later. Nonpharmacologic therapies are especially effective in reducing avoidance behaviors. The two classes of first-line medication treatments for panic disorder are the SSRIs and the benzodiazepines, and these agents are often used in combination.[106] Several TCA and MAO inhibitor antidepressants are also effective in treating panic disorder, but are reserved as second- or third-line options because of their clinical disadvantages compared with SSRIs. The heightened anxiety sensitivity common in panic disorder makes patients especially vulnerable to certain initial antidepressant side effects, such as anxiety and agitation. This is seen with most antidepressants, including SSRIs and TCAs, and is the reason why lower than usual starting doses of antidepressants are recommended in patients with panic disorder.

Selective Serotonin Reuptake Inhibitors

Among the SSRIs, paroxetine, sertraline, and fluoxetine are currently FDA approved for treating panic disorder. There is strong evidence that other SSRIs (fluvoxamine, citalopram, escitalopram) also are effective.[43,52] Several large controlled trials have demonstrated the superiority of paroxetine, sertraline, and fluoxetine over placebo in reducing the frequency of panic attacks, anticipatory anxiety, and associated depression.[116–119] Although low starting dosages are recommended (10 mg/day for paroxetine, 25 mg/day for sertraline, 5 to 10 mg/day for fluoxetine) to minimize side effects, higher doses are usually required for response. The recommended target dosage of paroxetine for panic disorder is 40 mg/day, since a fixed dose study found that 10 and 20 mg/day doses were not significantly effective.[119] Fixed-dose sertraline studies showed that the efficacy of 50 mg, 100 mg, and 200 mg/day doses was comparable; there was no consistent dose-response effect.[120] Therefore, 50 mg/day should be targeted as the minimum dose of sertraline that will be needed when treating panic disorder; higher doses may sometimes be required. The target dose of fluoxetine in panic disorder is 20 mg/day, and most patients are unlikely to require higher doses.[116] For citalopram, a 20- to 30-mg/day dosage range has been associated with better efficacy than 40 to 60 mg/day, whereas doses of 10 to 15 mg/day were ineffective.[43]

Response to SSRIs and other antidepressants in panic disorder occurs gradually, over the course of several weeks. Reduced frequency of panic attacks usually begins within 4 to 6 weeks. A trial period of 10 to 12 weeks should be allowed to fully assess response, and continued improvements may be seen over a treatment period of 6 months or longer.[106,110] Overall, the SSRIs are as effective as the TCAs in treating panic disorder, but they are better tolerated and may have a slightly faster onset of therapeutic effects.[110,121]

Benzodiazepines

The high-potency benzodiazepines, alprazolam and clonazepam, are FDA approved for treating panic disorder and are the most extensively studied agents of this class.[110,122,123] As previously described, new formulations of both of these agents (alprazolam XR, clonazepam Wafer) have been introduced specifically for use in panic disorder. Lorazepam is another high-potency agent that appears to be as effective as alprazolam and clonazepam.[110] Low-potency benzodiazepines such as diazepam were previously thought to be ineffective in treating panic disorder, but they can be effective if sufficiently high doses are used.[110]

Optimal benzodiazepine dosing is an important issue in panic disorder, because these individuals often need higher doses for response than patients with other anxiety disorders.[124] This may be related to reduced sensitivity of benzodiazepine binding sites in panic disorder.[6] An alprazolam dosage range of 4 to 6 mg/day is effective for most panic disorder patients, but others may require up to 10 mg/day for optimal response. An alprazolam plasma concentration ≥20 mg/L may be associated with greatest efficacy, but it is not routine to monitor alprazolam levels in clinical practice.[110] When clonazepam is used, the minimum effective dosage appears to be 1 mg/day, and most panic disorder patients do well in the range of 1 to 3 mg/day.

One problem with alprazolam use in panic disorder is that many patients experience breakthrough anxiety or panic attacks 3 to 5 hours after taking a dose because of its relatively short duration of action.[110] The total daily alprazolam dose usually needs to be taken in three or four, and sometimes five, divided doses to minimize this effect. The XR alprazolam formulation was developed to address this problem.[67] Alprazolam XR can be dosed QD or BID and is associated with minimal interdose anxiety. It may have a lower abuse liability than immediate-release alprazolam, but it is more expensive than generic alprazolam. Clonazepam is longer acting than regular alprazolam, and a twice-daily dosing schedule is usually sufficient. A switch to either clonazepam or alprazolam XR can be beneficial when breakthrough anxiety is a problem with immediate-release alprazolam.[122] Alprazolam XR is more expensive than generic clonazepam and probably offers no clinical advantage over clonazepam in most cases. Both forms of alprazolam are associated with more severe withdrawal symptoms than clonazepam, because clonazepam is longer acting and is eliminated from the body more gradually.[122] Panic disorder patients are especially sensitive to benzodiazepine withdrawal effects. For these reasons, clonazepam may be preferred over alprazolam in many panic disorder patients.[124]

Tricyclic Antidepressants, Monoamine Oxidase Inhibitors, and Other Antidepressants

TCAs were the first medications widely used in the treatment of panic disorder. Imipramine (Tofranil) and clomipramine (Anafranil) are as effective as alprazolam, but are less well tolerated.[107,123,125] One trial with desipramine (Norpramin) found that it improved panic disorder symptoms but it was not significantly different from placebo.[110] Well-conducted studies involving other TCAs are lacking. As indicated, especially low starting dosages of TCAs (10 mg/day) are needed to minimize initial anxiety-like side effects. Even so, many patients discontinue therapy because of poor tolerability. Imipramine should be slowly titrated up to the recommended target dosage of 100 mg/day.

Clomipramine appears to be more effective than other TCAs for panic disorder, perhaps because of its greater serotonergic effects.[125] The possibility of a therapeutic dosage window for clomipramine in panic disorder has been suggested, with dosages >80 mg/day being associated with a decreased chance of response.[125,126] Clomipramine seems to be most effective within the dosage range of 60 to 80 mg/day, which is relatively low but reasonably well tolerated. Patients who do not respond to clomipramine doses in this range are unlikely to benefit from further dose increases.

Among the MAO inhibitors, phenelzine (Nardil) is often heralded as being remarkably effective in the treatment of panic disorder, but this claim is based on studies that were conducted more than two decades ago in patients who would probably not even meet the current diagnostic criteria for panic disorder.[110] No recent MAO inhibitor studies are available to assess phenelzine's efficacy within the context of current treatment standards. Phenelzine may be extremely effective but it is generally an option of last resort for treatment-refractory cases because of the many clinical disadvantages of MAO inhibitors relative to other antidepressants (see Chapter 79, Mood Disorders I: Bipolar Disorders). Preliminary reports suggest that other newer antidepressants, including venlafaxine, nefazodone, mirtazapine, and escitalopram may also be beneficial in treating panic disorder.[52,110,124] These agents may be useful in patients who do not respond to SSRI therapy.

Miscellaneous Agents

Bupropion (Wellbutrin), buspirone, and trazodone are generally ineffective for panic disorder.[110] Trials of propranolol and clonidine have yielded mixed, but largely negative, results.[110] None of these agents are considered appropriate treatment options in panic disorder, although buspirone and pindolol have been effective in augmenting response to SSRI therapy.[124,127] Other medications that are reportedly effective in treating panic disorder include the anticonvulsants carbamazepine, oxcarbazepine, tiagabine, and valproate; the calcium channel blocker verapamil; the antipsychotic agent olanzapine; the antihistamine chlorpheniramine; the serotonin-3 receptor antagonist, ondansetron; and inositol.[110,124] More information is needed before any of these can be recommended for the treatment of panic disorder.

Nonpharmacologic Treatments

Cognitive and behavioral therapies (CBTs), including exposure treatment and relaxation training, are also established as being effective in panic disorder.[33,110] The cognitive theory of panic disorder is based on the observed heightened anxiety sensitivity in these patients and asserts that physical anxiety sensations are misinterpreted as being serious or life threatening and that these fears trigger a cycle of further worsening anxiety symptoms that finally progress to a panic attack. Reversing the cognitive component of this vicious cycle is an integral part of cognitive therapy and is important in producing lasting therapeutic effects of treatment.[110] Breathing retraining and exposure to fear cues are key components of behavioral therapy.

Some studies have found medications to be superior to CBTs in the treatment of panic disorder, whereas others report opposite results.[106,110] CBTs reportedly result in benefits that are maintained longer after therapy is stopped, and also have been effective in making benzodiazepine discontinuation easier.[33] Combining medication with CBTs can be useful, especially in patients with severe agoraphobia or those who only partially respond to either treatment modality used alone.[124,128]

Clinical Presentation and Differential Diagnosis of Panic Disorder

17. S.K., a 24-year-old female graduate student, presents to the ED complaining of chest pain, difficulty breathing, dizziness, and extreme nausea. She describes feeling "as if my head is going off in space and I am outside my body." She states that she has been under extreme stress lately with examinations, working too much, and constantly fighting with her roommate. S.K. fears that she has had a heart attack or stroke brought on by her stressful life. S.K. recently visited her family physician for the same symptoms; however, a complete physical examination and laboratory workup yielded no abnormalities, and she was advised to try to relax. She states that her first "attack" occurred out of the blue about 5 months ago while she was studying in the library and that she can never predict when they will happen. Since then, her symptoms have become more severe and frequent, and she has started skipping classes for fear they will return. S.K. denies any drug or alcohol use but states that she has suffered from depression in the past and was hospitalized for one severe episode 2 years ago. An ECG is performed and found to be normal. The physician's diagnosis is panic disorder with mild agoraphobia. What clinical features of panic disorder does S.K. display, and what are the important factors in the differential diagnosis of panic disorder?

S.K. exhibits many typical characteristics of panic disorder. As illustrated in this case, the first panic attack typically occurs without warning while the person is involved in a normal everyday activity and lasts 10 to 30 minutes. Panic attacks are extremely terrifying and usually leave the sufferer feeling anxious and convinced that something is medically wrong. As with S.K., it is not uncommon for persons to make ED visits following or during panic attacks, believing they have had a heart attack or other serious event. Unfortunately, panic disorder often is not recognized in primary care settings, and no medical cause for the symptoms can be identified. Faced with findings that they are apparently healthy, persons may make repeated ED visits and consult different doctors and specialists in an attempt to uncover a physical explanation for their frightening symptoms.

S.K. exhibits the following target symptoms of panic disorder: chest pain, shortness of breath, dizziness, abdominal distress, and depersonalization ("my head is going off in space, I am outside my body"). Mild agoraphobia is present since she has started limiting class attendance because of her panic attacks. Other factors consistent with a diagnosis of panic disorder include her young age, female gender, lack of abnormal physical findings, and absence of possible precipitating substances. This case also illustrates the association between onset of panic disorder and stressful life events, its common comorbidity with depression, and the frequent lack of recognition of panic disorder in primary care settings.

Because different substances or medical conditions can cause severe anxiety and panic, it is necessary to rule out these potential causes for panic disorder symptoms.[109] Notable triggers of panic attacks include caffeine, alcohol, nicotine, nonprescription cold preparations, cannabis, amphetamines, and cocaine.[109] Any medication that causes anxiety as a side effect can potentially precipitate panic attacks in predisposed individuals (see Table 76-1). Medical illnesses that can cause panic attacks include hyperthyroidism, hyperparathyroidism, pheochromocytoma, seizure disorders, and cardiac arrhythmias.[106] Panic disorder is also associated with higher-than-expected comorbidities with hypertension, mitral valve prolapse, asthma, coronary artery disease, peptic ulcer disease, Parkinson's disease, chronic pain syndromes, primary biliary cirrhosis, and irritable bowel syndrome.[110] In patients with comorbid medical conditions, panic disorder can worsen the physical illness.

Panic attacks also can occur in other anxiety disorders. However, in these cases, the panic attacks usually occur on exposure to a feared object or situation (in phobic disorders), an object of obsession (in OCD), or a stimulus associated with a traumatic stressor (in PTSD). S.K. reports that her panic attacks occur unexpectedly, and situationally bound or predisposed attacks are not evident; therefore, the features are consistent with panic disorder.

Treatment Selection for Panic Disorder, SSRI Dosing Issues, and Combination SSRI–Benzodiazepine Therapy

18. S.K. is referred to a psychiatrist who decides to initiate treatment with fluoxetine 20 mg Q AM. Three days later, S.K. calls the doctor complaining that her anxiety and panic attacks have greatly increased since she started taking fluoxetine. The psychiatrist prescribes alprazolam 0.5 mg (tablets) and instructs S.K. to take 1 tablet as needed for the anxiety. What factors should be considered in the selection of an initial medication treatment for panic disorder? Why is the prescribed treatment for S.K. inappropriate?

An SSRI, with or without concurrent benzodiazepine therapy, is appropriate first-line treatment for most panic disorder patients.[106,124] In patients like S.K. who have a history of depression, SSRIs may also help prevent depressive relapse. Patients with severe or distressing symptoms usually require concurrent benzodiazepine therapy, which provides quick relief from anxiety and panic attacks until the SSRI's therapeutic effects occur. At that time, usually after several weeks, the benzodiazepine can be gradually discontinued. An SSRI–benzodiazepine combination is currently the most commonly prescribed initial treatment for panic disorder and is superior in efficacy to initial monotherapy.[63] Although benzodiazepines are generally avoided in patients with a history of substance abuse, use of low doses for a limited time period may be appropriate for some such patients with disabling symptoms, as long as there is no current substance (especially alcohol) abuse.[86,124] Because of the levels of distress and impairment caused by S.K.'s panic disorder, combined SSRI–benzodiazepine therapy would have been the preferred initial treatment. Scheduled benzodiazepine dosing is preferred over as-needed dosing during initial therapy, so that panic attacks are prevented.[124] Because panic attacks generally last less than 30 minutes, they have usually passed by the time an as-needed benzodiazepine dose can take effect.

In choosing among SSRIs for the treatment of panic disorder, fluoxetine may be more likely to be anxiety provoking in some patients and there is less published evidence to support its use than for sertraline or paroxetine.[43] If fluoxetine is used, very low initial doses (5 to 10 mg/day) should be used; in S.K.'s case the prescribed 20-mg/day starting dose was much too high. Also, scheduled versus as-needed benzodiazepine dosing would have been the preferred. After 2 to 4 weeks, the benzodiazepine can be gradually discontinued while the SSRI therapy is continued and gradually titrated to the target effective dose. The potential for drug interactions must also be kept in mind when these SSRI–benzodiazepine combinations are used because certain SSRIs can inhibit benzodiazepine metabolism, leading to increased benzodiazepine side effects (see Benzodiazepine Drug Interactions).

Patient Counseling Information

Patients like S.K. who are beginning SSRI therapy for the treatment of panic disorder should be counseled about possible increased anxiety during the first 1 or 2 weeks of treatment, as well as other common SSRI side effects, including nausea, headache, and either insomnia or sedation. Because these are dose-related effects, patients should inform their clinician of any problems and a dosage reduction may be indicated. These adverse effects usually subside after 1 to 3 weeks of continued treatment. It also is important to inform patients that it may take several weeks before beneficial effects of antidepressant treatment are seen, and 6 to 12 weeks or longer may be required for full response. Patients receiving initial benzodiazepine therapy should be counseled about their relatively quick onset of effects to provide anxiolytic coverage during the initial weeks of SSRI therapy, as well as the likely limited duration of benzodiazepine therapy. Other pertinent counseling information for benzodiazepine treatment should also be included (see Question 6). The desired goals of therapy and likely duration of treatment should also be explained (see Question 20). Providing information about the nature of panic disorder, including reassurance that panic attacks are not life threatening, is also important. Many clinicians recommend that patients keep a "panic diary" in which they record frequency of panic attacks along with symptoms experienced during attacks.

Clinical Assessment and Goals of Therapy

19. **S.K. refuses to continue taking fluoxetine, so paroxetine is prescribed instead. After 1 week of paroxetine therapy, S.K. is still taking the initial dosage of 10 mg/day and is tolerating the medication well. The plan is to gradually increase the paroxetine to 40 mg/day over the next several weeks. S.K. is also taking alprazolam, 0.5 mg 2 to 3 times each day. What are the desired goals of treatment in this case and how can S.K.'s response to treatment be assessed?**

Five domains in panic disorder have been identified in which treatment outcomes should be assessed: frequency and severity of panic attacks, anticipatory anxiety, phobic avoidance behaviors, overall well-being, and illness-related disability in various areas (work, school, family).[110] The treatment goals in this case are first to stop S.K.'s panic attacks, then to reduce her anticipatory anxiety, followed by reversal of phobic avoidance.[61] These outcomes should enable her to attend class regularly and, secondarily, improve her overall functioning and quality of life.

Several different instruments have been used to assess outcomes of treatment in panic disorder.[61] In addition to the panic diary, others include the Fear Questionnaire, the Panic Appraisal Inventory, and the Panic Disorder Severity Scale. The latter is currently considered by many experts to be the most useful because it evaluates outcomes in all five identified target domains of panic disorder.[61,110]

Course and Duration of Therapy

20. **After 3 months of paroxetine therapy S.K. reports at her clinic appointment that she has had no panic attacks in the past month and that functioning has improved dramatically. She is currently taking 40 mg/day of paroxetine (two 20-mg tablets) and gradually stopped taking the alprazolam 3 to 4 weeks ago. S.K. reveals that she is going to class, making good grades, getting along with her roommate, and dating. S.K. is experiencing no significant side effects from paroxetine but complains that it is expensive and wonders how long she should continue taking it because she is doing so well. What is the recommended duration of treatment for panic disorder?**

Long-term medication trials in panic disorder support the recommendation that treatment should continue for at least 6 to 12 months after acute response.[110,129] The benefits of maintenance pharmacotherapy in preventing relapse are well documented. Maintenance treatment gives patients time to resume normal lifestyles and to re-establish daily activities following acute cessation of panic attacks. Effective maintenance doses of TCAs and benzodiazepines have been reported to be lower than those used during initial treatment, but whether this also applies to SSRI therapy is currently unknown.[106,110]

In this case, S.K.'s current paroxetine dosage of 40 mg/day is appropriate since this has been identified as the minimum effective dose for panic disorder. Paroxetine therapy should be continued at the current dosage for 3 to 6 more months. Use of a 40-mg paroxetine tablet instead of two 20-mg tablets each day can cut the drug expense in half. After a successful period of full remission, a trial of medication discontinuation may be attempted to determine whether continued treatment is necessary. Medication should not be stopped in patients who are experiencing stressful life events or substantial residual problems in any of the five domains. When medication is discontinued, it should be withdrawn gradually over several months regardless of which medication class is involved. The long-term course of panic disorder is variable, but an estimated 25% to 40% of patients relapse after medications are discontinued.[110] Because of the devastating impact that panic disorder can have, reinstitution of drug treatment is indicated if relapse occurs. Long-term treatment with antidepressants, and benzodiazepines if necessary, is generally successful in maintaining treatment benefits without detrimental effects or dosage escalations.[106] Panic disorder is accepted as an appropriate indication for long-term benzodiazepine therapy if it is necessary.

SOCIAL ANXIETY DISORDER AND SPECIFIC PHOBIAS
Classification and Diagnosis of Phobic Disorders

The DSM-IV category of phobic disorders includes two primary types: specific phobia (formerly called *simple phobia*) and social phobia (also called *social anxiety disorder*).[1] The term *social anxiety disorder* is more commonly used and is the term used in this text. These disorders involve fears that are excessive or unreasonable and lead to avoidance behavior to minimize anxiety. The DSM-IV criteria for phobic disorders are presented in Table 76-12.[1] The main difference between specific phobias and social anxiety disorder is that the former involves fear and avoidance of specific objects or situations, whereas the latter involves social situations.

Social Anxiety Disorder

In social anxiety disorder, there is an intense irrational fear of scrutiny or evaluation by others because of concerns about humiliation or being made to appear ridiculous.[1] The *generalized* type of social anxiety disorder refers to cases in which fears relate to most social situations (e.g., fear of general social interactions, speaking to people, attending social gatherings, dating), whereas the *nongeneralized* type involves more specific phobias.[1] Public speaking is by far the most common nongeneralized type; others include speaking to strangers, eating in public, and using public restrooms. A defining feature of either type is that the fears and anxiety are confined to social situations, and patients are usually symptom free when alone. The most common symptoms seen in social anxiety disorder include blushing, muscle twitching, and stuttering, in addition to other typical symptoms of anxiety. Panic attacks also may occur in either specific phobia or social anxiety disorder, on exposure to the feared object or situation. However, social anxiety disorder is differentiated from panic disorder and agoraphobia by involving the fear of humiliation and social scrutiny, rather than fear of having a panic attack.

The DSM-IV excludes a diagnosis of social anxiety disorder if the person fears public embarrassment due to some physical or medical condition. However, this criterion is controversial because it excludes social anxiety disorder that is due to certain socially stigmatizing conditions, such as Parkinson's disease, stuttering, obesity, and physical disfigurement or deformity.[1] These cases are sometimes referred to as *secondary social anxiety disorder*.

Specific Phobias

Specific phobias are classified into five subtypes: animal type (snakes, dogs, spiders), natural environment type (heights, water, storms), blood-injection type (blood, injury, medical procedures), situational type (flying, bridges, elevators), and others.[1] Exposure to the feared circumstance produces intense anxiety, sometimes to the degree of panic attacks, and avoidance of the stimuli is common. Significant impairment of functioning or marked distress must be present for a diagnosis of specific phobia to be warranted. For example, fear of flying might constitute specific phobia in a person whose job requires airplane travel, but it would not impair functioning in someone who never has occasion to fly.

Management of specific phobias traditionally has involved mere avoidance of the stimuli. Medications generally are not considered beneficial, but CBTs involving repeated exposure to the feared situation and systemic desensitization are very effective. Computer-generated, virtual environment desensitization (virtual reality) therapy has been used successfully to reduce fears associated with flying and heights. Benzodiazepines can effectively reduce anxiety associated with a phobic trigger, but can also interfere with the efficacy of exposure therapies.

Social Anxiety Disorder
Epidemiology and Clinical Course
The lifetime prevalence of DSM-IV social anxiety disorder is approximately 7%, which is lower than previous estimates of 13% to 14%.[19] The male:female prevalence ratio is approximately 2:3. Social anxiety disorder usually begins early in life, with a mean onset between the ages 14 and 16 years.[130] More than 50% of patients are affected before adolescence, and a history of shyness and behavioral inhibition throughout

---

Table 76-12 Diagnostic Criteria for Phobic Disorders

Social Anxiety Disorder (Social Phobia)

1. A marked and constant fear of one or more social situations in which the person is exposed to unfamiliar people or possible scrutiny by others and the person fears humiliation or embarrassment
2. Exposure to the situation provokes an immediate anxiety response
3. The person realizes the fear is excessive or unreasonable (not required in children)
4. The feared situation is avoided or endured with intense anxiety or distress
5. The fear or avoidance significantly interferes with the person's normal routine or activities or causes marked distress
6. In individuals less than 18 years of age, the duration of the fear is at least 6 months
7. The anxiety or phobic avoidance are not better accounted for by another psychiatric disorder (e.g., fear of having a panic attack, obsessions that accompany OCD, or trauma related to PTSD)

Specific Phobia

1. A marked and persistent fear of a specific object or situation that is excessive or unreasonable
2. Other criteria (2–7) that are listed above for social anxiety disorder

OCD, obsessive-compulsive disorder; PTSD, post-traumatic stress disorder.
Adapted from Reference 1.

childhood is common.[130] Unless effectively treated, the clinical course is often that of a chronic, unremitting, and lifelong disorder.

Comorbidity and Clinical Significance

Because social anxiety disorder usually begins during the teenage years, it can seriously interfere with development of normal social skills and abilities to form interpersonal relationships.[131] This can lead to functional disabilities that may persist for a lifetime. Social anxiety disorder can interfere with achievement of full academic and career potentials and is known to be associated with unemployment, lower levels of education, and dependence on public financial support systems.[19] Persons with social anxiety disorder are less likely to marry, and more than half report moderate to severe impairments in their abilities to carry out ordinary daily activities.[131]

Comorbidity in social anxiety disorder is high, with an estimated 70% to 80% of individuals having at least one other psychiatric disorder in their lifetime.[1,130] Common comorbid conditions include simple phobia, major depression, GAD, panic disorder, body dysmorphic disorder, and alcohol abuse. Because of its early onset, social anxiety disorder usually precedes the development of comorbid disorders. Alcohol commonly is used to decrease anxiety in social situations. The risk of suicide attempts is very high, especially in those with both social anxiety disorder and another comorbid psychiatric illness.[19]

Etiology and Pathophysiology

Social anxiety disorder is known to be a familial disease, but the relative contributions of genetic versus environmental influences have not been differentiated.[31] Early factors that may predispose to its development include anxious behavior modeling in parents and parental overprotection.[1] Shyness in children, which is associated with later development of social anxiety disorder, has been linked to a specific genetic polymorphism of the serotonin transporter promoter region.[132]

Biologic studies suggest that the generalized and nongeneralized types of social anxiety disorder may have different underlying pathophysiologies. Nongeneralized social anxiety disorder may mainly involve disturbances in noradrenergic system functioning, whereas there is substantial evidence for dopaminergic and serotonergic dysfunction in the generalized form.[133,134] Abnormally low dopamine neurotransmission in generalized social anxiety disorder is supported by findings of significantly decreased dopamine-2 receptor binding; markedly reduced dopamine transporter densities; low levels of the dopamine metabolite, homovanillic acid; high rates of social anxiety disorder in persons who later develop Parkinson's disease; and several reports of emergence of social anxiety disorder during antipsychotic treatment.[133,134] Social anxiety disorder appears to be unique among the anxiety disorders in its association with dopamine system abnormalities. Pharmacologic challenge studies suggest that serotonin type-2 receptors are hypersensitive in patients with social anxiety disorder, and neuroimaging studies have found specific neural circuits to be activated in this illness.[133]

Treatment of Social Anxiety Disorder

Early detection and treatment of social anxiety disorder are vital in reducing its lifelong functional consequences and may prevent development of comorbid disorders. Because of the very nature of the disorder, some sufferers are reluctant to seek treatment. Those who do seek help, even in psychiatric settings, are rarely diagnosed and treated appropriately.[130] Only in the past few years has pharmacotherapy become established as first-line therapy for social anxiety disorder. Nonpharmacologic treatments also can be very beneficial, and use of the two modalities may be complementary.

SELECTIVE SEROTONIN REUPTAKE INHIBITORS

As with many other anxiety disorders, SSRIs are considered the primary treatment option for most patients with social anxiety disorder.[130] Paroxetine was FDA approved for treating social anxiety disorder in 1999 and was the only medication with this official indication until sertraline and venlafaxine XR received approval in early 2003.[135–140] Fluvoxamine and escitalopram have also demonstrated efficacy in controlled clinical trials.[52,141] Open studies and case reports suggest that fluoxetine and citalopram can be effective in treating social anxiety disorder.[142,143] However, the only controlled fluoxetine trial found no difference in efficacy from placebo, although both groups showed significant response.[142]

Unlike patients with GAD and panic disorder, those with social anxiety disorder can usually tolerate standard antidepressant starting doses. Target effective SSRI doses for social anxiety disorder are within the normal antidepressant dosage ranges. The one fixed-dose study of paroxetine in social anxiety disorder found no overall difference in efficacy between 20, 40, and 60 mg/day.[135] Although some individuals may respond better to higher dosages, adequate time should be allowed at 20 mg/day before the dosage is increased. Response to SSRI treatment occurs gradually and an adequate medication trial to assess response should last at least 8 to 10 weeks. Many who experience minimal response at week 8 may show good response at week 12, and improvements have been found to continue throughout 16 weeks of treatment.[138,144]

OTHER ANTIDEPRESSANTS

The MAO inhibitors phenelzine and tranylcypromine also have demonstrated marked efficacy for social anxiety disorder but are reserved for SSRI nonresponders.[130] Before the advent of SSRIs, phenelzine was considered the mainstay of pharmacotherapy for social anxiety disorder. The typically effective dosage ranges are 60 to 90 mg/day for phenelzine and 30 to 60 mg/day for tranylcypromine.

The reversible monoamine oxidase-A inhibitors (RIMAs), moclobemide and brofaromine, which are currently unavailable in the United States, have shown mixed efficacy results in controlled studies.[130] Case reports and/or open studies suggest that other antidepressants, including nefazodone and bupropion, may be useful in treating social anxiety disorder, but controlled trials are needed to define their roles.[130] Imipramine is ineffective for social anxiety disorder, and TCAs are not among the recommended treatment options.[130,145]

BENZODIAZEPINES

The high-potency benzodiazepines, clonazepam and alprazolam, may also be useful in some patients with social anxiety disorder. Clonazepam was markedly efficacious in one controlled study, whereas alprazolam showed only modest efficacy over placebo.[130] The usual effective dosage ranges are 1 to 3 mg/day for clonazepam and 1 to 6 mg/day for alprazolam. In contrast to the antidepressants, benzodiazepines have a quicker onset of therapeutic effects and also can be used on an as-needed basis before stressful social situations. However, benzodiazepines can reduce the therapeutic effects of exposure therapy. Other disadvantages of the benzodiazepines include their lack of efficacy for many common comorbid psychiatric disorders, potential for abuse and dependence, and a potentially dangerous interaction with alcohol. Benzodiazepines are generally considered second-line therapy for social anxiety disorder, but in clinical practice they are commonly used on an as-needed basis in combination with SSRI therapy.

β-BLOCKERS AND OTHER MISCELLANEOUS AGENTS

β-Adrenergic receptor blockers reduce peripheral autonomic symptoms of anxiety, but they are not effective in treating generalized social anxiety disorder.[130] However, they are useful for nongeneralized social phobia involving performance-related situations.[58] Propranolol and atenolol are the two recommended agents and can be used on an as-needed basis to reduce performance anxiety. Small doses (10 to 80 mg of propranolol or 25 to 50 mg of atenolol) of either agent may be administered 1 to 2 hours before the performance to decrease symptoms such as tremors, sweating, and blushing. A test dose should be tried before the actual occasion to assess medication tolerability. β-Blockers are not recommended as monotherapy for the treatment of generalized social anxiety disorder. Buspirone does not appear to be effective as monotherapy for social anxiety disorder, but it has been successfully used to augment SSRI therapy.[36,130] Various other medications, including gabapentin, topiramate, tiagabine, ondansetron, clonidine, and augmentation with ropinirole and pramipexole, also have been reported to be effective in the treatment of social anxiety disorder, but their places in therapy are not yet clear.[130]

NONPHARMACOLOGIC TREATMENTS

Several studies have demonstrated CBTs to be comparable to medications in the treatment of social anxiety disorder.[145] The cognitive therapy component is aimed at changing the negative thought patterns such as expectations of performing poorly and overconcern about negative evaluation by others.[145] These negative expectations lead to increased apprehension and anxiety, which further impair performance abilities. The behavioral therapy component, as in other anxiety disorders, involves repeated exposure to the feared social situations and practice at performing in those situations. Cognitive-behavioral group therapies are especially beneficial in social anxiety disorder, because group members can practice social interactions with one another. Although medications may work faster, CBTs are thought to result in longer-lasting treatment gains.[145] Social skills training can also be beneficial in improving interpersonal communication skills.

Clinical Presentation of Social Anxiety Disorder

21. S.H., an 18-year-old man, is brought for psychiatric consultation by his mother who complains that her son is extremely shy. S.H. was referred to the psychiatrist by his primary care physician, who reports that S.H. is physically healthy. S.H.'s mother states that he is a very bright young man who made straight As in high school despite frequent absenteeism, but he has no friends and has never been on a date. S.H.'s mother says that during high school, S.H. never attended any school social functions and spent all of his time in his room working on his computer. Upon graduation from high school, he received a full scholarship to a community college but refused to go. When questioned by the psychiatrist, S.H.'s face turns bright red and his voice shakes when he speaks. S.H. admits that his behavior is not normal but says that he is afraid that he might do something stupid when he is around people and becomes extremely embarrassed when he has to talk to anyone. He has wanted to ask a certain girl for a date for 3 years but experienced severe anxiety attacks on the few occasions he has tried to approach her. S.H. is afraid of being turned down and believes that no girl would ever want to date someone like himself. The psychiatrist's diagnosis is social anxiety disorder. What clinical features of social anxiety disorder are present in S.H.?

S.H. exhibits many characteristic features of the generalized type of social anxiety disorder. S.H. admits that he does not like being around people for fear of embarrassment and he generally avoids social situations, which are classic traits of social anxiety disorder. His symptoms of blushing and shaking voice are also common in social anxiety disorder, as well as other typical anxiety symptoms such as palpitations, trembling, sweating, tense muscles, dry throat, hot/cold sensations, and a sinking feeling in the stomach. S.H. also displays hypersensitivity to rejection and low self-esteem, and he realizes that his behavior and fears are unreasonable. These symptoms and S.H.'s young age are consistent with a diagnosis of social anxiety disorder.

S.H.'s case illustrates the substantial disability that can result from this illness. S.H.'s anxiety disorder has deprived him of normal social development, making friends, dating, participating in social functions, and pursuit of higher education. Future impairments throughout S.H.'s life are likely to be significant unless his anxiety is treated successfully.

Treatment Selection for Social Anxiety Disorder

22. The physician decides to treat S.H. with medication and prescribes sertraline, 50 mg Q AM. Is the prescribed pharmacotherapy appropriate in this case?

Because S.H.'s generalized social anxiety disorder is severely impacting his life, medication treatment is indicated. The SSRIs are first-line therapy for treating social anxiety disorder, and sertraline is a good choice because it is FDA approved for this indication. Although not applicable in this case, sertraline is also effective for many of the other psychiatric disorders that are commonly seen in patients with social anxiety disorder. The sertraline starting dose of 50 mg/day is appropriate for S.H., and 50 mg increment dosage increases can be made every 4 weeks according to response, up to a maximum of 200 mg/day. In one flexible dose sertraline clinical trial, the average dose for responders was 150 mg/day.[138] Signs of response may be seen within 2 to 4 weeks, but 8 to 12 weeks is usually required for optimal results. If available, CBT also may be combined with pharmacotherapy for S.H.

Goals and Duration of Treatment

23. What are the goals of treatment in this case, and how can S.H.'s response to treatment be objectively assessed? How long should effective therapy be continued?

Three principle domains of treatment outcomes have been defined for social anxiety disorder: symptoms, functionality, and overall well-being.[61] It is recommended that efficacy assessments examine all three of these areas, because even if all anxiety symptoms disappear, treatment is not really clinically significant unless functioning also improves. The clinician-rated Liebowitz Social Anxiety Scale (LSAS) and the patient-rated Sheehan Disability Scale can be used for measuring improvements in the symptom and functional ability domains, respectively.[61] In S.H.'s case, the desired outcomes of treatment include reducing his fear and avoidance of social situations, enabling him to comfortably interact socially and attend college, and improving his overall quality of life.

Several studies have examined relapse rates after double-blind discontinuation of effective treatment in social anxiety disorder.[144–146] Based on their results, relapse appears to be very common. Long-term studies have shown that both sertraline and paroxetine prevent relapse of social anxiety disorder during continuation treatment.[136,138] Therefore, pharmacotherapy should be continued for at least 1 year after response.[130] After that time, a trial of gradual medication discontinuation may be attempted, accompanied by close monitoring for signs of relapse.

POST-TRAUMATIC STRESS DISORDER AND ACUTE STRESS DISORDER
Diagnostic Criteria

PTSD and acute stress disorder occur in people who have experienced a severely distressing traumatic event. These disorders are characterized by symptoms of intrusive re-experiencing, avoidance features, emotional numbing, and symptoms of autonomic hyperarousal.[1] PTSD has been recognized most commonly in war veterans and was referred to as "shell shock" after World War I. However, PTSD also occurs in persons exposed to events such as natural disasters, serious accidents, criminal assault, rape, physical or sexual abuse, and political victimization (refugees, concentration camp survivors, hostages). The trauma does not have to involve physical injury to the PTSD victim. Witnessing someone else being injured or killed, being diagnosed with a life-threatening illness, and experiencing the unexpected death of a loved one are common types of trauma that may lead to PTSD.[1]

The DSM-IV criteria for PTSD are presented in Table 76-13. PTSD is classified as having either an acute or delayed (after 6 months) onset in relation to the trauma; the latter is extremely rare.[1] Symptoms must persist for at least 1 month to meet the criteria for PTSD. *Acute stress disorder* is a separate diagnostic category in the DSM-IV and refers to cases in which symptoms last less than 1 month (but at least 2 days).[1] It involves many of the same clinical features as PTSD, but there is an additional requirement of peritraumatic dissociative symptoms (numbing, derealization, depersonalization, amnesia, feeling dazed). In both PTSD and acute stress disorder, the symptoms must be severe enough to interfere with some aspect of functioning.

Epidemiology and Clinical Course

PTSD was previously believed to affect approximately 1% of the general population, but recent studies reveal a much

---

Table 76-13 Diagnostic Criteria for PTSD

A. The person has experienced a traumatic event in which the individual witnessed, experienced, or was confronted with actual or threatened death, or serious injury to self or others and to which the person responded with intense fear, helplessness, or horror

B. The traumatic event is re-experienced persistently in some way (e.g., dreams, nightmares, flash backs, recurrent thoughts or images), or intense distress is experienced on exposure to stimuli associated with the traumatic event

C. Persistent avoidance of stimuli associated with the event and numbing of general responsiveness involving at least three of the following:
  1. Efforts to avoid thoughts, feelings, or conversations related to the trauma
  2. Efforts to avoid people, places, or activities that are reminders of the trauma
  3. Impaired recall of the traumatic event
  4. Decreased interest or participation in activities
  5. Feelings of detachment
  6. Restricted range of affect
  7. Sense of foreshortened future

D. Persistent symptoms of increased arousal (not present before the event) that include at last two of the following:
  1. Sleep disturbances
  2. Irritability or anger outbursts
  3. Difficulty concentrating
  4. Hypervigilance
  5. Exaggerated startle response

E. Duration of the disturbance (B, C, and D) of at least 1 month

F. The disturbance causes significant impairment in some aspect of daily functioning

PTSD, post-traumatic stress disorder.
Adapted from Reference 1.

---

higher lifetime prevalence of approximately 7% to 8%.[147] PTSD is twice as common in women than in men, although overall, men are exposed to trauma more often than women.[147] Rates of PTSD are expected to rise as the frequency of traumatic events throughout the world continues to increase. An estimated 80% to 90% of individuals in the United States today will experience at least one event during their lifetime that is traumatic enough to lead to PTSD.[147]

Most people who are exposed to a traumatic event do not develop PTSD; approximately 90% of individuals experience a normal acute stress response to trauma and fully recover.[147] Risk factors for the development of PTSD include experiencing assaultive violence, more severe and chronic traumas, a history of depressive or anxiety disorders, and experiencing dissociative or other intense symptoms during or soon after the trauma.[147,148] Previous exposure to trauma also increases the risk of developing PTSD after later traumas, and survivors of childhood sexual or physical abuse have been found to be especially vulnerable.[148,149] Among people exposed to various traumatic events, the overall conditional risks for PTSD are reported to be 6% for males and 13% for females.[147] In general, traumas involving personal assault (rape, combat) are associated with much higher conditional risks of developing PTSD than other types of trauma.

Most PTSD patients also suffer from other disorders at some point in their lifetime, including major depression, GAD, panic disorder, phobic disorders, and alcohol or other substance abuse.[147] Overall, 79% to 88% of those with PTSD have another lifetime psychiatric disorder, most commonly depression or substance abuse.[150,151] High rates of substance abuse and dependence in PTSD are related to attempts to self-medicate PTSD symptoms.[151] The suicide risk in PTSD is very high and comparable to that seen in major depression.[152] PTSD causes significant functional disability and has been associated with school failure, teenage pregnancy, unemployment, marital instability, legal problems, and impaired performance in the workplace.[152]

The course of PTSD is highly variable. Most patients who meet criteria for PTSD 1 month after trauma show spontaneous recovery within 6 to 9 months.[150] PTSD continues for years in a significant minority, estimated at 10% to 25%, and some sufferers experience a lifelong course of illness. The overall median duration of PTSD is reported to be approximately 2 years, but has been found to be four times longer in women (4 years) than in men (1 year).[150]

Etiology and Pathophysiology

Biologic studies have led to various findings in PTSD. The effects of stress on the brain have been a topic of intensive research. Apparently, psychological trauma, especially that which occurs early in life or is chronic in duration, can cause persistent changes in various aspects of brain functioning and in neurobiologic responses to stress.[153–155] Evidence of altered noradrenergic, serotonergic, glutaminergic, GABA system, neuroendocrine, substance P, and opioid system functioning has been found in PTSD.[16,153,156,157] Stress-induced hyperactivity of central noradrenergic systems is believed to lead to the generalized anxiety and autonomic hyperarousal associated with PTSD.[156] These symptoms also may be related to a supersensitivity of the HPA axis system in PTSD because affected patients have a blunted adrenocorticotrophic hormone response to CRF and decreased basal cortisol levels, as well as increased numbers of glucocorticoid receptors.[16,153] A portion of PTSD patients appear to have an abnormally sensitized serotonin system, and these patients may represent a neurobiologically distinct subgroup.[153,157]

Evidence also exists for dysregulation of the GABA and glutaminergic pathways in PTSD. One theory is that severe stress causes a down-regulation of the GABA system that results in excessive glutamate activity and overstimulation of N-methyl-D-aspartate receptors, which may exert a neurotoxic effect.[153] Numerous studies have found reduced hippocampal volumes in PTSD, which is a brain area involved in learning and memory that appears to be particularly vulnerable to the damaging effects of stress.[154] Neuropsychological tests show that reduced hippocampal volume is associated with cognitive and memory impairments in PTSD patients.[152,154] Functional neuroimaging studies in PTSD have found excessive activation of the amygdala and certain other brain areas in response to trauma-related stimuli.[153,158] Thus, the neurobiologic consequences of stress and trauma result in both structural and functional changes in the brain. Genetic factors also may play a role in influencing vulnerability to the damaging effects of stress.[158]

Treatment of PTSD

Both medications and CBTs are useful in treating PTSD. Non-pharmacologic therapies alone may be appropriate for initial treatment of mild PTSD cases, but pharmacotherapy, either alone or in combination with psychological therapies, is usually recommended for patients with moderate or severe illness.[148,152,159] When assessing various treatment options for PTSD, it is important to consider effects on all three core symptom clusters (re-experiencing/intrusive symptoms, avoidance/emotional numbing, hyperarousal symptoms). Not all PTSD treatments are effective for all of these major symptom domains.

The preferred first-line medications in PTSD are the SSRIs, but various other antidepressants may also be useful. Response to pharmacotherapy occurs very gradually, over 8 to 12 weeks or longer. Partial response at 12 weeks of treatment may be followed by full remission after several more months of therapy; therefore, an adequate time period should be allowed to fully determine response to a particular medication. However, lack of improvement after 4 weeks of therapy is unlikely to be effective with medication continuation, so alternate treatment strategies should be tried in these cases. Early treatment during the first 3 months that follow a trauma may prevent the development of chronic PTSD.[159]

Selective Serotonin Reuptake Inhibitors

Sertraline and paroxetine are currently the only FDA-approved medications for treating PTSD. Large controlled studies have demonstrated both of these agents are very effective and superior to placebo in reducing all three PTSD symptom clusters (re-experiencing, avoidance/numbing, and autonomic hyperarousal).[160–163] They also have beneficial effects on depression and general anxiety symptoms and have been associated with improvements in overall functioning as well as quality of life.[162,164] Fluoxetine also appears to be effective in treating PTSD in some patients, although study results have been mixed and a lack of significant effects on avoidance/numbing symptoms has been noted.[165–167] Male war veterans with longstanding combat-related PTSD have been noted to respond poorly to fluoxetine, compared with females and civilians, but this observation may apply to treatment of PTSD in general.[165,166] Citalopram and fluvoxamine have shown efficacy in the treatment of PTSD in open trials.[152]

Other Antidepressants

Several open studies and case reports suggest that nefazodone, mirtazapine, venlafaxine, and bupropion are also effective in treating the core symptoms of PTSD.[152,168–170] Although supporting evidence for these antidepressants is not as strong as for sertraline and paroxetine, they may be considered appropriate alternatives to the SSRIs in certain PTSD patients. The TCAs amitriptyline and imipramine and the MAO inhibitor phenelzine also have been found to be effective for PTSD in controlled trials, but these agents generally are not recommended because of their poor tolerability and safety profiles.[152,159] Because of the relatively high risk of suicide in PTSD, TCAs can be especially dangerous in this population. Trazodone has been beneficial in reducing PTSD symptoms in a small number of patients but is mainly used in low dosages (25 to 50 mg at bedtime) as a sedative agent in patients with sleep difficulties.[152]

Miscellaneous Agents

Various other medications have been used successfully in limited numbers of PTSD cases. The anticonvulsants carbamazepine, valproate, topiramate, tiagabine, gabapentin, oxcarbazepine, and lamotrigine have been reported to be markedly effective in certain patients and can be particularly useful for reducing irritability, impulsivity, and angry or violent outbursts.[171–174] Anticonvulsant therapy can also be effective for intrusive, re-experiencing, and hyperarousal symptoms. Atypical antipsychotic agents have been effectively used to treat PTSD-related psychotic symptoms (risperidone, clozapine, olanzapine) and sleep disturbances (olanzapine, quetiapine), but they do not appear to be useful for treating core PTSD symptoms.[159,175,176] The α_1-adrenergic antagonist, prazosin, was reported to decrease nightmares as well as other core symptoms in patients with combat-related PTSD.[177] Benzodiazepines are generally ineffective in treating PTSD, although they may be useful in managing sleep disturbances during the early weeks following trauma. Their use should be limited to short-term therapy in PTSD, as chronic use may have detrimental effects.[148,152]

Nonpharmacologic Treatments

Various types of psychosocial therapies have been used in the treatment of PTSD, including anxiety management training to help patients cope with stress, cognitive therapies, and exposure therapies.[152,159] Cognitive therapies seem to be most effective for symptoms of demoralization, guilt, and shame, whereas exposure therapies are better for reducing intrusive thoughts, flashbacks, and avoidance behaviors. Both cognitive and exposure therapies have been shown to be markedly and comparably effective in controlled PTSD trials, but exposure is probably more critical for optimal results.[152,159] Electroconvulsive therapy and the investigational procedure known as transcranial magnetic stimulation also have been effective in a small number of PTSD cases.[178]

Clinical Presentation of PTSD

24. **D.D. is a 42-year-old woman who was attacked and raped in the driveway of her home as she was getting out of her car 1 month ago. She did not seek medical treatment at the time and waited several days before reporting the incident to anyone, including her family. She presents to her physician complaining that she cannot sleep and that she is irritable, anxious, and depressed. When asked about any recent stressors in her life, she finally tells her doctor about the rape. D.D. has no history of psychiatric illness, admits that all of her symptoms have appeared since the attack, and says that she has never had any psychiatric problems until now. She states that she has nightly nightmares and becomes extremely anxious every time she comes home and gets out of her car at night (which she avoids doing when possible). She is startled when the phone rings or when someone approaches her unexpectedly, and she literally freezes if she sees a man who bears any physical resemblance to her attacker. D.D. also states that memories of the rape often flash through her mind for no reason, although she tries hard not to think about it. The assailant has not been caught, and D.D. feels extremely guilty for not promptly reporting the crime. Her symptoms are interfering significantly with her ability to work at her recep-**

tionist job and have put a strain on her marriage. **What clinical features of PTSD does D.D. display?**

Persons with PTSD often present with nonspecific complaints indicative of a generalized anxiety, depression, or substance use disorder. They may not realize or want to reveal an association between their symptoms and the trauma they have experienced. Careful evaluation by the clinician is required to elicit a pattern suggestive of PTSD. D.D. displays many target symptoms of PTSD, including re-experiencing (nightmares, recurrent memories), avoidance of the activity that reminds her of the trauma, and symptoms of increased arousal (sleep difficulties, irritability, exaggerated startle response). In addition, she is experiencing feelings of depression, distress, marital problems, and impairment in occupational functioning as a result of her symptoms. The lack of any previous psychiatric illness combined with the temporal relationship between the attack and her symptoms support the presence of PTSD as opposed to another anxiety or depressive disorder. Because her trauma occurred 1 month ago, her condition would be classified as acute-onset PTSD.

Treatment Selection and SSRI Dosing

25. **What factors are important in the selection of an initial treatment for D.D.?**

Because D.D. is exhibiting moderate to severe PTSD symptoms, pharmacotherapy is indicated. Medication treatment can also be combined with cognitive or behavioral therapies if they are available, but nonpharmacologic therapies alone are generally reserved for patients with mild symptoms. An SSRI is the preferred initial medication treatment for most PTSD patients.[157,159] Sertraline is an appropriate choice of treatment in this case and is FDA approved for PTSD. Low initial SSRI doses are recommended in PTSD, so sertraline can be started at 25 mg/day and gradually increased to the target dosage range of 100 to 150 mg/day, according to response and tolerability.[162,163] Regarding other SSRIs, studies suggest that a paroxetine dose of 20 mg/day is sufficient for most PTSD patients; higher doses have not been associated with better response.[160,161] In contrast, relatively high fluoxetine doses (40 to 60 mg/day) are usually required in PTSD, which may make this agent significantly more costly than treatment with either sertraline or paroxetine.[165] Persistent sleep complaints during the first month after a traumatic experience may predispose to chronic PTSD, so management of sleep disturbances is an important component of initial PTSD treatment.[152,179] Low-dose adjunctive trazodone (25 to 50 mg at bedtime) would be a good choice in this case because it is a safe, effective, and inexpensive sedative agent.

Even in the absence of formal CBTs, certain aspects of patient and family education are vital to the successful treatment of PTSD.[148,159] Providing information about the nature and treatability of PTSD and reassurance that many people experience similar reactions to trauma are important. The patient should be encouraged to talk with family and friends about the trauma, because repeated retelling of the traumatic event is therapeutic and can help facilitate recovery. Significant others need to understand the importance of listening and of being tolerant of the patient's emotional reaction and persistent preoccupation with his or her experience. Peer support groups are widely available and can be very beneficial in the recovery of trauma victims. Patients should be advised to try not to avoid things that remind them of the trauma, but rather to expose themselves to these situations as often as possible.

Clinical Assessment and Goals of Therapy

26. What are the goals of treatment in this case, and how can D.D.'s symptoms be objectively assessed?

The first goal of treatment of PTSD is to reduce the core symptoms of re-experiencing, avoidance, numbing, and hyperarousal. In D.D.'s case, these target symptoms include nightmares, intrusive memories, avoidance behaviors, irritability, startling easily, and sleep difficulties. Improvements should begin within the first 2 weeks and gradually continue over the course of 2 to 3 months. Secondary goals in this case include improving D.D.'s stress resilience, decreasing her work-and marriage-related disability, and improving her overall quality of life. Other general treatment goals in PTSD include decreasing detrimental behaviors (use of alcohol or substances, risky activities, violence) and treating any comorbid psychiatric conditions that may be present.

Several different rating scales have been developed to assess response to treatments in PTSD.[61] The most commonly used clinician-rated scales are the Clinician Administered PTSD Scale (CAPS) and the Treatment Outcome PTSD Scale (TOPS-8). CAPS is most often used in clinical PTSD trials, whereas TOPS-8 is shorter and easier to use in clinical practice. Patient-rated scales for evaluating PTSD symptoms include the Davidson Trauma Scale, and the Impact of Events Scale. The Sheehan Disability Scale is often used to assess functional impairment due to PTSD.

Course and Duration of Treatment

Good treatment response in PTSD is more likely to occur when treatment is begun within the first 3 months after the trauma.[152,159] There is no well established definition of response in PTSD, but a decrease in symptoms by 30% to 50%, along with substantial functional improvement, is commonly used in clinical trials. Full recovery during treatment of PTSD is fairly uncommon, and partial responders to either medication or psychosocial therapies may benefit from adding a trial of the other treatment modality. When an initial SSRI trial is ineffective, the patient may be switched to another SSRI or one of the other antidepressants that have been effectively used in PTSD.[159] Partial responders may benefit from the addition of a second medication, depending on which core symptoms predominate (see Pharmacotherapy of PTSD).

For patients who respond, treatment should be continued for an additional 6 to 12 months for acute cases (when symptoms were present <3 months before treatment) and 12 to 24 months for chronic cases (when symptoms lasted >3 months before treatment).[159] Long-term SSRI treatment can prevent relapse of PTSD, especially in those who show good response during the first 3 months of therapy.[164,165,180] When pharmacotherapy is discontinued, it should be withdrawn gradually over 1 to 3 months.

OBSESSIVE-COMPULSIVE DISORDER
Diagnostic Criteria

The DSM-IV criteria for OCD are presented in Table 76-14.[1] OCD is characterized by recurrent obsessions or compulsions, which are severe enough to be distressing, consume at least 1 hour a day, or significantly interfere with some aspect of functioning. An *obsession* is an intrusive or recurrent thought, image, or impulse that incites anxiety in the person and that cannot be ignored or suppressed voluntarily. The most common obsessions include germs and contamination; pathologic doubt; somatic concerns; need for order and symmetry; and religious, aggressive, or sexual thoughts.[181,182] A *compulsion* is a behavior or ritual that is performed in a repetitive or stereotypic way that is designed to reduce anxiety associated with obsessions or to prevent some future event or situation. However, the compulsions are not actually connected to the obsessions in any realistic way. Frequent compulsions include checking, cleaning, arranging symmetrically, ordering, hoarding, counting, and needing to ask questions or confess.[182] The obsessions and compulsions are unpleasant and disturbing to the sufferer and are not associated with pleasure or gratification. This feature distinguishes OCD from certain other detrimental behaviors (excessive gambling or shopping), which are often described as being "compulsive." Adults with OCD usually realize that their rituals are senseless and excessive at some point, but children may not make this distinction.[1]

OCD is a clinically heterogeneous disorder involving a wide range of symptoms. Five separate OCD symptom di-

---

Table 76-14 Diagnostic Criteria for OCD

A. The presence of either obsessions or compulsions:
   Obsessions:
   1. Recurrent and persistent ideas or thoughts are experienced, at some time during the disturbance, as intrusive and senseless
   2. The thoughts, impulses, or images are not simply excessive worries about real-life problems
   3. The person attempts to ignore or neutralize the ideas or thoughts with some other thought or action
   4. The person realizes the obsessions are the product of his or her own mind
   Compulsions:
   1. Repetitive and intentional behaviors or mental acts are performed in response to the obsession or according to rigid rules
   2. The behavior is designed to prevent or reduce distress or to prevent some dreaded event; however, the activity clearly is excessive and unrealistic to neutralize the situation
B. At some point during the disturbance, the person realizes that the obsessions and compulsions are excessive or unreasonable (not necessary in children)
C. The obsessions or compulsions cause marked distress, are time-consuming (>1 hr/day), or significantly interfere with some aspect of daily functioning
D. The content of the symptoms is not related to another psychiatric disorder, and the disturbance is not due to the direct effects of a substance, medication, or general medical illness

OCD, obsessive-compulsive disorder.
Adapted from Reference 1.

mensions have been defined: symmetry obsessions and repeating, counting, and ordering compulsions; contamination obsessions and cleaning compulsions; hoarding obsessions and compulsions; aggressive obsessions and checking compulsions; and sexual/religious obsessions and related compulsions. Although specific symptoms in an individual may change over time, they usually remain within the same dimension.[182] Hoarding and sexual/religious obsessions and compulsions appear to be less responsive to treatment than other types of symptoms.[183]

Epidemiology and Clinical Course

OCD once was thought to be a rare disorder, but epidemiologic studies reveal that it affects between 2% and 3% of the worldwide population.[1,184] The overall lifetime prevalence is slightly higher in women, but men tend to have an earlier onset of illness (between ages 6 and 15) than women (between ages 20 and 29).[1,27,184] Many patients report having mild symptoms for years before full OCD emerges, and an estimated one-third to one-half of patients have onset during childhood or adolescence. Prepubertal OCD is three times more common in boys than in girls.[27] Women with OCD often have worsening of symptoms during the premenstrual and postpartum periods, and onset or worsening of OCD during pregnancy appears to be fairly common.[94] Regardless of gender, the severity of illness usually worsens during stressful life periods.

The course and severity of OCD are highly variable and unpredictable, with some persons only mildly or intermittently affected and others suffering severely and constantly throughout their lifetime. The natural course of untreated OCD was followed for a 40-year period in a group of 144 patients.[185] Although 83% of patients were improved at the end of the follow-up period, only 20% experienced full remission. Two-thirds of patients continued to have some OCD symptoms, and a progressive deterioration was observed in 10%. Observational studies suggest that the long-term course of OCD may be improved substantially with appropriate treatment.[186,187] However, a portion of sufferers still experience a chronic and lifelong course.

It is no surprise that OCD can have seriously detrimental effects on functional abilities and quality of life. In large-scale surveys, OCD patients report that their symptoms significantly interfere with their abilities to socialize, study, work, make friends, and maintain good relationships with family and friends.[188] It is estimated that each person with OCD loses an average of 3 years' wages over his or her lifetime.[188] Quality-of-life ratings in OCD patients indicate marked impairments and are similar to those observed in patients with depression. Fortunately, treatment of OCD can be accompanied by significant improvements in quality of life and functional abilities.

Although several effective treatments are currently available for OCD, most patients do not seek treatment until the disorder is seriously affecting their lives. One study found that OCD patients waited an average of 7.5 years after the onset of OCD before seeking medical evaluation for their disorder.[188] This may be because most OCD patients realize that their symptoms are senseless, so they attempt to hide their disorder due to embarrassment. People with OCD often carry out their rituals in secret and may be very successful at concealing their symptoms from others. Initial treatment for OCD is commonly sought outside psychiatric settings, and the obsessive-compulsive symptoms are often missed.

Increased recognition that OCD is a biologic disorder for which effective treatments are available is needed among the general public as well as health care professionals. Four simple questions are recommended for screening for potential OCD[181]: Do you have to wash your hands over and over? Do you have to check things repeatedly? Do you have recurrent distressing thoughts that you cannot get rid of? Do you have to complete actions again and again or in a certain way? Clinicians in a variety of health care settings can incorporate these screening questions into their practice to use when possible signs of OCD are present. Health care providers should be prepared to provide education about the nature and treatability of OCD to suspected sufferers and to make appropriate treatment referrals in these cases.

Psychiatric Comorbidity and Obsessive-Compulsive Spectrum Disorders

As with other anxiety disorders, OCD often is accompanied by psychiatric comorbidity. Two-thirds of those with OCD develop major depression during their lifetime.[1,182] There is a higher-than-expected overlap of OCD with disorders such as specific and social phobias, GAD, panic disorder, schizophrenia, schizoaffective disorder, bipolar disorder, and eating disorders.[182] Identification of comorbid conditions with OCD is important because it can influence choice of treatments. Obsessive-compulsive personality disorder, which is classified as an Axis II disorder, occurs in a small percentage of OCD patients. Despite their name similarities, obsessive-compulsive personality disorder does not involve true obsessions and compulsions (which are senseless and distressing to the sufferer). Rather, it is a personality pattern characterized by rigid and inflexible preoccupation with rules, lists, order, and perfectionism.[1] Although these personality traits cause problems, the person with the personality disorder does not view his or her behavior as abnormal or unreasonable.

The relation between tic disorders and OCD is particularly striking. Tics occur in 20% to 30% of OCD patients and 5% to 7% have full Tourette's syndrome, whereas 35% to 50% of Tourette's patients exhibit OCD symptoms.[182] Individuals with OCD plus Tourette's syndrome are thought to represent a genetically and pathophysiologically distinct subtype of illness.[189] These patients are more likely to be male and tend to have an earlier age at OCD onset (before age 10), more severe symptoms, and poorer response to SSRIs than those with OCD alone.[190]

Another childhood neurologic disorder commonly associated with OCD is Sydenham's chorea. This is the neurologic variant of rheumatic fever, which is an autoimmune disease triggered by infection with group A β-hemolytic streptococcal pharyngitis. Recent reports describe children who developed sudden and severe tics and obsessive-compulsive symptoms after strep throat infections.[191,192] This condition is designated in the medical literature by the acronym PANDAS (pediatric autoimmune neuropsychiatric disorders associated with streptococcal infection), and it has been rapidly reversed by antibiotic or IV immunoglobulin treatment. The possibility of a PANDAS correlation should be considered in any child who develops abrupt onset of obsessive-compulsive symptoms, particularly those who have had pharyngitis within the past 6 months.

The term obsessive-compulsive spectrum disorder refers to a diverse collection of psychiatric conditions from various DSM-IV categories that have overlapping characteristics with OCD and involve recurrent or distressing thoughts and/or irresistible or repetitive behaviors.[193] These include somatoform disorders (body dysmorphic disorder, hypochondriasis), eating disorders (anorexia nervosa, bulimia nervosa, binge-eating disorder) and impulse control disorders (trichotillomania, pathologic gambling, compulsive nail biting, kleptomania, compulsive buying). Tourette's syndrome and autism are also often included in this spectrum of disorders. Some of these disorders, such as body dysmorphic disorder, have much higher comorbidities with OCD than others. Like OCD, many patients with these conditions have shown good response to treatment with serotonergic antidepressants such as clomipramine and SSRIs, sometimes preferentially over agents with mainly noradrenergic activity.[193] Examples include body dysmorphic disorder (preoccupation with an imagined or slight defect in appearance), compulsive buying, pathologic gambling, trichotillomania (recurrent impulses to pull out one's hair), binge-eating disorder, and bulimia nervosa.[193]

Etiology and Pathophysiology

A wealth of research has attempted to identify a specific biologic explanation for OCD. Because OCD displays such clinical heterogeneity, there may be several distinct etiologies for different subtypes of illness. One leading hypothesis has been that of serotonergic dysfunction, which is supported by the finding that the only effective medication treatments for OCD mainly influence serotonergic transmission.[194] However, the multitude of studies involving serotonergic challenges and other methods for assessing central serotonergic function in OCD have resulted in no conclusive answers, and the exact role of serotonin underlying OCD still has not been determined. It is interesting that naturally occurring animal models of OCD have been observed in dogs (canine acral lick) and birds (feather-picking disorder), and these conditions have been treated successfully with serotonin reuptake inhibitors.

More promising areas of OCD research involve functional brain imaging studies.[194] These techniques are used to assess regional metabolic activity in different areas of the brain. Studies in OCD patients have resulted in fairly consistent findings of abnormal hyperactivity (when compared with normal controls) in certain frontal lobe and basal ganglia regions, specifically the orbital frontal cortex, cingulate cortex, and head of the caudate nucleus.[194,195] Within individuals, the abnormal activation in these brain areas increases significantly during provocation of OCD symptoms, compared with what happens during nonprovoked or resting states.[195] Interestingly, these regional brain metabolic abnormalities normalize after successful treatment of OCD, and certain brain metabolism patterns may be associated with preferential response to SSRI versus CBTs.[194,196] These findings have led to one current hypothesis that OCD is

a neurologic disorder characterized by a hyperfunctioning circuit involving the aforementioned brain regions. In support, neurosurgical techniques that interrupt this circuit often are effective in the treatment of OCD. The mechanism of efficacy of the SSRIs for OCD may be related to desensitization of terminal serotonin autoreceptors in the orbitofrontal cortex, which enhances serotonin neurotransmission in this brain region.[194,195] Structural abnormalities also have been identified in OCD, including increased brain cortex and opercular volumes, decreased total white matter, and smaller pituitary gland size.[181,194] Specific types of cognitive dysfunction also have been found in OCD patients, including problems with nonverbal memory, visuospatial skills, and visual attention.[194] Impairments in memory functioning have been correlated with the aforementioned structural abnormalities in OCD.

In addition to biologic factors, twin and family studies provide evidence that genetic influences also are involved in the etiology of OCD.[31] Heredity appears to be most important in early-onset OCD cases (before age 18), because familial aggregation has not been observed in OCD cases with a later age at onset.[197] Several studies suggest an association between OCD and specific polymorphisms in the serotonin transporter, $5HT_{1D\beta}$ and $5HT_{2A}$ receptor genes, but others have failed to replicate these findings.[13,198] Other candidate gene research studies have linked OCD with functional polymorphisms in the cathechol O-methyltransferase and dopamine D4 receptor genes.[198]

Treatment of Obsessive-Compulsive Disorder

Both medications and behavioral therapies are effective in the treatment of OCD. Behavioral therapy is vitally important for OCD, and the combination of drugs plus behavioral therapy provides optimal treatment. All medications consistently effective in the treatment of OCD are potent inhibitors of serotonin reuptake. These include clomipramine, which is a TCA, and SSRIs: fluvoxamine, fluoxetine, paroxetine, and sertraline. All five of these medications are FDA approved for the treatment of OCD in adults, and all except paroxetine are indicated for use in children with OCD.

Clomipramine

Clomipramine was the first drug with proven efficacy in treating OCD, and it was considered the standard first-line treatment for several years until the SSRIs gained popularity. Many large well-controlled studies have documented that clomipramine is far superior to placebo and significantly improves OCD symptoms in approximately 60% to 70% of patients.[199–202] Although clomipramine is a TCA and differs structurally from imipramine by only a C-3 substituted chlorine group, it is unique among TCAs in its effectiveness for OCD. This distinct property is attributed to its more potent effects on serotonin reuptake inhibition compared with other TCAs. Clomipramine is often referred to as an SRI (serotonin reuptake inhibitor), not an SSRI (*selective* serotonin reuptake inhibitor) because its major active metabolite, desmethylclomipramine, is a potent inhibitor of norepinephrine reuptake. Clomipramine also blocks adrenergic, histaminergic, and cholinergic receptors similarly to other TCAs, resulting in an adverse effect profile similar to that of imipramine (see Chapter 79, Mood Disorders I: Major Depressive Disorders).

Although direct comparison studies have shown clomipramine to be similar in efficacy to various SSRIs in treating OCD, several meta-analyses have concluded that clomipramine is superior to SSRIs overall.[201–203] However, clomipramine is less well tolerated than SSRIs, and patients are more likely to discontinue clomipramine treatment because of side effects. Therefore, clomipramine is currently reserved as a second-line treatment option in OCD patients who do not respond adequately to SSRI therapy.[199,204] Details about the clinical use of clomipramine are discussed in Questions 32 through 34.

Selective Serotonin Reuptake Inhibitors

SSRIs are the only first-line medication treatments for OCD. Double-blind, placebo-controlled studies have documented the efficacies of fluvoxamine, fluoxetine, paroxetine, and sertraline in the treatment of OCD.[201,202,205–209] Citalopram and escitalopram also are likely to be effective, based on their SSRI activity, but there is limited information to support their use. There is no strong evidence that any one SSRI is more effective than the others in treating OCD, but some patients may respond to or tolerate one agent better than another.[43] The only controlled study to directly compare two different SSRIs in OCD found sertraline to be superior to fluoxetine in both response and remission rates, although both agents were significantly effective.[210] Usual SSRI starting dosages can be used in OCD, but at least 4 weeks should be allowed before exceeding the targeted minimally effective dosages (fluvoxamine 150 mg/day, fluoxetine 20 mg/day, paroxetine 40 mg/day, and sertraline 50 mg/day). Details about the clinical use of SSRIs in OCD are discussed in Questions 28 through 31.

Miscellaneous Agents and Augmentation Strategies

A wide variety of other medications have been tried in the treatment of OCD, with varying degrees of success. One controlled study supports results from previous open reports that venlafaxine can be very effective in the treatment of OCD.[211] Because venlafaxine is a potent inhibitor of both serotonin and norepinephrine reuptake, it may be viewed as being similar to clomipramine in mechanistic terms, but without the unwanted effects on cholinergic, α-adrenergic, or histamine receptors. The recent trial comparing venlafaxine with clomipramine in OCD found these agents to be comparably effective overall, but venlafaxine was better tolerated.[211] Preliminary results are available from another controlled study which found venlafaxine to be effective in 3 of 8 patients who had failed to respond to two previous SSRI trials.[204] Based on these findings, venlafaxine can be a reasonable choice for OCD patients who do not respond to first-line therapy.

Other than venlafaxine, none of the other miscellaneous agents studied in OCD have demonstrated impressive efficacy as monotherapy. However, several appear to be useful as augmentation therapy to boost response to SSRIs or clomipramine in partial responders to these agents.[204] The combination of an SSRI plus clomipramine is one such option for patients who show partial response, although attention must be paid to the potential drug interaction, which may lead to clomipramine toxicity (see Question 34).

Antipsychotic agents are among the most useful of the augmentation agents that have been examined in OCD. They may be particularly effective in patients with comorbid tic disorders, although recent reports suggest they can be equally effective in OCD patients without tics. Older typical antipsychotics, such as haloperidol and pimozide, have shown good efficacy in augmenting response to fluvoxamine in controlled trials (conducted before the dangerous interaction between pimozide and CYP 3A4 inhibitors such as fluvoxamine was identified). Recent reports have focused on newer atypical antipsychotics, since these agents are generally preferred over typical antipsychotics and are better tolerated.[199,204] Risperidone (2 to 4 mg/day), olanzapine (10 to 20 mg/day), and quetiapine (200 mg/day) have all been used successfully in treatment-resistant OCD to augment response to SSRIs, and their efficacy does not depend on the presence of tics.[204,212,213] It is interesting to note that atypical antipsychotics (risperidone, clozapine, olanzapine) have been reported to cause or worsen obsessive-compulsive symptoms in schizophrenic patients in a number of cases.[204] This effect is thought to be due to the antipsychotics' serotonin type-2 receptor antagonistic activity. When SSRI–antipsychotic combinations are used, attention must be paid to potential drug interactions between certain agents that may increase antipsychotic plasma levels and side effects, particularly extrapyramidal symptoms. Pimozide should not be used in combination with clomipramine, fluoxetine, sertraline, or fluvoxamine because of the potential for cardiac QT interval prolongation.

Pindolol is the only other augmenting agent for which efficacy is supported by a placebo-controlled study.[214] This trial involved treatment-resistant OCD patients and found pindolol (2.5 mg TID) to be most beneficial in patients who had shown partial response to SSRI therapy. Buspirone has been studied both as monotherapy and as augmentation therapy for OCD.[199] There are mixed findings regarding its efficacy, but controlled studies have been largely negative. Certain patients may benefit from relatively high buspirone doses (30 to 60 mg/day) as augmentation therapy. Case reports and open studies have reported other agents such as trazodone, L-triiodothyronine, gabapentin, clonidine, and lithium to be useful for augmenting response to SSRIs. However, controlled studies have demonstrated these agents to be ineffective.[199,204]

Benzodiazepines are generally not beneficial in treating OCD, although there are several reports of clonazepam being effective as adjunctive therapy or monotherapy.[199,204] Clonazepam appears to have serotonergic effects, which may explain its potential usefulness in OCD. This agent may be helpful in patients with prominent anxiety symptoms, but can also interfere with the effectiveness of CBT and should not be used concurrently. As discussed, fluvoxamine and fluoxetine can significantly increase serum levels of clonazepam.

The MAO inhibitor, phenelzine, was one of the first medications studied for OCD. Early case reports of its use were favorable, but more recent findings suggest that phenelzine is largely ineffective for OCD.[199,215] Although not available in the United States, several reports indicate that IV clomipramine can be rapidly effective in OCD patients who are nonresponsive to oral medications, including oral clomipramine.[199] A variety of other medications are reportedly effective in small numbers of cases of treatment-refractory OCD. These include tramadol, morphine, valproate, antiandrogen agents (cyproterone acetate, aminoglutethimide, triptorelin), and inositol.[199,204] Controlled trials are needed before any of these can be recommended, however.

Nonpharmacologic Treatments

COGNITIVE-BEHAVIORAL THERAPIES

CBT is an extremely important component of treatment for OCD and should be incorporated into the initial treatment plan whenever possible. CBT alone may be appropriate for mild OCD or in cases in which it is desirable to avoid medication (e.g., pregnancy, medical conditions). The combination of CBT and medication is generally superior to either treatment approach used alone.[181,216] Treatment gains achieved with CBT often are maintained long after its discontinuation, which is an advantage over pharmacotherapy.[181]

The cognitive therapy component of CBT is aimed toward changing the detrimental thought patterns in OCD and is most helpful for obsessions such as scrupulosity, moral guilt, and pathologic doubt. The behavioral therapy aspect, called exposure plus response prevention, involves exposure to feared objects or situations followed by prevention of the usual compulsive response. This type of therapy is most beneficial for patients with contamination fears, hoarding, and rituals involving symmetry, counting, or repeating. Because exposure plus response prevention is anxiety provoking and can be very distressing, many patients refuse to participate in it. Another barrier to its use is that trained cognitive-behavioral therapists are not always available. However, patients who do not have access to formal CBT can learn to carry out their own exposure therapy with the help of self-instructional manuals and computer-assisted programs that have been developed by leading medical experts in the field of OCD.[217]

NEUROSURGERY

Neurosurgical treatment of OCD has been practiced since the 1950s and is considered an option of last resort in treatment-refractory patients. Cingulotomy and capsulotomy are the most commonly used procedures. Indications for neurosurgery include OCD patients who are severely disabled from their obsessive-compulsive symptoms and who have failed on various treatments (drugs and behavioral therapies) that have been tried systematically for at least 5 years.[218] Reported success rates of neurosurgery in OCD range from 40% to 90% and complications, including potential infections, personality changes, cognitive impairment, and epilepsy, appear to be rare. A recent, long-term, follow-up study of patients who underwent neurosurgery during the 1970s found that therapeutic effects were maintained but that patients exhibited mild to moderate impairments in neuropsychological performance.[218] Permanent cognitive sequelae from neurosurgery may be more common than previously realized. A new neurosurgical procedure using an instrument called the gamma knife (anterior gamma capsulotomy) is being studied for treatment-refractory OCD. Preliminary results suggest good efficacy with improved short-and long-term safety compared with traditional neurosurgical techniques.[204]

Defining Response to Therapy

Response to medication treatment in OCD is gradual and often delayed. Initial improvements usually begin to appear within the first month, but maximal response may take as long as 5 to 6 months. An adequate period to assess response at lower medication dosages should be allowed before increasing to possibly unnecessary higher dosages. Patients who show unsatisfactory response to lower SSRI dosages by weeks 4 to 9 should have their dosages gradually increased to the manufacturer's recommended maximum, if necessary (see Question 28). A trial of 8 to 12 weeks at maximum medication dosages is recommended before determining response to a particular medication.

The primary goal of treatment in OCD is to decrease obsessions and compulsions to a level at which the person is able to function normally. Complete elimination of symptoms is rare with currently available treatments.[182] Most clinical trials in OCD define clinical response as a 25% to 35% reduction in Yale-Brown Obsessive-Compulsive Symptom Checklist (Y-BOCS) scores (see Question 27). Therefore, even those classified as responders may be left with 65% to 75% of their original symptoms, and this may or may not result in significant improvements in functioning or quality of life.

Strategies for Managing Partial Response and Nonresponse

Current estimates are that 60% to 70% of patients show at least moderate improvements in obsessive-compulsive symptoms during an initial (SSRI or clomipramine) medication trial, but only 10% exhibit marked response.[199] The remaining 20% to 30% derive minimal or no benefit from an initial trial and require further tactics. Approximately 20% of those who fail a first SSRI trial subsequently respond to another agent in this class; therefore, switching to a second SSRI is usually recommended as the next step before initiating a trial of clomipramine.[181] However, clomipramine can be extremely effective in SSRI nonresponders and it remains a useful treatment option despite its clinical disadvantages.

Partial responders to an initial SSRI trial may be better served by addition of one of the augmentation agents discussed in the previous section than by switching to a new medication. Also, inclusion of CBTs is important for optimizing treatment with any medication. Neurosurgery is an option for severe treatment-refractory cases. Predictors of poor response to treatment in OCD include poor insight, hoarding or sexual/religious dimension symptoms, prepubertal onset of illness, and presence of comorbid personality, mood, or eating disorders.

Clinical Presentation and Assessment

27. **R.G. is a 25-year-old woman whose husband complains that she spends 1.5 hours a day cleaning the stove and takes four showers each day. The unusual behavior began about 1 year ago after the birth of their son but has continued to worsen, and R.G.'s husband states that he cannot deal with her "odd habits" any more. R.G. recently lost her job as a secretary because of tardiness (it took her 3 hours to get ready for work) and spending too much time away from her desk in the ladies' room. R.G. admits that it is silly, but she has irresistible urges to make sure that both she and her surroundings are completely free of germs so that her child will not get sick. She also confines herself to one floor of their three-level house because she is afraid that she will fall down the stairs while carrying her son. R.G. also states that she constantly has "what if" thoughts about horrible things happening to her family, which are very disturbing. The physician's diagnosis is OCD. What clinical features of OCD does R.G. display, and how can her symptoms be objectively evaluated?**

R.G. displays many characteristic symptoms of OCD. The most commonly encountered clinical presentation of OCD involves patients with excessive fear of contamination with dirt, germs, or toxins, who repeatedly wash their hands or clean objects or their surroundings. These persons also typically avoid touching possibly dirty objects (e.g., doorknobs, money) or shaking hands with people. Another common clinical presentation is the OCD patient with pathologic doubt who constantly worries that something bad will happen because of his or her negligence. These people are afraid that they have failed to lock the door, turn off the stove, shut the refrigerator door, or secure the medicine cabinet from children. As a result, they continuously check and recheck their actions.

R.G. displays obsessions of contamination and pathologic doubt, and compulsions of excessive cleaning and washing. These symptoms are time-consuming, cause significant distress, and have led to her unemployment and marital difficulties. As seen in this case, most persons present with a mixture of various obsessions and compulsions. R.G. also realizes that her thoughts and behaviors are "silly," which most often is the case in OCD. This case also illustrates the onset of OCD during times of stressful or significant life events. Pregnancy, death of a relative, and marital discord have been identified as precipitating factors in the onset of OCD.[182,184]

The aforementioned Y-BOCS is a useful tool in the initial evaluation of those who present with symptoms of OCD and may be used in the objective assessment of R.G.'s symptoms. The Y-BOCS is a 10-item scale with a maximum possible score of 40; a score of >15 generally is considered to represent clinically significant obsessive-compulsive symptoms.[199] This scale is a standard tool for evaluating drug efficacy in OCD clinical trials and often is used in clinical practice to assess response to treatments. Other OCD assessment instruments include the National Institute of Mental Health Obsessive-Compulsive Scale, the Leyton Obsessional Inventory, and the self-rated Maudsley Obsessional-Compulsive Inventory. Special versions for use in children have been developed for the Y-BOCS and the Leyton Obsessional Inventory.

SSRI Treatment of OCD
SSRI Selection and Dosing

28. **Upon assessment, R.G.'s Y-BOCS score is found to be 33. Her physician prescribes fluvoxamine and instructs R.G. to take 100 mg Q AM for 1 week and then 200 mg Q AM thereafter. He also refers R.G. to a psychologist to receive CBT. Is this initial choice of therapy appropriate?**

SSRIs such as fluvoxamine are considered the best choice of initial pharmacotherapy for OCD. The primary differences between SSRIs involve pharmacokinetic properties and potential for drug interactions (see Chapter 79). Because there are no overall differences in efficacy among the four SSRIs approved for OCD, fluvoxamine is a suitable selection for R.G. However, the prescribed dosing instructions for R.G. are not appropriate. The initial recommended dosage for fluvoxamine in adults is 50 mg/day (25 mg in children), and it is best taken in the evening because it tends to be sedating. Thereafter, the dosage can be increased by 50-mg increments every 3 to 4 days according to patient tolerability, up to the initial targeted effective dose of 150 to 200 mg/day. Daily doses exceeding 100 mg should be given in two divided doses, based on fluvoxamine's elimination half-life of approximately 15 hours. A controlled-release fluvoxamine formulation that can be dosed once daily is under investigation.[219] This product has been reported to be better tolerated than regular fluvoxamine and possibly associated with a faster onset of therapeutic effects.

The optimal target dose of fluvoxamine in OCD has not been absolutely defined because no fixed-dose studies are available. In contrast, fixed-dose controlled trials have determined the minimum effective target doses for other SSRIs. For example, one study involving fluoxetine revealed no overall differences in efficacy between dosages of 20, 40, and 60 mg/day at study endpoint; however, patients taking the higher daily dosages experienced more adverse effects.[206] Although an earlier fluoxetine study found 40 mg and 60 mg doses to be more effective than 20 mg/day, this study only lasted 8 weeks so it is difficult to assess true differences in response. These findings are important because it was previously believed that fluoxetine dosages in the range of 60 to 80 mg/day were required for efficacy in OCD. Therefore, an adequate trial with 20 mg/day should be allowed before increasing the fluoxetine dose in OCD. Similar studies have determined the initial recommended target dosages for sertraline and paroxetine to be 50 and 40 mg/day, respectively. Using higher-than-necessary dosages can increase both adverse effects and medication costs, and these factors can lead to early termination of therapy.

Adjunctive Cognitive-Behavioral Therapy

The decision to include CBT in R.G.'s treatment plan is highly appropriate. The overall efficacy of these nonpharmacologic treatments is estimated to be 50% to 70% when used alone, and their use to complement pharmacotherapy is considered vital.[181] R.G.'s Y-BOCS score of 33 indicates a moderate to severe symptom severity, which provides further support for using a combined treatment approach. For R.G., exposure plus response prevention therapy might involve covering her hands with dirt and not allowing her to wash them for a certain time period. These behavioral techniques cause extreme anxiety and discomfort, which often lead to dropout from therapy or noncompliance with "homework assignments" (which involve continuation of the therapy principles outside the clinical setting), but are highly effective if the patient can adhere to treatment.

SSRI Adverse Effects and Patient Counseling

29. **What patient counseling information should be provided to R.G. in conjunction with the prescribed treatments?**

All OCD patients beginning treatment should be counseled that the medications do not work right away, that response occurs gradually, and that it may take several weeks before beneficial effects become noticeable. It is important to emphasize that maximum response may take 3 months or longer and that complete elimination of all symptoms is unlikely. It also is helpful to point out that a variety of other medication treatment options exist for those who do not respond adequately to an initial trial.

R.G. should be educated about possible fluvoxamine side effects, including nausea, sedation or insomnia, and headache. Medication should be taken with food to decrease these effects. Side effects are most common during the initial weeks of therapy, are usually dose related and often subside with continued treatment. Other aspects of SSRI therapy, including additional adverse effects and their management and drug–drug interactions, are discussed in Chapter 79. Patients should be encouraged to report any problems to their treatment provider. The importance of adhering to prescribed therapies, both pharmacologic and behavioral, also should be stressed.

30. **After 4 weeks, R.G. is taking fluvoxamine 200 mg QD and tolerating the medication well. She complains that she has not noticed much improvement and her Y-BOCS score is slightly decreased, at 30. R.G. has been to the cognitive-behavioral therapist twice but does not want to return because the therapy was so stressful. R.G. requests to be switched to another, more effective medication, and she also asks to be given some Xanax to help calm her anxiety during behavioral therapy sessions. What is the best course of action for R.G. at this point?**

Switching to another medication is not recommended at this point because not enough time has elapsed to assess fluvoxamine's efficacy. R.G. is tolerating fluvoxamine well and has shown a mild improvement, so this medication should be continued for at least another 4 weeks. Additional counseling information should be provided to R.G. to emphasize the gradual response to treatment in OCD. An increase in fluvoxamine dosage, up to 250 or 300 mg/day, may be considered after several more weeks, because some patients may respond better to higher dosages. If R.G.'s symptoms continue to cause significant functional impairment after 10 to 12 weeks of higher-dose fluvoxamine therapy, a change in treatment (e.g., switching to another SSRI or augmentation therapy) will be indicated.

R.G. should be encouraged to continue CBT to optimize the chance for successful treatment. An anxiety response is integral to the therapeutic benefits of behavioral therapies; since benzodiazepines can blunt this response, they may reduce their efficacy. Therefore, alprazolam should be avoided, and a temporary reduction in the intensity of behavioral therapy may be indicated instead. Fluvoxamine also can inhibit the CYP 3A4–mediated metabolism of alprazolam, resulting in more pronounced effects from a given dose.

Course and Duration of Therapy

31. **After 5 months of treatment, R.G. is happy to report that her OCD is much improved (Y-BOCS score of 11). She still has intermittent obsessions related to contamination and doubting, but they are less intense than before. She usually is able to resist urges to clean and wash excessively and is using the stairs in their home with only mild discomfort. Her previous employer has agreed to let her return to her secretarial position when she is ready and she plans to do so soon. R.G.'s husband is extremely pleased with her progress. Their primary question at this visit is whether treatment can be discontinued now because R.G. is doing so well. What recommendations should be provided regarding the long-term course of therapy for R.G.?**

This case illustrates a common outcome of OCD treatment, in which some symptoms persist (as evidenced by a Y-BOCS score of 11), but significant improvements in functioning occur. It is currently recommended that effective treatment for OCD be continued for at least 1 year after re-

sponse to reduce the risk of relapse. The effectiveness of maintenance pharmacotherapy in preventing relapse of OCD is well documented.[186,199] Therefore, continued drug treatment for at least 7 more months is indicated for R.G. Results from several studies suggest that decreased medication doses (with SSRIs and clomipramine) during maintenance therapy are comparably effective as full doses in preventing relapse.[199] If R.G. were experiencing any fluvoxamine-related problems, a decrease to the minimally effective dose (150 mg/day) during maintenance therapy might be recommended.

After a 1-year maintenance period, discontinuation of medication may be considered by carefully weighing the possible risks and benefits. When medication therapy for OCD is withdrawn, the dosage should be gradually decreased by approximately 25% every 1 to 2 months. Continuous monitoring for signs of relapse is required during this period. Gradual discontinuation also lessens the chance of the withdrawal syndrome that often occurs following abrupt discontinuation of SSRI or TCA therapy (see Chapter 79). Long-term or even lifelong maintenance pharmacotherapy usually is recommended after two to four severe relapses or three to four less-severe relapses.

Clomipramine Treatment
Dosing Guidelines

32. **K.T. is an 18-year-old Asian man who was diagnosed with OCD 2 years ago and also suffers from mild depression. His physician plans to start him on clomipramine therapy because he has failed previous trials with paroxetine and fluvoxamine. Is clomipramine an appropriate choice of therapy for this patient? What recommendations can be made regarding initiation of clomipramine treatment?**

Current guidelines recommend that clomipramine be reserved for OCD patients who fail at least two SSRI trials; therefore, its choice for this patient is appropriate. One precaution relevant to this case is that clomipramine, like other TCAs, is highly dangerous in overdose situations. Because K.T. is depressed, he should be evaluated carefully for any suicidal thoughts before starting clomipramine. If suicidal ideation is detected, it would be better to try another SSRI. This case also illustrates the common comorbidity of depression with OCD. Fortunately, most effective treatments for OCD fall into the antidepressant category, and drug treatment can be beneficial for both conditions. Nevertheless, the responses of depression and OCD to treatment are independent of one another so that depression may respond completely to a certain medication while OCD symptoms persist.[199]

Clomipramine should be initiated at a low dosage of 25 to 50 mg/day administered with meals. Divided daily doses are sometimes used initially to minimize side effects, but the total daily dose can be given at bedtime after dose titration. The pharmacokinetic parameters of clomipramine are comparable to other TCAs. Its average elimination half-life of 36 to 39 hours makes once-daily dosing appropriate.[220]

The clomipramine dosage should be increased to an initial target range of 150 to 200 mg/day over 2 to 4 weeks, guided by patient tolerability. The maximum recommended daily dosage of clomipramine is 250 mg/day because of the sharply increased risk of seizures (2.1% to 3.4%) with higher dosages as compared with the risk with dosages <250 mg/day (0.24% to

0.48%).[220] Longer duration of clomipramine therapy also may increase the risk of seizures. Clomipramine should be used with caution in persons with a history of seizures, head injury, or any other factors that might lower the seizure threshold.

Clomipramine Side Effects and Monitoring Guidelines

33. **What guidelines should be recommended for monitoring the outcomes (both therapeutic and adverse) of clomipramine therapy?**

Clomipramine is less well tolerated than the SSRIs and can cause a number of significant adverse effects, especially during the first few weeks of therapy. The most common side effects, reported in more than half of those taking clomipramine, include sedation, dry mouth, dizziness, and tremor.[220] Constipation, nausea, blurred vision, insomnia, and headache also occur frequently. K.T. should be advised that these are not serious effects and usually subside with continued treatment.

Many patients receiving long-term clomipramine (and other TCA) therapy gain substantial amounts of weight. As with the SSRIs, sexual dysfunction can be a problem in both men and women. In men, clomipramine can cause ejaculation abnormalities, which can impair fertility. Patients taking clomipramine also should be counseled about the additive CNS depressant effects with alcohol and to be cautious about the possible sedative effects while driving or performing other potentially hazardous activities.

As with other TCAs, an ECG should be performed before starting clomipramine in individuals at risk for heart disease and in pediatric patients. Elevations in liver enzymes have been observed frequently during the first 3 months of clomipramine treatment, and baseline liver function tests also should be obtained before initiating treatment. The liver enzyme changes are reversible upon discontinuation of clomipramine therapy.

No therapeutic range for plasma drug concentrations has been firmly established for clomipramine in OCD, but monitoring plasma levels may be clinically useful in certain patients to guide dosing and/or minimize drug toxicity. Clomipramine metabolism is highly variable from one person to the next, and it is difficult to accurately predict the resulting clomipramine level from any given dose. The initial hepatic metabolism of tertiary TCAs such as clomipramine involves demethylation through various isozymes, including CYP 1A2, CYP 2C19, and CYP 3A4.[221] The primary active metabolite (N-desmethylclomipramine) then undergoes CYP 2D6–mediated hydroxylation.

Although various studies have failed to find a correlation between clomipramine plasma level and clinical response, the ratio of clomipramine to N-desmethylclomipramine may be important.[222] Clomipramine is primarily serotonergic, whereas N-desmethylclomipramine is more noradrenergic; higher levels of N-desmethylclomipramine relative to clomipramine have been associated with poorer clinical response. Factors that impair the CYP 2D6–mediated elimination of N-desmethylclomipramine (concurrent medications that are potent CYP 2D6 inhibitors, CYP 2D6 poor metabolizers) may possibly decrease the efficacy of clomipramine by shifting the metabolic ratio in an undesired direction.

Asian patients such as K.T. have been found to have significantly decreased clearance of clomipramine and higher clomipramine:N-desmethylclomipramine ratios compared with whites, which may necessitate use of lower doses.[223] This is probably due to genetic polymorphism at either CYP 2C19 or CYP 2D6, which results in decreased metabolic capacity through these routes in the Asian population. Careful monitoring for possible signs of toxicity should accompany dose increases, and the clomipramine plasma level should be checked in those (Asian or otherwise) who show unexpected effects with usual doses. An opposite effect has been described in ultra-rapid CYP 2D6 metabolizers, in which unusually high clomipramine dosages may be required for therapeutic efficacy.

Clomipramine and Fluvoxamine Drug Interactions

34. **After 10 weeks of taking clomipramine 100 mg HS, K.T. has shown partial response. He continues to experience mild to moderate anticholinergic side effects and frequent daytime fatigue; his plasma clomipramine level is relatively high for the given dose at 450 ng/mL (clomipramine plus desmethylclomipramine). The physician decides to add fluvoxamine for augmentation effects. What potential drug interaction may be expected when fluvoxamine is added to clomipramine therapy, and how should this drug combination be monitored?**

Fluvoxamine is a potent inhibitor of CYP 1A2, CYP 3A4, and CYP 2C19 and can significantly increase the plasma level of any medication or substance that depends on these metabolic routes for elimination. Clinically important examples include clozapine, olanzapine, thioridazine, theophylline, caffeine, warfarin, mirtazapine, amitriptyline, imipramine, and clomipramine.[224] Based on the previously described metabolic pathways of clomipramine, any drug that affects its defined routes of metabolism may cause a significant interaction. Addition of fluvoxamine would be expected to decrease the metabolism of clomipramine to N-desmethylclomipramine and cause a significant increase in the clomipramine plasma level. This combination can be used, but must be accompanied by a substantial decrease in the clomipramine dosage (to 10 to 25 mg/day) to prevent potentially serious toxicity.[225] K.T. is already experiencing significant side effects, and he has a relatively high clomipramine level while taking a moderate clomipramine dosage. Fluvoxamine's metabolic inhibitory profile could theoretically shift the clomipramine: N-desmethylclomipramine ratio in the direction associated with better response.

Other medications that can increase clomipramine levels and cause toxicity include methylphenidate, haloperidol, fluoxetine, paroxetine, modafinil, valproic acid, and enalapril. Hepatic enzyme inducers such as carbamazepine, phenytoin, and phenobarbital can significantly decrease clomipramine plasma levels, possibly leading to decreased efficacy. Another potentially serious drug interaction with clomipramine is with MAO inhibitors. Although other TCAs can be used with caution in combination with MAO inhibitors, clomipramine has greater serotonergic effects than other TCAs, so its concurrent use with an MAO inhibitor is strictly contraindicated.[220] In addition, at least 2 weeks should be allowed between use of clomipramine and an MAO inhibitor. Last, any medications with marked sedative or anticholinergic activity can cause increases in these effects when coadministered with clomipramine.

Table 76-15 provides a list of resource organizations for people with anxiety disorders.

Table 76-15   Anxiety Disorders Resource Organizations

Anxiety Disorders Association of America
8730 Georgia Avenue, Suite 600
Silver Spring, MD 20910
(240) 485-1001
Website: www.adaa.org

The Anxiety Coach
1340 Remington Road, Suite D
Schaumburg, IL 60173
(847) 605-0453
Website: www.anxietycoach.com

Freedom From Fear
308 Seaview Ave.
Staten Island, NY 10305
(718) 351-1717
Website: www.freedomfromfear.org

Mental Help Net
570 Metro Place North
Dublin, OH 43017
Website: http://mentalhelp.net

National Mental Health Association
2001 N. Beauregard Street, 12th Floor
Alexandria, Virginia 22311
(800) 969-NMHA (6642)
Website: www.nmha.org/

Obsessive-Compulsive Foundation, Inc.
676 State Street
New Haven, CT 06511
(203) 401-2070
Website: www.ocfoundation.org

PTSD Alliance Resource Center
(877) 507-PTSD
Website: www.ptsdalliance.org

The Social Phobia/Social Anxiety Association
2058 E. Topeka Dr.
Phoenix, AZ 85024
Website: www.socialphobia.org

REFERENCES

1. American Psychiatric Association. Diagnostic and Statistical Manual of Mental Disorders, 4th Ed. Washington, DC: American Psychiatric Association, 1994.
2. Ninan PT. The functional anatomy, neurochemistry, and pharmacology of anxiety. J Clin Psychiatry 1999;60(Suppl 2):12.
3. Jetty PV et al. Neurobiology of generalized anxiety disorder. Psychiatr Clin North Am 2001;24:75.
4. Mohler H et al. A new benzodiazepines pharmacology. J Pharmacol Exp Ther 2002;300:2.
5. Low K et al. Molecular and neuronal substrate for the selective attenuation of anxiety. Science 2000;290:131.
6. Lydiard RB. The role of GABA in anxiety disorders. J Clin Psychiatry 2003;64(Suppl 3):21.
7. Iwata N et al. Relationship between a GABA $A_{\alpha6}$ Pro385Ser substitution and benzodiazepine sensitivity. Am J Psychiatry 1999;156:1447.
8. Cousins MS et al. GABA(B) receptor agonists for the treatment of drug addiction: a review of recent findings. Drug Alcohol Depend 2002;65:209.
9. Gavish M et al. Enigma of the peripheral benzodiazepines receptor. Pharmacol Rev 1999;51:629.
10. Gorman JM. New molecular targets for antianxiety interventions. J Clin Psychiatry 2003;64(Suppl 3):28.
11. Gorman JM et al. Neuroanatomical hypothesis of panic disorder, revised. Am J Psychiatry 2000;157:493.
12. Sanacora G et al. Increased occipital cortex GABA concentrations in depressed patients after therapy with selective serotonin reuptake inhibitors. Am J Psychiatry 2002;159:663.
13. Melke J. Serotonin transporter gene polymorphisms and mental health. Curr Opin Psychiatry 2003;16:215.
14. Zanardi R et al. Efficacy of paroxetine in depression is influenced by a functional polymorphism within the promoter of the serotonin transporter gene [Letter]. J Clin Psychopharmacol 2000;20:105.
15. Sullivan GM et al. The noradrenergic system in pathological anxiety: a focus on panic with relevance to generalized anxiety and phobias. Biol Psychiatry 1999;46:1205.
16. Koob GF. Corticotrophin-releasing factor, norepinephrine, and stress. Biol Psychiatry 1999;46:1167.
17. Yehuda R. Current status of cortisol findings in post-traumatic stress disorder. Psychiatr Clin North Am 2002;25:341.
18. Kessler RC et al. Lifetime and 12-month prevalence of DSM-III-R psychiatric disorders in the United States. Arch Gen Psychiatry 1994;51:8.
19. Lepine JP. The epidemiology of anxiety disorders: prevalence and societal costs. J Clin Psychiatry 2002;63(Suppl 14):4.
20. Greenberg PE et al. The economic burden of anxiety disorders in the 1990s. J Clin Psychiatry 1999;60:427.
21. Katon WJ, Walker EA. Medically unexplained symptoms in primary care. J Clin Psychiatry 1998;59(Suppl 20):15.
22. Wise MG, Griffies WS. A combined treatment approach to anxiety in the medically ill. J Clin Psychiatry 1995;56(Suppl 2):14.
23. Anon. Drugs that may cause psychiatric symptoms. Med Lett Drugs Ther 2002;44:59.
24. Kushner MG et al. Prospective analysis of the relation between DSM-III anxiety disorders and alcohol use disorders. Am J Psychiatry 1999;158:723.
25. Moller HJ. Anxiety associated with comorbid depression. J Clin Psychiatry 2002;63(Suppl 14):22.
26. Kessler RC et al. Impairment in pure and comorbid generalized anxiety disorder and major depression at 12 months in two national surveys. Am J Psychiatry 1999;156:1915.
27. Pigott TA. Gender differences in the epidemiology and treatment of anxiety disorders. J Clin Psychiatry 1999;60(Suppl 18):4.
28. Wittchen HU et al. DSM-III-R generalized anxiety disorder in the national comorbidity survey. Arch Gen Psychiatry 1994;51:355.
29. Brawman-Mintzer O. Pharmacologic treatment of generalized anxiety disorder. Psychiatr Clin North Am 2001;24:119.
30. Woodman CL et al. A 5-year followup study of generalized anxiety disorder and panic disorder. J Nerv Ment Dis 1999;187:3.
31. Hettema JM et al. A review and meta-analysis of the genetic epidemiology of anxiety disorders. Am J Psychiatry 2001;158:1568.
32. Borkovec TD. Psychotherapy for generalized anxiety disorder. J Clin Psychiatry 2001;62(Suppl 11):37.
33. Goisman RM et al. Psychosocial treatment prescriptions for generalized anxiety disorder, panic disorder, and social phobia, 1991-1996. Am J Psychiatry 1999;156:1819.
34. Hollister LO et al. Clinical uses of benzodiazepines. J Clin Psychopharmacol 1993;13(Suppl 6):1.
35. Uhlenhuth EH et al. International study of expert judgment on therapeutic use of benzodiazepines and other psychotherapeutic medications: IV. Therapeutic dose dependence and abuse liability of benzodiazepines in the long-term treatment of anxiety disorders. J Clin Psychopharmacol 1999;19(Suppl 2):23S.
36. Apter JT, Allen LA. Buspirone: future directions. J Clin Psychopharmacol 1999;19:86.
37. Mahmood I, Sahajwalla C. Clinical pharmacokinetics and pharmacodynamics of buspirone, an anxiolytic drug. Clin Pharmacokinet 1999;36:277.
38. Davidson JRT et al. Efficacy, safety, and tolerability of venlafaxine extended release and buspirone in outpatients with generalized anxiety disorder. J Clin Psychiatry 1999;60:528.
39. Dimitriou EC et al. Buspirone vs alprazolam: a double-blind comparative study of their efficacy, adverse effects and withdrawal symptoms. Drug Invest 1992;4:316.
40. Pecknold JC. A risk-benefit assessment of buspirone in the treatment of anxiety disorders. Drug Saf 1997;16:118.
41. Feiger AD et al. Gepirone extended-release: new evidence for efficacy in the treatment of major depressive disorder. J Clin Psychiatry 2003;64:243.
42. Stahl SM. Don't ask, don't tell, but benzodiazepines are still the leading treatments for anxiety disorder. J Clin Psychiatry 2002;63:756.
43. Lee KC et al. Beyond depression: evaluation of newer indications and off-label uses for SSRIs. Formulary 2002;37:240.
44. Rickels K et al. Antidepressants for the treatment of generalized anxiety disorder. Arch Gen Psychiatry 1993;50:884.
45. Pollack MH et al. Paroxetine in the treatment of generalized anxiety disorder: results of a placebo-controlled, flexible dosage trial. J Clin Psychiatry 2001;62:350.
46. Rocca P et al. Paroxetine efficacy in the treatment of generalized anxiety disorder. Acta Psychiatr Scand 1997;95:444.

47. Rickels K et al. Paroxetine treatment of generalized anxiety disorder: a double-blind, placebo-controlled study. Am J Psychiatry 2003;160:749.

48. Stocchi F et al. Efficacy and tolerability of paroxetine for the long-term treatment of generalized anxiety disorder. J Clin Psychiatry 2003;64:250.

49. Silverstone PH, Salinas E. Efficacy of venlafaxine extended release in patients with major depressive disorder and comorbid generalized anxiety disorder. J Clin Psychiatry 2001;62:523.

50. Montgomery SA et al. Effectiveness of venlafaxine, extended release formulation, in the short-term and long-term treatment of generalized anxiety disorder: results of a survival analysis. J Clin Psychopharmacol 2002;22:561.

51. Rickels K et al. Efficacy of extended-release venlafaxine in nondepressed outpatients with generalized anxiety disorder. Am J Psychiatry 2000; 157:968.

52. Waugh J, Goa KL. Escitalopram. A review of its use in the management of major depressive and anxiety disorders. CNS Drugs 2003;17:343.

53. Russell JM et al. Effect of concurrent anxiety on response to sertraline and imipramine in patients with chronic depression. Depress Anxiety 2001;13:18.

54. Fava M et al. Fluoxetine versus sertraline and paroxetine in major depression: tolerability and efficacy in anxious depression. J Affect Disord 2000;59:119.

55. Flament MF, Lane R. Acute antidepressant response to fluoxetine and sertraline in psychiatric outpatients with psychomotor agitation. Int J Psych Clin Pract 2001;5:103.

56. Fawcett J, Barkin RL. A meta-analysis of eight randomized, double-blind, controlled clinical trials of mirtazapine for the treatment of patients with major depression and symptoms of anxiety. J Clin Psychiatry 1998;59:123.

57. Ninan PT et al. Symptomatic and syndromal anxiety in chronic forms of major depression: effect of nefazodone, cognitive behavioral analysis system of psychotherapy, and their combination. J Clin Psychiatry 2002;63:343.

58. Bailly D. The role of β-adrenoceptor blockers in the treatment of psychiatric disorders. CNS Drugs 1996;5:115.

59. Beers MH. Explicit criteria for determining inappropriate medication use by the elderly. Arch Intern Med 1997;157:1531.

60. Llorca PM et al. Efficacy and safety of hydroxyzine in the treatment of generalized anxiety disorder: a 3-month double-blind study. J Clin Psychiatry 2002;63:1020

61. Ballenger JC. Treatment of anxiety disorders to remission. J Clin Psychiatry 2001;62(Suppl 12):5.

62. Stahl SM. Independent actions on fear circuits may lead to therapeutic synergy for anxiety when combining serotonergic and GABAergic agents. J Clin Psychiatry 2002;63:854.

63. Goddard AW et al. Early coadministration of clonazepam with sertraline for panic disorder. Arch Gen Psychiatry 2001;58:681.

64. Charney DS et al. Hypnotics and Sedatives. In: Hardman JG et al, eds. Goodman & Gilman's The Pharmacological Basis of Therapeutics, 10th Ed. New York: McGraw-Hill, 2001:399.

65. Schmider J et al. Relationship of in vitro data on drug metabolism to in vivo pharmacokinetics and drug interactions: implications for diazepam disposition in humans [Editorial]. J Clin Psychopharmacol 1996;16:267.

66. Bonate et al. Clonazepam and sertraline: absence of drug interaction in a multiple-dose study. J Clin Psychopharmacol 2000;20:19.

67. Klein E. The role of extended-release benzodiazepines in the treatment of anxiety: a risk-benefit evaluation with a focus on extended-release alprazolam. J Clin Psychiatry 2002;63(Suppl 14):27.

68. Liston HL et al. Drug glucuronidation in clinical psychopharmacology. J Clin Psychopharmacol 2001;21:500.

69. Hammerlein A et al. Pharmacokinetic and pharmacodynamic changes in the elderly. Clinical implications. Clin Pharmacokinet 1998;35:49.

70. Erstad BL, Meeks ML. Influence of injection site and route on medication absorption. Hosp Pharm 1993;28:853.

71. Fujita M et al. Changes of benzodiazepine receptors during chronic benzodiazepine administration in humans. Eur J Pharmacol 1999;368:161.

72. Rickels K et al. Psychomotor performance of long-term benzodiazepine users before, during, and after benzodiazepine discontinuation. J Clin Psychopharmacol 1999;19:107.

73. Gladsjo JA et al. Absence of neuropsychologic deficits in patients receiving long-term treatment with alprazolam-XR for panic disorder. J Clin Psychopharmacol 2001;21:131.

74. Hanlon JT et al. Benzodiazepine use and cognitive function among community-dwelling elderly. Clin Pharmacol Ther 1998;64:684.

75. Paterniti S et al. Long-term benzodiazepines use and cognitive decline in the elderly: the epidemiology of vascular aging study. J Clin Psychopharmacol 2002;22:285.

76. File SE et al. Conditions under which lorazepam can facilitate retrieval. J Clin Psychopharmacol 1999;19:349.

77. Bourin M et al. Alprazolam 0.125 mg twice a day improves aspects of psychometric performance in healthy volunteers. J Clin Psychopharmacol 1998; 18:364.

78. van Laar MW, Volkerts ER. Driving and benzodiazepine use. Evidence that they do not mix. CNS Drugs 1998;10:383.

79. Hemmelgarn B et al. Benzodiazepine use and the risk of motor vehicle crash in the elderly. JAMA 1997;278:27.

80. Ensrud KE et al. Central nervous system-active medications and risk for falls in older women. J Am Geriatr Soc 2002;50:1629.

81. Wang PS et al. Hazardous benzodiazepines regimens in the elderly: effects of half-life, dosage, and duration on risk of hip fracture. Am J Psychiatry 2001;158:892.

82. Bunney WE et al. Report of the Institute of Medicine committee on the efficacy and safety of Halcion. Arch Gen Psychiatry 1999;56:349.

83. Rothschild AJ et al. Comparison of the frequency of behavioral disinhibition on alprazolam, clonazepam, or no benzodiazepine in hospitalized psychiatric patients. J Clin Psychopharmacol 2000;20:7.

84. Jonas JM, Hearron AE. Alprazolam and suicidal ideation: a meta-analysis of controlled trials in the treatment of depression. J Clin Psychopharmacol 1996;16:208.

85. Smith WT et al. Short-term augmentation of fluoxetine with clonazepam in the treatment of depression: a double-blind study. Am J Psychiatry 1998; 155:1339.

86. Posternak MA, Mueller TI. Assessing the risks and benefits of benzodiazepines for anxiety disorders in patients with a history of substance abuse or dependence. Am J Addict 2001;10:48.

87. Rickels K et al. Pharmacologic strategies for discontinuing benzodiazepine treatment. J Clin Psychopharmacol 1999;19(Suppl 2):12S.

88. Rickels K et al. Trazodone and valproate in patients discontinuing long-term benzodiazepine therapy: effects on withdrawal symptoms and taper outcome. Psychopharmacol 1999;141:1.

89. Tanaka E. Clinically significant pharmacokinetic drug interactions with benzodiazepines. J Clin Pharm Ther 1999;24:347.

90. Greene DS et al. Coadministration of nefazodone and benzodiazepines: III. A pharmacokinetic interaction study with alprazolam. J Clin Psychopharmacol 1995;15:399.

91. Zevin S, Benowitz NL. Drug interactions with tobacco smoking. An update. Clin Pharmacokinet 1999;36:425.

92. The American Academy of Pediatrics Committee on Drugs. Use of psychoactive medication during pregnancy and possible effects on the fetus and newborn. Pediatrics 2000;105:880.

93. Weinberg MK, Tronick EZ. The impact of maternal psychiatric illness on infant development. J Clin Psychiatry 1998;59(Suppl 2):53.

94. Altshuler LL et al. Course of mood and anxiety disorders during pregnancy and the postpartum period. J Clin Psychiatry 1998;59(Suppl 2):29.

95. The American Academy of Pediatrics Committee on Drugs. Transfer of drugs and other chemicals into human milk. Pediatrics 2002;110:1030.

96. Weinbroun AA et al. A risk-benefit assessment of flumazenil in the management of benzodiazepines overdose. Drug Saf 1997;3:181.

97. Mathieu-Nolf M et al. Flumazenil use in an emergency department: a survey. Clin Toxicol 2001; 39:15.

98. Yonkers KA et al. Gender differences in pharmacokinetics and pharmacodynamics of psychotropic medication. Am J Psychiatry 1992; 149:587.

99. Matzke GR, Frye RF. Drug administration in patients with renal insufficiency. Minimizing renal and extrarenal toxicity. Drug Saf 1997;16:205.

100. Wan J et al. The elimination of diazepam in Chinese subjects is dependent on the mephenytoin oxidation phenotype. Br J Clin Pharmacol 1996; 42:471.

101. Hofmann B et al. Buspirone, a serotonin receptor agonist, increases CD4 T-cell counts and modulates the immune system in HIV-seropositive subjects. AIDS 1996;10:1339.

102. Chiaie RD et al. Assessment of the efficacy of buspirone in patients affected by generalized anxiety disorder, shifting to buspirone from prior treatment with lorazepam: a placebo-controlled, double-blind study. J Clin Psychopharmacol 1995;15:12.

103. Sramek JJ et al. Meta-analysis of the safety and tolerability of two dose regimens of buspirone in patients with persistent anxiety. Depression Anxiety 1999;9:131.

104. Sakr A, Andheria M. A comparative multidose pharmacokinetic study of buspirone extended-release tablets with a reference immediate-release product. J Clin Pharmacol 2001;41:886.

105. Clay PG, Adams MM. Pseudo-parkinson disease secondary to ritonavir-buspirone interaction. Ann Pharmacother 2003;37:202.

106. Gorman JM. A 28-year-old woman with panic disorder. JAMA 2001;286:450.

107. Lepola U et al. Sertraline versus imipramine treatment of comorbid panic disorder and major depressive disorder. J Clin Psychiatry 2003;64:654.

108. Roy-Byrne PP et al. Panic disorder in the primary care setting: comorbidity, disability, service utilization, and treatment. J Clin Psychiatry 1999; 60:492.

109. Ballenger JC. Panic disorder in the medical setting. J Clin Psychiatry 1997;58(Suppl 2):13.

110. American Psychiatric Association Practice Guidelines. Practice guideline for the treatment of patients with panic disorder. Am J Psychiatry 1998; 155:1.

111. Malizia AL et al. Decreased brain GABA$_A$-benzodiazepine receptor binding in panic disorder: preliminary results from a quantitative PET study. Arch Gen Psychiatry 1998;55:715.

112. Strohle A et al. Induced panic attacks shift gamma-aminobutyric acid type A receptor modulatory neuroactive steroid composition in patients with panic disorder. Arch Gen Psychiatry 2003; 60:161.

113. Goddard AW et al. Reductions in occipital cortex GABA levels in panic disorder detected with [1]H-magnetic resonance spectroscopy. Arch Gen Psychiatry 2001;58:556.

114. Cavallini MC et al. A segregation study of panic disorder in families of panic patients responsive to the 35% CO_2 challenge. Biol Psychiatry 1999;46:815.

115. Perna G et al. Antipanic drug modulation of 35% CO_2 hyperreactivity and short-term treatment outcome. J Clin Psychopharmacol 2002;22:300.

116. Michelson D et al. Efficacy of usual antidepressant dosing regimens of fluoxetine in panic disorder. Br J Psychiatry 2001;179:514.

117. Pollack M et al. Sertraline in the treatment of panic disorder: a flexible-dose multicenter trial. Arch Gen Psychiatry 1998;55:1010.

118. Pohl RB et al. Sertraline in the treatment of panic disorder: a double-blind multicenter trial. Am J Psychiatry 1998;155:1189.

119. Ballenger JC et al. Double-blind, fixed-dose, placebo-controlled study of paroxetine in the treatment of panic disorder. Am J Psychiatry 1998;155:36.

120. Sheikh JI et al. The efficacy of sertraline in panic disorder: combined results from two fixed-dose studies. Int Clin Psychopharmacol 2000;15:335.

121. Bakker A et al. SSRIs vs. TCAs in the treatment of panic disorder: a meta-analysis. Acta Psychiatr Scand 2002;106:163.

122. Moroz G, Rosenbaum JF. Efficacy, safety, and gradual discontinuation of clonazepam in panic disorder: a placebo-controlled, multicenter study using optimized dosages. J Clin Psychiatry 1999; 60:604.

123. Cross-National Collaborative Panic Study, second phase investigators. Drug treatment of panic disorder: comparative efficacy of alprazolam, imipramine, and placebo. Br J Psychiatry 1992; 160:191.

124. Zamorski MA, Albucher RC. What to do when SSRIs fail: eight strategies for optimizing treatment of panic disorder. Am Fam Physician 2002;66:1477.

125. Caillard V et al. Comparative effects of low and high doses of clomipramine and placebo in panic disorder: a double-blind controlled study. Acta Psychiatr Scand 1999;99:51.

126. Marcourakis T et al. Serum levels of clomipramine and desmethylclomipramine and clinical improvement in panic disorder. J Psychopharmacol 1999;13:40.

127. Hirschmann S et al. Pindolol augmentation in patients with treatment-resistant panic disorder: a double-blind, placebo-controlled trial. J Clin Psychopharmacol 2000;20:556.

128. Kampman M et al. A randomized, double-blind, placebo-controlled study of the effects of adjunctive paroxetine in panic disorder patients unsuccessfully treated with cognitive-behavioral therapy alone. J Clin Psychiatry 2002;63:772.

129. Mavissakalian MR, Perel JM. Duration of imipramine therapy and relapse in panic disorder with agoraphobia. J Clin Psychopharmacol 2002; 22:294.

130. Pollack MH. Comorbidity, neurobiology, and pharmacotherapy of social anxiety disorder. J Clin Psychiatry 2001;62(Suppl 12):24.

131. Stein MB. Disability and quality of life in social phobia: epidemiologic findings. Am J Psychiatry 2000;157:1606.

132. Arbelle S et al. Relation of shyness in grade school children to the genotype for the long form of the serotonin transporter promoter region polymorphism. Am J Psychiatry 2003;160:671.

133. Mathew SJ et al. Neurobiological mechanisms of social anxiety disorder. Am J Psychiatry 2001; 158:1558.

134. Schneier FR et al. Low dopamine D₂ receptor binding potential in social phobia. Am J Psychiatry 2000;157:457.

135. Liebowitz MR et al. A randomized, double-blind, fixed-dose comparison of paroxetine and placebo in the treatment of generalized social anxiety disorder. J Clin Psychiatry 2002;63:66.

136. Stein DJ et al. Efficacy of paroxetine for relapse prevention in social anxiety disorder. A 24-week study. Arch Gen Psychiatry 2002;59:1111.

137. Stein MB et al. Paroxetine treatment of generalized social phobia (social anxiety disorder): a randomized controlled trial. JAMA 1998;280:708.

138. van Ameringen MA et al. Sertraline treatment for generalized social phobia: a 20-week, double-blind, placebo-controlled study. Am J Psychiatry 2001;158:275.

139. Liebowitz MR et al. Efficacy of sertraline in severe generalized social anxiety disorder: results of a double-blind, placebo-controlled study. J Clin Psychiatry 2003;64:785.

140. Altamura AC et al. Venlafaxine in social phobia: a study in selective serotonin reuptake inhibitor non-responders. Int Clin Psychopharmacol 1999; 4:239.

141. Stein MB et al. Fluvoxamine treatment of social phobia (social anxiety disorder): a double-blind, placebo-controlled study. Am J Psychiatry 1999; 156:756.

142. Kobak KA et al. Fluoxetine in social phobia: a double-blind, placebo-controlled pilot study. J Clin Psychopharmacol 2002;22:257.

143. Bouwer C, Stein DJ. Use of the selective serotonin reuptake inhibitor citalopram in the treatment of generalized social phobia. J Affect Disord 1998; 49:79.

144. Stein DJ et al. Predictors of response to pharmacotherapy in social anxiety disorder: an analysis of 3 placebo-controlled paroxetine trials. J Clin Psychiatry 2002;63:152.

145. Fedoroff IC, Taylor S. Psychological and pharmacological treatments of social phobia: a meta-analysis. J Clin Psychopharmacol 2001;21:311.

146. Connor KM et al. Discontinuation of clonazepam in the treatment of social phobia. J Clin Psychopharmacol 1998;18:373.

147. Breslau N. The epidemiology of posttraumatic stress disorder: what is the extent of the problem? J Clin Psychiatry 2001;62(Suppl 17):16.

148. Ballenger JC et al. Consensus statement on posttraumatic stress disorder from the International Consensus Group on Depression and Anxiety. J Clin Psychiatry 2000;61(Suppl 5):60.

149. Widom CS. Posttraumatic stress disorder in abused and neglected children grown up. Am J Psychiatry 1999;156:1223.

150. Breslau N. Outcomes of posttraumatic stress disorder. J Clin Psychiatry 2001;62(Suppl 17):55.

151. Jacobsen et al. Substance use disorders in patients with posttraumatic stress disorder: a review of the literature. Am J Psychiatry 2001;158:1184.

152. Davidson JRT. Recognition and treatment of posttraumatic stress disorder. JAMA 2001;286:584.

153. Yehuda R. Biology of posttraumatic stress disorder. J Clin Psychiatry 2001;62(Suppl 17):41.

154. Bremnerr JD. Does stress damage the brain? Biol Psychiatry 1999;45:797.

155. Kaufman J, Charney DS. Neurobiological correlates of child abuse [Editorial]. Biol Psychiatry 1999;45:1235.

156. Southwick SM et al. Role of norepinephrine in the pathophysiology and treatment of posttraumatic stress disorder. Biol Psychiatry 1999;46:1192.

157. Friedman MJ. Future pharmacotherapy for posttraumatic stress disorder: prevention and treatment. Psychiatr Clin North Am 2002;25:427.

158. Shear MK. Building a model of posttraumatic stress disorder [Editorial]. Am J Psychiatry 2002; 159:1631.

159. Foa EB et al. Expert Consensus Guideline Series. Treatment of posttraumatic stress disorder. J Clin Psychiatry 1999;60(Suppl 16):4.

160. Marshall RD et al. Efficacy and safety of paroxetine treatment for chronic PTSD: a fixed-dose, placebo-controlled study. Am J Psychiatry 2001; 158:1988.

161. Tucker P et al. Paroxetine in the treatment of chronic posttraumatic stress disorder: results of a placebo-controlled, flexible-dosage trial. J Clin Psychiatry 2001;62:860.

162. Davidson JRT et al. Multicenter, double-blind comparison of sertraline and placebo in the treatment of posttraumatic stress disorder. Arch Gen Psychiatry 2001;58:485.

163. Brady K et al. Efficacy and safety of sertraline treatment of posttraumatic stress disorder. A randomized controlled trial. JAMA 2000;283:1837.

164. Rapaport MH et al. Posttraumatic stress disorder and quality of life: results across 64 weeks of sertraline treatment. J Clin Psychiatry 2002; 63:59.

165. Martenyi F et al. Fluoxetine versus placebo in posttraumatic stress disorder. J Clin Psychiatry 2002;63:199.

166. Hertzberg MA et al. Lack of efficacy of fluoxetine in PTSD: a placebo controlled trial in combat veterans. Ann Clin Psychiatry 2000;12:101.

167. Connor KM et al. Fluoxetine in posttraumatic stress disorder: randomized, double-blind study. Br J Psychiatry 1999;175:17.

168. Davis LL et al. Nefazodone treatment for chronic posttraumatic stress disorder: an open trial. J Clin Psychopharmacol 2000;20:159.

169. Canive JM et al. Bupropion treatment in veterans with posttraumatic stress disorder: an open study. J Clin Psychopharmacol 1998;18:379.

170. Connor KM et al. A pilot study of mirtazapine in posttraumatic stress disorder. Int Clin Psychopharmacol 1999;14:29.

171. Hertzberg MA et al. A preliminary study of lamotrigine for the treatment of posttraumatic stress disorder. Biol Psychiatry 1999;45:1226.

172. Malek-Ahmadi P. Gabapentin and posttraumatic stress disorder. Ann Pharmacother 2003;37:664.

173. Berlant J, van Kammen DP. Open-label topiramate as primary or adjunctive therapy in chronic civilian posttraumatic stress disorder: a preliminary report. J Clin Psychiatry 2002;63:15.

174. Ford N. The use of anticonvulsants in posttraumatic stress disorder: case study and overview. J Trauma Stress 1996;9:857.

175. Stein MB et al. Adjunctive olanzapine for SSRI-resistant combat-related PTSD: a double-blind, placebo-controlled study. Am J Psychiatry 2002; 159:1777.

176. Hamner MB et al. Quetiapine treatment in patients with posttraumatic stress disorder: an open trial of adjunctive therapy. J Clin Psychopharmacol 2003;23:15.

177. Raskind MA et al. Reduction of nightmares and other PTSD symptoms in combat veterans by prazosin: a placebo-controlled study. Am J Psychiatry 2003;160:371.

178. George MS. Transcranial magnetic stimulation: applications in neuropsychiatry. Arch Gen Psychiatry 1999;56:300.

179. Koren D et al. Sleep complaints as early predictors of posttraumatic stress disorder: a 1-year prospective study of injured survivors of motor vehicle accidents. Am J Psychiatry 2002;159:855.

180. Davidson J. Efficacy of sertraline in preventing relapse of posttraumatic stress disorder: results of a 28-week double-blind, placebo-controlled study. Am J Psychiatry 2001;158:1974.

181. Stein DJ. Obsessive-compulsive disorder. Lancet 2002;360:397.

182. Attiullah N et al. Clinical features of obsessive-compulsive disorder. Psychiatr Clin North Am 2000;23:469.

183. Mataix-Cols D et al. Use of factor-analyzed symptom dimensions to predict outcome with serotonin reuptake inhibitors and placebo in the treatment of obsessive-compulsive disorder. Am J Psychiatry 1999;156:1409.

184. Horwath E, Weissman MM. The epidemiology and cross-national presentation of obsessive-compulsive disorder. Psychiatr Clin North Am 2000;23:493.

185. Skoog G, Skoog I. A 40-year follow-up of patients with obsessive-compulsive disorder. Arch Gen Psychiatry 1999;56:121.

186. Koran LM et al. Efficacy of sertraline in the long-term treatment of obsessive-compulsive disorder. Am J Psychiatry 2002;159:88.

187. Mains G et al. Relapses after discontinuation of drug associated with increased resistance to treatment in obsessive-compulsive disorder. Int Clin Psychopharmacol 2001;16:33.

188. Hollander E. Obsessive-compulsive disorder: the hidden epidemic. J Clin Psychiatry 1997;58(Suppl 12):3.

189. Petter T et al. Clinical features distinguishing patients with Tourette's Syndrome and obsessive-compulsive disorder from patients with obsessive-compulsive disorder without tics. J Clin Psychiatry 1998;59:456.

190. do Rosario-Campos MC et al. Adults with early-onset obsessive-compulsive disorder. Am J Psychiatry 2001;158:1899.

191. Arnold P, Richter MA. Is obsessive-compulsive disorder an autoimmune disease? Can Med Assoc J 2001;165:1353.

192. Swedo SE et al. Pediatric autoimmune neuropsychiatric disorders associated with streptococcal infections: clinical description of the first 50 cases. Am J Psychiatry 1998;155:264.

193. Phillips KA. The obsessive-compulsive spectrums. Psychiatr Clin North Am 2002;25:791.

194. Stein DJ. Advances in the neurobiology of obsessive-compulsive disorder. Psychiatr Clin North Am 2000;23:

195. Saxena S, Rauch SL. Functional neuroimaging and the neuroanatomy of obsessive-compulsive disorder. Psychiatr Clin North Am 2000;23:563.

196. Saxena S et al. Differential brain metabolic predictors of paroxetine in obsessive-compulsive disorder versus major depression. Am J Psychiatry 2003;160:522.

197. Nestadt G et al. A family study of obsessive-compulsive disorder. Arch Gen Psychiatry 2000; 57:358.

198. Pato MT et al. Recent findings in the genetics of OCD. J Clin Psychiatry 2002;63(Suppl 6):30.

199. Hollander E et al. Pharmacotherapy for obsessive-compulsive disorder. Psychiatr Clin North Am 2000;23:643.

200. Clomipramine Collaborative Study Group. Clomipramine in the treatment of patients with obsessive-compulsive disorder. Arch Gen Psychiatry 1991;43:730.

201. Bisserbe JC et al. Double-blind comparison of sertraline and clomipramine in patients with obsessive-compulsive disorder. Eur Psychiatry 1997; 12:82.

202. Koran LM et al. Fluvoxamine versus clomipramine for obsessive-compulsive disorder: a double-blind comparison. J Clin Psychopharmacol 1996;16:121.

203. Ackerman DL, Greenland S. Multivariate meta-analysis of controlled drug studies for obsessive-compulsive disorder. J Clin Psychopharmacol 2002;22:309.

204. Hollander E et al. Refractory obsessive-compulsive disorder: state-of-the-art treatment. J Clin Psychiatry 2002;63(Suppl 6):20.

205. Greist JH et al. Double-blind parallel comparison of three dosages of sertraline and placebo in outpatients with obsessive-compulsive disorder. Arch Gen Psychiatry 1995;52:289.

206. Tollefson G et al. A multicenter investigation of fixed-dose fluoxetine in the treatment of OCD. Arch Gen Psychiatry 1994;51:559.

207. Mundo E et al. Multicentre, double-blind, comparison of fluvoxamine and clomipramine in the treatment of obsessive-compulsive disorder. Int Clin Psychopharmacol 2000;15:69.

208. Zohar J et al. Paroxetine versus clomipramine in the treatment of obsessive-compulsive disorder. Br J Psychiatry 1996;169:468.

209. Goodman WK et al. Treatment of obsessive-compulsive disorder with fluvoxamine: a multicentre, double-blind, placebo-controlled trial. Int Clin Psychopharmacol 1996;11:21.

210. Bergeron R et al. Sertraline and fluoxetine treatment of obsessive-compulsive disorder: results of a double-blind, 6-month treatment study. J Clin Psychopharmacol 2002;22:148.

211. Albert U et al. Venlafaxine versus clomipramine in the treatment of obsessive-compulsive disorder: A preliminary single-blind, 12-week, controlled study. J Clin Psychiatry 2002;63:1004.

212. McDougle C et al. A double-blind, placebo-controlled study of risperidone addition in serotonin reuptake inhibitor-refractory obsessive-compulsive disorder. Arch Gen Psychiatry 2000;57:794.

213. Denys D et al. Quetiapine addition to serotonin reuptake inhibitor treatment in patients with treatment-refractory obsessive-compulsive disorder: an open-label study. J Clin Psychiatry 2002; 63:700.

214. Dannon PN et al. Pindolol augmentation in treatment-resistant obsessive compulsive disorder: a double-blind placebo controlled trial. Eur Neuropsychopharmacol 2000;10:165.

215. Jenike MA et al. Placebo-controlled trial of fluoxetine and phenelzine for obsessive-compulsive disorder. Am J Psychiatry 1997;154:1261.

216. Simpson HB et al. Cognitive-behavioral therapy as an adjunct to serotonin reuptake inhibitors in obsessive-compulsive disorder: an open trial. J Clin Psychiatry 1999;60:584.

217. Marks IM et al. Home self-assessment of obsessive-compulsive disorder. Use of a manual and a computer-conducted telephone interview: two UK-US studies. Br J Psychiatry 1998;172:406.

218. Dougherty DD et al. Prospective long-term follow-up of 44 patients who received cingulotomy for treatment-refractory obsessive-compulsive disorder. Am J Psychiatry 2002;159:269.

219. Hollander E et al. A double-blind, placebo-controlled study of the efficacy and safety of controlled-release fluvoxamine in patients with obsessive-compulsive disorder. J Clin Psychiatry 2003;64:640.

220. Mosby. Mosby's Drug Consult. 13th ed. Elsevier Health Sci, 2003. Clomipramine hydrochloride.

221. Nielson K et al. The biotransformation of clomipramine in vitro, identification of the cytochrome P450s responsible for the separate metabolic pathways. J Pharmacol Exp Ther 1996;277: 1659.

222. Oesterheld J, Kallepalli BI. Grapefruit juice and clomipramine: shifting metabolic ratios. J Clin Psychopharmacol 1997;17:62.

223. Shimoda K et al. Pronounced differences in the disposition of clomipramine between Japanese and Swedish patients. J Clin Psychopharmacol 1999;19:393.

224. Christensen M et al. Low daily 10-mg and 20-mg doses of fluvoxamine inhibit the metabolism of both caffeine (cytochrome P4501A2) and omeprazole (cytochrome P4502C19). Clin Pharmacol Ther 2002;71:141.

225. Szegedi A et al. Combination treatment with clomipramine and fluvoxamine: drug monitoring, safety, and tolerability data. J Clin Psychiatry 1996;57:257.

226. Villikka K et al. Triazolam is ineffective in patients taking rifampin. Clin Pharmacol Ther 1997;61:8.

227. Backman JT et al. Concentrations and effects of oral midazolam are greatly reduced in patients treated with carbamazepine or phenytoin. Epilepsia 1996;37:253.

228. Furukori H et al. Effect of carbamazepine on the single oral dose pharmacokinetics of alprazolam. Neuropsychopharmacol 1998;18:364.

229. Dresser GK et al. Pharmacokinetic-pharmacodynamic consequences and clinical relevance of cytochrome P450 3A4 inhibition. Clin Pharmacokinet 2000;38:41.

230. Murphy A, Wilbur K. Phenytoin-diazepam interaction. Ann Pharmacother 2003;37:659.

231. Greenblatt DJ et al. Ketoconazole inhibition of triazolam and alprazolam clearance: differential kinetic and dynamic consequences. Clin Pharmacol Ther 1998;64:237.

232. Greenblatt DJ et al. Extensive impairment of triazolam and alprazolam clearance by short-term low-dose ritonavir: the clinical dilemma of concurrent inhibition and induction [Editorial]. J Clin Psychopharmacol 1999;19:293.

233. Ozdemir M et al. Interaction between grapefruit juice and diazepam in humans. Eur J Drug Metab Pharmacokinet 1998;23:55.

234. Zimordi K, Houston JB. Diazepam-omeprazole inhibition interaction: an in vitro investigation using human liver microsomes. Br J Clin Pharmacol 1996;42:157.

235. Samara EE et al. Effect of valproate on the pharmacokinetics and pharmacodynamics of lorazepam. J Clin Pharmacol 1997;37:442.

236. Guven H et al. Age-related digoxin-alprazolam interaction. Clin Pharmacol Ther 1993;54:42.

237. Herman RJ, Wilkinson GR. Disposition of diazepam in young and elderly subjects after acute and chronic dosing. Br J Clin Pharmacol 1996;42:147.

238. Kaplan GB et al. Single-dose pharmacokinetics and pharmacodynamics of alprazolam in elderly and young subjects. J Clin Pharmacol 1998;38:14.

CHAPTER 77

Sleep Disorders

Julie A. Dopheide, Glen L. Stimmel

"I wake to sleep, and take my waking slow. I learn by going where I have to go."

Theodore Roethke, *The Waking*

The human drive to sleep is strong and enduring. Most healthy people spend one-third of their lives asleep. Such a major part of life deserves full exploration and study. This chapter starts by reviewing the impact, epidemiology, and classification of disorders of the sleep/wake cycle. An overview of normal sleep physiology and neurochemistry precedes case discussions.

Societal Impact

The impact of sleep disorders on overall health, productivity, and quality of life has been increasingly appreciated. Sleep research shows that chronic insomnia, for example, can predict untreated illness or may contribute to injury and illness. Both mental and physical health are compromised by poor sleep patterns.[1-5]

In a study of 10,778 men and women age 35 to 59 years, poor sleepers were more than twice as likely as good sleepers to have ischemic heart disease in the following 6 years. Gastrointestinal (GI), renal, and musculoskeletal disorders and chronic pain are all associated with increased rates of sleep disturbance. Primary insomnia patients have impaired immune system function because of reduced natural killer cell activity.[4]

The *Diagnostic and Statistical Manual of Mental Disorders, Fourth Edition (DSM-IV)* field trial for sleep disorders documented high comorbidity of sleep complaints with psychiatric illness. For example, 77% of patients diagnosed with primary insomnia by a sleep specialist had a psychiatric disorder listed as a contributing factor.[3] Other studies confirm higher rates of depression, anxiety, social alienation, and diminished mental concentration in patients with primary sleep disorders (periodic limb movements during sleep [PLMS], obstructive sleep apnea, insomnia).[1,4,5] Insomnia and excessive daytime sleepiness in the elderly are leading predictors of institutionalization.[2]

Excessive sleepiness caused by a sleep disorder or sleep deprivation constitutes a serious public health hazard in health care workers, firefighters, policemen, and truck drivers.[6] An alert mind is crucial for maximum productivity in all occupations, particularly when driving is involved. Twenty percent of all drivers reportedly have fallen asleep at least once while driving, and at least 3% of all motor vehicle fatalities in the United States are attributable to driver sleepiness.[7] Motor vehicle accidents also tend to peak during the early morning (1 AM to 6 AM) and midafternoon (2 PM to 4 PM) hours—times when the circadian cycle for sleepiness is maximal.[6,7] Individuals with untreated sleep apnea or narcolepsy have a significantly greater risk of falling asleep at the wheel or on the job.[6,7]

The costs of untreated sleep disorders are increasingly well recognized. For example, insomniacs report 10 times more days of absence from work compared with those without insomnia. The direct cost of insomnia, which includes health care system use, prescription and nonprescription medication, and alcohol, is estimated at $13.9 billion for 1995.[8]

Epidemiology
Sleep Disorders

One in seven Americans has a longstanding sleep/wake disorder.[9] During the course of a year, approximately 30% of the population will experience insomnia, and approximately one-third of this group will consider the problem severe.[10] The term insomnia is used when it takes >30 minutes to fall asleep, when individuals awaken throughout the night and cannot immediately return to sleep, when individuals experience early-morning awakening, or when total sleep time is decreased to ≤6 hours. Insomnia is the most common sleep complaint, but the resulting daytime sleepiness, fatigue, or hypersomnia may become troubling after-effects. Insomnia is categorized into three general types: transient (lasting a few days), short-term (lasting ≤3 weeks), or chronic (persisting for >3 weeks).[10,11]

Major sleep disorders in order of decreasing prevalence are listed in Table 77-1.[1,9,12,13] Nightmares, nocturnal leg cramps, and snoring are other sleep disorders that tend to be more benign. Nightmares occur in 10% to 50% of children 3 to 5 years of age, and approximately 50% of adults have occasional nightmares, with 1% experiencing nightmares more than once a week. Primary snoring often can contribute to less restful sleep and can be a problem in 40% to 50% of men and women older than 65.[9]

Hypnotic Use

Behavioral interventions are the preferred treatment for insomnia because of well-established efficacy, absence of drug side effects, and sustained benefit over time.[14–16] Hypnotic medications are recommended when behavioral interventions fail or cannot be implemented.[14–16]

Prescribing trends have shifted away from benzodiazepine hypnotics toward antidepressants and newer nonbenzodiazepine hypnotics. From 1987 to 1996, prescriptions "to promote sleep" were studied from 2,790 office-based physicians across 24 specialties. Hypnotic drug prescriptions decreased by 53.7% over these 10 years, whereas antidepressant prescribing increased by 146%.[17] The increased use of drugs with significant sedating properties (e.g., the antidepressant trazodone) is based on a much lower propensity for substance abuse[15–17] compared with triazolam (Halcion) and zolpidem (Ambien).[18]

With aging, sleep typically changes in quality, partially because of sleep disruption secondary to chronic illnesses.[1,15,19] The elderly consume two to three times more hypnotics than the general population: 9% of elderly men and 12% of elderly women use hypnotics.[15,19]

The Sleep Stages
Normal Sleep

Each sleep stage serves a physiologic function and can be monitored in sleep laboratories by polysomnography. *Polysomnography* is the term used to describe three electrophysiologic measures: the electroencephalogram (EEG), the electromyogram (EMG), and the electro-oculogram (EOG). The pattern of brain waves, muscle tone, and eye movements can be used to categorize sleep as REM (rapid eye movement) sleep or NREM (nonrapid eye movement) sleep.[1,20]

NONRAPID EYE MOVEMENT SLEEP

Nonrapid eye movement (NREM) sleep is divided further into four stages with different quantities of time spent in each stage. Stage 1 is a transition between sleep and wakefulness known as *relaxed wakefulness* and generally comprises approximately 2% to 5% of sleep. Approximately 50% of total sleep time is spent in stage 2, which is rapid-wave (alpha) or lighter sleep. Stages 3 and 4 are slow-wave (delta) or deep sleep. Stage 3 occupies an average of 5% of sleep time, whereas stage 4 comprises 10% to 15% of sleep time in young, healthy adults. At sleep onset, the brain quickly passes through stage 1 and moves to stage 2. Muscle activity shuts down and brain waves become less active. After a brief REM period, the brain moves into slow-wave sleep (NREM stages 3 and 4) approximately 1 to 3 hours after a person falls asleep. The body continually moves through all of the sleep stages over the course of the night (Fig. 77-1). REM periods become longer and deep sleep lessens over the last half of the night.[20]

NREM sleep stages differ qualitatively as well as quantitatively. The function of stage 1 is to initiate sleep. Stage 2 provides rest for the muscles and brain through muscle atonia and low-voltage brain wave activity. Arousability from sleep is highest during stages 1 and 2. In contrast, it is difficult to awaken someone during stages 3 and 4, or delta sleep. Delta sleep, also known as restorative sleep, is enhanced by serotonin, adenosine, cholecystokinin, and interleukin (IL)-1. The ability of IL-1 to promote slow-wave sleep supports a widely held theory linking deep sleep to the augmentation of immune function. Some hormones (e.g., somatostatin, growth hormone) are released mainly during slow-wave sleep. Deep sleep is most abundant in infants and children and tends to level off at approximately 4 hours a night during adolescence.[20] At age 65, deep sleep accounts for only 10% of sleep and at age 75, it often is nonexistent.[19,20] Age-related in-

Table 77-1   Incidence of Major Sleep Disorders[1,29,30]

Sleep Disorder	Incidence
Insomnia	30–35%
Transient (few days)	
Short term (up to 3 wk)	
Chronic (>3 wk)	
PLMS (nocturnal myoclonus)	5–30%
RLS	5–15%
Sleep apnea	2–4%
Narcolepsy	0.06%
Primary snoring	45%

PLMS, periodic limb movements during sleep; RLS, restless legs syndrome.

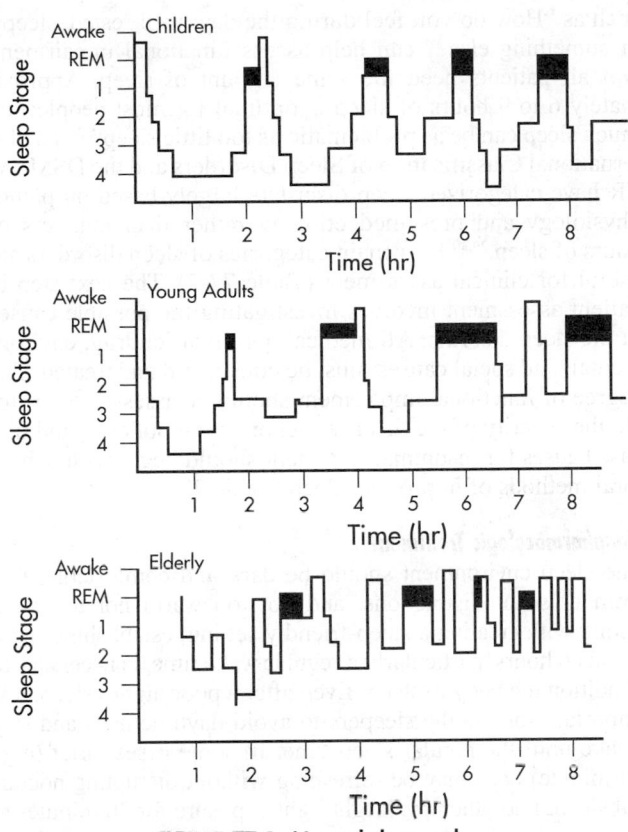

FIGURE 77-1 Normal sleep cycles.

creased awakenings, decreased deep sleep, and daytime sleepiness have been associated with increases in cortisol and the pro-inflammatory cytokine, IL-6.[19–22]

RAPID EYE MOVEMENT SLEEP

Whereas NREM sleep is necessary for rest and rejuvenation, the purpose of rapid eye movement (REM) sleep remains a mystery. REM sleep also is called *paradoxic sleep* because it has aspects of both deep sleep and light sleep. Body and brain-stem functions appear to be in a deep-sleep state as muscle and sympathetic tone drop dramatically. In contrast, neurochemical processes and higher cortical brain function appear active. Dreaming is associated closely with REM sleep, and when a person is awakened from REM, alertness returns relatively quickly.

Numerous physiologic functions are altered during REM. Breathing is irregular, consisting of sudden changes in both respiratory amplitude and frequency corresponding to bursts of REM. Temperature control is lost and the body temperature typically lowers. REM sleep brings on variability in heart rate, blood pressure (BP), cerebral blood flow, and metabolism. Cardiac output and urine volume decrease. Blood may become thicker as a result of autonomic instability and temperature changes.[23]

REM periods cycle approximately every 90 minutes throughout the night. Duration of REM increases in the last half of the night, becoming longer and more intense just after the time when body temperature is at its lowest, around 5 AM. Although the reason for the importance of REM sleep is unknown, it is clear that the human body needs REM. When de-

prived of REM, whether through poor sleep, drugs, or disease states, the brain and body try to catch up. REM rebound occurs, which may result in vivid dreams or an overall less restful sleep.[20,24]

Abnormal Sleep

Primary insomnia (difficulty sleeping not attributable to a drug, psychiatric disorder, or medical condition) can resemble a normal sleep pattern but may be associated with an increased time to fall asleep, multiple awakenings, or decreased total sleep time. Polysomnographic readings evaluating insomnia secondary to psychiatric disorders can be markedly different. In depressive disorders, decreased REM latency (i.e., the time from sleep onset to the appearance of REM) is a classic finding. Acute psychotic disorders feature prolonged global sleeplessness, with sleep onset latency, fragmented sleep, and decreased slow-wave sleep. Medical disorders (e.g., arthritis, cancer, infections) can be associated with significantly altered sleep-stage patterning. Uncontrolled pain can result in frequent awakenings, decreasing total sleep time. Oxygen saturation is at its lowest during REM sleep; therefore, less time in REM may be advantageous for patients with cystic fibrosis and other breathing disorders.[20,23]

Primary sleep disorders, including PLMS (synonymous with nocturnal myoclonus) may cause intermittent partial arousals out of stage 2 sleep and can impair the progress to slow-wave sleep. This may disrupt the quality of sleep and contribute to daytime impairment. Sleep apnea syndrome signals the brain to initiate multiple miniarousals in response to breathing cessation during sleep and therefore decreases the quality of sleep. Patients with narcolepsy may have the most unique pattern of sleep disruption because they fall almost immediately into REM sleep (instead of the usual 90-minute latency) and may experience an increased number of REM episodes.[1,12]

Although polysomnographic readings from sleep laboratories are interesting and can be useful diagnostic and assessment tools, they are neither routinely available nor are the costs routinely reimbursable by insurance companies. A thorough history of sleep problems obtained through patient interviews, along with both physical and psychiatric evaluations, are the most widely used methods of patient assessment. Although acknowledging the usefulness of clinical assessment, certain patients with more serious sleep problems such as sleep apnea, narcolepsy, or excessive daytime impairment should have sleep laboratory evaluations.

Neurochemistry of Sleep/Wake Cycle

Wakefulness-and Sleep-Promoting Neurochemicals

A basic understanding of brain neurochemistry is essential in understanding sleep disorders and the clinical use of hypnotics. Hypnotics exert their effects by modulating brain neurotransmitters and neuropeptides (e.g., serotonin, norepinephrine, acetylcholine, histamine, adenosine, and gamma-amino-butyric-acid [GABA]). The neuronal systems where neurotransmitters and neuropeptides act to control the sleep/wake cycle lie in the brain stem, hypothalamus, and basal forebrain, with connections in the thalamus and cortex. Noradrenergic, histaminergic, and acetylcholine-containing neurons promote wakefulness as they modulate cortical and subcortical neurons. Excitatory amino acids such as glutamate and stimulating neuropeptides (e.g., substance P, thyrotropin-releasing factor, corticotropin-releasing factor) also promote wakefulness.[24] Hypocretin 1 and 2 also known as orexin a and b are newly discovered neuropeptides that modulate the sleep/wake cycle. Hypocretin 1 and 2 are deficient in people with narcolepsy and primary hypersomnia.[25]

Wakefulness and sleep are antagonistic states competing for control of brain activity. Sleep takes over as the wakefulness-maintaining neuronal systems weaken and sleep-promoting neurons become active. Serotonin-containing neurons of the brain-stem raphe dampen sensory input and inhibit motor activity, promoting the emergence of slow-wave sleep.[20,24] Opiate peptides (e.g., enkephalin, endorphin) and GABA, an inhibitory neurotransmitter, also promote sleep.[24,26]

Drug-Induced Effects on Neurochemicals

The neurochemistry of sleep also can be understood by considering the effect of hypnotic drugs on specific neurotransmitters. GABA is facilitated when a benzodiazepine compound attaches to the benzodiazepine–chloride–ionophore complex and causes chloride channels to open and overexcited areas of the brain to be inhibited or calmed. GABA-facilitating hypnotics such as benzodiazepines induce sleep and decrease arousals between stages, providing more continuous stage 2 sleep. Unfortunately, benzodiazepines also may decrease stage 4 slow-wave sleep and suppress REM, leading to REM rebound upon abrupt discontinuation.[24,26,27] Some antihistamines promote sleep by blocking histamine-containing neurons involved in maintaining wakefulness. The excitatory effects of caffeine and other methylxanthines are attributed to their antagonism of adenosine receptors. Adenosine is a sleep-promoting neurotransmitter/ neuromodulator.[24]

Neurotransmitter alteration may or may not affect REM sleep. Drug-induced noradrenergic and serotonergic modulation usually decrease REM sleep. An increase in dopaminergic neurotransmission can increase wakefulness but has no direct effect on REM sleep.[24] By contrast, increased cholinergic neurotransmission triggers REM sleep.[12,24] Cortisol decreases REM sleep in young and old with unpredictable effects on slow-wave sleep and increased wakefulness in the old.[20–22] It is useful to think of the brain centers, neurochemicals, and neuropeptides involved as an interactive network regulating our sleep/wake cycle. Certainly, drugs or disease states that alter neurotransmission can have significant impact on the sleep/wake cycle. Sensory input (visual and acoustic) works with the internal network and signals brain centers to either wake or sleep. Thus, when it gets dark outside, the visual cue prepares the brain for sleep. Similarly, bright light serves to prepare the brain for wakefulness.[14,15,24,28]

Patient Assessment

Questions to Ask Patients

The first step in patient assessment is to determine whether the sleep problem is difficulty falling asleep, difficulty maintaining sleep, early-morning awakening, poor quality sleep, or excessive daytime sleepiness (EDS). Answers to the questions, "How long does it take you to fall asleep and how many hours do you sleep" should be compared with the patient's normal sleep pattern to determine how it varies. Questions

such as "How do you feel during the day: well rested, sleepy, or something else?" can help assess functional impairment. Not all patients need the same amount of sleep. Approximately 6 to 9 hours of sleep is optimal for most people: too much sleep can be as problematic as too little sleep.[6,20] The International Classification of Sleep Disorders and the DSM-IV-TR have categorized sleep disorders largely based on pathophysiology and presumed etiology rather than numbers of hours of sleep.[29,30] Four main categories of sleep disorders are useful for clinical assessment (Table 77-2). The next step in patient assessment involves investigating the possible causes of the sleep disorder. All medical, psychiatric, drug, environmental, and social causes must be considered and treated. The degree of functional impairment should be assessed to evaluate the severity of the disorder. After ruling out drug and disease causes for insomnia, treatment should begin with behavioral methods of improving sleep (Table 77-3).

Nonpharmacologic Treatment

The sleep environment should be dark and comfortable, free from noise or distractions, and not too warm nor too cold. Along with creating a sleep-friendly setting, establishing regular sleep hours, particularly a regular wake time, is necessary to condition the body to sleep. Even after a poor night's sleep, it is important for healthy sleepers to avoid daytime naps and stay awake until the regular sleep time. In some cases, brief (e.g., 20-minute) naps may be refreshing without disrupting nocturnal sleep. Phototherapy, bright light exposure for 30 minutes to 1 hour on awakening in the morning, is an additional tool that

Table 77-2 Classification of Sleep Disorders

Dyssomnias[a]

Intrinsic: Idiopathic insomnia, narcolepsy, sleep apnea, periodic limb movements during sleep
Extrinsic: Inadequate sleep fitness, substance-induced sleep disorder
Circadian rhythm sleep disorders: Jet lag, shift work, delayed sleep phase syndrome

Parasomnias[b]

Arousal: Confusional arousals, sleep walking, sleep terrors
Sleep/wake transition disorders: Sleep talking, nocturnal leg cramps
Associated with REM: Nightmares, sleep paralysis, impaired sleep-related penile erections
Other: Primary snoring, sudden infant death syndrome, sleep bruxism

Medical/Psychiatric/Substance-Induced Sleep Disorders

Associated with mental disorders: Mood disorders, anxiety disorders, psychotic disorders
Associated with neurologic disorders: Parkinson's disease, Huntington's disease, dementia
Associated with other medical disorders: Heart disease, renal insufficiency, pulmonary disease
Associated with a substance: Medication/substance abuse (e.g., phenylpropanolamine, cocaine)

Proposed Sleep Disorders

Menstrual-associated sleep disorder, pregnancy-associated sleep disorder, short or long sleeper

[a]Any sleep pattern that is abnormal (e.g., insomnia or excessive sleepiness).
[b]Any unusual behavior that emerges during sleep.
Adapted from References 29 and 30.

Table 77-3 Sleep Fitnessª Guide[1,14-16]

Keep the bedroom dark, comfortable, and quiet.

Keep a regular sleep schedule; awaken at the same time daily.

Avoid daytime naps even after a poor night of sleep.

Do not live in bed: the bedroom should be reserved for sleep and sex.

No eating, watching TV, or working in bed; it increases stress.

Turn the face of the clock aside to minimize anxiety about falling asleep.

If unable to sleep, get out of bed and do something to take your mind off sleeping.

Establish a pre-bedtime ritual to condition your body for sleep.

Relax before bedtime with soft music, mild stretching, yoga, or pleasurable reading.

Exercise early in the day before dinner to alleviate stress; avoid exercising right before bedtime.

Do not eat heavy meals before bedtime.

Do not take any caffeine (e.g., coffee, tea, candy, soda) in the afternoon.

Consult with a pharmacist, physician, or other primary care provider about your sleep problem because a physical or mental condition can cause poor sleep.

Prescribed medication and herbals can interfere with sleep.

ªAlso known as sleep hygiene.

can help set the circadian rhythm for regular sleep/wake cycles.[1,14,28] Healthy sleep often can be facilitated by avoiding problem-solving activities (e.g., finances, crossword puzzles), strenuous physical exercise, or exciting movies while in bed. Exercise early in the day can improve sleep fitness. Exercise should be completed before dinner time so that the body has a few hours to relax before it is time to sleep. Relaxation is the key to healthy sleep. If a sleeper finds himself or herself tossing or turning or worrying, it is time to get out of bed and stretch, read, or listen to soft music to relax. Health care practitioners should remind patients to avoid large meals at bedtime because the digestion of heavy meals can impair sleep. Last, chemicals that can disrupt sleep (e.g., alcohol, caffeine, other stimulants) should be eliminated when possible.[11,14,15]

Pharmacologic Treatment

When insomnia is severe and persistent, nondrug therapeutic interventions may not be sufficient, and hypnotic medication may be needed as an adjunct to behavioral strategies. Either benzodiazepine hypnotics or newer, benzodiazepine omega-1 selective hypnotics are first-line therapies because they offer significantly greater efficacy than over-the-counter (OTC) products, are safer than barbiturates, and are more effective compared with sedating antidepressants.[17,31]

Some patients need pharmacologic treatment for insomnia but do not seek treatment from their health care provider.[5,15,33] Alcohol and OTC sleep aids containing antihistamines are widely used to self-medicate insomnia, although the results are less than ideal.[2,15,31]

The ideal hypnotic has a rapid onset of effect (within 20 minutes, the natural time to fall asleep), helps the patient sleep throughout the night, does not cause daytime impairment, and has no abuse potential. Currently, there are no ideal hypnotics. Hypnotics that act at benzodiazepine receptors come closest to the ideal.[31,32] Available agents vary in onset, duration, and potential for daytime impairment mostly because of their individual pharmacokinetic profiles.[31-33] The selection of the appropriate hypnotic should consider the type of insomnia to be treated and the physiologic characteristics of the patient. For example, if someone cannot fall asleep but has no trouble staying asleep and wants no carry-over effect into the next day, a rapid-acting hypnotic with a short half-life and no active metabolites is desirable.[18,33,34]

Less common sleep disorders are treated with a variety of medications as well as some nondrug therapies. PLMS and restless legs syndrome can be improved with dopamine agonists, opioids, gabapentin or clonazepam.[35] Narcolepsy is best treated with planned naps, modafinil, stimulants, sodium oxybate, and/or some antidepressants.[1,12] Both sleep apnea and primary snoring can be worsened with central nervous system (CNS) depressants but usually improve with nondrug therapies such as continuous positive airway pressure (CPAP).[1,36] Sleep disturbances associated with medical and psychiatric diagnoses require special attention because a hypnotic can either improve or worsen the problem.[15,37,38]

DYSSOMNIAS

In a Normally Healthy Patient

Patient Assessment

1. E.P., a 31-year-old woman, is requesting a medication for treatment of her insomnia. She just returned to California from Hong Kong 2 days ago and is now having difficulty getting to sleep. When she arrived in Hong Kong, she went to sleep immediately at 4 PM and awoke at 3 AM. Her sleep pattern adjusted during her 6-week visit in Hong Kong, but on returning to California, it now takes her 2 to 3 hours to fall asleep. She has difficulty awaking in the morning and, as a result, sleeps past noon. She needs to be alert during the day to fulfill her obligations as a school teacher. What information provided by E.P. is important in the assessment of her insomnia? What additional information should be obtained from E.P. to assist in the assessment of her sleep disturbance?

E.P. describes a time-zone shift or disruption in circadian rhythm, which is a common cause of transient insomnia. Her major complaint is difficulty falling asleep, because she reports no trouble staying asleep or awakening too early. It is important for E.P. not to be sedated during the day because she is a teacher. Additional information needed from E.P. includes duration of insomnia, methods already tried to relieve insomnia and their efficacy, concurrent medications, coexisting medical or psychiatric problems, alcohol use, caffeine use, and current life stresses. E.P. should be advised that assessing all of the aforementioned information is necessary in treating her sleep problem.

2. In response to your additional questions, you learn that E.P. has no medical problems and takes no prescription medication. She has been taking pseudoephedrine at night for nasal stuffiness since returning from Hong Kong. She denies drinking alcoholic beverages and coffee but admits to recently increasing her tea intake to try to stay awake during the day. She denies a long history of insomnia, but adds, "I have not been able to sleep as well in my new apartment; I don't know why." What factors could be contributing to E.P.'s insomnia?

Several factors are contributing to E.P.'s type of insomnia, which can be classified as circadian rhythm sleep disorder related to jet lag. Her circadian rhythm has been disrupted because of travel, but she also takes a stimulating decongestant (i.e., pseudoephedrine) and drinks a caffeine-containing beverage (i.e., tea). In addition, she sleeps in new surroundings that may require time for adjustment. All these factors can contribute to her difficulty in falling asleep. Circadian rhythm sleep disorder results from a mismatch between the sleep/wake schedule required by a person's environment and the circadian sleep/wake pattern.

Nonprescription Sleep Aids

3. E.P. would like to purchase a nonprescription sleep medication. What would you recommend?

An individual risk-versus-benefit assessment is essential before recommending any medication, even OTC products. Most nonprescription sleep aids contain antihistamines such as diphenhydramine (Benadryl). The antihistamines can cause drowsiness and can help patients fall asleep. When single doses of either diphenhydramine 50 mg, triazolam 0.25 mg, ethanol 0.6 g/kg (2 to 4 drinks), or placebo were administered over 2 nights to volunteers, both diphenhydramine and triazolam (Halcion) produced comparable levels of sedation that differed from the nonsedative effects of ethanol and placebo.[39] The ability to cause sedation does not necessarily lead to hypnotic efficacy. Some patients do not feel well rested the next day after taking an antihistamine, and daytime residual effects are experienced by approximately 50% of patients.[31,39] This "hangover effect" can be significant and may be related to the lipid solubility and central histaminic (H_1) blockade of the antihistamine. Antihistamines with low lipid solubility (e.g., fexofenadine) do not cross the blood-brain barrier readily and do not cause sedation. Although diphenhydramine is the most common antihistamine found in nonprescription sleep medications, some preparations contain the antihistamines doxylamine or hydroxyzine. Tolerance may develop to the sedative effects of antihistamines after 1 to 2 weeks of continued use. Because of a high incidence of daytime sedation and risk of cognitive impairment[40] antihistamines are a poor choice for E.P., who is a teacher and must stay alert and functional throughout the day. Therefore, E.P.'s insomnia should be managed with behavioral interventions to promote sleep fitness before initiating any drug therapy.

Time-Zone Shift

4. Why is E.P. especially susceptible to the effects of time-zone shift (i.e., "jet lag"), and how might she avoid this problem in future travels?

Time-zone shift disrupts the natural circadian rhythm, which helps regulate sleep. E.P. traveled west, then east through multiple time zones. The severity of jet lag is related to the direction traveled and the number of time zones crossed. Individuals older than 50 years of age and those traveling eastward have more difficulty in adjusting their circadian rhythm to time-zone changes. Travelers should be made aware of the problem and should take steps to help their systems adjust. On arrival in the new time zone, travelers like E.P. should reset their watches and participate in activities corresponding to the new time. Staying active until the new time-zone bedtime and avoiding naps and stimulants can be helpful.

Short-to-intermediate-acting hypnotics (Table 77-4) may be used to induce and regulate sleep if the stay will be relatively short (<5 days) and if critical activities must be accomplished during the first 48 hours after arrival at the destination.[41] Long-acting hypnotics such as flurazepam (Dalmane) may prevent the traveler from awakening in the morning and should be avoided. Some hypnotic medications, especially the short half-life drug triazolam, can cause anterograde amnesia, which, on rare occasions, has been sufficiently severe to make the traveler unable to remember new information learned on the trip.

Patient Education

5. What information should be provided to E.P. about her sleep problem?

E.P. should be informed about the likely causes of her insomnia (i.e., jet lag, tea, pseudoephedrine, new surroundings). She also should understand that it may take 1 to 3 weeks for her system to readjust after traveling.[41] The importance of sleep fitness (see Table 77-3) should be emphasized. For E.P.,

Table 77-4 Pharmacokinetic Properties of Hypnotics Acting at Benzodiazepine Receptors[33,34,71]

Active Substance	Lipid Solubility	T_{max} (hr)	Onset (min)	Half-Life (hr)	Duration (hr)[a]
Zaleplon	Moderate	1.1	30	1.1	1–2
Zolpidem	Low	1–2	30	2.5	2–4
Triazolam	Moderate	1	15–30	2–5	2–4
Temazepam	Moderate	1.5–2.0	60–120	10–20	8–12
Estazolam	Low	2	60–120	10–20	10–15
Flurazepam					
Hydroxyethyl-	Low	1		2–3	
Aldehyde-	Low	1		1	
N-desalkyl-	Moderate	10	30–60	50–100	10–30
Quazepam	High	2	30	20–40	10–30
2-oxo	High	2	30	20–40	
N-desalkyl-flurazepam	Moderate	10	30–60	50–100	

[a]Time the patient feels the effects after a single dose; usually approximates half-life with multiple doses; individual variability exists; and tolerance may develop with continued use, lessening the duration.
T_{max}, time of maximum concentration.

it is necessary to pay particular attention to regulating her sleep cycle by making herself awaken at the same time each day and resisting daytime naps even after a poor night of sleep. This process, called chronotherapy, regulates the internal time clock. In addition, an hour of bright light in the morning can serve as an environmental stimulus, normalizing the circadian rhythm.[41] If E.P.'s insomnia persists despite adhering to the sleep fitness guidelines for several days, a prescription hypnotic may be necessary.

Melatonin

6. E.P. states she'd like to try melatonin for improved sleep but wonders whether it is safe and effective. What information is available on the safety and efficacy of melatonin for jet lag in E.P.?

Melatonin is a naturally occurring hormone secreted by the pineal gland, located in the center of the brain. The pineal gland is connected to the retina via a nerve pathway that runs through the suprachiasmatic nucleus of the hypothalamus, the body's circadian clock. The pineal gland produces melatonin (a byproduct of serotonin metabolism) only during the nocturnal phase of the circadian cycle and only in relative darkness. Exogenous melatonin has been promoted and studied as a treatment for circadian rhythm sleep disorders (e.g., jet lag, shift work sleep disorder, sleep/wake dysynchronization in the blind) and insomnia under the theory that rising melatonin levels "fool" the brain into sleep.[31,41]

Melatonin 0.5 to 10mg has been found effective for entraining the circadian rhythms in blind people[42] and for alleviating circadian rhythm sleep disorders in handicapped children.[43] Small controlled trials and uncontrolled data show efficacy for relieving symptoms of jet lag and associated insomnia when melatonin 0.5 to 5mg is taken 1 to 2 hours before bedtime.[31,41] In contrast, the largest randomized, double-blind trial of placebo and three regimens of melatonin (5 mg at bedtime, 0.5 mg at bedtime, and 0.5 mg at bedtime, and 0.5 mg taken on a shifting schedule) for jet lag found no difference in symptoms across all four groups.[44] Clearly, more studies are needed to assess efficacy for jet lag and associated insomnia. Melatonin may be useful for treating circadian rhythm sleep disorders as described above although, there is no comparative data with light therapy, behavioral interventions or hypnotics.[41] According to the International Consensus Conference on the Treatment of Insomnia, melatonin currently has no established place in the treatment of insomnia.[11] Consumers selecting melatonin should be advised that the safety and effectiveness of melatonin has not been clearly established and the purity of melatonin is not regulated by the FDA. Melatonin side effects include sleepiness, headache and nausea although usual doses of melatonin 0.5 to 5mg are described as well tolerated.[41] Melatonin use has been associated with reports of depression, liver disease, vasoconstrictive, immunologic and contraceptive effects.[31,41]

Short-Acting Hypnotics
TRIAZOLAM

7. Two weeks have passed and E.P. has questions about her new prescription for triazolam (Halcion) 0.25 mg Q HS PRN for sleep. She reports she was able to sleep better after reregulating her sleep cycle as previously recommended; however, new stresses at work prompted her to get a prescription to help her fall asleep on those occasional nights when it is difficult. Once she is asleep, she has no trouble staying asleep. What subjective and objective data in E.P.'s history make triazolam an appropriate selection for treatment of her insomnia?

E.P.'s insomnia seems to have changed from transient to short term (i.e., more than a few days but <3 weeks). Although the previously recommended sleep fitness guidelines were somewhat beneficial, her initial insomnia persisted and is aggravated by increased stress at work. Triazolam is appropriate for E.P.'s type of insomnia (i.e., occasional difficulty in falling asleep). It induces sleep rapidly because it reaches peak plasma concentrations in 30 minutes, and its ultrashort elimination half-life of 2 to 5 hours minimizes its likelihood of causing residual daytime sedation.[33,45] This is particularly important for E.P., who must be alert. Short-acting hypnotics such as triazolam may be used safely on an as-needed basis.

8. Subsequently, E.P. reported that the triazolam worked well for approximately 1 week, but then she noticed significant nervousness and even worse insomnia when she tried to discontinue its nightly use. Is it possible that triazolam may be causing E.P.'s worsening symptoms?

E.P.'s increased nervousness and enhanced difficulty falling asleep when she discontinued triazolam represent the phenomenon known as *rebound insomnia*. Rebound insomnia can occur after discontinuing the use of any benzodiazepine hypnotic, but it is particularly likely with triazolam because of its pharmacodynamic and pharmacokinetic properties.[45,46] Pharmacodynamically, triazolam has a high binding affinity to the benzodiazepine GABA chloride/ionophore receptor complex, which may be responsible for both hypnotic intensity and withdrawal difficulties.[27,31,45] Pharmacokinetically, triazolam's short half-life and rapid decrease in blood levels create the potential for the withdrawal symptoms of anxiety and insomnia. Triazolam is highly effective in inducing sleep when used on an as-needed basis. When used on consecutive days or nights, the risk of adverse effects may increase, including rebound insomnia upon drug discontinuation.[31,45]

9. What is E.P.'s risk of developing other CNS adverse effects from triazolam, and is this risk greater with triazolam than with other benzodiazepines?

CNS depression (drowsiness, dizziness, fatigue, or impaired coordination) was the most common adverse effect, occurring in 14.2% of patients taking triazolam 0.25 mg.[45,46] Triazolam can also cause new memory impairment (also known as anterograde amnesia), confusion, hyperexcitability states, suspiciousness, depression, and even reports of violent behavior and psychotic reactions.[46] The elderly, those taking doses ≥0.5 mg, those with underlying psychiatric disorders, and those who take alcohol with triazolam may be at increased risk for these adverse effects.[45,47] Alcohol does alter the area under the concentration-time curve of triazolam.[39] E.P. is 31 years old, a nondrinker, with no underlying psychiatric disorder, taking ≤0.25 mg of triazolam per dose; therefore, although she may experience additional adverse effects, she is not at high risk.

Considering all clinical data, triazolam has an increased incidence of CNS reactions when compared with other available benzodiazepine hypnotics, and the effects may be related to dose and duration of use.[45,47] Triazolam carries a strong recommendations for short-term treatment (7 to 10 days) with the lowest possible dosage (0.125 or 0.25 mg). Examination of efficacy and safety data on triazolam conclude that it is both safe and effective when 0.25 mg is used in nongeriatric individuals for ≤1 week.[45]

ZOLPIDEM AND ZALEPLON

10. **What alternatives to triazolam exist that offer a similar rapid onset and low risk of daytime sedation and can be administered safely over days to weeks if necessary?**

Zolpidem (Ambien) is an alternative to triazolam with similar pharmacokinetic parameters and corresponding clinical activity. Zolpidem is absorbed rapidly, reaches peak serum levels in 1 to 2 hours and is eliminated rapidly with an average half-life of approximately 2.5 hours. Both zolpidem and triazolam are metabolized by the oxidative cytochrome P450 isoenzyme 3A4; therefore, drug interactions should be considered when coadministered with 3A4 inhibitors. Zolpidem has no active metabolites and, like triazolam, it has a low risk of residual daytime sedation in recommended doses.[32,34,48] As stated earlier, E.P. must be alert during the day. The usual adult dose of zolpidem is 10 mg; elderly patients may be more sensitive to the sedating effects and should begin therapy with 5 mg.

Zolpidem is an imidazopyridine compound, structurally different from benzodiazepines. Despite its structural difference, zolpidem binds to the benzodiazepine–receptor complex much like medications with the chemical "benzodiazepine" structure.[32,34] Zolpidem is selective for the benzodiazepine (ω_1) receptor. All benzodiazepine compounds affect all three known benzodiazepine receptors and have varying degrees of anxiolytic, sedative, muscle relaxant, and anticonvulsant effects. Zolpidem's benzodiazepine$_1$-receptor selectivity imparts hypnotic efficacy with weaker anticonvulsant, anxiolytic, or muscle relaxant activity.[32,49]

Another alternative to triazolam for E.P. is zaleplon (Sonata) because it is least likely of all hypnotic agents to cause residual daytime sedation and it has the least effect on memory and psychomotor performance.[50,51] Zaleplon reaches peak plasma levels faster than zolpidem and has a shorter elimination half-life and duration of effect (see Table 77-4).[32] Zaleplon has no active metabolites; formation of its primary inactive metabolite is mediated by CYP 3A4.[51] Potential drug interactions with CYP 3A4 inhibitors require more careful monitoring. The usual adult dose of zaleplon is 10 mg, whereas the elderly should begin therapy with 5 mg.[50]

Similar to zolpidem, zaleplon is a nonbenzodiazepine agent that selectively binds to the benzodiazepine ω_1 receptor. This selectivity explains zaleplon's lower risk of causing amnesia, tolerance and dependence, potentiation of ethanol neurotoxicity, and impaired psychomotor performance compared with benzodiazepines.[34,50] These differences, coupled with its rapid time to peak effect and elimination half-life of 1 hour, allows zaleplon to be given during the night as long as there are 4 hours remaining in bed after dosing.[52]

An assessment of psychomotor performance, arousal, memory, and cognitive functioning with zaleplon dosed at 5, 4, 3, and 2 hours before awakening found no impairment. No

subjective or objective residual effects occurred when zaleplon was dosed between 2 and 5 hours before morning arousal.[53] The most common adverse effects with zaleplon include dizziness, headache, and somnolence. In dose escalation studies up to 60 mg, symptoms began to appear at approximately 30 minutes after dosing, peaked at 1 to 2 hours, and were no longer evident after 4 hours. Only the 30-and 60-mg doses of zaleplon produced pharmacodynamic effects that were clearly distinguishable from placebo.[54]

E.P. needs a medication that will hasten sleep onset, but needs no continued drug effect later in the night. Both zolpidem and zaleplon are useful alternatives for E.P. because of their efficacy for her sleep onset difficulty. Neither drug is useful for patients who also need increased total sleep time to treat frequent awakenings or early morning awakening.

11. **As an alternative to triazolam, zolpidem is prescribed instead of zaleplon because it has more postmarketing efficacy and safety data. What are other differences between triazolam and zolpidem that may be of clinical relevance to E.P.? Considering the differences between drugs and E.P.'s individual characteristics, what is an optimal dose of zolpidem for E.P.?**

Adverse effects with zolpidem occur in only 1% to 2% of patients given therapeutic doses and consist primarily of nausea, dizziness, and drowsiness.[48] More serious but rare central nervous system effects include delirium, nightmares, and hallucinations. The incidence of CNS adverse effects is increased with higher zolpidem doses, concomitant use of CYP 3A4 inhibitors, and drugs that displace zolpidem from protein binding sites. Elderly women also are more likely to experience adverse effects.[55] Tolerance and withdrawal reactions (including seizures) may be problematic at dosages higher than the recommended maximum of 20 mg/day.[49] A review comparing zolpidem and triazolam concluded that the two drugs have similar pharmacokinetic and pharmacodynamic effects in humans and that when given in equipotent doses they do not differ in efficacy, tolerability, residual effects, memory impairment, rebound insomnia, abuse potential, or other adverse effects.[56,57] The observation that zolpidem is both safe and effective for chronic insomnia (>3 weeks) at doses between 5 and 15 mg[58] suggests that E.P. is less likely to experience adverse CNS reactions when taking zolpidem for >10 days compared with triazolam.

Unlike benzodiazepines, zolpidem does not appear to alter sleep stages at usual dosages (5 to 10 mg); at higher dosages (20 mg), sleep stages are affected.[34] Because E.P. is a 31-year-old, otherwise healthy, woman with no previous hypnotic exposure, she should receive a zolpidem dose of 5 mg to take on an as-needed basis for insomnia, with counseling that 10 mg may be needed if 5 mg does not put her to sleep in 30 minutes.

12. **What other counseling should be provided to E.P. to ensure maximum benefit from zolpidem with low risk of adverse effects?**

Patient counseling is most effective when it is interactive. Interactive means both patient and practitioner are actively listening to each other while exchanging information. The practitioner should ask questions to verify patient understanding and to address specific patient concerns.[59] In this interaction with E.P., the importance of consistently adhering to sleep fitness guidelines, even though a prescription for zolpidem is available, should be emphasized. The practitioner should explain the directions and the rationale for selecting zolpidem (similar rapid onset and minimal daytime sedation with demonstrated safety during chronic use). The practitioner also needs to emphasize that zolpidem should be used occasionally, only short term, in the treatment of situational insomnia such as hers. The possible adverse effects of zolpidem (nausea, dizziness, sleepiness, and headache) should be explained, and E.P. should be encouraged to report both effectiveness and all adverse effects. E.P. should be instructed not to increase her dose on her own and to consult her health care practitioner before mixing zolpidem with any new medication. Alcohol should be avoided because of the potential for an intensified sedative effect. The practitioner should conclude the patient counseling by advising E.P. to call if she has any questions or concerns.

In a Medically Ill Patient
Insomnia and Effect on Sleep Stages

13. A.T., a 42-year-old woman with a 5-year history of hypothyroidism and a 2-year history of hypertension and chronic lower back pain, was just transferred from the intensive care unit (ICU) into a medical unit. Her cardiac status is considered "stable" 5 days post–myocardial infarction (MI). She is 5′9″ tall and weighs 72 kg. She is receiving aspirin (enteric-coated), levothyroxine, and felodipine. Her main complaint is insomnia, including difficulty falling asleep, difficulty maintaining sleep, and early-morning awakenings. A.T. reports insomnia for weeks before admission, which only worsened during the hospitalization. What type of insomnia does A.T. have and how might the insomnia affect her?

A.T.'s insomnia is considered chronic because she experienced it for weeks prior to hospital admission. It is severe because it involves difficulty falling asleep, maintaining sleep, and early-morning awakening. Careful monitoring and effective treatment of A.T.'s sleep disturbance is crucial as studies show disrupted sleep can increase the risk of another adverse cardiac event due to worsening autonomic instability and poor perfusion to the myocardium.[60]

Because normal sleep moves through all the stages of NREM and REM sleep in a continuous cycle, a patient deprived of continuous sleep may not receive enough time in each sleep stage. When stage 2 is diminished, muscles have insufficient opportunity to rest and rejuvenate. If NREM stages 3 and 4 are eliminated, immune function and the healing process can be disrupted. If REM sleep is deprived or excessive, neurotransmitter function may be altered and physiologic homeostatic processes are disrupted.[9,20,24]

Drug/Disease Etiologies

14. What individual drug/disease state factors will you assess in A.T. before developing a treatment plan?

Numerous medical disorders and primary sleep disorders are associated with difficulty falling asleep and maintaining sleep (Table 77-5).[2–4,8,9,12,60] First, A.T.'s pain management should be assessed for optimal efficacy. Acute post-myocardial infarction pain adds to A.T.'s chronic lower back pain. Fifty percent of patients with lower back pain experience poor sleep

Table 77-5 Potential Causes of Chronic Sleep Disorders[2,3–29,30]

Psychiatric Disorders

Anxiety disorders	Depressive disorders
Bipolar disorder	Psychotic disorders
Personality disorders	Somatoform disorders
Organic mental disorders	Substance abuse

Medical/Neurologic Disorders

Angina pectoris	Dementia
Bronchitis	Peptic ulcer disease
Chronic fatigue	Hyperthyroidism and hypothyroidism
Cystic fibrosis	Asthma
Huntington's disease	COAD
Parkinson's disease	Epilepsy
Hypertension	Gastroesophageal reflux
Arthritis	Renal insufficiency
Cardiac disease	Connective tissue disease
Chronic pain	
Cancer	

Sleep Disorders

RLS	Sleep apnea (obstructive or central)
PLMS (nocturnal myoclonus)	Primary snoring
Circadian rhythm sleep disorder (jet lag, shift work, delayed sleep phase)	Narcolepsy

Drugs Associated with Sleep Disturbance

INSOMNIA	HYPERSOMNIA
Alcohol	Alcohol
Bupropion	Benzodiazepines
Fluoxetine	Antihypertensives
Sertraline	Clonidine
MAO inhibitors	α-Adrenergic blockers
TCAs	ACE inhibitors
Thyroid supplements	β-Blockers
Calcium channel blockers	Anticonvulsants
Decongestants	Analgesics
Appetite suppressants	Chloral hydrate
Theophylline	Antipsychotics
Corticosteroids	Antihistamines
Dopamine agonists	Opioids

ACE, angiotensin-converting enzyme; COAD, chronic obstructive airway disease; MAO, monoamine oxidase; PLMS, periodic limb movements during sleep; RLS, restless leg syndrome; TCAs, tricyclic antidepressants.

patterns chronically.[4,61] Second, A.T. was just transferred out of the ICU. There is an alarmingly high rate of sleep deprivation in ICUs (20% to 60%) attributed to the continuous lighting, noise throughout the day and night, and constant interventions.[9,60] Sleep deprivation may prolong or worsen a disease process through diminished natural killer cell activity and decreased stages 3 and 4 of NREM sleep (when healing occurs).[2,23,60] Medications also may be contributing to A.T.'s insomnia (see Table 77-5). Levothyroxine can overstimulate the CNS if given in excessive doses[62]; therefore, A.T.'s thyroid status should be re-evaluated to make sure the thyroid dose is appropriate, especially given her post-MI status. Calcium channel blockers have been associated with occasional sleep disturbances; therefore, felodipine should be evaluated as a potential contributing factor.[38]

Another clue to a possible cause of A.T.'s sleep problem is her description of early-morning awakening, which could be related to hospital activity during these hours or to the presence of a major depressive disorder. A.T. requires psychiatric evaluation to rule out depression, which occurs in 33% to 88% of post-MI patients.[4,62] In general, patients with chronic illnesses are at increased risk of developing major depression, which typically presents with insomnia or hypersomnia. Interestingly, medical outcome studies of other chronic illnesses (cardiovascular, pulmonary, renal, neurologic disease) show a high prevalence of sleep disturbance even in those not suffering from depression.[4] Chronic insomnia related to multiple causes can be resistant to treatment; however, treatment of underlying causes increases the likelihood of insomnia resolution.

Comparing Available Hypnotics

15. **A.T.'s pain is now under control, her levothyroxine dose is appropriate, and felodipine-induced sleep disturbance, sleep-disordered breathing, restless legs syndrome, and PLMS have all been ruled out. A psychiatric evaluation finds that A.T. does not have major depression, but she is anxious about "life after a heart attack" and meets criteria for Primary Insomnia and Adjustment Disorder with Anxiety. She continues to have trouble falling asleep and staying asleep. She will be discharged in 2 days. The pain management team suggests an adjunctive medication with anxiolytic properties that may also help with sleep. Which hypnotic is best for A.T., considering her individual clinical characteristics?**

The ideal hypnotic for A.T. should act quickly and continue working throughout the night to provide her with uninterrupted sleep. A hypnotic that is not metabolized in the liver would have a lower potential for drug interactions and lessen the opportunity for systemic accumulation. However, if daytime drug concentrations are needed to calm anxiety, a hypnotic with slowly eliminated active metabolites may be desirable. The comparable doses of the hypnotic medications are listed in Table 77-6. When considering available hypnotic medications, differences in pharmacodynamic and pharmacokinetic properties (see Table 77-4) should be considered.

A nonselective benzodiazepine hypnotic is preferable in A.T. because of the need for anxiolytic properties in addition to hypnotic efficacy. ω_1 selective agents such as zolpidem and zaleplon are not effective antianxiety agents. Onset of effect is related to lipophilicity, receptor binding affinity, and time to maximum concentration.[33] Of the available benzodiazepines, midazolam (Versed) is the most lipophilic, reaching peak plasma concentrations within 45 minutes after intramuscular (IM) injection. It has the most rapid onset (5 to 15 minutes) and a short duration of action of approximately 2 hours (range, 1 to 6 hours)[63]. Midazolam's pharmacokinetic profile is optimal for rapidly inducing mild anesthesia with accompanying anterograde amnesia. For these reasons, it is used parenterally as a premedication for surgical procedures and orally as a premedicant for dental procedures.[63,64]

As a hypnotic, midazolam would be expected to induce sleep quickly, but not maintain sleep throughout the night, possibly resulting in rebound insomnia. Contrary to expectations, a comparative trial of midazolam 15 mg versus flurazepam 15 mg, flurazepam 30 mg, and placebo for 14 days in chronic insomnia showed no difference in sleep maintenance throughout the night and no rebound insomnia. The possible lower risk of rebound insomnia with midazolam when compared with triazolam may be related to triazolam's stronger binding affinity to the benzodiazepine–receptor complex.[27,65] Oral midazolam is not marketed for use as a hypnotic in the United States. Although an oral solution of midazolam has been used as a preprocedure medication, it is not an option for the treatment of A.T.'s insomnia.

The pharmacodynamic and pharmacokinetic properties of triazolam (Halcion) have already been presented. Its rapid onset is an advantage for A.T.; however, the duration of action would not be long enough to help A.T. stay asleep and it should not be used for >7 to 10 days because of the greater potential for adverse effects with prolonged use and the possibility of significant rebound insomnia on withdrawal.[45,65] A.T. may require a hypnotic for >7 to 10 days, which is the maximum duration for triazolam use.

Flurazepam (Dalmane) induces sleep within 15 to 45 minutes during chronic dosing. On the first night of use, however, flurazepam does not seem to induce sleep as well as triazolam. It has intermediate fat solubility but depends on plasma concentrations of its metabolite, desalkylflurazepam, for most of its activity.[65] Desalkylflurazepam concentrations take approximately 24 hours to accumulate and induce sleep. Studies show flurazepam maintains efficacy in sleep induction for at least 30 days; desalkylflurazepam has weak receptor binding affinity and a long half-life, resulting in gradual elimination from the system and little chance for rebound insomnia.[33,65] Desalkylflurazepam may accumulate during chronic dosing and can affect daytime cognition in some patients or compete for hepatic metabolism, resulting in altered levels of other hepatically metabolized medications.[33,65] Accumulation and daytime sedation can be therapeutic for some patients with daytime anxiety. A.T. has difficulty moving around during the day because of her chronic lower back pain, and oversedation from accumulation may impair her daytime functioning. Although flurazepam is a viable alternative, it is useful to explore other options.

Quazepam (Doral) is quite similar to flurazepam: both are hepatically metabolized to the same active metabolite, desalkylflurazepam. They have similar half-lives (30 to 100 hours) and can both accumulate under multiple dosing conditions, especially in the elderly, and in those with hepatic or renal impairment. Neither are associated with REM rebound on discontinuation.[33,66] However, quazepam and its minor active metabolite, 2-oxoquazepam, have considerably greater lipid solubility and thus a more rapid onset of effect (25 to 30 minutes) during the first night of use.[33,67] On subsequent nights,

Table 77-6 Hypnotic Dosing Comparison

Drug	Dose (mg)	Range (mg)
Midazolam (Versed)	15	10–30
Zaleplon (Sonata)	10	5–20
Zolpidem (Ambien)	10	5–20
Triazolam (Halcion)	0.25	0.125–0.25
Temazepam (Restoril)	15	7.5–30
Estazolam (ProSom)	1	1–2
Flurazepam (Dalmane)	15	15–30
Quazepam (Doral)	15	7.5–30

the difference in onset is insignificant. Quazepam and 2-oxoquazepam are specific for the benzodiazepine–ω_1 receptor and remain in the system for a significant time period (half-life $\approx$20 to 40 hours),[68] yet their relative contributions to the clinical effects of quazepam are not established clearly.[33,67] One study in both young and elderly patient populations noted less daytime drowsiness and psychomotor impairment in patients taking quazepam when compared with those on flurazepam.[69] Quazepam was safe and effective for 30 elderly insomniacs (mean age, 66 $\pm$ 4.5 years) over 10 days.[66] It has demonstrated efficacy given every other night as well.[70] The rapid onset and continued duration of effect throughout the night make quazepam an option for A.T. Quazepam and flurazepam are used infrequently due to the risk of daytime hangover effects.

Temazepam (Restoril) takes 1 to 2 hours to induce sleep. It has moderate fat solubility, similar to desalkylflurazepam, but it has a longer dissolution time. Temazepam takes 1.5 to 2 hours to reach peak plasma concentrations. Temazepam's longer dissolution time is because of its large drug particle size in a gelatin capsule. The European product formulation, consisting of a solution in a wax matrix, induces sleep in 30 minutes.[33,65] A potential advantage for using temazepam in A.T.'s case is its lack of hepatic metabolism and intermediate duration of action of 8 to 12 hours. It does not interfere with the metabolism of other hepatically metabolized drugs and it does not accumulate, minimizing the potential for daytime impairment.[33,67] The long onset of effectiveness may be of concern, although A.T. could take it 1 to 2 hours before bedtime to give it a chance to work.

Estazolam (ProSom) is similar to alprazolam (Xanax) and triazolam (Halcion) in chemical structure, because all are triazolobenzodiazepine derivatives. Pharmacokinetically, estazolam is more similar to temazepam. Estazolam reaches peak plasma concentration 1.5 to 2 hours after ingestion and is somewhat less fat soluble than temazepam. Like temazepam, estazolam induces sleep in 1 to 2 hours. Estazolam has an elimination half-life of 10 to 20 hours, also comparable with temazepam.[33,34] The difference is that estazolam is metabolized oxidatively in the liver and can accumulate in the elderly or in those with hepatic or renal impairment. Abrupt discontinuation can lead to transient rebound insomnia.[71] Estazolam has been studied mainly in patients with insomnia over a 7-day period. Efficacy and safety in chronic insomniacs are unknown.[72] Estazolam probably would not be a good choice for A.T., who suffers from chronic insomnia and may need a hypnotic for longer periods of time.

For A.T., the most appropriate choice is temazepam. Temazepam's advantages are intermediate activity, keeping her asleep throughout the night, and low risk of daytime impairment due to no known active metabolites.[72] On further discussion with A.T., who prefers to try behavioral interventions for anxiety reduction and sleep induction, temazepam 15 mg is prescribed on an as-needed basis. A.T. will be monitored regularly as an outpatient for efficacy and tolerability.

Dependence and Tolerance

16. As A.T. is preparing to leave the hospital, her daughter, B.T., expresses concerns about the potential for physical dependence on temazepam and the risk of A.T. becoming an addict. How would you respond to her concerns?

Fear of dependence and addiction to medications is a concern among the general public who, as a whole, are more health conscious. It seems that every television station has a "medical expert," every popular magazine has a "health section," and every famous person who has ever had a drug problem has his or her story reported on the evening news. Such publicity may increase the potential for confusion, erroneous impressions, and misinformation. For health care practitioners, it becomes even more crucial to provide sound drug information in common, easy-to-understand terms.

An example of the practitioner's response may be, "I'm glad you have expressed a concern; it gives us a chance to discuss temazepam therapy before your mother leaves the hospital. Temazepam has been prescribed for a medical reason, to improve your mother's sleep and to aid in her healing process. One therapeutic benefit of temazepam is an 8-hour duration of effect. Your mother will be able to sleep throughout the night so that she is well rested during the day. It also may decrease her anxiety over not sleeping, and that puts less stress on her heart.

The possible side effects of temazepam include sedation, unsteadiness, and dizziness. She should let her doctor know if she experiences any adverse effects. Right now, it is unclear how long your mother will be taking temazepam. Duration of therapy needs to be assessed on an ongoing basis. If your mother takes temazepam every night for more than 4 weeks, two things could happen: (1) she may develop a tolerance and it may not help her sleep anymore, or (2) her system may develop a dependence in which she may have worse insomnia if she does not take it. These two scenarios do not always occur and are not likely because your mother will be taking it on an as-needed basis. If one or the other does happen, some other intervention may be tried to help with her sleep, or the temazepam dose can be gradually decreased to prevent withdrawal problems. It is important to advise your mother to take the medication only as directed (no more or less), avoid alcohol, and report any decrease in effectiveness or adverse effects to her health care practitioner. Your mother, without a history of substance abuse, is not likely to become an addict. Although dependence is something to pay attention to, it is not the same as addiction and what matters is the functional ability of your mother while on and off the medication."

After discussing the information with B.T., the practitioner reviews the literature on benzodiazepine dependence and withdrawal. Epidemiologic data indicate that benzodiazepines are widely used by Americans primarily for brief periods of time, but are taken by a smaller number on a more long-term basis. Dependence can occur after continued use over 2 to 4 months.[73] Daily users for >1 year tend to be older, medically ill, and chronically dysphoric and have panic disorder or chronic insomnia. Most chronic use appears to be medically appropriate and does not lead to dose escalation or abuse. Among chronic dysphoric patients, the indications are less clear, and dose escalation is noted sometimes without notable therapeutic benefit. Benzodiazepines rarely are taken alone for pleasure, and generally are not likely to be abused. Among substance abusers, however, they frequently are taken as part of a polysubstance abuse pattern by alcoholics and narcotic, methadone, and cocaine users. In these groups, abuse is highly prevalent. Benzodiazepines are used to augment euphoria (narcotics and methadone users), to decrease anxiety and withdrawal symptoms (alcoholics), and to ease the "crash" from stimulant-induced euphoria (cocaine users).[73,74]

Physiologic dependence on benzodiazepines, resulting in a withdrawal and abstinence syndrome, develops usually after 2 to 4 months of daily use of the longer half-life benzodiazepines. There is some evidence that shorter half-life benzodiazepine use can result in physiologic dependence earlier (days to weeks) and may be associated with more withdrawal problems.[31,45] (See Table 77-4 for a comparison of pharmacokinetic properties of hypnotics.)

In Psychiatric Disorders
Stepwise Approach to Selecting a Hypnotic

17. P.H., a 35-year-old man, is hospitalized after a suicide attempt with an amphetamine and alcohol overdose 1 week ago. Before the overdose attempt, P.H. had been clean (i.e., abstinent) and sober for 2 years. He is diagnosed with major depression and organic mood disorder secondary to psychoactive substance abuse. His target symptoms include a 20-pound weight loss, low energy, social withdrawal, depressed mood, hopelessness, inability to experience pleasure, trouble falling asleep, and early-morning awakening. His medications include fluoxetine (Prozac), 20 mg QD; ranitidine (Zantac), 150 mg BID; and a multivitamin QD—all started 5 days ago. After completing your interview with P.H., you learn that he was doing well until 2 months ago when his significant other left him and he became increasingly depressed. He began to attend Alcoholics Anonymous groups more regularly, but his depression worsened. Two weeks before admission, he went on a drinking binge that led to the suicide attempt. P.H. reports feeling restless and sleeping only 3 to 4 hours a night. Use Table 77-7 to compare the clinically significant differences of available hypnotics and to demonstrate how such information can be used to develop patient-specific treatment plans. What is the best approach to solving P.H.'s sleep problem?

This stepped process serves as a useful guide for applying the information to an individual patient. Once the type of insomnia is known (difficulty falling asleep, difficulty maintaining sleep, early-morning awakening), possible causes must be identified and treated. Before a hypnotic is prescribed, behavioral interventions (i.e., sleep fitness) should be implemented. At step 3, if significant insomnia persists despite sleep fitness, a medication can be considered.

Step 4 lists factors to consider in the drug selection process. For example, agents with long-acting metabolites (flurazepam, quazepam) may accumulate or cause daytime hangover. Therefore, it is best to avoid flurazepam and quazepam in the elderly. If the hypnotic has no hepatic metabolism, it will not be subject to drug interactions with other agents that are hepatically metabolized. If insomnia is chronic and resistant to hypnotic treatment, or if low or no potential for abuse is desired (e.g., person with existing addictive disorder), trazodone or another sedating antidepressant may be selected.

Sleep Disturbance of Depression

18. What type of insomnia does P.H. have and how is it different from other types of insomnia?

P.H. has trouble falling asleep and early-morning awakening, and sleep time has decreased to 3 or 4 hours a night. He is diagnosed with major depression, and sleep difficulty is part of the disorder. The typical type of insomnia that is associated with depression generally is initial insomnia and early-morning awakening. P.H. has both.

The insomnia of depression probably is related to a dysregulation of neurotransmitters such as serotonin, norepinephrine, dopamine in addition to dysregulation of the hypothalamic-pituitary axis. All are involved in regulating mood and the sleep/wake cycle.[21,24] Neurotransmitter activity is modified by the effects of antidepressants on REM sleep. Most effective antidepressants (excluding nefazodone, trazodone, and bupropion) suppress REM, causing increased REM latency and decreased total REM time.[75–77] Indeed, REM sleep deprivation can elevate mood.[76] Depressed patients deliberately deprived of REM sleep have shown improvement in depressive symptoms. In addition to effects on REM, antidepressants redistribute slow-wave sleep to more physiologically natural patterns, with increased intensity in the first half of the night.[75] Sedating antidepressants with 5HT2 antagonist properties, such as trazodone, nefazodone, and mirtazapine, alleviate insomnia and improve sleep architecture.[77]

Causes: Psychiatric and Substance Abuse

19. What other factors may be contributing to insomnia in P.H.? How can his sleep problem be solved?

P.H. has been prescribed fluoxetine to treat his depression. Fluoxetine can cause insomnia in 10% to 20% of patients and should be dosed in the morning for this reason. P.H. also was abusing alcohol and stimulants before admission. Drug withdrawal and the lingering "abstinence syndromes" often are associated with insomnia, although sometimes hypersomnia is the predominant symptom.[73,78]

Treatment

The treatment for P.H.'s insomnia should begin with patient education. P.H. should be informed that >90% of depressed patients have some sleep disturbance, either too little or too much, and his sleep should improve after the depression clears (over 2 to 6 weeks). Sleep fitness counseling may be appropriate when P.H.'s depression begins to clear and he is more motivated to help himself sleep better. In the meantime, the potential contribution of fluoxetine to his restlessness or insomnia should be assessed by confirming that the drug is being dosed in the early morning to minimize this effect.

HYPNOTICS

Prescribing a hypnotic short term or a sedating antidepressant is recommended for depressed patients with insomnia because a good night's sleep can improve treatment adherence and daytime functioning until antidepressant effects become apparent.[77] Although trazodone is not thought to be a highly effective antidepressant, it has become the preferred adjunctive medication (50 to 200 mg) to induce sleep while awaiting the onset of the primary antidepressant's effect. All antidepressants, including selective serotonin reuptake inhibitors (SSRIs) such as fluoxetine, can improve sleep as the depression lifts; however, fluoxetine, bupropion, and monoamine oxidase inhibitors can all cause insomnia as well.

Hypnotics that act at benzodiazepine receptors are not recommended for P.H. because of his drug-abuse history. Non-

Table 77-7   Stepwise Approach to Selecting a Hypnotic for Insomnia

Step 1. Determine type of insomnia: DFA, DMS, EMA; duration.
Step 2. Consider possible etiologies: medical, psychiatric, drug; treat causes.
Step 3. Sleep fitness ineffective or only partially effective; significant insomnia persists.
Step 4. Assess type of patient: age, size, diagnosis, organ function, drug interactions, abuse potential.

Treatment Options	Type of Insomnia		
	DFA	DMS	EMA
Antidepressants	*Duration of therapy:* Chronic use in depressive diagnosis *Onset and duration of effects:* Intermediate to long onset *Pharmacokinetic considerations:* See individual antidepressant *Clinical considerations:* Substance abuse; treatment-resistant insomnia		*Duration of therapy:* Chronic use in depressive diagnosis *Onset and duration of effects:* Intermediate to long onset *Pharmacokinetic considerations:* See individual antidepressant *Clinical considerations:* Substance abuse; treatment-resistant insomnia
Chloral hydrate	*Duration of therapy:* Short-term use, 2–7 days *Onset and duration of effects:* Rapid onset; intermediate duration *Pharmacokinetic considerations:* Major metabolite, trichloroethanol, is active *Clinical considerations:* GI side effects; rapid tolerance; no EEG effects; drug interactions		
Estazolam		*Duration of therapy:* Short term and chronic *Onset and duration of effects:* Long onset; moderate duration *Clinical considerations:* Hepatic metabolism	
Flurazepam or quazepam	*Duration of therapy:* Short term and chronic *Onset and duration of effects:* Rapid onset; long duration *Pharmacokinetic considerations:* Active metabolite *Clinical considerations:* Efficacy long term	*Duration of therapy:* Short term and chronic *Onset and duration of effects:* Rapid onset, long duration *Pharmacokinetic considerations:* Active metabolite *Clinical considerations:* Efficacy long term	
Temazepam		*Duration of therapy:* Short term and chronic *Onset and duration of effects:* Long onset; moderate duration *Pharmacokinetic considerations:* No hepatic metabolism	
Zolpidem, zaleplon, or triazolam	*Duration of therapy:* Short-term use, 7–10 days *Onset and duration of effects:* Rapid onset; short duration *Pharmacokinetic considerations:* Short half-life *Clinical considerations:* Rebound insomnia; CNS side effects		

CNS, central nervous system; DFA, difficulty falling asleep; DMS, difficulty maintaining sleep; EEG, electroencephalogram; EMA, early-morning awakening; GI, gastrointestinal.

selective benzodiazepines can have a euphoriant effect, are cross-tolerant with alcohol, and are likely to be abused in patients with substance-abuse problems.[73,78] Abuse, dependence, and withdrawal reactions have been reported with ω_1 selective agents (zolpidem, zaleplon) therefore, neither are appropriate for P.H.[49,57]

If the clinician determines that fluoxetine treatment is preferred over nefazodone or mirtazapine, then trazodone may be added to alleviate insomnia.[77,78] The addition of trazodone to fluoxetine, bupropion, or monoamine oxidase inhibitors decreased time to sleep and increased duration of sleep but caused intolerable grogginess in a few patients who received fluoxetine. Tolerance did not develop to the sedative effects of trazodone.[77–79] The 5HT2 antagonist properties of trazodone at low dosages and its α-adrenergic blocking effects provide the rationale for its efficacy as a sedating agent[79,80]

ANTIDEPRESSANTS

20. What antidepressants other than trazodone are used in the treatment of insomnia? Discuss the pros and cons of using other sedating antidepressants for the treatment of insomnia in P.H.

Tricyclic antidepressants (TCAs) (e.g., amitriptyline, doxepin) were used to treat primary insomnia for years based on case reports describing efficacy in doses of 10 to 75 mg/night.[81] TCAs increase the risk of cardiovascular problems and anticholinergic side effects (see Chapter 79, Mood Disorders I: Major Depressive Disorders). In addition, no data indicate TCAs are as effective and safe as benzodiazepine hypnotics or trazodone.

For P.H., TCAs raise additional safety concerns. P.H. has a history of substance abuse and prior suicide attempts. Both are risk factors for future suicide attempts. TCAs are more toxic on overdose when compared with trazodone, and there are multiple reports of TCA plasma levels increasing to toxic levels when administered in combination with fluoxetine (see Chapter 79).

Switching to nefazodone or mirtazapine as antidepressants that offer more sedation is a reasonable consideration for P.H. Both have 5HT2 antagonist effects, which impart sedation, and they are safer than tricyclics in overdose.[77] However, nefazodone was recently linked with an increased risk of liver failure (approximately 1 in 250,000 to 300,000 patient-years of treatment), and for this reason mirtazapine may be preferred. Paroxetine (Paxil) is another option for treating both depression and insomnia in P.H. Paroxetine relieved insomnia for 15 primary insomnia patients over a 6-week, open, flexible-dose study.[82]

In the Elderly
Patient Assessment

21. S.B., a 78-year-old woman, just moved to a skilled nursing facility from her daughter's home because her family could not take care of her. She was unable to sleep at night and paced the house. Six weeks ago, she fell and broke a hip. She had a total hip replacement and uses a walker now. S.B. takes the following medications: salsalate 750 mg BID, lorazepam 0.25 mg TID, lisinopril 10mg QD, hydroxyzine 50 mg Q AM, and Senokot 1 tablet Q AM and Q HS. Zaleplon 10 mg Q HS has just been prescribed to treat insomnia, with the first dose to start tonight. What additional information is needed to evaluate S.B.'s sleep problem?

Thus far, it is unclear what type of insomnia S.B. suffers from: difficulty falling asleep, difficulty staying asleep, early-morning awakening, or just overall less restful sleep. Learning the type of insomnia helps to solve the problem. Next, as discussed in previous cases, there are many possible causes of sleep problems (e.g., disease states, medications, psychosocial factors, poor sleeping habits). The usual thorough evaluation is needed to understand the etiology of S.B.'s sleep disorder, after which her medication regimen can be optimized.

22. S.B. typifies the nursing home patient, struggling with medical problems and adjusting psychologically to new life situations. On review of the progress notes in the medical record, the consultant discovers S.B.'s type of insomnia is described as difficulty falling asleep and maintaining sleep. S.B. is charted as "sta-ble" medically, with satisfactory pain control and no major psychiatric diagnosis. The progress notes mention situational anxiety secondary to her move to the nursing home. Lorazepam (Ativan) was prescribed 3 days ago to treat the anxiety. No side effects had been documented in the medical record, but the nursing notes describe S.B. taking 2-hour naps two to three times a day and awakening two to three times nightly to urinate. What considerations are important for the assessment and treatment of insomnia in an elderly patient like S.B.?

Age-Related Effects on Sleep

S.B.'s age is an important consideration because sleep is qualitatively different in the elderly, but the need for sleep does not diminish. A circadian shift advance occurs whereby older individuals go to bed earlier and awaken earlier.[86] There are fewer cycles into slow-wave sleep and more frequent awakenings, which results in the experience of "lighter sleep."[14,15,19] The proportion of sleep time spent in REM does not appear to change significantly with aging, although there are some reports of increased time in the first cycle of REM with overall decrease in REM time.[19]

Chronic disease, depressed mood, poor perception of health, and the use of sedatives, but not age, were all associated with insomnia in one large, epidemiologic study of 6,800 individuals older than 65. Twenty-eight percent had insomnia at baseline, but nearly half (48%) did not report symptoms at follow-up 3 years later,[83] demonstrating that insomnia is not always persistent in the elderly. Persistent chronic medical illness (arthritis, cardiovascular disease, prostate problems) predicts persistent sleep disturbance.[2,9,15] Higher incidences of sleep-related respiratory disturbances and periodic leg movements in the elderly have been documented in several studies[35,84] and contribute to insomnia and excessive daytime sedation (EDS) in the elderly. EDS occurs in 7% to 30% of those older than 65; cardiovascular disease, dementia, excessive night-time awakenings, and sedating medications are factors associated with increased incidence of EDS.[15,19,84,85] All of these causes should be ruled out as contributors to poor sleep patterns in S.B.

Elderly individuals with chronic illness or social isolation report significantly more problems with sleep than those who are actively involved (e.g., club membership, religion, work) or have a close friend.[15,19] Anxiety and depression often are associated with insomnia, and the elderly tend to be more susceptible to anxieties and depression as they cope with bereavement, retirement, financial security, and social and functional losses. All of the aforementioned factors can contribute to poor sleep patterns in the elderly.[15,19] An often overlooked problem in the elderly is an alarmingly high rate of alcohol and drug abuse. Alcohol ingestion is associated with more fragmented, poor-quality sleep.[78] The observation that S.B. has several chronic medical conditions, has functional impairment, and has recently changed living environments all impact treatment decisions.

Fortunately for S.B., several studies document success with nonpharmacologic interventions to improve sleep in the elderly.[14,15] A controlled clinical trial in 78 older adults demonstrated that cognitive-behavioral therapy (CBT) emphasizing good sleep habits was more effective than temazepam in improving sleep as measured by sleep diaries. Polysomnography showed comparable efficacy between CBT and temazepam in improving sleep.[14] Of note is the observation that more than half of the patients screened and deemed eligible for the study (85/163) were excluded because of sleep apnea (40/163) medical or psychiatric conditions (17/163), or an inability to stop taking sedative-hypnotic agents (22/163). These exclusions exemplify the complex etiology of insomnia, the need for careful screening to rule out sleep apnea, and the reality of sedative-hypnotic dependence in a significant percentage of older adults.

Another study in 175 consecutive hospitalized elderly described how a nonpharmacologic sleep protocol (warm drink, massage, relaxation tapes) administered by nurses was effective for improving sleep and decreasing sedative-hypnotic use from 54% to 31% ($P < .002$). Back massage was useful in promoting sleep in a group of 24 critically ill men.[86] Light therapy administered in the evening by a visor for 30 minutes at 2,000 lux to 10 elderly women in the community improved sleep efficiency and decreased fatigue.[87] These nonpharmacologic interventions should be tried for S.B. in an effort to eliminate the risk of unsteady gait and excessive daytime cognitive impairment associated with any sedating medication.

Age-Related Effects on Hypnotic Disposition
PHARMACOKINETIC AND PHARMACODYNAMIC DIFFERENCES

Insomnia is not an easy problem to solve for most elderly patients because of the complex causes and potential risks of drug treatment. Risks can be minimized by consideration of the pharmacodynamic and pharmacokinetic differences in the way aged bodies respond to drugs. Pharmacodynamically, small amounts of drugs can elicit pronounced pharmacologic effects in the elderly, and pharmacokinetic differences greatly affect the amount of drug available at the receptor site.[67] Absorption of benzodiazepines can be decreased by diminished gastric acidity and decreased GI motility. The volume of distribution of a hypnotic drug can be affected because the elderly may have increased or decreased plasma proteins, depending on whether they have inflammatory disease or poor nutrition. Excessive fat stores can increase the volume of tissue into which lipophilic drugs redistribute.[67,88] Oxidative metabolism might be compromised in the elderly; however, results from several studies show no age-related change in oxidative metabolism.[89] Hypnotic drugs that undergo oxidative biotransformation (e.g., flurazepam, quazepam) probably accumulate more as a result of competition for hepatic metabolism and a decline in renal function than to inherent changes in oxidative metabolism. Elderly patients typically are on multiple drugs competing for metabolism in the liver. Excretion of more hydrophilic active metabolites can be slowed in the elderly secondary to a well-documented, age-related decline in renal function.[67,89]

OTHER DRUGS USED AS HYPNOTICS

23. What are the potential problems with S.B.'s current medication regimen, and what changes are needed?

S.B. is receiving lorazepam three times daily and hydroxyzine every morning. The hydroxyzine can exert intense, long-lasting sedation in the elderly and, when combined with multiple daily doses of lorazepam, is capable of inducing her frequent daytime naps.[90]One short nap during the day often is the norm for elderly people and usually does not impair nocturnal sleep, but multiple naps during the day could prevent S.B. from sleeping through the night.[19] Although lorazepam is not marketed as a hypnotic, it possesses sedative effects like all benzodiazepine compounds. Lorazepam does not undergo oxidative hepatic metabolism and interacts only with a few drugs. It has an intermediate elimination half-life of 10 to 20 hours, which could help S.B. maintain sleep, and it has no active metabolites.[67] Because S.B. currently is taking lorazepam for anxiety, a change in her dosing schedule from 0.25 mg three times daily to 0.25 mg every morning and 0.5 mg at bedtime may be useful in shifting daytime sedation more toward bedtime to help S.B. initiate sleep and maintain sleep throughout the night. Zaleplon can be discontinued because there is no need for it in combination with lorazepam. In addition, the starting dose is too high for an elderly individual (see Table 77-4). Neither zaleplon nor lorazepam may be needed at bedtime if behavioral interventions are successful. The risks of hydroxyzine (cognitive impairment due to central anticholinergic effects and excessive daytime sedation) outweigh its potential benefits for S.B. and it should be discontinued.

Rebound Insomnia and Withdrawal Symptoms

24. An attendant at a skilled nursing facility seeks assistance for one of his patients by presenting the following problem: "L.R. really has been complaining since his sleeping medication was changed. He is agitated, irritable, sweaty, and tosses and turns all night, barely sleeping. I have even noticed some BP and pulse fluctuations. He was taking flurazepam 15 mg Q PM for many years and approximately a week ago his new doctor discontinued the flurazepam and started zolpidem 5 mg. Do you think it could be due to the medication change?" What is causing L.R.'s symptoms?

L.R. is experiencing symptoms of benzodiazepine withdrawal. He took flurazepam every night for years and apparently developed a physical dependence. Withdrawal reactions are more common with short half-life benzodiazepines such as triazolam, but long half-life drugs such as flurazepam also can elicit withdrawal responses.[31,91]With long half-life drugs, the withdrawal symptoms typically occur later, 1 to 2 weeks after drug discontinuation. The lag time is due to the slow elimination of flurazepam. Zolpidem is cross-tolerant with benzodiazepines, including flurazepam. However, it could not prevent the withdrawal reaction because it was given in a significantly lower relative dose. In addition, zolpidem is metabolized and eliminated rapidly.

25. What therapeutic interventions should be initiated to manage L.R.'s withdrawal symptoms and rebound insomnia?

A slow, gradual dosage reduction is tolerated better by patients than immediate benzodiazepine discontinuation. Because L.R. is experiencing withdrawal symptoms, his nightly flurazepam should be restarted. Once the withdrawal symptoms (e.g., agitation, irritability, autonomic fluctuations, insomnia) are gone and L.R. is comfortable, his physician can discuss the gradual dosage reduction process with him. The gradual discontinuation of flurazepam in L.R. should begin by administering the flurazepam every other night. Subsequently, the flurazepam should be administered every few nights until L.R. no longer needs the medication. The withdrawal process may require several weeks. Unfortunately, the physical withdrawal he experienced may contribute to his becoming psychologically dependent on the flurazepam. L.R. needs reassurance, and he should be taught sleep-fitness guidelines.[73,91]

SLEEP APNEA
Clinical Presentation

26. O.R., a 56-year-old man, presents to an ambulatory care clinic complaining of chronic fatigue, low energy, excessive snoring, and overall less restful sleep. He describes his sleep: "It feels like I'm just skimming the surface of sleep, I'm tired all day, and my wife says my loud snoring and gasping to breathe keeps her awake." His symptoms have worsened over the past year and a half since early retirement. He has gained weight (5'10", 202 lb, body mass index [BMI] 29) and has developed hypertension since then. O.R.'s current BP reading is high, 140/90 mm Hg. Medications include hydrochlorothiazide 25 mg Q AM and aspirin 81 mg Q AM. What are the possible causes of O.R.'s sleep disorder, and why is it important for O.R. to have his problem evaluated in a sleep laboratory?

O.R. reports diminished sleep quality, excessive snoring, gasping for air, and weight gain. Although a number of causes could be responsible for O.R.'s symptoms, one of the most serious is sleep apnea. Sleep apnea is a neurologic disorder characterized by mini-episodes of cessation of breathing, which may occur 10 to 200 times an hour. The brain responds to these episodes with "mini-arousals," waking the individual to stimulate breathing.[1,36,92] These frequent mini-arousals prevent the individual from obtaining quality sleep by not allowing sufficient time in deep, slow-wave sleep, or REM. Obstructive sleep apnea (OSA), the most common type, may be induced when extra body weight (note O.R.'s weight gain) places pressure on the throat and uvula, narrowing the space into which air must travel; this results in the difficulty in breathing and excessive snoring. Biochemically, proinflammatory cytokines like C-reactive protein, tumor necrosis factor-α (TNF-α), and IL-6 have been associated with the pathogenesis of EDS and sleep apnea.[1,93]

Hypertension may be contributing to O.R.'s sleep difficulty. Several studies show an increased risk of sleep apnea in patients with hypertension, coronary artery disease, and cerebrovascular disease.[36,94,95] Although sleep apnea occurs in approximately 2% to 4% of the general population, mostly men, it occurs in up to 30% of patients with hypertension.[92] Treatment of OSA can improve BP control and lead to more restful sleep. Of note, OSA occurs in nonobese individuals and in all ages, including infants.[96] Sleep disordered breathing, including snoring is a significant risk factor for hypertension even in young individuals of normal weight.[94]

Overnight evaluation by polysomnography (i.e., EEG, EOG, EMG) in a sleep laboratory would confirm or rule out sleep apnea and allow distinction between OSA and the less common, central sleep apnea.[36,92] Central sleep apnea patients lack respiratory effort (the diaphragm does not move in attempt to take in air); they frequently gasp for air during the night.[92] Treatment of central sleep apnea requires continuous positive airway pressure (CPAP) as opposed to being alleviated through weight loss or anatomic manipulations. Central sleep apnea frequently occurs along with OSA.

Drug Treatment Considerations

27. Results from the sleep laboratory study clearly document O.R.'s problem as OSA. He experiences an average of 56 apneic episodes per hour. O.R.'s weight gain and inactivity probably contribute to the problem. Both are serious, potentially life-threatening conditions. Why should O.R.'s sleeping difficulties not be treated with a hypnotic medication?

Hypnotics, alcohol, or any CNS depressant can be deadly for sleep apnea patients and should not be prescribed for O.R. CNS depressants interfere with the mini-arousals required to stimulate breathing once it has stopped. In this case, the sleep laboratory study may have saved O.R. from a potential life-threatening breathing disorder that could have been exacerbated by a hypnotic with CNS depressant activity.

OSA can be treated by tracheostomy, nasal surgery, tonsillectomy, uvulopalatoplasty, and either nasal or orally administered CPAP.[1,92,97] Weight loss and CPAP therapy are the most effective treatments and must be maintained for continued therapeutic efficacy.[36,92] In CPAP, the patient wears a lightweight mask to bed each night and a constant flow of air is provided mechanically to prevent breathing cessation and to allow for more restful sleep Although CPAP is effective for both obstructive and central sleep apnea, the results are short lived and apneic episodes typically reappear when CPAP therapy is stopped. Preliminary studies in individuals with nocturnal bradycardia and sleep apnea show that insertion of a permanent cardiac pacemaker significantly improved bradycardia and sleep apnea.[98] More studies are needed. At this time, the best treatment for O.R.'s hypertension and sleep apnea is weight loss and CPAP.

28. If weight loss, surgery, and CPAP are all ineffective or impractical, what drug treatments are potentially effective for O.R.'s sleep apnea?

Modafinil is FDA approved to treat excessive daytime sleepiness caused by obstructive sleep apnea or shift work sleep disorder. For O.R., it is best used as an adjunct to CPAP at doses of 200-400 mg in the morning.[98a,b] Protriptyline, medroxyprogesterone, theophylline, and acetazolamide have been used successfully in small numbers of patients with sleep apnea.[99] Unfortunately, a decrease in apneic episodes is statistically significant, but not clinically significant for most patients.[92,99,100] Fluoxetine and paroxetine show promise in treating sleep apnea by increasing upper-airway patency during sleep.[100] To date, no clinically significant improvement has been documented with either agent.

NARCOLEPSY

Narcolepsy is an incurable neurologic disorder characterized by two main features: irrepressible sleep attacks and cataplexy. REM sleep episodes, known as *sleep attacks,* can intrude at any time during the narcoleptic's waking state. *Cataplexy* is the loss of muscle tone in the face or limb muscles and often is induced by emotions or laughter. Cataplexy can be subtle, where the patient is limp and not moving, or dramatic, where the narcoleptic collapses to the floor.[101] Hypnagogic hallucinations and sleep paralysis are other secondary symptoms not present in all narcoleptics. *Hypnagogic hallucinations* are perceptual disturbances (i.e., auditory, visual, tactile) that occur while experiencing a sleep attack. The patient may see objects, hear sounds, or feel sensations that are not occurring in reality. Sleep paralysis is a terrifying experience that may occur upon falling asleep or upon awakening. Patients are unable to move their limbs, to speak, or even breathe deeply. Fortunately, narcoleptics learn that sleep paralysis episodes are benign and brief (lasting <10 minutes).[12,101,102]

Symptoms of narcolepsy often begin at puberty, but patients usually are not diagnosed until years later, in their late teens or early 20s. Early symptoms consist of excessive daytime sedation and poor sleep quality. The sleep cycle becomes progressively more erratic with frequent bursts of REM and decreased regularity of deep or slow-wave sleep. Narcolepsy is thought to stem from genetic or early developmental abnormalities in catecholamine regulation within the brain.[12,101,102] Genetic research has further correlated narcolepsy with a disruption of the hypocretin receptor-2 gene (Hcrtr2).[12,25]

Comparing Treatments

Optimal treatment of narcolepsy involves treating both sleep attacks and cataplexy. Schedule II controlled substances methylphenidate (Ritalin) and dextroamphetamine (Dexedrine) were the first drugs used to treat narcolepsy, with 65% to 85% of patients deriving significant improvements in wakefulness.[12,101,102] The mechanism of action of methylphenidate and amphetamines is related to increasing neurotransmission of dopamine and norepinephrine. Modafinil (Provigil), a schedule IV controlled substance, is an effective treatment with less abuse potential. Its exact mode of action is not fully understood but it is thought to increase wakefulness through noradrenergic, α-adrenergic, GABA-modulating and hypocretin/orexin stimulating mechanisms.[103] In summary, these stimulating drugs decrease the number of sleep attacks, improve task performance, and increase the time to fall asleep, but cannot eliminate sleep attacks altogether.[12,101]

Cataplexy does not respond to psychostimulants or modafinil but can be lessened or even eliminated with low doses of antidepressants. TCAs imipramine and clomipramine were the first antidepressants used, but protriptyline, desipramine, and SSRIs (fluoxetine, sertraline, and paroxetine) are also demonstrated effective.[12,101,102] SSRIs and protriptyline offer the advantage of less daytime sedation, compared with TCAs. The effectiveness of antidepressants for treatment of cataplexy is related to REM-suppressant effects. Unfortunately, antidepressants are not effective in decreasing sleep attacks.[12,101]

Sodium oxybate (Xyrem), a salt form of the CNS depressant γ-hydroxybutyrate, is the only FDA-approved treatment for cataplexy. A 4-week controlled trial in 136 patients found that 6 to 9 g sodium oxybate solution per night given in divided doses (e.g., 450mg at bedtime then 450 mg 2 to 4 hours later) resulted in a significant decrease in cataplexy attacks and a decrease in daytime sleepiness.[104] Improved daytime wakefulness is an advantage compared with antidepressants. Adverse effects include nausea, headache, dizziness, and enuresis. Sodium oxybate can be administered safely with stimulants; however, co-administration with other CNS depressants, including hypnotic medication, is contraindicated because of the risk of respiratory depression.[12,102] Individuals taking sodium oxybate should take it on an empty stomach for maximum efficacy, and it should not be given to those with

sleep-disordered breathing, sleep apnea, or an alcohol or substance abuse disorder.[12,104] Because of a significant abuse potential, sodium oxybate is available only through restricted distribution, the Xyrem Success Program, by calling 1-866-997-3688 Orphan Medical (Xyrem package insert 2002). It is a schedule III controlled substance.[104,105]

METHYLPHENIDATE AND IMIPRAMINE

29. **G.B., a 23-year-old man with narcolepsy, is receiving methylphenidate long-acting (Ritalin LA) 60 mg Q AM and imipramine 75 mg Q HS to treat his narcolepsy and cataplexy. What are the potential risks of using both methylphenidate and imipramine to treat G.B.?**

Anorexia, stomach pain, nervousness, irritability, and headaches are common side effects of stimulant drugs.[12,102] Psychotic reactions also can occur in narcoleptic patients taking stimulants; however, these symptoms resolve when the stimulant is discontinued. Hypertension and abnormal liver function are more serious complications of long-term stimulant use. Stimulants, even at high dosages (e.g., 80 mg methylphenidate), usually do not bring a patient to a normal level of alertness, and sometimes nocturnal sleep is disrupted. To prevent stimulant-induced insomnia, doses should be taken before 3 PM. Unfortunately, tolerance may develop to the therapeutic effects of stimulants in some patients with narcolepsy.[12,101,102] Drug holidays sometimes can allow the patient to recapture therapeutic benefit. Nevertheless, it can be troubling for the patient when the drug stops working.

Imipramine, like all TCAs, can cause orthostatic hypotension, anticholinergic side effects, sedation, cardiac conduction changes, and periodic limb movements. In addition, G.B.'s imipramine therapy will be more complex because methylphenidate can inhibit the metabolism of imipramine, resulting in higher levels of imipramine.[106] G.B. should be monitored closely during the initiation of imipramine therapy and imipramine plasma levels should be assessed to minimize side effects and prevent toxicity. The optimal therapeutic plasma concentration of imipramine for treatment of cataplexy has not been established, but low doses clearly are effective and risk of toxicity from imipramine increases when serum imipramine concentrations are >300 ng/mL.

Modafinil

30. **G.B. develops intolerable nervousness, irritability, and nocturnal insomnia on methylphenidate as the dose is increased to 80 mg/day in attempt to further decrease sleep attacks. He asks about switching to modafinil (Provigil). Does modafinil offer any advantage for G.B.?**

Modafinil's relative efficacy to CNS stimulants has not been adequately assessed in controlled clinical trials; however, it has less potential for insomnia and adverse CNS reactions at recommended dosages between 200 and 400 mg/day administered in the morning.[12,102] It also has less abuse potential compared with stimulants and is a Schedule IV controlled substance. Headache was the only adverse experience rated significantly higher than placebo in 283 patients taking the recommended dose of either 200 or 400 mg/day of modafinil. Anorexia, nervousness, restlessness, and pulse and BP changes are dose-related side effects to discuss during counseling. The maximum tolerable single daily dose may be 600 mg/day, because 800 mg/day produced increased BP and pulse in one tolerability study.[107] Gradual dosage titration improves tolerability.

31. **What counseling should G.B. receive as he changes from methyphenidate to modafinil?**

People taking modafinil should receive counseling regarding the potential for drug interactions. Modafinil induces CYP 3A4 metabolism primarily in the gut; decreased levels of triazolam and ethinyl estradiol have been associated with modafinil co-administration.[108] In some cases, enzyme inhibition is possible. Modafinil's inhibition of CYP C19 is the proposed mechanism behind modafinil-associated clozapine toxicity.[109] Monitoring for drug interactions is more crucial since modafinil is increasingly used for other indications including daytime sleepiness associated with Parkinson's disease, fibromyalgia, sleep apnea, fatigue associated with multiple sclerosis and attention-deficit hyperactivity disorder (ADHD).[103,110,111]

Naps and Other Behavioral Interventions

32. **The benefits, possible risks, and importance of regular physician assessment have been explained to G.B., and he agrees to report efficacy and adverse effects to his primary care provider regularly. G.B.'s last imipramine level 2 weeks ago on the lower methylphenidate dose was 115 ng/mL, and G.B. is reminded to take the medicine at regular intervals along with daytime naps. Why are naps helpful in the treatment of G.B. and what other behavioral interventions are useful in treating narcolepsy?**

Strategically timed 15-to 20-minute naps taken at lunch and then again at 5:30 PM can be refreshing for narcoleptics and increase their time between sleep attacks. Narcolepsy support groups are available and may help G.B. better cope with such a life-changing chronic illness. It also is important for G.B. to avoid alcohol and to regulate his bedtime and wake-up time in the attempt to normalize his sleep habits.[12,101]

RESTLESS LEGS SYNDROME AND PERIODIC LIMB MOVEMENTS DURING SLEEP

Restless legs syndrome (RLS) is a condition characterized by unpleasant limb sensations occurring at rest, worsening at night, with an irresistible urge to move. Up to 15% of the population suffers from RLS while awake, and >80% of these also have PLMS.[35,112] PLMS, also known as *nocturnal* myoclonus, is best described as rhythmic extensions of the big toe and foot occurring every 5 to 90 seconds that may or may not be associated with flexions at the knee or hip level. Five or more movements per hour of sleep as recorded by EMG during polysomnography is considered pathologic. Depending on the severity, both RLS and PLMS contribute to insomnia and prevent restful sleep, and sufferers report impaired daytime functioning.[35,112]

RLS and PLMS can occur at any age but may be most common in the elderly. Sudden remissions, which may last for months or even years, are as difficult to explain as relapses, which appear without any apparent reason. Parkinson's disease, hypothyroidism, uremia, chronic bronchitis, iron deficiency, folate, B12 deficiency, and pregnancy are all associated with symptomatic RLS. The pathophysiology of both conditions involves dopaminergic neurotransmission because decreased D_2 receptor binding in the striatum of patients with RLS and PLMS has been documented.[35–112]

Treatment

Nonpharmacologic management includes reduction in caffeine and alcohol intake, regular exercise, and cessation of smoking.[35] Dopaminergic agents, benzodiazepines, opioids, and selected anticonvulsants have all demonstrated efficacy for RLS and PLMS. Drug selection is based on severity of symptoms, comorbid conditions, and tolerability.

Dopaminergic agonists including pergolide, pramipexole, ropinrole and cabergoline are effective in alleviating RLS for 70% to 100% of patients.[112] L-Dopa with carbidopa was the first dopaminergic agent to demonstrate efficacy. However, it is seldom recommended because of the finding that with chronic use, L-dopa treatment was associated with RLS earlier in the night (augmentation) and rebound RLS in the middle of the night. Bromocriptine 7.5mg/night is effective but causes excessive nausea, and CNS adverse events.[38] Pergolide (Permax) is the most well-studied dopaminergic agonist for RLS, effective at an average dose of 0.5 mg Q HS. Pergolide, bromocriptine and cabergoline are ergot derivatives with a significant risk of nausea, fibrosis and cardiac valvulopathy.[112–114] The toxicity risk of ergot derivatives increases with long-term use. RLS patients can require treatment for years, making ergots undesirable treatments for RLS. Pramipexole (Mirapex) and ropinrole (Requip) are nonergot drugs that stimulate both the D_2 and D_3 receptors. Preliminary evidence shows that pramipexole (0.375 to 1.5 mg/night) and possibly ropinrole at 0.5 to 1.5mg/night are more effective and better tolerated than pergolide. Dizziness, hypotension, nausea, daytime fatigue, and somnolence can occur with both agents; therefore, careful monitoring and counseling are needed. Pramipexole is eliminated renally; ropinrole is eliminated by hepatic metabolism via the CYP 1A2 isoenzyme. Careful dosage adjustment to control symptoms with tolerable side effects is important with the dopamine agonists. Insomnia is a potential problem with all dopaminergic agents and benzodiazepines may be necessary in combination to alleviate this symptom.[35,112]

Benzodiazepines, particularly clonazepam 0.5 to 2 mg and temazepam 7.5 to 30 mg, may be effective in relieving mild to moderate RLS. However, most studies have shown reduction in arousals from PLMS rather than elimination of movements. These agents should not be used if sleep apnea coexists because of respiratory depressant effects. The most common adverse effect with clonazepam is excessive daytime somnolence.[35] Agents with intermediate to long half-lives are preferred because agents with short half-lives (≤5 hours) may contribute to confusional states and nocturnal wandering in RLS patients.[115]

Opioids have been demonstrated effective; however, their use is limited because of side effects (constipation, sedation, nausea), dependence, and concern over addiction. Propoxyphene (65 to 130 mg) or codeine 30 mg may be useful in mild cases of RLS/PLMS for intermittent symptoms. Higherpotency agents, such as oxycodone 4.5 to 5 mg or methadone 5 to 10 mg, should be reserved for severe or resistant symptoms.[35] Opioids must be used with caution in those who have sleep apnea.[35]

Anticonvulsants are another potential treatment for RLS/PLMS without the insomnia of dopamine agonists or addiction potential of benzodiazepines or opioids. Carbamazepine 200 to 400 mg/day was found to be superior to placebo in one double-blind study and in small open trials.[35] Several open trials and one double-blind placebo-controlled study found gabapentin in divided doses of 900 to 3,000 mg/day to be effective, particularly when RLS occurs with pain.[35,116]

Tramadol, a central analgesic without the abuse potential of opioids, was found effective and well tolerated in 10 of 12 patients when given over 15 to 24 months in doses of 50 to 150 mg/day.[117] Magnesium supplementation of 12.4 mmol over 4 to 6 weeks was effective in significantly improving symptoms in 7 of 10 RLS/PLMS patients in one open trial.[119] Iron supplementation is recommended for RLS associated with iron deficiency.[35]

PEDIATRIC INSOMNIA

Behavioral interventions to promote sleep fitness (e.g., consistent bedtime and wake-time, pre-bedtime ritual) should be initiated during childhood and continued throughout adolescence to promote a lifetime of healthy sleep. One community survey of the parents of 987 children ages 5 to 12 years found a 27% incidence of bedtime resistance that was associated with inconsistent bedtime, falling asleep away from bed, fears, and psychiatric and medical conditions.[119]

Delayed sleep-phase syndrome, whereby the child or teen both stays up and awakens later than the sociologic norm (1 AM to 9 AM versus 10 PM to 6 AM) is more common in adolescents and may be physiologic in origin. Investigations on adolescent sleepiness find high rates of sleep deprivation with deleterious impact on functioning.[20,119]

33. Why is chloral hydrate used so frequently in children compared with other sedatives?

Chloral hydrate is the most extensively studied sedative agent in youth,[120,121] and there are several reasons for its widespread use: rapid onset, moderate duration, and lack of significant effects on the EEG. Chloral hydrate induces sedation and allows brain-wave assessment without drug interference.[122] When pharmacologic intervention is needed because behavioral interventions fail to promote sleep or a procedure requires sedation in a child, the question arises: Which drug is both safe and effective? Unfortunately, other sedative-hypnotics are not well studied in youth.[120]

The most common adverse effects of chloral hydrate administration are nausea, vomiting, or diarrhea, which can be minimized by giving the drug diluted or with food. Tolerance to the sedative effects develops rapidly over a 5-to 14-day period of continued use.[122] Chloral hydrate generally is void of cardiac and respiratory toxicity, but it has been linked to arrhythmias and even respiratory failure in children with compromised cardiac or respiratory systems. Therefore, it should not be used, or used only with extreme caution, in patients with severe cardiac or respiratory disorders.[121,123]

Therapeutic effects and known potential toxicities from chloral hydrate are associated with its two active metabolites: trichloroethanol and trichloroacetic acid. A single dose of trichloroethanol, the metabolite responsible for sedation, induces sedation within 30 minutes and has a usual duration of action of 4 to 8 hours, similar to its half-life of 8 to 11 hours in adults. The half-life can be longer (9 to 40 hours) in children, depending on the age and maturity of the patient. Trichloroacetic acid is a minor metabolite that does not achieve significant levels in most patients after a single dose. Upon multiple dosing, trichloroacetic acid can displace bilirubin or warfarin from albumin binding sites, potentially resulting in hyperbilirubinemia or hypoprothrombinemia.[121,124] The half-life of trichloroacetic acid is much longer (2 to 6 days), and this metabolite can accumulate under multiple dosing conditions.

Midazolam oral syrup (0.6 mg/kg dose of a 2 mg/mL solution) was used as a premedicant for children undergoing dental procedures in one pilot study.[125] Premedicant dosing of midazolam in children is generally recommended at a dosing range of 0.25 to 0.5 mg/kg with a maximum of 10 mg/dose. Metabolism occurs via the cytochrome CYP 3A4 isoenzyme with a half-life of 2.9 to 4.5 hours. Although more studies are needed, midazolam represents an alternative to chloral hydrate with fewer GI side effects, less potential for accumulation, and lower risk of cardiotoxicity.[65,125] Temazepam has also been used as a premedicant in children, but the long onset of effect requires dosing 1 to 2 hours before procedures.[120]

Melatonin at an average dose of 2 mg per night administered 1 hr before bedtime was effective and well-tolerated for 29 of 32 children age 9.6 ± 4.5yrs with chronic sleep initiation and sleep maintenance problems treated naturalistically over an average of 2.1 ± 2 months.[126]

When considering the best sedative for a child, it is useful to compare the advantages and disadvantages of available agents. Barbiturates (e.g., phenobarbital, pentobarbital) are sedating, but can have a higher incidence of cardiac, respiratory, and CNS depression than chloral hydrate or benzodiazepines.[123] Benzodiazepines have not been studied systematically in children, but there are some reports of paradoxic excitatory reactions, psychomotor impairment, and excessive sedation in young age groups.[120] Respiratory depression and altered EEG patterns can occur secondary to benzodiazepine therapy. An analysis of adverse sedation events in pediatric patients found that 60 of 95 cases resulted in death or permanent neurologic injury. Negative outcomes were associated with drug overdose, the use of multiple sedating medications, drug interactions, prescription/transcription errors, or inadequate monitoring and resuscitation of children undergoing sedation. Among chloral hydrate, barbiturates, ketamine, or benzodiazepines, there was no evidence that one drug or route of administration was associated with greater toxicity.[123]

The American Academy of Pediatrics considers chloral hydrate to be an effective sedative with a low incidence of acute toxicity when administered orally in the recommended dosage of 10 to 50 mg/kg (depending on the indication; see Chapter 93, Pediatric Considerations). Single or intermittent dosing is considered safe. Repetitive dosing is of concern because of the accumulation of the metabolites. Data are not available to establish the superiority of other sedatives with respect to safety and efficacy in children.[123] It comes down to the risk versus benefit of using a sedative, and each case should be considered individually. Any sedative should be used for the shortest period of time possible, with careful monitoring of respiratory, cardiac, and CNS functions.

FORMULARY MANAGEMENT OF HYPNOTICS

34. Balancing high-quality care with economic common sense is the responsibility of formulary managers in all health care organizations. The Pharmacy and Therapeutics Committee has decided that three hypnotics should be designated as first-line agents to promote the safe and effective treatment of insomnia. Other agents will require special permission for use. What factors should be involved in the selection of three first-line hypnotics?

Therapeutic efficacy, versatility, and patient tolerability should be foremost in identifying priority hypnotics for a health care system's core formulary. Adverse-effect profiles should be known and manageable. Another important factor is cost, which should be measured both directly (drug cost, frequency of health care utilization) and indirectly (functional ability and quality of life).[2] When balancing the clinical therapeutics against the economic realities of the available hypnotics, four factors should be considered: onset, duration of effect, metabolism, and cost (see Table 77-4 to review pharmacokinetic profiles).

A hypnotic with a rapid onset and short duration with no accumulation of active metabolites is advantageous for patients who only have difficulty falling asleep, because there is low or no risk of daytime impairment. Zolpidem (Ambien), zaleplon (Sonata), and triazolam (Halcion) fit this clinical profile. Compared with triazolam, zolpidem and zaleplon may be used in chronic insomnia, are associated with fewer adverse reactions on withdrawal, and do not appear to affect sleep stages at recommended doses.

The difference in residual sedation between zolpidem and zaleplon is significant enough to consider inclusion of both drugs on a formulary. A 10-mg dose of zaleplon is free of residual hypnotic or sedative effects when administered as little as 2 hours before waking in normal subjects, whereas residual effects are still present up to 5 hours after a 10-mg zolpidem dose.[54] Safety in elderly insomniacs has been established for all these short-acting agents (at recommended doses), but none has been studied in children. All three are expensive and no generics are available. If insomnia is effectively treated, however, costs may be decreased through decreased health care utilization, reduced work absenteeism, and improved quality of life.[2,8]

Chloral hydrate has a rapid onset and short-to-intermediate duration of action with no daytime hangover in patients with good hepatic function. Chloral hydrate has clinical usefulness in all age groups and, unlike other hypnotics, it is available in liquid, capsule, and suppository form, and is inexpensive. Chloral hydrate has been studied in all age groups. Disadvantages of chloral hydrate are its GI irritation, protein-binding interactions, and lack of usefulness for short-term or chronic insomnia.

Temazepam (Restoril) and estazolam (Prosom) have long onsets of action (1 to 2 hours) and intermediate duration (10 hours) of action. Temazepam offers several advantages over estazolam, however. It is not oxidized in the liver and does not compete for metabolism with other hepatically metabolized drugs nor accumulate with chronic use. In addition, temazepam has been studied in both young age groups as a premedication and in older age groups as a hypnotic. When dosed 1 to 2 hours before bedtime, it is useful in initiating and maintaining sleep.

Flurazepam (Dalmane) and quazepam (Doral) both are hepatically metabolized with long-acting active metabolites. Each is able to keep the patient asleep throughout the night and provide residual daytime sedation if needed for agitation or anxiety. They both maintain hypnotic efficacy over at least 30 days of continuous use. Quazepam has a faster onset the first night of use, but the difference is insignificant on subsequent nights. The disadvantage of both drugs include next-day cognitive impairment that may impact functioning.

In consideration of the available clinical and cost data, temazepam, zolpidem, and zaleplon should be considered priority hypnotics. Zolpidem initiates sleep effectively and maintains sleep for some. Zaleplon initiates sleep with the least risk of daytime hangover and can even be dosed during the night. Temazepam has a sufficient duration of action to benefit those with intolerable mid-night awakenings. Flurazepam should be available for select patients. However, it should not be considered as a first-line agent because of the risk of excessive cognitive and coordination impairment. Chloral hydrate should be available for occasional use in children when temazepam's long onset precludes its use as a preprocedure sedative. The disadvantages outweigh advantages for other available hypnotics. A review of any formulary decision should be conducted every 6 months to determine whether these selections need to be changed based on therapeutic outcome data.

REFERENCES

1. Vgontzas AN, Kales A. Sleep and its disorders. Annu Rev Med 1999;50:387.
2. Walsh J, Ustun TB. Prevalence and health consequences of insomnia. Sleep 1999;22(Suppl 3):S427.
3. Nowell PD et al. Clinical factors contributing to the differential diagnosis of primary insomnia and insomnia related to mental disorders. Am J Psychol 1997;154(10):1412.
4. Katz DA, McHorney CA. The relationship between insomnia and health-related quality of life in patients with chronic illness. J Fam Pract 2002;51(3):229.
5. Kapur VK et al. The relationship between chronically disrupted sleep and healthcare use. Sleep 2002;25(3):289.
6. Mitler MM et al. Sleep medicine, public policy and public health. In: Kryger MH et al, eds. Principles of Sleep Medicine, 3rd Ed. Philadelphia: WB Saunders, 2000:580.
7. Lyznicki JM et al. Sleepiness, driving and motor vehicle crashes. JAMA 1998;279(23):1908.
8. Walsh JK, Engelhardt CL. The direct economic costs of insomnia in the United States for 1995. Sleep 1999;22(Suppl 2):S386.
9. Shapiro CM, Dement WC. Impact and epidemiology of sleep disorders. Br Med J 1993;306:1532.
10. The Gallup Organization. Sleep in America: a national survey of U.S. adults [Commissioned by the National Sleep Foundation]. Princeton, NJ, 1995.
11. Stimmel GL, Dopheide JA. Sleep disorders: focus on insomnia. US Pharmacist 2000;25:69.
12. Mitler MM, Hayduk R. Benefits and risks of pharmacotherapy for narcolepsy. Drug Saf 2002;25(11):791.
13. Montplaiser J et al. Restless legs syndrome and periodic limb movement disorders. In: Kryger MH et al, eds. Principles of Sleep Medicine, 3rd Ed. Philadelphia WB Saunders, 2000:742.
14. Morin CM et al. Behavioral and pharmacological therapies for late-life insomnia: a randomized controlled trial. JAMA 1999;281(9):991.
15. Petit L et al. Non-pharmacological management of primary and secondary insomnia among older people: review of assessment tools and treatments. Age Ageing 2003;32:19.
16. Smith MT et al. Comparative meta-analysis of pharmacotherapy and behavior therapy for persistent insomnia. Am J Psychiatry 2002;159:5.
17. Walsh JK, Schweitzer PK. Ten-year trends in the pharmacological treatment of insomnia. Sleep 1999;22(3):371.
18. Rush CR et al. Acute behavioral effects and abuse potential of trazodone, zolpidem and triazolam in humans. Psychopharmacology 1999;144(3):220.

19. Bliwise DL. Normal aging. In: Kryger MH et al, eds. Principles of Sleep Medicine, 3rd Ed. Philadelphia: WB Saunders, 2000:26.
20. Carskadon MA, Dement WC. Normal human sleep: an overview. In: Kryger MH et al, eds. Principles of Sleep Medicine, 3rd Ed. Philadelphia, WB Saunders 2000:15.
21. Steiger A et al. Effects of hormones on sleep. Horm Res 1998;49:125.
22. Vgontzas AN et al. Impaired nighttime sleep in healthy old versus young adults is associated with eleveated plasma interleukin-6 and cortisol levels: physiologic and therapeutic implications. J Clin Endocrinol Metab 2003;88(5):2087.
23. Verrier RL et al. Cardiovascular physiology: central and autonomic regulation. In: Kryger MH et al, eds. Principles of Sleep Medicine, 3rd Ed. Philadelphia: WB Saunders, 2000:179.
24. Jones B. Basic mechanisms of sleep-wake states. In: Kryger MH et al, eds. Principles of Sleep Medicine, 3rd Ed. Philadelphia: WB Saunders, 2000:134.
25. Ebrahim IO et al. Hypocretin(orexin) deficiency in narcolepsy and primary hypersomnia. J Neurol Neurosurg Psychiatry 2003;74(1):127.
26. Lancel M. Role of GABA$_A$ receptors in the regulation of sleep: initial sleep responses to peripherally administered modulators and agonists. Sleep 1999;22(1):33.
27. Greenblatt DJ et al. Neurochemical and pharmacokinetic correlates of the clinical action of benzodiazepine hypnotics. Am J Med 1990;88(Suppl 3A):18S.
28. Terman M, Terman JS. Light treatment. In: Kryger MH et al, eds. Principles of Sleep Medicine, 3rd Ed. Philadelphia, WB Saunders, 2000:1258.
29. Thorpy MJ. Classification of sleep disorders. In: Kryger MH et al, eds. Principles of Sleep Medicine, 3rd Ed. Philadelphia: WB Saunders, 2000:547.
30. The Diagnostic and Statistical Manual of Mental Disorders, 4th Ed. Text Revised (DSMIV-TR) Washington, DC: American Psychiatric Association, 2000.
31. Wagner J et al. Beyond benzodiazepines: alternative pharmacologic agents for the treatment of insomnia. Ann Pharmacother 1998;32:680.
32. Terzano MG et al. New drugs for insomnia: comparative tolerability of zopiclone, zolpidem and zaleplon. Drug Saf 2003;26(4):261.
33. Greenblatt DJ. Benzodiazepine hypnotics: sorting the pharmacokinetic facts. J Clin Psychiatry 1991;52(Suppl 9):42.
34. Greenblatt DJ et al. Comparative kinetics and dynamics of zaleplon, zolpidem and placebo. Clin Pharmacol Ther 1998;64:553.
35. Tan EK, Ondo W. Restless legs syndrome: clinical features and treatment. Am J Med Sci 2000;319(6):397.
36. Flemons WW. Obstructive sleep apnea. N Engl J Med 2002;347(7):498.
37. Barthlen GM, Stacy C. Dyssomnias, parasomnias, and sleep disorders, associated with medical and psychiatric diseases. Mt Sinai J Med 1994;61(2):139.
38. Drugs that cause psychiatric symptoms. Med Lett Drugs Ther 2002;44:1134.
39. Roehrs T et al. Sedative effects and plasma concentrations following single doses of triazolam, diphenhydramine, ethanol and placebo. Sleep 1993;16(4):301.
40. Basu R et al. Sedative-hypnotic use of diphenhydramine in a rural, older adult, community-based cohort: effects on cognition. Am J Geriatr Psychiatry 2003;11:205.
41. Arendt J et al. Jet lag and sleep disruption. In: Kryger MH et al, eds. Principles of Sleep Medicine, 3rd Ed Philadelphia: WB Saunders, 2000:591.
42. Sack RL et al. Entrainment of free-running circadian rhythms by melatonin in blind people. N Engl J Med 2000;342(15):1070.
43. Jan MM. Melatonin for the treatment of handicapped children with severe sleep disorders. Pediatr Neurol 2000;23(3):229.
44. Spitzer RL et al. Jet lag: clinical features, validation of a new syndrome-specific scale, and lack of response to melatonin in a randomized, double-blind trial. Am J Psychiatry 1999;156:1392.
45. Bunney WE et al. Report of the institute of medicine committee on the efficacy and safety of Halcion. Arch Gen Psychiatry 1999;56:349.
46. Lader M. Rebound insomnia and newer hypnotics. Psychopharmacology 1992;108(3):248.
47. Wysowski DK, Barash D. Adverse behavioral reactions attributed to triazolam in the Food and Drug Administration's spontaneous reporting system. Arch Intern Med 1991;151:2003.
48. Holm K et al. Zolpidem: an update of its pharmacology, therapeutic efficacy and tolerability in the treatment of insomnia Drugs 2000;59:865.
49. Aragona M. Abuse, dependence, and epileptic seizures after zolpidem withdrawal: review and case report. Clin Neuropharmacol 2000;23:281.
50. Dooley M. et al. Zaleplon: a review of its use in the treatment of insomnia. Drugs 2000;60:413.
51. Troy SM et al. Comparison of the effects of zaleplon, zolpidem and triazolam on new memory, learning, and psychomotor performance. J Clin Psychopharmacol 2000;20:328.
52. Walsh JK et al. Lack of residual sedation following middle-of-the night zaleplon administration in sleep maintenance insomnia. Clin Neuropharmacol 2000;23:17.
53. Allen D. et al. The effects of single doses of CL284,846, lorazepam, and placebo on psychomotor and memory function in normal male volunteers. Eur J Clin Pharmacol 1993;45:313.
54. Danjou P et al. A comparison of the residual effects of zaleplon and zolpidem following administration 5 to 2 h before awakening. Br J Clin Pharmacol 1999;48:367.
55. Toner L et al. Central nervous system side effects associated with zolpidem treatment. Clin Neuropharmacol 2000;23:54.
56. Cavallaro R et al. Tolerance and withdrawal with zolpidem. Lancet 1993;342:374.
57. Lobo BL, Greene WL. Zolpidem: distinct from triazolam? Ann Pharmacother 1997;31:1408.
58. Rush CR, Griffiths RR. Zolpidem, triazolam, and temazepam: behavioral and subject-rated effects in normal volunteers. J Clin Psychopharmacol 1996;16:146.
59. Stimmel GL. How to counsel patients about depression and its treatment. Pharmacotherapy 1995;15(Pt 2):100S.
60. Verrier RL and Mittleman MA. Sleep-related cardiac risk. In Kryger MH et al. eds. Principles of Sleep Medicine, 3rd Ed. Philadelphia: WB Saunders, 2000:26.
61. Morin CM et al. Self-reported sleep and mood disturbance in chronic pain patients. Clin J Pain 1998;14(4):311.
62. Roose SP et al. Death, depression, and heart disease. J Clin Psychiatry 1991;52(Suppl 6):34.
63. Midazolam in American Hospital Formulary Service (AHFS). ASHP, 2003.
64. Vercellino CE. Preoperative medications and techniques of induction and maintenance. In: Barash PG, ed. Handbook of Clinical Anesthesia, 2nd Ed. Philadelphia: Lippincott, 1993:233.
65. Greenblatt DJ et al. Pharmacokinetic determinants of dynamic differences among three benzodiazepine hypnotics. Arch Gen Psychiatry 1989;46:326.
66. Roth TG et al. Hypnotic effects of low doses of quazepam in older insomniacs. J Clin Psychopharmacology 1997;17(5):401.
67. Greenblatt DJ et al. Clinical pharmacokinetics of anxiolytics and hypnotics in the elderly. Clin Pharmacokinet 1991;21(3):165.
68. Walmsley JK, Hunt MA. Relative affinity of quazepam for type 1 benzodiazepine receptors in brain. J Clin Psychiatry 1991;52(Suppl 9):15.
69. Dement WC. Objective measurements of daytime sleepiness and performance comparing quazepam with flurazepam in two adult populations using the multiple sleep latency test. J Clin Psychiatry 1991;52(Suppl 9):31.
70. Scharf MB. Feasibility of an every-other-night regimen in insomniac patients: subjective hypnotic effectiveness of quazepam, triazolam, and placebo. J Clin Psychiatry 1993;54(1):33.
71. Estazolam—a new benzodiazepine hypnotic.Med Lett Drugs Ther 1991;33(854):91.
72. Scharf MB et al. Estazolam and flurazepam: a multicenter, placebo-controlled comparative study in outpatients with insomnia. J Clin Pharmacol 1990;30:461.
73. Salzman C. Benzodiazepine dependency: summary of the APA task force on benzodiazepines. Psychopharmacol Bull 1990;26:61.
74. Dement WC. Overview of the efficacy and safety of benzodiazepine hypnotics using objective methods. J Clin Psychiatry 1991;52(Suppl):27.
75. Kupfer DJ et al. Antidepressants and sleep disorders in affective illness. Clin Neuropharmacol 1992;15(Suppl 1;Pt A):360A.
76. Vogel GW et al. Drug effects on REM sleep and on endogenous depression. In: Neuroscience and Biobehavioral Review. New York: Pergamon Press, 1990;14:49.
77. Thase ME. Antidepressant treatment of the depressed patient with insomnia. J Clin Psychiatry 1999;60(Suppl 17):28.
78. Christian-Gillin J, Drummond SPA. Medication and substance abuse. In: Kryger MH et al, eds. Principles of Sleep Medicine, 3rd Ed. Philadelphia: WB Saunders, 2000:1176. Philadelphia: WB Saunders, 2000:1176.
79. Jacobsen FM. Low-dose trazodone as a hypnotic in patients treated with MAOIs and other psychotropics: a pilot study. J Clin Psychiatry 1990;51(7):298.
80. Nierenberg A et al. Trazodone for antidepressant-associated insomnia. Am J Psychiatry 1994;151(7):1069.
81. Hauri P. Primary insomnia. In: Kryger MH et al, eds. Principles of Sleep Medicine. Philadelphia: WB Saunders, 1994:494.
82. Nowell PD et al. Paroxetine in the treatment of primary insomnia: preliminary clinical and electroencephalogram sleep data. J Clin Psychiatry 1999;60(2):89.
83. Foley DJ et al. Incidence and remission of insomnia among elderly adults: an epidemiologic study of 6,800 persons over three years. Sleep 1999;22(Suppl 2):S366.
84. Whitney CW et al. Correlates of daytime sleepiness in 4578 elderly persons: the cardiovascular health study. Sleep 1998;21(1):27.
85. Roberts RE et al. Prospective data on sleep complaints and associated risk factors in an older cohort. Psychosom Med 1999;61(2):188.
86. Richards KC. Effect of back massage and relaxation intervention on sleep in critically ill patients. Am J Crit Care 1998;7(4):288.
87. Cooke KM et al. The effects of evening light exposure on the sleep of elderly women expressing sleep complaints. J Behav Med 1998;21(1):103.
88. Wengel SP et al. Use of benzodiazepines in the elderly. Psychiatr Ann 1993;23(6):325.
89. Rudorfer MV. Pharmacokinetics of psychotropic drugs in special populations. J Clin Psychiatry 1993;54(Suppl 9):50.
90. Simons KJ et al. Pharmacokinetic and pharmacodynamic studies of the H$_1$-receptor antagonist hydroxyzine in the elderly. Clin Pharmacol Ther 1989;45:9.
91. Rickels K et al. Pharmacologic strategies for discontinuing benzodiazepine treatment. J Clin Psychopharm 1999;19(Suppl 2):12.
92. Kryger MH. Management of obstructive sleep apnea: overview. In: Kryger MH et al, eds. Principles of Sleep Medicine, 3rd Ed. Philadelphia: WB Saunders, 2000:940.
93. Yokoe T et al. Elevated levels of c-reactive protein and interleukin-6 in patients with obstructive sleep apnea syndrome are decreased by nasal continuous positive airway pressure. Circulation 2003;107(8):1129.
94. Bixler EO et al. Association of hypertension and sleep-disordered breathing. Arch Intern Med 2000;160(15):2289.
95. Bassetti C, Aldrich MS. Sleep apnea in acute cerebrovascular diseases: final report on 128 patients. Sleep 1999;22(2):217.

96. McNamara F et al. Obstructive sleep apnea in infants and its management with nasal continuous positive airway pressure. Chest 1999;116(1):10.
97. Smith PL et al. A physiologic comparison of nasal and oral positive airway pressure. Chest 2003; 123(3):689.
98. Garrigue S et al. Benefit of atrial pacing in sleep apnea syndrome. N Engl J Med 2002;346(6):404.
98a. Schwartz, JRL, Hirshkowitz M, Erman MK et al. Modafinil as adjunct therapy for daytime sleepiness in obstructive sleep apnea. Chest 2003;124: 2192–2199.
98b. Vastag B. Poised to challenge need for sleep, "Wakefulness Enhancer" rouses concerns. JAMA 2004;291(2):167–170.
99. Terra SG, Oberg KC. Medroxyprogesterone acetate in the treatment of obstructive sleep apnea. Ann Pharmacother 1997;31(6):776.
100. Kraiczi H et al. Effect of serotonin uptake inhibition on breathing during sleep and daytime symptoms in obstructive sleep apnea. Sleep 1999; 22(1):61.
101. Green P et al. Narcolepsy: signs, symptoms, differential diagnosis, and management. Arch Fam Med 1998;7(5):472.
102. Fry JM. Treatment modalities for narcolepsy. Neurology 1998;50(2 Suppl 1):S43.
103. Hogl B et al. Modafinil for the treatment of daytime sleepiness in Parkinson's disease: a double-blind, randomized, crossover, placebo-controlled polygraphic trial. Sleep 2002;25(8):905.
104. Cook H, Xyrem Multicenter study group. A randomized, double-blind, placebo-controlled multicenter trial comparing the effects of three doses of orally administered sodium oxybate with placebo

for the treatment of narcolepsy. Sleep 2002; 25(1):42.
105. Xyrem package insert Orphan Medical Minnetonka, MN. 2002.
106. Ritalin LA insert Novartis East Hanover, N.J. 2002.
107. Wong YN et al. A double-blind, placebo-controlled, ascending-dose evaluation of the pharmacokinetics and tolerability of modafinil tablets in healthy male volunteers. J Clin Pharmacol 1999;39(1):30.
108. Robertson P et al. Effect of modafinil on the pharmacokinetics of ethinyl estradiol and triazolam in healthy volunteers. Clin Pharm Ther 2002; 71(1):46.
109. Dequardo JR. Modafinil-associated clozapine toxicity. Am J Psych 2002;159(7):1243.
110. Black Jed. Modafinil has a role in management of sleep apnea. Am J Respir Crit Care Med 2003; 167:105.
111. Rammohan KW et al. Efficacy and safety of modafinil for the treatment of fatigue in multiple sclerosis: a two centre phase 2 study. J Neurol Neurosurg Psychiatry 2002;72(2):179.
112. Commella CL. Restless legs syndrome: treatment with dopaminergic agents. Neurology 2002;58(4 Suppl 1):87.
113. Bleumink GS et al. Pergolide-induced pleuropulmonary fibrosis. Clin Neuropharm 2002;25(5): 290.
114. Pritchett AM et al Valvular heart disease in patients taking pergolide. Mayo Clin Proc 2002; 77(12):1280.
115. Lauerma H. Nocturnal wandering caused by restless legs and short-acting benzodiazepines. Acta Psychiatr Scand 1991;83:492.

116. Garcia-Borreguero D et al. Treatment of restless legs syndrome with gabapentin: a double-blind, cross-over study. Neurology 2002;59(10):1573.
117. Lauerma H, Markkula J. Treatment of restless legs syndrome with tramadol. J Clin Psychiatry 1999; 60(4):241.
118. Hornyak M et al. Magnesium therapy for periodic leg movements-related insomnia and restless legs syndrome: an open pilot study. Sleep 1998; 21(5):501.
119. Blader JC et al. Sleep problems of elementary school children: a community survey. Arch Pediatr Adolesc Med 1997;151(5):473.
120. Coffey B. Review and update: benzodiazepines in childhood and adolescence. Psychiatr Ann 1993;23(6):332.
121. Kauffman RE et al. The use of chloral hydrate for sedation in children. Pediatrics 1993;92(3):471.
122. Kales A. Comparative effectiveness of nine hypnotic drugs: sleep laboratory studies. JAMA 1979;241:1692.
123. Cote CJ et al. Adverse sedation events in pediatrics: analysis of medications used for sedation. Pediatrics 2000;106(4):633.
124. Onks DL et al. The effect of chloral hydrate and its metabolites, trichloroethanol and trichloroacetic acid, on bilirubin-albumin binding. Pharmacol Toxicol 1992;71:196.
125. Haas DA et al. A pilot study of the efficacy of oral midazolam for sedation in pediatric dental patients. Anesth Prog 1996;43(1):1.
126. Ivaneko A et al. Melatonin in children and adolescents with insomnia: a retrospective study. Clin Pediatr 2003;42(1):51.

Schizophrenia

Jonathan P. Lacro

INTRODUCTION

Schizophrenia, a disease of the brain, is one of the most debilitating and emotionally devastating illnesses known to man. It is a chronic condition that frequently has devastating effects on many aspects of the patient's life and carries a high risk of suicide. Many experts consider schizophrenia to be the most severe expression of psychopathology, encompassing significant disruptions of thinking, perception, emotion, and behavior. Schizophrenia is usually a lifelong psychiatric disability. Family relationships, social functioning, and employment are frequently affected, and periodic hospitalizations are common. The management of schizophrenia involves multi-

ple strategies to optimize the patient's functional capacity, reduce the frequency and severity of symptom exacerbations, and reduce the overall morbidity and mortality from this disorder. Many patients require comprehensive and continuous care over the course of their lives.

The aim of this chapter is to provide a framework for the clinician to develop skills in schizophrenia management by considering the following: pathophysiology, assessment, clinical course, and treatment. Treatment is best designed and evaluated by combining information obtained from patient interviews, family or caregiver interviews, and data from previous medical records. Structured mental status examinations assist in evaluating clinical responses to pharmacotherapy. Although this chapter uses terminology based on mental status assessments, the reader is referred elsewhere for specific interviewing techniques.[1,2]

EPIDEMIOLOGY

In the United States, approximately 1% of the population develops schizophrenia during their lifetime. Although schizophrenia affects men and women with equal frequency, there are differences in the age of onset and course of illness. The onset of schizophrenia usually occurs during late adolescence or early adulthood, with men experiencing an earlier onset than women. Prevalence rates are similar throughout the world, but pockets of high prevalence have been reported in some areas. After adjusting for differences in diagnostic criteria for schizophrenia, similar prevalence rates across cultures have been observed.

ECONOMIC BURDEN

Mental disorders constitute a large part of the global burden of disease, with schizophrenia being among the greatest causes of disability in the United States and the world.[3] Unlike other chronic diseases such as diabetes and hypertension in which the onset generally occurs in late life, schizophrenia usually affects people when they are young and usually follows a chronic course that persists throughout the patient's lifetime. Most people with schizophrenia experience multiple hospitalizations and generally require social assistance. Even during relatively stable phases of their illness, most people with schizophrenia require support that ranges from a family member to day hospitalization. The total United States economic cost of schizophrenia in 1990 was estimated at $33 billion, including both direct and indirect costs. Direct costs include hospitalization, rehabilitation, professional services, medication, and office visits. Indirect costs include loss of productivity caused by illness, disability, premature death, and economic burden to families.[4] Schizophrenia accounts for approximately 2.5% of total annual health care costs in the United States. Persons afflicted by schizophrenia represent approximately 10% of this country's permanently disabled population; they consume 20% of Social Security benefit days; and, they occupy 25% of the hospital beds.[4,5]

ETIOLOGY (NEUROBIOLOGY)

Schizophrenia is a complex disorder with multiple causes. Partly because there is no consistent neuropathology or biomarkers of schizophrenia, current theories of the disorder have moved away from the view that it is a single entity and toward a conceptualization of schizophrenia as a collection of etiologically disparate disorders with common clinical features.[6,7] In this section, the genetic and environmental factors, neuroanatomic, and neurochemical features of schizophrenia are considered.

Genetic and Environmental Risk Factors

It has long been known that schizophrenia runs in families. First-degree biologic relatives of persons with schizophrenia have a tenfold greater risk of developing the disease than the general population.[8] The risk is highest (40% to 50%) in a monozygotic (identical) twin of a person with schizophrenia.[9,10] Because the concordance rate is not 100% in monozygotic twins, other nongenetic factors must contribute to the development of the disorder. Environmental factors such as prenatal difficulties (e.g., malnutrition in the first trimester of pregnancy or influenza in the second trimester), perinatal complications, and various nonspecific stressors may also influence the development of schizophrenia. Despite the overwhelming evidence that schizophrenia is an inherited illness, a single "schizophrenia gene" has not been found. Risk for schizophrenia is, to some extent, genetically transmitted and is probably determined by multiple genes. A recent review of the molecular genetics of schizophrenia cited linkage studies implicating chromosomes 6, 8, 10, 13, and 22.[11]

Neuroanatomy

Studies comparing the brains of individuals with schizophrenia with the brains of normal controls have uncovered a number of important differences. Although these studies suggest that anatomic and functional abnormalities are associated with schizophrenia, no single pathognomonic abnormality has been found consistently. In addition, localization of the site(s) responsible for the pathophysiology of schizophrenia remains elusive.

The most consistent structural finding seen among the many computed tomography (CT) and magnetic resonance imaging (MRI) studies in patients with schizophrenia has been enlarged ventricular spaces, particularly involving the lateral and third ventricles. In addition, there appears to be a relationship between brain asymmetry and the disease process.[12] When unilateral abnormalities have been reported, they have typically involved the left hemisphere.[12] As imaging technology has advanced, MRI studies in schizophrenia frequently have shown morphologic abnormalities involving the temporal lobes, frontal lobes, parietal lobes, and subcortical structures.[13–17] Findings include decreased neuronal volume and density, decreased synaptic connections, decreases in synaptophysin (a membrane protein of synaptic vesicles), and loss of microtubule associated protein and synaptosomal protein in certain regions of the cortex.[18,19] The lack of gliosis in association with the neuroantomic abnormalities in the brains of schizophrenia patients suggests that these changes occur neurodevelopmentally.[24] Functional imaging studies, such as positron emission tomography (PET), single photon emission computed tomography (SPECT), and functional magnetic resonance imaging (fMRI) have demonstrated alterations in either cerebral perfusion or glucose metabolism in frontal, temporal, and basal ganglia areas of the brain.[20–23] Additional attention has been directed toward the correlation of regional brain abnormalities with specific symptoms or subtypes of schizophrenia. Thus far, the most robust findings have been found in the relation between negative symptoms and the prefrontal cortex; positive symptoms and temporal lobes; and thought disorder and the planum temporale.[25]

In summary, neuroimaging studies have identified anatomic and functional abnormalities that affect different areas of the brain, particularly prefrontal and temporal areas, and that correspond with the impairments observed in schizophrenia.[26] Medial temporal structures are important for the processing of sensory information, and abnormalities in this area may explain distortions in the interpretation of external reality that are characteristic of schizophrenia. The prefrontal cortex is responsible for some of the complex and highly evolved human functions including the integration of information from other cortical areas. The prefrontal cortex is largely responsible for the regulation of working memory, which involves maintaining information in temporary memory while that information is used for executive functions. Hence, these abnormalities in prefrontal areas could explain the deficits in working memory and attention that are often present in schizophrenia. New theories of schizophrenia that have been proposed include the "cognitive dysmetria" theory (implicating the thalamus and its cortical and cerebellar connections), the "disconnection model" (implicating temporolimbic and prefrontal disconnections), and the "asynchronous neural firing" model.[27–29]

Neurochemistry

The discovery of the antipsychotic properties of chlorpromazine led to a fundamental understanding of the neurochemistry of schizophrenia. The finding that chlorpromazine and other antipsychotic drugs decrease dopamine activity by blocking specific postsynaptic receptors served as the foundation for the dopaminergic hypothesis of schizophrenia. Nearly all drugs that decrease dopamine activity decrease the positive symptoms of schizophrenia. Furthermore, the clinical efficacy of antipsychotic agents is roughly proportional to their affinity for a particular subtype of dopamine receptors, the D_2 receptor.[30,31] Although other classes of dopamine receptors have been identified (e.g., D_1, D_3, D_4), this close relationship to clinical potency exists only for the D_2 receptor subtype.[32] Indirect evidence supporting the dopamine hypothesis is found in the observation that dopamine agonists such as amphetamine, levodopa, methylphenidate, and other aminergic agents can worsen schizophrenia symptoms in some patients.[33–35] Although these observations indicate that manipulating the dopaminergic system can regulate the positive symptoms of schizophrenia, they do not directly implicate a central excess of dopamine as the sole cause of schizophrenia symptoms. This simplistic theory does not explain, for instance, cases of schizophrenia in which residual or negative symptoms predominate. The "hypofrontality theory" suggests that reduced or dysfunctional dopaminergic neurotransmission within the prefrontal cortex or mesocortical area of schizophrenic patients may be responsible for negative symptoms.[36,37] In addition to negative symptomatology, prefrontal dopaminergic dysfunction has been correlated with cognitive dysfunction, particularly in the area of working memory. It has also been proposed that a chronically low level of striatal dopamine release causes negative symptoms (caused by low levels of dopamine in the prefrontal cortex); the diminished dopamine release would lead to an upregulation of dopamine receptors, resulting in supersensitivity to phasic dopamine release in the context of environmental stressors (exhibited behaviorally as positive symptoms).[38] This theory explains why dopamine-blocking drugs would improve positive symptoms, but not negative symptoms.

Serotonin also seems to play a role in schizophrenia. Alteration in monoamine activity in the limbic circuit has been proposed as a possible link to the dopamine hypothesis of schizophrenia.[39] Serotonin receptors are abundant in mesocortical areas, and agonism at these receptor sites may have an inhibitory effect on dopaminergic receptors or dopamine release, possibly contributing to negative schizophrenia symptoms.

Another area of focus is the involvement of excitatory amino acids and the glutamate transmitter system in the pathogenesis of schizophrenia.[40] Decreased activation of N-methyl-D-aspartic acid (NMDA) or glutamate receptors may increase cortical dopamine release and produce a syndrome resembling schizophrenia. This hypofunctional NMDA-receptor theory was supported by findings of low glutamate levels in the cerebrospinal fluid of persons with schizophrenia and by the observation that phencyclidine, an NMDA antagonist, could produce florid psychosis.[41] In utero exposure to excitotoxins or viruses has been proposed as a possible mechanism for destruction of NMDA receptors within the brain. The clinical effect of neuronal destruction may not be expressed until late adolescence or early adulthood (when schizophrenic symptoms usually arise). γ-Aminobutyric acid (GABA), a major inhibitory amino acid, may act as a third link between the neuromodulation of glutamate and dopamine receptors. It has been suggested that GABA receptor function may be impaired within the prefrontal region, resulting in abnormal NMDA receptor concentrations.[42] It has also been proposed that an imbalance between NMDA, GABA, and dopamine (DA) receptors may cause the symptoms of schizophrenia. Studies examining the clinical effects of direct glycinergic agonists or inhibitors of glutamate uptake in persons with schizophrenia are needed to clarify the role of excitatory amino acid neurotransmission in this disorder.

Substantial progress has been made in neuropathologic and neuroanatomic studies of schizophrenia. Insights from physiologic imaging studies in living patients, studies of brain development and its genetic control, and pharmacologic studies using newer atypical antipsychotics are promising stepping stones that may lead to a better understanding of the pathogenesis of schizophrenia.

CLINICAL PRESENTATION
Historical Concept of Schizophrenia

Kraepelin[43] provided the first thorough description of the constellation of symptoms that make up schizophrenia, which he called "dementia praecox" (a syndrome of cognitive and behavioral deficits that tend to appear early in life). Kraepelin emphasized that dementia praecox generally followed a chronic course with no return to the premorbid level of functioning. Kraepelin also noted that no single pathognomonic symptom or cluster of symptoms served to characterize dementia praecox, an illness he considered so mysterious that he referred to it as a disorder whose causes were shrouded in "impenetrable darkness." Bleuler[44] concurred with Kraepelin's initial description of schizophrenia, although he suggested that some patients did recover and subsequently could lead productive lives. For Bleuler, the most important and fundamental feature was a fragmentation in the formulation and expression of thought, referring to it as "loosening of associations." Bleuler described the "4 A's" of schizophrenia, which include autism (preoccupation with internal stimuli), inappropriate affect (external manifestations of mood), loose associations (illogical or fragmented thought processes), and ambivalence (simultaneous, contradictory thinking). Thus, Bleuler focused on negative symptoms and thought disorganization rather than on the positive symptoms of schizophrenia such as delusions and hallucinations. Another important contribution to the defining features of schizophrenia was Schneider's "first-rank" symptoms[45] of schizophrenia that assisted the clinician in diagnosing schizophrenia. First-rank symptoms include delusions, auditory hallucinations, thought withdrawal, thought insertion, thought broadcasting, and experiencing feelings or actions that are under someone else's control. Schneider's first-rank symptoms provided the framework for the systematic diagnostic criteria used today in psychiatry.

Diagnosis and Differential Diagnosis

The *Diagnostic and Statistical Manual of the American Psychiatric Association,* text revision (DSM-IV-TR), is the latest edition of the guide for diagnosing and classifying schizophrenia and other psychiatric disorders. Compared with previous DSM editions, DSM-IV-TR has a greater emphasis on negative symptoms and the social and occupational dysfunction associated with schizophrenia.[10] Psychosis has many causes, and all must be excluded before the diagnosis of schizophrenia is made. In addition, a diagnosis can be made only if the DSM-IV-TR criteria are met (Table 78-1). Clinicians can misdiagnose psychotic patients when the diagnosis is based on presenting symptoms alone without regard to the longitudinal clinical course. An accurate diagnosis is important because treatments vary for psychoses with different origins. Schizophreniform disorder is similar to schizophrenia except that it lasts for >1 month but for <6 months. Brief psychotic disorder is diagnosed when positive symptoms present suddenly and are present for at least a day but for no longer than 1 month. After the episode subsides, premorbid functioning usually returns. Various personality disorders, including schizotypal, schizoid, and paranoid types also can resemble schizophrenia; however, these disorders lack the chronic thought disturbances seen in schizophrenia. Bipolar disorder, manic or depressive phase, and major depression can have psychotic features that usually are mood congruent. Negative symptoms of schizophrenia such as akinesia, anergy, apathy, and social withdrawal may resemble depression, but do not respond to antidepressant therapy. It is also important to differentiate extrapyramidal side effects of drugs, particularly akinesia seen with antipsychotic-induced parkinsonism, from the negative symptoms of schizophrenia. Common differential diagnoses are listed in Table 78-2.

Drug-induced psychosis is an important differential diagnosis when evaluating patients with schizophrenia-like symptoms. Illicit drugs may cause psychotic symptoms in any individual, but do not cause the illness of schizophrenia in persons without a predisposition to mental illness or an underlying psychiatric disorder. Drugs causing acute psychotic symptoms include amphetamines, cocaine, cannabis, phencyclidine (PCP or "angel dust"), lysergic acid diethylamide (LSD) and ketamine. In addition, anticholinergic delirium can occur if excessive doses or combinations of therapeutic agents with anticholinergic properties are prescribed. A urine toxi-

Table 78-1 DSM-IV-TR Criteria for Schizophrenia

A. Characteristic Symptoms

At least two of the following, each present for a significant portion of time during a 1-month period (or less if successfully treated):

1. Delusions
2. Hallucinations
3. Disorganized speech (e.g., frequent derailment or incoherence)
4. Grossly disorganized or catatonic behavior
5. Negative symptoms (i.e., affective flattening, alogia, or avolition)

Note: Only one "A symptom" is required if delusions are bizarre or hallucinations consist of a voice keeping up a running commentary on the person's behavior or thought, two or more conversations with each other.

B. Social/Occupation Dysfunction

For a significant portion of the time since the onset of the disturbance, one or more major areas of functioning such as work, interpersonal relationships, or self-care is markedly below the level achieved before the onset.

C. Duration

Continuous signs of the disturbance persist for at least 6 months. This 6-month period must include at least 1 month of symptoms (or less if successfully treated) that meet criterion A (i.e., active-phase symptoms) and may include prodromal and/or residual periods when the "A criterion" is not fully met. During these periods, signs of the disturbance may be manifested by negative symptoms or by two or more symptoms listed in "criterion A" present in an attenuated form (e.g., blunted affect, unusual perceptual disturbances).

D. Schizoaffective Disorder and Mood Disorder Exclusion

Schizoaffective disorder and mood disorder with psychotic features have been ruled out because either (1) no major depressive, manic, or mixed manic episodes have occurred concurrently with the active phase symptoms or (2) if mood episodes have occurred during active phase symptoms, their total duration has been brief relative to the duration of the active and residual periods.

E. Substance/General Medical Condition Exclusion

The disturbance is not due to direct physiologic effects of a substance (drug of abuse or medication) or a general medical condition.

F. Relationship to a Pervasive Development Disorder

If there is a history of autistic disorder or another pervasive development disorder, the additional diagnosis of schizophrenia is made only if prominent delusions or hallucinations also are present for at least a month (or less if successfully treated).

From Reference 10.

cology screen can help evaluate the contribution of substance abuse to psychosis, but because of the risk of false-negative results, the quality and progression of the presenting symptoms and physical findings also must be considered to make an accurate diagnosis. A particularly difficult problem is evaluating the cause of psychosis in a patient with schizophrenia and concurrent drug or alcohol abuse. Distinguishing between the two may not be possible until the patient becomes drug free and residual symptoms are assessed. There are some differences in the presentation of drug-induced psychosis and schizophrenia. For example, chronic stimulant abuse usually

Table 78-2   Differential Diagnosis for Schizophrenia (DSM-IV-TR)

Drug-Induced Psychoses

Amphetamine
Cocaine
Cannabis (marijuana)
Phencyclidine (PCP)
Lysergic acid diethylamide (LSD)
Anticholinergics

Primary Psychiatric Disorders

Brief psychotic disorder
Schizophreniform disorder
Bipolar affective disorder, manic type
Mood disorder with psychotic features

Personality Disorders

Schizotypal
Schizoid
Paranoid

does not present with a formal thought disorder. Cannabis psychosis may be differentiated from acute paranoid schizophrenia because patients with the former usually experience a subjective feeling of panic and retain insight into their problem.[46] Acute PCP ingestion can cause psychotic symptoms such as paranoia and acute catatonia, but other concomitant symptoms such as ataxia, hyperreflexia, nystagmus, and hypertension are not found in schizophrenia.

Target Symptoms

Schizophrenia is a complex disorder comprising different clusters of signs and symptoms. The characteristic symptoms of schizophrenia have often been conceptualized as falling into two broad categories: positive and negative (or deficit) symptoms. Positive symptoms can be further divided into two distinct groups, positive symptoms and disorganized symptoms. Positive symptoms include hallucinations (auditory, visual) and delusions (persecution, guilt, religion, mind control). Disorganized symptoms include disorganized speech, thought disorder (tangentiality, derailment, circumstantiality) and disorganized behavior (clothing, appearance, aggression, repetitive actions). Negative symptoms include affective flattening, decreased thought and speech productivity (alogia), loss of ability to experience pleasure (anhedonia), and decreased initiation of goal-directed behavior (avolition). Most patients with schizophrenia exhibit both positive and negative symptoms, although the dominance of one type over the other usually varies throughout the course of the illness. Younger patients tend to exhibit more positive symptoms, whereas in older patients negative symptoms predominate. Table 78-3 provides a glossary of commonly used terms in schizophrenia, and Table 78-4 lists positive and negative symptoms of schizophrenia.

Cognitive deficits, including problems with attention, memory, and concentration, are another frequently cited problem for people with schizophrenia. These impairments are common, affecting as many as 70% of individuals with schizophrenia.[47] The most consistently replicated deficits are

Table 78-3   Glossary of Commonly Used Terms in Schizophrenia

Affect: behavior (usually an expression of an emotion) that is observed by the interviewer. Common types of disturbances in affect include: *restricted*—mild decrease in range and intensity of the expression of emotion; *blunted*—significant decrease in intensity of the expression of emotion; *flat*—absence of expression of emotion; *inappropriate*—incongruency between patient's affect and mood or behavior; *labile*—abrupt shifts in expression of emotion.

Akathisia: syndrome consisting of subjective feelings of anxiety and restlessness, and objective signs of pacing, rocking, and an inability to sit or stand still for extended periods of time.

Akinesia: absence or decrease in voluntary movement; may be antipsychotic-induced (extrapyramidal side effects) or a manifestation of negative symptoms of schizophrenia.

Alogia: impoverished thinking usually manifested through speech and language deficits. Speech is brief and lacks spontaneity; replies to questions are very concrete (*poverty of speech*). *Poverty of content* refers to speech that is adequate in amount, but is of little substance (overly abstract), repetitive, or stereotyped.

Anergy: lack of energy.

Anhedonia: loss of interest or pleasure.

Avolition: an inability to initiate and sustain goal-directed activities. The patient may sit for extended periods of time and show minimal interest in participating in social or work-related activities.

Circumstantiality: a form of disorganized speech characterized by "talking in circles" or taking an unusually long length of time in answering a question or expressing one's point of view.

Delusions: a false belief that is firmly held in spite of evidence to refute the belief. The belief does not qualify as a delusion if it is a cultural or religious belief accepted by a group of individuals. Types of delusions include grandiose, persecutory, and somatic type.

Executive function: the ability to design and carry out a solution to a plan when the solution is not obvious. Loss of executive function presents as failure to learn from past experience, and failure to plan or organize life events.

Hallucination: a sensory perception (e.g., auditory, visual, somatic, tactile) experienced in the absence of external stimuli. Hallucinations may be recognized as false sensory perceptions in some, whereas others may believe that the experiences are reality based.

Loose associations: a form of disorganized, illogical speech characterized by unrelated words, phrases, and sentences used in a fashion that makes comprehension very difficult, if not impossible.

Mood: a pervasive and sustained emotion that is experienced by the patient. Examples include depressed, anxious, angry, or irritable mood.

Mood congruent delusions or hallucinations: delusions or hallucinations that are consistent with a mood or behavior (e.g., delusions/hallucinations of death, guilt, or punishment in the presence of a depressed mood).

Mood incongruent delusions or hallucinations: delusions or hallucinations that are not consistent with a mood or behavior (e.g., delusions/hallucinations of death, guilt, or punishment in the presence of mania).

Tangentiality: a form of disorganized speech in which answers are remotely or completely unrelated to questions, and patients' thoughts frequently shift in an unconnected fashion.

Thought broadcasting: a delusion that one's thoughts are being broadcast to others (e.g., a patient feels that others can read his or her mind).

Thought disorder: a general term often used to describe any type of abnormal thought process (e.g., delusion, loose association, conceptual disorganization).

Thought insertion: a delusion that one's thoughts are being inserted into one's mind by others.

Table 78-4 Positive and Negative Symptoms of Schizophrenia

Positive	Negative
Combativeness, agitation, and hostility	Psychomotor retardation
Tension	Affective flattening
Hyperactivity	Avolition
Hallucinations	Lack of socialization
Delusions	Alogia (poverty of speech)
Disorganized speech (loose associations, tangential, blocking)	Loss of emotional connectedness
	Loss of executive functions
Unusual behavior	

observed on tasks measuring attention, information processing speed, working memory, learning, and executive (i.e., frontal systems) functions.[48] These domains are not only commonly impaired in schizophrenia, but they are also strongly associated with functional outcomes (i.e., social and community functioning).[48] Although it is likely that the overall dysfunction observed in schizophrenia encompasses factors such as psychopathology, drug treatment, and social isolation, evidence suggests that cognitive impairments have a stronger relationship to the long-term functional outcome than positive symptoms.[48]

Typical Course and Outcome
Onset of Illness
The onset of the first psychotic episode may be abrupt or insidious, but the majority of individuals display some type of prodromal phase during which there is the slow and gradual development of a variety of signs and symptoms. Symptoms may include chronic somatic complaints such as headache, tinnitus, back and muscle pain, weakness, and digestive problems. Family and friends may eventually notice that the person has changed and is no longer functioning well in occupational, social, and personal activities (e.g., social withdrawal, loss of interest in school or work, deterioration of hygiene and grooming, unusual behavior, outbursts of anger). At this point, a patient may begin to develop an interest in abstract ideas, philosophy, the occult, or religion. Other prodromal signs and symptoms can include markedly peculiar behavior, abnormal affect, and strange perceptual experiences. Eventually, a symptom characteristic of the active phase (see Table 78-1, criterion A) appears, marking the disturbance as schizophrenia.

Typical Course
In contrast to the notion of an inevitable progressive deterioration in schizophrenia as proposed by Kraepelin, longitudinal studies of schizophrenia suggest that the course of illness is highly variable. The majority suffers from episodic exacerbations and remissions with some degree of residual symptoms.[43,49–51] Complete remission (i.e., a return to full premorbid functioning) is not common in this disorder. Of the patients who remain ill, some appear to have a relatively stable course, whereas others show a progressive worsening associated with severe disability. Reported remission rates range from 10% to 60%, and a reasonable estimate is that

20% to 30% of all schizophrenia patients are able to lead somewhat normal lives. About 20% to 30% of patients continue to experience moderate symptoms, and 40% to 60% of patients remain significantly impaired by their disorder for their entire lives. Early in the illness, negative symptoms may manifest as prodromal features. Subsequently, positive symptoms appear. Because these positive symptoms are particularly responsive to treatment, they typically diminish, but in many individuals negative symptoms persist between episodes of positive symptoms. As patients with schizophrenia age, the frequency and severity of acute episodes may decrease; however, negative symptoms may become more steadily prominent in some individuals, a state often referred to as *burn-out*.[49,50,52] The American Psychiatric Association Practice Guideline for the Treatment of Schizophrenia describe three phases of illness for the purpose of integrating treatment.[53] These phases are not always distinct or separate, but instead tend to overlap with each other. During the *acute phase*, patients suffer from floridly psychotic symptoms such as delusions and/or hallucinations, are severely disorganized, and usually require hospitalization. Negative symptoms become more severe during this phase as well. During the *stabilization phase*, acute symptoms gradually decrease in severity as the patient begins to stabilize. This stage may persist for as long as 6 months after the initial psychotic break. During this phase the individual is most vulnerable to relapse. During the *stable phase*, a level of functioning considered optimal for that individual patient is attained. Although complete resolution of symptoms is desired, many patients will never achieve this goal. Negative symptoms may persist and patients may experience nonspecific symptoms such as tension, anxiety, or mood instability during the stable phase.

Prognosis
Predictors of an improved long-term outcome in patients with schizophrenia include female gender, a positive family history of an affective disorder, a negative family history of schizophrenia, good premorbid functioning, higher IQ, married marital status, acute onset with precipitating stress, fewer prior episodes (both number and length), a phasic pattern of episodes and remissions (i.e., less residual symptoms), advancing age at onset, minimal comorbidity, paranoid subtype, and symptoms that are predominantly positive (delusions, hallucinations) and not disorganized (thought disorder, disorganized behavior).[53] Despite modern treatment advancements, schizophrenia remains a severe disease with a relatively poor outcome. Many patients experience repeated hospitalizations and exacerbations of symptoms; and, suicide attempts are relatively common. Individuals with schizophrenia have a 20% shorter life expectancy than the general population.[54] This is due in part, to an increased incidence of general medical illness (such as diabetes or cardiovascular disease) and suicide.[53] Patients with schizophrenia have approximately a 50% lifetime risk for a suicide attempt and as many as 9% to 13% may die because of a suicide attempt.[55]

TREATMENT
There is no cure for schizophrenia. The goal of any treatment program is to effectively alleviate the suffering of the patient (and caregivers) and to improve social and cognitive func-

tions. Many patients require comprehensive care and life-long treatment. Comprehensive care consists of pharmacologic, psychosocial, and rehabilitative treatment.

Role of Nonpharmacologic Interventions

Nonpharmacologic interventions are often combined with drug treatment and can provide additional benefits in such areas as relapse prevention, improved coping skills, better social and vocational functioning, and ability to function more independently. Interventions should be started as early as possible, even during the management of an acute episode. As a patient begins to stabilize during an acute episode, nonpharmacologic strategies can be implemented.[53] Individual therapy (e.g., supportive, insight oriented, reality oriented) can improve insight into the illness, improve medication adherence, teach ways to cope with medication side effects and stress, and help the patient identify early warning signs of relapse. Group therapy can enhance socialization skills. In patients who are less stable and who continue to exhibit negative symptoms, supportive therapy is generally more effective than group or other more complex, insight-oriented therapies. Family therapy is also important because family members need to learn ways to cope with such a devastating illness and how to be supportive of their loved one, while not being overly controlling. Vocational training can benefit patients who will likely need a significant amount of assistance in finding and maintaining long term employment.[61] Evidence-based practice guidelines for psychosocial treatment of schizophrenia now include interventions such as social skills training, cognitive/cognitive-behavioral therapy, family psychoeducation, and vocational rehabilitation.[56–60] For example, the Program for Assertive Community Treatment (PACT) is a team treatment approach designed specifically for patients with severe functional impairments who have avoided or not responded well to traditional outpatient mental health care and psychiatric rehabilitation services.[53] Persons served by PACT often have co-existing problems such as homelessness, substance abuse problems, or involvement with the judicial system. A key component of PACT is having a very high staff-to-patient ratio with the patient receiving individualized attention to the various nonpharmacologic strategies described above. PACT has been shown to reduce the rate and duration of psychiatric hospitalization and improve living conditions for patients with schizophrenia.[53]

Pharmacologic Interventions

Antipsychotics

CLASSIFICATION AND NOMENCLATURE OF THE ANTIPSYCHOTICS

Antipsychotics have been broadly classified into two groups. The older agents (i.e., those introduced in the United States before 1990) are referred to as *typical* or *conventional* antipsychotics or dopamine receptor antagonists, since their pharmacologic activity is attributed to the blockade of central dopamine receptors, particularly the D_2 receptor subtype. These agents have also been referred to as *major tranquilizers* and *neuroleptics*. The term major tranquilizer is inaccurate, since these agents—particularly the high-potency agents—can improve psychosis without sedating patients or making them tranquil. *Neuroleptic* is a more appropriate term and refers to the tendency of these drugs to cause neurologic side

effects, particularly extrapyramidal symptoms (EPS). Typical antipsychotics are further classified as high-or low-potency agents, based on their relative ability to block dopamine receptors. They can also be classed by chemical structure (phenothiazine and nonphenothiazine) and potential for common adverse effects (EPS, sedation, anticholinergic, and cardiovascular effects).[61,62] Examples of typical agents include haloperidol, fluphenazine, thiothixene, chlorpromazine and thioridazine.

Newer agents consist of clozapine, risperidone, olanzapine, quetiapine, ziprasidone and aripiprazole. They have been referred to as *atypical* or *serotonin-dopamine antagonists*. The latter term refers to the postsynaptic effects of these agents at $5-HT_{2A}$ and D_2 receptors. Some of the general characteristics that may be considered as features of atypical antipsychotic include an absence or decreased incidence of EPS, lack of effect on serum prolactin, greater efficacy for refractory schizophrenia, and greater activity against negative symptoms.[63] However, currently there are no widely accepted characteristics that define an "atypical" antipsychotic and clozapine is actually the only atypical agent which fulfills *all* of the criteria stated above. Recently, the term *second-generation antipsychotic* has also been proposed to describe this class of medications though there is no consensus on the nomenclature at the present time.[64]

MECHANISM OF DRUG ACTION

The specific mechanism of action of antipsychotics has not been elucidated, but most of the research attention has focused on postsynaptic blockade at dopamine D_2 and serotonin $5-HT_{2A}$ receptor sites. It is generally accepted that D_2 receptor antagonism plays a key role in the treatment of positive symptoms of schizophrenia as well as in the production of EPS and hyperprolactinemia-related side effects. Knowledge of the central dopamine pathways in the brain can be used as a model to understand the therapeutic and side effects of the antipsychotics. The central dopamine system is comprised of four tracts: mesolimbic, mesocortical, nigrostriatal, and tuberoinfundibular (Fig. 78-1). Drug action can be predicted if a clinician understands the function of each tract, along with the binding affinity of an agent for receptors located in the tract (Tables 78-5 and 78-6). Blockade of dopamine receptors in the mesolimbic tract is likely responsible for the reduction of positive symptoms of schizophrenia. Blockade of the other dopamine tracts is largely responsible for the adverse effects of antipsychotic treatment. The mesocortical tract is responsible for higher-order thinking and executive functions. Dopamine hypofunctioning in this area, either from the schizophrenia itself or by antipsychotic action, may be responsible for negative symptoms. The nigrostriatal tract modulates body movement. Antipsychotic-induced blockade in this area causes EPS. Lastly, antipsychotic-induced blockade of the dopamine tract in the tuberoinfundibular area of the anterior pituitary leads to hyperprolactinemia.[37] Ideally, selective dopaminergic blockade of the mesolimbic tract would be preferred. Unfortunately, typical antipsychotics block all four of these dopaminergic pathways. Studies have demonstrated that antipsychotic effects require a striatal D_2 receptor occupancy of 65% to 70%; D_2 receptor occupancy greater than 80% significantly increases the risk of EPS.[65,66] During chronic treatment with typical antipsychotic agents, between 70% and

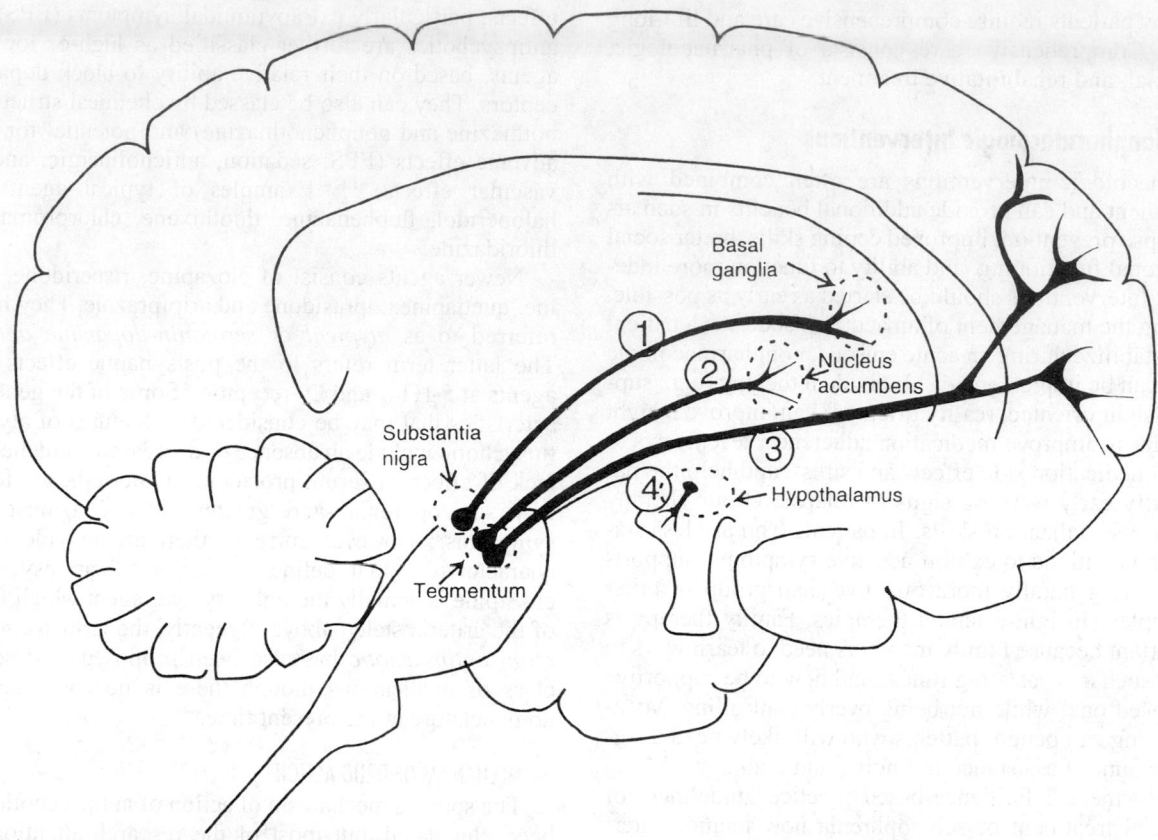

FIGURE 78-1 Four dopamine pathways in the brain. The neuroanatomy of dopamine neuronal pathways in the brain can explain both the therapeutic effects and the side effects of the known antipsychotic agents. (*1*) The nigrostriatal dopamine pathway projects from the substantia nigra to the basal ganglia, and is thought to control movements. (*2*) The mesolimbic dopamine pathway projects from the midbrain ventral tegmental area to the nucleus accumbens, a part of the limbic system of the brain thought to be involved in many behaviors, such as pleasurable sensations, the powerful euphoria of drugs of abuse, as well as delusions and hallucinations of psychosis. (*3*) A pathway related to the mesolimbic dopamine pathway is the mesocortical dopamine pathway. it also projects from the midbrain ventral tegmental area, but sends its axons to the limbic cortex, where it may have a role in mediating positive and negative psychotic symptoms or cognitive side effects of neuroleptic antipsychotic medications. (*4*) The fourth dopamine pathway of interest is the one that controls prolactin secretion, called the tuberoinfundibular dopamine pathway. It projects from the hypothalamus to the anterior pituitary gland.

Table 78-5 Neurotransmitter-Tract Function and Effect of Typical versus Atypical Antipsychotics

Neurotransmitter-Tract	Clinical Function	Typical Agent Effects	Atypical Agent Effects
Dopamine-nigrostriatal	Modulates EPS	Potent D_2 blockade causes EPS	Minimal EPS due to greater specificity for mesolimbic system
Dopamine-mesolimbic	Modulates arousal, memory, behavior	Effectively treats positive symptoms	Effectively treats positive symptoms
Dopamine-mesocortical	Modulates cognition, socialization, and other negative symptoms	Less effective for negative symptoms	Clozapine (possibly others) greater efficacy for negative symptoms; clozapine, risperidone (others?) may improve cognition
Dopamine-tuberoinfundibular	Regulates prolactin release	Increases prolactin release (dose related)	No increase in prolactin with clozapine, dose-related with risperidone, no significant increase with others
Serotonergic (5-HT2)	5-HT2 blockade reduces EPS, improves negative symptoms	Minimal affinity for 5-HT2 receptors	Greater affinity for 5-HT2 receptors

EPS, extrapyramidal side effects.
Adapted from References 37, 63, and 74.

Table 78-6 **Relative Receptor-Binding Affinities of Typical and Atypical Antipsychotic Agents**

Receptor	D₁	D₂	5-HT2	α₁	M₁	H₁
Typical Agents						
Chlorpromazine	–	+++	++	+++	+++	++
Fluphenazine	–	+++	+	+	–	–
Perphenazine	–	+++	++	++	–	++
Thioridazine	+	+++	++	+++	+++	+
Haloperidol	++	+++	+	+	–	–
Atypical Agents						
Clozapine	++	++	+++	+++	+++	+
Risperidone	–	+++	+++	+++	–	+
Olanzapine	++	++	+++	++	+++	++
Quetiapine	–	+	++	+++	+	+
Ziprasidone	+/–	++	+++	++	–	+
Aripiprazole	+	+++	++	++	–	+

D₁, dopamine subtype 1; D₂, dopamine subtype 2; 5-HT2, serotonin subtype 2; α1, alpha 1; M₁, muscarinic (cholinergic) subtype 1; H₁, histamine subtype 1.
–, none; +/–, unclear; +, minimal; ++, moderate; +++, high; ++++, very high.
Compiled from references 67, 128, and 164.

90% of D₂ receptors in the striatum are usually occupied.[67] Not surprisingly, all the typical antipsychotic agents have been observed to be effective in reducing positive symptoms of schizophrenia and they all can cause EPS.

In contrast to typical antipsychotic agents that affect all four dopamine tracts, atypical antipsychotics primarily affect dopamine tracts in the limbic system and have been termed *limbic-specific*.[37] For example, therapeutic doses of risperidone, olanzapine and ziprasidone produce greater than 70% occupancy at D₂ receptors.[68,69] However, attributing antipsychotic efficacy solely to D₂ receptor effects is an oversimplification since many patients will not respond to medication despite adequate D₂ occupancy.[65] Furthermore, low levels of D₂ striatal receptor occupancy (less than 70%) have been observed with therapeutic doses of clozapine and quetiapine. This may explain the low propensity of these agents to produce EPS, but also calls into question the minimum receptor occupancy necessary for antipsychotic efficacy as proposed for typical agents.[69,70]

Blockade of the 5-HT₂A receptors, a shared property of the atypical agents, has been investigated with regard to its significance in mediating antipsychotic effects.[73] At therapeutic doses most atypical agents occupy more than 80% of cortical 5-HT₂A receptors.[69,71,72] Blockade of 5-HT₂A receptors, independent of D₂ antagonism, has not been demonstrated to produce antipsychotic effects. However, it is postulated that a high 5-HT₂A to D₂ receptor affinity ratio may underlie the enhanced therapeutic efficacy and low propensity for EPS observed with atypical antipsychotics.[37] Serotonin is known to exert a regulatory effect on dopaminergic receptors or dopamine release, but the degree of control may vary depending on the pathway. Specifically, serotonin tonically inhibits dopamine release. Therefore, 5-HT₂A antagonism should enhance dopaminergic transmission. It has been proposed that the atypical properties of antipsychotics (efficacy against negative symptoms and low propensity to produce EPS) are due in part to augmentation of dopaminergic function via 5-HT₂A blockade in the mesocortical and nigrostriatal pathways and limbic specificity.[37,74] Aripiprazole is a new antipsychotic agent with unique effects at D₂ and 5-HT receptors. Specifically, this agent has partial agonist activity at D₂ and 5-HT₁A receptors and antagonist activity at serotonin 5-HT₂A receptors. Aripiprazole is a functional antagonist at D₂ receptors under hyperdopaminergic conditions but exhibits functional agonist properties under hypodopaminergic conditions.[75]

Antipsychotic drugs also affect other receptors, usually resulting in adverse effects rather than enhanced therapeutic response. For example, histamine-1 (H₁) blockade is responsible for sedation and possibly weight gain. Blockade of 5-HT₂C receptors may also play a role in the weight gain associated with some atypical agents. α₁-Adrenergic blockade causes orthostatic hypotension and plays a role in sexual dysfunction. Muscarinic-receptor blockade causes the classical anticholinergic effects such as dry mouth, blurred vision, constipation, and urinary retention. An understanding of the receptor-binding properties of the typical and atypical agents is helpful to predict their adverse effects profiles.[61,62,76] Properties of typical and atypical antipsychotics are listed in Tables 78-6 and 78-7.

EFFICACY

Typical antipsychotics are effective in reducing positive symptoms of schizophrenia during acute psychotic episodes and in preventing their recurrence in many patients.[77] These agents are less effective for treating negative symptoms. In fact, there is concern that typical agents may exacerbate negative symptoms by causing drug-induced akinesia. In general, all typical antipsychotic agents are believed to be equally effective when used in equivalent doses.

Clinical trials demonstrate that clozapine, risperidone, olanzapine, quetiapine, ziprasidone and aripiprazole are superior to placebo, and are at least as effective as typical antipsychotics for treatment of the positive and negative symptoms of schizophrenia.[75,79–86] In a meta-analysis of 52 randomized clinical trials comparing atypical agents (including clozapine,

Table 78-7   Relative Incidence of Antipsychotic Drug Adverse Effects

	Sedation	EPS	Anticholinergic	Orthostasis	Seizures	Prolactin Elevation	Weight Gain
Typical—Low Potency							
Chlorpromazine	++++	+++	+++	++++	+++	+++	++
Thioridazine	++++	++	++++	++++	++	+++	+++
Typical—High Potency							
Trifluoperazine	++	++++	++	++	+++	+++	++
Fluphenazine	++	+++++	++	++	++	+++	++
Thiothixene	++	++++	++	++	++	+++	++
Haloperidol	+	+++++	+	+	++	+++	++
Loxapine	+++	++++	++	+++	++	+++	+
Molindone	+	++++	++	++	++	+++	+
Atypicals							
Clozapine	++++	+	++++	++++	++++[c]	0	++++
Risperidone	+++	+[a]	++	+++	++	0 to +++[c]	++
Olanzapine	+++	+[b]	+++	++	++	+[c]	+++
Quetiapine	+++	+	++	++	++	0	++
Ziprasidone	++	+	++	++	++	0	+
Aripiprazole	++	+	++	++	++	0	+

[a]Very low at dosages <8 mg/day.
[b]With dosages <20 mg/day.
[c]Dose related.
0, no effect; +, very low; ++, low; +++, moderate; ++++, high; +++++, very high; EPS, extrapyramidal side effects.
Compiled from references 53, 119, 128, 135 and 164.

risperidone, quetiapine) with typical agents (haloperidol or chlorpromazine), Geddes and colleagues[87] found no difference in efficacy between these two drug classes if the dose of the typical agent was considered. Specifically, they argued that the apparent superiority of atypical antipsychotics (in terms of efficacy and drop-out rates) could be attributed to the use of excessive doses of typical agents (>12 mg/day haloperidol or equivalent). In contrast, two other meta-analyses concluded that the atypical agents have efficacy and tolerability advantages over typical agents that is independent of haloperidol dosages.[88,89] Davis and colleagues[89] concluded that available evidence demonstrates an efficacy advantage for some (clozapine, risperidone, olanzapine) but not all atypicals (quetiapine, ziprasidone and aripiprazole) when compared with typical agents. These authors suggest that the atypical agents are at least as efficacious as typical agents for positive symptoms and that atypical agents may be more efficacious in regard to negative and cognitive symptoms. This potential advantage of the atypical agents continues to be a source of much debate. On one hand, there are some who believe that atypical agents have a unique therapeutic effect on the primary negative symptoms, while others contend that this finding is actually a secondary effect on other related symptoms and disease manifestations.[78] Data on risperidone and olanzapine suggest a direct effect on primary negative symptoms that is independent of their effect on psychotic, depressive, or extrapyramidal symptoms.[90,91]

Nonantipsychotic Agents

BENZODIAZEPINES

Benzodiazepines are commonly added to antipsychotics and have been found to be useful in some studies for anxiety, agitation, global impairment and psychosis.[92] Adjunctive use

of benzodiazepines can spare the need for higher dosages of antipsychotics. However, some studies found that the benefits of benzodiazepines were sometimes not sustained.[53] Unfortunately, it is not possible to predict who will respond to adjunctive benzodiazepine treatment, and any potential benefit must be balanced against the risks of benzodiazepines. Common side effects of benzodiazepines include sedation, ataxia, cognitive impairment, and behavioral disinhibition. This latter effect can be a serious problem in those patients who are being treated for agitation. Withdrawal reactions, including psychosis and seizures, can significantly complicate management if a patient suddenly becomes noncompliant with benzodiazepine treatment. In addition, patients with schizophrenia are vulnerable to both abuse and addiction to benzodiazepines. For these reasons, the use of benzodiazepines should be limited to short trials (2 to 4 weeks in duration) for the management of severe agitation and anxiety.

LITHIUM

The use of lithium in schizophrenia has been investigated as monotherapy as well as an adjunctive treatment with antipsychotics. Studies evaluating the antipsychotic properties of lithium alone indicate that it has limited effectiveness as monotherapy in schizophrenia and may be harmful for some patients.[53] In combination with antipsychotics, lithium has been observed to improve psychosis, depression, excitement and irritability.[53,93,94] In general, adjunctive therapy with lithium may be considered in patients who have an inadequate response to an antipsychotic agent or in whom residual symptoms persist despite treatment. The dose of lithium should be sufficient to obtain a blood level in the range of 0.8 to 1.2 mEq/L. Patients should be monitored for adverse effects that are commonly associated with lithium (e.g., polyuria, tremor).

Reports of increased neurotoxicity from combined use of lithium and antipsychotic agents are inconclusive, and the risk appears to be no different with either medication used alone.[95]

ANTICONVULSANTS

Anticonvulsants such as carbamazepine and valproate are often prescribed in patients with schizophrenia. However, as with lithium, there is little support for the efficacy of these agents as monotherapy. Carbamazepine and valproate are most often prescribed as adjunctive treatment of psychosis, agitation, aggression, impulsivity and mood lability.[96,97] In general, the evidence to support the use of carbamazepine for schizophrenia is weak. Neppe[98] reviewed the literature and concluded that patients with nonresponsive psychosis and agitation, aggression, or "interpersonal difficulties" may benefit from the addition of carbamazepine. In a recent meta-analysis, Leucht and colleagues described a nonsignificant trend for a benefit from carbamazepine as an adjunct to antipsychotics.[96] An important consideration with carbamazepine is that the drug alters the metabolism of most antipsychotic agents, and dosage adjustment is often required. Carbamazepine should never be used concurrently with clozapine because of the additive risk of agranulocytosis.

Recent evidence indicates that valproate is being prescribed more frequently for schizophrenia and that the use of lithium and carbamazepine is declining.[99] This shift in utilization may reflect a more favorable side effect profile of valproate. In a recent investigation of hospitalized patients treated with risperidone and olanzapine for an acute exacerbation of schizophrenia, concurrent administration of divalproex resulted in earlier improvements in a range of psychotic symptoms.[100] Additional research is needed to confirm this finding. Dosages and target serum levels of carbamazepine and valproate are similar to those useful in the treatment of bipolar disorder (see Chapter 80, Mood Disorders II: Bipolar Disorders).

PROPRANOLOL

Propranolol, in combination with antipsychotic drugs, has been evaluated in nonresponders, with variable results. Potential explanations for the enhanced efficacy include a drug interaction leading to higher antipsychotic drug serum concentrations, relief of akathisia, or a primary improvement in psychosis. In addition, propranolol has improved chronic aggression in individuals with schizophrenia.[101] When used to treat aggression or to enhance the response to antipsychotic agents, high doses are needed. Propranolol is started at 40 to 80 mg twice a day and is increased every other day until intolerable adverse effects occur (systolic BP of <90 mm Hg or a heart rate <50 beats/minute). Dosages as low as 160 mg and as high as 1,920 mg have been effective; however, a reasonable trial usually is considered to be ≥240 mg/day for 2 months.[101,102]

GENERAL APPROACH TO TREATMENT AND THERAPEUTIC GOALS AT EACH PHASE

Because a diagnosis of schizophrenia cannot be made or monitored by laboratory or physical tests, the clinician must use target symptoms gathered from a patient interview and historic records to assess treatment response. A complete medical, psychiatric, and medication history, physical examination, laboratory panel (electrolytes; glucose; liver, renal, and thyroid function tests; complete blood count [CBC] with differential; urinalysis; urine toxicology screen), and electrocardiogram (ECG) should be obtained as soon as possible during the acute phase of illness or once the patient is cooperative (e.g., stable phase). A complete evaluation is needed to rule out other causes of psychosis, to identify co-morbid conditions requiring treatment, and to give guidance for selecting an antipsychotic and for determining the length of treatment.

Given the lack of insight that characterizes schizophrenia patients, collateral information should be gathered from the patient's relatives, friends, and significant others. Target symptoms (symptoms of schizophrenia) are specific for an individual patient, and they must be clearly identified and documented before and during the course of treatment to determine response to an intervention. Both specific treatment goals and the patient's previous baseline level of functioning should be clearly established at the onset of drug therapy. These data are used to give a direction for treatment and as a way of determining whether the outcome has been achieved. As stated earlier, schizophrenia is a chronic disease for which there is no cure. Most patients will have multiple relapses and experience residual symptoms between episodes during the course of their life. Realistically, treatment can decrease acute symptoms, decrease the frequency and severity of psychotic episodes, and optimize psychosocial functioning between episodes. Treatment is divided into three phases—*acute, stabilization,* and *stable*—with each phase using different drug and nondrug strategies to achieve the desired therapeutic outcome.

Prodromal Phase of the Relapse Process

Before the onset of the acute phase, there is usually a prodromal phase consisting of severe dysphoric symptoms, occasionally mild psychotic symptoms, and specific prodromal behaviors that can be typical for a particular patient. Family members and significant others should be educated about prodromal symptoms and what steps to take when these symptoms appear.

Acute Phase

During the acute phase of illness, patients are floridly psychotic and are usually hospitalized or placed in a supervised outpatient setting. The initial treatment goal is to calm agitated patients who may be physical threats to themselves or others. Medication is usually required to achieve this outcome, although nondrug interventions such as emotional support from the staff and use of quiet areas can also be helpful. An antipsychotic should be initiated as soon as feasible because prolonged psychotic episodes may be associated with a worsening of their course of illness.[103]

Selection of an Antipsychotic

The choice of a specific medication is usually based on a number of factors and is frequently more of an art than a science. Factors to be considered include experience with previous treatment (efficacy and side effects), the ease of attaining a therapeutic dose, available dosage forms, and formulary or cost considerations.

ANTIPYCHOTIC ADVERSE EFFECTS

An important factor in the selection of an antipsychotic is the potential risk for adverse events. Key adverse effects that differentiate the antipsychotics include EPS, anticholinergic side effects, cardiac effects, hyperprolactinemia, metabolic effects and sedation. Table 78-7 compares antipsychotic agents with regard to the risk of these adverse effects.

EPS is a broad term that describes several types of acute and chronic drug induced movement disorders. Acute dystonia, parkinsonism, and akathisia all occur early in treatment, whereas tardive dyskinesia (TD), tardive dystonia, and tardive akathisia have a late onset, usually after years of treatment. The acute forms of EPS usually develop soon after the initiation of antipsychotics, are dose-dependent and generally reversible soon after discontinuation of the offending agent.[104] It has been estimated that 60% of patients who receive typical antipsychotics develop some form of EPS acutely.[53] In general, typical agents are more likely to cause EPS than atypical agents when these medications are used at usual therapeutic doses. Among the six currently available atypical agents, clozapine and quetiapine are associated with the lowest risk for EPS. The increasing prescription of atypical antipsychotics (and decrease in use of the typical agents) has substantially reduced the problem of EPS. Similarly, the risk of antipsychotic-induced TD is suggested to be lower with atypical agents compared to typical agents. Most of the evidence documenting a decreased incidence of TD with atypical agents is derived from data and clinical experience with clozapine, risperidone, olanzapine and quetiapine.[105–108]

Anticholinergic effects are more significant with low-potency typical antipsychotics, and with the atypical agents, clozapine and olanzapine. Clinically, patients complain of constipation, urinary retention, and dry eyes, mouth, and throat. Dry mouth and throat can cause several additional problems, including dental caries and weight gain if thirst is satisfied with high sugar drinks. Oral fungal infections can also occur if gum or liquids with high sugar content are regularly consumed. The most serious complications from medications with anticholinergic properties are delirium and adynamic ileus.[109,110] Interestingly, clozapine causes significant hypersalivation despite its anticholinergic effects. The mechanism is unknown, but it may be caused by clozapine's augmentation of the adrenergic receptors that control salivation.[111] Drug therapy with benztropine, amitriptyline, and clonidine may alleviate hypersalivation, however these agents are not effective in all patients and when they are beneficial tolerance may develop. Even though anticholinergic effects are a minor problem with high-potency typical agents, some patients may still have problems when anticholinergic antiparkinsonian agents are added to treat EPS.

Antipsychotic drugs can cause a variety of cardiovascular complications, but the most common problem is orthostasis from α_1-adrenergic blockade. Low-potency typical agents and atypical antipsychotics pose the greatest risk for producing orthostatic hypotension. Orthostasis is most likely to occur during the first few days of treatment or when increasing the dose of medication. Although tolerance usually occurs within 4 to 6 weeks, orthostasis necessitates slow dose titration early in treatment for patients who are particularly prone to this side effect (e.g., elderly).

Tachycardia may occur as a result of the anticholinergic effects of antipsychotic medications on vagal inhibition, or secondary to orthostatic hypotension.[53] Clozapine produces the most pronounced tachycardia. If tachycardia is sustained or becomes symptomatic, low doses of a β-blocker such as atenolol or propranolol can be useful once an ECG has ruled out other medical causes.

ECG changes such as prolongation of the QT and PR intervals, ST-segment depression and T-wave flattening have been observed with antipsychotics.[112] The most clinically important of these potential changes is prolongation of the QTc interval (which is the QT interval adjusted for heart rate) and has drawn the attention of the U.S. Food and Drug Administration (FDA). QTc prolongation may lead to the development of ventricular tachyarrhythmias such as torsades de pointes and ventricular fibrillation, which can cause syncope, cardiac arrest, or sudden cardiac death. All antipsychotics have the potential to prolong the QTc interval to varying degrees. In 2000, Pfizer in consultation with the FDA, completed a study in which the QTc intervals of patients taking several antipsychotics, at usual therapeutic dosages and in the presence of a metabolic inhibitor, was compared (Fig. 78-2).[113] Thioridazine was shown to prolong the QTc interval at least 20 msec longer than haloperidol, risperidone, olanzapine or quetiapine. This led to a boxed warning on the FDA approved product labeling which states that thioridazine has been shown to prolong the QTc interval in a dose related manner and its use should be limited to patients who cannot be managed on other antipsychotics. In the same study, ziprasidone prolonged the QTc interval 5 to 15 msec longer than did haloperidol, risperidone, olanzapine, or quetiapine. Unlike thioridazine, the ziprasidone effects were not dose related. The exact point at which QTc prolongation becomes clinically dangerous is unclear. As most reported cases of torsades de pointes have appeared in individuals with a QT interval greater than 500 msec, discontinuation of the suspected offending agent has been recommended if the interval consistently exceeds 500 msec. It is important to note that no patients in this study had QTc intervals exceeding 500 msec or arrhythmias. Despite the fact that no increased risk of arrhythmia or sudden death has been demonstrated with ziprasidone, caution is warranted in patients with some types of cardiac disease and with an uncontrolled electrolyte disturbance. The co-prescription of ziprasidone with other drugs that prolong the QT interval should be avoided. Under most clinical circumstances, however, ziprasidone may be safely used without ECG monitoring or other special precautions.

Antipsychotic-induced hyperprolactinemia has come to the forefront because of differences found within the atypical agents. Before the introduction of the atypical agents, prolactin elevation was unavoidable since all typical antipsychotics elevate serum prolactin by blocking the tonic inhibitory actions of dopamine in the tuberoinfundibular tract.[114] Among the atypical agents, risperidone and, to a lesser extent, olanzapine produce a dose-related increase in prolactin levels that is equal to or greater than that seen with typical antipsychotics.[115,116] The remaining atypical agents have little impact on serum prolactin levels.[115] Hyperprolactinemia is of clinical importance because it may lead to galactorrhea, gynecomastia, amenorrhea, anovulation, impaired spermatogenesis, decreased libido and sexual arousal, and anorgasmia.[117] Interestingly the hyperprolactinemia is not always associated with clinical symptoms. For example, Kleinberg and

Mean Change in QTc from Baseline (steady state)

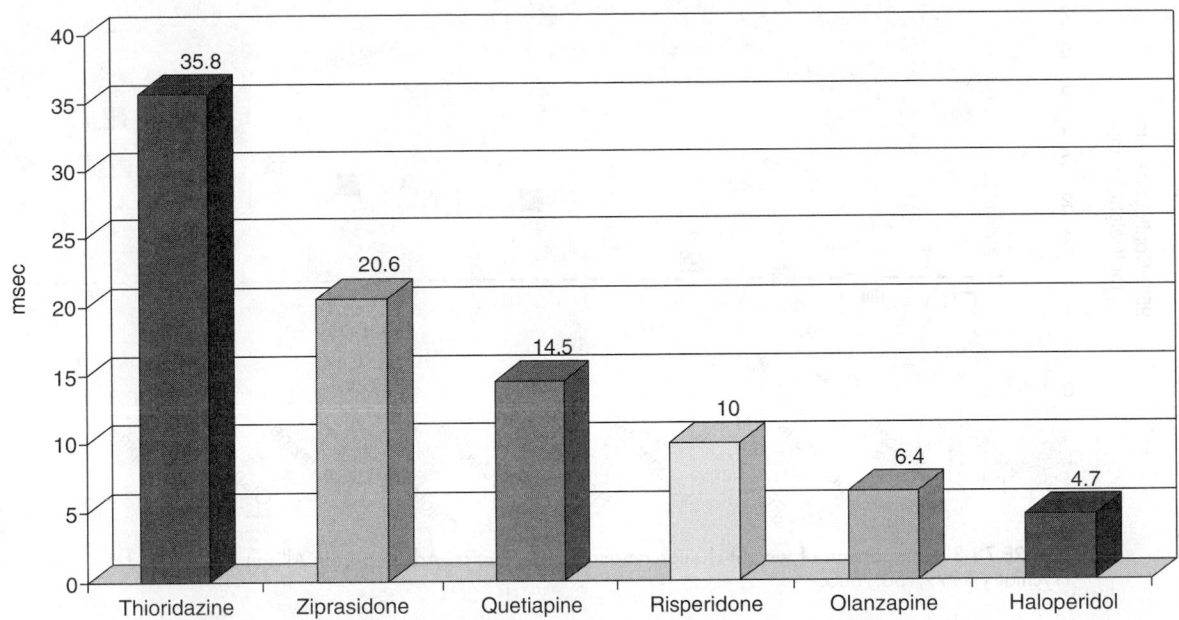

FIGURE 78-2 **Comparison of QTc changes with antipsychotics.** Adapted from Reference 113.

colleagues[116] failed to find an association between sexual dysfunction and risperidone-associated hyperprolactinemia. This may be a function of the multifactorial nature of sexual dysfunction or methodologic limitations in data collection. Patients often do not spontaneously report symptoms of sexual dysfunction and clinicians must remember to ask about these potential side effects.[115]

Weight gain is emerging as one of the most significant concerns associated with the use of antipsychotics, particularly among the atypical agents. The mechanism of antipsychotic-induced weight gain is unclear, but antagonism of histamine H_1 and serotonin $5-HT_{2C}$ receptors has been implicated.[118] Among the atypical agents, weight gain is most common with clozapine and olanzapine, lowest with ziprasidone and aripiprazole, and intermediate with risperidone and quetiapine.[119] In a meta-analysis, Allison and colleagues[120] found that the estimated weight gain at 10 weeks of therapy was greater with clozapine (4.45 kg) and olanzapine (4.15 kg) relative to risperidone (2.1 kg) and ziprasidone (0.04 kg), as illustrated in Figure 78-3. Moderate short-term weight gain has been demonstrated with quetiapine and is minimal with aripiprazole.[75,121] Similarly, clozapine and olanzapine have been implicated as having the largest effects on weight gain in long-term treatment.[121] The weight gain observed with clozapine and olanzapine does not appear to be dose dependent and tends to plateau between 6 and 12 months after treatment initiation.[122,123] However, other authors suggest that antipsychotic-associated weight gain plateaus within the first several months of treatment with risperidone, quetiapine and ziprasidone; yet can continue over several years for clozapine and olanzapine.[115] The issue of weight gain has important clinical implications as this has been linked with development of impaired glucose tolerance and type II diabetes, hyperlipidemia, and increased mortality.[53,124–127]

Sedation can occur with any antipsychotic agent; however, it is most pronounced with the low-potency typical agents and with clozapine and quetiapine. Sedation at the beginning of treatment may be desirable for anxious or aggressive patients. However, persistent sedation during long-term treatment may adversely affect daily functioning and quality of life. Most patients develop some tolerance to these sedating effects over time but it can be minimized by reducing the dose or by shifting administration to bedtime.

In all patients, the selection of a specific antipsychotic agent should be individualized. One of the best predictors of response is the patient's previous response to a specific antipsychotic, or a positive response in a first-degree relative. If a patient responded poorly to an antipsychotic in the past, an agent from a different chemical class should be prescribed. Also, if a patient has a particular aversion to an antipsychotic side effect, an appreciation for differences among the available antipsychotics in this regard would be helpful. Drugs with a similar side-effect profile should be avoided. Although all the antipsychotic agents have been shown to be efficacious during the acute phase of schizophrenia, atypical antipsychotics (with the exception of clozapine) have become the agents of first choice for the treatment of schizophrenia. The rationale for this practice is based on the lower risk of EPS and TD with the atypical agents. Adverse effects and their treatment is discussed in greater detail later in the chapter.

PHARMACOKINETICS AND DRUG INTERACTIONS

Dosing considerations also have a major influence on safe and effective antipsychtoic selections. Specific factors include the number of times a day a medication needs to be administered, the difference between a starting dose and a "target" therapeutic dose (i.e., titration required), and the risk for drug-drug interactions. The long average half-life (12 to 24 hours)

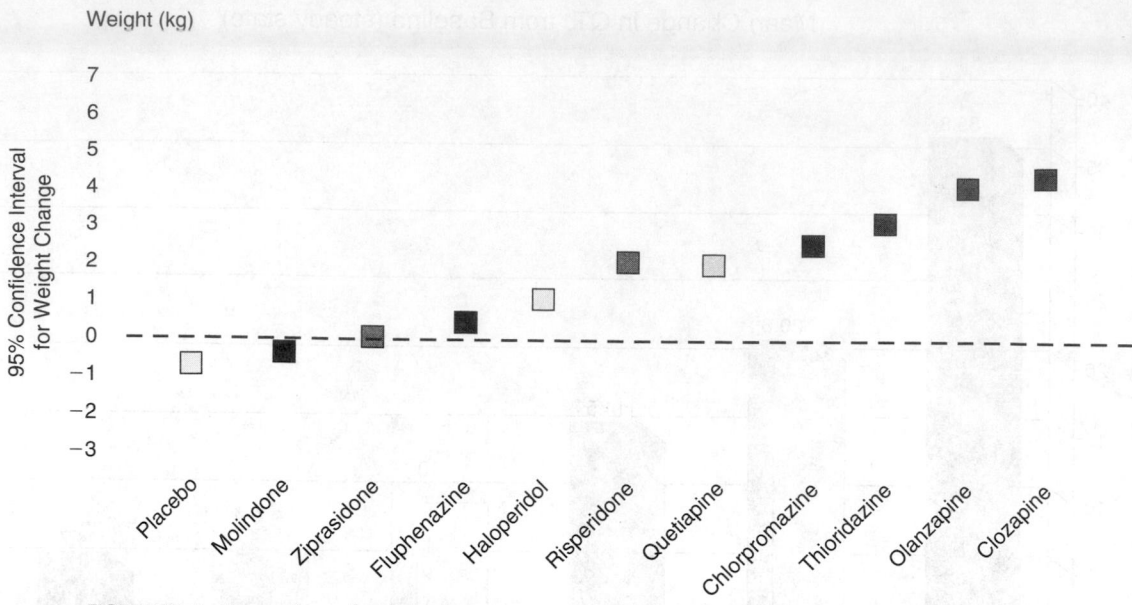

FIGURE 78-3 **Comparison of weight change among antipsychotics.** Adapted from Allison J et al. Am J Psychiatry 1999;156:1686.

and active metabolites of most oral antipsychotic drugs allow for once- to twice-daily dosing.[128] Most antipsychotics, with the exception of clozapine and ziprasidone, can be safely given once a day. Most antipsychotics achieve a steady-state concentration in 4 to 7 days, but it is important to understand that the onset of antipsychotic effect is not related to achieving steady state. Also, pharmacologic effects often persist for longer periods than plasma half-life information would imply. In some instances, treatment is initiated at a subtherapeutic dose and gradually titrated upward to an effective dose. This approach is taken to allow the patient to develop tolerance to adverse events such as sedation or orthostatic hypotension. In the case of acute agitation, antipsychotic doses are also often divided, despite the long half-lives of these drugs, so that the sedative effects are maintained over the day. Once a patient has been stabilized or has become tolerant to the adverse effects, the goal is to give medication once a day, usually at bed-

time. Bedtime dosing enhances medication adherence and concentrates ongoing adverse effects such as sedation at night.

Both pharmacokinetic and pharmacodynamic drug interactions can occur with antipsychotic agents. Cytochrome P450 enzymes, especially the 1A2, 2D6, and 3A4 isoenzymes, are responsible for the metabolism of many antipsychotics.[129] Induction or inhibition of these enzymes by other drugs may result in clinically important drug interactions. Table 78-8 summarizes the metabolic pathways for commonly used antipsychotic drugs. In the case of clozapine, serious complications such as seizures can occur when drug interactions cause serum concentrations of clozapine to rise significantly. Examples of drugs that have the potential to cause serious interactions with antipsychotics include: fluvoxamine (CYP 1A2 inhibitor); erythromycin, ketoconazole, and ritonavir (CYP 3A4 inhibitors); quinidine, risperidone, fluoxetine,

Table 78-8	Pharmacokinetic Comparisons of Antipsychotics		
Antipsychotic Agent	*Mean Half-Life (hr)*	*Major Cytochrome P450 Pathway*	*Plasma Concentration Range*
Chlorpromazine	8–35	2D6	Not well defined
Thioridazine	9–30	2D6	Not well defined
Perphenazine	8–21	2D6	Not well defined
Fluphenazine	14–24	2D6	0.2–2.8 μg/mL
Fluphenazine decanoate	8 days	2D6	0.2–2.8 μg/mL
Thiothixene	34	2D6	2–15 μg/mL
Haloperidol	12–36	2D6	4–12 ng/mL
Haloperidol decanoate	21 days	2D6	4–12 ng/mL
Clozapine	16	1A2, 3A4	350–420 μg/mL suggested
Risperidone	22	2D6	Not well defined
Olanzapine	30	1A2	>23.2 ng/mL @ 12 hours post dose
Quetiapine	7	3A4	Not well defined
Ziprasidone	4–5	3A4	Not well defined
Aripiprazole	75–94	2D6, 3A4	Not well defined

Compiled from references 128, 129, 164, 165, and 190.

and paroxetine (CYP 2D6 inhibitors); and cimetidine (multiple enzymes).[130] Conversely, inducers of drug metabolism such as carbamazepine (induces multiple enzymes) or cigarette smoking (induces CYP 1A2) can reduce the plasma concentrations of antipsychotic drugs. For example, carbamazepine has been shown to reduce plasma concentrations of haloperidol by 50%.[131] Cigarette smoking has been shown to increase the metabolism of clozapine and olanzapine.[129] Pharmacodynamic interactions may occur when medications with similar unwanted properties are concurrently prescribed. For example, concomitant use of low-potency typical agents or clozapine along with diphenhydramine or hydroxyzine may cause augmentation of anticholinergic effects. Pharmacodynamic drug interactions of greatest concern are those that can cause significant orthostatic hypotensive, anticholinergic effects, and sedation. Pharmacokinetic and dosing information for the antipsychotics are provided in Table 78-8 and 78-9.

PHARMACOECONOMIC CONSIDERATIONS

Although medication expenditures represent only a small portion of total resource utilization associated with the management of schizophrenia, concern exists about the cost of atypical antipsychotics and whether their relative advantages over typical agents are worth their increased cost.[132] Drug acquisition costs for atypical antipsychotics can be several 100-fold greater than typical antipsychotics. Most pharmacoeconomic studies with atypical antipsychotics show that these agents are at least cost-neutral and may offer cost advantages compared with traditional agents when total mental health costs are considered.[133] Depending on the individual study, the greater costs associated with atypical antipsychotics are offset by decreased hospital admissions, length of inpatient stay and outpatient visits. Hence, drug costs should not be the sole factor considered when selecting an antipsychotic. The selection of a medication should be individualized and factors such as efficacy, side effects, patient acceptance and total healthcare cost should be considered.

Initiation of Therapy and Dosage Forms

Pharmacotherapy during the acute phase is administered orally (as tablets or liquid concentrate) or intramuscularly (IM), depending on the patient's willingness to take medication, the risk of imminent harm, and the dosage form availability. Usually, antipsychotic therapy is administered orally. As a general rule, antipsychotic agents should be initiated and titrated over the first few days to an average effective "target" therapeutic dose unless the patient's physiologic status or history indicates that this dose may result in unacceptable adverse events.[134] After 1 week on the "target" dose, a modest dosage increase (within the recognized therapeutic range)

Table 78-9   Antipsychotic Relative Potency and Adult Dosing

Drug and Chemical Class	Dose Equivalence	Usual Starting Dose (mg/day)	Acute Phase Dosage (mg/day)	Maintenance/Stable Phase Dosage (mg/day)
Typical Agents Phenothiazines				
Aliphatic Type				
Chlorpromazine (Thorazine)	100	50–200	300–1,500[a]	150–800
Piperidine Type				
Thioridazine (Mellaril)	100	50–200	300–800	150–600
Piperazine Type				
Perphenazine (Trilafon)	10	4–16	32–64[a]	8–48
Trifluoperazine (Stelazine)	5	2–10	10–80	5–30
Fluphenazine (Prolixin)	2	2–10	5 80	2–20
Typical Agents—Nonphenothiazines				
Thioxanthene				
Thiothixene (Navane)	4	2–10	5–60[a]	5–30
Butyrophenone				
Haloperidol (Haldol)	2	2–10	5–100	2–20
Dibenzoxazepine				
Loxapine (Loxitane)	10	10–20	50–250[c]	25–100
Dihydroindolone				
Molindone (Moban)	10	25–75	25–225	25–100
Diphenylbutylpiperidone				
Pimozide (Orap)	1	1–2	10–30	2–6
Atypical Agents				
Risperidone (Risperdal)	2.0	1–2	2–16	2–8
Clozapine (Clozaril)	50	12.5–25	150–900	150–600
Olanzapine (Zyprexa)	5	5–10	10–20	10–20
Quetiapine (Seroquel)	75	50–100	300–750	400–600
Ziprasidone (Geodon)	60	40–80	80–200	80–160
Aripiprazole (Abilify)	7.5	10–15	10–30	15–30

[a]Dosages can be exceeded with caution, but high-dose therapy is rarely needed.
Compiled from References 53, 62, 128, 135, 164, and 166.

may be considered if minimal or no improvement has been observed. In instances in which symptoms improve after the dose is increased it may be difficult to know whether the response resulted from the dose change or from additional days on the drug. The duration of a therapeutic trial is 3 to 8 weeks in patients with little to no response, and 5 to 12 weeks in patients with a partial response.[134,135] Dosing recommendations for the antipsychotics are provided in Table 78-9.

Although all of the antipsychotics are available in oral formulations, only a few are available as injectables. Short-acting IM preparations of an antipsychotic may be preferred over oral medication if a patient is agitated and not likely to be cooperative. IM preparations bypass the gastrointestinal tract and first-pass metabolism and have a faster onset of action. For example, most IM antipsychotics reach a maximum plasma level within 30 to 60 minutes and patients usually experience substantial calming within 15 minutes.[136] Of the short-acting agents available for intramuscular use, most clinical experience has been with high-potency typical antipsychotic medications such as haloperidol or fluphenazine. Haloperidol and fluphenazine have the advantage of being calming without being sedating, but they can cause severe EPS. Some clinicians prefer low-potency agents such as chlorpromazine, because they are more sedating. Low-potency agents can also cause severe hypotension. High-potency agents can be given in larger doses because they have a lower risk of anticholinergic and cardiovascular complications than low-potency agents. In general, the use of oral typical agents has declined because of the neurologic risks. Studies have shown that intramuscular formulations of olanzapine and ziprasidone appear to be better tolerated than typical agents and are equally effective as haloperidol in the acute treatment of psychoses in patients with schizophrenia.[137,138] At the time of this writing, only the ziprasidone intramuscular formulation has been approved by the FDA.

If rapid tranquilization is required for a patient who is acutely agitated and exhibiting dangerous behavior, the combination of IM haloperidol and IM lorazepam appears to have better clinical efficacy than either treatment alone.[141] However, rapid tranquilization is not necessarily more effective than traditional dosing methods, and is associated with a greater incidence of acute side effects such as dystonic reactions.[142,143] Rapid tranquilization can be achieved when repeated IM injections of high-potency antipsychotics or benzodiazepines are given until the patient is either adequately calmed, a maximum recommended daily dose is reached, or dose-limiting adverse effects such as acute dystonia (antipsychotics), ataxia, or slurred speech (benzodiazepines) occur. The most commonly used regimen is haloperidol 2 to 5 mg combined with lorazepam 2 mg injected intramuscularly every 30 to 60 minutes to a maximum of three doses.[144] Patients should be monitored for severe adverse events, particularly those with medical or neurologic problems. Vital signs should be obtained before each injection and the dose should be held if clinically significant adverse effects occur.[143,145] The concept of rapid tranquilization should not be confused with rapid neuroleptization, which implies the use of very high loading dosages of antipsychotics (e.g., administering a series of closely spaced intramuscular doses over a period of hours) to produce a more rapid remission of psychotic symptoms.[144] The practice of rapid neuroleptization leads to a higher incidence of EPS without advantages of efficacy when compared with the administration of lower doses of the same drugs. Rapid neuroleptization is no longer recommended.[142]

Long-acting depot medications are not usually prescribed for acute psychotic episodes because these medications take months to reach a steady state concentration and they are eliminated very slowly.[53] Hence, it is difficult to correlate clinical effect with dosage, and it is extremely difficult to make dosage adjustments to manage side effects. However, long-acting depot medications can be useful for maintenance therapy in patients with a history of nonadherence to their oral medication and in those who prefer the convenience of long-acting or depot injections. In these situations, the oral form of available depot medications should be initiated first. If the oral form has been shown to be safe and effective, the patient can be converted to the depot form. At the time of this writing only fluphenazine and haloperidol are available as long-acting decanoate injections but promising 12-week and 52-week results have been reported for a long-acting depot formulation of risperidone.[146,147] Long-acting injectable risperidone appears to combine the most valuable features of an atypical antipsychotic (broadly efficacious and well tolerated) with those of injectable long-acting antipsychotics (improved bioavailability and assured medication delivery). This product is expected to receive FDA approval soon.

Factors to Consider When Evaluating a Poor Response

A large proportion of patients with schizophrenia do not have an adequate response to antipsychotic therapy. Inadequate response may be caused by inadequate dosing, poor adherence, or true resistance of their illness to antipsychotic treatment.[148] Some of these factors can be addressed. In some patients, the antipsychotic dose necessary to reduce symptoms cannot be reached because of intolerable side effects such as EPS, sedation or dizziness. As mentioned above, a therapeutic trial of 3 to 12 weeks at an optimal dosage may be necessary to evaluate the full benefit from an antipsychotic agent. Nonadherence with medications is a common obstacle in the management of schizophrenia, even under supervised settings. Blood level monitoring may be helpful to identify nonadherent patients as well as those in whom a pharmacokinetic factor may account for a poor response (e.g., poor drug bioavailability, rapid metabolizer, concomitant use of a metabolism-inducing agent). Therapeutic ranges of some antipsychotics are provided in Table 78-8.

A single definition of treatment resistance does not exist, but factors to consider include chronic or repeated hospitalizations, persistent positive symptoms, lack of improvement in negative symptoms, and breakthrough symptoms despite adherence to treatment.[148] Guidelines for determining treatment resistance has been proposed and include at least two prior drug trials of 4 to 6 weeks' duration at 400 to 600 mg chlorpromazine (or equivalent) with no clinical improvement, >5 years without a sustained period of good social or occupational functioning, and persistent psychotic symptoms.[148]

Clozapine has clearly demonstrated superiority to typical agents in treating refractory schizophrenia. In the pivotal study by Kane and colleagues,[149] 30% of clozapine-treated subjects versus 4% of chlorpromazine-treated subjects met criteria for response at 6 weeks. A review and meta-analysis of seven controlled trials compared clozapine with typical antipsychotics in treatment-resistant schizophrenia and found that clozapine was superior in terms of overall therapeutic response, EPS, and adherence rate.[150] However, similarly favorable response rates have not yet been seen with other atypical agents in treatment resistant schizophrenia. Risperidone and olanzapine have been most often studied in this regard. In a double-blind trial comparing risperidone with haloperidol in treatment refractory schizophrenia, a significantly greater response rate favoring risperidone was observed at week 4 but not at week 8.[151] In a 6-week clinical trial, only 7% of patients prospectively determined to be resistant to haloperidol responded to olanzapine; a rate that did not differ from chlorpromazine.[152] In general, atypical agents other than clozapine have not been consistently found to be as effective in treatment resistant schizophrenia.[153] Nevertheless, given the problems associated with clozapine (risk of agranulocytosis, burden of other side effects, and the requirement of hematologic monitoring), atypical agents should be tried before proceeding to clozapine in most patients.[148] However, some patients do not respond to clozapine following an adequate trial of at least 6 months at a therapeutic dose. In such situations, it is reasonable to prescribe the antipsychotic to which they had the historic best response. Augmentation strategies—such as the addition of mood stabilizers (lithium and valproate), benzodiazepines, propranolol, antidepressants, or another antipsychotic agent—may be attempted. However, the evidence basis for this approach is lacking.[153] Treatment guidelines recommend reserving augmentation strategies for patients who fail or cannot tolerate clozapine, although in practice these strategies are often tried before a trial of clozapine.[53,154]

Stabilization Phase

The goals of treatment during the stabilization phase of the illness are to reduce the likelihood of symptom exacerbation and develop a plan for long-term treatment.[53] The hope is that a patient will return to his or her premorbid level of functioning, although this is unlikely. Treatment should consist of a combination of pharmacologic and nonpharmacologic strategies. During the stabilization phase, treatment guidelines recommend that patients continue the same medication and dosage that they had received benefit from during the acute phase of illness. Treatment should be continued for at least 6 months.[53] During this period patients may ask for their antipsychotic medication dosages to be lowered or discontinued because of side effects or a lessening of the severity of their illness. In many instances, patients may follow through with these requests independent of medical advice. Patients should be monitored carefully for side effects such as sedation and EPS. In some cases, these side effects are tolerated during acute psychosis but are no longer acceptable once the patient is stabilized. Dose reductions in response to side effects should be done gradually to balance the risk of relapse (from an inadequate dose) and medication nonadherence (from unacceptable side effects). Extra caution is warranted in patients who are newly stabilized because they are highly susceptible to relapse.[53] When these patients experience adverse effects, it is more desirable to reduce the dosage in small increments rather than to switch to another antipsychotic agent since it is difficult to predict a patient's response to another drug and at least some response has been observed during the acute

phase. Conversion from a typical to an atypical antipsychotic would be a reasonable exception to this rule if EPS were present.

Another concern during the stabilization phase is that clinicians, patients and families may wrongly conclude that the antipsychotic stopped working if psychotic symptoms persist during this phase. For example, a patient may have suffered from hallucinations that were loud and derogatory before initiation of treatment; after 8 weeks of treatment, the voices might remain but become quieter and less demeaning. Because antipsychotics have been shown to provide gradual improvement over a period of months after the initial episode was treated, the current regimen should be continued.[155]

Several strategies have been proposed if a change in antipsychotic medication is necessitated by side effects or insufficient efficacy.[156] These include an *abrupt* switch (abrupt cessation of the current drug, with abrupt introduction of the new one at the expected therapeutic dose), a *gradual* switch (slow downward adjustment of the dosage of the current medication, with slow upward adjustment of the dosage of the new drug) or an *overlapping* switch (abrupt introduction of the new medication overlapping with the current medication, followed by downward adjustment of the dosage of the previous medication). None of these strategies has been demonstrated to be superior to another in terms of efficacy or safety, and the switch strategy depends on the clinical presentation.

Stable Phase

Treatment during the stable phase is designed to optimize functioning and minimize the risk and consequences of relapse. Antipsychotics are highly effective in preventing relapse. When developing a long-term strategy to prevent relapse and rehospitalization, the dose and type of antipsychotic, and the duration of therapy should be considered. Long-term pharmacotherapy reduces the risk of relapse in schizophrenic patients and also may reduce the risk of environmental-induced and stress-induced relapse relative to untreated patients.[157,158] The effectiveness of antipsychotics in remission prevention was demonstrated in studies in which stable patients were either continued on an antipsychotic or changed to placebo. In these studies, relapse rates were higher in patients who did not remain on an antipsychotic. Although results vary, approximately 70% of the patients who were switched to placebo experienced a relapse within 12 months. In contrast, only about 30% of drug-maintained patients had a relapse of their condition.[159] This supports the need for continuing antipsychotic treatment in patients after they have recovered from a psychotic episode.

Before the introduction of atypical antipsychotics, the goal of maintenance therapy with typical antipsychotics was to use the lowest effective dose so as to minimize the development of tardive dyskinesia. However, use of low doses may increase the risk for relapse and minimize the benefits of rehabilitation programs. The minimum effective dose varies for individual patients; however, analysis of several trials suggests that doses as low as 2.5 mg/day of oral fluphenazine or 2.5 to 12.5 mg every 2 weeks of fluphenazine decanoate can successfully maintain patients who are in a stable phase of their illness.[160–162] In addition to use of the lowest effective dosage, other strategies have been developed to reduce the cumulative exposure to typical antipsychotic drug therapy including the strategy of *intermittent* or *targeted* therapy.[162,163] In this approach, antipsychotic agents are tapered slowly and discontinued while in the stable phase of illness. Thereafter, the patient is evaluated regularly and restarted on medications at the first sign of decompensation. This strategy has theoretic merit because patients with schizophrenia usually do not experience abrupt recurrences. However, the patient and caregiver must be able to quickly detect prodromal symptoms and restart medication immediately to abort a recurrent acute psychotic episode. A study that compared the *low dose* and *targeted* therapy strategies with standard maintenance therapy found a greater use of rescue medication and increased numbers of relapses in the low-dose and targeted groups; however, only the targeted therapy group had increased rehospitalization rates. The low-dose group responded to temporary dose increases. The authors of this study concluded that about half of patients can be maintained on continuous low-dose antipsychotics and that targeted treatment should be reserved for those who otherwise refuse medication.[162] Studies of low-dose treatment were justified because of the TD liability with typical agents. Because it is generally accepted that the risk of TD is lower with atypical agents, the role of analogous low-dose strategies with these drugs is unclear.

There are no reliable predictors of relapse for an individual patient, but the following approach is recommended when determining length of therapy. All patients with schizophrenia should receive maintenance therapy for at least 1 year, unless antipsychotic agents are not tolerated or the diagnosis is uncertain. If a patient has only a single episode with predominately positive symptoms and is symptom free for 1 year after the acute episode, then discontinuation of the medication with careful follow-up can be considered.[53] Patients with a history of multiple episodes may be candidates for medication discontinuation after stability has been demonstrated for 5 years.[53] Lifelong treatment is indicated in patients who present a significant risk to themselves or to others when unmedicated.[53]

Treatment Adherence

Poor adherence with prescribed antipsychotic therapy is a significant problem in the long-term management of schizophrenia. Comprehensive reviews suggest that deviation (primarily underuse) from prescribed regimens occurs in about 50% of patients with schizophrenia.[167,168] During any phase of illness, nonadherence with maintenance antipsychotic therapy places patients at risk for exacerbation of psychosis, increased clinic and emergency room visits, and rehospitalization.[169,170] Nonadherence to prescribed regimens can also compromise patients' daily functioning and quality of life. Long-acting depot antipsychotics should be strongly considered for patients who have a history of nonadherence. In addition to assured medication delivery, another benefit of depot preparations is avoidance of potential bioavailability problems. Clinicians should suspect poor absorption if serum concentrations are much lower than expected for a given oral dose; however, factors such as nonadherence or drug-drug interactions must also be ruled out. Disadvantages of long-acting depot formulations include the time required to reach optimal dosing and the inability to immediately withdraw the drug if unpleasant side effects develop.[53,171] Because of this, patients should be converted to a depot form after confirmation that the oral dosage form is safe and effective.

CLINICAL PRESENTATION
Target Symptoms

J.C., a 22-year-old, single, unemployed man, was brought into the emergency department (ED) of a mental health hospital by the police after he was found running barefoot downtown dodging cars in subzero weather. In the ED, J.C. was extremely frightened, and stated, "they won't let me go."

History of Present Illness

J.C. is not a good historian. He is agitated easily and threatens the interviewer when asked questions regarding his illness. J.C. said he came to this city 5 years ago "to be the king of jazz music." He did not complete high school, has lost touch with his family and has been living at the Salvation Army for the past 3 years. He has no close friends, and does not trust most people. He hears voices of "dead people" who tell him he is worthless and "will be killed." He says, "The newscasters on the television are reading my mind and telling everyone my personal secrets." These problems and insomnia have been disturbing him for the past year.

Medical History

J.C. has no history of a previous psychiatric illness and has never been hospitalized. The administrator at the Salvation Army confirms that J.C. has been living at the facility for 3 years. His behavior has always been rather "odd and unusual," and has recently become more agitated. He does not get along with other tenants and staff and he has been unable to care for himself for the past year or so.

Psychosocial History

The hospital social worker reveals that J.C.'s mother was frequently hospitalized for unspecified psychotic episodes and his father was "never around." J.C. admits that he was somewhat of a "rebel" as a child; he has never held steady employment and relies on Social Security income and money from strangers to survive.

Physical Examination/Laboratory Tests

J.C. was given a complete physical examination, which was noncontributory. His laboratory tests, including CBC with differential, SMA-28 laboratory panel, and thyroid and liver function tests (LFTs) were within normal limits. The urine drug screen was negative, his neurologic examination was unremarkable, and no further tests were ordered.

Mental Status Examination

Appearance and Behavior: J.C. is a thin, disheveled-looking man with very poor hygiene, who appears much older than his stated age. He is extremely suspicious of the interviewer and his surroundings and continually asks, "Where am I, who are you, and what do you want?" He also is agitated easily. *Mood:*

J.C. is very anxious and worried, concerned that the "dead people" are going to track him down and "bury me alive." He hears these dead people talking to him. His affect is blunted, with a minimal range of reactivity to his emotions. *Memory:* Remote memory appears to be intact, although his immediate and short-term memory are difficult to assess because he is uncooperative. *Sensorium:* He is oriented to person, place, time, and situation. *Insight and Judgment:* Both are poor as evidenced by J.C.'s denial of his illness and need for treatment, and his behavior, which precipitated this admission. *Thought Process:* J.C. is very suspicious and exhibits loose associations such as "What are you doing to me? Don't you like my hat? Jazz musicians will save us all. You are with the FBI!" He appears to be responding to internal stimuli, mumbling to himself and answering his own questions.

Provisional Diagnosis
Schizophrenia, Paranoid Type

1. What target symptoms of schizophrenia are present in J.C.? How are target symptoms used to monitor treatment?

J.C. exhibits many of the classic Schneider's first-rank symptoms of schizophrenia, including auditory hallucinations (hearing voices from "dead people" telling him that he will be killed), delusions ("Jazz musicians will save us all. You are with the FBI. They will bury me alive."), and thought broadcasting ("The newscasters on the television are reading my mind."). Other target symptoms include agitation, suspiciousness, loose associations, poor grooming and hygiene, impaired sleep, decreased social skills, and impaired insight and judgment. These target symptoms will be the basis of assessing a change in clinical status and monitoring J.C.'s response to medications.

Diagnosis and Outcome

2. What other factors in J.C.'s history are consistent with the diagnosis of schizophrenia, and what is his prognosis?

Other factors that are consistent with schizophrenia in J.C. include onset of illness in early adulthood (typical age of onset is late adolescence to early 30s), a positive family history of psychiatric illness, inability to maintain steady employment and establish interpersonal relationships with others, and the apparent chronicity of the illness over the past year. His acute exacerbations of psychosis are also characteristic of schizophrenia. Because of J.C.'s young age at the time of his initial psychotic episodes, a positive family history for thought disorder, an unstable home environment, and a low premorbid level of functioning, his long-term prognosis is not good.

TREATMENT
Goals of Treatment

3. What are the specific treatment goals in J.C.?

The immediate treatment goal in J.C. is to reduce his agitation because he may be a physical threat to himself and others. Intermediate goals during the stabilization phase are to attenuate, or to eliminate, if possible, symptoms of psychoses

and the thought disorder. Long-term goals during the stable phase should include assisting J.C. in developing a psychosocial support system (e.g., caretakers, mental health workers, peer groups) to promote enhanced medication adherence and to enable him to live semi-independently and obtain possible part-time employment.

Role of Nonpharmacologic Therapy

4. Is nonpharmacologic therapy indicated for treatment of J.C.?

J.C. should be placed in an area of the hospital ward with low amounts of noise and stimulation until his agitation subsides. He needs careful observation by staff until he is fully assessed for the cause of his symptoms and his level of dangerousness. If the treatment team determines that he is very dangerous, he may need one-to-one supervision by an individual staff member. As his behavior calms, J.C. can receive more ward privileges and should begin to attend group therapy. Initial therapy focuses on issues such as "what is schizophrenia?" and "what are the ways to treat it?" Basic issues related to medication education are also discussed. These include symptoms that are improved with medication and recognition of common acute adverse effects. Socialization with other patients and staff should also be encouraged. As J.C. improves further, therapy and education can shift toward coping skills, stress management, recognition of prodromal symptoms of relapse, long-term adverse effects, and ways to enhance adherence to treatment. Family therapy should also be considered if J.C. allows contact to occur. Family therapy focuses on decreasing family stress surrounding the illness, family problem solving, and communication. If J.C. enters a stable phase after discharge from the hospital, other strategies such as psychosocial clubhouses to improve socialization, social skills training, and vocational rehabilitation can increase his quality of life and productivity.[53]

5. How should the staff and family members communicate most effectively with J.C., especially because he is paranoid?

Communication should be calm and nonjudgmental in an acutely psychotic and agitated patient. Open-ended questions should be used, with a switch to closed-ended questions if J.C. is unwilling to respond. His paranoid delusions should not be challenged directly because he will feel attacked and may become angry and more agitated. Instead of challenging the delusional thoughts, the clinicians should acknowledge that J.C. believes the "dead people" are real and that he is "the king of jazz," but that they do not share his belief. Direct eye contact should also be intermittent to avoid making the patient feeling threatened. If the patient is violent, they should be interviewed in the presence of another health care provider. The clinician must not react to the provocation of a threatening patient and should avoid using a loud voice or aggressive words. When interviewing a violent patient, questions should be focused on issues that need immediate attention, such as medication adherence before admission to the hospital, presence of medical conditions, and recent consumption of drugs and alcohol.[1,2] As J.C. calms he will likely be more cooperative with questions and assessments.

Efficacy of Pharmacotherapy and Predictors of Medication Response

6. What are predictors of response to antipsychotic agents in J.C.? Which of J.C.'s symptoms are most likely to respond to drug therapy?

J.C.'s positive symptoms of agitation, insomnia, auditory hallucinations, thought broadcasting, suspiciousness, loose associations, and poor hygiene and dress are most likely to respond to antipsychotic agents. His negative symptoms, including impaired judgment, poor insight into his illness, blunted affect, and poor socialization skills, may be *less* likely to respond to typical agents than to atypical antipsychotics.

Treating Acute Agitation

7. How should pharmacotherapy be used to treat the acute phase of schizophrenia in J.C., and what should be done first to manage his acute symptoms?

A fluphenazine (Prolixin) 5 mg IM injection can now be given to calm J.C., so further assessment can be completed. Fluphenazine (or haloperidol) is a good choice because it is a high-potency agent, has a rapid onset of action for agitation, and is available in a short-acting IM formulation. These are important features because J.C. is likely to refuse oral medications because of his paranoid symptoms (see Initiation of Therapy and Dosage Forms for a discussion of factors influencing drug selection). Also, high-potency agents have limited cardiovascular problems such as orthostasis allowing wider dose flexibility in extremely agitated patients. Lorazepam 1 to 2 mg orally or intramuscularly every 4 to 6 hours as needed may be given to J.C. to control ongoing agitation. Lorazepam is more appropriate than fluphenazine as an "as-needed" agent considering J.C. is at greater risk for developing acute dystonia from antipsychotic agents. As-needed medication should be available until J.C. is no longer aggressive for several consecutive days. If lorazepam alone does not calm J.C., an as-needed regimen of fluphenazine can be added.

Antipsychotic Selection During the Acute and Stabilization Phases

8. J.C. was given a single dose of lorazepam 2 mg IM. His agitation resolved after the first injection. What is the next medication decision needed for J.C., and what factors should be considered when selecting an antipsychotic for the acute and stabilization phases?

An antipsychotic prescribed at a dose reflective of the needs during the stabilization phase should also be started now. Olanzapine, 10 mg at bedtime, is an appropriate choice for pharmacologic treatment of schizophrenia in the acute phase. With the exception of clozapine, any of the other atypical agents would be appropriate choices as well.

Past experience with antipsychotics is also extremely important in predicting therapeutic success and selecting a regimen. J.C. does not have a past psychotropic medication history to guide drug selection. He also does not have a history of nonadherence, which would direct the choice toward a de-

pot product. A common starting dose for olanzapine is 10 mg/day. Antiparkinson agents are not indicated at this time.

Onset of Antipsychotic Action During the Acute and Stabilization Phases

9. When should J.C.'s target symptoms start to respond to olanzapine?

During the first week, often known as the *medicated cooperation stage,* J.C. should respond to the calming properties of the antipsychotic, and his symptoms of hostility, agitation, and insomnia should improve. During the next 2 to 6 weeks, the *improved socialization stage,* J.C. should begin to obey hospital rules, attend ward meetings, and generally become more sociable. Severely ill schizophrenic patients with chronic disease may never reach this stage. The *elimination of thought disorder stage* can occur within any time frame, but usually takes at least 2 to 3 weeks and up to several months to occur. During this stage, the core symptoms of schizophrenia such as delusions, hallucinations, and thought disturbance improve. It is important to give antipsychotics adequate time to work before unnecessarily escalating the dose and increasing the risk of adverse effects. If no improvement of J.C.'s core symptoms is observed after 3 weeks, then the dose should be increased slowly to 15 or 20 mg/day and the patient should be observed for another 3 to 4 weeks.

Duration of Therapy and Goal of Stable Phase Treatment

10. It is 6 months later. Most of J.C.'s symptoms have improved, he is residing in assisted living housing and working part-time at Goodwill Industries. Although he is not troubled by any side effects, he sees no point in continuing his medication. Should they be discontinued? What are current practice guidelines regarding long-term treatment?

J.C. clearly is responding well to olanzapine and has no side effects. Therefore, to minimize the risk of relapse, he should continue his current regimen for at least another 6 months. If his symptoms remain stable and he maintains good psychosocial functioning (e.g., continues work, keeps close contact with social workers, attends medication groups), discontinuation can be considered.

When J.C. has been stabilized for a total of approximately 1 year on olanzapine 10 mg every day, then the dose can be reduced by 20% every 3 to 6 months until it is discontinued or relapse occurs. If he exhibits recurrent target symptoms of schizophrenia or decompensation, then the dose should be increased to the previous effective dose (or medication restarted if it was discontinued). Because it is likely that J.C. will require lifelong antipsychotics, it is important to find the minimal effective dose to prevent recurrence, while minimizing the risk of adverse effects. J.C. is not a candidate for intermittent therapy during the stable phase. He is not a decanoate candidate because he is compliant with treatment.

Depot Antipsychotic Therapy
Indications

11. M.S., a 24-year-old man, was brought to the ED by the police because voices told him to strike his mother. His medical workup and urine drug screen were negative. M.S. has a diagnosis of schizophrenia, undifferentiated type, and has been hospitalized four times in the last 2 years secondary to poor adherence to his prescribed medication. He has had the same presentation on all previous hospitalizations. During his last hospitalization, M.S. was stabilized on thiothixene (Navane) 20 mg orally at bedtime without any signs of adverse effects. How can IM depot therapy decrease readmissions, and how do we determine if M.S. is a good candidate for IM depot therapy?

M.S.'s history suggests that he is a good candidate for depot therapy. He responds to typical antipsychotics, but relapses because of nonadherence. He should be able to tolerate higher-potency antipsychotics because he has tolerated moderate doses of thiothixene well. The patient should also be asked whether he is willing to take injections before proceeding with this strategy.

Conversion From Oral to Depot Therapy

12. How could M.S. be converted from oral therapy to depot therapy?

In patients such as M.S. who have never taken haloperidol or fluphenazine (the currently available long-acting depot forms of antipsychotics), an oral trial lasting several days to weeks is needed before conversion. The trial is necessary to ensure tolerability, to evaluate response, and when possible, to determine the minimum effective dose.

Various formulas to convert from oral formulations to the decanoates have been proposed, but no method has been proved clinically superior (discussed in the following section). Clinicians should strive to use the longest dosing interval between injections and minimize the duration of combination oral and depot therapy. Careful evaluation of both tolerance and response is required for several months after initiating depot therapy.

FLUPHENAZINE DECANOATE CONVERSION

After stabilizing the patient on oral fluphenazine, multiply the total daily fluphenazine oral dose by 1.2 and administer as fluphenazine decanoate intramuscularly every 1 to 2 weeks.[172] The decanoate dosing interval may be increased to every 3 weeks after 4 to 6 weeks of therapy because of fluphenazine accumulation.

Alternatively, 12.5 mg of fluphenazine decanoate can be administered intramuscularly every 1 to 2 weeks for every 10 mg (rounding to the nearest 10-mg increment) of oral fluphenazine per day (e.g., 25 mg/day orally rounded to 30 mg/day and given as 37.5 mg of decanoate).[173] There are no specific guidelines for the continuation of oral therapy after initiating the depot formulation; however, combination oral and IM therapy should be limited to the initiation period (1 to 4 weeks) or during times of decompensation.

HALOPERIDOL DECANOATE CONVERSION

Elderly patients or those stabilized on <10 mg of oral haloperidol per day should receive haloperidol decanoate in an IM dose that is 10 to 15 times the oral dose every 4 weeks. If higher oral doses are needed for stabilization, then the first decanoate dose should be 15 to 20 times the oral daily dose to a maximum of 450 mg.[174] The first injection of haloperidol decanoate should not exceed 100 mg; if more is required, the

balance of the dose can be given in an additional one to two injections (provided that there are no extrapyramidal symptoms) over 3 to 7 days. Because haloperidol accumulates, the monthly decanoate dose should be decreased every 3 to 4 months by 25% until a minimum effective dose is achieved. Most patients can be effectively managed with a maintenance dose of 50 to 200 mg every 4 weeks.[135] Guidelines for concomitant oral therapy remain unclear and should be based on response and adverse effects, with the goal of depot alone after the first month of treatment if the aforementioned strategy is used.[172]

Using these guidelines, M.S. should be converted from thiothixene 20 mg to 10 mg of oral haloperidol per day (see Table 78-9). Oral haloperidol should be continued alone for 1 week or longer until M.S. is stabilized. Once stabilization with oral haloperidol has occurred, haloperidol decanoate 100 mg IM can be administered. This can be followed with 50 mg IM 3 days later if no adverse effects are noted after the first injection. The total initial dose is 150 mg every 4 weeks (15 times the oral dose). A 200-mg total dose is also acceptable if the clinician believes the patient needs more drug. No oral medication is needed after the second injection and should only be given if M.S. shows signs of decompensation. M.S. should be monitored carefully for extrapyramidal side effects and response. M.S. should receive haloperidol decanoate 150 mg IM every 4 weeks with the dose adjusted according to response and tolerance; the dose can be decreased after 3 to 4 months because of drug accumulation.

LONG-ACTING RISPERIDONE FORMULATION

Specific guidelines for the conversion from the oral to the long-acting formulation of risperidone are not available. In published clinical trials, IM doses of 25, 50 or 75 mg have been administered at 2-week intervals.[146,147] Oral therapy of risperidone was continued for 2 to 3 weeks after the first IM injection and then discontinued.

Inadequate Response

13. J.H., a 33-year-old man, was diagnosed with chronic paranoid schizophrenia at age 21 and has been hospitalized 15 times because of his illness. He repeatedly presents in a paranoid and hostile state complaining of auditory hallucinations and paranoid delusions in which the police and the people in his apartment building are trying to kill him. His symptoms have prevented him from obtaining employment, and he has no close friends. He has been treated with fluphenazine 20 mg HS and perphenazine 48 mg HS, but has had only a partial response to each medication. After each discharge, J.H. stays out of the hospital for approximately 6 months, then relapses, even with good adherence. He currently is taking haloperidol 15 mg HS with only minimal improvement after 2 months of treatment. What can be done to improve his response?

J.H. meets criteria for treatment-resistant schizophrenia, and clozapine is the "gold standard" for the treatment of this type of patient.[148] Because of the risk of agranulocytosis, the burden of side effects, and the requirement of white blood cell monitoring associated with clozapine therapy, one of the other atypicals should be tried before proceeding to clozapine.[135,148]

Clozapine
Indications

14. J.H. did not respond to an adequate trial of quetiapine 400 mg BID and was just admitted to the hospital again. He is becoming increasingly isolated and paranoid. He has no other medical conditions and is taking only lorazepam 1 to 2 mg Q 4 to 6 hr PRN. His last dose of quetiapine was 2 days ago. Because of his refractory illness, J.H. is being considered for clozapine therapy. What are the advantages and disadvantages of clozapine therapy? What makes him a good candidate for clozapine?

Clozapine is approved by the U.S. FDA for treatment of resistant schizophrenia or when adverse effects such as TD and EPS preclude use of other antipsychotics. Clozapine is contraindicated in patients with a history of a myeloproliferative disorder or clozapine-induced agranulocytosis, or a current white blood cell (WBC) count of <3,500 mm³. Clozapine also should be used with caution in patients who cannot tolerate anticholinergic effects, in those at risk for drug-induced orthostasis, or in patients with significant renal or hepatic disease.[175] Because of J.H.'s progressive decline in social functioning and inadequate response to haloperidol, fluphenazine, perphenazine and quetiapine, clozapine should be considered.

Initiation of Therapy

15. How should clozapine be initiated in J.H.? What are its side effects and how should he be monitored?

Whenever possible, clozapine should be initiated when a patient is medication free. However, if the patient is too ill to be taken off all antipsychotic drugs before adding clozapine, the current medication can be discontinued after a therapeutic clozapine dose has been achieved. Alternatively, clozapine can be titrated upward while the first antipsychotic is slowly tapered downward. Whenever possible, high-potency antipsychotics should be the concurrent agent used during the clozapine titration to minimize additive adverse effects such as sedation, anticholinergic effects, and orthostasis. Benzodiazepines should not be used for early behavioral and anxiety control, because their combined use with clozapine can lead to respiratory or cardiac arrest.[53]

Clozapine can be started in an outpatient setting if patients are carefully monitored for tolerability, especially orthostasis. The starting dose is 12.5 to 25 mg once or twice a day with increases of 25 to 50 mg/day until a target dose is reached. Clozapine is given in divided doses. The optimal dose has not been specifically delineated although an initial target of 300 to 450 mg/day is reasonable based on clinical experience. The maximum daily dose is 900 mg, but titration should proceed slowly to such high doses, and only after adequate trials at lower doses. Response is based on improvement of individual target symptoms and can be monitored by psychometric rating scales (Table 78-10). In addition, the overall ability of a patient to function and care for oneself during clozapine therapy also should be considered.[176] Most patients improve significantly during the first 6 weeks, but some take longer. Although the exact length of an appropriate trial is unclear, 12 weeks is adequate for most clients; however, improvement may continue for 6 to 12 months after initiating therapy.[53,177,178]

Clozapine causes agranulocytosis in approximately 1% of patients, therefore baseline and weekly CBCs are required

Table 78-10 Common Rating Instruments for Schizophrenia and Antipsychotics
Psychosis
Brief Psychiatric Rating Scale (BPRS)
Positive and Negative Symptom Scale for Schizophrenia (PANSS)
Scale for Assessment of Positive Symptoms (SAPS)
Scale for Assessment of Negative Symptoms (SANS)
Movement Disorders—Tardive Dyskinesia
Abnormal Involuntary Movement Scale (AIMS)
Dyskinesia Identification System Condensed User Scale (DISCUS)
Movement Disorders—Parkinsonism
Simpson Angus Scale for Extrapyramidal Symptoms
Movement Disorders—Akathisia
Barnes Akathisia Scale

during treatment. Clozapine is automatically discontinued if a patient is noncompliant with the blood work. After 6 months of treatment, patients can be changed to biweekly WBC monitoring if their WBC counts are acceptable (≥3,000 mm³ and the absolute neutrophil count [ANC] is ≥1,500 mm³). If a patient takes clozapine for <6 months with no problems, but stops the drug for <1 month, WBC monitoring can restart where it was left off for a total of 6 months. If the break is >1 month, then an additional 6 months of weekly testing is needed.

If a patient is on clozapine for >6 months without a problem and takes a break for <1 year, the biweekly WBC monitoring can be reinstated when the drug is restarted. If the break is >1 year, then weekly WBC monitoring is needed for 6 months. At no time can WBC monitoring be discontinued.[179]

If baseline laboratory work is within normal limits and an informed consent is obtained, clozapine 25 mg at bedtime can be started in J.H. His clozapine dose should be increased by 25 to 50 mg every day until the dose is 300 mg/day, the minimum dose at which most patients respond. The doses should be split and given as 150 mg twice a day. Subsequently, clozapine should be increased incrementally according to the guidelines described above. If J.H. has no response to 300 mg after 4 to 8 weeks (based on a reduction in BPRS scores and global improvement), then the dose can be increased to 450 mg (150 mg three times daily). If response still is inadequate, then the dose can be increased slowly to a maximum of 900 mg/day. Careful monitoring for orthostasis, hyperthermia, and oversedation is needed, especially during early titration. Serum concentration monitoring can also help guide dose increases.

16. Four weeks after starting clozapine, J.H.'s WBC count drops to 4,000/mm³ from a baseline of 6,800/mm³. Two weeks later, he has a WBC count of 2,100/mm³ and an ANC of 980/mm³. What action, if any, should be taken?

[SI unit: WBC count, 4.0 and 3.1 × 10⁹/L, respectively]

The hematologic profile for clozapine is very different from that of other antipsychotic agents. The incidence of clozapine-induced agranulocytosis is at least 10 to 20 times greater than the incidence with typical antipsychotic medications.[175] The incidence increases with age and is higher among women.[180] Analysis of data from 150,409 patients followed by the Clozaril National Registry found agranulocytosis in 585 patients resulting in 19 deaths.[180] The risk of agranulocytosis is greatest early in treatment with most cases appearing during the first 3 months of treatment. After 6 months the risk for agranulocytosis decreases substantially but may occur in rare instances up to 5 years into treatment.[176,179] Trends in the weekly tests showing a continual decline in WBC count, even if it remains >3,000/mm^3, require careful attention. Guidelines for responding to reduction in WBC are described in Table 78-11.

Clozapine should be discontinued immediately, J.H. should be hospitalized, and hematologist and infectious disease specialists should manage his care. Granulocyte colony-stimulating factor (G-CSF) has been used successfully to manage clozapine-induced agranulocytosis.[181] Clozapine should not be reinstituted in J.H. because he has a very low ANC.

17. What pharmacotherapy options could be tried to improve J.H.'s response now that clozapine is contraindicated?

Sequential monotherapy trials with other atypical agents that he had not been previously exposed to may be initiated. Alternatively, strategies such as the combination of an antipsychotic and a mood stabilizer or another antipsychotic have been attempted. Because J.H. has no precautions or contraindications to an adjunctive trial of lithium, he is a candidate for a 1-month lithium trial along with an antipsychotic medication other than clozapine. The antipsychotic is selected

after reviewing his medication history and choosing the agent to which he had the best previous response. Lithium should be given at doses to achieve a target level of 0.8 to 1.2 mEq/L and continued for 1 month to allow the best chance for response. If the patient is unchanged at the end of 1 month, the lithium should be discontinued and another adjunctive agent tried for a 1-month trial.

Serum Concentration Monitoring

18. E.H., a 68-year-old woman who was diagnosed with chronic undifferentiated schizophrenia >30 years ago, requires maintenance therapy with antipsychotic drugs because she relapsed when her haloperidol dose was decreased to 10 mg/day. Currently, she is responding poorly to haloperidol 15 mg HS for 6 weeks despite good adherence to her therapy. She has moderate pseudoparkinsonism controlled by benztropine 1 mg BID. Why should a serum concentration of haloperidol be obtained before increasing E.H.'s dose of this drug?

Antipsychotic drug serum concentrations are not part of routine clinical care, but can be considered under the following circumstances[182]:

- Poor response to moderate doses after an adequate trial (dose and duration)
- Serious or unexpected adverse effects at moderate dosages
- Deterioration in a compliant and previously stable patient
- Use of higher-than-usual dosages
- Evaluating whether the lowest effective dose is used in maintenance therapy
- Children, elderly, and medically compromised patients with potentially altered pharmacokinetics

It is unnecessary and not cost-effective to obtain serum concentrations for antipsychotic drugs that do not have defined therapeutic ranges. Most studies describe haloperidol's therapeutic range to be between 5 and 12 ng/mL.[183,184] The recommended ranges for fluphenazine and thiothixene are 0.2 to 2.8 ng/mL and 2 to 15 ng/mL, respectively.[185–187] Evaluation of clozapine trials suggest an optimal concentration for clozapine is 350 to 420 ng/mL.[188,189] Greater response rates were observed in olanzapine-treated patients whose plasma concentrations were >23.2 ng/mL in blood samples collected 12 hours after the dose.[190] Samples should be collected 5 to 7 days after a fixed dose and 10 to 12 hours after the last dose for oral preparations. Two to three months should elapse before samples are collected in patients taking depot preparations.[182]

E.H. has received an adequate trial of haloperidol and has moderate antipsychotic-induced parkinsonism. To prevent exposure to higher-than-necessary doses, a serum haloperidol concentration is warranted before increasing the dose. The target serum concentration should be between 5 and 12 ng/mL.

ANTIPSYCHOTIC-INDUCED ADVERSE EVENTS AND THEIR TREATMENT
Acute Dystonia

Acute dystonia has the earliest onset of all the extrapyramidal symptoms. Most cases occur within the first few hours or days after initiation or after dose increase of antipsychotic medication. Dystonia is characterized by sustained muscle

Table 78-11 Guidelines for Response to Clozapine-Induced White Blood Cell Abnormalities

Do Not Initiate Clozapine

Initial WBC count <3,500/mm^3
History of myeloproliferative disorder
History of agranulocytosis related to clozapine

WBC <2,000/mm^3 or ANC <1,000/mm^3

Discontinue clozapine immediately
WBC and differential daily
Consider bone marrow aspiration
Protective isolation initiated if deficient granulopoiesis

WBC 2,000–3,000/mm^3 or ANC 1,000–1,500/mm^3

Discontinue clozapine
Check WBC with differential daily
Assess for signs of infection
Restart clozapine when:
  No signs of infection present
  WBC >3,000/mm^3 and ANC >1,500/mm^3
  Check WBC twice weekly until >3,500/mm^3

WBC Drops to 3,000–3,500/mm^3; >3,000/mm^3 over 1–3 weeks; Immature WBCs Present

Repeat WBC with differential
If repeated WBC between 3,000 and 3,500/mm^3 and ANC >1,500/mm^3
  Repeat WBC with differential twice weekly until >3,500/mm^3

ANC, absolute neutrophil count; WBC, white blood cell.
Compiled from references 53 and 179.

contractions. Common presentations of antipsychotic-induced dystonia include a sudden onset of brief or sustained abnormal postures, including tongue protrusion; oculogyric crisis (eyes rolling back into head); trismus (spasm of the jaw); torticollis (torsion of the neck); opisthotonos (arching of back); and unusual positions in the trunk, limbs, and toes. Laryngeal dystonias are the most serious and are potentially fatal. Risk factors for acute dystonia include younger age, male gender, high dosage of high-potency typical antipsychotics and previous history of dystonia.[53]

The exact pathophysiology of acute dystonia is uncertain. Conflicting theories describe either a hypodopaminergic or hyperdopaminergic state after an antipsychotic-induced blockade of postsynaptic dopamine receptors. Acute dystonia likely is caused by dysregulation of the dopamine system and imbalance between neurotransmitter systems after acute antipsychotic administration.[191]

19. **J.P., a 19-year-old man, was brought to the psychiatric ED because of assaultive behavior toward his mother. J.P. states he struck her because the devil told him to do it. Trifluoperazine 5 mg IM Q 4 to 6 hr PRN was started to control his assaultive behavior. He received four IM injections over 24 hours and was converted to 15 mg PO HS. On day 2 of the admission he complained of a stiff neck and protruding tongue. J.P. became very upset and wanted to leave the hospital and never take these medications again. No other medical conditions were noted. What evidence suggests that J.P. is experiencing an acute dystonia reaction?**

The sudden appearance of a stiff neck and a protruding tongue in J.P. is consistent with acute dystonia. In addition, J.P.'s young age, male gender, and use of a high-potency typical antipsychotic agent also place him at high risk for experiencing a dystonic reaction.

20. **How should acute dystonia be treated in J.P.?**

Acute dystonic reactions are sudden in onset, dramatic in appearance and can cause patients great distress. It requires immediate treatment. The initial goal of treatment is to relieve symptoms as soon as possible with either benztropine 1 to 2 mg or diphenhydramine 25 to 50 mg by IM injection. Although the intravenous (IV) route has a faster onset of action, it is not needed in J.P. because his reaction is not severe. If symptoms do not resolve within 15 to 30 minutes, then the dose should be repeated. If there are contraindications to the use of anticholinergic drugs, lorazepam 1 to 2 mg IM can be used. J.P. must be reassured that this is a temporary condition that can be prevented and treated. To prevent another reaction, J.P. should be given oral anticholinergic drugs in doses commonly used for pseudoparkinsonism for 2 weeks after this dystonic reaction.[191]

Parkinsonism

The clinical presentation of antipsychotic-induced parkinsonism includes bradykinesia or akinesia, which may be associated with decreased arm swinging, a masklike face, drooling, decreased eye blinking, and soft, monotonous speech; tremor, which is most commonly a rhythmic, resting tremor; and rigidity of the extremities, neck or trunk (most identifiable in the limbs as a "cogwheel" rigidity during passive motion).[191] Observable features of parkinsonian motor slowing are indistinguishable from slowness due to depression (e.g., motor retardation) or lack of motivation. Antipsychotic-induced parkinsonism has been estimated to occur in approximately 20% of patients treated with antipsychotic agents.[53] Symptoms can occur at any time, but usually develop within 4 weeks after antipsychotic initiation or a dose increase. It is generally accepted that advanced age, antipsychotic dose and potency and pre-existing extrapyramidal symptoms are the major risk factors of antipsychotic-induced parkinsonism.[192] The Simpson Angus Rating Scale is used commonly to assess the presence and severity of extrapyramidal symptoms (see Table 78-10).[193]

Antipsychotic-induced parkinsonism (as well as idiopathic Parkinson's disease) is thought to be due to postsynaptic dopamine-receptor blockade in the nigrostriatal system, leading to an imbalance between the dopaminergic and cholinergic systems. Reasons for the delay in onset between receptor blockade, which occurs within hours after initiating an antipsychotic, and development of symptoms are not well understood.[191]

Atypical antipsychotics are becoming the mainstay of the pharmacologic management of psychosis in patients vulnerable to developing antipsychotic-induced parkinsonism. The reduced parkinsonian liability of atypical antipsychotics has been associated with their limbic specificity, 5-HT$_{2A}$ blocking effects and in some cases less D$_2$ receptor blockade.[66,69,74]

Clinical Presentation

21. **S.B., a 46-year-old man, has a diagnosis of chronic undifferentiated schizophrenia and was treated with loxapine 50 mg TID with inadequate response. The dose cannot be increased because he becomes oversedated. Because of the incomplete response, S.B. was switched to haloperidol 5 mg Q AM and 10 mg HS. One week after the switch, S.B. returns to the clinic complaining of feeling "real slow." He has a bilateral hand tremor that improves when he picks up his coffee cup. Physical examination detected cogwheel rigidity in both arms, although it was worse on the right side. S.B. wants to be taken off this "bad" medication. What evidence suggests that S.B. has antipsychotic-induced parkinsonism?**

The onset of symptoms within 1 week of starting a new, high-potency typical antipsychotic is the first clue to the presence of extrapyramidal symptoms. The "slow feeling" perhaps is indicative of akinesia and S.B.'s bilateral tremor and cogwheel rigidity also are features of antipsychotic-induced parkinsonism.

Treatment

22. **What antiparkinsonian drug could be selected for S.B., if any?**

In mild cases of antipsychotic-induced parkinsonism, immediate intervention may not be required if the movement disorder is not bothersome to the patient. For troublesome cases, as experienced with S.B., the simplest intervention is to reduce the antipsychotic dose (haloperidol) to the lowest effective level. If dose reduction is not possible, then an antiparkinsonian agent can be added (Table 78-12).[191]

All anticholinergic antiparkinsonian agents are equally effective for antipsychotic-induced parkinsonism, although

Table 78-12 Agents to Treat Antipsychotic-Induced Parkinsonism and Akathisia

Medication	Equivalent Dose (mg)	Dose/Day (mg)
Anticholinergic		
Benztropine (Cogentin)[a]	0.5	2–8
Biperiden (Akineton)[a]	0.5	2–8
Diphenhydramine (Benadryl)[a]	25	50–250
Procyclidine (Kemadrin)	1.5	10–20
Trihexyphenidyl (Artane)	1	2–15
Dopaminergic		
Amantadine		100–300
Gabaminergic		
Diazepam (Valium)	10	5–40
Clonazepam (Klonopin)	2	1–3
Lorazepam (Ativan)[a]	2	1–3
Noradrenergic Blockers		
Propranolol (Inderal)		30–120

[a]Oral dose or intramuscular injection can be used.

there are differences in adverse effects and duration of action. Trihexyphenidyl is the least sedating, whereas diphenhydramine is the most sedating. Benztropine has the longest duration and can be used once or twice a day if needed, whereas the others have to be used three to four times a day. Benztropine 1 mg twice a day could be initiated for S.B. because he probably is too psychiatrically unstable to tolerate a reduction in the haloperidol dose. The tremor, rigidity, and akinesia should begin to resolve within the first few days of treatment. Alternatively, a switch to an atypical antipsychotic may negate the need for an antiparkinsonian drug in S.B.

23. **Once week later, all of S.B.'s acute symptoms of parkinsonism have disappeared. How long should benztropine be continued in S.B. now that his extrapyramidal symptoms are resolved?**

The long-term treatment of antipsychotic-induced parkinsonism with antiparkinsonian medication is controversial.[191] The World Health Organization published a consensus statement recommending that the prophylactic use of anticholinergic medication in patients receiving antipsychotics should be avoided or used only in cases where alternative strategies have failed.[194] For S.B., an attempt to taper and discontinue the antiparkinsonian treatment should be initiated 6 weeks to 3 months after symptoms resolve. Unfortunately, as many as 30% of patients chronically treated with typical antipsychotics will continue to experience parkinsonian symptoms.[67] If that should occur with S.B., he should be switched to an atypical agent.

RISKS OF LONG-TERM ANTICHOLINERGIC TREATMENT

24. **What risks are associated with long-term anticholinergic treatment?**

The risks of anticholinergics include constipation, dry mouth leading to dental caries, and blurred vision. They can also impair memory, especially in older patients. Some patients develop tolerance to these adverse effects, but others do not, even with chronic use. Patients sometimes abuse anticholinergic medications for their mood-elevating and hallucinogenic effects. Abuse may be confused with reluctance to discontinue antiparkinsonian medication because of the fear of recurrent extrapyramidal symptoms or ongoing symptoms.

25. **One week after the benztropine was started, S.B.'s psychiatric symptoms began to respond to the haloperidol, but he developed acute urinary retention. Reduction of the benztropine dose to 1 mg/day did not improve his urinary retention. What alternative treatments are available to manage S.B.'s pseudoparkinsonian symptoms that are without anticholinergic effects?**

S.B. is just beginning to gain benefit from his haloperidol; therefore, the haloperidol dose should not be reduced. Amantadine, an antiparkinsonian medication that directly stimulates postsynaptic dopamine receptors and restores the cholinergic and dopaminergic balance in the nigrostriatum, would be a reasonable alternative to benztropine in S.B. Amantadine is an option for patients who cannot tolerate or who respond poorly to anticholinergic drugs. It often is preferred in the elderly because of the lower incidence of cognitive impairment. The parkinsonian symptoms usually respond within 24 hours.

Amantadine 100 mg twice a day should be started in S.B. Benztropine also should be discontinued. He should be monitored to determine whether extrapyramidal symptoms reappear and whether his urinary retention problem is corrected. S.B. also should be monitored for the appearance of amantadine-associated, dose-related adverse effects such as tremor, slurred speech, ataxia, depression, hallucinations, rash, orthostatic hypotension, and insomnia. If he cannot tolerate amantadine, or if amantadine does not control his extrapyramidal symptoms, an atypical antipsychotic agent can be considered.

Akathisia

Akathisia is a syndrome consisting of subjective feelings of restlessness or the urge to move and an objective motor component expressed as a semipurposeful movement most often involving the lower extremities (pacing, rocking, and an inability to sit or stand in one place for extended periods of time). Akathisia is observed in approximately 20% to 25% of patients undergoing treatment with antipsychotics.[53] Akathisia is often extremely distressing to patients, is a common cause of medication nonadherence and, if allowed to persist, can produce dysphoria and possibly aggressive or suicidal behavior.[53] It is often difficult to distinguish from psychomotor agitation and worsening psychosis. Hence, the clinician must take care not to misdiagnose akathisia as an increase in antipsychotic dose could worsen this adverse event. It usually develops within days to weeks after initiating antipsychotic therapy.

The pathophysiology of akathisia is unclear but much attention has focused on two theories.[191] One theory states that the mesocortical postsynaptic DA blockade leads to increased locomotor activity. An alternate theory claims that akathisia is caused by DA antagonist-induced dysregulation of noradrenergic tracts that project from the locus ceruleus to the limbic system.

26. **J.P. was given a diagnosis of paranoid schizophrenia. His acute episode improved with trifluoperazine 15 mg HS, and he**

had no other dystonic reactions. Two weeks later he became increasingly agitated, began pacing the floor, was unable to sit or lie down for >10 minutes at a time, and subjectively had a feeling that he described as "I have ants in my pants." J.P. is observed rocking back and forth from one foot to the other while standing in line for his dinner. He has no symptoms of antipsychotic-induced parkinsonism. Should the dose of trifluoperazine be increased?

J.P.'s symptoms of rocking, pacing, agitation, and the inability to sit still are consistent with akathisia. Because his psychiatric symptoms have improved and the new symptoms developed within 2 weeks after the initiation of trifluoperazine, a diagnosis of akathisia is more probable than unresponsiveness to the antipsychotic medication. Therefore, the trifluoperazine dose should not be increased because it can worsen the akathisia.

27. **How should J.P.'s akathisia be managed?**

Akathisia is less responsive to treatment than are antipsychotic-induced parkinsonism and dystonia.[53] As an initial approach to manage his akathisia, a small reduction (5mg/day) in his trifluoperazine should be attempted. If symptoms of his psychosis return or if the akathisia persists, the addition of a β-blocking agent, an anticholinergic drug, or a benzodiazepine can be considered.[53,191] Propranolol would be a recommended agent since there is a suggestion that its efficacy and safety profile may be preferable compared with other agents.[195] Anticholinergic drugs would be an appropriate alternative if antipsychotic-induced parkinsonism is present. If his symptoms do not improve in response to a dosage reduction of his trifluoperazine within a week, J.P. should be started on propranolol 20 mg three times a day, and the dose should be increased by 20 mg every other day to a maximum of 120 mg, if necessary.[195] He has no contraindications to β-blocker therapy and does not have antipsychotic-induced parkinsonism; therefore, antiparkinsonian agents (see Table 78-12) are not preferred over propranolol. If the akathisia persists after a trial of propranolol 120 mg/day therapy for 1 week, benzodiazepines should be tried or he should be switched to an atypical antipsychotic.

Tardive Dyskinesia

TD is a syndrome characterized by involuntary choreoathetoid movements that occurs in individuals taking long-term antipsychotics. The face (tics, blinking, grimacing), tongue (chewing, protrusion, tremor, writhing), lips (smacking, pursing, puckering), neck and trunk (torsion and torticollis), and limbs (toe tapping, pill rolling, and writhing) are commonly involved. The movements may be choreiform (rapid, jerky, nonrepetitive), athetoid (slow, sinuous, continual) or rhythmic (stereotypic) in nature.

TD occurs in approximately 20% of patients who receive long-term treatment with typical agents.[104] The cumulative annual incidence is approximately 5% through the first 4 years of treatment in an adult who receives typical antipsychotic treatment.[196] Increasing age is the most consistently observed risk factor for the development of tardive dyskinesia.[197] The annual incidence rates of developing TD are three to five-fold greater in older patients compared to younger adults.[198,199] Other risk factors include higher mean daily and cumulative antipsychotic doses, and presence of extrapyramidal signs early in treatment.[198,199] Although there is some indication that the risk of TD may be higher in women, nonwhites, patients with affective psychiatric disorders, and patients taking concomitant anticholinergic agents, these findings are not consistently supported by available studies.[197]

For most patients, TD does not appear to be progressive or irreversible. The onset of symptoms tends to be subtle with a fluctuating course.[197] Most TD cases are relatively mild. However, a portion (5% to 10%) may develop a form of TD that is severe enough to impair functioning.[200] Severe oral dyskinesia may result in dental and denture problems that can progress to ulceration and infection of the mouth as well as muffled or unintelligible speech. Severe orofacial TD can impair eating and swallowing, which in turn could produce significant health problems. Gait disturbances due to limb dyskinesia may leave patients vulnerable to falls and injuries.

Although the exact cause of TD is unknown, dopaminergic hypersensitivity, disturbed balance between dopamine and cholinergic systems, dysfunction of γ-aminobutyric acid (GABA)ergic and noradrenergic systems and neurotoxicity via free radicals have been proposed.[104]

Clinical Presentation and Assessment

28. **C.M., a 31-year-old woman, was diagnosed with chronic paranoid schizophrenia 9 years ago. She responds to antipsychotic drugs, but has been hospitalized six times because of nonadherence to her medications. She has taken loxapine, haloperidol, and fluphenazine in the past and currently is being treated with trifluoperazine 25 mg HS (decreased from 30 mg 1 month ago). C.M. also has been taking trihexyphenidyl 2 mg TID for the past 5 years. Involuntary movements (including tongue protrusion, frequent blinking, and writhing movements of her legs) were noted during a recent evaluation. What data in C.M.'s history are consistent with TD?**

The 9 years of antipsychotic treatment and the symptoms of tongue protrusion, blinking, and writhing leg movements are consistent with TD. Long-term anticholinergic treatment (trihexyphenidyl) also may contribute to the development of C.M.'s abnormal movements.

29. **C.M. has no history of abnormal movements and currently has no extrapyramidal symptoms. What disorders or medications can produce symptoms similar to those of TD?**

Tourette's syndrome, dental problems, Huntington's or Sydenham's chorea, chorea of pregnancy, and systemic lupus erythematosus (SLE) are some of the disorders that have been associated with dyskinetic movements. Medications such as metoclopramide, amoxapine, bromocriptine, and levodopa/carbidopa also can cause TD. Spontaneous dyskinesia resembles TD but can occur in patients without previous exposure to antipsychotic medications.[197] This form of abnormal movement is noticeably more common in elderly patients. A baseline dyskinesia rating is essential before treating elderly patients with antipsychotic medications to avoid the potential diagnostic dilemma of differentiating spontaneous dyskinesia from antipsychotic-induced TD.

TD varies in severity and presentation and is reversible in many cases; therefore, rating scales are needed to standardize assessments (see Table 78-10). A temporal relationship between an antipsychotic dose change and movement severity should be evaluated when performing assessments. An increase in the antipsychotic dose can clinically suppress the symptoms, whereas a decrease in dose can transiently unmask the movements. For example, the movements C.M is exhibiting may have worsened as a result of the recent dose reduction in trifluoperazine. On the other hand, a dose increase may produce a temporary lessening of movement severity; which does not tend to persist. Patients taking long-term antipsychotics should be evaluated for TD by a well-trained clinician every 3 to 6 months using a standardized rating scale. Findings always should be documented in patient records to ensure continuity of care and medicolegal protection.

Management

30. **C.M. is diagnosed with antipsychotic-induced TD. How should C.M.'s TD be managed?**

Management of TD should focus first on prevention. That is, antipsychotic drugs must be reserved to treat conditions known to respond (e.g., psychotic disorders such as schizophrenia, major depression with psychotic features, schizoaffective disorder), and the total dose and duration of treatment should be minimized. Because C.M.'s long-term exposure to antipsychotics is the likely cause of her TD, discontinuation of her trifluoperazine would be the ideal treatment. Unfortunately, she has experienced multiple recurrent psychotic episodes and requires lifetime treatment with antipsychotics. Because of the reduced TD liability with atypicals, C.M. should be switched to an atypical agent.[105–108] It has been recommended that an atypical antipsychotic be used for mild TD symptoms, and that clozapine be considered when TD is severe or distressing to the patient.[105,135] Rapid reduction in the dose of trifluoperazine must be avoided to prevent severe withdrawal dyskinesias, but her dose should be slowly reduced as an atypical antipsychotic is titrated to the lowest effective dose. This will minimize her exposure to antipsychotic medications and her corresponding dyskinesia risk. Trihexyphenidyl should also be discontinued because of its possible contribution to TD. Because C.M. has already been diagnosed with TD, an evaluation of the risks and benefits of continued antipsychotic treatment must be discussed with her and documented in the chart.

31. **Are there other medications for treating TD?**

A number of other agents have been studied for their potential therapeutic effects on TD. Drugs that augment GABA neurotransmission (e.g., diazepam, clonazepam, valproic acid), adrenergic drugs (propranolol, clonidine) and free-radical scavengers (vitamin E) have all been used, with limited or inconsistent results.[196,201,202] These agents may be useful as adjunctive treatments when TD persists despite the use of atypical agents.

Neuroleptic Malignant Syndrome

32. **C.B., a 25 year-old man, was hospitalized with the diagnosis of schizophrenia, paranoid type, and was started on loxapine 25 mg HS. After 2 days of therapy, C.B. became rigid, appeared confused at times, and had a fever of 41°C. A diagnosis of neuroleptic malignant syndrome (NMS) was made. What features of this syndrome does C.B. have and how should it be treated?**

NMS is a rare, but potentially lethal, adverse effect associated with antipsychotic therapy. The risk of NMS appears to be lower for atypical agents than for typical agents.[128] However, cases of NMS have been linked to treatment with clozapine, risperidone, olanzapine, and quetiapine.[203]

NMS can occur hours to months after the initial drug exposure, and the mortality rate is reported to be as high as 20%.[53] The incidence is estimated at between 0.02% and 3.23% of patients taking typical antipsychotic drugs.[204] The cardinal features include muscular rigidity, hyperthermia, autonomic dysfunction, and altered consciousness. Extrapyramidal dysfunction (e.g., rigidity) and akinesia usually develop initially or concomitantly with a temperature elevation as high as 41°C. Autonomic dysfunction includes tachycardia, labile blood pressure (BP), profuse diaphoresis, dyspnea, and urinary incontinence. The patient's level of consciousness may vary from alert to mutism, stupor, and coma. Other neurologic findings include sialorrhea, dyskinesia, and dysphagia. Symptoms usually develop rapidly over 24 to 72 hours. Creatine kinase (CK), CBC, and LFTs are not diagnostic for NMS, but usually are increased.

C.B.'s fever of 41°C, rigidity, and confusion are consistent with NMS. C.B.'s loxapine should be discontinued and supportive measures initiated to treat hyperthermia and to prevent dehydration (e.g., antipyretics, a cooling blanket, and intravenous fluids).[205] Secondary complications such as pneumonia and renal failure should be managed as they develop.

If C.B.'s condition does not show a trend toward improvement or worsens after 1 to 3 days of observation and supportive therapy, a number of additional pharmacologic interventions should be considered.[205] NMS has been attributed to dopamine depletion caused by neuroleptic drug blockade of dopamine pathways in the basal ganglia and hypothalamus. For that reason, dopamine agonists such as amantadine or bromocriptine sometimes are beneficial. Dantrolene relaxes skeletal muscle and is specifically recommended for severe hyperthermia. C.B. should be started on dantrolene 50 mg four times daily and either bromocriptine 2.5 mg three times daily or amantadine 100 mg three times daily to accelerate reversal of his condition.[206] If he is unable to take oral medications, 1.25 to 1.5 mg/kg IV dantrolene should be used.

NMS is self-limiting and usually lasts 2 to 14 days after the oral antipsychotic is discontinued, or longer after discontinuation of depot medications. C.B.'s response to therapy can be assessed by frequently monitoring his vital signs and by measuring CK daily. After several weeks of recovery, treatment may be cautiously resumed with another atypical antipsychotic.[205,207]

Metabolic Effects

33. **L.A., a 45-year-old woman with chronic paranoid schizophrenia, had been managed successfully with haloperidol for many years. She subsequently developed tardive dyskinesia and was switched to olanzapine 20 mg HS. Before initiation of olanzapine 4 months ago, L.A. was 5'4" and weighed 132 lb. She has responded well to the olanzapine; however, she now weighs 148 lb. Can L.A.'s weight gain be attributed to olanzapine?**

Weight gain has been reported with typical antipsychotics, but even greater weight gain has been seen with atypical agents such as clozapine and olanzapine; and to a lesser extent, risperidone and quetiapine.[119-121] The cause of antipsychotic-induced weight gain is multifactorial and may include a change in food preferences, increased food or fluid intake, carbohydrate craving, or a lack of activity. Blockade of the histamine and 5-HT$_{2C}$ receptors are also contributory. H$_1$ blockade causes sedation that may produce inactivity. H$_1$ blockade may also increase weight by interfering with normal satiety signals from the gut, resulting in overeating. Evidence for a role of 5-HT$_{2C}$ antagonism is derived indirectly from appetite-suppressing drugs, such as fenfluramine that are thought to act via 5-HT$_{2C}$ agonism.[208]

L.A.'s weight gain should be taken seriously because it may contribute to medical conditions such as diabetes, hyperlipidemia, coronary artery disease, and hypertension.[209] A significant weight gain may cause her to have a poor self-image that may lead to treatment nonadherence. She should be enrolled in a weight management program. Switching L.A. to another antipsychotic with lower weight gain liability may be considered; however, this decision must be balanced against her current positive response to olanzapine.

34. How should the potential metabolic complications associated with antipsychotics be monitored?

Although the risk of TD appears to be significantly reduced with the use of atypical antipsychotics, there is concern regarding other long-term side effects with these agents including impaired glucose tolerance, type 2 diabetes, and hyperlipidemia.[115,124]

L.A. should be informed about these potential complications. The routine monitoring of weight, fasting glucose levels and lipid panels has been recommended and appropriate therapeutic options should be initiated if abnormalities are observed.[115,124] She should be encouraged to self-monitor her weight and report any significant weight fluctuations. Subjective evidence of a weight change may include a change in clothes or belt size. In addition, she should be routinely monitored for the presence of diabetic symptoms (e.g., polyuria, polydipsia) at every clinic visit.

Hepatic Dysfunction

35. **A.S., a 24-year-old woman, is brought to the hospital because of unusual behavior and violence toward her mother. The diagnosis for A.S. is schizophrenia, paranoid type, acute exacerbation. Quetiapine 25 mg BID was prescribed initially and the dose gradually increased until 200 mg TID was achieved. Her baseline laboratory tests (i.e., CBC with differential, a chemistry profile that included LFTs, and serum electrolytes) were within normal limits. The same tests were repeated 10 days after her psychosis was under evaluation. The aspartate aminotransferase (AST) and alanine aminotransferase (ALT) are now 2.5 times normal, but she has no GI complaints or medical problems. Should quetiapine be discontinued at this time?**

Benign elevations in LFTs (i.e., increases in AST or ALT less than two to three times normal) have long been reported early in the course of therapy with most antipsychotic drugs.[32,61,62] Such increases are not problematic; thus, none of the manufacturers of antipsychotic drugs is mandated by the FDA to suggest routine assessment of liver function.

A more specific hepatic complication, cholestatic jaundice, has been associated with antipsychotic agents. The phenothiazines, especially chlorpromazine, may be associated with cholestatic jaundice more often than the other agents. Most cases of antipsychotic drug-induced cholestatic jaundice develop within the first month of therapy.[61] The jaundice usually is preceded by prodromal symptoms of fever, chills, nausea, upper gastric pain, malaise, and pruritus. Discontinuation of the phenothiazine and symptomatic care are the primary modes of treatment because the cholestatic jaundice generally is self-limiting and usually resolves within 2 to 8 weeks. Occasionally, a more chronic course may develop. Once the signs and symptoms have resolved, an alternate class of antipsychotic, preferably a nonphenothiazine, should be prescribed.

The LFTs in A.S. are only modestly abnormal, and she is not experiencing symptoms of hepatotoxicity or cholestatic jaundice. Therefore, quetiapine should be continued. Routine laboratory monitoring of LFTs does not help to prevent drug-induced cholestatic jaundice; thus, no follow-up laboratory tests are required unless symptoms of hepatic dysfunction develop. Awareness and evaluation of A.S. for prodromal symptoms is the most appropriate action at this time.

Ocular Effects

36. Are there any additional baseline tests that should have been performed on A.S. before starting quetiapine?

The ocular effects of antipsychotic agents are well recognized and are generally of minor clinical consequence. Corneal and lens changes have been reported with several phenothiazines and thiothixene. Chlorpromazine is the most common cause, with the risk being greatest with long-term, high-dose exposure (1 to 3 kg lifetime dose).[62] The changes are visible only by slit lamp and vision is not impaired. When doses of 800 mg/day of thioridazine are exceeded, pigmentary retinopathy can occur and irreversible blindness is a possible outcome.

The ocular effects of quetiapine are different. Chronic quetiapine use in dogs resulted in cataracts, and lens changes have been observed after long-term use in humans. A causal relationship between quetiapine and cataracts in humans has not been demonstrated. Nonetheless, the FDA has recommended a baseline slit-lamp examination before starting quetiapine therapy or shortly thereafter and a repeat examination every 6 months thereafter.[210]

If A.S. has not yet had a slit-lamp evaluation, an ophthalmologist should evaluate her as soon as possible, and the result should be documented in her chart. A 6-month follow-up examination is also indicated. Quetiapine would probably be discontinued if lens changes were noted on any of the examinations.

Temperature Dysregulation and Dermatologic Effects

37. **N.M., a 27-year-old man, recently was diagnosed with undifferentiated schizophrenia and was stabilized with chlorpromazine 400 mg HS during a 3-month stay in an inpatient unit. N.M. has continued chlorpromazine 400 mg HS as an outpatient and has done so well that he is ready to return to work as a laborer at a construction site. What precautions should he take when working outside?**

N.M. should be advised to wear a hat when working outside, to drink fluids, to stay in the shade as much as possible, and to seek a cooler environment if he feels hot. This is because antipsychotics can cause temperature dysregulation, probably by inhibiting hypothalamic temperature regulation. The net result is poikilothermia (i.e., the normal body temperature cannot respond to heat or cold, and patients become hypothermic or hyperthermic, depending on the surrounding temperature).[211] The strong anticholinergic effects of N.M.'s chlorpromazine can impair cutaneous heat elimination and further exacerbate the problem. Olanzapine and clozapine also have strong anticholinergic properties, necessitating caution for patients exposed to excessive heat.

N.M. should also be advised to use a sunscreen with maximum SPF (sun protection factor), along with protective clothing. This is because chlorpromazine-induced photosensitivity can predispose him to severe sunburns. The tricyclic structure of some antipsychotic drugs absorbs ultraviolet rays, producing free radicals that damage skin. Chlorpromazine is the most common cause of photosensitivity, but it can occur with all phenothiazines and with thiothixene.[211]

Other dermatologic reactions can occur with antipsychotics, and N.M. should be advised to report any skin abnormalities to his physician. Dermatitis, presenting with a maculopapular rash on the face, neck, and upper chest occurs in approximately 5% of patients shortly after starting chlorpromazine. Localized or generalized urticaria also can develop. Antihistamines usually provide adequate relief, but the antipsychotic agent may have to be discontinued in severe cases. The rash rarely reappears after resumption of treatment.

Seizures

38. R.A., a 26-year-old woman recently diagnosed with chronic paranoid schizophrenia, is brought to the hospital after assaulting a neighbor. She presents in an acute psychotic state and has not calmed down since entering the hospital. She has struck two staff members on the psychiatric unit. R.A. has had generalized tonic-clonic seizures since age 14 and currently is taking carbamazepine 300 mg TID (serum concentration on admission is 8.2 mg/mL). R.A. has not been taking any antipsychotic medications and has been seizure free for 1 year. She needs acute treatment with an antipsychotic because of her dangerous behavior. How should an antipsychotic be initiated to treat her schizophrenia in light of her seizure disorder?

Antipsychotic drugs can lower the seizure threshold, producing seizures in patients who previously were seizure free. Seizures are most common with low-potency typical antipsychotics and clozapine.[53] Clozapine-induced seizures are dose-related. The seizure rate is approximately 1% at doses below 300 mg/day, 2.7% at doses between 300 and 600 mg/day, and 4.4% at doses above 600 mg/day.[212] Because R.A. is currently a danger to herself and to others, the benefits of antipsychotic treatment outweigh the risks. Strategies to minimize the risk of seizures should be employed and include slow dose titration, use of lowest effective doses, and concurrent administration of an antiepileptic drug (e.g. carbamazepine).[213]

Haloperidol, an agent with a low risk for causing seizures, is a good selection. An initial dose of 5 mg orally or 2.5 mg IM should be given immediately, and additional dosages should be carefully administered until the psychosis resolves or she is no longer dangerous. The decision to use scheduled or as-needed medications should be based on whether she remains dangerous after a few immediate doses and what the underlying cause of the psychosis is determined to be. Supplemental benzodiazepines may be used to avoid high doses of haloperidol. If necessary, R.A.'s carbamazepine dose should be adjusted to maintain good seizure control and serum concentrations should be monitored. Carbamazepine (and other enzyme-inducing antiepileptic drugs) can influence the hepatic metabolism of antipsychotic agents. R.A. should be monitored for recurrent symptoms of schizophrenia if her carbamazepine dosage is increased.

Sexual Dysfunction

39. K.J., a 24-year-old man with chronic paranoid schizophrenia, was rehospitalized for an acute exacerbation secondary to nonadherence with thioridazine 400 mg HS. During the medication history, it is discovered that he stopped taking thioridazine because he lost his interest in sex. When he tries to have intercourse, he experiences delayed ejaculation. About a week after stopping the thioridazine he is able to have a normal ejaculation. How does thioridazine contribute to K.J.'s sexual dysfunction?

Thioridazine is recognized as the most common cause of antipsychotic-induced sexual dysfunction.[214] Sexual side effects such as diminished libido, impaired arousal, and erectile and orgasmic dysfunction, however, have also been reported with both other typical agents and atypical agents.[115] The causes of antipsychotic-induced sexual dysfunction are related to a number of factors including hyperprolactinemia via dopamine blockade, α-adrenergic blockade, and anticholinergic and sedative effects.[215] Impaired sexual function has also been observed in untreated patients with schizophrenia, making the distinction between drug-induced and disease-induced symptoms difficult.[216] K.J.'s sexual dysfunction likely is related to the thioridazine because the symptoms resolved after he stopped the medication. Lowering the dose of thioridazine or converting him to another antipsychotic with less influence on sexual function may be helpful, although no reliable evidence is available to indicate which drugs are least likely to cause sexual dysfunction.

Considerations in Pregnancy

40. D.M., a 26-year-old woman, has a 6-year history of chronic undifferentiated schizophrenia that has been treated with chlorpromazine 400 mg HS. She is psychiatrically stable and was last hospitalized 2 years ago. When D.M. decompensates, she isolates herself, is unable to care for herself, does not eat properly, and does not maintain her grooming and hygiene. She just found out that she is 8 weeks pregnant. Should her chlorpromazine be continued and what are the risks if the medication is continued?

There are no consistently reported teratogenic changes with any of the antipsychotic drugs. Most of the available evidence on the use of antipsychotics during pregnancy has focused on typical antipsychotics. Among the typical antipsychotics, pooled results of large retrospective and small prospective controlled studies implicate an increased risk of congenital anomalies in patients treated with low potency phenothiazines, particularly when treated during the first trimester.[217] Guidelines have recommended that the use of antipsychotic medication during the first trimester should be minimized or avoided if possible, especially between weeks 6 and 10.[53] If an antipsychotic is necessary during this period, high-potency typical antipsychotics may be safer.[53] In addition to their teratogenic effects, there are other reasons to avoid low-potency antipsychotics. Low-potency agents can worsen constipation and cause orthostatic hypotension and uteroplacental insufficiency. Guidelines have also recommended that medications should be tapered 1 week before delivery to minimize neonatal complications such as dystonia, withdrawal dyskinesias, temperature dysregulation and irritability.[53]

Medication management should balance the needs of D.M. against those of her unborn child. D.M.'s schizophrenia has been stable for 2 years. Chlorpromazine should be discontinued because it is a low-potency phenothiazine and D.M. is currently in her first trimester. Because she is a danger to her-

self when ill, it is critical that treatment be initiated at the first evidence of decompensation. D.M. should be monitored by her clinician, family members, and caseworker at frequent intervals for reemergence of psychotic symptoms. If D.M. decompensates, treatment should be restarted with a nonphenothiazine, high-potency agent at the lowest possible dose (e.g., haloperidol or fluphenazine 2 to 5 mg at night). If D.M. does not respond to low-dose haloperidol or fluphenazine, or if she develops intolerable extrapyramidal side effects, then a lower-potency antipsychotic drug or an atypical agent can be selected. D.M.'s chart should include the following documentation: specific behaviors that necessitate treatment (danger to self, fetus, or others); goals of therapy (acute control of dangerous behavior or remission); dose, route of administration, schedule, and projected duration of treatment; obstetric history and other medications used during pregnancy; alcohol or illegal drug use; regular progress notes on response and need for continued treatment; and informed consent from the patient or guardian.

REFERENCES

1. Saddock BJ, Saddock VA. The doctor-patient relationship and interviewing techniques. In: Kaplan & Sadock's synopsis of psychiatry: behavioral sciences, clinical psychiatry. Philadelphia: Lippincott Williams & Wilkins, 2003:1.
2. Saddock BJ, Saddock VA. Psychiatric history and mental status examination. In: Kaplan & Sadock's synopsis of psychiatry: behavioral sciences, clinical psychiatry. Philadelphia: Lippincott Williams & Wilkins, 2003: 229.
3. Murray CJL, Lopez AD, eds. Global Burden of Disease. Cambridge, MA: Harvard University Press, 1996.
4. Rupp A, Keith SJ. The costs of schizophrenia. Assessing the burden. Psychiatr Clin North Am 1993; 16:413.
5. National Advisory Mental Health Council. Health care reform for Americans with severe mental illnesses: report of the National Advisory Mental Health Council. Am J Psychiatry 1993;150:1447.
6. Andreasen NC, Carpenter WT: Diagnosis and classification of schizophrenia. Schizophr Bull 1993;19:199.
7. Seaton BE, Goldstein G, Allen DN: Sources of heterogeneity in schizophrenia: the role of neuropsychological functioning. Neuropsychol Rev 2001; 11:45.
8. Kendler KS, Diehl SR. The genetics of schizophrenia: a current genetic-epidemiologic perspective. Schizophr Bull 1998;19:261.
9. Kendler KS, Robinett CD. Schizophrenia in the National Academy of Sciences-National Research Council Twin Registry: a 16-year update. Am J Psychiatry 1983;140:1551.
10. American Psychiatric Association. Diagnostic and Statistical Manual of Mental Disorders TR, 4th Ed. (DSM IV TR). Washington, DC: American Psychiatric Press, 2000.
11. Pulver AE: Search for schizophrenia susceptibility genes. Biol Psychiatry 2000;47:221.
12. Crow T et al. Schizophrenia as an anomaly of development of cerebral asymmetry: a postmortem study and a proposal concerning the genetic basis of the disease. Arch Gen Psychiatry 1989;46:1145.
13. Andreasen NC et al. Magnetic resonance imaging of the brain in schizophrenia. Arch Gen Psychiatry 1990;47:35.
14. Gur R et al. Magnetic resonance imaging in schizophrenia: I. Volumetric analysis of brain and cerebrospinal fluid. Arch Gen Psychiatry 1991;48:407.
15. Kelsoe JR et al. Quantitative neuroanatomy in schizophrenia: A controlled magnetic resonance imaging study. Arch Gen Psychiatry 1988;45:533.

16. Suddath RL et al. Temporal lobe pathology in schizophrenia: a quantitative magnetic resonance imaging study. Am J Psychiatry 1989;146:464.
17. Suddath RL et al. Anatomical abnormalities in the brains of monozygotic twins discordant for schizophrenia. N Engl J Med 1990;322:789.
18. Harrison PJ. On the neuropathology of schizophrenia and its dementia: Neurodevelopmental, neurodegenerative, or both? Neurodegeneration 1995; 4:1.
19. Bogrest B et al. Hippocampus-amygdala volumes and psychopathology in chronic schizophrenia. Biol Psychiatry 1991;33:239.
20. Kindermann SS et al. Review of functional magnetic resonance imaging in schizophrenia. Schizophr Res 1997;27:143.
21. Weinberger DR et al. Physiological dysfunction of dorsolateral prefrontal cortex in schizophrenia, I: Regional cerebral blood flow evidence. Arch Gen Psychiatry 1986;43:114.
22. Stevens AA et al. Cortical dysfunction in schizophrenia during auditory word and tone working memory demonstrated by functional magnetic resonance imaging. Arch Gen Psychiatry 1998;55:1097.
23. Mubrin Z et al. Regional cerebral blood flow patterns in schizophrenic patients. Cerebral Blood Flow 1982;3:43.
24. Roberts G. Is there gliosis in schizophrenia? Investigation of the temporal lobe. Biol Psychiatry 1987; 22:1459.
25. Andreasen NC et al. "Cognitive dysmetria" as an integrative theory of schizophrenia: A dysfunction in cortical-subcortical-cerebellar circuitry? Schizophr Bull 1998;24:203.
26. Herz MI, Marder SR. Neurobiology. In: Schizophrenia: comprehensive treatment and management. Philadelphia, Lippincott Williams & Wilkins, 2002:3.
27. Andreasen NC et al. Defining the phenotype of schizophrenia: cognitive dysmetria and its neural mechanisms. Biol Psychiatry 1999;46:908.
28. Weinberger DR: Neurodevelopmental Perspectives on Schizophrenia. In Bloom FE, Kupfer DJ, eds. Psychopharmacology: The Fourth Generation of Progress. New York, Raven Press, Ltd., 1995.
29. Green MF, Neuchterlein KH. Should schizophrenia be treated as a neurocognitive disorder? Schizophr Bull 1999;25:309.
30. Creese I et al. Dopamine receptor binding predicts clinical and pharmacological potencies of antischizophrenic drugs. Science 1976;192:481.
31. Seeman P et al. Antipsychotic drug doses and neuroleptic/dopamine receptors. Nature 1976;261:717.

32. Marder SR, van Kammen DP. Dopamine receptor antagonists. In: Kaplan H, Saddock B, eds. Comprehensive Textbook of Psychiatry VII. New York: Lippincott Williams & Wilkins, 1999:2356.
33. Davidson M et al. L-Dopa challenge and relapse in schizophrenia. Am J Psychiatry 1987;144:934.
34. Lieberman J et al. Methylphenidate challenge as a predictor of relapse in schizophrenia. Am J Psychiatry 1984;141:633.
35. Snyder S. Catecholamines in the brain as mediators of amphetamine psychosis. Arch Gen Psychiatry 1972;27:169.
36. Littrel RA et al. The neurobiology of schizophrenia. Pharmacotherapy 1996;16(6 Pt 2):143S.
37. Risch SC. Pathophysiology of schizophrenia and the role of newer antipsychotics. Pharmacotherapy 1996;116(Suppl 1 Pt 2):11S.
38. Davis KL et al. Dopamine in schizophrenia: A review and reconceptualization. Am J Psychiatry 1991;148:1474.
39. Joyce JN: The dopamine hypothesis of schizophrenia: Limbic interactions with serotonin and norepinephrine. Psychopharmacology 1993;112:S16.
40. Olney JW et al. Glutamate receptor dysfunction and schizophrenia. Arch Gen Psychiatry 1995;52:998.
41. Kim JS et al. Low cerebrospinal fluid glutamate in schizophrenia patients and new hypothesis on schizophrenia. Neurosci Lett 1980;20:379.
42. Akbarian S et al. Gene expression for glutamic acid decarboxylase is reduced without loss of neurons in prefrontal cortex of schizophrenics. Arch Gen Psychiatry 1995;52:528.
43. Kraepelin E. Dementia praecox and paraphrenia. Chicago: Chicago Medical Book, 1919. Barclay RM, translator.
44. Bleuler E. Dementia Praecox or the Group of Schizophrenias (1911). New York: International Press, 1950. Zinkin J, translator.
45. Schneider K. Clinical Psychopathology. New York: Grune & Stratton, 1959.
46. Thacore VR, Shukla SRP. Cannabis psychosis and paranoid schizophrenia. Arch Gen Psychiatry 1976;33:383.
47. Palmer BW et al. Is it possible to be schizophrenic and neuropsychologically impaired? Neuropsychology 1997;11:3437.
48. Green MF et al. Neurocognitive deficits and functional outcome in schizophrenia: Are we measuring the "right stuff"? Schizophr Bull 2000;26:119.
49. Bleuler M: The Schizophrenic Disorders: Long-Term Patient and Family Studies. New Haven: Yale University Press, 1978.

50. Huber G et al. Longitudinal studies of schizophrenic patients. Schizophr Bull 1980;6:592.

51. Ciompi L: Catamnestic long-term study on the course of life and aging of schizophrenics. Schizophr Bull 1980;6:608.

52. McGlashan TH, Fenton WS: Subtype progression and pathophysiologic deterioration in early schizophrenia. Schizophr Bull 1993;19:71.

53. American Psychiatric Association. Practice guideline for the treatment of patients with schizophrenia. Am J Psychiatry 1997;154(Suppl):1.

54. Newman SC, Bland RC: Mortality in a cohort of patients with schizophrenia: A record linkage study. Can J Psychiatry 1991;36:239.

55. Caldwell CB, Gottesman II. Schizophrenics kill themselves too: a review of risk factors for suicide. Schizophr Bull 1990;16:571.

56. Heinssen RK et al. Psychosocial skills training for schizophrenia: Lessons from the laboratory. Schizophr Bull 2000;26:21.

57. Beck AT, Rector NA: Cognitive therapy for schizophrenia patients. Harvard Ment Health Lett 1998;15:4.

58. Garety PA et al. Cognitive-behavioral therapy for medication-resistant symptoms. Schizophr Bull 2000;26:73.

59. Dixon L et al. Update on family psychoeducation for schizophrenia. Schizophr Bull 2000;26:5.

60. Cook JA, Razzano L: Vocational rehabilitation for persons with schizophrenia: Recent research and implications for practice. Schizophr Bull 2000; 26:87.

61. Janick PG et al. Principles and Practice of Psychopharmacotherapy. Baltimore: Williams & Wilkins, 1997:97.

62. Perry PJ et al. Psychotropic Drug Handbook. Washington: American Psychiatric Press, 1997.

63. Ames D et al. Advances in antipsychotic pharmacotherapy: clozapine, risperidone and beyond. Essent Psychopharmacol 1996;1:5.

64. Lohr JB, Braff DL. The value of referring to recently introduced antipsychotics as "Second Generation". Am J Psychiatry 2003;160:1371.

65. Nordstrom AL et al. Central D2 dopamine receptor occupancy in relation to antipsychotic drug effects: a double-blind PET study of schizophrenic patients. Biol Psychiatry 1993;33:227.

66. Kapur S et al. Relationship between dopamine D2 receptor occupancy, clinical response, and side effects: a double-blind PET study. Am J Psychiatry 2000;157:514.

67. Marder SR, Van Putten T. Antipsychotic medications. In: Schatzberg AF, Nemeroff CB, eds. The American Psychiatric Press Textbook of Psychopharmacology American Psychiatric Press, Washington DC, 1995:247.

68. Bench CJ et al. The time course of binding to striatal dopamine D2 receptors by the neuroleptic ziprasidone (CP-88,059-01) determined by positron emission tomography. Psychopharmacology (Berl) 1996;124:141.

69. Kapur S et al. Clinical and theoretical implications of 5-HT2 and D2 receptor occupancy of clozapine, risperidone and olanzapine in schizophrenia. Am J Psychiatry 1999;156:286.

70. Kapur S et al. A positron emission tomography study of quetiapine in schizophrenia: A preliminary finding of an antipsychotic effect with only transiently high dopamine D$_2$ receptor occupancy. Arch Gen Psychiatry 2000;57:553.

71. Nordstrom AL et al. D1, D2, and 5-HT2 receptor occupancy in relation to clozapine serum concentration: A PET study of schizophrenic patients. Am J Psychiatry 1995;152:1444.

72. Fischman AJ et al. Positron emission tomographic analysis of central 5-hydroxytryptamine2 receptor occupancy in healthy volunteers treated with the novel antipsychotic agent, ziprasidone. J Pharmacol Exper Therapeut 1996;279:939.

73. Meltzer HY. The role of serotonin in antipsychotic drug action. Neuropsychopharmacology. 1999;21(2 Suppl):106S.

74. SM Stahl. Antipsychotic agents. In: Essential Psychopharmacology: Neuroscientific Basis and Practical Applications. New York: Cambridge University Press, 2000;401.

75. Kane JM et al. Efficacy and safety of aripiprazole and haloperidol versus placebo in patients with schizophrenia and schizoaffective disorder. J Clin Psychiatry. 2002;63:763.

76. Casey DE. Side effect profiles of new antipsychotic agents. J Clin Psychiatry 1996;57(Suppl 11):40.

77. Lehman AF, Steinwachs DM. Translating research into practice: the Schizophrenia Patient Outcomes Research Team (PORT) treatment recommendations. Schizophr Bull 1998;24:1.

78. Marder SR, Meibach RC. Risperidone in the treatment of schizophrenia Am J Psychiatry 1994; 151:825.

79. Marder SR et al. The effects of risperidone on the five dimensions of schizophrenia derived by factor analysis: combined results of the North American trials. J Clin Psychiatry 1997;58:538.

80. Hoyberg OJ et al. Risperidone versus perphenazine in the treatment of chronic schizophrenic patients with acute exacerbations. Acta Psychiatr Scand 1993;88:395.

81. Tollefson GD et al. Olanzapine versus haloperidol in the treatment of schizophrenia and schizoaffective disorder and schizophreniform disorders: results of an international collaborative trial. Am J Psychiatry 1997;154:457.

82. Beasley CM Jr et al. Olanzapine versus placebo and haloperidol: acute phase results of the North American double-blind olanzapine trial. Neuropsychopharmacology 1996;14:111.

83. Arvanitis LA et al. Multiple fixed doses of "Seroquel" (quetiapine) in patients with acute exacerbation of schizophrenia: a comparison with haloperidol and placebo. Biol Psychiatr 1997;42:233.

84. Peuskens J, Link CG A comparison of quetiapine and chlorpromazine in the treatment of schizophrenia. Acta Psychiatr Scand 1997;96:265.

85. Goff DC et al. An exploratory haloperidol-controlled dose-finding study of ziprasidone in hospitalized patients with schizophrenia or schizoaffective disorder. J Clin Psychopharmacol 1998;18:296.

86. Daniel DG et al. Ziprasidone 80 mg/day and 160 mg/day in the acute exacerbation of schizophrenia and schizoaffective disorder: a 6-week placebo-controlled trial. Neuropsychopharmacology 1999; 20:491.

87. Geddes J et al. Atypical antipsychotics in the treatment of schizophrenia: systematic overview and meta-regression analysis. Br Med J 2000;321:1371.

88. Leucht S. Efficacy and extrapyramidal side-effects of the new antipsychotics olanzapine, quetiapine, risperidone, and sertindole compared to conventional antipsychotics and placebo: a meta-analysis of randomized controlled trials. Schizopr Res 1999;35:51.

89. Davis JM et al. A meta-analysis of the efficacy of second-generation antipsychotics. Arch Gen Psychiatry 2003;60:553.

90. Moller HJ. Neuroleptic treatment of negative symptoms in schizophrenic patients. Efficacy problems and methodological difficulties. Eur Neuropsychopharmacol 1993;3:1.

91. Tollefson GD, Sanger TM. Negative symptoms: a path analytic approach to a double-blind, placebo- and haloperidol-controlled clinical trial with olanzapine. Am J Psychiatry 1997;154:466.

92. Wolkowitz OM, Pickar D. Benzodiazepines in the treatment of schizophrenia: a review and reappraisal. Am J Psychiatry 1991;148:714.

93. Growe GA et al. Lithium in chronic schizophrenia. Am J Psychiatry 1979;136:454.

94. Small JG et al. A placebo-controlled study of lithium combined with neuroleptics in chronic schizophrenic patients. Am J Psychiatry 1975;132:1315.

95. Goldney RD, Spence ND. Safety of the combination of lithium and neuroleptic drugs. Am J Psychiatry 1986;143:882.

96. Leucht S et al. Carbamazepine augmentation for schizophrenia: how good is the evidence? J Clin Psychiatry. 2002;63:218.

97. McElroy SL et al. Sodium valproate: its use in primary psychiatric disorders. J Clin Psychopharmacol 1987;7:16.

98. Neppe VM. Carbamazepine in nonresponsive psychosis. J Clin Psychiatry 1988;49(Suppl 4):22.

99. Citrome L et al. Changes in use of valproate and other mood stabilizers for patients with schizophrenia from 1994 to 1998. Psychiatr Serv 2000; 51:634.

100. Casey DE et al. Effect of divalproex combined with olanzapine or risperidone in patients with an acute exacerbation of schizophrenia. Neuropsychopharmacology. 2003;28:182.

101. Sorgi PJ et al. Beta-adrenergic blockers for the control of aggressive behaviors in patients with chronic schizophrenia. Am J Psychiatry 1986; 143:775.

102. Lindstrom L, Persson E. Propranolol in chronic schizophrenia: a controlled study in neuroleptic treated patients. Br J Psychiatry 1980;137:126.

103. Wyatt RJ. Neuroleptics and the natural course of schizophrenia. Schizophr Bull 1992;17:325.

104. Casey DE. Neuroleptic-induced extrapyramidal syndromes and tardive dyskinesia. In, Hirsch SR, Weinberger DR, eds. Schizophrenia. Oxford, UK: Blackwell, 1995:546.

105. Casey DE. Tardive dyskinesia and atyipical antipsychotic drugs. Schizophr Res 1999; 35 (Suppl): 55-62.

106. Dolder CR, Jeste DV. Incidence of tardive dyskinesia with typical versus atypical antipsychotics in very high risk patients. Biol Psychiatry 2003; 53:1142.

107. Beasley CM et al. Randomized double-blind comparison of the incidence of tardive dyskinesia in patients with schizophrenia during long-term treatment with olanzapine or haloperidol. Br J Psychiatry 1999;174:23.

108. Jeste DV et al. Lower incidence of tardive dyskinesia with risperidone compared with haloperidol in older patients. J Am Geriatr Soc 1999;47:716.

109. Kane JM et al. Does clozapine cause tardive dyskinesia? J Clin Psychiatry 1993;54:327.

110. Janick PG et al. Principles and Practice of Psychopharmacotherapy. Baltimore: Williams & Wilkins, 1997:188.

111. Rogers DP, Shramko JK Therapeutic options in the treatment of clozapine-induced sialorrhea. Pharmacotherapy. 2000;20:1092.

112. Buckley NA, Sanders P. Cardiovascular adverse effects of antipsychotic drugs. Drug Saf 2000;23:215.

113. FDA Psychopharmacological Drugs Advisory Committee. 19 July 2000 Briefing Document for Ziprasidone HCl. Accessed from http://www.fda.gov/ohrms/dockets/ac/00/backgrd/3619b1a.pdf.

114. Petty R. Prolactin and antipsychotic medications: mechanism of action. Schizophr Res 1999;35:S67.

115. Wirshing DA et al. Understanding the new and evolving profile of adverse drug effects in schizophrenia. Psychiatr Clin North Am 2003;26:165.

116. Kleinberg DR et al. Prolactin levels and adverse events in patients treated with risperidone J Clin Psychopharmacol 1999;19:57.

117. Dickson RA, Glazer WM. Neuroleptic-induced hyperprolactinemia. Schizophren Res 1999;35:S75.

118. McIntyre RS et al. Mechanisms of antipsychotic-induced weight gain. J Clin Psychiatry 2001; 62(Suppl 23):23.

119. Tandon R. Safety and tolerability: how do newer generation "atypical" antipsychotics compare? Psychiatr Q 2002;73:297.

120. Allison DB et al. Antipsychotic-induced weight gain: a comprehensive research synthesis. Am J Psychiatry 1999;156:1686.

121. Sussman N. Review of atypical antipsychotics and weight gain. J Clin Psychiatry 2001;62(Suppl 23):5.

122. Henderson D et al. Clozapine: Diabetes mellitus, weight gain and lipid abnormalities: a five year naturalistic study. Am J Psychiatry 2000;157:975.

123. Kinon BJ et al. Long-term olanzapine treatment: weight change and weight-related health factors in schizophrenia J Clin Psychiatry 2001;62:92.

124. McIntyre RS, McCann SM, Kennedy SH. Antipsychotic metabolic effects: Weight gain, dia-

betes mellitus, and lipid abnormalities. Can J Psychiatry 2001;46:273.

125. Goldstein LE, Henderson DC. Atypical antipsychotics agents and diabetes mellitus. Prim Psychiatry 2000;7:65.

126. Melkersson KI, Hulting A-L, Brismar KE. Elevated levels of insulin, leptin, and blood lipids in olanzapine-treated patients with schizophrenia or related psychoses. J Clin Psychiatry 2000;61:742.

127. Fontaine KR et al. Estimating the consequences of antipsychotic induced weight gain on health and mortality rate. Psychiatry Res 2001;101:277.

128. Burns MJ. The pharmacology and toxicology of atypical agents. J Clin Toxicol 2001;39:1.

129. Ereshefsky L. Pharmacokinetics and drug interactions: update for new antipsychotics. J Clin Psychiatry 1996;57(Suppl 11):12.

130. Michalets EL. Update: clinically significant cytochrome P450 drug interactions. Pharmacotherapy 1998;18:84.

131. Jann MW et al. Effects of carbamazepine on plasma haloperidol levels. J Clin Psychopharmacol 1985;5:106.

132. Rice DP. The economic impact of schizophrenia. J Clin Psychiatry 1999;60(Suppl 1):4.

133. Hudson TJ et al. Economic evaluations of novel antipsychotic medications: a literature review. Schizophr Res 2003;60:199.

134. Mossum D. A decision analysis approach to neuroleptic dosing: insights from a mathematical model. J Clin Psychiatry 1997;58:66.

135. McEvoy JP et al. The expert consensus guideline series. Treatment of Schizophrenia, 1999. J Clin Psychiatry 1999;60(Suppl 11):1.

136. Milton GV, Jann MW. Emergency treatment of of psychotic symptoms: pharmacokinetic considerations for antipsychotic drugs. Clin Pharmacokinet 1995;28:494.

137. Brook S et al. Intramuscular ziprasidone compared with intramuscular haloperidol in the treatment of acute psychosis. J Clin Psychiatry 2000;61:933.

138. Daniel DG et al. Intramuscular ziprasidone 20mg is effective in reducing agitation associated with psychosis: a double-blind, randomized trial. Psychopharmacol 2001;155:128.

139. Breier A et al. A double-blind, placebo-controlled dose response comparison of intramuscular olanzapine and haloperidol in the treatment of acute agitation in schizophrenia. Arch Gen Psychiatry 2002;59:441.

140. Wright P et al. Double-blind, placebo-controlled comparison of intramuscular olanzapine and intramuscular haloperidol in the treatment of acute agitation in schizophrenia. Am J Psychiatry 2001; 158:1149.

141. Garza-Trevino ES et al. Efficacy of combinations of intramuscular antipsychotics and sedative-hypnotics for control of psychotic agitation. Am J Psychiatry 1989;146:1598.

142. Baldessarini R et al. Significance of neuroleptic dose and plasma level in pharmacological treatment of psychoses. Arch Gen Psychiatry 1988; 45:79.

143. Hillard JR. Emergency treatment of acute psychosis. J. Clin Psychiatry 1998;59(Suppl):57.

144. Altamura AC et al. Intramuscular preparations of antipsychotics: uses and relevance in clinical practice. Drugs 2003;63:493.

145. Dubin WR. Rapid tranquilization: antipsychotics or benzodiazepines? J Clin Psychiatry 1988; 49(Suppl):5.

146. Kane JM et al. Long-acting injectable risperidone: efficacy and safety of the first long-acting atypical antipsychotic. Am J Psychiatry 2003160:1125.

147. Martin SD et al. Clinical experience with the long-acting injectable formulation of the atypical antipsychotic, risperidone. Curr Med Res Opin 2003;19:298.

148. Conley RR, Kelly DL. Management of treatment resistance in schizophrenia. Biol Psychiatry 2001;50:898.

149. Kane J et al. Clozapine for treatment resistant schizophrenia. A double blind comparison with

chlorpromazine. Arch Gen Psychiatry 1988; 45.789.

150. Chakos M et al. Effectiveness of second-generation antipsychotics in patients with treatment-resistant schizophrenia: a review and meta-analysis of randomized trials. Am J Psychiatry 2001; 158:518.

151. Wirshing DA et al. Risperidone in treatment-refractory schizophrenia. Am J Psychiatry 1999; 156:1374.

152. Conley RR et al. Olanzapine compared with chlorpromazine in treatment-resistant schizophrenia. Am J Psychiatry 1998;155:914.

153. Pantelis C, Barnes TR. Drug strategies and treatment-resistant schizophrenia. Aust N Z J Psychiatry 1996;30:20.

154. Miller AL et al. The TMAP schizophrenia algorithms. J Clin Psychiatry 1999;60:649.

155. Robinson DG et al. Predictors of treatment response from a first episode of schizophrenia or schizoaffective disorder. Am J Psychiatry 1999, 156:544.

156. Ganguli R. Rationale and strategies for switching antipsychotics. Am J Health-Syst Pharm 2002; 59:S22.

157. Rifkin A. Pharmacologic strategies in the treatment of schizophrenia. Psychiatr Clin North Am 1993;16:351.

158. Kane JM. Treatment programme and long term outcome in chronic schizophrenia. Acta Psychiatr Scand 1990;358(Suppl):151.

159. Davis JM. Overview: maintenance therapy in psychiatry. I: Schizophrenia. Am J Psychiatry 1975;132:1237.

160. Marder SR et al. Low-and conventional-dose maintenance therapy with fluphenazine decanoate. Arch Gen Psychiatry 1987;44:518.

161. Hogarty GE et al. Dose of fluphenazine, familiarl expressed emotion, and outcome in schizophrenia: results of a two-year controlled study. Arch Gen Psychiatry 1988;45:797.

162. Schooler NR et al. Relapse and rehospitalization during maintenance treatment of schizophrenia. The effects of dose reduction and family treatment. Arch Gen Psychiatry 1997;54:453.

163. Herz MI et al. Intermittent versus maintenance medication in schizophrenia. Two-year results. Arch Gen Psychiatry 1991;48:333.

164. Marken PA, Stanislav SW. Schizophrenia. In: Koda-Kimble MA, Young LY, eds. Applied Therapeutics: The Clinical Use of Drugs. Baltimore: Lippincott, Williams & Wilkins, 2001;76.

165. Bristol Myers Squibb. Aripiprazole package insert. Princeton, NJ: 2003 May.

166. Woods SW. Chlorpromazine equivalent doses for the newer atypical antipsychotics. J Clin Psychiatry 2003;64:663.

167. Fenton WS et al. Determinants of medication compliance in schizophrenia: empirical and clinical findings. Schizophr Bull 1997;23:637.

168. Lacro JP et al. Prevalence of and risk factors for medication nonadherence in patients with schizophrenia: a comprehensive review of recent literature. J Clin Psychiatry 2002;63:892.

169. Weiden PJ, Olfson M. Cost of relapse in schizophrenia. Schizophr Bull 1995;21:419.

170. Terkelsen KG, Menikoff A. Measuring the costs of schizophrenia: implications for the post-institutional era in the US Pharmacoeconomics 1995; 52:173.

171. Barnes TR, Curson DA. Long-term depot antipsychotics. A risk-benefit assessment. Drug Saf 1994;10:464.

172. Ereshefsky L et al. Future of depot neuroleptic therapy: pharmacokinetic and pharmacodynamic approaches. J Clin Psychiatry 1984;45(5 Pt 2):50.

173. McEvoy GK, ed. American Hospital Formulary System Drug Information. Bethesda, MD: American Society of Hospital Pharmacists, 1998:1864.

174. McNeil Pharmaceutical. Haldol Decanoate package insert. Raritan, NJ: 2001 September.

175. Meltzer HY. New drugs for the treatment of schizophrenia. Psychiatry Clin North Am 1993;16:365.

176. Breier A et al. Clozapine treatment of outpatients: outcome and long-term response patterns. Hosp Comm Psychiatry 1993;44:1145.

177. Meltzer HY. Duration of a clozapine trial in neuroleptic-resistant schizophrenia. Arch Gen Psychiatry 1989;46:672.

178. Meltzer HY. Treatment of the neuroleptic-nonresponsive schizophrenic patient. Schizophr Bull 1992;18:515.

179. Novartis Pharmaceuticals. Clozapine package insert. East Hanover, NJ: 2002 February.

180. Alvir JMJ et al. Clozapine-induced agranulocytosis: incidence and risk factors in the United States. N Engl J Med 1993;329:162.

181. Gerson SL. G-CSF and the management of clozapine-induced agranulocytosis. J Clin Psychiatry 1994;55(Suppl 9B):139.

182. Preskorn SH et al. Therapeutic drug monitoring: principles and practice. Psychiatr Clin North Am 1993,16.611.

183. Volavka J et al. Plasma haloperidol levels and clinical effects in schizophrenia and schizoaffective disorder. Arch Gen Psychiatry 1995;52.

184. Van Putten T et al. Haloperidol plasma levels and clinical response: a therapeutic window relationship. Am J Psychiatry 1992;149:500.

185. Levison DF et al. Fluphenazine plasma levels, dosage, efficacy, and side effects. Am J Psychiatry 1995;152:765.

186. Mavroides M et al. Clinical relevance of thiothixene plasma levels. J Clin Psychopharmacol 1984;4:155.

187. Yesavage J et al. Correlation of initial thiothixene serum levels and clinical response. Arch Gen Psychiatry 1983;40:301.

188. Perry PJ et al. Clozapine and norclozapine plasma concentration and clinical response of treatment-refractory schizophrenic patients. Am J Psychiatry 1991;148:231.

189. Freeman DJ et al. Will routine therapeutic drug monitoring have a place in clozapine therapy? Clin Pharmacokinet 1997;32:93.

190. Perry PJ et al. Olanzapine plasma concentrations and clinical response: acute phase results of the North American Olanzapine Trial. J Clin Psychopharmacol 2001;21:14.

191. Holloman LC, Marder SR. Management of acute extrapyramidal effects induced by antipsychotic drugs. Am J Health-Syst Pharm 1997;54:2461.

192. Jeste DV, Naimark D. Medication-induced movement disorders. In: Tasman A, Kay J, Lieberman J, eds. Psychiatry. Philadelphia: WB Saunders, 1996:1304.

193. Simpson G, Angus JWS. A rating scale for extrapyramidal side effects. Acta Psychiatr Scand 1970;46(Suppl 221):11.

194. World Health Organization. Prophylactic use of anticholinergics in patients on long-term neuroleptic treatment: a consensus statement. World Health Organization heads of centres collaborating on WHO co-ordinated studies on biological aspects of mental illness. Br J Psychiatry 1990;156:412.

195. Fleischhacker WW et al. The pharmacological treatment of neuroleptic-induced akathisia. J Clin Psychopharmacol 1990;10:12.

196. Kane JM et al. Tardive dyskinesia: prevalence, incidence, and risk factors. J Clin Psychopharmacol 1988;8(4 Suppl):52S.

197. Kane JM et al. Tardive dyskinesia: a task force report to the American Psychiatric Association. Washington, DC: American Psychiatric Association, 1992.

198. Jeste DV et al. Risk of tardive dyskinesia in older patients. A prospective longitudinal study of 266 outpatients. Arch Gen Psychiatry 1995;52:756.

199. Woerner MG et al. Prospective study of tardive dyskinesia in the elderly: rates and risk factors. Am J Psychiatry 1998;155:1521.

200. Yassa R. Functional impairment in tardive dyskinesia: medical and psychosocial dimensions. Acta Psychiatr Scand 1989;80:64.

201. Boomershine KH et al. Vitamin E in the treatment of tardive dyskinesia. Ann Pharmacother 1999;33:1195.
202. Adler LA et al. Vitamin E treatment for tardive dyskinesia. Arch Gen Psychiatry 1999;56:836.
203. Farver DK. Neuroleptic malignant syndrome induced by atypical antipsychotics. Expert Opin Drug Saf 2003;2:21.
204. Caroff SN et al. Neuroleptic malignant syndrome. Med Clin North Am 1993;77:185.
205. Pelonero AL et al. Neuroleptic Malignant Syndrome: A Review. Psychiatr Serv 1998;49:1163.
206. Lazarus A. Therapy of neuroleptic malignant syndrome. Psychiatr Dev 1986;4:19.

207. Rosebush PI et al. Twenty neuroleptic rechallenges after neuroleptic malignant syndrome in 15 patients. J Clin Psychiatry 1989;50:295.
208. Garattini S et al. Reduction of food intake by manipulation of central serotonin: current experimental results. Br J Psychiatry 1989;155:41.
209. Must A et al. The disease burden associated with overweight and obesity. JAMA 1999;282:1523.
210. AstraZeneca Pharmaceuticals. Quetiapine Package Insert. Wilmington, DE: 2001.
211. Simpson CM et al. Adverse effects of antipsychotic drugs. Drugs 1981;21:138.
212. Devinsky O et al. Clozapine-related seizures. Neurology 1991;41:369.

213. Hummer M, Fleichhacker WW. Nonmotor side effects of novel antipsychotics. Curr Opin CPNS Invest Drugs 2000;2:45.
214. Kotin J et al. Thioridazine and sexual dysfunction. Am J Psychiatry 1976;133:82.
215. Meston CM, Frohlich PF. The neurobiology of sexual function. Arch Gen Psychiatry 2000;57:1012.
216. Aizenberg D et al. Sexual dysfunction in male schizophrenic patients. J Clin Psychiatry 1995;56:137.
217. Altshuler LL et al. Pharmacologic management of psychiatric illness during pregnancy: dilemmas and guidelines. Am J Psychiatry 1996;153:592.

CHAPTER 79

Mood Disorders I: Major Depressive Disorders

Patrick R. Finley, Lyle K. Laird, William H. Benefield, Jr.

We who squander our sorrows
How we look beyond them into the mournful passage of time
To see whether they might end

—Rainier Marie Rilke

INTRODUCTION

Depression is a common, chronic, and potentially debilitating illness that has tempered the human condition since the beginning of recorded history. The ancient Egyptians, for instance, wrote about depression more than 3,000 years ago. In the First Book of Samuel (dated about 700 BC), Saul, the King of Israel, is overcome by an "evil spirit" that causes him to feel "incapacitated, guilt-ridden and hopeless" leading ultimately to his suicide.[1]

Cultures throughout history have speculated on the origin of depression. The ancient Greeks thought depression was caused by an excess of bile. Hippocrates thoroughly described the condition as a somatic illness and is believed to have coined the term melancholia, which literally translates to "black bile." During the Middle Ages, depression, along with other psychiatric illnesses, was considered a punishment or an affliction from a vengeful God rather than actual illness. At that time, the church and society believed it to be a result of being weak-minded or sinful. Even today, many people suffering from a depressive episode carry the stigma of "having a nervous breakdown," and medications are viewed as a "crutch" to help cope with daily life. Through history, depression has affected the lives of many famous people, including Ludwig Van Beethoven, Meriwether Lewis, Abraham Lincoln, Charles Dickens, Winston Churchill, and Ernest Hemingway.[1]

Although many people experience "the blues" from time to time, the term *depression* is reserved in psychiatry to define a specific medical condition with distinctive biologic and pharmacologic implications. Similarly, the term *clinical depression* is liberally applied in popular culture to a condition that approximates the psychiatric diagnosis of major depression. In general, depressive disorders are an enormous health concern that are often misdiagnosed or undertreated. The physical and social dysfunction associated with depression is profound and is believed to outweigh many other chronic medical conditions, including hypertension, diabetes, and arthritis.[2] The Medical Outcomes Study, for instance, determined that the degree of impairment in depressed individuals is comparable to that seen in patients with chronic heart disease.[3] The financial ramifications of depression are tremendous and place an overwhelming burden on our society. In 1990, the estimated cost of depression in the United States was $43.7 billion annually, with most of these costs attributed to lost productivity and absenteeism in the workplace.[4]

Epidemiology

Since World War II, the lifetime incidence of depression has been rising steadily in studied populations.[5] Today, the annual incidence of mood disorders is estimated to range from 7% to 12% of the population, and approximately 1 in 10 adults will suffer from an episode of major depression during any 12-month period.[6] In 2003, results of a large national survey revealed a lifetime prevalence rate of major depression of 16.2%, and the 12-month prevalence rate was 6.6%.[7] Other studies from Europe and the United States have estimated the lifetime prevalence to be 5% to 12% in adult males and 9% to 26% in females.[8] Although the incidence of depression is remarkably similar across various races and ethnic groups, the illness may be slightly more common in lower socioeconomic classes.[9]

The onset of depression occurs most commonly in the late 20s, but there is a wide range and the first episode may actually present at any age. The observed peak onset for major depression in females is between 35 and 45 years of age and in males it occurs most commonly after age 55. One prevailing misconception is that depression is more common among elderly individuals.[10] Recent evidence suggests that the incidence is slightly lower in older persons than in the general population, but certain subtypes may be more common (e.g., melancholia, depression with psychotic features).[7,10]

Genetic factors may play a major role in the cause of depression. First-degree relatives (children, siblings, parents) of depressed individuals are 2.7 times more likely to have depression if one parent is afflicted, and 3.0 times more likely if both parents suffer from depression.[11] Concordance rates for monozygotic (identical) twins range from 54% to 65%, whereas dizygotic (fraternal) twins range from 14% to 24%.[12] Genetic factors also may predispose individuals to an earlier onset of depression (younger than 30 years of age).[13]

Alternatively, there is clear evidence that depression may occur as a result of stressful events (i.e., environmental factors) in one's life. These factors include a difficult childhood, pervasive low self-esteem, death of a loved one, loss of a job, and the end of a serious relationship. Depressive episodes are commonly attributed to such events unmasking mood disorders in genetically predisposed persons, but depression may also occur spontaneously in people lacking obvious environmental or genetic factors.

Diagnosis and Classification

The diagnosis and classification of depression have undergone many transformations since Emil Kraepelin's biologic model of the late 19th century. Kraepelin separated the functional psychoses into two groups: manic-depressive insanity and dementia praecox. Kraepelin's detailed descriptions of these two mental illnesses has laid the foundation for modern psychiatry.[14] In 2000, the American Psychiatric Association (APA) published refined, standardized criteria for diagnosing depressive disorders in the *Diagnostic and Statistical Manual of Mental Disorders,* Fourth Edition (DSM-IV-TR).[15] Depressive disorders are classified under Mood Disorders in DSM-IV-TR and include the following: major depressive disorder, single-episode or recurrent, dysthymic disorder, and depressive disorder not otherwise specified. See Table 79-1 for the classification of mood disorders.

As previously stated, a major depressive disorder may occur as a single episode but it is more commonly a recurrent event. Single episodes occur in 30% to 50% of individuals who experience major depression, whereas the remainder have multiple episodes in their lifetimes.[8] The frequency of

Table 79-1 **Classification of Mood Disorders**
I. Mood Disorders
A. Depressive Disorders
1. Major Depressive Disorder, Single Episode
2. Major Depressive Disorder, Recurrent
3. Dysthymic Disorder
4. Depressive Disorder Not Otherwise Specified
B. Bipolar Disorders
1. Bipolar Disorder, Single Episode
2. Bipolar Disorder, Recurrent
3. Cyclothymic Disorder
4. Bipolar Disorder Not Otherwise Specified
C. Secondary Mood Disorder due to Nonpsychiatric Medical Condition
D. Substance-Induced Mood Disorder
E. Mood Disorder Not Otherwise Specified

recurrent episodes is highly variable, with some people experiencing discrete episodes separated by many years of relatively normal mood (i.e., euthymia) and others experiencing residual symptoms between episodes that may never completely remit. The average number of episodes in the lifetime of individuals suffering from major depression is six, but the range is quite large.

Depressive disorders may be subclassified using cross-sectional symptom features, or specifiers, according to DSM-IV-TR.[15] For example, the phrase *with melancholic features* is used when patients possess primary neurovegetative symptoms, early-morning awakening, marked psychomotor agitation or retardation, and significant anorexia or weight loss. Melancholia is often a more severe form of depression and the cause is rather autonomous (i.e., lacking apparent environmental triggers).[16] It may also be less likely than other forms of depression to remit spontaneously. The phrase *with atypical features* is used when depressive symptoms include weight gain, hypersomnia, leaden paralysis, or rejection sensitivity. When hallucinations or delusions occur in patients who are primarily depressed, the phrase *with psychotic features* is applicable to the mood disorder. Other diagnostic specifiers used in DSM-IV-TR include *chronic, with catatonic features,* and *with postpartum onset.*

Dysthymic disorder is a type of depressive illness characterized by fewer symptoms than major depression, but the course is much more chronic with symptoms being present most of the time for at least 2 years. In practice, the distinction of major depression from dysthymia may be difficult to make and requires a detailed psychiatric history. Some patients may experience an episode of major depression superimposed on a history of dysthymia, a condition commonly known as *double depression.* The treatment for dysthymia has traditionally focused on psychotherapy, but recent evidence suggests that antidepressant medications may be effective as well.[17,18]

Differential Diagnosis

Symptoms of depression may be induced or exacerbated by numerous medical illnesses or medications (Tables 79-2 and 79-3). Consequently, DSM-IV-TR specifies that whenever an "organic cause" is temporally related to the onset of depres-

Table 79-2   Selected Medical Conditions That May Mimic Depression

Central Nervous System	Women's Health
Alzheimer's disease	Perimenopause
Cerebrovascular accident	Postpartum
HIV-associated dementia	Premenstrual dysphoric disorder
Multiple sclerosis	**Other**
Parkinson's disease	
Cardiovascular	Chronic fatigue syndrome
	Chronic pain syndrome
Cerebral arteriosclerosis	Fibromyalgia
Congestive heart failure	Irritable bowel syndrome
Myocardial infarction	Malignancies (various)
	Migraine headaches
Endocrine	Rheumatoid arthritis
	Systemic lupus erythematosus
Addison's disease	
Diabetes mellitus	
Hypothyroidism	

Table 79-3   Selected Medications That May Induce Depression

Cardiovascular Agents	Hormonal Agents
β-Blockers	Anabolic steroids
Clonidine	Corticosteroids
Methyldopa	Estrogen (?)
Procainamide	Progestins
Reserpine	Tamoxifen
Central Nervous System Agents	**Others**
	Indomethacin
Barbiturates	Interferon
Benzodiazepines (?)	Isotrotinoin
Chloral hydrate	Mefloquine
Ethanol	Narcotics
Phenytoin	

sive symptoms, the patient does not fit the criteria for major depression even if all other criteria are met.[15] The rationale for this stipulation is that if the medical illness is successfully treated or the offending agent is discontinued, the depressive illness will spontaneously resolve, eliminating the need for somatic intervention. Although lists of medical illnesses or medications are helpful, the clinician should be aware that the actual evidence demonstrating an association between depression and specific organic causes is often very limited and anecdotal. If a medication or condition is suspected of causing depression, the chronologic association should be investigated rigorously before other action is taken.

Clinical Presentation

For a diagnosis of major depressive disorder to be made, symptoms must be present for at least 2 weeks and must not be precipitated or influenced by a medical illness or medication (according to DSM-IV-TR criteria. Individuals must possess at least five symptoms, one of which is either depressed mood or anhedonia. The other seven symptoms are as follows:

1. Change in appetite
2. Change in sleep
3. Low energy
4. Poor concentration (or difficulty making decisions)
5. Feelings of worthlessness or inappropriate guilt
6. Psychomotor agitation or retardation
7. Thoughts of suicide

The diagnostic criteria also stipulate that the mood disturbance must cause marked distress or result in clinically significant impairment of social or occupational functioning. To distinguish depression from grief reactions or bereavement, it is also stipulated that the symptoms of major depression must persist for at least 2 months after the precipitating event. Table 79-4 lists the specific criteria for a diagnosis of major depressive disorder.

Although low energy and changes in sleep or appetite are present in most depressed patients, the clinical presentation of depression can be highly variable. Many patients, for example, will readily express profound sadness or hopelessness, but others can project a more anxious or irritable appearance. Psychomotor agitation may be apparent, featuring wringing of the hands, grimacing, pacing, or shouting. Conversely, psychomotor retardation can be evident, with slowed speech or thinking, soft monotone voice, or minimal facial expression. On occasion, psychotic symptoms (e.g., auditory hallucinations, persecutory delusions, somatic delusions of serious medical illness) may also occur.

Although the criteria for detecting major depression are exactly the same in the elderly population as in the general population, the presentation may be slightly different than in younger individuals. Elderly patients may be less likely to acknowledge sadness or melancholy and choose to dwell instead on somatic complaints such as headache, insomnia, joint pain, dizziness, or constipation.[19] As a result, clinicians are advised to consider the possibility of depression whenever a person presents with vague, chronic symptoms of physical illness and unclear etiology.

Table 79-4   Diagnostic Criteria for Major Depressive Disorder

A. At least five of the following symptoms have been present during the same 2-week period and represent a change from previous functioning. One of the symptoms must be either depressed mood or loss of interest/pleasure.
- Depressed mood most of the day, nearly every day
- Loss of interest in pleasurable activities most of the day, nearly every day
- Change in weight or appetite (increase or decrease) when not dieting
- Insomnia or hypersomnia nearly every day
- Fatigue or loss of energy nearly every day
- Diminished ability to think or concentrate, or indecisiveness
- Feelings of worthlessness or excessive or inappropriate guilt nearly every day
- Psychomotor agitation or retardation nearly every day
- Recurrent thoughts of death or suicidal ideation

B. Symptoms cause clinically significant distress or impairment in social, occupational, or other important areas of functioning.

C. Symptoms are not caused by an underlying medical condition or substance (e.g., medications or recreational drugs).

Pathophysiology

The biologic basis for depressive disorders has come a long way since Hippocrates first identified bile as a possible cause. Several modern theories addressing the origin of depression have evolved over the past three decades, focusing on neurotransmitter systems, including norepinephrine, serotonin, and dopamine. As unique antidepressant medications are developed and our understanding of the mechanisms of pharmacologic action improve, the neurotransmitter theories of depression will undoubtedly evolve.

In the past, the *monoamine hypothesis* proposed that decreased synaptic concentrations of norepinephrine and/or serotonin caused depression. The norepinephrine depletion theory was originally based on the observation that reserpine, which depleted catecholamine stores in the central nervous system (CNS), was capable of causing depression.[20,21] This theory evolved into the *permissive hypothesis* that emphasized a greater role for serotonin in promoting or "permitting" a decline in norepinephrine function. Specifically, this hypothesis suggests that a low concentration of serotonin, combined with elevated levels of norepinephrine, produced mania whereas low concentrations of both neurotransmitters precipitated depression. Antidepressants were therefore believed to relieve depression by inhibiting the reuptake of norepinephrine and/or serotonin from the synapse back up into the neuron.[22]

Although these theories were initially helpful in enhancing our understanding of how antidepressants worked, there were multiple reasons to suspect that other mechanisms and systems were involved. First of all, antidepressants were capable of blocking the reuptake of neurotransmitters almost immediately after administration, yet several weeks lapsed before therapeutic effects were evident (i.e., delayed onset).[23] Second, synaptic concentrations of biogenic amines are not always decreased in depressed individuals and can actually be higher than those seen in normal controls.[24] Last, antidepressants in development can work via other mechanisms, which do not involve relative increases in synaptic neurotransmitter concentrations (e.g., can block substance P or corticotropin-releasing factor).[25–27]

The *dysregulation hypothesis* has evolved in more recent times and suggests that depression, as well as other psychiatric disorders, is the result of a dysregulated neurotransmitter system. Specific criteria for dysregulation have been proposed as follows: (1) an impairment in the regulatory or homeostatic mechanisms, (2) an erratic basal output of the neurotransmitter system, (3) a disruption in normal periodicities (circadian rhythm), (4) a less selective response to environmental stimuli, (5) perturbation of the system resulting in a delayed return to baseline, and (6) restoration to efficient regulation through the use of pharmacologic agents.[28]

Regardless of the antidepressant mechanism of action, changes in the presynaptic and postsynaptic receptor densities (or sensitivities) have been described as being "down-regulated."[29] Changes include a decrease in postsynaptic β-adrenergic receptor sensitivity, along with alterations in the sensitivities of the α-adrenergic and serotonin receptor subtypes (5-HT$_{1A}$ and 5HT$_{2A}$). Newer, highly selective serotonin reuptake inhibitors (SSRIs), such as fluoxetine or sertraline, increase the efficiency of serotonergic neurotransmission. Although these medications may increase synaptic concentrations acutely (through reuptake blockade), the therapeutic effects are linked temporally with increased release of serotonin through down-regulation of presynaptic autoreceptors (5-HT$_{1A}$).[30–32]

Therefore, the dysregulation hypothesis incorporates the diversity of antidepressant mechanisms with the changes that occur over weeks in receptor sensitivities leading to down-regulation. The theory, in its simplest form, suggests that antidepressants repair or reset the equilibrium of the neurotransmitter system, similar to tripping a thermostat or restarting a computer when it locks up. This allows for a compensatory homeostatic change to occur in neuronal regulation by altering the sensitivity of norepinephrine and serotonin receptors. A more efficient signal-to-noise ratio of neurotransmitter results, the overall plasticity of the system improves, and eventually the clinical manifestations of depression resolve as well.

Today, emphasis continues to be placed on serotonin, norepinephrine, and dopamine neurotransmitters, and additional attention is also being paid to their differential effects on specific depressive symptoms. For instance, appetite, sleep, libido, motor function, anxiety, and aggression all appear to be influenced by serotonin transmission. Research evidence for serotonergic influence has demonstrated that the concentration of serotonin's primary metabolite (5-hydroxyindoleacetic acid, or 5-HIAA) is decreased in the cerebrospinal fluid (CSF) of depressed patients.[33] Low 5-HIAA concentrations have also been found in the CSF of patients attempting suicide and may have a role in triggering other violent activities.[34] Dietary depletion of L-tryptophan, a serotonin precursor, has induced relapse in depressed patients previously responsive to SSRIs.[35] Concentrations of serotonin in circulating platelets may have implications related to mood disorders as well (Fig. 79-1). In contrast, deficiencies in norepinephrine (and dopamine to some extent) are believed to mediate depressive symptoms such as anhedonia, energy, memory, and cognitive function.[36,37] Administration of α-methyl tyrosine (required for the synthesis of norepinephrine) has resulted in the return of depressive symptoms among patients previously treated successfully with noradrenergic antidepressants.[38] Ultimately, it is still felt that a common circuitry is influenced by the different neurotransmitters, resulting in the clinical manifestation of depression.[38]

Neuroendocrine Findings

Along with dysregulated neurotransmitter systems, neuroendocrine abnormalities may contribute to the development of depression. Depressed patients often have abnormal thyroid function tests (including low triiodothyronine [T$_3$] and/or thyroxine [T$_4$] levels).[39] They also may exhibit an abnormal response to challenge with thyroid-releasing hormone (TRH) consisting of a blunted or exaggerated thyroid-stimulating hormone (TSH) response.[40] Clinical hypothyroidism can also induce depressive symptoms, and thyroid supplementation can reverse this pathology, suggesting an indirect association between mood disorders and thyroid homeostasis.[41]

The hypothalamic-pituitary-adrenal (HPA) axis also may influence the manifestation of depression, with a relative hyperactivity of this system commonly reported in depressed individuals. Pituitary and adrenal glands are enlarged in depressed patients, the size of the hippocampus is reduced, and hypothalamic functions may be highly abnormal as well.[27] Concentrations of corticotropin-releasing factor (CRF) are of-

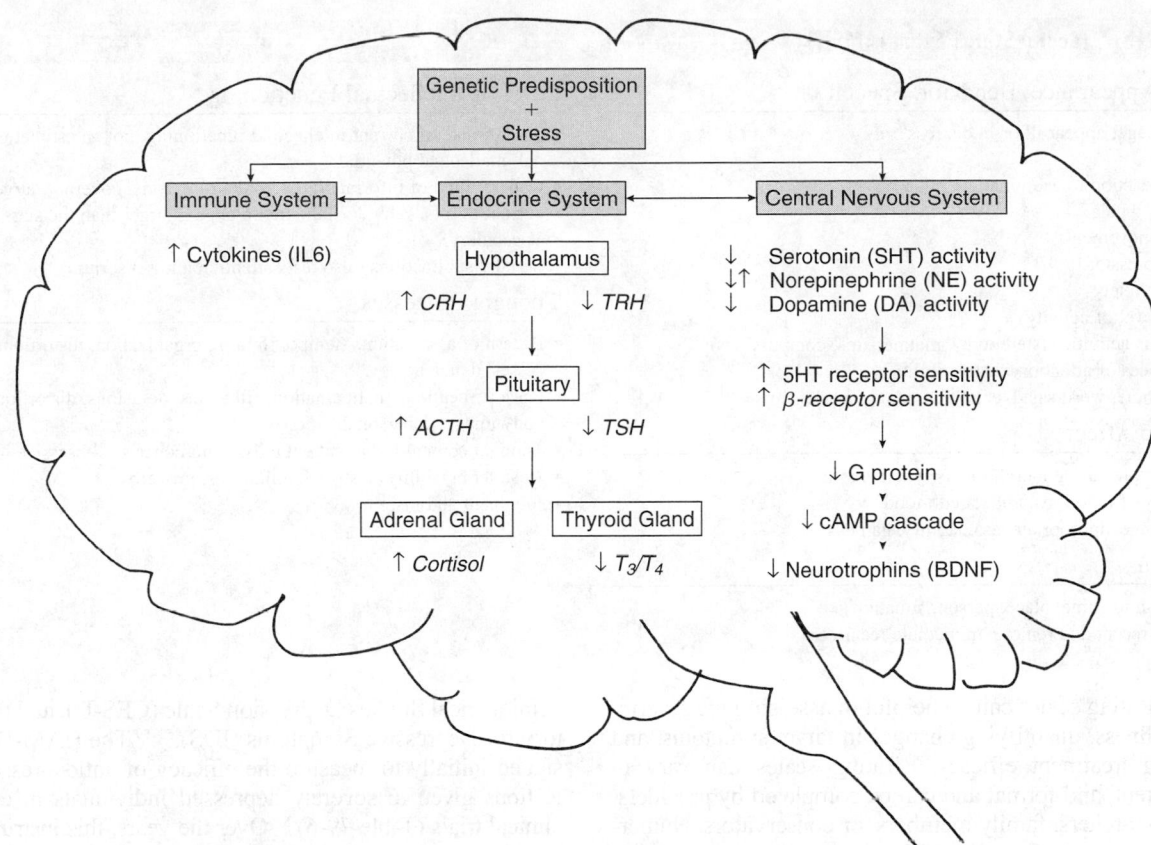

FIGURE 79-1 Influence of genetic and environmental factors upon the immune system, endocrine system, and central nervous system. © J.L. Corbitt, P.R. Finley 2003. CRH, corticotropin-releasing hormone (also known as CRF or corticotropin-releasing factor); TRH, thyrotrophin-releasing hormone; ACTH, adrenocorticotropic hormone; TSH, thyroid-stimulating hormone; T4/T3, thyroxine/triiodothyronine

ten elevated during depressive episodes and decline with the administration of antidepressant medications or electroconvulsive therapy (ECT).[42] Exogenous administration of CRF has elicited classic symptoms of depression in laboratory animals (including decreased appetite, anxiety, insomnia, and decreased libido).[43] In human subjects, medications that block postsynaptic corticosteroid receptors have also displayed antidepressant properties, as demonstrated with ketoconazole and mifepristone.[44,45] Because serotonin exerts a strong influence on the HPA axis (and vice versa), this may explain the efficacy of serotonin selective antidepressants. Activation of the postsynaptic serotonin receptors (5-HT$_2$) along the hypothalamic paraventricular nucleus can stimulate CRH-secreting neurons. Corticosteroids can modulate serotonin synthesis, metabolism, and reuptake as well.[27]

Imaging Studies

Imaging studies (including computed tomography [CT], magnetic resonance imaging [MRI], positron emission tomography [PET], and single-photon emission computed tomography [SPECT]) suggest that patients with depression have regional brain dysfunction, most often affecting the limbic structures and prefrontal cortex. Alterations in cerebral blood flow and/or metabolism in the frontal-temporal cortex and caudate nucleus are associated with common depressive symptoms such as dysphoria, anhedonia, hopelessness, and

flat affect.[46] Increased firing of the amygdala in the left hemisphere has been linked in PET studies with the future development of depression.[47] As subtypes of depression have been linked to different regional dysfunctions, a network hypothesis has begun to emerge which may lead to improvements in depression diagnosis and targeted treatments.[48]

Patient Assessment Tools

Pharmaceutical care in the depressed patient requires specialized knowledge of the illness and treatments, as well as refined interviewing skills. To obtain specific information about the target symptoms of depression and to assess the therapeutic impact of psychotropic medications, effective and productive interpersonal communication is vital. The structured mental status examination is an established systematic way of assessing a patient's mental health[49] (Table 79-5). Many functional domains are assessed in a mental status examination. Through this structured interview, the clinician has an observational basis for evaluating a patient's appearance, behavior, speech, mood, affect (i.e., outer manifestation of inner emotional states), sensorium, memory, and intellectual function. For a more detailed discussion of the mental status examination and specific psychiatric interviewing techniques, readers should refer to other sources.[50,51]

Behavioral rating scales have been used for many years in drug efficacy studies and are being used more often in the clin-

Table 79-5   Mental Status Exam (AMSIT)

General Appearance, Behavior, Speech

- Apparent age; appear ill or in distress?
- Dress
- General reaction to examination, negativism
- Posture and gait
- Unusual movements
- Facial expression
- Signs of anxiety
- General level of activity
- Repetitious activities (stereotypy, mannerisms, compulsions)
- Disturbances of attention: distractibility
- Speech: mute, word salad, echolalia, klang, neologisms

Mood and Affect

- Quality of prevailing mood; intensity and depth
- Constancy of mood, patient-stated mood
- Affect: range, appropriateness, lability, flatness

Sensorium

- Orientation for time, place, person, situation
- Memory: recent and remote, immediate recall

Level of Intellectual Functioning

- An estimate of current intellectual functioning, not an estimate of original intellectual potential
- General fund of information: presidents, oceans, governor, large cities, current events. Why does the moon appear larger than the stars?
- Vocabulary
- Serial 7 subtractions (also tests attention and sensorium)

Thought Processes

- Pattern of associations (tempo, rhythm, organization, distortions, excesses, deficiencies)
- False perceptions (hallucinations, illusions, delusions, distortions of body image, depersonalization)
- Thought content (what patient tells, main concerns, obsessive ideation)
- Abstracting ability (tests by similarities, proverbs)
- Judgment and insight

---

ical arena. Rating scales can be helpful in assessing the severity of mental illness, quantifying changes in target symptoms, and determining treatment efficacy.[52] Rating scales can vary in length, content, and format and can be completed by providers, patients, researchers, family members, or conservators. Numerous depression scales have been developed over the years, including the Hamilton Rating Scale for Depression (HAM-D), the Beck Depression Inventory (BDI), the Zung Depression Scale, the Hopkins Symptom checklist, the Montgomery Asberg Depression Rating Scale (MADRS), the Center for Epi-

demiological Studies Depression Scale (CES-D), and the Inventory for Depressive Symptoms (IDS).[53–59] The HAM-D was designed initially to measure the efficacy of antidepressant medications given to severely depressed individuals in controlled clinical trials (Table 79-6).[53] Over the years, this instrument has emerged as the gold standard of depression rating scales, although many clinicians are unaware of its limitations. For instance, the HAM-D was never designed for routine use in the general ambulatory care patient population and fails to address a number of target symptoms required for a DSM-IV-TR diag-

---

Table 79-6   Hamilton Depression Scale

For Each Item Check the Box Next to the Response that Best Characterizes the Patient

1. Depressed Mood (sadness, hopeless, helpless, worthless)	0 ❑	Absent
	1 ❑	These feeling states indicated only on questioning
	2 ❑	These feeling states spontaneously reported verbally
	3 ❑	Communicates feeling states non-verbally, i.e., through facial expression, posture, voice and tendency to weep
	4 ❑	Patient reports VIRTUALLY ONLY these feeling states in his or her spontaneous verbal and nonverbal communication
2. Feelings of Guilt	0 ❑	Absent
	1 ❑	Self-reproach, feels he has let people down
	2 ❑	Ideas of guilt or rumination over past errors or sinful deeds
	3 ❑	Presents illness as a punishment; delusions of guilt
	4 ❑	Hears accusatory or denunciatory voices and/or experiences threatening visual hallucinations
3. Suicide	0 ❑	Absent
	1 ❑	Feels life is not worth living
	2 ❑	Wishes he or she were dead or any thoughts of possible death to self
	3 ❑	Suicide ideas or gesture
	4 ❑	Attempts at suicide (only serious attempt rates 4)
4. Insomnia Early	0 ❑	No difficulty
	1 ❑	Complains of occasional difficulty falling asleep, i.e., more than one-half hour
	2 ❑	Complains of nightly difficulty falling asleep
5. Insomnia Middle	0 ❑	No difficulty
	1 ❑	Patient complains of being restless and disturbed during the night
	2 ❑	Waking during the night—any getting out of bed rates 2 *(except for purposes of voiding)*
6. Insomnia Late	0 ❑	No difficulty
	1 ❑	Waking in early hours of the morning but goes back to sleep
	2 ❑	Unable to fall asleep again if gets out of bed

Table 79-6 Hamilton Depression Scale—cont'd

7. Work and Activities	0 ☐	No difficulty
	1 ☐	Thoughts and feeling of incapacity, fatigue, or weakness related to activities; work or hobbies
	2 ☐	Loss of interest in activity; hobbies or work—either directly reported by patients, or indirect in listlessness, indecision and vacillation (feels he has to push self to work or activities)
	3 ☐	Decrease in actual time spent in activities or decrease in productivity, in hospital, rate 3 if patient does not spend at least 3 hours a day in activities or decrease in productivity, in hospital, rate 3 if patient does not spend at least 3 hours a day in activities (hospital job or hobbies), exclusive of ward chores
	4 ☐	Stopped working because of present illness, in hospital, rate 4 if patient engages in no activities except ward chores, or if patients fails to perform ward chores unassisted
8. Retardation (slowness of thought and speech; impaired ability to concentrate; decreased motor activity)	0 ☐	Normal speech and thought
	1 ☐	Slight retardation at interview
	2 ☐	Obvious retardation at interview
	3 ☐	Interview difficult
	4 ☐	Complete stupor
9. Agitation	0 ☐	None
	1 ☐	"Playing with" hands, hair, etc.
	2 ☐	Hand-wringing, nail-biting, hair-pulling, biting of lips
10. Anxiety Psychic	0 ☐	No difficulty
	1 ☐	Slight retardation at interview
	2 ☐	Obvious retardation at interview
	3 ☐	Interview difficult
	4 ☐	Complete stupor

11. Anxiety Somatic	0 ☐	Absent	Physiologic concomitants of anxiety, such as:
	1 ☐	Mild	Gastrointestinal (GI)—dry mouth, wind, indigestion, diarrhea, cramps, belching
	2 ☐	Moderate	Cardiovascular—palpitations, headaches
	3 ☐	Severe	Respiratory—hyperventilation, sighing
	4 ☐	Incapacitating	Sweating

12. Somatic Symptoms Gastrointestinal	0 ☐	None
	1 ☐	Loss of appetite but eating without staff encouragement; heavy feelings in abdomen
	2 ☐	Difficulty eating without staff urging; requests or requires laxatives or medication for bowels or medication for GI symptoms
13. Somatic Symptoms General	0 ☐	None
	1 ☐	Heaviness in limbs, back, or head, backaches, headache, muscle aches; loss of energy or fatigability
	2 ☐	Any clear-cut symptoms rates 2

14. Genital Symptoms	0 ☐	Absent	Symptoms such as: Loss of libido
	1 ☐	Mild	Menstrual disturbances
	2 ☐	Severe	

15. Hypochondriasis	0 ☐	Not present
	1 ☐	Self-absorption (bodily)
	2 ☐	Preoccupation with health
	3 ☐	Frequent complaints, requests for help, etc.
	4 ☐	Hypochondriacal delusions
16. Loss of Weight (answer only A or B)		A. When rating by history:
	0 ☐	No weight loss
	1 ☐	Probably weight loss associated with present illness
	2 ☐	Definite (according to patient) weight loss
		B. On weekly ratings by ward psychiatrist, when actual weight changes are measured:
	0 ☐	Less than 1 lb weight loss in week
	1 ☐	Greater than 1 lb weight loss in week
	2 ☐	Greater than 2 lb weight loss in week
17. Insight	0 ☐	Acknowledges being depressed and ill
	1 ☐	Acknowledges illness but attributes cause to bad food, climate, overwork, virus, need for rest, etc.
	2 ☐	Denies being ill at all

Investigator's Signature:

From Hamilton M. Development of a rating scale of primary depressive illness. Br J Soc Clin Psychol 1967;2:278.

nosis of major depression (e.g., low energy, poor concentration, reverse neurovegetative symptoms). The IDS has emerged recently as a more valuable instrument in the hands of primary care providers and can be completed within 10 to 15 minutes. It has been validated and used extensively in clinical and research settings and is available in a clinician-rated or patient-rated format. The BDI and Zung rating scales are other brief, patient-rated scales that are now routinely distributed to patients in waiting rooms and doctor's offices. Abbreviated versions of the IDS and CES-D have been recently developed, and this form of the CES-D, in particular, has served as a useful screening instrument among elderly populations[60] (Tables 79-7 and 79-8).

Table 79-7 Brief Inventory for Depressive Symptoms—Self-Report

NAME: _____   TODAY'S DATE:_____

Please circle the one response to each item that best describes you for the past seven days.

1. Feeling Sad:
   0   I do not feel sad.
   1   I feel sad less than half the time.
   2   I feel sad more than half the time.
   3   I feel sad nearly all of the time.
2. Feeling Irritable:
   0   I do not feel irritable.
   1   I feel irritable less than half the time.
   2   I feel irritable more than half the time.
   3   I feel extremely irritable nearly all of the time.
3. Feeling Anxious or Tense:
   0   I do not feel anxious or tense.
   1   I feel anxious (tense) less than half the time.
   2   I feel anxious (tense) more than half the time.
   3   I feel extremely anxious (tense) nearly all of the time.
4. The Quality of Your Mood:
   0   The mood (internal feelings) that I experience is very much a normal mood.
   1   My mood is sad, but this sadness is pretty much like the sad mood I would feel if someone close to me died or left.
   2   My mood is sad, but this sadness has a rather different quality to it than the sadness I would feel if someone close to me died or left.
   3   My mood is sad, but this sadness is different from the type of sadness associated with grief or loss.
5. Sleep During the Night:
   0   I do not wake up at night.
   1   I have a restless, light sleep with a few brief awakenings each night.
   2   I wake up at least once a night, but I go back to sleep easily.
   3   I awaken more than once a night and stay awake for 20 minutes or more, more than half the time.

Please complete *either* 6 *or* 7 (not both)
6. Decreased Appetite:
   0   There is no change in my usual appetite.
   1   I eat somewhat less often or lesser amounts of food than usual.
   2   I eat much less than usual and only with personal effort.
   3   I rarely eat within a 24-hour period, and only with extreme personal effort or when others persuade me to eat.
7. Increased Appetite:
   0   There is no change from my usual appetite.
   1   I feel a need to eat more frequently than usual.
   2   I regularly eat more often and/or greater amounts of food than usual.
   3   I feel driven to overeat both at mealtime and between meals.
8. Aches and Pains:
   0   I don't have any feeling of heaviness in my arms or legs and don't have any aches or pains.
   1   Sometimes I get headaches or pains in my stomach, back or joints but these pains are only sometime present and they don't stop me from doing what I need to do.
   2   I have these sorts of pains most of the time.
   3   These pains are so bad they force me to stop what I am doing.

9. Concentration/Decision Making:
   0   There is no change in my usual capacity to concentrate or make decisions.
   1   I occasionally feel indecisive or find that my attention wanders.
   2   Most of the time, I struggle to focus my attention or to make decisions.
   3   I cannot concentrate well enough to read and cannot make even minor decisions.
10. Energy Level:
   0   There is no change in my usual level of energy.
   1   I get tired more easily than usual.
   2   I have to make a big effort to start or finish my usual daily activities (for example, shopping, homework, cooking, or going to work).
   3   I really cannot carry out most of my usual daily activities because I just don't have the energy.
11. General Interest:
   0   There is no change from usual in how interested I am in other people or activities.
   1   I notice that I am less interested in people or activities.
   2   I find I have interest in only one or two of my formerly pursued activities.
   3   I have virtually no interest in formerly pursued activities.
12. Capacity for Pleasure or Enjoyment (excluding sex):
   0   I enjoy pleasurable activities just as much as usual.
   1   I do not feel my usual sense of enjoyment from pleasurable activities.
   2   I rarely get a feeling of pleasure from any activity.
   3   I am unable to get any pleasure or enjoyment from anything.
13. View of Myself:
   0   I see myself as equally worthwhile and deserving as other people.
   1   I am more self-blaming than usual.
   2   I largely believe that I cause problems for others.
   3   I think almost constantly about major and minor defects in myself.
14. View of My Future:
   0   I have an optimistic view of my future.
   1   I am occasionally pessimistic about my future, but for the most part I believe things will get better.
   2   I'm pretty certain that my immediate future (1–2 months) does not hold much promise of good things for me.
   3   I see no hope of anything good happening to me anytime in the future.
15. Thoughts of Death or Suicide:
   0   I do not think of suicide or death.
   1   I feel that life is empty or wonder if it's worth living.
   2   I think of suicide or death several times a week for several minutes.
   3   I think of suicide or death several times a day in some detail, or I have made specific plans for suicide or have actually tried to take my life.

Please review this test and write in this space _____ the numbers of the 3 items that were the most difficult to understand.

Which 3 items (questions) were the easiest to understand? _____

Thank you

Range 0–42   Score: _____

© 1995, A. John Rush, MD.

Table 79-8   Comparison of Selected Depression Rating Scales

Instrument	Minimal	Mild	Moderate	Severe
Hamilton (HAM-D)—17 item Clinician-rated	<7	7–17	18–24	>24
Beck Depression Inventory (BDI) Clinician-rated	<10	10–16	17–29	30–63
Beck Depression Inventory (BDI) Patient-rated	<10	10–15	16–23	>23
Inventory for Depressive Symptoms (IDS) Clinician-rated	<14	14–22	23–30	>30
Inventory for Depressive Symptoms (IDS) Patient-rated	<16	16–24	25–32	>32
Brief Inventory for Depressive Symptoms (BIDS) Patient-rated	<14	14–22	23–30	31–38

Although depression symptoms are clearly associated with many biochemical and endocrine anomalies, there are currently no useful laboratory tests that are routinely administered to aid the clinician in establishing a diagnosis of depression. For many years, the dexamethasone suppression test (DST) was used to confirm the diagnosis of depression, but now it is rarely indicated. The rationale for this test lies in the apparent inability of depressed patients to suppress cortisol concentrations after dexamethasone administration. The standard protocol consists of administering a 1-mg dose of dexamethasone at 11 PM and obtaining blood samples at 4 PM and 11 PM on the following day for the purpose of measuring subsequent cortisol concentrations. The results are considered abnormal (positive) if either of the two samples are >5 µg/dL. Studies have demonstrated that the DST is often more abnormal in older depressed subjects, and a meta-analysis concluded that a positive baseline DST was predictive of worse treatment outcomes.[61] Unfortunately, many medical conditions and medications may augment the cortisol response, resulting in a greater likelihood of false-positive findings. Furthermore, as many as half of depressed subjects may have a normal DST (i.e., manifesting in false negative findings). The APA Task Force on Laboratory Tests in Psychiatry has outlined some of the potential indications for the DST, and it may, in fact, be useful in certain clinical situations to confirm a diagnosis of depression.[62] However, in general, the DST is not recommended as a routine screening instrument at present.

Nondrug Therapies for Depression

The successful treatment of depression provides a most formidable challenge to modern medicine. In addition to the emotional turmoil and social disability that a depressed individual endures, the illness can have an affect on other disease states, slow the recovery process, or even promote complications.[63] Furthermore, the likelihood of future depressive episodes increases with each recurrence, dampening the patient's prognosis over time.

Although pharmacologic intervention has become the primary treatment modality for relieving depressive symptoms, the efficacy and suitability of other therapeutic options should not be overlooked. Under the influence of managed medical care, the role of medications has been overemphasized, and many patients may, in fact, fully recover from depression with less invasive or expensive means. A wide variety of other therapeutic interventions exist, including psychotherapy, ECT, light therapy, sleep deprivation, exercise, transcranial magnetic stimulation, vagus nerve stimulation and herbal remedies.

Psychotherapy

For the treatment of mild to moderate depression, psychotherapy has proved to be comparable to pharmacologic intervention and may actually be preferred by some patients.[64] For the acute treatment of severe depression, antidepressants appear to be more effective than psychotherapy with a more rapid onset of therapeutic action.[65] The beneficial effects of psychotherapy, on the other hand, may persist longer than medication-related benefits after the interventions have been formally discontinued. In addition, psychotherapy may be particularly beneficial for preventing relapse among patients who previously demonstrated a therapeutic response to antidepressants.[66] Overall, the combination of treatments is superior to either intervention alone, though the routine use of both modalities is often not feasible in today's health care environment.[65]

Several forms of psychotherapy are available (e.g., cognitive-behavioral therapy, psychodynamic therapy, interpersonal therapy), the descriptions of which are beyond the scope of this book. However, clinicians in the field are strongly encouraged to develop familiarity with general supportive counseling techniques that can serve to facilitate a therapeutic alliance and promote the recovery process.[67]

Electroconvulsive Therapy

ECT is a safe, rapid-acting, and highly effective therapeutic intervention that continues to suffer, ostensibly, from a poor public image. ECT was enormously popular during the 1940s and 1950s and was used without discretion to treat a wide variety of psychiatric conditions. This practice waned thereafter with the advent of effective psychotropic medications and with the accumulation of case reports describing fractures and severe cognitive impairment in treated patients. Since the

1950s, the ECT procedure has undergone considerable transformation and refinement.[68] Adjunctive medications are now routinely administered to prevent adverse effects and reduce morbidity (e.g., a short-acting barbiturate for general anesthesia, an anticholinergic agent to prevent bradycardia and dry excessive airway secretions, and succinylcholine to prevent fractures from tonic-clonic contractions). The electric stimulus itself is no longer applied in one steady current but now consists of a series of brief pulses that have been shown to decrease the severity of postictal headaches and memory impairment.

Fundamentally, ECT features the induction of generalized seizures through an electric current delivered by bilateral or unilateral electrode placement. Certain medications may raise seizure thresholds (benzodiazepines) or promote cognitive impairment (lithium) and should be discontinued before the procedure.[69] Adverse effects are generally minimal and consist mainly of transient anterograde amnesia (i.e., difficulty remembering events around the time of the procedure), retrograde amnesia, confusion, headaches, and muscle aches. Cardiovascular effects (e.g., ventricular arrhythmias, myocardial infarction [MI]) are the most ominous sequelae, but these events are actually quite rare.[70]

Many years of clinical experience have enabled clinicians to identify patient populations most likely to benefit from this intervention. Today, ECT is recommended for patients with treatment-resistant depression, severe vegetative depression, psychotic depression, and depression in pregnancy. Overall response rates are rather impressive, ranging from 70% to 90%, and ECT has the distinct advantage of inducing a therapeutic response within the first week or two of treatments.[71] The recommended frequency of ECT treatments is variable. Most institutions have used three sessions weekly to induce a therapeutic response acutely, although evidence suggests that twice-weekly sessions are better tolerated and more cost-effective.[72] The frequency of treatments thereafter (i.e., maintenance therapy) is unknown. Preliminary evidence suggests that a subsequent course of pharmacotherapy may prevent relapse while others have opined for continued ECT treatments of decreased frequency.[73,74]

Other Treatments

Other somatic interventions have also been used successfully to treat depression. Light therapy or phototherapy is particularly effective for relieving the irritability and malaise associated with seasonal affective disorder, a milder form of depression that has been attributed to decreases in natural sunlight found with seasonal variation.[75] Phototherapy is administered in the form of a light box delivering 1,500 to 10,000 lux over a period of 1 to 2 hours daily. It is generally very well tolerated, though case reports of mania have surfaced as with any other somatic intervention used for depression. Sleep deprivation may be an effective adjuvant to antidepressants and has also been studied as a remedy for premenstrual dysphoric disorder. The goal of sleep deprivation is to gradually advance sleep cycles by altering wake schedules, ultimately minimizing the duration of rapid eye movement (REM) sleep.[76]

Increased physical activity and sustained cardiovascular exertion increase serotonin concentrations, which also may help relieve depressive symptoms and improve self-esteem in all age groups. Although investigations examining the effectiveness of exercise for depression have met with mixed results, exercise can certainly improve cardiovascular fitness, regulate appetite and sleep patterns, and indicate a return to euthymic status.[77] Transcranial magnetic stimulation (TMS) is a noninvasive procedure involving the application of an electrical stimulus across the scalp, which ultimately generates an electrical field in the cerebral cortex.[78] Unlike ECT, TMS does not generate an actual seizure and is very well tolerated. Evidence of efficacy has been demonstrated in several investigations utilizing repetitive high frequency techniques, and imaging studies have shown functional improvements consistent with antidepressant properties. Vagus nerve stimulation is slightly more invasive, involving the placement of a subcutaneous electrical device that stimulates the left vagus nerve. Although preliminary investigations have been promising, evidence of efficacy is limited at the present time.[79] Certain herbal remedies may be effective as well and are discussed in Chapter 3, Herbs and Nutritional Supplements.

MAJOR DEPRESSIVE DISORDER
Diagnosis

1. A.R. is a 25-year-old woman who presents to the student health clinic for a routine physical examination. During her visit, A.R. states, "I've been feeling pretty down lately and just want to give up." Her physical examination is unremarkable, and all laboratory tests (complete blood count [CBC] with differential, chemistry panel, and thyroid function tests) are within normal limits. A β-human chorionic gonadotropin test is negative. Her medical history is noncontributory, she takes no medications other than an oral contraceptive, and she denies drinking alcohol or using other recreational substances.

When asked, A.R. states that she has had increasing periods of depressed mood over the past few months and often finds herself crying in the morning for no particular reason. She reports that she has no interest in her old hobbies (playing the piano, mountain biking, gardening). She is engaged to be married in 3 months but feels that she does not deserve to be a wife. Over the last 2 months, her appetite has decreased and she has lost 15 pounds. She feels overwhelmed about all of the plans that she needs to make for her wedding ('I don't even deserve a wedding this nice') and has difficulty sleeping, often waking in the middle of the night and being unable to fall back asleep. She has no energy during the day and finds it difficult to concentrate or make decisions. This is a major concern because she is a graduate student at the local university.

The mental status examination reveals an appropriately dressed female who appears sad but who is alert, coherent, and logical. Her affect is constricted, apprehensive, and sad. Mood is depressed, and she admits having suicidal ideation but no specific plans. She is oriented to person, place, and time but shows some recent memory deficits. Her intelligence is estimated to be above average. Concentration and abstractions (e.g., "don't cry over spilled milk" and "a rolling stone gathers no moss") are satisfactory. She denies hearing voices or other hallucinations. She has good insight and judgment into her illness. What signs and symptoms does A.R. have that support the diagnosis of major depressive disorder?

The target symptoms of depression are listed in Table 79-9 and can be recalled by the pneumonic *D-SIG-E-CAPS* or *DIG-SPACES*. Based on A.R.'s history, she describes a dysphoric or depressed mood as well as anhedonia (lack of interest in hobbies or pleasurable activities). In addition, she demonstrates frequent episodes of crying, decreased appetite (with an unintentional 15-pound weight loss), poor concentration, low energy, suicidal ideation, worthlessness, and inappropriate guilt ("I don't deserve to be a wife"). Her mental status examination is consistent with these target symptoms, revealing a constricted, sad affect (physical manifestation of inner emotional states) and frequent crying episodes during the interview.

Based on the DSM-IV-TR criteria, A.R. has major depressive disorder. Over the past 2 weeks, she has consistently exhibited at least five of the associated symptoms, one of which is depression or anhedonia. It does not appear that her symptoms are the result of any medical condition, medication, thought disorder, or uncomplicated bereavement. The anhedonia and vegetative symptoms (e.g., midnocturnal insomnia, decreased appetite, weight loss) are consistent with the depressive subtype of melancholia.

Suicide Assessment

2. What is the risk of A.R. hurting herself? How should suicidal ideation be assessed?

Patients with major depression should always be assessed for the presence of suicidal thoughts (e.g., "Are you thinking about hurting yourself?" "Do you ever feel like giving up?"). Suicide is viewed by the depressed patient as a remedy to insurmountable problems when all other options appear hopeless. Comments made by the patients alluding to suicide (e.g., "Life is not worth living anymore" or "I am leaving and may never see you again") should be taken seriously. Misunderstandings about suicidal ideation abound in the general public. Common myths include the ideas that people are more likely to commit suicide if asked about it, that people who attempt suicide are just looking for attention, or that suicide is usually attempted after a sudden traumatic event.

Several factors may place a person at greater risk for a suicide attempt. A detailed plan, for instance, suggests a serious intent and a higher risk for successful suicide. The clinician should be concerned if a change takes place in A.R.'s personality (e.g., giving away possessions, making a will, purchasing a firearm, asking about the lethal dose of medications). Other risks for suicide include living alone, having a physical illness, being unemployed, being 15 to 24 years of age or older than 65 years of age, having a history of alcohol/drug abuse, or having a family history of suicide.[80] Gender plays a

role as well, and women are much more likely to attempt suicide, but men are more often successful.

The management of patients who are potentially suicidal depends on the attendant risk, incorporating many of the factors just cited. For patients who are actively suicidal, hospitalization is often necessary and may even be facilitated against the patient's will in high-risk settings. Other lifesaving interventions include establishing close contact with the patient's family and health care provider, convincing the patient to contract for his or her safety, and avoiding antidepressants with a narrow therapeutic index (e.g., tricyclic antidepressants) or limiting the dispensed quantity to ≤10 days. Depressed patients surface in any health care environment, so all clinicians should have an emergency hotline or crisis telephone number at their disposal.

A.R. is at some risk for suicide, although she does not have a detailed plan at present. She should be monitored closely during the first few weeks of therapy by friends or family members. If her suicidal ideation becomes severe, A.R. should be admitted to a facility for her own safety. Unfortunately, it is not always possible to predict whether A.R. (or any depressed patient) will attempt to kill herself. Even with the most conservative precautions, a small percentage of patients succeed in their suicide attempts.

DRUG MANAGEMENT
Drug Selection: General Considerations

3. A.R. is diagnosed as follows: Axis I—Major Depressive disorder, single episode, with melancholic features; Axis II—none; Axis III—none. What drug options are available for A.R.'s depressive symptoms? What considerations should be made when selecting antidepressant therapy?

At present, 22 medications have received U.S. Food and Drug Administration (FDA) approval in the United States for the treatment of depression. They can be grouped together into four categories.

1. SSRIs
2. Tricyclic antidepressants (TCAs)
3. Monoamine oxidase (MAO) inhibitors
4. Miscellaneous (e.g., nefazodone, venlafaxine, bupropion, mirtazapine)

All the available antidepressants are equally effective in the general depressed patient population, with approximately 60% to 70% of patients responding to a therapeutic trial of a specific agent in controlled clinic studies (therapeutic response traditionally defined as a ≥50% drop in depression rating scores), and 30% to 40% achieving remission.[81] Similarly, all

Table 79-9	Depressive Disorder Target Symptom Mnemonic		
D	**SIG**	**E**	**CAPS**
Depressed mood	Sleep (insomnia or hypersomnia)	Energy loss	Concentration (loss)
	Interest (loss of, including libido)		Appetite (loss or gain)
	Guilt		Psychomotor (agitation or retardation)
			Suicide (ideation)

From Reference 77.

Table 79-10 Factors to Consider in Selecting an Antidepressant

- History of prior response (personal or family member)
- Safety in overdose
- Adverse effect profiles
- Patient age
- Concurrent medical/psychiatric conditions
- Concurrent medications
- Convenience (e.g., minimal titration, once-daily dosing)
- Cost
- Patient preference

the antidepressants possess the same delayed onset of therapeutic effects.

Because the response rates for all currently available antidepressants are comparable, other important considerations should influence the decision-making process (Tables 79-10 through 79-13). The first factor to consider is the patient's history of previous response. If this history is unavailable (or the patient has never received an antidepressant before), the clinician should inquire about the family history. If a first-degree relative had a successful course of antidepressant treatment with minimal adverse effects, that specific medication (or another from the same antidepressant class) would be a prudent choice for initiating therapy.

The potential impact of an antidepressant on concurrent medical conditions or disease states is often considered next. For example, certain antidepressants (e.g., TCA, mirtazapine) are associated with significant weight gain and would not be desirable choices for obese patients. Similarly, bupropion should be avoided in patients with a history of seizures, and venlafaxine may not be ideal for patients with hypertension. Many clinicians select an antidepressant by matching the patient's presenting symptoms to the side-effect profile of anti-

depressant medications. If a patient is particularly anxious, for instance, or unable to sleep, a more sedating antidepressant may be desirable (e.g., mirtazapine, nefazodone) and could relieve these presenting symptoms almost immediately. Conversely, some clinicians argue that if an antidepressant is clinically effective, it will relieve all target symptoms eventually, regardless of the adverse-effect profile. Nonetheless, tailoring antidepressant medications to a patient's presentation is a common practice that may minimize the initial side-effect burden and promote adherence.

Other important patient-specific factors to consider in the selection of an agent include safety in overdose, potential for drug interactions, ease of administration (once daily versus divided doses), necessity of titration practices, cost (to the patient/institution), and patient preference.

Because A.R. is a student, the clinician may wish to select an antidepressant that has minimal effects on alertness or cognitive function, such as an SSRI or a secondary amine from the TCA class (e.g., desipramine, nortriptyline). Of these two options, an SSRI may be preferred for A.R. because she is expressing suicidal thoughts and the TCAs are particularly dangerous in these situations.

Response Rates of Target Symptoms

4. A.R. is given a prescription for sertraline 50 mg QD PO and is asked to return to the clinic in 4 weeks for follow-up. How soon should A.R.'s target symptoms begin to resolve?

A similar delayed pattern of therapeutic response has been observed with all antidepressant medications. Traditionally, patients have been informed that approximately 4 to 6 weeks must elapse before they will experience any therapeutic benefit from medication. However, researchers in this field have been insisting in recent years that this conservative estimate is a result of standard drug efficacy studies ill-suited to answer

Table 79-11 Pharmacology of Antidepressant Medications

Medication	Serotonin	Norepinephrine	Dopamine	Bioavailability (Oral)	Protein Binding	Half-Life (in hours) (Active Metabolite)
SSRI						
Fluoxetine (Prozac)	++++	0/+	0	80%	95%	24–72 (146)
Sertraline (Zoloft)	++++	0/+	+	>44%	95%	26 (66)
Paroxetine (Paxil)	++++	+	0	64%	99%	24
Citalopram (Celexa)	++++	0	0	80%	<80%	33
Escitalopram (Lexapro)	++++	0	0	80%	56%	27–32
Tricyclics						
Desipramine (Norpramin)	+	++++	0/+	51%	90%	12–28
Nortriptyline (Pamelor)	++	+++	0	46–56%	92%	18–56
Amitriptyline (Elavil)	++++	++++	0	37–49%	95%	9–46 (18–56)
Imipramine (Tofranil)	+++	++	0/+	19–35%	95%	6–28 (12–28)
Doxepin (Sinequan)	+++	+	0	17–37%	68-85%	11–23
Others						
Bupropion (Wellbutrin)	0/+	+	+	>90%	85%	10–21
Venlafaxine (Effexor)	++++	+++	0	92%	25–29%	4 (10)
Nefazodone (Serzone)	+++	0	0	20%	99%	4–5 (4–18)
Mirtazapine (Remeron)	+++	++++	0	50%	85%	20–40

0, negligible; +, very low; ++, low; +++, moderate, ++++, high.

Table 79-12 **Adverse Effects of Antidepressant Medications**

Medication	Sedation	Agitation/Insomnia	Anticholinergic Effects	Orthostasis	GI Effects (Nausea/Diarrhea)	Sexual Dysfunction	Weight Gain
SSRI							
Fluoxetine (Prozac)	+	++++	0/+	0/+	++++	++++	+
Sertraline (Zoloft)	+	+++	0/+	0	+++	+++	+
Paroxetine (Paxil)	++	++	+	0	+++	++++	++
Citalopram (Celexa)	++	++	0/+	0	+++	++	+
Escitalopram (Lexapro)	+	++	0/+	0	+++	++	+
Tricyclics							
Desipramine (Norpramin)	++	+	++	+++	0/+	+	++
Nortriptyline (Pamelor)	++	+	++	++	0/+	+	++
Amitriptyline (Elavil)	++++	0/+	++++	++++	0/+	++	+++
Imipramine (Tofranil)	+++	0/+	+++	++++	0/+	++	++
Doxepin (Sinequan)	++++	0/+	++++	++++	0/+	++	++
Others							
Bupropion (Wellbutrin)	0	+++	+	0	+	0/+	0
Venlafaxine (Effexor)	++	++	+	0	+++	+++	+
Nefazodone (Serzone)	+++	+	+	++	++	0/+	0/+
Mirtazapine (Remeron)	++++	0	++	0/+	+	0/+	+++

0, negligible; +, very low; ++, low; +++, moderate; ++++, high.

Table 79-13 **Dosage Ranges and Costs of Antidepressant Medications**

Medication	Brand Name	Starting Dose (mg/day)	Maximum Dosage (mg/day)	Usual Dosage (mg/day)	Relative Cost[a]
SSRI					
Fluoxetine	Prozac	10	80	10–20 mg QD	$$$$[b]
Sertraline	Zoloft	25	200	50 mg QD	$$$$[c]
Paroxetine	Paxil	10	50	10–20 mg QD	$$$$[b,c]
Citalopram	Celexa	10	60	20 mg QD	$$$[c]
Escitalopram	Lexapro	5	20	10 mg QD	$$$[c]
TCA					
Desipramine	Norpramin	25	300	200 mg HS	$
Nortriptyline	Pamelor	10–25	150	100 mg HS	$
Others					
Nefazodone	Serzone	50	600	150 mg BID	$$$$
Bupropion	Wellbutrin	200	450	100 mg TID	$$$
Bupropion	Wellbutrin SR	150	400	150 mg BID	$$$$
Bupropion	Wellbutrin XL	150	450	300 QD	$$$$
Mirtazapine	Remeron	15	45	15–30 mg HS	$$$$[b,c]
Venlafaxine	Effexor	25	375	50 mg BID	$$$$
Venlafaxine	Effexor XR	37.5	225	150 mg QD	$$$$

[a]Based on average wholesale prices for usual therapeutic doses (April 2000).
[b]Also available in generic formulation at much lower cost.
[c]AWP reduced by approximately 50% if half-tablets prescribed (e.g., $^1/_2$ tab 100 mg Zoloft).
$, $0–25/month; $$, $25–50/month; $$$, $50–70/month; $$$$, >$70/month.

this question.[82] Often, for instance, patients begin to show signs of clinical response during the first 1 or 2 weeks of active treatment, but because the difference from placebo is assessed every 7 days and will not ordinarily achieve statistical significance until the third or fourth week, these patterns are misinterpreted to suggest that it may take a month or more for patients to improve. Some experts have contended, in fact, that trials uniquely designed to investigate the onset of therapeutic effect will conclusively show that patients exhibit initial improvement during the first 2 weeks of treatment.[83]

The pattern of patient response also can be generalized, with neurovegetative symptoms (e.g., altered sleep or appetite, decreased energy, excessive worrying and irritability) often the first to subside. The cognitive symptoms are slower to respond, and 3 to 4 weeks or more may elapse before improvements are evident. These symptoms include excessive guilt or pessimism, poor concentration, hopelessness or sadness, and decreased libido.

A.R. should be counseled concerning this anticipated delay in therapeutic response and advised that optimal improvement may take ≥4 weeks. If she is not aware of this time frame, she may stop the medication prematurely, prolonging her distress and further delaying the recovery process.

Selective Serotonin Reuptake Inhibitors
Adverse Effects

5. What are the most common side effects reported with SSRIs, and how should they be managed?

Although it is not accurate to say that SSRIs cause fewer side effects than TCAs, the adverse effects associated with this newer antidepressant class are generally milder and less likely to lead to discontinuation.[84] There also are generally fewer concerns with SSRIs and comorbid illnesses than one encounters with TCAs, suggesting that SSRIs may often be a better choice in medically complex patients.

As clinical experience has accumulated rapidly with the SSRIs, a distinct side-effect profile has emerged, consisting of gastrointestinal (GI) complaints, CNS disturbances, and sexual dysfunction.[85] All the SSRIs may induce nausea, but this tends to be a transient effect that diminishes after the first week or so of treatment. Typically, the SSRIs can cause some local GI irritation 1 to 2 hours after oral administration. For this reason, patients should always be advised to take the medication after a meal or snack, particularly during the first week of therapy. Nausea with SSRIs may also be mediated centrally through the stimulation of certain serotonin receptors ($5-HT_{3C}$) that activate the chemoreceptor trigger zone (CTZ).[86] Nausea triggered by this mechanism has a more delayed onset, corresponding to the accumulation of medication until steady-state dynamics are reached and often persists throughout the dosing interval. Patients who experience nausea mediated by CNS stimulation may be unable to tolerate this effect and often require dosage reduction or drug discontinuation.

SSRIs may also have transient and bothersome effects on bowel function. Unlike nausea, there does appear to be clinically relevant differences among SSRIs in this regard. Sertraline, fluoxetine, and citalopram have been associated with a 15% to 20% incidence of diarrhea.[85,87] Fortunately, the diarrhea often remits after 1 week or so of continued therapy and rarely requires an interruption of treatment. In contrast, paroxetine possesses a mild affinity for muscarinic receptors that can manifest as anticholinergic side effects such as constipation, dry mouth, or urinary hesitancy. This may discourage the use of paroxetine in patients with pre-existing constipation or those receiving other medications with anticholinergic potential.

SSRIs can have myriad effects on the CNS, with disturbances in sleep or disposition being a primary concern. Overall, the SSRIs appear to have significant effects on sleep architecture and may prolong the REM stage, resulting in less fitful sleep.[88] Although sleep disturbances are common with SSRIs, it should be emphasized that this is usually a transient phenomenon that occurs during the first week or two of treatment; sleep may actually improve from baseline once the antidepressant properties of the medications emerge.

Compared with older antidepressants, SSRIs generally are considered activating compounds, and there does appear to be a hierarchy among the individual agents. Fluoxetine, for example, is widely regarded as the most activating of the SSRIs, a property that may be desirable in anergic patients or undesirable in those who are agitated or have difficulty falling asleep.[89] For this reason, fluoxetine is usually administered in the morning after breakfast. However, it should be noted that fluoxetine is not necessarily activating for all patients. In fact, some find it to be slightly sedating or numbing. Daytime drowsiness can be experienced with fluoxetine, perhaps as a result of light, restless sleep. Sertraline, escitalopram and citalopram have also been associated with comparatively more insomnia than sedation but they are generally considered to be less activating than fluoxetine in this regard. The effects of paroxetine appear to be somewhat balanced, with approximately equal proportions of patients complaining of sedation and insomnia. Although sleep disturbances are common with SSRIs, it should be emphasized that this is usually a transient phenomenon during the first week or so of treatment and sleep actually improves for most patients over time.

Another type of CNS side effect reported with SSRIs involves the extrapyramidal system (EPS). SSRIs have been associated with EPS effects, consisting of akathisia, dystonias, and parkinsonian symptoms that are qualitatively identical to those commonly seen with high-potency antipsychotics. Fortunately, the reported incidence of EPS effects is much lower than with antipsychotic agents.[90] Although EPS reactions have been documented with all SSRIs, most case reports have featured paroxetine.[89] Because paroxetine has the highest affinity for serotonin receptors, this may lend support to the theory that these EPS effects are mediated through the indirect influence of serotonergic neurons on dopaminergic activity.[91] In certain areas of the brain, serotonin and dopamine appear to have an inverse relationship, whereby central stimulation of serotonin receptors results in a net decline in dopaminergic transmission.[92] Therefore, management of EPS effects induced by SSRI is identical with that of those precipitated by antipsychotics. Dystonias and parkinsonian side effects can be treated with anticholinergic agents and subsequent dosage reduction. Akathisia usually responds to a dosage decrease and/or administration of low-dose β-blockers.

The deleterious effects of SSRI on sexual function were overlooked in early clinical trials, but it is now known that they are very common and potentially profound consequences of SSRI treatment that can often lead to medication nonadherence or decrements in patient self-esteem.[93] In the medical literature, the reported incidence of sexual dysfunction ranges from 1.9% to 75%, reflecting the diversity of research methods (or lack thereof) used to detect this occurrence.[94,95] The actual incidence of SSRI-induced sexual dysfunction is approximately 30% to 50%, and it appears to be slightly more common in men.[93] Delayed ejaculation and anorgasmia are the most common complaints in male patients, whereas women have also reported difficulty achieving orgasms or notice a decrease in sexual activity altogether. This effect has actually been used to clinical advantage in men reporting premature ejaculation, but most patients find it undesirable.[96] All the SSRIs are commonly implicated with sexual dysfunction, but there are several indirect lines of evidence suggesting that paroxetine is the worst in this regard.[97,98] A double-blind, controlled investigation with fluoxetine, sertraline, and paroxetine found that paroxetine induced the greatest delay in orgasms (among men with premature ejaculation), but all three SSRIs had substantial effects that were significantly higher than fluvoxamine or placebo.[98]

6. **Are there any other adverse effects of SSRIs for A.R. to be aware of?**

In addition to GI, CNS, and sexual side effects, a variety of other, less common, adverse sequelae may jeopardize treatment. Dry mouth and headache occur with many antidepressants and, although these somatic complaints are prevalent in the general population, placebo-adjusted rates suggest that SSRIs may induce this phenomenon.[87] Increased sweating has also been reported with SSRIs and can be particularly uncomfortable or embarrassing.[99] Dosage reduction may help relieve this adverse effect, and α-blockers (e.g., terazosin, prazosin) and anticholinergic antidotes have been used as well (e.g., benztropine, scopolamine).[100,101] Bruxism, or teeth-grinding, can also be an unfortunate consequence of SSRI treatment, leading to chipped or cracked teeth and generally poor dentition.[102] Often, patients may not be aware of this nocturnal effect and complain merely of a dull, persistent headache during the morning hours. This, too, may be a dose-dependent side effect of all SSRIs, and several antidotes have been prescribed (e.g., buspirone, benzodiazepines).[103,104] In small retrospective studies and several case reports, SSRIs have been linked to dilutional hyponatremia or syndrome of inappropriate antidiuretic hormone (SIADH).[105,106] All the SSRIs (and venlafaxine) have been associated with this phenomenon, and elderly patients appear to be uniquely at risk.

The long-term effects of SSRIs on body weight are more variable and difficult to predict. It is worthwhile to recall that decreased appetite is one of the most common depressive symptoms and that a small weight gain after an antidepressant course may actually be viewed as a therapeutic effect of successful treatment. Early reports of weight loss with fluoxetine generated much optimism for the use of SSRI in obesity, but longitudinal studies found this to be a brief, transient phenomenon.[107] In recent times, all the SSRIs have been implicated with significant weight gain after long-term use, with paroxetine most often cited.[108,109] One long-term randomized controlled trial compared the effects of fluoxetine, sertraline and paroxetine on total body weight.[110] After 7 months of SSRI use, 25% of the patients receiving paroxetine gained a clinically significant amount of weight (defined as ≥7% increase in total body weight) compared with 7% with fluoxetine and 4% with sertraline. Long-term studies with citalopram and escitalopram suggest that 3% to 5% of patients will experience a significant weight gain. As weight gain may occur with any SSRI, it is best to monitor weight changes closely during long-term treatment and respond accordingly.

Dosage Titration

7. **A.R. calls the clinic 2 weeks later requesting a dosage increase. She reports that she has been taking 50 mg of sertraline every morning and has noticed considerable improvement in her sleep, appetite, and outlook ("Little things don't bother me so much anymore") but feels as if she could be doing better. She is less despondent but still feels as though her concentration could**

improve and admits that she has yet to resume her exercise regimen ("I still don't have the energy"). She asks you if she could increase her dosage. What changes would you make to her antidepressant regimen at this time?

It is very important to establish realistic expectations for treatment with antidepressants from the very beginning of therapy. Patients need to be informed of the anticipated course of antidepressant treatment and should be advised, for instance, that the onset of side effects usually precede that of therapeutic effects. Also, patients should be advised that, although antidepressants may relieve their acute symptoms and prevent relapse, they do not abolish environmental stressors, increase self-esteem, or reverse negative perceptions and emotions.

In regard to dosing and treatment response, one of the theoretical advantages of the SSRIs is that they appear to exhibit a flat dose-response curve, requiring less dosage titration than older agents. Fixed-dose studies with fluoxetine (20 mg/day), sertraline (50 mg), paroxetine (20 mg), citalopram (20 mg), and escitalopram (10 mg) support a flat dose-response relationship in the depressed, nonelderly adult population.[111–115] However, in practice many clinicians persist in rapidly increasing daily doses over the first few weeks in a fashion reminiscent of TCA prescribing practices.[116] For many patients, this aggressive treatment results in unnecessary expense and side effects, impeding medication adherence as well.

Fortunately, with the accumulation of clinical experience and extensive medical education, the average daily doses of SSRIs have crept down over the last few years to more reasonable figures. Some providers have found, in fact, that lower dosages of SSRIs may actually suffice (e.g., 10 mg/day of fluoxetine or paroxetine) if patients are informed of the delayed onset of therapeutic effects and are closely monitored for tolerance and response.[117] Because fixed-dose studies were rarely conducted with these lower dosages, it is difficult to endorse this practice empirically, but some experimental evidence shows that daily doses as small as 5 mg of fluoxetine are more effective than placebo and comparable to 20 mg in a significant segment of the depressed populace.[118]

For A.R., many factors must be considered before increasing her dosage. She has been receiving the medication for only 2 weeks, and the improvement she is exhibiting in neurovegetative symptoms may suggest that the resolution of cognitive symptoms is soon to follow. She should be reminded that the optimal effects of antidepressants may not be evident for 4 to 6 weeks. Furthermore, it is possible that the lack of improvement in her concentration and energy may be largely situational as the day of her wedding approaches. An increase in medication at this time would not necessarily address these environmental factors and would serve only to increase the side-effect burden. Therefore, a reasonable recommendation would be to continue with the current daily dose of 50 mg and to re-evaluate the medication's effects when she returns to clinic in 2 weeks.

8. **At the end of 4 weeks of treatment, A.R. is seen in the clinic and asked about side effects she has experienced. She recalls some mild nausea during the first week of treatment but continued to take the medication after breakfast (as directed) and noticed that this effect went away after approximately 3 or 4 days of therapy. She denies diarrhea, insomnia, or headache. Before**

leaving, she reluctantly admits that the only side effect she is experiencing is sexual. ("I love my fiancée but I have no interest in actually making love anymore.") How should this side effect be managed at this time?

From a clinician's standpoint, the detection and proper management of SSRI-induced sexual dysfunction can be one of the most important factors in ensuring medication adherence (Table 79-14). Clinicians may be uncomfortable asking patients about their sexual activities and satisfaction, but the high incidence of this side effect (and low likelihood of patients volunteering information) necessitates a thoughtful and direct approach. Some patients acknowledge sexual dysfunction but decide that the improvement in their mood and overall health outweighs limitations in sexual performance, but many others simply stop the medication if the side effect is never addressed.

It may be wise to advise patients that sexual function may change over time, depending on the type and etiology of sexual dysfunction experienced. Depression itself is associated with a decreased libido in at least 50% of untreated patients.[119] This symptom will most likely subside with a successful course of antidepressant treatment. Delayed ejaculation or anorgasmia, however, is usually an iatrogenic phenomenon with SSRIs and venlafaxine, often persisting and jeopardizing treatment. Because A.R. has been taking the medication faithfully for the first 4 weeks and the time course is consistent with the SSRI effects, it is unlikely that the condition will spontaneously remit now and some action must be taken.

Ordinarily, one of the first options in managing sexual dysfunction is to reduce the dosage, but this may precipitate a recrudescence of the original depressive symptoms in some patients. In A.R.'s case, she is taking a relatively low therapeutic dosage of sertraline, and a further decrease may be a risky proposition. An alternative solution for A.R.'s problem may be to recommend drug holidays. Small open-label studies with short-acting SSRIs (e.g., sertraline, paroxetine) suggested that if patients skipped their doses on Friday and Saturday, sexual function would return to normal on the weekends.[120,121] Although this method was reported to be successful, it may also promote nonadherence with medication and lead to increased risk of relapse.

If the patient has had a therapeutic response to the antidepressant, the next option in this setting is to consider antidotes to SSRI-induced sexual dysfunction, and the most popular treatment at present is bupropion. Clinical reports and uncontrolled investigations suggest that the addition of this antidepressant can be helpful for restoring sexual desire and may re-

---

Table 79-14 Management of SSRI-Induced Sexual Dysfunction

- Patience (may improve after 2 to 4 wk)
- Reduced dosage (if possible)
- Drug holidays (sertraline, paroxetine, citalopram, escitalopram only)
- Antidotes:
  - Bupropion 75–150 mg QD–BID
  - Sildenafil 50–100 mg QD PRN
  - Nefazodone 50–200 mg HS
  - Mirtazapine 7.5–15 mg HS
  - Cyproheptadine 4–12 mg PRN (1 hr prior)
  - Methylphenidate 2.5–5.0 mg QD
  - Others: yohimbine, amantadine, buspirone, gingko
- Change of antidepressants (e.g., bupropion, nefazodone, mirtazapine)

---

lieve delayed orgasm or anorgasmia as well.[122–124] A common dosing technique is to start with 150 mg of the sustained-release (SR) product daily. If unsuccessful, the dose can be increased to 150 mg SR twice daily after several days. Although open-label studies support bupropion for SSRI-induced sexual dysfunction, results of a recent small double-blind, placebo-controlled trial were less favorable.[125] Since bupropion has demonstrated efficacy in nondepressed patients suffering from sexual dysfunction and may provide antidepressant augmentation, it is still worthy of consideration.

From a mechanistic standpoint, sexual arousal and orgasm consititute a complex physiologic process, and it is not well understood how SSRIs induce adverse effects or how bupropion may provide relief. Some researchers have theorized that delayed ejaculation or orgasm is mediated by a stimulation of postsynaptic $5-HT_2$ or $5-HT_3$ receptors, whereas others suggest that the indirect effects of SSRIs on dopamine may be involved.[126] Additional theories point to the inhibitory effects of SSRIs on prolactin or nitric oxide synthetase (NOS).[126]

Other remedies have been prescribed for SSRI-induced sexual dysfunction. Recently, a large randomized, controlled trial examined the impact of sildenafil upon patients suffering from this side effect.[127] Overall, 54% of the male patients randomized to sildenafil found it be effective compared with a 4% response rate with placebo. Open-label trials of sildenafil in women experiencing SSRI-induced anorgasmia have also reported improvements, suggesting that controlled trials in this population are warranted.[128]

Cyproheptadine is an obscure antihistamine with potent antiserotonergic properties, which has also received some attention as a potential antidote. It has been used successfully for the treatment of SSRI-induced sexual dysfunction in doses of 4 to 12 mg just before intercourse.[129] Unfortunately, cyproheptadine is sedating and appears to have a limited role in this capacity. If it is used, one should never administer the medication on a regular schedule because reports of relapse in depressed patients have surfaced.[130] Amantadine, buspirone, and yohimbine have also been used successfully to reverse delayed ejaculation or decreased libido, but the evidence for efficacy is rather limited.[131–133] One small double-blind study compared the effects of amantadine with buspirone or placebo among depressed patients developing sexual dysfunction on antidepressants.[134] All three treatments improved sexual dysfunction to a comparable extent, and the only statistically significant finding was related to an increase in energy reported among patients receiving amantadine (versus placebo). An open-label trial of ginkgo biloba in men and women with sexual dysfunction reported very high success rates, but mixed results have been experienced in actual practice.[135] Nefazodone and mirtazapine are capable of blocking postsynaptic $5-HT_2$ receptors and theoretically may relieve ejaculatory difficulties, but controlled trials have not been conducted. Finally, stimulants such as methylphenidate or dextroamphetamine may increase libido in SSRI-treated patients, but the potential for dependence and abuse discourages their routine administration.[136]

The onset of A.R.'s decreased libido is consistent with the introduction of sertraline, and it appears, at this time, that her libido will not improve if she continues to take the SSRI. Because she is exhibiting some evidence of a therapeutic response, one would prefer to continue sertraline and discuss possible antidotes for sexual dysfunction with her. A.R. states that she would prefer to treat her problem with an herbal medication, and you recommend that she begin a 6-week trial of gingko biloba 60 mg twice a day.

Duration of Treatment

9. At 6 weeks, A.R. reports that her depressive symptoms are effectively in remission ("I feel like I have my old life back!"). Her energy has improved, she is doing well in her studies and looks forward, once again, to her wedding day. How long should A.R. continue taking the antidepressant?

According to the guidelines released by the Agency for Health Care Policy Research (AHCPR), antidepressant treatment can be broken down into three stages (Table 79-15).[137] The first stage, *acute treatment,* lasts approximately 12 weeks; during this time the clinician attempts to resolve the presenting symptoms and induce remission. The second stage is commonly called *continuation treatment* because the patient continues to receive the same antidepressant regimen that induced the initial treatment response and the clinician attempts to keep the acute symptoms in remission. The duration of continuation treatment is variable (4 to 9 months after initial treatment or response), but it is recommended that all patients suffering from major depression complete these first two stages. Therefore, the minimum duration of treatment is 7 months.

The third stage of treatment, *maintenance treatment* or prophylaxis, is not indicated for all patients, and the necessity of continuing medication beyond the first 7 months depends on many patient-specific factors. One must consider the number of previous episodes, family history of depression, patient's age, severity of presenting symptoms, response to therapy, and persistence or anticipation of environmental stressors. There are specific populations for whom indefinite pharmacologic treatment is advocated: (1) individuals with three or more previous episodes of major depression, (2) individuals older than 50 with two or more previous episodes, and (3) individuals older than 60 with one or more previous episodes.[137] Many experts believe that pharmacotherapy should also be continued indefinitely in all elderly people (older than 65 years) suffering from major depression, but research evidence to conclusively support this recommendation is currently lacking.[138,139]

Because A.R. is exhibiting a full therapeutic response to sertraline, the recommendation would be for her to continue with the effective dosage (50 mg/day) for at least 7 consecutive months.[137] At the end of this time frame, the clinician should sit down with the patient and review all the considerations that enter into the decision to continue treatment. Ultimately, the decision to continue antidepressant medications is left to the patient's judgment, and he or she should be well informed of the potential consequences of stopping treatment.

In the future, if A.R. decides to discontinue her antidepressant, she should be advised of potential withdrawal symptoms (Table 79-16). Abrupt discontinuation of chronic SSRI treatment (e.g., treatment >2 months) has been associated with dizziness, headache, anxiety, flulike symptoms, and paresthesias.[140] The onset of these symptoms is generally within 48 to 72 hours of stopping treatment, and effects may persist for ≥1 week. Withdrawal symptoms generally are mild and self-limiting but can be uncomfortable and alarming. Because of their relatively short half-life (and absence of long-acting metabolites), paroxetine, fluvoxamine, and venlafaxine have been associated with a more profound withdrawal presentation (than fluoxetine, sertraline, citalopram or escitalopram), but one should taper slowly off all antidepressant medications after an extended treatment course.

After A.R. has completed a full course of pharmacotherapy, it may be advisable to taper her sertraline over several weeks to minimize the risk of withdrawal, as well as to monitor for signs and symptoms of relapse. Although the risk of relapse is relatively low during the first month off medication, depressive symptoms often return during the second or third months, and the risk of relapse is highest during the first 6 months overall.[141]

Antidepressants in Pregnancy and Lactation

10. Eight months after starting her antidepressant, A.R. reports that she has continued to be symptom free and is now living happily with her husband. She has taken the sertraline faithfully each morning and is willing to do so for as long as it is prescribed ("I don't ever want to go through that again!"). She also reveals that she and her husband are thinking of starting a

Table 79-15 Duration of Antidepressant Treatment

Acute Treatment Phase:	3 mo
Continuation Treatment Phase:	4–9 mo
Maintenance Treatment Phase:	Variable

- Acute *and* continuation treatment recommended for all patients with major depressive disorder (i.e., minimal duration of treatment = 7 mo)
- Decision to prescribe maintenance treatment is based on the following.
  – Number of previous episodes
  – Severity of previous episodes
  – Family history of depression
  – Patient age (worse prognosis if elderly)
  – Response to antidepressant
  – Persistence of environmental stressors
- Indefinite maintenance treatment is recommended if any one of the following criteria are met.
  1. Three or more previous episodes (regardless of age)
  2. Two or more previous episodes and age older than 50 yr
  3. One or more and age older than 60 yr

Table 79-16 Discontinuation of Antidepressants

Withdrawal syndrome
- Worse with paroxetine, venlafaxine
- Symptoms: dizziness, nausea, paresthesias, anxiety/insomnia, flu-like symptoms
- Onset: 36–72 hr
- Duration: 3–7 days

Taper schedule (for patients receiving long-term treatment)
- Fluoxetine: generally unnecessary
- Sertraline: decrease by 50 mg every 1–2 wk
- Paroxetine: decrease by 10 mg every 1–2 wk
- Citalopram: decrease by 10 mg every 1–2 wk
- Escitalopram: decrease by 5 mg every 1–2 wk
- Venlafaxine: decrease by 25–50 mg every 1–2 wk
- Nefazodone: decrease by 50–100 mg every 1–2 wk
- Bupropion: generally unnecessary
- Tricyclics: decrease by 10%–25% every 1–2 wk

Note: Risk of relapse greatest 1 to 6 months after discontinuation.

family and asks if it is necessary to continue the medication through pregnancy. How should A.R. and her husband be counseled with regard to starting a family?

The risk for depression is substantial during pregnancy as well as the postpartum period.[142] Historically, patients have been informed that depression will spontaneously remit during pregnancy, but more recent evidence does not support this perception.[143] Before deciding to treat with an antidepressant during pregnancy, one should make a careful inventory of the benefits and risks. The consequences of maternal depression on the mother and fetus must be compared with potential risks of teratogenicity, growth impairment, and other adverse birth outcomes. One study reported that 50% of depressed women who stopped their antidepressant early in pregnancy experienced a relapse of their disorder by the end of the third trimester.[144] In addition to the mother's distress, depression during pregnancy may pose serious risks to the fetus, particularly if the mother's appetite is compromised. Neonatal studies have also shown that infants of mothers who became depressed during pregnancy were smaller at birth, with lower Apgar scores and manifest with more irritability and emotional problems.[145]

The attendant effects of antidepressants on the developing fetus have been difficult to predict or quantify. For obvious reasons, randomized controlled trials of potential teratogens are seldom conducted in expectant mothers, so study methods to assess fetal risk are less than ideal. From the evidence that has emerged, the overall risks to gestational development appear to be relatively minor with SSRIs, and they have all been given a Class C designation by the FDA for potential risks. Bupropion is the only antidepressant to have received a Class B rating, although this distinction is not necessarily predictive of safety.

Several studies have been published in recent years comparing the safety of TCAs, SSRIs, and known nonteratogens.[146–150] None of these investigations found a significant association between antidepressant medications and major birth defects. However, there has been evidence linking SSRIs with earlier delivery (and low birth weight) as well as neonatal adaptation difficulties.[150] One study compared the risk of mothers taking fluoxetine with expectant controls and discovered that women who continued the SSRIs into their third trimester were more likely to produce low-birth-weight infants (average birth weight of 188 g less than controls).[147] Children born to mothers receiving late-term fluoxetine were also more likely to have minor birth anomalies than mothers stopping fluoxetine after the first trimester (or controls). A retrospective comparison of TCAs to SSRIs reported a 0.9 week decrease in mean gestational age and a significant decrease in mean Apgar scores among those exposed to serotonergic agents (primarily fluoxetine).[150] A small controlled investigation recently (n = 40) examined the effects of fluoxetine and citalopram on CNS effects in newborns and found a significant increase in restlessness, tremor, shivering and hyperreflexia during the first four days of life (versus controls).[151] The study did not find any substantial difference in birthweight or preterm deliveries, but there was a significant decline in Apgar scores on average.

The effects of other SSRIs or newer antidepressants on newborns are not entirely clear. One prospective, multisite investigation featuring sertraline, paroxetine, and fluvoxamine failed to find an association between antidepressant use and prematurity or birth defects (behavioral effects were not assessed).[149] Placental passage of SSRIs appears to be incomplete, but research evidence suggests that fetal brain concentrations of the mother's antidepressant can approach 85% of maternal levels.[144] The developmental consequences of this finding are unknown.

From the limited data available, the risk of major birth defects appears not to be enhanced by TCAs or SSRIs. An association with minor defects or stunted growth cannot be discounted, however, as illustrated by evidence that has accrued with fluoxetine in particular. A prudent approach is to prescribe the lowest effecive dose, and one may also consider SSRIs with a shorter half-life to minimize exposure. More specific recommendations await further study.

For A.R., it is important to assess her risk for depression if she stops taking antidepressants. This was her first episode of depression (which occurred under stressful circumstances), and she does not have a strong genetic predisposition to mood disorders. If she is committed to starting a family, she may wish to consider being tapered off of the sertraline over several weeks just before conception. Once the medication has been discontinued and she appears to be psychiatrically stable, she may then stop the oral contraceptive.

11. What are the risks of continuing antidepressant medications during breast-feeding?

During the first few months after delivery, depressive symptoms are relatively common in new mothers, and treatment for mood disorders is often necessary. Approximately 70% of mothers report sadness or anxiety during the first month after delivery, and roughly 10% satisfy criteria for major depressive disorder.[144] Because breast-feeding is widely advocated in contemporary medical circles, the passive transfer of medication from mother to infant must be considered.

Studies with TCAs and SSRIs suggest that concentrations of antidepressants in breast milk are not negligible. However, subsequent concentrations in the infant's bloodstream are rarely substantial. Among the available agents, doxepin and fluoxetine have been associated with the highest concentrations in infants, and although the clinical or developmental consequences of this finding have not been elucidated, it has been recommended that these medications be avoided.[152] Recent studies with sertraline, paroxetine, and citalopram have reported that relatively low levels of exposure were evident from infant serum samples.[152,153] If an antidepressant is to be continued in a mother who is breast-feeding, the lowest dosage should be prescribed and the mother may wish to take the medication just before the infant's longest sleep period.

Drug Interactions

12. A.R. is not currently taking any prescription medications other than her antidepressant. She is concerned, however, that she may be prescribed medications over the course of her anticipated pregnancy and asked if there are any drug interactions for her to be aware of. Are there any significant drug interactions associated with sertraline?

There is a growing awareness of the potential for certain antidepressants (e.g., SSRIs, nefazodone) to inhibit the metabolism of other medications that are cleared through the cytochrome P450 system of isoenzymes (Table 79-17).[154] In general, these drug interactions are concentration dependent and most clinically relevant when the affected medication has

Table 79-17   **Drug Interactions of the Cytochrome P450 System**

Relative Rank	CYP1A2	CYP2C	CYP2D6	CYP3A
Offending Agent (inhibits enzyme)				
High	Fluvoxamine	Cyp2C19 Fluvoxamine Cyp2C9 Fluoxetine Fluvoxamine	Paroxetine Fluoxetine Duloxetine	Norfluoxetine Fluvoxamine Nefazodone
Moderate	Fluoxetine Paroxetine Sertraline (high dose)	Cyp2C19 Fluoxetine Sertraline	TCA Sertraline (high dose) Fluvoxamine	TCA (high dose)
Low	Escitalopram Citalopram Venlafaxine Nefazodone Bupropion Mirtazapine	Cyp2C19 Venlafaxine Cyp2C9 Sertraline	Escitalopram Citalopram Venlafaxine Nefazodone Bupropion	Sertraline Paroxetine Escitalopram Citalopram Mirtazapine
Other Inhibitors				
	Quinolones (ciprofloxacin, enoxacin, etc)	Modafinil (2C9, 2C19)	Fenfluramine	Macrolides (erythro, clarith)
	Macrolides (erythromycin, clarithromycin)	Cimetidine (2C19)	Yohimbine	Cimetidine
	Grapefruit juice	Omeprazole (2C19)	Methadone	Ca channel blockers (verapamil, diltiazem)
		Imidazoles (2C9, 2C19) (ketoconazole, fluconazole)	Quinidine	Imidazoles (ketoconazole, fluconazole)
			Celecoxib	Protease inhibitors Grapefruit juice
Other Inducers				
	Cigarettes Caffeine St. John's wort		Modafinil Phenytoin and phenobarbital; Carbamazepine Rifampin Prednisone Testosterone	St. John's wort
Affected Agent (increased concentration)				
	TCA-tertiary amines (imipramine, amitriptyline) Phenothiazines (chlorpromazine) Thiothixene Haloperidol Clozapine Olanzapine Caffeine Theophylline Propranolol Tacrine	Cyp2C19 TCA-tertiary amines (imipramine, amitriptyline) Citalopram Barbiturates Propranolol Omeprazole Cyp2C9 Bupropion Phenytoin Tolbutamide Warfarin NSAIDs	TCA-secondary amines (desipramine, nortriptyline) Fluoxetine Paroxetine Venlafaxine Nefazodone (m-CPP metabolite) Amphetamines Atomoxetine Risperidone Donepezil Codeine Hydrocodone Tramadol Dextromethorphan Chlorpheniramine β-Blockers (propranolol, metoprolol)	Fluoxetine Sertraline Venlafaxine Nefazodone Modafinil Quetiapine Ziprasidone Aripiprazole Buspirone Benzodiazepines (triazolam, alprazolam) Zolpidem Carbamazepine Donepezil Astemizole Cisapride CCB (verapamil, diltiazem, nifedipine) Sex hormones (estrogen) Corticosteroids Statins (lovastatin, simvastatin) Protease inhibitors Sildenafil

mcpp, XXX; NSAIDs, nonsteroidal anti-inflammatory drugs; TCA, tricyclic antidepressants.

a low therapeutic index, requires conversion to an active metabolite, or cannot be eliminated through other metabolic routes.[155] Important examples of affected medications include TCAs, calcium channel blockers, estrogen, theophylline, phenytoin, warfarin, triazolobenzodiazepines, and cisapride.

The SSRIs are potent inhibitors of the cytochrome P450 isoenzymes, but important differences exist among the individual agents in their affinity for the isoenzymes and for the specific metabolic pathways involved (see Table 79-17). For instance, the cytochrome P450 1A2 isoenzyme (or CYP 1A2) is most sensitive to the inhibitory effects of fluvoxamine, whereas fluoxetine and paroxetine have the highest affinity for CYP 2D6.[156] In comparison, sertraline citalopram, and escitalopram have the lowest potential for drug interactions but may still inhibit the metabolism of selected medications.[156–158]

Although in vitro affinities of antidepressants for the respective isoenzymes can be very helpful for predicting potentially dangerous drug combinations, there is wide interpatient variability in the susceptibility for these interactions. Much of this variability can be attributed to genetic polymorphism. With CYP 2D6, for example, approximately 5% to 10% of whites and 1% to 2% of Asians are considered poor metabolizers via this metabolic pathway (i.e., possess a nonfunctional variant of the enzyme); and the rest of these respective populations are regarded as extensive metabolizers.[159] However, genetic variation does not explain the unpredictable nature of the situation entirely.

One of the best examples of this variability can be found with desipramine, a secondary amine of the TCAs, which is metabolized almost exclusively through the CYP 2D6 pathway. In vitro affinities suggest that paroxetine would have the greatest impact on metabolism occurring via this route, but controlled investigations discovered that fluoxetine increased the plasma desipramine concentrations of adult volunteers by 350%, paroxetine by 125%, and sertraline by 20%.[160–162] One plausible explanation for this unexpected finding may be that therapeutic doses of fluoxetine are associated with much higher plasma concentrations than other SSRIs because of a smaller first-pass effect. Levels may also be higher at steady state because of the longer plasma half-life of fluoxetine and norfluoxetine compared with other SSRIs. It is also worth mentioning that even though sertraline had less of an impact on desipramine concentrations, two patients experienced a doubling of steady-state desipramine levels, emphasizing the wide variability in patient response.[162]

Nefazodone, fluvoxamine, and norfluoxetine have profound inhibitory effects on the CYP 3A4 isoenzyme, the most abundant family of isoenzymes found in the liver (and GI mucosa).[163] Serious drug interactions have been mediated through this pathway, the most notable involving cardiotoxicity and malignant ventricular arrhythmias precipitated by elevated concentrations of terfenadine, astemizole, and cisapride.[154] Another clinically significant interaction may occur when nefazodone is coadministered with the triazolobenzodiazepines (triazolam, alprazolam, and midazolam).[164,165] Concomitant administration of nefazodone and triazolam resulted in a fivefold increase in the half-life of the benzodiazepine, and nefazodone also has been associated with a doubling of steady-state alprazolam levels. Because these psychotropic medications are occasionally combined to manage anxiety

disorders or depression, clinicians are advised to empirically reduce the initial dosage of the triazolobenzodiazepines (75% with triazolam, 50% with alprazolam) in patients currently receiving nefazodone.[166]

Serotonin Syndrome

13. **What is serotonin syndrome, and is A.R. at risk for this interaction?**

Serotonin syndrome is a rare but potentially fatal interaction that has been precipitated by the combination of two or more drugs that enhance serotonin transmission.[167] The syndrome consists of a constellation of associated symptoms, including anxiety, shivering, diaphoresis, tremor, hyperreflexia, and autonomic instability (increased/decreased blood pressure (BP) and pulse rate).[168] Fatalities have been attributed to malignant hyperthermia.

With mild cases of serotonin syndrome, the symptoms ordinarily resolve 24 to 48 hours after the serotonergic agents have been discontinued. Supportive treatment is usually not necessary. For more severe reactions, various serotonergic antagonists, such as cyproheptadine, methysergide, and propranolol, have been used.[169–171] Dantrolene has been administered successfully to manage hyperthermia.[172]

Most case reports of serotonin syndrome (and most fatalities) have occurred with a combination of an MAO inhibitor and an SSRI, which is now considered an absolute contraindication. Other case reports involve the combination of an MAO inhibitor (or SSRI) and tryptophan, meperidine, tricyclics, dextromethorphan, and lithium.[167] One case of serotonin syndrome was reportedly induced by the combination of clomipramine with S-adenosylmethionine (SAMe).[173] Serotonin syndrome has been reported with concurrent administration of SSRIs as well. Theoretically, the combination of an SSRI with St. John's wort may precipitate this pharmacodynamic interaction also, but more recent evidence has suggested that the MAO inhibitory properties of the herbal preparation are minimal with therapeutic doses. Nonetheless, a case series of five older patients who developed symptoms reminiscent of serotonin syndrome has appeared in the literature and, given the degree of uncertainty that persists, this combination of antidepressant agents is best avoided.[174] The safety of combining an SSRI with certain migraine medications (e.g., sumatriptan) has not been elucidated, and clinicians are advised to avoid this combination if possible as well.

The combination of a phenylpiperazine (trazodone or nefazodone) with an SSRI may pose some concern because both classes of antidepressants augment serotonin activity in the CNS. Trazodone has been associated with serotonin syndrome in two incidences, one involving the coadministration of buspirone and the other associated with a concomitant MAO inhibitor.[168] However, in practice, trazodone has been commonly prescribed to patients receiving an SSRI for the treatment of insomnia, and no confirmed cases of serotonin syndrome have surfaced in the medical literature.[175] The combination of nefazodone with an SSRI also appears to be safe, although one should recall that the potential exists for a pharmacokinetic interaction because nefazodone may increase the plasma levels of any SSRI metabolized through the CYP 3A4 isoenzyme pathway (e.g., fluoxetine, sertraline, venlafaxine).

Refractory Depression

14. F.H. is a 55-year-old postmenopausal woman presenting to the women's health clinic who has reportedly suffered from multiple depressive episodes since the age of 30. She reports that she has been hospitalized on three different occasions. Although F.H. is unable to recall details of any specific antidepressant trials, her prescription record reveals treatment with imipramine (100 mg/day), nortriptyline (75 mg/day), diazepam (10 mg/day), and fluoxetine (20 mg/day for the last 8 weeks). Eventually, she recalls that imipramine made her "dizzy and left a strange taste in my mouth" and that diazepam made her "even more depressed." She says that the fluoxetine may be "helping a little bit but I feel so jumpy and irritable that no one can stand me." F.H. has grown rather despondent over her situation ("I almost feel like giving up"). What would be the next reasonable step for managing F.H.'s depressive illness?

Pooled results of clinical trials suggest that 60% to 70% of patients with major depression receiving an adequate trial of any antidepressant will have a therapeutic response, traditionally defined as at least a 50% reduction in depressive symptoms. However, for a patient who is severely depressed, a 50% reduction in symptoms still leaves him or her with significant psychopathology and associated disability. Consequently, there has been a strong movement in recent years to consider full remission as the preferred therapeutic endpoint.[81] Scientific support for this ideologic shift comes from long-term studies demonstrating that patients achieving remission are much less likely to suffer relapse. One longitudinal investigation found that patients with residual symptoms were three times more likely to suffer relapse during the 12 months after treatment than those who had remitted.[176] Although remission can be generally defined as the virtual absence of residual depressive symptoms, it can also be quantified with a corresponding threshold value on a depression rating scale (e.g., IDS <14; 17-item HAM-D <7).[81] As more clinical trials use these rigorous standards, it has become evident that approximately only 30% to 40% of patients receiving an adequate trial of an antidepressant actually achieve remission. Therefore, strident efforts are being made to make patients feel well and not merely better, and providers must undertake a thorough, rational, and perhaps aggressive approach to optimize treatment and achieve this goal.

For F.H., the first step would be to confirm her diagnosis and rule out potential medical explanations for her distress. Iatrogenic causes should also be explored, such as recent changes in her hormone replacement therapy. Persistent stressors or substance abuse patterns may be hindering her sustained recovery and should be addressed.

An assessment of F.H.'s attitude toward medication adherence is also vital, and her complete medical records should be obtained to verify the dose, duration, and results of previous antidepressant trials. It is critical to confirm that she received full therapeutic trials of all the antidepressants that she was prescribed before seeking other therapeutic options. A full therapeutic trial for the treatment of depression is considered to be a minimum of 4 weeks receiving a clinically effective dosage of medication. Although some improvement may be noted during the first 1 or 2 weeks of treatment, maximal response is rarely evident until 4 weeks of medication have been received. An open-label study with fluoxetine, for instance, randomized patients who were not fully responsive after 3 weeks of treatment (20 mg/day) to either continue with the original regimen or receive an increased dosage (60 mg/day) for 5 additional weeks.[178] At the end of the study period, 49% of the patients receiving 20 mg converted to full responders, suggesting that 3 weeks is an inadequate period to confidently assess patient response. Because 50% of the patients receiving 60 mg/day converted to full responders, it may also be inferred that dosage increases are not necessary in many patients.

Drug Selection
Venlafaxine

15. After a careful interview and workup, it was determined that F.H. is suffering from an acute episode of major depression with a probable history of dysthymia as well (i.e., double depression). She denies substance abuse, which is supported by a subsequent toxicology screen. From her medical chart and interview, it is confirmed that she received a therapeutic trial of nortriptyline and fluoxetine with inadequate clinical benefit. Her provider decides to start venlafaxine (37.5 mg SR preparation daily). Is this a reasonable choice?

Because 30% to 40 % of patients will effectively achieve remission and about 20% to 25% of patients will stop an antidepressant because of side effects, it is safe to say that *most* patients started on a given antidepressant ultimately need a significant adjustment or change to their original regimen.[179] Clinicians, therefore, are obligated to have a thorough understanding of several antidepressant medications and classes if they are to faciliate successful outcomes.

In F.H.'s case, she has previously failed a therapeutic trial of nortriptyline and is currently expressing vague suicidality, so an additional TCA would not be a reasonable choice (see full discussion of TCAs in the text that follows). Although she has also failed a fluoxetine trial, open-label studies have shown that 50% to 70% of patients who are unresponsive or intolerant of one SSRI will experience a therapeutic response to a different SSRI.[178,180,181] If a different SSRI is to be initiated, it may be wise to opt for one with less activating properties than fluoxetine (e.g., sertraline, paroxetine, citalopram, escitalopram). Alternatively, a medication from a different antidepressant class would possess the hypothetical benefit of a unique mechanism of action (e.g., venlafaxine, bupropion). Because F.H. is evidently experiencing much torment and despair, a sense of urgency may be perceived, justifying a different pharmacologic approach altogether.

Venlafaxine is the first member of a relatively new class of antidepressants known as serotonin norepinephrine reuptake inhibitors (SNRI). Duloxetine (Cymbalta), which possesses a very similar mechanism of action, has been recommended for FDA approval but was not yet available in the United States as this edition went to press.[182] Studies in severe melancholic depression and treatment-resistant depression suggest that venlafaxine is at least as effective as other antidepressants in these populations, and it has emerged in recent years as a valuable alternative agent.[183–185] At dosages less than 150 mg/day, venlafaxine's therapeutic effects are mediated primarily from the blockade of serotonin reuptake. Therefore, associated adverse effects at low dosages are qualitatively and quantitatively very similar to those found with SSRIs: GI distress, sleep disturbances, and sexual dysfunction. At higher dosages, effects on norepinephrine are observed, which distinguish venlafaxine from an SSRI in terms of adverse effects (e.g., causes hypertension) but may also confer additional therapeutic benefit.

Venlafaxine has a relatively brief plasma half-life (5 to 8 hours) and is demethylated to an active metabolite (*O*-desmethyl-venlafaxine) that has a short half-life as well (11 hours). Recently, an SR preparation was formulated that permits once-daily dosing, but clinicians should still be mindful of severe withdrawal reactions that may be associated with the abrupt discontinuation of either product. Venlafaxine is not a potent inhibitor of cytochrome P450 isoenzymes, so drug interactions are less of a concern than with certain SSRIs, but serotonin syndrome has been reported in patients receiving venlafaxine in combination with other serotonergic agents.[186]

For F.H., the choice of venlafaxine seems to be prudent. It is fairly safe in overdose, possesses a unique mechanism of action, and is generally less activating than fluoxetine (which had provoked some irritability in her). A starting dose of 37.5 mg is reasonable, and the extended-release (XL) preparation may improve her adherence. Baseline vitals should be recorded for F.H. and repeated when she achieves steady state as well as with every dosage change. In comparison to SSRIs, venlafaxine possesses a wide therapeutic range and ordinarily requires more dosage titration (which can increase resource utilization). Most patients respond to daily doses between 75 and 225 mg. Because F.H. is suffering from a relatively severe depression, it may be wise to increase her daily dose to 75 mg once she has exhibited good tolerance (i.e., after 4 to 7 days). In the event that F.H. has not exhibited a satisfactory response to 75 mg/day after 4 weeks, the dosage may be increased in increments of 37.5 to 75 mg every few weeks to a daily maximum of 225 mg. Although daily doses of the XL preparation above 225 mg are not recommended by the manufacturer, anecdotal success and relative safety have been reported for doses as high as 300 mg daily.[187]

Other Agents: Bupropion and Mirtazapine

16. Are there any other antidepressants to consider if F.H. fails her venlafaxine trial?

Bupropion is an aminoketone with a mechanism of action that is clearly different from that of any other antidepressant that has received FDA approval. The effects of bupropion on serotonin transmission are negligible, but it may act by enhancing dopamine or norepinephrine activity.[188] At therapeutic dosages, bupropion has an attractive adverse-effect profile, limited to occasional nausea and insomnia or jitteriness. Seizures, which were reported shortly after it was released in 1985, appear to be very unlikely with therapeutic dosing of bupropion, provided that patients are not predisposed (e.g., history of epilepsy or bulimia). Bupropion is one of the few antidepressants that may actually decrease appetite. A recent randomized, placebo-controlled investigation of bupropion in depressed obese patients observing caloric restriction found that bupropion was much more likely to induce significant weight loss than placebo.[189] After 26 weeks of treatment, 40% of the bupropion-treated patients lost >5% of their total body weight versus 16% with placebo. This weight loss was positively correlated with an improvement in depressive symptoms.

Bupropion is converted via the cytochrome P450 2B6 isoenzyme to an active metabolite (9 hydroxy-bupropion). Because of its short half-life (approximately 8 hours for the parent compound and 12 hours for the active metabolite), bupropion has historically been administered in divided doses, although a once-daily preparation was recently released (Wellbutrin XL). For the regular-release product, the recommended starting dose is 100 mg BID, increasing to 100 mg TID after at least 3 days. Individual doses must not exceed 150 mg and should be given at least 6 hours apart.[190] With the SR formulation, initial daily doses are 150 mg QD, increased to 150 mg BID by the fourth day at the earliest. Individual doses of bupropion SR can be as large as 200 mg, and divided doses should be given at least 8 hours apart.[191] For the XL formulation, the package insert recommends initiating at 150 mg QD and increasing to 300 mg QD as early as the fourth day. Maximum daily doses are 450 mg for regular and XL products and 400 mg SR.

Because bupropion does not have a strong inhibitory effect on cytochrome P450 isoenzymes, it does not pose a significant risk for drug interactions. One exception is with concurrent administration of bupropion with venlafaxine in which a depression augmentation study reported a threefold increase in venlafaxine levels after the addition of bupropion 150 mg daily.[124]

Mirtazapine is another novel antidepressant capable of modulating serotonin and norepinephrine activity through a complex mechanism of action. In vitro studies reveal that mirtazapine is an antagonist at presynaptic α_2-autoreceptors and postsynaptic 5-HT2 and 5-HT3 receptors.[192] In addition, it appears to possess some mild inhibitory properties at serotonin reuptake transporters. Therefore, the net effect of mirtazapine is to enhance serotonin and norepinephrine in a manner that is clearly distinct from any other antidepressants. In a comparative randomized trial with fluoxetine for moderate to severe depression, mirtazapine appeared to be much more effective than the SSRI after 4 weeks of treatment (58% responders versus 30% with the SSRI; $P < .05$), but the differences were no longer significant at 6 weeks (63% versus 54%; $P = .67$).[193]

The most common adverse effects experienced with mirtazapine are sedation and weight gain. Because mirtazapine has potent antihistaminergic effects, it is considered to be quite sedating. Anecdotally, it has been reported that higher daily doses of mirtazapine (≥ 30 mg) are less sedating than lower doses owing to an increase in noradrenergic effects. In addition to the substantial risk of increasing appetite and total body weight, mirtazapine has also been associated with significant increases in total cholesterol and triglycerides.[194] The recommended starting dosage is 15 mg at bedtime, and the therapeutic dosage ranges from 15 to 45 mg/day.[194] Data from controlled trials have demonstrated safety and efficacy in doses up to 60 mg daily.[193,195]

Irreversible MAO inhibitors may also be an alternative for patients who have failed multiple antidepressant trials. Like venlafaxine, TCAs, and mirtazapine, MAO inhibitors are believed to relieve depressive symptoms by enhancing the activity of multiple neurotransmitters, which may be desirable for refractory cases. Since serious drug and dietary interactions are encountered with MAO inhibitors, candidates for treatment should be chosen carefully; a full discussion of the clinical usefulness of MAO inhibitors can be found in the section on depression with psychotic features.

Antidepressant Augmentation

17. Three months later, F.H. reports that she feels less hopeless on venlafaxine XL (75 mg/day) and that her appetite has improved as well. However, she is still somewhat depressed and lethargic and attempts to increase her dosage have been limited by nausea and recurring insomnia. What pharmacologic options remain to help manage her refractory depression?

Because F.H. has obtained considerable relief from her venlafaxine trial but is experiencing dose-limiting side effects, one would prefer to add a second medication (i.e., augmentation therapy) rather than changing antidepressants at this time (Table 79-18). A reasonable next step would be to augment her current venlafaxine regimen with another medication such as lithium, bupropion, or thyroid hormone. Lithium augmentation in refractory depression has been well documented. In one report, all 8 nonresponsive patients in a group of 35 unipolar, depressed patients who had been treated for 3 weeks with various therapeutic doses of a TCA responded to lithium augmentation within 2 days.[196] Six of the eight patients subsequently were reported to have maintained the improvement. However, the short trial of the TCA in this study weakens its validity because the apparent response to the lithium simply may be a reflection of the antidepressant finally starting to work. Nevertheless, other reports of successful lithium augmentation of various antidepressants in refractory depression have been reported, including augmentation of fluoxetine or MAO inhibitors.[196–200] After supplementation with lithium, clinical improvement was noted after several days or in some instances after 1 to 6 weeks.[196] The lithium dosage used is generally within the range used to treat bipolar disorder. In one report, when serum lithium concentration dropped to 0.3 mEq/L, the depression relapsed and improved again when the dose of lithium was increased to achieve a serum level between 0.8 and 1.2 mEq/L.[198] As with the use of lithium therapy in bipolar disorder, all appropriate clinical monitoring parameters should be followed carefully (see Chapter 80, Mood Disorders II: Bipolar Disorders).

Because both lithium and venlafaxine are serotonergic, the patient should be monitored for symptoms of the serotonin syndrome. Predictors of response to lithium augmentation

Table 79-18 Partial Response to Antidepressant Treatment Augmentation Strategies (with SSRI)

Ensure completion of full therapeutic trial (4–6 wk).
Ensure optimal dose of antidepressant.
Consider combination therapies:
- Bupropion
- Lithium
- Thyroid supplements
- Pindolol (?)
- Buspirone
- Atypical antipsychotics
- Modafinil
- Lamotrigine

have been studied. An immediate and marked response to the addition of lithium is considered to be predictive of a good outcome.[201] Age, gender, number of prior antidepressant trials, type of preceding antidepressant, or mean serum lithium concentration did not predict outcome to lithium augmentation.[202]

Bupropion has also been used successfully as an augmenting agent for many years.[203,204] Patients receiving SSRIs who continue to complain of fatigue or lethargy are excellent candidates, and the combination treatment is usually well tolerated. A prospective, open-label trial of this approach recently reported that approximately half of the patients converted to therapeutic responders.[204] With F.H., one should be mindful that bupropion may increase her venlafaxine levels and hasten the return of GI and CNS effects.[124] Although the stimulating properties of bupropion may help relieve her lethargy, it may also exacerbate her insomnia.

An alternative to adding lithium or bupropion would be augmentation with thyroid hormone, such as triiodothyronine or L-thyroxine. In a randomized, double-blind, placebo-controlled study of 2 weeks' duration, 50 nonpsychotically depressed outpatients who had failed to respond to TCA therapy responded equally well to both lithium or T_3 augmentation.[205] In contrast, an earlier controlled study indicated that thyroid hormone was no more effective than an additional 4 weeks of TCA.[206] The fundamental theory behind the use of thyroid hormone involves evidence supporting a role for thyroid dysfunction in refractory depression (e.g., there are increased or decreased thyroid hormone levels that are associated with increased or decreased β-adrenergic receptors in various animal models).[207]

Although F.H.'s thyroid function tests are within normal limits, it is possible that she suffers from a subtle form of thyroid dysfunction, such as a subclinical hypothyroidism, because depressed patients are more likely to have such conditions.[208] Triiodothyronine (Cytomel) at a dosage of 25 mg/day can accelerate response to imipramine (as measured by the HAM-D) in depressed patients and may be considered for F.H.[209,210] Thyroxine, at a dosage of 0.1 mg/day, is another option.[211] The response to the thyroid supplementation should be noticeable within 3 weeks, much like that found when lithium is used to augment therapy. Whether T_3 is superior to T_4 is not resolved, although one study seemed to indicate that more patients respond to the former than to the latter.[212]

Among other options, pindolol is a unique β-blocker with intrinsic sympathomimetic properties that has received some attention as an augmenting agent.[213] Early open-label studies and one double-blind, controlled trial suggested that pindolol may enhance or accelerate the therapeutic effects of other antidepressants.[213–215] These benefits were attributed, in part, to the inhibitory effects that pindolol has on the 5-HT$_{1A}$ autoreceptor.[216] A more recent double-blind investigation enrolled 86 depressed patients in an effort to compare the antidepressant effects of pindolol with those of placebo.[217] Patients were randomized to a combination of fluoxetine (20 mg every day) plus pindolol (2.5 mg three times a day) or fluoxetine plus placebo. After 6 weeks of treatment, there was no statistical advantage to pindolol augmentation in terms of the onset or extent of antidepressant effect. A 3-week, single-blind, crossover followed the initial study phase, and again no benefits from the β-blocker were evident. Given the obvious discrepancies in study results, further research appears warranted to adequately assess whether pindolol enhances response to SSRIs or other antidepressant medications.

Early success with the anticonvulsant lamotrigine as add-on therapy for bipolar disorder has sparked interest in this agent for depression augmentation.[218,219] A small double-blind trial of lamotrigine in fluoxetine-treated patients with refractory unipolar and bipolar depression found that doses titrated up to 100 mg daily produced nonsignificant improvements in depressive symptoms and significant decreases in overall psychopathology.[220] Other medications have also been used successfully to augment a partial response to antidepressants, although rigorous research trials are currently lacking. These medications include buspirone, methylphenidate, dextroamphetamine, estrogen, pramipexole, and modafinil.[221–226]

The Elderly

18. **R.M., a 71-year-old man, is brought in to see a primary care provider by his daughter with whom he has been living since the death of his wife 6 months ago. His daughter reports that R.M. had been in good health until his wife's death and that since that time he has been keeping to himself, showing little interest in social activities. She reports that he used to be a happy, outgoing person but is now very irritable and becomes agitated over insignificant things. Over the past 4 months, he has lost approximately 12 pounds and has trouble falling asleep. He used to be a voracious reader but seems uninterested in current events now. He appears to be confused or preoccupied at times and is incapable of understanding new concepts. His only documented medical problem is benign prostatic hypertrophy (BPH), and current medications consist of a stool softener and bulk laxative. Today's physical examination is normal, and the laboratory examination is significant only for a mildly elevated prostate-specific antigen (PSA) of 10.0 ng/mL.**

On mental status examination, R.M. is perceived to be a thin, nervous, sad-appearing elderly man. He is oriented ×3. His response to questions is slow, and his volume of speech is reduced. Affect is sad. Mood is dysthymic. He shows mild impairments in his ability to think through problems and perform simple mathematical exercises. There is no evidence of delusions, hallucinations, or paranoia. He denies suicidal thoughts but feels hopeless at present and admits "there's no reason to live anymore." How does a depressive episode in late life, such as that in R.M., differ from an episode earlier in life?

Depression in late life is typically more difficult to recognize compared with depression in younger adults. Clinicians and patients may inappropriately attribute depressive symptoms to the "aging process" and minimize their significance. In addition, functional expectations are often lowered after retirement, making the degree of impairment difficult to evaluate. As medical comorbidities are also more common in the elderly, depressive symptoms may be overlooked or misinterpreted in the workup as well.[227]

In general, the elderly present with the same depressive target symptoms as younger adults, which is reflected in the fact that DSM-IV-TR diagnosis for major depression in adults is not specific for age. However, qualitatively, the presentation of depression among the elderly may be quite different.[228] For instance, older patients are more likely to present with psychomotor retardation and are less likely to acknowledge "depression" per se, preferring instead to dwell on somatic concerns (e.g., poor sleep, low energy, changes in bowel function, bodily aches and pains). They also are much less likely to share or admit suicidal thoughts, and because elderly men have the highest suicide success rate, an accurate assessment of depression and attendant risks is critical (see Drug Selection).[229]

19. **What is R.M.'s differential diagnosis? Should he receive antidepressant therapy?**

In assessing nonspecific behavioral and cognitive symptoms in the elderly, a careful differential diagnosis between medical and other psychiatric disorders is essential because numerous medical illnesses can mimic depressive symptoms. Anemia, malignancies, and endocrine abnormalities may all present in a manner similar to that in depressive illness and can be ruled out only with a careful line of questioning and systematic physical workup.

One of the more difficult differential diagnoses in this setting involves the distinction of depression from dementia.[230,231] Like depression, patients with dementia may present with apathy, poor memory or concentration, reduced facial expression, and lack of spontaneous interaction. The illnesses are often comorbid because 30% to 70% of patients with dementia suffer from major depression as well.[231] Some experts have suggested, in fact, that new-onset depression in elderly patients may actually be part of a prodrome toward the manifestation of Alzheimer's dementia (AD).[231,232] A longitudinal cohort study found that, among elderly patients suffering from an acute episode of major depression, 57% were ultimately diagnosed with AD within the next 3 years.[230] Diagnostically, there are three notable differences between dementia and depression: (1) the symptoms (slow and subtle changes with dementia, rapid with depression), (2) orientation (markedly impaired with dementia, intact with depression), and (3) principal CNS impairment (short-term memory with dementia, concentration with depression).

Drug Selection

A therapeutic trial of an antidepressant in a depressed individual with cognitive impairment may reverse the symptoms of the affective illness and restore functional capacity. Cognitive function may improve to some degree also. Moreover, because primary degenerative dementia is largely a diagnosis of exclusion, a successful trial of an antidepressant may help clarify the underlying pathologic condition and is strongly recommended in patients with a positive personal or family history of mood disorders. Patients with dementia, in fact, may benefit from antidepressant therapy even if they do not present with a major mood disorder.[233,234] Overlapping pathophysiology and neuroanatomic dysfunction in these two disorders might explain the efficacy of antidepressants for selected symptoms of degenerative dementia. Although R.M.'s physical examination and laboratory workup were normal, a therapeutic trial of an antidepressant is warranted based on his current depressive target symptoms.

Phenylpiperazines: Trazodone and Nefazodone

20. **The decision was made to treat R.M. with nefazodone. What advantages and disadvantages does nefazodone possess compared with other antidepressants?**

Nefazodone and trazodone belong to the phenylpiperazine class of antidepressants. The therapeutic effects of these medications are believed to result from a modification of serotonergic activity, but the presumed mechanism is clearly distinct from SSRIs. Nefazodone and trazodone are only modest inhibitors of serotonin reuptake but block postsynaptic serotonin receptors (5-HT$_2$) most avidly.[235] Although SSRIs are considered "activating" antidepressants in most patients, phenylpiperazines are relatively sedating compounds that may be preferred for depressed patients such as R.M., who are suffering from anxiety and insomnia.

Compared with TCAs, phenylpiperazines possess weak anticholinergic properties (which is advantageous in a patient with prostatic hypertrophy and constipation) and are unlikely to cause weight gain or sexual dysfunction.[236] Nefazodone and trazodone do not have pronounced effects on cardiac conduction, although there have been case reports of trazodone aggravating ventricular arrhythmias.[237] However, these cardiovascular effects do not appear to present a problem in R.M. based on his medical history.

Although R.M. is not suicidal, the safety of antidepressants in overdose is a major concern when treating the depressed elderly. Suicide is among the top 10 causes of death in individuals older than 65 years, and depressed older men who were recently widowed have the highest success rate for committing suicide among all demographic groups.[238] Both nefazodone and trazodone appear to be very safe in overdose, and there are no confirmed reports of fatalities with either drug when taken alone in supertherapeutic doses.[239,240]

The side effects most commonly reported with the phenylpiperazines are related to their sedating potential. Although trazodone is believed to be more sedating than nefazodone, both drugs may impair alertness and result in morning drowsiness ("hangover") even when administered at bedtime. Although early controlled clinical trials of trazodone demonstrated significant clinical benefit for treating depression (at dosages of 300 to 600 mg/day), many patients cannot tolerate the sedating properties of this agent, and its role in the clinical setting is now largely limited to routine use as a sedative-hypnotic (bedtime doses of 25 to 100 mg).[241,242]

Orthostatic hypotension is another potential side effect with the phenylpiperazines, and trazodone poses a higher risk in this regard as well.[243] In the elderly, orthostasis can be a major concern because of the risk of falls.[244] Fortunately, the orthostatic potential of trazodone (or nefazodone) is highest when plasma concentrations peak (i.e., 4 to 6 hours after ingestion), which generally occurs when patients are asleep. Nevertheless, elderly patients should be warned of this potential effect. Nonpharmacologic measures to minimize orthostatic hypotension include cautioning the patient to avoid rising from a lying or sitting position too quickly (i.e., arising slowly over at least a minute); maintaining adequate ambulation, hydration, and salt intake (unless contraindicated by cardiovascular disease [e.g., CHF]); and wearing support hose.

Nefazodone has been associated with rare, life-threatening liver failure with an approximate incidence of one case per 250,000 patient years.[166] Trazodone has been associated with a rare, painful, and idiosyncratic condition known as priapism (persistent abnormal erection of the penis). Although the reported incidence of priapism is 0.016% in men receiving trazodone, many practitioners believe that there is an underappreciation of this phenomenon; because this side effect can often result in surgical intervention and impotence, vigilance is advised.[245]

Based on nefazodone's pharmacologic properties and safety record, it appears to be an excellent choice in a patient such as R.M., who is experiencing agitation and insomnia. The dosing recommendations for the general population were originally to start at 100 mg twice a day and increase to a minimum of 300 mg daily (divided doses).[166] However, clinical experience suggests that this approach may be a bit aggressive and that the medication may be administered once daily at bedtime, potentially improving tolerability and adherence.[246] For elderly patients, the dosing recommendations are approximately half those of the general population, so a reasonable starting dosage for R.M. may be 50 mg at bedtime. If R.M. tolerates this initial regimen, his bedtime dose may be slowly advanced toward a minimal therapeutic dose in elderly patients of 100 to 150 mg/day.

Tricyclic Antidepressants (TCAs)

21. B.H. is an obese 52-year-old man suffering from his first episode of major depressive disorder. He has an 8-year history of congestive heart failure (CHF) (New York Heart Association [NYHA] functional class II) with an ejection fraction of 35% and atrial fibrillation. He is currently taking digoxin 0.25 mg PO QD and enalapril 10 mg PO BID. His CHF has been well controlled on this regimen, and he remains asymptomatic with regard to the CHF. His atrial fibrillation occurs about once every 6 months. All other laboratory parameters are within normal limits. His cardiologist works for a health maintenance organization (HMO) that requires that patients fail a TCA before other antidepressants (e.g., SSRIs) can be prescribed. How do the TCAs compare with the SSRIs in general, and is it reasonable for an HMO to enforce this policy?

For many years, the TCAs were the most popular class of medications used to treat depression. Over time, clinicians developed considerable confidence with the effectiveness of TCAs and familiarity with gradual dosage titration practices. The acquisition cost for TCAs is quite low, and there are some providers who continue to prefer this class of medication for the treatment of severe or melancholic depression.[247] TCAs continue to be prescribed for other indications as well (e.g., migraine prophylaxis, chronic pain). Unfortunately, TCAs possess a variety of adverse effects, ranging from bothersome (dry mouth, sedation, constipation) to serious (cardiovascular effects), which often prevent patients from receiving therapeutic doses of medication.[248] Patient adherence with prescribed medication may be compromised with TCAs as well.[249] This relatively high side-effect burden can also discourage clinicians from prescribing TCAs for elderly patients or those with certain medical conditions (e.g., benign prostatic hypertrophy, cardiac arrhythmias, narrow-angle glaucoma, dementia).

The discovery of SSRIs was heralded as a major breakthrough in the pharmacologic management of depressive symptoms, and collectively these medications have emerged as preferred agents for the treatment of depression.[250] Their popularity can be attributed to numerous advantages over older compounds, including a lower side-effect burden, safety in overdose, less dosage titration, once-daily administration, and patient preference. Results of a meta-analysis concluded that, although the overall efficacy of the two antidepressant classes was comparable, primary care patients receiving an SSRI were much less likely to discontinue therapy prematurely because of to side effects.[251] Although SSRIs are more expensive than TCAs, this additional cost may be offset by enhanced medication adherence rates and decreased relapse rates, as has been demonstrated in several pharmacoeconomic analyses.[250,252,253]

Side Effects

22. B.H.'s cardiologist is concerned about the effect of a TCA on his cardiac status. What are the general major adverse effects and toxicities of the TCAs, and how should these be managed?

The most common adverse effects of the TCAs are listed in Table 79-12. Anticholinergic effects are commonly encountered with the TCAs and may adversely effect adherence.[254] These side effects include dry mouth, blurred vision, constipation, and urinary retention. Although patients may develop tolerance to these effects, they may never disappear completely. Clinicians should be prepared to counsel patients about the appropriate way to manage these problems. Patients with dry mouth, for instance, may tend to drink excessive fluids to relieve discomfort. To minimize the inherent potential for weight gain with TCAs, patients should be advised to avoid caloric beverages and drink water or dietetic fluids instead. Sugarless gum or hard candy is often recommended as well.

TCAs also can be very sedating and are usually administered at bedtime to minimize functional impairments. Confusion or memory deficits also may occur with TCAs and can be particularly onerous in elderly patients. The secondary amines may be more tolerable in this regard, but all TCAs can impair concentration or alertness to some extent.

The impact of TCAs on cardiovascular function is a legitimate and serious concern. The most potentially dangerous adverse effect of the TCAs is their quinidine-like properties (type IA) on prolonging cardiac conduction through the His-Purkinje system. This, in conjunction with positive chronotropic and adrenergic-blocking properties of the TCAs, can lead to re-entry arrhythmias (e.g., torsades de pointes and other ventricular arrhythmias). In patients with pre-existing conduction defects and in overdose, there is a greater risk for cardiac arrhythmias.[255] Therefore, B.H. should receive a baseline electrocardiogram (ECG) before therapy.

Orthostatic hypotension is the most common and troublesome cardiovascular effect of the TCAs and MAO inhibitors and can result in significant morbidity and mortality.[256,257] Major clinical consequences of orthostatic hypotension include falls leading to bone fractures, lacerations, and even MI.[258] Patients with CHF, such as B.H., are at greatest risk for developing orthostatic hypotension.[259]

Imipramine and nortriptyline have been best studied with respect to their association with orthostatic hypotension. Amitriptyline, desipramine, doxepin, and clomipramine also are capable of producing it to varying degrees.[260–265] Although systematic comparisons of the propensity of the TCAs to cause orthostatic hypotension generally are lacking, the tertiary amines (e.g., imipramine) may cause more severe orthostatic hypotension than the secondary amines (e.g., nortriptyline), and research evidence supports the contention that nortriptyline has the lowest risk for causing orthostatic hypotension among TCAs.[255,266]

Antidepressants and Cardiac Disease

23. Will the choice of antidepressant affect B.H.'s arrhythmia?

Differences among antidepressants and antidepressant classes with regard to safety in cardiac disease are susbstantial. The SSRIs, in general, appear to be relatively safe in patients with a history of arrhythmias or recent MI.[267] In a placebo-controlled investigation, hospitalized patients with unstable cardiac disease were randomized to either sertraline or placebo.[268] Overall, both treatment arms were very well tolerated, and there was actually a lower risk of severe cardiac events reported in the sertraline group (versus placebo). Retrospective data suggest that SSRIs may be somewhat cardioprotective in depressed patients with heart disease, a benefit that might be explained by their ability to decrease platelet activation.[269,270]

TCAs increase heart rate, probably via intrinsic anticholinergic properties that increase sinus node activity. Clinically, this effect generally is not significant, especially in medically healthy, depressed patients.[271] However, it may be important in those with underlying conduction disease, coronary artery disease, or CHF. TCAs, when used at therapeutic dosages for the treatment of depression, decrease premature atrial and ventricular contractions in both depressed and nondepressed patients.[272,273] Antidepressants with class 1A antiarrhythmic activity (e.g., TCAs) also may have arrhythmogenic activity and thus increase the chances of ventricular arrhythmias and sometimes of sudden death. This effect on rhythm and conduction is believed to be related to the inhibitory effects of TCAs on the fast sodium channels and a decrease in Purkinje fiber action potential amplitude, membrane responsiveness, and slowed conduction.[273] Even nortriptyline, which is believed to be one of the safer TCAs in patients with heart disease, was associated with a greater risk for adverse cardiac events than paroxetine in a randomized controlled trial.[274]

Bupropion and mirtazapine appear unlikely to affect cardiac rhythm and induce arrhythmias in susceptible patients.[267] Bupropion, however, should be used with caution in patients with pre-existing hypertension because of potential increases in BP.[275] Its safety has not been well studied in patients with heart disease. Similarly, venlafaxine does not appear to be arrhythmogenic, but increases in BP may be seen with higher dosages (>150 mg daily) limiting its usefulness in certain patient populations.[187] The nonselective MAO inhibitors do not seem to affect rhythm significantly, although they generally do slow heart rate.[276] Other antidepressant medications such as trazodone, nefazodone, amoxapine, and maprtiline may affect rhythm and cause clinically significant arrhythmias.[267]

Plasma Concentration Monitoring

24. Are plasma concentrations clinically useful in monitoring antidepressant therapy? When should plasma antidepressant concentrations be obtained?

Attempts to demonstrate an association between plasma concentrations and therapeutic response for SSRIs, venlafaxine, and bupropion have been largely unsuccessful. In contrast to the newer agents, the serum concentration of some TCAs correlates well with clinical response. Nortriptyline exhibits a curvilinear effect, whereas imipramine demonstrates a sigmoidal relationship between serum levels and clinical response.[277,278] Maximum benefit of imipramine usually is associated with serum levels of imipramine plus its demethylated metabolite, desipramine, in excess of 250 ng/mL. The relationship between plasma concentration of desipramine and clinical response is less clear, but it appears that a linear relationship is likely.[279] The most controversy surrounds amitriptyline—studies have shown a linear relationship, a curvilinear relationship, and no relationship between serum concentration and outcome.[280–282]

The APA Task Force on the Use of Laboratory Tests in Psychiatry recommends plasma concentration monitoring when patients are elderly, not responding to therapy, nonadherent, experiencing adverse effects, or on multiple medications that may result in a possible drug interaction.[283] Plasma concentrations of imipramine, nortriptyline, and desipramine should be obtained after at least 1 week of a constant dosage when steady state has been achieved. Samples should be drawn 12 hours after the last dose has been administered. Routine therapeutic blood monitoring of other antidepressants is not recommended because information concerning their usefulness is limited; however, serum levels may be useful for evaluating adherence in some patients or ruling out serious toxicities.[284]

Other Medical Comorbidities
Diabetes

25. B.L. is a 43-year old woman who has become increasingly depressed over the past 4 months after the unexpected death of her father. She mentions that she was very upset immediately following his death, unable to sleep at night, and frequently crying at work. These symptoms have not abated in the months that have passed since that time. She is slightly obese and has always been 'borderline diabetic', but her blood sugar control has worsened since her father's death and she has subsequently gained 30 pounds (HbA$_{1c}$ = 8.2 last week, up from 6.1, 4 months ago). She is very upset that she has recently been diagnosed with type 2 diabetes and does not believe that she is capable of following the lifestyle modifications recommended. How strong is the association between depression and diabetes? Would an antidepressant be an appropriate treatment for her symptoms at this time and, if so, which agent(s) would be recommended?

The potential association of depression with diabetes has been discussed in the medical literature for over 300 years.[285] Results of a recent meta-analysis confirmed that diabetic patients are twice as likely to be suffering from depression than the general population, an association that appears to hold true for type 1 and type 2 diabetic illness.[286] Theories abound as to why diabetic patients become depressed, citing complex physiologic, psychological, and social factors, and a precise explanation has not been elucidated. Conversely, longitudinal studies have shown that depressed patients are twice as likely to develop type 2 diabetes with time, and in 80% to 90% of cases, the mood disorder preceded the metabolic condition.[287] It has also been established that depressed diabetic patients are much more likely to suffer long-term complications with

this metabolic disorder, and successful treatment of depression has been demonstrated to improve glycemic indices.[288–290]

Successful treatment of mood disorders in patients with diabetes is important for several reasons. Patients with depression or diabetes are at risk for cardiovascular illness, and successful antidepressant treatment, therefore, may substantially improve morbidity and mortality. Depressed patients are also much less likely to comply with treatment recommendations in general because of their hopelessness, cognitive impairment, and social isolation. As a result, they are three times more likely to stop taking their medications, leading to a worsening of other medical conditions.[291] Most depressed patients also report a change in their appetite at baseline, which may lead to a compromise in blood sugar control. Moreover, decreases in energy and motivation may sabotage diabetes treatment plans as well.

Although the number of clinical studies conducted with depressed diabetic patients is limited, antidepressants appear to possess the same efficacy rates for this particular comorbidity as previously found in the general population.[290] At the present time, there is not any evidence to suggest that one class of antidepressant is any more efficacious than another. Selection of an antidepressant in the diabetic population, therefore, rests largely on differences in adverse effect profiles and potential for drug interactions.

One important consideration in selecting an antidepressant is the potential impact of the agent on appetite, blood sugar control, and total body weight. Although research on the effects of antidepressants on glycemic control is preliminary and limited to rat populations, important differences appear to exist among antidepressants in regard to weight gain potential.[292] As discussed previously, the risk of clinically significant weight gain appears to be highest with mirtazapine, TCAs, and MAO inhibitors, and these medications should be avoided. Although SSRIs and venlafaxine may occasionally induce weight gain in susceptible patients (estimated incidence of 3% to 5%), this adverse effect appears to be of greatest concern with paroxetine (25% incidence). Since bupropion may cause appetite supression in some patients, there is a theoretical concern about hypoglycemia in diabetic patients, although case reports of this phenomenon are currently lacking. Other antidepressants, including nefazodone and trazodone, are less likely to adversely effect appetite and weight control.

Because one of the long-term complications of diabetes is sexual dysfunction, this potential side effect of antidepressants may also be worth considering. It should be emphasized, however, that erectile dysfunction and impotence are most commonly encountered by male diabetics. Thus, although the SSRI may impair sexual performance by delaying or preventing orgasm, this impairment occurs at a different stage of the sexual process and would not necessarily discourage use of SSRIs. Erectile problems are much less common with SSRIs, although this side effect has been reported to occur occasionally with TCAs and MAO inhibitors.

Pharmacokinetic drug interactions may also be a concern for certain antidepressants in diabetic patients. For instance, many of the oral antidiabetic agents are substrates for metabolism by the cytochrome P450 isoenzyme system. Inhibition of this metabolic step may precipitate a serious drug interaction by increasing plasma concentrations of the antidiabetic agents and enhancing hypoglycemic effects. Several of these agents are metabolized via the CYP 2C9 isoenzyme (e.g., tolbutamide, glyburide, glipizide, rosiglitazone), and the administration of certain SSRIs (e.g., fluoxetine or fluvoxamine) may potentiate their effects. Repaglinide and some of the sulfonylureas are metabolized via the CYP 3A4 isoenzyme, which may be inhibited by nefazodone, fluvoxamine, or norfluoxetine.

For B.L., the depressive symptoms she experienced after her father's death may be considered a natural response to this serious loss. Diagnostically, this is considered to be a grief reaction (or bereavement) if it occurs during the first 2 months after the event and does not necessarily require a course of antidepressant treatment. Because her symptoms have persisted for considerably longer, it is advisable that her depression receive serious attention (i.e., thorough assessment of psychiatric condition) and necessary treatment. Medical history, previous antidepressant trials, and concurrent use of other presciption medications should be investigated as well. If B.L. is amenable to an antidepressant, an SSRI that is unlikely to induce weight gain or potentiate drug interactions may be a prudent choice. Such agents would include sertraline, citalopram, or escitalopram.

Epilepsy

26. C.B., a 20-year-old woman, was recently diagnosed with major depressive disorder, single episode. Since the age of 8, she has also experienced complex partial seizures. Her seizures have been difficult to control in the past (at least six seizures per month), but her condition has improved recently (none for 8 months) on a combination of carbamazepine and gabapentin. Are there any special considerations with regard to antidepressant selection in this patient?

Although seizures are a relatively uncommon effect of antidepressant medications, they are frightening and serious when they occur. The overall risk of seizures with most antidepressants is quite low at therapeutic dosages, and, as a result, the precise risk is difficult to quantify with any statistical certainty.[293] Furthermore, the risk of new-onset seizures in the general population (i.e., not necessarily receiving antidepressants) is approximately 0.073% to 0.086% annually, suggesting the likelihood of occasional coincidental case reports.[294] Among the antidepressants marketed in the United States, imipramine may be the best studied, and the frequency of seizures was reported to be 0.1% among patients prescribed therapeutic dosages ($\leq$200 mg/day).[295]

Generally, it is believed that iatrogenic seizures are a dose-related phenomenon, so it is not surprising that most case reports of antidepressant seizures have involved overdose ingestions, most commonly with the TCAs. Seizures have been correlated to peak plasma concentrations of tricyclics (e.g., levels >1,000 ng/mL) and typically occur within 6 hours after the overdose.[296]

The specific antidepressant may also be of some importance, but one may wish to recall the methodologic difficulties inherent in estimating accurate figures. An older review cited amoxapine with the highest risk of seizures in overdose, followed by maprotiline and the TCAs (collectively).[297] Bupropion was withdrawn from the market in 1986 after the appearance of new-onset seizures in bulimic patients receiving

the antidepressant as part of a placebo-controlled trial (4 of 69 subjects).[298] After a re-examination of the original dosing recommendations, bupropion was released again in 1989, and a new SR preparation appeared in 1998. Among the 3,100 patients to receive the new preparation for up to 1 year, the cumulative seizure risk was 0.15%.[299] Although SSRIs have been associated with seizures in acute overdose, the comparative risk encountered with dosages in the therapeutic range has not been determined.

Because of C.B.'s seizure history, choosing a medication with a low risk of seizures is prudent. Bupropion, for instance, is contraindicated in patients with a pre-existing seizure disorder.[190] Because carbamazepine has a narrow therapeutic index and is metabolized by multiple isoenzymes within the cytochrome P450 system, antidepressants that may inhibit its clearance and raise plasma levels, such as nefazodone (CYP 3A4), fluoxetine (CYP 2D6), and paroxetine (CYP 2D6), should be avoided. Similarly, carbamazepine may induce the metabolism of certain TCAs, and it also possesses some of the cardiotoxic effects of these antidepressants (e.g., slowed conduction) further discouraging its use. Among the remaining alternatives, one may opt for an SSRI less likely to inhibit metabolic pathways (e.g., sertraline, citalopram) or venlafaxine.

AIDS

27. K.H., a 33-year-old HIV-positive woman, has been reasonably healthy over the past 2 years but recently developed AIDS after an episode of oral candidiasis. During the last few months, she has noticed a loss of interest in life, accompanied by decreased energy, easy fatigability, and difficulty concentrating (she has to read a sentence several times before she can comprehend its meaning). She also reports a depressed mood but denies suicidal ideation. Her current medications are zidovudine (Retrovir), lamivudine (Epivir), ritonavir (Norvir), and oral clotrimazole troche (Mycelex). After a thorough medical workup, other opportunistic infections have been ruled out. What precipitating factors may be contributing to K.H.'s current symptoms of depression?

Patients with terminal illnesses such as HIV/AIDS or certain cancers are faced with an extreme psychosocial stressor that can precipitate a depressive episode. Research evaluating the severity of emotional distress in persons with HIV has shown elevated anxiety, depression, social isolation, and suicidal ideation.[300] Chronic depression in AIDS patients has, in fact, been associated with an acceleration of the disease progression, as well as a significant reduction in the perceived quality of life (versus nondepressed HIV-infected controls).[301,302] K.H. currently is, or will be, confronted with a number of psychological issues, including fear of developing an opportunistic infection, chronic somatic preoccupations, debilitation, anger, possible death at a young age, and reactive depression.[303,304]

Although K.H.'s target symptoms (fatigue, decreased concentration, and depressed mood) may represent a depressive episode secondary to psychosocial stressors, her differential diagnosis also includes HIV-1–associated cognitive/ motor complex or dementia resulting from HIV disease (formally known as *AIDS dementia complex*).[305] HIV-associated dementia closely resembles the symptoms of a depressive disorder and is part of the Centers for Disease Control and Prevention classification system for HIV infection (category C).[306] Neoplasms and opportunistic infections of the CNS secondary to AIDS also can alter mental status. However, a thorough medical workup ruled out opportunistic infection in K.H.

28. Based on K.H.'s target symptoms, is she a candidate for antidepressant therapy? What considerations should be made when selecting antidepressant therapy for K.H.?

K.H. would benefit from antidepressant therapy to help ameliorate her target symptoms of decreased energy, lack of concentration, and depressed mood, regardless of whether it is a major depressive episode or direct HIV involvement within the CNS. However, several factors should be taken into account when selecting antidepressant medication in an HIV/AIDS patient. In general, comparative trials of SSRIs and TCAs have been associated with high dropout rates because of adverse effects, suggesting that HIV/AIDS patients may be more vulnerable to toxic effects or that lower doses of antidepressant medications should be used.[307,308]

Drug interactions can be a primary concern as well because several of the protease inhibitors undergo metabolic transformation via the cytochrome P450 system, primarily through the CYP 3A4 and CYP 2B6 isoenzymes. Therefore, nefazodone, fluvoxamine, and fluoxetine are best avoided. Among the alternatives, SSRIs and TCAs have demonstrated comparable efficacy in the depressed HIV/AIDS population, but the side-effect profile and burden of SSRIs may be more tolerable to these patients. Bupropion has become increasingly popular in depressed HIV/AIDS patients, and the activating properties may be attractive in this particular patient.[309] Inhibition of bupropion metabolism has been demonstrated with concurrent administration of ritonavir, efavirenz, and nelfinavir, however, which may restrict its use among certain patients.[310] Low-dose psychostimulants (e.g., methylphenidate, dextroamphetamine) also may be helpful because some limited evidence has demonstrated improved cognition and mood in AIDS patients.[311] For appetite stimulation, mirtazapine would also be a reasonable option in some AIDS patients, although the sedating potential should be carefully considered. An additional option may be ECT, which has been administered safely and effectively to the depressed AIDS population as well.[312]

Depression With Atypical Features (Atypical Depression)
Monoamine Oxidase Inhibitors

29. G.R., a 38-year-old, 73-kg woman, presents at the university outpatient psychiatric clinic with a chief complaint of extreme lethargy and depressed mood more days than not for the past 6 weeks. During this period, she has had trouble with sleeping too much and overeating (she says she has gained at least 10 pounds in this time frame). On interview, she also reports an intense fear of heights and consequently does not travel if it involves driving over a bridge or flying in an airplane. She reports that this episode seems to have started around the time of the break-up with her boyfriend, and she becomes extremely anxious and tearful in revealing this piece of her history. Her psychiatric history is consistent with at least two other similar depressive episodes, the first when she was 18 years old and the second occurring around age 25. She currently weighs 73 kg, and her physical examination and laboratory assessments are within

normal limits. In the past, she has exhibited a poor response to trials of fluoxetine and nortriptyline. During her last episode, she is noted to have responded to phenelzine 60 mg/day.

G.R.'s depressive illness manifests differently from that expected in most cases of depression. How is this depression of G.R. different from melancholic depression?

G.R. suffers from hysteroid dysphoria, more commonly known as atypical depression (Table 79-19). DSM-IV-TR now refers to it as depression with atypical features.[15] Clinically, atypical depression generally has been regarded as a fairly heterogenous group of depressive symptoms that represent a form of depressive illness. The term atypical depression first was used to describe patients with some symptoms of depression who experienced worsening of mood in the evening, lethargy, phobic and somatic anxiety, and emotional overreactivity to environmental events. These patients typically responded well to treatment with an MAO inhibitor.[313] Atypical depression also describes patients with phobic anxiety who may not have concurrent depression; those with a reversal of endogenous vegetative shifts in sleep, appetite, and diurnal variation in mood (i.e., hypersomnia, hyperphagia, and a mood that is good in the morning and progressively worsens through the day); and those with depression lacking endogenous symptoms.[314]

In studying atypical depression, one group of investigators has identified a set of explicit operational criteria for atypical depression (the "Columbia" criteria) based on the literature and their own clinical experience.[315] Briefly, the requirements are as follows: Patients must meet criteria for DSM depressive disorder; however, they are excluded if they have pervasive anhedonia (i.e., they have a mood reactivity or enjoy some activities or daily experiences). Furthermore, they must have at least two of the following: (1) hypersomnia, (2) leaden paralysis (profound lethargy), (3) hyperphagia, or (4) pathologic sensitivity to interpersonal rejection (rejection sensitivity). The features of atypical depression and melancholia are compared in Table 79-19.

G.R. reports a depressed mood, extreme lethargy, phobic avoidance of bridges or high places, and a recent problem with hypersomnia and hyperphagia with subsequent weight gain. She also seems to have a prominent rejection sensitivity regarding the relationship with her boyfriend.

Table 79-19 A Comparison of Atypical Depression and Melancholia

Feature	Atypical Depression	Melancholia
Onset	Teens (or younger)	Thirties (avg)
Gender	Females >>> males	Females > males
Course	Chronic	Episodic
Phenomenology		
Appetite/weight	Increased	Decreased
Sleep	Increased	Decreased
Energy	Low with leaden paralysis	Low
Reaction to rejection	Very sensitive	Indifferent
Treatment response	MAO inhibitor ≥ SSRI ≥ TCA	MAO inhibitor = TCA = SSRI

MAO, monoamine oxidase; SSRI, selective serotonin reuptake inhibitor; TCA, tricyclic antidepressant.

DOSAGE TITRATION

30. **What medication would you recommend for G.R.? Outline a dosage titration and treatment plan.**

For the treatment of depression, the modern pharmacologic era was ushered in by the discovery of iproniazid, an antitubercular medication and potent inhibitor of MAO.[316] Subsequent research with this MAO inhibitor ultimately led to the formulation of the biogenic amine hypothesis of depression, and it influenced antidepressant drug development for the next 20 years.

Although the MAO inhibitors, most notably phenelzine and tranylcypromine, were commonly prescribed for the treatment of depression in the 1970s and 1980s, their popularity has waned in recent years primarily because of the risks of serious drug–drug and drug–food interactions.[317] However, for the treatment of atypical depression, the MAO inhibitors are among the most effective pharmacologic agents available and are still prescribed for patients with this depressive subtype usually after failing an SSRI. Double-blind trials featuring MAO inhibitors versus TCAs have consistently demonstrated a superior response to the MAO inhibitors and a controlled trial comparing moclobemide with fluoxetine reported that the MAO inhibitor was superior as well.[318,319,320] Limited data comparing TCAs with SSRIs for atypical depression suggest that the two classes are comparable in efficacy, and both were superior to placebo.[321]

Because of G.R.'s positive response to phenelzine in the past, this choice of an antidepressant would be reasonable, but one should ask about the patient's previous experience with this medication (therapeutic effects, side effects, adherence, duration of treatment, and reason for discontinuation). If phenelzine is to be re-initiated, the starting dosage would be 30 mg/day (15 mg in morning and 15 mg at noon). This dosage should then be increased by 15 mg every week to a target dose of 60 mg/day by 14 days. Some investigators have recommended measuring platelet MAO activity and using this as an index of clinical outcome—the idea being that good response has been associated with MAO inhibition of at least 80%.[322] However, the availability of this laboratory parameter at most institutions is limited. G.R. should be carefully followed up clinically for resolution of target symptoms over a 4- to 6-week period. If further adjustments in his dosage are indicated, phenelzine may be increased by 15 mg/week to a maximum of 90 mg/day.

ADVERSE EFFECTS

31. **During this period of phenelzine therapy, G.R. should be monitored closely for suicidal ideation, especially because the MAO inhibitors are potentially lethal when taken in overdose. What adverse effects of the nonselective MAO inhibitors should be looked for in G.R. while she is being treated with phenelzine?**

Orthostatic hypotension, weight gain, edema, and sexual dysfunction are common during MAO inhibitor therapy.[323] As is the case with the TCAs, the nonselective MAO inhibitors can cause clinically significant postural decreases in BP. However, with the MAO inhibitors, the mechanism is thought to be a direct sympatholytic effect because both the lying and the standing systolic BP readings are decreased.[324,325] Phenelzine seems to cause orthostatic hypotension more commonly than does tranylcypromine.[326] Because the orthostatic hypotension appears to be dose related, a reduction in dosage may be helpful.[327] For more difficult cases, orthostatic hypotension has been managed pharmacologically by the addition of 25 mg/day of

triiodothyronine or initiation of fludrocortisone 0.025 to 0.05 mg once to twice a day.[328] Monitoring for BP changes as well as edema and serum electrolyte changes (e.g., hypokalemia) is paramount if these pharmacologic interventions are used. MAO inhibitor–induced weight gain may be managed by monitoring carbohydrate and fat intake. Edema can be treated by elevating the affected limbs and/or using a thiazide diuretic (e.g., hydrochlorothiazide 25 to 50 mg twice a day), with careful monitoring of other medications (e.g., serum lithium levels) for potential drug interactions.[328] Sexual dysfunction occurs in up to 20% of patients taking MAO inhibitors but may diminish and disappear spontaneously over time.[322,329] If necessary, it can be managed with bethanechol (Urecholine) at dosages up to 50 mg/day in both men and women.[323]

A switch into mania has been reported in up to 10% of patients with a history of bipolar disorder. Therefore, MAO inhibitors should be avoided in this population.[323] Although MAO inhibitors are not known as antimuscarinic medications, some patients complain of anticholinergic-like side effects, including blurred near vision and urinary retention. Dosage reduction may be helpful, but these effects may also diminish over time. Paresthesias also have been reported with the MAO inhibitors and can be treated with pyridoxine 50 to 150 mg/day.[330] The nonselective MAO inhibitors are not associated with proarrhythmic, antiarrhythmic, or contractility effects when used in therapeutic dosages.

DRUG–FOOD INTERACTIONS

32. **G.R. states that what she most fears is the "cheese reaction." What steps can be taken to avoid it?**

The "cheese reaction," also known as hypertensive crisis, is so named because it occurred in patients who were taking nonselective MAO inhibitors and ingested foods high in tyramine, a byproduct of tyrosine metabolism that is found in certain foods and beverages, such as aged cheese or Chianti wine (Table 79-20). When tyramine is ingested in the absence of an MAO inhibitor, it is rapidly metabolized by MAO in the GI tract before systemic absorption. In the presence of an MAO inhibitor, relatively high concentrations of tyramine may be achieved in circulation, resulting in the displacement of norepinephrine (and other catecholamines) from presynaptic storage granules. Norepinephrine surges out into the synapse, and as metabolic degradation is inhibited by the MAO inhibitor, a profound pressor response is triggered.[331] Systolic BP as high as 160 to 220 mm Hg and diastolic BP readings in the range of 100 to 130 mm Hg can occur.[332] The event is heralded by severe headache (occipital and temporal), stiff neck, flushing, a choking sensation, palpitations, diaphoresis, and nausea and vomiting. Hypertensive crisis can occur at any time after ingesting the tyramine-containing food and probably is not related to MAO inhibitor dosage or duration of therapy.[323] Reports of hypertensive crisis are sporadic and difficult to quantify. About 8% of phenelzine patients and 2% of tranylcypromine patients reported hypertensive reactions based on a chart review of 198 patients taking MAO inhibitors.[323] However, it is a relatively rare event and certainly is found less often than MAO inhibitor–related hypotension.

Patients who are to receive nonselectives should be reliable and willing to comply with food and medication restrictions. This adverse event can be minimized with a low-tyramine diet that begins several days before starting the MAO inhibitor and

Table 79-20	**Foods Containing Tyramine**

High Amounts of Tyramine[a]

Smoked, aged, or pickled meat or fish
Sauerkraut
Aged cheeses such as Swiss and cheddar
Yeast extracts
Fava beans

Moderate Amounts of Tyramine[b]

Beer
Avocados
Meat extracts
Red wines such as Chianti

Low Amounts of Tyramine[c]

Caffeine-containing beverages
Distilled spirits
Chocolate
Soy sauce
Cottage and cream cheese
Yogurt and sour cream

[a]May not consume.
[b]May consume in moderation.
[c]May consume.
Adapted from Shulman KI et al. Dietary restriction, tyramine, and the use of monoamine oxidase inhibitors. J Clin Psychopharmacol 1989;9:397.

continues for 3 to 4 weeks after stopping the MAO inhibitor. The severity of the cheese reaction is related to the amount of tyramine in any given food (i.e., 20 mg of tyramine can produce a severe hypertensive reaction), and the amount of tyramine can vary greatly in "high-tyramine food items."[333,334] Foods that absolutely should not be consumed with nonselective MAO inhibitors include aged cheeses, concentrated yeast extracts, fava beans, and sauerkraut.[335] Likewise, consumption of any food that has spoiled, is overripe, or has fermented, even if it is not found in the restricted list, should be avoided. Foods that typically contain tyramine and therefore should be avoided or consumed with caution when taking an MAO inhibitor are listed in Table 79-20.

33. How should an MAO inhibitor–induced hypertensive crisis be managed in G.R.?

A hypertensive crisis should be considered a medical emergency. In a hospital setting, general supportive measures are used, with attention to respiratory, metabolic, and cardiovascular systems. The urine should be acidified (e.g., with vitamin C) and IV α-blockers are often given (e.g., phentolamine [Regitine] 5 mg IV followed by 0.25 to 0.50 mg IV every 4 to 6 hours). On occasion, patients have also received prescriptions for nifedipine with instructions to carry the medication with them and administer a 10 mg sublingual dose (if necessary).[336]

DRUG–DRUG INTERACTIONS

34. What common drug–drug interactions are associated with the nonselective MAO inhibitors?

Several potentially fatal drug–drug interactions occur with this group of antidepressants. Like the reaction with tyramine, indirect sympathomimetics such as phenylpropanolamine and pseudoephedrine (common ingredients in over-the-counter cold preparations and diet pills) can cause a precipitous rise in

BP that can result in cerebrovascular accident. Meperidine (Demerol) can cause a life-threatening interaction with MAO inhibitors that is somewhat reminiscent of serotonin syndrome. This reaction is a result, in part, of the MAO inhibitor interfering with the degradation of the meperidine and is manifested by agitation, hyperthermia, and circulatory collapse.[337] Other narcotic analgesics do not appear to have this effect when combined with MAO inhibitors.

The potential for inducing serotonin syndrome with the combination of SSRIs and MAO inhibitors has been well chronicled. A washout period of at least 14 days should separate the use of an SSRI and an MAO inhibitor. Because fluoxetine (and its primary active metabolite norfluoxetine) has a much longer half-life, the recommended washout period is at least 5 weeks after discontinuing this particular SSRI.[338]

Depression With Psychotic Features (Psychotic Depression)

35. R.S., a 41-year-old man, is brought to the crisis stabilization unit (CSU) by the police because of extremely agitated behavior. His wife had called the police because R.S. was on the roof of their home with a gun shooting into the shingles. R.S. had worried for some time that the mortgage balance on the house was too large; now he was yelling that the house was "killing his spirit" and that he could not handle it any longer. He had told his wife that he was "inadequate as a provider" for her and their two children. In your interview with him at the CSU, he tells you that for the past week he has been hearing the voice of his deceased father telling him to kill himself after destroying the house. This has distressed him greatly. Of note, he recently was fired from his job as a computer analyst. His sleep is reported by his wife to be poor over the past month with difficulties in falling asleep as well as waking up during the night being unable to resume sleeping. His mood is depressed and he has lost 15 pounds in the past 2 weeks as a result of decreased appetite. His psychiatric history is positive for two past episodes of depression, one at age 22 and the other at age 35. Both episodes resolved after 8-week courses of imipramine 250 mg/day. He is diagnosed with major depressive disorder, recurrent, with psychotic features, and is admitted to the adjacent hospital for treatment. What features of psychotic depression are evident with R.S.?

Psychotic depression, also known as *delusional depression* or *depression with psychotic features,* is a type of affective illness (either unipolar or bipolar) in which the individual manifests with primary mood symptoms found in major depression and also demonstrates secondary psychotic features, such as delusions (fixed, false beliefs) and/or hallucinations (generally auditory). This disorder may be regarded as an extreme form of depression in which the individual's mood is so disturbed that perception is significantly impaired or distorted. Endocrine abnormalities and imaging studies strongly suggest that depression with psychotic features is distinct from unipolar depression, and there is evidence that it more closely resembles bipolar illness. Psychotic depression has been estimated to occur in at least 5% of the depression admissions to acute care hospitals in the United States, and it may be comparatively more common in the geriatric population.[339]

The delusions and hallucinations encountered with psychotic depression can be classified as either mood congruent or mood incongruent. Mood-congruent psychotic features imply that the psychosis is consistent with the depressive illness. In depression, mood-congruent delusions might include self-deprecatory thoughts, extreme feelings of guilt, sinfulness, or nihilistic ideation. Mood-incongruent psychotic features imply that the psychotic content is not consistent with the overall mood but, rather, is bizarre, much like that seen in schizophrenia. An example of mood-incongruent features may be a giggle or grin as a patient describes his or her misery and desire to commit suicide.

R.S. described mood-congruent hallucinations when he spoke of his dead father commanding him to kill himself. His ideas of being inadequate and not a good provider also are consistent with a mood-congruent delusion.

36. Why is it critical to resolve R.S.'s psychotic depression promptly? Why would ECT be preferred over pharmacotherapy for R.S.?

Psychotic depression is associated with much greater morbidity and mortality than other forms of major depression and also carries a higher risk of suicide than other types of depressive illness. This factor currently is a major concern in R.S.'s case because he has reported suicidal ideation. Psychotic depression is also fairly refractory to monotherapy.[340,341] Because of these two factors, ECT and combination treatment (i.e., antidepressant plus an antipsychotic) are considered first-line treatments for the disorder.[342] ECT has a success rate of 80% to 85% in this otherwise refractory form of depression and is the treatment of choice for R.S.

Antidepressant Plus Antipsychotic

37. If ECT is contraindicated in R.S. (or otherwise unavailable), how should his condition be treated?

If pharmacotherapy is used in R.S., the historical approach has been to prescribe an antipsychotic medication in addition to an antidepressant medication. The combination of an antipsychotic and an antidepressant has proved to be superior to either component alone in psychotic depression.[339] Several combination products are available that contain both an antipsychotic and an antidepressant, and, although these combination products probably work as well as the individual components, they are fixed-dose combinations and the dosage is more difficult to titrate than the dosages of the individual agents. In psychotic depression, as the psychosis lifts, it is reasonable to taper and discontinue the antipsychotic agent while maintaining the antidepressant medication for a full course of treatment.[343] Results of a recent investigation featuring fluoxetine and perphenazine demonstrated that the discontinuation of the antipsychotic agent after 5 weeks of combination treatment was not associated with high relapse rates.[343] If the antipsychotic drug is continued after the psychosis has lifted, the patient may be at greater risk for the neurotoxic effects of the antipsychotic (e.g., pseudoparkinsonism, tardive dyskinesia) as well as an increased side effect burden overall.

Individual Agents

Atypical antipsychotics, such as risperidone and olanzapine, are believed to possess some antidepressant properties, which has led researchers to consider their usefulness as monotherapy for this disorder.[344] There is still some controversy as to whether the atypical agents are relieving depressive symptoms or the negative symptoms of schizophrenia; however, their ability to block post-synaptic 5-HT$_2$ receptors is reminiscent of the principle pharmacologic actions of phenylpiperazines (e.g., trazodone and nefazodone), suggesting genuine antidepressant properties. Furthermore, their proven efficacy in treating bipolar disorder may suggest some clinical benefit in managing refractory depression or depression with psychotic features. At present, evidence supporting their use in psychotic depression is preliminary. The most rigorous trial compared the effects of risperidone with combination therapy with haloperidol and amitriptyline.[345] Although combination treatment did appear to be more efficacious, risperidone produced substantial declines in depression and general psychopathology. Several case reports suggest that the atypical antipsychotics are worthy of additional study.[346-348] High acquisition costs, substantial weight gain, and sedation are potential deterrents to their widespread use, however, in treating mood disorders.

An older option for treating psychotic depression is amoxapine, a metabolite of the antipsychotic loxapine (Loxitane). Amoxapine is an effective antidepressant medication that retains some of the dopamine-blocking activity of the parent compound. Some clinicians prefer amoxapine in psychotic depression because of these dual pharmacologic effects and because, as a single agent, it facilitates adherence.[349] Amoxapine is also effectively a fixed-dose preparation and thus has the inflexibility of not being able to titrate the antidepressant and antipsychotic independently. Like the fixed-dose combination products, amoxapine also would place the patient at some risk for developing adverse effects associated with antipsychotic medications (e.g., dystonia, pseudoparkinsonism, akathisia, neuroleptic malignant syndrome, galactorrhea, tardive dyskinesia) and is extremely dangerous in overdose situations.[350-352]

In summary, Table 79-21 offers seven points that everyone should know about depression.

Table 79-21 Patient Education

Seven Things That Everyone Should Know About Depression

- **Depression is NOT a personality flaw or a weakness of character.**
  Depression has been associated with a chemical imbalance in the nervous system, which can be easily corrected with antidepressant medications and associated counseling.
- **All antidepressants are equally effective.**
  Approximately 65% of patients receiving a therapeutic trial of any antidepressant medication will have a beneficial response.
- **Most patients receiving antidepressants will experience some side effect(s) initially.**
  Identify an accessible health professional who can answer your questions.
- **Antidepressants should be taken at the same time daily.**
  This will make it easier for you to remember to take the medication and may also minimize side effects.
- **The response to antidepressants is delayed.**
  Several weeks may pass before you begin to feel better and it may take 4 to 6 weeks before maximal benefits are evident.
- **Antidepressants must be taken for at least 6 to 9 months.**
  Even if you are feeling completely better, studies have shown that people who stop their medication during the first 6 months are much more likely to become depressed again.
- **Antidepressants are NOT addictive substances.**
  Antidepressants may elevate the moods of depressed individuals but they do not act as stimulants and are not associated with craving or other abuse patterns. However, if certain antidepressants are discontinued abruptly, mild withdrawal reactions may occur.

REFERENCES

1. Andreasen NC. The Broken Brain: The Biological Revolution in Psychiatry. New York: Harper & Row, 1984:36.
2. Ustun TB, Sartorius N, eds. Mental Illness in General Healthcare: An International Study. London: John Wiley & Sons, 1995.
3. Wells KB et al. The functioning and well-being of depressed patients. JAMA 1989;262:914.
4. Greenberg PE et al. The economic burden of depression in 1990. J Clin Psychiatry 1993;54:405.
5. The Cross-National Collaborative Group. The changing rate of major depression. JAMA 1992; 268:3098.
6. Narrow WE, Rae DS, Robbins LN, Regier DA. Revised prevalence estimates of mental disorders in the United States. Arch Gen Psychiatry 2002; 59:115.
7. Kessler RC et al. The epidemiology of major depressive disorder—results from the national comorbidity survey replication (NCS-R). JAMA 2003; 3095.
8. Hirschfeld RMA, Cross CK. Epidemiology of affective disorders. Arch Gen Psychiatry 1982;29:35.
9. Hollingshead AB, Redlich FC. Social Class and Mental Illness. New York: Wiley, 1958.
10. Kanowski S. Age-dependent epidemiology of depression. Gerontology 1994;40(Suppl 1):1.
11. Lieb R et al. Parental major depression and the risk of depression and other mental disorders in offspring: a prospective-longitudinal community study. Arch Gen Psychiatry 2002;59:365.
12. McGuffin P, Katz R. The genetics of depression and manic-depressive disorder. Br J Psychiatry 1989; 155:294.
13. Blehar MC et al. Family and genetic studies of affective disorders. Arch Gen Psychiatry 1988;4 5.289.
14. Kraepelin E. Manic Depressive Insanity and Paranoia. Edinburgh: ES Livingstone, 1921.
15. American Psychiatric Association. Diagnostic and Statistical Manual of Mental Disorders. 4th Ed. Text Revision. (DSM-IV-TR). Washington, DC: American Psychiatric Association; 2000.
16. Thase ME, Friedman ES. Is psychotherapy an effective treatment for melancholia and other severe depressive states? J Affect Disorder 1999;54:1.
17. Thase ME et al. A placebo-controlled, randomized clinical trial comparing sertraline and imipramine for the treatment of dysthymia. Arch Gen Psychiatry 1996;53:777.
18. Kocsis JH. Pharmacotherapy for chronic depression. Am J Psychol 2003;59:885.
19. Blazer D. Depression in the elderly. N Engl J Med 1989;320:164.
20. Schildkraut JJ. Neuropsychopharmacology and the affective disorders. N Engl J Med 1969;281:302.
21. Maas JW. Biogenic amines and depression. Arch Gen Psychiatry 1975;32:1357.
22. Prange AJ. L-tryptophan in mania: contribution to a permissive hypothesis of affective disorders. Arch Gen Psychiatry 1974;30:56.
23. Stahl SM. Basic psychopharmacology of antidepressants, part 1: antidepressants have seven distinct mechanisms of action. J Clin Psychiatry 1998;59(Suppl 4):5.
24. Schatzberg A, Rosenbaum A. Studies on MHPG levels as predictors of antidepressant response. McLean Hosp J 1980;6:138.
25. Kramer MS et al. Distinct mechanism for antidepressant activity by blockade of central substance p receptors. Science 1998;281:1640.
26. Gold PW, Drevets WC, Charney DS. New insights into the role of cortisol and the glucocorticoid receptor in severe depression. Biol Psychiatry 2002;52:381.
27. Nemeroff CB. New directions in the development of antidepressants: the interface of neurobiology and psychiatry. Hum Psychopharmacol 2002; 17(Suppl 1):13.
28. Siever LJ, Davis KL. Overview: toward a dysregulation hypothesis of depression. Am J Psychiatry 1985;142:1017.
29. Charney DS et al. Receptor sensitivity and the mechanisms of action of antidepressant treatment. Arch Gen Psychiatry 1981;381:1160.
30. Bonate PL. Serotonin receptor subtypes: functional, physiological, and clinical correlates. Clin Neuropharmacol 1991;14:1.
31. Palacios JM et al. Distribution of serotonin receptors. Ann NY Acad Sci 1990;600:36.
32. Stahl SM. Psychophsarmacology of Antidepressants. London: Martin Dunitz, Ltd, 1997.
33. Risch SC, Nemeroff CB. Neurochemical alterations of serotonergic neuronal systems in depression. J Clin Psychiatry 1992;53(Suppl 10):3.
34. Mann JJ et al. Serotonin and suicidal behavior. In: Witaker-Azmitia PM, Peroutka SJ, eds. The Neuropharmacology of Serotonin. Ann NY Acad Sci 1990;600:476–484.
35. Delgado PL et al. Serotonin function and the mechanism of antidepressant action. Arch Gen Psychiatry 1990;47:411.
36. Stahl SM. The psychopharmacology of energy and fatigue. J Clin Psychiatry 2002;63:7.
37. Miller HL et al Noradrenergic function and clinical outcome in antidepressant pharmacotherapy. Neuropsychopharmacology 2001;24:617.
38. Bremner JD et al. Regional brain metabolic correlates of alpha-methylparatyrosine-induced depressive symptoms: implications for the neural circuitry of depression. JAMA 2003;289:3125.
39. Morely JE, Shafer RB. Thyroid function screening in new psychiatric admissions. Arch Intern Med 1982;42:591.
40. Nemeroff CB, Evans DL. Thyrotropin-releasing hormone (TRH), the thyroid axis, and affective disorder. Ann NY Acad Sci 1989;553:304.
41. Fauci AS et al, eds. Principles of Internal Medicine, 14th Ed. New York: McGraw-Hill, 1998.
42. Banki CM et al. Cerebrospinal fluid corticotropin-releasing factor-like immunoreactivity in depression and schizophrenia. Am J Psychiatry 1987;144:873.
43. Gold PN, Rubinow DR. Neuropeptide function in affective illness corticotrophin releasing hormone and somatostatin as model systems. In: Meltzer HY, ed. Psychopharmacology: The Third Generation of Progress. New York: Raven, 1987:617.
44. Wolkowitz OM, Reus VI. Treatment of depression with antiglucocorticoid drugs. Psychosom Med 1999;5:698.
45. Belanoff JK et al. An open label trial of C-1073 (mifepristone) for psychotic major depression. Biol Psychiatry 2002;5:386.
46. George MS et al. SPECT and PET imaging in mood disorders. J Clin Psychiatry 1993;54:6.
47. Nemeroff CB. The neurobiology of depression. Sci Am 1998;278:42.
48. Mayberg HS. Modulating dysfunctional limbic-cortical circuits in depression: towards development of brain-based algorithms for diagnosis and optimised treatment. Br Med Bull 2003;65:193.
49. Detre TP et al. The assessment of the patient and examination, disposition and management. In: Detre TP et al, eds. Modern Psychiatric Treatment. New York: JB Lippincott, 1971:15.
50. Shea SC. Psychiatric Interviewing: The Art of Understanding, 2nd Ed. Philadelphia: WB Saunders, 1998.
51. Carlat DJ. The Psychiatric Interview: A Practical Guide. Baltimore: Lippincott Williams & Wilkins, 1999.
52. Fankhauser MP, German ML. Understanding the use of behavioral rating scales in studies evaluating the efficacy of antianxicty and antidepressant drugs. Am J Hosp Pharm 1987;44:2087.
53. Hamilton M. A rating scale for depression. J Neurol Neurosurg Psychiatry 1960;23:56.
54. Beck AT et al. An inventory for measuring depression. Arch Gen Psychiatry 1961;4:561.
55. Zung WK. A self-rating depression scale. Arch Gen Psychiatry 1965;12:63.
56. Derogatis LR et al. The Hopkins Symptom Checklist (HSCL): a self-report symptom inventory. Behav Sci 1974;19:1.
57. Montgomery SA, Asberg M. New depression scale designed to be sensitive to change. Br J Psychiatry 1979;134:382.
58. Radloff LS. The CES-D scale: a self-report depression scale for research in the general population. Appl Psychol Measurement 1977;1:385.
59. Rush AJ et al. The inventory for depressive symptomatology (IDS): preliminary findings. Psychiatr Res 1986;18:65.
60. Irwin M et al. Screening for depression in older adults. Arch Intern Med 1999;159:1701.
61. Ribeiro SCM et al. The DST as a predictor of outcome in depression: a meta analysis. Am J Psychiatry 1993;150(11):1618.
62. American Psychiatric Association Task Force on the Use of Laboratory Tests in Psychiatry. The dexamethasone suppression test: an overview of its current status in psychiatry. Am J Psychiatry 1987;144:1253.
63. Covinsky KE et al. Depressive symptoms and 3-year mortality in older hospitalized medical patients. Ann Intern Med 1999;130:563.
64. Schulberg H et al. Treating major depression in primary care practice: eight month clinical outcomes. Arch Gen Psychiatry 1996;53:913.
65. Keller MB et al. A comparison of nefazodone, the cognitive behavioral-analysis system of psychotherapy, and their combination for the treatment of chronic depression. N Engl J Med 2000;342:1462.
66. Arnow BA, Constantino MJ. Effectiveness of psychotherapy and combination treatment for chronic depression. J Clin Psychol 2003;59:893.
67. Brody DS et al. Strategies for counseling depressed patients by primary care physicians. J Gen Int Med 1994;9;569
68. Sadock BJ, Sadock VA. Synopsis of Psychiatry, 9th Ed. Baltimore: Lippincott Williams & Wilkins, 2003.
69. Persad E. Electroconvulsive therapy in depression. Can J Psychiatry 1990;35:175.
70. Abrams R. Electroconvulsive therapy in the medically compromised patient. Psychiatr Clin North Am 1991;14-871.
71. Devanand DP et al. Electroconvulsive therapy in the treatment-resistant patient. Psychiatr Clin North Am 1991;14:905.
72. Shapira B et al. Cost and benefit in the choice of ECT schedule. Br J Psychiatry 1998;172:44.
73. Sackheim HA et al. Continuation pharmacotherapy in the prevention of relapse following electroconvulsive therapy: a randomized controlled trial. JAMA 2001;285:1299.
74. Glass RM. Electronconvulsive therapy; time to bring it out of the shadows. JAMA 2001;285:1346.
75. Gross F, Gysin F. Phototherapy in psychiatry: clinical update and review of indications. Encephale 1996;22:143.
76. Wehr TA. Manipulations of sleep and phototherapy: nonpharmacological alternatives in the treatment of depression. Clin Neuropharmacol 1990;13:S54.
77. Lawlor DA, Hopker SW. The effectiveness of exercise as an intervention in the management of depression: systematic review and meta-regression analysis of randomized controlled trials. Br Med J 2001;322:763.
78. Gershon AA, Dannon PN, Grunhaus L. Transcranial magnetic stimulation in the treatment of depression. Am J Psychiatry 2003;160:835.
79. Trivedi MH. Treatment-resistant depression: new therapies on the horizon. Ann Clin Psychiatry 2003;15:59.
80. Kaplan HI, Saddock BJ, eds. Synopsis of Psychiatry. 9th Ed. Baltimore: Lippincott Williams & Wilkins, 2003.
81. Nierenberg AA, Wright EC. Evolution of remission as the new standard in the treatment of depression. J Clin Psychiatry 1999;60(Suppl 22):7.
82. Katz MM et al. Can the effects of antidepressants be observed in the first two weeks of treatment? Neuropsychopharmacology 1997;17:110.
83. Montgomery S. Are two week trials sufficient to indicate efficacy? Psychopharmacology Bull 1995; 31:41.

84. Hotopf M et al. Discontinuation rates of SSRIs and tricyclic antidepressants: a meta-analysis and investigation of heterogeneity. Br J Psychiatry 1997;170:120.

85. Edwards JG, Anderson I. Systematic review and guide to selective serotonin reuptake inhibitors. Drugs 1999;57:507.

86. Dubovsky SL. Beyond the serotonin reuptake inhibitors: rationale for the development of new serotonergic agents. J Clin Psychiatry 1994; 55(Suppl 2):34.

87. Preskorn SH. Comparison of the tolerability of bupropion, fluoxetine, imipramine, nefazodone, paroxetine, sertraline and venlafaxine. J Clin Psychiatry 1995;56(Suppl 6):12.

88. Vogel GW et al. Drug effects on REM sleep and on endogenous depression. Neurosci Biobehav Rev 1990;14:49.

89. Finley PR. Selective serotonin reuptake inhibitors: pharmacologic profiles and potential therapeutic distinctions. Ann Pharmacother 1994;28:1359.

90. Leo RJ. Movement disorders associated with selective serotonin reuptake inhibitors. J Clin Psychiatry 1996;57:449.

91. Lipinski JF et al. Fluoxetine-induced akathisia: clinical and theoretical implications. J Clin Psychiatry 1989;50:339.

92. Di Mascio M et al. Selective serotonin reuptake inhibitors reduce the spontaneous activity of dopaminergic neurons in the ventral tegmental area. Brain Res Bull 1998;46:547.

93. Gregorian RS, Golden KA, Bahce A, Goodman C, Kwong WJ, Khan ZM. Antidepressant-induced sexual dysfunction. Ann Pharmacother 2002;36: 1577.

94. Physicians' Desk Reference, 48th Ed. Montvale, NJ: Medical Economics Data, 1994:879.

95. Patterson WM. Fluoxetine-induced sexual dysfunction. J Clin Psychiatry 1993;54:71.

96. Lee HS et al. An open-label trial of fluoxetine in the treatment of premature ejaculation. J Clin Psychopharmacol 1996;16:379.

97. Modell JG et al. Comparative sexual side effects of bupropion, fluoxetine, paroxetine and sertraline. Clin Pharmacol Ther 1997;61:476.

98. Waldinger MD et al. Effect of SSRI antidepressants on ejaculation: a double-blind, randomized, placebo-controlled study with fluoxetine, fluvoxamine, paroxetine and sertraline. J Clin Psychopharmacol 1998;18:274.

99. Vida S, Looper K. Precision and comparability of adverse event rates of newer antidepressants. J Clin Psychopharmacol 1999;19:416.

100. Schatzberg AF, Cole JO, DeBattista C. Manual of clinical psychopharmacology, 4th Ed. Washington DC: American Psychiatric Publishing, 2003.

101. Mercadante S. Hyoscine in opioid-induced sweating. J Pain Symp Manage 1998;15:214.

102. Romanelli F et al. Possible paroxetine-induced bruxism. Ann Pharmacother 1996;30:1246.

103. Ellison JM, Stanziani P. SSRI-induced nocturnal bruxism in four patients. J Clin Psychiatry 1993; 54:432.

104. Rugh JD, Harlan J. Nocturnal bruxism and temporomandibular disorders. Adv Neurol 1988; 49:329.

105. Kirby D, Ames D. Hyponatremia and selective serotonin re-uptake inhibitors in elderly patients. Int J Geriatr Psychiatry 2001;16:484.

106. Arinzon ZH, Lehman YA, Fidelman ZG, Krasnyansky II. Delayed recurrent SIADH associated with SSRIs. Ann Pharmacother 2002;36:1175.

107. Levine LR et al. Use of a serotonin re-uptake inhibitor, fluoxetine, in the treatment of obesity. Int J Obes 1987;11(Suppl 3):185.

108. Sussman N, Ginsberg D. Weight gain associated with SSRIs. Primary Psychiatry 1998;1:28.

109. Richelson E. Weight gain on SSRIs: a paradox? Primary Psychiatry 1998;1:40.

110. Fava M, Judge R, Hoog SL, Nilsson ME, Koke SC. Fluoxetine versus sertraline and paroxetine in major depressive disorder: changes in weight with long-term treatment. J Clin Psychiatry 2000; 61:863.

111. Wernicke JF et al. Fixed dose fluoxetine therapy for depression. Psychopharmacol Bull 1987; 23:164.

112. Fabre LF. Sertraline safety and efficacy in major depression: a double-blind fixed-dose comparison with placebo. Biol Psychiatry 1995;38:592.

113. Dunner DL, Dunbar GC. Optimal dose regimen for paroxetine. J Clin Psychiatry 1992;53(Suppl 2):21.

114. Feighner JP. Fixed dose study of citalopram in depression (poster). American Psychiatric Association (annual meeting), 1997.

115. Burke WJ, Gergel I, Bose A. Fixed-dose trial of the single isomer escitalopram in depressed outpatients. J Clin Psychiatry 2002;63:331.

116. Cohen JS. Ways to minimize adverse drug reactions: individual doses and common sense are key. Postgrad Med 1999;106:163.

117. Finley PR et al. Case management of depression by clinical pharmacists in a primary care setting. Formulary 1999;34:864.

118. Wernicke JF et al. Low dose fluoxetine therapy for depression. Psychopharmacol Bull 1988; 24:180.

119. Casper RC, Redmond DE, Katz MM, Schaffer CB, Davis JM, Koslow SH. Somatic symptoms in primary affective disorder: presence and relationship to the classification of depression. Arch Gen Psychiatry 1985;42:1098.

120. Shen WW, Hsu JH. Female sexual side effects associated with selective serotonin reuptake inhibitors: a descriptive clinical study of 33 patients. Int J Psychiatry Med 1995;25:239.

121. Rothschild AJ. Selective serotonin reuptake inhibitor-induced sexual dysfunction: efficacy of a drug holiday. Am J Psychiatry 1995;152:1514.

122. Labbate LA, Pollack MH. Treatment of fluoxetine-induced sexual dysfunction with bupropion: a case report. Ann Clin Psychiatry 1994;6:13.

123. Ashton AK, Rosen RC. Bupropion as an antidote for serotonin reuptake inhibitor-induced sexual dysfunction. J Clin Psychiatry 1998;59:112.

124. Kennedy SH et al. Combining bupropion SR with venalafaxine, paroxetine or fluoxetine: preliminary report on pharmacokinetic, therapeutic, and sexual dysfunction effects. J Clin Psychiatry 2002;63:181.

125. Masand PS, Ashton AK, Gupta S, Frank B. Sustained-release bupropion for selective serotonin reuptake inhibitor-induced sexual dysfunction: a randomized, double-blind, placebo-controlled, parallel-group study. Am J Psychiatry 2001; 158:805.

126. Rosen RC, Lane RM, Menza M. Effects of SSRI on sexual function: a critical review. J Clin Psychopharmacol 1999;19:67.

127. Nurnberg HG et al. Treatment of antidepressant-associated sexual dysfunction with sildenafil. JAMA 2003;289:56.

128. Shen WW, Urosevich Z, Clayton DO. Sildenafil in the treatment of female sexual dysfunction induced by selective serotonin reuptake inhibitors. J Reprod Med 1999;44:535.

129. Aizenberg D et al. Cyproheptadine treatment of sexual dysfunction induced by serotonin reuptake inhibitors. Clin Neuropharmacol 1995;18:320.

130. Assalian P, Margolese HC. Treatment of antidepressant-induced sexual side effects. J Sex Marital Ther 1996;22:218.

131. Shrivastava RK et al. Amantadine in the treatment of sexual dysfunction associated with selective serotonin reuptake inhibitors. J Clin Psychopharmacol 1995;15:83.

132. Norden MJ. Buspirone treatment of sexual dysfunction associated with selective serotonin re-uptake inhibitors. Depression 1994;2:109.

133. Jacobsen FM. Fluoxetine-induced sexual dysfunction and an open-label trial of yohimbine. J Clin Psychiatry 1992;53:119.

134. Michelson D, Bancroft J, Targum S, Kim Y, Tepner R. Female sexual dysfunction associated with antidepressant administration: a randomized, placebo-controlled study of pharmacologic intervention. Am J Psychiatry 2000;157:239.

135. Cohen AJ, Bartlik B. Ginkgo biloba for antidepressant-induced sexual dysfunction. J Sex Marital Ther 1998;24:139

136. Delgado PL et al. Treatment strategies for depression and sexual dysfunction. J Clin Psychiatry 1999;17:15 [Monograph 1].

137. Depression Guideline Panel. Clinical Practice Guideline Number 5: Depression in Primary Care. Volume 2: Treatment of Depression. Rockville, MD: US Dept of Health and Human Services, Agency for Health Policy and Research 1993. AHCPR publication 93-0550.

138. Greden JF. Antidepressant maintenance medications: when to discontinue and how to stop. J Clin Psychiatry 1993;54(Suppl 8):39.

139. Alexopoulos GS et al. Recovery in geriatric depression. Arch Gen Psychiatry 1996;53:305.

140. Zajecka J et al. Discontinuation symptoms after treatment with serotonin reuptake inhibitors: a literature review. J Clin Psychiatry 1997;58:291.

141. Judd LL. The clinical course of unipolar major depressive disorders. Arch Gen Psychiatry 1997; 54:989.

142. Nonacs R, Cohen LS. Depression during pregnancy: diagnosis and treatment options. J Clin Psychiatry 2002;63 (Suppl 7):24.

143. Altshuler LL et al. Course of mood and anxiety disorders during pregnancy and the postpartum period. J Clin Psychiatry 1998;59(Suppl 2):29.

144. Lamberg L. Safety of antidepressant use in pregnant and nursing women. JAMA 1999;282:222.

145. Orr ST, Miller CA. Maternal depressive symptoms and the risk of poor pregnancy outcome: review of the literature and preliminary findings. Epidemiol Rev 1995;17:165.

146. Pastuszak A et al. Pregnancy outcome following first trimester exposure to fluoxetine. JAMA 1993;269:2246.

147. Chambers CD et al. Birth outcomes in pregnant women taking fluoxetine. N Engl J Med 1996;335:1010.

148. Nulman I et al. Neurodevelopment of children exposed in utero to antidepressant drugs. N Engl J Med 1997;336:258.

149. Kulin NA et al. Pregnancy outcome following maternal use of the new selective serotonin reuptake inhibitors. JAMA 1998;279:609.

150. Simon GE, Cunningham ML, Davis RL. Outcomes of prenatal antidepressant exposure. Am J Psychiatry 2002;159:2055.

151. Laine K, Heikkinen T, Ekblad U, Kero P. Effects of exposure to selective serotonin reuptake inhibitors during pregnancy on serotonergic symptoms in newborns and cord blood monoamine and prolactin concentrations. Arch Gen Psychiatry 2003;60:720.

152. Spigstet O, Hagg S. Excretion of psychotropic drugs into breast milk: pharmacokinetic overview and therapeutic implications. CNS Drugs 1998;9:111.

153. Wisner KL et al. Serum sertraline and n-desmethylsertraline levels in breast-feeding mother-infant pairs. Am J Psychiatry 1998;155:690.

154. Jefferson JJ. Drug interactions: friend or foe? J Clin Psychiatry 1998;59(Suppl 4):37.

155. Mitchell PB. Drug interactions of clinical significance with selective serotonin reuptake inhibitors. Drug Saf 1997;6:390.

156. Greenblatt DJ et al. Human cytochromes and some new antidepressants: kinetics, metabolism and some drug interactions. J Clin Psychopharmacol 1999;19(Suppl 1):23.

157. Gram LF et al. Citalopram: interaction studies with levomepromazine, imipramine and lithium. Ther Drug Monit 1993;15:18.

158. von Moltke LL et al. Escitalopram (s-citalopram) and its metabolites in vitro: cytochromes mediating the biotransformation, inhibitory effects, and comparison to r-citalopram. Drug Metab Dispos 2001;29:1102.

159. Jefferson JW, Griest JH. Brussel sprouts and psychopharmacology: understanding the cytochrome P450 system. Psychiatr Clin North Am 1996;3:205.

160. Crewe HK et al. The effect of selective serotonin re-uptake inhibitors on cytochrome P4502D6

(CYP2D6) activity in human liver microsomes. Br J Clin Pharmacol 1992;34:262.

161. Preskorn SH et al. Pharmacokinetics of desipramine coadministered with sertraline or fluoxetine. J Clin Psychopharmacol 1994;14:90.

162. Brosen K et al. Inhibition by paroxetine of desipramine metabolism in extensive but not in poor metabolizers of sparteine. Eur J Clin Pharmacol 1993;44:349.

163. Watkins PB. Noninvasive tests of CYP3A enzymes. Pharmacogenetics 1994;4:171.

164. Barbhaiya RH et al. Coadministration of nefazodone and benzodiazepines: II. A pharmacokinetic study with triazolam. J Clin Psychopharmacol 1995;15:320.

165. Green DS et al. Coadministration of nefazodone and benzodiazepines: III. A pharmacokinetic study with alprazolam. J Clin Psychopharmacol 1995;15:399.

166. Anon. Nefazodone prescribing information. Bristol-Myers Squibb Company: Princeton NJ, 2002.

167. Sporer KA. The serotonin syndrome—implicated drugs, pathophysiology and management. Drug Saf 1995;13:94.

168. Sternbach H. The serotonin syndrome. Am J Psychiatry 1991;148:705.

169. Lappin RI, Auchincloss EL. Treatment of serotonin syndrome with cyproheptadine. N Engl J Med 1994;331:1021.

170. Sandyk R. L-dopa induced 'serotonin syndrome' in a parkinsonian patient on bromocriptine. J Clin Psychopharmacol 1986;6:194.

171. Guze BH, Baxter LR. The serotonin syndrome: case responsive to propranolol. J Clin Psychopharmacol 1986;6:119.

172. Graber MA et al. Sertraline-phenelzine drug interaction: a serotonin syndrome reaction. Ann Pharmacother 1994;28:732.

173. Iruela LM et al. Toxic interaction of S-adenosylmethionine and clomipramine. Am J Psychiatry 1993;150:522.

174. Lantz MS, Buchalter E, Giambanco V. St. John's Wort and antidepressant drug interactions in the elderly. J Geriatr Psychiatry Neurol 1999;12:7.

175. Nirenberg AA et al. Trazodone for antidepressant-induced insomnia. Am J Psychiatry 1994;151:1069.

176. Paykel ES et al. Residual symptoms after partial remission: an important outcome in depression. Psychol Med 1995;25:1171.

177. Schweizer E et al. What constitutes an adequate antidepressant trial for fluoxetine? J Clin Psychiatry 1990;51:8.

178. Brown WA, Harrison W. Are patients who are intolerant to one serotonin selective reuptake inhibitor intolerant to another? J Clin Psychiatry 1995;56:30.

179. Bull SA, Hunkeler EM, Lee JY, Rowland CR, Williamson TE, Schwab JR, Hurt SW. Discontinuing or switching selective serotin-reuptake inhibitors. Ann Pharmacother 2002;36:578.

180. Thase ME, Ferguson J, Wilcox C. Citalopram treatment of paroxetine intolerant patients. Depress Anxiety 2002;16:128.

181. Calabrese JR, Londberg PD, Shelton MD, Thase ME. Citalopram treatment of fluoxetine-intolerant depressed patients. J Clin Psychiatry 2003; 64:562.

182. Kirwin JL, Goren JL. Duloxetine: an antidepressant that inhibits both norepinephrine and serotonin uptake. Formulary 2003;38:29.

183. Poirier MF, Boyer P. Venlafaxine and paroxetine in treatment resistant depression. Br J Psychiatry 1999;175:12.

184. Clerc GE et al. A double-blind comparison of venlafaxine and fluoxetine in patients hospitalized for major depression and melancholia. Int Clin Psychopharmacol 1994;9:139.

185. Thase ME, Entsuah MR, Rudolph RL. Remission rates during treatment with venlafaxine or selective serotonin reuptake inhibitors. Br J Psychiatry 2001;178:234.

186. Diamond S et al. Serotonin syndrome induced by transitioning from phenelzine to venlafaxine: four patient reports. Neurology 1998;51:274.

187. Anon. Effexor product labeling information. Philadelphia, PA: Wyeth Ayerst 2003.

188. Ascher JA et al. Bupropion: a review of its mechanism of antidepressant activity. J Clin Psychiatry 1995;56:395.

189. Jain AK, Kaplan RA, Gadde KM et al. Bupropion SR vs placebo for weight loss in obese patients with depressive symptoms. Obes Res 2002;10:1049.

190. Anon. Wellbutrin product labeling information. Research Triangle Park, NC: Burroughs Wellcome, 1989.

191. Anon. Wellbutrin SR product labeling information. GlaxoSmithKline: Research Triangle Park, NC, 2002.

192. De Boer T. The effects of mirtazapine on central noradrenergic and serotonergic neurotransmission. Int Clin Psychopharmacol 1995;10(Suppl 4):19.

193. Wheatley DP, van Moffaert M, Timmerman L, Kremer CM. Mirtazapine: efficacy and tolerability in comparison with fluoxetine in patients with moderate to severe major depressive disorder. J Clin Psychiatry 1998;59:306.

194. Anon. Remeron product labeling information. West Orange, NJ: Organon, 1996.

195. Guelfi JD, Timmerman L, Korgaard S. Mirtazapine versus venlafaxine in hospitalized severely depressed patients with melancholic features. J Clin Psychopharmacol 2001;21:425.

196. de Montigny C. Lithium induces rapid relief of depression in tricyclic antidepressant drug nonresponders. Br J Psychiatry 1981;138:252.

197. de Montigny C et al. Lithium carbonate addition in tricyclic antidepressant-resistant unipolar depression. Arch Gen Psychiatry 1983;40:1327.

198. Pope HG et al. Possible synergism between fluoxetine and lithium in refractory depression. Am J Psychiatry 1988;145:1292.

199. Price LH et al. Efficacy of lithium-tranylcypromine treatment in refractory depression. Am J Psychiatry 1985;142:619.

200. Bauer M, Dopfmer S. Lithium augmentation in treatment-resistant depression: meta analysis of placebo-controlled studies. J Clin Psychopharmacol 1999;19:427.

201. Nierenberg AA et al. After lithium augmentation: a retrospective follow-up of patients with antidepressant-refractory depression. J Affect Disord 1990;18:167.

202. Rybakowski J, Matkowski K. Adding lithium to antidepressant therapy: factors related to therapeutic potentiation. Eur Neuropsychopharmacol 1992;2:161.

203. Bodkin JA, Lasser RA, Wines JD, Gardner DM, Baldessarini RJ. Combining serotonin reuptake inhibitors and bupropion in partial responders to antidepressant monotherapy. J Clin Psychiatry 1997;58:137.

204. DeBattista C et al. A prospective trial of bupropion SR augmentation of partial responders and non-responders to serotonergic antidepressants. J Clin Psychopharmacol 2003;23:27.

205. Joffe RT et al. A placebo-controlled comparison of lithium and triiodothyronine augmentation of tricyclic antidepressants in unipolar refractory depression. Arch Gen Psychiatry 1993;50:387.

206. Gitlin MJ et al. Failure of T3 to potentiate tricyclic antidepressant response. J Affect Disord 1987; 13:267.

207. Bilezikian JP, Loeb JN. The influence of hyperthyroidism and hypothyroidism on alpha-and beta-adrenergic receptor systems and adrenergic responsiveness. Endocr Rev 1983;4:378.

208. Nemeroff CB et al. Antithyroid antibodies in depressed patients. Am J Psychiatry 1985;142:840.

209. Prange AJ et al. Enhancement of imipramine antidepressant activity by thyroid hormone. Am J Psychiatry 1969;126:457.

210. Wilson IC et al. Thyroid hormone enhancement of imipramine in non-retarded depression. N Engl J Med 1970;282:1063.

211. Stein D, Avni J. Thyroid hormones in the treatment of affective disorders. Acta Psychiatr Scand 1988;77:623.

212. Joffe RT, Singer W. A comparison of triiodothyronine and thyroxine in the potentiation of tricyclic antidepressants. Psychiatry Res 1990; 32:241.

213. Artigas F, Perez V, Alvarez E. Pindolol induces a rapid improvement of depressed patients treated with serotonin reuptake inhibitors. Arch Gen Psychiatry 1994;51:248.

214. Blier P, Bergeron R. Effectiveness of pindolol with selected antidepressant drugs in the treatment of depression. J Clin Psychopharmacol 1995; 15:217.

215. Berman RM et al. Effect of pindolol in hastening response to fluoxetine in the treatment of major depression: a double-blind, placebo-controlled trial. Am J Psychiatry 1997;154:37.

216. Hoyer D. 5-HT receptors: subtypes and second messengers. J Recept Res 1991;11:197.

217. Berman RM et al. The use of pindolol with fluoxetine in the treatment of major depression: final results from a double-blind, placebo-controlled trial. Biol Psychiatry 1999;45:1170.

218. Sporn J, Sachs G. The anticonvulsant lamotrigene in treatment-resistant manic-depressive illness. J Clin Psychopharmacol 1997;17:185.

219. Calabrese JR et al. Spectrum of activity of lamotrigene in treatment-refractory bipolar disorder. Am J Psychiatry 1999;156:1019.

220. Barbosa L, Berk M, Vorster M. A double-blind, randomized, placebo-controlled trial of augmentation with lamotrigene or placebo in patients concomitantly treated with fluoxetine for resistant major depressive episodes. J Clin Psychiatry 2003;64:403.

221. Jacobsen FM. Possible augmentation of antidepressant response with buspirone. J Clin Psychiatry 1991;52:217.

222. Stoll AL et al. Methylphenidate augmentation of serotonin selective reuptake inhibitors: a case series. J Clin Psychiatry 1996;57:72.

223. Masand PS, Anand VS, Tanquary JF. Psychostimulant augmentation of second generation antidepressants: a case series. Depression and Anxiety 1998;7:89.

224. Stahl SM. Augmentation of antidepressant by estrogen. Psychopharm Bull 1998;34:319.

225. Goldberg JF, Frye MA, Dunn RT. Pramipexole in refractory bipolar depression. J Clin Psychiatry 1999;156:798.

226. Markovitz PJ, Wagner S. An open-label trial of modafinil augmentation in patients with a partial response to antidepressant therapy. J Clin Psychopharmacol 2003;23:207.

227. Diagnosis and treatment of depression in late life: the NIH consensus development conference statement. Psychopharmacol Bull 1993;29:87.

228. Rothschild AJ. The diagnosis and treatment of late-life depression. J Clin Psychiatry 1996; 57(Suppl 5):5.

229. Duberstein PR et al. Suicide in widowed persons. Am J Geriatr Psychiatry 1998;6:328.

230. Reding M et al. Depression in patients referred to a dementia clinic: a three year prospective study. Arch Neurol 1985;42:894.

231. Meyers BS. The depression-dementia conundrum. Arch Gen Psychiatry 1998;55:102.

232. Green RC et al. Depression as a risk factor for alzheimer disease. Arch Neurol 2003;60:753.

233. Stokes PE. Current issues in the treatment of major depression. J Clin Psychopharmacol 1993; 13:2.

234. Cummings JL. Dementia and depression: an evolving enigma. J Neuropsych 1989;1:236.

235. Fontaine R. Novel serotonergic mechanisms and clinical experience with nefazodone. Clin Neuropharamcol 1993;16(Suppl 3):45.

236. Karniol IG et al. Comparative psychotropic effects of trazodone, imipramine, and diazepam in normal subjects. Curr Ther Res 1976;20:337.

237. Janowsky D et al. Ventricular arrhythmias possibly aggravated by trazodone. Am J Psychiatry 1983;140:796.

238. Blazer DG et al. Suicide in late life: review and commentary. J Am Geriatr Soc 1986;34:519.

239. Henry JA et al. Acute trazodone poisoning: clinical signs and plasma concentrations. Psychopathology 1984;17:77.

240. Davis R et al. Nefazodone: a review of its pharmacology and clinical efficacy in the management of major depression. Drugs 1997;53:608.

241. Brogden RN et al. Trazodone: a review of its pharmacological properties and therapeutic use in depression and anxiety. Drugs 1981;21:401.

242. Cohen LJ. Rational drug use in the treatment of depression. Pharmacotherapy 1997;17:45.

243. Van Zweiten P. Inhibition of the central hypotensive effect of clonidine by trazodone, a novel antidepressant. Pharmacology 1977;15:331.

244. Kantor SJ et al. The cardiac effects of therapeutic plasma concentration of imipramine. Am J Psychiatry 1978;135:534.

245. Warner MD et al. Trazodone and priapism. J Clin Psychiatry 1987;48:244.

246. Preskorn SH et al. Once-daily dosing of nefazodone for the treatment of depression in patients previously stabilized on twice-daily dosing. Paper presented at American Psychiatric Association Annual Meeting, 1997.

247. Perry PJ. Pharmacotherapy for major depression with melancholic features: relative efficacy of tricyclic versus selective serotonin reuptake inhibitor antidepressants. J Affect Disord 1996;39:1.

248. Katon W et al. Adequacy and duration of antidepressant treatment in primary care. Med Care 1992;30:67.

249. Sclar D et al. Antidepressant pharmacotherapy: economic outcomes in a health maintenance organization. Clin Ther 1994;16:715.

250. Schulberg HC et al. Treating major depression in primary care practice. Arch Gen Psychiatry 1998;55:1121.

251. MacGillivray S et al. Efficacy and tolerability of selective serotonin reuptake inhibitors compared with tricyclic antidepressants in depression treated in primary care: systematic review and meta-analysis. Br Med J 2003;326:1014.

252. Revicki DA et al. Cost-effectiveness of newer antidepressants compared with tricyclic antidepressants in managed care settings. J Clin Psychiatry 1997;58:47.

253. Simon GE et al. Initial antidepressant choice in primary care: effectiveness and cost of fluoxetine vs tricyclic antidepressants. JAMA 1996;275:1897.

254. Snyder SH. Antidepressants and the muscarinic acetylcholine receptor. Arch Gen Psychiatry 1977;34:236.

255. Cassem N. Cardiovascular effects of antidepressants. J Clin Psychiatry 1982;43:22.

256. Rabkin JG et al. Adverse reactions to monoamine oxidase inhibitors: II. Treatment correlates and clinical management. J Clin Psychopharmacol 1985;5:2.

257. Glassman AH. Cardiovascular effects of tricyclic antidepressants. Ann Rev Med 1984;35:503.

258. Thapa PB et al. Antidepressants and the risk of falls among nursing home residents. N Engl J Med 1998;339:875.

259. Glassman AH et al. The use of imipramine in depressed patients with congestive heart failure. JAMA 1983;250:1997.

260. Glassman AH et al. Clinical characteristics of imipramine-induced orthostatic hypotension. Lancet 1979;1:468.

261. Roose SP et al. Comparison of imipramine-and nortriptyline-induced orthostatic hypotension: a meaningful difference. J Clin Psychopharamcol 1981;1:316.

262. Kopera H. Anticholinergic and blood pressure effects of mianserin, amitriptyline, and placebo. Br J Clin Pharmacol 1978;5:29.

263. Nelson JC et al. Major adverse reactions during desipramine treatment: relationship to plasma drug concentrations, concomitant antipsychotic treatment, and patient characteristics. Arch Gen Psychiatry 1982;39:1055.

264. Veith RC et al. Cardiovascular effects of tricyclic antidepressants in depressed patients with chronic heart disease. N Engl J Med 1982;306:954.

265. DeWilde JE et al. Clinical trials of fluvoxamine vs chlorimipramine with single and three times daily dosing. Br J Clin Pharamcol 1983;15(Suppl):427.

266. Freyschuss U et al. Circulatory effects in man of nortriptyline, a tricyclic antidepressant drug. Pharmacologia Clin 1970;2:68.

267. Alvarez W, Pickworth KK. Safety of antidepressant drugs in the patient with cardiac disease: a review of the literature. Pharmacotherapy 2003;23:754.

268. Glassman AH et al. Sertraline treatment of major depression in patients with acute MI or unstable angina. JAMA 2002;288:701.

269. Sauer WH, Berlin JA, Kimmel SE. Selective serotonin reuptake inhibitors and myocardial infarction. Circulation 2001;104:1894.

270. Serebruany VL, O'Connor CM, Gurbel PA. Effect of selective serotonin reuptake inhibitors on platelets in patients with coronary artery disease. Am J Cardiol 2001;87:1398.

271. Bigger JT Jr et al. Cardiac antiarrhythmic effect of imipramine hydrochloride. N Engl J Med 1977;296:206.

272. Giardina EGV, Bigger JT Jr. Antiarrhythmic effect of imipramine hydrochloride inpatients with ventricular premature complexes with psychological depression. Am J Cardiol 1982;50:172.

273. Muir WW et al. Effects of tricyclic antidepressant drugs on the electrophysiological properties of dog Purkinje fibers. J Cardiovasc Pharmacol 1982;4:82.

274. Roose SP et al. Comparison of paroxetine and nortriptyline in depressed patients with ischemic heart disease. JAMA 1998;279:287.

275. Roose SP et al. Cardiovascular effects of bupropion in depressed patients with heart disease. Am J Psychiatry 1991;148:512.

276. Davidson J, Turnbull CD. The effects of isocarboxazid on blood pressure and pulse. J Clin Psychopharmacol 1986;6:139.

277. Asberg M, Cronholm B, Sjoqvist F, Tuck D. Relationship between plasma level and therapeutic effect of nortriptyline. Br Med J 1971;3:331.

278. Glassman AH et al. Clinical implications of imipramine plasma levels for depressive illness. Arch Gen Psychiatry 1977;34:197.

279. Nelson JC et al. Desipramine plasma concentrations and antidepressant response. Arch Gen Psychiatry 1982;39:1419.

280. Ziegler VE et al. Amitriptyline plasma levels and therapeutic response. Clin Pharmacol Ther 1976;19:795.

281. Moyes ICA et al. Plasma levels and clinical improvement—a comparative study of clomipramine and amitriptyline in depression. Postgrad Med J 1980;56:127.

282. Robinson DS et al. Plasma tricyclic drug levels in amitriptyline-treated depressed patients. Psychopharmacology 1979;63:223.

283. American Psychiatric Association Task Force. The use of laboratory tests in psychiatry: tricyclic antidepressants—blood level measurements and clinical outcome. An APA Task Force Report. Am J Psychiatry 1985;142:155.

284. Linder MW, Keck PE. Standards of laboratory practice: antidepressant drug monitoring. Clin Chem 1998;44:1073.

285. Willis T. Diabetes: A Medical Odyssey. New York: Tuckahoe, 1971

286. Anderson RJ, Freedland KE, Clouse RE, Lustman PJ. The prevalence of comorbid depression in adults with diabetes: a meta-analysis. Diabetes Care 2001;24:1069.

287. de Groot M et al. Association of depression and diabetes complications: a meta-analysis. Psychosom Med 2001;63:619.

288. Lustman PJ, Griffith LS, Clouse RE et al. Effects of nortriptyline on depression and glucose regulation in diabetes: results of a double-blind, placebo-controlled trial. Psychosom Med 1997;59:241.

289. Lustman PJ, Freedland KE, Griffith LS, Clouse RE. Fluoxetine for depression in diabetics: a randomized double-blind placebo-controlled trial. Diabetes Care 2000;23:618.

290. Lustman PJ, Clouse RE. Treatment of depression in diabetes: impact on mood and medical outcome. J Psychosom Res 2002;53:917.

291. DiMatteo MR, Lepper HS, Croghan TW. Depression is a risk factor for noncompliance with medical treatment: meta-analysis of the effects of anxiety and depression on patient adherence. Arch Intern Med 2000;160:2101.

292. Gomez R, Huber J, Tombini G, Barros HM. Acute effect of different antidepressants on glycemia in diabetic and non-diabetic rats. Braz J Med Biol Res 2001;34:57.

293. Lee KC, Finley PR, Alldredge BK. Risk of seizures associated with psychotropic medications: emphasis on new drugs and new findings. Expert Opin Drug Saf 2003;2:233.

294. Hauser WA, Kurland LT. The epidemiology of epilepsy in Rochester, Minnesota, 1935 through 1967. Epilepsia 1975;16:1.

295. Alldridge BK. Drug-induced seizures: controversies in their identification and management. Pharmacotherapy 1997;17:857.

296. Bigger JT Jr et al. Tricyclic antidepressant overdose: incidence of symptoms. JAMA 1977;238:135.

297. Wedin GP et al. Relative toxicity of cyclic antidepressants. Ann Emerg Med 1986;15:7.

298. Horne RL et al. Treatment of bulimia with bupropion: a multicenter controlled trial. J Clin Psychiatry 1988;49:262.

299. Dunner DL et al. A prospective safety surveillance study of bupropion sustained-release in the treatment of depression. J Clin Psychiatry 1998;59:366.

300. Atkinson JH Jr et al. Prevalence of psychiatric disorders among men infected with human immunodeficiency virus infection: a controlled study. Arch Gen Psychiatry 1988;45:859.

301. Leserman J et al. Progression to AIDS: the effects of stress, depressive symptoms and social support. Psychosom Med 1999;61:397.

302. Sherbourne CD et al. Impact of psychiatric conditions on health-related quality of life in persons with HIV infection. Am J Psychiatry 2000;157:248.

303. Beckett A, Rutan JS. Treating persons with ARCH and AIDS in group psychotherapy. Int J Group Psychother 1990;40:19.

304. Faulstich ME. Psychiatric aspects of AIDS. Am J Psychiatry 1987;144:551.

305. Perry AW. Organic mental disorders caused by HIV: update on early diagnosis and treatment. Am J Psychiatry 1990;147:696.

306. Revised Classification System for HIV infection. MMWR 1992;41:1.

307. Elliott AJ et al. Randomized, placebo-controlled trial of paroxetine versus imipramine in depressed HIV-positive outpatients. Am J Psychiatry 1998;155:367.

308. Rabkin JG, Wagner GJ, Rabkin R. Fluoxetine treatment for depression in patients with HIV and AIDS: a randomized, placebo-controlled trial. Am J Psychiatry 1999;156:101.

309. Currier MB, Molina G, Kato M. A prospective trial of sustained-release bupropion for depression in HIV-seropositive and AIDS patients. Psychosmatics 2003;44:120

310. Hesse LM et al. Ritonavir, efavirenz and nelfinavir inhibit CYP2B6 activity in vitro: potential drug interactions with bupropion. Drug Metab Dispos 2001;29:100.

311. Fernandez F, Levy JK, Galizzi H. Response of HIV-related depression to psychostimulants: case reports. Hospital and Community Psychiatry 1988;39:628.

312. Schaerf FW et al. ECT for major depression in four patients infected with human immunodeficiency virus. Am J Psychiatry 1989;146:782.

313. West ED, Dally PJ. Effect of iproniazid in depressive syndromes. Br Med J 1959;1:1491.

314. Paykel ES et al. Response to phenelzine and amitriptyline in sub-types of outpatient depression. Arch Gen Psychiatry 1982;39:1041.

315. Stewart JW et al. Atypical depression: a valid clinical entity? Psychiatr Clin North Am 1993;16:479.

316. Zeller EA et al. Influence of isonicotinic acid hydrazide and 1-isonicotinyl-2-isopropyl hydrazide on bacterial and mammalian enzymes. Experientia 1952;8:349.

317. Zisook S. A clinical overview of monoamine oxidase inhibitors. Psychosomatics 1985;26:240.

318. Ravaris CL et al. Phenelzine and amitriptyline in the treatment of depression. Arch Gen Psychiatry 1980;37:1075.

319. Davidson JRT et al. A comparison of phenelzine and imipramine in depressed inpatients. J Clin Psychiatry 1981;42:395.

320. Lonnquist J, Sihvo S, Syvalahti E, Kiviruusu O. Moclobemide and fluoxetine in atypical depression: a double-blind trial. J Affect Disord 1994; 32:169.

321. McGrath PJ et al. A placebo-controlled study of fluoxetine versus imipramine in the acute treatment of atypical depression. Am J Psychiatry 2000;157:344.

322. Robinson DS et al. Phenelzine and amitriptyline in the treatment of depression. Arch Gen Psychiatry 1978;35:629.

323. Rabkin JG et al. Adverse reactions to monoamine oxidase inhibitors. Part II. Treatment correlates and clinical management. J Clin Psychopharmacol 1985;5:2.

324. Murphy DL et al. Monoamine oxidase-inhibiting antidepressants: a clinical update. Psychiatr Clin North Am 1984;7:549.

325. Kronig MH et al. Blood pressure effects of phenelzine. J Clin Psychopharmacol 1983;3:307.

326. Salzman C. Clinical guidelines for the use of antidepressant drugs in geriatric patients. J Clin Psychiatry 1985;46:38.

327. Mallinger AG et al. Pharmacokinetics of tranylcypromine in patients who are depressed: relationship to cardiovascular effects. Clin Pharmacol Ther 1986;40:444.

328. Pollack MH, Rosenbaum JF. Management of antidepressant induced side effects: a practical guide for the clinician. J Clin Psychiatry 1987;48:3.

329. Mitchell JE, Popkin MK. Antidepressant drug therapy and sexual dysfunction in men: a review. J Clin Psychopharmacol 1983;3:76.

330. Stewart JW et al. Phenelzine-induced pyridoxine deficiency. J Clin Psychopharmacol 1984;4:225.

331. Haefely W et al. Biochemistry and pharmacology of moclobemide, a prototype RIMA. Psychopharmacology 1992;106:S6.

332. Davidson J et al. Practical aspects of MAO inhibitor therapy. J Clin Psychiatry 1984;45:81.

333. Sheehan DV et al. Monoamine oxidase inhibitors: prescription and patient management. Int J Psychiatry Med 1980;10:99.

334. Blackwell B et al. Hypertensive interactions between monoamine oxidase inhibitors and foodstuffs. Br J Psychiatry 1967;113:349.

335. Shulman KI et al. Dietary restriction, tyramine, and the use of monoamine oxidase inhibitors. J Clin Psychopharmacol 1989;9:397.

336. Clary C, Schweizer E. Treatment of MAOI hypertensive crisis with sublingual nifedipine. J Clin Psychiatry 1987;48:249.

337. Hansten PD, Horn JR. Drug Interactions Analysis and Management. Vancouver, WA: Applied Therapeutics, 1998.

338. Anon. Prozac product labeling information. Indianapolis: Dista Products Company, 1994.

339. Spiker DG et al. The pharmacological treatment of delusional depression. Am J Psychiatry 1985;142:430.

340. Glassman AH, Roose SP. Delusional depression. Arch Gen Psychiatry 1981;38:424.

341. Chan CH et al. Response of psychotic and nonpsychotic depressed patients to tricyclic antidepressants. J Clin Psychiatry 1987;48:197.

342. Kantor SJ, Glassman AH. Delusional depression: natural history and response to treatment. Br J Psychiatry 1977;131:351.

343. Rothschild AJ, Duval SE. How long should patients with psychotic depression stay on the antipsychotic medication? Am J Psychiatry 2003; 64:390.

344. Collaborative working group on clinical trial evaluations. Atypical antipsychotics for treatment of depression in schizophrenia and affective disorders. J Clin Psychiatry 1998;59(Suppl 12):41.

345. Muller-Siecheneder F et al. Risperidone versus haloperidol and amitriptyline in the treatment of patients with combined psychotic and depressive symptoms. J Clin Psychopharmacol 1998;18:111.

346. DeBattista C, Solvason HB, Belanoff J et al. Treatment of psychotic depression [Lletter]. Am J Psychiatry 1997;154:1625.

347. Lane HY, Chang WH. Risperidone monotherapy for psychotic depression unresponsive to other treatments. J Clin Psychiatry 1998;59:624.

348. Machi GS, Checkley SA. Olanzapine in the treatment of psychotic depression. Br J Psychiatry 1999;174:460.

349. Anton RF Jr et al. Amoxapine versus amitriptyline combined with perphenazine in the treatment of psychotic depression. Am J Psychiatry 1990; 147:1203.

350. Ayd F. Amoxapine side effects: an update. Int Drug Ther Newsl 1984;19:21.

351. Cooper DJ et al. The effects of amoxapine and imipramine on serum prolactin levels. Arch Intern Med 1981;141:1023.

352. Madakasira S. Amoxapine-induced neuroleptic malignant syndrome. Drug Intell Clin Pharm 1989;23:50.

CHAPTER 80

Mood Disorders II: Bipolar Disorders

Mary C. Borovicka, Raymond C. Love

Bipolar mood disorder is a chronic and progressive illness that produces significant morbidity and mortality for those afflicted. Based on a 1993 report prepared by the National Institute of Mental Health (NIMH) Advisory Council on the Cost and Treatment of Severe Mental Illness, bipolar patients typically spend one-fourth of their adult lives in the hospital and half of their lives disabled.[1]

Classification

Mood disorders are diagnosed using the criteria established in the *Diagnostic and Statistical Manual of Mental Disorders*, Fourth edition, Text Revision (DSM-IV-TR).[2] The clinician first examines and characterizes discrete episodes of mood disturbances that the patient has experienced. These are determined to be *major depressive episodes, manic episodes* (episodes of elevated mood), *mixed episodes* (with features of both depression and mania), or *hypomanic episodes*. Manic and hypomanic episodes (Table 80-1) are both characterized by a distinct period of abnormally and persistently elevated, expansive, or irritable mood.[3] However, the hypomanic episodes are less intense than the manic episodes. Manic episodes are severe enough to impair functioning (self-care, occupational, social), complicate a medical condition, result in psychotic features, or require hospitalization.[2]

Once the nature of past and current discrete episodes has been determined, an individual can be diagnosed as having a mood disorder. An individual who has experienced one or more episodes of depression, without past episodes of mania, is diagnosed as having a major depressive disorder. A person who has experienced one or more manic or mixed (criteria for both mania and depression are met) episodes with or without a depressive episode is diagnosed as having *bipolar I disorder*. An individual who has experienced one or more episodes of both hypomania and depression (without a history of manic or mixed episodes) is diagnosed as having *bipolar II disorder*.[2]

Bipolar disorder also is known as *manic-depressive disease*, a term originally coined by Kraepelin.[3] The diagnosis of a cyclothymic disorder is used for a person who has experienced at least 2 years of cycling mood characterized by numerous periods with hypomanic symptoms and separate periods with depressive symptoms that do not meet the criteria for a major depressive episode. *Bipolar disorder, not otherwise specified*, refers to disorders with features of mania or hypomania that do not meet the criteria for a specific bipolar disorder.[2]

The DSM-IV-TR also uses a series of descriptors called *specifiers* to further characterize the course of illness and the most recent type of episode experienced by the individual. Recent episodes are first classified as manic, mixed, or major depressive episodes. They may be described further in terms of severity (mild, moderate, severe), the presence of psychotic features (in partial or full remission), with or without catatonic features, or with onset during the postpartum period. Other specifiers convey information regarding the pattern of illness. For example, some individuals experience major depressive episodes at a characteristic time of the year (usually the winter) or switch from depression to mania during a particular season. The specifier "with seasonal pattern" applies only to the pattern of major depressive episodes. Other specifiers describe whether full recovery between episodes (i.e., with or without full interepisode recovery) occurs and

Table 80-1   DSM-IV TR Criteria for a Manic Episode*

1. A distinct period of abnormally and persistently elevated, expansive, or irritable mood, lasting at least 1 week (or of any duration if hospitalization is necessary).
2. During the period of mood disturbance, ≥3 of the following symptoms have persisted (4 if the mood is only irritable) and have been present to a significant degree:
   • Inflated self-esteem or grandiosity
   • Decreased need for sleep (e.g., feels rested after only 3 hours of sleep)
   • More talkative than usual or pressure to keep talking
   • Flight of ideas or subjective experience that thoughts are racing
   • Distractibility (i.e., attention too easily drawn to unimportant or irrelevant external stimuli)
   • Increase in goal-directed activity (either social, at work, at school, or sexually) or psychomotor agitation
   • Excessive involvement in pleasurable activities that have a high potential for painful consequences (e.g., the person engages in unrestrained buying sprees, sexual indiscretions, or foolish business investing)
3. The symptoms do not meet the criteria for a Mixed Episode.
4. The mood disturbance is sufficiently severe to cause marked impairment in occupational functioning or in usual social activities or relationships with others, or to necessitate hospitalization to prevent harm to self or others, or there are psychotic features.
5. The symptoms are not due to the direct physiologic effects of a substance (e.g., a drug of abuse, a medication, or other treatment) or a general medical condition (e.g., hyperthyroidism).

*A "manic syndrome" is defined as including criteria 1, 2, and 3. A "hypomanic syndrome" is defined as including criteria 1 and 2, but not 3 (i.e., no marked impairment). Maniclike episodes that are clearly caused by somatic antidepressant treatment (e.g., medication, electroconvulsive therapy, light therapy) should not count toward a diagnosis of bipolar I disorder.
Reprinted with permission from reference 2.

whether individuals experience rapid cycling (more than four episodes/year).[2]

The demonstration of rapidly alternating signs and symptoms of depression and mania such as those encountered in individuals with mixed mania or rapid cycling disorders can make diagnosis difficult. Accurate diagnosis often requires a longitudinal view of the course of illness.

Epidemiology and Cost Burden

Numerous epidemiologic studies have determined the lifetime rate of bipolar I disorder to be 0.8% to 1.6% of the adult population.[4–7] The prevalence of bipolar II disorder appears to be slightly less than bipolar I disorder at 0.5% or approximately 1.5 million people in the United States.[4] Epidemiologic studies in Europe have identified a prevalence rate ranging from 0.2% to 3.0% for bipolar II disorder using less strict diagnostic criteria. In fact, prevalence rates for the entire bipolar spectrum; which includes bipolar I and II disorder, cyclothymia, and hypomania, are noted to be higher when these less stringent criteria are used (2.6% to 6.4%).[8,9] There are no apparent gender differences in the occurrence of bipolar I disorder. This is in marked contrast to unipolar depression in which the gender ratio of females to males is about 2:1.[10] However, bipolar II disorder is more commonly seen in females.[10]

The familial nature of bipolar disorder has been well established. The concordance rate among monozygotic twin probands with bipolar disorder is approximately 75%. This contrasts with a rate of 27% in unipolar depression.[11]

The cost of bipolar illness has been reported to be $45 billion.[12] Direct costs accounted for 17% of the total, whereas the remaining 83% was due to indirect costs such as lost wages, suicide, institutional care, and caregiver burden.

Clinical Signs and Symptoms

A typical manic episode usually begins with a change in sleep patterns along with euphoria. Target symptoms typically include increased talkativeness, staying awake all night, and bursts of energy during which projects are begun but rarely completed. Mania often is characterized by thought disturbances. Patients may exhibit "flight of ideas" (rapid speech that switches among multiple ideas or topics) and delusions of grandeur (false beliefs of special powers, knowledge, abilities, importance, or identity). The behavior of manic patients is characterized as being intrusive, loud, intense, irritable, suspicious, and challenging. They often exercise poor judgment. For example, they may spend large sums of money in business deals that ultimately fail, become sexually promiscuous, take excessive risks, or fail to obey laws.

These symptoms usually develop gradually over several days to more than a week in three stages. *Stage I* is characterized by euphoria, labile affect, grandiosity, overconfidence, racing thoughts, increased psychomotor activity, and an increase in the rate and amount of speech. This stage corresponds to an episode of hypomania. *Stage II* features increasing irritability, dysphoria (a feeling of extreme discomfort and unrest), hostility, anger, delusions, and cognitive disorganization without apparent cause. Many patients progress no further than this stage. Others may proceed to stage III, in which the manic episode progresses to an undifferentiated psychotic state. Individuals in *stage III* experience terror and panic. Their behavior is bizarre and psychomotor activity is frenzied. They may experience hallucinations. They progress from disorganized thought patterns to incoherence and disorientation. Just as the manic episode gradually builds, it declines in a gradual manner. Psychotic symptoms usually resolve first, whereas irritability, paranoia, and excessive behavior continue. Gradually, remaining symptoms such as hyperverbosity, seductiveness, and dysphoria decrease.[13]

Course of Illness

The mean age of onset for bipolar disorder is 21 years.[4] There appears to be a peak onset between ages 15 to 19 years with another subsequent peak at ages 20 to 24 years.[14] Approximately 20% to 30% of new cases occur in children ages 10 to 15 years.[15,16] Patients may present initially with mania, hypomania, depression, or a mixed episode. However, 75% of patients report having had multiple episodes of depression before the development of a manic episode.[15] Misdiagnosis is common early in the illness with a startling 69% of patients reporting being misdiagnosed.[15] Furthermore, up to 26% reported visiting as many as five physicians before a correct diagnosis was made. Interestingly, although 70% of patients reported having at least one symptom of mania before diagnosis (erratic sleep, elevated mood, racing thoughts, pressured speech), only about 40% reported these symptoms to a physician.[15] There is a significant decrease in the new onset of bipolar disorder after 60 years of age.[14] A presentation of mania later in life should alert the clinician to an underlying medical problem as the possible cause.

An untreated episode of bipolar disorder may last for several months. Bipolar disorder is a recurrent illness; single episodes of mania occur in fewer than 10%.[2] Most individuals with this disorder suffer multiple episodes of mania, hypomania, or depression separated by periods of euthymia (normal mood) throughout the course of their lives. In the majority, mania occurs just before or immediately after a depressive episode.[2] There may be a 5- to 10-year period from the onset of illness until the first hospitalization or diagnosis.[14]

The course of illness for a given individual is characterized by episode length, length of euthymic intervals, frequency of relapse, severity of episodes, and predominant syndrome (mania, hypomania, or depression). These factors do not remain fixed throughout an individual's illness. For instance, individuals may experience episodes of dysphoria and depression before ever experiencing hypomania or mania. Often, the euthymic interval and cycle length decrease with additional episodes. Bipolar individuals can develop a course of alternating manic and depressive episodes without intervening euthymic episodes.

People diagnosed with either bipolar I or II disorder who experience shorter cycle lengths and who suffer from four or more episodes of depression, hypomania, mania, or a mixed episode in a year are identified as "rapid cyclers." Rapid cyclers account for 5% to 15% of bipolar individuals, and women make up 70% to 90% of patients with rapid cycling bipolar disorder.[2] Individuals with rapid cycling bipolar disorder often are refractory to conventional treatment and suffer significant morbidity and mortality because of their rapid changes in mood. They may have little or no euthymic period between manic and depressive episodes. This can have drastic family, social, and occupational consequences. The literature indicates that rapid cycling patients may be more likely than other bipolar patients to have hypothyroidism and that thyroid supplementation may exert a beneficial effect in this group.[17, 18] Conversely, one study determined rapid cycling patients in fact had normal thyroid indices.[19]

Unfortunately, despite adequate treatment, 73% of individuals with bipolar disorder relapse within 5 years. Furthermore, nearly half continue to experience significant mood symptoms between episodes, and less than 20% were euthymic or had minimal symptoms.[20]

Complications of Bipolar Illness

Patients with bipolar illness have higher rates of mortality from both natural and unnatural causes. Higher rates of natural mortality largely result from cardiovascular causes.[21] Suicide and excessive risk-taking behaviors during manic or hypomanic episodes also account for a high mortality rate in this group. Significant risk factors for suicide in bipolar patients include drug abuse, hospitalization for depression, age less than 35 years, a recent (within 2 years) hospitalization, previous suicide attempts, and a family history of affective disorders.[22,23] Overall mortality as well as deaths due to suicide or cardiovascular causes are significantly reduced in bipolar patients who are adequately treated.[20] Bipolar patients are especially prone to substance abuse. Approximately 60% of bipolar I patients have comorbid alcohol or substance abuse.[24] Rapid cyclers and those with dysphoric mania have the highest rates of concomitant substance abuse.[23] Individuals in a manic phase may engage in sexual indiscretions or risky sexual practices that expose them to sexually transmitted diseases.

The World Health Organization recently identified the top 10 causes of disability-adjusted life years in the world; bipolar disorder ranked sixth.[25] Individuals with bipolar disorder are likely to experience stress and upheaval in many areas of their lives, including relationships, employment, and finances. Eighty-eight percent of bipolar patients have been hospitalized once and 66% at least two times.[25] The stress resulting from manic and depressive episodes results in a two- to threefold increase in divorce rates. Patients often report having poor relationships with family members, and nearly 75% report that their family members have a limited understanding of bipolar illness.[15] Employment problems may result from bizarre, inappropriate, or unreliable behavior. In one study, 60% of patients reported being unemployed, 88% felt the disease affected how well they performed at work, and 63% felt that they were treated differently from their peers.[15] Financial and legal problems may result from excessive spending, involvement in schemes, substance abuse, and risk-taking behavior. Caregivers and family members may also suffer significant distress in caring for a relative with bipolar illness.[25]

Treatment Overview

Both the acute treatment of manic and depressive episodes and maintenance treatment for prophylaxis of future episodes require individualization. Lithium, valproate, or an atypical antipsychotic (olanzapine or risperidone) is recommended as monotherapy for the acute treatment of manic episodes.[14] Patients suffering from severe manic episodes and/or psychosis may benefit from combination therapy (e.g., lithium with an antipsychotic agent, or valproate with an antipsychotic).[14] Valproate and lithium are recommended first-line agents for rapid cycling mania; lamotrigine is reserved as a second-line agent.[14] The role of carbamazepine in rapid cycling is less clear. Recent practice guidelines[14] do not recommend the use of carbamazepine for rapid cycling; however, expert consensus guidelines[26] do recommend carbamazepine as a first-line agent in rapid cyclers with mixed or classic mania. Studies indicate that rapid cycling disorder is poorly responsive to monotherapy and that combination therapy is frequently required. Mixed or dysphoric mania may be treated with valproate or lithium.[14]

Some patients fail to respond to these first-line agents. In general, some reduction in the intensity and severity of symptoms should occur within the first week of therapy. If no response is seen within the first 1 to 2 weeks, another first-line agent (valproate, lithium, or an antipsychotic agent) may be added, or the patient may be switched to an alternative agent.[14,26] Second-line options are to add carbamazepine, oxcarbazepine, or an antipsychotic.[14] If a patient is already receiving an antipsychotic, then switching to another agent may be necessary. If a patient exhibits a partial resolution of symptoms in response to a first-line drug after 2 to 3 weeks of therapy, recommendations are to add valproate to a lithium regimen, or to add lithium to an anticonvulsant regimen.[26] If these options fail or are not feasible, the next preferred option is addition of carbamazepine. Lamotrigine and gabapentin also may be considered as alternatives if adjunctive therapy with carbamazepine fails.[26]

Sedative agents and antipsychotics are often used as adjunctive agents in the management of acute manic episodes. Benzodiazepines are a first-line adjunct when the objective is sedation or relief of accompanying anxiety symptoms. Antipsychotics are indicated when a patient experiences psychotic symptoms or if the episode is particularly severe.[14,26] Currently, the best evidence available indicates that olanzapine or risperidone are the antipsychotic agents of choice. However, these agents are available only in oral formulations. Severely agitated patients may be unable or unwilling to take medications orally, and an intramuscular antipsychotic may be necessary.

The treatment of acute depressive episodes in individuals with bipolar disorder differs from the treatment of major depressive disorder. In most cases, depressed individuals with bipolar disorder should be treated with a mood stabilizer in addition to an antidepressant, although some patients with milder episodes may respond to a mood stabilizer alone. In these cases, lithium or lamotrigine is the mood stabilizer of choice.[14,26] All antidepressants have the potential to switch a depressed patient into a manic episode (see Question 4). Many experts believe that bupropion, venlafaxine, and serotonin reuptake inhibitors are less likely to result in this switch.[26] Therefore, they are most commonly recommended as first-line treatments for bipolar individuals experiencing a major depressive episode.[14,26] Most experts prefer to avoid monoamine oxidase (MAO) inhibitors and tricyclic antidepressants (TCAs) in these patients.[26] Monotherapy with antidepressants must be avoided.

Mood stabilizers, including lithium and anticonvulsants, constitute the mainstay of maintenance pharmacotherapy. Bipolar disorder is a chronic disease that must be monitored carefully over time. Clinicians monitoring individuals with these disorders must familiarize themselves with patients' patterns of behavior and decompensation to intervene early in subsequent episodes. The trust built by long-term relationships may also prove useful in promoting adherence to prescribed regimens.[14] Nonadherence due to ambivalence, side effects, periodic lack of insight, or a reluctance to surrender the "high" of the manic episode is the major cause of relapse in this disorder.[14]

Mood disorders are associated with disturbances in sleep-wake and activity cycles. In addition to adherence with medication, individuals with these disorders should be advised to maintain regular patterns of daily activities. Regulation of sleep-wake, meal, exercise, and other schedules may prove useful. Alterations in sleep and other diurnal patterns may herald the onset of a mood episode. Prompt identification can lead to early recognition and treatment.[14]

CLINICAL ASSESSMENT
Clinical Presentation and Diagnosis

1. H.M., a 27-year-old man, is accompanied to the clinic by his wife, A.M. She had called the clinic before bringing H.M. and reported much of the following information. A.M. says that H.M. was doing well until about 3 weeks ago, when his niece was killed in an automobile accident. At the funeral, he borrowed some "nerve pills" from his cousin. Since then, H.M. has been acting increasingly "wild." He has been staying up later and later at night and often bursts into the bedroom at 2 or 3 AM and loudly awakens A.M. Sometimes, he presents her with expensive gifts, which they cannot afford. He often jumps on the bed and starts singing her love songs in a loud voice. A.M. notes that H.M. then almost always demands sex, after which he sleeps for a few hours and then loudly gets up and leaves the house.

H.M. recently has experienced problems at work, where he is a snack delivery truck driver. Over the last several weeks, he was noted to be loading his truck in a rapid and reckless manner. His boss received several reports that H.M. was driving in an unsafe manner and at high speed. Store owners called to complain that he was giving away free cases of snacks to customers. He often did not complete deliveries to the stores at the end of his route.

Last week, when his boss called to express concern over his behavior, H.M. said he was quitting his job. He wrote an illegible resignation note, which was at least 10 pages long, called an overnight air delivery service to deliver the note to his employer (who is located only 3 miles from his home), and then left the house before the driver arrived to pick it up. H.M. returned several hours later driving a brand new foreign car and wearing an expensive new suit, red cowboy boots, and a bright green hat with a large feather. He told A.M. that he had a new job, which was going to make him a millionaire.

Last night, she found a large sum of money in his pants pocket when emptying the clothes hamper. He did not come home at all, but he called her at 4 AM to tell her to pack for Dallas, where he was going to become the new head coach of the Dallas Cowboys.

Upon arriving at the clinic, H.M. insists, "I don't need no doc. I am supercalifragilistic!" He then bursts into song. He is dressed flamboyantly but needs a shave and shower. He gives the examiner (a stranger) a bear hug and has trouble sitting still, listening, or allowing others to talk. His speech is pressured and loud; he often fails to complete sentences or communicate entire ideas, and he is rhyming and punning. His mood obviously is elevated, but he becomes increasingly irritable throughout the examination. He insists he must get to Texas to sing the national anthem at a football game before the CIA can stop him; he then breaks down in tears. Within moments, he is again smiling and talking of money-making schemes. He is oriented to person and place, but thinks it is tomorrow. Intelligence seems average. When asked to interpret a proverb, H.M. becomes angry, throws a chair across the room, and yells, "Enough of this bull! Air Force One is waiting for me!" He then storms out of the office. How is H.M.'s presentation consistent with the diagnosis of a manic episode?

The hallmarks of a manic episode are changes in mood, behavior, and thought (see Table 80-1).[3] H.M. first demonstrates an elevated mood. He is exuberant and notes how great he feels. However, manic patients often demonstrate lability in their mood, and they may become irritable and easily frustrated, especially when challenged. H.M. becomes irritable and resentful when questioned by the examiner. His quick displays of sadness and anger further demonstrate the volatility of his mood.

H.M. displays behavior and speech typical of a manic patient. He has a reduced need for sleep, behaves recklessly, and is overactive. His speech is pressured, loud, and full of rhymes and puns, and he sings to express his emotion. As illustrated by H.M., the speech of manics may skip from topic to topic in a "flight of ideas." The behavior of manics often is characterized as being excessive and expansive. H.M. dresses flamboyantly, hugs his examiner, writes an unnecessarily lengthy letter of resignation, seeks an overnight courier service for local delivery, presents his wife with lavish gifts, and distributes merchandise to strangers.

Manic patients often are delusional. The delusions often are of a grandiose nature and deal with inflated abilities, self-importance, wealth, or special missions in life. H.M. makes unrealistic comments about his money-making schemes, his singing ability, his position as the coach of a professional football team, and his intended use of the presidential plane. Manic patients also may have delusions of a persecutory nature such as H.M.'s fear that the CIA is going to stop him.

Manic patients often are disorganized and do not complete tasks. They tend to skip from idea to idea and scheme to scheme. H.M. neglects his hygiene, fails to complete his deliveries, and neglects sending out his resignation letter. His speech reflects this disorganization.

2. **What differentiates H.M.'s signs and symptoms from those of schizophrenia?**

Many of H.M.'s signs and symptoms are consistent with schizophrenia. The distinction between a manic episode and a schizophrenic episode is difficult. Most often, mania is differentiated from schizophrenia based on the clinical course, premorbid history, and previous episodes. H.M. apparently has functioned well for most of his life, as evidenced by his ability to sustain a relationship (i.e., his marriage) and hold down a job. Most important, he has not displayed psychotic symptoms for more than a month or had a sustained (6-month) period in which he displayed psychiatric symptoms and experienced social or occupational dysfunction as required for a diagnosis of schizophrenia.[2]

Precipitating Factors

3. **What factors make H.M. vulnerable to the occurrence of a manic episode at this time?**

The median age of onset for bipolar disorder is 29 years of age in men and 34.5 years of age in women.[3] Thus, H.M. is at the age in which his disorder would be likely to first manifest itself. In addition, manic episodes are often precipitated by various psychosocial stressors, including changing jobs, moving, or the loss of a loved one.[27] The death of H.M.'s niece may have served as a predisposing factor for the development of a manic episode.

A variety of medications and clinical states can induce or precipitate manic episodes (Table 80-2). The most common drug causes of mania involve medications that affect monoamine neurotransmitters,[28] such as antidepressants and stimulants. Corticosteroids, anabolic steroids, isoniazid, levodopa, caffeine, and over-the-counter (OTC) stimulants can induce or aggravate mania. Sleep loss also can be a significant cause of mania.[27] A reduction in sleep after the death of his niece could have helped contribute to the development of H.M.'s manic episode.

4. **If the "nerve pills" borrowed by H.M. were antidepressants, could they have contributed to the development of his manic episode?**

The phenomenon of antidepressant-induced mania was first described with iproniazid, an antitubercular agent that is also an MAO inhibitor.[81] Since that time, several classes of antidepressants have been noted to precipitate switches from depression to mania including MAO inhibitors, TCAs, and heterocyclic antidepressants, and even selective serotonin reuptake inhibitors (SSRIs). Despite the purported risk, up to 78% of bipolar patients are treated with antidepressants, whereas only 56% receive mood stabilizers.[82] There are numerous case reports of induction of mania or hypomania with antidepressant treatment, but few controlled studies have been conducted. Switch rates for patients treated with TCAs in the absence of a mood stabilizer have been reported to be between 35% to 53%.[82-84] It is widely reported that newer antidepressants are associated with lower switch rates than TCAs or MAO inhibitors but few controlled trials validate this impression. In fact, two controlled studies reported low switch rates with bupropion and fluoxetine.[85,86] Because of the risk of antidepressant-induced "switching" in bipolar disorder, recommendations are to avoid antidepressant monotherapy for bipolar depressive episodes.[14] There is conflicting evidence regarding the protective role of mood-stabilizing agents against the development of mania when administered along with antidepressants.[82,83,87,88] Although antidepressants are associated with a switch to mania within a few weeks after their initiation, this could reflect a shortened (more rapid) depression-mania cycle rather than a precipitation of a manic episode.[84] This "cycle acceleration" phenomenon has been reported in up to 26% of bipolar patients treated with antidepressants.[84] It is plausible to consider an antidepressant with a mood stabilizer for patients with bipolar depression for the short-term, however the risks may outweigh the benefits if antidepressant treatment is continued long-term.[89] Antidepressant agents may have helped precipitate a manic episode in H.M. or shortened his cycle, moving him into an episode of mania from a pre-existing state of depression or normal mood.[84]

Treatment of Acute Mania

5. **Why does H.M. require treatment?**

Manic episodes have a number of severe complications. Left untreated, severe mania can result in confusion, fever, exhaustion, and even death. The impairment in judgment, the excesses, and the risk-taking that occur during manic episodes may devastate relationships, careers, and finances and lead to physical harm and loss of life. Manic individuals may engage in illegal activities or behave in a manner that results in a violation of the law. H.M. drives recklessly; may have lost his job; spends excessive amounts of money on gifts, clothing, and automobiles; and plans to participate in a variety of money-making schemes. He has acquired a great deal of cash suddenly, perhaps from withdrawing all of his family's savings or from some type of illegal enterprise.

Manic patients also may engage in risky sexual encounters, leading to infection with sexually transmitted diseases or HIV. Abuse of alcohol and drugs is common among these patients. Irritability, such as that demonstrated by H.M., can lead to

Table 80-2   Drugs Reported to Induce Mania

Antidepressants	Herbals
Monoamine oxidase inhibitors	St. John's wort
Tricyclic antidepressants	Ginseng
Bupropion	Ma-huang
Fluoxetine	Chromium piccolinate
Citalopram	**Stimulants**
Fluvoxamine	
Sertraline	Cocaine
Paroxetine	Methylphenidate
Nefazodone	Dexfenfluramine
Mirtazapine	Fenfluramine
Venlafaxine	Phentermine
Reboxetine	**Anticonvulsants**
Antipsychotics	
	Felbamate
Olanzapine	Gabapentin
Risperidone	Lamotrigine
Ziprasidone	Topiramate
Quetiapine	**Endocrine**
Flupenthixol	
Anxiolytics/Hypnotics	Corticosteroids
	Thyroid
Buspirone	Androgens
Alprazolam	Dehydroepiandrosterone (DHEA)
Triazolam	Testosterone patch
Miscellaneous	Leuprolide
	Antibiotic/Antiviral
Levodopa	
Amantadine	Efavirenz
Cimetidine	Trimethoprim-sulfamethoxazole
Tolmetin	Clarithromycin
Folate	Isoniazid
Pindolol	Erythromycin
Interferon-α	Amoxicillin
Donepezil	Ciprofloxacin
Tramadol	Ofloxacin
Guanfacine	Cotrimoxazole
Sibutramine	Metronidazole
Mannitol	
Omega-3 fatty acids	
Ifosfamide	

Compiled from references 28 through 80.

episodes of violence, resulting in potential harm to the patient or to others.

The goals of treatment are to reduce the severity, duration, and frequency of the current mood episode as well as to prevent recurrence of further episodes.

Valproate (Divalproex, Valproic Acid)

6.   What is the appropriate treatment for H.M.'s acute manic episode?

Depending on the type and severity of mania, agents considered to be first line for the treatment of mania include lithium, divalproex (an enteric-coated complex of valproic acid and sodium valproate in a 1:1 ratio), atypical antipsychotics (olanzapine or risperidone), or a combination of these agents.[14,26,90] Table 80-3 lists the treatment recommendations as summarized by three different groups. If an individual pre-

sents with euphoric (classic) mania or hypomania, reasonable first-choice agents include lithium, divalproex, or olanzapine. Carbamazepine, oxcarbazepine, and other atypical antipsychotics are reserved as second-line agents. If H.M. had a history of dysphoric or mixed bipolar disorder or had a contraindication to the use of lithium, divalproex or olanzapine would be preferred.[14,90]

Limited data are available regarding the management of rapid cycling bipolar disorder. Recommendations favor initiation of monotherapy with divalproex; lithium and lamotrigine are alternative agents.[14] However, most rapid cycling patients ultimately require combination therapy. These patients should also be evaluated and treated for hypothyroidism or substance abuse, both of which may trigger rapid cycling.[92] In addition, antidepressants may increase cycling and should be discontinued.[84] In a case of typical mania such as H.M. is experiencing, monotherapy with one of these agents—dival-

Table 80-3   Choice of Mood Stabilizer for Manic, Mixed, and Hypomanic Episodes

	APA	*TMAP*	*Expert Consensus*
Euphoric	Li or DVP or AAP	Li or DVP or OLZ	Li[a] or DVP
Mixed dysphoric	Li + AAP DVP + AAP	DVP or OLZ	DVP[a] or Li
Psychotic	Li + AAP DVP + AAP	Li or DVP or OLZ	DVP[a] or Li or AAP (OLZ or RIS)
Hypomania	Li or DVP or AAP	Li or DVP or OLZ	Li or DVP

[a]Drug of choice.
APA, American Psychiatric Association, Practice Guideline for the treatment of patients with bipolar disorder; TMAP, Texas Medication Algorithm Project; Expert Consensus: Expert Consensus Guidelines; Li, lithium; DVP, divalproex; AAP, atypical antipsychotic; OLZ, olanzapine; RIS, risperidone.
Adapted with permission from references 14, 26, and 90.

proex, lithium, or olanzapine—may be used as a first-line agent.[14,26,90] In the past, lithium was the gold standard first-line agent for mania, but its use may be limited by its narrow therapeutic index and side effect profile. However, some experts indicate that lithium remains the preferred mood stabilizer in euphoric mania.[26] More recently, the efficacy of divalproex in acute mania has been shown to be comparable to lithium, with approximately half of patients demonstrating at least a 50% reduction on the Schedule for Affective Disorders and Schizophrenia—Change Version (SADS-C), a standard for evaluating treatment response in bipolar disorder.[91] Divalproex may also be preferred in patients who have characteristics that may predict a poor response to lithium, such as substance abuse, a family history of treatment failure with lithium, rapid cycling or mixed manic episodes, or a course of illness in which a depressive episode is followed by a euthymic episode.[92] Divalproex was chosen for the management of H.M.'s mania because of comparable efficacy to lithium as well as the more rapid onset of effect of divalproex compared with that of lithium (5 to 7 days compared with about 14 days, respectively).[14]

DOSING AND MONITORING

7. How should divalproex therapy be initiated, and what baseline tests are necessary? How will H.M.'s response to therapy be monitored?

Divalproex is an acceptable first-line agent for H.M.'s euphoric mania and the treatment of choice for people who exhibit rapid cycling or present with mixed episodes.[14,90] The initial dose of divalproex sodium for H.M. should be 250 mg three times per day.[14] The dosage should then be increased by 250 to 500 mg every 2 to 3 days to obtain serum valproate levels between 45 and 125 μg/mL or a maximum dosage of 60 mg/kg.[93] The correlation between efficacy and serum concentrations is weak, although it appears that those who achieve a threshold level of at least 45 μg/mL are more likely to respond to therapy. If the need for control is acute, an oral loading regimen of divalproex sodium 20 mg/kg per day divided and given three or four times daily for 5 days can be initiated to rapidly attain serum valproic acid concentrations of >50 μg/mL.[94] Therapeutic serum concentrations occurred by day 2 (mean 89 ± 19 μg/mL) and symptom improvement was noted in the first 3 days. An alternate divalproex loading regimen of 30 mg/kg administered on the first and second days

followed by 20 mg/kg on the third to tenth days was compared to standard dose titration and found no differences in safety and tolerability between the two regimens.[95]

Before any valproic acid formulation is initiated, baseline laboratory tests, including a complete blood count (CBC) with differential and platelets, and liver function tests should be obtained. H.M.'s baseline weight and neurologic status should be recorded. In premenopausal females who have not undergone surgical sterilization, a baseline pregnancy test is warranted. Attention should be given to any medications that might be administered concurrently with valproic acid because interactions with aspirin, phenytoin, phenobarbital, lamotrigine, rifampin, warfarin, felbamate and carbamazepine are cited frequently (also see Chapter 54, Seizure Disorders).

Divalproex should decrease the severity and duration of H.M.'s current manic episode, may decrease the frequency of subsequent episodes, and can increase the normal mood interval between episodes. Once treatment has started, H.M. should be monitored for response of his initial target symptoms, including grandiosity, decreased need for sleep, pressured speech, distractibility, and impulsivity. Use of a rating scale (see Question 6) would provide an objective measure of response. Symptom improvement with divalproex therapy is noted in approximately 5 to 7 days.

SIDE EFFECTS

8. What are the potential side effects of divalproex therapy? How should H.M. be monitored for these possible effects?

H.M. should be monitored for potential dose-related adverse reactions of valproic acid, including various gastrointestinal (GI) complaints (nausea, diarrhea, dyspepsia, anorexia), sedation, ataxia, tremor, benign hepatic transaminase elevations, and thrombocytopenia. GI complaints may be mitigated by reducing the dosage, changing to an extended-release preparation, or administering an antacid or H$_2$-antagonist. Central nervous system (CNS) effects such as ataxia and sedation may respond to dosage reduction, although sedation may resolve with continued treatment. If tremor is bothersome or interferes with the patient's functioning, dosage reduction or the addition of a β-adrenergic blocker may provide relief. Small elevations in transaminases are considered benign; however, divalproex should be discontinued if elevations are more than two to three times the upper limit of normal. Alopecia may occur owing to chelation of zinc and selenium by valproate; supplementation of these trace elements may reduce the problem.[96]

Weight gain may be a serious and chronic problem and occurs in 44% to 57% of patients receiving divalproex.[97] It is particularly distressing and may contribute to nonadherence. Weight gain has been associated with valproic acid serum concentrations >125 μg/mL. Therefore, dosage reduction or a gradual switch to another agent are appropriate to allow for weight reduction, to reduce the risk of nonadherence, and to decrease the potential for medical complications associated with obesity.[96] Valproate-induced weight gain may also be related to the development of polycystic ovaries (PCO) or polycystic ovary syndrome (PCOS) in women.[97] PCO is defined as the presence of follicular cysts without endocrine or menstrual irregularities. PCOS differs in that ovulatory failure and hyperandrogenism define the syndrome, but the presence of actual cysts is not necessary. The clinical features associated with PCOS include menstrual irregularities, hirsutism, alopecia, insulin resistance, hyperlipidemia, and obesity. This syndrome was first reported in a group of epileptic patients treated with valproate.[98] One of the prevailing theories is that valproate-induced obesity may lead to hyperandrogenism and hyperinsulinemia resulting in the development of PCO or PCOS.[97] A causal relationship has not yet been determined; however, two recent studies in bipolar patients found higher rates of menstrual irregularities and hyperandrogenism in valproate-treated women compared with controls and those receiving lithium.[99,100]

There are a few case reports of valproate-induced hyperammonemia in psychiatric patients.[101,102] Although not a common adverse event, the incidence of hyperammonemia remains unknown. Symptom onset is reported to occur 1 to 2 weeks after initiation of divalproex. Patients may present with lethargy, somnolence, and delirium; some may progress to coma. Even with ammonia levels two to three times above normal or higher, liver indices usually remain normal. In patients with severe elevations of ammonia and those with related symptoms, reduction of divalproex dosage has been reported to result in a normalization of ammonia levels and symptom improvement.[102] More serious adverse events with divalproex include fulminant hepatic failure, agranulocytosis, and pancreatitis, all of which require termination of therapy.

Once divalproex therapy is begun, liver function tests, valproic acid serum levels, and CBCs with differential and platelets should be monitored at least monthly for the first 3 months and every 3 to 6 months thereafter.[14] Body weight should also be determined at baseline and monthly during therapy.

9. **H.M. was titrated to a total daily divalproex dosage of 2,500 mg/day. A routine complete blood cell count with differential and platelet count was ordered after 1 month. The following data were reported: white blood cell (WBC) count, 8.5 × 10³/mm³; hemoglobin, 14.5 g/dL; hematocrit, 43%; red blood cells (RBCs), 5.2 × 10⁶/mm³; neutrophils, 59%; lymphocytes, 27%; monocytes, 6%; eosinophils, 2%; basophils, 0.5%; and platelets, 75 × 10³/mm. What are the risk factors for developing valproic acid–induced thrombocytopenia?**

[SI units: WBC count, 8.5 × 10⁹/L (normal, 3.2 to 9.8); hemoglobin, 145 g/L (normal—male, 115 to 155); hematocrit, 0.43 l (normal—male, 0.39 to 0.49);

RBCs, 5.2 × 10¹²/L (normal—male, 4.3 to 5.9); neutrophils, 0.59 l (normal, 0.54 to 0.62); lymphocytes, 0.27 l (normal, 0.25 to 0.33); monocytes, 0.06 l (normal, 0.03 to 0.07); eosinophils, 0.02 l (normal, 0.01 to 0.03); basophils, 0.005 l (normal, 0 to 0.0075); platelets, 75 × 10⁹/L (normal, 130 to 400)]

Valproate-induced thrombocytopenia occurs rarely and is associated with higher dosages and serum levels.[103] Nevertheless, clinicians should educate patients to look for signs such as easy bruising or bleeding. In most cases, patients with thrombocytopenia remain asymptomatic and respond to a lowering of the dosage; therefore, complete discontinuation of the drug is often unnecessary.[104] H.M.'s dosage should be reduced, and his platelet count should be monitored closely. In addition, he should be observed for reemerging symptoms of mania.

SWITCHING FROM DIVALPROEX TO VALPROIC ACID

10. **If H.M.'s mania resolves on a stable dose of divalproex and he experiences no GI signs or symptoms, should he be maintained on divalproex or switched to a generic valproic acid preparation?**

Divalproex has delayed-release characteristics designed to reduce the GI upset and nausea experienced by many individuals taking valproic acid preparations. In one of the early studies examining GI tolerability of these preparations, Wilder and colleagues[105] found that 23 of 27 patients who could not tolerate valproic acid could tolerate divalproex. However, the high cost of divalproex compared with valproic acid has led several investigators to switch from divalproex to valproic acid in developmentally disabled patients who were already stabilized on divalproex. Cranor and colleagues[106] found no differences in seizure rates, GI complaints, use of laboratory tests, or nondrug costs following this drug interchange. They were able to switch 89% of patients successfully.

Similarly, Sherr and colleagues[107] found no differences in adverse upper GI side effects, seizure control, or severity of illness after switching patients from divalproex to valproic acid. Once H.M.'s dosage and psychiatric status have stabilized, he could be switched to the less expensive valproic acid preparation with appropriate monitoring.

Lithium
PRELITHIUM WORKUP

11. **C.N., a 21-year-old woman, was diagnosed with her first episode of mania 3 weeks ago. At that time, she was hospitalized and treated with lithium. C.N.'s manic episode was stabilized, and after 10 days she was discharged from the hospital. She was scheduled to see her outpatient psychiatrist for follow-up 1 week later but failed to show up for the appointment. Today, C.N. arrives at the emergency department at the request of her mother. C.N. is pulling her mom's hair and kicking wildly as she is pulled from the car. She can be heard screaming "The FBI is after me, Mom! You want them to find me, don't you? I would have made it out of the country if you hadn't gotten in the way! I was going to marry Prince Charles and become the new queen of England." Upon evaluation, C.N.'s mood is irritable, and she is pacing around the interviewer. She is dressed in a short skirt and high heels and is wearing an excessive amount of makeup and costume jewelry. During the interview, she interrupts the examiner, smiles, and says in a loud, provocative voice "Let's you and**

me get out of here!" Her mother states that after C.N. was discharged from the hospital, she lost her prescription and, within several days, stopped attending her classes at the local community college. She began staying out, playing her radio loudly, and driving in a reckless manner, finally hitting the side of the garage while pulling in this morning. What laboratory tests are required before initiating lithium therapy for C.N.?

Because lithium can affect many organ systems, baseline laboratory values must be established before therapy is initiated. These values will serve to determine whether future abnormal values are lithium related. Furthermore, various physiologic states may affect lithium's excretion or predispose one to lithium toxicity. In these cases, baseline laboratory tests are useful in determining the presence of factors that contraindicate the use of lithium or require an adjustment in dosage. As a young, healthy female, C.N.'s prescreening laboratory battery should include electrolytes, blood urea nitrogen, creatinine, urine-specific gravity, thyroid-stimulating hormone (TSH), thyroxine (T$_4$), and a WBC count (Table 80-4). Also, a pregnancy test should be obtained before starting therapy.

DOSING

12. C.N.'s baseline laboratory parameters were normal. How should treatment for C.N. be initiated?

Because C.N. has previously responded to lithium and does not have rapid cycling or mixed bipolar disorder, she is likely to respond to lithium again. Although any of the various strategies for calculating lithium dosage requirements could be used, it is simpler to begin C.N. at a dosage of 300 mg three times a day. This is an average starting dose for a healthy adult patient.

Patients experiencing an acute manic episode require higher lithium levels than are required during maintenance therapy. Therefore, the goal for the acute management of C.N. is a serum level between 0.5 and 1.2 mEq/L.[14] Because lithium is not immediately effective, C.N.'s level can be adjusted with the use of twice-weekly serum levels until the manic episode resolves. As she recovers and enters the maintenance phase of treatment, both C.N.'s lithium dosage and target lithium levels will require re-evaluation (see Question 28).

13. How long will it take to get the full effect of lithium?

Lithium has a slow onset of action, taking as long as 1 to 2 weeks to fully exert its therapeutic effects.[14] Therefore, it is appropriate to use an adjunctive medication to help reduce C.N.'s acute symptoms. Both benzodiazepines and antipsychotics have been used in this manner.[14] Either conventional or atypical (see Chapter 78, Schizophrenia) antipsychotics may be warranted as adjunctive therapy in acute mania when patients have hallucinations or delusions that are inconsistent with their mood (see Question 23).

SIDE EFFECTS

14. After 3 weeks of therapy, C.N. is demonstrating significant improvement in her sleep, impulsivity, delusions, and activity level. Her lithium level remains at 0.8 mEq/L. However, today she is complaining to the nursing staff that she has developed a hand tremor. Soon after her physician arrives to evaluate her, she asks to be excused so that she can go to the bathroom. How might C.N.'s presentation be related to her medication?

[SI unit: lithium, 0.8 mmol/L]

When considering side effect management early in lithium therapy, it becomes important to monitor lithium levels closely. When patients start to recover from acute mania, the rate of lithium clearance may decrease and patients may demonstrate an increase in lithium levels and worsening side effects (Table 80-5).[108] This does not seem to be the case with C.N. because her lithium level is within the accepted range for the management of acute mania.

C.N. is complaining of a hand tremor. She should be interviewed and examined to determine its origin. In this case, the likely medication-related cause for the complaint would be tremor secondary to lithium. Tremor occurs in 30% to 70% of those treated with lithium. Lithium-induced tremor, or intention tremor, is characteristically rapid, regular, and fine in amplitude. This is quite different from the resting, coarse, slow (4 to 7 cycles/ second) tremor at rest commonly seen in patients receiving antipsychotics. Often, this tremor occurs early in therapy and spontaneously resolves as therapy continues. Caffeine, anxiety, antidepressants, and adrenergic agents may worsen lithium-induced tremor.[109] The tremor is more

Table 80-4 Prelithium Workup

Baseline Determination[18,85]	Rationale
SrCr, BUN	Lithium is excreted renally.
Urine-specific gravity	Lithium may cause polyuria.
Electrolytes	Hyponatremia and dehydration lead to ↑ renal reabsorption of lithium and subsequent lithium toxicity; hypokalemia may ↑ the risk of lithium-induced cardiac toxicity.
ECG[a]	Lithium may worsen severe cardiac disease.
CBC with differential	Lithium may cause a 15–45% ↑ in the numbers of all WBC lines except basophils; lithium also may cause ↑ in platelet counts.
T$_4$, TSH	Lithium may induce hypothyroidism.
Glucose	Lithium may induce weight gain and complicate the presentation of diabetes mellitus.
Weight	Lithium may induce weight gain.
Lithium level	Manic patients may at times be poor historians.
Pregnancy test	Lithium is a potential teratogen.

[a]In patients with a history or at risk for cardiac disease.
BUN, blood urea nitrogen; CBC, complete blood count; ECG, electrocardiograph; SrCr, serum creatinine; TSH, thyroid-stimulating hormone; WBC, white blood cell.

Table 80-5   Side Effects of Lithium

Lithium Side Effect	Occurrence	Treatment Strategy
Cognitive effects	9%	Ensure that patient is not depressed; consider supportive therapy; differentiate from manic hyperacuity; lower dosage.
Fine tremor	15% but ↓ with time	May resolve with time; lower dosage; reduce caffeine intake; avoid tricyclic antidepressants, sympathomimetics; consider β-adrenergic blocking agents such as propranolol 40–160 mg/day
GI upset	33% in first 2 weeks	May resolve or improve with time; may be related to speed of rise of serum levels; consider divided doses or sustained-release preparations.
Diarrhea	6–20%	May be related to serum levels; reduce dosage.
Hypothyroidism	5–8%	Discontinue lithium or treat with levothyroxine.
Polyuria, polydipsia	36%	May be related to serum levels; reduce dosage; consider reducing frequency of administration; consider amiloride.
Weight gain	50–75%; average of 4 kg	Try to avoid polyuria and polydipsia and discourage use of high-calorie drinks; regular exercise; dietary consultation.
Worsening of dermatologic conditions	Follicular eruptions 33%	Consider reduction in dosage or discontinuation depending on severity of reaction; provide symptomatic treatment.

GI, gastrointestinal.

common in patients with higher serum levels and may be worse at times of peak serum levels.[14] If C.N. is not bothered by the tremor and suffers no impairment, treatment is not necessary. If the tremor becomes problematic, the lithium dosage may be reduced or β-adrenergic blocking agents can be added. Switching to a sustained-release lithium preparation may reduce peak serum levels and ameliorate tremors associated with the peak of absorption.[14] Because it is fairly early in treatment and C.N. has only a moderate lithium level, it is more reasonable to add propranolol 10 mg three times a day rather than to reduce the lithium dosage if an intervention is required. Propranolol usually is effective at dosages <160 mg/day.[110] C.N. also should be educated about her tremor and instructed to reduce her caffeine consumption.

In addition, C.N. should be asked about her trip to the bathroom during this clinic visit, because lithium may cause both diarrhea and polyuria. Its most prominent renal effect is interference with the action of antidiuretic hormone in the distal tubule of the kidney, resulting in nephrogenic diabetes insipidus.[111] With the lower serum levels of lithium commonly used today, the actual increase in urine volume may be as low as 20%; thus, a decrease in C.N.'s lithium dosage may help reduce polyuria if this is a problem. Urine output also has been correlated with troughs in lithium levels.[112] Although the advantages of once-daily administration of lithium are not universally accepted, switching a stabilized patient to this schedule with its lower trough levels also may help reduce urine volume.[14] If C.N. were to fail to respond to either of these interventions, either potassium supplementation or amiloride could be prescribed concurrently.[14] Amiloride appears to antagonize lithium's effects on free water clearance by reducing the entry of the ion into renal epithelial cells.

If C.N.'s trip to the bathroom was due to diarrhea, lithium should be evaluated as a possible cause because up to 20% of patients started on lithium experience diarrhea, epigastric bloating, and sometimes pain early in therapy.[112] Diarrhea from lithium is associated with high serum levels, once-daily dosing, and rapidly absorbed preparations; therefore, divided doses may help alleviate the problem. Use of lower doses and

switching to sustained-release preparations are alternative strategies that could be used. Sustained-release preparations can potentially lead to lower lithium levels in patients with rapid GI motility because the product must be present in the small intestine for several hours for maximal absorption to occur. If C.N. has diarrhea or polyuria, her fluid status and lithium levels should be monitored carefully. Dehydration leads to increased lithium reabsorption in the proximal tubule and could result in accumulation to toxic levels.

15. Should C.N. be switched to a sustained-release preparation of lithium?

Sustained-release dosage forms have often been used to aid in medication adherence and reduce side effects. Although standard lithium preparations are often administered three or four times per day, many clinicians prescribe them for once- or twice-daily administration. Sustained-release lithium is usually administered twice daily, results in lower peak levels, and may decrease side effects associated with high peak concentrations. Both lithium-induced tremor and gastric symptoms may respond to a change to sustained-release preparations.[14] Sustained-release lithium often results in higher trough levels of lithium, which could exacerbate polyuria. Sustained-release lithium is not particularly expensive, but it may cost several times more than generic lithium carbonate. If C.N. is no longer experiencing problems with tremor or GI side effects, she should be maintained on a standard preparation of lithium carbonate.

16. What should C.N. be told regarding potential renal damage from lithium?

C.N. should be informed that lithium can cause renal side effects; however, cases of irreversible kidney damage are relatively rare and have occurred mainly when patients have had pre-existing renal disease, have experienced episodes of lithium intoxication, or have been poorly monitored with regard to lithium levels.[113] Communication with her physician regarding situations that increase the risk of lithium toxicity (see Question 19) and cooperation with regular lithium and renal function monitoring can vastly reduce the risk of renal disease secondary to lithium therapy. Finally, C.N. must be informed that polyuria is not related to any of the more serious renal side effects.

PATIENT EDUCATION

17. **What does C.N. need to know about lithium before she is discharged?**

As with all drugs, C.N. should be instructed to disclose the medications she is taking to all health care professionals who provide care for her. She should be informed that dehydration, fever, vomiting, or sodium-restricted diets could lead to increases in her lithium level. Therefore, she needs to drink plenty of fluids and eat a diet consistent in its levels of sodium. C.N. should be instructed to contact her physician if she starts to experience any symptoms of lithium toxicity, including worsening tremor, slurred speech, muscle weakness or twitches, or difficulty walking.

C.N. also should be told to use caution in selecting OTC medications. Specifically, she should be warned to avoid routine use of preparations containing ibuprofen (Advil, Nuprin) or naproxen (Aleve), which can increase lithium levels.[114] C.N. should know that caffeine can sometimes be troublesome in patients taking lithium. On a short-term basis, caffeine can worsen lithium tremor; on a longer-term basis, it may lower lithium levels.[114] With regard to serum level monitoring, C.N. needs to know that lithium levels usually are drawn approximately 12 hours after a dose of lithium. If she is taking lithium in the evening and the morning, she should take her evening dose and then report for a blood sample to be drawn in the morning before taking her next dose.

TOXICITY

18. **One day, C.N.'s mother calls, concerned that C.N. has been complaining of nausea, vomiting, and diarrhea for several days. Her mother says that C.N. has taken her medications but has had little to eat or drink. Over the past few hours, C.N. has become confused and has developed a coarse tremor and slurred speech. It has been 4 months since C.N.'s lithium level has been checked. What action should be taken?**

There is a strong possibility that C.N. is suffering from lithium toxicity, which can occur acutely from an overdose or insidiously if excretion is reduced. *Mild toxicity* at levels <1.6 mEq/L usually includes feelings of apathy, lethargy, and muscle weakness accompanied by nausea and irritability. *Moderate toxicity* occurs between 1.5 and 2.5 mEq/L with symptoms progressing to coarse tremor, slurred speech, unsteady gait, drowsiness, confusion, muscle twitches, and blurred vision. *Severe toxicity* at levels >2.5 mEq/L can result in seizures, stupor, coma, and cardiovascular collapse. C.N. appears to be experiencing moderate lithium toxicity. She should be taken to the emergency department immediately, where stat laboratory tests, including a lithium level, electrolytes, and renal function, should be ordered. Intravenous solutions should be started to ensure that C.N. is hydrated adequately, and electrolyte abnormalities should be corrected promptly. Depending on the results of physical examination and laboratory tests, cardiac monitoring should be instituted.

Lithium levels must be interpreted with caution if they were drawn within 12 hours of lithium ingestion, because lev-els drawn sooner than 12 hours may appear falsely high. In contrast, levels that are drawn too soon may appear to be falsely low in individuals who have ingested large quantities of a sustained-release lithium formulation. Twelve-hour serum lithium levels >2.5 mEq/L, coma, shock, further deterioration, and failure to improve with conservative management are indications for dialysis. Although peritoneal dialysis has been instituted in cases of lithium intoxication, hemodialysis is preferred.[14]

HYPOTHYROIDISM

19. **After receiving lithium for 1 year, C.N. returns complaining that the lithium is slowing her down. She is tired and has gained weight in recent weeks and thinks that she is getting depressed. In the examining room, C.N. complains that the temperature is too cold. What is the most likely cause of C.N.'s complaints? What treatment should be instituted?**

C.N.'s symptoms are consistent with those of hypothyroidism. Lithium affects the incorporation of iodine into thyroid hormone, interferes with secretion of thyroid hormones, and may interfere with the peripheral degradation of T_4 to T_3 (triiodothyronine).[115] Depending on the criteria used, rates of lithium-induced hypothyroidism have been estimated to be between 5% and 35%.[114] Subclinical hypothyroidism with elevated levels of TSH may be present in an even larger number of patients taking lithium. Although it tends to occur early in the course of long-term lithium treatment, hypothyroidism can develop after many years of therapy. In fact, long-term treatment appears to be a risk factor for developing subclinical hypothyroidism. High dosages of lithium and pre-existing thyroid disease may be predisposing factors for lithium-induced hypothyroidism, which tends to occur more often in women than in men, as do other forms of hypothyroidism. Hypothyroidism also places patients at risk for rapid cycling bipolar disorder.

Thyroid function tests should be ordered to evaluate C.N.'s current symptoms. If she is found to be hypothyroid, discontinuation of therapy is not necessary. She should receive levothyroxine in doses that normalize her thyroid function tests. Even if she has an elevated TSH with normal levels of T_3 and T_4, treatment may help stabilize her course of illness, resolve her symptoms, and prevent breakthrough depressive symptoms.[115]

DRUG INTERACTIONS

20. **T.J., a 35-year-old man, is hospitalized and treated with lithium for a severe manic episode. He had a stable lithium level of around 0.80 mEq/L for several weeks, but his last two levels have dropped to 0.65 and 0.61 mEq/L, respectively, without any change in his drug therapy. T.J. insists that he is taking the medication as prescribed. The nursing staff believes that he is compliant with his medication but notes that he is spending more time off the ward and in the canteen. What factors could contribute to a decrease in T.J.'s lithium levels?**

[SI unit: lithium, 0.80, 0.65, and 0.61 mmol/L, respectively]

Drug interactions are a common cause of changes in lithium levels, but there have been no changes in T.J.'s regimen. Changes in formulation or brand may sometimes have an impact on lithium levels. However, lithium is relatively well absorbed and has a long elimination half-life, so this usually does not result in great changes in the 12-hour postdose lithium level. Occasionally, patients switched from lithium citrate to solid dosage forms experience small changes in lithium levels (Table 80-6).

In T.J.'s case, one should consider the ramifications of his visits to the canteen because diet can have a major influence on lithium excretion. If T.J. is consuming large amounts of caffeinated coffee or soft drinks or salty snacks in the canteen, these could be responsible for reductions in lithium levels. Both increases in dietary sodium and the ingestion of methylxanthines (e.g., caffeine, theophylline) can increase lithium clearance.[114]

Finally, acute mania can increase lithium clearance.[109] If T.J. were showing signs of a relapse, his decrease in lithium levels might be attributable to his return to a manic state.

LITHIUM IN PREGNANCY

21. **A.J., a 36-year-old woman, has been maintained successfully on lithium therapy for 5 years for bipolar disorder. She asks whether she should stay on lithium because she plans on becoming pregnant in the near future.**

Lithium has been associated with a variety of congenital malformations, including the rare cardiac malformation, Ebstein's anomaly.[97] There is considerable disagreement about the importance of lithium as a teratogen. Lithium was originally thought to increase the risk of Ebstein's anomaly 400 times; however, the risk is more likely one to eight times.[116] The estimated overall risk for congenital malformations is approximately 4% to 12% compared with 2% to 4% in controls.[116] Still, lithium is a pregnancy category D drug because of evidence of its risk to the human fetus. Because malformations of this type are most likely to occur in the first trimester of pregnancy, it is advisable for patients to discontinue lithium therapy, when possible, before conception and especially during the first trimester.

In addition to cardiac malformations, infants exposed to lithium have been reported to develop hypotonia, nephrogenic diabetes insipidus, and thyroid abnormalities.[97] Lithium administration during pregnancy increases the risk of premature delivery by a factor of two to three.[117] Thus, A.J. and her physician should discuss the individual risks involved in her case. In addition to the risks of teratogenicity, they must consider the harm that could result from the possible recurrence of episodes of mania or depression and the risks inherent in discontinuing lithium or switching to another antimanic

Table 80-6 Lithium Drug Interactions of Clinical Significance

Drugs That May Increase Lithium Levels

NSAIDs
Many NSAIDs have been reported to ↑ lithium levels as much as 50–60%. This probably is due to an enhanced reabsorption of sodium and lithium secondary to inhibition of prostaglandin synthesis.

Diuretics
All diuretics can contribute to sodium depletion. Sodium depletion can result in an ↑ proximal tubular reabsorption of sodium and lithium. Thiazide-like diuretics cause the greatest ↑ in lithium levels, whereas loop diuretics and potassium-sparing diuretics appear somewhat safer.

ACE inhibitors
ACE inhibitors and lithium both result in volume depletion and a reduction in glomerular filtration rate. This results in reduced lithium excretion.

Drugs That May Decrease Lithium Levels

Theophylline, caffeine
Theophylline and caffeine may ↑ renal clearance of lithium and result in a ↓ in levels in the range of 20%.

Acetazolamide
Acetazolamide may impair proximal tubular reabsorption of lithium ions.

Sodium
High dietary sodium intake promotes the renal clearance of lithium.

Drugs That Increase Lithium Toxicity

Methyldopa
Cases of sedation, dysphoria, and confusion due to the combined use of lithium and methyldopa have been reported.

Carbamazepine
Cases of neurotoxicity involving the combined use of lithium and carbamazepine have been reported in patients with normal lithium levels.

Calcium channel antagonists
Cases of neurotoxicity involving the combined use of lithium and the calcium channel blockers verapamil and diltiazem have been reported. Lithium does interfere with calcium transport across cells.

Antipsychotics
Cases of neurotoxicity (encephalopathic syndrome, extrapyramidal effects, cerebellar effect, EEG abnormalities) have been reported due to the combined use of lithium and various antipsychotics. The interaction may be related to ↑ in phenothiazine levels, changes in tissue uptake of lithium, and/or dopamine-blocking effects of lithium. Studies attempting to demonstrate this effect have yielded differing results.

Serotonin-specific reuptake inhibitors
Fluvoxamine and fluoxetine have been reported to result in an of toxicity when added to lithium. Sertraline has been reported to nausea and tremor in lithium recipients.

ACE, angiotensin-converting enzyme; EEG, electroencephalogram; NSAIDs, nonsteroidal anti-inflammatory drugs.

agent. Also, A.J. should be actively involved in the decision-making process.

If A.J. and her physician decide that she is to remain on lithium, her levels must be monitored closely during pregnancy and her dosage adjusted periodically. Glomerular filtration rate and lithium clearance both are elevated markedly in the second and third trimesters of pregnancy, resulting in a reduction in lithium levels and the possibility of breakthrough manic episodes.[109] Approximately 16 to 18 weeks after conception, screening tests, high-resolution ultrasound, and fetal echocardiography can be used to determine whether cardiac defects have developed.[97] If possible, A.J.'s physician should discontinue her lithium several days before delivery to minimize lithium levels in the newborn and to offset the reduction in lithium excretion that occurs after delivery.[109] In deciding when to discontinue lithium before delivery, A.J. and her physician should consider the increased risk of premature delivery due to the use of lithium.

If A.J. and her physician decide that she is to discontinue lithium, they must be prepared to deal with the risks of lithium discontinuation. Several cases of what are thought to be rebound manic episodes have resulted from the abrupt cessation of lithium therapy. If lithium is to be discontinued in A.J., it should be gradually reduced over 4 weeks.

22. A.J. did not use lithium throughout her pregnancy. Following delivery, A.J. and her physician decide to restart lithium. How soon can this take place?

Lithium can be restarted as soon as A.J.'s urine output is established and she is fully hydrated. However, this decision also may be affected by whether or not A.J. chooses to breast-feed her child because lithium does pass into the milk and is present in concentrations up to 24% to 72% of that found in the maternal blood.[97] Risks to the fetus include hypothyroidism, cyanosis, hypotonia, lethargy, and cardiac dysrhythmias. Hydration status must be closely monitored as lithium toxicity may develop during infantile illnesses. Thus, A.J. and her physician must discuss the advantages of breast-feeding versus the risks of exposing the newborn to lithium or withholding lithium during the postpartum period. A.J. should be informed that approximately 40% to 70% of bipolar women experience affective episodes after delivery.[97]

If A.J. chooses to breast-feed while taking lithium, she should consider using infant formula when the child becomes ill because febrile illness, vomiting, and diarrhea can increase the risk of lithium toxicity. She also should be instructed to contact her pediatrician if the infant experiences diarrhea, vomiting, hypotonia, poor sucking, muscle twitches, restlessness, or other unexplained changes in behavior or status.

Atypical Antipsychotics

23. D.W., a 34-year-old female singer and musician, recently experienced her fourth admission for a manic episode. She also suffers from psoriasis and asthma. A trial of lithium led to worsening of her psoriasis and unacceptable tremor, which interfered with her guitar playing. Use of β-blockers was not considered because of her asthma. She is currently receiving valproic acid. However, tremor has again become problematic. Furthermore, she is concerned about her appearance because she has begun to

experience weight gain and hair loss from the valproic acid. What other drugs are available for monotherapy of bipolar disorder?

Antipsychotics are used during the course of illness in up to 68% of patients with bipolar disorder. Recent evidence indicates that atypical antipsychotics are effective in the treatment of acute mania and have a more tolerable adverse effect profile compared with conventional agents. Several treatment algorithms list atypical antipsychotics as acceptable first-line choices for several types of mania (see Table 80-3). Atypical antipsychotics are effective in mania whether or not psychotic symptoms are present. In addition to being used as monotherapy, evidence also supports their use as adjunctive agents to mood stabilizers such as lithium, valproate, carbamazepine, and other anticonvulsants. Currently, olanzapine, risperidone, and quetiapine are approved by the FDA for the treatment of acute mania.

OLANZAPINE

Two short-term, randomized, double-blind, placebo-controlled trials confirmed the efficacy of olanzapine for the management of mania. The first found that 48.6% of olanzapine-treated patients had at least a 50% reduction in scores on the Young Mania Rating Scale, compared with 24.2% of placebo patients.[118] The second study reported a 65% response rate among olanzapine-treated patients.[119] Comparisons of olanzapine to lithium and valproate for acute mania show equal efficacy among these agents but greater side effects with olanzapine.[120, 121] Another trial reported that olanzapine was superior to valproate.[122] Olanzapine has also been studied as an adjunct to other mood stabilizers in acute mania. Zarate[123] evaluated patients receiving either olanzapine alone or olanzapine in combination with mood-stabilizing drugs and found that response rates were better for patients receiving the combination. In a study of patients partially responsive to lithium or valproate therapy, adjunctive olanzapine significantly improved response rates compared to olanzapine monotherapy (67.7% compared with 44.7%, respectively).[124] Case reports suggest that olanzapine augmentation of mood stabilizers may be effective for mixed bipolar states.[125] There are no direct comparisons between atypical antipsychotic agents. However, a 12 week retrospective study of risperidone, olanzapine, and clozapine found significant improvement on all regimens but no differences among them.[126] As expected, there was significantly more weight gain in the olanzapine group (16.1 lb) than with the risperidone group (7.8 lb). Clozapine and olanzapine appeared to cause similar increases in weight; however, the number of clozapine-treated patients was small.

Emerging data indicate that olanzapine also may be effective for the prophylaxis of bipolar disorder. In an open-label extension study, 113 patients were treated with olanzapine 5 to 30 mg daily for 49 weeks.[120,127] Lithium, fluoxetine, or benzodiazepines were added if necessary. Only 40% of patients remained on olanzapine monotherapy. Fluoxetine and lithium each were used in one-third of patients. Despite a dropout rate of 60%, the relapse rate over the year was 25.5%. Another long-term (43-week) open-label study of adjunctive olanzapine in treatment-resistant bipolar patients found improvement in 43% of patients.[128] However, on average, patients were receiving three other drugs; mood stabilizers and antipsychotics were the agents most commonly used.

Olanzapine 5 to 20 mg/day is effective, both as monotherapy and adjunctive therapy, for the management of acute mania and represents a reasonable choice for D.W. Treatment should be initiated at 10 mg/day and titrated as necessary for optimal response. Olanzapine also appears to be effective for the prophylaxis of mood episodes in bipolar patients, but further well-controlled studies are needed. The most frequently cited adverse effects of olanzapine are somnolence, weight gain, increased appetite, dry mouth, and slurred speech. D. W should be informed about the risk of developing diabetes. The development of diabetes mellitus is a serious concern with atypical antipsychotics, even in patients who have no personal or family history of diabetes. Therefore, routine monitoring for signs and symptoms is warranted.

RISPERIDONE

Risperidone is widely prescribed for the treatment of bipolar disorder and has proved to be effective for acute mania, both as monotherapy and as an adjunct to mood stabilizers. Early evidence of efficacy was provided by small open-label and retrospective studies.[129–132] These were followed by a larger, 6-week open-label study of 174 manic patients. Risperidone was added to existing mood stabilizer regimens for the majority of patients; 10% received risperidone monotherapy. The average risperidone dose was 4.9 mg/day. At 6 weeks, there were significant reductions in Young Mania Rating Scale Scores (YMRS, 26.3 to 5.7, P <.001), and some patients reported improvements in depressive symptoms as well. These trials were followed by two double-blind studies. In the first study, 45 acutely manic patients were treated with risperidone 6 mg/day, haloperidol 10 mg/day, or lithium 800 to 1,200 mg/day for 4 weeks.[133] At endpoint, all three treatment groups had significant improvements in manic symptoms compared with baseline, and no differences were noted between the groups. The second double-blind, controlled trial included 156 bipolar patients treated with either risperidone (up to 6 mg/day) with a mood stabilizer, or haloperidol (up to 12 mg/day) with a mood stabilizer, for 3 weeks.[134] Rating scale scores for both groups were significantly reduced compared with placebo, and no differences between the active treatment groups were found. Two 6-month, open-label trials reported continued improvements with risperidone over a 6-month period; relapse rates were 16% and 25%.[135,136]

Risperidone-associated mania has been reported in some patients; including some with no history of mania. Keck and colleagues[137] theorized that this might be a dose-related effect. Risperidone should be initiated at dosages no greater than 2 mg/day. Side effects, such as extrapyramidal symptoms, also tend to be related to higher dosages.

Based on short-term studies, risperidone is effective for the management of acute mania. More rigorous studies are needed to determine the role of rispderidone for prophylaxis of bipolar disorder, but open-label trials were positive. Risperidone, at dosages <6 mg/day, would be a reasonable first choice for antipsychotic therapy in D.W.; either as monotherapy or as an adjunct.

ZIPRASIDONE AND QUETIAPINE

Recently, a double-blind, placebo-controlled trial of ziprasidone in acute mania was published.[138] Two-hundred-seventy-four patients were included in the 3-week study. The results showed significant reductions in mania rating scale scores compared with placebo as early as day 2 and significant improvements in all ratings by day 7. Mean ziprasidone doses were 147 mg/day on day 2, and 138.1 mg/day and 130.1 mg/day during the second and third weeks, respectively. The most frequently cited adverse effects were somnolence, headache, dizziness, nausea, hypertonia, akathisia, insomnia, and dyspepsia. Most adverse effects were mild to moderate in severity. Based on these results, ziprasidone appears to be effective as monotherapy for the management of acute mania.

Quetiapine has not been as extensively studied as other atypical antipsychotics in bipolar disorder, but recently the FDA approved its use in acute mania. Case reports and open trials have shown positive results in this population.[139–141] Aripiprazole has been studied in acute mania and an FDA indication is expected soon.

CLOZAPINE

Clozapine has been studied in controlled and open trials and has been found to be more effective in mood disorders than in schizophrenia. When clozapine was used alone or in combination with other mood-stabilizing drugs, 71.2% of manic patients with bipolar disorder or schizoaffective disorder responded, compared with only 61.3% of patients with schizophrenia.[142] Also, patients with mixed or manic episodes were more likely to respond (response rates of 74% and 69%, respectively) than patients with unipolar, bipolar, or schizoaffective depression (51.7%).[142,143] Clozapine also is effective for managing treatment-resistant manic patients as well as for longer-term mood stabilization.[143–145] In treatment-resistant manic patients, clozapine is efficacious as monotherapy.[144] The evidence for clozapine efficacy in rapid cycling bipolar disorder is conflicting.[144,146] Clozapine must be initiated at a dosage no greater than 12.5 mg twice daily and increased by 25 to 50 mg per day. Thus, it could take longer than 1 week to reach therapeutic doses in a manic patient. Furthermore, clozapine's use is limited by the need for regular blood monitoring and the risk of side effects, including agranulocytosis, seizures, weight gain, sedation, anticholinergic effects, cognitive impairment, tachycardia, light-headedness, and sialorrhea. If clozapine therapy is interrupted, retitration is required to prevent orthostatic or syncopal episodes. The concomitant use of benzodiazepines with clozapine may add to the risk of respiratory depression and syncopal episodes. Clozapine should be reserved for only those patients who fail to respond to mood stabilizers, other atypical antipsychotic agents, or combinations of the two.

24. **What alternative agents are available for acute mania if lithium, valproate, or an atypical antipsychotic fails?**

Other Adjunctive Therapies

ANTICONVULSANTS

Many experts have suggested that carbamazepine represents the next logical choice for the management of acute mania when lithium, valproate and atypical antipsychotics fail.[26]

Only one placebo-controlled trial of carbamazepine in acute mania has been reported; the response rate of 63% was found. However, the trial had only 19 patients.[147] Trials comparing carbamazepine and lithium reported similar efficacy; however, the number of patients included was small and drop-out rates were high.[148,149] Carbamazepine was also found to have similar efficacy to chlorpromazine for mania.[150] One study reported efficacy of carbamazepine for rapid cycling bipolar disorder but subsequent studies failed to replicate this result.[151,152]

A recent review of combination therapies for bipolar disorder indicated that carbamazepine may be synergistic with either lithium or valproate for mania.[153] However, combination regimens may pose particular difficulties. The combination of carbamazepine and lithium may increase the risk of neurotoxicity, particularly in patients with pre-existing neurologic diseases. Therefore, the combination should be avoided in these patients. The combination of carbamazepine and valproate has a complex pharmacokinetic interaction. Carbamazepine is an inducer of the cytochrome P450 activity and can increase the metabolism of valproate, resulting in reduced serum concentrations and efficacy. Conversely, valproate may inhibit the metabolism of carbamazepine, leading to increased serum concentrations and adverse effects.

The initial dose of carbamazepine is 100 to 200 mg twice daily. The dose should be increased by 200 mg every 3 to 4 days until adequate serum levels have been reached.[14] Although no correlation between carbamazepine serum levels and response in bipolar disorder has been established, serum levels >12 μg/mL are associated with sedation and ataxia. Therefore, one should strive to reach serum levels in the range of 4 to 12 μg/mL.[14] Average daily doses for maintenance therapy range from 200 to 1,600 mg/day.

Carbamazepine adverse effects occur in up to 50% of patients.[14] Neurologic adverse effects including ataxia, blurred vision, diplopia, and fatigue are most frequently reported. Carbamazepine can cause adverse hematologic effects, including transient leukopenia and, more rarely, agranulocytosis, thrombocytopenia, and aplastic anemia. Carbamazepine therapy may also cause hyponatremia, skin rashes, elevation of liver enzymes, weight gain, and GI complaints. Women of childbearing potential should be tested for pregnancy because of the risk of teratogenicity, especially neural tube defects.

Before receiving carbamazepine, patients should undergo baseline laboratory testing, including a CBC with differential and platelets and liver function tests. Subsequent hematologic and liver function monitoring should be carried out every 2 weeks during the first 2 months of treatment and every 3 months thereafter (also see Chapter 54, Seizure Disorders).[14] During therapy, patients should be monitored for abnormal bleeding or petechiae, skin rashes, signs and symptoms of infection, and signs of hyponatremia such as mental status changes.

In addition to the above drug interactions, carbamazepine can induce the metabolism, and thereby reduce the effect, of a number of drugs including oral contraceptives, warfarin, theophylline, haloperidol, and TCAs. The concurrent use of erythromycin, cimetidine, fluoxetine, or calcium channel blockers may lead to increased levels of carbamazepine and unanticipated toxicity (see Chapter 54). Carbamazepine also has the ability to induce its own metabolism. This autoinduc-

tion effect may cause carbamazepine levels to decrease for up to 1 month after a dose adjustment is made.

Oxcarbazepine, a structural analog of carbamazepine, may be an option for the treatment of bipolar disorder. Oxcarbazepine has some advantages over carbamazepine. Drug level monitoring is not required and oxcarbazepine causes fewer drug interactions.[90] In addition, oxcarbazepine is not metabolized to an active epoxide metabolite; therefore, it may have fewer side effects than carbamazepine.

Other anticonvulsants studied in mania include lamotrigine, gabapentin, topiramate, and tiagabine. Initial open-label studies of lamotrigine in mania were promising, and there is only one published double-blind trial to date that showed a similar response between lamotrigine, lithium, and olanzapine.[154,155] The double-blind trial has been criticized for problems with study design. There are two unpublished trials of lamotrigine in mania, both of which are negative.[154] Currently, experts doubt that lamotrigine has any significant effect in acute bipolar mania.

Another anticonvulsant, gabapentin, has been studied in bipolar disorder. It is structurally similar to γ-aminobutyric acid, but its mechanism of action in bipolar disorder is unknown. Benefits of this medication include its renal route of elimination and an absence of significant drug interactions. Open trials and case reports suggest that adjunctive treatment with gabapentin may be effective in manic, hypomanic, and depressive states of bipolar disorder.[156-158] However, a more recent trial suggests that gabapentin may not be effective.[159] In a double-blind, placebo-controlled trial, gabapentin 900 to 3,600 mg/day was administered as an adjunct to mood stabilizers in patients with bipolar I disorder whose current episode was manic, hypomanic, or mixed. At 12 weeks, gabapentin failed to show any significant benefit over placebo. In fact, the placebo group did significantly better than the gabapentin-treated patients.

Topiramate, a monosaccharide derivative, is a novel anticonvulsant recently noted to have some beneficial effect in bipolar disorder.[160,161] An open trial of topiramate added to pre-existing mood-stabilizer therapy for bipolar disorder found that 52% of patients had a moderate to marked response over 16 weeks. The most commonly reported side effects included paresthesias, fatigue, somnolence, cognitive impairment, and reduced concentration.[160] In contrast to other mood stabilizers, topiramate has the added advantage of causing weight loss.[161] Double-blind, placebo-controlled trials of topiramate in bipolar disorder have yet to be published. Before topiramate can be recommended for routine use, more rigorous study is necessary.

Lastly, an open trial of zonisamide reported a 71% response rate in 24 bipolar patients.[162] Tiagabine failed to have any beneficial effect in an initial open trial.[163]

Despite the array of mood stabilizers, anticonvulsants, and antipsychotics available for the management of acute mania, large numbers of patients fail to respond to monotherapy, and combination therapy is becoming increasingly common.[153] The combination of lithium and valproic acid has been shown to be effective for incomplete responders and may be synergistic. Other potentially useful combinations include lithium and atypical antipsychotics, lithium and carbamazepine, valproate and atypical antipsychotics, and valproate and carbamazepine.

A combination to be avoided is carbamazepine and clozapine due to the increased risk of hematologic adverse effects.

VERAPAMIL

The calcium channel blocker, verapamil, has been evaluated for both treatment and prophylaxis of acute manic episodes at dosages of up to 480 mg/day.[164] Recent controlled trials failed to show a positive effect of verapamil in mania.[165,166]

Presently, verapamil may be considered an alternative agent in those who have failed other therapies. Nimodipine may hold particular promise for patients with extremely rapid fluctuations in mood.[14]

THYROID HORMONE

Patients with rapid cycling disorder might be candidates for adjunctive thyroid hormone treatment. A number of individuals with rapid cycling disorder have elevated levels of TSH and evidence of clinical or subclinical hypothyroidism.[167,168] On this basis, rapid cyclers have been medicated successfully with levothyroxine at dosages of 0.15 to 0.4 mg/day to achieve a free T_4 index above normal.[169] It has been suggested that low levels of T_4 may predispose a person to rapid cycling. Another hypothesis is that brain conversion of T_4 to T_3 is impaired in patients with rapid cycling.[169] Individuals who are rapid cyclers should be examined for physical and laboratory evidence of hypothyroidism. Even if no evidence is found, a trial of levothyroxine supplementation might be in order.

Benzodiazepines and Antipsychotics for Acute Agitation

25. M.B. is a 39-year-old man hospitalized for an acute manic episode. Although he has been started on lithium for his manic symptoms, he is becoming increasingly restless and irritable and is unable to sleep. What is an appropriate adjunctive treatment for M.B.?

Benzodiazepines and atypical or conventional antipsychotics are useful in treating agitation, irritability, and hyperactivity associated with acute manic episodes. Conventional antipsychotics have the disadvantage of causing extrapyramidal side effects (EPS), neuroleptic malignant syndrome, tardive dyskinesia, and anticholinergic side effects. On a longer-term basis, individuals with affective disorders such as bipolar disorder who receive conventional antipsychotics may be at a higher risk for developing tardive dyskinesia.[170] Atypical antipsychotics are associated with a lower risk of EPS and tardive dyskinesia.[171]

The use of atypical antipsychotics for acute agitation and aggression is becoming increasingly common, either as monotherapy or in combination with a benzodiazepine. Currently, ziprasidone is the only atypical antipsychotic available in an intramuscular (IM) dosage form. In doses of 10 to 20 mg, ziprasidone IM is effective for the management of psychotic agitation.[172] Also, olanzapine IM has been shown to be more effective than lorazepam IM in acutely agitated bipolar patients.[173] The use of IM injections is often unnecessary because many patients are willing to take liquid dosage forms. Risperidone is the only atypical antipsychotic available in a liquid preparation and when administered along with liquid lorazepam, it has been shown to be equally effective as

haloperidol IM with lorazepam IM for psychotic agitation.[174] The combined use of an antipsychotic with a benzodiazepine is often reserved for patients with psychotic agitation. Furthermore, benzodiazepine has been shown to allow reductions in the dosage of concomitantly administered antipsychotics.[175]

Intramuscular administration of typical antipsychotics, such as haloperidol, is common in the short-term management of agitated mania. The risk of tardive dyskinesia is low if long-term use is avoided. The newer IM atypical agents may be cost prohibitive. There is no reason to continue typical antipsychotics beyond the acute stage of bipolar disorder. These agents lack mood-stabilizing properties, increase the risk of bipolar depression, and are less effective than lithium for the management of core manic symptoms.[176,177] Patients who are treated with typical antipsychotics and have a continued need for antipsychotic therapy beyond the acute stage should be switched to an atypical agent.[178] However, the intramuscular depot forms of typical antipsychotics still have a role in bipolar disorder for those who are noncompliant with oral medication.[177]

The main concerns regarding the use of benzodiazepines for agitated mania are sedation and potential for abuse and addiction. Because adjunctive therapy is usually administered on an inpatient basis for a short period, abuse and addiction are unlikely to be important considerations.

M.B. is irritable and restless. Therefore, he should be started on lorazepam 2 mg orally with repeat doses being administered every 2 to 8 hours as needed to relieve his symptoms of insomnia, irritability, and restlessness.[175]

26. Fours hours after the first dose, there was little improvement in M.B.'s symptoms. Subsequently, he received a second dose of lorazepam 2 mg PO. The second dose appeared to provide little benefit, and his symptoms continued to escalate. The nursing staff began to suspect that M.B. might be cheeking the medication. How should M.B. be managed if he is unwilling to take oral medication?

Lorazepam has the added advantage of being available in intramuscular and liquid preparations. These dosage forms are more rapidly absorbed than the oral tablets and are beneficial when rapid sedation is required. Given M.B.'s symptom escalation and his refusal to take oral medication, lorazepam 2 mg IM every 2 to 8 hours as needed would be appropriate.[175] Once M.B. has stabilized and is more cooperative, the IM dose should be converted to an oral dosage form. The lorazepam should be tapered as M.B. begins to respond to lithium. If M.B. requires frequent and/or large doses of lorazepam, it is advisable to taper the benzodiazepine to prevent rebound agitation or irritability in the individual who is still in stage I or II of mania (see Clinical Symptoms).

Acute Bipolar Depression

27. H.C., a 31-year-old woman, was hospitalized for treatment of an acute manic episode 3 weeks ago. She was discharged 5 days ago on divalproex sodium 1,750 mg/day and olanzapine 15 mg QHS. Compared with her admission presentation, her behavior and speech had improved dramatically. However, she was still sleeping only 4 hours per night. Her parents called the mental health clinic to report that she has spent most of the day in bed for the last 2 days. She was sleeping most of this time. When out of bed, H.C. reportedly sat on the couch without moving for hours. She only nibbled at the food her parents offered her. She has no other signs or symptoms of physical illness and has not taken any additional medications, alcohol, or drugs of abuse to her parents' knowledge. On further questioning, they admit that she is intermittently tearful and expresses remorse for the "sins I committed when I was high." They also quote her as saying that she is "as low as I can go and I just want to die." They suspect she is suicidal. H.C.'s parents report that she is taking divalproex sodium and olanzapine as prescribed and that the last time she was this depressed lithium did not seem to help. Her valproate level on discharge was 80 μg/ml. What change in H.C.'s treatment should be instituted at this time?

Lithium

Acute bipolar depression is a recurring and chronic problem for many patients. The depression is often difficult to control and puts patients at significant risk for suicide. Until recently, little attention was paid to bipolar depression and little data is available regarding the best treatment options for these patients. Remission of depressive symptoms should be the primary goal for bipolar depression. A logical first step in the management of bipolar depression is to optimize the dose of the current mood stabilizer.[90] Although most studies of lithium for acute bipolar depression are nearly two decades old, this agent remains one of the drugs of choice.[14] In these older trials, approximately 79% of patients responded to lithium. However, in only 36% of patients was the response marked.[179] Higher serum lithium concentrations are associated with antidepressant activity in bipolar depression.[179]

Lamotrigine

Lamotrigine is also considered a first-line agent by some experts.[14] A double-blind, placebo-controlled trial of lamotrigine monotherapy in bipolar depression found that 51% of patients receiving lamotrigine 200 mg/day met criteria for response on the Hamilton Rating Scale for Depression (HAM-D), compared with 45% of those treated with lamotrigine 50 mg/day and 37% of placebo-treated patients.[180] The difference in response rates among the three groups did not reach statistical significance. However, a significant difference between both treatment groups and placebo was noted on the Montgomery-Asberg Depression Rating Scale (MADRS). A cross-over study of lamotrigine, gabapentin, and placebo reported response rates of 45%, 26%, and 19%, respectively.[181] An 18 month trial of lamotrigine, lithium, or placebo for prophylaxis of any mood episode in bipolar I patients found that both active treatments were equally effective and superior to placebo.[182] The time to a manic, mixed, or hypomanic episode was greater with lithium compared with placebo. Conversely, the time to a depressive episode was greater with lamotrigine than with placebo.

There are a few reports of patients who experienced increased cycling while taking lamotrigine.[180,181] The mood-stabilizing properties of lamotrigine are thought to result from its ability to stabilize neurons and reduce spontaneous discharges in a manner similar to other anticonvulsants in use for bipolar disorder.

Because H.C. did not respond to lithium during her past depressive episode, lamotrigine is a reasonable alternative agent to try for the current episode. The metabolism of lamotrigine is affected by the concomitant use of enzyme-inducing (e.g., carbamazepine) and enzyme-inhibiting drugs (e.g., valproate). Thus, the initial dose and titration schedule for lamotrigine must take into account these treatments. For patients receiving no inducers or inhibitors, the initial dose is 25 mg/day for 2 weeks, followed by 50 mg/day for 2 weeks, followed by 100 mg/day for 1 week. The target dose of lamotrigine is 200 mg/day. Patients receiving enzyme inducers should begin with 50 mg/day for 2 weeks, then 100 mg/day in two doses for 2 weeks. Thereafter, the dose can be increased by 100 mg/day every 1 to weeks to a target dose of 400 mg/day.

H.C. is taking valproate, which is known to inhibit the metabolism of lamotrigine. Therefore, the initial dose for H.C. is 25 mg every other day. The dose is increased in 2 weeks to 25 mg/day and may be increased further by 25 to 50 mg/day every 1 to 2 weeks to a target dose of 100 mg/day. In some patients, doses higher than the target dose may be useful. Dizziness, headache, ataxia, sedation, blurred vision, and GI disturbances are the most common side effects. Lamotrigine may cause a skin rash, especially when dosages are increased quickly or patients receive concomitant valproic acid. Lamotrigine-induced rash may progress to the life-threatening Stevens-Johnson syndrome. H.C. should be instructed to contact her physician immediately at the first sign of a skin rash.

Antidepressants

The combination of antidepressants along with mood stabilizers is yet another treatment option for depressed bipolar patients. Antidepressant augmentation of other mood-stabilizing agents seems safest in those with bipolar II disorder and most risky in those with rapid cycling disorder[81] (see Question 4). Recently published was a double-blind, placebo-controlled study of paroxetine, imipramine, or placebo as an adjunct to lithium.[183] This trial indicated that antidepressants offer no additional benefit to lithium, especially in patients with lithium levels >0.8 mEq/L. For those with lower lithium levels due to intolerance of higher doses, antidepressant treatment resulted in a significant improvement. In another trial, treatment with paroxetine or a mood stabilizer was added to an existing mood stabilizer regimen.[184] Both treatment groups exhibited a significant decrease in depressive symptoms over 6 weeks but there were more drop-outs in the additional mood stabilizer group owing to intolerability.

Maintenance Therapy of Bipolar Disorder

28. R.L., a 33-year-old man, has been treated for an episode of acute mania with lithium 600 mg BID for 3 weeks. He is no longer overtly manic. However, because R.L. may have had past episodes of depression and mania, his physician decides to institute prophylactic (maintenance) lithium therapy. What are the goals of maintenance lithium therapy for R.L.? How should he be monitored during this maintenance phase? How long should R.L. be maintained on lithium?

Lithium

Appropriate goals for maintenance therapy include an increase in the interval between episodes, a decrease in the frequency of episodes, and a reduction in the duration and severity of single episodes. Maintenance therapy with lithium clearly reduces the frequency and severity of mood episodes in patients with bipolar disorder. Goodwin and Jamison[185] have shown that in patients receiving maintenance lithium, only 34% relapsed, compared with 81% of patients receiving placebo. However, some studies indicate that lithium's effectiveness may be much lower. Naturalistic studies that followed patients on maintenance lithium indicate an episodic recurrence rate of 43% to 55%.[186,187] It is possible that these studies failed to identify patients with rapid cycling disorder who may have done poorly on lithium. Lithium therapy may have the added benefit of reducing mortality from suicide.[188] Conflicting results have been published recently regarding lithium's effectiveness for prevention of any mood episode in patients with bipolar I disorder.[182,189]

Target levels for maintenance therapy with lithium should be in the range of 0.5 to 0.8 mEq/L.[14] However, at least one study found that patients with lithium levels ranging from 0.4 to 0.6 mEq/L had relapse rates 2.6 times higher than patients with levels ranging from 0.8 to 1.0 mEq/L. Although these higher levels reduced the number of relapses, they also resulted in a higher incidence of side effects.[190]

In addition to determining appropriate maintenance lithium levels for R.L., this is an opportune time to consider whether once- or twice-a-day administration of lithium can improve adherence or side effects. During periods of dosage readjustment, R.L. will require monitoring of his lithium serum level every several days until it is stable. Once stabilized, the monitoring frequency can be reduced to no less than every 6 months but needs to be individualized.[14] If R.L. were to exhibit any of the risk factors that could predispose him to lithium toxicity (see Question 19) or if other medication changes were to occur, more frequent monitoring should be reinstituted temporarily.

While continuing on lithium, R.L. should be monitored periodically for thyroid function to detect lithium-related hypothyroidism. Also, renal function should be measured regularly to detect the development of conditions that might require an alteration in the lithium dosage and to ensure that any lithium effects on the kidney are detected early if they occur. These tests should be repeated approximately every 6 to 12 months.[14]

The decision to institute maintenance lithium therapy usually is made because of the severity of affective episodes and the belief that they will recur in the future. A period of successful maintenance therapy means that the individual is controlled, not cured, because most patients who are withdrawn from lithium relapse eventually. With each recurrent manic episode, the risk of experiencing subsequent and more frequent manic episodes increases. Furthermore, as individuals experience successive episodes, they tend to recover less completely and function at a diminished level between occurrences.[185] Because the goal is to prevent the trauma of repeated episodes and the deterioration that may accompany them, R.L. may require lithium for the remainder of his life.

Lithium Refractoriness

29. **P.B., a 42-year-old woman, has five previous hospitalizations for manic and/or depressive episodes. She has experienced approximately six severe mood swings in the past year, including**

episodes of depression and hypomania. Despite adequate plasma levels, she has not responded to a regimen that includes lithium and paroxetine. The addition of olanzapine 10 mg HS resulted in no further improvement. She now presents as depressed, with expressions of suicidal hopelessness about her condition, sleep disturbances, and poor appetite. Why is P.B. failing to respond to lithium?

There are several potential reasons for P.B.'s poor response. Poor adherence always must be considered as a potential reason for lithium failure; however, P.B. has an adequate level of lithium. If P.B. had been intermittently compliant in the past or if her therapy had been stopped, she might have developed a syndrome called *lithium discontinuation–induced refractoriness*. This phenomenon occurs in patients who once responded to lithium and then had their lithium discontinued. When an affective episode recurs, they fail to fully respond to lithium reintroduction. However, there is conflicting evidence regarding lithium refractoriness, and it is unclear how often this phenomenon occurs.[191,192] If P.B. had been having more and more breakthrough affective episodes gradually, she simply could have become tolerant to lithium. Thus, a careful review of P.B.'s history of adherence and the pattern of her affective episodes is necessary.

P.B. has another potential reason for nonresponse. She has had at least six affective episodes in the past year. Therefore, she is a rapid cycler. Approximately 70% to 80% of rapid cyclers have a poor response to lithium.[14]

Anticonvulsants

30. **Are any other mood stabilizers effective for maintenance of bipolar disorder?**

Because of the side effects of lithium, many patients become intolerant or unwilling to continue lithium therapy. Valproic acid and lamotrigine are reasonable alternatives that have shown efficacy in maintenance therapy.[182,193] Carbamazepine may also be an acceptable second-line agent for maintenance therapy, although it has not been rigorously studied.[14] Data with olanzapine for maintenance therapy of bipolar depression indicates that it, too, may be effective.[127,128] Patients should continue the regimen that was effective in resolving the acute episode, and many patients require combination therapy because of the high failure rates of monotherapy.[14,193]

Nonpharmacologic Therapies for Bipolar Disorder

31. **What is the role of psychotherapy in bipolar disorder?**

Although medication is the mainstay of treatment for bipolar disorder, psychotherapy is helpful in selected cases. Because early affective episodes may be precipitated by stressful life events, future episodes may be prevented if bipolar individuals and their families can learn to avoid or better cope with such stresses. Evidence suggests that later in the course of the illness, stress does not play a major role in precipitating individual episodes.[27]

Therapy may also help the family cope with the emotion and stress resulting from the disruption caused by a manic or depressive episode. Infidelity, unemployment, excessive bills, violent outbursts, reckless endangerment, lack of discretion, embarrassment, and fear concerning future episodes are among the issues with which a family must come to terms. Compliance with medication is another common issue that is addressed in therapy sessions because the issue of medication often turns into a struggle over who is in control. In addition, some patients must accept untoward effects or the fact that they will no longer experience their pleasant "highs."

Another nonpharmacologic therapy that should not be overlooked is electroconvulsive therapy. It has proved effective in manic episodes, depressive episodes, and prophylaxis, especially in pregnant individuals.[14]

REFERENCES

1. National Institutes of Mental Health. Key facts about mental illness. Rockville, MD: National Institutes of Mental Health, 1993.
2. American Psychiatric Association. Mood disorders. In: Diagnostic and Statistical Manual of Mental Disorder. Fourth Ed. Text Revision. Washington, DC: American Psychiatric Association, 2000:382.
3. Hamilton M. Mood disorders: clinical features. In: Kaplan HI, Sadock BJ, eds. Comprehensive Textbook of Psychiatry V. Baltimore: Williams & Wilkins, 1989:892. (need to update)
4. Robins LN, Regier DA, eds. Psychiatric Disorders in America: The Epidemiologic Catchment Area Survey. New York: Free Press;1991.
5. Kessler RC et al. Lifetime and 12-month prevalence of DSM-III-R psychiatric disorders in the US: results from the national comorbidity survey. Arch Gen Psychiatry 1994;51:8.
6. Weissman MM et al. Cross-national epidemiology of major depression and bipolar disorder. JAMA 1996;276:293.
7. Narrow WE et al. Revised prevalence estimates of mental disorders in the United States. Arch Gen Psychiatry 2002;59:115.
8. Angst J. The emerging epidemiology of hypomania and bipolar II disorder. J Affect Disord 1998;50:143.
9. Judd LL, Akiskal HS. The prevalence and disability of bipolar spectrum disorders in the US population: reanalysis of the ECA database taking into account the subthreshold cases. J Affect Disord 2003;73:123.
10. Evans DL. Bipolar disorder: diagnostic challenges and treatment considerations. J Clin Psychiatry 2000;61(Suppl 13):26.
11. Weissman MM, Smith AL. Epidemiology. In: Paykel ES, ed. Handbook of Affective Disorders, 2nd Ed. New York: Churchill Livingstone, 1992:111.
12. Wyatt RJ, Henter I. An economic evaluation of manic-depressive illness: 1991. Soc Psychiatry Psychiatr Epidemiol 1995;30:213.
13. Goodwin FK, Jamison KR. The manic-depressive spectrum. In: Manic-Depressive Illness. New York: Oxford University Press, 1990:74.
14. APA. Practice guidelines for the treatment of patients with bipolar disorder (revision). Am J Psychiatry 2002;159(4 Suppl):1.
15. Hirschfeld RM et al. Perceptions and impact of bipolar disorder: how far have we really come? Results of the national depressive and manic-depressive association 2000 survey of individuals with bipolar disorder. J Clin Psychiatry 2003;64:161.
16. Kupfer DJ et al. Demographic and clinical characteristics of individuals in a bipolar disorder case registry. J Clin Psychiatry 2002;63(2):121.
17. Bauer MS et al. Rapid cycling bipolar disorder. I. Association with grade I hypothyroidism. Arch Gen Psychiatry 1990;47:432.
18. Bauer MS, Whybrow PC. Rapid cycling bipolar disorder. II. Treatment of refractory rapid cycling with high-dose levothyroxine: a preliminary study. Arch Gen Psychiatry 1990;47:435.
19. Post RM. Et al. Rapid-cycling bipolar affective disorder: lack of relation to hypothyroidism. Psychiatry Res 1997;72(1):1.
20. Gitlin MJ. Swendsen J. Relapse and impairment in bipolar disorder. Am J Psychiatry 1995;152:1635.
21. Angst F et al. Mortality of patients with mood disorders: follow up over 34-38 yrs. J Affect Disord 2002;68:167.

22. Lopez P et al. suicide attempts in bipolar patients. J Clin Psychiatry 2001;62:963.
23. Tsai SY et al. Risk factors for completed suicide in bipolar disorder. J Clin Psychiatry 2002;63:496.
24. Nierenberg AA et al. Mood disorders and suicide. J Clin Psychiatry 2001;62(Suppl 25):27.
25. Woods SW. The economic burden of bipolar disorder. J Clin Psych 2000;61(Suppl 13):38.
26. Sachs GS et al. The expert consensus guidelines series: medication treatment of bipolar disorder 2000. Postgrad Med Special Report 2000(April):1.
27. Goodwin FK, Jamison KR. Course and outcome. In: Manic-Depressive Illness. New York: Oxford University Press, 1990:127.
28. Peet M. Drug-induced mania. Drug Saf 1995;12(2):146.
29. El-Mallakh RS. Buporpion manic induction during euthymia, but not during depression. Bipolar Disord 2001;3(3):159.
30. Fichtner C, Braun BG. Bupropion-associated mania in a patient with HIV infection [Letter]. J Clin Psychopharmacol 1992;12:366.
31. Berthier ML, Kulvisevsky J. Fluoxetine-induced mania in a patient with post stroke depression. Br J Psychiatry 1993;163:698.
32. Feder R. Fluoxetine-induced mania. J Clin Psychiatry 1990;51:524.
33. Benazzi F. Organic hypomania secondary to sibutramine-citalopram interaction. J Clin Psychiatry 2002;63(2):165.
34. Dorevitch A et al. Fluvoxamine-associated manic behavior: a case series. Ann Pharmacother 1993;27:1455.
35. Zaphiris HA et al. Probable nefazodone-induced mania in a patient with unreported bipolar disorder. Ann Clin Psychiatry 1996;8(4):207.
36. De Leon OA et al. Mirtazapine-induced mania in a case of poststroke depression [Letter]. J Neuropsych Clin Neurosci 1999;11(1):115.
37. Bhanji NH et al. Dysphoric mania induced by high-dose mirtazapine: a case for norepinephrine syndrome? Int Clin Psychopharmacol 2002;17(6):319.
38. Stoner SC et al. Possible venlafaxine-induced mania. J Clin Psychopharm 1999;19(2):184.
39. Gupta N. Venlafaxine-induced hypomanic switch in bipolar depression. Can J Psychiatry 2001;46(8):760.
40. Vieta E, Colom F et al. Reboxetine-induced hypomania. J Clin Psychiatry 2001;62(8):655.
41. Lindenmayer JP et al. Olanzapine-induced manic-like syndrome. J Clin Psychiatry 1998;59(6):318.
42. Fitz-Gerald MJ et al. Olanzapine-induced mania. Am J Psychiatry 1999;156(7):1114.
43. Koek RJ et al. Probable induction of mania by risperidone. J Clin Psychiatry 1996;57(4):174.
44. Diaz SF. Mania associated with risperidone use. J Clin Psychiatry 1996;57(1):41.
45. Lane HY et al. Mania induced by risperidone: dose related? J Clin Psychiatry 1998;59(2):85.
46. Lu BY, Lundgren R et al. A case of ziprasidone-induced mania and the role of 5-HT2A in mood changes induced by atypical antipsychotics. J Clin Psychiatry 2002;63(12):1185.
47. Atmaca M, Kuloglu M et al. Quetiapine-associated and dose-related hypomania in a woman with schizophrenia. Eur Psychiatry 2002;17(5):292.
48. Becker D, Grinber Y et al. Association between flupenthixol treatment and emergence of manic symptoms. Eur Psychiatry 2002;17(6):349.
49. Price WA, Prepubertal M. Buspirone-induced mania. J Clin Psychopharmacol 1989;9:150.

50. France RD, Krishnan KRR. Alprazolam-induced manic reaction. Am J Psychiatry 1984;141:1127.
51. Weilburg JB et al. Triazolam-induced brief episodes of secondary mania in a depressed patient. J Clin Psychiatry 1987;48:492.
52. Rego MD, Giller EL. Mania secondary to amantadine treatment of neuroleptic-induced hyperprolactinemia. J Clin Psychiatry 1989;50:143.
53. Hubain PP et al. Cimetidine-induced mania. Neuropsychobiology 1982;8:223.
54. Sotsky SM, Tossell JW. Tolmetin induction of mania. Psychosomatics 1984;25:626.
55. Kraus RP. Rapid cycling triggered by pindolol augmentation of paroxetine, but not with desipramine. Depression1996;4(2):92.
56. Monji A et al. A case of persistent manic depressive illness induced by interferon-alfa in the treatment of chronic hepatitis C. Psychosomatics 1998;39(6):562.
57. Benazzi F. Mania associated with donepezil. Int J Geriatr Psych 1998;13(11):814.
58. Watts BV et al. Tramadol-induced mania. Am J Psychiatry 1997;154(11):1624.
59. Horrigan JP et al. Guanfacine and secondary mania in children. J Affect Dis 1999;54(3):309.
60. Navarro V, Vieta E. et al. Mannitol-induced acute manic state. J Clin Psychiatry 2001;62(2):125.
61. Kinrys G. Hypomania associated with omega3 fatty acids. Arch Gen Psychiatry 2000;34(5);629.
62. Brieger P, Marencros A et al. Manic episode in an ifosfamide-treated patient. Gen Hosp Psychiatry 2000;22(1):52.
63. Nierenberg AA, Burt T et al. Mania associated with St. John's wort. Biol Psychiatry 1999;15(46):1707.
64. Gonzalez-Seijo JC et al. Manic episode and ginseng: report of a possible case. J Clin Psychopharm 1995;15(6):447.
65. Emmanuel NP et al. Use of herbal products and symptoms of bipolar disorder. Am J Psychiatry 1998;155(11):1627.
66. Koehler-Troy C et al. Methylphenidate-induced mania in a prepubertal child. J Clin Psychiatry 1986;47:566.
67. Bowden CL et al. Mania from dexfenfluramine. J Clin Psychiatry 1997;58(12):548.
68. Raison CL et al. Psychotic mania associated with fenfluramine and phentermine use. Am J Psychiatry 1997;154(5):711.
69. Hill RR et al. Secondary mania associated with the use of felbamate. Psychosomatics 1995;36(4):404.
70. Short C, Cooke L. Hypomania induced by gabapentin. Br J Psychiatry 1995;166:679.
71. Margolese HC, Beauclair L et al. Hypomania induced by adjunctive lamotrigine. Am J Psychiatry 2003;160(1):183
72. Jochum T, Bar KJ et al. Topiramate induced manic episode. J Neurol Neurosurg Psychiatry 2002;73(2):208.
73. Wada K, Yamada N et al. Corticosteroid-induced psychotic and mood disorders: diagnosis defined by DSM-IV and clinical pictures. Psychosomatics 2001;42(6):461.
74. Pope HG, Katz DL. Affective and psychotic symptoms associated with anabolic steroid use. Am J Psychiatry 1988;145:487.
75. Kline MD, Jaggers ED. Mania onset while using dehydroepiandrosterone. Am J Psychiatry 1999;156(6):971.
76. Weiss EL et al. Testosterone-patch-induced psychotic mania. Am J Psychiatry 1999;156(6):969.
77. Rachman M et al. Lupron-induced mania. Bio Psychiatry 1999;45(2):243.

78. Blanc J, Corbella B et al. Manic syndrome associated with efavirenz overdose. Clin Infect Dis 2001;33(2):270.

79. Abouesh A et al. Antimicrobial-induced mania (antibiomania): a review of spontaneous reports. J Clin Psychopharmacol 2002;22(1):71.

80. Abouesh A et al. Clarithromycin-induced mania. Am J Psychiatry 1998;155(11):1626.

81. Goodwin FK, Jamison KR. Medical treatment of acute bipolar depression. In: Manic-Depressive Illness. New York: Oxford University Press, 1990: 630.

82. Ghaemi SN et al. Diagnosing bipolar disorder and the effect of antidepressants: a naturalistic study. J Clin Psychiatry 2000;61:804.

83. Prien RF et al. Drug therapy in the prevention of recurrences in unipolar and bipolar disorders: report of the NIMH Collaborative Study Group comparing lithium carbonate, imipramine, and a lithium carbonate-imipramine combination. Arch Gen Psychiatry 1984;41:1095.

84. Altshuler LL, Post RM et al. antidepressant-induced mania and cycle acceleration: a controversy revisited. Am J Psychiatry 1995;152:1130.

85. Sachs GS et al. a double-blind trial of bupropion versus desipramine for bipolar depression. J Clin Psychiatry 1994;55:391.

86. Amsterdam JD et al. Efficacy and safety of fluoxetine in treating bipolar II major depressive episode. J Clin Psychopharmacol 1998;435.

87. Bottlender R et al. Mood stabilizers reduce the risk of developing antidepressant-induced maniform states in acute treatment of bipolar I depressed patients. J Affect Disord 2001;63:79.

88. Boerlin HL et al. Bipolar depression and antidepressant-induced mania: a naturalistic study. J Clin Psychiatry 1998;59:374.

89. Ghaemi SN et al. Effectiveness and safety of long-term antidepressant treatment in bipolar disorder. J Clin Psychiatry 2001;62:565.

90. Suppes T et al. Report of the Texas Consensus Conference Panel on Medication Treatment of Bipolar Disorder 2000. J Clin Psychiatry 2002; 62:288.

91. Bowden CL et al. Efficacy of divalproex vs lithium and placebo in the treatment of mania. JAMA 1994;271:918.

92. Moller HJ, Nasrallah HA. Treatment of bipolar disorder. J Clin Psychiatry 2003;64[Suppl 6]:9.

93. Bowden CL et al. Relation of serum valproate concentration to response in mania. Am J Psychiatry 1996;153:765.

94. Keck PE et al. Valproate oral loading in the treatment of acute mania. J Clin Psychiatry 1993; 54:305.

95. Hirschfel RM, Allen MH. Safety and tolerability of oral loading divalproex sodium in acutely manic bipolar patients. J Clin Psychiatry 1999; 60:815.

96. Bowden CL. Novel treatments for bipolar disorder. Exp Opin Invest Drugs 2001;10(4):661.

97. Ernst CL, Goldber JF. The reproductive safety profile of mood stabilizers, atypical antipsychotics, and broad-spectrum psychotropics. J Clin Psychiatry 2002;63[Suppl 4]:42.

98. Isojarvi JI, Laatikainen TJ. Polycystic ovaries and hyperandrogenism in women taking valproate for epilepsy. N Engl J Med 1993;329:1383.

99. O'Donovan C et al. Menstrual abnormalities and polycystic ovary syndrome in women taking valproate for bipolar mood disorder. J Clin Psychiatry 2002;63:322.

100. McIntyre RS, Mancini DA. Valproate, bipolar disorder and polycystic ovarian syndrome. Bipolar Disord 2003;5:28.

101. Eze E et al. Hyperammonemia and coma developed by a woman treated with valproic acid for affective disorder. Psychiatr Serv 1998;49(10):1358.

102. Panikkar GP, Gilman SM. Valproate-induced hyperammonemia in the psychiatric setting: 2 cases. J Clin Psychiatry 1999;60:557.

103. Allarakhia IN et al. Valproic acid and thrombocytopenia in children: a case-controlled retrospective study. Pediatr Neurol 1996;14:303.

104. Delgado MR et al. Thrombocytopenia secondary to high valproate levels in children with epilepsy. J Child Neurol 1994;9:311.

105. Wilder BJ et al. Gastrointestinal tolerance of divalproex sodium. Neurology 1983;33:808.

106. Cranor CW et al. Clinical and economic impact of replacing divalproex sodium with valproic acid. Am J Health-Syst Pharm 1997;54:1716.

107. Sherr JD, Kelly DL. Substitution of immediate-release valproic acid for divalproex sodium for adult psychiatric inpatients. Psychiatric Serv 1998;49(10):1355.

108. Goodwin FK, Jamison KR. Medical treatment of manic episodes. In: Manic-Depressive Illness. New York: Oxford University Press, 1990:603.

109. Goodwin FK, Jamison KR. Maintenance medical treatment. In: Manic-Depressive Illness. New York: Oxford University Press, 1990:665.

110. Gelenberg AJ et al. Lithium tremor. J Clin Psychiatry 1995;283.

111. Gitlin M. Lithium and the kidney: an updated review. Drug Saf 1999;20:231.

112. Mellerup ET. The side effects of lithium. Biol Psychiatry 1990;28:464.

113. Hetmar O et al. Lithium: long-term effects on the kidney. A prospective follow-up study ten years after kidney biopsy. Br J Psychiatry 1991;158:53.

114. Dunner DL. Drug interactions of lithium and other antimanic/mood-stabilizing medications. J Clin Psychiatry 2003;64(Suppl 5):38.

115. Kleiner J, Altshuler LL. Lithium-induced subclinical hypothyroidism: review of the literature and guidelines for treatment. J Clin Psychiatry 1999; 60:249.

116. Cohen LS et al. A reevaluation of risk of in utero exposure to lithium. JAMA 1994;271:146.

117. Troyer WA et al. Association of maternal lithium exposure and premature delivery. J Perinatol 1993;13:123.

118. Tohen M et al. Olanzapine versus placebo in the treatment of acute mania. Am J Psychiatry 1999;156:702.

119. Tohen M et al. Efficacy of olanzapine in acute bipolar mania: a double-blind, placebo-controlled study. Arch Gen Psychiatry 2000;57:841.

120. Berk M. Olanzapine compared to lithium in mania: a double-blind randomized controlled trial. Int Clin Psychopharmacol 1999;14:339.

121. Zajecka JM et al. A comparison of the efficacy, safety, and tolerability of divalproex sodium and olanzapine in the treatment of bipolar disorder. J Clin Psychiatry 2002;63:1148.

122. Tohen M et al. Olanzapine versus divalproex in the treatment of acute mania. Am J Psychiatry 2002;159:1011

123. Zarate CA. Clinical predictors of acute response with olanzapine in psychotic mood disorders. J Clin Psychiatry 1998;59(1):24.

124. Tohen M et al. Efficacy of olanzapine in combination with valproate or lithium in the treatment of mania in patients partially nonresponsive to valproate or lithium monotherapy. Arch Gen Psychiatry 2002;59(1):62.

125. Ketter TA et al. Rapid efficacy of olanzapine augmentation in nonpsychotic bipolar mixed states. J Clin Psychiatry 1998;59(2):83.

126. Guille C et al. A naturalistic comparison of clozapine, risperidone, and olanzapine in the treatment of bipolar disorder. J Clin Psychiatry 2000;61:638.

127. Sanger TM et al. Long-term olanzapine therapy in the treatment of bipolar I disorder: an open-label continuation phase study. J Clin Psychiatry 2001; 62:273:81.

128. Vieta E et al. Olanzapine as long-term adjunctive therapy in treatment-resistant bipolar disorder. J Clin Psychopharmacol 2001;21:469.

129. Ghaemi SN et al. Acute treatment of bipolar disorder with adjunctive risperidone in outpatients. Can J Psychiatry 1997;42:196.

130. Ghaemi SN et al. Long-term risperidone treatment in bipolar disorder: 6-month follow-up. Int Clin Psychopharmacol 1997;12:333.

131. Jacobsen FM. Risperidone in the treatment of affective illness and obsessive-compulsive disorder. J Clin Psychiatry 1995;56:423.

132. McIntytre RS et al. Risperidone treatment of bipolar disorder. Can J Psychiatry 1997;42:88.

133. Segal J et al. Risperidone compared with both lithium and haloperidol in mania: a double-blind randomized controlled trial. Clin Neuropharmacol 1998;21:176.

134. Sachs GS et al. Combination of a mood stabilizer with risperidone or haloperidol for treatment of acute mania: a double-blind comparison of efficacy and safety. Am J Psychiatry 2002;159:1146.

135. Vieta E et al. Risperidone safety and efficacy in the treatment of bipolar and schizoaffective disorders: results from a 6-month, multicenter, open study. J Clin Psychiatry 2001;62:818.

136. Vieta E et al. Risperidone in the treatment of mania: efficacy and safety results from a large, multicentre, open study in Spain. J Affect Disord 2002;72:15.

137. Keck PE et al. Clinical predictors of acute risperidone response in schizophrenia, schizoaffective disorder, and psychotic mood disorders. J Clin Psychiatry 1995;56(10):466.

138. Keck P et al. Ziprasidone in the treatment of acute bipolar mania: a three-week, placebo-controlled, double-blind, randomized trial. Am J Psychiatry 2003;160(4).741.

139. Ghaemi SN et al. The use of quetiapine for treatment-resistant bipolar disorder: a case series. Ann Clin Psychiatry 1999;11(3):137.

140. Vieta E et al. Quetiapine in the treatment of rapid cycling bipolar disorder. Bipolar Disorders 2002;4(5):535.

141. Zarate CA et al. Clinical predictors of acute response with quetiapine in psychotic mood disorders. J Clin Psychiatry 2000;61(3):185.

142. Zarate CA. Clozapine in severe mood disorders. J Clin Psychiatry 1995;56:411.

143. Banov MD et al. Clozapine therapy in refractory affective disorders: polarity predicts response in long-term follow-up. J Clin Psychiatry 1994; 55:295.

144. Calabrese JR et al. Clozapine for treatment-refractory mania. Am J Psychiatry 1996;153:759.

145. Suppes T et al. Clinical outcome in a randomized 1-year trial of clozapine versus treatment as usual for patients with treatment-resistant illness and a history of mania. Am J Psychiatry 1999;156:1164.

146. Suppes T et al. Clozapine treatment of nonpsychotic rapid cycling bipolar disorder: a report of three cases. Biol Psychiatry 1994;36:338.

147. Ballenger JC et al. Therapeutic effects of carbamazepine in affective illness: a preliminary report. Commun Psychopharmacol 1978;2:159.

148. Leher B et al. Carbamazepine versus lithium in mania: a double-blind study. J Clin Psychiatry 1987;48:89.

149. Small JG et al. Carbamazepine compared with lithium in the treatment of mania. Arch Gen Psychiatry 1991;48:915.

150. Okuma et al. Comparison of the antimanic efficacy of carbamazepine and chlorpromazine: a double-blind controlled study. Psychopharmacology 1979;66:211.

151. Post RM et al. Correlates of antimanic response to carbamazepine. Psychiatry Res 1987;21:71.

152. Denicoff KD et al. Comparative prophylactic efficacy of lithium, carbamazepine, and the combination in bipolar disorder. J Clin Psychiatry 1997;58:470.

153. Freeman MP et al. Mood stabilizer combinations: a review of safety and efficacy. Am J Psychiatry 1998;155:15.

154. Yatham LN. Third generation anticonvulsants in bipolar disorder: a review of efficacy and summary of clinical recommendations. J Clin Psychiatry 2002:63(4):275.

155. Berk M et al. Lamotrigine and the treatment of mania in bipolar disorder. Eur Neuropsychopharmacol 1999;9(Suppl 4):S119.

156. Young TL et al. Gabapentin as an adjunctive treatment in bipolar disorder. J Affect Dis 1999;55:73.

157. Schaffer CB et al. Gabapentin in the treatment of bipolar disorder. Am J Psychiatry 1997;154(2):291.
158. Ghaemi SN et al. Gabapentin treatment of mood disorders: a preliminary study. J Clin Psychiatry 1998;59(8):426.
159. Pande AC et al. Gabapentin in bipolar disorder: a placebo-controlled trial of adjunctive therapy. Bipolar Disord 2000;2(3 pt 2):249.
160. Marcotte D. Use of topiramate, a new anti-epileptic as a mood stabilizer. J Affective Disorders 1998;50:245.
161. Gordon A et al. Mood stabilization and weight loss with topiramate. Am J Psychiatry 1999;156:968A.
162. Kanba S et al. The first open study of zonisamide, a novel anticonvulsant, shows efficacy in mania. Prog Neuropsychopharmacol Biol Psychiatry 1994;18:707.
163. Grunze H et al. Tiagabine appears not to be efficacious in the treatment of acute mania. J Clin Psychiatry 1999;60:759.
164. Dubovsky SL et al. Calcium antagonists in mania: a double-blind study of verapamil. Psychiatry Res 1986;18: 309.
165. Janicak PG et al. Verapamil for the treatment of acute mania: a double-blind, placebo-controlled trial. Am J Psychiatry 1998;155(7):972.
166. Walton SA et al. Superiority of lithium over verapamil in mania: a randomized, controlled, single-blind trial. J Clin Psychiatry 1996;57:543.
167. Bommer M et al. Subclinical hypothyroidism in recurrent mania. Biol Psychiatry 1992;31:729.
168. Ananth J et al. Rapid cycling patients: conceptual and etiological factors. Neuropsychobiology 1993;27:193.
169. Bauer MS et al. Rapid cycling bipolar disorder. Treatment of refractory rapid cycling with high-dose levothyroxine: a preliminary study. Arch Gen Psychiatry 1990;47:435
170. Kane JM et al. Tardive dyskinesia: prevalence, incidence, and risk factors. J Clin Psychopharmacol 1988;52S.
171. Casey DE. Tardive dyskinesia and atypical antipsychotic drugs. Schizophrenia Res 1999;35 (Suppl):S61.
172. Brook S et al. Intramuscular ziprasidone compared with intramuscular haloperidol in the management of acute psychosis. J Clin Psychiatry 2000;61(12):933.
173. Meehan K et al. A double-blind, randomized comparison of the efficacy and safety of intramuscular injections of olanzapine, lorazepam, or placebo in treating acutely agitated patients diagnosed with bipolar mania. J Clin Psychopharmacol 2001; 21:389.
174. Currier GW et al. Risperidone liquid concentrate and oral lorazepam versus intramuscular haloperidol and intramuscular lorazepam for treatment of psychotic agitation. J Clin Psychiatry 2001;62(3):153.
175. Alderfer BS et al. Treatment of agitation in bipolar disorder across the life cycle. J Clin Psychiatry 2003;64(Suppl 4):3.
176. Tohen M et al. Antipsychotic agents and bipolar disorder. J Clin Psychiatry 1998;59(Suppl 1):38.
177. McElroy SL et al. Mania, psychosis, and antipsychotics. J Clin Psychiatry 1996;(Suppl 3):14.
178. Miller DS et al. Comparative efficacy of typical and atypical antipsychotics as add-on therapy too mood stabilizers in the treatment of acute mania. J Clin Psychiatry 2001;62(12):975.
179. Keck PE et al. New approaches in managing bipolar depression. J Clin Psychiatry 2003;64(Suppl 1):13.
180. Calabrese J et al. A double-bind placebo-controlled study of lamotrigine monotherapy in outpatients with bipolar I depression. J Clin Psychiatry 1999;60(2):79.
181. Frye MA et al. A placebo-controlled study of lamotrigine and gabapentin monotherapy in refractory mood disorders. J Clin Psychopharmacol 2000; 20:607.
182. Bowden CL et al. A placebo controlled 18-month trial of lamotrigine and lithium maintenance treatment in recently manic or hypomanic patients with bipolar I disorder. Arch Gen Psychiatry 2003;60:392.
183. Nemeroff CB et al. Double-blind, placebo-controlled comparison of imipramine and paroxetine in the treatment of bipolar depression. Am J Psychiatry 2001;158:906.
184. Young LT et al. Double-blind comparison of addition of a second mood stabilizer versus an antidepressant to an initial mood stabilizer for treatment of patients with bipolar depression. Am J Psychiatry 2000;157:124.
185. Goodwin FK, Jamison KR. Maintenance medical treatment. In: Manic-Depressive Illness. New York: Oxford University Press, 1990;665.
186. Harrow M et al. Outcome in manic disorders. Arch Gen Psychiatry 1990;47:665.
187. O'Connell RA et al. Outcome of bipolar disorder on long-term treatment with lithium. Br J Psychiatry 1991;159:123.
188. Tondo L et al. Lithium treatment and risk of suicidal behavior in bipolar disorder patients. J Clin Psychiatry 1998;59(8):405.
189. Bowden CL et al. A randomized, placebo-controlled 12 month trial of divalproex and lithium in treatment of outpatients with bipolar I disorder. Arch Gen Psychiatry 2000;57:481.
190. Gelenberg AJ et al. Comparison of standard and low serum levels of lithium for maintenance treatment of bipolar disorder. N Engl J Med 1989;321:1489.
191. Tondo L et al. Effectiveness of restarting lithium treatment after its discontinuation in bipolar I and bipolar II disorders. Am J Psychiatry 1997; 1543:548.
192. Coryell W et al. Lithium discontinuation and subsequent effectiveness. Am J Psychiatry 1998; 155:895.
193. Keck PE et al. Carbamazepine and valproate in the maintenance treatment of bipolar disorder. J Clin Psychiatry 2002;63(Suppl 10):13.

CHAPTER 81

Psychiatric Disorders in Children and Adolescents

Renée Spencer, Judy L. Curtis, Jay D. Sherr

The recognition and management of psychiatric disorders in children and adolescents are complicated by a number of issues. These issues include symptom interpretation, diagnostic difficulty, research limitations, environmental influences such as family dysfunction, and societal attitudes regarding psychiatric illness and medication usage in this population.

Symptoms must be assessed in light of the developmental level of the patient. The imaginative (or magical) thinking and temper tantrums that are developmentally normal for a 3-year-old child may represent significant symptomatology in a 10-year-old child. Elicitation of psychiatric symptoms, such as reports of hallucinations or depressive mood, depend on verbal communication skills, which also vary with developmental level. Therefore, the presentation of a psychiatric illness varies with age, developmental stage, psychosocial factors, and any cognitive delays or disabilities.

Environmental factors can influence the expression and severity of the psychiatric illness greatly. A dysfunctional family system may contribute significantly to the difficulties a child experiences. Although the child may be the identified patient, it often is as important to treat the entire family as it is to treat the child. Family therapy can be an integral component of the multimodal approach to treatment. Behavioral therapies often are used as components of the overall treatment plan. Behavioral treatment strategies may include training of adaptive behavior by using reinforcement to increase appropriate responses. Token economy systems (providing tokens such as poker chips for adaptive behavior, which are exchanged later to "buy" a desired item or activity) and checklists may be used to evaluate treatment and reward appropriate behavior. Diagnostic classifications from the *Diagnostic and Statistical Manual,* fourth edition (DSM-IV), are used throughout this chapter.[1]

Unlike other areas of psychiatry, research in psychopharmacology of pediatrics has lagged. Only recently have well-controlled medication studies been published. Before this, most of the literature has been filled with anecdotal case reports and open trials. Research has been hampered by a number of challenges. Diagnosis is not as reliable as that for adult psychiatric patients as a result of variability of presentation as discussed previously. Interpretation of study results is difficult because of the heterogeneity of the treatment groups.

Regulatory and legislative initiatives, some controversial, are also impacting pediatric drug research in all therapeutic areas. In the past, there has been less incentive to study drugs in children because the population, and therefore the financial return, is likely to be small. Federal policy initiatives recently have been developed to promote studies in pediatric populations. The Food and Drug Modernization Act (FDAMA) of 1997 offered pharmaceutical companies an additional 6 months of market exclusivity for products evaluated in children. In addition, the U.S. Food and Drug Administration (FDA) "Pediatric Rule" went into effect in April, 1999 and required pharmaceutical companies to provide safety and efficacy data in children on all new drug applications for agents with pediatric therapeutic value.[2] In October 2002, the courts ruled that the FDA did not have the authority to issue the Pediatric Rule and has barred the FDA from enforcing it. New legislation for mandatory pediatric drug testing may be forthcoming.

For additional information on the pathophysiology, presentation, and pharmacotherapy of the major psychiatric disorders, the reader is referred to the specific chapters of this text (e.g., Chapters 76, Anxiety Disorders; 77, Sleep Disorders; 78, Schizophrenia; 79, Mood Disorders I: Major Depressive Disorders; and 80, Mood Disorders II: Bipolar Disorders). Only the aspects of presentation and therapy for children and adolescents that differ from those seen in the usual adult psychiatric population are discussed here.

ATTENTION-DEFICIT HYPERACTIVITY DISORDER

The criteria for attention-deficit hyperactivity disorder (ADHD) (formerly known as *attention-deficit disorder*) include a developmentally inappropriate inability to maintain attention and/or hyperactivity–impulsivity. These symptoms must have persisted for at least 6 months; have an onset that causes impairment before age 7 years; cause significant distress or impairments in social or academic function; and be present in two or more settings.[1] The DSM-IV has included wording regarding workplace as well as academic functioning to facilitate diagnosis of ADHD in adults. Two groups (attention and hyperactivity-impulsivity) of nine symptoms each are used to categorize ADHD as predominantly inattentive type, predominantly hyperactive-impulsive type, and combined type.

Childhood ADHD

ADHD is the most common psychiatric disorder in children. DSM-IV estimates the prevalence rate in school aged-children to be 3% to 5%, with a male:female ratio of 4:1 in community surveys and 9:1 in clinical (inpatient) settings. Symptoms often begin as early as 3 years of age, although the child may not be brought in for treatment until entering school. The predominantly hyperactive-impulsive type may be twice as common in boys, whereas regardless of subtype, ADHD is likely underdiagnosed in girls.[3] ADHD is a familial disorder and twin studies show that heritability is high. The study of the genetics of ADHD is complicated by the comorbidity of depression, bipolar disorder, conduct disorder, and anxiety and learning disorder.[4]

A unifying theory of the neurobiology of ADHD remains obscure. Pregnancy complications, including toxemia, eclampsia, poor maternal health, duration of labor, fetal distress, low birth weight, and antepartum hemorrhage, are implicated in ADHD. Psychosocial adversity (e.g., family conflict, maternal psychopathology) is a common substrate in children with functional and emotional health problems and is commonly seen in ADHD families. Structural imaging studies show basal ganglia asymmetry defects.[5] Molecular genetic studies of variations in dopamine D_2 and D_4 receptor and dopamine transporter genes in ADHD patients have been encouraging but require additional substantiation.[6] Evidence suggests that circuits in the orbital frontal cortex and frontal-limbic pathways are underfunctioning. This is consistent with the fact that stimulants are the most efficacious drugs having actions to increase dopamine and norepinephrine.[7] Thus, biologic, psychosocial, and genetic insults all contribute to an increased liability for ADHD. Regardless of the cause or neurobiologic mechanism, stimulants decrease motor activity, increase coordination, and improve the child's ability to attend to task, thereby increasing learning potential and productivity.

Signs and Symptoms

1. **J.L., a physically healthy 5-year-old boy, is brought to his pediatrician by his mother, M.L., after a conference with his kindergarten teacher. The teacher told her that J.L. seldom completes an activity before moving on to the next one. His peers at school are starting to avoid him because he will not wait his turn. M.L. reports that her son often acts before thinking and has run into the street several times; he has not slowed down since he started to walk. On questioning, she reveals that trivial things like voices in another room or a truck passing by the window have always easily distracted him. During the brief initial examination, J.L. fidgets in his chair but otherwise appears attentive. What symptoms of ADHD are present in J.L.?**

J.L. exhibits the classic symptoms of ADHD, including impulsivity (acts before thinking, runs into the street, unable to wait his turn), hyperactivity (fidgets and is unable to slow down), and inattention (seldom completes activities, easily distracted). Peer rejection can have substantial impact on both social and academic development. His behavior has been longstanding, is severe enough to concern his teacher, and is inappropriate for his developmental level. In structured environments, his behavior may be near normal for a time. Symptoms are often most apparent in less supervised settings.

Treatment

2. **How should J.L. be treated?**

In contrast to other areas of child psychiatry, the literature on ADHD is extensive and well controlled. Stimulants have remained the drugs of choice since benzedrine was first tried in 1937 for hyperactive children. The goal of treatment is to minimize impairment in daily life functioning. As with any other psychiatric disorder in children, multiple therapeutic strategies should be used. Treatment should be comprehensive and multidisciplinary and include the parents, teachers, other primary care givers, and the treating clinician(s). A multimodal approach including parent training, educational and classroom adjustments, behavioral therapy as well as medications should be incorporated into the treatment plan. Stimulant medications are more effective than behavioral therapy alone on core ADHD symptoms, but the combination of stimulants and behavioral therapy appears to provide greater efficacy in other functioning domains such as social skills, academics, parent-child relations, oppositional behavior, and anxiety/depression.[8]

Double-blind, placebo-controlled trials have repeatedly shown that stimulants improve attention span and decrease hyperactivity and impulsivity in children with ADHD.[9] Stimulant response rates range from 65% to 75% compared with 5% to 30% for placebo.[10,11] Early stimulant trials demonstrated comparable efficacy among the four stimulant medications most often used clinically: methylphenidate, mixed amphetamine salts, dextroamphetamine, and pemoline. Some children respond favorably to one stimulant drug but less favorably or not at all to another. Pemoline (Cylert) is no longer recommended because, although effective, its use has been associated with life-threatening hepatic failure.[10]

Until recently, the major stimulants (methylphenidate, dextroamphetamine, and mixed amphetamine salts) were available as short- and intermediate-acting formulations. The immediate-release (IR), short-acting preparations provide a quick onset of action of less than 1 hour but offer a relatively brief 3- to 5-hour duration of behavioral effect, necessitating multiple daily doses to maintain improvement throughout the day. The slow-release (SR) or extended-release (ER), intermediate-acting formulations were developed using a wax-matrix or hydrophilic polymer controlled-release mechanism in an effort to decrease gastrointestinal (GI) side effects, delay peak plasma concentrations, and provide the benefits of once-daily dosing. They have a slightly longer duration of action but their slower rates of absorption delay their onset of effect. These SR/ER formulations have not been consistently comparable in effectiveness to IR preparations. Their slightly longer duration of action often does not extend long enough to cover the entire school day, whereas their slower onset can be problematic when a rapid effect is needed to improve early morning functioning at home or school. Several newer, long-acting products are now available that were designed to combine the properties of IR and SR/ER formulations in a single-delivery system to provide both rapid onset of action and sufficient duration of action to eliminate the need for mid-day dosing. Table 81-1 summarizes the distinguishing features among the most commonly used psychostimulant agents.

Methylphenidate (Ritalin) is the stimulant most commonly prescribed for hyperactive children. Methylphenidate is absorbed rapidly but incompletely, with a bioavailability of 10.5% to 52.5%. The plasma concentration peaks approximately 1.6 hours after an oral dose of IR methylphenidate. The rate, but not extent, of GI absorption of methylphenidate is increased with food, without affecting therapeutic response.[12] The serum half-life of IR methylphenidate is 2.5 to 3.5 hours, but serum levels do not correlate with response, and there is a large interindividual variation in serum levels on the same dose.[13] Although some studies find no significant difference in efficacy between the SR product (Ritalin SR) and IR methylphenidate,[14] others have found less efficacy with the SR product.[15] With the SR product, maximum methylphenidate concentrations are 20% lower and occur 1.5 hours later than with the immediate-release product. However, the area under the concentration time curve (AUC) is unchanged. The maximum cognitive benefits with IR methylphenidate are in the first 2 to 3 hours after dosing. It has been speculated that this time-response of cognitive benefit may be related to the rate of increase in blood, and subsequently to brain concentrations rather than the extent of absorption. This may be why some children appear to respond better to IR methylphenidate. The efficacy of SR methylphenidate lasts up to 8 hours.

The usual starting dose of methylphenidate IR is 5 mg in the morning. An additional dose may be added at noon, if necessary. Response should be rapid and may be seen within hours of the first dose, although usual practice is to wait at least 3 to 4 days to assess the dose. The dosage is titrated to achieve a maximum therapeutic response up to a maximum of 1 mg/kg or a total of 60 mg daily. Some children require a third dose at 4 PM if their behavior is unmanageable at home. The SR products may obviate the need for and can avoid the stigma of mid-day dosing, but the dosage forms that are available can make dose titration difficult for some patients. Children should be counseled not to chew any stimulant SR product because this can result in acute overdose.

Steadily decreasing serum concentrations may result in tolerance to methylphenidate efficacy.[16] In 2000, a novel methylphenidate dosage form, Concerta, an oral-release osmotic system (OROS), was approved by the FDA.[17] This tablet is composed of an immediate-release drug overcoat surrounding a semipermeable membrane, with two drug layers and an osmotically active component. In the GI tract, active drug is released via osmotic pressure through a laser-drilled hole in the membrane. The biologically inert membrane subsequently is eliminated in the stool. There is an initial serum peak concentration at 1 to 2 hours. Continued absorption results in maximum concentrations at approximately 6 to 8 hours. This results in a concentration-time profile that is similar to the peak concentrations observed with equal thrice-daily dosing of IR methylphenidate. In a 4-week placebo-controlled study comparing once-daily Concerta to three-times-daily methylphenidate, both active treatment arms demonstrated superior efficacy and tolerability when compared with placebo.[18] The two active treatments were similar with regard to efficacy and tolerability. A 1-year follow-up study showed that Concerta maintained efficacy without the emergence of new untoward effects.[19] Concerta is available in 18-mg, 27-mg, 36-mg and 54-mg tablets.[20] Dosing with Concerta may be initiated at 18 mg in the morning and titrated weekly to a maximum recommended daily dose of 54 mg. Prior titration on IR methylphenidate is not required.[21]

Metadate CD and Ritalin LA are the latest long-acting, modified-release methylphenidate formulations to gain FDA approval. They consist of two types of coated beads contained in a capsule. IR beads that provide an initial, rapid release of methylphenidate and ER polymer-coated beads that provide a continuous release of methylphenidate. Both agents produce biphasic plasma-time concentration profiles similar to methylphenidate IR given as two doses 4 hours apart; however, the two products are formulated with differing ratios of IR:ER methylphenidate beads. Metadate CD contains a 30:70 ratio of IR:ER methylphenidate beads, whereas Ritalin LA contains a 50:50 ratio of IR:ER methylphenidate beads. Initial dosing for each agent is 20 mg once daily administered before breakfast. Weekly dosage adjustments can be made up to a maximum daily dose of 60 mg administered as three of the 20-mg capsules once daily. High-fat meals delay the rate of absorption but do not affect the extent of absorption for both products.[22,23] Bioavailability studies indicate that Metadate CD and Ritalin LA may be sprinkled on applesauce; however, the beads should not be crushed or chewed to avoid acute overdose through destruction of the extended-release mechanism.

Pharmacokinetic data comparing the rate and extent of absorption of equivalent doses of Metadate CD and Concerta demonstrate equal AUC$_{total}$ for the two agents.[24] Measurements of methylphenidate plasma concentrations at 1.5, 3, and 4 hours after dosing were higher for Metadate CD than for Concerta, whereas plasma concentrations at 8, 10, and 12 hours were greater for Concerta.[24] The clinical significance of the earlier peaks found with Metadate CD remains to be determined. Preliminary data suggest greater efficacy of Metadate CD over Concerta at 1.5 to 7.5 hours post-dose,

Table 81-1   Characteristics of Commonly Prescribed Psychostimulants

Agent	Delivery System	Description	Strengths	Dosing Frequency	Maximum Daily Dose	Peak Concentration	Duration of Effect	Comments
Short-Acting Stimulants								
Ritalin, Methylin	IR tablet	MPH	5, 10, 20 mg	BID–TID	60 mg	1–2 hr	3–4 h	Generics available.
Focalin	IR tablet	D-MPH	2.5, 5, 10 mg	BID	20 mg	1–2 hr	4–5 h	SR product in development.
Dexedrine	IR tablet	DEX	5, 10 mg	BID–TID	40 mg	3 hr	3–5 h	Generics available.
Intermediate-Acting Stimulants								
Ritalin SR	Wax matrix SR tablet	MPH	20 mg	QD–BID	60 mg	4–5 hr	6–8 h	Generics available.
Methylin ER	hydrophilic polymer ER tablet	MPH	10, 20 mg	QD–BID	60 mg	4–5 hr	6–8 h	
Metadate ER	Wax matrix ER tablet	MPH	10, 20 mg	QD–BID	60 mg	4–5 hr	6–8 h	
Dexedrine Spansules	SR beads	Initial IR DEX followed by SR DEX	5, 10, 15 mg	QD–BID	40 mg	1st: 3 hr 2nd: 8 hr	5–8 h	May sprinkle capsule contents on applesauce—do not crush/chew.
Adderall	IR tablet	AMP	5, 10, 20, 30 mg	QD–BID	30 mg	3 hr	3–7 h	Longer duration at higher doses. Generics available.
Long-Acting Stimulants								
Metadate CD	Eurand Diffucaps Technology	30:70 ratio of IR: ER MPH beads	20 mg	QD	60 mg	1st: 1.5–3 hr 2nd: 4–6 hr	6–9 h	High-fat meal can delay absorption from IR portion of formulation resulting in delay of initial T_{max} of 1 hr. May sprinkle capsule contents on applesauce—do not crush/chew.
Ritalin LA	Spheroidal Oral Drug Absorption (SODAS)	50:50 ratio of IR:ER MPH beads	20, 30, 40 mg	QD	60 mg	1st: 1–2 2nd: 5–7 hr	8–10 h	High-fat meal can delay absorption. May sprinkle capsule contents on applesauce—do not crush/chew.
Concerta	Osmotic Release Oral System (OROS)	IR MPH coating (22%) with remainder delivered through laser drilled hole in tablet core	18, 27, 36, 54 mg	QD	54 mg	1st: 1–2 hr 2nd: 6–8 hr	12 h	MPH paste cannot be ground up and snorted, decreasing abuse potential. Tablet shell may appear in stool.
Adderall XR	Microtrol IR and controlled-release beads	50:50 ratio of IR:ER AMP beads	5, 10, 15, 20, 25, 30 mg	QD	30 mg	1st: 3 hr 2nd: 7 hr	10–12 h	High-fat meal can delay absorption and prolong T_{max} by 2.5 h. May sprinkle capsule contents on applesauce—do not crush/chew.

AMP, mixed amphetamine salts; DEX, dextroamphetamine; ER, extended release; IR, immediate release; MPH, methylphenidate; SR, sustained release.

roughly correlating with the earlier Metadate CD plasma-concentration peaks.[25] Also correlating with the plasma concentration profile, efficacy for Concerta was found to extend to 12 hours, whereas the efficacy of Metadate CD was no different from placebo at the 12 hour post-dose final evaluation.[25]

As the first once-daily, extended-release methylphenidate formulation on the market, the role of Concerta has been firmly established in the ADHD therapeutic armamentarium. However, the place in therapy of Metadate CD and Ritalin LA remains to be determined. Metadate CD may have greater efficacy at earlier time points compared to Concerta, although it may have a shorter duration of action. The shorter duration of action may be advantageous in children with insomnia or decreased appetite at bedtime but less advantageous for children who exhibit symptoms into the evening. Both Metadate CD and Ritalin LA may be sprinkled on applesauce, whereas Concerta tablets must be swallowed whole. Rates of absorption for Concerta seem less affected by food (high-fat breakfast) compared with Metadate CD and Ritalin LA. Although short delays in reaching T_{max} are observed with both Metadate CD and Ritalin LA when administered with high-fat meals, the clinical relevance of these delays and possible impact on onset of effect remain to be determined. The methylphenidate in Concerta is in the form of a paste that cannot be ground up and snorted; thus, Concerta has less abuse potential than Metadate CD and Ritalin LA. Although the pharmacokinetic profiles of the agents are roughly similar, technically they are not bioequivalent. Nevertheless, they each offer the advantage of once-daily dosing, which may improve compliance and minimize the problems associated with storing and administering controlled substances at school.

Methylphenidate dosages of 0.3 mg/kg per day improve performance on measures of cognitive function and task persistence.[26] There appears to be little additional benefit in cognitive function at 0.6 mg/kg per day, although there may be additional benefits in hyperactivity-impulsivity symptoms at higher dosages.[12] A decrease in cognitive performance has been noted at 1 mg/kg per day.[13] Methylphenidate significantly improves attention and ability to learn in the classroom and can produce long-lasting improvements in academic performance. Methylphenidate normalizes classroom behavior, improves peer interactions, and improves self-esteem and sense of control during therapy. A meta-analysis of 341 review articles found that the magnitude of symptom improvement was twice as large as improvements in IQ and achievement.[27] Nevertheless, individualized dosing with an emphasis on target symptoms and improvement in function (e.g., improved academic performance and peer relations) should remain the focus of therapy.

In J.L.'s case, a task-oriented checklist should be used at home to implement a behavioral program to help keep him on task, and he should be referred to a preschool with a more structured setting. In addition, Concerta 18 mg in the morning should be prescribed for J.L. Behavioral checklists focusing on specific target symptoms for both parents and teachers are important tools to assist in monitoring his response to therapy.[28,29] J.L. should be evaluated after one week and the dose titrated upward if needed.

SIDE EFFECTS

3. What potential side effects should be reviewed with M.L.?

The stimulants have been found to be generally safe and well tolerated. Common side effects associated with methylphenidate preparations (as well as the other stimulants) are insomnia, anorexia, headaches, nausea, abdominal pain, sadness, and irritability.[30] However, many side effects reported with stimulants occur at rates similar to placebo, and many are similar to symptoms of ADHD.[31] Most initial adverse effects are transient and diminish over a few weeks. Children often feel that stimulant medication helps them and are willing to continue therapy despite minor side effects.[32]

Other less common but more troublesome side effects that may occur with stimulant use include growth suppression, precipitation or exacerbation of tics, tachycardia and blood pressure changes. Although there is a potential for growth suppression in children taking stimulants, provision of "drug holidays" on the weekends and in the summer allow for catch-up growth for children in whom careful monitoring of height indicates growth suppression.[33] The growth suppression effects diminish in early adolescence.[34] Motor and vocal tics sometimes appear to be precipitated by the use of stimulants, especially in patients with a family history of tic disorders such as Gilles de la Tourette's syndrome. In fact, Tourette's syndrome is a comorbid condition known to present with ADHD. Approximately 7% of school-aged children with ADHD have tics or Tourette's syndrome, whereas up to 60% of children with Tourette's syndrome also have ADHD.[35]

Accumulating evidence suggests that most patients with ADHD and tics can be treated safely with stimulants.[36] Stimulant use in patients with tics requires careful monitoring for exacerbation of tics. Dose reduction or switching to another stimulant or class of medications are strategies used when tics are precipitated or exacerbated. Because of their dopamine agonist properties, methylphenidate and the other stimulants may worsen a pre-existing psychosis.[37] Stimulant use is generally avoided in patients with psychotic disorders. All the stimulants have been associated with statistically significant increases in blood pressure and heart rate though clinically important increases are less common. In children, monitoring for all the stimulant agents should include height, weight, blood pressure, and pulse. Routine laboratory monitoring is not required.

OTHER STIMULANTS

4. What other stimulants could be used to treat J.L.?

Both dextroamphetamine (Dexedrine, Dexedrine Spansules) and mixed amphetamine salts (Adderall, Adderall XR) are also effective in ADHD and could be selected based on clinician and patient preference. Methylphenidate is often prescribed as first-line treatment because it appears less likely to suppress appetite and cause insomnia compared with dextroamphetamine and mixed amphetamine salts.[10] Other less popular stimulant options include dexmethylphenidate (Focalin) and magnesium pemoline (Cylert). Methamphetamine hydrochloride (Desoxyn) and its SR product (Desoxyn Gradumet) are effective, but their use is limited because of concerns regarding abuse potential.

Dextroamphetamine is as effective as methylphenidate in ADHD.[38] The dosing strategy is similar to that used with methylphenidate. The usual starting dose is 2.5 mg at 8 AM, with the addition of a dose at noon if necessary; the peak effect occurs within 1 to 2 hours of dosing. Like methylphenidate, dextroamphetamine also is available as an SR product (Dexedrine Spansule). Three dosages are available. Although these SR dosage forms make it possible to change from IR to SR at the same total daily dose, as with methylphenidate, full therapeutic equivalence is controversial. There is some evidence that overall the adverse effects of dextroamphetamine occur more frequently and are more severe than those from methylphenidate.[9]

Adderall, a mixture of amphetamine and dextroamphetamine salts, is available in 5-, 10-, 20-, and 30-mg tablets. It is less studied in ADHD than the other stimulants, but some clinicians find a longer duration of effect after each dose compared to methylphenidate.[39,40] Adderall's duration of action appears dose-dependent, increasing with higher doses. Still, mid-day dosing may be required. Adderall XR is a modified-release product containing equal amounts of IR and ER beads. It is usually dosed once daily and produces a plasma-concentration time profile similar to an equivalent dose of Adderall administered twice daily 4 hours apart. Adderall XR is available in several strengths and can be initiated at 10 mg once daily in the morning. In addition, patients can be converted from Adderall to Adderall XR at the same total daily dose administered once daily. The contents of the XR capsule may be sprinkled on applesauce for children who have difficulty swallowing capsules but the beads should not be crushed or chewed. High-fat meals may delay the rate of absorption by 2.5 hours but do not affect the extent of absorption.[41] The exact clinical significance in the delay to T_{max} remains to be determined but concern exists that the onset of effect could also be delayed. Administering the dose before breakfast minimizes the delay in absorption associated with high-fat meals.

Dexmethylphenidate (Focalin) is the most recently approved stimulant product in the United States. It comprises only the D-enantiomer of racemic methylphenidate, which is thought to be the more pharmacologically active isomer. The safety and efficacy of dexmethylphenidate were demonstrated in three small, short-term clinical trials.[42] The agent appears similar in efficacy to methylphenidate when dosed at 50% of the total daily methylphenidate dose but does not appear to offer clinical advantages over methylphenidate with respect to tolerability, efficacy, or duration of action. Dosing is initiated at 2.5 mg BID with dose adjustments of 2.5 to 5 mg in weekly increments to a maximum daily dose of 20 mg. Given that many low-cost generic methylphenidate products are available, it is difficult to justify utilization of dexmethylphenidate (Focalin), which is more expensive and does not appear to demonstrate any clear advantage over methylphenidate.

Magnesium pemoline (Cylert) is comparable in efficacy to methylphenidate for the treatment of ADHD.[43] Unlike other stimulants, it is classified as a C-IV controlled substance. Pemoline is no longer recommended as a first-line therapy, however, owing to its association with life-threatening hepatic failure. The manufacturer indicates that 15 cases of acute hepatic failure have been reported to the FDA since 1975 when the drug was first marketed, 4 to 17 times the rate expected in the general population. Twelve of the cases resulted in liver transplantation or death, most within 4 weeks of onset of signs of liver failure. The package insert now contains a boxed warning recommending that baseline liver function tests and serum alanine aminotransferase (ALT or SGPT) concentra-

tions be monitored every 2 weeks. Cylert should be discontinued if serum ALT levels are more than twice normal.[44] It should not be initiated in patients with liver disease and should be discontinued in patients who show no significant clinical benefits after 3 weeks of completing the dose titration. Written informed consent from the patient or legal guardian is essential. The usual dosage range is from 18.75 to 112.5 mg/day usually as a single morning dose, although some children require an afternoon dose. Effects begin in 1 to 2 hours after a dose and can last up to 8 hours[45]; the half-life in children is 7 hours.[46] Adverse effects are similar to those seen with other stimulants with the exception of serious liver toxicity.

In summary, stimulants are the first line of pharmacotherapy for ADHD. However, response to each stimulant varies greatly and cannot be predicted. In one study of methylphenidate and dextroamphetamine, 25% of subjects responded positively to one drug after a poor response to the other.[47] In cases of poor initial response, a different stimulant should be tried before changing to another drug class.

5. **M.L. asks whether J.L. will "grow out" of his ADHD. What is the likelihood that pediatric patients will outgrow ADHD?**

The conventional wisdom is that children outgrow their ADHD as they enter puberty and that stimulant medications should be stopped at that time. However, a number of studies, which have looked at long-term outcome, do not support this assumption.[48] In one prospective study, symptoms persisted into adolescence (age 13 to 15) in 68% of patients.[49] Persistence into adulthood is discussed later.

DIET AND ALTERNATIVE MEDICINE

6. **J.L. has responded well to the combination of Concerta and the behavior checklist. His mother sends him off for his annual summer visit to his father and stepmother with his Concerta, 30 copies of his daily behavioral checklist to be completed by his father, and written instructions. One month later, J.L. returns with the full bottle of Concerta and 12 daily checklists in varying stages of completion; he reports that "they didn't let me eat any good stuff" as he bounces around the room. In a terse telephone discussion, his stepmother reports that she couldn't give J.L. "that poison" when proper management of his diet and giving him natural herbs could improve his behavior. What is the role of diet and alternative therapies in ADHD?**

Scientific evidence does not support the hypothesis that a food additive–free diet, such as the Feingold diet, improves behavior in most hyperactive children.[50] Controlled trials show no worsening of ADHD symptoms with sugar.[51] Some children may worsen with a specific food or additive, particularly tartrazine, a synthetic food dye. These may represent true food allergies but should be tested in a blinded fashion with the child. There is no evidence that megavitamin therapy is efficacious and it can result in toxicity. However, many parents are convinced that diet affects the child's behavior, and much has been written in the lay press about dietary treatment for the ADHD child. Although a diet restricting sugar and food additives probably will not improve the child's behavior, it may not be harmful if the restrictions are not severe and do not produce major conflicts between the parent and child.

The efficacy and safety of alternative or complementary medicine in the treatment of ADHD have not been systematically evaluated. Alternative treatments often include neurofeedback, homeopathy, herbal medicines, iron supplements, and other nutritional supplements. Use of herbal remedies is generally based on the traditional efficacy profile of an herb applied to the symptoms of ADHD. For example, sedating herbs such as chamomile, kava-kava, and valerian are used to target symptoms of hyperactivity, decreased concentration, and sleep difficulties associated with ADHD.[52] Similarly, gingko biloba is used in ADHD to improve concentration and attention because of its history in treating memory problems and to improve cognition.[52] Although anecdotal and empirical evidence is surfacing to support the efficacy of some alternatives,[53] further research is needed, especially in children, before they can be regarded as safe and effective treatments for ADHD.[54] In general, the use of more conventional treatments should be considered if alternative interventions prove unsuccessful.

NONSTIMULANT MEDICATIONS

7. J.L.'s parents read on the internet that the use of stimulants is associated with a greater likelihood of future substance abuse. They become fearful of continuing to use Concerta and insist on discontinuing treatment. What information might help put J.L.'s parents at ease? What nonstimulant medication options are available to treat J.L.?

Concerns exist that stimulant therapy for children and adolescents with ADHD may result in increased risk for subsequent substance use disorders. Recent studies have failed to demonstrate a link and add to the evidence from previous studies that also has not shown an association between stimulant use and later substance abuse. In one study, investigators followed 147 children with ADHD for 13 years to examine the impact of stimulant treatment during childhood and high school years and its risk for substance use, dependence, and abuse by young adulthood.[55] They found no association between stimulant treatment and an increased risk of later drug use, including stimulants and cocaine, among children with ADHD. A second study reviewed six long-term studies in which over 1,000 pharmacologically treated and untreated youths with ADHD were examined for later substance abuse disorder outcomes.[56] The results suggest that stimulant therapy in childhood is actually associated with a reduction in the risk for subsequent drug and alcohol disorders. Although these data are increasingly compelling, there is still a need for additional randomized controlled trials.

Atomoxetine (Straterra) is the first nonstimulant medication approved for the treatment of ADHD in children over 6 years old and adults. The exact mechanism by which it exerts it clinical effect is unclear, but atomoxetine is a selective presynaptic norepinephrine reuptake inhibitor. In animals studies, atomoxetine caused a threefold increase of both norepinephrine and dopamine in the prefrontal cortex, which is involved in attention and memory. Although atomoxetine increased the dopamine concentration in the prefrontal cortex, a similar effect was not found in the striatum or nucleus accumbens, suggesting that atomoxetine has less potential for abuse and motor impairment (e.g., tics). In comparison, methylphenidate caused a similar increase in norepinephrine and dopamine concentrations in the prefrontal cortex, but also demonstrated an increase in dopamine concentrations in the striatum and nucleus accumbens, providing support for the abuse potential of methylphenidate.[57]

Atomoxetine is rapidly and completely absorbed with a T_{max} of 1 hour. It is metabolized via the cytochrome P450 2D6 (CYP 2D6) enzyme system and excreted in the urine. Its plasma half-life varies in patients who are poor or extensive metabolizers. The half-life is 4 to 5 hours in patients who are CYP 2D6 extensive metabolizers and 19 to 24 hours in the 5% to 10% of patients who have a polymorphism of CYP2D6 and are poor metabolizers.

Four short-term, double-blind, randomized, placebo-controlled trials in over 750 children with ADHD demonstrated the safety and efficacy of atomoxetine dosed from 0.5 to 2 mg/kg/day.[58–60] Efficacy is similar for inattentive as well as hyperactive/impulsive symptoms. Overall atomoxetine is well tolerated with the most common adverse effects in children being abdominal pain, decreased appetite, nausea, vomiting, dizziness, and fatigue. The tolerability and efficacy of atomoxetine compared with methylphenidate are unclear since no adequately powered, controlled head-to-head studies have been conducted (though one is currently in progress). Like the stimulants, atomoxetine appears to be effective in approximately 70% of patients. A small open-label study showed no differences in efficacy or treatment discontinuation rates between atomoxetine and methylphenidate.[61] Vomiting and somnolence were more frequently reported with atomoxetine,[61] whereas insomnia has been more frequently reported with methylphenidate.[60] Additional head-to-head studies are needed to confirm these findings.

Mean height and weight percentiles declined in children treated with atomoxetine in open-label studies of 12 to 18 months.[62] Children taking the drug have had minor but statistically significant increases in blood pressure and pulse, which is consistent with taking a drug that increases overall noradrenergic tone. Monitoring should include height, weight, blood pressure, and pulse. As with the stimulants, interruption of therapy should be considered in patients who are not growing or gaining weight at an acceptable rate.

In children up to 70 kg, atomoxetine is initiated at doses of 0.5 mg/kg per day for a minimum of 3 days and then increased to a target dose of 1.2 mg/kg per day given as either a single morning dose or as evenly divided doses in the morning and late afternoon. No additional benefit was seen at doses >1.2 mg/kg per day. The maximum recommended daily dose is 1.4 mg/kg per day. Because poor metabolizers and extensive metabolizers showed only small differences in adverse events and efficacy, both populations are treated with the same dosing schedule. Dose adjustment is recommended for hepatic impairment and concomitant use of a strong CYP 2D6 inhibitor such as fluoxetine or paroxetine. Atomoxetine given once daily has not been directly compared with a twice-daily regimen of the drug, although the treatment effect size with once-daily dosing was similar to the treatment effect sizes with twice-daily dosing. An adequately sized direct comparison study is needed to establish the optimal frequency of administration. Atomoxetine may offer the advantage over the stimulants of continuous symptom relief. Despite atomoxetine's relatively short half-life of 4 to 5 hours, once-daily dosing in the morning was associated with effects that persisted into the evening. However, unlike the stimulants in which clinical effects can be observed immediately, symptom reduction with atomoxetine takes several days to observe. Atomoxetine is available as 5-, 10-, 18-, 25-, 40-, and 60-mg capsules and is not available in a liquid formulation.

The place of atomoxetine in the ADHD therapeutic armamentarium is still unclear. Advantages include the convenience of not being a controlled substance and its lack of abuse potential. It may also offer continuous symptom relief throughout the day and evening. Although data support its efficacy in ADHD, its long-term safety—particularly its effects on growth—remains to be determined. Also, data regarding atomoxetine's efficacy compared with stimulants are lacking. Additional studies are also needed to establish the optimal frequency of administration. From a cost perspective, atomoxetine is more expensive than the stimulants, including the newer extended-release formulations. It appears to be a reasonable alternative in patients who are intolerant to or failed to respond to stimulants or in patients who do not want to or should not take a controlled substance (e.g., in comorbid substance abuse disorders). Atomoxetine may provide particular benefit over the stimulants in patients with comorbid tics or anxiety.

If J.L.'s parents are not convinced that there is no link between stimulant use and future substance abuse, then atomoxetine should be recommended. For J.L.'s weight of 19 kg, dosing should be initiated at 10 mg in the morning and titrated after a minimum of 3 days to 25 mg in the morning.

Adulthood ADHD

8. **J.L.'s therapist arranges a meeting with M.L. (mother), F.L. (father), and S.L. (stepmother) to review J.L.'s progress, coordinate treatment, and provide consistency in both settings. During the course of the therapy session, M.L. reports that F.L. has "never taken responsibility for anything in his life" and is unable to hold a job for more than 6 months. He is unable to get along with his superiors or simply loses interest and quits. Although very intelligent, he dropped out of ninth grade because he was "always in detention." Both M.L. and S.L. report that F.L. often seems to act on impulse without thought toward the consequences, is unreliable, loses things easily, and never seems to complete anything. M.L. says that he is "just like a child, exactly like J.L." and that his behavior was a major reason for their divorce. S.L. admits that these things also are a problem within their relationship. What is the likelihood F.L. also has ADHD?**

ADHD can persist into adulthood. Follow-up studies indicate that this disorder may persist in 40% to 60% of children who are diagnosed with ADHD.[63] There is considerable comorbidity in adults with ADHD, including substance abuse (27% to 46%), anxiety disorders (up to 50%), and antisocial personality disorder (12% to 27%). Mood disorders occur in 15% to 20% of children with ADHD and may have a similar prevalence in adults.[64] The diagnosis of ADHD in adults can be difficult because the criteria state that evidence of the disorder must exist before age 7. Therefore, to make a diagnosis in F.L., who has not been previously diagnosed, requires a retrospective review of his behavior to determine whether the symptoms existed in childhood.[63,64] Rating scales, such as the Wender Utah Rating Scale or the Conners Rating Scale, may be used to help make the diagnosis. The Wender scale is a 61-item form that rates the memories of the adult patient with suspected ADHD. The diagnosis is made based on the scale and specific traits exhibited by the patient that are consistent with ADHD.

Adults with ADHD have traits similar to children with the disorder, which result in functional problems, including poor academic performance, conflicts with authority figures, marital disruption, frequent absenteeism, job changes, and low frustration tolerance.[50,63]

The treatment of ADHD in adults is not as well studied as for children, but it is essentially the same. Several studies have shown the efficacy of methylphenidate, atomoxetine, desipramine, bupropion, and possibly venlafaxine.[50,65,66] A clear history of early childhood onset of symptoms predicts a greater likelihood of response. Active substance abuse needs to be treated and a 1-month abstinence is recommended before starting ADHD pharmacotherapy. Methylphenidate has been studied in double-blind fashion in adults; efficacy is similar to that seen in children. Adults are more sensitive to both therapeutic and adverse effects compared with children, so similar absolute doses are commonly used. Stimulants remain a drug of choice in adults, although adults may require more frequent daily dosing and are more prone to medication abuse. Side effects are similar to those in children except for an increased risk of hypertension and tachycardia in adults.

Atomoxetine is the first nonstimulant approved by the FDA for treatment of ADHD in adults. Two identical 10-week double-blind trials in over 500 adults showed that atomoxetine (60 to 120 mg/day in divided doses) was superior to placebo in reducing ADHD symptoms.[66] Dosing in adults is initiated at 40 mg per day and increased after a minimum of 3 days to a target dose of 80 mg with a total maximum daily dose of 100 mg. It may be given as a single morning dose or as evenly divided doses in the morning and late afternoon. Constipation, dry mouth, urinary retention, and sexual dysfunction including erectile disturbance, impotence, and abnormal orgasm have been reported in adults. Comparison data with the stimulants are not available. Atomoxetine's place in therapy remains to be determined but it may be particularly useful in adults with a history of substance abuse in whom stimulants must be avoided.

Antidepressants offer advantages including once-daily dosing and efficacy in comorbid depression and anxiety. Anticholinergic side effects and lethality in overdose are more of a problem in adults than in children. One open study of bupropion found that 75% of patients had moderate or marked benefit and preferred bupropion to previous antidepressant or stimulant therapy. However, bupropion requires divided doses to minimize seizure risk, and its place in the therapy of ADHD awaits further controlled trials.

ADHD With Concurrent Depressive Symptoms

9. **R.J., a 9-year-old boy with ADHD, has also appeared depressed with episodes of withdrawal and crying spells over the past year. A trial of methylphenidate worsened his crying spells, and he became more nervous and irritable, although it did improve his ADHD somewhat. What alternative treatments are available?**

As illustrated by R.J., mood lability and anxiety (signs of depression in children) can be exacerbated by stimulants. In these children, the antidepressants may be preferable to the stimulants. Up to 15% to 20% of patients will not respond adequately to stimulants or develop intolerable side effects and should be considered for antidepressant therapy as well. The serotonin reuptake inhibitors are not useful in ADHD. The most studied tricyclic antidepressants (TCAs), imipramine (Tofranil) and desipramine (Norpramin), are superior to placebo but less effective than stimulants for ADHD. However, in the presence of comorbid anxiety disorder or depression, TCAs may offer improved efficacy.[67] Desipramine is effective at dosages up to 5 mg/kg per day, and there appears to be no relation between serum levels and response.[68] Unlike the stimulants, desipramine does not appear to suppress growth,[69] but there has been concern regarding its potential for cardiac toxicity based on several case reports of sudden death in children. However, review of the cases and available literature has brought into question whether there is a cause-and-effect association.[70] Ambulatory 24-hour electrocardiogram (ECG) monitoring of 71 children and adolescents taking desipramine showed no significant difference from normal controls.[71] Nevertheless, cardiac toxicity concerns have curtailed desipramine use in children. A family history of sudden death or early cardiac history and a patient history of cardiac disease may contraindicate use. Nortriptyline (Pamelor) is an alternative to desipramine.

In summary, vital signs and a baseline ECG are essential before TCAs are initiated. The ECG should be repeated during the dosage titration and maintenance therapy to ensure that the PR interval remains <200 msec, the QRS is <130% of baseline and <120 msec, and the QTc interval is <460 to 480 msec.[72]

The monoamine oxidase inhibitors clorgyline (no longer marketed) and tranylcypromine (Parnate) are as efficacious as dextroamphetamine in ADHD.[73] However, dietary restrictions may be difficult in children and adolescents. Bupropion (Wellbutrin) at dosages up to 6 mg/kg per day has shown some efficacy as early as the third day of therapy, but there are no direct comparative trials with stimulants.[74]

Clonidine (Catapres), an α-adrenergic agonist at 0.05 mg to 0.3 mg/day has been used with good efficacy in the hyperactive-impulsive type, but hypotension can be a problem.[50] A thorough cardiac history and ECG should precede initiation, and a history of syncope is a contraindication to its use. Sedation is the other major side effect of clonidine in these patients. Clonidine is a good alternative for the child with concurrent ADHD and Tourette's syndrome (see Question 30), but it is relatively contraindicated in a child with depressive symptoms because these may be worsened. In patients with a partial response to stimulants, it has become common to add clonidine. Despite a lack of controlled trials, clinical lore supports the combination. Four deaths have been reported to the FDA in patients taking this combination of drugs, although the relationship between the drugs and the deaths is unclear.[50] Regardless, high dosages of both clonidine and stimulants together should be used cautiously. Patients and care providers should be counseled on the danger of sudden discontinuation owing to the potential of serious hypertensive rebound. Guanfacine (Tenex) is an α-agonist with a longer half-life and causes less sedation and hypotension than clonidine. Open trials suggest it may be effective in some patients (e.g., ADHD with Tourette's whose tics worsen with stimulants, or patients who cannot tolerate clonidine), but controlled trials are lacking.

R.J. appears likely to benefit from an antidepressant. The methylphenidate is discontinued, and the following day vital signs, ECG, and liver enzymes are obtained. He is started on nortriptyline 25 mg at bedtime. Typical maintenance dosages are 25 to 75 mg/day often in two doses because of the short half-life in children younger than 16 years of age. Interindividual half-life variation as high as sevenfold makes subsequent serum level monitoring essential. Serum levels between 50 and 150 ng/mL are associated with efficacy while minimizing the risks of QTc interval widening.

DEPRESSIVE DISORDER IN CHILDREN AND ADOLESCENTS

Major depressive disorder (MDD) is one of the more common psychiatric illnesses in children and adolescents. The prevalence is almost 2% in children and 4% to 8% in adolescents.[3] The male:female ratio is equal in children but is approximately 1:2 by adolescence. Community samples document a cumulative incidence of approximately 20% by age 18. The risk of MDD is three times higher in children who have a parent with MDD.[75] Comorbid psychiatric diagnoses occur in at least 40% of young patients. Separation anxiety is the most common comorbid disorder in children, whereas adolescents are more likely to also suffer from conduct disorder, generalized anxiety, and substance abuse. Comorbid ADHD is common in both groups.[76]

The symptoms of depression vary depending on the age of the child.[77] In general, children with MDD express their illness as anxiety and somatic symptoms to a greater extent than adults. In infants, depression can be related to disruptions in the primary caregiver–infant interaction and manifests as feeding problems, lack of growth, sleep disruption, lethargy, irritability, and social withdrawal or apathy. This may be known as failure to thrive or psychosocial dwarfism.

In early childhood (ages 3 to 4), language skills may not have developed adequately to express mood. Symptoms in this age group include abnormal motor behavior or "acting-out" (e.g., hyperactivity, aggression, temper tantrums, and being in opposition to everything). Social withdrawal, separation problems, and eating or sleeping difficulties also can be seen.

In middle childhood (ages 5 to 8), depression can become more recognizable as low self-esteem issues, sadness, self-blame, and feelings of guilt, social withdrawal, accident proneness, somatic symptoms, lying, stealing, being contrary, and aggression. School problems may present as underachievement.

In late childhood (ages 9 to 12), symptoms include sadness, apathy, a sense of helplessness, anhedonia (lack of pleasure in normally enjoyable activities), anxiety, irritability, somatic symptoms, school problems, and inability to concentrate. At this age, suicidal ideation and attempts may appear.

By adolescence, depressive symptoms appear to be similar to those seen in adults. Symptoms include sleep and appetite disturbance, anhedonia, somatic symptoms, social withdrawal, antisocial behavior, and drug or alcohol abuse. Because adolescents are impulsive and tend to view the world in an all-or-none manner with the feeling that things will never change, the risk of suicide in youth is highest in this age group. Table 81-2 lists some of the risk factors associated with adolescent suicide attempts.[78]

As with adults, MDD is a serious, often chronic, condition.[79] Adults with a history of childhood depression are more likely to develop bipolar disorder than are patients with adult-onset depression. This suggests that childhood depression is a severe form of depression. In addition, the early presentation of MDD can result in interference in the development of age-dependent social and cognitive skills. Thus, early identification and treatment are vital in children, not only to relieve the suffering of this disabling illness but also to minimize adverse effects on developmental milestones that can result in long-lasting impairments in functioning.

Signs, Symptoms, and Risk Factors

10. **C.M., an 11-year-old girl, is referred to the outpatient clinic because of crying spells and school failure. She had been a friendly, well-behaved child who was active in gymnastics and was making good grades until about 1 year ago. At that time, she became withdrawn and irritable and began having crying spells. Her grades have suffered, and she dropped out of gymnastics. Over the past few months, her appetite has decreased, and she has lost 5 lb. C.M.'s mother also reports that she finds C.M. wandering around the house at night because she is unable to sleep. C.M.'s maternal aunt has had episodes of depression, including one suicide attempt. No significant psychosocial stressors (e.g., parental separation) are present. During the interview, C.M. tells the examiner that she is being evaluated "because I'm stupid" and that she wishes she could "go to sleep and never wake up." What symptoms and risk factors for depression are present in C.M.?**

Symptoms of depression exhibited by C.M. include low self-esteem ("I'm stupid"), decreased school performance, decreased appetite, sleep disturbance, irritability, crying spells, and suicidal ideation. The family history of depression places C.M. at higher risk for depression.

Treatment: Antidepressants

11. **What antidepressant medications are effective in treating depression in children and adolescents?**

It has been difficult to demonstrate antidepressant efficacy in children. Clinical trials with TCAs, the only available agents for decades, failed to prove efficacy. Small sample sizes, high placebo response rates, a high rate of comorbid conditions, and poor dosing have plagued studies. The high placebo response rate may reflect more rapid symptom fluctuation in children. An immature noradrenergic system may also contribute to a lower rate of response to the tricyclic medications, which are primarily noradrenergic. Emslie and colleagues[80] were the first to demonstrate the efficacy of antidepressants in children and adolescents. In their landmark placebo-controlled study, 56% of patients treated with fluoxetine (Prozac) 20 mg/day responded in contrast to 33% treated with placebo. Fluoxetine is the first selective serotonin reuptake inhibitor (SSRI) to gain FDA approval for treatment of depression in children and adolescents ages 7 to 17.

Until recently, SSRIs had been considered first-line therapy for children and adolescents with MDD because of their efficacy, safety, and mild side effects.[75] However, in 2003, the FDA, following in the footsteps of its British counterpart, warned that paroxetine may be linked to a possible increased rate of self-harming behaviors, including suicidal behavior in children and adolescents. As a result, the FDA recommended that the drug not be prescribed to this population for the treatment of MDD. Similar psychiatric adverse events in children were identified with venlafaxine use resulting in a package labeling warning against its use in children and adolescents. A chart review of 82 child and adolescent outpatients found psychiatric adverse events in 22% of cases.[81] The most common adverse events related to disturbances in mood. Psychiatric adverse events were not associated with one specific SSRI suggesting that this may be a class effect. Prospective longer-term studies are needed to evaluate the safety and efficacy of these agents in children and adolescents.

When an SSRI is used, the choice of agent is similar to that in adults and takes into account the symptom presentation of

---

Table 81-2   Risk Factors for Adolescent Suicide

Psychiatric Diagnosis	Genetic Predisposition
Mood disorders	Family history of mood disorders
Schizophrenia	Family history of suicide attempts
Conduct disorders	Family history of alcohol abuse
Substance abuse	**Other Factors**
Personality disorders (especially borderline and antisocial)	
Personality Traits	Biologic factors (serotonin and dopamine)
	"Contagion" effect (suicide clusters)
Aggression	Dysphoria regarding sexual orientation
Impulsiveness	
Hopelessness	
Psychosocial stressors	
Family dysfunction	
Parental loss	
Medical illness	
Lack of social supports	

Data from reference 73.

the patient, side effect profile of the SSRI, medical conditions, comorbid psychiatric conditions, concomitant drug use, and personal or family history of drug response. The presence of comorbidities may require alternative initial agents. For example, a child with depression and comorbid ADHD may benefit more from a TCA or bupropion than an SSRI.[75] Baseline laboratory tests are not required, and serum level monitoring is not useful except as a check of compliance or suspected overdose.[75] As of the time of this writing, children and adolescents should not be started on paroxetine or venlafaxine. When other SSRIs are used, these patients should be monitored for mood disturbances including hostility and suicidal ideation. The role of SSRIs for treating depression as well as other psychiatric disorders in children and adolescents remains to be determined.

TCAs are approved for the treatment of MDD in children 12 years of age and older. Although it has been a challenge to demonstrate the efficacy of TCAs in clinical trials, many children respond well in practice. TCAs remain useful for children who do not respond or are intolerant of selective serotonin reuptake inhibitors or have pertinent comorbid illnesses (e.g., ADHD). In addition, the severity of illness, socioeconomic status, and patient or family history of response are issues to be considered in selecting an antidepressant.

Of the TCAs, imipramine has been the best studied in children. The total plasma level (imipramine plus the active metabolite desipramine) seems to correlate with antidepressant response when in a therapeutic range of 125 to 225 ng/mL.[82,83] Serum concentrations >225 ng/mL have been associated with an increased risk of tachycardia and slowing of cardiac conduction. The serum concentrations of imipramine and its metabolites do not correlate with side effects, such as dry mouth, drowsiness, blurred vision, or tremors.[84] Imipramine is also the only TCA that is FDA approved for treatment of enuresis in children 6 years of age or older. Nortriptyline serum concentrations maintained in the range of 60 to 100 ng/mL are generally considered safe in children, but the effective therapeutic range is not well defined.[85]

Nonpharmacologic therapies (e.g., cognitive-behavioral therapy) are integral to treating children and adolescents with depression and are often used before and along with medication. Individuals predisposed to depression may be more reactive to negative life events, and psychotherapy plays an important role in youths having difficulty with maladaptive patterns of behavior and poor coping skills. If a child is unresponsive to nonpharmacologic measures and continues to display significant functional impairment at school or home, a trial of an antidepressant should be considered.

12. C.M.'s severe symptoms and functional impairment suggest she may benefit from an antidepressant. How should therapy be initiated and what monitoring parameters should be followed?

It is important to have clearly identified target symptoms in order to monitor efficacy. Expert consensus recommends serotonin reuptake inhibitors as first-line therapy.[75] Starting doses of SSRIs in children should be half those of adults with weekly increases as tolerated to an adequate dose. Older adolescents approaching 70 kg in weight may be started on adult dosages. After obtaining baseline vital signs and weight, C.M. is started on citalopram 10 mg each morning. Common dose-related side effects include nausea, sweating, headaches, dry

mouth, somnolence, insomnia, and impaired sexual function. Side effects are generally mild and transient, although impaired sexual functioning can be persistent. Once an adequate and tolerable dose is achieved, usually within 2 weeks, this regimen should be maintained at least 4 weeks to assess initial response. Except for lower initial dosages, administration is the same as that for adults. Typical adequate daily doses are citalopram 10 to 40 mg, fluoxetine 10 to 20 mg, paroxetine 10 to 50 mg, and sertraline 25 to 200 mg. Lower dosages are used more commonly in preadolescents. At the present time, clinical experience with escitalopram is quite limited and a usual dosing range has not been established in children.

If there is no response after 4 weeks of antidepressant treatment, a dose increase should be considered. Full response can take up to 10 weeks. With fluoxetine, the long half-life of the active metabolite norfluoxetine (7 to 19 days) results in accumulation of drug over at least 1 month. This should be considered before making dosage adjustments. Paroxetine is more sedating and mildly anticholinergic compared with other SSRIs. In children, behavioral activation can be more likely with the SSRIs and may result in silly, agitated, and impulsive acts, which need to be discriminated from mania and akathisia (drug-induced restlessness).[86] The minimum length of pharmacotherapy is one year.[87] Tapered discontinuation of citalopram, paroxetine, and sertraline is prudent to avoid an abrupt flulike discontinuation syndrome or symptoms resembling recurrence or relapse. This withdrawal syndrome does not occur with fluoxetine because of the long half-life of norfluoxetine.

Patients who do not respond to or cannot tolerate an SSRI may benefit from TCA therapy. Before starting a TCA, an ECG, pulse, blood pressure, and weight should be obtained. Therapy can begin with imipramine or desipramine 1 to 2 mg/kg per day or nortriptyline 1 mg/kg per day in two or more divided doses. Dosages can be increased gradually, generally at not more than 10 to 25 mg/day once or twice a week, titrating against tolerance to side effects. Symptom response pattern is similar to that seen in adults, with improvement in appetite and sleep seen before an improvement in mood. Full response may take 4 to 10 weeks. The usual daily dose for imipramine and desipramine is 2 to 5 mg/kg per day, and for nortriptyline, 1 to 3 mg/kg per day. Pulse, blood pressure, and ECG should be monitored routinely. The ECG should be repeated within several days of achieving dosages of 2.5 mg/kg per day for imipramine or desipramine, 1 mg/kg per day for nortriptyline and thereafter with dose increases of 50 to 100 mg/day. Regardless of the dosage, the ECG should be repeated if the pulse is irregular or exceeds 130 beats/minute. The dosage should be decreased or discontinued if the ECG shows a P-R interval >200 msec, a QRS interval >30% over baseline or >120 msec, or a QTc >460 to 480 msec.[72]

In children, the half-life of imipramine is 6 to 15 hours. Therefore, preadolescent children should receive imipramine in two or more divided daily doses to avoid peak-related side effects such as tachycardia. At steady state, plasma concentrations in younger children show a higher ratio of desipramine to imipramine compared with adults.[88] Older adolescents can receive an antidepressant in a single daily dose once they are at steady state. Imipramine is less protein bound in children than adults. Therefore, more free drug is available to bind to receptor sites. In addition, children have proportionally more lean body mass than adults; therefore, less drug distributes into fatty tissue. This may explain the observation that lower plasma concentrations are useful in children.

Adverse effects of TCAs in children are similar to those seen in adults. The risk for cardiotoxicity with TCAs can be minimized by repeated monitoring of pulse, blood pressure, and ECG. Children and adolescents tend to act impulsively. Therefore, the possibility of intentional overdoses should not be disregarded. The smallest fatal dose recorded in the literature is 8 mg/kg.[89]

BIPOLAR DISORDER IN CHILDREN AND ADOLESCENTS
Signs and Symptoms

13. V.L., a 15-year-old boy, is in his third psychiatric hospitalization. He has a long history of depressive symptoms (crying, sleep disturbance, depressed mood), conduct disorder symptoms (runaway, truancy, fighting), and alcohol abuse. Previous psychosocial interventions have failed, primarily because of V.L.'s chaotic home environment. During his second hospitalization, he was treated with fluoxetine, to which he responded with a significant reduction in depressive symptoms. He was discharged to a therapeutic group home, where he continued to do well until 3 weeks before this admission. At that time, he began staying up all night; became more irritable, hyperactive, and grandiose; and developed pressured speech. A diagnosis of bipolar disorder was made. What symptoms does V.L. display that are consistent with this diagnosis?

Symptoms of bipolar disorder in children and adolescents include silly, excited, hyperactive, irritable, paranoid, withdrawn, angry, or explosive behavior and affective lability.[90] Symptoms also can be very similar to those of adult bipolar disorder.[91,92] The adolescent may experience several depressive episodes before his first manic episode. The symptoms displayed by V.L. (e.g., irritability, hyperactivity, grandiosity, pressured speech, staying up all night) are consistent with those commonly associated with bipolar disorder.

Bipolar mood disorder was once perceived as rare in preadolescent children.[93] Although less common in preadolescent children than in adolescents, bipolar disorder is being diagnosed more often in children. The incidence of childhood bipolar disorder is controversial. Recent improvement in diagnostic criteria for both bipolar disorder and other childhood disorders are providing better diagnostic accuracy.[94–96] Further research on the specificity of symptoms is critically needed because diagnostic uncertainty can lead to a delay in appropriate and effective therapy. Children and adolescents appear more likely than adults to present with psychotic symptoms during manic episodes, resulting in potential misdiagnosis as schizophrenia.[97] It can also be misdiagnosed as ADHD. Up to 20% of adult bipolar patients report onset of symptoms during adolescence.[98] Children with a family history of affective disorders, especially bipolar disorder, are at higher risk for developing bipolar disorder.[99]

Treatment

14. How should V.L. be treated?

Lithium

Antidepressants are known to precipitate a switch from depression to mania.[100,101] As a result, the conversion of V.L.'s symptoms of depression to mania may represent a drug-induced mania. The first step is to discontinue fluoxetine. If this is not effective, lithium may be started. If V.L. responds to discontinuation of fluoxetine, future depressive episodes should be treated with a combination of lithium (or valproic acid) and an antidepressant to prevent the switch to mania.

Lithium is effective in children and adolescents with major affective disorders, including bipolar disorder and cyclothymic disorder.[102] Preliminary results from one study also suggest that lithium is effective in adolescents who suffer from both bipolar disorder and substance abuse because it reduces craving.[103] Therefore, lithium may be especially appropriate for V.L. who also has a history of alcohol abuse.

Lithium carbonate 30 mg/kg per day (0.8 mEq/kg per day) in three divided doses should be initiated in V.L. if he fails to respond to the discontinuation of fluoxetine. The dosage can be increased to obtain a serum concentration within the therapeutic range (0.6 to 1.2 mEq/L).[104] Administration with food decreases GI upset that commonly accompanies lithium therapy.

Overall, adverse effects with lithium therapy are less common in children than in adults.[105] Children appear to be more resistant to lithium-induced nephrotoxicity, perhaps because they tend to have better underlying renal function. No change in renal function was noted in one long-term study that followed up four children for 3 to 5 years.[106] However, proteinuria, polyuria, polydipsia, and a diabetes insipidus–like syndrome have been reported in children.[107] Therefore, urinalysis and serum creatinine concentrations should be monitored in children and adults alike. In addition, during summertime children receiving lithium should vigorously avoid situations that could lead to dehydration, which increases the risk of lithium-induced renal damage.

If V.L. is to be treated with lithium, thyroid-stimulating hormone should be monitored because lithium impairs thyroid function,[105] which could impair growth. In addition, lithium potentially can increase parathyroid hormone levels, leading to hypercalcemia, hypophosphatemia, and a decrease in calcium deposition in bone. Lithium itself can deposit in bone, especially in immature bone, and it redistributes out of bone very slowly only after the discontinuation of the drug. Although lithium does not appear to increase the risk of osteoporosis in adults, its effect on bone growth in children is inadequately studied.[106] Accurate growth charts should be maintained for pediatric patients such as V.L., and height and weight should be evaluated every 3 months. Lithium can exacerbate acne, an obvious concern for adolescents.[107] Lithium can cause some cognitive dulling, tremors, and weight gain, but these effects are usually considered minor compared with the disruptive consequences of manic episodes.

Valproic Acid

Valproic acid (e.g., divalproex sodium or Depakote) is now FDA approved for the treatment of bipolar disorder in adults, but no placebo-controlled studies are available in children or adolescents. Several case reports and two open trials support its efficacy in children.[108–112] When it is used, baseline liver function tests, complete blood counts, and coagulation tests should be obtained. Dosing usually begins at about 15 mg/kg per day, and clinical benefit has been seen at 10 to 60 mg/kg per day for children and 1,000 to 3,000 mg/day for adolescents. Because the correlation between serum levels and efficacy has not been well studied in bipolar youth, the therapeutic range used for seizures (50 to 100 μg/mL) is used. Common initial side effects include sedation and GI disturbances, which are usually mild and transient. Alopecia from valproic acid is less common and typically presents as mild thinning, which is transient. Mild weight gain, a particular concern for self-conscious adolescents, may respond to dieting. Serious liver toxicity has been a problem primarily in children younger than 2 years of age or in those taking other anticonvulsants. Thrombocytopenia is a dose-related side effect in adults and can occur in youth. Thus, baseline laboratory monitoring along with serum valproate levels should be obtained every 3 to 6 months. In longitudinal studies of seizure patients, 80% of women who received valproate before the age of 20 years developed polycystic ovaries, and 82% were subject to marked weight gain compared with controls.[113,114] These observations should be considered by clinicians and families before starting valproate in children, especially females.

Other Treatments

Carbamazepine, an anticonvulsant with proven efficacy in the acute and maintenance treatment of adults with bipolar disorder, is also considered a treatment option in children and adolescents, although no controlled studies in this population have been reported thus far. Newer third-generation anticonvulsants are of interest as mood stabilizers in adults as well as in children and adolescents. These include gabapentin, lamotrigine, and topiramate. Although initial case reports of gabapentin's efficacy in adults with bipolar disorder were promising, controlled studies have not supported these claims.[115,116] No controlled studies of gabapentin use in children or adolescents with bipolar disorder have been reported, but there are several case reports of aggressive behavior in children treated with gabapentin.[117–119] While lamotrigine may confer some benefit in adolescent bipolar depression, it cannot be recommended for use in children less than 16 years of age because of the risk of serious rashes, including Stevens-Johnson syndrome in about 1% of patients.[120] Lastly, the atypical antipsychotic agents including clozapine, olanzapine, risperidone, and quetiapine are being studied in both acute mania and maintenance treatment in adults with bipolar disorder. Initial reports in children and adolescents with bipolar disorder look promising.[121–123]

ANXIETY DISORDERS IN CHILDREN AND ADOLESCENTS

Anxiety disorders in children are common and very similar in presentation to those seen in adults. The diagnostic criteria are the same in all age groups for generalized anxiety disorder, panic disorder, obsessive-compulsive disorder (OCD), agoraphobia, social phobia, specific phobia, post-traumatic stress disorder, and anxiety disorder not otherwise specified. Separation anxiety disorder (SAD) is the only anxiety disorder that is specific to children.[1] Prevalence rates are 1.1% for social phobia, up to 3.5% for separation anxiety disorder, up to 4.6% for overanxious disorder (generalized anxiety), and up to 8.7% for all the anxiety disorders combined.[124,125]

Diagnosis of anxiety disorders is confounded by the developmental level of the child and the difficulty in obtaining accurate information from the parent or caregiver.[126] Further-

more, many anxiety disorders coexist with other psychiatric disorders, such as depression and ADHD.[124] Assessment of the child with an anxiety disorder must include a careful history of the onset of symptoms and any associated stressful events or situations. In addition, parent report instruments, self-rating scales, and clinician rating scales may help in determining the type and severity of the anxiety disorder.[124,125]

Treatment for anxiety disorders in children and adolescents usually involves a multimodal approach that includes behavioral treatment, psychotherapy, family therapy, and pharmacotherapy when appropriate. Pharmacotherapy should be used as an adjunct to behavioral treatment or psychotherapy not as a single intervention. The medications most commonly used are the TCAs and SSRIs. The SSRIs are effective in treating adults with anxiety disorders such as panic disorder, OCD, generalized anxiety, and social phobia. Evidence supports their use in children and adolescents as well,[127] and they have become the recommended first-line agents over the TCAs.[128] The benzodiazepines are recommended for short-term use only and may be used initially with a TCA or SSRI for a short time until the antidepressant takes effect.[124] Currently, there are no studies using bupropion, venlafaxine, or nefazodone in children. Very little information is available on the use of buspirone in children, but it appears ineffective in treating children with social phobia or panic disorder. β-Blocking agents are used in the adult population to control physical symptoms of anxiety, but little information exists on their use in children for this purpose. Antihistamines such as hydroxyzine are often stated to have anxiolytic effects, but there is no support for their use in children or adolescents. Furthermore, their side effects, including sedation, agitation, and cognitive problems, preclude their use as antianxiety agents in children.[128]

Separation Anxiety Disorder

SAD is characterized by excessive anxiety about separation from parents or important attachment figures. The child's developmental level must be taken into account for both avoidant disorder and separation anxiety because anxiety about strangers and separation is normal in preschool children. The criteria for diagnosis include three or more of the following: recurrent distress when separation from home or a major attachment figure occurs or is expected; excessive or unrealistic worry about harm to self or parents; persistent and excessive worry that an untoward event will lead to separation from an attachment figure (e.g., getting lost or kidnapped); refusal to attend school; reluctance to sleep alone or sleep away from home; excessively fearful of being alone or without major attachment figures at home; recurrent nightmares about separation; or physical symptoms including stomach aches, headaches, palpitations, and dizziness when separated from major attachment figures. School refusal may occur in up to 75% of children with SAD.[1,124,126]

Signs and Symptoms

15. **F.M., a 7-year-old boy, is brought to the clinic by his parents. F.M. has refused to go to school for the last 3 weeks and refuses to leave his mother. His mother complains of not being able to leave the house without her son. He constantly hangs onto her and follows her. During the examination, he sits on her lap.**

When she attempts to leave, he throws a temper tantrum and wraps himself around her legs, refusing to let go. He states he is afraid his mother will be killed and wants her in sight at all times. The diagnosis of SAD is made. What symptoms differentiate SAD from generalized anxiety disorder in F.M.?

SAD is more likely to present in a 7-year-old child than is generalized anxiety disorder (overanxious disorder). Refusal to go to school is common to both SAD and generalized anxiety disorder. However, children with SAD require frequent reassurance and are more likely to manifest marked self-consciousness, worry of future events, and worry of competence. Children with generalized anxiety disorder usually are older and do not cling to a parent or caregiver. F.M. exhibits four of the seven criteria as defined in the DSM-IV: school avoidance, fear of harm to his mother, excessive anxiety when she attempts to leave, and clinging behavior. A diagnosis of depression is ruled out because F.M. does not have a sleep disturbance and enjoys activities with family and friends.

Treatment

16. **What is the most appropriate treatment approach to F.M.'s problem?**

The treatment approach to a child or adolescent with an anxiety disorder requires an integrated approach using several treatment techniques. Initial intervention usually involves behavioral treatment that includes systematic desensitization, exposure and response conditioning, extinction, modeling, counter-conditioning, and family therapy.[124] Behavioral intervention requires the caregiver and child to participate in a behavioral treatment plan.[124,129] Initial behavioral treatment for F.M. and his family should include desensitization and relaxation in which each day F.M. is taken closer to his classroom and taught to relax when the first signs of anxiety occur. His mother should progressively distance herself from F.M. after he can successfully enter his classroom.

17. **F.M.'s parents ask if there is a drug that can be used to treat his separation anxiety. What pharmacologic options are available for F.M.?**

SSRIs and, less commonly, benzodiazepines or TCAs are used to treat separation anxiety and school refusal. The use of these drugs is based on sparse literature and few controlled studies. A recent multicenter study examining the effects of fluvoxamine in children and adolescents with social phobia, SAD, or generalized anxiety disorder showed a robust treatment response.[130] SSRIs have not been systematically studied in children with SAD but can be useful in reducing target symptoms.[124,131] There are four double-blind, controlled studies using imipramine or clomipramine to treat SAD and school refusal, and only one of these (performed in 1971) found imipramine to be superior to placebo in increasing school attendance. More recent studies have not shown superiority of the TCAs to placebo. Thus, TCA medications for anxiety disorders associated with school refusal is questionable, although clinical experience suggests that some children respond favorably.[124,129] Both chlordiazepoxide and clonazepam have been used in small open trials. Because of the potential for tolerance and dependence in children and adolescents, it is recommended that benzodiazepines be used for only short-term treatment if at all. More adequately controlled trials of benzodiazepine derivatives, antidepressant medications, and buspirone are needed to ascertain their effectiveness.[129] F.M.'s problem is treated best with the recommended behavioral therapy. If behavioral therapy proves unsuccessful, an SSRI should be considered. Currently, the literature to support the use of pharmacologic interventions is limited.

18. **What is the expected course of response to behavior treatment?**

Most children such as F.M. begin to respond to behavioral treatment in approximately 3 weeks and are able to attend school regularly shortly thereafter.

Obsessive-Compulsive Disorder

OCD exists in children at an estimated prevalence rate of 1% to 3.6%. The diagnostic criteria for children in the DSM-IV are the same as those for adults. In children, it is often difficult to distinguish between OCD and mild rituals and obsessions that occur in the normal development of the child, and symptoms vary considerably in their severity. There is considerable comorbidity with OCD in children. For example, at least 50% of children with Tourette's syndrome or tic disorders have obsessive-compulsive symptoms, and anxiety and mood disorders are also very common. Cognitive-behavioral therapy and pharmacologic agents have both proved useful in treating people with OCD.[132]

Signs and Symptoms

19. **R.D., a 10-year-old girl, is brought to the clinic by her parents who report that she is constantly washing her hands at home. She also spends at least 2 hours preparing for bed and must complete specific routines every night before going to sleep. She brushes her teeth at least 10 times daily, and her belongings all must be in the same place every night. She checks them repeatedly before she can lie down. Her teacher is very worried about her because she cannot complete school assignments. R.D. continually rewrites her schoolwork, even if it appears perfect to her teacher. R.D.'s routines and insistence on perfection are interfering greatly with normal functioning. She is late for school, cannot complete tasks, and has no friends. Her parents noticed these routines about 2 years ago, but they have become much worse over the last 6 months. R.D. is a well-developed child of average height and weight (72 lb), with hands that are chapped and rough. R.D. appears very anxious and asks to go to the bathroom, where she starts to wash her hands. The psychiatrist's diagnosis is OCD. What symptoms does R.D. display that are consistent with a diagnosis of OCD?**

R.D. displays symptoms commonly seen in adults and children with OCD. Most common target symptoms found by Swedo and colleagues[133] are excessive washing, bathing, or grooming (85%); repeated rituals (51%); excessive checking (46%); and rituals to remove contact with contaminants (23%). R.D. displays excessive washing, repeated rituals (bedtime activities), and excessive checking (redoing school work and checking her belongings).

Treatment

20. **What pharmacologic interventions should be initiated for R.D.?**

Clomipramine (Anafranil), fluoxetine (Prozac), fluvoxamine (Luvox), sertraline (Zoloft), and paroxetine (Paxil) are currently approved by the FDA for use in OCD. Of these, fluoxetine, fluvoxamine, and sertraline have FDA-approved indications for treatment of OCD in children. However, clomipramine is the most thoroughly studied agent in children, and several studies have shown it to be significantly superior to placebo. However, it carries with it all the side effects associated with TCAs (dry mouth, constipation, sedation, tremor) and a higher risk for seizures than SSRIs. Furthermore, clomipramine requires ECG monitoring. Serotonin reuptake inhibitors (fluoxetine, paroxetine, fluvoxamine, sertraline, and citalopram) are efficacious in treating adults with OCD and produce less serious side effects (nausea, headache, insomnia, agitation) than TCAs. Placebo-controlled trials (using fluoxetine, fluvoxamine, and sertraline), open studies and case reports suggest that SSRIs are as effective in treating OCD in children and adolescents as in adults.[134–141] The American Academy of Child and Adolescent Psychiatry recently published practice parameters for the treatment of OCD in children and adolescents and recommend making pharmacologic choices based on side effect profiles and potential for drug interactions.[132]

Based on the preceding information, R.D. should receive one of the SSRIs to treat her OCD. Sertraline is selected to treat R.D.'s OCD and should be initiated at 25 mg/day. The dosage may be increased by 25 mg/day at no less than a weekly interval. The maximum recommended daily dose for children and adults is 200 mg/day. The dosage should be increased gradually to minimize dose-related side effects.

21. R.D.'s parents are very concerned about "drugging" R.D. They specifically are concerned about side effects. What should they be told about sertraline?

It is very important that the parents be informed completely about the medication, its risks, and benefits because they are responsible for giving consent for use of the drug and ensuring R.D.'s compliance with therapy. The patient and caregivers need to be informed about the side effects, course of therapy, and expected outcomes. Sertraline is a serotonin reuptake inhibitor and has all the side effects commonly associated with that group of medications, including nausea, diarrhea, headache, insomnia, and tremor.[142] Generally, these medications are well tolerated by children, but the parents should watch for GI side effects, which often resolve with continued treatment. Full therapeutic effects may not be seen for 4 to 10 weeks.[132]

22. In 3 months, R.D. and her parents return to the clinic. She has been taking 75 mg of sertraline QD, and many of her OCD symptoms have resolved. She experienced some mild nausea, which disappeared with continuing therapy. If sertraline had failed to control her symptoms, what other alternatives are available?

Failure to respond to one SSRI does not mean that other drugs in the class would not be effective. It is recommended that at least 10 to 12 weeks elapse before switching medications in order to evaluate the full effects of an adequate trial. If after 3 months, the medication is ineffective, a trial of another SSRI is warranted. For individuals who do not respond to a single drug, combination therapy can be attempted. Risperidone and clonazepam have been effective in adults.[132] One open trial of seven children with OCD who did not respond to a single agent responded to the addition of clomipramine.[143]

SCHIZOPHRENIA IN CHILDREN AND ADOLESCENTS

Schizophrenia in children and adolescents is rare and difficult to diagnose. The lifetime prevalence rate for schizophrenia is between 1% and 1.9%, and the prevalence of schizophrenia in patients younger than 18 years of age is less than that of autism (0.04%). The DSM-IV defines childhood onset as occurring in those younger than 12 years of age and adolescent onset between the ages of 12 and 18 years.[1,144] Werry[145] defines *early-onset schizophrenia (EOS)* as occurring between the ages of 13 and 18 years and defines *very-early-onset schizophrenia (VEOS)* as occurring before 13 years of age. EOS and VEOS terminology are used in this discussion. The diagnoses of EOS and VEOS are based on the same criteria that are used for adults with schizophrenia.[1] Difficulty in diagnosis lies in the developmental level of the child and differentiation from autism and mood disorders.[145]

Diagnosis of schizophrenia is particularly difficult in children because symptoms (e.g., hallucinations) cannot be discerned until the child can communicate effectively. Normally developing young children may talk to unseen others ("imaginary" playmates), and imaginative or magical thinking is normal in young children. This may make diagnosis in a very young child or one who is severely developmentally delayed very difficult. Positive cognitive symptoms can be detected as early as 5 years of age, but below that age, their determination is questionable. Family history is an important risk factor in the development of schizophrenia. The incidence of schizophrenia in first-degree relatives of people with schizophrenia is 10% to 15%.[97] Careful consideration must be given to the diagnosis of schizophrenia because it is a serious disorder that carries with it considerable social stigma. Other disorders such as autism, mood disorders (especially bipolar disorder), schizoaffective disorder, and organic disorders must be ruled out.[145]

Certain clinical features of schizophrenia in children and adolescents are reported consistently in the literature. For example, EOS and VEOS occur predominantly in boys (2:1). Although a 3-year-old child and another at 5.7 years of age have been diagnosed as being schizophrenic, there does not appear to be enough information to specify a lower age limit for the diagnosis of schizophrenia. Onset of the illness usually is insidious in individuals with VEOS and EOS. Between 50% and 94% of patients with EOS and VEOS have premorbid abnormalities. These abnormalities include social withdrawal; odd personality; and delays in cognitive, motor, sensory, and social functioning. There are few studies that have looked at outcome of the disease in children. VEOS presumably follows a more chronic course. However, EOS is not always associated with a poor prognosis. Schizophrenia at any age of onset is a chronic condition,[97] although the course is variable. For example, some individuals display exacerbations and remissions, whereas others remain chronically ill. Some individuals have a relatively stable course, whereas others show progressive worsening.

Very-Early-Onset Schizophrenia
Target Symptoms

23. K.S., an 8-year-old boy, is admitted to an inpatient unit by his adoptive parents who have information about his biologic parents. Over the last several months before this hospitalization,

K.S. has become progressively difficult to handle. His parents report that he is very disruptive in school, and his teacher reports that he gives nonsensical answers to questions and talks to unseen people. Occasionally, he cries out "Stop hitting me!" and strikes out at the air. His parents have heard him talking to himself in his room, and he is afraid of "bad people" who are trying to hurt him. As a toddler, he often was withdrawn and was described as odd by caregivers.

Admission mental status reveals a somewhat unkempt child of normal weight (52 lb) and height. His speech is loose and tangential and centers around the "bad people" who he says will hurt him. When asked who the bad people are he states, "Well, you know, the guys on TV and at school, the food in the cafeteria is great, and my teacher is really happy." He makes good eye contact with the examiner, his mood is euthymic, and his affect is appropriate to the situation but mildly constricted. He is oriented to person and knows he is in a hospital. His intellect was not assessed formally but appears to be average for his age. What target symptoms of schizophrenia does K.S. display? What differentiates a diagnosis of schizophrenia from other psychiatric disorders in K.S.?

K.S. displays several target symptoms that are consistent with a diagnosis of schizophrenia. These symptoms include a mildly constricted affect (reduction in range and intensity of emotional expression), auditory and tactile hallucinations, and loose and tangential (disorganized, switching to unrelated or peripherally related topics) speech. Autism is less likely because K.S. has good speech development and maintained good eye contact with the examiner. It is more difficult to rule out mood disorders. The symptoms of early-onset bipolar disorder overlap considerably with schizophrenia, and patients with bipolar disorder have been misdiagnosed with schizophrenia.[97,145] K.S.'s premorbid personality (i.e., personality characteristics before onset of illness, including withdrawal and odd behavior) is consistent with schizophrenia.[97] As with all children and adolescents with psychosis, organic causes must be ruled out.[97] Because diagnosis is not clear cut, K.S. will require follow-up for many years to confirm this diagnosis.

Treatment

24. **What modes of therapy are available to K.S.?**

Psychosis in a child or adolescent is treated in the same way as in an adult. Treatment should involve a multimodal program aimed at treating K.S.'s specific symptoms and providing psychological and social support for the family.[97] The only specific treatment in schizophrenia is antipsychotic medication. The effectiveness of antipsychotic medications is well established in adults, but they are not well studied in children and adolescents.[146] Nevertheless, evidence of efficacy in the treatment of documented psychosis in children is sufficient to warrant the use of antipsychotic medications.

Antipsychotic medication can be broadly divided into two classes: conventional (typical) and atypical. The conventional or typical antipsychotic agents include high-potency and low-potency dopamine D_2 receptor blockers (e.g., haloperidol, chlorpromazine, respectively). The atypical antipsychotics (aripiprazole, clozapine, olanzapine, risperidone, quetiapine, and ziprasidone) share a common pharmacology; they block postsynaptic serotonin receptors (5-HT_2) more than dopamine (D_2) receptors.

Atypical antipsychotics have made a revolutionary difference in the treatment of chronic psychotic disorders and are now first-line therapy in adults (see Chapter 78, Schizophrenia); studies in youth are lacking. Although none is FDA approved for use in children, extensive data in adults, limited data in children and adolescents, and clinical experience support their use. Clozapine is the only antipsychotic that has improved the response profile in refractory patients (those who have failed to respond to other antipsychotics) and has been used successfully in EOS.[147] Clozapine use in VEOS is limited by the risk of agranulocytosis (and the need for regular blood monitoring) as well as sedation, weight gain and excessive drooling (sialorrhea). Compared with the traditional antipsychotics, youth treated with the atypical agents show fewer extrapyramidal symptoms (EPS) and negative symptoms (e.g., avolition, poverty of speech and thought; see Chapter 78 for a discussion of negative symptoms).

Although no traditional antipsychotic medication is superior to any other, side effect profiles differ, and these must be considered when a drug is selected. Currently, only two antipsychotic medications have been approved by the FDA for use in young children (haloperidol for children older than 3 years and chlorpromazine for children older than 6 months). Thioridazine was previously approved for use in children for behavioral problems, but labeling changes made in July 2000 restrict its use to patients with schizophrenia who have failed to respond to at least two trials of other agents. The labeling is silent on the age of schizophrenic patients that can be treated, but concerns about QTc prolongation and sudden death combined with the availability of other agents essentially make thioridazine use in children and adolescents obsolete. Thiothixene has been approved for use in children over the age of 12 and trifluoperazine for children older than 6 years of age.[148] There are no recommendations regarding the use of other antipsychotic medications in children. K.S. should be treated with an antipsychotic medication.

25. **What medication should be used to treat K.S. who weighs 52 lb?**

An atypical antipsychotic is indicated over a conventional agent for K.S. for several reasons. In general, atypical antipsychotics have a more tolerable side effect profile, especially lower EPS, an improved response of negative symptoms, and less risk of cognitive blunting. Furthermore, nonresponse to traditional antipsychotics in youth may be even higher than that seen in adults.[147] Risperidone, olanzapine, and quetiapine are potential initial medications for K.S. Because these agents have been available for a longer period of time, more data are available to support their safety and efficacy compared with the newer atypical agents aripiprazole and ziprasidone. Clozapine is reserved for treatment-refractory cases. A drug should be chosen based on the side effect profile, history of efficacy in the patient or family members, and cost.[97] K.S. is started on risperidone 0.5 mg twice a day.

Risperidone doses used to treat schizophrenia are 0.05 to 0.17 mg/kg per day and for olanzapine 0.15 to 0.41 mg/kg per day. Data on quetiapine are sparse. In one case report, a 14-year-old (unknown weight) who did not respond to risperidone or olanzapine, improved on quetiapine 200 mg/day.[149] Side effects common to the atypical agents include sedation, light-headedness, transient liver enzyme elevations, agitation, akathisia, mild tachycardia, and hypotension. Recommendations for baseline assessment are listed in Table 81-3.[97] Risperidone has more dose-related EPS than olanzapine, but these are rarely seen in children and, as in adults, are generally absent at dosages of less than 6 mg/day. In adults, the atypical agents are less likely than traditional antipsychotics to cause tardive dyskinesia. It is likely that this will hold true for children and adolescents.

Weight gain is a significant problem associated with atypical antipsychotic use. Kelly and colleagues[150] showed a body mass index increase in adolescents on risperidone for 6 months of 3.67 kg/m^2 versus 0.31 kg/m^2 for patients taking traditional antipsychotics. Weight gain from risperidone is generally modest. There are no studies quantifying weight gain in children on other atypical agents. In adults, clozapine and olanzapine cause more weight gain than risperidone, which can contribute to noncompliance. Furthermore, being overweight in adolescence has been related to obesity in adulthood, which can lead to significant morbidity and mortality. For example, some patients develop hyperlipidemia, and others have developed what appears to be drug-induced diabetes mellitus. There are three reports of rapid weight gain, liver enzyme elevations, and fatty liver infiltrates associated with risperidone.[151] Body weight should be monitored with all the atypical agents, and rapid weight gain warrants increased liver enzyme and blood glucose monitoring as well.

A trial of at least 6 weeks with adequate doses is necessary to gauge the effectiveness of a drug. However, it may be necessary to change medications earlier if the patient cannot tolerate the medication. K.S. is gradually titrated to risperidone 4 mg/day over 3 months, but his symptoms have improved only modestly. His tactile hallucinations are gone, but he continues to hear voices and his speech remains tangential; he also falls asleep several times a day. The decision is made to try a traditional antipsychotic.

Haloperidol, thiothixene, fluphenazine, thioridazine, and loxapine have been studied in children with psychotic disorders.[146] However, there is no evidence to suggest that any one traditional antipsychotic medication is more effective than any other. The high-potency antipsychotics (e.g., haloperidol, fluphenazine) cause a higher incidence of EPS, whereas lower-potency agents have higher anticholinergic, cognitive, and sedating effects.

Haloperidol should be started at a dosage of 0.05 to 0.15 mg/kg per day for children older than 3 years. This translates to a starting dose of 1 to 3 mg/day for K.S., who weighs about 24 kg. Therefore, he should be started on a 1-mg tablet orally two times a day. The dosage may be increased slowly, no more than 1 mg/day once or twice a week, until an initial response is seen. As with adults, it may take 4 to 6 weeks to see the full therapeutic effect of the antipsychotic.[146]

Patient Education

26. **K.S.'s parents are very concerned about giving him such a "strong" drug. What do they need to know about K.S.'s disease and the prescribed medication?**

It is essential that the parents be fully informed about K.S.'s disease and treatment. As with all treatment for a child, informed consent must be obtained initially and with each subsequent medication change. The parents and child should be aware of the potential risks and benefits of taking an antipsychotic medication.[146] Potential side effects need to be addressed, including the long-term side effects of tardive dyskinesia. The parents should look for and report certain side effects such as tremor, stiffness, restlessness, and abnormal involuntary movements.

27. **Seven hours after his first dose of haloperidol, K.S. comes to the nurse's station crying, with his head tilted to his left side. He states that it hurts and he obviously is in distress. What is the likely cause of this new problem being experienced by K.S.? How should K.S. be treated?**

K.S. is experiencing an acute dystonic reaction. These reactions are involuntary tonic muscle contractions that usually occur in the first few days after starting treatment, increasing the dose, or switching to a higher-potency antipsychotic medication. These reactions may be very frightening to the patient, but they are readily reversible and rarely serious. Occasionally, however, dystonic reactions may present as laryngospasm, which requires prompt treatment to avoid interference with respiration. Risk factors for dystonic reactions include youth, male gender and use of high-potency antipsychotics.[146] Dystonias are treated with diphenhydramine 1 mg/kg or benztropine 0.5 to 2 mg. The oral or intramuscular route of administration may be used, depending on the severity of the reaction. K.S. should be given diphenhydramine 25 mg intramuscularly because the onset of action is faster than oral administration and because K.S. is in pain and very distressed. Diphenhydramine has sedative properties as well that will help K.S. to relax. Alternatively, oral benztropine could have been started with haloperidol for the first few weeks of therapy to prevent the occurrence of a dystonia. Subsequently, the benztropine can be tapered off over a week. Tapering off anticholinergics prevents rebound cholinergic side effects (e.g., GI upset, diarrhea).

Withdrawal Dyskinesia and Re-emergence of Psychosis

28. **K.S.'s behavior stabilizes after 6 weeks of haloperidol therapy, and he is discharged to his parents' care with a plan to be seen monthly by the clinic psychiatrist. After 1 year, his parents tell the psychiatrist that K.S. is doing so well that they have stopped giving him his medication and do not intend to bring him again. Three weeks later, the family returns to the clinic. Some of K.S.'s disruptive behavior and paranoia have returned, and K.S. also is exhibiting repetitive movements of his tongue and lips. What has happened to K.S.?**

Table 81-3	Recommended Baseline Assessment for Antipsychotic Medications

Medical history (including seizures, liver and cardiac disease)
Weight, height, BP, pulse rate
Sleep and eating patterns
CBC, LFTs
Glucose
ECG (for pimozide and ziprasidone)
Abnormal movement assessment (using an established rating scale)

BP, blood pressure; CBC, complete blood count; ECG, electrocardiogram; LFTs, liver function tests.

It appears that K.S. is experiencing a withdrawal dyskinesia and re-emergence of his psychosis. Withdrawal dyskinesia is much more common in children than in adults and usually presents within 3 to 14 days after withdrawal of the drugs. It typically lasts a few days or weeks, but may last up to 32 weeks.[146] Individuals sensitive to EPS (e.g., K.S. had an acute dystonic reaction to a low dosage of haloperidol) may be at increased risk for developing tardive dyskinesia. It is the persistence of movements that differentiates withdrawal dyskinesia from tardive dyskinesia. Symptoms also must be distinguished from the re-emergence of stereotypes (persistent, inappropriate, mechanical repetition of movements) and mannerisms that may be present in psychotic, autistic, and mentally retarded children. A re-emergence of the psychosis, and behavioral problems presenting as irritability and aggression, can occur 1 to 2 weeks after the drug has been discontinued. Rebound autonomic symptoms, including insomnia, nightmares, sleep disturbances, and GI distress, also may occur.

K.S. has withdrawal dyskinesias because the movements appeared only after his treatment was discontinued. Stereotypic behavior is ruled out because K.S. did not exhibit these movements before or during drug treatment, and the movements in his tongue and lips are consistent with antipsychotic-induced dyskinesias. It also appears that he is becoming psychotic again. The use of neuroleptics in K.S. must be evaluated carefully and the risk of irreversible involuntary movements taken into consideration. K.S. has a chronic disease that will become progressively worse without treatment. A trial of olanzapine, quetiapine, aripiprazole, or ziprasidone should be considered. Regardless, he should be maintained on the lowest possible dosage of antipsychotic and monitored regularly for the emergence of drug-induced involuntary movements.

TOURETTE'S SYNDROME

Tourette's syndrome is a chronic familial disorder characterized by motor and phonic tics, as well as behavioral and emotional problems.[152] It was first described in a single patient by Itard in 1825 and then in nine patients by Gilles de la Tourette in 1885.[153] The syndrome, once thought to be rare, is now estimated to occur in 1 in 1,000 men and 1 in 10,000 women. The age of onset for the syndrome is from 2 to 15 years old, with a mean of 7 years old for the motor tics and 11 years old for the vocal tics.[154] Onset usually is gradual with one or several transient episodes followed by more persistent motor and phonic tics.[152] The anatomic location of tics can vary over time. Simple motor tics are seen in about 93% of individuals with Tourette's syndrome. Simple phonic or vocal tics such as grunts also are commonly reported (98%), with coprolalia (foul language) reported about 10% to 30% of the time.[1,154]

Tourette's syndrome is characterized by tics that are sudden, involuntary movements or sounds. The tics can be suppressed voluntarily with difficulty. Tics may be present during sleep and may wax and wane over time. Psychological stress tends to increase the intensity and frequency of tics.[153]

Behavioral symptomatology also is seen in Tourette's syndrome. Between 55% and 74% of individuals experience symptoms of OCD.[153,155] Approximately 50% of Tourette's patients also meet the criteria for ADHD.

Tourette's syndrome is considered a genetically determined neurologic disorder with an autosomal dominant pattern of inheritance.[153] Tourette's syndrome and OCD may represent different expressions of the same gene.[156] Although the exact pathophysiology is unknown, neuropathologic changes have been identified in some affected individuals. Brain imaging studies show changes in the basal ganglia, thalamus, and cortex.[152] Excessive dopamine also may play a role in the pathophysiology of Tourette's syndrome.[153]

Diagnosis

29. R.N., a 6-year-old boy, is referred to the Tourette's clinic by his pediatrician. R.N. has facial and phonic tics that have been evident for a few years but recently have become much worse. During his interview, R.N. demonstrates numerous tics characterized by blinking, eyebrow raising, and grimacing; he also shrugs his shoulders and shakes his head. Phonic tics include grunts and throat clearing. R.N. says that he is unable to stop moving and grunting and that he feels relieved when he moves. When asked to suppress the movements, he can, but only for a few minutes. A report from his teachers indicates that he often is disruptive in school, lacks focus, and does not appear to be able to pay attention for any length of time. His parents report that R.N.'s uncle and cousin also have similar movements. A diagnosis of Tourette's syndrome is made. What differentiates Tourette's syndrome from other movement disorders in R.N.?

Involuntary movements occur with other disorders such as dystonias, choreas, athetoid movements, and myoclonus. Dystonic movements are slow, twisting movements that occur with prolonged states of muscular tension. Choreiform movements are random, dancing, irregular, and nonrepetitive. Myoclonic movements are brief muscle contractions. Athetoid movements are slow, writhing movements most commonly seen in fingers and toes.[1] The diagnosis of Tourette's syndrome is made based on the presence of both motor and vocal tics,[1] the ability of the patient to suppress the tics, and an increasing urge to perform the tic followed by a sense of relief.[153]

R.N.'s movements and vocalizations are tics. They are rapid, recurrent, and sudden. He can suppress them, although for only a few minutes. R.N. also displays behavior that is consistent with ADHD, which commonly is seen in individuals with Tourette's syndrome. He is disruptive, lacks focus, and has trouble paying attention. His tics, behavior, and family history are consistent with the diagnosis of Tourette's syndrome.

Treatment

30. What pharmacologic treatments are available for R.N.?

Haloperidol (Haldol) and pimozide (Orap) have been the mainstay of treatment of Tourette's syndrome.[153,154] However, these drugs also cause serious side effects that result in medication discontinuation in up to 14% of patients.[155] Both of these medications suppress tics on a long-term basis at relatively low dosages: haloperidol 2 to 6 mg/day or pimozide 0.5 to 9 mg/day.[153,155] Side effects associated with haloperidol include all the extrapyramidal effects described with antipsychotic treatment. Pimozide also may cause cardiac complications, so periodic ECG monitoring is recommended.[153] A study conducted by Salle and colleagues[157] showed that pimozide was better tolerated by patients than haloperidol and appeared to be more efficacious.

The atypical antipsychotics may also be useful in the treatment of Tourette's syndrome. Risperidone is the most studied agent to date. Small controlled studies, open trials, and case reports indicate that risperidone suppresses tics in individuals with Tourette's syndrome with efficacy comparable to that of pimozide and clonidine.[158–162] Initial case reports and small trials with olanzapine, quetiapine, and ziprasidone indicate potential efficacy and the need for further study.[163–167] Clozapine has proved useful in a few individual case reports, but a double-blind crossover study of 12 individuals did not demonstrate clozapine's effectiveness in reducing tics, and low doses were associated with a worsening of tics in some individuals.[158]

Clonidine (Catapres), a centrally acting α-agonist, has been used to treat tics, attention deficits, and obsessive-compulsive symptoms seen in patients with Tourette's syndrome.[153,154,156,168] Clonidine appears to be effective in 40% to 60% of patients[153] and is well tolerated, with the most commonly reported side effect being sedation.[164] Another α-agonist, guanfacine (Tenex), also has been used to treat individuals with Tourette's syndrome and the coexisting attention-deficit disorder.[111] Guanfacine (0.5 to 4 mg/day) appears to have less hypotensive and sedative effects than clonidine. Attention-deficit symptoms were more likely to be decreased than tics in three open trials.

Antidepressants also have been used to treat Tourette's syndrome. Two retrospective studies show response of ADHD and tics in children treated with nortriptyline and desipramine.[169,170] Clomipramine, imipramine, fluvoxamine, fluoxetine, and citalopram have been used with equivocal results.[155,169,171] Other drugs that have been used with varying results include lithium, calcium channel blockers, naltrexone, and clonazepam.

31. R.N. is started on clonidine. R.N. weighs 51 lb. Why was clonidine selected for R.N.? What is the appropriate starting dose for him? What is the expected time course of therapeutic response?

The efficacy of clonidine in children with Tourette's syndrome and ADHD is less than that achieved with first line therapies for these conditions.[153,168] Nevertheless, because it is well tolerated and has fewer side effects than haloperidol or pimozide, it is often the first drug used in children with both Tourette's syndrome and ADHD. Haloperidol can cause tardive dyskinesia and other permanent involuntary movements, as well as pseudoparkinsonism and akathisia. Pimozide has the same side effects as the antipsychotic medications and may be cardiotoxic.[153] Furthermore, the antipsychotic agents are minimally effective in treating ADHD symptoms. The usual starting dose of clonidine in children with Tourette's syndrome is 0.05 mg once or twice a day, with administration of the initial dose at bedtime to minimize daytime sedation. If the initial dose is tolerated, it may be increased by 0.05 mg every 3 days until sedation or dizziness is noted. The usual tolerated dose is 5.5 μg/kg per day.[172] Improvement in symptoms may take up to several weeks. Based on his age and size, R.N.'s initial dose of 0.05 mg/day should be increased gradually to 0.15 mg/day as needed.

32. R.N. also is diagnosed with mild ADHD, but his parents are concerned about using stimulants for him because of his Tourette's syndrome. Can stimulants be used for children with both disorders?

The use of stimulants in children with coexisting ADHD and Tourette's syndrome is controversial because there are reports of stimulants provoking or exacerbating tics in children with or without a pre-existing tic disorder. However, Gadow and colleagues[36] showed no significant worsening of tics over a 2-year period in children with the two disorders when treated with methylphenidate. They also point out that the severity of tics wax and wane over time and much of the exacerbation of tics seen with stimulant use may have been the natural course of the disorder. Clonidine is a logical choice for initial treatment of R.N. because it can effectively treat both disorders. If it is not effective and hyperactivity is the prominent problem, stimulants may be given using the lowest effective dose and careful monitoring.[154] Nonstimulant medications may also be used. Atomoxetine is approved for use in ADHD and does not appear to exacerbate tics. TCAs, particularly imipramine and desipramine, have been used to control hyperactivity in children with ADHD. However, TCAs have prominent anticholinergic side effects and may be less effective than the stimulants.[173]

AUTISTIC DISORDER

Autistic disorder (autism) is a developmental disorder characterized by qualitative impairment in social interaction, verbal and nonverbal communication skills, and a restricted set of activities and interests.[1,174,175]

Approximately 75% of individuals with the diagnosis of autism are developmentally delayed,[1] and about 25% have a seizure disorder.[174] Autism usually is diagnosed before children are 36 months of age[1] and may be detectable as early as 18 months of age.[176] The incidence of autism is approximately 4 to 5 of every 10,000 children, and it is four to five times more common among males than among females. Females with autism may be more likely than males to have severe developmental delay.[1] Contrary to previous reports, autism is not linked to the upper socioeconomic class.[175]

The cause of autism is unknown, but studies of twins support a genetic component. Autism also is associated with medical disorders, such as the fragile X syndrome, tuberous sclerosis, and herpes encephalitis.[174–178] Neurochemical changes are evident in many people with autism. For example, serum concentrations of blood serotonin are increased in approximately 33% of autistic individuals, and dopamine metabolism may be altered.[175] The major metabolite of dopamine, homovanillic acid, was shown to be raised in the cerebrospinal fluid in children with autism in three different studies. Individuals with autism also may have neuroanatomical abnormalities, notably changes in the limbic system, amygdala, frontal lobe, cerebellum, hippocampus, and ventricle size. However, autism is a heterogeneous disorder, and these changes are nonspecific. There still is no known single anatomic abnormality associated specifically with autism.[175] Functionally, children with autism appear unable to integrate pieces of information into a coherent whole.[179]

The diagnosis of autistic disorder is made when criteria in each of three areas are met: impairment in social interaction, impairment in verbal and nonverbal communication, and a restricted pattern of activities and interests.[1]

The impairments in social interaction in autistic disorder are described as nonreciprocal. Autistic people do make eye contact, but it appears that they do not "connect" in a give-and-take manner. They have a markedly impaired awareness of others, especially the feelings of others (or even an awareness that others have feelings), and fail to develop peer relationships appropriate to their developmental level. They may also fail to seek comfort from caregivers when distressed.[175]

Impairments in nonverbal communication include an inability to use facial expressions or gestures to modulate communication and an inability to interpret facial expressions and body language of others. If speech develops, it may be abnormal in pitch, intonation, rate, and rhythm, and language may be stereotyped or idiosyncratic (e.g., repetitive use of a phrase, odd use of words). Autistic people do not appear to understand that language is a tool for communication. Many autistic children can say words and phrases; yet they do not use these for communication with other people.[175]

Individuals with autism display a restricted pattern of activities and interests. They may engage in stereotypic movements such as hand flapping and insist on sameness in the environment, exhibiting significant distress over small changes, such as moving their place at the dinner table. Autistic children may become preoccupied with a narrow interest, such as twirling a top, and imaginative play may be absent or markedly impaired.[175]

Signs and Symptoms

33. C.N., a 13-year-old boy, lives in a group home and attends a special school program for adolescents with developmental disabilities. C.N. does not interact much with his fellow students, teachers, and family. He prefers tasks that allow him to be alone and hits his head on walls, furniture, or the floor when the room is too noisy or he wants to be alone. C.N. engages in a bizarre ritual of self-restraint. He uses shoestrings and pieces of material to tie his hands together. He was described as a distant child who would not participate in family activities and was diagnosed as autistic at age 3. C.N. can use words and phrases to communicate his needs and desires. He also has good receptive skills for verbal information. C.N. hesitates to speak when spoken to and repeats what was said to him before responding. He has never been seen having a casual conversation and rarely initiates conversation. C.N.'s preferred activities include looking at magazines and doing math puzzles and problems. Although he has superior ability in mathematics, C.N. tests in the moderate range of mental retardation. C.N. is otherwise healthy and has no medical problems. He requires assistance with his activities of daily living. What characteristics of autistic disorder does C.N. have?

C.N. meets all three criteria. He is not involved with his family, other students, or teachers. Although he can verbally communicate, his ability to carry on or initiate a conversation is limited. C.N. has very few preferred activities. He prefers to be alone, read magazines, and work his puzzles. He also displays other features often seen in individuals with autism, such as hypersensitivity to noise and self-injurious behavior (hitting his head on floors and walls).

Treatment

34. What is the preferred method of treatment for C.N.'s autistic symptoms?

There is no cure or specific treatment for the symptoms of autism. Treatment should be individualized because of the wide variability of impairment. Typically, treatment involves an integrated approach that includes pharmacologic interventions, behavioral therapy, and special education. Behavioral approaches have proved the most successful, especially when integrated with appropriate educational programs.[180,181] In C.N.'s case, his self-injurious behavior is his way of telling his caregivers that he wishes to be alone or that the environment is too noisy. His treatment program should teach him a more appropriate way to communicate his need for a break. Ideally, he should not be allowed to escape his environment when he engages in self-injurious behavior. His attempts to hit his head should be blocked with a soft pillow or blanket. Because he has verbal skills, C.N. should be trained to state that he wants a break and then should be allowed to leave his environment when he appropriately communicates without injuring himself.

35. What psychopharmacologic intervention should be considered for C.N.? (Note: A previous drug trial with fluoxetine proved unsuccessful and resulted in worsening of behavior.)

Antipsychotic medications have been used widely in individuals with autism; of these, haloperidol has been studied most extensively. Low-dose haloperidol (0.25 to 4.0 mg/day) appears to be effective in reducing stereotypes (abnormal repetitive movements) and withdrawal in autistic children in placebo-controlled trials.[181] However, haloperidol carries the risk of EPS and tardive dyskinesia. The atypical antpsychotics also have been reported to be effective in reducing symptoms associated with autism. Although the risk for tardive dyskinesia still exists, it is much lower and there are fewer extrapyramidal side effects. Risperidone has the strongest evidence base supporting its efficacy and relative safety in autism. Numerous case reports, open trials, and two double-blind, placebo-controlled studies document the efficacy of risperidone in reducing repetitive behavior, aggression, anxiety, depression, and irritability.[182–189] The dose of risperidone used in the controlled trials ranged from 0.5 to 4 mg/day.[182,186] Mild, reversible withdrawal dyskinesias were noted.[187]

Three open trials and several case reports suggest that olanzapine may also be useful in treating people with autism.[190–193] The doses of olanzapine used were between 5 and 20 mg/day with an average of 8 mg/day. Weight gain was the most commonly reported side effect for both drugs, and sedation was common with olanzapine. One open trial used quetiapine in children and adolescents with autism. Quetiapine was poorly tolerated and did not improve symptoms associated with autism.[194]

Naltrexone also has been used to reduce symptoms of autism.[195] Two controlled studies using naltrexone found a modest improvement in behavioral symptoms but no improvement in learning or communication.[196,197] Stimulant medications may worsen withdrawal, stereotypes, and other repetitive behaviors, but they may help in individuals who display target symptoms of inattentiveness, distractibility, hyperactivity, and impulsivity.[175] In small double-blind, placebo-controlled studies, both oral[198] and transdermal[199] clonidine reduced irritability, stereotypy, hyperactivity, and inappropriate speech, and improved social relationships.

Gordon and colleagues[200] showed that clomipramine reduced the stereotypic, compulsive, and ritualized behaviors seen in individuals with autism in a double-blind, placebo-controlled trial. However, another placebo-controlled trial using clomipramine to treat behavioral symptoms in children with autism failed to show any difference between the clomipramine and placebo groups. Furthermore, serious side effects such as urinary retention, constipation, and behavioral worsening were reported.[201] Serotonin reuptake inhibitors (fluoxetine, fluvoxamine, sertraline, and paroxetine) have been reported to reduce repetitive behaviors and aggression and improve social interactions in case reports and open trials.[202–207] Only one double-blind, placebo-controlled trial has been performed with fluvoxamine in adults with autism. Of the 15 people treated with active drug, 8 had significant improvement in symptoms. None of those receiving placebo had any change in baseline symptoms.[200] The SSRIs have been reported to cause increased behavioral symptoms in some individuals with autism.[201–206]

Because of C.N.'s lack of response to fluoxetine and worsening behavior, the team decides to use risperidone. Risperidone should be initiated at a low dosage of 0.5 mg once a day and increased slowly because people with autism appear to respond to relatively low dosages of risperidone. The dosage can be increased up to 4 mg/day. His family and teachers should be advised to look for weight gain, EPS, and sedation. He should respond quickly to the medication, and reduction of stereotypic and ritualized behaviors should be seen in 1 to 2 weeks.

REFERENCES

1. American Psychiatric Association. Diagnostic and Statistical Manual of Mental Disorders, Fourth Ed. Washington, DC: American Psychiatric Association, 1994.
2. http://www.fda.gov/cder/pediatric/
3. Wolraich ML et al. Comparison of diagnostic criteria for attention-deficit hyperactivity disorder in a county wide-sample. J Am Acad Child Adolesc Psychiatry 1996;35:319.
4. Beiderman J. Attention deficit/hyperactivity disorder: a life-span perspective. J Clin Psychiatry 1998;59(Suppl 7):4.
5. Castellanos FX et al. Quantitative brain magnetic resonance imaging in attention-deficit hyperactivity disorder. Arch Gen Psychiatry 1996;53:607.
6. Zametkin AJ. The neurobiology of attention-deficit/hyperactivity disorder. J Clin Psychiatry 1998;59(Suppl 7):17.
7. Mercugliano M et al. Neurotransmitter alterations in attention deficit-hyperactivity disorder. Mental retardation and developmental disabilities. Res Rev 1995;1:220.
8. Jensen PS et al. Findings from the NIMH Multimodal Treatment Study of ADHD (MTA): implications and applications for primary care providers. J Dev Behav Pediatr 2001;22(1):60.
9. Green WH. Child & Adolescent Clinical Psychopharmacology, 3rd Ed. Philadelphia: Lippincott Williams & Wilkins, 2001:57.
10. Greenhill LL et al. Practice parameter for the use of stimulant medications in the treatment of children, adolescents, and adults. J Am Acad Child Adolesc Psychiatry 2002;41(2 Suppl):26S.
11. Cantwell DP. Attention deficit disorder: a review of the past 10 years. J Am Acad Child Adolesc Psychiatry 1996;35:978.
12. Gualtieri CT et al. Clinical studies of methylphenidate serum levels in children and adults. J Am Acad Child Psychiatry 1982;21:19.
13. Fitzpatrick PA et al. Effects of sustained-release and standard preparations of methylphenidate on attention deficit disorder. J Am Acad Child Adolesc Psychiatry 1992;31:226.
14. Anastopoulos AD et al. Stimulant medication and parent training therapies for attention deficit-hyperactivity disorder. J Learn Disabil 1991;24:210.
15. Dulcan MK. Using stimulants to treat behavioral disorders of children and adolescents. J Child Adolesc Psychophramacol 1990;1:7.
16. Swanson JM et al. Acute tolerance to methylphenidate in the treatment of attention deficit hyperactivity disorder in children. Clin Pharmacol Ther 1999;66:295.
17. Alza. Concerta package insert. Fort Washington, PA, August, 2000.
18. Swanson J. Initiating Concerta (OROS methylphenidate HCl) QD in children with attention-deficit hyperactivity disorder. J Clin Res 2000;3:59.
19. Wilens TE. Long-term ADHD treatment with OROS methylphenidate. Presented at the American Psychiatric Association Annual Meeting. May, 2000.
20. Wolraich ML. Evaluation of efficacy and safety of OROS methylphenidate HCl (MPH) extended release tablets, methylphenidate TID, and placebo in children with ADHD. Pediatr Res 2000;47(4):36A.
21. Swanson J et al. Initiating Concerta (OROS methylphenidate HCl) qd in children with attention-deficit hyperactivity disorder. J Clin Res 2000;3:59.
22. Metadate CD (methylphenidate HCl, USP) [package insert]. Rochester, NY: Celltech, Inc., 2002.
23. Ritalin LA (methylphenidate hydrochloride extended release capsules) [package insert]. East Hanover, NJ: Novartis Pharmaceuticals Corp., 2002.
24. Gonzales MA et al. Methylphenidate bioavailability from two extended-release formulations. Int J Clin Pharmacol Ther 2002;40(4):175.
25. Data on file, Celltech Americas, Inc., 2003.
26. Swanson JM et al. Methylphenidate hydrochloride given with or before breakfast: I. Behavioral, cognitive and electrophysiologic effects. Pediatrics 1983;72:49.
27. Swanson JM et al. Effect of stimulant medication on children with attention deficit disorder: a "review of reviews." Except Child 1993;60:154
28. Conners CK et al. Revision and restandardization of the Conners Teacher Rating Scale (CTRS-R): factor structure, reliability, and criterion validity. J Abnorm Child Psychology 1998;26:279.
29. Conners CK et al. The revised Conners' Parent Rating Scale (CPRS-R): factor structure, reliability, and criterion validity. J Abnorm Child Psychology 1998;26:257.
30. Greenhill LL. Attention-deficit hyperactivity disorder: the stimulants. Child Adolesc Psychiatr Clin North Am 1995;4:123.
31. Fine S et al. Drug and placebo side effects in methylphenidate-placebo trial for attention deficit hyperactivity disorder. Child Psychiatry Hum Dev 1993;24:25.
32. Bowen J et al. Stimulant medication and attention deficit-hyperactivity disorder. The child's perspective. Am J Dis Child 1991;145.291.
33. Mattes JA et al. Growth of hyperactive children on maintenance regimen of methylphenidate. Arch Gen Psychiatry 1983;40:317.
34. Vincent J et al. Effects of methylphenidate on early adolescent growth. Am J Psychiatry 1990;147:501.
35. Goldman LS et al. Diagnosis and treatment of attention-deficit/hyperactivity disorder in children and adolescents. JAMA 1998;279(14):1100.
36. Gadow KD et al. Long-term methylphenidate therapy in children with comorbid attention-deficit hyperactivity disorder and chronic multiple tic disorder. Arch Gen Psychiatry 1999;56:330.
37. Bloom AS et al. Methylphenidate-induced delusional disorder in a child with attention deficit disorder with hyperactivity. J Am Acad Child Adolesc Psychiatry 1988;27:88.
38. Elia J et al. Classroom academic performance: improvement with both methylphenidate and dextroamphetamine in ADHD boys. J Child Psychol Psychiatry 1993;34:785.
39. Faraone SV et al. Comparative efficacy of Adderall and methylphenidate in attention-deficit/hyperactivity disorder: a meta-analysis. J Clin Psychopharmacol 2002;22(5):468
40. Pliszka SR et al. A double-blind, placebo-controlled study of Adderall and methylphenidate in the treatment of attention-deficit/hyperactivity disorder. J Am Acad Child Adolesc Psychiatry 2000;39(5):619.
41. Tulloch SJ et al. SLI381 (Adderall XR), a two-component, extended-release formulation of mixed amphetamine salts: bioavailability of three test formulations and comparison to fasted, fed, and sprinkled administration. Pharmacotherapy 2002;22:1405.
42. Keating GM et al. Dexmethylphenidate. Drugs 2002;62(13):1899.
43. Conners CK et al. Pemoline, methylphenidate and placebo in children with minimal brain dysfunction. Arch Gen Psychiatry 1980;37:922.
44. Abbott Laboratories. Cylert\IR package insert. North Chicago: 1999 June.
45. Pelam WE et al. Pemoline effects on children with ADHD: a time-response by dose-response analysis on classroom measures. J Am Acad Child Adolesc Psychiatry 1995;34:1504.
46. Collier CP et al. Pemoline pharmacokinetics and long term therapy in children with attention deficit disorder and hyperactivity. Clin Pharmacokinet 1985;10:269.
47. Elia J et al. Methylphenidate and dextroamphetamine treatments of hyperactivity: are there true non-responders? Psychiatry Res 1991;36:141.
48. Hechtman L. Long-term outcome in attention-deficit hyperactivity disorder. Child Adolesc Psychiatry Clin North Am 1992;1:553.
49. Gittleman R et al. Hyperactive boys almost grown up. Arch Gen Psychiatry 1985;42:937.
50. American Academy of Child and Adolescent Psychiatry Official Action. Practice parameters for the assessment and treatment of children, adolescents and adults with attention-deficit/hyperactivity disorder. J Am Acad Child Adolesc Psychiatry 1997;36(10 Suppl):85S.
51. Wender EH et al. Effects of sugar on aggressive and inattentive behavior in children with attention deficit disorder with hyperactivity and normal children. Pediatrics 1991;88:960.
52. Chan E. The role of complementary and alternative medicine in attention-deficit hyperactivity disorder. Dev Behav Pediatr 2002;23(1S):S37.

53. Lyon MR et al. Effect of herbal extract combination *Panax quinquefolium* and gingko biloba on attention-deficit hyperactivity disorder: a pilot study. J Psychiatry Neurosci 2001;26(3):221.

54. Brue AW et al. Alternative treatments for attention-deficit/hyperactivity disorder: does evidence support their use? Altern Ther Health Med 2002;8:68, 72.

55. Barkley RA. Does the treatment of attention-deficit/hyperactivity disorder with stimulants contribute to drug use/abuse? A 13-year prospective study. Pediatrics 2003;111(1):97.

56. Wilens TE. Does stimulant therapy of attention-deficit/hyperactivity disorder beget later substance abuse? A meta-analytic review of the literature. Pediatrics 2003;111(1):179.

57. Bymaster FP et al. Atomoxetine increases extracellular levels of norepinephrine and dopamine in prefrontal cortex of rat: a potential mechanism for efficacy in attention deficit/hyperactivity disorder. Neuropsychopharmacology 2002;27(5):699.

58. Michelson D et al. Atomoxetine in the treatment of children and adolescents with attention-deficit/hyperactivity disorder: a randomized placebo-controlled, dose-response study. Pediatrics 2001; 108(5):E83.

59. Michelson D et al. Once-daily atomoxetine treatment for children and adolescents with attention deficit hyperactivity disorder: a randomized, placebo-controlled study. Am J Psychiatry 2002; 159(11):1896.

60. Spencer T et al. Results from 2 proof-of-concept, placebo-controlled studies of atomoxetine in children with attention-deficit/hyperactivity disorder. J Clin Psychiatry 2002;63:1140.

61. Kratochvil CJ. Atomoxetine and methylphenidate treatment in children with ADHD: a prospective, randomized, open-label trail. J Am Acad Child Adolesc Psychiatry 2002;41(7):776.

62. Strattera (atomoxetine HCl), package insert. Lilly Research Laboratories, 2003.

63. Spencer T et al. Adults with attention-deficit/hyperactivity disorder: a controversial diagnosis. J Clin Psychiatry 1998;59(Suppl 7):59.

64. Horning M. Addressing comorbidity in adults with attention-deficit hyperactivity disorder. J Clin Psychiatry 1998;59(Suppl 7):69.

65. Wender PJ. Attention-deficit hyperactivity disorder in adults. Psychiatr Clin North Am 1998;21:761.

66. Michelson D et al. Atomoxetine in adults with ADHD: two randomized, placebo-controlled studies. Biol Psychiatry 2003;53:112.

67. Spencer T et al. Pharmacotherapy of attention-deficit hyperactivity disorder across the life cycle. J Am Acad Child Adolesc Psychiatry 1996;35:409.

68. Rapoport JL. Antidepressants in childhood attention deficit disorder and obsessive-compulsive disorder. Psychosomatics 1986;27(Suppl):30.

69. Spencer T et al. Growth deficits in children treated with desipramine: a controlled study. J Am Acad Child Adolesc Psychiatry 1992;31:235.

70. Riddle MA et al. Another sudden death in a child treated with desipramine. J Am Acad Child Adolesc Psychiatry 1993;32:792.

71. Biederman J et al. A naturalistic study of 24 hour electrocardiographic recordings and echocardiographic findings in children and adolescents treated with desipramine. J Am Acad Child Adolesc Psychiatry 1993;32:805.

72. Daly JM et al. The use of tricyclic antidepressants in children and adolescents. Pediatr Clin North Am 1998;45:1123.

73. Zametkin AJ et al. Treatment of hyperactive children with monoamine oxidase inhibitors. I. Clinical efficacy. Arch Gen Psychiatry 1985;42:969.

74. Conners CK et al. Bupropion hydrochloride in attention deficit disorder with hyperactivity. J Am Acad Child Adolesc Psychiatry 1996;35:1314.

75. American Academy of Child and Adolescent Psychiatry Official Action. Practice parameters for the assessment and treatment of children, adolescents and adults with depressive disorders. J Am Acad Child Adolesc Psychiatry 1998;37(10 Suppl):63S.

76. Birmaher B et al. Childhood and adolescent depression: a review of the past 10 years. Part I. J Am Acad Child Adolesc Psychiatry 1996;35:1427.

77. Mitchel J et al. Phenomenology of depression in children and adolescents. J Am Acad Child Adolesc Psychiatry 1988;27:12.

78. Kupfer DJ. Summary of the national conference on risk factors for youth suicide. Report of the Secretary's Task Force Report on Youth Suicide. Vol 2. Washington, DC: US Department of Health and Human Services, 1989; DHHS publication no. (ADM) 89-1622:9.

79. Kovacs M. Presentation and course of major depressive disorder during childhood and later years of the life span. J Am Acad Child Adolesc Psychiatry 1996;35:705.

80. Emslie GJ et al. A double-blind, randomized, placebo-controlled trial of fluoxetine in children and adolescents with depression. Arch Gen Psychiatry 1997;54:1031.

81. Wilnes TE et al. A systematic chart review of the nature of psychiatric adverse events in children and adolescents treated with selective serotonin reuptake inhibitors. J Child Adoles Psychopharmacol 2003;13(2):143.

82. Puig-Antich J et al. Imipramine in prepubertal major depressive disorders. Arch Gen Psychiatry 1987;44:81.

83. Weller EB et al. Childhood depression: imipramine levels and response. Psychopharmacol Bull 1983; 19:59.

84. Preskorn SH et al. Plasma levels of imipramine and adverse effects in children. Am J Psychiatry 1983;140:1332.

85. Geller B et al. Pharmacokinetically designed double-blind placebo-controlled study of nortriptyline in 6-to 12-year-olds with major depressive disorder. J Am Acad Child Adolesc Psychiatry 1992;31:34.

86. Emslie GJ et al. Nontricyclic antidepressants: current trends in children and adolescents. J Am Acad Child Adolesc Psychiatry 1999;38:517.

87. Pine DS. Treating children and adolescents with selective serotonin reuptake inhibitors: how long is appropriate? J Child Adolesc Psychopharmacol 2002;12(3):189.

88. Weller EB et al. Steady-state plasma imipramine levels in prepubertal depressed children. Am J Psychiatry 1982;139:506.

89. Hayes TA et al. Imipramine dosage in children: a comment on "imipramine and electrocardiographic abnormalities in hyperactive children." Am J Psychiatry 1975;132:546.

90. Carlson GA. Classification issues of bipolar disorders in childhood. Psychiatr Dev 1984;4:273.

91. Reiss AL. Developmental manifestations in a boy with prepubertal bipolar disorder. J Clin Psychiatry 1985;46:441.

92. Potter RL. Manic-depressive variant syndrome of childhood. Clin Pediatr 1983;22:495.

93. Poznanski EO et al. Hypomania in a four-year-old. J Am Acad Child Psychiatry 1984;23:105.

94. Brumback RA et al. Mania in childhood II. Therapeutic trial of lithium carbonate and further description of manic-depressive illness in children. Am J Dis Child 1977;131:1122.

95. Gammon GD et al. Use of a structured diagnostic interview to identify bipolar disorder in adolescent inpatients: frequency and manifestations of the disorder. Am J Psychiatry 1983;140:543.

96. Strober M et al. Bipolar illness in adolescents with major depression. Arch Gen Psychiatry 1982; 39:549.

97. McClellan JM et al. A follow-up study of early onset psychosis: comparison between outcome diagnoses of schizophrenia, mood disorders, and personality disorders. J Aut Dev Disord 1993; 23:243.

98. Loranger AW et al. Age at onset of bipolar affective illness. Arch Gen Psychiatry 1978;35:1345.

99. Akiskal HS et al. Affective disorders in referred children and younger siblings of manic-depressives. Arch Gen Psychiatry 1985;42:996.

100. Geller B et al. Effect of tricyclic antidepressants on switching to mania and on the onset of bipolarity in depressed 6- to 12-year-olds. J Am Acad Child Adolesc Psychiatry 1993;32:43.

101. Venkataraman S et al. Mania associated with fluoxetine treatment in adolescents. J Am Acad Child Adolesc Psychiatry 1992;31:276.

102. Younes RP et al. Manic-depressive illness in children: treatment with lithium carbonate. J Child Neurol 1986;1:364.

103. Geller B et al. Early findings from a pharmacokinetically designed double-blind and placebo-controlled study of lithium for adolescents comorbid with bipolar and substance dependency disorders. Prog Neuropsychopharmacol Biol Psychiatry 1992;16:281.

104. Weller EB et al. Lithium dosage guide for prepubertal children: a preliminary report. J Am Acad Child Psychiatry 1986;25:92.

105. Alessi N et al. Update on lithium carbonate therapy in children and adolescents. J Am Acad Child Adolesc Psychiatry 1994;33:291.

106. Khandelwal SK et al. Renal function in children receiving long-term lithium prophylaxis. Am J Psychiatry 1984;141:278.

107. Lena B et al. The efficacy of lithium in the treatment of emotional disturbance in children and adolescents. In: Johnson FN et al, eds. Lithium in Medical Practice. Lancaster: MTP Press, 1978:79.

108. Pataki CS et al. Bipolar disorders: clinical manifestations, differential diagnosis, and treatment. In: Shafii M, Shafii SL, eds. Clinical Guide to Depression in Children and Adolescents. Washington, DC: American Psychiatric Press, 1992:269.

109. Vissleman JO et al. Antidysthymic drugs (antidepressants and antimanics). In: Werry JS, Aman MG, eds. Practitioner's Guide to Psychoactive Drugs for Children and Adolescents. New York: Plenum Publishing, 1993:239.

110. West SA et al. Open trial of valproate in the treatment of adolescent mania. J Child Adolesc Psychopharmacol 1994;4:263.

111. Mota-Castillo M et al. Valproate in very young children: an open case series with a brief follow-up. J Affect Disord 2001;67:193.

112. Wagner KD et al. An open-label trial of divalproex in children and adolescents with bipolar disorder. J Am Acad Child Adolesc Psychiatry 2002 ;41:1224.

113. Isojarvi JIT et al. Polycystic ovaries and hyperandrogenism in women taking valproate for epilepsy. N Engl J Med 1993;329:1383.

114. Isojarvi JIT et al. Obesity and endocrine disorders in women taking valproate for epilepsy. Ann Neurol 1996;39:579.

115. Frye MA et al. A placebo-controlled study of lamotrigine and gabapentin monotherapy in refractory mood disorders. J Clin Psychopharmacol 2000; 20:607.

116. Pande AC et al. Gabapentin in bipolar disorder: a placebo-controlled trial of adjunctive therapy. Gabapentin Bipolar Disorder Study Group. Bipolar Disord 2000;2(3 Pt 2):249.

117. Wolf R et al. Gabapentin toxicity in children manifesting as behavioral changes. Epilepsia 1995; 36:1203.

118. Lee DO et al. Behavioral side effects of gabapentin in children. Epilepsia 1996;37:87.

119. Tallian KB et al. Gabapentin associated with aggressive behavior in pediatric patients with seizures. Epilepsia 1996;37:501.

120. Kusumakar V et al. An open study of lamotrigine in refractory bipolar depression. Psychiatry Res 1997;72:145.

121. Soutullo CA et al. Olanzapine in the treatment of adolescent acute mania: a report of seven cases. J Affect Disord 1999;53:279.

122. Frazier JA et al. A prospective open-label treatment trial of olanzapine monotherapy in children and adolescents with bipolar disorder. J Child Adolesc Psychopharmacol 2001;11(3):239.

123. Delbello MP et al. A double-blind, randomized, placebo-controlled study of quetiapine as adjunc-

tive treatment for adolescent mania. J Am Acad Child Adolesc Psychiatry 2002;41(10):1216.

124. American Academy of Child and Adolescent Psychiatry Official Action. Practice parameters for the assessment and treatment of children and adolescents with anxiety disorders. J Am Acad Child Adolesc Psychiatry 1997;36(10 Suppl):69S.

125. Berstein GA et al. Anxiety disorders in children and adolescents: a review of the past 10 years. J Am Acad Child Adolesc Psychiatry 1996;35:1110.

126. Bernstein GA et al. Anxiety disorders of childhood and adolescence: a critical review. J Am Acad Child Adolesc Psychiatry 1990;30:519.

127. Fairbanks et al. Open fluoxetine treatment of mixed anxiety disorders in children and adolescents. J Am Acad Child Adolesc Psychiatry 1997;35:17.

128. Birmaher B et al. Pharmacologic treatment for children and adolescents with anxiety disorders. Pediatr Clin North Am 1998;45:1187.

129. Popper CW. Psychopharmacologic treatment of anxiety disorders in adolescents and children. J Clin Psychiatry 1993;54(Suppl 5):52.

130. The Research Unit on Pediatric Psychopharmacology Anxiety Study Group. Fluvoxamine for the treatment of anxiety disorders in children and adolescents. N Engl J Med 2001;26;344(17):1279.

131. Birhhmaher B et al. Fluoxetine for childhood anxiety disorders. J Am Acad Child Adolesc Psychiatry 1994;33:993.

132. American Academy of Child and Adolescent Psychiatry Official Action. Practice parameters for the assessment and treatment of children and adolescents with obsessive-compulsive disorder. J Am Acad Child Adolesc Psychiatry 1998;37(10 Suppl):27S.

133. Swedo SE et al. Obsessive-compulsive disorder in children and adolescents. Arch Gen Psychiatry 1989;46:335.

134. Robinson R. Obsessive-compulsive disorder in children and adolescents. Bull Menninger Clin 1998;62(4 Suppl A):A49.

135. March JS et al. Sertraline in children and adolescents with obsessive-compulsive disorder: a multicenter randomized controlled trial. JAMA 1998;280(20):1752.

136. Liebowitz MR et al. Fluoxetine in children and adolescents with OCD: a placebo-controlled trial. J Am Acad Child Adolesc Psychiatry 2002;41(12):1431.

137. Geller DA et al. Fluoxetine treatment for obsessive-compulsive disorder in children and adolescents: a placebo-controlled clinical trial. J Am Acad Child Adolesc Psychiatry 2001;40(7):773.

138. Cook EH et al. Long-term sertraline treatment of children and adolescents with obsessive-compulsive disorder. J Am Acad Child Adolesc Psychiatry 2001;40(10):1175.

139. Riddle MA et al. Fluvoxamine for children and adolescents with obsessive-compulsive disorder: a randomized, controlled, multicenter trial. J Am Acad Child Adolesc Psychiatry 2001;40(2):222.

140. Thomsen PH. Child and adolescent obsessive-compulsive disorder treated with citalopram: findings from an open trial of 23 cases. J Child Adolesc Psychopharmacol 1997;7(3):157.

141. Rosenberg DR. Paroxetine open-label treatment of pediatric outpatients with obsessive-compulsive disorder. J Am Acad Child Adolesc Psychiatry 1999;38(9):1180.

142. Roerig. Zoloft package insert. New York, 1997 October.

143. Figueroa Y et al. Combination treatment with clomipramine and selective serotonin reuptake inhibitors for obsessive-compulsive disorder in children and adolescents. J Am Acad Child Adolesc Psychiatry 1998;8:61.

144. Russel AT et al. The phenomenology of schizophrenia occurring in childhood. J Am Acad Child Adolesc Psychiatry 1989;28:399.

145. Werry JS. Child and adolescent (early onset) schizophrenia: a review in light of DSM-III-R. J Autism Dev Disord 1992;22:601.

146. Whitaker A et al. Neuroleptics in pediatric psychiatry. Psychiatr Clin North Am 1992;15:243.

147. Toren P et al. Use of atypical neuroleptics in child and adolescent psychiatry. J Clin Psychiatry 1998;59:644.

148. Realmuto GM et al. Clinical comparison of thiothixene and thioridazine in schizophrenic adolescents. Am J Psychiatry 1984;141:440.

149. Szigethy E et al. Quetiapine for refractory schizophrenia. J Am Acad Child Adolesc Psychiatry 1998;37:1127.

150. Kelly DL et al. Weight gain in adolescents treated with risperidone and conventional antipsychotics over six months. J Child Adolesc Psychopharmacol 1998;8:151.

151. Landau J et al. Is liver function monitoring warranted during risperidone treatment? J Am Acad Child Adolesc Psychiatry 1998;37:1007.

152. Cohen DJ. Developmental psychopathology and neurobiology of Tourette's syndrome. J Am Acad Child Adolesc Psychiatry 1994;33:2.

153. Sandor P. Gilles de la Tourette syndrome: a neuropsychiatric disorder. J Psychosom Res 1993; 37:211.

154. Robertson MM et al. Pharmacologic controversy of CNS stimulants in Gilles de la Tourette's syndrome. Clin Neuropharmacol 1992;15:408.

155. Robertson MM. The Gilles de la Tourette syndrome: the current status. Br J Psychiatry 1989; 154:147.

156. Golden GS. Tourette syndrome: recent advances. Pediatr Neurol 1990;8:705.

157. Salle FR et al. Relative efficacy of haloperidol and pimozide in children and adolescents with Tourette's disorder. Am J Psychiatry 1997;154: 1057.

158. Chappel et al. Future therapies of Tourette syndrome. Neurol Clin North Am 1997;15:429.

159. Scahill L et al. A placebo-controlled trial of risperidone in Tourette syndrome. Neurology 2003;60(7):1130.

160. Gaffney GR et al. Risperidone versus clonidine in the treatment of children and adolescents with Tourette's syndrome. J Am Acad Child Adolesc Psychiatry 2002;41(3):330.

161. Dion Y et al. Risperidone in the treatment of Tourette syndrome: a double-blind, placebo-controlled trial. J Clin Psychopharmacol 2002;22(1):31.

162. Bruggeman R et al. Risperidone versus pimozide in Tourette's disorder: a comparative double-blind parallel-group study. J Clin Psychiatry 2001; 62(1):50.

163. Bhadrinath BR. Olanzapine in Tourette syndrome. Br J Psychiatry 1998;172:366.

164. Budman CL et al. An open-label study of the treatment efficacy of olanzapine for Tourette's disorder. J Clin Psychiatry 2001;62(4):290.

165. Onofrj M et al. Olanzapine in severe Gilles de la Tourette syndrome: a 52-week double-blind crossover study vs. low-dose pimozide. J Neurol 2000;247(6):443.

166. Schaller JL et al. Quetiapine treatment of adolescent and child tic disorders. Two case reports. Eur Child Adolesc Psychiatry 2002;11(4):196.

167. Salle FR et al. Ziprasidone treatment of children and adolescents with Tourette's syndrome: a pilot study. J Am Acad Child Adolesc Psychiatry 2000;39(3):292.

168. Steingard R et al. Comparison of clonidine response in the treatment of attention-deficit hyperactivity disorder with and without comorbid tics. J Am Acad Child Adolesc Psychiatry 1993;32:350.

169. Spencer T. Nortriptyline treatment of children with attention-deficit hyperactivity disorder and tic disorder or Tourette's disorder. J Am Acad Child Adolesc Psychiatry 1993a;32:205.

170. Spencer T. Desipramine treatment of children with attention-deficit hyperactivity disorder and tic disorder or Tourette's disorder. J Am Acad Child Adolesc Psychiatry 1993b;32:354.

171. Bajo S et al. Citalopram and fluvoxamine in Tourette's disorder. J Am Acad Child Adolesc Psych 1999;38:230.

172. Erenberg G. Pharmacologic therapy of tics in childhood. Psychiatr Ann 1988;18:399.

173. Freeman RD. Attention deficit hyperactivity disorder in the presence of Tourette syndrome. Neurol Clin North Am 1997;15:441.

174. Baily AJ. The biology of autism. Psychol Med 1993;23:7.

175. Gillberg C. Autism and related behaviors. J Intellect Disabil Res 1993;37:343.

176. Baron-Cohen S et al. Can autism be detected at 18 months? The needle, the haystack and the CHAT. Br J Psychiatry 1992;161:839.

177. LeCoureur A. Autism: current understanding and management. Br J Hosp Med 1990;43:448.

178. Gillberg IC. Autistic syndrome with onset at age 31 years: herpes encephalitis as a possible model for childhood autism. Dev Med Child Neurol 1991;33:912.

179. Firth U. Autism. Explaining the Enigma. Cambridge, MA: Blackwell, 1989.

180. Kerbeshian J, Burd L. A clinical pharmacological approach to the treatment of autism. Habil Ment Healthcare News 1991;10:33.

181. Romanczyk RG et al. Schizophrenia and autism. In: Matson JL, Barrett RP, eds. Psychopathology in the Mentally Retarded, 2nd Ed. Needham Heights, MA: Allyn & Bacon, 1993:149.

182. McDougle CJ et al. A double-blind, placebo-controlled study of risperidone in adults with autistic disorder and other pervasive developmental disorders. Arch Gen Psychiatry 1998;55:644.

183. Dartnall NA et al. Brief report: two-year control of behavioral symptoms with risperidone in two profoundly retarded adults with autism. J Autism Dev Disord 1999;29:87.

184. Nicolson R et al. An open trial of risperidone in young autistic children. J Am Acad Child Adolesc 1998;37:372.

185. Horrigan JP, Barnhill LJ. Risperidone and explosive aggressive autism. J Autism Dev Dis 1997; 27:313.

186. McCracken JT et al. Risperidone in children with autism and serious behavioral problems. N Engl J Med 2002;347(5):314.

187. Malone RP et al. Risperidone treatment in children and adolescents with autism: short and long term safety and effectiveness. J Am Acad Child Adolesc Psychiatry 2002;41(2):140.

188. Masi G et al. Open trial of risperidone in 24 young children with pervasive developmental disorders. J Am Acad Child Adolesc Psychiatry 2001; 40(10):1206.

189. Masi G et al. Risperidone monotherapy in preschool children with pervasive developmental disorders. J Child Neurol 2001;16(6):395.

190. Potenza MN et al. Olanzapine treatment of children, adolescents, and adults with pervasive developmental disorders: an open-label pilot study. J Clin Psychopharmacol 1999;19:37.

191. Horrigan JP et al. Olanzapine in PDD. J Am Acad Child Adolesc Psychiatry 1997;36:1166.

192. Kemner C et al. Open-label study of olanzapine in children with pervasive developmental disorder. J Clin Psychopharmacol 2002;22(5):455.

193. Malone RP et al. Olanzapine versus haloperidol in children with autistic disorder: an open pilot study. J Am Acad Child Adolesc Psychiatry 2001;40(8):887.

194. Martin A et al. Open-label quetiapine in the treatment of children and adolescents with autistic disorder. J Child Adolesc Psychopharmacol 1999;9:99.

195. Campbell M et al. Treatment of autistic disorder. J Am Acad Child Adolesc 1996;35:134.

196. Feldman HM et al. Naltrexone and communication skills in young children with autism. J Am Acad Child Adolesc Psychiatry 1999;38:587.

197. Kolmen BK et al. Naltrexone in young autistic children: replication study and learning measures. J Am Acad Child Adolesc Psychiatry 1997;36: 1570.

198. Jaselskis CA et al. Clonidine treatment of hyperactive and impulsive children with autistic disorder. J Clin Psychopharmacol 1992;12:322.

199. Fankhauser MP et al. A double-blind, placebo-controlled study of the efficacy of transdermal clonidine in autism. J Clin Psychiatry 1992;53:77.

200. Gordon CT et al. A double-blind comparison of clomipramine, desipramine, and placebo in the treatment of autistic disorder. Arch Gen Psychiatry 1993;50:441.

201. Sanchez LE et al. A pilot study of clomipramine in young autistic children. J Am Acad Child Adolesc Psychiatry 1996;35:537.

202. Hossein S et al. fluoxetine in treatment of adolescent patients with autism: a longitudinal open trial. J Autism Dev Disord 1998;28:303.

203. Posey DJ et al. Paroxetine in autism. J Am Acad Child Adolesc Psychiatry 1999;38:111.

204. DeLong GR et al. Effects of fluoxetine treatment in young children with idiopathic autism. Dev Med Child Neurol 1998;40:551.

205. McDougle CJ et al. A double-blind, placebo-controlled study of fluvoxamine in adults with autistic disorder. Arch Gen Psychiatry 1996;53:1001.

206. Banford D et al. Selective serotonin re-uptake inhibitors for the treatment of perseverative and maladaptive behaviours of people with intellectual disability. J Intellect Disabil Res 1998;42:301.

207. Campbell M et al. Autism and aggression. In: Simeon JH, Ferguson HB, eds. Treatment Strategies in Child and Adolescent Psychiatry. New York: Plenum Publishing, 1990:77.

CHAPTER 82

Eating Disorders

Martha P. Fankhauser, Kelly C. Lee

OVERVIEW

Control of eating and maintenance of normal body weight are common problems in our society. For most of recorded history, it was fashionable and desirable to be overweight because it reflected wealth and the ability to survive if there were food shortages. However, with the abundance of food in developed countries during the past 75 years, eating has changed, with greater emphasis placed on eating well-balanced meals, physical fitness, and weight reduction. Public perception in the past three decades indicates that being successful, attractive, and desirable is related to being thin. Television programs, video tapes, articles, and books about dieting, weight loss products, and exercising have influenced society in the relentless pursuit of thinness. Despite the public and medical pressure to "stay fit," the incidence of obesity has doubled over the past two decades, particularly in children and adolescents.[1] A recent review of eating disorders and obesity, as well as recommendations for self-help books and websites related to eating disorders, can be found in the second edition of *Eating Disorders and Obesity: A Comprehensive Handbook.*[1]

The current worldwide epidemic of obesity may be secondary to overconsumption of high-fat, energy-rich foods; unhealthy snacking between meals; more food choices at restaurants, snack bars, and grocery stores; readily available inexpensive food 24-hours a day; larger sized portions of food and drinks; increased advertising of high-fat/carbohydrate foods and drinks; and the lack of physical activity. The addition of 20 to 30 kcal per day over a number of years can lead to significant weight gain; thus, energy intake and energy output through physical activity must be balanced for weight control.[1] The increase in the prevalence of obesity and negative health outcomes (i.e., diabetes, hyperlipidemia, cardiovascular disease) are major public health problems in industrialized countries. In addition, negative attitudes and discrimination toward obese individuals are recognized as important social problems.[1]

In Western societies, men have less pressure to be slim and to diet compared to young females (e.g., less media influences on dieting and exposure to abnormally thin body images). It is estimated that up to two-thirds of teenage women and one in six adult women in the United States diet each year.[1–3] Compared to men, women are twice as likely to report current dieting or a history of dieting. Adolescent girls often start dieting around 12 to 13 years and the rates increase between the ages of 12 and 16.[1] Dieting in males is more likely to be associated with participation in sports, gender identity conflicts, past obesity, and fear of medical complications than from any sociocultural pressures for dieting. Although some individuals use commercial weight loss programs based on nutritionally sound advice and supportive therapy that help teach healthy eating habits, others may turn to extreme diets, starvation, laxative and diuretic abuse, self-induced vomiting, extensive exercising, and diet pills to lose weight. Many "fad" diets provide inadequate nutrition, are medically dangerous, and result in rebound weight gain after dieting due to starvation-induced reduction in metabolic rate. Starvation or the lack of regular intake of food produces both physiologic and psychologic symptoms (i.e., anxiety, irritability, and distractibility), a preoccupation with food, a drive to eat, and binge eating behaviors.[1] Approximately one-third of obese individuals who go to weight loss clinics meet the diagnostic criteria for a binge-eating disorder. Restrictive dieting has not been shown to be effective for sustained weight-loss and may precipitate eating disorders.

Common weight loss behaviors include avoiding eating between meals, exercising, avoiding breakfast, selecting low-calorie foods, avoiding red meats, vegetarianism, counting calories, avoiding situations where food is offered, drinking water before eating, taking "natural" laxatives, smoking cigarettes, and not eating with family and friends. People without eating disorders appear to integrate cultural, behavioral, and chemical changes (release of chemicals from the stomach, intestine, and brain) to produce an appropriate perception of hunger or satiation and are more likely to maintain an ideal weight.

DEFINITIONS: EATING AND RELATED DISORDERS
Eating Disorders

Eating disorders should be considered a syndrome characterized by a cluster of symptoms that define the condition.[4-6] Anorexia nervosa, bulimia nervosa, binge eating, and obesity are examples of eating or metabolic disorders that evolve as a result of weight loss behaviors and are caused by a complex interaction of social, developmental, and biological factors.[4] Diagnosis of eating disorders is based on weight; engagement in weight loss behaviors (e.g., restricting or avoiding food, vomiting, laxative and diuretic abuse, use of appetite suppressants, overexercising); binge eating behaviors; abnormal attitudes and preoccupation with weight, shape, and food; and medical consequences.[5,6] Preoccupations with body weight and shape, food avoidance, and overeating are relatively "modern" clinical disorders and are found primarily in Westernized countries.

Ideal body weight can be measured by a number of calculations, but the body mass index (BMI) is most commonly used for assessing weight based on age and gender norms.[7-9] For calculations of BMI and guidelines for weight classes, see Table 82-1. Behaviors associated with each eating disorder are unique, but may overlap and occur throughout the individual's lifetime (Table 82-2 shows a comparison of eating

Table 82-1 Body Mass Index (BMI) and Guidelines for Weight Classes

Metric Conversion Formula Using Kilograms and Meters

$$BMI = \frac{\text{Weight in kilograms}}{\text{Height in meters}^2}$$

Nonmetric Conversion Formula Using Pounds and Inches

$$BMI = \frac{\text{Weight in pounds}}{\text{Height in inches}^2} \times 703$$

Weight Status	BMI	Obesity Class
Anorexia nervosa	≤17.5	
Underweight	<18.5	
Normal	18.5–24.9	
Overweight	25.0–29.9	
Obesity	30.0–34.9	I
	35.0–39.9	II
Extreme obesity	≥40	III

Adapted from reference 20.

Table 82-2 Comparison of Eating Disorders

	Anorexia Nervosa	Bulimia Nervosa	Binge Eating Disorder
Lifetime prevalence	0.5–1% females	1–3% females	Unknown
Prevalence rates			0.7–4% (community)
			15–50% (weight control programs
Female:male	10:1	10:1	1.5:1
Onset	Mid- to late adolescence (14–18 years)	Late adolescence or early adulthood	Late adolescence or early 20s
Dietary restriction	++	+	+
Bingeing	+	+++	++
Purging	++	+++	−
Crossover from AN to BN or vice versa	15%	~1%	N.A.
Subthreshold eating disorder	15%	20%	Unknown
Persistent disorder	10%	10%	Unknown
No clinical eating disorder after long-term followup (≤10 yr after referral)	50%	70%	Unknown
Death	10%	~1%	Unknown

AN, anorexia nervosa; BN, bulimia nervosa.
Adapted from references 1, 5 and 6.

disorders). The American Psychiatric Association's *Practice Guideline for the Treatment of Patients with Eating Disorders* provides diagnostic and treatment strategies for anorexia nervosa and bulimia nervosa.[10] Although effective therapies for eating disorders exist, many people do not seek treatment and up to 50% of cases are not recognized in clinical settings.[11]

Anorexia Nervosa

The term *anorexia* (the medical term for loss of appetite) was first used in 1873 by an English physician, Sir William Gull, who described a young woman with restrictive dieting and amenorrhea. When the focus on weight and thinness becomes pathologic and detrimental to the person's health (e.g., deficiency in essential amino acids, vitamins, minerals, and electrolytes; bone loss; depression; and cardiac changes) it is called *anorexia nervosa*. Criteria from the *Diagnostic and Statistical Manual of Mental Disorders*, Fourth Edition-Text Revision (DSM-IV-TR) are listed in Table 82-3.[6] Anorexia nervosa is defined by a BMI ≤ 17.5 kg/m². Because linear growth may be impaired in people with anorexia nervosa due to poor nutrition, adjustments to height and weight calculations must be made based on expected values for the age range.[1,2] Weight loss, a refusal to maintain a minimal normal weight for age and height, and amenorrhea are characteristic features of the disorder. Classic symptoms and attitudes include persistent and irrational fear of becoming overweight, a distorted perception of body image, and denial of the seriousness of the illness.

Anorexia nervosa is divided into two subtypes: restricting and binge eating/purging.[6] Weight loss is accomplished primarily by the reduction in total food intake (restriction), al-

though most will eventually try purging (i.e., misuse of laxatives and diuretics or self-induced vomiting) and use of excessive exercise to lose weight. Approximately 50% of women with anorexia nervosa develop bulimic symptoms; some women who initially have bulimic symptoms later develop anorexic symptoms.[10] Patients with anorexia can alternate between restricting and bulimic subtypes throughout their illness. Individuals with the binge eating/ purging type are likely to exhibit more impulse-control behaviors such as suicidal and self-harm behaviors, drug and alcohol abuse, mood lability, and increased sexual activity.[10,12]

Bulimia Nervosa

Bulimia, or binge eating (consuming a large amount of food over a short period), was first described in 1979 by Gerald Russell, a London psychiatrist, who observed that several of his anorectic patients went on eating binges. Bulimia was first recognized as a separate disorder from anorexia nervosa in the 1980 DSM-III. Originally, the criteria emphasized binge eating behaviors without the associated features of self-induced vomiting, laxative abuse, and preoccupation with shape and weight. Individuals with bulimia have a powerful urge to overeat in combination with a fear of becoming fat, thus they induce vomiting or abuse purgatives or both to get rid of ingested foods. One essential distinction from anorexia is that patients with bulimia nervosa usually maintain a normal weight.

The diagnostic criteria for bulimia nervosa have evolved over time to the most current DSM-IV-TR criteria (Table 82-4).[6] The characteristics of bulimia nervosa include binge eating along with inappropriate compensatory behaviors and methods to prevent weight gain that occur, on average, at least twice weekly for 3 months. Patients must satisfy all five criteria (Table 82-4) to be diagnosed with bulimia nervosa and may be further classified as either the purging or nonpurging type. Bulimia nervosa is divided into two specific subtypes: purging and nonpurging. Individuals with bulimia nervosa may use several methods to compensate for binge eating. Vomiting after binge eating (or purging) is the most common technique and is used by 80% to 90% of individuals with bulimia nervosa.[10] In comparison to nonpurging bulimics, those with purging behaviors have more anxiety about eating, a greater disturbance in body image, more self-injurious behaviors, and a higher incidence of comorbid anxiety, depression, and alcohol abuse.[1] Nonpurging forms of bulimia nervosa (such as excessive exercise or fasting), taking appetite suppressants or stimulants, and use of insulin for weight control in patients with diabetes mellitus may be related.[1]

Eating Disorder Not Otherwise Specified

A subset of individuals may have characteristics of anorexia nervosa and bulimia nervosa, but do not meet the complete diagnostic criteria of the disorder. In the DSM-IV-TR, these individuals are classified as having an "Eating Disorder Not Otherwise Specified" (ED-NOS), which also has been called an *atypical eating disorder.*[6] Subsyndromal or subclinical eating disorders have been found in 7% to 10% of young women.[13] Up to 50% of individuals presenting to eating disorder programs are given the diagnosis of ED-NOS because they fail to meet one DSM-IV-TR criteria (e.g., fewer than two eating binges per week for 3 months, <3 months of

---

Table 82-3 DSM-IV-TR Diagnostic Criteria for Anorexia Nervosa[6]

A. Refusal to maintain body weight at or above a minimally normal weight for age and height (e.g., weight loss leading to maintenance of body weight <85% of that expected; or failure to make expected weight gain during period of growth, leading to body weight <85% of that expected).

B. Intense fear of gaining weight or becoming fat, even though underweight.

C. Disturbances in the way that one's body weight or shape is experienced, undue influence of body weight or shape on self-evaluation, or denial of the seriousness of the current low body weight.

D. In postmenarchal females, amenorrhea (i.e., the absence of at least three consecutive menstrual cycles). (A woman is considered to have amenorrhea if her periods occur only following hormone [e.g., estrogen] administration.)

Specify type:

Restricting Type: during the current episode of anorexia nervosa, the person has not regularly engaged in binge eating or purging behavior (i.e., self-induced vomiting or the misuse of laxatives, diuretics, or enemas).

Binge Eating/Purging Type: during the current episode of anorexia nervosa, the person has regularly engaged in binge eating or purging behavior (i.e., self-induced vomiting or the misuse of laxatives, diuretics, or enemas).

Reprinted with permission from the Diagnostic and Statistical Manual of Mental Disorders, Fourth Edition, Text Revision. Copyright 2000 American Psychiatric Association.

Table 82-4 DSM-IV-TR Diagnostic Criteria for Bulimia Nervosa[6]

A. Recurrent episodes of binge eating. An episode of binge eating is characterized by both of the following:
  (1) eating, in a discrete period of time (e.g., within any 2-hour period), an amount of food that is definitely larger than most people would eat during a similar period of time and under similar circumstances
  (2) a sense of lack of control over eating during the episode (e.g., a feeling that one cannot stop eating or control what or how much one is eating)
B. Recurrent inappropriate compensatory behavior to prevent weight gain, such as self-induced vomiting; misuse of laxatives, diuretics, enemas, or other medications; fasting; or excessive exercise
C. The binge eating and inappropriate compensatory behaviors both occur, on average, at least twice a week for 3 months
D. Self-evaluation is unduly influenced by body shape and weight
E. The disturbance does not occur exclusively during episodes of anorexia nervosa

Specify type:
Purging Type: during the current episode of bulimia nervosa, the person has regularly engaged in self-induced vomiting or the misuse of laxatives, diuretics, or enemas
Nonpurging Type: during the current episode of bulimia nervosa, the person has used other inappropriate compensatory behaviors, such as fasting or excessive exercise, but has not regularly engaged in self-induced vomiting or the misuse of laxatives, diuretics, or enemas

Reprinted with permission from the Diagnostic and Statistical Manual of Mental Disorders, Fourth Edition, Text Revision. Copyright 2000 American Psychiatric Association.

amenorrhea).[10] Individuals who abuse weight reduction medications, take anabolic steroids, or use excessive exercise to lose weight and those with binge eating behaviors are diagnosed with ED-NOS. Extreme vegetarians or vegans may be a type of eating disorder due to their obsessive aversion to ingesting meat or animal by-products and strict avoidance of animal-derived foods. Cases of food refusal and undernutrition secondary to hypochondriasis may be an atypical eating disorder.[1] Individuals with a subsyndromal eating disorder are at risk for developing anorexia nervosa and bulimia nervosa and need professional help to reduce abnormal eating habits, food restriction, body-image distortion, and compulsive exercising.[10]

Binge Eating Disorder

Binge eating disorder is a proposed diagnostic entity in the DSM-IV-TR and is characterized by recurrent binge eating episodes unaccompanied by behaviors to prevent the weight gain, such as self-induced vomiting or laxative abuse.[6,10,14-16] The diagnostic criteria requires binge eating episodes that are associated with three (or more) of the following: eating very rapidly; eating until feeling uncomfortable; eating large amounts of food when not physically hungry; eating alone because of embarrassment about how much is eaten; and feeling disgusted, guilty, or depressed about overeating.[6,16] Binge eating episodes must occur at least 2 days a week for 6 months and cause significant distress about binge eating. In some individuals, binge eating may be triggered by dysphoric moods such as anxiety and depression, whereas others may feel "numb" or "spaced out" during the eating episode.[6,16] Binge

eating patients are more likely to overeat in response to negative emotional states, and obese binge eaters often eat in response to emotional stress.[16]

The onset of binge eating usually first occurs in late adolescence or in the early 20s and after a significant weight loss from dieting.[6] Binge eating is more common in women than men (approximately 1.5 times) and its estimated prevalence rate in the United States is between 2% and 5% of adult women.[14,17] A nighteating syndrome characterized by insomnia with evening hyperphagia has been recognized as a type of binge eating disorder.[1] Approximately 1.5% of the general population has nighteating syndrome and it is more common in obese individuals during periods of high stress. Nighttime eaters suffer from frequent awakenings and their snack intake is usually high carbohydrate-to-protein foods. During the night, they can consume more than 50% of their normal daily caloric intake.

Approximately 15% to 50% (average, 30%) of people in weight-control programs fit the criteria for a binge eating disorder; approximately one-third of these individuals are male.[6,10] Binge eating disorder may be a type of nonpurging bulimia nervosa or an overeating disorder, because this pattern of eating is found in both bulimia nervosa and in obesity.[18] Chronic, recurrent binge eating and dieting is associated with obesity that leads to significant morbidity and mortality.[19] Comorbid psychiatric disorders associated with binge eating disorder include anxiety, depression, obsessive-compulsive disorder, impulsive behaviors, substance-related disorders, and personality disorders (cluster B and C).[6,16]

Obesity

Obesity is not recognized as a psychiatric or eating disorder in the DSM-IV-TR, although individuals often have comorbid anxiety and depression, a history of "yo-yo" dieting (weight loss attempts followed by weight gain), binge eating behaviors, and obsessions about food and body weight.[18] Obesity is a chronic metabolic disorder that is determined by multiple biologic and environmental factors, a sedentary lifestyle, and a genetic predisposition. Obesity is defined as a BMI ≥ 30 kg/m^2, because statistics from life insurance companies indicate that obese individuals have increased morbidity and mortality compared with people with lower BMIs (see Table 82-1).[9,20] Obese patients (≥ 30 kg/m^2) have an estimated 50% to 100% increased mortality rate compared to patients with BMI in the range of 20 to 25 kg/m^2.[21,22] A BMI of 30 to 34.9 kg/m^2 is classified as class I or *mild obesity,* between 35 and 39.9 kg/m^2 as class II or *moderate obesity,* and 40 kg/m^2 or more as class III or *severe (morbid) obesity.*[23,24] People with a BMI range of 25 to 29.9 kg/m^2 are considered overweight and those >28 have an increased risk of developing chronic illnesses (e.g., musculoskeletal disorders, cardiovascular disease, diabetes). A BMI of 19 to 24.9 kg/m^2 is a healthy weight for most adults, and <18.9 kg/m^2 is considered underweight.

Waist circumference is another way of estimating obesity and abdominal fat content (and it is considered an independent predictor of increased risk in patients with BMI 25 to 34.9 kg/m^2).[9,20] High relative health risks are seen in patients with waist circumference >102 cm (40 inches) in men and >88 cm (35 inches) in women compared to patients with normal weight. Fat deposited around the waist appears to be more likely than fat on the hips or thighs to lead to health risks such as cardiovascular disease, insulin resistance, type 2 diabetes, hyperlipidemia, and increased blood pressure. The waist circumference may not be as predictive or helpful in patients with BMI ≥35 kg/m^2 and height ≤5 ft.[20] Men and women also deposit fat differently; men tend to store fat around their waist (i.e., apple shape) and women usually store fat around their hips and buttocks (i.e., pear shape). Waist:hip ratio (WHR) indicates regional fat distribution and increased health risk is seen in patients with high intra-abdominal fat (WHR >1 in men and >0.8 in women).[9] Skin-fold thickness can be used to assess body fat at various sites, but measurements may vary between observers and it does not provide information about intramuscular or abdominal fat.[9]

Body Dysmorphic Disorder

Several disorders are associated with overconcern about body shape and size (body image disturbance), but differ from standard eating disorders. For example, body dysmorphic disorder, a newly defined somatoform disorder, is characterized by a preoccupation with a defect in appearance or body shape that results in significant distress or impairment in functioning.[25,26] Individuals with body dysmorphic disorder are obsessed that some aspect of their appearance is deformed, not right in some way, or unattractive when the flaw is either nonexistent or minimal.[1] The disorder usually occurs first in adolescence, is equally common in men and women, and has a prevalence rate of 1% to 2% in the U.S. population.[26] Associated features include low self-esteem, fear of rejection, avoidant personality, depression, social anxiety and phobias, frequent checking of the "defect" in a mirror, measuring their body parts, excessive grooming, skin picking, use of cosmetics, camouflaging the defect, compulsive exercising or working out, body building, liposuction, and cosmetic surgery.[27,28] Individuals with body dysmorphic disorder may have poor insight, suicidal ideation, obsessive thoughts, and delusional thinking.[28,29] A majority of patients have ideas of reference that they think others are talking about their defect or are taking special notice of them because of their supposed defect.[1] A study comparing 45 women with anorexia or bulimia nervosa with 51 men and women with body dysmorphic disorder reported that those with eating disorders were mainly preoccupied with body shape and weight, whereas those with body dysmorphic disorder had more diverse physical complaints, had more negative self-evaluation, and higher public avoidance behavior because of their appearance.[30] Body dysmorphic disorder and some eating disorders (anorexia nervosa and bulimia nervosa) are considered a type of "obsessive-compulsive spectrum disorder"[31,32] and are responsive to serotonin-augmenting agents (e.g., fluoxetine, fluvoxamine, clomipramine).[1,27,28,31–36]

EPIDEMIOLOGY

The prevalence rates of anorexia nervosa, bulimia nervosa, binge eating, and obesity have increased over the past 50 years.[1,2] An estimated 5 million Americans have an eating disorder (i.e., anorexia nervosa, bulimia nervosa, binge eating disorder, and variations of disturbances in eating).[11] Eating disorders are more common in women (90% to 95% of cases are women, and lifetime male:female prevalence ratios range from 1:6 to 1:10).[10] Overall prevalence rates of eating disorders range from 1% to 4% in adolescent and young adult women.[10] Several studies have suggested that there may be a higher incidence of homosexuality among males with eating disorders.[10,37]

Anorexia Nervosa

The prevalence of anorexia nervosa has increased in industrialized societies where there is an abundance of food and where being thin is linked to attractiveness and success (e.g., United States, Canada, Europe, New Zealand, Australia, Japan, and South Africa).[1,10,11,38] Patients with anorexia nervosa are predominantly female (90% to 95% of cases), typically middle to upper-middle class, and white.[3] Lifetime prevalence rates among late adolescent and early adulthood females is 0.5% for narrowly defined and up to 4.1% for more broadly defined anorexia nervosa.[5,6,10] The incidence and prevalence of childhood-onset anorexia nervosa is not known. It is estimated that 19% to 30% of preadolescent cases with anorexia nervosa are male.[1–3,10] Homosexual orientation and premorbid obesity are risk factors for eating disorders among males.[1] There are no prevalence studies for men and for women who have characteristics of anorexia but do not meet the DSM-IV-TR criteria cut-off for weight loss. Common comorbid conditions associated with anorexia nervosa in both men and women include poor self-esteem, mood disorders (major depression, dysthymia, and bipolar), anxiety disorders (especially obsessive-compulsive disorders and social phobia), substance abuse, and personality disorders (cluster C spectrum, particularly avoidant personality disorder and obsessive-compulsive personality disorder).[1,3,10,39–41] Women who have recovered from anorexia nervosa are likely to have perfectionism, inflexible thinking, overly compliant behavior, social introversion, low self-esteem, as well as a continued drive for thinness and rigid eating habits.[1,17]

Bulimia Nervosa

The true prevalence of bulimia nervosa is not known because it is a secretive disorder and most patients appear to be within the standards of a healthy weight.[42] Furthermore, estimates of lifetime prevalence among women vary widely (1% to 4%) because most studies have examined selected populations such as high school or college students.[10,42] Male cases of bulimia nervosa are uncommon, whereas the ratio of binge eating disorder is more equivalent between genders.[1] One community-based study of bulimia nervosa reported a 1.1% lifetime prevalence for females and 0.1% for males.[43] Bulimia nervosa is 4 to 6 times more common than anorexia nervosa. Comorbid disorders associated with bulimia nervosa and binge eating include obesity, substance (alcohol, cocaine, nicotine) use disorders, personality disorders (cluster B and C spectrum, particularly borderline personality disorder and avoidant personality disorder, impulsive, and narcissistic personality), anxiety disorders (obsessive-compulsive disorder, panic disorder, and social phobia), mood disorders (major depression, dysthymia, and bipolar disorder), and impulse control disorders (compulsive buying, kleptomania, and self-mutilation).[10,16,19,39,41,44] Individuals who have recovered from bulimia nervosa often continue to have obsessional symptoms, abnormal eating behaviors, overconcern with body image, dysphoric mood, and low self-esteem.[1,17]

Obesity

Obesity is a major public health concern worldwide and is the leading cause of numerous medical conditions (e.g., cardiovascular disease, hypertension, dyslipidemia, diabetes, sleep apnea) and premature death.[9,20,23,24,45] Approximately 97 million adults in the United States are overweight or obese.[20] In recent years, the incidence of obesity (BMI $\geq$30 kg/m²) has been rising in industrialized countries, particularly in children and adolescents. According to the latest report from the National Health and Nutrition Examination Survey (NHANES) taken from data during 1999–2000, the age-adjusted prevalence of overweight and obesity increased by 8.6% and 7.6%, respectively.[46] During the same period, approximately 10.4% of 2- to 5-year-olds were overweight, 15.3% of 6- to 11-year-olds were overweight, and 15.5% of 12- to 19-year-olds were overweight,.[47] These figures can be compared to the overweight percentages of 7.2%, 11.3%, and 10.5% in the same age groups in the previous NHANES III report (data from 1988–1994).[48] In 1994, >50% of adults were considered overweight or obese and 20% of these patients had BMI $\geq$30 kg/m².[23] Obesity is more common in women (with higher rates in low socioeconomic status groups) and in those with diabetes mellitus.[10] In the recent NHANES report, obesity and overweight are more prevalent in non-Hispanic black women. The rate of class 3 obesity (BMI $\geq$40) was also highest among black women (6% versus 2.2% among all U.S. adults).[49] The economic impact of obesity in the United States in 1994 was estimated to be $68 billion for medical expenses and loss of income and ~$30 billion for diet programs and products.[50,51]

Adult obesity usually results from a steady weight gain from the mid-20s to between ages 50 and 59, when the prevalence of obesity peaks.[23] The increased prevalence of obesity with increasing age may be secondary to continued consumption of calories that is not expended because of reduction in daily exercise, reduction in the amount of energy the body needs for daily functions, and smoking cessation.[23]

ETIOLOGY AND PATHOPHYSIOLOGY

Eating behavior reflects an interaction between the individual's genetic makeup, physiologic state (e.g., balance of neurotransmitters and neuropeptides, metabolic state and rate, sensory receptors for smell and taste, condition of the gastrointestinal [GI] tract), and environmental factors (e.g., sight of the food, accessibility of food, ambient temperature, stress, social gatherings).[1,4,42] Cultural and religious beliefs and traditions about food also affect eating behaviors. Medical conditions, psychiatric disorders, medications, and substances (e.g., nicotine, central nervous system [CNS] stimulants) may influence appetite and eating behaviors as well.

Normally when a person has eaten an adequate amount of food, neurotransmitters or peptides in the brain signal the satiety centers in the hypothalamus and there is a reduced desire to eat. Because more bulimia patients starve themselves or use strict dieting between binges, their bodies may sense a "food-deprived state" and this changes brain chemistry to stimulate appetite.[42] When the "starving" person begins to eat, the brain neurotransmitters (e.g., serotonin) that normally turn off appetite may fail to work; thus, the person eats excessive amounts of food. Studies in patients with eating disorders have shown that the perceptions of hunger and satiety are abnormal in patients who binge and purge.[42]

The exact etiology and pathogenesis of anorexia nervosa is unknown, but it is likely a combination of familial, psychologic, sociocultural, and biologic factors.[1,3,4] Fluctuations in serotonin, dopamine, norepinephrine, leptin, neuropeptide Y, and cortisol levels modulate appetite, satiety, and eating behavior.[1,52] The neuropeptide, neurotransmitter, and hormonal disturbances found in anorexia nervosa are secondary to malnutrition and weight loss and appear to normalize after weight normalization and long-term recovery.[4,52]

There are many possible causes for obesity such as genetic predisposition, disturbances of hunger and satiety centers in the brain, endocrine abnormalities, environmental and cultural influences, socioeconomic status, medical conditions such as hypothyroidism, medications that stimulate appetite, and inactivity.[20,42] (See Table 82-5 for a list of medications and medical conditions that may cause weight gain.) Obese individuals tend to have more restrained eating (dieting with chronic caloric restriction) and lower levels of activity compared with persons with normal weight. This behavior can lead to lowered basal metabolic rates, less energy expenditure, and increased weight gain secondary to periodic overeating and binge eating.[18] A brief summary of biologic agents and their role in weight changes is presented in Table 82-6.

Individuals with mental illness are especially prone to development of medical conditions including obesity. Psychotropic medications including chlorpromazine, clozapine, and olanzapine cause significant weight gain.[53,55,58–60] Associated physiological changes may increase the risk of type 2 di-

---

Table 82-5 Medications and Medical Conditions That May Cause Weight Gain

Medications
Glucocorticoids (e.g., prednisone)
Insulin
Sulfonylureas (e.g., glyburide, glipizide)
Thiazolidinediones (e.g., pioglitazone, rosiglitazone)
Progestin-containing hormones (e.g., medroxyprogesterone)
Anastrozole
Antihistamines (e.g., diphenhydramine, cyproheptadine)
Mood stabilizers (e.g., lithium, valproic acid)
Antiepileptic drugs (e.g., carbamazepine, gabapentin, tiagabine)
Antipsychotics (e.g., chlorpromazine, thioridazine, clozapine, olanzapine)
Antidepressants (e.g., SRI,ᵃ TCA, MAOI, mirtazapine, nefazodone)
Protease inhibitors (e.g., ritonavir, indinavir)
Anxiolytics (e.g., zaleplon, alprazolam, buspirone)
α- and β-Blockers (e.g., terazosin, atenolol, propranolol)
Medical Conditions
Hypothyroidism
Diabetes mellitus
Chronic heart failure
Depression
Schizophrenia
Pregnancy

ᵃMechanism of action unclear.
MAOI, monoamine oxidase inhibitors; SRI, serotonin reuptake inhibitors; TCA, tricyclic antidepressants.
Adapted from references 53 and 213–217.

Table 82-6 Modulation of Neurotransmitters and Neuropeptides and Their Effects on Weight

	Modulation of Activity	Effect
Neurotransmitters		
Serotonin	Antagonism	Weight gain
Dopamine	Antagonism	Weight gain
Norepinephrine	Antagonism	Weight gain
Histamine	Antagonism	Weight gain
Glutamine	Agonism	Weight gain
Neuropeptides		
Cholecystokinin	Increased	Weight loss
Leptin	Increased	Weight loss
Neuropeptide Y	Increased	Weight gain
Peptide YY	Increased	Weight gain
Opioid	Agonism	Weight gain

Adapted from reference 59.

abetes mellitus.[54] Forty percent to 62% of patients with severe chronic mental illness are overweight before initiation of medication.[56,57] Contributing factors may include reduced access to medical care, lifestyle habits (decreased physical activity, poor diet), and economic issues that restrict participation in healthy living regimens.

Childhood obesity is unfortunate because typical weight reduction methods may not be successful and there is a greater negative psychologic impact on the child secondary to comments by his or her peers. It is known that children who are overweight will remain overweight as adults.[61] According to the recent NHANES, the prevalence of overweight among children, especially among non-Hispanic black and Mexican-American adolescents, has increased.[47] Although the cause for this increased prevalence is unclear, poor diet and lack of physical activity have been shown to be potential contributors.[62–64] As in adults, type 2 diabetes mellitus is a significant concern in overweight children.[65] The prevalence of type 2 diabetes mellitus in adolescents is <1%[66] but there has been an increased prevalence in ethnic minorities in the United States.[67] Treatment of childhood obesity should always be initiated as early as possible; most programs recommend a reduction in weight gain rather than weight loss.

Genetics

There is a genetic risk for anorexia nervosa, with higher rates among first-degree biologic relatives and higher concordance rates for monozygotic twins (approximately 55%) compared with dizygotic twins (approximately 5%).[1–3,10,69,70] A large epidemiological twin study found a strong genetic association between anorexia nervosa and bulimia nervosa, thus these eating disorders share a familial risk.[4,71] Comorbid mood disorders and an increased risk of mood disorders have been found among first-degree biologic relatives of individuals with the binge eating/purging type of eating disorder.[3,4] Eating disorders and excessive exercising have been linked to obsessive-compulsive personality disorder and to obsessive-compulsive disorder.[4,72–74] Patients with anorexia nervosa tend to have obsessive-compulsive personality traits, such as rigidity, per-

fectionism, perseverance, and restrained emotional expression.[73,74] Obsessional thinking and compulsive behaviors are commonly encountered with excessive exercising and eating disorders and a serotonergic deficiency has been implicated as a common biologic etiology.[75]

There is an increased frequency of bulimia nervosa, mood disorders, obsessive-compulsive disorders, and substance abuse and dependence among first-degree biologic relatives of patients with bulimia nervosa.[39,71,76] Twin studies show that monozygotic concordance rates for bulimia nervosa are higher than dizygotic twin rates, indicating a genetic risk for the disorder.[69] Women with bulimia tend to have a higher lifetime prevalence of affective disorder (43.5%), a positive history of alcohol or drug abuse (18.5%),[12,77] and a higher prevalence of psychologic, sexual, and physical abuse.[78] Studies with monozygotic twins raised apart suggest that genes may contribute to ~70% of the BMI, although family studies suggest a lower contribution (25% to 40%).[79–81] Genetic studies show that 80% of children with two obese parents are obese compared with 40% of children with one obese parent, and 10% of children with two normal-weight parents.[42] Genetic risks for obesity are associated with a higher "set-point" for appetite and food intake, which causes individuals to eat more before feeling full.

Hypothalamus Dysregulation

Neurobiologic theories of eating disorders have focused on dysregulation of the hypothalamic-pituitary-adrenal (HPA), hypothalamic-pituitary-gonadal (HPG), and hypothalamic-pituitary-thyroid (HPT) axes as well as dysregulation of neurotransmitters, neuropeptides, endogenous opioids, growth hormone, insulin, and leptin.[1,4,12,42,82] Alterations in hypothalamic functioning are associated with appetite changes, mood disorders, and neuroendocrine disturbances.[1,4,70] The hypothalamus is the major appetite and eating control center in the brain and is sensitive to a variety of facilitatory and inhibitory neurotransmitters and polypeptide neurohormones from the brain and GI tract.[1,42] Disruption of the ventromedial hypothalamus produces hyperphagia and obesity, whereas lesions of the lateral hypothalamus cause hypophagia and weight loss.[73] This suggests that there is a ventromedial "satiety" and lateral "feeding" center in the hypothalamus. The hypothalamus receives input from peripheral satiety sites (e.g., gastric and pancreatic peptides released secondary to food passing through the GI tract), from leptin that is produced by fat cells, and from the catecholamine and indoleamine neurotransmitter system in the brain.[1,4,83]

Neurotransmitters, neuropeptides, and hormones regulate the rate, duration, and size of meals as well as the type of food ingested (e.g., carbohydrates and protein).[4] Neuropeptide and hormone disturbances have been reported in anorexia nervosa and bulimia nervosa.[1,52] Starvation, psychologic stress, or chronic strenuous exercise increase the release of corticotropin-releasing hormone (CRH) and cortisol levels from the adrenal glands that inhibits feeding; stimulates motor activity; increases gluconeogenesis (to maintain blood glucose levels); and inhibits thyroid-stimulating hormone (TSH), thus decreasing T_4 and consequently T_3 production.[82] Dopamine, norepinephrine, and acetylcholine have been shown to directly stimulate CRH secretion, and serotonin activates the

HPA axis by stimulating the hypothalamic CRH and pituitary adrenocorticotropic hormone (ACTH) secretion.[84] Biologic studies of anorectic patients have found abnormalities of the HPA axis resulting in high CRH and cortisol levels, failure to suppress cortisol secretion after dexamethasone administration, low cerebrospinal fluid (CSF) norepinephrine levels (norepinephrine inhibits the CRH-inhibiting feeding effect), and a blunted ACTH response to CRH administration.[42,82,84] CRH administration to animals causes many of the same symptoms as anorexia nervosa (e.g., decreased feeding and sexual behavior, hypogonadism, hyperactivity).[52] When patients with anorexia nervosa are re-fed, the hypercortisolism generally resolves; thus, the HPA abnormalities are due to the stress of starvation.

The complete suppression of the HPG axis associated with anorexia causes amenorrhea in females (reduced estradiol, progesterone, and luteinizing hormone), diminished libido, and impotence in males (due to reduced testosterone).[84] Cortisol decreases the ability of sex steroids to act on the reproductive end-organs, which causes infertility and suppression of reproductive function (hypogonadism). Women with anorexia have a blunted luteinizing hormone and follicle-stimulating hormone response when challenged with synthetic gonadotropin-releasing hormones.[4] Once weight is restored to approximately 80% to 90% of ideal body weight, the pituitary-gonadal responsiveness may be restored, but menstruation may be delayed for months to several years. Because a certain accumulation of body fat is required for the onset of puberty and for menstruation, anorexic patients must gain enough weight to initiate the menstrual cycle. Serum leptin levels (released from fat tissue) must be at a certain level to maintain menstruation.[4] Weight loss and excessive exercise (when muscle mass is greater than body fat) causes prolonged amenorrhea, infertility, and lower bone density secondary to reduced plasma estradiol levels.[4]

During starvation, the HPT axis moves into a hypometabolic mode to conserve energy, and the peripheral conversion of T_4 to T_3 is reduced.[4] Low T_3 plasma levels lead to a conservation of muscular tissue during starvation and a decreased resting metabolic rate. Symptoms of the resulting hypothyroidism include bradycardia, cold intolerance, dry skin and hair, constipation, and hypercholesterolemia. The release of pituitary TSH is reduced (possibly due to increased cortisol activity), thus patients with anorexia may have normal values of T_4 and TSH and a reduced T_3 level. When anorexic patients gain back weight, T_3 levels may temporarily increase into the hyperthyroid range and TSH response to the administration of thyrotropin-releasing hormone (TRH) may be exaggerated.[4]

Neurotransmitter Dysregulation (Serotonin, Dopamine, and Norepinephrine)

Serotonin

Serotonin (5-hydroxytryptamine [5HT]) plays an important role in postprandial satiety, anxiety, sleep, mood, obsessive-compulsive, and impulse-control disorders.[1,4] Serotonin is synthesized from the essential amino acid, l-tryptophan, which must come from diet.[85] Under the influence of darkness, serotonin is metabolized in the pineal gland to melatonin, a major neuromodulator of sleep and reproductive function. Serotonin activity in the region of the medial hypo-

thalamus has an inhibitory effect on appetite and is responsible for satiety or the feeling of fullness after food intake.[74,75,85] Pharmacologic treatments that increase intrasynaptic serotonin or those that directly activate serotonin receptors cause satiety and reduce food consumption.[74] Injection of serotonin into the paraventricular nucleus in the hypothalamus suppresses eating and blocks norepinephrine-induced eating.[42] Antidepressants that inhibit serotonin reuptake into the presynaptic neurons (resulting in increased levels of serotonin in the synaptic cleft and increased postsynaptic serotonin$_{2C}$ activity), serotonin$_{2C}$ agonists (e.g., dexfenfluramine), and serotonin$_{1B/1D}$ agonists (e.g., sumatriptan) reduce appetite, increase satiety, and decrease food intake.[85]

Conversely, reduction of serotonergic activity in the CNS is associated with eating disorders, depression, anxiety disorders, and obsessive-compulsive disorder.[4,74,75] Low CSF 5-hydroxyindoleacetic acid (5-HIAA), the major metabolite of serotonin, is associated with aggressive, impulsive, and suicidal behavior and has been found in low-weight patients with anorexia nervosa and in patients with more frequent bingeing.[74] Diminished serotonin activity (either by tryptophan depletion or serotonin antagonists) can contribute to increased food intake and carbohydrate craving.[17,75] Dietary restriction of tryptophan has been shown to reduce brain serotonin synthesis, causing a deficiency state. The reduction in serotonin activity may up-regulate the appetite or satiety centers in the brain, thereby increasing the amount of food a person wants to eat. Agents that block postsynaptic serotonin activity (e.g., clozapine, olanzapine, risperidone, quetiapine, cyproheptadine, mirtazapine) can stimulate appetite and may cause weight gain.

Specific serotonin-receptor subtypes are involved in satiety and food intake. For example, agonists at the serotonin$_{1A}$ presynaptic receptor increase food intake, agonists at the serotonin$_{1B/1D/2A/2C}$ postsynaptic receptors decrease food intake, antagonists at the postsynaptic serotonin$_{2A/2C}$ stimulate appetite, and antagonists at the serotonin$_3$ receptor may decrease binge eating and self-induced vomiting.[75,85] Studies suggest that the postsynaptic serotonin$_{2C}$ receptor and/or the serotonin$_{1B}$ receptor (serotonin$_{1D\beta}$ in humans) play an important role in regulating appetite.[85–88] Fluoxetine, a serotonin reuptake inhibitor, has serotonin$_{2C/1B}$ agonist properties that cause anorexic effects.[75,89,90] Sibutramine, a mixed serotonin and norepinephrine reuptake inhibitor, increases postsynaptic serotonin$_{2C}$ activity as well as α_1- and β_1-adrenergic effects.[85]

A decreased responsivity of the postsynaptic serotonin$_{2A/2C}$ receptors after pharmacologic challenge studies with serotonin agonists (e.g., mCPP, fenfluramine, l-tryptophan) has been reported in patients with bulimia nervosa. Patients with anorexia nervosa also have a reduced CNS serotonergic responsiveness after pharmacologic challenges with different serotonergic agents (e.g., L-tryptophan, mCPP).[75] Weight-restored anorexic and recovered bulimic patients have an elevation of 5-HIAA in the CSF, and an increased response to serotonin challenges.[1,74]

Serotonin has an inhibitory effect on dopamine activity and its release is increased with motor activity. Excessive exercising and hyperactivity are found in many patients with eating disorders, particularly anorexia nervosa.[73] Physical exertion increases central serotonin synthesis and turnover that perpetuates reduced food intake and body weight.

Dopamine

Disturbances in dopamine activity and feedback regulation at different receptors have been postulated as a cause of anorexia nervosa.[74] Agents that increase dopamine activity (e.g., apomorphine, a dopamine agonist; L-dopa, a metabolic precursor of dopamine; and amphetamine, a releaser of dopamine from presynaptic stores) have been shown to have anorexic effects.[70] Dopamine agonists increase dopaminergic transmission and motor activity, which causes loss of appetite and hyperactivity; at higher doses these agents may cause psychosis (hallucinations and delusions) and repetitive/ stereotypical behaviors.[70] The CNS effects of dopaminergic agents occur in the cerebral cortex, in the reticular-activating system, and in the hypothalamic feeding center. The mesolimbic-mesocortical dopaminergic circuits are important for behavior reward and reinforcement and are involved with "addictive" behaviors.[70] Dopamine augmenting agents such as amphetamines are used for the treatment of exogenous obesity and may produce tolerance, dependence, and withdrawal reactions. Conversely, dopamine receptor antagonists such as clozapine, pimozide, and chlorpromazine may cause dysphoria and are often associated with causing weight gain. A blunted growth-hormone response to L-dopa has been reported in anorexia nervosa.[42] This indicates possible abnormalities in postsynaptic dopamine receptors, which may suppress the rewarding effects of food in patients with anorexia nervosa.

Norepinephrine

The hypothalamus is innervated by noradrenergic pathways, thus norepinephrine is involved in the regulation of eating behavior, the hypothalamic control of TRH secretion, CRH release, and gonadotropin secretion.[70] D-amphetamine, which inhibits the reuptake of norepinephrine, decreases hunger sensations and food intake. Injection of an α_2-adrenergic agonist into the paraventricular nucleus causes hyperphagia, with a preferential ingestion of carbohydrates, but stimulation of the β_2-adrenergic circuit in the perifornical hypothalamus inhibits feeding.[42] Low CSF norepinephrine levels have been found in anorectic patients who have regained weight within 15% of their normal body weight. Underweight anorexic patients have reduced peripheral and central sympathetic nervous system activity and exhibit hypotension, bradycardia, and hypothermia that is associated with low caloric intake and downregulation of the norepinephrine system.[4]

Abnormalities in leptin and β_3-adrenergic activity have been associated with obesity and diabetes.[45,91–93] The human β_3-adrenoceptor is involved in a feedback loop with leptin to regulate energy balance, lipolysis in adipocytes, serum insulin levels, and food intake.[94] The β_3-adrenoceptor is found in white and brown adipose tissue and helps regulate noradrenergic-induced changes in energy metabolism and thermogenesis.[91,93] Administration of leptin to obese mice (ob/ob) increases noradrenaline turnover in brown adipose tissue that promotes thermogenesis via the β_3-adrenergic receptor.[95] People with hereditary obesity or non–insulin-dependent diabetes mellitus may have abnormalities in the β_3-adrenoceptor or in leptin activity, signaling, or receptors.[90–93] A genetic variant of the β_3-adrenoceptor in humans has been associated with morbid obesity and non–insulin-dependent diabetes.[92] It is possible that some cases of obesity may be secondary to failure of the β_3-adrenoreceptor on brown adipocytes to respond appropriately to leptin-induced sympathetic activity.[95] β_3-Adrenergic receptor agonists are being studied to induce thermogenic activity and promote weight loss when combined with a calorie-restricted diet.[94]

Neuropeptide Dysregulation (Leptin, Neuropeptide Y, Peptide YY, and Opioid Peptides)

Leptin

Leptin, also known as ob protein and encoded by the ob gene, is produced by adipose tissue cells and secreted into systemic circulation.[1,4,52,96] Leptin enters the brain through a receptor-mediated transport system and acts in specific brain areas such as the hypothalamus to control food intake and regulate energy balance. The cloning of an obese gene in mice (ob/ob) indicates that a genetic predisposition or a mutation may reduce brain responsiveness to leptin activity resulting in increased feeding, decreased activity, and obesity. Treating obese mice with leptin decreases food intake, increases energy expenditure, and produces dramatic weight loss.[42] In several human families with a genetic mutation in the ob gene that causes low or undetectable levels of leptin, dramatic weight gain, and infertility have been identified.[83]

Leptin is thought to act as an afferent satiety signal in the brain to regulate body fat mass.[1,97,98] Leptin reduces food intake, decreases serum glucose and insulin levels, increases metabolic rate, and reduces body fat mass and weight by reducing neuropeptide Y activity.[83,97] Leptin serum levels are highly correlated with BMI and body fat,[98] and its secretion has a circadian rhythm and an oscillatory pattern similar to other hormones.[93,99] Leptin is supposed to signal the brain to stop eating, but the signal may not get through properly in some overweight people.[97] It has been postulated that some obese individuals may have partially resistant hypothalamic receptors or that there is a defect in the blood-brain barrier transport system for bringing leptin into the brain.[97,99,100] CSF leptin levels in some obese humans have been found to be much lower than expected compared to serum leptin levels which suggests that the brain uptake of leptin may be defective.[1] Leptin and leptin-like products currently are being investigated for weight reduction in obese patients and in overweight patients with non–insulin-dependent diabetes mellitus.[97] Whether exogenous leptin administration can enter the brain and be effective for obesity is not known.

Malnourished or underweight individuals with anorexia nervosa have reduced plasma and CSF leptin compared with normal weight controls.[96,98,101–103] When starvation occurs, decreased leptin levels play an important role in adaptive responses such as increasing neuropeptide Y (NPY) to stimulate appetite (see next section of this chapter). In anorexia, the production of leptin is decreased, which signals changes in metabolic responses associated with starvation (e.g., decreased fertility and procreation by lowering testosterone and luteinizing hormone concentrations, decreased thyroid hormones and thermogenesis, and increased stress hormones such as corticosterone and ACTH).[52,103,104] In anorexic patients, CSF leptin levels return to normal before full weight restoration and may contribute to difficulties in patients achieving and maintaining a normal weight.[4] In women with bulimia, serum leptin levels are correlated with body weight and are similar to normal controls.[4]

Women have more body fat than men and tend to have higher leptin levels.[1,4] The fat cells in the fatty tissues of women are different than men. Because adipocytes around a man's waist are larger and metabolically active, fat is released more readily when a man diets and exercises. In contrast, adipocytes that make up fatty tissues in the hips and buttocks of women are smaller and less metabolically active. Through evolution, this added fat may have been used as an extra energy store in case of pregnancy. Relative to men, women lose weight less easily because they have a lower resting metabolic rate, burn up less fat for a given amount of exercise, and have a lower thermogenic effect after eating food.

Neuropeptide Y and Peptide YY

NPY and peptide YY (PYY) are chemically related 36-amino-acid peptides and are two of the most potent stimulators of appetite.[1,96] Both enhance food intake in animals, possibly by causing hunger.[105] PYY is three times more potent in stimulating food intake than NPY.[4] Injection of NPY into the brain causes all of the features of leptin deficiency (e.g., hyperphagia and obesity).[100] Many of leptin's effects on food intake and energy expenditure are centrally mediated in the hypothalamus by neurotransmitters such as NPY.[83,97] NPY is a pancreatic polypeptide that increases both water and food intake when injected into the paraventricular nucleus of the hypothalamus.[42] NPY levels are high in the CSF of anorectic patients but are ineffective in overriding the appetite suppressant neurotransmitters and neuropeptides.[42,104] Leptin inhibits NPY, thereby decreasing food intake and increasing metabolic rate through the activation of β-adrenergic receptors.[96] Plasma leptin and CSF levels of NPY and PYY return to normal concentrations in women who have recovered from anorexia nervosa or bulimia nervosa.[96,102]

Opioid Peptides/Endorphins

Endogenous opiates play a role in food reward. Altered opioid activity may contribute to changes in feeding behavior, reproductive activity, and cortisol release.[4] β-Endorphin, an endogenous opiate peptide, stimulates feeding behavior in animals and humans and levels are highly correlated with body weight.[105] Underweight anorexic and some bulimic patients have reduced CSF β-endorphin concentrations that may contribute to changes in feeding behavior.[4] Dynorphin, an endogenous opioid receptor ligand, enhances feeding behavior and acts at the paraventricular nucleus in the hypothalamus.[42] Opioid agonists stimulate feeding, whereas opioid antagonists inhibit feeding.[106] For example, high doses of oral naltrexone or intravenous naloxone (opiate antagonists) reduce binge and purge frequency and food intake in people with bulimia nervosa.[106,107] However, naloxone and naltrexone are not recommended for the treatment of bulimia nervosa because naloxone is very short acting, requiring intravenous administration, and naltrexone works only in high doses that causes nausea, vomiting, and liver toxicity.

Miscellaneous Neurohormones and Peptides

Food intake and gastric emptying are regulated by the peripheral release of GI peptides such as cholecystokinin (CCK), glucagon, calcitonin, bombesin, and somatostatin, all of which inhibit feeding.[1,108] CCK is secreted by the gastrointestinal tract in response to food intake. CCK receptors in the paraventricular nucleus of the hypothalamus are involved with central regulation of feeding behavior. CCK induces satiety in animals and humans and delays gastric emptying, which decreases feeding and meal size. CCK stimulates serotonergic activity and serotonin stimulates CCK activity.[109] High levels of CSF CCK have been found in people with anorexia nervosa, whereas low levels are reported in patients with bulimia nervosa.[2,4,42] CCK levels have been shown to normalize in anorexic patients after partial weight restoration.[4]

Other hormones, neurotransmitters, and peptides involved in the regulation of hunger and satiety (e.g., histamine, oxytocin, vasopressin, galanin, CRH, melanocyte-stimulating hormone, hypocretin, and orexin) and lipotic action (e.g., growth hormone and dehydroepiandrosterone) are being investigated.[77,110] Histamine is involved in the regulation of appetite, and histamine$_1$ blocking agents (e.g., tricyclic antidepressants, antipsychotics, antihistamines) cause sedation and increase appetite in animals and humans.[88] Underweight patients with anorexia nervosa have abnormally high vasopressin levels (which controls free-water clearance from the kidney), reduced oxytocin levels (the effects of oxytocin are reciprocal to the effects of vasopressin), and increased growth hormone.[52] Patients with bulimia nervosa have normal CSF oxytocin levels but elevated CSF vasopressin levels.[4] Oxytocin is involved in the inhibition of food intake, promoting uterine contraction during delivery and postpartum lactation, and antagonizing vasopressin's effect on memory.[108] Levels of oxytocin and vasopressin return to normal after weight restoration in anorexics.[4] Galanin, a neuropeptide that stimulates fat intake, is low in patients with anorexia nervosa and may play a role in fat avoidance and food restriction.[1]

Growth hormone, a lipolytic hormone that acts at adipose tissue, reduces and redistributes body fat by releasing glycerol and free fatty acids into the circulation.[109] Growth hormone secretion is significantly lower in obese individuals, thus lipolysis is reduced. As people age, the secretion of growth hormone declines (it is estimated that 50% of people older than 65 have growth-hormone deficit).[109] Replacement doses of growth hormone have been suggested to treat obesity and to reverse body changes associated with aging. Dehydroepiandrosterone (DHEA), a steroid hormone intermediate in the pathway for the synthesis of testosterone, estrone, and estradiol, has been proposed as a possible therapeutic agent for the treatment of obesity.[110] DHEA has been shown to decrease hepatic fatty acid synthesis and reduce hyperglycemia and/or hyperinsulinemia in diabetic and obese (ob/ob) mice.[110] Human studies with DHEA are needed to determine its effectiveness as an antiobesity agent.

Psychologic Theories

Psychologic, psychodynamic, and cognitive theories have attempted to explain the emotional, perceptual, and phobic fears of eating disorders, but there are few studies evaluating the hypotheses.[1,10] Examples of psychologic and familial factors associated with anorexia nervosa include the fear and avoidance of sexuality and growth, failure of parents to encourage independence and self-expression, rigidity and overinvolvement of parents, and premorbid perfectionism and high-achieving characteristics.[10] Childhood sexual abuse or early sexual trauma may be a contributing factor in the etiology of eating disorders.[1]

Brain Changes

Once malnutrition occurs, the normal mechanisms for regulating eating behavior change and anorexia is perpetuated because of neurochemical dysregulation and, possibly, brain atrophy. Brain imaging studies have found generalized atrophy and/or ventricular dilation in patients with anorexia nervosa that reverse with weight gain.[4] Reduced regional cerebral blood flow in the temporal lobe has been reported in childhood-onset anorexia, indicating a possible functional abnormality of the brain.[111] Electroencephalograms (EEGs) of anorexic patients often show generalized abnormalities secondary to electrolyte, glucose, and fluid changes in the brain.[4] Morphologic brain changes (e.g., sulcal widening, enlarged ventricles) have been found on brain positron emission tomography (PET) and computed tomography (CT) scans in some bulimic patients. EEG changes (e.g., paroxysmal spike pattern) have been reported in some patients with bulimia nervosa, but brain wave changes usually are more disturbed with anorexia nervosa.[4]

INITIAL ASSESSMENT

A comprehensive evaluation of patients with eating disorders is essential in determining the diagnosis and selecting treatment options.[6,10,13,112] A psychiatric assessment is required to establish the diagnosis, to identify any comorbid psychiatric disorders, to determine the risk of suicide, and to evaluate psychosocial stressors.[10] Concurrent mood, anxiety, obsessive-compulsive, personality, and substance abuse disorders often accompany anorexia and bulimia nervosa and need to be identified. An interdisciplinary treatment team consisting of physicians, nurses, dietitians, and mental health professionals is recommended for the management of children and adolescents with eating disorders.[1,10,113]

A detailed weight history and growth chart are needed to detect the onset of an eating disorder.[10] Evaluation of eating behaviors, and purging helps identify patterns and factors that precede binge eating. Determining the frequency, type, and length of exercising identifies pathologic or excessive physical activity. Assessing body image beliefs and distortions, cultural attitudes about size and shape, and family attitudes toward appearance are important in determining perceptions and attitudes about appropriate weight. Menstrual cycle history and duration of amenorrhea identifies women with increased risk of osteopenia and osteoporosis. Males also develop osteopenia and osteoporosis and may have a lower bone density compared to females with anorexia nervosa.[1] Lowered libido and infertility are common due to diminished sex hormones, cessation of menstruation, and gonadal atrophy.[1] Diagnosis of comorbid psychiatric disorders (e.g., affective, anxiety, substance abuse, and personality disorders) and medical conditions (e.g., diabetes, thyroid abnormalities, inflammatory bowel disease) helps determine which management strategies should be used to correct an underlying condition.[10,41]

TREATMENT APPROACHES

A multifaceted treatment approach that addresses medical, dental, nutritional, psychiatric, and family needs is recommended for anorectic, bulimic, or obese patients.[1,3,10,11,42,114] Guidelines for the medical and psychiatric treatment of eating disorders have been published.[10,112] Because patients may be resistant or disinterested in treatment, family members or friends may initiate medical attention.[42] Interventions include education about the disorder, exercise, nutritional counseling, modification of eating behavior, psychotherapy, and pharmacotherapy. Obtaining the patient's cooperation in the program to establish healthy eating patterns is vital.[10,11] Most patients receive weekly outpatient assessments and therapy to monitor progress toward treatment goals over several months. Hospitalization is recommended for patients with severe anorexia nervosa who require life-saving intensive medical management, including refeeding.[10] Caloric intake, weight, urine output, serum electrolytes, heart rate, and blood pressure are monitored daily.[1,2] Indications for inpatient treatment include a 75% or less expected body weight, intractable purging, rapid weight loss, cardiac disturbances, severe electrolyte imbalances, psychosis, or suicide ideation.[10,11]

Residential eating disorder programs that specialize in the long-term treatment of eating disorders for those individuals that need more intensive therapy are available.[10] Relapse prevention requires long-term outpatient psychotherapy as well as psychopharmacologic agents when appropriate.[114]

Treatment of obesity generally does not involve hospitalization, although the patient's degree of overweight/obesity and its impact on quality of life is an important factor. Before recommending treatment, assessment of the BMI, waist circumference, presence of obesity-related diseases, risk factors for CHD and related conditions, and patient's motivation to lose weight should be assessed.[20] Patients should also be screened for medical conditions and/or medications that can increase the risk for obesity and these underlying factors should be corrected before recommending treatment.

ANOREXIA NERVOSA
Clinical Features

1. S.B., a 16-year-old girl, is referred to her physician because of a 30-lb weight loss over the past 6 months and amenorrhea for the past 9 months. She had a normal menarche at age 12 years and reached her maximum weight of 140 lb at age 11. S.B. is a star player on her high school tennis team and previously was involved in gymnastics as a child. Her current weight is 98 lb and height is 5′5″. S.B. feels that her weight is perfect, because it helps her move better on the tennis court, an opinion she believes is reinforced by her coach. S.B. rarely eats three meals a day and is on an extreme no-fat diet. She runs an average of 8 miles/day and practices tennis 2 to 3 hours/day after school. Despite her parent's concern about her weight, S.B. feels that if she gains weight, she will be fat and unable to play competitive tennis.

Upon further questioning, S.B. admits to a previous weight loss at around age 13 from 140 to 100 lb, which resulted in amenorrhea for >6 months. At that time, she was involved in gymnastics and was told she needed to lose weight to stay on the team. S.B. started exercising to burn off calories and skipping breakfast to lower her caloric intake. At times, she became dehydrated and had episodes of hypotension that resulted in dizzy spells. She also took "diet pills" that a friend gave her, which made her heart beat fast and caused insomnia. At times she had difficulty controlling her diet and would binge on foods that were "bad"; this usually only happened when she was under more stress at school and at home. During this time, S.B. was on the honor roll and involved in competitive gymnastics and tennis at her school. S.B. was referred by her school nurse to the school psychologist because of the noticeable weight loss. The psychologist recommended that she be evaluated by her pediatrician to receive treatment for an eating disorder. After this first episode of rapid weight loss and amenorrhea, S.B. was able to regain 25 lb and grew from 5'3" to 5'5" in a year. What characteristics does S.B. have that are related to anorexia nervosa? What are some typical clinical features and associated behaviors of patients with anorexia nervosa?

Anorexia nervosa, a condition of self-induced weight loss, is characterized by a BMI ≤17.5, weight loss of at least 15% of ideal body weight, a preoccupation with body weight and food, behaviors directed toward weight loss, intense fear of gaining weight, disturbances of body image, and amenorrhea.[6] S.B.'s BMI is 16.3 (98 lb ÷ (65 in.)^2 × 703), which fits the criteria for anorexia nervosa. The main clinical feature of anorexia nervosa is a morbid fear of becoming fat and losing control over eating.[6] Anorectic behaviors include restrictive dieting (e.g., drastically reducing the amount of food ingested, minimizing foods high in fat and carbohydrates, and vegetarianism), purging behaviors (e.g., self-induced vomiting and excessive use of laxatives or diuretics), and strenuous exercise. The anorectic person often has a starved, skeleton-like appearance that is caused by loss of subcutaneous fat tissue.[4] Associated behaviors include looking in mirrors to check for thinness, expressing concern about being fat, and preoccupation with food (e.g., collecting recipes, preparing elaborate meals, hiding or hoarding carbohydrate-rich foods, throwing away food, cutting food into small pieces, eating slowly). Personality traits include low self-esteem, sensitivity to rejection, perfectionism, competitiveness, an extreme sense of responsibility, excessive conformity, guilt, and an intolerance of angry feelings.[3] Sleep disturbances, depression, anxiety, phobias, social isolation, and sexual disinterest are commonly associated with anorexia nervosa. Anorexia nervosa has been considered a type of obsessive-compulsive disorder with obsessive thoughts about food and weight and compulsive acts or rituals to alleviate the thoughts or fears of being "fat."[1,4]

Course and Prognosis

2. How does the clinical course of S.B. resemble others with anorexia nervosa and what is her prognosis?

As illustrated by S.B., anorexia nervosa typically begins in adolescent girls between the ages of 13 and 18 years (mean age is 17 years; bimodal peaks occur at 13 to 14 and 17 to 18 years) and rarely occurs after age 40.[3] However, the incidence of anorexia nervosa has increased in prepubertal children due to overconcern and obsession about weight and dieting.[1–3,115] The onset of anorexia nervosa frequently is associated with a major change in life (e.g., leaving home for college) or after a stressful life event. Anorexia usually begins with significant food deprivation for a variety of reasons (e.g., dieting, stress, severe illness) along with strenuous physical exercising.[10] Most patients with anorexia nervosa are extremely overactive and obsessive about exercise routines to burn off calories and induce weight loss. Exercise is typically solitary and rigid, and patients feel guilty if they do not exercise. Individuals like S.B., who have occupational or athletic pressures to be thin

(e.g., gymnasts, figure skaters, long distance runners, ballet dancers, and models) are at increased risk for developing anorexia nervosa.[3,10,13] Among males, wrestlers, body builders, and runners appear to be at greatest risk for developing an eating disorder and for abusing anabolic steroids.[10]

The course and prognosis for anorexia nervosa is variable and individuals may only have a single episode, recurring cycles of weight loss and weight gain, or a chronic deteriorating course that may result in death.[1,2,114] Some individuals may be overweight initially, then develop anorexia nervosa when they start dieting, and later develop bulimia nervosa or obesity. Approximately 30% to 50% of patients with anorexia nervosa develop symptoms of bulimia during the course of their illness.[3,10] Approximately 45% to 50% of people with anorexia nervosa or bulimia nervosa recover completely, approximately 30% achieve a partial recovery, 20% to 25% are plagued with a long-term illness with no substantial change in symptoms, and <5% die.[1,2,4,10,11,39,116] Many patients who have recovered from anorexia nervosa continue to suffer from social phobias and generalized anxiety, obsessional thinking, compulsive behaviors, perfectionism, dysthymia, and depression.[4,10,17,39,116,117]

In severe weight loss cases, hospitalization is required to restore weight and correct electrolyte and fluid abnormalities. Those that require hospitalization have a higher rate of mortality (approximately 6% to 10%) secondary to suicide or from the physical effects of starvation, cardiac arrhythmias, or electrolyte imbalances.[116,118] The mortality rate of anorexia nervosa is approximately 0.56% per year, which is 12 times higher than the mortality rate in young women in the general population.[10,11,119] Recurrent depressive episodes and suicide have been reported in up to 5% of patients with chronic anorexia nervosa.[1,2,39] Patients with anorexia nervosa may have extreme anxiety, restlessness, and insomnia due to food deprivation.

Medical Complications

3. The physician treating S.B. is concerned about possible medical complications caused by her anorexia nervosa. What laboratory and other medical tests should be ordered when assessing S.B. for her anorexia nervosa? What are the most common laboratory abnormalities that you would expect to see and why do they occur?

Starvation can affect all major organ systems and results in serious laboratory, cardiac, bone, and brain abnormalities.[1,10,120] Self-induced vomiting, use of laxatives, diuretics, and enemas also can cause physiologic changes and abnormal laboratory tests (Table 82-7). Appropriate laboratory tests for evaluation of patients with anorexia nervosa include the following: complete blood count, urinalysis, electrolytes, lipid profile, serum albumin, amylase, renal function, liver function, thyroid function, electrocardiogram (ECG), and a bone density scan.[10] Follicle-stimulating hormone, luteinizing hormone, prolactin, and estradiol levels are ordered in females and testosterone levels in males.

In anorectic patients, the metabolic rate declines due to a loss of body mass that causes a reduction of T_3. Other abnormalities include elevated liver enzymes, increased lipid metabolism resulting in increased free fatty acids, hypoalbu-

Table 82-7　Medical Complications of Eating Disorders

Related to Weight Loss and Starvation

- **Cardiac**

Acrocyanosis (circulatory disorder in which hands and feet are cold, blue, and sweaty)

Arrhythmias (supraventricular premature beats or ventricular tachycardia)

Bradycardia

Dizziness or lightheadedness (from dehydration)

Electrocardiogram changes

   QT_c prolongation

   ST-segment depression

   T-wave inversion

Left ventricular changes (decreased mass and cavity size)

Mitral valve prolapse

Orthostatic hypotension (from dehydration)

Peripheral edema

Syncope

Tachycardia

- **Central Nervous System**

Anxiety symptoms

Brain imaging changes

   Cortical atrophy

   Decreased gray and white matter (MRI)

   Increased ventricular:brain ratio

   Ventricular enlargement

Cognitive impairment

Decreased attention and concentration

Depressed, irritable mood with suicidal thoughts

Electroencephalogram changes

   Diffuse abnormalities secondary to fluid and electrolyte changes

   Metabolic encephalopathy

Headache

Lethargy

Obsessional thinking about food, weight, metabolism, body image

Peripheral neuropathy

Seizures

- **Dermatologic**

Alopecia

Brittle nails

Dry skin and hair

Hair thinning

Lanugo (fine body hair)

Petechiae

Yellow skin (hypercarotenemia)

- **Endocrine/Metabolic**

Carbohydrate intolerance

Cold intolerance

Hyperamylasemia

Hypercortisolism

Hypoglycemia

Hypothermia

Hypothyroidism

Serum thyroxine (T_4)—in low-normal range

Triiodothyronine (T_3)—low

Impaired temperature regulation

Lipid abnormalities

Low basal metabolic rate

- **Fluid/Electrolyte/Renal**

Decreased glomerular filtration rate

Dehydration

Diuresis

Hypokalemia

Hypomagnesemia

Hyponatremia

Hypophosphatemia (especially on refeeding)

Hypozincemia

Ketonuria

Peripheral edema

Polyuria (from decreased renal concentration ability)

Renal dysfunction (dehydration and hypokalemia)

- **Gastrointestinal**

Abdominal pain

Abnormal bowel sounds

Abnormal taste sensation (zinc deficiency)

Bloating (abdominal distension with meals)

Constipation

Delayed gastric emptying

Gastric dilation (rapid refeeding)

Parotitis

- **Genitourinary**

Elevated blood urea nitrogen

Hypovolemic nephropathy

Impaired renal function (associated with chronic dehydration and hypokalemia)

Low glomerular filtration rate

Pitting edema

Renal calculi

- **Hematologic**

Anemia (normochromic normocytic)

Hypercholesterolemia

Leukopenia

Neutropenia

Thrombocytopenia

- **Hypoalbuminemia**

- **Increased liver enzymes**

- **Musculoskeletal**

Bone pain with exercise

Delayed linear growth

Fractures (from bone loss)

Muscle wasting, weakness, and aches

Myopathy

Osteopenia or osteoporosis (decreased bone density)

Short stature (arrested skeletal growth)

Stress fractures

- **Reproductive**

Amenorrhea

Arrested sexual development

   Atrophy of the breasts

   Delayed puberty

   Ovarian and uterine regression

   Regression in secondary sexual characteristics

Estrogen deficiency

Follicle-stimulating hormone (prepubertal levels)

Hypogonadism (men)

Infertility

Luteinizing hormone (prepubertal patterns)

Loss of libido

Oligomenorrhea

Pregnancy (low weight gain and low-birth-weight infant)

Testosterone deficiency (men)

- **Vitamin and Mineral Deficiencies**

Calcium

Iron

Zinc

Related to Purging (Vomiting and Laxative Abuse)

- **Cardiac**

Cardiomyopathy (from emetine toxicity from ipecac)

Mild ST changes

Continued

Table 82-7 **Medical Complications of Eating Disorders—cont'd**

• **Dental**	Pancreatic inflammation and enlargement (increase in serum amylase)
Calluses on the dorsum of the hand (from hand-induced vomiting)	Rectal prolapse
Dental caries (from acidic vomitus)	
Dental enamel erosion (from acidic vomitus)	• **Fluid/Electrolyte**
	Hypochloremia
• **Digestive/Gastrointestinal**	Hypokalemia
Abdominal pain and discomfort	Hypomagnesemia
Barrett esophagus	Hyponatremia
Constipation and decreased intestinal motility (from chronic laxative abuse)	Metabolic acidosis (laxative abuse)
Dehydration	Metabolic alkalosis (vomiting)
Delayed gastric emptying and motility	Elevated serum bicarbonate
Diarrhea (from laxative abuse and excessive hydration)	Hypochloremic alkalosis
Esophageal or gastric erosion and rupture (from vomiting)	Peripheral edema (cessation of laxative and diuretic abuse)
Esophagitis	
Gallstones	• **Neuropsychiatric**
Gastric dilation and rupture (from binge eating)	Fatigue and weakness
Hyperamylasemia	Mild cognitive disorder
Hypertrophy of salivary and parotid glands	Neuropathies
Mallory-Weiss tears	Seizures (related to large fluid shifts and electrolyte disturbances)

MRI, magnetic resonance imaging.
Adapted from reference 1, 3-6, 10, 11, and 118.

minemia, fasting hypoglycemia, and glucose intolerance. Hypokalemia due to emesis or chronic diarrhea following laxative abuse can cause skeletal and smooth muscle weakness, cardiac conduction abnormalities, arrhythmias, and possibly, cardiac arrest.[4] Amenorrhea may occur early in the illness before significant weight loss has occurred (i.e., when BMI is between 17 and 19) and can persist after weight gain, leading to infertility and bone loss.[13] The decrease in bone density correlates with the duration of amenorrhea in women with anorexia nervosa.[121] Bone loss and inadequate bone formation (i.e., osteopenia and osteoporosis) may be caused by calcium, vitamin, and micronutrient deficiencies; estrogen and testosterone deficiency; hypercortisolemia; insulinlike growth factor-I deficiency; and excessive exercise.[11,121,122] Bone density is correlated with caloric intake, fat mass, leptin levels, and BMI.[123] Studies have reported that young women with anorexia nervosa may have a bone density similar to menopausal women in the seventh and eighth decades of life.[121] Although body density may increase with weight recovery, osteopenia may be a permanent consequence of the disease, resulting in significant morbidity due to bone fractures.[121] In males, weight restoration leads to increased testosterone levels, but 10% to 20% may have some type of testicular abnormality secondary to prolonged starvation.[1]

Treatment
Medical Management

4. The laboratory tests for S.B. indicate that she has a low T_3, a mild anemia, an elevated blood urea nitrogen (BUN), hypokalemia, and hyponatremia. T-wave inversions and bradycardia are found on the ECG. Low estradiol and luteinizing hormone levels and reduced bone density on the bone scan are reported. S.B. has orthostatic hypotension from dehydration and is severely constipated. Physical examination reveals lanugo (fine body hair), dry skin and hair, and atrophy of the breasts. The physician recommends that S.B. be admitted to an inpatient program that specializes in eating disorders. Based upon the presentation of S.B., does this patient require hospitalization? What is the usual approach for correcting and monitoring these complications from anorexia nervosa?

Patients should be hospitalized for any of the following conditions: rapid weight loss of >15% of body weight, hypotension with a systolic blood pressure <90 mm Hg, bradycardia (heart rate, <50 beats/min), core body temperature <97°F, suicide ideation, medical complications, and nonresponsiveness to outpatient treatment (after 3 to 4 months).[10] S.B. should be hospitalized because of her medical complications of anorexia nervosa. Because the majority of medical complications associated with anorexia nervosa improve with nutritional rehabilitation, the first step in most eating disorder programs is to restore weight, rehydrate, and correct serum electrolytes under close medical supervision.[1,2,10,11] Vitamin and mineral deficiencies secondary to restricted dieting require supplementation of vitamins, minerals, and electrolytes (potassium, magnesium) along with nutritional refeeding. Parenteral or enteral nutrition is used for patients with severe undernutrition who are refractory to other methods of weight gain.[10] Rapid refeeding and weight gain are not recommended because they increase the risk of a "refeeding syndrome" characterized by gastric bloating, edema, cardiac changes, and congestive heart failure.[11] Initial caloric intake of 30 to 40 kcal/kg/day (1,000 to 1,600 kcal/day) with progressive increase up to 70 to 100 kcal/kg/day during the weight gain phase are usual standards for nutritional rehabilitation.[10] For the weight maintenance phase, intake of 40 to 60 kcal/kg/day is required to maintain growth in children and adolescents.[10]

Routine monitoring of laboratory tests (e.g., complete blood count and platelets, renal and hepatic function tests, electrolytes, BUN, urinalysis, ECG), weight, and vital signs is required to assess medical status.[3,10,120] Patients who are emaciated often have cognitive difficulties and psychologic changes that can interfere with their participation in behavioral and cognitive therapies.[42] Patients with a history of vomiting must be watched closely to prevent this compensatory behavior during hospitalization. Cardiac monitoring (e.g., blood pressure, pulse, ECG) is indicated to assess cardiac arrhythmias, ventricular tachycardia, or prolonged QT interval.[10,11]

Bone density studies at baseline and at 6- to 12-month intervals are recommended to assess lumbar spine bone density and to determine the risk of compression fractures.[121] Although weight restoration may reverse menstrual irregularities and pubertal delay, the catch up in height and reversal of bone loss may not always occur.[2] Prolonged amenorrhea (>6 months) has been associated with irreversible osteopenia (loss of bone density), greater risk of osteoporosis, a higher rate of spine and hip fractures, and infertility.[121]

Cognitive-Behavioral Therapy, Behavioral Therapy, and Family Therapy

5. S.B. and her family meet with a psychologist from the eating disorder's program to receive education about anorexia nervosa and to review treatment goals. At first, S.B. refuses to be admitted, but her parents strongly support a structured program because they argue and fight about her eating behaviors and excessive exercising. Because of the seriousness of her medical status, S.B. finally agrees to participate in therapy. What are the standard therapeutic approaches for patients with anorexia nervosa?

Anorexia responds to a variety of psychotherapeutic approaches that include individual, group, and family therapy.[1,10,42] Behavioral positive reinforcement programs (i.e., operant conditioning) and response-prevention techniques are very helpful in reducing destructive eating behaviors. Positive rewards, such as increasing social activities, visitations, and physical exercise, can be used when preset weight-gain goals are met. Those who use self-induced vomiting after eating can be observed for several hours after meals to prevent purging behavior. These techniques can be modified for both inpatient and outpatient programs to monitor progress toward treatment goals.

Cognitive-behavioral therapy (CBT) helps patients identify false thinking, distortions in processing and interpreting events, and their relationship to mood and behavior.[123] Patients are encouraged to evaluate thoughts and feelings related to eating, fears, anxiety, and control issues. Cognitive techniques are taught to help the person restructure his or her thought process, to improve problem-solving skills, and to better cope with life stresses. Cognitive therapy can help the person better understand his or her overvaluation of being thin and obsession with food.

Family counseling or therapy may be helpful in younger adolescents, particularly if family dynamics or unfair parental expectations are issues that increase stress.[10] Individual and family therapy provide opportunities to help patients understand themselves and their relationships with others.

Pharmacotherapy

6. S.B.'s mother asks the attending psychiatrist in the eating disorder's program about medications used for anorexia nervosa, because she feels that S.B. has been depressed and needs some type of treatment. The physician explains that psychotropic medications usually are not effective in treating the primary symptoms of anorexia nervosa until the person has gained at least 85% of their expected body weight. What are the goals of nutritional rehabilitation and potential side effects of refeeding? Are there any effective medications for anorexia nervosa? What treatment approaches are recommended?

The primary treatment for anorexia nervosa is to improve overall nutritional status, restore weight, restore gonadal function, and establish normal eating patterns.[10] Weight gain reduces the core symptoms of anorexia nervosa and improves dysphoric mood and obsessive-compulsive behaviors.[17] A minimum goal weight is approximately 90% of ideal weight for height using standard tables, but a final "healthy" goal weight is the weight at which normal ovulation and menstruation occurs.[10] Inpatient weight restoration programs can increase weight at a rate of 2 to 3 lb/week, whereas outpatient programs usually have lower weight goals of 0.5 to 1 lb/week. Guidelines for calorie intake and monitoring during refeeding can be found in the American Psychiatric Association's *Practice Guideline for the Treatment of Patients with Eating Disorders*.[10] Weight gain results in improvement in psychologic and medical complications associated with starvation and patients are more likely to participate and benefit from psychosocial treatments. Treatment should continue for at least 3 to 6 months after achieving the goal weight and until menstrual periods resume.[17] Cognitive and physiological abnormalities may persist for months after achieving the goal weight, thus abnormal eating behaviors and body-image distortions may return without a comprehensive treatment approach.[17]

Many pharmacologic agents have been tried in the acute treatment of anorexia nervosa, but none are more effective than a placebo. Various pharmacologic agents used to alleviate specific symptoms associated with anorexia nervosa are listed in Table 82-8. Malnourished patients may be prone to side effects of medications, and some antidepressant agents (e.g., tricyclic antidepressants) can increase the risk of dehydration, hypotension, arrhythmias, and seizures.[10] The pharmacokinetics of medications also can be altered in patients with anorexia nervosa due to changes in body fat and protein. For example, hypoalbuminemia can result in more free (unbound) drug and a decrease in body fat can reduce the volume of distribution of fat-soluble drugs, resulting in increased steady-state plasma levels.[123] Because of the increased risk of drug toxicity, any drug therapy should be started with very low doses that are titrated gradually based on adverse effects.

Serotonin-augmenting agents such as the *serotonin reuptake inhibitors* (SRIs) are more effective in the treatment of bulimia nervosa than in under-weight patients with anorexia nervosa.[3,10,124] Patients with reduced dietary tryptophan have low CSF serotonin, thus SRIs may not work due to low serotonin production and release.[17] After weight gain and adequate protein intake, SRIs are more likely to have a therapeutic effect in weight-restored anorexic patients. Antidepressants generally are reserved for patients with prominent depressive or obsessive-compulsive symptoms that persist after weight has been regained.[10] SRIs are considered the safest class of antidepressants and are the drugs of choice for comorbid anxiety, obsessive-compulsive-impulsive behaviors,

Table 82-8   Pharmacologic Treatment Approaches for Anorexia and Bulimia Nervosa

Indication	Medication
Severe constipation	Hydration, stool softeners, and bulk-forming laxatives
Decreased gastric motility	Metoclopramide (Reglan)—may cause extrapyramidal symptoms
Amenorrhea	Estrogen and progesterone combination therapy
Bone loss	Calcium 1,500 mg/day
	Multivitamin with minerals
	Vitamin D 400 IU/day
	Estrogen therapy (controversial; not always recommended because of negative studies in reversing bone loss)
	Exercise (nonstrenuous, aerobic, weight bearing)
Electrolyte depletion	Potassium supplements
Anxiety	Benzodiazepine (low dose before meals)
	Buspirone (BuSpar)
Bulimia nervosa, binge eating, depression, and obsessive-compulsive disorder	Serotonin-augmenting antidepressant:
	Citalopram (Celexa)
	Clomipramine (Anafranil)
	Escitalopram (Lexapro)
	Fluoxetine (Prozac)
	Fluvoxamine (Luvox)
	Paroxetine (Paxil)
	Sertraline (Zoloft)
Stimulation of appetite	Cyproheptadine (Periactin)

social phobia, and depression. SRIs are better tolerated than other classes of antidepressants (e.g., tricyclic antidepressants, monoamine oxidase inhibitors [MAOIs]).[10] Initial open trials with fluoxetine in anorexia nervosa reported improvement in weight gain and depressive symptoms, whereas others have found no benefit, particularly with lower weight subjects.[125] A 3-month study with citalopram in weight-restored anorexia nervosa demonstrated improvement in depression, obsessive-compulsive symptoms, impulsiveness and trait-anger compared to controls.[126] A 24-month, naturalistic, posthospital, prospective study with adjunctive fluoxetine showed no added benefit in patients with anorexia nervosa compared with a control group who did not receive adjunctive fluoxetine.[127] Recent studies with SRIs in hospitalized underweight patients with anorexia nervosa report minimal benefit in reducing symptoms and preventing hospitalization compared with a behaviorally oriented inpatient program.[128,129] A double-blind placebo-controlled study with weight-restored patients with restricting- and restricting-purging-type anorexia nervosa showed a reduced relapse rate after a 1-year trial of fluoxetine.[130] Subjects who continued to take fluoxetine for 1 year had a significant reduction in obsessive thoughts, anxiety, depression, and core eating disorder symptoms as well as a significant increase in weight.[130]

Antipsychotics, such as chlorpromazine and pimozide, were initially used to treat psychotic-like obsessional thinking, but there is no evidence that they are effective in anorexia nervosa.[2,17] Atypical antipsychotic agents with serotonin antagonist effects (i.e., olanzapine, quetiapine, risperidone) may exacerbate obsessive-compulsive disorder, worsen binge eating, and cause weight gain due to blockade of serotonin$_2$ receptors.[17] Cyproheptadine and amitriptyline (serotonin antagonists with antihistamine effects that increase appetite and promote weight gain) have been tried in anorexia nervosa with mixed results.[131] Nonbulimic anorexic patients may respond more positively to cyproheptadine (up to 32 mg/ day),

which can accelerate weight gain during the initial refeeding phase of treatment.[17] Lithium carbonate has been tried but has a narrow therapeutic range and may cause neurotoxicity at high plasma levels; it does not appear to be effective in increasing weight gain.[17] Naltrexone 100 mg twice a day has been tried in small studies to reduce bingeing and purging in anorexia and in cases of mixed anorexia/bulimia; however, larger studies are needed to confirm its efficacy in anorexia nervosa.[17] Tetrahydrocannabinol has not been useful to stimulate appetite in patients with anorexia nervosa and may worsen dysphoria.[17] Controlled trials of zinc supplementation have been conducted but results are mixed.[1]

Estrogen replacement is inadequate to increase bone density in patients with anorexia nervosa, particularly without weight restoration and normalization of body fat composition.[36,121,122] Calcium supplementation alone has not been shown to increase bone density in anorexia nervosa.[122] Newer agents used for the prevention of osteoporosis in postmenopausal women (e.g., alendronate, raloxifene) have not been studied in women with anorexia nervosa.[122] Adequate nutrition, weight gain, calcium and vitamin D supplementation, restoration of the regular menstrual cycle, and moderate weight-bearing aerobic exercise are currently the treatments of choice to maintain bone density.[121,122]

Other agents have been used to treat anorexia nervosa. Benzodiazepines (e.g., lorazepam 0.5 to 1.0 mg or oxazepam 15 to 30 mg) have been given before feeding to reduce anxiety symptoms, but these agents may cause CNS depression, dependence, and withdrawal reactions. Clonidine has not been found to increase weight or have therapeutic effects.[17] Metoclopramide and domperidone (dopamine$_2$ antagonists) have been investigated for increasing gastric emptying and reducing abdominal distension and bloating. One double-blind study with metoclopramide failed to confirm effectiveness in anorexia nervosa and there is concern about extrapyramidal reactions when these agents are used in high doses.[131]

BULIMIA NERVOSA
Clinical Features

7. R.G., a 21-year-old woman, has been on and off diets for the past 4 years since she started college. She constantly thinks about food and sometimes binge eats take-out meals at fast food restaurants late at night. The binge eating episodes have become very expensive and R.G. has started shoplifting and stealing money to support her "habit." Currently, R.G. has been binge eating at least three times a week over several months. She is beginning to gain weight even though she restricts food between bingeing episodes and induces vomiting afterwards to help control her weight. In the past she tried laxatives and diuretics to reduce calories, but she did not like the side effects of constipation and polyuria. R.G.'s eating disorder first began when she started college and was living in a dormitory with a self-serve cafeteria. She had always had difficulty controlling snacking between meals and would raid the refrigerator at night during high school. R.G. was constantly on diets and her weight sometimes fluctuated by 10 to 20 lb within several months. R.G. is very secretive about her binge eating and purging despite living in a sorority house at college. She plans the episodes late at night and often drives into the country to consume the food and to vomit. R.G. is scared of gaining weight, so she often does not eat for several days between the binge eating episodes. She has started smoking cigarettes and occasionally uses cocaine for its euphoric and appetite suppressant effects. What characteristics and behaviors of R.G. suggest that she may be suffering from bulimia nervosa?

Bulimia nervosa is often a chronic disorder with multiple episodes of relapse and remission, which begins in late adolescence or in early adult life between the ages of 15 and 24.[1,2,3,6,10] Bulimia may occur in normal weight, obese, or anorexic individuals. Binge eating usually is preceded by emotional factors (e.g., anxiety, depression, boredom, relationship or family problems) or a stressful life event.[10] Younger women tend to have family problems or are seeking independence from parents, whereas women older than age 20 are more likely to have marital or relationship difficulties preceding the onset of bulimia nervosa. Before the onset of the disorder, individuals may be overweight and report periods of severely restricting food intake, fasting, and using "fad" diets to lose weight.[1,2] Binge eating occurs when the person loses his or her control over food restriction and becomes "out of control" when consuming food. Before starting to binge eat, women can become sweaty, tachycardic, anxious, and tense, all of which may be related to starvation from dieting. During the bingeing episode, a sense of freedom and a reduction in anxiety or negative thoughts often is reported. Afterwards, the person may feel depressed, guilty, and anxious about gaining weight and try to reduce these negative emotions with the act of vomiting.

The course of the disorder may be intermittent, with periods of remission and recurrences of binge eating, or it may be chronic.[1,2,10,39] Between binges, individuals often diet rigorously, try to resist the urge to eat, and are fearful of weight gain. Over time, the frequency and severity of the binge eating increases and bulimia nervosa develops. Low self-esteem, anxiety, and guilt about binge eating, depression, impulsive behaviors, sexual conflicts, and problems with intimacy are commonly found in women with bulimia nervosa.[10] Follow-up studies have reported a 50% recovery rate after 5 to 10 years from initial presentation to clinics, but 20% continue to meet the diagnostic criteria for bulimia nervosa.[132] Approximately 5% of those with bulimia nervosa will later develop anorexia nervosa.[4]

Like R.G., binge eaters are secretive about their behaviors. They may plan ahead by hoarding and preparing food, buying food especially for the episode, or ordering large quantities of food from fast-food establishments. The type, amount, and nutritional content of food eaten vary widely depending on what food is available. High-calorie foods and sweets, such as cake and ice cream, are commonly ingested. The length of the binge eating episode may vary, with slower eating if the person is not disturbed, to stuffing food frantically into his or her mouth in a short period. Episodes usually last <2 hours but can vary from minutes to days. The number of binges per day may range from 1 to 6; some women have up to 10 to 20 episodes a day, each being terminated by self-induced vomiting. Bingeing may occur at any time of the day, but approximately one-third of binge eaters have a specific time, such as weekends, when they prefer to binge eat. The amount of food and calories eaten varies considerably, and ranges from 3 to 30 times the recommended daily allowance of calories.[1] Those who eat large quantities of food may exceed >20,000 kcal in a day and may binge at a slower rate by ingesting small quantities of fatty or carbohydrate-rich foods over several hours.[1] These individuals usually have higher body weights, use diuretics and appetite-suppressing medications, prepare food for a binge and/or eat all available food, and have nocturnal binges.

Many aspects of R.G.'s history are consistent with bulimia nervosa. She has a long history of secretive bingeing and purging and has used many other measures to offset possible weight gain. These have included fasting between binges, use of diuretics and laxatives, and cigarette smoking. She may have used cocaine to suppress her appetite, or it may reflect her attempt to compensate for depression that typically accompanies the condition.

8. What are the most common compensatory mechanisms used to prevent weight gain in patients with bulimia nervosa?

Most binge eaters end the episode because they become nauseated, full, or have discomfort.[6,10,42] Several strategies are used to reduce the fear of gaining weight. The most popular is to reduce the amount of calories absorbed from the food they have eaten by inducing vomiting (during or after binge eating) or restricting food (dieting) between binges.[42] Up to 80% to 90% of bulimic patients have induced vomiting after an episode of binge eating to decrease abdominal discomfort and to reduce the chance of gaining weight, and approximately 60% of patients regularly use self-induced vomiting. Initially, individuals may use a variety of methods to induce vomiting such as gagging themselves with their fingers, a toothbrush or a spoon. Later, individuals may be able to vomit without self-induction techniques.

Between 75% and 90% of binge eaters have abused laxatives during their illness but this method is less effective in controlling body weight. Approximately one-third of patients with bulimia nervosa use laxatives after binge eating to reduce absorption of the food. Laxatives act primarily on the large bowel to empty, but this occurs after food already has been absorbed in the small intestine. Excessive laxative intake may lead to electrolyte disturbances, particularly potassium deficiency. Approximately 60% have used over-the-counter (OTC) diet pills that may contain some form of laxative.

Some individuals may restrict food or starve between eating binges, use excessive exercise, and ingest appetite-suppressant products in an attempt to compensate for binge eating. A number of appetite-suppressing medications with sympathomimetic effects have addictive properties. Approximately 40% of binge eaters have used diuretics to lose weight, but this only loses fluid weight and is ineffective for reducing energy from food. Approximately 10% use prescription anorectic medications and at least 20% of bulimic patients abuse alcohol or drugs.

Misuse of diuretics and enemas, consuming syrup of ipecac to induce vomiting, or taking thyroid hormones are less frequently used methods to reverse binge eating effects. Approximately 50% of women diagnosed with bulimia nervosa regularly smoke cigarettes, which has been used to decrease appetite and weight gain.[44]

Medical Complications

9. R.G. has been experiencing constant headaches, muscle cramps, and fatigue for several days and feels she has the flu. She makes an appointment at the student health clinic and is evaluated by a nurse practitioner in a walk-in clinic. During the physical examination, the nurse notes abrasions on the top of her hand, hypertrophy of the salivary and parotid gland, and enamel loss on her teeth. R.G. is dehydrated and complains of chronic constipation. What signs and symptoms of bulimia nervosa are present on R.G.'s physical examination? What laboratory screening tests are recommended to rule out a medical diagnosis or medical complications from bulimia nervosa?

Individuals with bulimia nervosa are usually within their normal weight range; thus, medical complications, morbidity, and mortality associated with weight loss or obesity are less of a problem.[10] Common physiologic changes and abnormal laboratory tests associated with purging are listed in Table 82-7. Baseline laboratory tests often include the following: serum electrolytes, a complete blood count, liver and renal function tests, thyroid function tests, and an ECG.[10]

Purging behavior can produce electrolyte abnormalities (e.g., hypochloremia, hypokalemia, hyponatremia), fluid disturbances, and dehydration.[10,42] Metabolic alkalosis (elevated serum bicarbonate) is associated with loss of stomach acid through vomiting, and metabolic acidosis may occur secondary to diarrhea through laxative abuse. Hypokalemia occurs secondary to aldosterone secretion and increased potassium excretion from the kidneys, and through self-induced vomiting.[42] Electrolyte disturbances cause lethargy, weakness, and possibly, cardiac arrhythmias.

Permanent loss of dental enamel, especially on the front teeth, and dental cavities are common secondary to the effects of stomach acid.[42] Enlargement or inflammation of salivary glands (sialadenitis), particularly the parotid glands, from recurrent vomiting often is reported. Elevated serum amylase due to increases in salivary isoenzymes often results. Calluses or scars on the dorsal part of the hand secondary to trauma by the teeth (known as *Russell's sign*) is caused by repeated self-

induction of vomiting.[133] Individuals who chronically abuse syrup of ipecac to induce vomiting may develop myopathy (e.g., muscle weakness, aching, hyporeflexia, slurred speech) and/or cardiotoxicity (e.g., atrial premature contractions, supraventricular tachycardia, ventricular tachycardia, flattened or inverted T waves, prolonged QT and P-R intervals, changes in the QRS complex, decreased contractility, and cardiac arrest).[42] Ipecac contains a cardiotoxin that, in high doses, may cause permanent necrosis of heart fibers and interstitial edema.

Laxative abuse initially causes diarrhea, but continued use may result in rebound fluid retention and electrolyte disturbances. A withdrawal syndrome associated with discontinuation of laxatives is characterized by constipation, abdominal bloating and cramping, agitation, and feeling "sick." Diuretics or OTC slimming tablets cause electrolyte disturbances, particularly potassium deficiency. Fluid retention may result when long-term diuretic use is discontinued.

Approximately 40% of women with bulimia nervosa have irregular menstruation and 20% have amenorrhea. Menstrual disturbances usually cease when body weight is stabilized and when dangerous methods of weight control, including excessive exercise and intermittent starvation, are stopped.

Treatment
Medical Management

10. The nurse practitioner feels that R.G. may have bulimia nervosa based on the physical examination and laboratory tests (e.g., serum potassium of 3.0 mEq/L, BUN:creatinine ratio >30, volume depletion, scarring on the dorsum of the hand, and severe dental caries and enamel erosion). She confronts R.G. about her eating habits and recommends referral to a therapist and psychiatrist who have experience in eating disorders. R.G. finally confesses about how horrible she feels and asks for help. A plan is established that includes a psychiatrist, therapist, and nutritionist to manage the medical, psychologic, and nutritional aspects of treatment. What are the most common medical complications of bulimia nervosa with purging behaviors? How should physiologic complications be monitored and assessed?

Individuals who seek medical help may not tell their physician about their eating habits; thus, bulimia nervosa may be missed. Most patients with bulimia nervosa do not require hospitalization unless there is a medical or psychiatric indication such as severe depression with suicidal thoughts, severe concurrent drug or alcohol abuse, or a life-endangering medical problem (e.g., severe hypokalemia, metabolic alkalosis/acidosis, severe dehydration, acute pancreatitis, cardiomyopathy, cardiac arrhythmia).[10,17] Common medical complaints are GI problems (irritable bowel syndrome, spastic colon), gynecologic problems (menstrual irregularities), depression, or panic attacks. Those who seek treatment for bulimia nervosa have usually started inducing vomiting or taking purgatives, or both. Patients with self-induced vomiting should be monitored for esophageal tears; dehydration; metabolic alkalosis (hypochloremia and hypokalemia); elevated serum amylase (parotid gland enlargement); weakness and lethargy; cardiac arrhythmias; erosion of dental enamel or dental caries; and vitamin, electrolyte, and mineral deficiencies.[10] Correcting serum electrolyte abnormalities helps reduce the risk of medical complications such as cardiac arrhythmias. Individuals who abuse ipecac require monitoring of blood pressure (hypotension), heart rate (tachycardia), ECG to assess cardiac failure, and liver enzymes. An echocardiogram may be needed to diagnose cardiomyopathy.

Cognitive-Behavioral Therapy and Interpersonal Therapy

11. R.G. agrees to participate in an intensive outpatient eating disorder treatment program that is coordinated through the student health clinic. Her team feels that she will need help with self-esteem development, coping skills, and adherence with treatment, so they develop biweekly sessions to work on goals. What are the standard nonpharmacologic therapies for patients with bulimia nervosa or binge eating disorder?

Historically, psychoeducational groups, nutritional counseling, self-help manuals, and self-monitoring have all been used as first-line treatments for bulimia nervosa; Most patients, however, will benefit more from structured cognitive-behavioral therapy (CBT) approaches, requiring an average of 20 sessions over a 6-month period.[10,17,113,134] CBT and interpersonal psychotherapy (IPT) are useful in treating bulimia nervosa and binge eating disorder.[135–137] Time-limited IPT, up to 16 weeks, also has been shown to improve interpersonal problems and role transitions and reduces bulimic behaviors over the long term.[134,135] Reviews of psychologic and pharmacotherapy comparative studies for bulimia nervosa and binge eating disorders can be found elsewhere.[1]

Behavioral and cognitive techniques help individuals self-monitor their binge eating and purging episodes and document changes in mood and circumstances related to the binge-purge behavior.[11,134] CBT helps the person examine distortions in his or her thought processing and interpretation of events, and uses cognitive restructuring to change the way he or she thinks and reacts.[136] Several studies have reported that CBT or CBT in combination with antidepressants is more effective in reducing bulimic symptoms than giving antidepressant medications alone.[10,17,134,138,139] CBT has been reported to be more effective than supportive psychotherapy and the addition of an antidepressant may significantly improve depression and binge eating behaviors.[140] Psychoeducational approaches along with individual and group therapy are commonly used for CBT. Behavioral therapy is used to stop the binge eating and purging behaviors by restricting exposure to situations or cues that trigger a binge-purge episode, by finding alternative behaviors that are less destructive, and by delaying the purging response to eating. Response prevention techniques are used to prevent vomiting by placing an individual in a more restrictive environment or situation where it is very difficult to vomit.

Pharmacotherapy

12. The psychiatrist has several individual sessions with R.G. to assess the severity of the eating disorder and to rule out other psychiatric or medical disorders. R.G. has mild symptoms of depression that do not meet the criteria for a major depressive episode. Nicotine and cocaine help her mood, so R.G. wonders if an antidepressant would help her feel less anxious and reduce the urge to binge and purge. The psychiatrist agrees that the comorbid substance abuse, mild depression, anxiety symptoms, and obsessive-compulsive behaviors may respond to an antidepressant. What medications have been used to treat bulimia nervosa? How safe and effective are these agents, and how long should patients be maintained on treatment?

If medications are required, antidepressants are considered the drugs of choice for bulimia nervosa.[1,10,17] Bulimic patients do not need to be clinically depressed to benefit from treatment. Several short-term, double-blind, placebo-controlled studies have demonstrated that antidepressants are effective for reducing binge eating and vomiting episodes, although some classes such as tricyclic antidepressants and MAOIs have more adverse effects and may not be tolerated.[14,131,141,142] Antidepressants shown to be effective for bulimia nervosa or for binge eating include desipramine,[143–146] imipramine,[146–149] amitriptyline,[150] phenelzine,[151,152] isocarboxazid,[153] trazodone,[154] bupropion,[155] fluoxetine,[139,156–161] fluvoxamine,[162–165] sertraline,[166,167] and paroxetine.[168] Few long-term controlled studies have been done with antidepressants to evaluate if modifications in eating behaviors and weight are maintained over time. Fluoxetine and fluvoxamine combined with CBT was shown to be more effective than drug therapy alone in the treatment of binge eating disorder at 1-year follow-up based on BMI and eating disorder rating scales.[139] (See Chapter 79, Mood Disorders I: Major Depressive Disorders, for a complete review of antidepressant agents.)

Serotonin-augmenting agents are the most commonly prescribed antidepressants for bulimia nervosa and binge eating disorder and have a more favorable side effect profile in comparison to other classes.[17] Fluoxetine (up to 60 mg/day) has been shown to reduce the number of binge eating and vomiting episodes by approximately 70%, with complete recovery in 25% of patients, and to induce weight loss whether or not there are depressive symptoms.[159] Higher daily doses of fluoxetine (60 mg/d) may be superior to the standard antidepressant dose of 20 mg/d.[17] Nutritional counseling has been shown to be effective in bulimia nervosa and may have beneficial effects when combined with SRI treatment.[169]

Fluoxetine was approved by the Food and Drug Administration (FDA) in 1996 for the treatment of bulimia nervosa. Other SRIs (e.g., citalopram, escitalopram, fluvoxamine, paroxetine, sertraline, and venlafaxine) are alternative treatments for bulimia nervosa or binge eating disorder.[14,17] The efficacy and ideal dose of SRIs other than fluoxetine have not been established.[17] Fluvoxamine was studied in 72 patients with bulimia nervosa in a double-blind, randomized, placebo-controlled trial.[170] In patients who were treated successfully with inpatient psychotherapy, fluvoxamine significantly reduced self-rating and expert rating scales for symptoms of bulimia compared to placebo during a 19-week treatment course. Although there was a high dropout rate in the fluvoxamine group (38% versus 14% in placebo group), both the intent-to-treat and completer analyses showed improvement in the following primary outcome variables: Psychiatric Status Rating Scale for Bulimia Nervosa, number of binges in the previous 7 days, and Structured Interview for Anorexia and Bulimia Nervosa. Common side effects reported with SRIs include diarrhea, nausea, headache, insomnia, and sexual dysfunction. Bradycardia and hyponatremia have been reported with SRIs; thus, monitoring of heart rate, blood pressure, and serum electrolytes is recommended, particularly for patients who use diuretics or have purging behaviors.[107] See Table 82-8 for a list of pharmacologic approaches for symptoms or behaviors associated with bulimia nervosa.

A study evaluating naltrexone (an opiate antagonist) or imipramine versus placebo in normal weight bulimics and obese binge eaters reported that all three groups had a reduction in binge frequency without any significant differences in weight or mood.[149] D-fenfluramine, a serotonin-releasing agent with appetite suppressant properties, was found to be more effective than placebo in the treatment of binge eating disorder, but has been taken off the market due to reports of it causing cardiac valvular damage (i.e., aortic and mitral valve regurgitation) and pulmonary hypertension.[171] Bupropion is not recommended for the treatment of eating disorder patients due to reported risks of grand mal seizures in patients with bulimia nervosa.[155] Mood stabilizers (lithium), anticonvulsants (valproic acid, carbamazepine, gabapentin, lamotrigine, oxcarbazepine), and benzodiazepines (clonazepam) have not been studied in bulimia nervosa and are not recommended unless the person has an underlying cyclical mood disorder such as bipolar disorder. One placebo-controlled study of lithium in the treatment of bulimia nervosa found no evidence of effectiveness.[172] Topiramate, a novel antiepileptic agent, has been reported to decrease binge-eating episodes in an open-label trial in patients with binge-eating disorder.[173] Ondansetron, an antiemetic with serotonin$_3$ antagonist effects, was found to be more effective than placebo in reducing vomiting and binge eating in a 4-week trial in severely ill bulimic patients.[174]

Duration of antidepressant therapy is an important issue because patients treated for at least 6 months have a better long-term outcome than patients who receive shorter antidepressant trials.[141] Only 50% of patients achieve a complete remission following antidepressant treatment and a majority have relapses after the initial intervention has stopped.[17] Approximately one-third of patients may relapse with prophylactic antidepressant treatment.[17] A rapid relapse of binge eating behaviors has been reported when antidepressants are withdrawn in both bulimia nervosa and binge eating disorder.[141] In general, antidepressants should be prescribed for at least 6 months, and some patients may require long-term prophylactic antidepressant treatment.[17] Daily recordings of mood and binge eating behaviors, weekly weighings, and close monitoring may have their own therapeutic benefits as well.

OBESITY
Clinical Features

13. F.W., a 49-year-old African-American woman, is being evaluated at a chronic pain clinic for lower back and knee pain secondary to degenerative joint disease. F.W., 5'3" tall, weighs 230 lb, has a waist circumference of 40 inches, and is unable to move without significant joint and back pain. In the past 15 years she has developed diabetes, hypertension, and hyperlipidemia. F.W. is being treated for depression and perimenopausal symptoms. F.W.'s current medications include metformin, atenolol, atorvastatin, and paroxetine. How is obesity defined and assessed in a patient like F.W.? What common clinical features of obesity and risk factors are useful for determining the need for treatment in F.W.?

Obesity is an excessive accumulation of body fat secondary to poor appetite regulation and decreased energy metabolism. Appropriate treatment of the overweight/obese patient requires assessment of the degree of overweight and overall risk status. The best method to determine the degree of overweight/obesity is to measure the BMI, which is associated with total body fat content.[20] The waist circumference is an independent predictor of risk factors and morbidity and correlates to abdominal fat content. F.W.'s BMI is 40.7 (230 lb ÷ (63 in.)^2 × 703), which is in obesity class III (extreme obesity). To determine absolute risk and need for treatment of overweight/obesity, clinicians should be familiar with related diseases and other risk factors (Table 82-9).

Patients who are overweight/obese need to be monitored for other cardiovascular risk factors as recommended by the guidelines published by the National Cholesterol Education Program (NCEP) and the Sixth report of the Joint National Committee on Prevention, Detection, Evaluation and Treatment of High Blood Pressure (see Chapters 13 and 14 on Dyslipidemias, Atherosclerosis, and Coronary Heart Disease and Essential Hypertension). F.W. not only has increased BMI but her ethnicity may be a predisposing risk factor for developing obesity. In addition, the impact of F.W.'s current medications for her various chronic conditions and her limited mobility to participate in exercise regimens should be taken into consideration. Patient's motivation to lose weight is a significant predictor of success or failure in the weight management program. The willingness to participate in a regimen may depend on the past history of diets, social support at home and workplace, patient's understanding of the illness, time and financial burden.[20] Obesity is considered a chronic medical condition because it causes multiple physical com-

Table 82-9   Conditions That Increase the Risk Status in Overweight/Obese Patients

Disease Conditions	Risk for Disease Complications, Mortality
Coronary heart disease	Very high
Atherosclerotic disease	
Type 2 diabetes mellitus	
Sleep apnea	
Other Obesity-Related Diseases	
Gynecologic abnormalities	High
Osteoarthritis	
Gallstones and complications	
Stress incontinence	
Cardiovascular Risk Factors	
Cigarette smoking	Very high absolute risk if ≥2
Hypertension	risk factors
Increased LDL cholesterol	
Low HDL cholesterol	
Impaired fasting blood glucose	
Family history of premature CHD	
Age (men ≥45, women ≥55 or postmenopausal)	
Physical inactivity	
High serum triglycerides	

CHD, coronary heart disease; LDL, low density lipoprotein.
Adapted from reference 20.

plications.[9] The greater the degree of obesity, the harder it is for a person to lose weight permanently without medical and behavioral interventions. Major depressive disorder, anxiety disorders, and low self-esteem are common in obese patients due to social prejudice and discrimination in the work force.[18]

Course and Prognosis

14. **F.W. has steadily gained weight since her early 20s after the birth of her first child. She has always struggled with her weight and has three other siblings who are obese. She has gone on >15 diets to lose weight, but each time she stops the diet she regains even more weight. F.W. admits to overeating and, at times, uses laxatives and OTC diet pills to help her control her weight and appetite. What is the typical course and prognosis of obesity?**

Obesity is a chronic disease that can begin in childhood or adolescence and can be characterized by a slow and steady increase in body weight during adult life. The relationship between weight loss (unintentional or intentional) and mortality is uncertain; however, preliminary results suggest that the incidence rates for diabetes, hypertriglyceridemia, and decreased HDL levels were lower for patients who had surgically induced weight loss versus patients who had behavioral weight loss intervention.[175,176]

Overeating or binge eating along with restrictive dieting is a common occurrence among Americans and may be a chronic lifelong problem that leads to obesity. Recent studies have shown that 10% to 25% of obese people regularly engage in binge eating behavior and that the greater their weight, the more likely they are to be binge eaters[17]; at least 25% to 45% of obese individuals have symptoms that meet the criteria for binge eating disorder.[17,18,133] Unlike individuals with bulimia nervosa, obese binge eaters usually do not vomit or purge and may or may not restrict food intake between binge eating episodes. Obese binge eaters often have a preoccupation with their body shape and weight, but they have poor control of their eating habits. Women tend to be more concerned about their body shape and weight and are more likely to diet than men. More than 80% of people who lose weight gradually regain it; patients who continue on weight maintenance programs consisting of dietary, physical, and behavioral therapy have a better chance of not regaining weight than those who discontinue weight maintenance programs.[20]

Medical Complications

15. **The physician in the pain management clinic is very concerned about F.W.'s weight because of her current medical conditions and the likelihood of further complications during her lifetime. What are the most common medical conditions associated with obesity?**

Obesity has a tremendous impact on physiologic functioning and medical illnesses. Obese people tend to die young, and the more abdominal body fat, the greater the mortality. Obesity-related medical conditions in the United States result in 300,000 deaths per year and cost approximately $70 billion in health care costs.[177,178] Obesity is linked to many disabling diseases such as diabetes mellitus (non–insulin-dependent and insulin-resistant), pulmonary impairment (hypoventila-

tion, hypoxia, hypercapnia, and sleep apnea), gallbladder disease (gallstones and cholecystitis), cancers (colorectal, prostate, breast, cervical, endometrial, uterine, and ovarian), osteoarthritis (hips, knees, and back), gout, cardiac disease (shortness of breath, hypertension, stroke, congestive heart failure, and coronary heart disease), increased cholesterol and triglycerides (increased low-density lipoproteins and decreased high-density lipoproteins), dermatologic problems (intertrigo and stretching of skin), and menstrual irregularities (Table 82-10).[20,42] The Nurses Health Study showed that the risk of developing diabetes in women with BMI >35 was 60 times higher than the lowest risk group (BMI <22 kg/m^2).[179] It is estimated that >60% of type 2 diabetes mellitus cases are due to obesity.[50] Weight loss helps to control diseases associated with obesity and may even help prevent development of these diseases. Weight loss has been shown to be beneficial in lowering blood pressure, total cholesterol, LDL, TG, blood glucose in patients with diabetes mellitus type 2 and increasing HDL.[20]

Treatment
Medical Management

16. **The physician recommends that F.W. reduce her weight over the next 12 months to help improve the quality of her life, to reduce the associated morbidity from related medical conditions, and to prolong her life. What would be appropriate goals for weight loss with F.W.? What type of nutritional and exercise plan should be recommended for her weight loss intervention?**

Table 82-10	**Medical Complications of Obesity**
Cardiovascular	*Integument*
Hypertension	Venous stasis of legs
Congestive heart failure	Cellulitis
Cor pulmonale	Diminished hygiene
Varicose veins	Intertrigo, carbuncles
Pulmonary embolism	
Coronary artery disease	*Musculoskeletal*
	Immobility
Endocrine	Degenerative arthritis
Insulin resistance (Syndrome X)	Low-back pain
Type 2 diabetes mellitus	
Dyslipidemia	*Neurologic*
Polycystic ovarian syndrome/	Stroke
hyperandrogenism (F)	Idiopathic intracranial hypertension
Amenorrhea/infertility	Meralgia paresthetica
Gastrointestinal	
Gastroesophageal reflux disease	*Psychological/Psychosocial*
Hepatic steatosis	Depression/low self-esteem
Nonalcoholic steatohepatitis	Binge eating disorder
Cholelithiasis	Sexual dysfunction
Hernias	Work disability/social discrimination
Colon cancer	
	Respiratory
Genitourinary	Dyspnea and fatigue
Urinary stress incontinence	Obstructive sleep apnea
Hypogonadism (M)	Hypoventilation syndrome
Breast and uterine cancer	Pickwickian syndrome

Adapted with permission from Kushner RF, Weinsier RL. Evaluation of the obese patient: practical considerations. Med Clin North Am 2000;84(2):387.

According to the NHLBI guidelines, weight loss treatment should be initiated for patients who are overweight, who have increased waist circumference plus two or more risk factors, or are obese (BMI ≥30).[20] The general goals of weight loss and management are to prevent weight gain, reduce body weight, and maintain weight loss over a long period.[20] Treatment options to facilitate weight loss include moderate caloric restriction, medications (e.g., appetite suppressants, lipase inhibitors), physical activity, and behavior therapy. Obese patients (like F.W.) should strive to lose 10% of baseline weight at a rate of 1 to 2 lb/week with an energy deficit of 500 kcal/day over 6 months. Overweight patients should ideally lose 0.5 lb/week with an energy deficit of 300 to 500 kcal/day over 6 months. A low-calorie diet (LCD) consistent with NCEP Step 1 or Step 2 diet has been shown to be most effective. A low fat (LF) diet does not decrease weight unless total caloric intake is decreased. Total fat intake should account for 30% or less of total calories consumed per day.[20] Drastic caloric restriction is difficult to maintain and may lead to reduced metabolism and overeating due to hunger. Severe caloric restriction and rapid weight loss can be harmful and result in rebound binge eating behavior and weight gain.[134]

Increased physical activity can facilitate weight loss and is essential in preventing weight gain. Overweight children and adults should have at least 30 minutes of moderate-intensity physical exercise daily (with a gradual increment of increasing exercise by several minutes each day up to 30 minutes per day). Modest weight loss is beneficial, because even a small amount of weight loss, as little as 5%, is associated with significant improvements in health status.

Obese patients should be evaluated for hypothyroidism because it is a potential cause of weight gain. However, use of thyroid hormones to cause weight reduction in patients with normal thyroid function is not recommended.

Nonpharmacologic Therapy

17. F.W. has never participated in a behavior modification weight reduction or maintenance program. The physician recommends that she attend weekly social support meetings and learn more desirable behaviors for self-monitoring her diet and exercise. What types of nonpharmacologic therapies or programs are available for weight reduction and relapse prevention?

Behavioral modification programs using support groups, a balanced diet, and exercise are most effective for mild obesity (20% to 40% overweight).[42] Behavioral modification programs (e.g., nutritional education, exercise, cognitive restructuring, self-monitoring) are the most effective for overweight children and help motivate parents and children to alter their lifestyles.[20] Supportive family therapy is desirable, particularly for obese children. Obesity may be related to cultural attitudes, family eating behavior, and social events involving food. Relapse prevention should identify high-risk situations or events that may cause weight gain so that the person can learn new coping strategies to avoid overeating.

Due to the high demand by consumers, there are numerous types of weight loss programs, diets, and products that may or may not be effective. Individuals who want to lose weight frequently seek out popular structured programs (e.g., Jenny Craig, Weight Watchers). Other weight loss programs include low-fat, low-sodium, vegetarian, soy, Atkins, and Zone diets. Regardless of which weight loss program is chosen, patients should select a program that emphasizes the following: 1) counseling for lifestyle changes, 2) trained staff, 3) coping strategies for stressful times, 4) weight loss maintenance, and 5) flexible and appropriate food choices.[180]

Overall, a combination of low-calorie diet, behavioral modifications, and increased physical activity are most effective for reducing and maintaining weight loss. These measures must be attempted and maintained for at least 6 months before considering pharmacotherapy.[20]

Pharmacotherapy

18. F.W. asks the physician about medications that can help with weight loss. What is the current status of pharmacologic agents for obesity therapy? What are their mechanisms of action, efficacy, and potential side effects?

A comprehensive treatment approach to obesity includes a weight loss diet, exercise, supportive psychotherapy, and behavioral modification techniques. If indicated, medications such as an anorectic agent (to suppress hunger and appetite) or a GI lipase inhibitor (to reduce fat absorption) may be prescribed.[181] Weight loss is possible for most patients, but the main problem is that the vast majority of people regain the weight over time.[148] Obesity is a chronic, lifelong illness that may require long-term medication therapy. The National Task Force on the Prevention and Treatment of Obesity has published guidelines, potential benefits, and potential adverse effects of long-term pharmacotherapy in the management of obesity.[181] Medication should be considered only for patients with a BMI >30 kg/m² without risk factors or >27 kg/m² with an obesity-related risk factor (Table 82-9).[20] Anorectic medications or lipase inhibitors should not be considered a replacement for diet, behavioral modification, and exercise, but rather as add-on therapy.

The four main types of weight loss medications include agents that reduce energy intake (appetite suppressant), increase energy expenditure (increase metabolism), reduce absorption of nutrients and fat, and stimulate fat mobilization.[74,83] Medications used for the treatment of obesity in the United States are found in Table 82-11.

AMPHETAMINES AND SYMPATHOMIMETICS

Dextroamphetamine was first introduced in the 1930s for the treatment of narcolepsy, but later was found to decrease appetite and cause weight loss.[182] Amphetamines were initially prescribed for their appetite-suppressant effects in the 1950s and 1960s. Their mechanism of action is believed to involve an increase in norepinephrine and dopamine release from nerve terminals, leading to an activation of the hypothalamic feeding center ultimately suppressing appetite.[183] Amphetamines also increase thermogenesis secondary to their stimulating properties and behavioral activation. The enhancement of dopaminergic activity is believed to be responsible for amphetamine's rewarding, reinforcing, and addictive properties.[184] Because of their euphoric properties and risks of drug abuse, amphetamines are schedule II controlled agents and are not routinely used for weight loss.[185] Additional concerns with sympathomimetics are the potential for rebound binge eating, weight gain, lethargy, and depression when the

Table 82-11 **Medications Marketed or Used for the Treatment of Obesity**

Generic Name	Trade Name	Dosage	DEA Schedule or Class
Amphetamine/dextroamphetamine	Adderall	5–30 mg/day	II[a]
	Biphetamine	12.5–20 mg/day	II[a]
Benzphetamine hydrochloride	Didrex	25–50 mg one to three times daily	III
Dextroamphetamine			
Immediate release	Dexedrine	5–10 mg before meals	II[a]
Extended release	Dexedrine	10–30 mg AM	II[a]
Diethylpropion hydrochloride			
Immediate release	Tenuate	25 mg TID; 75 mg AM	IV
Controlled release	Tenuate Dospan	75 mg AM	IV
Ephedrine	Various products	20–60 mg/day	Over-the-counter
Fluoxetine	Prozac	20–60 mg AM	Prescription
Mazindol	Sanorex	1 mg TID; 2 mg AM	IV
Methamphetamine hydrochloride			
Immediate release	Desoxyn	2.5–5 mg before meals	II[a]
Extended release	Desoxyn	10–15 mg AM	II[a]
Orlistat	Xenical	120 mg TID	Prescription
Phendimetrazine tartrate	Bontril, Plegine, Prelu-2, X-Trozine	35 mg TID; 105 mg AM	III
Phenmetrazine	Preludin	25 mg BID-TID	II[a]
Phentermine			
Hydrochloride	Adipex-P, Fastin, Oby-Cap, Phentride	8 mg TID; 30–37.5 mg AM	IV
Resin	Ionamin	15–30 mg AM	IV
Sibutramine	Meridia	5–15 mg/day	IV

[a]High abuse potential, not recommended for routine or long-term use.
Adapted from references 11 and 83.

medication is stopped.[42] Other centrally active appetite suppressants that augment catecholamines (e.g., phentermine, mazindol, phendimetrazine, and diethylpropion) were developed for the treatment of obesity and may have a lower incidence and severity of CNS side effects compared with the amphetamines.[182]

OTHER SYMPATHOMIMETICS

OTC weight-loss products usually contain caffeine or sympathomimetics such as ephedrine that stimulate α- and β-adrenergic receptors, and possess anorectic and thermogenic properties.[186] Ephedrine (found in ephedra and ma huang) is included in several OTC and herbal products that promote their ability to increase energy expenditure, thus causing weight loss. In 1997, the FDA recommended limitations on ephedrine-containing dietary supplements (and in combination with other stimulants such as caffeine) due to many serious reports of adverse effects (e.g., stroke, seizures, and death).[186] Ephedra is more likely to cause adverse reactions than other herbs such as ginkgo and St. John's wort.[187] As of April 2004, the FDA has prohibited the sale of dietary supplements containing ephedrine alkaloids (ephedra). Phenylpropanolamine (PPA), a popular synthetic catecholamine that was widely found in OTC weight-loss products and decongestants, was voluntarily withdrawn in 2000.[188] PPA increased satiety by stimulating norepinephrine and dopamine release in the hypothalamic feeding center but studies found an increased risk of hemorrhagic stroke in women who took appetite suppressants containing more than 32 mg/day PPA.[189] These agents have produced modest short-term weight loss when combined with dietary programs but should not be used as monotherapy.[185] Sympathomimetic agents should be used only for those with obesity (i.e., BMI

>30 kg/m²) or in patients with medical risks such as type 2 diabetes mellitus and sleep apnea. Sympathomimetic agents are contraindicated in patients with hypertension and other cardiovascular diseases. The duration of treatment is controversial because long-term use of anorectic agents is generally not recommended. On the other hand, anorectic agents, in combination with a maintenance diet, an exercise program, behavioral modification instructions, and regular supportive group meetings, may prevent weight regain.[185]

SELECTIVE SEROTONIN REUPTAKE INHIBITORS

Serotonin- and/or norepinephrine-augmenting agents (e.g., serotonin or norepinephrine reuptake inhibitors) are the most effective agents for suppressing appetite drive and reducing weight. For obese binge eating patients, SRI antidepressants such as fluoxetine have been used successfully to reduce binge eating behavior, but this is not always associated with weight loss.[111] Several studies evaluating fluoxetine 60 mg daily[156,190–194] in obese individuals reported short-term weight loss (up to 6 months), but most patients regained the weight after 1 year.[124] The reason for the weight regain is unclear, but may relate to the development of tolerance or the lack of frequent follow-up visits.[124] Fluvoxamine was evaluated in overweight binge and nonbinge eaters and at lower doses (100 mg/day); it did not enhance weight loss, although binge eaters had a greater reduction in depressive symptoms.[195] Citalopram, the most selective inhibitor of serotonin reuptake, has been studied in severely obese subjects. At dosages of 60 mg/day, citalopram was found to have no significant benefit over placebo when added to a low-calorie diet.[196] Sertraline was compared to placebo in a study examining weight regain among subjects who had a weight loss of at least 10% of initial body weight.[197] Although sertraline initially resulted in additional weight loss during the first 6 weeks of treatment, there was no significant difference in regained weight between groups after one year. Antidepressants that have histamine$_1$ antagonist effects (i.e., tricyclic antidepressants) or block serotonin$_{2A/2C/\beta}$ receptors (e.g., mirtazapine) cause sedation and increase appetite and weight, and thus should not be used in obese patients.[88]

SEROTONIN-RELEASING AGENTS

Fenfluramine and dexfenfluramine, the dextro isomer of fenfluramine, resemble amphetamines chemically but are pharmacologically different.[198] Fenfluramine and dexfenfluramine act to increase serotonin activity by stimulating serotonin release into neuronal synapses. Fenfluramine often was combined with low doses of phentermine (fen-phen) after initial reports suggested that the combination had similar weight loss as monotherapy and that combining the two agents resulted in fewer cardiovascular and CNS adverse effects.[181] Fenfluramine and dexfenfluramine were voluntarily removed from the United States market in 1997 due to studies linking their usage to valvular heart disease and primary pulmonary hypertension.[199]

SEROTONIN/NOREPINEPHRINE REUPTAKE INHIBITORS

Sibutramine (Meridia), a prescription medication marketed for weight loss, is structurally related to amphetamines (β-phenylethylamine) and is classified as a schedule IV controlled agent.[200] Sibutramine and its two active metabolites inhibit the reuptake of serotonin and norepinephrine and, to a lesser extent, dopamine, therefore increasing concentrations of these neurotransmitters in the brain.[200–202] By increasing serotonin and norepinephrine activity, β-adrenergic, α-adrenergic, and serotonin$_{2A/2C}$ receptors are stimulated, which in turn causes a down-regulation of α- and β-adrenergic and serotonin receptors.[85,200] This promotes a sense of satiety and thus decreases appetite. A synergistic interaction between norepinephrine and serotonin has been shown to maximize reduction in food intake.[184,203] When a norepinephrine or serotonin reuptake inhibitor is given alone, food intake generally is not altered unless these agents are given in significantly higher dosages. Sibutramine has been shown to increase metabolic rate in animals for 6 hours after treatment via thermogenesis, but the studies performed thus far on humans are not definitive.[203] Sibutramine also is thought to cause a sympathetic stimulation of brown adipose tissue (thermogenesis to increase glucose utilization) via the β_3-adrenoceptors.[184,203]

In clinical studies, sibutramine (5 to 30 mg/day) caused a significant dose-related weight loss in obese patients.[200,201,204] In a fixed-dose 12-month study of obese subjects, those given a daily dose of 10 mg of sibutramine had an average weight loss of 4.8 kg. Those randomized to 15 mg daily experienced a weight loss of 6.1 kg. Subjects receiving placebo lost 1.8 kg.[204] Waist:hip ratios fell by 0.03 to 0.04 in patients treated with sibutramine 10 mg or 15 mg while no improvements in waist: hip ratios were found in the placebo-treated group. Improvements in total cholesterol levels, low-density lipoprotein, and plasma triglycerides also have been reported in sibutramine-treated groups.[201]

Continuous versus intermittent sibutramine treatment was compared in a randomized, double-blind, placebo-controlled study.[205] Overall weight loss at the end of the 48-week trial was comparable between the continuous and intermittent group (7.9 kg and 7.8 kg, respectively); the placebo-treated group experienced a 3.8 kg reduction in weight. Tolerability profiles were similar for the two active treatment groups. Sibutramine should always be combined with lifestyle modifications. In a one-year trial, women were randomized to receive sibutramine alone (drug only), sibutramine plus group lifestyle modification plus 1,200 to 1,500 kcal/day diet (drug plus lifestyle) or sibutramine plus group lifestyle modification plus 1,000 kcal/day diet for the first 4 months (combined treatment).[206] Patients who received lifestyle modification (drug plus lifestyle group and combined treatment group) had greater body weight loss than women who received sibutramine alone (drug only group). Sibutramine has been compared with dexfenfluramine in two clinical trials, and both agents exhibited similar rates of weight loss and adverse effects.[200] Sibutramine takes several weeks to have a clinical effect, which causes a slower weight loss than that seen with sympathomimetic agents.

Common adverse effects of sibutramine include headache, decreased appetite, dry mouth, constipation, and insomnia.[201,204] Other less common side effects include sweating, irritability, excitation, dizziness, insomnia, and increases in blood pressure and heart rate (increase in blood pressure by 1 to 3 mm Hg and in heart rate by 4 to 5 beats/min). Frequent blood pressure and pulse rate monitoring is recommended because these cardiovascular effects are believed to be dose-related. Sibutramine must be used cautiously in patients with high blood pressure and its use is not recommended in patients with heart disease, congestive heart failure, conduction disorders (arrhythmias), or stroke. Sibutramine is absolutely contraindicated in patients taking certain CNS medications that increase levels of norepinephrine or serotonin (e.g., MAOIs) and other centrally acting appetite suppressants. Precautions should be taken in patients who are coadministered lithium, antimigraine agents (e.g., sumatriptan, dihydroergotamine), and some opioid analgesics (e.g., tramadol, dextromethorphan). Drugs that inhibit liver enzymes (cytochrome P450 [CYP] 3A4), such as ketoconazole and erythromycin, can increase serum concentrations of sibutramine. Sibutramine is well absorbed and has high first-pass liver metabolism to produce two active metabolites, both with long elimination half-lives of 14 to 16 hours.[201] Initial dosing of sibutramine is 10 mg once daily with or without food (typically in the morning) and the dose can be increased to 15 mg once daily if needed. A 5-mg dose is available for patients who do not tolerate the recommended starting dose.

LIPASE INHIBITORS

Orlistat (Xenical), an FDA-approved weight loss medication, works to reduce dietary fat absorption by inhibiting GI (stomach and pancreas) lipase activity.[207,208] Orlistat is a hydrogenated derivative of lipstatin (a naturally occurring lipase inhibitor produced by *Streptomyces toxytricini*) that is a potent inhibitor of lipases and weak inhibitor of other intestinal hydrolases.[208] Gastric and pancreatic lipase are enzymes that play a pivotal role in the digestion of dietary fat (triglycerides). Before digestion and absorption of dietary fat is possible, each triglyceride molecule must be hydrolyzed by lipase enzymes into absorbable products—two fatty acid molecules and one 2-monoacylglycerol molecule. Orlistat inhibits lipase by binding to and inactivating the enzyme. Subsequently, triglycerides cannot be absorbed, and approximately 30% of ingested fat is excreted in the feces.[208] The therapeutic activity of orlistat takes place in the stomach and small intestine and effects are seen as soon as 24 to 48 hours after dosing.

Orlistat does not exert appetite suppressant effects, has no CNS effects, and has no systemic absorption.[208] It is most effective if combined with a reduced fat and calorie diet[207] and is indicated to reduce the risk of weight regain after prior weight loss. It also is indicated for obese patients with an initial BMI $\geq$30 kg/m^2 or $\geq$27 kg/m^2 in the presence of other obesity-related risk factors. Obese patients who received orlistat in conjunction with a low-calorie diet lost 8.4% of body weight in 6 months, compared with a 5.7% loss of body weight in patients on a diet plus placebo.[191] At the end of this 1-year trial, subjects receiving orlistat had a mean weight loss of 9% versus 5.8% in the placebo group.[207] In another 2-year study, weight loss was 8.8% (orlistat) and 5.8% (placebo) at 1 year, and at 2 years, the orlistat group had an average 7.6% weight loss from their initial weight compared with 4.5% for placebo.[209] At the end of the 2-year study, the group receiving orlistat plus a weight maintenance diet had significantly less weight gain and improved fasting low-density lipoprotein cholesterol and insulin levels compared with the placebo group. In a multicenter, European trial, patients who received orlistat 120 mg three times daily along with a hypocaloric diet had greater weight loss (10.2%) compared to placebo (6.1%) at the end of 1 year.[210] During the second year, patients who received orlistat gained less weight versus those switched to placebo ($P < 0.001$) while following a eucaloric diet.

The most common adverse effects associated with orlistat include GI problems (loose stools, oily spotting, flatus with discharge, fecal urgency, fatty/oily stools, increased defecation, fecal incontinence, bloating, and cramping).[209,211] The 1-year incidence rate of the most common adverse events reported were fatty/oily stool (31%), increased defecation (20%), and oily spotting (18%).[209] The most common non-GI problem was headache (6%). Side effects usually develop early in treatment and persist for 1 to 4 weeks, but occasionally last >6 months. Because GI adverse effects are worse with a high-fat diet, orlistat may enhance dietary compliance with a low-fat diet.[211]

Orlistat may reduce the absorption of fat-soluble vitamins (K, A, D, and E) and patients should take a multivitamin supplement that contains these vitamins.[208,212] The supplement should be taken once a day at least 2 hours before or after the administration of orlistat, such as at bedtime. Orlistat may interfere with vitamin K absorption and potentiate the bleeding effects of warfarin. Preliminary studies indicate that orlistat has very few clinically significant drug–drug interactions with commonly prescribed medications.[208,211] When used in diabetic patients, weight loss may be accompanied by improved control of diabetes, which requires a reduction in doses of diabetic medications, including insulin. Orlistat has additive effects when combined with lipid (cholesterol)-lowering agents such as pravastatin; thus, the dose can be reduced.[208] The dosage of orlistat in adults is 120 mg three times daily, during (or up to 1 hour after) each main meal containing fat. If a meal occasionally is missed or contains no fat, the dose may be omitted. Dosages exceeding 120 mg three times daily do not provide additional benefit.

MISCELLANEOUS AGENTS

Recent advances in pharmacological treatment of obesity have revealed positive experiences with several drugs normally used in other conditions. Bupropion SR in doses of 300 mg and 400 mg daily was found to produce a 7.2% and 10.1% decrease in baseline weight, respectively, compared to 5% weight reduction with placebo.[212] Topiramate is a second-generation antiepileptic agents which acts as an agonist at gamma-aminobutyric acid (GABA$_A$) receptors and as an antagonist at non-NMDA glutamate receptors. It has been shown to produce a dose-dependent weight loss between 1–8 kg and may also produce weight loss in patients with bipolar affective disorder.[59] In a 14-week, double-blind, placebo-controlled, flexible dose trial (25 to 600 mg/day; median dose, 212 mg/day), topiramate significantly reduced the BMI, weight and percent of total body fat (all secondary outcomes) in 61 patients with binge eating disorder.[213] The mean weight loss was 5.9 kg with topiramate versus 1.2 kg for placebo. Neither topiramate nor bupropion have been FDA approved for weight loss and both agents may cause significant adverse effects (See Chapter 79, Mood Disorders I: Major Depressive Disorders, and Chapter 54, Seizure Disorders, for full discussion of these products).

19. F.W. is willing to try a combination therapy of sibutramine and orlistat for weight reduction, but also has heard about the use of surgery to reduce the size of her stomach. When should surgical intervention be used? What are some complications related to the different types of surgical procedures?

Surgery

Surgery should be used only for morbidly obese individuals in whom behavioral or pharmacologic treatments have failed.[211] Surgical procedures used for severe (morbid) obesity (BMI $\geq$40 or $\geq$35 kg/m^2 with comorbid conditions) include gastric stapling or laparoscopic banding, gastric bypass, jaw-wiring, or suction lipectomy. For severely obese patients (>100% over normal weight), the most effective treatment is a surgical procedure to reduce the size of the stomach. Surgical procedures either reduce the absorptive surface of the GI tract resulting in malabsorption, or reduce the stomach volume so that the person feels full. Jejuno-ileal bypass (bypass of the duodenum and most of the jejunum) was first introduced more than 40 years ago and was popular in the 1970s in the United States. The operation resulted in many long-term complications (e.g., wound complications, severe metabolic disturbances, severe diarrhea, bloating, anal-rectal pain) and there was an increased death rate approximately 5 to 10 years after the surgery. This type of surgery is no longer performed and is considered an unsafe procedure. Alternative and less invasive surgeries have been tried to reduce energy intake and absorption. The insertion of a gastric balloon (called a *gastric bubble*) was used in the past but complications such as gastric ulcers, collapse of the bubble, and intestinal blockage have been reported; thus, this method is not used today.

Gastric bypass or gastroplasty (gastric reduction) are more commonly used today to reduce weight but are accompanied by complications such as nausea, stomach ulceration, stenosis, anemia, and cholelithiasis. Currently, vertical gastric stapling or banding via a laparoscope are the preferred methods of inducing weight loss as there are fewer complications in comparison to gastric bypass procedures.

REFERENCES

1. Eating Disorders and Obesity: A Comprehensive Handbook. 2nd Ed. New York: The Guildford Press, 2002.

2. Steiner H, Lock J. Anorexia and bulimia nervosa in children and adolescents: a review of the past 10 years. J Am Acad Child Adolesc Psychiatry 1998; 37:352.

3. Beresin E. Anorexia nervosa. Compr Ther 1997; 23:664.

4. Kay W. Strober M. The neurobiology of eating disorders. In: Charney DS et al., eds. Neurobiology of Mental Illness. New York: Oxford Press, 1999.

5. Halmi KA. Eating disorders. In: Sadock BJ, Sadock VA, eds. Kaplan & Sadock's Comprehensive Textbook of Psychiatry. 7th Ed. Philadelphia: Lippincott Williams & Wilkins, 2000.

6. American Psychiatric Association. Diagnostic and Statistical Manual of Mental Disorders. 4th Ed. Text Revised. Washington, DC: American Psychiatric Association, 2000.

7. Metropolitan Life Insurance Company. Statistical Bulletin of the Metropolitan Life Insurance Company. 1983;64:2.

8. Hammer LD et al. Standardized percentile curves of body-mass index for children and adolescents. Am J Dis Child 1991;145:259.

9. Willet WC et al. Guidelines for healthy weight. N Engl J Med 1999;341(6):427.

10. American Psychiatric Association. Practice Guideline for the Treatment of Patients With Eating Disorders. 2nd Ed. Am J Psychiatry 2000;7(1):1.

11. Becker AE et al. Eating disorders. N Engl J Med 1999;340(14):1092.

12. Holderness CC et al. Co-morbidity of eating disorders and substance abuse: review of the literature. Int J Eat Disord 1994;16:1.

13. Powers PS. Initial assessment and early treatment options for anorexia nervosa and bulimia nervosa. Psychiatr Clin North Am 1996;19(4):639.

14. Hudson JI et al. Antidepressant treatment of binge-eating disorder: research findings and clinical guidelines. J Clin Psychiatry 1996;57(Suppl 8):73.

15. de Zwann M et al. Binge eating disorder: clinical features and treatment of a new diagnosis. Harv Rev Psychiatry 1994;1:310.

16. Brewerton TD. Binge eating disorder: diagnosis and treatment options. CNS Drugs 1999;5:351.

17. Kaye WH, Walsh BT. Psychopharmacology of eating disorders. In: Davis KL et al., eds. Neuropsychopharmacology: The Fifth Generation of Progress. Philadelphia: Lippincott Williams & Williams, 2002.

18. Kaplan AS, Ciliska D. The relationship between eating disorders and obesity: psychopathologic and treatment considerations. Psychiatr Ann 1999; 29(4):197.

19. Brewerton TD et al. Comorbidity of axis I psychiatric diagnosis in bulimia nervosa. J Clin Psychiatry 1995;56:77.

20. Expert Panel on the Identification, Evaluation, and Treatment of Overweight in Adults. Clinical guidelines on the identification, evaluation, and treatment of overweight and obesity in adults: executive summary. Am J Clin Nutr 1998;68:899.

21. World Health Organization. Physical status: the use and interpretation of anthropometry. Report of a WHO Expert Committee. World Health Organ Tech Rep Ser 1995;854:1.

22. Troiano RP et al. The relationship between body weight and mortality: a quantitative analysis of combined information from existing studies. Int J Obes Relat Metab Disord 1996;20:63.

23. Flegal KM et al. Overweight and obesity in the United States: prevalence and trends, 1960–1994. Int J Obes Relat Metab Disord 1998;22:39.

24. World Health Organization. Obesity: preventing and managing the global epidemic: report of a WHO Consultation on Obesity, Geneva, June 3–5, 1997. Geneva: World Health Organization, 1998.

25. Phillips KA et al. A comparison study of body dysmorphic disorder and obsessive-compulsive disorder. J Clin Psychiatry 1998;59(11):568.

26. Hollander E, Aronowitz BR. Comorbid social anxiety and body dysmorphic disorder: managing the complicated patient. J Clin Psychiatry 1999;60 (Suppl 9):27.

27. Hollander E. Treatment of obsessive-compulsive spectrum disorders with SSRIs. Br J Psychiatry 1998;173(Suppl 35):7.

28. Phillips KA et al. Body image disturbance in body dysmorphic disorder and eating disorders: obsessions or delusions? Psychiatr Clin North Am 1995; 18(2):317.

29. Phillips KA. Body dysmorphic disorder: diagnosis and treatment of imagined ugliness. J Clin Psychiatry 1996;57(Suppl 8):61.

30. Rosen JC, Ramirez E. A comparison of eating disorders and body dysmorphic disorder on body image and psychological adjustment. J Psychosom Res 1998;44(304):441.

31. Phillips KA et al. Body dysmorphic disorder: an obsessive-compulsive spectrum disorder, a form of affective spectrum disorder, or both? J Clin Psychiatry 1995;56(Supp 4):41.

32. McKay D et al. Comparison of clinical characteristics in obsessive-compulsive disorder and body dysmorphic disorder. J Anxiety Disord 1997;11(4):447.

33. Phillips KA. Pharmacologic treatment of body dysmorphic disorder. Psychopharmacol Bull 1996; 32(4):597.

34. Phillips KA. An open study of buspirone augmentation of serotonin-reuptake inhibitors in body dysmorphic disorder. Psychopharmacol Bull 1996; 32(1):175.

35. El-Khatib HE, Dickey TO. Sertraline for body dysmorphic disorder. J Am Acad Child Adolesc Psychiatry 1995;34(11):1404.

36. Perugi G et al. Fluvoxamine in the treatment of body dysmorphic disorder (dysmorphophobia). Int Clin Psychopharmacol 1996;11(4):247.

37. Carlat DJ et al. Eating disorders in males: a report on 135 patients. Am J Psychiatry 1997;154:1127.

38. Klibanski A et al. The effects of estrogen administration on trabecular bone loss in young women with anorexia nervosa. J Clin Endocrinol Metab 1995;80:898.

39. Herzog DB et al. Comorbidity and outcome in eating disorders. Psychiatr Clin North Am 1996;19(4):843.

40. Braun DL et al. Psychiatric comorbidity in patients with eating disorders. Psychol Med 1994;24:859.

41. Wonderlich SA, Mitchell JE. Eating disorders and comorbidity: empirical, conceptual, and clinical implications. Psychopharmacol Bull 1997;33(3):381.

42. Halmi KA. Eating disorders: anorexia nervosa, bulimia nervosa, and obesity. In: Hales RE et al., eds. The American Psychiatric Press Textbook of Psychiatry. 3rd Ed. Washington, DC: American Psychiatric Press, 1999.

43. Garfinkel PE et al. Bulimia nervosa in a Canadian community sample: prevalence and comparison of subgroups. Am J Psychiatry 1995;152:1052.

44. Pomerleau CS. Co-factors for smoking and evolutionary psychobiology. Addiction 1997;92(4):397.

45. Kuczmarski RJ et al. Increasing prevalence of overweight among US adults: the National Health and Nutrition Examination Surveys, 1960 to 1991. JAMA 1994;272:205.

46. Flegal KM. Prevalence and trends in obesity among US adults, 1999-2000. JAMA 2002;288(14):1723.

47. Ogden CL et al. Prevalence and trends in overweight among US children and adolescents, 1999-2000. JAMA 2002;288(14):1728.

48. National Center for Health Statistics. Plan and operation of the Third National Health and Nutrition Examination Survey, 1988-1994. Vital Health Stat 1994;32:1.

49. Freedman DS. Trends and correlates of class 3 obesity in the United States from 1990 through 2000. JAMA 2002;288;14:1758.

50. Wolf AM, Colditz GA. Current estimates of the economic costs of obesity in the United States. Obes Res 1998;6:97.

51. Wolf AM, Colditz GA. The cost of obesity: the U.S. perspective. Pharmacoeconomics 1994;5:34.

52. Kaye WH et al. The role of the central nervous system in the psychoneuroendocrine disturbances of anorexia and bulimia nervosa. Psychiatr Clin North Am 1998;21(2):381.

53. Allison DB et al. Antipsychotic-induced weight gain: a comprehensive research synthesis. Am J Psychiatry 1999l;156:1686.

54. Wirshing DA et al. Novel antipsychotics and new onset of diabetes. Biol Psychiatry 1998;44:778.

55. Baptista T. Body weight gain induced by antipsychotic drugs. Acta Psychiatr Scand 1999;100:3.

56. Allison DB et al. The distribution of body mass index among individuals with and without schizophrenia. J Clin Psychiatry 1999;60:215.

57. Stanton JM. Weight gain associated with neuroleptic medication: a review. Schizophrenia Bull 1995;21:463.

58. Poyurovsky M et al. Olanzapine-induced weight gain in patients with first-episode schizophrenia: a double-blind, placebo-controlled study of fluoxetine addition. Am J Psychiatry 2002;159:1058.

59. Werneke U et al. Options for pharmacological management of obesity in patients treated with atypical antipsychotics. Int Clin Psychopharmacol 2002; 17:145.

60. Aquila R. Management of weight gain in patients with schizophrenia. J Clin Psychiatry 2002; 63(Suppl 4):33.

61. Serdula MK et al. Do obese children become obese adults? A review of literature. Prev Med 1993; 22:167.

62. Graunbaum JA et al. Youth risk behavior surveillance-United States, 2001. MMWR 2002;51:1.

63. Physical Activity and Health: A Report of the Surgeon General. Atlanta, GA: US Dept of Health and Human Services, Centers for Disease Control and Prevention, National Center for Chronic Disease Prevention and Health Promotion, 1996.

64. Goran MI, Treuth MS. Energy expenditure, physical activity and obesity in children. Pediatr Clin North Am 2001;48:931.

65. Fagot-Campagna A. Emergence of type 2 diabetes mellitus in children: epidemiologic evidence. J Pediatr Endocrinol Metab 2000;13(Suppl 6):1395.

66. Fagot-Campagna A et al. Diabetes, impaired fasting glucose, and elevated HbA1c in US adolescents: the Third National Health and Nutrition Examination Survey. Diabetes Care 2001;24:834.

67. Rosenbloom AL et al. Emerging epidemic of type 2 diabetes in youth. Diabetes Care 1999;22:345.

68. Karlson EW et al. Total hip replacement due to osteoarthritis: the importance of age, obesity, and other modifiable risk factors. Am J Med 2003; 114:93.

69. Hewitt JK. Behavior genetics and eating disorders. Psychopharmacol Bull 1997;33(3):355.

70. Gorwood P et al. Genetics and anorexia nervosa: a review of candidate genes. Psychiatr Genet 1998;8:1.

71. Lilenfeld LR et al. A controlled family study of anorexia and bulimia nervosa: psychiatric disorders in first-degree relatives and effects of proband comorbidity. Arch Gen Psychiatry 1998;55:603.

72. Davis C et al. The role of physical activity in the development and maintenance of eating disorders. Psychol Med 1994;24:957.

73. Davis C. Eating disorders and hyperactivity: a psychobiological perspective. Can J Psychiatry 1997; 42(2):168.

74. Kaye WH. Anorexia nervosa, obsessional behavior, and serotonin. Psychopharmacol Bull 1997; 33(3):335.

75. Wolfe BE et al. Research update on serotonin function in bulimia nervosa and anorexia nervosa. Psychopharmacol Bull 1997;33(3):345.

76. Lilenfeld LR et al. Psychiatric disorders in women with bulimia nervosa and their first-degree relatives: effects of comorbid substance dependence. Int J Eating Disord 1007;22:253.

77. Schuckit MA et al. Anorexia nervosa and bulimia nervosa in alcohol-dependent men and women and their relatives. Am J Psychiatry 1996;153:74.

78. Rorty M et al. Childhood sexual, physical, and psychological abuse in bulimia nervosa. Am J Psychiatry 1994;151:1122.

79. Bouchard C et al. Inheritance of the amount and distribution of human body fat. Int J Obes 1988;12:205.

80. Tambs K et al. Genetics and environmental contributions to the variance of the body mass index in a Norwegian sample of first-degree and second-degree relatives. Am J Hum Biol 1991;3:257.

81. Vogler GP et al. Influences of genes and shared family environment on adult body mass index assessed in an adoption study by a comprehensive path model. Int J Obes Relat Metab Disord 1995; 19:40.

82. Licinio J et al. The hypothalamic-pituitary-adrenal axis in anorexia nervosa. Psychiatry Res 1996;62:75.

83. Campfield LA et al. Strategies and potential molecular targets for obesity treatment. Science 1998;290:1383.

84. Laue L et al. The hypothalamic-pituitary-adrenal axis in anorexia nervosa and bulimia nervosa: pathophysiologic implications. Adv Pediatr 1991;38:287.

85. Blundell JE, Halford JCG. Serotonin and appetite regulation: implications for the pharmacological treatment of obesity. CNS Drugs 1998;6:473.

86. Baxter G et al. 5HT₂ receptor subtypes: a family re-united? Trends Pharmacol Sci 1995;13:21.

87. Curzon G et al. Appetite suppression by commonly used drugs depends on 5HT receptors but not on 5HT availability. Trends Pharmacol Sci 1998;13:21.

88. Stahl SM. Essential Psychopharmacology: Neuroscientific Basis and Practical Applications. 2nd Ed. New York: Cambridge University Press, 2000.

89. Stahl SM. Not so selective serotonin reuptake inhibitors. J Clin Psychiatry 1998;59:343.

90. Stahl SM. Neuropharmacology of obesity: my receptors made me eat it. J Clin Psychiatry 1998; 59:447.

91. Strosberg AD, Pietri-Rouxel F. Function and regulation of the β₃-adrenoceptor. Trends Pharmacol Sci 1996;17:373.

92. Strosberg AD. Association of β₃-adrenoceptor polymorphism with obesity and diabetes: current status. Trends Pharmacol Sci 1997;18:449.

93. Sinha MK, Caro JF. Clinical aspects of leptin. Vitam Horm 1998;54:1.

94. Arner P. Adrenergic receptor function in fat cells. Am J Clin Nutr 1992;55:228S.

95. Collins S et al. Role of leptin in fat regulation. Nature 1996;380:677.

96. Gendall KA et al. Leptin, neuropeptide Y, and peptide YY in long-term recovered eating disorder patients. Biol Psychiatry 1999;46(2):292.

97. Ferron F et al. Serum leptin concentrations in patients with anorexia nervosa, bulimia nervosa and non-specific eating disorders correlate with body mass index but are independent of the respective disease. Clin Endocrinol 1997;46:289.

98. Houseknecht KL et al. The biology of leptin: a review. J Anim Sci 1998;76:1405.

99. Considine RV et al. Serum immunoreactive-leptin concentrations in normal-weight and obese humans. N Engl J Med 1996;334:292.

100. Flier JS, Maratos-Flier E. Obesity and the hypothalamus: novel peptides for new pathways. Cell 1998;92:437.

101. Grinspoon S et al. Serum leptin levels in women with anorexia nervosa. J Clin Endocrinol Metab 1996;81:3861.

102. Mantzoros C et al. Cerebrospinal fluid leptin in anorexia nervosa: correlation with nutritional status and potential role in resistance to weight gain. J Clin Endocrinol Metab 1997;82:1845.

103. Nakai Y et al. Role of leptin in women with eating disorders. Int J Eat Disord 1999;26(1):29.

104. Ahima RS et al. Role of leptin in the neuroendocrine response to fasting. Nature 1996;382:250.

105. Ericsson M et al. Common biological pathways in eating disorders and obesity. Addict Behav 1996; 21(6):733.

106. de Zwann M, Mitchell J. Opiate antagonists and eating behavior in humans: a review. J Clin Pharmacol 1992;32:1060.

107. Marrazzi MA et al. Naltrexone use in the treatment of anorexia nervosa and bulimia nervosa. Int Clin Psychopharmacol 1995;10:163.

108. Rowland NE, Kalra SP. Potential role of neuropeptide ligands in the treatment of overeating. CNS Drugs 1997;6:419.

109. Gertner JM. Effects of growth hormone on body fat in adults. Horm Res 1993;40:10.

110. Berdanier CD et al. Is dehydroepiandrosterone an antiobesity agent? FASEB J 1993;7:414.

111. Gordon I et al. Childhood onset anorexia nervosa: towards identifying a biological substrate. Int J Eat Disord 1997;22:159.

112. Kreipe RE et al. Eating disorders in adolescents: a position paper of the Society for Adolescent Medicine. J Adolesc Health 1995;16:476.

113. Robin AL et al. Treatment of eating disorders in children and adolescents. Clin Psychol Rev 1998;18(4):421.

114. Pike KM. Long-term course of anorexia nervosa: response, relapse, remission and recovery. Clin Psychol Rev 1998;18:447.

115. Stice E et al. Risk factors for the emergence of childhood eating disturbances: a five-year prospective study. Int J Eat Disord 1999;25(4):375.

116. Eckert ED et al. Ten-year follow-up of anorexia nervosa: clinical course and outcome. Psychol Med 1995;25:143.

117. Pollice C et al. Relationship of depression, anxiety, and obsessionality to state of illness in anorexia nervosa. Int J Eat Disord 1997;21:367.

118. Neumarker KJ. Mortality and sudden death in anorexia nervosa. Int J Eat Disord 1997;21(3):205.

119. Sullivan PF. Mortality in anorexia nervosa. Am J Psychiatry 1995;152:1073.

120. Sharp CW, Freeman CPL. The medical complications of anorexia nervosa. Br J Psychiatry 1993; 162:452.

121. Grinspoon S et al. Mechanisms and treatment options for bone loss in anorexia nervosa. Psychopharmacol Bull 1997;33(3):399.

122. Powers PS. Osteoporosis and eating disorders. J Pediatr Adolesc Gynecol 1999;12(2):51.

123. Kleifield E et al. Cognitive-behavioral treatment of anorexia nervosa. Psychiatr Clin North Am 1996;19:715.

124. Mayer LE, Walsh BT. The use of selective serotonin reuptake inhibitors in eating disorders. J Clin Psychiatry 1998;59(Suppl 15):28.

125. Kaye WH et al. An open trial of fluoxetine in patients with anorexia nervosa. J Clin Psychiatry 1991;52:464.

126. Fassino S et al. Efficacy of citalopram in anorexia nervosa: a pilot study. Eur Neuropsychopharmacol 2002;12:453.

127. Strober M et al. Does adjunctive fluoxetine influence the post-hospital course of anorexia nervosa? A 24-month prospective, longitudinal follow-up and comparison with historical controls. Psychopharmacol Bull 1997;33:425.

128. Attia E et al. Does fluoxetine augment the inpatient treatment of anorexia nervosa? Am J Psychiatry 1998;155:548.

129. Ferguson CP et al. Are SSRI's effective in underweight anorexia nervosa ? Int J Eat Disord 1999; 25:11.

130. Kaye WH et al. Double-blind placebo-controlled administration of fluoxetine in restricting- and restricting-purging-type anorexia nervosa. Biol Psychiatry 2001;49:644

131. Kennedy SH, Goldbloom DS. Current perspectives on drug therapies for anorexia nervosa and bulimia nervosa. Drugs 1991;41(3):367.

132. Keel PK, Mitchell JE. Outcome in bulimia nervosa. Am J Psychiatry 1997;154:313.

133. Daluiski A et al. Russell's sign: subtle hand changes in patients with bulimia nervosa. Clin Orthop 1997;343:107.

134. Wilfley DE, Cohen LR. Psychological treatment of bulimia nervosa and binge eating disorder. Psychopharmacol Bull 1997;33(3):437.

135. Apple RF. Interpersonal therapy for bulimia nervosa. J Clin Psychol 1999;55(6):715.

136. Spangler DL. Cognitive-behavioral therapy for bulimia nervosa: an illustration. J Clin Psychol 1999; 55(6):699.

137. Peterson CB, Mitchell JE. Psychosocial and pharmacological treatment of eating disorders: a review of research findings. J Clin Psychol 1999; 55(6):685.

138. Goldbloom DS et al. A randomized controlled trial of fluoxetine and cognitive behavioral therapy for bulimia nervosa: short-term outcome. Behav Res Ther 1997;35(9):803.

139. Ricca V et al. Fluoxetine and fluvoxamine combined with individual cognitive-behavioral therapy in binge eating disorder: a one-year follow-up study. Psychother Psychosom 2001;70:298.

140. Walsh BT et al. Medication and psychotherapy in the treatment of bulimia nervosa. Am J Psychiatry 1997;154:523.

141. Agras WS. Pharmacotherapy of bulimia nervosa and binge eating disorder: longer-term outcomes. Psychopharmacol Bull 1997;33(3):433.

142. Jimerson DC et al. Medications in the treatment of eating disorders. Psychiatr Clin North Am 1996; 19(4):739.

143. Blouin J et al. Bulimia: independence of antibulimic and antidepressant properties of desipramine. Can J Psychiatry 1989;34:24.

144. Hughes PL et al. Treating bulimia with desipramine. Arch Gen Psychiatry 1986;43:182.

145. McCann UD, Agras WS. Successful treatment of nonpurging bulimia nervosa with desipramine: a double-blind, placebo-controlled study. Am J Psychiatry 1990;147:1509.

146. Barlow J et al. Treatment of bulimia with desipramine: a double-blind crossover study. Can J Psychiatry 1988;33:128.

147. Pope HG et al. Bulimia treated with imipramine: a placebo-controlled, double-blind study. Am J Psychiatry 1983;140:554.

148. Agras WS et al. Imipramine in the treatment of bulimia: a double-blind controlled study. Int J Eat Disord 1987;6:29.

149. Alger SA et al. Effect of a tricyclic antidepressant and opiate antagonist on binge eating behavior in normal weight bulimic and obese, binge-eating subjects. Am J Clin Nutr 1991;53:865.

150. Mitchell JE, Groat R. A placebo-controlled, double-blind trial of amitriptyline in bulimia. J Clin Psychopharmacol 1994;4:186.

151. Walsh BT et al. Treatment of bulimia with phenelzine. Arch Gen Psychiatry 1984;41:1105.

152. Walsh BT et al. Phenelzine vs. placebo in 50 patients with bulimia. Arch Gen Psychiatry 1988;45:471.

153. Kennedy SH et al. A trial of isocarboxazid in the treatment of bulimia nervosa. J Clin Psychopharmacol 1988;8:391.

154. Pope HG et al. A placebo-controlled study of trazodone in bulimia nervosa. J Clin Psychopharmacol 1989;9:254.

155. Horne RL et al. Treatment of bulimia with bupropion: a multicenter controlled trial. J Clin Psychiatry 1998;49:262.

156. Marcus MD et al. A double blind, placebo-controlled trial of fluoxetine plus behavior modification in the treatment of obese binge eaters and non-binge eaters. Am J Psychiatry 1990;147:876.

157. Fluoxetine Bulimia Nervosa Collaborative Study Group. Fluoxetine in the treatment of bulimia nervosa: a multicenter, placebo-controlled, double-blind trial. Arch Gen Psychiatry 1992;49(2):139.

158. Goldstein DJ et al. The Fluoxetine Bulimia Nervosa Collaborative Research Group. Long term fluoxetine treatment of bulimia nervosa. Br J Psychiatry 1995:166:660.

159. Goldstein DJ et al. Effectiveness of fluoxetine therapy in bulimia nervosa regardless of comorbid depression. Int J Eat Disord 1999;25:19.

160. Walsh BT et al. Fluoxetine for bulimia nervosa following poor response to psychotherapy. Am J Psychiatry 2000;157:1332.

161. Arnold LM et al. A placebo-controlled, randomized trial of fluoxetine in the treatment of binge-eating disorder. J Clin Psychiatry 2002;63:1028.

162. Gardiner HM et al. Fluvoxamine: an open pilot study in moderately obese female patients suffering from atypical eating disorders and episodes of bingeing. Int J Obesity 1993;17:301.

163. Ayuso-Gutierrez JL et al. Open trial of fluvoxamine in the treatment of bulimia nervosa. Int J Eat Disord 1994;15:245.

164. Fichter MM et al. Fluvoxamine in prevention of relapse in bulimia nervosa: effects on eating-specific psychopathology. J Clin Psychopharmacol 1996;16:9.

165. Hudson JL et al. Fluvoxamine in the treatment of binge-eating disorder: a multicenter placebo-controlled, double-blind trial. Am J Psychiatry 1998;155(12):1756.

166. Roberts JM, Lydiard RB. Sertraline in the treatment of bulimia nervosa [Letter]. Am J Psychiatry 1993;150:1753.

167. McElroy SL et al. Placebo-controlled trial of sertraline in the treatment of binge eating disorder. Am J Psychiatry 2000;157:1004.

168. Prats M et al. Paroxetine treatment for bulimia nervosa and binge eating disorder [Abstract 308]. Abstracts of the Sixth International Conference on Eating Disorders, New York, April 1994.

169. Beaumont PJV et al. Intensive nutritional counseling in bulimia nervosa: a role for supplementation with fluoxetine. Aust NZ J Psychiatry 1997; 31:514.

170. Fichter MM et al. Fluvoxamine in prevention of relapse in bulimia nervosa: effects on eating-specific psychopathology. J Clin Psychopharmacol 1996;16:9-18.

171. Stunkard A et al. d-fenfluramine treatment of binge eating disorder. Am J Psychiatry 1996;153:1455.

172. Hsu LKG et al. Treatment of bulimia nervosa with lithium carbonate: a controlled study. J Nerv Ment Dis 1991;179:351.

173. Shapira NA et al. Treatment of binge-eating disorder with topiramate: a clinical case series. J Clin Psychiatry 2000;61:368.

174. Faris PL et al. Effect of decreasing afferent vagal activity with ondansetron on symptoms of bulimia. Lancet 2000;355:792.

175. Williamson DF. Intentional weight loss: patterns in the general population and its association with morbidity and mortality. Int J Obes Relat Metab Disord. 1997;21(Suppl 1):S14.

176. Torgerson JS, Sjostrom L. The Swedish Obese Subjects (SOS) study—rationale and results. Int J Obes Relat Metab Disord 2002;25(Suppl 1):S2.

177. Calle EE et al. Body-mass index and mortality in a prospective cohort of U.S. adults. N Engl J Med 1999;341:1097.

178. Colditz GA. Economic costs of obesity and inactivity. Med Sci Sports Exerc 1999;31:S663.

179. Colditz GA et al. Weights as a risk factor for clinical diabetes in women. Am J Epidemiol 1990;132(3):501.

180. Choosing a safe & successful weight-loss program. US Department of Health and Human Services, Public Health Service, National Institutes of Health, National Institute of Diabetes & Digestive & Kidney Diseases, NIH Publication No. 94-3700, December, 1993.

181. National Task Force on the Prevention and Treatment of Obesity. Long-term pharmacotherapy in the management of obesity. JAMA 1996;276:1907.

182. Bray GA. Use and abuse of appetite-suppressant drugs in the treatment of obesity. Ann Intern Med 1993;119:707.

183. Aronne LJ. Modern medical management of obesity: the role of pharmaceutical intervention. J Am Diet Assoc 1998;98(Suppl 2):S23.

184. Heal DJ et al. Sibutramine: a novel anti-obesity drug. A review of the pharmacological evidence to differentiate it from d-amphetamine and d-fenfluramine. Int J Obes Relat Metab Disord 1998; 22(Suppl 1):S18.

185. Silverstone T. Appetite suppressants: a review. Drugs 1992;43:820.

186. Jequier E et al. Thermogenic effects of various β-adrenoceptor agonists in humans: their potential usefulness in the treatment of obesity. Am J Clin Nutr 1992;55:249S.

187. Bent S et al. The relative safety of ephedra compared with other herbal products. Ann Int Med 2003;138:468.

188. http://www.fda.gov/cder/drug/infopage/ppa/qa.htm. Access date: 8/21/02. FDA/Center for Drug Evaluation and Research. Questions and Answers: Safety of Phenylpropranolamine. 2000;November 6.

189. Morgenstern LB et al. Use of ephedra-containing products and risk for hemorrhagic stroke. Neurology 2003;60:132.

190. Pijl H et al. Effect of serotonin re-uptake inhibition by fluoxetine on body weight and spontaneous food choice in obesity. Int J Obes 1991; 15:237.

191. Darga LL et al. Fluoxetine's effect on weight loss in obese subjects. Am J Clin Nutr 1991;54:321.

192. Goldstein DJ et al. Fluoxetine: a randomized clinical trial in the treatment of obesity. Int J Obes Relat Metab Disord 1994;18:129.

193. Levin LR et al. Use of a serotonin re-uptake inhibitor, fluoxetine, in the treatment of obesity. Int J Obes 1987;11(Suppl 3):185.

194. Mitchell JE et al. Frequency and duration of binge-eating episodes in patients with bulimia. Am J Psychiatry 1981;138:835.

195. de Zwann M et al. Binge eating in overweight women. Compr Psychiatry 1992;33:256.

196. Szkudlarek J, Elsborg L. Treatment of severe obesity with a highly selective serotonin re-uptake inhibitor as a supplement to a low-calorie diet. Int J Obes Relat Metab Disord 1993;17:681.

197. Wadden TA et al. Sertraline and relapse prevention training following treatment by a very-low-calorie diet: a controlled clinical trial. Obes Res 1995;549.

198. Davis R, Faulds D. Dexfenfluramine: an updated review of its therapeutic use in the management of obesity. Drugs 1996;52:696.

199. McCann UD et al. Brain serotonin neurotoxicity and primary pulmonary hypertension from fenfluramine and dexfenfluramine: a systematic review of the evidence. JAMA 1997;278:666.

200. Luque CA, Rey JA. Sibutramine: a serotonin-norepinephrine reuptake-inhibitor for the treatment of obesity. Ann Pharmacother 1999;33:968.

201. Lean JEJ. Sibutramine—a review of clinical efficacy. Int J Obes Relat Metab Disorder 1997; 21(Suppl 1):S30.

202. Heal DJ et al. A comparison of the effects on central 5-HT function of sibutramine hydrochloride and other weight-modifying agents. Br J Pharmacol 1998;125:301.

203. Bray GA et al. Sibutramine produces dose-related weight loss. Obes Res 1999;7:189.

204. Weintraub M et al. Sibutramine in weight control: a dose-ranging, efficacy study. Clin Pharmacol Ther 1991;50:330.

205. Wirth A, Krause J. Long-term weight loss with sibutramine: A randomized controlled trial. JAMA 2001;286(11):1331.

206. Wadden TA et al. Benefits of lifestyle modification in the pharmacologic treatment of obesity: a randomized trial. Arch Intern Med 2001;161:218.

207. James W et al. A one-year trial to assess the value of orlistat in the management of obesity. Int J Obes 1997;21(Suppl):S24.

208. Guerciolini R. Mode of action of orlistat. Int J Obes 1997;21(Suppl):S12.

209. Sjostrom L et al. Randomized placebo-controlled trial of orlistat for weight loss and prevention of weight regain in obese patients. Lancet 1998; 352:167.

210. Davidson MH et al. Weight control and risk factor reduction in obese subjects treated for 2 years with orlistat: a randomized controlled trial. JAMA 1999; 281(3):235.

211. Heck AM et al. Orlistat, a new lipase inhibitor for the management of obesity. Pharmacotherapy 2000; 20(3):270.

212. Anderson JW et al. Bupropion SR enhances weight loss: a 48-wk double-blind, placebo-controlled trial. Obes Res 2002;10(7):633.

213. McElroy SL et al. Topiramate in the treatment of binge eating disorder associated with obesity: A randomized, placebo-controlled trial. Am J Psychiatry 2003;160:255.

214. Greenway FL. Surgery for obesity. Endocrinol Metab Clin North Am 1996;25:1005.

215. Taylor D, McAskill R. Atypical antipsychotics and weight gain—a systematic review. Acta Psychiatr Scand 2000;101:415.

216. Vanina Y et al. Body weight changes associated with psychopharmacology. Psychiatric Serv 2002; 53(7):842.

217. Fava M et al. Fluoxetine versus sertraline and paroxetine in major depressive disorder: changes in weight with long-term treatment. J Clin Psychiatry 2000;61(11):863.

CHAPTER **83**

Drug Abuse

Wendy O. Zizzo, Paolo V. Zizzo

ADDICTIVE DISEASE

Physical addiction or dependence occurs when repeated administration of a drug causes an altered physiologic state (neuroadaptation). Following neuroadaptation, a characteristic set of withdrawal symptoms occurs when the drug is abruptly discontinued. Psychological addiction or psychological dependence refers to a "behavioral pattern of drug use, characterized by overwhelming involvement with the use of a drug (compulsive use), the securing of its supply, and a high tendency to relapse after withdrawal."[1] Habituation is a state of either chronic or periodic drug use characterized by a desire (but not a compulsion) to continue using the drug, no tendency to increase the dose, and an absence of physical addiction despite some degree of psychological dependence.

These conditions collectively are now thought of as addictive disease. There is a different clinical syndrome associated with each drug, but all involve a chronic process with progressive deterioration of psychological and physiologic activity secondary to the habitual use of a drug. Although the neurochemistry of the addictive process is possibly the same for all drugs, the psychosocial and pharmacokinetic aspects vary from drug to drug. There is evidence, consistent with models established for alcoholism, that genetically inherited traits may result in expression of addictive disease when the person is exposed to certain drugs and other habituating psychic stimuli.[2–4]

The *DSM-IV* cites criteria for substance-related disorders and divides them into two groups: the substance use disorders (including criteria for distinguishing between substance dependence and abuse) and the substance-induced disorders (intoxication, withdrawal, and others).[5]

DRUG CULTURE

The drug-using population has developed colloquialisms referring to specific drugs as well as many of the aspects of their drug-using lives. Clinicians encountering unfamiliar expressions should simply ask the patient to explain any terms that are not mutually understood. Most patients are surprisingly willing to describe their drug use if they trust the clinician's ability to help them.

It is worthwhile to look at the business aspects of the illicit drug trade to gain some perspective on the accuracy of historical information provided by the patient. The supply of drugs to the illicit marketplace is subject to the demand for such commodities and obeys laws of economics just like other businesses. Nevertheless, there are some notable differences. There is no quality control at illicit drug laboratories such as that mandated by the Food and Drug Administration for legally sanctioned pharmaceutical manufacturers. Premarketing research for efficacy and safety is not of concern to illicit drug laboratories. The chemicals that the underground chemist must use to synthesize the desired products are to some degree controlled and monitored by the "narcs" (law enforcement officers, specifically plainclothes narcotics officers). As a particular drug synthesis process becomes known to law enforcement authorities, the sale of the required chemicals becomes restricted, and the illicit drug chemists will use alternate methods of synthesis, sometimes with unpredictable results. The dealer (drug seller) is generally attempting to maximize profits and may dilute the relatively expensive drug with cheaper sugars, local anesthetics, and other substances. Frequently, a cheaper or more readily available chemical is substituted for the one desired by the customer (e.g., ephedrine or phenylpropanolamine sold as amphetamine). Generally, substituted drugs are in the same pharmacologic class; otherwise, the customer would not obtain the desired psychic effect and would not purchase more drug from that dealer. Nor will a dealer wish to put any acutely toxic chemical in the drugs sold, because such an action discourages further purchases.

Despite a trend toward drugs of higher purity in the illicit marketplace, clinicians should be aware that the patients often do not really know which drug they have taken. Any history obtained from users concerning drug use should be substantiated by looking for the expected physical symptoms and obtaining appropriate laboratory studies. Any paraphernalia such as syringes or drug samples brought to the clinician may provide valuable evidence to explain a pathologic state. Needles should be considered infectious and should never be handled; they should be promptly discarded into appropriate needle disposal boxes.

URINE SCREENING

1. J.R., who is applying for a new job, has been told that his pre-employment physical will include a urine drug screen. He is worried because for the past 6 months he has been smoking one joint (i.e., cigarette) of marijuana per day, using cocaine twice per week, and drinking a half-pint of brandy to sleep on the days when he has been using cocaine. He last used these drugs 1 week ago. Now he wants to know if he can cleanse his urine of drugs in 2 days by drinking lots of water and exercising heavily. What is a reasonable answer to his question?

Drug users use several methods to avoid detection of illicit drugs in their urine. In addition to exercise and hydration, attempts at enhancing excretion include taking diuretics (attempted forced diuresis), drinking vinegar or cranberry juice and taking vitamin C (attempted pH manipulation for ion trapping of drugs in the urine and enhancing excretion), taking saunas (attempted hastening of drug elimination from fat stores), buying clean urine from a drug-free individual (assumes that the urine collection is unobserved so the switching of samples can be accomplished), and adding bleach, isopropanol, or salt (NaCl) to the urine sample (inactivates the enzymes used by the popular immunoassay "urine drug screen" systems). Most of these methods are derived from research literature describing the immunoassay techniques. While each of the above techniques may decrease the urinary concentration of a drug to some small degree, none of these methods will enhance the total body clearance of drug. Dehydration (e.g., from diuretics) may actually increase the effective drug concentration in the urine, allowing easier detection. Forced fluid administration, resulting in a greatly increased output of dilute urine, may cause a false-negative result for some very weakly positive urine samples, but dilution will not mask even a moderately positive sample.[6]

The immunoassay techniques used for drug detection are not 100% accurate. Several over-the-counter medications, foods, and workplace chemicals are cross-reactive and may produce false-positive results for certain intoxicating drugs.[7] For example, diphenhydramine in the urine can cause a false-positive result for methadone, phenylpropanolamine may test positive for amphetamine, and cloxacillin may test positive for benzodiazepines. Current product information should be studied for specific test systems, which are constantly being altered to minimize spurious results.

The use of the following drugs will result in positive urine tests from 1 to 4 days after the last dose: amphetamines, barbiturates (short-acting), cocaine (possibly up to 3 weeks for heavy users), hallucinogens, ethanol, and opioids (except methadone). Single or short-term use of marijuana can be detected in the urine even after 4 to 10 days; chronic use can be detected for 2 months or more. Methadone, phencyclidine, and phenobarbital will test positive in the urine for 1 to 2 weeks.

Drug testing does not pick up sporadic use that falls outside of these ranges, nor does it indicate chronicity of use. A positive test obtained by random screening is as likely to represent first-time use as it is chronic use.[8] Drug test results should be interpreted only by persons familiar with the laboratory technology and the pharmacokinetics of the drugs being tested.

Therefore, J.R.'s urine is likely to be positive only for marijuana when he is tested, assuming he uses no drugs in the meantime. Forced fluids and exercise will not affect his urinary drug tests.

OPIOIDS
Heroin

2. D.J., age 28, has been "fixing" (injecting) two "quarter bags" ($25 worth) of "junk" (heroin sold on the street) daily for about a month. This "run" (daily use) began when he met a new "connection" (drug supplier) at a party. D.J. describes a steady supply of "Mexican tar." He explains he began smoking the heroin but has now progressed to injecting. What is "Mexican tar"?

Over the past decade, there has been a dramatic shift in the heroin market in the United States. Southeast Asia, formerly the dominant supplier, has been replaced by South America, particularly in the East. However in the West, "Mexican tar" or "black tar" heroin from Mexico is the predominant form. The South American heroin (sold as a white powder) is frequently >90% pure, and this has resulted in increased availability of high-purity heroin from all sources. According to the Drug Enforcement Administration, the average purity for retail heroin from all sources in the year 2000 was 36.8% (compared to 26% in 1991 and 7% two decades ago).[9] This has led to a new, younger user population, who can smoke or snort this high-purity heroin and avoid the stigma and hazards associated with needle use. However, as the addiction progresses and the user's "habit" (amount used daily) increases, the user will often begin injecting the drug.

Traditionally, heroin has been sold in balloons containing 250 to 400 mg of powder. This quantity of heroin is often called a "dime" ($10) or "quarter" ($25) bag. Mexican tar, which looks and feels like sticky black roofing tar, is either sold raw as a sticky, 25-mg blob or as a "gumball," which is placed in the bottom or corner of a twisted or folded piece of plastic wrap or cellophane. This "gumball" is difficult for a dealer to discreetly "cut" (i.e., dilute with a cheap adulterant).

The increased availability of high-purity heroin has also been associated with a fall in price. This has led to significantly greater levels of heroin use nationwide. The number of heroin users in the United States has increased dramatically since the early 1990s, from an estimated regular user population of 630,000 in 1992 to 977,000 in 2002. In addition, the United States in the year 2002 had an estimated 514,000 occasional heroin users.[10]

Heroin Addiction

3. D.J. developed a "big habit" (tolerance developed, and his daily requirement of drug to maintain euphoria had increased). He could not "hustle" (obtain by any means) any more cash on a daily basis. When he tried "kicking" (abrupt cessation of drug use) the drug "cold turkey" (without any therapy for withdrawal symptoms), he became "dope sick" (typical heroin withdrawal symptoms), which was extremely unpleasant. He has been "chipping" (using only occasionally) since his withdrawal. Is D.J. "hooked" (addicted)?

Abstinence precipitated a withdrawal syndrome in D.J.; therefore, he is by definition physically addicted to heroin. The powerful ability of the drug to end the misery of withdrawal results in reinforcement to continue using the drug. D.J.'s ongoing desire to continue using heroin despite his inability to afford it and his all-day hustling constitutes a psychological dependence on heroin.

Noticeable physical dependence (demonstrated by the onset of an obvious withdrawal syndrome upon abstinence) is highly variable but usually is not apparent until after 2 to 4 weeks of daily use of heroin.

Opioid Withdrawal

4. D.J. arrives at the detoxification clinic 10 hours after his last dose of heroin. He is sweating and shaking and keeps yawning. Should he be treated for opioid withdrawal?

Six to 12 hours after the last dose of morphine or heroin (diacetylmorphine), the addict will develop symptoms of anxiety, hyperactivity, restlessness, and insomnia with yawning, sialorrhea, rhinorrhea, and lacrimation. There may also be profuse diaphoresis with concurrent shaking chills and pilomotor activity resulting in waves of gooseflesh of the skin (thus, the term "cold turkey"). Anorexia, nausea, vomiting, abdominal cramps, and diarrhea occur. Severe back pain may accompany muscle spasms that cause kicking movements ("kicking the habit"). These symptoms are most severe 48 to 72 hours after the last opioid dose. D.J. is exhibiting typical heroin withdrawal symptoms, and some therapy would be appropriate.

During withdrawal, the heart rate and blood pressure may be elevated. The levels of urinary 17-ketosteroids increase,[11] leukocytosis is common, and the failure to take in food and fluids, combined with vomiting, sweating, and diarrhea, can result in marked weight loss, dehydration, ketosis, and acid–base imbalance. Rarely, cardiovascular collapse has occurred during the peak phase of opiate withdrawal.

The more dramatic symptoms of heroin withdrawal subside after 5 to 10 days of abstinence even without treatment; however, a return to complete physiologic equilibrium may require months or longer.[12]

The character, severity, and time course of withdrawal symptoms that appear when an opioid drug is discontinued depend on many factors, including the particular opioid, total daily dose, interval between doses, duration of use, intent of drug use, and the health and personality of the user. Unlike the withdrawal symptoms from sedative-hypnotic drugs, opioid withdrawal symptoms are seldom life-threatening.

Withdrawal From Different Opioids

5. R.F. says he is addicted to methadone, but hours after his last dose he does not exhibit any signs of opioid withdrawal. Why is this reasonable?

Physiologic withdrawal symptoms from all opioid drugs are qualitatively similar but quantitatively different in onset, duration, and severity. Opioids with shorter durations of action tend to produce brief, intense abstinence syndromes, while those eliminated from the body at much slower rates produce prolonged but milder withdrawal syndromes. The abstinence syndrome of methadone is consistent with that expected for a long-acting opioid. Methadone withdrawal symptoms do not become apparent until 48 to 72 hours after the last dose. Although the symptoms are qualitatively similar to those of morphine and heroin, they are less severe overall but are most intense around the sixth day of abstinence. All observable symptoms except for persistent anorexia, insomnia, and lethargy subside and are minimal after 10 to 14 days of abstinence.[13] R.F. could be telling the truth, as his methadone withdrawal symptoms should not occur until 2 to 3 days after his last dose.

Iatrogenic Addiction

6. **J.B., a 21-year-old man who underwent bowel surgery, required morphine 10 mg subcutaneously Q 4 hr for 10 days. Is J.B. physically addicted to morphine?**

Mild symptoms of withdrawal, which may not even be recognized as such, will occur in patients who have received therapeutic doses of morphine several times daily for 1 or 2 weeks. If narcotic antagonists are administered, withdrawal symptoms can be precipitated in subjects who have been receiving four daily doses of morphine, methadone, or heroin after only 2 or 3 days.[14] Nevertheless, the percentage of patients who continue to seek opioids following the successful treatment of pain with narcotics is very small. The role of physical dependence in the development of compulsive heroin or morphine abuse is almost insignificant when one considers the extremely large number of patients who have received multiple daily doses of opiates during hospital stays lasting >2 or 3 days. Therefore, it would be extremely unlikely that J.B. would be psychologically dependent upon opiates, even though he most likely will experience mild withdrawal symptoms after terminating his morphine. These withdrawal symptoms are usually so mild that they seldom are attributed to opioid abstinence by the patient.

Medical Complications

7. **C.F., age 30, presented to the emergency department with violent shaking chills. She admitted that she was a heroin addict and was forced into "doing some cottons" because of an acute financial crisis. She now fears that she has "cotton fever." How should "cotton fever" be managed, and what other medical complications of heroin addiction might be suspected?**

When heroin is prepared for self-administration, cotton is used as a filter to trap adulterants; thus, some of the drug remains trapped in the cotton. These crude filters are saved, and when money or drug availability is poor, water or other solvents are added to the "old cottons" to extract any remaining drug for intravenous (IV) use. "Cotton fever" is an acute febrile reaction. The onset is within 30 minutes of injection, with shaking chills, diaphoresis, postural hypotension, tachycardia, and low-grade fever. These symptoms are initially suggestive of sepsis, but most of the symptoms resolve without treatment in 2 to 4 hours, with complete recovery in one day. In the past cotton fever was believed to be an allergic reaction to tiny cotton fibers injected with the drug, but a case report suggests that the causal agent is probably *Enterobacter agglomerans,* via a heat-stable endotoxin.[15] Cotton and cotton plants are heavily colonized with *E. agglomerans.*[16] C.F.

should have blood cultures performed and should be started on a regimen of empiric antibiotic therapy.

According to the Drug Abuse Warning Network (DAWN), heroin is consistently among the top three drugs reported in emergency department visits and drug-related deaths.[17,18] Bacterial endocarditis, sepsis, embolism, septic and aseptic abscesses, thrombophlebitis, cellulitis, and necrotizing fasciitis have also resulted from both improper sterilization of injection apparatus and needles and poor injection techniques.

The common practice of sharing "works" (needle and syringe) between friends has resulted in transmission of various infectious diseases. Chief among those is viral hepatitis, specifically the hepatitis C virus (HCV). Four million Americans were infected with HCV as of 1998, and at least 60% of the cases resulted from injection drug use. After 5 years of injecting, as many as 90% of injection drug users are infected with HCV.[19] According to the Centers for Disease Control and Prevention, in the United States, human immunodeficiency virus (HIV) infection due to injection drug use had an overall prevalence of 14% in women and 15% in men in 1997. The seroprevalence varies by region, however, with rates as high as 28% in the Northeast versus 3% in the West.[20] Other infectious diseases such as syphilis, tetanus, botulism, and malaria can be transmitted in a similar manner and should be considered when evaluating this patient.

Heroin Overdose

8. **T.F., age 21, was unconscious after an alleged "OD" (overdose) on "smack" (heroin). He had a decreased respiratory rate of four breaths per minute, cyanosis, symmetrically "pinned" (maximally miotic or pinpoint) pupils, and a slightly decreased blood pressure. He has one "fresh track" (needle puncture wound) and several "old tracks" (healed scars from needle puncture wounds) in the antecubital fossa area. What is the immediate treatment of choice in this patient?**

Immediate treatment includes airway management, cardiorespiratory support (ACLS if indicated), and opioid reversal with naloxone. Naloxone is a full opioid antagonist that rapidly reverses the respiratory depression and hypotension associated with overdose. The preferred route of administration is IV, but if access cannot be gained it may be given intramuscularly, subcutaneously or by endotracheal tube.[21]

Initial IV administration of 0.2 to 0.4 mg naloxone should be slow and should be discontinued if T.F. responds. There is no need to precipitate opioid withdrawal symptoms; the endpoint of naloxone therapy is a relative stabilization of the patient's vital signs. A naloxone-precipitated, sudden-onset withdrawal syndrome is more severe than the symptoms produced by abstinence alone. Repetitive doses should be given if the patient remains unresponsive, up to a total of 4 to 6 mg of naloxone. If the patient still has not responded, then another diagnosis should be quickly considered.[22] Overdose with buprenorphine, for example, may require much higher doses of naloxone.[23]

The duration of action of naloxone ranges from 20 to 60 minutes, depending on the dose and route of administration. Management of the methadone-overdosed patient will require serial dosing of naloxone every 20 to 60 minutes, since the toxic effects of this long-acting opiate recur. The patient must be carefully observed for about 6 hours following the termination of naloxone therapy to detect any reappearance of opioid intoxication. An IV infusion of naloxone may be appropriate if high doses are needed or if the patient has recurrent respiratory depression. Naloxone also has a very high therapeutic index. A single oral naloxone dose of 3,000 mg and IV doses of 80 to 100 mg have been tolerated with no reported side effects.[21] It does not produce tolerance or signs of physical dependence.[24,25]

Treatment of Opioid Dependence

9. A.X. has been addicted to heroin for 3 years but is tired of the street scene and wants to "get clean" (complete abstinence). He can no longer afford his growing daily habit but is not sure he can stop using opioids. He seems willing and determined to try anything. What treatments are available to him?

The ultimate goal of most detoxification programs is to transform the narcotic addict into a responsible, drug-free, emotionally stable, and productive member of society. Despite many claims, no program to date fulfils all of these goals. Furthermore, all programs either have a high recidivism rate or do not produce a drug-free state in the patient. Heroin addiction, or any other chronic compulsive form of drug abuse, is a symptom of a wide range of problems in the addictive disease patient. Therefore, no single treatment modality can be universally applied to all patients.

Treatment options may be loosely divided into either social model programs or medical model programs. Either model may be inpatient or outpatient based. Social model programs use a nonmedical approach to detoxification and ongoing recovery. Detoxification usually involves the "cold turkey" method of abrupt cessation of the opioid without supportive therapy. Medical model programs are based on pharmacotherapeutic treatment managed by medical professionals and additionally offer recovery-oriented counselling. One therapeutic approach involves opioid substitution for detoxification or maintenance. Currently methadone, levomethadyl acetate (formerly levo-alpha acetyl methadol [LAAM]), and buprenorphine are FDA approved for these indications.[26] Another approach involves symptomatic treatment of withdrawal. The mainstay of this approach is the α_2-agonist clonidine. A third approach employs rapid detoxification precipitated by an opioid antagonist under general anesthesia.

The Drug Addiction Treatment Act of 2000 allows qualified physicians to prescribe Schedule III, IV, and V medications approved for the treatment of opioid dependence in an office-based setting.[27] Currently only buprenorphine, a Schedule III medication, is approved for this indication.

With A.X.'s apparently strong psychological addiction to heroin (he does not know if he can live without opioids) and his desire to be abstinent, it would seem appropriate to attempt gradual detoxification with intensive psychosocial counselling, as opposed to maintenance therapy.

Substitution Pharmacotherapies for Opioid Dependence
Methadone Detoxification

10. A.X. starts a methadone detoxification program at a local methadone clinic. He claims to have a $100-a-day habit. What is the recommended methadone dose for starting treatment?

Methadone is a synthetic, fully addictive, orally acting opiate with a prolonged duration of action of 12 to 24 hours. Pharmacologically, it is qualitatively identical to morphine and other opioid analgesics.[28] Pioneered by Dole and Nyswander, methadone substitution was considered the treatment of choice for opioid addiction by many researchers by 1970.[29,30] It continues to be widely used today, but methadone has emerged as a drug of abuse and many deaths have resulted from its excessive use.[31]

The quality of illicit heroin is highly variable, as affected by the variables of the illicit marketplace. Methadone treatment units, like most large drug detoxification centers, send drug samples from the street to their contract laboratory (often it is the Drug Enforcement Administration's or local police department's crime laboratory) for both qualitative and quantitative analysis. By this evaluation, the currently available supply (which may vary from 0.5% to about 95% purity) has an average of 10% heroin. Usually 1 mg of methadone can substitute for 4 mg of morphine, 2 mg of heroin, or 20 mg of meperidine.[32] This addict reportedly uses $100/day or four "quarter bags" ($25) daily, each containing about 300 mg of powder, of which about 10% or 30 mg supposedly is heroin. Therefore, his total daily dose is about 120 mg of heroin, which is comparable to approximately 60 mg/day of methadone. Since a 20% daily reduction in dose is well tolerated with only a little discomfort, his initial methadone dose of 60 mg/day can be decreased on subsequent days to daily doses of 48 mg, 38 mg, 30 mg, 24 mg, 19 mg, 15 mg, 12 mg, 10 mg, and 8 mg on day 10. At that time the methadone can be discontinued. Most patients can be withdrawn completely from opioids in <10 days, but the actual clinical detoxification period varies. The patient should be observed for 2 to 3 days without medication, since the abstinence symptoms from methadone are not apparent for 48 to 72 hours after the last dose. The development of addiction to methadone apparently is not a problem within this withdrawal period, so the patient does not experience the greatly protracted abstinence symptoms associated with abrupt cessation of chronic methadone use.

Most clinicians do not discuss the dose of methadone with the patient. Objective evaluation of the appropriate dose of methadone for either detoxification or maintenance is best accomplished without the complication of patient bias concerning the "fairness" of a given dose. To facilitate administration of unrecognizable doses and to minimize diversion, the methadone dose is mixed into orange juice, which the patient must drink in the presence of the clinician.

Buprenorphine Detoxification

11. A.X. heard about a medication called buprenorphine that can be used instead of methadone. How might this medication be used for A.X.?

Buprenorphine, a synthetic partial opioid agonist, was approved by the FDA in October 2002 for the treatment of opioid dependence. It is a partial agonist at μ receptors, and in opioid-dependent patients it prevents withdrawal symptoms. However, at high doses buprenorphine can act as an antagonist and precipitate withdrawal. Due to its partial effects, it produces maximum "ceiling" analgesia with sublingual doses of 24 to 32 mg, a dosage equivalent to only 60 to 70 mg of oral methadone. This limits its use in the management of heroin addiction.

Buprenorphine has a long half-life due to its prolonged occupancy of μ receptors and produces a relatively mild withdrawal when discontinued. It is believed to be a safer alternative to methadone, as life-threatening respiratory depression is much less likely to occur than with a pure μ agonist, unless another central nervous system (CNS) depressant is taken concurrently. Most deaths involving buprenorphine have been caused by a combination of the drug with benzodiazepines.[26,33] Naloxone may not reverse respiratory depression caused by buprenorphine because of its prolonged occupancy of μ receptors.

Because buprenorphine is a Schedule III medication, it can be prescribed in an office-based setting under the Drug Addiction Treatment Act of 2000, as previously discussed. It is available as 2- and 8-mg tablets for sublingual use. The tablets contain buprenorphine hydrochloride alone or in combination with naloxone. The naloxone is poorly absorbed orally, and its presence in the combination tablets is to discourage the IV abuse of buprenorphine. When initiating buprenorphine, the first dose should not be given until ≥4 hours after the last dose of a short-acting opioid such as heroin, or 24 hours after a long-acting opioid such as methadone. Induction dosing should begin with 2 or 4 mg on the first day, which can be repeated every 2 to 4 hours if withdrawal symptoms subside and then reappear, up to a maximum of 8 mg. The dose can then be titrated the second day in 2- to 4-mg increments to a dose of 12 to 16 mg. Higher doses during induction may precipitate withdrawal symptoms. Most patients can be stabilized on 8 to 32 mg per day. Once stabilized, it may be possible to switch to alternate-day or three-times-a-week dosing schedules. The patient then can either be maintained on that dose or detoxified with tapering doses.[34]

Maintenance Therapy

12. A.X.'s friend B.P. also attends the methadone clinic but is on methadone maintenance. How is methadone used in maintenance therapy? Are there any maintenance alternatives?

During methadone maintenance, the addict is stabilized on a dose of methadone that will be sufficient to suppress heroin withdrawal symptoms for 12 to 24 hours without producing euphoria. Although methadone-maintained addicts often receive a daily methadone dose of >100 mg, the daily dose needed to prevent the onset of opioid withdrawal symptoms is generally <50 mg. The drug is administered in one daily oral dose to maintain daily contact with the patient. With the aid of daily counseling and rehabilitation, most clinicians attempt to eventually detoxify the patient from methadone as well.

The ultimate goal of methadone maintenance is controversial. By enabling addicts to escape from the illicit drug scene, review their present lifestyles, and reorient their goals, rehabilitation becomes possible. Early enthusiasm for methadone maintenance has now been tarnished by its use in the same abuse patterns as other opioids. Methadone is now a desired substitute for heroin among the addict population, even though the "high" it provides is generally considered inferior to that of heroin, codeine, and other opioids.

Whether rehabilitation occurs or is even possible is confused by the lack of clear and widely accepted goals of therapy. The addition of social objectives to the therapeutic medical goal of cessation of heroin self-administration further confuses the issue. Some people believe the patient must remain completely drug-free for life (including methadone) to consider the treatment program a success. Others see opioid addictive disease as a disorder in which some opioid (methadone for example) must always be administered to the addict to correct the underlying biochemical pathology before any social rehabilitation can occur.

Medical staffing problems and disruption of the patient's employment schedules brought about by the necessity for daily doses of methadone stimulated a search for alternative drugs to methadone. "Take home" dosing, allowing addicts to obtain more than a single day's dose of methadone for self-administration, has frequently led to drug diversion and heroin recidivism. A long-acting methadone homolog, levomethadyl acetate, is now available as a maintenance treatment agent to federally approved programs. Levomethadyl acetate is a synthetic opioid with a longer duration of action that allows for a three-times-per-week dosing schedule. The drug is hepatically metabolized into two long-acting metabolites with more potent opioid activity than the parent compound, which results in a delayed onset of action.[35] The delay in time to reach steady-state levels makes it more difficult to adjust the dose during the initial phase of treatment.

Levomethadyl acetate is generally started at a dose of 30 mg, with every-other-day dose adjustments of 5 to 10 mg depending on the patient's response. For patients already maintained on methadone, levomethadyl acetate can be substituted at a dosage 1.2 to 1.3 times the maintenance methadone dose, not to exceed 120 mg. The dose can then be adjusted in 5- to 10-mg increments every second or third day. Most patients stabilize on doses in the range of 50 to 90 mg three times a week.[35] Regulations prohibit take home dosages. Patients unable to come in for scheduled doses can be temporarily transferred to methadone. Maintenance with levomethadyl acetate has been shown to be as effective as methadone, but its use has been associated with prolonged-QT syndrome and arrhythmias and should therefore be reserved for patients in whom other treatments have failed.[36]

Another alternative for maintenance therapy is buprenorphine (see Question 11). As previously discussed, buprenorphine has the advantage of office-based availability, thus removing the stigma associated with attending a methadone clinic.

When levomethadyl acetate, buprenorphine, and high-dose methadone (60 to 100 mg) therapies were compared to low-dose methadone (20 mg),[37] all three therapies were effective in treating opioid dependence and were superior to low-dose methadone.

Pain Management

13. T.A., a 44-year-old man maintained on 120 mg daily of methadone, is in severe pain due to a fractured femur. What type of analgesic, and how much, can be used safely in this patient?

Because of tolerance to the analgesic effects of methadone, full therapeutic doses of analgesic opioids such as morphine, if indicated, should be used. In some cases, higher-than-usual doses and more frequent administration may be necessary. For

T.A., an initial dose of 10 mg of morphine might be used. The usual maintenance dose of methadone should be continued. Opioid withdrawal should be strictly avoided in this patient because it is associated with hypersensitivity to painful stimuli, followed by exaggerated catecholamine and anxiety responses. The partial antagonist/agonist narcotics pentazocine (Talwin), butorphanol (Stadol), buprenorphine (Buprenex), and nalbuphine (Nubain) should be avoided because their narcotic antagonist properties may precipitate opioid withdrawal symptoms when used in the methadone-maintained patient.

T.A.'s clinician at his methadone maintenance clinic should consult with the orthopedic surgeon and should attempt to maintain contact with T.A. during the hospital stay to ensure continuation of methadone maintenance therapy and support throughout a period with a high potential for relapse.

Methadone in Pregnancy

14. J.R., age 28, has been maintained on 100 mg methadone daily for the past year. She is now 8 months pregnant. What is the teratogenic potential of methadone?

Although many babies born to methadone-maintained mothers are premature by weight, methadone does not appear to be teratogenic, nor does it appear to have an adverse effect on mental development. Methadone-maintained women frequently have regular menstrual periods, ovulate, conceive, and have normal pregnancies. Heroin-addicted mothers, however, generally experience more problematic pregnancies because their lifestyle often predisposes them to a poor general state of health and precludes adequate prenatal medical care.[38] Infants born to heroin-addicted mothers may also be exposed to other substances (e.g., alcohol, cocaine, tobacco). These infants tend to be smaller, to weigh less at birth, and to be born prematurely compared to the children of women not using opiates.[39]

Neonatal Addiction

15. Since methadone crosses the placental barrier, will J.R.'s infant exhibit opioid withdrawal symptoms after birth?

Methadone crosses the placental barrier and can cause CNS and respiratory depression as well as opioid abstinence in the newborn. In one study, 50% of the infants born to methadone-maintained mothers exhibited withdrawal signs of twitching and irritability, and half of them required treatment. These withdrawal signs in the newborn may be delayed for up to 3 days.[40] J.R.'s infant will probably display some withdrawal symptoms such as irritability.

Withdrawal During Pregnancy

16. Why should methadone not be discontinued in J.R. despite its adverse effects on the fetus?

Since J.R. is in the eighth month of her pregnancy, she should probably be maintained on methadone to avoid precipitating a withdrawal syndrome. A structured methadone maintenance program that provides access to counseling and medical care is probably at least as beneficial to the pregnancy as the pharmacologic prevention of withdrawal. Lowering the maternal methadone dosage is associated with decreased incidence and decreased severity of neonatal withdrawal symptoms.[41] Therefore, the dose of methadone should be titrated

individually throughout the pregnancy. The neonate can be managed for either opioid-induced CNS depression or methadone withdrawal after delivery as needed.

Breast-Feeding

17. Should J.R. breast-feed her infant?

Methadone is excreted into the breast milk of methadone-maintained mothers. The quantities, though small, may be sufficient to cause some physical dependency in infants, and breast-feeding is not recommended.[42] J.R. should be encouraged to become drug-free if she wishes to breast-feed.

Treatment of Neonatal Addiction

18. What opioid withdrawal symptoms are likely to be manifested by J.R.'s infant, and how should they be managed?

Opioid withdrawal in the neonate manifests as a wide variety of nonspecific signs that might be compatible with numerous serious disorders of the newborn of a mother in poor health. In general, the most common withdrawal symptoms include restlessness, tremors, a high-pitched cry, hypertonicity, increased reflexes, regurgitation, tachypnea, diarrhea, and sneezing. Seizures are associated with but not necessarily caused directly by opioid withdrawal in the neonate.

Management of the neonate's opioid withdrawal syndrome entails careful attention to hydration with demand feeding and symptomatic care. Mild withdrawal symptoms need no therapy, but moderate to severe symptoms may require 14 or more days of treatment. Therapy of neonatal withdrawal should begin when symptoms occur. Prophylactic therapy is not recommended.

Symptoms of physiologic addiction are usually apparent within 48 hours of birth. At this time, treatment can be initiated. One of three medications is currently used to alleviate opioid withdrawal symptoms in the neonate. Phenobarbital is instituted in doses of 8 to 20 mg/kg in the first 24 hours, then tapered symptomatically, usually about 10% to 20% per day.[43] Diluted (i.e., 1:25) tincture of opium (DTO), which is preferred over the camphor-containing paregoric formulation, can be administered in a dose of 3 to 6 drops Q 3 to 6 hr as needed and adjusted to control withdrawal symptoms. Alternatively, DTO may be given at a dosage of 0.2 mL Q 3 hr and increased by 0.05 mL Q 3 hr until withdrawal symptoms are controlled. Paregoric (i.e., camphorated tincture of opium) may be given at the same dosages if used. The patient should be stabilized for 3 to 5 days, and then dosages should be gradually reduced over a 2-week period.[42] A combination of DTO and phenobarbital may be superior to either alone, resulting in shorter hospital stays and less severe withdrawal.[44] Neonatal addiction is an area still in need of much research.

J.R.'s infant initially feeds poorly and by day 2 becomes tremulous and extremely agitated. DTO is started at 0.2 mL Q 3 hr and eventually increased to 0.3 mL Q 3 hr to control the symptoms. This dosage is given for 3 days and then gradually tapered over 2 weeks.

Heroin Antagonist Treatments

19. A.J. is a surgeon seeking rehabilitation and reinstatement of his medical license following 5 years of meperidine abuse.

Why would the antagonist or "heroin blockade" approach to the treatment of opioid addiction be more appropriate for A.J. than methadone maintenance?

Purportedly, methadone (at a dose of 80 to 150 mg or more) blocks the euphoriant effects of other opioids without producing euphoria itself. This dose allegedly produces a high degree of cross-tolerance to other opioids so that it is extremely difficult to "get off" (obtain euphoria) with IV injection of other opioids. However, addicts have been able to obtain euphoria from doses of 60 to 100 mg of methadone. Furthermore, at lower maintenance doses of methadone that do not produce euphoria, addicts have been able to reach euphoric states through the concomitant IV administration of other opioids. Methadone in high blocking doses has become a secondary drug of abuse.

If opioid addiction results from a process of classical and instrumental conditioning and is positively reinforced by self-administration and drug-seeking behavior, then narcotic antagonists may break this addiction cycle. The narcotic antagonists naloxone and naltrexone can block the euphoriant effects of heroin and other opiates, prevent the development of physical dependence, and afford protection from opioid overdose deaths.

Of these two antagonists, only naltrexone appears to have any practical utility. Naloxone (Narcan) is impractical because of its short duration of action and its variable potency when taken orally. Naltrexone (Trexan) is orally active and provides a dose-related duration of opioid blockade. An oral dose of 100 mg of naltrexone will block opiate effects for 2 days, and 150 mg for 3 days. Thus, dosing on Monday, Wednesday, and Friday is possible and convenient for the patient. Patients selected for naltrexone therapy must be opioid free to avoid precipitation of withdrawal. For heroin or morphine addicts, a 4- to 7-day wait is recommended, while methadone addiction requires a 10- to 14-day wait. Patients who are highly motivated to abstain have been most successfully treated with this drug. A.J. is a good candidate for naltrexone therapy because of his desire to become rehabilitated and his need to remain drug-free despite continued access to opioids at work.

Ultra-Rapid Opiate Detoxification

20. **Before A.J. can start naltrexone therapy, he must undergo meperidine detoxification. Would rapid detoxification over a few hours be preferable to the more traditional detoxification methods for A.J.?**

Ultra-rapid opiate detoxification (UROD) has been advocated to shorten the opioid detoxification period by precipitating withdrawal with an opioid antagonist. UROD is performed under heavy sedation or general anesthesia so the patient does not consciously experience the acute withdrawal symptoms. The protocols for UROD vary in terms of the opioid antagonist, anesthetic agent, adjunctive medications, and duration of anesthesia. UROD has been performed as an outpatient or inpatient procedure, with costs ranging from $2,500 to $7,500.

No studies have yet compared UROD with other standard detoxification methods. There is little information regarding referral to ongoing treatment or relapse rates after UROD.[45] In addition, there is a risk of vomiting with aspiration when heavy sedation is used, and some studies have found a small but significant incidence of cardiovascular complications, including cardiac arrest and pulmonary edema.[46] Some patients have reported residual withdrawal symptoms over several days. UROD has been criticized for being simply a "quick fix" that fails to address the underlying behavior changes necessary for recovery. Additionally, it subjects patients to possible morbidity and mortality when there are safer established procedures. While the high cost of UROD will limit its accessibility, it may have a role for select patients who have failed other detoxification treatments.[47] More studies are needed to evaluate the risks and benefits of this approach. UROD would probably not be recommended as a first-line detoxification method for A.J.

Symptomatic Therapy of Opioid Withdrawal

21. **How can A.J.'s opioid withdrawal be managed symptomatically?**

As the heroin problem reached epidemic proportions in the late 1960s, outpatient treatment clinics integrated "street professionals" (ex-addicts) with "paper professionals" (pharmacists, physicians, nurses, psychologists). These individuals serve a large percentage of the addict population and are reasonably successful.

Programs like the Haight-Ashbury Drug Detoxification and Aftercare Project in San Francisco use nonnarcotic drugs to treat heroin withdrawal symptoms and emphasize psychosocial counseling and social-vocational rehabilitation. The four primary symptoms of opioid withdrawal are musculoskeletal aches and pains, anxiety, insomnia, and gastrointestinal disorders. A formulary of medications to treat these symptoms is established by first determining which of the nonnarcotic drugs are acceptable to the patient population. Of these, only those drugs that are associated with the highest therapeutic index and lowest addiction liability are included. Medications are dispensed on a daily basis along with counseling and medical monitoring. After 30 years of use, the medications originally selected remain the best of the numerous alternatives now available.[48]

Musculoskeletal aches and pains are managed individually. For bone or joint pain, a nonsteroidal anti-inflammatory drug (NSAID), such as ibuprofen 800 mg Q 8 hr with food, may be used. Muscle pain or cramps may be treated with a muscle relaxant such as methocarbamol 750 mg Q 6 hr.

Anxiety can be treated with clonidine (Catapres), which has been used for opioid detoxification since 1978. Noradrenergic outflow from the locus ceruleus is increased during opioid withdrawal and is blocked by administration of μ agonist opioids. Symptoms of opioid withdrawal, therefore, are partly due to excessive sympathetic activity in the locus ceruleus. Clonidine, a central α_2-adrenergic agonist, acts on presynaptic autoreceptors to inhibit locus ceruleus noradrenergic outflow during μ agonist opioid withdrawal, thereby significantly reducing anxiety. Clonidine is less effective at treating other target symptoms and therefore is best used in a multidrug regimen. Contraindications to clonidine include diastolic blood pressure <70 mm Hg, concurrent dependence on sedative-hypnotics, and clonidine hypersensitivity or previous intolerance.

A sublingual or oral test dose of 0.1 mg (0.2 mg for patients >91 kg) of clonidine is given: if diastolic blood pressure remains >70 mm Hg, additional doses may be instituted, usually as transdermal patches. Transdermal absorption of clonidine from patches (Catapres-TTS) avoids most of the problems encountered with oral therapy. The number of patches applied to a hairless area of the body (usually the upper back or scapular area) depends upon the patient's lean body weight: <50 kg, clonidine 5 to 7.5 mg (two or three TTS-1 patches); 50 to 91 kg, 10 mg (two TTS-2 patches or one TTS-2 and two TTS-1 patches), and >91 kg, 10 to 15 mg (two or three TTS-2 patches). Patients <73 kg should use two of the TTS-1 patches and one TTS-2 patch so that one TTS-1 patch can be removed in the event of hypotensive complications. Patches are left on for 7 days, are replaced with half the dosage during the second week, and then are discontinued.

Because transdermal delivery of clonidine requires 2 days to reach therapeutic levels, propoxyphene, either as 65-mg capsules as the hydrochloride or 100-mg tablets as the napsylate, is given at a dose of two Q 8 hr for the first 2 days. Oral clonidine is not used during these initial 2 days because of hypotensive complications.

For patients who cannot tolerate clonidine therapy, phenobarbital 30 mg or chlordiazepoxide 25 mg Q 4 to 6 hr may be used for anxiety; propoxyphene (65-mg capsules or 100-mg tablets, two Q 8 hr) can be given for pain; an NSAID can be given for bone or joint pain; and a muscle relaxant can be given for myalgias or cramps. Propoxyphene and antianxiety agents are continued for 14 days and then tapered off every other day over 1 week.

Insomnia is treated with trazodone 50 to 150 mg at bedtime. Alternatively, chloral hydrate 500 to 1,500 mg, flurazepam 30 to 90 mg, or doxepin 50 to 100 mg can be used. Flurazepam should be avoided if the patient has concurrent benzodiazepine dependence; chloral hydrate should not be used for patients receiving disulfiram. Three weeks of therapy is usually required.

Gastrointestinal hyperactivity can be managed using belladonna alkaloids with phenobarbital, two tablets Q 8 hr. Dicyclomine 20 mg Q 6 hr is an alternative. For nausea, prochlorperazine 10 mg or trimethobenzamide 300 mg orally Q 6 hr is used. In addition to suppressing diarrhea and abdominal cramping, the anticholinergic effects of these drugs alleviate the rhinorrhea, sialorrhea, diaphoresis, and lacrimation that occur during opioid withdrawal.

These average daily doses are evaluated daily and adjusted to the patient's needs. Polydrug abusers need individualized detoxification that may need to include additional therapy for alcohol, cocaine, or other drugs of abuse.

These therapeutic interventions have been effective for the population of heroin addicts treated at the Haight-Ashbury Clinic. For addict populations in different social, geographic, and cultural environments, these techniques may need to be modified.

A.J.'s blood pressure and drug history should be evaluated for clonidine therapy. Provided his diastolic blood pressure is >70 mm Hg after the clonidine test dose, he can receive the clonidine patches along with the other medications to treat his withdrawal symptoms, along with daily intensive psychosocial counseling.

SEDATIVE-HYPNOTICS

The sedative-hypnotics are a diverse group of compounds with broad clinical uses, including anesthesia, treatment of anxiety, and treatment of insomnia. Ethanol, also a sedative hypnotic agent, continues to be the most widely abused substance in the United States and is discussed in Chapter 84, Alcohol Abuse. Benzodiazepines, which have replaced barbiturates in clinical practice, have become the prototypical sedative-hypnotic drugs of abuse. Other abused sedative-hypnotic drugs include carisoprodol and γ-hydroxybutyrate (GHB). Carisoprodol, a nonscheduled skeletal muscle relaxant, has an active metabolite meprobamate, a sedative-hypnotic agent with known abuse potential.[49] GHB is a putative neurotransmitter abused for its euphoric and sedative-hypnotic effects.[50]

Onset of Sedative-Hypnotic Dependence

22. **During a year of therapy for anxiety, B.J. increased his dose of diazepam to two 10-mg tablets four times a day. Now he wants to stop using sedative drugs. Will he experience withdrawal symptoms if he suddenly discontinues diazepam?**

Withdrawal syndromes seen with sedative-hypnotics are similar to those seen with alcohol withdrawal. Patients who have been on long-term courses of therapeutic doses of these drugs often experience some withdrawal symptoms on abrupt discontinuation of therapy, a condition commonly referred to as long-term low-dose dependence. B.J. will likely experience withdrawal symptoms if he abruptly discontinues diazepam.

Abstinence Syndromes

23. **B.J. agrees that he is addicted to diazepam but is determined to be drug-free. On Friday he gives you the remainder of his tablets and proclaims that by Monday, "I'll be a new man!" Should you encourage him to pursue this course of action?**

Abstinence signs and symptoms may include insomnia, anxiety, and tremors of the upper extremities, muscular weakness, anorexia, nausea, and postural hypotension. They usually appear early. Postural hypotension may be of value in differentiating the abstinence syndrome from ordinary anxiety states. Generalized tonic-clonic seizures may occur as isolated seizures or as status epilepticus. The psychoses that develop resemble the delirium tremens produced by alcohol withdrawal and are usually characterized by disorientation, agitation, delusions, and hallucinations. During the delirium, hyperthermia and agitation may lead to exhaustion, rhabdomyolysis, cardiovascular collapse, or death. Abstinence from short-acting barbiturates and meprobamate produces symptoms that peak within 2 or 3 days. With long-acting sedatives, these symptoms take about a week to appear and are generally milder. Discontinuation of short-acting benzodiazepines (e.g., lorazepam, oxazepam, alprazolam, temazepam) results in the abrupt onset of withdrawal symptoms. Long-acting agents, and those with active metabolites, have a gradual onset of milder withdrawal symptoms compared to the short-acting agents. Withdrawal symptoms following chronic diazepam use typically appear after a week of abstinence.

B.J. has been taking twice the recommended upper limit of diazepam. It is likely that he will experience withdrawal, possibly including seizures, if he were to abruptly discontinue the diazepam. He should be encouraged for his desire to be drug-free, but his withdrawal from this medication should be medically managed. Furthermore, the decision to begin detoxification therapy over a weekend, when many clinics are closed, is not wise. He should undergo an initial physical examination and plan to be absent from his place of employment for at least a week to begin detoxification.

Treatment of Sedative Withdrawal

24. Would it be appropriate to encourage B.J. simply to reduce his diazepam dose by 10% per day until he is drug-free?

Treatment of sedative-hypnotic dependence focuses on preventing major symptoms and minimizing minor symptoms. The patient could probably be stabilized on any sedative-hypnotic and tapered slowly. However, many clinicians prefer phenobarbital for substitution withdrawal because it has a wide safety margin and long duration of action.[51] Avoidance of peaks and troughs of serum and brain levels by using a long-acting drug such as phenobarbital is desirable. Phenobarbital also is less likely to produce euphoria than most benzodiazepines and therefore has little to no street value.

The patient who is abusing sedative-hypnotics already has a strong association between the drug of choice and certain desired effects. Therefore, to minimize exacerbating addictive disease, the drug of abuse should never be used for detoxification. However, for patients with therapeutic dose dependence, an individualized taper of their drug over 6 to 12 weeks may be appropriate.[52]

The method of phenobarbital substitution involves calculating a replacement dose for the total daily dose of the sedative-hypnotic being abused. The calculation is based on phenobarbital equivalents, where 30 mg of phenobarbital is substituted for the following doses of sedative-hypnotics: alprazolam 0.5 to 1 mg, butalbital 100 mg, carisoprodol 350 mg, clonazepam 1 to 2 mg, diazepam 10 mg, ethanol 30 to 60 mL, lorazepam 2 mg, and temazepam 30 mg. If multiple sedative-hypnotics are being used, the totals for each drug and alcohol are summated. The total phenobarbital substitution dose should be given in divided doses, three or four times daily. Since the calculated dosage is an estimate based on patient history, which may be inaccurate, it is advisable to administer a test dose if the calculated replacement dose is >180 mg/day. The test dose, generally one-third the total dose, is given to the patient, who is then observed for 1 to 2 hours. The patient is observed for mitigation of withdrawal symptoms as well as signs of overmedication, such as somnolence or incoordination. Once an appropriate dose is determined, the patient is usually stabilized on that dose for 1 to 2 weeks. Following stabilization, an open-ended taper of phenobarbital is instituted, with dosages reduced by 30 mg Q 2 to 3 days as tolerated.[53]

B.J. has an addiction to diazepam, so it is a poor choice for tapering his dosage. Phenobarbital should be substituted for diazepam. His total dose of diazepam is 80 mg/day, so he should receive 240 mg of phenobarbital divided three or four times a day.

γ-Hydroxybutyrate

25. L.S. has been attending "raves" (all-night dance parties) every weekend for the past few months. She has been taking "liquid Ecstasy" at these parties and believes it is a safe drug because she heard it once was sold in health food stores. What drug is she likely taking, and what are the risks with its use?

γ-Hydroxybutyrate (GHB), commonly referred to as "liquid Ecstasy," has emerged as a potent "club drug." Once available as an over-the-counter nutritional supplement, primarily used by bodybuilders, it was removed from the retail market by the Food and Drug Administration in 1990 due to widespread reports of poisoning. GHB is structurally similar to GABA, although it does not appear to have direct action at the GABA receptors in usual doses. It is believed to be a neurotransmitter and causes increased release of dopamine and endogenous opioids, but its exact mechanism of action is not well understood.[50]

GHB has CNS depressant effects and is abused for its euphorigenic properties. It has a steep dose-response curve, and common adverse effects include dizziness, nausea, weakness, agitation, hallucinations, seizures, respiratory depression, and coma.[54] It effects are synergistic with alcohol.

Tolerance and physical dependence can occur with regular use, and a withdrawal syndrome has been seen in people who have taken high doses of GHB. Withdrawal symptoms may include muscle cramps, tremor, anxiety, insomnia, and delirium. Treatment of withdrawal using sedative-hypnotics remains unclear and should be reserved for severe cases.[50]

GHB may be misrepresented as a natural and safe hypnotic. The low therapeutic index and the unknown purity of illicit supplies, particularly when sold in solution, make this a potentially dangerous drug. Physical dependency is a possibility as well. L.S. should be educated about GHB's potential risks.

CENTRAL NERVOUS SYSTEM STIMULANTS

Cocaine

Cocaine is a naturally occurring alkaloid derived from the *Erythroxylon coca* plant, found mainly in the Andes Mountains of South America. Cocaine was first isolated in the 1800s and was a common ingredient in tonics and elixirs of the 1900s. The Harrison Narcotic Act of 1914 prohibited nonmedical use, and in 1970 it became a Schedule II controlled substance. Except for ethanol, tobacco, and cannabis, it is today the most frequently used drug of abuse. According to the 2001 National Household Survey on Drug Abuse, an estimated 27 million people in the continental United States have tried cocaine; 4 million people used cocaine within the previous year, and 1.7 million used cocaine at least once within a month before the survey.[55] Cocaine is a CNS stimulant and has vasoconstrictive and local anesthetic properties. Cocaine's stimulant effects are primarily due to blockade of reuptake of dopamine, norepinephrine, and serotonin. It also facilitates the release of dopamine and norepinephrine. This results in an overall increase in availability of neurotransmitters. Cocaine also has other indirect effects on neurophysiology, including effects on the endogenous opioid systems.[56,57] Cocaine is associated with compulsive use. The powerful reinforcing effects of cocaine have been identified as occurring in brain regions rich in dopaminergic nerve terminals.[56]

Dosage Forms and Routes of Administration

26. C.H. and his friends bought an "eight ball" (one eighth of an ounce) of "blow" (powdered cocaine). C.H. has only snorted cocaine, but one of his friends suggests they cook up some "rocks" to smoke. What are the distinctions between the various dosage forms and their respective routes of administration?

In the manufacture of cocaine, organic solvents are used to solubilize the alkaloidal bases from the leaves, which are then precipitated to form a sticky material, called "pasta" or "cocaine paste." The benzoylmethylecgonine (cocaine) in this "pasta" is separated from most of the other plant alkaloids, converted to the hydrochloride or other salts, precipitated, and dried. This product is the white cocaine hydrochloride powder usually seen in the illicit market. The final product is usually "stepped on" or "cut" (diluted) with various adulterants to increase profits for the dealers. According to the Drug Enforcement Administration, in 2001 the average purity of a kilogram of cocaine was 73%.[9] Cocaine is usually purchased on the illicit market in quantities of gram or ounce increments. The cost varies geographically. For example, in 2001, the price ranged from a low of $28 per gram in New York City to $150 per gram in New Orleans.[58]

Powdered cocaine is generally snorted. Usually 10 to 25 mg of powdered cocaine is placed on a mirror or flat surface, formed into a line, and then insufflated through a straw or rolled dollar bill. A typical low to moderate user may consume 1 to 3 g per week.

Cocaine powder may also be used for IV injection. The highly water-soluble powder is usually mixed with water and injected. When cocaine is injected simultaneously with heroin, this is known as a "speedball."

Cocaine hydrochloride melts at a high temperature, destroying much of its psychoactivity in the process. Therefore, it is inefficient to smoke cocaine hydrochloride in this form. The use of cocaine "freebase" became popular during the late 1970s, as this form of cocaine has a lower melting point and can therefore be smoked, producing an intense rush.

For freebase, the cocaine hydrochloride is dissolved into ethyl ether. When an alkali such as bleach (sodium hypochlorite) or sodium bicarbonate is added to this ethyl ether, the hydrochloride salt is cleaved from the free alkaloidal cocaine base. The sugars, salts, and some of the other water-soluble adulterants are precipitated out of solution, and the free alkaloidal base remains in the ethyl ether solution. When the ether is evaporated, the freebase of cocaine remains in a powder form. The synthesis of freebase is dangerous and the resultant product may contain residual organic solvents, thus making it highly volatile and putting the user at risk of burns.

In the mid-1980s a safer, easier method for extracting the cocaine base supplanted the traditional freebase process. In the manufacture of "crack," cocaine hydrochloride is dissolved in water. When alkali (bleach or sodium bicarbonate) is added to this aqueous solution, the free alkaloidal base ("crack") precipitates out while the salts and some adulterants stay in aqueous solution. The precipitate is commonly referred to as a "rock." The size of the rock varies but generally ranges from one tenth of a gram to a half a gram. Rocks can sell for $3 to $50, but prices generally range from $10 to $20.[9]

Both manufacturing methods produce cocaine free alkaloidal base of 90% or greater purity. Depending on the efficiency of the extraction process, 37% to 96% of the cocaine is recovered.[59,60] Smoking "crack" has surpassed snorting as the most common way to use cocaine.

Pharmacokinetics and Effects

27. C.H.'s friend gets some baking soda and water from the kitchen and proceeds to convert a few grams of their cocaine into "rock." After smoking a few "hits" (doses), C.H. feels euphoric, energized, and self-confident. Are these typical cocaine effects?

C.H. is indeed describing the euphoria associated with cocaine use. Cocaine generally produces a euphoriant action with a rapid onset and short duration. Snorting cocaine generally produces euphoria and stimulation within 2 minutes; smoking produces these effects within 6 to 8 seconds. Cocaine has a short elimination half-life of approximately 30 minutes due to its rapid metabolism by plasma esterases. Most of its metabolites are excreted in the urine within 24 hours.[61]

An initial relaxed, euphoric, gregarious, talkative, hyperactive state characterizes the "high" of cocaine. Additionally, the person may report increased interest in sexual matters, diminished short-term memory, periods of intense concentration on one limited subject, diminished hunger, hypervigilance, and a peculiar, slightly out-of-body sense of one's actions. Without additional doses of cocaine, these feelings usually resolve into a state of mild depression, fatigue, hunger, and sleepiness by 1 to 3 hours. Physiologic manifestations include mydriasis, sinus tachycardia, vasoconstriction with hypertension, bruxism, repetitive behavior, hyperthermia, and talkativeness.[61] After a few hours, continuous self-administration of cocaine will begin to progress from euphoria to dysphoria and hallucinosis and then to psychosis. Some users engage in nonstop binges of self-administration until psychological toxicity develops.

Adverse Effects

28. C.H. and his friends continue to smoke crack for the next 10 hours. C.H. decides to go out for a pack of cigarettes and collapses on the sidewalk outside his apartment. A passerby calls 911 and C.H. is rushed to the nearest emergency department in a semiconscious state. What has happened to C.H.?

Cocaine is the most frequently mentioned illicit substance in emergency department visits. In 2001 there were 193,000 reported cocaine-related visits to an emergency department in the United States.[62] The potential adverse effects associated with both acute and chronic use of cocaine are numerous and involve most organ systems in the body.

The cardiac complications associated with cocaine use include hypertension, arrhythmias, myocardial ischemia and infarction, dilated cardiomyopathy and hypertrophic cardiomyopathy, myocarditis, aortic dissection, and acceleration of atherosclerosis. These cardiac effects have occurred in individuals with and without underlying heart disease who have taken large or small doses by all routes of administration and may be associated with acute or chronic use. The cardiac events may occur before, during, or after other toxicities such as seizures and may be fatal. The mechanism of cocaine-induced myocardial infarction is most likely multifactorial, involving one or more of the following processes: coronary artery vasoconstriction, increased myocardial oxygen demand related to increased blood pressure and increased heart rate, increased platelet aggregation and thrombus formation, coronary vasospasm, and arrhythmia. The risk is greatest within the first hour following use.[63,64]

The medical management of acute coronary syndromes differs when cocaine is the cause. Specifically, nonselective β-blocker therapy (i.e., propranolol) is contraindicated, thrombolysis should be used with caution, and nitrates and benzodiazepines are part of first-line therapy.[22] In patients with cocaine-associated chest pain, a 12-hour observation period to rule out myocardial infarction or ischemia is probably sufficient before discharge from a medical facility.[65]

Cocaine has also been associated with cerebrovascular catastrophes. Stroke may occur as a result of increased blood pressure, vasoconstriction, or thrombosis. Intracranial hemorrhage and subarachnoid hemorrhage may occur more frequently in patients with underlying arteriovenous malformations or aneurysms.[66] Seizures are another CNS complication.

The route of cocaine administration also affects the nature of the adverse effects. For example, pulmonary complications, including pneumomediastinum, pneumothorax, pneumopericardium, acute exacerbation of asthma, diffuse alveolar hemorrhage, pulmonary edema, and "crack lung," are associated with smoking crack cocaine. Crack lung is a syndrome of acute pulmonary infiltrates associated with a spectrum of clinical and histologic findings.[67] Snorting cocaine may lead to perforation of the nasal septum because of the drug's local anesthetic and vasoconstrictive effects. IV use of cocaine has been associated with renal infarction, wound botulism, hepatitis, acquired immunodeficiency syndrome, bacterial endocarditis, sepsis, and other infectious complications.[68–71]

Medical management of acute cocaine intoxication in a conscious patient should include monitoring for hypertension, tachycardia, hyperthermia, mydriasis, hypertonicity, tremor, and altered mental status. In most cases, symptoms will begin within an hour of the last dose of cocaine and will resolve in 2 to 3 hours without treatment. If this symptom complex persists for >1 hour without improvement, or if the patient is unconscious, clinicians should be prepared to treat seizures, cardiac arrhythmias, myocardial infarction, cerebrovascular accident, rhabdomyolysis with metabolic acidosis and renal failure, cardiovascular collapse, and respiratory arrest. Most cocaine-related deaths are due to either cardiac arrhythmias or respiratory arrest within minutes of the last dose.

C.H. could be suffering from cardiovascular, cerebrovascular, or pulmonary complications due to his crack smoking. His emergency department workup should be thorough and directed by his symptoms.

Cocaine Addiction

29. **C.H. is released from the emergency department and returns home to find his friend with more crack. They resume smoking and binge for the next 4 days. They run out of drugs and money, and C.H. begins to "crash." In desperation he sells his skateboard to his neighbor for $20, buys another rock, smokes it, and feels good again. Is C.H. addicted?**

C.H. continues to use cocaine despite adverse consequences (emergency department visit), uses it compulsively, suffers withdrawal symptoms, and alleviates his symptoms with further use. He is indeed addicted.

Prolonged or heavy use of cocaine has been associated with the development of tolerance to some of its central effects. Tolerance to cocaine's euphoric effects has been shown to occur, but tolerance to its cardiovascular effects may be incomplete.[56] There is a withdrawal syndrome that may follow long-term or binge use. The initial, acute symptoms, referred to as the "crash," consist of depression, fatigue, craving, hypersomnolence, and anxiety. Anhedonia and hyperphagia soon follow. While most symptoms are mild and resolve within 1 to 2 weeks, the dysphoria and anhedonia may persist for weeks. These symptoms do not produce profound physiologic changes and are generally not life-threatening.[56]

Treatment of Addiction

30. **C.H. decides to get clean and seeks help from a detox clinic. What therapeutic options are available to him?**

Most cases of simple cocaine withdrawal do not require medical treatment. However, multiple pharmacologic therapies to facilitate abstinence from cocaine have been, and continue to be, under investigation. Most studies have yielded variable results, and to date no drug exists that is effective in treating cocaine dependence. Alleviation of post-cocaine dysphoria and craving may result from antidepressant alteration of dopamine receptors. Based on the "dopamine depletion hypothesis" that the "crash" results from decreased levels of brain dopamine activity, dopaminergic agents such as bromocriptine or amantadine have been studied. Methylphenidate (Ritalin) has been investigated as "maintenance treatment" to satisfy the cocaine addict's desire for further enhancement of mood; however, methylphenidate also can stimulate a powerful craving for the more intense euphoria of cocaine and has significant abuse potential. Various other treatments have been investigated, including naltrexone, disulfiram, anticonvulsants, and tyrosine.[72]

Because there are currently no drug therapies that are effective or approved by the Food and Drug Administration for the treatment of cocaine addiction, C.H. should receive psychosocial treatment, such as cognitive-behavioral therapy and relapse prevention.

Amphetamines

CNS stimulants have been used both with and without social acceptance for thousands of years. The Chinese prepared ephedrine-containing products from a plant they called Ma-Huang (*Ephedra vulgaris*).[73] People in East Africa and the Arabian peninsula chew the leaves of the khat bush (*Catha edulis*) for the stimulating effects of the alkaloid cathinone.[74] Caffeine is consumed worldwide in a usually socially acceptable manner in the form of coffee and cola soft drinks. CNS stimulation by amphetamine was reported in 1927.[75] The legal sanctions against widespread prescribing of amphetamines in the 1970s restricted their supply and fostered a black market thriving on the illicit production of methamphetamine powder ("speed," "meth," "crank," "crystal meth"). During the 1990s, California and the West Coast experienced a dramatic resurgence of methamphetamine-related hospital admissions, poison center calls, and law enforcement actions. According to the National Household Survey on Drug Abuse for 2001, 16 million Americans used amphetamines at some time in their lives, and 2.4 million had used amphetamines in the past year. Methamphetamine, the most commonly abused illicit type of amphetamine, was used by 9.6 million Americans at some time in their lives, and 1.3 million had used methamphetamine in the past year.[55]

Physical and Psychological Effects

31. **D.C., a college student, used speed this past weekend when partying with his friends. He has a midterm exam in 2 days and is too tired to study, so one of his friends suggests snorting some more speed and then hitting the books. Will this help overcome his fatigue?**

Methamphetamine produces CNS stimulation by enhancing the effects of norepinephrine, serotonin, and dopamine. This is accomplished by both blocking reuptake and stimulating release of these neurotransmitters. These effects are greater for dopamine and norepinephrine than for serotonin. Methamphetamine is metabolized in the liver, and its half-life is 6 to 15 hours.[76]

The powerful stimulating effects of amphetamine and methamphetamine have made their use popular among a wide variety of groups, including students, athletes, the military, dieters, and long-distance truck drivers. Initially, the user may experience wakefulness, euphoria, increased energy, the illusion of increased productivity, sociability, and decreased appetite. Continuous dosing, however, produces stereotypical grooming and other repetitive motions, bruxism, tremor, muscle twitching, mydriasis, hypertension, diaphoresis, elevated body temperature, periods of nausea and vomiting, dry mouth, weight loss, and malnutrition. Continued use over several days decreases productivity and is associated with disordered thoughts, paranoia, and psychosis. Tolerance develops very rapidly after continued use.

Illicit methamphetamine is commonly insufflated or injected, less commonly taken orally. In a pattern similar to that seen with smoking cocaine freebase, users are now freebasing methamphetamine and smoking it. Crystal methamphetamine, known as "crystal meth" or "ice," has become popular in Japan, Hawaii, and the West Coast of the United States. Heating the crystals and smoking the vapor, as with crack, is a common route of administration; however, snorting and IV administration are also used. Absorption is rapid after smoking "ice" and is accompanied by sympathetic stimulation similar to that produced by other forms of methamphetamine. Acute pulmonary edema has also been reported following inhalation.[77]

D.C. will probably be able to stay awake to study if he uses more methamphetamine. However, if he is up for too many days without sleep, his exam performance will likely suffer.

Adverse Effects and Toxicities

32. **D.C. finds speed very much to his liking and begins to use it daily. He goes many days at a time without sleeping or showering and starts losing weight because he seldom has an appetite. His friends start calling him a "tweaker." He believes his friends are working with the DEA and tapping his phone. What is happening to D.C.?**

D.C. is exhibiting classic signs of chronic methamphetamine abuse, which will likely progress if he continues using.

A "speed freak" or "tweaker" (methamphetamine user) is generally regarded even by other drug users as mentally unstable, aggressive, and emotionally labile, with unpredictable periods of violent, even homicidal, behavior.[78] Speed freaks characteristically develop complex paranoid delusional systems with hallucinations during extended periods of intoxication that may involve several sleepless days and nights of continuous methamphetamine administration. This "speed psychosis" may include tactile hallucinations such as formication, the sensation of something crawling under the skin. Initial attempts at reassuring, reality-oriented communication ("talking down") may be successful for an acute psychotic episode. However, an extremely agitated, anxious, psychotic user will often require administration of a benzodiazepine, such as diazepam or lorazepam. If psychosis persists, a high-potency neuroleptic, such as haloperidol, is preferred due to its minimal anticholinergic activity. Low-potency neuroleptics, with higher anticholinergic activity, may worsen symptoms of delirium and hyperthermia.[79]

The physiologic toxicity of stimulant drugs includes hypertension, stroke, seizures, hyperthermia, sexual dysfunction, dental caries, rhabdomyolysis, renal failure, cardiac arrhythmias and cardiomyopathies, myocardial infarction, and malnutrition.

The development of neurotoxicities involving dopaminergic and serotonergic neurons has been demonstrated in animals, but it is less clear if such toxicities develop in humans. While some studies have shown loss of dopamine transporters, resulting in slower motor function and decreased memory, there is evidence of recovery with protracted abstinence.[80]

Withdrawal and Treatment

33. **D.C. is arrested for assault following a bar fight. He is held in the county jail and is unable to post bail. What withdrawal symptoms might he experience during incarceration?**

D.C. will probably suffer intense cravings for methamphetamine and initial agitation, followed by fatigue and hypersomnolence.

A withdrawal state following acute cessation of chronic stimulant use is generally the same as that previously described for cocaine (see Question 29). As with cocaine, the "crash" is notable for marked fatigue, depression, and anhedonia. Most symptoms are mild and will resolve within 1 to 2 weeks, although anhedonia and depression may persist.

Clinical studies investigating treatments for methamphetamine dependence have borrowed from the experience studying cocaine treatments. There are currently no proven effective pharmacologic treatments for methamphetamine dependence. The most effective treatment so far appears to be cognitive-behavioral therapy.[81]

DISSOCIATIVE ANESTHETICS: PHENCYCLIDINE AND KETAMINE

Phencyclidine (phenylcyclohexylpiperidine) and ketamine are arylcycloalkylamine, dissociative, anesthetic agents. Phencyclidine (PCP) at one time was marketed as an IV anesthetic agent under the trade name of Sernyl.[82] Subsequent reports of postanesthetic dysphoric reactions caused the drug to be withdrawn in 1965. It was reintroduced in 1967 as Sernylan and marketed as a veterinary anesthetic until 1978, when the manufacture and sale of the drug became illegal. Ketamine is currently used clinically as an anesthetic in both animals and humans. Ketamine is shorter acting and somewhat less potent than PCP. Ketamine ("K," "Special K") is being used with increased frequency as a "club drug" and is sometimes misrepresented as MDMA (Ecstasy).

PCP first appeared on the street as the "PeaCe Pill" and "hog" in San Francisco and New York in 1966 and later as "angel dust" or "crystal."[83] The popular use of PCP was short-lived, presumably due to unexpected reactions encountered with its use. Subsequently, it reappeared as a substitute for a wide variety of street drugs (e.g., LSD, mescaline, peyote, psilocybin, THC, MDA, amphetamine, and cocaine). The initial adverse experiences with PCP may have been due to excessive doses. Smoking PCP allows for more careful titration of the dose than other routes of administration. Currently, the most common route of administration is smoking PCP that has been applied to parsley, marijuana ("dusted joint," "superweed"), or tobacco cigarettes. Oral, intranasal, and parenteral routes of administration are used by some. The combination of cocaine and PCP in a freebase smoking mixture is called "SpaceBase."

Phencyclidine

Phencyclidine Intoxication

34. J.R., age 18, is brought to the emergency department by police for violent, combative behavior. Friends claim he was smoking a "dusted joint" (PCP applied to a marijuana cigarette). He appears agitated, diaphoretic, and disoriented. His blood pressure is 160/100 mm Hg, pulse 130 beats/min, and temperature 101°F. He has vertical and horizontal nystagmus. Are these effects consistent with PCP intoxication?

J.R.'s symptoms are consistent with PCP intoxication. PCP and ketamine are noncompetitive antagonists of the N-methyl-D-aspartate (NMDA) receptor subtype of the major excitatory neurotransmitter, glutamate. The dose, route of administration, and serum concentration of phencyclidine all influence the pharmacologic effects of this drug and, thus, the symptoms of intoxication.[84,85] PCP in low doses causes inebriation, ataxia, changes in body image, numbness, and a dissociative feeling. Horizontal and/or vertical nystagmus is often present, and the anesthetic effect of the drug raises the pain threshold. Amnesia may occur following intoxication.

As the dose of PCP increases, the patient may manifest agitation, combativeness, catatonia, and psychosis. The action of PCP on the autonomic nervous system becomes more prominent and is characterized by a confusing combination of adrenergic, cholinergic, and dopaminergic effects. A hypertensive response is typically encountered. Tachycardia, tachypnea, and hyperthermia may also be noted in the moderately intoxicated patient.

The agitated, combative patient often has feelings of great strength. This combined with the anesthetic effect of PCP may result in serious injury because there is no pain sensation to stop the physical activity.

With large doses of PCP, marked CNS depression occurs and nystagmus may no longer be present. In addition to the physiologic effects noted earlier, respiratory depression, seizures, acidosis, and rhabdomyolysis may further compromise the patient's condition. Rhabdomyolysis, particularly in the presence of acidemia, can result in acute renal failure.[86] Opisthotonic posturing and muscular rigidity occur frequently in the severely intoxicated patient.

Medical Management of Intoxication

35. How should J.R. be treated?

There is no antidote to PCP, and treatment should be supportive. Environmental stimuli should be minimized. Even attempts to "talk down" the patient may trigger a combative response, and chemical restraints may be indicated. Benzodiazepines are useful in the management of the anxious, agitated patient with mild to moderate PCP intoxication. If patients are combative, psychotic, and dangerous to both themselves and the medical staff, haloperidol is effective.[87] Chlorpromazine should be avoided because there is a greater possibility of precipitating a hypotensive response or a seizure.

The other symptoms of PCP intoxication should be managed with supportive therapy. Hypertension may be managed with β-blockers or calcium channel blockers. Diazepam is a useful anticonvulsant for the management of PCP-induced seizures. Since extreme agitation, seizures, and hyperthermia can initiate rhabdomyolysis and secondarily cause myocardial, renal, or hepatic dysfunction, anxiolytics, neuroleptics, anticonvulsants, and cooling measures should be used as needed.

Management may also include attempts to increase elimination of PCP from the body. The urinary excretion of PCP is greatly enhanced when the urine is acidic (pH <5 to 6).[88] Although acidification of the serum and urine favors the formation of ionized PCP, which is more readily excreted by the kidney, only a small percentage of drug in the body is renally excreted. Thus, urinary acidification may increase the urinary concentration of PCP several-fold but will not decrease significantly the total amount of drug in the body. Since activated charcoal adsorbs PCP, it should prevent the intestinal reabsorption of this drug and promote its elimination.

Psychological and Prolonged Effects

36. J.R. is admitted for a 72-hour psychiatric evaluation. His history reveals that he is a chronic PCP abuser. What psychological adverse effects are associated with chronic use?

PCP administration can exacerbate existing schizophrenia or precipitate a schizophreniform psychosis that may last for several days or months. Psychotic states (flashbacks) can recur over a 30- to 40-day period despite abstinence from PCP use. These psychological disorders include autistic and delusional thinking, global paranoia, delusions of superhuman strength and invulnerability, as well as delusions of persecution and grandiosity. Behavior is extremely unpredictable: the patient may be cooperative one minute and violently assaultive the next.

Psychological dependence can result from chronic PCP use.[89] Animal studies have described a withdrawal syndrome, but it is unclear if a true withdrawal syndrome occurs in humans.[90] Long-term use has been associated with neurologic impairment, characterized by memory lapses and speech and visual disturbances. Depression, anxiety, and confusion have also been described. Chronic users often complain of feeling "spaced"; they may be irritable and antisocial and feel depersonalized and isolated from people. Prolonged depression may occur after PCP use is stopped.[91] Currently there are no pharmacologic treatments for PCP addiction.

HALLUCINOGENS

Hallucinogens can be categorized as indole alkylamines (e.g., lysergic acid diethylamide [LSD], psilocybin, and dimethyltryptamine) or phenethylamines (e.g., mescaline, 3,4-methylenedioxymethamphetamine [MDMA]). LSD is considered the prototype hallucinogen. While MDMA is classified as a phenethylamine, it has structural similarities to amphetamine and mescaline. It has been labeled an entactogen or empathogen because of its strong empathy-producing effects and mild hallucinogenic effects. The term "entactogen" can be translated as "a touching within." Hallucinogens are commonly referred to as psychedelics.

In 2001, >20 million Americans reported using LSD sometime in their lives, >1.5 million had used it in the past year, and 320,000 had used it in the past month. The popularity of MDMA (Ecstasy, X) has risen dramatically in recent years due in part to its use as a "club drug." In 2001 >8 million Americans reported using MDMA sometime in their lives, 3 million had used it in the past year, and 786,000 had used it in the past month.[55]

The usual pattern of use for hallucinogens is occasional self-administration for enhancement of recreational activities, such as dancing, or for "mind expansion." Certain individuals may develop psychological dependence and use hallucinogens in a more chronic and compulsive manner.

LSD

Effects

37. B.T. attended a dinner party with a few close friends and the host suggested they all "trip" (take LSD) after dinner. B.T. had no previous experience with LSD but was very excited to try it. She took a "hit" (dose) and her host told her she should cancel all plans for tomorrow. What can she expect?

Perhaps the most famous of all hallucinogens, LSD-25, was first synthesized by Albert Hofmann of Sandoz Laboratories in 1938. It was developed as an analeptic agent but produced significant uterine stimulation and caused experimental animals to become excited or cataleptic. Five years later, while resynthesizing LSD-25 for further pharmacologic testing, Dr. Hofmann experienced a restlessness that forced him to go home. This was followed by 2 hours of intense visual hallucinations of kaleidoscopic images and colors. Later he identified LSD-25 as a potent hallucinogen. Clinical experimentation produced hundreds of papers describing LSD as a drug that could facilitate psychotherapy, particularly in the management of addictive behavior. Widespread public self-experimentation with LSD for recreation and self-exploration, coupled with growing attention to adverse psychological consequences, led Sandoz to discontinue production of LSD-25 (as well as psilocybin, psilocin, and related congeners) in August 1965. The United States made LSD a Schedule I controlled substance in 1970 after the proliferation of illicit suppliers to meet the huge public demand for this drug.[92]

While the mechanism of action of classical hallucinogens is not fully understood, they appear to predominately act as agonists or partial agonists at serotonin (5-HT) receptors, specifically the 5-HT$_2$ receptor.[93] LSD, one of the most potent hallucinogens known, is active at doses of 25 to 250 μg. Most users take about 100 to 150 μg of LSD for a significant effect. This dose produces mild to moderate sympathomimetic effects, profound visual hallucinosis, and the sensation of disordered integration of sensory input. For example, sounds and music are perceived as visual imagery, odors are felt, and inanimate objects assume life-like qualities. In addition to these sensory-perceptual effects, psychic effects occur, such as depersonalization, dream-like feelings, and rapid alterations of affect. These are accompanied by somatic effects, including dizziness, nausea, weakness, tremor, and tingling skin.[94] These combined effects begin within an hour of ingestion of LSD and usually peak in intensity during the first 2 to 3 hours. After taking LSD, most people feel they have returned to a normal psychological state by 8 to 12 hours.

Within an hour after ingestion, B.T. will begin to experience altered sensations of her surroundings, in addition to some psychic and somatic effects.

Adverse Effects

38. After a few hours of "tripping," B.T. begins to think she will never return to a normal state. She fears she has "slipped over the edge" and begins to panic. What is happening to her?

The most frequently encountered adverse reaction associated with the hallucinogenic drugs is a mental state of acute anxiety and fear, typically referred to as a "bad trip." The hallucinogen experience is influenced by set (the user's mental state and expectations of drug effects) and setting (the environment in which drug use takes place, including the social conditions). Users may be able to calm themselves without outside intervention. The initial therapy of people undergoing a bad trip is frequently called "reality therapy" and consists of "talking down" the fear and panic. This consists of getting the person to a quiet, relaxed setting and helping him or her focus on explanations for the uncertainties that are causing the panic. This process also tends to reassure the person that he or she is in a safe physical environment and that the drug effects will diminish in a few hours. Most of these bad trips are resolved during the state of intoxication, but some last as long as 24 to 48 hours. Overall, these adverse psychological events occur in about 1% or less of trips taken.[95–98]

If the talk-down approach is not successful in resolving the panic, drug therapy can be considered. Sedation with an oral benzodiazepine (i.e., diazepam 5 to 20 mg) or an intramuscular benzodiazepine (i.e., lorazepam 2 mg) will frequently alleviate the panic. Supportive talking down should be continued because the benzodiazepine will not stop the trip; it will simply sedate the patient.[99,100] Haloperidol 2 to 5 mg intramuscularly may also be used in addition to benzodiazepines. Phenothiazines, specifically chlorpromazine, should not be used for initial management of bad trips because they may potentiate the panic and cause orthostatic hypotension, anticholinergic toxicity, or mental depression.[101,102] If mild sedation does not stop the panic reaction, or if the person requests that all hallucinogenic effects be stopped, a large dose of a benzodiazepine, orally or IV, can allow the patient to sleep through the rest of the effects.[103] For most of the hallucinogenic drugs, 6 to 12 hours is the maximum duration of action. Appropriate medical monitoring should accompany the benzodiazepine-induced sleep.

With regard to adverse physical effects, classical hallucinogens have a high margin of safety, although patients should be monitored for seizures or elevations in body temperature.

B.T. is experiencing a bad trip. Her friends should try to "talk her down," with reassurance that the effects of the drug will eventually wear off. If this approach is unsuccessful, she should be taken to the emergency room for pharmacologic treatment of her anxiety and panic.

Flashbacks and Long-Term Effects

39. **B.T.'s friends "talk her down," but she has heard that people sometimes have flashbacks after LSD use and is worried she will re-experience her bad trip. What are flashbacks? What are the long-term consequences of LSD use?**

The possibility of "brain damage" resulting from the use of hallucinogenic drugs has been difficult to establish because subtle changes in cognitive ability are difficult to document, and matched pair controls are usually impossible to arrange with certainty. A small percentage of persons who took many doses of hallucinogenic drugs (primarily LSD) during their late teens and early twenties became "acid burnouts" or "acid casualties." They have been characterized as chronic, undifferentiated schizophrenics. Although these individuals are socially disabled and treatment resistant, there is no evidence of a direct and singular drug etiology, and their psychological profile is the same as that of organic chronic, undifferentiated schizophrenics. The low frequency of occurrence of acid burn-out and the similarity of these cases to cases of organic schizophrenia suggest that the drug experience merely unmasked an underlying psychiatric condition.[104,105] Furthermore, the incidence of familial mental illness and pre-LSD psychopathology appears to be quite high in persons who developed longstanding psychosis after LSD use.[106,107] A singular personality type with a noncompetitive and eccentric nature seems to seek out hallucinogenic experiences and enjoy the effects, rather than the hallucinogenic drugs somehow changing a person biochemically into such a personality type.[108]

Hallucinogen persisting perceptual disorder (HPPD), commonly referred to as flashbacks, is characterized by recurrences of part or all of the hallucinogenic drug experiences following a period of normal consciousness in a person who used the drug previously. These events seem to occur more commonly in frequent users of hallucinogenic drugs. They may last from minutes to days or months (usually a few hours). The prevalence of flashbacks has been estimated to be 15% to 77%, but these figures seem high considering the many people who took 10 or fewer trips and have never experienced a flashback. Flashbacks are treated like acute drug-induced events.[100,109,110]

LSD and other classical hallucinogens have low addiction potential. There does not appear to be a clinically important withdrawal syndrome associated with their use. The rapid development of tolerance that occurs with these drugs may explain the intermittent use patterns commonly seen.

MDMA

Effects

40. **R.X. and her friend P.B. go to "raves" (all-night dance parties) every weekend and usually take Ecstasy (MDMA). R.X. says it makes her feel like "I love everyone around me," and P.B. likes to be able to "dance all night without getting tired." Are these effects common with MDMA?**

MDMA was patented by Merck Pharmaceuticals in 1914, but it was not until the 1950s that its use was examined in animal studies, when the U.S. Army Intelligence investigated it as a "brainwashing" agent. By the late 1970s a few therapists and psychiatrists began using the drug with reported success in patients with a wide range of conditions.[111] MDMA produces a very manageable and comfortable entactogenic effect, during which the person has a clear sensorium. The experience can be recalled in detail, and the insights gained during the session can be incorporated into normal life. The public gave several names to this drug, such as Ecstasy, XTC, Adam, and M&Ms. The media became aware of the anecdotal reports from both psychiatrists and people self-experimenting with MDMA. In 1985, the Drug Enforcement Administration made MDMA a Schedule I drug. Subsequently, supplies of the drug proliferated in the public illicit marketplace, and its popularity soared. In 2001, following successful lobbying by researchers interested in reinstituting MDMA in clinical practice, the FDA granted approval for a pilot study investigating the therapeutic use of MDMA in the treatment of posttraumatic stress disorder (PTSD).[112]

MDMA exerts its effects mainly by three neurochemical mechanisms: blockade of serotonin reuptake, stimulation of serotonin release, and stimulation of dopamine release.[113] The common psychological effects of MDMA intoxication include an overall heightened sense of empathy, interpersonal closeness, increased acceptance of others, and a powerful sense of well-being.[114] The experience is influenced by set and setting. The amphetamine-like side effects include mydriasis, tachycardia, sweating, increased energy and alertness, bruxism, nausea, and anorexia.[115] Users generally ingest MDMA in tablet form and the onset of action is usually after 30 to 60 minutes. Some users take a "booster" dose after 2 hours. The usual duration of action of MDMA is 4 to 6 hours and the half-life is approximately 8 hours. MDMA users in the "rave" scene often "stack" multiple doses, and polydrug use is common. The combined use of Ecstasy and LSD is referred to as "candy flipping."[113]

R.X.'s feelings of love for everyone are consistent with the empathogenic effects of MDMA, while P.B. is enjoying the amphetamine-like effects of increased energy to dance all night.

Adverse Effects

41. **Several hours after taking MDMA, P.B. is still dancing. She begins to feel hot and realizes she is profusely sweating. On her way to the bar for a drink, she begins to feel confused and collapses to the floor. Her friends witness her having a seizure and call 911. What is happening to P.B.?**

The "rave" scene, with its crowded conditions and often-high ambient temperatures, has unfortunately contributed to many adverse effects associated with MDMA ingestion. Due to their increased physical activity, the "ravers" may become dehydrated. Additionally, supplies of MDMA have been notoriously unreliable. Many other drugs have been misrepresented as MDMA, including other phenethylamines like MDA (3,4-methylenedioxyamphetamine) and PMA (paramethoxyamphetamine); amphetamine; cocaine; opiates; ketamine; and dextromethorphan. The common polydrug use practiced at "raves" compounds the problem. Dextromethorphan taken at high doses for its dissociative properties competes with MDMA for hepatic metabolism and its anticholinergic effects block perspiration, potentially leading to overheating.[111]

The most dangerous adverse physical effect of MDMA is hyperthermia. MDMA has a slight affinity for the 5-HT$_2$ receptor, and the increased body temperature may be the result of this activation.[113] The hyperthermia has led to rhabdomyolysis, and acute renal and hepatic failure, disseminated intravascular coagulation (DIC), and death. DIC has been the most common cause of death. Treatment of hyperthermia involves cooling measures and IV fluids. Benzodiazepines and dantrolene may be helpful. Other adverse physical effects may include hypertension, cardiac arrhythmias, convulsions, cerebrovascular accident, hepatitis, and hyponatremia.[115] While emergency room visits associated with MDMA continue to be relatively rare, they increased dramatically (over 2,000%) from 1994 to 2001.[116]

Adverse psychological effects are also possible, including anxiety, panic attacks, agitation, paranoia, and rarely psychosis. The treatment of these psychological adverse effects is the same as for those associated with the classical hallucinogens, including "talk down" therapy and benzodiazepine administration.

P.B. may be suffering from MDMA-induced hyperthermia and needs urgent medical evaluation.

Long-Term Effects

42. R.X. has read in the newspaper that MDMA is associated with "brain damage" and is worried that she has caused permanent damage to her brain. What are the long-term effects of MDMA?

Animal studies have consistently demonstrated long-term MDMA-induced serotonin depletion. This has been evidenced by lower levels of serotonin, decreased metabolite levels, lowered levels of tryptophan hydroxylase, and loss of serotonin reuptake transporters.[111] MDMA damages serotonin axonal projections; axonal resprouting and regeneration do occur, but it is unclear if these new projections are damaged. Despite this evidence of neurotoxicity, no associated functional changes have been demonstrated.[111,117]

Several retrospective studies in humans have claimed lowered cognitive performance in MDMA users compared with nonusers. These studies have serious methodologic flaws, including their retrospective design and failure to control for important confounding variables, such as other drug use and adulterant exposure and lifestyle factors.[111,117] Well-controlled prospective clinical trials are required to definitively establish any risk associated with MDMA ingestion.

MDMA does not appear to produce physical dependence, but some users may become psychologically dependent. Tolerance to the empathogenic effects develops rapidly and may last 24 to 36 hours. This may explain in part the more common practice of sporadic dosing of the drug.[114] No distinctive withdrawal syndrome has been described that would require pharmacologic treatment.

MARIJUANA

The psychoactive effects of the various derivatives of the *Cannabis* plant are due to the pharmacologic effects of all the cannabinoids; delta-9-tetrahydrocannabinol (THC) and cannabidiol (CBD) are the two most frequently studied as isolated compounds. There are many chemical constituents of the *Cannabis* plant, however, and the pharmacology of the crude plant extracts is similar to but different than the effects of the isolated chemical constituents.[118–122]

Marijuana is the most widely used illicit substance in the United States. In 2001, >83 million Americans reported using marijuana at some time in their lives, >21 million had used in the past year, and >12 million had used in the past month.[55] In the United States, the dried, chopped leaves and flowers of the *Cannabis* plant (nicknames: grass, pot, weed, green bud, chronic, mary jane) are rolled into a cigarette paper (marijuana cigarette, known as a joint or blunt; a "roach" is the butt of the marijuana cigarette) or smoked in a pipe or "bong." Each joint usually weighs 0.5 to 1 g, for a THC content of about 5 mg (very weak), 30 mg (average), or 100 mg (highest-quality sinsemilla).

There has been a dramatic increase in the potency of marijuana over the past two decades. Sold in quantities varying from fractions of ounces to kilograms ("kilo," "brick") on the consumer market, the typical leaf contains about 6% THC; carefully cultivated sinsemilla contains up to 13% THC.[9] The raw resin of the *Cannabis* plant can be pressed into cakes, balls, or sticks, called hashish ("hash," "temple balls"), which is smoked or eaten. Hashish may contain up to 12% THC. The oils can be extracted from the plant with organic solvents to produce "hash oil," perhaps the most potent *Cannabis* derivative, with THC concentrations of up to 60%.[123]

Researchers in cannabinoid neurobiology have discovered two cannabinoid receptors in the CNS: CB$_1$ and CB$_2$. In addition, two endogenous cannabinoids (endocannabinoids), arachidonic acid ethanolamide (anandamide) and 2-arachidonoylglycerol (2-AG), that act at the cannabinoid receptors have been discovered.[124]

Marijuana's therapeutic potential has been the center of much public controversy. Research on the effects of cannabinoids has led to several potential therapeutic uses, but the most promising appear to be in treating pain, relieving nausea and vomiting, and stimulating the appetite. A synthetic form of THC, dronabinol, is available as prescription tablets, but advocates of medicinal marijuana argue that inhalation allows for faster onset and easier titration of the dose. In addition, nauseated patients want to avoid the oral route of administration. Future research may focus on developing a safer delivery system that will be reliable, rapid, and safe.[124]

Effects

43. After school one day, P.H. is offered a "joint" by one of his friends. He smokes it and begins to feel light-headed and euphoric. He begins laughing at everything around him. Thirty minutes later he and his friend become very hungry ("the munchies") and eat several candy bars. Are these effects consistent with marijuana use?

Yes. The pharmacologic effects sought by most users of cannabis products are sedation, mental relaxation, euphoria, and mild hallucinogenic effects, and these effects are dependent upon set and setting. Other common effects that are usually perceived as pleasurable include silliness, subjective slowing of time, gregariousness, hunger, and mild perceptual changes of all the senses that engender an absorbing fascination with music, eating, and other sensual and sensory activities. The state of mind generated is referred to as "stoned," "high," "loaded," "wasted," and many other colloquial terms. Smoking marijuana typically causes a numbness and tingling of the extremities, light-headedness, loss of concentration, and a floating sensation in the first 3 or 4 minutes. Some of these effects are probably due to the hyperventilation associated with deep inhalation of the smoke (referred to as a "hit" or "toke") and breath holding to allow maximum absorption from the lungs. Over the first 10 to 30 minutes the user may experience tachycardia (possibly palpitations), mild diaphoresis, conjunctival injection, drying of the mouth, weakness, postural hypotension, periods of tremulousness, incoordination, and ataxia along with euphoria and the mental effects described above. These effects usually resolve by 1 to 3 hours and are followed by a 30- to 60-minute period of sleepiness before complete clearing and return to normal consciousness. Oral ingestion of cannabis products may delay the onset of effects by 45 to 60 minutes and prolong the duration.

Adverse Effects

44. P.H. smokes more marijuana with his friend. He liked it so much the first time, he decides to take several "hits" this time. He begins to think his friend is laughing at him and notices his heart is beating rapidly. He starts to panic. Is P.H.'s reaction due to the marijuana?

Consistent with its widespread use, marijuana was the second most frequently mentioned illicit substance in emergency department episodes, representing 18% of all drug-related episodes in the United States in 2001. There were >110,000 marijuana-related emergency department mentions in 2001.[17] Despite these numbers, there have been no documented cases of fatality in humans from marijuana overdose, and adverse effects tend to be self-limiting and often do not require medical treatment.

A syndrome consisting of anxiety, paranoia, depersonalization, disorientation, and confusion that can lead to panic states and incapacitating fear is perhaps the most frequently reported adverse effect of marijuana. Comforting reassurance ("talk down") and reducing stressful stimuli can alleviate this condition. Experienced users usually view these "paranoid flashes" as transient and unpleasant but manageable by constantly reaffirming to themselves that the paranoid thoughts are due to a drug effect, while exercising self-relaxation and calming techniques. The dysphoria and anxiety usually resolve in a few hours or less with such an approach. More severe incidents that evolve into panic reactions that are not resolved by sympathetic counseling may be relieved with oral benzodiazepine therapy in a dose equivalent to 5 to 10 mg of diazepam.

These adverse psychological reactions to cannabis products commonly occur with inexperienced users, high doses, concomitant use of other psychoactive drugs, and overtly stressful situations. Severe reactions requiring pharmacologic therapy are rare. Flashbacks from marijuana are reported only rarely, and the etiology is unexplained.[125–132] There is also some interesting evidence that persons who experience such psychotomimetic ("mimicking psychosis") reactions have a family history of schizophrenia (indicating a genetic predisposition to the disease) or have evidence of pre-existing psychiatric disease themselves.[133,134]

Adverse physical effects may include slowed psychomotor responses and short-term memory loss. Slowed psychomotor responses have been shown in certain groups of acutely intoxicated subjects and chronic users. Short-term memory loss is a frequently documented acute, reversible effect of marijuana intoxication as well.

The paranoid ideation and panic reaction of P.H. could certainly be due to the high dose and his inexperience with marijuana.

Long-Term Effects

45. P.H. continues to smoke marijuana daily. His parents discover his marijuana use and confront him, telling him it will make him stupid, unmotivated, and strung out, and may lead to the use of harder drugs. Are P.H.'s parents' concerns valid? What are possible long-term effects of marijuana use?

Chronic use of cannabis has been alleged to produce an "amotivational syndrome" characterized by apathy, lack of long-term goal achievement, inability to manage stress, and generalized laziness. There have even been suggestions that structural brain damage is associated with cannabis use.[135–139] Even granting the difficulty of designing unbiased epidemiologic studies for such multifaceted observations, the results of those studies have still been questioned. Other studies have failed to draw meaningful associations between cannabis use and any "amotivational syndrome."[140–145]

Cognitive impairment may occur after heavy marijuana use but appears to be reversible with abstinence.[146] Other concurrent drug use may also contribute to cognitive impairment associated with marijuana use.

The pulmonary complications of chronic heavy marijuana use are potentially significant. Pulmonary alveolar macrophage function and ciliary clearing of particulate matter from the airways is acutely impaired by smoking cannabis.[147] Chronic cough, laryngitis, hoarseness, bronchitis, and cellular changes typical of chronic tobacco smokers are reported in chronic cannabis smokers.[148–151] THC has been shown to be a potent bronchodilator. Both oral and smoked THC were shown to produce significant bronchodilation when given to healthy subjects. The bronchodilatory response in asthmatics given THC has been shown to be less vigorous.[67] Tolerance to these effects can develop after some weeks.[152] Epidemiologic studies have suggested an association between marijuana smoking and certain cancers (lung, head and neck); however, controlled studies have not established such a link.[153,154,155] *Aspergillus* has been found in marijuana samples obtained from street sales and is a possible infectious complication of marijuana use.[156] This is of particular concern in the immunocompromised patient, who may in fact be using marijuana for its medicinal value.

Tolerance to the psychoactive effects of marijuana does develop. Chronic users may not experience the full range of effects as new users unless they abstain for several days or weeks to regain initial sensitivity to the cannabis, and chronic users can tolerate large doses that generally are toxic to novices. Tolerance develops rapidly to both physiologic and psychological effects of cannabis. Dependence characterized by a physical withdrawal syndrome occurs after chronic high-dose use of cannabis. The withdrawal syndrome may involve irritability, restlessness, decreased appetite, sleep disturbance, sweating, tremor, nausea, vomiting, and diarrhea. Dysphoria and malaise similar to that experienced with influenza may also occur. Small doses of marijuana can alleviate the symptoms. The cumulative dose of cannabis and duration of use necessary to produce dependence have been quite variable. The withdrawal syndrome is generally mild and self-limiting, and pharmacologic treatments usually are not required.

Marijuana has been labeled as a "gateway drug," meaning that it will lead to the use of "harder" drugs, such as cocaine or heroin. Marijuana is the most widely used illicit drug, but use of drugs such as alcohol and tobacco often predates marijuana use. There have not been any conclusive studies demonstrating a causal link between marijuana use and subsequent other drug use.

P.H.'s parents' concerns are understandable but not entirely accurate. They should attempt to educate P.H. about the true risks involved with marijuana use, such as interference with studies, risk of pulmonary complications, and possible risk of dependence.

INHALANTS

The introduction of anesthetics (nitrous oxide, chloroform, and ether) to medicine in the early 1800s also promoted the widespread and popular recreational use of these inhalants for mind-altering recreational purposes. Gasoline and other petroleum distillates were also quickly abused and continue to be sporadically abused today. Glue sniffing became widespread in the late 1950s and experimentation with many other inhalants proliferated during the 1960s.[157]

In 2001 >18 million Americans reported using inhalants at some time in their lives, close to 2 million had used them in the past year, and >500,000 had used them in the past month. Highest past-year use and use in the month before occurred among 14- and 15-year-olds.[55] Abuse of inhalants is popular among children and adolescents because of their low cost, easy availability, rapid onset, and low threat of legal intervention. While marijuana is regarded by many to be the "gateway drug," more than half of young children who experiment with inhalants have not even tried marijuana.[158]

Males are much more likely to use inhalants than females, often by ratios as large as 10 to 1. In general, inhalant users are found in small groups within larger populations. These persons usually share common social, economic, or cultural backgrounds. Poor education, lack of social skills, and economic deprivation seem to be positively correlated with chronic solvent abuse in these populations. Solvent sniffers are often from families that are disorganized or lack an effective father figure. Solvent sniffers tend to exhibit emotional outbursts, passive-aggressive tendencies, antisocial behavior, social inadequacy, impaired judgment, and bashfulness. Poly-drug abuse is uncommon among younger solvent abusers. Even though relatively few appear to switch to other drugs of abuse, the manifestations of severe addictive disease are evident in these people.[159]

The two most commonly abused classes of inhalants are the volatile solvents (mostly hydrocarbons), and volatile nitrites (amyl, butyl, isobutyl, cyclohexyl). The fumes or vapors of these liquids, or paste in the case of glue, are directly inhaled (sniffed) out of their containers, or poured onto a rag, into a plastic bag, or merely cupped in the hands and inhaled. Aerosols and gaseous substances like nitrous oxide are also used to inflate a balloon and then inhaled out of the balloon by the user. Use of inhalants is commonly referred to as "huffing."

Even though other solvents certainly are abused, toluene has emerged as probably the most frequently sought solvent for abuse. Therefore, the medical complications of chronic solvent inhalation are most likely due to toluene, even though specific effects associated with other solvents have been identified. In general, solvent abusers have suffered neurologic damage such as severe dementia, cognitive impairment, cerebellar dysfunction, corticospinal tract dysfunction, oculomotor abnormalities, tremor, deafness, and hyposmia.[160] Sudden death from ventricular arrhythmias is reported with increasing frequency. It is likely that the "sensitization" of the myocardium to catecholamines is exacerbated by physical exercise, and fatal ventricular arrhythmias are stimulated.[161] Pulmonary complications, including hemorrhagic alveolitis in aerosol paint sniffers, have been reported.[162] Causes of death have included asphyxiation, sudden cardiac arrhythmias, aspiration of gastric contents, trauma (falls, drowning, hanging), and direct end-organ toxicity associated with specific solvents.[163]

Volatile Solvents

Effects

46. H.K., age 16, has been pouring degreasing solvents, gasoline, and paint thinners onto a rag and "huffing" the fumes to produce intoxication. What clinical presentation might be expected in this young man?

Volatile substances such as gasoline, kerosene, chloroform, alcohols, airplane glue, lacquer thinner, acetone (nail polish remover), benzene (nail polish remover, model cement), naphtha (lighter fluid), plastic cement, carbon tetrachloride, fluoride-based sprays, and liquid paper (i.e., White Out, usually containing 1,1,1-trichloroethane, also trichloroethylene and perchlorethylene) have all been abused.[164–181] Inhalation of these products produces a temporary stimulation and reduced inhibitions before the depressive CNS effects occur. Acute intoxication is associated with dizziness, slurred speech, unsteady gait, and drowsiness. Impulsiveness, excitement, and irritability may also occur. As the CNS becomes more deeply affected, illusions, hallucinations, and delusions develop. The user experiences an euphoric dreamy high culminating in a short period of sleep. Delirium with confusion, psychomotor clumsiness, emotional instability, and impairment of thinking are noticeable. The intoxicated state may last from minutes to an hour or more.

Acute Adverse Effects

47. **What acute adverse effects may H.K. experience from inhalation of these solvents?**

Complications may result from the effects of the solvents or other toxic ingredients such as lead in gasoline. Injuries to the brain, liver, kidney, bone marrow, and particularly the lungs can also occur and may be the effect of heavy exposure or hypersensitivity. Death occurs from respiratory arrest, cardiac arrhythmias, or asphyxia due to airway occlusion.

Chronic Adverse Effects

48. **What adverse effects could be expected from chronic exposure to the aliphatic hydrocarbons in the degreasing solvents and gasoline inhaled by H.K.?**

Model cements, rubber cements, adhesives, and paint thinners also contain aliphatic hydrocarbons (organic solvents) such as N-heptane, N-hexane, and gasoline. Chronic inhalation of a glue containing N-hexane has produced pain, tingling, and weakness in the legs with neurologic deficits that may last for a year or longer.[176] Excessive exposure to gasoline fumes has caused chronic pulmonary irritation, anemia, and neurologic problems. Gasoline can contain enough benzene to be hazardous to the formed elements in the blood and has been reported to cause chromosomal damage and leukemias in humans. Additionally, some types of gasoline contain the "antiknock" ingredient tetraethyl lead. Persons who inhale leaded gasoline, therefore, may experience symptoms of systemic lead poisoning. Permanent CNS damage has been known to follow the inhalation of large quantities of tetraethyl lead, including toxic psychosis from lead encephalopathy, cerebellar dysfunction, and a syndrome of ataxia, tremor, and encephalopathy.[177–180] Sudden death, presumably due to a fatal ventricular arrhythmia precipitated by sudden exercise, has been reported.[181]

Toxicity

49. **What toxicities are associated with the aromatic hydrocarbons in the gasoline, solvents, and paint thinner inhaled by H.K.?**

Aromatic hydrocarbons such as benzene, toluene, xylene, naphthalene, and styrene are volatile contents of gasoline, rubber cements, degreasers, adhesives, aerosols, and paint thinners. High concentrations of any aromatic hydrocarbon can cause coma and death. Benzene causes bone marrow aplasia, anemia, and necrosis and fatty degeneration of the liver and heart.[182,183]

Toluene is perhaps the most commonly abused solvent, and several pathologic problems have been associated with chronic toluene sniffing. With the notable exception of neurologic damage, these syndromes appear to be reversible when toluene inhalation is stopped. However, permanent morbidity and even mortality may occur, depending on the severity of the acute event. Permanent dysfunction of the cerebral cortical, cerebellar, auditory, pyramidal tract, brain stem, and peripheral nervous system have been documented.[184] A metabolic acidosis with elevated anion gap associated with renal tubular acidosis may complicate acute intoxication. Hyperchloremia, hypobicarbonatemia, and hypocalcemia also may occur, along with Fanconi's syndrome, hematuria, proteinuria, and pyuria. Rhabdomyolysis has been reported in several patients. Chronic gastrointestinal distress including hematemesis, neuropsychiatric symptoms, and skeletal muscle degeneration causing myalgias are common reasons for these patients to seek medical evaluation. There is also evidence that toluene is teratogenic.[185–187] Inhalation of xylene vapor is irritating to mucous membranes.

Nitrous Oxide

50. **N.H., a dentist, has been abusing nitrous oxide at work for 4 years and now reports numbness and tingling of his fingers and toes for a week. Is this a result of his nitrous oxide abuse?**

Nitrous oxide is an antagonist of the NMDA subtype of the glutamate receptor.[188] Hypoxia and asphyxia are the major toxic consequences of nitrous oxide abuse ("laughing gas," dental anesthetic, propellant for whipped-cream aerosols). This has led to death and permanent nerve damage from prolonged hypoxia when oxygen is not inhaled along with the gas.[189]

The effects of nitrous oxide on the liver and kidneys are usually assumed to be negligible. In the absence of hypoxia, there are few changes in other visceral organs. Although there have been reports of bone marrow depression and death following prolonged exposure to nitrous oxide, the primary problem associated with recreational use of this gas is neurotoxicity. Different patients have manifested progressive paresthesia, sensorimotor polyneuropathy, myelopathy, and encephalopathic delirium lasting up to 3 weeks after discontinuation of nitrous oxide inhalations. There have been reports that parenteral vitamin B_{12} may improve the nitrous oxide-induced neuropathy because nitrous oxide apparently inactivates vitamin B_{12}. Toxic byproducts of some consumer kits for the production of nitrous oxide from ammonium nitrate may produce respiratory distress.[190–192] Nitrous oxide has also caused chronic mental dysfunction as well as syncopal episodes. It may contribute to infertility, abortion, fetal malformations, and cancer. The effects of the gas will impair reaction time and judgment, causing a hazard if users try to drive or operate machinery.[157]

This dentist is likely to be experiencing the peripheral neuropathy typical of nitrous oxide abuse. He should stop inhaling nitrous oxide and should be referred to a neurologist for possible vitamin B_{12} and other therapy.

Volatile Nitrites

51. **P.A., age 32, presents to the substance abuse clinic for methamphetamine-related problems and is asked what other drugs he uses. He admits to occasional use of "poppers" to enhance sexual activity. What are "poppers," and what is the rationale for their popularity?**

The inhalation abuse of amyl nitrite and its analogs (i.e., butyl nitrite or alcohol, isobutyl nitrite or alcohol, cyclohexyl nitrite, and isoamyl alcohol) is widespread. Although amyl nitrite requires a prescription, and butyl and propyl nitrites have been banned, variants of these nitrites may still be purchased in some states as room deodorants or video head cleaners under trade names such as Rush, Bolt, Locker Room, Quick Silver, Aroma of Men, and Heart On. It appears that cyclohexyl nitrite is currently the most easily obtained nitrite. All of these products are collectively known as "poppers." The term comes from the "popping" noise made when an ampule of amyl nitrite is broken. They have been abused predominantly by urban male homosexuals because of their reputation as aphrodisiacs and enhancers of orgasm.

The major effect of nitrites is the relaxation of all smooth muscles in the body, including the blood vessels. This usually allows a greater volume of blood to flow to the brain. The onset of effects takes 7 or 8 seconds and the effects last about 30 seconds. There is a certain "rush" that may be followed by a severe headache, dizziness, and giddiness. Tolerance develops rapidly to the effects of the gas, although prolonged use may cause nitrite poisoning, vomiting, shock, or unconsciousness.[193]

Used medically to treat angina pectoris attacks since 1867, amyl nitrite abuse increased during the 1960s, resulting in its reclassification from an over-the-counter product to a prescription drug. The use of volatile nitrites has been reported to enhance orgasm and aid in intromission when used by male homosexuals during anal intercourse. Volatile nitrites relax intestinal and rectal smooth muscle, as well as the internal anal sphincter. Inhalation of volatile nitrites also may relax the external anal sphincter by causing general disinhibition and relaxation.[194–196] Vasodilation of the penile artery, leading to sustained erections, also occurs.[197]

Sensations of heightened intensity and increased duration of orgasm have been reported by persons who inhale volatile nitrites in conjunction with sexual activity. A reflex sympathetic nervous discharge, mediated by baroreceptor responses to hypotension, may add to the sympathetic discharge of orgasm to produce the sensation of a more powerful orgasm.

Medical Complications

52. **What medical complications might be expected in P.A. when he inhales volatile nitrites?**

The cardiovascular effects include profound vasodilation, resulting in hypotension and cutaneous flushing, which are followed by reflex vasoconstriction, tachycardia (due to sympathetic discharge), and transient electrocardiographic changes (inverted T waves and depressed ST segments). The actions of the volatile nitrites are more pronounced and short-lived than the effects of usual therapeutic doses of nitroglycerin. The hypotensive effect of these inhalants has caused syncope and subsequent trauma.

The CNS effects can include light-headedness, weakness, nausea, ataxia, delirium, headache (short-lived "nitrite headaches" or prolonged pulsatile headaches), syncope (following profound vasodilation), tolerance, sedation, and anesthesia.[198]

Methemoglobinemia rarely occurs following the usually inhaled doses of volatile nitrites, but there are several reports of significant methemoglobinemia and death following prolonged inhalation or ingestion of these products. Normocytic, normochromic anemia has been reported after industrial exposure.[199]

Irritation of the lungs, sinuses, and nasal passages can occur. Multiple cases of inflammatory sinusitis caused by pouring the liquid up the nose have occurred in the San Francisco Bay Area. A 30-year-old man died of cardiac arrest after drinking an isobutyl nitrite product. The oral ingestion of volatile nitrite products is dangerous because the user cannot titrate the dose as well as when it is inhaled.

P.A. is likely to experience light-headedness and headaches after inhaling volatile nitrites.

Acknowledgement
The authors acknowledge James F. Buchanan, Howard E. McKinney, Gregory N. Hayner, Darryl S. Inaba, Jeffery N. Baldwin, and Blaine Benson for their authorship of previous editions of this chapter. The authors also acknowledge Jeremiah Gonzales for his research assistance.

REFERENCES

1. Edwards G et al. Nomenclature and classification of drug-and alcohol-related problems: a WHO memorandum. Bull WHO 1981;59:225.
2. Milkman H, Sunderwirth S. Addictive processes. J Psychoactive Drugs 1982;14:177.
3. Dole VP. Addictive behavior. Sci Am 1980; December:138.
4. Busto U, Sellers EM. Pharmacokinetic determinants of drug abuse and dependence. Clin Pharmacokinet 1986;11:144.
5. American Psychiatric Association. Diagnostic and Statistical Manual of Mental Disorders, 4th ed. Washington, DC: American Psychiatry Press, 1994.
6. Morgan JP. Problems of mass urine screening for misused drugs. J Psychoactive Drugs 1984;16:305.
7. Allen LV, Stiles ML. Specificity of the EMIT drug abuse urine assay methods. Clin Toxicol 1981;18:1043.
8. Hayner G. Drugs of Abuse Testing. In: Traub S, ed. Basic Skills in Interpreting Laboratory Data, 2d ed. Bethesda: American Society of Health Systems Pharmacists, 1996;41.
9. United States Department of Justice, Drug Enforcement Agency. DEA Briefs and Background. Drug Trafficking in the United States. Online. Available

at: http://www.usdoj.gov/dea/concern/drug_traffickingp.html. Accessed March 3, 2003.
10. Guevara RE. United States Department of Justice, Drug Enforcement Agency. DEA Congressional Testimony, Dec. 12, 2002. United States Heroin Use. Online. Available at: http://www.usdoj.gov/dea/pubs/cngrtest/ct121202p.html. Accessed March 23, 2003.
11. Eiseman AJ et al. Urinary 17-ketosteroid excretion during a cycle of addiction to morphine. J Pharmacol Exp Ther 1958;124:305.
12. Martin WR. A homeostatic and redundancy theory of tolerance to dependence on narcotic analgesic. Proc Assoc Resp Nerv Mental Dis 1968;46:206.
13. Isbell H et al. Liability of addiction to 6-dimethylamino-4, 4-diphenyl-3-heptanone (methadone, amidone or 10820) in man. Arch Intern Med 1948;82:262.
14. Wikler A et al. N-allylnormorphine effects in single doses and precipitation of abstinence syndromes during addiction to morphine, methadone or heroin in man (post-addicts). J Pharmacol Exp Ther 1953;109:8.
15. Ferguson R et al. *Enterobacter agglomerans*-associated cotton fever. Arch Intern Med 1993;153:2381.

16. Rylander R, Ludholm M. Bacterial contamination of cotton and cotton dust and effects on the lungs. Br J Ind Med 1978;35:204.
17. Substance Abuse and Mental Health Services Administration, Office of Applied Studies. Emergency Department Trends From the Drug Abuse Warning Network, Preliminary Estimates January–June 2002, DAWN Series: D-22, DHHS Publication No. (SMA) 03-3779. Rockville, MD, 2002.
18. Substance Abuse and Mental Health Services Administration, Office of Applied Studies. Mortality Data from the Drug Abuse Warning Network, 2000, DAWN Series: D-19, DHHS Publication No. (SMA) 02-3633. Rockville, MD, 2002.
19. Centers for Disease Control. Recommendations for prevention and control of hepatitis C virus (HCV) infection and HCV-related chronic disease. MMWR 47 (RR-19), October 16, 1998.
20. Centers for Disease Control, National Center for HIV, STD and TB Prevention, Division of HIV/AIDS Prevention: HIV/AIDS Surveillance Report. US HIV and AIDS cases reported through December 2001, year-end edition; 13(2).
21. McEvoy GK et al., eds. AHFS Drug Information 2003. Bethesda, MD: American Society of Hospital Pharmacists; 2003:2088.

22. Albertson TE et al. TOX-ACLS: toxicologic-oriented advanced cardiac life support. Ann Emerg Med 2001;37:S78.

23. Jaffe JH, Martin WR. Opioid analgesics and antagonists. In: Gilman AG et al., eds. The Pharmacologic Basis of Therapeutics, 8th ed. New York: Pergamon Press 1990:485.

24. Hasbrouch JD. The antagonism of morphine anesthesia by naloxone. Anaesth Anal Curr Res 1971;50:954.

25. Jasinski DR et al. The human pharmacology and abuse potential of N-allylnormorphine (Naloxone). J Pharmacol Exp Ther 1967;157:420.

26. Abramowicz M, ed. Buprenorphine: An alternative to methadone. Medical Letter 2003;45:13.

27. Substance Abuse and Mental Health Services Administration, Center for Substance Abuse Treatment. Buprenorphine, Summary of Drug Addiction Treatment Act of 2000. Online. Available at: http://buprenorphine.samhsa.gov/titlexxxv.html. Accessed March 28, 2003.

28. Jaffe JH, Martin WR. Opioid analgesics and antagonists. In: Gilman AG et al., eds. The Pharmacological Basis of Therapeutics, 7th ed. New York: Macmillan, 1985:517.

29. Dole VP et al. A medical treatment for diacetylmorphine addiction. JAMA 1965;193:646.

30. Newman RG. Methadone treatment: defining and evaluating success. N Engl J Med 1987;317:447.

31. Newmeyer JA et al. Methadone for kicking and for kicks. Fourth National Conference on Methadone Treatment. San Francisco, 1972. National Association for the Prevention of Addiction to Narcotics. New York, 1972:461.

32. Jaffee JH. Drug addiction and drug abuse. In: Gilman AG et al, eds. The Pharmacological Basis of Therapeutics, 7th ed. New York: Macmillan, 1985:532.

33. Boatwright DE. Buprenorphine and addiction: challenges for the pharmacist. J Am Pharm Assoc 2002;42:432.

34. Wesson D et al. Buprenorphine in pharmacotherapy of opioid addiction: implementation in office-based medical practice. California Society of Addiction Medicine, 1999.

35. Ling W et al. Substitution pharmacotherapies for opioid addiction: from methadone to LAAM and buprenorphine. J Psychoactive Drugs 1994;26:119.

36. Schwetz B. From the Food and Drug Administration: Labeling changes for Orlaam. JAMA 2001; 285:2705.

37. Johnson RE et al. A Comparison of levomethadyl acetate, buprenorphine, and methadone for opioid dependence. N Engl J Med 2000;343:1290.

38. Bashore RA et al. Heroin addiction and pregnancy. West J Med 1981;134:506.

39. Little BB et al. Maternal and fetal effects of heroin addiction during pregnancy. J Reprod Med 1990; 35:159.

40. Ostrea EM et al. A study of factors that influence the severity of neonatal narcotic withdrawal. J Pediatr 1976;88:642.

41. Dashe JS et al. Relationship between maternal methadone dosage and neonatal withdrawal. Obstet Gynecol 2002;100:1244.

42. McEvoy GK et al., eds. AHFS Drug Information 2003. Bethesda, MD: American Society of Hospital Pharmacists, 2003:2042.

43. Rosen TS. Infants of addicted mothers. In: Farnoff AA, Martin RJ, eds. Neonatal-Perinatal Medicine. St. Louis: CV Mosby, 1987:1114.

44. Coyle MG et al. Diluted tincture of opium (DTO) and phenobarbital versus DTO alone for neonatal opiate withdrawal in term infants. J Pediatr 2002; 140:561.

45. Gowing L et al. Opioid antagonists under heavy sedation or anaesthesia for opioid withdrawal. Cochrane Review. In: The Cochrane Library, Oxford: Update Software. 2003; 1.

46. Stephenson J. Experts debate merits of 1-day opiate detoxification under anesthesia. JAMA 1997; 277:117.

47. O'Connor PG, Kosten TR. Rapid and ultrarapid opioid detoxification techniques. JAMA 1998; 279:229.

48. Galloway G, Hayner G. Haight-Ashbury Free Clinic Drug Detoxification Protocols, part 1: Opioids. J Psychoactive Drugs 1993;25:157.

49. Bailey DN, Briggs JR. Carisoprodol: an unrecognized drug of abuse. Am J Clin Pathol 2002; 117:396.

50. Galloway GP et al. Gamma-hydroxybutyrate: an emerging drug of abuse that causes physical dependence. Addiction 1997;92:89.

51. Smith DS, Wesson DR. Benzodiazepine dependency syndromes. J Psychoactive Drugs 1983; 15:85.

52. Brady K et al. Benzodiazepine and sedative abuse. In: Dunner DL, ed. Current Psychiatric Therapy. Orlando: WB Saunders, 1997.

53. Hayner G et al. Haight-Ashbury Free Clinics Drug Detoxification Protocols, part 3: benzodiazepines and other sedative-hypnotics. J Psychoactive Drugs 1993;25:331.

54. Centers for Disease Control. Multiple outbreak of poisonings associated with illicit use of gamma-hydroxybutyrate. MMWR 1990;39:861.

55. Substance Abuse and Mental Health Administration, Office of Applied Studies. National Household Survey on Drug Abuse, 2001. Rockville, MD: Department of Health and Human Services.

56. Gold MS, Miller NS. Cocaine (and crack): Neurobiology. In: Lowinson JH et al., eds. Substance Abuse: A Comprehensive Textbook, 3rd ed. Baltimore: Williams and Wilkins, 1997:166.

57. Kreek MJ. Goals and rationale for pharmacotherapeutic approach in treating cocaine dependence: insights from basic and clinical research. In: Tai B et al., eds. Medication Development for the Treatment of Cocaine Dependence: Issues in Clinical Efficacy Trials. NIDA Research Monograph 175. Rockville, MD: National Institute on Drug Abuse; 1997: 5. NIH Pub. No. 98-4125.

58. Office of National Drug Control Policy. Pulse Check: Trends in Drug Abuse, November 2001. Online. Available at: http://www.whitehousedrugpolicy.gov/publications/drugfact/pulsechk/fall2001/. Accessed March 23, 2003.

59. Siegel RK. Cocaine smoking. J Psychoactive Drugs 1982;14:313.

60. Washton AM et al. Crack: early report on a new drug epidemic. Postgrad Med 1986;80:52.

61. Warner EA. Cocaine abuse. Ann Intern Med 1993;119:226.

62. Substance Abuse and Mental Health Services Administration. Major Drugs of Abuse in ED Visits, 2001 Update. The DAWN Report. Rockville, MD, 2002.

63. Kloner RA, Rezkalla SH. Cocaine and the heart. N Engl J Med 2003;348:487.

64. Lange RA, Hillis LD. Cardiovascular complications of cocaine use. N Engl J Med 2001;345:351.

65. Weber JE et al. Validation of a brief observation period for patients with cocaine-associated chest pain. N Engl J Med 2003;348:510.

66. Levine SR, Welch KM. Cocaine and stroke. Stroke 1988;19:1003.

67. Tashkin DP. Airway effects of marijuana, cocaine, and other inhaled illicit agents. Curr Opin Pulm Med 2001;7:43.

68. Rapoport S et al. Wound botulism associated with parenteral cocaine abuse, New York City. MMWR 1982;31:87.

69. Sharff JA. Renal infarction associated with intravenous cocaine use. Ann Emerg Med 1984;13:1145.

70. Landesman SH et al. The AIDS epidemic. N Engl J Med 1985;312:521.

71. Richter RW. Medical Aspects of Drug Abuse. Hagerstown: Harper & Row; 1975.

72. McCance EF. Overview of potential treatment medications for cocaine dependence. In: Tai B et al., eds. Medication Development for the Treatment of Cocaine Dependence: Issues in Clinical Efficacy Trials. NIDA Research Monograph 175. Rockville,

MD: National Institute on Drug Abuse; 1997:36 NIH Pub. No. 98-4125.

73. Chen K. Ephedrine and related substances. Medicine (Baltimore) 1930;9:1.

74. Kalix P. Khat: scientific knowledge and policy issues. Br J Addict 1987;82:47.

75. Alles GA. The comparative physiological actions of all phenylisopropylamines. J Pharmacol 1927; 32:121.

76. Gorelick DA, Cornish JL. The pharmacology of cocaine, amphetamines, and other stimulants. In: Graham AW et al., eds. Principles of Addiction Medicine, 3rd ed. Chevy Chase: American Society of Addiction Medicine, 2003:175.

77. Nestor TA et al. Crystal methamphetamine-induced acute pulmonary edema: a case report. Hawaii Med J 1989;48:457.

78. Ellinwood EH. Assault and homicide associated with amphetamine abuse. Am J Psychol 1971; 127:1170.

79. Wilkins JN et al. Management of stimulant, hallucinogen, marijuana, phencyclidine, and club drug intoxication and withdrawal. In: Graham AW et al., eds. Principles of Addiction Medicine, 3rd ed. Chevy Chase: American Society of Addiction Medicine, 2003:673.

80. Volkow ND et al. Loss of dopamine transporters in methamphetamine abusers recovers with protracted abstinence. J Neurosci 2001;9:9414.

81. Department of Health and Human Services, National Institutes of Health. National Institute on Drug Abuse, Research Report Series. Methamphetamine Abuse and Addiction. NIH Pub. No. 02-4210. 2002.

82. Domino EF. History and pharmacology of PCP and PCP-related drugs. J Psychedelic Drugs 1980; 12:223.

83. Reed A, Kane AW. Phencyclidine (PCP): another illicit psychedelic drug. J Psychedelic Drugs 1972;5:8.

84. Aronow R et al. A therapeutic approach to the acutely overdosed PCP patient. J Psychedelic Drugs 1980;12:259.

85. McCarron MM et al. Acute phencyclidine intoxication: incidence of clinical findings in 1000 cases. Ann Emerg Med 1981;10:237.

86. Patel R, Connor G. A review of thirty cases of rhabdomyolysis associated renal failure among phencyclidine users. Clin Toxicol 1986;23:547.

87. Giannini AJ et al. Comparison of haloperidol and chlorpromazine in the treatment of phencyclidine psychosis. J Clin Pharmacol 1984;24:202.

88. Done AK et al. Pharmacokinetic basis for the diagnosis and treatment of acute PCP intoxication. J Psychedelic Drugs 1980;12:253.

89. Davis BL. The PCP epidemic: a critical review. Int J Addict 1982;17:1137.

90. Department of Health and Human Services. Phencyclidine (PCP) and Related Substances. Drug Abuse and Drug Abuse Research, Third Triennial Report to Congress, 1991.

91. Smith DE et al. The diagnosis and treatment of the PCP abuse syndrome. In: Petersen RC, Stillman RC, eds. Phencyclidine (PCP) Abuse: An Appraisal. Rockville: NIDA Research Monograph 21, DHHS publication no. (ADM) 85–728;1978:229.

92. Grinspoon L, Bakalar JB, eds. Psychedelic Reflections. New York: Human Science Press, 1983.

93. Glennon RA. Classical hallucinogens: an introductory overview. In: Lin GC, Glennon RA, eds. Hallucinogens: An Update. NIDA Research Monograph 146. Rockville, MD: National Institute on Drug Abuse, 1994:4.

94. Jacobs BL. How hallucinogenic drugs work. Am Scientist 1987;75:386.

95. Smart R et al. Unfavorable reactions to LSD: a review and analysis of available case reports. Can Med Assoc J 1967;97:1214.

96. Cohen S. A classification of LSD complications. Psychomatics 1966;7:182.

97. McGlothlin WH et al. LSD revisited: 10 year follow-up of medical LSD users. Arch Gen Psychiatry 1971;24:35.

98. Ungerleider JT et al. The dangers of LSD. An analysis of seven months' experience in a university hospital's psychiatric service. JAMA 1966; 197:389.

99. Taylor RL. et al. Management of "bad trips" in an evolving drug scene. JAMA 1970;213:422.

100. Strassman RJ. Adverse reactions to psychedelic drugs. J Nerv Ment Dis 1984;172:577.

101. Schwartz C. Paradoxical responses to chlorpromazine after LSD. Psychosomatics 1967;8:210.

102. Solursh L, Clement W. Use of diazepam in hallucinogenic drug crisis. JAMA 1968;205:644.

103. Hollister LE. Drug-induced psychiatric disorders and their management. Med Toxicol 1986;1:428.

104. Glass G, Bowers M. Chronic psychosis associated with long-term psychotomimetic drug abuse. Arch Gen Psychiatry 1970;23:97.

105. Glass G. Psychedelic drugs, stress, and the ego. J Nerv Ment Dis 1973;156:232.

106. Anastasopoulos G, Photiades H. Effects of LSD-25 on relatives of schizophrenic patients. J Ment Sci 1962;108:95.

107. Fink M et al. Prolonged adverse reactions to LSD in psychotic subjects. Arch Gen Psychiatry 1966;15:450.

108. McWilliams S, Tuttle R. Long-term psychological effects of LSD. Psychol Bull 1973;79:341.

109. Schick J et al. Analysis of the LSD flashback. J Psychedelic Drugs 1970;3:13.

110. Blumenfield M. Flashback phenomena in basic trainees who enter the U.S. Air Force. Milit Med 1971;136:39.

111. Grob CS. Deconstructing Ecstasy: the politics of MDMA research. Addiction Research 2000;8:549.

112. Doblin R. A clinical plan for MDMA (Ecstasy) in the treatment of post-traumatic stress disorder (PTSD): Partnering with the FDA. Multidisciplinary Association for Psychedelic Studies, 2002. Online. Available at: http://65.18.176.18/research/mdmaplan.html. Accessed March 12, 2003.

113. Malberg JE, Bonson KR. How MDMA works in the brain. In: Holland J, ed. Ecstasy: The Complete Guide. Rochester: Park Street Press, 2001:29.

114. Bravo GL. What does MDMA feel like? In: Holland J, ed. Ecstasy. The Complete Guide. Rochester: Park Street Press, 2001:21.

115. Henry JA, Rella JG. Medical risks associated with MDMA use. In: Holland J, ed. Ecstasy: The Complete Guide. Rochester: Park Street Press, 2001:71.

116. Substance Abuse and Mental Health Services Administration, Office of Applied Studies. Club Drugs, 2001 Update. The Drug Abuse Warning Network, The DAWN Report, 2002.

117. Baggott M, Mendelson J. Does MDMA cause brain damage? In: Holland J, ed. Ecstasy: The Complete Guide. Rochester: Park Street Press, 2001:110.

118. Clarke RC. Marijuana Botany. Berkeley: And/Or Press, 1981.

119. Mechoulam R. Marijuana chemistry. Science 1970;168:1159.

120. Turner CE et al. A review of the chemical constituents of Cannabis sativa L. Lloydia 1980;43:1.

121. El-Feraly FS, Turner CE. Alkaloids of Cannabis sativa leaves. Phytochemistry 1975;14:2304.

122. Turner CE. Chemistry and metabolism. In: Petersen RC, ed. Marijuana Research Findings: 1980. Rockville: NIDA Research Monograph. 31; June 1980.

123. Jones RT. Human effects: an overview. In: Petersen RC, ed. Marijuana Research Findings: 1980. Rockville: NIDA Research Monograph. 31; June 1980:54.

124. Watson SJ et al. Marijuana and medicine: assessing the science base: a summary of the 1999 Institute of Medicine report. Arch Gen Psychiatry 2000;57:547.

125. Brown A, Stickgold A. Marijuana flashback phenomenon. J Psychedelic Drugs 1976;8:275.

126. Weil AT. Adverse reactions to marijuana. N Engl J Med 1970;282:997.

127. Smith DE, Mehl C. An analysis of marijuana toxicity. Clin Toxicol 1970;3:101.

128. Weil AT et al. Clinical and psychological effects of marijuana in man. Science 1968;162:1243.

129. Tart CT. Marijuana: common experiences. Nature 1970;226:701.

130. Abruzzi W. Drug-induced psychosis. Int J Addict 1977;121:183.

131. Tennant FS et al. Psychiatric effects of hashish. Arch Gen Psychiatry 1972;27:133.

132. Weinberg D et al. Intoxication from accidental marijuana ingestion. Pediatrics 1983;71:848.

133. Thacore VR, Shulka SRP. Cannabis psychosis and paranoid schizophrenia. Arch Gen Psychiatry 1976;33:383.

134. Treffert DA. Marijuana use in schizophrenia: a clear hazard. Am J Psychiatry 1978;135:1213.

135. Kolansky H et al. Effects of marijuana on adolescents and young adults. JAMA 1971;216:486.

136. Kolansky H, Moore WT. Toxic effects of chronic marijuana use. JAMA 1972;222:35.

137. Campbell AMG et al. Cerebral atrophy in young marijuana smokers. Lancet 1971;2:1219.

138. Jones RT. Effects of marijuana on the mind. In: Tinklenberg JR, ed. Marijuana and Health Hazards. New York: Academic Press, 1975:115.

139. Brill NQ, Christie RL. Marijuana use and psychosocial adaptation. Arch Gen Psychiatry 1974;31:713.

140. Hannerz J, Hindmarsh T. Neurological and neuroradiological examination of chronic cannabis smokers. Ann Neurol 1983;13:207.

141. Co BT et al. Absence of cerebral atrophy in chronic cannabis users. JAMA 1977;237:1229.

142. Kuehnle J et al. Computed tomographic examination of heavy marijuana smokers. JAMA 1977;237:1231.

143. Rubin V, Comitas L. The clinical studies. In: Rubin V, Comitas L, eds. Ganja in Jamaica. The Hague: Mouton, 1975:81.

144. Stefanis C et al. Clinical and psychological effects of cannabis in long-term users. In: Braude MC, Szara S, eds. Pharmacology of Marijuana. New York: Raven Press, 1976:659.

145. Coggins WJ et al. Health status of chronic heavy cannabis users. Ann NY Acad Sci 1976;282:148.

146. Pope HG et al. Neuropsychological performance in long-term cannabis users. Arch Gen Psychiatry 2001;58:909.

147. Huber GL et al. Depressant effect of marijuana smoke on antibacterial activity of pulmonary alveolar macrophages. Chest 1975;68:769.

148. Henderson RL et al. Respiratory manifestations of hashish smoking. Arch Otolaryngol 1972;95:248.

149. Abramson HA et al. Respiratory disorders and marijuana use. J Asthma Res 1974;11:97.

150. Tennant FS et al. Medical manifestations associated with hashish. JAMA 1971;216:1965.

151. Waldman MM. Marijuana bronchitis. JAMA 1970;211:501.

152. Tashkin DP et al. Subacute effects of heavy marijuana smoking on pulmonary function in healthy men. N Engl J Med 1976;294:125.

153. Sidney S et al. Marijuana use and cancer incidence (California, United States). Cancer Causes Control 1997;8:722.

154. Zhang ZF et al. Marijuana use and increased risk of squamous cell carcinoma of the head and neck. Cancer Epidemiol Biomarkers Prev 1999;8:1071.

155. Fung M et al. Lung and aerodigestive cancers in young marijuana smokers. Tumori 1999;85:140.

156. Kagen SL. Aspergillus: an inhalable contaminant of marijuana. N Engl J Med 1981;304:483.

157. Schoener EP et al. Pharmacology of commonly abused drugs. In: The Society of Teachers of Family Medicine. Family Medicine Curriculum Guide to Substance Abuse. Kansas City: 1986:1.

158. Edwards RW, Oetting ER. Inhalant use in the U.S. In: Kozel N et al., eds. Epidemiology of Inhalant Abuse: An International Perspective. NIDA Research Monograph 148. Rockville, MD: National Institute on Drug Abuse, 1995:8.

159. Davies B et al. Progression of addiction careers in young adult solvent misusers. Br Med J 1985; 290:109.

160. Hormes JT et al. Neurologic sequelae of chronic solvent vapor abuse. Neurology 1986;36:698.

161. Boon NA. Solvent abuse and the heart. Br Med J 1987;March 21:722.

162. Engstrand DA et al. Pathology of paint sniffing lung. Forensic Toxicol 1986;7:232.

163. Anderson HR et al. Deaths from abuse of volatile substances: a national epidemiological study. Br Med J 1985;290:304.

164. Bass M. Sudden sniffing death. JAMA 1970; 212:2075.

165. Spencer JD et al. Halothane abuse in hospital personnel. JAMA 1976;235:1034.

166. Kaplan HG et al. Hepatitis caused by halothane sniffing. Ann Intern Med 1979;90:797.

167. Harris WS. Toxic effects of aerosol propellants on the heart. Arch Intern Med 1973;131:162.

168. Buie SE et al. Diffuse pulmonary injury following paint remover exposure. Am J Med 1986;81:702.

169. Strumann K et al. Methylene chloride inhalation: an unusual form of drug abuse. Ann Emerg Med 1985;14:903.

170. Miller L et al. Acute tubular necrosis after inhalation exposure to methylene chloride. Arch Intern Med 1985;145:145.

171. Tariot PN. Delirium resulting from methylene chloride exposure: case report. J Clin Psychiatry 1983;44:340.

172. Winek CL et al. Accidental methylene chloride fatality. Forensic Sci Int 1981;18:165.

173. Stewart RD, Hake CL. Paint-remover hazard. JAMA 1976;235:398.

174. King GS et al. Sudden death in adolescents resulting from the inhalation of typewriter correction fluid. JAMA 1985;253:1604.

175. Couri D, Nachtman JP. Toxicology of alcoholics, ketones, and esters: inhalation. In: Sharp CW, Brehm ML, eds. Review of Inhalants: Euphoria to Dysfunction. Washington, DC: NIDA Research Monograph. 15;1977:112.

176. Bruckner JV, Peterson RG. Toxicology of aliphatic and aromatic hydrocarbons. In: Sharp CW, Brehm ML. Review of Inhalants: Euphoria to Dysfunction. Washington, DC: NIDA Research Monograph. 15;1977:124.

177. Coulehan JL et al. Gasoline sniffing and lead toxicity in Navajo adolescents. Pediatrics 1983; 71:113.

178. Young RSK et al. Recurrent cerebellar dysfunction as related to chronic gasoline sniffing in an adolescent girl. Clin Pediatr 1977;16:706.

179. Hansen KS, Sharp FR. Gasoline sniffing, lead poisoning, and myoclonus. JAMA 1978;240:1375.

180. Robinson RO. Tetraethyl lead poisoning from gasoline sniffing. JAMA 1978;240:1373.

181. Bass M. Death from sniffing gasoline. N Engl J Med 1978;299:203.

182. Vigliani E, Forni A. Benzene and leukemia. Environ Res 1976;11:122.

183. Lazar RB et al. Multifocal central nervous system damage caused by toluene abuse. Neurology 1983;33:1337.

184. Streicher HZ et al. Syndromes of toluene sniffing in adults. Ann Intern Med NY 1981;94:758.

185. Fischman CM, Oster JR. Toxic effects of toluene: a new cause of high anion gap metabolic acidosis. JAMA 1979;241:1713.

186. Moss AH et al. Fanconi's syndrome and distal tubular acidosis after glue sniffing. Ann Intern Med 1980;92:69.

187. Aviado DM. Preclinical pharmacology and toxicology of halogenated solvents and propellants. In: Sharp CW, Brehm ML, eds. Review of Inhalants: Euphoria to Dysfunction. Washington, DC: NIDA Research Monograph. 15;1977:164.

188. Domino EF. The pharmacology of NMDA antagonists: psychotomimetics and dissociative

anesthetics. In: Graham AW et al., eds. Principles of Addiction Medicine, 3rd ed. Chevy Chase: American Society of Addiction Medicine, 2003:287

189. Helisten C. Nitrous oxide is a gas. Pharm Chem 1975;4(5):1.

190. Heyer EJ et al. Nitrous oxide: clinical and electrophysiologic investigation of neurologic complications. Neurology 1986;36:1618.

191. Sterman AB, Coyle PK. Subacute toxic delirium following nitrous oxide abuse. Arch Neurol 1983;40:446.

192. Messina FV, Wynne JW. Homemade nitrous oxide: no laughing matter. Ann Intern Med 1982; 96:333.

193. Nickerson M et al. Isobutyl Nitrite and Related Compounds. San Francisco: Pharm X, 1979.

194. Everett G. Effects of amyl nitrite ("poppers") on sexual experience. Med Aspects Human Sexuality 1972;6:146.

195. Gay GR, Sheppard C. Sex in the drug culture. Med Aspects Human Sexuality 1972;6:28.

196. Hollister L. Drugs and sexual behavior in man. Life Sci 1975;17:661.

197. Giannini AJ. The volatile agents. In: Miller NS, ed. Comprehensive Handbook of Drug and Alcohol Addiction. New York: Marcel Dekker, 1991:395.

198. Cohen S. The volatile nitrites. JAMA 1979;24: 2077.

199. Sharp CW, Stillman RC. Blush not with nitrites. Ann Intern Med 1980;92:700.

CHAPTER 84

Alcohol Abuse

Paul W. Jungnickel

ALCOHOL CONTENT AND DEFINITIONS

Ethyl alcohol (ethanol) is one of the few intoxicating drugs widely available for legal human consumption throughout most countries in the world (Table 84-1). Various beverages with a wide range of ethanol content are available, including light beer (2% to 4% ethanol); beer (4% to 6% ethanol); ale and special beers (up to about 12% ethanol); wine (10% to 20% ethanol); and distilled beverages such as whiskey, rum, cognac, and liqueurs (most 35% to 55% ethanol, some as high as 95% ethanol). These products are prepared by fermentation or a combination of fermentation and distillation. Beer and wine are prepared by yeast fermentation, which continues until the concentration of ethanol kills the yeast. The characteristic ethanol concentrations of the various beverages are determined by the type of yeast used in the fermentation. Beverages with higher concentrations of alcohol are prepared by distillation of wines and fermented grains, a process that concentrates the alcohol.

Proof typically refers to the alcohol content in distilled beverages. Proof is calculated by multiplying the ethanol concentration by two. Thus, 80-proof whiskey is 40% ethanol by volume; absolute (100%) ethanol is 200 proof. Several measures of alcohol are used commonly. A shot is 30 mL and a jigger is 45 mL. A fifth refers to one fifth of a gallon, which is 768 mL.

In the United States, many states have lowered the legal definition of drunkenness to 0.08% (80 mg/dL) blood alcohol concentration from the previous legal level of 0.1% (100 mg/dL). In some states, these reductions have been stimulated by federal legislation that requires states to lower their legal limit to 0.08% by October 1, 2003, or to lose federal highway construction funds.[1] In the medical literature, ethanol usually is expressed in mg/dL, although the Standard International (SI) units system, which expresses concentrations in mmol/L, is being used increasingly. The conversion used is (mg/dL) × (0.2171) = mmol/L. Thus, a blood ethanol level of 80 mg/dL is expressed as 17.4 mmol/L.[2]

Consumption, Consequences, and Costs

Although the overall use of alcohol has decreased in recent years, alcohol remains the most commonly used and socially accepted drug in the United States.[3] In terms of prevalence, a household survey of persons 18 and older found approximately 71% reported consuming alcohol at least once in the past year; approximately 75% of those 18 to 34 consumed alcohol, while use dropped to approximately 64% in those 35 or over.[4] Men are more likely than women to be drinkers, and to be heavier drinkers. For the total population, Whites are significantly more likely than Blacks or Hispanics to have consumed alcohol in the past year.

Although the use of alcohol is illegal in all 50 states for anyone under the age of 21, its use remains widespread among young people.[5] In fact, 82% of high school students have tried alcohol and 53% of high school seniors were current users (i.e., they had used it within the past month) in 1997.[6] Approximately 35% of high school seniors had engaged in binge drinking, defined as five or more drinks in a row, within the past 2 weeks. Alcohol abuse on college

Table 84-1   **Alcohol Content**

Product	Ethanol Content (%)
Light beer	2%–4%
Beer	4%–6%
Ales and special beers	≤12%
Wines	10%–20%
Distilled spirits (whiskey, rum, cognac)	35%–55% (some as high as 95%)

campuses is also a major concern. In a survey of college students, 84% reported some alcohol consumption, with 44% of students reporting binge drinking and 19% frequent binge drinking.[7] Binge drinking episodes per person per year increased by 17% (from 6.3 to 7.4) from 1993 to 2001. While binge drinking is most common in those aged 18 to 25, it also increased among those 26 and older.[8]

Epidemiologic data indicate that alcohol consumption is far from risk free and is widely associated with various health concerns.[9] Annually, alcohol use contributes to nearly 6 million nonfatal injuries at home, at play, or in public places.[10] As many as 18 million Americans show signs of alcoholism or alcohol dependence.[9] Fetal alcohol syndrome (FAS) is one of the most common known causes of birth defects with accompanying mental retardation, even though it is entirely preventable.[11] High-risk alcohol use also is associated with liver cirrhosis, cardiovascular disease, and various cancers, including mouth, throat, breast, and colorectal cancer.[12–15] Several alcohol-related behaviors (e.g., dependence, abuse, and heavier drinking) are associated with significantly greater risk for HIV infection.[16]

Perhaps the most serious health consequence of alcohol abuse is death.[17] Alcohol is closely connected to the four leading causes of accidental deaths in the United States: auto crashes, falls, drownings, and burns.[18] Nearly half (46%) of all fatal highway crashes involve alcohol; 16,792 people died from such crashes in 2000.[1] Binge drinking is strongly associated with alcohol-impaired driving.[8] In the workplace, up to 40% of industrial fatalities can be linked to alcohol consumption and alcoholism.[19]

As has been clearly demonstrated, alcohol is a major cause of premature death in the United States. In fact, misuse of alcohol contributes to approximately 100,000 deaths annually.[9] On average, people who die of alcohol-related causes lose 26 years from their normal life expectancy.[20] Deaths, injuries, and other negative consequences related to alcohol consumption also represent serious health problems for today's young people, with adolescents and young adults having a particularly high rate of alcohol-related mortality and morbidity.[21,22] With respect to morbidity, alcohol is the major cause of nonfatal crashes involving teenage drivers.[23] Moreover, the death rates in the United States for these age groups are dominated by causes associated with alcohol consumption. The number-one killer of teens and young adults is the alcohol-related traffic crash.[24] Alcohol use also is directly associated with homicides, suicides, and drownings (the other three leading causes of death among youth).[25]

The expensive and devastating costs of alcohol abuse are a matter of national concern.[26] In 1990, alcohol abuse and dependence cost about $98.6 billion, an increase of $28.3 billion from the 1985 estimate of $70.3 billion.[27] Specifically, alcohol abuse and dependency are costly to the nation in terms of reduced and lost productivity, medical resources used, treatment and rehabilitation, law enforcement, and motor vehicle accidents.[20] In 2000, the costs of alcohol related motor vehicle accidents alone had risen to $50.9 billion.[1]

For 1990, the direct costs of alcohol abuse amounted to $10.5 billion. Morbidity costs (i.e., the value of reduced or lost productivity due to illness) amounted to $36.6 billion, while mortality costs (i.e., the value of work years lost) amounted to $33.6 billion. Other alcohol-related costs (e.g., crime, motor vehicle crashes, FAS) amounted to $15.8 billion.[27] In addition, alcohol abuse generated a large demand on the nation's health care system.[14] Problem drinkers average four times as many days in the hospital as nondrinkers, primarily because of alcohol-related injuries. As many as 40% of all patients in general hospitals are there because of complications related to alcoholism.[20]

Alcohol abuse is a common problem that continues to present a significant challenge for health professionals. Clinicians can expect to routinely encounter patients with alcohol-related problems. By maintaining an accurate, current knowledge base concerning the issues surrounding alcohol use and abuse, health professionals will be equipped with the knowledge and skills necessary to address the issue when it arises in a professional situation. The importance of this issue is highlighted by the finding that <50% of primary care physicians correctly diagnosed alcohol abuse.[29]

PHARMACOKINETICS AND PHARMACOLOGY

When consumed in amounts typical of normal social drinking, the absorption of ethanol from the stomach, small intestine, and colon is complete; however, the rate is variable. Peak blood ethanol concentrations after oral doses in fasting subjects generally are reached in 30 to 75 minutes, but several factors can influence the rate and extent of absorption.[30] The most rapidly absorbed formulations are carbonated beverages containing 10% to 30% ethanol. In contrast, high concentrations of alcohol can produce vasoconstriction in the gastrointestinal (GI) mucosa, which results in slowed or even incomplete absorption of ethanol. Absorption of ethanol from the small intestine appears to be more rapid than any other part of the GI tract and does not depend on the presence or absence of food. Factors that control the rate of gastric emptying significantly control the rate of absorption by controlling the rate at which ethanol is delivered to the small intestine.[31,32] For example, beer or food in the stomach slows the absorption of ethanol, probably by slowing gastric emptying.

The level of intoxication achieved is not solely related to the plasma concentration. For any particular plasma concentration, greater cognitive impairment is seen during times when the plasma level is rising compared with when ethanol is primarily being eliminated. The degree of intoxication also appears to be directly related to the rate at which pharmacologically active plasma concentrations are attained.[33]

Ethanol is distributed throughout the body with reported volumes of distribution of 0.58 to 0.70 L/kg; calculations typically use an average volume of distribution of 0.65 L/kg. The alcohol dehydrogenase pathway (Fig. 84-1) is the major enzyme system responsible for alcohol metabolism in humans.

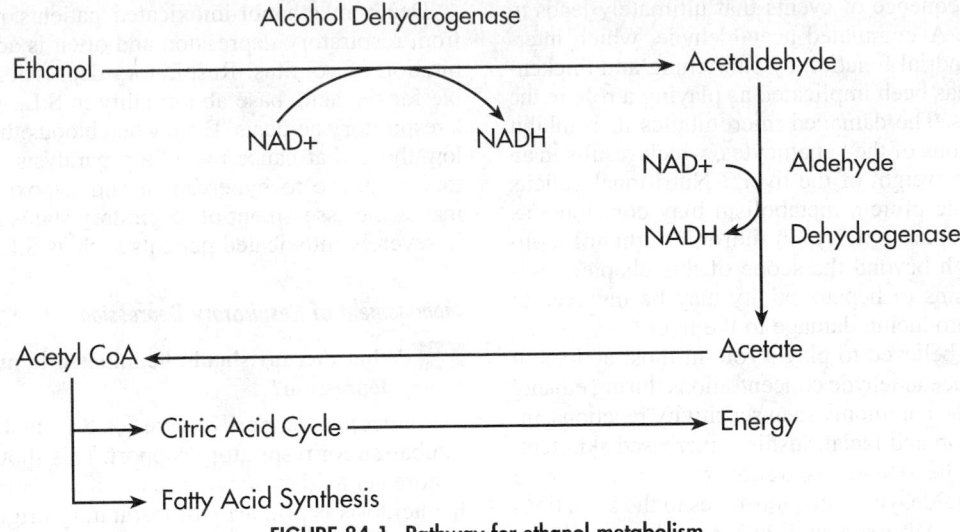

FIGURE 84-1 Pathway for ethanol metabolism.

Alcohol dehydrogenase is found in both the gastric mucosa and liver. The pathway involves conversion of ethanol to acetaldehyde via alcohol dehydrogenase, resulting in the reduction of nicotine-adenine-dinucleotide (NAD^+) to NADH. In the second step acetaldehyde is converted to acetate via the enzyme aldehyde dehydrogenase, which also reduces NAD^+ to NADH. These are the rate-limiting steps in ethanol metabolism, and this route becomes saturated when large amounts of ethanol deplete NAD^+.[34] Acetate ultimately is converted to carbon dioxide and water (see Fig. 84-1).

In some situations, a portion of the absorbed dose of ethanol does not appear to enter the systemic circulation, suggesting first-pass metabolism. The relative contribution of hepatic versus gastric alcohol dehydrogenase to this response continues to be debated.[35–37] Although gastric alcohol dehydrogenase has a lower affinity for ethanol compared with hepatic alcohol dehydrogenase, it may be capable of exerting modest metabolic effects at alcohol concentrations found in the stomach after a drink. The extent of first-pass extraction tends to decrease as the dose of alcohol increases. This is likely due to saturation of alcohol dehydrogenase, regardless of the source. Lower first-pass metabolism also has been found in alcoholics, women, the elderly, and Japanese subjects.[35,38] Gastric alcohol dehydrogenase also may play a role in the effect of food in reducing ethanol bioavailability. Food, by delaying gastric emptying, allows for more extensive gastric metabolism.

Ninety percent to 98% of a dose of ethanol is oxidized in the liver, with the remaining drug excreted unchanged in the alveolar air and by the kidneys. As the plasma ethanol level increases, hepatic alcohol dehydrogenase becomes saturated, resulting in increased unchanged excretion of alcohol. This results in a more intense odor of alcohol on the breath as the plasma ethanol concentration increases.

Ethanol metabolism formerly was described by zero-order kinetics; however, Michaelis-Menten and other nonlinear, concentration-dependent models are more accurate.[39–41] When plasma ethanol levels exceed 200 mg/dL, the alcohol dehydrogenase system becomes saturated. The metabolism of alcohol then tends to become nonlinear because of stimulation of cytochrome P-450 2EI, which produces metabolic tolerance to ethanol in chronic users.

The accepted average rate of ethanol oxidation commonly reported in the medical literature is 15 mg/dL per hour for men and 18 mg/dL per hour for women.[42] Although this rate still is widely used for both legal and medical purposes, other data suggest wide interindividual variability in ethanol metabolism. For example, wide differences in alcohol dehydrogenase activity have been demonstrated and attributed to heredity and other causes.[43,44] Chronic heavy drinkers frequently oxidize ethanol at twice the accepted rates, with their metabolic rates returning to baseline after a period of abstinence.[45] The rate of oxidation in chronic heavy drinkers also may increase with elevated blood ethanol levels.[46] In contrast, patients with end-stage liver disease may progress to the point at which they have almost no metabolic capacity. Thus, serial determinations of plasma ethanol concentrations are needed to evaluate pharmacokinetic parameters in a particular patient.

Because the enzymatic oxidation of ethanol to acetaldehyde (see Fig. 84-1) is accompanied by the reduction of NAD^+ to NADH and H^+, chronic ethanol use results in a reduction of the available supply of NAD^+ and an overproduction of NADH by the liver. This overproduction of NADH has been identified as one of the mechanisms contributing to ethanol hepatotoxicity.[47] To compensate for this, all the metabolic reactions in the liver try to convert NADH back to NAD^+. Several characteristic pathologic changes seen in alcoholics are the direct result of this hepatic redox state. Pyruvate, rather than being converted to glucose via gluconeogenesis, is reduced preferentially to lactate to generate NAD^+. This results in hypoglycemia in the absence of plentiful ingestion of dietary carbohydrate, a scenario that is likely in malnourished alcoholics. Hyperuricemia also occurs in chronic alcoholism, because uric acid excretion is inhibited by increased blood lactate levels.

Chronic alcohol use is associated with characteristic changes in the liver. Hyperlipidemia and fat deposition in the liver occur because of shunting of the excess hydrogen into fatty acid synthesis and direct oxidation of ethanol for energy instead of body fat stores being used for energy. Fatty liver is the first step in a sequence of events that ultimately leads to alcoholic cirrhosis. Accumulated acetaldehyde, which interferes with mitochondrial function by shortening and thickening microtubules, has been implicated as playing a role in the hepatotoxic process. The damaged microtubules then inhibit the secretory functions of the hepatocytes, which results in an increase in size and weight of the liver.[48] Nutritional deficits and impaired hepatic protein metabolism may contribute as mechanisms of hepatotoxicity in chronic ethanol consumers.[47,49] Although beyond the scope of this chapter, various other mechanisms of hepatotoxicity may be involved to various extents in producing damage to the liver.[50]

Acetaldehyde is believed to play a role in most actions of alcohol.[51] Elevated acetaldehyde concentrations during ethanol intoxication cause the commonly seen sensitivity reactions, including vasodilatation and facial flushing, increased skin temperature, increased heart and respiration rates, and lowered blood pressure. Acetaldehyde also contributes to the sensations of dry mouth and throat associated with bronchoconstriction and allergic-type reactions, as well as nausea and headache. These adverse effects mediated by acetaldehyde certainly have the potential to protect drinkers against the excessive ingestion of alcohol, but acetaldehyde also has the potential to produce euphoric effects that may reinforce alcohol consumption. Acetaldehyde also contributes to the increased incidence of GI and upper airway cancers that are seen with increased incidence in heavy consumers of alcohol and may also play a role in the etiology of liver cirrhosis.

Ethanol ingestion can depress the central nervous system (CNS) through all the different stages of anesthesia. Tolerance to this effect occurs after chronic use such that a blood ethanol level of 150 mg/dL will not produce apparent behavioral or neurologic dysfunction in persons who drink a pint or more of 80-proof liquor (or its equivalent in another beverage) daily for several years.

ACUTE ETHANOL INTOXICATION

Clinical Presentation

Toxicology

1. **S.L. is brought to the emergency department (ED) unresponsive except to noxious stimuli. Her friends report an evening of heavy drinking to celebrate her 21st birthday. Her respirations are 8 breaths/min and shallow. Blood pressure (BP) is 100/60 mm Hg, pulse is 100 beats/min, and temperature is 36°C. A stat arterial blood gas determination reveals a pH of 7.29 (normal, 7.36 to 7.44), PCO_2 of 52 mm Hg (normal, 35 to 45), and HCO_3^- of 19 mEq/L (normal, 21 to 27). Why is S.L.'s respiratory status of concern?**

[SI units: PCO_2, 6.9 kPa (normal, 4.7 to 6.0); HCO_3^-, 19 mmol/L (normal, 21 to 27)]

Ethanol can depress respirations by inhibiting the passive neuronal flux of sodium via a mechanism similar to that of general anesthetic agents.[52] The enzyme Na-K ATPase is inhibited, cyclic AMP concentrations are reduced, and γ-aminobutyric acid (GABA) synthesis is impaired. Ethanol is clearly a CNS depressant, and even the uninhibited behavior associated with its use is due to preferential suppression of inhibitory neurons. More global neuronal inhibition is seen at high ethanol concentrations.

Death in ethanol-intoxicated patients most often results from respiratory depression and often is accompanied by aspiration of vomitus. Respiratory depression also is responsible for the acid–base abnormality in S.L., which is primarily a respiratory acidosis. Even when blood ethanol levels are below those that cause medullary paralysis, a blunted respiratory response to hypercapnia and hypoxia is seen.[53,54] This makes the assessment of respiratory status a primary concern in severely intoxicated patients such as S.L.

Management of Respiratory Depression

2. **What therapy should be initiated to manage S.L.'s respiratory depression?**

Immediate supportive care for S.L. includes endotracheal intubation for respiratory support. This should be sufficient to restore her acid–base balance to within normal limits, because her acidosis is primarily of respiratory origin (pH 7.29, PCO_2 52 mm Hg). When metabolic acidosis is a significant component of the acid–base disturbance, it may be necessary to administer sodium bicarbonate. This should be done only in conjunction with appropriate respiratory support to prevent the development of hypercapnia. Analeptic agents such as doxapram (Dopram) and caffeine should not be used because they are ineffective and may cause seizures, arrhythmias, and hypertensive episodes.

S.L. was brought to the ED in a comatose state, and it is unknown whether she has ingested other drugs. She should be given a 1-mg dose of naloxone (Narcan) because alcohol intoxication often is complicated by co-ingestion of other drugs and because naloxone does not have respiratory depressant properties. This dose can be repeated at 2- to 3-minute intervals for up to 10 doses, depending on the patient's response and the clinician's index of suspicion for ingestion of respiratory depressants other than alcohol. Naloxone has been used to reverse alcohol-induced coma, to reverse clonidine-induced coma, to treat septic or cardiogenic shock, and to treat acute respiratory failure.[55–59] Although results have varied with naloxone use for these indications, which are not approved by the Food and Drug Administration (FDA), its use in these conditions is based on its postulated ability to reverse the effects of endogenous opiate-like agonists in the CNS. Use of naloxone generally would be safe in S.L. because, at her age, she is unlikely to have cardiovascular disease or other contraindications to naloxone use.

Serum Ethanol Concentration

3. **Thirty minutes later, the following laboratory results are reported: glucose, 49 mg/dL (normal, 70 to 110); sodium (Na), 142 mEq/L (normal, 135 to 147); potassium (K), 3.5 mEq/L (normal, 3.5 to 5.0); chloride (Cl), 104 mEq/L (normal, 95 to 105); HCO_3^-, 20 mEq/L (normal, 21 to 27); blood urea nitrogen (BUN), 18 mg/dL (normal, 5 to 22); creatinine, 0.9 mg/dL (normal, 0.6 to 1.1); and ethanol, 475 mg/dL. Based on the blood ethanol level, how severe is S.L.'s intoxication?**

[SI units: glucose, 2.7 mmol/L (normal, 3.9 to 6.1); Na, 142 mmol/L (normal, 135 to 147); K, 3.5 mmol/L (normal, 3.5 to 5.0); Cl, 104 mmol/L (normal, 95 to 105); HCO_3^-, 20 mmol/L (normal, 21 to 27); BUN, 6.4 mmol/L of urea (normal, 1.8 to 7.9); creatinine, 80 mmol/L (normal, 53 to 97); ethanol, 103 mmol/L]

Table 84-2 Blood Alcohol Relationship to Clinical Status

Blood Ethanol Concentration	Clinical Presentation[a]
50 mg/dL (0.05 mg%)	Motor function impairment observable
80 mg/dL (0.08 mg%)	Moderate impairment; legal definition of intoxication in most states[b]
450 mg/dL	Respiratory depression
500 mg/dL	LD$_{50}$ for ethanol

[a]Tolerance to alcohol varies among individuals.
[b]Some states define legal intoxication as 100 mg/dL (0.1 mg%)

The blood ethanol concentration generally correlates with the clinical presentation of the patient (Table 84-2), although tolerance varies among individuals. Impairment in motor function may become observable at levels of 50 mg/dL. Moderate motor impairment usually is seen at 80 mg/dL, which is the legal definition of intoxication in most states. Respiratory depression may occur with ethanol concentrations >450 mg/dL.[60] Therefore, the respiratory depression found in S.L. correlates well with the reported ethanol level of 475 mg/dL.

The accepted median lethal dose (LD$_{50}$) for ethanol in humans is a blood concentration of 500 mg/dL, although fatalities have been reported with ethanol concentrations ranging from 295 to 699 mg/dL.[61,62] Factors that may be associated with fatalities at lower ethanol concentrations include ingestion of other drugs, heart disease, and pulmonary aspiration. For example, patients who died of combined ethanol and barbiturate ingestions had a mean ethanol concentration of only 359 mg/dL.[62] Therefore, the clinician should order a toxicologic screening panel of S.L.'s urine to rule out possible concurrent drug ingestion.

In S.L.'s case, both the blood ethanol concentration and respiratory depression are indicative of severe intoxication.

Acute Management

4. After S.L.'s respiratory support needs are attended to, what other clinical conditions warrant attention?

Hypotension

Volume depletion resulting in hypotension often occurs in ethanol-intoxicated patients. Hypothermia also is a complication of severe intoxication and can contribute to hypotension. S.L.'s BP is not severely low and should normalize with fluid replacement and Trendelenburg bed positioning (i.e., foot of the bed is elevated such that the pelvis is higher than the head).

Hypoglycemia

As previously discussed, hypoglycemia most often occurs in conjunction with reduced carbohydrate intake. This situation is common in malnourished alcoholics but also might be particularly pronounced in S.L. if she were dieting. Because she is hypoglycemic, 50 mL of 50% glucose solution should be administered to her by intravenous (IV) push.

Other Treatment Modalities

5. What medical interventions can facilitate removal of ethanol from S.L.?

GI Decontamination

Gastric lavage may be useful if ingestion of other drugs is expected, or when the large consumption of alcohol is very recent. Activated charcoal absorbs ethanol poorly but should be administered when co-ingestion of other drugs is suspected.

Hemodialysis

Hemodialysis rapidly removes ethanol from the body,[63] but no clear guidelines exist regarding when it should be used. In uncomplicated cases, it has been suggested that dialysis be initiated when the blood ethanol concentration exceeds 600 mg/dL.[61] However, ventilatory assistance and good supportive care usually are sufficient for most cases because respiratory depression is the primary cause of death in ethanol intoxication. With good supportive care, dialysis would not be needed in a patient such as S.L. Dialysis may be considered if the patient cannot be stabilized or has other complicating factors, such as coexisting disease states or ingestion of other drugs.

The management of acute alcohol intoxication is summarized in Table 84-3.

Table 84-3 Acute Alcohol Intoxication: Symptoms and Treatment

Symptom	Cause	Treatment
Respiratory acidosis	Alcohol-induced respiratory depression; blunted response to hypercapnia and hypoxia	Endotracheal intubation for respiratory support
Coma	Alcohol-induced CNS depression; ingestion of other drugs	Gastric lavage, naloxone (Narcan) 1 mg, repeat every 2 to 3 minutes up to 10 doses, depending on response and suspicion of ingestion. Dialysis possible
Hypotension	Hypovolemia	IV fluid replacement
Hypoglycemia	Most often occurs in malnourished patients. Pyruvate is converted to lactate, rather than glucose, through gluconeogenesis.	50 mL 50% glucose by IV push

CNS, central nervous system; IV, intravenous.

ALCOHOL WITHDRAWAL

6. J.R., age 43, arrives at the ED by ambulance after a single-car vehicle accident. Police officers at the scene of the accident noticed a heavy odor of alcohol both in the car and on J.R.'s breath. Physical examination on admission reveals a probable fractured femur, which was confirmed by radiograph. His medical record indicates one prior hospitalization for alcohol-related seizures. When contacted by telephone, his wife reported that J.R. had been drinking heavily for the past 3 weeks and had missed several days of work. She also reported that about a year ago he had participated for a few weeks in an outpatient alcohol treatment program. His blood ethanol level on admission was 289 mg/dL. What are the immediate clinical concerns in J.R.?

[SI unit: blood ethanol, 63 mmol/L]

A high incidence of intoxication and alcohol abuse has been noted in patients who are seen in EDs and/or admitted to hospitals for both blunt or penetrating trauma; and alcohol-related trauma is seen in all age groups from adolescents to the elderly.[64–67] In cases when alcohol involvement is not as apparent as with J.R., patients seen in the ED or admitted to the hospital should be screened for alcohol abuse.

J.R.'s fractured femur should be evaluated and properly managed. However, a more important concern in J.R. is the evaluation and treatment of alcohol withdrawal. This occurs when a person who has been drinking for a long period either stops drinking or reduces the amount of ethanol consumed. Although individual reactions vary greatly, those who maintain higher ethanol blood levels for longer periods tend to have more severe withdrawal from alcohol.[68,69]

Signs and Symptoms

7. What signs and symptoms of alcohol withdrawal should be monitored in J.R.?

Although the hangover syndrome that follows a drinking episode may involve some component of acute withdrawal, it is not considered one of the four stages of true alcohol withdrawal (Table 84-4). Stage one generally begins within 6 to 8 hours after the blood ethanol level begins to fall. Typical symptoms reflect moderate autonomic hyperactivity and include tremulousness, anxiety, hyperreflexia, hypertension, tachycardia, diaphoresis, hyperthermia, nausea, vomiting, insomnia, and a craving for alcohol. Stage two begins in about 24 hours and lasts 1 to 3 days. It is characterized by auditory and visual hallucinations, anxiety, tremor, and varying degrees of the autonomic hyperactivity that is seen in stage one. Most patients remain lucid and oriented during this period. Approximately 4% of untreated patients progress to stage three, which involves grand mal seizures that occur from 7 to 48 hours after the drop in blood alcohol concentration. Isolated seizures can be experienced within a day or two after the onset of withdrawal. This stage also is referred to as "rum fits." Three to 5 days after the onset of withdrawal symptoms, about 5% of untreated patients experience stage four, which is known as delirium tremens (DTs). Fever of 40°C and untreated seizures during stage three are predictive for progression to DTs. Typical symptoms include confusion, illusions, hallucinations, agitation, tachycardia, diaphoresis, mydriasis, and fever. The estimated mortality associated with DTs is 5% to 15%, with mortality typically caused by aspiration, shock, hyperthermia, cardiac arrhythmias, infection, and trauma.[85,86]

The clinical diagnosis of uncomplicated alcohol withdrawal is often evident based on the patient's signs and symptoms but may be more difficult if other medical and psychiatric illnesses complicate the clinical presentation.[72] The fourth edition of the *Diagnostic and Statistical Manual of Mental Disorders* (DSM-IV) criteria for a diagnosis of alcohol withdrawal require patients to have at least two of the following symptoms after reduction or cessation of prolonged and heavy ingestion of alcohol: (1) autonomic hyperactivity; (2) increased hand tremor; (3) insomnia; (4) nausea or vomiting; (5) transient visual, tactile, or auditory hallucinations or illusions; (6) psychomotor agitation; (7) anxiety; and (8) grand mal seizures.[73] The DSM-IV further states that these symptoms must "cause clinically significant distress or impairment." The use of these criteria may assist in the diagnosis of alcohol withdrawal in more complicated cases, but they are far from infallible.

J.R. has been drinking heavily for several weeks and has had previously documented seizures. Both of these factors put him at risk for alcohol withdrawal that could be clinically serious. He should be monitored closely for symptoms of withdrawal and given treatment to prevent withdrawal symptoms.

Therapy

8. Twelve hours after admission, J.R. is noted to be sweating profusely, appears anxious and agitated, and demonstrates a coarse hand tremor. Shortly thereafter, he complains of nausea. His pulse is 130 beats/min. What treatment should be provided to J.R. for alcohol withdrawal?

Table 84-4 Stages of Ethanol Withdrawal

Stage	Onset After ↓ in Ethanol Blood Level	Clinical Features
I	≈6–8 hr	Moderate autonomic hyperactivity (anxiety, tremulousness, tachycardia, insomnia, nausea, vomiting, diaphoresis) and a craving for alcohol
II	≈24 hr	Autonomic hyperactivity with auditory and visual hallucinations lasting for 1–3 days. Most patients remain lucid and oriented.
III	≈1–2 days	About 4% of untreated patients develop grand mal seizures about 7–48 hr after ↓ in blood alcohol concentration.
IV	3–5 days	Delirium tremens (DTs) in ≈5% patients (confusion, illusions, hallucinations, agitation, tachycardia, hyperthermia). Estimated mortality associated with DTs is 5–15% attributed to arrhythmias, shock, infection, trauma, or aspiration.

Therapy for ethanol withdrawal should include supportive measures such as fluid and electrolyte management and thiamine (see Question #27).[72] Whereas patients with mild symptoms generally require only supportive care, those with more severe symptoms should be given benzodiazepines in doses sufficient to manage withdrawal symptoms.[72,74]

Benzodiazepines

Meta-analyses and evidence-based practice guidelines have established benzodiazepines as the drugs of choice for alcohol withdrawal because of their proven efficacy in managing withdrawal symptoms and preventing agitation and seizures.[74,76] Clinical experience with chlordiazepoxide (Librium), diazepam (Valium), and lorazepam (Ativan) is extensive, although all benzodiazepines appear to be equally effective when given in equivalent doses.[74] Most patients can be managed with high doses of oral benzodiazepines, although parenteral therapy may be required in more acutely agitated and combative patients. For example, an initial 10-mg IV dose of diazepam can be given, followed by an additional 5-mg dose every 5 minutes until the patient is calm. Comparable doses of chlordiazepoxide or lorazepam also may be used. For less severe cases, oral loading doses can be used. The dose of benzodiazepines should be carefully adjusted to provide effective anticonvulsant and sedative endpoints while avoiding the respiratory depression and hypotension that can result from excessive dosing.

Scheduled-dosage benzodiazepine therapy tapered over 3 to 5 days has long been the standard of practice for managing withdrawal symptoms. However, effective individualized therapy, triggered by patient symptoms, is easily accomplished by using a reliable and validated 10-item scale, the Clinical Institute Withdrawal Assessment-Alcohol, Revised (CIWA-Ar).[77] Use of this dosing strategy, compared with scheduled-dosage administration of chlordiazepoxide, resulted in equivalent control of alcohol withdrawal with a lower total chlordiazepoxide dose (100 mg versus 425 mg) and a shortened duration of therapy (9 hours versus 68 hours).[78] Another trial demonstrated similar results with oxazepam (Serax).[79] Symptom-triggered therapy appears to be advantageous in settings where unit staff are sufficiently trained in its use. In other settings, fixed-schedule therapy, with additional doses administered when symptoms are not controlled, may be preferable.

It has been argued that lorazepam should be the benzodiazepine of choice for the management of alcohol withdrawal because it has a shorter half-life (10 to 20 hours) and lacks active metabolites.[71] In contrast, both chlordiazepoxide and diazepam are oxidatively metabolized to active metabolites that have half-lives as long as 100 hours.[74] Thus, the shorter duration of action of lorazepam allows for easier dosage adjustment and prevention of excessive sedation, particularly in patients with significant liver disease; however, the longer duration of action of diazepam allows for a smoother withdrawal from alcohol. Another potential advantage of lorazepam is its predictable absorption after intramuscular (IM) administration, whereas both chlordiazepoxide and diazepam are erratically absorbed from IM sites, especially when administered gluteally (see also Chapter 76, Anxiety Disorders).

Other Drugs

Clonidine (Catapres) and β-blockers, particularly atenolol (Tenormin), may be used as ancillary therapy in the management of alcohol withdrawal and work by countering adrenergic responses.[74] Carbamazepine (Tegretol) is used widely in Scandinavia but infrequently in the United States. Further investigation is needed to establish the efficacy of this agent.[80] Phenothiazines may be useful in managing delirium, but these drugs lower the seizure threshold, may cause hypotension and extrapyramidal effects, and could exacerbate hyperthermia.[74] Sufficient doses of benzodiazepines can usually control the symptoms of psychosis that occur during withdrawal.

Since seizures are a significant complication, various anticonvulsant agents have been studied in the management of alcohol withdrawal. Divalproex sodium (Depakote) in a double-blind, placebo-controlled trial was at least as effective as benzodiazepine therapy in the management of alcohol withdrawal.[81] In another study, divalproex sodium compared to placebo, in patients who were treated with oxazepam administered in a symptom-triggered manner, resulted in less progression in severity of withdrawal symptoms ($P < 0.05$) and less use of oxazepam ($P < 0.033$).[82] Potential advantages of divalproex sodium over benzodiazepines include lack of abuse potential, pharmacologic synergy with alcohol, or CNS depressant effects.[82] The routine prophylactic use of phenytoin (Dilantin) has not been supported by clinical trials and likely has no benefit in managing alcohol withdrawal.[83–85] However, phenytoin may be of use in patients with focal neurologic deficits, head trauma, status epilepticus, or underlying seizure disorders.[86,87] Of course, appropriate anticonvulsant therapy should be provided to patients who develop seizures during withdrawal.

J.R. should be given supportive care and monitored for symptoms of alcohol withdrawal. Benzodiazepine therapy should be initiated with the symptom-trigger approach if the hospital staff is appropriately trained. Divalproex sodium is a possible alternative, but it has not been studied as extensively as benzodiazepine therapy.

CHRONIC ALCOHOLISM

Etiology

The etiology of chronic alcoholism has been attributed to genetic differences, psychosocial influences, and biochemical differences, but the precise role of each is unknown. Alcoholism does not occur in everyone who drinks, but chronic drinking is required to become an alcoholic. Some investigators have attributed the sole cause of alcoholism to psychosocial conditioning (the "nurture hypothesis").[88] However, over the past 40 years, several epidemiologic population surveys and biochemical studies have noted a genetic predisposition to alcoholism that possibly includes biochemical alterations in the metabolism of ethanol as well as neuropsychiatric differences in the behavioral response to ingestion of ethanol (the "nature hypothesis").[89]

Several lines of evidence provide support for the role of genetic influences. For example, the sons of male alcoholics have an incidence of alcoholism that is four times that of sons born to nonalcoholic men.[90] Several studies have identified similar genetic associations between alcoholism in offspring and parents of the same sex.[91] It also has been suggested that alcoholism is an X-linked recessive trait.[92] Although possible biochemical markers for alcoholism have been sought, no valid screening test has been developed to identify increased susceptibility to alcoholism.[93]

Diagnosis

Although most people seem to have an idea about what constitutes an alcoholic, creating a strict diagnostic profile for this disease has not been easy. This difficulty is highlighted by the greater prevalence of both harmful use or abuse of and dependence on alcohol when the DSM-IV criteria are used for diagnosis as compared with the *International Classification of Diseases,* 10th revision (ICD-10).[94] When using the DSM-IV, at least three of seven criteria must be met to establish a diagnosis of alcohol dependence.[95] From the limited information available about J.R., he meets the following four DSM-IV criteria:

1. Characteristic withdrawal syndrome for alcohol is present.
2. Previous efforts to decrease or control alcohol use have been unsuccessful.
3. Important social, occupational, or recreational activities are given up or reduced because of alcohol use (in J.R.'s case, missed work because of heavy drinking).
4. Alcohol is often consumed in larger amounts and over longer periods than was intended (e.g., J.R.'s heavy drinking for the past 3 weeks).

In addition, J.R. has had medical problems related to alcohol consumption (i.e., fractured femur and seizures). These problems, however, must be persistent or recurrent to meet this DSM-IV criterion.

9. **What are important considerations when discussing the diagnosis of alcoholism with J.R.?**

Most alcoholics are reluctant to reveal their disease and truly may believe they do not have a problem. Most attempt to maintain the appearance of a normal and reasonably successful life. Even patients such as J.R., who have been drinking continuously for several weeks, often deny they have a problem and argue they can control their alcohol consumption. Thus, when talking with patients who are in denial about their drinking problems, all objective data in support of this diagnosis (e.g., medical complications related to drinking) should be emphasized.

Some chronic alcoholics can consume the equivalent of one to two fifths of 80-proof liquor per day and still underreport the amount consumed. However, consumption of much less than this may represent alcoholism. The common social belief that one must drink every day to be an alcoholic is also not accurate; weekend or binge drinkers also may have alcoholism. The issue is not necessarily how much one drinks, but rather the loss of control that is associated with the consumption of alcohol despite clear evidence of adverse consequences. When questioning the patient about the amount consumed, the approach should be to start with large amounts and then work down. Many alcoholics are great confabulators and can counter each of the interviewer's subjective impressions. In confronting J.R., it is important to be firm in stressing the urgent need for treatment.

Treatment Programs

10. **What should be the role of "aftercare" for J.R.?**

After J.R. is successfully withdrawn from alcohol, he should be referred to an alcohol treatment program. The selection of the type of program depends not only on the seriousness of J.R.'s disease but also on his ability to pay for treatment, either from his own finances or through his insurance coverage. Participation in an Alcoholics Anonymous (AA) type of group during and after treatment should be recommended. J.R.'s success in the treatment program will be positively influenced by his willingness to acknowledge his alcoholism and active participation in his treatment program and in AA-type meetings.

The goal for J.R.'s successful recovery from alcoholism is complete abstinence from alcohol consumption. However, clinicians should understand that recovering patients will commonly relapse into periods of intoxication.[96] Although reports indicate some alcoholics can successfully resume limited consumption of alcohol, few alcoholics can evolve to stable moderate drinking.[97] Furthermore, many of the medical and psychiatric complications associated with years of heavy alcohol abuse can be exacerbated by resumption of alcohol use, even in limited amounts.[98] The duration of abstinence periods, reduction in alcohol use, and improvement in health and social functioning are reasonable alternative goals to complete alcohol abstinence in J.R.[98]

Disulfiram Aversion Therapy

Patient Selection

11. **Why would disulfiram (Antabuse) therapy not be appropriate for J.R.?**

The rationale behind aversion therapy (e.g., disulfiram) is based on the premise that patients will not drink ethanol because of the unpleasant and potentially life-threatening effects that occur when ethanol is co-ingested with disulfiram. Although several drugs can sensitize patients to ethanol, disulfiram is the only drug clinically used for this purpose in the United States. Case reports and open-label studies suggest disulfiram to be effective, but placebo-controlled trials have been inconclusive.[99] In the most rigorous and best controlled trial, no differences were found between placebo- and disulfiram-treated patients in rates of abstinence or length of time to first drink.[100] However, patients receiving active drug did drink less alcohol.

Patients most likely to benefit from disulfiram are those who desire to remain abstinent but have had periodic binge relapses. To be considered for disulfiram, patients must want to take the drug, must be socially stable and not depressed, and must have no medical contraindications to its use. Careful monitoring of compliance and adverse effects is essential in patients receiving disulfiram. Because J.R. is just initiating treatment for his alcoholism, disulfiram would not be appropriate at the present time, but it could be considered should he have problems with binge relapses and if he is willing to take the drug to deter drinking episodes.

Physiologic Response

12. J.R. successfully completes an outpatient treatment program but has difficulty maintaining abstinence. After his third relapse in 20 months, he requests treatment with disulfiram. What would be the physiologic response should J.R. consume ethanol while taking disulfiram?

Disulfiram blocks the enzyme aldehyde dehydrogenase; as a result, blood acetaldehyde concentrations increase by five- to 10-fold within 15 minutes after ethanol ingestion.[101] If he consumed alcohol, J.R. could expect the typical disulfiram–ethanol reaction (DER), characterized by peripheral vasodilation and associated with flushing, tachycardia, dyspnea, palpitations, and a throbbing headache. These symptoms generally are followed by nausea, persistent vomiting, thirst, diaphoresis, chest pain, and postural hypotension. Transient changes in the electrocardiogram (ECG) may include flattened T waves, ST-segment depression, and Q-T prolongation. J.R. typically would experience a period of weakness, dizziness, blurred vision, and confusion for 30 minutes to several hours, followed by several hours of sleep and recovery.

Symptomatic care usually is sufficient to manage a DER, unless it is complicated by cardiac arrhythmias, myocardial infarction, acute congestive heart failure, seizures, cerebral edema, or intracranial hemorrhage. The severity of the reaction is directly related to the dose of ethanol or disulfiram, or both. Anecdotal reports of DERs, however, have been associated with small exposures to unsuspected sources of alcohol, including the topical use of shampoo that contains beer.[102,103]

Dosage and Precautions

13. What would be a reasonable dose of disulfiram for J.R., and what precautions should accompany the use of this drug?

The usual adult regimen for disulfiram is 250 mg daily, although doses of 125 to 1,000 mg have been given based on patient response and adverse effects.[99] In using disulfiram, clinicians should be aware of serious harmful adverse effects associated with long-term use, including psychosis, peripheral neuropathy, hypercholesterolemia, hypertension, acetonemia, and hepatotoxicity.[104–107] Disulfiram may increase and prolong the effects of phenytoin (Dilantin), warfarin (Coumadin), isoniazid, and drugs metabolized by the mixed-function oxidase system.[99,108,109]

Thus, an appropriate dosage regimen for J.R. would be 500 mg/day for 2 weeks followed by 250 mg/day. J.R. should be cautioned to avoid all alcohol-containing products as well as occupational exposure to ethylene dibromide, and he should be tested for sensitivity to rubber or other thiram-containing products.[110,111] Because disulfiram can cause hepatitis, his liver function should be monitored periodically.[99] He should wear a medical alert bracelet indicating that he is taking disulfiram. Before starting disulfiram, J.R. should have abstained from alcohol for at least 12 hours and should be advised that DERs can occur for up to 14 days after disulfiram has been discontinued, because it may take this long for aldehyde dehydrogenase stores to be replenished.[101]

Other Drug Therapy

14. What other drug therapy approaches can be considered to help J.R. remain abstinent?

Although pharmacologic therapy of alcoholism continues to play a secondary role to psychosocial therapies, the development of new medications is based on the concept that addicting substances produce changes in brain pathways, including changes in neurotransmitter concentrations that remain long after a person ceases use of a substance. Alcohol affects various neurotransmitters, including dopamine, serotonin, GABA, and opioid peptides, all of which may have a role in controlling alcohol craving.[99,112]

Drugs that influence these various receptors produce many psychopharmacologic effects. Because alcohol dependence is often accompanied by psychiatric illness, drug therapy targeted at concomitant psychiatric conditions may be beneficial in managing alcoholism. In heavy drinkers without depression, selective serotonin-reuptake inhibitors have reduced alcohol consumption 15% to 20%,; and patients taking these drugs reported a reduced desire and liking for alcohol.[113–115] Unfortunately, the results in patients with diagnosed alcohol dependence have been more disappointing.[99]

Acamprosate

Acamprosate, an amino acid derivative, affects both GABA and excitatory amino acid (i.e., glutamine) transmission, but the precise mechanism of its action is not known.[116,117] It has been widely studied and used in Europe but is not available in the United States. Acamprosate appears to reduce craving for alcohol as a result of withdrawal. European clinical studies, measuring various therapeutic endpoints, have demonstrated modest efficacy for acamprosate.

Naltrexone

Naltrexone (ReVia), a μ-opioid (morphine-like) antagonist appears to reduce craving in patients who are abstinent and blocks the reinforcing effects of alcohol in patients who drink.[118,119] Although naltrexone is a narcotic antagonist with minimal agonist effects, the mechanism for its effects in managing alcoholism has not been established.[120] In meta-analyses and evidence-based reviews, naltrexone modestly alters drinking behavior in alcoholics, but benefits have not been consistent.[116–118,121,122] Naltrexone seems to reduce the amount of alcohol consumed and to have less of an effect on maintaining abstinence. The benefits and risks of long-term naltrexone therapy are unclear because most clinical studies lasted <12 weeks. Benefits observed during the initial 12-week treatment do not consistently persist after therapy is discontinued.[123]

Before initiation of naltrexone, patients should not have taken opioid drugs for at least 7 days. Common adverse effects of naltrexone include nausea (9.8%) and headache (6.6%).[124] Naltrexone can produce hepatocellular injury when given in excessive doses and should not be given to patients with clinically evident liver disease.[124] The recommended naltrexone dosage is 50 mg/day for up to 12 weeks.

In J.R.'s case, naltrexone may be a beneficial adjunct to his alcohol treatment program. Naltrexone appears to have some advantages over disulfiram, particularly with regard to safety.

However, additional studies are needed to define its true place in the management of alcoholism, including its use on a long term basis.

MEDICAL COMPLICATIONS OF CHRONIC ALCOHOLISM
Hepatitis

15. D.T., age 33, presents to the clinic with complaints of diminished appetite, weight loss, abdominal pain, and chills. She has an 8-year history of heavy drinking. She claims to drink several alcoholic beverages every evening with her husband and binge drinks on the weekends. Laboratory studies produced the following results: hemoglobin (Hgb), 10.3 g/dL (normal, 11 to 15); hematocrit (Hct), 31% (normal, 34% to 46%); mean corpuscular hemoglobin concentration (MCHC), 30 g/dL (normal, 34 to 36); mean corpuscular volume (MCV), 104 mm³ (normal, 80 to 100); platelets, 90 × 10³/mm³ (normal, 140 to 400); white blood cell (WBC) count, 2.8 × 10³/mm³ (normal, 4 to 11); serum folate, 3.8 ng/mL (normal, 7 to 18); serum vitamin B₁₂, 230 pg/mL (normal, >200); aspartate aminotransferase (AST), 235 IU/L (normal, 0 to 56); alanine aminotransferase (ALT), 127 IU/L (normal, 0 to 56); γ-glutamyl transpeptidase (GGT), 435 IU/L (normal, 8 to 78); alkaline phosphatase, 245 IU/L (normal, 40 to 143); total bilirubin, 3.4 mg/dL (normal, ≤1.2); albumin, 3.6 g/dL (normal, 3.5 to 5); BUN, 6 mg/dL (normal, 5 to 22); serum creatinine (SrCr), 0.6 mg/dL (normal, 0.6 to 1.1). What is the likely cause of D.T.'s symptoms based upon these data?

[SI units: Hgb, 103 g/L (normal, 110 to 150); Hct, 0.31 (normal, 0.34 to 0.46); MCHC, 0.30 g/L (normal, 0.34 to 0.36); MCV, 104 fL (normal, 80 to 100); platelets, 90 × 10¹¹/L (normal, 1.4 to 4.0); WBC count, 2.8 × 10⁹/L (normal, 4 to 10); serum folate, 8.6 nmol/L (normal, 16 to 40); serum vitamin B₁₂, 169 pmol/L (normal, >148); AST, 235 U/L (normal, 0 to 56); ALT, 127 U/L (normal, 0 to 56); GGT, 435 U/L (normal, 8 to 78); alkaline phosphatase, 245 U/L (normal, 40 to 143); total bilirubin, 58 mmol/L (normal, ≤21); albumin, 36 g/L (normal, 35 to 50); BUN, 2.1 mmol/L of urea (normal, 1.8 to 7.9); SrCr, 53 mmol/L (normal, 53 to 97)]

Hepatitis is part of a spectrum of liver disease that can occur in patients who consume large amounts of alcohol (Table 84-5). Fatty liver, or alcoholic steatosis, is the first stage of hepatotoxicity and is probably present in nearly all persons who consume ethanol in daily amounts of 20 to 40 g or more. Hepatitis develops in about 90% of alcoholics who have fatty livers if they continue to drink. Cirrhosis, the third and final stage of alcohol-induced liver toxicity, develops in 8% to 20% of patients with chronic alcoholism. It may follow acute symptomatic hepatitis or develop in patients without previously documented clinical hepatitis.[125,126]

The clinical presentation of alcoholic hepatitis varies considerably. Patients can be completely asymptomatic or can present with fulminant symptoms. The diminished appetite, weight loss, abdominal pain, and chills seen in D.T. are typical symptoms in patients with alcoholic hepatitis. Other symptoms include low-grade and/or spiking fevers, vomiting, jaundice, and GI bleeding. More serious complications can include esophageal varices, ascites, encephalopathy, splenomegaly, renal failure, and coagulopathies.[125,126] Patients with alcoholic hepatitis often exhibit anemia, leukocytosis or leukopenia, and thrombocytopenia. AST and ALT generally are elevated, although the AST is seldom more than five times the upper limit of normal, and the ALT concentration is usually less than half the AST value. The GGT level generally is elevated but does not correlate with the severity of the disease. The alkaline phosphatase and bilirubin levels also generally are elevated, reflecting cholestasis, which typically accompanies alcoholic hepatitis. In more severe cases, prothrombin time also may be elevated, reflecting reduced production of clotting factors by the liver. Significantly reduced serum albumin may reflect reduced hepatic synthetic function or malnutrition[127,128] (see also Chapter 29, Alcoholic

Table 84-5 Medical Complications of Chronic Alcoholism: Presentation and Treatment

Complication	Presentation	Treatment
Liver Disease		
• Progressive: fatty liver (steatosis), hepatitis, then cirrhosis	Varies from asymptomatic to fulminant. Anorexia, weight loss, abdominal pain, chills, fevers, vomiting, jaundice, GI bleeding, elevated AST and ALT, cholestatic changes, low albumin, high prothrombin time.	Abstinence to prevent progression; supportive care: bed rest, hydration, nutrition
Hematologic Complications		
• Megaloblastic anemia due to folate deficiency • Sideroblastic anemia and hemosiderosis due to deranged iron metabolism • Iron deficiency anemia due to poor diet and GI blood loss • Thrombocytopenia due to interference with platelet function and formation		Oral multiple vitamins, folic acid, iron sulfate (325 mg/day)

Table 84-5   Medical Complications of Chronic Alcoholism: Presentation and Treatment—cont'd

Complication	Presentation	Treatment
GI Effects		
• Diarrhea • Acute hemorrhagic, chronic and atrophic gastritis, may be due to *H. pylori* • Gastroesophageal reflux disease (GERD)	Acute abdominal pain, nausea, esophageal reflux, vomiting	Gastritis typically resolves a few days after discontinuing alcohol. Antacids, H₂-receptor antagonists, and proton pump inhibitors may provide pain and heartburn relief, and speed healing.
Pancreatitis		
• Heavy alcohol consumption is second most common cause (35% of cases) • Typically occurs after binge drinking	Severe abdominal pain radiating from the upper abdomen through to the back and flanks, nausea, vomiting, elevated lipase and amylase levels	Supportive care: NPO, parenteral analgesia, hydration and nutrition
Wernicke-Korsakoff Syndrome		
• A neurologic disorder caused by thiamine deficiency • Wernicke's encephalopathy can be precipitated by large glucose load. • Korsakoff's psychosis develops in 80% who survive but fail to recover in 48–72 hours. • A medical emergency	• Wernicke's: CNS depression (mental sluggishness, restlessness, confusion, coma), ambulation problems (wide-based, ataxic gait), ocular problems, hypothermia, hypotension, polyneuropathy • Korsakoff's: retrograde amnesia, anterograde amnesia, confabulation	Thiamine 100 mg by slow IV push before or concurrently with dextrose-containing fluids, then oral thiamine 50 to 100 mg/day
Cardiovascular Effects		
• Alcoholic cardiomyopathy after 10+ years of excessive alcohol leads to decreased contractile function. • Hypertension associated with >3 standard drinks/day • Arrhythmias can occur after heavy alcohol consumption.	Cardiomyopathy occurs between 30–60 years of age as low output failure	See Chapter 14, Essential Hypertension; Chapter 19, Heart Failure; and Chapter 20, Cardiac Arrhythmias
Endocrine Effects		
Hypogonadism due to reduced synthesis and increased metabolism of testosterone	• Women: amenorrhea, anovulation, hyperprolactinemia leading to infertility, spontaneous abortion, and impaired fetal growth and development • Men: loss of facial hair, gynecomastia, decreased muscle and bone mass, testicular atrophy, decreased libido, and sexual impotence	No treatment except discontinuation of alcohol
Myopathy		
A syndrome of muscle necrosis perhaps caused by direct toxicity of alcohol on muscle tissue	Ranges from asymptomatic to weakness, pain and swelling of muscles to frank rhabdomyolysis. Myoglobinuria and elevated MM fraction of creatine kinase.	Correct electrolyte abnormalities, maintain urine output, and use sodium bicarbonate to alkalinize the urine if myoglobin is present to prevent precipitation.
Neuropathy		
Autonomic and peripheral neuropathies are common; caused by neurotoxicity of alcohol.	Pain and weakness, but often asymptomatic	Discontinuation of alcohol; supportive care

CNS, central nervous system; GI, gastrointestinal; NPO, nothing by mouth.

Cirrhosis). D.T.'s symptoms and laboratory results are consistent with a diagnosis of alcoholic hepatitis.

16. **How should D.T.'s hepatitis be managed, and what is her prognosis?**

The cornerstone in the management of alcohol-induced liver disease is abstinence from alcohol. Although abstinence is sufficient to produce resolution of fatty liver, it may not be sufficient to produce clinical recovery in patients with alcoholic hepatitis. This is particularly true in severe cases or when complications are present.[129] Thus, even complete abstinence from alcohol does not ensure that a patient will survive an episode of alcoholic hepatitis.

General supportive care for patients with alcoholic hepatitis should include bed rest, correction of dehydration, appropriate dietary intake of carbohydrate and protein, and replacement of severe vitamin and mineral deficiencies (e.g., bicarbonate, calcium, chloride, magnesium, potassium, phosphate, sodium, vitamin A, folic acid, thiamine, vitamin B_{12}, iron, zinc).[125,130,131] Because D.T. does not have numerous complicating factors, her prognosis may be fairly good if she abstains from alcohol and receives appropriate supportive care.

17. **What specific drug therapy might be considered to treat D.T.'s alcoholic hepatitis?**

Insulin and glucagon, pentoxifylline, penicillamine, amlodipine (Norvasc), and colchicine have been studied in the management of alcoholic hepatitis, although further evaluation is needed.[48,126,132–134] A meta-analysis noted a lack of benefit from propylthiouracil in the management of alcoholic liver disease.[135]

Corticosteroids have been more widely studied, but varying results have produced controversy regarding their efficacy in alcoholic hepatitis. Furthermore, optimal doses have not been established. It has been suggested that corticosteroids reduce short-term mortality only when alcoholic hepatitis accompanied by hepatic encephalopathy occurs in patients without GI bleeding. This finding has been questioned, and it is unknown whether other subgroups of patients might benefit from corticosteroid therapy.[136] Data also are inconclusive regarding the long-term benefits of corticosteroids.[137] Corticosteroid therapy is not indicated in D.T. because no conclusive data support its effectiveness.

Hematologic Complications

18. **What is the explanation for D.T.'s abnormal hematologic values?**

Folate deficiency is the most common sign of malnutrition in chronic alcoholism, with about 30% of patients with severe alcoholism developing a megaloblastic anemia.[138–140] Several different causes account for folate deficiency in alcoholics. Most common are diets inadequate in sources of folate (i.e., green leafy vegetables, liver), impaired jejunal absorption of folate, decreased retention and storage of folate (which accompanies severe liver disease), acute effects of ethanol on tissue affinity of circulating folate, probable alteration of enterohepatic cycling of folate, and excretion of larger amounts of folate secondary to hemolysis.

People with chronic alcoholism also can experience derangements of iron metabolism that can produce both sideroblastic anemia and hemosiderosis. Sideroblastic anemia is a complex disorder that is due in part to deranged pyridoxine function and decreased enzyme activity involved with heme synthesis. Hemosiderosis is the accumulation of hemosiderin, a byproduct of phagocytic digestion of hematin that contains up to 37% iron. Iron deficiency anemia also is common in alcoholism and is due to inadequate dietary intake and, often, GI blood loss. Hemolytic anemia also can result from liver damage (see also Chapter 87, Anemias).

Several factors can make alcoholics more prone to bleeding. Alcohol can prolong bleeding times by interfering with platelet function, and it produces thrombocytopenia by suppressing platelet formation. As mentioned, alcohol-induced hepatotoxicity can diminish the production of vitamin K–dependent clotting factors by the liver.

In D.T.'s case, the increased MCV, low serum folate level, and normal vitamin B_{12} level are characteristic of a folate-deficiency, megaloblastic anemia. The low platelet count may be caused by the toxic effect of alcohol or it may be related to D.T.'s alcoholic hepatitis.

19. **How should D.T.'s anemia be managed?**

D.T.'s stool should be tested for occult blood to ensure that GI blood loss is not contributing to the anemia. This will determine whether an additional GI workup is necessary. D.T. should be given an oral multiple vitamin with folic acid daily along with ferrous sulfate 325 mg/day. This supplementation should be continued until it can be reasonably ensured that D.T. has stopped drinking and has resumed an adequate dietary intake.

Fetal Effects

20. **D.T. has no children but is planning to become pregnant. What effects could continued consumption of alcohol have on her fetus if she were to become pregnant?**

The characteristics of fetal alcohol syndrome (FAS) and fetal alcohol effects (FAE) are discussed in Chapter 47, Teratogenicity and Drugs in Breast Milk. The estimated incidence of FAS in the population as a whole ranges from 1 case per 700 to 2,000 live births. All reported babies with FAS have been born to mothers with chronic alcoholism who drank heavily throughout pregnancy, especially when mothers drank at least 150 g of ethanol per day. In prospective studies, FAS occurred in the offspring of alcohol-dependent women at rates ranging from 2.5% to 10%.[141,142] Both FAS and FAE have been observed in almost all ethnic groups and at various socioeconomic levels.

The most predictable consequence of prenatal exposure to alcohol is intrauterine growth retardation. The decrease in fetal growth is caused by alcohol itself and not by congeners present in alcoholic beverages. Alcohol appears to interfere with fetal growth by inducing hypoxia, which interferes with cellular processes (e.g., placental transport, protein synthesis) that require oxygen. Although alcohol exerts its greatest impact on fetal growth when consumed during the third trimester, teratogenic effects also have been correlated with first-trimester exposure to alcohol.[143] Thus, it is wise for women to avoid alcohol consumption throughout pregnancy.[143,144]

D.T. should delay pregnancy until she has abstained from alcohol. She should be told about the harmful effects of alcohol consumption on her fetus.

Gastritis and Ulcer Disease

21. R.K., age 45, sees his physician on a Monday morning with complaints of acute abdominal pain, nausea, vomiting, and diarrhea. He has been a heavy drinker for 15 years and binges on weekends. He denies that his drinking is a problem but entered an alcohol treatment program 4 years ago at the insistence of his wife and college-aged son. He resumed drinking within 2 weeks of completing the program. He has a 35 pack-year smoking history and currently smokes approximately 1.5 packs/day. What are the probable causes of R.K.'s GI distress?

Various GI disturbances have been attributed to chronic ethanol ingestion. Diarrhea is a common symptom in binge drinkers and may be related to an alteration in the intestinal cell morphology that interferes with the absorption of water and nutrients (e.g., amino acids, glucose, thiamine, folic acid, vitamin B_{12}, potassium, magnesium, phosphate, zinc).[145–147] This also may partially account for the significant malnutrition seen in many alcoholics.

Chronic alcohol ingestion can lead to acute hemorrhagic gastritis, chronic gastritis, and atrophic gastritis with hypochlorhydria, attributable to the injurious effects of alcohol on the GI mucosa.[50] A potential role for *Helicobacter pylori* in the pathogenesis of alcohol-related gastritis has not been supported because an inverse graded relationship has been noted between alcohol consumption and active infection with *H. pylori*.[148] The lower *H. pylori* incidence in heavier alcohol drinkers was attributed to alcohol's antibacterial effects against this organism. Despite the lower incidence of *H. pylori* infection in heavy drinkers, increased ammonia production by *H. pylori* may contribute to the development of gastritis in those who are infected.[149] Antibiotic therapy to eradicate *H. pylori* should therefore be considered in the management of chronic gastritis. (See Chapter 27, Upper Gastrointestinal Disorders.)

Although predisposition to peptic ulcers has been attributed to alcohol consumption, the increase in the risk of ulcer disease was small after controlling for cigarette smoking and other sociodemographic variables.[150] Alcohol also affects esophageal peristalsis and reduces lower esophageal sphincter pressure, which can contribute to gastroesophageal reflux disease (GERD) and lead to esophageal bleeding and stricture formation. In some patients, GERD, along with alcohol-induced impaired glottic reflexes, may result in aspiration and lung abscesses that typically occur during periods of alcoholic stupor[151,152] (see Chapter 27, Upper Gastrointestinal Disorders).

In R.K.'s case, alcohol-induced gastritis would seem to be a logical explanation for his symptoms, although peptic ulcer disease, alcoholic hepatitis, and/or pancreatitis (see Question 26) can present with similar symptoms.

22. A presumptive diagnosis of alcohol-induced gastritis is made for R.K. How should he be treated?

Gastritis induced by alcohol consumption typically resolves within a few days after ceasing alcohol consumption.

Antacids, H_2-receptor antagonists, and proton pump inhibitors may speed healing and provide rapid pain relief but generally are not required. R.K. should not receive any specific therapy at this time. If his symptoms persist, he should be tested for *H. pylori* and appropriately treated if he is infected (see Chapter 27, Upper Gastrointestinal Disorders).

H_2-Receptor Antagonist Interactions

23. R.K. receives a prescription for oral ranitidine (Zantac) 150 mg twice daily. What will happen if R.K. continues to drink while taking this drug?

H_2-receptor antagonists may inhibit gastric alcohol dehydrogenase, increase gastric emptying, and thereby reduce first-pass metabolism, which in turn increases blood alcohol concentrations and the chance of intoxication. Increases in blood alcohol concentrations have been highest in studies when small doses of ethanol (approximately 0.15 g/kg) were studied. The effect appears to be less pronounced at higher ethanol doses.[153] The available data do not support a clinically or socially significant ethanol interaction with H_2-receptor antagonists.[154] Because R.K. is a chronic drinker, he is unlikely to have a significant drug interaction. Proton pump inhibitors do not increase blood ethanol levels and may be better alternatives should R.K. require acid-suppressive therapy.[155–157]

Cancer

24. R.K.'s wife has heard that heavy alcohol use increases the risk of certain cancers. She knows that R.K., a smoker, already is at increased risk for cancer. What is the association of alcohol with carcinogenesis?

Excessive consumption of alcohol clearly increases the risk of developing cancer of the tongue, mouth, oropharynx, esophagus, liver, and breast.[145,158] Alcohol is not a true carcinogen, but it may act as a tumor "promoter" by chronically irritating membranes and by dissolving tobacco carcinogens, thus increasing mucosal concentrations in the mouth, pharynx, larynx, and esophagus.[145,146,159] A much higher incidence of these cancers has been noted in heavy drinkers who also smoke compared with those who do not smoke.[145] Various other mechanisms have been suggested by which alcohol could stimulate carcinogenesis, including the previously discussed role of acetaldehyde.[51,158]

R.K.'s drinking clearly increases his risk for cancer. If he stopped smoking but continued to drink, his cancer risk would be somewhat reduced.

Pancreatitis

25. R.K. presents to the ED 6 weeks later with more severe abdominal pain, which radiates from the upper abdominal area through to both flanks. He also has experienced nausea and vomiting for the past 12 hours. His wife reports that he has been on an alcohol binge over the past 4 days. Physical examination reveals a tender and distended abdomen. Laboratory results include a plasma amylase of 675 IU/L (normal, 0 to 130) and lipase of 1,045 IU/L (normal, 23 to 208). What is the likely cause of R.K.'s clinical symptoms?

[SI units: amylase, 675 U/L (normal, 0 to 130); lipase, 1,045 U/L (normal, 23 to 208)]

Heavy alcohol consumption now is the second most common cause of acute pancreatitis, accounting for 35% of cases.[160] Acute exacerbations typically occur after binge drinking episodes. Many years of alcohol abuse generally are required before an acute episode occurs, but other factors also must play a role in its development because only 5% of alcoholics develop pancreatitis. In most patients, alcoholic pancreatitis presents as an acute episode. Most often, this is superimposed on a chronic underlying pancreatic inflammation, while in a few patients acute pancreatitis probably develops in the absence of prior chronic disease. Hyperlipidemia, which often is present in patients with heavy alcohol consumption, also may contribute to the development of pancreatitis.[161]

Patients typically present with abdominal pain, often severe, that radiates from the upper abdomen through to the back or both flanks. As illustrated in R.K., the diagnosis generally is supported by serum amylase and lipase levels at the time patients present with abdominal pain. Lipase levels appear to be more sensitive and specific than amylase levels because lipase levels may remain elevated for several days, whereas amylase levels may quickly return to normal.[162] In addition, an elevated ratio of lipase to amylase may differentiate pancreatitis induced by alcohol from other forms of acute pancreatitis.[163]

In R.K., the severe radiating abdominal pain and elevated amylase, lipase, and lipase-to-amylase ratio all are indicative of acute pancreatitis. Pancreatitis also may have been the cause of the symptoms he experienced 6 weeks earlier.

26. **How should R.K. be treated?**

The appropriate management for R.K. is supportive therapy (e.g., NPO [nothing by mouth], parenteral analgesia, IV hydration or total parental nutrition if his nutritional status so dictates).[160] Nasogastric suction does not promote pain relief or reduce the length of hospital stays and should not be used in R.K. unless he develops ileus or severe vomiting. Various drugs, including cimetidine, have been used in the hope that they would reduce pancreatic stimulation, but they generally should not be used in patients such as R.K. because their effectiveness has not been demonstrated.

Wernicke-Korsakoff Syndrome

27. **T.W., age 58, is brought to the ED in a comatose state but responsive to pain. His family members report that he has been drinking heavily for the past few days and has consumed about a quart of bourbon daily for the past 11 years. Vital signs on admission include BP, 100/70 mm Hg; pulse, 120 beats/min; respiratory rate, 20 breaths/min; and rectal temperature 101.5°F. The electrocardiograph reveals atrial fibrillation. An IV line is established with 5% dextrose infusion; T.W. receives IV doses of 0.8 mg of naloxone, 100 mg of thiamine, and 50 mL of 50% dextrose. What are the potential causes of T.W.'s comatose state?**

Two potential causes of T.W.'s comatose state are acute ethanol intoxication and Wernicke's encephalopathy. Wernicke's encephalopathy is a neurologic disorder caused by thiamine deficiency and most commonly is encountered in patients with severe alcoholism. This condition is a medical emergency and carries an estimated 10% to 20% mortality rate. An abrupt onset and an evolving triad of symptoms that develop gradually over several days characterize the classic presentation of Wernicke's encephalopathy. However, classic Wernicke's encephalopathy is neither frequently nor consistently encountered in clinical practice. Typical symptoms include (1) CNS depression (e.g., mental sluggishness, restlessness, confusion, coma); (2) ambulatory difficulties (e.g., wide-based ataxic gait, vestibular paresis); and (3) ocular problems (e.g., horizontal nystagmus, conjugate gaze palsies, pupillary abnormalities, retinal hemorrhages, papilledema). In addition to this triad of symptoms, patients also may experience hypothermia, hypotension, and polyneuropathy.[145,164,165]

Chronic alcoholics, such as T.W., frequently are deficient in thiamine because of poor dietary intake. Because thiamine is a cofactor in glucose metabolism, thiamine deficiency, and consequently Wernicke's encephalopathy, can be precipitated by administration of a large glucose load. Therefore, parenteral thiamine (IM or slow IV push) should be administered before, or concurrently with, dextrose-containing IV fluids to known or suspected alcoholic patients. Subsequently, oral thiamine should be administered in a dosage of 50 to 100 mg/day to replenish thiamine stores.[164-166]

Korsakoff's psychosis develops in about 80% of patients with Wernicke's encephalopathy who survive but fail to recover in the first 48 to 72 hours. Characteristics of this condition include retrograde amnesia (inability to recall prior information) and anterograde amnesia (inability to assimilate new information). Confabulation (fabrication of stories) is typical in the early stages of this disease but frequently disappears during the later stages. About 25% to 50% of patients with Korsakoff's psychosis do not recover completely and may require long-term care.[165,166]

T.W.'s comatose condition could be caused by either acute ethanol intoxication or Wernicke's encephalopathy, and both possible diagnoses should be considered in developing his plan of care.

28. **Why was the therapy that T.W. received in the ED appropriate?**

Naloxone should be administered to all comatose patients such as T.W. to reverse the effects of possible opiate overdose in persons known to be substance abusers. For reasons previously described, IV thiamine was appropriate because T.W. has a long history of alcohol consumption. The 50% dextrose was administered to manage potential hypoglycemia, as previously discussed under acute ethanol intoxication.

Cardiovascular

29. **What cardiovascular effects of alcohol could account for T.W.'s sudden development of atrial fibrillation?**

Various beneficial and detrimental cardiovascular effects have been attributed to consumption of varying amounts of alcoholic beverages. In epidemiologic studies, light to moderate alcohol consumption (up to 2 drinks/day) has been associated with a reduced risk of myocardial infarction and sudden cardiac death,[167,168] although the results of some studies have suggested otherwise.[169] Alcohol increases high-density lipoprotein cholesterol, a factor that is inversely associated with coronary heart disease risk, and has an antithrombotic action.[170] Both of these effects may explain why light to moderate alcohol consumption is associated with a reduced cardiac risk, as well as a reduced risk of ischemic stroke.[171] In contrast, recent heavy alcohol consumption increases the risk of all major types of stroke.[171,172] Given the many severe adverse consequences of alcohol use, it appears unwise to advise nondrinkers to start consuming alcoholic beverages for possible modest cardiovascular benefits.

As previously mentioned, chronic alcoholics are frequently malnourished, and vitamin deficiencies may increase their risk of cardiovascular disease. Hyperhomocysteinemia is an independent risk factor for cardiovascular disease, and deficiencies of folic acid, vitamin B_6, and vitamin B_{12} are known causes of homocysteine elevations.[173] In addition to lowering homocysteine, folate has other potential cardiovascular benefits (e.g., antioxidant activity, effects on cofactor availability, direct interactions with the enzyme endothelial nitric oxide synthetase).[174] These findings seem to provide additional support for maintaining adequate nutritional status in heavy alcohol users, including vitamin supplementation as necessary. Since folate deficiency is common in chronic alcoholics, T.W.'s folate status should be a consideration in the workup of his cardiac problems.

Alcoholic cardiomyopathy is commonly seen in chronic alcoholics and apparently results from alterations in the contractile functions of the heart.[175] Of these individuals, about one third have a depressed cardiac ejection fraction.[176] Alcoholic cardiomyopathy usually becomes clinically apparent between the ages of 30 and 60 and typically requires at least 10 years of excessive alcohol consumption, but individuals consuming >90 g/day (seven or eight standard drinks) for 5 or more years are at increased risk.[175] In terms of symptomatology, this disease reflects low-output cardiac failure and cannot be differentiated from other dilated cardiomyopathies.

An increased prevalence of hypertension in alcoholics has been noted.[177] A daily alcohol consumption rate of three or more standard drinks seems to be the threshold for a consistent hypertensive response, although the threshold may be lower in older persons.[178] Possible mechanisms by which alcohol consumption may increase BP include (1) CNS imbalance; (2) impairment of the baroreceptors; (3) increased sympathetic activity; (4) stimulation of the renin-angiotensin-aldosterone system; (5) increased cortisol levels; (6) increased intracellular calcium with a resultant increase in vascular reactivity; (7) stimulation of the endothelium to release endothelin or inhibition of endothelium-dependent nitric oxide production; and (8) chronic subclinical alcohol withdrawal.[179]

Heavy alcohol consumption has been associated with an increased incidence of various cardiac conduction disturbances.[177,180] Heavy binge drinkers may present with a sudden onset of paroxysmal arrhythmias, including junctional tachycardia, premature ventricular or atrial contractions, atrial tachycardia, and ventricular tachycardia; however, atrial fibrillation and flutter are the two most commonly encountered arrhythmias.[181,182] These arrhythmias have been termed "holiday heart" when they appear in persons free of overt cardiomyopathies who appear in EDs after high alcohol consumption during holidays (e.g., New Year's Eve, St. Patrick's Day).[182] They have been attributed to various factors, including preclinical cardiomyopathy, electrolyte abnormalities (e.g., potassium, phosphate, magnesium), and conduction delays induced by alcohol and its metabolites. Renal tubular dysfunction frequently occurs during chronic alcohol abuse and produces electrolyte abnormalities that are reversible after 4 weeks of alcohol abstinence.[183] Obviously, such electrolyte disturbances may contribute to cardiac conduction defects.

In T.W.'s case, his recent heavy alcohol consumption may well have contributed to his development of atrial fibrillation.

30. How should T.W.'s atrial fibrillation be managed?

At present, no good data on the management of alcohol-related cardiac arrhythmias are available. Because many of these arrhythmias terminate within 24 to 48 hours, it seems wise to withhold therapy or limit therapy to a short course of β-blockers. Either approach could be considered appropriate for T.W. His serum electrolytes should be measured and replenished if deficiencies are found. Obviously, long-term treatment should be directed toward managing his alcoholism.[184]

Endocrine

31. R.R., age 47, is a malnourished street person who comes to the medical clinic complaining of pain, weakness, and swelling of his leg muscles, especially the calves. He also complains of recent loss of libido and sexual impotence. The findings on physical examination reveal a thin, unkempt man with loss of facial hair, gynecomastia, and testicular atrophy. He admits to drinking alcohol for the past 25 years. What signs and symptoms might suggest alterations of R.R.'s endocrine system due to alcohol abuse?

Various clinical features reflecting hypogonadism can occur in alcoholics. Changes seen in women may include amenorrhea, anovulation, luteal phase dysfunction, hyperprolactinemia, and ovarian pathology. Subsequent reproductive consequences may range from infertility and an increased risk of spontaneous abortion to impairment of fetal growth and development.[185]

In men, the hypogonadal features and changes that commonly are found are similar to those seen in R.R. They include loss of facial hair, gynecomastia, diminished muscle and bone mass, testicular atrophy, loss of libido, and sexual impotence. Alcohol may reduce testosterone by interfering with the testicular biosynthesis of testosterone and by inducing steroid reductases, which results in increased hepatic metabolism of testosterone. Alcohol may inhibit the pituitary release of luteinizing hormone, which is involved in testosterone biosynthesis.[145,186] At present, no treatment is effective for alcohol-induced hypogonadism, such as that seen in R.R., other than complete cessation of alcohol consumption. This may result in improvement in some patients.

Neuromuscular

32. How could R.R.'s complaints of weakness, pain, and swelling of the calf muscles be attributed to alcohol abuse?

Alcoholic myopathy is a syndrome of muscle necrosis that varies greatly in severity and occurs frequently in alcoholics. Initial presentation can range from frank rhabdomyolysis with myoglobinuria to asymptomatic, transient elevations of the

MM fraction of creatine kinase. More than 80% of all cases have been reported in men ages 40 to 60 years. When recurrent cases of myopathy occur, they almost always are associated with heavy drinking binges. When rhabdomyolysis occurs, acute tubular necrosis and subsequent renal failure, which may be fatal, will likely follow if it is not rapidly detected and treated. Evidence supports the contention that alcohol itself injures the skeletal muscle.[187] However, it has been hypothesized that some alcohol-associated myotoxicity could be due to ethanol induction of skeletal muscle cytochrome P450, which leads to the production of toxic metabolites of other compounds that injure the muscle.[188] Other factors such as crush injuries, seizures, or hypokalemia may also precipitate, or contribute to, rhabdomyolysis in alcoholics. Data also suggest that cardiomyopathy frequently is present in patients with skeletal muscular weakness.[189]

Autonomic and peripheral neuropathies are common in heavy drinkers and may produce weakness and muscular pain.[190] However, in many instances, alcoholic polyneuropathies may be asymptomatic and demonstrable only with electroneurographic testing.[191] Alcohol appears to be toxic to autonomic and peripheral nerves in a dose-dependent manner.

R.R.'s symptoms and drinking history are consistent with alcohol-induced myopathy, although neuropathy may be a contributing factor.

33. **Because alcoholic myopathy is suspected in R.R., how should he be evaluated and managed?**

An appropriate workup for R.R. includes testing of the urine for myoglobin because of its toxic effects on the kidney. His serum creatine kinase concentration should be measured and his renal function and urine output should be assessed. Appropriate management for R.R. includes correction of any electrolyte abnormalities, particularly potassium and magnesium. Appropriate urine output should be established and maintained. In addition, if myoglobin is found in the urine, IV sodium bicarbonate should be administered to maintain an alkaline urine, which will prevent deposition of myoglobin in the renal tubules. Of course, attempts should be made to have R.R. participate in an appropriate alcohol treatment program.

REFERENCES

1. Blincoe LJ et al. The Economic Impact of Motor Vehicle Crashes 2000. Washington, DC: US Department of Transportation, National Highway Traffic Safety Administration, 2002.
2. Lundberg GD et al. Now read this: the SI units are here. JAMA 1986;255:2329.
3. Department of Health and Human Services. Healthy People 2000: National Health Promotion and Disease Prevention Objectives. Washington, DC: U.S. Government Printing Office, 1991; DHHS publication no. (PHS)91-50212.
4. Office of Applied Studies. National Household Survey on Drug Abuse: Main Findings 1997. Rockville, MD: Substance Abuse and Mental Health Services Administration, 1999; DHHS publication no. (SMA)99-3295.
5. Klitzner M et al. Reducing underage drinking and its consequences. Alcohol Health Res World 1993;17:12.
6. National Institute on Drug Abuse. National Survey Results on Drug Use from the Monitoring the Future Study, 1975–1997. Washington, DC: U.S. Government Printing Office, 1998; NIH publication no. 98-4345.
7. Wechsler H. Alcohol and the American college campus: a report from the Harvard School of Public Health. Change 1996;July/August:20.
8. Naimi TS et al. Binge drinking among US adults. JAMA 2003;289:70.
9. McGinnis JM, Foege WH. Actual causes of death in the United States. JAMA 1993;270:32.
10. National Council on Alcoholism and Drug Dependence. NCADD Fact Sheet: Alcoholism and Alcohol-Related Problems. New York, 1990.
11. Day NL. The effects of prenatal exposure to alcohol. Alcohol Health Res World 1992;16:238.
12. Smart RG, Mann RE. Alcohol and the epidemiology of liver cirrhosis. Alcohol Health Res World 1992;16:217.
13. Arria AM, VanThiel DH. The epidemiology of alcohol-related chronic disease. Alcohol Health Res World 1992;16:209.
14. Center on Addiction and Substance Abuse. The Cost of Substance Abuse to America's Health Care System, Report 1: Medicaid Hospital Costs. New York: Columbia University, 1993.
15. Longnecker MP. Alcohol consumption in relation to risk of cancers of the breast and large bowel. Alcohol Health Res World 1992;16:238.
16. Stinson FS et al. Association of alcohol problems with risk for AIDS in the 1988 National Health Interview Survey. Alcohol Health Res World 1992; 16:245.
17. Office for Substance Abuse Prevention. Alcohol Practices, Policies and Potentials of American Colleges and Universities: A White Paper. Rockville, MD: The National Clearinghouse for Alcohol and Drug Information, 1991.
18. Cherpital CJ. The epidemiology of alcohol-related trauma. Alcohol Health Res World 1992;16:191.
19. Bernstein M, Mahoney JJ. Management perspectives on alcoholism: the employer's stake in alcoholism treatment. Occup Med 1989;4:223.
20. Institute for Health Policy, Brandeis University. Substance Abuse: The Nation's Number One Health Problem. Princeton, NJ: The Robert Wood Johnson Foundation, 1993.
21. Office for Substance Abuse Prevention. Too Many Young People Drink and Know Too Little About the Consequences. Rockville, MD: National Clearinghouse for Alcohol and Drug Information, 1991.
22. Roth RA. The impact of liquor liability on colleges and universities. J Coll Univ Law 1986;13:45.
23. Centers for Disease Control and Prevention. Morbidity and mortality weekly report: results from the national adolescent student health survey. JAMA 1989;261:2025.
24. National Highway Traffic Safety Administration. Fatal Accident Reporting System: 1987. Washington, DC: U.S. Department of Transportation, 1988.
25. National Commission on Drug-Free Schools. Toward a Drug-Free Generation: A Nation's Responsibility. Washington, DC: U.S. Department of Education, 1990.
26. Jackson VM et al. Measurement of social drinking: the need for specific guidelines. Health Values 1990;14:25.
27. Rice DP. The economic cost of alcohol abuse and alcohol dependence: 1990. Alcohol Health Res World 1993;17:10.
28. Moskowitz J. The primary prevention of alcohol problems: a critical review of the research literature. J Stud Alcohol 1989;50:54.
29. Wenrich MD et al. Do primary care physicians screen patients about alcohol intake using the CAGE questions? J Gen Intern Med 1995;10:631.
30. David DJ, Spyker DA. The acute toxicity of ethanol: dosage and kinetic nomograms. Vet Hum Toxicol 1979;21:272.
31. Oneta CM et al. First-pass metabolism of ethanol is strikingly influenced by the speed of gastric emptying. Gut 1998;43:612.
32. Jones AW et al. Effect of high-fat, high-protein, and high-carbohydrate meals on the pharmacokinetics of a small dose of ethanol. Br J Clin Pharmacol 1997;44:521.
33. Jones BM, Vega A. Cognitive performance measured on the ascending and descending limb of the blood alcohol curve. Psychopharmacology (Berl) 1972;23:99.
34. Hawkins RD, Kalant H. The metabolism of ethanol and its metabolic effects. Pharmacol Rev 1972; 24:67.
35. DiPadova C et al. Effects of fasting and chronic alcohol consumption on the first-pass metabolism of ethanol. Gastroenterology 1987;92:1169.
36. Ammon E et al. Disposition and first-pass metabolism of ethanol in humans: is it gastric or hepatic and does it depend on gender? Clin Pharmacol Ther 1996;59:503.
37. Brown AS et al. The effect of gastritis on human gastric alcohol dehydrogenase activity and ethanol metabolism. Aliment Pharmacol Ther 1995;9:57.
38. Seitz HK et al. Human gastric alcohol dehydrogenase activity: effect of age, sex, and alcoholism. Gut 1993;34:1433.
39. Wagner JG et al. Elimination of alcohol from human blood. J Pharm Sci 1976;65:152.
40. Wilkinson PK et al. Blood ethanol concentrations during and following constant-rate intravenous infusion of alcohol. Clin Pharmacol Ther 1976; 19:213.
41. Hammond KB et al. Blood ethanol: a report of unusually high levels in a living patient. JAMA 1973; 226:63.
42. Schumate RP et al. A study of the metabolic rates of alcohol in the human body. J Forensic Med 1967; 14:83.
43. Crabb DW et al. Alcohol sensitivity, alcohol metabolism, risk of alcoholism, and the role of alcohol and aldehyde dehydrogenase. J Lab Clin Med 1993;122:234.
44. Kopun M, Propping P. The kinetics of ethanol absorption and elimination in twins and supplementary repetitive experiments in singleton subjects. Eur J Clin Pharmacol 1977;11:337.
45. Mendelson JH et al. Effects of experimentally induced intoxication on metabolism of ethanol-1-C[14] in alcoholic subjects. Metabolism 1965;14:1255.
46. Adachi J et al. Comparative study on ethanol elimination and blood acetaldehyde between alcoholics and control subjects. Alcohol Clin Exp Res 1989; 13:601.

47. Lieber CS. Alcohol and the liver: 1994 update. Gastroenterology 1994;106:1085.

48. Lieber CS. Alcohol and the liver: 1984 update. Hepatology 1984;4:1243.

49. DeFeo P et al. Ethanol impairs post-prandial hepatic protein metabolism. J Clin Invest 1995;95:1472.

50. Lieber CS. Hepatic and other medical disorders of alcoholism: from pathogenesis to treatment. J Stud Alcohol 1998;59:9.

51. Eriksson CJP. The role of acetaldehyde in the actions of alcohol. Alcohol Clin Exp Res 2001;25:15S.

52. Melgaard B. The neurotoxicity of ethanol. Acta Neurol Scand 1983;67:131.

53. Kupari I et al. Acute effects of alcohol, beta blockade and their combination on left ventricular function and hemodynamics in normal man. Eur Heart J 1983;4:463.

54. Michiels TM et al. Naloxone reverses ethanol-induced depression of hypercapnic drive. Am Rev Respir Dis 1983;128:823.

55. Barros SR, Rodriguez GJ. Naloxone as an antagonist in alcohol intoxication. Anesthesiology 1981;54:174.

56. North DS et al. Naloxone administration in clonidine overdosage. Ann Emerg Med 1981;10:7.

57. Hackshaw KV et al. Naloxone in septic shock. Crit Care Med 1990;18:47.

58. Wright DJM et al. Naloxone in shock. Lancet. 1980;2:1360.

59. Tobin MJ et al. Effect of naloxone on breathing pattern in patients with chronic obstructive pulmonary disease with and without hypercapnia. Respiration 1983;44:419.

60. O'Neill S et al. Survival after high blood alcohol levels. Arch Intern Med 1984;144:641.

61. Sellers EM, Kalant H. Alcohol intoxication and withdrawal. N Engl J Med 1976;294:757.

62. Poikolainen K. Estimated lethal ethanol concentrations in relation to age, aspiration, and drugs. Alcohol Clin Exp Res 1984;8:223.

63. Jones AW, Hahn RG. Pharmacokinetics of ethanol in patients with renal failure before and after hemodialysis. Forensic Sci Int 1997;90:175.

64. Rivara FP et al. The effects of alcohol abuse on readmission for trauma. JAMA 1993;270:1962.

65. Rivara FP et al. The magnitude of acute and chronic abuse in trauma patients. Arch Surg 1993;128:907.

66. Rivara FP et al. A descriptive study of trauma, alcohol, and alcoholism in young patients. J Adolesc Health 1992;13:663.

67. Adams WL. Alcohol-related hospitalizations of elderly: prevalence and geographic variation in the United States. JAMA 1993;270:1222.

68. Isbell A et al. An experimental study of the etiology of "rum fits" and delirium tremens. Q J Stud Alcohol 1955;16:1.

69. Victor M, Adams RD. The effect of alcohol on the nervous system. Res Publ Assoc Res Nerv Ment Dis 1953;32:526.

70. Holloway HC et al. Recognition and treatment of acute alcohol withdrawal syndromes. Psychiatr Clin North Am 1984;7:729.

71. Bird RD, Makela EH. Alcohol withdrawal: what is the benzodiazepine of choice? Ann Pharmacother 1994;28:67.

72. Erstad BL, Cotugno CL. Management of alcohol withdrawal. Am J Health-Syst Pharm 1995;52:697.

73. American Psychiatric Association. Diagnostic and Statistical Manual of Mental Disorders (DSM-IV). Washington, DC: American Psychiatric Association, 1994:197.

74. Mayo-Smith MF. Pharmacological management of alcohol withdrawal: a meta-analysis and evidence-based practice guideline. JAMA 1997;278:144.

75. Holbrook AM et al. Meta-analysis of benzodiazepine use in the treatment of acute alcohol withdrawal. Can Med Assn J 1999;160:655.

76. Holbrook AM et al. Diagnosis and management of acute ethanol withdrawal. Can Med Assn J 1999;160:675.

77. Sullivan JT et al. Assessment of alcohol withdrawal: the revised Clinical Institute Withdrawal Assessment for Alcohol scale (CIWA-Ar). Br J Addict 1989;84:1353.

78. Saitz R et al. Individualized treatment for alcohol withdrawal: a randomized, double-blind controlled trial. JAMA 1994;272:519.

79. Daeppen JB et al. Symptom-triggered vs fixed-schedule doses of benzodiazepine for alcohol withdrawal: a randomized treatment trial. Arch Intern Med 2002;162:1117.

80. Castaneda R, Cushman P. Alcohol withdrawal: a review of clinical management. J Clin Psychiatry 1989;50:278.

81. Reoux JP et al. Divalproex sodium in alcohol withdrawal: a randomized double-blind placebo-controlled clinical trial. Alcohol Clin Exp Res 2001;25:1324.

82. Longo LP et al. Divalproex (Depakote) for alcohol withdrawal and relapse prevention. J Addictive Dis 2002;21:55.

83. Allredge BK et al. Placebo-controlled trial of intravenous diphenylhydantoin for short-term treatment of alcohol withdrawal seizures. Am J Med 1989;87:645.

84. Chance JF. Emergency department treatment of alcohol withdrawal seizures with phenytoin. Ann Emerg Med 1991;20:520.

85. Rathlev NK et al. The lack of efficacy of phenytoin in the prevention of recurrent alcohol-related seizures. Ann Emerg Med 1994;23:513.

86. Feussner JR et al. Computed tomography brain scanning in alcohol withdrawal seizures: value of neurological examination. Ann Intern Med 1981;94(Pt 1):519.

87. Wilbur R, Kulik FA. Anticonvulsant drugs in alcohol withdrawal: use of phenytoin, primidone, carbamazepine, valproic acid, and the sedative anticonvulsants. Am J Hosp Pharm 1981;38:1138.

88. Roe A. The adult adjustment of children of alcoholic parents raised in foster homes. Q J Stud Alcohol 1944;5:378.

89. Amark C. A study in alcoholism. Acta Psychiatr Neurol Scand 1951;70(Suppl):256.

90. Goodwin DW et al. Drinking problems in adopted and non-adopted sons of alcoholics. Arch Gen Psychiatry 1974;31:164.

91. Mendelson JH, Mello NK. Biologic concomitants of alcoholism. N Engl J Med 1979;301:912.

92. Spalt L. Alcoholism: evidence of an X linked recessive genetic characteristic. JAMA 1979;241:2543.

93. Rutstein DD, Veech RL. 2,3-Butanediol: an unusual metabolite in serum of severely alcoholic men during acute intoxication. Lancet 1983;2:534.

94. Grant BF. ICD-10 and proposed DSM-IV harmful use of alcohol/alcohol abuse and dependence. United States 1988: a nosological comparison. Alcohol Clin Exp Res 1993;17:1093.

95. American Psychiatric Association. Diagnostic and Statistical Manual of Mental Disorders (DSM-IV). Washington, DC: American Psychiatric Association, 1994:181.

96. O'Connor PB, Schottenfeld RS. Patients with alcohol problems. N Engl J Med 1998;338:592.

97. Helzer JE et al. The extent of long-term moderate drinking among alcoholics discharged from medical and psychiatric facilities. N Engl J Med 1985;312:1678.

98. Miller WR et al. Abstinence and controlled drinking in the treatment of problem drinkers. J Stud Alcohol 1977;38:986.

99. Swift RM. Drug therapy for alcohol dependence. N Engl J Med 1999;340:1482.

100. Fuller RK, Roth HP. Disulfiram for the treatment of alcoholism: an evaluation in 128 men. Ann Intern Med 1979;90:901.

101. Kitson TM. The disulfiram-ethanol reaction. J Stud Alcohol 1977;38:96.

102. Stoll D, King LE. Disulfiram-alcohol skin reaction to beer-containing shampoo. JAMA 1980;244:2045.

103. Kwentus J et al. Disulfiram in the treatment of alcoholism. J Stud Alcohol 1979;40:428.

104. Peachey JE et al. A comparative review of the pharmacological and toxicological properties of disulfiram and calcium carbimide. J Clin Psychopharmacol 1981;1:21.

105. Eneanya DI et al. The actions and metabolic fate of disulfiram. Ann Rev Toxicol 1981;21:575.

106. Bartle WR et al. Disulfiram-induced hepatitis: report of two cases and review of the literature. Dig Dis Sci 1985;20:834.

107. Bilbao JM et al. Filamentous axonopathy in disulfiram neuropathy. Ultrastruct Pathol 1984;7:295.

108. O'Reilly RA. Dynamic interaction between disulfiram and separated enantiomorphs of racemic warfarin. Clin Pharmacol Ther 1981;29:332.

109. Olesen OV. The influence of disulfiram and calcium carbimide on the serum diphenylhydantoin: excretion of HPPH in the urine. Arch Neurol 1967;16:642.

110. Yodaiken RE. Ethylene dibromide and disulfiram-a lethal combination. JAMA 1978;239:2783.

111. Webb PK et al. Disulfiram hypersensitivity and rubber contact dermatitis. JAMA 1979;241:2061.

112. Tinsely JA et al. Developments in the treatment of alcoholism. Mayo Clin Proc 1998;73:857.

113. Naranjo CA et al. The serotonin uptake inhibitor citalopram attenuates ethanol intake. Clin Pharmacol Ther 1987;41:266.

114. Naranjo CA et al. Fluoxetine attenuates alcohol intake and desire to drink. Int Clin Psychopharmacol 1994;9:163.

115. Naranjo CA, Bremner KE. Serotonin-altering medications and desire, consumption and effects of alcohol-treatment implications. EXS 1994;71:209.

116. Kranzler HR. Pharmacotherapy of alcoholism: gaps in knowledge and opportunities for research. Alcohol Alcoholism 2000;35:537.

117. Kranzler HR, Van Kirk J. Efficacy of naltrexone and acamprosate for alcoholism treatment: a meta-analysis. Alcohol Clin Exp Res 2001;25:1335.

118. Garbutt JC et al. Pharmacological treatment of alcohol dependence: a review of the evidence. JAMA 1999;281:1318.

119. Davidson D et al. Effects of naltrexone on alcohol self-administration in heavy drinkers. Alcohol Clin Exp Res 1999;23:195.

120. O'Mara NB, Wesley LC. Naltrexone in the treatment of alcohol dependence. Ann Pharmacother 1994;28:210.

121. Streeton C, Whelan G. Naltrexone, a relapse prevention maintenance treatment of alcohol dependence: a meta-analysis of randomized controlled trials. Alcohol Alcoholism 2001;36:544.

122. Modesto-Lowe V, Van Kirk J. Clinical uses of naltrexone: a review of the evidence. Exp Clin Pyschopharmacol 2002;10:213.

123. O'Malley SS et al. Six-month follow-up of naltrexone and psychotherapy for alcohol dependence. Arch Gen Psychiatry 1996;53:217.

124. Croop RS et al. The safety profile of naltrexone in the treatment of alcoholism: results from a multicenter usage study. Arch Gen Psychiatry 1997;54:1130.

125. Mezey E. Alcoholic liver disease: roles of alcohol and malnutrition. Am J Clin Nutr 1980;33:2709.

126. Pimstone NG, French SW. Alcoholic liver disease. Med Clin North Am 1984;68:39.

127. Maddrey WC. Alcoholic hepatitis: clinicopathologic features and therapy. Semin Liver Dis 1988;8:91.

128. Maddrey WC. Alcoholic hepatitis: pathogenesis and approaches to treatment. Scand J Gastroenterol 1990;25(Suppl 175):118.

129. Morgan MY. The treatment of alcoholic hepatitis. Alcohol Alcoholism 1996;31:117.

130. Kaysen GK, Noth RH. The effects of alcohol on blood pressure and electrolytes. Med Clin North Am 1984;68:221.

131. Russell RM. Vitamin A and zinc metabolism in alcoholism. Am J Clin Nutr 1980;33:2741.

132. Mendenhall CL et al. Short-term and long-term survival in patients with alcoholic hepatitis treated with oxandrolone and prednisolone. N Engl J Med 1984;311:1464.

133. Bird GL. Randomised controlled double-blind trial of the calcium channel antagonist amlodipine

in the treatment of acute alcoholic hepatitis. J Hepatol 1998;28:194.

134. Akriviadis E et al. Pentoxifylline improves short-term survival in severe acute alcoholic hepatitis: a double-blind, placebo-controlled trial. Gastroenterology 2000;119:1637.

135. Rambaldi A, Gluud C. Meta-analysis of propylthiouracil for alcoholic liver disease-a Cochrane Hepato-Biliary Group Review. Liver 2001;21:398.

136. Christensen E, Gluud C. Glucocorticoids are ineffective in alcoholic hepatitis: a meta-analysis adjusting for confounding variables. Gut 1995; 37:113.

137. Wrona SA, Tankanow RM. Corticosteroids in the management of alcoholic hepatitis. Am J Hosp Pharm 1994;51:347.

138. Larkin EC, Watson-Williams EJ. Alcohol and the blood. Med Clin North Am 1984;68:105.

139. Lindenbaum J, Roman MJ. Nutritional anemia in alcoholism. Am J Clin Nutr 1980;33:2727.

140. Halstead CH. Folate deficiency in alcoholism. Am J Clin Nutr 1980;33:2736.

141. Rosett HL, Weiner L. Alcohol and pregnancy: a clinical perspective. Ann Rev Med 1985;36:73.

142. Turner TB et al. Measurement of alcohol-related effects in man: chronic effects in relation to level of alcohol consumption. Johns Hopkins Med J 1977;141(Pt A):235.

143. Day NL. Prenatal exposure to alcohol: effect on infant growth and morphologic characteristics. Pediatrics 1989;84:536.

144. Burd L, Martsolf JT. Fetal alcohol syndrome: diagnosis and syndromal variability. Physiol Behav 1989;46:39.

145. West LJ et al. Alcoholism. Ann Intern Med 1984;100:405.

146. Burbige EJ et al. Alcohol and the gastrointestinal tract. Med Clin North Am 1984;68:77.

147. Hyumpa AM Jr. Mechanisms of thiamine deficiency in chronic alcoholism. Am J Clin Nutr 1980;33:2750.

148. Brenner H et al. Inverse graded relation between alcohol consumption and active infection with *Helicobacter pylori*. Am J Epidemiol 1999; 149:571.

149. Lieber CS. Gastric ethanol metabolism and gastritis: interactions with other drugs, *Helicobacter pylori* and antibiotic therapy (1957–1997)a review. Alcohol Clin Exp Res 1997;21:1360.

150. Chou SP. An examination of the alcohol consumption and peptic ulcer disease association-results of a national survey. Alcohol Clin Exp Res 1994;18:149.

151. Krumpe PE et al. Alcohol and the respiratory tract. Med Clin North Am 1984;68:201.

152. Adams HG, Jordan C. Infections in the alcoholic. Med Clin North Am 1984;68:179.

153. Fraser AG. Is there an interaction between H_2-antagonists and alcohol? Drug Metabol Drug Interact 1998;14:123.

154. Marshall JM. Interaction of histamine$_2$-receptor antagonists and ethanol. Ann Pharmacother 1994; 28:55.

155. Brown AS, Jame OF. Omeprazole, ranitidine, and cimetidine have no effect on peak blood ethanol concentrations, first-pass metabolism or area under the time-ethanol curve under real-life drinking conditions. Aliment Pharmacol Ther 1998;12:141.

156. Battiston L et al. Lansoprazole and ethanol metabolism: comparison with omeprazole and cimetidine. Pharmacol Toxicol 1997;81:247.

157. Jungnickel PW. Pantoprazole: a new proton pump inhibitor. Clin Ther 2000;22:1268.

158. Sietz HK et al. Alcohol and cancer. Recent Devel Alcoholism 1998;14:67.

159. Mufti SI et al. Alcohol, cancer and immunomodulation. Crit Rev Oncol Hematol 1989,9.243.

160. Steinberg W, Tenner S. Acute pancreatitis. N Engl J Med 1994;330:1198.

161. Cameron JL et al. Acute pancreatitis with hyperlipidemia: the incidence of lipid abnormalities in acute pancreatitis. Ann Surg 1973;177:483.

162. Gumaste V et al. Serum lipase: a better test to diagnose acute alcoholic pancreatitis. Am J Med 1993;92:239.

163. Tenner SM, Steinberg W. The admission serum lipase:amylase ratio differentiates alcoholic from nonalcoholic acute pancreatitis. Am J Gastroenterol 1992;87:1755.

164. Schenker S et al. Hepatic and Wernicke's encephalopathies: current concepts of pathogenesis. Am J Clin Nutr 1980;33:2719.

165. Reuler JB et al. Wernicke's encephalopathy. N Engl J Med 1985;312:1035.

166. Nakada T, Knight RT. Alcohol and the central nervous system. Med Clin North Am 1984; 68:121.

167. Albert CM et al. Moderate alcohol consumption and the risk of sudden cardiac death among U.S. male physicians. Circulation 1999;100:944.

168. Mukamal KJ et al. Roles of drinking pattern and type of alcohol consumed in coronary heart disease in men. N Engl J Med 2003;248:109.

169. Hart CL et al. Alcohol consumption and mortality from all causes, coronary heart disease, and stroke: results from a prospective cohort study of Scottish men with 21 years follow up. Br Med J 1999;318:1725.

170. Rubin R, Rand ML. Alcohol and platelet function. Alcohol Clin Exp Res 1994;18:105.

171. Hillbom M, Numminen H. Alcohol and stroke: pathophysiologic mechanisms. Neuroepidemiology 1998;17:281.

172. Hillbom M et al. Recent heavy drinking of alcohol and embolic stroke. Stroke 1999;30:2307.

173. Mangoni AA, Jackson SHD. Homocysteine and cardiovascular disease: current evidence and future prospects. Am J Med 2002;112:556.

174. Verhaar MC et al. Folates and cardiovascular disease. Arterioscler Thromb Vasc Biol 2002;22:6.

175. Piano M. Alcoholic cardiomyopathy: incidence, clinical characteristics, and pathophysiology. Chest 2002;121:1638.

176. Rubin E, Urbano-Marquez A. Alcoholic cardiomyopathy. Alcohol Clin Exp Res 1994;18:111.

177. Davidson DM. Cardiovascular effects of alcohol. West J Med 1989;151:430.

178. Wakabayashi I, Kobaba-Wakabayashi R. Effects of age on the relationship between drinking and atherosclerotic risk factors. Gerontology 2002; 48:151.

179. Grogan JR, Kochar MS. Alcohol and hypertension. Arch Fam Med 1994;3:150.

180. Segel LD et al. Alcohol and the heart. Med Clin North Am 1984;68:147.

181. Rich EC et al. Alcohol-related acute atrial fibrillation: a case-control study and review of 40 patients. Arch Intern Med 1985;145:830.

182. Ettinger PO et al. Arrhythmias and the "holiday heart": alcohol-associated cardiac rhythm disorders. Am Heart J 1978;95:555.

183. De Marchi S et al. Renal tubular dysfunction in chronic alcohol abuse-effects of abstinence. N Engl J Med 1993;329:1927.

184. Koskinen P, Kupari M. Alcohol and cardiac arrhythmias. Br Med J 1992;304:1394.

185. Mello NK, Mendelson JH. Neuroendocrine consequences of alcohol abuse in women. Ann NY Acad Sci 1989;562:211.

186. Noth RH, Walter RM Jr. The effects of alcohol on the endocrine system. Med Clin North Am 1984;68:133.

187. Urbano-Marquez A. The effects of alcoholism on skeletal and cardiac muscle. N Engl J Med 1989; 320:409.

188. Riggs JE. Alcohol-associated rhabdomyolysis: ethanol induction of cytochrome P450 may potentiate myotoxicity. Clin Neuropharmacol 1998; 21:363.

189. Fernandez-Sola J et al. The relationship of alcoholic myopathy to cardiomyopathy. Arch Intern Med 1994;120:529.

190. Monforte R et al. Autonomic and peripheral neuropathies in patients with chronic alcoholism: a dose-related toxic effect of alcohol. Arch Neurol 1995;52:45.

191. Vittadini G et al. Alcoholic polyneuropathy: a clinical and epidemiological study. Alcohol Alcoholism 2001;36:2001.

CHAPTER 85

Tobacco Use and Dependence

Robin L. Corelli, Karen Suchanek Hudmon

Long before Christopher Columbus traveled to the New World, tobacco use was widespread in the Americas—tobacco preparations were part of religious ceremonies for the Native Americans, and tobacco also was used medicinally. At that time, and for several subsequent centuries, little was known or suspected about the dangers of tobacco use. In retrospect, it is not surprising that these dangers were not recognized initially, because the more pressing health issues at that time were related to life-threatening, acute diseases as opposed to chronic diseases such as those imposed by tobacco. However, it is now well established that tobacco is a detrimental substance, and its use dramatically increases a person's odds of dependence, disability, and disease. As a major risk factor for a wide range of diseases, including cardiovascular conditions, cancers, and pulmonary disorders, *tobacco is the primary known pre-ventable cause of premature death in our society.* In 2000, an estimated 4.83 million people worldwide died prematurely from a tobacco-attributable disease.[1] Unless tobacco control efforts can reverse this trend, the number of annual deaths is likely to reach 10 million by the year 2030.[2]

Tobacco products are carefully-engineered formulations that optimize the delivery of nicotine, a chemical that meets the criteria for an addictive substance: (1) nicotine induces psychoactive effects, (2) it is used in a highly controlled or compulsive manner, and (3) behavioral patterns of tobacco use are reinforced by the pharmacologic effects of nicotine.[3] Although a variety of tobacco products are marketed, cigarettes are by far the most frequently used. Figure 85-1 depicts the shifts in per-capita consumption for the various tobacco products in the United States between 1880 and 2000.[4]

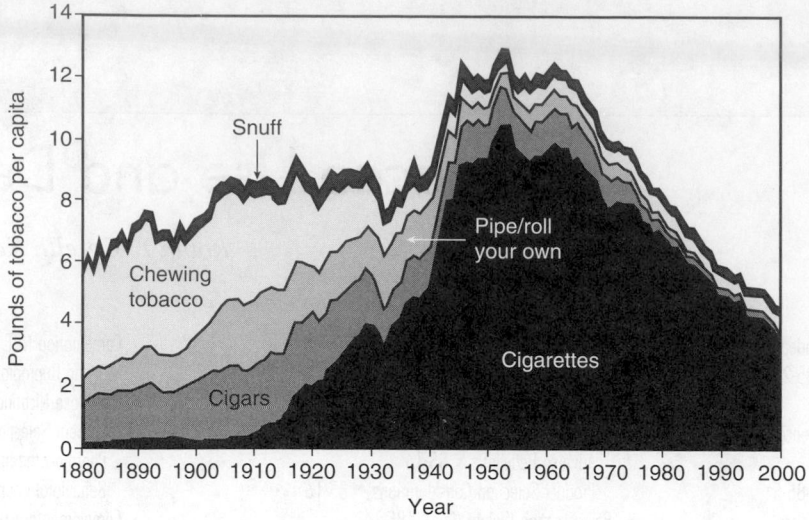

FIGURE 85-1 Adult per capita tobacco consumption, 1880 to 2000.[4] Adapted from NCI Smoking and Tobacco Control Monograph 8, 1997, p. 13. Data from U.S. Department of Agriculture. Reprinted with permission. Thun et al. Oncogene 2002;21:7307–7325.

During 1995 to 1999, smoking was responsible for approximately 440,000 premature deaths in the United States each year.[5] In addition to the harm imposed on users of tobacco, exposure to second-hand smoke results in an estimated 53,000 deaths each year.[6] Furthermore, enormous economic burden accompanies the morbidity and mortality results from tobacco use. Each pack of cigarettes smoked costs society $7.18 for associated medical care ($3.45) and productivity losses ($3.73), for a total of $157 billion in annual health-related economic losses.[5] Because of the enormous societal burden that it imposes, tobacco use and dependence should be addressed during each clinical encounter with all tobacco users.

Epidemiology of Tobacco Use and Dependence

Nicotine addiction is a form of chronic brain disease resulting from alterations in brain chemistry.[7,8] Dr. Alan Leshner, former director of the National Institute on Drug Abuse, defines drug addiction as "compulsive use, without medical purpose, in the face of negative consequences."[7] The addictive properties of nicotine are well documented.

In the United States, experimentation with cigarettes and the development of regular smoking typically occur during adolescence, with 88–89% of adult smokers having tried their first cigarette by 18 years of age,[9,10] and 71% of adult daily smokers having become regular smokers by age 18.[9] Because most teens who smoke at least monthly continue to smoke in adulthood,[9] tobacco-use trends among youth are a key indicator of the overall health trends for the nation.[11] According to the Centers for Disease Control and Prevention (CDC), the smoking prevalence among high school seniors rose during the 1990s, and peaked at 42.8% in 1999.[12] This worrisome trend identified an urgent need for tobacco prevention and cessation programs focused on younger age groups. More recently, the prevalence has decreased—in 2002, an estimated 26.7% of 12th graders had smoked one or more cigarettes in the past 30 days.[13]

Among adults, smoking prevalence varies by sociodemographic factors, including sex, race/ethnicity, education level, age, and poverty level. The CDC reported that in 2001, the percentage of current smokers (defined as having smoked 100 or more cigarettes during their lifetime and currently smoking every day or some days) was 22.8%; 25.2% of men and 20.7% of women were current smokers.[14] Table 85-1 summarizes the smoking prevalence estimates for various population subgroups, stratified by sex. In 2002, the highest median prevalence of current smoking was evident in Kentucky (32.6%), and West Virginia (28.4%). The lowest prevalence was in Utah (12.7%), California (16.4%), and Massachusetts (19.0%).[15]

Factors Contributing to Tobacco Use

Nicotine induces a variety of pharmacologic effects that lead to dependence. However, tobacco dependence is not simply a matter of nicotine pharmacology—it is a result of complex processes involving the interplay of environmental, physiologic, and pharmacologic factors that influence an individual's decision to use tobacco.[16] *Environmental factors* that contribute to tobacco use are numerous and varied; these include social events, exposure to tobacco advertising, access to tobacco products, social interactions, having family members and friends who use tobacco, and conditioned stimuli (e.g., smoking after a meal, while driving, or while drinking alcoholic beverages). *Physiologic factors,* such as pre-existing medical conditions (e.g., psychiatric co-morbidities) and one's genetic profile can predispose individuals to tobacco use. Notably, it has been estimated that approximately 50% of smoking is heritable.[17,18] *Pharmacologic factors* also contribute to tobacco use. The rapidity with which nicotine, the addictive component of tobacco, is absorbed and passes through the blood-brain barrier contributes to its addictive nature. After inhalation, nicotine reaches the brain in approximately 11 seconds.[19] As such, smokers experience nearly immediate onset of positive effects of nicotine, including pleasure, relief of anxiety, improved task performance, im-

Table 85-1 Percentage of Current Smokers[a] ≥18 Years by Selected Characteristics—National Health Interview Survey, United States, 2001[14]

Characteristic	Category	Men (n = 14,490)	Women (n = 18,836)	Total (n = 33,326)
Race/ethnicity[b]	White, non-Hispanic	25.4	22.8	24.0
	Black, non-Hispanic	27.7	17.9	22.3
	Hispanic	21.6	11.9	16.7
	American Indian/Alaska Native	33.5	31.7	32.7
	Asian[c]	18.5	6.3	12.4
Education[d]	0–12 years (no diploma)	32.2	23.3	27.5
	GED[e] (diploma)	47.9	47.7	47.8
	12 years (diploma)	29.3	23.4	26.1
	Associate degree	23.7	19.8	21.6
	Some college (no degree)	26.6	22.1	24.2
	Undergraduate degree	13.3	11.2	12.3
	Graduate degree	9.0	10.0	9.5
Age group (yr)	18–24	30.4	23.4	26.9
	25–44	27.3	24.5	25.8
	45–64	26.4	21.4	23.8
	≥65	11.5	9.2	10.1
Poverty level[f]	At or above	25.1	21.0	23.0
	Below	36.2	28.1	31.4
	Unknown	22.0	17.1	19.3
Total		**25.2**	**20.7**	**22.8**

[a]Persons who reported having smoked ≥100 cigarettes during their lifetime and who reported currently smoking every day or some days during the previous 30 days; excludes 301 respondents whose smoking status was unknown.
[b]Excludes 371 respondents of unknown, multiple, or other racial/ethnic categories.
[c]Excludes Native Hawaiians and other Pacific Islanders.
[d]Persons aged ≥25 years, excluding 316 persons with unknown number of years of education.
[e]General Educational Development.
[f]Calculated on the basis of U.S. Census Bureau 2000 poverty thresholds.

proved memory, mood modulation, and skeletal muscle relaxation.[20] These effects, mediated by alterations in neurotransmitter levels, reinforce continued use of nicotine-containing products.

Nicotine Pharmacology

Nicotine (*Nicotiana tabacum),* which is composed of a pyridine ring and a pyrrolidine ring, is one of the few natural alkaloids that exist in the liquid state. Nicotine is a clear, weak base (pK_a = 8.0) that turns brown and acquires the characteristic odor of tobacco after exposure to air.[16,21] In acidic media, nicotine is ionized and poorly absorbed; conversely, in alkaline media, nicotine is nonionized and well absorbed. Under physiologic conditions (pH = 7.3 to 7.5), approximately 31% of nicotine is nonionized and readily crosses cell membranes.[16] Given the relation between pH and absorption, the tobacco industry and pharmaceutical companies are able to titrate the pH of their tobacco products and nicotine replacement therapies to maximize the absorption potential of nicotine.[20,22]

Once absorbed, nicotine induces a variety of central nervous system, cardiovascular, and metabolic effects. Nicotine stimulates the release of several neurotransmitters, inducing a range of pharmacologic effects such as pleasure and reward (dopamine), arousal (acetylcholine, norepinephrine), cognitive enhancement (acetylcholine), appetite suppression (nor-epinephrine, serotonin), learning and memory enhancement (glutamate), mood modulation, and reduction of anxiety and tension (β-endorphin and GABA).[23] By stimulating the release of dopamine in the midbrain, nicotine activates the *dopamine reward pathway,* a network of nervous tissue in the middle of the brain that elicits feelings of pleasure in response to certain stimuli. Key structures of the reward pathway include the ventral tegmental area, the nucleus accumbens, and the prefrontal cortex (the area of the brain that is responsible for thinking and judgment). The neurons of the ventral tegmental area contain the neurotransmitter dopamine, which is released in the nucleus accumbens and in the prefrontal cortex. Immediately after inhalation, a bolus of nicotine enters the brain, stimulating the release of dopamine, which induces nearly immediate feelings of pleasure, along with relief of the symptoms of nicotine withdrawal. This rapid dose response reinforces repeated administration of the drug and perpetuates the smoking behavior.[20]

Chronic administration of nicotine has been shown to result in an increased number of nicotine receptors in specific regions of the brain[24]; this upregulation of receptors leads to the development of tolerance, a phenomenon by which repeated doses of a drug produce less of an effect than did the initial exposure. Chronic administration also leads to tolerance to the behavioral and cardiovascular effects of nicotine over the course of the day; however, tobacco users regain sensitivity to the effects of nicotine after overnight abstinence

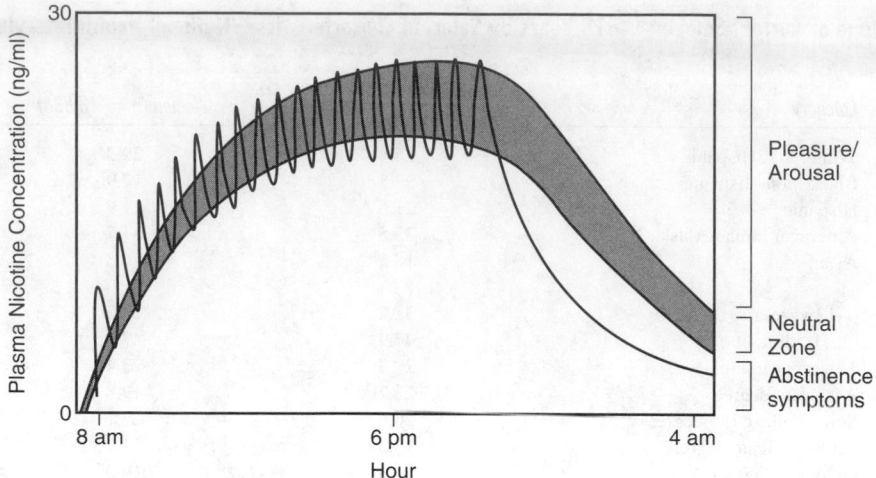

FIGURE 85-2 The nicotine addiction cycle throughout the day.[16] (Reprinted with permission from Benowitz NL. Med Clin North Am 1992;2:415.)

The saw-tooth line represents venous plasma concentrations of nicotine as a cigarette is smoked every 40 minutes from 8 AM to 9 PM.

The upper solid line indicates the threshold concentration for nicotine to produce pleasure or arousal.

The lower solid line indicates the concentrations at which symptoms of abstinence (i.e., withdrawal symptoms) from nicotine occur.

The shaded area represents the zone of nicotine concentrations (neutral zone) in which the smoker is comfortable without experiencing either pleasure/arousal or abstinence symptoms.

from nicotine, as shown in Figure 85-2.[16] Notably, after smoking the first cigarette of the day, the smoker experiences marked pharmacologic effects, particularly arousal. No other cigarette throughout the day produces the same degree of pleasure/arousal. For this reason, many smokers describe the first cigarette as the most important one of the day. Shortly after the initial cigarette, tolerance begins to develop. Accordingly, the threshold levels for both pleasure/arousal and abstinence rise progressively throughout the day as the smoker becomes tolerant to the effects of nicotine. With continued smoking, nicotine accumulates, leading to an even greater degree of tolerance. Late in the day, each individual cigarette produces only limited pleasure/arousal; instead, smoking primarily alleviates nicotine withdrawal symptoms. Lack of exposure to nicotine overnight results in resensitization of drug responses (i.e., loss of tolerance). Most dependent smokers tend to smoke a certain number of cigarettes per day (usually more than 10) and tend to consume 10 to 40 mg of nicotine per day to achieve the desired effects of cigarette smoking and minimize the symptoms of nicotine withdrawal.[16] Withdrawal symptoms include anger/irritability, anxiety, difficulty concentrating, drowsiness, fatigue, hunger/weight gain, impatience, and restlessness.[25] Tobacco users become adept at titrating their nicotine levels throughout the day to avoid withdrawal symptoms, to maintain pleasure and arousal, and to modulate mood.

Nicotine is extensively metabolized in the liver and to a lesser extent in the kidney and lung. Approximately 70% to 80% of nicotine is metabolized to cotinine, an inactive metabolite.[26] The rapid metabolism of nicotine ($t_{1/2}$ = 2 hours) to inactive compounds underlies tobacco users' need for frequent, repeated administration. The half-life of cotinine, however, is much longer ($t_{1/2}$ = 18 to 20 hours) and for this reason, cotinine commonly is used as marker of tobacco use as well as a marker for exposure to second-hand smoke.

Nicotine and other metabolites are excreted in the urine. Urinary excretion is pH dependent; the excretion rate is increased in acidic urine. Nicotine is excreted in breast milk and can be detected in the blood and urine of infants of nursing smokers.[20,21]

Assessment of Tobacco Use and Dependence

The American Psychiatric Association has published criteria for substance dependence in the *Diagnostic and Statistical Manual of Mental Disorders (DSM IV)*.[27] According to their definition, dependence exists if a patient reports that during the past year he or she experienced at least three of the seven characteristics shown in Table 85-2. A different method of determining dependence, commonly used in research and sometimes used in clinical practice to assess nicotine dependence, is the Fagerström Test for Nicotine Dependence (FTND; Table 85-3).[28] This six-item survey instrument can be completed by the patient or can be administered in an interview format. An individual's FTND scale score, which ranges from 0 to 10, is then computed as a sum of the responses to the six constituent items. In general, scores higher than 5 are considered indicative of substantial dependence. Modified versions of this scale are available for adolescents[29] and for spit tobacco users.[30]

The daily intake of nicotine can be estimated from a measured plasma cotinine level using the following equation[31]:

$$\text{Daily dose of nicotine (in mg)} = \text{plasma cotinine concentration (ng/mL)} \times 0.08.$$

Using this equation, an average cotinine concentration of 300 ng/mL (generally observed in a typical smoker) corresponds to a daily intake of 24 mg nicotine.[31] Because a smoker absorbs, on average, approximately 1 mg of nicotine per cigarette,[31,32] it can then be estimated that a plasma coti-

Table 85-2   DSM IV Criteria for Substance Dependence[27]

A maladaptive pattern of substance use, leading to clinically significant impairment or distress, as manifested by three (or more) of the following, occurring at any time in the same 12-month period:

1. Tolerance, as defined by either of the following:
   a. A need for markedly increased amounts of the substance to achieve intoxication or desired effect
   b. Markedly diminished effect with continued use of the same amount of substance
2. Withdrawal as manifested by either of the following:
   a. The characteristic withdrawal syndrome for the substance
   b. The same (or a closely related) substance is taken to relieve or avoid withdrawal symptoms
3. The substance is often taken in larger amounts or over a longer period than was intended.
4. There is a persistent desire or unsuccessful efforts to cut down or control substance use.
5. A great deal of time is spent in activities necessary to obtain the substance (e.g., driving long distances), use the substance (e.g., chain-smoking), or recover from its effects.
6. Important social, occupational, or recreational activities are given up or reduced because of substance use.
7. The substance use is continued despite knowledge of having a persistent or recurrent physical or psychological problem that is likely to have been caused or exacerbated by the substance (e.g., continued smoking despite previous myocardial infarction).

nine level of 300 ng/mL corresponds to a daily intake of approximately 24 cigarettes.

Drug Interactions with Smoking

It is widely recognized that the polycyclic aromatic hydrocarbons (PAHs) are responsible for most drug interactions with smoking.[33,34] PAHs, which are the products of incomplete combustion of tobacco, are found in appreciably large quanti-ties in tobacco smoke and are potent inducers of several hepatic cytochrome P450 microsomal enzymes (CYP1A1, CYP1A2, and possibly CYP2E1). Although other substances in tobacco smoke, including acetone, pyridines, benzene, nicotine, carbon monoxide, and heavy metals (e.g., cadmium), also might interact with hepatic enzymes, their effects appear to be less significant. Most drug interactions with tobacco smoke are pharmacokinetic, resulting from the induction of drug-metabolizing enzymes (especially CYP1A2) by compounds in tobacco smoke. Table 85-4 summarizes key interactions with smoking.[35]

Health Consequences of Tobacco Use

Smoking has a causal or contributory role in the development of a variety of medical conditions (Table 85-5).[3] In 2000, 8.6 million persons in the United States experienced an estimated 12.7 million smoking-attributable medical conditions.[36] Among current smokers, chronic bronchitis was the most common (49%) condition, followed by emphysema (24%). Among former smokers, the most prevalent condition was chronic bronchitis (26%), followed by emphysema (24%), and previous heart attack (24%). Lung cancer, the leading cause of cancer-related death for both men and women in the United States and a disease for which the 5-year survival rate is approximately 15%,[37] accounted for 1% of all smoking-attributable illnesses in current smokers and 2% in former smokers.[36] Cardiovascular disease is the primary cause of death among all United States deaths attributable to smoking.[5]

Exposure to second-hand smoke, which includes the smoke emanating from burning tobacco and that exhaled by the smoker, increases risk for fetal growth retardation and sudden infant death syndrome and predisposes individuals to lung and nasal sinus cancers, cardiovascular effects (heart disease mortality, acute and chronic coronary heart disease morbidity), and eye and nasal irritation.[6,38] In addition, children

Table 85-3   Fagerström Test for Nicotine Dependence[28]

Item	Patient Response Options	Coding[a]
1. How soon after you wake up do you smoke your first cigarette?	Within 5 minutes	3
	6–30 minutes	2
	31–60 minutes	1
	After 60 minutes	0
2. Do you find it difficult to refrain from smoking in the places where it is forbidden (e.g., in church, at the library, in cinema)?	Yes	1
	No	0
3. Which cigarette would you hate most to give up?	The first one in the morning	1
	Any other	0
4. How many cigarettes per day do you smoke?	10 or less	0
	11–20	1
	21–30	2
	31 or more	3
5. Do you smoke more frequently during the first hours after waking than during the rest of the day?	Yes	1
	No	0
6. Do you smoke if you are so ill that you are in bed most of the day?	Yes	1
	No	0

[a]Patient scale scores are computed as a sum of the constituent items; possible range is 0 to 10.

Table 85-4   Drug Interactions[a] With Smoking[34,35]

Drug/Class	Mechanism of Interaction and Effects
Benzodiazepines (diazepam, chlordiazepoxide)	Pharmacodynamic interaction: decreased sedation and drowsiness. May be caused by central nervous system stimulation by nicotine.
β-Blockers	Pharmacodynamic interaction: less effective antihypertensive and heart rate control effects. May be caused by nicotine-mediated sympathetic activation.
Caffeine	Increased metabolism (induction of CYP1A2); clearance increased by 56%. Caffeine levels may increase after cessation.
Chlorpromazine	Decreased area under the curve (36%) and serum concentrations (24%). Smokers may experience less sedation and hypotension and require higher dosages than nonsmokers.
Clozapine	Increased metabolism (induction of CYP1A2); plasma concentrations decreased by 28%.
Flecainide	Clearance increased by 61%; trough serum concentrations decreased by 25%. Smokers may require higher dosages.
Fluvoxamine	Increased metabolism (induction of CYP1A2); clearance increased by 25%; decreased plasma concentrations (47%). Dosage modifications not routinely recommended but smokers may require higher dosages.
Haloperidol	Clearance increased by 44%; serum concentrations decreased by 70%.
Heparin	Mechanism unknown but increased clearance and decreased half-life are observed. Smokers may require higher dosages.
Insulin	Insulin absorption may be decreased secondary to peripheral vasoconstriction; smoking may cause release of endogenous substances that antagonize the effects of insulin. Smokers may require higher dosages.
Mexiletine	Clearance (via oxidation and glucuronidation) increased by 25%; half-life decreased 36%.
Olanzapine	Increased metabolism (induction of CYP1A2); clearance increased by 40–98%. Dosage modifications not routinely recommended but smokers may require higher dosages.
Opioids (propoxyphene, pentazocine)	Pharmacodynamic interaction: by an unknown mechanism, decreased analgesic effect; higher dosages may be necessary in smokers.
Propranolol	Clearance (via side chain oxidation and glucuronidation) increased by 77%.
Oral contraceptives	Pharmacodynamic interaction: increased risk of risk of cardiovascular adverse effects (e.g., stroke, myocardial infarction, thromboembolism) in women who smoke and use oral contraceptives. Risk substantially increased in women who are both more than 35 years of age and heavy (≥15 cigarettes per day) smokers.
Tacrine	Increased metabolism (induction of CYP1A2); half-life decreased by 50%; serum concentrations threefold lower. Smokers may require higher dosages.
Theophylline	Increased metabolism (induction of CYP1A2); clearance increased by 58–100%; half-life decreased by 63%. Theophylline levels should be monitored if smoking is initiated, discontinued, or changed. Maintenance doses are considerably higher in smokers.

Table was adapted with permission from reference 35. Copyright 1999-2004 The Regents of the University of California, University of Southern California, and Western University of Health Sciences. All rights reserved.
[a]Light shaded rows indicate the most clinically-significant interactions.

who are exposed to second-hand smoke have an elevated risk for acute lower respiratory tract infections, asthma induction and exacerbation, chronic respiratory symptoms, and middle ear infections.[6] Recent evidence also suggests that second-hand smoke exposure is associated with pediatric dental caries.[39] Oral forms of tobacco (snuff, chewing tobacco) are associated with cancers of the mouth, throat, pharynx, larynx, and esophagus, as well as periodontal damage and oral leukoplakia.[40]

Benefits of Quitting

The 1990 Surgeon General's Report on the health benefits of smoking cessation describes numerous and substantial health benefits associated with quitting.[41] Benefits incurred soon after quitting (e.g., within 2 weeks to 3 months) include improvements in pulmonary function, circulation, and ambulation. Within 1 to 9 months of quitting, the ciliary function of the lung epithelial cells is restored; initially, this might result in increased coughing as the lungs clear excess mucus and tobacco smoke particulates. Smoking cessation results in measurable improvements in lung function[42] (see Chapter 24, Chronic Obstructive Pulmonary Disease, Fig. 24-1). Over time, patients experience decreased coughing, sinus congestion, fatigue, shortness of breath, and risk of pulmonary infection. One year after cessation, the excess risk of coronary heart disease is reduced to half that of continuing smokers. After 5 to 15 years, the risk of stroke is reduced to a rate similar to that of people who are lifetime nonsmokers, and 10 years after quitting, an individual's chance of dying of lung cancer is approximately half that of continuing smokers. In addition, the risk of developing mouth, throat, esophagus, bladder, kidney, or pancreatic cancer is decreased. Finally, 15 years after quitting, an individual's risk of coronary heart disease is reduced to a rate that is similar to that of people who have never smoked.[41] Smoking cessation also can lead to a

Table 85-5   Smoking-Related Diseases[3]

Cardiovascular diseases
  Aortic aneurysm
  Cerebrovascular disease
  Coronary heart disease
  Myocardial infarction
  Peripheral vascular disease
  Stroke
Cancers
  Causal role: lung, oral cavity, larynx, esophagus
  Contributory role: bladder, cervix, kidney, pancreas, stomach
Pulmonary diseases
  Asthma
  Chronic obstructive pulmonary disease
Pregnancy and perinatal complications
  Low birth weight
  Miscarriage/spontaneous abortion
  Preterm delivery
  Stillbirth
Reduced fertility
Cataract formation
Osteoporosis

Table 85-6   Methods for Treating Tobacco Use and Dependence: Estimates of Treatment Efficacy[48]

Treatment Method	Estimated odds ratio for tobacco abstinence (95% CI)	
	US PHS Guideline[46]	Cochrane Library[a]
Behavioral interventions		
Clinician intervention		
Physician advice to quit	1.3 (1.1–1.6)	1.69 (1.45–1.98)
Counseling by a physician[b]	2.2 (1.5–3.2)	1.44 (1.23–1.68)
Counseling by a non-physician	1.7 (1.3–2.1)	Not available
Format of smoking cessation counseling		
Self-help materials	1.2 (1.02–1.3)	1.24 (1.07–1.45)
Individual (face-to-face)	1.7 (1.4–2.0)	1.62 (1.35–1.94)
Group	1.3 (1.1–1.6)	1.97 (1.57–2.48)
By telephone (proactive)	1.2 (1.1–1.4)	1.56 (1.38–1.77)
Pharmacotherapy options		
First-line agents[c]		
Nicotine polacrilex gum	1.5 (1.3–1.8)	1.66 (1.52–1.81)
Nicotine lozenge/sublingual tablet	Not available	2.08 (1.63–2.65)
Nicotine transdermal patch	1.9 (1.7–2.2)	1.74 (1.57–1.93)
Nicotine oral inhaler	2.5 (1.7–3.6)	2.08 (1.43–3.04)
Nicotine nasal spray	2.7 (1.8–4.1)	2.27 (1.61–3.20)
Bupropion SR	2.1 (1.5–3.0)	1.97 (1.67–2.34)
Second-line agents[d]		
Nortriptyline	3.2 (1.8–5.7)	2.80 (1.81–4.32)
Clonidine	2.1 (1.4–3.2)	1.89 (1.30–2.74)

Reprinted with permission, American College of Physicians. Modified and updated to reflect current literature. The American College of Physicians-American Society of Internal Medicine is not responsible for the accuracy of the translation.
[a]Cochrane Database of Systematic Reviews. Available at www.cochrane.org/cochrane.
[b]Comparison group is physician advice only for Cochrane Library category. Comparison group is no intervention for USPHS Guideline category.
[c]Approved by the U.S. Food and Drug Administration as a smoking cessation aid; recommended by the USPHS guideline as a first-line agent for treating tobacco use and dependence.
[d]Not approved by the U.S. Food and Drug Administration as a smoking cessation aid; recommended by the USPHS Guideline as a second-line agent for treating tobacco use and dependence.

significant reduction in the cumulative risk of death from lung cancer, for both men and women.[43] Smokers who are able to quit by age 35 can be expected to live an additional 6 to 9 years compared with those who continue to smoke. Even individuals who postpone quitting until age 65 can incur up to 4 additional years of life compared with those who never quit.[44] Thus, it is never too late to quit and to incur subsequent benefits of quitting.

Tobacco Use and Dependence: Treatment Approaches

Most smokers quit without assistance, despite the fact that smokers who receive assistance are more likely to be successful in quitting.[45] For any patient who uses tobacco, the target goal is complete, long-term abstinence from all nicotine-containing products. Given the complexity of the tobacco-dependence syndrome and the constellation of factors that contribute to tobacco use (see previous text), treatment for addiction requires a multifaceted approach.[8] To assist clinicians and other specialists in providing cessation treatment to patients who use tobacco, the United States Public Health Service published the *Clinical Practice Guideline for Treating Tobacco Use and Dependence.*[46]

Clinicians can have an important impact on their patients' ability to quit. A meta-analysis of 29 studies[46] determined that compared with patients who do not receive an intervention from a clinician, patients who receive a tobacco cessation intervention from a physician clinician or a non–physician clinician are 2.2 and 1.7 times, respectively, more likely to quit (at 5 or more months after cessation). Although brief advice from a clinician has been shown to lead to an increased odds of quitting,[47] more intensive counseling yields more dramatic increases in quit rates.[46,47] Because the use of pharmacotherapy approximately doubles patients' chances of quitting,[46] when feasible and not contraindicated, cessation interventions should combine pharmacotherapy with behavioral counseling.[46] The estimated efficacies of various treatment strategies are shown in Table 85-6.[48] In prescribing or dispensing pharmacotherapy agents, clinicians can have a significant impact on a patient's likelihood of success by supplementing medication use with behavioral counseling, using the strategies described below.

Assisting Patients With Quitting
Behavioral Counseling Strategies
According to the Clinical Practice Guideline,[46] five key components make up the comprehensive counseling for tobacco cessation: (1) asking patients whether they use tobacco; (2) advising tobacco users to quit; (3) assessing patients' readiness to quit; (4) assisting patients with quitting; and (5) arranging follow-up care. These steps are referred to as the 5 A's and are described, in brief, below. Figure 85-3 can be used as a guide for structuring counseling interventions.

STEP One: ASK about Tobacco Use

➲ Suggested Dialogue

√ Do you ever smoke or use any type of tobacco?
– I take time to talk with all of my patients about tobacco use–because it's important

STEP Two: Strongly **ADVISE** to Quit

It is important to be sensitive, because patients might be defensive of their smoking. Project empathy in your voice; be understanding, not reprimanding.

➲ Suggested Dialogue

– It's important that you quit as soon as possible, and I can help you.
– I realize that quitting is difficult. It is the most important thing you can do to protect your health now and in the future. I have training to help my patients quit, and when you are ready I will work with you to design a specialized treatment plan.

STEP Three: ASSESS Readiness to Quit

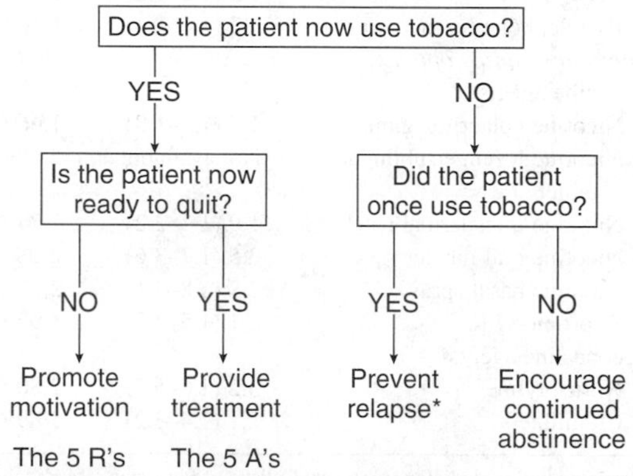

Does the patient now use tobacco?

YES → Is the patient now ready to quit?
 NO → Promote motivation — The 5 R's
 YES → Provide treatment — The 5 A's

NO → Did the patient once use tobacco?
 YES → Prevent relapse*
 NO → Encourage continued abstinence

* Relapse prevention interventions not necessary if patient has not used tobacco for many years and is not at risk for re-initiation.

Fiore MC, Bailey WC, Cohen SJ, et al. *Treating Tobacco Use and Dependence. Clinical Practice Guideline.* Rockville, MD: U.S. Department of Health and Human Services, Public Health Service, 2000.

Reprinted with permission from reference 35. Copyright © 1999-2003 The Regents of the University of California, University of Southern California, and Western University of Health Sciences. All rights reserved.

STEP Four: ASSIST with Quitting

√ **Assess Tobacco Use History**
• Current use: type(s) of tobacco used, brand, amount
• Past use:
 – Duration of tobacco use
 – Changes in levels of use recently
• Past quit attempts:
 – Number of attempts, date of most recent attempt, duration
 – Methods used previously–What did or didn't work? Why or why not?
 – Prior medication administration, dose, compliance, duration of treatment
 – Reasons for relapse

√ **Discuss Key Issues** (for the upcoming or current quit attempt)
• Reasons/motivation for wanting to quit (or avoid relapse)
• Confidence in ability to quit (or avoid relapse)
• Triggers for tobacco use
• Routines and situations associated with tobacco use
• Stress-related tobacco use
• Social support for quitting
• Concerns about weight gain
• Concerns about withdrawal symptoms

√ **Facilitate Quitting Process**
• Discuss methods for quitting: pros and cons of the different methods
• Set a quit date: more than 2–3 days away but less than 2 weeks away
• Recommend Tobacco Use Log
• Discuss coping strategies (cognitive, behavioral)
• Discuss withdrawal symptoms
• Discuss concept of "slip" versus relapse
• Provide medication counseling: compliance, proper use, with demonstration
• Offer to assist throughout the quit attempt

Evaluate the Quit Attempt (at follow-up)
√ • Status of attempt
• Inquire about "slips" and relapse
• Medication compliance and plans for discontinuation

STEP Five: ARRANGE Follow-up Counseling

√ Monitor patients' progress throughout the quit attempt. Follow-up contact should occur during the first week after quitting. A second follow-up contact is recommended in the first month. Additional contacts should be scheduled as needed. Counseling contacts can occur face-to-face, by telephone, or by e-mail. Keep patient progress notes.
√ Address temptations and triggers, discuss relapse prevention strategies.
√ Congratulate patients for continued success.

FIGURE 85-3 Tobacco Cessation Counseling Guidesheet. (Reprinted with permission from reference 35. Copyright © 1999-2004 The Regents of the University of California, University of Southern California, and Western University of Health Sciences. All rights reserved.)

Ask: Screening for tobacco use is crucial and should be a routine component of clinical care. The following question can be used to identify tobacco users: "Do you ever smoke or use any type of tobacco?" At a minimum, tobacco use status (current, former, never user) and level of use (e.g., number of cigarettes smoked per day) should be assessed and documented in the medical record.

Advise: All tobacco users should be advised to quit; the advice should be clear and compelling, yet delivered with sensitivity and a tone of voice that communicates concern and a willingness to assist with quitting. When possible, messages should be personalized by relating advice to factors such as a patient's health status, medication regimen, personal reasons for wanting to quit, or the impact of tobacco use on others. For example, "Ms. Pennick, I see that you now are on two different inhalers. It's important that you know that quitting smoking is the single most important treatment for your emphysema. I strongly encourage you to quit, and I would like to help you."

Assess: Key to the provision of appropriate counseling interventions is the assessment of a patient's readiness to quit.

Patients should be categorized as being either (a) not ready to quit in the next month; (b) ready to quit in the next month; (c) a recent quitter, having quit in the past 6 months; or (d) a former user, having quit more than 6 months ago.[46,49] This classification defines the clinician's next step, which is to provide counseling that is tailored to the patient's level of readiness to quit. As an example for a current smoker: "Mr. Martin, are you giving any serious consideration to quitting, maybe sometime in the next month?" The counseling interventions for patients who are ready to quit will be different from those for patients who are not considering quitting.

Assist: When counseling tobacco users, it is important that clinicians view quitting as a process that might take months or even years to achieve, rather than a "now or never" event. The goal is to promote "forward progress" in the process of change, with the target end-point being sustained abstinence.

When counseling *patients who are not ready to quit,* an important first step is to motivate the patient to start thinking about quitting and considering making a serious quit attempt sometime in the foreseeable future. Some patients who are not ready to quit truly might not believe that they need to quit; however, most will recognize the need to quit but simply are not ready to make the commitment to do so. Often, patients have tried to quit multiple times, and failed, and thus are too discouraged to try again. Strategies for working with patients who are not ready to quit involves promoting motivation to quit, and this can be accomplished by applying the "5 R's" [46] (Table 85-7) and by offering to work closely with the patient in designing a treatment plan. Although it might be useful to educate patients about the pharmacotherapy options, it is inappropriate to prescribe a treatment regimen for patients who are not ready to quit in the next month.

For patients who are ready to quit (i.e., in the next month), the goal is to work with the patient in designing an individualized treatment plan, addressing the key issues listed under the "Assist" component of Figure 85-3.[35] Except when contraindicated, patients should be encouraged to use pharmacotherapy (described below) in combination with a behavioral intervention. The first steps are to discuss the patient's tobacco use history, inquiring about levels of smoking, number of years smoked, methods used previously for quitting (what worked, what didn't, and why), and reasons for previous failed quit attempts. Clinicians should elicit patients' opinions about the different pharmacotherapies for quitting, and should work with patients in selecting the quitting methods (e.g., medications, behavioral counseling programs). While it is important to recognize that pharmaceutical agents might not be desirable or affordable for all patients, clinicians should educate patients

that medications, when taken correctly, can substantially increase the likelihood of quitting.

Patients should be advised to select a quit date that is more than 3 days but less than 2 weeks away. This timeframe provides patients with sufficient time to prepare for the quit attempt, including mental preparation, as well as preparation of the environment, such as by removing all tobacco products and ashtrays from the home, car and workspace and informing their family, friends, and coworkers about their upcoming quit attempt and requesting their support. Additional strategies for coping with quitting are shown in Table 85-8.[35] Patients should be counseled about coping with withdrawal symptoms (Table 85-9)[35] and medication use and compliance, and it is crucial to emphasize the importance of receiving behavioral counseling throughout the quit attempt. Finally, patients should be commended for taking important steps toward improving their health.

Arrange: Because patients' ability to quit increases when multiple counseling interactions are provided, arranging follow-up counseling is an important, yet typically neglected, element of treatment for tobacco dependence. Follow-up contact should occur soon after the quit date, preferably during the first week. A second follow-up contact is recommended within the first month after quitting.[46] Periodically, additional follow-up contacts should occur to monitor patient progress, to assess compliance with pharmacotherapy regimens, and to provide additional support.

Relapse prevention counseling should be part of every follow-up contact with patients who have recently quit smoking. When counseling recent quitters, it is important to address challenges in countering withdrawal symptoms (see Table 85-9)[35] and cravings or temptations to use tobacco. A list of strategies for key triggers or temptations for tobacco use are listed in Table 85-8.[35] Importantly, because tobacco use is a habitual behavior, patients should be advised to alter their daily routines; this helps to disassociate specific behaviors from the use of tobacco. Patients who slip and smoke a cigarette (or use any form of tobacco) or experience a full relapse back to habitual tobacco use should be encouraged to think through the scenario in which tobacco use first occurred and identify the trigger(s) for relapse. This process provides valuable information for future quit attempts.

Telephone Quit-Lines

Clinicians should become aware of local, community-based resources for tobacco cessation, including telephone quit-lines. When time or logistics do not permit comprehensive tobacco cessation counseling during a patient visit, clinicians are encouraged to apply a truncated 5 A's model, whereby they *Ask* about tobacco use, *Advise* tobacco users to quit, *Assess* readiness to quit, and then *refer* patients who are willing to quit to a telephone quit-line. Telephone services that provide tobacco cessation counseling have proliferated over the past decade; these services provide low-cost interventions that can reach patients who might otherwise have limited access to medical treatment because of geographic location or lack of insurance or financial resources. In clinical trials, telephone counseling services for smoking cessa-

---

Table 85-7 The 5 R's for Promoting Motivation to Quit[46]

- **Relevance.** Encourage patients to think about their reasons why quitting is important. Counseling should be framed such that it relates to the patient's risk for disease or exacerbation of disease, family or social situations (e.g., having children with asthma), health concerns, age, or other patient factors such as prior experience with quitting.
- **Risks.** Ask patients to identify specific negative health consequences of smoking, such as acute risks (shortness of breath, asthma exacerbations, harm to pregnancy, infertility), long-term risks (cancer, cardiac, and pulmonary disease) and environmental risks (promoting smoking among children by being a negative role model, effects of secondhand smoke on others, including children and pets).
- **Rewards.** Ask patients to identify the benefits that they anticipate from quitting, such as improved health, enhanced physical performance, enhanced taste and smell, reduced expenditures for tobacco, less time wasted or work missed, reduced health risks to others (fetus, children, housemates), and reduced aging of the skin.
- **Roadblocks.** Help patients to identify significant barriers to quitting and assist in developing coping strategies (see Table 85-8) for addressing each barrier. Common barriers include nicotine withdrawal symptoms (see Table 85-9), fear of failure, a need for social support while quitting, depression, weight gain, and a sense of deprivation or loss.
- **Repetition.** Continue to work with patients who are successful in their quit attempt. Discuss circumstances in which smoking occurred to identify the trigger(s) for relapse; this is part of the learning process and will be useful information for the next quit attempt. Repeat interventions when possible.

Table 85-8	**Cognitive and Behavioral Strategies for Tobacco Cessation**

Cognitive strategies

Focus on *retraining the way a patient thinks*. Often, patients mentally deliberate on the fact that they are thinking about a cigarette, and this leads to relapse. Patients must recognize that thinking about a cigarette doesn't mean they need to have one.

Review commitment to quit, focus on downside of tobacco	Remind oneself that cravings and temptations are temporary and will pass. Have patient announce, either silently or aloud "I want to be a nonsmoker, and the temptation will pass."
Distractive thinking	Deliberate, immediate refocusing of thinking toward other thoughts when cued by thoughts about tobacco use.
Positive self-talks, "pep-talks"	Saying "I can do this" and reminding oneself of previous difficult situations in which tobacco use was avoided with success.
Relaxation through imagery	Centering of mind toward positive, relaxing thoughts.
Mental rehearsal, visualization	Preparing for situations that might arise by envisioning how best to handle them. For example, a patient might envision what would happen if he or she were offered a cigarette by a friend—the patient would mentally craft and rehearse a response, and perhaps even practice it by saying it aloud.

Behavioral strategies

Involve *specific actions to reduce risk for relapse*. For maximal effectiveness, these should be considered before quitting, after determining patient-specific triggers for tobacco use. Following are some behavioral strategies for several common cues or triggers for relapse.

Stress	Anticipate upcoming challenges at work, at school, or in personal life. Develop a substitute plan for tobacco use during times of stress (e.g., deep breathing, take a break/leave the situation, call supportive friend or family member, self-massage, use nicotine replacement therapy).
Alcohol	Drinking alcohol can lead to relapse. The patient should consider limiting/abstaining from alcohol during the early stages of quitting.
Other tobacco users	Quitting is more difficult if the patient is around other tobacco users. This is especially difficult if there is another tobacco user in the household. During the early stages of quitting, patients should limit prolonged contact with individuals who are using tobacco. Ask co-workers, friends and housemates not to smoke or use tobacco in their presence.
Oral gratification needs	Have non–tobacco oral substitutes (gum, sugarless candy, straws, toothpicks, lip balm, toothbrush, nicotine replacement therapy, bottled water) readily available.
Automatic smoking routines	Anticipate routines associated with tobacco use and develop an alternative plan. Examples: *Morning coffee with cigarettes:* change morning routine, drink tea instead of coffee, take shower before drinking coffee, take a brisk walk shortly after awakening. *Smoking while driving:* remove all tobacco from car, have car interior detailed, listen to a book on tape or talk radio, use oral substitute. *Smoking while on the phone:* stand while talking, limit call duration, change phone location, keep hands occupied by doodling or sketching. *Smoking after meals:* get up and immediately do dishes or take a brisk walk after eating, call supportive friend.
Postcessation weight gain	Most tobacco users gain weight after quitting; most quitters gain less than 10 pounds, but there is a broad range of weight gain reported, with up to 10% of quitters gaining as much as 30 pounds.[46] Advise patient not to attempt to modify multiple behaviors at one time. If weight gain is a barrier to quitting, advise patient to engage in regular physical activity and adhere to a healthful diet (as opposed to strict dieting). Carefully plan and prepare meals, increase fruit and water intake to create a feeling of fullness, and chew sugarless gum or eat sugarless candies. Consider use of pharmacotherapy shown to delay weight gain (e.g., nicotine gum, bupropion).
Cravings for tobacco	Cravings for tobacco are temporary and usually pass within 5–10 minutes. Handle cravings through distractive thinking, take a break, change activities/tasks, take deep breaths, perform self-massage.

Adapted with permission from reference 35. Copyright 1999-2004 The Regents of the University of California, University of Southern California, and Western University of Health Sciences. All rights reserved.

tion have been shown to be effective in promoting quitting among the patients who use them,[50] and these positive results have been shown to translate into real-world effectiveness.[51] In addition, preliminary evidence suggests that that quit-lines also are effective for spit tobacco cessation.[52] The following website, created by the Tobacco Control Research Branch of the National Cancer Institute with contributions from other nationally recognized agencies and organizations, such as the CDC and the American Cancer Society, can be used to identify toll-free telephone quit-line services for each state in the United States: http://www.smokefree.gov/usmap.html.

Pharmacotherapy Options
All smokers who are trying to quit should be encouraged to use one or more FDA-approved pharmacologic aids for cessation; potential exceptions that require special consideration include medical contraindications, smoking fewer than 10 cigarettes per day, adolescence, and pregnancy or breastfeeding.[46] Currently, the FDA-approved, first-line agents[46] include five nicotine replacement therapy (NRT) dosage forms and sustained-release bupropion (bupropion SR). Pharmacologic agents that have not received FDA approval for smoking cessation but are recommended as second-line agents[46] include clonidine and nortriptyline.

Table 85-9 Postcessation Tobacco Withdrawal Symptoms Management

Symptoms	Cause	Duration	Relief
Chest tightness	Tightness is likely due to tension created by the body's need for nicotine or may be caused by sore muscles from coughing.	Few days	• Use relaxation techniques • Try deep breathing • Chew nicotine gum
Constipation, stomach pain, gas	Intestinal movement decreases for a brief period.	1–2 weeks	• Drink plenty of fluids • Add fruits, vegetables, and whole grain cereals to diet
Cough, dry throat, nasal drip	The body is getting rid of mucus, which has blocked airways and restricted breathing.	Few days	• Drink plenty of fluids • Avoid additional stress during first few weeks
Craving for a cigarette	Nicotine is a strongly addictive drug, and withdrawal causes cravings.	Frequent for 2–3 days; can happen for months or years	• Wait out the urge (which lasts only a few minutes) • Distract yourself • Exercise (take walks)
Difficulty concentrating	The body needs time to adjust to not having constant stimulation from nicotine.	Few weeks	• Plan workload accordingly • Avoid additional stress during first few weeks
Dizziness	The body is getting extra oxygen.	1–2 days	• Use extra caution • Change positions slowly
Fatigue	Nicotine is a stimulant.	2–4 weeks	• Take naps • Do not push yourself • Use nicotine replacement therapy
Hunger	Cravings for a cigarette can be confused with hunger pangs; sensation may result from oral cravings, or the desire for something in the mouth.	Up to several weeks	• Drink water or low-calorie liquids • Be prepared with low-calorie snacks
Insomnia	Nicotine affects brain wave function and influences sleep patterns; coughing and dreams about smoking are common.	1 week	• Avoid caffeine after 6 PM • Use relaxation techniques
Irritability	The body's craving for nicotine can produce irritability.	2–4 weeks	• Take walks • Try hot baths • Use relaxation techniques

Adapted with permission from reference 35. Copyright 1999-2004 The Regents of the University of California, University of Southern California, and Western University of Health Sciences. All rights reserved.

The first approved medication for smoking cessation was the nicotine gum, which was marketed in 1984. This later was followed by the nicotine transdermal patch (prescription-only formulation in 1991 and nonprescription formulations in 1996), the nicotine nasal spray in 1996, bupropion SR and nicotine nasal spray in 1996, the nicotine inhaler in 1997, and the nicotine lozenge in 2002. Each of these products has been shown to be effective in promoting smoking cessation.

First-Line Agents

NICOTINE REPLACEMENT THERAPY

NRT increases success for quitting by reducing the physical withdrawal symptoms associated with nicotine cessation while the patient focuses on modifying his or her behavior and coping with the psychological aspects of quitting. In addition, because the onset of action for NRT is not as rapid as that of nicotine obtained through smoking, patients become less accustomed to the nearly immediate, reinforcing effects of inhaled tobacco. A meta-analysis of 96 controlled trials of NRT showed that all products (gum, patch, inhaler, and nasal spray) result in statistically significantly improved abstinence rates when compared with placebo. Patients using NRT are 1.5 to 2 times more likely to quit smoking than are those receiving placebo.[53] Figure 85-4 depicts the concentration time curves for the various NRT products, compared with a cigarette and moist snuff (a form of spit tobacco). It can be seen that of the five NRT dosage forms, the nicotine nasal spray reaches its peak concentration most rapidly. The nicotine gum, lozenge, and oral inhaler have similar concentrations curves, and the nicotine transdermal patch has the slowest onset, but offers more consistent blood levels of nicotine over a much longer period of time. Dosing information, recommended duration of treatment, and adverse effects for the first-line agents are shown in Table 85-10.

Precautions

NRT should be used with caution in patients with underlying serious arrhythmias, those with serious or worsening angina pectoris and those with a recent (within 2 weeks) myocardial infarction (MI),[46] because nicotine may cause adverse cardiovascular effects by increasing the myocardial workload

Table 85-10 Pharmacotherapy Options

Product	Dosing	Duration	Adverse Effects
Nicotine Gum^OTC			
Nicorette *Generic Gum* 2 mg, 4 mg; regular, mint, orange	≥25 cigarettes/day: 4 mg <25 cigarettes/day: 2 mg Week 1–6: 1 piece Q 1–2 hr Week 7–9: 1 piece Q 2–4 hr Week 10–12: 1 piece Q 4–8 hr	Up to 12 wk	Mouth/jaw soreness, hiccups, dyspepsia, hypersalivation Effects associated with incorrect chewing technique: lightheadedness, nausea and vomiting, throat and mouth irritation
Nicotine Lozenge^OTC			
Commit 2 mg, 4 mg	1st cigarette ≤30 minutes after waking: 4 mg 1st cigarette >30 minutes after waking: 2 mg Week 1–6: 1 lozenge Q 1–2 hr Week 7–9: 1 lozenge Q 2–4 hr Week 10–12: 1 lozenge Q 4–8 hr	Up to 12 wk	Nausea, hiccups, cough, heartburn, headache, flatulence, insomnia
Nicotine Transdermal Patch^OTC/Rx			
Nicotrol Patch 5 mg, 10 mg, 15 mg 16-hour release	>10 cigarettes/day: 15 mg/day × 6 wk 10 mg/day × 2 wk 5 mg/day × 2 wk Not recommended for patients smoking ≤10 cigarettes per day	10 wk	Local skin reactions (erythema, pruritus, burning), headache
Nicoderm CQ 7 mg, 14 mg, 21 mg 24-hour release	>10 cigarettes/day: 21 mg/day × 6 wk 14 mg/day × 2 wk 7 mg/day × 2 wk ≤10 cigarettes/day: 14 mg/day × 6 wk 7 mg/day × 2 wk	8–10 wk	Local skin reactions (erythema, pruritus, burning), headache, sleep disturbances (insomnia) or abnormal/vivid dreams (associated with nocturnal nicotine absorption). May wear patch for 16 hours (remove at bedtime) if patient experiences sleep disturbances.
Generic Patch (formerly Habitrol) 7 mg, 14 mg, 21 mg 24-hour release	>10 cigarettes/day: 21 mg/day × 4 wk 14 mg/day × 2 wk 7 mg/day × 2 wk	8 wk	
Generic Patch (formerly Prostep) 11 mg, 22 mg 24-hour release	≤15 cigarettes/day: 11 mg/day ×6 wk >15 cigarettes/day: 22 mg/day × 6 wk	6 wk (no dose tapering)	
Nicotine Nasal Spray^Rx			
Nicotrol NS Metered spray 0.5 mg nicotine in 50 µL aqueous nicotine solution	1–2 doses/hr (8–40 doses/day) One dose = 2 sprays (one in each nostril); each spray delivers 0.5 mg of nicotine to the nasal mucosa. For best results, initially use at least 8 doses/day. Do not exceed 5 doses/hr or 40 doses/day	3–6 mo Gradually decrease usage over 3–6 mo	Nasal and/or throat irritation (hot, peppery, or burning sensation), rhinitis, tearing, sneezing, cough, headache
Nicotine Oral Inhaler^Rx			
Nicotrol Inhaler 10 mg cartridge delivers 4 mg inhaled nicotine vapor	6–16 cartridges/day; individualized dosing Initially, use at least 6 cartridges/day. Nicotine is depleted after 20 minutes of active puffing. Open cartridge retains potency for 24 hours.	Up to 6 mo	Mouth and/or throat irritation, unpleasant taste, cough, rhinitis, dyspepsia, hiccups, headache
Bupropion SR^Rx			
Zyban Sustained-release tablet	150 mg PO Q AM × 3 days, then increase to 150 mg PO BID Set quit date 1–2 weeks after initiation of therapy. Do NOT exceed 300 mg/day. Allow at least 8 hours between doses. Avoid bedtime dosing to minimize insomnia.	8–12 wk Maintenance up to 6 mo	Insomnia, dry mouth, nervousness, difficulty concentrating, rash, constipation, seizures (risk is 0.1%)

Adapted with permission from reference 35. Copyright 1999–2004 The Regents of the University of California, University of Southern California, and Western University of Health Sciences. All rights reserved. OTC, (over the counter) nonprescription product; Rx, prescription product.

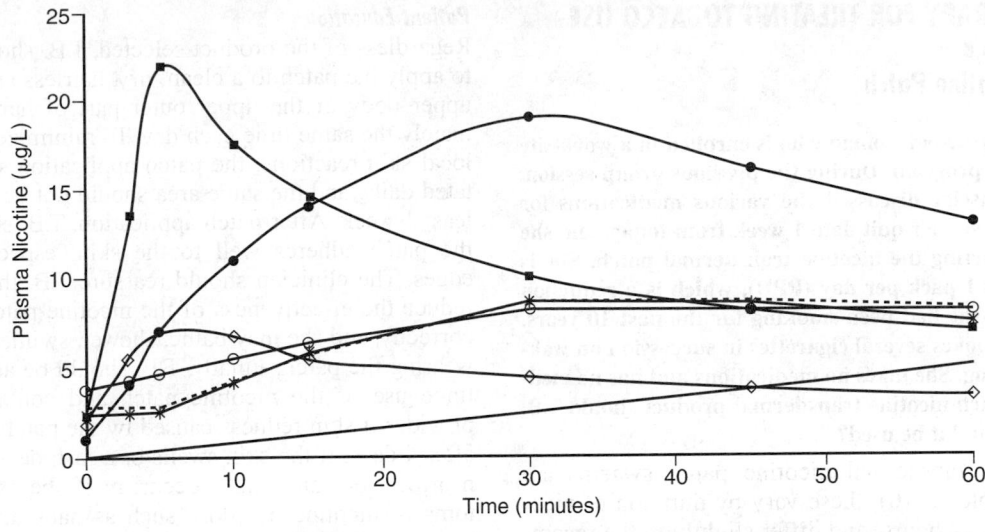

FIGURE 85-4 Plasma Nicotine Concentrations for Various Nicotine-Containing Products. (Reprinted with permission from reference 35. Copyright ©1999-2004 The Regents of the University of California, University of Southern California, and Western University of Health Sciences. All rights reserved. Plasma nicotine concentration curves derived from references 62, 78, and 126.)

through increased heart rate and blood pressure. Nicotine also may constrict coronary arteries, leading to cardiac ischemia.[54] However, the risks of NRT in patients with cardiovascular disease are small compared with the risks of continued smoking.[54,55]

NRT Use During Pregnancy

The FDA classifies nicotine as pregnancy risk category D, indicating that there is evidence of risk to the human fetus. Accordingly, none of the NRT formulations has received FDA approval for use in pregnancy. Although NRT may pose a risk to the developing fetus, the risk is arguably lower than the risks of continued smoking.[56] However, because it is assumed that NRT can cause fetal harm when administered during pregnancy, NRT should be reserved for women unable to quit using nonpharmacologic methods. If NRT is warranted, it is prudent to prescribe doses at the low end of the effective dose range and consider using formulations that provide intermittent rather than continuous drug exposure[46] (e.g., the nicotine gum, lozenge, nasal spray, or inhaler).

BUPROPION SR

Bupropion SR is an oral atypical antidepressant medication thought to affect the levels of brain neurotransmitters (e.g., dopamine, norepinephrine). By blocking neural dopamine or norepinephrine uptake in the central nervous system, bupropion decreases the craving for nicotine and

symptoms of withdrawal.[46] Similar to NRT, its use approximately doubles the long-term abstinence rate when compared with placebo.

Animal data suggest the absolute bioavailability of bupropion ranges from 5% to 20%. It undergoes extensive hepatic metabolism to three active metabolites; one of the metabolites, hydroxybupropion, is formed by the cytochrome P450 isoenzyme CYP2B6. Bupropion and its metabolites are eliminated in urine (87%) and feces (10%), with less than 1% being excreted unchanged in the urine. The half-life for bupropion is 21 hours, and its metabolites have a half-life range of 20 to 27 hours; steady-state plasma concentrations are reached within 5 and 8 days, respectively.[57]

Studies in healthy smokers suggest that bupropion may be safely used in combination with NRT. Bupropion is classified as pregnancy risk category B; it has not been studied in pregnant women and thus should be considered for use only when nonpharmacologic methods are ineffective.

Second-Line Agents

Although not FDA approved specifically for smoking cessation, the prescription medications clonidine and nortriptyline are recommended as second-line agents.[46] Lack of an FDA-approved indication for smoking cessation, as well as side effect profiles, currently prohibit these agents from achieving first-line classification.[46]

PHARMACOTHERAPY FOR TREATING TOBACCO USE AND DEPENDENCE
Transdermal Nicotine Patch

1. T.B. is a 32-year-old woman who is enrolled in a work-site smoking cessation program. During the previous group session, the cessation counselor discussed the various medications for cessation. T.B. has set her quit date 1 week from today, and she is interested in starting the nicotine transdermal patch. She is currently smoking 1 pack per day (PPD), which is a reduction from the $1\frac{1}{2}$ PPD she had been smoking for the past 10 years. T.B. reports she smokes several cigarettes in succession on wakening in the morning. She takes no medications and has no medical problems. Which nicotine transdermal product should T.B. select and how should it be used?

Four different transdermal nicotine patch systems are marketed (see Table 85-10); these vary by duration of nicotine release (16 or 24 hours) and differ slightly in the recommended dosing schedule. The efficacy of the transdermal nicotine patch is well documented, and all currently available nicotine patches significantly improve abstinence rates compared with placebo.[46,53] A meta-analysis of 34 randomized, double blind, placebo-controlled trials reported the odds ratio for abstinence (at $\geq$6 months) with nicotine patches versus placebo to be 1.74 (95% CI, 1.57 to 1.93).[53] The advantage of these systems lies in their simplicity of use, because they need to be applied only once daily. Three of the products (Nicoderm CQ and both generic formulations) are left on the skin continuously for 24 hours. The Nicotrol formulation, which provides continuous nicotine delivery over 16 hours, is applied in the morning and removed at bedtime. The transdermal formulations deliver nicotine more slowly than the gum, lozenge, nasal spray, and inhaler (see Fig. 85-4); however, the transdermal patch provides a more continuous blood nicotine level compared with the intermittent fluctuations in nicotine concentrations observed with the other NRT formulations. The 24-hour products have the theoretical advantage of continuous nicotine delivery throughout the night to provide coverage for early morning cravings, whereas the 16-hour patch may cause less sleep interference, insomnia, and vivid dreams.

Dosing
The manufacturers recommended dosages are listed in Table 85-10. In general, higher levels of smoking necessitate the use of higher-strength formulations and a longer duration of therapy. Patients with strong morning cravings for cigarettes might have better success with a 24-hour patch.[58] Ultimately, the starting dose, rate of tapering, and total duration of therapy must be individualized to the patient's baseline smoking levels, development of side effects (e.g., nausea, dyspepsia, nervousness, dizziness, sweating), and the presence or absence of withdrawal symptoms (see Table 85-9). T.B. currently smokes 20 cigarettes per day, and thus her starting dose should be at the higher end of the dosing range (e.g., 22 mg, 21 mg or 15 mg). Although published data suggest that the 16-hour and 24-hour formulations have comparable efficacy, because T.B. reports strong morning cravings for cigarettes, it is reasonable to initiate therapy with a 24-hour patch.

Patient Education
Regardless of the product selected, T.B. should be instructed to apply the patch to a clean, dry, hairless area of skin on the upper body or the upper outer part of her arm at approximately the same time each day. To minimize the potential for local skin reactions, the patch application site should be rotated daily, and the same area should not be used again for at least 1 week. After patch application, T.B. should ensure that the patch adheres well to the skin, especially around the edges. The clinician should reassure T.B. that water will not reduce the effectiveness of the nicotine patch if it is applied correctly, and she may bathe, shower, swim, or exercise while wearing the patch. Finally, T.B. should be advised to discontinue use of the nicotine patch and contact a health care provider if skin redness caused by the patch does not resolve after 4 days, if the skin swells or a rash develops; if irregular heartbeat or palpitations occur; or if she experiences symptoms of nicotine overdose such as nausea, vomiting, dizziness, diarrhea, sweating, weakness, and rapid heartbeat.

Product Selection Considerations
The primary advantage of the transdermal nicotine patch compared with other NRT formulations is that the patch is easy to use and conceal, releases a continuous dose of nicotine throughout the day, and requires administration once a day. As a result, patients who have difficulty adhering to regimens that require taking multiple doses of medications throughout the day or those who want a simplified regimen are likely to be more successful with the nicotine patch. Disadvantages of the patch include a high incidence (see text that follows) of skin irritation associated with the patch adhesives and the inability to acutely adjust the dose of nicotine to alleviate symptoms of withdrawal. Finally, patients with underlying dermatologic conditions (e.g., psoriasis, eczema, atopic dermatitis) should not use the patch, because they are more likely to experience skin irritation.[46]

Adverse Reactions

2. Ten days later, T.B. calls to complain of an itchy rash that she believes is caused by the nicotine patch. She noticed the rash yesterday when she removed the first patch from her left upper arm. This morning, after removing the second patch from her right upper arm, she noticed a similar rash. T.B. describes the skin on her right arm as slightly red but not swollen; the rash on her left arm has only a faint trace of pink discoloration. Her last cigarette was 2 days ago. How should T.B. be managed at this time?

The most common side effects associated with the nicotine patch are local reactions (erythema, burning, and pruritus) at the skin application site. These reactions, which tend to occur more commonly with the 24-hour products, are caused by skin occlusion or sensitivity to the patch adhesives. Rotating the patch application sites on a daily basis minimizes skin irritation; nonetheless, skin reactions to the patch adhesives occur in up to 50% of patch users. Fewer than 5% of patients discontinue therapy because of a skin reaction.[46] T.B. appears to be experiencing a mild skin reaction to the transdermal nicotine patch. She should be reassured that it is normal for the skin to appear erythematous for up to 24 to 48 hours after the patch is removed. T.B. can apply topical hydrocortisone cream (0.5% or 1%) or triamcinolone cream (0.5%) or can take an oral antihistamine for symptomatic treatment.[46] Because the rash on her left arm has nearly resolved, it is reasonable for T.B. to continue using the nicotine transdermal patch provided that the erythema is not too bothersome.

Other less common side effects associated with the transdermal nicotine patch include vivid or abnormal dreams, insomnia, and headache. Sleep disturbances are more commonly reported in patients using the 24-hour formulations and may be the result of nocturnal nicotine absorption. Patients using the 24-hour products should be instructed to remove the patch at bedtime if this side effect becomes troublesome.[59]

The clinician also should provide behavioral counseling support by asking T.B. about the current quit attempt. Appropriate issues to address include the following: her confidence in remaining tobacco free, situations in which she has been tempted to smoke and potential triggers for relapse, nicotine withdrawal symptoms, her social support system for quitting, and any other questions or concerns she might have. It is reasonable to review potential coping strategies (behavioral and cognitive; see Table 85-8) and schedule a future follow-up call. The clinician should commend T.B. for her decision to quit, should congratulate her for remaining tobacco free for 48 hours, and should reassure her that skin irritation is a common, yet generally manageable, complication with the nicotine patch.

Nicotine Gum

3. T.B. would like to discontinue the nicotine transdermal patch. She wants to know if the gum is an effective alternative.

Nicotine polacrilex gum is a resin complex of nicotine and polacrilin in a chewing gum base that allows for slow release and absorption of nicotine across the oral mucosa. The product is available as 2-mg and 4-mg strengths, in regular, mint, and orange flavors. The gum has a distinct, tobacco-like, slightly peppery, minty, or citrus taste and contains buffering agents (sodium carbonate and sodium bicarbonate) to increase the salivary pH to 8.5, which enhances the buccal absorption of nicotine. The amount of nicotine absorbed from each piece is variable, but approximately 1.1 mg and 2.9 mg of nicotine are extracted from the 2-mg and 4-mg gum formulations, respectively.[60] Peak plasma concentrations of nicotine are achieved approximately 30 minutes after chewing a single piece of gum and then slowly decline thereafter (see Fig. 85-4). Use of the nicotine gum improves long-term ($\geq$6 months) abstinence rates as evidenced by a recent meta-analysis of 51 studies that concluded that the odds of abstinence was 1.66 with the gum compared with placebo (95% CI, 1.52 to 1.81).[53]

Dosing

Table 85-10 outlines the manufacturer's recommended dosing schedule the nicotine gum. Individuals who smoke fewer than 25 cigarettes per day should use the 2-mg strength, and those smoking more should use the 4-mg strength. During the initial 6 weeks of therapy, patients should use 1 piece of gum every 1 to 2 hours while awake. In general, this amounts to at least 9 pieces of gum daily. The "chew and park" method described below allows for the slow, consistent release of nico-

tine from the polacrilin resin. Patients can use additional pieces of gum (to the daily maximum of 24 pieces per day) if cravings occur between scheduled doses. In general, patients who smoke a greater number of cigarettes per day will require more nicotine gum to alleviate their cravings than will patients who smoke fewer cigarettes per day. It is preferable to use the gum on a fixed schedule of administration, tapering over 1 to 3 months rather than using it "as needed" to control cravings.[46]

Patient Education

Proper chewing technique is crucial when using the nicotine gum. Patients should be instructed to chew the gum slowly until a peppery, minty, or citrus taste or a slight tingling sensation in the mouth is detected; this varies but generally occurs after about 15 chews. When the taste or tingling sensation is noted, the patient should "park" the gum between the cheek and gum to allow absorption of nicotine across the buccal mucosa. When the taste or tingling dissipates (generally after 1 to 2 minutes), the patient should resume chewing slowly. When the taste or tingle returns, the patient should stop chewing and park the gum in a different area in the mouth. Rotating the gum placement site within the mouth helps to decrease the incidence of oral irritation. The chew/park steps should be repeated until most of the nicotine is extracted; this generally occurs after 30 minutes and becomes obvious when chewing no longer elicits the characteristic taste or tingling sensation.

Patients should be warned that the absorption and therefore effectiveness of nicotine gum might be reduced by acidic beverages (e.g., coffee, juices, wine or soft drinks),[61] which transiently reduce the salivary pH. To prevent this interaction, patients should be advised not to eat or drink for 15 minutes before or while using the nicotine gum.

Adverse Reactions

The most common adverse reactions associated with use of the nicotine gum include jaw muscle fatigue, hypersalivation, mouth irritation, hiccups, and dyspepsia.[46] Many of these side effects can be minimized or prevented by using proper chewing technique. Because the nicotine polacrilin resin is more viscous than ordinary chewing gum, it is more likely to adhere to fillings, bridges, dentures, crowns, and braces. If excessive sticking or damage to dental work occurs, the patient should stop using the nicotine gum and consult a dentist. Patients should be warned that chewing the gum too rapidly may result in excessive release of nicotine leading to lightheadedness, nausea, vomiting, throat irritation, hiccups, and indigestion.

Product Selection Considerations

Advantages of nicotine gum include the fact that this formulation may be used to satisfy oral cravings and may delay weight gain.[46] For these reasons, the gum may be particularly beneficial for patients who have weight gain concerns or for patients who report boredom as a trigger for smoking. The gum also might be advantageous for patients who desire flexibility in dosing and prefer the ability to self-regulate nicotine levels to manage withdrawal symptoms. Some patients may find that the viscous consistency of the gum renders it difficult to use because it sticks to dental work. Others may find it difficult or socially unacceptable to chew the gum so frequently. Finally, to minimize adverse effects and derive maximal therapeutic benefit, it is imperative that patients use enough gum each day and utilize the correct chewing technique.

Nicotine Lozenge

4. **How does the nicotine lozenge differ from the nicotine gum?**

The nicotine polacrilex lozenge is a resin complex of nicotine and polacrilin in a sugar-free, light-mint-flavored lozenge. The product is available in 2-mg and 4-mg strengths which are meant to be consumed like hard candy or other medicinal lozenges (e.g., sucked and moved from side to side in the mouth until fully dissolved). Because the nicotine lozenge dissolves completely, it delivers approximately 25% more nicotine than does an equivalent dose of nicotine gum.[62] Like the nicotine gum, the lozenge also contains buffering agents (sodium carbonate and potassium bicarbonate) to increase salivary pH, thereby enhancing buccal absorption of the nicotine. Peak nicotine concentrations of nicotine with the lozenge are achieved after 30 to 60 minutes of use and then slowly decline thereafter (see Fig. 85-4). In a trial evaluating the formulation currently available in the United States, the nicotine lozenge approximately doubled the 12-month abstinence rates compared with placebo (16.4% versus 7.9%).[63] A recent meta-analysis of 3 studies using either the nicotine lozenge (nicotine polacrilin) or sublingual tablet (nicotine β-cyclodextrin complex; not available in the United States) concluded that the odds of abstinence at 6 or more months was 2.08 with the tablet/lozenge relative to placebo (95% CI, 1.63 to 2.65).[53]

Dosing

Unlike other NRT formulations, which use the number of cigarettes smoked per day as the basis for dosing, the recommended dosage of the nicotine lozenge is based on the time to first cigarette (TTFC). Some experts believe that the best indicator of nicotine dependence is the need to smoke soon after waking.[64] Based on this method, people who smoke their first cigarette of the day within 30 minutes of waking are considered more highly dependent on nicotine than those who smoke their first cigarette more than 30 minutes after waking. Because the nicotine polacrilin lozenge has been studied using the TTFC as a dosage selector, the product is licensed for use in the following manner: patients who smoke their first cigarette of the day within 30 minutes of waking should use the 4-mg strength lozenge, and patients who smoke their first cigarette of the day more than 30 minutes after waking should use the 2-mg strength lozenge. Patients are more likely to succeed if they use the lozenge on a fixed schedule rather than as needed. During the initial 6 weeks of therapy, patients should use 1 lozenge every 1 to 2 hours while awake. In general, this amounts to at least 9 lozenges daily. Patients can use additional lozenges (up to 5 lozenges in 6 hours or a maximum of 20 lozenges per day) if cravings occur between scheduled doses.

Patient Education

Similar to the gum, the nicotine lozenge is a specially formulated nicotine delivery system that must be used properly for optimal results. The lozenge should be allowed to dissolve slowly in the mouth; when nicotine is released from the polacrilin resin, a warm, tingling sensation may be experienced. The patient should occasionally rotate the lozenge to different areas of the mouth to reduce the potential for mucosal irritation. When used correctly, the lozenge should completely dissolve within 30 minutes. Patients should be counseled not to chew or swallow the lozenge, because this increases the incidence of gastrointestinal-related side effects.

Because the nicotine in the lozenge is dissolved in saliva and absorbed through the buccal mucosa, patients should be cautioned that the effectiveness of the nicotine lozenge may be reduced by acidic beverages such as coffee, juices, wine, or soft drinks. As recommended for the nicotine gum, patients should be advised not to eat or drink for 15 minutes before or while using the nicotine lozenge.

Adverse Reactions

In general, the nicotine lozenge is well tolerated. The most common side effects include nausea, hiccups, cough, dyspepsia, headache, and flatulence. Patients who use more than one lozenge at a time, continuously use one lozenge after another, or chew or swallow the lozenge are more likely to experience dyspepsia or hiccups.

Product Selection Considerations

The nicotine lozenge is similar to the nicotine gum formulation in that it may satisfy oral cravings and patients can self-titrate therapy to acutely manage withdrawal symptoms. Because the lozenge does not require chewing, many patients find this to be a more discrete nicotine delivery system. The disadvantages of the lozenge are the fact that it requires frequent dosing and the gastrointestinal side effects (nausea, hiccups, and heartburn) may be bothersome.

Postcessation Weight Gain

5. **T.B. is worried about gaining weight after she quits smoking. Is weight gain common after quitting and how can this be prevented?**

Most tobacco users gain weight after quitting. Studies suggest that most quitters gain fewer than 10 pounds, but there is a broad range of weight gain reported, with up to 10% of quitters gaining as much as 30 pounds.[46] In general, women tend to gain more weight than men. In a study of nearly 6,000 smokers who were followed up for 5 years after quitting, the average weight gain during the follow-up period was 19.2 pounds and 16.7 pounds among women and men, respectively.[65] For men and women, subgroups that are more likely to gain weight after quitting are African Americans, younger tobacco users (<55 years of age), and heavier tobacco users (those smoking more than 25 cigarettes per day).

The weight-suppressing effects of tobacco are well known. However, the mechanisms to explain why most successful quitters gain weight are not completely understood. Smokers have been found to have an approximately 10% higher metabolic rate compared with nonsmokers.[66] In some studies, higher caloric intakes were documented after cessation.[67,68] The increased caloric intake may result from an increase in appetite, improved sense of taste, or a change in the hand-to-mouth ritual through the substitution of tobacco with food.

The Clinical Practice Guideline[46] recommends that clinicians inform patients about the likelihood of weight gain as a result of quitting, but that patients should be advised against strict dieting while quitting. This should include a discussion about the greater health risks of continued tobacco use when compared with the modest weight gain associated with quitting. It is important for the clinician to stress that quitting tobacco use should be the patient's top priority.[46] In general, a patient is less likely to be successful if he or she attempts to change multiple behaviors at once. For this reason, strict dieting to prevent weight gain, especially early during the early stages of quitting, is generally not recommended. T.B. should be counseled that the average weight gain of less than 10 pounds is less detrimental to her overall health than is continued smoking. Because she is concerned about weight gain it is reasonable for the clinician to recommend that T.B. engage in some form of regular physical activity. Even modest physical activity (e.g., walking 30 minutes daily) has been found to attenuate the weight gain associated with smoking cessation.[68] Although strict dieting is not recommended, T.B. should carefully plan and prepare meals to avoid binge eating, increase her water intake to create a feeling of fullness, chew sugarless gum, and limit alcohol consumption. Furthermore, T.B. may consider pharmacotherapy known to delay weight gain such as bupropion SR or nicotine gum.[46]

Relapse Back to Smoking

6. **During a follow up contact, the clinician learns that T.B. smoked half a pack of cigarettes at a party over the weekend and has relapsed to her previous smoking levels after not having smoked for just over a month. How should the clinician respond?**

The clinician should thank T.B. for being honest about her smoking and should ask T.B. to discuss the circumstances during which the smoking occurred. At the time of her smoking, where was she, who was she with, how did she get access to cigarettes, and how was she feeling at the time? What, specifically, were the triggers for her relapse (e.g., alcohol, depression, friends who were smoking around her)? It is important that the clinician help the patient to use this information as part of the learning process, but it also is important to focus on the "positive," such as T.B.'s ability to have remained tobacco free for more than 1 month. After being smoke free for more than 4 weeks, most physical effects of nicotine withdrawal have completely resolved, and thus the relapse trigger for T.B. likely was psychological or situational and could be abated through application of effective coping techniques. After an informative discussion about the situation in which the smoking occurred, it is important that the clinician work with the patient in identifying strategies for avoiding relapse in the future (see Table 85-8).

Smoking and Cardiovascular Disease

7. **P.J. is a 62-year-old man admitted for an elective coronary artery bypass graft (CABG) procedure. His medical history is significant for angina, hypertension, dyslipidemia, peripheral vascular disease (PVD), and allergic rhinitis. He underwent a bilateral carotid endarterectomy procedure 2 years ago and had il-iac artery angioplasty with stent placement 5 years ago for PVD. P.J.'s social history is significant for tobacco use (1½ to 2 packs cigarettes/day) and alcohol (3 to 4 drinks per day). He is approximately 10 pounds overweight. His preoperative laboratory results are significant for a total cholesterol of 270 mg/dL (desirable, <200), low-density lipoprotein cholesterol count (LDL-C) of 163 mg/dL (optimal, <100), high-density lipoprotein cholesterol count (HDL-C) of 35 mg/dL (low, <40) and triglycerides of 350 mg/dL (normal, <150). His medications before admission include atenolol 50 mg QD, aspirin 81 mg QD, isosorbide dinitrate 20 mg TID, atorvastatin 10 mg QD, fluticasone nasal spray (50 μg/spray) 1 spray/nostril QD, and nitroglycerin 0.4 mg SL as needed. Which of P.J.'s chronic medical conditions may be caused or exacerbated by his tobacco use?**

[SI units: total cholesterol, 6.98 mmol/L; LDL-C, 4.22 mmol/L; HDL-C, 0.91 mmol/L; triglycerides, 3.95 mmol/L]

Considerable evidence suggests that cigarette smoking is a major cause of cardiovascular disease—responsible for more than 148,000 premature cardiovascular-related deaths each year.[5] Smoking is known to accelerate the process of atherosclerosis, leading to chronic cardiovascular disorders including coronary heart disease, cerebrovascular disease, peripheral vascular disease, and aortic aneurysm. In addition, smoking greatly elevates the risk for acute cardiovascular events, including sudden death, MI, stroke, and reocclusion of coronary or peripheral vessels after graft surgery or angioplasty.[69–71]

There are numerous plausible pathophysiologic mechanisms whereby tobacco smoking contributes to the development of cardiovascular disease. Oxidant gases and other compounds in tobacco smoke are believed to induce a hypercoagulable state characterized by increased platelet aggregation and thrombosis, which greatly increases the risk of MI and sudden death.[69,71] The carbon monoxide in smoke reduces the amount of oxygen available to tissues and organs, including myocardial tissue, and may reduce the ventricular fibrillation threshold.[69] Smoking may accelerate atherosclerosis through effects on serum lipids; smokers tend to have higher levels of total cholesterol, LDL-C and triglycerides but lower HDL-C than nonsmokers.[72] Smoking increases the levels of inflammatory mediators (C-reactive protein and fibrinogen) and homocysteine, which may contribute to the development and progression of atherosclerosis.[73] Finally, smoking stimulates the release of neurotransmitters (e.g., epinephrine, norepinephrine), which increase myocardial workload and induce coronary vasoconstriction leading to ischemia, arrhythmias, and sudden death.[69–71]

P.J.'s hospital admission for a CABG procedure for coronary heart disease and angina, as well as previous procedures for peripheral vascular disease (angioplasty with stent placement) and cerebrovascular disease (bilateral carotid endarterectomy), are all conditions associated with chronic tobacco use. His elevated total cholesterol, LDL-C, and triglycerides and reduced HDL-C levels are consistent with smoking-induced dyslipidemia. Cigarette smoking in combination with P.J.'s other established cardiovascular risk factors (hypertension, dyslipidemia) have synergistically increased his risk for serious cardiovascular disease.[69] Fortunately, the effects of smoking on lipids, coagulation, myocardial workload and coronary blood flow appear to be reversible, and P.J.'s risk of developing further cardiovascular-related complications will markedly decrease if he is able to quit smoking.[41,74,75] The clinician should approach this hospitalization as an opportunity to motivate and assist P.J. with quitting smoking.

8. The cardiothoracic surgeon has strongly advised P.J. to quit smoking. P.J. is willing to quit tobacco completely, but he is worried because he has tried to quit smoking "hundreds of times" and has never been able to quit for longer than 1 week. He expresses a desire for a medication to assist him during this quit attempt. He has tried the nicotine gum and transdermal patch during three previous quit attempts. He didn't like the gum because it made his jaw sore and stuck to his fillings. He had temporary success with the nicotine patch but found it to be less flexible than the gum. For example, when he needed extra nicotine during stressful situations he couldn't apply a second patch. What treatment alternatives are reasonable for P.J.?

P.J. has failed treatment with the nicotine gum and transdermal patch. First-line treatment options that he has not tried include the nicotine lozenge (see Question 4), nicotine nasal spray, nicotine inhaler, and bupropion SR.

Nicotine Nasal Spray

The nicotine nasal spray is an aqueous solution of nicotine available in a metered-spray pump for administration to the nasal mucosa. Each actuation delivers a metered 50 μL spray containing 0.5 mg of nicotine. Nicotine in the nasal spray is more rapidly absorbed than other NRT formulations, with peak nicotine concentrations achieved within 5 to 15 minutes after administration (see Fig. 85-4). Use of the nicotine nasal spray improves long-term ($\geq$5 months) abstinence rates as evidenced by a recent meta-analysis of four studies, which concluded that the odds of abstinence constituted 2.27 with the nasal spray compared with placebo (95% CI, 1.61 to 3.20).[53]

Dosing

A dose of nicotine (1 mg) is administered as two sprays, one (0.5 mg spray) in *each* nostril. The recommended initial regimen is 1 to 2 doses every hour while awake for 6 to 8 weeks. This may be increased, as needed, to a maximum recommended dosage of five doses per hour or 40 mg/day. For best results, patients should be encouraged to use at least eight doses per day during the initial 6 to 8 weeks of therapy because less frequent administration may be less effective. After 6 to 8 weeks, the dose should be gradually decreased over an additional 4 to 6 weeks.

Patient Education

Before using the nasal spray for the first time, the nicotine nasal spray pump must be primed. This is done by actuating the device into a tissue until a fine spray is visible (about 6 to 8 times). When administering a dose, the patient should tilt the head back slightly and insert the tip of the bottle into the nostril as far as is comfortable. After actuation of the pump, the patient should not sniff, swallow, or inhale through the nose because this increases the irritant effects of the spray. Patients should wait 5 minutes before driving or operating heavy machinery (because of the increased likelihood of tearing, coughing, and sneezing).

Adverse Reactions

Side effects commonly reported with the nicotine nasal spray include nasal and throat irritation (hot peppery sensation), sneezing, coughing, watery eyes and rhinorrhea. In clinical trials, 94% of patients report moderate-severe nasal irritation during the first two days of therapy; 81% of patients still reported mild-moderate nasal irritation after three weeks of therapy. Nasal congestion and transient alterations in taste and smell have also been reported.[46] Despite the high incidence of local adverse effects, with regular use during the first week, most patients become tolerant to the irritant effects of the spray.[76]

Product Selection Considerations

The primary advantage in using the nicotine nasal spray is the ability to rapidly titrate therapy to manage withdrawal symptoms. However, because nicotine from the spray more rapidly penetrates the central nervous system, there may be higher likelihood of developing dependence during treatment. The nicotine nasal spray has a dependence potential intermediate between tobacco products and other NRT products. About 15% to 20% of patients continue to use the nicotine nasal spray for longer periods than recommended (6 to 12 months), and 5% use the spray at higher doses than recommended.[46] Individuals with chronic nasal disorders (e.g., rhinitis, polyps, sinusitis) or severe reactive airway disease should not use the nicotine nasal spray because of the irritant effects of the spray. Exacerbation of asthma has been reported after use of the nicotine nasal spray.[77]

Nicotine Inhaler

The nicotine inhaler consists of a two-piece plastic device designed to deliver nicotine contained in individual cartridges. Each foil-sealed cartridge contains a porous plug with 10 mg of nicotine and 1 mg of menthol. Menthol is added to reduce the irritant effect of nicotine. Sharp plastic spikes found on the interior of both mouthpiece components pierce the protective foil covering on the cartridge, allowing the release of 4 mg of nicotine vapor following inhalation.

Given that the usual pack-a-day smoker repeats the hand-to-mouth motion up to 200 times per day or 73,000 times each year, it is not surprising that many smokers find they miss the physical manipulation of the cigarette and associated behaviors that go with smoking. The nicotine inhaler was designed to provide nicotine replacement in a manner similar to smoking while at the same time addressing the sensory and ritualistic factors that are important to many smokers.[78]

As a patient puffs on the inhaler, the nicotine vapor is delivered to the mouth and throat, where it is absorbed through the mucosa. Only a small amount (<5% of a dose) of nicotine reaches the lower respiratory tract.[79] With an intensive inhalation regimen (80 puffs over 20 minutes), about 4 mg of nicotine is delivered, and of that, 2 mg is absorbed.[80] Peak plasma nicotine concentrations with the inhaler are achieved after 30 to 45 minutes of use and then slowly decline thereafter (see Fig. 85-4). The efficacy of the nicotine inhaler has been evaluated in four controlled trials. Using meta-analysis, the odds of cessation was 2.08 with the inhaler compared with placebo (95% CI, 1.43 to 3.04).[53]

Dosing

During the initial 3 to 6 weeks of treatment, the patient should use one cartridge every 1 to 2 hours while awake. This should be increased, as needed, to a maximum of 16 cartridges per day. In clinical trials, most successful quitters used an average of 6 to 16 cartridges per day. The manufacturer recommends that each cartridge be depleted of nicotine by frequent continuous puffing over 20 minutes. The recommended duration of treatment is 3 months, after which patients may be weaned from the inhaler by gradual reduction of the daily dose over the following 6 to 12 weeks.

Patient Education
Patients should be instructed to inhale shallowly (as if puffing a pipe) to minimize the likelihood of throat irritation. When used correctly, 100 shallow puffs from the inhaler mouthpiece over 20 minutes approximates 10 puffs from one cigarette over 5 minutes.[78] The release of delivery of nicotine from the inhaler is temperature dependent and significantly reduced at temperatures below 59°F.[78] In cold conditions, patients should store the inhaler and cartridges in a warm place (e.g., inside pocket).[46] Conversely, under warmer conditions more nicotine is released per puff. However, nicotine plasma concentrations achieved using the inhaler in hot climates at maximal doses will not exceed levels normally achieved with smoking.[78]

As with other forms of NRT that are absorbed across the buccal mucosa, the effectiveness of the nicotine inhaler may be reduced by acidic foods and beverages, such as coffee, juices, wine, or soft drinks. Therefore, patients should be instructed not to eat or drink for 15 minutes before or while using the inhaler.

Adverse Reactions
The most common side effects associated with the nicotine inhaler include mouth/throat irritation (40%) and cough (32%).[46] Most patients rated cough and mouth and throat irritation symptoms as mild, decreasing with continued use. Other less common side effects are rhinitis, dyspepsia, hiccups, and headache. Adverse reactions necessitating discontinuation of treatment occurred in fewer than 5% of patients using the inhaler.

Product Selection Considerations
Patients who express a preference for therapy that can be easily titrated to manage withdrawal symptoms or one that mimics the hand-to-mouth ritual of smoking may find the nicotine inhaler to be an appealing option. Patients with underlying bronchospastic conditions should use the nicotine inhaler with caution because the nicotine vapor may be irritating and provoke bronchospasm.

Bupropion SR

Bupropion SR is a non-nicotine agent that inhibits the neuronal reuptake of dopamine and norepinephrine in the central nervous system. Although the exact mechanism of action in tobacco cessation is unknown, modulation of dopamine and norepinephrine (neurotransmitters believed to be important in maintaining nicotine dependence) may be responsible for reducing the cravings for tobacco and symptoms of withdrawal in patients receiving bupropion SR.[46] Clinical trials involving more than 5,000 patients have confirmed the effectiveness of bupropion SR as an aid to tobacco cessation. A recent meta-analysis of 16 trials concluded that the odds of abstinence at

6 or more months was 1.97 bupropion SR compared with placebo (95% CI, 1.67 to 2.34).[81]

Dosing
Treatment with bupropion SR should be initiated while the patient is still smoking, because approximately 1 week of treatment is necessary to achieve steady-state blood levels. Patients should set a target quit date that falls within the first 2 weeks of treatment, generally in the second week. The starting dose of bupropion SR is one 150-mg tablet each morning for the first 3 days. If the initial dose is tolerated, the dosage should be increased on the fourth day to the recommended maximum dosage of 300 mg/day (150 mg twice a day). Therapy should be continued for 7 to 12 weeks after the quit date; however, some patients might benefit from extended treatment. Whether to continue treatment with bupropion SR for periods longer than 12 weeks for smoking cessation must be determined for individual patients. In selected patients, maintenance treatment up to 12 months may be appropriate.[82]

Precautions
Bupropion is contraindicated in patients with a history of seizure disorders. Although seizures were not reported in the smoking cessation clinical trials, the incidence of seizures with the sustained-release formulation (Wellbutrin) used in the treatment of depression was 0.1% in patients without a previous history of seizures.[83] For this reason, bupropion is contraindicated or used with extreme caution in patients with a history of factors known to increase the risk of seizures, including a current or prior diagnosis of bulimia or anorexia nervosa, central nervous system tumors, serious head trauma, concurrent use of with medications known to lower the seizure threshold and in patients undergoing abrupt discontinuation of alcohol or sedatives, including benzodiazepines and patients with severe hepatic cirrhosis. Animal studies suggest that seizures may be related to the peak plasma concentration of bupropion[84], and as a precautionary measure, the manufacturer recommends that patients space the doses at least 8 hours apart and limit the total daily dose to no more than 300 mg.

Adverse Reactions
Adverse effects associated with bupropion therapy include insomnia (35% to 40%) and dry mouth (10%); these usually lessen with continued use. Taking the second daily dose in the early evening but no sooner than 8 hours after the first dose might reduce insomnia. Less common side effects include headache, nausea, tremors, and rash.

Product Selection Considerations
Bupropion SR may be the drug of choice for patients who prefer to take oral medications. Because bupropion SR is simple to use (twice daily oral dosing), this agent may be preferable for patients with regimen compliance concerns (e.g., those unable to consistently use short-acting NRT formulations that require multiple daily doses). Bupropion SR may be particularly beneficial for use in patients with coexisting depression or in individuals with a history of depressive symptoms during a previous quit attempt. Finally, bupropion SR can be used safely in conjunction with NRT, and data suggest that this combination might be slightly more effective than monotherapy with either agent.[85] Disadvantages of bupropion

SR include a high prevalence of insomnia and the need to carefully screen patients to prevent the rare complication of seizures.

P.J. has tried the nicotine gum and transdermal patch during previous quit attempts. Because he was intolerant to the nicotine gum (it stuck to his dental work), this form of NRT is not appropriate. P.J.'s experience with the transdermal patch suggests he may benefit from a short-acting NRT formulation that allows for active administration and titration of drug as need to alleviate symptoms of withdrawal. Other first-line therapies include the nicotine nasal spray, inhaler, and lozenge or bupropion SR. P.J. should not use the nicotine nasal spray because he has allergic rhinitis and may be more susceptible to the irritant effects of the spray. In addition, some data suggest that the bioavailability of nicotine is reduced in patients with rhinitis or the common cold.[86] Furthermore, the safety and efficacy of the nasal spray in patients with chronic nasal disorders have not been adequately studied. Reasonable choices for P.J. therefore include either bupropion SR or the nicotine lozenge or inhaler. Any of these three options are reasonable, and the choice of therapy should be dictated by P.J.'s individual preference. Alternatively, it is reasonable to consider combination NRT (see Question 10) using the transdermal patch to provide consistent basal nicotine levels with supplemental use of the nicotine lozenge or inhaler as needed to alleviate symptoms of withdrawal.

Safety of NRT in Patients with Cardiovascular Disease

9. **P.J. would like to try the nicotine inhaler. Is NRT safe for use in patients with cardiovascular disease?**

Nicotine activates the sympathetic nervous system leading to an increase in heart rate, blood pressure, and myocardial contractility. Nicotine may also cause coronary artery vasoconstriction.[54] These known hemodynamic effects of nicotine have led to doubts about the safety of using NRT in patients with established cardiovascular disease, particularly those with serious arrhythmias, unstable angina, or MI.

Soon after the nicotine patch was approved, anecdotal case reports in the lay press linked NRT (patch and gum) with adverse cardiovascular events (i.e., arrhythmias, MI, stroke). Since that time, several randomized, controlled trials have evaluated the safety of NRT in patients with cardiovascular disease including angiographically documented coronary artery stenosis, MI, stable angina and previous coronary artery bypass surgery or angioplasty.[55,87,88] The results of these trials suggest no significant increase in the incidence of cardiovascular events or mortality among patients receiving the nicotine patch when compared with placebo. However, because these trials specifically excluded patients with unstable angina, serious arrhythmias, and recent MI, the Clinical Practice Guideline recommends that NRT be used with caution among patients in the immediate (within 2 weeks) post-MI period, those with serious arrhythmias and those with serious or worsening angina due to a lack of safety data in these higher risk populations.[46]

NRT in patients with cardiovascular disease has been the subject of numerous reviews, and it is widely believed by experts in the field that the risks of NRT in this patient population are small in relation to the risks of continued tobacco use.[53,54,69,89,90] Although the use of NRT may pose some theoretical risk in a patient like P.J., cigarette smoking is far more hazardous to his health. Cigarettes, unlike NRT, deliver numerous toxins that induce a hypercoagulable state, reduce the oxygen carrying capacity of the blood, and adversely affect serum lipids. The amount of nicotine that P.J. will receive using the inhaler in the recommended doses will not exceed the amount he previously obtained from his 1- to 2-pack-per-day smoking habit. The clinician should strongly encourage pharmacotherapy, including NRT, during P.J.'s current quit attempt. Because P.J. is only 10 pounds overweight, the additional risk imposed by a modest weight gain after smoking cessation likely will not be of clinical significance, compared with that of continued smoking.

Patients Who Fail First-Line Therapy

10. **J.B. is a 60-year-old man referred to the pulmonary clinic for further evaluation and management of his chronic obstructive pulmonary disease (COPD). He complains of decreased exercise tolerance and has noted increasing shortness of breath (SOB) with minimal exertion (e.g., while golfing or climbing stairs). He currently uses an albuterol inhaler (90 μg/puff), 2 puffs Q 4 hours regularly for SOB. His medical history is otherwise unremarkable except for osteoarthritis controlled with acetaminophen 1 g TID and recently diagnosed mild benign prostatic hypertrophy. He currently smokes 1 pack of cigarettes a day. J.B. expresses an interest in smoking cessation but admits to numerous failed attempts. He has tried NRT (transdermal patch, gum, and inhaler), bupropion SR, acupuncture, and hypnotherapy with only short-term success. On physical examination, coarse breath sounds that clear after coughing are noted. His chest x-ray results are normal. Spirometry reveals a forced expiratory volume in 1 second (FEV_1) of 2.8 L (72% of predicted) and a forced vital capacity (FVC) of 4.1 L (81% of predicted). His FEV_1/FVC ratio is 68%.**

J.B. is concerned about his worsening pulmonary function and is committed to making another effort to quit. What treatment alternatives exist for patients failing first-line agents?

Smoking and COPD

COPD is a condition characterized by progressive airflow obstruction (caused by chronic bronchitis or emphysema) that is not fully reversible. The obstruction of airflow is caused by an abnormal inflammatory response of pulmonary tissue to inhaled toxins.[91,92] Respiratory symptoms associated with COPD include chronic cough, shortness of breath, and wheezing. COPD is the fourth leading cause of death in the United States with an estimated 16.4 million people afflicted with the disease.[92] The World Health Organization predicts that by 2020, COPD will be the third most common cause of death in the world. The marked increase in cigarette smoking and pollution in developing countries is believed to be a major factor behind this trend.[93] For a more detailed discussion see Chapter 24, Chronic Obstructive Pulmonary Disease.

Tobacco smoking is the single most important risk factor for COPD, accounting for an estimated 80% to 90% of the risk of developing COPD.[91,92,94] Medications (e.g., bronchodilators and anti-inflammatory agents) used to treat the symptoms of COPD have not been shown to alter the disease progression.[91,92] Smoking cessation is the only known treatment that positively influences the course of COPD.[91-93] J.B.'s pulmonary function tests indicate he has stage II (moderate) COPD[91]; given his worsening pulmonary symptoms, it is imperative that he stop smoking as soon as possible. J.B. should be advised that medications for COPD offer only limited symptomatic relief; the most important component of his treatment is smoking cessation. The clinician should work with J.B. in designing an individualized treatment plan.

Second-Line Agents
CLONIDINE

Clonidine is a centrally acting α_2-adrenergic agonist that reduces sympathetic outflow from the central nervous system. Clonidine is approved for use as an antihypertensive agent, but it is also effective in reducing the autonomic symptoms of both opioid and alcohol withdrawal. Studies of clonidine for smoking cessation have been inconsistent, but a recent meta-analysis concluded that clonidine was an effective agent for tobacco cessation with a pooled odds ratio for success with clonidine compared with placebo of 1.89 (95% CI, 1.30 to 2.74).[95] Dosages for tobacco cessation have ranged from 0.15 to 0.75 mg/day orally and 0.1 to 0.3 mg/day per day transdermally. The Clinical Practice Guideline recommends a starting dose of 0.1 mg twice daily or 0.1 mg/day transdermally, increasing by 0.10 mg/day per week as tolerated for up to 10 weeks.[46] The high incidence of side effects including dry mouth, sedation, dizziness, and constipation relegate clonidine as a second-line agent reserved for individuals who have failed or are intolerant of first-line agents.

NORTRIPTYLINE

Nortriptyline, a tricyclic antidepressant has demonstrated efficacy for smoking cessation in five long-term (6 to 12 month) studies with a 2.8 pooled odds ratio (95% CI, 1.81 to 4.32) of quitting compared with placebo.[81] The regimen used for treating tobacco dependence is 25 mg/day, increasing gradually to a target dosage of 75 to 100 mg/day, for approximately 12 weeks.[46] Because the half-life of nortriptyline is prolonged (up to 56 hours), therapy should be initiated at least 10 days before the quit date to allow it to reach steady-state concentrations at the target dose. The side effects most commonly observed with nortriptyline include sedation, dry mouth, blurred vision, urinary retention, light-headedness, and tremor. This drug should be used with caution in patients with underlying cardiovascular conditions because of the risk of arrhythmias and postural hypotension. Both clonidine and nortriptyline are available in generic formulations, and these agents may serve as less expensive alternatives for patients unable to afford NRT and bupropion SR.

Combination NRT

In recalcitrant quitters who have experienced numerous failed attempts using monotherapy, combination therapy may be appropriate. Combination NRT involves the use of a long-acting formulation (patch) in combination with a short-acting formulation (gum, lozenge, inhaler, or nasal spray). The long-acting formulation, which delivers relatively constant levels of drug, is used to prevent the onset of severe withdrawal symptoms, whereas the short-acting formulation, which delivers nicotine at a faster rate, is used as needed to control withdrawal symptoms that may occur during potential relapse situations (e.g., after meals, when stressed, or around other smokers). Although several small studies have found that the nicotine patch in combination with the inhaler,[96] gum,[97-99] or nasal spray[100] may be more effective than monotherapy, because of the increased risk of nicotine toxicity and lack of long-term safety data, this approach should be reserved for patients unable to quit using single-agent NRT.[46] Furthermore, clinicians should be aware that NRT products are not approved for dual use, and the optimal combinations, dosages, and duration of therapy for this more aggressive approach are unknown. Studies to date have used the 16-hour (15-mg) nicotine patch in combination with lower-dose short-acting NRT formulations (e.g., 2 mg gum).

NRT and Bupropion SR

The combination of bupropion SR and NRT has been evaluated in one controlled trial. Patients were randomized to either combination therapy with bupropion SR (150 mg twice daily for nine weeks) and the nicotine patch (21 mg tapered over 8 weeks), monotherapy with one of the two agents, or placebo.[85] In contrast to previous trials, the nicotine patches alone were only minimally more effective than placebo (1-year abstinence rates of 16.4% versus 15.6%, respectively). One-year abstinence rates were higher with combination therapy (35.5%) than with bupropion SR alone (30.3%), but the difference was not statistically significant.

High-Dose Nicotine Replacement Therapy

Plasma levels of nicotine achieved with NRT are generally much lower than those observed during regular smoking.[76,101] Given this incomplete level of nicotine replacement, it is possible that standard doses of NRT may be insufficient for some individuals, and in particular for moderate-to-heavy smokers. Studies using transdermal nicotine in doses up to 44 to 63 mg/day suggest that high-dose NRT is safe[101-103]; however, trials evaluating the effectiveness of high-dose NRT have yielded conflicting results. Some suggest that higher doses of NRT may be more effective in heavy smokers,[102,104,105] whereas others have demonstrated slight, but not statistically significant, improvements in cessation rates.[106,107] Despite the small number of trials that have evaluated high-dose NRT therapy, the results appear promising, and this approach may be particularly useful for refractory or heavier smokers who have been unable to quit using single-agent therapy or conventional-dose NRT.

Treatment Selection

Given the severity of J.B.'s condition, it is important to initiate treatment as soon as possible, assuming that J.B. is committed to quitting. His treatment should consist of pharmacotherapy in conjunction with behavioral counseling and appropriate follow up.

PHARMACOTHERAPY

The clinician should work with J.B. in selecting appropriate pharmacotherapy. As noted above, appropriate options would include the various NRT formulations or bupropion SR. Because of J.B.'s BPH, an agent with anticholinergic side effects like nortriptyline is not optimal. Clonidine may be considered but the risk of sedation and hypotension may be a problem in J.B. Thus, the best option for J.B., considering that he has failed using monotherapy (the nicotine patch, gum, and inhaler used independently), would be dual pharmacotherapy, such as the concurrent use of two NRT formulations or use of one NRT formulation in conjunction with bupropion SR.

BEHAVIORAL COUNSELING

Behavioral counseling (see Fig. 85-3) should begin with an accurate assessment of J.B.'s tobacco use history—type(s) of tobacco currently used, brand, and amount used; duration of use and changes in levels of use recently; and a thorough characterization of past quit attempts. This would include the number of attempts, the date and duration of the most recent attempt, methods used previously (what worked, what didn't, and why?), and an assessment of the appropriateness of previous medication choices, dosing, compliance, and duration of treatment. The clinician also should talk with J.B. about his reasons and motivations for wanting to quit, his confidence in his ability to quit, triggers for tobacco use, and routines and situations in which he typically smokes. It also would be helpful to discuss reasons why J.B. relapsed to smoking during past quit attempts, because this would provide useful insight into difficulties he might again encounter during the upcoming quit attempt. Examples of coping strategies for triggers and other situations that might be associated with smoking are shown in Table 85-8. In addition, the clinician should discuss appropriate use of the pharmacotherapy agents, the importance of compliance with the prescribed regimen, and the need for continued follow-up counseling throughout the quit attempt.[46] The first follow-up contact should occur during the first week after quitting. A second contact is recommended in the first month. Additional contacts should be scheduled as needed. Counseling can occur face to face, by telephone, or by e-mail. If J.B. has a spouse or significant other, this person should be invited to accompany J.B. to the counseling sessions.

Complementary Therapies

11. J.B. is worried about "taking more drugs" and asks whether one of the natural herbal products might be better for him than "prescription drugs."

Although many herbal and homeopathic products are available to help people quit smoking, data that support their safety and effectiveness are lacking. Most herbal preparations for smoking cessation contain lobeline, an herbal alkaloid with partial nicotine agonist activity. Although direct-to-consumer advertisements suggest that lobeline-containing preparations are safe and effective, a recent meta-analysis found no evidence to support the role of lobeline as an effective aid for smoking cessation.[108] Likewise, hypnosis[109] and acupuncture[110] have not been found to be effective treatments for smoking cessation.[46] Furthermore, patients should be cautioned that herbal cigarettes are not safe alternatives because they result in the inhalation of other toxins present in smoke. J.B. should be advised that the efficacy of the herbal therapies are not well established and use of these agents cannot be recommended at this time.

Drug Interactions With Smoking

12. M.K. is a new patient presenting to the pharmacy with a new prescription for Ortho Tri-Cyclen (norgestimate/ethinyl estradiol). The new patient history form completed by M.K. reveals that she is 32 years old, weighs 65 kg, and is 70 inches tall. She takes no prescription medications but occasionally uses loratadine 10 mg PRN for allergies and ibuprofen 400 mg PRN for dysmenorrhea. She has no significant medical history. Her father has hypertension and suffered a MI last year. Her mother has type 2 diabetes mellitus and dyslipidemia. Her social history is significant for tobacco use (1 PPD for 10 years); alcohol (1 glass of wine per night), and caffeine (5 to 6 cups of coffee daily). Are there any potential interactions with M.K.'s new prescription?

Smoking and Combined Oral Contraceptives

One of the most important, but often unrecognized, precautions to consider with oral contraceptive use is the potential interaction between tobacco smoke and estrogens in combination oral contraceptives. Estrogens are known to promote coagulation by altering clotting factor levels and increasing platelet aggregation. As described in Question 7, substances present in tobacco smoke, including oxidant gases and other products of combustion, induce a hypercoagulable state increasing the risk of acute cardiovascular events. Exposure to these factors (smoking and high levels of estrogen) in combination greatly increases the risk of thromboembolic and thrombotic disorders. Considerable epidemiologic evidence indicates that cigarette smoking substantially increases the risk of adverse cardiovascular events including stroke, MI, and thromboembolism in women who use oral contraceptive agents.[111] This risk is age related with an absolute risk of death from cardiovascular disease in oral contraceptive users who smoke—3.3 per 100,000 women aged 15 to 34 years compared with 29.4 per 100,000 women aged 35 to 44 years. To put this in perspective, the corresponding risk of death from cardiovascular disease in *nonsmoking* women who use oral contraceptives is much lower with a death rate of 0.65 per 100,000 women aged 15 to 34 years and 6.21 per 100,000 women aged 35 to 44 years.[112] Because of the increase risk of adverse cardiovascular events, experts generally believe that oral contraceptive use is contraindicated in women who are over 35 years of age *and* heavy smokers (15 or more cigarettes per day).[113,114] M.K. is 32 years of age and despite her heavy smoking status (20 cigarettes per day), oral contraceptive use is not contraindicated at this time. However, the clinician should strongly advise M.K. to quit smoking and assess her readiness to do so. M.K. should be informed that if she continues to smoke while using oral contraceptives, her risk of developing a blood clot, stroke, or heart attack will continue to increase over time. Her family history (father with recent MI and mother with diabetes and hyperlipidemia) suggests she may be genetically predisposed to cardiovascular disease and thus efforts to minimize preventable risk factors should be encouraged to reduce the likelihood that she will develop cardiovascular-related complications in the future.

Light Cigarettes

13. M.K. indicates she recently switched to "light" cigarettes and wonders if these are less likely to cause an interaction.

Cigarettes marketed as "light" and "ultra-light" are tobacco products designed to deliver reduced levels of tar, nicotine, and carbon monoxide. Contrary to popular belief, the tobacco in these products does not contain significantly reduced amounts of nicotine per cigarette. Indeed, in a study analyzing 32 of the top-selling American cigarettes (including regular, light, and ultra-light brands), the total nicotine content per cigarette was comparable among all varieties analyzed. For example, a Marlboro full-flavor cigarette contains only slightly more nicotine (10.9 mg per cigarette) than a Marlboro Light (10.6 mg per cigarette).[115] Light or ultra-light cigarettes deliver lower levels of tar, nicotine, and carbon monoxide through the incorporation of tiny ventilation holes in the filter that effectively "reduce" the yields as measured by a standardized testing method developed by the Federal Trade Commission (FTC).

Using the FTC method, tar, nicotine, and carbon monoxide levels are measured by a smoking machine calibrated to inhale 35 mL of smoke over 2 seconds every 60 seconds until the cigarette is smoked to a 23-mm (unfiltered brands) or 26-mm (filtered brands) butt length.[116] When light or ultra-light cigarettes are tested using the FTC method, room air is drawn through the perforations in the filter during the inhalation phase, diluting the amount of smoke in each puff. The less concentrated smoke yields significantly lower amounts of tar, nicotine, and carbon monoxide when measured by the smoking machine. For example, using the FTC method, the tar, nicotine, and carbon monoxide yields for Marlboro full flavor are 16 mg, 1.1 mg, and 14 mg per cigarette, respectively. The corresponding tar, nicotine, and carbon monoxide yields for Marlboro Light are 10 mg, 0.8 mg, and 11 mg per cigarette, respectively.[115]

However, smokers do not smoke cigarettes in the same manner that the machine does. Smokers can easily obstruct the filter ventilation holes with their lips or fingers, effectively delivering more concentrated smoke containing increased amounts of tar, nicotine and carbon monoxide. Depending on the smoking technique, the actual yield of tar, nicotine, and carbon monoxide might be similar or greater than that expected based on the reported machine test yields. As a result, the FTC method cannot be used to predict the tar, nicotine, and carbon monoxide exposure from a given cigarette for an individual under normal smoking conditions. This is due primarily to compensation—the tendency of smokers of lower rated cigarettes to alter their smoking technique to self-titrate their nicotine levels. Unfortunately, many smokers perceive light and ultra-light cigarettes to be safer than regular/full flavor cigarettes.[117] Rather than decreasing their nicotine intake, smokers who switch to light or ultra-light cigarettes often change their smoking behavior (obstruct filter vents, inhale deeper and/or longer) to attain levels of nicotine comparable to those obtained when smoking regular cigarettes.

After analysis of epidemiologic studies that failed to demonstrate a reduction in the risk of tobacco-related disease among reduced-yield cigarette smokers, the National Cancer Institute concluded that these products are not safe. The report further stated that, from a public health perspective, these products may pose an even greater risk if smokers are given the false impression that switching to light cigarettes is an acceptable alternative to smoking cessation.[116] M.K. should be informed that smoking light cigarettes does not reduce her risk for tobacco-related diseases and complications.

14. M.K. is not considering quitting smoking at this time and does not wish to discontinue her oral contraceptives because she is sexually active and needs a reliable form of birth control. She wonders if the new low-dose birth control pills are safer for smokers.

Combined oral contraceptives available in the United States contain estrogen in doses ranging from 20 to 50 μg of ethinyl estradiol. The results of in vitro studies have shown that oral contraceptives containing ≥50 μg of ethinyl estradiol induce greater procoagulatory effects than do preparations containing either 30 μg or 35 μg of ethinyl estradiol; formulations containing 20 μg of ethinyl estradiol appear to have little or no adverse effects on coagulation.[118] Early epidemiologic reports linking oral contraceptive use and severe cardiovascular events were largely observed in women using oral contraceptives containing ≥50 mg of ethinyl estradiol.[119] Since that time, manufacturers have reduced the dose of estrogen in oral contraceptives such that the majority of preparations available in the United States contain either 30 μg or 35 μg of ethinyl estradiol.[120]

In 2001, the U.S. Surgeon General stated that lower dose oral contraceptives may be associated with a reduced risk for coronary heart disease (CHD), compared with higher-dose formulations. Despite this conclusion, the report cautioned that heavy smokers who use oral contraceptives still have a greatly elevated risk for CHD.[121] Consistent with the Surgeon General's cautionary statement, a recent study found that women who smoked ≥25 cigarettes per day had a 20-fold higher risk of MI than nonsmoking women who used oral contraceptives. Interestingly, the elevated risk was independent of the dose of estrogen in the oral contraceptive; women using preparations containing ≥50 μg of estrogen were no more likely to experience a MI than were women using preparations containing <50 μg of estrogen. There was only one case involving the use of a preparation containing 20 μg of estrogen, and thus the safety of this dose could not be evaluated.[122]

M.K.'s prescribed oral contraceptive agent (Ortho Tri-Cyclen) is a triphasic formulation containing 35 μg of ethinyl estradiol in combination with weekly increasing doses of norgestimate (0.18 mg, 0.215 mg and 0.25 mg) throughout each monthly cycle. Although some clinicians recommend the use of low-dose (20 μg) estrogen preparations in smokers, the available evidence suggests that the prescribed regimen poses no additional risk in M.K. However, if M.K. increases her smoking levels to ≥25 cigarettes per day, some data suggest that her risk for a MI is increased.[122] The clinician should inform M.K. that currently there are no studies demonstrating a reduced risk of adverse cardiovascular events in smokers using oral contraceptives containing low doses (e.g. 20 μg) of estrogen. In the absence of data, only smoking cessation can be advocated to definitively reduce the risk of stroke, MI, and thromboembolism in women who use combined oral contraceptives.

Behavioral Counseling

Although M.K. is not considering quitting at this time, it is appropriate for the clinician to apply the 5 R's (see Table 85-7) to promote motivation to quit. This counseling should be relevant to M.K.'s situation and should highlight the risks of continued tobacco use, such as her elevated risk for thromboembolic and thrombotic disorders (associated with continued use of oral contraceptives). M.K. should be asked to think about the *rewards* of quitting and any potential *roadblocks* to quitting. At subsequent encounters the clinician should sensitively assess M.K.'s tobacco use status and motivation to quit and offer assistance with quitting when M.K. is ready. If M.K. decides to quit, it would be important to reassess her caffeine intake, because caffeine levels have been reported to increase by 56% in patients who quit smoking.[34]

FORMS OF TOBACCO
Spit Tobacco
Classification

15. T.M. is a 29-year-old man who presents to the clinic for evaluation of a painless "white patch" along his lower left gumline, which he noted several weeks ago while flossing his teeth. His social history is significant for the use of spit tobacco (consumes one can of Copenhagen moist snuff every 2 to 3 days), cigarettes (1 pack per week), and alcohol (one to two beers daily). T.M. reports he has "dipped" for the past 10 years but only recently started smoking "socially" in the evenings when out with friends. He is in otherwise excellent health and takes no medications. What is spit tobacco and how does it differ from cigarettes?

Spit tobacco, also known as smokeless tobacco, is a term used to describe forms of tobacco that are not burned and inhaled but rather held in the mouth to allow absorption of nicotine across the oral (buccal) mucosa. Spit tobacco products in the United States are broadly categorized as either chewing tobacco or snuff. Chewing tobacco, which is generally available in loose-leaf, plug, and twist formulations, is chewed or held in the cheek or lower lip. Snuff, which is commonly available as loose particles or sachets resembling mini-tea bags, has a much finer consistency and is generally held in the mouth and not chewed. Most snuff formulations in the United States are classified as moist snuff, and users place a small amount (a "pinch") between the cheek and gum (also known as dipping) and suck on the moist mass of tobacco for 30 minutes or longer. Dry snuff, which is generally sniffed or inhaled through the nostrils, is less commonly used.[123]

Epidemiology
According to the U.S. Department of Health and Human Services in 2002, an estimated 7.8 million Americans aged 12 years and older (3.3%) had used spit tobacco in the past month. Males (6.4%) were more likely than females (0.4%) to be current users.[124] The prevalence of spit tobacco use is highest among individuals between the ages of 18 and 25 and is substantially higher among American Indians, Alaskan Natives, residents of the southern United States, and persons living in in rural areas.[40,125]

Pharmacokinetics
Absorption of nicotine from chewing tobacco and snuff is pH-dependent, with more nicotine absorbed across the buccal mucosa under alkaline conditions. Spit tobacco manufacturers manipulate the nicotine content and pH of their products by adding alkaline buffering agents and changing the tobacco-processing methods to control the delivery of nicotine. For example, a "starter" formulation, such as Skoal Bandits has a lower nicotine content and is more acidic (pH = 5.4) to increase tolerability. Once dependence has been established, users generally advance to more alkaline, higher nicotine content products such as Skoal Fine Cut (pH = 7.6) and Copenhagen (pH = 8.6), which are capable of delivering higher levels of nicotine.[40] As depicted in Figure 85-4, the nicotine from spit tobacco is absorbed less rapidly than from cigarette smoke, and the peak levels generally occur after 20 to 30 minutes. Plasma levels of nicotine decline slowly even after removal of tobacco from the mouth because of the gradual release of nicotine from mucous membranes and the possible intestinal absorption of nicotine from swallowed tobacco.[126] Although the rate of nicotine absorption from cigarettes exceeds that from spit tobacco, the extent of absorption does not. In fact, regular spit tobacco users experience comparable exposure to nicotine and are as likely to develop physical dependence as are regular smokers.[40]

Health Consequences of Spit Tobacco Use

16. On examination, a superficial whitish lesion with moderate wrinkling of the tissue adjacent to the mandibular left canine and premolars is noted in T.M. In addition, there is localized gingival recession and moderate brown tobacco staining of the enamel surfaces. T.M. reports that he routinely places snuff between his lower left cheek and gum. He asks if the lesion might be cancerous and wonders if it's related to his spit tobacco habit. What are the health consequences of spit tobacco use?

Users of spit tobacco often believe this is a safe alternative to smoking cigarettes, because it is not inhaled. This is not true. All forms of tobacco are harmful. In addition to cosmetic concerns (e.g., halitosis, staining of teeth), the use of spit tobacco is associated with serious health effects,[40] including the following.

SOFT TISSUE ALTERATIONS/LEUKOPLAKIA
Spit tobacco users commonly develop an oral soft tissue condition called leukoplakia or "snuff dipper's lesion." These white-colored patches or plaques, which are observed in approximately 15% of chewing tobacco users and 60% of snuff users, generally develop at mucosal sites in contact with the tobacco.[127] Of concern is the fact that 3% to 6% of these lesions may transform into squamous cell carcinomas.[40] Fortunately, when users quit, the oral leukoplakia generally resolves within 6 weeks.[128]

PERIODONTAL EFFECTS
In addition to the soft tissue alterations noted above, regular users of spit tobacco are at significant risk for the development of gingival recession (complete or partial loss of the tissue covering the root of the tooth), caries and tooth abrasion. The loss of gingival tissue, observed in up to 27% of spit tobacco users, generally occurs at sites constantly exposed to tobacco.[127] The high sugar content found in many spit tobacco products in contact with exposed tooth root tissue might account for the increased incidence of dental caries in spit tobacco users.[40,127]

CANCER
The most serious consequence of spit tobacco use is an increased risk for oral and pharyngeal cancers. Spit tobacco contains high concentrations of numerous carcinogens, including nitrosamines, polycyclic aromatic hydrocarbons, and

radioactive polonium-210, which are in direct contact with mucosal tissues for prolonged periods.[123] The risk appears to be dose related with heavy, long-time users being more likely to develop oral cancer compared with nonusers.[40]

T.M. is presenting with an oral mucosal lesion commonly observed in spit tobacco users. His longstanding history of snuff use and characteristic white, wrinkled lesion appearing at a site where he habitually places snuff are consistent with leukoplakia. T.M. should be informed that the lesion is most likely caused by his chronic snuff use and he should be strongly advised to quit. With continued exposure to carcinogens present in spit tobacco, there is an increased risk that the leukoplakia will undergo malignant transformation. The presence of an identifiable tobacco-induced oral lesion may serve as a powerful motivator for a quit attempt. If he is able to quit snuff use, the gum tissue will likely normalize over a period of 6 weeks. If the lesion persists, he should be referred for a biopsy and further diagnostic evaluation. Finally, T.M. already has evidence of localized gingival recession, which increases his risk for serious periodontal disease and further dental-related complications. These periodontal problems will progress as long as he continues to use spit tobacco.

Treatment

17. T.M. relates that his new girlfriend is a "militant" non-smoker who is likely to stop seeing him if he doesn't quit. He is aware that tobacco is "bad for him" and is worried about developing oral cancer. He believes it will not be difficult to quit smoking because he smokes so little. He is more worried about stopping the use of snuff and wants to know if there are any medications to help him quit.

Despite the known health risks and high prevalence of spit tobacco use, there are limited evidence-based recommendations to guide clinicians in the treatment use spit tobacco use.[129] Ebbert and colleagues[125] recently reviewed the results of 14 randomized, controlled trials evaluating behavioral counseling and pharmacotherapy interventions for spit tobacco use; their findings are summarized below.

BEHAVIORAL THERAPY

Behavioral interventions including the use of self-help materials (written manuals, pamphlets, videotapes), brief (15- to 20-minute) counseling sessions, telephone support, oral examination with feedback, computerized gradual reduction of tobacco and use of non–tobacco oral substitutes (herbal and mint snuff, chewing gum) have been shown to significantly increase long-term (≥6 month) cessation rates (OR 1.7; 95% CI, 1.1 to 2.9) compared with control interventions. Interventions that incorporate an oral exam with clinician-delivered feedback to participants regarding oral lesions also have been shown to be associated with a greater odds of quitting (OR 2.9; 95% CI, 1.9 to 4.5).[125]

NICOTINE REPLACEMENT THERAPY

To date, the gum and transdermal patch are the only NRT formulations that have been evaluated in randomized controlled trials. Studies using the 15-mg nicotine patch for 6 weeks or the 21-mg patch with a tapering schedule over 10 weeks have been associated with modest increases in cessation rates (40.8%) at 6 months compared with placebo

(34.8%) [OR 1.3; 95% CI, 1.0 to 1.7].[125] The 2-mg gum formulation administered for 6 to 8 weeks appears to be less effective (31.4%) at 6 months compared with placebo (28.6%) [OR 1.1; 95% CI, 0.7 to 1.9].[125] Overall, the data suggest NRT might be effective in the treatment of spit tobacco use, but further studies are necessary to determine the optimal dose and duration of therapy.

BUPROPION SR

Bupropion SR (150 mg twice daily) has been evaluated in two small randomized, controlled trials. Following either a 7- or 12-week treatment course, subjects randomized to bupropion SR therapy were more likely to remain abstinent at 12 weeks (42.0%) than those receiving placebo (26.1%) [OR 2.1; 95% CI, 1.0 to 4.2).[125]

The Clinical Practice Guideline recommends that spit tobacco users receive the same interventions recommended for smokers.[46] Based on the available evidence, it appears that behavioral interventions are effective in the treatment of spit tobacco use. Limited data suggest that pharmacotherapy with bupropion SR or NRT is also effective. However, more research is necessary to determine whether combination therapy or higher dosages of NRT will provide improved cessation rates in spit tobacco users. T.M. should be provided with behavioral counseling tailored to his stage of readiness to quit—if he is ready to quit in the next 30 days, a treatment plan should be devised. If he is not ready to quit in the next 30 days, motivational counseling should be applied using the 5 R's (see Table 85-7). Because oral examination with patient feedback appears to increase abstinence rates, T.M. should be referred to a dental provider for additional monitoring and follow-up. T.M. has specifically asked about the use of pharmacotherapy as a cessation aid, and bupropion SR and NRT should be considered. T.M. should also be informed that a non–tobacco oral substitute (herbal and mint snuff) in combination with behavioral counseling is also effective.[125]

Cigars

18. R.N., a 35-year-old man who currently smokes 2 packs of cigarettes per day would like to know whether cutting down to 1 to 2 cigars/day is a safe alternative to cigarette smoking.

Cigars are conventionally defined as "*any roll of tobacco wrapped in leaf tobacco or in any substance containing tobacco.*"[130] The types of cigars available in the United States vary and include *little* cigars (shaped like cigarettes and weighing <1.3 g; *small* cigars or cigarillos (some with a plastic mouthpiece and weighing between 1.2 and 2.5 g); *regular* cigars (usually rolled to a tip on one end and banded; generally weighing between 5 and 17 g); and premium cigars (expensive, generally hand rolled and weighing >22 g).[131,132] Cigar tobacco is generally air cured and produces smoke with a more alkaline pH, which allows for buccal absorption of nicotine.

Cigar consumption has significantly increased over the past decade,[132] with 4.5% of men and 0.2% of women in the United States reporting they are current cigar smokers.[133] Some data suggest that the increased consumption is due to a greater prevalence of occasional cigar smoking by previous nonsmokers, particularly among those of higher socioeconomic status.[132] This trend is likely the result of enhanced marketing and promotional efforts by the tobacco industry; cigar advertisements often depict celebrities or athletes associating cigar smoking with glamour, affluence, and success. Increasing numbers of former cigarette smokers switching to cigars and experimentation among adolescents with cigar smoking may also play a role.[132]

Exactly how much nicotine an individual might obtain from a single cigar is difficult to determine or generalize, because cigar weight and nicotine content vary widely from brand to brand and from cigar to cigar. Most cigars range in weight from about 1 to 22 g; a typical cigarette weighs less than 1 g. The nicotine content of 10 commercially available cigars studied in 1996 ranged from 10 to 444 mg.[134] In comparison, standard U.S. cigarettes have a relatively narrow total nicotine content, ranging between 7.2 and 13.4 mg of nicotine per cigarette.[115] Relating these data, Henningfield and colleagues[134] concluded that it is possible for one large cigar to contain as much tobacco as an entire pack of cigarettes and deliver enough nicotine to establish and maintain dependence.

The adverse health effects of cigar smoking have been well described and include an increased risk of cancer of the lung, oral cavity, larynx, esophagus and pancreas. In addition, cigar smokers who inhale deeply are at increased risk for developing cardiovascular disease and COPD.[132] Cigarette smokers who switch to smoking only cigars decrease their risk of developing lung cancer, but their risk is markedly higher than if they were to quit smoking altogether.[132]

R.N. should be counseled that switching from cigarette smoking to low-level daily cigar smoking will not reduce his risk for developing a tobacco-related disease. The amount of nicotine delivered by 1 to 2 cigars per day is capable of sustaining his dependence on nicotine. In addition, former cigarette smokers are more likely to inhale deeply, which further increases the risk of cancer and cardiovascular and pulmonary disease. The clinician should strongly advise R.N. to quit smoking cigarettes and that switching to cigars is not a safe alternative.

Bidis and Clove Cigarettes

19. K.K. is a 16-year-old male who has been suspended from school after his third offense for smoking on campus. KK began experimenting with bidis and kreteks a few years ago and then started smoking cigarettes "socially" with his friends. For the past year he has been smoking about a half-pack of cigarettes per day. What are bidis and kreteks?

Bidis

Bidis are small, hand-rolled cigarettes imported to the U.S. primarily from India and other Southeast Asian countries. They consist of finely ground tobacco wrapped in a brown tendu or temburni leaf.[135] Bidis—similar in appearance to marijuana cigarettes—are readily available in tobacco shops and ethnic stores and via internet retailers in a variety of flavors (e.g., chocolate, vanilla, strawberry, cherry, mango, orange) and are becoming increasingly popular among younger smokers. In a 1999 survey of 642 urban adolescents in Massachusetts, 40% had smoked bidis at least once in the past, and 16% were current (e.g., had smoked more than one bidi in the last 30 days) bidis smokers. Among the reasons cited by teens for smoking bidis was the perception that bidis were better

tasting, less expensive, safer, and easier to purchase than traditional cigarettes.[135]

Although bidis contain less tobacco than standard cigarettes, studies have shown they produce substantial amounts of tar, nicotine, and carbon monoxide.[135-138] A study using standardized smoking machine testing methods found that bidis deliver three times the amount of carbon monoxide and nicotine and nearly five times the amount of tar found in standard cigarettes.[138] Because of the low combustibility of the tendu leaf wrapper, bidis must be puffed constantly to remain lit. As a result, bidi smokers inhale more frequently and more deeply, thereby markedly increasing the delivery of tar and other toxins.[135] Most bidis do not have a traditional filter tip, which further increases exposure to toxic constituents present in smoke. However, a filter does not confer added safety, as evidenced by a recent study that found that bidi cigarettes containing a filter actually delivered higher levels of tar, nicotine, and carbon monoxide when compared with unfiltered bidi brands. In this study, the filtered bidi cigarettes contained a small wad of cotton instead of the usual cellulose acetate filter found in American cigarettes. The investigators speculated that the inefficient cotton filter and the slightly larger size of the filtered bidi brands led to the observed higher yields of inhaled toxins.[137]

Although by law all packages of bidis sold in the United States must contain the Surgeon General warning about the hazards of smoking, spot checks in various retail outlets have shown that many of these products are not labeled with health warnings.[139] The absence of federally mandated warning labels may lead to the false impression that these products are safer than other forms of tobacco. However, studies in India have shown that bidi smokers have a comparable or greater risk of developing tobacco-related respiratory, cardiovascular, and neoplastic disease than cigarette smokers.[140]

Clove Cigarettes

Clove cigarettes or "kreteks" are cigarettes imported from Indonesia containing a mixture of approximately 60% to 70% tobacco and 30% to 40% minced cloves.[141] In Indonesia, where these are widely consumed, smokers typically do not inhale. In contrast, the typical clove cigarette smoker in the United States (age 17 to 30 years) inhales deeply and retains the smoke in the lungs, subsequently increasing the risk for potentially harmful effects. In smoking machine tests, clove cigarettes deliver twice as much nicotine, tar, and carbon monoxide as standard cigarettes.[141]

In addition to the hazards associated with smoking, clove cigarette use has been implicated in causing rare cases of hemorrhagic pulmonary edema, pneumonia, bronchitis, and hemoptysis.[141-143] It has been speculated that eugenol, a compound possessing local anesthetic properties and present in large quantities in clove cigarette smoke, might be toxic to pulmonary tissue. The anesthetic effects of eugenol also might place users at an increased risk of pulmonary aspiration resulting from an impaired gag reflex.[143]

There is concern among experts that use of alternate forms of tobacco (clove cigarettes, bidis) might serve as a "gateway" to regular cigarette smoking. That is, young smokers become dependent on the nicotine in candy-flavored cigarettes, later transferring their dependence to more conventional tobacco formulations such as cigarettes or spit tobacco.[144] K.K. began experimenting with bidis and clove cigarettes before he smoked cigarettes socially. It's difficult to know whether K.K.'s previous use of bidis and clove cigarettes led to regular cigarette smoking, but these products are capable of inducing and sustaining nicotine dependence.

Treatment of Adolescent Tobacco Use

20. Is K.K. an appropriate candidate for smoking cessation medications?

Nearly three fourths of ever-daily adolescent smokers have tried to quit, with females (77.6%) being more likely to try to quit than males (68.7%), and white adolescents (76.0%) being more likely than Hispanic adolescents (61.9%).[145] Despite a high prevalence of quit attempts, relapse rates are high among adolescent ex-smokers.[146] An estimated 50% of adolescent smokers have tried unsuccessfully to quit smoking by the age of 17.[147,148] Although adolescent smoking is a public health issue of much importance, there is a paucity of literature describing the effectiveness of methods for cessation in this population.[149,150]

Clinician-delivered smoking cessation interventions have a positive impact in adults and should be applied with adolescents to promote and sustain abstinence.[46] Although pharmacologic agents for cessation have been shown to be safe and effective in adults, less is known about their use in adolescents. As such, clinicians are encouraged use discretion when considering use of pharmacotherapy with patients less than 18 years of age. The Clinical Practice Guideline[46] suggests that because there is no evidence that bupropion SR or NRT is harmful for children or adolescents, their use may be considered when there is strong evidence of tobacco dependence and the adolescent is committed to quitting.

REFERENCES

1. Ezzati M, Lopez AD. Estimates of global mortality attributable to smoking in 2000. Lancet 2003; 362:847.
2. Peto R, Lopez A. Future worldwide health effects of current smoking patterns. In: Koop CE, Pearson CE, Schwartz MR, eds. Critical Issues in Global Health. San Francisco, CA: Jossey-Bass, 2001.
3. U.S. Department of Health and Human Services. The Health Consequences of Smoking: Nicotine Addiction. A Report of the Surgeon General. Washington DC: Government Printing Office, DHHS Publication No. (PHS) 88-8406, 1988.
4. Thun MJ et al. Tobacco use and cancer: an epidemiologic perspective for geneticists. Oncogene 2002;21:7307.
5. CDC. Annual smoking-attributable mortality, years of potential life lost, and economic costs—United States, 1995-1999. MMWR Morb Mortal Wkly Rep 2002;51:300.
6. National Cancer Institute. Health Effects of Exposure to Environmental Tobacco Smoke: The Report of the California Environmental Protection Agency. Smoking and Tobacco Control Monograph No. 10. Bethesda, MD: U.S. Department of Health and Human Services, National Institutes of Health, National Cancer Institute, NIH Publication No. 99-4645, 1999.
7. Leshner AI. Drug abuse and addiction are biomedical problems. Hosp Pract 1997:2.
8. Leshner AI. Science-based views of drug addiction and its treatment. JAMA 1999;282:1314.
9. U.S. Department of Health and Human Services. Preventing Tobacco Use among Young People: A Report of the Surgeon General. Atlanta, GA: U.S. Department of Health and Human Services, Public Health Service, Centers for Disease Control and Prevention, National Center for Chronic Disease Prevention and Health Promotion, Office on Smoking and Health, 1994.
10. Gilpin EA et al. Smoking initiation rates in adults and minors: United States, 1944-1988. Am J Epidemiol 1994;140:535.
11. U.S. Department of Health and Human Services. Healthy People 2010. Washington, D.C.: U.S. Department of Health and Human Services. 2000.
12. CDC. Trends in cigarette smoking among high school students—United States, 1991-2001. MMWR Morb Mortal Wkly Rep 2002;51:409.
13. Johnston LD et al. The Monitoring of the Future National Survey Results on Adolescent Drug Use: Overview of Key Findings, 2002. Bethesda, MD: National Institutes of Health, National Institute on Drug Abuse, NIH Publication No. 03-5374, 2003.
14. CDC. Cigarette smoking among adults—United States, 2001. MMWR Morb Mortal Wkly Rep 2003;52:953.
15. CDC. State-specific prevalence of current cigarette smoking among adults—United States, 2002. MMWR Morb Mortal Wkly Rep 2004;52:1277.
16. Benowitz NL. Cigarette smoking and nicotine addiction. Med Clin North Am 1992;76:415.
17. Sullivan PF, Kendler KS. The genetic epidemiology of smoking. Nicotine Tob Res 1999;1(Suppl 2): S51.
18. Li MD et al. A meta-analysis of estimated genetic and environmental effects on smoking behavior in male and female adult twins. Addiction 2003; 98:23.
19. Benowitz NL. Clinical pharmacology of inhaled drugs of abuse: Implications in understanding nicotine dependence. In: Chiang CN HR, ed. Research Findings on Smoking of Abused Substances, NIDA Research Monograph 99. Rockville, MD, 1990.
20. Benowitz NL. Nicotine addiction. Prim Care 1999;26:611.
21. Taylor P. Agents acting at the neuromuscular junction and autonomic ganglia. In: Hardman JG LL, ed. Goodman and Gilman's The Pharmacological Basis of Therapeutics. 10th Ed. New York: McGraw Hill, 2001.
22. Kessler DA. The control and manipulation of nicotine in cigarettes. Tob Control 1994;3:362.
23. Benowitz NL. The biology of nicotine dependence: from the 1988 Surgeon General's Report to the present and into the future. Nicotine Tob Res 1999;1(Suppl 2):S159.
24. Perry DC et al. Increased nicotinic receptors in brains from smokers: membrane binding and autoradiography studies. J Pharmacol Exp Ther 1999; 289:1545.
25. Hughes JR et al. Symptoms of tobacco withdrawal. A replication and extension. Arch Gen Psychiatry 1991;48:52.
26. Benowitz NL et al. Cotinine disposition and effects. Clin Pharmacol Ther 1983;34:604.
27. American Psychiatric Association. Diagnostic and Statistical Manual of Mental Disorders (DSM IV) (American Psychiatric Association. Diagnostic and Statistical Manual of Mental Disorders, Fourth edition (DSM-IV). Washington, DC, 2000.
28. Heatherton TF et al. The Fagerstrom Test for Nicotine Dependence: a revision of the Fagerstrom Tolerance Questionnaire. Br J Addict 1991;86:1119.
29. Prokhorov AV et al. Adolescent nicotine dependence measured by the modified Fagerström Tolerance Questionnaire at two time points. J Child Adol Subst Use 1998;7:36.
30. Severson HH, Hatsukami D. Smokeless tobacco cessation. Prim Care 1999;26:529.
31. Benowitz NL, Jacob P. Metabolism of nicotine to cotinine studied by a dual stable isotope method. Clin Pharmacol Ther 1994;56:483.
32. Benowitz NL, Jacob P. Daily intake of nicotine during cigarette smoking. Clin Pharmacol Ther 1984;35:499.
33. Schein JR. Cigarette smoking and clinically significant drug interactions. Ann Pharmacother 1995; 29:1139.
34. Zevin S, Benowitz NL. Drug interactions with tobacco smoking. An update. Clin Pharmacokinet 1999;36:425.
35. Rx for Change: Clinician-Assisted Tobacco Cessation. San Francisco, CA: The Regents of the University of California, University of Southern California, and Western University of Health Sciences, 1999-2003.
36. CDC. Cigarette smoking-attributable morbidity— United States, 2000. MMWR Morb Mortal Wkly Rep 2003;52:842.
37. American Cancer Society. Cancer Facts and Figures 2003. Available at: http://www.cancer.org/docroot/STT/content/STT_1x_Cancer_Facts__Figures_2003.asp. Accessed December 2, 2003.
38. Otsuka R et al. Acute effects of passive smoking on the coronary circulation in healthy young adults. JAMA 2001;286:436.
39. Aligne CA et al. Association of pediatric dental caries with passive smoking. JAMA 2003;289:1258.
40. Hatsukami DK, Severson HH. Oral spit tobacco: addiction, prevention and treatment. Nicotine Tob Res 1999;1:21.
41. U.S. Department of Health and Human Services. The Health Benefits of Smoking Cessation. A Report of the Surgeon General. U.S. Department of Health and Human Services, Public Health Service, Centers for Disease Control and Prevention and Health Promotion, Office on Smoking and Health. DSSH Publication No. (CDC) 90-8416, 1990.
42. Fletcher C, Peto R. The natural history of chronic airflow obstruction. Br Med J 1977;1:1645.
43. Peto R et al. Smoking, smoking cessation, and lung cancer in the UK since 1950: combination of national statistics with two case-control studies. Br Med J 2000;321:323.
44. Taylor DH et al. Benefits of smoking cessation for longevity. Am J Public Health 2002;92:990.
45. Zhu S et al. Smoking cessation with and without assistance: a population-based analysis. Am J Prev Med 2000;18:305.
46. Fiore MC et al. Treating Tobacco Use and Dependence, Clinical Practice Guideline. Rockville, MD: U.S. Department of Health and Human Services, Public Health Service; 2000.
47. Silagy C, Stead LF. Physician advice for smoking cessation. Cochrane Database Syst Rev 2001(2): CD000165.
48. Rigotti NA et al. Tobacco-control policies in 11 leading managed care organizations: progress and challenges. Eff Clin Pract 2002;5:130.

49. Prochaska JO, DiClemente CC. The transtheoretical approach: crossing traditional boundaries of therapy. Homewood, IL: Dow Jones-Irwin, 1984.

50. Ossip-Klein DJ, McIntosh S. Quitlines in North America: evidence base and applications. Am J Med Sci 2003;326:201.

51. Zhu SH et al. Evidence of real-world effectiveness of a telephone quitline for smokers. N Engl J Med 2002;347:1087.

52. Severson HH et al. A self-help cessation program for smokeless tobacco users: comparison of two interventions. Nicotine Tob Res 2000;2:363.

53. Silagy C et al. Nicotine replacement therapy for smoking cessation. Cochrane Database Syst Rev 2002(4):CD000146.

54. Benowitz NL, Gourlay SG. Cardiovascular toxicity of nicotine: implications for nicotine replacement therapy. J Am Coll Cardiol 1997;29:1422.

55. Joseph AM et al. The safety of transdermal nicotine as an aid to smoking cessation in patients with cardiac disease. N Engl J Med 1996;335:1792.

56. Dempsey DA, Benowitz NL. Risks and benefits of nicotine to aid smoking cessation in pregnancy. Drug Saf 2001;24:277.

57. GlaxoSmithKline. *Zyban package insert*. Research Triangle, NC March 2003.

58. Shiffman S et al. Comparative efficacy of 24-hour and 16-hour transdermal nicotine patches for relief of morning craving. Addiction 2000;95:1185.

59. Fant RV et al. Nicotine replacement therapy. Prim Care 1999;26:633.

60. Benowitz NL et al. Determinants of nicotine intake while chewing nicotine polacrilex gum. Clin Pharmacol Ther 1987;41:467.

61. Henningfield JE et al. Drinking coffee and carbonated beverages blocks absorption of nicotine from nicotine polacrilex gum. JAMA 1990;264:1560.

62. Choi JH et al. Pharmacokinetics of a nicotine polacrilex lozenge. Nicotine Tob Res 2003;5:635.

63. Shiffman S et al. Efficacy of a nicotine lozenge for smoking cessation. Arch Intern Med 2002;162:1267.

64. Heatherton TF et al. Measuring the heaviness of smoking: using self-reported time to the first cigarette of the day and number of cigarettes smoked per day. Br J Addict 1989;84:791.

65. O'Hara P et al. Early and late weight gain following smoking cessation in the Lung Health Study. Am J Epidemiol 1998;148:821.

66. Perkins KA et al. Acute effects of tobacco smoking on hunger and eating in male and female smokers. Appetite 1994;22:149.

67. Hatsukami D et al. Effects of tobacco abstinence on food intake among cigarette smokers. Health Psychol 1993;12:499.

68. Kawachi I et al. Can physical activity minimize weight gain in women after smoking cessation? Am J Public Health 1996;86:999.

69. Benowitz NL. Cigarette smoking and cardiovascular disease: pathophysiology and implications for treatment. Prog Cardiovasc Dis 2003;46:91.

70. Benowitz NL. The role of nicotine in smoking-related cardiovascular disease. Prev Med 1997;26:412.

71. Taylor BV et al. Clinical and pathophysiological effects of active and passive smoking on the cardiovascular system. Can J Cardiol 1998;14:1129.

72. Whitehead TP et al. The effects of cigarette smoking and alcohol consumption on blood lipids: a dose-related study on men. Ann Clin Biochem 1996;33:99.

73. Bazzano LA et al. Relationship between cigarette smoking and novel risk factors for cardiovascular disease in the United States. Ann Intern Med 2003;138:891.

74. van Domburg RT et al. Smoking cessation reduces mortality after coronary artery bypass surgery: a 20-year follow-up study. J Am Coll Cardiol 2000;36:878.

75. Thomson CC, Rigotti NA. Hospital- and clinic-based smoking cessation interventions for smokers with cardiovascular disease. Prog Cardiovasc Dis 2003;45:459.

76. Benowitz NL et al. Sources of variability in nicotine and cotinine levels with use of nicotine nasal spray, transdermal nicotine, and cigarette smoking. Br J Clin Pharmacol 1997;43:259.

77. Roth MT, Westman EC. Asthma exacerbation after administration of nicotine nasal spray for smoking cessation. Pharmacotherapy 2002;22:779.

78. Schneider NG et al. The nicotine inhaler: clinical pharmacokinetics and comparison with other nicotine treatments. Clin Pharmacokinet 2001;40:661.

79. Bergstrom M et al. Regional deposition of inhaled ^{11}C-nicotine vapor in the human airway as visualized by positron emission tomography. Clin Pharmacol Ther 1995;57:309.

80. Molander L et al. Dose released and absolute bioavailability of nicotine from a nicotine vapor inhaler. Clin Pharmacol Ther 1996;59:394.

81. Hughes JR et al. Antidepressants for smoking cessation. Cochrane Database Syst Rev. 2003(2):CD000031.

82. Hays JT et al. Sustained-release bupropion for pharmacologic relapse prevention after smoking cessation. a randomized, controlled trial. Ann Intern Med 2001;135:423.

83. Dunner DL et al. A prospective safety surveillance study for bupropion sustained-release in the treatment of depression. J Clin Psychiatry 1998;59:366.

84. Johnston AJ et al. Pharmacokinetic optimisation of sustained-release bupropion. Drugs 2002;62 Suppl 2:11.

85. Jorenby DE et al. A controlled trial of sustained-release bupropion, a nicotine patch, or both for smoking cessation. N Engl J Med 1999;340:685.

86. Lunell E et al. Relative bioavailability of nicotine from a nasal spray in infectious rhinitis and after use of a topical decongestant. Eur J Clin Pharmacol 1995;48:71.

87. Tzivoni D et al. Cardiovascular safety of transdermal nicotine patches in patients with coronary artery disease who try to quit smoking. Cardiovasc Drugs Ther 1998;12:239.

88. Nicotine replacement therapy for patients with coronary artery disease. Working Group for the Study of Transdermal Nicotine in Patients with Coronary Artery Disease. Arch Intern Med 1994;154:989.

89. Joseph AM, Fu SS. Safety issues in pharmacotherapy for smoking in patients with cardiovascular disease. Prog Cardiovasc Dis 2003;45:429.

90. McRobbie H, Hajek P. Nicotine replacement therapy in patients with cardiovascular disease: guidelines for health professionals. Addiction 2001;96:1547.

91. Fabbri LM et al. Global Strategy for the Diagnosis, Management and Prevention of COPD: 2003 update. Eur Respir J 2003;22:1. Available at: http://www.goldcopd.com/.

92. Pauwels RA et al. Global strategy for the diagnosis, management, and prevention of chronic obstructive pulmonary disease. NHLBI/WHO Global Initiative for Chronic Obstructive Lung Disease (GOLD) Workshop summary. Am J Respir Crit Care Med 2001;163:1256.

93. Barnes PJ. Chronic obstructive pulmonary disease. N Engl J Med 2000;343:269.

94. Mitchell BE et al. The adverse health effects of tobacco and tobacco-related products. Prim Care 1999;26:463.

95. Gourlay SG et al. Clonidine for smoking cessation. Cochrane Database Syst Rev 2000(2):CD000058.

96. Bohadana A et al. Nicotine inhaler and nicotine patch as a combination therapy for smoking cessation: a randomized, double-blind, placebo-controlled trial. Arch Intern Med 2000;160:3128.

97. Fagerström KO et al. Effectiveness of nicotine patch and nicotine gum as individual versus combined treatments for tobacco withdrawal symptoms. Psychopharmacology 1993;111:271.

98. Kornitzer M et al. Combined use of nicotine patch and gum in smoking cessation: a placebo-controlled clinical trial. Prev Med. 1995;24:41.

99. Puska P et al. Combined use of nicotine patch and gum compared with gum alone in smoking cessation: a clinical trial in North Karelia. Tob Control 1995;4:231.

100. Blondal T et al. Nicotine nasal spray with nicotine patch for smoking cessation: randomised trial with six year follow up. Br Med J 1999;318:285.

101. Lawson GM et al. Application of serum nicotine and plasma cotinine concentrations to assessment of nicotine replacement in light, moderate, and heavy smokers undergoing transdermal therapy. J Clin Pharmacol 1998;38:502.

102. Fredrickson PA, et al. High dose transdermal nicotine therapy for heavy smokers: safety, tolerability and measurement of nicotine and cotinine levels. Psychopharmacology 1995;122:215.

103. Benowitz NL et al. Suppression of nicotine intake during ad libitum cigarette smoking by high-dose transdermal nicotine. J Pharmacol Exp Ther 1998;287:958.

104. Dale LC et al. High-dose nicotine patch therapy. Percentage of replacement and smoking cessation. JAMA 1995;274:1353.

105. Tonnesen P et al. Higher dosage nicotine patches increase one-year smoking cessation rates: results from the European CEASE trial. Collaborative European Anti-Smoking Evaluation. European Respiratory Society. Eur Respir J 1999;13:238.

106. Jorenby DE et al. Varying nicotine patch dose and type of smoking cessation counseling. JAMA 1995;274:1347.

107. Hughes JR et al. Are higher doses of nicotine replacement more effective for smoking cessation? Nicotine Tob Res 1999;1:169.

108. Stead LF, Hughes JR. Lobeline for smoking cessation. Cochrane Database Syst Rev 2000(2):CD000124.

109. Abbot NC et al. Hypnotherapy for smoking cessation. Cochrane Database Syst Rev 2000(2):CD001008.

110. White AR et al. Acupuncture for smoking cessation. Cochrane Database Syst Rev 2002(2):CD000009.

111. Seibert C et al. Prescribing oral contraceptives for women older than 35 years of age. Ann Intern Med 2003;138:54.

112. Schwingl PJ et al. Estimates of the risk of cardiovascular death attributable to low-dose oral contraceptives in the United States. Am J Obstet Gynecol 1999;180(1 Pt 1):241.

113. Schiff I et al. Oral contraceptives and smoking, current considerations: recommendations of a consensus panel. Am J Obstet Gynecol 1999;180(6 Pt 2):S383.

114. World Heath Organization. Low dose combined oral contraceptives. In: Improving Access to Quality Care in Family Planning: Medical Eligibility Criteria for Contraceptive Use. 2nd ed. Geneva, Switzerland: World Health Organization, 2000:1.

115. Kozlowski LT et al. Filter ventilation and nicotine content of tobacco in cigarettes from Canada, the United Kingdom, and the United States. Tob Control 1998;7:369.

116. National Cancer Institute. Risks Associated with Low Machine-Measured Yields of Tar and Nicotine. Smoking and Tobacco Control Monograph No. 13. Bethesda, MD: U.S. Department of Health and Human Services, National Institutes of Health, National Cancer Institute, NIH Publication No. 02-5074, October, 2001.

117. Etter JF et al. What smokers believe about light and ultralight cigarettes. Prev Med 2003;36:92.

118. Fruzzetti F. Hemostatic effects of smoking and oral contraceptive use. Am J Obstet Gynecol 1999;180(6 Pt 2):S369.

119. U.S. Department of Health and Human Services. Women and Smoking. A Report of the Surgeon General. Atlanta, GA: U.S. Department of Health and Human Services, Centers for Disease Control and Prevention, National Center for Chronic Disease Prevention and Health Promotion, Office on Smoking and Health, 2001.

120. Petitti DB. Clinical practice. Combination estrogen-progestin oral contraceptives. N Engl J Med 2003;349:1443.

121. U.S. Department of Health and Human Services. The Health Consequences of Smoking: Cancer. A Report of the Surgeon General. Rockville, MD: Public Health Service, Office on Smoking and Health, DHHS Publication No. (PHS) 82-50179, 1982.

122. Rosenberg L et al. Low-dose oral contraceptive use and the risk of myocardial infarction. Arch Intern Med 2001;161:1065.

123. U.S. Department of Health and Human Services. The Health Consequences of Using Smokeless Tobacco. A Report of the Advisory Committee to the Surgeon General. NIH Publication No. 86-2874, 1986.

124. U.S. Department of Health and Human Services. Substance Abuse and Mental Health Services Administration. Results from the 2002 National Survey on Drug Use and Health: National Findings (Office of Applied Studies, NHSDA Series H-22, DHHS Publication No. SMA 03–3836). Rockville, MD, 2003.

125. Ebbert JO et al. Treatments for spit tobacco use: a quantitative systematic review. Addiction 2003; 98:569.

126. Fant RV et al. Pharmacokinetics and pharmacodynamics of moist snuff in humans. Tob Control 1999;8:387.

127. Taybos G. Oral changes associated with tobacco use. Am J Med Sci 2003;326:179.

128. Martin GC et al. Oral leukoplakia status six weeks after cessation of smokeless tobacco use. J Am Dent Assoc 1999;130:945.

129. Severson HH. What have we learned from 20 years of research on smokeless tobacco cessation? Am J Med Sci 2003;326:206.

130. U.S. Department of Agriculture. Tobacco Situation and Outlook Yearbook. Report TBS-2002. December 2002: U.S. Department of Agriculture, Market and Trade Economics Division, Economic Research Service, 2002.

131. Baker F et al. Health risks associated with cigar smoking. JAMA 2000;284(6):735.

132. National Cancer Institute. Cigars. Health Effects and Trends. Smoking and Tobacco Control Monograph No. 9. Bethesda, MD: U.S. Department of Health and Human Services, National Institutes of Health, National Cancer Institute, NIH Publication No. 98-4302, 1998.

133. Tomar SL. Trends and patterns of tobacco use in the United States. Am J Med Sci 2003;326:248.

134. Henningfield JE et al. Nicotine concentration, smoke pH and whole tobacco aqueous pH of some cigar brands and types popular in the United States. Nicotine Tob Res 1999;1:163.

135. CDC. Bidi use among urban youth—Massachusetts, March-April 1999. MMWR Morb Mortal Wkly Rep 1999;48:796.

136. Malson JL et al. Comparison of the nicotine content of tobacco used in bidis and conventional cigarettes. Tob Control 2001;10:181.

137. Watson CH et al. Determination of tar, nicotine, and carbon monoxide yields in the smoke of bidi cigarettes. Nicotine Tob Res 2003;5:747.

138. Rickert WS. Determination of yields of "tar", nicotine and carbon monoxide from bidi cigarettes: final report. Ontario, Canada: Labstat International, Inc., 1999.

139. Taylor TM, Biener L. Bidi smoking among Massachusetts teenagers. Prev Med 2001;32:89.

140. Gajalakshmi V et al. Smoking and mortality from tuberculosis and other diseases in India: retrospective study of 43000 adult male deaths and 35000 controls. Lancet 2003;362:507.

141. CDC. Illnesses possibly associated with smoking clove cigarettes. MMWR Morb Mortal Wkly Rep 1985;34:297.

142. American Medical Association. Evaluation of the health hazard of clove cigarettes. Council on Scientific Affairs. JAMA 1988;260:3641.

143. Guidotti TL et al. Clove cigarettes. The basis for concern regarding health effects. West J Med 1989;151:220.

144. CDC. Youth tobacco surveillance—United States, 2000. MMWR CDC Surveill Summ 2001;50(4):1.

145. CDC. Selected cigarette smoking initiation and quitting Behaviors Among High School Students—United States, 1997. MMWR Morb Mortal Wkly Rep 1998;47:386.

146. Prokhorov AV et al. Nicotine dependence, withdrawal symptoms, and adolescents' readiness to quit smoking. Nicotine Tob Res 2001;3:151.

147. CDC. Reasons for tobacco use and symptoms of nicotine withdrawal among adolescent and young adult tobacco users—United States, 1993. MMWR Morb Mortal Wkly Rep 1994;43:745.

148. Moolchan ET et al. A review of tobacco smoking in adolescents: treatment implications. J Am Acad Child Adolesc Psychiatry 2000;39:682.

149. Backinger CL et al. Adolescent and young adult tobacco prevention and cessation: current status and future directions. Tob Control 2003;12(Suppl 4):46.

150. Prokhorov AV et al. Adolescent smoking: epidemiology and approaches for achieving cessation. Paediatr Drugs 2003;5:1.

Anemias

Cindy O'Bryant, Dan Bestul

Definition

Anemia is a reduction in red cell mass. It often is described as a decrease in the number of red blood cells (RBCs) per mm^3 or as a decrease in the hemoglobin concentration in blood to a level below the normal physiologic requirement for adequate tissue oxygenation. The term *anemia* is not a diagnosis, but rather an objective sign of a disease. Diagnostic terminology for anemia requires the inclusion of the pathogenesis (e.g., megaloblastic anemia secondary to folate deficiency, microcytic anemia secondary to iron deficiency). An exact diagnosis is important to the understanding of the problem and to implement specific therapy to correct the anemia.

Pathophysiology

Anemia is a symptom of many pathologic conditions. It is associated with nutritional deficiencies and acute and chronic diseases; it also may be drug induced. Anemia may be caused by decreased red cell production, increased red cell destruction, or increased red cell loss. If the anemia is caused by decreased red cell production, it may be the result of disturbances in stem-cell proliferation or differentiation. Anemias caused by increased red cell destruction may be secondary to hemolysis, whereas increased red cell loss may be caused by acute or chronic bleeding. Anemias associated with acute blood loss, those that are iron related, and those caused by chronic disease comprise about 75% of all anemias.[1] Classifications of anemias according to pathophysiologic and morphologic characteristics are shown in Table 86-1.

Normally, RBC mass is maintained by feedback mechanisms that regulate levels of erythropoietin, a hormone that stimulates proliferation and differentiation of erythroid precursors in the bone marrow. Two types of erythroid precursors reside in the bone marrow: the BFUe (burst-forming unit, ery-

Table 86-1 Classifications of Anemia

Pathophysiologic (Classifies Anemias Based on Pathophysiologic Presentation)

Blood Loss

Acute: trauma, ulcer, hemorrhoids
Chronic: ulcer, vaginal bleeding, aspirin ingestion

Inadequate Red Blood Cell Production

Nutritional deficiency: B_{12}, folic acid, iron
Erythroblast deficiency: bone marrow failure (aplastic anemia, irradiation, chemotherapy, folic acid antagonists) or bone marrow infiltration (leukemia, lymphoma, myeloma, metastatic solid tumors, myelofibrosis)
Endocrine deficiency: pituitary, adrenal, thyroid, testicular
Chronic disease: renal, liver, infection, granulomatous, collagen vascular

Excessive Red Blood Cell Destruction

Intrinsic factors: hereditary (G6PD), abnormal hemoglobin synthesis
Extrinsic factors: autoimmune reactions, drug reactions, infection (endotoxin)

Morphologic (Classifies Anemias by Red Blood Cell Size [Microcytic, Normocytic, Macrocytic] and Hemoglobin Content [Hypochromic, Normochromic, Hyperchromic])

Macrocytic

Defective maturation with decreased production
Megaloblastic: pernicious (B_{12} deficiency), folic acid deficiency

Normochromic, normocytic

Recent blood loss
Hemolysis
Chronic disease
Renal failure
Autoimmune
Endocrine

Microcytic, hyperchromic

Iron deficiency
Genetic abnormalities: sickle cell, thalassemia

G6PD, glucose-6-phosphate dehydrogenase.

throid) and CFUe (colony-forming unit, erythroid). The BFUe is the earliest progenitor, which eventually develops into a CFUe. BFUe is moderately sensitive to erythropoietin and is under the influence of other cytokines (e.g., interleukin [IL]-3, granulocyte-macrophage colony-stimulating factor [GM-CSF]). In contrast, CFUe is highly sensitive to erythropoietin and differentiates into erythroblasts and reticulocytes. Normal endogenous levels of erythropoietin range from 10 to 20 U/L.[2] Ninety percent of erythropoietin is produced in the kidney; liver synthesis accounts for the remaining 10%. Reduced oxygen-carrying capacity is sensed by renal peritubular cells, and this stimulates release of erythropoietin into the bloodstream. Patients with chronic anemia may have a blunted response for the degree of anemia present or virtually no erythropoietin response because of renal insufficiency.

Detection

Signs and Symptoms

Signs and symptoms of anemia vary with the degree of RBC reduction as well as with the time interval over which it develops. Anemic patients may experience tissue hypoxia because of the decreased oxygen-carrying capacity of the reduced red cell mass. As a result, perfusion to nonvital tissues (e.g., skin, mucous membranes, extremities) is decreased to sustain tissue perfusion of vital organs (e.g., brain, heart, kidneys). This compensatory mechanism accounts for the skin pallor that can be noted in cases of severe anemia (hemoglobin [Hgb] <8 mg/dL). Uncorrected tissue hypoxia can lead to a number of complications in the central nervous, respiratory, and gastrointestinal (GI) systems. Changes in the blood hemoglobin concentration also lead to changes in the kidney tissue oxygen tension. The kidney responds to the hypoxemia by secreting erythropoietin, as discussed previously.[1,3]

In severe anemia, heart rate and stroke volume often increase in an attempt to improve the delivery of oxygen to tissues. These changes in heart rate and stroke volume may result in systolic murmurs, angina pectoris, high-output congestive heart failure, pulmonary congestion, ascites, and edema. Thus, anemia is generally not well tolerated in patients with cardiac disease.[4]

Anemia may be acute in onset or develop slowly. Slowly developing anemias may be asymptomatic initially or include symptoms such as slight exertional dyspnea, increased angina, fatigue, or malaise. The symptoms gradually increase as the anemia becomes more severe. Pallor of the skin and mucous membranes, jaundice, smooth or beefy tongue, cheilosis, and spoon-shaped nails (koilonychia) may be associated with severe anemia of different etiologies.

History

A thorough history and physical examination are essential because of the complexity of the pathologic conditions associated with anemia. A time line, which begins with the onset of symptoms (and surrounding events) and extends to current status, is important. Because longstanding anemias can indicate hereditary disorders, the family history should be noted. Past Hgb or hematocrit (Hct) determinations, transfusion history, as well as occupational, environmental, and social histories may be valuable. Finally, a medication history can help eliminate drug reactions or interactions as the cause of the anemia.

Physical Examination

On physical examination of a patient with anemia, pallor is most easily observed in the conjunctiva, mucous membranes, nail beds, and palmar creases of the hand. In addition, postural hypotension and tachycardia can be seen when hypovolemia (acute blood loss) is the primary cause of anemia. Patients with B_{12} deficiency may exhibit neurologic findings, which include changes in deep tendon reflexes, ataxia, and loss of vibration and position sense; all are consistent with nerve fiber demyelination. Patients with anemia from hemolysis may be slightly jaundiced from bilirubin release. Manifestations of hemorrhage can include petechiae, ecchymoses, hematomas, epistaxis, bleeding gums, blood in the urine, or blood in the stool.

Laboratory Evaluation

Even though anemia may be suspected from the history and physical examination, a full laboratory evaluation is necessary to confirm the diagnosis, establish its severity, and determine its cause. A list of the routine laboratory evaluations used in the workup for anemia are found in Table 86-2. The cornerstone of this evaluation is the complete blood count (CBC). Normal hematologic values can be found in Table 86-3. Females reach adult levels of Hct by late childhood. At puberty, males have a higher Hct secondary to stimulation of erythropoiesis by androgen hormones. The Hct also is increased in individuals living at altitudes above 4,000 feet in response to the diminished oxygen content of the atmosphere and blood.

The morphologic appearance of the RBC provides useful information about the nature of the anemia. Microscopic evaluation of the peripheral blood smear can detect the presence of macrocytic (large) RBCs, which usually are present when anemia results from a vitamin B_{12} or folic acid deficiency, or microcytic (small) RBCs, which usually are associated with iron deficiency anemia. Acute blood loss generally is associated with normocytic cells.

Together with the information gained from the history and physical examination, the routine laboratory evaluation can provide enough information to distinguish between the most common forms of anemia (Fig. 86-1). If the cause of the anemia is still not identified after routine evaluation, problems such as autoimmune disease, collagen vascular disease, chronic infection, endocrine disorders, or drug-induced destruction may be the cause. When uncertainty exists or an abnormal peripheral blood smear is noted, a bone marrow aspiration with biopsy is indicated.

There are many causes of anemia. This chapter is limited to the most common anemias managed with drugs. Hemolytic anemias are covered in Chapter 87, Drug-Induced Blood Disorders. Before proceeding, the reader should review the basic hematologic laboratory tests used to evaluate and monitor anemia (see Chapter 2:Interpretation of Clinical Laboratory Tests).

IRON DEFICIENCY ANEMIA

Iron deficiency is a state of negative iron balance in which the daily iron intake and stores are unable to meet the RBC and other body tissue needs.[5] The body contains approximately 3.5 g of iron, of which 2.5 g are found in Hgb. A significant amount of iron is stored as ferritin or aggregated ferritin (hemosiderin) in the reticuloendothelial cells of the liver, spleen, and bone marrow and by hepatocytes. Men have iron stores of 600 to 1,200 mg, whereas women have stores between 100 and 400 mg. Only a small fraction of iron is found in plasma (100 to 150 μg/dL), and most is bound to transferrin, the transport protein.

Despite the continuing turnover of RBCs, iron stores are well preserved because the iron is recovered and reutilized in

---

Table 86-2   Routine Laboratory Evaluation for Anemia Workup

Complete blood count (CBC): Hgb, Hct, RBC count, red cell indices (MCV, MCH, MCHC), WBC count (and differential)
Platelet count
Red cell morphology
Reticulocyte count
Bilirubin and LDH
Serum iron, TIBC, serum ferritin, transferrin saturation
Peripheral blood smear examination
Stool examination for occult blood
Bone marrow aspiration and biopsy[a]

[a]Performed in patients with abnormal peripheral blood smears.
Hct, hematocrit; Hgb, hemoglobin; LDH, lactic dehydrogenase; MCV, mean corpuscular volume; MCH, mean corpuscular hemoglobin; MCHC, mean corpuscular hemoglobin concentration; RBC, red blood cell; TIBC, total iron-binding capacity; WBC, white blood cell.

Table 86-3   Normal Hematology Values

Laboratory Test	Pediatric 1–15 yr	Adult Male	Adult Female
RBC (mm³)	4.7 ± 6	5.4 ± 0.7	4.8 ± 6
Hgb (g/dL)	13 ± 2	16 ± 2	14 ± 2
Hct (%)	40 ± 5	47 ± 5	42 ± 2
MCV (mm³)	80 ± 5	87 ± 7	90 ± 9
MCH (pg/cell)	33.5 ± 2	29 ± 2	34 ± 2
MCHC (g/dL)	31–36	31–36	31–36
Erythropoietin (mU/mL)	4–26	4–26	4–26
Reticulocyte count (%)	0.5–1.5	0.5–1.5	0.5–1.5
TIBC (mg/dL)	250–400	250–400	250–400
Fe (mg/dL)	50–120	50–160	40–150
Folate (ng/mL)	7–25	7–25	7–25
RBC Folate (ng/mL)		140–960	140–960
Fe/TIBC (%)	20–30	20–40	16–38
Vitamin B_{12} (pg/mL)	>200	>200	>200
Ferritin (ng/mL)	7–140	15–200	12–150

Fe, iron; Hgb, hemoglobin; Hct, hematocrit; MCH, mean corpuscular hemoglobin; MCV, mean corpuscular volume; RBC, red blood cell; TIBC, total iron-binding capacity.

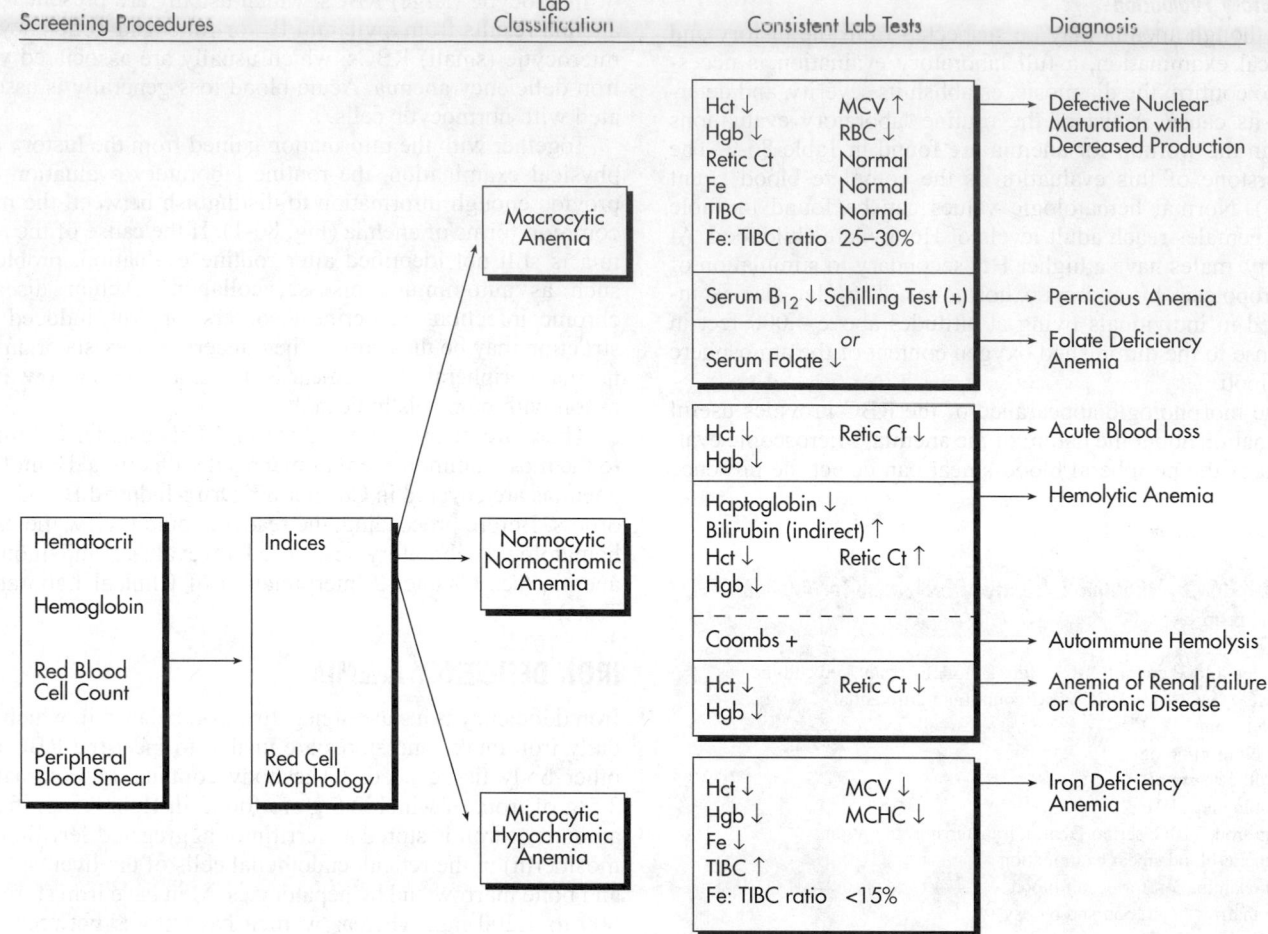

FIGURE 86-1 Laboratory diagnosis of anemia.

new erythrocytes. Only about 0.5 to 1 mg/day of iron is lost from urine, sweat, and the sloughing of intestinal mucosal cells that contain ferritin. Another 0.5 to 1 mg of iron is lost daily during menstruation. Pregnancy and lactation are other common sources of iron loss.

Individuals with normal iron stores absorb roughly 10% of ingested dietary iron. The average American diet contains 6 mg of elemental iron/1,000 Kcal. Thus, the average daily intake ranges between 10 and 12 mg, enough to replace the 1 mg lost daily (based on 10% absorption). However, for menstruating, pregnant, or lactating females, the daily iron intake requirement may be as high as 20 mg.

Iron is absorbed from the duodenum and upper jejunum by an active transport mechanism. Dietary iron, which is primarily in the ferric state, is converted to the more readily absorbed ferrous form in the acid environment of the stomach. It is the ferrous form that binds to transferrin for its journey to the bone marrow, where it is incorporated into the Hgb of mature erythrocytes.

A portion of the iron is bound to another protein, ferritin, which is important in the storage of iron. Ferritin circulates at concentrations that reflect total iron body stores.

GI absorption of iron is increased from the usual 10% to as much as 20% to 30% in iron deficiency states or when erythropoiesis occurs at a more rapid rate. Animal sources of iron

are better absorbed than plant sources. A gastrectomy or vagotomy may decrease the conversion of the ferric form of iron to the ferrous state, thereby diminishing iron absorption. In addition, certain foods and drugs can complex with iron, decreasing its absorption.

Anemia caused by iron deficiency is a common worldwide problem. Although there are many causes of iron deficiency anemia (Table 86-4), blood loss is considered one of the more common causes. Each milliliter of whole blood contains 0.5 mg of iron, whereas each milliliter of packed RBCs contains

Table 86-4 Iron Deficiency Anemia Causes
Blood Loss
Menstruation, gastrointestinal (e.g., peptic ulcer), trauma
Decreased Absorption
Medication (e.g., tetracycline), gastrectomy, regional enteritis
Increased Requirement
Infancy, pregnant/lactating females
Impaired Utilization
Hereditary, ↓ iron use

1 mg of iron. Common causes of chronic blood loss include peptic ulcer disease, hemorrhoids, ingestion of GI irritants, menstruation, multiple pregnancies, and multiple blood donations.

The increased amounts of iron required by pregnant or lactating women are hard to obtain through diet alone; thus, oral iron supplementation generally is necessary (see Chapter 46, Obstetrics). Although maternal iron usually provides term infants with enough stored iron for the first 6 months, infants 6 months to 3 years of age experience rapid growth and a three-fold increase in blood volume, which can increase the risk of iron deficiency. Premature infants have reduced iron stores and thus require replacement therapy. Supplementation of 10 to 15 mg/day of iron may be required for up to the first year of life. Maintenance iron therapy for normal older infants and children is roughly 1 to 2 mg/kg per day (not to exceed 20 mg/day). If iron deficiency develops in the pediatric patient, 3 to 6 mg/kg per day of elemental iron should be administered in two to three divided doses.[6] Table 86-5 provides a list of some available pediatric iron preparations.

Predisposing Factors

1. **D.G., a 35-year-old woman, is seen in the clinic. Her chief complaints include weakness, dizziness, and epigastric pain. She has a 5-year history of peptic ulcer disease, a 10-year history of heavy menstrual bleeding, and a 20-year history of chronic headaches. She has four children who are 1, 3, 5, and 7 years of age. D.G. is currently taking tetracycline 250 mg BID for acne, ibuprofen 400 mg PRN headaches, and frequent doses of antacids for GI distress. Her review of systems is positive for decreased exercise tolerance. Physical examination reveals a pale, lethargic, white female appearing older than her stated age. Her vital signs are within normal limits; her heart rate is regular at 100 beats/min. Her examination is notable for pale nail beds and splenomegaly.**

Significant laboratory results include the following: Hgb, 8 g/dL (normal, 14 to 18); Hct, 27% (normal, 40% to 44%); platelet count, 800,000/mm³ (normal, 130,000 to 400,000); reticulocyte count, 0.2% (normal, 0.5% to 1.5%); mean corpuscular volume (MCV), 75 m³ (normal, 80 to 94); mean corpuscular hemoglobin (MCH), 23 pg (normal, 27 to 31); mean corpuscular

Table 86-5 Iron Content of Liquid Iron Preparations[a,b]

Preparation	Trade Name	Iron Content (mg FE⁺⁺/mL)
Ferrous Sulfate		
Elixir (44 mg/mL)	Feosol	8.8
Drops (125 mg/mL)	Fer-in-Sol	25.0
Ferrous Gluconate		
Elixir (60 mg/mL)	Fergon	7
Ferrous Fumarate		
Suspension	Feostat	6.6

[a]There are other iron preparations that may be equally efficacious, and generic equivalents may be available.
[b]The listed preparations are not being endorsed.
FE, iron.

hemoglobin concentration (MCHC), 30% (normal, 33% to 37%); serum iron, 40 g/dL (normal, 50 to 160); serum ferritin, 9 ng/mL (normal, 15 to 200); total iron-binding capacity (TIBC), 450 g/dL (normal, 250 to 400); and 4+ guaiac stools (normal, negative).

Iron deficiency is determined to be the cause of D.G.'s anemia. An upper GI series with a small bowel follow-through are planned to evaluate her persistent epigastric pain. What factors predispose D.G. to iron deficiency anemia?

[SI units: Hgb, 80 g/L; Hct, 0.27; MCV, 75 fL; MCH, 23 pg; MCHC, 0.3; iron, 7.16 μmol/L; ferritin, 9 μg/L; TIBC, 80.87 μmol/L; platelets, 800 × 10⁹/L; reticulocyte, 0.002]

Several factors predispose D.G. to iron deficiency anemia. Her history of heavy menstrual bleeding and the 4+ stool guaiac indicate menstrual and GI sources of blood loss. The GI blood loss may be secondary to D.G.'s chronic use of nonsteroidal anti-inflammatory drugs and/or recurrent peptic ulcer disease.

Many women of childbearing age have a borderline iron deficiency that becomes more evident during pregnancy because of the increased iron requirements.[7,8] D.G. has given birth to four children. Therefore, her iron stores have been repeatedly taxed in recent years. In addition, absorption of dietary iron may be compromised by her use of antacids and tetracycline (see Question 6).

Signs, Symptoms, and Laboratory Tests

2. **What subjective or objective signs, symptoms, and laboratory tests are typical of iron deficiency in D.G.?**

D.G.'s constitutional symptoms of weakness and dizziness could be a result of her severe anemia. Generally, until the anemia is severe, such symptoms occur with equal frequency in the nonanemic population. The most important signs and symptoms of iron deficiency anemia are related to the cardiovascular system and are a reflection of the imbalance between the ongoing demands for oxygen against a diminishing oxygen supply. D.G.'s increased heart rate, decreased exercise tolerance, and pale appearance are consistent with tissue anoxia and the cardiovascular response that may be seen in iron deficiency anemia.

D.G.'s iron deficiency has advanced to symptomatic anemia. However, in patients who are not yet symptomatic, depletion of iron stores can be detected by measuring ferritin, the iron storage compound. Although ferritin is primarily an intracellular protein, serum concentrations of ferritin correlate closely with iron stores with only a few exceptions (e.g., liver disease and some malignancies).[9–12] A serum ferritin level <12 ng/mL is consistent with iron deficiency. An increased TIBC also can reflect depletion of storage iron, but it is less sensitive than serum ferritin. Thus, in iron deficiency, the serum ferritin concentration is low, whereas the TIBC is usually high; both of these parameters can be detected before the clinical manifestations of anemia are apparent. These abnormalities persist and worsen as the patient progresses to anemia as illustrated by D.G.'s values. If the bone marrow is examined at this time, hemosiderin granules (which contain approximately 25% to 30% of iron) would be absent. If the TIBC is low or normal, rather than high, in association with a low serum ferritin, other causes of anemia, such as malignancy, infections, or inflammatory disorders, should be considered. In these situations, further documentation (e.g., bone marrow examination) is necessary to determine the cause of the anemia.[13–15]

D.G.'s low serum iron, low serum ferritin, and elevated TIBC are typical of the laboratory findings associated with iron deficiency anemia. In addition to examining the absolute values reported for serum iron and TIBC, the ratio of the serum iron concentration to the TIBC (or the transferrin saturation ratio) should be determined [(S_{Fe}/TIBC) 100]. In iron deficiency, the transferrin saturation ratio falls below 15%. D.G.'s calculated transferrin saturation ratio (i.e., $40/450 \times 100\%$) is 8.9% and is consistent with iron deficiency anemia.

After the iron in the storage compartment is depleted, heme and hemoglobin synthesis are decreased. In severe iron deficiency, the RBCs become hypochromic (low MCHC) and microcytic (low MCV). Usually, the RBC indices do not become abnormal until the Hgb concentration falls to <12 g/dL in males or 10 g/dL in females. D.G.'s corpuscular indices indicate that her anemia is hypochromic and microcytic.

About 10% of iron-deficient patients experience neutropenia and either thrombocytopenia or thrombocytosis. Thrombocytosis can occur in 50% to 75% of patients with hypochromic anemia secondary to chronic blood loss. The thrombocytosis (e.g., 800,000 platelets) in D.G. returns to normal after adequate treatment with iron. The reticulocyte count provides an estimate of effective red cell production and is usually normal or low in iron deficiency anemia. D.G. has a reticulocyte count of 0.2% (normal, 0.5 to 1.5%), which also is compatible with iron deficiency anemia.

In the workup of a microcytic, hypochromic anemia, the stool should be examined for occult blood. D.G. has a 4+ stool guaiac, which suggests blood loss via the GI tract. Further diagnostic evaluations (e.g., endoscopy, GI films) are necessary to determine the underlying problem.

In summary, D.G.'s signs, symptoms, and laboratory findings all support the diagnosis of an iron deficiency anemia.

Iron Therapy
Oral Iron Dosing

3. How should D.G.'s iron deficiency be managed? What dose of iron should be given to treat D.G.'s iron deficiency anemia and for how long?

The primary treatment of D.G. should be directed toward control of the underlying causes of anemia, which in this case are many. D.G.'s iron stores are low because of GI blood loss, multiple childbirths, heavy menstrual flow, and perhaps, inadequate diet. Therefore, the cause of her GI blood loss should be corrected, her dietary intake should be analyzed and modified, and supplemental iron should be prescribed to replenish her stores and correct the anemia.

The usual adult dose of ferrous sulfate is 325 mg (1 tablet) administered three times daily, between meals. Actually, if no iron is being lost through bleeding, the required daily dose of elemental iron can be calculated using a formula that assumes that 0.25 g/dL per day is the maximal rate of hemoglobin regeneration.

Elemental iron (mg/day) = 0.25 g Hgb/100 mL blood/day
$$(5,000 \text{ mL blood})(3.4 \text{ mg Fe/1 g Hgb})$$
= 40 mg Fe/day/20% absorption (approximate absorption rate in iron-deficient states)
= 200 mg Fe/day
= 1,000 mg ferrous sulfate/day (ferrous sulfate contains 20% elemental iron)
= 325 mg TID ferrous sulfate

Product Selection

4. What are the differences between iron products? Which is the product of choice?

The ferrous form of iron is absorbed three times more readily than the ferric form. Although ferrous sulfate, ferrous gluconate, and ferrous fumarate are absorbed almost equally, each contains a different amount of elemental iron.[16,17] Table 86-6 compares the number of tablets of ferrous sulfate, gluconate, and fumarate required to provide a daily adult dose of 180 to 200 mg of elemental iron. If compliance is enhanced when the patient takes the smallest number of tablets, then ferrous sulfate or ferrous fumarate may be better choices.

PRODUCT FORMULATION

Product formulation is of considerable importance in product selection. Some believe that the more expensive, sustained-release (SR) iron preparations are inherently better. SR preparations fall into three groups: (1) those claimed to increase GI tolerance or decrease side effects, (2) those formulated to increase bioavailability, and (3) those with adjuvants claimed to enhance absorption. Because these products can be given once daily, increased compliance is an additional claim.

Anecdotal claims that SR iron preparations cause fewer GI side effects have not been substantiated by controlled studies. In fact, these products transport iron past the duodenum and proximal jejunum, thereby reducing the absorption of iron.[18] Therefore, poor absorption and poor hematologic responses may occur with ferrous sulfate SR capsules.

Adjuvants are incorporated into many iron preparations in an attempt to enhance absorption or decrease side effects. Several products contain ascorbic acid (vitamin C), which maintains iron in the ferrous state. Doses up to 1 g increase iron absorption by only 10%; however, smaller doses of vitamin C (e.g., 100 mg) do not significantly alter iron absorption.[19] Table 86-7 lists a number of combination products that contain a stool softener or vitamin C. It is unlikely that the small amount of vitamin C added to these products significantly enhances absorption enough to justify the significant increase in cost.

Table 86-6	Comparisons of Iron Preparations		
Preparation	**Dose (mg)**	**Fe⁺⁺ Content (mg)**	**% Fe**
Ferrous sulfate	325	65	20
Ferrous fumarate	300	99	33
Ferrous gluconate	300	35	11
Feosol tablets	200	60	20
Feostat chew tabs	100	33	33
Slow Fe (time released)	160	50	31

Table 86-7 **Combination Iron Products**

Drug	DOSS (mg)	Vitamin C (mg)	Fe⁺⁺ Content (mg)
Ferro-Grad 500 (Filmtabs)	0	500	105
Vitron C	0	125	66
Vitelle Irospan	0	150	65
Ferro DSS/Ferro-Sequel	100	0	50

DSS, dioctyl sodium sulfosuccinate; docusate sodium; Fe, iron.

Stool softeners are added to iron preparations to decrease the side effect of constipation. Generally, these combinations contain suboptimal doses of stool softener and are unwarranted. If constipation does develop, appropriate doses of stool softeners should be taken. It appears more rational to take iron supplements by themselves and to treat side effects as necessary.

In summary, D.G. should take the least expensive iron preparation containing ferrous sulfate, gluconate, or fumarate. In general, generic preparations of iron salts not in combination with adjuvant agents provide the best value.

Goals of Therapy

5. What are the goals of iron therapy? How should D.G. be monitored?

The goal of iron therapy is to normalize the Hgb and Hct concentrations and to replete iron stores. Initially, if the doses of iron are adequate, the reticulocyte count will begin to increase by the third to fourth day and peak by the seventh to tenth day of therapy. By the end of the second week of iron therapy, the reticulocyte count will fall back to normal.[20] The Hgb response is a convenient index to monitor in outpatients. Hematologic response is usually seen in 3 weeks with a 2 g/dL increase in hemoglobin and a 6% increase in the hematocrit. One can expect D.G.'s anemia to resolve in 1 to 2 months. However, iron therapy should be continued for 3 to 6 months after the hemoglobin is normalized to replete iron stores.[6,20,21] The duration of therapy is related to the absorption pattern of iron. During the first month of therapy, as much as 35 mg of elemental iron is absorbed from the daily dose. With time, the percentage of iron absorbed from the dose decreases, and by the third month of therapy, only 5 to 10 mg of elemental iron is absorbed.

Patient Information

6. What kind of information should be provided to D.G. upon dispensing oral iron? What can be done if she experiences intolerable GI symptoms (e.g., nausea, epigastric pain)?

Iron should be dispensed in a childproof container, and D.G. should be told to store it in a safe place away from children. Accidental ingestion of even small amounts (three to four tablets) of oral iron can cause serious consequences in small children.[22] (see Chapter 5, Managing Acute Drug Toxicity.) D.G. should be told that oral iron therapy produces dark stools. She should try to take her iron on an empty stomach because food, especially dairy products, decreases the absorption by 40% to 50%.[23,24]

Gastric side effects occur in 5% to 20% of patients and include nausea, epigastric pain, constipation, abdominal cramps, and diarrhea. Constipation does not appear to be dose related, but side effects such as nausea and epigastric pain occur more frequently as the quantity of soluble elemental iron in contact with the stomach and duodenum increases.[6,25]

To minimize gastric intolerance, oral iron therapy can be initiated with a single tablet of ferrous sulfate 325 mg/day; the dose is increased by increments of one tablet per day every 2 to 3 days until the full therapeutic dose of ferrous sulfate, 325 mg three times daily, can be administered[3,25] Other causes of epigastric pain (e.g., recurrent peptic ulcer disease, other GI diseases) also should be investigated.

D.G. also should be educated about potential drug interactions that may occur with iron therapy. Currently, she is taking antacids, which historically have not been recommended in combination with iron therapy. Antacids are thought to inhibit serum iron absorption by increasing the pH of the stomach and decreasing the solubility of ferrous salts.[26,27] Certain anions in antacids (carbonate and hydroxide) also are thought to form insoluble complexes when combined with iron. However, in a study evaluating the effect of antacids on iron absorption in patients with mild iron deficiency, Mylanta II (5 mL) given with 10 mg of iron did not significantly alter 2-hour iron levels relative to that achieved by a control dose.[28] In contrast, 1 g of $NaHCO_3$ decreased the 2-hour plasma ion concentration to 5% of the control level. Similarly, $CaCO_3$ 500 mg also decreased the 2-hour iron plasma level to only one-third of the control dose; $CaCO_3$ did not appear to affect iron absorption when it was incorporated into a multivitamin containing iron.[28] Although the issue remains controversial, this study indicates that a therapeutic dose of liquid antacid containing aluminum hydroxide and magnesium hydroxide does not significantly alter absorption of iron in mildly deficient adults. Although the clinical significance of the iron-antacid interaction remains to be established, D.G. should be advised to take her iron at least 1 hour before or 3 hours after the antacid dose.

D.G. also is taking tetracycline for the treatment of acne. Because the absorptions of both iron and tetracycline are decreased when administered concomitantly, the iron should be taken 3 hours before or 2 hours after the tetracycline dose.[29] Antacids also may impair the absorption of tetracycline; therefore, tetracycline should be separated from antacids by 1 to 2 hours.

Parenteral Iron Therapy
INDICATIONS

7. When would parenteral iron therapy be indicated for D.G.?

There are several indications for parenteral iron administration. Failure to respond to oral iron therapy would prompt a re-evaluation of D.G. Causes of oral therapy failure can include noncompliance, misdiagnosis (e.g., inflammation), malabsorption (e.g., sprue, radiation enteritis, duodenal or upper small intestine resection), and continuing blood loss equal to or greater than the rate of RBC production. Malabsorption can be evaluated by measuring iron levels every 30 minutes for 2 hours after the administration of 50 mg of ferrous sulfate. If her plasma iron levels increase by >50%, absorption is adequate. Besides failure to respond to oral therapy as one indication for parenteral iron administration, other indications include intolerance to oral therapy, required antacid therapy, or significant blood loss in patients refusing transfusion. All can warrant injectable iron therapy.[30] In D.G.'s case, if it was documented that she had malabsorption or required continued high-dose antacid therapy for her gastritis, she would be a candidate for injectable iron.

PREFERRED ROUTE

8. **What is the preferred route of parenteral iron administration?**

Iron can be given parenterally in the form of ferric gluconate (Ferrlecit), iron dextran (INFeD), and iron sucrose (Venofer). Iron dextran, the oldest of the parenteral iron agents, is Food and Drug Administration (FDA)-approved for the treatment of iron deficiency when oral supplementation is impossible or ineffective. In this particular formulation, iron is a complex of ferric hydroxide and dextran. Iron dextran can be administered undiluted intramuscularly or by very slow IV injection. Although not included in the labeling approved by the FDA, iron-dextran injection is commonly diluted in 250 to 1000 mL 0.9% NaCl and administered by IV infusion. IV administration is preferred to IM administration when muscle mass available for an IM injection is limited; when absorption from the muscle is impaired (e.g., stasis, edema); when uncontrolled bleeding is a risk (e.g., secondary to hemophilia, thrombocytopenia, anticoagulation therapy); and when large doses are indicated for therapy.

In a few instances, IM iron dextran is the preferred treatment (e.g., patients with limited IV access). In these cases, undiluted drug should be administered using a Z-track technique to avoid staining the skin. (The skin should be pulled laterally before injection; then the drug is injected and the skin is released to avoid leakage of dextran into the subcutaneous tissue.) IM iron dextran is absorbed in two phases. In the first 72 hours, 60% of the dose is absorbed, whereas the remaining drug is absorbed over weeks to months.[31]

Infusion rates of undiluted IV iron dextran should not exceed 50 mg (i.e., 1 mL) per minute. The upper limit of each daily dose is based on the patient's weight and should not be greater than 100 mg/day. Although the data are limited, total dose iron-dextran infusion is given in clinical practice[32–34] and has proved to be effective and convenient.[30] Infusions generally are given over 2 to 6 hours to minimize local pain and phlebitis.[6] The total dose method of administration may be associated with a higher prevalence of fever, malaise, flushing, and myalgias.

Ferric gluconate and iron sucrose, are parenteral iron formulations, which are FDA approved for the treatment of iron deficiency anemia in patients undergoing chronic hemodialysis and receiving supplemental erythropoietin.[35] Ferric gluconate may be administered undiluted as a slow IV injection (rate not to exceed 12.5 mg/minute) or as an IV infusion (125 mg ferric gluconate in 100 mL 0.9% NaCl over 1 hour). Likewise, iron sucrose may be administered undiluted as a slow IV injection (rate not to exceed 20 mg/minute) or as an IV infusion (dilute in a maximum of 100 mL 0.9% NaCl and infuse at a rate of 100 mg over 15 minutes). Iron requirements in these patients typically exceed 1 to 2 grams, and therefore multiple doses of ferric gluconate and iron sucrose are needed to achieve the total dose of iron.

DOSAGE CALCULATION

9. **How would you calculate a total dose of iron dextran for IV infusion that would be needed to achieve a normal hemoglobin value for D.G. and replenish her iron stores. How quickly should she respond?**

The total dose of iron dextran to be administered can be determined using the following equation:

$$\text{Iron (mg)} = [\text{Weight (pounds)} \times 0.3]\,\{100 - [100(\text{Hgb})/14.8]\}$$

where *Hgb* is the patient's measured hemoglobin (g/dL). The equation uses the person's weight (in pounds) and assumes that an Hgb of 14.8 g/dL is 100% of normal. Children weighing <30 pounds should be given 80% of the calculated dose because the normal mean Hgb in this population is lower.

For patients with anemia resulting from blood loss (e.g., hemorrhagic diatheses) or patients receiving chronic dialysis, the iron requirement is based on the estimate of iron contained in the blood lost. In this case, the following equation should be used:

$$\text{Iron (mg)} = \text{Blood loss (mL)} \times \text{Hct (the patient's measured Hct expressed as a decimal fraction)}$$

This formula assumes that 1 mL of normochromic blood contains 1 mg of iron.

After parenteral administration, iron dextran is cleared by the reticuloendothelial cells and processed. The iron is then released back into the plasma and bone marrow. Because the rate of iron incorporation into hemoglobin does not exceed that achieved by oral iron therapy, the response time is similar to that of oral iron therapy, and one can expect the Hgb to increase at a rate of 1.5 to 2.2 g/dL per week during the first 2 weeks and by 0.7 to 1.6 g/dL per week thereafter until normal values are attained.

SIDE EFFECTS

10. **What side effects can be expected from parenteral iron therapy?**

Anaphylactoid reactions can occur in <1% of patients treated with parenteral iron therapy.[6,32,35,36] This reaction is more commonly associated with iron dextran than with ferric gluconate and iron sucrose.[35,36] As a result, a 25-mg test dose of iron dextran should be given intramuscularly or by IV infusion over 5 to 10 minutes. If headache, chest pain, anxiety, or signs of hypotension are not experienced, the remainder of the dose can be administered parenterally. Nevertheless, delayed reactions (e.g., fever, urticaria, arthralgias, and lymphadenopathy) have occurred 24 to 48 hours after large doses of IV iron dextran and have lasted 3 to 7 days in 1% to 2% of patients.[37] A test dose is not indicated for ferric gluconate and iron sucrose because of the lower incidence of serious anaphylactoid reactions with these agents. Other side effects seen with parenteral iron agents include hypotension, nausea and vomiting, cramps, and diarrhea. Parenteral iron medications should not be mixed with or added to other medications or parenteral nutrition solutions for IV infusion.

MEGALOBLASTIC ANEMIAS

Megaloblastic anemia is a common disorder that may have several etiologies: (1) anemia associated with vitamin B_{12} deficiency; (2) anemia associated with folic acid deficiency; or (3) anemia caused by metabolic or inherited defects associated with decreased ability to utilize vitamin B_{12} or folic acid.[38,39]

Megaloblastosis results from impaired DNA synthesis in replicating cells and is recognized by a large immature nucleus. RNA and protein synthesis remain unaffected, and the cytoplasm matures normally. Megaloblastic changes can be observed microscopically in RBCs and in proliferating cells (e.g., in the cervix, skin, GI tract).[38]

Although the clinical effects of vitamin B_{12} and folic acid deficiencies may be different in various organ systems, they are similar in their effects on the hematopoietic system. Typically, macrocytic anemia develops slowly and can be identified by large, oval, well-hemoglobinized red cells; anisocytosis; and nuclear remnants. The reticulocyte count is low, and the bilirubin level is elevated. Thrombocytopenia is present, and the platelets are large. Leukopenia occurs with hypersegmentation of polymorphonuclear leukocyte nuclei. If biopsied, the bone marrow is markedly hypercellular. Nuclear immaturity is present, but the megaloblasts have normal maturation of the cytoplasm. Iron stores in the marrow are increased as a result of the intramedullary hemolysis. Symptoms include fatigue; exaggeration of pre-existing cardiovascular or pulmonary problems; a sore, pale, smooth tongue; diarrhea or constipation; and anorexia. Edema and urticaria also may be present.

Vitamin B_{12} Deficiency Anemia

Vitamin B_{12} Metabolism

Deficiency and poor utilization of vitamin B_{12} are two mechanisms for the development of megaloblastic anemia. Cobalamin (vitamin B_{12}) is naturally synthesized by microorganisms, and because humans are incapable of synthesizing vitamin B_{12}, it must be provided nutritionally. Although microorganisms found on roots and legumes of plants provide a source of vitamin B_{12} in vegetarian foods, animal protein is the primary dietary source of vitamin B_{12}. Meats richest in vitamin B_{12} include oysters, clams, liver, and kidney; moderate amounts of vitamin B_{12} are found in muscle meats, milk products, and egg yolks.[38]

The typical Western diet contains 5 to 15 μg/day of vitamin B_{12},[40,41] an amount sufficient to replace the 1 μg lost daily.[32] The total body stores of vitamin B_{12} range from 2,000 to 5,000 μg, much of which is stored in the liver.[42] Because body stores are extensive, 3 to 4 years are required before symptoms of vitamin B_{12} deficiency develop.

In the stomach, the vitamin B_{12} contained in food is released from protein complexes and bound to intrinsic factor, which protects the B_{12} from degradation by GI microorganisms. Intrinsic factor is essential for the absorption of vitamin B_{12}. Specific mucosal receptors in the distal small ileum allow for attachment of the intrinsic factor: B_{12} complex. B_{12} is then transferred to the ileal cell and finally to portal vein blood. The intrinsic factor mechanism is saturated by 1.5 to 3 μg of B_{12}; however, passive diffusion can occur when B_{12} is present in large quantities.

After vitamin B_{12} is absorbed, it is bound to specific β-globulin transport proteins, transcobalamin I, II, and III. Transcobalamin II is responsible for transporting B_{12} through cell membranes and delivering it to the liver and other organs; 50% to 90% of the total body stores of B_{12} are found in the liver. All three of the transport proteins prevent loss of B_{12} in the urine, sweat, and other body secretions. In the liver, vitamin B_{12} is converted to coenzyme B_{12}, which is essential for hematopoiesis, maintenance of myelin throughout the entire nervous system, and production of epithelial cells.[43,44]

Pathogenesis and Evaluation of Vitamin B12 Deficiency

Vitamin B_{12} deficiency may result from several etiologies: (1) decreased intake, absorption, transport, and utilization; or (2) increased requirements, metabolic consumption, destruction, and excretion. Strict vegetarians most frequently present with signs and symptoms of vitamin B_{12} deficiency. This population also can be iron deficient concurrently because iron is poorly absorbed from plant sources, and the microcytosis of iron-deficiency anemia can mask the vitamin B_{12} deficiency–induced macrocytic appearance of RBCs. Other causes of vitamin B_{12} deficiency include inadequate proteolytic degradation of vitamin B_{12} from protein, or congenital intrinsic factor deficiency. In addition, the gastric mucosa may be unable to produce intrinsic factor under conditions such as partial gastrectomy, autoimmune destruction (e.g., addisonian or juvenile pernicious anemia), or destruction of the gastric mucosa from caustic agents such as lye.[38]

Pernicious anemia results from the inability to absorb vitamin B_{12}. It may be caused by inherited atrophic gastropathy accompanied by reduced intrinsic factor and hydrochloric acid secretion, or it may be acquired as a result of gastrectomy, pancreatic disease, or malnutrition. Pernicious anemia occurs commonly in patients with thyrotoxicosis, Hashimoto's thyroiditis, vitiligo, rheumatoid arthritis, or gastric cancer. Less often, anti-intrinsic factor antibodies have been observed in the serum or gastric juices of some patients with pernicious anemia.

The onset of the pernicious anemia is insidious. Patients generally do not feel well for 6 to 12 months and often complain of at least two of the following triad of symptoms: weakness, sore tongue, and symmetric numbness or tingling in the extremities. The neurologic symptoms of vitamin B_{12} deficiency are associated with a defect in myelin synthesis and often are described as glove-stocking peripheral neuropathy or nonspecific complaints such as tinnitus, neuritis, vertigo, and headaches. Patients with neurologic symptoms have difficulty determining position and vibration sense and have an increase in deep tendon reflexes. These symptoms may progress to spastic ataxia, motor weakness, and paraparesis. However, no correlation exists between the extent of neurologic manifestations and the severity of anemia. Mental changes (dementia) may occur in severe cases. Anorexia, pallor, and dyspnea on exertion are bothersome symptoms that may overshadow the diagnostic triad.

Laboratory Evaluation

In general, the serum vitamin B_{12} level reliably reflects vitamin B_{12} tissue stores. The microbiologic and radioisotope dilution assays have variable normal ranges. False low vitamin B_{12} concentrations may be observed in patients with folic acid deficiency, transcobalamin I deficiency, multiple myeloma, or those who take very large doses of vitamin C. Falsely elevated vitamin B_{12} concentrations may be observed in patients with myeloproliferative diseases, hepatomas, autoimmune diseases, monoblastic leukemias, and histiocytic lymphomas.[45] In active liver disease, vitamin B_{12} liver stores can be released into the serum.[32] Thus, efflux of vitamin B_{12} may be identified by measuring serum methylmalonic acid and homocysteine levels.[40] These tests may assist in differentiating between folate and vitamin B_{12} deficiency. Once vitamin B_{12} therapy has been instituted, serum levels of these chemicals decrease if true vitamin B_{12} deficiency is present.[38]

The cause of vitamin B_{12} deficiency may be determined by the use of the Schilling test. Patients with pernicious anemia are not able to absorb vitamin B_{12} because intrinsic factor is not available for binding. The Schilling test evaluates vitamin B_{12} absorption in the following manner. A small tracer dose of radioactive vitamin B_{12} (0.5 to 2 μg of CN-[^{57}Co] Cbl) is given orally. Two hours later, unlabeled vitamin B_{12} (1 mg IM) is administered to saturate vitamin B_{12} serum-binding proteins. Urinary excretion of radioactive vitamin B_{12} reveals the degree of absorption. Urinary excretion of <5% (normal, 15% to 50%) is consistent with pernicious anemia. Renal insufficiency, low urine output, or incomplete urine collection can result in a falsely low vitamin B_{12} excretion.[46]

Some patients produce intrinsic factor but are still unable to absorb dietary vitamin B_{12}. Malabsorption can be caused by intestinal bacteria that usurp vitamin B_{12}, achlorhydria, pancreatic insufficiency, inadequate disassociation of vitamin B_{12} from proteins, or lack of intrinsic factor receptors secondary to ileal loops, bypass, or surgical resection.[47] A food Schilling test in which vitamin B_{12} is administered as a protein-bound form, can determine whether the patient is able to disassociate proteins from vitamin B_{12}.[39,48]

Pernicious Anemia
SIGNS, SYMPTOMS, AND LABORATORY FINDINGS

11. **C.L., a 60-year-old Scandinavian man, is seen by a private physician. C.L. has a 1-year history of weakness and emotional instability. He also complains of a painful tongue, alternating constipation and diarrhea, and a tingling sensation in both feet. Pertinent findings on physical examination include pallor, red tongue, loss of vibratory sense in the lower extremities, disorientation, muscle weakness, and ataxia.**

Significant laboratory findings include the following: Hgb, 9 g/dL (normal, 14 to 18); Hct, 29% (normal, 42% to 52%); MCV, 110 m³ (normal, 76 to 100); MCH, 38 pg (normal, 27 to 33); MCHC, 34% (normal, 33% to 37%); reticulocytes, 0.4 % (normal, 0.5% to 1.5%); poikilocytosis and anisocytosis on the blood smear; white blood cell (WBC) count, 4,000/mm³ (normal, 3,200 to 9,800); platelets, 105,000/mm³ (normal, 130,000 to 400,000); serum iron, 80 g/dL (normal, 50 to 160); TIBC, 300 g/dL (normal, 200 to 1,000); ferritin, 150 ng/mL (normal, 15 to 200); RBC folate, 300 ng/mL (normal, 140 to 460); serum vitamin B_{12}, 100 pg/mL (normal, 200 to 1,000); and <4% excretion on the Schilling test (normal, 15% to 50%). What signs, symptoms, and laboratory findings are typical of pernicious anemia in C.L.?

[SI units: Hgb, 90 g/L; Hct, 0.29; MCV, 110 fL; MCH, 38 pg; MCHC, 0.34; reticulocytes, 0.004; WBC count, 4 × 10⁹/L; platelets, 105 × 10⁹/L (normal, 250 to 400); iron, 14.38 μmol/L; TIBC, 53.91 μmol/L; ferritin, 150 μ/L; RBC folate, 679.8 nmol/L; vitamin B_{12}, 73.78 pmol/L]

C.L.'s signs and symptoms are classic for pernicious anemia. This disease occurs equally in both sexes (primarily in individuals of Northern European descent), with an average onset of 60 years. Pernicious anemia develops from a lack of gastric intrinsic factor production, which causes vitamin B_{12} malabsorption and, ultimately, vitamin B_{12} deficiency. C.L.'s signs and symptoms of vitamin B_{12} deficiency include painful red tongue, loss of vibratory sense in his lower extremities, vertigo, and emotional instability.

The elevated MCV suggests megaloblastic anemia. Folate and iron are two other factors that may affect the MCV and should be evaluated during the workup of a patient for anemia. In this case, C.L.'s folate and iron are normal, but his serum vitamin B_{12} level is low. The presence of poikilocytosis and anisocytosis observed in the blood smear represent ineffective erythropoiesis. Other cell lineages also may be affected in the bone marrow. Erythroid hypercellularity along with a decrease in the myeloid cells (leukocytes and platelets) increases the erythroid:myeloid ratio in C.L. The patient's low serum vitamin B_{12} levels and the low results obtained from the Schilling test are compatible with the diagnosis of pernicious anemia.

TREATMENT

12. **How should C.L.'s pernicious anemia be treated? How soon can a response be expected?**

C.L. should receive parenteral vitamin B_{12} in a dose sufficient to provide not only the daily requirement of approximately 2 μg, but also the amount needed to replenish tissue stores (about 2,000 to 5,000 μg; average, 4,000 μg). To replete vitamin B_{12} stores, cyanocobalamin 30 to 1000 μg is given intramuscularly in accordance with various regimens. C.L. may receive 100 μg of cyanocobalamin daily for 1 week, then 100 μg every other day for 2 weeks, followed by 100 μg every 3 to 4 days for 2 to 3 weeks. A monthly maintenance dose of cyanocobalamin 100 μg would then be required for the remainder of C.L.'s life. Another treatment option may be cyanocobalamin 1,000 μg once a week for 4 to 6 weeks followed by 1,000 μg per month for lifetime maintenance therapy.[49] IM or deep subcutaneous administration provides sustained release of vitamin B_{12} with better utilization compared with rapid IV infusion for the treatment of pernicious anemia. An intranasal cyanocobalamin gel (Nascobal) is available for maintenance therapy, after the patient has achieved hematologic remission.

With adequate vitamin B_{12} therapy, one can expect the following response. Neurologic symptoms should improve within 24 hours. However, with longstanding vitamin B_{12} deficiency, several months may pass before some symptoms are relieved; other symptoms may never resolve. Hematologic parameters should begin to improve within the first few days. The bone marrow becomes normoblastic within 48 hours, the reticulocyte count should peak around day 5 of therapy, and the Hct should return to normal in 1 to 2 months. Because the rapid production of RBCs may increase potassium demand, serum potassium should be monitored and potassium supplementation provided as necessary. Peripheral blood counts should be obtained every 3 to 6 months to evaluate the adequacy of therapy. If maintenance therapy is discontinued, pernicious anemia will recur within 5 years.

Oral Vitamin B₁₂

13. What factors affect the oral absorption of vitamin B_{12}? When is oral vitamin B_{12} therapy an effective alternative to parenteral therapy?

The amount of vitamin B_{12} that can be absorbed orally from a single dose or meal ranges from 1 to 5 μg; approximately 5 μg of vitamin B_{12} is absorbed daily from the average American diet. The percentage of vitamin B_{12} absorbed decreases with increasing doses. About 50% of a 1 to 2 μg dose of vitamin B_{12} is absorbed, whereas only about 5% of a 20μg dose is absorbed.[48] Doses of greater than 100 μg must be ingested to absorb 5 μg of vitamin B_{12}. Patients like C.L., who have pernicious anemia treated with combination preparations containing vitamin B_{12} and intrinsic factor, can become refractory to the therapy because antibodies form against intrinsic factor that is derived from hog mucosa. Therefore, preparations containing hog mucosal intrinsic factor are not recommended. Although intrinsic factor is necessary for optimal vitamin B_{12} absorption, oral therapy for pernicious anemia using high dosages of oral cyanocobalamin (1,000 to 2,000 μg) may be indicated in patients who refuse or cannot receive parenteral therapy.[50,51] Overall, oral vitamin B_{12} therapy cannot be recommended routinely for primary treatment because noncompliance or lack of response places the patient at substantial risk for significant neurologic damage. However, oral cyanocobalamin (1,000 to 2,000 μg) can also be used as maintenance therapy.[50–52] Patients receiving oral vitamin B_{12} therapy should be monitored more frequently to ensure compliance with therapy.

Anemias After Gastrectomy

14. F.M. has just undergone a total gastrectomy for recurrent nonhealing ulcers. What form(s) of anemia would be expected to develop in a postgastrectomy patient? Should F.M. receive prophylactic vitamin B_{12}?

Partial or total gastrectomy often results in anemia, particularly pernicious anemia, because the source of intrinsic factor is lost, and oral vitamin B_{12} absorption will be impaired.[38] The hematologic and neurologic abnormalities associated with B_{12} deficiency do not develop until existing vitamin B_{12} stores are depleted (about 2 to 3 years). Nevertheless, parenteral prophylactic vitamin B_{12} should be administered to this post–total gastrectomy patient. Because the vitamin B_{12} stores are not currently depleted, maintenance therapy, as discussed in Question 12, should be adequate for F.M.

Malabsorption of Vitamin B₁₂
SIGNS AND SYMPTOMS

15. P.G., a 55-year-old woman, complained of progressive confusion and lethargy 9 months ago. A CBC at that time revealed only mild leukocytosis. Today, she comes to the emergency department with a 4-week history of frequent (three to five per day) stools containing bright red blood. She reports continued lethargy, dizziness, ataxia, and paresthesias in her hands and feet.

Laboratory findings of interest include the following: Hgb, 12.8 g/dL (normal, 12 to 16); MCV, 90 m³ (normal, 76 to 100); iron, 150 μg/dL (normal, 50 to 160); iron/TIBC, 11% (normal, >15%); B₁₂, 94 pg/mL (normal, 200 to 1,000); folate, 21 ng/mL (normal, 7 to 25); hypersegmented polymorphonuclear leukocytes (PMNs); bilirubin, 3.0 mg/dL (normal, 0.1 to 1.0); and lactate dehydrogenase (LDH), 520 U/L (normal, 50 to 150). A subsequent bone marrow aspirate demonstrates megaloblastic erythropoiesis, giant metamyelocytes, and a low stainable iron. A barium swallow and follow-through show numerous jejunal and duodenal diverticuli. Jejunal and duodenal aspirates reveal aerobic and anaerobic bacterial overgrowth. Radioactive vitamin B_{12} urinary excretion from the Schilling test is <4% (normal, 15% to 20%). What signs, symptoms, and laboratory findings are typical for vitamin B_{12} deficiency in P.G.?

[SI units: Hgb, 120 g/L; MCV, 90 fL; iron, 25.87 μmol/L; B_{12}, 69.35 pmol/L; folate, 47.59 nmol/L; bilirubin, 51.3 μmol/L; LDH, 520 U/L]

The signs and symptoms in P.G. that are consistent with B_{12} deficiency include confusion, dizziness, ataxia, and paresthesias. Other signs and symptoms may be caused by other underlying conditions. For example, her lethargy may be the result of prolonged blood loss secondary to diverticulitis.

Notably, P.G. initially presented with a mild leukocytosis. Evaluation 9 months later shows a low Hgb, a low serum vitamin B_{12} level, and hypersegmented PMNs. The high LDH and bilirubin levels reflect intramedullary hemolysis of megaloblastic RBCs consistent with vitamin B_{12} deficiency, even though the MCV is within normal limits. The presence of megaloblastic erythropoiesis and giant metamyelocytes in the bone marrow also is consistent with vitamin B_{12} deficiency.

P.G.'s history of bloody stools and diverticuli suggests substantial long-term blood loss, which increased demand for iron and vitamin B_{12} to replace RBCs. Concurrent iron deficiency may mask megaloblastic changes in RBCs, which explains the suspiciously normal MCV (dimorphic anemia). The serum folate concentration is also falsely normal. Even though the RBC folate level is likely to be low, serum folate concentrations are normal because monoglutamated folates leak from cells into the serum in vitamin B_{12} deficient states.

TREATMENT

16. How should P.G.'s vitamin B_{12} deficiency be treated?

The cause of vitamin B_{12} malabsorption must be corrected before P.G. is given oral vitamin B_{12} therapy. The presence of diverticuli is not the cause of vitamin B_{12} malabsorption because diverticuli typically do not extend into the distal ileum. Instead, given P.G.'s medical history, the most likely cause of vitamin B_{12} malabsorption is bacterial usurpation of luminal vitamin B_{12}. P.G. should first be treated with a broad-spectrum antibiotic, such as tetracycline or a sulfonamide for 7 to 10 days. Thereafter, a repeat Schilling test should be normal, and P.G. can begin daily oral vitamin B_{12} supplementation to replenish her body stores. In this case, normal levels of intrinsic factor permit oral therapy. The recommended daily dose of vitamin B_{12} is 25 to 250 μg. Following antibiotic therapy, P.G. also should begin to absorb vitamin B_{12} in her diet.

Folic Acid Deficiency Anemia

Folic Acid Metabolism

Folate is abundant in virtually all food sources, especially fresh green vegetables, fruits, yeast, and animal protein. The average American diet provides 50 to 2,000 μg of folate per day; however, excessive or prolonged cooking (>15 minutes) in large quantities of water destroys a high percentage of the folate that is contained in food.[53,54] Human requirements for folate vary with age and depend on the rate of metabolism and cell turnover but are generally 3 μg/kg per day.[54] The minimum daily adult requirement of folate is 50 μg, but because absorption from food is incomplete, a daily intake of 200 μg is recommended. Folate requirements are increased in conditions in which the metabolic rate and rate of cellular division are increased (e.g., pregnancy, infancy, infection, malignancies, hemolytic anemia). The following are estimates of daily folate requirements based on age and growth demands: children, 3.3 μg/kg; infants, 16 to 32 μg; pregnant or lactating women, 400 to 800 μg.[54,55]

Dietary folic acid is in the polyglutamate form and must be enzymatically deconjugated in the GI tract to the monoglutamate form before it is absorbed. Once absorbed, the inactive dihydrofolate (FH_2) must be converted to active tetrahydrofolate (FH_4, folinic acid) by dihydrofolate reductase (DHFR).

In contrast to the large stores of vitamin B_{12}, the body's folate stores are relatively small (about 5 to 10 mg). Therefore, deficiency and subsequent megaloblastic anemia may occur within 3 to 4 months of decreased folate intake.

Predisposing Factors

Folate deficiency is most commonly associated with alcoholism, rapid cell turnover, and dietary deficiency. In alcoholics, the daily intake of the folate contained in food may be restricted or absent. In addition, enterohepatic recirculation of folate may be impaired by the toxic effect of alcohol on hepatic cells. Folate deficiency also may develop during the third trimester of pregnancy as a result of a marginal diet and the rapid metabolism of the fetus. Folate coenzymes are required for most metabolic pathways (Fig. 86-2). Therefore, folate deficiency will develop in any condition of rapid cellular turnover (e.g., hemolytic anemias, hemoglobinopathies, sideroblastic anemia, leukemias, lymphomas, multiple myeloma) or a diet lacking in folate (e.g., food faddism or a weight-loss diet). Folate deficiency also may occur with chronic hemodialysis, diseases that impair absorption from the small intestine (e.g., sprue, regional enteritis), extensive jejunal resections, and drugs that alter folate metabolism (e.g., trimethoprim, pyrimethamine, methotrexate, sulfasalazine, oral contraceptives, anticonvulsants).[38,56–58] Few patients have inborn errors of folate metabolism.[38,59]

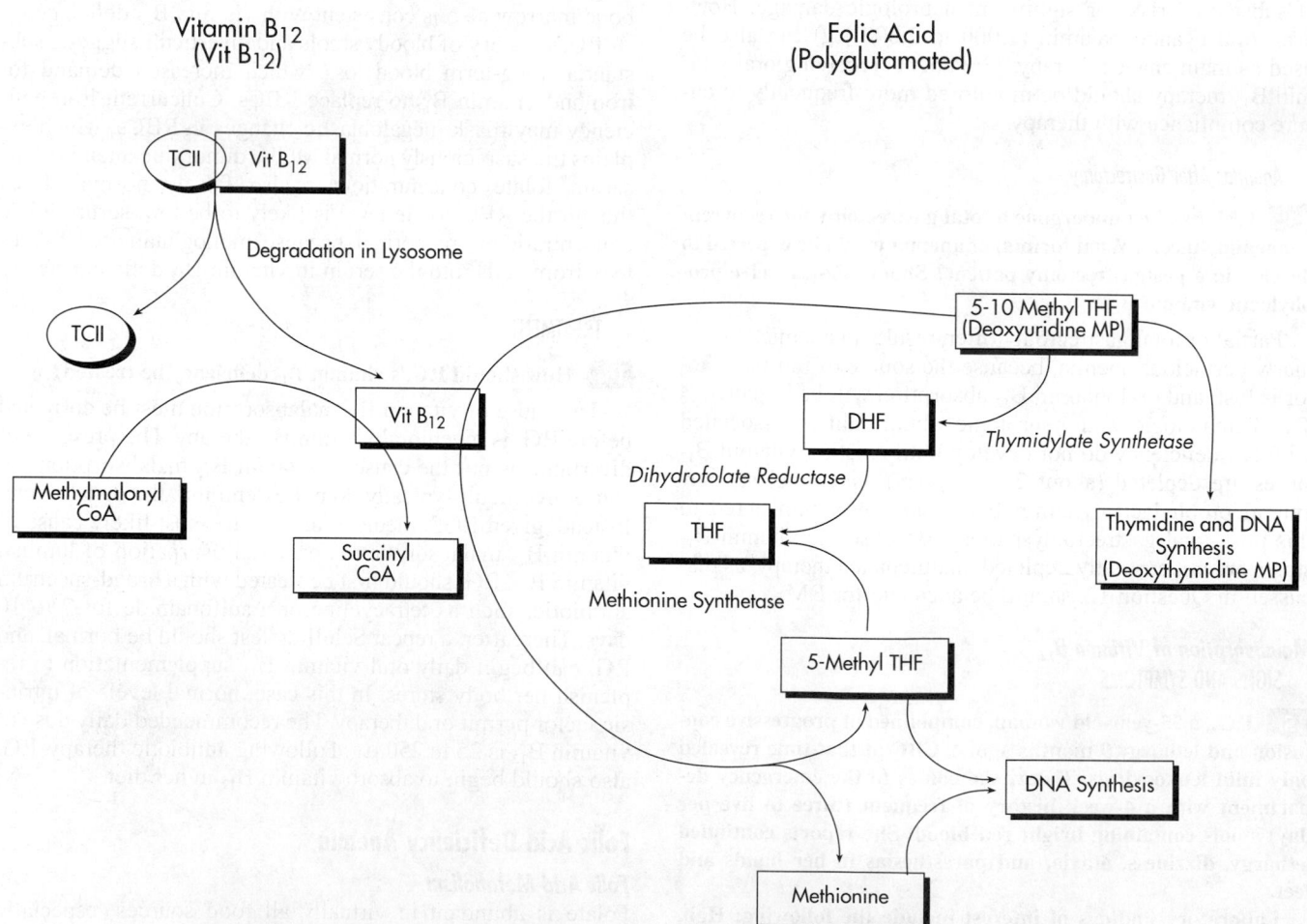

FIGURE 86-2 Intracellular metabolic pathways. Vitamin B_{12} and folic acid are both necessary for nucleic acid precursors used for DNA synthesis. DHF, dihydrofolate; MP, monophosphate; TCII, transcobalamine II; THF, tetrahydrofolate.

The evaluation of megaloblastic anemia must be thorough because indiscriminate use of "shotgun" hematinic therapy may be dangerous. Large doses of folate can partially reverse hematologic abnormalities caused by vitamin B_{12} deficiency; however, folate cannot correct neurologic damage caused by vitamin B_{12} deficiency. Therefore, folate deficiency absolutely must be differentiated from vitamin B_{12} deficiency before folate therapy is initiated. Otherwise, the progression of the neurologic sequelae of vitamin B_{12} deficiency can occur.

17. T.J., a malnourished-appearing woman in her second trimester of pregnancy, presents to the local health clinic for her regular checkup. She is a multiparous, 22-year-old woman who ran away from home when she was 16. T.J. has a 7-year history of excessive alcohol intake and has been using cocaine frequently for 3 years. She lives with her boyfriend and her 19-month-old daughter. During both pregnancies, T.J. lost 8 to 10 lbs during the first trimester secondary to nausea, vomiting, and anorexia. Her only complaints are dyspnea on exertion, palpitations, and diarrhea.

Pertinent laboratory values include the following: Hct, 25.5% (normal, 40% to 44%); MCV, 112 m³ (normal, 76 to 100); MCH, 34 pg (normal, 27 to 33); RBC, 1.1×10^6/mm³ (normal, 3.5 to 5.0); folate, 30 ng/mL (normal, in RBCs 140 to 960); serum vitamin B_{12}, 250 pg/mL (normal, 200 to 1,000); reticulocytes, 1% (normal, 0.5 to 1.5); platelets, 75,000/mm³ (normal, 130,000 to 400,000); WBC count, 2,000/mm³ (normal, 3,200 to 9,800) with hypersegmented PMNs; LDH, 450 U/L (normal, 50 to 150); and bilirubin, 1.5 mg/dL (normal, 0.1 to 1). T.J. is not taking any prescription medications. What factors make T.J. at risk for folate deficiency?

[SI units: Hct, 0.255; MCV, 112 fl. (normal, 76 to 100); MCH, 34 pg (normal, 27 to 33); RBC count, 1.1×10^{12}/L (normal, 3.5 to 5); folate, 67.98 nmol/L (normal, 317 to 2175); vitamin B_{12}, 184 pmol/L; folate, 184.45 pmol/ (normal, 150 to 750); reticulocytes, 0.01; platelets, 75×10^9/L (normal, 130 to 400); WBC count, 2×10^9/L; LDH, 450 U/L (normal, 50 to 150); bilirubin, 25.65 mmol/L (normal, 2 to 18)]

T.J. has had a history of risk factors for folate deficiency since she was 16. The diagnosis of folate deficiency is plausible, considering folate deficiency may develop in a matter of weeks to months. Like most folate-deficient patients, T.J. has more than one risk factor for folate deficiency. Cocaine and alcohol, together with multiparity complicated by anorexia, nausea, and vomiting, could lead to poor nutrition. Alcohol has toxic effects on the intestinal mucosa and interferes with folate utilization by the bone marrow.[60] T.J. should be asked specifically about her dietary habits and recent weight history. She may have a folate-poor diet for financial reasons or because she is overcooking her food. Alternatively, cocaine may be causing anorexia. The nutritional intake of people who abuse alcohol and drugs is often poor.

Diagnosis and Management

18. Which laboratory values support the diagnosis of folate deficiency? How should T.J. be managed and monitored?

T.J.'s laboratory values reflect macrocytic anemia (Hct, 25.5%; MCV, 112 μm³) with pancytopenia (reduced number of RBCs, WBCs, and platelets). Serum vitamin B_{12} concentrations reflect normal vitamin B_{12} stores, but folate stores are inadequate as exemplified by the low RBC folate concentration, pancytopenia, and macrocytic anemia.

Serum folate concentrations generally reflect folate balance over the past 3 weeks, although one balanced meal can raise serum levels and falsely elevate body stores. Tissue folate stores are more accurately reflected by the RBC polyglutamated folate content, which is approximately 10 to 30 times the corresponding serum folate concentrations.[61] Hemolysis or vitamin B_{12} deficiency causes leakage of monoglutamated folates from cell, thereby falsely elevating serum folate levels.[38,39]

T.J. should be counseled regarding her nutritional and social habits. Because the estimated total body folate store is only about 5 to 10 mg, 1 mg of folic acid given daily for 2 to 3 weeks should be more than adequate to replace her storage pool of folate. However, higher dosages (up to 5 mg) may be needed if absorption is compromised by alcohol or other factors.[62] Once stores are replenished, T.J. should continue folate supplements throughout her pregnancy and lactation period. She should be reassessed after the course of therapy to determine response to therapy and if the cause of the folate deficiency has been corrected. Supplementation with folic acid 1 mg/day may be required as long as risk factors are present. T.J.'s fetus is unlikely to develop folate deficiency because maternal folate is preferentially delivered to the fetus[57] (see Chapter 46).

T.J.'s response to therapy may be monitored by several different parameters. Although bone marrow aspirates are not obtained routinely, the RBC morphology should begin to revert back to normal within 24 to 48 hours after therapy is initiated, and hypersegmented neutrophils should disappear in the periphery in about 1 week. Serum chemistry and hemogram studies should begin to normalize within 10 days. The reticulocyte count should increase by day 2 to 3 and peak by day 10. LDH and bilirubin values should normalize in 1 to 3 weeks. Finally, the anemia should be corrected in 1 to 2 months. Once anemia is corrected, 0.1 mg of folate as a nutritional supplement should be adequate for maintenance treatment. If patients with underlying vitamin B_{12} deficiency are inappropriately treated with folate, neurologic sequelae will persist, and macrocytic anemia will improve but will not resolve completely.

SICKLE CELL ANEMIA
Pathogenesis

Sickle cell anemia is an inherited hemoglobin disorder characterized by a DNA substitution where the β-globin gene is located. Hemoglobin is a quaternary structure comprising two α-globin chains and two β-globin chains ($\alpha_2\beta_2$) in adults. The β-globin gene locus encodes several globin gene products during the course of development. These products result from transcription of the embryonic globin gene (ε), duplicated fetal genes (γ), and adult genes (σ and β). During fetal development, the γ-globin is the primary β-globin expressed, forming fetal hemoglobin (HbF or $\alpha_2\gamma_2$). Normally, the period from birth to approximately 3 to 6 months of age is marked by the replacement of γ-globin with β-globin, giving rise to the adult form of hemoglobin (HbA, $\alpha_2\beta_2$). Low levels of γ-globin persist throughout life, and HbF, present in F cells, may account for approximately 1% of the total hemoglobin content.[63,64] F cell numbers may increase in response to erythropoietic stress.[63] β^S represents the inheritance of the sickle β-globin gene.[62,63]

Sickle cell anemia results from a DNA substitution of thymidine for adenine in the glutamic acid codon forming a B6 valine instead of glutamic acid.[63–65] The hemoglobin produced from such a substitution has a more negative charge than normal HbA, and the deoxygenated state favors hemoglobin aggregation and polymerization, which forms sickled RBCs.[64,65] Sickled RBCs are more rigid and may become "lodged" when passing through microvasculature, resulting in vascular occlusions.

In addition, the sickled RBC surface contains rearranged aminophospholipids, and this alters the ability of the RBCs to initiate coagulation, adhere to vascular endothelium, and activate complement. These abnormal interactions with other cell types produce several complications such as anemia, vaso-occlusive episodes, multiorgan damage, and increased susceptibility to polysaccharide-encapsulated organisms.[64] For these reasons, much effort has been focused on neonatal diagnosis to reduce morbidity and mortality in children younger than 3 years of age.[66]

There is more than one inheritance pattern that results in abnormal hemoglobin polymerization. Patients with sickle cell anemia are homozygous, inheriting a sickle gene from each parent ($\alpha_2\beta_{2S}$), whereas patients with sickle cell trait are heterozygous and have inherited the sickle cell gene from one parent and the HbA gene from the other parent ($\alpha_2\beta^A\beta^S$). Other inheritance patterns include patients with a sickle cell gene and an HbC gene (where glutamic acid is substituted for lysine B6 [$\alpha_2\beta^S\beta^C$]). Finally, patients may inherit the sickle cell gene and the B-thalassemic gene ($\alpha_2\beta^S\beta^{Sthal}$), in which case the clinical course is less severe than with patients diagnosed with sickle cell anemia. Hematologic abnormalities are more commonly observed in patients with sickle cell anemia and less often in those with sickle cell hemoglobin C disease or sickle cell B_0-thalassemia.[63,64]

Laboratory Evaluation

Patients who have inherited the sickle cell gene can be diagnosed by electrophoretic procedures that separate different forms of hemoglobin. Fetal hemoglobin levels vary among patients. Often, an increase in the MCHC is used to predict the likelihood of polymer formation and vascular occlusion.

In the patient with sickle cell anemia, hematologic studies are informative. The WBC and platelet counts often are elevated, but the WBC differential is normal.[64] The reticulocyte count may range from 5% to 15%, and the MCV may be elevated. If MCV values are within the normal range, one must consider iron deficiency or B_0-thalassemia. Sickled cells may also be visually observed in poorly oxygenated blood of a patient with sickle cell anemia. In contrast, a patient with the SS trait should have normal RBC morphology and WBC, reticulocyte, and platelet counts. Sickled cells are rarely observed. In patients with sickle cell B_0 thalassemia, hematologic abnormalities vary depending on the amount of HbA present. This form may be difficult to distinguish from sickle cell anemia; RBC microcytosis may be the only differentiating parameter.[64]

Clinical Course and Management

Patients carrying the SS trait experience milder symptoms than those with sickle cell anemia. The kidney is the organ most commonly affected by microinfarction, which occurs in the renal medulla and impairs the kidney's ability to concentrate urine. During pregnancy, there is an increased frequency of urinary tract infections and hematuria, but vaso-occlusive events are uncommon. If they do occur, they usually are caused by hypoxic conditions resulting from excessive exercise or high altitudes.

Sickle cell hemoglobin C disease is usually associated with few clinical complications. These patients may have a normal physical examination with only splenomegaly. Patients are at risk for bacterial infections, and because of elevated hemoglobin levels, they may suffer from ocular, orthopedic, and pulmonary vaso-occlusive events.[64]

Unfortunately, the treatment of sickle cell anemia is largely directed toward prophylaxis against infections and supportive management of vaso-occlusive crises. The clinical course among patients with sickle cell disease is quite variable and difficult to predict. Some patients suffer from a multitude of health problems. Organs such as the kidneys, retina, spleen, and bones are frequent sites of vaso-occlusive events because these sites have a relatively low pH and oxygen tension. The health care professional often must manage complications such as pain, anemia, and infections, as well as cardiac, pulmonary, neurologic, hepatobiliary, obstetric/gynecologic, ocular, dermatologic, or orthopedic complications. The management of these complications is organ specific and aimed at supportive interventions.

Hemolytic Anemia

Hemolytic anemia is caused by splenic sequestration of abnormal RBCs. Sequestration reduces the RBC life span from 120 days to 15 to 25 days and elevates the reticulocyte count. Erythropoietin response is typically blunted for the degree of anemia, which may be a result of concurrent kidney dysfunction. Some patients may even experience aplastic anemia (bone marrow failure) when extensive hemolysis is accompanied by inadequate bone marrow response. However, it is usually self-limiting. Hemolytic anemia may also present in patients with glucose-6-phosphate dehydrogenase deficiency. Cardiac manifestations include high-output failure secondary to anemia. Management of the underlying anemia may include splenectomy following the first splenic sequestration event. Alternatively, patients may be managed with transfusions and careful observation.[64,65]

Infections

Infections occur more often in patients with sickle cell anemia because both the complement pathway and granulocyte function may be altered along with B-cell immunity. Also, impaired splenic function increases the risk for infection from polysaccharide-encapsulated bacteria such as *Streptococcus pneumoniae* and *Haemophilus influenzae*. Pneumonia caused by *S. pneumoniae,* mycoplasma, or viruses may worsen hypoxia, causing progression to vaso-occlusion and acute chest syndrome (chest pain in the presence of a local infiltrate on chest radiograph). Because of such complications, the prophylactic administration of penicillin has significantly reduced morbidity and mortality from pneumonia in children younger than 3 years of age. Pulmonary complications from pneumonia or vascular occlusion also can lead to right-sided heart failure. Other infectious conditions such as osteomyelitis from *Staphylococcus aureus* or *Salmonella ty-*

phimurium or urinary tract infections caused by *Escherichia coli* are common complications in patients with sickle cell anemia.[63–65] Because of the susceptibility of patients with sickle cell anemia to infections, antibiotic therapy should be instituted at the earliest sign of infection. Polyvalent pneumococcal vaccination of children between 6 and 12 months of age and a booster 6 to 12 months later has been recommended. Because sickle cell patients typically respond poorly, only 50% of patients will be protected by vaccination.[66]

Vascular Occlusion Episodes

Vascular occlusion episodes, or "sickle cell crises," cause severe pain and organ damage. The pain typically lasts 2 to 6 days and should be managed with narcotic analgesics (morphine or morphine derivatives). Narcotic addiction may occur over time but can be prevented by providing the patient with only a few days supply of analgesics following the crisis.[63,64]

Neurologic Complications

Neurologic complications are age dependent. Stroke most commonly occurs in the first decade of life, whereas intracerebral hemorrhage is a complication associated with adulthood. Approximately 50% of patients experience recurrent strokes within 3 years unless they are managed by RBC transfusion therapy. Therapeutic goals are aimed at maintaining the hemoglobin S level below 30%.[64]

Renal and Genital Complications

Renal and genital complications are common in sickle cell disease because the environment (hypoxic, acidotic, and hypertonic) predisposes the renal medulla or corpus cavernosum to infarction. Sequelae include reduced potassium excretion, hyperuricemia, hematuria, hyposthenuria, and renal failure. Patients with renal disease may have inappropriately low levels of erythropoietin as well, and men experiencing occlusion of the corpus cavernosum can experience acute or chronic priapism. Conservative management includes IV fluid administration and pain control. Refractory cases may require transfusions or surgery.[64,65]

Microinfarctions

Microinfarctions often produce ophthalmic, hepatic, orthopedic, and obstetric/gynecologic complications as well. The reader is referred to other references addressing these topics in more detail.[64,65]

Treatment for Frequent Vaso-occlusive Crises

Hemoglobin F has a protective effect against hemoglobin polymerization. Investigators have observed that patients with hemoglobin F levels >20% experience a relatively mild or benign course. Hydroxyurea has been found to increase hemoglobin F synthesis that may in turn decrease sickling of RBCs and the occurrence of clinical sequelae.[62,67,68] Hydroxyurea is used prophylactically in patients with recurrent moderate to severe vaso-occlusive crises but not in treatment of the crises. Studies have shown that increased levels of hemoglobin F synthesis to 15 to 20% may reduce the frequency of vaso-occlusive crises.[62,69] The use of hydroxyurea in the sickle cell population should be carefully weighed for risk versus benefit because this drug is a cytotoxic agent associated with bone marrow suppression. Patients taking hydroxyurea should have bone mar-

row studies performed before therapy and periodically during therapy.[70] Other adverse effects of hydroxyurea include GI effects (nausea/vomiting, diarrhea), dermatologic effects (macular papular rash, pruritus), and potential risk of developing a secondary neoplasm (leukemia) with prolonged use. The treatment dose of hydroxyurea for sickle cell anemia is 15 to 35 mg/kg per day. Several small clinical trials evaluating hydroxyurea with or without erythropoietin have shown variations in response to therapy. Large-scale clinical trials are needed to determine the efficacy of hydroxyurea with or without erythropoietin in the treatment of sickle cell anemia.[67,71] Other areas of potential promise for the treatment of sickle cell anemia include bone marrow transplantation and gene therapy.[63,72]

Clinical Assessment

19. J.T., a 28-year-old man with sickle cell anemia, presented to the emergency department with the chief complaint of rapid onset of abdominal pain and shortness of breath. Since infancy, J.T. has been severely incapacitated by his disease.

During early childhood, he experienced several episodes of acute pain, swelling of the hands and feet, and jaundice. Three years before this admission, J.T. required a left hip replacement secondary to bony infarctions. Recently, frequent blood transfusions have reduced the frequency of sickling crises.

Physical examination reveals J.T. as a thin black male in acute distress and with scleral icterus. He has a pulse of 110 beats/min, a respiratory rate of 18 breaths/min, and a temperature of 98.6°F. His lungs are clear, and cardiac auscultation reveals a hyperdynamic pericardium and a systolic murmur at the left sternal edge. Splenomegaly is noted, and a chest radiograph reveals only cardiomegaly.

A CBC is obtained. Notable results include the following: Hgb, 5.5 g/dL (normal, 4.7 to 6.1); Hct, 25% (normal, 42% to 52%); WBC count, 5,000/mm³ (normal, 3,200 to 9,800); platelets, 325,000/mm³ (normal, 130,000 to 400,000); reticulocyte count, 1% (normal, 0.5 to 1.5%); bilirubin, 5.8 mg/dL (normal, 0.1 to 1.0); serum creatinine (SrCr), 3.0 mg/dL (normal, 0.6 to 1.2); and blood urea nitrogen (BUN), 52 mg/dL (normal, 1 to 18). The peripheral blood smear shows target cells with an occasional sickled cell. What signs and symptoms are consistent with SSA? What is J.T.'s current complication?

[SI units: Hgb, 55 g/L; Hct, 0.25; WBC count, 5 × 10⁹/L; platelets, 325 × 10⁹/L; bilirubin, 99.18 μmol/L; SrCr, 265.2 μmol/L; BUN, 18.56 mmol/L urea]

Based on the presence of splenomegaly and anemia with target and sickled cells, J.T. currently is presenting with an acute splenic sequestration crisis. Splenomegaly rapidly evolves over several hours and is accompanied by progressive anemia. The low reticulocyte count is consistent with acute sequestration because a reticulocyte response would be expected if the anemia had developed in recent days. J.T.'s inadequate reticulocyte response may reflect rapid progression of the anemia or a blunted erythropoietin response secondary to compromised renal dysfunction. The hyperdynamic pericardium and systolic murmur are consistent with the high cardiac output required to deliver oxygen in an anemic state.

20. How should J.T. be managed?

J.T.'s signs and symptoms are serious enough to justify transfusion therapy. In addition, J.T. should be adequately hydrated, considering his elevated serum creatinine and BUN. Patients with sickle cell anemia often lose the ability to concentrate urine and may easily become dehydrated, which further contributes to sickling. Pain control also should be aggressively instituted for J.T.'s comfort and should be continued for a few days after hospital discharge (also see Chapter 9, Pain). Splenectomy may be indicated in instances of severe splenomegaly, repeated infarction, or pain in adults, and it is indicated when crises occur in children. Those patients with sickle cell anemia who are bedridden should be placed on chronic heparin therapy to prevent vascular occlusions and deep vein thrombosis.

ANEMIA OF CHRONIC DISEASE

Anemia of chronic disease (ACD) refers to a mild to moderate anemia associated with a number of disorders (e.g., rheumatoid arthritis [RA], systemic lupus erythematosus, chronic infections, chronic renal failure, acquired immunodeficiency syndrome [AIDS], neoplastic disease).[73] Because of the common occurrence of such conditions, ACD is encountered frequently and has been estimated to be the second most common anemia behind iron deficiency. Most often, ACD is a normochromic, normocytic anemia, although red cells may be hypochromic and microcytic in some patients. Serum iron and total iron-binding capacity are most often decreased, whereas iron stores (as reflected by serum ferritin), are usually normal or increased. Erythropoietin (EPO) levels in the serum may be increased, although not to an extent appropriate for the degree of anemia. This implicates bone marrow failure, in the setting of increased EPO, as the primary cause of the anemia associated with chronic diseases.[74]

Although the pathogenesis of ACD is not well understood, inflammatory cytokines such as interleukin-1 (IL-1), tumor necrosis factor-alpha (TNF-α), and gamma interferon (γ-IFN) are thought to play a major role by inhibiting burst forming units-erythroid (BFU-E) and colony forming units-erythroid (CFU-E).[74] Competition for EPO receptors by γ-IFN and IL-1 may possibly lead to EPO resistance.[75] IL-1 and TNF-α also inhibit hepatic and renal production of EPO, further contributing to the development of ACD. Inflammatory cytokines are directly correlated with the degree of anemia, and are often elevated in RA and other ACD-associated diseases.[74]

The management of mild to moderate ACD is usually focused on the underlying disease process. Anemia of chronic disease is not usually progressive or life-threatening, although it generally affects a patient's quality of life. Patients may require blood transfusions for symptomatic anemia. Unless a concurrent deficiency of vitamin B_{12}, folate, or iron exists, administration of vitamin supplements is not of value. Recombinant human EPO (rhEPO) has been used successfully to treat ACD in patients with RA, AIDS, and neoplastic diseases[74]; however medication costs can be significant and may outweigh benefits from the treatment of modest anemia.[75] Patients are less likely to respond to rhEPO if baseline serum EPO and inflammatory cytokine levels are elevated. Although serum iron often is decreased, reticuloendothelial iron stores are usually adequate, and treatment with iron has proved to be unsuccessful in most cases.[74]

Human Recombinant Erythropoietin Therapy

Human recombinant erythropoietin therapy (rhEPO; epoetin alfa) may be indicated for use in anemia associated with end-stage renal disease, AIDS, cancer, drug-induced anemia (chemotherapy and zidovudine therapy); in patients with low endogenous EPO levels; and with autologous blood transfusions for elective surgery. Previously, blood transfusions temporarily deterred symptomatic anemia of chronic disease; however, transfusion therapy is associated with risks such as hepatitis, viral infections, iron overload, and immunogenic reactions. Studies with rhEPO show that response is not only dose dependent but also dependent on the underlying cause of anemia.[76,77] Variables that may predict patient response are both patient specific and disease specific and are not always reliable. For example, response to rhEPO in chronic renal failure is dose related and can vary among patients with chronic renal failure. Repeated dose escalations may occur during therapy until a desirable hemoglobin response is achieved.[78] Approximately half of cancer patients respond to rhEPO.[79,80] Response in this population also is dose related, and therapeutic doses are most often higher in cancer patients than in renal failure patients.[77] Factors such as baseline Hct, transfusion requirement, and tumor type may influence response to rhEPO. Lower rhEPO response rates are seen in patients who have received intensive chemotherapy or radiotherapy.[77] In evaluating response to rhEPO, parameters such as increased serum ferritin, decreased transferrin saturation, increased corrected reticulocyte count, decreased transfusion requirements, and increased Hgb and Hct values have been used. Lack of response to rhEPO therapy in all patient populations is most commonly associated with iron deficiency.[76,77,81,82] The ability of rhEPO to stimulate the production of erythrocytes normal in both size and hemoglobin concentration is highly dependent on the availability of functional iron.[83]

Darbepoetin alfa is an erythropoiesis-stimulating protein that differs from rhEPO by the addition of two carbohydrate chains. The significance of the additional carbohydrate chains is an increased sialic acid content that improves biologic activity. The result is decreased clearance, and a serum half-life for darbepoetin alfa that is three times longer than that of rhEPO. The half-life is further increased when darbepoetin alfa is administered subcutaneously.[84,85] These kinetic differences allow darbepoetin alfa to be administered less frequently than rhEPO. Similar to rhEPO, hemoglobin response to darbepoetin is dose related. Most patients with chronic kidney disease[86,87] and more than half of cancer patients achieve the desired hemoglobin response with darbepoetin treatment.[88,89] Table 86-8 illustrates current therapeutic uses of rhEPO and darbepoetin alfa.

Renal Insufficiency–Related Anemia

21. K.S., a 35-year-old man with a 25-year history of diabetes mellitus, is diagnosed with renal failure and placed on hemodialysis three times weekly. One year later, K.S. is noted to have become increasingly transfusion dependent for correction of his anemia. Significant laboratory values include the following: Hgb, 7 g/dL (normal, 14 to 18); Hct, 26% (normal, 42% to 52%); ferritin, 360 ng/mL (normal, 15 to 200); and serum iron,

Table 86-8 Therapeutic Uses and Regimens for Recombinant Human Erythropoietin (rhEPO)[a]

| Anemia Pathogenesis[b] | Epoetin Alfa | | Darbopoetin Alfa | | Time to Respond (wk) | Overall Response Rate (%) |
	Dose (U/kg)[c]	Frequency	Dose (μg/kg)	Frequency		
AIDS	100	3×/wk			8–12	17–35
Chemotherapy-induced malignancy	150 or 40,000 units	3×/wk or once a week, respectively	2.25	Once a week	2–8	32–61[d] 48–83[e]
Renal insufficiency	50	3×/wk	0.45	Once a week	2–8	90–97

[a]Twelve- to sixteen-week course of rhEPO therapy.
[b]AIDS patients with endogenous erythropoietin levels <500 U/L.
[c]Moderate dose escalation is indicated if a partial response is observed after 4 to 8 weeks of therapy.
[d]Epoetin alfa.
[e]Darbepoetin alfa.

98 g/dL (normal, 50 to 160). In addition, K.S. complains of constant fatigue, poor appetite, and a low level of energy. What treatments are available to correct K.S.'s anemia?

[SI units: Hgb, 70 g/L; Hct, 0.26; ferritin, 1265.4 mmol/day; iron, 17.55 μmol/L]

Unlike the anemia associated with most chronic diseases, the hematocrit of patients with chronic renal failure often is markedly reduced. The cause of the anemia is complex but involves reduced erythropoietin production and a shortened RBC life span. In the past, these patients have been treated with transfusions and androgens.[90] Although effective, repeated transfusions cause complications such as iron overload, infections, reactions to leukocyte antigens, or the development of cytotoxic antibodies.

Since erythropoietin is secreted in the kidney in response to anoxia and is responsible for normal differentiation of RBCs from other stem cells, recombinant human erythropoietin is used to treat anemia in patients with renal failure who are undergoing hemodialysis, and K.S. is a candidate for this therapy. A dose-dependent rise in Hct is observed in patients with end-stage renal disease at a usual dosage range of epoetin alfa 50 to 100 units/kg three times weekly or darbepoetin alfa 0.45 μg/kg. However, patients like K.S. who have renal insufficiency appear to be predisposed to rhEPO-induced hypertension. Other adverse effects include functional iron deficiency preceded by an elevated reticulocyte count and a change in the rate of hematocrit rise.[91] Seizures also have been reported in approximately 5% of patients with end-stage renal disease[78] (also see Chapter 32, Chronic Renal Disease).

Malignancy-Related Anemia

22. T.K. is a 45 year-old female with non-Hodgkin's lymphoma diagnosed 2 months ago. She is being seen for her third of six cycles of chemotherapy. She complains of shortness of breath and fatigue when she walks up stairs. The only medication T.K. takes is ibuprofen 200 mg PRN for occasional headaches. Her CBC indicates the following: Hgb, 9.7 g/dL (normal, 12 to 16); Hct, 29% (normal, 40% to 44%); MCV, 90 m³ (normal, 81 to 99); MCHC, 30% (normal, 33% to 37%); serum erythropoietin, 29 U/L (normal, 4 to 26). The peripheral smear shows normochromic and normocytic RBCs. What is the most likely cause of T.K.'s anemia? What is the appropriate treatment?

T.K. appears to have malignancy-related anemia, which is often characterized as anemia of chronic disease or chemotherapy induced. This anemia is generally normocytic and normochromic and develops when a disease has persisted for >1 to 2 months. Generally, the anemia is mild or moderate, with a limited number of distinguishing characteristics. As with T.K., the anemia is often asymptomatic or mildly symptomatic (weakness, decreased exercise tolerance). RBC hypochromia may or may not be present, and RBC size is generally normal unless the patient has an underlying iron deficiency anemia. The reticulocyte count is usually low (if decreased bone marrow function is present) or within normal limits. Both the serum iron and TIBC are decreased, and transferrin saturation is usually less than normal.[92] Serum ferritin is a reliable measurement of iron stores in patients with chronic disease. Serum ferritin usually is increased but may be normal; if the anemia is caused by iron deficiency, ferritin values will be decreased. A bone marrow aspirate would reveal an elevated hemosiderin content. Factors that can influence the incidence of chronic anemia in patients with cancer are the type of malignancy, the stage and duration of disease, and the type, schedule and intensity of treatment, and history of prior myelosuppressive chemotherapy or radiation.[77] Although the prevalence of malignancy-related anemia is difficult to quantify, about 50% to 60% of patients with non-Hodgkin's lymphoma, multiple myeloma, or treatment for ovarian and lung cancer develop anemia that requires blood transfusions. The myelosuppressive and anemia-inducing effects of platinum agents (e.g., cisplatin, carboplatin), are well known.[93] These and other myelosuppressive agents are widely used in the treatment of many malignancies, and patients receiving therapy should be appropriately monitored for the development of anemia. Anemia of chronic disease does not respond to treatment with iron, vitamin B_{12}, or folic acid, unless there is an associated vitamin deficiency. Therapy is directed at treatment of the underlying disease, if possible.

In T.K.'s case, the clinician may choose from a number of anemia management options. For example, the current course of chemotherapy may be delayed to allow for hematologic recovery and resolution of anemia symptoms. Alternatively, an RBC transfusion may be given to relieve her symptoms and allow her to better tolerate chemotherapy. In addition, erythropoietic therapy with epoetin alfa or darbepoetin alfa also should be considered. Treatment with epoetin alfa or darbepoetin alfa increases Hct and Hgb, decreases the need for blood transfusions, and improves quality of life. In clinical studies, response rates are 50% to 60%. Therapy is very well tolerated, with most adverse events being attributable to chemotherapy or the underlying disease. Unlike in the chronic kidney disease population, hypertension is infrequently experienced in cancer patients.[94–97]

If treatment with epoetin alfa is desired for T.K., therapy can be administered at an initial dose of 150 U/kg subcutaneously three times a week.[96,98] Alternative dosing regimens, such as 10,000 U three times a week or 40,000 U once a week, have proved to be safe and effective in terms of hematopoietic, quality of life, and transfusion effects.[94,95] Response can be assessed initially by monitoring the reticulocyte count, which should peak by day 10 of treatment. A positive rhEPO response also can be predicted by observation of an increased serum ferritin, decreased transferrin saturation, or serum erythropoietin levels <200 IU/L.[99,100] Epoetin alfa usually is administered for a minimum of 4 weeks, although an increase in Hgb and Hct values should be noted after 2 to 4 weeks. If no hematopoietic response (increase in Hgb by 1 to 2 g/dL) is noted by the fourth to eighth weeks, an additional 4 to 8 weeks of therapy should be considered at an increased dose.[98] Common dose escalation schedules include 300 U/kg three times a week if initially treated with 150 U/kg three times a week dosing[96,98] or 60,000 U once a week if initially on 40,000 U once a week dosing.[95] The most common cause of nonresponse to erythropoietic therapy is iron deficiency. Functional iron deficiency occurs when iron stores are unable to be mobilized at a rate sufficient to satisfy the increased demand brought about by amplified bone marrow activity, which occurs with erythropoietic therapy.[98] Nonresponders should be evaluated for functional iron deficiency and supplemented with iron as appropriate at any point during erythropoietic therapy. For those who do not respond despite appropriate dose modifications, continuation of therapy for greater than 6 to 8 weeks is not beneficial.[101] Once hemoglobin and hematocrit parameters have increased sufficiently to relieve symptoms, the epoetin alfa dose should be reduced every 2 to 3 weeks until the lowest dose required to maintain these levels has been reached. In addition to laboratory monitoring, patients should be asked about their symptoms, such as fatigue and decreased exercise tolerance, and quality of life at frequent intervals while on therapy.

Darbepoetin alfa may also be a treatment option for T.K. Initial dosing of darbepoetin alfa is 2.25 μg/kg subcutaneously once a week.[97] Clinical studies of various doses administered every 2 weeks and every 3 weeks have also reported beneficial hematopoietic effects and decreased transfusion requirements[102,103] Response to therapy should be monitored in the same manner as epoetin alfa, with dose escalation to 4.5 μg/kg once a week considered after 6 weeks of therapy for nonresponders.[104]

AIDS-Related Anemia

23. J.M., a 37-year-old man, is currently calling his primary physician with complaints of acute worsening of shortness of breath and pounding in his chest. J.M. has a known history of AIDS and has had recent episodes of *Pneumocystis carinii* pneumonia (PCP) and cytomegalovirus (CMV) esophagitis. J.M. also has complained of frequent diarrhea. Trimethoprim-sulfamethoxazole was given intravenously for treatment of PCP; however, J.M. complained of fever while on maintenance therapy. J.M. is currently taking the following medications: dapsone 100 mg/day PO for PCP prophylaxis, ganciclovir 325 mg IV Monday through Friday for CMV prophylaxis, indinavir 800 mg PO Q 8 hr, lamivudine 150 mg PO BID, zidovudine 300 mg PO BID, fluconazole 100 mg/day PO PRN for thrush, and Imodium liquid 5 mL PRN for diarrhea.

The only remarkable findings on physical examination include a respiratory rate of 24 breaths/min and a heart rate of 120 beats/min. A chest examination reveals that J.M. is tachypneic and has bilateral dry rales. The Hickman catheter in the left subclavian vein appears dry and clean. Further workup of J.M.'s illness includes an unremarkable chest radiograph and negative cultures of the blood and sputum. The CBC includes normal WBC and platelet counts. Abnormal values include the RBC count of 3,300/mm³ (normal, 4,500 to 6,200), Hgb of 9.1 mg/dL, Hct of 28% (normal, 42% to 54%), and a CD4 of 387 cells/mm² (normal, 440 to 1,600). The morphology of the RBC was moderately anisocytic, normochromic, and normocytic. What factors can contribute to J.M.'s anemia?

[SI units: RBC count, 3.3×10^{12}/L (normal, 4.5 to 6.2); Hgb, 91 g/L; Hct, 0.28 (normal, 0.42 to 0.54)]

Anemia occurs in >70% of AIDS patients and correlates with the severity of the clinical syndrome.[105] In this patient population, anemia is a risk factor for early death.[106] Common symptoms such as fatigue, breathlessness, and difficulties in mental concentration may contribute to this patient population's decreased quality of life. Antibody responses against RBCs have been documented in AIDS patients,[107] although their role in the pathogenesis of AIDS has been challenged (see Chapter 69, Pharmacotherapy of Human Immunodeficiency Virus Infection, and Chapter 70, Opportunistic Infections in HIV-Infected Patients). Anemia occurs more often in patients with opportunistic infections (*Mycobacterium avium intracellulare, Cryptococcus neoformans,* and *Histoplasma capsulatum*), viruses (CMV, herpes simplex viruses type 1 and 2, and parvovirus B-19), or neoplasms.[108] Approximately 1% of all AIDS-related anemias are related to parvovirus and can be treated and reversed with IV gammaglobulin.[108,109] Enhanced production of cytokines, such as tumor necrosis factor-α, also may be correlated with hematologic abnormalities.[74] Anemia may be a consequence of various HIV drugs (e.g., zidovudine, zalcitabine, didanosine),[110–112] or other drugs often used to treat AIDS-associated illnesses (e.g., bone marrow suppressive chemotherapy, ganciclovir, trimethoprim-sulfamethoxazole, dapsone).[56] Kaposi's sarcoma and lymphoma, which impair normal bone marrow function, also can result in anemia in this population.

Iron stores in AIDS patients usually are adequate; yet, the characteristics of anemia are similar to those present in anemia of chronic disease: low serum iron and iron-binding capacity or an elevated serum ferritin. Vitamin B_{12} deficiency is a contributing cause to anemia in 15 to 30% of AIDS patients.[113–115] Vitamin B_{12} malabsorption may result from HIV-infected mononuclear cells within the lamina propia[116] or abnormal binding of vitamin B_{12} to transport proteins. Alterations in the utilization of vitamin B_{12} and folate[113,117] may place a patient at risk for hematologic toxicity of drugs such as zidovudine and trimethoprim. However AIDS patients generally do not respond to vitamin B_{12} supplementation.[118]

As illustrated by J.M., HIV-associated anemia has a characteristic RBC morphology, which is normochromic and normocytic. Mild anisocytosis and poikilocytosis also may be observed. Zidovudine-associated anemia is typically macrocytic.[2,110]

Erythropoiesis is often defective in AIDS patients, as reflected by an inappropriately low reticulocyte count and an increased or blunted erythropoietic response for the degree of anemia.[2,119] An ineffective erythropoietin response may be observed in some patients receiving zidovudine therapy as well.[2]

J.M. has many risk factors for anemia of chronic disease, including AIDS and its accompanying predisposition to malignancy and infection. He is also taking many medications (ganciclovir, zidovudine, and dapsone) that can induce anemia.

24. J.M.'s physician determines that J.M.'s endogenous erythropoietin level is 737 U/L (normal, 4 to 26). Is J.M. a candidate for rhEPO? How can you best predict response to rhEPO? What would an appropriate dosing regimen be to start treating J.M.?

Patients taking zidovudine who have baseline erythropoietin levels <500 IU/L experience a significantly higher rate of increase in Hct compared with patients with high baseline erythropoietin levels.[111] A patient who develops macrocytic anemia with moderate erythropoietin response (<500 IU/L) may require moderate transfusion support in response to zidovudine. A patient who develops normocytic anemia with a high erythropoietin response (>500 IU/L) may have substantial transfusion requirements.[120] A significant reduction in transfusion requirements has been observed in those patients with macrocytic anemia with moderate erythropoietin response who are given rhEPO 100 U/kg subcutaneously three times weekly. Therefore, rhEPO may be considered appropriate treatment for patients whose baseline erythropoietin level is ≤500 IU/L.

J.M.'s anemia is less likely to respond to rhEPO than that of patients who have endogenous erythropoietin levels <500 U/L. (Note: Although this level far exceeds normal, high values are often seen in anemias of chronic disease.) However, an rhEPO trial of therapy may be initiated at 100 U/kg subcutaneously three times weekly. J.M. should be followed up by evaluating his RBC indices in another 6 to 8 weeks. If he responds appropriately, the rhEPO dosage may be decreased to the lowest dose necessary to maintain RBC indices, to prevent symptoms or RBC transfusions. If J.M.'s response is marginal, the dose should be increased by 50 U/kg every 4 weeks until there is an increase in the hematocrit of 5% to 6%, a hemat-

ocrit of 36% is achieved, or a maximum dose of 300 U/kg is reached.[109] If J.M. does not respond to 300 U/kg, it is unlikely that he will benefit from further rhEPO therapy. Once-weekly dosing data suggest that epoetin alfa at a dose of 40,000 U/week is equally as effective as three times weekly dosing in improving HIV-related anemia.[106]

MULTIFACTORIAL ANEMIAS

25. P.W., a 33-year-old woman in her eighth month of pregnancy, complains of extreme lethargy at a routine obstetric visit. Her CBC was reported as follows: Hct, 28% (normal, 40% to 44%); Hgb, 9 g/dL (normal, 14 to 18); MCV, 90 m^3 (normal, 80 to 94); and reticulocytes, 0.5% (normal, 0.5% to 1.5%). Other laboratory results include the following: serum folate, 4 ng/mL (normal, 7 to 25); serum vitamin B_{12}, 400 pg/mL (normal, >200); serum iron, 40 g/dL (normal, 50 to 160); ferritin, 125 ng/mL (normal, 15 to 200), and TIBC, 440g/dL (normal, 250 to 400). A peripheral smear demonstrates both microcytic and macrocytic erythrocytes and hypochromia. P.W. admits that she has not been taking the prescribed iron and folate supplements regularly. Can the red cell indices be correlated with the peripheral smear? What other factors should be considered in the etiology of this mixed anemia?

[SI units: Hct, 0.28; Hgb, 90 g/L; MCV, 90 fL; folate, 9.06 nmol/L; vitamin B_{12}, 295.12 pmol/L; iron, 7.16 μmol/L; ferritin, 125 μg/L; TIBC, 78.8 μmol/L]

The combination of both macrocytic and microcytic RBCs offset each other to produce a normal MCV. The red cell indices reflect an average value and should only be considered as one of several diagnostic tools. Accordingly, a peripheral blood smear should be examined to ascertain RBC morphology and pathology. In this case, P.W. appears to have combined iron and folate deficiency anemia.

Many patients do not present with a single cause of anemia, and there are many examples of situations in which a mixed anemia occurs, including pregnancy. As previously discussed, iron and folate requirements increase during pregnancy. Folate deficiency anemia may occur by the third trimester.[121] P.W. requires folic acid 1 mg/day and ferrous sulfate 325 mg three times daily to treat her anemia. Hematologic laboratory parameters should be evaluated at the next visit to ensure compliance and appropriateness of therapy (also see Chapter 46).

Mixed anemia also can occur in patients with large-volume blood loss, chronic renal failure, cirrhosis, other liver diseases, and endocrine disorders.

Acknowledgment

We gratefully acknowledge Ann Bolinger, Jim Koeller, and Carla Van Den Berg for their contributions to this chapter.

REFERENCES

1. Bergin JJ. Evaluation of anemia. Postgrad Med J 1985;77:253.
2. Abels RI. Use of recombinant human erythropoietin in the treatment of anemia in patients who have cancer. Semin Oncol 1992;19(Suppl 8):29.
3. Dawson AA et al. Evaluation of diagnostic significance of certain symptoms and physical signs in anaemic patients. Br Med J 1969;4:436.
4. Duke M, Abelmann WH. The hemodynamic response to chronic anemia. Circulation 1969;39:503.
5. Finch CA, Huebers H. Perspectives in iron metabolism. N Engl J Med 1982;306:1520.
6. Antianemia drugs. In: McEvoy GK et al, eds. American Hospital Formulary Service Drug Information 03. Bethesda, MD: ASHP, 2003:1355.
7. Beal R. Hematinics: pathophysiological and clinical aspects. Drugs 1971;2:190.
8. Bentley DP. Iron metabolism and anemia in pregnancy. Clin Haematol 1985;14:613.
9. Lipschitz DA et al. A clinical evaluation of serum ferritin as an index of iron stores. N Engl J Med 1974;290:1213.
10. Jacobs A et al. Ferritin in serum: clinical and biochemical implications. N Engl J Med 1975;292:951.

11. Wheby MS. Effect of iron on serum ferritin levels in iron deficiency anemia. Blood 1980;55(1):138.

12. Harju E, Parkarinen A. The effect of iron treatment on serum ferritin concentrations and bone marrow stainable iron in iron deficient out—patients with gastritis, gastric ulcer and duodenal ulcer. J Int Med Res 1984;12:56.

13. Stojceski T et al. Studies on the serum iron-binding capacity. J Clin Pathol 1965;18:446.

14. Fairbanks VF. Iron deficiency: still a diagnostic challenge. Med Clin North Am 1970;54:903.

15. Beissner RS, Trowbridger AA. Clinical assessment of anemia. Postgrad Med 1986;80(6):83.

16. Brise H et al. Absorbability of different iron compounds. Acta Med Scand 1962;171(Suppl 376):23.

17. Ekenved G. Iron absorption studies: studies on oral iron preparations using serum iron and different radioiron isotope techniques. Scand J Haematol 1976;28(Suppl):7.

18. Middletown E et al. Studies on the absorption of orally administered iron from sustained-release preparations. N Engl J Med 1966;274:136.

19. Harju E, Lindberg H. Ascorbic acid does not augment the restoration effect of iron treatment for empty iron stores in patients after gastrointestinal surgery. Am Surg 1986;52(8):463.

20. Kellermeyer RW. General principles of the evaluation and therapy of anemias. Med Clin North Am 1984;68(3):533.

21. Bentley DP, Jacobs A. Accumulation of storage iron in patients treated for iron deficiency anemia. Br Med J 1975;2:64.

22. Saunders JR, Ferguson AW. Ferrous sulfate: danger to children. Br Med J 1977;1:57.

23. Grebe G et al. Effect of meals and ascorbic acid on the absorption of a therapeutic dose of iron as ferrous and ferric salts. Curr Ther Res 1975;17:382.

24. Norrby A. Iron absorption studies in iron deficiency. Scand J Haematol 1974;20(Suppl):5.

25. Hillman RS. Hematopoietic agents: growth factors, minerals and vitamins. In: Gilman AG et al, eds. Goodman and Gilman's: The Pharmacological Basis of Therapeutics, 10th ed. New York: McGraw-Hill, 2001:1487.

26. Ekenved G et al. Influence of a liquid antacid on the absorption of different iron salts. Scand J Haematol 1976;28(Suppl):65.

27. Hall G et al. Inhibition of iron absorption by magnesium trisilicate. Med J Aust 1969;2:95.

28. Kanazawa S et al. Removal of cobalamin analogue in bile by enterohepatic circulation of vitamin B_{12}. Lancet 1983;1:707.

29. Neuvonem P et al. Interference of iron with the absorption of tetracyclines in man. Br Med J 1970;4:532.

30. Kumpf NJ, Holland EG. Parenteral iron dextran therapy. DICP Ann Pharmacother 1990;24:162.

31. Will G. The absorption, distribution and utilization of intramuscularly administered iron-dextran: a radioisotope study. Br J Haematol 1968;14:395.

32. Halpin TC et al. Iron deficiency anemia in childhood inflammatory bowel disease: treatment with intravenous iron dextran. J Parenter Enteral Nutr 1982;6(1):9.

33. Reed MD. Use of intravenous iron dextran injection in children receiving total parenteral nutrition. Am J Dis Child 1981;135:829.

34. Auerbach M et al. Clinical use of the total dose intravenous infusion of iron dextran. J Lab Clin Med 1988;111:566.

35. Bailie GR et al. Parenteral iron use in the management of anemia in end stage renal disease patients. Am J Kidney Dis 2000;35:1.

36. Michael B et al for the Ferrlecit Publication Committee. Sodium ferric gluconate complex in hemodialysis patients: adverse reactions compared to placebo and iron dextran. Kidney Int 2002;61:1830.

37. Wallerstein RO. Intravenous iron dextran complex. Blood 1968;32:690.

38. Antony AC. Megaloblastic anemias. In: Hoffman R et al, eds. Hematology. Basic Principles and Practice, 3rd ed. New York: Churchill Livingstone, 1999:446.

39. Beck WS. Diagnosis of megaloblastic anemia. Annu Rev Med 1991;42;311.

40. Sullivan LW, Herbert V. Studies on the minimum daily requirement for vitamin B_{12}. N Engl J Med 1965;272:340.

41. Heyssel RM et al. Vitamin B_{12} turnover in man: the assimilation of vitamin B_{12} from natural food stuff by man and estimates of minimal daily dietary requirements. Am J Clin Nutr 1966;18:176.

42. Carmel R. Pernicious anemia. Arch Intern Med 1988;148:1712.

43. Hagedorn CH, Alpers DH. Distribution of intrinsic factor-vitamin B_{12} receptors in human intestine. Gastroenterology 1977;73:1019.

44. Hooper DC et al. Characterization of ileal vitamin B_{12} binding using homogeneous human and hog intrinsic factor. J Clin Invest 1973;52:3074.

45. Hsu JM et al. Vitamin B_{12} concentrations in human tissues. Nature 1966;210:1264.

46. Chanarin I, Waters DAW. Failed Schilling tests. Scand J Haematol 1974;12:245.

47. Murphy MF et al. Megaloblastic anaemia due to vitamin B_{12} deficiency caused by small intestinal bacterial overgrowth: possible role of vitamin B_{12} analogues. Br J Haematol 1986;62:7.

48. Nilsson-Ehle H et al. Low serum cobalamin levels in a population study of 70- and 75-year-old subjects. Dig Dis Sci 1989;34:716.

49. Watts DT. Vitamin B_{12} replacement therapy: how much is enough? Wis Med J 1994;93:203.

50. Lane LA et al. Treatment of vitamin B_{12}-deficiency anemia: Oral versus parenteral therapy. Ann Pharmacother 2002;36:1268.

51. Kuzminski AM et al. Effective treatment of cobalamin deficiency with oral cobalamin. Blood 1998;92:1191.

52. Vitamin B complex. In: McEvoy GK et al, eds. American Hospital Formulary Service Drug Information ASHP 03. Bethesda, MD: ASHP, 2003:3500.

53. Butterworth CE. The availability of food folate. Br J Haematol 1968;14:339.

54. Herbert V. Recommended dietary intakes (RDI) of folate in humans. Am J Clin Nutr 1987;45:661.

55. O'Neil-Cutting MA, Crosby WH. The effect of antacids on the absorption of simultaneously ingested iron. JAMA 1986;255(11):1468.

56. McKinsey DS et al. Megaloblastic pancytopenia associated with dapsone and trimethoprim treatment of 0 pneumonia in the acquired immunodeficiency syndrome. Arch Intern Med 1989;149:965.

57. Kornberg A et al. Folic acid deficiency, megaloblastic anemia and peripheral polyneuropathy due to oral contraceptives. Isr J Med Sci 1989;25:142.

58. Baker SJ et al. Vitamin-B_{12} deficiency in pregnancy and the puerperium. Br Med J 1962;16:1658.

59. Anon. Hereditary dihydrofolate reductase deficiency with megaloblastic anemia. Nutr Rev 1985;43:309.

60. Wesksler BB, Moore A. Anemia. In: Andreoli TE et al, eds. Cecil Essentials of Medicine, 2nd Ed. Philadelphia: WB Saunders, 1990:343.

61. Chanarin I. Megaloblastic anaemia, cobalamin, and folate. J Clin Pathol 1987:40;978.

62. Charache S et al. Effect of hydroxyurea on the frequency of painful crises in sickle cell anemia. N Engl J Med 1995;332:1317.

63. Stamatoyannopoulos JA. Future prospectives for treatment of hemoglobinopathies. West J Med 1992;157:631.

64. Embury SH, Vichinsky E. Sickle cell disease. In: Hoffman R et al, eds. Hematology. Basic Principles and Practice, 3rd Ed. New York: Churchill Livingstone, 1999:510.

65. Steinberg MH. Management of sickle cell disease. N Engl J Med 1999;340:1021.

66. John AB et al. Prevention of pneumococcal infection in children with homozygous sickle cell disease. Br Med J 1984;288:1567.

67. Goldberg MA et al. Treatment of sickle cell anemia with hydroxyurea and erythropoietin. N Engl J Med 1990;323:366.

68. Ferster A et al. Hydroxyurea for the treatment of severe sickle cell anemia: a pediatric clinical trial. Blood 1996;88:1960.

69. Rodgers GP et al. Augmentation by erythropoietin of the fetal-hemoglobin response to hydroxyurea in sickle cell disease. N Engl J Med 1993;328:73.

70. Hydroxyurea. In: McEvoy GK et al, eds. American Hospital Formulary Service Drug Information ASHP 03. Bethesda, MD: ASHP;2003:1012.

71. El-Hazmi MAF et al. On the use of hydroxyurea/erythropoietin combination therapy for sickle cell disease. Acta Haematol 1995;94:128.

72. Walters MC et al. Impact of bone marrow transplantation for symptomatic sickle cell disease: an interim report. Multicenter investigation of bone marrow transplantation for sickle cell disease. Blood 2000;95:1918.

73. Means RT, Krantz SB. Progress in understanding the pathogenesis of the anemia of chronic disease. Blood 1992;80:1639.

74. Krantz SB. Pathogenesis and treatment of the anemia of chronic disease. Am J Med Sci. 1994; 307:353.

75. Bertero MT, Caligaris-Cappio F. Anemia of chronic disorders in systemic autoimmune diseases. Haematologica 1997;82:375.

76. Naman A et al. Markers of masked iron deficiency and effectiveness of epo therapy in chronic renal failure. Am J Kidney Dis 1997;30:532.

77. Ludwig H. Epoetin in cancer-related anaemia. Nephrol Dial Transplant 1999;14(Suppl 2):85.

78. Eschbach JW et al. Recombinant human erythropoietin in anemic patients with end-stage renal disease: results of a phase III multicenter clinical trial. Ann Intern Med 1989;111:992.

79. Beguin Y. Prediction of response to optimize outcome of treatment with erythropoietin. Semin Oncol 1998;25(Suppl 7):27.

80. Ludwig H, Fritz E. Anemia of cancer patients: patient selection and patient stratification for epoetin treatment. Semin Oncol 1998;25(Suppl 7):35.

81. Weinberg ED. Iron therapy and cancer. Kidney Int 1999;55(Suppl 69):S131.

82. Cameron JS. Towards the millennium: a history of renal anaemia and the optimal use of epoetin. Nephrol Dial Transplant 1999;2(Suppl 14):10.

83. Cazzola M et al. Use of recombinant human erythropoietin outside of uremia. Blood 1997;89:4248.

84. Macdougall IC, Gray SJ, Elston O et al. Pharmacokinetics of novel erythropoiesis stimulating protein compared with epoetin alfa in dialysis patients. J Am Soc Nephrol 1999;10:2392.

85. Heatherington AC, Schuller J, Mercer AJ. Pharmacokinetics of novel erythropoiesis stimulating protein (NESP) in cancer patients: preliminary report. Br J Cancer 2001;84(Suppl 1):11.

86. Locatelli F, Olivares J, Walker R et al. Novel erythropoiesis stimulating protein for treatment of anemia in chronic renal insufficiency. Kidney Int 2001; 60:742.

87. Nissenson AR, Swan SK, Lindberg JS et al. Randomized, controlled trial of darbepoetin alfa for the treatment of anemia in hemodialysis patients. Am J Kidney Dis 2002;40:110.

88. Vansteenkiste J, Pirker R, Massuti B et al. Double-blind, placebo-controlled, randomized phase III trial of darbepoetin alfa in lung cancer patients receiving chemotherapy. J Natl Cancer Inst 2002;94:1211.

89. Smith RE, Jaiyesimi IA, Meza LA et al. Novel erythropoiesis stimulating protein (NESP) for the treatment of anaemia of chronic disease associated with cancer. Br J Cancer 2001;84(Suppl 1):24.

90. Neff MS et al. A comparison of androgens for anemia in patients on dialysis. N Engl J Med 1981;304:871.

91. Eschbach JW et al. Correction of the anemia of end-stage renal disease with recombinant human erythropoietin. N Engl J Med 1987;316:73.

92. Dallman PR et al. Prevalence and causes of anemias in the United States, 1976 to 1980. Am J Clin Nutr 1984;39(3):437.

93. Groopman JE, Itri LM. Chemotherapy-induced anemia in adults: incidence and treatment. J Natl Cancer Inst 1999;91:1616.

94. Demetri GD, Kris M, Wade J et al. Quality-of-life benefit in chemotherapy patients treated with epoetin alfa is independent of disease response or tumor type: results from a prospective community oncology study. J Clin Oncol 1998;16:3412.

95. Gabrilove JL, Cleeland CS, Livingston RB et al. Clinical evaluation of once-weekly dosing of epoetin alfa in chemotherapy patients: improvements in hemoglobin and quality of life are similar to three-times-weekly dosing. J Clin Oncol. 2001;19:2875.

96. Quirt I, Robeson C, Lau CY et al. Epoetin alfa therapy increases hemoglobin levels and improves quality of life in patients with cancer-related anemia who are not receiving chemotherapy and patients with anemia who are receiving chemotherapy. J Clin Oncol 2001;19:4126.

97. Vansteenkiste J, Pirder R, Massuti B et al. Double-blind, placebo-controlled, randomized phase III trial of darbepoetin alfa in lung cancer patients receiving chemotherapy. J Natl Cancer Inst 2002;94:1211.

98. Henry DH. Supplemental iron: a key to optimizing the response of cancer-related anemia to rHuEPO? The Oncologist 1998;3:275.

99. Amgen, Inc. Epogen (epoetin alfa) prescribing information (dated 1996 Nov). In: Physicians' Desk Reference, 52nd Ed. Montvale, NJ: Medical Economics Company, Inc, 1998:505.

100. Ortho Biotech Division. Procrit (epoetin alfa) prescribing information. Raritan, NJ; February 1997.

101. Rizzo JD, Lichtin AE, Woolf SH et al. Use of epoetin in patients with cancer: evidence-based clinical practice guidelines of the American Society of Clinical Oncology and the American Society of Hematology. Blood 2002;100:2303.

102. Glaspy J, Jadeja J, Justice G et al. Darbepoetin alfa administered every 1 or 2 weeks (with no loss of dose efficiency) alleviates anemia in patients with solid tumors [abstract]. Blood 2001;98:298a.

103. Kotasek D, Berg R, Poulsen E, Colowick A. Randomized, double-blind, placebo controlled, phase I/II dose finding study of Aranesp administered once every three weeks in solid tumor patients [abstract]. Blood 2000;96:294a.

104. Sabbatini P, Cella D, Chanan-Kahn A et al. NCCN Anemia Panel. Cancer and Treatment-Related Anemia. National Comprehensive Cancer Network Practice Guidelines in Oncology, vol.1, 2003.

105. Spivak JL et al. Serum immunoreactive erythropoietin in HIV-infected patients. JAMA 1989; 261:3104.

106. Claster S. Biology of anemia, differential diagnosis, and treatment options in human immunodeficiency virus infection. J Infect Dis 2002; 185:S105.

107. Donahue RE et al. Suppression of in vivo haematopoiesis following immunodeficiency virus infection. Nature 1987;326:200.

108. Henry DH. Experience with epoetin alfa and acquired immunodeficiency syndrome anemia. Semin Oncol 1998;25(Suppl 7):64.

109. Coyle TE. Hematologic complications of human immunodeficiency virus infection and acquired immunodeficiency syndrome. Med Clin North Am 1997;81:449.

110. Richman DD et al. The toxicity of azidothymidine (AZT) in the treatment of patients with AIDS and AIDS-related complex. N Engl J Med 1987; 317:192.

111. Fischl MA et al. A randomized controlled trial of a reduced daily dose of zidovudine in patients with the acquired immunodeficiency syndrome. N Engl J Med 1990;323:1009.

112. Schacter LP et al. Effects of therapy with didanosine on hematologic parameters in patients with advanced human immunodeficiency virus disease. Blood 1992;80:2969.

113. Beach RS et al. Altered folate metabolism in early HIV infection. JAMA 1988;259:519.

114. Harriman GR et al. Vitamin B12 malabsorption in patients with acquired immunodeficiency syndrome. Arch Intern Med 1989;149:2039.

115. Paltiel O et al. Clinical correlates of subnormal vitamin B12 levels in patients with the acquired immunodeficiency virus. Am J Hematol 1995; 49:318.

116. Burkes RL et al. Low serum cobalamin levels occur frequently in acquired immune deficiency syndrome and related disorders. Eur J Haematol 1987;38:141.

117. Tilkian SM et al. Altered folate metabolism in early HIV infection. JAMA 1988;259:3128.

118. Falguera M et al. Study of the role of vitamin B12 and folinic acid supplementation in preventing hematologic toxicity of zidovudine. Eur J Haematol 1995;55:97.

119. Camacho J et al. Serum erythropoietin levels in anaemic patients with advanced human immunodeficiency virus infection. Br J Haematol 1992;82:608.

120. Fischl M et al. Recombinant human erythropoietin for patients with AIDS treated with zidovudine. N Engl J Med 1990;322:1488.

121. Strieff R. Folic acid deficiency anemia. Semin Hematol 1970;7:23.

CHAPTER 87

Drug-Induced Blood Disorders

Larry D. Sasich, Sana R. Sukkari

OVERVIEW
Definitions

Drug-induced injuries of the blood are termed blood dyscrasias. In this chapter, blood dyscrasias refer to adverse effects that usually are not predictable; are not a direct extension of a drug's pharmacologic action; and occur in an unknown, though usually small, number of persons exposed to the agent in question. Thus, the decrease in white blood cell (WBC) count that is seen in many patients receiving marrow suppressant cancer chemotherapy would not be considered a blood dyscrasia, whereas the same reaction in someone receiving phenytoin for a seizure disorder would. Exceptions exist and are addressed as necessary. The four major types of drug-induced blood dyscrasias presented are (1) hemolytic anemia, (2) thrombocytopenia, (3) agranulocytosis/neutropenia, and (4) aplastic anemia. A consensus conference proposed standardized definitions and general criteria to assess the cause of drug-induced blood dyscrasias.[1] These definitions are discussed in the appropriate sections of the chapter. Older reports have used similar, although not necessarily identical criteria, and not all authors have adopted these standards.

Epidemiology

Accurate estimates of the incidence of drug-induced injuries, including drug-induced blood dyscrasias, are generally not obtainable. Controlled clinical trials provide incidence estimates of common adverse reactions; however, rare, serious events may not be detected because of the relatively small number of subjects exposed to drugs in clinical trials.

Adverse drug reaction reporting systems such as the Food and Drug Administration's (FDA) Medwatch program rely on spontaneous reports by health professionals and patients and do not capture all adverse events. Thus, spontaneous reports cannot provide a reliable numerator for calculating the incidence of adverse reactions. Likewise, prescription sales data used to approximate a denominator in an incidence calculation can only estimate the true number of persons exposed to a drug.

Underreporting is a widely recognized problem in postmarketing adverse reaction reporting systems. Studies have documented that only 10% to 15% of serious adverse reactions are reported.[2,3]

Spontaneous reporting systems by themselves do not give an accurate insight into the incidence of adverse drug reactions, and often spontaneous adverse event reporting rates are misinterpreted as the incidence of adverse reactions.

The FDA has addressed the misinterpretation of event reporting rates in some recent drug safety labeling changes. For example, thrombotic thrombocytopenic purpura (TTP) was not seen during clinical trials with the antiplatelet drug ticlopidine (Ticlid), but U.S. physicians reported approximately 100 cases between 1992 and 1997. Based on an estimated patient exposure of 2 to 4 million, and assuming an event reporting rate of 10% (the true rate is not known), the incidence of ticlopidine associated TTP may be as high as one case in every 2,000 to 4,000 patients exposed to the drug.[4]

Spontaneous reporting of suspected drug-induced blood dyscrasias is of greatest value in hypothesis generation and for the detection of new associations. Under certain specific conditions, spontaneous reports analyzed with prescription sales data can give a fairly accurate estimate of the relative and absolute risk. Calculating the risk using exposure data expressed in patient years may underestimate the risk for long-term treatment. For example, if the risk is highest during the first 3 months of treatment the denominator will include a major period of low risk. On the other hand, risk may be overestimated for short-term treatment when the number of prescriptions is probably a less inaccurate denominator.

Another problem concerns comparisons. Besides underreporting, selective reporting is a possibility. Thus, spontaneous reports are particularly vulnerable to bias when comparing risks with different drugs within a class or between drug classes. Comparative risk estimates, even though vital, are complicated when comparisons are made between old and new drugs. In situations when the risk is higher at the beginning of treatment, a population treated with a new drug will always contain a higher proportion of vulnerable patients than those who have tolerated an older drug over time. The best comparison in such cases is to include only first-time users in both groups.[5]

For these reasons, spontaneous reporting data must be interpreted with caution. Spontaneous reporting systems have been developed for signal generation and thus must sacrifice specificity for sensitivity. This can lead to possible false associations. Moreover, some well-known associations, such as heparin and thrombocytopenia, are not reported. Pharmacists' and other health professionals' spontaneous reporting of suspected drug-induced blood dyscrasia and other adverse drug events to the FDA is critical to the prompt identification of drug safety–related problems.

DRUG-INDUCED HEMOLYTIC ANEMIA

Drug-induced hemolysis refers to an increased rate of red cell destruction, caused directly or indirectly by a drug. Destruction can occur within the blood vessels (intravascular hemolysis) or outside the vascular space (extravascular hemolysis). Anemia develops when the rate of hemolysis exceeds the rate that bone marrow is capable of replacing destroyed cells.

Table 87-1 lists the mechanisms by which drugs induce red cell destruction. The first is by a direct toxic effect on cells as a result of genetically determined enzymopathies or hemoglobinopathies. The red blood cells (RBCs) of patients with these inherited abnormalities are predisposed to lysis when exposed to certain drugs or chemicals that would otherwise

Table 87-1	Mechanisms of Drug-Induced Hemolytic Anemia	
Hereditary RBC Defects	*Immunologic Destruction*
G6PD deficiency	Immune
Defects in glutathione metabolism	Autoimmune
Unstable hemoglobins	

G6PD, glucose 6-phosphate dehydrogenase; RBC, red blood cell.

not have any predictable toxic effect. Second, several drugs can elicit an immune response that results in destruction of normal RBCs; this occurs idiosyncratically (i.e., patients cannot be identified prospectively as being predisposed).

More than 70 drugs have been demonstrated to cause either positive direct antiglobulin tests (DATs) or immune hemolysis. Second- and third-generation cephalosporins, diclofenac, fludarabine, carboplatin, and β-lactamase inhibitors are among the drugs associated with severe or fatal hemolysis.[6]

Intravascular Hemolysis

Many drug-induced hemolytic anemias related to genetically determined red cell defects, as well as some classified as immune-mediated, are caused by destruction of RBCs within the vessels. Free hemoglobin, a potentially nephrotoxic substance, is released into the bloodstream. The amount of hemoglobin released from erythrocytes during extensive hemolysis overwhelms the mechanisms that usually are capable of efficiently removing hemoglobin (Hgb) from the circulation. Free Hgb initially binds tightly to haptoglobin, a circulating α-globulin. The resulting hemoglobin-haptoglobin complex is too large to be filtered at the glomerulus and is removed from the circulation by the fixed macrophages of the reticuloendothelial system. This occurs primarily in the liver, where the heme portion of the hemoglobin molecule is converted to bilirubin, iron is conserved, and serum levels of haptoglobin fall. Laboratory changes characteristic of hepatic hemoglobin and bilirubin metabolism after extravascular hemolysis, including hyperbilirubinemia and urobilinogenuria (see later discussion), also are observed. If the hemoglobin-binding capacity of haptoglobin is exceeded either by an acute, severe or ongoing hemolysis, some hemoglobin will be renally filtered.

The cells of the proximal tubule reabsorb hemoglobin, but as in the case of glucose, there is a threshold concentration beyond which free hemoglobin will spill into the urine. The reabsorbed hemoglobin is degraded to bilirubin and the iron is converted to ferritin and hemosiderin. Bilirubin may appear in the urine and, as the hemoglobin-injured tubular cells slough, so will hemosiderin. Hemoglobin not bound to haptoglobin or filtered at the glomerulus is metabolized to methemoglobin, the hemin moiety of which may then dissociate and bind to the circulating β-globulin, hemopexin. In severe hemolysis, the hemin moiety of methemoglobin binds with circulating albumin to form methemalbumin; serum hemopexin levels will decrease and methemalbumin will be detectable in the serum. Hemin dissociates from albumin and binds to newly synthesized hemopexin as depleted hemopexin supplies are replaced (Fig. 87-1).

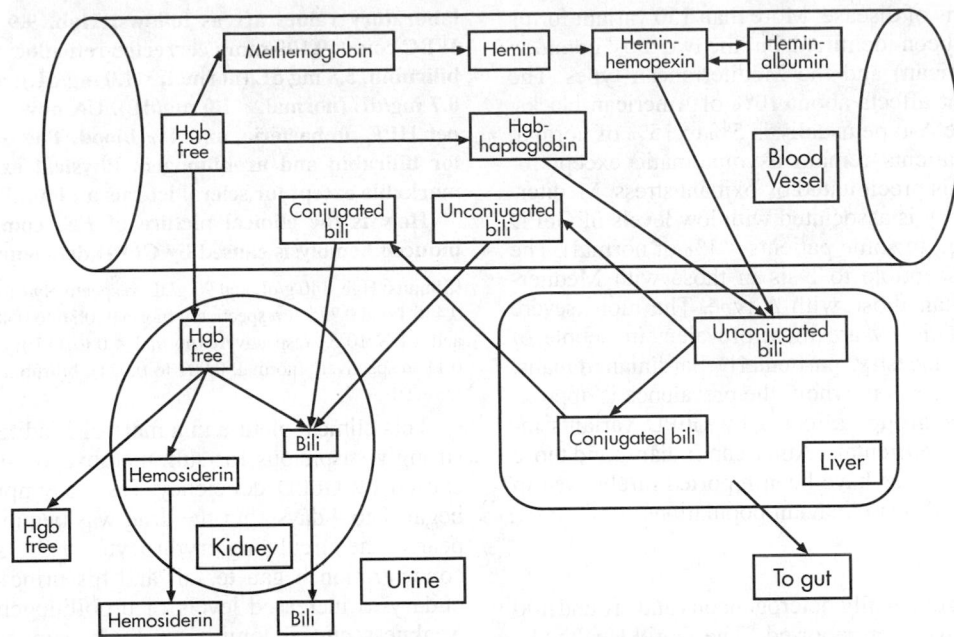

FIGURE 87-1 Intravascular hemolysis. See Figure 2-1 in Chapter 2, Interpretation of Clinical Laboratory Tests, for bilirubin metabolism after secretion into the gut.

Extravascular Hemolysis

Most immune-mediated drug-induced RBC destruction occurs extravascularly. Reticuloendothelial cells phagocytize the RBCs. The heme portion of hemoglobin is metabolized to unconjugated (indirect) bilirubin, which complexes loosely with albumin in the bloodstream and is transported to the liver where it is conjugated with glucuronic acid. When the increased rate of bilirubin formation exceeds the ability of the liver to conjugate it, the serum concentration of indirect bilirubin increases and clinical jaundice can result. The conjugated (direct) bilirubin is passed from the liver to the intestine where it is metabolized to urobilinogen. Most urobilinogen is excreted in the feces, but part is reabsorbed and enterohepatically recycled with some urobilinogen appearing in the urine (also see Fig. 2-1 in Chapter 2, Interpretation of Clinical Laboratory Tests).

Glucose-6-Phosphate Dehydrogenase Deficiency
Etiology
RBCs deficient in glucose-6-phosphate dehydrogenase (G6PD) are susceptible to hemolysis when exposed to certain oxidant drugs. The hexose monophosphate shunt in RBCs is responsible for maintaining glutathione in the reduced state. Glutathione is an antioxidant that prevents oxidation of hemoglobin to methemoglobin. NADPH is required to keep glutathione in the reduced state and G6PD is needed to reduce NADP to NADPH (Fig. 87-2). When RBCs are deficient in G6PD, the amount of NADPH is inadequate to keep glutathione in the reduced state, free radicals accumulate intracellularly, and the oxidation of hemoglobin to methemoglobin cannot be prevented. Heinz bodies (condensations of precipitated, denatured hemoglobin) appear in the RBCs. The now fragile cells are removed from the circulation (lysed) prematurely, primarily while passing through the splenic pulp. It is unclear whether methemoglobin contributes to Heinz body formation or is merely a concomitant occurrence. The degree of hemolysis is related both to the oxidant potential of the drug and the dose.[7]

Epidemiology
More than 200 million people are estimated to carry the trait for hereditary G6PD deficiency.[8] The disorder is sex-linked with transmission from mother to son. While the defect will be fully expressed in males, female heterozygotes have a mix of both normal and deficient RBCs and correspondingly less

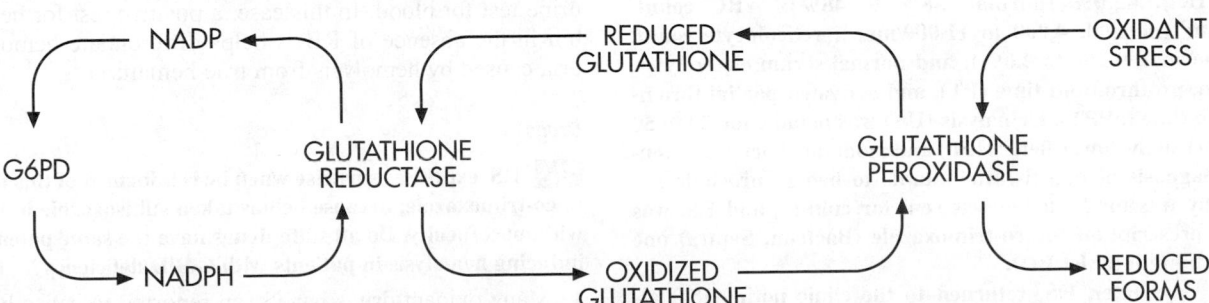

FIGURE 87-2 NADPH is required to keep glutathione in the reduced state, and G6PD is needed to reduce NADP to NADPH.

severe manifestations of disease. More than 150 variant forms of the enzyme have been identified, but the two most common are the A-type (African) and the Mediterranean types. The less severe A-variant affects about 10% of American blacks. G6PD activity in the A-type usually is 5% to 15% of normal. In this situation, patients remain asymptomatic except for episodes of hemolysis precipitated by oxidant stress. Mediterranean-type deficiency is associated with low levels of G6PD enzyme activity (e.g., in some patients <1% of normal). The RBCs are more susceptible to lysis in those with Mediterranean deficiency than those with A-type. The more severe forms of G6PD deficiency are most prevalent in people of Southern European ancestry, particularly Sardinian Italians, Greeks, and Kurdish Jews in whom the prevalence is approximately 50%.[9] Other groups affected by G6PD variants include Sephardic Jews, Orientals, American Indians, and those of Arabian ancestry. Cases have been reported rarely even in Western European and Scandinavian populations.

Classification

G6PD deficiency is genetically heterogeneous and around 400 different enzymes have been reported.[9] The World Health Organization (WHO) has established criteria to categorize different variant enzymes into five classes. Class I variants are associated with chronic nonspherocytic hemolytic anemia (CNSHA); class II variants have a G6PD activity of <10% of normal; class III variants have an activity of 10% to 60% of normal; class IV variants have near-normal activity and no clinical manifestations; and class V variants have increased activity.[10] The degree of hemolysis in all classes is related both to the degree of enzyme deficiency and the strength of the precipitating stimulus.

In the case of drugs, both the oxidant potential of the drug and the dose contribute to severity. Even topical administration of 1% silver sulfadiazine in a patient with extensive burns and 10% G6PD activity has resulted in significant RBC destruction.[11] Nondrug inducers of hemolysis include infection, diabetic ketoacidosis, unknown factors during the neonatal period, and ingestion of fava beans. Fava beans (*Vicia faba*), also known as broad beans, are a common dietary staple in some parts of the world and can cause severe hemolysis in some G6PD deficient patients.

Features

1. F.S., a 55-year-old, Italian American man, noted suprapubic pain and burning on urination. Laboratory data included the following values: Hgb, 14.0 g/dL (normal, 12 to 16 g/dL); hematocrit (Hct), 43.6% (normal, 38% to 48%); WBC count, 7,500/mm³ (normal, 4,000 to 11,000/mm³); reticulocyte count, 0.5% (normal, 0.2% to 2.0%); and normal serum electrolytes, bilirubin, prothrombin time (PT), and activated partial thromboplastin time (aPPT). Urinalysis (UA) was notable for 20 to 50 WBCs per high-power field (HPF) and moderate bacteria. A tentative diagnosis of cystitis attributable to benign prostatic hypertrophy was made, urine was sent for culture, and F.S. was given a prescription for co-trimoxazole (Bactrim, Septra) one double-strength tablet BID.

Four days later, F.S. returned to the clinic noting that although his original symptoms had resolved, he had begun feeling tired. He also noted that his urine had become dark. Current

laboratory values are as follows: Hgb, 9.9 g/dL; Hct, 32.5%; WBC count, 9,100/mm³; corrected reticulocyte count, 11%; total bilirubin, 3.8 mg/dL (normal, <1.0 mg/dL); and direct bilirubin, 0.7 mg/dL (normal, <1.0 mg/dL). UA now reveals 0 to 5 WBCs per HPF, no bacteria, and 4% blood. The urine also is positive for bilirubin and urobilinogen. Physical examination is unremarkable except for scleral icterus and a mild tachycardia.

How is the clinical picture of F.S. compatible with drug-induced hemolysis caused by G6PD deficiency?

[SI units: Hgb, 140 g/dL and 99 g/dL, respectively (normal, 120 to 160); Hct, 0.436 1 and 0.325 1, respectively (normal. 0.36 to 0.48); WBCs, 7.5 × 10⁹ L and 9.1 × 10⁹ L, respectively (normal, 4.0 to 11.0); reticulocytes, 0.005 and 0.11, respectively (normal, 0.001 to 0.024); bilirubin, 65 μmol/L (total), 12 (direct)]

This clinical picture in a male of Mediterranean descent is strongly suspicious for sulfamethoxazole-induced hemolysis caused by G6PD deficiency. F.S.'s asymptomatic hemolysis began 1 to 4 days after the drug was begun. Heinz bodies appear in the circulating erythrocytes. F.S.'s serum hemoglobin concentration began to fall and his urine became dark secondary to increased levels of urobilinogen. In severe cases, weakness and abdominal or back pain may occur and the urine may become nearly black (because of pyrolic substances produced from degradation of Heinz bodies). As F.S.'s levels of indirect bilirubin rise, he becomes icteric and a reticulocytosis develops as the body attempts to increase RBC production. In patients with class III deficiency, the hemoglobin will begin to rise toward normal in about 1 week as younger RBCs with greater G6PD activity replace the older, lysed ones. Even with continued drug ingestion, symptoms, if any, resolve and the appearance of the urine becomes normal. With class II deficiency, even the younger RBCs are destroyed and significant hemolysis with anemia continues unless the drug is stopped. A G6PD deficiency can be confirmed by assaying G6PD activity. In F.S.'s case, it is too early to determine with certainty the outcome if the drug were to be continued; the prudent course would be to discontinue the co-trimoxazole and substitute an appropriate nonoxidant agent. A cephalosporin or quinolone antibiotic are possible alternatives, but at this point, culture results should be available and can be used to guide therapy.

2. Why did F.S.'s urine test positive for blood when no RBCs were present?

The urine tests for blood are based on the ability to detect hemoglobin even after some or all of the RBCs have disintegrated and are no longer visible microscopically on HPF. Therefore, hemoglobin in the urine will result in a positive urine test for blood. In this case, a positive test for hemoglobin in the absence of RBCs helps differentiate hemoglobinuria caused by hemolysis from true hematuria.

Drugs

3. F.S. expresses surprise when he is informed of this reaction to co-trimoxazole, because he has taken sulfisoxazole in the past without difficulty. Do all sulfa drugs have the same potential for inducing hemolysis in patients with G6PD deficiency?

Many oxidant drugs have been reported to cause hemolysis in G6PD-deficient patients. In many cases, causality has not been well established. Several drugs, particularly antipyretic and antibiotic agents, have been implicated in causing hemolysis when, in fact, hemolysis may have been precipitated by the infections for which the drugs were prescribed. Other drugs have been implicated through the use of in vitro enzyme stability tests. The response of RBCs in this enzyme stability test does not necessarily correlate with significant in vivo hemolysis, and this test also fails to measure the effect of drug metabolites. The most reliable method of testing for hemolytic potency is to administer the drug in question to normal volunteers who have been infused with ^{51}Cr-labeled G6PD-deficient RBCs.

Drug-induced hemolysis in G6PD-deficient patients can be somewhat confusing. Sulfamethoxazole (Gantanol), alone or in combination as co-trimoxazole, causes hemolysis in class II deficiency, but class III deficient patients may be at low risk if the daily dose is 3.2 g or less.[12] Sulfisoxazole does not cause significant hemolysis at usually-prescribed doses. Therefore, F.S.'s hemolytic response to sulfamethoxazole, but not to sulfisoxazole, is consistent with existing data. Table 87-2 lists other drugs associated with significant hemolysis.

Management

4. **How should F.S.'s G6PD deficiency be treated?**

Other than discontinuation and avoidance of drugs and substances known to cause hemolysis, there is no specific therapy for G6PD deficiency. If hemolysis is severe, RBC transfusion may be necessary. The patient should be well hydrated to maintain a good urine flow to prevent or attenuate renal toxicity from hemoglobin. Vitamin E and oral selenium have been suggested as possible treatments for G6PD deficiency; however, neither has proven of value.[9] F.S. should be cautioned regarding his G6PD deficiency and the deleterious effects of certain drugs.

Immune Hemolytic Anemia

Drug molecules are potentially antigenic but are generally too small to elicit antibody production by themselves. They can, however, serve as haptens and be immunogenic when combined with some larger molecules (e.g., cell membranes, circulating proteins). Likewise, drug metabolites, particularly highly reactive metabolites, can act as haptens (e.g., penicillin and its penicilloyl by-product).[13] A metabolite of diclofenac has also been identified as a cause of acute immune hemolytic anemia.[14,15]

Table 87-2 Drugs and Chemicals Associated With Hemolysis in G6PD Deficiency

Acetanilid	Phenazopyridine	Sulfanilamide
Furazolidone	Phenylhydrazine	Thiazolsulfone
Isobutyl nitrate	Primaquine	Toluidine
Methylene blue	Sulfapyridine	Trinitrotoluene
Naphthalene	Sulfacetamide	Urate oxidase
Nitrofurantoin	Sulfamethoxazole	

G6PD, glucose 6-phosphate dehydrogenase.
From reference 7.

Coombs' Test (Antiglobulin Test)

5. **R.L., a 53-year-old man, is admitted with gas gangrene of the left leg. His leg was amputated below the knee, and he was given gentamicin 120 mg Q 8 hr and penicillin G 4,000,000 units Q 4 hr along with aggressive local care. On the ninth hospital day, his Hct was 30%, decreased from 41% 4 days previously. No signs of bleeding were found. Further evaluation revealed a corrected reticulocyte count of 8% (no baseline drawn), elevated indirect bilirubin, and a positive direct Coombs' test. What is the significance of a positive direct antiglobulin (DAT) or Coombs' test in R.L.?**

[SI units: Hct, 0.3 1 and 0.41 1, respectively; reticulocytes, 0.08 1]

The Coombs', or antiglobulin, test can detect both antibody coating of RBCs and circulating immunoglobulins directed against RBCs. A direct antiglobulin test (DAT) is the most important laboratory test in establishing immune hemolysis. The result of this test will direct further investigation. A positive DAT supports, but does not prove, an immune-mediated hemolytic process. The DAT detects IgG class immunoglobulin and complement or both on RBCs. As few as 100 to 200 molecules of IgG per RBC can be detected by the laboratory. The DAT may be negative even when the patient is hemolyzing, if there are <150 IgG molecules per RBC. Polyspecific antiglobulin serum must be used for the initial DAT to allow detection of both IgG and complement. If the DAT is positive, subsequent testing with monospecific anti-IgG and anti C3 should be performed. Positive anti-IgG or IgG + C3 indicates warm autoimmune hemolytic anemia. Positive anti-C3 only indicates either drug-induced hemolytic anemia or cold autoimmune hemolytic anemia.[16]

The DAT does not tell whether hemolysis is occurring, and, in fact, several drugs, including R.L.'s penicillin, are known to cause a positive test without significant RBC destruction.

Mechanisms

6. **How does penicillin cause hemolytic anemia? Why is R.L.'s penicillin a likely cause of his anemia?**

The three basic mechanisms by which drugs are thought to cause immunologic hemolytic anemia are (1) a high-affinity hapten-type reaction; (2) a reaction precipitated by low-affinity binding to RBCs, either via a low-affinity hapten-type reaction or by circulating immune complex formation, also known as an "innocent bystander reaction"; and (3) an autoimmune reaction (Table 87-3). Because R.L. is receiving 24 million units of penicillin per day, his hemolytic anemia is likely caused by penicillin.

HIGH-AFFINITY HAPTEN-TYPE REACTION: PENICILLIN

Penicillin is the prototype for the high-affinity hapten-type of immunologic drug-induced hemolytic anemia. Penicillin and penicillin metabolites bind strongly to the RBC membrane in dose-related fashion and are detectable on the cells of nearly all patients receiving >10 MU/day[17] or when penicillin blood levels are high (e.g., secondary to probenecid or diminished renal function). About 3% of patients receiving high-dose penicillin will produce IgG directed against the penicillin-membrane complex as detected by a positive Coombs' test.[18] Antibody-coated RBCs in a small number of cases are then recognized

Table 87-3 Drug-Induced Immunologic Hemolytic Anemia

Mechanism	Process	Common Drugs	Comment
High-affinity hapten-type reaction	Drug binds tightly to RBC membrane surface; immunoglobulins then form against the drug-membrane complex	Cephalosporins, penicillin, tetracycline	Penicillin is the classic prototype of this dose-related reaction
Low-affinity hapten-type reaction or immune complex formation	Drug binds to either (1) low-affinity specific antigenic loci on the cell membrane or (2) to circulating proteins to form an immune complex which adheres loosely to RBCs. Lysis via complement activation ensues	Acetaminophen, ASA, chlorpromazine, chlorpropamide, hydrochlorothiazide, INH, PAS, phenacetin, probenecid, quinidine, quinine, rifampin, sulfonamides	Subsequent to hemolysis, the drug or immune complex dissociates from RBC fragments, adheres to another RBC, and repeats the process. Small doses can cause large scale hemolysis. Quinidine is the prototype drug
Autoimmune reaction	Drug stimulates production of anti-RBC antibodies. Autoantibodies coat RBCs and extravascular lysis occurs	Levodopa, mefenamic acid, methyldopa, procainamide, ceftriaxone, cefotetan	Methyldopa is the prototype drug for autoimmune hemolysis

ASA, acetylsalicylic acid; INH, isoniazid; PAS, para-aminosalicylate sodium; RBC, red blood cell.

and destroyed in significant numbers extravascularly by the macrophages of the reticuloendothelial system, primarily in the spleen.[19] Other drugs reported to produce high-affinity hapten-type hemolysis, although much less frequently than penicillin, are tetracycline and tolbutamide.

First-generation cephalosporins (e.g., cephalothin) infrequently have been reported to cause immune hemolytic anemia. However, reports of severe, sometimes fatal immune hemolytic anemia associated with second- and third-generation cephalosporins have been increasing.[20] Among these, reports involving cefotetan are the most common.[21]

Of 43 cases of drug-induced immune hemolytic anemia that were referred to a single laboratory for investigation over 8 years, 38 were found to be caused by a cephalosporin (35 by cefotetan, 3 by ceftriaxone). Of the 38 cases, 11 (29%) resulted in fatal immune hemolytic anemia; 8 deaths were caused by cefotetan and 3 by ceftriaxone. The fatal cases were sometimes associated with either renal failure or disseminated intravascular coagulation, or both.[21]

The possibility of cefotetan-induced immune hemolytic anemia should be investigated in any patients (particularly healthy young women) who have received prophylactic cefotetan and experienced unexpected anemia after gynecologic or obstetric procedures.

Features

7. Has R.L.'s clinical course been consistent with penicillin-induced hemolytic anemia, and how quickly will the problem resolve once the drug is discontinued?

R.L.'s case is consistent with penicillin-induced hemolytic anemia. Anemia is subacute in onset, usually developing after 7 to 10 days of high-dose therapy. R.L.'s anemia developed after 9 days of treatment. In most but not all cases, no other signs suggest an allergic reaction, and other cell lines rarely are involved. R.L.'s laboratory values are typical of those seen in extravascular hemolysis. The DAT is strongly positive, and the indirect antiglobulin test (IAT) is positive only for penicillin. Hemolysis of decreasing severity may continue for some time after the drug is discontinued, probably because of cell-bound penicillin.

LOW-AFFINITY BINDING: QUINIDINE
Mechanisms

8. H.J. is a 63-year-old woman whose physician prescribed quinidine sulfate 200 mg QID yesterday for an "irregular heartbeat." She has taken quinidine for this problem in the past, but stopped taking it 6 months ago. She comes to the emergency department (ED) today with fever, chills, and shakes. H.J. is found to have an Hct of 24%, and her urine tests positive for blood. What drug-induced problem is compatible with this picture?

[SI unit: Hct, 0.24]

The second mechanism by which drugs cause immune hemolysis is through a low-affinity binding process. The classic explanation for this type of hemolysis involves the binding of the offending drug or drug metabolite to circulating serum proteins to form a complete antigen. Antibodies, usually IgM, are produced and combine with this antigen to create a circulating immune complex. This immune complex, in turn, is adsorbed onto the surface of an RBC, where it triggers activation of complement. The RBC is lysed and the immune complex, which has a low affinity for the cell membrane, dissociates and goes on to a second RBC to repeat the process. It is this "recycling" of the drug-antibody complex that explains why only small doses of drug are needed to cause large scale hemolysis in previously sensitized patients. Because antibodies are not directed against the cell itself, the RBC is destroyed as an innocent bystander, and this immune complex-mediated cell destruction has been termed an "innocent bystander reaction." The direct Coombs' test is positive only against complement because washing will remove the immune complexes from the cells.

H.J.'s quinidine is the prototype drug for the immune-complex form of immunologic hemolytic anemia. However, the innocence of the RBC in this reaction has been questioned.[22-25] An alternative explanation for findings in patients such as H.J. is the "low-affinity hapten." According to this hypothesis, the drug or a metabolite binds to a specific antigenic site on the cell membrane. It then forms a complete antigen or causes a conformational change in the membrane that reveals previously protected neoantigenic sites (sites that will not be recognized as "self" by the immune system). Antibodies directed against the new antigen are produced and bind to it, complement is activated, and cell lysis ensues. Because the drug has a relatively low affinity for its binding site, it is free to go on to another cell and repeat the process. Only cells with the particular drug-binding site would be able to form the drug-antigenic site-antibody complex needed to activate complement. The high degree of antigenic specificity inherent in this model applies to the immune destruction of WBCs and platelets as well as RBCs (see the following discussion) and helps explain why different drugs have a propensity to affect one cell line more frequently than others.[22]

Features

9. Why are H.J.'s symptoms more severe than those of R.L. with high-affinity hapten-type hemolysis?

The symptoms in hemolytic anemia are related to the degree of anemia produced (in relation to baseline blood count) and the severity or rapidity of hemolysis. Immune complex-mediated hemolysis frequently results in more rapid RBC destruction and more acute symptoms. Because the hemolysis is largely intravascular, large amounts of free hemoglobin may be released, resulting in hemoglobinuria and even acute renal failure caused by hemoglobin renal toxicity.

Management

10. How should H.J. be managed at this point?

The suspected causative agent, quinidine in this case, should be discontinued and an alternative agent substituted if necessary. A good urine flow should be maintained with or without urinary alkalinization to prevent or attenuate renal failure. RBC transfusion may be needed in symptomatic patients or in patients such as H.J. because of a significantly decreased Hct (e.g., H.J.'s hematocrit is 24%). Because immune complex hemolysis requires drug in the serum, it resolves soon after the drug is discontinued. An acute, severe RBC destruction can result from even a single dose of drug in a sensitized patient; therefore, this type of hemolysis should not be rechallenged. As always, patient education regarding the cause of this reaction and strict avoidance of quinidine are an important part of her therapy plan. (See Question 15 for a discussion of cross-sensitivity with quinine and Table 87-3 for other drugs associated with immune complex hemolysis.)

The fluoroquinolone antibiotic temafloxacin (Omniflox) was removed from the U.S. market in 1992 only 6 months after its approval because of frequent reports of serious hemolysis with or without organ system dysfunction. These adverse reactions were termed "temafloxacin syndrome." During this brief period an estimated 189,000 prescriptions were written for the drug.

The core structure of fluoroquinolones resembles that of quinine and quinidine, both of which are known to cause immune hemolytic anemia and thrombocytopenia. Other marketed fluoroquinolones with the same core structure have caused neither a comparable number nor a comparable spectrum of adverse reactions. Interestingly, the structure of temafloxacin most closely resembles that of trovafloxacin (Trovan), a fluoroquinolone that was withdrawn from European markets in June 1999 and whose use was severely restricted in the United States because of hepatotoxicity.[26,27]

A review of 95 cases of hemolysis associated with temafloxacin reported to the FDA found that renal dysfunction occurred in 57% of cases, 63% of which required dialysis.[28] Mean onset of symptoms (fever, chills, jaundice) was 6.4 days; patients who reacted to the first dose were significantly more likely to have taken quinolone antibiotics in the past, suggesting a typical anamnestic response and implying a cross-reactivity between temafloxacin and other quinolones.

The available data did not permit an estimate of the incidence rate for temafloxacin syndrome. Although an estimate of the number of prescriptions dispensed was available, information about samples given from physicians' offices was not reliable, and thus an accurate estimate of the denominator for patients exposed to temafloxacin was not possible. More importantly, there was uncertainty about the numerator for temafloxacin-associated events because of underreporting.

Autoimmune Reaction: Methyldopa

The third mechanism by which drugs cause immune RBC destruction is by an autoimmune process. Methyldopa (Aldomet) was once the most common cause of hemolysis via this mechanism, and most reported drug-induced autoimmune hemolysis cases have involved methyldopa. Because newer antihypertensive agents have largely supplanted methyldopa use, it is not clear whether this is still the case, at least in the United States. In addition, procainamide (Pronestyl) has been reported to cause this adverse reaction.[29]

The second- and third-generation cephalosporins are also associated with immune-mediated hemolytic anemia, particularly cefotetan (Cefotan) and ceftriaxone (Rocephin). In one report, ceftriaxone was implicated in 19 cases of immune hemolytic anemia involving 9 children and 10 adults. Six of the children and 3 of the adults died.[30]

Treatment of autoimmune hemolytic anemia consists of drug discontinuation and RBC transfusion if anemia is severe. Hemolysis resolves gradually over the following several weeks to months, but the antiglobulin test may remain positive for years. Despite the similarity of drug-induced autoimmune hemolytic anemia to the idiopathic variety, for which the role of corticosteroid therapy is well established, evidence supporting the use of steroids in patients with severe or life-threatening drug-induced autoimmune hemolysis is anecdotal at best.[31–35]

DRUG-INDUCED THROMBOCYTOPENIA

Cases of suspected drug-induced thrombocytopenia are frequently reported to spontaneous adverse drug reaction reporting systems.[36,37] Thrombocytopenia is defined as a decrease in platelet count to $<100,000/mm^3$.[1] Drugs can cause thrombocytopenia by three primary mechanisms: (1) immune-mediated suppression or destruction of platelets; (2) decreased production of platelets through direct suppression of thrombopoiesis; and (3), in the case of heparin, an apparently dose-related, non-immune direct effect on circulating platelets. It appears that immune platelet destruction occurs through reactions analogous to immunologic RBC destruction.

Most drugs causing thrombocytopenia appear to do so through immune mechanisms, although it has proven difficult to distinguish between immune and toxic effects on thrombopoiesis. Well over 100 drugs have been implicated as causes of thrombocytopenia, most in the form of case reports. It is often difficult to determine the cause of a low platelet count, particularly in acutely ill patients undergoing numerous procedures and receiving a large number of potentially platelet toxic drugs,[38] and errors in diagnosis can occur that may result in overreporting or underreporting, unnecessary discontinuation of treatment, or harmful continued exposure.[39]

George and colleagues[40] systematically reviewed all English-language reports on drug-induced thrombocytopenia. Articles describing thrombocytopenia caused by heparin were excluded from review. Case reports were also excluded from review for lack of evaluable data, platelet count of $\geq$100,000/mm³, use of cytotoxic or nontherapeutic agents, occurrence of dug-induced systemic disease, or occurrence of disease in children. For the 515 case reports meeting the inclusion criteria, a level of evidence for the drug as the cause of thrombocytopenia was assigned. The evidence supported a definite or probable causal role for the drug in 247 patient case reports (48%). Among the 98 drugs described in these reports, quinidine was mentioned in 38 reports, gold in 11, and trimethoprim-sulfamethoxazole in 10. Of the 247 patients described, 23 (9%) had major bleeding and 2 (0.8%) died of bleeding.

Suppressed Production: Thiazides
Mechanisms

11. J.Y., a 56-year-old man with mild hypertension, started taking hydrochlorothiazide 50 mg/day. Routine blood work at this time showed an adequate platelet estimate (>150,000/ mm³). The platelet estimate after 2 weeks of therapy was likewise normal. At a 1-month follow-up visit, however, J.Y.'s complete blood count (CBC) revealed a decreased platelet estimate, and a subsequent platelet count was 78,000/mm³. He reported no unusual bleeding, the physical examination was unremarkable, and the CBC was otherwise unchanged. Should the differential diagnosis include hydrochlorothiazide as a possible cause of J.Y.'s thrombocytopenia?

[SI units: platelet counts, $>1.5 \times 10^{11}$/L and 0.78×10^{11}/L, respectively]

Drugs should always be considered in evaluating blood dyscrasias. Thiazide diuretics as well as furosemide are known to be associated with thrombocytopenia. Drug-dependent antiplatelet antibodies have been identified in the serum of some patients with thrombocytopenia who also were taking thiazides,[41,42] suggesting an immune process. In most cases, however, antibodies are not demonstrable and marrow examination typically reveals decreased megakaryocytes, findings more consistent with suppression of platelet production. Thrombocytopenia recurs with rechallenge only after 1 to 4 weeks of drug administration, further supporting a nonimmune process. Although some cases of thiazide-induced thrombocytopenia may have an immunologic basis, the more common mechanism probably is one of direct marrow suppression.

Features

12. A bone marrow examination reveals only decreased megakaryocytes, and the initial workup fails to reveal other rea-

sons for a low platelet count. Is J.Y.'s clinical picture compatible with thiazide-induced thrombocytopenia?

J.Y.'s course to this point has been typical of thrombocytopenia caused by decreased thrombopoiesis. Onset is delayed and gradual rather than sudden and usually is not associated with fevers, rash, or other signs of immune reaction. The degree of platelet reduction frequently is mild, and without other risk factors, bleeding is relatively uncommon unless thrombocytopenia is severe.

Management

13. How should J.Y. be treated and monitored?

With discontinuation of hydrochlorothiazide, the platelet count would be expected to return to normal within about 2 weeks in J.Y. The drug should be discontinued and the platelet count should be monitored to verify resolution of the thrombocytopenia. J.Y. also should be monitored for signs of bleeding until recovery. For treatment of his hypertension, a suitable alternative agent should be prescribed. As always, J.Y. should be advised to avoid this drug in the future and to inform future caregivers of this reaction.

Acute and Chronic Effects of Alcohol

14. Why should J.Y. be advised to avoid alcohol?

Alcohol has a general marrow suppressant effect. Chronic use of alcohol results in a decreased rate of platelet production as well as reduced platelet survival. Thrombocytopenia unrelated to splenic sequestration of platelets occurs in up to 26% of alcoholics hospitalized for alcohol-related reasons[43,44] and 3% of "well" alcoholics.[45] In addition, acute alcohol intoxication can result in deficient platelet function.[46] The combination of thrombocytopenia and platelet dysfunction can result in significant bleeding complications. This situation would be further exacerbated by concomitant coagulopathy caused by alcoholic liver disease. In the patient with alcoholic thrombocytopenia, the platelet count begins to rise after several days of alcohol abstinence. By 5 to 21 days, the platelet count rises to well above baseline with one-third of patients overshooting to >450,000/mm³; in 1 to 3 additional weeks the platelet count returns to normal.[47]

No direct evidence supports that moderate alcohol intake would slow J.Y.'s recovery from hydrochlorothiazide-induced thrombocytopenia. Nevertheless, in view of the unfavorable effect of alcohol on platelet production, as well as the effect of acute ingestion on platelet function, it would seem prudent for him to abstain from excessive consumption of alcoholic beverages until platelet recovery is complete.

Immune Destruction: Quinine/Quinidine, Sulfamethoxazole/Sulfisoxazole, and Gemcitabine
Mechanisms and Features

15. K.B., a 65-year-old man, began taking quinine sulfate 300 mg HS for nocturnal leg cramps. He stopped taking the drug after 2 weeks when he read that stretching exercises might help. Three months later, with worsening cramps, he resumed taking the drug. The next morning he noted on his skin small, purple splotches that had not been present the evening before. This problem became worse throughout the day, particularly on his lower legs, causing him to seek medical attention. Upon questioning, he recalled experiencing a hot, flushed sensation shortly after taking the quinine dose but thought little of it. How might quinine be responsible for these events?

Quinine and quinidine are well-studied causes of drug-induced immune thrombocytopenia. When patients have been sensitized through previous exposure to the drug in question, constitutional symptoms such as warmth, flushing, chills, and headache can occur soon after the first dose. The platelet count falls precipitously, often to low levels, with bleeding (should it occur) commencing within hours or days of ingestion. Petechiae, purpura, and hemorrhagic oral bullae are common early signs, but patients can present with overt bleeding as the first indication of a drug reaction. Thrombocytopenia also can occur during initial exposure to drug, but this normally requires 7 to 10 days of therapy during which time antibodies are formed. Careful questioning of a patient with an acute reaction who denies having taken the drug before often will reveal previous drug use of which the patient was unaware. Exposure to the small amounts of quinine in tonic beverages is a typical example.

There have been a number of reports of quinine-induced hemolytic-uremic syndrome (HUS). It is an important cause of acute, often irreversible, renal failure. The clinical manifestations of HUS are inappropriate endothelial cell (EC) activations that lead to a procoagulant surface on ED, intravascular hemolysis, platelet aggregations, adhesions, and activations of white cells.[48]

Quinine is still frequently recommended for the treatment of nocturnal leg cramps, although safety and effectiveness for this use have not been established. At this time, there are at least 15 reports of quinine-HUS in the medical literature.[49] Gemcitabine (Gemzar), although unrelated to this particular patient, also has been associated with renal toxicity and at least 26 cases of gemcitabine-associated HUS.[50]

K.B.'s clinical and laboratory features are compatible with a low-affinity hapten-type reaction (see Immune Hemolytic Anemia). In patients with thrombocytopenia, quinine and quinidine-dependent antiplatelet antibodies have been shown to react with the GPIIb/IX or GPIIb/IIIa platelet membrane complex[51] and in some patients more than one antibody may be present. Similar findings with sulfamethoxazole and sulfisoxazole have been made.[52] A high degree of antibody specificity is indicated by the low cross-reactivity of quinine/quinidine and sulfamethoxazole/sulfisoxazole antibodies despite the structural similarities of the drugs.

Management

16. **How should K.B.'s acute reaction be treated?**

Treatment consists of drug discontinuation and support. The platelet count usually begins to rise within 3 to 4 days and returns to normal in 1 to 2 weeks as the drug and its metabolites are cleared from the body and platelet destruction stops. Because transfused platelets are destroyed rapidly if given during the acute process, their use is reserved primarily for control of active bleeding. Although the use of corticosteroids has not been demonstrated to either reduce bleeding or alter the course of the reaction, some recommend their use.[53] Rechallenge with the suspected drug can result in a potentially fatal reaction and should not be attempted for either di-

agnostic or therapeutic reasons except under the most extreme conditions. In the case of quinine/quinidine, sensitivity to one does not absolutely preclude use of the other because the antibodies are isomerically specific. Cross-reactivity has been documented[54]; thus, it would be prudent to avoid either substance. The patient should be advised of his serious drug "allergy" and warned to avoid that agent. In this case, K.B. also should be warned against consuming beverages that contain quinine.

Gold

17. **F.R. has been receiving gold injections weekly for the past 6 months, during which time her physician has been monitoring her platelet counts monthly. Believing that any problems should have appeared by now, she asks if she still needs these blood tests. What is a reasonable recommendation for F.R.?**

Thrombocytopenia has long been recognized as drug-induced dyscrasia associated with gold therapy.[55] Most patients have been taking the drug for several months, and in some cases the platelet count has fallen after gold was discontinued. Although gold-induced thrombocytopenia usually is subacute in onset and can occur within 1 month of a normal platelet count, its occurrence can be more gradual.[56] Most clinicians recommend monthly complete blood counts although the need for such frequent monitoring has been questioned.[57] The amount of gold administered, either in individual doses or total cumulative dose, does not seem to correlate with subsequent thrombocytopenia.[58] Increased megakaryocytes in the marrow,[59,60] and platelet-associated IgG or gold-dependent antiplatelet antibodies[61] indicate a probable mechanism of immune-mediated peripheral destruction. Patients with HLA-DR3 appear to be at increased risk. The ongoing risk of an adverse reaction should be explained to F.R. to enlist her continued cooperation with the drug monitoring regimen. Furthermore, F.R. should be monitored for other blood dyscrasias because gold salts can cause agranulocytosis and aplastic anemia, as well as thrombocytopenia.

Management

18. **If F.R. develops thrombocytopenia from her gold therapy, how should this problem be managed?**

Once gold has been discontinued, recovery from gold-induced thrombocytopenia is slow and frequently requires several months for complete resolution. This prolonged recovery period probably results from the persistence of gold within the body for long periods of time. For this reason, dimercaprol, a chelating agent, has been used to increase the rate of urinary gold elimination. Although dimercaprol may accelerate platelet recovery in some patients, clear proof of its efficacy is lacking. Corticosteroids in doses equivalent to about 60 mg/day of prednisone, with or without splenectomy, have been recommended. Successful use of immune globulin has been reported.[62] Anecdotal reports of numerous other approaches to gold-induced thrombocytopenia have been published. If F.R. develops thrombocytopenia, her gold treatments should be discontinued; the clinical situation will dictate whether dimercaprol and corticosteroids or both should be initiated.

Heparin
Mechanisms

19. M.U., a 65-year-old woman with a painful, swollen left leg, was admitted to the hospital to rule out deep vein thrombosis (DVT). A heparin infusion was begun after an appropriate loading dose. The diagnosis of DVT was confirmed by noninvasive venous testing and warfarin was started on the fourth day; the plan was to discontinue heparin after several days of heparin/warfarin overlap. Pain and swelling had resolved by the fourth day with bed rest, leg elevation, and anticoagulation. In the evening of the seventh day, M.U. experienced a recurrence of her symptoms despite an aPPT within the desired range and an INR of 2.2. Her platelet count, which had been 225,000/mm³ on admission, was now 54,000/mm³. Why is M.U.'s thrombocytopenia likely to be drug induced?

[SI units: platelet count, 2.25 and 0.54 10¹¹/L, respectively]

Heparin is the most common cause of drug-induced thrombocytopenia. Heparin can affect platelet counts by two separate mechanisms. Some patients experience a mild to moderate decrease in platelet count occurring early in therapy, which may resolve despite continued drug administration.[63] This appears to be caused by a direct platelet-aggregating effect of heparin leading to reversible platelet clumping and undercounting by electronic counters, which cannot distinguish between single platelets and platelet aggregates.[64] Counts rarely drop below 50,000/mm³, the phenomenon is transient, and complications are unlikely. This form of heparin-induced thrombocytopenia (HIT) is classified as HIT type I.

The more threatening form of HIT is less common and is classified as HIT type II. Heparin binds relatively weakly to platelets and forms a heparin/platelet factor 4 complex,[65,66] which either serves as a complete hapten or results in a conformational change that exposes membrane neoantigens that normally are concealed.[67,68] IgG directed against this complex causes platelet activation via the platelet Fc receptors. This type of HIT can lead to potentially devastating thromboembolic sequelae. Table 87-4 characterizes the two types of HIT.[69]

Heparin-dependent aggregation of donor platelets exposed to M.U.'s serum would help confirm the diagnosis of HIT. The most widely used is the platelet aggregation test, which measures the aggregation of normal donor platelets by patient serum or plasma with heparin. This test is simple, inexpensive, based on a technique that is in use in most hemostatic laboratories, and can provide a result within 2 to 3 hours. This test, when performed properly (the concentration of heparin and the quality of donor platelets used is important), is reportedly highly specific with a low incidence of false-positive results.[70,71] However, the test is not highly sensitive; that is, a negative test does not rule out HIT. A second test to detect heparin-dependent IgG antibodies, the 14C-labeled serotonin-release assay, is more sensitive but may not be as specific. One study used the test in 387 patients treated with unfractionated heparin or enoxaparin (Lovenox) after orthopedic surgery, including 12 patients suspected of having HIT.[72] Of the 20 who tested positive, only 6 actually had thrombocytopenia defined as a platelet count of <150,000/mm³ after > 5 days of therapy.

Incidence

20. How common is heparin-induced thrombocytopenia?

Although rates as high as 24% to 31% were reported initially,[73,74] reviews of subsequent prospective studies using full doses of heparin and defining thrombocytopenia as a platelet count of <100,000/mm³ found a 2.9% to 5.4% incidence with bovine source heparin and 1.1% to 2.7% with porcine heparin.[75] The reason for the apparent difference between the two sources of heparin has not been demonstrated clearly but may be related to differences in charge, degree of sulfation, or average molecular weights.

HIT appears to be more common with full-dose therapy, but it has been reported in all dose ranges. The incidence of thrombocytopenia with prophylactic heparin (5,000 U every 8 to 12 hours subcutaneously) is lower than with full-dose heparin. Thrombocytopenia has even been reported in association with heparin flushes (<500 U/day)[76] and heparin-coated pulmonary artery catheters.[77] Saline flushes be substituted for heparin flushes whenever possible to minimize this problem.[78]

The results of a double-blind, controlled trial in which 665 patients were randomized to either unfractionated heparin of low-molecular-weight heparin (LMWH) prophylaxis following elective hip surgery showed HIT occurred in 9 of 332 (2.7%) and 0 of 333 patients treated with LMWH.[79]

Features

21. How is the onset of M.U.'s thrombocytopenia typical of thrombocytopenia induced by heparin?

The thrombocytopenia caused by heparin usually occurs after 6 to 12 days of therapy. However, thrombocytopenia can occur much earlier, particularly in previously sensitized patients.[80] Thrombocytopenia can be profound, but in some cases platelet count may remain above 100,000/mm³ despite

Table 87-4 Characteristics of Type I and II Heparin-Induced Thrombocytopenia

	Type I	Type II
Frequency	10–20%	2–30%
Timing of onset	1–4 days	5–10 days
Nadir platelet count	100,000/μL	30,000–55,000/μL
Antibody mediated	No	Yes
Thromboembolic sequelae	None	30–80%
Hemorrhagic	None	Rarely
Sequelae management	Observe	Cessation of heparin, alternative anticoagulation, additional therapy

From reference 66.

relatively large decreases in total count.[81] Once heparin is discontinued, platelets usually return to normal over the course of 4 to 7 days although recovery can be delayed.

Thrombotic/Embolic Complications

22. What is the relationship between M.U.'s thrombocytopenia and the recurrence of her symptoms?

Heparin-induced thrombocytopenia can be complicated by the occurrence of embolic and thrombotic episodes.[81] Some patients with heparin-induced thrombocytopenia develop antibodies that deposit on vascular endothelial cells, creating a nidus for thrombus formation.[82] In others, the procoagulant properties of heparin-activated platelets may accelerate coagulation at sites of pre-existing thrombosis. The result is production or extension of thrombi in the venous or pulmonary circulation (i.e., "red clots"). Formation of large platelet aggregates (i.e., "white clots") in the arterial circulation results in stroke or arterial occlusion with or without secondary thrombus formation. The incidence of thromboembolic events as a complication of HIT has been reported as high as 75% to 88%.[80] Thromboembolic phenomena associated with heparin-induced thrombocytopenia can be difficult to distinguish from treatment failure and disease recurrence, particularly if the platelet count has not been monitored to determine that thrombocytopenia has occurred. Recognition of heparin-associated thrombosis/embolism is important because it is associated with significant morbidity and mortality. In addition, such a high degree of platelet activity can sometimes result in heparin resistance, probably caused by release of platelet factor 4 (antiheparin factor). In M.U.'s case, it is likely that heparin has induced thrombocytopenia and a resultant recurrence of her left leg thrombosis.

Management

23. How should M.U. be managed at this point?

There is no advantage to delaying warfarin therapy once the diagnosis of thrombosis has been established[83]; early warfarin use would allow discontinuation of heparin before the usual onset of heparin-induced thrombocytopenia. Warfarin was delayed in M.U.'s case, but because she is almost fully anticoagulated on warfarin after 4 days of overlap, the best approach is simply to discontinue the heparin. She should be monitored carefully for signs of pulmonary embolism or further extension of her DVT and observed for signs of bleeding. Surprisingly, bleeding is uncommon in this setting.

Unlike M.U., patients with HIT often are not yet fully stabilized with warfarin, and management decisions are not so easy. The full benefits of oral anticoagulants are delayed for several days, so they are not suitable for immediate treatment. Antiplatelet agents as well as dextran-40 have been used in this setting,[80] but while antiplatelet drugs may attenuate or stop further platelet aggregation, they are ineffective in treating either heparin-induced or underlying thrombotic disease and could worsen the risk of bleeding. Corticosteroids are not useful in this situation.

LMWHs are associated with a lower incidence of heparin-induced thrombocytopenia than standard heparin.[71] The manufacturer of enoxaparin (Lovenox) reports an incidence of 2% in preapproval trials as compared with 2.5% with standard hep-

arin.[84] There have been numerous anecdotal reports of successful use of various LMWH preparations to anticoagulate patients with thrombocytopenia caused by standard heparin. However, routine use of LMWH in patients with heparin-dependent antiplatelet antibodies is potentially hazardous. In vitro cross-reactivity and unfavorable clinical outcomes after substitution have been reported. The low-molecular-weight heparinoid, danaparoid, cross-reacts with standard heparin-dependent antibodies 0% to 19.6% of the time as compared with 25.5% to 94% cross-reactivity of various low-molecular-weight heparins (e.g., dalteparin and ardeparin).[85–88]

Anticoagulants have been developed for use when anticoagulation is required in patients exhibiting HIT. Ancrod (Viprinex), derived from the venom of the Malayan pit viper, is a defibrinogenating agent that reduces blood coagulability by degrading fibrinogen. It has produced favorable results in patients with heparin-induced thrombocytopenia when given in doses sufficient to decrease fibrinogen levels to as low as 50 to 100 mg/dL.[89,90] Ancrod is available in Canada for use in establishing and maintaining anticoagulation in heparin-intolerant patients who are undergoing cardiopulmonary bypass surgery. The drug has not gained approval in the United States.

Hirudin, a natural anticoagulant derived from the leech *Hirudo medicinalis,* inhibits coagulation by interfering with the activity of thrombin. Recombinant analogs of hirudin have been developed. The successful use of bivalirudin (Hirulog) in patients with heparin-induced thrombocytopenia have been published.[91–93] In October 1998, the FDA's Cardiovascular and Renal Advisory Committee voted not to recommended the approval of bivalirudin. The decision was based on two large multicenter trials with identical designs comparing bivalirudin to heparin in patients with unstable angina undergoing percutaneous transluminal angioplasty (PTCA). Despite a large number of patients, neither study—nor the two combined—demonstrated a significant difference between bivalirudin and heparin for the primary endpoint.[94]

Lepirudin (Refludan) is approved for anticoagulation in patients with HIT and associated thromboembolic disease to prevent further thromboembolic complications. Lepirudin is identical to natural hirudin except for substitution of leucine for isoleucine at the N-terminal end of the molecule and no sulfate group on the tyrosine at position 63.[95]

Thrombolytic agents have been used to simultaneously lyse heparin-induced venous and arterial thromboemboli while creating an anticoagulated state through fibrinogen degradation and production of fibrin/fibrinogen split products.[96,97] Thrombolytic therapy, however, is potentially dangerous in a severely thrombocytopenic patient and should be used only after careful consideration of both benefits and risks. Plasmapheresis[98,99] and plasma exchange[100] have each been used to remove heparin-associated IgG and hasten recovery.

Because transfused platelets meet the same fate as those of the patient, platelet transfusions are reserved for use in patients with active bleeding or at high risk for serious bleeding. Immune globulin 0.4 g/kg IV daily for 3 days has been used in heparin-induced thrombocytopenia unresponsive to platelet transfusions.[101] Immune globulin resulted in improved response to platelet transfusions.

Ticlopidine (Ticlid)/Clopidogrel (Plavix)-Associated Thrombotic Thrombocytopenic Purpura

Thrombotic thrombocytopenic purpura (TTP) is a life-threatening multisystem disease characterized by thrombocytopenia, microangiopathic hemolytic anemia, neurologic changes, progressive renal failure, and fever. The frequency of TTP is estimated to be 3.7 cases per million persons per year with mortality rates ranging from 10% to 20%. The cause of TTP is unknown; however, several drugs, including penicillin, antineoplastic chemotherapy agents, and oral contraceptives, have been associated with the syndrome.

The antiplatelet drug ticlopidine is associated with the development of TTP. A review of 60 cases from medical records, published case reports, and adverse events spontaneously submitted to the FDA found that ticlopidine had been prescribed for <1 month in 80% of the cases, and normal platelet counts had been found within 2 weeks of the onset of TTP in most patients. Mortality rates were higher among patients who were not treated with plasmapheresis (50% versus 24%; $P <$ 0.05). In these cases, the onset of ticlopidine-associated TTP was difficult to predict, despite close monitoring of platelet counts.[102]

A retrospective cohort study to determine the incidence and course of ticlopidine-associated TTP when the drug was used off-label found 9 cases in 43,322 patients who underwent a percutaneous coronary intervention and received a coronary stent during a 1-year period from 1996 to 1997. This equates to an incidence of 1 case per 4,814 patients (0.02%; 95% confidence internal, 1 case per 2,533 to 1 case per 10,541 patients treated). The mean time of ticlopidine treatment before the diagnosis of TTP was 22 days (range, 5 to 60 days). The case fatality rate was 21% (4 of 19), with all 4 deaths occurring in patients not treated with plasmapheresis. There were no deaths among the 13 patients who received plasmapheresis.[103]

Postmarketing surveillance has identified serious adverse drug reactions to ticlopidine, resulting in 259 deaths, with TTP accounting for 40 of the deaths. Ticlopidine's manufacturer revised the drug's professional product labeling in 1998 to include a black box warning describing an estimated incidence of ticlopidine-associated TTP of 1 in 2,000 to 1 in 4,000 patients.[104]

Clopidogrel (Plavix), like ticlopidine, is a thienopyridine derivative and is structurally identical to ticlopidine except for the addition of a carboxymethyl side group. Active surveillance by blood bank medical directors, hematologists, and the drug's manufacturer have identified cases of clopidogrel associated-TTP. Clinicians should be aware that TTP is a possibility with clopidogrel treatment.[105]

DRUG-INDUCED NEUTROPENIA
Definitions

Several terms are used to refer to abnormally low numbers of WBCs. The broadest description, leukopenia, simply describes a total WBC count of <3,000/mm³. Granulocytopenia describes a granulocyte count of <1,500 granulocytes/mm³ (including eosinophils and basophils), while neutropenia refers to a neutrophil count (segmented polymorphonucleocytes and band forms) of <1,500/mm³. Agranulocytosis is defined as a severe form of neutropenia with total granulocyte counts <500/mm³.[1] Unfortunately, authors use variable definitions when reporting drug-induced WBC dyscrasias. The term agranulocytosis has been used to describe granulocyte counts ranging from <100 to <1,000/mm³.

Epidemiology

Computerized information from Medicaid and managed care organization databases can be used as a tool for gaining epidemiologic information about adverse drug events. Using this method, Medicaid billing data from 1980 to 1984 in Minnesota, Michigan, and Florida were analyzed to identify patients with a hospital discharge diagnosis of agranulocytosis (the International Classification of Diseases or ICD-9 code used also included neutropenia).[106] Medical records of patients coded with this discharge diagnosis were then manually reviewed to exclude cases of recurrent or chronic neutropenia and those caused by cytotoxic or immunosuppressive therapy. Defining neutropenia as any neutrophil count below normal and using standard criteria for agranulocytosis, the study estimated incidences of 35.7 and 7.2 per million, respectively. Not surprisingly, the incidence in Florida, a state with an older population and therefore greater drug use, was higher than in the other states. Men were found to be at slightly higher risk than women, and blacks were at higher risk than whites. Incidence was highest in the 50- to 59-year-old age group. The Swedish adverse drug reaction reporting system, using data from their required ADR reporting system, quality assurance methods to confirm causality, and national drug sales data as an estimate of the at risk population, estimated an agranulocytosis incidence of 4.8 per million from 1985 to 1994.[5] Incidence was slightly higher in women and increased with age. Data from about 1980 to 1991 collected by the International Aplastic Anemia and Agranulocytosis Study (IAAAS) in Israel and Europe predicted an incidence of 3.4 cases per million.[107]

Agranulocytosis is the most common fatal adverse drug reaction, accounting for 26% of all drug-related deaths and 64% of deaths caused by blood dyscrasias in one series.[5] The mortality rate was about 30% according to reports in the 1960s and 1970s.[108] Another report using a diagnosis by exclusion methodology (similar to, but less stringent than the above U.S. study) demonstrated 16% mortality from drug-induced agranulocytosis at six hospitals from 1970 to 1989.[109] The IAAAS reported a 10% fatality rate. Reduced mortality in later reports likely is due to improvements in supportive care and treatment of infection. French investigators have noted that older individuals are overrepresented in all published series of agranulocytosis.[110]

Mechanisms

Drugs cause neutropenia by two basic mechanisms. One is immunologically mediated, either through peripheral destruction of circulating neutrophils or immune suppression of marrow precursors. The second is through a direct, toxic effect on marrow precursors.

Immune Versus Direct Mechanisms: Penicillins
MECHANISMS

24. **S.T. is a 54-year-old woman being managed for cellulitis. Nafcillin (Unipen) 2 g Q 4 hr IV was begun. WBC count was**

12,200/mm³ with 82% neutrophils, 3% band forms, 7% mono-cytes, and 8% lymphocytes. On the 13th day of therapy WBCs were 2,200/mm³ with 28% neutrophils and 5% bands. At this time, S.T. was experiencing no new symptoms and remained afebrile. Why might nafcillin be responsible for S.T.'s neutropenia?

Administration of penicillins, and to a lesser extent cephalosporins, in large doses for prolonged periods of time results in neutropenia in up to 15% of cases.[111] The problem occurs only rarely within the first week of therapy and is seen most often in patients receiving high doses of antibiotic for longer than 2 weeks.[112] Despite this apparent dose relationship, there is controversy regarding whether the neutropenia is immune-mediated or caused by toxic suppression of granulocyte development in the marrow. Some investigators have found drug- or metabolite-dependent antigranulocyte antibodies in patients receiving penicillin[113,114] and cephalosporins.[115] Serum from a patient with ceftriaxone-associated agranulocytosis suppressed in vitro proliferation of CFU-GM, an early WBC precursor.[116] These findings are similar to findings in some cases of drug-induced agranulocytosis where effects do not appear dose related. Others have demonstrated dose-dependent inhibition of granulocyte colony growth in vitro, and therefore believe that β-lactam–induced neutropenia is due to a direct toxic effect on granulopoiesis.[117] They suggest that antibodies frequently are present despite no identifiable granulocyte abnormalities.

Evidence indicates a potentially important role for reactive metabolites. Reactive metabolites are short lived and produced locally by cells, including neutrophils and neutrophil precursors in the marrow. It is suggested that in predisposed persons, certain drugs may be converted to reactive metabolites that may then go on to either directly damage precursor cells or cause formation of neoantigens, which would then initiate an immune response directed against the now altered cell.[118] The common finding of apparent maturation arrest of granulocyte precursors on marrow examination is compatible with either toxic suppression or an immune effect on precursors. Fever, rash, and eosinophilia in patients with penicillin-induced neutropenia imply an immune process in many cases despite an apparent dose-relationship. Overall, despite significant advances in our knowledge, it can be concluded that the mechanisms by which antibiotics cause neutropenia are heterogeneous, and that more study is needed in understanding these mechanisms. Few of the reports implicating >100 drugs as having caused neutropenia provide sufficient evidence to draw conclusions about mechanisms.

MANAGEMENT

25. How should S.T. have been monitored while receiving high doses of a drug known to be associated with neutropenia?

First, the need for high dosages of drug and long duration of therapy should be well established. In the case of antibiotics, many infections do not require maximum antibiotic dosage to achieve bacteriologic and clinical cure, and the incidence of neutropenia with short courses and more moderate amounts of drug is extremely low. One recommendation is to base drug dosage on body size, as is done in pediatric patients, rather than following the common practice of using standardized dosing for all adults.[119] Of course, doses should always be altered appropriately for impaired renal or hepatic function. The WBC count should be monitored carefully, particularly after the second week of therapy, and the patient should be observed for unexplained fevers and rashes.

26. How should S.T. be managed at this point?

The suspected offending drug, nafcillin in this case, should be discontinued and replaced by a structurally dissimilar agent if continued therapy is required. Structurally dissimilar antibiotics that are recommended for the treatment of *Staphylococcus aureus* or *Staphylococcus epidermidis* are vancomycin or a fluoroquinolone.[120]

S.T.'s WBC count would be expected to return to normal within several days. Although the neutropenia may resolve after merely decreasing the drug dose, this approach should be considered only if an alternative is unavailable. The patient should be monitored for fever or other signs of new or recurrent infection until the neutropenia has resolved. The precise course of action will be determined by the clinical situation. In S.T.'s case, the nafcillin was discontinued with subsequent hematologic recovery and without recurrence of the original infection.

Idiosyncratic Toxic Effect: Phenothiazines
MECHANISMS

27. J.K., a 34-year-old woman with schizophrenia, was found on routine blood testing to be moderately neutropenic. She started taking chlorpromazine (Thorazine) 8 weeks ago when she began hearing voices warning her that she was being followed by the CIA and that her brain had been bugged. Her chlorpromazine dose was quickly titrated up to 400 mg/day, which she has been taking for 6 weeks with a good clinical response. J.K. has no medical problems and takes no other medications. How likely is it that J.K.'s chlorpromazine is the cause of her neutropenia?

Phenothiazine derivatives are one of the most common causes of drug-induced neutropenia, chlorpromazine being the model drug.[121] The mechanism is one of toxic suppression of granulocyte production in the marrow of sensitive patients. Experiments using cultured bone marrow from normal patients as well as that of patients who had become neutropenic during chlorpromazine therapy have demonstrated an apparent drug effect on DNA synthesis resulting in defective granulocyte proliferation.[122] This appears to occur in at least one half of patients taking chlorpromazine, but the marrow of patients who do not become neutropenic is apparently able to compensate for this interference through proliferation of drug-resistant clones of committed stem cells. Patients who go on to develop neutropenia apparently do not have adequate compensatory mechanisms.

FEATURES

28. Why is J.K.'s presentation typical of phenothiazine-induced neutropenia?

As in J.K.'s case, the most common presentation of phenothiazine-induced neutropenia would be that of decreased numbers of neutrophils. Patients usually remain asymptomatic unless they become infected. Phenothiazine-induced neutropenia rarely occurs in <2 weeks or later than 10 weeks into therapy, although latent periods of ≥ 3 months have been reported. J.K.'s 6 weeks of chlorpromazine therapy certainly falls within this usual time frame, and her total dose of 10.8 g also is representative of the doses usually associated with chlorpromazine-induced neutropenia. A total cumulative dose of 10 to 20 g of chlorpromazine usually is required; neutropenia occurs only rarely in patients taking less than this amount of the drug. Patients who have developed neutropenia while taking high doses of chlorpromazine have subsequently been treated with reduced dosages uneventfully. Rechallenge with high doses again results in a delayed-onset fall in the neutrophil count. In addition, approximately 10% of patients taking chlorpromazine will experience a transient leukopenia, which resolves despite continuation of the drug.[123] Severe neutropenia is much less common; elderly females appear to be at increased risk. Most other phenothiazine derivatives, with the exception of promethazine (Phenergan), also have been reported to cause neutropenia, though none have been studied as extensively as chlorpromazine.

MANAGEMENT

29. **How should J.K. be managed at this point?**

Because J.K. is asymptomatic, no specific therapy is indicated at this time. Although it is possible that the neutropenia might resolve with a simple dose reduction of chlorpromazine, the most prudent course would be to withhold the drug completely until the WBC count returns to normal. Then, the patient could be restarted at a lower dose with close hematologic monitoring, or a neuroleptic agent with less propensity for marrow suppression could be substituted. Because the risk of agranulocytosis appears related to the absolute amount of phenothiazine given, a more potent agent or a nonphenothiazine neuroleptic should be chosen.

30. **How quickly should J.K.'s WBC count return to normal once chlorpromazine has been stopped?**

A peripheral hematologic response following the discontinuation of chlorpromazine will be delayed by 4 to 6 days but will then progress rapidly. In some cases, the increase in granulocytes may be preceded or accompanied by a monocyte increase, and myelocytes, metamyelocytes, and band forms may appear in relatively large numbers during the early recovery phase. The neutrophil and total WBC count then rapidly return to normal, sometimes with a WBC count "overshoot" into the 15,000 to 20,000/mm^3 range. Recovery usually is complete within about 2 weeks.

Colony-Stimulating Factors

31. **How can the rate of WBC recovery be hastened?**

There are numerous anecdotal reports in which patients with agranulocytosis or neutropenia caused by various drugs have been treated with the granulocyte colony-stimulating factor (G-CSF, filgrastim, Neupogen), and granulocyte-macrophage colony-stimulating factor (GM-CSF, sargramostim, Leukine, Prokine). It is difficult to determine the impact of intervention with CSFs on the clinical course or outcomes from case reports, and the expectation that granulocyte recovery will be hastened by precursor stimulation cannot be assumed. Variability in time to recovery is great

enough that increases occurring after CSFs are initiated could be attributable to the drug or they could represent the coincidental increases that would have been seen without any additional intervention. Likewise, it is difficult to determine whether patient outcomes would have been different had CSFs not been used.

A review of 70 reported cases of drug-induced agranulocytosis treated with G-CSF or GM-CSF found that peripheral granulocyte recovery time was 1.2 days with mild granulocytopenia, 2.6 days for moderate, and 5.8 days in the severe group.[124] No difference was noted between G-CSF (mean dose 4 μg/kg per day) and GM-CSF (mean dose 7 μg/kg per day). The mortality rate was 5%. The authors concluded that compared with previous published reports in which CSFs were not used, recovery time was faster and mortality was lower. These conclusions are limited by the use of historical controls and the biases inherent in such reviews. Clinicians are much more likely to report cases that are successes rather than failures.

Two randomized, controlled trials compared outcomes of treatment with or without CSFs in patients with febrile[125] and afebrile[126] neutropenia caused by cancer chemotherapy. In both studies, neutrophil recovery time was shortened but there were no differences in survival or duration of hospitalization. Although it may not be possible to extrapolate these results to the treatment of drug-induced neutropenia, it does appear that hastened white cell recovery does not necessarily result in improved clinical outcomes.

At present, therapeutic trials of CSFs are not appropriate as first-line treatment to hasten WBC recovery in drug-induced agranulocytosis or neutropenia. It should also be noted that significant complications related to CSF use for drug-induced agranulocytosis have been reported.[127]

Because J.K. currently is asymptomatic, use of CSFs is not indicated.

Clozapine (Clozaril), Olanzapine (Zyprexa)

32. **The possibility of using clozapine (Clozaril) to treat J.K. is discussed. Having suffered chlorpromazine-induced neutropenia, is J.K. at increased risk for neutropenia because of clozapine?**

Clozapine is a dibenzodiazepine neuroleptic that initially appeared to exhibit favorable adverse effect profile. However, in 1975, 16 cases of clozapine-induced neutropenia were reported in Finland.[128] Eight fatalities resulted when discovery of the neutropenia was delayed and clozapine was not promptly discontinued. In 1989, clozapine was approved for use in the United States for severely ill schizophrenic patients who were refractory to standard antipsychotic drug treatment. Initially the manufacturer made the drug available to patients only through a controversial, privately contracted distribution system that included mandatory weekly WBC counts and criteria for intensified monitoring and discontinuation of therapy. A national registry has continued to collect patient and blood count information since this system was discontinued in 1991, providing what may be the most complete postmarketing blood dyscrasia database for any drug available for general use.

The incidence of leukopenia reported in 99,502 patients treated with clozapine in the United States through 1994 was 2.95%.[129] Agranulocytosis occurred in 0.38% of cases and the death rate was reported as 0.012%. This is similar to the rates reported in the United Kingdom and Ireland, in which 2.9% of the patients developed neutropenia and 0.8% developed agranulocytosis, with fatal agranulocytosis occurring in 0.03% of patients.[130] The rate of agranulocytosis is lower than the originally estimated 1% to 2% and may be due, in part, to a 97% rate of compliance with the registry protocol for screening for previous blood dyscrasias, monitoring WBC counts weekly, and discontinuing therapy promptly if neutropenia develops. The 12 deaths that were reported represent a fatality rate of 3.2% of agranulocytosis cases, a number that compares favorably with the overall reported population-based rates discussed earlier. An earlier report of the first 11,555 U.S. patients indicated that the period of greatest risk during clozapine therapy is the first 6 months of therapy; only one case occurred after the first year and a half.[131] The risk of agranulocytosis increased with age and was higher in women.

In most but not all patients, agranulocytosis is preceded by a steady decline in WBCs over a period of at least 4 weeks. However, in 24% of cases leukopenia is not present within 8 days of development of agranulocytosis. Once clozapine is discontinued, recovery usually occurs within 2 weeks.

A history of clozapine-induced leukopenia may be a risk factor for hematologic reactions to olanzapine (Zyprexa). Canadian regulatory authorities have received 11 reports of hematologic reactions associated with olanzapine through July 2000. These reports described leukopenia, granulocytopenia, neutropenia, pancytopenia, or anemia in patients taking olanzapine. In 5 of 11 cases, the patient had a history of a hematologic reaction with clozapine.[132]

Marrow examination in patients with agranulocytosis reveals decreased myeloid precursors, and rechallenge has resulted in a more rapid WBC decline than in the initial episode.[133] An immune etiology is favored by the fact that no relationship exists between dose and falling white count. Serum taken from patients during clozapine-induced agranulocytosis was shown to suppress granulopoiesis and neutrophil function in vitro.[134] Clozapine or metabolites were not required, and neither clozapine nor its metabolites had an effect on this test system when normal serum was used. However, the reactive metabolite N-desmethylclozapine is produced by activated neutrophils in marrow.[135] Desmethylclozapine has been shown to suppress hematopoiesis in vitro at levels three to six times those achieved clinically.[136] It is unclear whether bone marrow suppression in vivo is due to covalent binding of metabolites to granulocyte precursors with formation of a hapten complex or neoantigen and subsequent initiation of a humoral or cellular immune response, to direct toxic suppression of precursors, or in some other as yet to be identified way. There may be more than one mechanism. It is not known what characteristics might predispose to neutropenia in a relatively small percentage of patients although an association between clozapine-induced agranulocytosis and certain histocompatibility antigens in some ethnic groups has been identified.[137]

J.K. is not at increased risk for clozapine-induced hematologic toxicity because there does not appear to be cross-reactivity between clozapine and other psychotropic agents, including chlorpromazine.[138,139] Clozapine, however, is not indicated for J.K. because she is not refractory to more typical neuroleptic therapy.

Immune Peripheral Destruction: Aminopyrine

33. What drugs cause acute onset agranulocytosis, and how might this reaction become manifested?

Several drugs have been associated with rapid onset, non–dose-related destruction of circulating granulocytes. Aminopyrine, an analgesic agent no longer available in many countries, has been extensively studied. Occurrence of neutropenia caused by aminopyrine appears to be completely unrelated to dose. Initial sensitization typically requires 7 to 10 days, but a reaction may occur with the first dose if the drug has been taken previously. The neutrophil count drops precipitously. Chills and high fever, malaise, weakness, headache, tachycardia, and even mild shock may occur as the contents of destroyed WBCs are released into the circulation. Necrotic lesions in the mouth and throat, oral abscesses, and bacteremia develop, and a fatal outcome can be expected if the drug is not discontinued. The granulocyte count returns toward normal within 6 to 8 days if the causative agent is discontinued promptly.

If a volunteer is given serum from a patient who previously has experienced aminopyrine neutropenia, no reaction will occur. If the volunteer subsequently is given a dose of aminopyrine, the WBC count falls. Conversely, a volunteer taking aminopyrine without incident will experience a drop in WBC count when infused with serum from a previous reactor.[140] This information, along with in vitro demonstration of antineutrophil antibodies in patients experiencing aminopyrine-induced agranulocytosis, supports an immune etiology for the reaction, probably of the low-affinity binding type.

Other drugs associated with immediate, non–dose related granulocyte lysis include dipyrone or metamizole (Novalgine) (an aminopyrine derivative),[141] several of the sulfa drugs, and antithyroid drugs.[142] Dipyrone remains available in many countries and is reported to be the most common drug sold to Mexican immigrants by illegal back room pharmacy shops in California near the U.S.-Mexican border, although the drug was withdrawn from the U.S. market in 1977.

DRUG-INDUCED APLASTIC ANEMIA

Aplastic anemia is defined as bicytopenia or pancytopenia with bone marrow trephine biopsy showing histologic evidence of decreased cellularity and absence of infiltration and significant fibrosis. Pancytopenia is defined by the presence of anemia (Hgb <10 g/dL), neutropenia, and thrombocytopenia. Bicytopenia is the presence of any two of these three abnormalities.[1] Diagnostic criteria also exist for cases of bicytopenia or pancytopenia with less definitive bone marrow findings. Drugs and chemicals are implicated in 25% to 50% of cases. Aplastic anemia is the rarest, most poorly understood and most serious of the drug-induced blood dyscrasias.

Mortality rates are high (approximately 10–40%). Although improvements in supportive care and primary treatment have increased survival rates,[143] clinical outcomes are influenced by patient age, severity of marrow suppression, and availability of well-matched marrow transplant donors. Survival figures are based on large series in which drug- or chemical-induced aplasia comprise a relatively small percentage of patients treated. Prognosis is worst for severely affected patients (severe bone marrow changes and meeting any two of the following three criteria: [1] neutrophils <500/mm³, [2] corrected reticulocytes <1%, or [3] platelets <20/mm³).

Historically, mortality at 1 to 2 years was estimated to be 80% to 90% in patients who were treated only with blood transfusions and antibiotics. Today, the most serious complication of aplastic anemia is the high risk of infection secondary to the absence of neutrophils; overwhelming bacterial sepsis and, especially, fungal infections are the most frequent causes of death.[144]

The underlying lesion is at the level of the pluripotent stem cell (PSC), before differentiation to committed stem cells. This is in contrast to reactions involving suppressed production of individual cell lines, in which drug-mediated effects are expressed at points distal to the PSC. The result is decreased or absent circulating RBCs, WBCs, and platelets with marrow hypoplasia and fatty replacement.

Our current understanding of the pathophysiology of aplastic anemia, including the mechanisms by which drugs cause it, remains incomplete despite recent advances in our understanding of hematopoiesis. Evidence points toward an autoimmune process (possibly with genetic predisposition) even in drug-induced cases where the primary insult to the PSC appears to be toxic in nature.[145–147] This view is supported by the efficacy of immunosuppressive therapy regardless of underlying cause and the similarity in clinical response between drug-induced and non–drug-related cases. Aplastic anemia caused by direct damage to the PSC and true immune-mediated marrow failure may be linked by the complex interactions between hematopoiesis and the lymphocyte/monocyte-produced cytokines that help modulate it.

Mechanisms

34. Why is chloramphenicol (Chloromycetin), an antibiotic with a broad spectrum of activity and excellent oral absorption, used so seldom?

Hundreds of cases of chloramphenicol-induced aplastic anemia have been reported since its introduction, with an estimated incidence of 1 in 20,000 to 30,000 patients. It is the only drug that has been well studied in this regard. The aplastic anemia is unpredictable and is not related to either dose or duration of use. The chemical structure of chloramphenicol contains a nitrobenzene ring whereas the closely related antibiotic thiamphenicol, a drug not clearly associated with aplastic anemia, does not. Unlike thiamphenicol, chloramphenicol inhibits DNA synthesis, and although conflicting information exists, cells from patients who have recovered from chloramphenicol-induced aplastic anemia may be more sensitive to this inhibition than normal.[148–152] Reduction of the nitrobenzene moiety produces a reactive nitrosometabolite, which affects DNA synthesis at low concentrations and in an irreversible manner.[153] In addition, two dehydrometabolites produced by enterobacteria in the colon have also been shown to be toxic to lymphocytes although less so than the nitroso byproduct.[154] These data suggest that rare patients may be predisposed, perhaps genetically, to chloramphenicol-induced aplasia mediated by one or more of these metabolites. The finding that this toxicity is confined primarily to the oral route of administration suggests the gut-derived metabolites may be

important.[155] However, the intravenous[156,157] and ocular[158,159] routes have also been implicated.

In addition to aplastic anemia, chloramphenicol also can cause an anemia that is dose related, predictable, and reversible. This anemia results from chloramphenicol-induced inhibition of iron utilization and clinically appears with reticulocytopenia, maturation arrest of committed precursors in all cell lines, increased serum concentration of iron, and increased total iron-binding capacity (TIBC). Anemia resulting from inhibited iron utilization with reticulocytopenia and elevated serum iron is not uncommon in patients receiving large doses of chloramphenicol. Discontinuation of the drug results in complete recovery.

Importance of a Careful History

35. P.D., a 62-year-old man, notes gradually increasing tiredness and lack of energy over the past month. He seeks medical help after unsuccessful self-medication with stress formula vitamins. His only other medical problem is osteoarthritis for which he has been taking diclofenac (Voltaren) 50 mg TID for the past 6 months, as well as aspirin on a PRN basis, generally 4 to 6 regular strength tablets daily. Physical examination is unremarkable except for pallor, several bruises on various parts of the body, and findings typical of osteoarthritis. However, a blood count reveals a Hgb of 6.2 g/dL, a corrected reticulocyte count of 0.5%, a WBC count of 1,800/mm³ with 50% neutrophils, and a platelet count of 35,000/mm³. Diagnostic considerations include drug-induced aplastic anemia. What additional information is needed before one can conclude that P.D.'s anemia probably is drug-induced?

[SI units: Hgb, 62 g/L; reticulocytes, 0.005 1; WBCs 1.8 × 10⁹/L; platelets 0.35 × 10¹¹/L]

Drug-induced aplastic anemia certainly is a possibility, but at this point the database is incomplete. Assuming this is indeed aplastic anemia, a more complete history would be necessary before one could implicate drugs as a causative factor. Many drugs and chemicals can cause marrow aplasia, which first becomes apparent long after the last exposure. The family history should be examined for family members who have experienced "blood problems" or sensitivity to drugs or substances. Social history also is important. Information such as types of present and past employment or military service can provide important clues regarding exposure to chemicals of which the patient may not be aware. An employee in a paint factory, for instance, may be exposed to any of several industrial chemicals known to cause aplastic anemia. A farmer could come in contact with various marrow-toxic insecticides. Finally, an exhaustive drug history is mandatory. Use of all drugs past and present, prescription and nonprescription, legal or illegal, regardless of route of administration, should be elicited and documented. This is, of course, true whenever one suspects drug-induced disease, but in the case of drug-induced aplastic anemia the relationship between exposure to the causative agent and disease onset often is not apparent, and only careful detective work will reveal a possible association. In one case, a child developed aplastic anemia from use of an herbal remedy 5 weeks before clinical presentation.[160] The product was analyzed with gas chromatography and mass spectrometry and found to contain unlabeled diclofenac and phenylbutazone, two drugs associated with aplastic anemia.

Features

36. A more complete history fails to reveal any additional pertinent information. Which of P.D.'s drugs is most likely to have caused this problem?

A number of commonly used drugs other than chloramphenicol have been associated with acquired aplastic anemia. These include nonsteroidal anti-inflammatory drugs (NSAIDs), sulfonamides, antithyroid drugs, antiepileptics and psychotropics, cardiovascular drugs, gold, penicillamine, and allopurinol.[142]

Felbamate (Felbatol) was approved in August 1993 for partial seizures with and without secondary generalization in adults and for Lennox-Gastaut syndrome in children. One year later, the FDA urged that patients be withdrawn from the drug unless felbamate's use was absolutely necessary because of 10 case reports of aplastic anemia. In all cases, patients had been on the drug for at least 2.5 months. Clinicians were cautioned that even close monitoring cannot protect against the occurrence of aplastic anemia.[161]

Three recently approved drugs, linezolid (Zyvox), ticlopidine (Ticlid), and interferon beta-1a (Avonex) have also been associated with the development of pancytopenia or aplastic anemia.

Linezolid is the first member of the oxazolidinone class of antibiotics and has rapidly become a widely used drug in the US. Three cases of dose-dependent reversible pancytopenia were observed after 2 weeks of linezolid treatment. These cases have features similar to those of the reversible form of chloramphenicol toxicity.[162] Warnings were added to the drug's professional product labeling cautioning that complete blood counts should be performed weekly in patients who receive linezolid, particularly in those who receive the drug for longer than two weeks, those with pre-existing myelosuppression, those receiving concomitant drugs that produce bone marrow suppression, or those with a chronic infection who have received previous or concomitant antibiotic therapy. Discontinuation of therapy with linezolid should be considered in patients who develop or have worsening myelosuppression.[163]

Ticlopidine-induced aplastic anemia has been reported in 57 patients. A direct effect on the PSC is the proposed mechanism of toxicity. There is no effective monitoring for preventing this adverse effect. Recombinant growth factors do not appear to shorten the neutropenic period.[164]

The professional product labeling for interferon beta-1a (Avonex) has been revised to warn of pancytopenia. Decreased peripheral blood counts in all cell lines, including pancytopenia and thrombocytopenia, have been reported from post-marketing experience Some cases of thrombocytopenia have had nadirs below 10,000/μL. Some cases reoccur with rechallenge. Patients using interferon beta-1a should be monitored closely for signs of these disorders.[165]

P.D.'s diclofenac has been associated with the development of aplastic anemia. The risk of aplastic anemia with diclofenac has been estimated to be 6.8 per million (about 1 in 150,000). Salicylates have also been linked with aplastic anemia in some[166] but not all[142] studies. Diclofenac is the most likely culprit among P.D.'s drugs, but aspirin cannot be ruled out.

37. What symptoms and signs in P.D. are typical of an initial presentation of aplastic anemia?

The symptoms of aplastic anemia at initial presentation usually are nonspecific and are directly related to deficiencies within the suppressed cell lines. Thus, P.D.'s pallor, tiredness, and lack of energy are due to anemia and his easy bruisability is due to thrombocytopenia. His bruisability has been exacerbated by use of aspirin. Many patients present with more severe symptoms. With severe anemia, high-output congestive heart failure, angina pectoris, or intermittent claudication may occur. Thrombocytopenia can result in petechiae, purpura, nose bleeds, oozing blood from the gums, or hemorrhage. Oral lesions, fever, and infection, or both secondary to leukopenia also may cause the patient to seek medical attention.

Although WBC counts typically are low at initial presentation in aplastic anemia, the degree of abnormality varies. Anemia is normochromic and either normocytic or macrocytic. The hemoglobin level ranges from 12 to as low as 3 g/dL. Because erythroid iron-consuming activity is low, serum iron and transferrin saturation usually are high, as are erythropoietin levels. Reticulocytes are low. The WBC count may be low normal or low, but absolute neutropenia almost always is present. P.D.'s WBC count of 1,800/mm^3 with 50% neutrophils (absolute neutrophil count = 1,800 × 50% = 900/mm^3) is compatible with this picture. Total lymphocyte count is affected least and may remain within normal limits until leukopenia becomes severe. Likewise, the platelet count may be near normal or, more commonly, severely depressed. The erythrocyte sedimentation rate (ESR) usually is elevated and, as previously noted, bone marrow is hypocellular with fatty replacement.

Management

38. Further evaluation, including bone marrow biopsy, confirms the diagnosis of aplastic anemia. No causes other than drugs are identified. How should P.D. be managed?

First and foremost, as is true in the management of most drug-induced diseases, all suspected causative agents should be discontinued. In this case, both diclofenac and aspirin should be stopped. In addition, supportive measures should be initiated as needed.

The approach to treatment is based first on severity of the disease. Patients with mild aplastic anemia have a relatively benign short-term prognosis and can be managed conservatively. There are two basic approaches to treating severe aplastic anemia; bone marrow transplant and immunosuppression.

Bone Marrow Transplantation

The treatment of choice for children and adults younger than 40 to 45 years of age is bone marrow transplant from an HLA-identical sibling donor if available. Overall long-term survival is achieved in 72% to 90% of cases this way.[167-169] Six-year survival of 82% was reported in one study that separately analyzed results in drug-induced cases.[170] Acute and chronic graft-versus-host disease (GVHD) is a frequent complication occurring in up to 80% and 50%, respectively, of transplant recipients.[171] A higher incidence makes success in older patients and those without well-matched donors less likely with this mode of therapy. GVHD was even reported in 4 of 33 transplants from genetically identical twins in one study,[172] a surprising finding, which supports the role of autoimmunity as part of the pathogenesis of this disease.

Immunosuppression

Immunosuppression is the treatment of choice for older patients and for young patients without suitable bone marrow donors. It has been suggested that this may also be appropriate for initial therapy in some patients who would otherwise be transplant candidates,[168] but this issue is controversial. Antithymocyte globulin (ATG) or antilymphocyte globulin (ALG) is administered daily for 8 to 10 days along with a corticosteroid (methylprednisolone 1 mg/kg per day or equivalent) to attenuate the adverse effects of the globulin. Addition of 3 months or more of cyclosporine to the regimen appears to be more effective than ATG or ALG alone.[173] It is postulated that the antilymphocyte activity of these agents results in immunosuppression and inhibited release of PSC-suppressant cytokines responsible for marrow failure. Although the optimum ATG regimen has not been determined, the manufacturer of the only ATG commercially available in the United States recommends a dose of 20 mg/kg per day for 8 to 14 days, followed by alternate-day therapy with the same dosage for up to another 14 days.[174] Symptoms of serum sickness are common and preexisting thrombocytopenia may be exacerbated, requiring platelet transfusions to continue therapy. An intradermal skin test of 0.1 mL of a 1:1,000 dilution of ATG along with a saline control is recommended before starting full-dose therapy.

Androgens

An alternative approach to treating aplastic anemia is to stimulate hematopoiesis. Considerable controversy exists regarding the use of androgenic steroids either alone or as an adjunct to ATG. Although most trials have failed to demonstrate clear benefit, numerous questions regarding patient selection, timing and duration of therapy, choice of agent, and dosing, any of which may affect results, have been raised.[175–177]

Colony-Stimulating Factors

Use of G-CSF and GM-CSF has increased neutrophil counts[178,179] and erythropoietin has increased red cell counts[180] in aplastic anemia. It appears that response, when it occurs, is limited primarily to a subset of patients with nonsevere depression of the cell line in question, and that the response lasts only as long as treatment continues. Interleukin-3 (IL-3) was reported to improve responsiveness to G-CSF in a patient who had not responded to G-CSF alone.[181] The authors speculate this may have been because of an IL-3–induced increase in the number of progenitor cells or an increased responsiveness of those cells to the colony-stimulating factor. One author noted a possible link between G-CSF use and subsequent development of myelodysplasia and leukemia in three children treated with G-CSF for severe aplastic anemia.[182] At this time, therapeutic trials of CSFs are not appropriate as first-line treatment of severe aplastic anemia.[183]

Because P.D.'s disease is not severe, discontinuing the drugs and transfusing RBCs are the only treatments indicated at this time. It is not possible to predict whether his blood counts will improve once the causative agents are discontinued.

DRUG-INDUCED AUTOIMMUNE PURE RED CELL APLASIA

Definitions

Pure red cell aplasia (PRCA) is a term used for a type of anemia that affects the erythroid cell line. PRCA is a rare condition that has been associated with autoimmune, viral, and neoplastic diseases as well as drug treatment. Other terms have been used to describe this particular marrow disorder such as erythroblastic hypoplasia, erythroplasia, erythroblastopenia, erythroid hypoplasia, and red cell agenesis. PRCA can be classified as: an acute self-limited type; a chronic type; and, either constitutional or acquired. PRCA was first described in 1922.[184,185]

Acquired PRCA may arise in association with thymoma, lymphoid cancer, or rheumatoid arthritis. It has also been attributed to drugs, particularly phenytoin, chlorpropamide, and isoniazid, or to infection with hepatitis B virus or parvovirus. PRCA due to neutralizing antibodies to erythropoietic proteins also has been described.[186–188]

Exogenous Epoetin and Pure Red Cell Aplasia

Endogenous human erythropoietin, a growth factor, is a glycosylated protein hormone that stimulates red cell production. It is produced mainly by the kidney and stimulates the division and differentiation of erythroid precursors in the bone marrow. Epoetin alfa, beta, and gamma are biosynthetic forms of the glycoprotein hormone erythropoietin. They have amino acid sequences identical to those of the endogenous hormone but different composition of the carbohydrate moieties.[189]

By the end of September 2002 there were 155 world wide reports of PRCA in patients treated with epoetin alfa (Eprex) confirmed by bone marrow aspirations. Of these, 112 reports had documented the presence of neutralizing antibodies with a high affinity and specificity against the protein moiety of epoetin. All but one of these cases were reported in patients with chronic renal failure.[190]

Patients who were diagnosed with PRCA before the introduction of epoetin therapy were rarely found to have antibodies against endogenous erythropoietin. One possibility is that a difference in the carbohydrate structure of exogenous epoetin and endogenous erythropoietin creates an epitope on the epoetin polypeptide to which an antibody binds, thereby inactivating not only epoetin but the endogenous hormone as well. However the anti-erythropoietin antibodies are not directed against the carbohydrate moiety on erythropoietin. Removal of the carbohydrate structure by enzymatic digestion had no effect on the antibody affinity for the erythropoietin protein.[187,188]

Other possibilities suggested as the cause of PRCA with epoetin alfa are the subcutaneous route of administration and a change in the stabilizer used in the final product formulation or both. Epoetin alfa is reported to be sensitive to physical stresses such as elevated temperature, exposure to light, or extreme shaking.[191] In December 2002, an important change in the prescribing information for the drug was made in the United Kingdom. The subcutaneous route is contraindicated for epoetin alfa use in patients with chronic renal failure.[190]

PRCA is suspected when an unexplained progressive drop in hemoglobin levels in the presence of low reticulocyte counts is detected. Treatment with epoetin must be discontinued immediately, and testing for erythropoietin antibodies and bone marrow aspiration should be performed. Patients with suspected PRCA should not be switched to another epoetin treatment.[192] Diagnosis of PRCA is usually confirmed when the bone marrow evaluation shows a virtual absence of redcell precursors. Patients diagnosed with epoetin-induced autoimmune PRCA are lifelong transfusion-dependent.[187,188]

REFERENCES

1. Benichou C, Celigny PS. Standardization of definitions and criteria for causality assessment of adverse drug reactions. Drug-induced blood cytopenias: report of an international consensus meeting. Nouv Rev Fr Hematol 1991;33:257.
2. Faich GA. Adverse-drug reaction monitoring. N Engl J Med 1986;314:1589.
3. Rogers AS et al. Physician knowledge, attitudes, and behavior related to reporting adverse drug events. Arch Intern Med 1988;148:1596.
4. Dear Doctor Letter from Russell H. Ellison, MD, Vice President, Medical Affairs, Roche Laboratories, Inc., August 1998.
5. Wilholm B-E, Emanuelsson S. Drug-related blood dyscrasias in a Swedish reporting system, 1985–1994. Eur J Haematol 1996;57(Suppl):42.
6. Wright MS. Drug-induced hemolytic anemias: increasing complications to therapeutic interventions. Clin Lab Sci 1999;12:115.
7. Beutler R. G6PD deficiency. Blood 1994;84:3613.
8. Beutler E. Glucose-6-phosphate dehydrogenase deficiency. N Engl J Med 1991;324:169.
9. Metha AB. Glucose-6-phosphate dehydrogenase deficiency. Postgrad Med 1994;70:871.
10. WHO Working Group. Glucose-6-phosphate dehydrogenase deficiency. Bull WHO 1989;67:601.
11. Eldad A et al. Silver sulphadiazine-induced haemolytic anaemia in a glucose-6-phosphate dehydrogenase-deficient burn patient. Burns 1991;17:430.
12. Markowitz N, Saravolatz LD. Use of trimethoprim-sulfamethoxazole in a glucose-6-phosphate dehydrogenase-deficient population. Rev Infect Dis 1987;9(Suppl 2):S218.
13. Levine BB, Ovary Z. Studies on the mechanism of the formation of the penicillin antigen: III. The N-(D-alpha-benzylpenicilloyl) group as an antigenic determinant responsible for hypersensitivity to penicillin. J Exp Med 1961;114:875.
14. Salama A et al. Autoantibodies and drug- or metabolite-dependent antibodies in patients with diclofenac-induced immune hemolysis. Br J Haematol 1991;77:546.
15. Bougie D et al. Sensitivity to a metabolite of diclofenac as a cause of acute immune hemolytic anemia. Blood 1997;90:407.
16. Wright MS, Smith LA. Laboratory investigation autoimmune hemolytic anemias. Clin Lab Sci 1999;12:119.
17. Levine BB, Redmond A. Immunochemical mechanisms of penicillin induced Coombs positivity and hemolytic anemia in man. Int Arch Allergy Appl Immunol 1967;31:594.
18. Petz LD, Garratty GM. Acquired Immune Hemolytic Anemias. New York, NY: Churchill Livingstone, 1980:279.
19. Nesmith LW, Davis JW. Hemolytic anemia caused by penicillin. JAMA 1968;203:27.
20. Garratty G. Immune cytopenia associated with antibiotics. Trans Med Rev 1993;7:255.
21. Garratty G et al. Severe immune hemolytic anemia associated with prophylactic use of cefotetan in obstetric and gynecologic procedures. Am J Obstet Gynecol 1999;181:103.
22. Packman CH, Leddy JP. Drug-related immune hemolytic anemia. In: Beutler E et al., eds. Hematology. 5th Ed. New York: McGraw-Hill, 1995:681.
23. Salama A, Mueller-Eckhardt C. Immune-mediated blood cell dyscrasias related to drugs. Semin Hematol 1992;29:54.
24. Salama A, Mueller-Eckhardt C. Immune-mediated blood cell dyscrasias related to drugs. Semin Hematol 1992;29:54.
25. Class FHJ. Immune mechanisms leading to drug-induced blood dyscrasias. Eur J Haematol 1996;57(Suppl):64.
26. The European Agency for the Evaluation of Medicinal Products. Public statement on Trovan/Turvel IV/Turvel IV (Trovafloxacin/Alatrofloxacin)—recommendation to suspend the marketing authorization in the European Union. June 15, 1999.

27. Food and Drug Administration. Public Health Advisory—Trovan (trovafloxacin/alatrofloxacin mesylate). June 9, 1999.
28. Blum MD, Graham DJ. Temafloxacin syndrome: review of 95 cases. Clin Infect Dis 1994;18:946.
29. Kleinman S et al. Positive direct antiglobulin tests and immune hemolytic anemia in patients receiving procainamide. N Engl J Med 1984;311:809.
30. Anonymous. Hemolysis from ceftriaxone. Med Lett Drugs Ther 2002;44:100.
31. Brandt NJ, Lund J. Methyldopa and haemolytic anaemia. Lancet 1966;1: 771.
32. Buchanan JG et al. Methyldopa and acquired haemolytic anaemia. Med J Aust 1966;2:700.
33. Hamilton M. Some aspects of the long-term treatment of severe hypertension with methyldopa. Postgrad Med J 1968;44:66.
34. Murad F. Immunohemolytic anemia during therapy with methyldopa. JAMA 1968;203:149.
35. Surveyor I et al. Autoimmune haemolytic anaemia complicating methyldopa therapy. Postgrad Med J 1968;44:438.
36. Pedersen-Bjergaard U et al. Thrombocytopenia induced by noncytotoxic drugs in Denmark 1968–91. J Intern Med 1996;239:509.
37. Wilholm BE, Emanuelsson S. Drug-related blood dyscrasias in a Swedish reporting system, 1985–1994. Eur J Haematol 1996;57(Suppl):42.
38. Bonfiglio M et al. Thrombocytopenia in intensive care patients: a comprehensive analysis of risk factors in 314 patients. Ann Pharmacother 1995;29:835.
39. Burnakis T. Inaccurate assessment of drug-induced thrombocytopenia: reason for concern. Ann Pharmacother 1994;28:726.
40. George JN et al. Drug induced thrombocytopenia: a systematic review of published case reports. Ann Intern Med 1998;129:886.
41. Nordquist P et al. Thrombocytopenia during chlorothiazide treatment. Lancet 1959;1:271.
42. Eisner EV, Crowell EB. Hydrochlorothiazide-dependent thrombocytopenia due to an IgM antibody. JAMA 1971;215:480.
43. Eichner ER, Hillman RS. The evolution of anemia in alcoholic patients. Am J Med 1971;50:218.
44. Cowan DH, Hines JD. Thrombocytopenia of severe alcoholism. Ann Intern Med 1971;74:37.
45. Eichner ER et al. Variations in the hematologic and medical status of alcoholics. Am J Med Sci 1972;263:35.
46. Haut MJ, Cowan DH. The effect of ethanol on hemostatic properties of human blood platelets. Am J Med 1974;56:22.
47. Cowan DH. Effect of alcoholism on hemostasis. Semin Hematol 1980;17:137.
48. Glynne P. Quinine-induced immune thrombocytopenic purpura followed by hemolytic uremic syndrome. Am J Kidney Dis 1999;33:133.
49. Crum NF, Gable P. Quinine-induced hemolytic-uremic syndrome. South Med J 2000;93:726.
50. Walter RB et al. Gemcitabine-associated hemolytic-uremic syndrome. Am J Kidney Dis 2002;40:E16.
51. Maguire RB et al. Recurrent pancytopenia, coagulopathy, and renal failure associated with multiple quinine-dependent antibodies. Ann Intern Med 1993;119:215.
52. Curtis BR et al. Antibodies in sulfonamide-induced immune thrombocytopenia recognize calcium-dependent epitopes on the glycoprotein IIb/IIIa complex. Blood 1994;84:176.
53. George JN et al. Thrombocytopenia due to enhanced platelet destruction by immunologic mechanisms. In: Beutler E et al., eds. Hematology. 5th Ed. New York: McGraw-Hill, 1995:1315.
54. Christie DJ et al. Structural features of the quinidine and quinine molecules necessary for binding of drug-induced antibodies to human platelets. J Lab Clin Med 1984;104:730.
55. Mettier SR et al. Thrombocytopenic purpura complicating gold therapy for rheumatoid arthritis. Blood 1948;3:1105.

56. Coblyn JS et al. Gold-induced thrombocytopenia: a clinical and immunogenetic study of twenty-three patients. Ann Intern Med 1981;95:178.
57. Comer M et al. Are slow-acting anti-rheumatic drugs monitored too often? An audit of current clinical practice. Br J Rheumatol 1995;34:966.
58. Adachi JD et al. Gold induced thrombocytopenia: 12 cases and a review of the literature. Semin Arthritis Rheum 1987;16:287.
59. Deren B et al. Gold-associated thrombocytopenia: report of six cases. Arch Intern Med 1974;134:1012.
60. Levin HA et al. Thrombocytopenia associated with gold therapy: observations on the mechanism of platelet destruction. Am J Med 1975;59:274.
61. Kosty MP et al. Thrombocytopenia associated with auranofin therapy: evidence for a gold-dependent immunologic mechanism. Am J Hematol 1989;30:236.
62. Goldstein R et al. Treatment of gold-induced thrombocytopenia by high-dose intravenous gamma globulin. Arthritis Rheum 1986;29:426.
63. Ansell J et al. Heparin induced thrombocytopenia: a prospective study. Thromb Haemost 1980;43:61.
64. Bell WR. Heparin-associated thrombocytopenia and thrombosis. J Lab Clin Med 1988;11:600.
65. Kelton JG et al. Immunoglobulin G from patients with heparin-induced thrombocytopenia binds to a complex of heparin and platelet factor 4. Blood 1994;83:3232.
66. Visentin GP et al. Antibodies from patients with heparin-induced thrombocytopenia/thrombosis are specific for platelet factor 4 complexed with heparin or bound to endothelial cells. J Clin Invest 1994;93:81.
67. Warkentin TE, Kelton JG. Heparin-induced thrombocytopenia. Prog Hemost Thromb 1991;10:1.
68. Anderson GM. Insights into heparin-induced thrombocytopenia. Br J Haematol 1992;80:504.
69. Brieger DB et al. Heparin-induced thrombocytopenia. J Am Coll Cardiol 1998;31:1449.
70. Kelton JG et al. Clinical usefulness of testing for a heparin-dependent platelet aggregating factor in patients with suspected heparin-associated thrombocytopenia. J Lab Clin Med 1984;103:606.
71. Chong BH et al. The clinical usefulness of the platelet aggregation test for the diagnosis of heparin-induced thrombocytopenia. Thromb Haemost 1993;69:344.
72. Warkentin TE. Heparin-induced thrombocytopenia in patients treated with low-molecular-weight heparin or unfractionated heparin. N Engl J Med 1995;332:1330.
73. Nelson JC et al. Heparin-induced thrombocytopenia. Arch Intern Med 1978;138:548.
74. Bell WR, Royall RM. Heparin-associated thrombocytopenia: a comparison of three heparin preparations. N Engl J Med 1980;303:902.
75. Schmitt BP, Adelman B. Heparin-associated thrombocytopenia: a critical review and pooled analysis. Am J Med Sci 1993;305:208.
76. Heeger PS, Backstrom JT. Heparin flushes and thrombocytopenia. Ann Intern Med 1986;105:143.
77. Laster JL et al. Thrombocytopenia associated with heparin-coated catheters in patients with heparin-associated antiplatelet antibodies. Arch Intern Med 1989;149:2285.
78. Garrelts JC. White clot syndrome and thrombocytopenia: reasons to abandon heparin i.v. lock flush solution. Clin Pharm 1992;11:797.
79. Warkentin TE et al. Heparin-induced thrombocytopenia in patients treated with low molecular weight heparin or unfractionated heparin. N Engl J Med 1995;1995:1330.
80. Laster J et al. Reexposure to heparin of patients with heparin-associated antibodies. J Vasc Surg 1989;9:677.
81. Warkentin TE et al. A 14-year study of heparin-induced thrombocytopenia. Am J Med 1996;101:502.
82. Cines DB et al. Immune endothelial-cell injury in heparin-associated thrombocytopenia. N Engl J Med 1987;316:581.

83. Hull RD et al. Heparin for 5 days as compared with 10 days in the initial treatment of proximal venous thrombosis. N Engl J Med 1990;322:1260.

84. Lovenox (enoxaparin) professional product labeling. Collegeville, PA: Rhone Poulenc, revised April 1995.

85. Gouault-Heilmann M et al. Low molecular weight heparin fractions as an alternative therapy in heparin-induced thrombocytopenia. Haemostasis 1987;17:134.

86. Chong BH et al. Heparin-induced thrombocytopenia: studies with a new low molecular weight heparinoid, Org 10172. Blood 1989;73:1592.

87. Ramakrishna R et al. Heparin-induced thrombocytopenia: cross-reactivity between standard heparin, low molecular weight heparin, dalteparin (Fragmin) and heparinoid, danaparoid (Orgaran). Br J Haematol 1995;91:736.

88. Vun CM et al. Cross-reactivity study of low molecular weight heparins and heparinoid in heparin-induced thrombocytopenia. Thromb Res 1996; 81:525.

89. Demers C et al. Rapid anticoagulation using ancrod for heparin-induced thrombocytopenia. Blood 1991;78:2194.

90. Yurvati AH et al. Heparinless cardiopulmonary bypass with ancrod. Ann Thorac Surg 1994;57:1656.

91. Chamberlin JR et al. Successful treatment of heparin-associated thrombocytopenia and thrombosis using Hirulog. Can J Cardiol 1995;11:511.

92. Schiele F et al. Use of recombinant hirudin as antithrombotic treatment in patients with heparin-induced thrombocytopenia. Am J Hematol 1995; 11:20.

93. Harenberg J et al. Anticoagulation in patients with heparin-induced thrombocytopenia type II. Semin Thromb Hemost 1997;23:189.

94. Pina I. FDA panel votes against approval for bivalirudin. Circulation 1999;99:1277.

95. Refludan (lepirudin) professional product labeling. March 1998. Berlex Laboratories, Montville, New Jersey.

96. Mehta DP et al. Heparin-induced thrombocytopenia and thrombosis: reversal with streptokinase a case report and review of literature. Am J Hematol 1991;36:275.

97. Murphy KD et al. The heparin-induced thrombocytopenia and thrombosis syndrome: treatment with intraarterial urokinase and systemic platelet aggregation inhibitors. Cardiovasc Interven Radiol 1996;19:123.

98. Nand S, Robinson JA. Plasmapheresis in the management of heparin-associated thrombocytopenia with thrombosis. Am J Hematol 1988;28:204.

99. Brady J et al. Plasmapheresis: a therapeutic option in the management of heparin-associated thrombocytopenia with thrombosis. Am J Clin Pathol 1991;96:394.

100. Bouvier JL et al. Treatment of serious heparin-induced thrombocytopenia by plasma exchange: report of 4 cases. Thromb Res 1988;51:335.

101. Frame JN et al. Correction of severe heparin-associated thrombocytopenia with intravenous immunoglobulin. Ann Intern Med 1989;111:946.

102. Bennett CL et al. Thrombotic thrombocytopenic purpura associated with ticlopidine. Ann Intern Med 1998;128:541.

103. Steinhuble SR et al. Incidence and clinical course of thrombotic thrombocytopenic purpura due to ticlopidine following coronary stenting. JAMA 1999;281:806.

104. Bennett CL et al. Thrombotic thrombocytopenic purpura associated with ticlopidine in the stetting of coronary artery stents and stroke prevention. Arch Intern Med 1999;159:2524.

105. Bennett CL et al. Thrombotic Thrombocytopenic purpura associated with clopidogrel. N Engl J Med 2000;342:1773.

106. Strom BL et al. Descriptive epidemiology of agranulocytosis. Arch Intern Med 1992;152:1475.

107. Kaufman DW et al. Drugs in the aetiology of agranulocytosis and aplastic anaemia. Eur J Haematol 1996;57(Suppl):23.

108. Reizenstein P, Edgard K. Mortality in agranulocytosis. Lancet 1974;2:293.

109. Julia A et al. Drug-induced agranulocytosis: prognostic factors in a series of 168 episodes. Br J Haematol 1991;79:366.

110. Kurtz J-E et al. Drug-induced agranulocytosis in older people: a case series of 25 patients [Letter]. Age Ageing 1999;28:325.

111. Neftel KA et al. Inhibition of granulopoiesis in vivo and in vitro by β-lactam antibiotics. J Infect Dis 1985;152:90.

112. Houmayouni H et al. Leukopenia due to penicillin and cephalosporin homologues. Arch Intern Med 1979;139:827.

113. Murphy MF et al. Demonstration of an immune-mediated mechanism of penicillin-induced neutropenia and thrombocytopenia. Br J Haematol 1983;55:155.

114. Salama A et al. Immune-mediated agranulocytosis related to drugs and their metabolites: mode of sensitization and heterogeneity of antibodies. Br J Haematol 1989;72:127.

115. Murphy MF et al. Cephalosporin-induced immune neutropenia. Br J Haematol 1985;59:9.

116. Rey D et al. Ceftriaxone-induced granulopoiesis related to a peculiar mechanism of granulopoiesis inhibition. Am J Med 1989;87:591.

117. Hauser SP et al. Effects of ceftazidime, a beta-lactam antibiotic, on murine haemopoiesis in vitro. Br J Haematol 1994;86:733.

118. Uetrecht JP. Reactive metabolites and agranulocytosis. Eur J Haematol 1996;57(Suppl):83.

119. Anonymous. Antibiotic-induced neutropenia [Editorial]. Lancet 1985;2:814.

120. Anonymous. The choice of antibacterial drugs. Med Lett Drugs Ther 1999;41;95.

121. Pisciotta AV. Immune and toxic mechanisms in drug-induced agranulocytosis. Semin Hematol 1973;10:279.

122. Pisciotta AV. Drug-induced agranulocytosis. Drugs 1978;15:132.

123. Pisciotta AV. Agranulocytosis induced by certain phenothiazine derivatives. JAMA 1969;208:1862.

124. Sprikkelman A et al. The application of hematopoietic growth factors in drug-induced agranulocytosis: a review of 70 cases. Leukemia 1994;12:2031.

125. Anaissie EJ et al. Randomized comparison between antibiotics alone and antibiotics plus granulocyte-macrophage colony-stimulating factor (Escherichia coli-derived) in cancer patients with fever and neutropenia. Am J Med 1996;100:17.

126. Hartmann LC et al. Granulocyte colony-stimulating factor in severe chemotherapy-induced afebrile neutropenia. N Engl J Med 1997;336:1776.

127. Demuynck H et al. Risks of rhG-CSF treatment in drug-induced agranulocytosis. Ann Hematol 1995; 70:143.

128. Amsler HA et al. Agranulocytosis in patients treated with clozapine: a study of the Finnish epidemic. Acta Psychiatr Scand 1977;56:241.

129. Honigfeld G. Effects of the clozapine national registry system on incidence of deaths related to agranulocytosis. Psychiatr Serv 1996;47:52.

130. Atkin K et al. Neutropenia and agranulocytosis in patients receiving clozapine in the UK and Ireland. Br J Psychiatr 1996;169:483.

131. Alvir JMJ et al. Clozapine-induced agranulocytosis: incidence and risk factors in the United States. N Engl J Med 1993;329:162.

132. Olanazpine (Zyprexa): suspected serious reactions. Can Adv Drug React Newslett 2000;10:85.

133. Pisciotta AV et al. On the possible mechanisms and predictability of clozapine-induced agranulocytosis. Drug Saf 1992;7(Suppl 1):33.

134. Pisciotta AV et al. Cytotoxic activity in serum of patients with clozapine-induced agranulocytosis. J Lab Clin Med 1992;119:254.

135. Maggs JL et al. The metabolic formation of reactive intermediates from clozapine, a drug associated with agranulocytosis in man. J Pharmacol Exp Ther 1996;275:1463.

136. Gerson SL et al. N-desmethylclozapine: a clozapine metabolite that suppresses haemopoiesis. Br J Haematol 1994;86·555.

137. Corzo D et al. The major histocompatibility complex region marked by HSP70-1 and HSP70-2 variants is associated with clozapine-induced agranulocytosis in two different ethnic groups. Blood 1995;86:3835.

138. Lieberman JA et al. Clozapine-induced agranulocytosis: non-cross-reactivity with other psychotropic drugs. J Clin Psychiatry 1988;49:271.

139. Bauer M, Mackert A. Clozapine treatment after agranulocytosis induced by classic neuroleptics. J Clin Psychopharmacol 1994;14:71.

140. Moeschlin S, Wagner K. Agranulocytosis due to the occurrence of leukocyte agglutinins. Acta Haematol 1952;8:29.

141. Hargis JB et al. Agranulocytosis associated with "Mexican aspirin" (dipyrone): evidence for an autoimmune mechanism affecting multipotential hematopoietic progenitors. Am J Hematol 1989; 31:213.

142. International Agranulocytosis and Aplastic Anemia Study. Risks of agranulocytosis and aplastic anemia: a first report of their relation to drug use with special reference to analgesics. JAMA 1986;256:1749.

143. Young NS, Barrett AJ. The treatment of severe acquired aplastic anemia. Blood 1995;85:3367.

144. Young NS. Acquired aplastic anemia. JAMA 1999; 282:271.

145. Young NS. The problem of clonality in aplastic anemia: Dr. Dameshek's riddle, restated. Blood 1992;79:1385.

146. Patton WN, Duffull SB. Idiosyncratic drug-induced haematological abnormalities. Drug Saf 1994;11:445.

147. Young NS. Autoimmunity and its treatment in aplastic anemia [Editorial]. Ann Intern Med 1997; 126:166.8.

148. Yunis AA et al. Chloramphenicol toxicity: pathogenetic mechanisms and the role of the p-NO2 in aplastic anemia. Clin Toxicol 1980;17:359.

149. Howell A et al. Bone marrow cells resistant to chloramphenicol in chloramphenicol-induced aplastic anemia. Lancet 1975;1:65.

150. Kern P et al. Bone-marrow cells resistant to chloramphenicol in chloramphenicol-induced aplastic anemia. Lancet 1975;1:1190.

151. Yunis AA et al. DNA damage induced by chloramphenicol and its nitroso derivative: damage in intact cells. Am J Hematol 1987;24:77.

152. Jimenez JJ et al. Chloramphenicol-induced bone marrow injury: possible role of bacterial metabolites of chloramphenicol. Blood 1987;70:1180.

153. Vincent PC. In vitro evidence of drug action in aplastic anemia. Blood 1984;49:3.

154. Lafarge-Frayssinet C et al. Cytotoxicity and DNA damaging potency of chloramphenicol and six metabolites: a new evaluation in human lymphocytes and Raji cells. Mutat Res 1994;320:207.

155. Yunis AA. Chloramphenicol toxicity: 25 years of research. Am J Med 1989;87:44.

156. Plaut ME, Best WR. Aplastic anemia after parenteral chloramphenicol: a warning renewed. N Engl J Med 1982;306:1486.

157. West BC et al. Aplastic anemia associated with parenteral chloramphenicol: a review of 10 cases including the second case of possible increased risk with cimetidine. Rev Infect Dis 1988;10:1048.

158. Fraunfelder FT, Bagby GC. Ocular chloramphenicol and aplastic anemia. N Engl J Med 1983; 308:1536.

159. Doona M, Walsh JB. Use of chloramphenicol as topical eye medication: time to cry halt. Br Med J 1995;310:1217.

160. Nelson L et al. Aplastic anemia induced by an adulterated herbal medication. Clin Toxicol 1995;33:467.

161. Food and Drug Administration. Recommendation for the immediate withdrawal of patients from treatment with Felbatol (felbamate). FDA Med Bull 1994;24:5.

162. Green SL et al. Linezolid and reversible myelo-suppression. JAMA 2001;285:1291.

163. Zyvox (linezolid) professional product labeling. Revised December 2002. Pharmacia, Kalamazoo, Michigan.

164. Symeonidis A et al. Ticlopidine-induced aplastic anemia: two new case reports, review, and meta-analysis of 55 additional cases. Am J Hematol 2002;71:24.

165. Avonex (interferon beta-1a) professional product labeling. Revised February 2003. Biogen, Cambridge, Massachusetts.

166. Baurnelou E et al. Epidemiology of aplastic anemia in France: a case-control study. I. Medical history and medication use. Blood 1993;81:1471.

167. Young NS. Autoimmunity and its treatment in aplastic anemia [Editorial]. Ann Intern Med 1997;126:1.

168. Paquette RL et al. Long-term outcome of aplastic anemia in adults treated with antithymocyte globulin: comparison with bone marrow transplantation. Blood 1995;85:283.

169. Dooney K et al. Primary treatment of acquired aplastic anemia: outcomes with bone marrow transplantation and immunosuppressive therapy. Ann Intern Med 1997;126:107.

170. Bacigalupo A et al. Bone marrow transplantation (BMT) versus immunosuppression for the treatment of severe aplastic anemia (SAA): a report of the EBMT SAA working party. Br J Haematol 1988;70:177.

171. Young NS, Barrett AJ. The treatment of severe acquired aplastic anemia. Blood 1995;85:3367.

172. Hinterberger W et al. Results of transplanting bone marrow from genetically identical twins into patients with aplastic anemia. Ann Intern Med 1997;126:115.

173. Frickhofen N et al. Treatment of aplastic anemia with antilymphocyte globulin and methylprednisolone with or without cyclosporine. N Engl J Med 1991;324:1297.

174. Atgam (lymphocyte immune globulin) Professional product labeling. Kalamazoo, MI: Upjohn Company, revised March 1993.

175. French Cooperative Group for the Study of Aplastic and Refractory Anemias. Androgen therapy in aplastic anemia: a comparative study of high and low-doses and of 4 different androgens. Scand J Haematol 1986;36:346.

176. Seewald TR et al. Successful treatment of severe refractory aplastic anemia with 3-B-etiocholanolone and nandrolone decanoate. Am J Hematol 1989;31:216.

177. Bacigalupo A et al. Treatment of aplastic anemia (AA) with antilymphocyte globulin (ALG) and methylprednisolone (Mpred) with or without androgens: a randomized trial from the EBMT SAA working party. Br J Haematol 1993;83:145.

178. Antin JH et al. Phase I/II study of recombinant human granulocyte-macrophage colony-stimulating factor in aplastic anemia of both acquired and myelodysplastic syndrome. Blood 1988; 72:705.

179. Kojima S et al. Treatment of aplastic anemia in children with recombinant human granulocyte colony-stimulating factor. Blood 1992;77:937.

180. Bessho M et al. Treatment of the anemia of aplastic anemia patients with recombinant human erythropoietin in combination with granulocyte colony-stimulating factor: a multicenter randomized controlled study. Eur J Haematol 1997;58:265.

181. Geissler K et al. Effect of interleukin-3 on responsiveness to granulocyte-colony-stimulating factor in severe aplastic anemia. Ann Intern Med 1992;117:223.

182. Kojima S et al. Myelodysplasia and leukemia after treatment of aplastic anemia with G-CSF [Letter]. N Engl J Med 1992;326:1294.

183. Marsh JCW et al. Haemopoietic growth factors in aplastic anaemia: a cautionary note. Lancet 1994;344:172.

184. Erslev AJ. Pure red cell aplasia. In: Beutler E et al., eds. Hematology. 5th Ed. New York: McGraw-Hill, 1995:448.

185. Lee GR. Anemia general aspects. In: Lee GR et al., eds. Wintrobe's Clinical Hematology. 1999: 897.

186. Wooltorton E. Epoetin alfa (Eprex): reports of pure red cell aplasia. Can Med Assoc J 2002; 166:480.

187. Bunn F. Drug induced autoimmune red cell aplasia [Editorial]. N Engl J Med 2002;346:522.

188. Casadevall N et al. Pure red cell aplasia after treatment with recombinant erythropoietin. N Engl J Med 2002;346:469.

189. McEvoy GK, ed. AHFS 2002 Drug Information. Bethesda, MD: American Society of Health-System Pharmacists Inc.

190. Committee on Safety of Medicines. Eprex (Epoetin Alfa) and pure red cell aplasia: contraindication of subcutaneous administration to patients with chronic renal disease. December 12, 2002.

191. J & J Eprex stability improvements planned in response to aplasia incidence. The Pink Sheet, September 16, 2002, page 24.

192. Important new safety information—Eprex (epoetin alfa): reports of pure red cell aplasia. Dear Healthcare Professional Letter. Toronto, Canada: Janssen-Ortho Inc. and Ortho Biotech, November 26, 2001.

NEOPLASTIC DISORDERS

Celeste Lindley
SECTION EDITOR

CHAPTER **88**

Neoplastic Disorders and Their Treatment: General Principles

Lisa Davis, Celeste Lindley

INTRODUCTION TO NEOPLASTIC DISEASES

Cancer (neoplasm, tumor, or malignancy) is not a single disease; rather, it is a group of diseases characterized by uncontrolled growth and spread of abnormal cells. Cancer cells do not respond to the normal processes that regulate cell growth, proliferation, and survival, and they cannot carry out the physiologic functions of their normal differentiated (mature) counterparts. Often, cancer cells are described as poorly differentiated or immature. Other characteristics of cancer cells include their ability to invade adjacent normal tissues and break away from the primary tumor (metastasize) and travel through the blood or lymph to establish new tumors (metastases) at a distant site. Their ability to stimulate the formation of new blood vessels (angiogenesis) and their endless replication potential further contribute to their continued growth and survival.[1] Cancers can arise in any tissue in the body and may be classified as benign or malignant. If malignant cancer cells are allowed to grow uncontrollably, they can eventually result in the death of the patient, whereas benign cancer cells cannot spread by tissue invasion or metastasize. Each year, the American Cancer Society (ACS) publishes the estimated number of new cases and number of cancer-related deaths. The National Cancer Institute (NCI) publishes cancer statistics that also include cancer risk, prevalence, and survival information.[2]

Cancer Statistics

The ACS estimates that 1 in 2 American men and 1 in 3 American women will eventually develop cancer and that approximately 1,334,100 new cases of cancer will be diagnosed in 2003.[3] The most common cancers and causes of cancer deaths in adult Americans are illustrated in Figure 88-1. The incidence of cancer and cancer-related deaths can be affected by

New Cancer Cases				Cancer Deaths			
Prostate	(33%)	Breast	(32%)	Lung and bronchus	(31%)	Lung and bronchus	(25%)
Lung and bronchus	(14%)	Lung and bronchus	(12%)	Prostate	(10%)	Breast	(15%)
Colon and rectum	(11%)	Colon and rectum	(11%)	Colon and rectum	(10%)	Colon and rectum	(11%)
Urinary bladder	(6%)	Uterine corpus	(6%)	Pancreas	(5%)	Pancreas	(6%)
Melanoma of skin	(4%)	Ovary	(4%)	Non-Hodgkin lymphoma	(4%)	Ovary	(5%)
Non-Hodgkin lymphoma	(4%)	Non-Hodgkin lymphoma	(4%)	Leukemia	(4%)	Non-Hodgkin lymphoma	(4%)
Kidney	(3%)	Melanoma of skin	(3%)	Esophagus	(4%)	Leukemia	(4%)
Oral cavity	(3%)	Thyroid	(3%)	Liver/intrahepatic bile duct	(3%)	Uterine corpus	(3%)
Leukemia	(3%)	Pancreas	(2%)	Urinary bladder	(3%)	Brain/ONS	(2%)
Pancreas	(2%)	Urinary bladder	(2%)	Kidney	(3%)	Multiple myeloma	(2%)
All other sites	(17%)	All other sites	(20%)	All other sites	(22%)	All other sites	(23%)
Men 675,300		Women 658,800		Men 285,900		Women 270,600	

FIGURE 88-1 Leading sites of new cancer cases and deaths in the United States, 2003, excluding basal and squamous cell skin cancers and in situ carcinomas except urinary bladder. ONS, other nervous system. (Data from reference 3.)

both age and ethnic background with the incidence greater in the elderly and African-American populations.[4] Other factors that may increase an individual's risk for developing a cancer include environmental and lifestyle factors, genetic predisposition, immunosuppression, and exposure to one or more potential carcinogens.[5]

Etiology

Cancers arise from the transformation of a single normal cell. An initial "event" causes damage or mutation to the cell's DNA. These events may include lifestyle, environmental, or occupational factors, as well as some medical therapies (e.g., cytotoxic chemotherapy, immunosuppressive therapy, or radiation therapy) and hereditary factors (Table 88-1). Currently, cigarette smoking is probably the most significant single factor that contributes to the development of cancers. The ACS estimates that tobacco use will be responsible for approximately 180,000 cancer deaths in 2003.[3] In addition, approximately one-third of expected cancer deaths in 2003 are thought to result from preventable causes such as physical inactivity, obesity, nutrition, and other lifestyle factors.[3,6]

Progress in our understanding about the development of cancer at the molecular level has led us to recognize that cancer is a genetic disease. Two gene classes, oncogenes and tumor-suppressor genes, play a major role in the pathogenesis of cancer. Damage to cellular DNA can result in mutations that lead to the development of oncogenes and loss or inactivation of tumor suppressor genes. Oncogenes are genes whose overactivity or presence in certain forms can lead to the development of cancer. Oncogenes arise from normal genes called proto-oncogenes through genetic alterations such as chromosomal translocations, deletions, insertions, and point mutations.

Growth and proliferation of normal cells are influenced by proteins, known as growth factors. When growth factors bind to receptors on the cell surface, they activate a series of enzymes within the cell that stimulate cell signaling pathways and gene transcription proteins in the nucleus, which encode

for proteins that regulate cell growth and proliferation. The coordination and integration of cellular signaling processes are referred to as signal transduction. Proto-oncogenes are responsible for encoding several components of signal trans-

Table 88-1 Carcinogens Associated With an Increased Risk of Cancer

Carcinogenic Risk Factor	Associated Cancer(s)
Environmental	
Ionizing radiation (radon gas emitted from soil containing uranium deposits)	Leukemia, breast, thyroid, lung
Ultraviolet radiation	Skin melanoma
Viruses	Leukemia, lymphoma, nasopharyngeal, liver, cervix
Occupational	
Asbestos	Lung, mesothelioma
Chromium, nickel	Lung
Vinyl chloride	Liver
Aniline dye	Bladder
Benzene	Leukemia
Lifestyle	
Alcohol	Esophagus, liver, stomach, oropharynx, larynx
Dietary factors	Colon, breast, gallbladder, gastric
Tobacco	Lung, oropharynx, pharynx, larynx, esophagus, bladder
Medical Drugs	
Diethylstilbestrol	Vaginal in offspring, breast, testes, ovary
Alkylating agents	Leukemia, bladder
Azathioprine	Lymphoma
Phenacetin	Bladder
Estrogens, tamoxifen	Endometrial
Cyclophosphamide	Bladder

duction pathways, including growth factors, growth factor receptors, signaling enzymes, and DNA transcription factors. Abnormal forms or excessive quantities of these stimulatory proteins disrupt normal cell growth-signaling pathways, leading to excessive growth and proliferation and, ultimately, a malignant transformation. For example, the epidermal growth factor receptor (EGFR) is a member of a family of type I receptor tyrosine kinases, which trigger cell signaling pathways that influence cell growth, proliferation, survival, tissue invasion, and metastases.[7] The family includes four related receptors: EGFR (also referred to as ErbB1 or HER1), ErbB2 (HER2, HER2/neu), ErbB3 (HER3), and ErbB4 (HER4). These receptor proteins are composed of an extracellular binding domain, a transmembrane segment, and an intracellular protein tyrosine kinase domain. In cancer cells, the receptors can become activated through receptor binding to the extracellular domain, resulting in heterodimerization (different members of the receptor family) or homodimerization (like members of the receptor family).[8]

Ligand-independent receptor dimerization can occur as well and is the principal form of activation of HER2, since HER2 does not bind to any known ligands.[9] The EGFR signaling pathway is depicted in Figure 88-2. Activation of the receptor protein tyrosine kinase leads to autophosphorylation of tyrosine and other intracellular substrates that initiate downstream cellular signaling events.[7] An important signaling route is the Ras-Raf-MAP kinase pathway, which regulates transcription of molecules that are associated with cell prolif-

eration, survival, and malignant transformation.[7] Other important routes for signaling include the phosphatidylinositol 3-kinase (PI3K)-protein-serine/threonine kinase Akt and the stress-activated protein kinase pathways.[7] EGFR is frequently overexpressed in human tumors, including cancers of the lung, head and neck, bladder, breast, ovary, prostate, colon, and glioblastoma.[7] Amplification of the HER2/neu gene or overexpression of the protein is present in 10 to 34% of invasive breast cancers.[10] Increased EGFR or HER2/neu expression in several cancers is associated with a more aggressive cancer growth pattern and poorer clinical outcome.[7]

Tumor-suppressor genes are normal genes that encode for proteins that suppress inappropriate cell division or growth. Gene losses or mutations of these genes can cause these proteins to become inactivated, eliminating the normal inhibition of cell division. Alterations in a third class of genes, DNA repair genes, are also implicated in cancer. DNA repair genes encode for proteins that correct errors that may arise during DNA duplication. Mutations in these genes further contribute to the accumulation of genetic changes that promote cancer progression.

Table 88-2 lists examples of genes frequently associated with human cancers. Multiple genetic mutations, including activation of oncogenes and loss or inactivation of tumor-suppressor genes within a cell, are necessary for malignant transformation.[11] Separate genetic changes are required for tumor invasion of normal tissues and metastases.

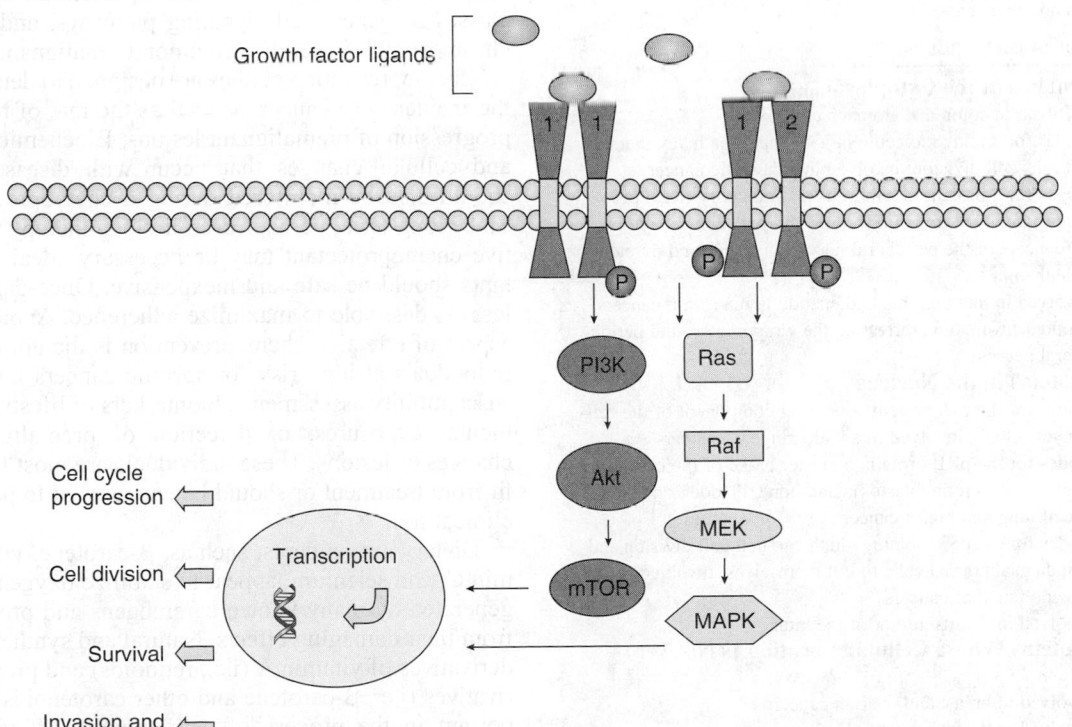

FIGURE 88-2 Epidermal growth factor signaling. Members of the ErbB receptor family become activated by dimerization. Ligand binding to the extracellular domain of epidermal growth factor receptor (EGFR) leads to receptor activation through homodimerization or heterodimerization with other ErbB receptors. Activation of the receptor tyrosine kinase results in tyrosine autophosphorylation and a series of phosphorylations of intracellular substrates that influence cell growth stimulatory signaling and other cellular activities.

Table 88-2   Some Genes Involved in Human Cancers[11]

Oncogenes

Genes for Growth Factors or Their Receptors

PDGF   Codes for platelet-derived growth factor; involved in glioma (a brain cancer)

erb-B   Codes for the receptor for epidermal growth factor; involved in glioblastoma (a brain cancer and breast cancer)

erb-B2   Also called *Her-2* or *neu;* codes for a growth factor receptor; involved in breast, salivary gland, and ovarian cancers

RET   Codes for a growth factor receptor; involved in thyroid cancer

Genes for Cytoplasmic Relays in Stimulatory Signaling Pathways

Ki-ras   Involved in lung, ovarian, colon, and pancreatic cancers

N-ras   Involved in leukemias

Genes for Transcription Factors That Activate Growth-Promoting Genes

c-myc   Involved in leukemias and breast, stomach, and lung cancers

N-myc   Involved in neuroblastoma (a nerve cell cancer) and glioblastoma

L-myc   Involved in lung cancer

Genes for Other Kinds of Molecules

Bcl-2   Codes for a protein that normally blocks cell suicide; involved in follicular B-cell lymphoma

Bcl-1   Also called *PRAD1;* codes for cyclin D1, a stimulatory component of the cell-cycle clock; involved in breast, head, and neck cancers

MDM2   Codes for an antagonist of the p53 tumor-suppressor protein; involved in sarcomas (connective tissue cancers) and others cancers

Tumor-Suppressor Genes

Genes for Proteins in the Cytoplasm

APC   Involved in colon and stomach cancers

DPC-4   Codes for a relay molecule in a signaling pathway that inhibits cell division; involved in pancreatic cancer

NF-1   Codes for a protein that inhibits a stimulatory (Ras) protein; involved in neurofibroma and pheochromocytoma (cancers of the peripheral nervous system) and myeloid leukemia

NF-2   Involved in meningioma and ependymoma (brain cancers) and schwannoma (affecting the wrapping around peripheral nerves)

Genes for Proteins in the Nucleus

MTS1   Codes for the p16 protein, a braking component of the cell-cycle clock; involved in a wide range of cancers

RB   Codes for the pRB protein, a master brake of the cell cycle; involved in retinoblastoma and bone, bladder, and small cell lung and breast cancer

p53   Codes for the p53 protein, which can halt cell division and induce abnormal cells to kill themselves; involved in a wide range of cancers

WT1   Involved in Wilms' tumor of the kidney

Genes for Proteins Whose Cellular Location Is Not Yet Clear

BRCA1   Involved in breast and ovarian cancers

BRCA2   Involved in breast cancer

VHL   Involved in renal cell cancer

Prevention
Chemoprevention

1. M.S., a 37-year-old woman, asks about taking antioxidant vitamins to reduce her risk of cancer. Her mother died several years ago of colon cancer, and she fears that she also will develop the disease. Does taking antioxidant vitamins alter the risk of cancer? What other measures might prevent cancer?

Cancer chemoprevention focuses on suppressing or reversing carcinogenesis in the early phases and preventing the development of invasive cancer. Also, much has been learned about the differences that exist among people and the interindividual variability in their inherited susceptibility to carcinogenic exposures.[12] This type of information will be useful in the design of a chemoprevention program that can be personalized for a specific individual. Chemoprevention strategies can be categorized as primary prevention (i.e., preventing cancer in a healthy individual at high risk), secondary prevention (i.e., preventing cancer in an individual with a premalignant lesion), or tertiary prevention (i.e., preventing a second primary cancer in an individual already cured of a prior malignancy).[13] Chemoprevention may involve treatment with nutrients or natural or synthetic chemicals that exert their protective effects by reversing the abnormal differentiation, inhibiting proliferation, or inducing apoptosis (programmed cell death) of premalignant cells.[14] Other agents can act to block the uptake of carcinogens into cells, inhibit the activation of pro-carcinogens by various enzymes, or directly detoxify activated carcinogens.[15] Specific phases of carcinogenesis that are current targets for chemoprevention include altered classes of genes, cell signaling pathways, and genetic (i.e., chromosomal) instability common to malignancies.[15,16]

Chemoprevention studies are designed to detect changes in the incidence of cancer, as well as the rate of regression and progression of premalignant lesions. Biochemical parameters and cellular changes that occur with disease progression should also be monitored during a chemoprevention study. Since long-term, perhaps even lifelong therapy with an effective chemoprotectant may be necessary, ideal chemoprotectants should be safe and inexpensive. Once-daily dosing (or less) is desirable to maximize adherence. Another important aspect of effective chemoprevention is the ability to identify individuals at high risk for specific cancers through genetic susceptibility assessments, biomarkers of lifestyle or environmental exposures, or detection of premalignant cellular changes or lesions. These individuals are most likely to benefit from treatment or should be encouraged to participate in a clinical trial.

Dietary antioxidants, such as, β-carotene, vitamin E, vitamin C, and selenium, appear to stabilize oxygen-free radicals generated by many known carcinogens and protect the body from their damaging effects. Natural and synthetic preformed derivatives of vitamin A (i.e., retinoids) and provitamin A derivatives (i.e., β-carotene and other carotenoids) are also important in the process of cell growth, differentiation, and apoptosis. Polyphenols, which are phenolic compounds found in green and black tea, are purported to have cancer-preventive effects. Epidemiologic studies evaluating dietary intake of these micronutrients have led investigators to believe that these compounds contribute to the lower incidence of cancer in some populations.[12,16] These studies led to a series of chemoprevention studies in high-risk populations, as well as public interest in dietary supplements. All of these micronutrients are being studied in chemoprevention trials, with a specific emphasis on preventing cancers of the lung, oral cavity, skin, gastrointestinal tract, and prostate. However, the results of such studies have been mixed. Findings from several large trials are described in Table 88-3.

The retinoids and β-carotene are among the agents most studied to date. Early trials of 13-*cis*-retinoic acid in patients with leukoplakia, a premalignant lesion of the oral cavity, showed that lesions regressed with therapy but recurred after the 13-*cis*-retinoic acid was discontinued.[13] Whether 13-*cis*-retinoic acid prevents the occurrence of secondary primary cancers in patients previously treated for head and neck cancer has been studied.[26] Although treatment was associated with an initial reduction in occurrence of a second malignancy, this effect diminished over time and with discontinuation of therapy.[13] Similar disappointing results were observed in randomized, placebo-controlled trials using β-carotene in smokers to prevent lung cancer. In fact, there appears to be a negative interaction between β-carotene and tobacco smoke.[17,18,19,20] Neither supplementation with β-carotene, retinol, α-tocopherol (vitamin E), alone or in combination, decreased the incidence of lung cancer in healthy individuals with no risk factors for lung cancer or in smokers or persons exposed to asbestos.[27] Furthermore, smokers who received pharmacologic dosages of β-carotene and retinol showed a higher risk of lung cancer and a greater likelihood of dying from lung cancer compared with smokers who received a placebo.[27] The role of other vitamin A derivatives, such as lycopene (a carotenoid derived from tomatoes), in cancer chemoprevention is being studied. In a study using selenium as chemoprevention for skin cancer, a secondary analysis showed a relative risk of colorectal cancer of 0.42 (95% CI, 0.18 to 0.95),[28] but the effect of selenium supplementation in populations who have a low selenium intake is unknown.[29]

Because these chemoprevention studies have failed to clearly define the benefit of dietary supplements, their widespread use is controversial. However, the use of these supplements would not be contraindicated in M.S. at standard recommended antioxidant dosages because they are relatively safe.[30] Smokers, however, should not take β-carotene or retinol supplements.

Table 88-3 Large, Randomized Chemoprevention Trials

Trial	Agents	Population	Duration of Intervention (yr)	End Points	Outcomes
Nutrients					
ATBC[18,19]	Vitamin E β-Carotene	Men with a history of smoking or a current smoker (n = 29,133)	6	Lung cancer	Negative: β-carotene showed no chemoprotective benefit with an increase in incidence and mortality; vitamin A showed no effect
CARET[17,20]	Vitamin A β-Carotene	Individuals with a history of smoking or a current smoker (n = 18,344)	4	Lung cancer	Negative: showed no chemoprotective benefit with an increase in incidence and mortality
Physician's Health Study[21]	β-Carotene	Male physicians with no significant medical history (n = 22,071)	12	Total cancer	Negative: showed no chemoprotective benefit on total cancer or lung, prostate, or colon cancer
SELECT[22]	Vitamin E Selenium	Men with no significant medical history	Ongoing	Prostate cancer	
Antiestrogens					
BCPT[23]	Tamoxifen	Women of higher-than-average risk of breast cancer (n = 13,000)	5.7	Breast cancer	Positive: reduced the risk of invasive and noninvasive cancers and the occurrence of estrogen receptorpositive tumors; tamoxifen received an indication for chemoprevention from the U.S. Food and Drug Administration
MORE[24]	Raloxifene	Postmenopausal women with osteoporosis (n = 7705)	3	Breast cancer	Positive: reduced the risk of invasive cancers
STAR[16]	Tamoxifen Raloxifene	Postmenopausal women at high risk for breast cancer (n = 22,000)	Ongoing	Breast cancer	
α-Reductase Inhibitors					
PCPT[25]	Finasteride	Men with no significant medical history	7 years	Prostate cancer	Positive: finasteride prevented or delayed the development of prostate cancer but was associated with greater risk of high-grade prostate cancer

Another option is to recommend that M.S. discuss the use of aspirin or another nonsteroidal anti-inflammatory drug (NSAID) with her primary health care provider. These agents potentially reduce the risk of colon cancer, although their benefit in the general population has not been established.[31] The action of cyclooxygenase may enhance the conversion of several procarcinogens into carcinogens, the production of oxygen free radicals, and otherwise stimulate cell proliferation.[14,15] In colorectal cancer cells and adenomatous polyps, elevated levels of cyclooxygenase-2 (COX-2) enzyme, messenger RNA and protein can be found and these are associated with increased proliferation and resistance to apoptosis.[14] In randomized, controlled clinical trials, aspirin, sulindac, and celecoxib have reduced the development of new or recurrent adenomas in high-risk patients.[31]

Finally, M.S. should be encouraged to modify her lifestyle in ways that reduce her overall risk of cancer. These include maintaining a healthful body weight, following a healthy diet, participating in a regular exercise program, avoiding tobacco and other known carcinogens, and avoiding or limiting alcohol consumption.

2. J.M., a 45-year-old woman, tells you that her twin sister was recently treated for breast cancer. She heard on the news that relatives of breast cancer patients are at higher risk for developing the disease and that there is now a drug that can prevent breast cancer. Should J.M. consider taking something to prevent breast cancer?

The Breast Cancer Prevention Trial (BCPT) of the National Surgical Adjuvant Breast Project (NSABP) enrolled 13,000 women who were at higher-than-average risk of developing breast cancer.[23] The trial demonstrated that the risk of invasive breast cancer was reduced by 49% in subjects treated with tamoxifen. During the 69-month follow-up period, 175 of the 6,599 women enrolled in the placebo arm developed invasive breast cancer, compared with 89 of the 6,576 women enrolled in the tamoxifen arm ($P < .00001$). Women in this trial received tamoxifen 20 mg/day orally for 5 years. It is important to note that women in the tamoxifen arm had a higher incidence of pulmonary embolism (relative risk, 3.01) and endometrial cancer (relative risk, 2.53). These risks were greatest in women older than 50. The results of this trial led the U.S. Food and Drug Administration (FDA) to approve tamoxifen for the prevention of breast cancer in high-risk women. Raloxifene, a new selective estrogen receptor modulator approved for prevention of osteoporosis, also has been shown to reduce the risk of invasive breast cancer in women with osteoporosis. Patients receiving raloxifene showed an increased risk of thromboembolic disease, but they did not show an increased risk of endometrial cancer in this single trial.[24] A randomized trial is currently ongoing to directly compare tamoxifen to raloxifene for the prevention of breast cancer.[16] Other agents, such as certain retinoids, COX-2 inhibitors, and epidermal growth factor receptor (EGFR) antagonists may prove useful in the future but require significant study.[12,32]

Because her sister developed breast cancer before menopause, J.M. may be at a higher-than-average risk for developing breast cancer and she may benefit from preventive therapy. J.M. should discuss the benefits and risks of chemoprevention with her primary health care provider.

Diet

Diet has been linked to the development of colon, prostate, and breast cancers. Worldwide, colon cancer is the third most common cancer in the Western world[33] but it is relatively uncommon in Africa and Asia, except Japan.[34] Epidemiologic studies show that the incidence of colon cancer in a population increases as individuals migrate from a low-incidence region to a high-incidence region, suggesting that diet or other environmental factors have an important impact on the etiology of colon cancer.[34] Western diets tend to contain more fat and less fiber compared with diets of low-incidence regions. However, randomized trials have been unable to show a benefit of high dietary fiber intake in reducing the recurrence of colorectal adenomas in people who have undergone resection of colorectal polyps.[12] Furthermore, the consequences of supplementing fiber in one's diet may produce confounding factors, such as decreased fat intake, decreased caloric intake, and even weight loss. Nevertheless, the American Cancer Society advocates a healthy diet that consists of vegetables, fruit, whole grains, and fiber and is low in fat and limits red meats.

Similar to the incidence of colon cancer, migrant studies suggest that diet, environmental, or social factors play a role in the cause of prostate cancer, particular in Asian men.[35] An increasing incidence of prostate cancer has been observed in Japan, which is thought to be associated with a shift toward a more Westernized diet.[35] In women, the risk of breast cancer is increased with obesity and physical inactivity, but an association with high-fat diet is less clear.[36] Furthermore, environmental or lifestyle factors influence the risk of breast cancer. For example, even moderate alcohol consumption has been associated with an increased risk of breast cancer.[37]

Sun Exposure

Most risk factors associated with skin cancer are uncontrollable variables, with the exception of sun exposure and other forms of ultraviolet radiation. The interaction between ultraviolet radiation and skin cancers is complex, since non-melanomas (e.g., basal cell and squamous cell carcinomas) are associated with total cumulative ultraviolet radiation exposure, whereas melanomas are associated with intermittent sun exposure.[38] The risk of melanoma is further increased in people who have a history of five or more severe sunburns in their lifetime, particularly during adolescence.[38] A rising incidence of melanoma skin cancers is thought to be due to excessive, intermittent sun exposures—particularly among individuals who travel to sunny regions during the winter—and to depletion of the ozone layer in the stratosphere.[38] Prevention is simply based on limiting sun exposure. The ACS guidelines recommend avoiding or limiting sun exposure from 10 AM to 4 PM when the ultraviolet rays are the strongest. Protective clothing, including a hat, sunglasses, and long-sleeved shirt and pants, and sunscreens are also advised to minimize exposure. The protective effects of sunscreens alone against melanoma, particularly for intentional sun exposure, is controversial.[39] To reduce the risk of skin cancer, individuals should be cautioned to limit direct sun exposure whenever possible.

Tumors

Growth

CELL CYCLE TRANSITION

Cancer cells, like normal cells, proceed through a specific and orderly set of events during cellular replication referred to as the cell cycle (Fig. 88-3). The cell cycle contains four phases (S, M, G_1, and G_2) of activity, each responsible for a different task necessary for cell division. During the first activity phase, the M phase, the cell undergoes mitosis, the process of cell division. After mitosis, the cell enters the first gap or resting phase (G_1). During the G_1 phase, the cell makes the enzymes necessary for DNA synthesis. The synthesis of DNA occurs during the next activity phase called the S phase. After the S phase, the cell enters a second gap phase (G_2). RNA and other proteins are synthesized during this gap phase to prepare for cell division during the M phase. The cells that complete mitosis may (1) continue to proceed through the cell cycle to divide again, (2) differentiate or mature into specialized cells and eventually die, or (3) enter a third resting phase called G_0.[40]

Proliferation of normal cells (or cell renewal) is under fine control to balance the loss of mature functional cells with the production of new cells. As mentioned, proto-oncogenes and tumor-suppressor genes provide the stimulatory and inhibitory signals, respectively, that regulate the cell cycle. The transition of cells through the cell cycle is an ordered, tightly-regulated process, which involves a series of checkpoints that assess these signals and the number and integrity of the cells.[40] *Cyclins,* a group of interacting proteins found in the nucleus, and cyclin-dependent kinases (CDKs), make up the molecular machinery that regulates passage of cells through various phases of the cell cycle. The cyclins combine with the CDKs to form complexes that act as molecular switches. A molecular switch allows the cell to move through a critical restriction point that occurs late in the G_1 phase to the S phase. If insufficient amounts of cyclins or CDKs are present during the G_1 phase, the cell will not enter the S phase to start cell division. Cells that pass through this point are irreversibly committed to the next phase of the cell cycle.[40] A decline in the level of the CDK complex signals the end of the phase.

The levels of cyclins and CDKs are influenced by several factors, such as transcription of cyclin genes, degradation of cyclins, activities of CDK inhibitors, and the transfer of phosphate groups to various proteins and enzymes. Cues from the cell's external environment are transmitted to the nucleus via growth factor receptor signaling pathways, which influence formation of cyclins and cyclin/CDK complexes. The complexes generate phosphate groups from molecules of adenosine triphosphate (ATP) and transfer them to a protein called

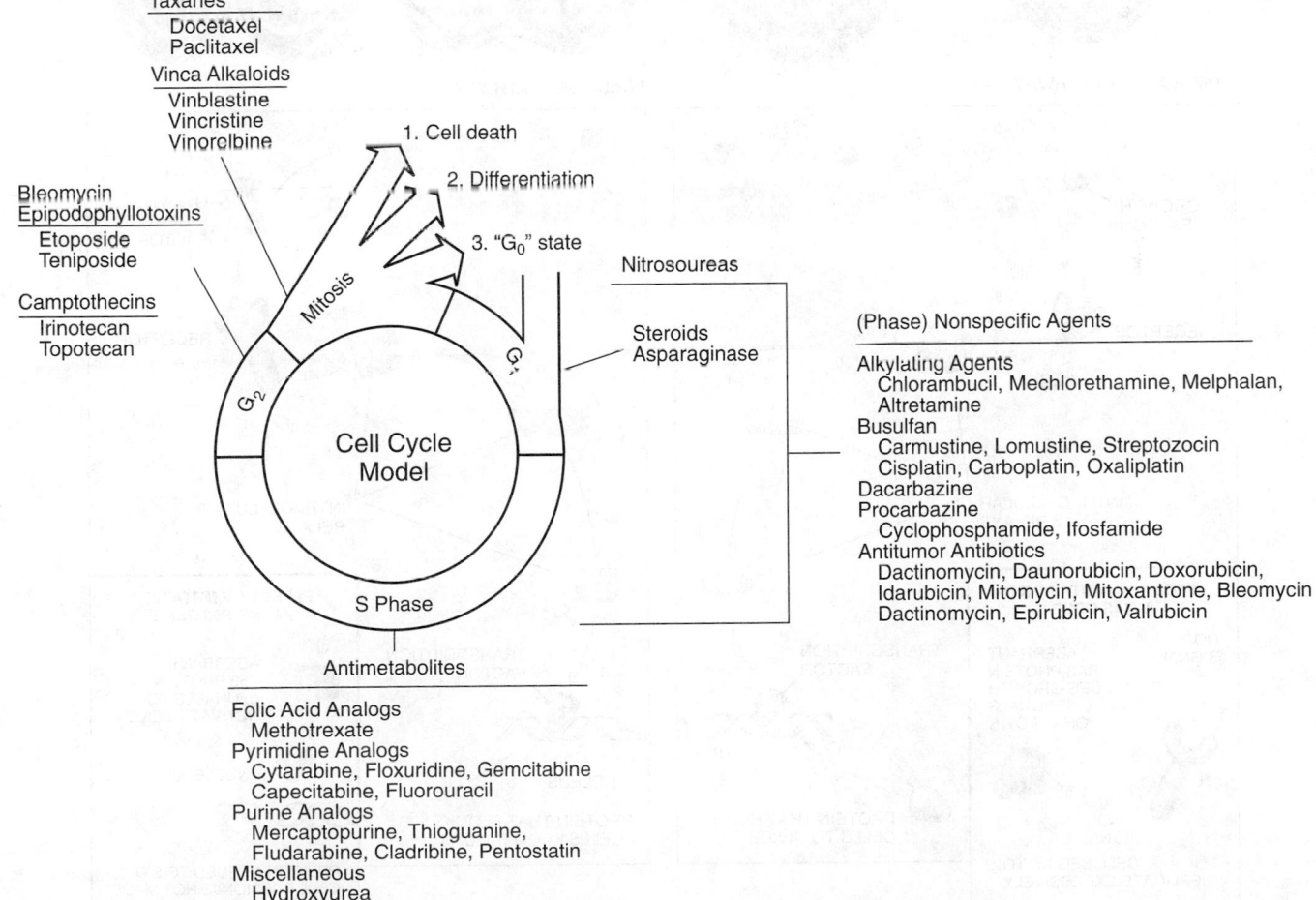

FIGURE 88-3 Cell cycle and effects of cytotoxic drugs on phases of the cell cycle.

a retinoblastoma protein (pRB). If the pRB acquires enough phosphate groups, it will release the transcription factors the cell needs to make proteins essential for a cell division. Naturally occurring CDK inhibitors block cell cycle progression in response to inhibitory growth signals.

In cancer cells, the regulation and function of cyclins, CDKs, and inhibitory proteins may be disrupted by a malignant transformation, or these proteins can undergo changes that cause a malignant transformation. Defects in these processes that are common in human cancers include deletion of the RB gene, a tumor suppressor gene that encodes for pRB, and dysregulation of the CDKs through over-activation of CDKs or loss of CDK inhibitors.[41] Without appropriate pRB regulation of cell cycle transition from G1 to S phase, excessive cell proliferation can occur. Loss or mutation of a second tumor suppressor gene, p53, is also common in human cancers, and is associated with the resistance of cancer cells to undergo cell cycle arrest or apoptosis (e.g., programmed

cell death). In normal cells, the p53 gene is responsible for temporarily arresting cell growth in response to biochemical or molecular damage until the damage can be repaired.[42] If the damage cannot be repaired, apoptosis is a normal cell suicide process that is initiated to prevent genetically damaged cells from growing uncontrollably. Figure 88-4 illustrates the normal stimulatory and inhibitory cell growth pathways and related effects of gene mutations on cell proliferation.

SURVIVAL

If the stimulatory and inhibitory growth signals do not program the cell to stop dividing, mechanisms such as apoptosis and senescence (aging) can help control excessive cell division. However, since abnormalities in the proto-oncogenes and tumor suppressor genes that regulate these processes are present in cancer cells, the balance between cell renewal and loss of mature (senescent) cells is disrupted. Also, cancer cells are less dependent on receiving stimulatory signals from ex-

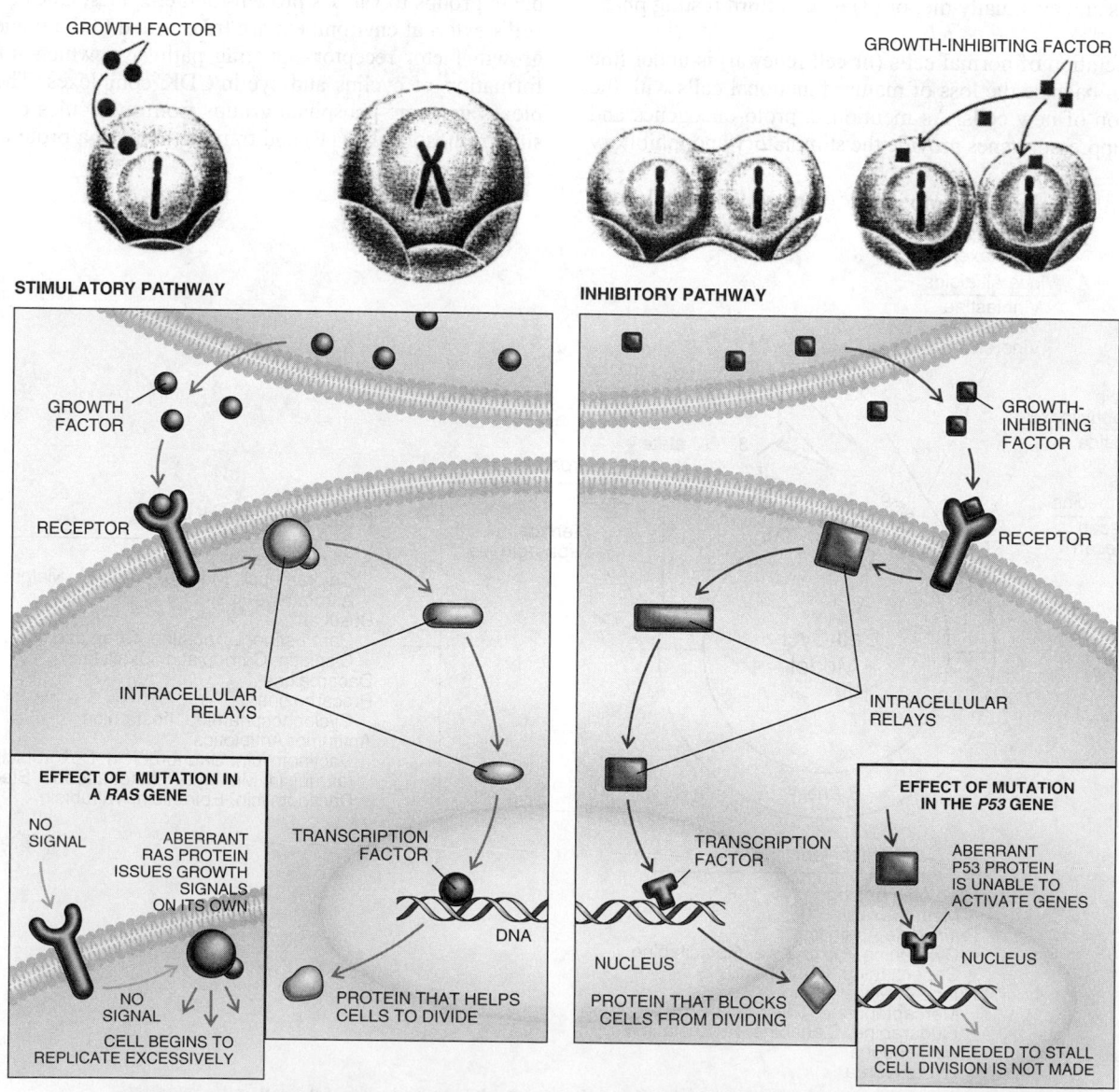

FIGURE 88-4 Normal stimulatory and inhibitory cell growth pathways and related effects of gene mutations on cell proliferation. (Reproduced with permission from reference 43).

ternal growth factors.[42] Furthermore, cancer cells possess unlimited replication potential, due to their ability to activate telomerase.[1,44] Telomerase is an enzyme that synthesizes sequences of telomeres, thereby enabling cells to proliferate endlessly. The expression of telomerase in most normal human cells is suppressed but it is reactivated in the majority of cancer cells.[42,44] Telomeres are repeats of DNA and DNA-binding proteins that form the ends of eukaryotic chromosomes.[44] Telomere loss occurs with each successive cell replication and after a critical length is reached, the cell undergoes irreversible growth arrest (replicative senescence).[44] Unlike normal cells, in which a finite telomere sequence regulates their life span, cancer cells are capable of immortality through their ability to maintain their telomeres indefinitely. Strategies to inhibit telomerase activity in cancer cells is one of many new molecular approaches that are being studied. Efforts are underway to target key genes, proteins, and receptors that facilitate cancer cell growth.

Spread

3. D.J., a 14-year-old boy, presented to the emergency department with a painful, swollen right leg. X-ray examination confirmed a fracture that appeared to be caused by a tumor mass in the bone. Biopsy confirmed osteogenic sarcoma. A routine chest x-ray study showed three nodules that were also believed to be malignant tumors. Does D.J. also have lung cancer? Are the tumors in D.J.'s lungs related to the sarcoma in his leg?

The tumor nodules in D.J.'s lung are most likely metastases from the sarcoma in his leg. The ability of cancer cells to disseminate and form metastases represents their most malignant characteristic. Unfortunately, tumor metastases to distant sites generally have a greater effect than the primary tumor on the frequency of complications and the patient's quality of life (see Complications of Malignancy). Metastases also have a greater effect than the primary tumor on mortality, with metastases associated with the majority of cancer-related deaths. Consequently, individuals diagnosed with metastases face a worse prognosis.

Cancer cells must develop new blood vessels to supply nutrients to the cells and to spread to distant sites (metastasize). In response to low oxygen supply (hypoxia) and other factors, the cancer cells and surrounding tissues secrete growth factors that stimulate the growth of the new blood vessels (or angiogenesis) from existing blood vessels in the surrounding normal host tissue. Although many growth factors secreted by the tumor can be considered angiogenic, vascular endothelial growth factor (VEGF), platelet derived growth factor (PDGF), and basic fibroblast growth factor (bFGF) are considered the most important for sustained endothelial cell growth. Once released by the tumor cells, these growth factors bind to receptors on the surface of endothelial cells of existing blood vessels and activate a series of intracellular relay proteins that transmit a signal to genes in the nucleus to produce factors required for new endothelial cell growth.[45] Once the older endothelial cells become activated by the growth factors, they begin making matrix metalloproteinase enzymes (MMPs). These enzymes destroy the extracellular matrix of the surrounding cells, allowing the older endothelial cells to invade the extracellular matrix and begin cell division.[45]

After cancer cells undergo angiogenesis, they must break away from the primary tumor and travel to other sites in the body to form metastases. Normally, cells adhere to both other cells and the extracellular matrix. The cell-to-cell adhesion molecules are called *cadherins,* and the cell-to-extracellular matrix molecules are called *integrins.* In cancer cells, these molecules are often absent, allowing tumor cells to easily move away from the primary tumor mass.

Once a tumor cells breaks off, it can move through the body to form metastatic sites. Two primary pathways, the blood vessels and the lymphatics, play a critical role in determining the location of metastatic sites (Table 88-4). A tumor cell can travel only to a distant site that receives blood or lymph from the primary site. Usually, tumor cells spread to the first capillary bed they encounter after their release from the primary tumor. If the primary site drains its blood supply into the vena cava, the cancer cells will reach the capillary bed in lung. Similarly, if the primary site drains its blood supply into the portal circulation, the cancer cells will reach the capillary bed in the liver. In addition, cancer cells can potentially pass through the first capillary bed they encounter and enter the arterial circulation. If malignant cells reach the arterial circulation, they can distribute to other organs and tissues throughout the body. Growth conditions (e.g., growth factors, physiologic conditions) within a tissue or organ also can determine the location of a metastatic site. After a cancer cell establishes a metastatic site, it must again undergo angiogenesis to ensure continued growth. Together, angiogenesis and hematogenous or lymphatic spread help cancer cells invade healthy tissues and increase morbidity and mortality associated with the disease.

Screening and Early Detection

Standardized screening tests can help identify disease in asymptomatic individuals (screening) or help diagnose a disease in symptomatic individuals (early detection). Ideally, a screening test should be quick and simple to maximize compliance with screening recommendations. The cancer

Table 88-4	Common Cancers and Sites of Metastases
Cancer	*Most Common Sites of Metastases*
Bladder	Pelvis, lymph nodes
Breast	
• Premenopausal	Lymph nodes, skin, lung, liver, bone, brain
• Postmenopausal	Lymph nodes, bone, soft tissue
Colon	Lymph nodes, liver, lung, adrenals, ovary, bone
Lung	
• Nonsmall cell	Lymph nodes, liver, bone, brain, adrenals
• Small cell	Lymph nodes, bone, liver, bone marrow, brain
Lymphomas	
• Hodgkin's disease lymphoma	Liver, spleen, stomach, bone marrow, lung
• Non-Hodgkin's	GI tract, bone marrow, liver, lung, CNS
Ovary	Peritoneum, lung
Prostate	Lymph nodes, bone, liver

CNS, central nervous system; GI, gastrointestinal.

screening tests recommended by the ACS meet four basic requirements: (1) there must be good evidence that the test is effective in reducing morbidity or mortality (e.g., effective treatment must be available for the screened disease), (2) the benefits of the test should outweigh its risks, (3) the costs of the test should be in balance with its presumed benefits, and (4) the test should be practical and feasible within the existing health care setting. Various professional organizations, including the ACS, regularly publish recommendations for cancer screening[3,46] (Table 88-5).

Table 88-5   **Guidelines for Screening Cancer**

	U.S. Preventative Task Force	American Cancer Society	National Comprehensive Cancer Network
Self-Examination			
Breast self-examination	Not recommended	≥20 yr: optional	≥20 yr: encouraged
Testicular self-examination	Not recommended (unless high risk)	Not recommended	Not recommended
Skin	High risk	Not recommended	Not recommended
Clinician Examination			
Clinical breast examination	Not recommended	20–39 yr: every 3 yr ≥40 yr: annually	20–39 yr: every 1–3 yr ≥40 yr: annually High risk: begin earlier and/or more frequently, depending on risk
Digital rectal examination	Not recommended	Colon: not recommended Prostate: if life expectancy ≥10 yr, ≥50 yr (normal risk) or ≥40-45 yr (high risk): annually	Not recommended
Pelvic examination	Not recommended	≥18 yr: annually	≥18 yr or within 3 years of onset of sexual activity: annually
Sigmoidoscopy	Recommended alone or in combination with FOBT: periodicity unspecified	Normal risk, ≥50 yr: every 5 yr, preferably with annual FOBT, as alternative to colonoscopy every 10 yr or double-contrast barium enema every 5 yr High risk: begin earlier than age 50 yr and/or more frequently	Normal risk, ≥50 yr: every 5 yr with annual FOBT, as alternative to colonoscopy every 10 yr or double-contrast barium enema every 5 yr High risk: begin earlier than age 50 yr and more frequently, depending on risk
Colonoscopy	Not recommended	Normal risk, ≥50 yr: every 10 yr as alternative to annual FOBT, sigmoidoscopy every 5 yr, or double-contrast barium enema every 5 yr High risk: begin earlier than age 50 yr and more frequently	Normal risk, ≥50 yr: every 10 yr with annual FOBT, as alternative to sigmoidoscopy every 5 yr, or double-contrast barium enema every 5 yr High risk: begin earlier than age 50 yr and more frequently, depending on risk
Laboratory Tests			
Stool guaiac	≥50 yr: periodicity unspecified	≥50 yr: annually High risk: begin earlier than age 50 yr: annually	≥50 yr: annually
Prostate specific antigen	Not recommended	If life expectancy ≥10 yr, ≥50 yr (normal risk) or ≥4045 yr (high risk): annually	Normal risk, life expectancy ≥10 yr, ≥50 yr: annually High risk, life expectancy ≥10 yr, ≥45 yr: annually
Pap smear	21 yr or within 3 years of onset of sexual activity if earlier: every 3 years Not recommended: age ≥65 if not high risk and if prior adequate recent screening with normal results	21 yr or within 3 years of onset of sexually activity if earlier: annually (regular Pap test) or every 2 yr (liquid-based Pap test) ≥30 yr: every 2 to 3 yr if 3 normal prior consecutive Pap test results ≥70 yr: optional if 3 or more normal prior consecutive Pap test results and no abnormal Pap test results in the last 10 yr	21 yr or within 3 years of onset of sexually activity if earlier: annually (regular Pap test) or every 2 yr (liquid-based Pap test) ≥30 yr: every 2 to 3 yr if 3 normal prior consecutive Pap test results ≥70 yr: optional if 3 or more normal prior consecutive Pap test results and no abnormal Pap test results in the last 10 yr
Mammogram	≥40 yr: every 1-2 yr, with or without CBE	≥40 yr: annually High risk: begin earlier than age 40 yr and/or have additional tests or more frequent testing	≥40 yr: annually High risk: begin earlier and/or more frequently, depending on risk

CBE, clinical breast examination; FOBT, fecal occult blood test.

Recommendations for cancer screening tests have been in existence for decades. As advances are made in screening techniques and the management of certain cancers, recommendations for cancer screening are updated as new information becomes available. Although the concepts of cancer screening and early cancer detection seem intuitively beneficial, particularly for cancers for which treatments are available, the acceptance of various cancer screening recommendations remains controversial.[47] The question that still needs to be answered is, "Will screening alter the natural history of the disease or simply detect the disease earlier without changing patient morbidity?" The NCI is following up more than 154,000 men and women who enrolled in the Prostate, Lung, Colorectal and Ovary (PLCO) Cancer Screening Trial to determine whether screening affects morbidity or mortality. One-half of participants undergo specific screening tests; the other half receives routine health care. Since the testing and follow-up occur over 16 years, the results will be unavailable for several years. Interestingly, cancer screening may not alter the mortality or morbidity associated with various cancers. Recent cancer statistics show that patients are still being diagnosed with potentially curable cancers late in the course of the disease, despite the introduction of these recommendations two decades ago.

As new information becomes available, the various professional organizations modestly change their cancer screening recommendations. Only minor changes have been made to the recommendations since the ACS first published their guidelines, because a newly discovered tumor marker or diagnostic procedure must first be validated as a screening test. New tests should fit the four basic requirements the ACS used to develop the current guidelines, including cost:benefit ratio. Because a new screening test could add substantial costs to an already stressed health care system, its costs, benefits, and risks should be evaluated thoroughly before it is recommended for routine use. Screening recommendations also accommodate patients who are at higher than-average risk for developing cancer due to genetic, environmental, and lifestyle factors.

Diagnosis and Staging

The histologic diagnosis of a tumor is the most important determinant of how a malignancy will be treated. This is because a tumor's histologic classification influences its natural history, pattern of progression, and responsiveness to treatment. A surgical biopsy or excision of the primary tumor, followed by a microscopic and a biochemical evaluation by a pathologist, can provide the most accurate histologic diagnosis. Thereafter, staging can begin.

4. **J.S. is diagnosed with breast cancer after a large breast mass was biopsied. Chemotherapy, radiation, and surgery all play an important role in the management of breast cancer. How does a clinician decide which treatment modalities are most appropriate for J.S.?**

The stage of the cancer, as well as the histologic diagnosis, significantly influences both the treatment and prognosis. Staging is the process that determines the extent or spread of the disease. For J.S., staging is crucial to guide therapy. If her disease is limited to her breast, surgery followed by radiation and/or chemotherapy or hormonal therapy would be recommended. However, if the cancer has spread beyond the breast,

surgery may not be recommended. J.S. should immediately consider systemic therapy (chemotherapy or endocrine therapy) if she has advanced disease.

Staging schemas have been developed for all major types of cancers. For solid tumors, the most widely used and accepted staging classification is the TNM system, which incorporates the size of the primary tumor (T), the extent of regional lymph node spread (N), and the presence or absence of metastatic spread to distant organs (M). Within each TNM category, the extent of cancer involvement is related to prognosis. Determining the stage of the cancer often requires tests that can physically or radiographically measure the size of the primary tumor (e.g., radiographs, computed tomography [CT] scans, or magnetic resonance imaging [MRI] scans), dissect and pathologically examine regional lymph nodes, and assess the patient for evidence of tumor spread. In addition, positron emission tomography [PET] scans are being used more frequently to help determine whether tissues contain cancerous cells. To find evidence of a metastatic site, clinicians perform tests that assess the most likely sites of tumor metastases (see Table 88-4) and they evaluate symptoms (e.g., pain) or signs (e.g., swelling, abnormal laboratory findings) that may indicate tumor involvement at a distant site.

An example of the TNM classification for solid tumors is shown in Table 88-6. Most solid tumor staging systems also incorporate the TNM classification into broader groups or stages to facilitate comparison between patient populations. Whereas

Table 88-6 Staging of Breast Carcinoma

TNM Classification[a]

Primary Tumor (T)

T1	Tumor ≤2 cm in greatest dimension
T2	Tumor >2 cm but not >5 cm in greatest dimension
T3	Tumor >5 cm in greatest dimension
T4	Tumor of any size with direct extension to chest wall or skin

Regional Lymph Nodes (N)

N0	No regional lymph node metastasis
N1	Metastasis to movable ipsilateral axillary lymph node(s)
N2	Metastasis to ipsilateral axillary lymph node(s) fixed to one another or other structures
N3	Metastasis to ipsilateral internal mammary lymph node(s)

Distant Metastasis (M)

M0	No distant metastasis
M1	Distant metastasis (includes metastasis to ipsilateral supra-clavicular lymph nodes)

Stage Grouping

Stage I	T1	N0	M0
Stage II_A	T0	N1	M0
	T1	N1	M0
	T2	N0	M0
Stage II_B	T2	N1	M0
	T3	N0	M0
Stage III_A	T0	N2	M0
	T1	N2	M0
	T2	N2	M0
	T3	N1, N2	M0
Stage III_B	T4	N0, N1, N2	M0
Stage III_C	Any T	N3	M0
Stage IV	Any T	Any N	M1

[a]See text for full explanation of TNM system of classification.
TNM, tumor-node-metastasis.

the TNM system adequately stages solid tumors, this staging system does not adequately stage hematologic malignancies, including leukemias, lymphomas, and multiple myelomas. Because hematologic malignancies occur in the blood cells and lymphatic tissues that are widely distributed throughout the body, the TNM staging system cannot sufficiently describe these diseases. To define the extent of disease, guide treatment, and provide prognostic information, specific staging systems have been developed for various hematologic malignancies. Examples of widely accepted staging systems for hematologic malignancies include the Rai system for chronic lymphocytic leukemia and the Ann Arbor system for lymphomas.

Staging systems for some tumors include other characteristics to further determine the stage and prognosis of the disease. These characteristics may include clinical signs or symptoms or biochemical characteristics of the tumor. For example, the staging system used for Hodgkin's disease includes a notation for constitutional symptoms (i.e., fever, night sweats, and weight loss). Studies indicate that these symptoms confer a poorer prognosis and could indicate the need for more intensive therapy. A subscript "B" (e.g., stage II_B) next to the stage indicates the patient has experienced these symptoms, whereas the subscript "A" indicates the patient has not experienced these symptoms.

Staging of the tumor is done at the time of initial diagnosis and periodically during treatment to assess the patient's response to therapy. Staging should also be repeated when (1) evidence shows that the cancer has either progressed during treatment or recurred following therapy to establish the most appropriate second-line therapy and (2) to enable measurement of response to that therapy.

Clinical Presentation

The initial signs and symptoms of malignant disease are variable and predominantly depend on the histologic diagnosis, the location (including metastases), and the size of the tumor. Pain secondary to compression, obstruction, and destruction of adjacent tissues and organs is the most common presenting symptom. Other common initial symptoms reported by patients with cancer include anorexia, weight loss, and fatigue. Table 88-7 lists the common signs and symptoms associated with specific cancers. Unfortunately, some symptoms may be obscured by a concomitant illness, such as chronic lung disease in patients with lung cancer. Whereas most tumors cause signs and symptoms early in the course of the disease, some cancers do not cause symptoms until late in the course of the disease and after significant tumor growth. In either of these circumstances, early diagnosis may be difficult. Thus, individuals at higher-than-average risk should be screened regularly to help detect early disease.

5. **P.N., a 59 year-old woman, presents with shortness of breath, fatigue, anorexia, weight loss, and abdominal pain and distention that have worsened significantly over the previous 3 weeks. An evaluation showed a large mass surrounding the head of her pancreas with biopsy results that confirmed pancreatic adenocarcinoma. The staging workup confirmed the presence of distant metastases. Her husband states that she was previously an active person, but that she most recently has been unable to dress herself or participate in normal daily activities. He states that she spends most of the day in bed. Will her activity level influence the type of treatment that she can receive?**

Table 88-7 Signs and Symptoms Associated With Common Cancers

Cancer	Local	Distant[a]
Bladder	Hematuria; bladder irritability; urinary hesitancy, frequency or urgency; dysuria; flank or pelvic pain	Edema of lower extremities and genitalia
Breast	Breast lumps; nipple retraction, dimpling, discharge; skin changes; axillary lymphadenopathy	Bone pain; elevated LFTs; hypercalcemia
Colorectal	Change in bowel habits; ↓ in stool caliber; occult bleeding; constipation	Elevated LFTs, CEA, and alkaline phosphatase; obstruction; hepatomegaly; perforation
Lung	New cough; hoarseness hemoptysis, dyspnea; unresolving pneumonias; chest wall pain; pain; dysphagia; effusion; tracheal obstruction	Anorexia; weight loss; elevated LFTs; bone pain, hypercalcemia; jaundice; lymphadenopathy; osteoarthropathy; neurologic (brain metastases and neuromuscular disorders); SIADH
Lymphomas	Painless lymphadenopathy	Fever; night sweats; weight loss; bone or retroperitoneal pain; hepatomegaly; splenomegaly; abnormal CBC
Melanoma	Change in size, color, or shape of a pre-existing nevus	Lymphadenopathy; elevated LFTs
Ovarian	Abdominal pain, discomfort, or enlargement; postprandial flatulence; vaginal bleeding; abdominal mass; urinary frequency; constipation, nausea; dyspepsia; early satiety	Peripheral neuropathies; pleural effusion; thrombophlebitis; elevated LFTs; abdominal distention or pain; Addison's or Cushing's syndrome
Prostate	Urinary hesitancy; nocturia; poor urine stream; dribbling; terminal hematuria	Bone pain; elevated acid phosphatase, PSA, and alkaline phosphatase
Testicular	Painless enlargement; epididymitis; gynecomastia; back pain; infertility/erectile dysfunction	Elevated HCG, α-fetoprotein, LD

[a]Local effects include those produced by the primary tumor, and distant effects include those associated with metastatic spread and paraneoplastic syndromes. Many cancers may not produce symptoms in the early stages, and diagnosis at that time is dependent on early detection and screening efforts.
CBC, complete blood count; CEA, carcinoembryonic antigen; HCG, β-human chorionic gonadotropin; LD, lactate dehydrogenase; LFTs, liver function tests; PSA, prostate-specific antigen; SIADH, syndrome of inappropriate antidiuretic hormone secretion.

The description of P.N.'s daily activities indicate that she has a relatively poor performance status. Performance status is a measure of the functional capacity of the patient and reflects a patient's ability to ambulate, care for him or herself, and carry out normal activities. For several tumors, a poor pretreatment performance status is associated with a decreased ability to tolerate treatment, decreased tumor response to treatment, and a worsened clinical outcome. In these cases, especially if the cancer is not known to respond well to treatment, a less aggressive treatment regimen may be recommended for patients with a poor performance status. For this reason, the performance status of a patient is important to assess at the time of staging evaluation and periodically during treatment. Different scales (i.e., Karnofsky score, Eastern Cooperative Oncology Group [ECOG]) can be used to determine performance status. The World Health Organization (WHO) performance scale is depicted in Table 88-8. Because P.N. has a WHO performance status of 3, her oncologist may recommend a less aggressive, less toxic treatment plan. Since other conditions could be responsible for her symptoms, however, P.N. should undergo a careful evaluation. Depression is a common problem in patients with cancer and, with treatment, can lead to improved patient outcomes.

6. G.D., a 68-year-old man, presents with lethargy, weakness, and nausea. His wife states that he does not take any medications and only occasionally consumes alcohol. He has smoked two packs of cigarettes per day for the past 45 years. Routine laboratory tests reveal a serum sodium (Na) of 129 mEq/L (normal, 135 to 147). His chest radiograph showed a large mass in his right lung, which is consistent with malignancy. Is the hyponatremia related to G.D.'s lung cancer?

[SI unit: Na, 129 mmol/L (normal, 135 to 147)]

G.D.'s hyponatremia is likely to be due to the syndrome of inappropriate antidiuretic hormone secretion (SIADH) caused by ectopic production of ADH (see Chapter 12, Fluid and Electrolyte Disorders) by his lung carcinoma. Although most signs and symptoms can be associated with the tumor, patients occasionally report symptoms or show clinical signs that are distant to the primary tumor site or metastases. These signs or symptoms, called paraneoplastic effects, are produced by substances secreted by the tumor. Table 88-9 lists some of the common paraneoplastic effects.

Complications of Malignancy

Cancer can have a profound effect on the patient's quality of life and his or her ability to tolerate appropriate therapy. For exam-

Table 88-8 World Health Organization (WHO) Performance Status Classification in Cancer

0	Able to carry out all normal activity without restriction
1	Restricted in physically strenuous activity but ambulatory and able to carry out light work
2	Ambulatory and capable of all self-care but unable to carry out work
3	Capable of only limited self-care; confined to bed or chair 50% or more of waking hours
4	Completely disabled; not capable of any self-care; confined to bed or chair

Table 88-9 Paraneoplastic Syndromes Associated With Cancers

Syndrome	Cancer
Dermatologic	
Sweet's syndrome	Hematologic malignancies and various carcinomas
Endocrine	
Addison's syndrome[a]	Adrenal carcinoma, lymphomas, and ovarian cancer
Cushing's syndrome[a]	Lung, thyroid, testicular, adrenal, and ovarian cancers
Hypercalcemia (not associated with bone metastases)[a]	Lung cancer
Syndrome of inappropriate antidiuretic hormone secretion	Lung and head and neck cancers
Hematologic/Coagulation	
Anemia[a]	Various cancers
Autoimmune hemolytic anemia[a]	Chronic lymphocytic leukemia, lymphomas, ovarian cancer
Disseminated intravascular coagulation[a]	Acute progranulocytic leukemia, lung and prostate cancers
Thrombophlebitis	Lung, breast, ovarian, prostate, and pancreatic cancers
Neuromuscular	
Dermatomyositis and polymyositis	Lung and breast cancers
Myasthenic syndrome (Eaton-Lambert syndrome)	Small cell lung, gastric, and ovarian cancers
Sensory neuropathies	Small cell lung and ovarian cancers

[a]This syndrome is discussed in more detail in other sections of this text. See the index.

ple, patients with malnutrition secondary to anorexia, mechanical obstruction, or pain may not tolerate some therapies because of significant physical debility. Tumor involvement of the liver, kidneys, or lungs also may complicate therapy by causing significant organ dysfunction and metabolic disturbances. In addition, compression or obstruction could produce a "mass effect" by impairing normal organ or tissue function and causing pain or other uncomfortable physical effects. Life-threatening physical effects that require immediate intervention include obstruction of the superior vena cava, spinal cord compression, and brain metastases. Common complications associated with specific cancers are illustrated in Chapter 90, Hematologic Malignancies, and Chapter 91, Solid Tumors.

TREATMENT

7. T.J., a 40-year-old man with no significant medical history, presents to his physician with complaints of abdominal pain, nausea and vomiting, weakness, and weight loss. On physical examination, he is noted to be slightly icteric, and the only significant laboratory abnormality is mild anemia (hemoglobin [Hgb], 11 g/dL [normal, 14 to 18], hematocrit [Hct], 33% [normal, 39% to 49%]). A CT scan of the abdomen reveals a mass present in the peripancreatic area that is suggestive of malignancy. T.J. is referred to a surgeon who explains that the first step in evaluating the mass is to obtain a tissue biopsy. T.J. asks the surgeon why he cannot remove all of the mass rather than take only part of it. He also wants to know whether this malignancy will be treated with surgery, radiation, chemotherapy, hormones, or immunotherapy. What is the basis for determining which cancer treatment modality is best suited for T.J.?

[SI units: Hgb, 110 g/L (normal, 140 to 180); Hct, 0.33 (normal, 0.39 to 0.49)]

Since a tissue diagnosis of malignancy has not been made, the appropriateness of more extensive surgery for T.J. can not be determined at this time. The choice of specific therapy depends not only on the histology and stage but also on the patient's predicted tolerance of the side effects and complications of the various treatment options. The goal of therapy should always be to cure the patient when possible. No matter what therapeutic options are under consideration, the likelihood of curing the patient is greater when the tumor burden is low. In most cases, either surgery or radiation therapy is the initial choice of therapy for localized tumors.

Surgery

Surgery is the oldest modality available to treat patients with cancer. With the recent advances in surgical techniques and an improved understanding of the patterns of tumor growth and spread, surgeons can now perform successful resections for an increasing number of patients. Surgery can play a significant role in preventing (e.g., removal of colonic polyps or cervical dysplasia), diagnosing, and staging various cancers (e.g., biopsy for histologic evaluation). Surgery may also be used to manage both localized and advanced tumors. When surgery provides definitive (i.e., curative) therapy for a localized tumor, the surgeon removes the tumor plus a margin of normal tissue surrounding the tumor. For extensive, localized tumors that cannot be completely removed, patients may undergo surgery to partially resect the tumor in an attempt to improve the likelihood that subsequent chemotherapy or radiation therapy may successfully kill the tumor. Cytoreductive surgery may be useful only if effective therapies are available to treat the residual disease. Patients with limited metastatic disease (e.g., one or a few metastases at a single site) also may benefit from surgical resection of the metastases if the primary tumor can be controlled with other treatments. Cytoreductive surgery for limited metastatic disease includes resecting pulmonary metastases for sarcomas, hepatic metastases for colorectal cancer, and solitary brain metastases. Patients with metastatic disease also can undergo surgery to relieve pain or improve functional abnormalities caused by the advanced tumor (e.g., gastrointestinal obstruction). Patients can undergo palliative surgery to improve their quality of life without prolonging survival. Thus, surgery plays a critical role in cancer treatment.

Radiation Therapy

Radiation therapy can be used to eradicate localized tumor masses. Not all cancers are sensitive to the lethal effects of radiation, so this modality has limited application in the treatment of some cancers. (Table 88-10) However, for others, radiation therapy provides potential advantages over surgery. For instance, radiation therapy could encompass a wider area

Table 88-10   Malignancies Frequently Treated With Radiation Therapy

Acute lymphocytic leukemia (CNS radiation)
Brain tumors
Breast cancer
Head and neck cancers, squamous cell
Lung cancer
• Non small-cell lung cancer
• Small cell lung cancer (CNS radiation and limited stage disease)
Lymphomas
Neuroblastoma
Prostate cancer
Rectal cancer
Testicular, seminoma

around the tumor and remove the tumor from regions of the body where surgery cannot safely reach. Radiation therapy also can be used when surgery could result in considerable disability or disfigurement. Radiation allows patients to receive treatment to multiple metastatic sites simultaneously. Unfortunately, the usefulness of radiation therapy can be limited by its toxic effects on normal tissues that surround the tumor, and these can be exacerbated if patients receive chemotherapy concomitantly or shortly after radiation therapy. Chemotherapy that follows completion of radiation therapy can produce a "recall" of local toxicity. Also, there is an established limit to the "dose" of radiation that can be delivered, depending on the type of tissue (e.g., bone, liver, brain) that is affected. Two methods are used most often to administer radiation to tumors. External-beam radiotherapy uses a radiation source (typically a supervoltage electrical machine) that is located a certain distance from the site of intended treatment. Brachytherapy involves placement of radioactive seeds, pellets, or needles within or close to the site of the tumor. Newer radiation therapy techniques, including intraoperative radiation, hyperfractionated radiation, stereotactic radiosurgery, intensity modulated radiation therapy (IMRT), computerized three-dimensional conformal treatment planning, and chemoradiosensitization (e.g., concomitant radiation-sensitizing chemotherapy), may reduce associated toxicities, enhance tumor responsiveness, and improve its clinical usefulness.[48]

Not all cancers can be cured by surgery or radiation therapy. Some patients have tumors that have already metastasized at the time of initial diagnosis, whereas others have tumors that could not be completely eradicated with treatment or have recurred some time after primary therapy with surgery or radiation therapy. In these circumstances, the tumor cells have been released from the primary tumor. Systemic treatments—including chemotherapy, endocrine therapy, signal transduction pathway inhibitors, antiangiogenic agents, and biologic response modifiers—generally offer the only hope of rendering the patient free of disease. Although chemotherapy was developed to treat advanced cancers, these agents are now used to treat many stages of malignant diseases.

Chemotherapy
Cytotoxic Chemotherapy

The era of cytotoxic chemotherapy can be traced to World War II, when an explosion of mustard gas produced bone marrow and lymphoid hypoplasia in seamen exposed to the gas.[49]

This incident led to the use of alkylating agents (derivatives of mustard gas) in the treatment of Hodgkin's disease and other lymphomas.[50]

MECHANISM OF ACTION

Classic cytotoxic chemotherapy kills cancer cells by damaging DNA, interfering with DNA synthesis, or otherwise inhibiting cell division. Chemotherapy agents have been classified by their effect on the cell cycle or their mechanism of action. Agents that affect the cell only during a specific phase of the cell cycle often are referred to as phase-specific agents or schedule-dependent agents. In contrast, agents that affect the cell during any phase of the cell cycle are often referred to as phase-nonspecific agents or dose-dependent agents (see Fig. 88-3). As the understanding of cancer biology continues to grow, other mechanisms of cytotoxicity have been identified for many chemotherapy agents.

The specific mechanisms of action for several chemotherapy agents are described in Table 88-11. Because most agents affect the cell cycle, their lethal effects are not realized until the cells proceed through the cycle. These drugs are most cytotoxic to tumor cells with a high growth fraction (see Tumors: Growth) and least cytotoxic to tumor cells arrested in the G_0 phase.

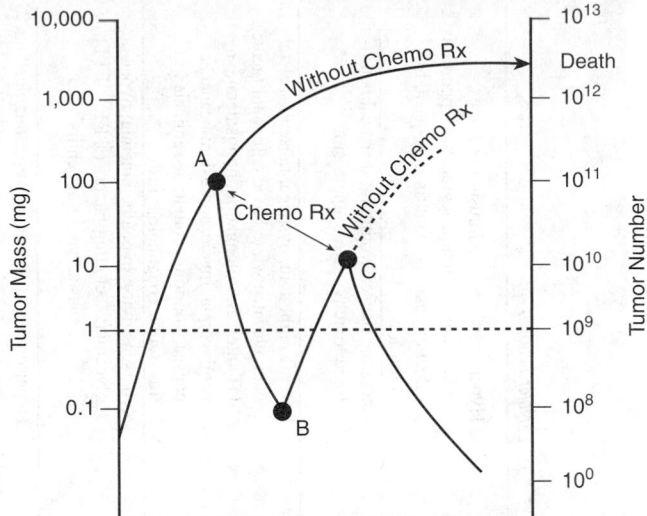

FIGURE 88-5 The growth rate of a tumor is initially very rapid and eventually slows as it approaches 10^{11} cells. Two trillion (2×10^{12}) cells or 2 kg of tumor is lethal to humans. An effective chemotherapy treatment given at point A will decrease the tumor number to point B. Regrowth of the tumor will occur during the recovery period until further chemotherapy is given at point C.

CELL KILL

Rodent studies done during the 1960s demonstrated that the number of tumor cells killed by the chemotherapy is proportional to the dose when the growth fraction is 100% (i.e., all cells are dividing) and the tumor cells are sensitive to the agent.[53,54] For example, if a dose of chemotherapy reduces the tumor burden from 10^{10} to 10^8 cells, the same dose administered when only 10^7 cells are present should reduce the tumor burden to 10^5 cells. This theory has become known as the cell-kill or log-kill hypothesis (Fig. 88-5).

FACTORS THAT INFLUENCE RESPONSE TO CHEMOTHERAPY

Unfortunately, in the clinical setting, tumor cells do not always decrease predictably with each successive course of chemotherapy. This is because the growth fraction of human tumors is not 100% and because the cell population is heterogeneous and some are resistant to chemotherapy. In patients with large tumors showing a plateau-like growth curve, the fraction of cells killed with each treatment is usually low. The ability of this model to adequately predict cell kill is also limited by the need to administer chemotherapy in cycles (e.g., every 2 or 3 or 4 weeks) to allow normal cells to recover from the toxic effects of chemotherapy. During the recovery period, tumor cells can start to replicate again. Therefore, successful treatment requires administration of the next course of therapy before the tumor has grown to its previous size. The objective of successive chemotherapy courses is a further decrease in size of tumor mass. Other factors that influence cell kill include dose intensity, schedule, drug resistance, tumor site, and a patient's performance status.

Dose Intensity

Unnecessary lengthening of the interval between successive courses of chemotherapy or decreasing the dose can negatively affect treatment outcomes. Evidence suggests that reducing a dose can cause treatment failure in patients with chemotherapy-sensitive tumors who are undergoing their first chemotherapy treatment.[55] Dose intensity equals the amount of chemotherapy administered per unit of time. In animal models, a low average dose intensity can markedly decrease the cure rate before it can significantly reduce the complete remission rate.[55] These models suggest that lower doses may eradicate the bulk of the tumor mass, but residual tumor cells left behind could ultimately be responsible for disease recurrence. A direct relationship between dose intensity and response rate also has been reported in several human tumors, including breast cancer, lymphomas, and advanced ovarian cancer.[56–59] Dose-dense treatment schedules have been designed to decrease the time period between chemotherapy administration based on the theory that this would be more effective in reducing the residual tumor burden between treatments than escalating doses.[60] Unfortunately, dose-intensive therapy has not consistently improved the overall cure rate of most solid tumors.

The dose intensity for most chemotherapy regimens is limited by the major dose-related toxicity, bone marrow suppression. To minimize this toxicity and administer higher doses, patients have received hematopoietic growth factors (see Chapter 89, Adverse Effects of Chemotherapy), autologous stem cell transplantations, and altered schedules of drug delivery.[61–63]

Schedule Dependency

The schedule of chemotherapy administration is also an important determinant of response. It influences dose intensity largely by affecting toxicity.[55] In some circumstances, changing the administration schedule can reduce the toxicity enough to allow patients to receive higher total doses or more frequent courses of therapy to increase the dose intensity. The optimal schedule is also influenced by the pharmacokinetics of the agent. For example, phase-specific agents can exert

Text continued on p. 88-23.

Table 88-11 Clinical Pharmacology of Chemotherapy Agents

Agents	Mechanism of Action	Pharmacokinetic Characteristics	Dosage Adjustment for Organ Dysfunction	Major Toxicities
Alemtuzumab (CamPath) Inj: 30 mg/mL	Monoclonal antibody; targets CD52 cell surface antigen; binding leads to lysis of CD52-positive leukemic cells.	$t^1/_2 \sim 12$ days; marked inter-patient variability.		Hypersensitivity and infusion reactions, myelosuppression/pancytopenia, opportunistic infection, nausea, vomiting, dyspnea, hypotension
Altretamine (Hexalen) Caps: 50 mg	Nonclassic alkylating agent. Metabolites generate reactive intermediates that cross-link DNA.	Bioavailability variable, probably due to extensive metabolism; $t^1/_{2\alpha} = 30$ min; $t^1/_{2\beta} = 4.7–13$ hr.		Anorexia; nausea, vomiting; diarrhea; neurologic toxicity; myelosuppression
Arsenic trioxide (Trisenox) Inj: 10 mg/mL	Metabolized to arsenic, which damages or degrades PML/RAR-alpha gene in leukemic cells; induces apoptosis in cancer cells.	Pharmacokinetics of trivalent arsenic (active species) not well described; $t^1/_{2\alpha} \sim 0.89$ hr, $t^1/_{2\beta} \sim 12$ hr.	Use with caution in renal dysfunction: effect of hepatic or renal dysfunction is unknown.	Fever, weight gain, dyspnea, musculoskeletal pain, elevated white blood cell count (acute); QT interval prolongation, hypokalemia, hyperglycemia, myelosuppression; headache, nausea, vomiting, cough; disseminated intravascular coagulation; rash
Asparaginase (Elspar) Inj: 10,000 IU/Vial	Enzyme; depletes essential amino acids and inhibits protein synthesis.	$t^1/_2 = 14–22$ hr; plasma clearance greatly accelerated in patients who develop hypersensitivity.		Hypersensitivity; hypoalbuminemia; hyperglycemia; ↓ clotting factors (↑ PT, ↑ PTT); ↑ LFTs; nausea/ vomiting; chills
Bevacizumab (Avastin) Inj: 25 mg/mL	Monoclonal antibody; inhibits development of new blood vessels (angiogenesis) by binding to and inhibiting vascular endothelial growth factor (VEGF) from interacting with receptors.	$t^1/_2 = 11–50$ days.		Hypertension; diarrhea, constipation; bleeding, thrombosis; gastrointestinal perforation; impaired wound healing; proteinuria; infusion reactions
Bexarotene (Targretin) Cap: 75 mg	Retinoid; selectively activates retinoid X receptors, which influence cell growth and differentiation.	Tmax ~ 2 hr; $t^1/_2 = 7$ hr, highly protein bound (>99%); high fat meals increase AUC by 35–48%; concentrations may be affected by CYP3A4 inhibitors or inducers.	Effect of hepatic or renal dysfunction is unknown; may need to hold or d/c if ↑ SGOT/SGPT/bilirubin ≥3 × ULN.	Lipid abnormalities (↑ LDL, triglycerides); nausea, asthenia, headache; dry skin, abdominal pain, peripheral edema; hypothyroidism; leukopenia
Bleomycin (Blenoxane) Inj: 15 mg/vial	Antitumor antibiotic; causes single- and double-strand breaks in DNA by generating free radicals.	$t^1/_{2\alpha} = 24$ min; $t^1/_{2\beta} = 2–4$ hr; longer $t^1/_2$ reported in patients with renal insufficiency; 45–70% excreted in urine in 24 hr	↓ if $Cl_{CR} <25$ mL/ min/m² in proportion with ↓.	Pulmonary toxicity; fever; skin changes: erythema, induration, hyperkeratosis, hyperpigmentation, peeling, and nail changes
Bortezomib (Velcade) Inj: 3.5 mg/vial	26S proteosome inhibitor; disrupts ubiquitin-proteosome pathway, leading to cancer cell growth delay or death.	$t^1/_2 = 9–15$ hr; protein binding 83%.	Effect of hepatic or renal dysfunction is unknown; clearance may be reduced in hepatic dysfunction.	Sensory peripheral neuropathy; hypotension; fever, asthenia, nausea, vomiting, diarrhea, constipation; thrombocytopenia
Busulfan (Myleran, Busulfex) Tab: 2 mg Inj: 60 mg/10 mL	Alkylating agent; forms reactive intermediates that cross-link DNA.	Well absorbed orally; metabolized extensively; no intact drug recovered in urine, but metabolites are excreted renally; 90% of dose cleared from plasma in 3 min.		Myelosuppression; pulmonary fibrosis; hyperpigmentation; suppression of testicular, ovarian, and adrenal function
Capecitabine (Xeloda) Tab: 150, 500 mg	Antimetabolite; prodrug metabolized to fluorouracil; incorporates into RNA and interferes with RNA function; inhibits thymidylate synthase and causes inhibition of DNA synthesis.	$t^1/_2 = 0.75$ hr; 35% protein bound; C_{max} and AUC varies >85%.		Nausea/vomiting; stomatitis; hand-foot syndrome; bone marrow suppression; anorexia

Drug	Mechanism	Pharmacokinetics	Dosage Adjustment	Toxicities
Carboplatin (Paraplatin) Inj: 50, 150, 450 mg/vial	Nonclassic alkylating agent; binds to DNA to form interstrand cross-links and adducts.	$t^1/_{2\alpha} = 12–24$ min; $t^1/_{2\beta} = 1.3–1.7$ hr; $t^1/_{2\gamma} = 22–40$ hr; $\geq 90\%$ excreted in urine.	↓ if $Cl_{CR} <60$ mL/min or use methods described by Egorin or Calvert.[51,52]	Myelosuppression (especially thrombocytopenia); nausea/vomiting
Carmustine (BiCNU) Inj: 100 mg/vial	Alkylating agent; metabolites generate, reactive intermediates that cross-link DNA.	>30% metabolite excreted in urine; $t^1/_2 = 5$ min; good CSF penetration.	↓ may be necessary if a patient has ↓ bone marrow reserve.	Delayed myelosuppression; nausea/vomiting; pulmonary fibrosis; hepatotoxicity; renal toxicity
Cetuximab (Erbitux) Inj	Monoclonal antibody; inhibits cell proliferation by preventing activation of the epidermal growth factor receptor (EGFR).	$T^1/_2 = 41–213$ hr; intrinsic clearance approximately 25% lower in females.		Anaphylactic/anaphylactoid reactions; acneiform skin rash; asthenia; nausea/vomiting
Chlorambucil (Leukeran) Tab: 2 mg	Alkylating agent; forms reactive intermediates that cross-link DNA.	Oral bioavailability 70–80%, reduced by 10–20% if ingested with food; rapidly metabolized to inactive metabolites and active phenylacetic acid mustard; $t^1/_2 = 1.5–2$ hr (parent) 2.5 hr (active metabolite); <1% excreted unchanged in urine in 24 hr.		Myelosuppression; pulmonary fibrosis
Cladribine (Leustatin) Inj: 10 mg/vial	Antimetabolite; following intracellular phosphorylation, causes inhibition of enzymes that impair DNA synthesis; impairs DNA repair.	$t^1/_{2\alpha} = 35$ min; $t^1/_{2\beta} = 6.7$ hr.	Effect of renal or hepatic disease unknown.	Myelosuppression; fever; immunosuppression (B and T cells); acute tubular necrosis; neurotoxicity (paraparesis, quadraplegia); rash
Cisplatin (Platinol) Inj: 10, 50 mg/vial	Nonclassic alkylating agents; binds to DNA to form interstrand cross-links and adducts.	$t^1/_{2\alpha} = 20–30$ min; $t^1/_{2\beta} = 60$ min; $t^1/_{2\gamma} = 24$ hr; >90% excreted in urine.	↓ or discontinue for renal dysfunction.	Nephrotoxicity; nausea/vomiting; peripheral neuropathy; ototoxicity; hypomagnesemia; visual disturbances (rare)
Cyclophosphamide (Cytoxan) Inj: 100, 200, 500, 1,000, 2,000 mg/vial Tab: 25, 50 mg	Alkylating agent; metabolite generates reactive intermediates that cross-link DNA.	Oral bioavailability 100%; must be activated in liver by microsomal enzymes to active compounds and toxic metabolites; 22% of parent and 60% of metabolites excreted in urine; $t^1/_2 = 3–10$ hr; 6.5–≥8 hr (alkylating activity).		Myelosuppression; hemorrhagic cystitis; nausea/vomiting; alopecia; cardiomyopathy (rare); "allergic" interstitial pneumonitis; SIADH
Cytarabine (Cytosar) Inj: 100, 500, 1,000, 2,000 mg/vial	Antimetabolite; incorporates into DNA and causes termination of DNA chain elongation and inhibition of DNA polymerase.	Metabolized by deamination primarily in liver, 8% parent and 72% as metabolite excreted unchanged in urine; $t^1/_{2\alpha} = 1.6–20$ min; $t^1/_{2\beta} = 9–111$ min.		Myelosuppression; nausea/vomiting; stomatitis; fever; rash; intrahepatic cholestasis, ↑ LFT and bilirubin (rare)
Cytarabine liposomal (DepotCyt) Inj: 50 mg/5 mL]		Intrathecal: biphasic elimination profile, $t^1/_{2\beta} = 100–263$ Hr.		Intrathecal: chemical arachnoiditis (headache, nausea, vomiting, fever); increased risk of neurotoxicity with spinal/brain irradiation or chemotherapy
Dacarbazine (DTIC-Dome) Inj: 50 μg/vial	Nonclassic alkylating agent; metabolite causes methylation of nucleic acids; causes direct DNA damage and inhibits purine synthesis.	Extensively metabolize to active compound; 50% parent and 9–18% major metabolite excreted in urine; some hepatobiliary excretion; $t^1/_{2\alpha} = 3$ min; $t^1/_{2\beta} = 41$ min.	↓ may be required for moderate to severe hepatic or renal dysfunction.	Myelosuppression; nausea/vomiting; myalgias; fever; malaise; headache; pain at injection site; photosensitivity; fatal hepatic vein occlusion (rare)
Dactinomycin (Cosmegen) Inj: 500 μg/vial	Antitumor antibiotic; intercalates into DNA and inhibits RNA and protein synthesis.	Urinary excretion 20% fecal excretion 14%; $t^1/_{2\beta} = \geq 36$ hr.		Myelosuppression, nausea, vomiting, diarrhea; mucositis; alopecia; hepatotoxicity; vesicant if extravasated

Continued

Table 88-11 Clinical Pharmacology of Chemotherapy Agents—cont'd

Agents	Mechanism of Action	Pharmacokinetic Characteristics	Dosage Adjustment for Organ Dysfunction	Major Toxicities
Daunorubicin (Cerubidine) Inj: 20 mg/vial	Antitumor antibiotic, intercalates to DNA double helix; topoisomerase II–mediated DNA damage; produces oxygen-free radicals.	Extensive binding to tissues; know routes of elimination account for only 50–60% of dose; extensively metabolized by liver; $t^1/_{2\alpha} = 40$ min; $t^1/_{2\beta} = 45$–55 hr; 20–30% biliary excretion; 14–23% excreted in urine as parent and metabolites.	↓ if very severe hepatic dysfunction; 75% if severe renal dysfunction.	Myelosuppression, mucositis; alopecia cumulative cardiac toxicity; dose-related acute ECG changes; severe tissue damage if extravasated
Daunorubicin, liposomal (Daunoxome) Inj: 50 mg/vial	Antitumor antibiotic; intercalates into DNA double helix; topoisomerase II–mediated DNA damage; produces oxygen-free radicals.		↓ with hepatic dysfunction: 75% if bilirubin 1.2–3.0; 50% if bilirubin >3.0.	
Denileukin diftitox (Ontak) Inj: 300 μg/2 mL	Diphtheria toxin fusion protein; interacts with IL-2 receptor on leukemia and lymphoma cells; induces cell death via inhibition of cell protein synthesis.	$t^1/_{2\alpha} = 2$–5 min; $t^1/_{2\beta} = 70$–80 min; Vd = 0.06–0.08 L/kg; development of anti-denileukin diftitox antibodies increases systemic clearance 2 to 3-fold.		Hypersensitivity reaction; vascular leak syndrome (hypotension, edema, hypoalbuminemia); fluike syndrome, nausea, vomiting, fever, chills, asthenia; diarrhea, dehydration; rash; thrombosis.
Docetaxel (Taxotere) Inj: 40 mg/mL	Taxane; promotes microtubule assembly and arrests cell cycle in G_2 and M phases.	$t^1/_{2\alpha} = 4$ min; $t^1/_{2\beta} = 36$ min; $t^1/_{2\gamma} = 11$ hr; Cl 21 L/hr/m²; Vd = 113 L.	Discontinue treatment if bilirubin > ULN; SGOT/SGPT >1.5 × ULN or alkaline phosphatase >2.5 × ULN.	Peripheral edema; bone marrow suppression; hypersensitivity reaction
Doxorubicin (Adriamycin, Rubex) Inj: 10, 20, 50, 100, 150, 200 mg/vial	Antitumor antibiotic; intercalates into DNA double helix; topoisomerase II–mediated DNA damage; produces oxygen-free radicals.	Extensive binding to tissues; known routes of elimination only account for 50–60% of dose; extensively metabolized by liver; $t^1/_{2\alpha} = 40$ min; $t^1/_{2\beta} = 45$–55 hr; 20–30% biliary excretion; 14–23% excreted in urine as parent and metabolites.	↓ if hepatic dysfunction: 100% if bilirubin ≤1.2; 50% if bilirubin 1.2–3.0; 25% if bilirubin >3.0.	Myelosuppression; mucositis; nausea/vomiting; alopecia; cumulative cardiac toxicity; dose-related acute ECG changes; severe tissue damage if extravasated
Doxorubicin, liposomal (Doxil) Inj: 20 mg SDV	Antitumor antibiotic; intercalates into DNA double helix; topoisomerase II–mediated DNA damage; produces oxygen-free radicals.		↓ if hepatic dysfunction: 50% if bilirubin 2.0–3.0; 25% if bilirubin ≥3.	
Epirubicin (Ellence) Inj: 50 mg/25 mL, 200 mg/100 mL	Anthracycline antitumor antibiotic; intercalates into DNA double helix; topoisomerase II–mediated DNA damage; produces oxygen-free radicals.	$T^1/_{2\alpha} = 3$min, $t^1/_{2\beta} = 2.5$ hr, $t^1/_{2\gamma} = 33$ hr; protein binding 77%; epirubicin or metabolite excretion in bile (35%) or urine (20%); plasma clearance reduced 35% in females ≥70 years.	↓ dose by 50% for bilirubin 1.2–3 mg/dL or AST 2–4 × ULN; ↓ dose 5% for bilirubin > 3 mg/dL or AST > 4 ×ULN; may need ↓ dose with serum creatinine >5 mg/dL.	Myelosuppression; nausea, vomiting, diarrhea, mucositis, alopecia; cumulativ dose-related cardiomyopathy, acute ECG changes; severe tissue damage (if extravasated);
Estramustine (Emcyt) Cap: 140 mg	Endocrine therapy and alkylating agent; probably impairs mitotic spindle formation.	Milk ↓ absorption; readily dephosphorylated absorption to estradiol and estrone congeners.		Estrogenic effects; cardiovascular (edema, thrombophlebitis, pulmonary embolus); nausea/vomiting; diarrhea; gynecomastia; mild ↑ LFT

Drug	Mechanism of Action	Pharmacokinetics	Dose Adjustment	Toxicity
Etoposide (VePesid) Inj: 100 mg/5 mL Cap: 50 mg	Epipodophyllotoxin; produces DNA strand breaks by inhibiting topoisomerase II; arrests cells in late S or early G_2 phase.	Oral bioavailability 37-67% (average 50%); 30-40% excreted rapidly in the urine (70% of excreted drug is unchanged); terminal $t_{1/2}$ = 6-8 hr; 6-15% excreted in bile; >2% excreted in feces.	↓ if renal dysfunction in proportion to ↓ in CL_{Cr}.	Myelosuppression; nausea/vomiting; alopecia; mucositis; hypotension (related to rapid infusion); hypersensitivity reactions; fever; bronchospasm
Floxuridine (FUDR) Inj: 500 mg/vial	Antimetabolite; incorporates into RNA and interferes with RNA function; inhibits thymidylate synthase and inhibits DNA synthesis.	$t_{1/2}$ = 20 min; >90% hepatically metabolized.	Adjustments are made depending on clinical hematologic, and GI toxicity.	Mucositis; myelosuppression; nausea/vomiting; diarrhea; skin changes
Fludarabine (Fludara IV) Inj: 50 mg/vial	Antimetabolite; inhibits ribonucleotide reductase and DNA polymerase causing inhibition DNA synthesis.	Undergoes rapid dephosphorylation to F-ara-A; terminal $t_{1/2}$ F-ara-A 8 hr; terminal $t_{1/2}$ F-ara-ATP 15 hr.		Myelosuppression; neurotoxicity; peripheral neuropathy; pulmonary toxicity; nausea/vomiting; immunosuppression
Fluorouracil Inj: 500 mg/vial	Antimetabolite; incorporates into RNA, interferes with RNA function; inhibits thymidylate synthase and inhibits DNA synthesis.	$t_{1/2}$ = 6-20 min; ≥90% hepatically metabolized.	Adjustments are made depending on clinical, hematologic, and GI toxicity.	Mucositis; diarrhea, myelosuppression; dermatologic, nausea/vomiting
Gefitinib (Iressa) Tab: 250 mg	Epidermal growth factor receptor (EGFR) tyrosine kinase inhibitor; inhibits intracellular phosphorylation of tyrosine kinases signaling pathways.	Mean bioavailability = 60%; peak plasma concentrations 3-7 hr; $t_{1/2}$ ~ 48 hr; Vdss = 1400 L; plasma protein binding = 90%; hepatically metabolized; excretion in feces (86%) with renal elimination <4% of administered dose.	Effect of hepatic impairment unknown, although studies in patients with liver abnormalities did not reveal altered Pharmacokinetics.	Diarrhea, rash, acne, nausea/vomiting, dry skin; pulmonary toxicity (acute dyspnea, cough, fever, interstitial lung disease); eye pain, corneal ulcer
Gemcitabine (Gemzar) Inj: 200 mg/vial or 1,000 mg/10 mL	Antimetabolite; inhibits ribonucleotide synthesis reductase and inhibits DNA synthesis.	Parameters dependent on infusion; $t_{1/2}$ = 32-94 min or 245-638 min; V = 50 L/m² or 370 L/m².		Bone marrow suppression; flu-like syndrome; nausea/vomiting; edema
Gemtuzumab ozogamicin (Mylotarg) Inj: 5 mg/20 mL	Monoclonal antibody; linked to a calicheamicin cytotoxic derivative; targets CD33 antigen on leukemic blast cells; binding introduces cytotoxic into cells, causing DNA strand breakage and cell death.	$T_{1/2}$ calicheamicin ~ 45 hr (total) and 100 hr (unconjugated); $t_{1/2}$ antibody ~ 72 hr; probably undergoes hepatic metabolism but metabolic studies have not been performed.	Effect of hepatic or renal dysfunction unknown; use in patients with bilirubin >2 mg/dL has not been studied.	Myelosuppression (severe); hypersensitivity and infusion reactions; pulmonary events (dyspnea, pleural effusion, pulmonary infiltrates, acute respiratory distress syndrome); hepatotoxicity; nausea/vomiting
Hydroxyurea (Hydrea) Cap: 500 mg	Antimetabolite; inhibits ribonucleotide reductase and inhibits DNA synthesis.	T_{max} = 2 hr; 80% excreted in urine in 12 hr.		Myelosuppression; stomatitis; nausea/vomiting; diarrhea; rash
Ibritumomab tiuxetan (Zevalin) Inj: 10 mg/10 mL, 50 mg/50 mL	Monoclonal antibody; Yttrium-90 (Y-90)-linked antibody directed against the CD20 antigen on malignant B lymphocytes; binds to antigen and releases radiation (β particles) which induces cell damage and death.	Mean effective $t_{1/2}$ for Y-90 = 30 hr; median of 7.2% of injected radioactivity recovered in urine over 7 days; Y-90 β particle decay $t_{1/2}$ = 64 hr.	↓ dose for platelet count 100,000-149,000 cells/mm².	Infusion reactions (hypotension, angioedema, hypoxia, bronchospasm); asthenia, chills, nausea; myelosuppression; see also rituximab
Idarubicin (Idamycin) Inj: 5, 10 mg/vial	Antitumor antibiotic; intercalates into DNA double helix; topoisomerase II-mediated DNA damage; produces oxygen-free radicals.	Terminal $t_{1/2}$ = 15-18 hr.		Myelosuppression; mucositis; anorexia; nausea/vomiting; diarrhea; fever; alopecia

Continued

Table 88-11   Clinical Pharmacology of Chemotherapy Agents—cont'd

Agents	Mechanism of Action	Pharmacokinetic Characteristics	Dosage Adjustment for Organ Dysfunction	Major Toxicities
Imatinib mesylate (Gleevec) Tab: 100 mg, 500 mg	Tyrosine kinase inhibitor; inhibits kinases for Bcr-Abl, platelet-derived growth factor (PDGF), c-kit, and stem cell factor, thereby inhibiting cell proliferation and inducing apoptosis.	Mean bioavailability = 98%; Cmax 2–4 hr; $t^1/_2$ of imatinib (= 18 hr) and major metabolite (= 40 hr); plasma protein binding = 95%; hepatically metabolized via CYP3A4; eliminated as unchanged drug in feces (20%) and urine (5%); interpatient variability in clearance = 40%; susceptible to alterations in clearance with CYP3A4 inducers and inhibitors.	Effect of hepatic or renal impairment unknown; patients with serum creatinine >2 × ULN not studied.	Fluid retention, edema; nausea/vomiting, diarrhea, rash, fatigue, muscle cramps, musculoskeletal pain; intra-tumoral bleeding; myelosuppression, hepatic toxicity
Irinotecan (Camptostar) Inj: 20 mg/mL	Camphothecin; inhibits DNA-strand religation by binding topoisomerase I-DNA complex.	$t^1/_2$ = 6 hr; 36–68% protein bound.		Diarrhea; cholinergic syndrome; myelosuppression
Isofamide (Ifex) Inj: 1, 3 g/vial	Alkylating agent; metabolites generates reactive intermediates that cross-link DNA.	Parameters are dose and schedule dependent; 60–80% excreted in urine as unchanged drug or metabolite within 72 hr.	Adjustments may be necessary based on clinical response.	Myelosuppression; hemorrhagic cystitis (should be administered with MESNA); nephrotoxicity; neurotoxicity; anorexia; nausea/vomiting; alopecia
Lomustine (CeeNu) Cap: 10, 40, 100 mg	Nonclassic alkylating agent; metabolites generates reactive intermediates that cross-links DNA.	Well absorbed orally; $t^1/_2$ of metabolites = 16–48 hr; 50% metabolites excreted in urine within 24 hr.	↓ may be required for patients with ↓ bone marrow reserves.	Myelosuppression; nausea/vomiting; nephrotoxicity; pulmonary infiltrates/fibrosis; hepatotoxicity
Mechlorethamine (Mustargen) Inj: 10 mg/vial	Alkylating agent; forms reactive intermediates that cross-link DNA.	Rapid metabolism; <0.01% unchanged drug excreted in urine; 50% of metabolites excreted in urine within 24 hr.		Myelosuppression; nausea/vomiting; sterility, menstrual irregularities; local irritant/vesicant (if extravasated)
Melphalan (Alkeran) Tab: 2 mg Inj: 50 mg/vial	Alkylating agent; forms intermediates that cross-link DNA.	Oral absorption erratic and incomplete (30%); not actively metabolized but spontaneous chemical degradation; $t^1/_2$ = 90 min; 10–15% excreted in urine within 24 hr.	↓ if renal dysfunction: 50% dose for BUN >30 mg/dL or creatinine >1.5 mg/dL.	Myelosuppression; pulmonary fibrosis
Mercaptopurine (Purinethol) Tab: 50 mg	Antimetabolite; metabolites incorporated into DNA or RNA and inhibit purine synthesis.	Oral absorption highly variable; $t^1/_2$ = 20–60 min; elimination primarily hepatic.	↓ if hepatic or renal dysfunction.	Myelosuppression; anorexia, nausea, vomiting; hepatic toxicity (biliary stasis)
Methotrexate Tab: 2.5 mg Inj: 25, 50, 100, 200, 250, 1,000 mg/vial	Antifolate; inhibits dihydrofolate reductase and depletes reduced folates and inhibits DNA synthesis.	Oral absorption appears to be better with smaller doses; exhibits interpatient bioavailability; "third space" collections of fluid may provide a reservoir for drug accumulation; $t^1/_{2\alpha}$ = 1.5–3.5 hr; $t^1/_{2\beta}$ = 8–15 hr; 90% dose excreted in urine within 24 hr.	↓ or discontinue if renal dysfunction; monitor serum methotrexate levels with ↓renal function or fluid accumulation.	Myelosuppression; nephrotoxicity; hepatotoxicity; mucositis, pulmonary toxicity; neurotoxicity
Mitoxantrone (Novatrone) Inj: 20, 25, 30 mg/vial	Antitumor antibiotic; intercalates into DNA double helix; topoisomerase II-mediated DNA damage; produces oxygen-free radicals.	$t^1/_{2\alpha}$ = 10 min, $t^1/_{2\beta}$ = 6 hr; $t^1/_{2\gamma}$ = 2 days; <10% excreted in the urine.		Myelosuppression; cumulative cardiac toxicity (total dose >100 mg); ↑ risk with prior anthracycline therapy; nausea/vomiting; mild stomatitis

Drug	Mechanism of Action	Pharmacokinetics	Dosing Adjustments	Toxicities
Oxaliplatin (Eloxatin) Inj: 50 mg/10 mL, 100 mg/20 mL	Nonclassic alkylating agent; binds to DNA to form interstrand cross-links and adducts.	$t\frac{1}{2}\alpha$ = 0.43 hr, $t\frac{1}{2}\beta$ = 15.8 hr, $t\frac{1}{2}\gamma$ = 391 hr; Vd ultrafilterable platinum = 440 L; extensive and irreversible plasma protein binding (>90%); nonenzymatically biotransformed; renal primary route of elimination: 54% at 5 days.	Use caution in patients with renal impairment.	Anaphylactic/anaphylactoid reactions; peripheral sensory neuropathy, sensitivity to cold, jaw spasm, dysphagia; nausea/vomiting, diarrhea, fatigue; pulmonary fibrosis
Paclitaxel (Taxol) Inj: 30 mg/vial	Taxane; promotes microtubule assembly and arrests cell cycle in G_2 and M phases.	<10% excreted in urine; liver and biliary primary routes of elimination; $t\frac{1}{2}\alpha$ = 0.3 hr; $t\frac{1}{2}\beta$ = 1.3–8.6 hr.	↓ for severe neutropenia (following prior therapy), severe peripheral neuropathy or hepatic dysfunction.	Hypersensitivity reactions (premedications recommended); cardiac disturbances; sensory neuropathy; myalgia; arthralgia; myelosuppression
Pegaspargase (Oncaspar) Inj: 3750 IU/5 mL	Enzyme; depletes essential amino acids and inhibits protein synthesis.	$t\frac{1}{2}$ ~ 3.24 days in patients with hypersensitivity to l-asparaginase, $t\frac{1}{2}$ ~ 5.69 days in non-hypersensitive patients.		Hypersensitivity; hypoalbuminemia; hyperglycemia; ↓ clotting factors (↑ PT, ↑ PTT; ↑ LFTs; nausea/vomiting; chills
Pentostatin (Nipent) Inj: 100 mg/vial	Antimetabolite; inhibits adenosine deaminase and subsequent DNA and RNA synthesis.	90% excreted in urine; $t\frac{1}{2}\alpha$ = 11–85 min; $t\frac{1}{2}\beta$ = 5–15 hr (longer in patients with ↓ renal function).	↓ for renal dysfunction: Cl_{CR} <60 mL/min.	Myelosuppression; immunosuppression; lethargy; seizures; conjunctivitis; rash; nausea/vomiting; renal dysfunction (rare)
Procarbazine (Matulane) Cap: 50 mg	Nonclassic alkylating agent; prodrug, metabolite causes methylation of nucleic acids; causes direct DNA damage and inhibits purine synthesis.	Oral dose well absorbed; 70% excreted in urine as active metabolite.	↓ for renal dysfunction: SrCr >2.0 or bilirubin >3.0.	Myelosuppression; nausea/vomiting; neurotoxicity; sterility; pulmonary hypersensitivity; ↓ with drugs metabolized by phase I enzymes, sympathomimetic drugs and tyramine-rich foods; disulfiram-like reaction with alcohol
Rituximab (Rituxan) Inj: 100 mg/10 mL, 500 mg/50 mL	Monoclonal antibody; lyses B cells by recruiting immune effectors.	$t\frac{1}{2}$ variable.		Tumor lysis; hypersensitivity reactions; mucocutaneous reactions; lymphopenia
Streptozocin (Zanosar) Inj: 1,000 mg/vial	Alkylating agent; forms reactive intermediates that cross-links DNA.	$t\frac{1}{2}\alpha$ = 5–15 min; $t\frac{1}{2}\beta$ = 35 min; 60–72% excreted in urine within 4 hr.	↓ may be required in patients with renal dysfunction.	Renal toxicity-dose related; nausea/vomiting; myelosuppression; abnormal glucose tolerance; hepatotoxicity
Temozolomide (Temodar) Caps: 5, 20, 100, 250 mg	Nonclassic alkylating agent; metabolite causes methylation of nucleic acids; causes direct DNA damage.	Rapidly and completely absorbed; food reduces the rate and extent of absorption; spontaneously hydrolyzed to an active form and metabolite; temozolomide $t\frac{1}{2}$ = 1.8 hr; mean apparent Vd = 0.4 L/kg; elimination primarily in urine (≈38% of a total radioactive dose recovered over 7 days).	Cl_{CR} 36–130 mL/min/m² has no effect on temozolomide clearance; ↓ dose may be required for moderate to severe hepatic or renal dysfunction.	Myelosuppression; nausea/vomiting, constipation, diarrhea; fatigue; headache; myalgias; fever; ↑ LFTs
Teniposide (Vumon) Inj: 50 mg/ampule	Epipodophyllotoxin; produces DNA strand breaks by inhibiting topoisomerase II; arrests cells in late S or early G_2 phases.	4–12% excreted in urine; terminal $t\frac{1}{2}$ = 6–10 hr; ↑ hepatic enzymes correlate with ↓ clearance.	Adjustments may be necessary for hepatic dysfunction.	Myelosuppression; hypotension; nausea, vomiting; secondary leukemia
Thioguanine Tab: 40 mg	Antimetabolite; interrupts purine synthesis and inhibits RNA and DNA synthesis.	Oral absorption incomplete and ↓ with food; clearance is mainly hepatic with methylation of parent drug to inactive metabolites; $t\frac{1}{2}\alpha$ = 15 min; $t\frac{1}{2}\beta$ = 11 hr.	No adjustment necessary.	Myelosuppression; stomatitis; hepatotoxicity (↑ alkaline phosphatase and ↑ direct bilirubin); nausea/vomiting

Continued

Table 88-11 Clinical Pharmacology of Chemotherapy Agents—cont'd

Agents	Mechanism of Action	Pharmacokinetic Characteristics	Dosage Adjustment for Organ Dysfunction	Major Toxicities
Thiotepa Inj: 15 mg/vial	Alkylating agent; forms reactive intermediates that cross-link DNA.	Metabolized to TEPA; 15% of TEPA excreted in urine within 24 hr; $t^1/_{2\alpha}$ = 7.5 min; $t^1/_{2\beta}$ = 109 min.	↓ may be required for patients with ↓ bone marrow reserve.	Myelosuppression; nausea/vomiting
Topotecan (Hycamtin) Inj: 10 mg/mL	Camptothecin; inhibits DNA-strand religation by binding toposomerase I-DNA complex.	$t^1/_2$ = 2–3 hr; 35% protein bound; 30% excreted in urine.	↓ renal dysfunction: 0.75 mg/m² if Cl_{CR} 20–39 mL/min.	Bone marrow suppression; nausea/vomiting; diarrhea; alopecia
Tositumomab (Bexxar) Inj: 35 mg/2.5 mL, 225 mg/16.1 mL	Monoclonal antibody; iodine-131 (I-131)-linked antibody directed against the CD20 antigen on malignant B lymphocytes; binds to antigen and induces apoptosis, complement- and/or antibody-depended cytotoxicity; ionizing radiation induces cell damage and death.	Total body clearance influenced by high tumor burden, extent of splenomegaly and bone marrow involvement; I-131 eliminated in urine (98% of administered dose); I-131 β and γ particle decay $t^1/_2$ = 8.04 days.	Effect of renal or hepatic impairment unknown; renal dysfunction may delay elimination of I-131.	Hypersensitivity reactions; myelosuppression; hypothyroidism; nausea/vomiting, abdominal pain, diarrhea; myelodysplastic syndrome, acute leukemia
Trastuzumab (Herceptin) Inj: 440 mg/ 30 mL	Monoclonal antibody; inhibits proliferation of human tumor cells that express HER2 proto-oncogene.	$t^1/_2$ = 5.8 hr; Vd = 44 mL/kg.		Carciomyopathy; diarrhea; nausea/vomiting; hypersensitivity reaction
Tretinoin (Vesanoid) Cap: 10 mg	Retinoid; decreases proliferation and induces maturation of acute promyelocytic leukemia cells.	$t^1/_2$ = 0.5–2 hr with initial dosing; induces own metabolism with continued dosing; protein binding >95%; hepatically metabolized; >63% of tretinoin and metabolites recovered in the urine in 3 days; 31% eliminated in the feces over 6 days.	Effect of hepatic or renal impairment unknown.	Headache, fever, fatigue, malaise; lipid abnormalities (↑ LDL, triglycerides); ↑ LFTs; dry skin/mucous membranes; bone pain; nausea/vomiting; rash; retinoic acid syndrome (fever, dyspnea, weight gain, pulmonary infiltrates, fever, pleural/pericardial effusion); leukocytosis; benign intracranial hypertension
Valrubicin (Valstar) Inj: 200 mg/5 mL	Anthracycline antitumor antibiotic; intercalates into DNA double helix; topoisomerase II-mediated DNA damage; produces oxygen-free radicals.	Almost completely excreted in the instillate following direct instillation into the bladder; metabolism during 2-hr instillation period is negligible; low but variable systemic exposure with bladder administration.	Avoid in patients with small bladder capacity unable to tolerate 75 mL fluid instillation.	Urinary frequency, urgency; hematuria, dysuria; bladder pain, urinary incontinence
Vinblastine (Velban) Inj: 10 mg/vial	Vinca alkaloid; reversibly inhibits mitosis; binds to microtubule protein, tubulin and ultimately inhibits formation.	Primarily metabolized and excreted in bile; 10% excreted in feces; $t^1/_{2\alpha}$ = 4.5 min.	↓ if hepatic dysfunction: >50% if bilirubin >3.0.	Myelosuppression; neurotoxicity (rare); vesicant (if extravasated)
Vincristine (Oncovin) Inj: 1, 2, 5 mg/ vial; 2-mg pre-filled syringe	Vinca alkaloid; reversibly inhibits of mitosis; binds to microtubule protein, tubulin and ultimately inhibiting formation of mitotic spindles.	$t^1/_{2\alpha}$ = <1 min; $t^1/_{2\beta}$ = 7.4 min; $t^1/_{2\gamma}$ = 164 min.		Neurotoxicity (primarily distal neuropathy that affects sensory and motor abilities); autonomic neuropathies (high dosages); SIADH; vesicant (if extravasated)
Vinorelbine (Navelbine) Inj: 10 mg/1 mL; 50 mg/5 mL	Vinca alkaloid; reversibly inhibits mitosis; binds to microtubule protein, tubulin and ultimately inhibits formation of mitotic spindles.	<20% excreted in urine; $t^1/_{2\alpha}$ = 2–6 min; $t^1/_{2\beta}$ = 1.9 hr.		Leukopenia; neurotoxicity; ↓ DTR; vesicant (if extravasated)

BUN, blood urea nitrogen; Cl_{CR}, creatinine clearance; CSF, cerebrospinal fluid; DTR, deep tendon reflexes; GI, gastrointestinal; LFT, liver function tests; PT, prothrombin time; PPT, partial thromboplastin time; SrCr, serum creatinine; $t^1/_{2\alpha}$, α half-life; $t^1/_{2\beta}$, β half-life; $t^1/_{2\gamma}$, γ half-life; SIADH, syndrome of inappropriate antidiuretic hormone secretion.

their cytotoxic effects only when the cell is in a particular phase of the cell cycle. If a phase-specific agent with a short half-life is administered by intravenous bolus, a significant number of tumor cells will probably not cycle through the vulnerable phase of the cell cycle during exposure to the agent. Comparatively, the same agent administered by frequent intravenous bolus or continuous infusion could expose more cells to the agent during the vulnerable phase. New attempts to improve cytotoxicity include administering agents during certain times of the day (called *chronomodulation*). Theoretically, administration of chemotherapy at certain times based on the circadian rhythm can improve cell kill. Although studies evaluating chronomodulation for colorectal cancer and endometrial cancer have shown that this approach can reduce toxicity and permit higher doses of chemotherapy, it does not appear to significantly improve patient survival when compared to standard therapy.[64,65]

Drug Resistance

8. **B.C. is a 39-year-old man with an aggressive non-Hodgkin's lymphoma (NHL). At the time of diagnosis, B.C. had enlarged cervical lymph nodes, dyspnea, and a large mediastinal mass noted on chest x-ray examination. Chemotherapy was initiated with the CHOP regimen, which consists of cyclophosphamide, doxorubicin, vincristine, and prednisone. After the first course of chemotherapy, B.C.'s lymphadenopathy was greatly reduced. Chest x-ray examination repeated after the second course of therapy showed marked improvement. When he returned for his fourth cycle of chemotherapy, recurrent lymphadenopathy was noted and the chest radiograph confirmed enlargement of the mediastinal mass. Why is B.C.'s cancer growing despite continued chemotherapy, and how should his treatment be altered?**

Most likely B.C.'s cancer is now growing because the tumor has become resistant to the chemotherapy; therefore, it would be wise to discontinue the CHOP regimen. Biochemical resistance to chemotherapy is the major impediment to successful treatment with most cancers.[55] Resistance can occur de novo in cancer cells or develop during cell division as a result of mutation.[55] In 1979, a proposed mathematical model predicted that tumor cells mutate to drug resistance at a rate related to the genetic instability of the tumor.[66] Thus, the probability that a tumor mass will contain resistant clones is related to both the rate of mutation and the size of the tumor. Many specific mechanisms now have been identified by which cancer cells resist the activity of cytotoxic agents (Table 88-12).

Some cell lines that become resistant to a single chemotherapy agent may also be resistant to structurally unrelated cytotoxic compounds. This phenomenon is called pleiotropic drug resistance or multidrug resistance (MDR).[67] Cell lines that display this type of resistance generally are resistant to natural product cytotoxic agents such as the vinca alkaloids, antitumor antibiotics, epipodophyllotoxins, camptothecins, and taxanes. The primary mechanism believed to be responsible for MDR is an increase in p-glycoprotein in the cell membrane. This protein mediates efflux of the chemotherapy agent, causing a decreased accumulation of drug within the cell (the site of drug activity).[67] Other transport proteins have been implicated in resistance to chemotherapy, as well.[68]

Table 88-12   Possible Mechanisms of Anticancer Drug Resistance

Mechanism	Chemotherapy Agents
Improved proficiency in repair of DNA	Cisplatin, cyclophosphamide, melphalan, mitomycin, mechlorethamine
↓ in drug activation	Cytarabine, doxorubicin, fluorouracil, mercaptopurine, methotrexate, thioguanine
↑ in drug inactivation	Cytarabine, mercaptopurine
↓ in cellular uptake of drug	Methotrexate, melphalan
↑ in efflux of drug (multidrug resistance)	Doxorubicin, daunorubicin, etoposide, vincristine, vinblastine, teniposide, docetaxel, paclitaxel, vinorelbine
Alternative biochemical pathways	Cytarabine, fluorouracil, methotrexate
Alterations in target enzymes (DHFR, topoisomerase II)	Fluorouracil, hydroxyurea, mercaptopurine, methotrexate, thioguanine, etoposide, teniposide, doxorubicin, daunorubicin, idarubicin

Drugs that are known to inhibit P-glycoprotein (e.g., verapamil, cyclosporine, quinidine) have been investigated as potential adjunctive therapies to reduce resistance. Unfortunately, the dosages of the agents required to inhibit P-glycoprotein have been associated with significant morbidity. Studies of newer agents that are more potent and specific inhibitors of P-glycoprotein are underway.[67,69] These agents can inhibit P-glycoprotein-mediated drug efflux, but whether their clinical use with chemotherapy will improve patient outcomes is still unknown. A second type of MDR is mediated by altered binding to topoisomerase II, an enzyme that promotes DNA strand breaks in the presence of anthracyclines and epipodophyllotoxins.[70] Because of the likelihood of MDR, B.C. should receive a chemotherapy regimen that does not include chemotherapy agents inactivated by the MDR mechanism. An alternative regimen such as high-dose methotrexate with leucovorin rescue would be appropriate because this regimen is effective against NHL and is not affected by the MDR gene.

Tumor Site

The cytotoxic effects of chemotherapy agents are related to the time the tumor is exposed to an effective concentration of the agent (i.e., concentration X time [C X T]). The dosage regimen, including the dose, infusion rate, route of administration, and lipophilicity, can influence the concentration-time product. Other factors, such as tumor size and location, can also critically affect an agent's cytotoxicity. As tumors grow larger, their degree of vascularity lessens, making it more difficult for agents to penetrate the entire tumor mass. Tumors located in sites of the body with poor drug penetration (e.g., the brain) may not receive a sufficient concentration to provide effective kill.

Combination Chemotherapy

9. **K.K. has advanced Hodgkin's disease and is to begin chemotherapy today with the ABVD (adriamycin, bleomycin, vinblastine, and dacarbazine) regimen. She is reluctant because of her fear of side effects. She asks if, rather than receiving all four drugs today, she could receive just one and if it does not work then try another one?**

CHOICE OF AGENTS

Although single-agent chemotherapy can cause significant early regressions of Hodgkin's disease, acute lymphocytic leukemia, and adult NHL, most tumors show only a partial response of a very short duration to single-agent therapy. Recognition that single-agent chemotherapy rarely produced prolonged remission led to the simultaneous use of multiple chemotherapy agents. In Hodgkin's disease, the use of combination chemotherapy results in long-term, disease-free survival for >60% of patients. If K.K. were to receive single-agent therapy, her disease would not be cured. Combination chemotherapy is absolutely recommended to provide her with the best chance for long-term, disease-free survival. She should be reassured that appropriate measures, including prophylactic antiemetic therapy, will be taken to reduce her chances of both acute and chronic toxicities.

Combination chemotherapy provides broader coverage against resistant cell lines within the heterogeneous tumor mass. Several principles provide the basis for selecting the agents to be included in a chemotherapy regimen:

- Only agents with demonstrable single-agent activity against the specific type of tumor should be used in combination therapy.
- All agents in the regimen should have different mechanisms of action.
- Agents should not have overlapping toxicities so that the severity and duration of acute and chronic toxicities are minimized.
- All agents in the regimen should be used in their optimal dose and schedule.

Table 88-13 lists examples of commonly used combination chemotherapy regimens.

APPLICATIONS

It has been estimated that >500,000 patients are candidates for chemotherapy each year in the United States alone. Although effective chemotherapy regimens are not available for all cancers, many patients with advanced malignancies may benefit from this modality. Chemotherapy has cured a fraction of patients with each of the advanced tumors listed in

Table 88-13 Commonly Used Chemotherapy Regimens[a]

Acronym	Agents	Dose/Schedule	Cycle
Breast Cancer			
CMF	Cyclophosphamide[71]	500 mg/m² IV days 1 and 8	Q 28 days
	Methotrexate	40–60 mg/m² IV days 1 and 8	
	Fluorouracil	600 mg/m² IV days 1 and 8	
	Or		
	Cyclophosphamide[71]	100 mg/m² PO days 1–14	Q 28 days
	Methotrexate	40–60 mg/m² IV days 1 and 8	
	Fluorouracil	600 mg/m² IV days 1 and 8	
Herceptin-tax	Trastuzumab (Herceptin)[72]	4 mg/kg IV week 1, then 2 mg/kg IV Q wk	Q 21 days
	Paclitaxel	175 mg/m² IV over 3 hr day 1	
CAF	Cyclophosphamide[73]	100 mg/m² PO days 1–14	Q 28 days
	Doxorubicin (Adriamycin)	30–50 mg/m² IV days 1 and 8	
	Fluorouracil	500 mg/m² IV days 1 and 8	
	Or		
	Cyclophosphamide[74]	400 mg/m² IV day 1	Q 21 days
	Doxorubicin (Adriamycin)	40 mg/m² IV day 1	
	Fluorouracil	400 mg/m² IV day 1	
	Or		
	Cyclophosphamide[75]	500 mg/m² IV day 1	Q 21 days
	Doxorubicin (Adriamycin)	50 mg/m² IV day 1	
	Fluorouracil	500 mg/m² IV day 1	
AC	Doxorubicin (Adriamycin)[76]	60 mg/m² day 1	Q 21 days
	Cyclophosphamide	600 mg/m² day 1	
Colorectal Cancer			
IFL	Irinotecan[77]	125 mg/m² IV day 1	Q wk for 4 weeks, repeated Q 6 wk
	Fluorouracil	500 mg/m² IVP day 1	
	Leucovorin	20 mg/m² IVP day 1	
FOLFIRI	Irinotecan[78]	180 mg/m² IV day 1	Q 2 wk
	Leucovorin	400 mg/m² IV day 1	
	Fluorouracil	400 mg/m² IVP day 1	
	Fluorouracil	2.4–3 gm/m² 46-hr IV infusion day 1	
FOLFOX4	Oxaliplatin[79]	85 mg/m² IV day 1	Q 2 wk
	Leucovorin	200 mg/m² IV day 1 and 2	
	Fluorouracil	400 mg/m² IVP day 1 and 2	
	Fluorouracil	600 mg/m² 22-hr IV infusion day 1 and 2	

Table 88-13   Commonly Used Chemotherapy Regimens[a]—cont'd

Acronym	Agents	Dose/Schedule	Cycle
Colorectal Cancer—cont'd			
FU/leucovorin	Flourouracil[80]	370 mg/m² /day IVP days 1–5	Q 28 days × 2 then Q 35 days
	Leucovorin	20 mg/m² /days 1–5 immediately followed by FU	
	Or		
	Fluorouracil[81]	600 mg/m² IVP at 1 hr after starting leucovorin infusion	Q wk × 6 wk
	Leucovorin	500 mg/m² IV over 2 hr	
	Or		
	Fluorouracil[82]	435 mg/m² IVP days 1–5	Q 4–5 wk
	Leucovorin	20 mg/m² IVP days 1–5	
Gastric Cancer			
ECP	Epirubicin[83]	50 mg/m² IV day 1	Q 21 day
	Cisplatin	60 mg/m² IV day 1	
	Fluorouracil	200 mg/m² /d continuous IV infusion up to 6 mo	
FAM	Fluorouracil[84]	600 mg/m² IV days 1, 8, 29, and 36	Q 8 wk
	Doxorubicin (Adriamycin)	30 mg/m² IV days 1 and 29	
	Mitomycin	10 mg/m² IV day 1	
EAP	Etoposide[85]	120 mg/m² IV days 4, 5, and 6	Q 21–28 days
	Doxorubicin (Adriamycin)	20 mg/m² IV days 1 and 7	
	Cisplatin	40 mg/m² IV days 2 and 8	
Ovarian Cancer			
CP	Cyclophosphamide[86]	750 mg/m² IV day 1	Q 21 days
	Cisplatin	75 mg/m² IV day 1	
CT	Paclitaxel[86]	135 mg/m² IV over 3 or 24 hr day 1	Q 21 days
	Cisplatin	75 mg/m² IV	
Carbo-tax	Paclitaxel[87]	135 mg/m² IV over 24 hr or 175 mg/m² over 3 hr, day 1	Q 21 days
	Carboplatin	Targeted by Calvert equation to AUC 7.5 IV	
Testicular Cancer			
BEP	Bleomycin[88]	30 units IV weekly for 12 weeks	Q 21 days
	Etoposide	100 mg/m² IV days 1–5 IV	
	Cisplatin	20 mg/m² IV days 1–5	
EP	Etoposide[89]	100 mg/m² IV day 1–5	Q 21 days
	Cisplatin	20 mg/m² IV days 1–5	
Bladder Cancer			
M-VAC	Methotrexate[90]	30 mg/m² IV days 1, 15, and 22	Q 28 days
	Vinblastine	3 mg/m² IV days 2, 15, and 22	
	Adriamycin (Doxorubicin)	30 mg/m² IV day 2	
PC	Paclitaxel[91]	200 mg/m² over 3 hr day 1	Q 21 days
	Carboplatin	Targeted by Calvert equation to AUC 5.0 after paclitaxel day 1	
Small Cell Lung Cancer			
EP or PE	Cisplatin[92]	25 mg/m² /day IV days 1–3	Q 21–28 days
	Etoposide	100 mg/m² /day IV days 1–3 + radiation therapy	
Non–Small Cell Lung Cancer			
EP or PE	Cisplatin[93]	100 mg/m² IV day 1	Q 21 days
	Etoposide	80 mg/m² IV days 1–3	
	Or		
	Cisplatin[94]	60 mg/m² IV day 1	Q 21–28 days
	Etoposide	120 mg/m² IV days 4, 6, and 8	
Carbo-tax	Paclitaxel[95]	225 mg/m² IV over 3 hr, day 1	Q 21 days
	Carboplatin	Targeted by Calvert equation to AUC 6 IV	
EC	Etoposide[96]	100–120 mg/m² IV days 1–3	Q 21–28 days
	Carboplatin	300–325 mg/m² IV day 1	
Gemcitabine-Cis	Gemcitabine[95]	1,000 mg/m² IV days 1, 8, and 15	Q 28 days
	Cisplatin	100 mg/m² IV day 1	
Docetaxel-Cisplatin	Docetaxel[95]	75 mg/m² IV day 1	Q 21 days
	Cisplatin	75 mg/m² IV day 1	

Continued

Table 88-13   Commonly Used Chemotherapy Regimens"—cont'd

Acronym	Agents	Dose/Schedule	Cycle
Head and Neck Cancer			
CF	Cisplatin[97]	100 mg/m² IV day 1	Q 21–28 days
	Fluorouracil	1,000 mg/m²/day CIV days 1–5	
Lymphomas			
Non-Hodgkin's Lymphomas			
CHOP	Cyclophosphamide[98]	750 mg/m² IV day 1	Q 21 days
	Doxorubicin (Hydroxyl Daunorubicin)	50 mg/m² IV day 1	
	Vincristine (Oncovin)	1.4 mg/m² IV day/(max 2 mg)	
	Prednisone	100 mg/m²/day PO days 1–5	
CHOP-Rituximab	Cyclophosphamide[99]	750 mg/m² IV day 1	Q 21 days
	Doxorubicin	50 mg/m² IV day 1	
	Vincristine	1.4 mg/m² IV day 1 (max 2 mg)	
	Prednisone	40 mg/m² PO days 1–5	
	Rituximab	375 mg/m² IV day 1	
MACOP-B	Methotrexate[100]	400 mg/m² IV weeks 2, 6, and 10	Only 1 cycle
	Leucovorin	15 mg PO every 6 hours for 6 doses starting 24 hr after methotrexate	
	Doxorubicin (Adriamycin)	50 mg/m² IV weeks 1, 3, 5, 7, 9, and 11	
	Cyclophosphamide	350 mg/m² IV weeks 1, 3, 5, 7, 9, and 11	
	Vincristine (Oncovin)	1.4 mg/m² IV weeks 2, 4, 6, 8, 10, and 12	
	Prednisone	75 mg PO daily, tapered over last 15 days	
	Bleomycin	10 units/m² IV weeks 4, 8, and 12	
ESHAP	Etoposide[101]	40 mg/m² IV days 1–4	Q 21–28 days
	Methylprednisolone	500 mg IV days 1–5	
	Cisplatin	25 mg/m²/day CIV days 1–4	
	Cytarabine	2,000 mg/m² IV day 5 immediately following completion of etoposide and cisplatin	
Hodgkin's Disease			
MOPP	Mechlorethamine[102]	6 mg/m² IV days 1 and 8	Q 28 days
	Vincristine (Oncovin)	1.4 mg/m² days 1 and 8	
	Prednisone	40 mg/m² PO days 1–14, cycles 1 and 4	
	Procarbazine	100 mg/m² PO days 1–14	
ABVD	Doxorubicin (Adriamycin)[103]	25 mg/m² IV days 1 and 15	Q 28 days
	Bleomycin	10 mg/m² IV days 1 and 15	
	Vinblastine	6 mg/m² IV days 1 and 15	
	Dacarbazine	375 mg/m² IV days 1 and 15	
Multiple Myeloma			
VAD	Vincristine[104]	0.4 mg/m²/day CIV days 1–4	Q 28 days
	Doxorubicin (Adriamycin)	9 mg/m²/day CIV days 1–4	
	Dexamethasone	40 mg/m² PO days 1–4, 9–12, and 17–20	
MP	Melphalan[105]	0.25 mg/kg/day PO days 1–4	Q 42 days
	Prednisone	2 mg/kg/day PO days 1–4	

"Original citations should be consulted for dosage adjustments due to toxicity or underlying organ dysfunction.
CIV, continuous intravenous infusion; IV, intravenous; IVP, intravenous push; PO, by mouth.

Table 88-14. Chemotherapy may also prolong survival or provide symptomatic relief for many additional patients who cannot be cured.

Primary Chemotherapy

Chemotherapy is the primary treatment modality used for hematologic malignancies, as well as a number of solid tumors that have metastasized at the time of diagnosis or have recurred at metastatic sites after initial therapy. Chemotherapy is frequently used in different ways during the course of an individual's malignancy (Fig. 88-6). Primary chemotherapy can be either curative or palliative, depending on the specific type of tumor. The term "induction chemotherapy" is used to describe chemotherapy that is used as a first step toward shrinking the cancer and in evaluating the cancer's response to treatment. These patients may receive additional chemotherapy in an attempt to successfully eradicate the tumor. Additional chemotherapy is often referred to as secondary chemotherapy, second-line chemotherapy, or salvage chemotherapy. Induction chemotherapy can also refer to the initial treatment of patients who present with hematologic malignancies (e.g., acute leukemia). After successful induction chemotherapy, patients usually receive postremission therapy to improve their chances of long-term survival. Postremission therapy can in-

Table 88-14 Tumors That Respond to Chemotherapy

Advanced Tumors That Can Be Cured with Chemotherapy

Choriocarcinoma	Wilms' tumor
Acute lymphocytic leukemia	Embryonal rhabdomyosarcoma
Testicular cancer	Peripheral neuroepithelioma
Acute myelogenous leukemia	Neuroblastoma
Hodgkin's disease	Small cell lung cancer (limited
Non-Hodgkin's lymphoma	stage)
(especially high-grade	Hairy cell leukemia
lymphomas)	

Chemotherapy as Adjuvant Therapy With Curative Intent

Breast cancer (stages I–III)	Ewing's sarcoma
Colorectal cancer	Wilms' tumor
(stages II and III)	Osteosarcoma
	Ovarian cancer

Chemotherapy as Neoadjuvant Therapy With Potential Curative Intent

Soft tissue sarcoma	Head and neck cancer
Anal cancer	Non–small cell lung cancer
Breast cancer (locally advanced)	(stage III$_A$)
Esophageal cancer	Osteosarcoma
Cervical cancer	Bladder cancer

Advanced Tumors in Which Chemotherapy May Prolong Survival or Palliate Symptoms

Bladder cancer	Endometrial cancer
Chronic myelogenous leukemia	Adrenocortical carcinoma
Multiple myeloma	Medulloblastoma
Gastric carcinoma	Prostate cancer
Cervical carcinoma	Insulinoma
Soft tissue sarcoma	Breast cancer
Head and neck cancer	Colorectal cancer
Osteogenic sarcoma	Non–small cell cancer
Pancreatic cancer	Melanoma

clude consolidation, intensification, and maintenance treatment phases.

Adjuvant Chemotherapy

10. **F.R., a 36-year-old woman with no other medical problems, recently underwent a lumpectomy and radiation therapy for breast cancer. She has been told that the cancer is all gone; however, she also is told that she should now receive 6 months of chemotherapy. She knows that chemotherapy will cause her to vomit, lose her hair, gain weight, and place her at risk for life-threatening infections. Why would chemotherapy be recommended now when she is disease free?**

Some patients may have unrecognized micrometastases or residual disease after primary treatment. These patients have a high probability of disease recurrence, even though the primary treatment may have successfully removed all visual evidence of the primary tumor. To eradicate any undetectable tumor, the patient could receive systemic therapy after initial curative surgery (or radiation therapy). Systemic chemotherapy administered after primary therapy is referred to as *adjuvant chemotherapy*. Because the tumor burden is relatively low at this time, chemotherapy should immediately follow primary therapy. For adjuvant therapy to provide any benefit, the risk of recurrence must be high, and effective agents must be available to eradicate the tumor. Adjuvant therapy is considered standard treatment in management of breast and colorectal cancer, but it also has benefited selected patients with ovarian cancer, Ewing's sarcoma, Wilms' tumor, and other malignancies.[55] (Also see Chapter 91, Solid Tumors.) Because it is impossible to predict which patients have unrecognized disease, it is difficult to determine which patients should receive adjuvant therapy. To help with these decisions, clinicians frequently consider histologic and cytogenetic characteristics of the primary tumor that are associated with high risk of relapse. Unfortunately, some patients who may never relapse will undergo adjuvant chemotherapy.

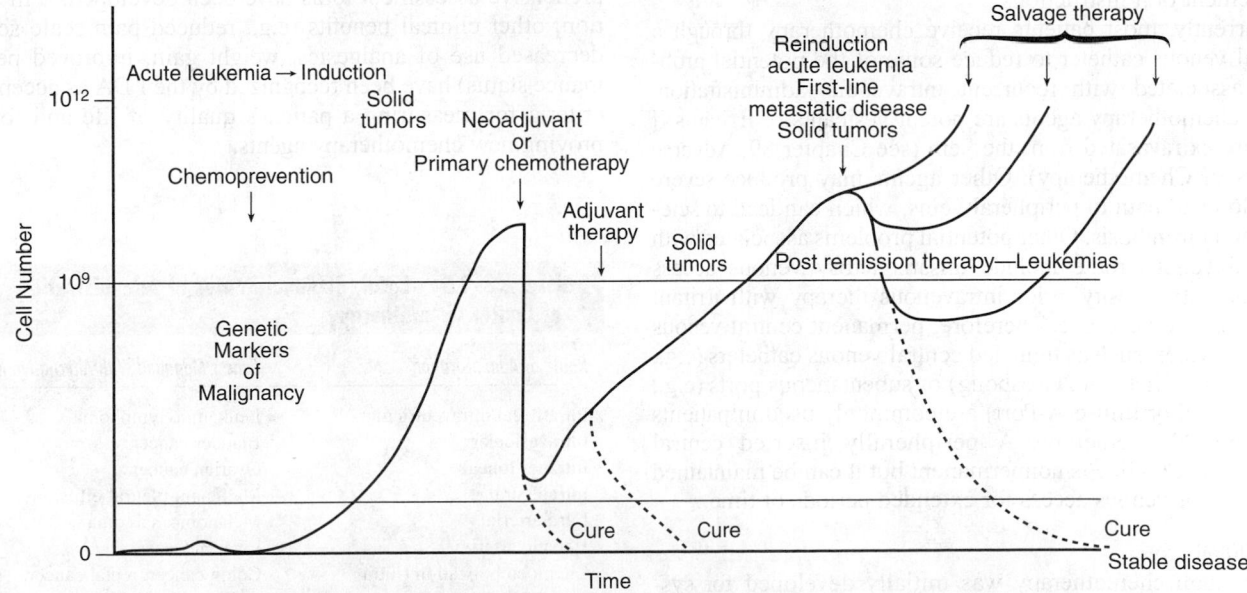

FIGURE 88-6 Chemotherapy during various phases of malignancy. Cell kill hypothesis.

Neoadjuvant Chemotherapy

Neoadjuvant chemotherapy has been used to describe the initial treatment for patients who present with locally advanced tumors (e.g., large tumors or those that are impinging on surrounding vital structures) that are unlikely to be cured with primary surgery or radiation therapy. The objective is to reduce the tumor mass with chemotherapy or hormonal therapy and to increase the likelihood of eradication by subsequent surgery or radiation therapy. Neoadjuvant therapy also can lessen the amount of radical surgery or radiation therapy that the patient needs, which can preserve cosmetic appearances and function of the surrounding normal tissues. Unfortunately, the tumor can be resistant to the primary chemotherapy and continue to grow, making surgery even more difficult. Patients may also experience toxicities that delay surgery or impair postsurgical healing. Locally advanced tumors in which neoadjuvant chemotherapy has been shown to improve survival rates include stage III_A non–small cell lung cancer, stage III breast cancer, sarcomas, esophageal cancers, laryngeal cancer, bladder cancer, and osteogenic sarcoma.[55]

Administration
SYSTEMIC

Systemic chemotherapy is most commonly administered by the intravenous route, either as an intravenous bolus injection (generally <15 minutes), a short infusion (15 minutes to several hours), or a continuous infusion (lasting 24 hours to several weeks). Some systemic chemotherapy agents can be administered by the oral route, whereas other agents can be administered by the intramuscular or subcutaneous route. No matter which route of administration is selected for therapy, the individual administering the chemotherapy should be able to proficiently administer the agent by the chosen route and be aware of the most common acute and chronic toxicities associated with the chemotherapy. All aspects of drug administration should be discussed with the patient before starting chemotherapy, including any adverse events they may experience during or after the injection and throughout therapy. Printed patient educational materials are recommended to supplement oral instructions.

Currently, most patients receive chemotherapy through a central venous catheter to reduce some of the potential problems associated with recurrent intravenous administration. Some chemotherapy agents are potent vesicants or irritants if they are extravasated from the vein (see Chapter 89, Adverse Effects of Chemotherapy). Other agents may produce severe irritation and pain to peripheral veins, which can lead to sclerosis and thrombosis. Other potential problems associated with the intravenous route include unsatisfactory venous access secondary to obesity, prior intravenous therapy with irritant drugs, or advanced age. Therefore, permanent central venous access devices, such as tunneled central venous catheters (e.g., the Broviac, Hickman, Groshong) or subcutaneous ports (e.g., Port-A-Cath or Infuse-A-Port) are commonly used in patients receiving chemotherapy. A peripherally inserted central catheter (PICC) line is nonpermanent but it can be maintained and used for venous access for extended periods of time.

REGIONAL

Although chemotherapy was initially developed for systemic use, techniques have been developed to locally administer agents to specific sites of the body affected by the tumor. Tumors commonly managed by localized administration techniques are listed in Table 88-15. Regional or local chemotherapy allows high concentrations of agents to be achieved at the site of the tumor while reducing systemic exposure and subsequent toxicity. On the other hand, undetectable metastases at distant sites may not be exposed to the chemotherapy, allowing continued growth of the tumor mass.

Assessing Response to Therapy

A very important step in the process of treating a patient with chemotherapy is to assess his or her response to treatment. The assessment should evaluate the chemotherapy's antitumor and toxic effects, as well as its effect on the patient's overall quality of life and survival. Re-evaluation should occur at regularly scheduled intervals during treatment and should include a physical examination, laboratory tests, and repeat diagnostic tests (radiologic or other tests such as bone marrow biopsy, bronchoscopy) used to stage the patient. Usually, only tests that previously were positive for the tumor are repeated unless new signs or symptoms suggest additional metastases.

Several standard criteria are used to define the patient's response to treatment (Table 88-16). The use of standardized criteria in clinical trials evaluating new therapies is especially important because it helps define the potential use of new therapies compared with standard treatments. Criteria used to assess the antitumor effects include direct measures of the tumor size, duration of response, and patient survival.[106] Parameters used to assess the toxic effects include the incidence and severity of specific toxicities. Standardized toxicity grading scales used to assess toxicity associated with a chemotherapy agent include scales provided by the World Health Organization, the NCI, and the ECOG.[107,108]

Because the toxicities associated with many chemotherapy agents are potentially severe, it is important to evaluate the risk of the treatment in relation to the potential benefit. The benefits of a treatment regimen should outweigh the negative effects it has on the physical, mental, and social well-being of the patient. To monitor a patient's quality of life, several comprehensive assessment tools have been developed.[109] In addition, other clinical benefits (e.g., reduced pain scale scores, decreased use of analgesics, weight gain, improved performance status) have been recognized by the FDA as acceptable criteria for measuring a patient's quality of life and for approving new chemotherapy agents.

Table 88-15   Local/Regional Routes of Administration of Cancer Chemotherapy

Route of Administration	Cancer Managed With Alternative Route
Intrathecal/intraventricular	Leukemia, lymphoma
Intravesicular	Bladder cancer
Intraperitoneal	Ovarian cancer
Intrapleural	Malignant pleural effusions
Intra-arterial	Melanoma, sarcoma
Hepatic artery	Liver metastases
Chemoembolization (intra-arterial or intravenous)	Colon cancer, rectal cancer, carcinoid, liver metastases

Table 88-16 Response Criteria for Evaluating Effects of Chemotherapy

Complete Response

Disappearance of all clinical evidence of active disease for at least 4 weeks. No new lesions may appear during this period.

Partial Response

>50% reduction in sum of products of two perpendicular diameters of all measured tumors for at least 4 weeks. No tumor or metastasis may show progression and no new lesions may appear.

Stable Disease

<50% reduction or 25% ↓ in the sum of the product of two perpendicular diameters of all measured lesions; no appearance of new lesions; and no deterioration of the performance status for a minimum of 4 weeks.

Disease Progression

Reappearance of a lesion after complete response, appearance of any new lesions or an ↑ of ≥25% in the product of the two perpendicular diameters of any measurable lesion.

Disease-Free Survival

Time from documentation of complete response until disease relapse or death.

Overall Survival

Time from treatment until time of death.

Table 88-17 Clinically Useful Tumor Markers

Tumor Marker	Cancers Commonly Associated With Increased Markers
CA-19-9	Pancreatic
CA-15-3	Breast
CA-27-29	Breast
Neuron-specific enolase	Neuroblastoma, small cell lung cancer
α-Fetoprotein	Liver
CA-125	Ovarian, testicular—nonseminoma
Carcinoembryonic antigen	Colon, lung
Human chorionic gonadotropin	Trophoblastic, testicular
β_2-Microglobulin	Multiple myeloma
Prostate-specific antigen	Prostate

firmatory tests and as part of follow-up care to detect recurrent disease. In most cases, tumor markers lack specificity for the tumor, and they could be elevated with other disease states. Patients who have elevated levels of a tumor marker at initial diagnosis should have elevated levels with disease recurrence. Other techniques used to detect very low levels of recurrent cancer in leukemias and lymphomas (e.g., minimal residual disease) include real-time quantitative PCR (RT-PCR) analysis of immunoglobin or gene arrangements or chromosome aberrations in cells.[111] By detecting cancer recurrence at its earliest state, treatments may be more successful.

12. Describe other agents used to treat cancer beyond those that are considered cell-cycle specific or non-cell cycle specific.

Endocrine Therapy

Endocrine therapy can be used to treat several common cancers, including breast, prostate, and endometrial cancers, which arise from hormone-sensitive tissues (Table 88-18). These tumors grow in response to endogenous hormones that trigger growth signals by binding to specific receptors located on a cell membrane or within the cytoplasm of a cell. Current endocrine therapies inhibit tumor growth by blocking the receptors or by eliminating the endogenous hormone feeding the tumor. (Note: Interruption of hormonal secretion also can be achieved through surgical removal of hormonal producing organs.) Unfortunately, not all tumors arising from hormone-sensitive tissues respond to endocrine manipulation. Lack of response could be associated with hormone-resistant tumor cells or inadequate suppression of the endogenous feeding hormones.[112]

Signal Transduction Pathway Inhibitors

By understanding the mechanisms by which cancer cells exhibit unregulated growth, immortality, and possess the ability to invade tissues and metastasize[1], it has been possible to design drugs that inhibit these processes. The EGFR, HER2/neu, and VEGF signaling pathways can be blocked by monoclonal antibodies that inhibit receptor tyrosine kinase activation by binding to the extraceullar domain. Small molecules that directly inhibit tyrosine kinase activation by competing with ATP for binding to the intracellular tyrosine kinase domain have been developed, as well.[7] A potential advantage of targeting the tyrosine kinase activity of the

11. G.K. is a 67 year-old woman who was recently diagnosed with metastatic bladder cancer. Her symptoms include widespread pain, anorexia, and fatigue. She began receiving a combination chemotherapy regimen and has received three cycles of treatment. A recent CT scan of her abdomen showed marked shrinkage at several sites of tumor and her pain has decreased. How long should she continue to receive chemotherapy?

Since G.K.'s tumor is responding well to treatment, she should continue to receive therapy as long as her tumor is responding and she does not experience intolerable or life-threatening treatment-related toxicities. For some cancers (e.g., non–small cell lung cancer), continued administration of chemotherapy after a certain number of treatment cycles is not associated with further benefit to patients; however, chemotherapy is continued in most situations until the cancer stops responding.

TUMOR MARKERS

Tumor markers are biochemical indicators commonly found in abnormally high concentrations with a cancer. The ideal tumor marker should be produced and released primarily by the cancer cells (or by other tissues in response to the tumor) at levels proportional to the tumor mass. Surgical removal of the tumor or a therapeutic response to chemotherapy or radiation therapy should cause the level of the marker to decline. In addition, the ideal tumor marker should be detectable at very low levels, so tumors may be detected at sizes smaller than conventional diagnostic tests such as radiographs or CT scans permit.[110] Few tumor markers fulfill these criteria sufficiently to be clinically useful as the sole screening or diagnostic test (Table 88-17). These markers are primarily used as con-

Table 88-18 Endocrine Therapy Used for Hormone-Sensitive Tumors

Class	Drug	Dosage	Side Effects	Indication
Antiestrogens	Tamoxifen	10–20 mg PO BID 60 mg PO daily	Disease flare, hot flashes, nausea, vomiting, edema, thromboembolism, endometrial cancer	Breast
	Toremifene			
	Fulvestrant	250 mg IM Q mo		
Aromatase inhibitors	Anastrazole	1 mg PO daily	Hot flashes, nausea, fatigue, insomnia, increased risk of bone fractures	Breast
	Letrozole	2.5 mg PO daily		
	Exemestane	25 mg PO daily		
	Aminoglutethimide	250 mg PO 4 times daily with hydrocortisone 40 mg PO daily	Lethargy, rash, postural dizziness, ataxia, nystagmus, nausea	Breast, prostate
LHRH analogs[a]	Leuprolide	7.5 mg SQ Q 28 days	Amenorrhea, hot flashes, nausea	Breast, prostate
	Goserelin	3.6 mg SC Q 28 days		
	Triptorelin	3.75 mg IM Q 28 days		
Antiandrogens	Flutamide	250 mg PO TID	Gynecomastia, hot flashes, breast tenderness, hepatic dysfunction, diarrhea	Prostate
	Bicalutamide	50 mg PO daily		
	Nilutamide	300 mg PO daily for 30 days, then 150 mg PO daily		
Progestins	Medroxyprogesterone acetate	400–1,000 mg IM Q wk	Weight gain, hot flashes, vaginal bleeding, edema, thromboembolism	Breast, prostate
	Megestrol acetate	10–40 mg PO 4 times daily		Anorexia
Estrogens	Ethynylestrradiol	1 mg PO TID	Nausea/vomiting, fluid retention, hot flashes, anorexia, thromboembolism, hepatic dysfunction	Breast
	Conjugated estrogens	2.5 mg PO TID		
Androgens	Fluoxymestrone	10 mg PO BID	Deepening voice, alopecia, hirsutism, facial/truncal acne, fluid retention, menstrual irregularities, cholestatic jaundice	Breast

[a]Leuprolide and triptorelin also available in extended release/depot formulations.

receptor should be the ability to inhibit cells that do not overexpress the receptor on their surface or have mutated forms of the receptor that results in its activation. The first commercially available receptor tyrosine kinase inhibitor was imatinib mesylate, also known as STI-571. Imatinib mesylate specifically inhibits the Abl and c-KIT kinases, and platelet-derived growth factor receptors α and β.[113] This agent is active against chronic myelogenous leukemia, gastrointestinal stromal tumors, and is under investigation for other malignancies that are dependent on the activity of the Bcr-Abl or c-KIT tyrosine kinases.

Inhibition of the 26S proteosome, which is responsible for the intracellular degradation of ubiquinated proteins, can induce apoptosis in a wide variety of cancer cell lines.[114] VEGF, bFGF, MMPs, and receptor tyrosine kinases that are activated in endothelial cells subsequent to endothelial cell activation are also targets for antiangiogenic agents. Unlike most cytotoxic chemotherapeutic agents, bone marrow suppression is not a frequent dose-limiting side effect of signal transduction pathway inhibitors. Because of their mechanism of action, their effects are exerted primarily through inhibition of cell growth rather than through direct cytotoxicity. However, occasionally significant tumor regression is observed. Based on current knowledge, treatment regimens that incorporate use of these agents and cytotoxic drugs are most likely to have the greatest impact on patient outcomes in cancer treatments. Recent treatment advances in these targeted approaches are summarized in Table 88-19.

Biologic Response Modifiers

Biologic response modifiers used to treat cancers include the administration of organic substances such as proteins, antibodies, cells, and genes. Therapy with these agents can be used to kill cancer cells or to bolster the host's defense mechanisms. An individual's immune system plays a crucial role in determining the risk of developing cancer. Normally, an intact immune system can protect the host against malignant cells and infectious pathogens, but current evidence shows that individuals with "weakened" immune systems face an increased risk of developing cancer. For example, individuals with AIDS face an increased risk of developing lymphomas compared with the normal population. Other individuals with weakened immune systems, including neonates and the elderly, also face an increased risk of developing cancer. Bolstering an individual's immune system could help prevent or treat a malignancy. Some evidence shows that malignancies can undergo spontaneous regression, especially during periods of immune activation (i.e., an acute bacterial infection).[119] Current biologic response modifiers aim to bolster an individual's immune response, as well as provide a direct cytotoxic effect.

Gene Therapy

Gene therapy represents a potential treatment modality in which a functioning gene is inserted into a cell to correct a metabolic abnormality or to introduce a new function. In cancer, the goal of gene therapy is to inactivate an oncogene or to replace a missing or mutant tumor-suppressor gene. The major difficulty with gene therapy lies with the selective insertion into tumor cells located in the human body. Currently, gene therapy involves the transfer of a gene into cells outside of the body (ex vivo) with subsequent reinfusion of the infected cells into the body. The reinfused cells can then perform functions such as stimulating the immune response, increasing tumor recognition, or increasing the survival of immune cells.

Table 88-19   Molecular Approaches in Cancer Therapy[117,126]

Cancer Feature	Molecular Targets	Therapeutics
Oncogene activation leading to self-sufficient growth signaling through excessive Ras protein or kinase activity	Abl, EGF receptor, Erb-B2, and Src kinases	Anti-EGF antibodies;[7] growth factor receptor tyrosine kinase inhibitors[7]
	Ras proteins	Farnesyl transferase inhibitors;[100] antisense oligonucleotides[120]
	PKC-α, Raf, and cyclin-dependent kinases	Ras/Raf signaling inhibitors;[101] mTOR inhibitors[122], cyclin-dependent kinase modulators[121]; antisense oligonucleotides[120]
Resistance to apoptosis; loss of tumor suppressor genes or function	APC, AT, DCC, RB, and p53 genes; Bcl-2; death receptor ligands (TNFα, Fas ligand, TNF-related apoptosis-inducing ligand [TRAIL]); nuclear factor (NF)-κB	Gene therapy to restore normal suppressor gene function; antisense oligonucleotides[120]; proteosome inhibitors[118]; NF-κB inhibitors;[114] TRAIL receptor agonists
Lack of senescence (cell aging) in tumor cells	Telomerase	Telomerase inhibitors[44]
Angiogenesis	Endothelial cell growth factors (VEGF, bFGF, PDGF, EGF)	Anti-VEGF/VEGFR antibodies[123]; VEGF receptor tyrosine kinase inhibitors[124,125]
	Newly formed vasculature (neovasculature) of actively growing tumors	Flavone acetic acid derivatives,[125] tubulin-binding agents[124,125]
	Endothelial cell integrin receptors	$\alpha_v\beta_3$, $\alpha_v\beta_5$ antagonists[124,125]
Metastases	Metalloproteases	Protease inhibitors[115,124,125]

Another gene-based therapy involves the use of antisense antinucleotides, which are short pieces of single-stranded DNA or RNA that are designed to interact with complementary mRNA and block the synthesis of the corresponding protein.[120] Thus, the action of a specific gene can be inhibited. Clinical availability of these applications is likely in the future.

Research for biologic response modifiers that target molecular changes associated with carcinogenesis is proceeding at a rapid rate. Commercially available biologic response modifiers used for treatment include interleukins, interferons, and monoclonal antibodies. Considerable progress has been made in identifying clinically useful monoclonal antibodies against cancer. Advances are being made in vaccine therapy, as well.

Interferon-Alfa

The first recombinant cytokine to become available for the treatment of cancer was interferon-alfa. This interferon affects tumor cells through several different mechanisms, including (1) a direct antiproliferative effect; (2) an immunomodulatory effect on natural killer cells, T cells, B cells, and macrophages; (3) an induction of tumor cell antigens; and (4) a differentiating effect on tumor cells. Interferons also possess antiangiogeneic effects.[45] Current studies show that interferon-alfa has antitumor effects against several human malignancies.[127] Interferon-alfa is sometimes given in combination with radiation therapy, other biologic response modifiers, or chemotherapy agents.

Interleukin-2

Interleukin (IL)-2 is a recombinantly produced lymphokine that has numerous immunoregulatory functions. In normal cells, IL-2 stimulates both T-and B-cell proliferation and differentiation.[128] The idea to use IL-2 to treat cancer arose from the observation that lymphoid cells incubated with IL-2 developed the capacity to lyse tumor cells (lymphokine-activated killer [LAK] cells).[129,130] This observation led to the development of some adoptive immunotherapies. Initial studies showed that patients with advanced tumors, such as renal cell carcinoma and melanoma, experienced tumor regression after receiving IL-2. Subsequent studies using high dosages of IL-2 also reported responses in similar patient populations with advanced disease.[130-132] High-dose IL-2 therapy is accompanied by significant, dose-related toxicity. The most serious toxicities (hypotension, pulmonary edema, oliguria, increased bilirubin) occur secondary to a diffuse capillary leak that develops during IL-2 therapy. These signs usually resolve promptly after discontinuing therapy.

HANDLING OF CYTOTOXIC DRUGS
Impact on the Pharmacy

13. The administrator of a health plan recently has announced that two medical oncologists will be joining the professional staff. In the past, patients were referred to outside oncologists, and no cytotoxic drugs were prepared or administered at the clinics. What implications will the addition of these physicians have on the pharmacy department?

The new oncologists will affect three areas of the pharmacy department: the budget, the policies and procedures for safe drug handling, and the staff education program. The pharmacy department will need to increase their budget to accommodate the additional personnel and to purchase new equipment, supplies, supportive care medicines, and chemotherapy agents. To estimate the projected increase in the budget, a pharmacist should meet with the oncologists to discuss the anticipated volume of chemotherapy orders, the chemotherapy agents they are likely to prescribe, and supportive care medicines they plan to use. All new chemotherapy agents and supportive care medicines (e.g., antiemetic therapy, analgesics) should be added to the health plan formulary. In addition, the pharmacist should determine the projected use of investigational agents, clinical pharmacy services that will be needed, and any plans to develop an ambulatory infusion program. The department must create new policies and procedures to ensure safe handling of chemotherapy agents by all personnel. These should be conveyed to all personnel through a new staff education program, because safe handling of chemotherapy agents can significantly decrease the risk of medication errors and injuries.

Medication Errors

In recent years, several unfortunate chemotherapy-related medication errors that resulted in death or permanent disability have been highly publicized. These devastating events have brought significant attention to the entire drug use process in oncology and have identified several factors that appear to contribute to the risk (Table 88-20). In particular, the use of abbreviations, verbal orders, multiple-day regimens, poor-quality carbon orders, poor facsimile medication orders, and incorrect references have contributed to a number of reported medication errors. Several groups have responded to the problem by issuing policy recommendations to minimize such errors.[133–136]

Risks

14. What are the potential risks of handling cytotoxic drugs, and what resources are available to assist the director and the pharmacy staff in the development of policies and procedures?

For almost two decades, the potential hazards of chemotherapy agents have received considerable attention. Many of these agents are carcinogenic, teratogenic, or mutagenic in animal models and in humans at therapeutic doses.[137–140] The danger to health care personnel handling such agents results from both the inherent toxicities of the

agents and the extent to which the workers are exposed during drug handling.[141] Various studies have attempted to assess the effect of occupational exposure to hazardous drugs by health care workers. These studies included measurements of urine mutagenicity, chromosomal damage, drug absorption, and, most recently, the level of contamination that occurs in the work areas used for drug preparation and administration.[141–151] Although somewhat controversial, the documentation of urine mutagenicity or chromosomal damage was thought to be a direct result of cytotoxic exposure. Other reports correlate reproductive and birth defect risks in pregnant workers handling cytotoxic drugs.[150,152] Results of these reports together with the toxicities observed in patients receiving therapeutic doses led the American Society of Hospital Pharmacists to conclude that "health care workers exposed to hazardous drugs during their work may be absorbing these drugs and may be at risk for adverse outcomes."[141]

In response to the concerns regarding occupational exposure to hazardous drugs, several groups have published guidelines for the safe handling of these agents in the workplace (i.e., storage, preparation, administration, and disposal).[141,153,154] These documents can be helpful to the pharmacy department when developing policies and procedures.

Policies and Procedures

15. What specific policies and procedures are necessary, and what other departments should be consulted during the development and implementation of the handling guidelines?

Policies must be developed that address the entire scope of potential occupational exposures within the workplace. These policies should include (1) a worker's "right to know" of po-

Table 88-20 Factors That May Increase the Risk of Medication Errors Involving Chemotherapy

Contributing Factor	Recommendation
Verbal orders	Do not accept; accept only written signed orders. If not possible have two health professionals accept verbal orders, have written policy regarding verbal orders.
Multiple-day drug courses (e.g., etoposide 50 mg/m² × 5)	Use standardized order forms or format. Order should clearly state total dose to be administered each day and actual dates of administration (e.g., etoposide 50 mg/m²/ day = 100 mg per day on 3/1, 3/2, 3/3, 3/4, and 3/5/00). Orders should also explicitly state infusion guidelines, other specific instructions (e.g., administer 30 min after antiemetic) and other pertinent patient information such as body surface area, weight, height, and age.
Trailing zeros following decimal points (example, 50.0 mg) or the decimal point may be lost or overlooked on carbon or fax copies	Do not permit trailing zeros. Leading zeros before decimal points should be required (example, 0.5 mg) so that the decimal point will not be overlooked.
Orders written by prescribers unfamiliar with chemotherapy	Require orders to be written by appropriately credentialed practitioners.
Use of abbreviations	Only approved generic names should be used when ordering chemotherapy or documenting regimens in patient records
Wide variability in chemotherapy doses that may be appropriate for different disease states or combinations	Educate all practitioners involved in the chemotherapy use process (physicians, nurses, pharmacists) regarding commonly used regimens and make printed or electronic resources to verify doses and regimens readily available. Institutional dosing guidelines are recommended.
Inappropriate interpretation of orders	Two pharmacists should verify orders at the point of entry and nurses should reverify before administration. All practitioners should be instructed to resolve all questions before dispensing or administration.
Labeling errors	Labels should be double-checked and include all pertinent information including route of administration. Syringe labels should be directly attached to the syringe.
Poor communication or confusion regarding chemotherapy	Written institutional policies and procedures should address every aspect of the chemotherapy use process, including ordering, preparing, dispensing, administration, and documentation.

tential hazards; (2) an education and training program for workers involved with hazardous drug handling; (3) a quality assurance program to monitor adherence to safe handling procedures; and (4) guidelines for workers attempting to conceive a child, who become pregnant, or who are nursing.

Specific procedures that outline the appropriate handling of hazardous agents during all aspects of institutional storage, use, and disposal should be developed. These procedures should include guidelines that outline the appropriate (1) storage in the receiving and storeroom areas, (2) preparation and administration of parenteral formulations, (3) manipulation and dispensing of oral and topical formulations, (4) clean-up of spills, (5) management of acute exposures, and (6) disposal of hazardous agents and supplies used to prepare and dispense chemotherapy. If the oncology program includes ambulatory infusion or home care components, procedures should also be developed for the appropriate handling and disposal of these products in the home.

Other departments that may be affected by these guidelines include the medical staff, nursing, housekeeping (in the clean up of spills and equipment), maintenance (upkeep of equipment), and the receiving area (where cytotoxic drugs may be received from suppliers). The institutional safety office and legal staff also should be consulted to help devise the policies and procedures.

Necessary Equipment and Supplies

16. **What equipment and supplies are necessary for handling hazardous drugs?**

Various equipment and supplies can minimize occupational exposure in the health care workplace by protecting both the worker and the environment. All handling guidelines recommend that manipulations (e.g., reconstitution, admixing) of hazardous drugs be done in a class II biologic safety cabinet (BSC) to provide maximum protection for the worker and the work environment. However, reports of measurable levels of chemotherapy agents found in work areas despite the use of BSCs has renewed concerns regarding worker safety.[154] It is not clear how the work areas became contaminated, although the very low vapor pressure of cyclophosphamide at room temperature may result in the release of particles too small to be retained by the high-efficiency particulate air filters within the BSC. Additional research will be required to assess whether other chemotherapy agents vaporize under similar circumstances and subsequently expose individuals in the work area. Workers also should wear gloves (one or two pairs) and a disposable, closed-front gown of lint-free, low-permeability fabric with a solid front, long sleeves, and knit cuffs. In addition, only syringes and intravenous sets with Luer-Lok fittings should be used. Final products (e.g., syringes, intravenous bags or bottles) should be placed in sealable containers such as zipper-closure plastic bags and clearly labeled as a hazardous drug. Other supplies that may be necessary for the sterile product preparation area include plastic-back paper liners for the bottom surface of the BSC and 0.2-mm hydrophobic filters.

The disposal of hazardous waste also requires specific receptacles, which should be placed in all areas where workers handle these drugs. Disposal of these agents should follow institutional and/or state and local regulations. Materials for the clean up of spills (e.g., absorbent material, plastic bags or containers, protective garments) also must be kept in all areas where hazardous drugs are stored, prepared, or administered.

REFERENCES

1. Hanahan D, Weinberg RA. The hallmarks of cancer. Cell 2000;100:57.
2. National Cancer Society Surveillance, Epidemiology, and End Results (SEER) Home Page. URL: http://seer.cancer.gov. [Accessed 2003 Mar 16].
3. American Cancer Society. Cancer Facts & Figures 2003. Atlanta, GA: American Cancer Society, 2003.
4. Ries LAG et al, eds. SEER Cancer Statistics Review, 1975-2000. National Cancer Institute. Bethesda, MD: National Cancer Institute, 2003. URL: http://seer.cancer.gov/csr/1975_2000. [Accessed 2003 Jul 9].
5. Tucker MA. Epidemiology of cancer: epidemiologic methods. In: DeVita VT et al, eds. Cancer: Principles and Practice of Oncology, 6th Ed. Philadelphia: Lippincott Williams & Wilkins, 2001:219.
6. Calle EE et al. Overweight, obesity, and mortality from cancer in a prospectively studied cohort of U.S. adults. N Engl J Med 2003;348:1625.
7. Mendelsohn J, Baselga J. Status of epidermal growth factor receptor antagonists in the biology and treatment of cancer. J Clin Oncol 2003;21:2787.
8. Ross JS et al. The Her-2/neu gene and protein in breast cancer 2003: biomarker and target of therapy. Oncologist 2003;8:307.
9. Olayioye MA. Update on HER-2 as a target for cancer therapy: intracellular signaling pathways of ErbB2/HER-2 and family members. Breast Cancer Res 2001;3:385.
10. Stern DF et al. p185, a product of the *neu* protooncogene, is a receptorlike protein associated with tyrosine kinase activity. Mol Cell Biol 1986;6:1729.
11. Weinberg R. How cancer arises. an explosion of research is uncovering the long-hidden molecular underpinnings of cancer-and suggesting new therapies. Sci Am 1996;9:62.
12. Sabichi AL et al. Frontiers in cancer prevention research. Cancer Res 2003;63:5649.
13. Hong WK et al. Cancer chemoprevention in the 21st century: genetics, risk modeling, and molecular targets. J Clin Oncol 2000;18:9S.
14. Hong WK, Sporn MB. Recent advances in chemoprevention of cancer. Science 1997;278:1073.
15. Steele VE. Current mechanistic approaches to the chemoprevention of cancer. J Biochem Mol Biol 2003;36:78.
16. Lippman SM, Hong WK. Cancer prevention science and practice. Cancer Res 2002;62:5119.
17. Omenn GS et al. Effects of a combination of beta carotene and vitamin A on lung cancer and cardiovascular disease. N Engl J Med 1996;334:1150.
18. The α-tocopherol, β-carotene cancer prevention study group. The effect of vitamin E and β-carotene on the incidence of lung cancer and other cancers in male smokers. N Engl J Med 1994;330:1029.
19. Albanes D et al. Alpha-tocopherol and beta-carotene supplements and lung cancer incidence in the alpha-tocopherol, beta-carotene cancer prevention study: effects of base-line characteristics and study compliance. J Natl Cancer Inst 1996;88:1560.
20. Omenn GS et al. Risk factors for lung cancer and for intervention effect in CARET, the beta-carotene and retinol efficacy trial. J Natl Cancer Inst 1996;88:1550.
21. Hennekens CH et al. Lack of effect of long-term supplementation with beta carotene on the incidence of malignant neoplasms and cardiovascular disease. N Engl J Med 1996;334:1145.
22. Klein EA. Clinical models for testing chemopreventative agents in prostate cancer and overview of SELECT: the Selenium and Vitamin E Cancer Prevention Trial. Recent Results Cancer Res 2003;163:212.
23. Fisher B et al. Tamoxifen for prevention of breast cancer: report of the National Surgical Adjuvant Breast and Bowel Project P-1 Study. J Natl Cancer Inst 1998; 90:1371.
24. Cummings SR et al. The effect of raloxifene on risk of breast cancer in postmenopausal women. Results from the MORE randomized trial. JAMA 1999;281:2189.
25. Thompson IM. The influence of finasteride on the development of prostate cancer. N Engl J Med 2003;349:213.
26. Benner SE et al. Prevention of second primary tumors with isotretinoin in squamous cell carcinoma of the head and neck: long-term follow-up. J Natl Cancer Inst 1994;86:140.
27. Caraballoso M et al. Drugs for preventing lung cancer in healthy people. Cochrane Database Syst Rev 2003;2:CD002141.
28. Clark LC et al. Effects of selenium chemoprevention in patients with carcinoma of the skin. A randomized controlled trial. Nutritional Prevention of Cancer Study Group [published erratum appears in JAMA 1997;277:1520] JAMA 1997;276:1957.
29. Lippman SM et al. Cancer chemoprevention: promise and progress. J Natl Cancer Inst 1998;90:1514.
30. Seifried HE et al. The antioxidant conundrum in cancer. Cancer Res 2003;63:4295.

31. Herendeen JM, Lindley C. Use of NSAIDs for the chemoprevention of colorectal cancer. Ann Pharmacother 2003;37:1664.

32. Harris RE et al. Breast cancer and nonsteroidal anti-inflammatory drugs: prospective results from the Women's Health Initiative. Cancer Res 2003;63:6096.

33. Parkin DM et al. Estimates of the worldwide incidence of 25 major cancers in 1990. Int J Cancer 1999;80:827.

34. Skibber JM et al. Cancer of the colon. In: DeVita VT et al, eds. Cancer: Principles and Practice of Oncology, 6th Ed. Philadelphia: Lippincott Williams & Wilkins, 2001:1216.

35. Carroll PR et al. Cancer of the prostate. In: DeVita VT et al, eds. Cancer: Principles and Practice of Oncology, 6th Ed. Philadelphia: Lippincott Williams & Wilkins, 2001:1418.

36. Chlewboski RT. Reducing the risk of breast cancer. N Engl J Med 2000;343:191.

37. Hamajima N et al. Alcohol, tobacco and breast cancer—collaborative reanalysis of individual data from 53 epidemiological studies, including 58,515 women with breast cancer and 95,067 women without the disease. Br J Cancer 2002;18:1234.

38. Gilchrest BA. The pathogenesis of melanoma induced by ultraviolet radiation. N Engl J Med 1999;340:1341.

39. Christensen D. Data still cloudy on association between sunscreen use and melanoma risk. J Natl Cancer Inst 2003;95:932.

40. Park MT, Lee SJ. Cell cycle and cancer. J Biochem Mol Biol 2003;36:60.

41. Sherr CJ. Cancer cell cycles. Science 1996;274:1672.

42. Hahn WC, Weinberg RA. Rules for making human tumor cells. N Engl J Med 2002;347:1593.

43. Sukumar S et al. A transforming rans gene in tumorigenic guinea pig cell lines initiated by diverse chemical carcinogens. Science 1984;223:1197.

44. Hahn WC. Role of telomeres and telomerase in the pathogenesis of human cancer. J Clin Oncol 2003;21:2034.

45. Rundhaug JE. Matrix metalloproteinases, angiogenesis, and cancer. Clin Cancer Res 2003;9:551.

46. National Comprehensive Cancer Network Guidelines for Detection, Prevention, and Risk of Cancer. © National Comprehensive Cancer Network, Inc. 2001, 202, 2003. URL: http://www.nccn.org/physician_gls/f_guidelines.html [Accessed 25 September 2003].

47. Clark R. Principles of cancer screening. H. Lee Moffitt Cancer Center Research Institute. Cancer Control Journal 1995;2(6). URL: http://www.moffitt.usf.edu/pubs/ccj/. [Accessed 2003 Jul 11].

48. Heron DE et al. Radiation medicine innovations for the new millennium. J Natl Med Assoc 2003;95:55.

49. Hersh SM. Chemical and biological warfare: America's hidden arsenal. New York: Bobbs Merril, 1968.

50. Marshall EK Jr. Historical perspectives in chemotherapy. In: Goldin A, Hawking IF, eds. Advances in Chemotherapy. Vol. 1. New York: Academic Press, 1964:1.

51. Calvert AH, Egorin MJ. Carboplatin dosing formulae: gender bias and the use of creatinine-based methodologies. Eur J Cancer 2002;38:11.

52. Calvert AH et al. Carboplatin dosage: prospective evaluation of a simple formula based on renal function. J Clin Oncol 1989;7:1748.

53. Skipper HE et al. Experimental evaluation of potential anticancer agents: XII. On the criteria and kinetics associated with "curability" of experiment leukemia. Cancer Chemother Rep 1964;35:1.

54. Skipper HE. Reasons for success and failure in treatment of murine leukemias with the drugs now employed in treating human leukemias. Cancer Chemotherapy. Vol 1. Ann Arbor, MI: University Microfilms International, 1978:1.

55. Chu E, DeVita JT Jr. Principles of cancer management: chemotherapy. In: DeVita VT Jr et al, eds. Cancer: Principles and Practice of Oncology, 6th Ed. Philadelphia: Lippincott Williams & Wilkins, 2001:289.

56. Wood WC et al. Dose and dose intensity of adjuvant chemotherapy for stage II, node-positive breast carcinoma. N Engl J Med 1994;330:1253.

57. Bezwoda WR et al. Treatment of Hodgkin's disease with MOPP chemotherapy: effect of dose and schedule modification on treatment outcome. Oncology 1990;47:29.

58. DeVita VT Jr et al. The chemotherapy of lymphomas: looking back, moving forward. The Richard and Hinda Rosenthal Foundation Award Lecture. Cancer Res 1987;47:5810.

59. Repetto L et al. The impact of received dose intensity on the outcome of advanced ovarian cancer. Eur J Cancer 1993;29A:181.

60. Citron ML et al. Randomized trial of dose-dense versus conventionally scheduled and sequential versus concurrent combination chemotherapy as postoperative adjuvant treatment of node-positive primary breast cancer: first report of Intergroup Trial C9741/Cancer and Leukemia Group B Trial 9741. J Clin Oncol 2003;21:1431.

61. Valley AW. New treatment options for managing chemotherapy-induced neutropenia. Am J Health Syst Pharm 2002;59:S11.

62. Richard S, Schuster MW. Stem cell transplantation and hematopoietic growth factors. Curr Hematol Rep 2002;1:103.

63. Hawkins TE, Juttner CA. Blood cell transplantation. Curr Opin Oncol. 1995;7:122.

64. Mormont MC, Levi F. Cancer chronotherapy: principles, applications, and perspectives. Cancer 2003;97:155.

65. Gallion HH et al. Randomized phase III trial of standard timed doxorubicin plus cisplatin versus circadian timed doxorubicin plus cisplatin in stage III and IV or recurrent endometrial carcinoma: a Gynecologic Oncology Group Study. J Clin Oncol 2003;21:3808.

66. Goldie JH, Coldman AJ. A mathematic model for relating the drug sensitivity of tumors to the spontaneous mutation rate. Cancer Treat Rep 1979;63:1727.

67. Gottesman MM. Mechanisms of cancer drug resistance. Annu Rev Med 2002;53:615.

68. Leonard GD et al. The role of ABC transporters in clinical practice. Oncologist 2003;8:411.

69. Thomas H, Coley HM. Overcoming multidrug resistance in cancer: an update on the clinical strategy of inhibiting p-glycoprotein. Cancer Control 2003;10:159.

70. Pessina A et al. Altered DNA-cleavage activity of topoisomerase from WEHI-3B leukemia cells with specific resistance to ciprofloxacin. Anticancer Drugs 2001;12:441.

71. Jonat W et al. Goserelin versus cyclophosphamide, methotrexate, and fluorouracil as adjuvant therapy in premenopausal patients with node-positive breast cancer: the Zoladex Early Breast Cancer Research Association Study. J Clin Oncol 2002;20:4628.

72. Slamon DJ et al. Use of chemotherapy plus a monoclonal antibody against HER2 for metastatic breast cancer that overexpresses HER2. N Engl J Med 2001;344:783.

73. Bull JM et al. A randomized comparative trial of Adriamycin versus methotrexate in combination drug therapy. Cancer 1978;41:1649.

74. Tranum B et al. Adriamycin in combination for the treatment of breast cancer. Cancer 1978;41:2078.

75. Smalley R et al. A comparison of cyclophosphamide, Adriamycin, 5-fluorouracil (CAF) and cyclophosphamide, methotrexate, 5-fluorouracil, vincristine, prednisone (CMFVP) in patients with metastatic breast cancer. Cancer 1977;40:625.

76. Biganzoli L et al. Doxorubicin and paclitaxel versus doxorubicin and cyclophosphamide as first-line chemotherapy in metastatic breast cancer: The European Organization for Research and Treatment of Cancer 10961 multicenter phase III trial. J Clin Oncol 2002;20:3114.

77. Saltz LB et al. Irinotecan plus fluorouracil and leucovorin for metastatic colorectal cancer. Irinotecan Study Group. N Engl J Med 2000;343:905.

78. Andre T et al. CPT-11 (irinotecan) addition to bi-monthly, high-dose leucovorin and bolus and continuous-infusion 5-fluorouracil (FOLFIRI) for pretreated metastatic colorectal cancer. GERCOR. Eur J Cancer 1999;35:1343.

79. Rothenberg ML et al. Superiority of Oxaliplatin and Fluorouracil-Leucovorin Compared With Either Therapy Alone in Patients With Progressive Colorectal Cancer After Irinotecan and Fluorouracil-Leucovorin: Interim Results of a Phase III Trial. J Clin Oncol 2003;21:2059.

80. Poon MA et al. Biochemical modulation of fluorouracil: evidence of significant improvement of survival and quality of life in patients with advanced colorectal carcinoma. J Clin Oncol 1989;7:1407.

81. Petrelli N et al. The modulation of fluorouracil with leucovorin in metastatic colorectal carcinoma: a prospective randomized phase III trial. J Clin Oncol 1989;7:1419.

82. Poon MA et al. Biochemical modulation of fluorouracil with leucovorin: confirmatory evidence of improved therapeutic efficacy in advanced colorectal cancer. J Clin Oncol 199;9:1967.

83. Waters JS et al. Long-term survival after epirubicin, cisplatin and fluorouracil for gastric cancer: results of a randomized trial. Br J Cancer 1999;80:269.

84. MacDonald JS et al. 5-fluorouracil, doxorubicin, and mitomycin (FAM) combination chemotherapy for advanced gastric cancer. Ann Intern Med 1980;93:533.

85. Preusser P et al. Phase II study with the combination etoposide, doxorubicin, and cisplatin in advanced measurable gastric cancer. J Clin Oncol 1989;7:1310.

86. McGuire WP et al. Cyclophosphamide and cisplatin compared with paclitaxel and cisplatin in patients with stage III and stage IV ovarian cancer. N Engl J Med 1996;334:1.

87. McGuire WP, Ozols RF. Chemotherapy of advanced ovarian cancer. Semin Oncol 1998;25:340. Erratum in: Semin Oncol 1998;25:707.

88. Bokemeyer C et al. First-line high-dose chemotherapy compared with standard-dose PEB/VIP chemotherapy in patients with advanced germ cell tumors: a multivariate and matched-pair analysis. J Clin Oncol 1999;17:3450.

89. Motzer RJ et al. Etoposide and cisplatin adjuvant therapy for patients with pathologic stage II germ cell tumors. J Clin Oncol 1995;13(11):2700.

90. Sternberg CN et al. Preliminary results of M-VAC (methotrexate, vinblastine, doxorubicin and cisplatin) for transitional cell carcinoma of the urothelium. J Urol 1985;133:403.

91. Vaughn DJ et al. Paclitaxel plus carboplatin in advanced carcinoma of the urothelium: an active and tolerable outpatient regimen. J Clin Oncol 1998;16:255.

92. Evans WK et al. VP-16 and carboplatin in previously untreated patients with extensive stage small cell lung cancer. Br J Cancer 1988;58:464.

93. Goldhirsch A et al. Cis-dichlorodiammineplatinum (II) and VP 16-213 combination chemotherapy for non-small cell lung cancer. Med Pediatr Oncol 1981;9:205.

94. Dhingra HM et al. Chemotherapy for advanced adenocarcinoma and squamous cell carcinoma of the lung with etoposide and cisplatin. Cancer Treat Rep 1984;68:671.

95. Schiller JH et al. A randomized phase III trial of four chemotherapy regimens for advanced non-small-cell lung cancer. N Engl J Med 2002; 346:92.

96. Pronzato P et al. Carboplatin and etoposide as outpatient treatment of advanced non-small-cell lung cancer. Chemotherapy 1994;40:144.

97. Kish JA et al. A randomized trial of cisplatin (CACP) + 5-fluorouracil (5-FU) infusion and CACP + 5-FU bolus for recurrent and advanced squamous cell carcinoma of the head and neck. Cancer 1985;56:2740.

98. Armitage JO et al. Predicting therapeutic outcome in patients with diffuse histiocytic lymphoma

treated with cyclophosphamide, adriamycin, vincristine, and prednisone (CHOP). Cancer 1982;50: 1695.

99. Coiffier B et al. CHOP chemotherapy plus rituximab compared with CHOP alone in elderly patients with diffuse large-B-cell lymphoma. N Engl J Med 2002;346:235.

100. Klimo P, Connors JM. MACOP-B chemotherapy for the treatment of diffuse large cell lymphoma. Ann Intern Med 1985;102:596.

101. Velasquez VS et al. ESHAP—an effective chemotherapy regimen in refractory and relapsing lymphoma: a 4-year follow-up study. J Clin Oncol 1994;12:1169.

102. DeVita VT Jr et al. Combination chemotherapy in the treatment of advanced Hodgkin's disease. Ann Intern Med 1970;73:881.

103. Santoro A et al. Alternating drug combinations in the treatment of advanced Hodgkin's disease. N Engl J Med 1982;306:770.

104. Barlogie B et al. Effective treatment of advanced multiple myeloma refractory to alkylating agents. N Engl J Med 1984;310:1353.

105. Alexanian R et al. Combination chemotherapy for multiple myeloma. Cancer 1972;30:382.

106. Therasse P et al. New guidelines to evaluate the response to treatment in solid tumors. J Natl Cancer Inst 2000;92:205.

107. Cancer Therapy Evaluation Program, Common Terminology Criteria for Adverse Events (CTCAE) Version 3.0, DCTD, NCI, NIH, NDDS. March 31, 2003 (http://ctep.cancer.gov), Publish Date: June 10, 2003.

108. Oken MM, Creech RH, Tromey DC et al : Toxicity and response criteria of the Eastern Cooperative Oncology Group. Am J Clin Oncol 1982;5:649.

109. Cella D. Advances in quality of life measurements in oncology patients. Semin Oncol 2002;29(3 Suppl 8):60.

110. Perkins GL. Serum tumor markers. Am Fam Physician 2003;68:1075.

111. van der Velden VH. Detection of minimal residual disease in hematologic malignancies by real-time quantitative PCR: principles, approaches, and laboratory aspects. Leukemia 2003;17:1013.

112. Ali S, Coombs RC. Endocrine-responsive breast cancer and strategies for combating resistance. Nat Rev Cancer 2002;2:101.

113. Mauro MJ et al. STI571: A Paradigm of New Agents for Cancer Therapeutics. J Clin Oncol 2002;20:325.

114. Mitchell BS. The Proteasome—An Emerging Therapeutic Target in Cancer. N Engl J Med 2003;348:2597.

115. Hidalgo M, Eckhardt SG. Development of matrix metalloproteinase inhibitors in cancer therapy. J Natl Cancer Inst 2001;93:178.

116. Scappaticci FA. Mechanisms and future directions for angiogenesis-based cancer therapies. J Clin Oncol 2002;20:3906.

117. Oliff A, Gibbs JB, McCormick F. New molecular targets for cancer therapy: investigators are exploiting the characteristic molecular abnormalities of cancers in new approaches to treatment. Sci Am 1996;275:144.

118. Yamamoto Y, Gaynor RB. Therapeutic potential of inhibition of the NF-κB pathway in the treatment of inflammation and cancer. J Clin Invest 2001;107:135.

119. Mihich E. Historical overview of biologic response modifiers. Cancer Invest 2000;18:456.

120. Stephens AC, Rivers RP. Antisense oligonucleotide therapy in cancer. Curr Opin Mol Ther 2003;5:118.

121. Senderowicz AM. Novel small molecule cyclin-dependent kinases modulators in human clinical trials. Cancer Biol Ther 2003;2(4 Suppl 1):S84.

122. Hidalgo M, Rowinsky E. The rapamycin-sensitive pathway as a target for cancer therapy. Oncogene 2000;19:6680.

123. Dvorak HF. Vascular permeability factor/vascular endothelial growth factor: a critical cytokine in tumor angiogenesis and a potential target for diagnosis and therapy. J Clin Oncol 2002;20:4368.

124. Rosen L. Antiangiogeneic strategies and agents in clinical trials. Oncologist 2000;5(suppl 1):20.

125. Rak J, Kerbel RS. Prospects and progress in the development of anti-angiogenic agents. In: Rosenberg SA, ed. Principles and Practice of Biologic Therapy of Cancer Updates. Philadelphia: Lippincott Williams & Wilkins, 2002;3:1.

126. Garrett WD, Workman P. Discovering novel chemotherapeutic drugs for the third millennium. Eur J Cancer 1999;35:2010.

127. Kirkwood J. Cancer immunotherapy: the interferon-alpha experience. Semin Oncol 2002;29(3 Suppl 7):18.

128. Atkins MB. Interleukin-2: clinical applications. Semin Oncol 2002;29(3 Suppl 7):12.

129. Lotze MT et al. In vitro growth of cytotoxic human lymphocytes IV: lysis of fresh and cultured autologous tumor by lymphocytes cultured in T cell growth factor (TCGF). Cancer Res 1981; 41:4420.

130. Rayner AA et al. Lymphokine-activated killer (LAK) cell phenomenon: analysis of factors relevant to the immunotherapy of human cancer. Cancer 1985;55:1327.

131. Rosenberg SA et al. A progress report on the treatment of 157 patients with advanced cancer using lymphokine-activated killer cells and interleukin-2 or high-dose interleukin-2 alone. N Engl J Med 1987;316:889.

132. Rosenberg SA et al. Treatment of 283 consecutive patients with metastatic melanoma or renal cell cancer using high-dose bolus interleukin 2. JAMA 1994;271:907.

133. American Society of Health-System Pharmacists. ASHP guidelines on preventing medication errors with antineoplastic agents. Am J Health-System Pharm 2002;59:1649.

134. American Society of Clinical Oncology. American Society of Clinical Oncology statement regarding the use of outside services to prepare or administer chemotherapy drugs. J Clin Oncol 2003;21:1882.

135. Cohen MR et al. Preventing medication errors in cancer chemotherapy. Am J Health-Syst Pharm 1996;53:737.

136. Attilio RM. Caring enough to understand: the road to oncology medication error prevention. Hosp Pharm 1996;31:17.

137. Berk PD et al. Increased incidence of leukemia in polycythemia vera associated with chlorambucil therapy. N Engl J Med 1981;304:441.

138. Stephens JD et al. Multiple congenital abnormalities in a fetus exposed to 5-fluorouracil during the first trimester. Am J Obstet Gynecol 1980; 137:747.

139. Benedict WF et al. Mutagenicity of cancer chemotherapeutic agents in the Salmonella/microsome test. Cancer Res 1977;37:2209.

140. Rieche K. Carcinogenicity of antineoplastic agents in man. Cancer Treat Rev 1984;11:39.

141. ASHP technical assistance bulletin on handling cytotoxic and hazardous drugs. Am J Hosp Pharm 1990;47:1033.

142. Finley RS et al. Pharmacy practice issues in oncology. In: Finley RS, Balmer CM, eds. Concepts in Oncology Therapeutics, 2nd Ed. Bethesda, MD: American Society of Health-System Pharmacists, 1998.

143. Anderson RW et al. Risk of handling injectable antineoplastic agents. Am J Hosp Pharm 1982;39: 1881.

144. Falck K et al. Mutagenicity in urine of nurses handling cytostatic drugs. Lancet 1979;1:1250.

145. Waksvik H et al. Chromosome analyses of nurses handling cytostatic agents. Cancer Treat Rep 1981; 65:607.

146. Chrysotomou A et al. Mutation frequency in nurses and pharmacists working with cytotoxic drugs. Aust N Z Med 1984;14:831.

147. Hirst M et al. Occupational exposure to cyclophosphamide. Lancet 1984;1:186.

148. Venitt S et al. Monitoring exposure of nursing and pharmacy personnel to cytotoxic drugs: urinary mutation assays and urinary platinum as markers of absorption. Lancet 1984;1:74.

149. Connor TH et al. Surface contamination with antineoplastic agents in six cancer treatment centers in Canada and the United States. Am J Health-Syst Pharm 1999;56:1427.

150. Selevan SH et al. A study of occupational exposure to antineoplastic drugs and fetal loss in nurses. N Engl J Med 1985;333:1173.

151. Baker ES, Connor TH. Monitoring occupational exposure to cancer chemotherapy drugs. Am J Health-Syst Pharm 1996;53:2713.

152. Hemminki K et al. Spontaneous abortions and malformations in the offspring of nurses exposed to anesthetic gases, cytostatic drugs and other potential hazards in hospitals, based on registered information outcome. J Epidemiol Community Health 1985;39:141.

153. National Study Commission on Cytotoxic Exposure. Recommendations for handling cytotoxic agents. 1987.

154. AMA Council on Scientific Affairs. Guidelines for handling parenteral antineoplastics. JAMA 1985; 253:1590.

CHAPTER 89

Adverse Effects of Chemotherapy

Celeste Lindley

Chemotherapy agents are toxic not only to cancer cells but also to various host tissues and organs. The adverse effects of chemotherapy can be classified as common and acute toxicities, specific organ toxicities, and long-term complications. Common and acute toxicities generally include adverse effects that occur as a result of inhibition of host cell division. Host tissues most susceptible to chemotherapy include tissues with renewal cell populations, such as lymphoid tissues, bone marrow, and epithelium of the gastrointestinal (GI) tract and skin. Some other common and acute toxicities (e.g., nausea and vomiting, hypersensitivity reactions) frequently occur in patients shortly after chemotherapy. Specific organ toxicities often are attributed to a unique uptake of the chemotherapy agent by the organ or a selective toxicity of the agent to the organ. Long-term complications are toxicities that occur months to years after chemotherapy. These categories of toxicities can overlap. For example, many specific organ toxicities are evident within days following treatment, whereas other specific organ toxicities are not evident until months after

treatment. Despite the overlapping definitions, this classification system provides some framework to discuss the adverse effects associated with chemotherapy.

The toxicities associated with chemotherapy are the most important factors limiting the use of potentially curative doses. Therefore, all discussions regarding the benefits of chemotherapy agents must include a discussion of toxicities associated with their use. Concerns regarding the toxicities of chemotherapy include the incidence, predictability, severity, and reversibility of the adverse effects. Although the incidence and predictability may be well defined in specific patient populations, the incidence often varies depending on individual susceptibility. In addition, the specific chemotherapy agent, dose intensity, and treatment duration can influence the incidence of several adverse effects. Unfortunately, the specific adverse effects that an individual patient will experience can be difficult to predict. Because several toxicities do have well-defined characteristics, clinicians treating patients with chemotherapy should be aware of the most common adverse effects.

Clinicians should also be aware of patient-specific factors, such as the stage of disease, concomitant illnesses, and concurrent medications, that could cause signs or symptoms that mimic the adverse effects associated with chemotherapy. Many patients have significant disease involvement and impairment of organ function because of the malignant cells. In addition, most patients with cancer commonly receive many other medications, including antibiotics and analgesics that can cause additional adverse effects. When the patient reports a new symptom, it may be difficult to determine whether it is secondary to chemotherapy, concurrent medications, or disease progression. Therefore, the clinician needs to be aware of the presentation, management, and prevention of the most common toxicities that could affect patients receiving chemotherapy.

COMMON AND ACUTE TOXICITIES
Hematologic Toxicities
Effects of Chemotherapy on Bone Marrow

The bone marrow contains a population of pluripotent stem cells capable of self-renewal and differentiation into any mature blood cell. At some point, their progeny commit to either the myeloid or the lymphoid cell line. The myeloid stem cell further commits to developing into an erythrocyte, megakaryocyte, granulocyte, or monocyte. After committing to a particular cell line, bone marrow precursor cells undergo a series of divisions (mitosis) to increase the number of cells. The cells then undergo several developmental stages to mature and differentiate into their final forms and leave the bone marrow (postmitotic). The total time required for a cell to pass through the mitotic and postmitotic pool under normal resting conditions is approximately 10 to 14 days. This process is regulated by several cytokines; although many cytokines have been identified, only a few are now produced through recombinant DNA technology. These growth factors can expand the mitotic pool and accelerate maturation and differentiation. Ultimately, these growth factors decrease the total time spent in these stages to approximately 5 to 7 days.

The development and circulating life span of hematopoietic cell lines determines the severity of the depression of that cell line (nadir) and the time course of peripheral cytopenias. Because red blood cells (RBCs) survive approximately 120 days in the peripheral blood, clinically significant anemia is not likely to occur if RBC production is impaired for a short period of time. Instead, anemia usually develops slowly after several courses of chemotherapy. In contrast, platelets survive approximately 10 days and granulocytes survive approximately 6 to 8 hours. This is why granulocytopenia generally occurs before thrombocytopenia, but both granulocytopenia and thrombocytopenia may be observed after the first or subsequent courses of chemotherapy. The depression of peripheral blood cells following chemotherapy can help determine the dosage, concurrent chemotherapy, and route of administration for subsequent courses. Life-threatening granulocytopenia or thrombocytopenia often necessitates some action to minimize the risk of adverse effects with additional chemotherapy. In the past, clinicians usually reduced the dose of the myelosuppressive agent. However, the availability of colony-stimulating factors (CSFs) and interleukin-11 (oprelvekin) provides an alternative approach to preventing severe neutropenia or thrombocytopenia following myelosuppressive chemotherapy.

MYELOSUPPRESSION

1. J.T., a 45-year-old, 59-kg man with no significant past medical history, presents to the University Hospital with complaints of cough and shortness of breath (SOB). Chest radiograph reveals a lesion in the right upper lobe; bronchoscopy washings and cytologic examination are positive for small cell lung cancer. A workup for metastases is negative. J.T. is diagnosed with limited small cell lung cancer. His physicians plan to initiate radiation therapy to the right upper lobe with concurrent chemotherapy, to include carboplatin targeted to an area under the concentration-time curve (AUC) of 5 mg/mL per min on day 1, topotecan 0.5 mg/m^2 daily on days 1 through 3, and etoposide 100 mg/m^2 per day PO on days 4 through 6. Discuss with J.T. the toxicities that might be expected to occur with this regimen. What effects on the bone marrow can be anticipated and how might they clinically appear in J.T.? What factors can influence the incidence and severity of these adverse effects? When can J.T. expect these effects to occur?

Although several toxicities are commonly associated with carboplatin (Paraplatin), topotecan (Hycamtin), and etoposide (Vepesid), the most predictable and dangerous toxicity associated with this regimen is myelosuppression. This chemotherapy regimen can significantly affect any cell line, including RBCs, neutrophils, and platelets, and the cytopenias can cause significant morbidity or mortality. Decreased RBCs can cause anemia, and patients usually present with fatigue and decreased exercise tolerance. Low neutrophil counts can cause neutropenia, which significantly increases a patient's risk for bacterial infections. Moreover, reduced platelets can cause thrombocytopenia, which can cause bleeding from the GI and genitourinary tracts. Decreases in non-neutrophil granulocytes and monocytes are not associated with clinically significant consequences.

Both patient- and agent-related factors can significantly influence the degree of cytopenia a patient faces after chemotherapy. Agent-related factors include chemotherapy agent, dose intensity, and the schedule of administration. In addition, the effects of concurrent chemotherapy may intensify the individual myelosuppressive effect of a specific agent. Host factors that specifically affect the cellularity of the bone marrow compartment also influence the degree of cytopenia. They include: [1]

1. Patient age. Younger patients are better able to tolerate certain doses of an agent than elderly patients because they have a more cellular marrow with a decreased percentage of fat.
2. Bone marrow reserve in relation to the amount of involvement by a particular neoplastic process (e.g., fibrosis and tumor cells, including leukemic cells in the marrow).
3. The degree of compromise from previous chemotherapy, radiation therapy, or both. Prior chemotherapy and radiation therapy to fields involving marrow-producing bone reduce bone marrow reserves.
4. The patient's nutritional status. The greater the degree of negative nitrogen balance, with its associated loss of weight, the less tolerant the patient is likely to be.

5. The liver's or kidneys' ability to metabolize and/or excrete the compounds administered.

These factors, along with the pharmacokinetics of the stem cells, can help clinicians predict the severity and duration of cytopenia observed following therapy.

With most agents, the patient's white blood cell (WBC) and platelet counts begin to fall within 5 to 7 days, reach a nadir within 7 to 10 days, and recover within 14 to 26 days. Phase-specific chemotherapy agents, such as the plant alkaloids and antimetabolites, cause a fairly rapid onset of cytopenia that recovers faster than the cytopenias occurring after treatment with phase-nonspecific agents, such as alkylating agents and antitumor antibiotics. For poorly understood reasons, nitrosureas typically produce severe, delayed neutropenia and thrombocytopenia 4 to 6 weeks after therapy. Other agents that exhibit this pattern include mitomycin and mechlorethamine. All these chemotherapy agents exert their cytotoxic effects during the resting phase of the cell cycle. When resting, damaged cells enter a growth phase, and the delayed cytopenias become evident. Unfortunately, these agents can cause two neutropenic nadirs; the first nadir occurs at the conventional time expected for phase-nonspecific agents and the second nadir occurs approximately 4 to 6 weeks after therapy. Many combination regimens that use these agents recommend 6-week cycles to avoid treatment before the second nadir. Most other myelosuppressive regimens recommend dosing intervals of 3 to 4 weeks to allow the bone marrow time to recover.

All the agents included in J.T.'s regimen have marked myelosuppressive activity. J.T. should be carefully counseled to contact his physician or report to the emergency department (ED) if he experiences signs or symptoms of an infection (including fever) or bleeding. Typically, these symptoms occur 10 to 14 days after the first day of chemotherapy.

Prevention

2. About 9 days after the first course of chemotherapy, J.T. developed a severe sore throat and fever. He was admitted to the hospital and treated with intravenous (IV) antibiotics. At the time, his WBC count was 300/mm³. His fever resolved after 3 days, and all cultures were negative for bacterial growth. It is now 3 weeks after chemotherapy, and he is scheduled to receive a second course. Should he receive the same doses he was given initially?

In the past, the chemotherapy doses would have been reduced (usually by 25%) for all subsequent cycles for any patient who experienced febrile neutropenia. Although a dose reduction can clearly cause less neutropenia, it can also compromise the response and survival of patients with chemotherapy-sensitive tumors. Because J.T.'s cancer (i.e., limited-stage small cell lung cancer), is both chemosensitive and potentially curable, a dosage reduction is undesirable. To minimize the risk of neutropenia with future therapy, CSFs can be administered to J.T. to prevent potential complications associated with neutropenia.

The prophylactic administration of CSFs can be used to protect against the myelosuppressive effects of chemotherapy. Two CSFs, granulocyte colony-stimulating factor (G-CSF [filgrastim]) and granulocyte-monocyte colony-stimulating factor (GM-CSF [sargramostim]), are available in the United States. These products were approved by the Food and Drug Administration (FDA) in 1991 to enhance neutrophil recovery after chemotherapy. A pegylated long-acting form of filgrastim, pegfilgrastim, was approved by the FDA in February 2002. Pegfilgrastim was developed with the aim of providing the same pharmacologic benefit as filgrastim while offering the advantage and convenience of fewer injections. Evidence-based clinical practice guidelines for the use of CSFs have been developed by the American Society of Clinical Oncology.[1,2] These guidelines recommend primary prophylaxis for all patients receiving chemotherapy regimens that have been previously reported to cause an incidence of ≥40% of febrile neutropenia. A CSF used in these patients can reduce the need for hospitalizations and broad-spectrum antibiotics. Because the regimen J.T. received does not typically produce a 40% incidence of febrile neutropenia, a CSF was not recommended for him after his first course of chemotherapy. Because J.T. did experience febrile neutropenia and he has a potentially curable malignancy, a CSF is indicated with subsequent courses of chemotherapy to prevent additional febrile episodes.

3. **How are CSFs dosed to prevent chemotherapy-induced neutropenia?**

The recommended initial dose of filgrastim (G-CSF) is 5 μg/kg per day as a single daily subcutaneous (SC) injection, and the recommended initial dose of sargramostim (GM-CSF) is 250 mg/m² per day as an SC injection. Because the recommended dose of G-CSF is expressed in μg/kg and GM-CSF in μg/m², it is helpful to keep in mind that a dose in μg/m² can be divided by 40 to obtain a rough estimate of the equivalent dose in μg/kg. Changing the units for GM-CSF shows the recommended initial dose of GM-CSF (6 μg/kg) is roughly equivalent to that of G-CSF (5 μg/kg). The ASCO guidelines state that rounding the dose of either agent to the nearest vial size may enhance patient convenience and reduce cost without clinical detriment. Because commercially available vials contain either 300 or 480 μg of G-CSF, patients <75 kg should receive 300 μg daily and patients >75 kg should receive 480 μg daily.[3] Because of differences in commercially available vial sizes, the weight breakpoint for GM-CSF is slightly different; patients who weigh ≥60 kg should receive 500 μg daily and patients who weigh <60 kg should receive 250 μg daily.

The ASCO guidelines also recommend a shorter duration of treatment than the manufacturer. The manufacturer recommends that therapy with filgrastim or sargramostim continue until the patient's neutrophil count exceeds 10,000 cells/mm³ after the expected chemotherapy nadir. This is based on the observation that the neutrophil count falls roughly 50% after discontinuing a CSF. However, the risk of bacterial infection is highest in patients with neutrophil counts of <500 to 1,000/mm³; patients with neutrophil counts >500 to 1,000/mm³ are not thought to be at high risk for developing bacterial infections. Thus, many clinicians elect to discontinue CSFs when the neutrophil count reaches 2,000 to 4,000/mm³ following the chemotherapy nadir. This reduces the number of treatment days and the cost associated with therapy without placing the patient at excessive risk for bacterial infections. The ASCO guidelines support this recommendation to discontinue CSFs earlier.

The introduction of pegfilgrastim to the U.S. market occurred after the most recent ASCO Guidelines for the use of CSFs. However, there is little doubt that the next revision will contain a recommendation for pegfilgrastim for prevention of chemotherapy-induced neutropenia. Two pivotal, randomized, blinded multicenter phase III trials have evaluated the efficacy of single dose pegfilgrastim in the prevention of chemotherapy-induced neutropenia in patients with high-risk stage II, stage III, and stage IV breast cancer.[4,5] The patients (n = 310)[4] (n = 157)[5] received four cycles of doxorubicin 60 mg/m^2 and docetaxel 75 mg/m^2 chemotherapy on day 1 of each cycle and were randomized to either single-dose pegfilgrastim on day 2 or filgrastim 5 μg/kg/day from day 2 until the ANC was >10 × 10^9/L or for a maximum of 14 doses. In one study, the pegfilgrastim was a 6-mg fixed dose[5] and in the other study the pegfilgrastim dose was based on weight (100 μg/kg).[4] The primary endpoint was duration of severe grade IV neutropenia (neutrophil count <0.5 × 10^9/L) in cycle 1. Secondary endpoints included the degree of ANC nadir, time to recovery, incidence of grade IV neutropenia and incidence of febrile neutropenia. In these phase III breast cancer trials, no significant difference in duration of grade IV neutropenia was seen between the pegfilgrastim and filgrastim groups (1.7 versus 1.8 days, respectively,[4] and 1.8 versus 1.6 days, respectively[5]). The incidence of severe neutropenia after chemotherapy was similar in the pegfilgrastim and filgrastim arms. In patients treated with pegfilgrastim, the incidence of febrile neutropenia over four cycles of chemotherapy in the two pivotal phase III trials[4,5] was lower than in the patients treated with filgrastim. In the larger of the trials, this difference was clinically significant (P .029). The time to ANC recovery was defined as the time from chemotherapy administration until the ANC increased to >2 × 10^9/L. In the larger phase III trial,[4] the mean was 9.3 days in the pegfilgrastim group compared with 9.7 days in the filgrastim group. In all studies, pegfilgrastim has been well tolerated. From these data, it appears clear that a single 6-mg dose of pegfilgrastim is at least equivalent to daily subcutaneous injections of filgrastim and clearly offers advantages with respect to convenience and patient comfort. Therefore, it may represent the treatment of choice and is quickly becoming the community standard for prevention of febrile neutropenia in patients whose chemotherapy is likely to produce an incidence of febrile neutropenia of ≥40%.

In summary, J.T. should be given either G-CSF 300 μg/day or GM-CSF 250 μg/day SC beginning the day after his last dose of chemotherapy. Treatment should continue until the neutrophil count exceeds 2,000 to 4,000/mm^3. Alternatively, J.T. could receive a single 6 mg injection of pegfilgrastim the day after chemotherapy administration. Aside from high cost and inconvenience, the only negative effect of G-CSF therapy is mild transient bone pain. Bone pain is most commonly experienced when patients begin to recover peripheral blood cells following their nadir. The proposed mechanism suggests the stimulatory effect of G-CSF on granulopoiesis causes the pain. Most patients commonly report pain in bone marrow–rich areas, such as the sternum. They should be advised that the bone pain experienced during marrow recovery is normal and usually is relieved with analgesic agents.

Treatment

4. **If J.T. was not given G-CSF and presented with febrile neutropenia, would G-CSF therapy be helpful?**

Because the duration of neutropenia is the most significant prognostic factor in patients with established febrile neutropenia, the major benefit of CSFs is their ability to reduce the duration of neutropenia. CSFs accelerate hematopoiesis by expanding the mitotic pool of committed progenitor cells and shortening the time spent in the postmitotic pool from 6 days to 1 day. If CSFs reduced the duration of neutropenia in patients who present with febrile neutropenia, then morbidity, mortality, and cost should be significantly reduced.

The ability of CSFs to reduce the duration of neutropenia in patients with established febrile neutropenia has been addressed in numerous randomized, double-blind, placebo-controlled trials.[1,2,6,7] The combined data for G-CSF and GM-CSF reveal minimal to moderate benefit in reducing hospital stays. Furthermore, several groups have questioned whether all patients with febrile neutropenia require hospitalization.[8–10] Although CSFs do appear to hasten neutrophil recovery, the true cost-benefit associated with the use of these products in established febrile neutropenia remains to be determined. The ASCO currently does not support routine use of CSFs in patients with febrile neutropenia, although they do recognize that certain patients with febrile neutropenia and prognostic factors predictive of clinical deterioration (e.g., pneumonia, fungal infection, sepsis syndrome) may benefit from use of CSFs.

5. **Fourteen days after his fourth course of chemotherapy, J.T.'s platelet count is 7,000/mm^3. Although he has no evidence of bleeding, the clinician decides to administer a prophylactic platelet transfusion. Would oprelvekin (Neumega) be helpful in preventing the need for further platelet transfusions?**

Oprelvekin (Neumega) is indicated to prevent severe thrombocytopenia and reduce the need for platelet transfusions following myelosuppressive chemotherapy in patients with nonmyeloid malignancies at high risk for developing severe thrombocytopenia. Because carboplatin has a cumulative myelosuppressive effect on platelet precursors, J.T. is at risk for developing severe thrombocytopenia with future courses of chemotherapy. In a randomized, double-blind clinical trial, oprelvekin reduced the need for platelet transfusions in about 20% of patients who were similar to J.T. The recommended dose is 50 μg/kg per day SC until the postnadir platelet count is >50,000/mm^3 or up to 21 days following chemotherapy.[11] Because only about 20% of patients respond to oprelvekin, J.T. may still require additional platelet transfusions. In addition, the cost-benefit ratio of oprelvekin (cost per day, $120) compared with platelet transfusions has not been demonstrated in clinical trials. Based on current evidence, J.T. should not receive oprelvekin at this time.

Anemia and Erythropoietin

6. **Is erythropoietin useful in cancer patients with anemia?**

Anemia usually is not a dose-limiting toxicity commonly associated with chemotherapy, because RBCs survive approximately 120 days. Chemotherapy predominantly affects RBCs by causing anisocytosis and macrocytosis. These effects are related to inhibition of DNA synthesis, and they predominantly occur following treatment with antimetabolites, including folic acid analogs, hydroxyurea, purine antagonists, and pyrimidine antagonists. Anemia commonly does not accompany these changes in RBC size. In addition, chemotherapy-induced effects on RBCs are rarely the sole factor contributing to the low hemoglobin (Hgb) levels that necessitate a RBC transfusion.

Nevertheless, anemia commonly occurs in cancer patients secondary to the primary disease. The exact mechanism by which this anemia occurs is not well understood. Impaired erythrocyte response to erythropoietin (possibly mediated by IL-1 and tumor necrosis factor [TNF] release associated with malignant disease), reduced hematopoietic precursors caused by chemotherapy and/or radiation therapy, and disrupted marrow architecture caused by invasion of malignant cells may all play a role. Erythropoietin can ameliorate anemia associated with cancer and chemotherapy, reduce the need for transfusions, and enhance the patient's quality of life.[3,12–14] Because of its high cost, erythropoietin generally is reserved for patients who require RBC transfusions, have symptoms of anemia, or whose downward trend in hemoglobin/hematocrit counts suggests that intervention will be required to avoid transfusion. Intervention is generally indicated in patients whose hemoglobin level is ≤11g/dL.

Recombinant human erythropoietin (r-HUEPO, Epoietin alpha) is approved for use in cancer patients receiving chemotherapy. The recommended starting dose for r-HUEPO is 150 U/kg three times per week, which is significantly higher than the recommended dose for anemia of renal failure. Many clinicians choose to administer a standard dose of 10,000 U consistent with the vial size. Alternatively, 40,000 U once weekly has also been shown to be effective.[15] These initial doses should be given for 4 weeks. If the Hgb increases <1 g/dL then the dose should be increased to 300 U/kg three times weekly or 60,000 U once weekly. Up to 8 weeks of treatment may be required to significantly decrease transfusion requirements. Only about 50% of patients respond (i.e., reduce their requirement for transfusion or report a significant decrease in symptoms) to erythropoietin, so patients who do not respond positively within 8 to 12 weeks should discontinue therapy. Since pretreatment erythropoietin levels do not consistently correlate with the rate and likelihood of response, clinicians cannot predict which patients will respond to therapy.[16] Adverse effects, such as hypertension, seizures, and angina, which can occur in patients with renal failure following a rapid dose escalation or normalization of hematocrit, have not been observed in patients with cancer. Therefore, erythropoietin may provide a safe and effective treatment for cancer- or chemotherapy-associated anemia.

Darbepoetin alfa (Aranesp) is an erythropoiesis-stimulating protein closely related to erythropoietin that is produced in Chinese hampster ovary cells by recombinant DNA technology. It stimulates erythropoiesis by the same mechanism as erythropoietin. Darbepoetin was recently approved for the treatment of anemia associated with cancer chemotherapy and it is distinguished from erythropoietin by its approximately threefold longer half-life and greater biologic potency. This allows for an extended dosing interval relative to erythropoietin. Two dose-finding studies in 429 patients found that darbepoetin alfa 1.5 μg/kg, once per week, achieved the same mean hemoglobin change from baseline as that of recombinant human erythropoietin dosed at 150 U/kg, three times a week. At a dose of 3 mg/kg weekly, darbopoetin alpha elicited a hematopoietic response after 2 weeks similar to that produced by recombinant human erythropoietin 40,000 to 60,000 U

once per week. Studies are ongoing with darbepoetin to identify the appropriate dose for a Q 3-week dosing interval.[17,18]

Epoetin alfa and darbepoetin alfa are currently indicated only for patients actively receiving chemotherapy; however, recent evidence suggests that cancer patients experiencing anemia associated with their underlying disease may benefit from therapy.[19] The reduced need for transfusion therapy should be balanced with the cost and inconvenience of erythropoietin therapy for anemia.

Chemotherapy and Coagulation

7. **What effect does chemotherapy have on blood coagulation?**

Patients with cancer can develop bleeding or thrombosis after chemotherapy. Most patients receiving chemotherapy commonly develop bleeding secondary to thrombocytopenia caused by bone marrow suppression.

Bleeding can also occur after treatment with L-asparaginase (Elspar), which can inhibit the synthesis of fibrinogen and other specific coagulation factors produced by the liver under the influence of vitamin K.[20,21] L-Asparaginase has a widespread effect on protein synthesis, and many plasma protein factors are depressed shortly after treatment with this agent. A patient receiving L-asparaginase can often show a prolonged prothrombin time (PT) and partial thromboplastin time (PTT). However, bleeding or thrombosis occurring as a direct result of changes in coagulation factors has not been frequently reported or conclusively documented. Coagulation factors may return to normal levels with continued administration of the agent, which suggests that the impairment of protein synthesis created by L-asparaginase is partially overcome by the liver. Specific treatment of prolonged PT and PTT with coagulation factors, fibrinogen, or vitamin K is not indicated.

THROMBOTIC EVENTS

Thrombotic events have been associated with the administration of chemotherapy.[22] Evidence of intravascular coagulation from plasma fibrinopeptide A, a specific activation peptide of fibrinogen, has been reported after starting chemotherapy.[23] Conversely, a decrease in fibrinolytic activity reflected by a decrease in functional plasminogen activator also has been reported.[23] Other protein abnormalities associated with thrombosis, including a decrease in the anticoagulant proteins C and protein S (free and total),[24,25] have occurred after chemotherapy. Deficiencies of these proteins have been reported to result in spontaneous thrombosis. Although chemotherapy can potentially increase a patient's risk of thrombosis, the underlying disease can also affect risk.

Assessing the risk of thrombosis from administration of chemotherapy is complicated by the fact that many cancers are associated with an increased incidence of thrombosis. This is particularly true in tumors of the GI tract and acute promyelocytic leukemia. Trousseau[26] first reported an increased incidence of venous thrombosis in patients with cancer, but many investigators have since confirmed the relationship of multiple or migratory venous thrombosis in up to 15% of patients with cancer.[27] Up to one-third of apparently healthy adults who develop otherwise unexplained deep vein thrombosis eventually prove to have a malignancy.[28,29]

Removal of the tumor often causes thrombotic episodes to disappear. Although warfarin or low-molecular-weight heparin therapy is indicated, thrombosis associated with cancer is often resistant to anticoagulant therapy.

Initiating treatment for acute promyelocytic leukemia commonly is associated (i.e., up to 85%) with disseminated intravascular coagulation.[30] The lysed tumor cells appear to release procoagulant materials following chemotherapy. Although most patients receive heparin to minimize their risk of coagulation, some investigators have reported excellent results in patients treated almost entirely with blood product support (fibrinogen and/or antithrombin III) without heparin.[26] With the exception of acute promyelocytic leukemia, no general guidelines are recommended to prevent thrombosis associated with cancer or chemotherapy.

Other factors may cause patients to develop thrombosis. Most patients receiving cancer chemotherapy often have multiple other illnesses that could predispose them to developing thrombosis. In addition, surgical procedures and bed rest can increase the risk of thrombosis. Clinicians should maintain a high index of suspicion when a patient with cancer presents with signs or symptoms of thrombosis.

Gastrointestinal Tract Toxicities

The GI tract may be second only to the bone marrow in its susceptibility to toxic effects produced by chemotherapy. GI toxicities include nausea and vomiting, oral complications, esophagitis, and lower bowel disturbances.

Nausea and Vomiting

Nausea and vomiting are common and serious toxicities associated with most chemotherapy agents. Chemotherapy agents, their metabolites, or neurotransmitters may stimulate dopamine or serotonin receptors in the GI tract, the chemoreceptor trigger zone, or the central nervous system (CNS) that ultimately act on the vomiting center. Emesis most commonly occurs on the first day of chemotherapy and often persists for several days thereafter.[31] Most patients who receive chemotherapy require antiemetics before chemotherapy and after chemotherapy for several days to control these symptoms. The most appropriate antiemetic regimen is based on patient-and agent-specific factors.(see Chapter 8, Nausea and Vomiting).

Complications of the Oral Cavity

Complications of the oral cavity include mucositis (or stomatitis), xerostomia (dry mouth), infection, and bleeding. Approximately 40% of patients treated with chemotherapy develop oral complications, and virtually all patients who receive radiation therapy to the head and neck develop oral complications.[32] These toxicities occur because of the nonspecific effects of chemotherapy on cells undergoing rapid division, including the cells of the mouth that undergo rapid renewal with a turnover time equal to 7 to 14 days. Chemotherapy reduces the renewal rate of the basal epithelium and can cause mucosal atrophy, as well as glandular and collagen degeneration.[33] Radiation therapy to the head and neck also causes mucosal atrophy by decreasing cell renewal. Radiation can also cause fibrosis of the salivary glands, muscles, ligaments, and blood vessels and damage to the taste buds.[34]

The combined effects of chemotherapy and radiation therapy on the oral mucosa can also cause infection and bleeding in the oral cavity. Infection and bleeding occurs when treatment causes bone marrow suppression, including thrombocytopenia and neutropenia. Because the oral mucosa is highly vascular and frequently traumatized, bleeding occurs commonly with low platelet counts. In addition, chemotherapy and neutropenia can alter the extensive microbial flora harbored in the oral cavity, thus leading to oral infections. Unfortunately, oral complications often compound one another. For example, xerostomia can accelerate the development of mucositis as well as the formation of dental caries and local infection. Mucositis can clearly predispose the oral cavity to local bleeding and infection, as well as sepsis. In addition, all these oral complications can cause varying degrees of discomfort and adversely affect the patient's ability to eat, which potentially can lead to a compromised nutritional status. Topical treatments of oral complications are summarized in Table 89-1.

XEROSTOMIA

8. **J.B. is a 55-year-old man with newly diagnosed, locally advanced head and neck cancer. Neoadjuvant chemotherapy with cisplatin, methotrexate (MTX), and fluorouracil (fluorouracil), followed by a 2-week course of radiation therapy (200 rads/day for three cycles) and surgical resection of persistent residual disease are planned. A review of systems suggests that J.B. has poor oral hygiene, and a decision is made to consult the dental department of the University Hospital before initiating radiation and chemotherapy. Is J.B. at risk for developing oral complications of chemotherapy? Is there anything that should be done at this point to decrease his risk?**

J.B. is at high risk for several of the oral complications previously described. Xerostomia is one of the most frequent side effects of radiation therapy to the head and neck and occurs secondary to radiation-induced changes to the salivary glands. Evidence supports a direct relationship between the dose of radiation to the salivary glands and the extent of glandular changes.[34] In most patients treated with <6,000 rads, radiation-induced changes to the salivary glands are reversible within 6 to 12 months after the end of therapy. However, J.B. also will be receiving chemotherapy agents (i.e., MTX, fluorouracil) that can cause xerostomia and enhance the toxicity to the salivary glands. Clinically, xerostomia has been caused by as little as two to three radiation doses of 200 rads.[34]

Damage to the salivary glands causes various effects, including a loss of salivary buffering capacity, lower salivary pH, no mechanical flushing, and decreased salivary IgA. In addition, xerostomia can alter the sense of taste, causing some patients to lose their ability to differentiate between sweet and salty foods and others to report a bitter taste. Xerostomia also commonly causes caries. Caries and decalcification may become severe enough to compromise tooth integrity and cause fracture. Because saliva is no longer available to help clear bacteria from the mouth, xerostomia also predisposes patients to infection secondary to the increases in oral bacteria. Administering a chemoprotectant before chemotherapy or radiation therapy may help reduce these adverse effects.

Amifostine (Ethyol), an organic thiophosphate chemoprotectant agent, is approved to reduce the incidence of moderate

Table 89-1   Topical Medications for Oral Complications of Chemotherapy and/or Radiation Therapy

Problem	Products	Use
Xerostomia	Pilocarpine 5-mg tablet +	1–2 tablets TID to QID
	Saliva substitutes and/or	Rinse or spray PRN
	Sugar-free hard candy; sugar-free gum; ice chips	PRN
Mucositis	Dyclonine HCL 0.5% or 1% solution	Swish and expectorate 5–15 mL Q 2–3 hr PRN
Generalized	or	
	Viscous lidocaine 2% solution	Swish and expectorate 5–15 mL Q 2–3 hr PRN
	or	
	Diphenhydramine capsules (125 mg) +	Swish and expectorate 5–15 mL Q 2–3 hr PRN
	Dyclonine 1% 30 mL +	
	Nystatin 1 mL and ≤120 mL Maalox	
	or	
	Diphenhydramine + nystatin + hydrocortisone (various formulations)	Swish and expectorate 5–15 mL Q 2–3 hr PRN
	or	
	Sucralfate suspension (8 tablets in 40 mL sterile water plus 40 mL 70% sorbitol; shake well and add water to 120 mL)	Swish and expectorate 5–15 mL Q 2–3 hr PRN
	or	Dissolve candy in mouth PRN
	Capsaicin candy[31]: Combine sugar, corn syrup, water, cornstarch, butter, and salt in 2-quart saucepan; cook over medium heat, stirring constantly to 256° on candy thermometer; remove from heat; stir in vanilla and cayenne pepper; pull taffy until light in color and stiff; pull into 1/2-inch long strip; cut with scissors into 1-inch pieces	Apply to affected dried area Q 2–3 hr; not to be used in the presence of an infection
Localized	Benzocaine in orabase	Apply to affected area with gauze sponge and hold in place with pressure for 30 min; do not remove formed clots
Local bleeding (gingival)	Topical thrombin solution	
Mucosal surface bleeding	Aminocaproic acid	Swish and spit 250 mg Q 4 hr for up to 12 hr
General infection	Chlorhexidine gluconate 0.12% oral rinse	Rinse BID after breakfast and at HS for 30 sec; do not swallow
Prevention and treatment of oral candidiasis	Nystatin oral suspension	Rinse and swallow (if tolerated) 500,000–1,000,000 units TID to QID
	or	
	Clotrimazole troche 10 mg	Dissolve 1 tablet 5 times/day
Prevention of caries	Acidulated fluoride rinse	Rinse daily for 1 min with 5–10 mL; do not swallow; switch to neutral fluoride if mucositis is present
	or	
	Neutral fluoride rinse	Rinse daily for 1 min with 5 mL; do not swallow; switch back to acidulated fluoride rinse when mucositis resolves
	or	
	Stannous fluoride gel 0.4%	Brush daily at HS; swish for 30 sec; spit out and rinse
	or	
	Sodium fluoride gel 1.1%	Brush daily at HS; swish for 30 sec; spit out and rinse

to severe xerostomia in patients undergoing postoperative radiation treatment for head and neck cancer when the radiation port includes a substantial portion of the parotid glands. A randomized, clinical trial demonstrated that the incidence of xerostomia was reduced by about 30% in patients receiving 200 mg/m² as a 3-minute IV infusion 15 to 30 minutes before each fraction of radiation. Recent guidelines published by ASCO support the use of amifostine to reduce the incidence of acute and late toxicity in patients receiving fractionated radiation therapy for head and neck cancer.[36] Unfortunately, amifostine cannot prevent xerostomia from occurring in all patients.

If xerostomia occurs, treatment can stimulate existing salivary flow and replace lost secretions. Relatively low doses of systemically administered pilocarpine (5 to 10 mg orally three times daily) may stimulate salivary flow and produce clinically significant benefits in patients with postradiation xerostomia.[37,38] Dose-related adverse effects include cholinergic effects such as sweating, rhinitis, headache, nausea, and abdominal cramps. Sucrose-free hard candy and sugar-free chewing gum can also stimulate salivation, but these treatments are typically considered oral comfort agents. Saliva substitutes can also provide oral comfort to patients with xerostomia. Commercially available saliva substitutes generally are recommended for use before meals and at bedtime. They are available in several formulations, including sprays, rinses, and chewing gums. Patients who find one product or formulation unacceptable or unsuccessful may benefit from experimenting with other formulations or product lines. Studies have shown that salivary substitutes containing carboxymethylcellulose or hydroxyethylcellulose are more effective in relieving dryness than water- or glycerin-based solutions.[39,40] Other treatment modalities attempt to prevent the complications associated with xerostomia.

Prevention of radiation-induced caries is best accomplished by aggressively using fluorides.[41] Generally, acidulated fluorides are the most effective, although neutral fluorides may be more acceptable to patients with mucositis. Patients are instructed to rinse daily for 1 minute with 5 to 10 mL of a fluoride rinse. Stannous fluoride gels 0.4% or sodium fluoride gel 1.1% tooth brushing agents may be also be used by patients to minimize their risk of caries. Meticulous attention to oral hygiene with regular dental checkups and avoidance of sucrose is essential to minimize the development of caries.

In general, a dentist should see patients who will be receiving radiation therapy to the head and neck or chemotherapy agents with a high risk of oral complications before starting therapy. This includes patients with hematologic malignancies who will most likely experience severe myelosuppression for prolonged periods. Oral evaluation before therapy, intervention to eliminate potential sources of infection or irritation, and preventive measures taken during therapy can dramatically decrease the frequency of oral complications.[42] Given J.B.'s risk factors, a dental examination is indicated before initiating therapy.

MUCOSITIS/STOMATITIS

9. J.B. successfully completed his first 2-week course of combined chemotherapy and radiation therapy; however, 3 days into his second 2-week cycle, he complains of generalized burning, discomfort, and pain on the ventral surface of his tongue. On clinical observation, both the ventral surface of his tongue and the floor of his mouth appear erythematous, and several discrete lesions are present in both areas. What is the most likely explanation for J.B.'s new onset of symptoms? What treatment is indicated at this time?

J.B.'s symptoms are consistent with therapy-related mucositis. As discussed earlier, this complication occurs as a nonspecific effect of chemotherapy agents and radiation therapy on the basal epithelium of the mouth. Nonkeratinized mucosa is affected most often. Thus, the buccal, labial, and soft palate mucosa; the ventral surface of the tongue; and the floor of the mouth are the most common sites of involvement. Although lesions are usually discrete initially, they often progress to produce large areas of ulceration. The lesions typically do not progress outside the mouth, but they may extend to the esophagus and involve the entire GI tract. Signs and symptoms generally occur about 5 to 7 days after chemotherapy or at almost any point during radiation therapy. The antimetabolites (e.g., MTX, fluorouracil, and cytarabine) and the antitumor antibiotics are the chemotherapy agents that most commonly produce direct stomatotoxicity. Lesions generally regress and resolve completely in approximately 1 to 3 weeks, depending on their severity.

Patients with mucositis can present with various symptoms, but patients often complain of pain so severe that parenteral opioid analgesics are required for relief. Other signs or symptoms include decreased ability to eat and speak and local or systemic infections. Bacterial, fungal, or viral infections can occur. Although different microbial agents can cause a characteristic lesion, the lesion's appearance usually does not always correlate with the infectious agent. This particularly occurs in patients with neutropenia who cannot mount a full inflammatory response. In these individuals, the clinical appearance of an infected lesion may be muted relative to the presence or number of pathogens. Under normal conditions, the mucosa provides a natural barrier to the entry of normal oral flora, but the broken mucosa allows pathogens access to the bloodstream. The patient could develop life-threatening infection or sepsis in addition to a local infection. After assessing the complications associated with mucositis, the patient should be treated to minimize discomfort and morbidity.

Treatment

Treatment of mucositis is palliative. Topical anesthetics, including viscous lidocaine or dyclonine hydrochloride 0.5 or 1%, often are recommended. Equal portions of kaolin, diphenhydramine, and magnesium- or aluminum-containing antacids may be used for their anesthetic and astringent properties. Many institutions may compound mouthwash products containing these ingredients as well as antibiotics, nystatin, or corticosteroids. Corticosteroids provide anti-inflammatory properties, and the antibiotics and antifungals provide antibacterial or antifungal properties. Other topical agents used to treat oral mucositis discomfort include capsaicin and sucralfate. When applied to the skin or mucous membranes, capsaicin, a component of chili peppers, produces a burning pain and ultimately desensitizes pain receptors.[35] Oral application via a candy formulation has been shown to significantly decrease pain in patients with mucositis.[35] Sucralfate suspension may provide some benefit by coating the lesion and reducing discomfort. All of these topically applied products are only used for symptom control, and data supporting superior efficacy of one product over another in relieving pain are lacking.

All the topical anesthetic-type preparations are recommended for use as "swish-and-spit" preparations. Generally, 5 to 10 mL are used three to six times a day. The longer the patient can hold the solution in the mouth, the longer the contact, and, theoretically, the better the symptom relief. Therefore, patients should be advised to hold and swish the solution around the mouth for as long as possible before spitting it out. Other treatment options include topical benzocaine in Orabase and ice chips. For small localized lesions, ointments such as benzocaine in Orabase may be applied to the affected area after it is dried with a sponge. Patients may also find ice chips soothing. Unfortunately, most patients require systemic analgesics to alleviate the pain.

Gelclair is a bioadherent oral gel containing polyvinylpyrollidone and sodium hyaluronate (but no alcohol or anesthetic agent). It provides an adherent barrier over the mucosal surfaces, thereby shielding oral lesions from the effect of food, liquids, and saliva.[43] Although clinical data are scant, an uncontrolled open-label study has been conducted in 30 hospice patients with oral lesions (only three of whom had chemotherapy-related mucositis).[44] Oral pain scores were recorded at baseline, 5 to 7 hours after application, and between 7 and 10 days after daily use was begun. All patients reported a substantial reduction in oral discomfort within 5 to 7 hours of initial treatment, and 87% reported improvement in pain associated with eating and drinking within 1 week. Benefit continued for more than 3 hours after each dose in most patients.

J.B. appears to have a mild case of stomatitis/mucositis at this time; however, the lesions may progress over the next several days. Appropriate treatment may include the use of any of the topical products listed in Table 89-1. Table 89-2 lists additional guidelines for managing stomatitis.

Prevention

10. **Could J.B.'s mucositis have been prevented?**

Specific measures to reduce the incidence or severity of chemotherapy-induced mucositis have received some attention in the past few years. Historically, treatment of chemotherapy-and radiation-induced mucositis has been aimed at reducing symptoms once they occur and avoiding further trauma to the oral mucosa. Cryotherapy has been marginally effective in reducing the severity of chemotherapy-induced mucositis.[45] Ice chips are placed in the mouth 5 minutes before chemotherapy begins and retained for 30 minutes. Theoretically, this will reduce blood flow to the mouth, thereby protecting the dividing cell population from toxins.

Glutamine is an important substrate for rapidly proliferating tissue. In two randomized trials, oral glutamine supplementation was associated with a reduction in the severity and duration of oral pain after chemotherapy.[46,47] In one trial of bone marrow transplant (BMT) recipients, glutamine significantly reduced the severity and duration of oropharyngeal mucositis in those who had received autologous transplants, but not in those who had received allogeneic transplants.[47] In contrast, glutamine failed to prevent mucositis in two trials of patients receiving standard-dose fluorouracil-based chemotherapy.[48,49]

Chlorhexidine gluconate 0.12% (Peridex, PerioGard) also may reduce the frequency and severity of mucositis infection.[50,51] Unfortunately, not all studies have shown a benefit.

Table 89-2 Guidelines for the Management of Stomatitis

1. Remove dentures to prevent further irritation and tissue damage.
2. Maintain gentle brushing of teeth with a soft toothbrush.
3. Avoid mouthwashes or rinses that contain alcohol because they may be painful and cause drying of the mucosa. Consider normal saline or sodium bicarbonate.
4. Lubricants, such as artificial saliva, may loosen mucus and prevent membranes from sticking together. Avoid mineral oil and petroleum jelly because they can be aspirated.
5. Apply local anesthetics for localized pain control, especially before meals (may add an antacid or an antihistamine). Systemic analgesics may be required to control pain associated with severe mucositis.
6. Ensure that adequate hydration and nutrition are maintained:
   - Eat a bland diet, avoiding spiced, acidic, and salted foods.
   - Avoid rough food; process in a blender if necessary.
   - Use sugar-free gum or sugar-free hard candy to stimulate salivation and facilitate mastication.
   - If necessary, provide intravenous support.
   - Avoid extremely hot or cold foods.
   - Use shakes with nutritional supplements or ice cream.

This solution should be used twice daily as a rinse. Side effects include occasional burning (which is thought to be caused by the product's alcohol content and can be reduced by diluting it with water) and superficial brown tooth staining, which polishes off easily. Chlorhexidine may reduce the frequency and severity of mucositis by eliminating microorganisms in the oral cavity. Growth factors may also provide some benefit by eliminating microorganisms in the mouth. Preliminary and anecdotal data suggest that some growth factors may positively modify mucositis in myelosuppressed patients with cancer.[52]

Despite these prophylactic measures, no methods have a proven effect, so most patients still develop this complication.

Reducing the dose of radiation or chemotherapy decreases the incidence and severity of symptoms, but doing so comes at the risk of compromising treatment outcomes. Stomatitis remains the dose-limiting toxicity for several chemotherapeutic regimens.

Esophagitis

Chemotherapy and radiation therapy also may damage the mucosa lining the esophagus. Although dysphagia is a common symptom reported by patients with esophagitis, other causes of dysphagia should be ruled out. Because patients receiving myelosuppressive chemotherapy could develop infectious esophagitis, bacterial, viral, and fungal cultures should be completed to rule this out before starting treatment for esophagitis. Symptomatic management of esophagitis is similar to the management of mucositis. Other treatment modalities, including behavioral modifications and other medications (e.g., H_2-receptor antagonist, antacids, and proton pump inhibitors) may also help reduce esophageal irritation and improve comfort. Patients with severe esophagitis should be carefully monitored to ensure adequate oral hydration and nutritional intake and instructed to avoid acidic or irritating foods. Symptoms should resolve in 1 to 2 weeks once the bone marrow recovers.

Lower GI Tract Complications

Lower GI tract complications associated with chemotherapy include malabsorption, diarrhea, and constipation. These complications may be related to structural changes that occur to the GI tract after chemotherapy or radiation therapy. Several investigators noted villus atrophy and cessation of mitosis within crypts in patients and animals treated with combination chemotherapy.[53–55] Other investigators noted swelling and dilation of mitochondria and endoplasmic reticulum and shortening of the microvilli. These or other changes to the small and large bowel may cause decreased absorption of medications that are primarily absorbed in the upper portion of the small intestine. Decreased absorption has been documented with several drugs with narrow therapeutic indexes, including phenytoin, verapamil, and digoxin following chemotherapy.[56–58] Patients receiving medications for concurrent illnesses should be carefully monitored for new signs or symptoms of adverse effects.

Chemotherapy-induced intestinal changes also may be responsible for diarrhea, which frequently occurs with regimens containing irinotecan, high-dose cytarabine, or fluorouracil. Unlike diarrhea, constipation is rare. Only the vinca alkaloids, which produce colicky abdominal pain, constipation, and adynamic ileus caused by autonomic nerve dysfunction (see Neurotoxicity), may cause chemotherapy-induced constipation. Unfortunately, the true incidence of diarrhea and constipation associated with chemotherapy is difficult to discern because many medications (e.g., opioid analgesics, antiemetics, antacids) and settings (e.g., immobility) commonly associated with cancer and chemotherapy can cause these symptoms as well.

DIARRHEA

11. B.G., a 60-year-old woman with recurrent colorectal cancer refractory to fluorouracil, is beginning her first course of irinotecan 125 mg/m^2 weekly for 4 weeks followed by a 2-week rest period. What instructions should she receive regarding the management of diarrhea should she experience this complication?

Irinotecan (Camptosar) can cause severe diarrhea both early and late in the course of chemotherapy. The early- and late-onset diarrhea appears to be mediated by different mechanisms. Early-onset diarrhea (within 24 hours after treatment) may be mediated by parasympathetic stimulation. Patients often report other cholinergic symptoms, such as rhinitis, increased salivation, miosis, lacrimation, diaphoresis, flushing, and abdominal cramping as well. These symptoms may be prevented or managed with atropine IV or SC 0.25 to 1 mg. Late-onset diarrhea (generally occurring >24 hours after treatment) can be prolonged leading to dehydration, electrolyte imbalances, and significant morbidity. Patients should promptly receive loperamide (Imodium) 4 mg with the first episode of diarrhea and repeat doses equal to 2 mg every 2 hours until 12 hours have passed without a bowel movement.[59] For patients who do not respond to initial therapy, some clinicians recommend higher doses equal to 4 mg every 2 hours. Fluid and electrolyte replacement should also be administered, if necessary. With the potential severe complications associated with irinotecan-associated diarrhea, prompt treatment cannot be overemphasized.

If a patient fails to respond to adequate doses of loperamide, the somatostatin analog, octreotide (Sandostatin), may be used to manage the diarrhea. A randomized trial comparing loperamide with octreotide in patients with acute leukemia or those undergoing bone marrow transplantation found loperamide to be more effective.[60,61] Nevertheless, some evidence does show that octreotide can be used to successfully manage diarrhea associated with fluorouracil and other high-dose chemotherapy regimens.[62,63] Octreotide produces antisecretory activity in the gut and promotes the absorption of sodium, chloride, and water from luminal content. Patients should receive doses ranging from 100 to 2,000 μg SC three times daily.[63] Although responses seem to correlate with octreotide dose, more studies are needed to determine the optimal dose. Based on current evidence, octreotide should be limited to second-line therapy for chemotherapy-associated diarrhea.

Dermatologic Toxicities

Dermatologic toxicities associated with chemotherapy include alopecia, hypersensitivity reactions, extravasations, and hyperpigmentation. Toxicities, including alopecia, nail changes, dry skin, and blistering, occur when chemotherapy agents reduce or inhibit mitosis in the epidermis and nail matrix. Other chemotherapy agents can cause various skin reactions when they interact with ultraviolet (UV) light or radiation. Dermatologic toxicities also can occur when chemotherapy agents with vesicant properties extravasate from the veins into surrounding soft tissue. In addition, some chemotherapy agents produce specific skin eruptions, nonspecific eruptions, or "rashes" by unknown mechanisms. Several reviews serve as excellent references.[64-66]

Alopecia
PATHOGENESIS

12. C.W., a 45-year-old woman with recently diagnosed breast cancer, had a lumpectomy, which is to be followed by 20 courses of radiation therapy to the affected breast. She will also receive chemotherapy to minimize her risk of recurrence. She is in the clinic today to receive the first of 6 cycles of cyclophosphamide, doxorubicin, and fluorouracil (CAF regimen). Although C.W. had minimal problems with surgery, she particularly fears receiving combination chemotherapy. You start counseling C.W. about the most common toxicities by reviewing the likelihood and management of myelosuppression, nausea, and vomiting. C.W. is appropriately attentive as you discuss these issues with her; however, her overriding concern is whether or not she will lose her hair. Is C.W.'s concern typical of most cancer patients? How would you respond?

C.W.'s concern regarding hair loss is typical of cancer patients starting chemotherapy. In fact, several investigators have reported that hair loss ranks second only to nausea and vomiting as a patient's greatest fear. Because hair bulb cells replicate every 12 to 24 hours, the cells are susceptible to various chemotherapy agents. Normally, hair follicles independently move cyclically through phases of growth (anagen), involution or transition (catagen), and rest (telogen). Although most persons normally lose about 100 scalp hairs a day, patients with cancer can lose substantially more. Because approximately 85% to 90% of hair follicles are in the anagen phase, chemotherapy agents may partially or completely inhibit mitosis or impair metabolic processes in the hair matrix. These effects can cause a thinned or weakened hair shaft or failure to form hair. Even mild trauma, such as normal hair grooming or rubbing the head on a pillow, can fracture the thinned hair shaft and cause hair loss. Hair loss usually begins 7 to 10 days after one treatment, with prominent hair loss noted within 1 or 2 months. Other terminal hairs, such as beards, eyebrows, eyelashes, axillary, and pubic hair can be affected; however, these effects are somewhat variable, depending on the rate of mitosis and the percentage of hairs in the anagen phase.[64-66]

C.W. should be informed about the expected onset of hair loss, and she should be reassured that alopecia caused by chemotherapy is reversible. She can expect her hair to begin regenerating 1 to 2 months after therapy is completed. The color and texture of her hair may be altered; the new hair may be lighter, darker, or curlier as it regrows. Agents most commonly associated with severe alopecia are listed in Table 89-3.

PREVENTION

Several interventions have been proposed to prevent scalp hair loss during chemotherapy. These procedures attempt to prevent chemotherapy agents from circulating to the hair follicles with either an occlusive scalp tourniquet or an ice cap that produces a localized hypothermia and vasoconstriction. These

Table 89-3 Single Agents Associated With Alopecia Pigmentation Changes and Nail Disorders

	Frequent	Occasional
Alopecia[a]	Cyclophosphamide	Mechlorethamine
	Ifosfamide	Thiotepa
	Fluorouracil	Methotrexate
	Dactinomycin	Vinblastine
	Daunorubicin	Vincristine
	Doxorubicin	Etoposide
	Bleomycin	Carmustine
	Vindesine	Hydroxyurea
	Paclitaxel	Cytarabine
	Irinotecan	Topotecan
	Epirubicin	Gemcitabine
	Docetaxel	
Pigmentation	Busulfan	Cyclophosphamide
	Fluorouracil	Methotrexate
	Doxorubicin	Dactinomycin
	Bleomycin	Daunorubicin
	Epirubicin	Hydroxyurea
		Ifosfamide
		Thiotepa
Nail		Cyclophosphamide
		Fluorouracil
		Daunorubicin
		Doxorubicin
		Bleomycin
		Hydroxyurea
		Epirubicin
		Docetaxel
		Paclitaxel

[a]Degree and onset of alopecia depend on dose, schedule of administration, rate and route of delivery, and various combinations of agents.

interventions should be initiated before chemotherapy is begun and maintained for several hours after the time of peak concentration. Recognizing that such devices create a refuge for tumor cells, these procedures are contraindicated in patients with hematologic malignancies and in others at risk for scalp metastases. Although these scalp devices were manufactured and marketed by several U.S. companies for several years, the FDA did not review them until the early 1990s. They became concerned that the safety and efficacy of these devices had not been substantiated by adequate clinical data[67-71] and requested evidence or data to address the following concerns:

- The potential for scalp metastases posed by the use of these devices
- The potential for reducing agent circulation to other anatomic sites beyond the scalp, such as the skull and possibly the brain
- The effectiveness of these devices in preventing hair loss and how specific cytotoxic doses and other variables affected the results achieved

To date, no company has come forward with clinical evidence supporting the safety and effectiveness of these devices. Although they are no longer commercially available, there are other ways to induce scalp hypothermia or create a scalp tourniquet. The questions of safety and efficacy raised by the FDA should be discussed with patients seeking infor-

mation about these devices and hair preservation techniques.[67-71]

C.W.'s concern is a legitimate one expressed by many patients with cancer, not just patients with breast cancer. Unfortunately, she is likely to experience near or complete hair loss, depending on the thickness of her hair and its growth rate. She should be told how to minimize the effect of alopecia on her appearance through the use of hair pieces or stylish head scarves, turbans, or hats. She also should be referred to volunteer groups and organizations that can help her through this difficult time. For example, several small private businesses have been started by former patients who distribute or sell various hair coverings. Hair pieces are tax deductible as a medical expense and are covered by some health insurance policies. If C.W. thinks she will use a hair piece, she should be advised to select a wig before hair loss begins. Other resources include the American Cancer Society's rehabilitation program called "Look Good Feel Better," which was developed to assist women compensating for hair loss and skin changes during cancer treatment. Also, the American Cancer Society Hot-Line (1-800-395-LOOK) can help C.W. find volunteer beauticians and cosmetologists who help women look and feel more comfortable with changes in their appearance caused by chemotherapy, including dry, discolored, or blotching skin; discolored nails; and alopecia. (See Table 89-4 for other resources for breast cancer patients.)

Table 89-4 Information and Toll-Free Hotlines for Cancer Support

Toll-Free Hotlines

The American Cancer Society's (ACS) National Toll-Free Hotline: 800-ACS-2345

The American College of Radiology (ACR): 800-648-8900

The American Society of Plastic and Reconstructive Surgeons: 800-635-0635

Breast Settlement Information Line: 800-887-6828

The FDA Breast Implant Hotline: 800-532-4440

National Bone Marrow Transplant Link: 800-546-5268

The National Cancer Institute (NCI): 800-4-CANCER

The National Cancer Information Service (NCI): 800-4-CANCER

The National Consumer Insurance Helpline (HIAA): 800-942-4242

The National Council Against Health Fraud: 800-821-6671

The National Lymphedema Network: 800-541-3259

PDQ (Physicians Data Query): 800-4-CANCER

The Susan Komen Alliance Treatment and Information Line: 800-462-9273 [800-I'M AWARE]

The Susan G. Komen Breast Cancer Foundation: 800-462-9273 [800-I'M AWARE]

The Y-ME National Organization for Breast Cancer Information and Support's National Toll-free Hotline: 800-221-2141[a]

Organizations for Information and Support

Cancer Care, Inc., and the National Cancer Care Foundation: 212-221-3300

Cancer Research Council: 301-654-7933

The Chemotherapy Foundation: 212-213-9292

The Health Insurance Association of America (HIAA): 202-866-6244

The National Alliance of Breast Cancer Organizations (NABCO): 212-719-0154

The National Breast Cancer Coalition: 202-296-7477

The National Coalition for Cancer Survivorship: 505-764-9956

[a]A support line for husbands.

Skin and Nail Changes

13. Besides alopecia, what other skin or nail changes should C.W. anticipate?

Several skin and nail changes have been associated with chemotherapy, which C.W. may find disturbing. Fortunately, the major consequences of these toxicities are cosmetic and they usually resolve within 6 to 12 months after discontinuing chemotherapy.

NAIL CHANGES

The growth of fingernails and toenails is arrested in a manner similar to hair growth. A reduction or a cessation of mitotic activity in the nail matrix causes a horizontal depression of the nail plate. Within weeks, these pale horizontal lines ("Beau's lines") begin to appear in the nail beds. They are most commonly seen in patients receiving chemotherapy for ≥6 months. These growth arrest lines move distally as the nail grows and normally disappear from the fingernails in approximately 6 months. Some other nail pigmentation changes that can occur following therapy with cyclophosphamide, fluorouracil, daunorubicin, doxorubicin, and bleomycin are less well understood.[72–79] Brown or blue lines deposit as horizontal or vertical bands in the nails. These lines are seen more commonly in dark-skinned patients.[78] Like Beau's lines, these pigmentation lines generally grow out with the nail.

DERMATOLOGIC PIGMENT CHANGES

Dermatologic pigment changes are among the most common and least well understood side effects of chemotherapy. Hypopigmentation has been reported occasionally in patients receiving chemotherapy, but hyperpigmentation is most frequently reported. Usually, hyperpigmentation is not associated with an identifiable cause or systemic toxicity. It usually occurs following treatment with a wide variety of chemotherapy agents, including antitumor antibiotics, alkylating agents, and antimetabolites. Most agents cause a diffuse, generalized hyperpigmentation, but the pigmentation changes may also be localized, involving only the mucous membrane, hair, or nails. Busulfan, cyclophosphamide, fluorouracil, dactinomycin, and hydroxyurea are examples of specific agents that can cause widespread cutaneous hyperpigmentation.[80–85] Patients receiving busulfan may also experience an addisonian-like syndrome consisting of diffuse cutaneous hyperpigmentation, weakness, weight loss, and diarrhea. Unfortunately, pulmonary fibrosis is more common in patients with this type of hyperpigmentation.[66] Usually, the pigmentation normalizes when busulfan is discontinued. Despite extensive evaluation, no endocrine abnormalities consistent with Addison's disease have been documented with busulfan.

Various chemotherapy agents may cause significantly diverse patterns of hyperpigmentation. A peculiar serpiginous hyperpigmentation can occur over veins used to administer fluorouracil and bleomycin.[79–87] Some investigators have attributed this phenomenon to a subclinical phlebitis. Hyperpigmentation has also been noted over pressure points after the use of bleomycin. Patients receiving hydroxyurea often show hyperpigmentation more prominently in traumatized areas. Bleomycin may also cause peculiar linear or flagellate streaks of hyperpigmentation. Because of their characteristic location and appearance, these streaks may result from scratching during therapy; however, attempts to reproduce these lesions iatrogenically have not been successful. Thiotepa has been reported to cause hyperpigmentation in areas of skin occluded by bandages, which may be caused by secretion of thiotepa in sweat.[88] Interestingly, skin contact with thiotepa has been reported to cause hypopigmentation.[89] Topical contact with mechlorethamine and carmustine also has caused hyperpigmentation.[90,91] Although hyperpigmentation reactions commonly affect the skin, some rare reactions are noted in hair. Methotrexate can cause hyperpigmented banding of light-colored hair. This phenomenon has been described in a patient receiving intermittent high-dose methotrexate and has been referred to by some investigators as the "flag sign" of chemotherapy.[92] To minimize a patient's concern regarding these pigment changes, they should receive counseling before treatment.

As previously stated, pigment changes that occur in patients receiving chemotherapy are basically a cosmetic concern. It is important to anticipate these distressing side effects and educate patients in appropriate cases. At this time, C.W. should receive counseling, explaining that these side effects may occur because she will be receiving several agents that have been implicated in producing both diffuse, as well as localized, cutaneous nail hyperpigmentation. She should be reassured that pigment changes usually resolve with time.

HAND–FOOT SYNDROME

Some patients receiving chemotherapy may develop tender, erythematous skin on the palms of their hands and sometimes on the soles of their feet. Patients may also complain of tingling, burning, or shooting sensations in their hands or feet usually not described as painful. These signs and symptoms may resolve after several days, or they may progress to bullous lesions that can desquamate. This reaction is referred to as *chemotherapy-associated acral erythema* or *the palmar-plantar erythrodysesthesia syndrome.* Agents reported to cause this reaction include cytarabine, fluorouracil, doxorubicin, methotrexate, capecitabine, and hydroxyurea.[65,66] Most of the reported cases involve patients with leukemia receiving bone marrow transplants or blood products or patients receiving continuous infusions or large doses of the chemotherapy agents previously listed. No specific therapy exists for hand–foot syndrome. Typically, the offending agent is discontinued at least until recovery occurs.

ACNEIFORM–ERYTHEMATOUS RASH

The most common toxicities reported with the new epidermal growth factor receptor (EGFR) inhibitors are skin related and are probably due to inhibition of the tyrosine kinase pathways in EGFR-dependent tissues. Several EGFR inhibitors are currently in clinical development. These include small molecule tyrosine kinase inhibitors that target the intracellular domain of the EGFR (e.g., gefitinib, Iressa; AstraZeneca Pharmaceuticals LP, Wilmington, DE and OSI-774), and monoclonal antibodies that target the extracellular domain (e.g., IMC-C225 and ABX-EGF), as well as pan-EGFR inhibitors that target more than one receptor (e.g., CI-1033 and GW572016). Skin effects associated with treatment with gefitinab have consisted of a characteristic acnelike or erythematous rashes primarily in the facial area. The rashes were predominantly grade 1 or 2 in severity, sometimes associated with dry skin and itching, did not worsen over time, and completely resolved without sequelae when the drug was discontinued. No patients discontinued treatment because of rash at the recommended dose of 250 mg/day. Steroid creams, topical or systemic antibiotics (such as the ones used for teenage acne), topical or systemic antihistamines (e.g., diphenhydramine) and occasionally retinoid creams have all been used to manage gefitinib-related skin changes. All these agents have demonstrated activity in some patients, but none has worked consistently in all. Therefore, if one agent is not successful, alternative agents may be tried.

DRY SKIN

Many chemotherapy agents (especially bleomycin, hydroxyurea, and fluorouracil) can cause dry skin with fine scaling on the surface. Normally, sebaceous and sweat glands provide lipids, lactates, and other products that contribute to the pliability and moisture retention of the stratum corneum. In patients receiving chemotherapy, the dry skin may be caused by the cytostatic effect of chemotherapy agents on sebaceous and sweat glands. Topical application of emollient creams may provide some symptomatic relief of this dryness.

Interactions With Radiation Therapy

14. **C.W. recently completed her course of total breast radiation therapy. She also plans to leave for a 1-week vacation in Florida 3 days after this clinic visit. Are there any interactions between radiation therapy and sunlight exposure with chemotherapy agents? Are there any specific precautions C.W. should take, or signs and symptoms of toxicity that she should know about?**

The interactions between chemotherapy and radiation therapy or UV light (from both external beam and natural sources) can be divided into radiation enhancement, radiation recall, photosensitivity reactions, and sunburn reactivation (Table 89-5). Several excellent reviews are available that describe each of these interactions in great detail. A discussion of the important principles of the interaction between radiation therapy and chemotherapy follows.[64-66]

A synergistic interaction between a small number of chemotherapy agents and radiation therapy results in an en-

hanced radiation effect. This may be caused by an agent's ability to interfere with radiation repair. Radiation therapy can alter the molecular structure of DNA, but excision repair allows cells to remove small damaged portions of one strand of DNA and insert new bases using the other strand as a template. This repair mechanism requires several enzymes, including DNA polymerase. Chemotherapy agents may interfere with some of the enzymes and synthetic mechanisms needed to rejuvenate damaged cells. Although the synergistic effects of radiation therapy and chemotherapy are often exploited therapeutically for the treatment of solid tumors, these reactions can inadvertently cause undesirable reactions in nonneoplastic tissues, such as the skin, esophagus, lung, and GI tract. The skin is the most common target of radiation reactions. These reactions can produce severe tissue necrosis, which can compromise organ function and delay or mandate discontinuation of future treatment courses.

These reactions may be further classified as either radiation enhancement or radiation recall reactions. The primary distinction between radiation enhancement reactions and radiation recall reactions lies in the temporal relationship between radiation therapy and chemotherapy. Generally, enhancement reactions occur when chemotherapy is given concurrently or within 1 week of radiation therapy. In comparison, recall reactions occur several weeks to years after radiation therapy, when a chemotherapy agent causes an inflammatory reaction in tissues previously treated with radiation. Radiation recall is independent of previous, clinically apparent radiation damage. Not surprisingly, the chemotherapy agents that have been associated with radiation recall reactions are the same as those that cause radiation enhancement reactions. Agents most commonly associated with these reactions include the antitumor antibiotics dactinomycin, epirubicin, and doxorubicin; however, other agents, such as bleomycin, fluorouracil, capecitabine, hydroxyurea, methotrexate, etoposide, vinblastine, and paclitaxel, also may cause radiation reactions. Chemotherapy may also interact with UV light to cause similar reactions.

Because ultraviolet light has sufficient energy to cause photochemical changes in biologic molecules, chemotherapy agents can interact with UV light. The subsequent reactions are usually less severe than reactions that occur with radiation therapy, and they may be caused by a different mechanism. Photosensitivity reactions, defined as enhanced erythema responses to UV light, have been reported with dacarbazine, fluorouracil, methotrexate, and vinblastine. Methotrexate may also reactivate sunburns, causing a similar, but less severe reaction compared with the radiation recall reactions described previously. The reaction may be more severe than the initial sunburn, resulting in severe blisters, and it usually occurs only in patients who receive large doses of methotrexate. Although the precise incidences of photosensitivity reactions caused by chemotherapy agents are unknown, they may be more common than generally believed. For example, photosensitivity may account for many of the erythematous periodic rashes attributed to allergy.

C.W. received doxorubicin and fluorouracil, both of which can interact with radiation therapy. Although not commonly reported, doxorubicin also may cause some increased erythema in the specific area of skin treated with radiation. Because C.W. may have an increased risk for a photosensitivity

Table 89-5	Chemotherapy and Radiation Reactions	
Radiation Enhancement Reactions		
Bleomycin	Doxorubicin	Hydroxyurea
Dactinomycin	Fluorouracil	Methotrexate
Etoposide		
Radiation Recall Reactions		
All of the above plus		
Vinblastine	Epirubicin	Capecitabine
Etoposide	Paclitaxel	
Reactions With Ultraviolet Light		
Phototoxic reactions		
Dacarbazine	Thioguanine	Methotrexate
Fluorouracil	Vinblastine	Mitomycin
Reactivation of sunburn		
Methotrexate		

reaction, she should be advised to avoid direct exposure to the sunlight for several days to a week after chemotherapy. Although no data exist regarding the efficacy of sunscreens in this patient population, C.W. should be advised to use a protective sunscreen with a high sun protective factor (SPF) when she cannot avoid sun exposure. Furthermore, she should periodically assess her skin's reaction to the sun with intermittent periods of rest and observation throughout the day.

15. How will C.W. know if she has a radiation reaction? How should she be managed if such a reaction occurs?

If C.W. has a radiation reaction, she will experience "easy burning" and erythema or redness, followed by dry desquamation. With a more severe reaction, small blisters (vesicles) and oozing can develop. Necrosis with persistent painful ulceration may also occur in more severe cases. Postinflammatory hyperpigmentation or depigmentation may follow. The severity of the reaction can help determine the best treatment option.

Treatment options may vary, depending on the severity of the reaction. Milder cases can be treated with topical steroids in an emollient cream base and cool wet compresses. Unfortunately, necrosis and ulcers are notoriously difficult to treat because radiated skin does not heal well. Ulcers are often treated with surgical debridement to keep the ulcer clean. Even when the ulcers are clean, exudation and bacterial contamination may be persistent. Radiation reactions that occur in tissues other than the skin (e.g., the lungs, esophagus, GI tract) often are managed with oral corticosteroids, although data regarding the efficacy of these agents in ameliorating the symptoms or reducing the extent of damage are lacking. If C.W. experiences any of these signs or symptoms, she should immediately seek medical attention.

Irritant and Vesicant Reactions

16. C.W. complained of pain and burning at the injection site immediately following the administration of her third course of IV chemotherapy with cyclophosphamide, doxorubicin, and fluorouracil. She described the sensation as being distinctly different from the mild discomfort she had experienced with previous chemotherapy. Physical examination of the injection site revealed mild erythema and slight induration. What types of local reactions can occur after the administration of chemotherapy?

Several distinct types of local reactions (ranging from transient local irritation to severe tissue necrosis of the skin, surrounding vasculature, and supporting structures) have been reported following chemotherapy[93,94] (Table 89-6). Some of these reactions (particularly those associated with anthracyclines) may be caused by local hypersensitivity reactions. These reactions usually are characterized by immediate local burning, itching, and erythema. Some patients may also experience a "flare" reaction along the length of the vein used for treatment. Hypersensitivity reactions usually are self-limited and subside within a few hours. Administration of the antihistamine, diphenhydramine, before the next course of chemotherapy may reduce the severity or duration of hypersensitivity reactions.[95,96] More severe reactions, including irritation of the vein (or phlebitis) caused by the irritant properties of an agent or a diluent, can occur following chemotherapy.

Table 89-6	Chemotherapeutic Drugs Reported to Produce Local Toxicities
Potential Vesicants	
Dactinomycin	Plicamycin
Daunorubicin	Streptozocin
Doxorubicin	Vinblastine
Idarubicin	Vincristine
Mechlorethamine	Paclitaxel
Mitomycin	Oxaloplatin
Potential Irritants	
Carmustine	Etoposide
Cisplatin	Mitoxantrone
Dacarbazine	Melphalan
Vinorelabine	Vindesine
Drugs That Produce Local Hypersensitivity Reactions	
Daunorubicin	Mechlorethamine
Doxorubicin	Docetaxel
Idarubicin	

Local reactions resulting from the extravasation of agents with vesicant or irritant properties may be more severe. All agents with vesicant properties potentially can produce these devastating reactions. Agents known to bind to DNA (i.e., the anthracyclines) have the propensity to produce the most severe damage. Treatment with a chemotherapy agent with these properties may produce phlebitis and pain, and extravasations may cause local irritation or soft tissue ulcers, depending on the amount, agent, and concentration extravasated. In addition, there is no clear agreement regarding the vesicant potential of many chemotherapy agents, and various references may categorize agents differently based on their vesicant or irritant properties. Initially, it may be impossible to distinguish a local irritant reaction from a vesicant extravasation; therefore, if an agent with vesicant or irritant properties has been administered, the reaction should be treated as a potential extravasation.

Patients who experience an extravasation can show a range of different signs or symptoms. Infiltration of a vesicant into tissue often produces a severe burning sensation that may persist for hours. However, in some cases no immediate symptoms or signs are evident. In the days to weeks that follow, the skin overlying the extravasation site may become reddened and firm. The redness may gradually diminish or progress to ulceration and necrosis. Histologically, inflammatory cells rarely are observed in either human tissue samples or experimental animal models.[97,98]

17. What factors increase the risk of extravasation, and what administration techniques and precautions can minimize these risks?

Several factors have been associated with an increased risk of extravasation and subsequent tissue damage following administration of chemotherapy. Risk factors include (1) generalized vascular disease commonly found in elderly and debilitated patients or in patients who have undergone frequent venipuncture and treatment with irritating chemotherapy (the latter causes venous fragility and instability or decreased local blood flow); (2) elevated venous pressure, which typically occurs in patients with an obstructed superior vena cava or venous drainage after axillary dissection; (3) prior radiation therapy to the injection site; (4) recent venipuncture in the same vein; and (5) use of injection sites over joints, which increases the risk of needle dislodgement.[99,100] In addition, tissue damage may be more severe if extravasation occurs in areas with only a small amount of subcutaneous tissue (e.g., the back of the hand or wrist) because wound healing is more difficult and exposure of deeper structures, such as the tendons, is increased.[96] Also, in an experimental model, the size and healing times for skin ulcers increased with the volume and concentration of doxorubicin administered.[101] These risks have led to the increased use of indwelling central catheters in patients receiving vesicant chemotherapy.

Extravasations of agents with vesicant properties can produce devastating tissue damage that can potentially cause loss of an extremity or death. To prevent significant morbidity or mortality, major emphasis must be placed on prevention. All caretakers who administer agents with vesicant or irritant properties should be skilled in IV drug administration and receive special instruction before administering these agents. The patient also must be told how agent administration should feel and to report immediately any change in sensation, including pain, burning, or itching. Recommendations to reduce the risk of local complications during cytotoxic agent administration are outlined in Table 89-7.

18. The oncology nurse believes that the doxorubicin may have extravasated during C.W.'s chemotherapy administration. How should this be managed? Do management guidelines differ for other vesicant agents?

Immediate management of a potential vesicant extravasation should include stopping the injection if all of the agent has not been administered. Various other recommended measures may minimize vesicant exposure and subsequent tissue damage (Table 89-8). These include application of cold compresses to the extravasation site and elevation of the extremity. Warm compresses are recommended for vinca alkaloids and epipodophyllotoxins.[93,94] Specific antidotes thought to inactivate the extravasated agent have been suggested; however, many of these antidotes are based on observations in few patients or animal models, and their effectiveness, in many cases, is unsubstantiated. Some have suggested that antidotes recommended in some guidelines may actually worsen tissue damage (e.g., sodium bicarbonate for doxorubicin). Recommended treatments for suspected extravasation of vesicant agents are outlined in Table 89-9.[93,94]

Because doxorubicin skin damage may be related to the formation of toxic free oxygen radicals, a free radical scavenger may prevent ulceration. Dimethylsulfoxide (DMSO) is a potent free radical scavenger that penetrates all tissue planes. In pig and rat models, topical DMSO has decreased doxorubicin-induced skin ulcers.[103] Several series of case reports and a single-arm clinical study have reported that topical application of DMSO can safely and effectively manage an extravasation with an anthracycline.[104–109] DMSO also has been reported to be beneficial in patients with mitomycin extravasations.[108]

Table 89-7   Guidelines for Administration of Cytotoxic Agents[89,90,92]

Administration of chemotherapy should be performed only by persons familiar with its toxic effects.

The site of infusion is selected with consideration of visualization of the vessel, its size, and potential damage if extravasation occurs in the following order of preference: forearm > dorsum of the hand > wrist > antecubital fossa.

- Limbs with compromised circulation (e.g., invading neoplasm, axillary dissection, severe bruising) should not be used.
- The lower extremities should not be used.
- Pre-existing IV lines should not be used because the site may already have occult vein or tissue irritation or phlebitis.

A 23-or 25-gauge scalp vein ("butterfly") needle is inserted into the vein. Only 1 venipuncture should be performed on a vein to avoid leakage.

The wings of the needle should be lightly taped in place with care not to obscure the injection site so that it may be visualized during injection.

Test the integrity of the IV line by injecting a small volume of saline solution and withdrawing a small amount of blood. If extravasation of the saline is obvious, select another vein or a site proximal on the same vein to avoid upstream leakage.

Administer the drug at the recommended rate (preferably through the tubing of an IV running by gravity to assess for back pressure).

During the administration, question the patient about discomfort, check for blood return by aspirating the syringe gently, observe the continuous flow of the running IV, and visualize the IV site frequently. If the patency of the line is in doubt at any time, the injection should be stopped and an alternate site selected.

After administration, the IV line should be flushed with at least 10 mL of saline or other IV fluid to flush the needle and tubing of all drug.

If multiple drugs are to be given, the IV should be flushed between each drug.

Apply pressure with sterile gauze for 3–4 minutes after the needle is removed. Inspect the site before applying a bandage.

IV, intravenous.

Table 89-8   Suggested Procedures for Management of Suspected Extravasation of Vesicant Drugs[89,90,92]

1. Stop the injection immediately, but do not remove the needle. Any drug remaining in the tubing or needle, as well as the infiltrated area, should be aspirated.
2. Contact a physician as soon as possible.
3. If deemed appropriate, instill an antidote in the infiltrated areas (via the extravasated IV needle if possible).
4. Remove the needle.
5. Apply ice to the site and elevate the extremity for the first 24 to 48 hr (if vinca or podophyllotoxin, use warm compresses).
6. Document the drug, suspected volume extravasated, and the treatment in the patient's medical record.
7. Check the site frequently for 5–7 days.
8. Consult a surgeon familiar with extravasations early so that he or she can periodically review the site, and if ulceration begins, the surgeon can rapidly assess if surgical debridement or excision is necessary.

Table 89-9   Recommended Extravasation Antidotes[a]

Class/Specific Agents	Local Antidote Recommended	Specific Procedure

Alkylating Agents
  Cisplatin[a]
  Oxaloplatin
  Mechlorethamine
	1/6 or 1/3 M solution sodium thiosulfate	Mix 4–8 mL 10% sodium thiosulfate USP with 6 mL of sterile water for injection, USP for a 1/6 or 1/3 M solution. Into site, inject 2 mL for each mg of mechlorethamine or 100 mg of cisplatin extravasated.

Mitomycin-C	Dimethylsulfoxide 50–99% (w/v)	Apply 1–2 mL to the site Q 6 hr for 14 days. Allow to air-dry; do not cover.

DNA intercalators
  Doxorubicin
  Daunorubicin
	Cold compresses
	Dimethylsulfoxidle 50–99% (w/v)
		Apply immediately for 30–60 min for 1 day.
		Apply 1–2 mL to the site Q 6 hr for 14 days. Allow to air dry; do not cover.

Vinca alkaloids
  Vinblastine
  Vincristine
	Warm compresses
	Hyaluronidase
		Apply immediately for 30–60 min, then alternate off/on every 15 min for 1 day.
		Inject 150 U into site.
		Apply immediately for 30–60 min, then alternate off/on every 15 min for 1 day.

Epipodophyllotoxins[a]
  Etoposide
  Teniposide
	Warm compresses
	Hyaluronidase
		Inject 150 U into site.
		Dilute 150 U in 3 mL NS; inject locally into site.

Paclitaxel	Hyaluronidase	

[a]Treatment indicated only for large extravasations (e.g., doses one-half or more of the planned total dose for the course of therapy).
NS, normal saline; w/v, weight per volume.
Reprinted with permission from reference 93.

Hypersensitivity Reactions

All cancer chemotherapy agents except altretamine, the nitrosureas, and dactinomycin, have produced at least an isolated instance of a hypersensitivity reaction.[102–110] All types of hypersensitivity reactions can occur with chemotherapy agents, although type 1 is the most common reaction documented following chemotherapy. Type 1 hypersensitivity reactions occur when an antigen interacts with IgE bound to a mast cell membrane, causing degranulation of mast cells. Major signs and symptoms of type 1 reactions include urticaria, angioedema, rash, bronchospasm, abdominal cramping, and hypotension. Although many reactions associated with chemotherapy agents probably are immunologically mediated, other mechanisms may cause type 1 reactions. Other mechanisms include the degranulation of mast cells and basophils through a direct effect on the cell surface that releases histamine and other vasoactive substances. Activation of the alternative complement pathway also can release vasoactive substances from mast cells. When non–IgE-mediated mechanisms account for the symptoms of a type 1 reaction, it is called an *anaphylactoid reaction.*

Many of the type 1 hypersensitivity reactions produced by chemotherapy agents appear to be mediated by non-IgE mechanisms. Although there is little research on the mechanism of these reactions, two features suggest that they are not mediated by IgE. First, many reactions occur after the first dose. This is in contrast to immunologic reactions that require prior exposure (i.e., one must be sensitized before becoming hypersensitized). In addition, certain symptoms or symptom complexes are more diagnostic of immunologically mediated disorders. These symptoms include urticaria, angioedema, bronchospasm, laryngeal spasm, cytopenias, arthritis, mucositis, vasculitic syndromes, and vesicular dermatitis. If a patient did not experience any of these symptoms after the first dose, he or she most likely did not experience an immunologically mediated hypersensitivity reaction.

Although the spectrum of symptoms and their severity varies widely in the case reports, most hypersensitivity reactions that occur with chemotherapy agents are classified as grade 1 (transient rash, mild) or grade 2 (mild bronchospasm, moderate) by the National Cancer Institute (NCI) Common Toxicity Criteria. Furthermore, a patient who has had a reaction to an agent safely can receive future courses of chemotherapy if he or she receives appropriate premedication. For example, appropriate premedication allows many (>60%) patients who have previously experienced a hypersensitivity reaction secondary to paclitaxel to continue therapy; this also reduces the incidence of hypersensitivity reactions associated with short duration of infusion (i.e., 3 hours). (See Table 89-10 for NCI common toxicity criteria.) Other chemotherapy agents can commonly cause hypersensitivity reactions after the first and subsequent doses of chemotherapy.

Chemotherapy agents most frequently reported to produce hypersensitivity reactions and their characteristic reactions are listed in Table 89-11. Unfortunately, most valuable information stems from patient series and case reports and often provides conflicting and contradictory information, particularly with respect to incidence, severity, characteristic symptoms, time course, and the success of rechallenge. If a patient experiences a hypersensitivity reaction and the clinician opts to continue therapy with this regimen, a full review of all of the relevant literature as well as manufacturer's data is advised. Several excellent reviews are available to assist in this effort.[92,100]

Some newer chemotherapy agents, such as rituximab (Rituxan) and trastuzumab (Herceptin), can cause more hypersensitivity reactions than the traditional chemotherapy agents. This is because these agents are genetically engineered humanized monoclonal antibodies containing foreign proteins that can trigger the reaction. During the first infusion with trastuzumab, approximately 40% of patients experience a symptom complex, mild to moderate in severity, which con-

Table 89-10   **National Cancer Institute Common Toxicity Criteria**

Toxicity[a]	Grade 0	Grade 1	Grade 2	Grade 3	Grade 4
Hematologic					
WBC	≥4.0	3.0–3.9	2.0–2.9	1.0–1.9	<1.0
Platelets	WNL	75.0–normal	50.0–74.9	25.0–49.9	<25.0
Hgb g/100 mL	WNL	10.0–normal	8.0–10.0	6.5–7.9	<6.5
g/L	WNL	100–normal	80–100	65–79	<65
mmol/L	WNL	6.2–normal	4.95–6.2	4.0–4.9	<4.0
Granulocytes/bands	≥2.0	1.5–1.9	1.0–1.4	0.5–0.9	<0.5
Lymphocytes	≥2.0	1.5–1.9	1.0–1.4	0.5–0.9	<0.5
Hematologic (other)	None	Mild	Moderate	Severe	Life-threatening
Hemorrhage (Clinical)	None	Mild, no transfusion	Gross, 1–2 units transfusion per episode	Gross, 3–4 units transfusion per episode	Massive, >4 units transfusion per episode
Infection	None	Mild, no active treatment	Moderate, PO antibiotic	Severe, IV antibiotic, antifungal, or hospitalization	Life-threatening
Gastrointestinal					
Nausea	None	Can eat reasonable intake	Intake significantly but can eat	No significant intake	—
Vomiting	None	1 episode in 24 hr	2–5 episodes in 24 hr	6–10 episodes in 24 hr	>10 episodes in 24 hr or requiring parenteral support
Diarrhea	None	↑ of 2–3 stools/day over pretreatment	↑ of 4–6 stools/day or nocturnal stools, or moderate cramping	↑ of 7–9 stools/day or incontinence, or severe cramping	↑ of ≥10 stools/day or grossly bloody diarrhea, or need for parenteral support

IV, intravenous; PO, orally; WBC, white blood cell; WNL, within normal limits.

sists of chills and/or fever. These symptoms usually do not recur with subsequent injections.[146] In comparison, approximately 80% of patients receiving rituximab may experience an infusion-related reaction ranging from fever, chills, and rigors to severe reactions (7%) characterized by hypoxia, pulmonary infiltrates, adult respiratory distress syndrome, myocardial infarction, ventricular fibrillation, or cardiogenic shock with the first dose. Approximately 40% of patients receiving rituximab develop infusion-related reactions with subsequent infusions (5% to 10% severe).[145] Treatment of these reactions follows the recommendations for treatment of hypersensitivity reactions that occur with more traditional agents.

Recommended treatment of hypersensitivity reactions is reviewed in Table 89-12. If a patient develops a severe type 1 hypersensitivity reaction to any chemotherapy agent, the treatment should be stopped. If a structural analog or another agent in the same chemical class is an effective treatment for the same cancer, subsequent therapy should use the analog or other agent to minimize the risk of future reactions. If the reaction is mild or moderate, the patient may continue with the same chemotherapy if treatment is preceded by methods to prevent or minimize hypersensitivity reactions. General rec-

ommendations for preventing anaphylactoid reactions are found in Table 89-11. Although the true type 1 anaphylactic reactions seldom are circumvented by preventive measures, pretreatment with antihistamines and corticosteroids may reduce the incidence and severity of type 1 anaphylactoid reactions caused by roentgenographic contrast agents.[150,151] Despite evidence showing pretreatment with prednisone and diphenhydramine causes a significant decrease in the frequency and severity of anaphylactoid reactions, the effect of H_2-receptor antagonists and ephedrine remains controversial. Because the success of these preventive measures depends on the cause of the reaction (immunologic or anaphylactoid), the aforementioned characteristics of type 1 reactions should be used to assess the underlying pathogenesis. In addition, other chemicals present in the formulation or other agents administered concomitantly with the chemotherapy may cause the hypersensitivity reaction. Potential allergens included in the diluent or formulation of chemotherapy agents include Cremophor EL (present in paclitaxel and teniposide) and benzyl alcohol (present in the parenteral form of methotrexate and cytarabine). Recognizing potential allergens can significantly affect treatment of the current reaction and minimize the risk of future reactions.

Table 89-11 Cancer Chemotherapeutic Agents Commonly Causing Hypersensitivity

Drug	Frequency	Risk Factors	Manifestations	Mechanism	Comments
L-Asparaginase[110-114]	10–20%	Increasing doses; interval (weeks to months) between doses; IV administration; history of atopy/allergy; use without prednisone 6-MP and/or vincristine	Pruritus, dyspnea, agitation, urticaria, angioedema, laryngeal spasm	Type I	Substitute PEG-L-asparaginase, but up to 32% may demonstrate mild hypersensitivity
Paclitaxel[115,116]	Up to 10% first or second dose	None known	Rashes, dyspnea, bronchospasm, hypotension	Nonspecific release of mediators; ? Cremophor	Premedicate with diphenhydramine corticosteroids, and H$_2$-receptor antagonists
Teniposide[117-122]	6–40%; can occur with first dose	Increasing doses or number of doses; young age/leukemia	Dyspnea, wheezing, hypotension, rash, facial flushing	Type I versus nonspecific; ? Cremophor	Etoposide may be substituted in some cases; decrease rate of infusion
Cisplatin[123-128]	Up to 20% intravesicular 5–10% systemic; case reports of hemolytic anemia	Increasing number of doses Anemia: None known	Rash, urticaria, bronchospasm Anemia: Hemolytic anemia	Type I Anemia: Type III	Carboplatin may be substituted in some cases but cross-reactivity has been reported
Procarbazine[129-134]	Up to 15% case reports	None known	Urticaria Pneumonitis	Type I Type III	All patients rechallenged have prompt return of symptoms
Anthracyclines[135-141]	1–15% depending on anthracycline	None known	Dyspnea, bronchospasm, angioedema	Unknown; ? nonspecific release	Cross-reactivity documented, but incidence and likelihood unknown
Bleomycin[142-144]	Common	Lymphoma	Fever (up to 42°C), tachypnea	Endogenous pyrogen release	Not technically classified as HSR; premedicate with acetaminophen and diphenhydramine
Rituximab[145]	First treatment 80%; subsequent treatments 40%	Female gender, pulmonary infiltrates, CLL or mantle cell lymphoma	Fevers, chills, occasional nausea, urticaria, fatigue, headache, pain, pruritis, bronchospasm, SOB, angioedema, rhinitis, vomiting, ↓ BP, flushing	Unknown; ? related to manufacturing process	Stop or ↓ infusion rate by 50%; provide supportive care with IV fluids, acetaminophen, diphenhydramine, vasopressors PRN
Trastuzamab[146]	First treatment 40%; subsequent treatments rare	None known	Chills, fever, occasional nausea/vomiting; pain, rigors, headaches, dizziness, SOB, ↓ BP, rash, asthenia	Unknown, ?, related to manufacturing process	Manage with acetaminophen, diphenhydramine, meperidine
Docetaxel[147]	0.9% with premedication	None known	↓ BP, bronchospasm, rash, flushing, pruritus, SOB, pain, fever, chills	Unknown	Premedicate with acetaminophen, dexamethasone, and diphenhydramine
Doxorubicin[148] liposomal	6.8%	None known	Flushing, SOB, angioedema, HA, chills, ↓ BP	Unknown, ? related liposomal components	Stop infusion; restart at a lower rate
Daunorubicin[149] liposomal	13.8%	None known	Back pain, flushing, chest tightness	Unknown, ? related liposomal components	Stop infusion; restart at a lower rate

Type I: Antigen interaction with IgE bound to mast cell membrane causes degranulation. Drug binding to mast cell surface causes degranulation. Activation of classic or alternative complement pathways produces anaphylatoxins. Neurogenic release of vasoactive substances. Type III: Antigen–antibody complexes form intravascularly and deposit in or on tissues.
BP, blood pressure; CLL, chronic lymphocytic leukemia; HA, headache; HSR, hypersensitivity reaction; 6-MP, 6-mercaptopurine; PEG-l-asparaginase, pegaspargase; SOB, shortness of breath.

Table 89-12 Prophylaxis and Treatment of Hypersensitivity Reactions From Antitumor Drugs

Prophylaxis

IV access must be established.

BP monitoring must be available.

Premedication

Dexamethasone 20 mg PO and diphenhydramine 50 mg PO 12 and 6 hr before treatment, then the same dose IV immediately before treatment

Consider addition of H_2-antagonist with similar schedule

Have epinephrine and diphenhydramine readily available for use in case of a reaction.

Observe the patient up to 2 hr after discontinuing treatment.

Treatment

Discontinue the drug (immediately if being administered IV).

Administer epinephrine 0.35–0.5 mL IV Q 15–20 min until reaction subsides or a total of 6 doses is administered.

Administer diphenhydramine 50 mg IV.

If hypotension is present that does not respond to epinephrine, administer IV fluids.

If wheezing is present that does not respond to epinephrine, administer nebulized albuterol solution 0.35 mL.

Although corticosteroids have no effect on the initial reaction, they can block late allergic symptoms. Thus, administer methylprednisolone 125 mg (or its equivalent) IV to prevent recurrent allergic manifestations.

BP, blood pressure; IV, intravenous; PO, orally.

SPECIFIC ORGAN TOXICITIES

Neurotoxicity

Cytarabine and L-Asparaginase

19. A.L., a 39-year-old woman with acute lymphoblastic leukemia, has been admitted to the hospital for induction chemotherapy. Cytarabine 5 g Q 12 hr for eight doses, vincristine 2 mg IV push weekly, prednisone 100 mg/day, L-asparaginase 15,000 U/day for 14 days, and allopurinol 300 mg/day are ordered. Laboratory data obtained on admission include a WBC count of 120,000/mm³ (normal, 3,200 to 9,800), with 9% neutrophils (normal, 54% to 62%), 11% lymphocytes (normal, 25% to 33%), and 80% blasts and a uric acid of 7.5 mg/dL (normal, 2 to 7). On day 3, A.L. is confused and she has difficulty performing a finger-to-nose neurologic examination. After 3 weeks, she complains of numbness in her hands and feet. In addition, the clinician notes an eyelid lag and ataxia. A.L. also complains of severe constipation. What is the possible cause of A.L.'s mental status? Should chemotherapy be continued?

[SI unit: uric acid, 446 mmol/L]

High dosages of cytarabine (>1 g/m² in multiple doses) are associated with CNS toxicity in 15% to 37% of patients.[152,153] These neurotoxicities are dose and schedule related. Doses exceeding 18 g/m² per course increase the frequency of neurotoxicity. Older patients are more susceptible than younger patients, and the prevalence seems higher in subsequent versus initial courses of therapy. As illustrated by A.L., neurotoxicity may become evident within a few days after treatment with cytarabine, and most commonly, the neurotoxicity is manifested by a generalized encephalopathy with symptoms such as confusion, obtundation, seizures, and coma. Cerebral dysfunction, presenting as ataxia, gait and coordination difficulties, dysmetria (inability to arrest muscular movement when desired and lack of harmonious action between muscles when executing voluntary movement), also is commonly observed in patients receiving high-dose cytarabine therapy. These neurologic symptoms at least partially resolve over days to weeks after discontinuation of therapy. Other neurologic toxicities reported with cytarabine include progressive leukoencephalopathy and chemical meningitis. Leukoencephalopathy typically presents with progressive personality and intellectual decline; dementia; hemiparesis; and, sometimes, seizures. Chemical meningitis can occur with intrathecal administration of cytarabine (see Chapter 90, Hematologic Malignancies). These neurotoxicities also can occur following treatment with other chemotherapy agents, including L-asparaginase.

L-Asparaginase often causes encephalopathy, which presents most commonly as lethargy and confusion.[154] Severe cerebral dysfunction occurs occasionally, and patients may present with stupor, coma, excessive somnolence, disorientation, hallucination, or severe depression. Symptoms can occur early (within days of administration of L-asparaginase) or late depending on the treatment schedule.[155,156] The acute syndrome usually clears rapidly, but the delayed syndrome may last several weeks.

A.L.'s symptoms most likely are the result of CNS toxicity caused by both cytarabine and L-asparaginase. A decision regarding further treatment with these agents is complicated because decreasing the dose of cytarabine and/ or L-asparaginase could compromise the likelihood of a complete remission. Although L-asparaginase–induced CNS neurotoxicities are usually reversible, high-dose cytarabine cerebellar toxicity may not be. Therefore, the clinician can opt to continue treating A.L. with modified doses.

Other Agents

20. What other chemotherapy agents produce CNS toxicity?

Other agents that produce CNS toxicities include methotrexate, fluorouracil, interferon-alfa, fludarabine, carmustine, hexamethylmelamine, procarbazine, and ifosfamide (Table 89-13).

METHOTREXATE

Methotrexate causes little or no neurotoxicity when administered orally or intravenously in the usual doses; however, high-dose IV methotrexate (usually >1 g/m²) can occasionally cause acute encephalopathy. Similar to the encephalopathy caused by other agents, the encephalopathy that occurs following therapy with methotrexate is usually transient and reversible. Other patients may develop a progressive leukoencephalopathy following high-dose IV methotrexate. The risk of leukoencephalopathy increases with higher cumulative doses of methotrexate and concomitant cranial radiation therapy.[157–159] Similar to intrathecal cytarabine, intrathecal methotrexate can cause a chemical meningitis. In addition, intrathecal methotrexate can less commonly cause myelopathy and paraplegia (see Chapter 90). Patients receiving intrathecal therapy or high-dose methotrexate should be carefully monitored for signs and symptoms associated with neurotoxicity.

Table 89-13   Neurotoxicity of Selected Chemotherapeutic Agents

Encephalopathy	Acute Encephalopathy	Chronic Syndrome	Cerebellar Neuropathy	Peripheral Neuropathy	Cranial Neuropathy	Autonomic (IT Dose)	Arachnoiditis Syndrome	Strokelike	SIADH
Alkylating Agents									
Cyclophosphamide									+
Ifosfamide	+		+	+	+				
Thiotepa		+					+		
Cisplatin	+		++	++					
Oxaliplatin				++					
Altretamine	+		+	++					
Procarbazine	++		+	+					
Antimetabolites									
Fluorouracil			++	+	+				
Fludarabine	+		+						
Cytarabine	+	+					+		
Methotrexate	+	+	+				+	+	
Plant Alkaloids									
Vinca alkaloids				++		++			+
Vincristine									
Vinblastine									
Vinorelabine									
Taxanes				+					
Paclitaxel									
Docetaxel									
Miscellaneous									+
Asparginase	++	+							

+, reported but appears rare; ++, common in some cases and may present a clinical problem.
SIADH, syndrome of inappropriate secretion of antidiuretic hormone.

FLUOROURACIL

Fluorouracil can cause acute cerebellar dysfunction characterized by the rapid onset of gait ataxia, limb incoordination, dysarthria, and nystagmus.[160,161] Cerebellar dysfunction occurs in approximately 5% to 10% of patients receiving fluorouracil and occurs with all treatment schedules in common use. A more diffuse encephalopathy presenting as headache, confusion, disorientation, lethargy, and seizures can also occur after therapy with fluorouracil. These symptoms can be reversed if fluorouracil is discontinued or the dose is reduced. Other neurotoxicities observed with fluorouracil include rare reports of optic neuropathy and decreased vision. As with methotrexate, patients should be carefully monitored for signs and symptoms associated with neurotoxicity.

INTERFERON-ALFA

Interferon-alfa can cause a neurologic complex characterized by headache and encephalopathy (weakness, confusion, lethargy). The symptoms occur in one-third of patients receiving interferons and can cause severe reactions in 10%. Severe reactions can cause coma, obtundation, major depression, and suicidal behavior. The symptoms typically begin after several weeks of therapy. Elderly patients receiving high dosages may be more susceptible to these effects. The symptoms may be dose-limiting and usually resolve within 3 weeks after dose attenuation or discontinuation of therapy. If further treatment is warranted, treatment may later be resumed at a lower dosage.[162,163]

FLUDARABINE

Fludarabine (Fludara) can cause severe neurotoxicity when used at dosages >90 mg/m² for 5 to 7 days.[162–165] Symptoms include altered mental status, photophobia, amaurosis (blindness that usually is temporary without change in the eye itself), generalized seizures, spastic or flaccid paralysis, quadriparesis, and coma. In addition, some patients die despite discontinuing therapy. Fortunately, this neurotoxicity does not usually occur with the current recommended dosage of 25 mg/m² per day for 5 days. Only few and mild neurologic symptoms are typically reported with the current recommended dosages, although they can still cause severe neurotoxicity[165,166] and optic demyelination.[167] Patients with signs or symptoms suggestive of significant neurotoxicity should receive a neurologic examination and if warranted, therapy should be discontinued.

CARMUSTINE AND OTHER ALKYLATING AGENTS

Carmustine and other alkylating agents cause little or no neurotoxicity in the usual IV doses, but higher dosages can increase the incidence of these adverse effects. Carmustine (BiCNU) produces encephalopathy associated with confusion or seizures if the dose exceeds 600 to 800 mg/m².[168] Concurrent cranial radiotherapy and intracarotid administration may increase the risk of neurotoxicity.[169,170] Other alkylating agents reported to produce CNS toxicity include ifosfamide,[171,172] procarbazine,[173] altretamine,[174] and cisplatin.[175–180] These agents have been associated with encephalopathy that manifests as confusion, lethargy, and in some instances, psychosis and depression. When a patient presents with any signs or symptoms of neurotoxicity, they should receive a neurologic examination followed by a dose reduction or discontinuation of therapy.

Peripheral Nerve Toxicity

21. **What is causing A.L.'s numbness?**

Paresthesia (numbness and tingling) involving the feet and hands (or both) is an early subjective symptom of vincristine (Oncovin) neurotoxicity, which often appears within the first few weeks of therapy. This peripheral nerve toxicity commonly is bilateral and symmetric and is often referred to as a "stocking-glove" neuropathy. Symptoms initially consist of paresthesias, loss of ankle jerks, and depression of deep tendon reflexes. Areflexia (absent reflexes) typically occurs in about 50 to 70% of patients treated with a cumulative dose that exceeds 6 to 8 mg. Paresthesias can also commonly occur in patients receiving vincristine. Although older patients appear to be more susceptible to paresthesias than younger ones, almost all complain of paresthesias following combination chemotherapy that incorporates vincristine or vinblastine (Velban). Pin and temperature sensory loss is usually more pronounced than vibration and proprioception sensory loss. Patients also may display motor weakness with a foot drop or muscle atrophy. Motor weakness can become the most disabling symptom associated with vincristine neurotoxicity and can occasionally cause muscle wasting. Although some patients develop muscle atrophy, true muscle weakness seldom occurs after treatment with vincristine. Stumbling and falling that can occur with this peripheral neuropathy is not usually caused by muscle weakness; instead, it occurs in the dark when patients lose proprioception because they lack visual orientation. These complications are either partially or completely reversible, but recovery often takes several months.[181,182]

22. **What other agents may cause similar complaints of numbness?**

Other agents that often share the peripheral nerve toxicity of vincristine include vinblastine (Velban), vinorelbine (Navelbine), cisplatin (Platinol), etoposide (Velesid), oxaliplatin (Eloxatin), paclitaxel (Taxol), and docetaxel (Taxotere). Other agents that may cause peripheral nerve toxicity include agents commonly associated with CNS toxicity. Unlike the vinca alkaloids, most of the agents listed cause numbness only and not a loss of reflexes, paresthesias, or weakness. These side effects generally are not dose limiting and are reversible on discontinuation of the agents. Several reviews provide detailed references for this information.[179,180]

Oxaliplatin (Eloxatin) also causes a unique peripheral neuropathy, which is characterized by transient acute dysesthesias triggered by a cold sensation.[183] With cumulative dosing, a more typical peripheral neuropathy occurs that is usually reversible several months after the drug is discontinued. Dose modifications for neurotoxicity in patients receiving oxaliplatin 85 mg/m^2 every 2 weeks have been developed.[183] For cold-related dysethesias and paresthesias that are nonpersistent, no dose modification is recommended. However, for paresthesias associated with pain complaints or functional impairment, the recommendation is to stop therapy until improvement or recovery occurs and restart with a reduced dose of 75 mg/m^2.[183]

Cranial Nerve Toxicity

23. **What is the significance of A.L.'s lid lag?**

Cranial nerve toxicity occurs in 1% to 10% of patients receiving vinca alkaloids. Most patients present with ptosis or ophthalmoplegia.[184,185] This toxicity probably occurs after damage to the third cranial nerve. Toxicity to other cranial nerves may cause trigeminal neuralgia, facial palsy, depressed corneal reflexes, and vocal cord paralysis.[186] Other nerve toxicities associated with the vinca alkaloids include jaw pain that can occur after the first or second injection[186]; the pain usually resolves spontaneously and does not recur with subsequent doses. Several of the cranial nerve toxicities, especially with vincristine, may be dose limiting with evidence showing an increased prevalence associated with increasing doses. A.L.'s eyelid lag probably is caused by vincristine.

24. **Do other chemotherapy agents produce cranial nerve toxicity?**

Ifosfamide, vinblastine, cisplatin, and several experimental chemotherapy agents have been reported to cause cranial neuropathies. Intra-arterial administration of chemotherapy agents may increase the risk of encephalopathy and cranial neuropathies.[179,180]

Ototoxicity, characterized by a progressive, high-frequency, sensorineural hearing loss, commonly occurs with cisplatin.[187,188] Most likely, cisplatin has a direct toxic effect on the cochlea. Ototoxicity occurs more frequently at higher dosages, worsens with concurrent cranial radiation therapy, and appears to be more pronounced in children. The reversibility of cisplatin ototoxicity is questionable. At some centers, routine audiometric tests are performed in patients receiving cisplatin; and as a result, these centers have a greater percentage of patients with documented decreases in audio acuity than others. Early cessation of cisplatin may result in greater hearing improvement. Although ototoxicity appears to be a major toxicity associated with cisplatin, it is not commonly cause by other platinum analogs. For example, only 8 out of 710 (1.1%) patients who received carboplatin experienced clinical hearing deficits, mainly tinnitus.[189] If ototoxicity is suspected, a hearing test should be performed and therapy discontinued if alternate treatments are available.

Autonomic Neuropathy

25. **What is the cause of A.L.'s constipation, and how might this problem have been prevented?**

Vincristine, as well as vinblastine, commonly causes an autonomic neuropathy. The earliest symptoms (colicky abdominal pain with or without constipation) are reported by one-third to one-half of patients receiving these agents.[184,185] The constipation can sometimes be troublesome causing severe constipation that can progress to, or include, adynamic ileus. Prophylactic laxatives are recommended on a regular basis for patients receiving vincristine and vinblastine. Stimulant laxatives such as the senna derivatives or bisacodyl (Dulcolax) are believed to be the most effective agents. Stool softeners also may be used concurrently. Unfortunately, there is no compelling evidence that laxatives prevent constipation. Other less frequent manifestations of autonomic dysfunction associated with vinca alkaloids include bladder atony with urinary retention, impotence, and orthostatic hypotension.[190,191] Patients should be monitored carefully for these signs or symptoms and receive appropriate management following diagnosis.

Cardiac Toxicities
Doxorubicin

26. **D.A., a 35-year-old man with stage IV Hodgkin's disease, is receiving CHOP (cyclophosphamide 750 mg/m² day 1, doxorubicin 50 mg/mm³ IV day 1, vincristine 2 mg IV day 1, and prednisone 100 mg PO days 1 to 5) and concurrent radiation therapy to a large mediastinal mass. He comes to the clinic to receive his fifth cycle of CHOP and complains of tachycardia, SOB, and a nonproductive cough. Physical examination reveals neck vein distention, pulmonary rales, and ankle edema. What is the most likely cause of D.A.'s current symptoms?**

D.A. is experiencing symptoms of congestive heart failure (CHF) most likely caused by doxorubicin therapy. Doxorubicin (Adriamycin, Rubex), an anthracycline antibiotic, can cause a dose-dependent cardiomyopathy that generally occurs with repeated administration. Doxorubicin causes myocyte damage by a mechanism that differs from its cytotoxic effect on tumor cells. Because myocytes stop dividing in infancy, they presumably would not be affected by an agent whose cytotoxicity relies on actively cycling cells. Many mechanisms have been proposed to explain the cardiac toxicity associated with doxorubicin.[192,193]

D.A.'s presentation is fairly typical of doxorubicin-induced cardiomyopathy, although he has no significant risk factors usually associated with CHF. The total cumulative dose of doxorubicin is the most clearly established risk factor for the CHF.[194–196] Patients such as D.A. who are receiving bolus doses of doxorubicin at the standard 3-week interval face little risk of CHF until a total dose of 450 mg/m² to 550 mg/m² has been reached. After a patient has received a total dose ≥550 mg/m², the risk of CHF rises rapidly. Patients receiving <550 mg/m² of doxorubicin face a 0.1% to 1.2% risk of developing CHF. Comparatively, patients receiving ≥550 mg/m² face a risk that rises more or less linearly; the probability of CHF in patients receiving a total dose of 1,000/m² may be nearly 50%.[196]

Other factors that could increase D.A.'s risk of developing doxorubicin cardiomyopathy include mediastinal radiation therapy, pre-existing cardiac disease, hypertension, and age. Young children, as well as older patients, are likely to experience CHF at a lower cumulative dose. Concurrent chemotherapy agents (e.g., cyclophosphamide, etoposide, mitomycin, melphalan, trastuzumab, paclitaxel, vincristine, bleomycin) may also potentiate doxorubicin cardiac toxicity.[197] When patients receive paclitaxel (Taxol) and doxorubicin, the risk of cardiac toxicity appears to be related to the sequence and proximity of the infusions. In a pharmacokinetic study, paclitaxel increased the AUC of doxorubicin and its active metabolite, doxorubicinol, when paclitaxel administration immediately preceded doxorubicin. Therefore, the infusions should be separated by 24 hours. The relationship between risk factors and the total cumulative dose of doxorubicin is strong enough to warrant guidelines restricting the total cumulative dose of doxorubicin to 450 mg/m² in patients with one or more identified risk factors (high-risk patients) and to 550 mg/m² in patients without risk factors (low-risk patients).

It is unusual that D.A., a 35-year-old man who has received only 200 mg/m² of doxorubicin, would be presenting with symptoms of CHF. However, mediastinal radiation therapy, cyclophosphamide, or undiagnosed cardiac disease may have contributed to this unfortunate event. In addition, Hodgkin's disease involving the myocardium may be responsible for this presentation.

27. **Is routine cardiac monitoring recommended in patients receiving doxorubicin?**

Prevention of cardiomyopathy is achieved primarily by limiting the total cumulative dose. Unfortunately, limiting the total dose cannot entirely prevent the cardiomyopathy for two reasons. First, individual tolerance to doxorubicin varies such that cardiotoxicity may occur before the arbitrary dose limit; second, some clinical situations warrant exceeding the dose limit to achieve positive chemotherapeutic outcomes.

Early efforts to prevent cardiomyopathy focused on monitoring systolic time intervals, QRS voltage loss, or ST-T segment changes on an electrocardiogram (ECG). However, these changes were too nonspecific or occurred too late to be useful; serial echocardiography has some usefulness in children.[198,199] Other current state-of-the-art monitoring for anthracycline cardiomyopathy includes radionuclide ventriculography (RNV) and endomyocardial biopsy. The use of radionuclide ventriculography (also referred to as radionuclide cardiac angiography; gated blood pool imaging; multiple gated acquisition [MUGA]) for early detection of doxorubicin-induced cardiac dysfunction has been investigated extensively.[200] RNV can accurately detect functional cardiac status, but it is not particularly sensitive in detecting patients who have early myocyte damage. Augmenting the RNV with exercise appears to give a more accurate picture of functional cardiac reserve. Because myocyte damage usually occurs days to weeks after treatment with doxorubicin, the RNV should be obtained just before, rather than just after, a course of the agent. Although guidelines vary, most institutions recommend obtaining an RNV before starting therapy with doxorubicin. Additional RNVs should be obtained when a patient shows signs or symptoms of CHF or when the patient receives cumulative doses >450 mg/m² in low-risk patients or >350 mg/m² in high-risk patients if additional doses are planned. Most guidelines recommend stopping doxorubicin or obtaining an endomyocardial biopsy when an absolute decrease in the RNV exceeds 10% to 20%, the RNV is <40%, or the RNV fails to increase >5% with exercise.[197] ASCO currently recommends frequent cardiac monitoring after doses >400 mg/m².[36] The study should be repeated after patients receive >500 mg/m² and with every additional dose of 50 mg/m². The guidelines published by ASCO support the recommendations to discontinue therapy when patients show clinical signs or symptoms of CHF or if the left ventricular ejection fraction decreases below institutional normal limits.[36]

Endomyocardial biopsies along with a quantitative assessment of morphologic changes provide the most specific evaluation of myocardial damage induced by anthracyclines. Progressive myocardial pathology is graded on a scale (the Billingham Score) of 0 (no change from normal) to 3 (diffuse cell damage in >35% of total number of cells with marked change in cardiac ultrastructure).[193] The prevalence of abnormal RNVs and the appearance of signs and symptoms of CHF correlate with biopsy scores. Usually, a significant change in cardiac function is not seen with scores <2 to 2.5. Several investigators have evaluated the predictive value of this technique. With a score of 2, a patient has less than a 10% chance of developing heart failure if 100 mg more of doxorubicin is given.[201–203]There are occasional false-negative biopsies, and fatal CHF has been encountered in at least one patient with a relatively normal (1.0) biopsy score.[204] The most significant risk associated with endomyocardial biopsy is perforation of the right ventricle with associated tamponade; this occurs rarely and depends largely on the experience of the operator.

In summary, RNV and endomyocardial biopsy are complementary procedures that when used together along with clinical evaluation can provide a degree of confidence in predicting tolerance to additional doxorubicin dosing. The endomyocardial biopsy provides a distinct advantage by allowing early myocyte damage to be appreciated before the RNV changes or the patient shows signs or symptoms of CHF.

Other Agents

28. **How do the other members of the anthracycline class compare with doxorubicin in terms of cardiotoxicity and clinical usefulness?**

DAUNORUBICIN

Daunorubicin differs structurally from doxorubicin only by hydroxylation of the fourteenth carbon. Unlike doxorubicin, daunorubicin is primarily used to treat hematologic malignancies, such as acute nonlymphocytic leukemia. During its initial clinical evaluations 25 years ago, clinicians lacked a good understanding of the dose-schedule/toxicity relationships for daunorubicin, and it became known on some hospital wards as "the red death." Doxorubicin became favored to treat solid tumors because daunorubicin caused excessive mucositis and myelosuppression when patients received antileukemic dosages to treat solid tumors. Since then, clinical trials have given clinicians a better understanding of daunorubicin's side effects and how to provide better supportive care when it is used to treat these tumors. Now, daunorubicin safely produces clinical responses in patients with Hodgkin's disease, non-Hodgkin's lymphomas, melanoma, sarcomas, lung carcinomas, breast carcinomas, and GI tract carcinomas.[205] In randomized trials comparing daunorubicin and doxorubicin, daunorubicin caused less mucositis and a lower incidence of colonic damage and perforation.[206] However, cardiac toxicities are similar for both drugs, although somewhat higher cumulative doses of daunomycin are typically tolerated.[207] Risk factors for CHF appear to be the same, and similar assessments should be undertaken to monitor for cardiotoxicity.

IDARUBICIN

Idarubicin (Idamycin) is an anthracycline that is approved for the treatment of acute leukemias. Although idarubicin appears less cardiotoxic than doxorubicin in animal models[208]

and daunorubicin in some early clinical trials,[209–211] other studies show equivalent myelosuppressive doses can cause cardiotoxicity comparable to that of doxorubicin and daunorubicin.[212,213] Until additional studies adequately define the cumulative dose associated with cardiotoxicity, patients receiving idarubicin should be routinely monitored for signs and symptoms of CHF.

EPIRUBICIN

Epirubicin (Ellence) is another anthracycline approved by the FDA for adjuvant therapy of breast cancer after surgical resection. Like the other anthracyclines, epirubicin can cause a dose-dependent, potentially fatal CHF. CHF occurs in 1.6% of patients receiving 700 mg/m^2 and in 3.3% of patients receiving 900 mg/m^2. Risk factors for cardiotoxicity include a history of cardiovascular disease, prior or concomitant radiation therapy to the mediastinum or pericardium, previous therapy with other anthracyclines or mitoxantrone or concomitant use of other cardiotoxic medications. Cumulative doses should not exceed 900 mg/m^2, which could result in toxicity.[214] Patients receiving epirubicin should receive cardiac monitoring with continued therapy to minimize the risk of severe CHF.

MITOXANTRONE

Mitoxantrone (Novantrone) is an anthracenedione that is structurally similar to the anthracyclines. Typically, patients receive one-fifth the dose of doxorubicin or 12 to 14 mg/m^2 every 3 weeks. The important risk factors for mitoxantrone cardiotoxicity include a history of mediastinal radiation, cardiovascular disease, and anthracycline exposure. Predicting mitoxantrone cardiotoxicity is similar to that of doxorubicin and daunorubicin. In patients without risk factors, the risk for cardiotoxicity does not begin to rise significantly until patients receive about 160 mg/m^2. This dose is equivalent to about 800 mg/m^2 of doxorubicin. For patients who have received doxorubicin (mean cumulative dose, 239 mg/m^2), the risk starts to rise when the cumulative mitoxantrone dose reaches about 100 mg/m^2.[215–217] The guidelines suggested for monitoring doxorubicin-induced cardiotoxicity should be followed with mitoxantrone therapy to minimize the risk for CHF.

Prevention

29. **Can CHF be prevented by the use of a different dose or dosing schedule or by agents that protect the myocardium?**

Altering the dose schedule of doxorubicin to more frequent, smaller doses while maintaining dose intensity has consistently resulted in reduction of cardiotoxicity without obvious compromise of antitumor effects.[218–223] Several reports suggest that peak plasma levels, as well as cumulative dose, have an important relationship to doxorubicin cardiotoxicity. Low doses of doxorubicin administered weekly or prolonged continuous IV infusions (48 to 96 hours) can be relatively cardiac sparing, allowing higher cumulative doses to be administered. In a retrospective, uncontrolled study of 1,000 patients receiving weekly doxorubicin, a total dose of 900 to 1,200 mg/m^2 of doxorubicin given in weekly fractions had the equivalent cardiotoxicity of 550 mg/m^2 given in every-3-week fractions.[219] Although well-designed studies comparing cardiac toxicity following bolus doses with fractionated therapy or continuous infusion are lacking, treatment that incorporates these alternative schedules should be considered in patients with pre-existing risk factors or patients who will be receiving total doses of more than 450 to 550 mg/m². The concurrent use of drugs that might minimize the risk of cardiotoxicity without compromising efficacy can be considered as well.

Dexrazoxane (Zinecard) is a chemoprotectant that reduces the incidence and severity of cardiomyopathy. It is indicated in women with metastatic breast cancer who have received a cumulative doxorubicin dose of 300 mg/m². It may do so by chelating iron and impairing the subsequent generation of a singlet oxygen by doxorubicin. The ability of dexrazoxane to prevent or reduce the incidence and severity of doxorubicin-induced cardiomyopathy was demonstrated in three placebo-controlled clinical trials. Patients who started on dexrazoxane only after receiving 300 mg/m² of doxorubicin had the same clinical benefit as patients who started on dexrazoxane with their initial doses of doxorubicin. Unfortunately, dexrazoxane can cause some myelosuppression and thereby compromise tolerance to full doses of chemotherapy. The recommended dosing ratio of dexrazoxane:doxorubicin is 10:1 slow IV push 30 minutes before starting doxorubicin.

Currently, the ASCO guidelines do not support the routine use of dexrazoxane in patients unless there is a plan to continue doxorubicin beyond a total cumulative dose that exceeds 300 mg/m². Although the FDA approved the use of dexrazoxane only for patients with metastatic breast cancer, the ASCO guidelines currently suggest its use in all patients receiving total cumulative doses exceeding 300 mg/m². Because dexrazoxane may decrease tumor responses, clinicians should carefully weigh the risk:benefit ratio.[36,224] Clinical trials are evaluating the benefits of dexrazoxane in children and patients receiving other anthracyclines. Some evidence supports the use of dexrazoxane in patients receiving epirubicin.[225,226]

Another unusual approach to protecting against doxorubicin cardiotoxicity focuses on delivering anthracycline encapsulated in liposomes.[227,228] To date, experience with high cumulative doses of these formulations is too limited to document whether cardiac toxicity is reduced.

Management

30. **How should doxorubicin- or other anthracycline-induced CHF be managed clinically?**

Anthracycline-induced CHF presents similarly to other forms of biventricular CHF. It occurs between 0 to 231 days after the last dose of doxorubicin (mean, 33 days). Anthracycline-induced CHF should be treated with diuretics, activity restriction, inotropic agents, and vasodilators. Unfortunately, these measures often are ineffective. The clinical course varies, with some patients showing stable disease and others showing improvement. Before cardiotoxicity was a widely recognized toxicity, the course of anthracycline-induced CHF was characterized by a rapid progression that generally led to death in a few weeks. Now, anthracycline therapy is promptly discontinued after patients initially present with signs and symptoms, if not sooner. Consequently, the high fatality rates and failed responses to conventional therapy reported in the older literature may not hold true. Treatment should focus on improving a patient's quality of life.

Other Cardiac Toxicities

31. **What other chemotherapy agents have been associated with cardiac toxicities?**

Electrocardiographic changes have been observed during or after treatment with doxorubicin, other anthracyclines, cisplatin, etoposide, paclitaxel, cyclophosphamide, and mechlorethamine. Most commonly, ECG changes involve ST-T segment changes, decreases in voltage, T-wave flattening, and atrial and ventricular ectopy. Other ECG abnormalities may be seen as well. Most studies suggest that arrhythmias occur in 6% to 40% of patients receiving bolus doxorubicin.[229] Paclitaxel also caused significant arrhythmias and conduction defects in phase I and II trials[230]; most patients developed sinus bradycardia. All other chemotherapy agents occasionally cause a rhythm disturbance, but these are limited to a few scattered reports and should not be considered clinically significant. Therapy should not be discontinued unless the patient develops a serious cardiac arrhythmia.

FLUOROURACIL (FU)

Fluorouracil has been associated with angina pectoris and myocardial infarction. Angina may occur in 1.6% to 18%[231–233] of patients receiving fluorouracil and appears to occur with an increased incidence in patients with a history of ischemic cardiomyopathy or in patients receiving 5-day infusions. Angina has been associated with both initial and subsequent courses. Although ischemia occurs most frequently during continuous infusion, it occasionally is delayed 3 to 18 hours after fluorouracil administration and has been reported after an oral dose. The cause of fluorouracil cardiotoxicity is uncertain. Direct myocyte damage is suggested from animal studies; however, human studies suggest that coronary artery spasm is the most likely cause of angina. Because the chest pain associated with fluorouracil responds to nitrates, this problem could be theoretically managed prophylactically or therapeutically with long-acting nitrates or calcium channel blockers.[231] Other agents (including vincristine, vinblastine, etoposide, paclitaxel, and bleomycin) can cause chest pain or infarction based on case reports in the literature.[197]

ALKYLATING AGENTS

Myocardial necrosis rarely has been reported with alkylating agents, including cyclophosphamide, ifosfamide, busulfan, and mechlorethamine. Typically, cardiotoxicity occurs when patients receive high doses, such as the doses used for bone marrow ablation. Pericarditis and hemorrhagic myocardial necrosis also have been reported in these cases. Risk factors are similar to those associated with doxorubicin and daunorubicin; however, a clear relationship between dose and cardiac dysfunction has not been demonstrated consistently in all case reports.[187]

TRASTUZUMAB (HERCEPTIN)

Signs and symptoms of CHF such as dyspnea, increased cough, peripheral edema, S₃ gallop, and reduced ejection fraction have been reported in 3% to 7% of patients receiving trastuzumab single-agent therapy. Five percent of these patients had New York Heart Association class III or IV heart failure.[146] The incidence increases to 11% when patients concurrently receive paclitaxel and to 28% when patients concurrently receive cyclophosphamide and doxorubicin.[234] Current evidence suggests that the combination of trastuzumab and doxorubicin is contraindicated. Trastuzumab-associated cardiac toxicity does not appear to be dose related, and it usually responds to standard medical treatment or discontinuation of the drug.[235] Before and periodically during treatment with trastuzumab, patients should undergo cardiac evaluation to assess left ventricular ejection fraction. Therapy should be discontinued if patients develop a clinically significant decrease in left ventricular function. Guidelines for formal assessment of cardiac function and recommendations for management have been proposed.[235]

Nephrotoxicity
Cisplatin (Platinol-AQ)

32. T.J., a 58-year-old man with nonresectable head and neck cancer, is being treated with cisplatin 100 mg/m^2 on day 1 and fluorouracil 1 g/m^2 per day for 5 days. He presents today for the third cycle of this regimen. A 24-hour urine for creatinine collected by T.J. at home revealed a creatinine clearance (Cl$_{Cr}$) of 75 mL/min, down from 110 mL/min at baseline. Other abnormalities include serum magnesium (Mg) of 1.2 mEq/L (normal, 1.6 to 2.2mg/dL); all other electrolyte values are within normal range. Is cisplatin responsible for T.J.'s decreased glomerular filtration rate (GFR) and serum magnesium levels?

[SI units: Cl$_{Cr}$, 1.25 mL/sec; Mg, 0.6 mmol/L]

Cisplatin, a heavy-metal complex, is widely used clinically because it has activity against various solid tumors. The major dose-limiting toxicity of cisplatin is nephrotoxicity, and various renal and electrolyte disorders, both acute and chronic, have been associated with cisplatin. In the early 1970s, before the need for vigorous hydration was recognized, cisplatin often caused acute renal failure. Today, with the use of vigorous hydration, acute renal failure is uncommon; however, tubular dysfunction and decreased GFR remain problematic.

Morphologic damage is greatest in the straight segment of the proximal renal tubules where the highest concentration of platinum occurs. Acute and cumulative renal tubular damage have been demonstrated by increased urinary excretion of proximal tubular enzymes such as β_2-microglobulin, alanine aminopeptidase, and N-acetyl glucosamine. Increases in proximal tubular enzymes correlate well with urinary excretion of protein and magnesium as well as decreased reabsorption of salt and water in the proximal tubules. T.J. has hypomagnesemia, which is the most common electrolyte abnormality caused by cisplatin. Hypomagnesemia appears to be dose related, but it can occur after a single treatment. Despite replacement with oral magnesium, renal losses of magnesium and decreased serum magnesium levels can persist for months or even years after completion of cisplatin therapy. Hypocalcemia and hyponatremia occur less frequently. The cause of these electrolyte abnormalities is thought to be similar to that of hypomagnesemia in that a proximal tubular defect occurs that interferes with reabsorption of these electrolytes.[236,237]

Chronic renal toxicity associated with cisplatin presents as a decrease in the GFR. Published reports suggest that the GFR decreases by 12% to 25% in most patients receiving multiple courses.[236–239] The decrease appears to be persistent and only partially reversible. An increase in serum creatinine or a decrease in creatinine clearance does not necessarily reflect the decline in GFR. More sensitive measures of renal function, such as radioisotope clearance, may better characterize the changing GFR, but they are not widely available at most institutions. Nonetheless, the renal function of patients receiving cisplatin therapy should be evaluated because dosage reductions may be necessary if the creatinine clearance decreases. Methods that estimate creatinine clearance based on serum creatinine should be avoided, especially in patients with borderline renal function, because poor correlation has been demonstrated in some cancer patient populations. In addition, changes in creatinine clearance are not always reflected by changes in serum creatinine in these patients. Until a more sensitive and specific determinant of GFR becomes widely available, creatinine clearance should be determined using a 12- to 24-hour urine collection for creatinine.

T.J.'s decreased GFR and low serum magnesium likely are caused by cisplatin therapy. Although a dose reduction of cisplatin generally is not recommended for creatinine clearances in this range, the clinician should provide T.J. with adequate and aggressive hydration to prevent cisplatin nephrotoxicity. In addition, T.J. should receive an oral magnesium supplement, although diarrhea usually limits the use of the oral route when large doses are necessary. IV administration should be used if it is required. Typically, therapy begins with 5 g of MgSO$_4$ (40 mEq) in 500 mL of fluid infused over 5 hours followed by measurement of serum magnesium levels and repeated courses, as necessary. Patients should undergo frequent measurements of their electrolytes, including magnesium, to minimize potential complications.

PREVENTION

33. What measures should be taken to prevent cisplatin nephrotoxicity in T.J.?

Several measures have been used to minimize or prevent cisplatin-induced nephrotoxicity, including hydration with saline, mannitol, and prophylactic magnesium. The patient should be vigorously hydrated with 2 to 3 L of normal saline over 8 to 12 hours to maintain a urine output of 100 to 200 mL/hour for at least 6 hours after treatment with cisplatin.[240–242] A loop diuretic such as furosemide may be required in elderly patients to eliminate excess sodium or in patients with compromised cardiac reserve, but these diuretics should not be used routinely to prevent nephrotoxicity. Mannitol (25 to 50 g) should be administered just before chemotherapy to prevent cisplatin-induced renal artery vasoconstriction, which can increase the concentration of platinum in the renal tubules.[242,243] Most patients may also benefit from prophylactic magnesium supplementation. Patients who received prophylactic magnesium 16 mEq IV daily during a 5-day course of cisplatin followed by 60 mEq orally (20 mEq three times daily) between courses experienced less nephrotoxicity compared with those who received no supplements in a prospective trial of 16 patients with testicular carcinoma.[244]

Although most of these preventive measures can adequately minimize the risk of nephrotoxicity, amifostine (Ethyol), an organic thiophosphate that is a chemoprotectant, is also available. It is indicated for reducing the cumulative renal toxicity associated with repeated administration of cisplatin in patients with advanced ovarian cancer. Amifostine's mechanism is based on the assumption that oxygen-free radicals generated by cisplatin and radiation therapy are toxic to normal cells. It preferentially enters normal cells where it generates an active thiol metabolite, which scavenges the free radicals. A pivotal clinical trial demonstrated that pretreatment with amifostine significantly reduced grade 4 neutropenia, nephrotoxicity, and neurotoxicity. There was no evidence that amifostine interfered with the antitumor activity of cisplatin or cyclophosphamide.[245] This trial, along with several others suggests that amifostine may be able to prevent other toxicities associated with chemotherapy, including neurotoxicity, neutropenia, and ototoxicity. The ASCO guidelines currently support the use of amifostine for the prevention of nephrotoxicity and neutropenia; its use to prevent ototoxicity or neurotoxicity is not supported.[36,246]

The recommended dosage of amifostine is 910 mg/m² administered once daily as a 15-minute IV infusion starting 30 minutes before chemotherapy. Because amifostine can cause significant hypotension, all antihypertensives should be discontinued 24 hours before treatment. In addition, patients should receive IV saline and remain in the Trendelenburg position during the infusion. If a patient experiences significant decreases in systolic blood pressure or signs or symptoms of hypotension during the infusion, treatment with amifostine should be stopped temporarily. In most cases, the systolic blood pressure returns to near normal in 5 minutes. Any patient who appears hypotensive or dehydrated should not receive amifostine. Additional adverse reactions include infusion-related flushing, fever or chills, dizziness, hiccups, sneezing, and severe nausea and vomiting.[36,246] Using amifostine in combination with traditional preventive measures may significantly reduce the incidence of cisplatin-induced nephrotoxicity.

34. At what point would cisplatin therapy be discontinued in a patient with a diminished GFR?

Guidelines to modify the dosage of cisplatin in patients with decreased renal function are available. Most suggest a 50% dosage reduction when the GFR decreases to 30 to 60 mL/minute and discontinuation when the GFR falls to <10 to 30 mL/minute (Table 89-14).[237] Percentage dose reductions

---

Table 89-14 Chemotherapeutics Requiring Dosage Modification in Renal Failure

Drug	>60 mL/min	30–60 mL/min	10–30 mL/min
Bleomycin	NC	75%	75%
Cisplatin	NC	50%	Omit
Cyclophosphamide	NC	NC	NC
Methotrexate	NC	50%	Omit
Mitomycin	NC	75%	75%
Nitrosureas	NC	Omit	Omit
Topotecan	NC	NC	25%

Carboplatin Dosing Recommendation

Calvert Equation

Dose (mg) = Target AUC (mg/mL × min) × [GFR (mL/min) % 25]

Suggested Target AUC for Adults

  Single agent, untreated 7 mg/mL/min

  Single agent, previously treated 5 mg/mL/min

  Combination chemotherapy 4.5 mg/mL/min

NC, no change.

---

generally refer to the recommended dose for a specific cancer in a given combination chemotherapy regimen. Because the cisplatin dose ranges from 50 mg/m² to 150 mg/m², the precise dose for a patient with a GFR of <60 mL/minute must be individualized to the situation. If the tumor responds to carboplatin, substitution should be considered because it does not cause nephrotoxicity. The dose of carboplatin also must be modified in patients with decreased GFRs because it is primarily excreted by the kidneys. To help calculate the dose for carboplatin, the manufacturer provides recommendations in their product information insert.

Other Nephrotoxic Agents

35. What other chemotherapy agents can cause nephrotoxicity? What are the clinical consequences of nephrotoxicity produced by these agents?

PROXIMAL TUBULE DYSFUNCTION

Other agents reported to cause renal tubular defects include streptozocin, lomustine (CCNU), carmustine (BCNU), plicamycin, and ifosfamide.[225,226] Nephrotoxicity appears to be related to the total cumulative dose for streptozocin, BCNU, CCNU, and plicamycin. Comparatively, a clear relationship between dosage and renal tubular toxicity with ifosfamide has not been established; however, the renal abnormality associated with high doses of bolus ifosfamide did lead to the use of fractionated doses. Plicamycin also infrequently causes signs of nephrotoxicity when patients receive doses used for the management of hypercalcemia associated with their cancer.[236,237] Most patients show signs and symptoms consistent with proximal tubular dysfunction.

The primary renal lesion associated with each of these agents occurs in the proximal renal tubule, and patients show several electrolyte imbalances, such as loss of protein, glucose, bicarbonate, and potassium. Serum creatinine, bicarbonate, potassium, urinary pH, protein, and glucose should be monitored closely in patients receiving these agents. Because the reversibility of the lesions varies among clinical reports and a significant number of patients who develop renal toxicity with these agents require dialysis,[236,237] patients should discontinue treatment with these agents if they show any changes in serum creatinine or electrolytes.

HEMOLYTIC UREMIC SYNDROME

The antitumor antibiotic mitomycin has been associated with a hemolytic uremic syndrome.[236,237] This often fatal syndrome most commonly occurs after several courses of therapy, but patients may develop symptoms earlier in the course of therapy. Signs and symptoms include abrupt onset of microangiopathic hemolytic anemia, increasing serum creatinine, increased fibrin degradation products, thrombocytopenia, and hypertension. The syndrome also has been associated with combination chemotherapy (bleomycin, cisplatin, and vincristine[248] or bleomycin, cisplatin, and methotrexate[249]) and with carboplatin alone.[250] Early recognition and prompt treatment with plasmapheresis and hemodialysis may be beneficial.[247]

METHOTREXATE

36. J.R., a 15-year-old boy with osteogenic sarcoma of the right knee, was treated with amputation of his right leg. His leg is now healed and chemotherapy consisting of high-dose methotrexate, leucovorin rescue, doxorubicin, dactinomycin, bleomycin, cisplatin, and ifosfamide is planned. The dose of methotrexate is 15 g/m² administered over 3 hours. What precautions are necessary to prevent the renal and other toxicities associated with high-dose methotrexate therapy in J.R.?

Methotrexate normally is not nephrotoxic, although 90% of the agent is excreted unchanged in the urine; however, acute tubular obstruction may occur with high-dose methotrexate if appropriate precautions are not taken. Acute tubular obstruction is caused by secondary tubular precipitation of methotrexate, which is poorly soluble at a pH <7.0. To prevent this occurrence, preventive measures should be planned for J.R., including brisk diuresis to produce urine outputs in the range of 100 to 200 mL/hour for at least 24 hours after the administration of high-dose methotrexate and urinary alkalinization. A urine pH >7.0 usually can be ensured by administration of 25 to 50 mEq/L sodium bicarbonate. Acetazolamide, a carbonic anhydrase inhibitor, promotes urinary bicarbonate excretion and is used by some clinicians at doses of 500 mg two to four times daily to assist in maintaining a urinary pH >7.0. J.R.'s urine output and pH must be monitored closely to prevent acute tubular obstruction associated with high-dose methotrexate therapy.[236,237]

If J.R. has any existing renal insufficiency, methotrexate excretion will be decreased significantly, and he may suffer greater bone marrow suppression and GI side effects because of prolonged exposure to high serum methotrexate levels. Therefore, it is important to ensure that appropriate leucovorin rescue is initiated within 48 hours after the high-dose methotrexate infusion. In addition, intrapatient and interpatient variability in methotrexate clearance is considerable, particularly with high doses of methotrexate therapy. Renal excretion of methotrexate is a complex process involving glomerular filtration, tubular reabsorption, and secretion. Concentrations of methotrexate obtained within 24 hours after the infusion often are not predictive of concentrations at 48 hours. Therefore, methotrexate concentrations between 24 and 48 hours must be monitored in J.R. and in all patients receiving high-dose therapy. Methotrexate levels are necessary to optimize leucovorin rescue (see Chapter 91, Solid Tumors). However, leucovorin rescue does not affect the renal toxicity of methotrexate. Acute tubular obstruction associated with high-dose methotrexate therapy can be prevented only by appropriate attention to optimal urinary output before and for at least 24 hours after high-dose methotrexate administration and urinary alkalization.

IFOSFAMIDE (IFEX)

37. J.R. also is receiving ifosfamide. What unique bladder toxicity occurs with ifosfamide that requires attention before its administration?

Pathogenesis
Ifosfamide, a structural analog of cyclophosphamide belonging to the oxazaphosphorine class of antitumor alkylating agents, which must be activated by the mixed-function oxidase system of the liver. The oxazaphosphorines are a reactive species capable of interacting with nucleic acids and cellular materials to cause cell damage and death. The 4-hydroxy metabolite spontaneously liberates acrolein in many sites throughout the body, and acrolein is responsible for oxazaphosphorine urotoxicity. Both ifosfamide and cyclophosphamide produce cystitis characterized by tissue edema and ulceration followed by sloughing of mucosal epithelial cells, necrosis of smooth muscle fibers and arteries, and culminating in focal hemorrhage. The selective urotoxicity of oxazaphosphorine occurs because the bladder contains a low concentration of thiol compounds (glutathione, cysteine), which can react with and neutralize many reactive chemicals by virtue of their nucleophilic sulfhydryl groups. Because the metabolic activation of ifosfamide proceeds more slowly than the metabolic activation of cyclophosphamide, the dosages of ifosfamide are three to four times higher than the dosages of cyclophosphamide. This may explain the higher incidence of urotoxicity associated with ifosfamide.

Clinical Presentation
Patients with oxazaphosphorine-induced hemorrhagic cystitis initially go through an asymptomatic stage characterized by complaints of brief episodes of painful urination, frequency, and hematuria. The symptoms may subside over a period of several days or weeks after discontinuing the agent. The course of oxazaphosphorine-induced hemorrhagic cystitis usually is relatively benign, although death from massive refractory hemorrhage has occurred. Factors that may predispose J.R. to hemorrhagic cystitis include IV administration, large doses, and his young age.

Prevention
Forced hydration is the primary method used to prevent hemorrhagic cystitis in patients treated with cyclophosphamide therapy. Theoretically, hydration flushes the toxic metabolites out of the bladder so that insufficient contact time is available to set up the tissue reaction. The more urotoxic agent ifosfamide was introduced to the market with a uroprotective agent called *mesna* (Mesnex). Mesna liberates free thiol groups in the bladder, which can neutralize the oxazaphosphorine metabolite. When administered in an appropriate dosing schedule, mesna can prevent the bladder toxicity completely.

The manufacturer and ASCO currently recommend a parenteral mesna dose of 20% weight/weight (w/w) of the ifosfamide dose (<2.5 g/m²) given intravenously at zero, 4, and 8 hours after ifosfamide (total of 60% w/w).[36] The goal is to maintain mesna levels within the urinary tract for some time after treatment with ifosfamide to provide adequate uroprotection. Repeated administration is required because mesna has a short elimination half-life (<1 hour), especially compared with the relatively long half-life of ifosfamide. If patients receive a continuous infusion of ifosfamide, clinicians fear that patients may not receive adequate uroprotection with this divided dose regimen. Therefore, for patients receiving a continuous infusion of ifosfamide ASCO guidelines recommend a 20% w/w IV bolus of mesna followed by a 40% w/w continuous infusion for 12 to 24 hours after the end of the ifosfamide infusion.[36] This regimen ensures that mesna remains in the bladder for an extensive amount of time following the end of the ifosfamide infusion.

Various other mesna dosing guidelines are clinically used, but no trials have compared the different regimens. One author suggests that a total mesna dose equivalent to 17% w/w of the ifosfamide dose was just as effective in preventing urotoxicity as the 60% w/w dose.[251] Many investigators use a 1:1 w/w dose of mesna to ifosfamide when administered by continuous infusion. Unfortunately, the dosing guidelines become less well defined when patients receive higher dosages of ifosfamide (>2.5 g/m²).

The lack of data and the unique pharmacokinetic properties of ifosfamide have caused some concerns about the current dosing guidelines. The pharmacokinetics of ifosfamide are dose dependent.[252] The elimination half-life associated with doses of 2.5 g/m² is 6 to 8 hours, whereas the elimination half-life associated with doses of 3.5 to 5 g/m² is 14 to 16 hours. The current recommendations for mesna administration provide protection for approximately 12 hours after an IV bolus thus, with higher dosages of ifosfamide, mesna should be infused beyond the recommended 8 hours after ifosfamide to maintain bladder protection. Furthermore based on pharmacokinetic data of ifosfamide and mesna following continuous infusion and clinical evidence of hematuria developing 1 to 2 days after the end of a combined ifosfamide and mesna infusion, mesna infusions should be continued for some period of time following discontinuation of ifosfamide.[253] Also, there is concern that the 4-hour dosing interval may be inadequate to maintain sufficient mesna levels within the bladder. Although most of the mesna dose after IV administration is eliminated within 4 to 6 hours, the data demonstrate that elimination rates (mg/kg per hour) are highest in the first 2 hours after IV administration.[254,255] To ensure maximum protection against urotoxicity, ASCO currently recommends more frequent or prolonged mesna dosage regimens.[32] Indeed, several clinicians opt to administer mesna by continuous infusion to avoid the need for frequent bolus dosing. Because ifosfamide and mesna are compatible in solution, combined continuous infusion allows patients to conveniently receive uroprotection.

Another question concerns the influence of micturation on the efficacy of mesna uroprotection. Several authors have suggested that the frequency of mesna doses be adjusted based on frequency and amount of micturation.[256,257] Although forced hydration has been the mainstay for prevention of cyclophosphamide-induced hemorrhagic cystitis, it is unnecessary and potentially disadvantageous when mesna is administered with ifosfamide or cyclophosphamide. This is because forced hydration can increase micturation and increase the evacuation of mesna from the bladder.

An oral formulation of mesna is not commercially available, but the IV formulation can be given orally. The oral bioavailability of mesna is approximately one-half that of IV mesna. Therefore, patients should receive two times the standard IV dose if they receive mesna orally. The manufacturer recommends an oral regimen of 40% w/w of the ifosfamide bolus dose 2 hours before and 4 and 8 hours after ifosfamide.[258] Others have recommended that a dose also be given with the ifosfamide dose. Several centers administer the first dose of mesna intravenously followed by oral doses at 4 and 8 hours, particularly in the outpatient clinic setting.[36] All patients receiving cyclophosphamide should receive saline diuresis or forced saline diuresis to protect urothelial tissue. When patients receive cyclophosphamide for a bone marrow transplant, they should receive mesna in conjunction with saline diuresis because the higher dosages used in this situation can produce significantly more of the urotoxic metabolites than conventional dosing. These recommendations are currently supported by the ASCO consensus guidelines[36] (see Chapter 92, Hematopoietic Cell Transplantation).

38. **If J.R. develops hemorrhagic cystitis, how should it be treated?**

Once hemorrhagic cystitis develops, the chemotherapy agent causing the disorder must be discontinued and vigorous hydration started. If gross hematuria occurs, a large-bore catheter should be inserted to avoid obstruction of the urethra by clots. Some clinicians also use continuous silver nitrate irrigation, local instillation of formalin, or electrocauterization of bladder blood vessels. If these measures fail, surgical intervention may be necessary to divert urine flow away from the bladder.

Pulmonary Toxicities

39. **J.A., a 67-year-old man with an 8-year history of chronic lymphocytic leukemia (CLL), was treated intermittently for 7 years with chlorambucil and prednisone. About 1 year ago, increasing lymphadenopathy was noted and a biopsy revealed that his CLL had transformed to large-cell lymphoreticular lymphoma. (This transformation is called Richter's syndrome.) At that time, he was started on a chemotherapy regimen of cyclophosphamide, doxorubicin, vincristine, prednisone, and bleomycin (CHOP-Bleo), and his disease stabilized. Three weeks after his ninth course, he developed dyspnea, a nonproductive cough, and fever. Chest radiograph showed diffuse bilateral infiltrates; his respiratory rate (RR) was 36 breaths/ min; and his arterial blood gases (ABGs) were pH, 7.50 (normal, 7.35 to 7.45); PO_2, 62 (normal, 80 to 100 mm Hg); PCO_2, 28 (normal, 35 to 45 mm Hg); and an O_2 saturation of 92% (normal, 95% to 98%). What are the possible causes of his new pulmonary findings?**

J.A. is at risk for several processes that could produce diffuse pulmonary infiltrates and dyspnea. He undoubtedly is immunosuppressed secondary to both his lymphoma and the chemotherapy; therefore, J.A. has an increased risk for infection (e.g., *Pneumocystis carinii* or cytomegalovirus [CMV]). In addition, his lymphoma now may be resistant to the therapy, and the infiltrates may represent progression of the disease. Pulmonary infiltrates also may represent toxicity resulting from one or more of the chemotherapy agents he has received. Further diagnostic workup is necessary to establish the cause.

40. **A bronchoscopy with bronchoalveolar lavage and a biopsy with pathologic and microbiologic evaluations were performed. Bacterial, fungal, and viral cultures were negative, and the biopsy revealed inflammation and fibrosis with no evidence of lymphoma. These results are highly suggestive of agent-induced pulmonary damage. (Note: If the results of the bronchoscopy had not been helpful in establishing a diagnosis, an open-lung biopsy would have been recommended.) Which of the agents that J.A. received are associated with pulmonary toxicity, and what other factors may have increased his risk of pulmonary toxicity?**

Many chemotherapy agents have been associated with pulmonary toxicity (Table 89-15). According to the list, J.A. has

Table 89-15   Chemotherapy-Induced Pulmonary Toxicity

Drug	Histopathology	Clinical Features	Treatment/Outcome
Aldesleukin[259]	Capillary leak, pulmonary edema	*Clinical presentation.* ↓ BP, fever, SOB, anorexia, rash, mucositis	Stop infusion; provide supportive care to cause a quick resolution of symptoms.
Bleomycin[260–268]	Interstitial edema and hyaline membrane formation; mononuclear cell infiltration pneumonitis with progression to fibrosis; eosinophilic infiltrations seen in patients with suspected hypersensitivity-type reactions	Cumulative dose-related toxicity with risk increasing substantially with total dose >450 mg or 200 mg/m²; may occur during or after treatment *Clinical presentation:* cough, fever, dyspnea, tachypnea, rales, hypoxemia, bilateral infiltrates, dose-related ↓ in diffusing capacity	Recovery if bleomycin is discontinued while symptoms and radiologic changes still minimal; progressive and usually fatal if symptoms severe. Avoid cumulative doses >200 mg/m²; monitor serial pulmonary function tests. Discontinue therapy if diffusing capacity ≤40% of baseline, FVC <25% of baseline, or if any signs or symptoms suggestive of pulmonary toxicity occur. Steroids may be helpful if toxicity is result of hypersensitivity.
Busulfan[272]	Pneumocyte dysplasia; mononuclear cell infiltrations; fibrosis	Does not appear to be dose-related, but no cases reported with total doses <500 mg *Clinical presentation:* insidious onset of dyspnea, dry cough, fever, tachypnea, rales, hypoxemia diffuse linear infiltrate, ↓ in diffusing capacity	Fatal in most patients; progressive despite discontinuation of busulfan. High-dose steroids (50–100 mg prednisone daily) have been helpful in a few cases.
Carmustine[268–271]		Dose-related; usually occurs with doses >1,400 mg/m² *Clinical presentation:* dyspnea, tachypnea, dry hacking cough, bibasilar rales, hypoxemia, interstitial infiltrates; spontaneous pneumothorax has been reported	May continue to progress after carmustine discontinued. No evidence that steroids improve or alter incidence. High mortality rate if symptoms severe. Serial pulmonary function studies recommended. Total cumulative dose should not exceed 1,400 mg/m².
Chlorambucil[273]	Pneumocyte dysplasia; fibrosis	Usually occurs after at least 6 months of treatment with total cumulative doses of >2 g *Clinical presentation:* dyspnea, dry cough, anorexia, fatigue, fever, hypoxemia, bibasilar rales, localized infiltrates progressing to diffusing involvement of both lung fields	Fatal in most cases despite discontinuation of chlorambucil and treatment with high-dose steroids.
Cyclophosphamide[270,271]	Endothelial swelling, pneumocyte dysplasia, lymphocyte infiltration fibrosis	Does not appear to be schedule- or dose-related and may occur after discontinuation *Clinical presentation:* progressive dyspnea, fever, dry cough, tachypnea, fine rales, ↓ diffusing capacity and restrictive ventilatory defect, bilateral interstitial infiltrates	Clinical recovery reported in about 50% of patients within 1–8 wk if therapy stopped. Some of these patients received steroid therapy; however, others have died despite steroid therapy. Occasionally, therapy has been restarted without recurrence.
Cytarabine[274]	Pulmonary edema	*Clinical presentation:* tachypnea, hypoxemia, interstitial/alveolar infiltrates	Not always fatal.
Gemcitabine[275]	Pulmonary edema	Dyspnea was reported in 23% of patients; severe dyspnea in 3%; dyspnea occasionally accompanied by bronchospasm (<2% of patients); rare reports of parenchymal lung toxicity consistent with drug-induced pneumonitis	Treatment is supportive care measures. Symptoms resolve and are usually not seen with rechallenge.
Fludarabine[276]	Interstitial infiltrates, alveolitis, centrilobular emphysema	*Clinical presentation:* fever, dyspnea, cough, hypoxia; onset 3–28 days after third or fourth course; bilateral infiltrates and effusions	Resolves spontaneously over several weeks with or without corticosteroids.
Melphalan[273]	Pneumocyte dysplasia	Not dose-related *Clinical presentation:* dyspnea, dry cough, fever, tachypnea, rales, pleuritic chest pain, hypoxemia	Most patients die because of progressive pulmonary disease. Most reported cases occurred while patients were receiving concomitant prednisone therapy. Usually progresses rapidly

Table 89-15   Chemotherapy-Induced Pulmonary Toxicity—cont'd

Drug	Histopathology	Clinical Features	Treatment/Outcome
Methotrexate[277-281] _Delayed_	Nonspecific changes; occasional fibrosis	No evidence that dose related; daily or weekly schedules more likely to cause toxicity than monthly dosing _Clinical presentation:_ headache, malaise prodrome, dyspnea, dry cough, fever, hypoxemia, tachypnea, rales, eosinophilia, cyanosis in up to 50% of patients, interstitial infiltrates, ↓ diffusing capacity, restrictive ventilatory defect	Most patients recover within 1–6 wk (some may have persistent infiltrates or ↓ pulmonary function parameters). Steroids may produce more rapid resolution. May resolve despite continuation of methotrexate, but discontinuation may speed resolution. Rarely fatal.
Noncardiac pulmonary edema _Pleuritic chest pain_	Acute pulmonary edema	Occurs very rarely 6–12 hr after PO or IT methotrexate Not related to other methotrexate toxicities or serum levels; may not occur with each course of therapy _Clinical presentation:_ right sided chest pain, occasional pleural effusion or collapse of lung, thickened pleural densities	Fatal in 2 of 3 reported cases. Resolved wtihin 3 days in 1 case. Usually resolves within 3–5 days.
Mitomycin[273,281]	Similar to bleomycin	_Clinical presentation:_ dyspnea, dry cough, basilar rales, hypoxemia, bilateral interstitial or finely nodular infiltrates, ↓ diffusing capacity	Fatal in ≈50% of cases. Complete resolution reported in some patients, including some who received steroid therapy.
Procarbazine[282,283]	Hypersensitivity pneumonitis with eosinophilia and interstitial fibrosis	_Clinical presentation:_ nausea, fever, dry cough, dyspnea within a few hours of ingestion, bilateral interstitial infiltrates, and pleural effusion	Rapid resolution after discontinuation.
Vinblastine[229]	Hyperplasia, dysplasia, interstitial edema, and fibrosis	Associated with concomitant treatment with mitomycin _Clinical presentation:_ acute respiratory distress, bilateral infiltrates	Initial improvement with subsequent progression.

BP, blood pressure; FVC, forced vital capacity; IT, intrathecal; SOB, shortness of breath.

received three agents with potential pulmonary toxicity, including chlorambucil, cyclophosphamide, and bleomycin. Factors that may increase the risk of agent-induced pulmonary toxicity are listed in Table 89-16. Because J.A. has received three potentially pulmonary toxic agents and because of his advanced age, he is at increased risk for pulmonary toxicity.

Among the chemotherapy agents, bleomycin most commonly causes pulmonary toxicity. Although several forms

Table 89-16   Factors Associated With Increased Risk of Chemotherapy-Induced Pulmonary Toxicity

Risk Factor	Drug(s)
Total cumulative dose	Bleomycin, carmustine
Age	Bleomycin
Oxygen therapy	Bleomycin, cyclophosphamide, mitomycin
Irradiation to lungs	Bleomycin, busulfan, carmustine, mitomycin
Concurrent therapy with other drugs	Bleomycin, carmustine, cyclophosphamide, methotrexate, mitomycin, vinblastine
Pre-existing pulmonary disease	Carmustine
Tobacco use	Carmustine

Adapted from reference 285.

have been reported, the most frequent is interstitial pneumonitis followed by pulmonary fibrosis.[260,261,273,281,285] Patients generally present with a nonproductive cough and dyspnea. Clinicians may detect only fine crackling bibasilar rales that often progress to coarse rales. The chest radiograph may be normal in the early stages, but patients can develop bilateral alveolar and interstitial infiltrates. ABGs show hypoxia, and pulmonary function tests generally show a progressive fall in the diffusing capacity without a significant decrease in the forced vital capacity.[273] The most significant factor associated with the development of pulmonary toxicity is the cumulative dose of bleomycin. At total doses <400 mg, less than 10% of patients may develop pulmonary toxicity. When the cumulative dose reaches 450 to 500 mg, the dose-related effect becomes more prominent. The incidence may be lower when patients receive bleomycin by a continuous infusion.[262] A rarer, hypersensitivity reaction produces fever, eosinophilia, and diffuse infiltrates, and this pulmonary toxicity is not dose related. The mortality associated with bleomycin pulmonary toxicity is about 50%.[273,281,285] If bleomycin is discontinued while symptoms are minimal and before pulmonary function has decompensated significantly, the damage may not progress. In contrast, patients with prominent physical and radiographic findings generally die because of pulmonary complications. Other chemotherapy agents can potentially exacerbate the pulmonary toxicity associated with bleomycin.

Less commonly, chlorambucil and cyclophosphamide induce pulmonary toxicities similar to bleomycin. Chlorambucil-induced lung damage appears to be dose related because most cases have occurred in patients who received a total dose exceeding 2 g over >6 months.[273] In most instances, patients died of severe interstitial pulmonary fibrosis. Cyclophosphamide pulmonary toxicity does not appear to be related to the dosage regimen. Approximately 50% to 65% of patients improve clinically after discontinuing therapy. If a patient presents with signs or symptoms consistent with pulmonary toxicity, the patient should undergo a diagnostic workup after discontinuing therapy.

41. **Why are routine pulmonary evaluations indicated in patients like J.A. who receive bleomycin or other pulmonary toxic agents?**

Because a dose-related decrease in diffusing capacity has been observed in patients receiving bleomycin before the onset of clinical symptoms, routine baseline and serial pulmonary function studies are recommended.[263] Bleomycin therapy should be withheld if the diffusing capacity falls below 40% of the baseline value, if the forced vital capacity falls below 75% of the baseline value, or if patients develop any signs or symptoms of pulmonary damage.[273] Some practitioners also recommend limiting the total cumulative dose to 450 mg or less. Specific screening is not routinely recommended for patients receiving other pulmonary toxic agents; however, if patients develop any symptoms or clinical findings, therapy should be withheld until the cause can be determined.

Management

42. **How should J.A.'s agent-induced pulmonary toxicity be managed?**

The most effective way to manage pulmonary toxicity is to prevent it. However, if pulmonary toxicity becomes evident, all responsible agents (in J.A.'s case: bleomycin, chlorambucil, and cyclophosphamide) should be discontinued and the patient should receive symptomatic support based on his physical condition (e.g., oxygen). As illustrated by J.A., other treatable causes of pulmonary infiltrates (e.g., infection) also should be ruled out. Unfortunately, in many cases, pulmonary toxicity is irreversible and progressive, and effective treatments are unavailable. Corticosteroids often are administered but probably are effective only in cases in which hypersensitivity caused the pulmonary damage. Nevertheless, because other effective treatments are lacking, a trial of steroids generally is indicated for all patients; if steroids are discontinued, they must be tapered carefully to avoid clinical deterioration.

Hepatotoxicity

43. **J.D. has received two courses of chemotherapy with cytarabine and daunorubicin. Before chemotherapy was started, his liver function tests (LFTs) and coagulation studies were within normal limits. His current laboratory values include the following: aspartate aminotransferase (AST), 204 U/L (normal, 8 to 46); alanine aminotransferase (ALT), 197 U/L (normal, 7 to 46); lactate dehydrogenase (LDH), 795 U/L (normal, 100 to 190); alkaline phosphatase, 285 U/L (normal, 25 to 100); bilirubin, 1.2 mg/dL (normal, <1.5); and PT, 13.1 seconds (normal, 11 to 16). Why could J.D.'s chemotherapy be responsible for these laboratory abnormalities?**

[SI units: AST, 3.4 mkat/L; ALT, 22.98 mkat/L; LDH, 13.25 mkat/L; alkaline phosphatase, 4.75 mkat/L; bilirubin, 20.52 mmol/L]

Elevated LFTs occur frequently in cancer patients and their causes are listed in Table 89-17. Other signs and symptoms include jaundice, nausea, vomiting, abdominal pain, and rarely, encephalopathy. Patients should receive an extensive workup to determine whether they require any immediate attention for tumor involvement of the liver or possible infection. In addition, patients should discontinue any nonessential medications that can potentially cause hepatotoxicity. The clinician may also need to consider discontinuing chemotherapy because some agents may cause the hepatotoxicity observed.

Several chemotherapy agents, including cytarabine given to J.D., have been associated with hepatocellular damage (Table 89-18). The agents most commonly associated with

Table 89-17 Common Causes of Elevated LFTs in Patients With Cancer

Primary or metastatic tumor involvement of the liver
Hepatotoxic drugs (e.g., cytotoxics, hormones [estrogens, androgens], antiemetics [phenothiazines], antimicrobials [rifampin, isoniazid])
Infections (e.g., hepatic candidiasis, viral hepatitis)
Parenteral nutrition
Allopurinol
Portal vein thrombosis
Paraneoplastic syndrome
History of liver disease

LFTs, liver function tests.

Table 89-18 Hepatotoxicity From Antineoplastic Drugs

Drug/Schedule	Prevalence	Type
Asparaginase[292–294]		
Daily	Frequent	Hepatocellular fatty metamorphosis
Carmustine[295–296]		
Weekly bolus	Common	Hepatocellular
Daily × 3	Common	
Bolus	Infrequent	
Cytarbine[297]		
Daily	Common	Cholestatic
Decarbazine		
Daily × 5	Infrequent	Hepatocellular
Bolus		
Etoposide[300]		
High dose	Common with high dose	Hepatocellular
Lomustine[298,299]	Infrequent	
Mercaptopurine[303,304]		
Daily	Common	Cholestatic
High dose		Hepatocellular
Methotrexate[305,306]		
Daily	Common	Hepatocellular
Weekly bolus	Rare	Hepatocellular
High dose	Uncommon	Hepatocellular
Mitomycin[307]		
High dose	Infrequent	Veno-occlusive disease
Plicamycin[308,309]		
Daily × 5	Common	Hepatocellular
Streptozocin[310]		
Bolus	Common	Hepatocellular
Thioguanine[311]		
Daily	Rare	Veno-occlusive disease
Epirubicin	Infrequent	Hepatocellular

Table 89-19 **Chemotherapeutics Requiring Dose Modification in Hepatic Dysfunction**

Bilirubin	AST	Adriamycin	Daunorubicin	Vincristine Vinblastine Etoposide	Methotrexate	5-Fluorouracil
<1.5	<60	100%	100%	100%	100%	100%
1.5–3.0	60–80	50%	75%	50%	100%	100%
3.1–5.0	>180	25%	50%	Omit	100%	100%
5.0		Omit	Omit	Omit	75%	100%
					Omit	Omit

Paclitaxel-CALGB Recommendations for Dosing in Patients With Liver Dysfunction

	AST >2 × ULN and Bilirubin ≤1.5	<135 mg/m²
	Bilirubin = 1.6–3.0	≤75 mg/m²
	Bilirubin ≥3.1	≤50 mg/m²

Epirubicin

	Bilirubin 1.2–3.0 AST 2–4 × ULN	↓ dosage by 50%
	Bilirubin .3 or AST ≥4 × ULN	↓ dosage by 75%

AST, aspartate aminotransferase; CALGB, cancer and leukemia group B; ULN, upper limit of normal.

hepatotoxicity include asparaginase, carmustine, cytarabine, mercaptopurine, and streptozocin. Both methotrexate and mithramycin have caused hepatotoxicity when given on a daily schedule; however, if they are given on an intermittent basis, the incidence of toxicity decreases significantly.[305,306,308,309] These drugs come in contact with the liver by entering the liver's blood supply; the liver uniquely receives a dual blood supply from the portal and superior mesenteric veins. The liver can detoxify or inactivate noxious substances and metabolizes many chemotherapeutic agents as well. When chemotherapy agents undergo metabolism, they may damage the metabolic processes in the liver. The exact mechanisms by which chemotherapy agents cause hepatotoxicity are unknown, but most agents probably cause hepatic damage by (1) interfering with the mitochondrial function of the hepatocyte, (2) depleting hepatic glutathione stores, (3) eliciting hypersensitivity reactions, (4) decreasing bile flow, or (5) causing phlebitis of the central hepatic vein to produce veno-occlusive disease.[312] All patients receiving potentially hepatotoxic chemotherapy should undergo routine monitoring to minimize their risk of long-term complications.

Several laboratory tests can provide markers of liver structure and function. Serum transaminases, alkaline phosphatase, and bilirubin levels should be monitored routinely in patients receiving hepatotoxic chemotherapy. Although these laboratory indices are sensitive indicators of liver injury, they are nonspecific for the type of liver disease and do not necessarily correlate with hepatic function. Serum levels of proteins produced by the liver such as ferritin, albumin, prealbumin, or retinol-binding protein also may be helpful in assessing liver function. Once the patient shows evidence of hepatotoxicity, the clinician needs to determine how to manage the patient's cancer.

The decision to continue or discontinue chemotherapy in patients with apparent hepatic dysfunction can be difficult. If the chemotherapy is the suspected cause, therapy should be withheld until LFTs are within normal ranges. The clinician should also consider alternative (nonhepatotoxic) chemother-

apy for future treatment. In addition, agents that are cleared predominantly via the liver may require dosage adjustments and should be administered cautiously (Table 89-19).

J.A.'s therapy is likely responsible for his elevated liver enzymes. Therefore, costly workup should be deferred to allow recovery of liver function. Recovery should occur within 2 weeks of chemotherapy. If full recovery does not occur, further therapy (agents and/or doses) may require modifications.

LONG-TERM COMPLICATIONS OF CHEMOTHERAPY
Second Malignancies After Chemotherapy
Acute Nonlymphocytic Leukemia

44. T.D., a 60-year-old woman, was diagnosed with epithelial carcinoma of the ovary stage 1, 6 years before this admission. She underwent a total abdominal hysterectomy, bilateral salpingo-oophorectomy, and omentectomy. Pathologic features suggested that she may be at a high risk for recurrent disease and that adjuvant therapy could be beneficial. Consequently, T.D. received a course of melphalan 0.2 mg/kg per day PO for 5 days Q 4 weeks for 10 courses. On this admission, she has no evidence of ovarian cancer; however, she has complaints of increasing fatigue, fever, and chills. A peripheral blood smear shows a WBC count of 120,000/mm³ with a differential of >90% leukemic blasts, a bone marrow examination confirms acute nonlymphocytic leukemia (ANLL). Subsequent cytogenetic analysis revealed abnormalities of chromosomes 5 and 7. What factors support the diagnosis of chemotherapy-associated acute leukemia in T.D.?

Acute leukemia has been associated with chemotherapy used to treat hematologic malignancies, solid tumors, and nonmalignant diseases.[313] It usually occurs 3 to 4 years after the patient finishes chemotherapy.[314] Myelodysplastic syndrome (preleukemia changes) commonly occurs in 50% of patients before overt acute leukemia.[315,316]Although all alkylating agents can cause acute leukemia, melphalan appears to be the most potent leukemogenic agent in this class; other classes of chemotherapy agents do not appear to carry as significant a risk. Large doses, continuous daily dosing, prolonged treatment periods, age >40 years, and concomitant radiation therapy may increase the risk of developing acute leukemia. Several additional factors may increase a patient's risk of developing acute leukemia.[317-320]

ANLL also has been reported after combination chemotherapy that involves topoisomerase inhibitors including teniposide, etoposide, and antracyclines.[321] These leukemias usually occur sooner, and myelodysplasia does not usually occur before the leukemia. Other characteristics include FAB M4 or M5 classification and chromosomal abnormalities involving chromosome 11q23. Cumulative risks of 4% to 12% have been reported with a higher prevalence observed in children treated with relatively high doses of teniposide and other agents with or without radiation therapy for acute lymphocytic leukemia. It is unclear what role other chemotherapy agents and radiation played in these reports. Nonetheless, combination chemotherapy with epipodophyllotoxins confers some risk of leukemia. This is an important area for research given the widespread use of these agents for many curable diseases.

Evidence that chemotherapy can cause secondary lymphoid malignancies, particularly non-Hodgkin's lymphoma (NHL), is also strong. Immunosuppression from the disease and its treatment rather than the particular chemotherapy agent may be the primary cause of NHL. Other secondary malignancies can occur after chemotherapy as well. Solid tumors have been associated with superficial bladder cancer in patients treated with daily oral cyclophosphamide and bone sarcoma has occurred after treatment with alkylating agents.[323] The secondary solid tumors in patients treated with other chemotherapy agents is considered coincidental.[291,323,324]

T.D.'s ANLL probably occurred secondary to her previous melphalan therapy. The chemotherapy agent, as well as the time course for her acute leukemia, is consistent with alkylating agent-induced malignancies. In addition, cytogenetic abnormalities occur in >90% of those patients who have received chemotherapy or radiation therapy and have subsequently developed therapy-related myelodysplastic syndrome or acute nonlymphocytic leukemia.[316] Chromosomes 5 and 7 are involved in almost 90% of cases with cytogenetic abnormalities.[325] Deletions of all or part of chromosomes 5 and 7 in T.D. strongly support the diagnosis of chemotherapy-associated acute leukemia rather than de novo leukemia.

THERAPY AND PROGNOSIS

45. **Are the therapy and prognosis of T.D. with treatment-associated ANLL similar to those of patients with de novo ANLL?**

Therapy of patients with treatment-associated ANLL compares poorly with that of patients with de novo leukemia. Complete remissions with standard cytarabine and daunorubicin regimens are obtained in less than half of patients with treatment-associated ANLL compared with a complete remission rate of 70% to 80% in patients with de novo leukemia[326,327] (see Chapter 90). High-dose cytarabine produced remissions in 10 of 11 patients with acute nonlymphocytic leukemia secondary to chemotherapy in one series.[328] However, most series reported a lower response rate, with responses of short duration and a median survival of only 3 to 4 months. Isolated case reports suggest that bone marrow transplantation may benefit younger patients and those with human leukocyte antigen (HLA) identical donors.[329,331]

The best "treatment" of therapy-associated ANLL is prevention. In patients like T.D. with curable malignancies, avoiding the use of alkylating agents is strongly encouraged. Efforts to eliminate alkylating agents from regimens used to treat patients with curable disease are ongoing. Although the choice of melphalan for adjuvant treatment of T.D.'s ovarian cancer was not inappropriate at the time, she would be far less likely to receive melphalan today.

Fertility and Teratogenicity
Effects on Oogenesis

46. **C.L., a 32-year-old woman with recently diagnosed stage II breast cancer, underwent a lumpectomy and external-beam radiation therapy and is scheduled to begin adjuvant chemotherapy with cyclophosphamide, doxorubicin, and fluorouracil (CAF). C.L. was married 12 months before her diagnosis and wishes to have children. What are C.L.'s prospects for fertility following adjuvant chemotherapy?**

Chemotherapy is potentially gonadotoxic in humans. Ovarian biopsies taken from women treated for cancer demonstrate loss of ova and follicular elements.[332,333] This injury is evident even in prepubertal females treated for cancer.[334,335] Ova die or become nonfunctional by direct injury to the ova or by indirect injury resulting from loss of supporting follicular cells. If the damage to the follicular elements is extensive and irreversible, fertility is impaired even if the ova are spared.

Agent-induced injury to ova and follicular elements reduces ovarian estrogen and progesterone secretion in menstruating women. This causes the hypothalamus and pituitary to secrete more follicle-stimulating hormone (FSH) and luteinizing hormone (LH), which in turn increase follicular recruitment and the number of follicles vulnerable to chemotherapy agents. If the gonadal toxicity is severe and/or prolonged, permanent ovarian failure can occur secondary to depletion of ova and follicles. However, recovery of some of the affected follicles often occurs, and this may be manifested by irregular menses or delayed recovery of menses. If the ova are spared and follicular cells recover sufficiently, ovulation and pregnancy may occur, but premature ovarian failure is inevitable in most women treated with large doses of gonadotoxic agents given over long periods.

Prepubertal girls have a greater reserve of primary follicles and because their ovaries are not producing estrogen and progesterone, increases in FSH and LH with resultant recruitment of follicular elements do not occur. For this reason, prepubertal girls can tolerate large doses without apparent effects even if the pathology previously described occurs. The gonadal effects of chemotherapy in women and girls are described in several reviews.[334,335]

C.L. is going to receive one of the alkylating agents, which are the most potent gonadotoxic agents. Cyclophosphamide is well known for producing infertility in men and women and gonadal failure even in children. The effect is influenced strongly by the total dose of cyclophosphamide and the patient's age at the onset of chemotherapy. Nearly 100% of women over 29 years of age develop amenorrhea when the mean total dose is 20.8 g/m^2. The same consequence can be expected in women 30 to 39 years of age who receive 7.55 g/m^2 and in women 40 years of age and older who receive 3.25 g/m^2. Depending on the exact dose of cyclophosphamide in the CAF regimen planned, C.L. may or may not fall into a dose range that would be expected to produce permanent amenorrhea.

The clinician also must consider that a synergistic gonadotoxic effect has been reported when doxorubicin is combined with cyclophosphamide. The onset of amenorrhea may occur at half the total dose of cyclophosphamide after therapy with doxorubicin and cyclophosphamide than after treatment with cyclophosphamide, methotrexate, and fluorouracil. Fluorouracil is unlikely to play any role in producing ovarian failure. Aside from the alkylating agents, the only chemotherapy agents with strong evidence of gonadal toxicity include vinblastine, etoposide, and cisplatin. Several excellent reviews discuss the doses of chemotherapy agents, used both alone and in combination, and specific incidences of associated gonadotoxicity, as well as the prevalence of temporary and permanent amenorrhea.[336–338]

C.L. will most likely experience amenorrhea along with the signs and symptoms of menopause as estrogen and progesterone production diminish during chemotherapy. C.L. may recover from chemotherapy-induced amenorrhea months to years after completion of her therapy. Recovery may be manifested as amenorrhea interspersed with normal menstrual periods. Pregnancy is possible during periods of normal menstruation because ovulation does occur in most instances. However, premature menopause is inevitable. Because the greatest risk of pregnancy exists early in the course of chemotherapy, C.L. should be counseled to practice birth control while receiving chemotherapy. Since oral contraceptives are contraindicated in breast cancer patients, barrier methods (i.e., diaphragm, condoms, spermicide) should be advised.

Effects on Spermatogenesis

47. **J.K., a 25-year-old man with recently diagnosed stage IV Hodgkin's lymphoma, will receive systemic chemotherapy. What effect does systemic chemotherapy have on male gonadal function?**

The primary gonadal toxic effect of chemotherapy agents in males is a progressive dose-related depletion of the germinal epithelium lining the seminiferous tubule.[339,340] The clinical manifestations of germinal depletion include a marked reduction in testicular volume and azoospermia. The Leydig cells responsible for testosterone production remain morphologically intact, although mild functional impairment occurs rarely. The major toxicity of chemotherapy in men is loss of reproductive capacity. During treatment, libido and sexual activity may decline, but most men report a return to pretreatment sexual function after chemotherapy.[339,340]

Of the chemotherapy agents, alkylating agents most commonly are associated with azoospermia. Progressive dose-related oligospermia occurs in men receiving chlorambucil,[341,342] cyclophosphamide,[343,344] nitrogen mustard, busulfan, procarbazine, and nitrosureas; procarbazine appears to be the most gonadotoxic alkylating agent in men. Doxorubicin, vinblastine, cytarabine, and cisplatin also have been associated with azoospermia,[345] and doxorubicin appears to have a synergistic toxic effect in men when given with cyclophosphamide similar to that previously described in women. Phase-specific agents, such as antimetabolites and plant alkaloids, seem unlikely to produce azoospermia when used alone but may play a minor role in combination chemotherapy regimens.

In contrast to oogenesis, in which women are born with a full complement of ova, spermatogenesis occurs in a continuous cycle of regeneration, differentiation, and maturation beginning in the second month of embryogenesis and continuing through old age. Although different chemotherapy agents appear to exert more damage to germ cells in specific phases of spermatogenesis in animal models, in humans, gonadotoxic agents generally are used in large enough doses to affect varying proportions of maturing sperm cells in any stage of development. This has two realistic implications. The first is that because spermatogenesis must start at the beginning after agent-induced azoospermia occurs, the length of recovery is prolonged, usually lasting at least 2 to 3 years. The second is that the relationship of age to the development of azoospermia is far less clear than the relationship of age to ovarian suppression. Although conventional wisdom holds that prepubertal males are less likely to be affected by chemotherapy agents than adult males, the reserve of primitive sperm cells in male children is far less than it is in adults. Therefore, the spermatogenesis potential in prepubertal testes may make them more vulnerable to cytotoxic damage than those of adults. A review of the literature regarding the effects of chemotherapy administered to male children concluded that agents and regimens known to be toxic in men should be considered toxic in young boys.[336] Short of a testicular biopsy, the damage cannot be detected until puberty.

The two diseases most likely to affect young men who are concerned with their fertility are Hodgkin's disease and testicular cancer. The two treatment regimens for advanced Hodgkin's disease are (1) mechlorethamine, vincristine, prednisone, and procarbazine (MOPP) and (2) doxorubicin, bleomycin, vinblastine, and dacarbazine (ABVD) (see Table 88-10 in Chapter 88, Neoplastic Disorders and Their Treatment). Of the two, ABVD is considered equally efficacious and less toxic. In a comparison of these treatment regimens, azoospermia occurred in 100% of MOPP-treated patients versus 35% of those receiving ABVD. Furthermore, spermatogenesis nearly always recovered in the ABVD-treated patients.[345] This is consistent with information regarding the potential of mechlorethamine and procarbazine to produce testicular germ cell depletion when compared with the agents included in the ABVD regimen. This information may be important in planning treatment for young men with Hodgkin's disease who are concerned about preservation of fertility after treatment of their curable malignancy.

A similar scenario exists in patients about to start on chemotherapy for testicular cancer. Evidence to date suggests that chemotherapy-induced azoospermia that follows treatment with vinblastine, bleomycin, and cisplatin for nonseminomatous testicular carcinoma is reversible within 2 to 3 years in approximately 50% of patients treated and that those who recover spermatogenesis are capable of impregnating their partners.[346,347] In this particular patient population, it is important to recognize that retroperitoneal lymph node dissection, which results in retrograde ejaculation, as well as cryptorchidism, which predisposes to infertility, may contribute to the lack of full recovery of fertility potential.

48. **Aside from the use of chemotherapy agents with less gonadal toxicity, are there means of circumventing infertility in young patients receiving chemotherapy?**

Sperm/gamete cryopreservation should be considered in males. A major limitation of this approach has been the finding of diminished sperm counts, sperm volume, and sperm motility in young males affected with Hodgkin's disease and testicular cancer before combination chemotherapy is initiated.[348,349] Although published studies suggest that the quantity and motility of sperm are important determinants of successful artificial insemination, pregnancies have been reported.[350,351] Thus, sperm banking should be considered even in oligospermic males.

Oocyte and embryo cryopreservation now are feasible options for young women about to undergo cytotoxic chemotherapy. Even in the face of chemotherapy-induced ovarian failure, in vitro fertilization of an ovum, and implantation into the endometrium with proper hormonal support can successfully accommodate a term pregnancy.[352,353] This may be an option for C.L. described in Question 46.

In both genders, it has been hypothesized that gonadal toxicity from chemotherapy could be decreased by inhibiting spermatogenesis or follicular development during chemotherapy. Methods used to suppress gonadal function have included administration of testosterone in men,[354] oral contraceptives in women,[355] and gonadotropin-releasing hormone analogs (LHRH analogs) in both men and women.[336,355,356] Unfortunately, none of these approaches has proved effective despite encouraging preliminary results in experimental animal and human studies.

Teratogenicity

49. **If C.L. or J.K. regain fertility after their planned combination chemotherapy regimens, are they at risk for producing offspring with congenital abnormalities or an excess risk of cancer?**

Most of the agents used to treat cancer are designed specifically to interfere with DNA synthesis, cellular metabolism, and cell division. Thus, there is reason to suspect that they may cause mutation of ova or spermatocytes exposed to these effects. The actual outcomes of pregnancies in survivors of cancer are published as case reports, small series, and retrospective case series. Nearly 1,600 children have been born to 1,078 patients previously treated for malignancy in childhood or as adults. A review of the published information suggests no evidence that spontaneous abortion, genetic disease, or congenital anomalies occurs more frequently in the progeny of cancer survivors. Similarly, there does not appear to be an increased risk of malignancy in the offspring of patients treated for cancer.[336] The likely explanation for this is that ova and sperm cells affected by chemotherapy usually are killed. The risk of producing an abnormal offspring thus would be highest at the time of ongoing germ cell exposure. Men and women should be explicitly discouraged from conception during chemotherapy. In general, adults surviving cancer should be advised to wait ≥2 years after completion of therapy before attempting to parent a child; this allows time for elimination of damaged germ cells. This also provides time to assess the likelihood of the necessity for further treatment that would have grave consequences, particularly in the case of female patients.

REFERENCES

1. American Society of Clinical Oncology. Recommendations for use of hematopoietin colony-stimulating factors: evidence-based clinical practice. Guidelines. J Clin Oncol 1994;12:2471.
2. American Society of Clinical Oncology Home Page. Available at: http://www.asco.org. Accessed March 12, 1999.
3. Doweiko JP, Goldberg MA. Erythropoietin therapy in cancer patients. Oncology 1991;5:31.
4. Citron ML et al. Randomized trial of dose-dense versus conventionally scheduled and sequential versus concurrent combination chemotherapy as postoperative adjuvant treatment of node-positive primary breast cancer: First report of intergroup trial C9741/Cancer and Leukemia Group B Trial 9741. J Clin Oncol 2003;21:1431.
5. Holmes FA et al. Blinded, randomized, multicenter study to evaluate single administration pegfilgrastim once per cycle versus daily filgrastim as an adjunct to chemotherapy in patients with high-risk stage II or stage III/IV breast cancer. J Clin Oncol 2002;20:727.
6. Mayordomo JI et al. Decreasing morbidity and cost of treating febrile neutropenia by adding G-CSF and GM-CSF to standard antibiotic therapy: results of a randomized trial. Proc Am Soc Clin Oncol 1993;12:437.
7. Pekka Riikonen et al. rh GM-CSF in the treatment of fever and neutropenia: a double-blind, placebo-controlled study in children with malignancy. Proc Am Soc Clin Oncol 1993;12:443.
8. Tomaik A et al. Duration of intravenous (IV) antibiotic and hospital stay for patients with febrile neutropenia after chemotherapy: experience of Ottawa Regional Cancer Centre. Proc Am Soc Clin Oncol 1993;12:435.
9. Rolston K et al. Outpatient treatment of febrile episodes in low-risk neutropenia cancer patients [Abstract]. Proc Am Soc Clin Oncol 1993;12:436.
10. El-Dairy W, Morris L. High cost of hospital admissions for cancer patients at low risk to develop complications from febrile neutropenia [Abstract]. Proc Am Soc Clin Oncol 1993;12:461.
11. Neumega package insert. Cambridge, MA: Genetics Institute, Inc., 1998 June.
12. Abels RI, Rudnick SA. Erythropoietin: evolving clinical applications. Exp Hematol 1991;19:842.
13. Oster W et al. Erythropoietin for the treatment of anemia of malignancy associated with neoplastic bone marrow infiltration. J Clin Oncol 1990;8:956.
14. Platanias LC et al. Treatment of chemotherapy-induced anemia with recombinant human erythropoietin in cancer patients. J Clin Oncol 1991;9:2021.
15. Gabrilove JL et al. Once-weekly dosing of epoetin alfa is similar to three-times weekly dosing in increasing hemoglobulin and quality of life [Abstract]. Proc Am Soc Clin Oncol 1999;18:573a.
16. Glaspy J et al. Impact of therapy with epoetin alfa on clinical outcomes in patients with nonmyeloid malignancies during cancer chemotherapy in community oncology practice. Procrit Study Group [Abstract]. J Clin Oncol 1997;15:1218.
17. Glaspy JA et al. Darbepoetin alfa administered every 1 or 2 weeks (with no loss of dose efficiency) alleviates anemia in patients with solid tumors [abstr]. Blood 2001;98:298a.
18. Glaspy JA et al. Darbepoetin alfa given every one or two weeks alleviates anaemia associated with cancer chemotherapy. Br J Cancer 2002 Jul 29(87)(3):268–276.
19. Henry DH. Recombinant human erythropoietin for the treatment of anemia in patients with advanced cancer. Semin Hematol 1993;30(4 Suppl 6):12.
20. Whitecare JP Jr et al. L-Asparaginase. N Engl J Med 1970;282:732.
21. Ramsay NKC et al. The effect of L-asparaginase on plasma coagulation factors in acute lymphoblastic leukemia. Cancer 1977;40:1398.
22. Levine MN et al. The thrombogenic effect of anticancer agent therapy in women with stage II breast cancer. N Engl J Med 1988;318:404.
23. Ruiz MA et al. The influence of chemotherapy on plasma coagulation and fibrinolytic systems in lung cancer patients. Cancer 1989;63:643.
24. Rogers JS II et al. Chemotherapy for breast cancer decreases plasma protein C and protein S. J Clin Oncol 1988;6:276.
25. Kaufman PA et al. Autologous bone marrow transplantation and factor XII, factor VII, and protein C deficiencies: report of a new association and its possible relationship to endothelial cell injury. Cancer 1990;66:515.
26. Trousseau A. Phlegmasia alba dolens. Clinique medicale de L'Hotel-Dieu de Paris. London: The New Sydenham Society, 1865;3:94.
27. Sack GH Jr et al. Trousseau's syndrome and other manifestations of chronic disseminated coagulopathy in patients with neoplasms: clinical, pathophysiologic, and therapeutic features. Medicine 1977;56:1.
28. Aderka D et al. Idiopathic deep vein thrombosis in an apparently healthy patient as a premonitory sign of occult cancer. Cancer 1986;57:1846.
29. Goldberg RJ et al. Occult malignant neoplasm in patients with deep venous thrombosis. Arch Intern Med 1987;147:251.
30. Goldberg MA et al. Is heparin administration necessary during induction chemotherapy for patients with acute promyelocytic leukemia? Blood 1987;69:187.
31. Lindley CM. Incidence and duration of chemotherapy-induced nausea and vomiting in an outpatient cancer population. J Clin Oncol 1989;7:1142.
32. Sonis ST et al. Oral complications in patients receiving treatment for malignancies other than of the head and neck. J Am Dent Assoc 1978;97:468.

33. Lockhart PB, Sonis ST. Alterations in the oral mucosa caused by chemotherapy agents. J Dermatol Surg Oncol 1981;7:1019.

34. Eneroth CM et al. Effects of fractionated radiotherapy on salivary gland function. Cancer 1972;30:1147.

35. Berger A et al. Oral capsaicin provides temporary relief for oral mucositis pain secondary to chemotherapy/radiation therapy. J Pain Symptom Manage 1995;10:243.

36. Hensley ML et al. American Society of Clinical Oncology clinical practice guidelines for the use of chemotherapy and radiotherapy protectants. J Clin Oncol 1999;17(10):3333.

37. LeVeque FG et al. A multicenter, randomized, double-blind, placebo-controlled, dose-titration study of oral pilocarpine for treatment of radiation-induced xerostomia in head and neck cancer patients. J Clin Oncol 1993;11:1123.

38. Johnson JT et al. Oral pilocarpine for post-radiation xerostomia in patients with head and neck cancer. N Engl J Med 1993;329:390.

39. Donatsky O et al. Effect of saliment on parotid salivary gland secretion and on xerostomia caused by Sjogren's syndrome. Scand J Dent Res 1982;90:157.

40. Klestov AC et al. Treatment of xerostomia: a double-blind trial of 108 patients with Sjogren's syndrome. Oral Surg Oral Med Oral Pathol 1981;51:594.

41. Keys HM, McCasland JP. Techniques and results of a comprehensive dental care program in head and neck cancer patients. Int J Radiat Oncol Biol Phys 1976;1:859.

42. Sonis ST et al. Pretreatment oral assessment. J Natl Cancer Inst 1990;9:29.

43. Gelclair Drug Information, Cell Pathways, Inc. (www.cellpathways.com/2_GELCLAIR/gelclair.html).

44. Innocenti M, Moscatelli G, Lopez S. Efficacy of gelclair in reducing pain in palliative care patients with oral lesions: Preliminary findings from an open pilot study (letter). J Pain Symptom Manage 2002;24:456.

45. Mahood D et al. Inhibition of fluorouracil-induced stomatitis by oral cryotherapy. J Clin Oncol 1991;9:449.

46. An derson PM, Schroeder G, Skubitz KM. Oral glutamine reduces the duration and severity of stomatitis after cytotoxic cancer chemotherapy. Cancer 1998;83:1433.

47. Anderson PM et al. Effect of low dose oral glutamine on painful stomatitis during bone marrow transplantation. Bone Marrow Transplant 1998;22:339.

48. Okuno SH et al. Phase III controlled evaluation of glutamine for decreasing stomatitis in patients receiving fluorouracil (fluorouracil)-based chemotherapy. Am J Clin Oncol 1999;22:258.

49. Jebb SA et al. 5-fluorouracil and folinic acid-induced mucositis: No effect of oral glutamine supplementation. Br J Cancer 1994;70:732.

50. Ferretti GA et al. Chlorhexidine in prophylaxis against oral infections and associated complications in patients receiving bone marrow transplantation. J Am Dent Assoc 1987;114:292.

51. Ferretti GA et al. Chlorhexidine prophylaxis for chemotherapy and radiotherapy-induced stomatitis: a randomized, double-blind trial. Oral Surg Med Oral Pathol 1990;69:331.

52. Gabrilove JL et al. Effect of granulocyte colony-stimulating factor on neutropenia and associated morbidity due to chemotherapy for transitional-cell carcinoma of the urothelium. N Engl J Med 1988;318:1414.

53. Shaw MT et al. Effects of cancer, radiotherapy and cytotoxic agents on intestinal structure and function. Cancer Treat Rev 1979;6:141.

54. Wurth MA, Musacchila XJ. Mechlorethamine effects on intestinal absorption in vitro and on cell proliferation. Am J Physiol 1973;225:73.

55. Roche AC et al. Correlation between the histological changes and glucose intestine absorption following a single dose of 5-fluorouracil. Digestion 1970;3:195.

56. Kuhlmann J et al. Effects of cytostatic agents on plasma levels and renal excretion of B-acetyl-digoxin. Clin Pharmacol Ther 1981;30:519.

57. Finchman R, Stoccelius D. Decreased phenytoin levels in chemotherapy therapy. Ther Agent Monit 1984;6:302.

58. Kuhlmann J et al. Verapamil plasma concentrations during treatment with cytostatic agents. J Cardiovasc Pharmacol 1985;7:1003.

59. Camptostar (irinotecan hydrochloride for injection) package insert. Kalamazoo, MI: Pharmacia & Upjohn Company, 1999 March.

60. Geller RB et al. Randomized trial of loperamide versus dose escalation of octreotide acetate for chemotherapy-induced diarrhea in bone marrow transplant and leukemia patients. Am J Hematol 1995;50(3):167.

61. Casincu S et al. Octreotide versus loperamide in the treatment of fluorouracil-induced diarrhea: a randomized trial. J Clin Oncol 1993;11(1):148.

62. Petrelli NJ et al. Bowel rest, intravenous hydration, and continuous high-dose infusion of octreotide acetate for the treatment of chemotherapy-induced diarrhea in patients with colorectal carcinoma. Cancer 1997;72(5).1543.

63. Casincu S et al. Control of chemotherapy-induced diarrhoea with octreotide in patients receiving 5-fluorouracil. Eur J Cancer 1992;28(20-3):482.

64. Hood AF. Cutaneous side effects of cancer chemotherapy. Med Clin North Am 1986;70:187.

65. DeSpain JD. Dermatologic toxicity of chemotherapy. Semin Oncol 1992;19:501.

66. Dunagin WG. Dermatologic toxicity. In: Perry MC, Yarbro JW, eds. Toxicity of Chemotherapy. Orlando: Grune & Stratton, 1984.

67. Claudia Seipp. Alopecia. In: De Vita VT et al, eds. Cancer: Principles and Practice of Oncology, 4th Ed. Philadelphia: JB Lippincott, 1993.

68. Middleton J et al. Failure of scalp hypothermia to prevent hair loss when cyclophosphamide is added to doxorubicin and vincristine. Cancer Treat Rep 1985;69:373.

69. Wheelock JB et al. Ineffectiveness of scalp hypothermia in the prevention of alopecia in patients treated with doxorubicin and cisplatin combinations. Cancer Treat Rep 1984;68:1387.

70. Seipp CA. Scalp hypothermia: indicators for precaution [Letter]. Oncol Nurs Forum 1983;10:12.

71. Camp Sorrell D. Scalp hypothermia devices: current status. ONS News 1991;7:1.

72. Jessen RT et al. Cutaneous and other complications of cyclophosphamide: a brief review. Rocky Mt Med J 1978;75:204.

73. Faulkson G, Schulz EJ. Skin changes in patients treated with 5-fluorouracil. Br J Dermatol 1962;74:229.

74. Harrison BM, Wood CBS. Cyclophosphamide and pigmentation. Br Med J 1972;2:352.

75. DeMarinis M et al. Nail pigmentation with daunorubicin therapy. Ann Intern Med 1978;89:516.

76. Priestman TJ, James KW. Adriamycin and longitudinal pigmented banding of fingernails. Lancet 1975;1:1337.

77. Rothberg H et al. Adriamycin (NSC-123127) toxicity: unusual melanotic reaction. Cancer Chemother Rep 1974;58:749.

78. Pratt CB, Shanks EC. Hyperpigmentation of nails from doxorubicin. JAMA 1974;228:460.

79. Shetty MR. Case of pigmented banding of the nail caused by bleomycin. Cancer Treat Rep 1977;61:501.

80. Adrian RM et al. Mucocutaneous reactions to neoplastic agents. CA Cancer J Clin 1980;30:143.

81. Ma HK et al. Actinomycin D in the treatment of methotrexate-resistant trophoblastic tumours. J Obstet Gynaecol Br Commonw 1971;78:166.

82. Kennedy BJ et al. Skin changes secondary to hydroxyurea therapy. Arch Dermatol 1975;111:183.

83. Harrold BP. Syndrome resembling Addison's disease following prolonged treatment with busulfan. Br Med J 1966;1:463.

84. Kyle RA et al. A syndrome resembling adrenal cortical insufficiency associated with long-term busulfan (Myleran) therapy. Blood 1961;18:497.

85. Delmonte L, Jukes TH. Folic acid antagonists in cancer chemotherapy. Pharmacol Rev 1962;14:91.

86. Hrushesky WJ. Serpentine supravenous fluorouracil hyperpigmentation. JAMA 1976;236:138.

87. Fernandez-Obregon AC et al. Flagellate pigmentation from intrapleural bleomycin. A light microscopy and electron microscopy study. J Am Acad Dermatol 1985;13:464.

88. Horn TD et al. Observations and proposed mechanisms of N,N',N"-triethylenethiophosphoramide (Thio-TEPA)-induced hyperpigmentation. Arch Dermatol 1989;125:524.

89. Harben DJ et al. Thiotepa-induced leukoderma. Arch Dermatol 1979;115:973.

90. Vonderheid EC. Topical mechlorethamine chemotherapy. Int J Dermatol 1984;23:180.

91. DeVita VT et al. Clinical trials with 1,3-Bis (2-chloroethyl)-1-nitrosourea, NSC-409962. Cancer Res 1965;25:1876.

92. Wheeland RG et al. The flag sign of chemotherapy. Cancer 1983;51;1356.

93. Dorr RT. Pharmacologic management of vesicant chemotherapy reactions. In: Dorr RT, Von Hoff DD, eds. Cancer Chemotherapy Handbook, 2nd Ed. East Norwalk, CT: Appelton & Lange, 1993.

94. Gallina C, Ellen J. Practical guide to chemotherapy administration for physicians and oncology nurses. In: De Vita VT et al, eds. Cancer: Principles and Practice of Oncology, 4th Ed. Philadelphia: JB Lippincott, 1993.

95. Vogelzang NJ. "Adriamycin flare": a skin reaction resembling extravasation. Cancer Treat Rep 1979;63:2067.

96. Souhami L, Feld R. Urticaria following intravenous doxorubicin administration. JAMA 1978;240:1624.

97. Luedke DW et al. Histopathogenesis of skin and subcutaneous injury induced by adriamycin. Plast Reconstr Surg 1979;63:463.

98. Rudolph R et al. Skin ulcers due to adriamycin. Cancer 1976;38:1087.

99. Ignoffo RJ, Friedman MA. Therapy of local toxicities caused by extravasation of cancer chemotherapy agents. Cancer Treat Rev 1980;7:17.

100. Rudolph R, Larson DL. Etiology and treatment of chemotherapy agent extravasation injuries: a review. J Clin Oncol 1987;5:1116.

101. Rudolph R et al. Experimental skin necrosis produced by adriamycin. Cancer Treat Rep 1979;63:529.

102. Weiss RB. Hypersensitivity reactions. Semin Oncol 1992;19:458.

103. Desao MH, Teres D. Prevention of doxorubicin-induced skin ulcers in the rat and pig with dimethyl sulfoxide (DMSO). Cancer Treat Rep 1982;66:1371.

104. Bertelli G et al. Dimethyl sulfoxide and cooling after extravasation of antitumor agents. Lancet 1993;341:1098.

105. Lawrence HJ, Goodnight SH. Dimethyl sulfoxide and extravasation of anthracycline agents [Letter]. Ann Intern Med 1983;98:1026.

106. Olver IN et al. A prospective study of topical dimethyl sulfoxide for treating anthracycline extravasation. J Clin Oncol 1988;6:1732.

107. Ludwig CU et al. Prevention of cytotoxic agent-induced skin ulcers with dimethyl sulfoxide (DMSO) and alpha-tocopherol. Eur J Cancer Clin Oncol 1987;23:327.

108. Alberts DS, Dorr RT. Case Report: Topical DMSO for mitomycin C-induced skin ulceration. Oncol Nurs Forum 1991;19:693.

109. Van Slotten-Harwood K, Aisner J. Treatment of chemotherapy extravasation: current status. Cancer Treat Rep 1984;7-8:939.

110. Weiss RB. Hypersensitivity reactions. In: Perry MC, ed. The Chemotherapy Source Book. Baltimore: Williams & Wilkins, 1992:555.

111. Evans WE et al. Anaphylactoid reactions to *Escherichia coli* and *Erwinia asparaginase* in children with leukemia and lymphoma. Cancer 1982; 49:1378.

112. Clavell LA et al. Four-agent induction and intensive asparaginase therapy for treatment of childhood acute lymphocytic leukemia. N Engl J Med 1986;315.657.

113. Rausen AR et al. Superiority of L-asparaginase combination chemotherapy in advanced acute lymphocytic leukemia of childhood. Randomized comparative trial of combination versus solo therapy. Cancer Clin Trials 1979;1:137.

114. Land VJ et al. Unexpectedly high incidence of allergic reactions with high dose (HD) weekly asparaginase (ASP) consolidation (cons) therapy (Rx) in children with newly diagnosed non-T, non-B acute lymphoblastic leukemia (ALL): a Pediatric Oncology Group (POG) study [Abstract]. Proc Am Soc Clin Oncol 1989;8:215.

115. Swenerton K et al. Taxol in relapsed ovarian cancer: high vs. low and short vs. long infusion: a European-Canadian study coordinated by the NCI Canada Clinical Trials Group [Abstract]. Proc Am Soc Oncol 1993;12:256.

116. Weiss RB et al. Hypersensitivity reactions from Taxol. J Clin Oncol 1990;8:1263.

117. O'Dwyer PJ et al. Hypersensitivity reactions to teniposide (VM-26): an analysis. J Clin Oncol 1986;4:1262.

118. Hayes FA et al. Allergic reactions to teniposide in patients with neuroblastoma and lymphoid malignancies. Cancer Treat Rep 1985;69:439.

119. Carstensen H et al. Hypersensitivity reactions to teniposide in children. J Clin Oncol 1987;5:1491.

120. Canal P et al. Phase I/pharmacokinetic study of intraperitoneal teniposide (VM 26). Eur J Cancer Clin Oncol 1989;25:815.

121. O'Dwyer PJ, Weiss RB. Hypersensitivity reactions induced by etoposide. Cancer Treat Rep 1984;68:959.

122. Tucci E, Pirtoli L. Etoposide-induced hypersensitivity reactions. Report of two cases. Chemioterapia 1985;4:460.

123. Anderson T et al. Chemotherapy for testicular cancer: current status of the National Cancer Institute combined modality trial. Cancer Treat Rep 1979;63:1687.

124. Denis L. Anaphylactic reactions to repeated intravesical instillation with cisplatin. Lancet 1983;1:1378.

125. Getaz EP et al. Cisplatin-induced hemolysis. N Engl J Med 1980;302:334.

126. Levi JA et al. Haemolytic anemia after cisplatin treatment. Br Med J 1981;282:2003.

127. Bacha DM et al. Phase I study of carboplatin (CB-DCA) in children with cancer. Cancer Treat Rep 1986;70:865.

128. Allen JC et al. Carboplatin and recurrent childhood brain tumors. J Clin Oncol 1987;5:459.

129. Glovsky MM et al. Hypersensitivity to procarbazine associated with angioedema, urticaria, and low serum complement activity. J Allergy Clin Immunol 1976;57:134.

130. Eyre HJ et al. Malignant glioma: a randomized trial of radiotherapy plus BCNU, procarbazine, or DTIC: a SWOG study [Abstract]. Proc Am Soc Clin Oncol 1982;1:180.

131. Brunner KW, Young CW. A methylhydrazine derivative in Hodgkin's disease and other malignant neoplasms. Ann Intern Med 1965;63:69.

132. Lokich JJ, Moloney WC. Allergic reaction to procarbazine. Clin Pharmacol Ther 1972;13:573.

133. Jones SE et al. Hypersensitivity to procarbazine (Matulane) manifested by fever and pleuropulmonary reaction. Cancer 1972;29:498.

134. Ecker MD et al. Procarbazine lung. Am J Roentgenol 1987;131:527.

135. Arnold DJ, Stafford CT. Systemic allergic reaction to adriamycin. Cancer Treat Rep 1979;63:150.

136. Solimando DA, Wilson JP. Doxorubicin-induced hypersensitivity reactions. Agent Intell Clin Pharm 1984;18:808.

137. Collins JA. Hypersensitivity reaction to doxorubicin. Agent Intell Clin Pharm 1984;18:402.

138. Etcubanas E, Wilbur JR. Uncommon side effects of adriamycin (NSC-123127). Cancer Chemother Rep (Part 1) 1974;58:757.

139. Crowther D et al. Management of adult acute myelogenous leukaemia. Br Med J 1973,1:131.

140. Mathe G et al. Phase II trial of THP-Adriamycin (pirarubicin), the most efficient and least toxic anthracycline in breast cancer. In: Kuemmerle H-P, ed. Advances in Experimental and Clinical Chemotherapy. Landsberg, Germany: Ecomed, 1988.

141. Tan CTC et al. Phase I trial of rubidzone (NSC 164011) in children with cancer. Med Pediatr Oncol 1981;9:347.

142. Rosenfelt F et al. A fatal hyperpyrexial response to bleomycin following prior therapy: a case report and literature review. Yale J Biol Med 1982;55:529.

143. Leung W-H et al. Fulminant hyperpyrexia induced by bleomycin. Postgrad Med J 1989;65:417.

144. Bochner BS, Lichtenstein LM. Anaphylaxis. N Engl J Med 1991;324:1785.

145. Rituxan (rituximab) package insert. San Francisco, CA: Genetech, Inc., 1999 July.

146. Herceptin (trastuzamab anti her 2 monoclonal antibody) package insert. San Francisco: Genetech, 1998 Sept.

147. Taxotere package insert. [Table] Collegeville, PA: Rhone-Poulenc Rorer Pharmaceuticals, Inc, 1996 October.

148. Doxil package insert. [Table] Menlo Park, CA: SEQUUS Pharmaceuticals, Inc, 1997 May.

149. DaunoXome package insert. [Table] San Dimas, CA: NexStar Pharmaceuticals, Inc, 1996.

150. Greenberger PA et al. Pretreatment of high-risk patients requiring radiographic contrast media studies. J Allergy Clin Immunol 1981;67:185.

151. Greenberger PA et al. Emergency administrations of radio contrast media in high-risk patients. J Allergy Clin Immunol 1986;77:630.

152. Baker WJ et al. Cytarabine and neurologic toxicity. J Clin Oncol 1991;9:679.

153. Graves T, Hooks MA. Agent-induced toxicities associated with high-dose cytosine arabinoside infusions. Pharmacotherapy 1989;9:23.

154. Pratt CB et al. Low dose asparaginase treatment of childhood acute lymphocytic leukemia. Am J Dis Child 1971;121:406.

155. Weiss HD et al. Neurotoxicity of commonly used chemotherapy agents. N Engl J Med 1974;297:127.

156. Ohnuma T et al. Biochemical and pharmacological studies with asparaginase in man. Cancer Res 1970;30:2297.

157. Allen JC, Rosen G. Transient cerebral dysfunction following chemotherapy for osteogenic sarcoma. Ann Neurol 1978;3:441.

158. Bleyer WA, Griffin TW. White matter necrosis mineralizing microangiopathy, and intellectual abilities in survivors of childhood leukemia: associations with central nervous system radiation and methotrexate therapy. In: Gilbert HA, Kagan AR, eds. Radiation Damage to the Nervous System. New York: Raven Press, 1980.

159. Allen JC et al. Leukoencephalopathy following high-dose IV methotrexate chemotherapy with leucovorin rescue. Cancer Treat Rep 1980;64:1261.

160. Moertel CG et al. Cerebellar ataxias associated with fluorinated pyrimidine therapy. Cancer Chemother Rep 1964;41:15.

161. Lynch HT et al. "Organic brain syndrome" secondary to 5-fluorouracil toxicity. Dis Colon Rectum 1981;24:130.

162. Intron A (interferon alpha-2b recombinant for injection) package insert. Kenilworth, NJ: Schering Corporation, 1997 March.

163. MacDonald DR. Neurotoxicity of chemotherapeutic agents. In: Perry MC, ed. The Chemotherapy Source Book, 2nd Ed. Baltimore: Williams & Wilkins, 1996.

164. Warrell RP, Berman E. Phase I and II study of fludarabine phosphate in leukemia: therapeutic efficacy with delayed central nervous system toxicity. J Clin Oncol 1986;4:74.

165. Chun HG et al. Central nervous system toxicity of fludarabine phosphate. Cancer Treat Rep 1986; 70:1225.

166. Puccio CA et al. A loading/continuous infusion schedule of fludarabine phosphate in chronic lymphatic leukemia. J Clin Oncol 1991;9:1562.

167. Merkel DE et al. Central nervous system toxicity with fludarabine. Cancer Treat Rep 1986;70:1449.

168. Phillips GL et al. Intensive 1, 3-bis (2-chloroethyl)-1-nitrosourea (BCNU) monochemotherapy and autologous marrow transplantation for malignant glioma. J Clin Oncol 1986; 4:639.

169. Shapiro WR, Green SB. Re-evaluating the efficacy of intra-arterial BCNU. J Neurosurg 1987; 66:313.

170. Mahaley MS Jr et al. Central neurotoxicity following intracarotid BCNU chemotherapy for malignant gliomas. J Neurooncol 1986;3:297.

171. Watkin SW et al. Ifosfamide encephalopathy: a reappraisal. Eur J Cancer Clin Oncol 1989;25: 1303.

172. Merimsky O et al. Ifosfamide-related acute encephalopathy: clinical and radiological aspects. Eur J Cancer 1991;27:1188.

173. Brunner KW, Young CW. A methylhydrazine-derivative in Hodgkin's disease and other malignant neoplasms: therapeutic and toxic effects studied in 51 patients. Ann Intern Med 1965; 63:69.

174. Weiss RB. The role of hexamethylmelamine in advanced ovarian carcinoma treatment. Gynecol Oncol 1981;12:141.

175. Gerritsen van der Hoop R et al. Incidence of neuropathy in 395 patients with ovarian cancer treated with or without cisplatin. Cancer 1990;66:1967.

176. Legha SS, Dimery IW. High dose cisplatin administration without hypertonic saline: observation of disabling neurotoxicity. J Clin Oncol 1985;3: 1373.

177. Cersosimo RJ. Cisplatin neurotoxicity. Cancer Treat Rev 1989;16:195.

178. Thompson SW et al. Cisplatin neuropathy: clinical, electrophysiologic, morphologic, and toxicologic studies. Cancer 1984;54:1269.

179. Weiss RB, Vogelzang NJ. Miscellaneous toxicities. In: De Vita VT, Cancer: Principles and Practice of Oncology, 4th Ed. Philadelphia: JB Lippincott, 1993.

180. MacDonald DR. Neurotoxicity of chemotherapy agents. In: Perry MC, ed. The Chemotherapy Source Book. Baltimore: Williams & Wilkins, 1992:666.

181. Sandler SG et al. Vincristine-induced neuropathy: a clinical study of fifty leukemic patients. Neurology 1969;19:367.

182. Casey EG et al. Vincristine neuropathy: clinical and electrophysiological observations. Brain 1973;96:69.

183. Gamelin E et al. Clinical aspects and molecular basis of oxaliplatin neurotoxicity: current management and development of preventive measures. Semin Oncol 2002;29:25.

184. Sandler SG et al. Vincristine-induced neuropathy: a clinical study of fifty leukemic patients. Neurology (Minn) 1969;19:367.

185. Albert DM et al. Ocular complications of vincristine therapy. Arch Ophthalmol 1967;78:709.

186. Holland JF et al. Vincristine treatment of advanced cancer: a cooperative study of 392 cases. Cancer Res 1973;33:1258.

187. Granowetter L et al. Enhanced cisplatinum neurotoxicity in pediatric patients with brain tumors. J Neurooncol 1983;1:293.

188. Schaefer SD et al. Ototoxicity of low-and moderate-dose cisplatin. Cancer 1985;56:1934.

189. Canetta R et al. Carboplatin, the clinical spectrum to date. Cancer Treatment Rev 1985;12(A):125.

190. Carmichael SM et al. Orthostatic hypotension during vincristine therapy. Arch Intern Med 1973;126:290.

191. Gottlieb RJ et al. Vincristine-induced bladder atony. Cancer 1971;28:674.

192. Allen A. The cardiotoxicity of chemotherapy agents. In: Perry MC, ed. The Chemotherapy Source Book. Baltimore: Williams & Wilkins, 1992:582.

193. Alexander J et al. Serial assessment of doxorubicin cardiotoxicity with quantitative radionuclide angiography. N Engl J Med 1979;300:278.

194. Tan C et al. Adriamycin—an antitumor antibiotic in the treatment of neoplastic diseases. Cancer 1973;32:9.

195. Lefrak EA et al. A clinicopathologic analysis of adriamycin cardiotoxicity. Cancer 1973;32:302.

196. Von Hoff DD et al. Risk factors for doxorubicin induced CHF. Ann Intern Med 1977;62:200.

197. Allen A. The cardiotoxicity of chemotherapy agents. Semin Oncol 1992;19:529.

198. Bloom K et al. Echocardiography in adriamycin cardiotoxicity. Cancer 1978;41:1265.

199. Biancaniello T et al. Doxorubicin cardiotoxicity in children. J Pediatr 1980;97:45.

200. Steinberg JS, Wasserman AG. Radionuclide ventriculography for evaluation and prevention of doxorubicin cardiotoxicity. Clin Ther 1985;7:660.

201. Bristow MR. Toxic cardiomyopathy due to doxorubicin. Hosp Pract 1982;17:101.

202. Bristow MR et al. Dose-effect and structure-function relationships in doxorubicin cardiomyopathy. Am Heart J 1981;102:709.

203. Bristow MR et al. Efficacy and cost of cardiac monitoring in patients receiving doxorubicin. Cancer 1982;50:32.

204. Bristow MR et al. Doxorubicin cardiomyopathy: evaluation by phonocardiography, endomyocardial biopsy, and cardiac catheterization. Ann Intern Med 1978;88:168.

205. Von Hoff DD. Use of daunorubicin in patients with solid tumors. Semin Oncol 1984;11(Suppl 3):23.

206. Yates J et al. Cytosine arabinoside with daunorubicin or adriamycin for therapy of acute myelocytic leukemia. A GALGB study. Blood 1982; 60:454.

207. Von Hoff DD et al. Daunomycin-induced cardiotoxicity in children and adults. Am J Med 1977;62:200.

208. Cassaza AM. Effects of modifications in position 4 of the chromophore or in position 4′ of the amino sugar on the antitumor activity and toxicity of daunorubicin and doxorubicin. In: Crooke ST, Reich SD, eds. Anthracyclines: Current Status and New Developments. New York: Academic Press, 1980:403.

209. Hurteloup P, Ganzina F. Clinical studies with new anthracyclines: epirubicin, idarubicin, esorubicin. Agents Exp Clin Res 1986;12:233.

210. Hurteloup P et al. Phase II trial of idarubicin (4-demethoxydaunorubicin) in advanced breast cancer. Eur J Cancer Clin Oncol 1989;25:423.

211. Villani F et al. Evaluation of cardiac toxicity of idarubicin (4-demethoxydaunorubicin). Eur J Clin Oncol 1989;25:13.

212. Tan CT et al. Phase I and clinical pharmacological studies with 4-demethoxydaunorubicin (Idarubicin) in children with advanced cancer. Cancer 1987;47:2990.

213. Feig SA et al. Determination of the maximum tolerated dose of idarubicin when used in a combination chemotherapy program of reinduction childhood ALL at first marrow relapse and a preliminary assessment of toxicity compared to that of daunorubicin: a report from the Children's Cancer Study Group. Med Pediatr Oncol 1992; 20:124.

214. Ellence package insert. Kalamazoo: Pharmacia & Upjohn Company, 1999 Sept.

215. Crossley RJ. Clinical safety and tolerance of mitoxantrone. Semin Oncol 1984;11(Suppl 1):54.

216. Posner LE et al. Mitoxantrone: an overview of safety and toxicity. Invest New Agents 1985;3:123.

217. Henderson IC et al. Randomized clinical trial comparing mitoxantrone with doxorubicin in previously treated patients with breast cancer. J Clin Oncol 1989;7:560.

218. Weiss AJ et al. Studies on adriamycin using a weekly regimen demonstrating its clinical effectiveness and lack of cardiac toxicity. Cancer Treat Rep 1976;60:813.

219. Weiss AJ. Studies on cardiotoxicity and antitumor effect of doxorubicin administered weekly. Cancer Treat Symp 1984;3:91.

220. Jain KK et al. A randomized comparison of weekly (Arm I) vs monthly (Arm II) doxorubicin in combination with mitomycin C in advanced breast cancer [Abstract]. Proc Am Soc Clin Oncol 1983;2:206.

221. Torti FM et al. Reduced cardiotoxicity of doxorubicin delivered on a weekly schedule. Assessment by endomyocardial biopsy. Ann Intern Med 1983;99:745.

222. Valdivieso M et al. Increased therapeutic index of weekly doxorubicin in the treatment of non-small cell lung cancer: a prospective, randomized study. J Clin Oncol 1984;2:207.

223. Lum BL et al. Doxorubicin: alteration of dose scheduling as a means of reducing cardiotoxicity. Agent Intell Clin Pharm 1985;19:259.

224. Zinecard package insert. Kalamazoo, MI: Pharmacia & Upjohn Company, 1996 April.

225. Seymour L, Bramwell V, Moran LA. Use of dexrazoxane as a cardioprotectant in patients receiving doxorubicin or epirubicin chemotherapy for the treatment of cancer. The Provincial Systemic Treatment Disease Site Group. Cancer Prev Control 1999;3:145.

226. Seymour L, Bramwell V, Moran LA. Use of dexrazoxane as a cardioprotectant in patients receiving doxorubicin or epirubicin chemotherapy for the treatment of cancer. The Provincial Systemic Treatment Disease Site Group. Cancer Prev Control 1999;3:145.

227. Rahman A et al. Doxorubicin-induced chronic cardiotoxicity and its protection by liposomal administration. Cancer Res 1982;42:1817.

228. Herman EH et al. Prevention of chronic doxorubicin cardiotoxicity in beagles by liposomal encapsulation. Cancer Res 1983;43:5427.

229. Wortman JE et al. Sudden death during doxorubicin administration. Cancer 1979;44:1588.

230. Rowinsky EK et al. Cardiac disturbances during the administration of Taxol. J Clin Oncol 1991;9:1704.

231. Labianca R et al. Cardiac toxicity of 5-fluorouracil: A study on 1,083 patients. Tumor 1982; 68:505.

232. Eskilsson J et al. Adverse cardiac effects during induction chemotherapy treatment with cisplatin and 5-fluorouracil. Radiother Oncol 1988;13:41.

233. Pottage A et al. Fluorouracil cardiotoxicity. Br Med J 1978;6112:547.

234. Cobleigh MA. Her-2-Neu as a target for breast cancer therapy. 34th Annual ASCO meeting:3-7.

235. Keefe DL. Trastuzumab-associated cardiotoxicity. Cancer 2002;95:1592.

236. Patterson WP, Reams GP. Renal and electrolyte abnormalities due to chemotherapy. In: Perry MC, ed. The Chemotherapy Source Book. Baltimore: Williams & Wilkins, 1992:648.

237. Patterson WP, Reams GP. Renal toxicities of chemotherapy. Semin Oncol 1992;19:521.

238. Fjeldborg P et al. The long-term effect of cisplatin on renal function. Cancer 1986;58:2214.

239. Macleod PM et al. The effect of cisplatin on renal function in patients with testicular tumors. Clin Radiol 1988;39:190.

240. Ries F, Klastersky J. Nephrotoxicity induced by cancer chemotherapy with special emphasis on cisplatin toxicity. Am J Kidney Dis 1986;8:368.

241. Finley RS et al. Cisplatin nephrotoxicity: a summary of preventative interventions. Agent Intell Clin Pharm 1985;19:362.

242. Pera MF et al. Effects of mannitol or furosemide diuresis on the nephrotoxicity and physiological disposition of cis-dichlorodiammineplatinum-(II). Cancer Research 1979;39:1269.

243. Ries F, Klastersky J. Nephrotoxicity induced by cancer chemotherapy with special emphasis on cisplatin toxicity. Am J Kidney Dis 1986;8:368.

244. Willox JC et al. Effects of magnesium supplementation on testicular cancer patients receiving cisplatin: a randomized trial. Br J Cancer 1986;54:12.

245. Kemp G et al. Amifostine pretreatment for protection against cyclophosphamide-induced and cisplatin-induced toxicities: results of a randomized control trial in patients with advanced ovarian cancer. J Clin Oncol 1996;14:201.

246. Ethyol (amifostine) for injection package insert. Palo Alto, CA: ALZA Pharmaceuticals, 1999 June.

247. Fields S, Lindley CM. Thrombotic microangiopathy associated with chemotherapy: case report and review of the literature. DICP Ann Pharmacother 1989;23:582.

248. Angiola G et al. Hemolytic-uremic syndrome associated with neoadjuvant chemotherapy in the treatment of advanced cervical cancer. Gynecol Oncol 1990;39:214.

249. Gradishar WJ et al. Chemotherapy-related hemolytic-uremic syndrome after the treatment of head and neck cancer: a case report. Cancer 1990;66:1914.

250. Walker RW et al. Carboplatin-associated thrombotic microangiopathic hemolytic anemia. Cancer 1989;64:1017.

251. Scheef W et al. Controlled clinical studies with an antidote against the urotoxicity of oxazaphosphorines: preliminary results. Cancer Treat Rep 1982; 18:1377.

252. Samuels ML et al. Large-dose bleomycin therapy and pulmonary toxicity: a possible role of prior radiotherapy. JAMA 1976;235:1117.

253. Klein HO et al. High-dose ifosfamide and mesna as continuous infusion over five days—a phase I/II trial. Cancer Treat Rev 1983;10(Suppl A):167.

254. Ormstad K. Pharmacokinetics and metabolism of sodium 2-mercaptoethanesulfonate in the rat. Cancer Res 1983;43:333.

255. Brock N et al. Studies of the urotoxicity of oxazaphosphorine cytostatics and its prevention. 2. Comparative study of the uroprotective efficacy of thiols and other sulfur compounds. Eur J Cancer Clin Oncol 1981;17:1155.

256. Shaw IC, Graham MI. Mesna—a short review. Cancer Treat Rev 1987;14:67.

257. Finn GP et al. Protecting the bladder from cyclophosphamide with mesna [Letter]. N Engl J Med 1986;314:61.

258. Goren MP et al. Pharmacokinetics of an intravenous-oral versus intravenous-mesna regimen in lung cancer patients receiving ifosfamide. J Clin Oncol 1998;16:616.

259. Proleukin (aldesleukin injection) package insert. Emeryville, CA: Chiron Corporation, 1994.

260. Weiss RB, Muggia FM. Cytotoxic agent-induced pulmonary disease: update 1980. Am J Med 1980; 68:259.

261. Blum RH et al. A clinical review of bleomycin—a new chemotherapy agent. Cancer 1973;31:903.

262. Sikic BI et al. Improved therapeutic index of bleomycin when administered by continuous infusion in mice. Cancer Treat Rep 1978;62:2011.

263. Comis RL et al. Role of single breath carbon monoxide diffusing capacity in monitoring the pulmonary effects of bleomycin in germ cell tumor patients. Cancer Res 1979;39:5076.

264. Goldiner PL et al. Factors influencing postoperative morbidity and mortality in patients treated with bleomycin. Br Med J 1978;1:1664.

265. Hakkinen PJ et al. Nyperoxia, but not thoracic x-radiation potentiates bleomycin and cyclophosphamide-induced lung damage in mice. Am Rev Respir Dis 1982;126:281.

266. Tryka AF et al. Differences in effects of immediate and delayed hyperoxia exposure on bleomycin-induced pulmonary injury. Cancer Treat Rep 1984;68:759.

267. Einhorn L et al. Enhanced pulmonary toxicity with bleomycin and radiotherapy in oat cell cancer. Cancer 1976;37:2414.

268. Durant JR et al. Pulmonary toxicity associated with bischloroethylnitrosurea (BCNU). Ann Intern Med 1979;90:191.

269. Schreml W et al. Progressive pulmonary fibrosis during combination chemotherapy with BCNU. Blut 1978;36:353.

270. Skarin AT et al. The treatment of advanced non-Hodgkin's lymphoma (NHL) with bleomycin, adriamycin, cyclophosphamide, vincristine and prednisone. Blood 1977;49:759.

271. Holoye PY et al. Pulmonary toxicity in long-term administration of BCNU. Cancer Treat Rep 1976;60:1691.

272. Wilson KS et al. Fatal pneumothorax in "BCNU lung." Med Rad Oncol 1982;10:195.

273. Ginsberg SJ, Comis RL. The pulmonary toxicity of chemotherapy agents. In: Perry MC, Yarbro JW, eds. Toxicity of Chemotherapy. Orlando: Grune & Stratton, 1984.

274. Haupt HM et al. Ara-C lung: noncardiogenic pulmonary edema complicating cytosine arabinoside therapy of leukemia. Am J Med 1981; 70:256.

275. Gemzar package insert [Table]. Indianapolis, IN: Eli Lilly, Inc., 1996 May.

276. Hurst PG et al. Pulmonary toxicity associated with fludarabine monophosphate. Invest New Agents 1987;5:207.

277. Wall MA et al. Lung function in adolescents receiving high-dose methotrexate. Pediatrics 1979; 63:741.

278. Zusman J et al. Rapid resolution of "methotrexate lung" with preoperative steroids [Abstract]. Proc Am Assoc Cancer Res 1979;20:412.

279. Lascari AD et al. Methotrexate-induced sudden fatal pulmonary reaction. Cancer 1977;40:1393.

280. Walden PAM et al. Pleurisy and methotrexate treatment. Br Med J 1977;2:867,

281. Muggia FM. Pulmonary toxicity of antitumor agents. Cancer Treat Rev 1983;10:221.

282. Jones SE et al. Hypersensitivity to procarbazine (Mutalane) manifested by fever and pleuropulmonary reaction. Cancer 1972;29:498.

283. Lokich JJ. Allergic reaction to procarbazine. Clin Pharmacol Ther 1972;13:573.

284. Konits PH et al. Possible pulmonary toxicity secondary to vinblastine. Cancer 1982;50:2771.

285. Stover DE. Pulmonary toxicity. In: De Vita VT et al, eds. Cancer: Principles and Practice of Oncology, 5th Ed. Philadelphia: Lippincott-Raven, 1997;2729.

286. Bauer KA et al. Pulmonary complications associated with combination chemotherapy programs containing bleomycin. Am J Med 1983;74:557.

287. Oliner H et al. Interstitial pulmonary fibrosis following busulfan therapy. Am J Med 1961;31:134.

288. White DA et al. Chemotherapy-associated pulmonary toxic reactions during treatment for breast cancer. Arch Intern Med 1984;144:953.

289. Konits PH et al. Possible pulmonary toxicity secondary to vinblastine. Cancer 1982;50:2771.

290. Aronin PA et al. Prediction of BCNU pulmonary toxicity in patients with malignant gliomas: an assessment of risk factors. N Engl J Med 1980; 303:183.

291. Zarrabi MH. Association of non-Hodgkin's lymphoma (NHL) and second neoplasms. Semin Oncol 1980;7:340.

292. Pratt CB et al. Duration and severity of fatty metamorphosis of liver following L-asparaginase therapy. Cancer 1971;28:361.

293. Ohnuma T et al. Biochemical and pharmacological studies with L-asparaginase in man. Cancer Res 1970;30:2297.

294. Oettgen HF et al. Toxicity of E. coli L-asparaginase in man. Cancer 1969;25:253.

295. DeVita VT et al. Clinical trials with 1,3-Bis (2-chloroethyl)-1-nitrosurea, NSC-79037. Cancer 1965;25:1876.

296. Takvorian T et al. Single high-dose of BCNU with autologous bone marrow (ABM). Proc Am Soc Clin Oncol 1980;21:341.

297. Slavin RE et al. Cytosine arabinoside-induced gastrointestinal toxic alterations in sequential chemotherapy protocols. Cancer 1978;42:1747.

298. Fosch PJ et al. Hepatic failure in a patient treated with DTIC for malignant melanoma. J Cancer Res Clin Oncol 1979;95:281.

299. Ceci G et al. Fatal hepatic vascular toxicity of DTIC: is it really a rare event? Cancer 1988;61: 1988.

300. Johnson D et al. Etoposide-induced hepatic injury: a potential complication of high-dose therapy. Cancer Treat Rep 1983;67:1023.

301. Hoogstraten B et al. CCNU and bleomycin in the treatment of cancer: a Southwest Oncology Group Study. Med Pediatr Oncol 1975;1:95.

302. Hoogstraten B et al. CCNU (1,(2-chloroethyl)-3-cyclohexyl-1-nitrosurea, NSC-79037) in the treatment of cancer. Cancer 1973;32:38.

303. Einhorn M et al. Hepatotoxicity of 6-mercaptopurine. JAMA 1964;188:802.

304. Clark PA et al. Toxic complications of treatment with 6-mercaptopurine: two cases with hepatic necrosis and intestinal ulceration. Br Med J 1960;1:393.

305. Dahl MGC et al. Methotrexate hepatotoxicity in psoriasis—comparison of different dosage regimens. Br Med J 1972;1:654.

306. Podugiel BJ et al. Liver injury associated with methotrexate therapy for psoriasis. Mayo Clin Proc 1973;48:787.

307. Lazarus HM et al. Veno-occlusive disease of the liver after high-dose mitomycin C therapy and autologous bone marrow transplantation. Cancer 1982;49:1789.

308. Kennedy BJ. Metabolic and toxic effects of mithramycin tumor therapy. Am J Med 1970;49:494.

309. Perlia CP. Mithramycin treatment of hypercalcemia. Cancer 1970;25:389.

310. Schein PS et al. Clinical antitumor activity and toxicity of streptozotocin (NSC-85998). Cancer 1974;34:993.

311. Gill RA et al. Hepatic veno-occlusive disease caused by 6-thioguanine. Ann Intern Med 1982;96:58.

312. Woodley PV. Hepatic and pancreatic damage produced by cytotoxic agents. Cancer Treat Rev 1983;10:17.

313. Dorr FA, Coltman CA Jr. Second cancers following chemotherapy therapy. Curr Probl Cancer 1985;9:1.

314. Casciato DA, Scott JL. Acute leukemia following prolonged cytotoxic agent therapy. Medicine (Baltimore) 1979;58:32.

315. De Gamont A et al. Preleukemic changes in cases of non-lymphocytic leukemia secondary to cytotoxic therapy: analysis of 105 cases. Cancer 1986;58:630.

316. Kantarjian HM et al. Therapy-related leukemia and myelodysplastic syndrome: clinical, cytogenic, and prognostic features. J Clin Oncol 1986;4:1748.

317. Tucker MA et al. Leukemia after therapy with alkylating agents for childhood cancer. J Natl Cancer Inst 1987;78:459.

318. Kaldor JM et al. Leukemia following chemotherapy for ovarian cancer. N Engl J Med 1990;332:1.

319. Kaldor JM et al. Leukemia following Hodgkin's disease. N Engl J Med. 1990;322:7.

320. Kyle RA, Gertz MA. Second malignancies after chemotherapy. In: Perry MC, ed. The Chemotherapy Source Book. Baltimore: Williams & Wilkins, 1992:689.

321. Pedersen-Bjergaard J et al. Increased risk of myelodysplasia and leukaemia after etoposide, cisplatin, and bleomycin for germ-cell tumors. Lancet 1991;338:359.

322. Reference deleted in proofs.

323. Tucker MA et al. Bone sarcomas linked to radiotherapy and chemotherapy in children. N Engl J Med 1987;317:588.

324. Stegman R, Alexanian R. Solid tumors in multiple myeloma. Ann Intern Med 1979;90:780.

325. Le Beau MM et al. Clinical and cytogenetic correlations in 63 patients with therapy-related myelodysplastic syndromes and acute non-lymphocytic leukemia: further evidence for characteristic abnormalities of chromosomes no. 5 and 7. J Clin Oncol 1986;4:325.

326. Pedersen-Bjergaard J et al. Acute non-lymphocytic leukemia, preleukemia, and acute myeloproliferative syndrome secondary to treatment of other malignant diseases. Clinical and cytogenetic characteristics and results of in vitro culture of bone marrow and HLA typing. Blood 1981; 57:712.

327. Bloomfield CD et al. Treatment-induced acute non-lymphocytic leukemia (t-ANLL): response to cytarabine-anthracycline therapy [Abstract]. Blood 1982;60(Suppl 1):152.

328. Preisler HD et al. Therapy of secondary acute non-lymphocytic leukemia with cytarabine. N Engl J Med 1983;308:21.

329. Marmont AM et al. Bone marrow transplantation for secondary (therapy-related) acute non-lymphoblastic leukaemia: report of a case associated with adoptive beta-thalassemia. Bone Marrow Transplant 1987;2:91.

330. Geller RB et al. Successful marrow transplantation for acute myelocytic leukemia following therapy for Hodgkin's disease. J Clin Oncol 1988; 6:1558.

331. Brusamolino E et al. Treatment-related leukemia in Hodgkin's disease: a multi-institution study of 75 cases. Hematol Oncol 1987;5:83.

332. Belohorsky B et al. Comments on the development of amenorrhea caused by Myleran in cases of chronic myelosis. Neoplasma 1960;7:397.

333. Sobrinho LG et al. Amenorrhea in patients with Hodgkin's disease treated with chemotherapy agents. Am J Obstet Gynecol 1971;109:135.

334. Himelstein-Braw R et al. Influence of radiation and chemotherapy on the ovaries of children and abdominal tumors. Br J Cancer 1977;36:269.

335. Nicosia SV et al. Gonadal effects of cancer therapy in girls. Cancer 1985;55:2364.

336. Chapman RM. Gonadal toxicity and teratogenicity In: Perry MC, ed. The Chemotherapy Source Book. Baltimore: Williams & Wilkins, 1992:710.

337. Myers SE, Schilsky RL. Prospects for fertility after cancer. Semin Oncol 1992;19:597.

338. Griffin JE, Wilson JD. Disorders of the testes and male reproductive tract. In: Wilson JD, Foster DW, eds. Williams Textbook of Endocrinology. Philadelphia: WB Saunders, 1985:259.

339. Monesi V. Spermatogenesis. In: Austin CR, Short RV, eds. Reproduction in Mammals. Book 1: Germ Cells and Fertilization. Oxford: Cambridge University Press, 1972:1.

340. Meistrich ML. Critical components of testicular function and sensitivity to disruption. Biol Reprod 1986;34:17.

341. Miller DG. Alkylating agents and human spermatogenesis. JAMA 1971;217:1662.

342. Cheviakoff S et al. Recovery of spermatogenesis in patients with lymphoma after treatment with chlorambucil. J Reprod Fertil 1973;33:155.

343. Fairley KF et al. Sterility and testicular atrophy related to cyclophosphamide therapy. Lancet 1972;1:568.

344. Buchanan JD et al. Return of spermatogenesis after stopping cyclophosphamide therapy. Lancet 1975;2:156.

345. Vivani S et al. Gonadal toxicity after combination chemotherapy for Hodgkin's disease: comparative results of MOPP vs ABVD. Eur J Cancer Clin Oncol 1985;21:601.

346. Drasga RE et al. Fertility after chemotherapy for testicular cancer. J Clin Oncol 1983;1:179.

347. Nijman JM et al. Gonadal function after surgery and chemotherapy in men with stage II and III nonseminomatous testicular tumors. J Clin Oncol 1987;5:651.

348. Fossa SD et al. Recovery of impaired pretreatment spermatogenesis in testicular cancer. Fertil Steril 1990;54:493.

349. Einhorn LH, Donahur J. Cis-diammine-dichloro-platinum, vinblastine and bleomycin combination chemotherapy in disseminated testicular cancer. Ann Intern Med 1977;87:293.

350. Lange PH et al. Fertility issues in the therapy of nonseminomatous testicular tumors. Urol Clin North Am 1987;14:731.

351. Berthelsen JG, Skakkebaek NE. Sperm counts and serum follicle-stimulating hormone levels before and after radiotherapy and chemotherapy in men with testicular germ cell cancer. Fertil Steril 1984;41:281.

352. Tournage H et al. In vitro fertilization techniques with frozen-thawed sperm: a method for preserving the progenitive potential of Hodgkin's patients. Fertil Steril 1991;55:443.

353. Davis OK et al. Pregnancy achieved through in vitro fertilization with cryopreserved semen from a man with Hodgkin's lymphoma. Fertil Steril 1990;53:377.

354. Redman J et al. Prospective, randomized trial of testosterone cypionate to prevent sterility in men treated with chemotherapy for Hodgkin's disease: preliminary results. In: Proceedings of the 14th International Cancer Congress, Budapest. Basel: S. Karger, 1986.

355. Chapman RM, Sutcliffe SB. Protection of ovarian function by oral contraceptives in women receiving chemotherapy for Hodgkin's disease. Blood 1981;58:849.

356. Johnson DH et al. Effect of luteinizing hormone-releasing hormone agonist given during combination chemotherapy on post-therapy fertility in male patients with lymphoma: preliminary observations. Blood 1985;65:832.

CHAPTER 90

Hematologic Malignancies

Adult: R. Donald Harvey III, John M. Valgus; Pediatric: Mark T. Holdsworth

HEMATOLOGIC MALIGNANCIES: ADULT DEFINITIONS AND CLASSIFICATION

Cancers arising from hematopoietic cells and lymphoid tissue are termed *hematologic malignancies* and include leukemias, lymphomas, plasma cell disorders, and myeloproliferative disorders. Compared with other cancers, they are relatively rare (<10% of all newly diagnosed cancers) and accounted for approximately 58,300 deaths in the United States in 2002.[1] Chemotherapy is the primary treatment for most cases of hematologic malignancies because they are usually disseminated at the time of diagnosis. Focal treatment with surgery and/or radiation therapy is not commonly used to manage these cancers. Compared with solid malignancies, the growth rate of most hematologic malignancies is rapid, and aggressive combination chemotherapy regimens can provide high response rates and cures. Complex supportive care regimens are often needed in conjunction with chemotherapy because of multiple disease symptoms and toxicities associated with chemotherapy. The hematologic malignancies also serve as the most common experimental laboratory models of cancer growth, biology, and treatment effects. In addition, advances in delineating molecular targets and improved disease detection continue to lead to changes in therapeutic approaches.

Leukemias

Leukemias are hematologic malignancies that are derived from cytogenetic alterations in hematopoietic cells. Biologically, they originate in the bone marrow before disseminating to systemic tissues. Leukemias are classified based on the cell of origin (myeloid or nonlymphocytic and lymphocytic) and clinical course. Myeloid leukemias include disorders of granulocytes, monocytes, erythrocytes, and platelets. Lymphocytic leukemias include disorders of B and T lymphocytes. Leukemias are further classified as acute or chronic.

Acute leukemia is characterized by the expansion and differentiation arrest of immature hematopoietic cells. This expansion causes large numbers of early progenitor cells (blasts) to appear in the bone marrow. Leukemic blasts develop a growth advantage that leads to failure of the bone marrow to produce adequate numbers of functional mature blood cells. The immature blast cells generally retain some features that indicate their origin from the hematopoietic lineage. If the blasts have lymphoid features, the leukemia is classified as *acute lymphocytic leukemia* (ALL). If the blasts have myeloid features, the leukemia is classified as *acute myeloid leukemia* (AML). Clinical and laboratory distinction of AML from ALL is illustrated in Table 90-1. AML and ALL can be distinguished based on morphologic examination of the bone marrow and peripheral blood, along with special cytochemical stains, surface membrane phenotyping, and chromosomal analysis. Acute leukemias appear suddenly and progress very rapidly. Death due to infection or bleeding occurs within weeks to months if the patient is not effectively treated.

Chronic leukemias follow a more insidious onset and course than acute leukemias and are associated with proliferation of more mature hematopoietic cells. Chronic lymphocytic leukemia (CLL) is characterized by overproduction of mature lymphocytes. Chronic myeloid (or granulocytic)

Table 90-1 Distinction of Acute Myeloid from Acute Lymphocytic Leukemia

	AML	ALL
Clinical Features		
Age	Commonly adults	Commonly children
Lymphadenopathy	Rare	Common
CNS involvement	Unusual	5%
Cytochemical Stains		
Myeloperoxidase	Positive	Negative
Periodic acid (Schiff)	Negative (except M$_6$)	Positive
Other Studies		
Surface markers	Myeloid	Lymphoid
CALLA	No	In early pre-B lineage ALL
Tdt	Absent	Present
Gene Arrangement Studies		
T-cell receptor	Absent	Present in T-cell ALL
Immunoglobulin	Absent	Present in B-cell ALL
Common Cytogenic Abnormalities		
	t(9,22)	t(9,22)
	t(8,21)	t(4,11) null cell ALL
	t(15,17) in AML-M$_3$	t(8,14) B-cell Burkitt's type
	5q-, 7q-	t(ll,14) B-cell
	Inv 16 in AML-M$_4$Eo	t(1,19) B-cell

ALL, acute lymphocytic leukemia; AML, acute myelogenous leukemia; CALLA, common ALL antigen; CNS, central nervous system.

leukemia (CML or CGL) is associated with overproduction of mature neutrophils or granulocytes. Deposition of these cells in various organs as well as high numbers in vascular spaces have profound and unique consequences that are discussed in subsequent cases. Other less common chronic leukemias include hairy cell leukemia and chronic myelomonocytic leukemia. Patients with chronic leukemias also often have decreased production of red blood cells (RBCs) and platelets. Although patients with chronic leukemias may survive for years with suppressive therapies, these disorders are curable in only a fraction of patients who are candidates for immune-based approaches using chemotherapy and progenitor cell replacement (see Chapter 92, Hematopoietic Cell Transplantation).

Lymphomas

The lymphomas are a heterogeneous group of hematologic malignancies that originate in lymphoid tissues. A lymphoma may arise within single or multiple lymph nodes or in extranodal sites commonly involving the lymphoid tissue of the gastrointestinal (GI) tract, central nervous system (CNS), or numerous other sites. The two major types of lymphomas are Hodgkin's disease (HD) and non-Hodgkin's lymphomas (NHL) (Table 90-2). It is estimated that these hematologic malignancies account for >60,000 new cases annually, with seven times as many patients affected by NHL compared with HD.[1] NHLs represent a spectrum of diseases marked by different pathologic features, natural history, response to treat-

Table 90-2   **Comparison of Hodgkin's Disease and Non-Hodgkin's Lymphoma**

Characteristic	Hodgkin's Disease	Non-Hodgkin's Lymphomas Low Grade	Intermediate-High Grade
Site(s) of origin	Nodal	Extranodal (≈10%)	Extranodal (≈35%)
Nodal distribution	Axial (centripetal)	Centrifugal	Centrifugal
Nodal spread	Contiguous	Noncontiguous	Noncontiguous
CNS involvement	Rare (<1%)	Rare (<1%)	Uncommon (<10%)
Hepatic involvement	Uncommon	Common (>50%)	Uncommon
Bone marrow involvement	Uncommon (<10%)	Common (>50%)	Uncommon (<20%)
Marrow involvement adversely affects prognosis	Yes	No	Yes
Curable by chemotherapy	Yes	No	Yes

CNS, central nervous system.

ment, and prognosis. NHLs have been divided into categories based on cell of origin (B or T), histology (low, intermediate, or high grade), immunophenotypic characteristics, cytogenetic abnormalities, and natural history. The main classification systems used for NHLs are the Working Formulation (WF) and the Revised European-American Classification of Lymphoid Neoplasms (REAL). The WF classification is based on the morphology and clinical behavior of the disease; the REAL classification has been advocated because it also incorporates immunophenotypic and molecular characteristics. Further classification of all neoplastic diseases of myeloid and lymphoid tissues by the World Health Organization (WHO) beyond the 1994 REAL system is currently ongoing, with the goal of removing arbitrary clinical groupings of lymphoid neoplasms from clinical practice and relying on more complete information (including morphology, immunophenotype, cytogenetic features, and clinical features) to guide prognosis and therapy.[2] The additional information included with further classification will ideally provide insight into the biologic diversity of each type of lymphoma and assist with therapeutic decisions.[3,4]

Plasma Cell Disorders

Plasma cell disorders include a group of neoplasms that arise from antibody-secreting B cells that overproduce excessive amounts of a monoclonal immunoglobulin or part of a monoclonal immunoglobulin (light chains). If the monoclonal protein is in the IgM subclass, the disease is called Waldenström's macroglobulinemia, and the malignant cells are called plasmacytoid lymphocytes. If the monoclonal protein is in the IgG (70% of cases) or IgA (20% of cases) subclass or if only monoclonal light chains are present in blood, the disease is called multiple myeloma and the malignant cells are called plasma cells.[5] High monoclonal immunoglobulin concentrations can be found in conditions other than multiple myeloma or Waldenström's macroglobulinemia, such as monoclonal gammopathy of undetermined significance (MGUS) or amyloidosis. However, the amount of immunoglobulin produced with multiple myeloma or Waldenström's macroglobulinemia generally exceeds the amount produced with other conditions. Excessive amounts of protein cause a number of clinical manifestations including hyperviscosity and renal dysfunction. If plasma cells infiltrate the bone marrow, a decreased produc-

tion of RBCs and platelets occurs. Multiple myeloma is the most common plasma cell disorder, accounting for 14% of all hematologic malignancies.[1]

ACUTE MYELOID LEUKEMIA
Signs and Symptoms

1.   **D.M., a 35-year-old woman, presented to the emergency department with increasing fatigue and fever. This past week, a peripheral blood smear (complete blood count [CBC]) revealed a white blood cell (WBC) count of 80,000/mm³ (normal, 4,000 to 11,000) with a differential of >90% leukemic blasts (normal, 0%), a hematocrit (Hct) of 31% (normal, 40% to 44%), and a platelet count of 46,000/mm³ (normal, 150,000 to 400,000). A bone marrow aspirate and biopsy confirmed the diagnosis of AML (FAB-M2, myeloid with maturation; 60% blasts, myeloperoxidase positive; CD13- and CD33-positive). All serum chemistry values were within normal limits, with the exception of the following: potassium (K), 3.2 mEq/L (normal, 3.5 to 5.5); phosphorus, 5.5 mg/dL (normal, 2.5 to 4.5); and lactic dehydrogenase (LD), 3,000 mU/mL (normal, 30 to 120). Physical examination was unremarkable except for a perirectal cellulitis. Which signs and symptoms exhibited by D.M. are consistent with AML?**

[SI units: WBC count, 80 × 10⁹/L (normal, 4 to 11) with differential >0.9 leukemic blasts (normal, 0); Hct, 0.31 (normal, 0.40 to 0.44); platelets 46 × 10⁹/L (normal, >150); K, 3.2 mmol/L (normal, 3.5 to 5.5); phosphorus, 5.5 mmol/L (normal, 2.5 to 4.5); LD, 3000 (normal, 30 to 120)]

D.M.'s symptoms of increasing fatigue and fever of 1 week's duration are consistent with a rapid reduction in RBCs leading to anemia (Hct, 31%) and a low neutrophil count leading to infection (perirectal cellulitis). Although her WBC count is high, the differential reveals that >90% are "blasts," which are immature, nonfunctional cells of myeloid or lymphoid origin. Circulating blast cells typically are not present in chronic leukemias or mild to moderate infection. However, blasts may be observed on the peripheral smear in patients with anemia associated with primary bone marrow dysfunction (myelodysplastic syndromes). They also are present in patients with severe infection, stress, or trauma and in those with CML in "transformation" to acute leukemia. D.M.'s platelet count is also low. Collectively, these are often the presenting signs and symptoms of acute leukemia.

D.M.'s symptoms are consistent with either AML or ALL. However, patients with ALL also commonly present with lymphadenopathy and hepatosplenomegaly. It is important to distinguish between these two disorders, because treatment regimens differ significantly. AML is far more common in adults than in children. (For a complete discussion of ALL, see Acute Lymphoblastic Leukemia of Childhood.)

Classification and Diagnosis

For a definitive diagnosis of AML to be made, the bone marrow aspirate must contain more than 20% leukemic blast cells. A normal bone marrow aspirate would typically contain less than 5% blasts. Eight major variants of AML are defined by the French-American-British (FAB) classification system based on morphologic characteristics (Table 90-3). Cells of myeloid origin commonly contain myeloperoxidase enzymes and express surface markers CD13, CD33, CD14, and CD15. Specific clonal chromosomal abnormalities are associated with several AML subtypes. These aberrations include gains or losses of whole chromosomes on the long (q) or short (p) arms of chromosomes, as well as a variety of structural rearrangements (e.g., translocations, inversions, insertions). A number of cytogenetic abnormalities in AML have suggested molecular-clinical syndromes, which are now being analyzed at the genetic level. The translocation t(15;17)(q22;q12) is the cytogenetic hallmark of acute promyelocytic leukemia (AML-M3). This translocation splits the retinoic acid receptor gene on chromosome 17 and blocks expression of retinoic acid-controlled genes required for cell differentiation. Treating patients with acute promyelocytic leukemia with all-*trans* retinoic acid (ATRA, tretinoin) has caused complete morphologic responses. This example shows how defining cytogenetic or chromosomal abnormalities in acute leukemia can be critical to understanding its pathophysiology and identifying optimal treatments. Currently, three chromosomal abnormalities are recognized as being associated with a good prognosis[6,7]: t(8;21), t(15;17), and inv 16; several chromosomal abnormalities and others have been associated with a relatively poor prognosis including inv 3, del 5, del 5q, del 7, and del 7q, trisomy 8, and complex (three or more unrelated cytogenetic abnormalities) cytogenetics. These chromosomal findings are increasingly being used to guide treatment decisions. For example, patients with cytogenetic findings associated with a poor prognosis may be considered for more aggressive postremission therapy such as high-dose chemotherapy with stem cell support (i.e., transplantation). Other poor prognostic signs in AML include age older than 60 years at the time of diagnosis, a pre-existing hematologic disorder (e.g., myelodysplastic syndrome), prior exposure to a chemotherapy agent (e.g., a secondary leukemia), and poor baseline performance status.

D.M. has FAB-M2 (myelomonocytic) AML. Approximately 10 to 20% of patients with FAB-M2 acute leukemia have a translocation of t(8;21)(q22;q22).[6] This translocation usually is seen in young patients like D.M. and is associated with a favorable response to therapy, although overall survival is not clearly better than average. D.M.'s bone marrow has been sent for cytogenetic analysis; however, results will not be available for several days. Although the cytogenetic analysis will not alter recommendations for induction therapy for D.M., these findings, in combination with other prognostic features, do influence postremission therapy recommendations.

Treatment
Goal of Therapy

2. What is the goal of treatment, and what type of therapy is indicated for D.M. at this time?

The leukemic cells populating D.M.'s blood are abnormal and incapable of fighting infection. Their rapid proliferation also is suppressing RBC and megakaryocyte production in the bone marrow. D.M. is at substantial risk for both life-threatening infections and bleeding complications. The goal of the

Table 90-3 Classification of Acute Myeloid Leukemia (AML)[a]

Designation	Name	Predominant Cell Type	Cytogenetics	Frequency (%)	Morphology
M$_0$	Undifferentiated myeloblastic				No maturation of myeloblasts
M$_1$	Undifferentiated myelocytic	Myeloblasts	t(9;22) + 8 del(5), del(7)	2–3	Minimal maturation of myeloblasts
M$_2$	Myelocytic	Myeloblasts, promyelocytes, myelocytes	t(8;21) + 8 del(5), del(7)	20	Prominent maturation of myeloblasts
M$_3$	Promyelocytic	Hypergranular promyelocytes	t(15;17)	25–30	Promyelocytic
M$_3$ variant					Promyelocytic in marrow; atypical monocytes in blood
M$_4$	Myelomonocytic	Promyelocytes, myelocytes, promonocytes, monocytes	t(4;11), t(9;11) + 8 del(5), del(7)	8–15	Myelomonocytic
M$_4$Eo			inv(16)		With atypical eosinophils
M$_{5a}$	Monoblastic	Monoblasts	t(9;11) + 8 del(5), del(7)		Monoblastaic
M$_{5b}$	Differentiated monocytic	Monoblasts, promonocytes, monocytes		20–25	Promonocytic
M$_6$	Erythroleukemia	Erythroblasts	+ 8 del(5), del(7)	5	Erythroblastic
M$_7$	Megakaryocytic	Megakaryocytes		1–2	Megakaryoblastic

[a]French-American-British (FAB) classification system.

initial chemotherapy is to clear the bone marrow and peripheral blood of all blast cells in the hope that normal blood cell components can regenerate.

Induction Therapy

Standard induction chemotherapy for AML includes an anthracycline (either daunorubicin or idarubicin) and cytarabine, an antimetabolite. One commonly used regimen includes idarubicin 12 mg/m^2 per day on days 1 to 3 as an intravenous (IV) bolus injection plus cytarabine 100 mg/m^2 per day as a continuous intravenous infusion on days 1 to 7. This combination (7 + 3) is one of the most successful chemotherapy regimens used in the treatment of AML, with complete response rates of 60% to 80%.[6] Continuous infusions of cytarabine are preferred because these regimens produce higher response rates than bolus injections during induction therapy.[8,9] Using higher doses of cytarabine by increasing the number of days of therapy to 10, doubling the daily dose to 200 mg/m^2, and using high-dose cytarabine (0.5 to 6.0 g/m^2 per day) has not shown consistent improvements in complete remission rates or survival.[10] Adding etoposide for 7 days may increase complete response rate, response duration, and survival in patients younger than 55.[11] However, other investigators have not shown a benefit with the addition of etoposide to the standard 7 + 3 induction regimen.[12]

If a patient presents with a very high WBC count, he or she may experience complications associated with hyperviscosity of the blood (e.g., ringing ears, stroke, blindness, or headache as a result of impaired oxygen delivery to the CNS, pulmonary infarction). Because it may take several days for cytarabine and idarubicin to substantially decrease the WBC count, the patient may receive hydroxyurea 2 to 4 g orally or undergo leukapheresis to quickly reduce the WBC count.

TRETINOIN AND ARSENIC TRIOXIDE FOR ACUTE PROMYELOCYTIC LEUKEMIA

3. Would induction therapy for other FAB subtypes of AML differ from that described previously?

Induction therapy is standard for all types of AML, with one exception: FAB-M3 or acute promyelocytic leukemia (APL). APL is uniquely characterized by the t(15;17) translocation that fuses the PML gene on chromosome 15 to the retinoic acid receptor alpha (RAR alpha) gene on chromosome 17. Severe coagulopathy is also common in patients with APL at the time of diagnosis or during induction therapy. Myeloperoxidase and procoagulant substances released from granules contained within the leukemia cells cause these complications. As discussed previously, tretinoin or ATRA induces promyelocyte differentiation and maturation.[13] In clinical trials, ATRA has induced complete remissions in approximately 90% of patients with APL.[14] Serial bone marrow aspirations after initiation of ATRA therapy demonstrate progressive differentiation without hypoplasia.[14–16] Unfortunately, ATRA typically induces brief remissions. A number of trials have investigated combination treatment with chemotherapy and ATRA.[17,18] Current evidence supports the use of concurrent ATRA plus conventional chemotherapy for induction, with ATRA starting 2 days before chemotherapy. In addition, postremission therapy should include at least two cycles of an anthracycline-based regimen.[18,19] Maintenance therapy with intermittent ATRA has been shown to decrease the relapse rate.[17,20]

ATRA therapy, though avoiding life-threatening myelosuppression, can produce significant toxicities, including the retinoic acid syndrome (RAS), which manifests as fever, weight gain, respiratory distress, lung infiltrates, pleural or pericardial effusion, hypotension, and acute renal failure.[21] If RAS develops, corticosteroid therapy (dexamethasone 10 mg twice a day for at least 3 days) should be initiated.[22] In patients receiving concurrent ATRA and chemotherapy, ATRA may be stopped if the patient has received ATRA for at least 20 days or if symptoms of RAS are life threatening or not improving with dexamethasone. Patients with leukocytosis seem to be more likely to experience RAS. Concurrent use of chemotherapy and ATRA has been reported to reduce the likelihood of RAS.[22] ATRA also causes dryness of the lining of the mouth, rectum, and skin; hair loss; skin rash; blepharon conjunctivitis; corneal erosions; muscle weakness; nail changes; depression; elevated liver enzymes; and high cholesterol. Despite the risk of serious complications and death during induction therapy, the long-term disease-free survival rate of patients with APL is superior compared with other AML subtypes. Approximately 75% of patients who receive ATRA-based induction and maintenance therapy are alive 3 to 5 years after diagnosis.[20]

Arsenic trioxide (ATO) has also been evaluated in the treatment of patients with APL. Recent clinical trials have confirmed that ATO is highly effective for the treatment of patients with relapsed APL, with complete remission rates up to 85%.[23] Preliminary results suggest no benefit to adding ATRA to ATO in this setting; however, future studies will determine whether ATO in combination with other strategies will yield superior outcomes.[24] There are several clinically significant adverse effects associated with ATO use. QT-interval prolongation and torsades de pointes have been reported in a small number of patients and warrant careful monitoring and management. Signs and symptoms of RAS were also reported, suggesting that this syndrome is not specific to therapy with ATRA and may be more appropriately referred to as APL syndrome. The monitoring and management of APL syndrome with ATO are the same as with ATRA. Coagulopathy, leukocytosis, neuropathy, nausea and vomiting, cough, headache, rash, hypokalemia, and hyperglycemia have also been frequently reported with ATO therapy and should be monitored appropriately.

COMPLICATIONS OF INDUCTION THERAPY

Tumor Lysis Syndrome

4. Twenty-four hours after D.M.'s induction chemotherapy was initiated, the following laboratory values were obtained: WBC count, 28,000/mm^3 (normal, 4 to 11); K, 5.3 mEq/L (normal, 3.5 to 5.5); phosphorus, 6.0 mg/dL (normal, 2.5 to 5.5); uric acid, 9.8 mg/dL (normal, 2.5 to 8); calcium, 6.0 mg/dL (normal, 9.0 to 11.5), and creatinine, 1.6 mg/dL (normal, 0.8 to 1.2). Why have these laboratory values changed so suddenly? Could they have been minimized or prevented? How should these metabolic disturbances be managed?

[SI units: WBC count, 58 × 10^9/L; K, 5.3 mmol/L; phosphorus, 1.94 mmol/L; uric acid, 582.9 mmol/L (normal, 148.7 to 475.84); calcium, 1.5 mmol/L (normal, 2.25 to 2.875); creatinine, 141.44 μmol/L (normal, 88.4 to 176.8)]

D.M. presented with a very high number of peripheral blasts. Consequently, chemotherapy resulted in rapid lysis of the blast cells and the release of their cellular contents into the blood. A hypercellular bone marrow with a very high number of blast cells can also lead to rapid lysis of the blast cells. The release of cellular contents can produce a tremendous metabolic burden on the kidneys. Several metabolic abnormalities that can lead to renal failure and electrocardiographic (ECG) abnormalities may occur (Table 90-4). As the tumor cells lyse, hyperuricemia often develops owing to the breakdown of purines that are released. Patients can present with tumor lysis syndrome (TLS), but most commonly, TLS occurs 12 to 24 hours after chemotherapy is initiated. TLS may occur after therapy for other malignancies, particularly in those with a high tumor burden such as high-grade lymphomas and ALL. TLS rarely occurs after therapy for solid tumors.

Before chemotherapy is initiated, leukopheresis to reduce D.M.'s peripheral WBC count may minimize TLS. Leukopheresis is not routinely done unless the patient is experiencing symptoms of hyperviscosity. Patients should receive IV hydration (2 to 3 L/day) beginning 24 to 48 hours before chemotherapy to (1) maintain renal perfusion, (2) optimize the solubility of tumor lysis products, and (3) compensate for fluid losses due to fever or vomiting. Alkalinization of the urine also may reduce or prevent uric acid from precipitating in the renal tubules and collection ducts by maintaining the urate in its ionized state. However, increased pH may increase the risk of precipitating calcium phosphate in both soft tissue and kidney tubules and aggravate hypocalcemia.[25]

Allopurinol should be started before chemotherapy to minimize the complications of TLS. The recommended dosage is 300 to 600 mg/day. D.M.'s serum uric acid and electrolytes should be monitored at least two to three times a day for 24 to 48 hours after initiating chemotherapy. If severe abnormalities occur, more aggressive measures should be initiated. Allopurinol may be discontinued if the serum uric acid is within normal limits and the WBC count is low. Rasburicase, a newly developed recombinant urate oxidase product, can also be used as prophylaxis in patients who are at high risk of developing TLS or for the treatment of patients who present with or develop TLS. Rasburicase acts as a catalyst in the enzymatic oxidation of uric acid to allantoin, which is 5 to 10 times more soluble than uric acid and undergoes rapid renal excretion. The recommended dose of rasburicase for both the prevention and treatment of TLS is 0.2 mg/kg per dose. Rasburicase results in a rapid reduction in serum uric acid (within 4 hours of administration) and is generally well tolerated.[26] Most of the clinical data for rasburicase is in the pediatric population; however, data from compassionate use trials suggest that rasburicase is equally effective in adults.[27,28] Although rasburicase has demonstrated excellent efficacy and tolerability, its optimal role in the prevention and management of hyperuricemia in adults remains to be defined because of cost considerations and lack of randomized trial comparison data with other interventions.

Although D.M.'s serum potassium was low on admission, it has increased significantly as a result of tumor cell lysis. For this reason, replacement potassium therapy is not recommended before chemotherapy in patients in whom TLS is highly likely. In extreme circumstances, dialysis may be required to correct severe metabolic and electrolyte disturbances associated with TLS.

Myelosuppression

5. D.M. received allopurinol therapy and aggressive hydration throughout her induction chemotherapy. The metabolic abnormalities gradually resolved as her WBC count declined and tumor lysis diminished. What other complications may occur during induction therapy. Can they be treated?

Patients receiving cytarabine and idarubicin induction therapy develop profound anemia, granulocytopenia (e.g., WBC count, $<100/mm^3$) and thrombocytopenia ($<20,000$ platelets/ mm^3) shortly after therapy is initiated that persists for 21 to 28 days. All infectious complications must be considered life-threatening in severely immunocompromised patients like D.M. (see Chapter 68, Prevention and Treatment of Infections in Neutropenic Cancer Patients).

Filgrastim (granulocyte colony-stimulating factor [G-CSF]) and sargramostim (granulocyte-macrophage colony-stimulating factor [GM-CSF]) stimulate leukemic cells as well as normal granulocyte precursors in vitro; however, several studies have demonstrated that these agents, when used as an adjunct to AML chemotherapy, are safe and do not adversely affect disease outcome.[29–32] Most studies have demonstrated that CSFs can modestly decrease the length of profound neutropenia and sometimes reduce the incidence of infection-related morbidity, the duration of systemic antibiotics and antifungals, and decrease the number of days of hospitalization. Guidelines published by the American Society of Clinical Oncology recommend that patients older than 55 are most likely to benefit from CSF administration after completion of induction chemotherapy.[33] Despite the impact on short-term complications, administration of CSFs after induction chemotherapy does not appear to have an impact on the rate of complete remissions or the long-term outcomes of the disease.

Severe thrombocytopenia may result in bleeding episodes that range in severity from oozing gums to massive GI hemorrhage. Serious bleeding complications usually can be avoided if patients receive platelet transfusions when their platelet counts decrease to $<10,000/mm^3$ or when patients experience bleeding. Currently, there are no data to support the use of interleukin (IL)-11 (oprelvekin) or other investigational thrombopoietic agents in this setting. Because D.M. is premenopausal, she has a significant risk of excessive vaginal bleeding if she begins menstruating while she is thrombocytopenic. The menstrual cycle may be suppressed with daily, uninterrupted oral contraceptives or progesterone (e.g., medroxyprogesterone 10 to 20 mg/day orally). If spotting occurs, dosages should be increased until bleeding stops. After D.M.'s platelet count returns to normal, suppressive therapy can be discontinued.

Other common drug-induced complications that may occur during induction therapy include nausea and vomiting, mu-

Table 90-4	Complications Associated with Acute Tumor Lysis Syndrome
Hypocalcemia	Renal failure
Hyperkalemia	Electrocardiogram changes
Hyperphosphatemia	Metabolic acidosis
Hyperuricemia	

cositis, fever, and skin rash (see Chapter 8, Nausea and Vomiting, and Chapter 89, Adverse Effects of Chemotherapy).

Postremission Therapy
Rationale

6. After completion of her induction chemotherapy, D.M.'s WBC count fell to <100/mm³ and her platelet count fell to 5,000/mm³. She received platelet transfusions approximately every 2 to 3 days to prevent bleeding complications. On day 9, she developed a fever of 38.8°C. She was started immediately on empiric, broad-spectrum antibiotic therapy, which resolved her fever. On day 29, her WBC count was 5,600/mm³ with a normal differential, and her platelet count was 168,000/mm³. She received packed RBC transfusions on two separate occasions when her Hct fell to <30%. A repeat bone marrow aspirate showed no evidence of persistent leukemia, and D.M. was told that her leukemia was in remission. Nevertheless, her oncologist recommended additional chemotherapy and D.M. questions why this is necessary. Is postremission therapy necessary, and if so, what therapeutic options are available to D.M.?

Although >60% of patients treated for AML achieve complete remission after induction therapy, the median duration of the remission is only about 12 to 18 months and only 20% to 40% of patients have a disease-free survival exceeding 5 years.[10] Short remissions have been attributed to proliferation of clinically undetectable leukemic cells. Thus, the rationale for administering chemotherapy after remission is to eradicate these residual cells.

In AML, postremission therapy (also referred to as *consolidation therapy*) includes two to four cycles of chemotherapy. Clinical trials have shown that high-dose postremission therapy results in a higher percentage (30% to 40%) of long-term (>2 to 5 years) disease-free survivors than either no or low-dose postremission chemotherapy.[34,35] Postremission therapy regimens usually include high dose cytarabine alone or in combination with one or more agents such as mitoxantrone, idarubicin, or etoposide. Patients 60 years of age and older or those with comorbid disease may not be able to tolerate this intensive postremission therapy. In these circumstances, the risk of life-threatening toxicity may outweigh the potential benefits of postremission chemotherapy. Allogeneic bone marrow transplantation also has been studied in the postremission treatment of AML and is addressed in Chapter 92, Hematopoietic Cell Transplantation.

Administration of chemotherapy (thioguanine, methotrexate) and biologics (IL-2) for a prolonged period has been investigated to see if it can prolong survival. This is often referred to as maintenance therapy. With the exception of APL, maintenance chemotherapy has not been shown to improve survival in patients with AML.

High-Dose Cytarabine

7. D.M does not have any siblings that would be a compatible donor for an allogeneic stem cell transplant. Consequently, her oncologist recommends three courses of high-dose cytarabine as postremission therapy while an unrelated compatible donor is sought. One week after she was declared to be in remission, D.M. is readmitted to the hospital to receive cytarabine 3 g/m² Q 12 hr, over 3 hours, on days 1, 3, and 5. What are the potential acute

and delayed toxicities associated with high-dose cytarabine, and how can these effects be prevented?

At conventional dosages of 100 to 200 mg/m² per day, adverse effects associated with cytarabine include myelosuppression, fever, and skin rashes. Occasionally, liver enzymes rise transiently. The side effect profile for high-dose cytarabine (HiDAC) (>1g/m² per day), however, is very different and can produce major cerebellar, ocular, and skin toxicities.[36–38]

CEREBELLAR TOXICITY
Cerebellar toxicity occurs in approximately 10% of patients receiving HiDAC therapy. See Chapter 89 for details regarding cytarabine-induced cerebellar toxicity.

OCULAR TOXICITY
Ocular toxicity results from damage to corneal epithelium, when cytarabine penetrates the epithelium through the anterior chamber of the eye or tears. Symptoms include conjunctivitis, excessive lacrimation, "burning" ocular pain, photophobia, and blurred vision. Artificial tears (2 drops every 4 to 6 hours) administered concurrently with high-dose cytarabine generally prevents these symptoms. Corticosteroid eyedrops should be used if symptoms of conjunctivitis occur.[39]

DERMATOLOGIC TOXICITY
Dermatologic toxicity may be manifested as a rash covering most of the body (similar to that seen with conventional doses) or plantar-palmar erythema. Desquamation of the palms and soles can occur with plantar-palmar erythema causing significant pain and allowing for pathogenic organisms to enter the body.

ACUTE LEUKEMIA IN THE ELDERLY

8. Would recommendations for induction and postremission therapy differ if D.M. were elderly (60 years of age or older)?

The incidence of AML gradually increases with age; with the median age of affected patients between 65 to 70 years. Several clinical trials have shown lower complete remission rates, and reduced disease-free and overall survival in patients older than 55 years. The reason for this is most likely multifactorial including a decreased tolerance to chemotherapy, comorbidities, and compromised organ function, as well as inherent biologic differences between AML in the elderly and in younger patients.[40] Poor prognostic factors more common in the elderly include a history of preleukemic syndrome (myelodysplastic syndrome), poor cytogenetic abnormalities, high expression of multidrug-resistant glycoprotein MDR1, and prior radiation therapy or chemotherapy.[41] Whether the elderly should receive aggressive chemotherapy is often debated.[42] Two studies have evaluated a standard induction regimen versus alternatives of low-dose or palliative chemotherapy.[43,44] Both studies demonstrated superior prolonged survival in the standard therapy arms at the cost of increased treatment related mortality. It must be taken into consideration, though, that these studies were performed approximately 20 years ago and that improvements in supportive care may significantly improve the treatment related mortality observed in these studies. Nevertheless, many oncologists believe aggressive therapy is warranted in most elderly patients given the rapid progression of the disease and certain death within weeks if the disease is not treated.

The decision of postremission therapy is a difficult decision in elderly patients because they have a higher risk of morbidity and mortality and, more importantly, no clinical trials have demonstrated the benefit of postremission therapy specifically in the elderly. The intensity of the regimens often must be attenuated because there is risk of serious toxicities. This is particularly true with HiDAC therapy due to the increased risk of cerebellar toxicity in the elderly. Studies have shown that postremission therapy with low-dose cytarabine (100 mg/m^2 by continuous infusion for 5 days) is as effective as high-dose cytarabine and better tolerated in elderly patients.[34]

Refractory or Resistant AML

9. A.W., a 65-year-old man, is 30 days post induction therapy with 7 + 3. His neutrophil count has been <200/mm^3 since day 12. Bone marrow biopsy reveals 60% blasts, confirming the diagnosis of refractory AML. What are treatment options for A.W. at this time?

Given the decreased efficacy and tolerability of myelosuppressive chemotherapy in the elderly, novel immunotherapeutic approaches are being developed. Recently, gemtuzumab ozogamicin, a humanized anti-CD33 antibody coupled to calicheamicin, an anthracycline-like toxin, was approved for relapsed or refractory AML in patients 60 and older who are not considered candidates for further cytotoxic chemotherapy.[45] CD33 is a cluster differentiation antigen present on the majority of blast cells, but not on hematopoietic stem cells. The conjugation of an anthracycline to the anti-CD33 antibody targets the delivery of the toxin to the CD33-positive blast cells. A total of 142 patients participating in open-label trials were treated with gemtuzumab 9 mg/m^2 on days 1 and 15.[45] Gemtuzumab provided an overall response rate of 30%. Myelosuppression and thrombocytopenia appear to be of longer duration compared to conventional chemotherapy regimens in this setting; however, it is associated with less nonhematologic side effects such as mucositis, nausea and vomiting, and alopecia. Infusion-related adverse events such as rigors, chills, and fever are common and are severe in approximately 30% of patients. This drug may be a reasonable alternative to additional chemotherapy for A.W.

CHRONIC MYELOID LEUKEMIA
Signs and Symptoms

10. P.D., a 61-year-old white woman, recently sought medical attention for increasing fatigue, weight loss, and fevers. Her CBC showed a WBC count of 60,000/mm^3 with 90% neutrophils, Hct of 30%, and a platelet count of 900,000/mm^3. The only pertinent physical finding was splenomegaly. A bone marrow aspirate revealed a hypercellular marrow with less than 5% blasts. Cytogenetic analysis confirmed a diagnosis of Philadelphia chromosome–positive CML. Explain P.D.'s high WBC counts. What are the possible clinical consequences of these abnormal values?

[SI units: WBC count, 60 × 10^9/L with 0.9 neutrophils; Hct, 0.3, platelets 900 × 10^9/L]

Chronic myeloid leukemia is a myeloproliferative disorder characterized by unregulated stem cell proliferation in the bone marrow and an increase in mature granulocytes in the peripheral blood. Common clinical symptoms on presentation include fatigue, fever, anorexia, and weight loss. Approximately 50% to 70% of patients present with a leukocyte count >100,000/mm^3. Symptoms of hyperleukocytosis and hyperviscosity include priapism, headaches, tinnitus, and cerebrovascular accidents. On physical examination, the most common abnormal finding is splenomegaly, which results from increased activity of the reticuloendothelial system to remove increased white blood cells. Although these symptoms are common, approximately 30% to 40% of patients are asymptomatic at presentation, and initial suspicion for CML is based solely on an abnormal complete blood count.[46]

Clinical Course and Prognosis

11. What is the expected disease progression for P.D. and others with newly diagnosed CML?

The natural history of CML can be divided into three distinct phases: chronic phase, accelerated phase, and blastic phase. Early in the disease (chronic phase), patients exhibit leukocytosis and associated symptoms as described earlier. Bone marrow examination and peripheral blood smear reveal <5% immature blast cells.[47] The duration of the chronic phase may range from a few months to many years. Because symptoms may be nonspecific and relatively minor, CML may remain undiagnosed until patients progress into more advanced stages. The annual transition rate from chronic phase to accelerated phase is 5% to 10% in the first 2 years and 20% in subsequent years. Common signs and symptoms suggestive of this transition include increased leukocytosis, anemia, increased splenomegaly, fever, and bone pain.

During the second phase of the disease, the accelerated phase, leukocytosis progresses (despite therapy), and an increased number of immature leukocytes (blasts) appear in the peripheral blood. Patients often report significant symptoms. The accelerated phase generally lasts <6 weeks. The final phase of the disease (blastic phase or blast crisis) is characterized by a predominance of immature cells. Bone marrow examination of the peripheral blood at this time reveals >30% blasts.[47] During this phase, CML is indistinguishable from AML with the exception of cytogenetics. In blast crisis, patients often experience bone pain, fatigue, worsening anemia, infections, and bleeding complications. The blast phase is often refractory to conventional induction regimens for AML, and median survival is approximately 5 months.[46] Because less than 5% blast cells are present in P.D.'s bone marrow, she is in the chronic phase of the disease.

12. What is the significance of the finding of the Philadelphia chromosome?

The cytogenetic hallmark of CML is the Philadelphia chromosome, which is present in over 90% of cases. Cytogenetic analysis reveals a translocation of chromosomes 9 and 22 t(9;22) (q34;q11).[48] This translocation creates a new protein (BCR-ABL) that has unregulated tyrosine kinase activity. The three major mechanisms that have been implicated in the malignant transformation by unregulated tyrosine kinase include abnormal cell cycling, inhibition of apoptosis, and increased proliferation of cells.[48] Identifying the Philadelphia chromosome helps to confirm the diagnosis of CML and helps with monitoring the efficacy of treatment.

Treatment

13. What therapy is appropriate for P.D.?

In newly diagnosed patients who present with very high leukocyte counts (>100,000/mm^3), the initial goal of therapy is to reduce leukocytosis and its related symptoms.[47] Hydroxyurea is still the most common agent used for leukocyte reduction. Treatment is initiated with 2 g/day orally, and the dosage is titrated to a WBC count of <20,000/mm^3. A small dosage decrease often permits a considerable rise in leukocyte count in 1 or 2 days. Hydroxyurea is well tolerated and is relatively free of nonhematologic side effects.

The ultimate goal of therapy for CML is to cure patients of their disease. The only curative therapy for CML to date is allogeneic bone marrow transplantation. The best results are achieved with HLA-matched related donors; however, HLA-matched unrelated donor transplants in select patients can also yield favorable long-term disease-free survival rates.[49] When patients are transplanted during the blast phase, only 10% to 20% survive >5 years. If patients are transplanted during the chronic phase, 50% to 60% are disease free at 5 years.[50] The highest rate of prolonged disease-free survival occurs in younger patients who undergo transplantation within 1 year of initial diagnosis during the chronic phase.[51] For patients who will be receiving a bone marrow transplant, hydroxyurea is the agent of choice for initial cytoreduction. This is mostly due to its relatively rapid onset of action, excellent tolerability profile, and lack of adverse effect on bone marrow transplantation outcomes. Several reports have demonstrated that interferon (IFN)-alfa may have deleterious effects on transplantation outcomes.[52,53] There is currently no information on the effect of prior imatinib administration on transplantation outcomes.

Since most patients newly diagnosed with CML are not transplant candidates because of their age and lack of a suitable donor, alternative therapies must be considered. When cure is not an option, the primary goals of therapy are to prolong survival, prevent progression of disease, and attain a complete hematologic and/or cytogenetic remission. The definition of a complete hematologic response is a reduction in leukocyte count to less than 10,000/mm^3 and platelet count to less than 450,000/mm^3. A cytogenetic response is defined by the percentage of cells in metaphase that are positive for the Philadelphia chromosome in the bone marrow (Table 90-5).

Interferon-Alfa

Until recently, the combination of IFN-alfa and low-dose cytarabine was the standard of care in patients with newly diagnosed CML in chronic phase who were not transplant candidates. IFN, when compared with other available therapies such as hydroxyurea or busulfan in a large meta-analysis, was superior in terms of cytogenetic remission and overall 5-year survival.[54] The addition of low-dose cytarabine to IFN has resulted in improved survival compared with IFN alone.[55] In a large, nonrandomized trial from the MD Anderson Cancer Center, the degree of cytogenetic response had a profound correlation with survival.[56] Thus, monitoring the cytogenetic response provides a superior surrogate endpoint compared with monitoring the hematologic response alone.

Imatinib

In May of 2001, the Food and Drug Administration approved imatinib mesylate (Gleevec) for the treatment of patients with CML. Imatinib is a tyrosine kinase inhibitor that occupies the adenosine triphosphate binding site of several tyrosine kinase molecules and prevents phosphorylation of substrates that are involved in regulating the cell cycle. Imatinib was initially tested in patients with chronic-phase CML who were refractory to or intolerant of IFN-based therapy. Ninety-eight percent of patients receiving 300 mg or more per day of imatinib achieved a complete hematologic response, whereas 31% of patients at the same dose achieved a major cytogenetic response.[57] Imatinib has also shown efficacy in accelerated and blastic phase CML.[58,59] These impressive results set the stage for the pivotal IRIS trial, which compared imatinib with the combination of IFN-alfa plus low-dose cytarabine in patients with newly diagnosed CML in the chronic phase. A total of 1,106 patients were randomly assigned to either imatinib (400 mg orally daily) or the combination of IFN (gradual titration to target dose of 5 million U/m^2 per day) and cytarabine (begun after maximum tolerated dose of IFN achieved at 20 mg/m^2 per day for 10 days per month with a maximum daily dose of 40 mg subcutaneously).[60] For patients on imatinib, the dose could be escalated to 400 mg BID if no hematologic response was seen within 3 months or if no cytogenetic response was seen within 12 months. All the primary and secondary end points of the trial including rates of complete hematologic remission, major and complete cytogenetic response, and freedom from progression to the accelerated-phase or blast crisis-demonstrated superiority of imatinib over IFN plus cytarabine (Table 90-6). Estimated survival rates at 18 months between the two arms were not significantly different (97.2% versus 95.1% for imatinib and IFN–cytarabine, respectively $P = 0.16$). This lack of difference is most likely due to a large percentage of patients (89%) in the IFN–cytarabine arm who crossed over to the imatinib arm due to lack of efficacy or intolerance to therapy. In addition to superior efficacy, imatinib was very well tolerated. The most common toxicities reported with imatinib are superficial edema,

Table 90-5	**Definition of Cytogenetic Response in Chronic Myeloid Leukemia**
Cytogenetic Response[a]	Philadelphia (Ph) Chromosome–Positive Cells (%)
Complete	0
Partial	1–35
Minor	36–65
Absent	>65

[a]Major response is defined as complete or partial responses.

Table 90-6	**Response Rates in IRIS Trial**	
Response	% Imatinib (N = 553)	% IFN plus Cytarabine (N = 553)
Complete hematologic	95.3 (93.2–96.9)	55.5 (51.3–59.7)
Major cytogenetic	85.2 (81.9–88.0)	22.1 (18.7–25.8)
Complete cytogenetic	73.8 (69.9–77.4)	8.5 (6.3–11.1)
Partial cytogenetic	11.4 (8.9–14.3)	13.6 (10.8–16.7)

IFN, interferon.

nausea, muscle cramps, and rashes. Only 12% of patients in the imatinib arm discontinued therapy due to adverse events compared with 33% in the IFN–cytarabine arm. This landmark trial clearly showed the superiority of imatinib over IFN–cytarabine in the treatment of patients with newly diagnosed CML in chronic phase and also showed the potential promise of molecularly targeted therapies for the treatment of oncologic disorders in general. Based on these results, imatinib is now considered the new frontline standard of care for patients with CML in chronic phase.

Although the superior response rates with imatinib are clear, these results raise several controversies in the management of patients with CML as well as several practical issues with imatinib therapy. Controversies in CML management include the following:

- With the possibility of improved overall survival with imatinib, do clinicians need to rethink which patients to refer to transplant?
- At what point, if any, should one consider stopping imatinib in patients with a long-term (>5 years) cytogenetic remission?
- What is the proper therapy in patients who do not respond to or relapse on imatinib therapy?

Practical management strategies for issues such as dosing, management of toxicities, and possible drug interactions have been reviewed extensively elsewhere.[61] It is hoped that more mature data from the IRIS trial, results from ongoing clinical trials, and more experience will help answer these and other controversies in the near future.

CHRONIC LYMPHOCYTIC LEUKEMIA
Signs and Symptoms

14. **B.R., a 63-year-old man, recently presented to his family physician with a persistent cough. A routine CBC revealed a Hgb of 13.8 g/dL with normal indices, a WBC count of 34,000/mm³ with 80% lymphocytes, and a platelet count of 175,000/mm³. Physical examination and chest radiograph were unremarkable, and he was afebrile. Blood pressure was 120/70 mm Hg, heart rate 70 beats/min, and respiratory rate 20 breaths/min. He was prescribed azithromycin for presumptive mycoplasma pneumonia and scheduled for a return visit in 2 weeks. At that time, his CBC results were Hgb, 13.8 g/dL with normal indices; WBC count, 32,000/mm³ with 82% lymphocytes; and platelets, 168,000/mm³. Physical examination was unchanged and his cough had resolved. B.R. was referred to a hematologist for evaluation of his persistent lymphocytosis. What is the most likely cause of persistent lymphocytosis in B.R.?**

[SI units: Hgb 138 g/L (normal, 135 to 175); WBC count, 34 × 10⁹/L with 0.8 lymphocytes and 32 × 10⁹/L with 0.82 lymphocytes, respectively (normal WBC 4.5 to 10 with 0.15 to 0.5 lymphocytes); platelets, 175 × 10⁹/L and 168 × 10⁹/L (normal 150 to 440)]

Causes of lymphocytosis (>5,000 lymphocytes/mm³ in peripheral blood) include infectious mononucleosis, pertussis, acute infectious lymphocytosis (viral and other infections), CLL, and ALL. Examination of the peripheral blood lymphocyte morphology by an experienced hematologist or pathologist may be helpful in distinguishing these disorders. Patients with ALL commonly have lymphoblasts in the peripheral blood, and patients with other disorders, including mononucle-

osis, have a high percentage of atypical lymphocytes. Because B.R. has no fever or systemic symptoms of infection and lymphocytes in the peripheral blood are mature, he most likely has CLL. Bone marrow aspiration, biopsy, and cell surface markers are required to determine the definitive diagnosis.

Staging and Prognosis

15. **Bone marrow examination reveals normal cellularity with >30% of nucleated cells lymphocytes. The immunophenotype indicates peripheral blood lymphocytes are predominately B cells and are positive for CD5, CD19, and CD20. A diagnosis of CLL is confirmed. What is the usual presentation and prognosis of CLL? What treatment is indicated at this time?**

CLL is a monoclonal neoplastic disorder of slowly proliferating, long-lived lymphocytes that are immunologically incompetent. CLL is the most common type of leukemia in adults, and it occurs twice as often in men as in women. The median age at diagnosis is 62, and 90% of patients are over 50.[62] Like B.R., approximately 25% of patients are asymptomatic at initial presentation, and many are diagnosed by routine CBCs. Survival is variable and depends on the stage of disease at diagnosis. CLL is staged based on peripheral lymphocyte counts; enlargement of lymph nodes, liver, and spleen; and presence of anemia and/or thrombocytopenia. B.R. has very-early-stage disease because his only finding is absolute lymphocytosis. The prognosis for patients with early-stage disease is good, with a median survival of >11 years.[63] Table 90-7 illustrates the two most commonly used staging systems for CLL and associated prognoses.

Studies have demonstrated that no clear advantage exists in treating asymptomatic patients with early-stage disease and early treatment may be detrimental; therefore, B.R. should be observed at this time.[62,64] As CLL progresses, B.R. will become less able to produce immunoglobulins, and his lymphocytes will become more resistant to apoptosis (programmed cell death).[65] Vaccination against infection at this stage has been suggested; however, a small number of studies demonstrate a blunted and delayed antibody response in patients with CLL, and there is no evidence that vaccination reduces the incidence and severity of infections.[65–67]

Treatment

16. **B.R. returns to the hematologist every 3 months and does well for about 2 years. At that time, physical examination reveals enlargement of cervical, inguinal, and axillary lymph nodes; hepatomegaly; and splenomegaly. His lymphocyte count has increased from 32,000/mm³ 6 months ago to 68,000/ mm³ today. His Hgb is 11.7 g/dL, and his platelet count is 140,000/ mm³. Is treatment now indicated?**

[SI units: lymphocyte count, 32 × 10⁹/L and 68 × 10⁹/L, respectively; Hgb, 117 g/L; platelets, 140 × 10⁹/L]

B.R.'s CLL has obviously progressed based on the enlarged lymph nodes, hepatomegaly, splenomegaly, and progressive lymphocytosis (doubling of count in <6 months). Other indications for initiating treatment include recurrent infections or the development of anemia or thrombocytopenia that is not immune mediated.[68] Treatment should be initiated at this time to prevent further deterioration of B.R.'s hematologic and immune functions.

Table 90-7 **Classification of Chronic Lymphocytic Leukemia**

Binet Classification

		Median Survival		
Stage	Blood Counts		Involved Areas	Years
A	Hb 10 g/dL and platelets >100 × 10⁹/L		<3	12
B	Hb 10 g/dL and platelets >100 ×10⁹/L		>3	7
C	Hb 10 g/dL or platelets <100 × 10⁹/L or both		Any number	2

Rai Classification

		Median Survival	
Stage	Modified Stage	Description	Years
0	Low risk	Lymphocytosis	>10
I/II	Intermediate risk	Lymphocytosis+ lymphadenopathy + splenomegaly ± hepatomegaly	7
III/IV	High risk	Lymphocytosis + anemia + thrombocytopenia	2–4

Adapted from reference 62.

Initial Therapy
CHLORAMBUCIL

Historically, initial treatment of CLL has included chlorambucil. However, newer agents with improved response rates are replacing it as initial therapy. Approximately 70% of previously untreated patients will respond satisfactorily to chlorambucil but few will achieve complete remissions of their disease.[62,63] A variety of daily and intermittent dosing schedules have been used, with similar response rates seen. Daily therapy usually consists of chlorambucil 6 to 14 mg/day orally and treatment is continued until signs and symptoms diminish or toxicity is seen.[69,70] At that time, maintenance dosages may be given for up to 3 years.[65,71] Intermittent therapy usually consists of 0.7 mg/kg given over 2 to 4 days and repeated every 3 weeks until the disease stabilizes. Many variations of these regimens produce similar response rates. Once therapy is initiated, patients require frequent monitoring of blood counts and physical findings. The chlorambucil dosage must be adjusted to maximize benefit while preventing serious toxicities.

FLUDARABINE

Comparisons of single-agent fludarabine with chlorambucil and combination chemotherapy regimens has demonstrated an improvement in complete response rates and progression-free survival, but not overall survival.[72,73] Regimens of 25 to 30 mg/m² for 5 days monthly produce response rates of 60% to 90% in untreated patients with 35% complete response.[65] Acute toxicities are generally mild, but profound lymphopenia and infections can occur necessitating prophylaxis in patients with advanced disease, renal dysfunction, an absolute neutrophil count <1,000/mm³, and prior chemotherapy treatment.[74] Patients with a creatinine clearance <80 mL/min are more likely to develop hematologic toxicities and infectious complications earlier in the course of therapy.[75]

COMBINATION CHEMOTHERAPY REGIMENS

A combination of corticosteroids and chlorambucil may be useful in patients requiring a rapid reduction in lymphadenopathy or in patients with immune complications such as autoimmune hemolytic anemia or thrombocytopenia. However, complete response rates and overall survival are not improved over single-agent chlorambucil, and the risk of infectious complica-

tions is increased.[62,64] Currently, most recommendations do not include corticosteroids as empiric initial therapy.[62,63] Response rates seen with chlorambucil led to investigations with multi-agent regimens that most commonly include some combination of cyclophosphamide, doxorubicin, vincristine, and prednisone. No survival difference between single-agent chlorambucil and these regimens has been consistently shown, and regimen-related toxicities are increased.[63,65]

The combination of rituximab and fludarabine has demonstrated improvements in complete response rates, but with more hematologic and infectious toxicity.[76] Rituximab 50 mg/m² was given on day 1 over 4 hours, followed by 325 mg/m² on day 4 on the first cycle only when infusional toxicities and elevated lymphocyte counts are seen in patients with CLL.[77] Further cycles were given as 375 mg/m² on day 1, and all fludarabine regimens were 25 mg/m² on days 1 to 5. In 51 patients, concurrent administration of the two agents was superior to sequential administration (rituximab given after six cycles of fludarabine) and there was a 47% complete response rate. Overall survival could not be fully assessed after 23 months of follow-up. Neutropenia occurred in 76% of patients during the first cycle, and a documented opportunistic infection was seen in eight patients throughout the evaluation.

The addition of cyclophosphamide to fludarabine has produced complete response rates in 66% of untreated patients in one small trial, and a large phase III evaluation is currently ongoing comparing single-agent fludarabine with the combination.[78] It is important to note that no combination therapy has yet demonstrated improvements in progression-free or overall survival compared with single-agent fludarabine or chlorambucil; however, it is clearly associated with more toxicity. Improvements in complete response rates and supportive care will translate into superior overall outcomes as the clinical trial data mature.

Alemtuzumab

17. **B.R. receives six cycles of fludarabine as initial CLL therapy. After the third, he has complete regression of his lymphadenopathy and hepatosplenomegaly, and his lymphocyte count decreases to 8,000/mm³. B.R. comes to clinic 2 years after completion of fludarabine and a CBC is obtained that reveals the following: WBC**

count 55,000/mm³ with 70% lymphocytes, a Hgb of 10 g/dL, and a platelet count of 90,000/mm³. On physical examination, B.R. is found to have some cervical, inguinal, and axillary lymphadenopathy with no palpable splenomegaly, and he complains of excessive fatigue and fever. A 2-month trial of pulse chlorambucil is tried with no change in WBC count, lymphadenopathy, or symptoms. What therapies may be helpful in B.R. at this point?

[SI units: WBC count, 55 × 10⁹/L; Hgb 100 g/L; platelets, 80 × 10⁹/L]

Second-line therapies in CLL should generally be chosen based on criteria similar to those used for initial management. Single-agent chlorambucil and fludarabine are widely used in salvage therapies, but rarely produce significant durable responses. Re-treatment with fludarabine may produce responses in up to 50% of patients whose initial response was >1 year.[62] Because of low toxicity and CD20 expression on CLL cells, single-agent rituximab has been evaluated in the salvage setting. Overall, disappointing results have been seen (no complete responses and partial responses ranging from 0% to 36%), and phase I trials of dose escalation (up to 2,250 mg/m²) to assess percentage and duration of response were halted because of expense.[79] Alemtuzumab, a monoclonal antibody directed against CD52, has been approved for use in patients who have been exposed to alkylating agents and have failed fludarabine. It is administered as 3 mg IV, and, if tolerated, 10 mg IV on day 2, increased to a goal of 30 mg IV three times weekly. Infusion reactions—including rigors, fever, rash, and dyspnea—are common and require pretreatment with acetaminophen and diphenhydramine. The response rate in a heavily pretreated advanced-stage population was 33% with a median survival of 16 months.[80] Hematologic toxicity is common with 70% and 52% of patients experiencing neutropenia and thrombocytopenia, respectively. Lymphopenia is severe after alemtuzumab treatment. Therefore, prophylaxis against *Pneumocystis carinii* pneumonia with trimethoprim/sulfamethoxazole DS BID three times per week and viral infections (herpes simplex and cytomegalovirus) with famciclovir (or equivalent) 250 mg BID are required upon initiation of alemtuzumab therapy. Prophylaxis should be continued for 2 months after completion of therapy or until the CD4 count is ≥200 cells/μL, whichever occurs later. In consultation with his oncologist, B.R. decides to pursue alemtuzumab therapy.

Infectious Complications

18. Six weeks after the initiation of alemtuzumab, B.R. complains of progressive shortness of breath and fever. Upon questioning, he reveals he quit taking his trimethoprim/sulfamethoxazole and famciclovir because "he felt fine." Chest radiograph reveals bilateral infiltrates. B.R. is admitted to the hospital for further evaluation and treatment. A CBC reveals a WBC count of 22,000/mm³ with 80% lymphocytes and an absolute neutrophil count of 800/mm³, Hgb of 11 g/dL, and platelet count of 70,000/mm³. Quantification of serum immunoglobulins reveals profound hypogammaglobulinemia. What are the possible causes of B.R.'s pneumonia and what treatment is indicated?

[SI units: WBC count, 22 × 10⁹/L; Hgb 110 g/L; platelets, 70 × 10⁹/L]

Infections in advanced CLL are common and present predominantly as bacterial infections of the sinuses and lungs, although viral and fungal infections are seen in approximately 13% and 5% of cases, respectively.[81,82] Since B.R. is receiving alemtuzumab, the possibility of opportunistic infections in-

cluding cytomegalovirus, herpes viruses, mycobacteria, *Listeria monocytogenes,* and *Pneumocystis carinii* must be considered in addition to etiologies seen in advanced CLL and febrile neutropenia. Broad-spectrum antimicrobials are indicated and a thorough work-up for opportunistic etiologies is warranted. The use of supplemental intravenous immune globulin is controversial, particularly in the setting of acute infection. However, in patients with recurrent serious infections requiring hospitalization, low dose supplementation (250 mg/kg every 4 weeks) to maintain IgG values of ≥500 mg/dL appears to be justified.[83,84]

NON-HODGKIN'S LYMPHOMA
Clinical Presentation

19. R.G., an otherwise healthy 39-year-old woman, presents with complaints of swollen lymph nodes and occasional fevers and night sweats. Physical examination reveals marked supraclavicular and inguinal lymphadenopathy and a large abdominal mass. Biopsy of a supraclavicular lymph node confirms a diagnosis of diffuse large B-cell lymphoma. How does this type of lymphoma differ from other types of NHL?

Lymphomas are a heterogeneous group of disorders that arise from malignant transformation of cells of lymphoid origin. A lymph node consists of anatomic and functional compartments, such as follicular (germinal) centers, follicular mantle, and interfollicular and medullary areas (Fig. 90-1). The growth pattern of lymphoma is described as nodular or follicular when enlarged follicles predominate. When the normal architecture of the lymph node is totally replaced by a uniform population of neoplastic lymphocytes, the growth pattern is described as diffuse. Other cytologic features, such as the neoplastic cell type (including size and appearance), are also determined because it helps establish the specific subtype of NHL and aids in making treatment recommendations.[85]

A number of different classification systems have been used to classify this diverse group of malignancies. Clinically, the WF classification has historically been the system most commonly used; however, differences in prognosis in certain molecular subtypes have necessitated newer classification schemes.[4,86] The WF characterizes lymphomas based on their morphology and clinical behavior. In the WF classification, NHLs are divided into three broad groups. Low-grade lym-

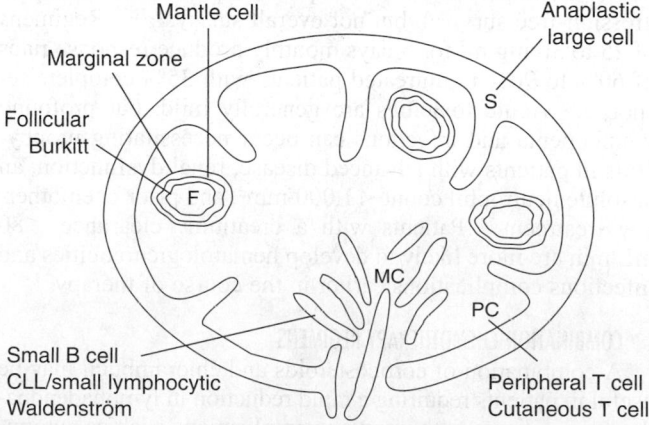

FIGURE 90-1 Sites of origin of malignant lymphomas in a lymph node according to anatomic and functional compartments of the immune system. CLL, chronic lymphocytic leukemia; F, follicles, or germinal centers; MC, medullary cords; PC, paracortex, or interfollicular areas; S, sinuses.

phomas include small cleaved cells with follicular or nodular growth patterns. These lymphomas tend to be more indolent in their natural history and patients typically survive for prolonged periods with minimal symptoms, although they cannot be cured with conventional therapy. In contrast, high-grade lymphomas tend to include larger cells with diffuse growth patterns. These lymphomas spread rapidly to other organs and result in death within weeks to months if untreated. However, these lymphomas are often very responsive to chemotherapy, with approximately 60% to 90% of patients cured after treatment with combination chemotherapy, depending on the extent

of disease at presentation.[87] Intermediate-grade lymphomas have an intermediate natural history and prognosis. R.G. has diffuse large B-cell lymphoma, which is an intermediate-grade lymphoma and among the most common of the NHLs.

Whereas previous classification systems were based on morphology and clinical behavior, the Revised European-American Lymphoma (REAL) classification incorporates morphology, immunophenotype (B cell, T cell, T/NK cell), cytogenetics, and clinical information.[88] All lymphoid malignancies, including lymphocytic leukemias, are included in the REAL classification system. (A comparison of the WF and REAL classification

Table 90-8 Comparison of the Working Formulation with the REAL Classification

	Revised European-American Classification	
Working Formulation	B-Cell Neoplasms	T-Cell Neoplasms
Low Grade		
Small lymphocytic consistent with CLL	B-cell CLL/PLL/SLL	T-cell CLL/PLL
	Marginal zone/MALT	LGL
	Mantle cell	ATL/L (chronic and smoldering)
Plasmacytoid	Lymphoplasmacytic-immunocytoma	
	Marginal zone/MALT	
	B-cell CLL/PLL/SLL	
Follicular, predominately small cleaved cell	Follicle center, follicular, grade I	
	Mantle cell	
	Marginal zone/MALT	
Follicular, mixed small cleaved and large cell	Follicle center, follicular, grade II	
	Marginal zone/MALT	
Intermediate Grade		
Follicular, large cell	Follicle center, follicular, grade III	
Diffuse, small cleaved cell	Mantle cell	T-cell CLL/PLL
	Follicle center, diffuse small cell	LGL
	Marginal zone/MALT	ATL/L
		Angioimmunoblastic
		Angiocentric
Diffuse, mixed small and large cell	Large B-cell lymphoma (rich in T cells)	Peripheral T-cell, unspecified
	Follicle center, diffuse small cell	ATL/L
	Lymphoplasmacytoid	Angioimmunoblastic
	Marginal zone/MALT	Angiocentric
	Mantle cell	Intestinal T-cell lymphoma
Diffuse, large cell	Diffuse large B-cell lymphoma	Peripheral T-cell, unspecified
		ATL/L
		Angioimmunoblastic
		Angiocentric
		Intestinal T-cell lymphoma
High Grade		
Large-cell immunoblastic	Diffuse large B-cell lymphoma	Peripheral T-cell, unspecified
		ATL/L
		Angioimmunoblastic
		Angiocentric
		Intestinal T-cell
		Anaplastic large cell
Lymphoblastic	Precursor B-lymphoblastic	Precursor T-lymphoblastic
Small noncleaved cell		
Burkitt's	Burkitt's	
Non-Burkitt's	High-grade B-cell	Peripheral T-cell, unspecified
	Burkitt-like diffuse large B-cell	

ATL/L, adult T-cell lymphoma; CLL, chronic lymphocytic leukemia; LGL, large granular lymphocyte leukemia; MALT, mucosa-associated lymphoid tissue; PLL, prolymphocytic leukemia; SLL, small lymphocytic lymphoma.
Adapted from reference 87.

systems is illustrated in Table 90-8.) With the additional information included in the REAL classification system, newer clinical groupings (indolent, aggressive, and highly aggressive tumors) were defined that recognized entities not included in the WF (Table 90-9). More recently, the WHO classification of lymphomas, which is based on the REAL system, has been proposed.[2] The WHO classification system advocates removal of clinical groupings because distinct biologic characteristics of specific diseases may be lost when grouped with other lymphomas based on clinical behavior alone. However, the WF and REAL classifications remain the most common reporting systems for prognosis and treatment decisions.

The most common clinical presentation of lymphoma is painless enlargement of one or more lymph nodes. Fever, night sweats, and weight loss are constitutional symptoms that are frequently initial symptoms of lymphoma as well.[87] R.G. did report increased swelling in her lymph nodes, occasional fever, and night sweats. R.G.'s tumor burden as measured by lymphadenopathy is large, which is not uncommon in patients with aggressive lymphomas.

Staging and Prognosis

The Cotswold/Ann Arbor staging system is commonly used to define the extent of disease in patients with lymphomas (Table 90-10). In general, stage I and II disease is referred to as limited disease and may be managed with external-beam radiation and a short course of combination chemotherapy.[89] Of patients with NHL, 80% present with advanced-stage disease (stage III or IV). The clinical and morphologic classifications and the stage of disease are important considerations when making treatment decisions. R.G. has disease on both sides of her diaphragm (stage III) and an aggressive lymphoma; therefore, she will require treatment with systemic chemotherapy.

Risk factors and survival for patients with aggressive NHL were identified by the International Non-Hodgkin's Lymphoma Prognostic Factors Project (Table 90-11). The International Prognostic Index (IPI) predicts the survival and relapse free survival after standard chemotherapy for NHL based on age, performance status, stage, lactic dehydrogenase (LDH), and extranodal involvement.[90] The IPI is increasingly used to identify patients likely to benefit from more aggressive therapeutic approaches such as high-dose chemotherapy with hematopoietic cell support.

Treatment
Aggressive and Highly Aggressive Lymphomas

20. R.G. received combination chemotherapy consisting of cyclophosphamide, doxorubicin, vincristine, and prednisone (CHOP). Is this considered standard therapy?

Patients like R.G. who have aggressive NHL require prompt treatment with combination chemotherapy. Although many different regimens have been investigated using a wide variety of drugs, doses, and schedules, the CHOP regimen has emerged as the gold standard. A large multi-institutional trial involving approximately 900 patients reported that remission rates and overall survival at 3 years did not differ significantly for patients receiving CHOP, MACOP-B, m-BACOD, or Pro-MACE-CytaBOM (Table 90-12). However, patients receiving CHOP reported fewer severe toxicities and fatalities.[91]

21. R.G. has a complete response to CHOP chemotherapy demonstrated by restaging studies performed after her third and sixth cycle of CHOP. Every 3 months she has a follow-up examination for disease recurrence. At her 15-month follow-up visit, she has radiographic evidence of disease recurrence in her ab-

---

Table 90-9   Clinical Grouping of Currently Recognized Non-Hodgkin's Lymphomas

B-Cell Neoplasms	T- and NK-Cell Neoplasms
Indolent Lymphomas (Untreated Survival Measured in Years)	
Indolent Disseminated Lymphomas/Leukemias	
B-cell CLL/SLL/PLL	T-cell CLL/PLL
Lymphoplasmacytic lymphoma/immunocytoma	Large granular lymphocyte leukemia
Splenic marginal zone lymphoma/SLVL	
Hairy cell leukemia	
Plasmacytoma/myeloma	
Indolent Extranodal Lymphomas	
Extranodal marginal zone/MALT lymphomas	Mycosis fungoides
Indolent Nodal Lymphomas	
Nodal marginal zone B-cell lymphoma	
Follicle center lymphoma	
Mantle cell lymphoma	
Aggressive Lymphomas (Untreated Survival Measured in Months)	
Diffuse large B-cell lymphoma variants	Anaplastic large-cell lymphoma
	Peripheral T-cell lymphomas
Highly Aggressive Acute Lymphomas/Leukemias (Untreated Survival Measured in Weeks)	
Precursor B-lymphoblastic leukemia/lymphoma	Precursor T-lymphoblastic lymphoma/leukemia
	Blastic NK-cell lymphoma
Burkitt's lymphoma	Adult T-cell lymphoma/leukemia (HTLVI+)

CLL, chronic lymphocytic leukemia; HTLVI, human T-cell leukemia virus type I; MALT, mucosa-associated lymphoid tissue; PLL, prolymphocytic leukemia; SLL, small lymphocytic lymphoma; SLVL, splenic lymphoma with villous lymphocytes.
Adapted from reference 87.

Table 90-10   Cotswold (Ann Arbor) Classification for the Staging of Non-Hodgkin's Lymphoma and Hodgkin's Lymphoma

Stage I:	Disease involvement of a single lymph node region (I) or lymphoid structure (e.g., spleen, thymus) or a single localized extranodal organ or site (I_E)
Stage II:	Disease involvement of two or more lymph node regions on the same side of the diaphragm (II); localized contiguous involvement of one extranodal organ or site and lymph node region on the same side of the diaphragm (II_E)
Stage III:	Disease involvement of lymph node regions on both sides of the diaphragm (III); may also be accompanied by localized involvement of an extralymphatic organ or site (III_E) or by involvement of the spleen (III_S), or both (III_{SE})
	III_1: indicates with or without involvement of splenic, hilar, celiac, or portal nodes
	III_2: indicates involvement of para-aortic, iliac, or mesenteric nodes
Stage IV:	Diffuse or disseminated disease involvement of one or more extranodal organs or tissues, with or without associated lymph node enlargement

Designations Applicable to Any Stage Disease

A	Asymptomatic
B	Symptomatic: weight loss >10% of body weight, unexplained fever with temperature >39°C (100.4°F), and night sweats
X	Designates bulky disease as >⅓ widening of the mediastinum or >10 cm maximum dimension of nodal mass
E	Involvement of a single extranodal site that is contiguous or proximal to the known nodal site.

Staging should be identified as clinical stage (CS) or pathologic stage (PS).

Adapted from reference 87.

domen. **What treatment options are available to R.G. at this time?**

Patients who respond to initial CHOP therapy and then suffer relapse should be given non–cross-resistant combination chemotherapy regimens such ESHAP (etoposide, methylprednisolone, high-dose cytarabine, and cisplatin), DHAP (dexamethasone, high-dose cytarabine, and cisplatin), or ICE (ifosfamide/mesna, carboplatin, and etoposide). Approximately 40% to 60% of patients who experience relapse after CHOP chemotherapy will have a complete response to a salvage chemotherapy regimen.[91,92] Studies have shown that patients who demonstrate chemosensitivity, defined as a complete or partial response to two cycles of a salvage regimen, benefit from high-dose chemotherapy with stem cell support.[93,94]

22. **How does treatment differ for highly aggressive NHL?**

Highly aggressive NHLs progress very rapidly and usually involve the CNS early in the course of the disease.[87,95] Patients treated with regimens such as CHOP may progress between cycles of chemotherapy. Therefore, regimens more similar to those used to treat ALL are used because they provide more continuous exposure to more intensive chemotherapy. These regimens also must include CNS prophylaxis with intermittent intrathecal methotrexate or cytarabine.[96]

Indolent Lymphoma
CLINICAL PRESENTATION

23. **D.J. is a 23-year old man who had a persistent toothache that led to extraction of an impacted wisdom tooth and biopsy of lymphoid tissue underlying the cavitary lesion. Pathologic examination revealed follicle center, follicular, grade 1 lymphoma (WF follicular, predominantly small cleaved cell). He was otherwise asymptomatic. A complete physical examination and other staging procedures revealed positive bone marrow biopsies. What are appropriate treatment options at this time?**

Low-grade/indolent lymphomas are slow-growing malignancies and therefore do not respond to traditional cytotoxic chemotherapy as well as the other NHLs do. However, the

Table 90-11   Risk Factors and Survival According to the International Non-Hodgkin's Lymphoma Prognostic Factors Project

All Patients	Patients <60 Years of Age
Age ≥60 years of age	LDH > normal
LDH > normal	Performance status ≥2
Performance status ≥2	Ann Arbor stage III or IV
Ann Arbor stage III or IV	
Extranodal involvement >1 site	

Risk Group	# of Risk Factors	5-Year Survival Rate (%)
Patients of All Ages		
Low	0, 1	73
Low-intermediate	2	51
High-intermediate	3	43
High	4, 5	26
Patients ≤60 Years of Age		
Low	0	83
Low-intermediate	1	69
High-intermediate	2	46
High	3	32

LDH, lactate dehydrogenase.
Adapted from reference 90.

Table 90-12   Comparison of Standard CHOP With Three Intensive Chemotherapy Regimens for Advanced Non-Hodgkin's Lymphoma

Regimen	6-Year Overall Survival (%)	Fatal Toxicities (%)
CHOP	33	1
m-BACOD	36	5
ProMACE-CytaBOM	34	3
MACOP-B	32	6

Adapted from reference 91.

progression of the disease is typically very slow, and patients often survive for 7 to 10 years after diagnosis.[97] Most experts advocate treating these patients only after they become symptomatic. This approach does not adversely affect the duration of survival as long as treatment is initiated at the onset of symptoms.[98,99] Patients with bulky disease or systemic symptoms should be treated immediately. Although D.J. has bone marrow involvement (stage IV disease), he is currently asymptomatic. Therapy is not indicated at this time.

TREATMENT

24. D.J. remains asymptomatic for 3 years. At this time, he develops abdominal and splenic lymphadenopathy, night sweats, and weight loss over a 2-month period. What treatment options are available for D.J.?

The choice of initial treatment for symptomatic patients is controversial and includes single-agent chemotherapy with chlorambucil, cyclophosphamide, a purine analog (cladribine or fludarabine), interferon-alfa, or combination chemotherapy. Treatment is usually initiated with an oral alkylating agent because these agents are safe, convenient, and inexpensive compared with other chemotherapy agents. Although fludarabine and combination chemotherapy regimens produce higher response rates than oral alkylating agents, a long-term survival advantage has not been demonstrated.[100,101] Typically, patients respond to first-line treatment for a median period of approximately 18 to 24 months. When the disease progresses, re-treatment with the initial agent or one of the other listed treatment options are used as second-line therapy. Unfortunately, response rates and duration of response decrease with each successive treatment.[87]

25. D.J. is 6 years out from his initial diagnosis and has received intermittent oral alkylating agents and, most recently, fludarabine. His disease was stable during the most recent course of fludarabine, which ended 2 months ago. However, in the past 2 months, he has experienced progression of his disease. The decision is made to administer rituximab to D.J. What efficacy and toxicities are seen with the administration of rituximab?

Rituximab is a chimeric anti–CD20 antibody that is thought to produce its antineoplastic action through antibody-dependent cytotoxicity or by interfering with signal transduction pathways and inducing apoptosis.[102,103] CD20 is a cell-surface antigen commonly found on normal and malignant B lymphocytes. Forty to fifty percent of patients with relapsed and refractory, low-grade, CD20-positive B-cell NHLs respond to rituximab.[104]

Rituximab is administered in the outpatient setting as a weekly infusion of 375 mg/m² for 4 consecutive weeks. The first infusion should be administered at a rate of 50 mg/hour and can be escalated in increments of 50 mg/hour every 30 minutes to a maximum of 400 mg/hour. Subsequent infusions can be administered at a rate of 100 mg/hour and increased to 400 mg/hour as tolerated.[105] An infusion-related symptom complex consisting of fever, chills, and rigors occurs in most patients during the first rituximab infusion leading to the recommendation to premedicate with diphenhydramine and acetaminophen. Other less common infusion-related symptoms include nausea, urticaria, fatigue, headache, pruritus, bronchospasm, angioedema, and hypotension. These reactions generally occur within 30 minutes to 2 hours from the start of the infusion and resolve by slowing or interrupting the infusion. Another side effect associated with rituximab is TLS (tumor lysis syndrome), which occurs mostly in patients with a high number of circulating tumor cells.[106]

Impressive response rates with single-agent rituximab in refractory/relapsed indolent B-cell lymphomas in addition to in vitro data showing synergy between rituximab and chemotherapy have led to clinical trials investigating its use in combination with chemotherapy. Impressive results have been reported in previously untreated indolent NHL as well as in elderly patients with aggressive CD20-positive NHLs.[107–109] Ninety-five percent of patients with indolent lymphoma had a response to six cycles of rituximab–CHOP, and 74% remained in remission 2.5 years after initiation.[108] Long-term follow-up is required to assess durability of responses in indolent lymphoma.

Radioimmunoconjugates are monoclonal antibodies linked to radioisotopes that target CD20-positive cells and deliver local radiation therapy. Ibritumomab tiuxetan and iodine-131 (I¹³¹) tositumomab have been used in relapsed patients who have received prior chemotherapy. Patients are candidates if they have <25% bone marrow involvement due to significant hematologic toxicity. Response rates range from 57% to 74% with 15% to 34% complete responses.[110] Rituximab is used before imaging with indium-111 ibritumomab tiuxetan to clear circulating lymphoma cells. This is done to provide a better view of biodistribution of the antibody. Dosimetric images are collected over the next 2 to 3 days to ensure low levels of distribution to potential target organs (lung, liver, bowel) before administration of the therapeutic yttrium-90–ibritumomab tiuxetan on day 7. For I¹³¹ tositumomab, patients should receive saturated solution of potassium iodide (2 drops orally three times/day) at least 24 hours before the dosimetric dose; this should be continued for 14 days after the therapeutic dose. For dosimetry, unlabeled tositumomab over 1 hour at a dose of 450 mg is administered followed by 5 millicuries (mCi) of I¹³¹ labeled to 35 mg of tositumomab given over 20 minutes. Gamma camera images are obtained on the dosimetry day and 2 other days in the following week to determine patient-specific I¹³¹ doses to deliver a total body radiation dose of 75 cGy. The therapeutic dosing consists of the same unlabeled tositumomab infusion followed by the patient-specific activity of I¹³¹ (in millicuries) labeled to 35 mg of tositumomab as a 20-minute infusion. Because of concerns of low-level radiation exposure to contacts, patients receiving either agent should be counseled to wash their hands thoroughly after using the toilet, avoid sharing utensils or cups, clean up spilled urine and dispose of body fluid-contaminated material (flush in toilet or place in plastic bag in household trash) for up to 7 days after administration.[111] Hematologic toxicity can occur 7 to 9 weeks after administration with a median duration of neutropenia and thrombocytopenia of approximately 3 weeks. Secondary malignancies may be a concern over the long term.

HODGKIN'S DISEASE
Clinical Presentation and Prognosis

26. C.L. is a 45-year-old woman who presented with chief complaints of fever, night sweats, cough, and a 10-lb weight loss. Chest x-ray examination revealed a mediastinal mass and a computed tomography (CT) scan of the abdomen showed multiple enlarged lymph nodes in the perisplenic and inguinal areas. Bone marrow biopsy was positive for lymphoma cells. Biopsy of an inguinal node revealed nodular sclerosis Hodgkin's disease with Reed-Sternberg cells. Is this a typical presentation of Hodgkin's disease? What is C.L.'s prognosis?

Hodgkin's disease can occur at any age and represents <1% of all cancers in the United States. Presentation can be limited to a single lymph node or to a extralymphatic organ or site or it can involve multiple lymph nodes and extralymphatic organs. The WHO classification of Hodgkin's lymphoma is shown in Table 90-13. Nodular sclerosis classic Hodgkin's lymphoma is the most common subtype and represents about two-thirds of cases of Hodgkin's lymphoma. The Cotswold staging system for lymphomas is shown Table 90-10.[112] C.L. has disease above and below the diaphragm and bone marrow involvement; therefore, she has stage IV disease. She has also been experiencing constitutional symptoms (i.e., fever, night sweats, and weight loss), which are designated by the letter *B* in the staging system. Hodgkin's disease is one of the few malignancies that is typically curable even in the advanced stages. The 20-year disease-free survival rate is >60%.[113]

Treatment

27. C.L. is scheduled to begin chemotherapy with the ABVD (doxorubicin, bleomycin, vinblastine, and dacarbazine) regimen. Is this the most appropriate treatment?

Two 4-drug combination chemotherapy regimens have demonstrated equivalent long-term survival rates for patients with advanced Hodgkin's disease. These regimens are the MOPP (mechlorethamine, vincristine, procarbazine, and prednisone) regimen originally reported in the early 1970s and the ABVD regimen developed about a decade later. Although efficacy appears equivalent for these regimens, the MOPP regimen is associated with a higher risk of severe emesis, myelosuppression, secondary leukemias, and other cancers. Therefore, the ABVD regimen is currently the preferred regimen by most clinicians. Hybrid regimens using alternating or sequential variations of the MOPP and ABVD regimens have also been evaluated. However, these varied regimens do not show a clear advantage compared with standard ABVD or MOPP.[114] In addition, a higher frequency of secondary leukemias has been associated with the hybrid regimens.[115–117] Hodgkin's disease is a chemotherapy-sensitive disease, and administration of full doses is critical. Unnecessary dosage attenuation can compromise the ability to achieve a cure. Cycles of ABVD are given every 28 days, and all patients should continue treatment for two cycles beyond documentation of complete remission for a total of six to eight cy-

cles. Traditionally, all subclasses of Hodgkin's lymphoma have been treated in a similar fashion and this remains the standard of care. Recent reports suggest that lymphocyte-predominant Hodgkin's disease (LPHD), due to the overexpression of CD20, may benefit from therapy with rituximab.[118] The role of rituximab in the treatment of LPHD remains to be determined, and these patients should be referred to ongoing clinical trials.

Relapsed Disease

28. C.L. achieved a complete remission and received a total of six courses of full-dose ABVD. Three years after completion of chemotherapy, a routine follow-up chest radiograph revealed enlarged lymph nodes, which were subsequently found to be recurrent disease. What treatment should C.L. receive?

Because it has been more than 1 year since she completed chemotherapy, data support re-treatment with the same regimen (i.e., ABVD). If C.L. fails to respond to ABVD, salvage regimens such as MOPP, EPOCH (etoposide, prednisone, vincristine, cyclophosphamide, and doxorubicin) or ICE (ifosfamide, carboplatin, and ctoposide) could be considered.[114,119] Alternatively, she could be evaluated for high-dose chemotherapy with stem cell support. Data suggest that up to 50% of patients with refractory disease may achieve a durable complete response after high-dose chemotherapy with stem cell support.[114]

MULTIPLE MYELOMA
Clinical Presentation

29. T.B. is a 59-year-old man who presents with complaints of low back pain increasing over the past month and fatigue. He has been self-medicating his back pain with over-the-counter nonsteroidal anti-inflammatory drugs (NSAIDs), but has achieved little relief. Plain films of the spine show a compression fracture at the L1 level. Further workup reveals a hemoglobin of 9 g/dL (normal, 13.5 to 17.5), a serum calcium of 10 mg/dL (normal, 8.5 to 10.2), and a serum creatinine of 2.4 mg/dL (normal, 0.8 to 1.4). Serum and urine electrophoresis are obtained and reveal a monoclonal protein typed as IgG lambda (λ) of 8.8 g/dL (normal, 0.5 to 1.6); IgA is 0.008 g/dL (normal, 0.04 to 0.4); and IgM is 0.025 g/dL (normal, 0.03 to 0.2). A 24-hour urine collection showed 5.2 g total protein excreted, with 77% Bence Jones proteins. A serum β_2-microglobulin was 4.5 mg/L (normal, 1.1 to 2.5). Bone marrow biopsy reveals 47% plasma cells. Skeletal survey shows additional lesions in the skull and ribs. A diagnosis of multiple myeloma (MM) stage IIIB is made. Is this presentation consistent with the diagnosis of MM?

[SI units: Hgb, 90 g/L (normal, 135 to 165); calcium 2.5 mmol/L (normal, 2.13 to 2.55); creatinine 212.2 micromol/L (normal, 70.7 to 123.8); IgG 0.088 g/L (normal, 0.005 to 0.016); IgA 0.00008 g/L (normal, 0.0004 to 0.004); IgM 0.00025 g/L (normal, 0.0003 to 0.002); β_2-microglobulin 0.0045 g/L (normal, 0.0011 to 0.0025)]

MM is a malignancy of fully differentiated B lymphocytes called *plasma cells*. Proliferation and accumulation of plasma cells leads to excessive antibody (immunoglobulin) production. A variety of clinical manifestations can be seen and are related to immunoglobulin production, plasma cell infiltration, and immune deficiency. Of patients who develop MM,

Table 90-13	WHO Classification of Hodgkin's Lymphoma

Nodular lymphocyte-predominant Hodgkin's lymphoma
Classic Hodgkin's lymphoma
    Nodular sclerosis
    Mixed cellularity
    Lymphocyte depletion
    Lymphocyte-rich

55% are male and 98% are 40 or older.[1,5] The disease occurs twice as often in African Americans compared with Whites.[120]

T.B. presents with a number of the classic features of MM. Bone pain and skeletal disease are common and occur when plasma cells infiltrate the bone and secrete osteoclast-activating factor and other cytokines. Plain radiographic films often show osteopenia and/or multiple osteolytic bone lesions (punched-out areas on radiographs). Hypercalcemia and pathologic fractures often accompany the osteolytic lesions associated with this disease. Plasma cells can infiltrate the bone marrow and lead to a normocytic normochromic anemia in up to 70% of patients. Comparatively, neutropenia and thrombocytopenia are rarely present at the time of diagnosis. Hypercalcemia, bone lesions, and anemia directly correlate with tumor mass and prognosis.[121] Renal dysfunction is generally attributable to deposition of κ or λ light chains of immunoglobulin in the distal tubule and up to 50% of patients have or will develop renal insufficiency with the disease.[122] In most patients with MM, only light chains are found in the urine. Myelomas that overproduce light chains are most commonly associated with renal dysfunction. Renal dysfunction can be further complicated by dehydration secondary to hypercalcemia, the use of NSAIDs for pain relief, and the use of contrast dyes in radiographic evaluation. Another feature that may accompany MM is hyperviscosity syndrome, more commonly seen with IgA subtype.[5] Hyperviscosity causes CNS, renal, cardiac, and pulmonary symptoms and complications. Plasmapheresis may be used emergently to alleviate life-threatening cases. Patients may develop recurrent infections due to depressed production of other immunoglobulin classes, leading to an inability to opsonize bacteria.

Staging and Prognosis

Plasma cell disorders comprise a spectrum of disorders that range from MGUS to MM. Differential diagnoses for all plasma cell disorders are shown in Table 90-14. T.B. clearly meets the criteria for MM. The prognosis for patients diagnosed with myeloma depends on the initial stage of disease. Median survival ranges from 5 years for patients with stage I disease to 2 years for patients with stage III disease.[5] The presence of renal dysfunction (A versus B subclassification) significantly worsens the prognosis. An elevated β2-microglobulin (a light chain protein expressed on all nucleated cells) is also associated with a worse prognosis, regardless of the type of therapy administered. T.B. has stage IIIB disease (Table 90-15).

Treatment
Initial Therapy

30. **The decision is made to begin systemic chemotherapy with VAD (vincristine, doxorubicin [Adriamycin], and dexamethasone). What advantages and disadvantages does VAD have compared with other regimens?**

Patients who meet the diagnostic criteria for MM and are symptomatic are candidates for systemic chemotherapy (Table 90-16). Oral melphalan and prednisone was the first regimen to show significant activity in myeloma. The combination produces response rates of 50% to 60%; however, complete responses are uncommon (3% to 5%) and median sur-

---

Table 90-14 Diagnostic Criteria for Plasma Cell Disorders

Multiple Myeloma (MM)

Major criteria:
1. Plasmocytoma on tissue biopsy
2. Bone marrow plasmacytosis with ≥30% plasma cells
3. Monoclonal immunoglobulin spike on serum electrophoresis: IgG >3.5 g/dL. IgA >2 g/dL light chain excretion on urine electrophoresis ≥1g/24 hr

Minor criteria:
1. Bone marrow plasma cells 10–30%
2. Monoclonal immunoglobulin spike present, but less than levels defined above
3. Osteolytic bone lesions
4. Suppressed uninvolved immunoglobulins (IgM <0.05 g/dL, IgA <0.1 g/dL, IgG <0.6 g/dL)

The diagnosis of myeloma generally requires a minimum of one major and one minor criterion (1 + 1 not considered sufficient) or three minor criteria that must include 1 + 2

Indolent Myeloma

Criteria as for myeloma with the following limitations:
1. Absent or only limited bone lesions (≤3 lytic lesions), no compression fractures
2. Immunoglobulin levels: IgG <7 g/dL, IgA <5 g/dL
3. No symptoms or associated disease features: Karnofsky performance status >70%, hemoglobin >10 g/dL, serum calcium normal, serum creatinine <2 mg/dL, no infections

Smoldering Myeloma

Criteria as for indolent myeloma with additional constraints:
1. No bone lesions
2. Bone marrow plasma cells 10–30%

Monoclonal Gammopathy of Undetermined Significance (MGUS)

1. Paraprotein levels: IgG ≤3.5 g/dL, IgA ≤2 g/dL, Bence Jones protein ≤1 g/24 hr
2. Bone marrow plasma cells <10%
3. No bone lesions
4. No symptoms

Adapted from reference 5.

---

vival as sole therapy is only 30 to 36 months[5,120] Combination regimens containing multiple alkylating agents, vinca alkaloids, anthracyclines, and corticosteroids have improved response rates and shortened the time to response but have failed to influence overall survival[5,123,124] Patients who are not candidates for hematopoietic cell transplantation (see below) usually receive oral melphalan (or other alkylating agent) and prednisone as initial therapy. VAD is preferred over alkylating agent-containing regimens in transplantation candidates because of its lower myelotoxicity, which improves stem cell collection. Also, if a rapid response is required because of significant symptomatic disease, VAD is preferred. Alternatively, single-agent dexamethasone has shown response rates similar to those of melphalan and prednisone but inferior to those of VAD.[125] One disadvantage of VAD is the requirement of continuous infusion vincristine and doxorubicin over a 4-day period. Replacing conventional doxorubicin with doxorubicin liposome and giving vincristine on day 1 only has been shown to be as effective as infusional VAD in one study and is more convenient.[126]

Table 90-15   Myeloma Staging System

Stage	Criteria	Measured Myeloma Cell Mass (Cells × 10^{12}/m²)

I	All of the following:
	 1. Hemoglobin value >10 g/dL
	 2. Serum calcium normal (≤12 mg/dL)
	 3. On radiograph, normal bone structure or solitary bone plasma-cytoma only
	 4. Low monoclonal immunoglobulin production
	    A. IgG value <5 g/dL
	    B. IgA value <3 g/dL
	    C. Urine light chain
	    Monoclonal protein on electrophoresis <4 g/24 hr
		<0.6

II	Fitting neither stage I nor stage III	0.6–1.2 (intermediate)

III	One or more of the following:
	 1. Hemoglobin value <8.5 g/dL
	 2. Serum calcium >12 mg/dL
	 3. Advanced lytic bone lesions
	 4. High monoclonal immunoglobulin production
	    A. IgG value >7 g/dL
	    B. IgA value >5 g/dL
	    C. Urine light chain
	    Monoclonal protein on electrophoresis >12 g/24 hr
		>1.2 (high)

Subclassification

A = Relatively normal renal function (serum creatinine value <2.0 mg/dL).
B = Abnormal renal function (serum creatinine value ≥2.0 mg/dL).

Examples

Stage IA = Low cell mass with normal renal function.
Stage IIIB = High cell mass with abnormal renal function.

Adapted from reference 5.

Table 90-16   Multiple Myeloma Treatment Regimens

Regimen	Agents	Comments
Initial Therapy		
MP	Melphalan 8–10 mg/m² PO QD, days 1–4 Prednisone 60 mg/m2 PO QD, days 1–4 Repeat cycle every 28–42 days	Should be given on empty stomach due to variable absorption when administered with food
VAD	Vincristine 0.4 mg/day continuous intravenous infusion (CIV), days 1–4 Doxorubicin 9 mg/m²/day CIV, days 1–4	Should be administered through an indwelling central venous catheter to reduce extravasation risk
Dexamethasone	Dexamethasone 40 mg PO QD, days 1–4, 9–12, 17–20 Repeat cycle every 28 days	
Pulse dexamethasone	Dexamethasone 20 mg/m² PO QD, days 1–4, 9–12, 17–20 Repeat cycle every 35 days	
DVD	Doxorubicin liposome 40 mg/m² mg IV once, day 1 Vincristine 2 mg IV once, day 1 Dexamethasone 40 mg PO QD, days 1–4 Repeat cycle every 28 days	
Thalidomide +/–dexamethasone	Thalidomide 200–400 mg PO QD with or without Dexamethasone 40 mg PO QD, days 1–4, 9–12, 17–20	Should be given in evening to minimize sedation. Titration at 50–100 mg increments weekly to achieve target dose improves tolerability; may also be used as salvage therapy.
Salvage Therapy		
Bortezomib	Bortezomib 1.3 mg/m² IV once, days 1, 4, 8, 11 Repeat cycle every 21 days	Dose reduction to 1 mg/m² may be necessary in patients with peripheral neuropathies
DTPACE	Dexamethasone 40 mg PO QD, days 1–4 Thalidomide 400 mg PO QD at night Cisplatin 10 mg/m²/day CIV days 1–4 Doxorubicin 10 mg/m²/day CIV days 1–4 Cyclophosphamide 400 mg/m²/day CIV days 1–4 Etoposide 40 mg/m²/day CIV days 1–4	Thromboembolic events with thalidomide are increased in combination with doxorubicin and require prophylactic anticoagulation.

DTPACE, high-dose dexamethasone, thalidomide, and 4-day continuous infusion of cisplatin, doxorubicin, cyclophosphamide, and etoposide; DVD, doxorubicin liposome, vincristine, dexamethasone; VAD, vincristine, doxorubicin (Adriamycin), and dexamethasone.

Thalidomide has also been evaluated as a single agent and in combination with dexamethasone for previously untreated patients.[127,128] The mechanism of action is unclear but may be angiogenesis inhibition and/or reduction in cytokines that stimulate myeloma cell growth. Doses of thalidomide have ranged from 200 to 800 mg daily in the evening, with most patients tolerating a 200-mg titration every 2 weeks. Dose-related toxicities include sedation, constipation, thrombosis, and neuropathies, which often preclude increases above 400 mg daily. Responses to single-agent thalidomide were seen in 36% of patients treated; in combination with dexamethasone, response rates increase to 64% to 72%. Single-agent use in relapsed or refractory patients shows similar efficacy; however, patients over 65 years old may not respond as frequently as younger ones.[129,130] Because of teratogenic effects, thalidomide is available only through a restricted distribution program, and patients must be thoroughly counseled about contraception. Thalidomide with or without dexamethasone is an initial alternative to melphalan/prednisone in patients who have cytopenias and/or are not candidates for hematopoietic cell transplantation.

Hematopoietic Cell Transplantation

Efforts to improve the outcome of MM treatment have led to the investigation hematopoietic cell transplantation using high-dose chemotherapy regimens with autologous stem cell support and nonmyeloablative regimens with allogeneic support. Randomized comparisons of high-dose chemotherapy with autologous stem cell support and conventional chemotherapy in previously untreated patients younger than 65 years old have been conducted.[131–134] All patients received two to six cycles of conventional chemotherapy before randomization to high-dose or standard chemotherapy. Most trials have reported higher response rates and improved survival in patients randomized to receive high-dose chemotherapy with stem cell support. Younger age, chemosensitive disease, and fewer pretransplant therapies have emerged as important predictive factors for response to high-dose chemotherapy.[131–134] Despite flaws in study design, high-dose chemotherapy is generally regarded as the current treatment of choice for patients with MM who achieve complete responses following initial therapy.[135] The use of nonmyeloablative allogeneic transplant regimens in myeloma represents a potential curative option in patients with complete responses after autologous transplants. Nonmyeloablative regimens are generally associated with fewer regimen-related toxicities than full allogeneic transplants but maintain a graft-versus-tumor effect to eradicate residual disease (see Chapter 92, Hematopoietic Cell Transplantation). Initial limited clinical trial results have been encouraging in high-risk heavily treated patients, but infectious complications and graft-versus-host disease may limit widespread use of this approach.[136,137] T.B. will receive four cycles of VAD and be evaluated for high-dose chemotherapy with autologous stem cell support.

Supportive Care
Bisphosphonates

31. Zoledronic acid 4 mg IV over 15 minutes every 28 days is ordered for T.B. What is the rationale for bisphosphonate therapy in the presence of a normal serum calcium? What benefits and toxicities are associated with bisphosphonate therapy?

The efficacy of intravenous pamidronate and zoledronic acid for the prevention of skeletal fractures in myeloma patients with osteolytic bone lesions has been established and guidelines for their use developed.[138] Equivalent efficacy with monthly infusion has been shown with pamidronate 90 mg and zoledronic acid 4 mg. Zoledronic acid can be given over 15 minutes, whereas pamidronate is given over 2 hours. Higher doses and shorter infusion times have been associated with renal damage. In addition, in patients with baseline creatinine values of <3 mg/dL, no adjustment in dose or infusion rate is necessary with either agent. Use of either agent in patients with baseline creatinine values of ≥3 mg/dL has not been fully established. Patients who have creatinine elevations of ≥0.5 mg/dL following a normal baseline value on bisphosphonates should have therapy withheld until renal function returns to baseline.[138] Hypocalcemia, myalgias, arthralgias, and flulike symptoms may be seen with bisphosphonate therapy. Currently, pamidronate is available generically and costs much less than zoledronic acid; however, a reduced infusion time with zoledronic acid reduces clinic time for patients and treatment centers.[138]

Relapsed and Refractory Disease

32. T.B. receives four cycles of VAD and has no response. What other therapies may offer benefit for his myeloma? If he has a response to another treatment, what, if any, maintenance therapy should he receive?

Treatment options for relapsed and refractory MM include thalidomide with or without dexamethasone, bortezomib, and multiple-agent chemotherapy (see Table 90-16). Bortezomib acts by inhibiting the proteosome, a multi-enzyme complex responsible for regulation of proteins that promote cell survival, stimulate growth, and reduce susceptibility to programmed cell death. It is given as a 1.3 mg/m² intravenous push twice weekly (at least 72 hours apart) for 2 weeks every 21 days up to 8 cycles. Dexamethasone 20 mg on the day of and after bortezomib may be added in patients who do not respond after two cycles. Common toxicities include sensory neuropathies (37%), thrombocytopenia (43%), nausea (64%), diarrhea (51%), and vomiting (36%). Dose reductions or omissions may be necessary for thrombocytopenia and neuropathies. In a phase II trial in patients treated with at least two prior therapies (including high-dose chemotherapy with autologous stem cell support), the response rate was 35% after 24 weeks of therapy with a median time to progression of 7 months.[139]

Results with single-agent thalidomide and few overlapping toxicities led to interest in combination therapy with conventional chemotherapy earlier in the course of disease. A regimen of two cycles of high-dose dexamethasone, thalidomide, and a 4-day continuous infusion of cisplatin, doxorubicin, cyclophosphamide, and etoposide (DTPACE) given 4 to 6 weeks apart was evaluated in relapsed patients treated with two prior regimens who also remained candidates for autologous stem cell transplantation.[140] Treatment was delayed or reduced for neutrophil counts <1,000/μL or platelet counts <100,000/μL. An overall response rate of 48% was seen in patients able to receive full doses of therapy for both cycles. Significant differences were seen in both complete and partial response rates for patients receiving <100% of scheduled doses. Thromboembolic events necessitated anticoagulant prophylaxis during the study and neutropenia, thrombocytopenia, nausea, and sensory neuropathies were seen in 65%, 37%, 21%, and 13% of patients, respectively. DTPACE represents an effective regimen in patients who can tolerate significant cytopenias and remain eligible for transplantation.

HEMATOLOGIC MALIGNANCIES: PEDIATRIC

ACUTE LYMPHOBLASTIC LEUKEMIA OF CHILDHOOD

The two most common types of childhood leukemia are acute lymphoblastic leukemia (ALL) and acute myelogenous leukemia (AML), with the former accounting for 75% of cases and the latter for approximately 19%. ALL is the most common childhood cancer, accounting for approximately 30% of all malignancies in children.[141] Approximately 2,400 new cases of childhood ALL occur each year in the United States, with an estimated incidence of 34 cases per million in children less than 15 years old.[141]

A distinct peak incidence occurs at ages 2 to 3 years for ALL (>80 cases/million), then decreases substantially for 8 to 10 year olds (20 cases/million). A higher incidence of ALL is seen in White children than in Black children. This racial difference is most apparent in the 2- to 3-year-old age group, with a nearly threefold greater incidence rate for White children. Over the past 20 years, the incidence rate of ALL in U.S. children has increased by approximately 0.9% per year. These incidence figures are derived from the Surveillance, Epidemiology and End Results Program (SEER), which collects data from nine tumor registries throughout the United States.[141] The nine registries account for approximately 13% of the U.S. population. Total U.S. incidence is then estimated by applying the SEER data to the total population size. It is unknown how reflective the SEER data are of the true U.S. incidence, and/or if certain unmonitored regions may have significantly different rates of disease.

Before the early 1970s, ALL was a fatal illness; most children did not survive >2 to 3 months after diagnosis. Today, >80% of children will achieve prolonged survival with antileukemic therapy, and the majority will be cured.[141,142] New innovations in therapy for ALL are now focusing on additional refinements in therapy to further improve upon survival and to decrease the long-term morbidity associated with the therapeutic components of current treatment regimens.

Etiology

The etiology of ALL is unknown; however, several interesting associations have been discovered. A high incidence of leukemia was found among survivors of the atom bomb explosion in Japan during World War II, and those closest to the epicenter of the blast were at greatest risk.[143,144] Leukemia also occurs in children exposed to radiation *in utero*.[145] Other factors that have been suggested to cause ALL include exposure to electromagnetic fields, pesticides, maternal use of alcohol, contraceptives, and cigarette smoking.[146–149] Viruses have not been proved to cause childhood ALL.[150]

Evidence supporting an association between ALL and electromagnetic field exposure is currently inadequate.[141,151] In particular, the incidence of childhood ALL has not in-

creased markedly over the past 40 years during a time when electricity use has seen a large increase.[152] Clusters of leukemia cases that occur over certain time frames and around certain places may represent merely instances of statistic coincidence.[153] Because the incidence of childhood ALL in the United States has increased moderately over the past 20 years and because the SEER program samples data only from a small portion of the U.S. population and excludes several geographic regions, it is unclear whether significant variations in childhood ALL incidences across the nation may be related to certain environmental factors.

Pathophysiology

The pathophysiology of ALL involves the replacement of normal bone marrow elements with an accumulation of immature lymphoid cells. The essential lesion in ALL is a stabilization of a transit cell in the lymphocyte differentiation process. Many factors are involved in the control of normal cellular proliferation. Leukemia may represent a disruption in one or more of the normal relationships within the cell proliferation pathway, such as an abnormal response to lymphoid cell growth factors.[154]

With the availability of classification systems of lymphoblasts based on morphology, immunology, and cytogenetics, it has become clear that ALL is a heterogeneous disease. This is especially true with regard to cytogenetic abnormalities. The immunologic heterogeneity results from leukemic transformation at various stages of lymphocyte differentiation. As discussed later, these classifications have important prognostic value.

Clinical Presentation

The signs and symptoms of ALL are nonspecific, and many are shared with other childhood diseases such as juvenile rheumatoid arthritis (JRA). This occasionally leads to a child with ALL being mistakenly treated with corticosteroids for JRA. As a general rule, children should not be treated with chronic corticosteroids without first performing a CBC and/or a bone marrow aspirate. These signs and symptoms reflect the uncontrolled growth and differentiation of the leukemic clone and the resulting deficiency in normal bone marrow elements: namely neutrophils, RBCs, and platelets. Frequent clinical findings include fever (61%), bleeding (48%), and bone pain (23%).[155] Bone pain is believed to be the result of hypercellular bone marrow and infiltration of leukemic lymphoblasts into pain-sensitive structures such as the periosteum. Although bone pain may be severe, it quickly resolves once chemotherapy is initiated. On physical examination, many patients have lymphadenopathy (50%), splenomegaly (63%), and/or hepatosplenomegaly (68%).[155]

A CBC will demonstrate that at least 59% of patients have a normal or low WBC count; the remainder have elevated counts.[155] The WBC differential reveals a low percentage of neutrophils and bands and a marked lymphocytosis. Lymphoblasts may be present in the peripheral blood even with a low WBC count (e.g., 2,000 to 4,000/mm^3), but they are more likely when the WBC count is elevated.[155] A normochromic, normocytic anemia along with thrombocytopenia is present in most patients.[155]

A bone marrow aspirate and biopsy usually are necessary to confirm the diagnosis of ALL. Occasionally, in patients with elevated WBC counts, the diagnosis can be confirmed by studies of lymphoblasts in the peripheral blood. The diagnosis of ALL is made when at least 25% of lymphoid cells in the bone marrow are blasts.[156] Most ALL patients have far greater than 25% blasts, and many have complete replacement of bone marrow with lymphoblasts. Once a child is diagnosed with ALL, it is important to determine the various characteristics that influence treatment decisions and the prognosis.

Prognostic Variables

Clinical Variables

Certain clinical and laboratory findings that are present at diagnosis are important to predict a child's prognosis and to classify his or her risk stratification. Children with ALL are classified by their risk of relapse into one of the following categories: low, intermediate, or high risk. It is important to stress that much debate continues over which variables most strongly influence patient outcome. A recent workshop agreed that the most important risk-defining features of childhood ALL are age and initial WBC count.[157] However, several ongoing investigations are likely to further refine what constitutes different ALL risk populations.

WHITE BLOOD CELL COUNT

The initial WBC count is considered to be among the most important predictors of outcome in childhood ALL. Its importance as a prognostic feature often is retained after the adjustment for other important prognostic criteria.[156] Children with the highest WBC counts at presentation have the short-est duration of complete remissions.[158–163] There appears to be a linear relationship between the duration of remission and the WBC count at presentation (Fig. 90-2). Although exactly where the demarcation line for predicting a good or a poor prognosis is unknown, an initial WBC count >50,000/mm³ generally is associated with a poor prognosis.[157]

AGE

Patients younger than 1 year or older than 9 years of age at diagnosis tend to have worse prognoses.[157] At least one trial has demonstrated that more intensive therapy may overcome the adverse prognostic factor of adolescent age.[164] These investigators reported that young adults (16 to 21 years of age) with ALL have an event-free survival of approximately 60% at 6 years, which is similar to that of patients 10 to 15 years of age, and superior to that achieved in most trials of older adults.[164] Age is the most ominous predictor of prognosis with regard to infants, a group in which survival is exceedingly poor compared with other age groups.[165–168] For this group, even with intensified chemotherapy regimens, long-term disease-free survival is usually <50%.

GENDER

Patient gender also has been shown to be an important prognostic factor in several studies.[163,169,170] Testicular relapse is responsible for a somewhat worse prognosis in males, but it is not thought to completely account for the better prognosis of females. However, occult testicular disease usually is not ruled out when males experience relapse. Another factor that may be of importance is the inherent ability of males to tolerate higher doses of chemotherapy.[171] Greater therapy tolerance

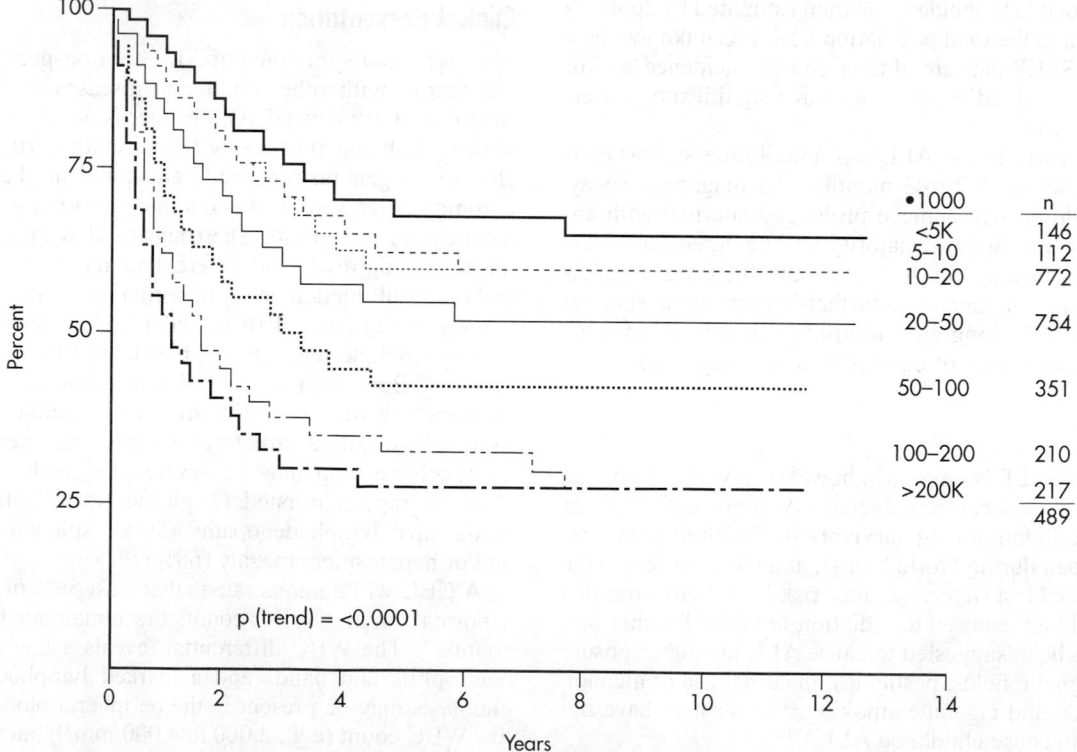

•1000	n
<5K	146
5–10	112
10–20	772
20–50	754
50–100	351
100–200	210
>200K	217
	489

p (trend) = <0.0001

FIGURE 90-2 Percentage of Children with ALL in Continuous Complete Remission Stratified According to Their WBC Count at the Time of Diagnosis. (Reprinted with permission of Wiley-Liss, a division of John Wlley and Sons, Inc. Hammond D et al. Medical and Pediatric Oncology. Wiley-Liss, 1986;14:125.)

in males suggests the need to use the maximum tolerated dose intensity to produce the same therapeutic effect achieved in females at lower doses. This finding may be due to a gender difference in the metabolism of certain chemotherapy agents.[172] Whether current improvements in the treatment of childhood ALL have nullified the adverse prognostic association of male gender has recently been reevaluated. A large series examined the outcome in >2,000 patients treated over >30 years. Females had significantly better outcomes than males in the early era, and although prognosis improved for both genders, an approximate 10% event-free survival advantage in females remained during the modern era (73.4% versus 63.5%). After accounting for differences in immunophenotype and DNA index between genders, these differences were no longer present. It was noted that males were significantly more likely to have T-cell ALL, and there was a trend for them to have a less favorable DNA index, thus indicating that these factors may be responsible for the adverse prognostic factor of male gender.[173]

RACE

Although Blacks have a lower incidence of ALL, several studies have shown that Black children appear to have a higher relapse rate than White children.[141,174–176] Data from the SEER program demonstrate a 5-year survival rate of 64% versus 78% for Black and White children, respectively. The differences in outcome for Blacks appears to be the result of a more severe form of ALL in this patient population.[176] A recent trial with more intensive therapy failed to show a worse outcome in Black children.[177]

MORPHOLOGY

Cells with the L1 morphology are the most common in childhood ALL and are associated with the best prognosis. Cells with L3 morphology are consistent with B-cell leukemia and Burkitt's lymphoma. Although historically associated with a poor prognosis, B-cell leukemia prognosis now has improved greatly with the advent of short-term, very intensive chemotherapy.[178,179] The L2 morphology has been associated with a poor prognosis in several studies.[180–182] Patients tend to have a worse outcome when >10% of their leukemic lymphoblasts have the L2 subtype.[180] However, other studies have not found the L2 morphology to be an important independent predictor of prognosis.[158,183]

Immunologic Variables

ALL is classified into different immunologic subsets based on cell surface markers and/or antigens present on the leukemic lymphoblasts at diagnosis. These can be categorized as cells of B-cell and T-cell origin. The B-cell lineage is further classified into various subtypes through the use of monoclonal antibodies. These subtypes reflect the various stages of differentiation at which leukemia may develop. Approximately 20% of children with ALL have leukemia with a T-cell lineage[184,185] and 1% to 2% of patients have leukemia with a mature B-cell origin.[185,186] Using more sophisticated diagnostic techniques, the majority of patients who were previously classified as non–T-, non–B-cell ALL (null-cell ALL) now are known to have leukemia of a more immature B-cell lineage.[187–189] Most patients with B-cell lineage ALL (80%) have cells that are positive for the common ALL antigen (CALLA)

on their surface[190,191]; this is referred to as common ALL. An additional marker, cytoplasmic immunoglobulin, has been used to further determine the level of differentiation of leukemic cells of the B-cell lineage. Intermediate cells of the B-cell lineage (pre-B cells) possess this marker, but more immature cells (early pre-B cells) do not.[189,192] More than 60% of children with ALL have a leukemia of the early pre-B subtype and approximately 20% have a leukemia of pre-B cells.

Mature B-cell ALL traditionally has been associated with a poor prognosis,[189,193,194] although, as mentioned previously, modern chemotherapy treatment has produced a marked improvement in overall survival in recent years.[178,179] Although differences in outcome have been noted among the B-cell subtypes,[189] when other prognostic factors are considered and when effective therapy is used, these differences may no longer be evident.[169,195,196] At present, immunologic features that differentiate B-cell precursor, T-cell, and mature B-cell ALL are thought to be clinically important because different types of chemotherapeutic strategies are employed for these three immunophenotypes.[142,179]

Patients with T-cell ALL have several distinguishing features, including a greater likelihood of being older males with high initial WBC counts and the presence of a mediastinal mass and/or initial leukemic involvement of the CNS.[197,198] Patients with T-cell ALL historically have had a decreased survival, although more intensive treatment is improving their outcomes.[158,199,200] Because T-cell ALL occurs in older children with high initial WBC counts, it is unclear whether this immunologic classification is an independent predictor of prognosis.[155,158] It recently has been demonstrated that T-cell lymphoblasts are less efficient at polyglutamating methotrexate, because these cells have lower concentrations of the methotrexate–polyglutamate synthesizing enzyme, folylpolyglutamate synthetase.[201] This has been proposed as a possible explanation for the relative chemotherapy resistance and the need for increased methotrexate dose-intensity in patients with T-cell ALL.[142]

Patients with ALL may present with a mixed-cell lineage disease, containing lymphoblasts that also express myeloid antigens. Expression of myeloid antigens is not thought to be an important prognostic factor in predicting the risk of relapse.[142]

Cytogenetic Variables

Advances in chromosomal analysis have improved the understanding of ALL biology. Abnormalities in either chromosome number (ploidy) and structure of the leukemic clone have been found in 60% to 75% of ALL cases.[142] Many of these abnormalities appear to have prognostic importance.[142,202] Ploidy is represented by the DNA index. A value of 1.0 indicates a normal number of chromosomes and a value >1.0 indicates an increased number of chromosomes by a multiplication factor of the normal chromosome number. Children with leukemia blasts containing >50 chromosomes (DNA index >1.16, hyperdiploid) appear to have an increased probability of continuous complete remission versus patients with leukemia blasts containing a diploid chromosome complement or with a DNA index <1.16.[202] Approximately 30% of ALL cases have a DNA index >1.16.[203] Patients whose ALL cells are hyperdiploid also tend to have other favorable prognostic features.[202] Children with hyperdiploid ALL may have a more favorable prognosis owing to their increased sensitivity to chemotherapy. An in vitro study of hyperdiploid versus nonhyperdiploid ALL revealed that those cells with a higher DNA index were more sensitive to antimetabolites (e.g., mercaptopurine) and asparaginase.[204] It also has been demonstrated recently that B-precursor hyperdiploid ALL cells contain more reduced folate carriers than diploid B-precursor blasts. Hyperdiploid cells were noted to have elevated levels of gene expression for these carriers, which may account for the higher levels of methotrexate polyglutamates noted in these cells as compared with patients with B-precursor diploid ALL.[205,206]

Translocations are the most common structural abnormalities occurring in leukemic cells[207] and occur in approximately 75% of childhood ALL cases.[208] Certain translocations are associated with treatment failure and relapse.[142] The translocations most commonly associated with treatment failure are the MLL rearrangements [t(4;11), t(11;19), and t(1;11)] and the BCR-ABL fusion transcript (t9;22, Philadelphia chromosome).[209] In particular, children with the Philadelphia chromosome appear to represent a population at very high risk of relapse. This translocation occurs in approximately 2% to 5% of childhood ALL cases. A recently published review compared the outcome of 30 patients with this translocation from a group of 1,322 children enrolled on ALL studies. This study demonstrated a 4-year event-free survival estimate of only 20% for children with the Philadelphia translocation versus 76% in those without it. This difference remained regardless of patient age, initial WBC count, or rapidity of response to therapy. Most patients with this translocation who were event-free survivors underwent bone marrow transplantation during their first remission.[210] A second case series of 61 children with Philadelphia chromosome–positive ALL identified early treatment response as a strong independent predictor of outcome in these patients. In this latter trial, 65% of these patients had a good initial response and a lower risk of treatment failure with either intensive chemotherapy or bone marrow transplantation when compared with the poor initial responders (event-free survival = 55 versus 10%, respectively).[211]

Using more sensitive (polymerase chain reaction [PCR]-based) methods than available with classic cytogenetic techniques, the previously unrecognized TEL/AML1 rearrangement (t12;21, ETV6-CBFA2 fusion transcript) has now been identified as the most commonly occurring (in approximately 18% of patients) translocation in childhood ALL. This translocation is associated with a patient age between 1 and 10 years, and most are precursor B-cell type and nonhyperdiploid. It has been shown that the TEL/AML1 translocation is an independent predictor of good prognosis. However, recently it has been reported that relapses tend to occur later in these patients, thus necessitating a long follow-up to determine the ultimate impact of this translocation.[208] At present, reducing the intensity of chemotherapy for children with this translocation is not recommended.[208]

The prognostic value of the main clinical variables often can be explained by cytogenetic abnormalities. For instance, most infants have rearrangements of the MLL gene, and this abnormality, as well as the Philadelphia chromosome, occurs more often in adolescents and adults.[142] In addition, two cytogenetic abnormalities associated with improved outcome (hyperdiploidy and the TEL-AML translocation) are found mainly in the 1- to 9-year age group.

Once a patient achieves complete remission, abnormalities of both ploidy and structure are not evident in the patient's recovered bone marrow by morphologic assessment, although a leukemic cell burden as large as 10^{10} may remain.[212] However, new techniques based on PCR assays can detect minimum residual disease (MRD) in many patients.[212] If relapse does occur, the leukemic cell cytogenetic characteristics are usually identical to those observed at diagnosis.[207]

Early Response
An additional factor of prognostic importance in childhood ALL is that of early response to therapy. Several investigations have noted that early response, as measured by either clearance of blasts from the peripheral blood or morphologic bone marrow remission (e.g., <5% bone marrow blasts) on day 7 or 14 of therapy, is predictive of long-term disease-free survival. In a review of 15 trials, early response was an independent prognostic factor in each of the studies.[213] Response was most commonly measured based on morphologic evaluation of day 14 bone marrow results, and it appeared that assessment of early response was more sensitive with bone marrow studies. Children who were slow early responders were 2.7 times more likely to have an adverse event than those with more rapid clearance of blasts. Interestingly, the rapidity of response maintained its prognostic significance within different strata delineated by the initial WBC count, providing further evidence that this variable is an important independent marker of prognosis. The rapidity of response is an intuitive marker of treatment sensitivity. However, the use of morphologic criteria to assign responder status will still include many patients with a significant disease burden. It is important to note that such tests of bone marrow burden may represent a dilute sample or a decrease in marrow cellularity and may not reflect the total leukemia burden in the body. It is estimated that these measures of early response may detect up to 25% of children at risk for early relapse.[213]

Minimum Residual Disease
Several investigators have examined the prognostic value of detecting MRD in bone marrow samples through the use of sophisticated PCR-based assays. A variety of lymphoblast characteristics, including gene fusion transcripts, immunophenotype, and antigen receptor gene rearrangements may be relied on for minimal disease detection in children with ALL. Although specific fusion transcripts can be relied on as PCR targets in only one-third of childhood ALL cases, clonal antigen receptor gene rearrangements occur in virtually all cases.[212] Using various techniques, approximately 50% of children with ALL are MRD positive at the completion of induction therapy, and roughly 45% of these patients will experience a relapse. The association for a negative test for MRD at the completion of induction therapy appears stronger because it has a negative predictive value of 92.5% and a positive predictive value of 44.5% at this time point. In patients positive for MRD, there is a continuous decrease in MRD during the months of chemotherapy treatment. Persistence of MRD beyond 4 to 6 months or re-emergence of MRD is almost always predictive of future relapse. It is now established that the presence of MRD is an important prognostic factor, regardless of the patient's initial WBC count or age at presentation.[212] At the time of this writing, monitoring of

MRD had not yet become standard practice in the management of childhood ALL, and it is unclear how MRD detection will be used in the design or decision making of future childhood ALL treatment protocols.

Additional Variables

Several additional variables may determine the prognosis of children with ALL. A complete discussion of these factors is beyond the scope of this text, but a few of these deserve brief mention. In addition to having an increased risk for developing ALL, children with Down's syndrome are at a slightly greater risk of treatment failure. Their adverse outcome has been ascribed to an excess of therapy-related toxicities, especially associated with high-dose methotrexate.[214] One variable that has not been traditionally listed as a prognostic factor is that of nutritional status. Although this usually is not an important variable in the United States and in developed nations, it may be a significant factor in Third World countries, which are home to the majority of the world's children. It has been reported in several trials that the outcome in childhood ALL is significantly worse for malnourished patients. In at least one trial, the most important predictor of relapse was malnutrition.[215] This may be related to a decrease in patient tolerance to chemotherapy in malnourished children. A malnutrition prevalence rate of up to 50% for children with ALL in Third World countries has been reported. When compared with socioeconomic status, malnutrition was more closely related to prognosis than was poverty. It appears that height for age is a more reliable predictor of prognosis than weight for age, suggesting that chronic stunting is more important than acute wasting in malnourished patients.[215]

All these prognostic variables can be used to assign patients to various categories based on their risk of relapse. These categories are important in determining the therapy that patients should receive. Although there is considerable agreement regarding the importance of certain variables in assigning patients to a defined risk group (e.g., age, initial WBC, DNA index, translocations), institutions that treat ALL differ in their definitions of what constitutes high-, intermediate-, and low-risk patients. This makes it difficult to compare treatment results from different institutions or treatment groups. Last, newer prognostic variables, especially rapidly evolving cytogenetic prognosticators, complicate the comparisons of treatment regimens over time.

Treatment

Remission Induction Therapy

ALLOPURINOL INTERACTION

33. J.B. is a 4-year-old Hispanic boy presenting with a 2-week history of an upper respiratory tract infection and a 1-week history of otitis media. His symptoms have worsened and he now presents with a nosebleed and fatigue. Physical examination reveals appreciable pallor and hepatosplenomegaly. A CBC with differential reveals a normochromic, normocytic anemia with a Hct of 15.7% (normal, 39% to 49%), Hgb of 5.7 g/dL (normal, 14 to 18), WBC count of 4,300/mm³ (normal, 3,200 to 9,800), and platelet count of 13,000/mm³ (normal, 150,000 to 400,000). A differential on the WBC count reveals 82% lymphocytes (normal, 30% to 40%), 7% neutrophils (normal, 50% to 60%), and 11% lymphoblasts (normal, 0%). Based on these findings, a bone marrow biopsy is performed, which reveals 95% lymphoblasts. A diagnosis of ALL is made. The ALL is morphologically an L1 type, and the immunologic class is early pre-B cell. Analysis of the chromosomes reveals the TEL-AML1 translocation and a DNA index of 1.0. The chest radiograph does not reveal a mediastinal mass, and a lumbar puncture shows that there are no leukemic lymphoblasts in the cerebrospinal fluid (CSF). J.B. is hydrated and alkalinized and treated with oral allopurinol 200 mg/m² per day, with a plan to institute induction therapy the next day. (For a discussion of the use of allopurinol in induction chemotherapy for the prevention of TLS, see Acute Nonlymphocytic Leukemia: Complications of Induction Therapy.) Within a few days, J.B. will be treated with several drugs for his leukemia. Do any of the agents that are likely to be used in J.B. exhibit significant drug interactions with allopurinol?

[SI units: Hct, 0.157 (normal, 0.39 to 0.49); Hgb, 57 g/L (normal, 140 to 180); WBC count, 4.3 × 10⁹/L (normal, 3.2 to 9.8) with 0.82 lymphocytes (normal, 0.3 to 0.4), 0.07 neutrophils (normal, 0.5 to 0.6), 0.11 lymphoblasts (normal, 0); and platelets, 13 × 10⁹/L (normal, 150 to 400)]

Xanthine oxidase, the enzyme inhibited by allopurinol, also converts mercaptopurine to 6-thiouric acid.[216] Thus, allopurinol may markedly increase the plasma concentrations of oral mercaptopurine by inhibiting first-pass metabolism, and this may lead to toxicity.[217] Although this is a potentially serious drug interaction, it is usually irrelevant for most patients with ALL because these agents are rarely used together. Allopurinol usually is employed early in the first week of induction therapy, and patients do not receive mercaptopurine until they finish induction therapy.

34. What is the goal of the induction therapy that J.B. will receive? Which agents should be used to achieve this goal?

GOAL OF INDUCTION

The goal of induction therapy is complete remission (i.e., the inability to detect leukemic cells in the peripheral blood or the bone marrow by morphologic microscopic evaluation). J.B.'s peripheral blood values must be within the normal range and the bone marrow must reveal <5% lymphoblasts.[218] This definition also assumes the absence of lymphoblasts in the CSF. Although these findings indicate an adequate response to chemotherapy, they do not indicate a cure. Most patients have a total of 10¹² cells at diagnosis, and successful induction regimens reduce this cell load by 99% to 10⁹.[219,220] Therefore, continuation of therapy will be required for J.B. to further reduce the leukemic cell population and to increase his chances of long-term survival. Without continuation of therapy, the majority of patients with ALL will relapse within 1 to 2 months.[221,222]

INDUCTION COMBINATION CHEMOTHERAPY

The agents most commonly used in remission induction therapy are vincristine (Oncovin), prednisone (Deltasone), asparaginase (Elspar), and daunorubicin (Cerubidine). The prednisone dose is not routinely tapered at the end of induction treatment.[223,224] (See Chapter 88: Table 88-13.)

No chemotherapy drug meets the criteria of an ideal agent (i.e., toxic to leukemic cells only and active in all phases of the cell cycle). Prednisone, vincristine, and asparaginase come closest to this ideal in terms of activity primarily against lymphocytic leukemia, because none of these agents is myelosuppressive to normal marrow elements. To improve the success in attaining complete remission, additional agents have been added to vincristine, prednisone, and asparaginase (see Table 88-13). The most frequently used additional agent is an anthracycline, such as daunorubicin or doxorubicin. Use of at least a three-drug induction regimen is the current standard of care for children at low or intermediate risk of relapse and results in improvements in both the remission rate and duration versus less intensive therapy.[225–229] Currently, a four-drug regimen, or an even more intensive induction regimen consisting of more than four drugs, and often of a duration of >4 weeks, is used for children at high risk of relapse, as with adult ALL patients.[223,230–233]

If complete remission is not achieved with three agents by the end of induction, patients are treated with additional agents (e.g., an additional 2 to 4 weeks of daunorubicin and prednisone; initiation of cytarabine with additional asparaginase; vincristine and prednisone for 1 to 2 weeks).[126] Because this occurs rarely, there is no consensus about the most effective agents or schedules when a complete remission has not been attained by the end of the induction period. Most such patients have a decreased survival and a higher relapse rate.[234]

Intensive induction treatment has benefits for the majority of children with ALL. This treatment strategy supports the hypothesis of Goldie and Coldman,[235] that intensification of early treatment may decrease the chance that drug resistance will develop and may therefore potentially increase the proportion of long-term relapse-free survivors. Although J.B. has a DNA index of 1.0, based on his age, initial WBC count, and translocation, he is a patient with a low–intermediate risk of relapse. A three-drug induction regimen consisting of vincristine, prednisone, and asparaginase is recommended to optimize his chances for long-term, disease-free survival.[236,237]

Vincristine Toxicity

35. J.B. is discharged from the hospital during the second week of induction chemotherapy. Results of his CBC and differential indicate that he is responding well to his chemotherapy (i.e., WBC count 2,600/mm³, neutrophils 69%, lymphocytes 22%, platelets 229,000/m³, Hct 28.6%, and blasts 0). However, during the third week of induction chemotherapy, J.B. develops severe abdominal pain. It is discovered that he has not had a bowel movement in 6 days. J.B. also has been exhibiting "acting out" behaviors in recent days. How might these symptoms be explained?

[SI units: WBC count, 2.6×10^9/L; neutrophils, 0.69; lymphocytes, 0.22; platelets, 229×10^9/L; Hct, 0.286; blasts, 0]

The use of vincristine is associated with an autonomic neuropathy, which may substantially reduce GI motility[238]; in severe cases, paralytic ileus may result. Constipation often is accompanied by colicky abdominal pain, which may be quite distressing.[239] These symptoms usually become apparent 3 to 10 days after drug administration and usually resolve over several days. Prophylactic use of a stool softener (docusate [Colace]) and/or laxative (senna [Senokot]) may lessen the severity of J.B.'s constipation and facilitate defecation and should have been instituted soon after the first dose of vincristine.

J.B.'s emotional changes are likely the result of the prednisone he is receiving. Emotional lability, sleep disturbances, depressed mood, and listlessness have occurred during corticosteroid therapy in children with ALL.[240] These behavioral changes can be quite disruptive and parents should be prepared for them in advance. Behavioral disturbances resolve within 2 weeks after prednisone discontinuation.[240]

CNS Preventive Therapy

36. In addition to the aforementioned drugs, J.B. also receives intrathecal (IT) chemotherapy for CNS prophylaxis with methotrexate, cytarabine (Cytosar-U), and hydrocortisone (Solu-Cortef) at the beginning (week 1) and end (week 4) of induction therapy. What is the purpose of IT chemotherapy? What are the various treatments available for CNS preventive therapy? What determines which one is chosen for J.B.?

PURPOSE

The purpose of IT or CNS preventive therapy is to decrease the chance of relapse within the CNS and increase J.B.'s chance of long-term survival. Before CNS preventive therapy was routine, the CNS was the most common site of leukemic relapse and predicted bone marrow relapse.[241,242] Patients at greatest risk for CNS relapse include those with very high initial WBC counts, T-cell ALL, and infants.[66,243] However, all patients with ALL are at risk for CNS relapse; it is known that one of the largest incremental improvements in disease-free survival took place after the routine use of CNS preventive therapy.[142] Because many antileukemic agents do not distribute well into the CSF, it appears to function as a sanctuary site for leukemic lymphoblasts. The aim is to eradicate any CNS leukemic lymphoblasts present at diagnosis and to prevent the emergence of a relapse within the CNS.

CNS PREVENTIVE THERAPY OPTIONS

All centers treating childhood ALL use some form of CNS preventive therapy, although different regimens are used. The first successful CNS prophylaxis treatments were 2,400 cGy of craniospinal radiation with or without IT methotrexate, which markedly reduced the CNS relapse rate.[244,245] To avoid the myelosuppression and reductions in spinal growth due to craniospinal irradiation, the standard CNS preventive therapy was modified to 2,400 cGy of cranial irradiation along with IT methotrexate. However, cranial irradiation has remained problematic owing to adverse effects such as decreased intellectual function, dysfunctions of the neuroendocrine system, and poorer psychosocial functioning.[246–250] As a result, clinicians have sought alternative, potentially safer forms of CNS preventive therapy. For example, lower doses (1,800 cGy) of cranial irradiation were combined with IT methotrexate to reduce the CNS effects.[243,251] The 1,800-cGy dose has proved to be equivalent to 2,400 cGy in preventing CNS relapse,[251] and the results of a long-term follow-up study indicate mild, but diffuse, deficits in information processing in patients receiving 2,400 cGy of cranial irradiation but not in patients treated with 1,800 cGy. This suggests that the lower radiation dose reduces neuropsychological morbidity.[252] Other approaches include periodic injections of triple IT chemotherapy (methotrexate, cytarabine, and hydrocortisone) or IT methotrexate, and intermediate-dose methotrexate with IT methotrexate.[113–256]

Because patients differ in their risk of developing CNS leukemia, CNS preventive therapy should be tailored accordingly. It has been demonstrated that children with low- and intermediate-risk ALL have equivalent CNS protection rates with either cranial radiation or IT chemotherapy, as long as adoquutely intensive systemic therapy is provided.[254,257,258] Patients at low or intermediate risk of relapse may be treated with either triple IT chemotherapy or IT methotrexate, depending on the institutional protocol.[254,257] Some high-risk children who are early responders to chemotherapy and who do not have CNS disease on presentation may also obtain adequate CNS protection with IT methotrexate alone.[259] Currently, most patients with T-cell disease still receive cranial radiation therapy as a component of their CNS preventive therapy, although with current intensive systemic therapy a radiation dose of 1,200 cGY appears to provide adequate CNS protection.[142]

INTRATHECAL CHEMOTHERAPY: CHRONIC ADVERSE EFFECTS

The chronic toxicities of IT chemotherapy are now being determined. When examined for effects on growth, triple IT chemotherapy demonstrated no effect on the final height achieved by children in contrast to a reduced final height in patients receiving cranial irradiation.[260] Limited evidence suggests that IT chemotherapy may be associated with some neuropsychological deficits. At least one study of patients receiving IT chemotherapy without cranial irradiation has demonstrated deficits in higher-order cognitive function tasks as well as learning disabilities in mathematics.[261] Another recent study has demonstrated that children who were treated with IT chemotherapy before age 5 years had deficits in the cerebellar-frontal brain subsystem and in neuropsychological performance.[262] It is unclear whether these deficits will translate into significant long-term consequences for these children.

Dosage

37. J.B. is at a low risk for CNS relapse and the decision is made to treat him with the triple IT combination. What doses of IT chemotherapy should J.B. receive?

High chemotherapy concentrations can be attained within the CSF with relatively low doses because the CSF volume of distribution is small in contrast to the peripheral plasma volume (140 versus 3,500 mL).[263,264] Drug exposure also is maximized by the longer half-life of most drugs in the CSF.[265] The approach used for IT dosing differs from systemic administration, which is based on body weight or body surface area. CSF methotrexate concentrations appear to correlate better with patient age than size.[266] As seen in Figure 90-3, the CSF

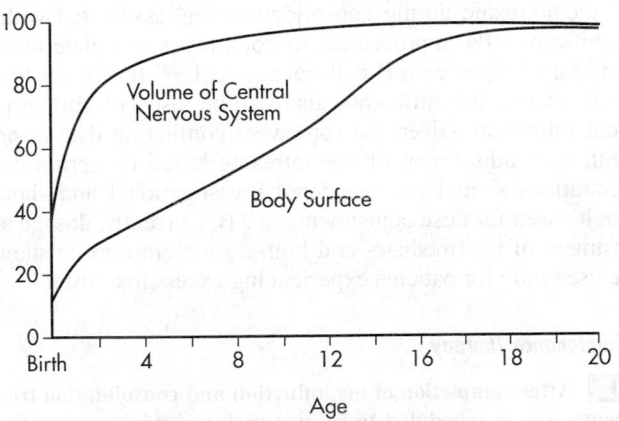

FIGURE 90-3 Relationship Between Body Surface Area and CNS Volume as a Function of Age. CNS volume increases at a more rapid rate than body surface area, reaching adult volume by 3 years of age. (Reprinted with permission from PRR Inc. Oncology 1991;5:107.)

volume in children approaches that of an adult by the age of 3 years. Because CSF volume does not correlate with body surface area, IT doses based on body size result in subtherapeutic concentrations in young children and potentially toxic concentrations in older children and adults. The age-based dosing regimens shown in Table 88-14 are less neurotoxic and are associated with a lower rate of CNS relapse than doses based on size.[267] Using this dosing regimen, J.B.'s dose of IT methotrexate should be 12 mg. The doses of IT cytarabine and hydrocortisone will be 24 and 12 mg, respectively. These latter doses are also based on age, but no literature exists to support how they were derived. Nevertheless, empiric evidence supports their efficacy.[254]

PRECAUTIONS

38. J.B.'s triple IT chemotherapy is to be administered on the same day as his vincristine dose. Are there any special precautions that should be taken when these medications are administered in close proximity?

Inadvertent IT administration of vincristine is almost uniformly fatal,[268–270] although there is one report of a patient in whom death was prevented.[271] Despite widespread educational efforts and numerous precautionary measures used by the pharmaceutical industry in recent years, deaths from the inadvertent IT administration of vincristine continue to be reported.[272] The clinical course in patients mistakenly given IT vincristine typically has progressed from backache and headache on day 1, muscle weakness (generalized) on day 2, apnea on day 5, loss of evidence of electroencephalographic activity by days 7 to 9, and death on day 12.[268] To avoid the tragedy of IT vincristine administration, vincristine should be admixed separately from IT medications, specially labeled, and preferably delivered to the patient area for IV infusion after the administration of IT medications.

Acute Adverse Effects

39. J.B. develops severe nausea and vomiting following his triple IT chemotherapy treatment. Is this common following IT chemotherapy? What can be done to decrease this toxicity for future IT chemotherapy treatments?

Several acute toxicities have been reported following IT chemotherapy. Acute arachnoiditis may occur 12 to 24 hours after injection, resulting in headaches, nausea, vomiting, and various other signs of increased intracranial pressure.[273] Severe symptoms occurred in 4 of 91 children receiving combination IT chemotherapy.[274] IT methotrexate alone produces these side effects in 38% of cases.[275] Fortunately, these reactions are usually self-limiting and can be reduced by use of doses based on patient age.[267]

Nausea and vomiting due to IT chemotherapy is usually mild to moderate in severity.[276] The emetogenic effect of IT chemotherapy is likely the result of direct contact between the chemotherapy and the chemoreceptor trigger zone. IV ondansetron (a 5-HT$_3$ antagonist) at a dose of 0.15 mg/kg before and 3 to 4 hours after IT chemotherapy can significantly reduce the incidence and severity of nausea and vomiting secondary to triple IT chemotherapy.[276] Without antiemetic protection, only 22% of children receiving IT chemotherapy had no vomiting. With the addition of ondansetron, complete protection from vomiting rose to 69%.[276] The efficacy of ondansetron is consistent with animal data demonstrating that 5-HT$_3$ antagonists administered directly into the brain stem can block the emetic response of systemically administered chemotherapy.[277] (Also see Chapter 8, Nausea and Vomiting.)

Rarely, a form of methotrexate neurotoxicity resulting in either paraplegia or necrotizing leukoencephalopathy may occur.[278–280] Leukoencephalopathy is associated with cranial irradiation given before or during IT therapy.[280] The preservatives in the chemotherapy diluents (methylhydroxylbenzoate and benzyl alcohol) rather than the chemotherapy agents are thought to be responsible for the paraplegia. This emphasizes the importance of diluting IT chemotherapy with a preservative-free diluent.[278] In addition, acute seizures associated with IT methotrexate have been reported. It also has been shown that methotrexate can increase the CSF concentration of homocysteine, as a consequence of decreased CSF folate. It is known that homocysteine can be metabolized to excitatory neurotransmitters that are agonists of the *N*-methyl-D-aspartate (NMDA) receptor, leading to seizures.[281,282] It is possible that known NMDA receptor antagonists (e.g., dextromethorphan) may decrease the risk of seizures in patients who develop this toxicity.[282]

Consolidation Therapy

40. J.B. had bone marrow aspirations performed at day 15 and at the completion of induction treatment on day 29; both indicated a complete morphologic remission. After completion of the induction phase, J.B. was scheduled to receive an intensified phase of chemotherapy known as *consolidation therapy*. What is the purpose of consolidation treatment, and what are some examples of effective regimens for this phase of treatment?

Consolidation or early intensification is a period of dose-intensive chemotherapy following induction therapy. This phase of treatment has proved to be an important strategy for the prevention of relapse in children with ALL and has helped produce event-free survival of approximately 80% in low-risk childhood ALL.[142,283] To date, the optimum consolidation regimen has yet to be determined. However, a few interesting findings from investigations of consolidation therapy will be briefly mentioned. A comparison between methotrexate 1 g/m² intravenously (intermediate-dose methotrexate) and low-dose (180 mg/m² divided into six doses) oral methotrexate revealed an approximate 4.4% increase in continuous complete remission with the higher-dose regimen.[283] This study is considered to be one of the pivotal trials demonstrating the superiority of higher-dose methotrexate in childhood ALL.[142] Although this difference was statistically significant, it may not have been clinically significant because leukoencephalopathy also occurred in 4.5% of children treated with the higher-dose regimen, compared with 0.6% of those treated with low-dose methotrexate. Although this study was not designed to examine differences in gender, female patients failed to benefit from the higher-dose regimen. This study also has been criticized for using the same leucovorin dosage with both methotrexate regimens, because it is known that a lower-dose oral regimen without leucovorin may produce similar RBC concentrations to that achievable with higher-dose methotrexate with leucovorin.[284]

A second trial evaluating the addition of either intensified asparaginase or cytarabine to intermediate-dose methotrexate in standard-risk ALL patients failed to show any incremental benefit in event-free survival over that achievable with methotrexate alone, although the cytarabine regimen did result in an increase in both infectious morbidity and hospitalizations.[237] Some examples of state-of-the-art consolidation regimens are provided in Chapter 88: Table 88-15.[233,236,237,283]

METHOTREXATE CONCENTRATION MONITORING

41. J.B. receives consolidation therapy with intermediate-dose methotrexate. His methotrexate serum concentrations are monitored after the administration of each dose of methotrexate during this phase of therapy. Why is monitoring of serum concentrations important when giving this dose of methotrexate? Are methotrexate concentrations important in predicting the outcome of ALL therapy?

After dose-intensive methotrexate therapy, concentration monitoring is crucial to establish the dose of leucovorin and the duration of hydration and alkalinization needed to prevent systemic methotrexate toxicity.[285] Before serum methotrexate concentrations were routinely monitored after high-dose methotrexate, severe GI desquamation and myelosuppression led to fatalities in as many as 6% of patients.[286] Methotrexate concentrations are measured approximately 24 hours after completion of the methotrexate infusion and repeated daily until the concentration falls below the toxic threshold of 0.05 μmol/L. Patients who have unexpectedly high concentrations after high-dose methotrexate may require higher doses of leucovorin and prolonged hydration and alkalinization to circumvent methotrexate toxicity.[285] (See the Pediatric Tumors: Osteosarcoma section of Chapter 91, Solid Tumors, for details on monitoring methotrexate concentrations and dosing leucovorin.)

Investigators have evaluated the influence of serum concentrations of methotrexate on the outcome of ALL patients.[286,287] These studies have determined that children with higher methotrexate clearance values appear to be at higher risk of relapse, and suggest that concentration monitoring also may play a role in enhancing the long-term survival of these patients.[287] However, when follow-up was extended, the survival advantage reported in one of these studies was lost.[287,288] A subsequent investigation of individualized chemotherapy versus standard dosing based on body surface area also demonstrated that concentration monitoring and subsequent dose adjustment of methotrexate during consolidation was associated with a significant 10% improvement in continuous complete remission for children with B-cell lineage ALL.[231] It remains to be seen whether this difference also will be lost with further patient follow-up. Given the somewhat conflicting data at present, dose adjustment of methotrexate based on serum concentrations should be considered investigational and should not be used for dose adjustments in J.B. Currently, dosage adjustment of intermediate- and high-dose methotrexate should be used only for patients experiencing excess toxicity.

Maintenance Therapy

42. After completion of his induction and consolidation treatments, J.B. is scheduled to receive maintenance (continuation) treatment for 2.5 years. His parents question why treatment will be of such a long duration and ask whether this is necessary because J.B. is already in remission. **What is the purpose of J.B.'s maintenance or continuation treatment for ALL? Which agents should be used in J.B. for this phase of therapy?**

PURPOSE

The purpose of maintenance or continuation treatment is to sustain the complete remission achieved from induction chemotherapy. Early trials have shown that without maintenance treatment, the majority of ALL patients relapse within 1 to 2 months.[221,222] It must be stressed that patients who have successfully responded to induction and consolidation therapy may still have a high leukemic cell burden (although undetectable), which must be eradicated by additional treatment. This is supported by the results of bone marrow biopsies from patients who have experienced relapse after several months to years of treatment. The cytogenetic characteristics of the leukemic cells in relapsed patients are identical to those at the time of diagnosis.[289,290] Maintenance therapy also is supported by the results of MRD studies, which demonstrate that some amount of measurable leukemic cells are still present months after the completion of induction therapy.[212]

CHEMOTHERAPY REGIMENS

Drugs that are effective during induction therapy cannot, by themselves, prolong remission during maintenance therapy.[156] However, other agents are effective in sustaining a complete remission. Two of the most effective drugs are mercaptopurine (Purinethol) and methotrexate.[226,291,292] Methotrexate is most effective and least toxic when administered intermittently, usually on a weekly basis in oral doses of 20 mg/m² per week. Mercaptopurine is effective and well tolerated orally when dosed daily, usually at a dose of 50 to 75 mg/m² per day.

Other agents have been added to, or used in place of, standard maintenance therapy with mercaptopurine and methotrexate to improve remission duration and to increase a patient's chances for long-term survival. These more aggressive maintenance regimens include intermittent pulses of vincristine and prednisone, intensification phases with etoposide (Vepesid) and cytarabine, intermediate dose methotrexate, and rotational combinations of various agents.[158,199,223,293,294] The value of these additional agents and more aggressive dosing schemes is controversial.[294] Impressive improvements in disease-free survival are achieved with several of these regimens, especially in patient populations with a high risk of relapse.[223,224] There is evidence that monthly pulses of vincristine and prednisone offer advantages (lower bone marrow and testicular relapse rates) in standard-risk patients as well.[295] Currently, many of the modern treatment regimens for childhood ALL have intensified induction and consolidation phases, and sometimes include a reinduction and/or a delayed intensification phase within the first 6 months.[232,233,236,237,283] Following this early intensive treatment schema, these newer protocols use a less intensive maintenance therapy consisting of methotrexate and mercaptopurine in combination with periodic IT chemotherapy treatments, either with or without intermittent vincristine/prednisone pulses.[232,233,236,237,283] It is unclear which of these regimens is best because risk criteria used to assign patients to various maintenance treatment arms within these protocols have varied among investigators.

The available evidence suggests that a patient like J.B. with standard-risk ALL will benefit from use of daily mercaptopurine 50 to 75 mg/m² orally and weekly methotrexate 20 mg/m² orally, intramuscularly, or intravenously along with periodic pulse therapy with vincristine 1.5 mg/m² for 1 day and prednisone 40 mg/m² orally for 7 days every 4 weeks. In addition, IT chemotherapy should be repeated every 8 to 12 weeks.

Potential Problems

43. After 6 weeks of maintenance therapy with the aforementioned regimen, J.B. has an absolute neutrophil count (ANC) that has ranged between 2,000 and 3,500 cells/mm³ for >6 weeks. Other CBC findings also are within normal limits. Should any changes in his maintenance therapy be considered at this time? Are there any potential problems with mercaptopurine and methotrexate that could explain his ANC values and that might increase his risk of treatment failure?

Diurnal variation of methotrexate concentration and marked interpatient variability in absorption and metabolism of mercaptopurine have been described, which may explain the varied response among patients to standard doses.[296–298] Most patients are able to tolerate full doses of mercaptopurine, which is inactivated by the enzyme thiopurine methyltransferase (TPMT). It is known that approximately 89% to 94% of patients have high TPMT activity, whereas 6% to 11% have intermediate activity, and 0.3% have deficient activity. Patients with deficient TPMT activity develop severe and even fatal toxicity with standard mercaptopurine doses and require very low doses (approximately 10 mg/m² three times per week) for avoidance of profound myelosuppression.[299,300]

Patients receiving half doses of these agents have shorter remission durations[301]; however, those who tolerate maximal protocol dosages also may be at greater risk of relapse.[171] Patients who are able to tolerate maximal doses without significant myelosuppression may require even higher doses than are recommended in some protocols. Investigations, including studies of intracellular concentrations of active metabolites, have not found the pharmacokinetics of mercaptopurine nor methotrexate to be predictive of outcome in children with ALL.[302–304] However, one of these trials did demonstrate that dose intensity of mercaptopurine was a significant predictor of event-free survival.[302] Because bioavailability is a concern for both agents and because some patients, particularly males, may be able to tolerate high dosages without toxicity, doses often are adjusted upward based on the degree of leukopenia. Some protocols allow for dosage increases of methotrexate or mercaptopurine every 4 to 6 weeks to maintain a target ANC in the range of 300 to 2,000/mm³.[302,302] This usually is accomplished by alternately increasing the doses of mercaptopurine and methotrexate by 25%.

For J.B., this means an increase in mercaptopurine from 50 mg/day to a daily schedule alternating 50 mg with 75 mg, or an increased methotrexate dose from 20 to 25 mg/week. Although parenteral administration of methotrexate is logical, it does not consistently improve the results of therapy.[304,305] To assess whether J.B. is receiving an adequate dose, weekly WBC counts are essential. This allows one to accurately appraise the adequacy of his dose and to follow his disease status to ensure that remission is continuing. If an inadequate degree of myelosuppression is demonstrated, J.B.'s compliance should be investigated, because decreased compliance is a frequent problem in the therapy of childhood ALL.[306–308] A recent investigation found improved compliance with evening administration of mercaptopurine.[306]

Duration of Therapy

44. **How long should J.B.'s maintenance therapy be continued?**

Most centers treat children with ALL for 2.5 to 3 years, which includes the length of induction therapy.[309,310] Extending maintenance treatment to 5 or 6 years adds no benefit.[309,310] Other data suggest that a shorter duration of 18 months may be adequate for girls, but not for boys.[311] Most patients who experience relapse do so during therapy or within the first year of completing therapy. After the second year of therapy and for every year thereafter, relapses become much less common but are occasionally observed. Some centers are exploring whether more intensive treatment protocols could decrease the duration of maintenance treatment, because the optimal duration is based on less aggressive protocols. Until there is more conclusive evidence regarding the duration of ALL maintenance therapy, patients with J.B.'s characteristics should receive chemotherapy for 2.5 to 3 years.

High-Risk ALL
LONG-TERM SEQUELAE

45. **N.B. is a 12-year-old Hispanic boy with a 4- to 5-week history of an enlarging right-sided neck mass. On physical examination, he is found to have a 6 × 3-cm right neck mass with extension to the nape of the neck. A chest radiograph indicates an anterior mediastinal mass. The CBC reveals a WBC count of 62,000/mm² (43% lymphoblasts, 27% neutrophils, and 27% lymphocytes), Hct of 41.5%, and platelet count of 83,000/mm³. Other pertinent laboratory results are urate of 15.1 mg/dL and LDH of 1,636. A bone marrow biopsy confirms the diagnosis of ALL and shows that 85% of the bone marrow is replaced by leukemic lymphoblasts. The leukemic cells are T cells and their DNA index is 1.0. A lumbar puncture reveals a few cells within the CSF that are terminal deoxynucleotidal transferase (TdT) negative, but are rather suspicious.**

N.B. is started on rasburicase 0.2 mg/kg/day for 1 to 3 days instead of allopurinol and hydration and alkalinization. Based on his age, initial WBC count, and leukemic cell type, N.B. is judged to have high-risk ALL and is begun on an intensive protocol. The induction regimen consists of six drugs, including prednisone 40 mg/m² per day PO on days 1 to 29; vincristine 1.5 mg/m² intravenously weekly for 5 weeks; cyclophosphamide (Cytoxan) 1 g/m² on day 1 and 600 mg/m² on day 22; doxorubicin (Adriamycin) 50 mg/m² on day 1; cytarabine 100 mg/m² per day via continuous infusion for 5 days starting on day 22; and asparaginase 10,000 units/m² intramuscularly on days 27, 29, and 31. Triple IT therapy consists of methotrexate 15 mg, cytarabine 30 mg, and hydrocortisone 15 mg administered weekly for 6 weeks. Why was rasburicase used instead of standard TLS (tumor lysis syndrome) preventive strategies?

Despite the standard prophylactic regimen for TLS, some high-risk patients may develop urate nephropathy. Patients with a significant elevation in uric acid and/or renal dysfunction may not derive significant early benefit from the standard regimen, which is designed to prevent the formation of addi-

tional uric acid and to aid in its excretion. Significant elevations in uric acid and/or renal dysfunction may even delay the initiation of chemotherapy. Rasburicase is a recombinant form of urate oxidase, the enzyme that catalyzes the conversion of uric acid to the more water soluble allantoin. Rasburicase produces a dramatic reduction in uric acid within 4 hours of administration. Uric acid is often reduced below the normal range, and additional daily doses are not necessary if uric acid normalizes and remains within normal limits. Given N.B.'s significantly elevated uric acid, he is at significant risk for TLS and is a good candidate for initial management with rasburicase. Rasburicase obviates the need for both allopurinol and hydration and alkalinization.[312]

46. **N.B. achieves a complete remission based on the results of a bone marrow specimen on day 29. His parents are concerned about the doxorubicin, because they have heard about heart problems with this drug. His protocol includes significant doses of this agent throughout his treatment plan. They ask about the likelihood for cardiac toxicity, what might be done to screen for it, and whether any preventive strategies exist that might be of value. What is the natural history, recommended screening tools, and preventive strategies for anthracycline cardiotoxicity in children? Is there evidence that corticosteroids used in the treatment of childhood ALL have the potential for long-term sequelae?**

The relationship between cumulative anthracycline dose and cardiotoxicity is well established; a dramatic increase in congestive heart failure (CHF) is observed at cumulative doses >450 mg/m².[142,313] However, because this is a median dose for cardiotoxicity, limiting the total dose to this threshold will not protect all patients. In children, although some early reports suggested reversibility, subsequent follow-up data confirm a worsening of CHF over time.[314–317] Late-occurring cardiotoxicity (i.e., years following completion of chemotherapy) has been reported in children.[314,318] One of these studies used a very sensitive echocardiography technique and reported that the majority of patients had either abnormal contractility or afterload.[318] The other study used a less sensitive echocardiography technique and reported a lower prevalence of cardiotoxicity, although the rate of abnormalities was shown to increase substantially with longer patient follow-up.[318] It is currently unclear what the long-term risk of CHF is in children. Close patient follow-up is important for early detection, although currently used screening tools such as echocardiography detect only functional damage and have not demonstrated value in preventing CHF. Newer nuclear medicine probes currently are showing some promise in the early detection of anthracycline-induced cardiotoxicity and may be used in the future for identifying children before the development of functional deficits.[319] Studies support the efficacy of dexrazoxane (Zinecard), an intracellular iron chelator, in the prevention of anthracycline-induced CHF in adults.[320,321] Because of a decreased antitumor response in dexrazoxane-treated patients in one of these trials, this agent was subsequently studied at a reduced dose and has been approved for use only in women with breast cancer after a cumulative anthracycline dose of 300 mg/m². The results of one small trial in children demonstrated a decreased risk of cardiotoxicity and improved tolerance of higher cumulative anthracycline doses for patients receiving dexrazoxane.[322] However, left ventricular ejection fraction did decline in both groups with higher cumulative anthracycline doses. It is unclear to what extent dexrazoxane may circumvent the long-term risk of anthracycline-induced CHF in children. It may be that some degree of long-term cardiotoxicity or CHF risk in children is unavoidable when an anthracycline is used. Because anthracyclines are an important component of many ALL treatment protocols and have figured significantly into the improved survival rates achieved in high-risk patients in recent years, the benefits seem to outweigh the risks in these patients at present. Although N.B. will be monitored closely for the occurrence of cardiac deterioration, there is currently no proven way to completely eliminate the risk of cardiotoxicity, although restricting children to a cumulative dose of <300 mg/m^2 has resulted in a low frequency of late occurring cardiotoxicity.[323]

Many survivors of childhood ALL therapy are found to have decreased bone mineral density.[324–327] This has been attributed to both corticosteroids and cranial radiation therapy. A significant number of patients (up to 38%) also developed osteonecrosis during therapy, although lesions were often asymptomatic and improvement and/or resolution often occurred.[326] An increased risk of fractures during chemotherapy also has been reported in children with ALL.[325] The long-term risks of osteoporosis in survivors of childhood ALL are unknown, but do argue in favor of close monitoring as well as optimization of mineral supplementation.

47. After an intensive consolidation phase, N.B. is scheduled to receive a rotational maintenance therapy consisting of 10 separate 9-week cycles of chemotherapy. Each 9-week cycle will consist of the following: cytarabine/cyclophosphamide, followed by vincristine/doxorubicin/prednisone/mercaptopurine, then followed by cytarabine/teniposide (Vumon). Asparaginase at a dose of 25,000 U/m^2 intramuscularly also will be given weekly for the first 20 weeks of maintenance therapy. Is this the usual dose of asparaginase? What is the value of asparaginase in patients with T-cell leukemia?

This dosage of asparaginase is higher than that usually used in the treatment of ALL (6,000 to 10,000 units/m^2). However, a recent trial of patients with T-cell ALL employed an intensive induction and consolidation phase, followed by an intensive maintenance phase.[200] During the maintenance phase, half of these patients were also randomized to receive asparaginase 25,000 units/m^2 intramuscularly every week for 20 doses. This trial demonstrated a significant improvement in continuous complete remission at 4 years for those who received the additional high-dose asparaginase therapy (68 versus 55%) and provided evidence that patients with T-cell ALL may achieve long-term remission rates similar to that of other ALL immunologic subtypes.

48. Two weeks following his vincristine/doxorubicin/prednisone/mercaptopurine and 5 days following his fifth dose of asparaginase, N.B. develops severe abdominal pain and hyperglycemia. N.B. has been having normal bowel movements and does not have abdominal distention. The serum amylase is markedly elevated to 450 IU/L (normal, 111–296). Which agent is likely responsible for N.B.'s abdominal pain? What other complications are associated with this chemotherapy agent?

Pancreatitis

Pancreatitis has been noted in children following the administration of asparaginase.[328] As illustrated by N.B., this often presents as abdominal pain accompanied by an elevated serum amylase and hyperglycemia. Insulin may be required to control the hyperosmotic, nonketotic hyperglycemia that may result.[329,330] The pancreatitis is occasionally severe, and fatalities have been reported.[331] Unfortunately, the serum amylase may not predict whether patients will develop acute fatal pancreatitis.[191] N.B.'s pancreatitis secondary to asparaginase makes further treatment with this agent inadvisable. Because this reaction is not a hypersensitivity reaction, further therapy with the *Erwinia* form of asparaginase also is not recommended. N.B. may be treated with supportive care and insulin therapy. He should recover fully and be able to receive further chemotherapy.

Hypersensitivity Reactions

Hypersensitivity reactions are common, occurring in 20% to 35% of patients; they are usually mild. The mild reactions generally present as urticarial eruptions.[329] Premedication does not appear to prevent subsequent reactions in most patients.[332] Severe anaphylactoid reactions may occur and can be fatal.[333] Clinical reactions correlate better with asparaginase-specific IgG rather than IgE antibodies, and severe hypersensitivity reactions can be explained in most instances by complement activation.[334,335]

Anaphylactoid reactions appear to be less common when asparaginase is administered intramuscularly.[336,337] This is because the slow absorption of asparaginase after IM administration results in delayed, less severe acute reactions. Because these reactions can be delayed, prolonged monitoring is recommended after IM asparaginase.[338] Most serious hypersensitivity reactions tend to occur after the patient has received several doses.

A significant number of patients receiving asparaginase as a component of ALL treatment test positive for anti–asparaginase antibodies, and antibody concentrations are significantly greater in patients who experience a hypersensitivity reaction.[332] Patients who are receiving asparaginase also may develop "silent" immune clearance, resulting in rapid clearance of asparaginase from the plasma (similar to patients with hypersensitivity) but without an allergic reaction.[209,339–341] Such patients may not obtain benefit from asparaginase and may be at greater risk of treatment failure.[342] The prevalence of silent allergy to asparaginase is unknown, and it has been suggested that a routine assay for asparagine depletion is needed to identify patients who have this allergy.[342] Because premedication usually does not prevent future reactions and because of the possibility that patients who exhibit hypersensitivity may derive no benefit from asparaginase, it appears that the best course of action is to switch patients from the *Escherichia coli* preparation to an alternate asparaginase preparation.

Preparations

Asparaginase is available from two natural sources, *E. coli* and *Erwinia* . Because these two preparations may not be cross-reactive, the *Erwinia* product may be substituted for the *E. coli* product when hypersensitivity reactions occur and further dosing is planned.[343] However, cross-reactions occur in 17% to 26% of patients.[224,344] Because of the shorter half-life of the *Erwinia* product, some dosage increase of *Erwinia* asparaginase may be necessary to mimic the activity of the

E. coli product.[142,342,345] The incidences of hypersensitivity reactions are equivalent for these two preparations.[343]

Asparaginase also is available as an altered form known as *PEG-asparaginase* (Oncaspar). This agent is formed by covalently linking monomethoxy-polyethylene glycol (PEG) to *E. coli* asparaginase. PEG-asparaginase has a prolonged half-life of 5.8 days compared with 1.2 days for *E. coli* asparaginase and appears to be safe and effective even in patients with prior reactions to *E. coli* and *Erwinia* asparaginase.[346] The prolonged half-life allows for less frequent (i.e., every 2 week) dosing of PEG-asparaginase than for the natural-source asparaginase products (i.e., three times a week).[340]

Asparaginase compounds derived from different *E. coli* strains may differ in both enzyme activity and half-life. At least one study has reported an unexpected mortality rate in childhood ALL associated with an assumption of equivalence among different *E. coli* asparaginase preparations.[347]

Asparaginase-Induced Coagulation Disorders

Asparaginase is known to cause decreases in albumin, fibrinogen, and α-and β-globulins owing to its effects on general protein synthesis, which can result in inhibition of the synthesis of various clotting factors.[348,349] Asparaginase also may produce abnormalities in the coagulation-inhibiting and fibrinolytic system, along with deficiencies in antithrombin III and plasminogen.[348,349] This complex series of events can result in coagulopathies, occasionally leading to cerebral hemorrhage or infarction.[224,348–350] Although monitoring of markers of both the coagulation-inhibiting and fibrinolytic system have been suggested to identify patients at risk for severe coagulation disturbances,[348] no prospective studies have documented the ability of screening to decrease the risk of this complication.

TENIPOSIDE

49. During N.B.'s maintenance treatment with teniposide (Vumon) and cytarabine, he develops flushing, chills, urticaria, and hypotension. This reaction responds to discontinuation of the teniposide infusion and administration of IV diphenhydramine. Is this reaction common with epipodophyllotoxins such as teniposide? Is it possible for N.B. to receive additional teniposide or etoposide?

Hypersensitivity Reactions

Hypersensitivity reactions—usually characterized by flushing, chills, and occasionally, bronchospasm and hypotension—are common following both teniposide and etoposide. One study of 108 children reported that approximately 50% of patients receiving these agents repeatedly experienced a hypersensitivity reaction.[351] Reports from analysis of a literature search encompassing 2,250 patients documents a 3.5% incidence of hypersensitivity reactions in patients receiving teniposide.[352] These reactions appear to be more common in children with neuroblastoma and brain tumors (accounting for 45% to 82% of reactions) than in patients with other malignancies.[352,353] The higher incidence of hypersensitivity in the smaller report is attributed to repeated epipodophyllotoxin exposure during prolonged therapy.[351] This report also noted a higher incidence in patients receiving teniposide versus etoposide and noted that 42% reacted to

teniposide alone, whereas only 12% reacted to etoposide alone. Fortunately, <2% of scheduled doses were discontinued due to severe reactions.[351] This trial also demonstrated that the risk of hypersensitivity reactions increased with the total cumulative dose up to an eventual plateau for both of these agents. These reactions may not become manifest until the infusion is complete.

A study comparing teniposide with its excipient (Cremophor) found that although the drug led to basophil degranulation in a dose-dependent fashion, the excipient did not, suggesting that these reactions occur due to teniposide itself.[354] However, other investigators have noted that these reactions were Cremophor-like, and that most patients subsequently were able to tolerate etoposide (which does not contain this excipient).[355] Also of interest is that, for patients who develop a hypersensitivity reaction to an epipodophyllotoxin, rechallenge is less successful with teniposide than for etoposide.[351–353,356] It would be best to convert N.B. to etoposide rather than to rechallenge him with teniposide. He should be premedicated with antihistamines with or without corticosteroids and closely monitored for signs of hypersensitivity. The etoposide conversion dose is twice the dose of teniposide.

50. Are there any other significant long-term risks from this maintenance regimen?

Secondary Acute Myelogenous Leukemia

Patients with childhood ALL who are receiving epipodophyllotoxins appear to be at increased risk for developing secondary AML,[357] which is unresponsive to standard AML therapy.[357] No definitive data exist to predict an individual patient's risk for developing secondary AML, but rate estimates published by several investigators report a cumulative risk at 6 years of 3.8% to 12.4%, and a relative risk of 3.4% to 39.4%.[357–359] The higher risk values have been associated with higher doses and more frequent administration of epipodophyllotoxins.[358,359] However, a recent analysis of secondary AML from 12 different clinical trials using epipodophyllotoxins failed to identify a relationship between cumulative dose and risk of secondary leukemia.[360] Another recent trial failed to identify altered etoposide pharmacokinetics in patients who developed secondary AML.[361] Since epipodophyllotoxins carry a significant risk of secondary AML, these agents are currently not used in most childhood ALL treatment regimens.

Relapsed ALL

51. After 1 year of continuation therapy, N.B. undergoes a routine lumbar puncture. Analysis of the CSF indicates the presence of numerous lymphoblasts. A CBC reveals the following: Hct of 29.5%, platelet count of 120,000/mm³, and WBC count of 5,300/mm³ with 45% lymphocytes, 50% neutrophils, and 5% bands. A bone marrow biopsy confirms relapsed ALL, with 53% lymphoblasts. Would routine bone marrow biopsies of N.B. have allowed for early detection of N.B.'s relapse and an increased chance for long-term survival? What are N.B.'s chances of achieving a second remission and long-term survival? Which treatments could be used in N.B. in an attempt to attain

a complete remission and improve his chances of long term survival?

[SI units: Hct, 0.295; platelets, 120 × 10⁹/L; WBC count, 5.3 10⁹/L with 0.45 lymphocytes, 0.50 neutrophils, and 0.05 bands]

N.B. is asymptomatic at the time of relapse, as are most patients experiencing a relapse of ALL. Most of these patients are diagnosed by routine bone marrow biopsies and/or lumbar punctures.[362] Routine bone marrow biopsies identify some bone marrow relapses before they become evident on a CBC (as with N.B.), but it has not been demonstrated that earlier identification of bone marrow relapse by morphologic criteria makes an impact on long-term survival. In the future, recognition of MRD with molecular probes may change the prognostic value of routine bone marrow examination.

N.B.'s chances of achieving a second remission with salvage chemotherapy are good. Approximately 80% to 85% of relapsed patients attain a second complete remission with further chemotherapy.[362–365] Unfortunately, however, bone marrow relapse in childhood ALL is associated with poor long-term survival.[362–368] Only 6% to 29% of patients with bone marrow relapse may be rendered disease free for 2 years after relapse.[366–368] Allogeneic bone marrow transplantation for ALL in relapse results in a 10% to 20% long-term leukemia-free survival.[369] However, better results with bone marrow transplantation are possible after a second remission has been achieved. Studies of children with ALL receiving allogeneic bone marrow transplantation in second remission report 5-year disease-free survival rates of 40% and 64%.[370–372] These results are superior to those of chemotherapy in patients like N.B.[370,373,374] However, no randomized trials have established that bone marrow transplantation is superior to chemotherapy for children with ALL in second remission, and some of the reported advantages with transplantation may be due to selection bias.[370] Autologous bone marrow transplantation does not appear to be superior to chemotherapy for children with ALL in second remission.[370,375] Unfortunately, one report of bone marrow transplantation has noted an extremely poor event-free survival rate (3% at 5 years) with all postrelapse treatment strategies for children with a bone marrow relapse within 2 years of diagnosis.[370] N.B.'s family should be offered the option of a bone marrow transplant if testing determines that he has an acceptable bone marrow donor match. However, because N.B. has incurred an early relapse, he and his family should be apprised of the lower chance for long-term success of any of the available therapeutic options.

Agents used in salvage regimens are similar to those used in high-risk ALL regimens. In general, treatment usually consists of an intensive three- or four-agent induction regimen of vincristine, prednisone, and daunorubicin with or without asparaginase. This is accompanied by radiation therapy to sites of local relapse (e.g., testis, CNS) and IT chemotherapy.[374,377,378] After this regimen has been completed, the patient may continue with courses of intensification therapy and continuation therapy as well as IT therapy.[377,378] N.B. already has been treated with many different chemotherapeutic agents. Therefore, the regimen selected should include agents to which N.B. has had little or no exposure. This theoretically increases his chances of maintaining a second remission. For example, a regimen that includes doxorubicin, asparaginase,

and cyclophosphamide appears most appropriate for N.B. If N.B. fails to respond to the initial reinduction attempt, high-dose cytarabine (3 g/m² every 12 hours for four doses) in conjunction with standard-dose asparaginase may be used to induce a remission. This approach has been demonstrated to be successful in approximately 40% of patients. However, the median duration of second remission was only 3 months.[376]

PEDIATRIC NON-HODGKIN'S LYMPHOMA

Lymphomas account for approximately 10% of all childhood malignancies, and they are less common in children than in adults. Children younger than 16 years of age account for only 3% of all lymphoma cases. The malignancy can occur in any lymphoid cell at any level of differentiation and appears to be a consequence of a genetic alteration. Considerable progress has been made in the treatment of children with NHL, and currently approximately 80% are cured.[377]

Classification

Numerous classification systems for NHL exist, and there is considerable variation in terminology among these systems.[378–382] Pediatric NHLs are best classified using histopathology, which divides them into three different categories: lymphoblastic, B-cell, and anaplastic large-cell lymphomas.[383,384] This is a narrower range of histologic types than in adults.

Lymphoblastic lymphomas account for approximately 30% of childhood NHLs, B-cell for about 50%, and large-cell for the remainder.[377] The lymphoblastic lymphomas are usually immature T cells that are histologically identical to the cells of ALL. The distinction between lymphoblastic lymphoma and ALL is made on the basis of bone marrow involvement, with ALL being diagnosed if there is >25% bone marrow infiltration. This distinction is made by the amount of bone marrow infiltration that is present at the time of diagnosis. B-cell lymphomas may be further divided into Burkitt's, Burkitt's like and large B cell lymphomas. Anaplastic large-cell lymphomas may be T cell or null cell in origin. Other lymphomas often included in this category but which do not possess all of the features of large-cell lymphomas are immunoblastic lymphomas and Ki-1 anaplastic lymphomas.

Clinical Presentation

Pediatric patients with NHL may present with a number of different symptoms, many of which are related to the cell type of NHL. In general, these symptoms differ from those in adults because of the propensity of pediatric NHLs to be extranodal in origin in contrast to the common nodal presentation of adult NHL.[377] Patients with lymphoblastic lymphoma commonly present with a mediastinal mass or pleural effusions.[377] They also may have pain, dyspnea, or swelling of the face and upper arms if superior vena cava obstruction is present. Lymphoblastic lymphoma also has a predilection for the bone marrow and the CNS.[385,386] Lymphadenopathy in patients with lymphoblastic lymphoma tends to be supradiaphragmatic. Patients with B-cell NHL typically present with an abdominal tumor, abdominal pain, an alteration in bowel function, and possibly nausea and vomiting.[387] In addition, many patients with B-cell NHL present with bone marrow involvement.[388] Lymphadenopathy in these patients typically occurs below the diaphragm in the inguinal or iliac area. Anaplastic large-cell lymphomas may involve the gut or unusual sites such as the lung, skin, face, or CNS.[377]

Staging

Several staging systems for pediatric NHLs are used.[387] Most include four or more stages, with stage I being a single tumor and higher stages including cases with more than one anatomic site involved. The highest stage usually refers to patients with bone marrow or CNS involvement. The main predictor of outcome in pediatric patients with NHL is tumor burden at presentation.[389,390] Serum concentrations of several different molecules, particularly serum LDH and IL-11R, help clinicians estimate tumor burden.[387,389–391]

Treatment

Lymphoblastic (T Cell)

The primary treatment for all stages and histologic types of pediatric NHL is combination chemotherapy because it is a generalized disease at the time of diagnosis.[377] A wide variety of chemotherapy agents have activity in childhood NHL. Two of the most effective protocols studied in lymphoblastic lymphoma are the German BFM and the Memorial Sloan-Kettering LSA_2L_2 protocols[392,393] (see Table 90-16). Both protocols use an intensive scheme of multiagent chemotherapy administered in two- or four-drug rotational combination cycles for a treatment duration of approximately 2 years. Patients with lymphoblastic lymphoma require a longer treatment duration ($\geq$18 months) than patients with B-cell or large-cell lymphoma. These chemotherapy plans are similar to those used in the treatment of ALL and are designed to deliver continuous or weekly therapy. All patients with lymphoblastic lymphoma are given CNS preventive therapy, regardless of stage.

Long-term disease-free survival with the LSA_2L_2 protocol is approximately 60% to 80% for patients with advanced-stage disease and even higher for patients with early-stage disease.[394] Few patients with lymphoblastic lymphoma present with limited disease (stages I and II), thus making it difficult to conduct adequate studies in this patient population. Attempts to shorten the duration of therapy for patients with limited-stage disease have been unsuccessful, although less intensive therapy is administered to patients with early-stage disease on some protocols.[377] For advanced-stage lymphoblastic lymphoma (stages III and IV), some evidence indicates that the LSA_2L_2 regimen may be inferior. It has been demonstrated in the Institut Gustave-Roussy (IGR) protocol that the addition of high-dose methotrexate to the LSA_2L_2 regimen appears to improve survival for patients with advanced-stage disease.[377] The latest BFM protocol has also achieved an impressive 5-year event-free survival rate of 95%, with no significant difference between stage III (91%) and stage IV (94%) patients.[392]

B Cell

The main differences between the treatment of lymphoblastic and B-cell lymphoma are the use of more agents in the former and a shorter treatment duration and more frequent use of methotrexate in the latter. The trend in the treatment of B-cell lymphomas has been toward using short-duration, intensive therapy with alkylating agents in conjunction with high-dose antimetabolite therapy (e.g., methotrexate, cytarabine). Chemotherapy is administered in rapid succession with limited recovery from neutropenia (i.e., ANC $\geq$500) between cycles. Patients with localized B-cell lymphomas respond as adequately to a 4-drug regimen as they do to a 10-drug regimen.[393]

Evidence suggests that a 6-month course is as efficacious as the previously used 18-month course for patients with localized B-cell lymphomas.[255] Studies indicate that even 6 months of chemotherapy may be unnecessary for patients with limited-stage disease, as it has been demonstrated that maintenance treatment offered no additional benefit after 9 weeks of combination chemotherapy.[377] Current protocols for children with limited-stage, B-cell disease have now limited chemotherapy to two to three cycles with excellent results. Some patients with limited-stage disease may not require CNS preventive therapy.

The treatment strategies useful in advanced-stage lymphoblastic lymphoma have resulted in lower failure-free survival rates for patients with advanced-stage, B-cell lymphomas.[393,394] With the addition of high-dose methotrexate, ifosfamide, etoposide, and high-dose cytarabine to the standard regimen, patients with stage III disease are now achieving survival rates comparable to those of patients with limited-stage disease. Patients with bone marrow disease also benefit from these intensive therapeutic strategies and have achieved impressive survival rates of approximately 80%.[377] Currently, patients with advanced-stage disease are treated with a total of six to eight cycles of chemotherapy, and these treatment protocols achieve superior results to those of a much longer duration (e.g., 1 to 2 years) used previously.[377,396,397]

Large Cell

Large-cell lymphomas have responded well to both types of regimens.[377,393,398,399] Thus, the use of the shorter, less complicated, B-cell protocols is appropriate. Patients who fail to respond may be treated with additional courses of their prescribed protocol in hopes of eventually inducing a response. Patients who relapse may be reinduced with intensive chemotherapy, but their prognosis for long-term survival is unfavorable.

Lymphoblastic Lymphoma

Treatment

ACUTE TREATMENT

52. D.B., a 16-year-old girl, presents with a history of shortness of breath and chest pain for 3 weeks before admission. A mediastinal mass is found, and a biopsy confirms a lymphoblastic (T-cell) lymphoma. A chest radiograph reveals a right pleural effusion. Laboratory values show the following: erythrocyte sedimentation rate (ESR), 35 (normal, 0 to 20); WBC count, 22,000/mm³ (normal, 4,500 to 11,000), uric acid 7 mg/dl and LDH, 1259 U/L (normal, 280 to 540). The bone marrow, CNS, and abdomen are negative for lymphoma. How should D.B. be managed acutely? Besides chemotherapy, what types of adjunctive therapies should be initiated to minimize the acute effects of treatment?

Given D.B.'s shortness of breath and chest pain, it is likely that her mediastinal mass may be obstructing the superior vena cava. To alleviate this obstruction, the most appropriate course of action is to decrease the tumor mass by initiating chemotherapy as soon as possible. Radiation therapy offers no additional benefit in patients such as D.B., with a tumor like NHL, which is highly responsive to chemotherapy.[400] Because of the high cell kill that will result from the initial chemotherapy treatment, uric acid nephropathy is also possible. However, the risk of this complication is probably greater in patients with B-cell NHL in whom the fraction of cells in S phase is higher.[401,402]

Alkaline diuresis and allopurinol should be instituted before chemotherapy to prevent this complication (see Acute Lymphoblastic Leukemia of Childhood). Because D.B. has a pleural effusion, fluids may collect in this third space, resulting in weight gain and decreased urine output. Thus, in addition to placement of a chest tube with suction, D.B. should be given diuretics to maintain an adequate urine output. To minimize intravascular volume depletion and maintain electrolyte balances, fluid input and output, body weight, and electrolyte panels should be monitored daily. These values should be used to make appropriate adjustments in D.B.'s electrolyte and fluid balance.

ADVERSE EFFECTS

53. **D.B. is treated with a combination chemotherapy regimen designed from experience with the two most effective regimens used to date: the BFM and LSA$_2$L$_2$ treatment programs. She is to receive induction therapy for 1 month (one cycle): cyclophosphamide 1,000 mg/m² on day 1; weekly vincristine 1.5 mg/m² (maximum, 2.0 mg) on days 1, 8, 15, and 22; daunorubicin 60 mg/m² intravenously on days 12 and 13; and prednisone 40 mg/m² per day (divided into three-times-daily dosing) on days 1 to 28 with doses decreasing to 0 on days 29 to 35. Which acute adverse effects is D.B. likely to experience with these agents? How can they be monitored, minimized, and treated?**

Several toxicities are expected with the four chemotherapy agents used. For vincristine, both constipation and neuropathy are likely to appear during or following the 4 weeks of therapy.[238] Constipation can be prevented or minimized by use of stool softeners with or without a laxative.[403] Neuropathy may be painful (especially when jaw pain occurs) but can be managed with mild analgesic regimens consisting of NSAIDs and/or acetaminophen with codeine. Both toxicities are self-limiting and are not reasons to discontinue or decrease the dosage of vincristine unless neuromuscular toxicity, as evidenced by motor weakness, develops.

Prednisone is likely to increase D.B.'s appetite and may cause gastritis, although divided doses will help decrease stomach upset. In addition, prednisone-induced behavioral disturbances are not uncommon.[240]

Unlike prednisone and vincristine, both daunorubicin and cyclophosphamide produce significant myelosuppression. Leukopenia is the primary sign, with the nadir occurring in approximately 8 to 14 days and recovery occurring by approximately day 21 after administration. To allow for bone marrow recovery, additional treatment with myelosuppressive chemotherapy will not be given for about 2 to 3 weeks after administration.

Hemorrhagic cystitis may occur with cyclophosphamide, but it usually is associated with high-dose therapy or with prolonged administration, which D.B. is not receiving. Vigorous IV hydration to maintain urine output of approximately 50 to 100 mL/m² per hour should reduce the risk of this toxicity at this dose. Because most of the induction regimen will be administered on an outpatient basis, patients and/or parents should be instructed to report signs or symptoms of infection (e.g., febrile episodes) immediately so that proper treatment may be instituted as soon as possible. To decrease the risk of hemorrhagic cystitis, parents should be instructed to report whether patients are not urinating regularly after cyclophosphamide.

Nausea and vomiting are likely to be induced by both doxorubicin and cyclophosphamide.[404] D.B.'s chemotherapy regimen includes a corticosteroid (prednisone), which may provide some antiemetic activity.[405] However, to maximize tolerance to her chemotherapy, D.B. should receive a potent antiemetic. Ondansetron may be used in this setting and is more effective than metoclopramide when either is combined with a corticosteroid.[406] Ondansetron also has a safety profile that is superior to that of metoclopramide in children.[407–409] Although ondansetron is synergistic with corticosteroids, D.B. may not require additional amounts because prednisone already is included in her chemotherapy regimen. Furthermore, ondansetron alone (0.15 mg/kg intravenously every 4 hours × 3) has been shown to be efficacious against cyclophosphamide-induced emesis.[410] If necessary, an additional dose of a corticosteroid (e.g., dexamethasone 0.25 to 0.5 mg/kg once) may be added to the antiemetic regimen without changing the prednisone dosage.

CNS Prophylaxis

54. **What is the importance of CNS prophylaxis for D.B., and what type of treatment regimen is typically used?**

All pediatric patients with lymphoblastic lymphoma should receive some form of CNS prophylaxis. Although lymphoblastic lymphoma rarely presents with CNS involvement, as illustrated by D.B., it was a common site of relapse before CNS prophylaxis was included as a routine part of the chemotherapy regimen.[385,386] Recurrence of NHL within the CNS is rare when intrathecal methotrexate and/or cytarabine are given.[390,393] D.B. will be treated with triple intrathecal therapy consisting of methotrexate, hydrocortisone, and cytarabine every other week for eight doses for her initial phase of treatment.

Myelosuppression and Hematopoietic Recovery

55. **After completion of initial therapy, the chemotherapy plan for D.B. consists of a continuation regimen of ten 9-week treatment cycles. Each 9-week cycle includes the following sequence of agents: (1) cytarabine 150 mg/m² per day by continuous IV infusion 72 hours and cyclophosphamide 75 mg/m² by slow IV push Q 12 hr for six doses (during cytarabine infusion); (2) vincristine 2.0 mg/m² (maximum, 2 mg) IV push one dose, doxorubicin 30 mg/m² intravenously over 15 minutes one dose, and both prednisone 120 mg/m² per day PO and mercaptopurine 300 mg/m² per day PO divided TID for 5 days; and (3) teniposide 150 mg/m² by IV infusion over 45 minutes and cytarabine 300 mg/m² IV push following teniposide, repeated 3 days later. A repeat**

triple IT treatment also will be given during the teniposide/cytarabine sequence. Each cycle will be separated by approximately 3 weeks to allow for hematopoietic recovery. How should D.B.'s hematopoietic recovery be monitored, and what guidelines may be used to determine when it is appropriate for her to receive the next sequence of a treatment cycle?

D.B.'s hematopoietic recovery should be monitored weekly throughout the continuation phase with WBC and differential, platelet, and RBC counts. Hematopoietic recovery may be considered adequate for the next treatment if the absolute neutrophil count is $\geq$500/mm^3 and platelets have recovered to 100,000/mm^3. An ANC of <1,000/mm^3 may sometimes lead to delayed myelosuppression with subsequent treatments, leading some clinicians to use an ANC of $\geq$1,000/mm^3 as the threshold for initiating the next chemotherapy treatment.

Modification for Delayed Recovery

56. D.B. has received six of the ten 9-week treatment cycles and has done well, with no severe drug toxicities or signs of recurring NHL. After her last treatment with vincristine, doxorubicin, prednisone, and mercaptopurine, her WBC count was slow to recover. Her ANC was 200/mm^3 2 weeks later, and this caused a 1-week delay in the next treatment (teniposide and cytarabine). What modifications should be made with her next 4-day treatment sequence?

Delayed recovery after repeated courses of myelosuppressive chemotherapy is common. The myelosuppressive agents in this four-drug regimen, which have likely resulted in delayed recovery, are doxorubicin and mercaptopurine. Because dose intensity is known to be an important factor in the treatment of chemotherapy responsive tumors such as lymphoma, attempts should be made to maintain dose intensity whenever possible. Use of a CSF (e.g., filgrastim) may allow for a more prompt recovery from neutropenia and should be considered in this patient before reducing the chemotherapy dose. If filgrastim is unsuccessful, dosages of doxorubicin and/or mercaptopurine should be reduced by 25% in subsequent treatments.

REFERENCES

1. American Cancer Society (ACS). Estimates of new cancers for the year 2002. Available at: http://www.cancer.org/downloads/STT/Cancer-Facts&Figures2002TM.pdf. Accessed July, 2003.
2. Harris NL et al. World Health Organization classification of neoplastic diseases of the hematopoietic and lymphoid tissues: Report of the Clinical Advisory Meeting—Airlie House, Virginia, November 1997. J Clin Oncol 1999;17:3835.
3. Armitage JO et al. New approaches to classifying non-Hodgkin's lymphomas: clinical features of the major histologic subtypes. J Clin Oncol 1998;16:2780.
4. Koeppen H, Vardiman JW. New entities, issues and controversies in the classification of malignant lymphoma. Semin Oncol 1998;25:421.
5. Munshi NC et al. Plasma cell neoplasms. In: DeVita VT et al., eds. Cancer. Principles and Practice of Oncology, 6th Ed. Philadelphia: Lippincott Williams & Wilkins, 2001:2465.
6. Lowenberg B et al. Acute myeloid leukemia. N Engl J Med 1990;341:1051.
7. Visani G et al. The prognostic value of cytogenetics is reinforced by the kind of induction/consolidation therapy in influencing the outcome of acute myeloid leukemia-analysis of 848 patients. Leukemia 2001;15:903.
8. Frei E et al. Dose schedule and antitumor studies of arabinosylcytosine. Cancer Res 1967;29:1325.
9. Rai KR et al. Treatment of acute myelocytic leukemia: a study by cancer and leukemia group B. Blood 1981;58:1203.
10. Scheinberg DA et al. Acute Leukemias. In: DeVita VT et al., eds. Cancer. Principles and Practice of Oncology, 6th Ed. Philadelphia: Lippincott Williams & Wilkins, 2001:2404.
11. Bishop JF et al. Etoposide in acute nonlymphocytic leukemia. Blood 1990;75:27.
12. Hann IM et al. Randomized comparison of DAT vs. ADE as induction chemotherapy in children and younger adults with acute myeloid leukemia. Results of the Medical Research Council's 10th AML Trial. Blood 1997;89:2311.
13. Brietman TR et al. Terminal differentiation of human promyelocytic leukemic cells in primary culture in response to retinoic acid. Blood 1981;57:1000.
14. Fenaux P et al. Effect of all transretinoic acid in newly diagnosed acute promyelocytic leukemia.

Results of a multicenter randomized trial. European APL 91 Group. Blood 1993;82:3241.
15. Warrell RP et al. Differentiation therapy of acute promyelocytic leukemia with tretinoin (all-transretinoic acid). N Engl J Med 1991;324:1385.
16. Castaigne S et al. All-*trans* retinoic acid as a differentiation therapy for acute promyelocytic leukemia: I. Clinical results. Blood 1990;76:1704.
17. Fenaux P et al. A randomized comparison of all transretinoic acid (ATRA) followed by chemotherapy and ATRA plus chemotherapy and the role of maintenance therapy in newly diagnosed acute promyelocytic leukemia. Blood 1999;94:1192.
18. Sanz MA et al. High molecular remission rate and low toxicity with modified AIDA protocol omitting cytarabine and etoposide from treatment of newly diagnosed PML-RAR-alpha positive acute promyelocytic leukemia. Blood 1999;94:4015.
19. Estey E et al. Treatment of newly diagnosed acute promyelocytic leukemia without cytarabine. J Clin Oncol 1997;15:483.
20. Tallman MS et al. All-transretinoic acid in acute promyelocytic leukemia. N Engl J Med 1997;337:1021.
21. Tallman MS et al. Clinical description of 44 patients with acute promyelocytic leukemia who developed the retinoic acid syndrome. Blood 2000;95:90.
22. DeBotton SD et al. Incidence, clinical features, and outcome of all transretinoic acid syndrome in 413 cases of newly diagnosed acute promyelocytic leukemia. Blood 1998;92:2712.
23. Soignet SL, et al. United States multicenter study of arsenic trioxide in relapsed acute promyelocytic leukemia. J Clin Oncol 2001;19:3852.
24. Raffoux E, et al. Combined treatment with arsenic trioxide and all-transretinoic acid in patients with relapsed acute promyelocytic leukemia. J Clin Oncol 2003;21:2326.
25. Flombaum CD. Metabolic emergencies in the cancer patient. Semin Oncol 2000;27:322.
26. Pui C-H, et al. Recombinant urate oxidase for the prophylaxis or treatment of hyperuricemia in patients with leukemia or lymphoma. J Clin Oncol 2001;19:697.
27. Pui C-H, et al. Recombinant urate oxidase (rasburicase) in the prevention and treatment of malignancy-associated hyperuricemia in pediatric and

adult patients: results of a compassionate-use trial. Leukemia 2001;10:1505.
28. Bosly A, et al. Rasburicase (recombinant urate oxidase) for the management of hyperuricemia in patients with cancer: report of an international compassionate use study. Cancer 2003;98:1048.
29. Souza LM et al. Recombinant human granulocyte-colony stimulating factor: effects on normal and leukemic myeloid cells. Science 1986;232:61.
30. Dombret H et al. A controlled study of recombinant human granulocyte colony-stimulating factor in elderly patients after treatment for acute myelogenous leukemia. N Engl J Med 1995;332:1678.
31. Stone RM et al. Granulocyte-macrophage colony-stimulating factor after initial chemotherapy for elderly patients with primary acute myelogenous leukemia. N Engl J Med 1995;332:1671.
32. Rowe JM et al. A randomized placebo-controlled phase III study of granulocyte-macrophage colony-stimulating factor in adult patients (>55 to 70 years of age) with acute myelogenous leukemia: a study of the Eastern Cooperative Oncology Group. Blood 1995;86:457.
33. Ozer H et al. 2000 Update of recommendations for the use of hematopoietic colony-stimulating factors: Evidence-based, clinical practice guidelines. J Clin Oncol 2000;18:3558.
34. Mayer RJ et al. Intensive postremission chemotherapy in adults with acute myeloid leukemia. N Engl J Med 1994;331:896.
35. Tallman MS et al. Evaluation of intensive postremission chemotherapy for adults with acute nonlymphocytic leukemia using high-dose cytosine arabinoside with L-asparaginase and amsacrine with etoposide. J Clin Oncol 1987;5:918.
36. Graves T, Hooks MA. Drug-induced toxicities associated with high-dose cytosine arabinoside infusions. Pharmacotherapy 1989;9:23.
37. Herzig RH et al. Central nervous system toxicity with high-dose cytosine arabinoside. Semin Oncol 1985;12(Suppl 3):233.
38. Ritch PS et al. Ocular toxicity from high-dose cytosine arabinoside. Cancer 1983;51:430.
39. Higa GM et al. The use of prophylactic eye drops during high-dose cytosine arabinoside therapy. Cancer 1991;68:1691.
40. Leith CP et al. Acute myeloid leukemia in the elderly: assessment of multidrug resistance (MDR) and cytogenetics distinguishes biologic subgroups

with remarkable distinct responses to standard chemotherapy. A Southwest Oncology Group Study. Blood 1997;89:3323.

41. Hiddemann W et al. Management of acute myeloid leukemia in elderly patients. J Clin Oncol 1999: 17;3569.

42. Stone RM et al. The difficult problem of acute myeloid leukemia in the older adult. CA Cancer J Clin 2002:52;363.

43. Tilly H et al. Low-dose cytarabine versus intensive chemotherapy in the treatment of acute nonlymphocytic leukemia in the elderly. J Clin Oncol 1990;7:272.

44. Lowenberg B et al. On the value of intensive remission induction chemotherapy in elderly patients of 65+ years with acute myeloid leukemia: a randomized Phase III study of the European Organization for Research and Treatment of Cancer leukemia Group. J Clin Oncol 1989;7:1268.

45. Sievers EL et al. Efficacy and safety of gemtuzumab ozogamicin in patients with CD33-positive acute myeloid leukemia in first relapse. J Clin Oncol 2001:19;3244.

46. Garcia-Manero GS et al. Chronic myelogenous leukemia: a review and update of therapeutic strategies. Cancer 2003;98:437.

47. Anonymous. Chronic myelogenous leukemia (PDQ) treatment-health professionals. CancerNet website. Available at: http://www.nci.nih.gov/cancerinfo/pdq/treatment/CML/healthprofessional/. Accessed September 1, 2003.

48. Sawyers CL. Chronic myeloid leukemia. N Engl J Med 1999;340:1330.

49. McGlave P. Unrelated donor transplant therapy for chronic myelogenous leukemia. Hematol Oncol Clin N Am 1998;12:93.

50. Pasweg JR et al. Related donor bone marrow transplantation for chronic myelogenous leukemia. Hematol Oncol Clin N Am 1998;12:81.

51. Silver RT et al. An evidence based analysis of the effects of busulfan, hydroxyurea, interferon, and allogeneic bone marrow transplantation in treating the chronic phase of CML: developed by the American Society of Hematology. Blood 1999;94:1517.

52. Beelan DW, et al. Prolonged administration of interferon-alpha in patients with chronic-phase Philadelphia chromosome-positive chronic myelogenous leukemia before allogeneic bone marrow transplantation may adversely affect transplant outcome. Blood 1995;85:2981.

53. Giralt SA, et al. Effect of prior interferon alfa therapy on the outcome of allogeneic bone marrow transplantation for chronic myelogenous leukemia. J Clin Oncol 1993;11:1055.

54. Chronic Myeloid Leukemia Trialists' Collaborative Group. Interferon alfa versus chemotherapy for chronic myeloid leukemia: a meta-analysis of seven randomized trials. J Nat Cancer Inst 1997;89:1616.

55. Guilhot F et al. Interferon alfa-2b combined with cytarabine versus interferon alone in chronic myelogenous leukemia. N Engl J Med 1997;337:223.

56. Kantarjian HM et al. Prolonged survival in chronic myelogenous leukemia after cytogenetic response to IFN-α therapy. Ann Intern Med 1995;122:254.

57. Druker BJ et al. Efficacy and safety of a specific inhibitor of the bcr-abl tyrosine kinase in chronic myeloid leukemia. N Engl J Med 2001;344:1031.

58. Talpaz M et al. Imatinib induces durable hematologic and cytogenetics responses in patients with accelerated phase chronic myeloid leukemia: results of a phase 2 study. Blood 2002;99:1928.

59. Sawyers CL et al. Imatinib induces hematologic and cytogenetics responses in patients with chronic myelogenous leukemia in myeloid blast crisis: results of a phase II study. Blood 2002;99:3530.

60. O'Brien SG et al. Imatinib compared with interferon and low-dose cytarabine for newly diagnosed chronic-phase chronic myeloid leukemia. N Engl J Med 2003;348:994.

61. Deininger M, et al. Practical management of patients with chronic myeloid leukemia receiving imatinib. J Clin Oncol 2003;21:1637.

62. Cheson BD. The chronic lymphocytic leukemias. In: DeVita et al., eds. Cancer. Principles and Practice of Oncology, 6th Ed. Philadelphia: Lippincott Williams & Wilkins, 2001:2447.

63. Kay NE et al. Chronic lymphocytic leukemia. Hematology (Am Soc Hematol Educ Program) 2002:193.

64. Anonymous. Chemotherapeutic options in chronic lymphocytic leukemia: a meta-analysis of the randomized trials. CLL Trialists' Collaborative Group. J Natl Cancer Inst 1999;91:861.

65. Pangalis GA et al. B-chronic lymphocytic leukemia: practical aspects. Hematol Oncol 2002;20:103.

66. Morrison VA. The infectious complication of chronic lymphocytic leukemia. Semin Oncol 1998; 25:98.

67. Larson DA, Tomlinson LJ. Quantitative antibody studies in man III: antibody response in leukemia and other malignant lymphomata. J Clin Invest 1953;32:317.

68. Cheson BD et al. National Cancer Institute-sponsored Working Group guidelines for chronic lymphocytic leukemia: revised guidelines for diagnosis and treatment. Blood 1996;12:4990.

69. Knospe WH et al. Bi-weekly chlorambucil treatment of chronic lymphocytic leukemia. Cancer 1974;33:555.

70. Sawitsky A et al. Comparison of daily versus intermittent chlorambucil and prednisone therapy in the treatment of patients with chronic lymphocytic leukemia. Blood 1977;50:1049.

71. Jaksic B, Brugiatelli M. High dose chlorambucil vs intermittent chlorambucil plus prednisone for treatment of B-CLL–IGCI CLL-01 trial. Nouv Rev Fr Hematol 1988;30:437.

72. Johnson S et al. Multicentre prospective randomized trial of fludarabine versus cyclophosphamide, doxorubicin, and prednisone (CAP) for treatment of advanced stage chronic lymphocytic leukemia. Lancet 1996;347:1432.

73. Rai KR et al. Fludarabine compared with chlorambucil as primary therapy for chronic lymphocytic leukemia. N Engl J Med 2000;343:1750.

74. Anaissie EJ et al. Infections in patients with chronic lymphocytic leukemia treated with fludarabine. Ann Intern Med 1998;129:559.

75. Martell RE et al. Analysis of age, estimated creatinine clearance and pretreatment hematologic parameters as predictors of fludarabine toxicity in patients treated for chronic lymphocytic leukemia: a CALGB (9011) coordinated intergroup study. Cancer Chemother Pharmacol 2002;50:37.

76. Byrd JC et al. Randomized phase 2 study of fludarabine with concurrent versus sequential treatment with rituximab in symptomatic, untreated patients with B-cell chronic lymphocytic leukemia: results from Cancer and Leukemia Group B 9712 (CALGB 9712). Blood 2003;101:6.

77. Winkler U et al. Cytokine-release syndrome in patients with B-cell chronic lymphocytic leukemia and high lymphocyte counts after treatment with an anti-CD20 monoclonal antibody (rituximab, IDEC-C2B8). Blood 1999;94:2217.

78. O'Brien SM et al. Results of the fludarabine and cyclophosphamide combination regimen in chronic lymphocytic leukemia. J Clin Oncol 2001;19:1414.

79. Mavromatis B and Cheson BD. Monoclonal antibody therapy of chronic lymphocytic leukemia. J Clin Oncol 2003;21:1874.

80. Keating MJ et al. Therapeutic role of alemtuzumab in (Campath-1H) in patients who have failed fludarabine: results of a large international study. Blood 2002;99:3554.

81. Tsiodras S et al. Infection and immunity in chronic lymphocytic leukemia. Mayo Clin Proc 2000;75: 1039.

82. Perkins JG et al. Frequency and type of serious infections in fludarabine-refractory B-cell chronic lymphocytic leukemia and small lymphocytic lymphoma. Cancer 2002;94:2033.

83. Weeks JC et al. Cost effectiveness of prophylactic intravenous immune globulin in chronic lymphocytic leukemia. N Engl J Med 1991;325:81.

84. Chapel H et al. Immunoglobulin replacement in patients with chronic lymphocytic leukaemia: a comparison of two dose regimens. Br J Haematol 1994;88:209.

85. Hoffbrand AV, Pettit JE, eds. Color Atlas of Clinical Hematology, 2nd Ed. London; Baltimore: Mosby Wolfe, 1994.

86. Rosenberg SA. Classification of lymphoid neoplasms. Blood 1994;84:1359.

87. Armitage JO et al. Non-Hodgkin's lymphomas. In: DeVita et al., eds. Cancer. Principles and Practice of Oncology, 6th Ed. Philadelphia: Lippincott Williams & Wilkins, 2001:2256.

88. Harris NL et al. A revised European-American classification of lymphoid neoplasms: a proposal from the International Lymphoma Study Group. Blood 1994;84:1361.

89. Miller TP et al. Chemotherapy alone compared with chemotherapy plus radiotherapy for localized intermediate and high-grade non-Hodgkin's lymphoma. N Engl J Med 1998;339:21.

90. The International Non-Hodgkin's Lymphoma Prognostic Factors Project. A predictive model for aggressive non-Hodgkin's lymphoma. N Engl J Med 1993;329:987.

91. Fisher RI et al. Comparison of a standard regimen (CHOP) with three intensive chemotherapy regimens for advanced non-Hodgkin's lymphoma. N Engl J Med 1993;328:1002.

92. Velasquez WS et al. ESHAP: an effective chemotherapy regimen in refractory and relapsing lymphoma: a 5-year follow-up study. J Clin Oncol 1994;12:1169.

93. Moskowitz CH et al. Ifosfamide, carboplatin, and etoposide: a highly effective cytoreduction and peripheral-blood progenitor-cell mobilization regimen for transplant-eligible patients with non-Hodgkin's lymphoma. J Clin Oncol 1999;17:3776.

94. Shipp MA et al. International consensus conference on high-dose therapy with hematopoietic stem cell transplantation in aggressive non-Hodgkin's lymphoma: report of the jury. J Clin Oncol 1999;17:423.

95. Skarin AT, Dorfman DM. Non-Hodgkin's lymphomas: current classification and management. CA Cancer J Clin 1997;47:351.

96. Magrath IT. Management of high-grade lymphoma. Oncology (Huntington) 1998;12(10 Suppl 8):40.

97. Cheson BD. Current approaches to therapy for indolent non-Hodgkin's lymphoma. Oncology (Huntington) 1998;12(10 Suppl 8):25.

98. Brice P et al. Comparison in low-tumor burden follicular lymphomas between an initial no-treatment policy, prednimustine, and interferon alfa: a randomized study from the Groupe d'Etude des Lymphomes Folliculaires. J Clin Oncol 1997; 15:110.

99. Coiffier B. Towards a cure in indolent lymphoproliferative disease? Eur J Cancer 1995;31A:2135.

100. Klasa R et al. Randomized phase III study of fludarabine phosphate versus cyclophosphamide, vincristine, and prednisone in patients with recurrent low-grade non-Hodgkin's lymphoma previously treated with alkylating agent or alkylator-containing regimen J Clin Oncol 2002;20: 4649.

101. Hagenbeck A et al. Fludarabine versus conventional CVP chemotherapy in newly diagnosed patients with stages III and IV low grade malignant non-Hodgkin's lymphoma [Abstract 1294]. Proceedings of the American Society of Clinical Oncology, 1998.

102. Harjupaa A et al. Rituximab (anti-CD20) therapy of B-cell lymphomas: direct complement killing is superiour to cellular effector mechanisms. Scand J Immunol 2000;51:634.

103. Demidem A et al. Chimeric anti-CD20 (IDEC-C2b8) monoclonal antibody sensitizes a B-cell lymphoma line to cell killing by cytotoxic drugs. Cancer Biother Radiopharm 1997;12:177.

104. McLaughlin P et al. Rituximab chimeric anti-CD20 monoclonal antibody therapy for relapsed

indolent lymphoma: half of patients respond to a four-dose treatment program. J Clin Oncol 1998;16:2825.

105. Rituxan (Rituximab) prescribing information. IDEC Pharmaceuticals Corporation, Genentech Inc., 2002.

106. Byrd JC et al. Rituximab therapy in hematologic malignancy patients with circulating blood tumor cells: association with increased infusion related side effects and rapid blood tumor clearance. J Clin Oncol 1999;17:791.

107. Coiffier B et al. Rituximab (anti-CD20 monoclonal antibody) for the treatment of patients with relapsing or refractory aggressive lymphoma: a multicenter phase II study. J Clin Oncol 1998; 92:1927.

108. Czuczman MS et al. Treatment of patients with low-grade B-cell lymphoma with the combination of chimeric anti-CD20 monoclonal antibody and CHOP chemotherapy. J Clin Oncol 1999;17:268.

109. Coiffier B et al. CHOP chemotherapy plus rituximab compared with CHOP alone in elderly patients with diffuse large-B-cell lymphoma. N Engl J Med 2002;346:235.

110. Cheson BD. Radioimmunotherapy of non-Hodgkin's lymphoma. Blood 2003;101:391.

111. Dillman RO. Radiolabeled anti-CD20 monoclonal antibodies for the treatment of B-cell lymphoma. J Clin Oncol 2002;20:3545.

112. Carbone PP et al. Report of the committee on Hodgkin's disease staging. Cancer Res 1971;31:1860.

113. Advani RJ, Horning SJ. Treatment of early stage Hodgkin's disease. Semin Oncol 1999;26:270.

114. Diehl V et al. Hodgkin's Disease. In DeVita VT et al., eds. Cancer. Principles and Practice of Oncology, 6th Ed. Philadelphia: Lippincott Williams & Wilkins, 2001:2339.

115. Andrieu JM, Colonna P. Are ABVD and MOPP/ABV truly equivalent for treating Hodgkin's disease at advanced stages? J Clin Oncol 1998;16:2283.

116. Engert A et al. Treatment of advanced Hodgkin's lymphoma. Standard and experimental approaches. Semin Oncol 1999;36:282.

117. Duggan DB et al. Randomized comparison of ABVD and MOPP/ABV hybrid for the treatment of advanced Hodgkin's disease: report of an Intergroup trial. J Clin Oncol 2003;21:607.

118. Ekstrand BC, et al. Rituximab in lymphocyte-predominant Hodgkin disease: results of a phase 2 trial. Blood 2003;101:4285.

119. Moskowitz CH et al. A 2-step comprehensive high-dose chemoradiotherapy second-line program for relapsed and refractory Hodgkin disease: analysis by intent to treat and development of a prognostic model. Blood 2001;97:616.

120. Barlogie B et al. Biology and therapy of multiple myeloma in 1996. Semin Hematol 1997;34:67.

121. Bataille R, Harousseau JL. Multiple myeloma. N Engl J Med 1997;336:1657.

122. Goldschmidt H et al. Multiple myeloma and renal failure. Nephrol Dial Transplant 2000;15:301.

123. Oken MM et al. Comparison of melphalan and prednisone with vincristine, carmustine, melphalan, cyclophosphamide and prednisone in the treatment of multiple myeloma. Cancer 1997;78:1561.

124. Anonymous. Combination chemotherapy versus melphalan plus prednisone as treatment for multiple myeloma: an overview of 6,633 patients from 27 randomized trials. Myeloma Trialists' Collaborative Group. J Clin Oncol 1998;16:3832.

125. Alexanian R et al. Primary dexamethasone treatment of multiple myeloma. Blood 1992;80:887.

126. Hussein MA et al. A phase II trial of pegylated liposomal doxorubicin, vincristine, and reduced-dose dexamethasone combination therapy in newly diagnosed multiple myeloma patients. Cancer 2002;95:2160.

127. Rajkumar S et al. Combination therapy with thalidomide plus dexamethasone for newly diagnosed myeloma. J Clin Oncol 2002;20:4319.

128. Weber D, et al. Thalidomide alone or with dexamethasone for previously untreated multiple myeloma. J Clin Oncol 2003;21;16.

129. Singhal S et al. Antitumor activity of thalidomide in refractory multiple myeloma. N Engl J Med 1999;341:1565.

130. Mileshkin L, et al. Multicenter phase 2 trial of thalidomide in relapsed/refractory multiple myeloma: adverse prognostic impact of advanced age. Blood 2003;102:69.

131. Ferman JP et al. High-dose therapy and autologous peripheral blood stem cell transplantation in multiple myeloma: up-front or rescue treatment? Results of a multicenter sequential randomized trial. Blood 1998;92:3131.

132. Attal M et al. A prospective randomized trial of autologous bone marrow transplantation and chemotherapy in multiple myeloma. N Engl J Med 1996;335:91.

133. Lenhoff S et al. Impact on survival of high-dose therapy with autologous stem cell support in patients younger than 60 years with newly diagnosed multiple myeloma: a population-based study. Blood 2000;95:7.

134. Child JA et al. High-dose chemotherapy with hematopoietic stem-cell rescue for multiple myeloma. N Engl J Med 2003;348:1875.

135. Hahn T et al. The role of cytotoxic therapy with hematopoietic stem cell transplantation in the therapy of multiple myeloma: an evidence-based review. Biol Blood Marrow Transplant 2003;9:4.

136. Kroger N et al. Autologous stem cell transplantation followed by a dose-reduced allograft induces high complete remission rate in multiple myeloma. Blood 2002;100:755.

137. Badros A et al. Improved outcome of allogeneic transplantation in high-risk multiple myeloma patients after nonmyeloablative conditioning. J Clin Oncol 2002;20:1295.

138. Berenson JR et al. American Society of Clinical Oncology clinical practice guidelines: the role of bisphosphonates in multiple myeloma. J Clin Oncol 2002;20:3719.

139. Richardson PG et al. A phase 2 study of bortezomib in relapsed, refractory myeloma. N Engl J Med 2003;348:2609.

140. Lee C-K et al. DTPACE: an effective, novel combination chemotherapy with thalidomide for previously treated patients with myeloma. J Clin Oncol 2003;21:2732.

141. Ries LAG et al., eds. Cancer incidence and survival among children and adolescents: United States SEER Program 1975–1995. Bethesda MD: National Cancer Institute, SEER Program, 1999. NIH publication no. 99-4649.

142. Pui C-H, Evans WE. Acute lymphoblastic leukemia. N Engl J Med 1998;332:605.

143. Bizzozero OJ, Jr et al. Radiation-related leukemia in Hiroshima and Nagasaki, 1946–64: I. Distribution, incidence and appearance in time. N Engl J Med 1966;274:1095.

144. Folley JH et al. Incidence of leukemia in survivors of the atomic bomb in Hiroshima and Nagasaki, Japan. Am J Med 1952;13:311.

145. Morgan KZ. Radiation-induced health effects. Science 1977;195:344.

146. Van Steensel-Moll HA et al. Are maternal fertility problems related to childhood leukemia? Int J Epidemiol 1985;14:555.

147. Stjernfeldt M et al. Maternal smoking during pregnancy and risk of childhood cancer. Lancet 1986;1:1350.

148. London SL et al. Exposure to residential electric and magnetic fields and risk of childhood leukemia. Am J Epidemiol 1991;134:923.

149. Greenberg RS, Shuster JL. Epidemiology of cancer in children. Epidemiol Rev 1985;7:22.

150. Wyke J. Principles of viral leukemogenesis. Semin Hematol 1986;23:189.

151. Michaelson SM. Household magnetic fields and childhood leukemia: a critical analysis. Pediatrics 1991;88:630.

152. Pool R. Is there an EMF-cancer connection? Science 1990;249:1096.

153. Lewis MS. Spatial clustering in childhood leukemia. J Chronic Dis 1980;33:703.

154. Miller DR. Childhood acute lymphoblastic leukemia: 1. Biological features and their use in predicting outcome of treatment. Am J Pediatr Hematol Oncol 1988;10:163.

155. Miller DR. Acute lymphoblastic leukemia. Pediatr Clin North Am 1980;27:269.

156. Margolin JF, Poplack DG. Acute lymphoblastic leukemia. In: Pizzo PA, Poplack DG, eds. Principles and Practice of Pediatric Oncology. Philadelphia: Lippincott-Raven, 1997:409.

157. Smith M et al. Uniform approach to risk classification and treatment assignment for children with acute lymphoblastic leukemia. J Clin Oncol 1996;14:18.

158. Kalwinsky DK et al. Clinical relevance of lymphoblast biological features in children with acute lymphoblastic leukemia. J Clin Oncol 1985;3:477.

159. Simone JV et al. Initial features and prognosis in 363 children with acute lymphocytic leukemia. Cancer 1975;36:2009.

160. Sather HN. Statistical evaluation of prognostic factors in ALL and treatment results. Med Pediatr Oncol 1986;14:158.

161. Bleyer WA et al. The staging of childhood acute lymphoblastic leukemia: strategies of the Children's Cancer Study Group and a three-dimensional technique of multivariate analysis. Med Pediatr Oncol 1986;14:271.

162. Mastrangelo R et al. Report and recommendations of the Rome Workshop concerning poor-prognosis acute lymphoblastic leukemia in children: biologic bases for staging, stratification, and treatment. Med Pediatr Oncol 1986;14:191.

163. Robison L et al. Assessment of the interrelationship of prognostic factors in childhood acute lymphoblastic leukemia. Am J Pediatr Hematol Oncol 1980;2:3.

164. Nachman J et al. Young adults 1621 years of age at diagnosis entered on Children's Cancer Group acute lymphoblastic leukemia and acute myeloblastic leukemia protocols: results of treatment. Cancer 1993;71(Suppl):3377.

165. Silverman LB et al. Intensified therapy for infants with acute lymphoblastic leukemia: results from the Dana-Farber Cancer Institute Consortium. Cancer 1997;80:2285.

166. Pui C-H, Evans WE. Acute lymphoblastic leukemia in infants. J Clin Oncol 1999;17:438.

167. Lauer SJ et al. Intensive alternating drug pairs after remission induction for treatment of infants with acute lymphoblastic leukemia: a Pediatric Oncology Group pilot study. J Pediatr Hematol Oncol 1998;20:229.

168. Reaman GH et al. Treatment outcome and prognostic factors for infants with acute lymphoblastic leukemia treated on two consecutive trials of the Children's Cancer Group. J Clin Oncol 1999;17:445.

169. Hammond D et al. Analysis of prognostic factors in acute lymphoblastic leukemia. Med Pediatr Oncol 1986;14:124.

170. Lanning M et al. Superior treatment results in females with high-risk acute lymphoblastic leukemia in childhood. Acta Paediatr 1992; 81:66.

171. Hale JP, Lilleyman JS. Importance of 6-mercaptopurine dose in lymphoblastic leukaemia. Arch Dis Child 1991;66:462.

172. Lilleyman JS et al. Childhood lymphoblastic leukemia: sex difference in 6-mercaptopurine utilization. Br J Cancer 1984;49:703.

173. Pui C-H et al. Sex differences in prognosis for children with acute lymphoblastic leukemia. J Clin Oncol 1999;17:818.

174. Kalwinsky DK et al. Variation by race in presenting clinical and biologic features of childhood acute lymphoblastic leukaemia: implications for treatment outcome. Leuk Res 1985;9:817.

175. Sklo M et al. The changing survivorship of white and black children with leukemia. Cancer 1978;42:59.

176. Walters TR et al. Poor prognosis in negro children with acute lymphoblastic leukemia. Cancer 1972;29:210.

177. Pui C-H et al. Outcome of treatment for childhood cancer in black as compared with white children: the St. Jude Children's Research hospital experience, 1962 through 1992. JAMA 1995;273:633.

178. Reiter A et al. Favorable outcome of B-cell acute lymphoblastic leukemia in childhood: a report of three consecutive studies of the BFM group. Blood 1992;80:2471.

179. Patte C. Non-Hodgkin's lymphoma. Eur J Cancer 1998;34:359.

180. Miller DR et al. Prognostic implications of blast cell morphology in childhood acute lymphoblastic leukemia: a report from the Children's Cancer Study Group. Cancer Treat Rep 1985;69:1211.

181. Lilleyman JS et al. The clinical significance of blast cell morphology in childhood lymphoblastic leukemia. Med Pediatr Oncol 1986;14:144.

182. Miller DR et al. Prognostic importance of morphology (FAB classification) in childhood acute lymphoblastic leukemia. Br J Haematol 1981; 48:199.

183. van Eyes J et al. The French-American-British (FAB) classification of leukemia. The Pediatric Oncology Group experience with Lymphocytic leukemia. Cancer 1986;57:1046.

184. Gupta S, Good RA. Markers of human lymphocyte subpopulations in primary immunodeficiency and lymphoproliferative disorders. Semin Hematol 1980;17:1.

185. Brouet JC et al. The use of B and T membrane markers in the classification of human leukemias, with special reference to acute lymphoblastic leukemia. Blood Cells 1975;1:81.

186. Brouet JC, Seligmann M. The immunological classification of acute lymphoblastic leukemias. Cancer 1978;42:817.

187. Cossman J et al. Induction of differentiation in the primitive B-cells of common, acute lymphoblastic leukemia. N Engl J Med 1982;307:1251.

188. Nadler LM et al. Induction of human B-cell antigens in non-T-cell acute lymphoblastic leukemia. J Clin Invest 1982;70:433.

189. Crist WM et al. Immunologic markers in childhood acute lymphocytic leukemia. Semin Oncol 1985;12:105.

190. Pesando JM et al. Leukemia-associated antigens in ALL. Blood 1979;34:1240.

191. Ritz J et al. A monoclonal antibody to human acute lymphoblastic leukemia antigen. Nature 1980;283:583.

192. Pullen DJ et al. Southwest Oncology Group experience with immunological phenotyping in acute lymphocytic leukemia of childhood. Cancer Res 1981;41:4802.

193. Magrath IT et al. Bone marrow involvement in Burkitt's lymphoma and its relationship to acute B-cell leukemia. Leuk Res 1979;4:33.

194. Flandrin G et al. Acute leukemia with Burkitt's tumor cells: a study of six cases with special reference to lymphocyte surface markers. Blood 1975;45:183.

195. Look AT. The emerging genetics of acute lymphoblastic leukemia: clinical and biological implications. Semin Oncol 1985;12:92.

196. Lampert F et al. Acute lymphoblastic leukemia: current status of therapy in children. Recent Results Cancer Res 1984;93:159.

197. Bowman WP et al. Cell markers in lymphomas and leukemias. In: Stollerman GH, ed. Advances in Internal Medicine. Chicago: YearBook Medical Publishers, 1980;25:391.

198. Sallan SE et al. Cell surface antigens: prognostic implications in childhood acute lymphoblastic leukemia. Blood 1980;55:395.

199. Steinherz PG et al. Improved disease-free survival of children with acute lymphoblastic leukemia at high risk for early relapse with the New York regimena new intensive therapy protocol: a report from the Children's Cancer Study Group. J Clin Oncol 1986;4:744.

200. Amylon MD et al. Intensive high-dose asparaginase consolidation improves survival for pediatric patients with T cell acute lymphoblastic leukemia and advanced stage lymphoblastic lymphoma: a Pediatric Oncology group study. Leukemia 1999;13:335.

201. Rots MG et al. Role of folylpolyglutamate synthetase and folylpolyglutamate hydrolase in methotrexate accumulation and polyglutamylation in childhood leukemia. Blood 1999;93:1677.

202. Look AT et al. Prognostic importance of blast cell DNA content in childhood acute lymphoblastic leukemia. Blood 1985;65:1079.

203. Secker-Walker LM et al. Cytogenetics of acute lymphoblastic leukaemias in children as a factor in the prediction of long-term survival. Br J Haematol 1982;52:389.

204. Kaspers GJL et al. Favorable prognosis of hyperdiploid common acute lymphoblastic leukemia may be explained by sensitivity to antimetabolites and other drugs: results of an in vitro study. Blood 1995;85:751.

205. Zhang L et al. Reduced folate carrier gene expression in childhood acute lymphoblastic leukemia: relationship to immunophenotype and ploidy. Clin Cancer Res 1998;4:2169.

206. Belkov VM et al. Reduced folate carrier expression in acute lymphoblastic leukemia: a mechanism for ploidy but not lineage differences in methotrexate accumulation. Blood 1999;93:1643.

207. Look AT. The cytogenetics of childhood leukemia: clinical and biological implications. Pediatr Clin North Am 1988;35:723.

208. Borkhardt A et al. Biology and clinical significance of the TEL/AML1 rearrangement. Curr Opin Pediatr 1999;11:33.

209. Capizzi RL et al. L-Asparaginase: clinical, biochemical, pharmacological and immunological studies. Ann Intern Med 1971;74:893.

210. Uckun FM et al. Clinical significance of Philadelphia chromosome positive pediatric acute lymphoblastic leukemia in the context of contemporary intensive therapies. A report from the Children's Cancer Group. Cancer 1998;83:2030.

211. Schrappe M et al. Philadelphia chromosome-positive (Ph+) childhood acute lymphoblastic leukemia: good initial steroid response allows early prediction of a favorable treatment outcome. Blood 1998;92:2730.

212. Foroni L et al. Investigation of minimal residual disease in childhood and adult acute lymphoblastic leukaemia by molecular analysis. Br J Haematol 1999;105:7.

213. Gaynon PS et al. Early response to therapy and outcome in childhood acute lymphoblastic leukemia. A review. Cancer 1997;80:1717.

214. Dordelmann M et al. Down's syndrome in childhood acute lymphoblastic leukemia: clinical characteristics and treatment outcome in four consecutive BFM trials. Leukemia 1998;12:645.

215. Gomez-Almaguer D et al. Nutritional status and socio-economic conditions as prognostic factors in the outcome of therapy in childhood acute lymphoblastic leukemia. Int J Cancer 1998;11:52.

216. Elion GB et al. Relationship between metabolic rates and antitumor activities of thiopurines. Cancer Res 1963;23:1207.

217. Zimm S et al. Inhibition of first pass metabolism in cancer chemotherapy: interaction of 6-mercaptopurine and allopurinol. Clin Pharmacol Ther 1983;34:810.

218. Bisel HF. Criteria for the evaluation of response to treatment in acute leukemia. Blood 1956;11:676.

219. Skipper HE, Perry SE. Kinetics of normal and leukemic leukocyte populationsrelevance to chemotherapy. Cancer Res 1970;30:1883.

220. Hart JS et al. The mechanism of induction of complete remission in acute myeloblastic leukemia in man. Cancer Res 1969;29:2300.

221. Frei E III. Progress in treatment for the leukemias and lymphomas. Cancer 1965;18:1580.

222. Lonsdale D et al. Interrupted vs continued maintenance therapy in childhood leukemia. Cancer 1975;336:342.

223. Rivera GK et al. Improved outcome in childhood acute lymphoblastic leukaemia with reinforced early treatment and rotational combination chemotherapy. Lancet 1991;337:61.

224. Clavell LA et al. Four-agent induction and intensive asparaginase therapy for treatment of childhood acute lymphoblastic leukemia. N Engl J Med 1986;315:657.

225. Vietti TJ et al. Vincristine, prednisone and daunomycin in acute leukemia of childhood. Cancer 1971;27:602.

226. Aur RJA et al. Childhood acute lymphocytic leukemia: study VIII. Cancer 1978;42:2123.

227. Pinkel D. Treatment of acute leukemia. Pediatr Clin North Am 1976;23:117.

228. Ortega JA et al. L-Asparaginase, vincristine, and prednisone for induction of first remission in acute lymphocytic leukemia. Cancer Res 1977;37:535.

229. Simone JV. Factors that influence haematological remission duration in acute lymphocytic leukemia. Br J Haematol 1976;32:465.

230. Gaynon PS et al. Improved therapy for children with acute lymphoblastic leukemia and unfavorable presenting features: a follow-up report of the Childrens Cancer Group study CCG-106. J Clin Oncol 1993;11:2234.

231. Evans WE et al. Conventional compared with individualized chemotherapy for childhood acute lymphoblastic leukemia. N Engl J Med 1998; 338:499.

232. Reiter A et al. Chemotherapy in 998 unselected childhood acute lymphoblastic leukemia patients. Results and conclusions of the multicenter trial ALL-BFM 86. Blood 1994;84:3122.

233. Sackmann-Muriel F et al. Treatment results in childhood acute lymphoblastic leukemia with a modified ALL-BFM'90 protocol: lack of improvement in high-risk group. Leuk Res 1999; 23:331.

234. Miller DR. Prognostic factors in childhood lymphoblastic leukemia. J Pediatr 1974;87:672.

235. Goldie JH et al. Rationale for the use of alternating non cross resistant chemotherapy. Cancer Treat Rep 1982;66:439.

236. Tubergen DG et al. Improved outcome with delayed intensification for children with acute lymphoblastic leukemia and intermediate presenting features: a Children's Cancer Group phase III trial. J Clin Oncol 1993;11:527.

237. Harris MB et al. Consolidation therapy with antimetabolite-based therapy in standard-risk acute lymphocytic leukemia of childhood: a Pediatric Oncology Group study. J Clin Oncol 1998;16: 2840.

238. Kaplan RS, Wiernik PH. Neurotoxicity of antineoplastic drugs. Semin Oncol 1982;9:103.

239. Legha SS. Vincristine neurotoxicity: pathophysiology and management. Med Toxicol 1986;1:421.

240. Drigan R et al. Behavioral effects of corticosteroids in children with acute lymphoblastic leukemia. Med Ped Oncol 1992;20:13.

241. Price RA, Johnson WW. The central nervous system in childhood leukemia: I. The arachnoid. Cancer 1973;31:520.

242. Evans AE et al. The increasing incidence of central nervous system leukemia in children. Cancer 1970;26:404.

243. Bleyer WA, Poplack DG. Prophylaxis and treatment of leukemia in the central nervous system and other sanctuaries. Semin Oncol 1985;12:131.

244. Aur RJA et al. A comparative study of central nervous system irradiation and intensive chemotherapy early in remission of childhood acute lymphocytic leukemia. Cancer 1972;29:381.

245. Aur RJA et al. Central nervous system therapy and combination chemotherapy of childhood lymphocytic leukemia. Blood 1971;37:272.

246. Hill JM et al. A comparative study of the long term psychosocial functioning of childhood acute lymphoblastic leukemia survivors treated by intrathecal methotrexate with or without cranial radiation. Cancer 1998;82:208.

247. Brouwers P et al. Long-term neuropsychological sequelae of childhood leukemia: correlation with CT brain scan abnormalities. J Pediatr 1985; 106:723.

248. Meadows A et al. Declines in IQ scores and cognitive dysfunction in children with acute lymphocytic leukemia treated with cranial irradiation. Lancet 1981;1:1015.

249. Oliff A et al. Hypothalamic-pituitary dysfunction following CNS prophylaxis in acute lymphocytic leukemia: correlation with CT scan abnormalities. Med Pediatr Oncol 1979;7:141.

250. Pizzo P et al. Neurotoxicities of current leukemia therapy. Am J Pediatr Hematol Oncol 1979;1:127.

251. Nesbit ME Jr et al. Presymptomatic central nervous system therapy in previously untreated childhood acute lymphoblastic leukemia: comparison of 1800 rad and 2400 rad. A report for Children's Cancer Study Group. Lancet 1981;1:461.

252. Halberg FE et al. Prophylactic cranial irradiation dose effects on late cognitive function in children treated for acute lymphoblastic leukemia. Int J Radiat Oncol Biol Phys 1991;22:13.

253. Haghbin M et al. Treatment of acute lymphoblastic leukemia in children with "prophylactic" intrathecal methotrexate and intensive systemic therapy. Cancer Res 1975;35:807.

254. Sullivan MP et al. Equivalence of intrathecal chemotherapy and radiotherapy as central nervous system prophylaxis in children with acute lymphatic leukemia: a Pediatric Oncology Group Study. Blood 1982;60:948.

255. Freeman AT et al. Comparison of intermediate-dose methotrexate with cranial irradiation for postinduction treatment of acute lymphocytic leukemia in children. N Engl J Med 1983; 308:477.

256. Komp DM et al. CNS prophylaxis in acute lymphoblastic leukemia. Cancer 1982;50:1031.

257. Tubergen DG et al. Prevention of CNS disease in intermediate-risk acute lymphoblastic leukemia: comparison of cranial radiation and intrathecal methotrexate and the importance of systemic therapy: a Children's Cancer Group report. J Clin Oncol 1993;11:520.

258. Tsurusawa M et al. Improvement in CNS protective treatment in non-high-risk childhood acute lymphoblastic leukemia: report from the Japanese Children's Cancer and Leukemia Study Group. Med Pediatr Oncol 1999;32:259.

259. Nachman J et al. Response of children with high-risk acute lymphoblastic leukemia treated with and without cranial irradiation: a report from the Children's Cancer Group. J Clin Oncol 1998; 16:920.

260. Katz JA et al. Final attained height in patients successfully treated for childhood acute lymphoblastic leukemia. J Pediatr 1993;123:546.

261. Brown RT et al. Chemotherapy for acute lymphocytic leukemia: cognitive and academic sequelae. J Pediatr 1992;121:885.

262. Lesnik PG et al. Evidence for cerebellar-frontal subsystem changes in children treated with intrathecal chemotherapy for leukemia: enhanced data analysis using an effect size model. Arch Neurol 1998;55:1561.

263. Collins JM. Regional therapy: an overview. In: Poplack DG et al., eds. The Role of Pharmacology in Pediatric Oncology. Boston: Martinus Nijhoff, 1987:125.

264. Poplack DG et al. Pharmacologic approaches to the treatment of central nervous system malignancy. In: Poplack DG et al, eds. The Role of Pharmacology in Pediatric Oncology. Boston: Martinus Nijhoff, 1987:125.

265. Poplack DG et al. Pharmacology of antineoplastic agents in cerebrospinal fluid. In: Wood JH, ed. Neurobiology of Cerebrospinal Fluid. New York: Plenum Press, 1980;2:561.

266. Bleyer WA. Clinical pharmacology of intrathecal methotrexate: II. An improved dosage regimen derived from age-related pharmacokinetics. Cancer Treat Rep 1977;61:1419.

267. Bleyer WA et al. Reduction in central nervous system leukemia with a pharmacokinetically derived intrathecal methotrexate dosage regimen. J Clin Oncol 1983;1:317.

268. Shepherd DA et al. Accidental intrathecal administration of vincristine. Med Pediatr Oncol 1978;5:85.

269. Bain PG et al. Intrathecal vincristine: a fatal chemotherapeutic error with devastating central nervous system effects. J Neurol 1991;238:230.

270. Solimando DA, Wilson JP. Prevention of accidental intrathecal administration of vincristine sulfate. Hosp Pharm 1982;17:540.

271. Dyke RW. Treatment of inadvertent intrathecal injection of vincristine. N Engl J Med 1989;321:1270.

272. Fernandez CV et al. Intrathecal vincristine: an analysis of reasons for recurrent fatal chemotherapeutic error with recommendations for prevention. J Pediatr Hematol Oncol 1998;20:587.

273. Geiser CF et al. Adverse effects of intrathecal methotrexate in children with acute leukemia in remission. Blood 1975;45:189.

274. Sullivan MP et al. Combination intrathecal therapy for meningeal leukemia: two versus three drugs. Blood 1977;50:471.

275. Sullivan MP et al. Remission maintenance for meningeal leukemia: intrathecal methotrexate vs. intravenous bis-nitrosourea. Blood 1971;38:680.

276. Holdsworth MT et al. Assessment of emetogenic potential of intrathecal chemotherapy and response to prophylactic treatment with ondansetron. Support Care Cancer 1998;6:132.

277. Higgins GA et al. 5-HT$_3$ receptor antagonists injected in the area postrema inhibit cisplatin-induced emesis in the ferret. Br J Pharmacol 1989;97:247.

278. Saiki JG et al. Paraplegia following intrathecal chemotherapy. Cancer 1972;29:370.

279. Gagliano R, Costani J. Paraplegia following intrathecal methotrexate: report of a case and review of the literature. Cancer 1976;37:1663.

280. Rubinstein LJ et al. Disseminated necrotizing leukoencephalopathy: a complication of treating central nervous system leukemia and lymphoma. Cancer 1975;35:291.

281. Quinn CT et al. Methotrexate, homocysteine, and seizures [Letter]. J Clin Oncol 1998;16:393.

282. Quinn CT, Kamen BA. A biochemical perspective of methotrexate neurotoxicity with insight on non-folate rescue modalities. J Invest Med 1996; 44:522.

283. Mahoney DH et al. Intermediate-dose intravenous methotrexate with intravenous mercaptopurine is superior to repetitive low-dose oral methotrexate with intravenous mercaptopurine for children with lower-risk B-lineage acute lymphoblastic leukemia: a Pediatric Oncology Group phase III trial. J Clin Oncol 1998;16:246.

284. Kamen BA et al. Oral versus intravenous methotrexate: another opinion. J Clin Oncol 1998;16:2283.

285. Crom WR, Evans WE. Methotrexate. In: Evans WE et al., eds. Applied Pharmacokinetics: Principles of Therapeutic Drug Monitoring. Vancouver, WA: Applied Therapeutics, 1992:29.

286. Borsi JD, Moe PJ. Systemic clearance of methotrexate in the prognosis of acute lymphoblastic leukemia in children. Cancer 1987;60:3020.

287. Evans WE et al. Clinical pharmacodynamics of high-dose methotrexate in acute lymphocytic leukemia: identification of a relation between concentration and effect. N Engl J Med 1986; 314:471.

288. Evans WE et al. Reappraisal of methotrexate clearance as a prognostic factor in childhood acute lymphocytic leukemia [Abstract]. Proc Amer Assoc Canc Res 1989;30:241.

289. Wright JJ et al. Gene rearrangements as markers of clonal variation and minimal residual disease in acute lymphoblastic leukemia. J Clin Oncol 1987;5:735.

290. Secker-Walker LM et al. Bone marrow chromosomes in acute lymphoblastic leukemia: a long-term study. Med Pediatr Oncol 1985;7:371.

291. Freireich EJ et al. The effect of 6-mercaptopurine on the duration of steroid induced remission in acute leukemia: a model for evaluation of other potentially useful therapy. Blood 1963;21:699.

292. Holland JV, Glidewell OA. Chemotherapy of acute lymphocytic leukemia of childhood. Cancer 1972;30:1480.

293. Niemeyer CM et al. Comparative analysis of treatment programs for childhood acute lymphoblastic leukemia. Semin Oncol 1985;12:122.

294. Rivera GK, Mauer AM. Controversies in the management of childhood acute lymphoblastic leukemia: treatment intensification, CNS leukemia, and prognostic factors. Semin Hematol 1987;24:12.

295. Bleyer WA et al. Monthly pulses of vincristine and prednisone prevent bone marrow and testicular relapse in low-risk childhood acute lymphoblastic leukemia: a report of the CCG-161 study by the Children's Cancer Study Group. J Clin Oncol 1991;9:1012.

296. Ferrazzini G et al. Diurnal variation of methotrexate disposition in children with acute leukaemia. Eur J Clin Pharmacol 1991;41:425.

297. Kato Y et al. Dose-dependent kinetics of orally administered 6-mercaptopurine in children with leukemia. J Pediatr 1991;119:311.

298. Lennard L, Lilleyman JS. Variable mercaptopurine metabolism and treatment outcome in childhood lymphoblastic leukemia. J Clin Oncol 1989;7:1816.

299. Andersen JB et al. Pharmacokinetics, dose adjustments, and 6-mercaptopurine/methotrexate drug interactions in two patients with thiopurine methyltransferase deficiency. Acta Paediatr 1998;87:108.

300. McLeod HL et al. Analysis of thiopurine methyltransferase variant alleles in childhood acute lymphoblastic leukaemia. Br J Hematol 1999;105:696.

301. Pinkel D et al. Drug dosage and remission duration in childhood lymphocytic leukemia. Cancer 1971;27:247.

302. Relling MV et al. Prognostic importance of 6-mercaptopurine dose intensity in acute lymphoblastic leukemia. Blood 1999;93:2817.

303. Balis FM et al. Pharmacokinetics and pharmacodynamics of oral methotrexate and mercaptopurine in children with lower risk acute lymphoblastic leukemia: a joint Children's Cancer Group and Pediatric Oncology Branch study. Blood 1998;92:3569.

304. Pearson ADJ et al. The influence of serum methotrexate concentrations and drug dosage on outcome in childhood acute lymphoblastic leukaemia. Br J Cancer 1991;64:169.

305. Chessels JM et al. Oral methotrexate is as effective as intramuscular in maintenance therapy of acute lymphoblastic leukemia. Arch Dis Child 1987;62:172.

306. Lau RCW et al. Electronic measurement of compliance with mercaptopurine in pediatric patients with acute lymphoblastic leukemia. Med Pediatr Oncol 1998;30:85.

307. Festa RS et al. Therapeutic adherence to oral medication regimens by adolescents with cancer. I. Laboratory assessment. J Pediatr 1992;120: 807.

308. Kamen BA et al. Methotrexate and folate content of erythrocytes in patients receiving oral vs intramuscular therapy with methotrexate. J Pediatr 1984;104:131.

309. Land VJ et al. Long term survival in childhood acute leukemia: "late" relapses. Med Pediatr Oncol 1979;7:19.

310. Nesbit ME et al. Randomized study of 3-years versus 5 years of chemotherapy in childhood acute lymphoblastic leukemia. J Clin Oncol 1983;1:308.

311. Medical Research Council Working Party on Leukaemia in Childhood. Duration of chemotherapy in childhood acute lymphoblastic leukemia. Med Pediatr Oncol 1982;10:511.

312. Pui C-H et al. Recombinant urate oxidase for the prophylaxis or treatment of hyperuricemia in patients with leukemia or lymphoma. J Clin Oncol 2001;19:697.

313. Von Hoff DD et al. Risk factors for doxorubicin-induced congestive heart failure. Ann Intern Med 1979;91:710.

314. Lewis AB et al. Recovery of left ventricular function following discontinuation of anthracycline chemotherapy in children. Pediatrics 1981;68:67.

315. Goorin AM et al. Congestive heart failure due to adriamycin cardiotoxicity: its natural history in children. Cancer 1981;47:2810.

316. Goorin AM et al. Initial congestive heart failure, six to ten years after doxorubicin chemotherapy for childhood cancer. J Pediatr 1990;116:144.

317. Steinherz L et al. Delayed anthracycline cardiac toxicity. In: DeVita VT et al., eds. Cancer: Principles and Practice of Oncology. Philadelphia: J.B. Lippincott, 1991;5:1.

318. Lipshultz SE et al. Late cardiac effects of doxorubicin therapy for acute lymphoblastic leukemia in childhood. N Engl J Med 1991;324:808.

319. Carrio I et al. Indium-111-antimyosin and iodine-123-MIBG studies in early assessment of doxorubicin cardiotoxicity. J Nucl Med 1995;36:2044.

320. Speyer JL et al. ICRF-187 permits longer treatment with doxorubicin in women with breast cancer. J Clin Oncol 1992;10:117.

321. Swain SM et al. Congestive heart failure (CHF) after doxorubicin-containing therapy in advanced breast cancer patients treated with or without dexrazoxane (ICRF-187, ADR-529). Proc Am Soc Clin Oncol 1996;15:536.

322. Wexler LH et al. Randomized trial of the cardioprotective agent ICRF-187 in pediatric sarcoma patients treated with doxorubicin. J Clin Oncol 1996;14:362.

323. Nysom K et al. Relationship between cumulative anthracycline dose and late cardiotoxicity in childhood acute lymphoblastic leukemia. J Clin Oncol 1998;16:545.

324. Arikoski P et al. Reduced bone mineral density in long-term survivors of childhood acute lymphoblastic leukemia. J Pediatr Hematol Oncol 1998;20:234.

325. Atkinson SA et al. Bone and mineral abnormalities in childhood acute lymphoblastic leukemia: influence of disease, drugs and nutrition. Int J Cancer 1998;11:35.

326. Ojala AE et al. Osteonecrosis during the treatment of childhood acute lymphoblastic leukemia: a prospective MRI study. Med Pediatr Oncol 1999;32:11.

327. Warner JT et al. Relative osteopenia after treatment for acute lymphoblastic leukemia. Pediatr Res 1999;45:544.

328. Haskell CM et al. L-asparaginase: therapeutic and toxic effects in patients with neoplastic disease. N Engl J Med 1969;281:1028.

329. Capizzi RL et al. L-asparaginase [Abstract]. Annu Rev Med 1970;21:2433.

330. Faletta JM et al. Nonketotic hyperglycemia due to prednisone (NSC-10023) following ketotic hyperglycemia due to L-asparaginase (NSC-109229) plus prednisone. Cancer Chemother Rep 1972;56:781.

331. Land VJ et al. Toxicity of L-asparaginase in children with advanced leukemia. Cancer 1972;30:339.

332. Woo MH et al. Anti-asparaginase antibodies following E. coli asparaginase therapy in pediatric acute lymphoblastic leukemia. Leukemia 1998; 12:1527.

333. Zubrod CG. The clinical toxicities of L-asparaginase in treatment of leukemia and lymphoma. Pediatrics 1970;45:555.

334. Fabry U et al. Anaphylaxis to L-asparaginase during treatment for acute lymphoblastic leukemia in childrenevidence of a complement-mediated mechanism. Pediatr Res 1985;19:400.

335. Cheung N-KV et al. Antibody response to Escherichia coli L-asparaginase: prognostic significance and clinical utility of antibody measurement. Am J Pediatr Hematol Oncol 1986;8:99.

336. Nesbit M et al. Evaluation of intramuscular versus intravenous administration of L-asparaginase in childhood leukemia. Am J Pediatr Hematol Oncol 1979;1:9.

337. Lobel JS et al. Methotrexate and asparaginase combination chemotherapy in refractory acute lymphoblastic leukemia of childhood. Cancer 1979;43:1089.

338. Spiegel RJ et al. Delayed allergic reactions following intramuscular L-asparaginase. Med Pediatr Oncol 1980;8:123.

339. Capizzi RL. Asparaginase revisited. Leuk Lymphoma 1993;10(Suppl):147.

340. Capizzi RL, Holcenberg JS. Asparaginase. In: Holland JF, ed. Cancer Medicine, 3rd Ed. Philadelphia: Lea & Febiger, 1993:796.

341. Ohnuma T et al. Biochemical and pharmacological studies with asparaginase in man. Cancer Res 1970;30:2297.

342. Ettinger LJ. Asparaginases: where do we go from here? J Pediatr Hematol Oncol 1999;21:3.

343. Dellinger CT, Miale TD. Comparison of anaphylactic reactions to asparaginase derived from Escherichia coli and from Erwinia cultures. Cancer 1976;38:1843.

344. 204. Evans WE et al. Anaphylactoid reactions to Escherichia coli and Erwinia asparaginase in children with leukemia and lymphoma. Cancer 1982;49:1378.205.

345. Nowak-Gottl U et al. Changes in coagulation and fibrinolysis in childhood acute lymphoblastic leukaemia re-induction therapy using three different asparaginase preparations. Eur J Pediatr 1997;156:848.

346. Kurtzberg J et al. The use of polyethylene glycol-conjugated L-asparaginase in pediatric patients with prior hypersensitivity to native L asparaginase [Abstract]. Proc Am Soc Clin Oncol 1990;9:219.

347. Liang D-C et al. Unexpected mortality from the use of E. coli L-asparaginase during remission induction therapy for childhood acute lymphoblastic leukemia: a report from the Taiwan Pediatric Oncology Group. Leukemia 1999;13:155.

348. Urban C, Sager WD. Intracranial bleeding during therapy with L-asparaginase in childhood acute lymphocytic leukemia. Eur J Pediatr 1981; 137:323.

349. Saito M et al. Changes in hemostatic and fibrinolytic proteins in patients receiving L-asparaginase therapy. Am J Hematol 1989;32:20.

350. Cairo MS et al. Intracranial hemorrhage and focal seizures secondary to use of L-asparaginase during induction therapy of acute lymphocytic leukemia. J Pediatr 1980;97:829.

351. Kellie SJ et al. Hypersensitivity reactions to epipodophyllotoxins in children with acute lymphoblastic leukemia. Cancer 1991;67:1070.

352. O'Dwyer PJ et al. Hypersensitivity reactions to teniposide (VM-26): an analysis. J Clin Oncol 1986;4:1262.

353. Hayes FA et al. Allergic reactions to teniposide in patients with neuroblastoma and lymphoid malignancies. Cancer Treat Rep 1985;69:439.

354. Nolte H et al. VM-26 (teniposide)-induced hypersensitivity and degranulation of basophils in children. Am J Pediatr Hematol Oncol 1988;10:308.

355. Siddall SJ et al. Anaphylactic reactions to teniposide. Lancet 1989;1:394.

356. Hudson MM et al. Acute hypersensitivity reactions to etoposide in a VEPA regimen for Hodgkin's disease. J Clin Oncol 1993;11:1080.

357. Pui C-H et al. Secondary acute myeloid leukemia in children treated for acute lymphoid leukemia. N Engl J Med 1991;325:1682.

358. Smith MA et al. Report of the Cancer Therapy Evaluation Program Monitoring Plan for secondary acute myeloid leukemia following treatment with epipodophyllotoxins. J Natl Cancer Inst 1993;85:554.

359. . Hawkins MM et al. Epipodophyllotoxins, alkylating agents, and radiation and risk of secondary leukaemia after childhood cancer. Br Med J 1992;304:951.

360. Smith MA et al. Secondary leukemia or myelodysplastic syndrome after treatment with epipodophyllotoxins. J Clin Oncol 1999;17:569.

361. Relling MV et al. Etoposide and antimetabolite pharmacology in patients who develop secondary acute myeloid leukemia. Leukemia 1998;12:346.

362. Rivera G et al. Recurrent childhood lymphocytic leukemia: clinical and cytokinetic studies of cytosine arabinoside and methotrexate for maintenance of second hematologic remission. Cancer 1978;42:2521.

363. Ekert H et al. Poor outlook for childhood acute lymphoblastic leukemia with relapse. Med J Aust 1979;2:224.

364. Amadori S et al. Combination chemotherapy for marrow relapse in children and adolescents with acute lymphocytic leukemia. Scand J Haematol 1981;26:292.

365. Amato KR et al. Combination chemotherapy in relapsed childhood acute lymphoblastic leukemia. Cancer Treat Rep 1984;68:411.

366. Baum E et al. Prolonged second remission in childhood acute lymphocytic leukemia: a report from the Children's Cancer Study Group. Med Pediatr Oncol 1983;11:1.

367. Rivera GK et al. Intensive treatment of childhood acute lymphoblastic leukemia in first bone marrow relapse. N Engl J Med 1986;315:273.

368. Culbert SJ et al. Remission induction and continuation therapy in children with their first relapse of acute lymphoid leukemia: a Pediatric Oncology Group Study. Cancer 1991;67:37.

369. Champlin R, Gale RP. Acute lymphoblastic leukemia: recent advances in biology and therapy. Blood 1989;73:2051.

370. Wheeler K et al. Comparison of bone marrow transplant and chemotherapy for relapsed childhood acute lymphoblastic leukaemia: the MRC UKALL X experience. Br J Haematol 1998;101:94.

371. Sanders JE et al. Marrow transplantation for children with acute lymphoblastic leukemia in second remission. Blood 1987;70:324.

372. Brochstein JA et al. Allogeneic marrow transplantation after hyperfractionated total body irradiation and cyclophosphamide in children with acute leukemia. N Engl J Med 1987;317:1618.

373. Barrett AJ et al. Bone marrow transplants from HLA-identical siblings as compared with chemotherapy for children with acute lymphoblastic leukemia in a second remission. N Engl J Med 1994;331:1253.

374. Butturini A et al. Which treatment for childhood acute lymphoblastic leukemia in second remission? Lancet 1987;1:429.

375. Borgmann A et al. Autologous bone-marrow transplants compared with chemotherapy for children with acute lymphoblastic leukaemia in a second remission: a matched-pair analysis. Lancet 1995;346:873.

376. Harris RE et al. High-dose cytosine arabinoside and L-asparaginase in refractory acute lymphoblastic leukemia: the Children's Cancer Group experience. Med Pediatr Oncol 1998;30:233.

377. Magrath IT. Malignant non-Hodgkin's lymphomas in children. In: Pizzo PA, Poplack DG, eds. Principles and Practice of Pediatric Oncology. Philadelphia: Lippincott Williams & Wilkins, 2002:661.

378. Nathwani BW et al. Malignant lymphoma, lymphoblastic. Cancer 1976;38:964.

379. Bennett HM et al. Classification of non-Hodgkin's lymphomas. Lancet 1974;1:1295.

380. Lennert K et al. The histopathology of malignant lymphoma. Br J Haematol 1975;31(Suppl):193.

381. Lukes RJ et al. New approaches to the classification of the lymphomata. Br J Cancer 1975;31(Suppl 2):1.

382. National Cancer Institutesponsored study of classifications of non-Hodgkin's lymphomas. Summary and description of a working formulation for clinical usage. Cancer 1982;49:2112.

383. Magrath IT. Lymphocyte differentiation pathways: an essential basis for the comprehension of lymphoid neoplasia. J Natl Cancer Inst 1981;67:501.

384. Magrath IT. Malignant lymphomas. In: Levine AS, ed. Cancer in the Young. New York: Masson, 1982:473.

385. Wanatabe A et al. Undifferentiated lymphoma, non-Burkitt's type: meningeal and bone marrow involvement in children. Am J Dis Child 1973;125:57.

386. Hutter JJ et al. Non-Hodgkin's lymphoma in children. Correlation of CNS disease with initial presentation. Cancer 1975;36:2132.

387. Magrath IT. Burkitt's lymphoma. In: Mollander D, ed. Diseases of the Lymphatic System: Diagnosis and Therapy. Heidelberg: Springer-Verlag, 1983:103.

388. Magrath IT et al. Bone marrow involvement in Burkitt's lymphoma and its relationship to acute B-cell leukemia. Leuk Res 1980;4:33.

389. Magrath IT et al. Prognostic factors in Burkitt's lymphoma: importance of total tumor burden. Cancer 1980;45:1507.

390. Magrath IT et al. An effective therapy for both undifferentiated (including Burkitt's) lymphomas and lymphoblastic lymphomas in children and young adults. Blood 1984;63:1102.

391. Wagner DK et al. Soluble interleukin II receptor levels in patients with undifferentiated and lymphoblastic lymphomas. J Clin Oncol 1987;5:1262.

392. Reiter A, et al. Intensive ALL-type therapy without local radiotherapy provides a 90% event-free survival for children with T-cell lymphoblastic lymphoma: a BFM group report. Blood 2000;95:416.

393. Anderson JR et al. The results of a randomized therapeutic trial comparing a 4-drug regimen (COMP) with a 10-drug regimen (LSA²-L²). N Engl J Med 1983;308:559.

394. Bogusawska-Jaworska J et al. Evaluation of the LSA²-L² protocol for treatment of childhood non-Hodgkin's lymphoma. A report from the Polish Children's Leukemia/Lymphoma Study Group. Am J Pediatr Hematol Oncol 1984;6:363.

395. Meadows AT et al. Similar efficacy of 6 and 18 months of therapy with four drugs (COMP) for localized non-Hodgkin's lymphoma of children: a report from the Children's Cancer Study Group. J Clin Oncol 1989;7:92.

396. Patte C et al. The Societe Francaise d'Oncologie Pediatrique LMB89 protocol: highly effective multiagent chemotherapy tailored to the tumor burden and initial response in 561 unselected children with B-cell lymphomas and L3 leukemia. Blood 2001;97:3370.

397. Reiter A et al. Improved treatment results in childhood B-cell neoplasms with tailored intensification of therapy: a report of the Berlin-Frankfurt-Munster group trial NHL-BFM 90. Blood 1999;94:3294.

398. Weinstein HJ et al. APO therapy for malignant lymphoma of large cell "histiocytic" type of childhood: analysis of treatment results for 29 patients. Blood 1984;64:422.

399. Murphy SB et al. Non-Hodgkin's lymphomas of childhood: an analysis of the histology, staging, and response to treatment of 338 cases at a single institution. J Clin Oncol 1989;7:186.

400. Mott MG et al. Adjuvant low dose radiation in childhood T cell leukaemia/lymphoma (report from the United Kingdom Children's Cancer Study Group, UKCCSG). Br J Cancer 1984;50:457.

401. Murphy SB et al. Correlation of tumor cell kinetic studies with surface marker results in childhood non-Hodgkin's lymphoma. Cancer Res 1979;39:1534.

402. Hirt A et al. Differentiation and cytokinetic analysis of normal and neoplastic lymphoid cells in B and T cell malignancies of childhood. Br J Haematol 1984;58:241.

403. Dorr RT, Von Hoff DD, eds. Vincristine Sulfate. Cancer Chemotherapy Handbook, 2nd Ed. Norwalk, CT: Appleton & Lange, 1994:951.

404. Tortorice PV, O'Connell MB. Management of chemotherapy-induced nausea and vomiting. Pharmacotherapy 1990;12:129.

405. Mehta P et al. Methylprednisolone for chemotherapy-induced emesis: a double-blind randomized trial in children. J Pediatr 1986;108:774.

406. Roila F. Ondansetron plus dexamethasone compared to the `standard' metoclopramide combination. Oncology 1993;50:163.

407. Bryson JC. Clinical safety of ondansetron. Semin Oncol 1992;19(Suppl 15):26.

408. Terrin BN et al. Side effects of metoclopramide as an antiemetic in childhood cancer chemotherapy. J Pediatr 1984;104:138.

409. Howrie DL et al. Metoclopramide as an antiemetic agent in pediatric oncology patients. Drug Intell Clin Pharm 1986;20:122.

410. Cubeddu LX et al. Antagonism of serotonin S3 receptors with ondansetron prevents nausea and emesis induced by cyclophosphamide-containing chemotherapy regimens. J Clin Oncol 1990;8:1721.

Solid tumors include the malignancies that initially present as discrete masses. They arise from malignant transformations of cells within virtually any organ system except the hematopoietic system. Solid tumors are far more common than hematologic malignancies and represent the major causes of cancer-related morbidity and mortality. Depending on the specific type of cancer and its stage, surgery, radiation, chemotherapy, immunotherapy, and hormonal manipulation all play important roles in patient management. The types of solid tumors that occur in adult versus pediatric populations are distinctively different. Specific tumors commonly treated with drug therapy are included in this chapter.

ADULT TUMORS

BREAST CANCER
Premenopausal Women
Risk Factors

1. **B.W., a 37-year-old woman, is found to have a 2.2-cm mass in the upper, outer quadrant of her left breast during routine screening mammography. Biopsy of the mass reveals infiltrating ductal carcinoma. Physical examination is unremarkable, and she has no complaints. All laboratory values, including the complete blood count (CBC) and liver function tests (LFTs), are within normal limits and a chest radiograph is negative. Her family history is significant in that her mother died of breast cancer at age 42, and her 44-year-old sister had a breast tumor removed about 5 years ago. B.W. reports that she had her first menstrual cycle at age 10 and has had regular periods since that time. She is married but has never been pregnant. What is the incidence of breast cancer in premenopausal women? Did any factors place B.W. at an increased risk of developing breast cancer?**

Overall, breast cancer is the most common cancer in women in the United States and accounts for 31% of their cancers.[1] Approximately 1 in 8 women will develop breast cancer with the greatest risk occurring after age 65.[2] For women 35 years of age or younger, the chance of developing breast cancer is <1%; however, a strong family history of breast cancer increases the relative risk.[3,4]

Some cases of familial breast cancer, especially those occurring in premenopausal women, have been linked to specific breast cancer susceptibility genes, BRCA-1 and BRCA-2. Persons who are carriers of these genes have an increased risk of breast, ovarian, and prostate cancers. Women like B.W. who have a positive family history and who are carriers of the gene have an 85% chance of developing breast cancer and a 60% chance of developing ovarian cancer by age 70.[3,4] The risk is not this significant in women who are carriers and who do not have a positive family history. Genetic testing is available; however, if a woman chooses to have such testing, appropriate genetic counseling and psychologic support should be made available.[5]

The optimal medical intervention for women who are carriers but who have no evidence of the disease is not known. Prophylactic bilateral mastectomy and oophorectomy are options, but these procedures are not completely effective in preventing cancer.[6] Despite this strong relationship, it is also important to realize that BRCA gene mutations account for only 5% to 10% of all cases of breast cancer. Several additional factors have been associated with an increased risk of developing breast cancer (Table 91-1). Nulliparous women like

Table 91-1 Risk Factors Associated With Development of Breast Cancer
Strong Risk Factors
History of breast cancer in the contralateral breast
Family history of breast cancer, especially in first-degree relatives
Benign breast "cancer" (i.e., atypical hyperplasia)
Early menarche, late menopause
Late first pregnancy greater than no pregnancy
Advancing age
Possible Risk Factors
Obesity
High-fat diet
Long-term use of exogenous estrogens
Alcohol

B.W. also have a higher incidence of breast cancer than women who have had one or more pregnancies, but age at first pregnancy appears to be an even more important determinant. One study indicated that the risk of developing breast cancer was substantially higher in women whose first pregnancy was after age 30, compared with those whose first pregnancy was before age 18. Early menarche also has been associated with an increased risk of breast cancer.[7]

Screening

2. **Is routine screening mammography recommended for B.W. because of her increased risk of breast cancer? Is it recommended for all women?**

Women with a positive family history often are instructed to begin screening at an earlier age.[1] Several different guidelines for breast cancer screening are available. Although strong evidence of benefit is lacking, it generally is agreed that women should perform monthly breast self-examinations. Annual examination for breast cancer performed by a health care provider is recommended for all women older than 40 years of age.

Nearly 75% of breast cancers occur in women older than 50 years of age. All screening guidelines recommend that women in this age group have annual mammography but disagree over the role of mammography screening in women age 40 to 49. Meta-analyses reveal the risk reduction from mammography screening does not differ substantially by age, although absolute benefits are lower in women younger than age 50 compared with women aged 50 and older.[8] For this reason, the American Cancer Society updated their recommendations to include annual mammography screening beginning at age 40.[8]

It is not clear how long screening should be continued. Women older than 70 years of age are at increased risk for developing breast cancer; however, no randomized trials have evaluated the merits of annual mammography in this group. The American Cancer Society states there is no chronologic age at which screening should stop, emphasizing that as long as a woman is in good health she is likely to benefit from annual mammography.

Surgery

3. **After receiving the results of the biopsy, B.W. undergoes a partial mastectomy, full axillary lymph node dissection, and local radiation therapy. A tissue sample of the tumor is estrogen-**

and progesterone-receptor negative; human epidermal growth factor receptor-2 (erB-2 or HER-2/neu) is positive; and 4 of 20 lymph nodes are positive for tumor involvement. Is partial mastectomy as effective as more extensive surgical procedures such as modified radical mastectomy? Is radiation indicated following surgery?

Historically, radical mastectomy (removal of the breast, axillary lymph nodes, and pectoralis muscles) and modified radical mastectomy (radical mastectomy with preservation of the pectoralis muscles) have been the standard surgical procedures used for primary breast cancer. However, the psychologic and cosmetic effects of breast loss can be substantial. This has led to increased use of more conservative surgical procedures such as lumpectomy, partial mastectomy, and evaluation of axillary lymph nodes utilizing lymph node mapping with sentinel lymph node biopsy. Lumpectomy consists of gross removal of the tumor without attention to margins; a partial mastectomy includes excision of the tumor with clean surgical margins. Evaluation of the axilla through the use of the sentinel lymph node, the lymph node first reached by the lymph draining the tumor, is becoming more routine in the hands of an experienced surgeon, reducing the number of patients who require axillary lymph node dissection.[9] Early trials evaluating conservative procedures without treatment of the remaining breast tissue or axillary lymph nodes reported high failure rates. Failures presented primarily as recurrences in the remaining breast tissue or axilla.[10–12] Postoperative radiation therapy reduces the risk of local recurrence. Several randomized trials have indicated no difference in survival between patients undergoing conservative surgery (e.g., partial mastectomy) followed by local radiation therapy and those treated with radical surgery.[10–12]

Adjuvant Therapy

4. **B.W. recalls that her sister also received chemotherapy after her surgery for breast cancer. She now questions whether she should receive any additional therapy and what the chances are that she has been cured. What factors determine the need for adjuvant systemic therapy following surgery, and what are the indications for administering adjuvant chemotherapy or hormonal therapy?**

The benefit of systemic adjuvant therapy is directly related to the likelihood of disease recurrence. Size of the primary tumor, presence and number of involved axillary lymph nodes, HER-2/neu oncogene amplification, nuclear or histologic grade, and the presence of hormone receptors (estrogen and/or progesterone) appear to be the most important factors that predict prognosis.[13,14] Additional potential prognostic factors include tumor growth fraction (S-Phase) and ploidy (DNA content).[13] Intense research in this area is ongoing.

The single most important factor that predicts recurrence of breast cancer in patients like B.W., whose tumor is initially small and localized, is the presence and extent of lymph nodes positive for cancer. Women with positive lymph nodes (stage II disease) have a 40% to 60% chance of being cured with surgery alone. Women with negative lymph nodes (stage I disease) have a 70% to 90% chance of cure with surgery alone. Therefore, B.W., who has four positive nodes, negative hormone receptors, and positive HER-2/neu, would be considered at high risk for recurrence.[13,14]

Trials of systemic adjuvant therapy in women with breast cancer began in the 1960s. These trials originally focused on patients with stage II disease; however, recognizing the significant rate of disease recurrence in patients with stage I disease, later trials included stage I patients as well. Many trials evaluating the effects of systemic adjuvant chemotherapy, endocrine therapy, and combined chemoendocrine therapy have been conducted over the past 40 years. Since many of the individual trials have included relatively small numbers of patients, multiple patient subsets, or different therapeutic strategies, a series of meta-analyses have been performed by the Early Breast Cancer Trialists' Collaborative Group.[15,16] The most recent meta-analysis reviewed data from 133 randomized clinical trials conducted worldwide, which included 75,000 women with stages I and II breast cancer. The overview concluded that appropriate use of cytotoxic chemotherapy and hormonal therapy can reduce the rate of death by as much as 27%[15] and 47%,[16] respectively. The proportional reduction in risk of death in stages I and II is approximately equivalent; however, the absolute survival difference is greater in stage II patients who would have a higher risk of recurrence. B.W.'s risk of recurrence is approximately 50%, so systemic adjuvant therapy would be expected to improve her absolute chance of cure by approximately 10%.

Treatment recommendations for patients with stages I and II breast cancer continue to evolve.[17–19] The earliest guidelines were based on menopausal status (if unknown, based on age older than or younger than 50 years) and the presence of involved axillary lymph nodes at the time of the initial surgery. The results of these early studies demonstrated conclusively that premenopausal women, particularly those with four or more positive lymph nodes, who received chemotherapy had significant prolongation in disease-free and overall survival compared with untreated controls. These trials also demonstrated that postmenopausal women treated with adjuvant endocrine therapy, such as tamoxifen or anastrozole, had significant improvement in disease-free and overall survival compared with untreated controls. Thus, chemotherapy was recommended for premenopausal women and endocrine therapy for postmenopausal women.

The significance of menopausal status for adjuvant therapy is related to hormone receptors in the primary tumor. Whereas most premenopausal women are hormone receptor negative, most postmenopausal women are hormone receptor positive. Endocrine therapy is most likely to benefit women with positive hormone receptors. In early studies, hormone receptor assays were not available and menopausal status served as a surrogate marker of hormone receptor positivity. Although current adjuvant treatment guidelines retain the categories of premenopause and postmenopause, they also incorporate hormone receptor status.

The most recent adjuvant therapy guidelines hail from the Seventh International Conference on Adjuvant Therapy of Primary Breast Cancer held in St. Gallen, Switzerland, in February 2001.[18] The St. Gallen treatment recommendations are based on the presence of tumor in axillary lymph nodes and menopausal and hormone receptor status (Table 91-2).

The most important feature for determining baseline prognosis is the nodal status. For node-negative patients, two patient populations have been defined based on prognostic factors that define risk of disease recurrence. Minimal/low risk

Table 91-2 Adjuvant Systemic Treatment for Patients With Operable Breast Cancer

Risk Group	Premenopausal	Postmenopausal
Endocrine-Responsive		
Node-negative, minimal/low risk	Tamoxifen or none	Tamoxifen or none
Node-negative, average/high risk	Ovarian ablation (or GnRH analog) + tamoxifen [±chemotherapy[a]], or	Tamoxifen or
	Chemotherapy + tamoxifen [±ovarian ablation (or GnRH analog)] or Tamoxifen, or	Chemotherapy + tamoxifen[a]
	Ovarian ablation (or GnRH analog)	
Node-positive	Chemotherapy + tamoxifen[a] [±ovarian ablation (or GnRH analog)], or	Chemotherapy + tamoxifen[a]
	Ovarian ablation (or GnRH analog) + tamoxifen [±chemotherapy[a]]	or tamoxifen
Endocrine-Nonresponsive		
Node-negative, minimal/low risk	Not applicable	Not applicable
Node-negative, average/high risk	Chemotherapy[b]	Chemotherapy[b]
Node-positive	Chemotherapy[b]	Chemotherapy[b]

Brackets indicate questions pending answers from ongoing clinical trials. Regarding gonadotropin releasing hormone (GnRH), research was conducted using goserelin.
[a]The addition of chemotherapy is considered an acceptable option based on evidence from clinical trials. Considerations about a low relative risk, age, toxic effects, socioeconomic implications, and information at the patient's preference might justify the use of tamoxifen alone. For patients with endocrine-responsive disease, whether tamoxifen should be started concurrently with chemotherapy or delayed until the completion of chemotherapy must awaits the results of ongoing trials.
[b]For patients with endocrine-nonresponsive disease, questions of timing, duration, agent, dose, and schedules of chemotherapy are subjects for research studies.
Reprinted with permission from the American Society of Clinical Oncology from reference 18.

includes patients with estrogen receptor and/or progesterone receptor positive tumors and all of the following: tumors ≤2 cm in diameter, histologic and/or nuclear grade 1, and age 35 years or older. Average/high-risk patients includes patients with estrogen receptor and/or progesterone receptor positive tumors and at least one of the following: tumor >2 cm, histologic and/or nuclear grade 2 or 3, or age younger than 35 years. Node-positive patients are considered high risk. Distinguishing therapy for elderly patients, performed in previous editions of the conference, was not believed to be useful for treatment determinations. Consideration of the risks, including undesired toxic effects, with potential benefits, including a reduction in the absolute risk of relapse and competing causes of morbidity and mortality, are now to be applied to each group.

RECOMMENDED REGIMENS

5. **Based on these guidelines and the estrogen receptor negativity of her tumor, B.W.'s physician recommends that she receive adjuvant cytotoxic chemotherapy. What regimens are currently recommended?**

B.W. has several poor prognostic characteristics associated with her disease, including the presence of positive lymph nodes, negative hormone receptors, and positive erB-2. The erB-2 oncogene has undergone extensive study as both a prognostic and a predictive factor in early stage breast cancer.[14,20–22] The gene encodes for a growth factor receptor, and its overexpression correlates with a poor prognosis and predicts an improved likelihood of response to an anthracycline-containing regimen. Additionally, the use of anthracycline-based regimens led, on average, to improved treatment results compared to non-anthracycline based regimens in node-positive breast cancer.[15] For this reason, B.W. should probably receive a doxorubicin-containing regimen.

A large study of >3,000 high-risk women evaluated escalating doses of doxorubicin and the addition of paclitaxel. Patients were initially randomized to receive cyclophosphamide plus either 60, 70, or 90 mg/m² of doxorubicin for four cycles. After completion, they were again randomized to receive either paclitaxel 250 mg/m² every 2 weeks for four courses or no further therapy. Increasing the dose of doxorubicin did not appear to influence treatment outcomes; however, the addition of paclitaxel resulted in a significant reduction of the rate of recurrence and the rate of death.[23]

Although there was no benefit to the increased doxorubicin dose, the role of dose-density was also hypothesized to be important in the adjuvant setting. Dose-density refers to the administration of drugs with a shortened intertreatment interval. A clinical trial evaluating more than 2,000 female breast cancer patients with node-positive disease revealed that dose-dense chemotherapy of doxorubicin and cyclophosphamide every 2 weeks, either sequentially or concurrently with paclitaxel, resulted in improved disease-free and overall survival compared to conventional dosing every 3 weeks.[24] These two trials evaluating the addition of a taxane[23] and utility of dose-dense therapy,[24] respectively, represent the most significant improvements in the adjuvant therapy of breast cancer in the past 25 years. Therefore, it is recommend that B.W. receive dose-dense doxorubicin and cyclophosphamide followed by paclitaxel.

ENDOCRINE THERAPY

6. **Should B.W. receive adjuvant endocrine therapy in addition to chemotherapy?**

Since B.W.'s tumor was negative for hormone receptors, endocrine therapy is not indicated. However, in premenopausal women with positive hormone receptors, combined chemoendocrine therapy may be beneficial. Results of the meta-analysis found that ovarian ablation in patients younger than 50 years of age was as effective as chemotherapy in reducing recurrence and mortality.[25] However, this is an indirect comparison of results of trials employing ovarian ablation to those using combination chemotherapy. The report of this meta-analysis has stimulated renewed interest in the value of endocrine therapy (ovarian ablation, tamoxifen, or luteinizing hormone–releasing hormone [LHRH] analogs) in premenopausal women. Combination chemotherapy often produces permanent ovarian failure in premenopausal women and evidence exists that this is associated with a favorable prognosis.

If B.W.'s tumor had been hormone receptor positive, chemoendocrine therapy would have been indicated. In the meta-analysis, chemoendocrine therapy was associated with the greatest reduction in risk of death in women ages 50 to 69 years.[15,16] Consequently, chemoendocrine therapy is now recommended for postmenopausal hormone receptor positive patient subgroups, representing a significant shift in adjuvant treatment of breast cancer over the past decade.

Adjuvant tamoxifen is the classical standard care for the endocrine therapy of breast cancer. Subsequently, anastrozole was shown to be significantly better than tamoxifen in the adjuvant setting, with an improvement in the disease-free survival rate at 3 years of 91% compared with 89% in the tamoxifen group.[26] Additionally, anastrozole was superior to tamoxifen in terms of a lower risk for endometrial cancer, thrombotic events, and hot flashes.[27] However, anastrozole was associated with more bone fractures and musculoskeletal disorders (arthritis or arthralgias). Despite these positive results, the current recommendations from the American Society of Clinical Oncology Working Group is to use anastrozole only in postmenopausal women with a hormone-receptor positive tumor who have a contraindication to the use of tamoxifen.[19] This recommendation was made because results of the anastrozole trial are still premature; only a small percentage of the study participants have been followed for 5 years, the time point at which the maximum benefit of tamoxifen has been evaluated. Had B.W. been estrogen receptor positive, she would not have received anastrozole because aromatase inhibitors have not been evaluated in premenopausal women and are contraindicated outside of a clinical trial in this population.

Metastatic Disease
Prognosis

7. Approximately 7 months after completing adjuvant chemotherapy, B.W. begins experiencing back pain that is partially relieved by ibuprofen 400 mg PRN. Since the pain was temporally related to moving some furniture in her living room, she did not seek medical attention. Five days after the onset of the back pain her husband noted that she was "sleepy" and mildly confused. He contacted her physician who suggested she come to the clinic immediately. Physical examination was negative for lymphadenopathy or breast masses, and chest and abdominal examinations were unremarkable. Pertinent laboratory values were as follows: calcium (Ca), 15 mg/dL (normal, 9.0 to 11.5 mg/dL); phosphorus, 4.2 mg/dL (normal, 2.5 to 4.5 mg/dL); sodium (Na), 138 mEq/L (normal, 136 to 145 mEq/L); potassium (K), 4.3 mEq/L (normal, 3.5 to 5.5 mEq/L); albumin, 3.0 g/dL (normal, 3.5 to 5.5 g/dL); alkaline phosphatase, 580 mU/mL (normal, 15 to 70 mU/mL); aspartate aminotransferase (AST), 258 mU/mL (normal, 5 to 20 mU/mL); and alanine aminotransferase (ALT), 96 mU/mL (normal, 5 to 24 mU/mL). The complete blood count (CBC) was within normal limits. Spinal cord radiographs revealed several lytic vertebral lesions consistent with metastatic carcinoma, but a myelogram did not show any evidence of spinal cord compression.

B.W. is admitted to the hospital for acute management of hypercalcemia (see Chapter 12, Fluid and Electrolyte Disorders) and restaging of her breast cancer to determine the extent of tumor spread. A bone scan shows positive uptake in the spine and right scapula and a liver scan reveals two small nodules consistent with metastatic disease. A computed tomography (CT) scan of the brain is negative. Is any further assessment of the disease stage necessary at this time? What is the prognosis now that B.W.'s disease has metastasized?

[SI units: Ca, 3.75 mmol/L (normal, 2.25 to 2.88); phosphorus, 1.36 mmol/L (normal, 0.81 to 1.45); Na, 138 mmol/L (normal, 136 to 145); K, 4.3 mmol/L (normal, 3.5 to 5.5); albumin, 30 g/L (normal, 35 to 55); alkaline phosphatase, 580 U/L (normal, 15 to 70); AST, 258 U/L (normal, 5 to 20); ALT, 96 U/L (normal, 5 to 24)]

The purpose of documenting all sites of disease involvement is to enable the evaluation of the effect of treatment and to identify any disease sites that may require immediate therapy to avoid life-threatening complications (e.g., brain metastases). B.W. has documented disease in the liver and bones. Other common sites of disease are the remaining breast tissue, bone marrow, and the lungs. Since her CBC is normal, further examination of the bone marrow is not necessary at this time; however, a chest radiograph should be ordered to rule out involvement of the lungs.

Metastatic breast cancer is rarely curable. After metastatic disease is documented, survival may range from a few months to several years, depending on the site(s) and number of metastases as well as the rate of tumor growth (which may be assessed by the disease-free interval). The median duration of survival after recurrence is approximately 2 years. Multiple sites of metastatic disease, a relatively short disease-free interval (<1 year), liver involvement, negative estrogen and progesterone receptors at the time of diagnosis, and premenopausal status all confer a poor prognosis for B.W.

Treatment
COMBINATION AND SINGLE-AGENT CHEMOTHERAPY

8. What treatment options are available for B.W. at this time?

B.W. has tumor in both the liver and bones, and systemic therapy is necessary to simultaneously treat both disease sites. Bone and soft tissue metastases tend to have a better prognosis and are more likely to respond to endocrine therapy. However, she is unlikely to respond to endocrine manipulations such as hormonal therapy or oophorectomy because her tumor is hormone receptor negative and she is premenopausal. Liver metastases do not respond well to hormonal therapy. Patients like B.W. who are symptomatic and unlikely to benefit from hormonal therapy should receive combination chemotherapy.

Most antitumor agents have some degree of activity against breast cancer, a tumor generally considered to be chemosensitive.[28–32] Several combination regimens that have been widely used in advanced breast cancer are listed in Chapter 88.

Response rates to combination chemotherapy regimens in metastatic disease in patients who have not received prior chemotherapy are high (approximately 50% to 80%). Unfortunately, the response rates to chemotherapy in patients who have had prior exposure to chemotherapy are low. Although doxorubicin is considered one of the most active agents against breast cancer, the overall response rate to chemotherapy in patients who have had prior doxorubicin is only 20% to 30%. The taxanes, paclitaxel and docetaxel, are approved for treatment of breast cancer after failure of combination chemotherapy for metastatic disease or relapse within 6 months of adjuvant chemotherapy. Prior therapy should have included an anthracycline, unless clinically contraindicated. Sixty percent response rates to single-agent paclitaxel (250 mg/m²) and docetaxel (100 mg/m²) have been reported in patients who developed metastatic disease 12 or more months following adjuvant chemotherapy with cyclophosphamide, methotrexate, and 5-fluorouracil (CMF) or cyclophosphamide, Adriamycin (doxorubicin), and fluorouracil (CAF).[33,34]

B.W. had received an anthracycline-containing regimen followed by paclitaxel in the adjuvant setting only a few months before the relapse of her breast cancer. This suggests that her disease is resistant to these drugs. Consequently, further therapy with these drugs is unlikely to produce a significant response. Now that she has metastatic disease and she has a HER-2/neu positive tumor, she would be a candidate for trastuzumab in combination with chemotherapy. In the largest trial of trastuzumab in patients with HER-2/neu-positive untreated metastatic breast cancer, trastuzumab plus chemotherapy prolonged the median time to disease progression and median response duration, increased the overall response rate, and improved overall survival time.[35] The greatest improvement was seen in patients receiving the combination of trastuzumab and paclitaxel. Since B.W. has already received paclitaxel, regimens consisting of other active agents with trastuzumab such as vinorelbine is a reasonable choice for B.W. at this time. Weekly trastuzumab and vinorelbine resulted in an 84% response rate in patients receiving this regimen as first-line therapy for metastatic disease.[36] An additional option would be the use of docetaxel in combination with trastuzumab, since several clinical trials have reported that approximately 20% of patients who have received prior treatment with paclitaxel will respond to single-agent docetaxel. Thus, the combination of trastuzumab and docetaxel would also be a possible alternative for B.W.

SPINAL CORD COMPRESSION

9. **If B.W.'s myelogram had indicated impending spinal cord compression, what therapy would have been appropriate?**

Bone pain in patients with breast cancer without evidence of epidural spinal cord compression should be treated first with systemic chemotherapy, as suggested for B.W. Radiation therapy may be added later if systemic treatment is not effective in relieving symptoms. Compression of the spinal cord by expansion of the tumor or fracture of the vertebrae can result in paralysis and anal sphincter dysfunction. If a potential compression is impending, high-dose steroids (e.g., dexamethasone 10 mg every 6 hours orally or IV then titrated for maximum response) should be initiated immediately followed by radiation therapy. Steroids decrease edema and inflammation around the tumor mass and contribute to pain relief. In some instances, steroid therapy also may produce some cytotoxic effect.[37,38]

Postmenopausal Women
Hormonal Therapy
ESTROGEN AND PROGESTERONE RECEPTORS

10. **M.L., a 68-year-old woman with breast cancer, underwent a modified radical mastectomy followed by radiation therapy 7 years ago. At that time she had been postmenopausal for approximately 10 years, and her tumor was documented to have high concentrations of both estrogen and progesterone receptors. She remained disease-free until recently when she was found to have bone metastases in her left scapula and several ribs. No other sites of disease involvement were identified. Her only symptom is shoulder pain. Would it be appropriate to treat M.L. with endocrine therapy at this time?**

Breast cancer is one of the few human tumors that may be very sensitive to hormonal manipulations; however, it is also well recognized that only a subset of patients with breast cancer respond to the various endocrine therapies. Patients with tumors that are potentially endocrine-sensitive can be identified by measuring estrogen and progesterone receptors in the tumor tissue. Patients whose tumors are positive for both estrogen receptors (ER+) and progesterone receptors (PR+) have a much higher response rate to endocrine therapy than patients without either receptor (approximately 70% versus 10%). Patients with ER+, PR− tumors have an intermediate response rate (30%).[39] Patients with endocrine-responsive tumors also are reported to have longer disease-free intervals after initial surgery, such as M.L. experienced.[39,40] In addition, they may have a longer survival after the documentation of metastatic disease. M.L.'s tumor was strongly ER+ and PR+ and she had a long disease-free interval (7 years); therefore, she is likely to respond to endocrine therapy.

Endocrine Therapy and Bisphosphonates

11. **M.L. starts letrozole 2.5 mg PO QD and zoledronic acid 4 mg IV monthly. Is this a reasonable approach?**

Hormonal agents, including antiestrogen (e.g., tamoxifen, toremifene) and aromatase inhibitors (e.g., anastrozole, letrozole), are equally effective for the initial treatment of endocrine-responsive breast cancer. However, until recently antiestrogens were generally considered first-line endocrine therapy. Trials have now shown that the aromatase inhibitors, anastrazole and letrozole, are just as efficacious as tamoxifen as initial therapy and generally are better tolerated.[41,42]

Following the initiation of endocrine therapy, it usually takes 4 to 6 weeks before the therapeutic response can be assessed. In patients like M.L. with only bone metastases, assessment may be difficult because it may take 4 to 6 months to re-ossify the involved bones. In such cases, the decision to continue therapy may be based on the lessening of bone pain and disease stabilization (i.e., no new metastatic sites).

Bone metastases occur frequently in metastatic breast cancer and they are associated with significant pain, hypercalcemia, and fracture. Current guidelines support the use of bisphosphonates in women with radiographic evidence of bony metastases.[43] In these patients, pamidronate has been shown to significantly reduce pain, hypercalcemia, and pathologic fractures.[44] More recently, zoledronic acid 4 mg was shown to be as effective and well tolerated as pamidronate 90 mg in the treatment of osteolytic and mixed bony metastases in patients with advanced cancer or multiple myeloma.[45] The advantage of zoledronic acid over pamidronate is that therapy can be administered as a 15-minute infusion versus a 2-hour infusion. Therefore, M.L. should begin zoledronic acid therapy.[43]

DISEASE PROGRESSION

12. Over the next 18 months, M.L. continues letrozole therapy and has a complete resolution of her shoulder pain with considerable improvement of the radiographs and no appearance of new lesions. She is now experiencing left hip pain and a bone scan documented new metastatic disease. What therapy should be considered at this time?

M.L. had a good initial response to letrozole, so she is likely to respond again to another type of endocrine therapy. Exemestane is an irreversible nonsteroidal aromatase inhibitor that has been shown to be effective as second line therapy.[46] Tamoxifen, an antiestrogen, could also be utilized. The nonsteroidal aromatase inhibitors (anastrazole, letrozole, and exemestane) inhibit the conversion of androgens to estrogens and have far greater selectivity and potency than the previously recommended aromatase inhibitor, aminoglutethimide. The major advantage of these drugs is their improved toxicity profile, which is limited to mild nausea, hot flashes, and fatigue. Also, supplemental corticosteroids are not required as they were with aminoglutethimide. Megestrol can be considered as a third-line hormonal therapy in doses of 160 to 320 mg daily. Radiation therapy also may provide M.L. with palliative relief of pain. If M.L. had rapidly worsening disease involving a visceral organ, such as the liver, or if she had not responded well to prior endocrine therapy, cytotoxic chemotherapy may have been more appropriate.

COLON CANCER
Screening

13. E.R., a 55-year-old man, is undergoing his first physical examination in >10 years because he has noted a change in his bowel habits recently. His father died of colorectal cancer 2 months ago. E.R. questions whether his risk is increased and if there is anything that he can do to prevent colon cancer or decrease his risk of dying from it.

Colorectal cancer is the second leading cause of cancer deaths in the U.S. adult population.[1] Multiple risk factors are well recognized and include family history; age older than 50 years; high-fat, low-fiber diet; obesity; chronic inflammatory bowel disease; and a personal history of colorectal polyps or cancer. Several hereditary syndromes are recognized that place persons at an extremely high risk, such as hereditary nonpolyposis colorectal cancer (HNPCC or Lynch's syndrome) and familial adenomatous polyposis (FAP).[47] The American Society of Clinical Oncology currently recommends genetic testing for those at high risk.[48]

Evidence suggests that continuous aspirin or other nonsteroidal anti-inflammatory drug (NSAID) use may prevent the development of colorectal cancer by inhibiting cyclooxygenase (COX-2) expression.[49] Presumably, COX-2 acts as a tumor promotor in the intestine. In fact, celecoxib, a COX-2 inhibitor, is approved as an oral adjunct to usual care in patients with FAP because it was shown to reduce the number

and size of colorectal polyps in these patients.[50] Large-scale, prospective clinical trials evaluating aspirin and classic NSAIDs have revealed promising results,[51] and trials with the newer selective COX-2 inhibitors are ongoing. Other potential preventive measures include calcium supplementation[52] and a high-fiber diet.[53]

Since E.R. is older than 50 years of age and has a family history of colorectal cancer, he should undergo screening. In addition, he also has symptoms (i.e., change in bowel habits) that heighten suspicion. Current screening recommendations for colorectal cancer include fecal occult blood testing and, depending on risk, sigmoidoscopy or total colonic examination.[54]

Fecal Occult Blood Testing

14. What methods to detect fecal occult blood (FOBT) are available, and are there any advantages of one method over another?

Fecal occult blood testing increases the diagnosis of colorectal cancer to early stage disease and has been associated with a 30% reduction in colorectal cancer mortality.[54] Of the three methods used, the guaiac test is the most common, simple, and inexpensive, although newer methods may be more sensitive and specific. The guaiac test is a colorimetric test in which guaiac dye is oxidized to a bluish quinone compound in the presence of a peroxidase (e.g., hemoglobin). Foods, other substances, and medical conditions that contain or produce peroxidase activity may yield false-positive readings (Table 91-3). Conversely, large amounts of ascorbic acid may produce false-negative guaiac test results.

A second method is a quantitative test based on fluorometry of heme-derived porphyrin. During intestinal transit, hemoglobin is broken down to porphyrin. The third method is an immunochemical test (e.g., HemeSelect) that uses antiserum to human hemoglobin to detect blood in the feces. This test is very sensitive and specific; however, it does lose sensitivity if

Table 91-3 Causes of Positive Fecal Guaiac Test
Foods With Peroxidase Activity
Broccoli
Cauliflower
Turnips
Horseradish
Cabbage
Potatoes
Cucumbers
Mushrooms
Artichokes
Medications That Interfere With Fecal Blood Testing
Steroids
NSAIDs
Reserpine
Common Causes of Blood in the Stool
Colorectal cancer
Colorectal polyps
Diverticulitis
Hemorrhoids
Fissures
Proctitis
Inflammatory bowel disease

the bleeding is from the proximal colon because bacteria alter the globin.[55] The immunochemical test eliminates the need for dietary restrictions; however, there is a 24-hour delay in reading the results because an extract needs to be prepared from the stool sample. Red meat should be eliminated from the diet for 3 days before occult blood is tested using the guaiac methods and for 4 days before testing using methods based on heme-derived porphyrins.[56] Approximately 2% of persons older than 50 years of age will have a positive FOBT. Of these, 10% will be diagnosed with cancer, 30% with polyps, and the remaining 60% will have false-positive results.

PROGNOSIS

15. E.R.'s fecal occult blood tests are positive on specimens obtained on 2 consecutive days. Sigmoidoscopy revealed a 2.5-cm mass, and a biopsy of the lesion is interpreted as adenocarcinoma of the colon. Surgical resection of the mass and regional lymph nodes is performed. The tumor is confined to the bowel wall, although four regional lymph nodes show evidence of tumor involvement. Distant metastases of the tumor are not evident at this time, and his colon cancer is staged as Dukes C2. E.R.'s physical examination is otherwise unremarkable and all laboratory values are within normal limits except for an elevated lactate dehydrogenase (LDH) and a carcinoembryonic antigen (CEA) level of 647 ng/mL (normal, <5 ng/mL) before the surgical procedure. What is the prognosis for stage C2 colon cancer? Could earlier detection have improved the prognosis?

When colorectal cancer is diagnosed in the early stages, it is curable with surgical intervention and >90% of patients survive 5 years. The 5-year survival rate declines to 30% to 40% in patients like E.R. with stage C disease. The Dukes staging system is most commonly used for colon cancer. Stage A indicates penetration into but not through the bowel wall. Stage B indicates penetration through the bowel wall, and stage C indicates lymph node involvement. Patients with early-stage colorectal cancer often are asymptomatic; therefore, intensive screening programs as just described are advocated to reduce the mortality of this disease. Sixty percent to 90% of patients with metastatic and recurrent colorectal cancer have elevated CEA or CA-19-9 levels. Levels are elevated in relation to the stage and extent of disease, the degree of tumor differentiation, and the site of metastases. If the CEA level is elevated at the time of initial diagnosis, as in E.R., it can be monitored after surgical resection of the tumor for evidence of recurrent disease.[57]

Treatment
Adjuvant Therapy

16. All evidence of tumor is removed, and E.R.'s CEA level declines. Therefore, the surgery may be considered potentially curable. Should E.R. receive any additional therapy at this time?

Tumor recurrence is a significant problem associated with stage C colon and rectal cancers, with up to 60% of all surgically treated patients eventually having local recurrences.[58,59] Causes of these relapses may include peritoneal seeding caused by exfoliation of tumor cells in the colonic lumen and spillage during surgery. Most tumor recurrences are secondary to either disease spread to the regional lymph nodes or extension of the tumor into the bowel wall, with subsequent

hematogenous dissemination. Metastasis to the liver via hematogenous spread (through the portal circulation) is the most common site of disease spread beyond the regional lymph nodes and occurs in 50% of patients with invasive disease.[60] Lung metastases (without liver metastases) occur rarely and generally are associated with lesions in the lower rectum.

Because of the significant relapse rate in patients with stage C and high-risk stage B colon cancer, adjuvant chemotherapy has been extensively studied and shown to improve disease-free survival (DFS) in those patients, such as E.R., who have had "potentially curative surgery."[61–64] Currently, fluorouracil (FU) plus leucovorin given for 6 months is effective in reducing disease recurrence,[61–64] improving 3-year DFS by 10% to 15%. The shorter 6-month regimens with FU and leucovorin currently have greater acceptance than the 12-month regimens. Toxicities, such as leukopenia, severe diarrhea, and stomatitis, are associated with these regimens. In summary, adjuvant chemotherapy is recommended for all patients with stage C disease and for high-risk patients with stage B disease. E.R. begins adjuvant therapy with FU and leucovorin 3 weeks after surgery. The regimen consists of FU 425 mg/m^2 per day plus leucovorin 20 mg/m^2 for 5 consecutive days repeated every 4 weeks for 6 months.

Follow-Up Care

17. Within 6 months after surgery, E.R.'s CEA level has fallen to <2.5 ng/mL and he completes the adjuvant therapy without serious sequelae. What follow-up care is recommended at this time?

E.R. continues to be at significant risk for developing recurrent disease. If recurrences are detected early, it is possible to cure them with additional surgery. In most cases, patients with early recurrences are asymptomatic; therefore, an active follow-up program is necessary to detect them, including history, physical examination, and CEA levels every 3 months for the first 3 years, then every 6 months for 2 years, and then annually.[57] Colonoscopy is repeated annually for several years and then every 3 to 5 years. He should receive a chest radiograph annually or when prompted by an elevated CEA or symptoms. Additional tests, such as abdominal and pelvic CT scans and liver function chemistries, should be done if routine tests are abnormal or if symptoms are suggestive of recurrent disease.[57]

Recurrent Disease
Rising Carcinoembryonic Antigen Level

18. Eighteen months after completing adjuvant chemotherapy, E.R. returns for routine follow-up; his CEA levels are elevated. What is the significance of a rising CEA level?

Although widespread serum CEA level monitoring is not an efficient way to screen for colorectal cancer in the general population, a rising CEA level in a patient with a history of colorectal cancer may be the first indication of recurrent disease if the patient had an elevated CEA level at the time of original diagnosis. Generally, the CEA level is measured every 2 to 4 months for 3 years and then every 6 months for 2 years.[57] More than 50% of patients who have recurrent disease also have elevated CEA levels.

Chemotherapy

19. On a routine follow-up visit several months later, a CT scan of E.R.'s abdomen shows that the disease in his colon has recurred and the liver CT shows two discrete nodules that are consistent with metastatic disease; however, E.R. is feeling well and has no symptoms suggestive of metastases. What is the role of further chemotherapy now that E.R. has recurrent disease?

Various approaches using chemotherapy have been employed to manage patients with advanced colorectal cancer. These include single-agent therapy (fluorouracil, irinotecan, oxaliplatin, capecitabine), combination chemotherapy, and hepatic intra-arterial administration of chemotherapy agents to treat localized liver metastases. Factors that appear to influence response include the sites and extent of metastases, and the patient's performance status.

FLUOROURACIL

The lack of active agents in the treatment of colorectal cancer in the past has resulted in extensive investigations of fluorouracil (FU) and FU-based combinations. Multiple doses and schedules of administration of 5-FU have been investigated. The most promising systemic regimen thus far is the biochemical modulation of FU with the reduced folate, leucovorin.[65–67] Fluorouracil exerts its cytotoxic activity by inhibiting thymidylate synthase, which ultimately results in the inhibition of DNA synthesis. In vitro tests have shown that by increasing the intracellular concentration of a reduced folate, the formation of a stable complex of the FU metabolite (FUMP), the reduced folate, and the thymidylate synthase will be favored, thus augmenting the cytotoxicity of FU by blocking further steps toward DNA synthesis.[64–67] Numerous FU and leucovorin regimens (variations in schedule, dose, and route of administration) have been studied in metastatic colorectal cancer, and some have been associated with improved survival when compared with untreated controls. A French study evaluated a monthly regimen of intravenous leucovorin 20 mg/m² plus bolus FU 425 mg/m² for 5 days every 4 weeks versus a bimonthly regimen of intravenous leucovorin 200 mg/m² as a 2-hour infusion followed by a 5-FU bolus of 400 mg/m² and a 22-hour continuous infusion of FU 600 mg/m² for 2 consecutive days every 2 weeks.[68] The bimonthly regimen that included the continuous infusion FU was more effective and less toxic than the monthly regimen; however, there was no evidence of increased survival. A meta-analysis of the randomized clinical trials confirmed the benefit of continuous infusion administration over bolus administration of FU.[69] Tumor response and overall survival was significantly higher in patients receiving FU by continuous infusion than in patients receiving FU by bolus administration. Grade 3 or 4 hematologic toxicity was more frequent in patients assigned to FU bolus, whereas hand-foot syndrome was more frequent in patients who received FU by continuous infusion.[69]

IRINOTECAN

Irinotecan, a semisynthetic derivative of the natural alkaloid camptothecin, inhibits topoisomerase I function by binding to the DNA-topoisomerase cleavable complex. Irinotecan became commercially available based on its activity as second-line therapy for patients previously treated for colorectal cancer with FU.[70,71] The demonstrated benefits for irinotecan as second-line therapy led to the evaluation of the combination of FU, leucovorin, and irinotecan (IFL) as first-line therapy.[72,73] Two phase III trials showed the superiority of the new combination regimen IFL over FU and leucovorin (IFL) alone; median survival significantly improved. However, diarrhea was more significant in the regimens containing irinotecan,[72,73] and when the FU was administered as a continuous infusion with irinotecan,[73] there was more toxicity than with FU alone. More serious toxicity, including an unexpected number of deaths occurring within the first 60 days of therapy was identified in another trial involving IFL.[74] These data were evaluated by a panel of experienced investigators who determined that the death rate was not excessive. Nevertheless, they recommended close monitoring, holding therapy in the presence of unresolved drug-related toxicity, and aggressive use of antidiarrhea medications and antibiotics.[74]

OXALIPLATIN

Oxaliplatin is a new third-generation cisplatin analog with significant activity against advanced colorectal cancer and in vitro synergistic action with FU. Various doses, schedules, and combinations have been evaluated. Oxaliplatin 85 to 130 mg/m² administered IV plus FU as a 2-hour infusion followed by a 22-hour continuous infusion and leucovorin (referred to as FOLFOX) has produced response rates of 11% to 15% in patients previously treated with IFL for refractory metastatic colorectal cancer.[75–77] This finding resulted in FDA approval of oxaliplatin for use in combination with FU and leucovorin as second-line therapy of patients with colorectal cancer previously treated with irinotecan, FU, and leucovorin. Several trials have assessed the impact of FOLFOX as first-line therapy for metastatic colorectal cancer; it was recently approved as a first-line agent in combination with infusional FU and leucovorin.[78,79]

Unlike cisplatin, oxaliplatin does not cause significant nephrotoxicity or hearing loss. Neurotoxicity (peripheral neuropathy plus cold sensory dysesthesias) occurs and peripheral neuropathy is associated with the cumulative dose. Cold sensory dysesthesias commonly occur early in treatment and are completely reversible after treatment withdrawal.[80]

ORAL FLUOROPYRIMIDINES

Several pharmaceutical manufacturers are vigorously pursuing the development of orally administered fluoropyrimidines that maintain or improve the effectiveness of intravenous FU. Administration of oral fluoropyrimidines may mimic the pharmacokinetics of continuous infusion FU. Capecitabine, a fluoropyrimidine carbonate, is the only oral fluorinated pyrimidine commercially available for the treatment of metastatic colorectal cancer. Capecitabine's pharmacologic advantage is that it passes through the intestine as an intact molecule and is thereafter converted to fluorouracil by thymidine phosphorylase in tumor cells. Since levels of the activating enzyme are higher in tumor cells than normal cells, capecitabine is intended to provide selective improvement in the therapeutic index of FU.[81]

The effectiveness of capecitabine has been compared with bolus FU and leucovorin[82,83] in two large phase III trials but not with FU administered by infusion. As first line chemotherapy for metastatic colorectal cancer, capecitabine yielded higher objective response rates and equivalent median time to progression and overall survival as FU/leucovorin. Additionally, patients experienced lower rates of diarrhea, stomatitis, nausea, and severe neutropenia with capecitabine than FU/leucovorin, but a higher rate of hyperbilirubinemia and hand-foot syndrome. Phase II trials of capecitabine with irinotecan and oxaliplatin in patients with advanced disease indicate that the combinations produce response rates similar to those expected with FU/leucovorin delivered by infusion in combination with these agents.[84,85] Ongoing phase III trials in advanced disease and the adjuvant setting will further define the role of capecitabine combined with irinotecan or oxaliplatin in the treatment of colorectal cancer. Currently, capecitabine is indicated as first-line treatment for patients with metastatic colorectal cancer when treatment with fluoropyrimidine therapy alone is preferred. Documented interactions have resulted in the warning that patients receiving concomitant capecitabine and oral coumarin-derivative anticoagulant therapy should have their anticoagulant response (INR or prothrombin time) monitored frequently to adjust the anticoagulant dose.

Hepatic Metastases

Surgical resection, if possible, is the most effective treatment modality for potential long-term survival in colorectal patients with liver metastases. However, because the liver is the most common site of metastatic colorectal cancer, many patients could potentially benefit from effective therapy for hepatic metastases. These tumors derive most of their blood supply from the hepatic artery, and direct administration of effective anticancer drugs into the hepatic artery provides high drug concentrations to the area of tumor involvement.[86] Hepatic intra-arterial administration of FU, FUDR, or other chemotherapeutic agents also has been extensively studied in patients with metastases confined to the liver.

Hepatic Intra-Arterial Chemotherapy

20. **J.D. is a 59-year-old patient with metastatic colorectal cancer limited to a single 2- to 3-cm nodule in his liver. He underwent a laparotomy during which the hepatic artery was canalized and an Infusaid pump implanted. No additional sites of metastases were observed. He subsequently received a continuous hepatic arterial infusion of FUDR 0.2 mg/kg per day for 14 days every 28 days. What are the characteristics of a drug administered by this route? Does this method of drug delivery produce increased antitumor effects over conventional intravenous infusions?**

Optimal characteristics for a drug to be administered by this method should include the following: (1) efficacy against colorectal carcinoma, (2) high extraction by the liver, and (3) rapid clearance of the drug once it reaches systemic circulation. Therefore, FUDR is a logical agent because 95% of the dose is extracted by the liver and it has a half-life of approximately 20 minutes when it does reach the systemic circulation.

Initial uncontrolled trials using intrahepatic FUDR reported response rates of 29% to 88%, suggesting that this mode of therapy may be superior to conventional systemic therapy.[86,87] Several randomized trials of intravenous versus hepatic intra-arterial FUDR administration have been completed. Intra-arterial FUDR consistently produced significantly higher response rates (complete plus partial responses) than intravenous administration (40% to 60% versus 10% to 20%); however, survival has not been improved with intrahepatic chemotherapy alone in the major trials. A recent trial using intrahepatic FUDR and dexamethasone plus systemic FU and leucovorin compared to systemic FU and leucovorin alone resulted in a 2-year survival advantage for the combination of intrahepatic and systemic chemotherapy.[88] To date, no trials have been reported using intrahepatic chemotherapy and systemic irinotecan or oxaliplatin combinations.

FUDR TOXICITY

21. **Are the toxicities produced by intra-arterial FUDR similar to those commonly associated with intravenous FUDR? What follow-up monitoring is recommended?**

Toxicities associated with FUDR (and FU) therapy depend on the dose, route, and schedule of administration. When administered by intravenous bolus injections each week, the dose-limiting toxicity is usually myelosuppression. However, when the dose is given as a continuous intravenous infusion over several days, the dose-limiting toxicities are mucositis and diarrhea. If these toxicities begin during therapy, the decision may be made to discontinue the infusion before completion to avoid life-threatening toxicity. Nausea and vomiting associated with FU or FUDR are dose related and generally only mild to moderate in severity. Dermatologic changes are more commonly associated with continuous infusion therapy and include alopecia, onycholysis, acral erythema (erythema of the hands and feet), and dermatitis.

In contrast, the dose-limiting toxicities associated with intra-arterial infusions are generally hepatic or gastrointestinal in nature. Cumulative FUDR-associated hepatobiliary toxicity, which can progress to biliary sclerosis and liver failure, has been related both to the total dose administered and the duration of therapy.[89] The initial sign of hepatic toxicity is usually an elevation of alkaline phosphatase and when this occurs, the dosage should be reduced or treatment interrupted until normalization occurs. Failure to do so may result in severe jaundice, chemical cholecystitis and eventual biliary sclerosis.[89,90] Patients also may experience transient increases in AST and LDH. Gastritis and gastric ulcers also have been associated with intra-arterial FUDR therapy. This probably is related to inadvertent perfusion of the gastric artery.

Before initiating therapy, E.R. should have a baseline CT scan of the liver and LFTs. Physical examination and LFTs should be repeated before and after each course of therapy. Although myelosuppression is unusual following intra-arterial FUDR, E.R. also should have a CBC done periodically. Serum chemistries also should be evaluated before each course.

Embolization

22. **Is chemo-embolization the same technique as intra-arterial chemotherapy? Would E.R. benefit from this therapy? Is E.R. a candidate for chemo-embolization?**

Embolization is a technique that involves deliberate obstruction of the artery that supplies blood to the tumor site. This procedure produces tumor necrosis, but also necrosis of the organ in which the tumor is located. Because the liver has a dual blood supply, a tumor can be embolized through the hepatic artery while the parenchyma is sustained by portal venous inflow. Chemo-embolization combines intra-arterial chemotherapy with obstruction of the vasculature, thereby prolonging the exposure of the tumor to the drug. Typical complications include pain; elevated liver enzymes; and rarely, infection, adhesions, infarctions, and abscesses. Patients who are candidates for this type of therapy include people like E.R. whose tumors are confined to the liver. Although this type of therapy is promising, it is not clear if survival is significantly improved.[91]

LUNG CANCER
Clinical Presentation

23. H.H., a 57-year-old, white woman with a 6-month history of weight loss and increasing fatigue, recently noted shortness of breath (SOB) and fever. She also complains of joint pain in her knees and elbows and has noted a change in her fingers and nails over the past several months. Physical examination is significant for swelling and tenderness over her knees and elbows as well as hypertrophy and clubbing of the distal joints of both hands. A chest radiograph and CT scan reveals a central mass causing obstruction of the middle right lobe as well as mediastinal lymphadenopathy. Bronchoscopy washings and cytology were positive for small cell lung carcinoma. H.H. denied exposure to any environmental or occupational carcinogens but did admit to a 40-pack/year history of cigarette smoking. Are H.H.'s symptoms typical of those associated with lung cancer?

Signs and symptoms associated with lung cancer depend on the size and location of the tumor and degree of spread outside of the lungs. The most common symptoms at presentation are those associated with the primary tumor and include cough, wheezing, chest pain, hemoptysis, and dyspnea.[92,93] However, because many patients have other medical problems, such as chronic obstructive airway disease related to cigarette smoking, the worsening of these symptoms may go unnoticed for a period or may be attributed to other smoking-related illnesses. A large tumor may result in obstruction, leading to fever and other evidence of pneumonia.

Regional spread to lymph nodes and other structures within the thorax may result in dysphagia, superior vena cava obstruction, pleural effusion, and hoarseness. Patients with distant metastatic spread may have findings associated with the site of disease involvement. For example, if the tumor has spread to the liver, patients are likely to have elevated LFTs, or if they have brain metastases, severe headache, neurologic impairment, or seizures may be present.

In addition, lung cancers often are associated with distant or paraneoplastic syndromes. Almost one-third of patients with lung cancer present with anorexia and weight loss.[92,93] Hypertrophic osteoarthropathy, with inflammation of the outer covering of bones and clubbing, can cause pain, tenderness, and swelling over the affected bones such as that experienced by H.H. This often mimics bone metastases (bone scans also may be positive); however, further studies will reveal no evidence of direct tumor involvement of the bones. Other paraneoplastic syndromes commonly seen in patients with lung cancer include ectopic Cushing's syndrome and the

syndrome of inappropriate antidiuretic hormone secretion (SIADH). Characteristically, paraneoplastic syndromes improve after successful treatment of the tumor.

Prevalence and Risk Factors

24. How common is lung cancer and what factors place H.H. at risk?

The American Cancer Society estimates that 169,400 new cases of lung cancer will be diagnosed in 2003. Although the World Health Organization recognizes that there are >10 types of primary pleuropulmonary malignancies, four major types of carcinomas account for up to 95% of all lung cancers.[92,93]

The relative prevalence of the four major types are as follows: epidermoid carcinoma (also called squamous cell carcinoma), 30%; adenocarcinomas, 25% to 40%; large cell carcinomas, 15%; and small cell carcinomas, 15%.[92,93] Commonly, the first three are grouped together and referred to as non–small cell lung cancers (NSCLC) because they are similar in prognosis and response to therapy.

Cigarette smoking is the predominant cause of lung cancer worldwide, and the risk appears to increase with the number of cigarettes smoked each day.[94] Approximately 75% to 80% of lung cancer cases are attributable to smoking.[94] Although the risk of developing any type of lung cancer increases with cigarette smoking, the relative risk of small cell lung cancer (SCLC) is among the highest.[93] Therefore, patients such as H.H. who have a long history of cigarette smoking have the highest risk of developing lung cancer relative to any other population. Other risk factors for lung cancer include exposure to passive smoke (i.e., nonsmokers who live with smokers); pipe and cigar smoking; and exposure to asbestos, radon, or other occupational carcinogens such as heavy metals, chloromethyl ether, and arsenic.[95,96]

Prevention and Screening

25. What are the current recommendations for prevention and screening for early detection of lung cancer in patients like H.H.?

By far, the most important intervention for preventing lung cancer is to avoid or cease smoking and to avoid secondary smoke whenever possible. Antioxidants and β-carotene have no protective effect, and in at least two large trials, there was an increase in lung cancer in persons receiving β-carotene.[97,98] Secondary analysis in a trial of selenium for the prevention of skin cancer revealed a significant reduction in the occurrence of lung cancer,[99] but definitive trials are still in progress.

Unfortunately, no specific recommendations for lung cancer screening have affected overall mortality. In the early 1970s, the National Cancer Institute (NCI) launched three studies evaluating sputum cytology and chest radiography as lung cancer screening tests. Patients at the Johns Hopkins Hospital in Baltimore and Memorial Sloan-Kettering Cancer Center in New York received annual chest radiography, and every 4 months their sputum cytology was evaluated. At the Mayo Clinic, the control group received only standard medical advice and the treatment group was screened as just described. Even though cancers were detected earlier, the overall mortality rates in the two groups did not differ significantly.[100,101]

Since the time of these studies, the quality of diagnostic testing has been substantially enhanced and there are many new, more effective therapies; therefore, new screening studies, especially for high-risk populations are underway. Spiral computed tomography (CT) is a promising but unproven technology for lung cancer screening.[102] Ongoing trials will better determine its role in the evaluation of patients at high-risk for lung cancer.

SMALL CELL LUNG CANCER VERSUS NON–SMALL CELL LUNG CANCER

26. How do treatment and prognoses for SCLC and NSCLC differ?

The natural history and response to treatment of patients with SCLC and NSCLC differ significantly. Therefore, it is extremely important to establish a histologic diagnosis before contemplating treatment. In general, the NSCLCs are less likely to metastasize early in the course of the disease and are less sensitive to chemotherapy than SCLCs. In contrast, SCLC progresses rapidly, but is sensitive to many chemotherapeutic agents.

Surgery is curative only in early stages of NSCLC.[92] Radiation therapy may be considered an alternative for patients who are poor surgical risks. Radiotherapy also is used as an adjuvant therapy to surgery to treat NSCLC characterized by large tumors or extensive lymph node involvement; however, no survival advantage has been observed with the addition of radiation therapy.[103] In advanced stages of NSCLC, overall response rates to combination chemotherapy are 20% to 40%, with fewer than 5% of patients achieving a complete response.[104,105] The highest response rates for chemotherapy in NSCLC have been achieved with regimens using cisplatin or carboplatin combined with etoposide, paclitaxel, docetaxel, vinorelbine, and gemcitabine.

SCLC is staged as "limited" (stages I to III) or "extensive." Limited-stage disease is confined to one hemithorax and can be encompassed within one radiation port. Because SCLC disseminates early in the disease, surgery is almost never indicated. The only exception is the rare patient who presents with very early stage disease. Such patients may benefit by resection of the tumor followed by combination chemotherapy. Overall, the use of combination chemotherapy regimens for SCLC has increased median survival by fourfold to fivefold.[93] In disease limited to the thoracic cavity, optimal chemotherapy regimens produce response rates of 85% to 95%, with 50% to 60% of patients achieving a complete response. Although many patients initially respond to therapy, most eventually relapse and die from their SCLC. The median duration of survival is 12 to 16 months and the 2-year DFS rate is usually 15% to 20% for patients with limited disease. Response rates are somewhat lower for patients with disease outside the thoracic cavity and the median survival is only 7 to 11 months. The 2-year DFS for these patients is <2%.[93]

Small Cell Lung Cancer
Staging

27. What information, in addition to the histologic type, is necessary before H.H.'s treatment can be initiated?

Before initiating therapy, the stage of H.H.'s disease should be evaluated. This will help establish a prognosis and identify tumor lesions that can be monitored to evaluate the response to therapy. Staging also will assist in determining if H.H. will benefit from radiation therapy in addition to chemotherapy. Because the tumor node metastasis (TNM) staging factors do not appear to correlate with survival, a simple two-stage system is used for SCLC. Limited disease is defined as that confined to one hemithorax and the regional lymph nodes, whereas extensive disease is that which extends beyond the thorax. Staging procedures should include a thorough workup of any areas that are suspicious for tumor involvement, a chest radiograph and CT scans, a CBC, LFTs, physical examination of the liver, and a neurologic examination. In addition, H.H.'s physiologic and performance status should be assessed to determine her ability to tolerate the aggressive chemotherapy and possible radiation therapy. This includes evaluation of her nutritional, cardiac, and pulmonary status. Renal and hepatic function also should be evaluated to determine if chemotherapy elimination is normal.

Cancer Cachexia

28. Results of H.H.'s staging procedures determined that she had limited-stage SCLC. However, her body weight is 25% below her ideal weight and her serum albumin is 3.0 g/dL (normal, 3.5 to 4.5 g/dL). H.H. states that she has little appetite and has not been eating much for several months. Her oncologist is concerned because chemotherapy is likely to worsen H.H.'s anorexia. Are H.H.'s anorexia and weight loss related to her cancer? Should chemotherapy be withheld until the anorexia is corrected? Can anything be done to stimulate her appetite?

[SI units: albumin, 30 g/L (normal, 35 to 45)]

Malnutrition is a common complication of cancer. Weight loss and poor nutritional status do not necessarily correlate with tumor histology, disease stage, or absolute caloric intake. The syndrome of cancer cachexia is complex and multifactorial and, ultimately, effective therapy for the tumor results in successful treatment of the cachexia. Therefore, H.H. should receive chemotherapy.

CAUSES
Cancer cachexia has many causes and is common in cancer, occurring in up to 80% of patients with gastrointestinal tumors and 60% of those with lung cancer at the time of diagnosis. The most obvious causes include mechanical alterations caused by the tumor mass or complications from treatment that result in the loss or failure of organ function (e.g., liver, GI tract), infections, or tissue damage (e.g., stomatitis, esophagitis). Frequently, patients with cancer have taste alterations, such as a decreased tolerance to sweetness, an aversion to meat, and an increase in the tolerability of salty and sour foods.[106,107] These taste abnormalities usually resolve following effective treatment of the tumor. Psychologic factors also can cause or contribute to anorexia in the cancer patient. Emotional stress can stimulate the release of catecholamines, which have a negative effect on appetite. Depression and food aversions that were learned during emetogenic chemotherapy also influence appetite.

Cancer cachexia cannot always be readily attributed to reduced caloric intake secondary to these factors. Even in advanced disease, the tumor mass is only a small percentage of the patient's total body weight, and it is unlikely that it competes with the host for sources of energy to the point of starvation. Changes in plasma protein concentrations and alterations in metabolic rates also occur in cancer patients.[108] Current biological evidence supports theories that center on the immune effects of cancer as etiological factors in the development of primary cachexia.[109] Cytokines are the most frequently implicated mediators of cachexia.[110] Tumor necrosis factor, interleukin-1, interleukin-6, interferon, and 24K proteoglycan have all been identified as cytokines that contribute to the cachectic process.[110] Cachectin (also called tumor necrosis factor [TNF]) is reported to cause anorexia and to alter the activity of adipocyte lipogenic enzymes.[111]

MANAGEMENT

Calorie supplements and alternate feeding methods may play a supportive role when anorexia, nausea, and vomiting limit administration of appropriate treatment for the underlying malignancy. High-dose megestrol acetate increases appetite and produces weight gain in cancer patients. Tchekmedyian and others reported significant weight gain in patients with advanced breast cancer who received 480 to 1,600 mg/day orally. Weight gain occurred regardless of pretreatment weight, response of the breast cancer, or the extent of disease spread.[112] Megestrol acetate or one of its metabolites may exert an effect at the cellular level to enhance appetite and metabolic activity.[113] Dronabinol or delta-9-tetrahydrocannabinol (Marinol) can stimulate appetite and weight gain in patients with AIDS.[114] The doses of dronabinol used in these trials (5 to 10 mg twice daily) are lower than those used for chemotherapy-induced emesis, and side effects were rare. Hydrazine sulfate is thought to augment appetite and retard weight loss through the inhibition of phosphoenolpyruvate kinase. However, controlled trials have failed to demonstrate any benefit.[115,116]

Chemotherapy: Small Cell Lung Cancer
Combination Chemotherapy

29. **H.H. is to start a chemotherapeutic regimen of cisplatin 100 mg/m² IV on day 1 and etoposide 100 mg/m² IV on days 1 through 3. The chemotherapy is to be repeated every 28 days. She also will receive radiation therapy to the area of tumor involvement. Is H.H. likely to benefit from the addition of other cytotoxic agents to her regimen?**

Although combination chemotherapy is clearly superior to single-agent therapy in the treatment of SCLC, there are no major differences between several combination chemotherapy regimens that have been widely studied when compared for response rate or survival.[117] Most current first-line regimens include cisplatin or carboplatin in combination with etoposide. Other active agents for SCLC include topotecan, paclitaxel, docetaxel, ifosfamide, cyclophosphamide, teniposide, doxorubicin, vincristine, and methotrexate.

Cisplatin has only modest activity as a single agent in SCLC patients who have failed prior therapy. However, its synergistic activity with etoposide in experimental systems has led to the evaluation of this combination in many human tumors, including SCLC. Early trials of the cisplatin and etoposide regimen in patients with refractory SCLC produced

encouraging reports and led to its evaluation as first-line therapy.[118] Carboplatin appears to be as efficacious as cisplatin and is frequently used in combinations.

Etoposide Capsules

30. **Can oral etoposide be substituted for the intravenous administration of this drug, and if so, are equivalent dosages used?**

Clinical trials in patients with SCLC have demonstrated that combination regimens containing oral etoposide produce results comparable with those achieved with the intravenous formulation.[119] Because the bioavailability of etoposide capsules is approximately 50%, the recommended oral dose is double the intravenous dose rounded to the nearest 50 mg.

However, because of the severe nausea and vomiting that can be caused by the cisplatin given on day 1, H.H. should receive the first dose of etoposide IV to avoid vomiting the capsules. If her vomiting is controlled by day 2, she can take the remaining doses orally. H.H. should contact her physician immediately if she experiences any vomiting.

More protracted schedules (2 to 3 weeks) of daily oral etoposide have shown activity in previously treated and newly diagnosed patients with SCLC; however, it is not known whether this schedule is superior to the schedule that H.H. will receive.[120,121]

Follow-Up Care

31. **How should H.H. be monitored during therapy?**

Approximately 80% of patients respond to initial chemotherapy for SCLC. Because this is a chemosensitive disease, people typically show evidence of response within days. Follow-up care of a patient receiving chemotherapy should include the following: (1) assessment of chemotherapy-associated toxicities (e.g., mucositis, CBC, renal function, electrolytes) so that appropriate interventions may be initiated; (2) regular re-evaluation of renal, hepatic, and bone marrow function to assess the patient's ability to tolerate further treatment; and (3) assessment of the antitumor effects of the treatment.

Myelosuppression (i.e., granulocytopenia, thrombocytopenia) is generally only moderate with cisplatin-etoposide regimens; however, the addition of radiation therapy is likely to increase its severity. Therefore, H.H. should have her CBC monitored weekly once therapy begins. Because nephrotoxicity is the usual dose-limiting toxicity of cisplatin, renal function must be evaluated.

Chest radiographs and CT scans should be repeated after every two to three courses of therapy to assess antitumor effects. Therapy should be continued if the tumor is responding to treatment and discontinued or changed if there is evidence of tumor progression.

Duration of Therapy and Prophylactic Irradiation

32. **After six courses of this regimen, repeat chest radiographs and CT scans reveal no evidence of residual tumor in H.H. A repeat bronchoscopy is also negative. Is additional treatment indicated?**

Despite the high recurrence rate for patients with SCLC who achieve a complete response, no current evidence supports prolonged administration of chemotherapy after complete response is achieved. Long-term survival rates appear to be similar for patients who receive 4 to 6 months of treatment and those who receive 12 to 24 months.[93] In addition, patients who receive a shorter duration of chemotherapy exposure are less likely to suffer major toxicities. Unfortunately, after disease recurrence, response rates to second-line therapy are only 20% to 40% with few complete responses; the median survival is only a few months. Today, the topoisomerase inhibitors topotecan or irinotecan, and the taxanes, paclitaxel or docetaxel, gemcitabine or vinorelbine are the most widely used second-line agents.

At least 20% to 25% of patients with SCLC eventually develop brain metastases, which produce significant morbidity. Clinical trials have demonstrated that prophylactic cranial irradiation significantly reduces the incidence of subsequent brain metastases in patients achieving a complete remission following chemotherapy.[122] Therefore, prophylactic cranial irradiation is recommended for patients such as H.H. who attain a complete response. She also may require antiemetics to alleviate nausea.

Non–Small Cell Lung Cancer

33. M.D., a 62-year-old man, was recently diagnosed with stage IV adenocarcinoma of the lung. His past medical history is not significant, and he is otherwise in good health. What are the current treatment recommendations?

Although NSCLC is less chemosensitive than SCLC, evidence gathered over the past decade substantiates that combination chemotherapy therapy improves median survival from 16 weeks to 26 weeks and enhances 1-year survival rates by 10% over the best supportive care. The American Society of Clinical Oncology now recommends two to eight cycles of platinum-based combination chemotherapy for patients with stage IV disease and good performance status (Eastern Cooperative Oncology Group [ECOG] 0, 1, and possibly, 2).[105] The most widely used first-line regimens include carboplatin or cisplatin plus either paclitaxel, docetaxel, vinorelbine, or gemcitabine. Some newer regimens also incorporate three of these agents. Response is generally re-evaluated after two cycles of chemotherapy, and if a response or stable disease is noted, treatment is continued for up to eight cycles. If disease progression is evident, second-line therapy with agents not previously received or palliative radiation therapy is recommended. One-year survival rates range from 25% to 40% using these newer regimens.

The novel tyrosine kinase inhibitor that acts on epidermal growth factor receptors, gefitinib, was approved by the FDA under the accelerated approval program as a single-agent treatment for patients with NSCLC who failed prior platinum and docetaxel regimens. The approval was based on the results of a study of 216 patients with NSCLC where the response rate was 10.6% with a median duration of response of 7 months.[123] The response rate was highly variable in certain subgroups, with women, those with adenocarcinoma, and nonsmokers having higher response rates. Importantly, no advantage has been shown in clinical trials by adding gefitinib to platinum-based chemotherapy; therefore, it is not indicated in this setting.

For patients with unresectable stage III disease, there have now been at least 10 major multi-institutional trials in which patients were randomized to treatment with thoracic radiation with or without platinum-based chemotherapy. There is a statistically significant survival advantage for the combined modality therapy.[124]

OVARIAN CANCER
Clinical Presentation and Risk Factors

34. C.R., a 50-year-old woman, presents to her family physician complaining of vague abdominal pain over the last several weeks. A detailed history revealed that she had experienced increasing abdominal girth without significant weight gain and a change in her usual bowel habits. The abdominal and pelvic ultrasound reveal a 6- to 10-cm mass, and her serum CA-125 antigen is significantly elevated. C.R. is then referred to a surgical gynecologist who performs a total abdominal hysterectomy and bilateral salpingo-oophorectomy. Pathologic examination of the mass determined it to be epithelial carcinoma of the ovary. The large intra-abdominal mass and numerous peritoneal tumor implants were resected during surgery; however, several small (<0.5 cm) tumor implants were not resectable. What factors are associated with an increased risk of ovarian cancer? Are C.R.'s symptoms consistent with ovarian cancer?

Ovarian cancer is the fifth most common cause of cancer and cancer deaths in women.[1] Postmenopausal women (50 to 75 years) are most likely to develop carcinoma of the ovary, whereas germ cell neoplasms are more common in younger women. Other factors that appear to increase the risk of ovarian cancer include positive family history, nulliparity or a low number of pregnancies, first child after age 35, prolonged use of ovulation-inducing drugs, and increasing age.[125] There can also be a genetic predisposition to ovarian cancer, which can be related to hereditary breast cancer. Genetic mutations in the BRCA1 and BRCA2 genes may play a role in the development of ovarian cancer.[48]

As in C.R.'s case, patients with early stages of ovarian cancer may be relatively asymptomatic. The patient's only complaint may be vague abdominal symptoms, and she may not seek medical attention until symptoms become significantly worse. Unfortunately, ovarian carcinoma usually has extended beyond the pelvis at the time of diagnosis. Pain, abdominal distention, and vaginal bleeding are the most common symptoms in patients with advanced disease.[125] Other symptoms may include weight loss, nausea, or a change in bowel or bladder habits if the tumor mass is compressing adjacent structures.

Detection and the Papanicolaou Test

35. C.R. is surprised by the diagnosis and questions why the cancer was not diagnosed earlier. She has always had routine annual physical and gynecologic examinations that included the Papanicolaou (Pap) test.

Although the Pap test is the single most successful screening test used in gynecology, it is not useful for detecting ovarian cancer.[125,126] The dramatic decrease in invasive cancers along with a 70% reduction in mortality confirms the efficacy of the Pap test as a screening tool for uterine cervical cancer.[126,127]

Although the pelvic examination is the most common method of screening for ovarian cancer, it has a low sensitivity; for every 10,000 examinations, approximately one tumor is detected.[128] Laparoscopy should not be used as a diagnostic tool for ovarian carcinoma because of the potential for spilling malignant cells into the peritoneal cavity and spreading the disease.[125]

Ovarian cancer has a low prevalence (13.8/100,000); however, women with a family history have increased risk for developing the disease. Ovarian masses may become large before they are detected because the ovaries are suspended by ligaments in a large spacious pelvic cavity. At the time of diagnosis, 75% of women with ovarian cancer have evidence of spread beyond the ovaries, and in 60%, the cancer has spread beyond the pelvis.[125] The high incidence of ovarian cancer in women with a family history emphasizes the need for an effective screening program.

Abdominal ultrasounds produce a high number of false positives, even in high-risk populations. Andolf and others used ultrasound as an adjunct to pelvic examination in 801 women ages 40 to 71 years who presented with gynecologic complaints. There were 163 patients with abnormal ultrasounds and further workup revealed only two endometrial cancers and one borderline ovarian cancer. They concluded that ultrasound does not have a role in screening for ovarian cancer.[129] Transvaginal ultrasonography produces clearer images than abdominal scanning and more accurately identifies intrapelvic disease. Currently, neither test is recommended for screening women in the general populations. Although no data indicate their value as screening tests, annual rectovaginal pelvic examinations, CA-125 determination, and transvaginal ultrasonography are often performed in high-risk women.

CA-125 is a monoclonal antibody that reacts to a tumor-specific antigen. It is the most promising of the monoclonal antibodies, but unfortunately lacks sensitivity in detecting early ovarian cancer in that it is elevated in various nonmalignant states. Elevated CA-125 levels become more sensitive as the clinical stage of ovarian cancer advances: 50% for stages 1 and 2 and 90% for stages 3 and 4.[130,131]

Chemotherapy

36. Following surgery, C.R. is advised that she should receive chemotherapy to eradicate the remaining tumor cells. Which antineoplastic drugs are effective in advanced ovarian carcinoma?

Single agents that have exhibited activity in the treatment of advanced ovarian cancer include cisplatin, paclitaxel, docetaxel, topotecan, gemcitabine, and altretamine. The most commonly used first-line regimen is carboplatin plus paclitaxel. An initial trial evaluating the role of paclitaxel in newly diagnosed ovarian cancer reported an overall response rate of 73% for patients receiving the cisplatin and paclitaxel combination versus 60% for patients receiving the standard cisplatin and cyclophosphamide regimen.[132] Overall survival for the paclitaxel regimen was 38 months versus 24 months for the cyclophosphamide regimen. Subsequent trials substituted carboplatin for cisplatin to improve the toxicity profile and the ease of administration. A trial involving 840 patients reported that response rates and median time for recurrence-free survival were similar for the paclitaxel plus carboplatin and the paclitaxel plus cisplatin treatment arms.[133] Nonhematologic toxicity was greatest in the cisplatin-containing arm and thrombocytopenia was more common with the carboplatin-containing arm. An international workshop of ovarian cancer experts concluded that the benefits of carboplatin plus paclitaxel, in terms of reduced toxicity, justified its widespread adoption at this time.[134]

Recurrent Disease

37. After six courses of paclitaxel and carboplatin, C.R. has no remaining evidence of ovarian cancer. Planned follow-up included repeat serum CA-125 levels and CT scans at 3-month intervals. Six months after completing chemotherapy, the CA-125 level was increased and a CT scan of the abdomen revealed several new masses. Should C.R. receive more paclitaxel and carboplatin therapy at this time?

Patients with disease that recurs within 6 months after treatment are unlikely to benefit from additional therapy with the first-line agents.[135] Therefore, it is most appropriate to treat C.R.'s cancer with a drug that has a different mechanism of action and, hopefully, a different pattern of resistance. Topotecan, a topoisomerase I inhibitor, has activity in patients whose disease has progressed after receiving platinum-based regimens. Response rates range from 14% to 25%.[136,137] The recommended dose is 1.5 mg/m² daily as a 30-minute infusion for 5 consecutive days; this course is repeated every 21 days. The major toxicity associated with topotecan is myelosuppression.

Other alternative, second- and third-line regimens include altretamine, liposomal doxorubicin,[138] gemcitabine,[139] oral etoposide,[140] and intraperitoneal chemotherapy.

Intraperitoneal Chemotherapy

38. What is the role of intraperitoneal chemotherapy in ovarian cancer?

Ovarian carcinoma is usually limited to the peritoneal cavity. Commonly, tumor plaques are attached to the underside of the diaphragm as well as to the exterior of other organs within the abdominal cavity. Even following meticulous surgical removal of the tumor, there is nearly always some residual disease. Thus, intraperitoneal instillation of chemotherapeutic agents allows drug delivery directly to the site of the tumor and produces higher concentrations of drug at the tumor than could be attained by systemic administration. Although drug delivery to the tumor is primarily by surface diffusion, agents that are then absorbed systemically from the peritoneum also reach the tumor via capillary flow.[141] Intraperitoneal cisplatin has been the most widely studied intraperitoneal drug in both the adjuvant and metastatic setting.[141,142] A randomized trial in previously untreated stage III ovarian cancer with minimal disease following surgery compared cisplatin 100 mg/m² IV with the same intraperitoneal dose in conjunction with intraperitoneal cyclophosphamide 600 mg/m².[143] Median survival was significantly longer and moderate to severe toxicities were fewer in the intraperitoneal group. A similar trial compared standard intravenous cisplatin and paclitaxel to intraperitoneal carboplatin followed by intravenous carboplatin and paclitaxel; again, the intraperitoneal arm had an improved outcome of approximately 25%.[144] Although the evidence from the randomized trials of intraperitoneal chemotherapy have revealed modest improvements in outcomes—such as progression-free survival and, when assessed, overall survival—it is still not considered standard of care. This is most likely due to concerns about the toxicity of the specific regimens evaluated, which included higher rates of GI, metabolic, and hematologic toxicities. Toxicities associated with intraperitoneal administration include chemical peritonitis, fibrosis, and pain. In addition to intraperitoneal chemotherapy, drugs or radioisotopes occasionally are injected into the peritoneal cavity to control malignant ascites. Such instillation provides symptomatic relief with minimal treatment-related toxicity.

BLADDER CANCER
Clinical Presentation and Risk Factors

39. B.B., a 65-year-old man, presented with complaints consistent with cystitis, including burning and pain on urination. Urinalysis reveals no white blood cells (WBCs) or bacteria and 10 red blood cells (RBCs)/high-power field (HPF). B.B. is a textile worker who smokes cigarettes but does not drink alcohol. He is referred to a urologist for cystoscopy, and the biopsy is consistent with multifocal, transitional cell carcinoma of the bladder, grade 3. What factors placed B.B. at risk for bladder cancer?

Risk factors for bladder cancer include age older than 60 years, male gender, occupational exposure to chemical carcinogens (aryl amines, including organic chemical, aniline dye, rubber, and paint industries), cigarette smoking, drugs (oral cyclophosphamide and phenacetin), and chronic urinary tract infections.[145] Because the whole uroepithelium is chronically exposed to carcinogens excreted in the urine, these cancers tend to recur in multiple sites even after surgical resection. B.B.'s male gender, long career as a textile worker, coupled with his significant history of cigarette smoking, place him at increased risk of bladder cancer.

The only symptom many patients experience before diagnosis is bladder irritation; in women, this may be mistaken for interstitial cystitis. Microscopic or gross hematuria is often the finding that prompts the patient to seek medical intervention. Patients with more extensive tumors may experience flank pain, constipation, or lower extremity edema.

Treatment
Intravesical Therapy

40. Further workup establishes that B.B. has superficial disease. He undergoes transurethral endoscopic resection (TURB) and fulguration (tumor is charred and then scraped with a curet). Is further therapy indicated at this time?

Although resection is highly effective in eradicating existing lesions, 30% to 85% of patients eventually develop new lesions.[146] B.B.'s tumor is also grade 3 (poorly differentiated) and multifocal, which further increase his risk for recurrence.[147] Adjuvant intravesical therapy (instillation into the urinary bladder) is recommended for high-risk patients to reduce the risk of recurrence. This route places high concentrations of the drug into direct contact with the bladder mucosa and can delay or prevent progression of disease (which could require cystectomy or systemic chemotherapy).[148] The limited systemic absorption of intravesicular therapy also minimizes the risk of serious systemic toxicities.

Drugs that have been used intravesicularly include thiotepa, doxorubicin, valrubicin, mitomycin, and Bacillus Calmette-Guerin (BCG).[149] The few randomized studies that have been conducted suggest that BCG is superior to doxorubicin,[150] but definitive studies have not established superiority of BCG over mitomycin. Valrubicin, a derivative of doxorubicin, is the newest agent marketed for treatment of superficial carcinoma of the bladder. In one report, 29% of patients refractory to BCG demonstrated complete response to valrubicin therapy.[151] BCG is accepted as the standard therapeutic intervention for carcinoma inside of the bladder and for prophylaxis of tumor recurrence in superficial bladder cancer.[150] Some patients experience a dose-limiting local irritation following BCG therapy, which presents as dysuria, hematuria, and increased urinary frequency. Approximately 6% of patients experience severe systemic effects, including fever, chills, and joint pain. Other systemic effects following intravesical therapy are rare; however, myelosuppression is seen in approximately 20% of patients receiving thiotepa. Chemical cystitis is also a common toxicity following both mitomycin and doxorubicin therapy, with some patients experiencing contact dermatitis in the urogenital area.

The agents usually are diluted in sterile saline or water and administered via catheter into an empty bladder; patients are asked to retain the dose for 2 hours. Doses used are 30 to 60 mg of thiotepa, 20 to 80 mg of doxorubicin, 800 mg of valrubicin, or 20 to 60 mg of mitomycin C, each diluted in 60 to 75 mL. BCG is given in a dose of 120 mg in sterile saline. Of the seven substrains of BCG, the TICE, RIMV (Rotterdam Institute of Veterinary Medicine), Pasteur, Japanese, Connaught, and Armand Frappeir strains appear to be effective, whereas the Glaxo strain appears to be relatively ineffective.[152] Although schedules vary, they generally consist of an initial weekly induction phase that lasts 6 weeks followed by monthly maintenance instillations for up to 12 months.

Metastatic Disease

41. Six months after starting adjuvant BCG, B.B. is found to have recurrent, metastatic disease (stage IV) involving his lungs and liver. What is the incidence of disease dissemination and what type of treatment should B.B. receive?

Approximately 40% of patients with bladder cancer develop metastatic disease during their clinical course. The most common sites of disease spread are the lymph nodes, liver, lung, and bone. Follow-up histories, physical examinations, and assessments should focus on these areas. Once the disease disseminates to a distant site, the prognosis is poor and the focus of treatment is to reduce symptoms and prolong survival. Combination chemotherapy with regimens such as methotrexate, vinblastine, doxorubicin, cisplatin (M-VAC); cisplatin plus FU; or other investigational therapies may be considered if the patient can tolerate aggressive therapy. Results from a randomized trial comparing M-VAC with single-agent cisplatin in advanced bladder cancer show a significant advantage with M-VAC in both response rate and median survival time.[153] The outpatient regimen of paclitaxel and carboplatin is active and well tolerated, with partial response rates of approximately 50%.[154,155] The combination of cisplatin and gemcitabine can also be considered in the metastatic setting. In a trial of 400 patients that were chemotherapy naïve, the combination of gemcitabine and cisplatin was associated with a higher response rate and less toxicity, including significantly less neutropenic sepsis and grade III/IV mucositis, compared to MVAC.[156] Because bladder cancer with distant metastases is considered an incurable disease, patients should be encouraged to participate in clinical trials whenever feasible.

MELANOMA
Treatment

42. B.C., a 35-year-old white man, has worked for the past 12 years as a landscaper in south Florida. Two years before this admission he had undergone surgical resection of a stage I malignant melanoma. He underwent a wide excision of the area, but because he did not have lymphadenopathy, the regional lymph nodes were not dissected. B.C. now presents with complaints of enlarging, painful lymph nodes in his groin, and physical examination reveals several enlarged inguinal nodes and hepatomegaly. A lymph node biopsy confirms recurrence of malignant melanoma and LFTs as follows: AST, 190 IU/L (normal, 5 to 35 IU/L); ALT, 165 IU/L (5 to 45 IU/L); and bilirubin, 2.2 mg/dL (2 to 18 mg/dL). Is chemotherapy indicated for B.C. who has metastatic malignant melanoma?

[SI units: AST, 190 U/L; ALT, 165 U/L; bilirubin, 37.62 mmol/L]

Today, melanoma accounts for only 3% of all cancer diagnoses in the United States; however, in the year 2003 the lifetime risk of an American developing invasive melanoma was 1 in 82. This represents the most dramatic increase in incidence of any of the neoplastic diseases. Melanoma can occur in adults of all age groups and predominantly affects whites. The precise cause of melanoma is unknown; however, epidemiologic studies suggest that sunlight is the most important factor in its pathogenesis.[157] Melanocytes, the normal precursor cells, are found in the skin and other peripheral sites and synthesize melanin, which protects against ultraviolet damage. Various growth factor receptors, binding proteins, and other surface antigens have been identified on the surface of melanocytes at different stages during their transformation to malignant melanoma cells. Research is now focused on elucidation of the role of these antigens in the malignant transformation and their potential as targets for therapeutic interventions.

Cutaneous melanoma can arise on any surface of the skin and is perhaps the most visible of malignancies; therefore, it can be detected in asymptomatic persons. Early detection and recognition of melanoma are essential for possible cure. Occasionally, melanomas develop in noncutaneous tissues (e.g., the retina). The most critical factor in determining the prognosis following surgical removal of a melanoma is the vertical extension of the lesion into the skin and subcutaneous tissue; those that extend into the subcutaneous fat have a high rate of tumor recurrence and a grave prognosis. Once the melanoma has metastasized, surgery is no longer a therapeutic option.

To date, the results of chemotherapy in the treatment of melanoma have been disappointing. Single agents that have demonstrated modest activity (approximately 20%) include alkylating agents such as dacarbazine, carboplatin, carmustine, temozolomide, and cisplatin. However, most responses are only partial, and the duration of response is generally only 3 to 6 months. Over the past 30 years numerous combination chemotherapy regimens have been used but have not consistently demonstrated differences in response or survival.[158,159] No combination regimen has yet been proven to be superior to dacarbazine alone.

Tamoxifen was initially added to many combination chemotherapy regimens for melanoma because estrogen receptors are present on some melanoma cells. A randomized trial comparing dacarbazine alone with dacarbazine plus tamoxifen reported a higher response rate (28% versus 12%) and a longer survival (48 versus 29 weeks) for patients receiving tamoxifen.[160] The addition of tamoxifen to the three-drug combination regimen of cisplatin, carmustine, and dacarbazine (i.e., the Dartmouth regimen) showed high response rates in phase II studies, but a phase III trial of the three drugs with and without tamoxifen showed no benefit with the addition of tamoxifen; the response rates were 20% to 30% in both treatment arms.[161] In other nonrandomized trials, the impact of tamoxifen has been controversial. Thus, the strength of the evidence does not support the use of tamoxifen in combination with cisplatin-containing chemotherapy for the treatment of melanoma.[162]

For several reasons, melanoma has been one of the most widely studied tumors in the area of immunotherapy. Commonly, melanoma cells express surface antigens that can be targeted by specific immunotherapy (e.g., monoclonal antibodies) and these surface antigens enhance recognition by the host's own immune system. The latter is supported by the lymphocytic infiltrates commonly observed in tumor biopsies. In addition, melanoma and its normal precursor cells, melanocytes, require growth factors for proliferation. Although melanocytes require exogenous growth factors, melanoma cells (at least sometimes) produce their own. This may explain, in part, the progressive nature of malignant melanomas. The interferons, interleukin-2 (IL.-2), and vaccines are biologic therapies that have been most widely studied in the treatment of melanoma. Other biologic therapies that have been added to IL-2 but have not improved response rates or durable remissions include monoclonal antibodies, active immunotherapy by vaccination, and adoptive immunotherapy using tumor-infiltrating lymphocytes or lymphokine-activated killer (LAK) cells.

Early studies using interferon-α (INF-α) demonstrated overall response rates of 8% to 22%, with survival durations and time to progression of disease approximating that produced by cytotoxic chemotherapy regimens.[163] In many cases, it may take 3 to 6 months for patients to achieve the maximum response to interferon. Patients most likely to respond include those with only cutaneous or pulmonary disease who have small tumor burdens. The optimal dose of interferon in melanoma has not been clearly defined; similar responses have been reported for doses ranging from 10 million units/m^2 per day to 50 million units/m^2 every other day.

Initial studies using high-dose IL-2 either alone or in combination with LAK cells produced overall response rates of only 10% to 20%. Importantly, about 5% of patients responded completely, most of whom have been maintained for many years.[164–166] Partial responses are typically brief.

Several different preparations of IL-2 have been used in clinical trials and variations in administration (on a per meter squared or per kilogram of body weight basis) as well as the use of different unit standards has caused some confusion. The World Health Organization has now defined international units.[167] In the case of the commercially available aldesleukin (Proleukin, Chiron Therapeutics, Inc), a milligram, which had previously been defined as equivalent to 3 million Cetus units, is now defined as equivalent to 18 million international units. Attention to the formulation and units is crucial to ensure the use of appropriate dosages.

Regimens using high doses of IL-2 (e.g., 600,000 IU/kg every 8 hours for 15 days) have been associated with considerable dose-related toxicities.[168] Most of these can be included in a "diffuse capillary leak syndrome" characterized by intravascular volume depletion, oliguria, and edema of all major organs resulting in multiorgan dysfunction. Once therapy is discontinued, the capillary leak and related toxicities resolve quickly. During therapy, fluid balance must be carefully and frequently evaluated and intravenous hydration administered cautiously. Early administration of vasopressors is usually necessary when patients receive high-dose therapy to maintain systemic perfusion and enhance urinary output. Patients also require H_2-receptor antagonists to prevent gastritis, and premedication with acetaminophen and an NSAID (e.g., indomethacin) to prevent fever and chills associated with IL-2 administration. Meperidine is usually effective in attenuating chills when they occur. Concurrent with resolution of widespread edema, desquamation and intense pruritus often are observed, which can be managed with emollients. Corticosteroids should not be given because they may attenuate the immunomodulatory effects of IL-2. Even though patients receiving single-agent IL-2 do not become neutropenic, a high incidence of staphylococcal bacteremia also has been observed.

Active specific immunotherapy (vaccination) uses tumor-associated antigens to induce an immune response against melanoma. Both autologous and allogeneic vaccines have been studied, with the allogeneic vaccines, Melacine (made from whole cell lysates of two melanoma cell lines) and CancerVax (made from three allogeneic irradiated melanoma cell lines) being the two agents that are the closest to obtaining FDA approval. Prolonged survival has been noted with Melacine in patients with stage IIB disease and in advanced disease when combined with interferon.[169,170] An ongoing phase III trial in patients with stage III malignant melanoma is comparing Melacine plus standard dose interferon alfa to single-agent high-dose interferon-α therapy. CancerVax has been tested in clinical trials since 1984, with a randomized trial of patients with completely resected stage IV melanoma recently completed. The 5-year overall survival rates were 39% for patients receiving the vaccine versus 19% for patients not receiving the vaccine.[171] Results from ongoing, randomized phase III studies for both vaccines will provide further rationale for the approval of these agents.

Combinations of chemotherapy and biologics (also known as chemoimmunotherapy or biochemotherapy) have been evaluated against chemotherapy alone for metastatic disease. Four studies comparing dacarbazine (DTIC) and IFN-α with DTIC alone have shown conflicting results.[172] However, a meta-analysis of 20 randomized trials that compared single-agent dacarbazine to combination chemotherapy with or with-

out immunotherapy found that the combination of dacarbazine and interferon-α found a tumor response rate 53% greater than that seen with dacarbazine alone, although there was no difference in overall survival.[173] IL-2 has been combined with cisplatin in several phase II trials[174,175] with encouraging response rates, but data supporting an improvement in survival are lacking. A recent single-institution randomized trial of chemotherapy and biochemotherapy demonstrated a doubling of objective response rates and time to progression but no advantage for overall survival.[176] This was supported by the report of three phase III randomized trials evaluating the use of biochemotherapy, where there was no overall benefit of adding biochemotherapy to current regimens.[177-179] Therefore, the current data for biochemotherapy do not support its adoption as standard therapy.

PROSTATE CANCER
Etiology and Risk Factors

43. **J.D., a 65-year-old African American man, was diagnosed with prostate carcinoma 18 months ago. At that time, he underwent a radical prostatectomy and was found to have stage B2 disease (confined to the prostate). Before surgery, his prostate-specific antigen (PSA) was 25 ng/mL (normal, <4.0 ng/mL). At a regular follow-up examination, J.D.'s only complaint is mild backache, which he attributes to strain. Now, his PSA is 100 ng/mL and a CT scan of the pelvis shows several enlarged lymph nodes consistent with metastatic prostate cancer. Bone scan reveals blastic lesions in the lumbar region of the spine. J.D. is otherwise asymptomatic. His only other medical problems are a 20-year history of essential hypertension and evidence of early congestive heart failure. What are J.D.'s risk factors for prostate cancer?**

Although adenocarcinoma of the prostate is the most common malignancy in adult males in the United States, specific risk factors (other than male gender and increasing age) have not been identified. The median age at diagnosis is 66 and the disease is rare before the age of 40. The highest incidence worldwide is in African-American men, which is 1.7 times that of white men in the United States.[1] Unfortunately, the mortality rate in African-American men is 2.4 times that of white men.

The cause of prostate cancer is unknown. Regional variation in incidence worldwide suggests that environmental factors may have a role.[180] Nationalized males have incidence rates that are intermediate between those born in the United States and those who have remained in their native country, which also suggests that environmental factors contribute. Textile workers and others exposed to industrial chemicals may have a higher risk. Increased risk also has been linked to high-fat diets. High levels of testosterone also have been implicated in prostate cancer development.[180] Support for a hormonal etiology includes the hormone dependence of prostate cancer, the absence of prostate cancer in eunuchs, and the increased incidence in male populations with higher testosterone levels. An increased risk of prostate cancer in patients with benign prostatic hyperplasia has been suggested, although others have not observed this association. Lifetime risk of prostate cancer is 16% if one first-degree relative has prostate cancer compared with 8% if there is no family history.

Conclusive evidence that widespread screening and early detection of prostate cancer improves survival is lacking. Screening leads to earlier diagnosis and most agree that screening for prostate cancer has led to the recent declines in prostate cancer mortality. Since PSA is specific to the prostate and not specific for cancer, it is not a sensitive screening tool when used alone. Furthermore, several situations can falsely elevate PSA. Finasteride reportedly doubles the PSA, and prostate manipulation, biopsy, and the digital rectal examination increase the PSA as well. Nevertheless, the routine evaluation of PSA in men older than 50 years of age has become the standard of care.

Adjuvant Therapy

44. **Could J.D. have received adjuvant therapy for his localized prostate cancer after his radical prostatectomy?**

The role of adjuvant therapy is to extend the cure rate of traditional therapies such as radical prostatectomy, external beam radiotherapy, or watchful waiting. In a compilation of three international trials involving more than 8,000 patients with a median follow-up of more than 3 years, there was a 42% reduction in the risk of objective progression with the administration of adjuvant bicalutamide 150 mg daily compared to placebo (13.8% versus 9.0%) when administered as an adjuvant to treatment intended to be curative for prostate cancer.[181] The side effects were largely treatment related and included primarily gynecomastia and breast tenderness. It is too early to determine if there is a difference in overall survival.

The rationale for adjuvant bicalutamide for localized prostate cancer is based on a trial in which bicalutamide monotherapy was compared to castration in patients with locally advanced/node positive prostate cancer. Pooled data from two open label studies involving patients with T3/T4 prostate cancer found no difference in the overall survival or time to progression after a median follow-up of 6.3 years in patients receiving either bicalutamide 150 mg daily or castration (orchiectomy of 3.6 mg goserelin acetate every 28 days).[182] However, there were statistically significant benefits in the bicalutamide group in two quality of life parameters: sexual interest and physical capacity. This trial led to the evaluation of bicalutamide in earlier stage disease. Since J.D. has localized disease, monotherapy with bicalutamide 150 mg daily is an appropriate alternative to no therapy in the adjuvant setting.

Staging

45. **Is J.D.'s disease still considered stage B2?**

No. Stage B2 disease is confined to the prostate, and from the CT scan J.D. now has obvious spread to the pelvic lymph nodes and bone (stage D2). The stage of the disease determines the most appropriate therapy. Whereas stage B usually is treated with surgery (radical prostatectomy) or radiation therapy, the mainstay of treatment for symptomatic stage D prostate cancer is hormonal manipulation. It is becoming increasingly more common to use hormonal therapy for patients with stage D2 disease even before symptoms develop. Recent combined androgen deprivation trials demonstrate a survival advantage for stage D2, asymptomatic, young, good performance status, minimal disease patients treated with hormone therapy, suggesting that early initiation of treatment may be appropriate.[183]

Treatment

46. **Does J.D.'s disease require therapy at this time?**

J.D. has advanced disease and is experiencing symptoms that could progress, causing him considerable pain and loss of neurological function if left untreated. Hormonal manipulation that reduces testosterone to levels consistent with castration is the mainstay of pharmacotherapy for advanced symptomatic prostate cancer. Testosterone deprivation is effective against prostate cancer cells because the growth of both normal and malignant prostate tissue depends on it.

Multiple hormonal manipulations can be employed, including (1) ablation of androgen sources, (2) inhibition of testosterone production, and (3) interference of testosterone binding at its receptor site.

Testosterone is produced by the testicles in response to pituitary follicle-stimulating hormone (FSH) and luteinizing hormone (LH) and also by metabolic conversion of androgens produced by the adrenal glands. Testosterone is converted by α-reductase enzymes to dihydrotestosterone, the major intracellular androgen, which then binds to a specific cytoplasmic receptor protein. The receptor-dihydrotestosterone complex is then translocated into the prostatic nucleus where it binds to and activates DNA to induce the production of messenger RNA. Messenger RNA then codes for proteins essential for the metabolic functions of the prostate cells, including prostate cancer cells.

Therapeutic options for J.D. at this time include (1) orchiectomy; (2) LHRH analogs (e.g. leuprolide, goserelin), which decrease FSH and LH synthesis and production, which in turn decrease testosterone production; (3) an antiandrogen (e.g., flutamide, bicalutamide, nilutamide), which inhibits dihydrotestosterone binding to its receptor; or (4) combined androgen blockade, using both an LHRH analog and an antiandrogen.

Choice of Therapy

47. **Which therapy would be the most appropriate choice for J.D. at this time?**

BILATERAL ORCHIECTOMY

Bilateral orchiectomy is considered by many to be the therapy of choice because it permanently removes the primary source of testosterone production (95%) with few surgical complications. Orchiectomy does cause impotence (as do all forms of testosterone ablation) and patients may suffer from hot flashes; however, the need for regular long-term administration of drugs that have potential side effects is avoided.[184] Nevertheless, some patients find this procedure unacceptable.

LHRH ANALOGS

Leuprolide (Lupron) and goserelin (Zoladex) are LHRH analogs. Like LHRH itself, they stimulate the release of FSH and LH by the pituitary, which increases the production of testosterone. Thus, when therapy is initiated, there is an initial testosterone surge (during the first 10 to 14 days), which can transiently worsen symptoms such as pain (i.e., flare reactions). Some clinicians choose to initiate short-term antiandrogen therapy before or together with the LHRH agonist and to continue the antiandrogen for about a month. This method is intended to reduce the possibility for the flare reaction. Over several weeks, the LHRH receptors in the pituitary are down-regulated by the continuous onslaught of synthetic LHRH, and there is a decline in the release of LH. Ultimately, the levels of FSH, LH, and testosterone become profoundly suppressed.

In a large trial comparing leuprolide with diethylstilbestrol (DES), response rates were equivalent and there was less toxicity in the leuprolide group.[185] Leuprolide and goserelin are long-acting formulations that can be administered as monthly, every-3-months, or every-4-months injections. The efficacy of leuprolide and goserelin appears to be similar, although large-scale comparative trials have not been completed. Long-term use of LHRH agonists is associated with anemia, fatigue, and osteoporosis. Therapy with either drug is continued until the disease progresses (i.e., new metastatic sites). Many experts advocate continuing androgen deprivation with these agents for the duration of the patient's life, even after disease progression and the addition of chemotherapy.

ANTIANDROGENS

Monotherapy with antiandrogens such as flutamide, bicalutamide, and nilutamide has been evaluated in previously untreated patients in a small number of trials.[186] The most studied antiandrogen for monotherapy in the metastatic setting is bicalutamide.[186] When compared to castration, bicalutamide was associated with a statistically decreased time to treatment failure, time to objective progression, and increased risk for death, but there was no statistical difference in survival.[187] Another trial comparing bicalutamide to flutamide plus goserelin found no difference in outcomes.[188] Patients treated with bicalutamide alone were assigned to castration if they progressed. The use of bicalutamide alone in the metastatic setting remains investigational until results from several trials mature. The most common antiandrogen-related adverse effects include gynecomastia, hot flashes, GI disturbances, breast tenderness, and liver function abnormalities. Because antiandrogens do not directly reduce testosterone levels, patients often can maintain sexual potency.

COMBINED HORMONAL BLOCKADE

The rationale for combination hormonal therapy is to interfere with multiple hormonal pathways to completely eliminate androgen action. In clinical trials, combination hormonal therapy, sometimes also referred to as maximal androgen deprivation or total androgen blockade, has been used. The combination of LHRH analogs or orchiectomy with antiandrogens is the most extensively studied combined androgen deprivation approach. A meta-analysis comparing combined hormonal blockade with conventional medical or surgical castration failed to show any additional survival benefit associated with maximal androgen blockade.[189] However, several individual trials have shown benefit in progression-free survival and overall median survival.[190,191] Thus far, studies have demonstrated a major benefit in patients with minimal disease.[190,192]

Combined androgen blockade (e.g., leuprolide plus flutamide) or orchiectomy plus nilutamide would be appropriate choices given J.D.'s minimal disease and good performance status.

Monitoring Therapy

48. **J.D. started leuprolide 22.5 mg IM q 3 months and flutamide 250 mg TID. How should his response to therapy be monitored?**

Blastic bone lesions heal slowly and have been shown to persist even when biopsy documents absence of disease. Therefore, a repeat bone scan would not be a useful indicator of response; however, it may be used to rule out new lesions or progressive disease. If bony lesions improve, it may take up to 6 months for resolution on the bone scan because of the slow rate of bone remodeling in elderly men.

Measurement of PSA is the most useful tool to follow response to therapy. Because the serum half-life of PSA is only 2 to 4 days, serial measurements provide a rapid indication of tumor status. It also is less expensive and more sensitive than imaging techniques (e.g., CT scans, bone scans). Control of symptoms, such as pain and maintenance of quality of life, are important outcome indicators in this disease and should be monitored frequently.

Second-Line Therapies

49. **Following initiation of treatment, J.D.'s PSA level fell to 20 ng/mL and remained stable for the next 18 months. During this time, he had no clinical evidence of disease progression. However, his most recent clinic visit revealed an increase in his PSA level to 75 ng/mL and a repeat bone scan and pelvic CT showed some progression. Is a change in therapy warranted at this time?**

Various second-line hormonal therapies have been studied. If J.D. had been receiving an LHRH agonist alone, a testosterone level could be checked to ensure castrate levels had been achieved. If castrate testosterone levels (<20 ng/dL) are not achieved, then an orchiectomy or addition of an antiandrogen are options.[193] Since J.D. was receiving combined androgen blockade, a trial of antiandrogen withdrawal should be initiated. This approach produces symptomatic improvement and objective signs of tumor regression and/or a decrease in PSA in up to 35% of patients.[194] This is likely because of a mutation in the androgen receptor and a change in the selectivity or activation of the receptor that allows antagonists to act as agonists. Therefore, J.D.'s flutamide should be discontinued. The addition of an aromatase inhibitor, such as aminoglutethimide or ketoconazole, is also a reasonable choice. Because J.D. is not experiencing progressive symptoms at this time, the benefits of additional therapy with either aminoglutethimide or ketoconazole probably do not outweigh the potential risks and complications of treatment and its associated costs.

AMINOGLUTETHIMIDE

Aminoglutethimide inhibits the desmolase enzyme complex in the adrenal gland thereby preventing synthesis of all adrenally derived steroids. Therefore, concurrent physiologic replacement of glucocorticoids is essential, and mineralocorticoid replacement may be necessary in selected patients. Therapy usually is initiated with 250 mg twice a day and gradually increased to 250 mg four times a day as the patient tolerates therapy. Responses to aminoglutethimide may take up to 4 to 6 weeks. Approximately 50% of patients experience adverse effects, which may include central nervous system (CNS) effects (lethargy, ataxia, dizziness) and a morbilliform, pruritic rash that is self-limiting and usually resolves within 5 to 8 days with continued therapy.

KETOCONAZOLE

Ketoconazole, an imidazole antifungal agent, interferes with both adrenal and testicular steroidogenesis. In doses of 400 mg every 8 hours, response is rapid and adverse effects include GI intolerance, impotence, gynecomastia, transient increases in liver function tests, weakness, lethargy, and skin pigmentation. Concurrent physiologic replacement of glucocorticoids also is recommended.

Cytotoxic Chemotherapy

50. J.D.'s metastatic disease continues to progress. Would cytotoxic chemotherapy be beneficial at this time?

Almost all patients with metastatic prostate cancer initially treated with androgen deprivation will develop progressive disease within 2 to 3 years. The term androgen independent prostate cancer describes the situation in which a patient has a documented castrate testosterone level and progressive disease. These patients typically have a median survival of 6 months.

Despite extensive testing of both single agents, combination chemotherapy regimens, and combination chemotherapy/hormonal regimens, no currently approved antineoplastic agent or combinations prolong survival in patients with advanced prostate cancer.[195] This may be because most chemotherapy trials have been done in patients with hormone-refractory prostate cancer when the expected resistance rate is high. Mitoxantrone combined with prednisone is an FDA approved regimen for the treatment of androgen independent prostate cancer.[196] The response is typically manifested as objective tumor regression (partial response rates up to 30%), PSA declines, pain relief, and a delay in bone scan progression. Other possible chemotherapeutic regimens include estramustine in combination with an antimicrotubule such as vinblastine,[197] paclitaxel,[198] or docetaxel.[199]

TESTICULAR CANCER
Clinical Presentation

51. M.W., a 26-year-old man, noted painless swelling of his left testicle approximately 2 or 3 weeks before seeing his family physician. Physical examination reveals an indurated mass located in the lower pole of the left testicle. Epididymitis is ruled out because of the location. Laboratory evaluation reveals the following: α-Fetoprotein (AFP) is 300 ng/mL (normal, <40), β-human chorionic gonadotropin (β-hCG) (<5 IU/L) is negative, and LDH is 43 U/L. He is referred to a urologist who performs a radical inguinal orchiectomy and a nerve-sparing retroperitoneal lymph node dissection. M.W. has two positive nodes and the pathology report reveals embryonal carcinoma. Following orchiectomy, the AFP declines exponentially; a metastatic workup, including chest radiograph and CT scan of the abdomen and pelvis, reveals no evidence of disease. Is this a typical presentation of testicular cancer?

[SI units: AFP, 300 and 270 mg/L, respectively (normal, <40); LDH, 43 U/L]

Testicular cancer is the most common malignancy in men between ages 15 and 35 years. M.W.'s presentation is typical in that the cancer presents as a painless swelling in one gonad. The cause of testicular cancer is unknown, but approximately 10% of patients have a history of cryptorchidism.[200] Other possible risk factors include race (the incidence is much lower among African-American males) and family history.[201]

Histologic Classification

52. Does histologic classification provide a clinical basis for therapeutic decisions?

Germinal neoplasms are divided into seminomas and various other types known collectively as nonseminomatous germ cell tumors (Table 91-4).

Seminomas arise from malignant transformations of spermatocytes, whereas nonseminomas arise from transformation of germ cells of placental origin. Although treatment of advanced disease is similar, seminoma is exquisitely sensitive to radiation and therefore early stages of the disease are more frequently treated with radiotherapy.[201] Determination of the most appropriate therapy depends on both the histology and stage of the disease. Because M.W. has a nonseminoma (i.e., embryonal carcinoma), initial radiation is not indicated.

Staging

53. What is the stage of M.W.'s disease?

Stage I disease is limited to the testes; stage II disease involves the testes and lymph nodes; and stage III disease includes all metastatic tumors. Following orchiectomy, a metastatic workup was completed to rule out spread of the disease. This workup should include chest radiograph, CT evaluation of retroperitoneal lymph nodes, and assessment of decline in the tumor markers following orchiectomy. Because M.W. has two positive lymph nodes, his disease is classified as stage II.

Treatment
Adjuvant Chemotherapy

54. M.W. is diagnosed with stage II disease. Following surgery, the AFP declined exponentially. Is adjuvant chemotherapy indicated at this time?

Table 91-4 Histologic Classification of Primary Tumors of the Testes

Germinal Neoplasms
Seminoma
Embryonal carcinoma
Teratoma
Choriocarcinoma
Yolk sac tumor
Nongerminal Neoplasms
Specialized gonadal stromal neoplasms (e.g., Leydig cell tumor)
Gonadoblastoma
Miscellaneous (e.g., adenocarcinoma, carcinoid, mesenchymal)

Approximately 30% of patients like M.W. (<6 positive nodes) whose disease is apparently completely resected (AFP declined following lymph node dissection) ultimately experience relapse, and adjuvant chemotherapy (two cycles of a platinum-based regimen) dramatically reduces this risk.[202,203] However, if patients do not receive adjuvant chemotherapy and are monitored closely for early detection of relapse, the chance of cure following aggressive induction of chemotherapy remains high (>80%).[202]

Metastatic Disease

55. It is decided that M.W. will not receive adjuvant therapy at this time. Instead, he will be followed by a monthly history, physical examination, and AFP for the first year, every 2 months during the second year, and every 6 months thereafter. After 4 months M.W. is lost to follow-up. He returns to his urologist 1 year later with complaints of abdominal discomfort and shortness of breath. A chest radiograph reveals multiple nodules in the lung, and an abdominal CT reveals a 6- to 10-cm mass. His AFP is 360 ng/mL and the β-hCG is 290 ng/mL. Is chemotherapy indicated at this time?

[SI unit: AFP, 360 mg/L]

M.W. now has metastatic testicular cancer and should receive systemic chemotherapy. For many years the combinations of either cisplatin, vinblastine, and bleomycin or cisplatin, etoposide plus bleomycin have produced responses in almost all men and complete responses in 60% to 80% of patients.[204–206] A randomized trial demonstrated a higher long-term survival rate for patients who had received the regimen containing etoposide in this subset of poor-risk patients, and this combination is most widely used today.[206]

Before initiating chemotherapy, pulmonary function tests, an audiogram, and a 24-hour urinary creatinine clearance are obtained. M.W. is hydrated with intravenous D5/0.45 sodium chloride and chemotherapy is initiated with cisplatin 20 mg/m^2 per day for 5 days; etoposide 100 mg/m^2 on days 1 to 5; and bleomycin 30 units on days 2, 9, and 16. Courses are repeated every 21 days. Because M.W. has poor-risk disease (i.e., nonseminomatous, extragonadal disease) he should receive a minimum of four courses.

MONITORING THERAPY

56. How should M.W. be monitored for therapeutic and toxic responses to chemotherapy?

Response to chemotherapy would be demonstrated by a reduction in the size of the abdominal mass, a reduction in the size and number of pulmonary nodules, and a steady decrease in the AFP and β-hCG without any other evidence of disease progression. CT scans, chest radiographs, and tumor markers are typically re-evaluated after every second course of therapy.

The most significant toxicities associated with this regimen include myelosuppression and the nephrotoxicity and neurotoxicity associated with cisplatin. A CBC with differential and platelet count should be performed once weekly until the myelosuppression has resolved and just before the next course. Serum creatinine, blood urea nitrogen (BUN), and electrolytes (including potassium and magnesium) should be monitored daily during chemotherapy and weekly thereafter. If evidence of toxicity appears, more intense monitoring may

be recommended. Weekly symptom analysis and physical examination should include assessment for cisplatin neurotoxicity and other chemotherapy-associated toxicities. To assess bleomycin lung toxicity, baseline pulmonary function tests should be performed before the first course and after every second or third course.

57. M.W.'s AFP and β-hCG drop dramatically after his first course of chemotherapy and less so after his second course; however, they appear to plateau at an AFP of 170 ng/mL and β-hCG of 200 ng/mL after the third course. There is no evidence of tumor on the abdominal CT scan or chest radiograph. Should the fourth and fifth cycles of chemotherapy be administered?

[SI unit: AFP, 170 mg/L]

ENDOCRINE THERAPY

The plateau of the tumor markers confirms that M.W.'s disease is not continuing to regress after chemotherapy. First-line, cisplatin-based combination chemotherapy cures 70% of patients with disseminated germ cell tumors.[200] The remaining 30% of patients are candidates for salvage chemotherapy at the time of relapse or disease progression. Additional cycles of chemotherapy with the same regimen are unlikely to produce further tumor regression and normalization of the tumor markers. Because he had an initial good response to cisplatin therapy, it is reasonable to continue cisplatin in this circumstance.[200] M.W. could receive salvage chemotherapy with cisplatin 20 mg/m^2 per day for 5 days, vinblastine 0.11 mg/kg on days 1 and 2, and ifosfamide 1.2 g/m^2 per day for 5 days. As a single agent, ifosfamide produces responses in approximately 22% of patients with refractory germ cell tumors.[207] In patients like M.W., the combination of ifosfamide with cisplatin and vinblastine has produced a 36% complete response rate with a median duration of remission of 34 months. Mesna should be administered concurrently with ifosfamide to prevent hemorrhagic cystitis.

The response and long-term survival rates reported with both first-line and salvage chemotherapy for testicular cancer are considerably higher than for most solid tumors. Because of the likelihood of long-term survival, efforts are now focused on minimizing the long-term sequelae of chemotherapy (e.g., secondary malignancies, sterility).

Alternatively, at the time it was recognized that M.W.'s AFP and β-hCG plateaued, high-dose chemotherapy and autologous stem cell support could have been considered. This approach has resulted in encouraging complete response rates and durable remissions in 40% to 60% of patients.[208]

PEDIATRIC TUMORS
STATISTICS

In the United States, more children between 1 and 14 years of age die of cancer than any other disease.[209] Yet, many common pediatric cancers that had low cure rates before the advent of chemotherapy now have 5-year survivals >70%. Acute leukemias are the most common malignancies of childhood (Table 91-5), whereas the solid tumors discussed in this chapter each represent 3% to 7% of all childhood malignancies.[210] Many common pediatric solid tumors are uncommon in adults. Likewise, many tumors common in adults occur infrequently in children. In general, sarcomas and embryonal tu-

Table 91-5 Relative Incidence of Malignancies in Children 0 to 14 Years of Age

Malignancy	Relative Incidence (%)
Acute lymphoblastic leukemia	23.2
Central nervous system	20.7
Neuroblastoma	7.3
Non-Hodgkin's lymphoma	6.3
Wilms' tumor	6.1
Hodgkin's lymphoma	5.0
Acute myeloid leukemia	4.2
Rhabdomyosarcoma	3.4
Retinoblastoma	2.9
Osteosarcoma	2.6
Ewing's sarcoma	2.1
Other histologic types	16.4

Adapted from Gurney JG et al. Incidence of cancer in children in the United States. Cancer 1995;75(8):2186. Copyright 1995 American Cancer Society. Reprinted by permission of Wiley-Liss, Inc., a subsidiary of John Wiley & Sons, Inc. Based on National Cancer Institute Surveillance, Epidemiology, and End Results data from 1974–1989. Total incidence, 133.3 per million children.

mors are common in children, whereas carcinomas predominate in adults.

Small Round Cell Tumors

Several pediatric malignancies present as small round cell tumors, making morphologic diagnosis by traditional light microscopy more difficult. The most challenging diagnostic problems are the less typical forms of these diseases. The list commonly includes peripheral primitive neuroectodermal tumors, extraosseous Ewing's sarcoma, extranodal lymphoma, rhabdomyosarcoma, metastatic neuroblastoma, and some bone sarcomas.[211] Problems involved with diagnosing these tumors have stimulated the development of newer techniques aimed at detecting tumor-specific antigens or chromosomal aberrations. This information may prove useful in identifying prognostic subgroups as well as tumor types in children and adults with cancer. Identification of the t(11;22) chromosomal translocation in both peripheral primitive neuroectodermal tumors and Ewing's sarcomas has resulted in the classification of both into the Ewing's sarcoma family of tumors.[212]

Genetics

Similar to adult cancers, the association of many pediatric cancers with chromosomal aberrations or genetic defects is well confirmed. Examples[211,213] include the association of Wilms' tumor with congenital malformations, acute lymphoblastic leukemia with Down syndrome, and the association of some pediatric cancers with loss of the p53 or retinoblastoma genes. The latter two are tumor suppressor genes.

Carcinogens

The role of carcinogens in pediatric cancer is probably less prominent than in adults because of the long latency periods required. However, carcinogens are implicated in the etiology of some childhood cancers.[214] Postnatal exposure to ionizing radiation is associated with acute leukemias, chronic myelogenous leukemia, and solid tumors such as brain, thyroid, bone, and other sarcomas.[213,214] Treatment of pediatric malignancies with alkylators is associated with an increased risk of leukemias.[215] Etoposide and teniposide are associated with an increased risk of secondary acute myelogenous leukemia.[216] Treatment of childhood acute lymphoblastic leukemia, especially in those younger than 5 years of age who received irradiation, results in an increased risk of CNS neoplasms, leukemia, lymphoma, and other neoplasms later in life.[217] The only well-documented prenatal carcinogen is DES, which is associated with an increased risk of vaginal or cervical cancer in offspring.[218]

Patient Age

Patient age can be a factor in pediatric cancers and their treatment. Neuroblastoma is the most common malignancy in infants; however, an infant's prognosis is typically better than a child's. This is apparently due to the biology of the disease in this age group.[219] In contrast, infants with acute lymphoblastic leukemia tend to have a worse prognosis than older children.[220] The biology and location of rhabdomyosarcoma are often different in younger and older children, with younger children having the better overall survival.[221]

Similarly, age may be a consideration with regard to the toxicity of treatments. Children may have increased susceptibility to toxicity from irradiation relative to adults. Normal organ development may be disrupted; the skeletal system and, in children younger than 4 years old, the brain are particularly susceptible.[214,219] Prepubertal children may have a decreased risk of fertility problems from chemotherapy,[214] and conversely, children appear to have a greater risk for anthracycline cardiovascular toxicity than adults.[222]

Multi-Institutional Research Groups

With the exception of a few pediatric oncology centers, most treatment centers do not have enough patients with specific diagnoses to scientifically establish the efficacy of therapeutic regimens within a reasonable time frame. Thus, most centers join the Children's Oncology Group (COG), the largest pediatric multi-institutional research group in the United States and Canada. Through this mechanism, clinical trials often can be finished over 3 to 4 years, allowing for more rapid progress in the treatment of pediatric cancers. With the number of childhood cancer survivors increasing, research is focusing on reducing the long-term risks and complications of treatment modalities. It is important to determine which patients are at greatest risk from their cancer and to stratify treatments such that the minimum treatment to produce cure is given when the prognoses are good, and maximal treatment is given when the potential benefits outweigh the risks. Progress is already being made in this direction, and the future holds promise, especially with rapid gains in our understanding of the biology of cancers.

NEUROBLASTOMA

Neuroblastoma develops in immature cells of sympathetic nervous system origin.[223] It is the most common extracranial tumor of childhood, representing 7.3% of all childhood cancers.[210] The median age at diagnosis is 22 months; 36% occur in children younger than 1 year of age, and 79% before 4 years of age.[223] Sixty-five percent of neuroblastomas are abdominal (half of these adrenal) and 20% are thoracic.[223]

Neuroblastoma often presents as a fixed, hard, abdominal mass noted on physical examination by the family or physician without any other signs or symptoms, although other findings may be present depending on the location of the primary tumor and metastases. For example, gastrointestinal fullness, discomfort, or dysfunction can occur. Other less common but characteristic signs include proptosis with periorbital ecchymoses, increased-renin hypertension, secretory diarrhea with increased vasoactive intestinal peptide, respiratory distress, nerve root compression, opsomyoclonus, and unilateral ptosis.[224] The most common sites of metastases are the bone marrow, bone, liver, and skin.[223]

The catecholamine metabolites vanillylmandelic acid (VMA) and homovanillic acid (HVA) are elevated in the urine of 90% of neuroblastoma patients.[225,226] Because infants have a better prognosis than older children with neuroblastoma, efforts have been made to screen infants using urinary concentrations of VMA and HVA.[227,228] To date, these efforts have resulted in the diagnosis of more infants with good-risk disease, but have not reduced the number of older children diagnosed with poor-risk disease.

Two older staging systems have been combined into an international staging system (Table 91-6).[229] Forty-three percent of infants (younger than 1 year) and 78% of children have stages 3 or 4 disease at the time of diagnosis.[223] Two-year disease-free survival (DFS) for patients with stages 3 or 4 is 10% to 30%; for patients with stages 1, 2, or 4S, it is 75% to 90%.[223] A large number of prognostic factors have been identified and are discussed elsewhere.[230] Patients are stratified for treatment based on age, stage, N-myc amplification, Shimada histology, and diploidy. The Children's Oncology Group guidelines divide patients into three risk levels (Table 91-7).[217] Note that infants have better outcomes for the same stage of disease and stage 4S has a significant incidence of spontaneous regression or regression with minimal treatment.[224,232–234]

In the past, treatment for higher-risk disease has included cisplatin, etoposide, cyclophosphamide, and doxorubicin, with or without vincristine, as seen in the NCCN guidelines.[235] If chemotherapy was used for lower-risk disease, cyclophosphamide and doxorubicin were used, with cisplatin and etoposide added for poor responders.[236,237]

In current U.S. clinical trials, patients with low-risk disease are typically treated with surgery. Progression or recurrence may be treated with surgery again, unless unresectable, in which case chemotherapy is used. Two to four courses of

chemotherapy may be used with initial surgery if organ or life-threatening symptoms are present. Intermediate-risk disease is treated with surgery and four or eight courses of chemotherapy (Table 91-8) for favorable or unfavorable histology disease. Chemotherapy for low- or intermediate-risk patients avoids cisplatin to reduce nephrotoxicity and ototoxicity, limits the total doxorubicin dose to avoid cardiac toxicity, limits the total etoposide dose to reduce the risk of secondary acute myelogenous leukemia, and avoids ifosfamide to eliminate Fanconi's renal syndrome. Radiation therapy is only used for poor responders.

Therapy for high-risk disease generally involves a first surgery for biopsy, aggressive chemotherapy (Table 91-9), second-look surgery for residual tumor resection, either additional aggressive chemotherapy or high-dose chemotherapy with progenitor cell rescue, and then radiation to the tumor bed. High-dose chemotherapy with progenitor cell rescue has raised 2-year, progression-free survival to 49% from historic values of 10% to 20%; however, relapses may occur later, with 7-year progression-free survival of only 26%.[238] Evidence suggests that survival can be improved (46% versus 29% 3-year postchemotherapy disease-free survival) for pa-

---

Table 91-7 Children's Oncology Group Neuroblastoma Risk Groups

Low Risk
All stage 1 patients
Patients >1 year, 2A or 2B, and N-myc not amplified, or amplified but with favorable histology
Infants <1 year and stages 2A, 2B, or 4S with N-myc not amplified, favorable histology and hyperdiploidy

Intermediate Risk
Patients >1 year old at diagnosis with stage 3, N-myc not amplified, and favorable histology
Infants with stages 4S and N-myc not amplified, and either diploidy or unfavorable histology
Infants with stage 3 or 4 and N-myc not amplified

High Risk
Infants with stages 3 or 4 and N-myc amplified
Patients >1 year with stage 2A or 2B, N-myc amplified, and unfavorable histology
Patients >1 year with stage 4, or stage 3 and N-myc amplified, or stage 3 and N-myc not amplified but unfavorable histology

Adapted from reference 231.

Table 91-6 International Neuroblastoma Staging System (Abbreviated)

Stage 1	Local tumor with complete gross excision
Stage 2A	Unilateral localized tumor with incomplete gross excision
Stage 2B	Unilateral localized tumor, complete or incomplete excision, with ipsilateral nonadherent lymph node spread
Stage 3	Involves both sides of the midline
Stage 4	Distant lymph node or organ involvement
Stage 4S	Infants less than 1 year of age with localized primary tumor (stage 1 or 2) with dissemination limited to liver, skin and/or <10% of bone marrow

Adapted from reference 229.

Table 91-8 Sequence of Chemotherapy Combinations Used in U.S. Intergroup Low- and Intermediate-Risk Neuroblastoma

Clinical Trials[a]
Carboplatin, etoposide
Carboplatin, cyclophosphamide, doxorubicin
Cyclophosphamide, etoposide
Carboplatin, doxorubicin, etoposide
Cyclophosphamide, etoposide
Carboplatin, cyclophosphamide, doxorubicin
Carboplatin, etoposide
Cyclophosphamide, doxorubicin

[a]Generally the first four courses are used in patients with favorable histology disease, and all eight for patients with unfavorable histology.

Table 91-9 Sequence of Chemotherapy Combinations Used in U.S. Intergroup Trials for High-Risk Neuroblastoma Patients*a*

1. Cisplatin, etoposide
2. Vincristine, doxorubicin, cyclophosphamide
3. Ifosfamide, etoposide
4. Carboplatin, etoposide
5. Cisplatin, etoposide
6. Ifosfamide, etoposide
7. Vincristine, doxorubicin, cyclophosphamide
8. Cisplatin, etoposide
9. Vincristine, doxorubicin, cyclophosphamide
10. Carboplatin, etoposide

*a*Combinations 6–10 may be skipped if the patient is ready to proceed to high-dose chemotherapy with progenitor cell rescue after the first 5 combinations.

tients with higher-risk disease if standard-dose or high-dose chemotherapy is followed by six cycles of 13-cis-retinoic acid 80 mg/m[2] given orally twice daily for 14 days of each 28-day cycle.[239] Typical conditioning regimens preceding progenitor cell rescue include carboplatin and etoposide with either cyclophosphamide or melphalan, or thiotepa and cyclophosphamide. Total body irradiation may also be used.

Clinical Presentation and Diagnosis

58. H.K. is a 2-year-old girl with a 3-month history of constipation and progressive abdominal distention. She has a decreased appetite, 1-week history of vomiting, and is pale and tired. She has a large retroperitoneal mass and multiple bilateral enlarged inguinal lymph nodes. Her hemoglobin is 5.1 g/dL (normal, 11 to 14 g/dL); the WBC count, differential, and platelets are within normal limits. Serum sodium, potassium, chloride, creatinine, and glucose are within normal limits. LDH is 6,144 U/L (normal, 322 to 644 U/L), and albumin is 2.3 g/dL (normal, 3.5 to 5.0 g/dL). Urine HVA is 570 μg/mg creatinine (normal, <26 μg/mg); VMA, 31 μg/mg creatinine (normal, <11 μg/mg). Biopsies of the abdominal mass and bone marrow are positive for neuroblastoma. The lymph nodes are negative for neuroblastoma. Scans are negative for other sites of disease. Which of these signs, symptoms, and laboratory results are consistent with a diagnosis of neuroblastoma?

[SI units: hemoglobin (Hgb), 51 g/L (normal, 110 to 140); LDH, 6,144 U/L (normal, 322 to 644)]

Virtually all of H.K.'s findings are consistent with neuroblastoma. However, the low hemoglobin and albumin and high LDH are not specific for this cancer. In addition to the biopsy, the elevated urine VMA and HVA (catecholamine metabolites) are most helpful in confirming the diagnosis of neuroblastoma. Neuroblastomas can contain malignant (neuroblastoma) and benign (ganglioneuroma) cells within the same tumor, which is referred to as ganglioneuroblastoma.[223] In H.K., biopsies of the bone marrow, lymph nodes, and primary tumor are necessary to demonstrate the presence or absence of neuroblastoma at more than one site for staging purposes.

Treatment

59. What stage of disease does H.K. have? What treatment will she receive?

H.K.'s abdominal disease with distant bone marrow involvement indicates stage 4 disease. Considering her age and disease stage, H.K. has a high risk of dying from her disease. Therefore, she is started on chemotherapy consisting of cisplatin (40 mg/m[2] per day on days 1 through 5) and etoposide (100 mg/m[2] per dose every 12 hours on days 1 through 3). Subsequent courses will contain vincristine, cyclophosphamide, and doxorubicin; ifosfamide and etoposide; carboplatin and etoposide; and a repeat of the cisplatin and etoposide.

60. H.K. is 81.5 cm tall, weighs 11.65 kg, and has a body surface area of 0.5 m[2]. She starts cisplatin and etoposide with hydration fluids of 5% dextrose with 0.45% sodium chloride at 62.5 mL/hr. Urine output is 4 mL/kg per hour. How does monitoring of H.K.'s chemotherapy differ from that of an adult?

Monitoring Vital Signs for Etoposide

Although prevention and monitoring of toxicities to chemotherapy agents in children follow the same basic rules as in adults, there are some differences. When monitoring vital signs for hypotensive reactions to etoposide, normal blood pressure will be lower (ninetieth percentile 106/68 mm Hg for a 2-year-old girl) and the pulse higher (mean, 120 beats/min for a 2-year-old) than in adults.[240] It is important to have baseline vital signs so that hypotension or tachycardia will be recognized.

Monitoring Hydration for Cisplatin

In adults receiving cisplatin, hydration is often standardized with 1 to 2 L of intravenous fluids given before the drug, 1 to 2 L with the drug, and continuous hydration for at least 24 hours after the dose.[241] In children, hydration volumes should be calculated based on size. To decrease the risk of cisplatin nephrotoxicity, most pediatric protocols recommend intravenous fluids at twice maintenance rates to maintain urine outputs of at least 2 mL/kg per hour. The Children's Oncology Group (COG) calculates maintenance fluids as 1,500 mL/m[2] per 24 hours, so H.K. should receive 3,000 mL × 0.5 m[2] = 1,500 mL over 24 hours (62.5 mL/hr). H.K.'s measured urine output is 4 mL/kg per hour, which should be adequate to prevent nephrotoxicity. Weight should also be monitored throughout cisplatin administration to ensure fluid balance. Acute weight gain may require diuretics to prevent overhydration, and weight loss may indicate dehydration with impending reduction of urine output that could lead to acute nephrotoxicity. Increased intravenous fluids would help prevent the latter.

Adjustment of Creatinine Clearance to Adult Size

61. H.K.'s measured creatinine clearance (Cl$_{Cr}$) is 39 mL/min. Should her cisplatin be withheld or the dose adjusted because of low creatinine clearance?

[SI unit: Cl$_{Cr}$, 0.65 mL/sec]

Often cisplatin is not administered when the creatinine clearance is <50 mL/min per 1.73 m[2].[242] H.K.'s creatinine clearance of 39 mL/min appears to be low, but it is reported for the patient's size (i.e., 39 mL/min per 0.5 m[2]). Guidelines for dosing drugs cleared by glomerular filtration are based on creatinine clearance for normal adult body size, 1.73 m[2]. Therefore, it is important to correct H.K.'s creatinine clearance to adult body size.[243] Multiplying by 1.73/0.5, her creatinine clearance is 135 mL/min per 1.73 m², so this is not a reason to withhold cisplatin. One precaution is that the accuracy of serum creatinine and creatinine clearance in assessing renal function during cisplatin therapy in children has been questioned.[244]

Partial Response

62. H.K. obtains a partial response to the aforementioned regimen with reduction of urine VMA and HVA concentrations and a 50% decrease in the size of the primary tumor in the abdomen. Second-look surgery is performed to debulk the tumor, and pathology results indicate that the residual tumor contains 95% mature (benign) ganglioneuroma cells, but neuroblastoma cells are still present. What further treatment is available for H.K.?

Stem Cell Transplant

The best chance for prolonged disease-free survival (DFS) for H.K. is dose-intensive chemotherapy combined with autologous peripheral blood stem cell rescue. Although long-term DFS has not been improved in all trials, 2- to 3-year DFS is significantly better with intensive chemotherapy and autologous stem cell rescue.[230] The plan for H.K. is to proceed to high-dose chemotherapy with an autologous stem cell rescue. If a complete response is achieved, she would then receive 6 months of cis-retinoic acid therapy.

Treatments Based on Disease Biology

With rapid advances in neuroblastoma biology being made, future alternatives may include biologic treatments. Two treatments that are in clinical trials are anti-GD2 ganglioside monoclonal antibodies and deferoxamine (Desferal).[245–249] The GD2 ganglioside is a cell surface antigen commonly expressed on neuroblastoma cells. The monoclonal antibody directed against it can stimulate both complement-dependent and antibody-dependent cellular cytotoxicity against the tumor cells. Iron is necessary for enzyme activity in human cell lines and microorganisms. Lack of iron may specifically inhibit ribonucleotide reductase, an enzyme important for DNA synthesis. Deferoxamine binds intracellular iron and increases its excretion, resulting in growth inhibition of neuroblastoma cells, which are relatively sensitive to deferoxamine.[249] Deferoxamine has shown activity for removing neuroblastoma cells from autologous bone marrow grafts,[246] and has shown activity alone[247] or with chemotherapy[248] in neuroblastoma patients. A third agent entering clinical trials is iodine-131-metaiodobenzylguanidine (^{131}I-MIBG), a compound that delivers radiation directly to catecholamine-secreting cells such as neuroblastoma. Pilot studies have used ^{131}I-MIBG as part of the conditioning regimen prior to stem cell rescue in neuroblastoma patients.[250] Although clinical trials with these agents are in progress, a published trial has demonstrated improved survival for high-risk patients in complete response who are postchemotherapy and receive cis-retinoic acid.[239] This agent is thought to promote differentiation of the cancer cells.

WILMS' TUMOR

Wilms' tumor, also known as nephroblastoma, is a kidney tumor composed of various kidney cell types at different stages of maturation.[251] Approximately 6% of all childhood cancers are Wilms' tumor, making it the most common intra-abdominal tumor of childhood.[210] The peak incidence occurs at 3 years of age.[252] Wilms' tumor frequently presents as an asymptomatic abdominal mass, although malaise and/or pain may be reported.[251] Hematuria and high renin hypertension each occur in approximately 25% of patients. Metastases, when present at diagnosis, most commonly involve the lung (80%) or the liver (15%).

The relationship of genetic factors to Wilms' tumor is demonstrated by the approximately 1.5% of Wilms' tumor patients who have family members with the disease, and the approximately 10% who have aniridia, hemihypertrophy, or genitourinary anomalies.[251] Chromosomal aberrations at 11p13 and 11p15, known respectively as WT1 and WT2, are thought to be losses of tumor suppressor genes that occur in nonfamilial Wilms' tumor. The familial syndrome is probably related to unidentified genes.[251]

Overall, Wilms' tumor has an excellent prognosis. Treatment is based on disease stage following surgical resection or debulking, and favorable histology versus focal or diffuse anaplasia. A simplified description of the staging is as follows: stage I is limited to the kidney and can be completely removed surgically; stage II is extended beyond the kidney but can be completely excised; stage III is characterized by residual tumor confined to the abdomen; stage IV is distant metastases; and stage V is bilateral disease.[253] Metastases are present in only 15% of patients at diagnosis, and even these patients have relatively good prognoses. Four-year, relapse-free survival rates from the third National Wilms' Tumor Study (NWTS-3) range from 75% for stage IV with favorable histology to 55% for stage IV with unfavorable histology, although it may be as low as 17% for patients with diffuse anaplasia.[253,254] Survival is approximately 90% for stage I patients regardless of histology.

Clinical Presentation and Treatment

63. B.N. is a 34-month-old boy who is pale, irritable, and has had abdominal complaints with decreased bowel movements and reduced oral intake for 2 weeks. He has played less than normal for the last 4 weeks. B.N.'s blood pressure has intermittently been as high as 146/87 mm Hg (normal, ninetieth percentile, 106/69). His Hgb is 7.9 g/dL (normal, 11.5 to 13.5) and his erythrocyte sedimentation rate is 139 mm/hr (normal, <10). B.N. has a history of hypospadias and left hydronephrosis. Scans show a right kidney mass extending through the capsule plus two distant metastases in the peritoneum. Chest radiography shows one nodule in the lung also. Pathology from a biopsy sample shows favorable histology Wilms' tumor. What is the current treatment for Wilms' tumor?

The series of five National Wilms' Tumor Studies have sought to progressively minimize toxicities from radiation and chemotherapy while maintaining the excellent cure rate. The fourth National Wilms' Tumor Study Group (NWTS-4) study demonstrated that intermittent, higher doses of dactinomycin allowed higher dose intensity with less myelosuppression than lower doses given daily for 5 days. Using greater dose intensity and dose density, 6 months of therapy was shown to be as effective as 15 months of therapy given the traditional way.[255] There were also fewer clinic visits, with estimated costs reduced by 50%.[255,256] The fifth NWTS study (ongoing) is using surgery followed by 18 to 24 weeks of chemotherapy, with the drugs determined by the stage and histology (Table 91-10). Abdominal radiation therapy is used for stage II disease with unfavorable histology (focal or diffuse anaplasia) or stages III or IV with any histology; pulmonary radiation is used for stage IV disease if the chest radiograph is positive for metastases. For stage V patients, or those with inoperable tumors, surgery can be delayed until chemotherapy reduces the tumor size.

Dosing Chemotherapy in Infants

64. **Are there any special precautions for dosing chemotherapy in B.N.?**

The NWTS-2 noted an excessive number of toxic deaths in good-prognosis infants, and this resulted in a dosing change.[257] After chemotherapy doses were decreased by 50%, severe hematologic toxicity, toxic deaths, and pulmonary and hepatic complications were reduced.[258] Importantly, no decrease in therapeutic effect was noted. Reduction of chemotherapy doses in infants may be a consideration for other pediatric cancers as well.[259–261] Reasons for increased toxicity may include altered pharmacokinetics or organ sensitivity as well as the larger body surface area per kilogram relative to older children and adults.[257] In NWTS-5, dosages of chemotherapy agents for children <30 kg are converted from mg/m^2 to mg/kg. By assuming the average 1-m^2 child weighs 30 kg, one can divide the dose/m^2 by 30 and arrive at a dose/kg to be used in dosing calculations. This adjustment lowers the dose by 20% to 50% in children who weigh <15 kg. In NWTS-5, infants less than 12 months of age receive doses that are further reduced by halving the mg/kg dose.

Interaction of Chemotherapy With Radiation

65. **Are there any dosing precautions required because of potential interactions between B.N.'s treatments?**

Table 91-10 National Wilms' Tumor Study V Treatment Regimens by Stage and Histology

Stages I and II, Favorable Histology; Stage I, Focal or Diffuse Unfavorable Histology:
1. Surgery followed by 18 weeks of vincristine and dactinomycin

Stage III, Favorable Histology; Stages II and III, Focal Anaplasia:
2. Surgery followed by 24 weeks of vincristine, dactinomycin, and doxorubicin, with abdominal radiation. *Stage IV, Favorable Histology or Focal Anaplasia:* add pulmonary radiation if chest radiograph shows metastases

Stage II or III, Diffuse Anaplasia; Stages I to III Clear Cell Sarcoma of the Kidney (Unfavorable Histology):
3. Surgery followed by 24 weeks of vincristine, doxorubicin, etoposide, and cyclophosphamide with mesna, abdominal radiation. *Stage IV, Diffuse Anaplasia or Clear Cell Sarcoma of the Kidney:* add pulmonary radiation if chest radiograph is positive for metastases

Stage V:
4. Biopsy followed by neoadjuvant vincristine, dactinomycin, and doxorubicin, then complete resection or debulking followed by more chemotherapy and if a poor response, radiation therapy; more aggressive treatment if unfavorable histology (10%)

Stages I–IV, Rhabdoid Tumor (Unfavorable Histology):
5. Surgery followed by 24 weeks of carboplatin, etoposide, and cyclophosphamide with mesna, abdominal radiation

Another drug-related problem that may arise in B.N. is the interaction of dactinomycin and doxorubicin with radiation therapy.[262–266] Two effects have been reported. One is acute enhancement of radiation effects, and the other is recurrence (recall) of radiation effects up to several weeks later, especially to skin and mucous membranes. Because B.N. is to receive abdominal and lung irradiation during his chemotherapy treatment, concurrent doses of dactinomycin and doxorubicin will need to be reduced by 50% or held if wet desquamation of the skin occurs. In many of the Ewing's sarcoma and rhabdomyosarcoma protocols, dactinomycin or doxorubicin is stopped during concurrent radiation treatments.

Doxorubicin Cardiotoxicity in Pediatrics

66. **When B.N. receives lung irradiation for his metastases, how will it affect the doxorubicin he is scheduled to receive?**

Although it is well known that mediastinal irradiation can increase the risk of anthracycline-induced cardiac toxicity,[267] the only adjustment for B.N. would be temporary reduction of doxorubicin doses as described in Question 65. The total doxorubicin dose for his protocol is already limited to no more than 5 mg/kg (150 mg/m^2 in larger children). In earlier Wilms' tumor studies, the risk of congestive heart failure was 4.4% at 20 years, or up to 17.4% in patients that relapsed and received more doxorubicin.[268] Thus, cardiovascular toxicity may develop as long as 20 years after the end of therapy, with an apparent decrease in left ventricular wall thickness and increased ventricular afterload, probably related to inadequate numbers of myocytes.[269–271] These reports emphasize the need to minimize chemotherapy in good-prognosis patients, as the Wilms' tumor studies are doing. New recommendations include better standardization of cardiac monitoring and continuation of monitoring for life in survivors of childhood cancer who receive cardiotoxic agents.[272,273]

Dactinomycin Hepatotoxicity

67. **B.N. is to receive vincristine 0.05 mg/kg weekly for 10 weeks; doxorubicin 1.5 mg/kg on weeks 3 and 9; 1 mg/kg on weeks 15 and 21; and dactinomycin 0.045 mg/kg on weeks 0, 6, 12, 18, and 24. During the third week of treatment, his ALT is elevated to 78 U/dL (normal, 7 to 56). Is this related to his drug therapy?**

Early in the NWTS-4, an increased incidence (14.3%) of severe hepatotoxicity (elevation of AST and/or ALT 10 times normal with or without ascites) was reported with the pulse-intensive dactinomycin doses (0.060 mg/kg per single dose) in patients receiving no abdominal radiation.[274] Subsequently, dactinomycin doses were reduced. Still, the incidence of hepatotoxicity in patients receiving the newer 0.045-mg/kg pulse doses (3.7%), as well as those receiving the standard 0.015 mg/kg per day for 5 days (2.8%), remained elevated relative to the NWTS-3 results (0.4%), which used 0.015 mg/kg per day for 5 days.[275] The reasons for the increased hepatotoxicity are not known. Liver function usually returns to baseline within 1 to 2 weeks after discontinuation of chemotherapy. Chemotherapy was restarted in some patients, although frequently at lower doses or without dactinomycin. B.N. should be monitored closely in case his liver enzymes continue to rise, especially since he will receive abdominal radiation treatments. If his ALT rises to two to five times normal, or his total bilirubin is 3 to 5 mg/dL, doses of all three of his drugs should be reduced by 50%. If his ALT or bilirubin rises above two to five times normal, the drugs should be withheld until laboratory values return to the aforementioned range.

OSTEOSARCOMA

Osteosarcoma is a malignant bone tumor that occurs most commonly in children in the second decade of life.[276] It occurs most frequently in the metaphyseal ends of the distal femur, proximal tibia, or proximal humerus, but it can occur in the flat bones as well.[277] The age range and bones involved suggest a malignant response associated with the normal childhood growth spurts.[276]

The most common manifestation at diagnosis is pain at the site, which can sometimes be present for several weeks to months.[276] Clinically detectable metastases are present in 15% to 20% of patients, usually in the lungs but occasionally in bone.

If surgery alone is used for treatment, 80% of patients will die within 5 years of recurrent metastatic disease, indicating subclinical micrometastases at the time of diagnosis.[277,278] Although surgery is the main treatment of the primary tumor, chemotherapy is used to prevent development of metastases. Drugs frequently used for osteosarcoma include high-dose methotrexate,[279] cisplatin,[280,281] doxorubicin,[282] ifosfamide,[283] carboplatin, and etoposide.[284] The tumor is relatively resistant to radiation therapy, which is usually reserved for cases in which local control cannot be achieved surgically.[276,285] When chemotherapy is used with surgery, long-term (2 to 5 years) DFS estimates typically range from 50% to 75%.[277,278,286]

68. G.C. is an 18-year-old man with a 2- to 3-month history of left shoulder pain. A tumor is found on radiograph, and biopsy confirms a high-grade conventional osteosarcoma of the left proximal humerus. No apparent metastases are found with CT and bone scans. G.C. begins neoadjuvant chemotherapy consisting of high-dose methotrexate alternating with cisplatin and doxorubicin. Two cycles of this chemotherapy will be given before his surgery, after which he will receive two additional cycles with all three drugs and two more without the cisplatin. What is the goal of chemotherapy? What is the role of presurgical (neoadjuvant) chemotherapy in G.C.?

Because G.C.'s osteosarcoma is in his proximal humerus, the surgeon can remove the primary tumor using one of the various operations that have been described elsewhere.[276] Limb salvages typically work well in the upper extremities, with fewer complications than when they are used for lower extremities. Because osteosarcoma patients usually die from metastases, the goal of the chemotherapy is to eradicate micrometastases. Neoadjuvant chemotherapy of osteosarcoma was developed to treat micrometastases while waiting for limb salvage surgeries to be arranged, performed, and healed. Neoadjuvant therapy may also facilitate limb-sparing surgery by shrinking the tumor; it also allows histologic grading of the response to initial chemotherapy at surgery, a prognostic factor for risk of relapse. There is no convincing evidence to date that DFS is better for patients who receive neoadjuvant chemotherapy relative to those who receive only adjuvant therapy.[285,287]

Prognostic Factors

69. At surgery, G.C.'s tumor shows excellent histologic response, with 99% necrosis. At diagnosis, his LDH was 684 IU/L (normal, 322 to 644 IU/L). Both of these factors indicate that G.C. is a good-risk patient. How do prognostic factors affect the choice of therapy in osteosarcoma?

Conventional staging systems do not correlate well with prognosis for most bone cancers. Clinically apparent metastases or a location that does not allow complete surgical removal of the primary tumor are associated with a poor prognosis.[285] Newer surgical techniques and treatments have improved the outlook, with 20% to 30% of these patients cured with neoadjuvant chemotherapy and surgery of the primary tumor and metastases.[284,288] Patients with these poor prognostic factors continue to be less likely to benefit from conventional surgery and chemotherapy. Therefore, newer investigational treatments are considered for poor-risk patients. Current proposals include the combination of topotecan and cyclophosphamide, or trastuzumab (Herceptin)[289] for patients with HER-2/neu positive disease. Other potential prognostic factors have been identified; however, few of these factors have been used to stratify patients to different treatment regimens.[285] One exception is the histologic grade of the tumor at surgery. In current studies, patients with >95% tumor necrosis after two cycles of neoadjuvant chemotherapy are considered good risk and are treated with standard chemotherapy like G.C. is receiving. Patients whose tumors have less necrosis at surgery are considered to be standard risk, and efforts are being made to increase their response rates by using higher cumulative doses of doxorubicin with dexrazoxane as a cardioprotectant. Dose escalation of ifosfamide is also being considered for standard-risk patients.

Delayed Clearance After High-Dose Methotrexate

70. After reconstructive surgery using a vascularized fibula graft, G.C. restarts his chemotherapy. During his fourth cycle of chemotherapy, after high-dose methotrexate is given, G.C.'s peak methotrexate concentration is 1,300 μmol/L and the 72-hour concentration is 0.22 μmol/L (normal, <0.1 μmol/L at 72 hours). Recorded urine-specific gravities are <1.015, urine pHs are >6.5, and urine output is >2 mL/kg per hour, all meeting the guidelines to reduce the risk of methotrexate-induced nephrotoxicity. However, his creatinine has increased from 0.9 to 1.1 mg/dL (normal, 0.5 to 1.2 mg/dL). Leucovorin rescue (15 mg IV every 6 hours) is continued. What potential problems could be causing his retention of methotrexate?

Accumulations of protein-containing "third-space" fluids such as pleural effusion and ascites, or GI obstruction, may retain methotrexate and cause slow terminal excretion.[290–292] Many drugs interact with methotrexate. Cisplatin reportedly reduces the excretion of methotrexate, especially at cumulative doses >300 mg/m².[293] G.C. has received four doses of 120 mg/m² of cisplatin, so this could be a cause of reduced methotrexate excretion in him. He has not received concomitant nephrotoxins such as aminoglycosides or amphotericin B. Weak organic acids such as salicylates, ketoprofen, or trimethoprim-sulfamethoxazole (TMP-SMX) can compete with methotrexate for renal tubular secretion.[294,295]

Although G.C.'s serum creatinine appears to be the same that it was at diagnosis (1.1 mg/dL), serum creatinine is not always a good indicator of renal function, so it is possible that G.C. has suffered some renal damage that is not apparent from his serum creatinine concentrations.[244] A measured creatinine clearance was 176 mL/minute per 1.73 m² at diagnosis, and a repeat at this point is 106 mL/min per 1.73 m². Even measured creatinine clearance may not always be accurate when compared with ⁵¹Cr-EDTA measurement of glomerular filtration rate.[244] Although the reduced renal clearance may be contributing, it is not clear why G.C. is retaining methotrexate; future courses of methotrexate will need close monitoring.

Leucovorin Rescue

71. **How long should leucovorin be administered to G.C.?**

Cytotoxic effects of methotrexate depend on concentration and duration of exposure.[296] Many high-dose methotrexate protocols continue leucovorin rescue until serum methotrexate concentrations are 0.1 μmol/L, which would be expected to occur approximately 72 hours after a 12-g/m² dose infused over 4 hours. Because G.C. has delayed clearance with persistence of low methotrexate levels past 72 hours, prevention of GI and bone marrow cytotoxicity may require continuation of leucovorin rescue until methotrexate concentrations are <0.01 to 0.05 μmol/L.[292] For G.C., methotrexate concentrations did not fall below 0.1 μmol/L until 108 hours after his dose, thus leucovorin was continued 24 hours past that. Other considerations may be important in other patients receiving leucovorin rescue. Because of the competitive nature of leucovorin rescue, higher leucovorin doses may be needed for patients with methotrexate concentrations above the usual range at a specified time after the dose.

Crom and Evans have published a figure that helps identify patients who are at high risk of methotrexate toxicity if given the usual low doses of leucovorin rescue[291] (Fig. 91-1). Using their guidelines, if G.C.'s methotrexate concentrations had remained between 1 and 5 μmol/L 42 hours after the beginning of the infusion, recommendations would include increasing the dose of the leucovorin to 30 mg/m² every 6 hours until methotrexate concentrations fall below 1 μmol/L. A rough guideline for normal methotrexate concentrations after a 12-g/m² dose is infused over 4 hours would be as follows: 1,000 μmol/L for the peak, 10 μmol/L at 24 hours, 1 μmol/L at 48 hours, and 0.1 μmol/L at 72 hours. If concentrations exceed 1 μmol/L and are above these normal values, it is appropriate to look at Crom and Evans guidelines or those in the protocol to determine if higher doses of leucovorin are needed. Oral leucovorin administration should not be used when the patient has emesis or requires larger doses (>50 mg), which are often poorly absorbed.[291]

RHABDOMYOSARCOMA

Rhabdomyosarcoma is the most common soft tissue sarcoma of childhood, occurring in 3.4% of all children with cancer.[210] The two most common histologic types are embryonal and alveolar. Embryonal rhabdomyosarcoma cells resemble striated muscle and occur most frequently in young children with involvement in the head and neck or genitourinary tract. Alveolar rhabdomyosarcoma cells resemble lung parenchymal

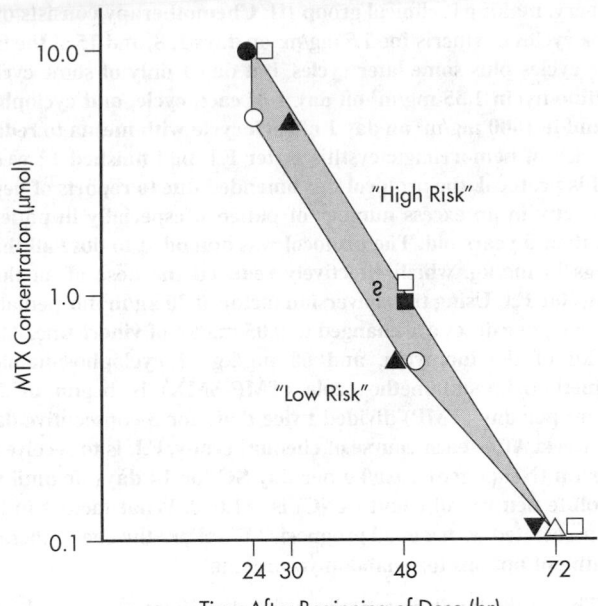

FIGURE 91-1 **Composite semilogarithmic plot of serum methotrexate (MTX) concentrations that have been proposed to identify patients at "high risk" to develop toxicity from high-dose MTX if conventional low-dose leucovorin is administered.** Data obtained from reports of (▲) Evans,[297] (△) Tattersal,[298] (●) Isacoff,[299] (○) Isacoff,[300] (□) Nirenberg,[301] (■) Stoller,[302] and (▼) Rechnitzer.[303] (Reprinted from Evans WE et al. Applied Pharmacokinetics: Principles of Therapeutic Drug Monitoring. 3rd Ed. Vancouver, WA: Applied Therapeutics Inc., 1992.)

cells and occur more frequently in older children or adolescents with involvement of the trunk or extremities. Generally, patients with alveolar rhabdomyosarcoma have a poorer prognosis than patients with the embryonal type. The clinical presentation of rhabdomyosarcoma varies with its location.

Treatment combines surgery, irradiation, and chemotherapy. Complete surgical removal is often difficult given its locations and infiltrative characteristic. However, since good local control improves the prognosis,[221] irradiation is used to achieve this. Combination chemotherapy is necessary because the 5-year survival with local control alone is 10% to 30%. Vincristine, dactinomycin, and cyclophosphamide (VAC regimen) have been used extensively to treat rhabdomyosarcoma.[221] Other agents producing responses include doxorubicin,[304] ifosfamide,[305] etoposide,[306] cisplatin,[307] dacarbazine,[308] and methotrexate.[309] Melphalan (Alkeran) has little activity in heavily pretreated patients (8% partial responses), but previously untreated patients respond well (77% partial responses).[310] The Intergroup Rhabdomyosarcoma Study III had a 3-year, progression-free survival of 67% using chemotherapy with local treatment.[311] Results of the fourth study indicate a 76% failure-free survival for nonmetastatic patients.[312]

Clinical Presentation and Prognostic Factors

72. **F.J. is a 2-year-old girl with a rapidly enlarging mass on the lateral head of the gastrocnemius muscle in the right calf. F.J. has no other complaints. Bone marrow and scans are negative for metastatic disease. The diagnosis is embryonal rhabdomyosarcoma, stage III (unfavorable site and >5 cm mass). Initial expectations were that gross residual tumor would remain after the**

surgery, making it clinical group III. Chemotherapy consists of 3-week cycles of vincristine 1.5 mg/m² on days 1, 8, and 15 of the first four cycles plus some later cycles, but day 1 only of some cycles, dactinomycin 1.35 mg/m² on day 1 of each cycle, and cyclophosphamide 1800 mg/m² on day 1 of each cycle with mesna to reduce the risk of hemorrhagic cystitis. After F.J. had finished 12 weeks of this protocol, the protocol was amended due to reports of hepatotoxicity in an excess number of patients, especially in patients less than 3 years old. The protocol was amended to dose all three drugs in mg/kg, which effectively reduced the dose of all three drugs for F.J. Using the conversion factor of 30 kg/m² for pediatric patients, her doses are changed to 0.05 mg/kg of vincristine, 0.045 mg/kg of dactinomycin, and 60 mg/kg of cyclophosphamide. Trimethoprim-sulfamethoxazole (TMP-SMX) is begun at 150 mg/m² per day (TMP) divided twice daily for 3 consecutive days per week. After each course of chemotherapy, F.J. is to receive filgrastim (Neupogen) 5 μg/kg per day SC for 14 days or until the absolute neutrophil count (ANC) is >1,000. What factors in F.J. are associated with a good prognosis? What are the chemotherapy treatment options for rhabdomyosarcoma?

The embryonal histopathologic classification has a better prognosis than the alveolar one, although there is evidence that the primary tumor site is more important than the histology.[221,313,314] The primary site affects resectability, route of spread, and how early the diagnosis is made. The Intergroup Rhabdomyosarcoma Studies (IRS) have used a clinical grouping system (groups I to IV), which is based on spread of the disease and extent of resection. This system has been useful because of its correlation with prognosis; complete surgical removal and lack of metastases both correlate with good prognosis.[221] The fourth and fifth IRS studies are comparing the clinical grouping system to a TNM staging system similar to that used in adult cancers.

In rhabdomyosarcoma, the tumor site is one important part of the T rating in the staging system. F.J.'s tumor involves an unfavorable site, and is greater than 5 cm, making it stage III. Although her tumor was expected to be clinical group III, after a good response to neoadjuvant chemotherapy, a complete resection was performed, making it clinical group I. This suggests that she has an 80% to 90% chance of 3-year survival based on the IRS-II, IRS-III, and IRS-IV results.[221,311,312] The IRS-V study currently in progress classifies patients as having low-, intermediate-, or high-risk disease. Low-risk includes patients with embryonal rhabdomyosarcoma at favorable sites, or at unfavorable sites with no more than microscopic residual tumor. Intermediate-risk patients have the embryonal subtype with gross residual tumor; metastatic disease if they are younger than 10 years of age; or the alveolar subtype without metastatic disease. High-risk patients include those with metastatic alveolar disease or those who are at least 10 years old with metastatic embryonal disease.

Chemotherapy for many of the low-risk patients is limited to vincristine and dactinomycin. Most intermediate-risk patients are treated with vincristine, dactinomycin, and high doses of cyclophosphamide. High-risk patients are candidates for trials with newer drugs such as irinotecan. If the patient responds to the new agent(s) given at the beginning of treatment, the new treatment is continued along with vincristine, dactinomycin, and cyclophosphamide. F.J. is in the low-risk group; however, her large tumor justifies adding high-dose cyclophosphamide to the vincristine and dactinomycin. Since radiation to her leg would stop bone growth, and her surgical margins were tumor-free, no radiation is being administered.

TMP-SMX PROPHYLAXIS AND FILGRASTIM FOR MYELOSUPPRESSION

73. What are the reasons for treating F.J. with TMP-SMX and filgrastim?

F.J.'s VAC regimen (vincristine, dactinomycin, and cyclophosphamide) was associated with a high incidence of neutropenic fevers even during the pilot studies. Because of the frequency of severe myelosuppression, TMP-SMX is used until 6 months after chemotherapy for prophylaxis against *Pneumocystis carinii,* an opportunistic pathogen. Filgrastim is used to minimize neutropenia so that the chemotherapy dose intensity can be maintained. The benefit of using a post-nadir ANC of 1,000 as an endpoint for filgrastim therapy is unknown.

RENAL FANCONI'S SYNDROME WITH IFOSFAMIDE

74. F.J.'s mother read on the internet about a patient with rhabdomyosarcoma who had received vincristine, ifosfamide, and etoposide and was cured. She wants to know why that regimen is not being used for her daughter?

The IRS-IV results for local/regional disease (intermediate risk) demonstrated no advantages of vincristine, ifosfamide, and etoposide or vincristine, dactinomycin, and ifosfamide over the standard vincristine, dactinomycin, and cyclophosphamide treatment.[312] Additionally, the ifosfamide-containing regimens caused more toxicity. Ifosfamide has been associated with renal Fanconi's syndrome, a proximal tubular defect that is characterized by wasting of electrolytes, glucose, and amino acids, as well as renal tubular acidosis and an increased serum creatinine. Data suggest that the risk of Fanconi's syndrome is increased in children who are younger than 3 years old; have received total doses >72 to 100 g/m²; have hydronephrosis, a single kidney, or an elevated serum creatinine; or have received previous platinum therapy.[315–318] During each course of her chemotherapy, F.J. develops ketonuria, however, this is not a toxicity of her chemotherapy. Ketonuria is caused by her mesna therapy, which has been reported to routinely cause false-positive ketone tests.[319]

REFERENCES

1. American Cancer Society. Cancer Facts and Figures—2003. Atlanta, GA: American Cancer Society, 2003.
2. Feuer EJ et al. The lifetime risk of developing breast cancer. J Natl Cancer Inst 1993;85:892.
3. Ford D et al. Risks of cancer in BRCA1-mutation carriers. Breast Cancer Linkage Consortium. Lancet 1994;343:692.
4. Struewing JP et al. The risk of cancer associated with specific mutations of BRCA1 and BRCA2 among Ashkenazi Jews. N Engl Med 1997;336:1401.
5. Frank TS et al. The pros and cons of genetic testing for breast and ovarian cancer risk. Int J Fertil 1999;44(3):139.
6. Schrag D et al. Life expectancy gains from cancer prevention strategies for women with breast cancer and BRCA1 or BRCA2 mutations. JAMA 2000;283(5):617.

7. Armstrong K et al. Assessing the risk of breast cancer. N Engl J Med 2000;342(8):564.

8. Smith RA et al. American Cancer Society Guidelines for Breast Cancer Screening: Update 2003. CA Cancer J Clin 2003;53:141.

9. Viale G et al. Intraoperative examination of axillary sentinel lymph nodes in breast carcinoma patients. Cancer 1999;85:2433.

10. Hermann RE et al. Results of conservative operations for breast cancer. Arch Surg 1985;120:746.

11. Veronesi U et al. Comparing radical mastectomy with quadrantectomy, axillary dissection and radiotherapy in patients with small cancers of the breast. N Engl J Med 1981;305:6.

12. Fisher B et al. Five-year results of a randomized clinical trial comparing total mastectomy and segmental mastectomy with or without radiation in the treatment of breast cancer. N Engl J Med 1985;312:666.

13. McGuire WL et al. Prognostic factors and treatment decisions in axillary node negative breast cancer. N Engl J Med 1992;326:1765.

14. Andrulis IL et al. Neu-erbB-2 amplification identifies a poor-prognosis group of women with node-negative breast cancer. J Clin Oncol 1998;16:1340.

15. Early Breast Cancer Trialists' Collaborative Group. Polychemotherapy for early breast cancer: an overview of the randomized trials. Lancet 1998; 352:930.

16. Early Breast Cancer Trialists' Collaborative Group. Tamoxifen for early breast cancer: an overview of the randomized trials. Lancet 1998;351:1451.

17. NIH. National Institutes of Health consensus development conference statement: adjuvant therapy for breast cancer. November 1–3, 2000. www.nih.gov. Bethesda, Maryland.

18. Goldhirsch A et al. Meeting highlights: International Consensus Panel on the treatment of primary breast cancer. J Clin Oncol 2001;19(18):3817.

19. Winer EP et al. American Society of Clinical Oncology Technology Assessment working group update: use of aromatase inhibitors in the adjuvant setting. J Clin Oncol 2003;21(13):2597.

20. Muss HB et al. c-erbB-2 expression and response to adjuvant therapy in women with node-positive early breast cancer. N Engl J Med 1994;330:1260.

21. Mehta RR et al. Plasma c-erb-2 levels in breast cancer patients: prognostic significance in predicting response to chemotherapy. J Clin Oncol 1998; 16(7):2409.

22. Gusterson BA et al. Prognostic importance of c-erbB-2 expressions in breast cancer. J Clin Oncol 1992;10(7):1049.

23. Henderson IC et al. Improved outcomes from adding sequential paclitaxel but not from escalating doxorubicin dose in an adjuvant chemotherapy regimen for patients with node-positive primary breast cancer. J Clin Oncol 2003;21(6):976.

24. Citron ML et al. Randomized trial of dose-dense versus conventionally scheduled and sequential versus concurrent combination chemotherapy as postoperative adjuvant treatment of node-positive primary breast cancer: first report of intergroup trial C9741/Cancer and Leukemia Group B trial 9741. J Clin Oncol 2003;21(7):1431.

25. Baum M et al. Early Breast Cancer Trialists' Collaborative Group. Ovarian ablation in early breast cancer: overview of the randomized trials. Lancet 1998;348:1189.

26. Anastrozole alone or in combination with tamoxifen versus tamoxifen alone for adjuvant treatment of postmenopausal women with early breast cancer: First results of the ATAC randomized trial. Lancet 2002;359:2131.

27. Sainsbury R, on behalf of the ATAC Trialists' Group. Beneficial side-effect profile of anastrozole compared with tamoxifen by additional 7 months of exposure data: a safety update from the ATAC trial. Breast Cancer Res Treat 2002;76(Suppl 1):156.

28. Hortobagyi GN. Developments in chemotherapy of breast cancer. Cancer 2000;88:3073.

29. Henderson IC. Chemotherapy for metastatic disease. In: Harris JR et al., eds. Breast Diseases. 2nd Ed. Philadelphia: JB Lippincott, 1991:604.

30. Johnson SA et al. Vinorelbine: an overview. Cancer Treat Rev 1996;22:127.

31. Michaud LB et al. Risks and benefits of taxanes in breast and ovarian cancer. Drug Saf 2000;23:401.

32. Fossati R et al. Cytotoxic and hormonal treatment for metastatic breast cancer: a systematic review of published randomized trials involving 31,510 women. J Clin Oncol 1998;16:3439.

33. Eisenhauer EA, Vermorken JB. The taxoids: comparative clinical pharmacology and therapeutic potential. Drugs 1998;55(1):5.

34. Valero V. Docetaxel as single-agent therapy in metastatic breast cancer: clinical efficacy. Semin Oncol 1997;24(4 Suppl 13):S13.

35. Slamon DJ et al. Use of chemotherapy plus a monoclonal antibody against HER2 for metastatic breast cancer that over expresses HER2. N Engl J Med 2001;344(11):783.

36. Burstein HJ et al. Clinical activity of trastuzumab and vinorelbine in women with HER2-overexpressing metastatic breast cancer. J Clin Oncol 2001; 19(10):2722.

37. Rodriques M, Dinapoli RP. Spinal cord compression with special reference to metastatic epidural tumors. Mayo Clin Proc 1980;55:442.

38. Gilbert RW et al. Epidural spinal cord compression from metastatic tumor: diagnosis and treatment. Ann Neurol 1978;3:40.

39. McGuire WL. Hormone receptors: their role in predicting prognosis and response to endocrine therapy. Semin Oncol 1978;5:428.

40. Singhakowinta A et al. Estrogen receptor and natural course of breast cancer. Ann Surg 1983;183:84.

41. Nabholtz JM et al. Anastrozole is superior to tamoxifen as first-line therapy for advanced breast cancer in postmenopausal women: results of a North American Multicenter Randomized trial. J Clin Oncol 2000;18(22):3758.

42. Mouridsen H et al. Phase III study of letrozole versus tamoxifen as first-line therapy of advanced breast cancer in postmenopausal women: analysis of survival and update of efficacy from the International Letrozole Breast Cancer Group. J Clin Oncol 2003;21(11):2101.

43. Hilner BE et al. American Society of Clinical Oncology guideline on the role of bisphosphonates in breast cancer. J Clin Oncol 2000;18(6):1378.

44. Hortobagyi G et al. Long-term prevention of skeletal complications of metastatic breast cancer with pamidronate. J Clin Oncol 1998;16(6):2038.

45. Rosen LS et al. Zoledronic acid versus pamidronate in the treatment of skeletal metastases in patients with breast cancer or osteolytic lesions or multiple myeloma: a phase III, double-blind, comparative trial. Cancer 2001;7:377.

46. Lonning PE et al. Activity of exemestane in metastatic breast cancer after failure of nonsteroidal aromatase inhibitors: a phase II trial. J Clin Oncol 2000;18(11):2234.

47. Lynch HT, de la Chapelle A. Hereditary colorectal cancer. N Engl J Med 2003;348:919.

48. American Society of Clinical Oncology. Statement of the American Society of Clinical oncology: genetic testing for cancer susceptibility. J Clin Oncol 1996;14(5):1730.

49. Subongkot S et al. Selective cyclooxygenase-2 inhibition: a target in cancer prevention and treatment. Pharmacotherapy 2003;23:9.

50. Steinbach G et al. The effect of celecoxib, a cyclooxygenase-2 inhibitor, in familial adenomatous polyposis. N Engl J Med 2000;342:1946.

51. Baron JA. A randomized trial of aspirin to prevent colorectal adenomas. N Engl J Med 2003;348:891.

52. Baron JA et al. Calcium supplements for the prevention of colorectal adenomas. N Engl J Med 1999;340:101.

53. Howe GR et al. Dietary intake of fiber and decreased risk of cancers of the colon and rectum: evidence from the combined analysis of 13 case-control studies. J Natl Cancer Inst 1992;84:1887.

54. Ransohoff DF, Lang CA. Screening for colorectal cancer with the fecal occult blood test: a background paper. American College of Surgeons. Ann Intern Med 1997;126:811.

55. Adams EC, Layman KM. Immunochemical confirmation of gastrointestinal bleeding. Ann Clin Lab Sci 1974;4:343.

56. Feinberg EJ et al. How long to abstain from eating red meat before fecal occult blood tests. Ann Intern Med 1990;113:403.

57. Benson AB et al. 2000 update of American Society of Clinical Oncology colorectal cancer surveillance guidelines. J Clin Oncol 2000;18:3586.

58. Willett CG et al. Failure patterns following curative resection of colonic carcinoma. Ann Surg 1984; 200:685.

59. Eisenberg B et al. Carcinoma of the colon and rectum: the natural history review in 1704 patients. Cancer 1982;49:1131.

60. Weiss L et al. Hematogenous metastatic patterns in colonic carcinoma: an analysis of 1541 necropsies. J Pathol 1986;150:195.

61. Efficacy of adjuvant fluorouracil and folinic acid in colon cancer. International Multicentre Pooled Analysis of Colon Cancer Trials investigators. Lancet 1995;345(8955):939.

62. O'Connell M et al. Prospectively randomized trial of postoperative adjuvant chemotherapy in patients with high-risk colon cancer. J Clin Oncol 1998;16:295.

63. Brown ML et al. Adjuvant therapy for stage III colon cancer: economics returns to research and cost-effectiveness of treatment. J Natl Cancer Inst 1994;86:424.

64. Mamounas EP et al. Comparative efficacy of adjuvant chemotherapy in patients with Dukes' V vs Duke's C colon cancer: results from four NSABP adjuvant studies (C01,C02,C03,C04). Proc Am Soc Clin Oncol 1996;15:205.

65. Poon MA et al. Biochemical modulation of fluorouracil: evidence of significant improvement of survival and quality of life in patients with advanced colorectal carcinoma. J Clin Oncol 1989;7:1407.

66. Petrelli N et al. The modulation of fluorouracil with leucovorin in metastatic colorectal carcinoma: a prospective randomized phase III trial. J Clin Oncol 1989;7:1419.

67. Poon MA et al. Biochemical modulation of fluorouracil with leucovorin: confirmatory evidence of improved therapeutic efficacy in advanced colorectal cancer. J Clin Oncol 1991;9:1967.

68. Efficacy of intravenous continuous infusion of fluorouracil compared with bolus administration in advanced cancer: Meta-analysis Group in Cancer. J Clin Oncol 1998;16:301.

69. de Gramont A et al. Randomized trial comparing monthly low-dose leucovorin and fluorouracil bolus with bimonthly high-dose leucovorin and fluorouracil bolus plus continuous infusion for advanced colorectal cancer: a French intergroup study. J Clin Oncol 1997;15:808.

70. Cunningham D et al. Randomised trial of irinotecan plus supportive care versus supportive care alone after fluorouracil failure for patients with metastatic colorectal cancer. Lancet 1998;352:1413.

71. Rougier P et al. Randomised trial of irinotecan versus fluorouracil by continuous infusion after fluorouracil failure in patients with metastatic colorectal cancer. Lancet 1998;352:1407.

72. Saltz LB et al. Irinotecan plus fluorouracil and leucovorin for metastatic colorectal cancer. Irinotecan Study Group. N Engl J Med 2000;343:905.

73. Douillard JY et al. Irinotecan combined with fluorouracil compared with fluorouracil alone as first-line treatment for metastatic colorectal cancer: a multicentre randomized trial. Lancet 2000;355:1041.

74. Rothenberg ML et al. Mortality associated with irinotecan plus bolus fluorouracil/leucovorin: summary findings of an independent panel. J Clin Oncol 2001;19:3801.

75. Rothenberg ML et al. Superiority of oxaliplatin and fluorouracil-leucovorin compared with either therapy alone in patients with progressive colorectal cancer after irinotecan and fluorouracil-leucovorin: interim results of a phase III trial. J Clin Oncol 2003;21:2059.

76. Tournigand C et al. FOLFIRI followed by FOLFOX versus FOLFOX followed by FOLFIRI in metastatic colorectal cancer: Final results of a phase III study [Abstract]. Proc Am Soc Clin Oncol 2001;20:124.

77. Garay CA et al. Randomized trial of bolus plus infusional 5-FU/leucovorin (LV5FU2) with/without oxaliplatin (FOLFOX4) after sequential flouropyrimidine and CPT-11 in the treatment of advanced colorectal cancer [Abstract]. Proc Am Soc Clin Oncol 2003;22:1019.

78. Giacchetti S et al. Phase III multicenter randomized trial of oxaliplatin added to chronomodulated fluorouracil-leucovorin as first-line treatment of metastatic colorectal cancer. J Clin Oncol 2000;18(1):136.

79. Golberg RM et al. N9741: oxaliplatin or CPT-11 + 5-fluorouracil (5-FU)/leucovorin or oxaliplatin+ CPT-11 in advanced colorectal cancer. Initial toxicity and response data from a GI intergroup study. Proc Am Soc Clin Oncol 2002;21:511.

80. Wiseman LR et al. Oxaliplatin: a review of its use in the management of metastatic colorectal cancer. Drugs Aging 1999;14:459.

81. Budman DR et al. Preliminary studies of a novel oral fluoropyrimidine carbamate: capecitabine. J Clin Oncol 1998;16(5):1795.

82. Twelves C et al. Capecitabine improves medical resource use compared with 5-fluorouracil plus leucovorin in a phase III trial conducted in patients with advanced colorectal carcinoma. Eur J Cancer 2001;37:597.

83. Hoff PM et al. Comparison of oral capecitabine versus intravenous fluorouracil plus leucovorin as first-line treatment in 605 patients with metastatic colorectal cancer: results of a randomized phase III study. J Clin Oncol 2001;19:2282.

84. Scheithauer W et al. Randomized multicenter phase II trial of two different schedules of capecitabine plus oxaliplatin as first-line treatment of advanced colorectal cancer. J Clin Oncol 2003;21(7):1307.

85. Borner MM et al. A randomized phase II trial of capecitabine (CAP) and two different schedules of irinotecan (IRI) in first-line treatment of metastatic colorectal cancer (MCC) [Abstract]. Proc Am Soc Clin Oncol 2003;22:1068

86. Breedis C, Young C. The blood supply of neoplasms in the liver. Am J Pathol 1954;30:969.

87. Rougier P et al. Hepatic arterial infusion of floxuridine in patients with liver metastases from colorectal carcinoma: long-term results of a prospective randomized trial. J Clin Oncol 1992;10:1112.8.

88. Kemeny N et al. Hepatic arterial infusion of chemotherapy after resection of hepatic metastases from colorectal cancer. N Engl J Med 1999; 341:2039.

89. Hohn DC et al. Biliary sclerosis in patients receiving hepatic arterial infusion of floxuridine. J Clin Oncol 1985;3:98.

90. Kemeny N et al. Sclerosing cholangitis after continuous hepatic artery infusion of FUDR. Ann Surg 1985;202:176.

91. Kato T et al. Targeted cancer chemotherapy with arterial microcapsule chemoembolization: review of 1013 patients. Cancer Chemother Pharmacol 1996;37(4):289.

92. Ginsberg RJ et al. Non-small cell lung cancer. In: DeVita VT et al., eds. Cancer: Principles and Practice of Oncology. 6th Ed. Philadelphia: Lippincott, Williams & Wilkins, 2001:925.

93. Murren J et al. Small cell lung cancer. In: DeVita VT et al., eds. Cancer: Principles and Practice of Oncology. 6th Ed. Philadelphia: Lippincott, Williams & Wilkins, 2001:983.

94. National Academy of Sciences. Environmental Tobacco Smoke: Measuring Exposures and Assessing Health Effects. Appendix D. Washington, DC: National Academy Press, 1986.

95. Speizer FE. Overview of the risk of respiratory cancer from airborne contaminants. Environ Health Perspect 1986;70:9.

96. Omenn GS et al. Contribution of environmental fibers to respiratory cancer. Environ Health Perspect 1986;70:51.

97. The Alpha-Tocopherol, Beta Carotene Cancer Prevention Study Group. The effect of vitamin E and beta carotene on the incidence of lung cancer and other cancers in male smokers. N Engl J Med 1994;330:1029.

98. Omenn GS et al. Effects of a combination of beta-carotene and vitamin A on lung cancer and cardiovascular disease. N Engl J Med 1996;334: 1150.

99. Clark LC et al. Effects of selenium supplementation for cancer prevention in patients with carcinoma of the skin. A randomized controlled trial. Nutritional Prevention of Cancer Study Group. JAMA 1996;276:1957.

100. Berlin NI et al. The National Cancer Institute Cooperative Early Lung Cancer Detection Program: results of the initial screen (prevalence). Early lung cancer detection: introduction. Am Rev Respir Dis 1984;13:545.

101. Maras PM et al. Lung cancer mortality in the Mayo Lung Project: impact of extended follow-up. J Natl Cancer Inst 2000;92(16):1308.

102. Swensen SJ et al. Lung cancer screening with CT: Mayo Clinic experience. Radiology 2003; 226(3):756.

103. PORT Meta-analysis Trialists Group. Postoperative radiotherapy in non-small cell lung cancer: systematic review and meta-analysis of individual patient data from randomized controlled trials. Lancet 1998;352:257.

104. Non-Small Cell Lung Cancer Collaborative Group. Chemotherapy in non-small cell lung cancer: a meta-analysis using updated data on individual patients from 52 randomized clinical trials. Br Med J 1995;311:899.

105. American Society of Clinical Oncology: Clinical practice guidelines for the treatment of unresectable non-small cell lung cancer. J Clin Oncol 1997;15:2996.

106. Carson JAS et al. Taste acuity and food attitudes of selected patients with cancer. J Am Diet Assoc 1977;70:361.

107. DeWys WD. Changes in taste sensation and feeding behavior in cancer patients: a review. J Hum Nutr 1978;32:447.

108. Terrell M et al. Plasma protein synthesis in experimental cancer compared to paraneoplastic conditions, including monokine administration. Cancer Res 1987;47:5825.

109. Dunlop RJ, Campbell CW. Cytokines and advanced cancer. J Pain Sympt Manage 2000; 20:214.

110. Tisdale MJ. Biology of cancer cachexia. J Natl Cancer Inst 1997;89:1763.

111. Beutler B et al. Identity of tumor necrosis factor and the macrophage-secreted factor cachectin. Nature 1985;316:552.

112. Tchekmedyian NS et al. High-dose megestrol acetate. JAMA 1987;257:1195.

113. Aisner J et al. Studies of high-dose megestrol acetate: potential applications in cachexia. Semin Oncol 1988;15:88.

114. Struwe M et al. Effect of dronabinol on nutritional status in HIV infection. Ann Pharmacother 1993; 27:827.

115. Loprinzi CL et al. Randomized placebo-controlled evaluation of hydrazine sulfate in patients with advanced colorectal cancer. J Clin Oncol 1994;12:1121.

116. Loprinzi CL et al. Placebo controlled trial of hydrazine sulfate in patients with newly diagnosed non- small-cell lung cancer. J Clin Oncol 1994;12:1126.

117. Bunn PA, Carney DN. Overview of chemotherapy for small cell lung cancer. Semin Oncol 1997;24(2 Suppl 7):S69.

118. Evans WK et al. Etoposide (VP-16) and cisplatin: an effective treatment for relapse of small cell lung cancer. J Clin Oncol 1985;3:65.

119. Clark PI. Current role of oral etoposide in the management of small cell lung cancer. Drugs 1999;58(Suppl 3):17.

120. Johnson DH et al. Prolonged administration of oral etoposide in patients with relapsed or refrac-

tory small-cell lung cancer: a phase II trial. J Clin Oncol 1990;8:1613.

121. Clark PI. Prolonged administration of single agent etoposide in patients with untreated small cell lung cancer [Abstract]. Proc Am Soc Clin Oncol 1990;9:226.

122. Glantz MJ et al. Prophylactic cranial irradiation in small cell lung cancer: rationale, results, and recommendations. Semin Oncol 1997;24:477.

123. Pritchard RS et al. Chemotherapy plus radiotherapy compared with radiotherapy alone in the treatment of locally advanced, unresectable, non-small-cell lung cancer: a meta analysis. Ann Intern Med 1996;125:723.

124. Kris MG et al. A phase II trial of ZD1839 ('Iressa') in advanced non-small cell lung cancer (NSCLC) patients who had failed platinum-and docetaxel-based regimens [Abstract]. Proc Am Soc Clin Oncol 2002;21:292.

125. NIH Consensus Development Panel on Ovarian Cancer. Screening, treatment, and follow-up. JAMA 1995;273:491.

126. Averette HE et al. Screening in gynecologic cancers. Cancer 1993;72:1043.

127. Koss LG. Cervical (PAP) smear. Cancer 1993;71: 1406.

128. Creasman WT, DiSaia PJ. Screening in ovarian cancer. Am J Obstet Gynecol 1991;165:7.

129. Andolf E et al. Ultrasound examination for detection of ovarian carcinoma in risk groups. Obstet Gynecol 1990;75:106.

130. Zurawski VR Jr et al. An initial analysis of preoperative serum CA-125 levels in patient with early stage ovarian carcinoma. Gynecol Oncol 1988; 30:7.

131. Jacobs I, Bast RC Jr. The CA-125 tumor associated antigen: a review of literature. Hum Reprod 1989;4:1.

132. McGuire WP et al. Cyclophosphamide and cisplatin compared with paclitaxel and cisplatin in patients with stage III and stage IV ovarian cancer. N Engl J Med 1996;334:1.

133. Ozols RF et al. Randomized phase III study of cisplatin (CIS)/paclitaxel (PAC) versus carboplatin (CARBO)/PAC in optimal stage III epithelial ovarian cancer (OC): Gynecologic Oncology Group Trial (GOG 158) [Abstract 1273]. Proc Am Soc Clin Oncol 1999;18:356a.

134. Berek JS et al. Advanced epithelial ovarian cancer. Ann of Oncol 1999;10(Suppl 1):87.

135. Markman M et al. Second-line platinum therapy in patients with ovarian cancer previously treated with cisplatin. J Clin Oncol 1991;9:389.

136. ten Bokkel Huinick WB et al. Topotecan versus paclitaxel for the treatment of recurrent epithelial ovarian cancer. J Clin Oncol 1997;15:2183.

137. Herzog TJ. Update on the role of topotecan in the treatment of recurrent ovarian cancer. Oncologist 2002;7(Suppl 5):3.

138. Muggia FM et al. Phase II study of liposomal doxorubicin in platinum and paclitaxel refractory epithelial ovarian cancer. J Clin Oncol 2000;18: 3093.

139. Lund B et al. Phase II study of gemcitabine in previously treated ovarian patients. J Natl Cancer Inst 1994;86:1530.

140. Rose PG et al. Prolonged oral etoposide as second-line therapy for platinum-resistant and platinum-sensitive ovarian carcinoma: a Gynecologic Oncology Group Study. J Clin Oncol 1998; 16:405.

141. Markman M. Intraperitoneal antineoplastic agents for tumors principally confined to the peritoneal cavity. Cancer Treat Rev 1986;13:219.

142. Brenner DE. Intraperitoneal chemotherapy: a review. J Clin Oncol 1986;4:1135.

143. Alberts DS et al. Intraperitoneal cisplatin plus intravenous cyclophosphamide versus intravenous cisplatin plus intravenous cyclophosphamide for stage III ovarian cancer. N Engl J Med 1996; 335:1950.

144. Markman M et al. Phase III trial of standard-dose intravenous cisplatin plus paclitaxel versus moderately high-dose carboplatin followed by intra-

venous paclitaxel and intraperitoneal cisplatin in small-volume stage III ovarian carcinoma: an Intergroup study of the Gynecologic Oncology Group, Southwestern Oncology Group, and Eastern Cooperative Oncology Group. J Clin Oncol 2001;19:1001.

145. Lamm DL, Torti. Bladder cancer. CA Cancer J Clin 1996;46:93.

146. Heney NM et al. TA and T1 bladder cancer: occasion, recurrence and progression. Br J Urol 1982; 54:152.

147. Batts CN. Adjuvant intravesical therapy for superficial bladder cancer. Ann Pharmacother 1992; 26:1270.

148. Jaske G et al. Stage T_1, grade 3 transitional cell carcinoma of the bladder: an unfavorable tumor? J Urol 1987;137:39.

149. Herr HW. Intravesical therapy. Hematol Oncol Clin North Am 1992;6:1.

150. Lamm DL et al. A randomized trial of intravesical doxorubicin and immunotherapy with Bacille Calmette-Guerin for transitional-cell bladder carcinoma of the bladder. N Engl J Med 1991;325: 1205.

151. Steinberg G et al. Efficacy and safety of valrubicin for the treatment of Bacillus Calmette-Guerin refractory carcinoma of the bladder. J Urol 2000; 165:761.

152. Brosman SA, Lamm DL. The preparation, handling and use of intravesical bacillus Calmette-Guerin for the management of stage T_a, T_1, carcinoma-in-situ and transitional cell cancer. J Urol 1990;144:313.

153. Loehrer PJ et al. A randomized comparison of cisplatin alone or in combination with methotrexate, vinblastine, and doxorubicin in patients with metastatic urothelial carcinoma: a cooperative group study. J Clin Oncol 1992;10(7):1066.

154. Vaughn DJ et al. Paclitaxel plus carboplatin in advanced carcinoma of the urothelium: an active and tolerable outpatient regimen. J Clin Oncol 1998; 16(1):255.

155. Redman BG et al. Phase II trial of paclitaxel and carboplatin in the treatment of advanced urothelial carcinoma. J Clin Oncol 1998;16(5):1844.

156. Von der Maase H et al. Gemcitabine and cisplatin versus methotrexate, vinblastine, doxorubicin, and cisplatin (MVAC) in advanced or metastatic bladder cancer: results of a large, randomized, multinational, multicenter, phase III study. J Clin Oncol 2000;17:3068.

157. Koh HK. Cutaneous melanoma. N Engl J Med 1991;325:171.

158. Anderson CM et al. Systemic treatments for advanced cutaneous melanoma. Oncology 1995; 9(11):1149.

159. Chapman PB et al. Phase III multicenter randomized trial of the Dartmouth regimen versus dacarbazine in patients with metastatic melanoma. J Clin Oncol 1999;17(9):2745.

160. Cocconi G et al. Treatment of metastatic malignant melanoma with dacarbazine plus tamoxifen. N Engl J Med 1992;327:516.

161. Rusthoven JJ et al. A randomized, double-blind, placebo-controlled trial comparing the response rates of carmustine, dacarbazine, and cisplatin with and without tamoxifen in patients with metastatic melanoma. National Cancer Institute of Canada Clinical Trials Group. J Clin Oncol 1996;14(7):2083.

162. Rusthoven JJ. The evidence of tamoxifen and chemotherapy as treatment for metastatic melanoma. Eur J Cancer 1998;34(Suppl 3):S31.

163. Agarwala SS, Kirkwood JM. Interferons in melanoma. Curr Opin Oncol 1996;8(2):167.

164. Atkins MB et al. High-dose recombinant interleukin 2 therapy for patients with metastatic melanoma: analysis of 270 patients treated between 1985 and 1993. J Clin Oncol 1999;17(7): 2105.

165. Atkins MB et al. High-dose recombinant interleukin-2 therapy in patients with metastatic melanoma: long-term survival update. Cancer J Sci Am 2000;6(Suppl 1):S11.

166. Rosenberg SA et al. Treatment of 283 consecutive patients with metastatic melanoma or renal cell cancer using high-dose bolus interleukin 2. JAMA 1994;271 (12): 907.

167. Gearing AJH, Thorpe R. The international standard for human interleukin-2: calibration by international collaborative study. J Immunol Meth 1988; 114:3.

168. Siegal JP, Puri RK. Interleukin-2 toxicity. J Clin Oncol 1991;9:694.

169. Sondak VK et al. Adjuvant immunotherapy of resected, intermediate-thickness, node-negative melanoma with an allogenic tumor vaccine: overall results of a randomized trial of the Southwest Oncology Group. J Clin Oncol 2002;20(8):2058.

170. Vaishampayan U et al. Active immunotherapy of metastatic melanoma with allogeneic melanoma lysates and interferon alfa. Clin Cancer Res 2002;8:3696.

171. Hsueh EC et al. Prolonged survival after complete resection of disseminated melanoma and active immunotherapy with a therapeutic cancer vaccine. J Clin Oncol 2002;20(23):4549.

172. Anderson CM et al. Systemic treatments for advanced cutaneous melanoma. Oncology 1995; 9(11):1149.

173. Huncharek M et al. Single-agent DTIC versus combination chemotherapy with or without immunotherapy in metastatic melanoma: a meta-analysis of 3273 patients from 20 randomized trials. Melanoma Res 2001;11(1):75.

174. Demchak PA et al. Interleukin-2 and high-dose cisplatin in patients with metastatic melanoma: a pilot study. J Clin Oncol 1991;9(10):1821.

175. Flaherty LE et al. A phase II study of dacarbazine and cisplatin in combination with outpatient administered interleukin-2 in metastatic malignant melanoma. Cancer 1993;71(11):3520.

176. Eton O et al. Sequential biochemotherapy versus chemotherapy for metastatic melanoma: results from a phase III randomized trial. J Clin Oncol 2002;20(8):2045.

177. Atkins MB et al. A prospective randomized phase III trial of concurrent biochemotherapy with cisplatin, vinblastine, dacarbazine (CVD), IL-2 and interferon alpha-2b versus CVD alone in patients with metastatic melanoma (E3695): An ECOG-coordinated intergroup trial. Proc Am Soc Clin Oncol 2003;22:ab2847.

178. Keilholz U et al. Dacarbazine, cisplatin and IFN-a2b with or without IL-2 in advanced melanoma: Final analysis of EORTC randomized phase III trial 18951. Proc Am Soc Clin Oncol 2003; 22:ab2848.

179. Del Vecchio M et al. Multicenter phase III randomized trial of cisplatin, vindesine and dacarbazine (CVD) versus CVD plus subcutaneous interleukin-2 and interferon-alpha-2b in metastatic melanoma patients. Proc Am Soc Clin Oncol 2003;22:ab2847.

180. Pienta KJ, Esper PS. Risk factors for prostate cancer. Ann Intern Med 1993;118:793.

181. See WA et al. Bicalutamide as immediate therapy either alone or as adjuvant to standard care of patients with localized or locally advanced prostate cancer: First analysis of the early prostate cancer program. J Urol 2002;168:429.

182. Iversen P et al. Bicalutamide monotherapy compared with castration in patients with nonmetastatic locally advanced prostate cancer: 6.3 years of follow-up. J Urol 2000;164:1579.

183. Medical Research Council Prostate Cancer Working Party Investigators Group. Immediate versus deferred treatment for advanced prostatic cancer: initial results of the Medical Research Council Trial. Br J Urol 1997;79(2):235.

184. DiPaola RS et al. State-of-the-art prostate cancer treatment and research. NJ Med 2001;98:23.

185. Leuprolide Study Group. Leuprolide versus diethylstilbestrol for metastatic prostate cancer. N Engl J Med 1984;311:1281.

186. Boccardo F. Hormone therapy of prostate cancer: is there a role for antiandrogen monotherapy? Crit Rev Oncol Hem 2000;35:121.

187. Tyrrell CJ et al. A randomized comparison of 'Casodex' (bicalutamide) 150 mg monotherapy versus castration in the treatment of metastatic and locally advanced prostate cancer. Eur Urol 1998;33:447.

188. Boccardo F et al. Bicalutamide monotherapy versus flutamide plus goserelin in prostate cancer: updated results of a multicentre trial. Eur Urol 2002;42:481.

189. Prostate Cancer Trialists' Collaborative Group. Maximum androgen blockade in advanced prostate cancer: an overview of the randomized trials. Lancet 2000;355:1491.

190. Crawford ED et al. A controlled trail of leuprolide with and without flutamide in prostatic carcinoma. N Engl J Med 1989;321:419.

191. Janknegt RA et al. Orchiectomy and nilutamide or placebo as treatment of metastatic prostatic cancer in a multinational double-blind randomized trial. J Urol 1993;15:2928.

192. Garnick MB. Hormonal therapy in the management of prostate cancer: from Huggins to the present. Urology 1997;49:5.

193. Oefelein MG, Cornum R. Failure to achieve castrate levels of testosterone during luteinizing releasing hormone agonist therapy: the case for monitoring serum testosterone and a treatment decision algorithm. J Urol 2000;164:726.

194. Kelly WK et al. Steroid hormone withdrawal syndromes: pathophysiology and clinical significance. Urol Clin North Am 1997;24:421.

195. Goodin S et al. State-of-the-art treatment of metastatic hormone refractory prostate cancer. Oncologist 2002;7(4):360.

196. Tannock IF et al. Chemotherapy with mitoxantrone plus prednisone or prednisone alone for symptomatic hormone-resistant prostate cancer: a Canadian randomized trail with palliative end points. J Clin Oncol 1996;14:1756.

197. Hudes GR et al. Phase II study of estramustine and vinblastine, two microtubule inhibitors, in hormone refractory prostate cancer. J Clin Oncol 1992;10:1754.

198. Hudes G et al. Phase II study of weekly paclitaxel by 1-hour infusion plus reduced-dose oral estramustine in metastatic hormone-refractory prostate carcinoma. Proc Am Soc Clin Oncol 2001;20:175a.

199. Petrylak DP et al. Phase I trial of docetaxel with estramustine in androgen independent prostate cancer. J Clin Oncol 1999;17:958.

200. Richie JP. Detection and treatment of testicular cancer. CA Cancer J Clin 1993;43:151.

201. Hellerstedt BA, Pienta KJ. Testicular cancer. Curr Opin Oncol 2002;12(3):260.

202. Williams SD et al. Immediate adjuvant chemotherapy versus observation with treatment at relapse in pathological stage II testicular cancer. N Engl J Med 1987;317:1433.

203. Kondagunta GV, Motzer RJ. Adjuvant chemotherapy for stage II nonseminomatous germ-cell tumors. Semin Urol Oncol 2002;20(4):239.

204. Wozniak AJ et al. A randomized trial of cisplatin, vinblastine, and bleomycin versus vinblastine, cisplatin, and etoposide in the treatment of advanced germ cell tumors of the testis: a Southwest Oncology Group Study. J Clin Oncol 1991;9:70.

205. DeWit R et al. Four cycles of BEP versus an alternating regimen of PVB and BEP in patients with poor prognosis metastatic testicular nonseminoma: a randomized trial of the EORTC Genitourinary Tract Center Cooperative Group. Br J Cancer 1995;71:1311.

206. Williams SD et al. Treatment of disseminated germ-cell tumors with cisplatin, bleomycin, and either vinblastine or etoposide. N Engl J Med 1987;316:1435.

207. Miller K et al. Salvage chemotherapy with vinblastine, ifosfamide, and cisplatin in recurrent seminoma. J Clin Oncol 1997;15:1427.

208. Brown ER et al. Long-term outcome of patients with relapsed and refractory germ cell tumors treated with high-dose chemotherapy and autologous bone marrow rescue. Ann Intern Med 1992; 117:124.

209. Jemal A et al. Cancer statistics, 2003. CA Cancer J Clin 2003;53:5.

210. Gurney JG et al. Incidence of cancer in children in the United States. Cancer 1995;75:2186.

211. Triche TJ, Sorensen PHB. Molecular pathology of pediatric malignancies. In: Pizzo PA, Poplack PG, eds. Principles and Practice of Pediatric Oncology. 4th Ed. Philadelphia: Lippincott, Williams & Wilkins, 2002:161.

212. Delattre O et al. The Ewing family of tumors—a subgroup of small-round-cell tumors defined by specific chimeric transcripts. N Engl J Med 1994; 331:294.

213. Plon SE, Malkin D. Childhood cancer and heredity. In: Pizzo PA, Poplack PG, eds. Principles and Practice of Pediatric Oncology. 4th Ed. Philadelphia: Lippincott, Williams & Wilkins, 2002:21.

214. Dreyer ZE et al. Late effects of childhood cancer and its treatment. In: Pizzo PA, Poplack PG, eds. Principles and Practice of Pediatric Oncology. 4th Ed. Philadelphia: Lippincott, Williams & Wilkins, 2002:1431.

215. Tucker MA et al. Leukemia after therapy with alkylating agents for childhood cancer. J Natl Cancer Inst 1987;78:459.

216. Pui CH et al. Acute myeloid leukemia in children treated with epipodophyllotoxins for acute lymphoblastic leukemia. N Engl J Med 1991;325: 1682.

217. Neglia JP et al. Second neoplasms after acute lymphoblastic leukemia in childhood. N Engl J Med 1991;325:1330.

218. Melnick S et al. Rates and risks of diethylstilbestrol-related clear-cell adenocarcinoma of the vagina and cervix: an update. N Engl J Med 1987; 316:514.

219. Reamon GH, Bleyer A. Infants and adolescents with cancer: special considerations. In: Pizzo PA, Poplack DG, eds. Principles and Practice of Pediatric Oncology. 4th Ed. Philadelphia: Lippincott, Williams & Wilkins, 2002:409.

220. Crist W et al. Clinical and biologic features predict a poor prognosis in acute lymphoid leukemias in infants: Pediatric Oncology Group study. Blood 1986;67:135.

221. Wexler HL et al. Rhabdomyosarcoma and the undifferentiated sarcomas. In: Pizzo PA, Poplack DG, eds. Principles and Practice of Pediatric Oncology. 4th Ed. Philadelphia: Lippincott, Williams & Wilkins, 2002:939.

222. Von Hoff DD et al. Daunomycin induced cardiotoxicity in children and adults. Am J Med 1977;62:200.

223. Brodeur GM, Maris JM. Neuroblastoma. In: Pizzo PA, Poplack DG, eds. Principles and Practice of Pediatric Oncology. 4th Ed. Philadelphia: Lippincott, Williams & Wilkins, 2002:895.

224. Castleberry RP. Biology and treatment of neuroblastoma. Pediatr Clin North Am 1997;44:919.

225. Laug WE et al. Initial urinary catecholamine metabolite concentrations and prognosis in neuroblastoma. Pediatrics 1978;62:77.

226. LaBrosse EH et al. Urinary excretion of 3methoxy-4-hydroxymandelic acid and 3-methoxy- 4-hydroxy-phenylacetic acid by 288 patients with neuroblastoma and related neural crest tumors. Cancer Res 1980;40:1995.

227. Woods WG et al. Screening for neuroblastoma is ineffective in reducing the incidence of unfavorable advanced stage disease in older children. Eur J Cancer 1997;33:2106.

228. Yamamoto K et al. Spontaneous regression of localized neuroblastoma detected by mass screening. J Clin Oncol 1998;16:1265.

229. Brodeur GM et al. Revisions of the international criteria for diagnosis, staging and response to treatment. J Clin Oncol 1993;11:1466.

230. Weinstein JL et al. Advances in the diagnosis and treatment of neuroblastoma. Oncologist 2003; 8:278.

231. Http://www.cancer.gov/cancerinfo/pdq/treatment/neuroblastoma/healthprofessional/ Accessed February 25, 2003.

232. Evans A et al. Do infants with Stage IV-S neuroblastoma need treatment? Arch Dis Child 1981;56:271.

233. McWilliams NB. IV-S neuroblastoma: treatment controversy revisited. Med Pediatr Oncol 1986; 14:41.

234. Stokes SH et al. Stage IV-S neuroblastoma—results with definitive therapy. Cancer 1984;53. 2083.

235. O'Reilly R et al. NCCN pediatric neuroblastoma practice guidelines. Oncology 1996;10:1813.

236. Hartman O et al. Very high-dose cisplatin and etoposide in children with untreated advance neuroblastoma. J Clin Oncol 1988;6:44.

237. Green AA et al. Sequential cyclophosphamide and Adriamycin for induction of complete remissions in children with disseminated neuroblastoma. Cancer 1982;48:2310.

238. Philip T et al. 1070 myeloablative megatherapy procedures followed by stem cell rescue for neuroblastoma: 17 years of European experience and conclusions. Eur J Cancer 1997;33:2130.

239. Matthay KK et al. Treatment of high-risk neuroblastoma with intensive chemotherapy, radiotherapy, autologous bone marrow transplantation, and 13-cis-retinoic acid. N Engl J Med 1999;341: 1165.

240. Phoon C. Cardiology. In: Johnson KB, ed. The Harriet Lane Handbook. 13th Ed. St. Louis: Mosby, 1993:101.

241. Bristol Laboratories Oncology Products. Platinol-AQ package insert. Evansville, IN: January 1991.

242. McEvoy GK et al., eds. AHFS Drug Information 93. Bethesda, MD: American Society of Hospital Pharmacists, 1993:543.

243. D'Angio R et al. Creatinine clearance: corrected versus uncorrected [Letter]. Drug Intell Clin Pharm 1988;22:32.

244. Womer RB et al. Renal toxicity of cisplatin in children. J Pediatr 1985;106:659.

245. Ozkaynak MF et al. Phase I study of chimeric human/murine anti-ganglioside GD2 monoclonal antibody (ch14.18) with granulocyte-macrophage colony-stimulating factor in children with neuroblastoma immediately after hematopoietic stem-cell transplantation: a Children's Cancer Group study. J Clin Oncol 2000;18:4077.

246. Skala JP et al. Deferoxamine as a purging agent for autologous bone marrow graft in neuroblastoma. Prog Clin Biol Res 1992;377:71.

247. Donfrancesco A et al. Effects of a single course of deferoxamine in neuroblastoma patients. Cancer Res 1990;50:4929.

248. Donfrancesco A et al. D-CECaT: a breakthrough for patients with neuroblastoma. Anticancer Drugs 1993;4:317.

249. Becton DL, Bryles P. Deferoxamine inhibition of human neuroblastoma viability and proliferation. Cancer Res 1988;48:7189.

250. Yanik GA et al. Pilot study of iodine-131-metaiodobenzylguanidine in combination with myeloablative chemotherapy and autologous stem-cell support for the treatment of neuroblastoma. J Clin Oncol 2002;20:2142.

251. Grundy PE et al. Renal tumors. In: Pizzo PA, Poplack DG, eds. Principles and Practice of Pediatric Oncology. 4th Ed. Philadelphia: Lippincott, Williams & Wilkins, 2002:865.

252. Breslow NE et al. Age distribution of Wilms' tumor: report from the National Wilms' Tumor Study. Cancer Res 1988;48:1653.

253. D'Angio GJ et al. Treatment of Wilms' tumor: results of the third National Wilms' Tumor Study. Cancer 1989;64:349.

254. Http://www.cancer.gov/cancerinfo/pdq/treatment/wilms/healthprofessional/ Accessed February 25, 2003.

255. Green DM et al. Comparison between single-dose and divided-dose administration of dactinomycin and doxorubicin for patients with Wilms' tumor: a report from the National Wilms' Tumor Study Group. J Clin Oncol 1998;16:237.

256. Green DM et al. Effect of duration of treatment on treatment outcome and cost of treatment for Wilms' tumor: a report from the National Wilms' Tumor Study Group. J Clin Oncol 1998;16:3744.

257. Jones B et al. Toxic deaths in the second National Wilms' Tumor Study. J Clin Oncol 1984;2:1028.

258. Morgan E et al. Chemotherapy-related toxicity in infants treated according to the second National Wilms' Tumor Study. J Clin Oncol 1988,6.51.

259. Woods WG et al. Life-threatening neuropathy and hepatotoxicity in infants during induction therapy for acute lymphoblastic leukemia. J Pediatr 1981; 98:642.

260. Allen JC. The effects of cancer therapy on the nervous system. J Pediatr 1978;93:903.

261. Reaman G et al. Acute lymphoblastic leukemia in infants less than one year of age: a cumulative experience of the Childrens Cancer Study Group. J Clin Oncol 1985;3:1513.

262. D'Angio GJ et al. Potentiation of x-ray effects by actinomycin D. Radiology 1959;73:175.

263. Tan CTC et al. The effect of actinomycin D on cancer in childhood. Pediatrics 1959;24:544.

264. Donaldson SS et al. Adriamycin activating a recall phenomenon after radiation therapy. Ann Intern Med 1974;81;407.

265. Greco FA et al. Adriamycin and enhanced radiation reaction in normal esophagus and skin. Ann Intern Med 1976;85:294.

266. Phillips TL, Fu KK. Acute and late effects of multimodal therapy on normal tissues. Cancer 1977;40:489.

267. Merrill J et al. Adriamycin and radiation-synergistic cardiotoxicity. Ann Intern Med 1975;82:122.

268. Green DM et al. Congestive heart failure after treatment for Wilms' Tumor: a report from the National Wilms' Tumor Study Group. J Clin Oncol 2001;19:1926.

269. Goorin AM et al. Initial congestive heart failure, six to ten years after doxorubicin chemotherapy for childhood cancer. J Pediatr 1990;116:144.

270. Lipshultz SE et al. Late cardiac effects of doxorubicin therapy for acute lymphoblastic leukemia in childhood. N Engl J Med 1991;324:808.

271. Steinherz LJ et al. Cardiac toxicity 4 to 20 years after completing anthracycline therapy. JAMA 1991;266:1672.

272. Steinherz LJ et al. Guidelines for cardiac monitoring of children during and after anthracycline therapy: report of the Cardiology Committee of the Childrens Cancer Study Group. Pediatrics 1992;89:942.

273. Jakacki RI et al. Comparison of cardiac function tests after anthracycline therapy in childhood. Cancer 1993;72:2739.

274. Green DM et al. Severe hepatic toxicity after treatment with single-dose dactinomycin and vincristine. Cancer 1988;62:270.

275. Green DM et al. Severe hepatic toxicity after treatment with vincristine and dactinomycin using single-dose or divided-dose schedules: a report from the National Wilms' Tumor Study. J Clin Oncol 1990;8:1525.

276. Link MP et al. Osteosarcoma. In: Pizzo PA, Poplack DG, eds. Principles and Practice of Pediatric Oncology. 4th Ed. Philadelphia: Lippincott, Williams & Wilkins, 2002:1051.

277. Goorin AM et al. Osteosarcoma: fifteen years later. N Engl J Med 1985;313:1637.

278. Link MP et al. The effect of adjuvant chemotherapy on relapse-free survival in patients with osteosarcoma of the extremity. N Engl J Med 1986;314: 1600.

279. Pratt C et al. High dose methotrexate used alone and in combination for measurable primary and metastatic osteosarcoma. Cancer Treat Rep 1980; 64:11.

280. Ochs JJ et al. Cis-dichlorodiammineplatinum (II) in advanced osteogenic sarcoma. Cancer Treat Rep 1978;62:239.

281. Baum ES et al. Phase II study of cis-dichlorodiammineplatinum (II) in childhood osteosarcoma:

Children's Cancer Study Group report. Cancer Treat Rep 1979;63:1621.

282. Cortes EP et al. Doxorubicin in disseminated osteosarcoma. JAMA 1972;221:1132.

283. Marti C et al. High-dose ifosfamide in advanced osteosarcoma. Cancer Treat Rep 1985;69:115.

284. O'Reilly R et al. NCCN pediatric osteosarcoma practice guidelines. Oncology 1996;10:1799.

285. Jenkin R et al. Osteosarcoma: an assessment of management with particular reference to primary irradiation and selective delayed amputation. Cancer 1972;30:393.

286. Meyers PA et al. Chemotherapy for nonmetastatic osteogenic sarcoma: the Memorial Sloan-Kettering experience. J Clin Oncol 1992;10:5.

287. Goorin AM et al. Presurgical chemotherapy compared with immediate surgery and adjuvant chemotherapy for nonmetastatic osteosarcoma: Pediatric Oncology Group study POG-8651. J Clin Oncol 2003;21:1574.

288. Pastorino U et al. The contribution of salvage surgery to the management of childhood osteosarcoma. J Clin Oncol 1991;9:1357.

289. Meyers P et al. Expression of HER2/c-erb-2 correlates with event-free-survival in patients with osteosarcoma [Abstract]. Proc Am Soc Clin Oncol 1999;18:554a.

290. Evans WE, Pratt CB. Effect of pleural effusion on high-dose methotrexate kinetics. Clin Pharmacol Ther 1978;23:68.

291. Crom WR, Evans WE. Methotrexate. In: Evans WE et al., eds. Applied Pharmacokinetics. 3rd Ed. Philadelphia: Lippincott, Williams & Wilkins, 1992:29.

292. Evans WE et al. Pharmacokinetics of sustained serum methotrexate concentrations secondary to gastrointestinal obstruction. J Pharm Sci 1981;70:1194.

293. Crom WR et al. The effect of prior cisplatin therapy on the pharmacokinetics of high-dose methotrexate. J Clin Oncol 1984;2:655.

294. Hansten PD, Horn JR, eds. Drug Interactions Analysis and Management. St. Louis, MO: Facts & Comparisons, 1999:69.

295. Gerrazzini G et al. Interaction between trimethoprim-sulfamethoxazole and methotrexate in children with leukemia. J Pediatr 1990;117:823.

296. Pinedo HM, Chabner BA. Role of drug concentration, duration of exposure and endogenous metabolites in determining methotrexate cytotoxicity. Cancer Treat Rep 1977;61:709.

297. Evans WE et al. Pharmacokinetic monitoring of high-dose methotrexate: early recognition of high-risk patients. Cancer Chemother Pharmacol 1979;3:161.

298. Tattersall MHN et al. Clinical pharmacology of high-dose methotrexate (NSC-740). Cancer Chemother Rep 1975;6(Pt 3):25.

299. Isacoff WH et al. High-dose methotrexate therapy of solid tumors; observations relating to clinical toxicity. Med Pediatr Oncol 1976;2:319.

300. Isacoff WH et al. Pharmacokinetics of high-dose methotrexate with citrovorum factor rescue. Cancer Treat Rep 1977;61:1665.

301. Nirenberg A et al. High dose methotrexate with CF rescue: predictive value of serum methotrexate concentrations and corrective measures to avert toxicity. Cancer Treat Rep 1977;61:779.

302. Stoller RC et al. Use of plasma pharmacokinetics to predict and prevent methotrexate toxicity. N Engl J Med 1977;297:630.

303. Rechnitzer C et al. Methotrexate in the plasma and cerebrospinal fluid of children treated with intermediate dose methotrexate. Acta Paediatr Scand 1981; 70:615.

304. Tan C et al. Adriamycin—an antitumor antibiotic in the treatment of neoplastic diseases. Cancer 1973;32:9.

305. Miser JS et al. Ifosfamide with mesna uroprotection and etoposide: an effective regimen in the treatment of recurrent sarcomas and other tumors of children and young adults. J Clin Oncol 1987;5:1191.

306. Chard RL Jr et al. Phase II study of VP-16-213 in childhood malignant disease: a Children's Cancer Study Group report. Cancer Treat Rep 1979;63:1755.

307. Crist W et al. Intensive chemotherapy including cisplatin with or without etoposide for children with soft-tissue sarcomas. Med Pediatr Oncol 1987;15:51.

308. Finkelstein JZ et al. 5-(3,3-dimethyl-triazeno) imidazole-4-carboxamide (NSC-45388) in the treatment of solid tumors in children. Cancer Chemother Rep 1975;59:351.

309. Bode U. Methotrexate as relapse therapy for rhabdomyosarcoma. Am J Pediatr Hematol Oncol 1986; 8:70.

310. Horowitz ME et al. Phase II testing of melphalan in children with newly diagnosed rhabdomyosarcoma: a model for anticancer drug development. J Clin Oncol 1988;6:308.

311. Crist W et al. The Third Intergroup Rhabdomyosarcoma Study. J Clin Oncol 1995;13:610.

312. Crist W et al. Intergroup Rhabdomyosarcoma Study-IV: results for patients with nonmetastatic disease. J Clin Oncol 2001;19:3091.

313. Crist WM et al. Prognosis in children with rhabdomyosarcoma: a report of the Intergroup Rhabdomyosarcoma Studies I and II. J Clin Oncol 1990; 8:443.

314. Rodary C et al. Prognostic factors in 281 children with non-metastatic rhabdomyosarcoma (RMS) at diagnosis. Med Pediatr Oncol 1988;16:71.

315. Raney B et al. Renal toxicity in patients receiving ifosfamide/mesna on intergroup rhabdomyosarcoma study (IRS)-IV Pilot regimens for gross residual sarcoma [Abstract]. Proc Am Soc Clin Oncol 1993;12:418.

316. Rossi R et al. Unilateral nephrectomy and cisplatin as risk factors of ifosfamide-induced nephrotoxicity: analysis of 120 patients. J Clin Oncol 1994;12:159.

317. Suarez A et al. Long-term follow-up of ifosfamide renal toxicity in children treated for malignant mesenchymal tumors: an International Society of Pediatric Oncology report. J Clin Oncol 1991; 9:2177.

318. Skinner R et al. Risk factors for ifosfamide nephrotoxicity in children. Lancet 1996;348:578.

319. Yehuda AB et al. False positive reaction for urinary ketones with mesna [Letter]. Drug Intell Clin Pharm 1987;21:547.

CHAPTER 92

Hematopoietic Cell Transplantation

Jeannine S. McCune, Laura L. Winter, Suzanne D. Day

Overview

Hematopoietic cell transplantation (HCT) is defined broadly as the infusion of hematopoietic stem cells into a patient to treat disease and/or restore normal hematopoiesis and lymphopoiesis. Originally, this procedure developed from allogeneic bone marrow transplantation (BMT) as potentially curative therapy for diseases involving the bone marrow or immune system.[1,2] These early allogeneic BMTs involved administration of a myeloablative preparative regimen, which was followed by true "transplantation" of bone marrow from one individual to another.[1,2] Bone marrow contains pluripotent stem cells and post-thymic lymphocytes, which are responsible, respectively, for long-term hematopoietic reconstitution, immune recovery, and its associated graft-versus-host disease (GVHD).[3] Subsequently, the "dose-intensity" concept for cancer treatment (see related information in Chapter 88, Neoplastic Disorders and Their Treatment: General Principles) was expanded to using myeloablative preparative regimens followed by autologous HCT. *Autologous HCT,* or infusion of a patient's own hematopoietic stem cells, allows for the administration of higher doses of chemotherapy, radiation, or both to treat the malignancy.[4] In the setting of autologous

HCT, the hematopoietic stem cells "rescue" the patient from otherwise dose-limiting hematopoietic toxicity. The recognition of graft-versus-tumor (GVT) effect, which is proposed to be exerted by cytotoxic T lymphocytes in the donor stem cells led to investigations with nonmyeloablative transplantations (NMT), in which less toxic preparative regimens are used with the hope of expanding the availability of HCT to those recipients whose medical condition or age prohibits use of myeloablative regimens.[5–7]

The combination of chemotherapy and/or radiation administered before infusion of hematopoietic stem cells is referred to as the *preparative* or *conditioning regimen.* In the setting of an allogeneic HCT, the preparative regimen is designed to suppress the recipient's immunity, eradicate residual malignancy, or to create space in the marrow compartment. A myeloablative or nonmyeloablative preparative regimen may be used with allogeneic HCT; only myeloablative preparative regimens are used for autologous HCT. The basic schema for myeloablative preparative regimens with an allogeneic graft is illustrated in Figure 92-1. Myeloablative preparative regimens involve administration of near-lethal doses of chemotherapy and/or radiation, which are generally followed by a 1- to 2-day

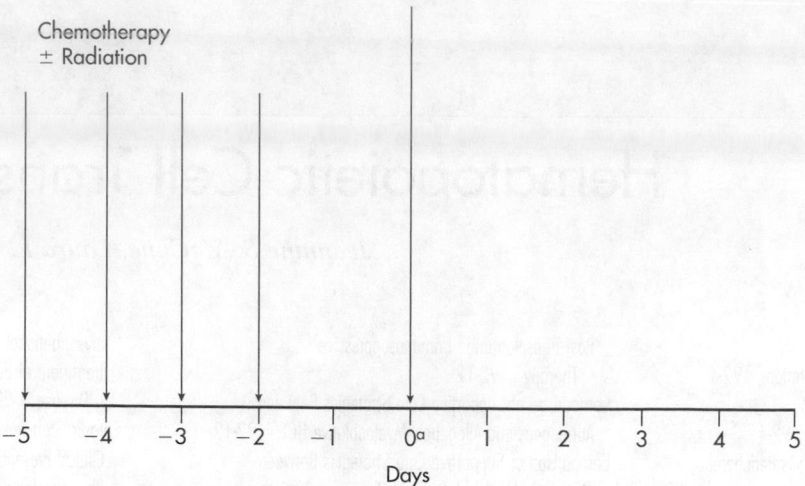

FIGURE 92-1 Basic schema for myeloablative hematopoietic cell transplant. ᵃDay 0 = bone marrow, peripheral blood progenitor cell, or umbilical cord blood infusion.

rest and then infusion of stem cells.[1,2] For most chemotherapy-based regimens, the rest period is necessary to allow for elimination of toxic metabolites from the chemotherapy that could damage infused cells. After chemotherapy and radiation, a period of pancytopenia lasts until the infused stem cells re-establish functional hematopoiesis. This process is called *engraftment* and commonly is defined as the point at which a patient can maintain a sustained absolute neutrophil count (ANC) of >500 cells/mm³ and a sustained platelet count of ≥20,000/mm³ lasting ≥3 consecutive days without transfusions.[8] The median time to engraftment is a function of several factors, including the source of stem cells with peripheral blood progenitor cells (PBPC), which can result in earlier engraftment than bone marrow[9–15] (Fig. 92-2). Myeloablative preparative regimens have significant regimen-related toxicity and morbidity and thus are usually limited to healthy, younger (i.e., usually less than 50 years) patients.[16] Alternatively, non-myeloablative transplantations, also referred to as nonablative stem cell transplantations or "mini-transplants," are being performed with the hope of curing more patients with cancer by increasing the availability of HCT with less regimen-related toxicity and by using the GVT effect. In the year 2000, NMT represented approximately 25% of allogeneic HCTs.[17]

Hematopoietic cell transplantation was previously referred to as BMT. The term HCT more aptly describes this procedure as, in addition to bone marrow, stem cells may be obtained from the PBPC and umbilical cord blood. For the purpose of an HCT, the key properties of the hematopoietic stem cells are their ability to engraft, the speed of engraftment, and the durability of engraftment.[3] Transplantation with peripheral blood progenitor cells (PBPCT) has essentially replaced BMT as autologous rescue after myeloablative preparative

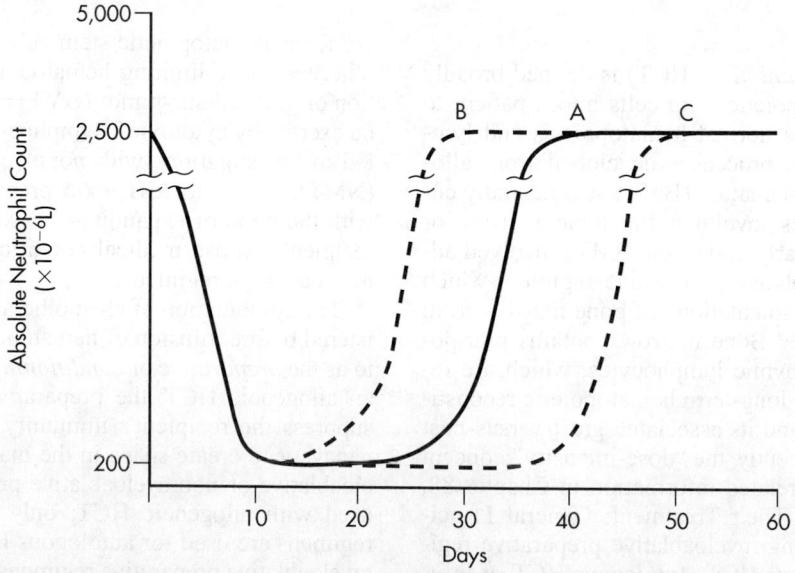

FIGURE 92-2 Time to engraftment. *A,* Bone marrow infusion without complications or hematopoietic growth factors. *B,* Accelerated engraftment with peripheral blood progenitor cells (PBPCs), and/or combination of autologous bone marrow with hematopoietic growth factors. *C,* Delayed engraftment caused by infection, purged bone marrow, and/or inadequate dose of hematopoietic stem cells.

regimens and is being increasingly used in the allogeneic setting.[17] Cord blood stem cell transplantation (CBT), a form of allogeneic HCT, is currently restricted to select pediatric and adult recipients because of the limited number of stem cells obtained from the umbilical cord blood and the necessary cell dose that is associated with adequate engraftment.[18,19]

The type of HCT performed depends on a number of factors, including type and status of disease, availability of a compatible donor, patient age, performance status, and organ function. Characteristics of autologous and allogeneic transplantation, with either myeloablative or nonmyeloablative preparative regimens, are compared in Table 92-1. Many diseases have been treated with autologous or allogeneic HCT and are listed in Table 92-2.[17,20–25] Modifications to the basic schema for HCT are necessary based on the immunologic source (i.e., allogeneic or autologous) and the anatomic source (i.e., bone marrow, PBPC, or umbilical cord blood) of stem cells infused. The number of autologous transplants exceeds the number of allogeneic transplantations performed each year. In 2000, approximately 25,000 autologous HCTs were performed worldwide compared with 15,000 allogeneic HCTs.[17] The number of autologous HCTs performed has decreased because of a dramatic decline in the use of this procedure for breast cancer; this decline is due to the equivocal benefits of HCT relative to standard-dose chemotherapy in this patient population.[17,22] The number of allogeneic HCTs has reached a plateau since 1998, most likely because of the limited availability of suitable donors, the limited success to date with HLA-disparate donors, and the increasing availability of targeted therapies for diseases that were traditionally treated with HCT (e.g., imatinib for newly diagnosed chronic-phase chronic myelogenous leukemia).[17,26]

Table 92-1 Comparison of Hematopoietic Cell Transplantation

| | Myeloablative | | Nonmyeloablative |
| | Autologous | Allogeneic | Allogeneic |
Risk[a]			
Relapse after HCT	+++	+	+
Rejection	–	+	++
Delayed engraftment	++	+	+
Graft-versus-host disease	–	+	++
Infection	+	++ to +++[b]	++ to +++[b]
Transplant-related morbidity	+	+++	++
Transplant-related mortality	+	++	+
Cost of procedure	++	+++	++ to +++

[a]Risk also varies depending on underlying disease, patient characteristics, and previous medical history.
[b]Risk of infection increases with prolonged immunosuppression and/or chronic graft-versus-host disease.

Table 92-2 Indications for Myeloablative HCT[20–25,326]

	Established Role	Promising/Experimental	Equivocal
Allogeneic			
Nonmalignant	Aplastic anemia	Sickle cell anemia	
	Homozygous β-thalassemia	Severe leukocyte adhesion deficiency	
	Severe combined immunodeficiency disease	X-linked agammaglobulinemia	
	Wiskott-Aldrich syndrome	Common variable immunodeficiency	
	Fanconi's anemia		
	Infantile osteopetrosis		
Malignant	AML	Agnogenic myeloid metaplasia	
	ALL	CLL (young patients only)	
	CML	Multiple myeloma	
	Intermediate and high-grade NHL	Myelodysplastic syndrome	
Autologous			
Malignant	Intermediate and high-grade NHL	Multiple myeloma	Metastatic breast cancer
	Adults with AML (if they lack suitable allogeneic donors)	Neuroblastoma	AML in pediatric patients
	Relapsed or refractory HD	Ovarian cancer	Small-cell lung cancer
	Testicular cancer	Low-grade lymphomas	
		Rhabdomyosarcoma	

[a]Timing relative to diagnosis and other therapies may vary.
AML, acute myelogenous leukemia; CLL, chronic lymphocytic leukemia; CML, chronic myelogenous leukemia; HCT, hematopoietic cell transplant; HD, Hodgkin's disease; NHL, non-Hodgkin's lymphoma.

Autologous Hematopoietic Cell Transplantation

The defining characteristic of autologous HCT is that the donor and the recipient are the same individual. Consequently, pretransplantation and post-transplantation immunosuppression is unnecessary. Autologous hematopoietic cells must be obtained (i.e., harvested) before the myeloablative preparative regimen is administered and subsequently stored for administration after the preparative regimen. Essentially, these hematopoietic cells are administered as a rescue intervention to re-establish bone marrow function and avoid long-lasting, life-threatening marrow aplasia that results from the myeloablative preparative regimen.[27] In addition, autologous hematopoietic cells obtained during complete remission are an alternative to allogeneic HCT for the treatment of acute leukemias in patients who cannot receive an allogeneic HCT because of their age or limitations in finding a suitable donor.[28]

Indications for Autologous HCT

1. P.J., a 46-year-old man, has diffuse large-cell B-cell non-Hodgkin's lymphoma (NHL) in first relapse after a complete remission of 1 year's duration. An 80% reduction in measurable disease is noted after two cycles of dexamethasone, high-dose cytarabine, and cisplatin (DHAP) salvage chemotherapy. P.J.'s bone marrow biopsy and lumbar puncture are negative for malignant cells. Is a myeloablative preparative regimen with autologous HCT indicated for P.J.? If so, should hematopoietic cells be obtained from bone marrow or peripheral blood?

Autologous HCT is used to treat a variety of malignancies (see Table 92-2); NHL and multiple myeloma are the most common indications for this procedure and represent over one-third of all autologous HCT.[17] Patients with NHL are more frequently treated with an autologous HCT than with an allogeneic HCT because autologous HCT has equivalent or superior survival to allogeneic HCT.[29,30] Also, autologous HCT circumvents the need for histocompatible donors, is associated with lower mortality due to HCT, and is not restricted by age to patients younger than 50 years.[16] In addition, the usefulness of NMT is currently being evaluated for the treatment of NHL because of the potential advantages of a graft-versus-lymphoma effect and of using stem cells unexposed to prior cytotoxic chemotherapy.[5-7]

The most appropriate patient population and timing for autologous HCT in the treatment of NHL are being defined. A significant percentage of patients with aggressive NHL are cured with conventional chemotherapy alone. Adding autologous HCT to initial combination chemotherapy does not improve outcomes in patients with aggressive NHL.[31-33] However, retrospective analyses of some of these trials[31,33] suggested that the International Prognostic Index[34] may identify a subset of patients who may benefit from the addition of autologous HCT to initial combination chemotherapy. The primary eligibility criterion for autologous HCT is relapsed disease that is chemotherapy sensitive.[32,35] Data from several retrospective and prospective phase II studies support this recommendation; however, only one randomized, controlled trial has been conducted.[35] Autologous BMT, compared with conventional chemotherapy with DHAP, resulted in a 5-year event-free survival of 46% and 12%, respectively ($P = .001$).

Overall 5-year survival was 53% in the BMT group and 32% in the conventional chemotherapy patients ($P = .038$). Prospective studies comparing preparative regimens, stem cell mobilization techniques, and stem cell source (i.e., BMT versus PBPCT) are not available; however, autologous PBPCT has become the standard of care, most likely owing to the improved outcomes with PBPCT in other disease settings.[32] Relative to chemotherapy-sensitive disease, survival is improved with autologous HCT in a smaller number of patients with chemotherapy-resistant relapse or patients with refractory disease who do not respond to chemotherapy.[32]

P.J. has minimal residual disease that has demonstrated chemotherapy sensitivity (i.e., he had a partial response to chemotherapy).[35] His long-term prognosis will be improved with autologous PBPCT rather than further conventional chemotherapy, as described above.[35] Thus, autologous PBPCT is indicated.

Harvesting Autologous Bone Marrow

2. What is the best way to harvest and preserve harvested stem cells?

Autologous hematopoietic stem cells are obtained or harvested from bone marrow or peripheral blood. Because the harvest occurs before administering the preparative regimen, autologous hematopoietic cells must be cryopreserved and stored for future use.[36] Dimethylsulfoxide (DMSO) is the cryopreservative commonly used to protect hematopoietic cells from damage during freezing and thawing. When infused into the patient, DMSO can be associated with side effects, including nausea and vomiting, arrhythmias, and a temporary unpleasant odor lasting approximately 24 to 36 hours.[37] After collection, autologous hematopoietic cells may be purged using various techniques to minimize tumor contamination or to enrich the hematopoietic cell composition. "Negative purging" techniques bathe the hematopoietic cells in either chemotherapy or monoclonal antibodies in an attempt to eradicate remaining tumor cells.[38] "Positive selection" techniques involve running the autologous product through a device (i.e., a column) in an attempt to separate the earliest hematopoietic progenitor cells from the malignant cells or committed progenitor cells.[39] An example of positive selection is the use of CD34 antigen in a column as a marker to select out the earliest hematopoietic progenitor cells.

The technique for harvesting autologous hematopoietic cells varies based on the anatomic source (i.e., bone marrow or peripheral blood). Harvesting bone marrow entails a surgical procedure in which marrow is obtained from the iliac crests. At the time of infusion, the autologous bone marrow is thawed and then infused into the patient in the same manner as a blood transfusion. Historically, autologous hematopoietic cells obtained from the bone marrow were used after myeloablative preparative regimens. Recently, autologous PBPC use has increased and has essentially replaced bone marrow in many transplant centers. In 2000, over 95% of autologous HCTs in adults and 80% in children used PBPC as the source of hematopoietic cells.[17] Peripheral blood was first advocated as a means of obtaining hematopoietic cells in patients when bone marrow was difficult to harvest (e.g., patients with bone marrow involvement of the disease or those treated with pelvic irradiation).[40] Relative to a bone marrow graft, PBPCT results in more rapid neutrophil and platelet recovery, fewer platelet transfusions, fewer days of IV antibiotics, and a shorter duration of hospitalization.[9,10] Thus, the shift to the use of PBPC over bone marrow for autologous HCT is primarily because of the more rapid engraftment and decreased health care resource use. These and other potential advantages or differences between autologous BMT and PBPCT are outlined in Table 92-3.

Mobilization and Collection of Autologous Peripheral Blood Progenitor Cells

3. For PBPC mobilization, P.J. received one dose of cyclophosphamide 4,000 mg/m² IV on day 1, followed by filgrastim 10 μg/kg per day SC beginning on day 2 and continuing through completion of apheresis. Twelve days after receiving cyclophosphamide, P.J.'s WBC count recovered to 3,000/mm³ and apheresis was begun. An adequate number of stem cells are collected after two apheresis sessions are processed and then stored. What was the rationale for administering filgrastim and cyclophosphamide? What determines the duration of apheresis?

[SI units WBC 3,000 × 10⁶ cells/L]

Peripheral blood progenitor cells are obtained by administering a mobilizing agent(s) followed by apheresis; this is an outpatient procedure similar to dialysis.[41] Hematopoietic growth factors (HGFs) alone or in combination with myelosuppressive chemotherapy are used for mobilization of PBPC.[42] The HGF granulocyte-macrophage colony-stimulating factor (sargramostim, Leukine) and granulocyte colony-stimulating factor (filgrastim, Neupogen) are used as mobilizing agents for PBPC collection.[13] The most frequently used filgrastim doses for PBPC mobilization in cancer patients are in the range of 5 to 16 μg/kg per day, administered subcutaneously, with higher doses (>10 μg/kg per day) of filgrastim yielding more PBPC cells.[42,43] The highest values of mobilized progenitor cells are observed 5 to 6 days after mobilization with filgrastim alone.[42]

The combination of chemotherapy with HGF enhances PBPC mobilization relative to HGF alone.[42,44] In addition to treating the underlying malignancy, this approach lowers the risk of tumor cell contamination and the number of apheresis collections required, but there is a greater risk of neutropenia and thrombocytopenia than the use of HGF alone.[42] Examples of chemotherapy regimens used for PBPC mobilization include: cyclophosphamide 4 g/m² IV,[45] cyclophosphamide 4 g/m² on day 1 and etoposide 200 mg/m²/day IV days 1 to 3 (CE), or paclitaxel 200 mg/m² IV day 1 and cyclophosphamide 3 g/m² IV day 2.[46] When used with chemotherapy, filgrastim may be superior to sargramostim for PBPC mobilization,[44] although confirmatory data are needed. The HGF is initiated 24-hours after completion of chemotherapy. Apheresis begins when the peripheral white blood cell (WBC) count begins to recover and the HGF is continued until apheresis is complete.[40,42]

Apheresis is continued daily until the target number of PBPC per kilogram of the recipients' weight is obtained. For adult recipients, the number of cells infused that express the CD34 antigen (i.e., CD34⁺ cells) correlates with time to engraftment.[46–49] The CD34 antigen is expressed on 1% to 4% of human marrow cells. It is expressed on virtually all unipotent and multipotent colony-forming cells and on precursors of colony-forming cells but not on mature peripheral blood cells.[50] In adults, the minimal number of CD34⁺ cells needed for an autologous PBPCT to produce complete (i.e., white blood cell [WBC], red blood cell [RBC], and platelet) engraftment is not well defined, but it may be in the range of 2 × 10⁶ CD34⁺ cells/kg of recipient weight.[49] A shorter time to recovery of platelet counts and less supportive care requirements are needed with infusion of ≥5 × 10⁶ CD34⁺ cells/kg of recipient weight; thus, this is the target number of CD34⁺ cells recommended to be obtained with apheresis.[46–49] More intensive prior chemotherapy or radiation therapy is associated with a lower yield of CD34⁺ cells. In addition, lower yield is associated with administration of stem cell toxic drugs such as carmustine and melphalan, which should not be used for mobilizing chemotherapy.[42] There is a paucity of information regarding the parameters associated with engraftment in children undergoing an autologous PBPCT.[51] After apheresis, the cells are cryopreserved, stored, thawed, and infused into the patient as described for autologous bone marrow.[40]

Myeloablative Preparative Regimens

4. What are the goals and characteristics of agents used for myeloablative preparative regimens in patients like P.J?

The primary goal of the high-dose, myeloablative preparative regimen is to eradicate residual malignancy. Because the donor and recipient are genetically identical, there is no need to induce immunosuppression. Consequently, if radiation is

Table 92-3 Comparison of Source of Hematopoietic Cells in Autologous HCT: Bone Marrow versus Peripheral Blood

	Bone Marrow	Peripheral Blood
Duration of neutropenia	++	+
Duration of thrombocytopenia	++	+
Transfusion support needs	++	+
Number of hematopoietic cells collected/infused	+	++
Duration of hospitalization	++	+
Early complications	++	+
Late complications[a]	?	?
Tumor contamination of hematopoietic cell product[b]	++	+
Cost of procedure	+++	++

[a]Limited comparative data on long-term complications.
[b]Clinical relevance of differences in tumor contamination for certain diseases under evaluation

used in conjunction with high-dose chemotherapy and hematopoietic cell support, it is because radiation has inherent activity against the tumor being treated (e.g., lymphoma). Combination chemotherapy with multiple alkylating agents comprises the most common high-dose regimens before autologous HCT. Alkylating agents are used because they exhibit a steep dose-response curve for various malignancies and are characterized by dose-limiting bone marrow suppression.[4] Ideally, if combinations of antineoplastics are used, they should have nonhematologic toxicities that do not overlap and are not life-threatening. Examples of common myeloablative regimens used with stem cell support are illustrated in Table 92-4.

Complications of Autologous HCT

5. What complications must be anticipated as a consequence of autologous HCT? How can these be minimized? How can treatment be provided in an outpatient setting?

The most common cause of death after autologous HCT is the primary disease. The more concerning toxicities of the preparative regimen are infection and organ failure each occurring in less than 5% of the patients.[17] Because autologous HCT is not complicated by profound immunosuppression or GVHD, supportive care strategies vary from allogeneic HCT in the early and later recovery periods. Isolation and use of laminar air flow (LAF) rooms are unnecessary, although many centers continue to provide care for patients undergoing autologous HCT in HEPA-filtered rooms. The use of autologous PBPCT is associated with shorter periods of neutropenia and less need for clinical resources. Thus, some transplant centers have developed programs that incorporate outpatient care into the initial recovery; these programs also offer cost savings to the payer for health services.[52,53] Successful outpatient care during administration of a myeloablative preparative regimen and the neutropenic period requires careful development and implementation of the necessary supportive care strategies to prevent or minimize infection; chemotherapy-induced nausea and vomiting, pain, and bleeding along with admission criteria for more severe complications. Use of prophylactic oral antibiotics and once-daily IV antibiotics to prevent or treat

uncomplicated febrile neutropenia have facilitated outpatient care and prevented many patients from being hospitalized.[54] In addition, outpatient care during autologous HCT demands that transplantation centers have appropriate resources, facilities, and staff to provide 24-hour patient care coverage. Patients undergoing outpatient care must meet eligibility criteria, including the availability of caregivers 24 hours a day and housing within close proximity to the HCT center.

Hematopoietic Growth Factors After Autologous PBPC Infusion

6. After 10 days of rest, P.J. is admitted for his autologous BMT. He receives a myeloablative preparative regimen with cyclophosphamide, carmustine, and etoposide (CBV) with an autologous PBPC graft. An order is written to begin filgrastim 5 μg/kg/day SQ, beginning on day 0 and continuing until the ANC has recovered to 500/mm³ for 2 consecutive days. What is the rationale for filgrastim in P.J. following the transplant procedure?

[SI units: ANC 500 × 10⁶ cells/L]

Autologous HCTs, regardless of the stem cell source, are associated with profound aplasia due to the myeloablative preparative regimen. Aplasia typically lasts 20 to 30 days after an autologous BMT and 7 to 14 days after an autologous PBPCT.[9] (see Fig. 92-2) During this period of aplasia, patients are at high risk for complications such as bleeding and infection. Filgrastim and sargramostim exert their effects by stimulating the proliferation of committed progenitor cells and, once engraftment occurs, hematopoietic recovery may be accelerated.

Several factors need to be considered when discussing the role of HGF in accelerating engraftment after HCT. First, the anatomic source of hematopoietic cells predicts the degree of benefit, with the greatest benefit observed in enhancing neutrophil recovery and decreased associated resources in the setting of autologous BMT. The benefits of the HGF have been shown in several large multicenter, randomized, double-blind, placebo-controlled trials.[55–57] The majority of the trials suggest HGF administration is associated with a shorter time to neutrophil engraftment (by 4 to 7 days), less infectious complications, and shorter hospitalization after autologous BMT.[55,56,58] Survival is equivalent in those who received a HGF or a placebo.[55,57]

Table 92-4 Representative Myeloablative Preparative Regimens Used in HCT

Type of HCT	Disease State	Regimen	Dose/Schedule
Allogeneic[115]	Hematologic malignancies[a]	CY/TBI	CY 60 mg/kg/day IV on 2 consecutive days before TBI 1,000–1,575 rads fractionated over 1–7 days
Allogeneic[327]	Aplastic anemia	CY	CY 60 mg/kg/day IV on 4 consecutive days (–5, –4, –3, –2)
Allogeneic Autologous[21,115,116]	Acute and chronic leukemias	Bu/CY	Bu: adult—1 mg/kg/dose PO Q 6 hr × 16 doses Children <7 yr—37.5 mg/m² PO Q 6 hr × 16 doses CY 50 mg/kg/day IV QD × 4 days after Bu or 60 mg/kg/day IV QD × 2 days after Bu
Autologous[35]	Non-Hodgkin's lymphoma	BEAC (carmustine/etoposide/cytarabine/cyclophosphamide)	Carmustine 300 mg/m²/day IV × 1, day –6 Etoposide 200 mg/m²/day IV × 4, days –5, –4, –3, –2 Cytarabine 200 mg/m²/day IV BID × 4, days –5, –4, –3, –2) CY 35 mg/kg/day IV × 4, days –5, –4, –3, –2 ± mesna 50 mg/kg/day IV × 4, days –5, –4, –3, –2

[a]Includes acute myelogenous leukemia, acute lymphocytic leukemia, chronic myelogenous leukemia, non-Hodgkin's lymphoma, and Hodgkin's disease.
Ara-C, cytarabine; BCNU, carmustine; Cy, cyclophosphamide; HCT, hematopoietic cell transplantation; TBI, total body irradiation.

Although some studies in the autologous PBPCT setting note more rapid neutrophil recovery after HGF use, others report no difference in infection rates and minimal decreases in associated resource use such as the duration of hospitalization.[56,58–60] In addition, sargramostim administration had no benefit (i.e., neutrophil and platelet engraftment) over placebo after autologous PBPCT in one trial.[61] Concern remains that platelet engraftment will be delayed by a HGF in patients who received a PBPCT with a low CD34[+] count (i.e., <2.5 × 10[6]/kg).[47] Although clinical practice guidelines for HGF support their use after both autologous BMT and PBPCT, pharmacoeconomic analyses are needed to further evaluate the true benefit of HGFs after autologous PBPCT.

Filgrastim often is used preferentially for this indication in clinical practice. The reason most commonly cited for using filgrastim is the desire to avoid febrile reactions associated with sargramostim, which complicate interpretation of febrile neutropenia. Although sargramostim or filgrastim theoretically may stimulate proliferation of leukemia myeloblasts, no evidence to date suggests that the incidence of leukemia relapse is higher in patients who receive these HGFs after autologous or allogeneic HCT.[62,63] This may be due to the fact that patients with leukemia usually are in remission at the time of HCT. Thus, the population of residual leukemia cells probably is minimal.

Although both filgrastim and sargramostim successfully hasten neutrophil recovery, neither agent stimulates platelet production or augments platelet recovery.[55,56] This is an important consideration because thrombocytopenia is often a cause of prolonged hospitalization in the HCT patient. Successful engraftment of all hematopoietic cell lines likely will require combinations of growth factors that work in concert to augment hematopoiesis. However, erythropoietin (Epogen, Procrit) and interleukin (IL)-11 (Neumega) have only been used experimentally in the HCT patient. At this time, there is no established role for either agent in the care of these patients.

In summary, P.J. is undergoing autologous PBPCT for the treatment of a lymphoid malignancy. Thus, either sargramostim or filgrastim is an acceptable option for accelerating engraftment. Whether the addition of either agent will reduce infection and other clinically relevant outcomes is debatable.[43] A complete blood cell (CBC) count with differential should be obtained daily. Filgrastim should be continued until neutrophil recovery is achieved.

Allogeneic Hematopoietic Cell Transplantation

Allogeneic HCT involves the transplantation of hematopoietic cells obtained from a donor's bone marrow, peripheral blood, or umbilical cord blood to a patient. Unless the donor and the patient are identical twins (referred to as a *syngeneic HCT*), they are dissimilar genetically. Allogeneic transplantation offers the potential for a GVT effect in which immune effector cells from the donor recognize and eliminate residual tumor in the recipient.[5] GVHD is caused by the activation of donor lymphocytes leading to immune damage to the skin, gut, and liver in the recipient. Histocompatibility differences between the donor and recipient necessitate post-transplantation immunosuppression after allogeneic HCT because considerable morbidity and mortality are associated with graft rejection and GVHD. Thus, to understand the application of and complications after allogeneic HCT, a working knowledge of immunology and the major histocompatibility complex (MHC) (referred to as *human leukocyte antigen* [HLA] in humans) is necessary; a detailed review of this topic can be found elsewhere.[64] (Also see related information in Chapter 35, Solid Organ Transplantation.)

Eligibility criteria for allogeneic HCT vary between institutions. Having a matched sibling donor is no longer a requirement for allogeneic HCT as improved immunosuppressive regimens and the National Marrow Donor Program have allowed an increase in the use of unrelated or related matched or mismatched HCT.[65] Normal renal, hepatic, pulmonary, and cardiac functions are necessary for eligibility at most centers. Historically, patients older than 55 were excluded from allogeneic HCT because they were more likely to succumb to transplantation-related complications.[1,2] However, many centers are now considering patients up to 65 years, basing their selection criteria on physiologic rather than biologic age.

Indications for Allogeneic HCT

7. **B.S., a 22-year-old man, has acute myelogenous leukemia (AML) in first remission after induction chemotherapy with standard doses of cytarabine and daunorubicin and consolidation with high-dose cytarabine. HLA typing performed on family members has identified a fully HLA-matched sibling donor. B.S. returns to clinic today for a pretransplantation workup. At this time, his physical examination is noncontributory, bone marrow aspirate and biopsy reveal favorable cytogenetics, and a lumbar puncture is negative for leukemic infiltrates. All laboratory values are within normal limits. A bone marrow biopsy reveals <5% blasts. B.S. has a normal electrocardiogram and normal cardiac wall motion study, renal and hepatic function, and pulmonary function tests. Is an allogeneic HCT indicated for B.S.?**

B.S. has a diagnosis of AML, which is one of the most common indications for allogeneic HCT.[17] The primary indications for allogeneic HCT include treatment of otherwise fatal diseases of the bone marrow or immune system (see Table 92-2). The optimal role and timing of allogeneic HCT in contrast to other therapies remains controversial,[66] especially because treatment options for AML have increased.[67] An advantage of allogeneic HCT over chemotherapy is a decreased incidence of leukemia relapse, since patients in first complete remission who receive an HLA-matched HCT from a sibling have a less than 20% risk of relapse.[41,68] The lower risk of relapse is due to the use of the myeloablative preparative regimen and the GVT effect mediated by the donor immune system. The major disadvantage of allogeneic myeloablative HCT is an increased incidence of early mortality caused by regimen-related toxicities, GVHD, and infectious complications that result from profound immunosuppression (see Question 9).[41,68] Nonetheless, allogeneic HCT has been advocated for eligible young (under 55-years) patients with AML in early first remission if there are histocompatible donors.[69]

This recommendation to perform an allogeneic HCT early in the course of AML is based on diminishing efficacy of HCT later in the course of the disease. In adult patients with AML in first remission, four large studies have evaluated allogeneic HCT in those patients with an HLA-matched sibling donor and randomized the remaining patients to autologous HCT or chemotherapy.[70–73] Disease-free survival after autologous HCT was superior[70,73] or equivalent[71,72] to chemotherapy in two trials; however, up to 45% of those randomized to autologous HCT did not receive a transplant. Similarly, allogeneic HCT had similar[71,72] or improved disease-free survival when compared with chemotherapy.[70] Higher early mortality in the HCT arms (particularly those undergoing an allogeneic HCT) and a higher incidence of relapse in chemotherapy-treated patients equalized overall survival between transplant arms. The association of cytogenetics with response to the three different treatment arms has been evaluated; however, conflicting results have been obtained perhaps due to the small numbers of patients within each category.[73,74] For older patients or patients who do not have an appropriate allogeneic donor, the decision to proceed with conventional chemotherapy in first remission appears clear. The key issue for young patients with an available HLA-matched sibling donor, such as B.S. has, is whether to undergo an allogeneic HCT at the time of first remission or first relapse.[28] Unfortunately, no trials have addressed this question. Data from the International Bone Marrow Transplant Registry (IBMTR) indicated that 60% of patients with AML in first remission who received a matched sibling allogeneic HCT have a 3-year probability of survival; survival decreases to 44% in those in second or subsequent remission.[17] The 3-year probability of survival for recipients of unrelated HCT in first or second remission are 40% and 37%, respectively.[17] Current research efforts focus on retrospective analysis of completed trials to identify subsets of patients (e.g., those with unfavorable cytogenetics) who may respond favorably to allogeneic HCT transplantation and the use of novel preparative regimens in hopes of improving the outcome of allogeneic HCT.[74,75]

B.S. is eligible for allogeneic HCT by virtue of his diagnosis and the availability of a histocompatible donor. In addition, he meets age and organ-function eligibility requirements and is in complete remission with minimal residual disease. The decision regarding timing of allogeneic HCT compared with other therapies must be made weighing the aforementioned risks and benefits. B.S. can either undergo allogeneic HCT now or receive consolidation chemotherapy and delay HCT until early in his first relapse.

Histocompatibility

8. How does histocompatibility influence the risks for graft rejection and graft-versus-host reactions in patients like B.S. who undergo an allogeneic HCT?

The tissue transplanted in allogeneic HCT is immunologically active, and thus there is potential for bidirectional graft rejection.[1,2,76] In the first scenario, cytotoxic T cells and natural killer (NK) cells belonging to the host (recipient) recognize MHC antigens of the graft (donor hematopoietic cells) and elicit a rejection response. In the second scenario, immunologically active cells in the graft recognize host MHC antigens and elicit an immune response. The former is referred to as host-versus-graft disease and the latter as graft-versus-host disease (GVHD). Host-versus-graft effects are more common in solid organ transplantation. When host-versus-graft effects occur in allogeneic HCT, they are referred

to as graft failure, which results in ineffective hematopoiesis (i.e., adequate ANC and/or platelet counts were not obtained). Therefore, an essential first step for patients eligible for HCT is finding an HLA-compatible graft with an acceptable risk of rejection and GVHD.

Rejection is least likely to occur with a syngeneic donor, meaning that the recipient and host are identical (monozygotic) twins. Identical twins occur spontaneously in nature in approximately 1 in 100 births; thus, it is unlikely that a patient would have a syngeneic donor. In those patients without a syngeneic donor, initial HLA typing is conducted on family members because the likelihood of complete histocompatibility between unrelated individuals is remote. Siblings are the most likely individuals to be histocompatible within a family. However, because each offspring inherits only one parental haplotype, the chance for complete histocompatibility occurring in an individual with only one sibling is 25%.[1,2] Approximately 40% of patients with more than one sibling have an HLA-identical match.[1,2]

Determination of histocompatibility between potential donors and the patient is completed before allogeneic HCT.[64] Initially, HLA typing performed using blood samples and compatibility for class I MHC antigens (HLA-A, HLA-B, and HLA-C), is determined through serologic and DNA-based testing methods.[77] In vitro reactivity between donor and recipient can also be assessed in mixed-lymphocyte culture, a test used to measure compatibility of the MHC class II antigens (HLA-DR, HLA-DP, HLA-DQ).[77] Currently, most clinical and research laboratories are also performing molecular DNA typing using polymerase-chain reaction methodology to determine the HLA allele sequence.[77] A donor–recipient pair with different HLA antigens (i.e., "antigen mismatched") always have different alleles, whereas pairs with the same allele always have the same antigen and are termed "matched." However, some pairs have the same HLA antigen but have different alleles and are thus "allele mismatched."[78]

Lack of an HLA-matched sibling donor can be a barrier to allogeneic HCT. The use of alternative sources of allogeneic hematopoietic cells, such as related donors mismatched at one or more HLA-loci, or phenotypically (i.e., serologically) matched unrelated donors has been evaluated.[65] Establishment of the National Marrow Donor Program has helped increase the pool of potential donors for allogeneic HCT.[65] Through this program, an HLA-matched unrelated volunteer donor might be identified. Recipients of an unrelated graft are more likely to experience graft failure and acute GVHD relative to recipients of a matched-sibling donor.[79] Thus, work is ongoing to identify factors that predict graft failure or GVHD to improve the availability and safety of unrelated donor transplants.[80] (See Graft Failure section below.)

The preparative regimen or GVHD prophylaxis may be altered based on the mismatch between the donor and recipient. The risk of graft failure decreases with better matches, such that those with a class I (i.e., HLA-A, B, or C) antigen mismatch have the highest risk of rejection compared with those with just one class I allele mismatch who have a minimal risk. Graft failure does not appear to associated with mismatch at a single class II antigen or allele.[78] GVHD, both acute and chronic, and survival have also been associated with disparity for class I and II antigens and alleles.[81,82]

Harvesting, Preparing, and Transplanting Allogeneic Hematopoietic Stem Cells

9. What methods can be used to harvest stem cells from B.S.'s histocompatible sibling and prepare them for transplant? Are there any advantages to the use of bone marrow, peripheral blood, or umbilical cord blood as a source for stem cells?

BONE MARROW

The technique of obtaining allogeneic hematopoietic stem cells varies according to the anatomic site (i.e., bone marrow, peripheral blood, or umbilical cord blood) from which the cells are being harvested. Allogeneic bone marrow is obtained from the donor under spinal or general anesthesia in the operating room under sterile conditions on day 0 of BMT.[1,2] Multiple aspirations of marrow are obtained from the anterior and posterior iliac crests until a volume with a sufficient number of hematopoietic cells is collected (e.g., 600 to 1,200 mL of bone marrow). The bone marrow then is processed to remove fat or marrow emboli and is usually immediately infused intravenously into the patient like a blood transfusion. The marrow may need additional processing if the donor and recipient are ABO incompatible, which occurs in up to 30% of HCTs. RBCs may need to be removed before infusion into the recipient to prevent immune-mediated hemolytic anemia and thrombotic microangiopathic syndromes.[83]

PERIPHERAL BLOOD PROGENITOR CELLS

When obtaining allogeneic hematopoietic cells from peripheral blood, the compatible donor first undergoes mobilization therapy with a HGF to increase the number of hematopoietic cells circulating in the peripheral blood.[84] The most commonly used regimen to mobilize allogeneic (healthy) donors is a 4- to 5-day course of filgrastim, 10 to 16 µg/kg per day, administered subcutaneously, followed by leukapheresis on the fourth or fifth day when peripheral blood levels of CD34+ cells peak.[85] An adequate number of hematopoietic cells is usually obtained with one to two apheresis collections, with the optimal number of CD34+ collected being 5 to 8 × 10^6 cells/kg of recipient body weight.[86,87] Higher cell doses have been associated with not only more rapid engraftment, but also fewer fungal infections and improved overall survival.[88] Hematopoietic cells obtained from the peripheral blood are processed like bone marrow–derived stem cells and may be infused immediately into the recipient or frozen for future use. Allogeneic donation of PBPC has a similar level of physical discomfort to bone marrow donation; however, PBPC donation leads to quicker recovery.[87] The donor may experience musculoskeletal pain, headache, mild increases in hepatic enzyme or lactate dehydrogenase levels due to filgrastim administration and hypocalcemia due to citrate accumulation, which decreases ionized calcium concentrations during apheresis.[84,89]

The use of allogeneic PBPC is increasing; in the year 2000, 40% of allogeneic HCTs performed worldwide used PBPC as the sources of hematopoietic cells rather than bone marrow.[17] In HLA-matched sibling donors, retrospective comparison suggested that PBPC infusions were associated with quicker engraftment[15,90] and with similar costs to BMT.[91] Transplantation with PBPC in HLA-matched sibling donors results in quicker neutrophil and platelet engraftment, with equivalent or higher rates of acute and chronic GVHD with PBPCT relative to BMT in several randomized clinical trials.[11–14] Similar trends have been found with unrelated donors.[92,93] Allogeneic PBPC grafts contain approximately 10 times more T and B cells than bone marrow grafts. Because these cells survive long-term, lymphocytes subsets are higher and the rate of severe infections after engraftment is lower in PBPCT.[94] However, there has also been significant concern that the greater T- and B-cell content of PBPCT could increase the risk of acute and/or chronic GVHD. The relative risk of acute and chronic GVHD after PBPCT were 1.16 and 1.53, respectively, compared with BMT ($P < .006$ for both), with a 66% higher risk of clinically extensive chronic GVHD with PBPCT.[95]

UMBILICAL CORD BLOOD

The use of allogeneic hematopoietic cells from umbilical cord blood (UCB) is increasing in recipient's age ≤20 years.[17] Transplantation with UCB offers an alternative stem cell source to those patients who do not have an acceptable matched related or unrelated donor. When allogeneic hematopoietic cells are obtained from UCB, the cord blood is obtained from a consenting donor in the delivery room after birth and delivery of the placenta.[96] The cord blood is then processed as described earlier, a sample is sent for HLA typing, and the cord blood is frozen and stored for future use. Numerous UCB registries exist with the goal of providing alternative sources of allogeneic stem cells.[97] Functional hematopoietic progenitor and stem cells can be found in UCB cryopreserved for up to 15-years; however, their ability to successfully engraft in a patient is unknown.[98] Case series have shown that UCB transplantation, from a related or unrelated donor, is effective in children with cancer and non-malignant conditions.[99,100] Retrospective comparisons of BMT to UCB transplant have been conducted in recipients of grafts from unrelated[101,102] and related[103] donors. Engraftment is slower in UCB transplants, with a lower risk of GVHD and similar survival rates relative to a BMT.[101–103] In children, engraftment is related to the dose of nucleated cells with an optimal dose of approximately 2 × 10^7 nucleated cells per kilogram of recipient body weight.[19] This raises the question as to whether a UCB transplant can provide enough nucleated cells to adequately engraft within an adult. In adults who do not have a related or unrelated donor for bone marrow or PBPC donation, a UCB transplant is feasible when at least 1 × 10^7 nucleated cells per kilogram of recipient body weight are administered.[18]

In summary, it is most reasonable to harvest PBPC from B.S.'s sibling to use for B.S. myeloablative transplant.

T-CELL DEPLETION

10. What are the risks and benefits of removing T cells from the donor bone marrow before its infusion into the recipient? If bone marrow is harvested from B.S.'s sibling, should T cells be removed?

Immunocompetent T lymphocytes may be depleted from the donor bone marrow ex vivo before infusion (referred to as *T-cell–depleted hematopoietic cells*) into the recipient as a means of preventing GVHD.[36] Depletion of T lymphocytes in donor hematopoietic cells is completed ex vivo using physical (e.g., density gradient fractionation) and/or immunologic (e.g., CAMPATH-1 monoclonal antibody against human CD52) methods.[104] Functional recovery of T cells in the recipient is delayed, and the risk of Epstein-Barr virus–associated lymphoproliferative disorders is higher with the use of T-cell–depleted bone marrow.[104] T-cell–depleted grafts reduce the incidence of GVHD,[104] but graft failure is more common. Before T-cell depletion, graft failure rates with a myeloablative BMT ranged from 1% to 5% but were as high as 50% to 80% with the use of T-cell–depleted bone marrow.[105,106] The higher relapse rates with T-cell–depleted BMT are discussed in the section, Graft-versus-Tumor Effect. Data are evolving regarding the use of selective T-cell depletion in hopes of reducing GVHD while maintaining the GVT effect.[107] Donor lymphocyte infusion in patients who suffer relapse after receiving a T-cell–depleted BMT also is under study.[108]

Presently, it is not clear which patients should receive a T-cell–depleted bone marrow or PBPC. Thus, B.S. should not receive a T-cell–depleted preparation of his donor PBPC, unless he is participating in a clinical trial evaluating the risks and benefits of T-cell depletion.

Graft-versus-Tumor Effect

11. What is the graft-versus-tumor effect? Which tumors are most responsive to this effect?

Initial clinical evidence of a graft-versus-tumor (GVT) effect came from the observation that patients with GVHD had lower relapse rates compared with those who did not.[109,110] This suggests a GVT effect due to the donor lymphocytes. Further support for a GVT effect is the higher rate of leukemia relapse after T-cell–depleted BMT, in part due to the reduction in GVHD and concomitant loss of GVT effect.[104,111] The effectiveness of donor lymphocyte infusions in patients who experienced relapse after allogeneic HCT also suggests a GVT effect. Lymphocytes are collected from the peripheral blood of the donor and administered to the recipient. Eradication of the recurrent malignancy is due to either specific targeting of the tumor antigens or to GVHD, which may affect cancer cells preferentially. Different illnesses vary in their responsiveness to donor lymphocyte infusions, with CML and acute leukemias being the most and least responsive, respectively.[112] Patients with certain solid tumors (e.g., renal cell carcinoma) also appear to benefit from a GVT effect.[113] These data gave rise to the use of nonmyeloablative preparative regimens, which are discussed later in this chapter.

Preparative Regimens for Allogeneic HCT
MYELOABLATIVE PREPARATIVE REGIMENS

12. What is the rationale for using myeloablative preparative regimens for patients like B.S. who are to receive an allogeneic HCT? What types of regimens are used and what is recommended for B.S.?

The combination of chemotherapy and/or radiation used in allogeneic HCT is referred to as the preparative or conditioning regimen. The initial rationale for high-dose myeloablative preparative regimens was similar to that discussed under "Autologous HCT" in this chapter. Specifically, infusion of stem cells circumvents dose-limiting myelosuppression, maximizing the potential value of the steep dose-response curve to alkylating agents and radiation,[4] suppressing the host immune system, and creating space in the marrow compartment to facilitate engraftment.[1,2] The preparative regimen is designed to eradicate immunologically active host tissues (lymphoid tissue and macrophages) and to prevent or minimize the development of host-versus-graft reactions. In contrast, a myeloablative preparative regimen may not be necessary if a histocompatible allogeneic HCT is performed on a patient with a poorly functioning immune system (e.g., severe combined immunodeficiency disease [SCID]).[114] In the absence of a functioning immune system, the likelihood of a host-versus-graft reaction to histocompatible donor hematopoietic cells is small. Similarly, patients undergoing syngeneic transplantation do not require immunosuppressive preparative regimens before HCT because the donor and the patient are genetically identical.[1,2] Thus, the preparative regimen is tailored to the primary disease and to HLA compatibility between the recipient–donor pair.

Examples of common preparative regimens for allogeneic HCT are shown in Table 92-4.[21,35,115,116] Most allogeneic preparative regimens for the treatment of hematologic malignancies contain either cyclophosphamide or radiation, or both. The combination of cyclophosphamide and total body irradiation (TBI) was one of the first preparative regimens used and is still used widely today.[1,2] This regimen is immunosuppressive and has inherent activity against hematologic malignancies (e.g., leukemias, lymphomas). TBI has the added advantage of being devoid of active metabolites that might interfere with the activity of donor hematopoietic cells. In addition, TBI eradicates residual malignant cells at sanctuary sites such as the central nervous system. Modifications of the cyclophosphamide–TBI preparative regimen include replacing TBI with other agents (e.g., busulfan) and adding other chemotherapeutic or monoclonal agents to the existing regimen. These measures are designed to minimize the long-term toxicities associated with TBI (e.g., growth retardation in children, cataracts) or to provide additional antitumor activity, respectively. In the case of a mismatched allogeneic HCT with a substantially increased chance of graft rejection, antithymocyte globulin (ATG) may also be added to the preparative regimen to further immunosuppress the recipient.

The optimal myeloablative preparative regimen for allogeneic HCT is challenging to study because several indications for HCT (e.g., SCID, thalassemia) are rare enough that it is not feasible or is cost-prohibitive to conduct clinical trials that are adequately powered to detect clinically relevant differences. However, the long-term outcomes of busulfan/cyclophosphamide (BU/CY) and cyclophosphamide/total body irradiation (CY/TBI) in patients with AML and CML—the more common indications for allogeneic HCT—have been compared in a meta-analysis of four clinical trials.[117] Equivalent rates of long-term complications were present between the two preparative regimens, except for a greater risk of cataracts with CY/TBI and alopecia with BU/CY. Overall and disease-free survival rates were similar in patients with CML, whereas there was a trend for improved disease-free survival with CY/TBI in AML patients. Thus, the preparative regimen can be tailored to the primary disease and to the HLA compatibility.

Based on these data, the CY/TBI preparative regimen is preferred for B.S.

NONMYELOABLATIVE PREPARATIVE REGIMENS

13. Describe the rationale for nonmyeloablative preparative regimens. Is B.S. a candidate for such a regimen?

The regimen-related toxicity of a myeloablative preparative regimen (Table 92-5) limits the use of HCT to younger patients who have minimal comorbidities. Most patients diagnosed with cancer are elderly, and thus myeloablative HCT cannot be offered to a substantial portion of these patients.[118] The concept of donor immune response having a GVT effect gave rise to the theory that a strongly immunosuppressive but not myeloablative preparative regimen (i.e., a nonmyeloablative transplantation or NMT) may result in a state of chimerism in which the recipient and donor are co-existing.[119] The toxicity and efficacy of NMT are also being evaluated in patients with nonmalignant conditions, such as congenital immunodeficiency, who are not eligible for a myeloablative HCT.[120]

A nonmyeloablative preparative regimen allows for development of mixed chimerism (defined as 5% to 95% peripheral donor T cells) between the host and recipient to allow for a GVT effect as the primary form of therapy (Fig. 92-3). Chimerism is evaluated to monitor disease response and engraftment at varying time points after NMT. Chimerism is assessed within peripheral blood T cells and granulocytes and bone marrow using conventional (e.g., using sex chromosomes for opposite sex donors) and molecular (e.g., variable number of tandem repeats) for same sex donors. The methods used to characterize chimerism after HCT are reviewed elsewhere.[121]

The nonmyeloablative regimen does not completely eliminate host normal and malignant cells. The donor cells eradicate residual host hematopoiesis, and the GVT effects generally occur after the development of full donor T-cell chimerism.[122] After engraftment, mixed chimerism should be present as evidenced by the ability to detect both donor- and recipient-derived cells. Thus, if the graft is rejected, autologous recovery should promptly occur. The intensity of immunosuppression required for engraftment depends on the immunocompetence of the recipient histocompatibility, and the composition of the HCT.[123] More intensive regimens that are required for engraftment in the setting of unrelated-donor or HLA-mismatched related HCT have recently been termed "reduced-intensity" myeloablative transplants.[123] After chimerism develops, donor–lymphocyte infusion can be safely administered in patients without GVHD to eradicate malignant cells.

Nonmyeloablative preparative regimens typically consist of a purine analog (e.g., fludarabine) in combination with an alkylating agent or low-dose TBI.[120,124,125] Adverse effects are decreased because of the lower-intensity preparative regimen. Thus, patients who were not healthy or young enough to receive a myeloablative preparative regimen could undergo a nonmyeloablative preparative regimen. However, the risk of GVHD remains with NMT. Therefore, GVHD prophylaxis, though different from that used with myeloablative regimens, is still necessary, as is follow-up for infectious complications.[126,127]

Presently, NMT is not indicated as first-line therapy for any malignant or nonmalignant conditions and therefore is not an option for B.S. Clinical research over the past 6-years has focused on developing preparative regimens with acceptable toxicity that are capable of achieving mixed chimerism.[128] Currently, NMT should only be conducted in the setting of a clinical trial. NMT is being evaluated for cancers sensitive to a GVT effect (e.g., CML, AML), in older patients or for those with comorbidities who would not be able to tolerate a myeloablative HCT.[7,123,129,130]

Table 92-5 Common Toxicities Associated With Myeloablative Allogeneic HCT

Early	Late
Nausea, vomiting, diarrhea	Increased susceptibility to infections
Mucositis	Endocrine disorders (hypothyroidism, infertility, growth retardation)
Hemorrhagic cystitis	
Veno-occlusive disease	Secondary malignant neoplasms
Renal dysfunction	Chronic GVHD
Cardiotoxicity	Cataracts
Pneumonitis	
Graft rejection	
Acute GVHD	

GVHD, graft-versus-host disease; HCT, hematopoietic cell transplantation.

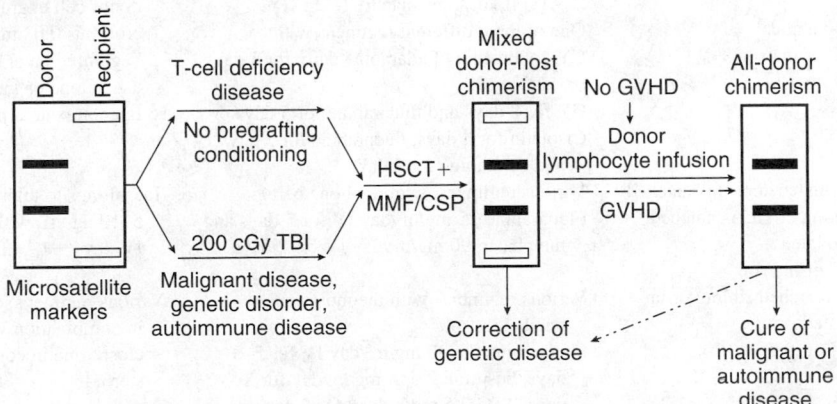

FIGURE 92-3 Nonmyeloablative allogeneic hematopoietic cell transplantation. (CSP, cyclosporine; GVHD, graft-versus-host disease; HSCT, hematopoietic stem cell transplantation; MMF, mycophenolate mofetil; TBI, total body irradiation.)

There is a paucity of data regarding the optimal source of hematopoietic stem cells after NMT. Most case series have combined data from peripheral blood progenitor and marrow grafts (Table 92-6). Some data suggests that, compared with bone marrow grafts, PBPC is associated with more favorable outcomes, such as quicker engraftment, earlier T-cell chimerism, longer progression-free survival, and lower risk of graft rejection.[131,132]

Post-Transplantation Immunosuppressive Therapy

14. What is the rationale for immunosuppressive therapy after an allogeneic HCT? What is recommended for B.S.?

After infusion of hematopoietic cells, immunosuppressive therapy is administered to prevent or minimize GVHD. Patients receiving syngeneic transplants or a T-cell–depleted histocompatible allogeneic transplant generally do not receive post-transplantation immunosuppressive therapy. In the former, the donor and the patient are genetically identical and GVHD should not be elicited. In the latter, the volume of donor T cells infused into the patient usually is insufficient to elicit a significant graft-versus-host reaction.[104,133] Numerous immunosuppressive agents given alone or in combination have been evaluated for the prevention of GVHD. Commonly used regimens after myeloablative HCT include cyclosporine or tacrolimus administered with a short course of low-dose methotrexate.[134] Corticosteroids may also be used to prevent GVHD but are more commonly used to treat GVHD. In allogeneic HCT recipients without GVHD, immunosuppressive therapy is slowly tapered and discontinued over 6 months to 1 year because of immunologic tolerance.[1,2] GVHD prophylaxis

varies between a myeloablative and nonmyeloablative HCT. Over time, the immunologically active tissue between host and recipient become tolerant of one another and cease recognizing the other as foreign. In contrast, solid organ transplant recipients usually continue immunosuppressive therapy for the duration of the recipient's life.

Thus, B.S. should receive cyclosporine or tacrolimus administered with a short course of methotrexate for post-transplantation immunotherapy. This combination regimen will lower the risk of GVHD after his allogeneic HCT with a myeloablative preparative regimen.

Comparison of Supportive Care Strategies Between Autologous and Allogeneic Myeloablative HCT

15. How do supportive care strategies used for myeloablative preparative regimens with an autologous graft differ from those described for an allogeneic graft?

Supportive care strategies common to patients receiving a myeloablative preparative regimen, regardless if an autologous or allogeneic HCT, include use of indwelling central venous catheters; blood product support; and pharmacologic management of chemotherapy-induced nausea and vomiting (CINV), mucositis, and pain. These similarities are a function of the adverse drug reactions (ADRs) that occur as a result of administering high-dose, myeloablative chemotherapy.

The supportive care diverges because of the different needs for immunosuppression with an autologous and allogeneic HCT. Allogeneic HCT patients experience an initial period of pancytopenia followed by a more prolonged period of im-

---

Table 92-6 Representative Nonmyeloablative Preparative Regimens Used in Allogeneic HCT

Disease State	Donor	Preparative Regimen	Post-Transplantation Immunosuppression
Hematologic malignanacies[128]	HLA-matched or mismatched unrelated PBPC or marrow	Fludarabine 30 mg/m²/day IV on 3 consecutive days (–4, –3, –2), TBI 2 Gy as single fraction on day 0	Cyclosporine 6.25 mg/kg PO BID, days –3 to day +100 with taper from day +100 to +180 Mycophenolate mofetil 15 mg/kg PO BID, day +0 to +40 with taper from day +40 to +90
Metastatic renal cell[124]	0–1 HLA mismatched sibling PBPC	CY 60 mg/kg/day IV on 2 consecutive days (–7, –6), fludarabine 25 mg/m²/day IV on 5 consecutive days (–5, –4, –3, –2, –1) + ATG if HLA mismatch	Cyclosporine 3 mg/kg/day IV (6 mg/kg/day PO BID if tolerated), started day –4 and tapered based on the speed and degree of donor cell engraftment
Lymphoid malignancies[7]	HLA-identical PBPC or marrow	One of three different regimens with: CY, followed by fludarabine daily for 3 days or CY for 2 days and fludarabine for 5 days or Cisplatin for 4 days, fludarabine for 3 days, and cytarabine for 2 days	Tacrolimus 0.03 mg/kg/day IV, started day –2, beginning taper day 90 if no GVHD present; used alone or in combination with methotrexate 5 mg/m²/day day +1, +3, +6
Various[328]	HLA-matched or mismatched sibling or HLA-matched unrelated PBPC or marrow	Various regimens, with final one being: Fludarabine 25 mg/m²/day IV for 5-days and melphalan 90 mg/m²/day IV for 2 days	Tacrolimus to maintain blood concentration of 5–10 ng/mL with methotrexate 5 mg/m²/day IV days +1, +3, +6, +11
Various[131]	HLA-matched sibling or unrelated PBPC or marrow	Various regimens, with the most common one being: Fludarabine 25–30 mg/m²/day IV for 5–6 days, busulfan 2 or 4 mg/kg/day for 2 days, ATG 2.5 mg/kg/day for 5 days	Various regimens: cyclosporine, cyclosporine in combination with methotrexate or cyclosporine in combination with corticosteroids

ATG, antithymocyte globulin; CY, cyclophosphamide; GVHD, graft-versus-host disease; HCT, hematopoietic cell transplantation; PBPC, peripheral blood progenitor cells; TBI, total body irradiation.

munosuppression, which substantially increases the risk of bacterial infections, but more importantly, fungal, viral, and other opportunistic infections.[135] The risk of infection increases as additional immunosuppressive therapy is incorporated to prevent or treat GVHD. Supportive strategies designed to minimize infection during immunosuppression are essential after allogeneic HCT (see Infectious Complications section in text that follows).

Comparison of Supportive Care Strategies Between Allogeneic Myeloablative and Nonmyeloablative HCT

16. How do supportive care strategies used for myeloablative and nonmyeloablative preparative regimens with an allogeneic graft differ?

A direct comparison of the toxicities with a myeloablative and nonmyeloablative preparative regimen is difficult because NMT is offered only to patients who are not candidates for myeloablative allogeneic HCT. These preparative regimens differ substantially in terms of the chemotherapy agents used (see Tables 92-4 and 92-6) and the degree of myelosuppression. NMT may have a different time pattern of infectious complications and has a similar incidence and severity of acute GVHD; however, comparisons between the preparative regimens is challenging because of the differences in the pre-HCT health of the recipients.[123] Clinical research within NMT is focusing on designing optimal preparative regimens with acceptable efficacy and toxicity (i.e., mixed chimerism, disease response). Thus, more variability is seen for immunosuppression after a NMT than for that following a myeloablative HCT (see Table 92-6).

Dose Calculations in Obesity

17. K.M. is a 36-year-old woman with CML in chronic phase. After her initial diagnosis, a successful search for an unrelated 6/6 HLA–matched allogeneic donor was conducted. K.M. is being admitted for myeloablative allogeneic BMT. Orders for K.M.'s preparative regimen are written as follows: height, 162 centimeters; actual body weight (ABW), 80 kg; ideal body weight (IBW = 54 kg; body surface area (BSA), 1.85 m²; body mass index (BMI), 30.5 kg/m²; busulfan, 16 mg/kg total dose to be administered over 4 days (1 mg/kg per dose PO Q 6 hr for 16 doses, days –9, –8, –7, and –6). Cyclophosphamide 50 mg/kg IV to be administered on days –5, –4, –3, and –2. Day –1 is a "rest" day, followed by infusion of bone marrow on day 0. Which weight should be used to calculate doses of K.M.'s preparative regimen?

K.M.'s ABW is 48% over her ideal body weight. She is considered obese since her ABW is 30% greater than her ideal body weight and her BMI is between 27 to 35 kg/m². Obesity has numerous effects on the pharmacokinetic disposition of medications; unfortunately, there is a paucity of data regarding the effects of obesity on the clinical outcomes of anticancer agents. The risk associated with inaccurate dosing of the preparative regimen for a myeloablative HCT leaves a particularly challenging situation since using a weight that is too high can cause lethal toxicity and one that is too low could result in inadequate marrow ablation or disease eradication.

Few studies have evaluated the association of body weight and outcome to preparative regimens for myeloablative

HCT.[130–138] Differing conclusions regarding optimal dose adjustment of oral busulfan were made from two small case series, with 16 and 20 patients, respectively.[136,137] Busulfan's apparent oral clearance (CL/F) expressed in relation to adjusted ideal body weight (AIBW) or body surface area (BSA) was similar in normal (BMI of 18 to 27 kg/m²) and obese patients in a case series of 279 adolescent and adults undergoing HCT.[138] Thus, routine dosing of oral busulfan based on AIBW or BSA does not require a specific accommodation for obesity.

K.M.'s busulfan dose should not be based on her ABW because it does not accurately correct for her obesity and may predispose her to hepatic veno-occlusive disease (VOD). Her initial busulfan doses should be based on IBW or BSA.

Complications Associated With HCT

18. What is the nature of the toxicities associated with myeloablative preparative regimen that must be anticipated in K.M.? Are they similar to those anticipated after standard-dose chemotherapy?

Myelosuppression is a frequent dose-limiting toxicity for antineoplastics when administered in conventional doses used to treat cancer. However, because myelosuppression is circumvented with hematopoietic rescue in the case of patients receiving HCT, the dose-limiting toxicities of these myeloablative preparative regimens are nonhematologic (i.e., extramedullary) in nature. The toxicities vary with the preparative regimen used.

Most patients undergoing HCT experience toxicities commonly associated with chemotherapy (e.g., alopecia, mucositis, nausea and vomiting, infertility). (Also see related information in Chapter 89, Adverse Effects of Chemotherapy.) However, these toxicities are magnified in the HCT population. For example, mucositis often is severe enough to warrant airway protection, preclude oral intake, and require IV opioids for pain control. Table 92-5 depicts a range of toxicities that can occur after myeloablative preparative regimen for HCT, and Figure 92-4 depicts the time course for complications after HCT. Specific toxicities are discussed in detail in the following sections.

Busulfan Seizures

19. In addition to her preparative regimen, the following supportive care agents and monitoring parameters are prescribed for K.M: on the day of admission (day –10), administer a phenytoin loading dose (10 to 15 mg/kg) orally in divided doses (300, 300, and 400 mg Q 3 hr). Continue 300 mg PO daily from days –9 to –6. Busulfan pharmacokinetic blood sampling is to occur after dose 1 to a target busulfan concentration at steady state (Css) greater than 900 ng/mL. Begin normal saline hydration 3,000 mL/m²/day 4 hours before cyclophosphamide and continue for 24 hours after the last cyclophosphamide dose. Mesna to be given concurrently with cyclophosphamide as 10% of the cyclophosphamide dose administered intravenously (IV) 30 minutes before starting cyclophosphamide dose, then as 100% of cyclophosphamide dose administered as a continuous IV infusion over 24 hours after each dose of cyclophosphamide. Beginning on day –5, weigh patient twice daily, check fluid input and urinary output every 4 hours, and monitor urine for RBCs daily until 24 hours after the last cyclophosphamide dose. If urine output

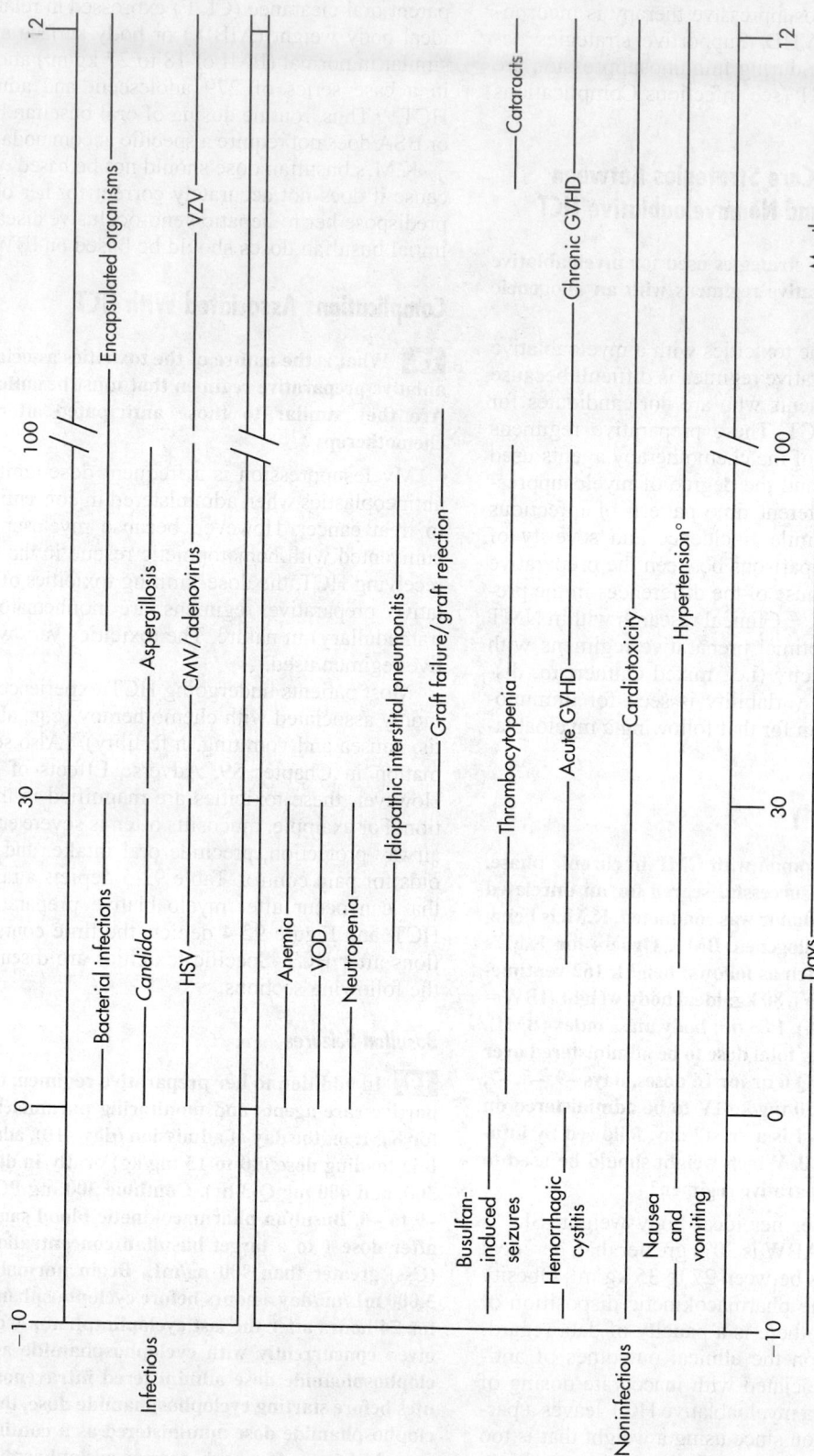

FIGURE 92-4 Complications after hematopoietic cell transplantation by time. [a]Patients undergoing myeloablative allogeneic HCT only. CMV, cytomegalovirus; GVHD, graft-versus-host disease; HSV, herpes simplex virus; VOD, veno-occlusive disease; VZV, varicella-zoster virus.

drops below 300 mL over 2 hours, administer an IV bolus of 250 mL normal saline and give furosemide 10 mg/m², not to exceed 20 mg IV. What is the rationale for these supportive care therapies and monitoring parameters prescribed for K.M. as they relate to busulfan therapy?

Seizures have been reported in both adult and pediatric patients receiving high-dose busulfan for HCT preparative regimens.[139,140] Busulfan is highly lipophilic and crosses the blood–brain barrier with an average CSF:plasma ratio of 0.95 after administration of high doses.[141] Neurotoxicity appears to be dose related, and the incidence of seizures is significantly higher in children with an elevated CSF:plasma ratio.[141] Although the exact incidence of busulfan-induced neurotoxicity is unknown, 7.5% of 96 children experienced seizures during or within 24-hours of completing busulfan.[139]

Anticonvulsants are used to minimize the risk of seizures. Anticonvulsants are begun shortly before busulfan, with the loading dose completed at least 6 hours before the first busulfan dose. Most centers monitor phenytoin concentrations after 2 days of dosing, particularly when using an oral regimen. Oral loading and maintenance regimens are generally sufficient because target concentrations of 10 to 20 μg/mL can be achieved by the peak time of seizure risk. If patients are experiencing significant vomiting or are having difficulty maintaining therapeutic phenytoin concentrations, IV phenytoin should be substituted for oral doses. Benzodiazepines such as lorazepam or clonazepam have also been used for seizure prophylaxis during high-dose busulfan therapy before HCT.[142] Antiseizure medications are usually discontinued 24 to 48 hours after administration of the last dose of busulfan. Seizures can still occur despite the use of prophylactic anticonvulsants and usually do not result in permanent neurologic deficits.

Adaptive Dosing of Busulfan

20. What dosing strategies can be used to minimize busulfan toxicities?

The considerable interpatient variability in the clearance of both oral and IV busulfan, along with the identified concentration–effect relationships, has led to the adaptive dosing of busulfan. The clearance of Busulfex (IV busulfan) exhibited interpatient variability adjusted for weight with a coefficient of variation (CV, standard deviation/mean) of 25% in 59 patients.[143] There is similar variability with oral busulfan, with a CV of CL/F adjusted for actual body weight (mL/min per kilogram) of 21% in 279 adult patients, the largest patient population analyzed for busulfan pharmacokinetics.[138] Weight, disease, and age are factors that may influence the clearance of oral busulfan.[138] Busulfan CL/F is enhanced in young children (≤4 years old) compared with adults and older children (>10 years old).[144]

Adjusting the busulfan dose to achieve a target concentration appears to minimize the toxicities of the BU/CY regimen, particularly VOD while improving engraftment and relapse rates.[145–147] The pharmacodynamic relationships are briefly reviewed; more complete reviews of these relationships after oral busulfan administration are available elsewhere.[148,149] When reviewing pharmacodynamic data with busulfan, close attention should be taken in their interpretation because of the potential changes in the concentration–effect relationships between busulfan C_{SS} and outcome with each patient population and with each preparative regimen. Most studies have shown a pharmacodynamic relationship in patients receiving the BU/CY preparative regimens. Data are also represented as area under the plasma concentration time curve (AUC) or C_{SS}; data are easily converted to C_{SS} (C_{SS} = AUC divided by the dosing interval). One must also pay close attention to the units used in these studies. Results are expressed as μM-min or ng/mL; an AUC of 1,500 μM-min is roughly equivalent to a C_{SS} of 1,025 ng/mL based on busulfan's molecular weight of 246.

Hepatic VOD was observed more frequently in patients receiving BU/CY with a busulfan C_{SS} >925 to 1,025 ng/mL. In BU/CY regimens, busulfan C_{SS} >600 ng/mL favor engraftment, although contradictory data exist. Higher busulfan concentrations (C_{SS} >900 ng/mL) were associated with lower relapse rates in adult CML patients receiving BU/CY before HLA-matched grafts, without unacceptable rates of VOD. Thus, a busulfan C_{SS} >900 ng/mL is targeted for K.M. because she has CML.

An intravenous busulfan product, Busulfex, was FDA approved in February 1999 in combination with cyclophosphamide as a preparative regimen before allogeneic HCT for CML. The FDA-approved dose is 0.8 mg/kg IV every 6 hours for 16 doses, which is similar to the oral busulfan dose of 1 mg/kg with a mean fraction absorbed (F) of 90%.[148] Recent data with Busulfex in combination with either cyclophosphamide or fludarabine suggest that therapeutic drug monitoring may be needed.[150] In addition, the product labeling states "high busulfan area under the plasma concentration versus time curve (AUC) values (>1,500 μM-min) may be associated with an increased risk of developing hepatic VOD)" which has caused many HCT centers to institute therapeutic drug monitoring after Busulfex is administered.

Hemorrhagic Cystitis

21. What is the rationale for these supportive care therapies and monitoring parameters prescribed for K.M. as they relate to cyclophosphamide therapy?

In HCT patients receiving cyclophosphamide, moderate to severe hemorrhagic cystitis occurs in 4% to 20% receiving hydration alone.[151] The putative bladder toxin is acrolein, a metabolite of cyclophosphamide.[152] Consequently, a variety of preventive measures are taken to lower the risk of hemorrhagic cystitis in HCT patients receiving cyclophosphamide. The methods used include forced hydration with normal saline or D₅ normal saline 3,000 mL/m² per day, continuous bladder irrigation with normal saline 200 to 1,000 mL/hour via a three-way Foley catheter, and/or concomitant use of the uroprotectant, mesna. ASCO Guidelines for the Use of Chemotherapy and Radiotherapy Protectants recommends the use of mesna plus saline diuresis or forced saline diuresis to lower the incidence of urothelial toxicity with high-dose cyclophosphamide in the setting of HCT.[153]

In three randomized controlled clinical trials, the efficacy of mesna has been compared with forced hydration with or without the addition of continuous bladder irrigation for prevention of cyclophosphamide-induced hemorrhagic cystitis in HCT patients.[151,154,155] Although the interpretation of their results is complicated by varying definitions of hematuria, all three studies report similar or lower rates of hematuria (of any grade or severity) in mesna-treated patients.[151,154,155] However, this difference was statistically significant in only two of these studies.[154,155] It is important to note that hematuria or hemorrhagic cystitis can occur despite the use of any of these methods.[151,154,155] Thus, the decision to use one method over another will depend on the relative merits of the various methods, whether the patient will be receiving cyclophosphamide as an inpatient or outpatient, and the preference of the HCT center personnel.

Disadvantages of Foley catheter irrigation include intensive nursing time, patient dissatisfaction, and a higher incidence of microbiologically detected urinary tract infections.[155] Furthermore, Foley trauma itself can cause mild hematuria, which can confuse the diagnosis of cyclophosphamide-induced hemorrhagic cystitis.[155] Concern that was initially posed regarding delayed engraftment in mesna-treated patients[154] has not been borne out in subsequent randomized trials.[151,155] Also, a cost analysis comparing Foley bladder irrigation with mesna demonstrated very little difference between the two methods when total costs, including urine cultures and laboratory tests, were compared.[155]

The optimal mesna dose with high-dose cyclophosphamide in preparation for myeloablative HCT is unknown. A variety of different regimens have been used, including intermittent bolus dosing (mesna dose 20% to 40% of cyclophosphamide dose, administered for three or four doses) or continuous infusion regimens (mesna 80% to 160% of cyclophosphamide dose).[151,154,155] To date, there have been no randomized, comparative trials evaluating the most effective dose or method of administration. Mesna should be continued for 24 to 48 hours after the last cyclophosphamide dose, such that mesna is present within the bladder to donate free thiol groups at the same time as the urotoxic metabolite acrolein. After IV administration of mesna, most of it (i.e., 60% to 100%) is excreted within the urine over 4 hours.[156] Cyclophosphamide has an average half-life of 7 hours after administration of 60 mg/kg,[157] and acrolein may be present within the urine for 24 to 48 hours after cyclophosphamide administration.[158]

Thus, K.M. is receiving hydration with normal saline and mesna, administered as a continuous infusion, to minimize her risk of hemorrhagic cystitis due to cyclophosphamide. K.M. should also be monitored for any RBC present in the urine along with her urinary output to allow for rapid intervention if hemorrhagic cystitis occurs.

Chemotherapy-Induced Gastrointestinal Effects

22. What other end-organ toxicities must be watched for? Should any medications be ordered for K.M. to prevent and treat the gastrointestinal effects associated with myeloablative therapy?

Preparative regimens for myeloablative HCT result in other end-organ toxicities such as renal failure[159] and idiopathic pneumonia syndrome.[160] In addition, recipients of myeloablative preparative regimens are at risk for severe gastrointestinal toxicity, specifically chemotherapy-induced nausea and vomiting (CINV) and mucositis. In this population, CINV can be due to administration of highly emetogenic chemotherapy over several days, the administration of total body irradiation, and also poor control of CINV prior to consideration for HCT. Thus, patients such as K.M. who are undergoing a myeloablative HCT should be treated with a serotonin antagonist plus a corticosteroid.[161] Higher doses of serotonin antagonists may be necessary in the patient population[161,162]; however, few randomized trials have been conducted in this area and most of the information comes from case series.[162] Recent data suggest that ondansetron may increase cyclophosphamide clearance in breast cancer patients undergoing a myeloablative HCT[163,164]; however, further work is needed to identify the clinical implications of this finding because, to date, cyclophosphamide concentrations have not been consistently associated with clinical outcomes in patients undergoing a myeloablative HCT.[165,166] In patients who do not have thrombocytopenia, electropuncture may also be beneficial when used in conjunction with antiemetics.[167] In addition, severe mucositis may require parenteral opioid analgesics for pain relief[168] and total parenteral nutrition to prevent the development of nutritional deficits (see Chapter 9, Pain, and Chapter 37, Adult Parenteral Nutrition).

Myelosuppression and Growth Factor Use

23. An order is written to begin filgrastim on day 0 and to continue administration until the ANC has recovered to 500/mm³ for 2 consecutive days. Is this therapy appropriate for K.M.?

[SI units: ANC 500×10^6 cells/L]

Primary administration of the HGFs filgrastim and sargramostim accelerate neutrophil recovery and lower costs after allogeneic HCT with a bone marrow or umbilical cord graft.[169,170] Fear of exacerbating GVHD by stimulating macrophage production (hence, tumor necrosis factor [TNF], a cytokine implicated in the pathogenesis of GVHD) initially limited the use of sargramostim. Enhanced GVHD has been reported with sargramostim after allogeneic BMT in a small number of patients.[171] In contrast, other trials have failed to substantiate this concern.[62,63] In a phase III trial, patients receiving sargramostim after allogeneic HCT experienced more rapid neutrophil recovery, less severe mucositis, and fewer days in the hospital compared with patients receiving placebo.[169] No difference in the incidence of GVHD, relapse, or survival was observed among groups. Filgrastim also has been evaluated in the allogeneic setting and has hastened neutrophil recovery without increasing the incidence of GVHD.[172]

The use of HGFs after infusion of allogeneic PBPC is controversial. Administration of HGFs may not provide further acceleration of hematopoietic recovery after PBPC infusion because large numbers of progenitor cells can be obtained and the number of progenitor cells correlate with hematopoietic recovery in the this setting. However, hematopoietic recovery may be hindered by proliferation of stem and progenitor cells by HGFs being concomitantly administered with methotrexate, which is used after myeloablative allogeneic HCTs for GVHD prophylaxis.[27] There is concern that HGFs will increase the risk of GVHD as filgrastim administration after PBPC is associated with abnormal antigen-presenting cell function and T-cell reactivity.[173–175] Nevertheless, preliminary data indicate that filgrastim accelerates neutrophil recovery compared with placebo in patients receiving PBPCT with no differences in the incidence of acute GVHD, although the trials were not powered to address this specific issue.[176,177] The ASCO Guidelines do not specifically recommend filgrastim in regard to allogeneic PBPC, but state that HGFs "are recommended to help mobilize PBPC and after PBPC infusion" without consideration for the donor type.[43] K.M. is receiving a bone marrow graft, and thus can receive filgrastim starting on day 0.

Veno-Occlusive Disease of the Liver

24. **K.M.'s pretransplantation admission laboratory values are within normal limits. Her weight on admission is 80 kg. During the first 5 days after marrow infusion, K.M.'s weight begins to increase by approximately 0.5 kg/day, her inputs exceeding her outputs by about 500 to 1,000 mL/day, and she is mildly febrile with an axillary temperature of 38°C. Blood and urine cultures are all negative. On day +6 her weight is 85 kg. Laboratory values drawn on day +7 are significant for a total bilirubin of 1.5 mg/dL, an aspartate aminotransferase (AST) of 40 U/L (normal, 0 to 45), and an alkaline phosphatase of 120 U/L (normal, 30 to 120). By day +10, K.M. is complaining of midepigastric and right upper quadrant pain and a liver that is tender to palpation. Over the next few days, K.M. begins to look icteric. Her liver function tests continue to rise slowly, until day +18 when they reach the following peak values: total bilirubin 5.0 mg/dL (normal, 0.1 to 1), AST 150 U/L, and alkaline phosphatase 180 U/L. On day +18, K.M.'s weight is 90 kg. "Rule out VOD of the liver" is included on her problem list in the medical record. What is VOD?**

[SI units: total bilirubin, 25.65 and 85.5 μmol/L, respectively; AST, alkaline phosphatase, same as above]

Hepatic VOD (veno-occlusive disease) is a life-threatening complication that may occur secondary to preparative regimens or radiation used in myeloablative HCT with an autologous or allogeneic HCT or in nonmyeloablative HCT.[128,178,179] Considerable variability exists in the incidence of VOD, with larger case series suggesting the incidence ranges from 5.3% to 54%.[179,180] Although the pathogenesis is not understood completely, several mechanisms have been proposed. The key event appears to be endothelial damage caused by the preparative regimen. Since recent studies have shown that the primary site of the toxic injury is the sinusoidal endothelial cells, the term "sinusoidal obstruction syndrome (SOS)" has been proposed in place of "VOD."[181] The endothelial damage initiates the coagulation cascade, induces thrombosis of the hepatic venules, and eventually leads to fibrous obliteration of the affected venules.[180] The cardinal histologic features are marked sinusoidal fibrosis, necrosis of pericentral hepatocytes, and narrowing and eventual fibrosis of central veins.[181] In patients with VOD, early microscopic changes include subendothelial swelling leading to several physiologic changes, including narrowing of hepatic venules and necrosis of centrizonal hepatocytes.[180]

CLINICAL PRESENTATION

25. **What signs and symptoms in K.M. are consistent with a diagnosis of VOD?**

The signs and symptoms associated with VOD are hyperbilirubinemia (≥2 mg/dL), weight gain (>5% above baseline), hepatomegaly, azotemia, elevated alkaline phosphatase, ascites, elevated AST, and encephalopathy.[182] Insidious weight gain exceeding 5% of baseline usually is the first manifesta-

tion of impending VOD, occurring in over 90% of patients within 3 to 6 days after marrow infusion.[179] Weight gain is caused by sodium and water retention, as evidenced by decreased renal sodium excretion. This usually is distinguished from cyclophosphamide-induced syndrome of inappropriate secretion of antidiuretic hormone by the time course relative to administration of the preparative regimen. Hyperbilirubinemia, which also occurs in virtually all patients, follows the onset of weight gain and usually appears within 10 days after hematopoietic cell infusion. In over half of the patients, the peak bilirubin concentration is >6 mg/dL. Other liver function test abnormalities usually occur after hyperbilirubinemia and include elevations in AST and alkaline phosphatase. Ascites, right upper quadrant pain, and encephalopathy lag behind changes in liver function tests and develop within 10 to 15 days after infusion of hematopoietic cells.[179]

A clinical diagnosis of VOD is made when two of the following features occur within the first 20 days of HCT: (1) hyperbilirubinemia (total serum bilirubin >2 mg/dL), (2) hepatomegaly or right upper quadrant pain, and (3) sudden weight gain.[179] To make a clinical diagnosis of VOD, the features listed previously must occur without other causes of post-transplantation liver failure, including GVHD, viral hepatitis, fungal abscesses, and drug reactions. A clinical diagnosis can be confirmed histologically via liver biopsy.

In summary, the signs and symptoms consistent with VOD in K.M. include insidious weight gain, hyperbilirubinemia, and right upper quadrant pain. The onset and timing of these signs and symptoms are consistent with VOD and occurred without other causes of hepatic toxicity.

PREVENTION AND TREATMENT

26. **What is the likelihood that K.M. will recover from her VOD? How should she be treated?**

The overall mortality for patients who develop VOD is approximately 50% and is correlated with the onset and severity of disease.[179,182] For example, patients with early weight gain, severely elevated bilirubin and/or AST, or encephalopathy are more likely to die of VOD when compared with patients with mild elevations of liver function tests and no encephalopathy.[182] Mortality for patients with severe VOD exceeds 90% and usually is accompanied by multiorgan system failure.[179]

Several case series have focused on identifying risk factors and algorithms predicting VOD risk in hopes of preventing this condition or its progression through early treatment.[183] Although various risk factors have been identified, their association is variable and conflicting reports of their association can be found. Risk factors identified before administration of the preparative regimen include a mismatched or unrelated graft, cyclophosphamide administration, increased transaminases before HCT, and a history of hepatitis.[180] The administration of intravenous immunoglobulin (IVIG) does not appear to be associated with VOD after BMT.[184] Interpatient variability in the metabolism and clearance of the chemotherapy used within the preparative regimen may also be associated with a poor outcome, although the relationships vary within the various preparative regimens.[148,185] The association of VOD with busulfan concentrations is discussed in Adaptive Dosing of Busulfan in this chapter. Preliminary data suggest that IV busulfan may be associated with a lower risk of VOD, although more data are needed.[186] More recently, VOD risk has been associated with elevated concentrations of a metabolite of cyclophosphamide, carboxyethylphosphoramide mustard (CEPM), in patients receiving the CY/TBI preparative regimen.[166] Elevations in plasminogen activator inhibitor-1 antigen have been associated with the occurrence and severity of VOD and may also be used as a diagnostic marker for VOD.[187]

In addition, pharmacologic methods to prevent VOD have been evaluated. Although initial data were positive, VOD is not prevented by pentoxifylline, which is thought to inhibit production of TNF-α from monocyte-macrophages.[188,189] Prostaglandin E_1 (PGE$_1$) appeared promising initially but further data demonstrated considerable toxicity.[190] Results of clinical trials evaluating low-dose unfractionated heparin or low-molecular-weight heparin as VOD prophylaxis have not been consistent. The efficacy of ursodiol combined with unfractionated heparin is equivalent to heparin alone; thus, the use of this combination is not recommended as prophylaxis for VOD.[191,192] Single-agent ursodiol (600 mg/day PO) has been associated with a lower incidence of VOD,[193,194] or with a lower frequency of total serum bilirubin > 3 mg/dL.[195] Ursodiol, which is a bile acid, has also been associated with a decreased incidence of severe acute GVHD and a greater 1-year survival relative to placebo.[195] However, more evidence is needed because this finding has not been consistent.[194] Based on these data, the use of single-agent ursodiol, at a dose of 600 mg PO daily, is recommended for VOD prophylaxis.

The mainstay of treatment for established VOD is supportive care aimed at sodium restriction, increasing intravascular volume, decreasing extracellular fluid accumulation, and minimizing factors that contribute to or exacerbate hepatotoxicity and encephalopathy. Thus, volume expanders such as albumin and colloids may be used to maintain intravascular volume; spironolactone may be used to minimize extravascular fluid accumulation; and protein restriction and lactulose may be used if encephalopathy develops. Unfortunately, improved outcomes with these measures have not been confirmed. In addition, avoidance of central nervous system–active drugs, if possible, helps provide an accurate assessment and interpretation of the patient's mental status.

Because mortality after development of severe VOD exceeds 90%[179] and available treatment options are limited, investigational alternatives are being sought. Although positive data emerged from a pilot study, recombinant human tissue plasminogen activator (rh-TPA) with heparin has not proved beneficial for the treatment of established severe VOD.[196] Defibrotide, an investigational new drug, has shown promising results in the treatment of VOD.[197–199] Defibrotide, a ribonucleotide, has antithrombotic, anti-ischemic, and thrombolytic activity without producing significant systemic anticoagulation. In a compassionate-use trial of 88 patients with severe VOD and associated organ dysfunction, 36% of patients had complete resolution of VOD and 35% survived past day 100 after HCT.[199] Numerous predictors of survival were observed. Younger patients and those who received an autologous graft were more likely to have better outcomes, whereas those who received a busulfan-based preparative regimen had worse outcomes. A decrease in plasminogen activator inhibitor-1 concentrations and serum creatinine during defibrotide treatment predicted better survival as well. A prospective phase II study of defibrotide (25 versus 40 mg/kg/day) is ongoing.

Since K.M. does not meet the criteria for severe VOD, she should be managed conservatively with fluid restriction and spironolactone. Her signs and symptoms should resolve over the next 2 weeks. Because she has mild VOD, she has a 50% chance of recovering completely without sequelae.

Graft Failure

27. E.R. is a 65-year-old woman diagnosed with AML in first remission. After her initial diagnosis, a successful search for a completely HLA matched unrelated donor was conducted. E.R. will receive a nonmyeloablative allogeneic HCT using PBPC. E.R.'s preparative regimen orders are written as follows: fludarabine 30 mg/m² per day on days −4, −3 and −2 and 2 Gy total body irradiation on the day of PBPC infusion with postgrafting cyclosporine and mycophenolate mofetil.

It now is day +40, and E.R.'s CBC reveals the following: WBC count, <0.1 cells/mm³ (normal, 3,200 to 9,800); no granulocytes or monocytes detected on differential; platelets 18,000/mm³ (normal, 130,000 to 400,000), and Hct, 22% (normal, 33% to 43%). A bone marrow biopsy reveals a hypocellular bone marrow with no evidence of leukemic infiltrates. What is E.R. experiencing and how should she be treated?

[SI units: WBC, <0.1 cells/L platelets, 18 × 10⁹ cells/L Hct, 0.22]

Engraftment usually is evident within the first 30 days in patients undergoing a NMT with this preparative regimen; however, rejection can occur after initial engraftment.[6] Because E.R. has no evidence of engraftment by day +40, she most likely is experiencing primary graft failure.

Graft rejection is defined as the lack of functional hematopoiesis after HCT[1,2] and is classified as primary graft failure (failure to engraft) or graft failure. With a myeloablative preparative regimen, primary graft failure is more likely to occur after autologous HCT. In these patients, the likelihood of graft failure is increased with intense prior chemotherapy, residual malignancy in grafts from patients with leukemias or lymphomas, or use of ex vivo purging methods. In myeloablative allogeneic HCT, graft rejection is less common because the donor PBPC or marrow is unmanipulated and free from the toxic effects of prior chemotherapy.[1,2] However, a delicate balance between host and donor effector cells is necessary, and residual host-versus-graft effects may lead to graft rejection. The incidence of graft rejection is higher in patients with aplastic anemia and in patients undergoing HCT with histoincompatible marrow or T cell–depleted marrow.[1,2] Graft rejection is uncommon in leukemia patients receiving myeloablative preparative regimen with a histocompatible allogeneic donor.

Therapeutic options for the treatment of graft rejection or graft failure are limited. A second HCT is the most definitive therapy, although the toxicities are formidable.[200] Graft rejection is best managed with immunosuppressants such as antithymocyte globulin. Primary graft failure occasionally can be treated successfully using hematopoietic growth factors, although patients who received purged autografts are less likely to respond.[201,202]

E.R. has primary graft failure. Although she has no evidence of residual leukemia, she has a history of extensive prior chemotherapy and has received an allogeneic NMT. The role of a second NMT is not well studied, and E.R. is not a candidate for a myeloablative preparative regimen followed by an allogeneic graft. Thus, a trial of filgrastim 5 µg/kg per day is an option. E.R.'s hematopoietic function should be monitored with daily CBCs and a bone marrow biopsy every 2 weeks. Two to three weeks of therapy often is necessary before engraftment is noted.

Graft-versus-Host Disease

GVHD is divided into two forms (i.e., acute or chronic) based on clinical manifestations and an arbitrarily designated time relative to day 0 of HCT. GVHD can occur after allogeneic HCT regardless of the preparative regimen used. The vast majority of the data regarding the prevention and treatment of GVHD have been obtained after myeloablative preparative regimens. Therefore, this section refers only to trials conducted in recipients of a myeloablative allogeneic HCT.

Acute GVHD is a clinical syndrome affecting primarily the skin, liver, and gastrointestinal (GI) tract and usually occurs in the first 100 days after allogeneic HCT. In contrast, chronic GVHD can affect almost any organ system, closely resembles several autoimmune diseases, and usually occurs after day 100.

Immune-mediated destruction of tissues, a hallmark of GVHD, disrupts the integrity of protective mucosal barriers and thus provides an environment that favors the establishment of opportunistic infections. The combination of GVHD and infectious complications are leading causes of mortality for allogeneic HCT patients.

Acute Graft-versus-Host Disease
RISK FACTORS

28. M.P., a 22-year-old, 70-kg man, undergoes a one-antigen mismatched allogeneic HCT from his sister for the diagnosis of CML in chronic phase. After a preparative regimen of cyclophosphamide and TBI, the following immunosuppressive regimen is ordered: cyclosporine 1.5 mg/kg IV Q 12 hr from days –1 until tolerating oral medications, then switch to cyclosporine (Neoral) 4 mg/kg PO Q 12 hr until day +50. Methotrexate 15 mg/m² IV on day +1, then 10 mg/m² day +3, +6, and +11. What factors are associated with an increased risk of acute GVHD?

The single most important factor associated with the development of GVHD is the degree of histocompatibility between donor and recipient. Clinically relevant grade II–IV acute GVHD occurs in 20% to 50% of HLA-matched sibling grafts and 50% to 80% of HLA-mismatched sibling or HLA-identical unrelated donors.[203] The pathophysiology for acute GVHD in the setting of well-matched grafts is unclear.[204] In addition, the onset of acute GVHD is earlier and severity is increased in mismatched grafts relative to matched grafts and also in matched unrelated donors relative to matched sibling donors.[79,205] Other factors that consistently increase the risk of developing acute GVHD include increasing recipient or donor age (older than 20 years), female donor to a male recipient, and previous recipient infections with herpes virus.[79,203] T-cell depletion and receipt of an umbilical cord blood graft lower the risk of acute GVHD.[101–104,133]

M.P. is receiving allogeneic bone marrow from a female sibling donor that is mismatched at one HLA antigen. These two factors increase his risk of developing acute GVHD.

CLINICAL PRESENTATION

29. On day +14, the time at which engraftment occurred, M.P. is noted to have a diffuse macular papular rash on his arms, hands, and front trunk. He does not have diarrhea, and his liver function tests are within normal limits. At the onset of his rash, M.P.'s empiric antibiotics are changed from cefepime to imipenem. Despite the change in antibiotics, M.P.'s rash persists. How is M.P.'s presentation consistent with acute GVHD?

The primary targets of immune-mediated destruction of host tissue by donor lymphocytes in acute GVHD are the skin, liver, and GI tract.[203] Acute GVHD of the skin usually manifests as a diffuse maculopapular rash that starts on the palms of the hands or soles of the feet or behind the ears. In more severe cases, skin GVHD can progress to a generalized total body erythroderma, bullous formation, and skin desquamation.[1,2] In patients with acute GVHD of the GI tract, persistent nausea and anorexia may be early signs.[206] Watery or bloody diarrhea also occurs, which can result in electrolyte abnormalities, dehydration, or ileus in severe cases. Clinical manifestations of liver GVHD include, primarily, elevated bilirubin but may also include increased alkaline phosphatase and hepatic transaminases, which can progress to fulminant hepatic failure. Acute GVHD usually is not evident until the time of engraftment, when donor lymphoid elements begin to proliferate. The skin usually is the first organ to be involved. The onset of liver or GI GVHD usually lags behind the onset of skin GVHD by approximately 1 week and infrequently occurs without skin GVHD.[1,2]

Acute GVHD must be distinguished accurately from other causes of skin, liver, or GI toxicity in the HCT patient. For example, a maculopapular rash, which may occur as a manifestation of an allergic reaction to antibiotics, usually begins on the trunk or upper extremities and rarely presents on the palms of the hands or soles of the feet. Diarrhea can be caused by chemotherapy, radiation, infection, or antibiotic therapy. However, diarrhea caused by the preparative regimen is rarely bloody and usually resolves within 3 to 7 days after discontinuation of drugs and radiation. Diarrhea caused by infectious agents such as *Clostridium difficile* or CMV should be distinguished from GVHD. Liver GVHD must be distinguished primarily from VOD and, to a lesser extent, hepatitis induced by drugs, blood products, or parenteral nutrition. Although liver function test abnormalities between these syndromes are similar, liver GVHD rarely is associated with insidious weight gain or right upper quadrant pain. A tissue biopsy of the affected organ in conjunction with clinical evidence is the only way to definitively diagnose acute GVHD. Acute GVHD is associated with characteristic histologic changes to affected organs.[1,2] A staging system based on clinical criteria is used to grade acute GVHD. The severity of organ involvement is determined first (Table 92-7), and then an overall grade is established based on number and extent of involved organs (Table 92-8).[1,2]

M.P. developed a rash at the time of engraftment that could have been consistent with either an antibiotic-induced rash or acute GVHD. Although it was appropriate to change antibiotics, the fact that M.P.'s rash did not improve is suggestive of acute GVHD. M.P.'s rash is present on 36% of his body, but because there are no signs of GI or liver involvement at this time, M.P. is likely to have grade I GVHD (see Tables 92-7 and 92-8).

Table 92-7   Proposed Clinical Staging of Graft-versus-Host Disease According to Organ System

Stage	Skin	Liver	Intestinal Tract
+	Maculopapular rash <25% of body surface	Bilirubin 2–3 mg/dL	>500 mL/day diarrhea
+ +	Maculopapular rash 25–50% body surface	Bilirubin 3.1–6 mg/dL	>1,000 mL/day diarrhea
+ + +	Generalized erythroderma	Bilirubin 6.1–15 mg/dL	>1,500 mL/day diarrhea
+ + + +	Generalized erythroderma with bullous formation and desquamation	Bilirubin >15 mg/dL	>2,000 mL/day diarrhea or severe abdominal pain with or without ileus

Reprinted with permission from Thomas ED et al. Bone-marrow transplantation. N Engl J Med 1975;292:895. Copyright © 2003 Massachusetts Medical Society. All rights reserved.

Table 92-8   Overall Clinical Grading of Severity of Graft-versus-Host Disease

Grade	Degree of Organ Involvement
I	+ to + + skin rash; no gut involvement; no liver involvement; no decrease in clinical performance
II	+ to + + + skin rash; + gut involvement or + liver involvement (or both); mild decrease in clinical performance
III	+ + to + + + skin rash; + + to + + + gut involvement or + + to + + + + liver involvement (or both); marked decrease in clinical performance
IV	Similar to grade III with + + to + + + + organ involvement and extreme decrease in performance status

Reprinted with permission from Thomas ED et al. Bone-marrow transplantation. N Engl J Med 1975;292:895. Copyright 2003 Massachusetts Medical Society. All rights reserved.

IMMUNOSUPPRESSIVE PROPHYLAXIS

30. Why did M.P. receive prophylactic immunosuppressive therapy with cyclosporine and methotrexate?

GVHD is a leading cause of morbidity and mortality after allogeneic HCT. Thus, efforts have focused on identifying prophylactic measures for GVHD, with two approaches having been taken. The first and most common method is to administer post-transplantation immunosuppressive therapy that successfully minimizes GVHD risk but is also associated with toxicity. The second approach involves T-cell depletion, which was more fully discussed in the "T-Cell Depletion" section above.

Initially, acute GVHD was prevented with single-drug therapy using antithymocyte globulin (ATG), cyclophosphamide, methotrexate, or cyclosporine.[207–209] ATG binds nonspecifically to mononuclear cells and depletes hematopoietic progenitor cells in addition to lymphocytes; consequently, ATG is rarely used for fear of a high incidence of graft failure.[207] In most patient populations, randomized comparative trials have documented the superiority of combination immunosuppressive therapy for cyclophosphamide, methotrexate, or cyclosporine.[210,211] However, in patients with acute leukemia who are at high risk of relapse, combination immunosuppression was associated with an early decrease in mortality from acute GVHD but an increase in late mortality due to an increased incidence of leukemic relapse.[211] This is most likely due to the GVT effect mediated in conjunction with acute GVHD, since an inverse relationship between

Table 92-9   Regimens of Prophylaxis of Acute GVHD

Drug	Dosing Examples
Single Agent	
Methotrexate[1,2]	15 mg/m² IV, day +1 10 mg/m² IV, days +3, +6, +11
ATG[207]	15 mg/kg every other day for 6 doses
Cyclosporine[208]	1.5 mg/kg IV or 6.25 mg/kg (Sandimmune) PO Q 12 hr, days –1 to +50, then taper 5% per week and discontinue by day +180
Combination Therapy	
Cyclosporine/ short-term methotrexate[209]	Same doses as listed for single agents
Tacrolimus/ short-term methotrexate[134]	Tacrolimus 0.03 mg/kg/day continuous IV infusion or 0.12 mg/kg/day PO BID Methotrexate as above
Cyclosporine/ methotrexate/ prednisone[215]	Cyclosporine 5 mg/kg/day IV continuous infusion, day –2 to +3, then 3–3.75 mg/kg IV until day +35; then 10 mg/kg/day (Sandimmune) PO, dose adjusted to cyclosporine concentrations (via RIA) of 200–600 ng/mL. Taper by 20% Q 2 wk; then discontinue by day +180 Methotrexate 15 mg/m² IV day +1, 10 mg/m² IV day +3, +6 Methylprednisolone 0.5 mg/kg/day IV, day +7 until day +14, then 1 mg/kg/day IV until day +28, then prednisone 0.8 mg/kg/day PO until day +42, then taper slowly and discontinue by day +180

ATG, antithymocyte globulin; GVHD, graft-versus-host disease.

acute GVHD and leukemic relapse has been observed.[5] Patients with acute leukemias at high risk for relapse may receive single-agent prophylaxis for acute GVHD because the development of some acute GVHD may facilitate a GVT effect.

A variety of two- and three-drug combination immunosuppressive regimens have been used for prophylaxis against GVHD (Table 92-9). Methotrexate, cyclosporine or tacrolimus, and corticosteroids are the agents most commonly incorporated into combination immunosuppressive regimens. Although the most widely published regimen is short-course methotrexate plus cyclosporine (Seattle regimen),[209] there is no national consensus with regard to the most effective regimen. Methotrexate is administered up to day +11, although the incidence of acute GVHD is reduced when the duration of therapy is increased (59% compared with 25% incidence with methotrexate administered to day +102).[212] The combination of tacrolimus and short-course methotrexate has been compared with cyclosporine plus short-course methotrexate in patients undergoing allogeneic HCT using HLA-matched siblings[213,214] and unrelated donors.[134] Recipients of matched-sibling grafts treated with tacrolimus had a lower incidence of grade II to IV acute GVHD but a similar incidence of chronic GVHD.[213] Overall survival was lower in the tacrolimus group as a result of more toxic deaths in patients with advanced-stage disease; however, a higher number of advanced stage disease patients in the tacrolimus/methotrexate group make the results of this trial somewhat difficult to determine.[213]

Subsequently, the IBMTR conducted a matched control study that suggested that the survival difference between the two arms was in fact due to the imbalance in the underlying risk factors.[214] In patients receiving HLA-matched or slightly mismatched unrelated grafts, those given tacrolimus had a lower incidence of grade II to IV acute GVHD, a similar incidence of chronic GVHD and similar disease-free and overall survival rates.[134] Patients with advanced hematologic malignancies were excluded from this study. Both regimens are currently used in allogeneic HCT after myeloablative preparative regimens. Several studies have compared triple-drug with two-drug immunosuppression. The incidence of acute GVHD has been similar or lower with triple-drug regimens, but infectious complications are higher and overall survival is similar to two-drug regimens.[215,216] Three-drug immunosuppression regimens are still being evaluated and are used mainly in mismatched or unrelated allogeneic HCT, where the risk of acute GVHD is increased.

M.P. received acute GVHD prophylaxis with a two-drug regimen of short-course methotrexate and cyclosporine. This regimen is effective for the prophylaxis of acute GVHD in CML patients undergoing allogeneic HCT.[217]

31. **What principles are used in dosing medications used for acute GVHD prophylaxis?**

Although the various combination immunosuppressive regimens vary slightly by drug, dose, and combination, several guidelines are consistent throughout all the regimens. First, cytotoxic agents used in combination for prophylaxis of acute GVHD (e.g., methotrexate, cyclophosphamide) are withheld or given in reduced doses if mucositis or myelosuppression is severe.[209,215] Methotrexate for GVHD prophylaxis can delay engraftment, increase the incidence and severity of mucositis and cause liver function test elevations. The methotrexate dose is reduced in the setting of renal or liver impairment.[204]

The calcineurin inhibitors (i.e., cyclosporine, tacrolimus) should be initiated before or immediately after donor cell infusion (day −1 or 0) when used for GVHD prophylaxis. This schedule is recommended because of the known mechanism of action of cyclosporine (see Chapter 35, Solid Organ Transplantation), which entails blocking the proliferation of cytotoxic T cells by inhibiting production of helper T-cell–derived IL-2. Administering cyclosporine before the donor cell infusion allows inhibition of IL-2 secretion to occur before a rejection response has been initiated.

Cyclosporine usually is administered intravenously until the GI toxicity from a myeloablative preparative regimen has resolved (e.g., for 7 to 21 days).[209] This is because GI effects of the preparative regimen (e.g., CINV, diarrhea) and GVHD affect the oral absorption of microemulsion cyclosporine and may result in inconsistent blood concentrations.[218] Most centers have switched the standard oral formulation of cyclosporine to the new microemulsion formulation, Neoral, or to other new generic microemulsion formulations that have improved bioavailability. When the old formulation is used (i.e., Sandimmune) a ratio of 1:4 is commonly used when converting IV therapy to oral. With the Neoral formulation, a ratio of 1:2 or 1:3 is used. The most common ratio used when converting tacrolimus from IV to oral is 1:4. Different conversion ratios for IV to oral regimens may be used when patients are receiving concomitant medications that affect cytochrome P450 3A or P-glycoprotein, which are involved in the metabolism and transport of the calcineurin inhibitors (e.g., itraconazole). Thus, careful monitoring for drug interactions with the calcineurin inhibitors is warranted.[219]

The dose of cyclosporine or tacrolimus is adjusted based on serum drug levels and the serum creatinine (SrCr) concentration. Doses usually are reduced by 50% if the SrCr concentration doubles above baseline and are withheld for SrCr concentrations >2 mg/ dL.[209,217] Although the calcineurin inhibitors do not contribute to myelosuppression, common adverse effects to these agents include neurotoxicity, hypertension, and/or nephrotoxicity (which may lead to an impaired clearance of methotrexate).

When corticosteroids are added to combination immunosuppressive regimens, they usually are withheld until engraftment is expected (7 to 14 days after marrow infusion). Administering corticosteroids earlier in the post-transplantation period (e.g., day 0) paradoxically increases the incidence of GVHD when used in combination with methotrexate and cyclosporine.[220] Corticosteroids are associated with several adverse effects, including infectious complications, hyperglycemia and an increased incidence of hypertension when used in combination with a calcineurin inhibitor.

Tapering schedules for cyclosporine or tacrolimus and corticosteroids vary widely between institutions. The general goal is to keep calcineurin inhibitor doses stable to day +50, and then slowly taper with the intent of discontinuing all immunosuppressive agents by 6 months after HCT. By this time, immunologic tolerance has developed, and patients no longer require immunosuppressive therapy.

ADAPTIVE DOSING OF CALCINEURIN INHIBITORS

32. **On day +18, a cyclosporine level is drawn right before the morning dose and is reported to be 150 ng/mL (by radioimmunoassay [RIA]). Why are cyclosporine levels being obtained for M.P.?**

The role of pharmacokinetic monitoring of cyclosporine in HCT patients is not well defined. An association between cyclosporine concentrations and acute GVHD was not found in early studies; however, other studies have suggested that cyclosporine trough concentrations less than 200 ng/mL are associated with an increased risk of acute GVHD.[221,222] Pharmacokinetic monitoring may play a more important role in minimizing the risk of cyclosporine-induced nephrotoxicity. Cyclosporine trough concentrations >400 ng/mL (via RIA and high-pressure liquid chromatography assay) are associated with a higher incidence of nephrotoxicity in some series.[223] However, it is important to note that cyclosporine-induced nephrotoxicity can occur despite low or normal concentrations of cyclosporine and may be a consequence of other drug- or disease-related factors known to influence the development of nephrotoxicity (e.g., genetic risk factors, concurrent use of other nephrotoxic agents, sepsis).

Thus, it is reasonable to adjust doses to maintain cyclosporine trough concentrations between 200 to 400 ng/mL in patients undergoing allogeneic HCT with a myeloablative preparative regimen. Recommendations for dose adjustments should be based on cyclosporine concentrations and SrCr concentration. Dosage adjustments should be made for SrCr, regardless of cyclosporine concentration, as recommended previously. No standard dosage adjustment schedule exists, but most centers adopt their own standardized approach. M.P. has a normal SrCr, and his cyclosporine level is <200 ng/mL. Therefore, his cyclosporine dosage should be increased.

Pharmacokinetic monitoring of tacrolimus is more defined in terms of target concentrations. In general, desired trough concentrations are in the range of 5 to 15 ng/mL. Tacrolimus concentrations >20 ng/mL have been associated with increased risk of toxicity, primarily nephrotoxicity.[224,225] Adjustments in tacrolimus dosing for increased SrCr should be made in a manner similar to that described for cyclosporine.

INVESTIGATIONAL THERAPIES FOR PROPHYLAXIS

33. **What other therapies have been proposed for the prophylaxis of acute GVHD?**

The role of intravenous immunoglobulin (IVIG) in the prevention of GVHD is controversial. Two large studies noted a relationship between administration of immunoglobulins and a decreased prevalence of acute GVHD, with the most benefit observed in patients younger than 20 years of age.[226,227] Administration of immunoglobulin throughout the first year after allogeneic HCT has not reduced post-transplantation complications or chronic GVHD and may actually impair humoral immunity.[228] Given the multitude of other factors that influence the development of acute GVHD, it is unlikely that minimal differences between products would result in major differences in the incidence of acute GVHD. Although patients with acute GVHD have been shown to have increased levels of circulating TNF-α, two clinical trials evaluating pentoxifylline as a means of decreasing circulating TNF-α levels and thereby preventing GVHD have not shown beneficial effects.[188,229] Investigational agents being considered for prophylaxis of acute GVHD include high-affinity IL-2 receptor antibodies (i.e., daclizumab, basiliximab), mycophenolate mofetil (MMF), sirolimus, CTLA4Ig and monoclonal antibodies against CD40 ligand, and GLAT.[204,230,231] The role of these agents is yet to be defined.

TREATMENT OF ESTABLISHED ACUTE GRAFT-VERSUS-HOST DISEASE

34. **On day +19, the suspicion of acute skin GVHD is confirmed by biopsy. On the same day, M.P. experiences 1,000 mL of diarrhea over the next 24 hours and is noted to have a biliru-** bin of 2.8 mg/dL. He is started on methylprednisolone 35 mg IV Q 6 hr. What is the rationale for methylprednisolone therapy in M.P.?

[SI units: total bilirubin = 48 μmol/L]

The most effective way to treat GVHD is to prevent its development. Once GVHD has presented, only 40% of patients respond to corticosteroids, which are the first-line therapy for treatment of established disease.[232] In addition, patients with mild to moderate (grades I to III) acute GVHD who respond to initial therapy have a significantly better survival advantage when compared to patients with severe acute GVHD disease that does not respond to initial therapy. Patients who do not respond to therapy or have ongoing severe GVHD usually die from a combination of GVHD and infectious complications.[233]

When treating acute GVHD, corticosteroids are generally tapered based on response. The rate at which tapering occurs depends on the patient. Patients who develop acute GVHD or who experience flares of existing GVHD during a tapering trial will have to have their dosages increased or tapered more slowly as tolerated.

Because M.P. has objective evidence of established acute GVHD, he was given systemic corticosteroids at the first sign of progressive disease. This was appropriate because single-agent corticosteroids are considered the therapy of choice for established acute GVHD.[232] Corticosteroids indirectly halt the progression of immune-mediated destruction of host tissues by blocking macrophage-derived IL-1 secretion. IL-1 is a primary stimulus for helper T-cell–induced secretion of IL-2, which in turn is responsible for stimulating proliferation of cytotoxic T lymphocytes (see Chapter 35). The recommended dosage of methylprednisolone for the treatment of established acute GVHD is 2 mg/kg per day, given intravenously or orally in four divided doses for a minimum of 14 days, followed by a tapering schedule that is determined by response.[233] The dosage of methylprednisolone in M.P. (35 mg intravenously every 6 hours) is approximately 2 mg/kg/day and thus is consistent with these recommendations. Comparative trials suggest no advantage to higher dosage of corticosteroids (i.e., 10 mg/kg per day) compared with 2 mg/kg per day as initial treatment of acute GVHD.[234] Nonetheless, high-dose pulse therapy with IV methylprednisolone 20 to 60 mg/kg per day or 500 mg/m^2 every 6 hours followed by a rapid taper has been advocated.[235]

Other therapies that have been used to treat established acute GVHD include ATG 15 to 30 mg/kg per day intravenously daily or every other day for 3 to 10 doses,[233] cyclosporine 3 mg/kg per day intravenously or 12.5 mg/kg per day orally (Sandimmune),[233] and murine monoclonal antibody (OKT$_3$) 5 mg/day intravenously for 14 days.[236] Single-agent therapy and combination therapy also have been used, although a high incidence of death resulting from infection is seen when more than two agents are used, most likely because of enhanced immunosuppression.[235] Cyclosporine is used to treat established GVHD only in patients who did not receive cyclosporine as part of their prophylactic regimen. In addition, cyclosporine levels do not correlate with response in the setting of acute GVHD.[235] If a patient fails to respond to one drug, switching to another agent for rescue therapy occasionally is successful. However, response rates to salvage therapy for acute GVHD are low.[237]

New agents directed against blocking the accelerated cytokine cascade are under investigation for the treatment of established acute GVHD. These include anti–IL-2 receptor monoclonal antibody, monoclonal anti–TNF-α antibody, and soluble TNF receptor and humanized anti–CD3 monoclonal antibody.[238–240] The most effective dose, timing, or combination of these new therapies still is unknown.

M.P. should be evaluated for response to methylprednisolone after 4 to 7 days. If his acute GVHD has improved or stabilized, he should be continued on therapy at this dose for a total of 14 days. If M.P. responds to therapy, his steroid dose should be tapered slowly over a minimum of 1 month, and he should be monitored for any evidence of recurrent GVHD. If GVHD flares during his steroid taper (as evidenced by worsening skin reactions, increased bilirubin, or increased diarrhea volume), the dose should be increased again until his disease is stable, with the subsequent taper initiated at a slower rate. If M.P. fails to respond to first-line therapy with methylprednisolone, he should receive salvage therapy with ATG, OKT$_3$, or an investigational drug on protocol. Extracorporeal photochemotherapy with ultraviolet A radiation and a photosensitizing agent (e.g., psoralen) have shown benefit in treating cutaneous GVHD.[241]

Chronic Graft-versus-Host Disease
CLINICAL PRESENTATION

35. **M.P. was successfully treated for his acute GVHD, is no longer taking corticosteroids, and currently is tapering his cyclosporine. On day +200, M.P. comes to clinic for follow-up after a 2-week vacation in Florida. On examination, M.P. is found to have a mild skin rash on his arms and legs, hyperpigmentation of the tissue surrounding the eyes, and white plaque-like lesions in his mouth. He also is complaining of dry eyes. Laboratory tests reveal an increased alkaline phosphatase and total bilirubin concentration. What is the most likely cause of M.P.'s findings?**

Chronic GVHD is the most common late complication of allogeneic HCT, which occurs in 30% to 70% of long-term survivors of myeloablative allogeneic HCT.[242,243] In addition, chronic GVHD is the major cause of nonrelapse mortality and morbidity.[76,244,245] Chronic GVHD occurs in approximately 45% of patients undergoing allogeneic HCT and is unrelated to the regimen used for prophylaxis of acute GVHD.[207–210,215]

In recipients of HLA-identical grafts, an increased incidence of chronic GVHD is associated with grades II to IV acute GVHD, female donor to a male recipient, increasing donor or recipient age, transfusion of donor buffy coat and the use of PBPC (see previous section on Peripheral Blood Progenitor Cells for discussion of allogeneic PBPC and GVHD risk). Recipients of a graft from an unrelated donor have a higher incidence of chronic GVHD.[242,244] The most important risk factors for developing extensive chronic GVHD are a prior diagnosis of acute GVHD and the use of corticosteroids at day 100.[246]

The time course for the onset of chronic GVHD follows three typical patterns: progressive, quiescent, or de novo.[247,248] Progressive chronic GVHD evolves directly from acute GVHD, with no resolution of acute disease in between. This form of chronic GVHD carries the worst prognosis.[249] Quiescent chronic GVHD appears slowly after a period of complete resolution of acute GVHD, and de novo late-onset chronic GVHD occurs spontaneously with no history of acute GVHD. Chronic GVHD tends to occur during or shortly after tapering of the 6-month duration cyclosporine used for preventing acute GVHD.[250] Therefore, the efficacy of extending the duration of cyclosporine from 6 months to 24 months has been studied in patients who experienced acute GVHD or had chronic GVHD of the skin at day 80, when the cyclosporine taper usually is ongoing.[251] Unfortunately, there were no significant differences in the rate of developing chronic GVHD, transplant-related mortality, or overall survival.[251]

The clinical course of chronic GVHD is multifaceted, involving almost any organ in the body. Because of its diffuse nature, chronic GVHD is not graded by organ system and instead is described as limited or extensive, based on the extent of involvement. Limited chronic GVHD is characterized by localized skin or liver involvement. Extensive chronic GVHD is characterized by extensive skin or hepatic involvement, mucosal changes, and/or involvement of any other organ system. Signs and symptoms of chronic GVHD in various organ systems are listed in Table 92-10.

The signs and symptoms of chronic GVHD in M.P. include a rash in sun-exposed areas of the skin, hyperpigmentation of tissues surrounding his eyes, white plaquelike lesions in the mouth, dry mucous membranes, and increased alkaline phosphatase and total bilirubin levels. These symptoms appeared after a period of complete resolution of acute GVHD. Thus, M.P. has limited-involvement, quiescent chronic GVHD.

Table 92-10	**Signs and Symptoms of Chronic GVHD[329]**
Affected Organ	**Clinical Manifestations**
Skin	Rash, hypopigmentation or hyperpigmentation, erythema, alopecia, sclerosis, or scleroderma with joint contractures if severe, lichen planus lesions
Eyes	↓ tear formation, dry eyes, burning, photophobia
GI Tract	↓ saliva production, dry mouth leading to cracking or fissure formation, change in taste sensation, diarrhea and abdominal pain, fat malabsorption, chronic malnutrition, web formation
Liver	Increased LFTs, histologic changes consistent with combined hepatocellular injury and cholestasis
Lungs	Nonproductive cough, wheezing, bronchospasm, diffuse interstitial pneumonitis, restrictive or obstructive abnormalities on PFTs
Bone Marrow	Eosinophilia, thrombocytopenia, antibody formation and subclass distribution
Musculoskeletal	Myalgias, arthralgias, clinical picture resembling systemic lupus erythematosus or rheumatoid arthritis
Miscellaneous	Circulating autoantibodies (antinuclear antibody, rheumatoid factor, positive direct Coombs' test)

GI, gastrointestinal; GVHD, graft-versus-host disease; LFTs, liver function tests; PFTs, pulmonary function tests.

PHARMACOLOGIC MANAGEMENT

36. M.P. is started on prednisone 1 mg/kg PO QD for the treatment of his chronic GVHD. His cyclosporine taper is stopped, and the dosage is raised to therapeutic concentrations. Is this therapy rational? What other agents are available to treat chronic GVHD?

There is no specific prophylactic therapy for chronic GVHD.[244] The mainstay of therapy for chronic GVHD is long-term immunosuppressive therapy. Although oral prednisone, azathioprine, procarbazine, and cyclophosphamide all have been used, prednisone, azathioprine, and cyclosporine have emerged as the most commonly used agents with the best efficacy and toxicity profiles. M.P. was started on single-agent prednisone for chronic GVHD. This is a reasonable decision because single-agent immunosuppressive therapy is the treatment of choice for standard-risk (i.e., limited involvement quiescent or de novo chronic GVHD) patients. The use of combination immunosuppressive therapy in this setting with prednisone and azathioprine resulted in a higher incidence of nonrelapse mortality and lower survival than with prednisone alone.[252] However, if M.P. fails to respond to prednisone alone or if he had presented initially with progressive or extensive chronic GVHD, combination therapy with prednisone and cyclosporine would be a reasonable alternative.[248] For high-risk patients, specifically those with thrombocytopenia associated with chronic GVHD, the combination of cyclosporine and prednisone has resulted in higher survival and lower nonrelapse mortality when compared with prednisone or cyclosporine alone.

When used alone or in combination, the dosage of prednisone for the treatment of chronic GVHD is 1 mg/kg per day, administered orally in divided doses for 30 days. After 30 days, the dosage is converted slowly to alternate-day therapy by increasing the "on-day" and decreasing the "off-day" dose until a total of 2 mg/kg per day on alternate days is administered.[248,252] Once the alternate-day conversion has occurred, the patient is tapered slowly to the final dosage of 1 mg/kg every other day. Alternate-day therapy is preferred to minimize adrenocortical suppression.[248,252] The dosage of azathioprine to treat chronic GVHD, alone or in combination, is 1.5 mg/kg per day.

Other therapies may be required for patients considered to be at high risk for developing chronic GVHD (defined as patients with GVHD that progresses from acute GVHD or the presence of thrombocytopenia). Cyclosporine in combination with prednisone in an alternating sequence has a similar incidence of transplant-related mortality and overall survival compared with prednisone alone.[253] However, the two-drug combination has a lower disease-free survival with a slight reduction in avascular necrosis (13% for two-drug combination versus 22% for prednisone alone, $P = .04$).[253] The dosage of cyclosporine (Sandimmune) is 6 mg/kg orally every 12 hours every other day, alternating with prednisone 1 mg/kg orally every other day.[253] When using the microemulsion formulations of cyclosporine (Neoral), lower doses may be used because of improved bioavailability.

Thalidomide, a sedative hypnotic with immunosuppressive properties, can be used as salvage therapy for chronic GVHD, although data supporting its clinical benefit are equivocal.[254]

In addition, the adverse effects of thalidomide complicate therapy (e.g., neurotoxicity, neutropenia, constipation).[255,256] Because of its adverse effects, escalation to the desired dose of 800 mg/day could not be achieved in most patients receiving thalidomide with cyclosporine and prednisone.[256] No clinical benefit, even if full doses of thalidomide could be attained, was apparent with the addition of thalidomide to a variety of immunosuppressants (i.e., cyclosporine and prednisone, corticosteroids, or calcineurin inhibitors).[255,256]

Once immunosuppressive therapy is initiated, 1 to 2 months may pass before an improvement in clinical symptoms is noted; therapy usually is continued for 9 to 12 months. If after this time there has been resolution of signs and symptoms of chronic GVHD, immunosuppressive therapy can be tapered slowly. If a flare-up of chronic GVHD occurs during the tapering schedule or after therapy is discontinued, immunosuppressive therapy is restarted. Other potential approaches for patients who are refractory to initial therapy include etanercept, infliximab, mycophenolate mofetil and tacrolimus, tacrolimus alone, extracorporeal photochemotherapy, acitretin, clofazimine, or hydroxychloroquine.[244,257]

When immunosuppressive therapy is administered for long periods, the patient must be monitored closely for chronic toxicity. Blood counts should be monitored routinely in patients on azathioprine because hematologic toxicity resulting in infection and bleeding may occur. Cushingoid effects, aseptic necrosis of the joints, and diabetes can develop with long-term corticosteroid use. Other severe complications include a high incidence of infection with encapsulated organisms and atypical pathogens such as *P. carinii* pneumonia, CMV, and herpes zoster. Cyclosporine therapy is associated with nephrotoxicity, neurotoxicity, and hypertension, although these effects are minimized with an alternate-day schedule.

ADJUVANT THERAPIES

37. Suggest some adjuvant therapies that should be instituted in a patient like M.P. with chronic GVHD.

Patients being treated for chronic GVHD should receive trimethoprim-sulfamethoxazole for prophylaxis of *P. carinii* and also encapsulated organisms, such as *Streptococcus pneumoniae* and *Haemophilus influenzae*. Ensuring optimal prophylactic antibiotics in chronic GVHD patients is critical since infection is primarily the cause of death during treatment.[257] In addition, the use of artificial tears and saliva may improve lubrication and decrease the occurrence of cracking and fissures in mucous membranes. If nutritional intake is poor, consultation with a clinical nutritionist and use of oral nutritional supplementation may be advisable. Also, patients should be instructed to apply sunscreens to exposed areas whenever prolonged sun exposure is anticipated. Liver function abnormalities have been improved by up to 30% with the use of ursodiol as bile acid displacement therapy.[193–195] Calcium supplements, estrogen replacement, or other antiosteoporosis agents should be considered in women or other patients at risk for fracture or bone loss while receiving prolonged regimens with immunosuppressant therapy.[258] Last, patient education regarding the delay in improvement of symptoms, anticipated duration of therapy, and importance of compliance with oral immunosuppressive therapy is essential.

Infectious Complications

Opportunistic infections are a major source of morbidity and mortality after myeloablative and nonmyeloablative HCT. Three major periods of infectious risks have been described (see Fig. 92-4). During the early period pre-engraftment, particularly for patients undergoing myeloablative HCT, the primary pathogens are aerobic bacteria and herpes simplex virus (HSV). Chemotherapy-induced mucosal damage serves as a portal of entry for many organisms into the bloodstream such as *Streptococcus viridans* and aerobic Gram-negative bacteria. *Staphylococcus* is also a predominant organism because all patients undergoing HCT have indwelling IV central catheters. HSV rarely occurs now with the routine use of antiviral prophylaxis. Systemic and oral candidiasis may occur during this period. Respiratory viruses such as respiratory syncytial virus, influenza, adenovirus, and parainfluenza are being increasingly recognized as pathogens causing pneumonia, particularly during community outbreaks of infection with these organisms.[259] To reduce potential exposure of HCT recipients to such respiratory viruses, visitors and staff members with respiratory signs and symptoms of a viral illness may not be allowed direct contact with patients.

A potential advantage of NMT (nonmyeloablative transplantation) is the relative nontoxicity associated with the preparative regimen compared with myeloablative HCT. Frequently, NMT regimens do not result in true neutropenia,[6] and the incidence of mucositis during the early period is reduced compared with myeloablative HCT.[127] In a matched controlled study designed to assess the incidence of bacterial and fungal infections after NMT compared with myeloablative HCT, investigators noted a significantly reduced incidence of bacteremia (9% versus 27%) during the first 30 days post-transplantation in the NMT group.[127] Moreover, episodes of infection attributable to mucositis in the first 30 days were significantly fewer (2% versus 14%) in the NMT group.

The second or middle period of infectious risk occurs after engraftment to post transplantation day +100. Although bacterial infections may still occur, pathogens such as CMV, adenovirus, and *Aspergillus* are common during this period. Interstitial pneumonitis is a common manifestation of infection and can be caused by several infectious agents, including CMV, adenovirus, *Aspergillus* and *P. carinii*. Immune suppression resulting from acute GVHD and corticosteroids may contribute to the risk of such infections during this period. Therefore, patients undergoing NMT who experience GVHD and are treated with corticosteroids can be expected to have a similar risk for infection as those undergoing myeloablative HCT during this time period.[127] Invasive fungal infections over the first year after HCT occur at a similar rate in patients with NMT when compared with historical controls receiving a myeloablative preparative regimen.[126]

During the late period (after day +100), the predominant organisms are the encapsulated bacteria (e.g., *S. pneumoniae, H. influenzae, Neisseria meningitidis*), fungi, and varicella-zoster virus (VZV). The encapsulated organisms commonly cause sinopulmonary infections. The risk of infection during this late period is increased in patients with chronic GVHD as a result of prolonged immunosuppression.

Because of the morbidity associated with these opportunistic infections in HCT recipients, optimal pharmacotherapy for preventing and treating infections in this patient population is critical. In 2000, the Centers for Disease Control and Prevention (CDC) published guidelines for preventing these infections among HCT recipients.[8] These guidelines were constructed from available data by an expert panel from the CDC, the Infectious Disease Society of America, and the American Society for Blood and Marrow Transplantation. The guidelines provide a comprehensive review of the data regarding prevention of opportunistic infections in HCT recipients. The review below incorporates information from the CDC guidelines and also provides an update on the pharmacotherapy of opportunistic infections for all types of HCT (i.e., myeloablative autologous, myeloablative allogeneic and nonmyeloablative allogeneic HCT recipients).

Prevention and Treatment of Bacterial and Fungal Infections

38. S.D. is a 26 year-old woman with Ph$^+$ acute lymphocytic leukemia (ALL) in her first complete remission who is admitted for allogeneic myeloablative HCT. The following orders are written: Admit to a room with a positive-pressure high-efficiency particulate air (HEPA) filter. Flush double-lumen Hickman catheter per protocol. Immunosuppressed patient diet as tolerated. Begin fluconazole 400 mg PO Q 24 hr, acyclovir 800 mg PO Q 12 hr on admission. Begin ceftazidime 2 g IV Q 8 hr with first fever when ANC <500/mm³. Transfuse 2 units of packed RBCs for hematocrit <25% and 1 unit of single-donor platelets when <20,000/mm³. What is the rationale for these supportive measures?

As a result of disease-related immunosuppression, intensive preparative regimens, and/or post-transplantation immunosuppressive therapy, patients undergoing allogeneic HCT require careful vigilance for regimen-related toxicities and intensive supportive care directed toward maintaining an adequate CBC, preventing or treating infection, and providing adequate nutrition.

Placement of a semipermanent double-lumen or triple-lumen central venous catheter (e.g., Hickman, Groshong, Broviac, Neostar) is mandatory in all patients. The need for prolonged administration of chemotherapy, blood products, antibiotics, parenteral nutrition, and adjunctive medications such as immunoglobulin therapies preclude the use of peripheral access sites that require frequent rotation. In addition, the use of central venous catheters allows delivery of maximum concentrations of all medications into an area of high blood flow, a measure that can reduce administration time and minimize daily fluid infusion.

After administration of the preparative regimen and preceding successful engraftment, allogeneic myeloablative HCT patients undergo a period of pancytopenia that can last from 2 to 6 weeks. During this time, patients may require multiple transfusions with RBCs and platelets. Packed RBCs and platelets usually are given for a hematocrit <25% and platelets <10,000 or 20,000/mm³, respectively.[1,2] Transfusions with multiple blood products put patients at risk for blood product–derived infection (e.g., CMV, hepatitis). In addition, sensitization to foreign leukocyte HLA antigens (i.e., alloimmunization) can cause immune-mediated thrombocytopenia. Thus, blood product support in the myeloablative allogeneic HCT patient must incorporate strategies that reduce the risk of viral infection and alloimmunization. Methods used include minimizing the number of pretransplant infusions, use of single-donor rather than pooled-donor blood products, irradiating blood products, or filtering blood products with leukocyte-reduction filters.

Given the reduced intensity of the preparative regimen, NMT patients may or may not experience neutropenia and generally have reduced requirements for blood products. In fact, many centers perform NMT in the outpatient setting and admit patients to the hospital only if they have complications requiring more intensive management.

Several measures are recommended to minimize the risk of infection in autologous and allogeneic myeloablative HCT patients. Private reverse isolation rooms equipped with positive-pressure HEPA filters and adherence to strict handwashing techniques reduce the incidence of bacterial and fungal infections.[8] To reduce exposure to exogenous sources of bacteria in immunosuppressed patients, low-microbial diets are instituted on hospital admission, and visitors are not allowed to bring plants or flowers into the patient's room. In addition, patients are encouraged to maintain good oral hygiene because the mouth can be a focus of bacterial and fungal infections. The mouth should be kept clean by using frequent (four to six times daily) mouth rinses with sterile water, normal saline, or sodium bicarbonate.[8] Brushing or flossing teeth is avoided during periods of thrombocytopenia and neutropenia. Other measures designed to reduce the risk of infection include aggressive use of antibacterial, antifungal, and antiviral therapy—both prophylactically and for treatment of documented infection.

Antibiotics with a broad Gram-negative spectrum may be instituted prophylactically once the patient becomes neutropenic, or empirically after the patient is neutropenic and experiences a first fever. S.D. will be receiving ceftazidime empirically when she becomes neutropenic and has her first fever. Alternatively, some HCT centers prescribe a prophylactic fluoroquinolone (e.g., ciprofloxacin) on admission for HCT and then switch to a broad-spectrum IV antibiotic such as ceftazidime when the patient is neutropenic and experiences a first fever. Fluoroquinolones significantly reduce the incidence of Gram-negative bacteremia, however, they do not make an impact on the number of days with fever or on mortality in these patients.[8] Concerns regarding quinolone use in the prophylactic setting during HCT include the emergence of resistant organisms and an increased risk of streptococcal infection.[8,260] The incidence of streptococcal infection due primarily to *S. viridans* is increasing during HCT, and prompt, aggressive treatment of these infections is warranted because of their morbidity (e.g., streptococcal shock syndrome).[8,261] Prophylactic antibiotics (e.g., penicillin, vancomycin) have been studied; however, because of their lack of efficacy in preventing streptococcal infections and concern over antibiotic-resistant bacteria, their use is not recommended.[8] The antibacterial prophylactic regimens vary substantially among HCT centers. At a minimum, broad-spectrum IV antibiotics should be initiated or added at the time of the first neutropenic fever under the treatment guidelines endorsed by the Infectious Disease Society of America practice guidelines for management of fever of unknown origin in the neutropenic host.[8,262] (Also see Chapter 68, Prevention and Treatment of Infections in Neutropenic Cancer Patients.)

Finally, S.D. is to be given fluconazole 400 mg/day because prophylactic use of this agent until day +75 after transplantation has been shown to decrease the incidence of systemic fungal infection and death caused by fungal infection compared with placebo in patients undergoing BMT.[263,264] Of note, use of prophylactic fluconazole by most HCT centers has led to increasing reports of breakthrough infections with resistant fungi.[265,266] In the setting of a persistent fever during neutropenia after HCT despite use of broad-spectrum antibiotics, amphotericin B is substituted for fluconazole to maximize antifungal coverage. (See Chapter 70, Opportunistic Infections in HIV-Infected Patients, for a complete discussion of the use of antimicrobials and antifungal therapy in the immunocompromised host.)

Another azole antifungal agent, itraconazole, has better in vitro activity against fungi that are resistant to fluconazole (e.g., *Aspergillus* and some *Candida* species). A randomized clinical trial demonstrated that itraconazole (200 mg IV Q 24 hr or oral solution 200 mg BID) was more effective than fluconazole (400 mg/day) for long-term prophylaxis of invasive fungal infections after allogeneic HCT; itraconazole was associated with more frequent gastrointestinal side effects (e.g., nausea, vomiting).[267] Patient education should be provided regarding the importance of compliance with the unpleasant tasting itraconazole solution and the necessity of maintaining plasma concentrations >500 ng/mL for effective prophylaxis.[266]

Prevention of Herpes Simplex Virus and Varicella-Zoster Virus

39. **On routine screening before transplantation, S.D. is found to be HSV and VZV seropositive. How will this affect her management?**

Before engraftment, patients who are HSV antibody seropositive before HCT are at high risk for reactivation of their HSV infection (e.g., 43% to 70% of HSV-seropositive patients undergoing myeloablative allogeneic HCT experience reactivation).[268,269] Acyclovir is highly effective in preventing HSV reactivation, and thus prophylactic acyclovir is commonly used in HSV-seropositive patients who are undergoing an allogeneic or autologous HCT.[8] Dosing regimens for prophylactic acyclovir vary widely; acyclovir is given at 250 mg/m^2 IV Q 12 hr, whereas oral doses of acyclovir range between 600 and 1,600 mg/day with 200 mg PO TID being a commonly used dose.[8] The recommended duration of acyclovir prophylaxis is also controversial, but most centers continue therapy until between day +30 and day +180 after transplantation. Valacyclovir, a prodrug of acyclovir with improved bioavailability, may allow for adequate serum concentrations to prevent HSV in patients with mucositis or gastrointestinal GVHD.[270] Typically, valacyclovir is administered as 500 mg PO Q 12 hr in the prophylactic setting.[271,272] In addition, VZV-seropositive patients are at risk for developing herpes zoster, particularly in the late period (3 to 6 months) after HCT.[270] Prophylactic acyclovir also reduces the risk of VZV reactivation.[273] The appropriate duration of VZV prophylaxis is controversial[8]; some centers continue therapy through the period of greatest risk for reactivation (6 months to 1-year post-transplantation) in all patients, and others reserve treatment for those who are more severely immunosuppressed.

In contrast, patients who are HSV or VZV seronegative rarely develop primary HSV or VZV infection; therefore, prophylactic acyclovir is not warranted. If HSV does occur, lesions usually appear on the oral mucosa, nasolabial mucous membranes, or genital mucocutaneous area and can be managed with treatment doses of acyclovir.

Because S.D. is HSV and VZV seropositive, she is at risk for reactivating these infections and will be given prophylactic acyclovir.

Prevention of Cytomegalovirus Disease

40. S.D. is also CMV seropositive. What is the significance of this finding and what measures can be taken to prevent reactivation of CMV?

CMV infection is common after allogeneic HCT, and the associated morbidity and mortality are high. Allogeneic HCT patients are at greater risk for CMV disease than autologous HCT recipients primarily because autologous HCT patients more efficiently reconstitute their immune system after transplantation. However, autologous HCT recipients who are CMV seropositive before HCT are at risk for CMV infection, and prophylaxis should be considered in selected patients.[8,274] Two CMV syndromes may occur. CMV infection is usually asymptomatic and occurs when replication of CMV is noted primarily in body fluid such as the blood (viremia), bronchoalveolar fluid, or urine (viruria). CMV disease is symptomatic and occurs when CMV invades an organ or tissue. The most common types of CMV disease after allogeneic HCT are pneumonia and gastritis. A CMV infection substantially increases the risk for developing invasive CMV disease. Strategies to prevent CMV infection have resulted in dramatic reductions in the incidence of CMV infection and disease.

Primary CMV can be prevented in the CMV-seronegative recipient by avoiding exposure to the virus. This can be accomplished by transplanting PBPC or bone marrow from CMV-seronegative donors and infusing CMV-negative blood products. However, HCT from a CMV-seronegative donor into a CMV-seronegative recipient and exclusive use of blood products from CMV-seronegative donors are not always possible. Therefore, other strategies, such as the use of filtered blood products (leukopoor), prophylactic antiviral therapy, IVIG, or a combination of these, may be used.

Antiviral drugs are the mainstay of preventing secondary CMV or its reactivation in the seropositive recipient. Prophylactic IVIG has had mixed results and is not recommended for preventing CMV among HCT recipients.[8,228,275] Use of ganciclovir to prevent CMV is the standard of care after allogeneic HCT, with two primary methods of choosing when prophylaxis is initiated—universal prophylaxis or pre-emptive prophylaxis. With universal prophylaxis, ganciclovir administration begins at the time of engraftment and continues until approximately day +100 in allogeneic recipients who are CMV seropositive or in a seronegative recipient receiving a CMV-positive graft. This strategy significantly decreases the incidence of CMV infection and disease compared with placebo, although mortality is not decreased.[276] Prophylactic ganciclovir therapy is associated with neutropenia in 30% of patients, which contributes to an increased risk of invasive bacterial and fungal infections.[276,277] Neutropenia associated with ganciclovir therapy may lead to interruptions in antiviral therapy or necessitate administration of filgrastim daily or several times per week to maintain adequate neutrophil counts.

Pre-emptive therapy, also called risk-adjusted therapy, has evolved as the most commonly used strategy for preventing CMV disease after allogeneic HCT.[270,278] The ability to detect early reactivation of CMV using shell vial cultures, assays of blood for CMV antigens (such as pp65) or viral nucleic acids using polymerase chain reaction (PCR) allow for rapid and selective initiation of ganciclovir therapy in patients at highest risk for developing CMV disease.[279–281] In a randomized trial, antigenemia-based pre-emptive therapy has similar efficacy in preventing CMV disease as universal ganciclovir prophylaxis,[277,282] and pre-emptive therapy has also been associated with a significant reduction in CMV mortality.[283–285] Pre-emptive strategies typically use an induction course of ganciclovir 5 mg/kg IV Q 12 hr for 7 to 14 days followed by a maintenance course of 5 mg/kg IV daily until 2 or 3 weeks after the last positive antigenemia result or until day +100 after HCT.[8] The ability to selectively administer ganciclovir based on detection of CMV reactivation ensures that only patients at highest risk for developing CMV disease are exposed to the potential toxicity of ganciclovir and thus reduces overall cost.[270]

Foscarnet may be given as an alternate to ganciclovir to prevent CMV disease, although its use is complicated by nephrotoxicity and electrolyte wasting.[285,286] Oral valacyclovir at a dose of 2 g QID has shown efficacy equal to that of IV ganciclovir in the prevention of CMV in CMV-seropositive allogeneic HCT recipients.[287] Autologous HCT recipients who are CMV seropositive pre-HCT should receive antiviral treatment pre-emptively as outlined above.[8,274] Similarly, data regarding the risk of CMV infection and disease in patients undergoing NMT are emerging. Since host T cells may persist in the peripheral blood for up to 6 months after NMT, it has been postulated that their presence may provide protection against early CMV disease. A matched controlled study comparing the incidence and outcome of CMV infection between myeloablative and nonmyeloablative HCT demonstrated that although the time of CMV antigenemia onset was similar between the groups, fewer patients post-NMT developed CMV disease in the early period.[288] It is interesting that the overall 1-year incidence of CMV disease was similar between groups, indicating that patients undergoing NMT have an increased risk for developing late CMV disease (>100 days after transplantation) compared with their myeloablative counterparts.[288] For this reason, it is recommended that NMT patients should receive pre-emptive antiviral therapy and should be monitored for development of CMV antigenemia for 1 year after transplantation.[288,289]

S.D.'s absolute neutrophil count recovers to >1,000 cells/μL on day +20, and on day +32 her weekly surveillance blood sample is positive for CMV by PCR. Pre-emptive ganciclovir therapy is initiated at 5 mg/kg IV every 12 hours. After 3 weeks of therapy, S.D.'s surveillance samples are negative and ganciclovir is discontinued. Weekly surveillance sampling continues until day +100. If surveillance samples again become positive for CMV by PCR, ganciclovir therapy should be re-instituted.

Diagnosis and Treatment of Aspergillus Infection
RISK FACTORS

41. A.W., a 60-kg, 165-cm, 15-year-old boy, is day +79 after a matched, unrelated nonmyeloablative PBPC transplantation for acute lymphocytic leukemia (ALL) in his third complete remission. He presents to the clinic for evaluation of a temperature of 102.3°F and a 3-day history of a nonproductive cough. Significant medical history includes skin and gut GVHD (which is stable on his current regimen of cyclosporine, mycophenolate mofetil, and prednisone) and congestive heart failure thought to be secondary to anthracycline exposure. A.W. has chronic low-grade nausea and magnesium wasting necessitating daily IV hydration with magnesium supplementation. Relevant laboratory values are as follows: Na, 138 mEq/L (normal, 135 to 147); K, 4.2 mEq/L (normal, 3.5 to 5.0); Cl, 100 mEq/L (normal, 95 to 105); CO_2, 23 mEq/L (normal, 22 to 28); blood urea nitrogen (BUN), 18 mg/dL (normal, 8 to 18); SrCr, 0.8 mg/dL (normal, 0.6 to 1.2); total bilirubin, 0.6 mg/dL (normal, 0.1 to 1); Mg, 1.5 mg/dL (normal, 1.6 to 2.4); WBC count, 3,500/mm³ (normal, 3,200 to 9,800); platelets, 78,000/mm³ (normal, 130,000 to 400,000); ANC, 1810 cells/L (normal, >1,700); and Hgb, 10.8 g/dL (normal, 12 to 15). He was CMV and HSV seropositive before HCT. Oral medications include cyclosporine 275 mg Q 12 hr; mycophenolate mofetil 900 mg Q 12 hr; prednisone 60 mg Q AM and 12.5 mg Q PM (tapering); co-trimoxazole 160 mg/800 mg BID on Monday and Tuesday; fluconazole 400 mg daily; valacyclovir 500 mg BID; digoxin 0.125 mg Q 12 hr; enalapril 10 mg Q 12 hr and a One a Day Plus vitamin daily.

On physical examination, A.W. is a chronically ill-appearing child with moon facies, dry skin with thickened areas, a pleural friction rub and thinning hair. Blood cultures, a urinalysis, and a chest x-ray are obtained. Chest x-ray revealed several small cavitary lesions worrisome for fungal disease. A.W. is admitted for further workup and management of presumed *Aspergillus* infection. What risk factors does A.W. have for developing infection with aspergillus?

[SI units: Na, 138 mmol/L; K, 4.2 mmol/L; Cl, 100 mmol/L; CO_2, 23 mmol/L; BUN, 6.43 mmol/L; SrCr, 71 μmol/L; total bilirubin, 10.26 μmol/L; Mg, 0.61 mmol/L; WBC count, 3, 500 × 10⁶ cells/L; platelets, 78 × 10⁹ cells/L; ANC, 1,810 × 10⁶ cells/L; Hgb, 108 g/L]

An increasing cause of morbidity and death after allogeneic and autologous HCT are invasive mold infections (e.g., *Aspergillus* species, *Fusarium* species, Zygomycetes, and *Scedosporium* species).[265] This trend is largely because (1) bacterial and viral infections are more effectively prevented (as described above) and (2) fluconazole prophylaxis reduced the incidence of candidemia and candida-related mortality.[263–265,290,291] Infections with the *Aspergillus* species are the most common mold infections.[265] The incidence of invasive aspergillosis (IA) has risen over the past decade. The annual incidence of IA was 10.5% among allogeneic and 5.3% among autologous HCT recipients in the 1998.[265]

Several risk factors for developing invasive fungal disease have been identified.[290,291] Given that neutrophils are critical for host defense against fungal infections, prolonged neutropenia is considered the single most important predictor of development of invasive fungal infections at all time points after HCT.[266,290]

GVHD, both acute and chronic, and treatment with corticosteroids are also important risk factors for developing invasive fungal infection, particularly late-onset (i.e., day +40 to +100 after transplantation) aspergillosis.[290,291] Neutrophil dysfunction as a result of GVHD and treatment with corticosteroids is assumed to be the principal mechanism for this in-

crease in risk.[292] Lastly, although widespread use of fluconazole (400 mg/day) prophylaxis since the early 1990s has led to a significant decline in the morbidity and mortality associated with invasive candidiasis in BMT recipients,[291] the incidence of infections due to fluconazole-resistant *Candida* species, such as *C. krusei* and *C. glabrata* as well as the incidence of IA has increased substantially as a result of this practice.[290,293,294]

A.W. is receiving corticosteroid treatment for GVHD and is taking fluconazole as antifungal prophylaxis. These factors increase his risk for developing invasive aspergillosis.

TREATMENT

42. **A.W. undergoes a bronchoalveolar lavage in an attempt to identify the organism responsible for his infection. Pathologic examination of the fluid obtained reveals septate, branching hyphae, and results from a culture of the fluid confirm a diagnosis of *Aspergillus fumigatus* infection. CT scans confirm the presence of lung nodules but are negative for any other sites of disease. A.W. is started on amphotericin B lipid complex (Abelcet) at 300 mg IV daily. How is aspergillosis usually diagnosed and what are the acceptable alternatives for treating this infection?**

In practice, the ability to definitively diagnose, and thus appropriately treat IA, is quite challenging. Although early diagnosis and institution of aggressive antifungal therapy may reduce the high mortality rate of patients with IA, rapid diagnosis is difficult and relies on obtaining tissue or fluid from an infected site.[295] Although the lower respiratory tract is frequently the primary focus of infection, *Aspergillus* may invade blood vessels and spread hematogenously to other organs including the brain, liver, kidneys, spleen, and skin.[296] Head, chest, abdomen, and pelvic CT scans are performed to assess the extent of disease as the findings may influence management and overall prognosis. Also, the medical condition of many HCT recipients prohibits obtaining a biopsy of the infected tissue; some biopsies suffer from low specificity for detecting *Aspergillus*. Moreover, *Aspergillus* grows slowly in culture.[296] With these techniques, many clinicians have adopted the European Organization for Research and Treatment of Cancer's (EORTC) criteria for diagnosis of proven, probable, and possible IA (Table 92-11).[297]

Promising newer diagnostic techniques including detection of fungal nucleic acids using PCR and detection of a component of the aspergillus cell wall called galactomannan (GM) using an enzyme-linked immunosorbent assay (EIA) are being developed.[298,299] An *Aspergillus* Galactmannan enzyme immunoassay (GM-EIA) was FDA approved in spring of 1999[300]; prospective screening for GM allows for earlier diagnosis than conventional diagnostic criteria based on data in European allogeneic HCT recipients.[301] Currently, GM-EIA may be considered in a neutropenic HCT recipient when IA is suspected or as a surveillance tool during the at-risk period (e.g., days 60 to 100).

ANTIFUNGALS

Outcomes for IA patients, particularly after HCT, are poor, with approximately 20% of IA patients alive after 1 year.[290] Outcomes depend not only on the use of intensive antifungal therapy, but also on recovery of the host's immune system and reduction of immune suppression.[295,302] In fact, studies have

Table 92-11 Diagnostic Criteria for Fungal Infections

Type of infection	Description
• Proven invasive fungal infections	
Deep tissue infections	Histopathologic or cytopathologic examination showing hyphae or yeast cells from needle aspiration or biopsy specimen with evidence of associated tissue damage; *or* positive culture result for sample obtained by sterile procedure from normally sterile and clinically or radiographically abnormal site consistent with infection, excluding urine and mucous membranes
Fungemia	Blood culture that yields fungi, excluding *Aspergillus* species and *Penicillium* species other than *Penicillium marneffei*, or *Candida* species accompanied by temporally related clinical signs and symptoms compatible with relevant organism
• Probable invasive fungal infections	At least 1 host factor criterion and 1 microbiologic criterion plus 1 major or 2 minor clinical criteria from abnormal site consistent with infection (see below)
• Possible invasive fungal infections	At least 1 host factor criterion plus 1 microbiologic or 1 major (or 2 minor) clinical criteria from abnormal site consistent with infection

Host Factor Criteria

- ANC < 500 cells/mm^3 for >10 days
- Persistent fever for >96 hr despite broad-spectrum antibiotics
- Temperature >38°C and any of the following:
  Prolonged neutropenia in past 60 days
  Use of immunosuppressive agents in past 30 days
  History of fungal infection
- Signs/symptoms of GVHD
- Prolonged use of corticosteroids in past 60 days

Microbiologic Criteria

- Positive culture or microscopic evaluation for fungi from sputum, BAL fluid samples, or sinus aspirate
- Positive findings of cytologic or direct microscopic examination for fungal elements in sterile body fluid samples
- Positive result of blood culture for *Candida* species

Clinical Criteria

Major
- CT imaging demonstrating halo sign, air crescent sign, or cavity within area of consolidation
- Radiologic evidence of invasive infection in sinuses or CNS

Minor
- Symptoms of lower respiratory tract infection (cough, chest pain, hemoptysis, dyspnea); physical finding of a pleural rub; any new infiltrate not fulfilling major criterion
- Upper respiratory symptoms (nasal discharge, stuffiness); maxillary tenderness
- Focal neurologic symptoms and signs including seizures, hemiparesis, and cranial nerve palsies; mental status changes; meningeal irritation findings

ANC, absolute neutrophil count; BAL, bronchoalveolar lavage; CNS, central nervous system; CT, computed tomography; GVHD, graft-versus-host disease.
From Ascioglu S. Defining opportunistic invasive fungal infections in immunocompromised patients with cancer and hematopoietic stem cell transplants: an international consensus. Clin Infect Dis 2002; 34:7–14.

found that the single most important predictor of mortality for IA in the allogeneic HCT recipients is high total doses of corticosteroids.[302]

Traditionally, conventional amphotericin B (c-AmB) at a minimum dose of 1 mg/kg per day has been the gold standard antifungal therapy for any IA infection. Depending on the severity of the underlying immune suppression, complete and partial response rates for single agent c-AmB range from 28% to 51%; however, 65% of responders eventually die of their infection.[295] In addition, toxicity associated with c-AmB is significant and frequently limits dose and duration of therapy. (Refer to Case 43 for further discussion of amphotericin toxicity). Recently, newer agents including liposomal derivatives of amphotericin B, broad-spectrum triazoles, and a new class of antifungals called the echinocandins have become available. These alternatives offer a promising spectrum of therapeutic options for fungal disease.

Since the mid 1990s, three liposomal formulations of amphotericin have been developed that may be used in place of c-AmB to manage fungal disease and for empiric therapy in neutropenic patients at high risk for nephrotoxicity. These include amphotericin B lipid complex (Abelcet, ABLC), liposomal amphotericin B (Ambisome, L-Amb) and amphotericin B colloidal dispersion (Amphotec, ABCD). (Refer to Chapter 68, Prevention and Treatment of Infections in Neutropenic Cancer Patients, for a complete review of these products.) Practice guidelines are available for the use of these agents for treatment of fungal infections in HCT patients.[303] Overall, studies of single-agent liposomal formulations of amphotericin B for patients with IA who have failed or are intolerant to c-Amb therapy reveal response rates in the range of 23% to 71%, regardless of the agent used. However, no randomized studies have confirmed that these liposomal formulations result in better outcomes compared with c-Amb for the treatment of IA.[302] Various doses of the liposomal formulations were given in these trials, most commonly 5 mg/kg per day for ABLC and L-Amb and 4 to 6 mg/kg per day for ABCD. Although lower doses, particularly of L-Amb (1 to 3 mg/kg per day) have been studied for empirical use in neutropenic patients with persistent fever, it remains to be determined whether such doses are efficacious in the treatment of IA.[304,305] A notable difference between the liposomal formulations and c-Amb described is the decreased risk for nephrotoxicity when liposomal products are used.

An additional factor that limits widespread use of the liposomal products is their high cost compared with c-Amb. ABLC and ABCD are approximately 15 times more expensive than c-Amb, whereas L-Amb is 30 times more expensive when compared with doses used to treat IA. Drug acquisition cost should be balanced with the potentially greater cost of managing c-Amb nephrotoxicity in the hospital. A recent pharmacoeconomic evaluation comparing hospital costs for neutropenic patients with persistent fever treated with L-Amb or c-Amb revealed that overall costs were significantly higher for patients receiving L-Amb.[306] Furthermore, this difference in cost was principally attributable to the higher acquisition cost of L-Amb. Thus, establishing cost-effective strategies for the appropriate use of these agents is imperative. Most HCT centers have developed criteria for appropriate use based on the patient's risk for nephrotoxicity and the severity of the infection being treated.

Two newer broad-spectrum triazoles have been licensed for the treatment of fungal infections in patients who fail or are intolerant of amphotericin B therapy. Itraconaozle (Sporonox) was the first to become available. In a compassionate use trial in patients with aspergillosis unresponsive to amphotericin B, 27% of patients were found to have a complete response to itraconazole and another 35% experienced improvement in their infection.[307] Patients in this trial who had undergone HCT had responses similar to those patients who were less immunocompromised. Itraconazole is available for both oral and intravenous use. Unfortunately, oral itraconazole exhibits erratic absorption, and the IV formulation is complicated by the risk of precipitation of the drug in the IV line.[295]

More recently, voriconazole (Vefend) has been approved by the FDA for treatment of fungal infections unresponsive to alternative agents. An advantage of voriconazole is its 96% oral bioavailability, which makes this oral drug an attractive and less expensive alternative. Voriconazole has been compared directly with c-Amb for treatment of primary IA.[308] The primary objective of this trial was to demonstrate the noninferiority of voriconazole compared with c-Amb after 12 weeks of therapy in patients with definite or probable IA. Patients received either voriconazole 6 mg/kg IV Q 12 hr × 2 doses followed by 4 mg/kg IV Q 12 hr for at least 7 days at which point they could switch to oral voriconazole 200 mg Q 12 hr or c-Amb 1 to 1.5 mg/kg per day. Patients who couldn't tolerate or failed to respond to initial therapy could receive alternate licensed antifungal therapy (itraconazole, liposomal formulations of amphotericin B). Of 144 evaluable patients who received voriconazole, 76 (52.8%) had either a complete or partial response compared with 42 of 133 (31.6%) patients treated with c-Amb. The median duration of therapy for patients treated with voriconazole was 77 days and 52 of 144 patients switched to an alternate antifungal drug. In contrast, the median duration of therapy for patients receiving c-Amb was 10 days and 107 of 133 patients switched to another agent (most commonly a liposomal derivative of amphotericin B). In addition, the survival rate in the voriconazole group was 70.8% compared with 57.9% in the c-Amb group. The authors concluded that voriconazole was not inferior to c-Amb in the treatment of IA. In fact, initial therapy with voriconazole appeared to be superior to initial therapy with c-Amb.

Finally, extensive research using a novel class of antifungals called the echinocandins in the treatment of fungal disease is underway. Echinocandins have a novel target for their antifungal activity, β-1,3 glucan synthase, an enzyme that produces an important component of the fungal wall. Of this class, caspofungin (Cancidas) is the first such product licensed for use. It is indicated for treatment of IA refractory to alternate therapy. Caspofungin may be administered only IV because its oral bioavailability is <2%.[309] An open-label, noncomparative trial evaluated the efficacy of caspofungin in 69 patients with IA who had not responded to or were intolerant of a minimum of 7 days of standard antifungal therapy.[309] Patients received 70 mg IV on day 1 of therapy followed by 50 mg IV daily. Of the 63 evaluable patients, 26 (43%) had a favorable response to treatment. When outcomes were assessed in patients who had received a minimum of 7 days of therapy, 26 of 52 patients (50%) had a favorable response. To date, there have been no randomized controlled trials comparing caspofungin with amphotericin B products for the treatment of IA.

In summary, the spectrum of agents available to manage IA has expanded greatly in the past few years. Although it remains to be determined which agent(s) will ultimately lead to the best outcomes, the similar efficacy profiles of the liposomal formulations of amphotericin B, itraconazole, voriconazole, and caspofungin allow clinicians to tailor therapy to the individual patient based on response, tolerability, and cost.

ANTIFUNGAL TOXICITIES

43. **Despite premedication with acetaminophen and diphenhydramine, A.W. experiences significant chills and rigors with his Abelcet infusions. In addition, he is having daily temperatures exceeding 39°C. On day 5 of therapy, morning laboratory tests reveal a SrCr of 1.4 mg/dL, K of 2.7 mEq/L and Mg of 1.4 mg/dL. What expected adverse reactions of conventional amphotericin B–based therapy does A.W. demonstrate?**

[SI units: SrCr, 123.8 µmol/L; K, 2.7 mmol/L; Mg, 0.57 mmol/L]

The most troublesome side effect of amphotericin B therapy is nephrotoxicity. Depending on the definition of renal toxicity used, up to 80% of patients receiving c-Amb will experience an episode of altered renal function during treatment.[310] The mechanisms of amphotericin B nephrotoxicity are complex and may involve vasoconstriction resulting in cortical ischemia and a subsequent decrease in GFR as well as tubular defects in acid secretion. Several risk factors for nephrotoxicity have been identified. Notably, concomitant administration of other nephrotoxic agents, such as aminoglycosides, cyclosporine, cisplatin, or radiocontrast dye, significantly increases risk. Concomitant cyclosporine administration was found to be the most significant risk factor for developing severe nephrotoxicity in HCT patients.[310] Additional risk factors include longer mean duration of amphotericin B therapy, history of chronic renal disease, male gender, and a mean daily dose ≥35 mg.[311]

Liposomal derivatives of amphotericin B were developed with the specific intent of reducing nephrotoxicity. Indeed, each of the liposomal products has demonstrated significantly lower incidences of renal toxicity compared with c-Amb.[303,304,312–314] Furthermore, patients treated with c-Amb who experience nephrotoxicity and who are then switched to a liposomal formulation frequently show improvement in renal function. It is difficult to determine the true incidence of nephrotoxicity associated with the liposomal derivatives because most trials evaluate their use in patients who have received prior c-Amb therapy. In addition, many trials do not control for other factors known to reduce the risk of nephrotoxicity including salt loading and fluid boluses administered before c-Amb infusions. However, clinical experience supports the reduced incidence of nephrotoxicity with these products, and they are recommended as first-line therapy for patients at high risk for nephrotoxicity or in whom baseline renal function is impaired.

Additional toxicities of c-Amb include infusion-related reactions (fever, chills, rigors, hypotension, hypoxia), electrolyte wasting, nausea, and anemia. Generally, premedications such as acetaminophen, diphenhydramine, meperidine, and/or hydrocortisone are administered before each dose to ameliorate these infusion-related events with variable degrees of success. Moreover, patients may become tolerant to these effects over time. There appears to be a reduced incidence of infusion-related reactions when liposomal products are used. Electrolyte wasting, especially potassium and magnesium, secondary to amphotericin B therapy (either conventional or liposomal) can be significant and persist well beyond discontinuation of the drug. Most patients require daily potassium and magnesium supplementation, particularly if they require prolonged amphotericin therapy.

LENGTH OF ANTIFUNGAL THERAPY AND COMBINATION ANTIFUNGAL THERAPY

44. In response to A.W.'s rise in SrCr, his physician elects to discontinue Abelcet and begin voriconazole 6 mg/kg IV Q 12 hr × 2 doses followed by 4 mg/kg IV Q 12 hr and caspofungin 70 mg IV on day 1 and 50 mg IV QD thereafter. What side effects should be monitored for with this new regimen and what is the rationale for combination therapy for A.W.? How long should A.W. receive antifungal therapy for his aspergillosis?

Common toxicities reported with voriconazole to date include infusion-related, transient visual disturbances (blurred vision, altered color perception, photophobia, visual hallucinations), skin reactions (rash, pruritus, photosensitivity), elevations in hepatic transaminases and alkaline phosphatase, nausea, and headache.[308,315,316] Caspofungin appears to have fewer adverse events. Most commonly, mild to moderate infusion reactions and headache have been reported. In addition, a smaller number of patients have experienced dermatologic reactions related to histamine release (flushing, erythema, wheals). Caspofungin therapy has also been associated with elevations in hepatic transaminases in approximately 6% of patients.[309] A.W. should be monitored for changes in liver function and counseled regarding the potential visual side effects of voriconazole.

Data regarding combination therapy with newly available triazoles, echinocandins, and polyenes in patients with fungal disease are lacking. However, in vitro data suggest combinations of voriconazole with caspofungin or caspofungin with polyenes may be synergistic.[317,318] Furthermore, no evidence of antagonism among these agents has been demonstrated in vitro. Given the overall poor prognosis of IA in severely immunosuppressed patients, many practitioners are treating patients with combination therapy known to be synergistic in vitro to maximize the chance of response. Thus, voriconazole in combination with caspofungin is a reasonable alternative for A.W., particularly considering the degree of toxicity he is experiencing with Abelcet therapy.

Finally, the optimum duration of appropriate antifungal therapy for treating IA is unknown.[302] The appropriate duration largely depends on the individual's reconstitution of their immune system and their response to antifungal treatment. Most clinicians continue aggressive antifungal therapy until the infection has stabilized radiographically and may continue with less aggressive "maintenance" therapy (such as single-agent oral voriconazole) until the degree of immune suppression is decreased. In general, it is not uncommon to require several months of antifungal therapy to manage IA.

Prevention of Pneumocystis carinii Pneumonia

45. A.W. is receiving co-trimoxazole, 1 single-strength tablet PO BID on Mondays, Wednesdays, and Fridays. What is the rationale for its use in A.W.?

Pneumocystis is a common cause of infection after allogeneic HCT and has a high mortality rate if left untreated (see Chapter 70, Opportunistic Infections in HIV-Infected Patients, for description, diagnosis, and treatment). *Pneumocystis carinii* pneumonia (PCP) prophylaxis is routine after allogeneic HCT. Data are lacking as to the best regimen in HCT and current practices primarily are based on the pediatric cancer literature. Most centers administer co-trimoxazole for PCP prophylaxis.[8] Dapsone or aerosolized pentamidine are alternatives for patients who are allergic to sulfa drugs or who do not tolerate co-trimoxazole.

PCP most commonly occurs after engraftment. Therefore, co-trimoxazole usually is begun after the counts have recovered to ANC >1,000 cells/mm[3]. However, some centers administer co-trimoxazole throughout the neutropenic period. Because of the myelosuppressive effects of co-trimoxazole, this practice is approached with some caution and, although not proven, may delay or prevent engraftment. It is common for co-trimoxazole prophylaxis to be held back after engraftment if WBC or platelet counts fall unexplainably. This occurs more often in patients receiving ganciclovir for CMV prophylaxis or methotrexate for GVHD prophylaxis. Rash may occur secondary to the sulfa component in co-trimoxazole and require its discontinuation. Co-trimoxazole usually is avoided on days of methotrexate administration because of the ability of sulfonamides to displace methotrexate from plasma binding sites and decrease renal methotrexate clearance, resulting in higher methotrexate concentrations. Prophylaxis usually is continued for 6 months to 1 year after transplantation.

Autologous HCT recipients with underlying hematologic malignancies (e.g. lymphoma, leukemia) are also at risk.[8] The routine use of PCP prophylaxis after autologous HCT is controversial and practices vary widely among centers. Autologous HCT patients do not receive post-transplant immunosuppression. Thus, their risk of developing PCP is lower. PCP prophylaxis is often used after autologous HCT for NHL, Hodgkin's disease, multiple myeloma, and lymphocytic leukemias because of the immunosuppressive nature of the underlying disease. PCP prophylaxis is not generally used after autologous transplantation for breast cancer.

Issues of Survivorship After Hematopoietic Cell Transplantation

46. H.O. is a 32-year-old woman who received a BU/CY preparative regimen and an HLA-matched sibling BMT for treatment of CML in chronic phase at age 21. H.O. received her BMT over 10 years ago, is disease free, and has not had chronic GVHD for 9-years. Her only medication is one multivitamin tablet PO QD. What issues of cancer survivorship are of concern to H.O.?

A greater proportion of cancer patients are surviving their cancer diagnosis without evidence of their primary malignancy, but they are at risk for long-term physical and emotional sequelae of their cancer treatments.[319] These sequelae are of paramount importance to HCT recipients because 5-year disease-free survival after HCT is increasing and the myeloablative preparative regimens put them at high risk for long-term toxicities.[203,320] HCT recipients are also at risk for diseases common in the general population.[320]

Mortality for HCT recipients is higher than the general population, with the principal causes of death being relapse, GVHD, infection, a secondary malignant neoplasm, and end-organ failure.[321] Immune function can take over 2 years to recover, even without immunosupressants.[320] Treatment of GVHD exacerbates immune system defects, necessitating prophylaxis for and vigilant monitoring for infectious complications. Fevers should be rapidly assessed and treated within HCT survivors to prevent a fatal infection. Recipients of HCT also lose protective antibodies to vaccine-preventable diseases. Therefore, HCT survivors need to be re-vaccinated for selected infectious diseases and with due consideration for the risk of vaccination. The CDC and European Group for Bone Marrow Transplantation have issued recommendations for immunization for HCT recipients, which have been summarized by Goldberg and colleagues.[322]

Survivors of HCT have a threefold higher risk for secondary malignant neoplasms.[320,321,323] Long-term impairment of end-organ function may be due to the preparative regimen, infectious complications (either autologous or allogeneic grafts) and post-transplantation immunosuppression (allogeneic grafts only).[324] Endocrine dysfunction is common, with hypothyroidism occurring in up to 25% of adults owing to total body irradiation.[324] Adrenal insufficiency can also result from long-term corticosteroids used to treat GVHD. Infertility is commonly observed after myeloablative HCT because of the high doses of alkylating agents and radiation administered. Frequently, men become azoospermic and chemically-induced menopause develops in women. However, pregnancies have occurred after HCT. Up to 60% of HCT recipients have osteopenia, most likely resulting from gonadal dysfunction and corticosteroid administration; avascular necrosis due to corticosteroids can also occur.[324] In addition, a significant portion (15% to 40%) of HCT survivors have pulmonary toxicity with variable symptoms (e.g., restrictive, chronic obstructive lung disease) and multiple causes.[324] Hepatitis infections can occur in HCT recipients, with the prevalence of chronic hepatitis C ranging from 5% to 70% in long-term HCT survivors.[325] Because of this, cirrhosis and its complications may become an important late complication of HCT.[192,325] Hepatic dysfunction can also result from iron overload, which may occur secondary to multiple PRBC transfusions administered during aplasia after myeloablative preparative regimens and before HCT.[192] Alopecia is a common late effect with BU/CY, as are cataracts with CY/TBI.[117]

H.O. should be routinely monitored for signs of relapse and chronic GVHD. To lower the risk of infectious complications, she should be counseled to obtain prompt medical care for fevers or signs of an infection, and she should be re-vaccinated if she has not done so since receiving her myeloablative HCT. Thorough evaluation of end-organ function, including renal, hepatic, thyroid, and ovarian function, should be assessed at regular intervals. In addition, her bone mineral density should be determined, and H.O. should be counseled on preventive measures for osteopenia (e.g., calcium supplementation). In addition to standard cancer screening tests, H.O. should be closely monitored for secondary malignant neoplasms.[320]

REFERENCES

1. Thomas ED et al. Bone-marrow transplantation (part 1). N Engl J Med 1975;292:832.
2. Thomas ED et al. Bone-marrow transplantation (part 2). N Engl J Med 1975;292:895.
3. Schmitz N, Barrett J. Optimizing engraftment—source and dose of stem cells. Semin Hematol 2002;39:3.
4. Eder JP et al. A phase I-II study of cyclophosphamide, thiotepa, and carboplatin with autologous bone marrow transplantation in solid tumor patients. J Clin Oncol 1990;8:1239.
5. Appelbaum FR. Haematopoietic cell transplantation as immunotherapy. Nature 2001;411:385.
6. McSweeney PA et al. Hematopoietic cell transplantation in older patients with hematologic malignancies: replacing high-dose cytotoxic therapy with graft-versus-tumor effects. Blood 2001;97:3390.
7. Khouri IF et al. Transplant-lite: induction of graft-versus-malignancy using fludarabine-based nonablative chemotherapy and allogeneic blood progenitor-cell transplantation as treatment for lymphoid malignancies. J Clin Oncol 1998;16:2817.
8. Guidelines for preventing opportunistic infections among hematopoietic stem cell transplant recipients. MMWR Recomm Rep 2000;49:1.
9. Schmitz N et al. Randomised trial of filgrastim-mobilised peripheral blood progenitor cell transplantation versus autologous bone-marrow transplantation in lymphoma patients. Lancet 1996;347:353.
10. Smith TJ et al. Economic analysis of a randomized clinical trial to compare filgrastim-mobilized peripheral-blood progenitor-cell transplantation and autologous bone marrow transplantation in patients with Hodgkin's and non-Hodgkin's lymphoma. J Clin Oncol 1997;15:5.
11. Bensinger WI et al. Transplantation of bone marrow as compared with peripheral-blood cells from HLA-identical relatives in patients with hematologic cancers. N Engl J Med 2001;344:175.
12. Schmitz N et al. Transplantation of mobilized peripheral blood cells to HLA-identical siblings with standard-risk leukemia. Blood 2002;100:761.
13. Couban S et al. A randomized multicenter comparison of bone marrow and peripheral blood in recipients of matched sibling allogeneic transplants for myeloid malignancies. Blood 2002;100:1525.
14. Mohty M et al. Chronic graft-versus-host disease after allogeneic blood stem cell transplantation: long-term results of a randomized study. Blood 2002;100:3128.
15. Champlin RE et al. Blood stem cells compared with bone marrow as a source of hematopoietic cells for allogeneic transplantation. IBMTR Histocompati-

bility and Stem Cell Sources Working Committee and the European Group for Blood and Marrow Transplantation (EBMT). Blood 2000;95:3702.

16. Little MT, Storb R. History of haematopoietic stem-cell transplantation. Nat Rev Cancer 2002;2:231.

17. Report on state of the art in blood and marrow transplantation. IBMTR/ABMTR Newsletter 2002;9:1.

18. Laughlin MJ et al. Hematopoietic engraftment and survival in adult recipients of umbilical-cord blood from unrelated donors. N Engl J Med 2001;344:1815.

19. Gluckman E. Hematopoietic stem-cell transplants using umbilical-cord blood. N Engl J Med 2001;344:1860.

20. Gross TG et al. Pediatric hematopoietic stem cell transplantation. Hematol Oncol Clin North Am 2001;15:795.

21. Woods WG et al. A comparison of allogeneic bone marrow transplantation, autologous bone marrow transplantation, and aggressive chemotherapy in children with acute myeloid leukemia in remission: a report from the Children's cancer group. Blood 2001;97:56.

22. Farquhar C et al. High dose chemotherapy and autologous bone marrow or stem cell transplantation versus conventional chemotherapy for women with early poor prognosis breast cancer Cochrane Database Syst. Rev. 2003(1):CD003142.

23. Guardiola P et al. Allogeneic stem cell transplantation for agnogenic myeloid metaplasia: a European Group for Blood and Marrow Transplantation, Societe Francaise de Greffe de Moelle, Gruppo Italiano per il Trapianto del Midollo Osseo, and Fred Hutchinson Cancer Research Center Collaborative Study. Blood 1999;93:2831.

24. Witherspoon RP et al. Hematopoietic stem-cell transplantation for treatment-related leukemia or myelodysplasia. J Clin Oncol 2001;19:2134.

25. MacNeil M, Eisenhauer EA. High-dose chemotherapy: is it standard management for any common solid tumor? Ann Oncol 1999;10:1145.

26. O'Brien SG et al. Imatinib compared with interferon and low-dose cytarabine for newly diagnosed chronic-phase chronic myeloid leukemia. N Engl J Med 2003;348:994.

27. Anderlini P, Champlin R. Use of filgrastim for stem cell mobilisation and transplantation in high-dose cancer chemotherapy. Drugs 2002;62(Suppl 1):79.

28. Appelbaum FR. Who should be transplanted for AML? Leukemia 2001;15:680.

29. Ratanatharathorn V et al. Prospective comparative trial of autologous versus allogeneic bone marrow transplantation in patients with non-Hodgkin's lymphoma. Blood 1994;84:1050.

30. Rizzo JD 1998 Summary Data from International Bone Marrow Transplant Registry/Autologous Bone Marrow Transplant Registry. ABMTR Newsletter 1998;5:4.

31. Santini G et al. VACOP-B versus VACOP-B plus autologous bone marrow transplantation for advanced diffuse non-Hodgkin's lymphoma: results of a prospective randomized trial by the non-Hodgkin's Lymphoma Cooperative Study Group. J Clin Oncol 1998;16:2796.

32. Hahn T et al. The role of cytotoxic therapy with hematopoietic stem cell transplantation in the therapy of diffuse large cell B-cell non-Hodgkin's lymphoma: an evidence-based review. Biol Blood Marrow Transplant 2001;7:308.

33. Haioun C et al. Survival benefit of high-dose therapy in poor-risk aggressive non-Hodgkin's lymphoma: final analysis of the prospective LNH87-2 protocol—a groupe d'Etude des lymphomes de l'Adulte study. J Clin Oncol 2000;18:3025.

34. A predictive model for aggressive non-Hodgkin's lymphoma. The International Non-Hodgkin's Lymphoma Prognostic Factors Project. N Engl J Med 1993;329:987.

35. Philip T et al. Autologous bone marrow transplantation as compared with salvage chemotherapy in relapses of chemotherapy-sensitive non-Hodgkin's lymphoma. N Engl J Med 1995;333:1540.

36. Jones R, Burnett AK. ACP Broadsheet No 134: December 1992. How to harvest bone marrow for transplantation. J Clin Pathol 1992;45:1053.

37. Rowley SD, Hematopoietic stem cell cryopreservations. In: Thomas ED et al, eds. Hematopoietic Cell Transplantation. Malden, MA: Blackwell Science, 1999:481.

38. Yeager AM et al. Autologous bone marrow transplantation in patients with acute nonlymphocytic leukemia, using ex vivo marrow treatment with 4-hydroperoxycyclophosphamide. N Engl J Med 1986;315:141.

39. Shpall EJ et al. Transplantation of enriched CD34-positive autologous marrow into breast cancer patients following high-dose chemotherapy: influence of CD34-positive peripheral-blood progenitors and growth factors on engraftment. J Clin Oncol 1994;12:28.

40. To LB et al. The biology and clinical uses of blood stem cells. Blood 1997;89:2233.

41. Champlin RE et al. Treatment of acute myelogenous leukemia. A prospective controlled trial of bone marrow transplantation versus consolidation chemotherapy. Ann Intern Med 1985;102:285.

42. Kanz L, Brugger W. Mobilization and ex vivo manipulation of peripheral blood progenitor cells for support of high-dose cancer therapy. In: Thomas ED et al, eds. Hematopoietic Cell Transplantation. Malden, MA: Blackwell Science, 1999:455.

43. Ozer H et al. 2000 update of recommendations for the use of hematopoietic colony-stimulating factors: evidence-based, clinical practice guidelines. American Society of Clinical Oncology Growth Factors Expert Panel. J Clin Oncol 2000;18:3558.

44. Weaver CH et al. Mobilization of peripheral blood stem cells following myelosuppressive chemotherapy: a randomized comparison of filgrastim, sargramostim, or sequential sargramostim and filgrastim. Bone Marrow Transplant 2001;27(Suppl 2):S23.

45. To LB et al. Single high doses of cyclophosphamide enable the collection of high numbers of hemopoietic stem cells from the peripheral blood. Exp Hematol 1990;18:442.

46. Weaver CH et al. An analysis of engraftment kinetics as a function of the CD34 content of peripheral blood progenitor cell collections in 692 patients after the administration of myeloablative chemotherapy. Blood 1995;86:3961.

47. Bensinger W et al. Factors that influence collection and engraftment of autologous peripheral blood stem cells. J Clin Oncol 1995;13:2547.

48. Schulman KA et al. Effect of CD34(+) cell dose on resource utilization in patients after high dose chemotherapy with peripheral-blood stem-cell support. J Clin Oncol 1999;17:1227.

49. Gianni AM. Where do we stand with respect to the use of peripheral blood progenitor cells? Ann Oncol 1994;5:781.

50. Berenson RJ et al. Engraftment after infusion of CD34+ marrow cells in patients with breast cancer or neuroblastoma. Blood 1991;77:1717.

51. Figueres E et al. Analysis of parameters affecting engraftment in children undergoing autologous peripheral blood stem cell transplants. Bone Marrow Transplant 2000;25:583.

52. Meisenberg BR et al. Outpatient high-dose chemotherapy with autologous stem-cell rescue for hematologic and nonhematologic malignancies. J Clin Oncol 1997;15:11.

53. Rizzo JD et al. Outpatient-based bone marrow transplantation for hematologic malignancies: cost saving or cost shifting? J Clin Oncol 1999;17:2811.

54. Gilbert C et al. Sequential prophylactic oral and empiric once-daily parenteral antibiotics for neutropenia and fever after high-dose chemotherapy and autologous bone marrow support. J Clin Oncol 1994;12:1005.

55. Gisselbrecht C et al. Placebo-controlled phase III trial of lenograstim in bone-marrow transplantation. Lancet 1994;343:696.

56. Greenberg P et al. GM-CSF accelerates neutrophil recovery after autologous hematopoietic stem cell transplantation. Bone Marrow Transplant 1996;18:1057.

57. Rabinowe SN et al. Long-term follow-up of a phase III study of recombinant human granulocyte-macrophage colony-stimulating factor after autolo-

gous bone marrow transplantation for lymphoid malignancies. Blood 1993;81:1903.

58. Klumpp TR et al. Granulocyte colony-stimulating factor accelerates neutrophil engraftment following peripheral-blood stem-cell transplantation: a prospective, randomized trial. J Clin Oncol 1995;13:1323.

59. Spitzer G et al. Randomized study of growth factors post-peripheral-blood stem-cell transplant: neutrophil recovery is improved with modest clinical benefit. J Clin Oncol 1994;12:661.

60. Cortelazzo S et al. Granulocyte colony-stimulating factor following peripheral-blood progenitor-cell transplant in non-Hodgkin's lymphoma. J Clin Oncol 1995;13:935.

61. Legros M et al. rhGM-CSF vs placebo following rhGM-CSF-mobilized PBPC transplantation: a phase III double-blind randomized trial. Bone Marrow Transplant 1997;19:209.

62. De Witte T et al. Recombinant human granulocyte-macrophage colony-stimulating factor accelerates neutrophil and monocyte recovery after allogeneic T-cell-depleted bone marrow transplantation. Blood 1992;79:1359.

63. Powles R et al. Human recombinant GM-CSF in allogeneic bone-marrow transplantation for leukaemia: double-blind, placebo-controlled trial. Lancet 1990;336:1417.

64. Erlich HA et al. HLA DNA typing and transplantation. Immunity 2001;14:347.

65. Davies SM et al. Engraftment and survival after unrelated-donor bone marrow transplantation: a report from the national marrow donor program. Blood 2000;96:4096.

66. Estey EH. Treatment of Acute Myelogenous Leukemia. Oncology 2002;16:343.

67. Sievers EL et al. Efficacy and safety of gemtuzumab ozogamicin in patients with CD33-positive acute myeloid leukemia in first relapse. J Clin Oncol 2001;19:3244.

68. Appelbaum FR et al. Bone marrow transplantation or chemotherapy after remission induction for adults with acute nonlymphoblastic leukemia. A prospective comparison. Ann Intern Med 1984;101:581.

69. Lowenberg B et al. Acute myeloid leukemia. N Engl J Med 1999;341:1051.

70. Zittoun RA et al. Autologous or allogeneic bone marrow transplantation compared with intensive chemotherapy in acute myelogenous leukemia European Organization for Research and Treatment of Cancer (EORTC) and the Gruppo Italiano Malattie Ematologiche Maligne dell'Adulto (GIMEMA) Leukemia Cooperative Groups. N Engl J Med 1995;332:217.

71. Cassileth PA et al. Chemotherapy compared with autologous or allogeneic bone marrow transplantation in the management of acute myeloid leukemia in first remission. N Engl J Med 1998;339:1649.

72. Harousseau JL et al. Comparison of autologous bone marrow transplantation and intensive chemotherapy as postremission therapy in adult acute myeloid leukemia. The Groupe Ouest Est Leucemies Aigues Myeloblastiques (GOELAM). Blood 1997;90:2978.

73. Burnett AK et al. Randomised comparison of addition of autologous bone-marrow transplantation to intensive chemotherapy for acute myeloid leukaemia in first remission: results of MRC AML 10 trial. UK Medical Research Council Adult and Children's Leukaemia Working Parties. Lancet 1998;351:700.

74. Slovak ML et al. Karyotypic analysis predicts outcome of preremission and postremission therapy in adult acute myeloid leukemia: a Southwest Oncology Group/Eastern Cooperative Oncology Group Study. Blood 2000;96:4075.

75. Matthews DC et al. Phase I study of (131)I-anti-CD45 antibody plus cyclophosphamide and total body irradiation for advanced acute leukemia and myelodysplastic syndrome. Blood 1999;94:1237.

76. Devine SM et al. Recent advances in allogeneic hematopoietic stem-cell transplantation. J Lab Clin Med 2003;141:7.

77. Mickelson E, Petersdorf EW. Histocompatibility. In: Thomas ED et al, eds. Hematopoietic Cell

Transplantation. Malden, MA: Blackwell Science, 1999:28.

78. Petersdorf EW et al. Major-histocompatibility-complex class I alleles and antigens in hematopoietic-cell transplantation. N Engl J Med 2001;345:1794.

79. Weisdorf DJ et al. Allogeneic bone marrow transplantation for chronic myelogenous leukemia: comparative analysis of unrelated versus matched sibling donor transplantation. Blood 2002;99:1971.

80. Anasetti C et al. Improving availability and safety of unrelated donor transplants. Curr Opin Oncol 2000;12:121.

81. Morishima Y et al. The clinical significance of human leukocyte antigen (HLA) allele compatibility in patients receiving a marrow transplant from serologically HLA-A, HLA-B, and HLA-DR matched unrelated donors. Blood 2002;99:4200.

82. Sierra J, Anasetti C. Hematopoietic transplantation from adult unrelated donors. Curr Opin Organ Transplant 2003;8:99.

83. Sniecinski I, O'Donnell MR. Hemolytic complications of hematopoietic cell transplantation. In: Thomas ED et al, eds. Hematopoietic Cell Transplantation. Malden, MA: Blackwell Science, 1999:674.

84. Siena S et al. Therapeutic relevance of CD34 cell dose in blood cell transplantation for cancer therapy. J Clin Oncol 2000;18:1360.

85. Tjonnfjord GE et al. Characterization of CD34+ peripheral blood cells from healthy adults mobilized by recombinant human granulocyte colony-stimulating factor. Blood 1994;84:2795.

86. Brown RA et al. Factors that influence the collection and engraftment of allogeneic peripheral-blood stem cells in patients with hematologic malignancies. J Clin Oncol 1997;15:3067.

87. Rowley SD et al. Experiences of donors enrolled in a randomized study of allogeneic bone marrow or peripheral blood stem cell transplantation. Blood 2001;97:2541.

88. Bittencourt H et al. Association of CD34 cell dose with hematopoietic recovery, infections, and other outcomes after HLA-identical sibling bone marrow transplantation. Blood 2002;99:2726.

89. Bolan CD et al. Controlled study of citrate effects and response to i.v. calcium administration during allogeneic peripheral blood progenitor cell donation. Transfusion 2002;42:935.

90. Guardiola P et al. Retrospective comparison of bone marrow and granulocyte colony-stimulating factor-mobilized peripheral blood progenitor cells for allogeneic stem cell transplantation using HLA identical sibling donors in myelodysplastic syndromes. Blood 2002;99:4370.

91. van Agthoven M et al. Cost analysis of HLA-identical sibling and voluntary unrelated allogeneic bone marrow and peripheral blood stem cell transplantation in adults with acute myelocytic leukaemia or acute lymphoblastic leukaemia. Bone Marrow Transplant 2002;30:243.

92. Ringden O et al. Peripheral blood stem cell transplantation from unrelated donors: a comparison with marrow transplantation. Blood 1999;94:455.

93. Remberger M et al. No difference in graft-versus-host disease, relapse, and survival comparing peripheral stem cells to bone marrow using unrelated donors. Blood 2001;98:1739.

94. Storek J et al. Immune reconstitution after allogeneic marrow transplantation compared with blood stem cell transplantation. Blood 2001;97:3380.

95. Cutler C et al. Acute and chronic graft-versus-host disease after allogeneic peripheral-blood stem-cell and bone marrow transplantation: a meta-analysis. J Clin Oncol 2001;19:3685.

96. Broxmeyer HE, Smith FO. Cord blood stem cell transplantation. In: Thomas ED et al, eds. Hematopoietic Cell Transplantation. Malden, MA: Blackwell Science, 1999:431.

97. Reed W et al. Comprehensive banking of sibling donor cord blood for children with malignant and nonmalignant disease. Blood 2003;101:351.

98. Broxmeyer HE et al. High-efficiency recovery of functional hematopoietic progenitor and stem cells from human cord blood cryopreserved for 15 years. Proc Nat Acad Sci 2003;100:645.

99. Kurtzberg J et al. Placental blood as a source of hematopoietic stem cells for transplantation into unrelated recipients. N Engl J Med 1996;335:157.

100. Rubinstein P et al. Outcomes among 562 recipients of placental-blood transplants from unrelated donors. N Engl J Med 1998;339:1565.

101. Barker JN et al. Survival after transplantation of unrelated donor umbilical cord blood is comparable to that of human leukocyte antigen-matched unrelated donor bone marrow: results of a matched-pair analysis. Blood 2001;97:2957.

102. Rocha V et al. Comparison of outcomes of unrelated bone marrow and umbilical cord blood transplants in children with acute leukemia. Blood 2001;97:2962.

103. Rocha V et al. Graft-versus-host disease in children who have received a cord-blood or bone marrow transplant from an HLA-identical sibling. Eurocord and International Bone Marrow Transplant Registry Working Committee on Alternative Donor and Stem Cell Sources. N Engl J Med 2000;342:1846.

104. Ho VT, Soiffer RJ. The history and future of T-cell depletion as graft-versus-host disease prophylaxis for allogeneic hematopoietic stem cell transplantation. Blood 2001;98:3192.

105. Powles RL et al. Mismatched family donors for bone-marrow transplantation as treatment for acute leukaemia. Lancet 1983;1:612.

106. Martin PJ et al. Graft failure in patients receiving T cell-depleted HLA-identical allogeneic marrow transplants. Bone Marrow Transplant 1988;3:445.

107. Nimer SD et al. Selective depletion of CD8+ cells for prevention of graft-versus-host disease after bone marrow transplantation. A randomized controlled trial. Transplantation 1994;57:82.

108. Drobyski WR et al. T-cell depletion plus salvage immunotherapy with donor leukocyte infusions as a strategy to treat chronic-phase chronic myelogenous leukemia patients undergoing HLA-identical sibling marrow transplantation. Blood 1999;94:434.

109. Weiden PL et al. Antileukemic effect of graft-versus-host disease in human recipients of allogeneic-marrow grafts. N Engl J Med 1979;300:1068.

110. Weiden PL et al. Antileukemic effect of chronic graft-versus-host disease: contribution to improved survival after allogeneic marrow transplantation. N Engl J Med 1981;304:1529.

111. Marmont AM et al. T-cell depletion of HLA-identical transplants in leukemia. Blood 1991;78:2120.

112. MacKinnon S. Who may benefit from donor leucocyte infusions after allogeneic stem cell transplantation? Br J Haematol 2000;110:12.

113. Childs RW. Nonmyeloablative allogeneic peripheral blood stem-cell transplantation as immunotherapy for malignant diseases. Cancer J 2000;6:179.

114. Pinkel D. Bone marrow transplantation in children. J Pediatr 1993;122:331.

115. Clift RA et al. Marrow transplantation for patients in accelerated phase of chronic myeloid leukemia. Blood 1994;84:4368.

116. Vassal G et al. Is 600 mg/m2 the appropriate dosage of busulfan in children undergoing bone marrow transplantation? Blood 1992;79:2475.

117. Socie G et al. Busulfan plus cyclophosphamide compared with total-body irradiation plus cyclophosphamide before marrow transplantation for myeloid leukemia: long-term follow-up of 4 randomized studies. Blood 2001;98:3569.

118. Balducci L, Extermann M. Cancer and aging. An evolving panorama. Hematol Oncol Clin North Am 2000;14:1.

119. Johnson PW and Orchard K. Bone marrow transplants. Br Med J 2002;325:348.

120. Slavin S et al. Nonmyeloablative stem cell transplantation and cell therapy as an alternative to conventional bone marrow transplantation with lethal cytoreduction for the treatment of malignant and nonmalignant hematologic diseases. Blood 1998;91:756.

121. Bryant E, Martin PJ. Documentation of engraftment and characterization of chimerism following hematopoietic cell transplantation. In: Thomas ED et al, eds. Hematopoietic Cell Transplantation. Malden, MA: Blackwell Science, 1999:197.

122. Childs R et al. Engraftment kinetics after nonmyeloablative allogeneic peripheral blood stem cell transplantation: full donor T-cell chimerism precedes alloimmune response. Blood 1999;94:3234.

123. Champlin R et al. Nonmyeloablative preparative regimens for allogeneic hematopoietic transplantation. Biology and current indications. Oncology (Huntingt) 2003;17:94.

124. Childs R et al. Regression of metastatic renal-cell carcinoma after nonmyeloablative allogeneic peripheral-blood stem-cell transplantation. N Engl J Med 2000;343:750.

125. Nagler A et al. Allogeneic peripheral blood stem cell transplantation using a fludarabine-based low intensity conditioning regimen for malignant lymphoma. Bone Marrow Transplant 2000;25:1021.

126. Fukuda T et al. Risks and outcomes of invasive fungal infections in recipients of allogeneic hematopoietic stem cell transplants after nonmyeloablative conditioning. Blood 2003;102:827.

127. Junghanss C et al. Incidence and outcome of bacterial and fungal infections following nonmyeloablative compared with myeloablative allogeneic hematopoietic stem cell transplantation: a matched control study. Biol Blood Marrow Transplant 2002;8:512.

128. Niederwieser D et al. Low-dose total body irradiation (TBI) and fludarabine followed by hematopoietic cell transplantation (HCT) from HLA-matched or mismatched unrelated donors and postgrafting immunosuppression with cyclosporine and mycophenolate mofetil (MMF) can induce durable complete chimerism and sustained remissions in patients with hematological diseases. Blood 2003;101:1620.

129. Horowitz MM et al. Graft-versus-leukemia reactions after bone marrow transplantation. Blood 1990;75:555.

130. Storb R. Mixed allogeneic chimerism and graft-versus-leukemia effects in acute myeloid leukemia. Leukemia 2002;16:753.

131. Michallet M et al. Allogeneic hematopoietic stem-cell transplantation after nonmyeloablative preparative regimens: impact of pretransplantation and posttransplantation factors on outcome. J Clin Oncol 2001;19:3340.

132. Maris M et al. Nonmyeloablative hematopoietic stem cell transplants using 10 HLA antigen matched unrelated donors for patients with advanced hematologic malignancies. American Society of Hematology 2002;100;275a.

133. Martin PJ et al. Effects of in vitro depletion of T cells in HLA-identical allogeneic marrow grafts. Blood 1985;66:664.

134. Nash RA et al. Phase 3 study comparing methotrexate and tacrolimus with methotrexate and cyclosporine for prophylaxis of acute graft-versus-host disease after marrow transplantation from unrelated donors. Blood 2000;96:2062.

135. Wingard JR. Infections in allogeneic bone marrow transplant recipients. Semin Oncol 1993;20:80.

136. Kasai M et al. Toxicity of high-dose busulfan and cyclophosphamide as a preparative regimen for bone marrow transplantation. Transplant Proc 1992;24:1529.

137. Schuler U et al. Busulfan pharmacokinetics in bone marrow transplant patients: is drug monitoring warranted? Bone Marrow Transplant 1994;14:759.

138. Gibbs JP et al. The impact of obesity and disease on busulfan oral clearance in adults. Blood 1999;93:4436.

139. Vassal G et al. Dose-dependent neurotoxicity of high-dose busulfan in children: a clinical and pharmacological study. Cancer Res 1990;50:6203.

140. Grigg AP et al. Busulphan and phenytoin. Ann Intern Med 1989;111:1049.

141. Vassal G et al. Pharmacokinetics of high-dose busulfan in children. Cancer Chemother Pharmacol 1989;24:386.

142. Tran HT et al. Individualizing high-dose oral busulfan: prospective dose adjustment in a pediatric population undergoing allogeneic stem cell transplantation for advanced hematologic malignancies. Bone Marrow Transplant 2000;26:463.

143. Busulfex Product Information 1999.

144. Gibbs JP et al. Age-dependent tetrahydrothiophenium ion formation in young children and adults receiving high-dose busulfan. Cancer Res 1997;57:5509.

145. Dix SP et al. Association of busulfan area under the curve with veno-occlusive disease following BMT. Bone Marrow Transplant 1996;17:225.

146. Bolinger AM et al. Target dose adjustment of busulfan using pharmacokinetic parameters in pediatric patients undergoing bone marrow transplantation for malignancy or inborn errors. Blood 1997;90:374a.

147. Radich JP et al. HLA-matched related hematopoietic cell transplantation for CML chronic phase using a targeted busulfan and cyclophosphamide preparative regimen. Blood 2003;

148. McCune JS et al. Plasma concentration monitoring of busulfan: does it improve clinical outcome? Clin Pharmacokinet 2000;39:155.

149. Slattery JT, Risler LJ. Therapeutic monitoring of busulfan in hematopoietic stem cell transplantation. Ther Drug Monit 1998;20:543.

150. Grochow LB. Parenteral busulfan: is therapeutic monitoring still warranted? Biol Blood Marrow Transplant 2002;8:465.

151. Shepherd JD et al. Mesna versus hyperhydration for the prevention of cyclophosphamide-induced hemorrhagic cystitis in bone marrow transplantation. J Clin Oncol 1991;9:2016.

152. Cox PJ. Cyclophosphamide cystitis—Identification of acrolein as the causative agent. Biochem Pharmacol 1979;28:2045.

153. Hensley ML et al. American Society of Clinical Oncology clinical practice guidelines for the use of chemotherapy and radiotherapy protectants. J Clin Oncol 1999;17:3333.

154. Hows JM et al. Comparison of mesna with forced diuresis to prevent cyclophosphamide induced haemorrhagic cystitis in marrow transplantation: a prospective randomised study. Br J Cancer 1984;50:753.

155. Vose JM et al. Mesna compared with continuous bladder irrigation as uroprotection during high-dose chemotherapy and transplantation: a randomized trial. J Clin Oncol 1993;11:1306.

156. James CA et al. Pharmacokinetics of intravenous and oral sodium 2-mercaptoethane sulphonate (mesna) in normal subjects. Br J Clin Pharmacol 1987;23:561.

157. Ren S et al. Pharmacokinetics of cyclophosphamide and its metabolites in bone marrow transplantation patients. Clin Pharmacol Ther 1998;64:289.

158. Fleming RA et al. Urinary elimination of cyclophosphamide alkylating metabolites and free thiols following two administration schedules of high-dose cyclophosphamide and mesna. Bone Marrow Transplant 1996;17:497.

159. Cohen EP. Renal failure after bone-marrow transplantation. Lancet 2001;357:6.

160. Bilgrami SF et al. Idiopathic pneumonia syndrome following myeloablative chemotherapy and autologous transplantation. Ann Pharmacother 2001;35:196.

161. Gralla RJ et al. Recommendations for the use of antiemetics: evidence-based, clinical practice guidelines. American Society of Clinical Oncology [published erratum appears in J Clin Oncol 1999 Dec;17(12):3860]. J Clin Oncol 1999;17:2971.

162. Perez EA et al. Antiemetic therapy for high-dose chemotherapy with transplantation: report of a retrospective analysis of a 5-HT(3) regimen and literature review. Support Care Cancer 1999;7:413.

163. Gilbert CJ et al. Pharmacokinetic interaction between ondansetron and cyclophosphamide during high-dose chemotherapy for breast cancer. Cancer Chemother Pharmacol 1998;42:497.

164. Cagnoni PJ et al. Modification of the pharmacokinetics of high-dose cyclophosphamide and cisplatin by antiemetics. Bone Marrow Transplant 1999;24:1.

165. McCune JS, Slattery JT. Pharmacological Considerations of Primary Alkylators. In: Andersson B, Murray D, eds. Clinically Relevant Resistance in Cancer Chemotherapy. Boston: Kluwer Academic Publishers, 2002:323.

166. McDonald GB et al. Cyclophosphamide metabolism, liver toxicity, and mortality following hematopoietic stem cell transplantation. Blood 2003;101:2043.

167. Weiger WA et al. Advising patients who seek complementary and alternative medical therapies for cancer. Ann Intern Med 2002;137:889.

168. Stiff P. Mucositis associated with stem cell transplantation: current status and innovative approaches to management. Bone Marrow Transplant 2001;27(Suppl 2):S3.

169. Nemunaitis J et al. Phase III randomized, double-blind placebo-controlled trial of rhGM-CSF following allogeneic bone marrow transplantation. Bone Marrow Transplant 1995;15:949.

170. Lee SJ et al. Efficacy and costs of granulocyte colony-stimulating factor in allogeneic T-cell depleted bone marrow transplantation. Blood 1998;92:2725.

171. Zander AR et al. High dose cyclophosphamide, BCNU, and VP-16 (CBV) as a conditioning regimen for allogeneic bone marrow transplantation for patients with acute leukemia. Cancer 1987;59:1083.

172. Masaoka T et al. Recombinant human granulocyte colony-stimulating factor in allogeneic bone marrow transplantation. Exp Hematol 1989;17:1047.

173. Nemunaitis J et al. Phase I/II trial of recombinant human granulocyte-macrophage colony-stimulating factor following allogeneic bone marrow transplantation. Blood 1991;77:2065.

174. Nemunaitis J et al. rhGM-CSF after allogeneic bone marrow transplantation from unrelated donors: a pilot study of cyclosporine and prednisone as graft-versus-host disease prophylaxis. Leuk Lymphoma 1993;10:177.

175. Volpi I et al. Postgrafting administration of granulocyte colony-stimulating factor impairs functional immune recovery in recipients of human leukocyte antigen haplotype-mismatched hematopoietic transplants. Blood 2001;97:2514.

176. Bishop MR et al. A randomized, double-blind trial of filgrastim (granulocyte colony-stimulating factor) versus placebo following allogeneic blood stem cell transplantation. Blood 2000;96:80.

177. Przepiorka D et al. Controlled trial of filgrastim for acceleration of neutrophil recovery after allogeneic blood stem cell transplantation from human leukocyte antigen-matched related donors. Blood 2001;97:3405.

178. Horn B et al. Veno-occlusive disease of the liver in children with solid tumors undergoing autologous hematopoietic progenitor cell transplantation: a high incidence in patients with neuroblastoma. Bone Marrow Transplant 2002;29:409.

179. McDonald GB et al. Veno-occlusive disease of the liver and multiorgan failure after bone marrow transplantation: a cohort study of 355 patients. Ann Intern Med 1993;118:255.

180. Strasser SI, McDonald GB. Gastrointestinal and hepatic complications. In: Thomas ED et al, eds. Hematopoietic Cell Transplantation. Malden, MA: Blackwell Science, 1999:627.

181. DeLeve LD et al. Toxic injury to hepatic sinusoids: sinusoidal obstruction syndrome (veno-occlusive disease). Semin Liver Dis 2002;22:27.

182. Jones RJ et al. Venoocclusive disease of the liver following bone marrow transplantation. Transplantation 1987;44:778.

183. Bearman SI et al. Venoocclusive disease of the liver: development of a model for predicting fatal outcome after marrow transplantation. J Clin Oncol 1993;11:1729.

184. Sullivan KM et al. Intravenous immunoglobulin and the risk of hepatic veno-occlusive disease after bone marrow transplantation. Biol Blood Marrow Transplant 1998;4:20.

185. Slattery JT et al. Conditioning regimen-dependent disposition of cyclophosphamide and hydroxycyclophosphamide in human marrow transplantation patients. J Clin Oncol 1996;14:1484.

186. Kashyap A et al. Intravenous versus oral busulfan as part of a busulfan/cyclophosphamide preparative regimen for allogeneic hematopoietic stem cell transplantation: decreased incidence of hepatic venoocclusive disease (HVOD), HVOD-related mortality, and overall 100-day mortality. Biol Blood Marrow Transplant 2002;8:493.

187. Lee JH et al. Plasminogen activator inhibitor-1 is an independent diagnostic marker as well as severity predictor of hepatic veno-occlusive disease after allogeneic bone marrow transplantation in adults conditioned with busulphan and cyclophosphamide. Br J Haematol 2002;118:1087.

188. Clift RA et al. A randomized controlled trial of pentoxifylline for the prevention of regimen-related toxicities in patients undergoing allogeneic marrow transplantation. Blood 1993;82:2025.

189. Holler E et al. Increased serum levels of tumor necrosis factor alpha precede major complications of bone marrow transplantation. Blood 1990;75:1011.

190. Bearman SI et al. A phase I/II study of prostaglandin E1 for the prevention of hepatic venocclusive disease after bone marrow transplantation. Br J Haematol 1993;84:724.

191. Park SH et al. A randomized trial of heparin plus ursodiol vs. heparin alone to prevent hepatic veno-occlusive disease after hematopoietic stem cell transplantation. Bone Marrow Transplant 2002;29:137.

192. Arai S et al. A systematic approach to hepatic complications in hematopoietic stem cell transplantation. J Hematother Stem Cell Res 2002;11:215.

193. Essell JH et al. Ursodiol prophylaxis against hepatic complications of allogeneic bone marrow transplantation. A randomized, double-blind, placebo-controlled trial. Ann Intern Med 1998;128:975.

194. Ohashi K et al. The Japanese multicenter open randomized trial of ursodeoxycholic acid prophylaxis for hepatic veno-occlusive disease after stem cell transplantation. Am J Hematol 2000;64:32.

195. Ruutu T et al. Ursodeoxycholic acid for the prevention of hepatic complications in allogeneic stem cell transplantation. Blood 2002;100:1977.

196. Bearman SI et al. Treatment of hepatic venocclusive disease with recombinant human tissue plasminogen activator and heparin in 42 marrow transplant patients. Blood 1997;89:1501.

197. Richardson PG et al. Treatment of severe veno-occlusive disease with defibrotide: compassionate use results in response without significant toxicity in a high-risk population. Blood 1998;92:737.

198. Chopra R et al. Defibrotide for the treatment of hepatic veno-occlusive disease: results of the European compassionate-use study. Br J Haematol 2000;111:1122.

199. Richardson PG et al. Multi-institutional use of defibrotide in 88 patients after stem cell transplantation with severe veno-occlusive disease and multisystem organ failure: response without significant toxicity in a high-risk population and factors predictive of outcome. Blood 2002;100:4337.

200. Wolff SN. Second hematopoietic stem cell transplantation for the treatment of graft failure, graft rejection or relapse after allogeneic transplantation. Bone Marrow Transplant 2002;29:545.

201. Nemunaitis J et al. Use of recombinant human granulocyte-macrophage colony-stimulating factor in graft failure after bone marrow transplantation. Blood 1990;76:245.

202. Vose JM et al. The use of recombinant human granulocyte-macrophage colony stimulating factor for the treatment of delayed engraftment following high dose therapy and autologous hematopoietic stem cell transplantation for lymphoid malignancies. Bone Marrow Transplant 1991;7:139.

203. Tabbara IA et al. Allogeneic hematopoietic stem cell transplantation: complications and results. Arch Intern Med 2002;162:1558.

204. Goker H et al. Acute graft-vs-host disease: pathobiology and management. Exp Hematol 2001;29:259.

205. Beatty PG et al. Marrow transplantation from related donors other than HLA-identical siblings. N Engl J Med 1985;313:765.

206. Wu D et al. Persistent nausea and anorexia after marrow transplantation: a prospective study of 78 patients. Transplantation 1998;66:1319.

207. Weiden PL et al. Anti-human thymocyte globulin (ATG) for prophylaxis and treatment of graft-versus-host disease in recipients of allogeneic marrow grafts. Transplant Proc 1978;10:213.

208. Deeg HJ et al. Cyclosporine as prophylaxis for graft-versus-host disease: a randomized study in patients undergoing marrow transplantation for acute nonlymphoblastic leukemia. Blood 1985; 65:1325.

209. Storb R et al. Methotrexate and cyclosporine compared with cyclosporine alone for prophylaxis of acute graft versus host disease after marrow transplantation for leukemia. N Engl J Med 1986; 314:729.

210. Ramsay NK et al. A randomized study of the prevention of acute graft-versus-host disease. N Engl J Med 1982;306:392.

211. Storb R et al. Methotrexate and cyclosporine versus cyclosporine alone for prophylaxis of graft-versus-host disease in patients given HLA-identical marrow grafts for leukemia: long-term follow-up of a controlled trial. Blood 1989;73:1729.

212. Sullivan KM et al. Graft-versus-host disease as adoptive immunotherapy in patients with advanced hematologic neoplasms. N Engl J Med 1989;320:828.

213. Ratanatharathorn V et al. Phase III study comparing methotrexate and tacrolimus (prograf, FK506) with methotrexate and cyclosporine for graft-versus-host disease prophylaxis after HLA-identical sibling bone marrow transplantation. Blood 1998;92:2303.

214. Horowitz MM et al. Tacrolimus vs. cyclosporine immunosuppression: results in advanced-stage disease compared with historical controls treated exclusively with cyclosporine. Biol Blood Marrow Transplant 1999;5:180.

215. Chao NJ et al. Cyclosporine, methotrexate, and prednisone compared with cyclosporine and prednisone for prophylaxis of acute graft-versus-host disease. N Engl J Med 1993;329:1225.

216. Bacigalupo A et al. Prophylactic antithymocyte globulin reduces the risk of chronic graft-versus-host disease in alternative-donor bone marrow transplants. Biol Blood Marrow Transplant 2002; 8:656.

217. Storb R et al. Marrow transplantation for chronic myelocytic leukemia: a controlled trial of cyclosporine versus methotrexate for prophylaxis of graft-versus-host disease. Blood 1985;66:698.

218. Schultz KR et al. Effect of gastrointestinal inflammation and age on the pharmacokinetics of oral microemulsion cyclosporin A in the first month after bone marrow transplantation. Bone Marrow Transplant 2000;26:545.

219. Trotter JF. Drugs that interact with immunosuppressive agents. Semin Gastrointest Dis 1998;9:147.

220. Storb R et al. What role for prednisone in prevention of acute graft-versus-host disease in patients undergoing marrow transplants? Blood 1990;76: 1037.

221. Yee GC et al. Serum cyclosporine concentration and risk of acute graft-versus-host disease after allogeneic marrow transplantation. N Engl J Med 1988;319:65.

222. Schmidt H et al. Correlation between low CSA plasma concentration and severity of acute GvHD in bone marrow transplantation. Blut 1988;57:139.

223. Hows JM et al. Use of cyclosporin A in allogeneic bone marrow transplantation for severe aplastic anemia. Transplantation 1982;33:382.

224. Wingard JR et al. Relationship of tacrolimus (FK506) whole blood concentrations and efficacy and safety after HLA-identical sibling bone marrow transplantation. Biol Blood Marrow Transplant 1998;4:157.

225. Przepiorka D et al. Relationship of tacrolimus whole blood levels to efficacy and safety outcomes after unrelated donor marrow transplantation. Biol Blood Marrow Transplant 1999;5:94.

226. Winston DJ et al. Intravenous immune globulin for prevention of cytomegalovirus infection and interstitial pneumonia after bone marrow transplantation. Ann Intern Med 1987;106:12.

227. Sullivan KM et al. Immunomodulatory and antimicrobial efficacy of intravenous immunoglobulin in bone marrow transplantation. N Engl J Med 1990;323:705.

228. Sullivan KM et al. A controlled trial of long-term administration of intravenous immunoglobulin to prevent late infection and chronic graft-vs.-host disease after marrow transplantation: clinical outcome and effect on subsequent immune recovery. Biol Blood Marrow Transplant 1996;2:44.

229. Attal M et al. Prevention of regimen-related toxicities after bone marrow transplantation by pentoxifylline: a prospective, randomized trial. Blood 1993;82:732.

230. Basara N et al. Mycophenolate mofetil for the prophylaxis of acute GVHD in HLA-mismatched bone marrow transplant patients. Clin Transplant 2000;14:121.

231. Simpson D. Drug therapy for acute graft-versus-host disease prophylaxis. J Hematother Stem Cell Res 2000;9:317.

232. Lazarus HM et al. Prevention and treatment of acute graft-versus-host disease: the old and the new. A report from the Eastern Cooperative Oncology Group (ECOG). Bone Marrow Transplant 1997;19:577.

233. Deeg HJ et al. Treatment of human acute graft-versus-host disease with antithymocyte globulin and cyclosporine with or without methylprednisolone. Transplantation 1985;40:162.

234. Van Lint MT et al. Early treatment of acute graft-versus-host disease with high- or low-dose 6-methylprednisolone: a multicenter randomized trial from the Italian Group for Bone Marrow Transplantation. Blood 1998;92:2288.

235. Neudorf S et al. Prevention and treatment of acute graft-versus-host disease. Semin Hematol 1984; 21:91.

236. Gratama JW et al. Treatment of acute graft-versus-host disease with monoclonal antibody OKT3. Clinical results and effect on circulating T lymphocytes. Transplantation 1984;38:469.

237. Weisdorf D et al. Treatment of moderate/severe acute graft-versus-host disease after allogeneic bone marrow transplantation: an analysis of clinical risk features and outcome. Blood 1990;75:1024.

238. Massenkeil G et al. Basiliximab is well tolerated and effective in the treatment of steroid-refractory acute graft-versus-host disease after allogeneic stem cell transplantation. Bone Marrow Transplant 2002;30:899.

239. Kobbe G et al. Treatment of severe steroid refractory acute graft-versus-host disease with infliximab, a chimeric human/mouse antiTNFalpha antibody. Bone Marrow Transplant 2001;28:47.

240. Carpenter PA et al. A humanized non-FcR-binding anti-CD3 antibody, visilizumab, for treatment of steroid-refractory acute graft-versus-host disease. Blood 2002;99:2712.

241. Greinix HT et al. Extracorporeal photochemotherapy in the treatment of severe graft-versus-host disease. Leuk Lymphoma 2000;36:425.

242. Remberger M et al. Risk factors for moderate-to-severe chronic graft-versus-host disease after allogeneic hematopoietic stem cell transplantation. Biol Blood Marrow Transplant 2002;8:674.

243. Beatty PG et al. Marrow transplantation from HLA-matched unrelated donors for treatment of hematologic malignancies. Transplantation 1991; 51:443.

244. Ratanatharathorn V et al. Chronic graft-versus-host disease: clinical manifestation and therapy. Bone Marrow Transplant 2001;28:121.

245. Zecca M et al. Chronic graft-versus-host disease in children: incidence, risk factors, and impact on outcome. Blood 2002;100:1192.

246. Wagner JL et al. The development of chronic graft-versus-host disease: an analysis of screening studies and the impact of corticosteroid use at 100 days after transplantation. Bone Marrow Transplant 1998;22:139.

247. Shulman HM et al. Chronic graft-versus-host syndrome in man. A long-term clinicopathologic study of 20 Seattle patients. Am J Med 1980; 69:204.

248. Sullivan KM et al. Chronic graft-versus-host disease in 52 patients: adverse natural course and successful treatment with combination immunosuppression. Blood 1981;57:267.

249. Wingard JR et al. Predictors of death from chronic graft-versus-host disease after bone marrow transplantation. Blood 1989;74:1428.

250. Storb R et al. Methotrexate and cyclosporine for graft-vs.-host disease prevention: what length of therapy with cyclosporine? Biol Blood Marrow Transplant 1997;3:194.

251. Kansu E et al. Administration of cyclosporine for 24 months compared with 6 months for prevention of chronic graft-versus-host disease: a prospective randomized clinical trial. Blood 2001;98:3868.

252. Sullivan KM et al. Prednisone and azathioprine compared with prednisone and placebo for treatment of chronic graft-v-host disease: prognostic influence of prolonged thrombocytopenia after allogeneic marrow transplantation. Blood 1988; 72:546.

253. Koc S et al. Therapy for chronic graft-versus-host disease: a randomized trial comparing cyclosporine plus prednisone versus prednisone alone. Blood 2002;100:48.

254. Vogelsang GB et al. Thalidomide for the treatment of chronic graft-versus-host disease. N Engl J Med 1992;326:1055.

255. Arora M et al. Randomized clinical trial of thalidomide, cyclosporine, and prednisone versus cyclosporine and prednisone as initial therapy for chronic graft-versus-host disease. Biol Blood Marrow Transplant 2001;7:265.

256. Koc S et al. Thalidomide for treatment of patients with chronic graft-versus-host disease. Blood 2000;96:3995.

257. Vogelsang GB. How I treat chronic graft-versus-host disease. Blood 2001;97:1196.

258. Stern JM et al. Bone density loss during treatment of chronic GVHD. Bone Marrow Transplant 1996;17:395.

259. Bowden RA. Respiratory virus infections after marrow transplant: the Fred Hutchinson Cancer Research Center experience. Am J Med 1997;102:27.

260. Engels EA et al. Efficacy of quinolone prophylaxis in neutropenic cancer patients: a meta-analysis. J Clin Oncol 1998;16:1179.

261. Tunkel AR, Sepkowitz KA. Infections caused by viridans streptococci in patients with neutropenia. Clin Infect Dis 2002;34:1524.

262. Hughes WT et al 2002 guidelines for the use of antimicrobial agents in neutropenic patients with cancer. Clin Infect Dis 2002;34:730.

263. Goodman JL et al. A controlled trial of fluconazole to prevent fungal infections in patients undergoing bone marrow transplantation. N Engl J Med 1992;326:845.

264. Slavin MA et al. Efficacy and safety of fluconazole prophylaxis for fungal infections after marrow transplantation: a prospective, randomized, double-blind study. J Infect Dis 1995;171:1545.

265. Marr KA et al. Epidemiology and outcome of mould infections in hematopoietic stem cell transplant recipients. Clin Infect Dis 2002;34:909.

266. Cornely OA et al. Evidence-based assessment of primary antifungal prophylaxis in patients with hematologic malignancies. Blood 2003;101:3365.

267. Winston DJ et al. Intravenous and oral itraconazole versus intravenous and oral fluconazole for long-term antifungal prophylaxis in allogeneic hematopoietic stem-cell transplant recipients. A multicenter, randomized trial. Ann Intern Med 2003;138:705.

268. Saral R et al. Acyclovir prophylaxis of herpes-simplex-virus infections. N Engl J Med 1981; 305:63.

269. Selby PJ et al. The prophylactic role of intravenous and long-term oral acyclovir after allogeneic bone marrow transplantation. Br J Cancer 1989;59:434.

270. Ljungman P. Prevention and treatment of viral infections in stem cell transplant recipients. Br J Haematol 2002;118:44.

271. Vusirikala M et al. Valacyclovir for the prevention of cytomegalovirus infection after allogeneic stem cell transplantation: a single institution retrospective cohort analysis. Bone Marrow Transplant 2001;28:265.

272. Dignani MC et al. Valacyclovir prophylaxis for the prevention of Herpes simplex virus reactivation in recipients of progenitor cells transplantation. Bone Marrow Transplant 2002;29:263.

273. Steer CB et al. Varicella-zoster infection after allogeneic bone marrow transplantation: incidence, risk factors and prevention with low-dose aciclovir and ganciclovir. Bone Marrow Transplant 2000;25:657.

274. Holmberg LA et al. Increased incidence of cytomegalovirus disease after autologous CD34-selected peripheral blood stem cell transplantation. Blood 1999;94:4029.

275. Bass EB et al. Efficacy of immune globulin in preventing complications of bone marrow transplantation: a meta-analysis. Bone Marrow Transplant 1993;12:273.

276. Goodrich JM et al. Ganciclovir prophylaxis to prevent cytomegalovirus disease after allogeneic marrow transplant. Ann Intern Med 1993;118:173.

277. Boeckh M et al. Cytomegalovirus pp65 antigenemia-guided early treatment with ganciclovir versus ganciclovir at engraftment after allogeneic marrow transplantation: a randomized double-blind study. Blood 1996;88:4063.

278. Zaia JA. Prevention of cytomegalovirus disease in hematopoietic stem cell transplantation. Clin Infect Dis 2002;35:999.

279. Boeckh M et al. Plasma polymerase chain reaction for cytomegalovirus DNA after allogeneic marrow transplantation: comparison with polymerase chain reaction using peripheral blood leukocytes, pp65 antigenemia, and viral culture. Transplantation 1997;64:108.

280. St George K et al. A multisite trial comparing two cytomegalovirus (CMV) pp65 antigenemia test kits, biotest CMV brite and Bartels/Argene CMV antigenemia. J Clin Microbiol 2000;38:1430.

281. Nichols WG et al. High risk of death due to bacterial and fungal infection among cytomegalovirus (CMV)-seronegative recipients of stem cell transplants from seropositive donors: evidence for indirect effects of primary CMV infection. J Infect Dis 2002;185:273.

282. Boeckh M et al. Successful modification of a pp65 antigenemia-based early treatment strategy for prevention of cytomegalovirus disease in allogeneic marrow transplant recipients. Blood 1999;93:1781.

283. Schmidt GM et al. A randomized, controlled trial of prophylactic ganciclovir for cytomegalovirus pulmonary infection in recipients of allogeneic bone marrow transplants: The City of Hope-Stanford-Syntex CMV Study Group. N Engl J Med 1991;324:1005.

284. Goodrich JM et al. Early treatment with ganciclovir to prevent cytomegalovirus disease after allogeneic bone marrow transplantation. N Engl J Med 1991;325:1601.

285. Ljungman P et al. Results of different strategies for reducing cytomegalovirus-associated mortality in allogeneic stem cell transplant recipients. Transplantation 1998;66:1330.

286. Reusser P et al. Randomized multicenter trial of foscarnet versus ganciclovir for preemptive therapy of cytomegalovirus infection after allogeneic stem cell transplantation. Blood 2002;99:1159.

287. Winston DJ et al. Randomized comparison of oral valacyclovir and intravenous ganciclovir for prevention of cytomegalovirus disease after allogeneic bone marrow transplantation. Clin Infect Dis 2003;36:749.

288. Junghanss C et al. Incidence and outcome of cytomegalovirus infections following nonmyeloablative compared with myeloablative allogeneic stem cell transplantation, a matched control study. Blood 2002;99:1978.

289. Mohty M et al. High rate of secondary viral and bacterial infections in patients undergoing allogeneic bone marrow mini-transplantation. Bone Marrow Transplant 2000;26:251.

290. Marr KA et al. Invasive aspergillosis in allogeneic stem cell transplant recipients: changes in epidemiology and risk factors. Blood 2002;100:4358.

291. De La Rosa GR et al. Risk factors for the development of invasive fungal infections in allogeneic blood and marrow transplant recipients. Transpl Infect Dis 2002;4:3.

292. Clark RA et al. Defective neutrophil chemotaxis in bone marrow transplant patients. J Clin Invest 1976;58:22.

293. Wingard JR et al. Increase in *Candida krusei* infection among patients with bone marrow transplantation and neutropenia treated prophylactically with fluconazole. N Engl J Med 1991; 325:1274.

294. Wingard JR et al. Association of *Torulopsis glabrata* infections with fluconazole prophylaxis in neutropenic bone marrow transplant patients. Antimicrob Agents Chemother 1993;37:1847.

295. Patterson TF et al. Invasive aspergillosis. Disease spectrum, treatment practices, and outcomes. I3 Aspergillus Study Group. Medicine (Baltimore) 2000;79:250.

296. Soubani AO, Chandrasekar PH. The clinical spectrum of pulmonary aspergillosis. Chest 2002;121: 1988.

297. Ascioglu S et al. Defining opportunistic invasive fungal infections in immunocompromised patients with cancer and hematopoietic stem cell transplants: an international consensus. Clin Infect Dis 2002;34:7.

298. Kretschmar M et al. Galactomannan enzyme immunoassay for monitoring systemic infection with Aspergillus fumigatus in mice. Diagn Microbiol Infect Dis 2001;41:107.

299. Raad I et al. Polymerase chain reaction on blood for the diagnosis of invasive pulmonary aspergillosis in cancer patients. Cancer 2002;94:1032.

300. Platelia B-R. *Aspergillus* EIA package insert 2003.

301. Maertens J et al. Use of circulating galactomannan screening for early diagnosis of invasive aspergillosis in allogeneic stem cell transplant recipients. J Infect Dis 2002;186:1297.

302. Marr KA et al. Aspergillosis. Pathogenesis, clinical manifestations, and therapy. Infect Dis Clin North Am 2002;16:875.

303. Quilitz RE et al. Practice guidelines for lipid-based amphotericin B in stem cell transplant recipients. Ann Pharmacother 2001;35:206.

304. Prentice HG et al. A randomized comparison of liposomal versus conventional amphotericin B for the treatment of pyrexia of unknown origin in neutropenic patients. Br J Haematol 1997;98:711.

305. Wingard JR et al. A randomized, double-blind comparative trial evaluating the safety of liposomal amphotericin B versus amphotericin B lipid complex in the empirical treatment of febrile neutropenia. L Amph/ABLC Collaborative Study Group. Clin Infect Dis 2000;31:1155.

306. Cagnoni PJ. Liposomal amphotericin B versus conventional amphotericin B in the empirical treatment of persistently febrile neutropenic patients. J Antimicrob Chemother 2002;49(Suppl 1):81.

307. Stevens DA, Lee JY. Analysis of compassionate use itraconazole therapy for invasive aspergillosis by the NIAID Mycoses Study Group criteria. Arch Intern Med 1997;157:1857.

308. Herbrecht R et al. Voriconazole versus amphotericin B for primary therapy of invasive aspergillosis. N Engl J Med 2002;347:408.

309. Stone EA et al. Caspofungin: an echinocandin antifungal agent. Clin Ther 2002;24:351.

310. Luber AD et al. Risk factors for amphotericin B-induced nephrotoxicity. J Antimicrob Chemother 1999;43:267.

311. Harbarth S et al. The epidemiology of nephrotoxicity associated with conventional amphotericin B therapy. Am J Med 2001;111:528.

312. Walsh TJ et al. Amphotericin B lipid complex for invasive fungal infections: analysis of safety and efficacy in 556 cases. Clin Infect Dis 1998;26:1383.

313. White MH et al. Amphotericin B colloidal dispersion vs. amphotericin B as therapy for invasive aspergillosis. Clin Infect Dis 1997;24:635.

314. Wingard JR. Efficacy of amphotericin B lipid complex injection (ABLC) in bone marrow transplant recipients with life-threatening systemic mycoses. Bone Marrow Transplant 1997;19:343.

315. Walsh TJ et al. Voriconazole compared with liposomal amphotericin B for empirical antifungal therapy in patients with neutropenia and persistent fever. N Engl J Med 2002;346:225.

316. Denning DW et al. Efficacy and safety of voriconazole in the treatment of acute invasive aspergillosis. Clin Infect Dis 2002;34:563.

317. Perea S et al. In vitro interaction of caspofungin acetate with voriconazole against clinical isolates of *Aspergillus* spp. Antimicrob Agents Chemother 2002;46:3039.

318. Lewis RE, Kontoyiannis DP. Rationale for combination antifungal therapy. Pharmacotherapy 2001;21:149S.

319. Kiss TL et al. Long-term medical outcomes and quality-of-life assessment of patients with chronic myeloid leukemia followed at least 10 years after allogeneic bone marrow transplantation. J Clin Oncol 2002;20.2334.

320. Antin JH. Clinical practice. Long-term care after hematopoietic-cell transplantation in adults. N Engl J Med 2002,347.36.

321. Thomas ED. Does bone marrow transplantation confer a normal life span? N Engl J Med 1999;341:50.

322. Goldberg SL et al. Vaccinations against infectious diseases in hematopoietic stem cell transplant recipients. Oncology (Huntingt) 2003;17:539.

323. Kolb HJ et al. Malignant neoplasms in long-term survivors of bone marrow transplantation. Late Effects Working Party of the European Cooperative Group for Blood and Marrow Transplantation and the European Late Effect Project Group. Ann Intern Med 1999;131:738.

324. Socie G et al. Nonmalignant late effects after allogeneic stem cell transplantation. Blood 2003;101: 3373.

325. Strasser SI, McDonald GB. Hepatitis viruses and hematopoietic cell transplantation: a guide to patient and donor management. Blood 1999;93:1127.

326. Lennard AL, Jackson GH. Stem cell transplantation. Bmj 2000;321:433.

327. Storb R et al. Allogeneic marrow grafting for treatment of aplastic anemia. Blood 1974;43:157.

328. Giralt S et al. Melphalan and purine analog-containing preparative regimens: reduced-intensity conditioning for patients with hematologic malignancies undergoing allogeneic progenitor cell transplantation. Blood 2001;97:631.

329. Atkinson K et al. Consensus among bone marrow transplanters for diagnosis, grading and treatment of chronic graft-versus-host disease. Committee of the International Bone Marrow Transplant Registry. Bone Marrow Transplant 1989;4:247.

Pediatric Considerations

Sherry Luedtke, Mark Haase, Michelle Condren

MEDICATION ADMINISTRATION ISSUES IN CHILDREN

Children represent >25% of the population and receive an average of three prescription medications before 5 years of age. Establishing safe and effective therapeutic regimens for children is challenging due to the lack of FDA indications and dosing guidelines for this population, limited evidence based medicine, and the lack of appropriate dosage formulations. It is estimated that 60% of drugs do not have approval by the Food and Drug Administration (FDA) for use in children, and even fewer have approval for use in infants. Although most of our current laws governing FDA approval of drugs are the result of pediatric tragedies (e.g., thalidomide, sulfanilamide), it was not until the 1990s that legislation was considered to encourage research in pediatrics. In 1994 manufacturers were asked to evaluate available pediatric data and if possible, seek a labeling change. If data were not available, the drug labeling was required to state that "safety and effectiveness in pediatric patients have not been established." This voluntary approach failed to produce a significant increase in drugs with pediatric labeling. As a result, the Rule was revised. The 1998 FDA Pediatric Rule *required* new drugs and biologicals to be studied in children. While the Pediatric Rule was under discussion, the FDA Modernization Act of 1997 (FDAMA) was enacted. FDAMA provided a 6-month patent extension as an incentive for manufacturers to conduct pediatric research. The Best Pharmaceuticals for Children Act (BPCA), approved in January 2002, reauthorizes FDAMA through 2007 and also allows the FDA to request studies of a selected list of already marketed drugs. The role the FDA has taken to encourage manufacturers to pursue pediatric labeling is not without controversy. The Pediatric Rule was contested and overthrown in October 2002 when it was concluded that the FDA did not have the authority to enforce the rule. BCPA remains in effect and plans are underway to pass legislation that would give the FDA authority to enforce the Pediatric Rule. While some manufacturers will take advantage of the BCPA incentive program, it is likely that the use of drugs in children will continue to be based primarily on clinical experience instead of clinical trials. Unfortunately, this approach continues to place our most fragile patients at potential risk.

This chapter focuses on general principles guiding pediatric pharmacotherapy for common pediatric disorders and highlights select diseases, which are unique to pediatrics.

Medication Error Prevention

Children are at significant risk for medication errors, which occur at rates 3 times that reported in adults. Of these medication errors, up to 19% have been reported as being preventable.[1] Reasons for the high rate of medication errors relative to adults include lack of appropriate dosing information and/or guidelines, the need to compound oral dosage forms or dilute commercially available formulations, and the miscalculation of doses.

Drug Administration
Oral Medications

A young child or infant often needs to be restrained to facilitate accurate and rapid administration. It is best accomplished with two adults; one gently restraining the child and the other administering the medication. An alternative is to wrap or swaddle the child (restraining arms and legs) using a blanket or large towel (Fig. 93-1). Liquid medications are most easily administered to the back cheek of the infant in 1- to 2-mL amounts, using an oral syringe. Household teaspoons should not be used to measure medications because teaspoons are of variable sizes and can hold from 3 to 8 mL of a liquid. The administration device (cup, syringe, or dropper) packaged with the medication product provides the most accurate measurement.

Crushed tablets or capsule contents mixed in small amounts (1 to 2 teaspoons) of food (e.g., chocolate pudding, applesauce, ice cream, jelly, chocolate syrup) offer an alternative to liquid formulations. Methods of improving the taste of liquid dosage formulations include refrigeration of liquids, use of flavoring agents, and use of "chasers" (i.e., following the dose with a popsicle or flavored soda). Although medications may be delivered in small amounts (10 to 15 mL) of liquid in a bottle (juice, milk, formula), doses should not be diluted into an entire scheduled feeding or prepared ahead in batches in anticipation of future administration. Limiting the volume more likely facilitates delivery of the entire dose and adding the medication to a feeding bottle immediately before delivery minimizes the potential of drug instability. Knowledge about drug–food interactions also should be considered before recommending the addition of drugs to feeding formulations. Fortunately, most children are able to swallow tablets when they reach 5 to 8 years of age. Duplicate supplies of medication should be provided to the caregiver when mid-day doses are required for children who attend school or childcare in the event a dose is dropped. Children of all ages should be encouraged and praised for their cooperation in taking their medicine. Rewards, gold stars, or stickers may be useful to gain cooperation in an older child.

Ear, Nose, and Eye Drops

The administration of otic, ophthalmic, and nasal medications to infants and young children often necessitates different administration techniques than those for adults. Otic medications should be instilled by pulling the auricle down and out in infants and young children, whereas older children should have the auricle of the ear held up and back to straighten the canal. During the instillation of nose and eye drops, positioning of infants and toddlers such that the head is lower than the rest of the body is advantageous because the forces of gravity assist in dispersing the medication. This can be achieved by laying the infant across a bed with the shoulders projecting over the edge of the bed. Restraint is often required during delivery of ophthalmic products to avoid injury to the eye caused by sudden movement of the infant (Fig. 93-2).

To minimize fear and improve cooperation during instillation of drops, caregivers should explain the procedure to the

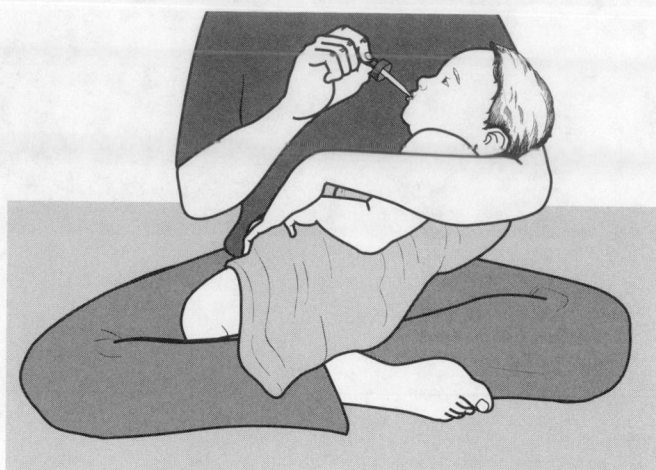

FIGURE 93-1 Administration of oral liquid medication to a young child. (1) Premeasure the medication and have it within reach. (2) Hold the child in your lap, placing one of the child's arms behind your back and both of the child's legs between your legs. Restrain the child's other arm securely with your nondominant arm. (3) Tilt the child's head back slightly, pressing gently on the child's cheeks to open the mouth. Using your dominant hand, aim the dropper or syringe between the rear gum and cheek. Administer small amounts of medication (1 to 2 mL) at a time, making sure the baby swallows.

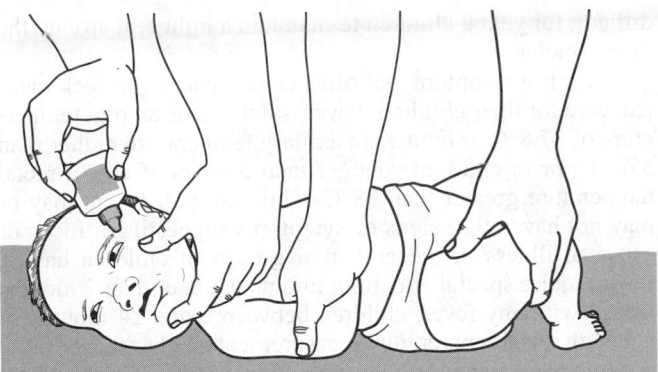

FIGURE 93-2 Administering eye drops to a young child. (1) Place the child on a flat surface. Enlist the help of a second adult to restrain the child or swaddle the child as described in Figure 93-1. (2) Holding the child's head steady, gently pull the eyelids apart. Administer the medication as directed.

child as simply as possible. It is best to warm the medication in your hand for a few minutes before administration; even a product stored at room temperature can feel very cold inside the ears or nose.

INFANT CARE
Teething

The growth and development of teeth begin as early as the sixth week of embryonic life. Calcification of the enamel and dentin begins at 4 months of gestation. Normal eruption of primary or deciduous teeth rarely begins before 4 to 5 months of age and usually is completed by 36 months of age.[2] Although premature infants usually experience delayed eruption of their deciduous teeth, their first tooth appears (based on postconceptual age) at the same time as term infants.[3] A significant number of term infants, however, do not erupt teeth until the end of the first year; and delayed eruption of all teeth may indicate systemic or nutritional disturbances (e.g., hypothyroidism, hypopituitarism, rickets).[2] Early eruption is less common and also associated with medical conditions (e.g., hyperthyroidism, precocious puberty, and long-term steroid therapy).

Normal Eruption of Primary Teeth
Signs and Symptoms

1. C.J., a 6-month old, has become increasingly irritable and has been waking up four to five times a night. She also seems to be drooling excessively and biting on hard objects constantly. A brief examination of C.J.'s mouth shows red and tender gums. No teeth are present, and C.J. is afebrile. Her mother is concerned that C.J.'s teething has caused a secondary illness. Are these symptoms unusual?

C.J.'s regular sleeping pattern has been disturbed by symptomatic teething. As the teeth penetrate the gums, the site may become tender; this process also may be associated with increased salivation. Bacterial invasion through a break in the tissue or under a gingival flap covering the teeth may cause inflammation and edema, but "teething" does not cause systemic disturbances.[4] In general, teething has been associated with restlessness, increased salivation, thumb sucking, gum rubbing, and decreased appetite.

Treatment

2. What course of treatment can be suggested for C.J.?

GENERAL MANAGEMENT

Gentle irrigation with water often relieves the inflammation around a gum flap. A topical anesthetic applied with a cotton-tipped applicator may be rubbed gently on the mucous membranes overlying the erupting tooth. Alcohol-free products containing 7.5% benzocaine for infants older than 4 months of age should be recommended. Some examples include Orajel Baby Gel and Orabase Baby Analgesic Teething Gel.[5] Long-term use of local anesthetics is not recommended. Topical anesthetics containing lidocaine are not recommended for the symptomatic relief of teething because infants may absorb significant amounts of lidocaine, which can lead to systemic toxicity.

Other palliative measures include having the child chew on a blunt, firm object or cracked ice wrapped in a soft cloth to hasten tooth eruption and relieve pain. Rubber teething rings of various shapes may be beneficial, but trauma from the teething ring can lead to angular cheilitis.[6] In addition, water-containing rings should be avoided because these can become contaminated with bacteria.

Ibuprofen and acetaminophen are commonly prescribed for younger children to relieve pain associated with the eruption of primary dentition. Ibuprofen, with its anti-inflammatory activity and duration of 6 to 8 hours, may be especially helpful at bedtime. Pediatric dosage recommendations should be strictly followed. Topical aspirin should never be used because it can cause oral chemical burns.

Diaper Rash
Etiology

Diaper dermatitis is commonly encountered in pediatric practice, occurring in up to 35% of infants at any given time. Although the pathogenesis of diaper dermatitis is not well defined, a number of factors (e.g., chemical irritants, friction, bacteria) have been associated with skin inflammation in the diaper area.

Both skin wetness and pH have been implicated in diaper dermatitis, although the impact of wetness appears to be greater than that of pH. Overhydration of the skin increases the permeability of low molecular weight compounds and exacerbates the effects of friction.[7] Cloth diapers covered with plastic pants or disposable diapers with plastic outer linings can cause irritation by decreasing air circulation and increasing moisture in the diaper area.[8] Other potential irritants include residual chemicals or laundry detergents in the diaper (cloth or disposable), or a soap, medication, or lotion that has been applied directly to the infant's skin. A persistent diaper rash may represent fungal or bacterial infection.[8]

Clinical Presentation

Four clinical presentations of dermatitis are associated with diaper wear:

1. A mild, scaling rash in the perianal area
2. A sharply demarcated confluent erythema
3. Ulceration distributed through the diaper area
4. A beefy red confluent erythema with satellite lesions, vesiculopustular lesions, and diffuse involvement of the genitalia

Treatment

3. K.G., a 3-month-old infant, has had a severe "diaper rash" for the past 4 days. It is confined to the diaper area, it is very inflamed and tender, and vesicular satellite lesions are present on the periphery of the main erythematous area. K.G.'s mother uses only cloth diapers and has not changed soap or her normal pattern of diaper care since K.G. was born. Based on the clinical appearance of the rash and its duration, the clinician prescribed clotrimazole 1% cream and gave K.G.'s mother instructions for treatment. Why was clotrimazole prescribed? How should diaper rash be treated and prevented?

K.G.'s rash is consistent with a candidal infection, which typically is beefy red and associated with vesicular satellite lesions. Presence of a rash for >3 days and diffuse involvement of the genitalia and inguinal folds also are characteristic of this form of diaper rash. K.G.'s rash can be treated with clotrimazole or miconazole cream applied to the inflamed area four times daily until it has resolved. Nystatin ointment can be applied, but it may not be as effective as the imidazole antifungals because of increasing rates of resistance of candida species to nystatin.

General treatment measures include removal of the stool and urine by gentle rinsing with plain water; baby wipes containing alcohol will sting and should be avoided until the rash has resolved. A good protective agent containing zinc oxide or petrolatum (e.g., Desitin) should be applied with each diaper change to act as a barrier to irritants and seal out moisture. Alternatively, powdered protective agents, such as cornstarch or talc, can be used to minimize friction. Powders should be used cautiously because the infant may aspirate the particles and develop a chemical pneumonia.[9] Powders should be shaken into the diaper or applied close to the body, away from the baby's face. Although many believe that cornstarch is a culture media for *C. albicans,* this has not been substantiated[10]; therefore, its use appears to be both safe and effective.

Other prevention and treatment measures should include the following:

1. Change the diaper as soon as it is wet or at least every 2 to 4 hours during the day.
2. Keep the diaper area clean (e.g., nightly baths until resolved).
3. Use super absorbent disposable diapers at night.
4. Expose the diaper area to air as often as possible.
5. Dry the diaper area completely before a new diaper is put on.
6. For cotton diapers, use a bacteriostatic agent in the diaper pail and rinse water or employ a diaper service to ensure that diapers are sterile.
7. Apply a low-potency topical corticosteroid such as 0.5% to 1% hydrocortisone twice daily for up to 1 week when severe inflammation is present.[11]

Fever

Normal body temperature varies throughout the day, peaking in late afternoon or early evening. Body temperature can be measured rectally, orally, axillary (under the arm), and tympanically. Rectal temperatures are most reliable in infants younger than 3 months of age. Oral measurements are not appropriate in children younger than age 3 years because it is difficult for young children to maintain a tight seal around the thermometer.

Fever is a symptom that often causes parents to seek medical care for their children. Fever is defined as an oral temperature of 37.8°C or higher, an axillary temperature higher than 37.2°C, or in children younger than 5 years of age, a rectal temperature greater than 38°C. Children with fevers may or may not have other signs or symptoms suggesting a focus or cause of illness. In general, four groups of children having fever require special attention: infants younger than 2 months of age with any fever; children between 6 and 24 months of age with rectal temperature measurements higher than 38.9°C accompanied by abnormal white blood cell (WBC) counts; all children with temperature measurements of 41.0°C or higher; and children with fever who are immunocompromised or have been diagnosed with asplenia.[12]

Clinical Presentation

Fever in children younger than 2 months of age is not predictive of the degree of illness. Clinical manifestations of a serious infection often are subtle and nonspecific. Therefore, any child younger than 2 months of age who develops a fever (e.g., rectal temperature >100°F) requires a complete evaluation by a physician that may include blood culture, urinalysis, and lumbar puncture. Antibiotic therapy is usually initiated while awaiting the results of the studies.

Children between 6 and 24 months of age with a temperature greater than 38.9°C and WBC counts less than 5,000/mm^3 or greater than 15,000/mm^3 are at an increased risk for bacteremia. Blood cultures, lumbar puncture, urinalysis, and chest radiograph should be considered on an individual basis to help determine the cause of infection.

Immunocompromised children are at risk of developing gram-negative or gram-positive sepsis. Children with functional or anatomic asplenia are at an increased risk for fulminant infection caused by *Streptococcus pneumoniae,* Salmonella species, *Escherichia coli,* and other Gram-negative organisms. Febrile children with these disorders should receive prompt antibiotic therapy.

Temperature elevations >41°C commonly are associated with bacterial disease. Children of any age who develop a fever >41°C should be evaluated for bacteremia and meningitis.

4. R.B. is a 12-month-old, 10-kg baby boy. His mother calls to request advice about the treatment of a fever in R.B. She states that R.B. was well until yesterday afternoon when he felt warm to her touch. For the past 24 hours, he has remained warm and is fussy and less active. A rectal temperature taken 15 minutes ago was 39°C. Although the pediatrician said that R.B. only has a viral infection, she is worried that R.B.'s temperature will continue to rise and that he might have a seizure. Are R.B.'s mother's concerns valid? How should R.B.'s febrile illness be treated?

Risk of Febrile Seizures

Febrile seizures occur in approximately 2% to 4% of children between the ages of 6 months and 5 years who have temperature elevations >38°C.[13] The etiology and pathogenesis are unknown, but the temperature and the rate of temperature increase appear to be important factors.[14] In addition, genetics appears to have an influence because febrile seizures occur with greater frequency among family members.[13] There are two types of febrile seizures: simple and complex. Simple febrile seizures last <15 minutes and do not have significant focal features. Complex febrile seizures have a longer duration, occur in series, and are associated with focal changes. Typically, febrile seizures occur within the first 24 hours of a febrile episode.[13] Although R.B. is in the age group at greatest risk for having a febrile seizure, he has been febrile for more than 24 hours and it is unlikely that a seizure will occur during this illness.

Treatment

ANTIPYRETIC THERAPY

Acetaminophen is the most common antipyretic agent used in children. The usual oral or rectal dose is 10 to 15 mg/kg per dose administered every 4 to 6 hours as needed to a maximum of 65 mg/kg per day. Other alternatives include aspirin or ibuprofen.

Aspirin 10 to 15 mg/kg per dose can be administered orally or rectally. However, salicylic acid may accumulate with repeated dosing when using the upper range of this guideline.[15] Aspirin therapy is not recommended for treatment of fever in children or adolescents with chickenpox, gastroenteritis or respiratory viral infections because of its association with Reye's syndrome.[16] Reye's syndrome, a rare illness affecting otherwise healthy children, consists of acute noninflammatory encephalopathy, hepatic dysfunction, and various metabolic derangements. Reye's syndrome is associated with a 10% to 40% mortality rate, although these numbers have decreased in recent years because of early diagnosis and aggressive therapy.[16,17]

Ibuprofen is administered as 5 to 10 mg/kg per dose orally every 6 to 8 hours as needed to a maximum of 40 mg/kg per day. Ibuprofen is as effective as acetaminophen as an antipyretic and is associated with a low incidence of adverse effects.[18,19] Although renal failure has been reported after ibuprofen use in children,[20,21] the risk of renal impairment is small with short-term use and not any greater than with acetaminophen.[19,21]

Acetaminophen or ibuprofen would be effective in lowering R.B.'s fever. Acetaminophen typically is considered to be a first-line drug in children. Dosing errors have occurred when teaspoonful quantities of acetaminophen infant drops (80 mg/0.8 mL) were given instead of the liquid formulation (160 mg/5 mL) or when regular strength tablets (325 mg) have been substituted for chewable children's tablets (160 mg). Caretakers should be questioned about the dosage form of acetaminophen they have at home, concurrent use of any other products containing acetaminophen, and whether cumulative doses are within the recommended range. Ibuprofen is an alternative in R.B. because adverse effects are limited when used for antipyresis. Ibuprofen is available in two liquid formulations (infant drops, 50 mg/1.25 mL; children's suspension, 100 mg/5 mL) and two chewable tablet dosage formulations (50 mg, 100 mg); caution should be used to avoid dosing errors. While some practitioners may alternate acetaminophen and ibuprofen during the day, no data are available to support the efficacy or safety of combination therapy. Aspirin, because of its association with Reye's syndrome, should be avoided in pediatric patients with viral infections.

Cough and Cold

The second most common diagnosis in children is viral upper respiratory infection or the common cold.[22] Children with a cold often present with sore throat, nasal congestion, rhinorrhea, sneezing, cough, and irritability.

Clinical Presentation and Treatment

5. J.K. is a 3-month-old female who began having nasal congestion, rhinorrhea, and cough yesterday. She has had no fever and is eating well, but did not sleep well last evening. J.K.'s mother called her pediatrician and was told that J.K. most likely has a cold caused by a virus. How can J.K.'s symptoms be treated?

A cool mist humidifier can increase the amount of moisture in room air and decrease irritation in the upper airway when humidity is low. Saline nose drops followed by bulb suctioning can help to clear the nasal passages in J.K. who is younger than 6 months old.[22] It is especially important to do this before feedings. If a topical nasal decongestant is needed, phenylephrine is preferred over oxymetazoline and xylometazoline, which are associated with toxicity in children younger than 6 years of age because of case reports of sedation, convulsions, insomnia, and coma.[23,24] Nasal decongestants should be limited to 3 to 5 days to prevent rebound hyperemia.

Orally administered decongestants such as pseudoephedrine or phenylephrine may be beneficial if topical therapy is ineffective; however, they may cause sleeplessness, irritability, or tachycardia. Antihistamines are not effective for rhinorrhea caused by the common cold and should not be recommended. Antitussives should not be used if the child's cough is productive, but may be useful if the cough is dry and interfering with activities or sleep.[22] Cough suppressant formulations for children often contain dextromethorphan or diphenhydramine. Expectorants such as guaifenesin are not effective and evidence is insufficient to support the use of vitamin C, zinc, or echinacea in children for treatment or prevention of the common cold.

Over-the-counter products for upper respiratory symptoms are numerous and present a difficult challenge to parents when trying to make an appropriate selection. Products containing single ingredients are preferred to help minimize the chance for adverse effects.

Constipation

Constipation, affecting approximately 3% of pre-school children and up to 2% of school-age children,[25] can be defined as a stool frequency of less than 3 per week or occurrence of pain on defecation (signifying hard stools).[25] Beyond the neonatal period, constipation is most commonly idiopathic or functional and may be due to a diet low in fiber, lack of time or routine for toileting, or passage of a painful stool resulting in a fear of defecating. Stool retention over time may result in soiling or encopresis.

Clinical Presentation and Treatment

6. R.J., a 2-year-old boy, has had abdominal pain for several weeks. On average he has 1 stool weekly and he cries each time due to pain. After obtaining a thorough history and performing a physical examination, the physician determines that R.J. has functional constipation. What treatment measures should be taken to relieve and prevent R.J's constipation?

Before maintenance therapy can be started, disimpaction is necessary. While no controlled studies compare efficacy of the oral and rectal routes, oral therapy is preferred because it is less invasive and may achieve better adherence.[25,26] Options for oral disimpaction include mineral oil, polyethylene glycol, and bisacodyl. Rectal medications include phosphate soda enemas, glycerin suppositories in infants, and bisacodyl suppositories in older children. After disimpaction, maintenance therapy is initiated to promote regular stool production and prevent re-impaction. This is achieved by a combination of behavioral, dietary, and medication therapies. Dietary interventions include adequate fluid and fiber intake. Medications include mineral oil, lactulose, or sorbitol and should be titrated to produce 1 to 2 soft stools daily. Stimulant laxatives may be used intermittently.

Vomiting and Diarrhea

Vomiting and diarrhea are two commonly encountered complaints in pediatric practice. Most cases are self-limited, but severe cases can result in serious complications, such as dehydration, metabolic disturbances, and even death. Infants and young children are particularly prone to more severe complications.

Pathogenesis and Presentation of Vomiting

Vomiting or emesis is defined as forceful expulsion of GI contents through the mouth or nose; nonforceful expulsion of GI contents is considered regurgitation. In newborns, regurgitation of small amounts of breast milk or formula after feeding, especially when burping, is common. In most cases, regurgitation usually resolves by 1 year of age and rarely causes a problem.[27,28] Extensive evaluation of regurgitation is not needed in a child who is growing well. Other causes of vomiting during the newborn period include pyloric stenosis, gastroesophageal reflux, overfeeding, food intolerance, and GI obstruction. Beyond the neonatal period, the most common cause of vomiting is infection.

Conditions causing emesis in older infants and children range from viral gastroenteritis to more severe illnesses, such as bowel obstruction or head injury, that require immediate medical attention (Table 93-1).[27,28] Acute vomiting also may result from medication or toxic ingestions. Vomiting in infants and children also can be caused by central nervous system (CNS) disease (e.g., intracranial tumors), metabolic disease (e.g., urea cycle disorder), inflammatory bowel disease, and ulcers. In teenagers, migraine, pregnancy, and psychological disorders such as bulimia have been associated with vomiting.

Pathogenesis and Presentation of Diarrhea

Diarrhea refers to an increase in frequency, volume, or liquidity of stool when compared to normal bowel movements. In developing countries, diarrhea is a common cause of death. In the United States, approximately 38 million cases of diarrhea will occur, resulting in approximately 2 to 4 million physician visits, 220,000 hospitalizations, and approximately 400 deaths annually.[29]

Acute diarrhea is abrupt in onset and usually lasts a few days with most cases having a viral etiology. (Infectious diar-

Table 93-1 Causes of Vomiting in Infants and Children[27,28]

Causes	Other Signs and Symptoms
Drug Induced	
Cancer chemotherapy	Nausea
Narcotics	
Theophylline/ Aminophylline	
Antibiotics	
Alcohol	
Anesthetics	
Metabolic or Endocrine Disorders	Alteration in behavior
Infectious Diseases	Fever
Otitis media	Symptoms of otitis media
Meningitis	Stiff neck, toxic appearance
Appendicitis	Abdominal pain
Urinary tract infection/ pyelonephritis	Dysuria, frequency and urgency in older children
Viral or bacterial gastroenteritis	Diarrhea
Mechanical Obstruction	
Bowel obstruction	Abdominal distention, green emesis
Pyloric stenosis	Projectile nonbilious vomiting Abdominal pain
Inflammatory	
Pancreatitis	
Inflammatory bowel	Diarrhea
PUD	Black or red vomitus
Psychologic	
Chemotherapy	
Bulimia	
Miscellaneous	
Gastroesophageal reflux	Usually self-limited; indications for evaluation include recurrent pneumonia, poor growth, GI blood loss, dysphagia, or heartburn
↑ Intracranial pressure	Mental status alternation
Head injury/trauma	History of trauma, mental status changes
Food or milk intolerance or allergy	Irritability, loose stool, blood in stool

GI, gastrointestinal; PUD, peptic ulcer disease.

rhea is discussed in Chapter 62, Infectious Diarrhea and management of viral gastroenteritis is in the following section). Diarrhea is considered chronic if it lasts longer than 2 weeks. Chronic diarrhea is caused by a variety of problems including malabsorption, inflammatory disease, alteration of intestinal flora, milk or protein intolerance, and drugs.[30]

Infants and children are at high risk for morbidity and mortality secondary to diarrhea for several reasons. Dehydration can occur easily as acute net intestinal fluid losses are relatively much greater in young children than in adults. This may be due to inefficient transport systems in the developing intestine. In addition, the percent of total body water in children is higher than in adults; thus, they are more susceptible to body fluid shifts. Total body water changes from 80% of total body weight in premature infants to 70% in term infants and 60% in adults.[31] Finally, the renal capacity to compensate for fluid and electrolyte imbalances in the infant is limited compared with an adult's.[32]

VIRAL GASTROENTERITIS

7. J.R., a 15-month-old male infant, began vomiting this morning but has not had a fever or diarrhea. Upon questioning, you discover that many children attending day care with J.R. are experiencing vomiting, diarrhea, and low-grade temperatures. How should J.R.'s vomiting be treated?

Routine use of antiemetics for acute vomiting in children is not recommended because the effectiveness of antiemetics in viral gastroenteritis has not been demonstrated and side effects commonly are reported. In addition, antiemetics may delay the diagnosis of a treatable illness.[33–35]

Parents should be educated about the signs and symptoms of serious illness that warrant medical attention. A pediatrician should be contacted if a child is toxic appearing or has unusual behavior, abdominal pain or distention, red or black vomitus, or signs of an ear infection. In addition, a pediatrician should be called if there is a history or suspicion of toxic ingestion or head trauma. Fever may accompany vomiting in viral gastroenteritis. A physician should be notified of any fever occurring in a neonate; in older infants and children, a change in fever pattern or prolonged fever also warrants seeking medical attention.

When communicating information regarding a vomiting child, it is helpful if the parents have knowledge of the child's fluid intake along with the frequency of vomiting and urination. It is easy to overestimate the amount of vomitus. To estimate volume, one tablespoon makes a spot four inches wide and a quarter-cup makes a spot approximately 8 inches wide.

Vomiting associated with gastroenteritis usually resolves in 24 to 48 hours. The most important treatment during this period is fluid and electrolyte replacement (see Question 9). Infants are particularly susceptible to the development of fluid and electrolyte abnormalities.

J.R.'s vomiting should be managed by withholding food or drink for 2 to 4 hours and administering an oral electrolyte replacement solution (ORS). Even in the vomiting child, oral hydration therapy can be successful if given in small volumes.[33,35] Every 5 to 10 minutes, 5 to 10 mL should be administered, increasing the volume gradually as tolerated. If vomiting recurs, the practitioner should continue to administer ORS.[36] ORS should only be abandoned in children with intractable vomiting, as well as those in shock, loss of consciousness, or with bowel obstruction.[24,25] More than 90% of infants will tolerate oral hydration when small amounts are given frequently. Using a spoon or oral syringe to administer the fluid may be more effective than using a nipple or cup. As dehydration is corrected, the frequency of vomiting typically decreases. Once rehydration is achieved, fluids other than ORS and a diet appropriate for age may be started.[35,36]

Assessment of Dehydration

8. On the second day of illness, J.R. develops a mild fever and diarrhea that has increased in frequency and water content. How can the severity of J.R.'s diarrhea be assessed? Should he be hospitalized for intravenous (IV) fluid replacement, or can he be treated on an outpatient basis?

To determine whether IV fluid replacement is needed, consider the following questions:

1. Does the child have any of the following signs and symptoms of severe dehydration? A depressed fontanel (useful up to 6 months of age), sunken eyes, dry mucus membranes, crying without tears, a diminished urine output, a fever without perspiration, or thirst?
2. Are a large number of copious stools still being produced?
3. Is there a risk of dehydration from inadequate monitoring, or is the parent unable to care for the child? Specific inquiries should be made about the number and consistency of stools in children with diarrhea.
4. Are other signs and symptoms present, such as lethargy, severe emesis, or a history of convulsions, that preclude management at home?

Estimating the degree of dehydration is particularly valuable in assessing the patient with diarrhea; weight loss is a good criterion. A 5% weight loss is considered mild dehydration, up to 10% is considered moderate, and greater than 10% is severe or life-threatening dehydration. (See Chapter 97, Pediatric Nutrition, for a discussion on IV replacement therapy in children with 10% or more dehydration.)

Oral Replacement Therapy

9. Upon questioning, it is determined that J.R. is not dehydrated. What recommendations can be made regarding the management of J.R. on an outpatient basis?

The object of therapy is to prevent significant dehydration and restore or maintain adequate hydration and electrolyte balance. Mild to moderate diarrhea without dehydration generally is managed at home by continued age-appropriate feeding. Stool losses may be replaced by using an ORS containing glucose.[36] Glucose provides a caloric source and enhances the absorption of salt and water in the small intestine by mechanisms that usually are unimpaired in many toxin-induced diarrheas. Previously, parents were instructed to prepare salt and sugar solutions at home; frequent errors in preparing the solutions led to problems in fluid and electrolyte balance. Homemade remedies do not contain appropriate compositions of electrolytes and should not be used.[31] Commercially available oral glucose–electrolyte solutions (e.g., Pedialyte) have been designed to enhance absorption of glucose and sodium and should be used in infants and young children. Gatorade is an alternative for older children. Carbonated beverages and fruit juice have inadequate sodium to replace diarrhea losses. Rehydration and maintenance solutions can be made more palatable with sugar-free flavorings (e.g., Kool-Aid, Crystal Lite).

The World Health Organization (WHO) promotes the use of an oral replacement solution (WHO formula) containing sodium (90 mEq/L), potassium (20 mEq/L), bicarbonate (30 mEq/L), chloride (80 mEq/L), and 2.5% glucose for the widespread management of acute diarrhea in Third World countries. WHO formula has a 90% successful rehydration rate for all forms of diarrhea. It contains a high concentration of sodium because sodium loss is associated with secretory diarrhea (e.g., cholera). Malabsorptive diarrheas, such as rotavirus infections, have much lower sodium concentrations (<40 mEq/L); thus, the commercially available oral replacement solutions are effective. Glucose is added to oral electrolyte solutions to enhance glucose-coupled sodium transport, but concentrations greater than 3% may actually impair sodium absorption. At this level, the glucose-coupled sodium transport system is saturated and any additional glucose acts as an osmotically active solute in the bowel lumen. The electrolyte content of commonly used oral solutions is provided in Table 93-2.

10. How should J.R. be managed if his diarrhea causes mild to moderate dehydration? Can oral hydration be utilized in J.R.? When should oral feeding be re-instituted?

ORS may also be used to treat mild to moderate dehydration. Children may be managed at home depending on the parent's ability and the child's cooperation. Oral replacement is contraindicated in the presence of shock with inability to drink; persistent vomiting; and stool losses exceeding 100 mL/kg per hour making oral replacement impractical.

The American Academy of Pediatrics recommends that ORS containing 75 to 90 mEq/L of sodium (e.g., Rehydralyte) be used for rehydration in situations of mild to moderate dehydration caused by diarrhea. Volumes equal to estimated fluid deficit (usually 40 to 50 mL/kg) should be given over approximately 4 hours. The patient should be reassessed and, once rehydrated, solutions containing 40 to 60 mEq/L of sodium (e.g. Pedialyte, Infalyte) should be used for maintenance hydration. For each diarrhea stool, an additional 10 mL/kg of oral electrolyte solution should be given. Fluid should be initially administered in small amounts (5 to 10 mL) and increased as tolerated. Breast milk or formula should be given as tolerated.[35]

Reinstitution of Oral Feedings

In the past, feeding has been delayed because of the malabsorption that typically occurs during and after diarrhea. However, the malabsorption is self-limiting and substantial amounts of carbohydrate, protein, and fat can still be absorbed. The reinstitution of a regular diet does not affect mild diarrhea and can be beneficial.[35-37] Parents are encouraged to continue feeding their children using age-appropriate, carbohydrate-rich foods within 24 hours. Advantages of continued feeding during diarrhea include prevention of protein and energy deficits, maintenance or repair of intestinal mucosa, promotion of recovery of brush border membrane disaccharidases, and sustained breast-feeding.[35-37] Although lactose intolerance has been reported, experts agree that most children with mild diarrhea can tolerate full-strength animal milk, animal milk–based formula, and breast milk.[35] If the child is lactose intolerant, a lactose-free formula may be substituted for 2 to 6 weeks until GI lactase returns.

Drug Therapy

11. What medications can be recommended for the treatment of diarrhea in children?

Medications play a minor role in the treatment of acute infantile diarrhea because most episodes are self-limiting. Antibiotics should be used only when systemic bacteremia is suspected; when immune defenses are compromised; or when a persistent enteric infection is sensitive to antibiotics.[33,35] In general, antidiarrheal preparations are not recommended for infants or children because they have little effect on acute diarrhea, are associated with side effects, and direct attention away from the use of oral hydration therapy.[33,35-37] Drugs that alter GI motility should be avoided, especially in children with high fever, toxemia, or bloody mucoid stools, because they may worsen the clinical course of the bacterial infection. Adsorbents, such as Kaopectate, adsorb bacterial toxins and water and improve the symptoms of diarrhea by producing more formed stools, but they do not decrease the duration of diarrhea or fluid and electrolyte losses. Kaopectate also can adsorb nutrients, enzymes, and antibiotics (especially with prolonged use).[33,35-37]

GASTROESOPHAGEAL REFLUX

Gastroesophageal reflux (GER) is a common disorder, with 50% to 67% of infants experiencing recurrent vomiting and regurgitation during the first 4 months of life.[38] Most reflux in infants is primarily caused by transient relaxations of the lower esophageal sphincter (LES). Other reasons infants may be predisposed to having reflux include: slumped (such as in a car seat) or supine positioning; a liquid diet that exceeds the volume capacity of the stomach, and in premature infants, a decrease in peristaltic activity.[39] Fortunately, 80% of cases of reflux in infants are benign and resolve by 18 months of age.[40] GER in older children runs a course that is similar to adults. Infants and young children may also have underlying conditions, predisposing them to reflux (e.g., neurologic disorders, hiatal hernia). Possible complications of untreated GER include strictures secondary to esophagitis, GI hemorrhage, aspiration leading to chronic respiratory disease, and apnea. Death has occurred secondary to aspiration, malnutrition, or prolonged apnea.

Clinical Presentation

The most common symptom of GER in infants is vomiting or regurgitation. Other nonspecific signs and symptoms include failure to thrive (FTT), recurrent pneumonia, apnea, dysphagia, reactive airway disease, apparent life-threatening events (ALTE), hematemesis, and anemia.[41] Diagnostic evaluation is generally not indicated in healthy infant with functional GER

Table 93-2   Oral Electrolyte Solutions[29,35]

Solution	Sodium (mmol/L)	Potassium (mmol/L)	Carbohydrate (mmol/L)	Osmolality
Rehydration				
Rehydralyte	75	20	140	310
WHO formula	90	20	111	310
Maintenance				
Infalyte (Ricelyte)	50	25	70	200
Pedialyte	45	20	140	250
Resol	50	20	111	270
Home Remedies				
Apple juice	3–5	32	690	730
Gatorade	20	3	255	330
Ginger ale	3	1	500	540
Chicken broth	250	8	—	500
Cola	2	—	690	730

presenting as recurrent vomiting.[42] Empiric management of these infants can be recommended once other causes of vomiting are eliminated. Further diagnostic evaluation is indicated to confirm GER in infants and children presenting with additional symptoms such as FTT, irritability, ALTE, or respiratory problems to confirm that GER is the cause.[42] The gold standard diagnostic evaluation for GER is esophageal pH monitoring, while the use of endoscopy and biopsy is indicated to diagnose the presence of esophagitis.[42] Barium contrast radiography may be indicated if anatomical abnormalities, such as strictures or pyloric stenosis, are suspected.[42]

Treatment

GER usually resolves spontaneously in infants by 18 months of age and therefore therapy is aimed at relieving symptoms and maintaining normal growth.[42] Therapy is aimed at healing esophagitis and preventing complications in infants and children with pathologic GER so that surgery can be avoided.[42] Infants and young children with underlying neurological problems (e.g., cerebral palsy) are unlikely to have spontaneous resolutions of GER and frequently require aggressive anti-reflux therapies and surgical intervention.

Positional and Dietary Measures

12. S.B., a 3-month-old, 6-kg, 60-cm male infant, has a 2-week history of regurgitation after each feeding. The pediatrician noted that S.B. had not gained weight since his last visit 1 month earlier. The presumptive diagnosis is FTT secondary to GER, and S.B. was referred to a pediatric gastroenterologist. The gastroenterologist admitted S.B. to the hospital and confirmed the diagnosis using 24-hour pH monitoring. How should S.B. be managed initially?

Because S.B. does not have life-threatening complications, he should be treated conservatively. Dietary and positional measures should be tried first. Dietary measures include thickening his foods with rice cereal and feeding smaller volumes more frequently. Occasionally, infants with milk protein allergies can present similarly, thus a change to a hypoallergenic formula may be warranted. Positional therapy consists of maintaining the infant in a semiupright position 24 hours a day to promote clearance of acid from the esophagus and to minimize reflux after meals. S.B. should be kept at a 60° angle while sitting and a 30° position at night. Infants with milder cases of GER can be managed successfully by dietary measures alone and by propping them upright during and 1 hour after feedings.[43] Although placing infants prone during sleep significantly reduces reflux, the greater risk of sudden infant death syndrome (SIDS) in infants younger than 12 months of age outweighs the benefits of such positioning.[42]

Drug Therapy

13. Four weeks after instituting positional and dietary measures, S.B. continues to vomit and still has not been gaining weight. Upon physical examination, the gastroenterologist notes bilateral wheezes; endoscopy rules out esophagitis. What would be the next step of therapy?

There is no evidence that pharmacologic therapy alters the course of disease in the management of infants with uncomplicated GER.[42] However, if an infant with uncomplicated GER continues to have recurrent vomiting, a therapeutic trial of a prokinetic agent may be warranted to reduce the number of episodes of vomiting. In infants or children who present with nonspecific symptoms or complications, such as S.B., the addition of acid suppression therapy or prokinetic therapy is warranted even in the absence of documented esophagitis.[42] When esophagitis is present, acid suppression is always recommended to aid in the healing process.[42] The various agents to treat infant GER are listed in Table 93-3.

Table 93-3 Oral Drugs Used to Treat GER in Infants[41–59]

Agent	Mode of Action	Oral Dosage
Acid Suppressing Agents		
Antacids (aluminum/ magnesium hydroxide)	Neutralizes acid;	0.5–1.0 mL/kg/dose before and after feeding(max, 15 mL/dose)
Proton Pump Inhibitors	↓ acid secretion via inhibition of gastric hydrogen-potassium adenosine triphosphatase	
Omeprazole		1 mg/kg/day div QD–BID
Lansoprazole		0.5–1.6 mg/kg/day QD
H₂ Receptor Antagonists	Blocks H₂-receptors; ↓ acid secretion	
Cimetidine		40 mg/kg/day div QID
Famotidine		1 mg/kg/day div BID
Nizatidine		10 mg/kg/day div BID
Ranitidine		5–0 mg/kg/day div TID–QID
Prokinetic Agents		
Bethanechol	Cholinergic agent; stimulates peristalsis ↑ ↑ LES pressure; ↑gastric emptying; ↑ colonic motility ↑gastric emptying; ↑ LES pressure; augments esophageal clearance	0.1–0.2 mg/kg/dose QID given 30–60 min before feeding and HS
Cisapride		0.8 mg/kg/day div QID
Metoclopramide		0.1–0.2 mg/kg/dose QID given 30 min before feeding and HS
Surface Active Agents		
Sucralfate	Forms paste and adheres to damaged esophageal mucosa	40–80 mg/kg/day div QID

GER, gastroesophageal reflux; LES, lower esophageal sphincter.

ACID SUPPRESSANT AGENTS

Antacids

Antacid therapy is not recommended for management of GER in infants and infants treated with aluminum containing antacids accumulate blood levels of aluminum sufficient to cause osteopenia and neurotoxicity.[41,44] Information on the use of other types of antacids in infants is limited; however, they can provide short-term relief of symptoms in older children and adults.

Proton Pump Inhibitors

Proton pump inhibitors (PPIs) are superior to histamine receptor antagonists (H$_2$RA) in relieving symptoms and healing in infants, young children, and adults with significant esophagitis.[45,46] PPIs control both basal and meal-stimulated acid secretion, which may in part be a reason for their improved efficacy. The incidence of adverse effects in children is similar to that reported in adults; however studies on their long term safety have yet to be performed.[45,46] Omeprazole and lansoprazole are available in extended-release capsules, which may be opened and sprinkled on soft foods; lansoprazole is also available as granules for an oral suspension. Suspension formulations for both drugs have been extemporaneously compounded, developed, and evaluated for stability.[48] Doses of PPIs may need to be titrated to achieve appropriate acid suppression as guided by pH probe follow-up evaluation.

Histamine Receptor Antagonists

Histamine receptor antagonists (H$_2$RA) reduce histamine-stimulated acid secretion but have limited effects on acid secretion by meals and other stimuli. In randomized controlled trials, H$_2$RAs in infants and children relieved symptoms and healed esophageal tissue.[49,50] However, tolerance to the acid suppressant activity of H$_2$RAs over a relatively short time ($<$30 days)[51,52] may limit their role for long-term management of esophagitis.

PROKINETIC AGENTS

Metoclopramide and domperidone improve gastric emptying, increase LES pressure, enhance esophageal clearance, and accelerate transit time in the small bowel; however, data are insufficient to support their use for the management of GER. The prokinetic drug cisapride is no longer available in the United States but can be obtained in a limited access protocol for children in whom conventional therapy has failed.[42] Domperidone has been studied more extensively than metoclopramide in infant GER but it also is not available in the United States.[54] Metoclopramide, a dopamine antagonist with cholinergic and serotonergic effects, accelerates gastric emptying and transit time without stimulating secretions. Use of metoclopramide in managing GER in children has mixed results on vomiting and esophageal pH[54–57]; it has also been associated with CNS effects (e.g., restlessness, drowsiness, extrapyramidal reactions) and rare reports of gynecomastia and galactorrhea.[58]

Bethanechol is a cholinergic agonist that has been reported to reduce vomiting episodes in infants with GER.[59–61] Its role in managing GER is limited due to the potential induction of bronchospasm and stimulation of gastric acid secretion. Administration of bethanechol requires extemporaneous compounding for young infants.

SURFACE ACTIVE AGENTS

Sucralfate (see Chapter 27, Upper Gastrointestinal Disorders) in one study was of equal efficacy compared with cimetidine for use in esophagitis.[62] However, evidence supporting its use for this condition is limited due to the concern about the use of aluminum containing products in infants.

Acid suppression therapy and the use of a prokinetic agent may be considered for the management of S.B. There are two approaches to acid suppression therapy in children who have complications from GER: a "step up" approach in which treatment is initiated with an H$_2$RA followed by the use of a PPI if no improvement occurs versus the "step down" approach which involves the initiation of a PPI to gain control, followed by an H$_2$RA for maintenance therapy.[42] There is no evidence supporting the preferential use of one H$_2$RA or PPI versus another.

The effectiveness of acid suppression for managing symptoms is not as well documented in children as it for healing esophagitis, however, it is believed to play a useful role for symptom control, particularly those respiratory in nature.[42] Of the prokinetic agents, metoclopramide is the agent of choice for S.B. at a dose of 0.6 mg (0.1 mg/kg per dose) four times daily, 30 minutes before meals and at bedtime. This dose can be adjusted based on his response.

Treatment should be continued for at least 3 to 4 months, although the optimal duration of therapy is unknown. If S.B. requires drug therapy to control symptoms of GER beyond 18 months to 2 years of age, surgery should be considered because GER is unlikely to resolve spontaneously after this age.[40] Surgery may be considered earlier if he fails medical therapy or if he develops an esophageal stricture, apnea, or recurrent respiratory disease.[40,42]

SEDATION AND ANALGESIA

Sedation

Conscious Sedation

Sedation often is needed for children who must undergo diagnostic or therapeutic procedure or when placed in an intensive care setting. Table 93-4 lists characteristics of drugs commonly used to produce conscious sedation. In general, the intravenous administration of drugs provides rapid onset of action and sedation should be used continuously when administered intravenously. The absorption of intramuscularly, rectally, or orally administered sedatives can be variable, especially in infants and young children.[63]

14. A.J., a 3-year-old, 15-kg girl, is admitted for evaluation of abdominal mass. A computed tomography scan is ordered. What regimen should be used to sedate A.J.?

The ideal sedative should be easy to administer, have a rapid and predictable onset, have minimal adverse effects, and have a duration of action that approximates the duration of many common medical procedures. Chloral hydrate, barbiturates, narcotic analgesics, benzodiazepines, and anesthetic agents such as propofol and ketamine have been used in pediatric patients to facilitate short duration diagnostic procedures. Although chloral hydrate often is thought to be an ideal hypnotic agent, it has not been tested extensively for toxicity or efficacy.[64] Several years ago, chloral hydrate was thought to have potential carcinogenicity and genotoxicity.[65] These con-

Table 93-4   Drugs Commonly Used for Conscious Sedation[67]

Drug	Dosage[a]	Onset of Action	Duration	Comments
Chloral hydrate	25–100 mg/kg (max, 1 g/dose to a total of 2 g) *Route:* PO, PR	20–30 min	Unpredictable	Rapidly metabolized to active metabolite trichloroethanol; paradoxical excitation may occur; hyperbilirubinemia has been associated with chloral hydrate (repeated doses) in premature infants and neonates
Diazepam (Valium)	*IV:* 0.04–0.3 mg/kg (max: 10 mg) *PO:* 0.2–0.3 (max: 10 mg)	*IV:* 2–3 min *PO:* 30–45 min	2–6 hr	May burn when given IV (lipid soluble); do not use small veins; infuse IV over 3 min and at most 5 mg/min; potentiates the effect of narcotics and barbiturates
Fentanyl (Sublimaze)	*IV:* 1–2 µg/kg (up to 100 µg/dose) *PO:* 5–15 µg/kg (max: 400 µg)	*IV:* 1–1.5 min *IM:* 7–8 min *PO:* 5–15 min	*IV:* 30–60 min *IM:* 1–2 hr *PO:* 1–2 hr	Infuse IV over 3–5 min; effects potentiated by benzodiazepines; Oralet available in 200-, 300-, and 400-µg doses Max dose is 400 µg. Only about 25% of dose of Actiq is absorbed from the oral mucosa
Lorazepam (Ativan)	*IV:* 0.05 mg/kg *PO:* 0.02–0.1 mg/kg	*IV:* 2–5 min *IM:* 15–30 min *PO:* 30–60 min	6–24 hr	Infuse IV over 2–3 min, not to exceed 2 mg/min; potentiates the effect of narcotics and barbiturates
Meperidine (Demerol)	*IV:* 0.5–1.5 mg/kg *SC/IM:* 1–2 mg/kg (max, 100 mg/dose) See combination drugs below for Demerol/Phenergan/Thorazine dosage	*IV:* 1–5 min *SC/IM:* 10 min	*IV:* 1–2 hr *SC/IM:* 2–4 hr	Metabolite (normeperidine) has neurotoxic effect; accumulation of normeperidine may result in central nervous system manifestation; caution in patients with renal impairment after high or repeated doses; infuse IV dose over 3–5 min
Midazolam (Versed)	*IV:* 0.05–0.1 mg/kg *Intranasal:* 0.2–0.3 mg/kg *PO:* 0.25–0.5 (max: 20 mg)	*IV:* 1–3 min *IM:* 10–15 min *Intranasal:* 5 min *PO:* 5–10 min	*IV:* 30–60 min *IM:* 2–6 hr *Intranasal:* 40–75 min *PO:* 30–90 min	3–4 times potency of diazepam; potentiates the effect of narcotics; infuse IV dose over 1–2 min
Morphine	*IV:* 0.05–0.1 mg/kg	*IV:* 1.0–2.5 min	1–2 hr	Maximal respiratory depression occurs within 7 min; effect potentiated by benzodiazepines; infuse IV dose over 3–5 min
Pentobarbital (Nembutal)	*PO/PR/IM:* 2–6 mg/kg (max, 100 mg/dose) *IV:* 1–3 mg/kg in increments of 1 mg/kg (max: 100 mg/dose)	*PO/PR:* 15–60 min *IM:* 10–25 min *IV:* 1–2 min	*PO/PR:* 1–4 hr *IM:* 30–60 min *IV:* 15–20 min	IV administration over at least 1 min or not to exceed 50 mg/min
Propofol (Diprivan)	*IV:* ≥2.5 mg/kg × 1 7.5–15 mg/kg/hr	*IV:* 30 sec after bolus	3–10 min, longer with prolonged use	Titrate to desired effect; lower dosages required when used with narcotics; metabolic acidosis with fatal cardiac failure has been reported in children
Combination drugs Demerol/ Phenergan/ Thorazine	*IM:* Demerol: 2 mg/kg (up to 50 mg) Phenergan: 1 mg/kg (up to 12.5 mg) Thorazine: 1 mg/kg (up to 12.5 mg) *IV:* 1/2 of IM dose	*IM:* 10–15 min *IV:* 5–10 min	2–5 hr	Infuse IV dose over 5 min; hypotension can occur with rapid IV infusion; may be mixed in the same syringe
Ketamine	*IV:* 0.5–2 mg/kg *IM:* 3–7 mg/kg *PO:* 6–10 mg/kg	*IV:* 30 sec *IM:* 10–15 min *PO:* 30 min	*IV:* 1–2 hr *IM:* 3–4 hr	Can result in hallucinogenic emergence reactions; less common in younger patients, can be decreased by concurrent BZDP use; can cause ↑ bronchial secretions

[a]Use low end of the dose if combined with another agent(s).

cerns surfaced because chloral hydrate is a metabolite of trichloroethylene, an industrial solvent and cleaning fluid, which induced cancer in rodents. Although the extrapolation of animal data to humans is theoretical, the possible carcinogenicity of chloral hydrate was alarming to clinicians who have used the drug for many years without evidence of problems.[64] The American Academy of Pediatrics (AAP) believes that many practitioners are familiar with the use of chloral hydrate and that it is an effective agent with a low incidence of toxicity. There is a greater concern by the AAP that a sudden switch by practitioners to an agent that they are less familiar with might pose a greater risk than a theoretical risk of carcinogenesis.[66] Although it is unreasonable to ban a drug like chloral hydrate based on limited animal data, practitioners should become increasingly familiar with other sedating agents, especially for situations when chloral hydrate fails to produce the desired effect. The risks of chloral hydrate in pediatric patients needs further study.

The usual chloral hydrate dose is 25 to 100 mg/kg per dose to a maximum total dose of 1 g for infants and 2 g for older children.[67] Most children respond to 50 to 75 mg/kg; however, dose requirements can vary.[66,68–70] Repetitive dosing of chloral hydrate to maintain prolonged sedation in infants and children during mechanical ventilation is not recommended because its pharmacologically active metabolites can accumulate and cause excessive CNS depression and other complications.[64,66] Chloral hydrate may be particularly useful for sedating infants and children in situations in preparation for electroencephalogram and pulmonary function tests.

Pentobarbital induces sedation in children more rapidly than chloral hydrate and has shorter duration of action. A lower mg/kg dose of pentobarbital is needed in older patients than younger infants and children. Intravenous pentobarbital should be given in 1 mg/kg increments to minimize risk of respiratory depression.[71,72] In clinical trials, pentobarbital has compared favorably to chloral hydrate for sedation before imaging studies.[73,74] Paradoxical reactions (e.g., excitation and hyperactivity) can occur with barbiturates; however, the administration of a narcotic (e.g., morphine) to the excited child can convert the reaction to a peaceful sedation.

Morphine, fentanyl, and meperidine can provide both sedation and analgesia in patients undergoing painful procedures (e.g., bone marrow biopsy). However, because analgesic effects occur at lower doses than those required for sedation, narcotics rarely are used alone for sedation. Oral fentanyl (Oralet) in doses of 200, 300, and 400 μg is available for use in presurgical sedation. Fentanyl oral lozenge (Actiq) is available in 200, 400, 600, 800, 1200, and 1600 μg strengths for the child to suck on the flavored lozenge until he or she falls asleep.[75] Comparisons of oral transmucosal fentanyl to oral midazolam in premedication sedation have shown mixed results,[76,77] and some clinicians question the associating of drug therapy with candy-like preparations. Narcotic analgesics can induce respiratory depression (especially when combined with benzodiazepines), however, the respiratory depression can be reversed by naloxone.[78,79]

Benzodiazepines (lorazepam, diazepam, and midazolam) can induce sedation, hypnosis, muscle relaxation, amnesia, and can decrease anxiety in patients undergoing procedures.[78,79] These benzodiazepines usually are administered intravenously before the procedure, although midazolam also has produced successful sedation when administered intranasally.[80] Flumazenil, a specific benzodiazepine antagonist, can be used for complete or partial reversal of the sedative effects of benzodiazepines.[81]

The combination of meperidine (Demerol), promethazine (Phenergan), and chlorpromazine (Thorazine), (also known as DPT or pedi cocktail) when administered as an IM injection produces sedation in a majority of patients. This particular combination was less effective and associated with more adverse effects than the oral combination of ketamine with midazolam.[82] In one study, approximately 70% of patients were sedated for ≥7 hours.[83] Therefore, patients receiving DPT should be monitored closely for several hours. Other combination regimens include fentanyl and midazolam, meperidine and pentobarbital, and morphine and various benzodiazepines. These combinations also have been associated with adverse effects and a prolonged duration of action.[78]

Propofol, an anesthetic agent, as a sedative in elective pediatric procedures appears safe for short term sedation. It is as efficacious as other sedative regimens, and is associated with shorter recovery times and hospital stays.[84–86] However, transient hypotension and severe respiratory depression may occur, so appropriate monitoring is essential.[86]

As a result of prolonged sedation with agents such as DPT and opioid/benzodiazepine combinations, and because propofol administration generally requires anesthesiology support, ketamine has been investigated as a sedative agent for procedures in children. Ketamine, a dissociative anesthetic, has proven to be an effective adjunct to benzodiazepines,[87] and has compared favorably to benzodiazepines and opioid/benzodiazepine and other combinations.[82,88,89] Adverse effects associated with ketamine include increased bronchial secretions, hypertension and increased muscle tone. Older children may experience emergence phenomenon with hallucinations or vivid and disturbing dreams. This emergence reaction may be attenuated by concurrent benzodiazepine administration.[88]

Available data do not indicate that one particular sedative combination is superior to another. The choice and dosage of medication(s) usually depend on the type of procedure and the degree of sedation required. Other important considerations include the age of the patient and their clinical condition, location of the procedure, and the cardiopulmonary resuscitation expertise of the staff administering the agents. For A.J., several of the regimens discussed above could be considered. Provided there is adequate anesthesiology support, propofol would be a good choice given its safety profile during short term procedures and the rapid recovery time associated with its use. Ketamine alone or in combination with benzodiazepines, chloral hydrate, pentobarbital or opioid/benzodiazepine (i.e., fentanyl/midazolam) combinations would be appropriate choices as well. Serious adverse events do not appear to be related to medication class or route of administration, though there is an association with adverse outcome when three or more medications are used.[90] Any previous history of successful sedation also can be helpful in the selection of sedation for a patient. The patient should be monitored closely during and after the procedure, and adequate personnel and resuscitation equipment should be readily available.[91]

Intensive Care Unit Sedation

15. **M.P., a 5-year-old boy, is admitted to the pediatric intensive care unit (ICU) for sepsis. He currently is intubated and appropriately paralyzed by medication. What are the considerations when sedating critically ill patients such as M.P.?**

Children who require mechanical ventilation commonly receive medication to induce sedation to facilitate ventilator manipulations without resistance from the patient. In children who receive drugs to induce paralysis, adequate sedation is particularly important to avoid the fear associated with being aware but unable to move.

Critically ill patients often require constant sedation; therefore, scheduled administration (not PRN) of medication or continuous infusions of medication are recommended. Intermittent administration results in peak and trough effects, whereas continuous infusions provide a more constant serum concentration and more constant sedation. However, incompatibility with other IV medications often can be a problem with continuous IV infusions. IM administration of sedation medications should be avoided because of injection pain and erratic absorption in critically ill patients. Medication to induce sedation can be administered orally, but oral administration often is impractical. Clinicians must be diligent in ensuring that sedation for critically ill children is adequate. In one study, even though a majority of recollections were positive, 66% of children receiving morphine and midazolam remembered the PICU, many recalled pain, and that they were scared and could not sleep.[92]

Narcotic analgesics and benzodiazepines are the most commonly used agents for sedation in the ICU. When these drugs are administered repeatedly, the drugs and their metabolites can accumulate and result in adverse consequences especially in patients with impaired hepatic and/or renal function. Repeated doses of chloral hydrate can result in the accumulation of active metabolites and the development of hyperbilirubinemia in newborns or respiratory depression and hypotonia in infants. Normeperidine, an active metabolite of meperidine, can cause seizures in patients with renal impairment after high or repeated doses.

In recent years, propofol has become popular in the ICU. This agent has a rapid onset of action and quick recovery from sedation once discontinued. Propofol has no analgesic effects and is best combined with a narcotic when used after a painful procedure. Adequate sedation is usually achieved with a bolus dose followed by a continuous infusion titrated to effect.[93] Side effects include hypotension in compromised patients, dose-dependent respiratory depression, and myoclonus and seizure activity. Serious and fatal events with prolonged use of propofol have been reported in children[94-98]; however, a direct link between these events and propofol has not been substantiated.[98] If propofol is to be used as a continuous infusion

in the PICU, close monitoring of acid base and clinical status of the patient are warranted. If prolonged mechanical ventilation is required, it may be more appropriate to use agents such as opioids and benzodiazepines.

Children who receive repeated doses of agents for sedation may develop tolerance and require larger doses to achieve the desired effect. In addition, pediatric patients who receive narcotics or benzodiazepines for several days to weeks are at risk for developing symptoms of drug withdrawal.[99,100] Agents used for long-term sedation should never be discontinued abruptly. Problems associated with acute withdrawal can be minimized by decreasing infusion rates 10% to 20% per day or by converting to long-acting oral narcotics and benzodiazepines like methadone and lorazepam.

16. S.C., a 7-year-old boy, is admitted to the hospital after being hit by a car while riding his bicycle. He sustained multiple fractures and has just returned from surgery after an open reduction and internal fixation of his left femur and left humerus. He is tearful and states that he is in a lot of pain. What classes of pain medication are available for use in children? What problems can be anticipated after the use of analgesics in children?

NARCOTIC ANALGESICS

The use of morphine, meperidine, and fentanyl to treat moderate to severe pain in pediatric patients is well documented and Table 93-5 lists characteristics of common analgesics.

Morphine is one of the most commonly used agents. The elimination and clearance of morphine in children older than 5 months of age is similar to that in adults. Neonates demonstrate decreased clearance of morphine and a longer elimination half-life when compared with older infants and children.[101] In neonates, the prolonged half-life may allow for adequate pain control when using intermittent bolus doses. When morphine is administered intermittently, however, older

---

Table 93-5   Analgesic Agents Used in Children[67]

Product	Initial Dose	Comments
Nonopioid		
Acetaminophen	10–15 mg/kg/dose Q 4–6 hr	No anti-inflammatory effect
Salicylates	10–15 mg/kg/dose Q 4–6 hr	Associated with Reye's syndrome; has anti-inflammatory effect
NSAIDs		
Ibuprofen	5–10 mg/kg/dose Q 6–8 hr	Gastritis with prolonged use
Naprosyn	5–7 mg/kg/dose Q 8–12 hr	
Ketorolac	*Adults:* 15–30 mg IM/IV Q 6 hr	Increased risk of bleeding if high doses are used for >5 days
	Children: Not well established; 0.4–1mg/kg IM/IV Q 6 hr; do not exceed adult dose	
Opioids		
Codeine	0.5–1.0 mg/kg/dose Q 4–6 hr (*Adults:* 30–60 mg/dose)	Frequently combined with acetaminophen
Fentanyl	1–2 μg/kg/dose IV/IM (*Adults:* 50–100 μg/dose)	Chest wall rigidity, especially after rapid IV administration
	Infusion: 3–10 μg/kg/hr	
Meperidine	*IV/IM:* 1.0–1.5 mg/kg Q 2–4 hr	Active metabolite has neurotoxic effect; avoid in renal failure
	PO: 1–2 mg/kg Q 3–4 hr (*Adults:* 50–100 mg/dose)	
Morphine	*IV:* 0.05–0.1 mg/kg/dose Q 2–4 hr	When changing to sustained release formulation, give daily dose as 2–3 divided doses
	IM: 0.1–0.2 mg/kg Q2–4 hr	
	PO: 0.2–0.5mg/kg Q 4–6 hr	
	IV infusion: 0.05–0.1 mg/kg/hr	

IM, intramuscular; IV, intravenous; NSAID, nonsteroidal anti-inflammatory drug; PO, oral.

infants and children will require a shorter dosing interval (e.g., every 2 to 3 hours). This frequent dosing schedule has led to an increased use of continuous IV morphine infusion, patient-controlled analgesia (PCA), and epidural infusion.

Meperidine is useful for treatment of rigors postoperatively or after amphotericin B infusion, but offers no analgesic advantages over other opioids such as morphine, fentanyl, or hydromorphone.[101] In addition, meperidine is associated with dysphoria and can precipitate seizures secondary to the accumulation of its active metabolite, nor-meperidine.

Fentanyl, a popular analgesic because of its rapid onset and short duration of action, is most often administered as a continuous or epidural infusion for the management of postoperative pain. It also is administered as an intermittent bolus for short procedures. Fentanyl is highly lipophilic and rapidly penetrates the blood brain barrier. Because it has a larger volume of distribution in neonates, infants, and toddlers, higher dosages may be needed to achieve a desired effect. Also, repeated fentanyl dosing or continuous infusion can lead to accumulation of drug.[101]

Codeine often is administered in combination with acetaminophen to treat mild to moderate pain. Although codeine can be administered intramuscularly, it offers no advantage over the IM administration of morphine or meperidine.

NON-NARCOTIC ANALGESICS

Acetaminophen, salicylates, or nonsteroidal anti-inflammatory drugs (NSAIDs) commonly are used for mild to moderate pain (see Table 93-5.) Salicylates and NSAIDs are useful for bone pain and pain associated with inflammation and can result in an opioid sparing effect. Because of its association with Reye's syndrome, aspirin is not used routinely in children. Ketorolac (Toradol) is the only NSAID available parenterally.[101,102]

ADVERSE EFFECTS

At equipotent doses, all narcotic analgesic agents will cause a similar degree of respiratory depression and constipation. Nausea and vomiting occur secondary to stimulation of the chemoreceptor trigger zone in the brain. Fentanyl produces less sedation than meperidine and morphine. Morphine can produce peripheral vasodilation, which can lead to significant hypotension in hypovolemic patients. Meperidine should be avoided in patients with renal failure because accumulation of its metabolite, normeperidine, has been associated with seizures. The most serious side effect after administration of opioid analgesics is respiratory depression. Infants younger than 3 months of age are particularly susceptible because of their immature blood brain barrier and decreased clearance of narcotics.[101] Patients receiving concomitant therapy with benzodiazepines or barbiturates may be at increased risk for cardiorespiratory side effects.

Adverse effects associated with epidural administration of morphine include nausea, pruritus, urinary retention, and late respiratory depression. Although late respiratory depression appears to be less common in children than adults, respiratory status should still be monitored carefully for up to 12 hours after administration of morphine.

Side effects associated with salicylates and NSAIDs are minimal although gastritis may occur, especially after prolonged use. NSAIDs also have been associated with renal toxicity.

TOLERANCE AND DRUG WITHDRAWAL

Tolerance may occur in some children receiving several days of narcotic therapy resulting in the need for an increased dose to produce the same pain relief. If the patient continues to have reason for pain, doses should be adjusted accordingly. If narcotics are being used for sedation, an alternative agent should be considered.[103]

When opioids are discontinued abruptly after continued use for more than 7 to 10 days. Symptoms of withdrawal can be managed by slowly tapering the drug over several days, or switching to a long-acting oral agent such as methadone. Phenobarbital also can be used to minimize the agitation associated with withdrawal.[103–105]

Analgesia

Inadequate pain control in children usually is the result of inaccurate pain assessment or misconceptions about pain. During the past 30 years, much attention has been placed on the undertreatment of pain experienced by infants and children. In addition, clinical studies have documented that pain experienced by children is treated less aggressively than adult pain.[106] As the effects of pain on psychologic, physiologic, and endocrine systems have become better understood, there has been an increased emphasis on ensuring adequate pain control in pediatric patients.[101]

Administration Schedules

The choice of drug, dose, frequency, and route of administration must be individualized. As-needed dosing schedules are undesirable because patients must endure and/or complain about pain before receiving analgesia. Generally, less medication is needed to prevent the return of pain than to control it. Therefore, scheduled (around the clock) administration of pain medications is preferred over a "PRN" schedule for administration. Continuous IV infusion and scheduled administration of pain medication maintain more constant blood levels and minimizes peak (sedation) and trough (return of pain) effects.

PCA, which allows the patient to administer small bolus doses of analgesia, is an alternative to continuous IV infusion and scheduled administration regimens. PCA eliminates the time between pain perception and relief and gives the patient control over pain therapy. PCA in children and adolescents is safe and effective.[101] Children as young as 6 years of age can be taught to use PCA devices, although the age of children capable of understanding the concept of PCA will vary.[107] In some instances nurses or parents (especially when providing palliative care) are allowed to activate analgesia for the patients who are too young or unable to activate the pump themselves.[102] However, if parents are to be allowed to participate, education on the appropriate and safe activation of the PCA pump should be provided to them and their actions should be closely supervised by nursing personnel. A low-dose continuous infusion combined with PCA has the added benefit of providing baseline pain relief, especially while the patient is sleeping, but can contribute to increased side effects such as hypoxia.[101]

Routes of Administration

Typically, pain medication is administered intravenously, intramuscularly, or orally. The IV route provides the most rapid onset of action. When medication is administered intramuscularly, children may deny pain to avoid injections. When changing from parenteral to oral route, bioavailability and absorption need to be considered. Sustained-release oral formulations may be useful in children with chronic pain, but use of such products often is limited by the ability of the patient to swallow whole tablets and tablet strengths.

Anesthesia also can be achieved through the administration of local anesthetics (e.g., bupivacaine, lidocaine) or narcotics (e.g., morphine, fentanyl). Epidural administration of analgesics can provide pain relief for long periods of time with minimal sedation in children of all ages.[101,107] The transdermal fentanyl patch also offers a unique approach to pain control, and may be useful in children with severe cancer pain.[101] Patches have limited use in young patients since they cannot be cut to deliver smaller doses.

17. Z.Z., a 15-month-old, 10-kg boy, has been receiving fentanyl continuous infusion for 3 weeks for pain and sedation during mechanical ventilation. The infusion has been decreased from 10 μg/kg/hr to 1 μg/kg/hr over the past 5 days. Because Z.Z. has been successfully extubated and will be transferred to the ward in the morning, the fentanyl drip must be discontinued. Is Z.Z. at risk for narcotic withdrawal? What can be done if Z.Z. develops signs and symptoms of withdrawal?

The risk of fentanyl withdrawal is associated with the total dose and duration of the infusion. When the total fentanyl dose is >1.5 mg/kg or the duration of infusion has exceeded 5 days, approximately 50% of patients could experience opioid withdrawal symptoms. When the total fentanyl dose is >2.5 mg/kg or the duration of infusion is >9 days, almost all patients will experience withdrawal.[100] Z.Z. has been receiving fentanyl for 3 weeks; therefore, his risk of withdrawal symptoms is very high.

The fentanyl infusion for Z.Z. should be decreased by 10% every 6 hours, and then converted to an oral narcotic. Once Z.Z. is established on an oral regimen, it can be decreased by 10% to 20% a day. Z.Z. should be monitored for withdrawal symptoms, which usually occur within 24 hours of abrupt discontinuation or dosage reduction. Symptoms of opioid withdrawal include neurologic excitation (irritability, insomnia, tremors, seizures), GI dysfunction (nausea, vomiting, diarrhea), and autonomic dysfunction (sweating, fever, chills, tachypnea, nasal congestion, and rhinitis).[100] If Z.Z. develops withdrawal symptoms, the narcotic agent should be increased to the previously tolerated dose. Clonidine may be a useful adjunct to help prevent symptoms of withdrawal.[106]

TOPICAL ANESTHETICS

18. M.M., a 3-year-old boy, is brought to the emergency department (ED) by his parents for repair of a facial laceration. The physician in the ED orders TAC solution for repair of M.M.'s wound. M.M.'s father is concerned about using TAC because it contains cocaine. What alternatives are available?

TAC solution is a topical anesthetic containing tetracaine, adrenaline (epinephrine), and cocaine that is used for minor procedures such as laryngoscopy, bronchoscopy, and suturing of minor lacerations. Tetracaine and cocaine are potent local anesthetics. Adrenaline and cocaine have vasoconstrictive effects, helping to decrease bleeding and systemic absorption of the solution. TAC typically is supplied as tetracaine 0.5% to 1%, epinephrine 1:2,000, and cocaine 4% to 11.8%. Solutions with low concentrations of cocaine are as effective and less costly.[107]

Local infiltration of anesthetics (e.g., lidocaine) for wound repair often is painful and has the potential to distort wound edges. Although TAC solution is not typically associated with pain, topical anesthetics result in better patient acceptability and more cooperative patients.[108,109]

TAC is not effective when applied to intact skin, and accidental or deliberate applications of the solution to mucosal membranes or burn wounds have resulted in CNS effects including seizures and death. Therefore, TAC should not be used on mucosal surfaces, burns, or large wounds (>10 cm) because of the potential for absorption. TAC also should not be administered to areas where vasoconstriction may compromise vascularity (e.g., ear lobes, tip of nose, digits, penis) and should not be used in patients with a history of seizures or cardiac arrhythmias.

The following guidelines should be used to ensure the safety and efficacy of TAC[110]:

- Determine allergy history
- Thoroughly clean wound and surrounding tissue
- Saturate a sterile gauze pad or cotton ball with TAC solution (children, 0.05 mL/kg; maximum, 3 mL) and cover wound surface
- Let stand for 10 to 20 minutes
- Check for loss of pain sensation before wound repair

Other important considerations include parental acceptance of the solution and the period between TAC application and the repair procedure. If adequate analgesia is not achieved after proper application of TAC or wound repair is delayed, TAC solution may be reapplied to a maximum total dose of 3 mL. However, to avoid exposure to excessive amounts of cocaine, supplemental lidocaine infiltration may be a better alternative than reapplication of TAC.

Because of the high cost of TAC and concern about the cocaine component, other preparations have been evaluated for use as local anesthetics in wound repair. LAT (lidocaine 4%, adrenaline 1:2,000, and tetracaine 0.5%), is less expensive and equally effective in providing anesthesia for facial, scalp, and other lacerations when compared with TAC.[111] Other compounded products used for facial and scalp laceration repair include tetraphen (tetracaine 1% with phenylephrine 5%) and prilophen (3.56% prilocaine and phenylephrine 0.99%). These alternatives are applied in the same manner as TAC; eliminate the need for a controlled substance (i.e., cocaine) to be incorporated into its formulations.[111,112]

19. K.M., a 6-year-old girl, comes to the cancer clinic for IV and intrathecal chemotherapy. Her mother was instructed to apply EMLA at home to facilitate the procedure. Should EMLA be administered? If K.M.'s mother forgets to apply EMLA at home, what alternatives are available?

EMLA topical anesthetic cream, containing 2.5% lidocaine and 2.5% prilocaine, safely and effectively used as a transdermal local reduces pain associated with venipuncture and appears to produce analgesia comparable to that of lidocaine infiltration without requiring an injection.[113,114] EMLA should be applied to intact skin about 1 hour before the procedure. Adverse effects of EMLA include local reactions, which usually resolve spontaneously within 1 to 2 hours; allergic reactions to lidocaine or prilocaine; and a very rare systemic reaction of methemoglobinemia.[113]

EMLA also has been evaluated for use in procedure related pain (e.g., IV cannulation, lumbar puncture). Children receiving EMLA as pre-medication to lumbar puncture reported significantly less pain than those receiving placebo, and EMLA-treated infants seem to have less pain, crying, and tenderness around the vaccination site.[115–117] Fear of the procedure itself is not likely to be reduced significantly with the use of EMLA.[117]

If K.M.'s mother forgets to apply EMLA 1 hour before her scheduled appointment, local anesthesia can be induced within 10 minutes of application using a product marketed as Numby Stuff. This product uses the principles of iontophoresis to deliver a topical solution of 2% lidocaine and 1:100,000 epinephrine with the aid of a battery-powered dose-controlling unit. A mild electrical current delivers the lidocaine and epinephrine directly into the target tissue and thereby produces dermal anesthesia. Lidocaine and epinephrine are positively charged and delivered by the iontophoretic system from the positive electrode. Numby Stuff is well tolerated and is as effective as EMLA.[114,118,119] The use of this product has been associated with the development of urticaria under the electrode, burning sensations, and paresthesias. Another alternative to EMLA for patient K.M. is ELA-max (4% or 5% lidocaine in a liposomal delivery system), a quicker onset of action after application (30 minutes for ELA-max 5% versus 60 minutes for EMLA).[117,120]

HEMOLYTIC UREMIC SYNDROME

Hemolytic uremic syndrome (HUS) is the most common cause of renal failure in children. It is characterized by microangiopathic hemolytic anemia, thrombocytopenia, and acute renal failure. HUS typically occurs several days to 2 weeks after an episode of gastroenteritis, upper respiratory tract infection, or acute flu-like illness. HUS is classified into diarrhea-associated (D+) and non–diarrhea-associated (atypical or D−) illness. Diarrhea-associated HUS is more frequent, has seasonal variation, and occurs primarily between 6 months and 4 years of age. It most often is associated with E. coli (usually subtype O157:H7) that produces a vero-cytotoxin similar to the shigatoxin produced by Shigella species. Pathologically, WBC activation and endothelial cell injury in the kidney lead to fibrin deposition and platelet adherence to vessel walls. Glomerular lumens are swollen and occluded resulting in renal insufficiency. Red blood cells (RBCs) and platelets are damaged by the fibrin strands as they pass through the narrowed vessels. Abnormalities in coagulation involving prostacyclin-thromboxane axis and von Willebrand factor have been implicated in the pathogenesis of thrombocytopenia.[121,122]

The shiga-toxin–producing E. coli (STEC) is spread by contaminated and/or undercooked food and through person-to-person contact. In 1993, a single outbreak of STEC (subtype O157:H7) associated with hamburgers from a fast food chain caused over 600 cases of diarrhea, 151 hospitalization, 45 cases of HUS, most in children, and 3 deaths.[123] As a result, all ground beef should be well cooked until juices run clear and are no longer pink. E. coli O157:H7 outbreaks also have been associated with unpasteurized milk and juices,

fresh produce, alfalfa sprouts, home made beer, venison, lettuce, and contaminated swimming and drinking water.[124,125] Although E. coli O157:H7 is by far the most common etiology, other bacteria and viruses have been implicated in D+ HUS, including Shigella dysenteriae type 1, Salmonella, Campylobacter, Yersinia, Pseudomonas, Bacteroides, Aeromonas, Coxsackie, influenza, and Epstein-Barr.[126] Atypical HUS may be inherited or caused by oral contraceptives, cyclosporine, or cancer chemotherapeutic agents. It also has been seen after pregnancy, Kawasaki's disease, or bone marrow transplant.[121,126] Atypical disease has been increasingly associated with pneumococcal infections.[50] The estimated prevalence of HUS in the United States ranges from 0.3 to 10 per 10,000 children; children with non–diarrhea-associated HUS appear to have a worse prognosis.[127]

20. How can STEC infection be prevented?

The risk of STEC infection can be minimized by using the following guidelines.

1. Wash all fresh food thoroughly.
2. Remove the outer leaves of lettuce and greens.
3. Cook chicken and ground meats until all pink is gone and juices run clear.
4. Cook fish until it is opaque and flakes easily.
5. Do not drink unpasteurized milk, milk products, or juices.
6. Do not eat raw eggs.
7. Wash hands with soap and water after using the bathroom, changing diapers, before eating, and after handling raw meat, poultry, or seafood.[41,51]

Clinical Presentation

21. R.H., a 14-month-old, 9.4 kg girl, has been increasingly irritable and lethargic over the past 24 hours. The sudden appearance of dark urine 24 hours ago and significantly decreased urine output in the past 12 hours caused her mother to bring her in for evaluation. Her recent medical history is significant for 3 days of gastroenteritis with blood which resolved 2 days before the onset of her present symptoms. R.H.'s diet includes breast milk and table food; her mother states that she fed R.H. hamburger earlier in the week.

On physical examination, R.H. is pale, somnolent, and has small purple bruises over her arms and legs. Significant laboratory results reveal the following: partial thromboplastin time (PTT), 26 seconds (normal, 25 to 35 seconds); hemoglobin (Hgb), 7.6 g/dL (normal, 11.8 g/dL); hematocrit (Hct), 22.5%(normal, 36%); WBC, 15,100 cells/mm³ (normal, 6,000 –17,500cells/mm³); platelet count, 44,000 cells/mm³ (normal, 150,000 –400,000 cells/mm³); reticulocytes, 4.7%(normal, 0.5 –1.5%); blood urea nitrogen (BUN), 60 mg/dL (normal, 5 to 18 mg/dL); serum creatinine (SrCr), 3.9 mg/dL (normal, 0.3 to 0.7 mg/dL); potassium (K), 5.4 mEq/L (normal, 3.5 to 5.5 mEq/L); urinalysis, 3+ protein and 3+ blood; blood smear, schistocytes (fragmented RBCs); factor V and VIII within normal limits; fibrinogen within normal limits; and fibrin split within normal limits. R.H. is admitted to the hospital with a diagnosis of HUS. Which signs, symptoms, and laboratory tests are consistent with HUS in R.H.?

[SI units: Hgb 1.178 mmol/L (normal 1.829); Hct, 0.225 (normal 0.36); platelet count, 44 × 10⁹/L (normal 150 to 400); WBC, 15.1 × 10⁹/L (normal 6 to 17.5); reticulocytes, 0.047 (normal 0.005 to 0.015); BUN, 21.42 mmol/L (normal 1.8 to 6.4); SiCi, 344.8 μmol/L (normal 26.5 to 61.9); K, 5.4 mmol/L (normal, 3.5 to 5.5)]

R.H. exhibits many signs and symptoms associated with HUS. Her lethargy, irritability, change in mental status, and pale color are symptoms of anemia. The dark color of her urine is indicative of hemolysis and renal damage; other signs of renal damage include anuria and hypertension. The purpura (i.e., bruises) on her arms and legs are evidence for thrombocytopenia.

R.H.'s laboratory abnormalities also help confirm a diagnosis of HUS. The low hemoglobin and hematocrit are consistent with anemia, whereas the high reticulocyte count and presence of schistocytes indicate hemolysis. Nephropathy in R.H. is manifested by proteinuria and elevations in BUN and creatinine. The hyperkalemia is a sign of both nephropathy and hemolysis. Finally, normal coagulation studies, absence of fibrin split products, and normal levels of clotting factors and fibrinogen indicate that R.H., like many children with HUS, does not have active disseminated intravascular coagulation (DIC) at initial presentation.

Treatment

22. On admission, R.H. is given intravenous fluids at half maintenance without potassium and nifedipine 2 mg (0.2 mg/kg) PO Q 4 to 6 hr PRN for hypertension. However, her urine output decreased significantly and peritoneal dialysis was initiated within 24 hours. How should R.H. be managed? What is the role of antibiotic therapy?

Therapeutic approaches aimed at modifying the acute phase of HUS have been unsuccessful, and supportive care is the only widely accepted form of treatment. Therapy for R.H. should be directed at managing complications associated with HUS, including fluid and electrolyte imbalance, anemia, thrombocytopenia, renal failure, hypertension, and seizures. Antimotility agents should be avoided because, in addition to having little if any clinical benefit, they may increase morbidity.[124,133] The value of using antibiotics to treat E. coli O157:H7 infections is questionable and may increase the rate of progression to HUS.[134,135] The rate of HUS was increased in children with diarrhea caused by E. coli O157:H7 who were treated with either trimethoprim/sulfamethoxazole or beta lactam antibiotics.[136] As a result, until conclusive data indicate otherwise, antibiotics should be avoided.[137]

Correction of Hemostatic and Electrolyte Imbalances

R.H.'s hemostatic and electrolyte imbalances need to be corrected first. Packed RBCs are recommended in severe anemia (Hct <15%) or if the patient is symptomatic from anemia. Infusion of platelets should be limited to those patients with active bleeding and those requiring surgery or central line placement as platelets may exacerbate platelet aggregation and thrombus formation.[57] R.H. should not receive potassium in IV fluids, and her electrolytes should be monitored frequently. If peritoneal dialysis is not initiated, R.H. may require potassium lowering therapy. Blood pressure elevations should be treated with nifedipine, and seizures should be treated initially with benzodiazepines, followed by phenobarbital or phenytoin if they cannot be controlled.[138]

23. What other modes of therapy have been used to treat HUS in children?

Many treatments have been evaluated in HUS, but few have demonstrated an impact on outcome. Antiplatelet agents have been used in an attempt to decrease the formation of platelet thrombi on damaged endothelium and to secondarily limit renal damage.[139] Aspirin and dipyridamole have been used singly or in combination, but studies have not demonstrated clinical efficacy.[140–142]

Heparin has been used in attempt to prevent further fibrin deposition in the kidneys, thereby limiting progression of nephropathy. Although anticoagulants may be beneficial in the small subgroup of children with HUS who have active DIC, they do not affect the outcome of most children with HUS.[141–143]

It was hoped that streptokinase and urokinase might limit the renal damage in HUS by lysing fibrin in renal blood vessels. Although these drugs should hasten resolution of nephropathy in HUS, they do not improve prognosis.[144]

Plasmapheresis has been attempted, but is not a well-established treatment for HUS.[139] It theoretically increases prostacyclin production by replacing a plasma factor that stimulates release of vascular prostacyclin or by removing an inhibitor of prostacyclin synthesis. Increased prostacyclin levels may decrease platelet aggregation in renal capillaries, thereby improving renal function indirectly.[145] Exchange transfusion and fresh frozen plasma (FFP) were thought to benefit children with HUS by normalizing prostacyclin synthesis, but two prospective studies evaluating the use of FFP in patients with HUS found no effect on the course, pathology, or outcome of the disease.[146,147] Corticosteroids have been evaluated in HUS but do not appear to dramatically improve outcome.[148] A vaccine for E. coli O157:H7 has been investigated, as has a toxin binding agent, but neither have been approved for use.[149,150]

IDIOPATHIC THROMBOCYTOPENIC PURPURA

Idiopathic thrombocytopenic purpura (ITP) in children generally is an acute, self-limited, benign disease with spontaneous remission occurring in approximately 80% of cases within 6 months of diagnosis whether treated or not.[128] Chronic ITP evolves from the acute form in approximately 25% of cases, although <10% of these are clinically significant.[129,130] Mortality rates are low, and most deaths can be attributed to intracranial hemorrhage, which occurs in <1% of children with platelet counts <10,000/mm³.[128] Some experts feel the incidence of hemorrhage may be overestimated.[131] The social and psychologic effects that occur secondarily to restriction of normal childhood physical activity constitute the primary forms of morbidity.

The etiology of ITP in children is unknown. ITP is thought to be triggered by a viral infection that induces formation of antigen–antibody complexes. These complexes adhere to platelets resulting in increased platelet consumption by the reticuloendothelial system (RES). The chronic form, which is similar to adult ITP, may be due to production of autoantibodies to platelet antigens.[128,132]

Clinical Presentation

24. J.T., a 3-year-old, 15-kg, previously healthy girl, presents with a 3-week history of increased bruising and repeated nosebleeds after an episode of gastroenteritis. Physical examination is remarkable for generalized petechiae and scattered bruising. Her Hgb, Hct, WBC count and differential, and peripheral smear are within normal limits, but the platelet count is 10,000/mm³ (normal, 250,000 to 350,000/mm³). She is admitted to the hospital with a diagnosis of acute ITP. Which signs, symptoms, and laboratory tests in J.T. are consistent with ITP?

[SI unit: platelet count, 10×10^9/L (normal, 250 to 350)]

Diagnosis of ITP is based on clinical presentation, complete blood count (CBC), and examination of peripheral smear.[129] As illustrated by J.T., children with acute ITP classically present with a sudden appearance of purpura or petechiae within 6 weeks of the onset of a viral infection. Approximately 25% of children with acute ITP have epistaxis (nosebleeds), 5% have hematuria, and <4% have massive purpura or retinal hemorrhages. Diagnosis of ITP is confirmed by presence of thrombocytopenia with no apparent cause. The marked decrease in J.T.'s platelet count to <25,000 cells/mm³ with a normal CBC is indicative of ITP.

Treatment

25. How should J.T. be managed initially?

Hospitalization is indicated for children with life-threatening bleeding regardless of the platelet count. J.T. can be managed conservatively because she is not massively hemorrhaging. Medical treatment is indicated in the two groups of children thought to be at highest risk for intracranial hemorrhage: (1) children with platelet counts <20,000 cells/mm³ who have moderate mucous membrane bleeding and (2) children with platelet counts <10,000 cells/mm³ with minor purpura.[129] If J.T.'s platelet count were higher, some clinicians would delay treatment because the risk of spontaneous, severe bleeding is low if platelet counts remain >30,000/mm³. Also, clinicians may not treat children like J.T. who are not massively hemorrhaging or bleeding internally, regardless of the platelet count, since the incidence of catastrophic hemorrhage is very low.[131,151]

Splenectomy

The treatment of choice is controversial because the mortality rate is low, the rate of spontaneous remission is high, and data for different therapies are inconsistent.[129] The only therapeutic modality with undisputed efficacy is splenectomy because the major site of platelet phagocytosis and antibody formation is removed. However, because splenectomy is a major surgical procedure leaving a child at risk for serious infection, and treatment with IV gamma globulin (IVIG) therapy or high-dose steroids is associated with good results, many clinicians reserve splenectomy for children with resistant cases of ITP.[129,130]

26. What treatments are available for acute ITP?

Observation, splenectomy, glucocorticoids, IVIG, and anti-D immune globulin have been used to treat acute ITP. Platelet transfusions are ineffective because infused platelets are removed rapidly by the reticuloendothelial system.

Glucocorticoids

Glucocorticoids have been used as treatment for acute ITP for many years, but their benefits and indications are controversial.[128] Glucocorticoids may decrease the duration of thrombocytopenia by inhibiting platelet phagocytosis and they also may lower the risk of hemorrhage by increasing capillary integrity.

The efficacy of glucocorticoids has been disputed. First, not all studies have shown that steroids induce a more rapid rise in platelet levels than would occur spontaneously. Second, there is not enough evidence to support the claim that steroids increase capillary integrity. Also, indications for using steroids vary among clinicians. However, most agree that high-dose glucocorticoids should be considered if the patient's platelet count is <50,000/mm³ with severe bleeding, <20,000/mm³ with mucous membrane bleeding, or <10,000/mm³ with minor purpura.[129]

The optimal steroid regimen for acute ITP has not been determined. Prednisone dosages of 4 mg/kg for 7 days followed by a taper until day 21 or methylprednisolone 30 to 50 mg/kg/day for 7 days produce platelet recovery similar to IVIG.[152–154] More recently, a short course of prednisone at 4 mg/kg/day for 4 days has been shown to be effective at increasing platelet counts above 20,000/mm³, although 41% required retreatment at 1 month.[155] The risks of using steroids are low because they are used for a short period. Behavioral abnormalities, weight gain, acne, and GI upset have been reported in children receiving high-dose glucocorticoid therapy.

Anti-D Immune Globulin

Anti-D immune globulin (anti-D) is a polyclonal antiserum against the Rh(D) antigen of RBCs that was first licensed to prevent hemolytic disease of newborns caused by Rh isoimmunization. Anti-D has been considered as a treatment option for ITP because it has a lower cost and shorter infusion time (15 minutes) compared to IVIG. It has the greatest efficacy in D antigen–positive patients and is thought to increase platelet counts in ITP by binding to Rh-positive erythrocytes. This leads to removal of the sensitized RBCs by the spleen, allowing the antibody-coated platelets to survive.[156] Most patients experience a mild, transient hemolysis.

A randomized trial comparing anti-D to two doses of IVIG and high-dose prednisone in the treatment of acute ITP in patients with platelet counts <20,000/mm³ found that anti-D (25 μg/kg per day for 2 days) took longer to increase platelet counts to >20,000/mm³ and >50,000/mm³.[152] As a result, anti-D has been considered third-line therapy. A trial in 20 Rh-positive children with acute or chronic ITP found that larger doses (mean, 60 μg/kg) of anti-D caused a greater increase in platelet counts than previously reported.[153] In addition, another trial using 45 to 50 μg/kg of anti-D was as effective as IVIG, with times to platelet counts of 20,000 and 40,000/mm³ and length of hospitalization the same.[157] Randomized trials are under way to compare the efficacy of higher-dose anti-D to traditional therapies used in ITP. While anti-D appears at least as safe and maybe as effective as IVIG, serious adverse events may occur.[158,159]

Intravenous Gamma Globulin

IVIG is commonly used therapy for acute ITP. IVIG induces a rapid rise in platelet counts, and this action may prevent hemorrhage. An advantage of IVIG is that it induces a more rapid increase in platelet levels than glucocorticoids or no therapy.[153] However, while platelet counts typically increase more quickly with IVIG treatment,[153] similar platelet recovery times have been attained with higher doses of corticosteroids (methylprednisone 30 to 50 mg/kg/day for 7 days).[154]

The mechanism of action of IVIG in ITP has been studied extensively. It is thought to work by blocking phagocytosis of antibody-coated platelets by the reticuloendothelial system or by eliminating circulating immune complexes and microbial antigens.[128] Adverse reactions to IVIG usually are mild and related to the rate of administration. Reactions may include flushing, chills, fever, headache, dizziness, diaphoresis, and nausea and can be minimized by stopping the infusion or decreasing the infusion rate. Hypotension, dyspnea, myalgias, joint pain, and abdominal pain also have been reported. Anaphylactic reactions have been reported in patients with IgA deficiency. Another consideration is the relatively high cost of IVIG therapy.

IVIG or high-dose glucocorticoids are reasonable treatments for J.T. because she is at high risk for bleeding. On the other hand, some clinicians might elect to withhold therapy and monitor J.T. closely.

DOSING

27. **The hematologist decides to treat J.T. with IVIG and orders Gammagard 15 g IV Is this regimen optimal for J.T.?**

IVIG regimens of 400 mg/kg/day for 2 to 5 days, 1 g/kg for one dose, and a single infusion of 800 mg/kg have been effective in the treatment of ITP.[152,157] Proper IVIG administration can reduce the incidence of side effects. Headaches, nausea, chills, fever, and hypotension may be avoided by infusing IVIG slowly.[160] Premedication with an antipyretic or an antihistamine also may help minimize these adverse reactions.[160,161] Other side effects include cutaneous rashes and local reactions at the injection site. Recommended infusion rates differ for each of the commercially available preparations. To avoid an inflammatory response, infusions of IVIG should begin at a low rate and be increased as tolerated.

J.T.'s dose of IVIG is 1 g/kg for one dose and should be effective, however, the optimal dose of IVIG to treat ITP is unknown. The 15-g dose should be infused over several hours. The infusion should be initiated at a rate recommended by the manufacturer of the IVIG. To minimize adverse effects, 200 mg acetaminophen (13 mg/kg per dose) and 15 mg diphenhydramine (1 mg/kg per dose) can be administered 30 to 60 minutes before starting the IVIG infusion. Epinephrine and hydrocortisone should be readily available in the event of an anaphylactic reaction.

Goals of Therapy

28. **What are the goals of therapy?**

The ultimate goal of therapy is induction of remission. If remission does not occur, therapy is aimed at maintenance of hemostatic platelet levels and prevention of catastrophic hemorrhage. Unfortunately, severe internal bleeding has occurred in patients despite treatment with steroids or IVIG. Another goal of therapy is to avoid performing a splenectomy, which would put the child at an increased risk for infection.[129]

Prognosis

29. **What is J.T.'s prognosis?**

J.T.'s prognosis is good, much better than the prognosis of adults with ITP.[129] Only 10% to 20% of children will fail to achieve remission within 6 months of diagnosis.[162] Children with chronic ITP will enter remission slowly over a period of years or after a splenectomy.[129] Although early institution of nonsurgical treatments for acute ITP can decrease morbidity and mortality, they probably cannot prevent the development of chronic ITP.[129]

Chronic Idiopathic Thrombocytopenic Purpura

30. **J.T.'s platelet count rose to 260,000/mm³ after she received the IVIG, and her counts have remained within normal limits for the past year. J.T. appears to be in remission. If she had developed chronic ITP, how would she have been managed?**

[SI unit: platelet count, 260×10^9/L]

Chronic ITP is defined as thrombocytopenia lasting for longer than 6 months. There are different approaches to the treatment of chronic ITP, but all agree that splenectomy should be delayed to allow for spontaneous remission as long as hemostatic platelet counts are maintained and the child remains asymptomatic.[129]

IVIG, glucocorticoids, or anti-D can be used to maintain adequate platelet counts or control symptoms before a splenectomy.[129] IVIG sometimes is cited as the treatment of choice for chronic ITP because it has relatively few side effects. Repeated doses of IVIG (0.8 to 1 g/kg) or anti-D (50 to 75 µg/kg) may be required to maintain hemostatic platelet counts.[130] Dexamethasone at doses of 20 mg/m² did not prove to be effective in chronic ITP.[163] As a result of adverse events such as exacerbation of thrombocytopenia, delayed bone growth, and also a lack of effectiveness,[158] long-term steroid use is discouraged. Other modalities (e.g., plasmapheresis, danazol, α-interferon, azathioprine [Imuran], cyclophosphamide [Cytoxan], vincristine [Oncovin], vinblastine [Velban], 6-mercaptopurine) have been attempted for children with steroid or IVIG resistant chronic ITP, but data are insufficient to support their routine use.[129]

Splenectomy is effective in 70% of children with chronic ITP and is indicated in symptomatic children with platelet counts that have remained below 30,000/mm³ for 12 months.[129,130] A good response to IVIG could be predictive of good response to splenectomy.[164,165] Steroids or IVIG can be given before splenectomy to obtain platelet counts that will maintain hemostasis during surgery.[129] Children should be immunized with Hib, pneumococcal, and meningococcal vaccines at least 2 weeks before an elective splenectomy. Therefore, if J.T. develops chronic ITP, she could receive a repeat course of IVIG with booster doses to maintain hemostasis; a second line of therapy would be steroids or anti-D. Splenectomy and immunosuppressive drugs would be considered last resorts.

Finally, parents should be educated to avoid medications with antiplatelet effects (e.g., aspirin, dipyridamole, nonsteroidal anti-inflammatory drugs) in children with ITP. Parents also should be instructed to monitor their child's physical activity to avoid any trauma that could precipitate life-threatening hemorrhage.

NEPHROTIC SYNDROME

Nephrotic syndrome in children (typically characterized by proteinuria, hypoalbuminemia, edema, hypercholesterolemia) is a common reason for referral of children to pediatric nephrologists.[166,167] Overall, it is still a relatively rare pediatric disorder with an incidence of 2 to 7 cases per 100,000 children under 18 years of age.[166,167] This idiopathic nephrotic state can present as minimal change nephrotic syndrome or focal segmental glomerular sclerosis. Minimal change disease is in part characterized by normal glomeruli on microscopic analysis.[168,169] It is by far the more common manifestation in children, with more than 75% of those younger than 12 years of age having this type of nephritic syndrome.[167,169]

In minimal change disease, a loss in charge selectivity of the glomerular membrane barrier, which allows large plasma proteins such as albumin and immunoglobulins to be filtered into the urine that would otherwise be reabsorbed.[169] The etiology is complex, and has not been fully characterized, but T-lymphocyte dysfunction may play a role in the pathogenesis of nephrotic syndrome.[170]

Clinical Presentation

31. **GG, a previously healthy 4 year-old, 21-kg boy, has been noted by his mother to have swelling in his face, especially his eyes the past several mornings. The facial swelling disappears during the day, but at night his feet and lower legs are swollen. Physical examination reveals normal vital signs but is significant for mild facial puffiness, and 2–3+ pitting edema of the lower extremities. Laboratory analysis reveals the following: urinalysis significant for 4+ protein (normal, negative or trace); specific gravity, 1.029 (normal, 1.002 to 1.030); serum albumin, 1.6 g/dL (normal, 3.9 to 5 g/dL); and serum cholesterol 296 mg/dL (normal, 109 to 189 mg/dL); the rest of the chemistry results are within normal limits. What signs and symptoms are consistent with nephrotic syndrome?**

[SI units: albumin, 16 g/L (normal, 39 to 50), serum cholesterol, 7.7 mmol/l (normal, 2.8 to 4.8)]

G.G. presents with typical findings of nephrotic syndrome. Edema of the face early in the day, and lower extremities at night is a result of the loss of oncotic pressure caused by hypoalbuminemia. Other manifestations of this complication can include swelling of the scrotum, which can lead to testicular torsion. Decreased oncotic pressure can also result in abdominal pain due to decreased perfusion to the splanchnic capillary bed.

The main laboratory finding in nephrotic syndrome is proteinuria. Levels of proteinuria associated with nephrotic syndromes have been quantified as >50 mg/kg/24 hr and 3.5 g/1.73 m²/day, but have also been generally been described as "heavy proteinuria" or proteinuria that is significant enough to result in the four major clinical findings in nephrotic syndrome.[166,167,169] GG has 4+ protein in his dipstick urinalysis (≥2000 mg/dl), which is significant. If the dipstick protein is persistently elevated (≥1+), a spot urine analysis, using the first morning void, may be done to assess the protein/creatinine ratio (Pr/Cr). If the Pr/Cr is abnormal (normal for children younger than 2 years of age is <0.2 mg Pr/1 mg Cr), a complete workup should be pursued, including history and other pertinent tests.[166]

Serum albumin levels of less than 2 g/dL will likely result in visible edema. Serum cholesterol and triglyceride are often elevated. Reasons for this are not entirely clear, but may be due to decreased catabolic capacity of the liver, and also increased production.[167] Other laboratory abnormalities can include hypocalcemia, hyperkalemia, and hyponatremia. Patients with idiopathic minimal change disease do not usually present with gross hematuria, hypertension, or renal dysfunction.

Treatment

32. **G.G. is eventually diagnosed with nephrotic syndrome. How should he be managed initially? What nonpharmacologic interventions can be considered?**

Patients with nephrotic syndrome have an increased total body sodium due to increased retention, even in the presence of low serum levels and decreased intravascular volume.[166,167,169] Therefore, sodium restriction is important. Although it is not practical to set a sodium limit in children, a "no-added salt" diet is usually recommended in which family support and participation is crucial. Many institutions will provide patients with examples of foods that are low in sodium, such as fresh beef or chicken, certain cheeses, and fresh vegetables, among others. Patients may eat the normal recommended daily allowance of protein, as protein restriction does not consistently decrease proteinuria or impact the progression of renal disease.[166,167]

High-dose corticosteroids are first-line therapy. One regimen is prednisone 2 mg/kg/day or 60 mg/m²/day (80 mg/day maximum) for 4 weeks, and then switched to 2 mg/kg/day or 40 mg/m²/day every other day and tapered over another 4 weeks. Some data support a longer regimen of 6 weeks of every day therapy followed by 6 weeks of every other day therapy. Although long-course therapy may result in a higher rate of remissions, side effects are more common and the overall benefit is not always significant.[166,167] Long-term, high-dose corticosteroid regimens are associated with a number of adverse effects, and parents must be properly educated (Table 93-6).[166,167]

33. **How is G.G.'s response to steroid therapy determined?**

Most children with minimal change disease respond within weeks of initiating corticosteroids. Remission is defined as negative or trace protein for at least 3 consecutive days on dipstick urinalysis.[166] Of patients who respond, 60% to 80% will

Table 93-6 Complications of Corticosteroid Therapy[166,167]	
CNS	***Gastrointestinal***
Depression	Gastric irritation
Steroid psychosis	Ulcer
Behavioral changes/mood lability	Increased appetite
Pseudotumor cerebri	
Endocrine/Metabolic	***Miscellaneous***
Growth retardation	Immune suppression
Osteoporosis	Cataracts
Avascular necrosis	Cushingoid features
Diabetes	Hypertension
Weight gain/fluid retention	Night sweats

have multiple relapses, defined as >2+ proteinuria for 3 consecutive days or 3–4+ proteinuria with edema. Relapses are treated with high dose prednisone until the urine is protein free for 3 days. Prednisone is then tapered over 4 to 6 weeks using alternate day therapy.[166]

34. What options exist for patients with frequent relapses or for those who are steroid dependent or resistant?

More than 50% of children with nephrotic syndrome will have relapses. Frequent relapse is been defined as ≥2 relapses in the first 6 months after initial response or ≥4 relapses in any 1 year period. Steroid dependency occurs when there are 2 consecutive relapses during steroid tapering or relapse within 14 days of steroid discontinuation. Steroid resistance is described as a failure to achieve remission after 4 weeks of every day high dose therapy followed by 4 weeks of alternate day therapy.[166] Several studies have investigated patient characteristics that predict relapses in nephrotic patients. One study found that patients who responded within 1 week of therapy and did not present with hematuria were less likely to have frequent relapses in the first year.[171] Another examined 467 relapses in 121 patients over a 20 year follow-up period: children who relapsed within 1 year or who had short remissions before relapse were more likely to have subsequent relapses.[172] Yap and colleagues found that an initial remission time of 9 or more days and concurrent upper respiratory tract infections were predictive of steroid dependency.[173] Age at onset of disease, gender, and race were not associated with risk in any of the studies.

In difficult to manage patients, high-dose alternate day regimens tapered to monthly intravenous pulse doses of methylprednisolone at 30 mg/kg (maximum, 1 g) have been used.[166,167] Such patients should be under the care of a pediatric nephrologist and should be monitored for infusion reactions like hypertension. Cytotoxic drugs are reserved for patients who do not respond to steroids after multiple courses or in those whom side effects have become intolerable. Cyclophosphamide at 2 mg/kg/day for 8 to 12 weeks has produced long remissions, often resulting in decreased use or even no requirement for steroids.[166,174] Other agents such as chlorambucil, cyclosporine, and levamisole are also effective in inducing remission, with chlorambucil proving as effective as cyclophosphamide. Relapses tend to occur shortly after cyclosporine and levamisole are discontinued.[166,167,174,175] Any time cytotoxic agents are utilized, patients must be monitored for bone marrow suppression. Other potential problems that must be discussed with the family before initiation of these agents include the possibility of malignancy, infertility, alopecia, increased infection risk, and hemorrhagic cystitis with cyclophosphamide.

35. What other complications are possible in children with nephrotic syndrome?

Nephrotic syndrome can lead to a hypercoagulable state. Many factors are thought to contribute to this problem including increased factor V and VIII, increased fibrinogen and decreased coagulation inhibitors such as antithrombin III. In addition, platelet activity is elevated.[169] This alteration in hemostasis can lead to life-threatening events in children,[176,177] although such events are less common than in adults.[169] Antiplatelet or anticoagulant agents are recommended in patients who have a history of a thromboembolic event.[166] In addition, diuretics must be administered with caution in patients with a history of an event.

Children with nephrotic syndrome have an increased risk of infection secondary to alterations in circulating immune globulins, cellular immunity, and chemotaxis. Cellulitis and spontaneous bacterial peritonitis occur at higher rates in this population; children with albumin <1.5 g/dl are thought to be at greatest risk.[178] Encapsulated organisms such as *Streptococcus pneumoniae* and gram negative rods like *Escherichia coli* are the most frequent causes of bacterial infection. Prophylactic antibiotics have been used during active relapse, but efficacy in preventing peritonitis has not been shown, and there is no consensus among pediatric nephrologists on how to manage the infection risk in these patients.[166,179] Patients should receive standard vaccination using the childhood immunization schedule. The pneumococcal conjugate vaccine (Prevnar) or the pneumococcal polysaccharide vaccine (Pneumovax) should be administered to children with nephrotic syndrome if they were not immunized as infants.[166,180] Live viral vaccines are appropriate for these patients, but must not be given while receiving high dose corticosteroids or other immunosuppressive therapy. Varicella vaccine has been studied in nephrotic patients and is safe and effective.[166,181]

Hyperlipidemia is a common complication of nephritic syndrome, but it usually resolves spontaneously in steroid responsive patients. Lipid levels may remain elevated in steroid resistant patients and, if diet intervention has no impact, many lipid lowering agents are available. While only bile acid sequestrants are FDA approved for use in pediatric patients, hepatic 3-methylglutaryl coenzyme A reductase inhibitors (statins) have been evaluated in children.[182,183] Therapy with statins appears to significantly reduce total cholesterol and low density lipoprotein (LDL) and triglycerides, but has no documented impact on disease progression. Statin therapy may have beneficial effects on arterial endothelium.[184]

Renal protein excretion may be decreased by angiotensin converting enzyme inhibitors (ACE-I). Long term benefit in children with nephrotic syndrome is not known. ACE-I should be given with caution, especially during initial steroid therapy because of the risk of hypotension, resulting in an increased risk of thrombosis.[166]

36. What is the prognosis of children with nephrotic syndrome?

In minimal change disease, mortality is approximately 2%, mostly due to peritonitis or thrombotic complications. The majority of patients will be steroid responsive, but will likely have multiple relapses over several years. Considering all categories of nephrotic syndrome in children, 20% will sustain remission, 50% will have relapses in any 5-year follow-up period, and the remaining 30% will develop nephrosis. Half of this last group can attain remission with combination therapy of prednisone and cytotoxic drugs if they have minimal change disease.[167]

REFERENCES

1. Kaushal R et al. Medication errors and adverse drug events in pediatric inpatients. JAMA 2001;285:2114.
2. Johnson D, Tinanoff N. Development and developmental anomalies of the teeth. In: Behrman Re et al., eds. Textbook of Pediatrics. 16th Ed. Philadelphia: WB Saunders, 2000:1108.
3. Golden NL et al. Teething age in prematurely born infants. Am J Dis Child 1981;135:903.
4. Wake M et al. Teething and tooth eruption in infants: a cohort study. Pediatrics 2000;106:1374.
5. Sims KM. Oral pain and discomfort. In: Handbook of Nonprescription Drugs. 13th Ed. Washington, DC: American Pharmaceutical Association, 2002:654.
6. Skoglund RR. Teething ring cheilitis. Cutis 1984;34:362.
7. Berg RW et al. Association of skin wetness and pH with diaper dermatitis. Pediatric Dermatol 1994; 11(1):18.
8. Jordon WE. Relationship of diapers to diaper rashes. J Pediatr 1980;96:957.
9. Mofenson HC et al. Baby powder—a hazard. Pediatrics 1981;68:265.
10. Leyden JJ. Corn starch, Candida albicans and diaper rash. Pediatr Dermatol 1984;1:322.
11. Sires UI, Mallory SB. Diaper dermatitis: how to treat and prevent. Postgrad Med 1995;98(6):79.
12. Jaffe D. Assessment of the child with fever. In: Rudolph AM, ed. Rudolph's Pediatrics. 21st Ed. New York: McGraw-Hill, 2002:889.
13. Warden CR et al. Evaluation and management of febrile seizures in the out-of-hospital and emergency department settings. Ann Emerg Med 2003; 41:215.
14. Applegate MS, Lo W. Febrile seizures: current concepts concerning prognosis and clinical management. J Fam Pract 1989;29:422.
15. Yip L et al. Concepts and controversies in salicylate toxicity. Emerg Med Clinic North Am 1994; 12(2):351.
16. Glasgow JF, Middleton B. Reye's syndrome—insights on causation and prognosis. Arch Dis Child 2001;85:351.
17. Delay ED et al. Reye's syndrome in the United States from 1981 through 1997. N Engl J Med 1999;340:1377.
18. Wilson JT et al. Single dose, placebo-controlled comparative study of ibuprofen and acetaminophen antipyresis in children. J Pediatr 1991;119:803.
19. Lesko SM, Mitchell AA. The safety of acetaminophen and ibuprofen among children younger than two years old. Pediatrics 1999;104:e39.
20. Lesko SM, Mitchell AA. An assessment of the safety of pediatric ibuprofen: a practitioner-based randomized clinical trial. JAMA 1995;273:929.
21. Lesko SM, Mitchell AA. Renal function after short-term ibuprofen use in infants and children. Pediatrics 1997;100:954.
22. Katcher ML. Cold, cough, and allergy medications: uses and abuses. Pediatr Rev 1996;17:12.
23. Soderman P et al. CNS reactions to nose drops in small children. Lancet 1984;1:573.
24. Dunn C et al. Coma in a neonate following single intranasal dose of xylometazoline. Eur J Pediatr 1993;152:541.
25. Felt B et al. Guideline for the management of pediatric idiopathic constipation and soiling. Arch Pediatr Adolesc Med 1999;153:380.
26. Baker SS et al. Constipation in infants and children: evaluation and treatment. A medical position statement of the North American Society for Pediatric Gastroenterology and Nutrition. J Pediatr Gastroenterol Nutr 1999;29:612.
27. Li UK, Stevenson RJ. Common symptoms and signs of gastrointestinal disorders. In: Rudolph AM, ed. Pediatrics. 20th Ed. Norwalk, CT: Appleton and Lange, 1996:1027.
28. Ulsher M. Major symptoms and signs of digestive tract disorders. In: Behrman RE, ed. Nelson Textbook of Pediatrics. Philadelphia: WB Saunders, 2000:1101.
29. Gastanaduy AS, Begue RE. Acute gastroenteritis. Clin Pediatr 1999;38:1.
30. Leung AKC, Robson WLM. Evaluating the child with chronic diarrhea. Am Fam Phys 1996;53(2):635.
31. Leighton L. Body composition, normal electrolyte concentrations, and the maintenance of normal volume, tonicity and acid base metabolism. Pediatr Clin North Am 1990;37:241.
32. Blackburn P. Dehydration and fluid replacement. In: Reisdorf EJ et al., eds. Pediatric Emergency Medicine. Philadelphia: WB Saunders;1993:108.
33. Snyder JD. Evaluation and treatment of diarrhea. Semin Gastro Dis 1994;5:47.
34. Anquist KW et al. Diagnostic delay after dimenhydrinate use in vomiting children. Can Med Assoc J 1991;145:965.
35. American Academy of Pediatrics Practice Guideline: the management of acute gastroenteritis in young children. Pediatrics 1996;97(3):424.
36. Murphy MS. Guidelines for managing acute gastroenteritis based on a systematic review of published research. Arch Dis Child 1998;79(3):279.
37. Armon K et al. An evidence and consensus based guideline for acute diarrhoea management. Arch Dis Child 2000l;85:132.
38. Nelson SP et al. Prevalence of symptoms of gastroesophageal reflux during infants: a pediatric practice-based survey. Pediatric Practice Research Group. Arch Pediatr Adolesc Med 1997;151:569.
39. DeMeester TR et al. Biology of gastroesophageal reflux disease: pathophysiology relating to medical and surgical treatment. Ann Rev Med 1999;50:469.
40. Nelson SP et al. One-year follow-up of symptoms of gastroesophageal reflux during infancy. Pediatric Research Group. Pediatrics 1998;102:E67.
41. Wooodard-Knight L et al. Aluminum absorption and antacid therapy in infancy. J Paediatr Child Health 1992;28:257.
42. Rudolph CD et al. North American Society for Pediatric Gastroenterology and Nutrition. Guidelines for evaluation and treatment of gastroesophageal reflux in infants and children: recommendations of the North American Society for Pediatric Gastroenterology and Nutrition. J Pediatr Gastroenterol Nutr 2001;32(S):S1.
43. Marcon MA. Advances in the diagnosis and treatment of gastroesophageal reflux disease. Curr Opin Pediatr 1997;9(5):490.
44. Tsou VM et al. Elevated plasma aluminum levels in normal infants receiving antacids containing aluminum. Pediatrics 1991;87:148.
45. Hassall E et al. and the International Pediatric Omeprazole Study Group. Omeprazole for treatment of chronic erosive esophagitis in children: a multicenter study of efficacy, safety, tolerability and dose requirements. J Pediatr 200;137:800.
46. Abdulllah B et al. Long-term management of moderate/severe peptic esophagitis in children/adolescents: H2blocker vs proton pump inhibitor (PPI) [Abstract]. Gatroenterology 1998;114:A51.
47. Chiba N et al. Speed of healing and symptom relief in grade II to IV gastroesophageal reflux disease: a meta-analysis. Gastroenterology 1997;112:1798.
48. DiGiacinto JL et al. Stability of suspension formulations of lansoprazole and omeperazole stored in amber colored plastic oral syringes. Ann Pharmacother 2000;34(5):600.
49. Cucchiara S et al. Cimetidine treatment of reflux esophagitis in children: an Italian multicentric study.. J Pediatr Gastroenterol Nutr 1989;8:150.
50. Simeone D et al Treatment of childhood peptic esophagitis: a double-blind placebo controlled trial of nizatidine. J Pediatr Gastroenterol Nutr 1997; 25:51.
51. Hyman PE et al. Tolerance to intravenous ranitidine. J Pediatr 1987;110:794.
52. Nwokolo CU et al. Tolerance during 29 days of conventional dosing with cimetidine, nizatidine, famotidine, or ranitidine. Aliment Pharmacol Ther 1990;4(1):29.
53. Grill BB et al. Effects of domperidone therapy on symptoms and upper gastrointestinal motility in infants with gastroesophageal reflux. J Pediatr 1985;106:311.
54. Leung C, Lai W. Use of metoclopramide for the treatment of gastroesophageal reflux in infants and children. Curr Ther Res 1984;36:911.
55. De Loore I et al. Domperidone drops in the symptomatic treatment of chronic paediatric vomiting and regurgitation. A comparison with metoclopramide. Postgrad Med J 1979;55:40.
56. Machida HM et al. Metoclopramide in gastroesophageal reflux of infancy. J Pediatr 1988;112:483.
57. Bellissant E et al. The triangular test to asses the efficacy of metoclopramide in gastroesophageal reflux. Clin Pharmacol Ther 1997;61:377.
58. Putnam PE et al. Tardive dyskinesia associated with use of metoclopramide in a child. J Pediatr 1992;121:983.
59. Euler AR. Use of bethanechol for the treatment of gastroesophageal reflux. J Pediatr 1980;96:321.
60. Sondheimer JM et al. Bethanechol treatment of gastroesophageal reflux in infants: effect on continuous esophageal pH records. J Pediatr 1984;104:128.
61. Levi P et al. Bethanechol versus antacids in the treatment of gastroesophageal reflux. Helv Paediatr Acta 1985;40:349.
62. Arguelles-Mart F et al. Sucralfate versus cimetidine in the treatment of reflux esophagitis in children. Am J Med 1989;86:73.
63. Besunder JB et al. Principles of biodisposition in the neonate: a critical evaluation of the pharmacokinetic-pharmacodynamic interface (part 1). Clin Pharmacokinet 1988;14:189.
64. Steinburg AD. Should chloral hydrate be banned? Pediatrics 1993;92(3):442.
65. Smith MT. Chloral hydrate warning. Science 1990;250:359.
66. Committee on Drugs and Committee on Environmental Health, AAP. Use of chloral hydrate for sedation in children. Pediatrics 1993;92:471.
67. Taketomo KC et al., eds. Pediatric Dosage Handbook. 9th Ed. Hudson, OH: LexiComp, 2002.
68. Napoli KL et al. Safety and efficacy of chloral hydrate sedation in children undergoing echocardiography. J Pediatr 1996;129(2):287.
69. McCarver-May DG et al. Comparison of chloral hydrate and midazolam for sedation of neonates for neuroimaging studies. J Pediatr 1996;128(4):573.
70. Hollman GA. Chloral hydrate versus midazolam sedation for neuroimaging studies [Letter]. J Pediatr 1996;129(6).
71. Strain JD et al. Intravenously administered pentobarbital sodium in sedation in pediatric CT. Radiology 1986;161:105.
72. Strain JD et al. IV Nembutal: safe sedation for children undergoing CT. AJR 1988;151:975.
73. Chung T et al. The use of oral pentobarbital sodium (Nembutal) versus oral chloral hydrate in infants undergoing CT and MR imaging—a pilot study. Pediatr Radiol 2000;30:332.
74. Ziegler MA et al. Is administration of enteric contrast media safe before abdominal CT in children who require sedation? Experience with chloral hydrate and pentobarbital. AJR 2003;180:13.
75. Streisand JB et al. Absorption and bioavailability of oral transmucosal fentanyl citrate. Anesthesiology 1991;75:223.
76. Howell TK et al. A comparison of oral transmucosal fentanyl and oral midazolam for premedication in children. Anaesthesia 2002;57:778.
77. Klein EJ et al. A randomized, clinical trial of oral midazolam plus placebo versus oral midazolam plus oral transmucosal fentanyl for sedation during laceration repair. Pediatrics 2002;109(5):894.
78. Yaster M et al. Midazolam-fentanyl intravenous sedation in children: case report of respiratory arrest. Pediatrics 1990;86:463.
79. Krauss B, Green SM. Sedation and analgesia for procedures in children. N Engl J Med 2000;342(13):938.
80. Latson LA et al. Midazolam nose drops for outpatient echocardiography sedation in infants. Am Heart J 1991;121(1):209.
81. Shannon M et al. Safety and efficacy of flumazenil in the reversal of benzodiazepine-induced conscious sedation. J Pediatr 1997;131:582.

82. Auden SM et al. Oral ketamine/midazolam is superior to intramuscular meperidine, promethazine, and chlorpromazine for pediatric cardiac catheterization. Anesth Analg 2000;90:299.

83. Nahata MC et al. Adverse effects of meperidine, promethazine and chlorpromazine for sedation in pediatric patients. Clin Pediatr 1985;24:558.

84. Hertzog JH et al. Prospective evaluation of propofol anesthesia in the pediatric intensive care unit for elective oncology procedures in ambulatory and hospitalized children. Pediatrics 2000;106(4):742.

85. Havel CJ et al. A clinical trial of propofol vs midazolam for procedural sedation in a pediatric emergency department. Acad Emerg Med 1999; 6:989.

86. Hertzog JH et al. Propofol anesthesia for invasive procedures in ambulatory and hospitalized children: experience in the pediatric intensive care unit. Pediatrics 1999;103:E30.

87. Parker RI et al. Efficacy and safety of intravenous midazolam and ketamine as sedation for therapeutic and diagnostic procedures in children. Pediatrics 1997;99(3):427.

88. Wathen JE et al. Does midazolam alter the clinical effects of intravenous ketamine sedation in children? A double-blind, randomized, controlled, emergency department trial. Ann Emerg Med 2000;36(6):579.

89. Kennedy RM et al. Comparison of fentanyl/midazolam with ketamine/midazolam for pediatric orthopedic emergencies. Pediatrics 1998;102(4):956.

90. Cote CJ et al. Adverse sedation events in pediatrics: analysis of medications used for sedation. Pediatrics 2000;106(4):633.

91. Committee on Drugs, AAP. Guidelines for monitoring and management of pediatric patient during and after sedation for diagnostic and therapeutic procedures. Pediatrics 1992;89:1110.

92. Playfor S et al. Recollection of children following intensive care. Arch Dis Child 2000;83:445.

93. Reed et al. A pharmacokinetically based propofol dosing strategy for sedation of the critically ill, mechanically ventilated pediatric patient. Crit Care Med 1996;24:1473.

94. Hanna JP et al. Rhabdomyolysis and hypoxia associated with prolonged propofol infusion in children. Neurology 1998:50:301

95. Cray SH et al. Lactic academia and bradyarrhythmia in a child sedated with propofol. Crit Care Med 1998;26(12):2087.

96. Strickland RA, Murray MJ. Fatal metabolic acidosis in a pediatric patient receiving an infusion of propofol in the intensive care unit: Is there a relationship? Crit Care Med 1995;23(2):405.

97. Parke TJ et al. Metabolic acidosis and fatal myocardial failure after propofol infusion in children: five case reports. Br Med J 1992;305:613.

98. Sulsa GM. Propofol toxicity in critically ill pediatric patients: show us the proof [Editorial]. Crit Care Med 1998;26(12):1959.

99. Fonsmark L et al. Occurrence of withdrawal in critically ill sedated children. Crit Care Med 1999;27(1):196.

100. Katz R et al. Prospective study on the occurrence of withdrawal in critically ill children who receive fentanyl by continuous infusion. Crit Care Med 1994;22(5):763.

101. Berde CB, Sethna NF. Analgesics for the treatment of pain in children. N Engl J Med 2002;347(14):1094.

102. Sutters KA et al. Comparison of morphine patient-controlled analgesia with and without ketorolac for postoperative analgesia in pediatric orthopedic surgery. Am J Orthop 1999;28:351.

103. Ananad KJS et al. Opioid tolerance and dependence in infants and children. Crit Care Med 1994;22;334.

104. Tobias JD et al. Outpatient therapy of iatrogenic drug dependency following prolonged sedation in the pediatric intensive care unit. Intens Care Med 1994:20:504.

105. Yaster M et al. The management of opioid and benzodiazepine dependence in infants, children and adolescents. Pediatrics 1996;98(1):135–40.

105. Tobias JD, Tolerance, withdrawal, and physical dependence after long-term sedation and analgesia of children in the pediatric intensive care unit. Crit Care Med 2000;28(6):2122.

106. Hoder EL et al. Clonidine in neonatal narcotic abstinence syndrome. N Engl J Med 1981;305:1284.

106. Schechter NL. The undertreatment of pain in children: an overview. Pediatr Clin North Am 1989; 36:781.

107. Cassady JF et al. A randomized comparison of the effects of continuous thoracic epidural analgesia and intravenous patient-controlled analgesia after posterior spinal fusion in adolescents. Reg Anesth Pain Med 2000;25:246.

107. Vinci RJ, Fish SS. Efficacy of topical anesthesia in children. Arch Pediatr Adolesc Med 1996;150(5): 466.

108. Berde CB. Toxicity of local anesthetics in infants and children. J Pediatr 1993;122:S14.

109. Bonadio WA et al. Half-strength TAC topical anesthetic. Clin Pediatr 1988;10:495.

110. Cannon CR et al. Topically applied tetracaine, adrenaline and cocaine in the repair of traumatic wounds of the head and neck. Otolaryngol Head Neck Surg 1989;100:78.

111. Smith GA et al. New non-cocaine-containing topical anesthetics compared with tetracaine-adrenaline-cocaine during repair of lacerations. Pediatrics 1997;100(5):825.

112. Yaster M et al. Local anesthetics in the management of acute pain in children. J Pediatr 1994; 124(2):165.

113. Kumar AR et al. Methemoglobinemia associated with a prilocaine-lidocaine cream. Clin Pediatr 1997;36(4):239.

114. Galinkin JL et al. Lidocaine iontophoresis versus eutectic mixture of local anesthetics (EMLA) for IV placement in children. Anesth Analg 2002; 94(6):1484.

115. Cassidy KL et al. A randomized double-blind, placebo-controlled trial of the EMLA patch for the reduction of pain associated with Intramuscular injection in four to six-year-old children Acta Paediatr 2001;90(11):1329.

116. Uhare M. A eutectic mixture of lidocaine and prilocaine for alleviating vaccination pain in infants. Pediatrics 1993;92:719.

117. Friedman PM et al. Topical anesthetics update: EMLA and beyond. Dermatol Surg 2001;27(12): 1019.

118. Ashburn MA et al. Iontophoretic administration of 2% lidocaine HCl and 1:100,000 epinephrine in humans. Clin J Pain 1997;13:22.

119. Zempsky WT et al. Lidocaine iontophoresis for topical anesthesia before intravenous line placement in children. Pediatrics 1998;132(6):1061.

120. Chen BK, Eichenfield LF. Pediatric anesthesia in dermatology surgery: when hand-holding is not enough. Dermatol Surg 2001;27(12):1010.

121. Pickering LK et al. Hemolytic-uremic syndrome and enterohemorrhagic Escherichia coli. Pediatr Infect Dis J 1994;13:459.

122. Ray PE, Liu XH. Pathogenesis of shiga toxin-induced hemolytic uremic syndrome. Pediatr Nephrol 2001;16:823.

123. Bell BP et al. A multi-state outbreak of Escherichia coli O157:H7-associated bloody diarrhea and hemolytic uremic syndrome from hamburgers. JAMA 1994;272:1349.

124. Begue REet al. Escherichia coli and the hemolytic-uremic syndrome. South Med J 1998;91:798.

125. Trachtman H, Christen E. Pathogenesis, treatment, and therapeutic trials in hemolytic uremic syndrome. Curr Opin Pediatr 1999;11:162.

126. Grimm PC, Ogborn MR. Hemolytic uremic syndrome: the most common cause of acute renal failure in childhood. Pediatr Ann 1994;23(9):505.

127. Siegler RL. The hemolytic uremic syndrome. Pediatr Nephrol 1995;42:1505.

128. Di Paola JA, Buchanan GR. Immune thrombocytopenic purpura. Pediatr Clin North Am 2002; 49(5):911.

129. George JN et al. Idiopathic thrombocytopenic purpura: a practice guideline developed by explicit methods for the American Society of Hematology. Blood 1996;88:3.

130. Blanchette V. Childhood chronic immune thrombocytopenic purpura. Blood Rev 2002;16:23.

131. Bolton-Maggs PHB et al. The nontreatment of childhood ITP (or "the art of medicine consists of amusing the patient until nature cures the disease"). Semin Thromb Hemost 2001;27(3):269.

132. Gillis S. The thrombocytopenic purpuras: recognition and management. Drugs 1996;51(6):942.

133. Cimolai N et al. Risk factors for the progression of Escherichia coli O157:H7 enteritis to hemolytic-uremic syndrome. J Pediatr 1990;116:589.

134. Pavia AT et al. Hemolytic-uremic syndrome during an outbreak of Escherichia coli O157:H7 infections in institutions for mentally retarded persons: clinical and epidemiologic observations. J Pediatr 1990; 116:544.

135. Proulx F et al. Randomized, controlled trial of antibiotic therapy for Escherichia coli O157:H7 enteritis. J Pediatr 1992;121:299.

136. Wong CS et al. The risk of the hemolytic-uremic syndrome after antibiotic treatment of Escherichia coli O157:H7 infections. N Engl J Med 2000; 342(26):1930.

137. Boyce TG et al. Escherichia coli O157:H7 and the hemolytic-uremic syndrome. N Engl J Med 1995;333:364.

138. Siegler RL. The hemolytic uremic syndrome. Pediatr Clin North Am 1995;42(6):1505.

139. von Baeyer H. Plasmapheresis in thrombotic microangiopathy-associated syndromes: review of outcome data derived from clinical trials and open studies. Ther Apher 2002;6(4):320.

140. O'Reyan S et al. Aspirin and dipyridamole therapy in the hemolytic-uremic syndrome. J Pediatr 1980; 97:473.

141. Bergstein JM. Anticoagulant therapy in human renal disease. Int J Pediatr Nephrol 1981;2:1.

142. Monnens L et al. "Active" intravascular coagulation in the epidemic form of hemolytic-uremic syndrome. Clin Nephrol 1982;17:284.

143. Coalthard MG. An evaluation of treatment with heparin in the haemolytic-uraemic syndrome successfully treated by peritoneal dialysis. Arch Dis Child 1980;55:393.

144. Jones RWA et al. End-arterial urokinase in childhood hemolytic-uremic syndrome. Kidney Int 1981;20:723.

145. Gillot A. Plasmapheresis as a therapeutic measure in hemolytic-uremic syndrome in children. Klin Wochenschr 1983;61:363.

146. Loriat C et al. Treatment of childhood haemolytic-uraemic syndrome with plasma. A multicenter randomized controlled trial. Pediatr Nephrol 1988; 2:279.

147. Rizzoni G et al. Plasma infusion for hemolytic uremic syndrome in children: results of a multicenter controlled trial. J Pediatr 1988;112:284.

148. Perez N et al. Steroids in the hemolytic uremic syndrome. Pediatr Nephrol 1998;12:101.

149. Konadu EY et al. Investigational vaccine for Escherichia coli O157: Phase I study of O157 O-specific polysaccharide-Pseudomonas aeruginosa recombinant exoprotein A conjugates in adults. J Infect Dis 1998;177:383.

150. Armstrong GD et al. A phase I study of chemically synthesized verotoxin (shiga-like toxin) Pk-trisaccharide receptors to chromosorb for preventing hemolytic uremic syndrome. J Infect Dis 1995;171:1042.

151. Nugent DJ. Childhood immune thrombocytopenic purpura. Blood Rev 2002;16:27.

152. Blanchette V et al. Randomised trial of intravenous immunoglobulin G, intravenous anti-D and oral prednisone in childhood acute immune thrombocytopenic purpura. Lancet 1994;344:703.

153. Blanchette VS et al. A prospective, randomized trial of high-dose intravenous immune globulin G therapy, oral prednisone therapy and no therapy in childhood acute thrombocytopenic purpura. J Pediatr 1993;123:989.

154. Albayrak D et al. Acute idiopathic thrombocytopenic purpura: a comparative study of very high

oral doses of methylprednisolone and intravenously administered immune globulin. J Pediatr 1994;125:1004.

155. Carcao MD et al. Short-course oral prednisone therapy in children presenting with acute immune thrombocytopenic purpura (ITP). Acta Paediatr 1998;(Suppl 424):71.

156. Freiberg A, Mauger D. Efficacy, safety and dose response of intravenous anti-D immune globulin (WinRho SDF) for the treatment of idiopathic thrombocytopenic purpura in children. Semin Hematol 1998;35(1):23.

157. Tarantino MD et al. Treatment of childhood acute immune thrombocytopenic purpura with anti-D immune globulin or pooled immune globulin. J Pediatr 1999;134(1):21.

158. Sandler SG. Intravenous Rh immune globulin for treating immune thrombocytopenic purpura. Curr Opin Hematol 2002;8(6):417.

159. Gaines AR. Acute onset hemoglobinemia and/or hemoglobinuria and sequelae following Rh$_o$(D) immune globulin intravenous administration in immune thrombocytopenic patients. Blood 2000;95(6):2523.

160. NIH Consensus Conference. Intravenous immunoglobulin: prevention and treatment of disease. JAMA 1990;264(24):3189.

161. Ryan ME. Adverse effects of intravenous immunoglobulin therapy. Clin Pediatr 1996;35(1):23.

162. Bolton-Maggs PHB. Idiopathic thrombocytopenic purpura. Arch Dis Child 2000;83:220.

163. Borgna-Pignatti C et al. A trial of high-dose dexamethasone therapy for chronic idiopathic thrombocytopenic purpura in childhood. J Pediatr 1997;130(1):13.

164. Hemmila MR et al. The response to splenectomy in pediatric patients with idiopathic thrombocytopenic purpura who fail high-dose intravenous immune globulin. J Pediatr Surg 2000;35(6):967.

165. Holt D et al. Response to intravenous immunoglobulin predicts splenectomy response in children with immune thrombocytopenic purpura. Pediatrics 2003;111(1):87.

166. Hogg RJ et al. Evaluation and management of proteinuria and nephrotic syndrome in children: recommendations from a pediatric nephrology panel established at the National Kidney Foundation Conference on Proteinuria, Albuminuria, Risk, Assessment, Detection, and Elimination (PARADE). Pediatrics 2000;105(6):1242.

167. Roth KS et al. Nephrotic syndrome: pathogenesis and management. Pediatr Rev 2002;23(7):237.

168. Schapner HW, Robson AM. Nephrotic syndrome: minimal change disease, focal glomerulosclerosis, and related disorders. In: Schrier RW, Gottschalk CW, eds. Diseases of the Kidney, 6th Ed. Boston: Little, Brown, and Company, 1997:64.

169. Orth SR, Ritz E. The nephrotic syndrome. N Engl J Med 1998;338(17):1202

170. Warshaw BL. Nephrotic syndrome in children. Pediatr Ann 1994;23(9):495.

171. Constantinescu AR et al. Predicting first-year relapses in children with nephrotic syndrome. Pediatrics 2000;105(3):492.

172. Takeda A et al. Prediction of subsequent relapse in children with steroid-sensitive nephrotic syndrome. Pediatr Nephrol 2001;16:888.

173. Yap HK et al. Risk factors for steroid dependency in children with idiopathic nephrotic syndrome. Pediatr Nephrol 2001;16:1049.

174. Mendoza SA, Tune BM. Management of the difficult nephrotic patient. Pediatr Clin North Am 1995;42(6):1459.

175. Durkan AM et al. Immunosuppressive agents in childhood nephrotic syndrome: a meta-analysis of randomized controlled trials. Kidney Int 2001;59:1919.

176. Silva JMP et al. Premature acute myocardial infarction in a child with nephrotic syndrome. Pediatr Nephrol 2002;17:169.

177. Lin CC et al. Thalamic stroke secondary to straight sinus thrombosis in a nephrotic child. Pediatr Nephrol 2002;17:184.

178. Hingorani SR et al. Predictors of peritonitis in children with nephrotic syndrome. Pediatr Nephrol 2002;17:678.

179. Shroff A et al. Prevention of serious bacterial infections in new-onset nephrotic syndrome: a survey of current practices. Clin Pediatr 2002;41:47.

180. Policy statement: Recommendations for the prevention of pneumococcal infections, including the use of pneumococcal conjugate vaccine (Prevnar), pneumococcal polysaccharide vaccine, and antibiotic prophylaxis (RE9960). Pediatrics 2000;106(2):362.

181. Alpay H et al. Varicella vaccination in children with steroid-sensitive nephrotic syndrome. Pediatr Nephrol 2002;17:181.

182. Sanjad SA et al. Management of hyperlipidemia in children with refractory nephrotic syndrome: the effect of statin therapy. J Pediatr 1997;130(3):470.

183. Saland JM et al. Dyslipidemia in pediatric renal disease: epidemiology, pathophysiology, and management. Curr Opin Pediatr 2002;14:197.

184. Dogra GK et al. Statin therapy improves brachial artery endothelial function in nephrotic syndrome. Kidney Int 2002;62:550.

CHAPTER 94

Neonatal Therapy

Donna M. Kraus, Jennifer Tran Pham

The rational use of medications in neonates depends on an appreciation of both the physiologic immaturity and the developmental maturation that influence neonatal drug disposition and pharmacologic effects. Much progress has been made to decrease neonatal mortality and to increase survival of more premature and lower-birth-weight newborns. Neonates, particularly those of extremely low birth weights, pose a pharmacotherapeutic challenge to the clinician. The alterations of body composition, weight, size, and physiologic and pharmacokinetic parameters that occur with normal growth and maturation during the first few months of life are greater than at any other time. Although the amount of neonatal drug information is increasing, the overall lack of well-designed pharmacokinetic and pharmacodynamic studies still hinders the clinical use of many drugs in this population. This is especially true for newborns of the lowest birth weights (<750 g).

The term *therapeutic orphans*,[1] which was coined >30 years ago to describe the lack of medications labeled for use in children, unfortunately still is applicable today.[2] Although the number of medications under development for children has significantly increased over recent years, 71% of new molecular entities approved by the U.S. Food and Drug Administration (FDA) do not have pediatric drug labeling.[3] In addition, practical issues such as technical problems of drug delivery and a lack of suitable dosage formulations further complicate neonatal pharmacotherapeutics.

This pediatric dilemma led to the passage of the FDA Modernization Act of 1997.[4] This federal legislation offered incentives (in the form of a 6-month drug patent extension) to pharmaceutical companies to conduct pediatric research. The Best Pharmaceuticals for Children Act of 2002 reauthorizes the use of these incentives and provides a process to increase pediatric studies for medications that are no longer "on patent."[5] In addition, this law specifically includes neonates, as a population that should be studied. These and other regulations, plus the establishment of the Pediatric Pharmacology Research Unit Network by the National Institutes of Child Health and Human Development,[3] will increase pediatric drug studies, enhance the neonatal labeling of medications, and lead to more rationale use of medications in neonates. Until that time, the clinical use of drugs in neonates presents unique therapeutic challenges for the clinician.

Terminology

An understanding of common neonatal terminology is important because every newborn is evaluated and classified at birth according to birth weight, gestational age, and intrauterine growth status. These factors influence patient outcome and long-term prognosis.[6] Common neonatal terminology is listed in Table 94-1. Pharmacokinetic parameters, pharmacodynamics, and dosing recommendations often are specified according to these terms.

Neonatal Monitoring Parameters

Many pharmacotherapeutic monitoring parameters used in adults also are used in neonates. However, normal values for neonates may differ. To adequately monitor pharmacotherapy in neonates, one must be aware of the differences in normal vital signs and laboratory parameters. For example, neonates have higher heart rates (HR) and respiratory rates (RR) and lower blood pressures (BP) compared with adults. Appropriate texts should be consulted for neonatal normal values when providing comprehensive pharmacy care.[7,8]

The physiologic transitions from intrauterine to extrauterine life may influence disease states and drug disposition. For example, the change from fetal to adult circulation results in an increase in perfusion of organs that are responsible for the elimination of drugs. The developmental changes in absorption, distribution, metabolism, and excretion affect drug disposition and, ultimately, neonatal drug dosing. This chapter focuses on applied therapeutics for common neonatal disease states and the safe and effective use of drugs in the neonate.

NEONATAL PHARMACOKINETICS
Drug Absorption
Gastrointestinal Absorption

Numerous developmental factors, including gastric acidity, gastric emptying time, intestinal integrity and motility, and bacterial colonization may influence the absorption of enterally administered drugs during the neonatal period. Neonates, especially preterm newborns, have a decreased capacity to secrete gastric acid compared with adults.[9] This relative lack of gastric acid output may be referred to as relative achlorhydria or

Table 94-1 Common Neonatal Terminology[6,8]

Term	Definition
Gestational age	*By Dates:* The number of weeks from the onset of the mother's last menstrual period until birth
	By Examination: Assessment of gestational maturity by physical and neuromuscular examination; gestational age estimates the time from conception until birth
Postnatal age	Chronologic age after birth
Postconceptional age	Gestational age plus postnatal age
Corrected age	Postconceptional age in weeks minus 40; represents postnatal age if neonate had been born at term (40 weeks' gestational age)
Preterm	<38 weeks' gestational age at birth
Term	38–42 weeks' gestational age at birth
Post-term	≥43 weeks' gestational age at birth
Extremely low birth weight	Birth weight <1 kg
Very low birth weight	Birth weight <1.5 kg
Low birth weight	Birth weight <2.5 kg
Small for gestational age	Birth weight below 10th percentile for gestational age
Appropriate for gestational age	Birth weight between 10th and 90th percentiles for gestational age
Large for gestational age	Birth weight above 90th percentile for gestational age

hypochlorhydria. Although the exact maturational pattern of gastric acid secretion needs more clarity, a biphasic pattern in term infants usually is described. At birth, the pH of gastric contents is neutral owing to the presence of residual amniotic fluid. (Amniotic fluid is swallowed regularly during intrauterine life.) In term infants, acid output begins within minutes after birth and gastric pH decreases to 1.5 to 3 within a few hours. Gastric acidity then decreases (pH increases) over the next 10 days; subsequently, basal acid output gradually rises. The maturational pattern of acid secretion in term infants is different in preterm neonates. Gastric acid rarely is present in the fetal stomach before 32 weeks' gestation, and the early decrease in gastric pH usually is not seen or may be delayed in preterm neonates. Hypochlorhydria with a basal pH >4.0 is present in approximately 20% of preterm neonates 1 to 2 weeks of age. After 6 weeks of life, gastric pH falls to <4.[10] Although gastric acid production correlates with postnatal age, extrauterine factors (e.g., initiation of enteral feedings) appear to be responsible for the stimulation of gastric acid output.[10] In general, gastric acidity is lower during the neonatal period, and adult values for maximal acid output are not reached until 2 years of age.[9,11]

Both gastric and duodenal pH affect drug ionization and absorption.[11,12] Generally, an acidic environment favors absorption of acidic drugs because these drugs will be un-ionized and therefore more lipid soluble. Basic drugs, however, will be mostly ionized in an acid environment. As a result, basic drugs in an acidic environment are hydrophilic and less well absorbed. Likewise, an acidic drug in an alkaline environment also will be primarily in the ionized form and less well absorbed. Therefore, the hypochlorhydria (i.e., relatively alkaline gastric pH) in neonates can result in decreased bioavailability of acidic drugs (e.g., phenobarbital, phenytoin), as well as increased bioavailability of weakly basic drugs or acid-labile drugs (e.g., penicillin, ampicillin, erythromycin) compared with that in adults.[11,13]

Because most drugs are absorbed in the small intestine, gastric emptying time plays an important role in both the rate and the degree of drug absorption. During the neonatal period, gastric emptying time can be prolonged up to 6 to 8 hours and may not attain adult values until 6 to 8 months of age.[11] The rate of gastric emptying is affected by gestational age, disease states, and dietary intake. Prematurity, respiratory distress syndrome (RDS), congenital heart disease, and ingestion of long-chain fatty acids prolong gastric emptying time. The rate of gastric emptying is increased with consumption of human milk and hypocaloric feedings but is unaffected by osmolality and posture. A prolonged gastric emptying time may delay drug absorption, resulting in a longer time to reach maximal serum drug concentrations and a decrease in the peak concentration.

Motility of the small intestine is irregular in both neonates and young infants,[13] making it difficult to predict the time for peak absorption or the extent of absorption of enterally administered drugs. In addition, the immature or altered permeability of the intestinal mucosa, which may result in increased drug absorption, actually may be more important than both gastric emptying time and intestinal motility.[14] Osmolality also may influence gastrointestinal (GI) tract integrity and absorption, particularly in preterm infants.[13] Enteral administration of drugs or solutions with high osmolalities may destroy GI tract integrity and increase the risk of necrotizing enterocolitis (NEC) in neonates.

Drug absorption in the neonate also can be affected by other factors. For example, the reduced rate of bile acid synthesis and pancreatic secretions in preterm neonates may decrease the absorption of fat-soluble vitamins D and E.[12,13,15] Absorption of these vitamins may be reduced further by cholestasis, and water-soluble forms of these vitamins may be necessary. Short-bowel syndrome (which may occur as a result of NEC) may decrease the intestinal surface area available for drug absorption and result in decreased drug bioavailability. Changes in bacterial colonization of the GI tract during the neonatal period can influence the fate of conjugated forms of drugs excreted in bile. The high activity of β-glucuronidase in the neonatal intestinal lumen results in hydrolysis of drug glucuronide conjugates and potentially alters the disposition of the parent drug or its metabolite.[11,13]

During the neonatal period, drugs such as phenobarbital, digoxin, and sulfonamides are absorbed at a slower rate but the total amount absorbed is similar to that of older children.[14] In contrast, the total absorption of drugs such as phenytoin, acetaminophen, carbamazepine, and rifampin is decreased in neonates.[11,13,15]

Rectal Absorption

The routine use of the rectum for administration of drugs such as aminophylline has been discouraged because of erratic drug absorption and toxicities.[13] With the proper drug and dosage formulation, however, the rectum can be an important alternative route for drug administration with rapid and efficient absorption.[11,13] For example, rectal administration of diazepam solution for injection produces serum concentrations similar to those from intravenous (IV) administration.[16] This route is therapeutically important in the neonate with seizure activity in whom rapid IV access is not available.

Intramuscular Absorption

Many physiologic factors, as well as physicochemical characteristics of drugs, influence intramuscular (IM) absorption.[11–13] During the first few days of life, both the rate and the amount of IM absorption may be reduced due to the relatively decreased muscle blood flow, higher percentage of water in muscle mass, and diminished strength of muscular contractions.[11] The amount of both muscle and subcutaneous (SC) tissue in the newborn is directly proportional to gestational age. The low muscle mass to total body mass ratio in neonates can result in decreased absorption of an intramuscularly administered drug because absorption is influenced by the surface area of the muscle that comes into contact with the injected medication. In addition, the degree of muscle activity, which directly affects the rate of drug absorption from both IM and SC injections, can be greatly decreased in the severely ill, immobile, or paralyzed neonate.[11–13] Adequate perfusion of the injection site also is required for systemic absorption to occur. Blood supply to muscles may be compromised in the critically ill neonate with low cardiac output or hypotensive states such as patent ductus arteriosus (PDA), sepsis, or RDS.[12,17] Drugs that more commonly may be administered intramuscularly to neonates include vitamin K, aminoglycosides, phenobarbital, and penicillins.[8,12]

Percutaneous Absorption

Percutaneous absorption is increased in neonates (especially in preterm newborns) because of decreased thickness of the stratum corneum, increased skin hydration, and increased ratio of surface area per kilogram body weight.[11-13] Because the epidermis is barely present before 34 weeks' gestational age, preterm newborns (especially those less than 2 weeks' postnatal age) are at greatest risk for percutaneous drug absorption. After 2 to 3 weeks' postnatal age, the epidermis of the preterm newborn histologically matures to that seen at term.[18] Although the epidermis of a term neonate is functionally intact, the epidermis continues to develop through 4 months of age. The newborn's ratio of skin surface area to body weight is approximately three times that of an adult. Therefore, for the same percutaneous dose, a neonate absorbs three times more drug per kilogram than an adult. In addition, occlusive dressings or an interruption in the integrity of the skin (e.g., abrasion) increases the amount of drug absorbed percutaneously. Various toxicities have been described in neonates after topical administration of iodine, hexachlorophene, boric acid, salicylic acid, alcohol, epinephrine, corticosteroids, and triple antibiotic (bacitracin, neomycin, polymyxin B) spray.[18]

The increased percutaneous absorption of drugs in preterm newborns has potential therapeutic implications.[18] For example, transdermal theophylline, administered as a gel with an occlusive dressing, produces therapeutic serum concentrations in preterm newborns who are 30 weeks or less gestational age and 20 days or less postnatal age. Clinical application of transdermal drug delivery in preterm newborns appears promising and may avoid problems associated with other routes of administration. However, transdermal drug delivery is limited by the normal maturation of the epidermis, and drug absorption decreases with increasing postnatal age and in newborns older than 32 weeks' gestational age.[18]

Drug Distribution

Drug distribution, the process of drug partition among various body organs, fluids, and tissues, depends on pH, composition and size of body compartments (e.g., total body water, intracellular and extracellular water, and adipose tissue mass), protein binding, membrane permeability, and hemodynamic factors such as cardiac output and regional blood flow.[19]

Water Compartments
Total body water, as a percentage of body weight, is increased in the newborn (especially the preterm neonate) and decreases with increasing age. The total body water of a preterm, 1-kg newborn is 80% and that of a term newborn is 75%. These values are much higher than those of a 3-month old (60%) or an adult (55%).[20] Newborns also have an increase in extracellular water as a percentage of body weight, and an increase in the extracellular water to intracellular water ratio. Extracellular water decreases from approximately 40% at term to approximately 20% at 3 months of age.[20] The higher total body water and extracellular water in newborns typically result in larger volumes of distribution (Vd) for water-soluble drugs (Table 94-2).[8,12,21,22] In addition, the Vd for water-soluble drugs that distribute to the extracellular water compartment (e.g., gentamicin) roughly parallels extracellular water as a percentage of body weight. Because the Vd in newborns usually is larger for water-soluble drugs, larger mg/kg loading doses of these agents are needed in neonates, particularly preterm newborns, to achieve initial drug concentrations similar to that of an adult. As the neonate grows and matures, total body water and extracellular water decrease, causing the Vd for water-soluble drugs and therefore mg/kg loading doses to decrease with increasing age.

Adipose Tissue
Compared with the adult, the neonate has much less adipose tissue. A preterm newborn is composed of only 1% to 2% fat, whereas a term neonate is approximately 15% fat.[20] Neonatal adipose tissue also contains more water. The decreased amount of adipose tissue and the higher water content in the newborn may decrease the Vd for fat-soluble drugs (e.g., diazepam). Because of the smaller Vd for fat-soluble or lipophilic drugs, smaller mg/kg loading doses should be administered in neonates.

Protein Binding
In general, neonatal protein binding of drugs is decreased compared with adults (see Table 94-2). The decrease in plasma protein binding is a result of several factors, including a lower concentration of binding proteins (e.g., albumin, lipoproteins, α_1-acid glycoprotein, and β-globulins); the presence of fetal albumin, which has decreased affinity for drugs; a lower plasma pH, which can decrease protein binding of acidic drugs; and the presence of endogenous substances (e.g., bilirubin and free fatty acids) or transplacentally ac-

---

Table 94-2 Pharmacokinetics of Selected Drugs in Neonates and Adults[8,12,21,22]

Drug	Plasma t½ (hr) Neonates	Adults	Vd (L/kg) Neonates	Adults	% Protein Bound Neonates	Adults
Caffeine	40–230	3–7	1.0	0.5–0.6	N/A	30–40
Diazepam	25–100	20–30	1.8–2.1	1.6–3.2	84–86	94–98
Digoxin	20–80	25–50	4–10	7	14–26	23–40
Gentamicin	3–12	1.5–3	0.4–0.7	0.2–0.3	<10	<10
Indomethacin	15–30	4–10	0.35–0.53	0.15–0.26	95–98	90–95
Morphine	5–14	2–4	1.7–4.5	2.4–4.2	18–22	33–37
Phenobarbital	40–400	50–180	1.0	0.6–0.7	28–43	45–50
Phenytoin	15–105	15–30	1.0	0.6–0.7	70–90	89–93
Theophylline	20–60	6–12	1.0	0.45	36–50	50–65
Vancomycin	6–12	5-8	0.48–0.97	0.3–0.7	N/A	30–55

N/A, not available; t½, half-life; Vd, volume of distribution.

quired interfering substances (e.g., hormones and pharmacologic agents) that may compete for protein-binding sites.[11,23] Decreased protein binding (increased free fraction) has been described in neonates for many drugs, including ampicillin, carbamazepine, diazepam, lidocaine, penicillin, phenobarbital, phenytoin, propranolol, salicylic acid, sulfonamides, and theophylline.[11,12,23] Total plasma protein concentration, as well as the affinity of albumin for acidic drugs, increases with age and approaches adult values at 10 to 12 months.[12] Therefore, as the newborn grows and matures, protein binding also increases.

A decrease in protein binding may result in an increased Vd, increased free (unbound) fraction, or increased free concentration of a drug. Drugs that have an increased Vd may require larger mg/kg loading doses in neonates to attain the same total serum concentration as that of an adult. However, for a given total serum concentration, the increased free fraction will result in a higher free concentration. The increased free concentration may result in increased therapeutic or toxic effects. For example, protein binding of theophylline in term newborns (36%) is decreased compared with adults (56%).[24] The commonly accepted total theophylline serum concentration of 10 to 20 µg/mL in adults produces free theophylline serum concentrations of 4.4 to 8.8 µg/mL in adults but 6.4 to 12.8 µg/mL in newborns (i.e., approximately 1.5 times the adult free concentrations). Pharmacologic and toxic effects of drugs are related to the free concentration (i.e., the amount of drug that can pass through membranes and reach the receptor). Therefore, the total theophylline serum concentration range used in adults (10 to 20 µg/mL) could result in toxicities if applied to the neonatal population. In neonates, a total theophylline serum concentration of approximately 7 to 14 µg/mL would produce free concentrations comparable with those seen with total concentrations of 10 to 20 µg/mL in adults.[24] Likewise, the decreased protein binding of phenytoin in neonates and resultant increased free fraction suggests that total phenytoin therapeutic serum concentrations in newborns should be 8 to 15 µg/mL rather than the 10 to 20 µg/mL as accepted in adults.

Decreased protein binding also may be a result of endogenous or exogenous substances displacing highly protein-bound drugs from protein-binding sites. Higher concentrations of free fatty acids in neonates may be responsible for the decreased protein binding of diazepam, propranolol, salicylates, and valproic acid.[23] In addition, bilirubin may displace acidic drugs, such as phenytoin, from albumin-binding sites. A positive correlation between total bilirubin concentrations and free fraction of phenytoin has been described. Unbound phenytoin was reported as 11% in normal newborns, but approximately 20% in neonates when bilirubin concentrations were 20 mg/dL.[25]

Some drugs (e.g., sulfonamides) or free fatty acids can displace bilirubin from albumin-binding sites, facilitating the deposition of unconjugated bilirubin in the brain. This condition, known as *kernicterus* or *bilirubin encephalopathy,* may produce neurologic injury and cell death and is frequently fatal. Survivors experience central hearing loss, ataxia, and choreoathetosis.[26] The displacement of bilirubin from albumin-binding sites depends on several factors, including pH; the affinity of albumin for the drug and bilirubin; and the individual molar concentrations of the drug, bilirubin,

and albumin. Preterm newborns may be at an increased risk for bilirubin displacement because of lower albumin concentrations, decreased albumin affinity for bilirubin, lower pH, and higher bilirubin concentrations (secondary to overproduction or decreased hepatic glucuronide conjugation). To displace bilirubin, a specific molar concentration of a drug is necessary to occupy a critical portion of the reserve albumin. Generally, if the molar concentration of a drug is much lower than the molar concentration of albumin, displacement of bilirubin from albumin-binding sites is unlikely.[12,27] For example, highly protein-bound drugs such as furosemide, indomethacin, and cardiac glycosides can be administered to neonates without fear of displacing bilirubin from albumin (even though some of them are potent displacers of bilirubin) because they achieve low plasma concentrations.[12] In contrast, ceftriaxone can significantly displace bilirubin off albumin-binding sites and therefore should be avoided in the presence of hyperbilirubinemia.[28,29] Sulfonamides are associated with the development of kernicterus, and therefore generally are avoided in infants younger than 2 months of age. However, not all sulfonamides have the same ability to displace bilirubin. Therapeutic concentrations of trimethoprim-sulfamethoxazole do not alter albumin's capacity to bind bilirubin, and this drug occasionally is used in neonates if no reasonable alternative antibiotic exists.[30]

Other Factors

Decreased skeletal muscle mass and alterations in tissue affinity, membrane permeability, and hemodynamics also may influence drug distribution in neonates. The increased permeability of the central nervous system (CNS) to certain lipophilic drugs, such as phenytoin, may be due to the composition of the immature brain (lower myelin content) and the higher cerebral blood flow as compared with adults.[11] The increased permeability of drugs into neonatal tissues, such as the CNS or red blood cells (e.g., digoxin, theophylline), also may contribute to the increased Vd observed in newborns.[19]

Metabolism

Most drugs are lipophilic and require biotransformation into more water-soluble substances before they can become inactivated and eliminated from the body. Biotransformation (i.e., metabolism) of drugs is catalyzed by specific enzymes. Drug-metabolizing enzyme activity is ultimately determined by an individual's underlying genetic makeup (pharmacogenetics); however, it is also greatly influenced by developmental and environmental factors. Thus, the clinically observed rate of enzyme activity and metabolism of a specific drug depends on a patient's genetic constitution, age, development, race, and gender; environmental and nutritional influences; and concomitant drug exposure and disease states.[31] Although biotransformation may take place at various sites (e.g., plasma, skin, GI tract, lungs, and kidney), it typically occurs in the liver with subsequent elimination of metabolites via the kidneys, lungs, or biliary tract. Hepatic biotransformation may include phase I (oxidation, reduction, hydrolysis, and demethylation) and phase II reactions (conjugation with sulfate, glucuronide, glycine, glutathione, and hippurate; acetylation; and methylation).[32] In general, hepatic metabolism is reduced in the neonate because of decreases in hepatic blood flow, cellular uptake of drugs, hepatic enzyme capacity, and biliary excretion. Hepatocellular uptake and intrahepatic transport of drugs may be decreased at birth because of reduced concentrations of the hepatocyte acceptor proteins Y and Z. This may result in decreased hepatic clearance for capacity-limited drugs (i.e., drugs with low extraction ratios and low intrinsic clearance).[11,12] Concentrations of acceptor proteins significantly increase during the first 10 days of life.[12,32]

Phase I Biotransformation Reactions

Phase I biotransformation reactions are significantly reduced in the newborn but increase with both gestational and postnatal age.[11] Maturation of enzyme activity (phase I and phase II) occurs at different ages for different metabolic pathways, may be regulated by endogenous hormones (e.g., growth hormone or corticosteroids), and may be substrate specific. The development of isoenzymes, presence of endogenous competitive substrates, and in utero or postnatal induction of hepatic enzymes may alter the maturation of drug metabolism.

The major group of enzymes responsible for phase I biotransformation reactions are the cytochromes P450.[33] Cytochrome P450 enzymes catalyze the biotransformation of many lipophilic drugs and endogenous substances. These enzymes are actually a "superfamily" of heme-containing proteins that exist as many different isoforms (i.e., isoenzymes). Cytochrome P450 isoenzyme nomenclature uses the root symbol CYP, followed in order by (1) an Arabic number to denote the gene family, (2) an upper case letter to designate a subfamily of highly related genes, and (3) another Arabic number to identify the individual isoenzyme within the subfamily. Seventeen human CYP gene families have been described. The most important gene families involved in human drug metabolism include CYP1, CYP2, and CYP3.[34] Table 94-3 lists important drug-metabolizing enzymes, their known developmental pattern, and important neonatal substrates.[33] It is important to remember that isoenzymes may catalyze more than one type of biotransformation reaction, and the metabolism of certain drugs may be catalyzed by more than one isoenzyme. For example, CYP1A2 catalyzes the 3-demethylation and 8-hydroxylation of theophylline. However, theophylline 8-hydroxylation may also be catalyzed by CYP2E1 and CYP3A4. In preterm and newborn infants with low CYP1A2 activity, the contribution to 8-hydroxylation by CYP2E1 and CYP3A4 may become important. However, in general, decreased isoenzyme activity results in decreased drug clearance. Clinical examples of decreased drug metabolism in neonates according to specific phase I biotransformation reactions are described in the following sections.

Oxidation

In term newborns, activity of cytochrome P450 enzymes and NADPH-cytochrome-C-reductase is approximately 50% of the adult value.[35] This decreased oxidative capacity results in a reduced clearance of some drugs (e.g., diazepam, phenobarbital, phenytoin, valproic acid, theophylline, indomethacin, and metronidazole), particularly in the first few weeks of life.[11,32] Compared with other enzyme systems, maturation of oxidative reactions occurs rapidly after birth. For example, in term newborns hydroxylation of phenytoin and phenobarbital matures as early as 2 to 4 weeks' postnatal age.[32] In preterm infants, however, the rapid postnatal maturation of hydroxylation is delayed. Hydroxylation of theophylline is related primarily to postconceptional age and approaches adult values by 40 weeks' postconceptional age.[36] In general, oxidative biotransformation pathways have one-third to one-half the adult activity at birth but increase to two to five times that of an adult by 1 year postnatal age.

Hydrolysis

Hepatic and plasma esterase activity is reduced in neonates, especially preterm newborns, and reaches adult values within 10 to 12 months.[11] The decreased esterase activity results in reduced elimination of ester anesthetics such as procaine, tetracaine, and cocaine. This may explain the increased effects

---

Table 94-3 Important Neonatal Phase I Drug-Metabolizing Enzymes, Substrates, and Known Developmental Patterns

Enzyme	Neonatal Substrates	Known Developmental Pattern
CYP1A2	Acetaminophen, caffeine, theophylline, warfarin	Not present to an appreciable extent in human fetal liver. Adult levels reached by 4 months of age and may be exceeded in children 1 to 2 years of age. Activity slowly declines to adult levels, which are attained at the conclusion of puberty. Gender differences in activity are possible during puberty.
CYP2C9 CYP2C19	Phenytoin, S-warfarin; Diazepam, phenytoin, propranolol	Not apparent in fetal liver. Inferential data using phenytoin disposition as a nonspecific pharmacologic probe suggest low activity in first week of life, with adult activity reached by 6 months of age. Peak activity (as reflected by average values for V_{max}, which are 1.5- to 1.8-fold adult values) may be reached at 3 to 4 years of age and declines to adult values at the conclusion of puberty.
CYP2D6	Captopril, codeine, propranolol	Low to absent in fetal liver but uniformly present at 1 week of postnatal age. Poor activity (approximately 20% of that in adults) at 1 month of postnatal age. Adult competence attained by approximately 3 to 5 years of age.
CYP3A4	Acetaminophen, alfentanil, carbamazepine, cisapride, diazepam, erythromycin, lidocaine, midazolam, theophylline, verapamil, R-warfarin	Low activity in the first month of life, with approach toward adult levels by 6 to 12 months of postnatal age. Pharmacokinetic data for CYP3A4 substrates suggest that adult activity may be exceeded between 1 and 4 years of age. Activity then progressively declines, reaching adult levels at the conclusion of puberty.
CYP3A7	Dehydroepiandrosterone sulfate, ethinylestradiol, triazolam	Functional activity in fetus is approximately 30 to 75% of adult levels of CYP3A7.

Modified with permission from reference 33.

and cardiorespiratory depression seen in newborns exposed to local anesthetics.

Demethylation

The dealkylation pathway for some drugs (e.g., diazepam and lidocaine) may be less impaired than the hydroxylation pathway at birth.[11] In contrast, the N-demethylation pathways of theophylline are greatly reduced in comparison with hydroxylation.[36] Maturation of theophylline N-demethylation occurs at 55 weeks' postconceptional age and lags behind the maturation of the oxidation pathways seen at 40 weeks' postconceptional age. Despite the earlier maturation of theophylline hydroxylation, theophylline clearance is not increased significantly until the N-demethylation pathway matures.[36] Clearances of other drugs such as diazepam, morphine, and meperidine also are affected by low N-demethylation activity.

Phase II Reactions

Most phase II reactions are decreased in the newborn (Table 94-4).[33] Sulfation, however, is more developed than other conjugation reactions because sulfotransferase activity may approximate adult values at birth (e.g., estrogen sulfotransferase).[32] Methylation also is functional at birth, as demonstrated by the ability of both term and preterm newborns to methylate theophylline to caffeine. Methyltransferase activity is known to be present even in the fetus because methylation is required for synthesis of pulmonary surfactant. In contrast, acetylation of sulfonamides via N-acetyl-transferase 2 (NAT2) is decreased in neonates, especially preterm newborns.[32] Other drugs such as hydralazine that are eliminated via acetylation have decreased hepatic clearance in the neonate. In fact, almost all infants younger than 2 months of age are phenotypically slow acetylators. This is in contrast to 50% of 4- to 7.5-month-old infants and 62% of 7.5- to 11-month-old infants being phenotypically fast acetylators.[33]

Glucuronide Conjugation

Uridine diphosphate (UDP)-glucuronosyltransferase (UGT) activity is significantly reduced at birth and generally reaches adult levels by 6 to 18 months of age.[33] However, at least 10 different UGT isoforms exist, and adult levels of UGT metabolism may be reached at different ages for different substrates (drugs).[37] As a result of the decreased UGT activity, metabolism is significantly decreased in the neonate for compounds that undergo glucuronidation (e.g., chloramphenicol, morphine, lorazepam, corticosteroids, bilirubin, and trichloroethanol [the active metabolite of chloral hydrate]). Toxic effects of these agents may be seen unless doses are decreased appropriately. Reduced glucuronidation with resultant accumulation of chloramphenicol was responsible for the toxic symptoms of the "gray baby syndrome" (i.e., cardiovascular collapse and shock).

The effects of decreased glucuronidation may not be as dramatic for drugs that have alternate metabolic pathways because a shift to a more mature pathway may occur. For example, in neonates, the decreased glucuronidation of acetaminophen is partially offset by an increase in acetaminophen-sulfate conjugation. This change to sulfation only partially compensates for decreased glucuronidation because acetaminophen half-life is still prolonged in the newborn.[12]

Glycine Conjugation

Glycine conjugation is decreased in newborns but increases to adult levels by approximately 8 weeks of age. In adults, benzyl alcohol (a preservative) is converted to benzoic acid (benzoate), which then is detoxified in the liver through conjugation with glycine to form hippuric acid. Because neonates have a decreased capacity to conjugate p-amino benzoate and benzoate with glycine, benzoic acid can accumulate in newborns given excess benzyl alcohol or benzoic acid.[38] Accumulation of benzoic acid results in the "gasping syndrome," which consists of multiple-organ system failure, severe metabolic acidosis, and gasping respirations. This potentially fatal syndrome is associated with cumulative benzyl alcohol doses ≥99 mg/kg in preterm neonates.[39] As recommended by the FDA, drugs containing the preservatives benzyl alcohol or benzoic acid should not be used in neonates.[40] The use of preservative-free IV solutions, diluents, and medications is advised.

Table 94-4 Important Neonatal Phase II Drug-Metabolizing Enzymes, Substrates, and Known Developmental Patterns

Enzyme	Neonatal Substrates	Known Developmental Pattern
N-acetyltransferase-2 (NAT2)	Caffeine, clonazepam, hydralazine, procainamide, sulfamethoxazole	Some fetal activity present by 16 weeks. Virtually 100% of infants between birth and 2 months of age exhibit the slow metabolizer phenotype. Adult phenotype distribution reached by 4 to 6 months of postnatal age, with adult activity present by approximately 1 to 3 years of age.
Thiopurine methyltransferase	Azathioprine, mercaptopurine, thioguanine	Levels in fetal liver are approximately 30% of those in adult liver. In newborn infants, activity is approximately 50% higher than in adults, with a phenotype distribution that parallels that in adults. In Korean children, adult activity appears at approximately 7 to 9 years of age.
Glucuronosyltransferase (UGT)	Acetaminophen, chloramphenicol, morphine, valproic acid	Ontogeny is isoform specific as reflected by pharmacokinetic data for certain pharmacologic substrates (e.g., acetaminophen or chloramphenicol). In general, adult activity as reflected from pharmacokinetic data seems to be achieved by 6 to 18 months of age.
Sulfotransferase	Acetaminophen, bile acids, chloramphenicol, cholesterol, dopamine, polyethylene glycols	Ontogeny (based on pharmacokinetic studies) seems to be more rapid than that for UGT; however, it is substrate specific. Activity for some isoforms (e.g., that are responsible for acetaminophen metabolism) may exceed adult levels during infancy and early childhood.

Modified with permission from reference 33.

Induction of Enzymes

Maturation of hepatic enzymes can be influenced by in utero or postnatal exposure to enzyme-inducing agents.[32] Neonatal enzymes may have a faster and greater response to inducing agents compared with adults. Hydroxylation and glucuronidation pathways are especially affected.[11] For example, the plasma half-life of diazepam is 40 to 100 hours in preterm neonates and 20 to 45 hours in term neonates, but only 11 to 18 hours in neonates briefly exposed to the enzyme-inducing drug, phenobarbital.[41,42] This shortened diazepam half-life is a result of an increase in the hydroxylation and conjugation pathways. Because phenobarbital can induce UDP-glucuronosyltransferase (and therefore glucuronide conjugation), it sometimes is used to treat neonatal unconjugated hyperbilirubinemia. Antenatal corticosteroid administration, which commonly is used to promote fetal lung maturation, also can induce postnatal metabolism of both theophylline and metronidazole.[11]

Other Effects

Decreased cardiac output, respiratory distress, decreased liver perfusion, or hypoxia may further decrease neonatal hepatic enzymatic activity.[11] Decreased phenobarbital clearance has been demonstrated in asphyxiated neonates.[43]

Renal Elimination

Glomerular filtration, tubular secretion, and tubular reabsorption are decreased in preterm and term newborns compared with adults. Because most drugs and metabolites are eliminated renally, clearance generally is decreased in neonates. As a result, maintenance doses of drugs that are eliminated renally must be decreased. Although overall renal function increases with age, the maturational rates of individual physiologic functions vary. For example, glomerular filtration matures several months before tubular secretion, and factors increasing tubular reabsorption mature after tubular secretion. Because renal elimination depends on the balance of filtration, secretion, and reabsorption, predictions of renal clearance of drugs eliminated by more than one of these mechanisms may be difficult in the maturing neonate.

Glomerular Filtration

At birth, glomerular filtration rate (GFR) is significantly decreased. The GFR for term newborns is 2 to 4 mL/minute, or approximately 10 to 20 mL/minute per 1.73 m². For preterm newborns, GFR is only 0.7 to 0.8 mL/minute or approximately 0.5 % of an adult.[44] In term newborns, GFR increases markedly after birth, doubling by 1 to 2 weeks' postnatal age. Despite the continued increase postnatally, GFR is only 50 mL/minute per 1.73 m² at 2.5 weeks' postnatal age[45] and does not reach adult values until 3 to 5 months' postnatal age.

In preterm neonates, postnatal development of GFR is delayed and a lower GFR persists beyond the first few months of life, especially in very low-birth-weight newborns 30 weeks' gestational age or younger. Even at a corrected postnatal age of 9 months (i.e., 18 months' postconceptional age), GFR is significantly decreased in very low-birth-weight infants compared with term infants of the same postconceptional age.[45] Although the exact age at which GFR matures in very low-birth-weight infants is not known, a normal GFR should not be assumed in older preterm infants even up to 1 to 2 years postnatal age.

Serum creatinine (SrCr) concentrations in all neonates are elevated at birth, reflecting maternal concentrations. In healthy newborns greater than 30 weeks' gestational age, serum creatinine steadily decreases throughout the first week of life to approximately 0.4 mg/dL. SrCr concentrations in very low-birth-weight infants born at 30 weeks or less gestational age are significantly higher than their term counterparts, even at a corrected postnatal age of 9 months.[45]

Clearance of drugs primarily eliminated by glomerular filtration (e.g., digoxin, vancomycin, and the aminoglycosides) is well correlated with GFR. Therefore, maturation of GFR must be considered when developing dosing guidelines for these medications. For example, both vancomycin clearance and gentamicin clearance correlate with postnatal age, weight, and creatinine clearance (Cl_{Cr}), as well as postconceptional age.[46–50] Therefore, guidelines that incorporate these patient factors are more likely to result in therapeutic serum concentrations in the developing neonate. An example of neonatal gentamicin dosing guidelines[51,52] that are used commonly is given in Table 94-5.

Other conditions such as asphyxia, decreased cardiac output, renal disease, or indomethacin therapy may further decrease GFR and drug clearance during the perinatal period.[53–55] The hypoxia, hypercarbia, hypotension, and decreased cardiac output that occur during asphyxia cause significant decreases in GFR. In addition, compensatory mechanisms such as an increased formation of renovascular constricting prostaglandins may aggravate this condition further.[44] Therefore, dosage regimens of renally eliminated drugs should be empirically decreased in severely asphyxiated neonates. Dosage reduction before the initiation of indomethacin therapy also is necessary because significant elevations of aminoglycoside and digoxin serum concentrations have resulted with concomitant indomethacin therapy.[54,55] For example, a 50% dosage reduction of digoxin is recommended in preterm infants receiving indomethacin.[55]

In contrast, an increase in dosage may be required for drugs (e.g., thiazide and loop diuretics) that depend on GFR for sufficient intraluminal concentrations and pharmacologic effect. A diminished diuretic response may be seen in preterm neonates, particularly during the first month of life. Because

Table 94-5 Gentamicin Dosing Guidelines for Neonates and Infants			
Postconceptional Age (wk)	Postnatal Age (days)	Dose (mg/kg/dose)	Interval (hr)
≤29 or significant asphyxia	0–28	2.5	24
	>28	3.0	24
30–36	0–14	3.0	24
	>14	2.5	12[a]
≥37	0–7	2.5	12
	>7	2.5	8

[a]Use 18 to 24 hours if birth weight ≤1,200 g and postnatal age <28 days.[52]
Adapted with permission from Young TE, Mangum OB. Neofax '96: A Manual of Drugs Used in Neonatal Care. 9th ed. Raleigh, NC: Acorn Publishing, Inc., 1996:30. A more recent version of this table appears in the 2000 edition of Neofax. The 2000 version includes extended-interval dosing of gentamicin.

furosemide is less dependent on GFR, it is the preferred diuretic in neonates.

Tubular Secretion

Tubular secretion is approximately 20% to 30% of adult values at birth and matures more slowly than GFR. Despite a doubling over the first 7 days of life, tubular secretion does not reach adult values until 30 to 40 weeks' postnatal age. By 1 year of age, tubular secretion is 10 times higher than at birth.[11,12]

Therefore, in neonates, a decreased clearance is seen for drugs that are eliminated by proximal tubular secretion (e.g., furosemide, penicillins, thiazides, atropine, and morphine). Tubular secretion, however, can be enhanced in the immature kidney after continued exposure to certain drugs. Substrate stimulation of tubular secretory pathways and subsequent increases in elimination (and therefore dosing requirements) have been reported for penicillin, ampicillin, and dicloxacillin.[12,56]

Tubular Reabsorption

Tubular reabsorption, a passive process that is concentration dependent, is decreased in the neonate owing to the decreased GFR and reduced filtrate load.[11] The low urinary pH seen in neonates results in an increase in reabsorption of weak acids (decreased clearance) and a decrease in reabsorption of weak bases. In addition, the normal diurnal variation in urine pH is not present until 2 years postnatal age.[11]

Clinical Relevance to Dosing

Decreased enzyme activity and renal function in neonates result in a decreased clearance and prolonged half-life for many drugs (see Table 94-2). Because drug clearance determines the maintenance dose, mg/kg/day dosages must be reduced in neonates, particularly preterm neonates, to avoid toxicities. As biotransformation reactions and renal function mature, daily dosages subsequently must be increased with age to prevent subtherapeutic concentrations. Because of these dynamic changes, periodic clinical assessment and therapeutic drug monitoring are extremely important in neonates.

RESPIRATORY DISTRESS SYNDROME

RDS is a major cause of morbidity and mortality in preterm neonates, affecting approximately 50,000 infants in the United States each year.[57] This clinical syndrome is characterized by respiratory failure with atelectasis, hypoxemia, decreased lung compliance, small airway epithelial damage, and pulmonary edema. The principle cause of RDS is pulmonary surfactant deficiency. Pulmonary surfactant decreases the surface tension at the air/fluid interface in the alveoli and prevents alveolar collapse. Surfactant also facilitates the clearance of pulmonary fluid, prevents pulmonary edema, and stabilizes alveoli during aeration. At birth, the clearance of residual fetal lung fluid is accompanied by an increase in pulmonary blood flow, which facilitates the transition from fetal to adult circulation.[58,59]

In the fetus, endogenous cortisol stimulates the synthesis and secretion of pulmonary surfactant at 30 to 32 weeks' gestational age.[60] However, sufficient amounts of pulmonary surfactant for normal lung function are not present before 34 to 36 weeks' gestation.[61] Therefore, the incidence and severity of RDS increase as gestational age decreases. RDS occurs in <20% to 30% of neonates born at 30 to 31 weeks' gestational age, but in 50% of neonates born at 26 to 28 weeks' gestational age.[58]

Without adequate amounts of surfactant, the surface tension within the alveoli is so great that the alveoli collapse (atelectasis), resulting in poor gas exchange (e.g., hypoxemia, hypercapnia). Low lung compliance also results and large inspiratory pressures are needed to aerate the lungs. Unfortunately, the extremely compliant neonatal chest wall makes it difficult to create the large negative inspiratory pressures necessary to open the alveoli. This results in an increased work of breathing and alterations of ventilation and perfusion (V/Q mismatch).[58,59]

Aeration of the surfactant-deficient lung also results in the cyclic collapse and distention of bronchioles with resultant bronchiolar epithelial injury and necrosis. This epithelial damage causes pulmonary edema by allowing fluid and proteins to leak from the intravascular space into the air spaces and interstitium of the lung. The necrotic epithelial debris and proteins then form fibrous hyaline membranes.[59] Hyaline membranes and pulmonary edema further impair gas exchange. The term hyaline membrane disease has been used to describe the presence of these fibrous membranes. However, because hyaline membrane disease is not specific to surfactant deficiency, the term *respiratory distress syndrome* (RDS) is preferred.

The inadequate oxygenation and ventilation and increased work of breathing caused by RDS may result in the need for assisted positive-pressure ventilation. Complications of RDS may be related to mechanical ventilation and include the following: pulmonary barotrauma (e.g., pneumothorax, pulmonary interstitial emphysema), intraventricular hemorrhage (IVH), patent ductus arteriosus (PDA), retinopathy of prematurity, and chronic lung disease or bronchopulmonary dysplasia (BPD).[59] (Also see Bronchopulmonary Dysplasia.)

Clinical Presentation

1. L.D., an 800-g male, was precipitously born at 27 weeks' gestational age to a 38-year-old gravida 6 para 5 female. Apgar scores were 5 at 1 minute and 7 at 5 minutes. One hour after birth, L.D. appears cyanotic and has retracting respirations with grunting and nasal flaring. HR is 160 beats/min and RR is 65 breaths/min. An arterial blood gas (ABG) on 100% oxygen by nasal cannula is as follows: pH, 7.26; PCO_2, 50 mm Hg; PO_2, 53 mm Hg; and base deficit, 7. Arterial to alveolar oxygen tension ratio (a/A) is <0.2. L.D. is intubated immediately and placed on positive-pressure–assisted ventilation. A catheter is inserted in his umbilical artery for frequent ABG monitoring, and an umbilical vein catheter is inserted for central venous access. L.D.'s chest radiographc shows moderate hyaline membrane disease. Ampicillin 50 mg/kg Q 12 hr and gentamicin 2.5 mg/kg Q 24 hr are ordered IV to rule out sepsis. What risk factors does L.D. have for RDS? What signs and laboratory data are consistent with RDS?

[SI units: PCO_2, 6.67 kPa; PO_2, 7.1 kPa]

L.D.'s risk factors for RDS are prematurity and male gender. Other risk factors include gestational diabetes, cesarean section with no labor, second-born twins, perinatal asphyxia, and maternofetal hemorrhage.[58,59,62] Clinical signs and laboratory data consistent with RDS in L.D. include tachypnea (RR, 65 breaths/min); cyanosis, retracting respirations, grunting, nasal flaring, hypoxemia (PO_2, 53 mm Hg); hypercapnia (PCO_2, 50 mm Hg); and a mixed respiratory and metabolic acidosis.[50,59,62] Clinical manifestations classically present within the first 6 hours of life.[62]

Tachypnea, the first sign of respiratory distress, is an attempt to compensate for the inadequate ventilation, hypercapnia, and acidosis. L.D.'s retracting respirations (the use of intercostal, subcostal, suprasternal, or sternal accessory muscles) reflect the increased work of breathing necessary to maintain ventilation. His nasal flaring decreases resistance during inspiration and increases oxygenation. Grunting is the result of forceful exhalation against a partially closed glottis in an effort to prolong expiration and maximize oxygenation. Grunting also increases intrathoracic pressure during expiration in an attempt to stabilize the alveoli and prevent atelectasis. L.D.'s cyanosis, hypoxemia, hypercapnia, and mixed respiratory and metabolic acidosis are consequences of inadequate oxygenation and poor ventilation and are consistent with RDS.[58,59]

Prevention

2. **What maternal treatment might have prevented RDS in L.D.?**

RDS may be prevented if pregnancy can be prolonged long enough for fetal lungs to mature or if production of pulmonary surfactant can be accelerated in utero. Premature labor can be suppressed pharmacologically with drugs that inhibit uterine contractions (tocolytic agents). Tocolytic agents such as the β-adrenergic agonists (e.g., ritodrine, terbutaline) and magnesium sulfate may be administered parenterally to stop uterine activity. Therapy then may be continued with oral β-agonists.[63,64] (See Chapter 46, Obstetrics.)

Maternal administration of glucocorticoids can accelerate fetal lung maturation and decrease the incidence and severity of RDS. L.D.'s mother should have been considered a candidate for antenatal corticosteroids, unless immediate delivery was anticipated. A meta-analysis of 15 antenatal maternal corticosteroid trials with >3,400 participants demonstrated a significant reduction in RDS along with significant decreases in NEC, IVH, and neonatal death, regardless of the infant's gender and race. Furthermore, there was no evidence of an increased incidence of fetal, neonatal, or maternal infection, or fetal death associated with the use of antenatal steroids. The incidence of BPD, however, was not affected, and the decrease in RDS was not significant for newborns greater than 34 weeks' gestational age.[65]

To encourage consideration of antenatal corticosteroids, the National Institutes of Health (NIH) formed a consensus panel to evaluate the use of antenatal corticosteroids for fetal lung maturation.[64] The panel recommended administration of antenatal steroids in all pregnant women at high risk for premature delivery. Because the effects of antenatal steroids had not been shown to last beyond 7 days, many centers repeated the course of steroids every 7 days until 34 weeks' gestation. Even though the potential benefits and risks of repeated courses were essentially unknown, multiple-course antenatal

steroids became widespread, with usage ranging from 85% to 98%.[66] Recent studies found a decrease in birth weight and head circumference, and an increase in neonatal sepsis and death associated with multiple-course antenatal steroids.[67,68] Investigation by a second NIH consensus panel resulted in a recommendation that a single course of antenatal corticosteroids be considered for all pregnant women between 24 and 34 weeks gestation who are at risk of preterm delivery within 7 days; repeat courses of antenatal steroids are not routinely recommended and should be reserved for patients enrolled in randomized controlled trials.[69]

Betamethasone injection 12 mg IM every 24 hours for two doses or dexamethasone injection 6 mg IM every 12 hours for four doses are the only two NIH-recommended regimens to accelerate lung maturation.[64,69] Fetal lung maturity can be assessed by measuring certain components (e.g., lecithin, sphingomyelin) of lung surfactant found in amniotic fluid. A ratio of lecithin to sphingomyelin greater than 2 indicates functionally mature fetal lungs and a decreased risk for RDS.[59] Meta-analyses have shown that although both betamethasone and dexamethasone decrease the incidence of RDS, only betamethasone decreases neonatal mortality and the risk for periventricular leukomalacia.[70,71]

Maternal administration of glucocorticoids increases the production of fibroblast-pneumocyte factor, which stimulates the biosynthesis of surfactant in type II pneumocytes. This mimics the physiologic response of fetal lungs to the increased cortisol production that normally begins at 30 to 32 weeks' gestation.[60] Certain obstetric conditions may stress the fetus and stimulate adrenal activity and corticosteroid release in utero, thereby enhancing fetal lung maturity. For example, an unusually low incidence of RDS occurs in neonates born prematurely to mothers with hypertension, infection, cardiovascular disease, hemoglobinopathies, heroin addiction, premature rupture of membranes >48 hours, and decreased placental function.[59,61] Antenatal steroids also improve postnatal responsiveness to exogenous surfactant administration.[62,64,72] Administration of thyrotropin-releasing hormone (TRH) in combination with antenatal steroids was initially thought to enhance fetal lung maturation, decrease the incidence of RDS, and decrease the incidence of BPD. Unfortunately, these effects were not supported in a recent meta-analysis.[64,73] In fact, prenatal TRH increased neonatal ventilation usage, lowered 5-minute Apgar scores, and was associated with poorer 12-month outcomes. Therefore, antenatal use of TRH cannot be recommended.

Treatment
Surfactant Therapy

3. **What treatments should be initiated for L.D.?**

Before L.D. is treated for RDS, other causes of respiratory distress must be ruled out. Infections, for example (particularly group B streptococcal [GBS] sepsis or pneumonia), often present with respiratory distress. Because it is difficult to distinguish between RDS and infection, all infants with severe RDS should receive antibiotics. L.D. was started empirically on antibiotics, and a complete evaluation of possible sepsis should be performed.

Exogenous surfactant should be administered intratracheally to L.D. as soon as possible. Surfactant is the most comprehensively studied new therapy in neonatal medicine.[72,74] Until the late 1980s, oxygen supplementation, mechanical ventilation, fluid restriction, and supportive care were the general treatment measures for RDS. Because RDS primarily is a consequence of surfactant deficiency, the administration of exogenous surfactant should decrease the severity of RDS and the risk of death.[75]

Human surfactant is synthesized and secreted by type II alveolar epithelial cells of the lung. It contains 70% to 80% phospholipids, approximately 10% neutral lipids, and approximately 10% proteins.[61] The major surface-active component is dipalmitoylphosphatidylcholine (DPPC), also known as *colfosceril* or *lecithin*. However, this phospholipid slowly adsorbs to the air/fluid interface in the alveoli. Other phospholipids, such as phosphatidylcholine and phosphatidylglycerol, and four surfactant apoproteins (SP-A, SP-B, SP-C, and SP-D) enhance spreadability and surface adsorption.[61,72,76] Adsorption and surface spreading of the surfactant in the alveoli are important determinants of surface-tension activity. SP-A may also help regulate alveolar surfactant reuptake and metabolism.[61]

Three types of exogenous surfactants have been evaluated clinically: natural, modified natural, and synthetic. Natural surfactants are derived from bovine or porcine lung-lipid or lavage extracts, or from human amniotic fluid. Modified natural surfactants are lung-lipid extracts supplemented with phospholipids or other components.[72] Currently, four surfactant products are commercially available for clinical use in the United States: Exosurf (colfosceril palmitate) is synthetic, Survanta (beractant) is a modified natural, and Infasurf (calfactant) and Curosurf (poractant alfa) are natural surfactants. Only three products have FDA approval for the prevention (i.e., prophylaxis) of RDS (Exosurf, Survanta, Infasurf); all four products are indicated for the treatment (i.e., rescue therapy) of RDS.[77–80]

Exosurf is protein free and contains synthetic DPPC (84%), cetyl alcohol to enhance surface activity, and tyloxapol (an emulsifier) to facilitate spreading and adsorption.[62,72] It does not contain SP-A, SP-B, or SP-C. Survanta is prepared by mincing bovine lung, which contains lung surfactant and phospholipids from lung cells. During the extraction process, cholesterol is removed and synthetic DPPC is added to improve surface activity. Surfactant apoprotein B (SP-B), which is thought to be the most critical protein for surfactant activity, is removed with cholesterol. As a result, Survanta contains only trace amounts of SP-B (<0.5% of total protein). Ninety-nine percent of the protein in Survanta is SPC.[81,82]

In contrast, Infasurf is extracted from washings of newborn calves' lungs; therefore it contains less contaminating lung-cell components. No synthetic DPPC is added to Infasurf. Forty percent of the protein in Infasurf is SP-B and 60% is SP-C. Curosurf is extracted from washings of pigs' lungs and is purified by liquid-gel chromatography to remove neutralized lipids such as cholesterol. As with Infasurf, no synthetic DPPC is added to Curosurf.[83] It is composed of 99% lipids and 1% apoproteins (SP-B [30%] and SP-C [70%]). Neither Survanta, Infasurf, nor Curosurf contain SP-A.[81–83]

Other comparisons between these four products are listed in Table 94-6.[77–80]

PHARMACOLOGIC AND LONG-TERM EFFECTS

4. **What are the effects of exogenously administered surfactant in RDS?**

Oxygenation and lung compliance rapidly and markedly improve after the administration of surfactant. Supplemental oxygen and mechanical ventilation can be reduced significantly. The increased lung compliance and decreased need for high inspiratory pressures result in a dramatic decrease in the incidence of pneumothorax and pulmonary interstitial emphysema. Survival in treated infants increases by approximately 40% regardless of birth weight or gestational age, and neonatal mortality from RDS is decreased to approximately 20%.[75] Other complications of RDS such as severe BPD, IVH, and PDA have not been decreased consistently with surfactant therapy. Although the severity of retinopathy of prematurity was decreased with the use of exogenous surfactants, overall incidence was unchanged.[75]

NUMBER OF DOSES

5. **At 2 hours of age, 4 mL/kg of Survanta was administered to L.D. intratracheally. Within 1 hour, oxygenation improved and the FiO$_2$ was weaned from 100% to 80%. Six hours later, the ABGs revealed the following: pH, 7.36; PCO$_2$, 45 mm Hg; PO$_2$, 80 mm Hg; base deficit, 2; and O$_2$ saturation of 94% on the following ventilator settings: FiO$_2$, 0.73; IMV, 40; PiP, 18; and PEEP, +3. The a/A ratio is <0.2. Should another dose of Survanta be administered?**

[SI units: PCO$_2$, 6.0 kPa; PO$_2$, 10.7 kPa]

Because the response to a single dose usually is transient, more than one dose of surfactant is needed. Response to surfactant therapy can be variable, especially in preterm newborns <750 g.[77] Reasons for nonresponse include surfactant inhibition by proteins that have leaked into the alveolar spaces, inactivation of surfactant by inflammatory mediators (i.e., free oxygen radicals, proteases), presence of conditions such as pulmonary edema that can decrease surfactant effectiveness, or poor delivery of surfactant to the alveoli (due to atelectasis). The degree of responsiveness to surfactant also decreases with increasing postnatal age.[72,82]

Although the indications for subsequent doses of surfactant have varied in investigational studies, persistence of respiratory failure is the major clinical indicator for retreatment. A second dose of Survanta should be given to L.D. because he still requires mechanical ventilation with relatively high inspiratory pressures and supplemental oxygen (FiO$_2$ ≥0.3) to maintain an arterial PO$_2$ ≥50 mm Hg and oxygen saturation of 90%. Also, most clinicians would agree that an a/A ratio of <0.2 is an indication for repeat dosing.[75] Although meta-analyses have shown a reduction in the incidence of neonatal death and pneumothorax associated with multiple surfactant doses, other large trials have not reported any additional advantage with more than two doses of Exosurf or Infasurf.[84,85] In practice, despite these conflicting findings, most infants receive an average of two surfactant doses. Further studies evaluating the need for retreatment, including specific timing and indications, are required.

Table 94-6 Comparison of Currently Marketed Surfactant Products[77-80]

Variable	Calfactant (Infasurf)	Poractant (Curosurf)
Type and source	Natural surfactant, calf lung wash	Natural surfactant, porcine lung mince extract
Phospholipids	Natural DPPC with mixed phospholipids	Natural and DPPC and mixed phospholipids
Proteins	Calf proteins SP-B and SP-C	Porcine proteins SP-B and SP-C
Dispersing and adsorption agents	Proteins SP-B and SP-C	Proteins SP-B and SP-C
Recommended dose	3 mL/kg (phospholipids 105 mg/kg)	Initial dose: 2.5 mL/kg (phospholipids 200 mg/kg); Repeat dose: 1.25 mL/kg (phospholipids 100 mg/kg)
Indications	Prophylaxis and rescue therapy	Rescue therapy
Criteria for prophylaxis	Premature infants <29 weeks' gestational age at high risk for RDS	Not approved
Recommended regimen for prophylaxis	Give first dose ASAP after birth, preferably within 30 minutes; repeat every 12 hours up to a total of three doses if infant still remains intubated or repeat as early as 6 hours up to a total of four doses if infant still remains intubated and requires FiO_2 ≥0.3 with PaO_2 ≤80 mm Hg	Not approved
Criterion for rescue therapy	Infants ≤72 hours of age with confirmed RDS who require endotracheal intubation	Infants with confirmed RDS who require endotracheal intubation
Recommended regimen for rescue therapy	Give first dose ASAP after RDS diagnosed, repeat every 12 hours up to a total of three doses if infant still remains intubated or repeat as early as 6 hours up to a total of four doses if infant still remains intubated and requires FiO_2 ≥0.3 with PaO_2 ≤80 mm Hg	Give first dose ASAP after RDS diagnosed, repeat every 12 hours up to a total of three doses if infant still remains intubated and requires mechanical ventilation with supplemental oxygen
Recommended administration technique	Administer through side-port of ETT adapter via ventilator, divide dose into 2 aliquots with position change OR through disconnect ETT via 5-French catheter, divide dose into 4 aliquots with position change	Administer through disconnected ETT via 5-French catheter, divide dose into 2 aliquots with position change
Formulation	Suspension	Suspension
Storage	Refrigerate 2 to 8°C; protect from light	Refrigerate 2 to 8°C; protect from light
Volume/vial	6 mL	1.5 mL, 3 mL
Special instructions	Gentle swirling of the vial may be necessary for redispersion; warming to room temperature is **not** necessary; do not shake	Warm to room temperature before use, do not shake
Stability	If warmed to room temperature <24 hours, unopened, unused vials may be returned once to refrigerator; single-use vial contains no preservative, discard unused portion	If warmed to room temperature for <24 hours, unopened, unused vials may be returned only once to refrigerator; single-use vial contains no preservative, discard unused portion
Cost per vial	$732 (6 mL)[a]	$312 (1.5 mL), $611 (3 mL)[a]

PROPHYLACTIC ADMINISTRATION

6. **Could prophylactic administration of surfactant have prevented RDS in L.D.?**

Prophylactic administration of surfactant may reduce the incidence and severity of RDS, but does not always prevent the disease.[59,75] Theoretically, the first dose of surfactant could be given before the newborn's first breath or before positive-pressure ventilation.[75,82] This would avoid the early lung injury seen in RDS that may interfere with surfactant distribution, bioavailability, and effectiveness.[72] However, this strategy increases the cost of care because newborns who may never go on to develop RDS would be intubated and treated unnecessarily.[62,72,84] In addition, delivery room treatment may interfere with resuscitation and stabilization of the neonate.[82]

Although prophylactic surfactant has been associated with significant reductions in the incidence of pneumothorax and mortality, the incidence of BPD, PDA, and IVH have not been reduced.[75,82] In addition, pulmonary hemorrhage may be increased (see Question 7). Therefore, the use of prophylactic surfactant therapy remains controversial. To date, prophylactic

use of surfactant (given within 1 hour of birth) has not been compared with very early rescue surfactant treatment (administered within 2 hours of birth). However, when prophylactic surfactant was compared with rescue treatment (2 to 6 hours after birth) in infants with gestational ages of 27 to 32 weeks, no difference in the incidence of BPD, death, severe IVH (grade ≥3), or duration of mechanical ventilation was found.

In summary, surfactant treatment should be administered as soon as clinical signs of RDS appear.[86] Early rescue therapy avoids progression of the disease and the potential for decreased surfactant effectiveness. Prophylactic administration in the delivery room (i.e., administration within 10 to 15 minutes after birth) should be reserved for extremely premature neonates who are at the highest risk for RDS.[75,82,86]

COMPLICATIONS

7. **What complications of surfactant treatment is L.D. at risk of developing?**

The most common adverse effects of surfactant therapy are related to the method of administration.[82] During administra-

Table 94-6 Comparison of Currently Marketed Surfactant Products[77-80]

Variable	Colfosceril (Exosurf)	Beractant (Survanta)
Type and source	Synthetic	Modified natural surfactant, bovine lung mince extract
Phospholipids	Synthetic DPPC (hexadecanol and DPPC)	Natural and supplemented DPPC and mixed phospholipids
Proteins	None	Bovine proteins SP-B and SP-C
Dispersing and adsorption agents	Cetyl alcohol, tyloxapol	Proteins SP-B and SP-C
Recommended dose	5 mL/kg (DPPC 67.5 mg/kg)	4 mL/kg (phospholipids 100 mg/kg)
Indications	Prophylaxis or rescue therapy	Prophylaxis or rescue therapy
Criteria for prophylaxis	Birth weight <1,350 g with risk for RDS; birth weight >1,350 g with evidence of lung immaturity	Birth weight <1,250 g or evidence of surfactant deficiency
Recommended regimen for prophylaxis	Give first dose ASAP after birth; give second and third doses 12 and 24 hours later to all who remain on ventilator	Give first dose ASAP after birth, preferably within 15 min; repeat as early as 6 hours up to a total of four doses if infant still remains intubated and requires FiO_2 ≥0.3 with PaO_2 ≤80 mm Hg
Criterion for rescue therapy	Infants with confirmed RDS who require endotracheal intubation	Infants with confirmed RDS who require endotracheal intubation
Recommended regimen for rescue therapy	Give first dose ASAP after RDS diagnosed; give second dose 12 hours later to all who remain on ventilator	Give first dose ASAP after RDS diagnosed, preferably by 8 hours postnatal age; repeat as early as 6 hours up to a total of four doses if infant still remains intubated and requires FiO_2 ≥0.3 with PaO_2 ≤80 mm Hg
Recommended administration technique	Administer through side port of ETT adapter via ventilator, divide dose into 2 aliquots with position change	Administer through disconnected ETT via 5-French catheter, divide dose into 4 aliquots with position change
Formulation	Lyophilized powder	Suspension
Storage	Room temperature	Refrigerate 2 to 8°C; protect from light
Volume/vial	8 mL (after reconstitution)	4 mL, 8 mL
Special instructions	Reconstitute with 8 mL of preservative-free Sterile Water for Injection, follow mixing procedures carefully; do not shake vigorously, use gentle shaking or swirling	Warm to room temperature before use; do not shake
Stability	Stable up to 12 hours after reconstitution; single-use vial contains no preservative, discard unused portion	If warmed to room temperature for <8 hours, unopened, unused vials may be returned only once to refrigerator; single-use vial contains no preservative, discard unused portion
Cost per vial	$732 (8 mL)[b]	$460 (4 mL), $832 (8 mL)[a]

[a]Average wholesale price 2003 Red Book.
[b]Average wholesale price 2002 Red Book.
ASAP, as soon as possible; DPPC, dipalmitoylphosphatidylcholine; ETT, endotracheal tube; FiO_2, fractional inspired oxygen; PaO_2, partial pressure of oxygen; RDS, respiratory distress syndrome.

tion, bradycardia and oxygen desaturation may occur secondary to vagal stimulation and airway obstruction.[77-80,82] These adverse events may temporarily require surfactant administration to be discontinued and ventilator support to be increased. Mucous plugging with obstruction, BP changes, and altered electroencephalogram (EEG) tracings also may occur.[82] Airway obstruction may be decreased by delivering surfactant as a continuous intratracheal infusion over 10 to 20 minutes via an infusion pump.[87]

Surfactant therapy may increase the risk of pulmonary hemorrhage. Although the exact mechanism is unknown, surfactant may increase pulmonary blood flow through the ductus arteriosus, increase pulmonary microvascular pressures, and cause hemorrhagic pulmonary edema.[75] Although an earlier meta-analysis reported the incidence of pulmonary hemorrhage to be nearly doubled after prophylactic synthetic surfactant therapy (Exosurf), a recent meta-analysis did not find a significant difference in the incidence of pulmonary hemorrhage between natural and synthetic surfactants.[74] The benefits of surfactant therapy, however, far outweigh the increased risk of pulmonary hemorrhage.

Neonates given surfactant may be at a greater risk for apnea requiring methylxanthine treatment. Because surfactant-treated neonates can be weaned from ventilator support sooner, they may display apnea more easily.[75] Individual trials with natural surfactants have suggested an increased incidence of sepsis and NEC (necrotizing enterocolitis), but most studies have not validated these findings.[75] No difference in the incidence of NEC or apnea treated with methylxanthines was noted between products in three comparative trials (Exosurf versus Survanta, Infasurf versus Exosurf, Infasurf versus Survanta).[81,88,89] One study found a significantly higher incidence of sepsis in infants treated with Exosurf (17%) compared with Infasurf (12%).[89]

PRODUCT SELECTION

8. Are there any advantages of one surfactant product over the other?

Not enough data exist to label one commercially available product superior to the other. Although several studies have compared two products, no study has compared all four products. In a randomized, comparative trial, Survanta-treated neonates responded more rapidly (i.e., oxygen and ventilator pressures were able to be decreased sooner) than those who received Exosurf. In addition, pneumothorax was significantly lower in the Survanta-treated infants (9% compared with those who received Exosurf [15%]).[88] No significant differences occurred in BPD, mortality, or secondary outcomes (e.g., pulmonary hemorrhage, PDA, NEC, sepsis, apnea, IVH, and retinopathy of prematurity).

In a randomized, double-blind trial of Infasurf and Survanta, Infasurf-treated infants required significantly less supplemental oxygen and mean airway pressures (MAP) during the acute phase of respiratory distress.[81] However, the duration of mechanical ventilation and the use of supplemental oxygen for the rest of the hospital stay were not significantly different between the two groups. The number of infants requiring four doses of surfactant was significantly less in the Infasurf-treated group. In addition, the Infasurf group also had a longer dosing interval, indicating that Infasurf may have a longer duration of effect. The incidence of death, BPD, and secondary outcomes, including pneumothorax were not significantly different between the two groups.[81]

Infasurf was also compared with Exosurf in a randomized, double-blinded trial. Similar to the previous trial, infants treated with Infasurf had lower requirements for oxygenation and MAP for the first 72 hours compared with those treated with Exosurf. In addition, infants treated with Infasurf had a significantly lower incidence of pneumothorax than those treated with Exosurf. As with the other two comparative trials, the incidence of BPD, death, and secondary outcomes were not significantly different between the two groups.[89]

In a randomized trial of Curosurf and Survanta, Curosurf-treated infants required significantly less supplemental oxygen and mechanical ventilation than infants treated with Survanta during the acute phase of RDS.[83] These improvements were significant for up to 24 hours after treatment. Pneumothorax tended to be higher in the Survanta-treated infants (5 of 40 versus 2 of 33); however, a significant difference was not detected because of the small sample size. The overall duration of mechanical ventilation and total time of oxygen therapy, mortality, the incidence of BPD, and other secondary outcomes were not significantly different between the two groups.

Based on these four comparative trials, the naturally derived surfactants appear to have a faster onset of action than synthetic surfactant (Exosurf), and both Infasurf and Curosurf may have a longer duration of effect than Survanta. The increased incidence of pneumothorax was observed only with synthetic surfactant (Exosurf). The incidence of BPD, death, and other secondary outcomes are not different between natural, modified natural, and synthetic surfactants.[81,83,88,89]

Surfactant should be administered by qualified physicians with the presence of nursing and respiratory therapy personnel.[90] Because Exosurf comes with various size endotracheal tube adapters, neonates do not need to be disconnected from the ventilator during administration.[77] Neonates receiving Survanta or Curosurf need to be disconnected from the ventilator before surfactant administration.[78,80] As a result, clinicians will transiently increase both Fio2 and peak inspiratory pressures before disconnecting the ventilator. These higher settings and interruption from the ventilator may be avoided, however, if Survanta is given through a neonatal suction valve. This method is equally effective, simpler, and possibly safer than methods with ventilator disconnection.[91] Infasurf, on the other hand, has the advantage of flexible administration techniques. It can be administered intratracheally via a catheter passed through the endotracheal tube with brief interruptions in ventilation (as with Survanta and Curosurf) or via a side-port adapter into the endotracheal tube without disconnecting the ventilator (as with Exosurf).[79]

Because Survanta, Infasurf, and Curosurf are all derived from natural sources, they contain proteins that are potentially antigenic. Thus, theoretically, they may cause an immunologic response. However, there are no reports of Survanta-, Infasurf-, or Curosurf-induced hypersensitivity reactions.[75] Surfactant products are expensive and are commercially available only in single-use vials (see Table 94-6).

The availability of a second size vial for Survanta (4 mL, 8 mL) and Curosurf (1.5 mL, 3 mL) may make these product more cost-effective.[92]

Diuretics

9. **What is the role of diuretics in the management of RDS?**

The therapeutic role of diuretics in RDS is controversial. In the natural course of RDS, an abrupt diuresis (urine output >80% of fluid intake) occurs within the first 48 to 72 hours of life. This diuresis is followed by an improvement in pulmonary function, which is thought to be due to a decrease of alveolar or interstitial pulmonary fluid. Before surfactant was commercially available, neonates who did not have this diuresis (or had it after 72 hours) were more likely to develop BPD.

ROUTINE USE

Routine early administration of furosemide to pharmacologically mimic the natural course of RDS may facilitate diuresis and weaning from mechanical ventilation. Although diuretics do not decrease the incidence of BPD or mortality, infants receiving early (prophylactic) therapy of furosemide had a greater increase in urine output, decrease in ventilator MAPs, and improvement in oxygenation compared with infants not receiving furosemide.[62] However, infants receiving prophylactic furosemide had hemodynamic instability and a greater postnatal weight loss. Furthermore, long-term use of furosemide can result in hypercalciuria, renal calcifications, and other electrolyte imbalances (e.g., hyponatremia, hypochloremia, and hypokalemia).[62] Finally, treatment with furosemide may promote patency of the ductus arteriosus, which may further worsen pulmonary edema.[93] Therefore, routine administration of diuretics in RDS is not indicated.[62]

SELECTIVE USE

Because pulmonary edema is present in RDS, furosemide occasionally is administered to enhance lung fluid elimination and decrease pulmonary edema. If L.D. had signs of pulmonary edema with compromised pulmonary function (e.g., hypoxemia and hypercapnia), furosemide 1 mg/kg IV push could be given.

BRONCHOPULMONARY DYSPLASIA
Definition and Incidence

10. J.T. is an 80-day-old, 2-kg, female ex-preemie born at 25 weeks' gestation. Her medical history includes RDS, episodes of sepsis and pneumonia, and chronic parenteral hyperalimentation. J.T. has also failed extubation numerous times and is currently requiring mechanical ventilation with an FiO_2 of 0.5. Current vital signs are as follows: RR, 60 breaths/min; HR, 150 beats/min; BP, 80/55 mm Hg; O_2 saturation, 90%. On physical examination, J.T. has intercostal and subcostal retractions, shallow breathing, and an expiratory wheeze. Bilateral diffuse haziness with lung hyperinflation, focal emphysema (with bleb formation), atelectasis, and irregular fibrous streaks are seen on chest radiograph. J.T. is currently receiving enteral feedings with a standard preterm 20-cal/oz formula at 40 mL Q 3 hr. Based on the aforementioned findings, the diagnosis of BPD (bronchopulmonary dysplasia) is made. What risk factors for BPD does J.T. have? What is the pathogenesis of BPD? What clinical signs and laboratory evidence of BPD are apparent in J.T?

BPD is the most common form of chronic pulmonary disease in infants. The disease develops in newborns who require supplemental oxygen and positive-pressure ventilation for RDS or other primary lung disorders. BPD is defined as a chronic lung disease associated with supplemental oxygen dependency (>21% FiO_2) at 28 days of life and at 36 weeks' postconceptional age with clinical signs of respiratory distress.[94] BPD is a significant cause of infant morbidity and mortality. Approximately 7,500 new cases of BPD occur in the United States each year.[95] The incidence of BPD is inversely related to gestational age and birth weight. Infants with birth weights <700 g have as high as an 85% risk of developing BPD compared with a 5% risk in infants with birth weights >1,500 g.[96] J.T. has two of the most important risk factors for BPD, low birth weight and decreased gestational age. She is also at risk for BPD due to mechanical ventilation, oxygen toxicity, and fluid excess (160 mL/kg per day). Other risk factors include male sex, white ethnicity, and persistent PDA.[97]

Pathogenesis and Clinical Manifestations

The cause of BPD appears to be multifactorial. Lung immaturity, surfactant deficiency, oxygen toxicity, barotrauma/volutrauma, and inflammation all play important roles. Premature infants, especially those less than 26 weeks' gestation, are at a higher risk for BPD due to lung immaturity.[98] Surfactant deficiency (which causes severe RDS) and the immature parenchymal structure of the lung and chest wall contribute to the development of BPD. Oxygen therapy, which causes a release of free oxygen radicals, is directly associated with the pathogenesis of BPD. Prolonged exposure to high oxygen concentrations and free oxygen radicals causes tissue damage, alveolar-capillary leaks, and atelectasis with resultant impaired gas exchange and pulmonary edema.[98] This may lead to the chronic pulmonary fibrotic changes seen in infants with BPD. In term infants, the lungs contain antioxidant enzymes that help protect the lung from damage produced by free oxygen radicals. However, in preterm infants, the concentration of antioxidant enzymes may be low or absent. Therefore, premature infants are more susceptible to develop BPD than term infants.

Barotrauma secondary to positive-pressure ventilation is also a major factor in the pathogenesis of BPD, independent of oxygen toxicity.[98] Barotrauma is caused by repetitive distention of the terminal airways during mechanical ventilation. This results in disruption of the epithelium and an increase in capillary permeability to proteinaceous fluid. The severity of lung injury is related to the amount of positive peak pressure used. Volutrauma is also involved in the pathogenesis of BPD and is caused by high tidal volume ventilation and overdistention. Volutrauma may be due to unusually high peak inflation pressures compared with lung compliance. The combined iatrogenic insults of oxygen toxicity and barotrauma/volutrauma, both inflicted on an immature lung over a period of time, can worsen lung damage.

The inflammatory process in the lung is activated by oxygen toxicity, barotrauma/volutrauma, or other injury. This results in the attraction and activation of leukocytes (e.g., neutrophils, macrophages), which may cause further release of inflammatory mediators, elastase, and collagenase.[95] Elevated levels of elastase and collagenase can destroy the elastin and collagen framework of the lung. α_1-Proteinase inhibitor, a major defense against elastase activity, may be inactivated by free oxygen radicals. Therefore, the combined elevated levels of elastase and the decreased activity of α_1-proteinase inhibitor may enhance lung injury and lead to the development of BPD. Infants who are going to develop BPD also have elevated levels of cytokines such as platelet-activating factor (PAF), leukotrienes, tumor necrosis factor (TNF), and fibronectin.[98] These agents combined with the activated leukocytes cause significant lung damage with breakdown of capillary endothelial integrity and capillary leakage. Furthermore, the increased fibronectin levels found in tracheal aspirate samples of infants with early BPD may predispose them to develop pulmonary fibrosis.[98]

Infection and nutrient deficiency may also play a role in the pathogenesis of BPD. Pathogens such as *Ureaplasma, Chlamydia,* or cytomegalovirus (CMV) may cause chronic infection and contribute to the development of BPD. Studies have shown direct correlations between *Ureaplasma* colonization and the presence of BPD.[98] Deficiencies in nutrients such as vitamin A (retinol) or trace elements such as zinc, copper, and selenium (which are integral components of the antioxidant enzyme structure), may also play a role in the pathogenesis of BPD.

BPD is characterized by tachypnea with shallow breathing, intercostal and subcostal retractions, and expiratory wheezing as demonstrated in J.T. Other signs and symptoms include rales, rhonchi, cough, airflow obstruction, airway hyperreactivity, increased mucus production, hypoxemia, and hypercarbia.[95,96] J.T.'s chest radiograph shows evidence of BPD, including focal emphysema (with bleb formation), atelectasis, bilateral diffuse haziness (interstitial thickening) with increased expansion of the lungs (hyperinflation), and irregular fibrous streaks. Mucous plugging, sepsis, and pneumonia can also develop in BPD infants on chronic mechanical ventilation. Infants with severe BPD eventually develop cardiovascular complications such as pulmonary hypertension, cor pulmonale, systemic hypertension, and left ventricular hypertrophy. In addition to chronic respiratory and cardiovascular complications, infants with BPD have significant growth, nutritional, and neurodevelopmental problems.

Management

11. What nonpharmacologic and therapeutic agents should be used to manage BPD in J.T.?

The medical management of infants with BPD includes supplemental oxygen therapy, mechanical ventilation, fluid restriction, nutritional management, and various pharmacologic interventions. Supplemental oxygen administered via mechanical ventilation, continuous positive airway pressure, or nasal cannula should be provided to maintain an oxygen saturation of 93 to 96% and prevent hypoxemia.[97] Fluids should be restricted to 120 to 130 mL/kg per day to prevent congestive heart disease and pulmonary edema. Because infants with BPD have a 25% increase in caloric expenditure (due to the increased work of breathing), hypercaloric formulas (e.g., 24 or 27 cal/oz) may be used to optimize calories while restricting fluid intake.[95] If this increased energy is not provided, infants are at risk for developing a catabolic state that places them at higher risk for developing BPD (inadequate nutrition may potentiate the toxic effects of oxygen toxicity and barotrauma). The goal of nutritional therapy is to produce weight gains of 10 to 30 g/day, which can usually be accomplished by providing 140 to 160 kcal/kg per day.[95,98] If infants do not tolerate enteral feedings, parenteral alimentation should be substituted until the GI tract becomes more functional. Because J.T. is on a 20-cal/oz formula, switching her to a hypercaloric formula (i.e., 24 or 27 cal/oz) would help optimize her weight gain. Her fluids should be restricted to 240 to 260 mL/day (120 to 130 mL/kg per day).

Pharmacologic Therapy

The treatment of BPD consists of multiple-drug therapy, which includes diuretics, bronchodilators, and corticosteroids. Despite the advancement of drug therapy, none of these drugs has been shown to reverse pulmonary damage in infants with BPD. Instead, they are used primarily to reduce clinical symptoms and to improve lung function. Pharmacologic therapy and dosage regimens for the management of BPD are shown in Table 94-7.[8,95,97,99]

Diuretics

Infants with BPD are particularly prone to pulmonary edema due to cardiogenic and noncardiogenic factors. Left ventricular failure may superimpose the already existing right ventricular failure. Pulmonary vascular permeability is increased due to the disruption of the alveolar-capillary unit and causes an increased amount of fluid in the interstitium. Although the precise mechanism in the treatment of BPD is unknown, diuretics help reduce interstitial lung water. In addition, diuretics lower pulmonary vascular resistance and improve gas exchange, thereby reducing oxygen requirements. Among the diuretics available, furosemide is the drug of choice because of its potent diuretic effect. It acts by blocking the reabsorption of chloride in the ascending loop of Henle. In addition, it also increases lymphatic flow and plasma oncotic pressure, and decreases pulmonary interstitial edema. The use of furosemide in infants with BPD has been associated with short-term improvement in lung compliance and oxygenation, decreased total pulmonary resistance, and facilitation in ventilator weaning.[95,100] However, chronic use of furosemide can result in increased urinary losses of chloride, potassium, and sodium and may result in hypochloremia, hypokalemia, and hyponatremia. Furthermore, volume depletion, hypercalciuria, nephrocalcinosis, osteopenia, and ototoxicity may also occur.[95] Excessive fluid loss or hypochloremia may result in metabolic alkalosis and worsen respiratory acidosis. Some of

Table 94-7 Pharmacologic Management of Bronchopulmonary Dysplasia[8,95,97,99]

Drug Therapy	Dosage Regimen
Diuretics	

Chlorothiazide	*Neonates and infants <6 months:*
	  PO: 20–40 mg/kg/day in two divided doses; maximum dose: 375 mg/day
	Infants >6 months:
	  PO: 20 mg/kg/day in two divided doses; maximum dose: 1 g/day

Furosemide	PO: 1–4 mg/kg/dose 1–2 times/day IV: 1–2 mg/kg/dose Q 12–24 hr Nebulized: 1mg/kg/dose diluted to a final volume of 2 mL with NS (use IV form)
Hydrochlorothiazide/Spironolactone	PO: 1–2 mg/kg/dose Q 12 hr (dose based on hydrochlorothiazide)
Systemic Bronchodilators	
Caffeine citrate	*Loading dose:* 20 mg/kg (10 mg/kg as caffeine base) IV over 30 min *Maintenance dose:* 5 mg/kg/dose (2.5 mg/kg/dose as caffeine base) Q 24 hr; start 24 hr after loading dose; may administer IV (over 10 min) or PO (use IV form)
Theophylline	*Loading dose:* 5 mg/kg IV or PO *Maintenance dose:* 2–3 mg/kg/dose Q 8–12 hr IV or PO
Inhaled Bronchodilators	
Albuterol	0.02–0.04 mL/kg/dose of 0.5% solution (0.1–0.2 mg/kg/dose) diluted to 1–2 mL NS; give via nebulization Q 4–6 hr or PRN; minimum dose: 0.1 mL (0.5 mg); maximum dose: 1 mL (5 mg)
Cromolyn sodium	20 mg (2 mL) via nebulization Q 6–8 hr; may need up to 2–4 weeks for response to occur
Ipratropium bromide	0.13–0.4 mL/kg/dose of 0.02% solution (0.026–0.08 mg/kg/dose) diluted to 2–2.5 mL NS; give via nebulization Q 6–8 hr; do not exceed 0.9 mL (0.18 mg) per dose
Metaproterenol	0.01–0.02 mL/kg/dose of 5% solution (0.5–1 mg/kg) diluted to 1.5–2 mL NS; give via nebulization Q 6 hr or PRN; minimum dose: 0.1 mL (5 mg); maximum dose: 0.3 mL (15 mg)

IV, intravenous; NS, normal saline; PO, oral; PRN, as needed.

those adverse effects may be reduced by using alternate-day furosemide therapy or nebulized furosemide.[100] Both of these regimens were not associated with electrolyte imbalances and were shown to significantly increase lung compliance and decrease pulmonary resistance.[100]

Thiazide diuretics (e.g., hydrochlorothiazide) in combination with a potassium-sparing diuretic (e.g., spironolactone) have also been shown to improve lung function and decrease oxygen requirements with increased diuresis.[95,100] Although less potent than furosemide, the combination of these two diuretics can reduce the incidence of hypokalemia commonly associated with loop or thiazide diuretics. Adverse effects commonly seen with a combination of a thiazide and spironolactone include hyponatremia, hyperkalemia or hypokalemia, hypercalciuria, hyperuricemia, hyperglycemia, azotemia, and hypomagnesia.[95] Various diuretics and dosage regimens are listed in Table 94-7.

Generally, infants are initially treated with furosemide but are changed to a combination diuretic (spironolactone/hydrochlorothiazide) if long-term treatment is needed to avoid adverse effects. Suggested indications for initiating furosemide therapy include the following: (1) 1-week-old infants with early BPD and ventilator dependency, (2) infants with stable BPD who significantly worsen due to fluid overload, (3) infants with chronic BPD who do not improve, and (4) infants requiring an increased fluid intake to provide adequate calories.[98]

Because J.T. has chronic BPD and is not improving (i.e., she has not been able to be weaned off the ventilator), furosemide 1 mg/kg every 12 hours should be initiated. J.T. should be monitored for electrolyte disturbances while on furosemide. Electrolyte supplements such as potassium chloride or sodium chloride may be required to prevent hypokalemia, hyponatremia, and hypochloremia.

12. J.T. is started on furosemide 2 mg Q 12 hr. One week later, she still requires high ventilatory settings and is unable to be weaned from the ventilator. What other therapeutic agents may be considered to treat J.T.'s BPD?

Systemic Bronchodilators

Methyxanthines (theophylline, caffeine) have been used extensively in infants with BPD because of a direct bronchodilating effect. Methylxanthines can also improve diaphragmatic and skeletal muscle contractility and act as mild diuretics (see section on Apnea of Prematurity, later in this chapter). Improvement in skeletal muscle contractility may improve functional residual capacity, which can help facilitate ventilator weaning. Both theophylline and caffeine reduce pulmonary resistance and increase lung compliance.[95] Unfortunately, most studies in infants with BPD have only evaluated the short-term benefits of methylxanthines in improving lung function; long-term outcome studies are needed.[97]

If J.T. is started on theophylline, a loading dose of 5 mg/kg followed by a maintenance dose of 2 mg/kg every 8 hours is recommended (see Table 94-7). J.T. should be monitored for adverse effects, including tachycardia, gastroesophageal reflux, vomiting, diarrhea, agitation, and seizures. Caffeine may be preferred because of its fewer side effects and wider therapeutic index. However, caution should be taken to ensure that the dosing reflects the salt form of the caffeine prescribed (e.g., caffeine base or caffeine citrate).[99] Therapeutic serum concentrations for theophylline and caffeine are not well defined for BPD. However, most clinicians target the upper range cited for apnea of prematurity (see Apnea of Prematurity).

Inhaled Bronchodilators

Infants in the early stages of BPD generally have airway hyperactivity and smooth muscle hypertrophy. They are also at higher risk for bronchoconstriction due to increased airway resistance secondary to hypoxia. Therefore, the use of bronchodilators may be helpful in these infants. β_2-Agonists, such as albuterol or metaproterenol, have been shown to provide short-term improvements (duration of 4 hours) in lung compliance and pulmonary resistance due to bronchial smooth muscle relaxation.[95] However, inhaled bronchodilators are not effective in all infants with BPD. Infants in the late stages of BPD may have severe pulmonary damage and fibrotic changes. Only half of these infants demonstrate a decrease in pulmonary resistance after albuterol therapy.[101] Although β_2-agonists are more potent bronchodilators than theophylline or caffeine, their adverse effect profile, which includes cardiovascular side effects (e.g., tachycardia, hypertension), limit their use. In addition, tolerance may develop with prolonged administration.[95] Therefore, inhaled bronchodilators should be reserved for infants who clearly demonstrate improvements during therapy. Currently, there are no well-designed studies evaluating chronic use of inhaled bronchodilators for the treatment of BPD. Further studies evaluating the efficacy and safety of long-term inhaled bronchodilator therapy are needed.

Inhaled anticholinergics such as ipratropium bromide have produced short-term benefits (duration ≥ 4 hours) in infants with BPD by improving pulmonary function.[97,102] These drugs work by preventing the action of acetylcholine at the muscarinic cholinergic receptor site, thereby interfering with vagally mediated bronchoconstriction. Anticholinergics relax bronchial smooth muscle and decrease mucus secretion. Inhaled anticholinergics are generally reserved for those infants who fail or who are intolerant to albuterol, or as an adjunct to albuterol if clinical improvement is not seen.[95] The combined therapy of albuterol and ipratropium may be more effective than either drug alone.[95,97,102] The adverse effect profile of ipratropium is minimal because the drug is poorly absorbed.

Cromolyn prevents the release of inflammatory mediators from mast cells. In a limited number of reports, inhaled cromolyn sodium provided some beneficial effects in the treatment of BPD; however, effects may not be seen until 2 to 4 weeks of therapy.[97,100] Cromolyn should not be used during acute episodes of bronchoconstriction because it does not have acute bronchodilating effects. Further studies evaluating the efficacy and safety of cromolyn in the management of BPD are required before routine use can be recommended.

A major problem with inhaled bronchodilators is their method of administration and drug delivery. Inhaled bronchodilators can be given by jet or ultrasonic nebulization or via a metered-dose inhaler.[100] For ventilator-dependent infants receiving metered-dose inhalers, the metered-dose inhaler is connected to an adapter that is attached to the ventilator circuit and endotracheal tube (ETT). Metered-dose inhalers can also be given through bag ventilation via the ETT. For

LIVERPOOL
JOHN MOORES UNIVERSITY
AVRIL ROBARTS LRC
TEL 0151 231 4022

nonventilated infants, the metered-dose inhaler can be given using a spacer/AeroChamber and a face mask.

Compared with metered-dose inhalers, nebulization of inhaled bronchodilators has several disadvantages. Loss or inefficient delivery of drug and cooling of the inspired oxygen mixture may occur with nebulization. In several studies in neonates, metered-dose inhalers with a spacer provided more efficient delivery of inhaled bronchodilators and greater improvements in oxygenation and ventilation.[103] In addition, metered-dose inhalers are less expensive than nebulization. Therefore, the use of metered-dose inhalers with an appropriate spacing device is preferred for most infants. Various products and dosage regimens can be found in Table 94-7.

Corticosteroids

Corticosteroids, particularly dexamethasone, have been used extensively for the treatment of BPD. Mechanisms of action of corticosteroids include (1) reduction of polymorphonuclear leukocyte migration to the lung; (2) reduction of lung inflammation; (3) inhibition of prostaglandin, leukotriene, TNF, and interleukin (IL) synthesis; (4) reduction of elastase production; (5) stimulation of surfactant synthesis; (6) reduction of vascular permeability and pulmonary edema; (7) enhancement of β-adrenergic receptor activity; (8) reduction of pulmonary fibronectin (which can reduce the risk of interstitial fibrosis); and (9) stimulation of serum retinol concentrations.[95,100,104] Treatment with dexamethasone (initiated ≥7 days of life) in infants with documented BPD or with clinical signs and chest radiograph findings consistent with BPD reduces the release of inflammatory mediators, improves pulmonary mechanics and clinical status, facilitates weaning from mechanical ventilation, and decreases the duration of oxygen therapy.[95,98,100,104–106] In most studies, dexamethasone therapy was not shown to significantly reduce the duration of hospitalization or improve survival in infants with BPD.[95,100,104,106,107]

Systemic dexamethasone is associated with many serious short-term adverse effects including: hyperglycemia, increased BP, hypertrophic cardiomyopathy, GI bleeding, intestinal perforation, pituitary-adrenal suppression, bone demineralization, poor weight gain, and increased risk of infection.[95,98,100,104,108] Serious long-term adverse effects have also been identified in preterm infants who receive systemic corticosteroids. Two recent reviews (which assessed infants at ≥1 year) reported an increase in the incidence of cerebral palsy, neurodevelopmental delay, and motor dysfunction in preterm infants who received systemic steroids for the prevention and treatment of BPD.[109,110]

Because of the short-term and long-term adverse effects, the American Academy of Pediatrics (AAP) does not recommend the use of steroids for the prevention and treatment of BPD in preterm infants.[111] Systemic corticosteroids should be reserved for preterm neonates enrolled in randomized, double-blind, controlled trials; long-term neurodevelopmental assessment is highly encouraged. In general, the clinical use of systemic steroids should be limited to exceptional circumstances (e.g., an infant on maximal ventilatory and oxygen support) where the benefits may outweigh the risks. The AAP advises that parents should be fully informed about the short- and long-term adverse effects of systemic corticosteroids.[111] In situations where steroids are felt to be essential, some centers have delayed treatment until the infant reaches a postnatal age of >28 days. A lower dose and shorter duration of therapy may also be considered. One dosing regimen that has been used includes dexamethasone 0.1 mg/kg/day in two divided doses for 3 days followed by 0.05 mg/kg/day given once a day for 3 days.

Inhaled steroids such as beclomethasone dipropionate, flunisolide, dexamethasone, fluticasone, and budesonide have also been used for the treatment and prevention of BPD.[98,100,112] Infants receiving inhaled steroids for the treatment of BPD may have a reduction in oxygen requirements and duration of mechanical ventilation, and improvement in lung mechanics.[98,100,111,112] However, the onset of clinical improvements may be delayed compared with systemic steroids. In contrast, the preventative use of inhaled steroids has not been shown to decrease the incidence of BPD or the duration of mechanical ventilation and oxygen therapy; however the use of systemic steroid may be decreased.[113] Adverse effects of inhaled steroids reported in BPD infants are less common than with systemic steroids.[114] These include mild adrenal suppression, bronchospasm, tongue hypertrophy, and oral candidiasis.[112,115] High-dose inhaled fluticasone (500 μg every 12 hours for 2 weeks) has also been associated with moderately severe pituitary-adrenal suppression in very low-birth-weight infants.[116] The infant's mouth should be cleaned after each use of inhaled steroid to minimize complications such as oral thrush. As with inhaled bronchodilators, administration is a therapeutic problem with these medications. The amount of drug delivered to the infant can vary from 0.02 (by jet nebulizer) to 14.2% (by metered-dose inhaler with an aerochamber).[104] Further studies evaluating the optimal dose, duration of therapy, route of administration, time of initiation, most appropriate preparation, and long-term adverse effects of corticosteroids are needed.

Long-Term Sequelae

13. Six months have passed, and J.T. is now 6 months old (corrected age), 5 kg, and ready for discharge. Over the past several months, ventilation requirements slowly decreased and J.T. was eventually extubated. However, she still requires supplemental oxygen at an FiO$_2$ of 30%, ⅛ L/min via nasal cannula to maintain an oxygen saturation of 93% to 95%. Discharge medications include multivitamins with iron 0.5 mL Q 12 hr; spironolactone/hydrochlorothiazide suspension, 5 mg Q 12 hr; sodium chloride solution, 2 mEq Q 8 hr; nebulized albuterol (0.5% solution), 0.25 mL Q 6 hr; and beclomethasone metered-dose inhaler (42 μg per actuation), 2 puffs Q 12 hr. What are the long-term complications of BPD that can be expected in J.T.?

Infants with BPD have little pulmonary reserve and are therefore at higher risk for developing frequent respiratory exacerbations. BPD places J.T. at risk for recurrent infections of the lower respiratory tract and she may require frequent hospitalizations during the first year for bronchiolitis and pneumonia.[96] Approximately 50% of all children with BPD require hospitalization for respiratory exacerbations during the first 2 years of life.[96] Respiratory syncytial virus is a common cause of respiratory distress (airway obstruction, mucus plugging, and airway edema) and recurrent atelectasis. With time, most preterm survivors with BPD have an improvement in pulmonary function due to lung growth; however, many continue to have airway hyperreactivity. Infants with severe BPD can also develop pulmonary hypertension, cor pulmonale, systemic hypertension, and left ventricular hypertrophy.

In addition to pulmonary and cardiovascular complications, J.T. may be at risk for developing bone demineralization and rickets. Very low-birth-weight infants are born with inadequate stores of vitamin D. In general, these premature infants may not receive an adequate intake of vitamin D, either parenterally or through their diet. Most very low-birth-weight infants will require prolonged parenteral nutrition, which may cause cholestasis or hepatic failure. Prolonged cholestasis or chronic hepatic congestion due to heart failure may cause malabsorption of calcium and vitamin D. In addition, furosemide may exacerbate calcium deficiencies by causing hypercalciuria. These combined factors may result in bone demineralization and rickets. As mentioned previously, infants with BPD usually have a high catabolism and increased oxygen consumption due to an increased work of breathing and chronic hypoxia. Inadequate nutritional support may negatively affect weight gain, growth, and long-term outcome of BPD.

Neurologic and developmental abnormalities such as learning disabilities, speech delays, vision and hearing impairment, and poor attention span can also occur in infants with BPD.[97] BPD itself is not an independent risk factor for neurologic abnormality; related factors include birth weight, gestational age, and socioeconomic status.[95,98] Long-term follow-up evaluations at 1 to 3 years of age in infants previously treated with dexamethasone revealed an increase in neurodevelopmental abnormalities such as cerebral palsy.[98,109] However, it is not known if these abnormalities were due to an adverse effect of dexamethasone on brain development or to an improved survival of infants who may already be at risk for developing these abnormalities.

Mortality rates for infants with severe BPD range from 30% to 40%.[97] Approximately 80% of deaths associated with BPD occur during initial hospitalization and are due to respiratory failure, sepsis, pneumonia, cor pulmonale, and congestive heart failure.[97]

Prevention

14. What preventive measures could have been used to decrease the incidence of BPD in J.T.?

Prevention of prematurity and other etiologic factors of RDS is the most effective means of preventing BPD. The administration of antenatal steroids to mothers before delivery decreases the incidence of RDS and, potentially, BPD. Exogenous surfactant therapy also reduces the incidence of RDS, but not the incidence of BPD. Early administration of dexamethasone (initiated < 96 hours of life) in preterm infants reduces pulmonary inflammation and lung injury, decreases the incidence of BPD and oxygen requirements, improves lung function, and facilitates weaning from the ventilator.[95,104,107,108] However, early dexamethasone therapy has also been associated with an increased risk of infection, gastrointestinal bleeding, intestinal perforation, hypertrophic cardiomyopathy, growth failure and of greatest concern, neurological impairment and cerebral palsy.[107,108] Because of the inconsistent improvements in outcome and mortality, and the lack of long-term follow-up data, early dexamethasone therapy is not recommended for routine use.[111] Clinicians should weigh the potential benefits versus the risks of early dexamethasone therapy for the prevention of BPD.

As mentioned previously, one of the causes of BPD includes the lack of micronutrients such as vitamin A. Vitamin A deficiency can predispose infants to BPD due to impaired lung healing, increased susceptibility to infection and loss of cilia, and decreased number of alveoli.[117,118] Premature infants, especially very low-birth-weight infants, are at greatest risk due to low body stores, inadequate intake during feedings, and decreased enteral absorption of vitamin A. Although some studies have shown beneficial effects of vitamin A (IM retinyl palmitate 2,000 or 4,000 IU every other day for 28 days) in the prevention of BPD, other studies have failed to confirm these findings.[117] The difference in results may be due to the populations studied (e.g., race, birth weight), prior surfactant and dexamethasone therapy, and the amount of vitamin A intake. A higher dose of vitamin A (IM retinyl palmitate 5,000 IU three times a week for 4 weeks) significantly decreased the incidence of BPD or death by 11%.[118] Vitamin A appears to be a relatively safe drug; the incidence of adverse effects were similar between the treated and control groups. Despite the beneficial findings in this latest study, further studies evaluating the efficacy, safety, and optimal dosage regimen of vitamin A for the prevention of BPD are needed before routine use is recommended.

Optimization of nutritional support may also help prevent the development of BPD because proper nutrition helps promote lung maturation, growth, and repair. Excessive fluid administration should be avoided because it may lead to BPD. Fluid restriction was shown to decrease both the incidence of BPD and mortality.[100] In addition, the early use of high-frequency ventilation in infants may decrease the severity and incidence of BPD.[95]

PATENT DUCTUS ARTERIOSUS
Pathogenesis

Several major differences between adult and fetal circulation exist. To understand the pathophysiology and clinical manifestations of PDA, fetal circulation and the cardiovascular changes that occur at birth are reviewed.

Fetal Circulatory Anatomy
The fetus has three unique circulatory structures that differ from the adult: (1) the ductus venosus, which permits blood to bypass the liver; (2) the foramen ovale, which allows blood to pass from the right atrium into the left atrium; and (3) the ductus arteriosus, the structure that connects the pulmonary artery to the descending aorta and allows blood to bypass the lungs (Fig. 94-1).[119]

In addition to these structural differences, vascular resistance and pressure play important roles in determining the pathway of fetal circulation. For example, the relative hypoxia that occurs in utero causes pulmonary vasoconstriction. Pulmonary vasoconstriction, along with compression of pulmonary blood vessels by unexpanded fetal lung mass, results in a high pulmonary vascular resistance and decreased pulmonary blood flow. This decreased pulmonary blood flow is

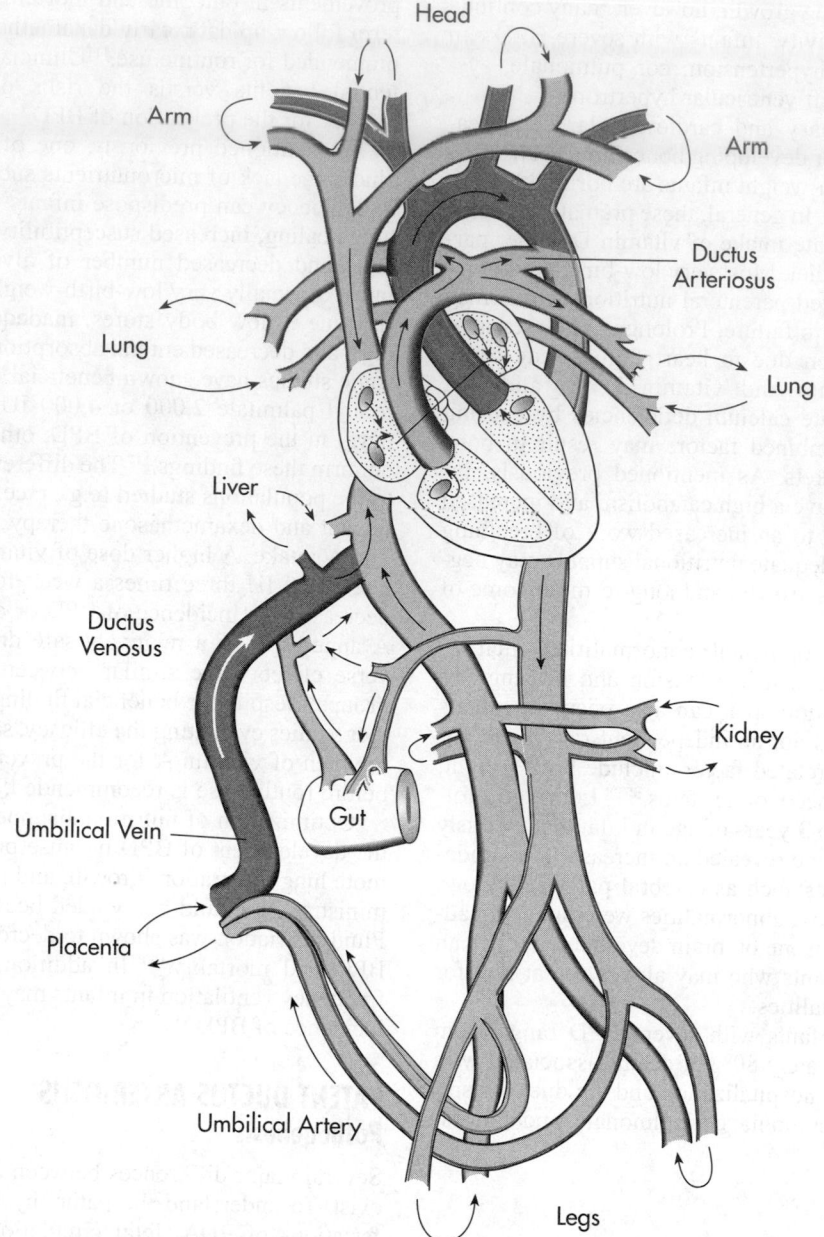

FIGURE 94-1 Fetal circulation. (Modified with permission from Bernstein D. The fetal to neonatal circulatory transition: the fetal circulation. In: Behrman RE et al, eds. Nelson Textbook of Pediatrics, 16th Ed. Philadelphia: WB Saunders, 2000:1341.)

acceptable in utero because the lungs essentially are nonfunctional. Large amounts of blood, however, must be pumped through the placenta where gas exchange occurs.

Fetal Circulation

Maximally oxygenated blood (PO_2, 30 to 35 mm Hg) flows from the placenta to the fetus through the umbilical vein (see Fig. 94-1). Approximately 50% of the umbilical venous blood is shunted away from the liver through the ductus venosus and directed into the inferior vena cava. Blood from the inferior vena cava and superior vena cava then enters the right atrium. Most of the blood from the inferior vena cava, which is well oxygenated, is directed in a straight pathway across the right

atrium through the foramen ovale directly into the left atrium. It then enters the left ventricle through the mitral valve and is pumped into the vessels of the head and forelimbs. Thus, the fetal brain is preferentially perfused with blood containing a higher amount of oxygen. Deoxygenated blood returning from the head region via the superior vena cava enters the right atrium and is directed through the tricuspid valve into the right ventricle, where it then is pumped into the pulmonary artery. Most of this blood is diverted through the ductus arteriosus into the descending aorta and then through the two umbilical arteries to the placenta. A small percentage of the blood flows to the lower extremities and then is returned to the heart via the inferior vena cava.[119]

Changes at Birth

At birth, major circulatory changes result from umbilical cord clamping, aeration and expansion of the lungs, and an increase in arterial Po_2. These changes are important in the transition from fetal to adult circulation. When the umbilical cord is clamped, blood flow decreases through the ductus venosus, which then closes within 3 to 7 days. Clamping of the umbilical cord also results in a twofold increase in systemic vascular resistance. This increase in systemic vascular resistance increases aortic, left ventricular, and atrial pressures and cardiac output. Pulmonary pressures and blood flow also change. After the neonate's first breath, the lungs expand, oxygenation improves, and pulmonary vascular resistance immediately drops. This increases pulmonary blood flow, causing a decrease in pulmonary artery, right ventricle, and right atrium pressures.[119]

If hypoxia occurs after delivery, pulmonary vasoconstriction results and the neonate may develop pulmonary hypertension with a persistence of fetal circulation. This is termed persistent pulmonary hypertension of the newborn or persistent fetal circulation. Oxygenation of these neonates is extremely difficult because of the pulmonary vasoconstriction and resultant decreased pulmonary blood flow. Systemic alkalization (through hyperventilation and the use of sodium bicarbonate) and inotropic support often are necessary.[119] Severe cases may require extracorporeal membrane oxygenation.

Closure of the Foramen Ovale

Because of the decreased right atrium pressure and increased left atrium pressure that occur after birth, blood attempts to flow down the pressure gradient from the left atrium through the foramen ovale into the right atrium. This is in the opposite direction from what occurs in fetal life. The small valvelike flap that lies over the foramen ovale on the left side of the atrial septum closes over the foramen ovale opening when the pressure in the left atrium exceeds the pressure in the right atrium. Closure of this flap prevents further flow through the foramen ovale. As long as the pressure in the left atrium is higher than the right atrium, the foramen ovale remains functionally closed, until it closes anatomically.

Closure of the Ductus Arteriosus

Closure of the ductus arteriosus is more complex and depends on many factors. In utero, patency of the ductus arteriosus is maintained through the combined vasodilatory effects of a low Po_2 and high concentrations of prostaglandins, particularly prostaglandin E_2 (PGE_2).[120] Prostacyclin (PGI_2) also plays a role in maintaining ductal patency.[120,121] After birth, the smooth muscles of the ductus arteriosus constrict as arterial oxygenation increases and concentrations of placentally derived prostaglandins, particularly PGE_2 decrease.[121] In utero, Po_2 of the ductal blood is 18 to 28 mm Hg, whereas after birth in a term neonate, it is approximately 100 mm Hg. Normally, the ductus arteriosus of a term neonate functionally closes within the first few days of life (i.e., in 82% of infants within 48 hours of life and in 100% of infants within 96 hours of life).[120] Anatomic closure of the ductus occurs within 2 to 3 weeks of life.[121] When the ductus arteriosus fails to close, it is called *patent ductus arteriosus* (PDA). In a term neonate, a PDA beyond the first few days of life generally is permanent. It usually is secondary to an anatomic defect in the wall of the ductus arteriosus and requires surgical ligation. In contrast, a PDA in a preterm neonate may persist for weeks and still undergo spontaneous closure.

When a PDA is present, the direction and amount of shunting through this opening are determined by the pressure between the systemic and pulmonary circulation. Usually, blood flows from the aorta into the pulmonary circulation. Because systemic vascular resistance and aortic pressure are increased, and pulmonary vascular resistance and pulmonary artery pressure are decreased after birth, blood pumped from the left ventricle into the aorta flows from the aorta (a high-pressure area) through the PDA and into the pulmonary artery (a lower-pressure area). This flow is called *left-to-right shunting* and is in contrast to the right-to-left shunting that occurs through the PDA during fetal life.

Although the persistence of a PDA is pathologic, it is necessary for the survival of patients with cyanotic congenital heart disease while awaiting corrective or palliative cardiac surgery. These patients have congenital cardiac defects that depend on the ductus arteriosus to maintain cardiac output and systemic perfusion (e.g., coarctation of the aorta, aortic stenosis, and hypoplastic left heart syndrome) or to provide pulmonary blood flow and maintain systemic oxygenation (e.g., pulmonary artery atresia or severe stenosis and tricuspid atresia). Patency of the ductus arteriosus can be maintained pharmacologically with a continuous infusion of alprostadil (PGE_1). The initial starting dose of alprostadil is 0.05 to 0.1 μg/kg per minute and may be increased every 15 to 30 minutes up to 0.2 μg/kg per minute until achievement of clinical response. Infusion doses up to 0.4 μg/kg per minute have also been used by several centers. Alprostadil infusion should be reduced to the lowest effective dose once patency of the ductus arteriosus is achieved.[8,122]

Clinical Presentation

15. T.S. is a 750-g female who was born at 25 weeks' gestational age to a 22-year-old gravida 2 para 1 female. One hour after birth, T.S. developed symptoms of RDS and two doses of Survanta were given within the first 24 hours of life. After the second dose of Survanta, T.S.'s respiratory function greatly improved and no further doses of Survanta were required. On the third day of life, the nurse noticed that T.S. had tachycardia, a systolic murmur, a hyperactive precordium, and a widened pulse pressure. Her lungs sounded "wet". In addition, the nurse noted that T.S.'s combined IV fluid rates total 160 mL/kg per day instead of the desired fluid intake of 120 mL/kg per day. Current vital signs are as follows: HR, 190 beats/min; RR, 65 breaths/min; BP, 55/23 mm Hg; and O_2 saturation, 89%. ABGs include pH, 7.22; Pco_2, 55 mm Hg; Po_2, 77 mm Hg; base deficit, 10. Ventilator support is increased to compensate for T.S.'s deteriorating respiratory status. Echocardiography is performed and shows a moderate-size PDA with significant left-to-right shunting. The chest radiograph shows pulmonary edema and an enlarged heart. What risk factors for PDA does T.S. have?

[SI units: Pco_2, 7.33 kPa; Po_2, 10.3 kPa]

T.S. has two major risk factors for developing a symptomatic PDA: prematurity and RDS. The occurrence of a PDA is inversely proportional to gestational age and birth weight. The incidence of PDA is approximately 45% in premature infants with a birth weight of <1,750 g but can be as high as 80% in premature infants with a birth weight of <1,200 g.[121] In contrast, the incidence of PDA in term infants is only 0.04%.[120] Preterm neonates are at a higher risk for PDA than term newborns because the smooth muscle of the immature ductus is more sensitive to the dilatory effects of prostaglandins and less sensitive to the constrictive effects of increased oxygen tension. In addition, circulating concentrations of PGE_2 are often elevated in premature infants due to the decreased pulmonary metabolism of prostaglandins.[120] These factors contribute to the delayed closure of the ductus arteriosus in premature infants. With advanced gestation, the ductus is less responsive to the relaxant effects of prostaglandins and is more sensitive to the constricting effects of oxygen.[120,123]

RDS also increases the risk for PDA. Exogenous surfactant, especially prophylactic use, also may increase the risk of symptomatic PDA.[123,124] PDA can further complicate the course of RDS.[123,125] T.S.'s course is typical of a preterm neonate with resolving RDS. T.S.'s pulmonary function improved after surfactant administration. Consequently, pulmonary vascular resistance decreased and the degree of left-to-right shunting across the ductus arteriosus increased, causing a deterioration in respiratory status. In addition, the excess fluid that T.S. received is an iatrogenic factor that may have increased the shunting across the PDA, aggravating the degree of pulmonary congestion.[123]

16. How is T.S.'s presentation consistent with that of PDA?

T.S.'s clinical presentation is due to the increased pulmonary blood flow, decreased systemic perfusion, and left-ventricular volume overload that resulted from the shunting of left-ventricular cardiac output through the PDA into the lungs. To compensate for the inadequate peripheral perfusion, HR increases. This results in an increase in cardiac output and a greater left-to-right shunt through the PDA, creating a vicious cycle. The widened pulse pressure (the difference between systolic and diastolic pressures, 32 mm Hg) is a result of diversion of aortic blood flow through the PDA, which is causing the bounding pulses. The systolic murmur, which is not always present, is the result of turbulent blood flow through the ductus arteriosus occurring as the pulmonary vascular resistance decreases. Tachycardia, hyperactive precordium, and a continuous murmur are results of the left-to-right shunting through the ductus arteriosus during systole.[121]

17. What are the potential complications of this hemodynamically significant PDA in T.S.?

The increased pulmonary blood flow and resultant pulmonary edema will worsen T.S.'s respiratory disease and increase the need for ventilatory support. The higher ventilatory settings (increase in MAP and FiO_2) place T.S. at risk for developing BPD. If the PDA is left untreated, T.S. may develop congestive heart failure secondary to an increased left ventricular end diastolic volume. A hemodynamically significant PDA also places T.S. at risk for IVH and NEC.[123]

Treatment

18. How should PDA be managed in T.S.?

The initial medical management for T.S.'s symptomatic PDA is supportive care, which includes fluid management (e.g., fluid restriction and diuretic therapy), correction of anemia, and treatment of hypoxia and acidosis. Although excessive fluid administration may increase the risk of PDA, fluid restriction alone is unlikely to result in ductal closure. T.S.'s fluid intake should be restricted to 100 to 120 mL/kg per day (approximately 80% of total fluid maintenance requirements) to avoid worsening of her pulmonary edema and to prevent congestive heart failure.[121,123] Furosemide 1 mg/kg IV push should also be given to T.S. immediately to treat her pulmonary edema (see Question 9). In addition to fluid management, correction of anemia is important. Low concentrations of hemoglobin result in an increased cardiac output, which may worsen the infant's cardiac function. Anemia not only increases the demand of left ventricular output to ensure adequate oxygen delivery to the tissues, but may also increase the magnitude of the left-to-right shunt by decreasing the resistance of blood flow through the pulmonary vascular bed.[123] Maintaining a hematocrit level of >40% to 45% is often recommended.[121] Because of T.S.'s gestational age, birth weight, and size of PDA, it is unlikely that she will respond to these general measures alone. Therefore, T.S. will require treatment with indomethacin. Indomethacin nonspecifically inhibits prostaglandin synthesis, thereby eliminating the vasodilator effects of the PGE series on the ductus arteriosus. Unfortunately, not every infant who is treated with indomethacin will respond with constriction of the ductus arteriosus; therefore, surgical ligation of the PDA may be required for T.S. Ligation generally is reserved for neonates who do not respond to indomethacin therapy or those in whom indomethacin therapy is contraindicated (see Question 20).[123]

Indomethacin

19. What is the dose of indomethacin and what route should be used for its administration?

The treatment of choice for T.S. is pharmacologic therapy with IV indomethacin. Enteral indomethacin is less effective than IV indomethacin. This reduced effectiveness may be due to the formulation of the suspension and decreased, erratic, enteral absorption.[126]

A large interpatient variability of indomethacin pharmacokinetics occurs in preterm neonates. Serum concentrations do not correlate consistently with therapeutic or adverse effects.[126] Furthermore, the optimal therapeutic serum concentration is not yet defined. Although many dosage regimens have been reported, dosing guidelines from the National Collaborative Study are commonly used.[125] Three indomethacin doses are given in 12-to 24-hour intervals, with the first dose equal to 0.2 mg/kg IV in all neonates. Because indomethacin clearance is directly proportional to postnatal age, the second and third doses are determined by postnatal age at initiation of indomethacin therapy.[121] If onset of treatment was at less than 2 days postnatal age, neonates receive 0.1 mg/kg per dose; if initiation of therapy occurred at 2 to 7 days postnatal age, neonates receive 0.2 mg/kg per dose; and if therapy began more than 7 days postnatal age, neonates receive 0.25 mg/kg per dose. Second and third doses are administered at 12- to 24-hour intervals. No specific guidelines exist regarding which patients receive every-12-hour versus every-24-hour dosing; however, the individual dosing interval generally is determined by the neonate's urine output.[121] If urine output remains >1 mL/kg per hour after an indomethacin dose, then the next dose may be given in 12 hours. If urine output is <1 mL/kg per hour but >0.6 mL/kg per hour, then the dosing interval may be extended to 24 hours.

Other indomethacin dosing regimens have been evaluated more recently for the treatment of PDA in preterm infants. An initial dose of 0.2 mg/kg followed by either 0.1 mg/kg or 0.2 mg/kg for two doses at 12- to 24-hour intervals has been used. In a study measuring serum concentrations, higher doses of indomethacin were required in older neonates (i.e., >10 days postnatal age).[127] This may be due to an increased indomethacin clearance in these infants. Because rapid IV administration of indomethacin can vasoconstrict the mesenteric arteries and renal vascular beds, longer infusion rates of 20 to 30 minutes are recommended. Continuous infusion of indomethacin appears to further decrease the adverse effects, but additional studies are needed.[123]

Response to indomethacin therapy can be determined by assessing the clinical signs of PDA such as tachycardia, widened pulse pressure, bounding pulses, heart murmur, and the ability to wean ventilator support. In certain cases, echocardiography may be performed to confirm closure of a PDA.

MONITORING THERAPY

20. **What clinical and laboratory data should be monitored during T.S.'s indomethacin therapy?**

Before initiating indomethacin therapy, T.S. should receive an echocardiogram to rule out ductal-dependent congenital heart disease and to confirm the presence of a PDA. In addition, a serum creatinine and blood urea nitrogen (BUN) should be obtained from T.S. before indomethacin therapy because nephrotoxicity is the most common adverse effect. Infants receiving indomethacin can develop transient oliguria with increased serum creatinine. This occurs as a result of indomethacin-induced decreases in renal blood flow and GFR.[125] Dilutional hyponatremia may occur secondary to either decreased urine output or decreased free water diuresis due to increased antidiuretic hormone activity.[122] Treatment of hyponatremia should be aimed at decreasing free water intake through fluid restriction rather than by sodium supplementation. Typically, renal function normalizes within 72 hours after the last dose of indomethacin.[122] In general, indomethacin therapy is contraindicated in neonates with renal failure, urine output <0.6 mL/kg per hour, or serum creatinine ≥1.8 mg/dL.[125] Although furosemide has been reported to decrease indomethacin-induced nephrotoxicity without affecting PDA, more studies are needed to confirm these findings.[128] In addition, serum concentrations of aminoglycosides, digoxin, and other renally eliminated drugs should be monitored carefully. Indomethacin therapy may decrease renal drug clearance and cause accumulation of these agents.[129]

A platelet count should also be obtained from T.S. before therapy because indomethacin may decrease platelet aggregation. Thrombocytopenia (platelet count, <50,000/mm^3) is a contraindication to indomethacin therapy.[122,125] In cases of thrombocytopenia, indomethacin may be withheld temporarily until platelets can be transfused. Other potential contraindications to indomethacin therapy include active bleeding and clinical evidence of NEC because GI bleeding, perforation, and NEC have been reported with indomethacin use.[123] These GI effects may be related to decreases in intestinal blood flow usually seen with rapid IV infusions. Grades II to IV IVH also is frequently quoted as a contraindication to indomethacin therapy; however, indomethacin treatment probably is not associated with progression of IVH. In fact, prophylactic treatment with indomethacin may be associated with a decrease in the incidence of severe IVH (grades III and IV).[123,124]

Ibuprofen

Because of the adverse effects of indomethacin, other prostaglandin inhibitors such as ibuprofen have been studied for the closure of the ductus arteriosus. Results indicate that ibuprofen is as effective as indomethacin and causes significantly less of a decrease in renal, mesenteric and cerebral blood flow.[130] Intravenous ibuprofen has been studied using an initial dose of 10 mg/kg followed by two doses of 5 mg/kg given at 24-hour intervals. Despite these promising results, most studies did not include sufficient numbers of extremely premature infants (<28 weeks gestational age). Therefore, additional studies evaluating the therapeutic and adverse effects of ibuprofen are needed. At this time, intravenous ibuprofen is not commercially available in the United States.

21. **When is the best time to initiate indomethacin for symptomatic treatment of PDA?**

Conflicting data exist on when to initiate indomethacin therapy for the treatment of symptomatic PDA. Some centers may opt to treat within the first 2 to 3 days of life (early symptomatic PDA) when infants initially present with clinical signs of PDA (i.e., murmur, widened pulse pressures, tachycardia). Others may not treat until clinical signs of congestive heart failure are present (late symptomatic PDA; 7 to 10 days of life).[124] Both indomethacin treatment strategies (early and late) significantly decrease the incidence of PDA, but both cause significant transient reduction of urine output and serum creatinine elevation. In some studies, infants receiving early treatment of indomethacin had significant reductions in the incidence of BPD and NEC and the need for surgical ligation.[124] In contrast, one study found that final PDA closure rates and the need for surgical ligation were comparable in early versus late indomethacin-treated neonates. In fact, spontaneous closure was observed in 43% of the late treatment group, which may indicate unnecessary treatment in the early group. In addition, renal adverse effects and ventilatory requirements were higher in the infants treated early.[131] Thus, early administration of indomethacin should not be used routinely.

RECURRENCE

22. **T.S. completes a course of indomethacin 0.16 mg IV Q 12 hr × 3 doses. The physicians were able to decrease T.S.'s ventilator support within the first 12 to 24 hours after starting indomethacin treatment. After 3 to 4 days of gradual and consistent ventilator weaning, the ventilator settings could not be decreased further. Over the next 2 to 3 days, T.S.'s respiratory status deteriorates and she requires increased ventilator support. T.S. now has tachycardia, a widened pulse pressure, bounding pulses, and a hyperactive precordium. Repeat echocardiogram shows a small-to moderate-size PDA. Current data include**

the following: BUN, 10 mg/dL; SrCr, 1.1 mg/dL; sodium (Na), 134 mEq/L; potassium (K), 4.9 mEq/L; chloride (Cl), 97 mEq/L; urine output, 2.3 mL/kg per hour; fluid intake, 130 mL/kg per day; and platelets, 180,000/mm³. Why did PDA recur in T.S.?

[SI units. BUN, 3.6 mmol/L of urea; SrCr, 97.2 μmol/L; Na, 134 mmol/L; K, 4.9 mmol/L; Cl, 97 mmol/L; platelets, 180 × 10⁹/L]

Successful closure of the PDA with indomethacin occurs in 70% to 90% of infants; however, ductal reopening or recurrence can occur in 20% to 35% of infants who initially respond to indomethacin.[120,132] Recurrence of PDA occurs especially in lower-birth weight infants.[132] Several reasons might explain T.S.'s transient response to indomethacin. Recurrence of PDA is inversely proportional to gestational age; the incidence of ductal reopening is significantly higher in infants ≤26 weeks' gestational age compared with infants born ≥27 weeks' gestation (37% versus 11%, respectively).[133] The higher recurrence in younger-gestational-age neonates may be due to resumption of PGE₂ production after indomethacin serum concentrations decline and heightened sensitivity of the immature ductus arteriosus to the dilating effects of PGE.[123,132] This is particularly important in ventilator-dependent patients such as T.S. because mechanical ventilation increases circulating vasodilating prostaglandins.[120] Furthermore, the rate of ductal reopening is independent of indomethacin serum concentrations but appears to be related to the timing of indomethacin therapy, postnatal age, and the amount of fluid intake 24 hours before indomethacin treatment.[133] The rate of recurrence is lower in infants who were treated with indomethacin within the first 48 hours of life compared with those receiving treatment after 7 days of life.[123] Because anatomic closure of a PDA may be delayed for a couple of weeks, it is not surprising that the ductus arteriosus reopened in T.S. after her initial response to indomethacin.[123]

Although controversial, prolonged indomethacin therapy may prevent recurrences and allow for permanent closure of the ductus arteriosus. Several prolonged treatment regimens have been successful in preventing ductal reopening.[123,132] One such regimen (indomethacin 0.2 mg/kg per dose IV every 12 hours for three doses, followed by 0.2 mg/kg per dose ever 24 hours for five doses) was able to significantly decrease the recurrence of PDA in neonates <1,500 g from 47 to 10% without increasing toxicity. The need for surgical ligation also was decreased significantly.[132] However, some studies report an increased mortality in infants receiving prolonged therapy (seven doses) compared with those receiving the short course (three doses).[123] Furthermore, other investigators found a significantly higher PDA closure rate in the short-course group (initial, 0.2 mg/kg then 0.1 mg/kg for two doses, each given at 12-hour intervals). The prolonged course (0.1 mg/kg per dose every 24 hours for seven doses) had a higher incidence of NEC and urea retention, and a longer duration of oxygen therapy.[134] Therefore, the optimal duration of indomethacin therapy and dosing regimen need to be identified.

23. Should indomethacin be given to T.S. again? Can future recurrences be prevented?

T.S. remains ventilator dependent and is at increased risk for developing BPD. Because she has no contraindications to indomethacin therapy, a second course should be given. To prevent further recurrences, an additional five doses of indomethacin (0.1 to 0.2 mg/kg per dose every 24 hours) may be given to T.S. after she completes the standard three-dose regimen.[132,134] If the PDA fails to respond to this prolonged regimen or if it recurs again after an initial response, and T.S. remains ventilator dependent, surgical ligation most likely will be required to permanently close the PDA.

PROPHYLACTIC ADMINISTRATION

24. Could prophylactic indomethacin have prevented the development of a symptomatic PDA?

Prophylactic indomethacin therapy is defined as the administration of indomethacin to infants who have echocardiographic evidence but no clinical signs of PDA. Only 40% of infants with severe RDS and echocardiographic evidence of PDA during the first day of life go on to develop a hemodynamically significant PDA. Therefore, 60% of infants would be treated unnecessarily if prophylactic indomethacin was given on day 1 of life.[123] Prophylactic use of indomethacin for the prevention of PDA significantly decreases the incidence of PDA and IVH (grades III and IV)[124,135] and the need for surgical ligation.[124] Unfortunately, most studies have not been able to show that prophylactic ductal closure with indomethacin decreases the incidence of death, BPD, or NEC.[124,135] In fact, infants receiving prophylactic therapy had a higher incidence of NEC (when studies were evaluated individually),[135] oliguria, and elevated serum creatinine.[124,135] Therefore, routine prophylactic administration is not warranted. Preterm neonates, particularly those at high risk for developing a large PDA (e.g., extremely-low-birth-weight neonates), should be treated as soon as clinical signs appear.

Prophylactic ibuprofen therapy (administered at <24 hours of life) has been reported to significantly increase ductal closure rate without increasing IVH, NEC, or mortality or decreasing renal function.[136,137] However, one study was terminated early due to three cases of severe hypoxemia and pulmonary hypertension that occurred in ibuprofen-treated infants.[136] Early administration of ibuprofen (i.e., <6 hours of life in this study versus <24 hours of life in other studies) may have prevented the decrease in pulmonary vascular resistance that normally occurs shortly after birth. Additional studies are needed before routine use of prophylactic ibuprofen therapy can be recommended.

NECROTIZING ENTEROCOLITIS
Pathogenesis and Classification

25. C.D., an 11-day-old, female neonate, was born at 28 weeks' gestational age with a birth weight of 908 g. Her postnatal course has been complicated by RDS, sepsis, and PDA for which she required intubation and mechanical ventilation, two doses of Survanta, a 7-day course of ampicillin and gentamicin, and indomethacin. Enteral feedings with a standard preterm 24-cal/oz formula were started on day 7 of life at 5 mL Q 3 hr (44 mL/kg per day). Feedings were increased by 5 mL/feed on days 8 through 10 to 20 mL/feed Q 3 hr on day 10 of life (176 mL/kg per day). This morning C.D. developed a distended abdomen, bloody stools, multiple episodes of apnea that required reintubation and assisted ventilation, and metabolic acidosis. ABG results revealed the following: pH, 7.20; Pco$_2$, 47 mm Hg, and Po$_2$, 55 mm Hg. An abdominal radiograph revealed pneumatosis intestinalis (the presence of gas in the intestinal submucosa). C.D. is to take nothing by mouth (NPO), and gentamicin 2.5 mg/kg IV infusion Q 24 hr and ampicillin 50 mg/kg IV push Q 12 hr are restarted. What clinical signs of NEC does C.D. have? What is the pathogenesis of NEC and what risk factors for NEC does C.D. have?

NEC, a type of acute intestinal necrosis, is the most common life-threatening nonrespiratory condition, affecting 1,200 to 9,600 newborns in the United States each year.[138] Approximately 62% to 94% of NEC occurs in premature infants, however, NEC can infrequently occur in full-term neonates.[138,139] NEC occurs in 3% to 15% of neonatal intensive care unit (ICU) admissions and has a mortality rate of 25% to 30%; approximately 25% of survivors develop long-term complications.[139,140] The age of onset of NEC is inversely related to gestational age and birth weight; the greater the gestational age of the infant at birth, the sooner the onset of NEC. Although NEC is less common in term infants, it usually develops within 3 to 4 days of age. In contrast, infants born ≤30 weeks' gestation develop NEC at a mean postnatal age of 20 days. Thus, preterm infants are at a risk for NEC for a longer period of time.[138,140] Although C.D. is extremely premature, she developed NEC early (at 11 days of age), most likely due to the aggressive advancement of feedings (see following discussion).

C.D. has several clinical signs of NEC, including abdominal distention, bloody stools, apnea, metabolic acidosis, and pneumatosis intestinalis on abdominal radiograph. Gastric retention of feedings, respiratory distress, occult blood in stools, lethargy, temperature instability, thrombocytopenia, and neutropenia also may occur. NEC may progress to bowel perforation, peritonitis, sepsis, disseminated intravascular coagulopathy (DIC), and shock. On abdominal radiograph, the presence of gas in the intestinal mucosa or in the portal venous system is diagnostic of NEC, and free air in the abdomen is observed with bowel perforation. Although these radiographic findings confirm the diagnosis of NEC, a lag time may occur between the initial clinical signs of NEC and radiologic confirmation.[139]

NEC can evolve slowly over a period of 24 to 48 hours, from a clinically benign course to an advanced stage of shock, peritonitis, and widespread intestinal necrosis. Although NEC can affect any part of the GI tract, most of the disease is confined to the ileum and colon.[141] A staging system, which categorizes severity according to systemic, intestinal, and radiologic signs, has been developed to permit a more consistent evaluation and treatment of patients.[142] Stages IA and IB NEC includes neonates and infants with suspected disease or "rule out" NEC. These patients may have mild GI problems such as emesis and increased gastric residuals, temperature instability, apnea, bright red blood from rectum, or a mild ileus. Infants with stages IIA and IIB have definite NEC and usually present with abdominal distention, bloody stools, and the presence of pneumatosis intestinalis on radiograph. Infants with stage IIB may also develop metabolic acidosis and thrombocytopenia. C.D.'s presentation is most consistent with stage IIB NEC. Infants with stages IIIA and IIIB (advanced disease) are severely ill with clinical signs, including peritonitis, ascites, shock, severe metabolic and respiratory acido-

sis, and DIC. Those with stage IIIB have intestinal perforation.

The exact pathogenesis of NEC is unknown but appears to be multifactorial. Most likely, NEC results from the effects of intestinal bacteria and other factors on injured intestinal mucosa (Fig. 94-2). Inflammatory mediators such as PAF, TNF-α, and IL-1β and IL-8 may also contribute to mucosal damage.[143] The neonatal intestinal mucosa is prone to injury for the following reasons: (1) increased permeability to potentially harmful substances, such as bacteria and proteins; (2) decreased immunologic host defenses, including low concentrations of IgA in intestinal mucosa; and (3) decreased nonimmunologic defenses, such as decreased concentrations of proteases and gastric acid. In addition, numerous factors (both prenatal and postnatal) can cause injury to the neonatal intestinal mucosa and increase the risk for NEC.[141] Prenatal maternal factors include eclampsia, prolonged rupture of membranes, fetal distress, maternal cocaine use, and cesarean section. Postnatal factors include prematurity, low birth weight, ischemia/hypoxemia, asphyxia, hypotension, respiratory distress, apnea, malnutrition, infection, hemodynamically significant PDA, congenital GI anomalies, cyanotic heart disease, toxins, hyperosmolar substances (e.g., feedings, medications), rapid advancement of enteral feedings, exchange transfusions, and the presence of umbilical catheters.[140–142,144] However, the most significant clinical risk factor for NEC is prematurity.[138,142]

C.D. has several risks for developing NEC, which include prematurity (gestational age of 28 weeks), extremely low birth weight (908 g), history of infection, and RDS requiring mechanical ventilation. Furthermore, C.D. was not only given a hyperosmolar formula (24 cal/oz instead of 20 cal/oz), but her feedings were advanced aggressively. These two factors may also contribute to the development of NEC. Approximately 90% to 95% of infants with NEC have received enteral feedings.[145] Rapid advancements in the volume of feeds increases the risk of NEC. Feedings should be increased by ≤10 to 20 mL/kg per day; increases ≥20 mL/kg per day can place the infant at risk for NEC.[145] C.D. was started at 44 mL/kg per day and increased by 44 mL/kg per day. If C.D. were appropriately fed, she would have reached full feedings in 7 to 14 days instead of 4 days. Last, the presence of PDA and the use of indomethacin for the treatment of PDA may also have contributed to NEC in C.D. Her PDA or the use of indomethacin may have caused a decrease in mesenteric blood flow with resultant ischemia and intestinal mucosal injury.[140]

Treatment
General Management

26. How should C.D. be managed?

Significant abdominal distention may compromise respiratory function and blood flow to the intestines. Therefore, as soon as NEC is suspected, feedings should be stopped immediately and an orogastric tube with low intermittent suction placed to decompress the abdomen. C.D.'s vital signs and abdominal circumference should be closely monitored for disease progression. A complete blood count (CBC) and platelet count should be obtained frequently to monitor for neutropenia and thrombocytopenia. Blood, urine, and stool cultures

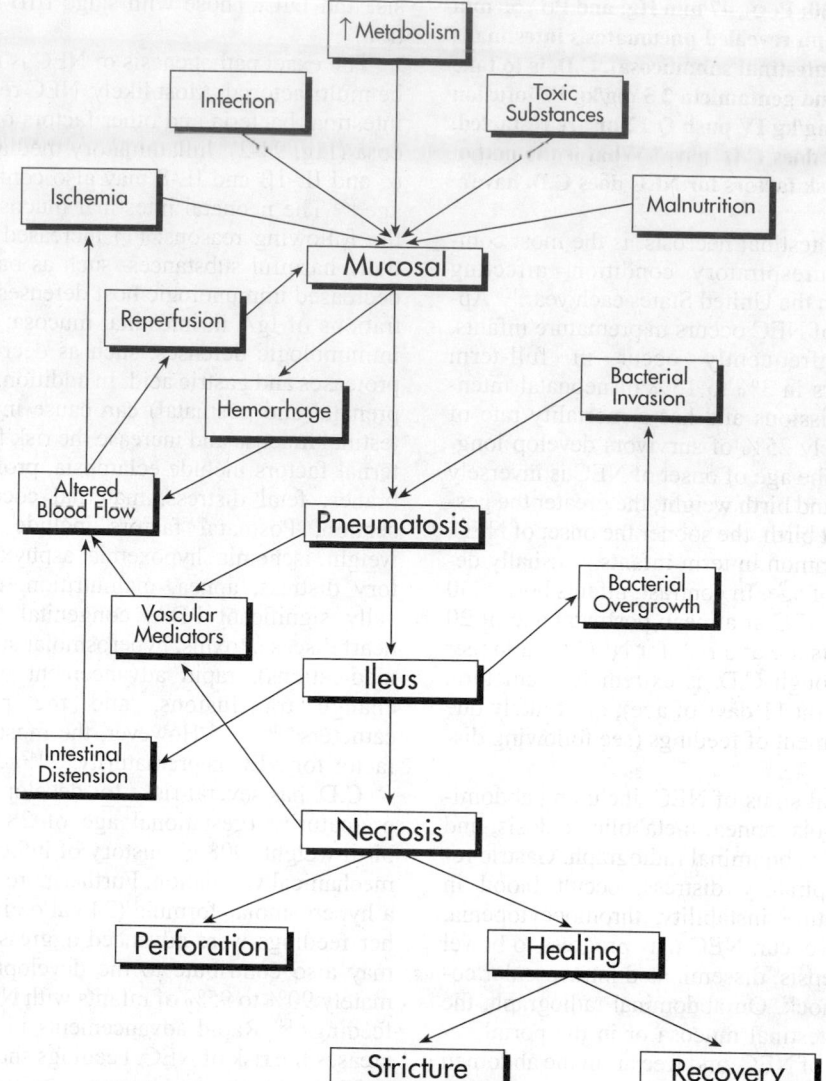

FIGURE 94-2 Necrotizing enterocolitis (NEC). This schematic is a composite of the theories about factors believed to be involved in the pathogenesis of NEC. The progression of this disease is denoted in large type. The factors believed to initiate or propagate the disease process are in smaller type. (Reproduced with permission from Crouse DT. Necrotizing enterocolitis. In: Pomerance JJ, Richardson CJ, eds. Neonatology for the Clinician. Norwalk, CT: Appleton & Lange, 1993:364.)

should be obtained, and parenteral antibiotics should be started as soon as possible. In infants with stage I NEC, antibiotic therapy is usually given for 3 days pending culture results and clinical signs. Once the diagnosis of NEC is ruled out, antibiotics may be discontinued.[142] Enteral feedings can then be initiated slowly. However, if the diagnosis of NEC is made, antibiotics are continued and parenteral nutrition is initiated at that time. Infants require 7 to 14 days of bowel rest (NPO). The length of antibiotic therapy and bowel rest in infants with documented NEC (stages II or III) is determined by the severity of systemic illness (e.g., metabolic acidosis, thrombocytopenia). C.D. has stage IIB disease and needs to be NPO (nothing by mouth) for at least 10 to 14 days and will require total parenteral nutrition during that time. Infants with stage III disease may also require fluid resuscitation, administration of inotropic agents such as dopamine and dobutamine, and surgical intervention.[140]

Antibiotics

27. **C.D. just completed a 7-day course of ampicillin and gentamicin, is it appropriate to restart these antibiotics?**

The selection of antibiotics for NEC depends on the common microorganisms observed in an individual neonatal unit and their sensitivities. Many organisms have been implicated in NEC, including Enterobacteriaceae (e.g., *Escherichia coli, Klebsiella* species), *Pseudomonas, Staphylococcus aureus* (in rare cases, methicillin-resistant), *Staphylococcus epidermidis, Clostridium,* enteroviruses, and rotaviruses.[139,142,144]For most cases of NEC, treatment with a broad-spectrum penicillin, such as ampicillin, and an aminoglycoside (e.g., gentamicin) is appropriate.

However, in some nurseries, *S. epidermidis* is the most common cause of neonatal nosocomial infections. Increases in *S. epidermidis*–associated NEC also have been reported.

Therefore, vancomycin and an aminoglycoside may be used as routine treatment in some nurseries or in specific patients at risk for *Staphylococcus* infections (e.g., neonates with central catheters or prolonged ICU stays). Vancomycin may be more appropriate than ampicillin because vancomycin has coverage against methicillin-resistant *S. epidermidis,* as well as enterococcal and streptococcal species. Because C.D. has been hospitalized for more than a week, vancomycin and gentamicin may be more appropriate, especially if her neonatal ICU has a high incidence of staphylococcal nosocomial infections. C.D. should be treated with parenteral antibiotics for 10 to 14 days.

Other antibiotic combinations used to treat NEC include cefotaxime and vancomycin, and cefotaxime and ampicillin. The combination of cefotaxime and vancomycin has been shown to prevent severe peritonitis and death in <2,200-g birth weight neonates with NEC, whereas gentamicin and ampicillin have not. Suppression of aerobic fecal floral by the combination of cefotaxime and vancomycin, but not by ampicillin and gentamicin, may explain these findings.[146]

ENTERAL ANTIBIOTICS

28. The neonatologist would like to give gentamicin 2.5 mg/kg via the orogastric tube Q 12 hr in addition to parenteral antibiotics. Is there any added benefit to adding enteral gentamicin to the current parenteral antibiotic regimen?

Enteral administration of aminoglycosides does not prevent GI perforation or change the course of NEC. In addition, enteral aminoglycosides can be absorbed systemically in neonates with NEC, via the inflamed intestinal mucosa.[142] Systemic absorption may significantly increase the serum concentrations of concomitantly administered parenteral aminoglycosides. Therefore, routine enteral administration of antibiotics such as gentamicin is not warranted for C.D. In select patients and during NEC epidemics, however, prophylactic administration of enteral aminoglycoside antibiotics or vancomycin decreases the incidence of NEC. Unfortunately, prophylactic use of these antibiotics has been associated with the emergence of resistant organisms, which limits their systemic use.[147] Systemic absorption of enterally administered vancomycin also can occur through inflamed intestinal mucosa.

ADDITIONAL ANTIBIOTICS

29. Two days later, C.D. develops peritonitis with ascites, hypotension, metabolic acidosis, neutropenia, and disseminated intravascular coagulation. IV fluids and dopamine are administered for the hypotension, fresh frozen plasma and whole blood are given to treat the coagulopathy, and morphine 0.05 mg/kg IV push Q 4 hr PRN is started for pain control. Free air in the abdomen is observed on abdominal radiograph. Blood and urine cultures have had no growth for 48 hours. What additional antimicrobial coverage should be provided?

Peritonitis secondary to intestinal perforation may be polymicrobial, involving both aerobes and anaerobes. Therefore, an antimicrobial agent with anaerobic activity should be added to C.D.'s current regimen.[140] The two most commonly used agents are clindamycin and metronidazole. Empiric anaerobic coverage in the treatment of NEC without perforation is controversial.[139] Routine use of clindamycin in the treatment of NEC has not decreased the incidence of intestinal gangrene or perforation. In addition, it has been associated with an increased incidence of abdominal strictures.[148]

Prognosis

30. C.D. is taken urgently to the operating room and 10 cm of necrotic ileum is removed along with the ileocecal valve. What long-term nutritional problems is C.D. likely to develop?

C.D. is at risk of developing short-bowel syndrome, a condition of malabsorption and malnutrition that results from surgical removal of a significant portion of the small intestine. The most important factors that determine short-bowel syndrome are the length of the remaining small intestine and the presence of the ileocecal valve. Because C.D. has had a majority of her ileum and her ileocecal valve removed, she most likely will suffer from short-bowel syndrome.

Because the terminal ileum is an important site for absorption of vitamins, trace minerals, and nutrients, C.D. will be at risk for decreased absorption of these substances. C.D. also will have a faster GI transit time and diarrhea because her ileocecal valve was removed. (The ileocecal valve plays a major role in controlling intestinal transit time.) Absorption of enterally administered medications also may be decreased in patients with short-bowel syndrome. As C.D. starts to receive most of her nutrition enterally, she should be monitored for fat malabsorption and other nutritional deficiencies (e.g., deficiencies in vitamins A, B_{12}, D, E, and K), and supplemented accordingly.[149]

Prevention

31. What could have been done to prevent NEC in C.D.?

Several interventions may decrease the incidence of NEC. Enteral feedings in preterm infants can be withheld for several weeks and parenteral nutrition initiated. Intestinal priming (i.e., using a small amount of full-strength formula or breast milk to stimulate GI mucosal development) in addition to parenteral nutrition can improve feeding tolerance and increase GI motility.[150] Because breast milk provides antibodies, growth factors, and cellular immune factors, it may reduce the incidence of NEC. In contrast, the use of hyperosmolar formulas or medications can cause osmotic injury to the bowel and may result in NEC. Maternal steroids (commonly used to accelerate fetal lung maturation) can decrease the incidence of NEC due to a maturational effect on the microvillous membranes. Strict infection control measures, such as preventing fecal and oral spread of bacterial pathogens after epidemic outbreaks, also decrease the incidence of NEC.[144]

NEONATAL SEPSIS AND MENINGITIS
Pathogenesis and Clinical Presentation

32. J.E., a 28-week gestation, 850-g male, was born to a mother with prolonged rupture of membranes (>72 hours). The newborn's mother is febrile with a white blood cell count (WBC) of $20 \times 10^3/mm^3$ and differential of 70% segmented neutrophils, 20% bands, 7% lymphocytes, and 3% monocytes. J.E. had Apgar scores of 4 at 1 minute and 3 at 5 minutes after birth.

Mechanical ventilation was instituted and J.E. was admitted to the neonatal ICU. Vital signs upon admission were as follows: HR, 190 beats/min; temperature, 35.8°C; and BP, 56/33 mm Hg. Blood and urine cultures are pending. Significant laboratory data include the following: WBC, 3,000 cells/mm³ with a differential of 50% segmented neutrophils, 30% bands, 15% lymphocytes, and 5% monocytes; platelets, 75,000/mm³. What is the etiology and pathogenesis of neonatal sepsis? What risk factors for sepsis does J.E. have? What clinical signs and laboratory evidence of sepsis are apparent in J.E.?

[SI units: WBC, 3,000 × 10⁶ cells/L with 0.5 neutrophils, 0.3 bands, 0.15 lymphocytes, and 0.05 monocytes; platelets, 75 × 10⁹/L]

Bacterial sepsis significantly contributes to neonatal morbidity and mortality. Neonates, especially preterm newborns, are at increased risk for infections and should be considered immunocompromised. The neonate's decreased immune function (e.g., immature function of neutrophils, lower amounts of immunoglobulin) also results in a reduced ability to localize infections. Once a tissue site becomes infected, bacteria can spread easily, resulting in disseminated disease. In addition, the lack of opsonic antibodies in preterm infants such as J.E. increases the susceptibility to infections caused by bacteria with polysaccharide capsules (e.g., group B streptococcus, *E. coli, Haemophilus influenzae* type B).[151]

The incidence of neonatal sepsis varies from 1 to 10 cases per 1,000 live births, but is higher in low-birth-weight neonates.[151] In very-low-birth-weight infants with prolonged hospitalization, the incidence increases to 300 per 1,000 very-low-birth-weight infants.[152] Risk factors (as demonstrated in J.E.) include prematurity, low birth weight, male gender, and predisposing maternal conditions (e.g., prolonged rupture of membranes, maternal fever, elevated maternal WBC or left shift, chorioamnionitis, and urinary tract infection).[152,153] Despite treatment, mortality rates for neonatal sepsis can be as high as 30% to 50%, with the highest mortality observed in newborns <1,500 g.[154,155] Meningitis occurs as a complication of bacterial sepsis in 10% to 30% of septic neonates[154,155] and has a mortality rate of 20% to 50% depending on the pathogen.[152]

Common Pathogens

The fetal environment within the amniotic membranes is normally sterile until the onset of labor and delivery. Once the membrane is ruptured, the infant may be at risk for colonization of microorganisms from the maternal genital tract. Many of these organisms do not cause infection in the mother but may be detrimental to the infant. Early-onset neonatal sepsis (i.e., sepsis that presents during the first 5 to 7 days of life) usually is caused by organisms acquired from the maternal genital tract. The most common pathogens found in early-onset neonatal sepsis are group B streptococcus and *E. coli*. Other primary pathogens include *Listeria monocytogenes, Enterococcus,* and other Gram-negative bacilli (e.g., *H. influenzae, Klebsiella pneumoniae*). Late-onset sepsis (sepsis presenting after 5 to 7 days postnatal age) usually is caused by these primary organisms or by nosocomial pathogens, such as coagulase-negative staphylococci (particularly *S. epidermidis*), *S. aureus, Pseudomonas* species, anaerobes, and *Candida* species.[153,154,156,157] The major risk factor for nosocomial septicemia is the presence of IV catheters (umbilical and central).[158] Other risk factors include low birth weight, prolonged

hospital stay, prior antibiotic use, parenteral hyperalimentation, lipid emulsion, invasive procedures, and the presence of other indwelling devices (e.g., endotracheal tubes, ventriculoperitoneal shunts).[152,157,159]

Over the past two decades, coagulase-negative staphylococcus such as *S. epidermidis* has emerged as the most common pathogen for late-onset neonatal nosocomial septicemia, causing 55% to 58% of cases.[158,160] This emergence is most likely due to the increased survival of extremely premature neonates with a resultant prolonged hospital stay and an increase in the associated risks of infection (i.e., placement of umbilical and central venous catheters and arterial lines, use of hyperalimentation and intralipid). More disturbing, however, is the reported persistence of coagulase-negative staphylococcal bacteremia, despite appropriate treatment in low-birth-weight neonates without central venous catheters.[161]

Neonatal sepsis may present with nonspecific or subtle signs especially in very-low-birth-weight infants.[152,159] The most common signs are poor feeding, temperature instability, lethargy, or apnea.[152,155] Other signs of neonatal sepsis include glucose instability (hypoglycemia or hyperglycemia), tachycardia, dyspnea or cyanosis, tachypnea, diarrhea, vomiting, feeding intolerance, abdominal distension, metabolic acidosis, and abnormal WBC.[152,159] Clinical signs and laboratory evidence of neonatal sepsis observed in J.E. include tachycardia (HR, 190 beats/minute), hypothermia (temperature 35.8°C), neutropenia (WBC, 3 × 10³/mm³), a left shift in the differential, and thrombocytopenia (platelets, 75,000/mm³). Hypothermia is more common than fever in neonatal sepsis, especially in preterm newborns. However, if fever is present, it is strongly associated with bacterial infection. Neutropenia, especially with a left shift (as seen in J.E.) can be a sign of WBC depletion from bone marrow due to overwhelming sepsis. An elevated WBC also can indicate a neonatal infection, but may be less specific.[159] Late signs of neonatal infection include jaundice, hepatosplenomegaly, and petechiae.[152] A bulging fontanelle, posturing, or seizures would indicate meningitis, although these CNS signs are not always present when meningitis exists.

Bacterial meningitis should always be considered in infants with neonatal sepsis. The definitive diagnostic method for bacterial meningitis is lumbar puncture. Lumbar puncture should be performed in infants with a positive blood culture, abnormal neurologic signs, an elevated WBC or left shift, or the presence of bacterial antigen in the urine.[162] The cerebrospinal fluid (CSF) should be tested with Gram's stain, cell counts with differential, glucose and protein levels, and bacterial culture. Neonatal CSF cell counts are difficult to interpret because values may overlap with normal neonatal values. The diagnosis of neonatal sepsis is confirmed by isolation of the pathogen from blood, urine, CSF, or other body sites. Latex agglutination tests that detect antigens (e.g., bacterial cell-wall fragments) of group B streptococcus, *E. coli, S. pneumonia, N. meningitidis,* and *H. influenzae* type B in body fluids can facilitate a prompt diagnosis, especially in patients who previously were treated with antibiotics.[163]

Treatment of Sepsis
Antibiotic Selection

33. What antibiotic regimen should be prescribed for J.E.?

Empiric treatment with appropriate IV antibiotics must be initiated immediately in J.E. Significant morbidity or fatality would occur if antibiotics were withheld until a diagnosis was confirmed by culture results (in 24 to 72 hours). This is especially true in patients in whom meningitis is suspected. The initial empiric antibiotic treatment of choice for early-onset neonatal sepsis and meningitis is ampicillin plus an aminoglycoside. These antibiotics are used because they (1) are bactericidal against the common neonatal pathogens; (2) penetrate into the CNS; (3) are relatively safe; and (4) have proven clinical efficacy. If group B streptococcus is suspected, antibiotic therapy should be switched to high-dose penicillin G. Penicillin is preferred over ampicillin because of its higher activity against group B streptococcus.[156]

Therefore, ampicillin 45 mg every 12 hours IV plus an aminoglycoside (e.g., gentamicin 2 mg every 24 hours IV) should be started in J.E. for suspected neonatal sepsis and possible meningitis. Meningitic doses of ampicillin should be used in J.E. until meningitis can be ruled out. Ampicillin is active against group B streptococci, group D streptococci, *Listeria,* and most strains of *E. coli.* Aminoglycoside antibiotics (e.g., gentamicin or tobramycin) usually are active against Gram-negative bacilli. In addition, aminoglycosides may provide synergy with ampicillin against *Listeria* and group B streptococci.[153] Selection of the specific aminoglycoside should be determined by antibiotic resistance patterns within the neonatal ICU. Amikacin should be reserved for Gram-negative organisms resistant to gentamicin and tobramycin. Aminoglycoside regimens need to be designed to achieve safe and therapeutic serum concentrations (gentamicin and tobramycin peak 6 to 8 μg/mL, trough <2 μg/mL; amikacin peaks 20 to 30 μg/mL, troughs <10 μg/mL).[8,49]

In some nurseries, a third-generation cephalosporin (e.g., cefotaxime [Claforan] or ceftriaxone [Rocephin]), instead of an aminoglycoside, is added to ampicillin for initial empiric treatment of early-onset neonatal sepsis and meningitis.[153,156] The spectrum of activity of these third-generation cephalosporins includes many Gram-negative organisms and group B streptococci. However, third-generation cephalosporins do not have sufficient activity against *Listeria* or group D streptococci. Therefore, these agents must be used in combination with ampicillin for empiric neonatal therapy. As previously mentioned, ceftriaxone should be avoided in neonates with hyperbilirubinemia due to bilirubin displacement from albumin binding sites. Ceftriaxone has also been associated with sludging in the gall bladder and cholestasis.[8] Hence, cefotaxime is the preferred cephalosporin for neonatal use.

The third-generation cephalosporins have advantages over the aminoglycosides, including better CNS penetration, the elimination of serum concentration measurements, and less nephrotoxicity. However, these cephalosporins do not significantly improve clinical or microbiologic endpoints compared with the standard ampicillin and gentamicin regimen. Furthermore, extensive use of the third-generation cephalosporins in neonatal ICUs may lead to rapid emergence of resistant Gram-negative bacilli (e.g., *Enterobacter cloacae, Pseudomonas aeruginosa,* and *Serratia* species) and vancomycin resistance in enterococci. In contrast, gentamicin has not been associated with rapid development of these resistant strains.[156] Thus, combinations such as ampicillin and cefo-

taxime should be reserved for the following situations: (1) neonatal ICUs where aminoglycoside resistance to Gram-negative enteric bacilli is of concern, (2) neonatal ICUs where serum concentrations of aminoglycosides cannot be measured, and (3) specific neonates in whom aminoglycoside therapy could be of concern (e.g., neonates with known renal failure).[156]

Therapy for late-onset sepsis or meningitis is directed toward nosocomial pathogens plus the primary pathogens of early-onset infection (see Question 32). Selection of initial antibiotic therapy should consider the specific neonatal ICU's nosocomial pathogen and antibiotic resistance patterns, as well as the neonate's risk factors, clinical condition, and previous antibiotic therapy.[164] Coagulase-negative staphylococcus is now the most common pathogen of late-onset neonatal nosocomial septicemia. Because of the high incidence of methicillin-resistant coagulase-negative staphylococci (as high as 80% in some neonatal ICUs),[164] vancomycin has been used as the drug of choice for empiric therapy for suspected late-onset neonatal sepsis. However, widespread use of vancomycin has led to the emergence of vancomycin-resistant enterococci. Therefore, the routine use of vancomycin as empiric therapy for nosocomial neonatal sepsis should be discouraged. Two retrospective studies have shown that highly selective use of vancomycin for neonatal coagulase-negative staphylococci septicemia results in low morbidity and mortality while significantly reducing vancomycin use.[160,165] Guidelines for the selective use of vancomycin should be tailored according to individual neonatal ICU's nosocomial pathogens, susceptibility patterns, and patient risk factors, clinical condition, and antibiotic history. Therefore, if J.E. had a central venous catheter and presented with a late-onset sepsis, initial antibiotic therapy should include an aminoglycoside (for Gram-negative coverage) plus either an antistaphylococcal penicillin (e.g., nafcillin or methicillin) or vancomycin (for activity against *S. aureus* and *S. epidermidis*). Vancomycin is used in place of the antistaphylococcal penicillin in neonatal units with methicillin-resistant *S. aureus* and for selective use to cover *S. epidermidis* (a coagulase-negative staphylococcus) as outlined previously.[156,164] If *Pseudomonas* infection is suspected, an antipseudomonal penicillin such as piperacillin, ticarcillin, or mezlocillin combined with an aminoglycoside should be used for their synergistic bacterial activity. For systemic fungal infections, amphotericin B (with or without flucytosine) is considered to be the initial treatment of choice.[155] Because uncommon organisms are not suspected in J.E., the regimen of ampicillin 45 mg IV every 12 hours plus gentamicin 2 mg IV every 24 hours is appropriate.

Dosage and Route of Administration

Dosage regimens for the antimicrobial agents commonly used in neonates[8,51,52,166,167] are listed in Tables 94-5 and 94-8. Dosing guidelines for tobramycin and netilmicin are the same as gentamicin (see Table 94-5). The IV route is preferred for treatment of all septic neonates. If the IV route is not available, the IM route can be used in neonates with sufficient muscle mass, adequate peripheral perfusion, and a normal, stable coagulation status. Oral administration almost never is used in serious neonatal infections because GI drug absorption is extremely variable during this age. Meningitic doses of antibiotics should be used for the treatment of any seriously

Table 94-8   Antibiotic Dosage Regimens for Neonates: Dosages and Intervals of Administration

Drug	Weight <1,200 g[52] 0–4 Weeks[a] (mg/kg)	Weight 1,200–2,000 g 0–7 Days[a] (mg/kg)	>7 Days[a] (mg/kg)	Weight >2,000 g 0-7 Days[a] (mg/kg)	>7 Days[a] (mg/kg)
Ampicillin					
Meningitis	50 Q 12 hr	50 Q 12 hr	50 Q 8 hr	50 Q 8 hr	50 Q 6 hr
Other diseases	25 Q 12 hr	25 Q 12 hr	25 Q 8 hr	25 Q 8 hr	25 Q 6 hr
Cefazolin	20 Q 12 hr	20 Q 12 hr	20 Q 12 hr	20 Q 12 hr	20 Q 8 hr
Cefotaxime	50 Q 12 hr	50 Q 12 hr	50 Q 8 hr	50 Q 12 hr	50 Q 8 hr
Ceftazidime	50 Q 12 hr	50 Q 12 hr	50 Q 8 hr	50 Q 12 hr	50 Q 8 hr
Ceftriaxone	50 Q 24 hr	50 Q 24 hr	50 Q 24 hr	50 Q 24 hr	75 Q 24 hr
Chloramphenicol	22 Q 24 hr	25 Q 24 hr	25 Q 24 hr	25 Q 24 hr	25 Q 12 hr
Clindamycin	5 Q 12 hr	5 Q 12 hr	5 Q 8 hr	5 Q 8 hr	5 Q 6 hr
Erythromycin	10 Q 12 hr	10 Q 12 hr	10 Q 8 hr	10 Q 12 hr	13.3 Q 8 hr
Methicillin					
Meningitis	50 Q 12 hr	50 Q 12 hr	50 Q 8 hr	50 Q 8 hr	50 Q 6 hr
Other diseases	25 Q 12 hr	25 Q 12 hr	25 Q 8 hr	25 Q 8 hr	25 Q 6 hr
Metronidazole	7.5 Q 48 hr	7.5 Q 24 hr	7.5 Q 12 hr	7.5 Q 12 hr	15 Q 12 hr
Mezlocillin	75 Q 12 hr	75 Q 12 hr	75 Q 8 hr	75 Q 12 hr	75 Q 8 hr
Oxacillin	25 Q 12 hr	25 Q 12 hr	25 Q 8 hr	25 Q 8 hr	37.5 Q 6 hr
Nafcillin	25 Q 12 hr	25 Q 12 hr	25 Q 8 hr	25 Q 8 hr	37.5 Q 6 hr
Penicillin G					
Meningitis	50,000 units Q 12 hr	50,000 units Q 12 hr	75,000 units Q 8 hr	50,000 units Q 8 hr	50,000 units Q 6 hr
Other diseases	25,000 units Q 12 hr	25,000 units Q 12 hr	25,000 units Q 8 hr	25,000 units Q 8 hr	25,000 units Q 6 hr
Piperacillin	75 Q 12 hr	75 Q 12 hr	75 Q 8 hr	75 Q 8 hr	75 Q 6 hr
Ticarcillin	75 Q 12 hr	75 Q 12 hr	75 Q 8 hr	75 Q 8 hr	75 Q 6 hr
Vancomycin	15 Q 24 hr[b]	20 Q 24 hr	15 Q 12 hr	15 Q 12 hr	15 Q 8 hr

[a]Postnatal age.

[b]If weight <750 g and postnatal age <14 days, use 10.0 to 12.5 mg/kg every 24 hours.

Adapted with permission from Nelson JD, Bradley JS. Nelson's Pocket Book of Pediatric Antimicrobial Therapy. 14th ed. Philadelphia: Lippincott Williams & Wilkins, 2000:16; incorporating references 8, 167.

ill neonate until meningitis is excluded by negative CSF cultures.

Extended-interval aminoglycoside dosing (also known as once-daily dosing or single-daily dosing) has been widely used in the adult population. Aminoglycoside antibiotics display concentration-dependent killing of bacteria. Rationale for the use of extended-interval aminoglycoside dosing include the following: (1) enhancement of bacterial killing by providing a higher peak serum concentration to minimal inhibitory concentration (MIC) ratio, (2) provision of a prolonged postantibiotic effect, and (3) minimization of adaptive postexposure microbial resistance.[168] Recent meta-analyses of clinical studies in adults indicate that extended-interval aminoglycoside dosing appears to have similar efficacy without increased toxicity compared with traditional multiple daily dosing.[169] In addition, extended-interval aminoglycoside dosing can reduce costs associated with drug wastage, administration time, and therapeutic monitoring.[170]

Because of these beneficial effects, the use of extended-interval aminoglycoside dosing has been studied in the pediatric population. Most studies have included term or near-term newborns (i.e., gestational age 34 weeks or greater).[168] As expected, the use of extended-interval aminoglycoside dosing resulted in higher peak and lower trough serum concentrations in these neonates compared with traditional multiple-daily dosing. However, neonatal studies have not established optimal regimens to achieve the best peak serum concentration to MIC ratio. In addition, few studies have in-

cluded preterm neonates. Furthermore, most studies in neonates used extended-interval aminoglycoside dosing for short periods of time, for example during the workup to rule out neonatal sepsis (i.e., 72-hour duration). Studies describe only a few neonates who received extended-interval aminoglycoside dosing to actually treat documented neonatal infections. Other neonatal-specific factors, such as the neonate's immature immune function and a potential decreased postantibiotic effect, have not been adequately addressed. Therefore, large, well-designed studies evaluating the clinical efficacy and safety of extended-interval aminoglycoside dosing for the treatment of infections in neonates are required before routine use can be recommended.

Once a pathogen is isolated, the antimicrobial susceptibilities should be evaluated and the drug therapy modified appropriately. Blood, CSF, or urine cultures should be repeated to document bacterial sterilization after 24 to 48 hours of appropriate therapy. J.E. should be evaluated carefully for the development of serious bacterial complications such as meningitis, osteomyelitis, abscess formation, or endocarditis.[153]

Duration of Therapy

As long as there is no evidence of meningitis or other focal infection (e.g., abscess formation), the duration of therapy for most systemic bacterial infections is 7 to 10 days (or approximately 5 to 7 days after significant clinical improvement). Antibiotic therapy may need to be continued for 14 to 21 days if the neonate's clinical response is slow or if multiple organ systems are involved [155] If cultures are negative at 72 hours and the infant does not have any clinical or laboratory signs of sepsis, antibiotics can be discontinued. In neonates presenting with signs of severe infection followed by improvement after initiation of antibiotics, therapy may be continued despite negative cultures.

Treatment of Meningitis

34. **How should J.E. be treated if meningitis is suspected?**

Antibiotic Selection

The major pathogens causing neonatal sepsis also are the primary pathogens that cause neonatal meningitis. Seventy-five percent of neonatal meningitis is caused by group B streptococcus and *E. coli*; *L. monocytogenes* is the third most common organism.[155] Initial empiric antibiotic therapy of choice consists of ampicillin plus an aminoglycoside.[152] Ampicillin plus a third-generation cephalosporin (cefotaxime or ceftriaxone) may be used empirically for early-onset neonatal meningitis in situations as outlined previously for early-onset neonatal sepsis (see Question 33). In addition, because of their greater CSF penetration compared with the aminoglycosides, the combination of a third-generation cephalosporin with ampicillin may be preferred when the CSF Gram stain indicates a Gram-negative infection. Initial empiric antibiotic treatment of late-onset meningitis should follow guidelines similar to those for late-onset sepsis with consideration of nosocomial as well as primary pathogens (see Question 33). As with neonatal sepsis, once an organism is recovered from the CSF, the most appropriate antibiotic is selected based on susceptibility.

Duration of Therapy

If CSF cultures are positive, repeat CSF cultures should be obtained daily or every other day in J.E. to document when the CSF becomes sterilized. The duration of therapy for neonatal meningitis depends on the clinical response and duration of positive CSF cultures after therapy is initiated. Appropriate antibiotics should be continued for a minimum of 14 days after the CSF is sterilized. This is equivalent to a duration of antibiotic therapy for a minimum of 21 days for Gram-negative organisms and at least 14 days for Gram-positive pathogens.[152,155] As a general rule, it takes longer to sterilize the CSF of neonates infected by Gram-negative enteric bacilli (72 hours) than those infected by Gram-positive bacteria (36 to 48 hours).[152] Although surgical placement of a ventricular reservoir for intraventricular administration of an antibiotic (usually an aminoglycoside) has been used to treat meningitis not responding to IV antimicrobial therapy, the Neonatal Meningitis Cooperative Study group reported no beneficial effect of this method of administration in infants with Gram-negative meningitis. In fact, infants treated with intraventricular gentamicin had a threefold increase in mortality rate compared with infants treated solely on IV antibiotics.[155] (See Chapter 58, Central Nervous System Infections.)

Intravenous Immune Globulin

35. **On day 2 of life, J.E.'s blood culture is reported as positive for group B streptococcus. His current vital signs are as follows:**

HR, 135 beats/min; temperature, 37°C; and BP, 59/40 mm Hg. Laboratory data include the following: WBC, 7,000 cells/mm³ with a differential of 53% segmented neutrophils, 15% bands, 25% lymphocytes, and 7% monocytes; platelets, 150,000/mm³. J.E.'s ventilatory settings are slightly improved. What is the role of intravenous immune globulin (IVIG) in a patient like J.E.?

[SI units: WBC, $7,000 \times 10^6$ cells/L with 0.53 neutrophils, 0.15 bands, 0.25 lymphocytes, and 0.07 monocytes; platelets, 150×10^9/L]

Rationale

Neonatal humoral immunity is provided primarily by transplacental transport of maternal IgG to the fetus. Active transfer starts at 17 weeks' gestation and increases with gestational age. By 33 weeks' gestation, fetal IgG levels are equal to maternal IgG.[171] Therefore, neonates born before 33 weeks' gestation have very low IgG concentrations. In addition, because of the neonate's poor antibody response to antigenic stimuli, these low concentrations of IgG can decrease further during the first few weeks of life.[172] Low IgG concentrations, as well as a lack of microorganism-specific antibodies, and opsonic antibody activity against the polysaccharide capsules of certain bacteria (i.e., group B streptococcus, *E. coli*, and *H. influenzae*) significantly contribute to the neonate's increased susceptibility to infections.[172] Exogenous administration of IVIG may correct low IgG serum concentrations and improve neonatal host defenses. Therefore, administration of IVIG has been proposed for the prevention and treatment of neonatal infections.

Efficacy

The efficacy of IVIG as an adjunct to antimicrobial therapy for the prevention and treatment of neonatal sepsis has been assessed in numerous studies. However, comparisons between studies are difficult because of differences in study design, sample size, dosage regimens (dose and duration of therapy), specific product used, pathogen-specific antibodies, lot-to-lot variability, inclusion criteria, and outcome measures. In addition, studies assessing IVIG for treatment of neonatal sepsis differ in the specific infecting organism and the rates and severity of infection.[151] Despite these differences, several meta-analyses have been conducted to try to summarize the data evaluating the effectiveness of IVIG for prophylaxis and treatment of neonatal sepsis.

An early evaluation of published articles assessing prophylaxis of IVIG concluded that its effectiveness depended on the pathogen-specific antibody activity of the individual product used. Other evaluations have found encouraging results or no clear evidence of benefit for preterm infants.[151] In a recent systematic review of 19 studies (representing approximately 5,000 preterm infants) prophylactic IVIG was associated with a significant, but very small reduction in sepsis (3%) and serious infections (4%). However, NEC, IVH, length of hospital stay, and mortality were not significantly affected.[173] Therefore, the use of prophylactic IVIG is of marginal clinical benefit and thus cannot be routinely recommended.

Few studies have evaluated IVIG as adjunctive treatment with antibiotics for treatment of neonatal sepsis. In a recent Cochrane review of 13 studies of suspected or proven infections in >500 neonates, IVIG treatment was associated with reductions in length of hospitalization (for term infants) and mortality. However the reduction in mortality for clinically suspected infections was of borderline significance.[174] Owing to the lack of power of this meta analysis, further studies are needed to determine the effectiveness of IVIG for the treatment of suspected or proven neonatal infections. Clinically, the routine use of IVIG for suspected or proven infections cannot be recommended. However, IVIG may be considered for select patients with proven infections.

Large, well-designed, prospective studies are required to determine the optimal IVIG dosage regimen, including dose per kilogram, number of doses, and timing of treatment. Studies of the cost-effectiveness of IVIG are also needed. Unlabeled or low concentrations of antibodies against the primary pathogens of neonatal sepsis may limit the use of commercial IVIG preparations. However, the use of preselected lots of IVIG that possess antibodies against specific neonatal pathogens may be of benefit. Other immunologic agents, such as monoclonal antibodies and hyperimmune immunoglobulin preparations, may be more effective and currently are being investigated.

Initiation of Therapy

At this time, routine use of IVIG for all newborns to prevent or treat neonatal sepsis is not indicated.[151,172] However, treatment with IVIG should be considered in septic neonates who are not responding to standard antibiotic treatment and supportive care.[151] Because J.E. has responded to antibiotic therapy, as evidenced by his improvement in vital signs, WBC, differential, platelet count, and ventilatory settings, IVIG would not be indicated.

Dosing, Administration, and Adverse Effects

36. IVIG 500 mg/kg IV push weekly for four doses has been ordered for J.E. because of prescriber preference. How should IVIG be administered and what should be monitored for adverse effects?

The optimal dose of IVIG has not been established. The National Institute of Child Health and Human Development (NICHD) study used prophylactic doses of 900 mg/kg for neonates 501 to 1,000 g and 700 mg/kg for neonates 1,001 to 1,500 g to attain IgG serum concentrations of 700 mg/dL.[175] Doses were repeated every 2 weeks. Trough concentrations after the first dose were ≥700 mg/dL in approximately 50% of the neonates. Only 13% of neonates had all trough concentrations at or above the target concentration during the study period.[175] These findings suggest that the clinical use of these doses or even slightly higher doses would be adequate. However, the optimal total IgG serum concentration for treatment or prophylaxis of neonatal sepsis has not been established. In addition, the amount of specific immunoglobulins directed against the primary neonatal pathogens may be more important. Although many dosing regimens have been studied,[151,172,175] doses of 500 to 1,000 mg/kg are commonly used. Some institutions repeat treatment every 2 weeks.[151] Doses ≥1,000 mg/kg may not be more effective and may have toxic effects. Suppression of opsonophagocytosis and decreased bacterial clearance have been reported with high-dose IVIG in neonatal animal models.[176]

Although the dose of IVIG prescribed for J.E. is reasonable, IVIG should *never* be administered via IV push. Rapid IV administration may result in significant adverse effects.

Administration rates for IVIG are product specific and most neonatal doses should be infused intravenously over 2 to 6 hours. Because anaphylaxis can occur, slower initial infusion rates are recommended. In this case, the specific IVIG product used in J.E.'s neonatal ICU should be identified, and an appropriate rate in the package insert should be consulted for proper administration rates. Neonates receiving IVIG should be monitored routinely for adverse effects such as tachycardia, dyspnea, hypotension, hypertension, fever, flushing, irritability, tremors, restlessness, and emesis.[175] These reactions may be related to the rate of infusion and generally resolve when the infusion rate is decreased or when the infusion is discontinued temporarily. In the NICHD study, the overall rate of NEC in the IVIG group (12%) was not statistically higher than in the control group (9.5%). However, a significantly greater number of NEC cases occurred during phase 2 of the study in the IVIG group (12%) compared with placebo (8.3%).[175] Therefore, because of the potential association with NEC, indiscriminate use of IVIG is not warranted. Other adverse effects may be identified as neonatal investigations continue with IVIG use.

CONGENITAL INFECTIONS
TORCH Titers

37. S.Y., a 2,000-g female, was born at 34 weeks' gestational age by vaginal delivery. She was born at another institution and transferred to your hospital on day 3 of life. S.Y.'s birth was complicated by prolonged rupture of membranes >72 hours, a difficult labor and delivery, and fetal distress requiring a fetal scalp monitor. On physical examination, S.Y. is an extremely irritable newborn with RR of 60 breaths/min. Several vesicular skin lesions located on the scalp and around the eyes are noted. Conjunctivitis also is present. S.Y. is placed on supplemental oxygen and ABGs are obtained. Blood, CSF, and urine were cultured for bacteria and fungus and S.Y. was started on ampicillin 75 mg IV Q 12 hr and gentamicin 4.5 mg IV Q 24 hr to rule out sepsis. Antimicrobial therapy will not be altered until culture results are available. What other tests and/or information are needed for S.Y. at this time?

Certain bacteria, viruses, and protozoa can cause fetal infections that may result in fetal death, congenital anomalies, serious CNS sequelae, intrauterine growth retardation, or preterm birth.[177] The primary organisms that cause these infections can be remembered by the acronym, TORCH: *t*oxoplasmosis; *o*ther (i.e., syphilis, gonorrhea, hepatitis B, listeria); *r*ubella; *c*ytomegalovirus; *h*erpes simplex. Because of the potential severity of these diseases, newborns who display any signs of infection (e.g., irritability, fever, thrombocytopenia, hepatosplenomegaly) need to be evaluated for these intrauterine and perinatally acquired infections. The diagnosis of each of these infections should be considered separately. A complete infectious disease workup should include specific antibody titer measurements to the suspected organisms rather than sending a single serum sample for TORCH titer measurement.[177,178]

Primary clinical manifestations and treatment[8,177–182] for selected congenital infections are listed in Table 94-9. The clinical signs of these infections may overlap, and concurrent infection with two or more microorganisms is possible. The

Table 94-9   Selected Congenital and Perinatal Infections in the Neonate[177–182]

Organism	Primary Clinical Manifestations	Treatment of Proven or Highly Probable Disease
Herpes simplex[a,b]	Cutaneous vesicles, keratoconjunctivitis, microcephaly, CNS infection, hepatitis, pneumonitis, prematurity, respiratory distress, sepsis, convulsion, chorioretinitis	*Acyclovir:* 20 mg/kg Q 8 hr IV × 14–21 days *Ocular Involvement:* Acyclovir IV plus topical therapy: 1–2% trifluridine, 1% iododeoxyuridine, or 3% vidarabine
Toxoplasmosis	Chorioretinitis, ventriculomegaly, microcephaly, hydrocephaly, intracranial calcifications, ascites, hepatosplenomegaly, lymphadenopathy, jaundice, anemia, mental retardation	Sulfadiazine 100 mg/kg/day in two divided doses PO for 1 year *AND* pyrimethamine 1 mg/kg/day for 2–6 months followed by 1 mg/kg QOD to complete 1-year therapy *AND* folinic acid (leucovorin) 5–10 mg three times/week
Treponema pallidum[a]	*Early:* Osteochondritis, periostitis, hepatosplenomegaly, skin rash (maculopapular or vesiculo-bullous), rhinitis, meningitis, IUGR, jaundice, hepatitis, anemia, thrombocytopenia, chorioretinitis *Late:* Hutchinson's triad (interstitial keratitis, eighth-nerve deafness, Hutchinson's teeth), mental retardation, hydrocephalus, saddle nose, mulberry molars	Aqueous crystalline penicillin G × 10–14 days IV (preferred) or IM: ≤7 days postnatal age: 50,000 units/kg Q 12 hr >7 days postnatal age: 50,000 units/kg Q 8 hr *OR* Procaine penicillin G 50,000 units/kg/day IM Q 24 hr × 10–14 days
Hepatitis B[c]	Prematurity; usually asymptomatic; long-term effects include chronic hepatitis, cirrhosis, liver failure, hepatocellular carcinoma	*Perinatal Exposure (maternal HbsAg-positive):* HBIG 0.5 mL IM and hepatitis B vaccine IM (different IM sites) within 12 hours after birth; repeat hepatitis B vaccine at 1 and 6 months
Rubella	*Early:* IUGR, retinopathy, hypotonia, hepatosplenomegaly, thrombocytopenic purpura, bone lesions, cardiac effects *Late:* Hearing loss, mental retardation, diabetes *Rare:* Myocarditis, glaucoma, microcephaly, hepatitis, anemia	Supportive care
Cytomegalovirus	Petechiae, hepatosplenomegaly, jaundice, prematurity, IUGR, increased liver enzymes, hyperbilirubinemia, anemia, thrombocytopenia, interstitial pneumonitis, microcephaly, chorioretinitis, intracranial calcifications *Late:* Hearing loss, mental retardation, learning and motor abnormalities, visual disturbances	IV ganciclovir (under investigation)
Neisseria gonorrhoeae[a]	Ophthalmia neonatorum, scalp abscess, sepsis, arthritis, meningitis, endocarditis	*Nondisseminated (including ophthalmia neonatorum):* Ceftriaxone 25–50 mg/kg IV or IM × 1 (maximum dose: 125 mg); alternative for ophthalmic neonatorum: cefotaxime 100 mg/kg IM or IV × 1; use saline eye irrigations for ophthalmia neonatorum *Disseminated:* Ceftriaxone 25–50 mg/kg IV or IM Q 24 hr; cefotaxime 25–50 mg/kg IV or IM Q 12 hr Duration of therapy: • Arthritis or septicemia: 7 days • Meningitis: 10–14 days Use cefotaxime if hyperbilirubinemic

[a]See Chapter 65, Sexually Transmitted Diseases.
[b]See Chapter 72, Viral Infections.
[c]See Chapter 73, Viral Hepatitis.
CNS, central nervous system; HBIG, hepatitis B immune globulin; HbsAg, hepatitis B surface antigen; IM, intramuscular; IUGR, intrauterine growth retardation; IV, intravenous; QOD, every other day.

detection of congenital infections often is difficult because many neonates are asymptomatic at birth. Therefore, prenatal maternal screening and accurate evaluation of maternal history for risk factors are very important. Other organisms that can cause congenitally acquired infections include human immunodeficiency virus (HIV), human parvovirus, varicella-zoster virus, and measles virus.[177,178]

When congenital infections are suspected, appropriate diagnostic tests for each suspected organism should be performed. Viral cultures of the urine, oropharynx, nasopharynx, stool, and conjunctiva and a complete maternal history along with the results of recent maternal vaginal cultures also should be obtained.[177,178] Measurements of IgM levels specific for each possible organism under consideration are also rec-

ommended. S.Y. has signs of a congenital infection (i.e., respiratory distress, skin rash, and conjunctivitis). Because of the nature of S.Y.'s skin rash (i.e., vesicular), infection with the herpes simplex virus (HSV) should be highly suspected. Skin vesicles, conjunctiva, oropharynx, nasopharynx, rectum, urine, and CSF should be cultured for HSV and other organisms known to cause congenital infections.[178,183,184] Rapid diagnostic testing using tissue scrapings from vesicles and fluorescein-conjugated monoclonal HSV antibody can also be performed.[178,184] Other appropriate tests for the diagnosis and workup of suspected congenital infections also should be performed (e.g., liver enzymes, prothrombin time, partial thromboplastin time, EEG, computed tomography [CT] scan, or magnetic resonance imaging [MRI]).[177,178]

Congenital Herpes

38. Upon investigation it is discovered that S.Y.'s mother has genital herpes. This infection is her first known genital HSV episode and was accompanied by fever and headache. S.Y.'s mother had herpes genital lesions present during the vaginal delivery of S.Y. What are risk factors for HSV infection in S.Y.? What interventions could have lowered S.Y.'s risk for HSV?

The incidence of neonatal HSV infection is approximately 1 in 3,000 live births resulting in an estimated 1,500 to 2,200 new cases each year in the United States.[184] Neonatal HSV may be acquired in utero by either transplacental or ascending vaginal and cervical infections, perinatally via passage through a birth canal with active herpes lesions, or postnatally.[178] Most congenital HSV infections (90%) are acquired during passage through the birth canal in the intrapartum period, whereas 5% are acquired transplacentally, and 5% postnatally through close contact.[183] Ascending infections are more likely to occur with prolonged rupture of membranes. Factors that increased the risk of HSV in S.Y. include primary maternal infection during delivery, prolonged rupture of membranes, presence of active lesions at vaginal birth, and use of a fetal scalp monitor during active herpes infection.[178] The most important of these risk factors is primary maternal genital HSV infection at the time of delivery. Neonates born vaginally to these women are 10 times more likely to develop HSV infections than neonates born vaginally to women with recurrent HSV infection (33% to 50% risk of HSV versus 3% to 5%).[182] Identification of newborns at high risk for HSV is difficult, however, because most women who give birth to HSV-infected neonates have asymptomatic or unrecognized HSV infection at the time of delivery. These women also have negative histories for HSV genital infection.

In women with active genital herpes lesions, delivery by cesarean section can reduce the newborn's exposure to HSV lesions and therefore decrease the risk of perinatal transmission. Prolonged rupture of membranes, however, can lessen the protective effect of cesarean delivery by increasing the risk of an ascending HSV infection. Therefore, cesarean section cannot prevent all cases of neonatal HSV. In fact, as many as 20% to 30% of infants with congenital HSV infection are delivered by cesarean section.[183] In S.Y.'s case, delivery by cesarean section may have decreased S.Y.'s risk for HSV infection, especially if performed before or shortly (within 4 to 6 hours) after the rupture of membranes.[183]

Treatment

39. Cultures for HSV and other organisms have been obtained from S.Y. as described in Question 37. Why should therapy be initiated before culture results are available?

Neonatal HSV infections can result in significant morbidity and mortality. Given S.Y.'s signs of infection and risk factors, she should be treated as a case of probable HSV infection until culture results confirm the diagnosis. Three patterns of neonatal HSV infection can occur: (1) disseminated infection (multiple organ involvement) with or without encephalitis; (2) localized CNS infection; and (3) localized infection of the skin, eyes, or mouth (SEM). Approximately 25% to 30% of newborns are symptomatic on the first day of life. Most infants present with SEM disease; however, 60% to 70% progress to disseminated disease or CNS infection.[183] S.Y. has several signs of disseminated infection, including irritability, respiratory distress, and skin vesicles. Other signs of disseminated disease include seizures, coagulopathy, jaundice, and shock. Neonates with CNS disease usually present at 10 to 14 days of life with temperature instability, hypotonia, lethargy, or seizures.[178] Morbidity and mortality for neonatal HSV infections are extremely high if left untreated but can be decreased with appropriate treatment. Even with treatment, disseminated infections have the worst prognosis with a mortality rate of 57%.[183] Mortality rates for CNS disease are 15%, and approximately two-thirds of these infants will have neurologic abnormalities; mortality from SEM disease is essentially zero.[178,184] Early treatment also is important because it can halt the progression of less severe SEM infections to more severe forms (i.e., encephalitis and disseminated disease).

Intravenous acyclovir is the antiviral of choice for the treatment of neonatal HSV infection.[182] The recommended acyclovir dose is 60 mg/kg per day in three divided doses given intravenously for a minimum of 14 days. A longer duration (21 days) is recommended for the treatment of CNS or disseminated HSV disease.[182] Since acyclovir is primarily excreted via the kidneys, the dose must be reduced in neonates with renal dysfunction (e.g., SCr >0.8 mg/dL). These neonates should receive 20 mg/kg per dose administered every 12 to 24 hours, depending on serum creatinine.[185] S.Y. should receive acyclovir 40 mg IV every 8 hours (60 mg/kg per day) for a minimum of 14 days plus topical antiviral ophthalmic therapy (see Table 94-9). Liver enzymes, serum creatinine, BUN, and CBC should be monitored for adverse effects of acyclovir. Phlebitis at the injection site also may occur.[8]

Recurrence of mucocutaneous HSV is common and is associated with neurologic sequelae if it occurs more than three times during the first 6 months of life.[182] In a small, phase I/II trial, oral acyclovir suppressive therapy (300 mg/m² per dose given three times daily for 6 months), initiated after completion of 10 days of acyclovir treatment for neonatal SEM disease, prevented cutaneous recurrences of HSV.[186] However, approximately 50% of the infants developed neutropenia while receiving suppressive acyclovir therapy. A larger study comparing different acyclovir suppressive dosage regimens and the effects on neurologic outcome of infants is needed.

Other Congenital Infections
Toxoplasmosis

Congenital toxoplasmosis, an infection caused by the protozoan organism, *Toxoplasma gondii*, usually results from maternal ingestion of uncooked meat or contact with infected cats. In the United States, 400 to 4,000 cases of congenital toxoplasma infection are reported yearly.[179] The only mode of human-to-human transmission is transplacental. The rate of transmission is highest during the later stages of pregnancy. However, if infection occurs earlier in gestation, the infant will develop a more severe form of infection. Most newborns infected with *T. gondii* are asymptomatic. The most common manifestation of *T. gondii* infection in neonates is chorioretinitis. These infants may develop permanent visual loss.[179]

Other clinical symptoms are listed in Table 94-9. Maternal treatment with spiramycin (currently investigational) can be administered to the infected mother to help reduce vertical transmission of *T. gondii*. If the diagnosis of an in utero toxoplasmosis infection is made, treatment of both the mother and the fetus reduces the sequelae in the infant. Therapy includes sulfadiazine and pyrimethamine. Folinic acid (leucovorin) is given to decrease potential toxic effects of pyrimethamine.[179,187]

Syphilis

Syphilis is caused by a spirochete, *Treponema pallidum,* and can be acquired by direct contact with ulcerative, denuded lesions of the mucous membranes or skin of the infected person. Vertical transmission of congenital syphilis can either occur transplacentally or during delivery by contact of the newborn with genital lesions. In fact, the rate of transmission can be as high as 100% during the secondary stage of the disease.[182] Forty percent of pregnancies in women with untreated early syphilis result in spontaneous abortion, stillbirth, nonimmune hydrops, premature delivery, and perinatal death.[182] Clinical manifestations of congenital syphilis are divided into two syndromes, early (occurring before 2 years of life) and late (occurring after 2 years). The most classic presentations of congenital syphilis are bone lesions, hepatosplenomegaly, erythematous maculopapular rash (primarily on the hands and feet), and rhinitis ("snuffles"). Other clinical manifestations are listed in Table 94-9. Parenteral penicillin G is the preferred treatment and is the only drug that has documented efficacy for the treatment of congenital syphilis. If >1 day of therapy is missed, the entire course must be restarted.[182]

Hepatitis B Virus

Unlike other congenital infections (e.g., toxoplasmosis, syphilis), hepatitis B virus (HBV) infection is rarely transmitted transplacentally, especially if infection occurs during the first or second trimesters. However, the rate of transmission can be as high as 60% if infection occurs in the third trimester.[181] Most infants with HBV are infected around the time of birth as a consequence of exposure to maternal HBV-positive genital tract secretions and blood.[181] Newborns with HBV infection are usually asymptomatic initially, but the majority (91%) can become chronic carriers of HBsAg. Many of these infants develop long-term sequelae such as chronic hepatitis, cirrhosis, and hepatocellular carcinoma. Neonatal chronic carrier rates of HBV can be significantly decreased to 0% to 14% with the combined use of hepatitis B vaccination and hepatitis B immune globulin (HBIG).[181] Owing to these beneficial effects, the Centers for Disease Control and Prevention (CDC) recommends that all newborn infants should be immunized with hepatitis B vaccination regardless of the mothers' hepatitis status (see Chapter 95, Immunizations).

Rubella

Rubella was a common viral illness affecting humans; however, with the advent of vaccines, the prevalence of rubella has significantly decreased. The virus crosses the placenta and infects the fetus, resulting in spontaneous abortion, stillbirth, or birth defects known as congenital rubella syndrome (CRS). The rate of congenital infection is highest during the first trimester (80%), but transmission can also occur at any time of pregnancy.[178] CRS is characterized by hearing loss, cataracts, and congenital heart disease (primarily PDA [patent ductus arteriosus] and pulmonary artery stenosis); intrauterine growth retardation also commonly occurs. Other clinical findings of CRS are listed in Table 94-9. In a 20-year follow-up study, ocular disease (i.e., cataracts, retinopathy, glaucoma) was found to affect approximately 80% of infants with CRS.[178] Currently, there are no effective antiviral medications for the treatment of CRS; therefore, it is important to provide universal immunization with rubella vaccination to all children.[182]

Cytomegalovirus Infection

CMV is the most common cause of congenital infection affecting approximately 40,000 infants each year.[188] Transmission of CMV can occur transplacentally at any stage of pregnancy or during delivery. The rate of transmission from the mother to the fetus is much higher in mothers with primary CMV infection (40% to 50%) than in those with recurrent infection (<1%).[188] CMV infection can also be transmitted through breast milk or close contact.[178] Approximately 10% of the infants with CMV infection are symptomatic at birth (i.e., 90% are asymptomatic).[188] The most common manifestations of CMV infection in symptomatic infants less than 2 weeks of age are petechiae, hepatosplenomegaly, jaundice, and prematurity.[178] Mortality rates in severely affected infants can be as high as 30%, and most infants surviving the infection have permanent damage such as visual deficits, hearing loss, seizure disorders, and learning and motor disabilities.[178,188] Currently there is no proven effective antiviral therapy for congenital CMV infection. Treatment with IV ganciclovir is under investigation for infants with symptomatic CMV infection.[178,188]

APNEA

Pathogenesis

Apnea in neonates is a life-threatening condition that occurs more frequently in premature newborns and newborns of lower birth weights. Only 7% of infants 34 to 35 weeks' gestational age have apnea.[189] In contrast, the incidence of apnea has been reported to be 78% in infants 26 to 27 weeks' gestational age and 84% in infants with birth weights <1,000 g.[189] Although several definitions exist,[190,191] clinically significant apnea may be defined as cessation of breathing for ≥15 seconds, or less if accompanied by bradycardia (HR <100 beats/minute), significant hypoxemia, or cyanosis.[192–194] Pallor or hypotonia also may occur.

In neonates, apnea may be caused by a severe underlying illness, drugs, or prematurity itself (Fig. 94-3). Appropriate patient history, physical examination, and laboratory tests must be evaluated to rule out other causes of apnea before the diagnosis of apnea of prematurity can be made.[192,193] It is especially important to rule out sepsis before apnea of prematurity is presumed. If an etiology other than prematurity is identified, therapy would be directed toward that specific cause. For example, antibiotics would be used to treat neonatal sepsis with secondary apnea.

Apnea of prematurity is classified into three types: central, obstructive, and mixed. Approximately 40% of apneic episodes are of central origin (i.e., no respiratory effort), 10% are due to obstruction, and 50% are due to both (i.e., mixed

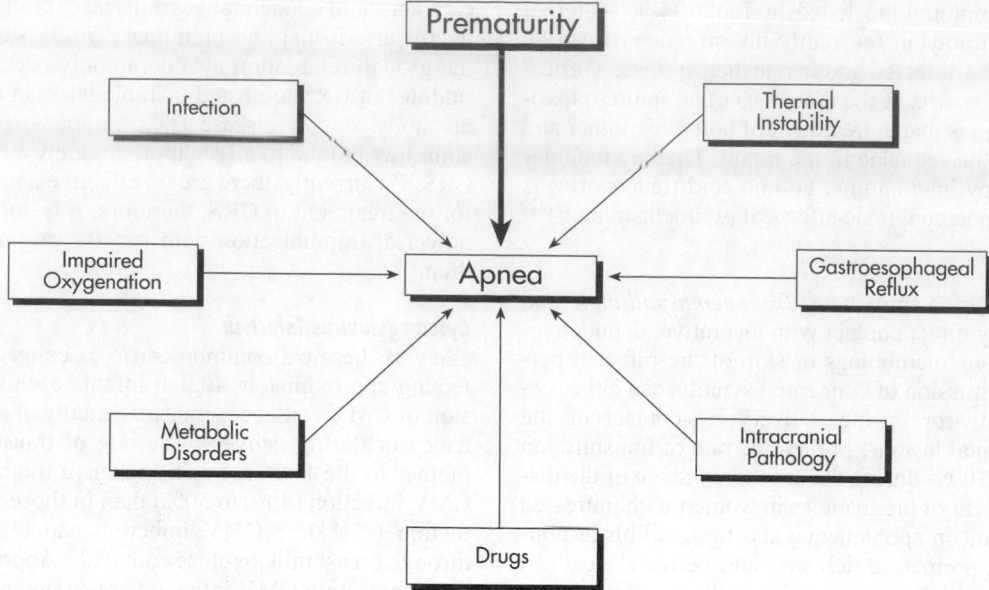

FIGURE 94-3 Causes of apnea in the neonate. (Reproduced with permission from Martin RJ et al. Pathogenesis of apnea in preterm infants. J Pediatr 1986;109:738.)

events).[195] Although these terms imply separate mechanisms, recent investigations suggest that obstruction/airway closure is important in all three types (even "central").[189] Treatment of apnea of prematurity includes the use of supplemental oxygen, gentle tactile stimulation, environmental temperature control, oscillation water beds, methylxanthines, nasal continuous positive airway pressure, and positive-pressure ventilation.[192,193]

Treatment
Methylxanthines

40. S.M., a premature male newborn of 29 weeks' gestational age, had a birth weight of 995 g. On day 2 of life, he develops seven episodes of apnea followed by bradycardia with HR as low as 85 beats/min. These episodes last 20 to 30 seconds in duration and require administration of oxygen and tactile stimulation. Three prolonged episodes required bag and mask ventilation. Between apneic spells the newborn appears well; physical examination and laboratory tests are normal for gestational age. Appropriate cultures are drawn for a septic workup and ampicillin and gentamicin are initiated. The decision is made to begin aminophylline. What is the rationale for the use of methylxanthines in apnea of prematurity and what dosing considerations must be addressed?

RATIONALE
Methylxanthine therapy generally is initiated for apnea of prematurity when apneic episodes are frequent (e.g., more than three episodes), prolonged (e.g., duration >20 to 30 seconds), or severe in nature (e.g., accompanied by significant bradycardia or cyanosis) or are not controlled by nonpharmacologic means (e.g., gentle tactile stimulation, environmental temperature control, or oscillation water beds). This infant's apneic episodes are frequent, prolonged, and severe, and therefore will require pharmacologic intervention.

Methylxanthines, specifically theophylline and caffeine, are widely accepted as the initial pharmacologic approach for the treatment of idiopathic apnea of prematurity.[193,196] These agents decrease apneic episodes via both central and peripheral effects. Methylxanthines stimulate the medullary respiratory center and increase receptor responsiveness to carbon dioxide. This results in an increase in respiratory drive and minute ventilation.[193,196] Central stimulatory effects may be mediated by adenosine receptor blockade. Adenosine is a known inhibitor of respiration, and both theophylline and caffeine competitively inhibit adenosine at the receptor level.[197] Other central effects, such as alteration of sleep-awake patterns, also may be important.[198] Peripherally, methylxanthines increase diaphragmatic contractility, decrease diaphragmatic fatigue, and improve respiratory muscle contraction.[196,199,200] In addition, methylxanthines increase catecholamine release and metabolic rate. This may improve cardiac output and oxygenation, lessen hypoxic episodes, and decrease apneic spells.

DOSING CONSIDERATIONS
Several developmental pharmacokinetic and pharmacodynamic factors need to be considered when dosing theophylline in neonates. Protein binding of theophylline is decreased in term newborns (36%) compared with adults (65%).[24] The decreased protein binding along with an increased tissue distribution results in a larger Vd of theophylline in neonates (see Table 94-2). This larger Vd results in larger loading-dose requirements to attain similar serum concentrations.

Theophylline clearance in preterm newborns (17.6 mL/hour per kilogram) is much slower than that observed in young children 1 to 4 years of age (100 mL/hour per kilogram).[24] As a result, smaller theophylline maintenance doses are required in neonates. Theophylline clearance increases dramatically during the first year of life, approaching adult values at 55 weeks' postconceptional age.[36] Theophylline clearance and therefore maintenance doses increase with increasing postconceptional age. Adjustment of maintenance doses is especially important in infants 40 to 50 weeks' postconceptional age when the greatest maturational changes in theophylline clearance occur.[36]

In adults, theophylline is eliminated primarily via hepatic metabolism by C-8 oxidation to 1,3-methyluric acid (39% of a dose) and by N-demethylation to 3-methylxanthine (16%) and 1-methyluric acid (20%).[201] Small amounts of theophylline are eliminated unchanged in the urine (13%) and 6% of the dose is N-methylated to caffeine.[201,202] In contrast, the primary route of theophylline elimination in neonates is renal excretion of unchanged drug (55%).[36] Hepatic metabolism of theophylline (especially N-demethylation) is decreased in the neonate. Lower amounts of theophylline are eliminated by C-8 oxidation to 1,3-methyluric acid (24%) and by N-demethylation to 3-methylxanthine (1.4%) and 1-methyluric acid (8.2%).[36] As in adults, theophylline is methylated to caffeine in the neonate. The neonate's decreased demethylation pathway, however, results in a decrease in caffeine elimination and significant serum caffeine accumulation. On average, serum caffeine concentrations can be 40% of the serum theophylline concentration.[36] The theophylline-derived caffeine may contribute to the pharmacologic and toxic effects seen in neonates receiving theophylline. After 50 weeks' postconceptional age, the theophylline-derived serum caffeine concentrations become insignificant.

The generally accepted therapeutic range of theophylline for apnea of prematurity is 6 to 12 μg/mL. This range is lower than that which is normally accepted for the treatment of asthma (10 to 20 μg/mL) for several reasons: (1) the higher free fraction of theophylline found in neonates results in a higher free concentration at any given total concentration; (2) there is a significant accumulation of the unmeasured active metabolite, caffeine; and (3) a different mechanism of action for theophylline is being exploited for apnea (i.e., central stimulation versus bronchodilation for asthma). Although some neonates may respond to theophylline serum concentrations as low as 2.8 μg/mL,[198] most require concentrations in the generally accepted therapeutic range.[203]

DOSING AND ADMINISTRATION

Although oral aminophylline and theophylline are considered to be well absorbed in the neonate, many neonates initially have feeding problems when apnea and bradycardia are present. Therefore, S.M. should initially receive IV therapy, and an oral nonalcoholic solution can be used when S.M. is stable and tolerating oral feedings. It should be remembered that depending on the specific product used, aminophylline is 80% to 85% theophylline.

An aminophylline IV loading dose of 6 to 7 mg/kg (4.8 to 5.6 mg/kg of theophylline) will produce theophylline levels of approximately 6.4 to 7.5 μg/mL. Most centers use initial maintenance doses of aminophylline in the range of 1 to 2 mg/kg per dose given every 8 to 12 hours, with the lower doses in this range used in younger, more premature infants. For IV administration in neonates, aminophylline should be diluted to 1 mg/mL and infused over 20 to 30 minutes.[8] An aminophylline maintenance dose for S.M. of 1 mg/kg per dose every 8 hours should produce steady-state theophylline serum concentrations in the midtherapeutic range. Lower

doses for S.M., as recommended by the FDA guidelines (theophylline 1 mg/kg every 12 hours for preterm neonates less than 24 days postnatal age),[204] will result in serum concentrations below 5 μg/mL in most infants less than 40 weeks' postconceptional age.[205] Concomitant drug therapy and disease states (e.g., hepatic or renal dysfunction) also should be taken into consideration when selecting initial theophylline doses.

41. **S.M. was given aminophylline 6 mg (6 mg/kg of aminophylline, 4.8 mg/kg theophylline) as an IV loading dose over 20 minutes. Maintenance doses of 1 mg Q 8 hr have been ordered. Describe your pharmacotherapeutic monitoring plan for S.M. Include monitoring parameters for efficacy and toxicity and duration of therapy.**

The goal of methylxanthine therapy in the treatment of apnea of prematurity is to decrease the number of episodes of apnea and bradycardia. Continuous monitoring of HR and RR is required for proper evaluation. The time, duration, and severity of episodes; activity of the infant; and any necessary intervention performed should be documented. Relationships between the apneic episodes and the feeding schedule and volume of feeds, as well as the dosing schedule of theophylline (e.g., trough), should be examined.

Apnea of prematurity usually resolves by 37 weeks' postconceptional age; however, it may persist in some infants up to or beyond 40 weeks' postconceptional age.[206] In general, the younger the gestational age of the infant at birth, the older the postconceptional age at cessation of apnea. Apnea of prematurity frequently persists beyond 36 weeks' postconceptional age in infants born at 28 weeks' gestational age or less, and persists beyond 40 weeks' postconceptional age in 22% of infants born at 24 weeks' gestational age.[206] Therefore, methylxanthine therapy usually is discontinued at 35 to 37 weeks' postconceptional age provided that the infant has not been having apneic spells.[193] Infants that require therapy for longer periods of time may be discharged home on methylxanthines with apnea monitors.

Toxicities noted in neonates include tachycardia, agitation, irritability, hyperglycemia, feeding intolerance, gastroesophageal reflux, and emesis or occasional spitting up of food. Tachycardia is the most common toxicity and usually responds to a downward adjustment of the theophylline dose. Tachycardia may persist for 1 to 3 days after dosage reductions owing to the decreased elimination of theophylline-derived caffeine. Seizures also have been reported with accidental overdoses. Methylxanthine toxicity can be minimized with careful dosing and appropriate monitoring of serum concentrations. Serum theophylline concentrations should be monitored 72 hours after initiation of therapy or after a change in dosage. Serum concentrations of theophylline also should be measured if the infant experiences an increase in the number of apneic episodes, signs or symptoms of toxicity, or a significant increase in weight. In asymptomatic neonates, once steady-state levels are obtained, theophylline concentrations may be monitored every 2 weeks.

42. **S.M. now is 3 weeks old (32 weeks' postconceptional age) and weighs 1,100 g. His septic workup was negative. Currently, S.M. has several apneic spells per day, which respond to tactile stimulation; his apneic episodes have not required ventilatory assistance. S.M. receives 1 mg aminophylline IV Q 8 hr, and his**

trough theophylline level this morning was 5.7 µg/mL. The medical team is considering switching S.M.'s theophylline therapy to caffeine because of possible improved benefits. How does caffeine compare with theophylline with regard to its pharmacokinetics, efficacy, and toxicity? What treatment should be selected?

PHARMACOKINETICS

The plasma clearance of caffeine is considerably lower and the half-life is extremely prolonged in the premature newborn (see Table 94-2). The low clearance is a reflection of the decreased neonatal hepatic metabolism and a resultant dependence of elimination on the slow urinary excretion. In the preterm neonate, the amount of caffeine excreted unchanged in the urine is 85%, compared with <2% in adults. Adult urinary metabolite patterns are seen by 7 to 9 months of age.[207] The half-life of caffeine decreases with increasing postconceptional age[208] and plasma clearance reaches adult levels after 3 to 4.5 months of life.[209] As a result of the maturational changes, doses usually need to be adjusted after 38 weeks' postconceptional age and dosing intervals need to be shortened to 8 hours after 50 weeks' postconceptional age.[208]

EFFICACY, TOXICITY, AND DOSING

Comparative studies have found similar efficacy for theophylline and caffeine in the control of apnea of prematurity.[196,210] Caffeine, however, may have some advantages over theophylline, including a wider therapeutic index. Adverse effects such as tachycardia, CNS excitation, and feeding intolerance are reported more frequently with theophylline than with caffeine. The prolonged half-life of caffeine in premature neonates results in less fluctuation in plasma concentrations and permits the use of a 24-hour dosing interval. Because the half-life is prolonged and dosing requirements do not change quickly over time, caffeine serum concentrations can be monitored less frequently. Loading doses of 10 mg/kg of caffeine base (20 mg/kg of caffeine citrate), followed 24 hours later by maintenance doses of 2.5 mg/kg (5 mg/kg caffeine citrate) given daily will maintain plasma caffeine concentrations in the therapeutic range (5 to 20 µg/mL).[196] Loading doses of caffeine citrate are recommended to be given IV over 30 minutes using a syringe infusion pump. Maintenance doses can be administered IV over 10 minutes or given orally.[99] Because of the longer half-life, infants receiving caffeine must be monitored for a longer period of time (e.g., for 7 to 10 days) for adverse effects if toxicities occur and for efficacy once the medication is discontinued. Another disadvantage of caffeine is its high cost. Although infants who are unresponsive to theophylline may respond to caffeine,[211] S.M.'s theophylline therapy presently is not optimized; his serum concentration is <6 µg/mL. S.M. appears to have partially responded to theophylline and may benefit from an increase in the dose with resultant therapeutic serum concentrations. S.M.'s aminophylline dose should be increased to 1.5 mg every 8 hours to achieve serum concentrations of approximately 8 µg/mL. Caffeine may have several advantages over theophylline. Now that a preservative-free caffeine citrate product is available in the United States,[99] its use is increasing. It is important to remember that another IV caffeine product is marketed in the United States as the sodium benzoate salt. Benzoic acid has been associated with the gasping syndrome and also may displace bilirubin from albumin binding sites.[39,40] Because of these toxicities, the caffeine sodium benzoate product should not be used in neonates.

Other Agents

43. S.M.'s dose of theophylline has been optimized and theophylline serum concentrations now are 12.4 µg/mL. S.M. continues to have apneic episodes. What other pharmacologic agents can be used?

Doxapram, an analeptic agent, has been shown to be as effective as theophylline for the treatment of apnea of prematurity.[212,213] Because of the limited number of investigations and uncertain side effects, however, doxapram should be restricted to patients who are refractory to methylxanthine therapy.[196] In addition, the IV preparation commercially available in the United States contains 0.9% benzyl alcohol and should be used with caution. Although doses are not well defined, a loading dose of 2.5 to 3 mg/kg given IV over 15 to 30 minutes followed by a 1 mg/kg per hour continuous infusion has been recommended.[196] Doses may be increased by 0.5 mg/kg per hour increments to a maximum dose of 2.5 mg/kg per hour.[196] Lower doses have been used in infants receiving concomitant methylxanthine therapy with approximately 50% responding to IV doxapram doses of 0.5 mg/kg per hour.[214] A few studies have administered doxapram enterally; however, bioavailability in preterm newborns is not well defined[196,215] and routine use of oral doxapram cannot be recommended.[216] Side effects associated with doxapram include the following: cardiovascular problems such as increased BP (usually with doses >1.5 mg/kg per hour)[214] and second-degree atrioventricular heart block with prolonged QT interval[217]; GI disturbances such as abdominal distention, regurgitation, increased gastric residuals, and vomiting; and CNS adverse effects such as increased agitation, excessive crying, jitteriness, irritability, disturbed sleep, and seizures. Further studies of doxapram are needed to better delineate its adverse effects and to help define its safety and efficacy for the treatment of apnea of prematurity.

PERIVENTRICULAR-INTRAVENTRICULAR HEMORRHAGE
Pathogenesis

44. M.C., a 3-day-old male infant, was born at 28 weeks' gestation with a birth weight of 980 g. He was intubated shortly after birth for respiratory distress and last night developed a pneumothorax. This morning, M.C. required a blood transfusion because of a significant drop in hematocrit. Hypotension, hypotonia, and decreased responsiveness now are noted on physical examination. An ultrasound of the infant's head was ordered to confirm the suspicion of an intraventricular bleed. What factors are associated with an increased risk for the development of periventricular-intraventricular hemorrhage (PV-IVH)?

PV-IVH is a significant cause of death in premature newborns and is one of the most common serious neurologic injuries that occurs during the neonatal period. The incidence and severity of PV-IVH is inversely related to gestational age, with the highest frequency occurring in the most immature neonates.[218] PV-IVH occurs in approximately 3% of healthy, term newborns; in >20% of premature newborns <1,500 g birth weight; and in >60% of preterm infants <700 g birth weight.[219,220]

The most common site of origin of the hemorrhage is the periventricular germinal matrix, a highly vascularized cellular region that contains neuronal precursor cells. This vascular network, which is prominent at 26 to 34 weeks' gestational age, contains poorly supported blood vessels that are fragile and vulnerable to injury.[218] Most factors associated with an increased risk of PV-IVH alter cerebral blood flow or arterial BP, which results in damage to these vessels. M.C. has two risk factors that are strongly associated with PV-IVH: prematurity and acute respiratory failure requiring mechanical ventilation.[218] Other associated risk factors include pneumothorax (which M.C. also has), hypotension, hypertension, hypoxia, hypercapnia, asphyxia, acidosis, rapid volume expansion, coagulation defects, infusion of hyperosmolar substances (e.g., sodium bicarbonate), hypernatremia, hyperglycemia, seizures, PDA, heparin use, tracheal suctioning, and inadvertent noxious stimulation.[218–221] The use of low-dose heparin in umbilical catheter infusions (1 unit/mL) may not increase the risk of PV-IVH, but larger studies are required.[222]

Common signs and symptoms of PV-IVH include hypotension, hypotonia, a drop in hematocrit, and a decrease in responsiveness as illustrated by M.C. Apnea, oculomotor disturbances, areflexia, tonic posturing, flaccid quadriparesis, seizures, and death also may occur.[223] Prognosis for normal neurologic development in survivors depends on location and severity of the bleed. Mild hemorrhages (grade I, isolated germinal matrix hemorrhage and grade II, hemorrhage extending into normal-size ventricles) have a better prognosis, but may result in cognitive deficits such as reading disabilities or other learning problems. Approximately 10% of infants with mild hemorrhages develop a major disability, such as spastic diplegia. Infants with moderate (grade III, hemorrhage extending into enlarged ventricles) or severe hemorrhages (grade IV, intraparenchymal hemorrhage) do worse with an increase in major motor (e.g., spastic hemiparesis, quadriplegia) and intellectual deficits. Infants with moderate and severe bleeds also are more likely to develop posthemorrhagic hydrocephalus and seizure activity. Those with severe hemorrhage have a higher mortality rate.[218]

Treatment

45. How is PV-IVH managed and what therapies have been investigated to prevent PV-IVH?

Management and prevention of PV-IVH include the reduction or elimination of known risk factors. Because prematurity is a major risk factor, prevention of premature birth is the most effective way to eliminate PV-IVH. However, antenatal tocolytic agents such as maternal β-sympathomimetics and indomethacin have been shown to increase the incidence of IVH in infants.[220,221] Other antenatal pharmacologic agents (magnesium sulfate, phenobarbital, vitamin K, and corticosteroids) have been investigated to reduce PV-IVH, but only antenatal corticosteroids are currently recommended.[64,218,220,221] Antenatal maternal corticosteroids significantly reduce the incidence and severity of PV-IVH (as well as the incidence of RDS and infant mortality).[64,220] Corticosteroids may prevent PV-IVH by stabilizing or promoting maturation of the endothelium of the fragile blood vessels of the germinal matrix.[218,221] Because even partial courses of maternal corticosteroids are beneficial, M.C may have benefited from prompt

treatment of his mother with corticosteroids as soon as the risk for preterm delivery was identified (see previous section, Respiratory Distress Syndrome).[64,219,221]

To prevent PV-IVH after birth, wide variations in BP and cerebral blood flow, abnormalities in serum osmolality and blood gases, and noxious stimulations should be avoided. Several postnatal pharmacologic agents, including phenobarbital, indomethacin, ethamsylate, vitamin E, and pancuronium have been investigated for the prevention of PV-IVH.[218] At present, none of these are widely accepted for routine use in newborn infants. Of the agents studied, low-dose indomethacin offers the best potential for PV-IVH prophylaxis.[220,224] A multicenter, randomized, placebo-controlled trial using indomethacin (0.1 mg/kg per dose IV at 6 to 12 hours after birth and every 24 hours for two additional doses) significantly lowered the incidence and severity of IVH in neonates of 600 to 1,250 g birth weight.[224] Postnatal low-dose indomethacin therapy also significantly lowered the incidence of IVH in infants whose mothers received antenatal corticosteroid therapy.[225]

Indomethacin, a cyclooxygenase inhibitor, may prevent IVH by reducing the synthesis of vasodilating prostanoids and prostaglandins. This results in a decrease in baseline cerebral blood flow and changes in cerebral blood flow modulation. Inhibition of cyclooxygenase also may decrease formation of harmful free radicals. Because indomethacin lowers cerebral blood flow, concerns about increased risks of cerebral ischemic injury and neurodevelopmental handicaps exist. One follow-up study conducted at 36 months of corrected age showed that low-dose indomethacin did not result in any adverse cognitive or motor outcomes.[225] Although this appears promising, further long-term follow-up investigations are needed before the use of low-dose indomethacin in premature infants can be recommended universally.[219,221]

NEONATAL SEIZURES
Pathogenesis and Diagnosis

46. F.H., a term female newborn (weight 3.5 kg), has a history of perinatal asphyxia. Apgar scores were 2 and 4 at 1 and 5 minutes, respectively. Forty-eight hours after birth, F.H. begins to have rhythmic clonic twitching of the right hand, repetitive chewing movements, fluttering of the eyelids, and occasional pendular movements of the extremities that resemble swimming motions. What interventions should be initiated immediately for F.H.?

Seizure activity may be difficult to recognize in the term or premature neonate. Because of the immaturity of the cortex, neonatal seizures rarely are generalized tonic-clonic events, but can be clonic (focal or multifocal), tonic (focal or generalized), myoclonic (focal, multifocal, or generalized), or subtle in nature.[226] Subtle seizures include activities such as abnormal oral-buccal-lingual movements; ocular movements; swimming, pedaling, or stepping movements; and occasionally apnea.[223] In addition, autonomic nervous system signs such as changes in HR, BP, respirations, skin color, oxygenation, salivation, or pupil size may occur.[227] Clinical neonatal seizures may or may not be associated with EEG changes.[227]

Neonatal seizure activity is a common manifestation of a life-threatening underlying neurologic process (Table 94-10)

Table 94-10 Causes of Neonatal Seizures

Metabolic

Hypoxic-ischemia (i.e., asphyxia)
   Hypoxia
   Hypoglycemia
   Hypocalcemia
Hypoglycemia
   Intrauterine growth retardation
   Infant of a diabetic mother
   Glycogen storage disease
   Galactosemia
   Idiopathic
Hypocalcemia
   Hypomagnesemia
   Infant of a diabetic mother
   Neonatal hypoparathyroidism
   Maternal hyperparathyroidism
   High phosphate load
Other electrolyte imbalances
   Hypernatremia
   Hyponatremia

Cerebrovascular Lesions (other than trauma)

Cerebral infarction (thrombotic versus embolic) ischemic versus
   hemorrhagic
Cortical vein thrombosis

Trauma

Subarachnoid hemorrhage
Intracranial hemorrhage
Subdural/epidural hematoma
Intraventricular hemorrhage

Infections

Bacterial meningitis
Viral-induced encephalitis

Congenital infections
   Herpes
   Cytomegalovirus
   Toxoplasmosis
   Syphilis
   Coxsackie meningoencephalitis
   AIDS
Brain abscess

Brain Anomalies (i.e., cerebral dysgenesis from either congenital or acquired courses)

Drug Withdrawal or Toxins

Prenatal substance: methadone, heroin, barbiturate, cocaine, etc.
Prescribed medications: propoxyphene, isoniazid
Local anesthetics
Bilirubin

Hypertensive Encephalopathy

Amino Acid Metabolism

Branched-chain amino acidopathies
Urea-cycle abnormalities
Nonketotic hyperglycinemia
Ketotic hyperglycinemia

Pyridoxine Dependency

Familial Seizures

Neurocutaneous syndromes
Tuberous sclerosis
Incontinentia pigmenti
Autosomal-dominant neonatal seizures

Selected Genetic Syndrome

Zellweger syndrome
Neonatal adrenal leukodystrophy
Smith-Lemli-Opitz syndrome

Adapted with permission from reference 227.

and therefore initial efforts may not include antiepileptic drug therapy. Definitive treatment is directed toward specific identified etiologies. The acute evaluation of neonatal seizures includes assessment of the infant's airway, breathing, and circulation and a review of the infant's history, physical examination, and laboratory studies. Every neonate with seizure activity should have a bedside determination of glucose; laboratory determinations of serum electrolytes, including sodium, BUN, glucose, calcium (Ca), and magnesium (Mg); blood gases; bilirubin; and an infectious disease workup, including CBC with platelets, blood culture, urine culture, lumbar puncture with CSF analysis (cell count, protein, glucose), and CSF culture.[223,226] Treatment with antiepileptic drugs is indicated after correction of known electrolyte abnormalities. Antiepileptic drug therapy can be initiated (after correction of hypoglycemia) while laboratory test results are pending.

If the aforementioned tests do not reveal any abnormalities, an EEG, metabolic disease workup (e.g., serum ammonia, lactate, pyruvate; serum and urine amino and organic acids), and screening of blood and urine for drugs can be performed.[223,226,227] Intrauterine infections that are associated with congenital neurologic abnormalities and seizures can be identified by obtainment of TORCH titers (see Question 37). Cranial ultrasounds, CT scans, and MRIs may be obtained to identify infarcts, hemorrhages, calcifications, or cerebral malformations that may cause seizure activity.[223,228]

47. **The physician assesses F.H. as having adequate ventilation and circulation. She establishes an IV line and sends blood samples for electrolytes, Ca, and Mg. A Chemstrip reveals a blood glucose of 20 mg/dL. What is your assessment and recommendation at this time?**

Hypoglycemia appears to be the cause of F.H.'s seizure activity. Hypoxic ischemic encephalopathy (secondary to asphyxia), however, is the most common cause of neonatal seizures. Hypoxic ischemic encephalopathy can be associated with metabolic abnormalities such as hypoglycemia, hypocalcemia, and hyponatremia (due to inappropriate secretion of antidiuretic hormone). Hypocalcemia may also be accompanied by hypomagnesemia.[227] Hypoglycemia is defined as a whole blood glucose <20 mg/dL for premature infants and <30 mg/dL for term infants during the first 72 hours of life and <40 mg/dL for any neonate after 72 hours of age. In clinical practice, however, a glucose <40 mg/dL in a neonate of any age would be treated.[229]

F.H. should receive an IV bolus dose of 7 to 14 mL (2 to 4 mL/kg) of dextrose 10% (200 to 400 mg/kg) given over 2 to 3 minutes, followed by a continuous infusion of dextrose 10% at an initial dose of 12.6 to 16.8 mL/hour (6 to 8 mg/kg per minute or 3.6 to 4.8 mL/kg per hour).[228] Serum glucose should be monitored and the dextrose infusion should be titrated as needed. If hypoglycemia persists, possible causes such as islet tumor of the pancreas, adrenal insufficiency, and inborn errors of metabolism should be investigated. Corticosteroids, glucagon, and diazoxide have been used to treat persistent hypoglycemia.[229]

Treatment of Hypocalcemia and Hypomagnesemia

48. The physician administers 10 mL (1 g) of 10% dextrose solution IV and starts an IV infusion of glucose at 8 mg/kg per minute. A repeat Chemstrip reveals a blood glucose of 80 mg/dL, but F.H. continues to have seizure activity. F.H.'s laboratory results come back with the following results: Na, 137 mEq/L; K, 4.3 mEq/L; CO_2, 22 mEq/L; Cl, 104 mEq/L; BUN, 7 mg/dL; SrCr, 0.7 mg/dL; glucose, 25 mg/dL; Mg, 1.0 mEq/L; and Ca, 5 mg/dL. What should be done next to control F.H.'s seizures?

[SI units: Na, 137 mmol/L; K, 4.3 mmol/L; CO_2, 22 mmol/L; Cl, 104 mmol/L; BUN, 2.5 mmol/L of urea; SrCr, 61.9 μmol/L; glucose, 1.4 mmol/L; Mg, 0.5 mmol/L; Ca, 1.25 mmol/L]

F.H. also has hypocalcemia and hypomagnesemia, both of which may cause seizure activity. Neonatal hypocalcemia is defined as a serum calcium <7.5 mg/dL in preterm and <8 mg/dL in term infants[227] or an ionized serum calcium <3 mg/dL.[228] Hypomagnesemia (defined as a serum magnesium <1.5 mEq/L) is rare but may coexist with hypocalcemia. Hypomagnesemia should be suspected when hypocalcemia cannot be corrected despite large doses of calcium.[230]

F.H. should receive calcium gluconate 700 mg (200 mg/kg) given slowly intravenously as a 10% solution[227] and magnesium sulfate 25 to 50 mg/kg per dose (0.2 to 0.4 mEq/kg per dose) intramuscularly as a 50% solution or intravenously as a dilute solution (maximum concentration, 100 mg/mL) admin-

istered over 2 to 4 hours.[8] Doses of calcium gluconate and magnesium sulfate may be repeated based on serum determinations. If IV calcium is administered too quickly, vasodilation, hypotension, bradycardia, and cardiac arrhythmias may occur. Calcium gluconate may be administered intravenously at a maximum rate of 50 mg/ minute while monitoring HR, BP, and electrocardiogram (ECG).[8] To avoid IV extravasation with resultant severe dermal necrosis, calcium salts should be administered through a properly working IV line, and the IV site should be monitored for signs of infiltration.

Treatment With Antiepileptic Drugs

49. Despite normalization of her laboratory tests, F.H. continues to have seizure activity. Phenobarbital 35 mg IV push over 1 minute is administered. Ten minutes later, F.H. continues to have intermittent seizure activity. Describe a pharmacotherapeutic plan to control F.H.'s seizure activity.

Phenobarbital is the initial antiepileptic drug of choice for neonatal seizures; phenytoin and lorazepam usually are considered the second and third drugs of choice.[231] Because of the large Vd of phenobarbital in neonates (approximately 1 L/kg), large initial loading doses of 20 mg/kg are required to produce therapeutic serum concentrations (Table 94-11). Because F.H. received only 10-mg/kg dose (35 mg) of phenobarbital, an additional 10 mg/kg should be given now. Phenobarbital should be administered IV at a rate of ≤1 mg/kg per minute,[8] so a 35-mg dose should be given over at least 10 minutes, not over 1 minute. Rapid administration of phenobarbital may cause respiratory depression, apnea, or hypotension. If F.H. continues to have seizure activity after a total phenobarbital loading dose of 20 mg/kg, additional 5- to 10-mg/kg loading doses may be given every 15 to 20 minutes as needed up to a total loading dose of 40 mg/kg. Ventilatory support may be required when using these higher doses, and serum phenobarbital concentrations should be monitored. Phenobarbital's therapeutic effect of controlling neonatal seizures plateaus at serum concentrations of 40 μg/mL; adverse effects increase at higher serum concentrations.[232]

Table 94-11 Pharmacotherapy of Neonatal Seizures[a]

Drug	Loading Dose	Maintenance Dose	Therapeutic Concentration
Phenobarbital	*IV:* Initial: 20 mg/kg then 5–10 mg/kg Q 15–20 min if needed until total load of 40 mg/kg	*IV PO:* Initial: Premature: 3 mg/kg/day Term: 4 mg/kg/day May need to ↑ to 4–5 mg/kg/day by 2–4 weeks of therapy	20–40 μg/mL
Phenytoin	*IV:* 15–20 mg/kg	*IV:* Initial: 5 mg/kg/day May need to ↑ to ≥10 mg/kg/day by 2–4 weeks of therapy	8–15 μg/mL
Lorazepam	*IV:* 0.05–0.1 mg/kg	May repeat doses if needed Q 10–15 min	—
Diazepam	*IV:* 0.1–0.3 mg/kg	May repeat doses if needed Q 10–15 min	—
Pyridoxine	*IV:* 50–100 mg	*IV PO:* 20–50 mg/day; ↑ dose PRN with age	—
Paraldehyde	*Rectal:* 0.3 mL/kg; dilute 2:1 with mineral oil	May repeat dose if needed in 4–6 hours	—
Valproic acid	*PO:* 20 mg/kg	*PO:* 10 mg/kg/dose Q 12 hr	40–50 μg/mL

[a]See text for comments on appropriate IV administration and monitoring.
IV, intravenous; PO, oral.

If seizure activity is not controlled in F.H. (despite optimal phenobarbital loading doses), a phenytoin loading dose of 70 mg (20 mg/kg) should be administered IV at a rate ≤0.5 mg/kg per minute.[8,226] Rapid IV administration of phenytoin may cause cardiac arrhythmias, bradycardia, or hypotension. Phenytoin also may cause severe damage to tissues if extravasation occurs. Therefore, BP, HR, ECG, and the IV site of infusion should be monitored. Recently, fosphenytoin, the diphosphate ester salt of phenytoin, became available in the United States for IV and IM use in adults.[8] Fosphenytoin is a water-soluble prodrug of phenytoin that undergoes conversion by plasma and tissue esterases to phenytoin, phosphate, and formaldehyde. Fosphenytoin has several advantages over phenytoin. Because of its greater water solubility, the IV preparation does not contain propylene glycol, and thus fosphenytoin may have less cardiovascular adverse effects associated with IV administration. Unlike phenytoin, fosphenytoin's more neutral pH also allows for IM administration. Unfortunately, appropriate clinical studies of fosphenytoin in neonates have not yet been conducted. Unanswered concerns about the neonatal handling of formaldehyde also exist. Currently, routine use of fosphenytoin in neonates cannot be recommended. Studies assessing the safety, efficacy, and optimal dosing are needed.

Lorazepam or diazepam may be used to treat F.H.'s seizures if they are unresponsive to phenobarbital and phenytoin.[233,234] Although lorazepam offers the advantage of a longer duration of effect than diazepam, the use of either agent (especially in combination with phenobarbital) may cause respiratory and CNS depression. RR, BP, and HR should be monitored. Both IV preparations contain propylene glycol and benzyl alcohol. Although these substances have been reported to cause toxicities in newborns, the actual amount administered when using appropriate benzodiazepine doses is minimal and should not pose a significant risk.[233] Doses of lorazepam should be diluted with an equal volume of D_5W, normal saline, or sterile water for injection before IV use and administered slowly over 2 to 5 minutes. The relatively high concentration of diazepam injection (which results in <0.1-mL doses) and its physical incompatibility with most diluents, make it impractical to use in small neonates. As a result, lorazepam has become the preferred benzodiazepine in many neonatal ICUs.

If F.H. continues to have seizure activity, IV pyridoxine, rectal paraldehyde, or oral valproic acid should be considered.[227,235] Oral carbamazepine, primidone, or lamotrigine have also been used to treat neonatal seizures in limited numbers of patients.[226,236] Pyridoxine is a cofactor required for the synthesis of the inhibitory neurotransmitter gamma-aminobutyric acid (GABA). Patients with pyridoxine dependency require higher amounts of pyridoxine for proper GABA synthesis. Pyridoxine dependency is a rare disorder but should be considered in neonates with seizure activity unresponsive to antiepileptic drug therapy. Supplementation of pyridoxine is required for life in these patients.[227]

Antiepileptic Drug Maintenance Doses

50. F.H.'s seizure activity stopped after receiving a total loading dose of 105 mg of phenobarbital and 70 mg of phenytoin. A serum phenobarbital concentration of 35 μg/mL and a phenytoin concentration of 17 μg/mL were measured 1 hour after the phenytoin loading dose (2 hours after the last phenobarbital loading dose). How should maintenance doses of antiepileptic drugs be instituted in F.H.?

It is not surprising that F.H. required both phenobarbital and phenytoin to control her seizures. Although phenobarbital and phenytoin are equally effective, neonatal seizures are controlled in <50% of neonates with either agent alone. When both agents are used together, neonatal seizures are controlled in approximately 60% of neonates.[237]

F.H. should be placed on maintenance doses of both phenobarbital and phenytoin because both drugs were needed to control her seizure activity. Because the half-life of phenobarbital is prolonged in neonates (about 100 to 150 hours), maintenance doses can be instituted 24 hours after the loading dose at 3 to 4 mg/kg per day[227,238] as a single daily dose (see Table 94-11). Although this newborn is term, she should receive a lower dose of phenobarbital (2.5 to 3 mg/kg per day) because of her history of asphyxia. Asphyxiated neonates have a decrease in phenobarbital clearance and therefore require lower maintenance doses than nonasphyxiated neonates to achieve similar phenobarbital serum concentrations.[43] Maintenance doses of phenytoin (3 to 4 mg/kg per day given in divided doses every 12 hours) may be initiated 12 to 24 hours after the loading dose. Serum concentrations of these agents should be monitored periodically because maintenance-dose requirements will increase with time (usually by the second to fourth week of therapy).[238] This may be due to a normal maturation of hepatic enzyme systems with age or induction of P450 enzymes. In neonates, oral phenytoin is poorly absorbed and should be avoided in the acute setting. A routine 25% increase in the dose is needed when converting IV phenytoin to oral to attain similar serum concentrations. In addition, after 2 to 4 weeks of age, dosing intervals of every 8 hours may be needed.

The optimal duration of anticonvulsant treatment of neonatal seizures has not been clearly established. Typically, anticonvulsants are continued for approximately 6 months in neonates with persistently abnormal neurological exams. Because of the potential long-term toxicities of these medications and the low risk of seizure recurrence, anticonvulsants are generally discontinued prior to discharge if the neonate's neurological exam and EEG are normal.[239] However, the duration of anticonvulsant medications should be individualized.

NEONATAL ABSTINENCE SYNDROME

A disturbing incidence of maternal substance abuse and associated obstetric and neonatal complications exists.[240–242] Drugs such as alcohol, opiates, barbiturates, and benzodiazepines readily cross the placenta and may induce fetal dependency. In addition to neonatal abstinence syndrome (NAS), other problems seen in infants of addicted mothers must be recognized to optimize patient care. In utero exposure to drugs of abuse may have serious short-and long-term consequences on fetal growth, physiologic functions, and neurologic development. The use of cocaine during pregnancy may cause complications such as fetal distress, preterm labor, spontaneous abortion, abruptio placentae, stillbirths, or congenital malformations and may place the infant at a higher risk for IVH and NEC.[241,243] Intrauterine growth retardation and sudden infant death syndrome have been associated with heroin, methadone, and cocaine abuse during pregnancy.[241,242] Neonatal systolic hypertension, abnormal thyroid function, hyperbilirubinemia, thrombocytosis, and increased platelet aggregation have been reported with maternal methadone use.[241] The increase of polydrug abuse during pregnancy also may complicate treatment.

Although environmental, familial, and neonatal coexisting factors (such as prematurity and low birth weight) need to be considered, investigations assessing neurobehavioral development suggest that drug-exposed infants may be at a greater risk for certain learning, developmental, and behavioral problems.[240,241] For example, infants born to narcotic-dependent mothers may have later difficulties with short-term memory, attention, concentration, and general processing of perception. Delayed language development has been noted for methadone- and cocaine-exposed infants. Hyperactivity, aggressiveness, impulsiveness, uncontrollable temper, and other behavioral problems have been reported in follow-up studies of infants of drug-dependent mothers.[240,241] Investigations that control for confounding factors are needed to fully assess the long-term neurobehavioral outcomes of drug-exposed infants and the long-term effects of currently recommended therapies.[244]

Clinical Presentation

51. A.K., a 38-week gestation, 2,000-g, small-for-gestational-age female, was born to a gravida 3 para 2 mother with a history of frequent heroin use during pregnancy. A.K.'s mother was enrolled in a methadone maintenance program 1 month ago, and her last dose of methadone was 12 hours before delivery. On further questioning, A.K.'s mother admits to the continued use of heroin and occasional use of crack cocaine. Her last "fix" was 3 hours before delivery. On the first day of life, A.K. became restless, irritable, and tachypneic and displayed spontaneous tremors and a high-pitched cry. A.K. developed vomiting and diarrhea on day 2 of life after starting feedings with a standard formula. Although A.K. frequently would suckle on her fist, she was not able to suckle properly while feeding. A.K.'s drug screen was positive for cocaine, opiates, and methadone. What clinical symptoms of neonatal drug abstinence does A.K. demonstrate? How do the onset, severity, and duration of NAS vary with various commonly abused substances?

Symptoms of drug withdrawal occur in 50% to 90% of infants born to narcotic-dependent mothers, with a higher incidence for methadone (70% to 90%) compared with heroin (50% to 75%).[241] NAS is a generalized disorder characterized by CNS hyperirritability (e.g., hyperactivity, irritability, high-pitched or prolonged cry, hyperreflexia, fist sucking, abnormal sleep pattern, tremor, myoclonic jerks, and rarely, seizures); respiratory difficulties (e.g., stuffy nose, rhinorrhea, respiratory distress, tachypnea, respiratory alkalosis, and apnea); GI dysfunction (e.g., regurgitation, drooling, vomiting, diarrhea, hyperphagia, uncoordinated suck and swallow reflex, and poor feeding); and vague autonomic symptoms (e.g., sneezing, yawning, hiccups, sweating, lacrimation, hyperthermia or hypothermia, and skin mottling).[240–242,244]

The onset, severity, and duration of NAS may be influenced by many factors, including the specific drug(s) abused, duration of drug exposure, time and amount of the mother's last dose before delivery, elimination of the drug by the infant, and the gestational age of the infant at birth.[242,244–246] Preterm infants display a less severe abstinence syndrome compared with term infants, possibly because of their CNS immaturity or a decreased total in utero drug exposure.[245] Neonatal methadone withdrawal may be more severe than heroin withdrawal and is associated with a higher incidence of seizures (10% to 20%).[241] Withdrawal from non-narcotic drugs usually is less severe, but can also be associated with seizures.[247] Typically, the cocaine-exposed newborn is hypertonic when alert, irritable, and tremulous. Infants may display decreased interactive behavior, disorganized sleeping and feeding patterns, abnormal cry patterns, seizures, and may be intermittently lethargic. These symptoms are considered to be signs of cocaine toxicity rather than withdrawal.[242,247,248]

The onset of narcotic drug withdrawal ranges from minutes after delivery to 2 weeks of age, with most symptoms appearing within 72 hours.[242,244] Withdrawal from methadone, however, may be delayed in some infants, with symptoms presenting as late as 2 to 4 weeks of age.[241] Similarly, symptoms of barbiturate withdrawal can appear as late as 10 to 14 days.[244,246] The long elimination half-life of these abused substances contributes to the delayed onset of drug withdrawal (and possibly a greater duration of symptoms). Major symptoms of opiate withdrawal usually continue for 2 to 3 weeks, but subacute signs may persist for 2 to 6 months.[242,244,247] In mild cases, significant symptoms may subside within a week. Maternal polydrug abuse, as seen in A.K., may result in biphasic patterns or recurrence of abstinence syndrome.[244]

A.K.'s presentation is consistent with neonatal narcotic abstinence syndrome. However, clinical manifestations of NAS are similar to other serious neonatal diseases. Disorders such as infection (sepsis, meningitis), metabolic abnormalities (hypoglycemia, hypocalcemia, hypomagnesemia, hypothermia), endocrine dysfunction (adrenal insufficiency, hyperthyroidism), and CNS abnormalities (hemorrhage and anoxia) must be ruled out before specific neonatal abstinence therapy is begun.[242,247] Failure to recognize and treat the aforementioned diseases would have dire consequences for A.K. A.K. also may be at risk for hepatitis and sexually transmitted diseases, including HIV. Therefore, an accurate maternal history or testing also should be performed.

Treatment

52. What initial therapy is recommended for A.K.'s narcotic withdrawal symptoms.

Supportive Care

Because pharmacologic therapy may prolong A.K.'s hospital stay or expose her to unnecessary adverse effects, initial treatment should include nonpharmacologic measures directed at decreasing sensory stimulation. Provision of a quiet, dark, warm environment, gentle handling, and swaddling can be beneficial. Use of a pacifier for non-nutritive, excessive sucking also may help. Hypercaloric formulas (24 cal/oz) should be given as frequent small feedings to supply the additional calories that these infants require (150 to 250 cal/kg per day).[247] Changes in severity of symptoms, vital signs, sleeping and feeding patterns, and weight loss or gain should be monitored. Successful management of 40% to 50% of symptomatic infants can be accomplished with supportive care alone.[242] In addition, most infants who are exposed to cocaine as the primary drug of abuse can be managed successfully without pharmacologic intervention.[242]

Monitoring and Indications for Pharmacologic Treatment

An abstinence scoring system should be used to more objectively assess symptoms of withdrawal and the need for pharmacologic treatment or dosage adjustment. The abstinence scoring sheet lists common signs and symptoms of neonatal opiate withdrawal. The infant is monitored and a number score that indicates severity is assigned to each observed symptom. A "total score" is calculated for each 2- or 4-hour observation period and is used to initiate, increase, decrease, or discontinue pharmacologic therapy.[242] Standardized scoring systems currently are used for all neonates regardless of gestational age; however, one study suggests the need for development of specific scoring systems for preterm newborns.[245] In general, indications for pharmacologic treatment include seizures; excessive weight loss or dehydration due to diarrhea, vomiting, or poor feeding; severe hyperactivity, irritability, tremors, or tachypnea that interferes with feeding; inability to sleep; and significant hypothermia or hyperthermia.[241,247]

A.K. should be monitored closely and, if her symptoms are not controlled with supportive care, pharmacologic therapy is indicated. Pharmacologic therapy is needed in approximately 60% to 90% of infants with NAS.[249] The most common agents used to treat neonatal narcotic or CNS depressant withdrawal are phenobarbital, paregoric (camphorated tincture of opium), diluted tincture of opium, and diazepam. The choice of agent depends on the specific nursery, the predominant symptoms displayed, and the substance of abuse. For example, diazepam would be the preferred agent in neonatal withdrawal from maternal benzodiazepine abuse. Doses of these agents should be initiated at lower amounts and titrated upward to a dose that controls withdrawal symptoms but does not produce toxicity. Once A.K. is symptom free for 3 to 5 days, the dose should be decreased gradually by 10% to 20% per day with close patient monitoring. The goals of pharmacologic therapy are to control the symptoms of withdrawal and wean the patient completely off therapy.

53. A.K.'s laboratory tests were within normal limits and other diseases have been ruled out. Her symptoms have worsened despite supportive care and pharmacologic therapy for NAS is initiated. Phenobarbital was started on day 3 of life with an IV dose of 10 mg Q 12 hr for four doses, followed by 3 mg Q 8 hr. This morning's phenobarbital serum concentration was 27 µg/mL. A.K. is less irritable today (day 6 of life) and no longer is tachypneic. Her tremors have decreased significantly and she no longer has a high-pitched cry. She continues to have significant diarrhea and is feeding poorly. A.K. has not gained weight in the past 4 days. Evaluate A.K.'s therapy. What are your recommendations?

Phenobarbital

Phenobarbital is the drug of choice for NAS due to nonnarcotic (e.g., barbiturate, alcohol) and polydrug abuse[242,246] and because it is a second-line agent for treatment of seizures due to withdrawal. Phenobarbital is effective in approximately

50% of neonates exposed to methadone in utero, but it is effective in approximately 90% of infants exposed to multiple drugs in utero.[247,250] Phenobarbital is especially useful (as demonstrated in A.K.) for controlling symptoms of CNS hyperirritability.[242] GI symptoms of withdrawal, however, do not respond well to phenobarbital. A.K. received the proper phenobarbital total loading dose (20 mg/kg) and maintenance therapy (4.5 mg/kg per day). The recommended loading dose is 15 to 20 mg/kg and can be given as a single dose or in divided doses.[246] A single IV, IM, or oral loading dose may be given when rapid control of symptoms is desired. However, single loading doses may be associated with CNS and respiratory depression (e.g., sedation, apnea, or an increase in periodic breathing). Maintenance doses range from 2 to 6 mg/kg per day.[242] Doses should be adjusted according to symptoms, and serum concentrations should be monitored to avoid toxicity. High dosages of phenobarbital may result in oversedation and impairment of the suck reflex. Other disadvantages of phenobarbital include development of tolerance to the sedative effects, induction of drug metabolism, and oral availability as an elixir containing 14% to 25% alcohol.[246,247] The therapeutic serum concentration for control of withdrawal symptoms has not been clearly identified; however, 20 to 30 µg/mL has been suggested.[244,246] Although A.K.'s serum phenobarbital concentration is within the normal range, she continues to have diarrhea and has not gained weight. Because GI symptoms do not respond well to phenobarbital, an alternative agent (preferably a narcotic) should be selected.

Narcotic Agents

Because paregoric (0.4 mg/mL anhydrous morphine), tincture of opium (10 mg/mL morphine), morphine, and methadone are narcotics, they may have a physiologic advantage over non-narcotics in the treatment of neonatal opiate withdrawal syndrome.[244] In addition, the constipating side effects of narcotics may be advantageous when diarrhea is part of withdrawal symptoms. Although any narcotic theoretically could be used, most studies assessing opioid treatment have used paregoric. Paregoric is easy to administer and controls withdrawal symptoms in 90% of infants. In comparative studies, paregoric improved sucking coordination, nutrient ingestion, and weight gain better than diazepam or phenobarbital. Infants treated with paregoric also may have a lower incidence of seizure episodes than those treated with phenobarbital or diazepam. Unfortunately, large doses of paregoric often are needed and the duration of treatment usually is longer than with other agents.[242,247] In addition to opium alkaloids, paregoric contains unwarranted compounds such as antispasmodics (noscapine, papaverine), camphor (a CNS stimulant that is eliminated slowly), high concentrations of alcohol (44% to 46%), anise oil, benzoic acid, and glycerine. Because some of these substances may have adverse effects on the newborn, a 25-fold dilution of tincture of opium with water (final concentration 0.4 mg/mL morphine) now is preferred.[247] The dilution of tincture of opium is free of unnecessary ingredients and has a lower alcohol concentration. It is stable for 2 weeks after dilution.[246] For term infants, the dose of paregoric (or a 25-fold dilution of tincture of opium) is 0.1 mL/kg or 2 drops/kg (0.04 mg/kg morphine)[247] given orally with feedings every 3 to 4 hours until control of withdrawal symptoms. A.K.'s dose may be initiated at 0.2 mL/dose (or 4 drops/dose) and titrated upward as needed by 0.1 mL/kg per dose every 3 to 4 hours until withdrawal symptoms are controlled. Once symptoms are controlled for 3 to 5 days, the dosage can be tapered gradually (keeping the same dosing interval).[247] A.K. also should be monitored for signs of overtreatment such as hypotonia, lethargy, irregular respirations, and bradycardia.[242]

The use of oral morphine to control neonatal withdrawal symptoms has not been well studied; however, oral preparations of 2 and 4 mg/mL may be used.[247] Oral morphine preparations contain less alcohol than paregoric and do not contain unwanted additives. Parenteral morphine has been used in infants to treat narcotic withdrawal seizures unresponsive to antiepileptic agents[251] and vasomotor collapse secondary to heroin withdrawal.[247] Parenteral morphine, however, may contain sodium bisulfite and phenol, substances that have been associated with adverse effects in newborns when given at higher doses.[247] Parenteral morphine may be used if A.K. is unable to take oral medications and a narcotic agent is desired. Methadone also may be used, but the prolonged elimination half-life (26 hours) makes tapering the dosage difficult. Initial methadone doses of 0.05 to 0.1 mg/kg given every 6 hours are recommended. Doses may be increased by 0.05 mg/kg per dose until control of withdrawal symptoms. Methadone can be administered every 12 to 24 hours once signs of withdrawal are controlled and can be discontinued once doses are weaned down to 0.05 mg/kg per day.[247]

Diazepam, Chlorpromazine, and Clonidine

Diazepam (0.3 to 0.5 mg/kg given every 8 hours) has been used to control the CNS hyperactivity associated with neonatal narcotic withdrawal symptoms.[241] However, diazepam may be less effective than paregoric or phenobarbital in treating symptoms of NAS.[250] Adverse effects, which may be related to prolonged elimination and accumulation of diazepam and metabolites, can limit the drug's usefulness (e.g., depression of the suck reflex, sedation, late-onset seizures, and bradycardia).[244] In addition, the parenteral formulation contains substances (benzyl alcohol, sodium benzoate, ethanol, propylene glycol) known to cause problems in the newborn (see Question 49).[247]

Chlorpromazine (0.5 to 0.7 mg/kg given every 6 hours) controls the CNS and GI symptoms of neonatal withdrawal.[244] Disadvantages of chlorpromazine include a wide spectrum of pharmacologic effects such as cerebellar dysfunction, decreased seizure threshold, prolonged elimination in the neonate (half-life, 3 days), hypothermia, hematologic problems such as eosinophilia, and lack of long-term studies on behavioral outcomes.[244,247] As a result, chlorpromazine rarely is used to treat NAS.

Clonidine is commonly used in adults to treat narcotic withdrawal symptoms. One pilot study in neonates (n = 7) used oral clonidine at an initial single dose of 0.5 to 1 μg/kg. Doses were then increased slowly over 1 to 2 days to 3 to 5 μg/kg per day divided every 4 to 6 hours.[252] Clonidine controlled most neonatal methadone withdrawal symptoms except for poor sleeping. Hypotension and other cardiac adverse effects did not occur. Transient mild metabolic acidosis, however, was reported in two patients. Mean duration of clonidine treatment (13 days) was shorter than phenobarbital treatment (27 days) in a retrospective comparative group. Further clinical trials are needed before clonidine can be routinely recommended for treatment of NAS.

A.K. should receive long-term follow-up to monitor for potential developmental problems. Because A.K. is at risk for recurrence of drug withdrawal, her parents should receive information on recognition of symptoms. Her parents will need instructions of how to care for this drug-exposed infant as well as counseling for drug addiction.

SEDATION AND PARALYSIS DURING VENTILATION
Pharmacology and Monitoring Parameters

54. M.M., a 42-week-gestation (post-term), 3,500-g male, is born with a history of meconium-stained amniotic fluid. At birth, meconium was removed by suction from M.M.'s nose and mouth. M.M. was tachypneic (RR, 80 breaths/min) and cyanotic and had decreased peripheral perfusion. His Apgar score at 1 minute was 5. M.M. was intubated shortly after delivery and his trachea was suctioned to remove meconium. Immediate ABGs, obtained while M.M. was intubated and ventilated with an Ambu bag at 60 breaths/min and 100% oxygen, revealed the following: pH, 7.18; PCO_2, 55 mm Hg; and PO_2, 50 mm Hg. M.M.'s clinical condition and ABG results (acidosis, increased PCO_2, and hypoxia) were consistent with persistent pulmonary hypertension of the newborn and appropriate tests confirmed the diagnosis. He currently is receiving mechanical ventilation using hyperoxia and hyperventilation to achieve a target PCO_2 of 30 mm Hg and pH of 7.5. M.M. had been "fighting the ventilator" and pancuronium bromide 0.35 mg IV every 30 to 60 minutes as needed for spontaneous movement was initiated. M.M.'s other medications are ampicillin and gentamicin to rule out sepsis, and dopamine, dobutamine, and sodium bicarbonate for his persistent pulmonary hypertension of the newborn. After evaluating M.M.'s paralysis therapy, what medications should be started immediately for him?

[SI units: PCO_2, 7.33 kPa, 4.0 kPa, respectively; PO_2, 6.7 kPa]

Neonates with severe lung disease (e.g., RDS, persistent pulmonary hypertension of the newborn, pneumonia) may require mechanical ventilation with high ventilatory settings (high rates or pressures). Ineffective mechanical ventilation results when neonates fight the ventilator (i.e., spontaneously breathe asynchronously or out of phase with mechanical ventilation). Advancements in ventilator technology (e.g., synchronized ventilation or patient-triggered ventilation) may help decrease asynchronized breathing. However, sedation generally is indicated when high ventilator settings are used or when patients fight the ventilator after ventilator adjustments. Paralysis usually is reserved for cases when sedation alone does not improve the effectiveness of mechanical ventilation. Typically, paralysis is required in severely ill, hypoxic neonates such as M.M. Paralysis increases chest wall compliance and allows for adequate oxygenation and ventilation.[253,254] It also decreases oxygen consumption, improves blood gases, and may decrease the risk for pneumothorax.[253,255] In addition, paralysis of neonates with persistent pulmonary hypertension of the newborn (like M.M.) indirectly decreases right-to-left shunting through the ductus arteriosus and foramen ovale and results in increased oxygenation.[256]

Pancuronium bromide causes skeletal muscle paralysis by competitively blocking acetylcholine at postsynaptic nicotinic cholinergic receptors located on the muscle fiber (motor endplate) of the neuromuscular junction.[255,257] At normal clinical doses, pancuronium has minimal ganglionic blocking effects and possesses little histamine-releasing activity.[255,257] Onset of effect occurs within minutes and duration, which typically lasts 30 to 60 minutes following a single dose, increases with incremental dosing. Like pancuronium, vecuronium is also a nondepolarizing neuromuscular blocking agent commonly used in neonates.[8] Each agent may offer certain advantages in specific neonatal patients. Pancuronium is primarily eliminated via the kidneys (60%). Thus, without a dosage adjustment, patients with decreased renal function will have a prolongation of pancuronium's neuromuscular blocking effect. Vecuronium, however, is excreted primarily via biliary elimination (50%) and therefore, dosage reduction in hepatic (but not renal) dysfunction is required. M.M.'s dose of pancuronium is appropriate. Pancuronium and vecuronium can be dosed at 0.05 to 0.1 mg/kg every 30 to 60 minutes IV as needed for spontaneous movement. Some neonates will require a continuous infusion, using doses of either agent of 0.02 to 0.05 mg/kg per hour. Many factors (e.g., serum electrolytes, acid/base balance, concomitant medications) can affect the duration of action of neuromuscular blocking agents and dosage needs to be individualized.[8]

The greatest danger of using any neuromuscular blocking agent is inadvertent disconnection from the ventilator with resultant apnea. When paralytic agents are initiated, adjustments in ventilator settings usually are required to avoid hypoventilation. Clinically important adverse effects include tachycardia and fluid retention with significant edema.[255,258] Although pancuronium usually does not have a significant effect on BP,[258] hypertension[259] and occasional reports of hypotension[260] (usually in marginally hypovolemic neonates) have been reported. Ventilatory settings, blood gases, spontaneous movements, daily weights, fluid intake and output, HR, and BP should be monitored. If tachycardia becomes serious, another nondepolarizing neuromuscular blocking agent with fewer cardiovascular effects, such as vecuronium, can be used.

Paralysis, as well as intubation and mechanical ventilation, may be extremely stressful to the neonate. Neuromuscular blocking agents do not possess any analgesic, sedative, or amnestic effects.[255,257] Therefore, sedation therapy should be instituted as soon as possible in M.M. Neonates and even premature newborns have the anatomic structures and physiologic capacity to sense pain.[261,262] Because clinical symptoms of pain may go undetected in paralyzed neonates, a sedative/analgesic such as morphine may be preferred for sedation. In fact, preliminary data suggest that poor neurologic outcomes may occur less frequently in mechanically ventilated neonates who receive continuous low-dose morphine infusions compared with those who receive infusions of midazolam or placebo.[263] In addition, administration of analgesics for painful procedures may be easily forgotten when neonates are sedated with nonanalgesics such as phenobarbital, benzodiazepines, or chloral hydrate. Because paralysis will mask the clinical symptoms of seizures,[255] M.M. should be monitored carefully for rhythmic fluctuations in HR, BP, ECG, and oxygenation. These rhythmic changes may indicate seizure activity in a paralyzed neonate and, if observed, EEG testing is indicated.[264] The EEG also may be monitored in paralyzed newborns who are at high risk for seizure activity (e.g., asphyxiated neonates). Alternatively, some clinicians advocate routine sedation with phenobarbital

(rather than morphine), which also would treat any clinically inapparent seizure activity.

Morphine usually is administered by slow IV push over 1 to 2 minutes at initial doses of 0.05 to 0.1 mg/kg every 2 to 4 hours.[265] The dose is then titrated according to clinical symptoms. A continuous morphine infusion may be preferred for patients with persistent pulmonary hypertension or in infants requiring intermittent morphine doses every 2 hours or less. Clinically, a bolus infusion of 0.05 mg/kg can be given, followed by a continuous infusion at an initial dose of 0.02 mg/kg per hour (20 μg/kg per hour). The infusion should be carefully titrated. Morphine clearance in neonates, especially premature neonates, is greatly reduced but increases with postconceptional age.[266] Adverse effects of morphine include hypotension, decreased GI motility, respiratory depression, tolerance, and physiologic dependence with prolonged use. The use of morphine in neonates may be limited by histamine release and the development of hypotension.

Fentanyl, a synthetic opiate with less histamine-releasing activity and fewer cardiovascular effects, may be used as an alternative agent. Fentanyl is 50 to 100 times more potent than morphine, but has a shorter duration of action and therefore usually is administered by continuous IV infusion (0.5 to 2 μg/kg per hour).[8,267] Continuous infusion of fentanyl, however, may be associated with a greater development of tolerance and physical dependence compared with intermittent morphine administration.[268,269] Continuous fentanyl infusions of 5 and 9 or more days have been associated with a >50% and a 100% chance, respectively, of developing withdrawal symptoms,[270] and withdrawal has been reported after as few as 3 days.[271]

At this time, recommendations for M.M. should include the addition of morphine as a sedative agent (initial bolus infusion of 0.18 mg, followed by a continuous infusion starting at 0.07 mg/hour [70 μg/hour]) and an ocular lubricant to prevent corneal abrasions. Neuromuscular blocking agents prevent blinking, and corneal abrasions may occur. Because tolerance to opiates develops, the morphine dose will need to be increased with continued use. Determination of adequate sedation is difficult in paralyzed infants, but increases in HR and BP or decreases in oxygenation may indicate inadequate sedation. M.M. may also require additional sedation/anxiolytic therapy with benzodiazepines such as lorazepam or midazolam. Diazepam is not a preferred agent for sedation in neonates due to its long half-life and accumulation of its active metabolite (N-desmethyldiazepam).

Drug/Disease Interactions

55. Morphine and an ocular lubricant (as an ophthalmic ointment applied to both eyes Q 6 hr PRN) were added to M.M.'s therapy. On day 2 of life, M.M. continues on mechanical ventilation with hyperoxia and hyperventilation. His ABG is pH, 7.5; PCO_2, 30 mm Hg; and PO_2, 55 mm Hg. M.M. continues to receive IV ampicillin, gentamicin, dopamine, dobutamine, sodium bicarbonate, and pancuronium. What factors may influence the neuromuscular blocking effect of pancuronium in M.M.? What adjustments to his dosing schedule should be made?

[SI units: PCO_2, 4.0 kPa; PO_2, 7.33 kPa]

Both alkalosis and gentamicin may potentiate the neuromuscular blocking effects of pancuronium in M.M.[255] Although alkalosis may potentiate and acidosis may antagonize the effects of pancuronium, the opposite effects have been reported with vecuronium.[255] Pancuronium already is being dosed in M.M. on an "as-needed" basis. Monitoring for spontaneous movement should continue, and a longer required dosing interval may be noted. If gentamicin then is discontinued or pH is normalized, the duration of effect may shorten. Other factors such as electrolyte status, disease states, and other medications may influence the pharmacodynamics of neuromuscular blocking agents.[255] For instance, renal or hepatic impairment (such as cholestasis) may result in accumulation of drug or active metabolite (3-hydroxypancuronium) and a prolonged effect.

Toxicity

56. **Sodium bicarbonate, dobutamine, and dopamine were discontinued on day 3 of life. On day 4 of life, M.M.'s antibiotics were discontinued after culture results ruled out infection. On Friday (day 5 of life), pancuronium was discontinued and M.M. remained intubated. Concerns about morphine "addiction" resulted in the discontinuation of morphine and the initiation of chloral hydrate 250 mg NG Q 4 hr for sedation. On Monday morning, M.M. was noted to have severe lethargy, decreased deep tendon reflexes, and respiratory depression requiring an increase in ventilator settings. Bowel sounds were absent and M.M. had marked abdominal distention. Is M.M. experiencing prolonged paralysis from pancuronium? What is your assessment of this situation?**

Administration of opiates for sedation or analgesia does not cause addiction.[272] The term addiction should be used only to describe complex behavioral patterns characterized by a preoccupation with obtainment of a drug (drug-seeking behavior) and compulsive drug use. Prolonged administration of opiates may cause tolerance (i.e., a decreased effect after repeated administration of the original dosage or an increasing dosage requirement to attain the original effect) or physical dependence. Physical dependence requires the continued administration of a medication to prevent symptoms of withdrawal. Although symptoms of withdrawal may occur when opiates are discontinued, careful weaning of the opiate and appropriate monitoring of symptoms using an abstinence scoring method will lessen withdrawal severity. Opioids may be weaned in <72 hours when low to moderate doses have been used for <1 week. Typically, the dose is decreased by 25% to 50% initially (and by 20% subsequently) every 6 to 8 hours. If opioids are used for >1 week, smaller decreases in doses, a longer total weaning time, and conversion to an oral agent usually are required.[272] In M.M.'s case, IV morphine could have been continued for sedation or an appropriate oral agent could have been used if normal bowel function was apparent.

Disuse atrophy, muscle weakness, joint contractures, and prolonged paralysis have been reported after discontinuing neuromuscular blocking agents.[255] Prolonged neuromuscular blockade may be more common in patients with renal or hepatic dysfunction or with the use of continuous infusion, pro-

longed therapy, or certain concomitant medications. In particular, prolonged paralysis may be seen after discontinuation of steroidally based neuromuscular blocking agents (e.g., pancuronium, vecuronium) when these agents have been administered with corticosteroids.[273] In this case, M.M. did not have any apparent renal or hepatic disease, was treated with intermittent "as-needed" doses, received short-term paralysis, and did not receive corticosteroids. Therefore, M.M. would be at a low risk for developing prolonged paralysis after discontinuation of pancuronium.

The most likely cause of M.M.'s current symptoms is chloral hydrate intoxication. The recommended initial dose of chloral hydrate for prolonged sedation in neonates is 10 to 30 mg/kg per dose given every 6 to 8 hours on an as-needed basis.[274] Although some clinicians recommend 20 to 40 mg/kg per dose every 4 to 6 hours as needed (80 to 240 mg/kg per day),[265] toxicity has been reported in a term infant with persistent pulmonary hypertension of the newborn receiving doses of 44 to 50 mg/kg every 6 hours (176 to 200 mg/kg per day).[274] M.M. received approximately 70 mg/kg per dose every 4 hours around the clock for 3 days.

Chloral hydrate is metabolized quickly in erythrocytes and the liver by alcohol dehydrogenase to trichloroethanol, an active metabolite. Trichloroethanol is metabolized to trichloroacetate and to trichloroethanol glucuronide in the liver and renally eliminated. The conversion of chloral hydrate to trichloroethanol may not be as rapid in neonates,[275] and both chloral hydrate and trichloroethanol may be responsible for the sedative effects seen in neonates.[276] The parent drug (chloral hydrate) may be responsible for the immediate short-term sedative effects, whereas trichloroethanol may be responsible for long-term effects. The short duration of sedation (2 hours) necessitates frequent repeated dosing that unfortunately results in accumulation of the active metabolite, trichloroethanol, and toxic effects. The half-life of trichloroethanol is prolonged in preterm (40 hours) and term neonates (28 hours).[275] Because trichloroethanol may accumulate, chloral hydrate should be used only on an as-needed basis for long-term sedation in neonates. The lower end of the recommended dosage range should be used for preterm newborns, and all neonates, especially those who require frequent repeated doses, should be monitored for toxic effects.

Toxicities of chloral hydrate include CNS, respiratory, and myocardial depression; gastric irritation; adynamic ileus; cardiac arrhythmias; hypotension; renal impairment; bladder atony; and direct hyperbilirubinemia.[274] Although M.M. is showing signs of CNS depression (lethargy, decreased deep tendon reflexes), respiratory depression (increased ventilator settings), and GI effects (absent bowel sounds, abdominal distention), a physical examination and appropriate laboratory tests should be performed to identify other known toxicities (e.g., serum BUN and SrCr to detect renal impairment). In addition, other causes of M.M.'s current condition also should be ruled out (e.g., sepsis, meningitis, intracranial hemorrhage, metabolic disorder). Chloral hydrate should be discontinued and trichloroethanol serum concentrations determined, if available. Supportive care should be given and severe toxicities may require exchange transfusions.[274]

USE AND ADMINISTRATION OF MEDICATIONS
Drug Formulation Problems

57. What problems are encountered with the use of commercially available medications in the neonate?

The lack of appropriate enteral and parenteral formulations results in many unique problems of drug use and administration in the neonatal population.

Lack of Nonsolid Enteral Dosage Formulations

Many drugs used in neonates and infants are not commercially available in an enteral liquid dosage form, including acetazolamide, captopril, clonazepam, rifampin, and spironolactone. For some medications, such as caffeine citrate, the liquid injectable form can be given enterally. Otherwise, extemporaneous powder formulations or liquid preparations must be made from the solid dosage forms.[8,277]

Little information exists regarding the preparation and stability of extemporaneous formulations.[278] Formulations intended for neonates should limit the use of pharmaceutical adjuvants, unnecessary ingredients (e.g., flavoring agents for drugs administered via nasogastric tubes), and other substances that would increase osmolality.

Inappropriate Concentrations

Most drugs are formulated for use in the adult population. As a result, the available concentrations of liquid formulations will result in appropriate volumes for adult doses, but extremely small volumes for the doses required by neonates. Frequently, these volumes are too small to accurately measure (i.e., <0.1 mL). Therefore, dilutions of commercially available injections (e.g., aminophylline, digoxin, morphine, phenobarbital) are necessary to accurately measure the small doses required by neonates. Proper diluents and dilutional techniques must be ensured because inappropriate dilutions are a common source of potentially fatal medication errors (Table 94-12).[265,279] In addition, the sterility and stability of these diluted injections need to be documented before being used in neonates.[278]

Hypertonicity

In the neonate, parenteral and enteral administration of hypertonic medications may result in severe adverse effects.[280,281] NEC and IVH have been associated with IV administration of hyperosmolar drugs, such as radiographic contrast media or sodium bicarbonate. Infusions of hypertonic medications directly into the umbilical or portal vein have resulted in severe hepatic injury. In addition, enteral administration of hyperosmolar medications and feedings have been associated with NEC.[280,281] Therefore, appropriate dilutions of hypertonic medications should be made before administration to neonates.

Pharmaceutical Adjuvants

Ingredients used for the enhancement of bioavailability, stability, taste, or appearance of medications can cause adverse effects in neonates.[282] Preservatives such as benzyl alcohol or methylparaben may displace bilirubin from albumin binding sites.[23] Benzyl alcohol also may cause the potentially fatal "gasping syndrome" (discussed previously in the Neonatal Pharmacokinetics, Metabolism section). Propylene glycol, a

---

Table 94-12 Potential Errors in Drug Administration Techniques

Factors Involving Drug (Dose) Preparation

Inappropriate dilutions

Similarity in appearance of dose units

Loss of potentially large amounts of drug dose in the dead space of a syringe or infusion Y site

Unsuitable drug formulations for administration

Unlabeled or undesirable ingredients in dosage forms

Undesirable drug concentrations and/or osmolalities

Errors in interpreting drug orders and/or dose calculations

Factors Involving IV Drug Administration

Loss of drug consequent to routine changing of IV sets

Reduction in serum concentrations for drugs with rapid plasma clearance that are infused slowly

Extreme ↑ in plasma concentrations consequent to rapid infusion of drugs with small central compartment Vd

Delayed infusion of total dose when IV line is not flushed

Inadvertent admixture of drugs by the manual IV retrograde method

Large distance between the site of drug infusion into an IV line and the insertion of the line into the patient

Potential loss of large-volume doses in the overflow syringe with the IV retrograde technique

Possible loss of drug because of binding to IV tubing

Use of large intraluminal diameter tubing for small patients

Infiltrations not detected by pump alarms

Infusion of multiple medications/fluids at different rates by means of a common "hub"

Oscillations in fluid/dose rate of potent medications infused with piston-type pumps

Factors Involving Other Routes of Drug Administration

Loss of delivery (NG tube dead space) or from oral cavity

Leakage of drug from IM or SC injection site

Expulsion of drug from the rectum

Misapplication to external sites (i.e., ophthalmic ointment in young infants)

Reproduced with permission from Blumer JL, Reed MD. Principles of neonatal pharmacology. In: Yaffe SJ, Aranda JV, eds. Pediatric Pharmacology: Therapeutic Principles in Practice. 2nd Ed. Philadelphia: WB Saunders, 1992;168.
IM, intramuscular; IV, intravenous; NG, nasogastric; SC, subcutaneous; Vd, volume of distribution.

---

solubilizing agent, may cause several toxicities in neonates, including hyperosmolality, lactic acidosis, seizures, CNS and respiratory depression, hypotension, and arrhythmias.[282] Emulsifiers, such as Polysorbate 20 and Polysorbate 80, have been associated with hypotension, renal dysfunction, hepatotoxicity, and death in low-birth-weight infants.[283] Sorbitol, a poorly absorbed sweetener, may cause osmotic diarrhea, intestinal gas, bloating, and abdominal pain when administered enterally in large doses. A report of sorbitol-induced pneumatosis intestinalis in a child underscores the serious consequence of receiving multiple liquid medications containing sorbitol.[284] Unfortunately, these undesired substances are currently not required by law to be listed in the package insert of oral medications.[282] The safety of pharmaceutical adjuvants should be examined thoroughly before these substances are used in the neonatal population. In addition, further studies are required to identify other pharmaceutical ingredients that may be potentially toxic to the neonate.

Drug Administration

58. D.S., a 4-day-old female neonate born at 30 weeks' gestational age with a current weight of 1,200 g, has a birth history of prolonged rupture of membranes and a difficult delivery. Her current problems include rule out sepsis and apnea of prematurity. D.S. receives the following: ampicillin, 60 mg IV Buretrol Q 12 hr at 2 AM and 2 PM (100 mg/kg per day); gentamicin, 3.6 mg IV Buretrol Q 24 hr at 7 AM (3 mg/kg per day); aminophylline, 1.2 mg IV Buretrol Q 12 hr at 10 AM and 10 PM (2 mg/kg per day); and dextrose, 5% NaCl 0.2% with KCl 1.8 mEq/day and calcium gluconate 250 mg/day at 6 mL/ hr. Gentamicin serum concentrations were obtained today (day 4 of antibiotic therapy) and reported as a trough of 1.2 μg/mL at 6:50 AM and a peak of 2.8 g/mL at 8 AM. Using standard pharmacokinetic equations you calculate a Kd of 0.037 hr-1, half-life of 18.7 hours, and Vd of 1.8 L/kg. What should be done next for D.S.?

Serum concentrations of aminoglycosides and other drugs can be affected significantly by the IV-drug delivery system.[285,286] The low IV infusion rates required by neonates significantly delay drug delivery, especially if medications are administered via volumetric chamber devices (e.g., Buretrol or Metriset) or via the Y-site injection port distal to the patient. Even when factors such as injection site, infusion rate, drug volume, and tubing diameter are considered, actual drug delivery may be delayed up to 2 hours using volumetric chamber devices.[285] If aminoglycosides are administered by Y-site injection, peak concentrations can be decreased by a mean of 2.5 μg/mL and delayed by 1.5 hours compared with IV sy-ringe pump administration.[287] Trough concentrations, however, are not significantly affected. As a result of inappropriate administration methods, a larger Vd and prolonged half-life would be calculated, as demonstrated in D.S.

D.S.'s unbelievably large Vd should lead to suspicion of the method of drug administration. At this time, no dosage change can be recommended for D.S. Serum aminoglycoside concentrations should be repeated after an appropriate IV administration method is instituted. This method should include the use of a neonatal syringe pump, low-volume IV tubing, and drug injection into the port most proximal to the neonate.[285,286]

Other potential neonatal IV drug administration errors are listed in Table 94-12. Additional problems include significant overdoses resulting from the unintended delivery of residual drug from the hub or needle of syringes (i.e., dead spaces), and underdosages due to trapping of medications in IV filters.[265,279] In addition, the neonate's limited ability to tolerate excess fluid prohibits drug delivery via IV riders or "piggybacks," which would significantly increase fluid administration. Neonates also require special IV rates of drug infusion (i.e., mg/kg per minute) to avoid significant adverse effects. Appropriate references should be consulted for drug-specific methods and rates of infusion, appropriate final concentrations, and other special neonatal considerations.[8]

Acknowledgment
The authors would like to acknowledge Dr. Fotini Hatzopoulos for her contribution to a previous edition of this chapter.

REFERENCES

1. Shirkey H. Editorial comment: therapeutic orphans. Pediatrics 1999;104:583.
2. Gilman JT, Gal P. Pharmacokinetic and pharmacodynamic data collection in children and neonates. a quiet frontier. Clin Pharmacokinet 1992;23-1
3. Wilson JT. An update on the therapeutic orphan. Pediatrics 1999;104:585.
4. Pediatric studies of drugs, Section 111, FDA Modernization Act of 1997, Public Law 105-115, 105th Congress of the United States.
5. Best Pharmaceuticals for Children Act, Public Law, 107-109, 107th Congress of the United States.
6. Fletcher MA. Physical assessment and classification. In: Avery GB et al, eds. Neonatology: Pathophysiology and Management of the Newborn, 5th Ed. Philadelphia: Lippincott Williams & Wilkins, 1999:301.
7. Avery GB et al. Neonatology: Pathophysiology and Management of the Newborn, 5th Ed. Philadelphia, PA: Lippincott Williams & Wilkins, 1999:1501.
8. Taketomo CK et al. Pediatric Dosage Handbook, 10th Ed. Hudson, OH: Lexi-Comp, 2003.
9. Yahav J. Development of parietal cells, acid secretion, and response to secretagogues. In: Lebenthal E, ed. Human Gastrointestinal Development. New York: Raven Press, 1989:341.
10. Hyman PE et al. Gastric acid secretory function in preterm infants. J Pediatr 1985;106:467.
11. Morselli PL. Clinical pharmacology of the perinatal period and early infancy. Clin Pharmacokinet 1989;17(Suppl 1):13.
12. Besunder JB et al. Principles of drug disposition in the neonate. A critical evaluation of the pharmaco kinetic-pharmacodynamic interface. Part I. Clin Pharmacokinet 1988;14:189.
13. Radde IC. Mechanisms of drug absorption and their development. In: Radde IC, MacLeod SM, eds. Pediatric Pharmacology and Therapeutics. St. Louis: Mosby-Year Book, 1993:16.
14. Heimann G. Enteral absorption and bioavailability in children in relation to age. Eur J Clin Pharmacol 1980;18.43.
15. Stewart CF, Hampton EW. Effect of maturation on drug disposition in pediatric patients. Clin Pharm 1987;6:548.
16. Seigler RS. The administration of rectal diazepam for acute management of seizures. J Emerg Med 1990;8:155.
17. Wu PYK et al. Peripheral blood flow in the neonate. 1. Changes in total, skin, and muscle blood flow with gestational and postnatal age. Pediatr Res 1980;14:1374.
18. Barrett DA, Rutter N. Transdermal delivery and the premature neonate. Crit Rev Ther Drug Carrier Syst 1994;11:1.
19. Radde IC. Growth and drug distribution. In: Radde IC, Macleod SM, eds. Pediatric Pharmacology and Therapeutics. St. Louis: Mosby-Year Book, 1993:43.
20. Friis-Hansen B. Water distribution in the foetus and newborn infant. Acta Paediatr Scand 1983; 305(Suppl):7.
21. Morselli PL et al. Clinical pharmacokinetics in newborns and infants. Clin Pharmacokinet 1980; 5:485.
22. Besunder JB et al. Principles of drug disposition in the neonate. A critical evaluation of the pharmacokinetic-pharmacodynamic interface. Part II. Clin Pharmacokinet 1988;14:261.
23. Radde IC. Drugs and protein binding. In: Radde IC, Macleod SM, eds. Pediatric Pharmacology and Therapeutics. St. Louis: Mosby-Year Book, 1993:31.
24. Aranda JV et al. Pharmacokinetic aspects of theophylline in premature newborns. N Engl J Med 1976;295:413.
25. Rane A et al. Plasma protein binding of diphenylhydantoin in normal and hyperbilirubinemic infants. J Pediatr 1971;78:877.
26. Cashore WJ. Hyperbilirubinemia. In: Pomerance JJ, Richardson CJ, eds. Neonatology for the Clinician. Norwalk: Appleton & Lange, 1993:231.
27. Robertson A, Brodersen R. Effect of drug combinations on bilirubin-albumin binding. Dev Pharmacol Ther 1991;17:95.
28. Martin E et al. Ceftriaxone-bilirubin-albumin interactions in the neonate: an in vivo study. Eur J Pediatr 1993;152:530.
29. Stutman HR et al. Potential of moxalactam and other new antimicrobial agents for bilirubin-albumin displacement in neonates. Pediatrics 1985;75:294.
30. Springer C, Eyal F. Pharmacology of trimethoprim-sulfamethoxazole in newborn infants. J Pediatr 1982;100:647.
31. Kearns GL. Pharmacogenetics and development: are infants and children at increased risk for adverse outcomes? Curr Opin Pediatr 1995;7:220.
32. Radde IC, Kalow W. Drug biotransformation and its development. In: Radde IC, Macleod SM, eds. Pediatric Pharmacology and Therapeutics. St. Louis: Mosby-Year Book, 1993:57.
33. Leeder JS, Kearns GL. Pharmacogenetics in pediatrics: implications for practice. Pediatr Clin North Am 1997;44:55.
34. de Wildt SN et al. Cytochrome P450 3A: ontogeny and drug disposition. Clin Pharmacokinet 1999; 37:485.
35. Aranda JV et al. Hepatic microsomal drug oxidation and electron transport in newborn infants. J Pediatr 1974;85:534.
36. Kraus DK et al. Alterations in theophylline metabolism during the first year of life. Clin Pharmacol Ther 1993;54:351.

37. de Wildt SN et al. Glucuronidation in humans: pharmacogenetic and developmental aspects. Clin Pharmacokinet 1999;36:439.

38. LeBel M. Benzyl alcohol metabolism and elimination in neonates. Dev Pharmacol Ther 1988;11:347.

39. Gershanik J et al. The gasping syndrome and benzyl alcohol poisoning. N Engl J Med 1982;307. 1384.

40. Food and Drug Administration. Benzyl alcohol may be toxic to newborns. FDA Drug Bull 1982;12:10.

41. Morselli PL et al. Diazepam elimination in premature and term infants and children. J Perinat Med 1973;1:133.

42. Sereni F et al. Induction of drug metabolizing enzyme activities in the human fetus and in the newborn infant. Enzyme 1973;15:318.

43. Gal P et al. The influence of asphyxia on phenobarbital dosing requirements in neonates. Dev Pharmacol Ther 1984;7:145.

44. Radde IC. Renal function and elimination of drugs during development. In: Radde IC, Macleod SM, eds. Pediatric Pharmacology and Therapeutics. St. Louis: Mosby-Year Book, 1993;87.

45. Vanpee M et al. Renal function in very low birthweight infants: normal maturity reached during early childhood. J Pediatr 1992;121:784.

46. Rodvold KA et al. Bayesian forecasting of serum vancomycin concentrations in neonates and infants. Ther Drug Monit 1995;17:239.

47. Rodvold KA et al. Pharmacokinetics and administration regimens of vancomycin in neonates, infant and children. Clin Pharmacokinet 1997;33:32.

48. Rodvold et al. Prediction of gentamicin concentrations in neonates and infants using a bayesian pharmacokinetic model. Dev Pharmacol Ther 1993; 20:211.

49. Kildoo C et al. Developmental pattern of gentamicin kinetics in very low birthweight (VLBW) sick infants. Dev Pharmacol Ther 1984;7:345.

50. Kasik JW et al. Postconceptional age and gentamicin elimination half-life. J Pediatr 1985;106:502.

51. Young TE, Mangum OB. Neofax '96: A Manual of Drugs Used in Neonatal Care, 9th Ed. Raleigh, NC: Acorn Publishing, 1996:30.

52. Prober CG et al. The use of antibiotics in neonates weighing less than 1200 grams. Pediatr Infect Dis J 1990;9:111.

53. Friedman CA et al. Gentamicin disposition in asphyxiated newborns: relationship to mean arterial pressure and urine output. Pediatr Pharmacol 1982;2:189.

54. Zarfin Y et al. Possible indomethacin-aminoglycoside interaction in preterm infants. J Pediatr 1985; 106:511.

55. Koren G et al. Effects of indomethacin on digoxin pharmacokinetics in preterm infants. Pediatr Pharmacol 1984;4:25.

56. Hook JB, Hewitt WR. Development of mechanisms for drug excretion. Am J Med 1977;62:497.

57. Notter RH. Lung surfactants. In: Lenfant C, ed. Lung Biology in Health and Disease. New York: Marcel Dekker, 2000:233.

58. Whitsett JA et al. Acute respiratory disorders. In: Avery GB et al, eds. Neonatology: Pathophysiology and Management of the Newborn, 5th Ed. Philadelphia: Lippincott Williams & Wilkins, 1999:485.

59. Hagedorn MI et al. Respiratory diseases. In: Merenstein GB, Gardner SL, eds. Handbook of Neonatal Intensive Care, 4th Ed. St. Louis: Mosby-Year Book, 1999:437.

60. Stark AR, Frank ID. Respiratory distress syndrome. Pediatr Clin North Am 1986;33:533.

61. Jobe AH. Lung development. In: Fanaroff AA, Martin RJ, eds. Neonatal-Perinatal Medicine: Diseases of the Fetus and Infant, 6th Ed. St. Louis: Mosby-Year Book, 1997:991.

62. Martin RJ, Fanaroff AA. The respiratory distress syndrome and its management. In: Fanaroff AA, Martin RJ, eds. Neonatal-Perinatal Medicine: Diseases of the Fetus and Infant, 6th Ed. St. Louis: Mosby-Year Book, 1997:1018.

63. Goldenberg RL, Rouse DJ. Medical progress: prevention of premature birth. N Engl J Med 1998; 339:313.

64. National Institutes of Health (NIH) Consensus Development Panel. Effect of corticosteroids for fetal maturation on perinatal outcomes. JAMA 1995; 273:413.

65. Crowley PA. Antenatal corticosteroid therapy: a meta-analysis of the randomized trials, 1992–1994. Am J Obstet Gynecol 1995;173:322.

66. Aghajafari F et al. Multiple courses of antenatal corticosteroids: a systematic review and meta-analysis. Am J Obstet Gynecol 2001;185:1073.

67. French H et al. Repeated antenatal corticosteroids: size at birth and subsequent development. Am J Obstet Gynecol 1999;180:114.

68. Vermillion ST et al. Neonatal sepsis and death after multiple courses of antenatal betamethasone therapy. Am J Obstet Gynecol 2000;183:810.

69. National Institutes of Health Consensus Development Panel. Antenatal corticosteroids revisited: repeat courses- National Institute of Health Consensus Development Conference Statement, August 17-18, 2000.

70. Ballard PL, Ballard RA. Scientific basis and therapeutic regimens for use of antenatal glucocorticoids. Am J Obstet Gynecol 1995;173:254.

71. Baud O et al. Antenatal glucocorticoid treatment and cystic periventricular leukomalacia in very premature infants. N Engl J Med 1999;341:1190.

72. Hallman M et al. The fate of exogenous surfactant in neonates with respiratory distress syndrome. Clin Pharmacokinet 1994;26:215.

73. Crowther CA et al. Prenatal thyrotropin-releasing hormone for preterm birth. Cochrane Database Syst Rev, The Cochrane Library 2003;1:CD000019.

74. Halliday H. Synthetic or natural surfactants. Acta Pediatr 1997;86:233.

75. Walti H, Monset-Couchard M. A risk-benefit assessment of natural and synthetic exogenous surfactants in the management of neonatal respiratory distress syndrome. Drug Saf 1998;18:321.

76. Curley AE, Halliday HL. The present status of exogenous surfactant for the newborn. Early Hum Dev 2001;61:67.

77. GlaxoWellcome Inc. Exosurf neonatal for intratracheal suspension package insert. Research Triangle Park, NC: 1998 January.

78. Ross Products Division, Abbott Laboratories Inc. Survanta intratracheal suspension package insert. Columbus, OH: 1999 October.

79. Forest Pharmaceuticals, Inc. Infasurf intratracheal suspension package insert. St. Louis, MO: 2002 December.

80. Dey. Curosurf intratracheal suspension package insert. Napa, CA: 2002 March.

81. Bloom BT et al. Comparison on Infasurf (calf lung surfactant extract) to Survanta (beractant) in the treatment and prevention of respiratory distress syndrome. Pediatrics 1997;100:31.

82. Kattwinkel J. Surfactant: evolving issues. Clin Perinatol 1998;25:17.

83. Speer CP et al. Randomised clinical trial of two treatment regimens of natural surfactant preparations in neonatal respiratory distress syndrome. Arch Child 1995;72:F8.

84. Soll RF. Surfactant therapy in the USA: trials and current routines. Biol Neonate 1997;71(Suppl 1):1.

85. Kattwinkel J et al. High-versus low-threshold surfactant retreatment for neonatal respiratory distress syndrome. Pediatr 2000;106:282.

86. Gortner L et al. Early versus late surfactant treatment in preterm infants of 27 to 32 weeks' gestational age: a multicenter controlled clinical trial. Pediatrics 1998;102:1153.

87. Sitler CG et al. Pump administration of exogenous surfactant: effects on oxygenation, heart rate, and chest wall movement of premature infants. J Perinatol 1993;13:197.

88. Vermont-Oxford Neonatal Network. A multicenter, randomized trial comparing synthetic surfactant with modified bovine surfactant extract in the treatment of neonatal respiratory distress syndrome. Pediatrics 1996;97:1.

89. Hudak ML et al. A multicenter randomized, masked comparison trial of natural versus synthetic surfactant for the treatment of respiratory distress syndrome. J Pediatr 1996;128:396.

90. American Academy of Pediatrics. Committee on Fetus and Newborn. Surfactant replacement therapy for respiratory distress syndrome. Pediatrics 1999;103:684.

91. Zola EM et al. Comparison of three dosing procedures for administration of bovine surfactant to neonates with respiratory distress syndrome. J Pediatr 1993;122:453.

92. Tran JH, Raju TNK. Cost-analyses from repackaging of expensive drugs: An example using an exogenous surfactant preparation [Abstract]. Pediatr Res 1999;40:220A.

93. Green TP et al. Furosemide promotes patent ductus arteriosus in premature infants with the respiratory distress syndrome. N Engl J Med 1983; 308:743.

94. Jobe AH, Bancalari E. NICHD/NHLBI/ORD workshop summary: bronchopulmonary dsyplasia. Am J Respir Crit Care Med. 2001;163:1723.

95. Davis JM, Rosenfeld WN. Chronic lung disease. In: Avery GB et al, eds. Neonatology: Pathophysiology and Management of the Newborn, 5th Ed. Philadelphia: Lippincott Williams & Wilkins, 1999:509.

96. Abman SH, Groothius JR. Pathophysiology and treatment of bronchopulmonary dysplasia. Pediatr Clin North Am 1994;41:277.

97. Farrell PA, Fiascone JM. Bronchopulmonary dysplasia in the 1990s: a review for the pediatrician. Curr Probl Pediatr 1997;27:133.

98. Hansen T, Corbet A. Chronic lung disease: bronchopulmonary dysplasia. In: Taeusch HW, Ballard RA, eds. Avery's Diseases of the Newborns, 7th Ed. Philadelphia: WB Saunders, 1998:634.

99. Mead Johnson & Company. Cafcit Injection and Oral Solution package insert. Bedford, OH: 2003, May.

100. Barrington KJ, Finer NN. Treatment of bronchopulmonary dysplasia: a review. Clin Perinatol 1998;25:177.

101. De Boeck K et al. Response to bronchodilators in clinically stable 1-year-old patients with bronchopulmonary dysplasia. Eur J Pediatr 1998; 157:75.

102. Brundage KL et al. Bronchodilator response to ipratropium bromide in infants with bronchopulmonary dysplasia. Am Rev Respir Dis 1990;142: 1137.

103. Ward RM, Lugo RA. Drug therapy in the newborn. In: Avery GB et al, eds. Neonatology: Pathophysiology and Management of the Newborn, 5th Ed. Philadelphia: Lippincott Williams & Wilkins, 1999:1363.

104. Bancalari E. Corticosteroids and neonatal chronic lung disease. Eur J Pediatr 1998;157(Suppl 1): S31.

105. Halliday H et al. Moderately early (7-14 days) postnatal corticosteroids for preventing chronic lung disease in preterm infants. Cochrane Database Syst Rev, The Cochrane Library 2003;1:CD001144.

106. Halliday HL et al. Delayed (>3 weeks) postnatal corticosteroids for chronic lung disease in preterm infants. Cochrane Database Syst Rev, The Cochrane Library 2003;1:CD001145.

107. Halliday HL et al. Early postnatal (<96 hours) corticosteroids for preventing chronic lung disease in preterm infants. Cochrane Database Syst Rev, The Cochrane Library 2003;1:CD001146.

108. Garland JS et al. A three-day course of dexamethasone therapy to prevent chronic lung disease in ventilated neonates: a randomized trial. Pediatrics 1999;104:91.

109. Barrington KJ. The adverse neuro-developmental effects of postnatal steroids in the preterm infant: a systematic review of RCTs. BioMed Central Pediatr 2001;1:1.

110. Doyle LW, Davis PG. Postnatal corticosteroids in preterm infants: systematic review of effects on mortality and motor function. J Paediatr Child Health 2000;36:101.

111. American Academy of Pediatrics. Committee on Fetus and Newborn. Canadian Paediatric Society.

Fetus and Newborn Committee. Postnatal corticosteroids to treat or prevent chronic lung disease in preterm infants. Pediatrics 2002;109:330.

112. Avent ML et al. The role of inhaled steroids in the treatment of bronchopulmonary dysplasia. Neonatal Network 1994;13:63.

113. Shah V et al. Early administration of inhaled corticosteroids for preventing chronic lung disease in ventilated very low birth weight preterm neonates. Cochrane Database Syst Rev 2003: 1:CD001969.

114. Shah SS et al. Inhaled versus systemic corticosteroids for preventing chronic lung disease in ventilated very low birth weight preterm neonates. Cochrane Database Syst Rev 2003:1:CD002058.

115. Cole CH et al. Early inhaled corticosteroid therapy to prevent bronchopulmonary dysplasia. N Engl J Med 1999;340:1005.

116. Ng PC et al. Pituitary-adrenal suppression in preterm, very low birthweight infants after inhaled fluticasone propionate treatment. J Clin Endocrinol Metab 1998;83:2390.

117. Shenai JP. Vitamin A supplementation in very low birthweight neonates: rationale and evidence. Pediatrics 1999;104:1369.

118. Tyson JE et al. Vitamin A supplementation for extremely-low-birth-weight infants. N Engl J Med 1999;340:1962.

119. Berstein D. The fetal to neonatal circulatory transition. In: Behrman RE et al, eds. Nelson Textbook of Pediatrics, 16th Ed. Philadelphia: WB Saunders, 2000:1341.

120. Hammerman C. Patent ductus arteriosus: clinical relevance of prostaglandins and prostaglandin inhibitors in PDA pathophysiology and treatment. Clin Perinatol 1995;22:457.

121. Brook MM, Heymann MA. Patent ductus arteriosus. In: Emmanouilides G et al, eds. Moss and Adam's Heart Disease in Infants, Children, and Adolescents, 5th Ed. Baltimore: Williams & Wilkins, 1995:746.

122. Bell SG. Neonatal cardiovascular pharmacology. Neonatal Network 1998;17.7.

123. Clyman RI. Patent ductus arteriosus in the premature infant. In: Taeusch HW, Ballard RA, eds. Avery's Diseases of the Newborn, 7th Ed. Philadelphia: WB Saunders, 1998:699.

124. Clyman RI. Recommendations for the postnatal use of indomethacin: an analysis of four separate treatment strategies. J Pediatr 1996;128:601.

125. Gersony WM et al. Effects of indomethacin in premature infants with patent ductus arteriosus: results of a national collaborative study J Pediatr 1983;102:895.

126. Clyman RI. Medical treatment of patent ductus arteriosus in premature infants. In: Long WA, ed. Fetal and Neonatal Cardiology. Philadelphia: WB Saunders, 1990:682.

127. Shaffer CL et al. Effect of age and birth weight on indomethacin pharmacodynamics in neonates treated for patent ductus arteriosus. Crit Care Med 2002;30:343.

128. Brion LP, Campbell DE. Furosemide in indomethacin-treated infants—systematic review and meta-analysis. Pediatr Nephrol 1999;133:212.

129. Gal P, Gillman JT. Drug disposition in neonates with patent ductus arteriosus. Ann Pharmacother 1993;27:1383.

130. Pham JT, Carlos MA. Current treatment strategies of symptomatic patent ductus arteriousus. J Pediatr Health Care 2002;16:306.

131. Van Overmeire B al. Early versus late indomethacin treatment for patent ductus arteriosus in premature infants with respiratory distress syndrome. J Pediatr 2001;138:205.

132. Hammerman C, Aramburo MJ. Prolonged indomethacin therapy for the prevention of recurrences of patent ductus arteriosus. J Pediatr 1990;117:771.

133. Weiss H et al. Factors determining reopening of the ductus arteriosus after successful clinical closure with indomethacin. J Pediatr 1995; 127:466.

134. Tammela O et al. Short versus prolonged indomethacin therapy for patent ductus arteriosus in preterm infants. J Pediatr 1999;134:552.

135. Fowlie PW. Prophylactic indomethacin: systematic review and meta-analysis. Arch Dis Child 1996;74:F81.

136. Gournay V et al. Pulmonary hypertension after ibuprofen prophylaxis in very preterm infants. Lancet 2002;359:1486.

137. De Carolis MP et al. Prophylactic ibuprofen therapy of patent ductus arteriosus in preterm infants. Eur J Pediatr 2000;159:364.

138. Stoll BJ. Epidemiology of necrotizing enterocolitis. Clin Perinatol 1994;21:205.

139. Crouse DT. Necrotizing enterocolitis. In: Pomerance JJ, Richardson CJ, eds. Neonatology for the Clinician. Norwalk: Appleton & Lange, 1993:363.

140. Berseth CL, Abrams SA. Special gastrointestinal concerns. In: Taeusch HW, Ballard RA, eds. Avery's Diseases of the Newborn. Philadelphia: WB Saunders, 1998:965.

141. Pierro A. Necrotizing enterocolitis: pathogenesis and treatment. Br J Hosp Med 1997;58:126.

142. Walsh MC, Kliegan RM. Necrotizing enterocolitis: treatment based on staging criteria. Pediatr Clin North Am 1986;33:179.

143. Edelson MB et al. Circulating pro-and counterinflammatory cytokine levels and severity in necrotizing enterocolitis. Pediatrics 1999;103:766.

144. Boccia D et al. Nosocomial necrotising enterocolitis outbreaks: epidemiology and control measures. Eur J Pediatr 2001;160:385.

145. McKeown RE et al. Role of delayed feeding and of feeding increments in necrotizing enterocolitis. J Pediatr 1992;121:764.

146. Scheifele DW et al. Comparison of two antibiotic regimens for neonatal necrotizing enterocolitis. J Antimicrob Chemother 1987;20:421.

147. Bury RG, Tudehope D. Enteral antibiotics for preventing necrotizing enterocolitis in low birthweight or preterm infants. Cochrane Database Syst Rev, The Cochrane Library 2003;1:CD000405.

148. Faix RG et al. A randomized trial of parenteral clindamycin in neonatal necrotizing enterocolitis. J Pediatr 1988;112:271.

149. Vanderhoof JA. Short bowel syndrome in children and small intestinal transplantation. Pediatr Clin North Am 1996;43:533.

150. Thureen PJ, Hay WW. Early aggressive nutrition in preterm infants. Semin Neonatol 2001;6.403.

151. Perez EM, Weisman LE. Novel approaches to the prevention and therapy of neonatal bacterial sepsis. Clin Perinatol 1997;24:213.

152. Cole FS. Bacterial infections of the newborn. In: Taeusch HW, Ballard RA, eds. Avery's Diseases of the Newborn, 7th Ed. Philadelphia: WB Saunders, 1998:490.

153. Smith JB. Bacterial and fungal infections of the neonate. In: Pomerance JJ, Richardson CT, eds. Neonatology for the Clinician. Norwalk: Appleton & Lange, 1993:185.

154. Philip AGS. The changing face of neonatal infection: experience at a regional medical center. Pediatr Infect Dis J 1994;13:1098.

155. Freij BJ, McCracken GH. Acute infections. In: Avery GB et al, eds. Neonatology Pathophysiology and Management of the Newborn, 5th Ed. Philadelphia: WB Saunders, 1999:1189.

156. McManus MC. Prudent selection of antimicrobials for neonatal sepsis. Am J Health-Syst Pharm 1996;53:1956.

157. Baltimore RS. Neonatal nosocomial infections. Semin Perinatol 1998;22:25.

158. Gaynes RP et al. Nosocomial infections among neonates in high-risk nurseries in the United States. Pediatrics 1996;98:357.

159. Faranoff AA et al. Incidence, presenting features, risk factors and significance of late onset septicemia in very low birthweight infants. Pediatr Infect Dis J 1998;17:593.

160. Krediet TG et al. Clinical outcome of cephalothin versus vancomycin therapy in the treatment of coagulase-negative Staphylococcal septicemia in neonates: relation to methicillin resistance and

mec A gene carriage of blood isolates. Pediatrics 1999;103(3). URL: http://www.pediatrics.org/cgi/content/full/103/3/e29.

161. Patrick CC et al. Persistent bacteremia due to coagulase-negative staphylococci in low birthweight neonates. Pediatrics 1989;84:977.

162. Harvey D et al. Bacterial meningitis in the newborn: a prospective study of mortality and morbidity. Semin Perinatol 1999;23:218.

163. Norris CMR et al. Aseptic meningitis in the newborn and young infant. Am Fam Physician 1999; 59:2761.

164. Payne NR et al. Selecting antibiotics for nosocomial bacterial infections in patients requiring neonatal intensive care. Neonatal Network 1994; 13:41.

165. Matrai-Kovalskis Y et al. Positive blood cultures for coagulase-negative Staphylococci in neonates: does highly-selective vancomycin usage affect outcome? Infection 1998;26:85

166. Nelson JD, Bradley JS. Nelson's Pocket Book of Pediatric Antimicrobial Therapy, 14th Ed. Philadelphia: Lippincott Williams & Wilkins, 2000:16.

167. Fanos V, Dall'Agnola A. Antibiotics in neonatal infections: a review. Drugs 1999;58:405.

168. Kraus DM et al. Efficacy and tolerability of extended-interval aminoglycoside administration in pediatric patients. Pediatr Drugs 2002;4:469.

169. Rodvold KA et al. Single daily doses of aminoglycosides. Lancet 1997;350:1412.

170. Parker SE, Davey PG. Once-daily aminoglycoside administration in gram-negative sepsis. PharmacoEconomics 1995;7:393.

171. Schelonka RL, Infante AJ. Neonatal immunology. Semin Perinatol 1998;22:2.

172. Jenson HB, Pollock BH. Meta-analyses of the effectiveness of intravenous immune globulin for prevention and treatment of neonatal sepsis. Pediatrics 1997;99(2). URL: http://www.pediatrics.org/cgi/content/full/99/2/e2.

173. Ohlsson A, Lacy JB. Intravenous immunoglobulin for preventing infection in preterm and/or low-birth-weight infants. Cochrane Database Syst Rev, The Cochrane Library 2003:1:CD000361.

174. Ohlsson A, Lacy LB. Intravenous immunoglobulin for suspected or subsequently proven infection in neonates. Cochrane Database Syst Rev, The Cochrane Library 2003:1:CD001239.

175. Faranoff AA et al. A controlled trial of intravenous immune globulin to reduce nosocomial infections in very-low-birth-weight infants. N Engl J Med 1994;330:1107.

176. Weismann LE, Lorenzetti PM. High intravenous doses of human immune globulin suppress neonatal group B streptococcal immunity in rats. J Pediatrics 1989;115:445.

177. Gotoff SP. Pathogenesis and epidemiology. In: Behrman RE et al, eds. Nelson Textbook of Pediatrics, 16th Ed. Philadelphia: WB Saunders, 2000:538.

178. Burchett SK. Infections: viral infections. In: Cloherty JP, Stark AR, eds. Manual of Neonatal Care, 4th Ed. Philadelphia: Lippincott-Raven, 1998:239.

179. Beazley DM, Egerman RS. Toxoplasmosis. Semin Perinatol 1998;22:332.

180. Hollier LM, Cox SM. Syphilis. Semin Perinatol 1998;22:323.

181. Cowles TA, Gonik B. Perinatal infections. In: Fanaroff AA, Martin MJ, eds. Neonatal-Perinatal Medicine: Diseases of the Fetus and Infant, 6th Ed. St. Louis: Mosby-Year Book, 1997:327.

182. American Academy of Pediatrics. Pickering LK, ed. 2000 Red Book: Report of the Committee on Infectious Diseases, 25th Ed. Elk Grove Village, IL: American Academy of Pediatrics, 2000.

183. Riley LE. Herpes simplex virus. Semin Perinatol 1998;22:284.

184. Jacobs RF. Neonatal herpes simplex virus infections. Semin Perinatol 1998;22:64.

185. Kimberlin DW et al. Safety and efficacy of high-dose intravenous acyclovir in the management of neonatal herpes simplex virus infections. Pediatrics 2001;108:230.

186. Kimberlin D et al. Administration of oral acyclovir suppressive therapy after neonatal herpes simplex virus disease limited to the skin, eyes, and mouth: results of a Phase I/II trial. Pediatr Infect Dis J 1996;15:247.

187. Guerina NG. Infections: toxoplasmosis. In: Cloherty JP, Stark AR, eds. Manual of Neonatal Care, 4th Ed. Philadelphia: Lippincott-Raven, 1998: 318.

188. Brown HL, Abernathy MP. Cytomegalovirus infection. Semin Perinatol 1998;22:260.

189. Poets CF et al. Epidemiology and pathophysiology of apnoea of prematurity. Biol Neonate 1994;65:211.

190. Barrington K, Finer N. The natural history of the appearance of apnea of prematurity. Pediatr Res 1991;29:372.

191. Consensus Statement. National Institutes of Health Consensus Development Conference on Infantile Apnea and Home Monitoring, Sept. 29 to Oct. 1, 1986. Pediatrics 1987;79:292.

192. Martin GI. Infant apnea. In: Pomerance JJ, Richardson CJ, eds. Neonatology for the Clinician. Norwalk: Appleton & Lange, 1993:267.

193. Miller MJ, Martin RJ. Apnea of prematurity. Clin Perinatol 1992;19:789.

194. Martin RJ et al. Pathogenesis of apnea in preterm infants. J Pediatr 1986;109:733.

195. Finer NN et al. Obstructive, mixed, and central apnea in the neonate: physiologic correlates. J Pediatr 1992;121:943.

196. Aranda JV et al. Drug treatment of neonatal apnea. In: Yaffe SJ, Aranda JV, eds. Pediatric Pharmacology: Therapeutic Principles in Practice. Philadelphia: WB Saunders, 1992:193.

197. Darnall RA. Aminophylline reduces hypoxic ventilatory depression: possible role of adenosine. Pediatr Res 1985;19:706.

198. Myers TF et al. Low-dose theophylline therapy in idiopathic apnea of prematurity. J Pediatr 1980;96:99.

199. Kritter KE, Blanchard J. Management of apnea in infants. Clin Pharm 1989;8:577.

200. Lopes JM et al. The effects of theophylline on diaphragmatic fatigue in the newborn. Pediatr Res 1982;16:355A.

201. Tang-Lui DDS et al. Nonlinear theophylline elimination. Clin Pharmacol Ther 1982;31:358.

202. Tang-Lui DD, Reigelman S. Metabolism of theophylline to caffeine in adults. Res Commun Chem Pathol Pharmacol 1981;34:371.

203. Muttitt SC et al. The dose response of theophylline in the treatment of apnea of prematurity. J Pediatr 1988;112:115.

204. Hendeles L et al. Revised FDA labeling guideline for theophylline oral dosage forms. Pharmacotherapy 1995;15:409.

205. Kraus DM et al. Pharmacokinetic evaluation of two theophylline dosing methods for infants. Ther Drug Monit 1994;16:270.

206. Eichenwald EC et al. Apnea frequently persists beyond term gestation in infants delivered at 24 to 28 weeks. Pediatrics 1997;100:354.

207. Aldridge A et al. Caffeine metabolism in the newborn. Clin Pharmacol Ther 1979;25:447.

208. LeGuennec JC et al. Maturational changes of caffeine concentration and disposition in infancy during maintenance therapy for apnea of prematurity: influence of gestational age, hepatic disease, and breast-feeding. Pediatrics 1985;76:834.

209. Aranda JV et al. Maturation of caffeine elimination in infancy. Arch Dis Child 1979;54:946.

210. Larsen PB et al. Aminophylline versus caffeine citrate for apnea and bradycardia prophylaxis in premature neonates. Acta Paediatr 1995;84:360.

211. Davis JM et al. Use of caffeine in infants unresponsive to theophylline in apnea of prematurity. Pediatr Pulmonol 1987;3:90.

212. Eyal F et al. Aminophylline versus doxapram in idiopathic apnea of prematurity: a double-blind controlled study. Pediatrics 1985;75:709.

213. Peliowski A, Finer NN. A blinded, randomized, placebo-controlled trial to compare theophylline and doxapram for the treatment of apnea of prematurity. J Pediatr 1990;116:648.

214. Barrington KJ et al. Dose-response relationship of doxapram in the therapy for refractory idiopathic apnea of prematurity. Pediatrics 1987;80:22.

215. Tay-Uyboco J et al. Clinical and physiological responses to prolonged nasogastric administration of doxapram for apnea of prematurity. Biol Neonate 1991;59:190.

216. Papageorgiou A, Bardin CL. The extremely-low-birth-weight infant. In Avery GB et al, eds. Neonatology: Pathophysiology & Management of the Newborn, 5th Ed. Philadelphia: Lippincott Williams & Wilkins, 1999:445.

217. De Villiers GS et al. Second-degree atrioventricular heart block after doxapram administration. J Pediatr 1998;133:149.

218. Papile LA. The central nervous system, part five: intracranial hemorrhage. In: Fanaroff AA, Martin RJ, eds. Neonatal-Perinatal Medicine: Diseases of the Fetus and Infant, 6th Ed. St. Louis: Mosby-Year Book, 1997:891.

219. Hill A. Intraventricular hemorrhage: emphasis on prevention. Semin Pediatr Neurol 1998;5:152.

220. Wells JT, Ment LR. Prevention of intraventricular hemorrhage in preterm infants. Early Hum Dev 1995;42:209.

221. Roland EH, Hill A. Intraventricular hemorrhage and posthemorrhagic hydrocephalus: current and potential future interventions. Clin Perinatol 1997;24:589.

222. Chang GY et al. Heparin and the risk of intraventricular hemorrhage in premature infants. J Pediatr 1997;131:361.

223. Moe P, Paige PL. Neurologic disorders. In: Merenstein GB, Gardner SL, eds. Handbook of Neonatal Intensive Care, 4th Ed. St. Louis: Mosby-Year Book, 1998:571.

224. Ment LR et al. Low-dose indomethacin and prevention of intraventricular hemorrhage: a multicenter randomized trial. Pediatrics 1994;93:543.

225. Ment LR et al. Neurodevelopmental outcome at 36 months' corrected age of preterm infants in the multicenter indomethacin intraventricular hemorrhage prevention trial. Pediatrics 1996;98:714.

226. Hill A, Volpe JJ. Neurological and neuromuscular disorders. In: Avery GB et al, eds. Neonatology: Pathophysiology & Management of the Newborn, 5th Ed. Philadelphia: Lippincott Williams & Wilkins, 1999:1231.

227. Scher MS. Seizures in the newborn infant: diagnosis, treatment, and outcome. Clin Perinatol 1997;24:735.

228. Morrison A. Neonatal seizures. In: Pomerance JJ, Richardson CJ, eds. Neonatology for the Clinician. Norwalk: Appleton & Lange, 1993:411.

229. Haymond MW. Hypoglycemia in infants and children. Endocrinol Metab Clin North Am 1989; 18:221.

230. Stafstrom CE. Neonatal seizures. Pediatr Rev 1995;16:248.

231. Massingale TW, Buttross S. Survey of treatment practices for neonatal seizures. J Perinatol 1993; 13:107.

232. Gilman JT et al. Rapid sequential phenobarbital treatment of neonatal seizures. Pediatrics 1989; 83:674.

233. Deshmukh A et al. Lorazepam in the treatment of refractory neonatal seizures: a pilot study. Am J Dis Child 1986;140:1042.

234. McDermott CA et al. Pharmacokinetics of lorazepam in critically ill neonates with seizures. J Pediatr 1992;120:479.

235. Gal P et al. Valproic acid efficacy, toxicity, and pharmacokinetics in neonates with intractable seizures. Neurology 1988;38:467.

236. Singh B et al. Treatment of neonatal seizures with carbamazepine. J Child Neurol 1996;11:378.

237. Painter MJ et al. Phenobarbital compared with phenytoin for the treatment of neonatal seizures. N Engl J Med 1999;341:485.

238. Painter MJ et al. Phenobarbital and phenytoin in neonatal seizures: metabolism and tissue distribution. Neurology 1981;31:1107

239. Levene M. The clinical conundrum of neonatal seizures. Arch Dis Child Fetal Neonatal Ed 2002;86:F75.

240. Ostrea EM at al. The infant of the drug-dependent mother. In: Avery GB et al, eds. Neonatology: Pathophysiology and Management of the Newborn, 5th Ed. Philadelphia: Lippincott Williams & Wilkins, 1999:1407.

241. Rosen TS. Infants of addicted mothers. In: Fanaroff AA, Martin RJ, eds. Neonatal-Perinatal Medicine: Diseases of the Fetus and Infant, 6th Ed. St. Louis: Mosby-Year Book, 1997:672.

242. Weiner SM, Finnegan LP. Drug withdrawal in the neonate. In: Merenstein GB, Gardner SL, eds. Handbook of Neonatal Intensive Care, 4th Ed. St. Louis: Mosby-Year Book, 1998:129.

243. Plessinger MA, Woods JR. Cocaine in pregnancy: recent data on maternal and fetal risks. Obstet Gynecol Clin North Am 1998;25:99.

244. Levy M, Spino M. Neonatal withdrawal syndrome: associated drugs and pharmacological management. Pharmacotherapy 1993;13:202.

245. Doberczak TM et al. Neonatal opiate abstinence syndrome in term and preterm infants. J Pediatr 1991;118:933.

246. Tran JH. Treatment of neonatal abstinence syndrome. J Pediatr Health Care 1999;13:295.

247. American Academy of Pediatrics, Committee on Drugs. Neonatal drug withdrawal. Pediatrics 1998;101:1079.

248. Greenglass EJ. The adverse effects of cocaine on the developing human. In: Yaffe SJ, Aranda JV, eds. Pediatric Pharmacology: Therapeutic Principles in Practice. Philadelphia: WB Saunders, 1992:598.

249. Coyle MG et al. Diluted tincture of opium (DTO) and phenobarbital versus DTO alone for neonatal opiate withdrawal in term infants. J Pediatr 2002;140:561.

250. Theis JGW et al. Current management of the neonatal abstinence syndrome: a critical analysis of the evidence. Biol Neonate 1997;71:345.

251. Wijburg FA et al. Morphine as an anti-epileptic drug in neonatal abstinence syndrome. Acta Paediatr Scand 1991;80:875.

252. Hoder EL et al. Clonidine treatment of neonatal narcotic abstinence syndrome. Psychiatry Res 1984;13:243.

253. Stark AR et al. Muscle relaxation in mechanically ventilated infants. J Pediatr 1979;94:439.

254. Crone RK, Favorito J. The effects of pancuronium bromide on infants with hyaline membrane disease. J Pediatr 1980;97:991.

255. Buck ML, Reed MD. Use of nondepolarizing neuromuscular blocking agents in mechanically ventilated patients. Clin Pharm 1991;10:32.

256. Carlo WA et al. Assisted ventilation and complications of respiratory distress. In: Fanaroff AA, Martin RJ, eds. Neonatal-Perinatal Medicine: Diseases of the Fetus and Infant, 6th Ed. St. Louis: CV Mosby, 1997:1028.

257. Taylor P. Agents acting at the neuromuscular junction and autonomic ganglia. In: Hardman JG et al, eds. Goodman and Gilman's The Pharmacological Basis of Therapeutics, 9th Ed. New York: McGraw-Hill, 1996:177.

258. Greenough A et al. Investigation of the effects of paralysis by pancuronium on heart rate variability, blood pressure and fluid balance. Acta Paediatr Scand 1989;78:829.

259. Cabal LA et al. Cardiovascular and catecholamine changes after administration of pancuronium in distressed neonates. Pediatrics 1985;75:284.

260. Piotrowski A. Comparison of atracurium and pancuronium in mechanically ventilated neonates. Intensive Care Med 1993;19:401.

261. Menon G et al. Practical approach to analgesia and sedation in the neonatal intensive care unit. Semin Perinatol 1998;22:417.

262. Abu-Saad HH et al. Assessment of pain in the neonate. Semin Perinatol 1998;22:402.

263. Anand KJS et al. Analgesia and sedation in preterm neonates who require ventilatory support:

results from the NOPAIN trial. Arch Pediatr Adolesc Med 1999;153:331.

264. Goldberg RN et al. Detection of seizure activity in the paralyzed neonate using continuous monitoring. Pediatrics 1982;69:583.

265. Zenk KE. Practical pharmacology for the clinician caring for the newborn. In: Pomerance JJ, Richardson CJ, eds. Neonatology for the Clinician. Norwalk: Appleton & Lange, 1993:59.

266. Scott CS et al. Morphine pharmacokinetics and pain assessment in premature newborns. J Pediatr 1999;135:423.

267. Roth B et al. Analgesia and sedation in neonatal intensive care using fentanyl by continuous infusion. Dev Pharmacol Ther 1991;17:121.

268. Norton SJ. After effects of morphine and fentanyl analgesia: a retrospective study. Neonatal Network 1988;7:25.

269. Arnold JH et al. Changes in the pharmacodynamic response to fentanyl in neonates during continuous infusion. J Pediatr 1991;119:639.

270. Katz R et al. Prospective study on the occurrence of withdrawal in critically ill children who receive fentanyl by continuous infusion. Crit Care Med 1994;22:763.

271. Lane JC et al. Movement disorder after withdrawal of fentanyl infusion. J Pediatr 1991;119:649.

272. Anand KIS, Arnold JH. Opioid tolerance and dependence in infants and children. Crit Care Med 1994;22:334.

273. Watling SM, Dasta JF. Prolonged paralysis in intensive care unit patients after the use of neuromuscular blocking agents: a review of the literature. Crit Care Med 1994;22:884.

274. Anyebuno MA, Rosenfeld CR. Chloral hydrate toxicity in a term infant. Dev Pharmacol Ther 1991;17:116.

275. Mayers DJ et al. Chloral hydrate disposition following single-dose administration to critically ill neonates and children. Dev Pharmacol Ther 1991;16:71.

276. Mayers DJ et al. Sedative/hypnotic effects of chloral hydrate in the neonate: trichloroethanol or parent drug? Dev Pharmacol Ther 1992;19:141.

277. Nahata MC, Hipple TF. Pediatric Drug Formulations, 4th Ed. Cincinnati, OH: Harvey Whitney Books Company, 2000.

278. Nahata MC. Lack of pediatric drug formulations. Pediatrics 1999;104:607.

279. Blumer JL, Reed MD. Principles of neonatal pharmacology. In: Yaffe SV, Aranda JV, eds. Pediatric Pharmacology: Therapeutic Principles in Practice, 2nd Ed. Philadelphia: WB Saunders, 1992:164.

280. Ernst JA et al. Osmolality of substances used in the intensive care nursery. Pediatrics 1983;72:347.

281. White KC, Harkavy KL. Hypertonic formula resulting from added oral medications. Am J Dis Child 1982;136:931.

282. American Academy of Pediatrics, Committee on Drugs. "Inactive" ingredients in pharmaceutical products: update (subject review). Pediatrics 1997;99:268.

283. Balistreri WF et al. Lessons from the E-Ferol tragedy. Pediatrics 1986;78:503.

284. Duncan B et al. Medication-induced pneumatosis intestinalis. Pediatrics 1997;99:633.

285. Nahata MC. Intravenous infusion conditions: implications for pharmacokinetic monitoring. Clin Pharmacokinet 1993;24:221.

286. Roberts RJ. Issues and problems associated with drug delivery in pediatric patients. J Clin Pharmacol 1994;34:723.

287. Nahata MC et al. Effect of infusion methods on tobramycin serum concentrations in newborn infants. J Pediatr 1984;104:136.

CHAPTER 95

Pediatric Immunizations

Sherry Luedtke, Michelle Condren, Mark Haase

The use of immunizations to control common childhood infectious diseases has been one of the most important medical developments to date. Children are now routinely immunized against 13 infectious diseases (Table 95-1). As a result, cases of diphtheria, tetanus, mumps, measles, rubella, polio, and *Haemophilus influenzae type b* are at record-low levels.[1] Despite the availability of immunizations, many preschoolers in the United States lack adequate protection.[2] In one survey, only 74% of children ages 19 to 35 months had completed the required 4:3:1:3 vaccination series (four doses diphtheria/tetanus/pertussis [DTP], three doses polio, one dose measles/mumps/rubella [MMR], and three doses *H. influenzae type b* conjugate vaccine [HbCV]). An estimated 1 million or more children require additional vaccine doses to be completely protected.[3]

Health care providers play a vital role in clarifying misconceptions and educating parents and health care practitioners about the importance of proper and complete immunizations. Any contact with a pediatric patient represents an opportunity to promote immunization. Every medication history should include a complete immunization history, and the child's vaccination card should be used to detect any deficiency in immunization status.[1,4–8]

GUIDELINES
Schedule for Immunizations

1. K.C., a 1-month-old baby girl, is brought to the clinic for a scheduled well-baby visit. K.C.'s mother inquires about immunizations for her daughter. What are the current recommendations for immunizing pediatric patients? When should these immunizations be given to K.C.?

The goal of pediatric immunization is to prevent specific infectious diseases and their sequelae. For maximum effectiveness, a vaccine must be administered to the susceptible population before anyone has been exposed to the pathogen. However, the age at which immunizations are administered to specific individuals depends on several factors (e.g., age-specific risks of the disease, risks of complications, presence of maternal antibodies transferred through the placenta, maturity of the immune system). Usually, immunizations are administered at the youngest age that the child is able to develop an adequate antibody response.

The recommended childhood and adolescent immunization schedule for 2003 is shown in Table 95-1. This schedule is published annually in *Morbidity and Mortality Weekly Reports* by the Center for Disease Control (CDC) and is available on-line through their website (http://www.cdc.gov/mmwr) Immunization schedules can be adjusted to meet individual needs and may begin at any time of the year.[9] Vaccines should not be administered at intervals shorter than that recommended to achieve maximal immunity benefits. The CDC also has developed an administration schedule for children and adolescents who begin their immunizations late or who are >1 month behind in their immunizations along with minimal intervals between doses (Tables 95-2 and 95-3) for the administration of various vaccines.[9] An interruption or delay in the recommended schedule does not interfere with the final immunity gained.

2. K.C.'s mother was hepatitis B-surface antigen (HbsAg) negative before delivery, and her baby received Engerix-B shortly after birth. When should K.C. receive her next immunization for hepatitis B?

Hepatitis B virus (HBV) can be transmitted via exposure to contaminated blood (e.g., blood products, medical instruments, needles used in intravenous drug abuse or tattooing), exposure to body fluids (e.g., sexual intercourse), and transplacentally from a HbsAg-positive mother. The prevention of HBV maternal transmission to an infant is important because acute disease can progress to a chronic carrier state, which can lead to chronic liver disease and primary hepatocellular carcinoma. Children acquiring HBV infection before 5 years of age are at an especially high risk of developing chronic infection.[10]

Table 95-1 Recommended Childhood and Adolescent Immunization Schedule[a]—United States, 2003

Vaccine	Birth	1 mo	2 mo	4 mo	6 mo	12 mo	15 mo	18 mo	24 mo	4–6 yr	11–12 yr	13–18 yr
Hepatitis B[b]	Hep #1 only if mother HBsAg(+)		HepB #2			HepB #3					HepB series	
Diphtheria, Tetanus, Pertussis[c]			DTaP	DTaP	DTaP		DTaP			DTaP	Td	
Haemophilus influenzae Type b[d]			Hib	Hib	Hib	Hib						
Inactivated Polio			IPV	IPV		IPV				IPV		
Measles, Mumps, Rubella[e]						MMR #1				MMR #2	MMR #2	
Varicella[f]						Varicella					Varicella	
Pneumococcal[g]			PCV	PCV	PCV	PCV			PCV	PPV		
Hepatitis A[h]											HepA series	
Influenza[i]					Influenza (yearly)							

Range of recommended ages / Catch-up vaccination / Preadolescent assessment

Vaccines below this line are for selected populations

[a]Indicates the recommended ages for routine administration of currently licensed childhood vaccines, as of December 1, 2002, for children through age 18 years. Any dose not given at the recommended age should be given at any subsequent visit when indicated and feasible. ▓ Indicates age groups that warrant special effort to administer those vaccines not given previously. Additional vaccines may be licensed and recommended during the year. Licensed combination vaccines may be used whenever any components of the combination are indicated and the vaccine's other components are not contraindicated. Providers should consult the manufacturers' package inserts for detailed recommendations.

[b]**Hepatitis B vaccine (HepB).** All infants should receive the first dose of HepB vaccine soon after birth and before hospital discharge; the first dose also may be given by age 2 months if the infant's mother is HBsAg-negative. Only monovalent HepB vaccine can be used for the birth dose. Monovalent or combination vaccine containing HepB may be used to complete the series; 4 doses of vaccine may be administered when a birth dose is given. The second dose should be given at least 4 weeks after the first dose except for combination vaccines, which cannot be administered before age 6 weeks. The third dose should be given at least 16 weeks after the first dose and at least 8 weeks after the second dose. The last dose in the vaccination series (third or fourth dose) should not be administered before age 6 months. *Infants born to HbsAg-positive mothers* should receive HepB vaccine and 0.5 mL hepatitis B immune globulin (HBIG) within 12 hours of birth at separate sites. The second dose is recommended at age 1–2 months. The last dose in the vaccination series should not be administered before age 6 months. These infants should be tested for HbsAg and anti-HBs at 9–15 months of age. *Infants born to mothers whose HbsAg status is unknown* should receive the first dose of the HepB vaccine series within 12 hours of birth. Maternal blood should be drawn as soon as possible to determine the mother's HbsAg status; if the HbsAg test is positive, the infant should receive HBIG as soon as possible (no later than age 1 week). The second dose is recommended at age 1–2 months. The last dose in the vaccination series should not be administered before age 6 months.

[c]**Diphtheria and tetanus toxoids and acellular pertussis vaccine (DTaP).** The fourth dose of DTaP may be administered at age 12 months provided that 6 months have elapsed since the third dose and the child is unlikely to return at age 15–18 months. **Tetanus and diphtheria toxoids (Td)** is recommended at age 11–12 years if at least 5 years have elapsed since the last dose of Td-containing vaccine. Subsequent routine Td boosters are recommended every 10 years.

[d]*Haemophilus influenzae* **type b (Hib) conjugate vaccine.** Three Hib conjugate vaccines are licensed for infant use. If PRP-OMP (PedvaxHIB® or ComVax® [Merck]) is administered at age 2 and 4 months, a dose at age 6 months is not required. DTaP/Hib combination products should not be used for primary vaccination in infants at age 2, 4, or 6 months but can be used as boosters following any Hib vaccine.

[e]**Measles, mumps, and rubella vaccine (MMR).** The second dose of MMR is recommended routinely at age 4–6 years but may be administered during any visit provided that at least 4 weeks have elapsed since the first dose and that both doses are administered beginning at or after age 12 months. Those who have not received the second dose previously should complete the schedule by the visit at age 11–12 years.

[f]**Varicella vaccine.** Varicella vaccine is recommended at any visit at or after age 12 months for susceptible children (i.e., those who lack a reliable history of chickenpox). Susceptible persons aged ≥13 years should receive 2 doses given at least 4 weeks apart.

[g]**Pneumococcal vaccine.** The heptavalent **pneumococcal conjugate vaccine (PCV)** is recommended for all children aged 2–23 months and for certain children aged 24–59 months. **Pneumococcal polysaccharide vaccine (PPV)** is recommended in addition to PCV for certain high-risk groups. See *MMWR* 2000;49(No. RR-9):1–37.

[h]**Hepatitis A vaccine.** Hepatitis A vaccine is recommended for children and adolescents in selected states and regions, and for certain high-risk groups. Consult local public health authority and *MMWR* 1999;48(No. RR-12):1–37. Children and adolescents in these states, regions, and high-risk groups who have not been immunized against hepatitis A can begin the hepatitis A vaccination series during any visit. The two doses in the series should be administered at least 6 months apart.

[i]**Influenza vaccine.** Influenza vaccine is recommended annually for children aged ≥6 months with certain risk factors (including but not limited to asthma, cardiac disease, sickle cell disease, HIV, and diabetes, and household members of persons in groups at high risk (see *MMWR* 2002;51[No. RR-3]:1–31), and can be administered to all others wishing to obtain immunity. In addition, healthy children aged 6–23 months are encouraged to receive influenza vaccine if feasible because children in this age group are at substantially increased risk for influenza-related hospitalizations. Children aged ≤12 years should receive vaccine in a dosage appropriate for their age (0.25 mL if 6–35 months or 0.5 mL if ≥3 years). Children aged ≤8 years who are receiving influenza vaccine for the first time should receive 2 doses separated by at least 4 weeks.

Additional information about vaccines, including precautions and contraindications for vaccination and vaccine shortages, is available at http://www.cdc.gov/nip or at the National Immunization information hotline, telephone 800-232-2522 (English) or 800-232-0233 (Spanish). Copies of the schedule can be obtained at http://www.cdc.gov/nip/recs/child-schedule.htm. Approved by the **Advisory Committee on Immunization Practices** (http://www.cdc.gov/nip/acip), the **American Academy of Pediatrics** (http://www.aap.org), and the **American Academy of Family Physicians** (http://www.aafp.org).

Table 95-2 Catch-up Schedule for Children Aged 4 Months–6 Years

| Dose One (Minimum Age) | Minimum Interval Between Doses | | | |
	Dose One to Dose Two	Dose Two to Dose Three	Dose Three to Dose Four	Dose Four to Dose Five
DTaP (6 wks)	**4 wk**	**4 wk**	**6 mo**	**6 mo**[a]
IPV (6 wks)	**4 wk**	**4 wk**	**4 wk**[b]	
HepB[c] (birth)	**4 wk**	**8 wk** (and 16 weeks after first dose)		
MMR (12 mo)	**4 wk**[d]			
Varicella (12 mo)				
Hib[e] (6 wk)	**4 wk:** if 1st dose given at age <12 mo **8 wk (as final dose):** if 1st dose given at age 12–24 mo **No further doses needed:** if 1st dose given at age ≥15 mo	**4 wk**[f]: if current age ≥12 mo **8 wk (as final dose)**[f]: If current age ≥12 mo and 2nd dose given at age <15 mo **No further doses needed:** if previous dose given at age ≥15 mo	**8 wk (as final dose):** this dose only necessary for children aged 12 mo–5 yr who received 3 doses before age 12 mo	
PCV[g] (6 wk)	**4 wk:** if 1st dose given at age <12 mo and current age <24 mo **8 wk (as final dose):** if 1st dose given at age ≥12 mo or current age 24–59 mo **No further doses needed:** for healthy children if 1st dose given at age ≥24 mo	**4 wk:** if current age <12 mo **8 wk (as final dose):** if current age ≥12 mo **No further doses needed:** for healthy children if previous dose given at age ≥24 mo	**8 wk (as final dose):** this dose only necessary for children aged 12 mo–5 yr who received 3 doses before age 12 mo	

[a]**Diphtheria and tetanus toxoids and acellular pertussis vaccine (DTaP):** The fifth dose is not necessary if the fourth dose was given after the fourth birthday.
[b]**Inactivated Polio (IPV):** For children who received an all-IPV or all-OPV series, a fourth dose is not necessary if third dose was given at age ≥4 years. If both OPV and IPV were given as part of a series, a total of 4 doses should be given, regardless of the child's current age.
[c]**Hepatitis B vaccine (HepB):** All children and adolescents who have not been vaccinated against hepatitis B should begin the hepatitis B vaccination series during any visit. Providers should make special efforts to immunize children who were born in, or whose parents were born in, areas of the world where hepatitis B virus infection is moderately or highly endemic.
[d]**Measles, mumps, and rubella vaccine (MMR):** The second dose of MMR is recommended routinely at age 4–6 years, but may be given earlier if desired.
[e]**Haemophilus influenzae type b (Hib):** Vaccine is not recommended generally for children aged ≥5 years.
[f]**Hib:** If current age is <12 months and the first 2 doses were PRP-OMP (PedvaxHIB or ComVax [Merck]), the third (and final) dose should be given at age 12–15 months and at least 8 weeks after the second dose.
[g]**Pneumococcal conjugate vaccine (PCV):** Vaccine is not recommended generally for children aged ≥5 years.

Table 95-3 Catch-up Schedule for Children Aged 7–18 Years

| Minimum Interval Between Doses | | |
Dose One to Dose Two	Dose Two to Dose Three	Dose Three to Booster Dose
Td: **4 wk**	**Td:** **6 mo**	**Td:**[a] **6 mo:** if 1st dose given at age <12 mos and current age <11 yrs **5 yr:** if 1st dose given at age ≥12 mos and 3rd dose given at age <7 yrs and current age ≥11 yrs **10 yr:** if 3rd dose given at age ≥7 yrs
IPV[b]: **4 wk**	**IPV**[b]: **4 wk**	
HepB: **4 wk**	**HepB:** **8 wk** (and 16 wk after 1st dose)	
MMR: **4 wk**		
Varicella[c]: **4 wk**		**IPV**[b]

[a]**Tetanus toxoid:** For children aged 7–10 years, the interval between the third and booster dose is determined by the age when the first dose was given. For adolescents aged 11–18 years, the interval is determined by the age when the third dose was given.
[b]**Inactivated Polio (IPV):** Vaccine is not recommended generally for persons aged ≥18 years.
[c]**Varicella:** Give 2-doses series to all susceptible adolescents aged ≥13 years.

All pregnant women should be tested for HbsAg and infants born to HbsAg-positive mothers should receive their first vaccine dose within 12 hours of birth.[11] Subsequent vaccine doses should be administered at age 1 to 2 months if the mother is HbsAg negative and again at age 6 months (see footnotes to Table 95-1). Hepatitis B immunoglobulin (HBIG) should be administered as soon as possible for infants born to HbsAg-positive mothers. If the mother's HbsAg status is unknown, the infant should be also immunized within 12 hours of birth. In-fants born to HbsAg-negative mothers should begin their immunization series before hospital discharge, but more flexibility in scheduling is possible. All unimmunized children should receive hepatitis B vaccine to initiate protection before high-risk behaviors begin.[9]

Two hepatitis B (HepB) vaccines are currently available for use in the United States. Recombivax-HB and Engerix-B are yeast-derived recombinant vaccines administered as a three-dose series. Adolescents and adults also should follow a three-dose schedule at 0, 1, and 6 months apart. As an option, adolescents may receive a two-dose schedule of the adult formulation of Recombivax-HB.[9] Dialysis patients and other immunocompromised patients may require a fourth dose if the anti-HBs level is <10 mLU/mL 2 months after the third dose.[12] Antibody screening following immunization is only recommended in high-risk groups. Dosage recommendations depend on whether the patient is in a high-risk group, which vaccine is used, and the patient's age.[13] Hepatitis B vaccine is combined with *Haemophilus influenzae* type b vaccine in Comvax. PEDIARIX is a combination of DTaP, hepatitis B, and IPV. Monovalent vaccines are preferred for the initial vaccination, however, combination vaccines may be used to complete the series after 6 weeks of age.[9,14]

K.C.'s immunization against hepatitis B at birth was appropriate based on current national guidelines, and hepatitis immune globulin (HBIG) was not needed because her mother is HbsAg negative. K.C. can receive her subsequent doses of hepatitis B vaccine according to the schedule in Table 95-1. Either formulation may be used because the immune response from a course using different vaccines is comparable to that of a full series using a single vaccine.[14,15]

Contraindications

3. K.C. returns at 2 months of age for another well-baby visit. She is alert, healthy, and growing appropriately. K.C. is scheduled to continue her primary immunization series. What immunizations should K.C. receive at this visit? K.C. has been exposed to a viral upper respiratory tract infection. Should her immunizations be delayed?

Misconceptions about contraindications and precautions for immunization often result in missed opportunities to provide needed immunizations. True contraindications to both live and killed vaccines include acute, severe febrile illness; history of anaphylaxis to the vaccine or vaccine components; and history of a severe reaction to an immunization. Immunization should not be delayed in a child who has a minor illness (e.g., upper respiratory tract infection, otitis media, diarrhea) with or without low-grade fever. Family history of seizures, allergies, and sudden infant death syndrome are not contraindications. Immunization of a child with a history of anaphylaxis to a vaccine or vaccine component should be withheld until the child has undergone desensitization.[16] Preterm infants should be immunized according to their chronologic age for all vaccines, with the exception of hepatitis B vaccination which may require modification of timing of immunization in infants <2 kg.[16–18a]

Contraindications to live attenuated virus vaccines and live bacterial vaccines include allergic reaction to previous exposure to vaccine components, immunosuppression (e.g., immunosuppressive therapy, immunodeficiencies), encephalopathy, recent administration of blood products, and pregnancy (although the risk in pregnancy is largely theoretical). Pooled blood products (e.g., immunoglobulins, packed red blood cells, platelet transfusions) can impair the immune response to a live vaccine because these products contain antibodies, which can prevent an infant's immune system from mounting an adequate response. The impairment of an immune response to an immunization varies depending upon the type and amount of blood product administered and immunizations may need to be delayed for up to 12 months if pooled blood products have been administered recently.[19] If there is a question about immune response, antibody titers can be obtained to determine if a patient needs to be re-immunized.[15]

Because K.C. does not have any contraindications, she can continue her active immunization series at this visit. She should receive her first doses of diphtheria, tetanus, pertussis, inactivated polio, *H. influenzae type b*, and pneumococcal vaccines.

Adverse Effects

4. K.C.'s mother is very concerned about the potential adverse effects of vaccines. How should parents evaluate the balance between the benefits against the risks of immunizations?

Immunizations have had a dramatic impact on several once common childhood infections. For example, smallpox has been eradicated from the world, polio is moving toward global eradication, and invasive *H. influenzae type b* disease among children has declined 95%.[20] However, vaccines have potential side effects that often cause concern for parents.

Adverse reactions to inactivated vaccines include pain at the injection site (also see Question 8) and fever within 48 to 72 hours of administration. In contrast, adverse effects from live attenuated vaccines occur 7 to 10 days after immunization, after the virus has replicated and the immune system has responded. Adverse reactions to live attenuated vaccines mimic the symptoms of disease. Transient rash occurs in 5% of patients receiving MMR immunizations, and a mild varicella-like rash (median of five lesions) occurs in fewer than 5% of patients receiving the varicella vaccine. Syncope, usually occurring within 30 minutes of immunization, has been reported.[21] Although anaphylactic reactions to vaccines are rare, an allergic reaction may occur as a result of specific allergy to the vaccine itself or to trace components in the vaccine (e.g., preservatives, antibiotics). Children with egg allergy can receive vaccines produced in chick-embryo-fibroblast tissue culture (e.g., measles, rubella, mumps) because the risk for serious reaction to these vaccines in egg-allergic children is very low.[22–24] MMR should be used cautiously in individuals with a history of a severe reaction to gelatin, which is a stabilizer in the MMR vaccine. Trace amounts of streptomycin, bacitracin, and neomycin are present in oral polio virus vaccine (OPV), IPV, and MMR; therefore, these vaccines should not be administered to individuals with a history of an anaphylactic reaction to these antibiotics.[25]

Overall, vaccinations are safe, especially when compared with the risks of the diseases that these vaccines prevent, and the safety of immunizations are scrutinized continually. In response to concerns about vaccine safety, the National Vaccine Injury Compensation Act mandated an ongoing review of evidence regarding the possible adverse effects of vaccines and established a no-fault injury compensation program for selected vaccines.[20,25,26]

PERTUSSIS

Pertussis ("whooping cough"), an infectious disease caused by *Bordetella pertussis,* is characterized by a paroxysmal cough with a whoop-like, high-pitched inspiratory noise, vomiting, and lymphocytosis. It is a highly communicable infection, which can affect 90% of infants and young children in non-immunized households, and is associated with serious sequelae. An estimated 0.3% to 14% of patients with pertussis experience encephalopathy, 0.6% to 2% have permanent neurologic damage, and about 0.1 to 4% die.[27] This serious childhood infection has been mitigated with the availability of a pertussis vaccine, which commonly is administered in combination with diphtheria and tetanus vaccines (i.e., DTP). The efficacy of the DTP vaccines against pertussis after primary immunization (three doses) is greater than 80%.[28,29] Protection increases to 90% after the last booster (age 4 to 6 years) then decreases over the next 12 years, after which protection is minimal.[30]

Despite the availability of an effective vaccine and a high rate of vaccine coverage, reports of pertussis continue to rise.[31] Decreased immunity in adolescents and adults is believed to contribute to this problem. It is estimated that 12% of adult patients with a cough lasting longer than two weeks have pertussis.[32] Although the illness is typically mild in adults and adolescents, they serve as a source of transmission to unprotected infants. Administration of a booster vaccine to young adults could be one added approach in an effort to eradicate pertussis. Currently, the pertussis vaccine is administered only to children up to 7 years of age because of concern about the incidence and severity of adverse reactions. The importance of pertussis immunization was reinforced when epidemic outbreaks of whooping cough occurred in England, Japan, and Sweden after many people discontinued pertussis immunization.[27]

The association of serious adverse events with whole cell pertussis vaccine generated considerable controversy on whether the risk/benefit ratio was sufficient to warrant immunization. As a result, vaccines containing whole cell pertussis have been replaced with acellular pertussis. Despite a much more favorable adverse effect profile, the diphtheria, tetanus, and acellular pertussis (DTaP) vaccine is still contraindicated in any child experiencing an anaphylactic reaction or encephalopathy within 7 days of immunization with DTaP which cannot be attributed to another cause.[33] In addition, careful consideration of subsequent doses should be given to infants experiencing a temperature 105°F (not resulting from another cause) or persistent, inconsolable crying lasting >3 hours within 48 hours after the administration of a pertussis-containing vaccine.[33] The pertussis component of the DTaP vaccine should be eliminated (i.e., continue vaccination with DT) in any child experiencing collapse or a hypotonic-hyporesponsive episode. If an evolving neurological disorder is present, pertussis immunization should be deferred until the problem has been fully evaluated. Pre-existing stable neurologic conditions (e.g., well-controlled seizures), are not contraindications because the benefits of pertussis immunization outweigh the risks.[15] A family history of seizures or other CNS disorder is not a contraindication.

The recommended schedule for DTaP immunization is shown in Table 95-1. Acetaminophen or ibuprofen should be administered at regular intervals for 24 hours after immunization to minimize the possibility of postvaccination fever and pain associated with the local reaction.

Five DTaP vaccines (ACEL-IMUNE, Infanrix, Certiva, Tripedia, and Daptacel) are approved for use. The combination product of DTaP-HepB-IPV (PEDIARIX) is approved for the primary vaccination series. If possible, the same DTaP product should be used for all five doses because information with respect to immunity, safety, and efficacy when interchanging vaccines is not available.[14,15] However, if the product information is unknown or unavailable from prior vaccination, any licensed DTaP vaccine may be used to complete the vaccination series.[14,15,21]

POLIO

Polio is an infectious disease caused by a highly contagious enterovirus. It can strike at any age but primarily affects children younger than 3 years of age (more than 50% of cases). The disease causes paralysis, which is almost always permanent. The three identified serotypes of poliovirus are transmitted person to person by direct fecal-oral contact or indirect exposure to infectious saliva, feces, or contaminated water. After household exposure, 90% of susceptible contacts become infected. The poliovirus enters through the mouth and then multiplies in the throat and intestines. Once established in the intestines, poliovirus can enter the bloodstream and invade the central nervous system. As it multiplies, the virus destroys nerve cells which cannot be regenerated, and as a result, muscles no longer function because of the lack of electrical stimuli from affected nerve cells. The muscles of the legs are affected more often than arm muscles; however, trunk muscles and muscles of the thorax and abdomen also increasingly can be affected, ultimately resulting in quadriplegia. The polio virus also can attack the motor neurons of the brainstem and thereby cause difficulty in speaking, swallowing, and breathing.

Immunity to polio can be achieved following natural infection with poliovirus; however, infection by one serotype of the poliovirus does not protect an individual against infection with the other two types. Immunity also can be achieved through immunization, and the development of effective vaccines to prevent paralytic polio was one of the major medical breakthroughs of the 20th century. Since the advent of the trivalent oral polio vaccine (OPV) and inactivated polio vaccine (IPV), the incidence of paralytic poliomyelitis has been reduced dramatically. Inspired by the success of the smallpox initiative, a global poliomyelitis eradication initiative has been initiated by the World Health Assembly. As a result of exclusive use of OPV, the Americas, Europe, and the Western Pacific regions have been certified free of indigenous wild poliomyelitis. However, the possibility for importation of wild virus still exists unless worldwide eradication is achieved. To prevent a polio epidemic in the United States, high levels of immunization for children during the first year of life are essential.

5. K.C.'s mother is surprised when the nurse brings in a polio injection because her son received an oral form of the vaccine when he was a baby. Why is KC receiving a different form of polio vaccine than her older brother received?

Until recently, the OPV or Sabin vaccine has been the vaccine of choice in the United States. Its advantages include low cost and ease of administration. OPV induces lifelong immunity similar to that observed after natural infection. In addition, OPV provides a high level of gut immunity, thus preventing the carrier state. Finally, the fecal shedding of vaccine virus after Sabin vaccine administration is an effective way to immunize or boost the pre-existing immunity in close contacts.[34] Despite these benefits, OPV carries the risk of vaccine-associated paralytic polio (VAPP), especially after the first dose. In the United States, 8 to 10 cases of VAPP occur each year. The current overall rate of paralytic disease is approximately 1 case per 2.4 million doses distributed, or 1 case per 1.4 million doses for immunologically normal children receiving OPV for the first dose.[35] The risk of VAPP is higher for immunocompromised patients, especially those with B-lymphocyte disorders (e.g., agammaglobulinemia, hypogammaglobulinemia).[36]

In contrast to OPV, the Salk vaccine (IPV) has not been associated with VAPP or other reactions. Enhanced potency IPV (IPOL, POLIOVAX), with an improved immunogenic response, has been available in the United States since 1987.[37] IPV provides the same systemic immunity as OPV. Although inferior to OPV, IPV induces some immunity of the gastrointestinal tract mucosa.[38] Intestinal immunity improves when two doses of OPV follow the first two doses of IPV.[39] Unfortunately, IPV is administered only by injection.

There has been great debate over which immunization, OPV or IVP, should be used in the United States. OPV is necessary for global eradication and should be used in countries endemic for poliovirus. However, because of the reduced threat of wild poliovirus, the risks associated with OPV have become less acceptable. In 1997, the ACIP provided three options for poliovirus vaccination: sequential use of IPV and OPV, OPV alone, and IPV alone.[40] In 1999, as the global polio initiative progressed and the likelihood of importing wild polio into the United States greatly decreased, the Advisory Committee on Immunization Practices (ACIP) modified the polio vaccination recommendations to include only an all-IPV schedule. Based on these revised recommendations, all children will receive four doses of IPV (ages 2 months, 4 months, 6 to 18 months, and 4 to 6 years).[41] Currently, OPV may be used only in special circumstances such as vaccination to control outbreaks of paralytic polio, unvaccinated children traveling in <4 weeks to areas endemic for polio, and children of parents who reject the number of vaccine injections (these children should receive IPV for the first two doses followed by OPV for doses three and four).[41] This revised strategy provides protection against poliomyelitis while minimizing the possibility of VAPP among OPV recipients as well as household and community contacts. IPV is the only poliovirus vaccine that should be used in patients with an immunodeficiency disorder, those receiving immunosuppressive chemotherapy, or children living with a person who is known or suspected to have these conditions.

6. A 28-year-old patient is planning extensive travels through the African continent and is concerned about polio because she had not been immunized as a child. What would be a prudent immunization schedule for her if her trip includes travel to a polio-endemic area?

Routine poliovirus vaccination of persons older than 18 years of age is not necessary in the United States because they are at minimal risk of exposure. Vaccination, however, should be considered for adults at high risk of polio exposure (e.g., travel to an area endemic for polio, close contact with children who will be receiving OPV, close contact with patients who

may be excreting wild polioviruses, work that requires handling poliovirus specimens). IPV is the vaccine of choice because adults have a higher incidence of vaccine-associated paralytic polio (VAPP) than children. Ideally, non-immunized persons anticipating exposure should receive two doses of IPV, administered 4 to 8 weeks apart followed by a third dose 6 to 12 months later. If exposure is likely in less than 8 weeks, two doses of IPV should be administered at least 4 weeks apart. If this patient's travel must be undertaken on short notice, the patient and physician must weigh the risk of OPV use against the risk of infection abroad. Adults who have completed a primary series of OPV or IPV may receive another dose of OPV or IPV before travel. In domestic outbreaks of polio, OPV is routinely given to adult contacts because the risk of natural disease is much greater than the risk of paralysis from OPV. Pregnancy is not a contraindication to OPV immunization when protection is needed (i.e., during an epidemic).

HAEMOPHILUS INFLUENZAE TYPE b

Haemophilus influenzae type b (Hib) was the most common cause of bacterial meningitis and a leading cause of serious, systemic bacterial diseases in children younger than 5 years of age until an effective vaccine was added to the routine immunization schedule.[42–44] The mortality rate associated with Hib meningitis was approximately 5%, with neurologic sequelae observed in 25% to 35% of survivors.[45,46] Epiglottitis, cellulitis, septic arthritis, osteomyelitis, pericarditis, and pneumonia also were commonly caused by *H. influenzae*. Although *H. influenzae* are commonly associated with otitis media and respiratory tract infections, type b strains account for only 5% to 10%.[47]

7. K.C. will be attending day care. Which of the available Hib immunizations should be administered to K.C.?

The first Hib polysaccharide vaccine was capable of eliciting an adequate immune response in children older than two years of age; however, the immune response in children 18 to 23 months of age only responded partially and a booster dose was required at 24 months of age[48,49] The polysaccharide vaccine was replaced by conjugate Hib vaccines to improve the immune response in younger children. It has led to a 95% reduction in the incidence of Hib disease in children younger than 5 years of age.[20] The four currently available Hib polysaccharide conjugate vaccines (HbCV) are as follows: Hib diphtheria toxoid conjugate vaccine or PRP-D (ProHIBiT), Hib meningococcal protein conjugate vaccine or PRP-OMP (PedvaxHIB), Hib tetanus toxoid conjugate vaccine or PRP-T (ActHIB, OmniHIB), and Hib diphtheria CRM197 protein conjugate vaccine or HbOC (HibTITER).[20] Like the original polysaccharide vaccine, immunogenicity of the conjugate vaccines are age dependent (i.e., older children have an improved immune response).[45,50] These four conjugated vaccines have been approved for use in infants, the group at highest risk for *H. influenzae* infection.[51,52] The HbCV immunization series requires a priming series followed by a booster dose at 12 to 18 months. PRP-OMP (PedvaxHIB) follows a slightly different priming series schedule compared to the other HbCVs; the primary series is administered at 2 and 4 months of age in contrast to the schedule of 2, 4, and 6 months primary series for the other vaccines. Ideally, the primary series should be completed with the same HbCV; however, there are data to support the interchangeability of the products for the priming and booster doses.[15,53] If PRP-OMP (PedVaxHIB) is used in a priming series with another HbCV, the number of doses necessary to complete the series for the other product should be administered.[15,53] K.C. could be immunized with any of these four Hib immunizations.

The number of doses of HbCV vaccine needed in older infants and children is dependent upon their age at presentation. Children who begin HbCV at 7 to 11 months of age should receive a primary series of two doses of a HbOC-, PRP-T-, or PRP-OMP-containing vaccine followed by a booster dose at 12 to 18 months of age administered at least 2 months after the previous dose. Children ages 12 to 15 months should receive a primary series of one dose followed by a booster dose 2 months later. If a child reaches 15 months of age without receiving HbCV, only one dose is necessary. HbCV is not indicated in children older than 5 years of age unless special circumstances place a child at an increased risk of infection.[5,51] The ACIP suggests considering immunization of children over 5 years of age who have functional asplenia, sickle cell anemia, or HIV infection.

Availability of HbCV for infants and children has dramatically reduced the incidence of invasive Hib infections. K.C. should start her primary series with a HbCV approved for young infants.

COMMON PARENT CONCERNS

8. K.C.'s mother is very concerned about the pain associated with immunization and the number of injections K.C. is to receive at each office visit. Can anything be done to minimize the pain associated with immunization injections? Can any of the immunizations be given together in the same syringe to minimize the number of injections?

The pain associated with injection of immunizations is typically brief and often more upsetting for the parent than the child. However, the need for multiple injections can result in an unhappy baby, especially by the third or fourth injection. Administration of an oral sucrose solution during the injection may help alleviate pain.[54,55] Topical anesthetics containing prilocaine and lidocaine can reduce pain and crying associated with immunization, however, high cost and the time required between application and injection have limited the use of these agents. More importantly, the use of topical anesthetics do not seem to modify the fear of injection or post-immunization discomfort.[56]

Ideally, pediatricians and parents would like to be able to deliver all needed vaccines with the fewest number of injections. Combination preparations (e.g., DTaP with HbCV; DTap with HepB and IPV; HepB with HbCV) are available to reduce the number of injections and may be used after 6 weeks of age.[14] If combination products are not used, the vaccines should be administered at different sites. If more than one injection must be administered in the same limb, the thigh is the preferred location because of the greater muscle mass.[56]

9. Some opponents to immunizations have raised the questions of whether immunizations can cause autism or weaken a child's immune system. What are the bases for these concerns?

Some parents are concerned that the MMR vaccine may cause autism. Due to a rise in the incidence of autism as well as the development of autistic symptoms around the time of vaccination, it was suggested that MMR vaccination may cause autism.[58,59] However, multiple epidemiologic studies have shown no correlation between vaccination and the development of autism.[57,59,60]

A survey conducted by the National Network for Immunization Information Steering Committee found that 25% of parents believe that administering "too many" immunizations at one time can weaken a child's immune system.[61] While children now receive as many as 20 immunizations by 2 years of age, the number of antigens they are exposed to is far less than children received in the 1980s. It is estimated that only 0.1% of the immune system would be affected if 11 immunizations are given simultaneously.[62] Current studies do not support the hypothesis that multiple immunizations weaken the immune system.

VARICELLA VACCINE

10. A working mother of two children learned there has been a case of chickenpox at their elementary school. Can her children be immunized against this infection?

Varivax, a live attenuated vaccine against varicella-zoster (chickenpox) is the first herpes virus vaccine to be widely tested in healthy and high-risk children and adults.[63–65] Chickenpox is a highly contagious, mild childhood disease in healthy children, but it can be severe and even fatal, especially in the immunocompromised patient. Unusual complications, such as severe bacterial superinfections, Reye's syndrome, and other encephalopathics, are worth preventing with an immunization program. Before the vaccine was available, approximately 4 million cases of chickenpox were reported annually, with 4,000 to 9,000 hospitalizations and 100 deaths. Historically, 55% of varicella-related deaths occur in adults, many of whom are infected by exposure to unvaccinated preschool-aged children with typical cases of varicella.[66]

Although most children with chickenpox have a self-limited disease lasting 4 to 5 days, there are many direct and indirect costs. Direct costs include nonprescription and prescription (e.g., acyclovir) medications used to treat the illness, whereas indirect costs are those associated with missed work to be home to care for an ill child.[67] It is likely that universal immunization to prevent chickenpox will be less costly than universal treatment with oral acyclovir, even if a two-dose schedule is used for maximal protection.[68]

In healthy children, the vaccine has been efficacious in preventing varicella.[69] In the immunocompromised patient, a low clinical attack rate has been observed. Although the vaccine may not entirely prevent chickenpox from occurring, one of its effects may be to modify the disease. In the Collaborative Varicella Vaccine Study sponsored by the National Institutes of Health, a seroconversion rate of only 85% after a single dose was observed in adults, compared with 95% in healthy children and 90% in children with leukemia.[70] Therefore, two doses generally are given to adults. In addition, the vaccine also may be given to healthy varicella-susceptible children, such as those described in this case who already have been exposed. Chickenpox can be prevented if vaccine is administered within 3 days of exposure, and might be prevented within 5 days.[71] If the exposure does not cause infection, the vaccination will provide protection for future exposures.

The primary concern regarding the varicella vaccine is the potential for breakthrough varicella (BV) occurring in children previously vaccinated with live varicella vaccine. There is fear that BV could become more severe as the time from immunization increases. However, breakthrough cases occurring up to 8 years after vaccination are reported to be clinically mild with one-sixth fewer total vesicular lesions and a shorter duration of illness when compared to natural varicella infection.[72] The most common adverse effect associated with vaccine administration is rash. Transmission of the virus from the vaccine has been documented in only 3 of 15 million doses administered, all of which occurred in the presence of a vesicular rash post-vaccinaton.[73] Salicylates should not be used for 6 weeks after administration of the varicella vaccine because of the association between chickenpox and Reye's syndrome. Other analgesics that do not contain salicylic acid are acceptable.

The varicella virus vaccine is included in the Recommended Childhood Immunization Schedule to be administered after the first birthday.[9,73] A single dose of the vaccine is recommended for children 12 months to 12 years of age who lack a reliable history of varicella infection; two injections 4 to 8 weeks apart are recommended for children who are 13 years old.[9,73] The CDC strongly recommends immunizations in susceptible adolescents and adults who are at high risk of acquiring the infection, including working or living in environments in which transmission of virus is likely (e.g., households with young children, college attendance).[73]

Varicella vaccine is generally not recommended in children who have cellular immunodeficiencies, but can be used in those with impaired humoral immunity.[73] The vaccine should be avoided in children with symptomatic HIV, but may be considered in asymptomatic or mildly symptomatic patients.[73] Although the vaccine is not licensed for routine use in children with acute lymphocytic leukemia, immunization is available for patients enrolled in specific research protocols.

Additional studies are yet to be undertaken to determine the need for booster doses. Studies are under way to evaluate the safety and efficacy of a quadrivalent vaccine that includes the varicella vaccine and MMR. At this time, Varivax may be administered at the same time as MMR but at separate injection sites.

11. What is the role of varicella immune globulin (VZIG) in children who have been exposed to chickenpox? What is the recommended dosage of VZIG?

VZIG (prepared from plasma of healthy volunteer donors with high VZV titers) can decrease the incidence of varicella in selected individuals. It is not useful for treatment of varicella or herpes zoster. VZIG is distributed by the American Red Cross and can prevent clinical varicella if administered within 72 to 96 hours of exposure. Exposure is usually defined as direct contact, substantial exposure, and brief contact. Direct contact with an infected person or continuous household exposure carries the greatest risk of infection.

VZIG is recommended for individuals at high risk for serious complications following exposure to varicella. Those at risk include immunocompromised children or adults (e.g., acquired or congenital immunodeficiency, immunosuppressive therapy, cancer) and premature infants <28 weeks' gestation or <1,000 g at birth. Pregnant women who have not had chickenpox are at high risk of severe varicella complications (e.g., disseminated infection, pneumonia, death) and should receive VZIG within 72 hours of exposure of varicella. Neonates born to women with symptoms of varicella within five days before and two days after delivery should receive VZIG regardless of whether or not the mother received VZIG.

VZIG is administered intramuscularly at a dose of 125 U/10 kg of body weight up to a maximum of 625 U. The minimum dose is 125 U, and fractional doses are not recommended. Protection is thought to last approximately three weeks. To limit the need for VZIG in the hospital setting, all susceptible personnel (including health professional students) should be immunized with varicella virus vaccine.[74]

MEASLES/MUMPS/RUBELLA

12. At 15 months, K.C. (Question 1) is scheduled to receive her MMR (a combination vaccine containing live attenuated measles, mumps, and rubella viruses). K.C.'s mother, who has never received MMR, is pregnant with her third child. Should K.C.'s immunization be delayed because of her mother's pregnancy? Should K.C.'s mother be immunized?

Measles

Measles is a highly contagious and previously common disease of childhood. Symptoms include high fever, rash, cough, rhinitis, and conjunctivitis. Complications, although uncommon, may include pneumonia and encephalitis. Live attenuated measles virus vaccine produces a benign infection that is thought to produce lifelong immunity. When the measles vaccine was first licensed in 1963, a single dose was administered at age 9 months. In 1965, the age of immunization was increased to 12 months because of primary vaccine failure in younger children. In 1976, the age of immunization was raised to 15 months because of greater vaccine efficacy in children older than 15 months of age.[75]

Despite the availability of the vaccine, measles is responsible for approximately 10% of deaths among children younger than 5 years of age in developing countries. The United States is currently in its third attempt to eliminate measles infection. The most significant decrease in the incidence of measles occurred when children were required to receive the vaccine before entering school.[76] During the 1985–1988 epidemic, most measles transmission occurred in areas documenting 95% immunization rates, indicating that some children fail to respond adequately to the initial vaccine dose.[77] As a result, a two-dose schedule was implemented in 1989 and adopted by 41 states and the District of Columbia. During the 1989–1991 measles resurgence, most of the cases reported occurred in non-vaccinated, preschool-age children. This realization prompted an effort to improve immunization coverage in young children. Current surveillance data indicate that up to 47% of reported cases are the results of international importation of measles with the remaining cases occurring as outbreaks in school-age children who did not receive a second dose of a measles-containing vaccine.[78]

Recommendations to prevent measles include administration of the first dose of MMR at age 12 to 15 months followed by a second dose of MMR at entrance to grade school (age 4 to 6 years).[9,15,19] During an epidemic outbreak, infants can be immunized at age 6 to 9 months with single-antigen measles, followed by a dose of MMR at age 12 months and a dose of MMR at age 4 to 6 years; older children should receive an additional vaccine dose.[15,76,79] For adult immunization, one dose of a measles-containing vaccine also should be administered to persons born in or after 1957 unless they have a medical contraindication, documentation of at least one dose of a live measles containing vaccine, or acceptable evidence of immunity. Adults should receive a second dose of MMR if they were born between 1963–1967, previously vaccinated with killed measles vaccine, are students in post-secondary institutions, work in health care facilities, travel internationally, or were recently exposed to a measles outbreak.[62] Persons born after 1968 should receive one dose of a measles-containing vaccine.[19,80]

Mumps

Mumps immunization remains controversial in childhood because mumps illness in children rarely produces complications. Meningoencephalitis generally is a benign meningitis, and post-infectious encephalitis, a serious complication, is extremely rare (1/6,000). Deafness, commonly considered a risk of mumps, occurs rarely (1/15,000) and usually is unilateral. Orchitis primarily is a complication in infected adult males. Controversy exists because vaccination at 12 to 15 months of age may not protect male children into their adult years. Although administration of a second dose of MMR at age 4 to 6 years may provide longer protection, current immunization practices are aimed at eliminating the mumps virus from the pool of young children, thereby minimizing the exposure of non-immunized adults.[80] The mumps virus vaccine temporarily suppresses the reaction to tuberculin skin tests. Therefore, tuberculin skin testing should be performed before, simultaneously with, or six weeks after administration of the vaccine.

Rubella

Rubella is a common childhood infection that often is misdiagnosed because its signs and symptoms vary widely. The most common symptoms include post-auricular and suboccipital lymphadenopathy, arthralgia, transient erythematous rash, and low fever. The most important consequences of rubella occur in pregnant women and include abortions, miscarriages, still births, and fetal anomalies. This is especially true if the infection occurs during the first trimester. Preventing congenital rubella through elimination of the viral pool is the primary objective of rubella immunization programs because approximately 10% to 20% of women of child-bearing age have not acquired natural immunity.

Live rubella virus vaccination is recommended for all children at 12 to 15 months of age. Immunization and/or rubella antibody titer screening of women at premarital examinations and postpartum also is recommended. Women of childbearing age receiving the rubella vaccine should use contraception for at least 28 days after immunization.[85] Antibody titers should be measured 3 months after immunization to evaluate anti-body response in individuals who have received blood products or immunoglobulin within 8 weeks of immunization because the latter may inhibit antibody stimulation.[82,83]

Previously, when rubella immunization was administered to women who were unknowingly pregnant, approximately 10% of fetuses acquired congenital rubella infection. The current RA27/3 vaccine was reformulated in 1979 and has reduced the risk of fetal infection dramatically.[79,84] Data from the U.S. Rubella Vaccine in Pregnancy Registry and the U.K. National Congenital Rubella Surveillance Programme found no evidence of congenital rubella syndrome in 680 women who were inadvertently administered rubella vaccine three months before or during pregnancy.[85] Current recommendations are to avoid pregnancy for 28 days following vaccination with a rubella containing vaccine due to the theoretical risk of contracting disease from the vaccine.[85]

K.C.'s mother should have rubella antibody titers measured. If she does not have natural immunity to rubella, she should receive MMR postpartum. Because the vaccine presents no risk to non-immunized close contacts, K.C. should receive MMR vaccination at this visit.

TETANUS TOXOID AND RABIES VACCINE

13. **A.R., a 9-year-old boy, presents to the emergency department 3 hours after being bitten by a neighbor's dog. He has two deep lacerations and one puncture wound on his right hand. The wounds are cleaned and he is given amoxicillin-clavulanic acid. The neighbor claims that the dog has been vaccinated against rabies but has no proof. The county health department is notified, and the dog is placed in quarantine. A.R.'s immunizations are up to date (verified by card) and his last tetanus shot (DTP) was 4 years ago. Should A.R. receive tetanus immunoglobulin (TIG) or tetanus toxoid (Td)? What is the role of rabies immunoglobulin (RIG) and rabies vaccine in animal bites?**

Tetanus (lockjaw) is a highly fatal, noncommunicable disease that is most notably manifested by generalized, board-like muscular rigidity. It results from wounds (including animal bites) infected by *Clostridium tetani,* an anaerobic, gram-positive rod that exists in nature as an extremely resistant spore. All clinical features of tetanus are produced by an exotoxin; the organism itself causes no disease.[86,87] There is no natural immunity to tetanus. Prophylaxis can be achieved by actively stimulating antibody formation against the toxin through immunization with Td. Passive immunity can be achieved by administrating TIG. Because his immunizations are up to date and it has been less than 5 years since his last dose of tetanus, A.R. does not need to receive Td or TIG.[86,87]

Rabies is an important concern in any patient presenting with an animal bite. Wild animals (e.g., bats, skunks, squirrels, coyotes, raccoons) serve as reservoirs for rabies and may infect domestic animals. All wild animals should be considered rabid until proven otherwise. In the United States, domestic dogs and cats have a low incidence of rabies but must be quarantined for 7 to 10 days and monitored for signs and symptoms of rabies unless proof of vaccination is available.

Infection with rabies virus produces an acute illness with rapid, progressive encephalitis. Once the onset of symptoms occurs, the prognosis is extremely poor and thus emphasis is placed on prevention. Following exposure, rabies prophylaxis includes passive immunization with RIG (20 U/kg) as soon as possible and active immunization with rabies vaccine on days 0, 3, 7, 14, and 28.[88,89] Because the dog that attacked A.R. was a family pet and in good health, A.R. does not need to receive rabies prophylaxis at this time. Postexposure prophylaxis will need to be initiated immediately if the dog develops any sign of rabies.[87–91]

PNEUMOCOCCUS

14. **The pneumococcal, influenza, and hepatitis A vaccines have been added to the pediatric immunization schedule. What is the role of the pneumococcal and influenza vaccines in children? Should all children receive these vaccines?**

In the United States, *Streptococcus pneumoniae* (pneumococcus) is responsible for approximately 3,000 cases of meningitis, 500,000 cases of pneumonia, and 7 million cases of otitis media.[92] Children younger than 2 years of age and adults older than 65 years are at highest risk for developing pneumococcal infections. The risk for disseminated pneumococcal infections is increased by some underlying medical conditions (heart failure, chronic obstructive pulmonary diseases), chronic liver disease (e.g., cirrhosis), functional or anatomic asplenia (e.g., sickle cell disease, splenectomy), and acquired or inherited immunosuppressive conditions (e.g., HIV, cancer, immunosuppressive therapy). *S. pneumoniae* is a common pathogen in children with HIV, often presenting as one of the first manifestations of HIV infection.

There are two pneumococcal vaccines in use: the original polysaccharide vaccine (Pneumovax) and the new conjugate pneumococcal vaccine (Prevnar). Pneumovax contains 23 purified capsular polysaccharide antigens of *S. pneumoniae*. Unfortunately, antibody response to the polysaccharide vaccine is poor or inconsistent in children younger than two years of age. In addition, the antigens included in Pneumovax protect against strains that typically cause adult disease. The conjugate pneumococcal vaccine (Prevnar) was developed to improve immunogenicity and efficacy in infants and toddlers. This vaccine protects against the seven strains of pneumococcus that cause 80% of all pneumococcal invasive disease in children younger than 6 years of age. The ACIP recommends use of the conjugate vaccine for all children up to 23 months of age and any child younger than 5 years of age who is at high risk of pneumococcal disease.[92] The use of the polysaccharide vaccine is recommended in addition to the conjugate vaccine for certain high-risk children (e.g., sickle cell anemia).[92]

Immunocompromised patients typically have an unreliable response to vaccines, but because of the potential benefits, the pneumococcal vaccines should be administered. Some studies have found transient elevation of plasma HIV levels after pneumococcal vaccination, although this has not been associated with decreased patient survival.[93,94] To maintain immunity, revaccination with the 23 valent polysaccharide vaccine is recommended after 3 years in high-risk children younger than 10 years of age and after 5 years in older patients.

INFLUENZA

The influenza vaccine is currently recommended for anyone older than 6 months of age who is at increased risk for complications secondary to influenza. The CDC also recommends that healthy children 6 to 23 months of age be vaccinated with influenza vaccine because this population is at increased risk for influenza-related hospitalizations.[9,95] Additional target groups for the influenza vaccine include the following:

- People older than 65 years of age
- Residents of chronic care facilities
- Adults and children with chronic pulmonary or cardiovascular disorders, diabetes mellitus, renal dysfunction, hemoglobinopathies, or immunosuppression
- Children younger than 18 years of age receiving aspirin therapy (because of an increased risk of Reye's syndrome after influenza)
- Women in the second or third trimester of pregnancy during influenza season
- Household members and care providers in close contact with high-risk patients
- People 50 to 64 years of age with high-risk conditions

Each year, the influenza vaccine includes three inactivated influenza virus strains (usually two type A and one type B) thought to be circulating in the United States during the upcoming winter. The vaccine is available as both a split- and whole-virus preparation. The split-virus vaccine is used in children younger than 12 years of age to decrease the likelihood of a febrile reaction. Immunocompetent children and young adults typically develop high post-vaccination antibody titers. Elderly patients and some people with chronic disorders have lower antibody titers and may remain susceptible to influenza despite vaccination.[9,95]

Influenza vaccine should be administered annually for adequate protection. Children younger than nine years of age require two doses of the split-virus vaccine administered one month apart to achieve adequate antibody response. However, if these children received influenza vaccination in a previous season, only one dose is required. One dose of the split-virus vaccine is indicated for children 9 to 12 years of age and a single dose of whole-cell vaccine is used for anyone older than 12 years of age. Influenza vaccine contains a small amount of egg protein and historically has been contraindicated in patients with a severe egg allergy. However, there is evidence that even patients with severe egg allergies can safely receive the influenza vaccine.[96,97]

A live attenuated trivalent intranasal influenza vaccine (Flumist) is available for use in health people 5 to 49 years of age. After administration, recipients become infected with attenuated virus strains, which stimulate both local IgA and circulating IgG antibodies.[98–101] Although the health and economic benefits of protecting targeted groups of adults from influenza are well documented, the cost-effectiveness of routine immunization for children is not known at this time.

HEPATITIS A

Viral hepatitis can be caused by at least six hepatotrophic viruses (identified by letters A through G) and can present as either an acute or chronic illness (see Chapter 73, Viral Hepatitis). Typically, the course of hepatitis A includes an incubation phase, an acute hepatitis phase, and a convalescent phase. Symptoms often include fever, malaise, anorexia, nausea, abdominal discomfort, and jaundice. Clinical illness typically lasts 1 to 2 months. More than 70% of older children and adults have symptomatic infection, but just as many children younger than 6 years of age are asymptomatic. Asymptomatic children serve as a source of infection, especially for household or other close contacts.

About one third of hepatitis A cases occur in children younger than 5 years of age.[102] Among all reported cases, the most common source of infection is household or sexual contact, followed by day care attendance or employment, international travel, and food or waterborne outbreak.

The ACIP recommends routine vaccination of children 2 years of age and older in communities with an average incidence of ≥20 cases per 100,000 population (during years of 1987–1997).[103] The committee also recommends routine vaccination be considered people who live in states, counties, or other communities in which the average annual incidence is between 10 and 20 cases per 100,000 population. Vaccination programs targeting toddlers and young children are important because children are often asymptomatic and unwittingly transmit the virus to adolescents and adults. In addition, data suggest a "herd effect" when vaccination of children is widespread.[104] A program aimed exclusively at toddlers in an endemic area reduced the prevalence of hepatitis A by >90%, not only in the 2- to 4-year-old vaccine recipients, but in all age groups.

Havrix and Vaqta are two hepatitis A vaccines with adult and pediatric formulations. Both of these vaccines are indicated for adults and children 2 years of age or older. Two doses are recommended, the second dose should be administered 6 to 12 months after the initial dose (see Chapter 7: Viral Hepatitis). The pediatric formulations of each product are indicated for those 2 to 18 years of age and contain half the antigen of adult formulations.

PEDIATRIC IMMUNIZATIONS FOR IMMUNOCOMPROMISED PATIENTS

15. B.R. is a 15-month-old boy who is HIV positive and lives with foster parents taking care of two other immunocompromised children. He is taking zidovudine 180 mg/m^2 PO QID, didanosine 120 mg/m^2 PO BID, TMP-SMX 75 mg/m^2 PO BID three times weekly, and intravenous immunoglobulin (IVIG) 400 mg/kg once monthly. His recent CD-4 T-lymphocyte counts were 976 g/L (23%). Currently, he is asymptomatic and has not received any immunizations. What immunizations are recommended for immunocompromised children and their close contacts?

Immunocompromised patients include those with acquired or congenital immunodeficiencies, leukemia, lymphoma, generalized malignancies, as well as patients receiving cancer chemotherapy or other immunosuppressive agents. The regularly scheduled inactivated vaccines should be administered to all immunocompromised children, although an adequate immune response cannot be guaranteed. The administration of live virus vaccines had been contraindicated in all immunosuppressed patients because of the possibility of infection from uncontrolled viral replication; however, the risk of disease may outweigh the risk of vaccination in some immunocompromised children. Patients receiving high-dose corticosteroids (>2 mg/kg/day of prednisone or its equivalent) for >2 weeks should not receive live attenuated vaccines for

at least three months after the discontinuation of the corticosteroid. In HIV-infected patients, concerns also include the possibility of increased HIV replication. Although the clinical significance is unclear, transient increased viremia from immune activation has been reported in HIV-infected adults after a booster dose of tetanus toxoid.[15,105,106]

IPV is the polio immunization recommended for all children and is of even greater importance for children known to be immunocompromised. OPV has been administered to asymptomatic HIV-infected children without problems; however, use of IPV eliminates the potential risk of VAPP to the patient as well as spread of vaccine virus to close contacts who may be immunocompromised. IPV also should be used when polio immunization is indicated for household members or other close contacts of immunocompromised children.[15,63,65]

MMR is a live virus vaccine and should not be administered to severely immunocompromised patients.[107] Since the risk of developing illness from the vaccine is low, MMR can be administered to HIV patients who are not severely immunocompromised (as determined by age-appropriate CD4 lymphocyte counts and percentage).[19,106,108] Response to the vaccine declines as HIV progresses; therefore, susceptible individuals should be vaccinated as soon after diagnosis as possible.[19] HIV infected infants should be vaccinated at 12 months of age with a second dose administered 1 month later rather than waiting to give the booster dose at 5 years of age.[9] To reduce the risk of measles, mumps, and rubella infection in immunocompromised patients, susceptible close contacts of these patients should be vaccinated with MMR. HIV-infected infants often receive monthly IVIG infusions to prevent overwhelming bacterial infections; therefore, MMR vaccine should be administered 2 weeks before initiating IVIG to minimize interference with vaccine response.[19] Since immunocompromised patients may have diminished antibody responses, immunoglobulin (IG) should be administered after exposure to measles infection unless IVIG has been administered within the past 3 weeks. In severely immunocompromised patients, supplemental doses of IVIG may also be considered. For children with leukemia, MMR vaccine may be administered 3 months after the last dose of chemotherapy.[19]

In the past, the varicella vaccine was contraindicated in immunocompromised children including those with primary or acquired immunodeficiencies. However, asymptomatic and mildly symptomatic HIV infected children have experienced safe and effective responses to the vaccine. Given the risks associated with varicella and herpes zoster infections in HIV infected children, varicella vaccine should be considered for asymptomatic or mildly symptomatic HIV-infected children in CDC class N1 or A1 with age-specific CD4+ T-lymphocyte percentages >25%.[73] Varicella vaccine continues to be contraindicated to patients with cellular immunodeficiencies.

Information regarding the immunization of transplant patients receiving immunosuppressive agents is limited. The re-immunization of children after bone marrow transplant (BMT) is controversial and different transplant centers have different approaches. Re-immunization with inactivated vaccines including diphtheria, tetanus, *Haemophilus influenzae*, pneumococcus, hepatitis B, influenza, polio, and hepatitis A has been suggested starting at 12 months after transplant using modified dosing regimens.[109] Some practitioners recommend serologic evaluation before re-immunization, while others re-immunize all BMT patients. Yearly influenza vaccination is strongly recommended in BMT patients. MMR and varicella vaccines are contraindicated before 24 months after the transplant.[109] MMR may be administered after 24 months if patients are immunocompetent, while administration of varicella vaccine in immunocompetent patients post-BMT is currently limited to research protocols.[109] Children undergoing solid-organ transplantation should receive MMR and varicella vaccinations at least one month before transplantation with serological evaluation one year after the tranplant.[109–112] Serological evaluation and re-immunization before transplantation, if indicated, is recommended in children previously vaccinated with MMR and varicella vaccines.[109]

In summary, although B.R.'s ability to mount an antibody response cannot be determined, he should receive all inactivated vaccines as scheduled including pneumococcal and influenza vaccinations. B.R. and his close contacts should be immunized against polio with IPV. Since he is asymptomatic and has an adequate CD4 lymphocyte count for his age, varicella and MMR vaccines should be considered. Unfortunately, his monthly administration of IVIG may compromise his ability to respond to the MMR and varicella vaccines.[19,113] If BR is exposed to chickenpox or measles, passive prophylaxis with VZIG and IG, respectively, should be instituted if it has been more than 3 weeks since his last dose of IVIG.

SMALLPOX

16. A.L. is a healthy 2-year-old boy who is current with his immunizations. He lives in the Middle East with his father, an officer in the U.S. Army who recently was immunized against smallpox. Should A.L. be immunized against smallpox at this time?

Smallpox is caused by the variola virus and the infection is described as a macular rash that develops first on the face and extremities and progresses to papules, vesicles, and finally pustules that cause significant scarring. Patients will remain contagious until scabs are shed. Mortality rates >30% have been reported during previous smallpox outbreaks, but certain variants of smallpox approach 100% mortality.[114]

Routine vaccination for smallpox was discontinued in 1972, and the last natural case of smallpox occurred in Somalia in 1977. With the achievement of worldwide eradication, smallpox was no longer a public health concern. However, the looming threat of bioterrorism and concerns that stockpiles of smallpox virus may be in terrorist hands has returned smallpox to public consciousness.

Smallpox vaccine itself does not contain variola, but rather a related virus, vaccinia, in live form. Effective protection is provided with a single dose of smallpox vaccine, but antibodies decline significantly over a 5- to 10-year period. Controversy exists whether the benefits of population immunity to smallpox outweigh the vaccine's risks. The administration of the smallpox vaccine has been associated with cardiovascular toxicity, death, encephalitis, progressive vaccinia, eczema vaccinatum, and generalized rash. Moreover, the accidental self-inoculation to the eyes, face, or other sites is of concern.[114] Patients with chronic skin conditions, especially atopic dermatitis, are at increased risk for eczema vaccinatum, which can be fatal. The extrapolation of data from the late 1960s concludes that 40 persons per million immunized could experience serious or life-threatening complications. Data suggest that successful immunization can be achieved with 5- and 10-fold dilutions of the vaccine, which may help decrease the severity of adverse reactions.[115]

There has been much debate regarding the best policy for protection of the public. Major proposals include mass immunization, voluntary immunization, and surveillance and containment.[114] Mass immunization has received support because this method would best prevent spread of disease, and terrorists are less likely to attack an area known to have a high level of immunity. However, such a large campaign would deplete existing supplies of vaccine quickly, and vaccinia immune globulin (VIG) would not be available in quantities needed to treat the expected number of patients experiencing severe adverse effects. In addition, models devised to assist in the development of immunization policy suggest that vaccination of the general public would only be beneficial in the event of a large attack or if multiple attacks are likely.[116] Supporters of voluntary immunization suggest that each person should determine whether they should be vaccinated. Voluntary pre-exposure vaccination reduces the likelihood that smallpox could be used effectively as a weapon. In addition, the management of non-immunized patients in the event of an attack would be easier in this scenario.[117] However, the general public and the medical community need better understandings of potential problems and complications associated with vaccinia immunizations.[118]

The American Academy of Pediatrics and the CDC recommend a plan that entails isolation of infected persons, identification and immunization of contacts, and immunization of health care responders who would be caring for infected persons.[119] Much of the rationale for this plan is based on the fact that protection can be provided to non-immune exposed individuals if the vaccine is delivered within 3 to 4 days, and symptoms can be alleviated if vaccine is given within 1 week of exposure. Until a safer vaccine is developed, until more VIG is available for use, and if the threat of a terrorist attack with smallpox virus is considered likely, this method for protection of the public has been recommended.[114] A.L. should not receive the smallpox vaccine at this time. Current recommendations are to vaccinate only children who are exposed to an infected person. Future studies evaluating the safety and immunogenicity of current and newly developed smallpox vaccines should include children.[114]

REFERENCES

1. Centers for Disease Control and Prevention. National, state, and urban area vaccination coverage levels among children aged 19–35 months—United States, January–December 1995. MMWR 1997; 46:176.
2. Kum-Nji P et al. Immunization status of hospitalized preschool children: risk factors associated with inadequate immunization. Pediatrics 1995;96:434.
3. Centers for Disease Control and Prevention. Status report on the childhood immunization initiative: national, state, and urban area vaccination coverage levels among children aged 19–35 months, July 1996–June 1997. MMWR 1998;47(6):108.
4. Wood D et al. Knowledge of the childhood immunization schedule and of contraindications to vacci-

nate by private and public providers in Los Angeles. Pediatr Infect Dis J 1996;15:140.

5. Schaffer SJ et al. Immunization status and birth order. Arch Pediatr Adolesc Med 1995;149:792.

6. Watson MA et al. Inadequate history as barrier to immunization. Arch Pediatr Adolesc Med 1996; 150:135.

7. Moneymaker CS et al. Missed opportunities to immunize in public, private and military primary care settings in Norfolk, VA [Abstract]. Pediatr Res 1996;39:96A.

8. Zell E et al. Reliability of vaccination cards and parent-derived information for determining immunization status: lessons from the 1994 national health interview survey (NHIS) provider record check (PRC) study. Pediatr Res 1997;41:101A.

9. Committee on Infectious Diseases Recommended Childhood and Adolescent Immunization Schedule—United States, 2003. Pediatrics 2003;111:212.

10. Margolis HS et al. Hepatitis B: evolving epidemiology and implications for control. Semin Liver Dis 1992;11:84.

11. Centers for Disease Control and Prevention. Protection against viral hepatitis: recommendations of the Immunization Practices Advisory Committee (ACIP). MMWR 1990;39:5.

12. Hollinger FB. Factors influencing the immune response to hepatitis B vaccine, booster guidelines and vaccine protocol recommendations. Am J Med 1989;87(S-3A):36S.

13. Immunization Practices Advisory Committee (ACIP). Hepatitis B virus: a comprehensive strategy for eliminating transmission in the United States through universal childhood vaccination. MMWR 1991;40:1.

14. Advisory Committee on Immunization Practices. Combination vaccines for childhood immunizations. MMWR 1999;48(RR-5):1.

15. Advisory Committee on Immunization Practices. General recommendations on immunization. MMWR 2002;51(RR-2):1.

16. Advisory Committee on Immunization Practices (ACIP). Hepatitis B virus: a comprehensive strategy for eliminating transmission in the United States through universal childhood vaccination. MMWR 1991;40:1.

17. Centers for Disease Control and Prevention. Immunization of adolescents: recommendations of the Advisory Committee on Immunization Practices, the American Academy of Pediatrics, the American Academy of Family Physicians, and the American Medical Association. MMWR 1996;4:RR-13.

18. American Academy of Pediatrics. Hepatitis B. In: Pickering LK, ed. 2000 RedBook: Report of the Committee on Infectious Disease. 25th ed. Elk Grove Village, IL: American Academy of Pediatrics, 2000:297.

18a. American Academy of Pediatrics. Recommendations for immunization of preterm and low birth infants. Pediatrics 2003;112:193.

19. Centers for Disease Control and Prevention. Measles, mumps, and rubella—vaccine use and strategies for elimination of measles, rubella, and congenital rubella syndrome and control of mumps: recommendations of the Advisory Committee on Immunization Practices (ACIP). MMWR 1998; 47(RR-8):1.

20. Centers for Disease Control and Prevention. Progress toward elimination of Haemophilus influenzae type b disease among infants and children—United States, 1987–1995. JAMA 1996;276(19):1542.

21. Braun MM et al. Syncope after immunization. Arch Pediatr Adolesc Med 1997;151:255.

22. Kemp A et al. Measles immunization in children with clinical reactions to egg protein. Am J Dis Child 1990;144:33.

23. Fasano MB et al. Egg hypersensitivity and adverse reactions to measles, mumps, rubella vaccine. J Pediatr 1992;120:878.

24. James JM et al. Safe administration of the measles vaccine to children allergic to eggs. N Engl J Med 1995;332:1262.

25. Centers for Disease Control and Prevention. Update: vaccine side effects, adverse reactions, contraindications and precautions. Recommendations

of the Advisory Committee on Immunization Practiced (ACIP). MMWR 1996;45:RR-12.

26. Smith M. National childhood vaccine injury compensation act. Pediatrics 1988;82(2):264.

27. Katz SL. Controversies in immunization. Pediatr Infect Dis J 1987;6:607.

28. Hinman AR, Koplan JP. Pertussis and pertussis vaccine: reanalysis of benefit and costs. JAMA 1984;251:3109.

29. Centers for Disease Control and Prevention. Pertussis vaccination: use of acellular pertussis vaccines among infants and young children. Recommendations of the Advisory Committee on Immunizations practices (ACIP). MMWR 1997; 46:RR-7.

30. Bass JW, Wittler RR. Return of epidemic pertussis in the United States. Pediatr Infect Dis J 1994;13:343.

31. Centers for Disease Control and Prevention. Pertussis vaccination: acellular pertussis vaccine for reinforcing and booster use. Supplementary ACIP statement. MMWR 1992;41(1):1.

32. Nenning ME et al. Prevalence and incidence of adult pertussis in an urban population. JAMA 1996;275(21):1772.

33. Centers for Disease Control and Prevention. Use of diphtheria toxoid-tetanus toxoid-acellular pertussis vaccine in a five dose series. MMWR 2000;49(RR-13):1.

34. Ogra PL, Faden HS. Poliovirus vaccine: live or dead. J Pediatr 1986;108:1031.

35. National Immunization Program, Department of Health and Human Services. Epidemiology and Prevention of Vaccine-Preventable Diseases, Poliomyelitis. Atlanta, GA: Centers for Disease Control and Prevention, 2001.

36. Sutter RW, Prevots DR. Vaccine associated paralytic poliomyelitis among immunodeficient persons. Infect Med 1994;190:41.

37. Faden H et al. Comparative evaluation of immunization with live attenuated and enhanced-potency inactivated trivalent poliovirus vaccines in childhood: systemic and local immune responses. J Infect Dis 1990;162:1291.

38. Onorato IM et al. Mucosal immunity induced by enhanced-potency inactivated and oral polio vaccines. J Infect Dis 1991;163:1.

39. Modlin JF et al. Humoral and mucosal immunity in infants induced by three sequential inactivated poliovirus vaccine-live attenuated poliovirus vaccine immunization schedules. J Infect Dis 1997; 175(Suppl 1):S228.

40. Centers for Disease Control and Prevention. Poliomyelitis prevention in the United States: introduction of a sequential vaccination schedule of inactivated poliovirus vaccine followed by oral poliovirus vaccine. Recommendations of the Advisory Committee on Immunizations Practices (ACIP). MMWR 1997;46:RR-3.

41. Centers for Disease Control and Prevention. Recommendations of the Advisory Committee on Immunization Practices: revised recommendations for routine poliomyelitis vaccination. MMWR 1999; 48(27):590.

42. Fraser DW. Haemophilus influenza in the community and the home. In: Sell SH, Wright PF, eds. Haemophilus influenzae: Epidemiology, Immunology, and Prevention of Disease. New York: Elsevier Science, 1982:11.

43. Schlech W et al. Bacterial meningitis in the United States, 1978 through 1981. JAMA 1985;253:1749.

44. Dajani AS et al. Systemic Haemophilus influenzae disease: an overview. J Pediatr 1979;98:355.

45. Taylor HG et al. Intellectual, neuropsychological, and achievement outcomes in children six to eight years after recovery from Haemophilus influenzae meningitis. Pediatrics 1984;74:198.

46. Peltoa H et al. Prevention of Haemophilus influenzae type b bacteremic infections with the capsular polysaccharide vaccine. N Engl J Med 1984; 310:1566.

47. Anonymous. Polysaccharide vaccine for prevention of Haemophilus influenzae type b disease. JAMA 1985;253:2630.

48. Black SB et al. Efficacy of Haemophilus influenzae type b capsular polysaccharide vaccine. Pediatr Infect Dis 1988;7:149.

49. Harrison LH et al. Haemophilus influenzae type b polysaccharide vaccine: an efficacy study. Pediatrics 1989;84(2):255.

50. Lepow ML et al. Safety and immunogenicity of Haemophilus influenzae type b diphtheria toxoid conjugate vaccine (PRP-D) in infants. J Infect Dis 1987;156:591.

51. American Academy of Pediatrics Committee on Infectious Diseases. Haemophilus influenzae type b conjugate vaccines: update. Pediatrics 1989; 84(2):386.

52. Food and Drug Administration approval of use of Haemophilus b conjugate vaccine for infants. MMWR 1990;39(39):698.

53. Centers for Disease Control and Prevention. Notice to readers: recommended childhood immunization schedule—United States, 1998. MMWR 1998; 47(01):8.

54. Allen KD et al. Sucrose as an analgesic agent for infants during immunization injections. Arch Pediatr Adolesc Med 1996;150:270.

55. Lewindon PJ et al. Randomised controlled trial of sucrose by mouth for the relief of infant crying after immunization. Arch Dis Child 1998;78:453.

56. Uhari M et al. A eutectic mixture of lidocaine and prilocaine for alleviating vaccination pain in infants. Pediatrics 1993;92:719.

57. Wakefield AJ et al. Ileal-lymphoid-nodular hyperplasia, non-specific colitis, and pervasive developmental disorder in children. Lancet 1998;351:637.

58. Madsen KM et al. A population-based study of measles, mumps, and rubella vaccination and autism. N Engl J Med 2002;347:1477.

59. Taylor B et al. Autism and measles, mumps, and rubella vaccine: no epidemiological evidence for a causal association. Lancet 1999;353:2026.

60. Taylor B et al. Measles, mumps, and rubella vaccination and bowel problems or developmental regression in children with autism: population study. BMJ 2002;324:393.

61. Offit PA et al. Addressing parents' concerns: do multiple vaccines overwhelm or weaken the infant's immune system? Pediatrics 2002;109:124.

62. Centers for Disease Control. Clarification: Vol 51, No.40 Recommended Adult Immunization Schedule—United States, 2002 2003. MMWR 2003; 52:345.

63. Centers for Disease Control and Prevention. Prevention of varicella. Recommendations of the Advisory Committee on Immunization Practices. MMWR 1996;45:RR-11.

64. Gershon AA. Live attenuated varicella vaccine. Pediatr Ann 1984;13:653.

65. Arbeter AM et al. Immunization of children with acute lymphoblastic leukemia with live attenuate varicella vaccine without complete suspension of chemotherapy. Pediatrics 1990;85(3):338.

66. Centers for Disease Control and Prevention. Varicella-related deaths among adults—United States 1997. MMWR 1997;46(19):409.

67. Lieu AT et al. The cost of childhood chickenpox: parents' perspective. Pediatr Infect Dis J 1994;13:173.

68. Lieu TA et al. Cost-effectiveness of a routine varicella vaccination program for US children. JAMA 1994;271(5):375.

69. Weibel RE et al. Live attenuated varicella virus vaccine—efficacy trial in healthy children. N Engl J Med 1984;310:1409.

70. Gershon A et al. NIAID Varicella Vaccine Collaborative Study Group: live attenuated varicella vaccine in immunocompromised children and healthy adults. Pediatrics 1986;78:757.

71. Arbeter AM et al. Varicella vaccine studies in healthy children and adults. Pediatrics 1986;78:748.

72. Bernstein HH et al. Clinical survey of natural varicella compared with breakthrough varicella after immunization with live attenuated oka/Merke varicella vaccine. Pediatrics 1993;92(6):833.

73. Centers for Disease Control and Prevention. Prevention of varicella: updated recommendations of the Advisory Committee on Immunization Practices (ACIP) MMWR 1999;48(RR06):1-5.

74. Centers for Disease Control and Prevention. Varicella zoster immune globulin for the prevention of chickenpox. MMWR 1984;33:84.

75. Markowitz LE et al. Duration of live measles vaccine-induced immunity. Pediatr Infect Dis 1990; 9:101.

76. Robbins KB et al. Low measles incidence: association with enforcement of school immunization laws. Am J Public Health 1981;71:270.

77. Gustafson TL et al. Measles outbreak in a fully immunized secondary-school population. N Engl J Med 1987;316:771.

78. Centers for Disease Control and Prevention. Measles outbreak among internationally adopted children arriving in the United States, February-March 2001. MMWR 2002;51(49):1115.

79. Bernstein DI et al. Fetomaternal aspects of immunization with RA 27/3 live attenuated rubella virus vaccine during pregnancy. J Pediatr 1980;97:467.

80. American Academy of Pediatrics Committee on Infectious Disease. Measles: reassessment of the current immunization policy. Pediatrics 1989;84(6): 1110.

81. Reference deleted from text.

82. Landes RD et al. Neonatal rubella following postpartum maternal immunization. J Pediatr 1980;97:465.

83. Centers for Disease Control and Prevention. Rubella prevention recommendation of the immunization practices advisory committee. MMWR 1990;39:RR-15.

84. Balfour HH et al. RA 27/3 rubella vaccine: a four-year follow up. Am J Dis Child 1980;134:350.

85. Centers for Disease Control and Prevention. Notice to Readers: Revised ACIP Recommendation for avoiding pregnancy after receiving a rubella-containing vaccine. MMWR 2001;50(49):1117.

86. American Academy of Pediatrics. Tetanus In: Pickering LK, ed. 2000 RedBook: Report of the Committee on Infectious Disease. 25th Ed. Elk Grove Village, IL: American Academy of Pediatrics, 2000:563.

87. Centers for Disease Control and Prevention (CDC). Tetanus: United States 1987 and 1988. MMWR 1990;39:37.

88. American Academy of Pediatrics. Rabies. In: Pickering LK, ed 2000 Red Book: Report of the Committee on Infectious Diseases. 25th Ed. Elk Grove Village, IL; American Academy of Pediatrics, 2000:475.

89. Centers for Disease Control and Prevention. Human rabies prevention—United States, 1999 recommendations of the Advisory Committee on Immunization Practices (ACIP). MMWR 1999;48(RR-1):1.

90. Griego RD et al. Dog, cat and human bites: a review. J Am Acad Dermatol 1995:1019.

91. Centers for Disease Control and Prevention (CDC). Rabies postexposure prophylaxis—Connecticut 1990–1994. MMWR 1996;45:232.

92. Centers for Disease Control and Prevention. Preventing pneumococcal disease among infants and children: recommendations of the Advisory Committee on Immunization Practices (ACIP). MMWR 2000;49:RR-9.

93. Brichacek B et al. Increased plasma HIV-1 burden following antigenic challenge with pneumococcal vaccine. J Infect Dis 1996;174:1191.

94. Katzenstein TL et al. Assessment of plasma HIV RNA and CD4 counts after combined Pneumovax and tetanus toxoid vaccination: no detectable increase in HIV replication 6 weeks after immunization. Scand J Infect Dis 1996;28:239.

95. Centers for Disease Control and Prevention and Control of Influenza. Recommendations of the Advisory Committee on Immunization Practices (ACIP). MMWR 2001;59(RR04):1

96. Murphy KR et al. Safe administration of influenzae vaccine in asthmatic children hypersensitive to egg proteins. J Pediatr 1985;106:931.

97. James JM et al. Safe administration of influenza vaccine to patients with severe allergy. J Pediatr 1998;133(5):624.

98. Belshe RB et al. The efficacy of live attenuated, cold-adapted, trivalent, intranasal influenza virus vaccine in children. N Engl J Med 1998;338:1405.

99. Edwards KM et al. A randomized controlled trial of cold-adapted and inactivated vaccines for the prevention of influenza A disease. J Infect Dis 1994;169:68.

100. Nichol KL et al. Effectiveness of live, attenuated intranasal influenza virus vaccine in healthy, working adults. JAMA 1999;282:137.

101. Belshe RB et al. Efficacy of vaccination with live attenuated, cold-adapted, trivalent, intranasal influenza virus vaccine against a variant (A/Sydney) not contained in the vaccine. J Pediatr 2000; 136(2):168.

102. National Immunization Program, Department of Health and Human Services. Epidemiology and Prevention of Vaccine Preventable Diseases. Hepatitis A. Atlanta, GA: Centers for Disease Control and Prevention, 2001.

103. Centers for Disease Control and Prevention. Prevention of hepatitis A through active or passive immunization: recommendations of the Advisory Committee on Immunization Practices (ACIP). MMWR 1999;48(RR-12):1.

104. Dagan R et al. National hepatitis A (HAV) immunization program aimed exclusively at toddlers in an endemic country resulting in >90% reduction in morbidity rate in all ages. Paper presented to IDSA 40th Annual Meeting, Chicago, IL, 2002.

105. Recommendations of the Advisory Committee on Immunization Practices (ACIP). Use of vaccines and immune globulins for persons with altered immunocompetence. MMWR 1993;42(RR-4):1.

106. McLaughlin M et al. Live virus vaccines in human immunodeficiency virus-infected children: a retrospective survey. Pediatrics 1988;82:229.

107. Committee on Pediatric AIDS. Evaluation and medical treatment of the HIV-exposed infant. Pediatrics 1997;99(6):909.

108. Stanley SK et al. Effect of immunization with a common recall antigen on viral expression in patients infected with human immunodeficiency virus type 1. N Engl J Med 1996;334:1222.

109. American Academy of Pediatrics. Immunizations in special clinical circumstances. In: Pickering LK, ed. 2000 RedBook: Report of the Committee on Infectious Disease. 25th ed. Elk Grove Village, IL: American Academy of Pediatrics, 2000:56.

110. Huzly D et al. Routine immunizations in adult renal transplant recipients. Transplant 1997;63:839.

111. Gershon AA. Immunizations for pediatric transplant patients. Kidney Int 1993;44:S87.

112. Furth SL et al. Immunization practices in children with renal disease: a report of the North American Pediatric Transplant Cooperative Study. Pediatr Nephrol 1997;11:443.

113. American Academy of Pediatrics Committee on Infectious Diseases. Recommended timing of routine measles immunizations for children who have recently received immune globulin preparations. Pediatrics 1994;93:682.

114. American Academy of Pediatrics Committee on Infectious Diseases. Small pox vaccine policy statement. Pediatrics 2002;110(4):841.

115. Frey SE et al. Clinical responses to undiluted and diluted smallpox vaccine. J Engl J Med 2002; 346(17):1265.

116. Bozette SA et al. A model for smallpox-vaccination policy. N Engl J Med 2003;348(5).

117. Bicknell WJ. The case for voluntary smallpox vaccination [Editorial]. N Engl J Med 2002; 346(17):1323.

118. Blendon RJ et al. The public and the smallpox threat. N Engl J Med 2003;348:5.

119. Centers for Disease Control and Prevention. Vaccinia (smallpox) vaccine: recommendations of the Advisory Committee on Immunization Practices (ACIP), 2001. MMWR 2001;50(RR-10):1.

CHAPTER 96

Pediatric Infectious Diseases

Ann M. Bolinger, Nicholas Blanchard

Infectious diseases account for the vast majority of annual visits to the pediatrician. Acute febrile illnesses, either viral or bacterial, occur in children on average six to eight times a year. For this reason, the management of pediatric infectious diseases remains a significant component of care.

Several host and microbial factors contribute to the relatively high incidence of infectious diseases in pediatric patients. Deficiencies in both cellular and humoral immunity have been described in the immediate newborn period as well as in the first several years of life (Table 96-1).[1] Concentrations of all the immunoglobulins (IgG, IgM, IgD, IgE, and IgA) are diminished at birth, particularly in the premature neonate.[2] Although some immunoglobulin G (IgG) is transferred to the newborn from the mother via the placenta, this is generally a short-lived effect that dissipates during the first year of life. Deficits in complement and C-reactive protein decrease opsonization, and the phagocytic and intracellular killing functions of neutrophils and macrophages are depressed. The microbial naivety of children also has a significant impact on their ability to fight infection. Potential pathogens are able to colonize and cause clinical infection more readily in newborns and infants because the full complement of normal flora bacteria has not been fully developed. Children begin acquiring their own immunity to organisms by becoming exposed to antigens, developing an immune response, and generating lasting-memory immunity cells.

Children are increasingly exposed to potential pathogens at an earlier age, placing them at greater risk of infection. Approximately 60% of households with children younger than 6 years of age have a single working parent or both parents employed outside of the home.[3] As a result, more children are attending day care and school environments, where they are more likely to come in contact with an infected child or caregiver.

Bacterial and viral pathogens that most commonly affect pediatric patients are summarized in Table 96-2.[4] The age of the child, as well as the site of infection, implicate different potential pathogens; however, there is significant overlap. *Streptococcus pneumoniae, Moraxella catarrhalis,* and *Haemophilus influenzae* are the most common pathogens. Antimicrobial therapy in pediatric patients almost always includes an agent that is active against these organisms—especially when the organism is unknown. Many different viruses cause respiratory infections in children, but these are not cultured clinically because treatments are not readily available. Respiratory syncytial virus (RSV), a common viral pathogen that causes respiratory tract infection in pediatric patients, is an exception. An agent for prophylaxis of RSV, as well as one for treatment, is available to use in high-risk children.[5]

Table 96-1   Immunologic Parameters in Infants, Children, and Adults

	Birth	1 Month	1 Year	5 Years	Adult
Average white blood cell count (cells/mm³)	18,100	10,800	10,600	8,500	7,400
Average neutrophil count (cells/mm³)	8,500	2,700	2,900	8,500	7,400
Average lymphocyte count (cells/mm³)	4,300	6,000	6,400	3,200	3,700
Average serum immunoglobulin G concentration (mg/dL)	1,100	650	800	900	1,000
Average serum immunoglobulin M concentration (mg/dL)	15	80	140	150	200
Average serum immunoglobulin A concentration (mg/dL)	3	35	140	120	230
Average complement C³ concentration (mg/dL)	—	110	130	140	130
Average complement C⁴ concentration (mg/dL)	—	25	25	25	30

Compiled from reference 1.

Table 96-2   Common Viral and Bacterial Pathogens Associated With Specific Pediatric Infectious Diseases

	Otitis Media	Sinusitis	Pharyngitis	Bronchiolitis	Croup Syndrome
Viral					
Parainfluenza	+	+	++	++	+++
Influenza	++	+	++		++
Adenovirus	+	+	+++	+	+
Rhinovirus		++	+		+
RSV	+++	+	+	+++	+
Coronavirus		++			+
Enterovirus	+	+	+++		+
EBV			++		
Bacterial					
S. pneumoniae	+++	+++	+		
S. pyogenes	+	+	+++		
S. aureus		+^{b}	+		+^{b}
H. influenzae	++	++	++		+^{b}
M. catarrhalis	++	++			
C. diphtheriae			+		+
Oral anaerobes		+^{a}	+		
M. pneumoniae	+	+	+	+	+

^{a}Mostly isolated to chronic infections.
^{b}Most common bacterial pathogens, but are rare overall. *S. aureus* is more common than *H. influenzae* as a cause of bacterial tracheitis, but *H. influenzae* is more common as cause for supraglottitis.
+++, most common pathogens; ++, common pathogens; +, occasional pathogens; EBV, Epstein-Barr virus; RSV, respiratory syncytial virus.
Adapted with permission from the University of Kentucky College of Pharmacy Office of Continuing Education Independent Study Program entitled Pediatric Pharmacotherapy.

OTITIS MEDIA

Otitis media, inflammation of the middle ear, is diagnosed more than 5 million times per year in the United States and occurs in >75% of all children by the age of 2 years.[6,6B] It is one of the most common childhood illnesses, accounting for approximately 31 million visits to physicians annually. The diagnosis of otitis generally is treated with an antibiotic despite the absence of substantial evidence in support of antibiotic therapy.[6B] Approximately half of all prescriptions written for children in this country are for the treatment of otitis media—at a cost of $3.8 billion annually.[7,8]

The middle ear is the anatomic location of the hearing apparatus. It is separated from the outer ear canal by the tympanic membrane (eardrum) and drains into the nasopharynx via the eustachian tubes. The presence of a dull, red, bulging, tympanic membrane that shows no movement during insufflation (application of slight changes in air pressure in the ear canal) or otoscopic examination is diagnostic of acute otitis media. Otitis media peaks between 6 months and 3 years of age and is thought to be most likely due to eustachian tube obstruction and secondarily due to the decreased immunocompetence present in young children. Eustachian tube dysfunction has been associated with upper respiratory tract infections and allergies.[9–11] Some children may have three or four infections per year, whereas others suffer from continuous "chronic" otitis media for prolonged periods (>3 months). Viruses cause most otitis media infections; however, it is difficult to distinguish viral from bacterial etiology based solely on clinical presentation and otoscopic examination.[10]

Clinical Presentation and Classification

1. M.G., a 10-month-old, 22-lb boy, is brought to the emergency department (ED) with a history of increased irritability but no fever over the last 2 days. He has been waking up crying at night and is refusing to drink from a bottle. He lives at home with both parents; his mother smokes tobacco in the house. M.G. attends daycare 5 days a week and has had one previous episode of left ear otitis media 3 months ago treated with amoxicillin/clavulanate 45 mg/kg per day (amoxicillin) BID for 10 days. When M.G. was evaluated after the completion of antibiotics, he still had an accumulation of serous fluid behind the tympanic membrane but no signs of an acute infection. Physical examination revealed a red, inflamed, opaque, and bulging right tympanic membrane. On gentle air insufflation, the tympanic membrane is immobile and extremely painful. The left ear has an accumulation of serous fluid behind the tympanic membrane, but is not red or bulging and is mobile and causes no pain on air insufflation. A tympanogram of the left ear indicates fluid in the middle ear. M.G.'s immunizations are up to date. He lives in a community known to have >50% of *H. influenzae* and >95% of *M. catarrhalis* isolates producing β-lactamase. How would you classify the diagnosis of otitis media in M.G. based on the presenting symptoms, history, and physical examination?

Otitis media is a general term that describes inflammation of the middle ear. For purposes of treatment, there are four basic diagnostic categories: acute otitis media (AOM), otitis media with effusion (OME), chronic otitis media, and recurrent otitis media.[11] The infection in M.G.'s right ear represents the most common and clearly defined classification, AOM. As seen in M.G., symptoms of AOM develop suddenly and usually include a history of ear pain and irritability, with or without fever. Patients may also experience nasal congestion, coughing, loss of appetite, vomiting, and discharge from the ear. On otoscopic examination, the tympanic membrane (TM) is found to be poorly mobile, bulging, and opaque or yellow due to the accumulation of fluid and pus in the middle ear. Inflammation causes the TM to be red; immobility during insufflation indicates fluid accumulation behind the membrane in the middle ear.

Evaluation of M.G's left ear suggests OME. Fluid is visualized behind the TM and there is decreased mobility, but air insufflation does not elicit pain. A tympanogram measures impedance of the TM and is used to determine the presence of fluid in the middle ear. Although tympanograms can be helpful in identifying middle ear effusions, the test requires special equipment. M.G. has a history of otitis media in the left ear, treated 3 months ago. Fluid remains in the middle ear for up to 1 month after therapy in 40% of children.[8] Effusion after acute otitis media generally is not treated because it resolves spontaneously within 3 months in 90% of patients.[8] However, in M.G.'s case, the effusion in the left ear persists and requires further evaluation.

Chronic otitis media, or OME lasting >3 months, can present with signs and symptoms similar to those of AOM or with subtle changes in balance, lack of speech development, and hearing loss.[12] Recurrent otitis media generally is defined as three episodes of AOM within a 6-month period or four or more episodes within 1 year.[6] If M.G. develops another episode of AOM within the next 3 months or two more infections in the next 9 months, the diagnosis of recurrent otitis media would be appropriate. Environmental factors such as childcare attendance, second-hand smoke exposure, and pacifier use may increase the incidence of AOM.[13,14] Exclusive breast feeding for 3 to 6 months can decrease the incidence of AOM by as much as 13%, with effects lasting up to 12

months.[15] M.G. also has had two middle ear infections in the first year of life, another prognostic sign that he may develop recurrent otitis media.[16]

Microbiology

2. What are the most likely organisms causing M.G.'s middle ear infection?

S. pneumoniae, H. influenzae, and *M. catarrhalis* account for nearly 70% of all bacterial otitis media infections.[8] Other organisms such as *Staphylococcus aureus,* group A *Streptococcus,* and Gram-negative rods also can cause otitis media.[8] Gram-negative rods such as *Escherichia coli* may occur in newborns with otitis media; however, middle ear infection in this population is rare and generally is managed as a possible sepsis (see Chapter 94, Neonatal Therapy). Although other atypical organisms such as *Chlamydia trachomatis* and *Mycoplasma pneumoniae* have been isolated from middle ear fluid, these pathogens are not common.[21] It is important to recognize that up to 50% of acute otitis media cases are viral infections, which will resolve regardless of antibiotic therapy.[8] However, it is difficult to determine whether M.G. has viral or bacterial disease based on the clinical presentation. Although M.G. has been immunized against *H. influenzae* type b, most otitis media caused by *H. influenzae* is nontypable (90%), and the vaccine does not confer protection against nontypable strains. Use of the heptavalent pneumococcal conjugate vaccine (PCV) has been associated with a decrease in otitis media episodes.[17] Influenza vaccination has been shown to decrease the incidence of otitis media by 28% to 36% during influenza season.[18] *Tympanocentesis* (a procedure in which the tympanic membrane is punctured and an aspirate of middle ear fluid is obtained) is not done routinely because it is both painful and expensive.

In AOM, antibiotic therapy effective against the most common organisms, *S. pneumoniae, H. influenzae,* and *M. catarrhalis,* is prescribed empirically.[19] It is important to be aware of the local resistance patterns for these pathogens. Antibiotic-resistant strains of *H. influenzae* and *M. catarrhalis* have become more prevalent. These two organisms produce β-lactamase enzymes, inactivating β-lactam antibiotics that are not β-lactamase stable (Table 96-3). The increased prevalence of drug-resistant *S. pneumoniae* (DRSP) is also of concern.[8,21] This organism has developed multiple mechanisms of resistance to commonly used antibiotics such as erythromycin, TMP-SMX, and β-lactams.[22] The mechanism of *S. pneumoniae* resistance is a genetic alteration in the penicillin-binding protein that decreases the affinity of β-lactam antibiotics for the target site, not β-lactamase production. Therefore, use of high dose amoxicillin to ensure adequate drug levels can overcome many of the resistant pneumococci.[23]

Treatment
Antibiotics

Antimicrobial treatment of otitis media is controversial. The first, most important decision to make is whether drug therapy truly is indicated. Traditional management recommended by the American Academy of Pediatrics (AAP) and the Centers for Disease Control and Prevention (CDC) supports the empiric use of antibiotics. However, meta-analyses of antibiotics

Text continued on p. 96-9.

Table 96-3 Oral Antibiotics for the Treatment of Common Pediatric Infectious Diseases

Antibiotic	Dose	Spectrum[a]					β-Lactamase Stable	Compliance Factor Ratings[b]	Side Effects/ Comments	Refrigeration Required
		S. aureus	S. pneumonia	H. influenzae	M. catarrhalis	Group B β-Hemolytic Strep				
Penicillins										
Penicillin VK,[c] Penicillin V	250 mg = 400,000 units of Penicillin G. 25–50 mg/kg/day divided Q 6 hr (max, 3 g/day)	+	+++	—	—	+++	—	1	Allergy, drug fever, eosinophilia, interstitial nephritis, CNS toxicity; ↓ dose in renal failure	
Penicillinase-Resistant Penicillins										
Dicloxacillin[d]	25–50 mg/kg/day divided Q 6 hr	+++	+++	—	—	+++	+++	1	Mild GI symptoms, diarrhea	
Cloxacillin[e]	50–100 mg/kg/day divided Q 6 hr	+++	+++	—	—	+++	+++	1	Mild GI symptoms, diarrhea	
Broad-Spectrum Penicillins										
Amoxicillin[f]	Standard dose: 20–40 mg/kg/day divided BID to TID. High dose: 80–90 mg/kg/day divided BID	+	+++	++	+	+++	—	2	↓ dose in renal failure; good activity against Salmonella; poor activity against Shigella	Preferred
Amoxicillin-clavulanate[g]	25–45 mg/kg/day divided BID	+++	+++	+++	+++	+++	+++	2	GI distress; take with food; do not give two of the 250 mg amoxicillin/125 mg clavulanate at one time; may result in GI toxicity	Yes
Ampicillin[h]	50–100 mg/kg/day divided Q 6 hr	+	+++	++	+	+++	—	1	Useful in treatment of Shigella; fair to good activity against Salmonella	
Cephalosporins (All Adjusted in Renal Failure)										
1st Generation										
Cephalexin (Keflex)[i]	25–50 mg/kg/day divided Q 6 hr	+++	+++	+	+	+++	+	2	GI distress, dizziness, fatigue, headache, neutropenia, rash, ↑ AST, false-positive test for urinary reducing substances	Yes

Drug	Dose							Adverse Effects	
Cephradine (Velosef, Anspor)ʲ	25–50 mg/kg/day divided Q 6 hr	+++	+++	+	+++	+	2	GI distress, pseudomembranous colitis, rash, joint pains, transient leukopenia or neutropenia, ↑ hepatic enzymes or bili	
Cefadroxil (Duricef)ᵏ	30 mg/kg/day divided Q 12 hr	+++	+++	+	+++	+	3	Allergy, GI distress, transient neutropenia, pruritus	Yes
2nd Generation									
Cefaclor (Ceclor)ˡ	20–40 mg/kg/day divided Q 8–12 hr	+	+++	++	+++	+	3	GI distress, eosinophilia, pruritus, positive Coombs, false-positive test for urinary glucose, serum sickness	
Loracarbef (Lorabid)ᵐ	15 mg/kg/day divided Q 12 hr	++	+++	+++	+++	++	3	GI distress, eosinophilia, pruritus, positive Coombs, false-positive test for urinary glucose	Preferred
Cefuroxime axetil (Ceftin)ⁿ	30 mg/kg/day divided Q 12 hr (40 mg/kg/day for otitis)	+++	+++	+++	+++	++	1	Minor GI complaints	Preferred
3rd Generation									
Cefixime (Suprax)ᵒ	8 mg/kg/day divided Q 12–24 hr	+	++	+++	+++	+++	3	GI distress	Yes
Cefpodoxime (Vantin)ᵖ	10 mg/kg/day divided Q 12 hr	++	+++	+++	+++	+++	3	GI distress, ↑ hepatic enzymes, allergy, dizziness, ↓ leukocytes, eosinophilia	Yes
Cefdinir (Omnicef)ᵠ	14 mg/kg/day divided Q 12–24						3	GI distress, serum sickness ↑ hepatic enzymes headache, rash	No

continued

Table 96-3 Oral Antibiotics for the Treatment of Common Pediatric Infectious Diseases—cont'd

Antibiotic	Dose	Spectrum						Compliance Factor Ratings	Side Effects/Comments	Refrigeration Required
		S. aureus	S. pneumonia	H. influenzae	M. catarrhalis	Group B β-Hemolytic Strep	β-Lactamase Stable			
Cephalosporins (All Adjusted in Renal Failure)—cont'd										
3rd Generation—cont'd										
Cefprozil (Cefzil)	30 mg/kg/day divided Q 12 h	+++	+++	++	+++	+++	+++	3	GI distress, ↑ hepatic enzymes, dizziness	Yes
Ceftibuten (Cedax)	9 mg/kg/day	+	+	++	++	+++	+++	1	Headache, dizziness, GI distress, eosinophilia, ↑ hepatic enzymes, ↑ BUN	Yes
Macrolides										
Erythromycin	30–50 mg/kg/day divided Q 6 hr. Infants less than 4 months of age: 20–40 mg/kg/day divided Q 6 hr	+	+++	+	++	+++	+++	1	Absorption not affected by food; avoid in hepatic failure; GI distress, diarrhea; drug interactions with theophylline, carbamazepine, digoxin, cyclosporine	
Clarithromycin (Biaxin)	15 mg/kg/day divided BID	+	+++	++	++	+++	+++	2	GI side effects less than erythromycin; drug interactions include ↑ theophylline and carbamazepine concentrations	No

Drug	Dose								Yes/No	Side Effects/Comments
Azithromycin (Zithromax)	10 mg/kg on day 1, followed by 5 mg/kg on days 2–5	+	++	++	+++	+++		1	Yes	GI side effects less than erythromycin; drug interactions include ↑ theophylline and carbamazepine concentrations
Others										
TMP-SMX[v]	6–12 mg TMP/30–60 mg SMX/kg/day divided Q 12 hr	+	+++	+++	+++	–	+++	3	No	Not in patients less than 2 months (kernicterus); mild GI symptoms, skin rash, thrombocytopenia (rare), neutropenia (rare); ↑half-life of phenytoin
Erythromycin-sulfisoxazole[w] (Pedizole)	40 mg/kg/day of erythromycin divided Q 6–8 hr	++	+++	+++	+++	+++	+++	1	Yes	Same as erythromycin; also, neutropenia, agranulocytosis, thrombocytopenia, aplastic anemia, allergy, GI distress, crystalluria
Metronidazole[x]	15–35 mg/kg/day divided Q 6 hr	–	–	–	–	–	+++	1		Anaerobic infections, C. difficile colitis, alcohol intolerance, GI distress, metallic or unpleasant taste
Tetracycline[y]	25–50 mg/kg/day divided Q 6 hr. **Use only in patients older than 9 years.**	++	+	+	++	+++	+++	1	No	Depressed bone growth, discolor teeth, enamel hypoplasia, photosensitivity, GI distress, esophageal ulceration
Doxycycline[z]	2–4 mg/kg/day divided Q 12 hr on day 1, then half dose Q 24 hr. **Use only in patients older than 9 years.**	++	+	+	+++	+++	+++	2		Depressed bone growth, discolor teeth, enamel hypoplasia, photosensitivity, GI distress, esophageal ulceration

Table 96-3 Oral Antibiotics for the Treatment of Common Pediatric Infectious Diseases—cont'd

Antibiotic	Dose	Spectrum[a]							Compliance Factor Ratings[c]	Side Effects/ Comments	Refrigeration Required
		S. aureus	S. pneumonia	H. influenzae	M. catarrhalis	Group B β-Hemolytic Strep	β-Lactamase Stable				
Others—cont'd											
Clindamycin[aa]	20–30 mg/kg/day divided Q 6–8 hr	+++	+++	—	+	+++	+++		2	C. difficile diarrhea, allergy, minor ↑ in hepatocellular enzymes, neutropenia, thrombocytopenia	
Rifampin[bb]	H. influenzae: 20 mg/kg/day QD × 4 days N. meningitis: 20 mg/kg/day divided BID × 2 days	+++	++	+++	++	+++	+++		2	Resistance develops rapidly; rash, GI distress, increased hepatic enzymes discolors body fluids (urine, tears, sweat) many drug interactions	

[a] +++, good; ++, average; +, minimal; —, none.
[b] FR, factor ratings; 1, less favorable; 2, average; 3, more favorable.
[c] Penicillin VK available as 15, 250, 500 mg tablets; 125, 250 mg/5 mL suspension; Penicillin V available as 250, 500 mg tablets; 125, 250 mg/5 mL suspension.
[d] Dicloxacillin available as 250, 500 mg capsules; 62.5 mg/5 mL suspension.
[e] Cloxacillin available as 250, 500 mg capsules; 125 mg/5 mL suspension.
[f] Amoxicillin available as 250, 500 mg capsules; 125, 250 mg chewable tablets; 125, 250 mg/5 mL suspension.
[g] Amoxicillin-clavulanate available as chew tabs: 200 mg amoxicillin/28.5 mg clavulanate; 250 mg amoxicillin/62.5 mg clavulanate; 400 mg amoxicillin/57 mg clavulanate; suspension: 125 mg amoxicillin/31.25 mg clavulanate/5 mL; 200 mg amoxicillin/28.5 mg clavulanate/5 mL; 400 mg amoxicillin/57 mg clavulanate/5 mL; 600 mg amoxicillin/42.9 mg clavulanate/5 mL.
[h] Ampicillin available as 250, 500 mg capsules; 125, 250 mg/5 mL suspension.
[i] Cephalexin available as 250, 500 mg capsules; 125, 250 mg/5 mL suspension.
[j] Cephradine available as 250, 500 mg capsules; 125, 250 mg/15 mL suspension.
[k] Cefadroxil available as 50 mg, 1 g capsules; 125, 250, 500 mg/5 mL suspension.
[l] Cefaclor available as 250, 500 mg capsules; 125, 187.5, 250, 375 mg/5 mL suspension.
[m] Loracarbef available as 200 mg pulvules; 100 mg/5 mL suspension.
[n] Cefuroxime axetil available as 125, 250, 500 mg tablets; 125 mg/5 mL suspension.
[o] Cefixime available as 200, 400 mg tablets; 100 mg/5 mL suspension.
[p] Cefpodoxime available as 100, 200 mg capsules; 50, 100 mg/5 mL suspension.
[q] Cefdinir available as 300 mg capsules, 125 mg/5 mL suspension.
[r] Cefprozil available as 250, 500 mg tablets; 125, 250 mg/mL suspension.
[s] Erythromycin available as Estolate: 125, 250 mg/5 mL suspension; ethylsuccinate available as 200, 400 mg/5 mL suspension; base available as 400 mg tablets; stearate available as 250, 500 mg tablets.
[t] Clarithromycin available as 250, 500 mg tablets; 125, 250 mg/5 mL suspension.
[u] TMP-SMX, trimethoprim-sulfamethoxazole. Regular strength tablets: 80 mg TMP/400 mg SMX; double-strength tablets: 160 mg TMP/800 mg SMX; suspension: 40 mg TMP/200 mg SMX/5 mL.
[v] Erythromycin-sulfisoxazole available as 200 mg erythromycin + 600 mg sulfisoxazole/5 mL.
[w] Metronidazole available as 250, 500 mg tablets.
[x] Tetracycline available as 250, 500 mg capsules.
[y] Doxycycline available as 50, 100 mg capsules and tablets; 25 mg/5 mL suspension; 50 mg/5 mL syrup.
[aa] Clindamycin available as 75, 150, 300 mg capsules; 75 mg/5 mL suspension.
[bb] Rifampin available as 150, 300 mg capsules; suspension can be compounded.
AST, aspartate transaminase; BUN, blood urea nitrogen; CNS, central nervous system; GI, gastrointestinal.

versus placebo indicate that about 80% of AOM cases resolve spontaneously within 1 week compared with about 94% of antibiotic recipients.[6B] In one study of 315 children (6 months to 10 years of age) who presented with acute otitis media, immediate antibiotic treatment provided symptomatic benefit mainly after the first 24 hours, when symptoms already were resolving. For some children experiencing a mild acute otitis, a wait-and-see approach seems reasonable and should reduce the use of antibiotics for acute otitis media substantially.[6C] Recommendations for treatment are usually based on the relative risk of DRSP or the likelihood of a complicated case of AOM. Risk factors for DRSP include age <2 years, geographic location, daycare attendance, antibiotic use within the last month, and recurrent AOM. All other children are considered low risk. In a low-risk, nontoxic-appearing child, 24 to 48 hours of observation with adjuvant analgesic therapy is a reasonable option (Table 96-4). If an antibiotic is to be prescribed, amoxicillin is recommended as the first-line agent in penicillin-nonallergic patients because it is inexpensive, has few side effects, and targets the most common pathogens.

Most clinicians advocate a stepped approach to the antimicrobial therapy of AOM (see Table 96-4). In low-risk children, the standard amoxicillin dose should be tried initially. In children at high risk for DRSP, an increase in the empiric treatment dose of amoxicillin to 80 to 90 mg/kg per day (high-dose amoxicillin) is recommended.[24] If the initial antibiotic regimen does not reduce symptoms within 3 days, then a change in therapy should be considered. Alternative therapy should be effective against β lactamase–producing *H. influenzae* and *M. catarrhalis* as well as *S. pneumoniae*. Antibiotics that meet these criteria include the following: amoxicillin/clavulanate, cefdinir, cefpodoxime, cefuroxime axetil and ceftriaxone. If DRSP is also a concern, high-dose amoxicillin/clavulanate using the newer formulation, Augmentin ES (600 mg/5 mL) is recommended.[25] This formulation provides 90 mg/kg of amoxicillin with 6.4 mg/kg clavulanate.[26] Alternatively, standard-dose amoxicillin/clavulanate (45 mg of amoxicillin/kg per day) using the older formulation in combination with standard-dose amoxicillin (45 mg/kg per day) can be used to keep the clavulanate dosage at <10 mg/kg per day. Pneumococcal surveillance data have documented increasing resistance to SMX-TMP, cefaclor and Azithromycin, which should be used only as alternative first-line agents in low-risk, penicillin-allergic patients.[24] Patients failing standard dose amoxicillin are likely to have TMP-SMX–resistant infections.

3. Why was (or was not) amoxicillin/clavulanate a good choice for the treatment of M.G.'s AOM 3 months ago?

M.G. is considered to be "high risk" for DRSP because he is <2 years of age and attends daycare. He also lives in a community known to have a relatively high resistance pattern,

Table 96-4 AOM Treatment Recommendations [23,24,28]

Low-Risk Children (>2 years, no antibiotic use in prior month, no history of recurrent otitis media)

	Recommended	Alternatives
First-line treatment First episode of AOM or recurrence >1 month after previous AOM	Standard-dose amoxicillin[a] or Observation for 24–48 hours. Treat if symptoms persist.[b]	TMP/SMX Azithromycin
Second-line treatment Clinical failure after 48–72 hours of treatment or recurrence <1 month from previous AOM	High-dose amoxicillin[b] or High-dose amoxicillin/clavulanate[c]	Cefdinir Cefpodoxime Cefuroxime axetil

High-Risk Children (<2 years old, antibiotic use in the prior month, history of recurrent otitis media)

	Recommended	Alternatives
First-line treatment First episode of AOM Or recurrence>1 month after previous AOM	High-dose amoxicillin[c]	Cefdinir Cefpodoxime Cefuroxime axetil Cefprozil IM ceftriaxone[e]
Second-line Treatment Clinical failure after 48–72 hours of treatment Or recurrence <1 month from previous AOM	High-dose amoxicillin/clavulanate[d]	

[a]Standard dose amoxicillin is 40 to 45 mg/kg per day divided BID.
[b]Observation is not recommended for ill-appearing child.
[c]High-dose amoxicillin is 80 to 90 mg/kg per day divided BID or TID.
[d]High-dose amoxicillin/clavulanate is 80 to 90 mg/kg of amoxicillin with 6.4 mg/kg per day of clavulanate divided BID (use newer formulations or combination with amoxicillin).
[e]Most efficacious if three doses are used.

with >50% of *H. influenzae* and 95% of *M. catarrhalis* strains producing β-lactamase enzymes. Since it is likely that amoxicillin would be ineffective against these resistant strains, the choice of amoxicillin/clavulanate as initial therapy for treatment of AOM in M.G. was appropriate. In communities where *H. influenzae* β-lactamase resistance is <30% to 40%, but the risk of DRSP exists, high-dose amoxicillin would be recommended as initial therapy for AOM for a "high risk" child. Standard-dose amoxicillin could be considered for a child <2 years of age who lives in a community known to have a low incidence of DRSP. A single dose of 50 mg/kg of ceftriaxone has been shown to be as effective as 10 days of amoxicillin/clavulanate and is approved for use in AOM caused by penicillin-susceptible pneumococcus.[27] Although such a treatment strategy seems appealing, especially in patients prone to poor compliance, some clinicians feel that a three-dose regimen is more appropriate.[28]

4. **What would be the recommended antibiotic treatment for M.G.'s current episode of otitis media?**

M.G. presents with two separate problems that need to be treated; AOM in his right ear and a chronic asymptomatic middle ear effusion in his left ear.

ACUTE OTITIS MEDIA

M.G.'s right ear AOM can be treated using the guidelines outlined in Table 96-4. There is no single oral antibiotic agent that eliminates all pathogens. Oral amoxicillin continues to be the first-line antimicrobial agent for treating uncomplicated AOM; dosing depends on whether the patient is considered to be at low risk or high risk for DRSP.[24] Second-line treatment must be explored if amoxicillin therapy fails after 3 days. In choosing the best alternative antibiotic, a systematic, individualized approach allows flexibility while optimizing therapeutic outcome. The first consideration must be based on efficacy against the major pathogens (*S. pneumoniae, H. influenzae,* and *M. catarrhalis*). This eliminates the natural penicillins, penicillinase-resistant penicillins, tetracyclines, rifampin, and erythromycin. Second, side effect profiles of effective agents should be evaluated. In the past, amoxicillin/clavulanate was associated with significant diarrhea. This is much less of a problem with the new formulations of amoxicillin/clavulanate. Cefixime (Suprax) and oral cefuroxime (Ceftin) can also cause diarrhea, and erythromycin/sulfisoxazole (Pediazole) has a high incidence of gastrointestinal (GI) upset. It is important to keep in mind that most antibiotics have side effects, and the clinician and patient must agree on which are the most tolerable. The third consideration should focus on compliance with therapy. Amoxicillin, amoxicillin/clavulanate, cefprozil (Cefzil), TMP-SMX, and cefuroxime axetil (Ceftin) are dosed twice a day; azithromycin, cefpodoxime (Vantin) and cefdinir (Omnicef) can be dosed once a day. Erythromycin/sulfisoxazole and cefaclor require every 6- to 8-hour dosing. Children often find erythromycin/sulfisoxazole suspensions and cefuroxime axetil to have a bad taste, whereas cefaclor has been favored in taste evaluations.[29] Cefixime (Suprax), loracarbef (Lorabid), and TMP-SMX do not require refrigeration. The cost of amoxicillin and TMP-SMX is much less than the newer cephalosporins and amoxicillin/clavulanate.

Considering M.G.'s known community resistance patterns, past history of response to amoxicillin/clavulanate and time period of >1 month since antibiotics have been used, amoxicillin/clavulanate would be a good choice to treat his current AOM. In view of the community resistance patterns, other alternatives include cefdinir (Omnicef), cefpodoxime (Vantin), cefprozil (Cefzil), cefuroxime (Ceftin), loracarbef (Lorabid), or a single intramuscular (IM) injection of ceftriaxone. Traditionally, treatment for AOM has been for 10 to 14 days, but no data support this length of treatment over shorter courses of 3 to 5 days[27,30,31] A 10-day course of therapy for children at high risk of recurrence or complications (e.g., age <2 years, recurrent otitis media, perforated eardrum, recent antibiotic treatment, craniofacial abnormalities, hearing loss, impaired immune system) is recommended, and a 5-day course of treatment for all other children. Because M.G. is only 10 months old, he should be treated for 10 days with a follow-up appointment at the end of therapy to assess his response.

CHRONIC OTITIS MEDIA WITH EFFUSION

Chronic OME, which is representative of the process occurring in M.G.'s left ear, should be treated if the effusion persists for >3 months after the AOM infection.[32] The pathogens that typically cause the chronic infection are the same as for AOM, except that there should be higher suspicion of resistant organisms. A systematic approach, similar to the one described for AOM, should be taken when evaluating antibiotic therapy for chronic OME. Ceftriaxone has not been evaluated for chronic otitis media and is not a therapeutic option at this time. Middle ear effusions that do not resolve after a second course of antibiotic therapy should be evaluated for more aggressive adjunctive therapy or surgical placement of tympanostomy tubes. In M.G., the treatment strategies for the infections in both ears overlap and a single drug (amoxicillin/clavulanate) can be used.

The efficacy of antibiotic therapy should be evaluated in M.G. by observing him for resolution of presenting symptoms, such as irritability, anorexia, and waking at night. Otoscopic examination of the ears in 2 weeks should provide direct evidence of infection resolution, particularly in the left ear, which was asymptomatic. Monitoring for side effects and toxicity of amoxicillin/clavulanate should focus on any GI complaints such as vomiting and diarrhea, or any dermatologic reaction, such as rash (see Table 96-3). Compliance with the medication regimen is essential for optimal results.

Adjunctive Therapy

5. **What adjunctive therapies might be beneficial in M.G.?**

Analgesics and antipyretics are appropriate to relieve the symptoms of ear pain and fever. Acetaminophen (10 to 15 mg/kg per dose every 4 to 6 hours) or ibuprofen (5 to 10 mg/kg per dose every 6 to 8 hours) can be administered as needed. Ibuprofen can be particularly useful at night because of its long duration of action.

The role of decongestants and antihistamines in the treatment of otitis media remains controversial. Multiple clinical studies have failed to demonstrate any benefit of oral or topical decongestants in the treatment of AOM.[28] Decongestants and antihistamines may help prevent otitis media in infants and children who have a significant allergic component that contributes to upper airway congestion. M.G. does not have a history of allergies and his episodes are not seasonal; thus, antihistamines and decongestants are not indicated.

Limited research has suggested that oral corticosteroids in conjunction with oral antibiotic therapy resolve middle ear effusions more effectively than antibiotics alone.[33,34] The use of corticosteroids is not without risk, and many experts do not recommend the use of oral corticosteroid for OME because of possible severe side effects.

Prophylaxis

Antimicrobial prophylaxis only is of small benefit, reducing recurrences by one episode per year.[33] The benefit of prophylaxis, therefore, must be weighed against the risk of promoting resistance. For this reason, prophylaxis should only be considered for children at high risk of recurrence, such as those with less than three documented episodes of AOM within a 6-month period or more than four episodes within 1 year. Prophylaxis should begin immediately after completion of antibiotic therapy and continue for up to 3 months or for the time the increased risk of recurrent otitis media (i.e., presence of effusion) diminishes. Data regarding use of intermittent antibiotic prophylaxis at the onset of upper respiratory infection are inconclusive. Options for prophylaxis include amoxicillin or sulfisoxazole at one-half the standard daily dose.[19,20] Surgical placement of tympanostomy tubes reduces the frequency of recurrent AOM and is an alternative to antibiotic prophylaxis.

Complications and Sequelae

Although hearing loss is the most common complication of otitis media, a variety of other conditions may occur as secondary complications. These include meningitis, subdural and extradural abscesses, and focal encephalitis. For these reasons, otitis media, whether treated with antibiotics or not, should be followed appropriately by the patient's clinician.

SINUSITIS
Acute Sinusitis
Clinical Presentation

6. P.L., a 4-year-old, 16-kg boy is seen at the pediatrician's office with complaints of headache, runny nose, cough, and a new onset of fever. His mother states that he has had a decreased appetite and that she has noticed that he has very bad breath. He has had a cold for 2 weeks but there has been an increase in nasal secretions that have changed from clear to a greenish-yellow appearance. P.L. has a history of recurrent otitis media; his last episode 6 months ago resolved when treated with a 10-day course of amoxicillin/clavulanate (Augmentin). He is taking no medications and has no history of allergies. On physical examination, P.L. is found to have a temperature of 102.6°F (oral), maxillary tenderness, purulent green-yellow nasal discharge, and a mildly erythematous throat without evidence of exudates. His ear examination is normal. Laboratory tests indicate a white blood cell (WBC) count of 17,000/mm³ with 82% neutrophils, 10% lymphocytes, 5% monocytes, and 3% eosinophils. Sinus radiographs indicate bilateral opaque maxillary sinuses, suggestive of sinusitis. P.L. also lives in a community known to have >50% of H. *influenzae* and >95% of M. *catarrhalis* isolates producing β-lactamase. What clinical observations in P.L. suggest that he may have sinusitis?

Acute sinusitis is a common heath problem, affecting more than 37 million people a year. Although a child's sinuses are not fully developed until age 20, children can still suffer from a sinus infection. Sinusitis is difficult to diagnose in children because respiratory infections are common in this population and symptoms can be subtle. P.L. has several distinct features of acute sinusitis. The history of an upper respiratory infection with cough that has persisted for 2 weeks; increased nasal discharge, which has changed from a clear to green-yellow color; and halitosis suggest the possibility of a secondary bacterial sinus infection.[35] In some cases, nasal discharge may be clear and nonpurulent. The fever and decreased appetite are suggestive of systemic illness. P.L. has a headache, a common symptom of sinusitis in adults but often not present in pediatric patients until after 6 years of age.[36] Maxillary tenderness and the bilateral opaque maxillary sinuses on radiography suggest maxillary sinus involvement; P.L.'s erythematous throat is most likely caused by postnasal mucous drip from the sinuses and nasopharynx. Although WBC counts are not routinely needed or obtained for the diagnosis of sinusitis, P.L. has an elevated WBC count with a predominance of neutrophils, suggesting a bacterial infection.

Microbiology

7. What pathogens are most likely to be causing sinusitis in P.L.?

An acute bacterial infection of the sinus cavities is often preceded by a viral upper respiratory tract infection or allergy attack. Immune deficiency, asthma and gastroesophageal reflux (GERD) may also predispose children to sinusitis. While viruses cause inflammation of the sinuses, the pathogenic organisms of acute sinusitis are similar to that of AOM, with S. *pneumoniae*, H. *influenzae*, and M. *catarrhalis* responsible for most of the bacterial infections.[37] Obtaining sinus cultures requires direct aspiration of the sinus cavity. Since sinus cultures do not usually correlate with pathogens that are causing the problem, this painful procedure is avoided unless a patient has repeated infections.[36]

Treatment
ANTIBIOTIC THERAPY

8. What treatment options are available for P.L., and which are recommended?

Because the pathophysiology and microbiology of sinusitis and otitis media are similar, treatment options discussed in Questions 3 and 4 also pertain to therapy for P.L. The sinusitis in P.L. can be treated with any oral antibiotic that is effective against S. *pneumoniae*, H. *influenzae*, and M. *catarrhalis*. Watchful waiting may be appropriate for a child who does not appear to have systemic illness (fever, elevated WBC). Amoxicillin is currently the drug of choice for acute sinusitis in a non–penicillin-allergic patient. Resistance patterns must also be considered when prescribing antibiotics. P.L. lives in a community with a high incidence of β-lactamase–producing

H. influenzae and *M. catarrhalis;* amoxicillin, therefore, may be ineffective as initial therapy. Antibiotic selection must be individualized as described in the treatment of otitis media and should include an assessment of efficacy, adverse effects, compliance factors, and cost. P.L. has a history of recurrent otitis media; a detailed drug history from P.L.'s mother may elicit information that could help guide antibiotic selection for his current sinus infection. P.L. was treated with amoxicillin/clavulanate for his last episode of otitis media, which has not recurred for 6 months; therefore, it may be a reasonable choice for the treatment of his current sinusitis. Treatment can be discontinued after 10 to 14 days if a complete response has been observed. However, any residual signs or symptoms such as nasal discharge (clear or purulent), cough, fever, or headaches mandate an additional 7 to 10 days of antibiotic therapy.[37]

ADJUVANT THERAPY

9. **What is the role of adjuvant therapy in P.L.?**

In patients with a significant allergic history and nasal congestion, decongestants and antihistamines can reduce congestion and the risk of secondary bacterial sinusitis.[37] P.L. has no history of allergies, and the current episode was associated with a preceding upper respiratory tract infection. Therefore, antihistamines would not be of benefit in the treatment of P.L.'s sinusitis. Intranasal steroids have not been found to be of benefit in patients with sinusitis.[38,39] Nasal sprays containing decongestants are also of limited value; products containing naphazoline are contraindicated in children <6 years of age.[40] Saline nasal drops or spray can be used to help promote drainage of secretions. Acetaminophen, ibuprofen, and warm compresses will help to reduce facial pain.

Chronic Sinusitis
Antibiotic Therapy

10. **Four months later, P.L. returns to the clinic with similar complaints and a history of continuous nasal discharge and cough for the last 3 months. Although he initially responded to therapy (3 weeks of amoxicillin/clavulanate 45 mg/kg per day), P.L.'s symptoms reappeared 1 week after discontinuation of antibiotic therapy and have progressively worsened. What should be considered when selecting an antibiotic for P.L. at this visit?**

When sinusitis recurs frequently or symptoms last >12 weeks, it is classified as chronic. P.L. has chronic sinusitis with persistent symptoms of nasal discharge, cough, and headaches. Chronic sinusitis is often caused by allergies or a mixture of bacteria including organisms, such as *S. aureus, Streptococcus pyogenes, nontypable H. Influenzae, M. catarrhalis,* or anaerobes.[34] It is also possible that P.L. has developed a chronic infection with a resistant organism or an allergic fungal sinusitis.[41]

The antimicrobial agent selected for P.L. should be effective against both the typical and atypical organisms described previously. Amoxicillin/clavulanate (Augmentin) has the most comprehensive staphylococcidal and anaerobic activity of the broad-spectrum oral antibiotics and may be preferred based on efficacy.[36] However, P.L. has previously been treated with amoxicillin/clavulanate for 21 days and now presents with a recurrence of his sinusitis. A careful medication history

should be obtained to assess his adherence to the previous amoxicillin/clavulanate therapy.

11. **P.L.'s parents describe a period of 10 days during which P.L. was at his grandparents' house and the medicine was not refrigerated. How does this information affect the choice of an antimicrobial for P.L. at this time?**

Amoxicillin/clavulanate loses some of its potency if left at room temperature for 4 hours and up to 90% of its potency if left unrefrigerated for 48 hours.[42] Lack of refrigeration is likely to have had a negative impact on the effectiveness of the previous treatment. Based on this information, it may be appropriate to prescribe another 21-day course of amoxicillin/clavulanate for P.L. with additional patient counseling on the proper storage and administration of this medication. Likewise, it may be prudent to switch to an antibiotic that does not require refrigeration, especially if P.L. is likely to be at his grandparents' home during this time. Cefixime (Suprax) does not require refrigeration, but it may be only marginally effective against *S. aureus* and *S. pneumoniae.*[43] Cefprozil (Cefzil), cefpodoxime (Vantin), and cefuroxime (Ceftin) can be given every 12 hours, but all of these antibiotics require refrigeration. TMP-SMX can be stored at room temperature but is not effective against *S. pyogenes* and is less palatable than amoxicillin/clavulanate or cefixime. Amoxicillin without clavulanate would not be effective against β-lactamase–producing organisms, and cefaclor has been associated with treatment failures with β-lactamase–producing *M. catarrhalis* and *H. influenzae.*[44] Loracarbef has limited data in the treatment of sinusitis but does not require refrigeration and can be given every 12 hours. Clarithromycin and azithromycin could also be considered. It is often difficult to make the "most appropriate" antibiotic selection but, based on efficacy, amoxicillin/clavulanate and loracarbef seem to be the best options for P.L. Cefpodoxime, cefuroxime, and cefprozil would also be reasonable options.

PHARYNGITIS
Clinical Presentation

12. **T.R. is a 14-year-old, 52-kg boy with a severe sore throat and fever. He states that the sore throat developed yesterday afternoon and was extremely painful when he woke up this morning. He is an otherwise healthy 8th grader with no history of allergies. Several of his classmates have been absent from school with sore throats over the last several weeks. T.R. has two younger brothers, ages 5 and 8; the 8-year old had "strep throat" 2 weeks ago. On physical examination, T.R.'s throat is erythematous with exudative patches. He has a fever of 102°F (oral) and a respiratory rate of 30 breaths/minute. Laboratory results indicate a positive streptococcal rapid antigen test of the throat. What is the likelihood that T.R. has a bacterial, rather than a viral, pharyngitis?**

Differentiation between viral and bacterial pharyngitis is difficult because many of the signs and symptoms overlap. Bacterial pathogens account for approximately 30% of pediatric pharyngitis cases. Several features of T.R.'s presentation are suggestive of bacterial pharyngitis. T.R. describes a history of a family member treated for bacterial pharyngitis as well as several friends at school with sore throats (which is suggestive of an epidemic). Epidemic outbreaks of bacterial or viral pharyngitis in the community should be taken into consideration when evaluating patients with pharyngitis. The rapid onset of symptoms, an associated high fever, and the classic exudative patches in the throat all suggest bacterial infection; however, these findings also can be associated with viral etiologies. Rapid streptococcal antigen detection tests (RADT) are throat swab tests that identify the presence of group A streptococcal antigens. This screening test provides results in a few minutes to several hours but is positive in only approximately 85% of cases of streptococcal pharyngitis.[44,45] The positive RADT in T.R. indicates a bacterial etiology, with high probability. RADTs have a low incidence of false-positive results, and since the test cannot detect other kinds of bacteria, a negative result does not confirm a nonbacterial infection. In patients with a negative RADT, a throat culture should be obtained to confirm or rule out a diagnosis of bacterial pharyngitis.[46] Because T.R. has a positive RADT as well as a history and physical examination suggestive of streptococcal pharyngitis, throat culture is not necessary and antimicrobial treatment should be initiated.

Microbiology

13. What common causative organisms could be responsible for T.R.'s pharyngitis?

T.R. has a clinical presentation highly suggestive of a bacterial etiology, but viruses cause pharyngitis in 40% of cases.[46] Adenovirus and enterovirus are the most common cause, but parainfluenza, influenza, and Epstein-Barr viruses also can cause pharyngitis (see Table 96-2). In children <2 years of age, most pharyngitis is of viral etiology. Viral pharyngitis is usually self-limited and therapy is largely symptomatic. If T.R. did have viral pharyngitis, oral analgesics such as acetaminophen and ibuprofen could be used to relieve the pain and fever; aspirin should be avoided during acute viral infections because of concern about Reye's syndrome. Topical anesthetic sprays also can provide symptomatic pain relief but will not reduce fever and require frequent administration.

Group A β-hemolytic streptococci (GABHS), also known as *S. pyogenes,* is the most common bacterial organism in children 5 to 15 years of age. The RADT specifically identifies GABHS antigen and is highly suggestive of GABHS pharyngitis when the screening test is positive, as it is in T.R. Other less common causes of bacterial pharyngitis are listed in Table 96-2. Diphtheria should be considered only in unimmunized or immigrant patients. Approximately 20% of asymptomatic children are long-term carriers of GABHS.[47]

Complications of Group A β-Hemolytic Streptococci Infection

14. Why should antimicrobial therapy be prescribed to treat T.R.'s bacterial pharyngitis?

Bacterial pharyngitis can be a self-limiting infection that usually resolves in several days without treatment; however, important suppurative, toxin-mediated and nonsuppurative sequelae can be avoided by use of antibiotics. Suppurative complications include peritonsillar abscess, cervical lymphadenitis, otitis media, mastoiditis, and sinusitis.[48] Data suggest that the virulence patterns of GABHS are significant in the development of suppurative complications. GABHS is classified by M types: M-1, M-3, and M-18 isolates have been associated with an increased incidence of invasive disease.[49] GABHS is associated with the cytolytic toxins, streptolysin S and O. Streptolysin O induces persistently high antibody titers and is a useful marker of GABHS infection and its nonsuppurative complications.

Scarlet fever is an example of a toxin-mediated complication of GABHS, although it has become nearly nonexistent in the United States. An invasive streptococcal infection associated with shock and organ failure has also been reported. This streptococcal toxic-shock syndrome affects people of all ages, most of whom do not have underlying diseases.[50] Toxin-mediated illnesses occur after pharyngitis in a small percentage of the population.

Nonsuppurative complications, or delayed antibody-mediated diseases of GABHS infections, include acute rheumatic fever. Acute rheumatic fever causes chronic progressive damage to the heart and its valves; it was a leading cause of death in children until 1960. If untreated, GABHS pharyngitis develops into rheumatic fever in 0.3% of children and 3% of adults. The incidence of rheumatic fever in the United States has declined over the last several decade due to antibiotic treatment of streptococcal infections or a change in streptococci virulence.[51] Developing countries have an increased incidence of acute rheumatic fever, with up to 40% of reported cases occurring in these areas. Certain GABHS serotypes (M-3, M-5, M-18, M-19, and M-24) have been implicated in the pathogenesis of acute rheumatic fever.[52] Rheumatic fever can be prevented if antibiotic treatment is initiated within 9 days from onset of symptoms.[53,54]

Poststreptococcal glomerulonephritis (PSGN) is now an uncommon immunologic complication of GABH infection. Immune complexes formed from streptococcal antigen, antibodies and complement are trapped in the glomeruli of the kidneys causing inflammation with resultant inefficient filtering, decreased renal function and hypertension. Symptoms of PSGN develop within 10 days of pharyngitis or 3 weeks after a group A streptococcal skin infection. PSGN usually resolves spontaneously after several weeks to months although in adults it can progress to chronic renal failure. Adequate antibiotic treatment of known GABHS infection is thought to decrease the incidence of PSGN.[48]

Antibiotic treatment of T.R.'s GABHS pharyngitis will rapidly reduce his symptoms and decrease transmission of the infection to others. In addition, treatment with appropriate antibiotics will prevent complications, including acute rheumatic fever and PSGN.

Treatment
Antibiotic Therapy

15. What antibiotic is most appropriate for treatment of T.R.'s pharyngitis? How long should he be treated?

GABHS is exquisitely sensitive to all β-lactam antibiotics.[55] Penicillin has long been the treatment of choice because of its low side effect profile and cost. Penicillin BID regimens are as effective as QID regimens for the treatment of

GABHS pharyngitis; however, many clinicians are hesitant to prescribe twice-daily penicillin because minor noncompliance may render the therapy ineffective, and the cost difference between twice-daily versus three-or-four-times-daily regimens is minimal.[56,57] When oral penicillin is not dependable, a single dose of IM benzathine penicillin G is acceptable. All the macrolide antibiotics (e.g., erythromycin, azithromycin, clarithromycin, roxithromycin) commonly are prescribed for respiratory tract infections; however, azithromycin generally is not used as first-line therapy for pharyngitis due to group A streptococci. Nevertheless, the 5-day regimen of one daily dose of azithromycin is a viable option.[58] A macrolide or clindamycin should be given to patients with a history of penicillin allergy; however, many would prescribe a first-generation cephalosporin in the presence of a poorly documented penicillin allergic history. In patients allergic to both penicillins and cephalosporins, erythromycin has been considered the alternative agent of choice, largely based on cost. Until recently, resistance of groups A streptococci to macrolide antibiotics has been rare in the United States. However, a sudden outbreak of erythromycin-resistant group A streptococci (48% of isolates) in Pittsburgh schoolchildren between October 2000 and May 2001 has raised the question of whether culture and sensitivity testing should precede the use of erythromycin for the routine treatment of pharyngitis.[58B,58C] T.R. has no drug allergies; therefore, oral penicillin it is the most cost-effective therapy for his GABHS pharyngitis.

T.R. should take oral penicillin for 10 days. Pharyngitis symptoms typically resolve after 24 to 48 hours of therapy, but therapy should be continued for the full 10 days to reduce the risk of subsequent rheumatic fever. Shorter courses of therapy have high relapse rates, which may be associated with an increased risk of rheumatic fever.[57] Since clinical trials to evaluate the direct effect of treatment-course duration on rheumatic fever reduction need to evaluate very large numbers of patients; a definitive answer to this issue of short-course antibiotic regimens is not likely to be available anytime soon.

Prophylaxis of Household Members

16. What efforts should be made to eradicate GABHS from T.R.'s household?

GABHS pharyngitis is highly contagious, and it is not surprising that two cases have been documented in T.R.'s household during the last 2 weeks. Up to 25% of people are thought to be asymptomatic carriers of GABHS.[59] Although it is possible to acquire pharyngitis from an asymptomatic carrier, it is more common to acquire the infection from a person with symptoms. Carriers should be diagnosed and treated when there is a family history of rheumatic fever or a community outbreak of rheumatic fever or if a family member experienced more than three episodes of documented GABHS pharyngitis within 12 months. Routine prophylaxis of households with multiple cases of GABHS pharyngitis is not necessary. To identify a carrier, throat swabs should be taken from all household members during a time when everyone is symptom-free. All culture-positive individuals should be treated with a course of penicillin. If eradication of GABHS

has not been achieved with two successive courses of penicillin, rifampin 20 mg/kg per day (maximum, 300 mg) once a day or in two daily divided doses for the last 4 days of the penicillin treatment can be prescribed to eradicate this organism from the upper respiratory tract.[60,61]

ACUTE RHEUMATIC FEVER
Clinical Presentation and Diagnosis

17. Three days later, C.R. (T.R.'s 8-year-old brother) complains of joint pain in his knees and wrists. He has a fever of 102°F (oral) and a nonpruritic rash with distinct disklike borders on his thighs and stomach. On physical examination, C.R. has a respiratory rate of 24 breaths/min, a heart rate of 120 beats/min, and a mitral valve regurgitation murmur; his knees are inflamed, hot, and painful. His medical history is significant for pharyngitis diagnosed 2 weeks ago and treated with a 10-day course of TMP-SMX. Laboratory tests indicate an erythrocyte sedimentation rate (ESR) of 120 mm/hr, a WBC count of 28,700 cells/mm³, and an antistreptolysin O (ASO) titer of 845 Todd units. A chest radiograph shows a normal heart size and no pulmonary edema. What signs and symptoms does C.R. have that support the diagnosis of acute rheumatic fever?

The American Heart Association guidelines for the diagnosis of acute rheumatic fever include major and minor criteria. In addition to evidence of a previous streptococcal infection, diagnosis requires two major Jones' criteria or one major plus two minor Jones' criteria (Table 96-5).[62,63] C.R. has a history of presumed GABHS pharyngitis treated with TMP-SMX. TMP-SMX is ineffective against GABHS; therefore, C.R. remained at risk for acute rheumatic fever despite antimicrobial therapy. Documentation of a recent GABHS infection is important for the diagnosis of acute rheumatic fever, but it is not elicited in approximately 50% of cases.[62] C.R. has several major criteria diagnostic of acute rheumatic fever, including polyarthritis, erythema marginatum, and carditis (detected by a new murmur with tachycardia). He also has several of the minor criteria: fever, increased ESR, and leukocytosis. The ASO titer is also a useful marker of a nonsuppurative complication of GABHS. C.R. does not have congestive heart failure as evidenced by the normal heart size on chest radiograph and the lack of other symptoms such as edema, lethargy, tachypnea, and tachycardia. Symptoms of acute rheumatic fever usually occur 1 to 5 weeks (average 19 days) after GABHS pharyngitis. Acute rheumatic fever is rare in children under 4 years of age, peaks at age 8, and occurs most often between the ages of 6 and 15 years.[64]

Treatment

18. What pharmacologic treatment should be considered for C.R.'s acute rheumatic fever?

Antimicrobial therapy should be instituted in C.R. While antibiotics will not modify an attack of acute rheumatic fever, a 10-day course of oral penicillin is recommended to eradicate any GABHS remaining in the patient. Appropriate alternative antibiotics (see Question 15) should be used in penicillin-allergic patients.

C.R. should also receive anti-inflammatory therapy to treat the acute inflammatory manifestations of rheumatic fever.[65]

Table 96-5 The Modified Jones Criteria for the Diagnosis of Acute Rheumatic Fever

Clinical Findings	Description
Major Manifestations	
Carditis	Carditis usually manifests as a valvulitis and is associated with a systolic or diastolic murmur; myocarditis and pericarditis in the absence of a murmur are not likely
Polyarthritis	Frequently in the larger joints and migratory in nature; classically responds to salicylates within 48 hours
Chorea	Involuntary movements of the trunk or extremities that tend to have a delayed appearance
Erythema marginatum	The rash is a rare occurrence and is transitory and migrant; the lesions are nonpruritic, round with a pale center, and occur mostly on the trunk
Subcutaneous nodules	Firm, painless nodules develop over bony surfaces such as the elbows and knees; they move freely and are not inflamed; most often seen in patients with carditis
Minor Manifestations	
Arthralgia	Arthralgia is a joint pain without evidence of inflammation, which would be arthritis
Fever	A temperature of at least 39°C that usually occurs early in the course of the disease
Elevated erythrocyte sedimentation rate (ESR)	$\uparrow$ acute-phase reactant that is relatively nonspecific
Elevated C-reactive protein	$\uparrow$ acute-phase reactant that is more specific than ESR
Prolonged PR interval	Nonspecific finding suggestive of carditis; does not predict development of chronic heart disease
Evidence of Antecedent Group A Streptococcal Infection	
(+) Throat culture	Does not differentiate between acute infection and carrier state; only positive in approximately 25% of acute rheumatic fever patients
(+) Rapid streptococcal antigen screen	Does not differentiate between acute infection and carrier state; relatively specific but lacks sensitivity; negative results need to be confirmed with culture
Elevated or rising antibody titers	A $\geq$2 dilution $\uparrow$ in titers is suggestive of recent infection; Antistreptolysin O and Anti-DNase B are the most common; Antistreptolysin O titers >320 Todd units and Anti-DNase titers >240 Todd units generally are considered elevated in children

Aspirin at dosages of 100 mg/kg per day divided every 6 hours dramatically reduces all manifestations of the disease with the exception of chorea. Trough salicylate concentrations should be maintained in the range of 20 to 25 mg/dL. Drug therapy should continue until signs and symptoms of rheumatic fever are resolved (6 to 8 weeks) and the ESR normalizes (<20 mm/hour)[66] The use of corticosteroids is controversial. Some experts believe that prednisone should be used in acute rheumatic fever patients with moderate to severe pericarditis (i.e., cardiomegaly, heart failure, third-degree heart block).[65] However, corticosteroids to prevent or reduce the risk of heart valve lesions were not beneficial according to a Cochrane review.[67] Digoxin, diuretics (furosemide, spironolactone), afterload reduction (e.g., angiotensin-converting enzyme inhibitor), oxygen, bed rest and sodium and fluid restriction may be considered for patients with heart failure.

Prophylaxis

19. **What advice should C.R. be given regarding antibiotic prophylaxis?**

C.R. has a 75% chance of having a recurrence of rheumatic fever in the absence of long-term antibiotic prophylaxis.[64,68] Therefore, long-term penicillin prophylaxis should be initiated either as benzathine penicillin IM injections every 4 weeks (3 weeks in areas where rheumatic fever is endemic) or daily oral penicillin.[69] Prophylactic antibiotic regimens for acute rheumatic fever patients and recommendations for penicillin-allergic patients are summarized in Table 96-6 and ex-

Table 96-6 Prophylactic Antibiotic Regimens for Acute Rheumatic Fever Patients

Long-Term Antibiotic Prophylaxis for the Prevention of Secondary Rheumatic Fever or Heart Disease

Benzathine penicillin G 1.2 million units IM Q 3–4 wk
or
Penicillin V 125–250 mg PO Q 12 hr (125 mg <60 lb >250 mg)
or
Sulfadiazine or sulfisoxazole 500–1,000 mg QD (500 mg <60 lb >1,000 mg)
or
Erythromycin 250 mg Q 12 hr

Prophylaxis for Endocarditis in Patients with Rheumatic Fever or Heart Disease Already Receiving Long-Term Secondary Prophylaxis

Dental, oral, and upper respiratory procedures
Azithromycin or clarithromycin 15 mg/kg PO 1 hr before procedure (max dose, 500 mg)
or
Clindamycin PO or IV, 20 mg/kg 1 hr before procedure (max dose, 300 mg)
or
Cephalexin or cefadroxil 50 mg/kg PO 1 hr before procedure (max dose, 2 g)
Genitourinary and gastrointestinal procedures
Vancomycin IV, 20 mg/kg (max dose, 1 g) *and* gentamicin IV 1.5 mg/kg (max dose, 120 mg) both given within 30 min of starting procedure

tensively presented in Chapter 59, Endocarditis. Although an increased incidence of allergic reactions associated with IM penicillin injections has been suspected, clinical studies have not been able to document an increased risk.[70] Benzathine penicillin IM can improve compliance; however, young children such as C.R. often are reluctant to receive repeated IM injections, and oral therapy may be preferred. Rheumatic fever patients without evidence of carditis should receive prophylaxis for 5 years or until 21 years of age, whichever is longer. Rheumatic fever patients with carditis, but without valvular disease, should receive prophylaxis for at least 10 years or well into adulthood, whichever is longer. Patients with carditis and persistent valve disease should receive life-long prophylaxis.[68] Since C.R. presented with carditis, the duration of his prophylaxis will be determined by the presence, or absence, of persistent valvular disease.[67] C.R. should be educated about the need for secondary antibiotic prophylaxis before minor surgical procedures or instrumentation if evidence of rheumatic heart disease (valvular damage) is present. Secondary prophylaxis with antibiotics during increased-risk procedures should be initiated with an antimicrobial agent other than a penicillin because C.R. is taking long-term penicillin prophylaxis.

BRONCHIOLITIS
Clinical Presentation

20. S.M. is a 14-month-old, 11-kg girl who presents with difficulty breathing, congestion, fever, and decreased appetite. She has a 3-day history of fussiness and low-grade fever. Yesterday, she developed mild wheezing, cough, and a fever of 101°F (rectal). She has a history of reactive airway disease (RAD) that responds to nebulized albuterol and cromolyn. On physical examination, S.M. is in moderate respiratory distress. She has decreased breath sounds and expiratory wheezes bilaterally, intercostal retractions, a respiratory rate of 50 breaths/min, and a heart rate of 130 beats/min. Laboratory tests indicate the following: venous blood gas pH, 7.35; PCO_2, 56 mm Hg; PO_2, 50 mm Hg; and a pulse oximetry reading of 90% oxygen saturation. Her WBC count is 15,100/mm³, with 22% neutrophils, 69% lymphocytes, and 9% monocytes. A nasal swab for RSV is positive. What presenting signs and symptoms are suggestive of bronchiolitis in this patient and which are important in assessing the severity of disease?

S.M. has several typical presenting signs and symptoms of bronchiolitis. Her history of a previous upper respiratory tract infection, as evidenced by the congestion and fever, is common in infants that develop bronchiolitis. The differentiation between bronchiolitis and an acute exacerbation of RAD is difficult, and the two diseases can occur concurrently. Wheezing, tachypnea, hypoxia, and hypercapnia occur frequently with both diseases; however, fever and leukocytosis are not common in RAD. S.M. also has a positive RSV swabbing of the nares, which is suggestive of RSV bronchiolitis infection (see also Chapter 72, Viral Infections).

Respiratory distress or difficulty is classified based on signs and symptoms, and these typically range from mild to moderate to severe. Important parameters to assess when evaluating the severity of disease include respiratory rate, oxygenation, carbon dioxide retention, lung auscultation, and the use of respiratory accessory muscles (Table 96-7). S.M. has an elevated respiratory rate (50 breaths/minute), which is contributing to the poor oxygenation and CO_2 retention. S.M.'s venous blood gas results are not useful in evaluating the oxygenation, but are still helpful in determining her acid–base and CO_2 status. The pulse oximetry provides adequate evaluation of S.M.'s oxygenation status without the need for an arterial blood gas determination. S.M. has a low oxygenation of 90% by oximetry, indicating moderate hypoxia. The elevated CO_2 of 56 mm Hg indicates moderate CO_2 retention. Lung auscultation findings of decreased breath sounds and expiratory wheezing suggest moderate respiratory distress because they are present throughout the entire expiratory phase, but not during both inspiration and expiration. Intercostal muscle retractions indicate that S.M. is using her diaphragmatic muscles to assist her respirations more than usual and are suggestive of moderate to severe respiratory difficulty. Based on the data provided, S.M. appears to be in moderate respiratory distress. However, these clinical signs and symptoms should be monitored frequently because S.M. could easily develop severe respiratory distress.

Table 96-7 Classification of Pediatric Respiratory Distress

	Mild	Moderate	Severe
Respiratory rate (breath/min)			
6 mo–1 yr	35–45	45–55	>55
>1-5 yr	25–35	35–45	>45
>6 yr	20–30	30–40	>40
Color	Normal-pink	Pink-pale	Pale-gray-blue
Dyspnea	None or with exertion	With exertion	At rest
Lung auscultation	Equal inspiratory and expiratory phases, ↓ breath sounds, end expiratory phase wheezing	Inspiratory phase > expiratory phase, dull breath sounds, entire expiratory phase wheezing	Inspiratory phase < expiratory phase, few or no breath sounds, inspiratory and expiratory phase wheezing if breath sounds present
Accessory muscle use	None	Intercostal and subcostal retractions	Also subclavicular retractions
Oxygenation (PO_2)	Normal (O_2 saturation >95%)	Low-normal (O_2 saturation 90–95%)	↓ (O_2 saturation <90%)
Ventilation (PCO_2)	Normal	↑ (PCO_2 <35 mm Hg)	↓ (PCO_2 >45 mm Hg)

Treatment
Bronchodilators

21. Would inhaled bronchodilators be beneficial in improving S.M.'s respiratory status?

The efficacy of bronchodilators, such as β-agonists, in infants with bronchiolitis and croup is controversial. The controversy is based on the decreased pharmacologic effect of β-agonists in infants younger than 18 months of age and on the underlying pathophysiology of viral upper respiratory tract infections. Early data suggested that β-agonists did not produce significant bronchodilation in infants.[71,72] These studies suffered from the absence of an objective measure of bronchodilation in this patient population, which cannot produce reliable incentive spirometry data. Efforts to objectively measure infant lung function with whole-body plethysmography have failed to demonstrate a benefit of β-agonists in this age group.[73] However, several studies have documented subjective improvement in clinical symptoms with the use of inhaled β-agonists in infants with bronchiolitis, which may justify a therapeutic trial.[74,75]

S.M. may be a candidate for a trial of inhaled β-agonist bronchodilator therapy because she has a history of RAD that responds to albuterol nebulizations. Acute viral respiratory infections can trigger RAD in predisposed patients such as S.M. A trial of albuterol or a similar β-agonist should be initiated at 0.10 to 0.15 mg/kg per dose, given as often as every 30 minutes if needed, to improve respiratory status.[74,75] If a response is not observed within 6 hours, the benefits of continuing β-agonist nebulization therapy should be re-evaluated. The indiscriminate use of inhaled β-agonists is not recommended because not all patients benefit, and there have been reports of deterioration in respiratory status and oxygenation in infants with bronchiolitis who received these agents.[76,77] These reactions may be related to the osmolality and pH of the nebulization solution.[78–80]

Adjunctive Therapies

22. What drug therapy can be used for the treatment of RSV bronchiolitis in S.M.?

RIBAVIRIN
Ribavirin therapy can be associated with clinical deterioration and the cost of therapy is considerable (see Chapter 72, Viral Infections).

OTHER THERAPY
Bronchiolitis is a viral infection and antibiotics are not indicated unless signs and symptoms of a secondary bacterial infection are present. S.M. has an elevated WBC count, but there is not a predominance of neutrophils that would be suggestive of bacterial infection; thus, her infection is likely to be caused by RSV. Bronchodilators such as ipratropium[81,82] and theophylline[83,84] have been investigated in small clinical trials, but the outcomes have been discouraging.

Corticosteroids do not have a defined role in the treatment of bronchiolitis. Although a few studies evaluating corticosteroids in patients with bronchiolitis have indicated potential benefit,[85,86] others have found no value.[87–89] The lack of well-controlled clinical trials in terms of patient selection, concurrent therapies, and assessment criteria has made interpretation of the studies difficult. Perhaps the most important issue when considering the use of corticosteroids in bronchiolitis is whether the patient has pre-existing RAD.[90] The use of corticosteroids in patients such as S.M., who present with RAD in conjunction with bronchiolitis, may be beneficial, particularly when used in combination with β-agonists.[85] The appropriate corticosteroid regimen has not been firmly established, but methylprednisolone 2 to 4 mg/kg per day or dexamethasone 0.4 to 0.6 mg/kg per day for 1 to 4 days may be used. Infants with bronchiolitis who do not have pre-existing RAD should not receive corticosteroids.

CROUP
Clinical Presentation

23. R.G., a 9-month-old, 8-kg boy, is brought to the ED because of difficulty in breathing. His parents state that R.G. has a mild cold and was fussy earlier in the evening with a decreased appetite. Around 2 AM, his parents heard a noisy, barking cough and found R.G. in his crib having trouble breathing. They noticed that his lips were turning blue and decided to bring him to the ED. The parents state that the baby seemed to get a little better during the drive to the hospital. On physical examination, R.G. is found to be in moderate respiratory distress with a respiratory rate of 60 breaths/min, heart rate of 150 beats/min, and a temperature of 101°F (axillary). He has stridor at rest with intercostal retractions and mild wheezing in the lower lung fields. WBC is 5,100/mm³. Signs of cyanosis have not been present during the ED visit. What is a likely cause of R.G.'s breathing problem?

Croup, a contagious viral infection of the upper and lower respiratory tract, typically occurs in children age 6 months to 6 years of age. It is characterized by waking at night with difficulty in breathing (especially when inhaling), a barking cough, hoarseness or stridor, and fever.[91] More precisely, croup refers to a subglottic inflammatory disease usually of viral origin. Several viruses (e.g., parainfluenza virus, influenza A and B, adenovirus, RSV, measles virus) have been associated with the development of croup. Some differentiate between spasmodic, or recurrent, croup and laryngotracheitis because spasmodic croup may have an allergic component and may improve independent of treatment; however, others consider both to be simply manifestations of a single disease.[99B] Croup often begins with a common cold, but as the viral infection spreads, the lining of the larynx and trachea swell leading to significant airway compromise, especially in young children. Symptoms are most severe during the first 2 nights and the illness resolves in 4 to 7 days. Cool night air can temporarily decrease the swelling of the larynx and improve symptoms. Children often improve during the day, only to become worse again in the middle of the night. If croup repeats itself, it is likely to be spasmodic croup caused by allergies or viral infection; patients with spasmodic croup do not usually have a fever. R.G. has several symptoms consistent with a diagnosis of croup.

Treatment

24. What supportive therapies may benefit R.G.?

The emergency management of croup should begin with an evaluation of the extent of airway obstruction and the need for supplemental oxygen. Since nonbacterial croup often is a self-limiting disease that can spontaneously resolve in many patients, treatment generally is supportive and based on the severity of symptoms. High humidity appears to be beneficial for many patients with croup; however, convincing evidence of efficacy is lacking. Humidifiers or cool mist vaporizers theoretically reduce drying in the upper airway and ease breathing. Children should be kept calm to minimize oxygen demand and respiratory muscle fatigue. Heart rate, respiratory rate and pulse oximetry should be monitored closely for signs of hypoxemia.

Several pharmacologic alternatives (e.g., nebulized epinephrine, corticosteroids) are available to treat patients who have moderate croup symptoms.

Racemic Epinephrine

Moderate to severe croup symptoms such as stridor, tachypnea, and cough respond well to 0.25 to 0.5 mL of a 2.25% solution of racemic epinephrine mixed in 3 mL of saline and administered via nebulizer.[92] The mixture of D and L isomers causes adrenergic stimulation, resulting in local vasoconstriction of the laryngeal and tracheal tissues and decreased mucosal edema.[93–95] Doses may be required every 20 to 30 minutes for children with severe symptoms and every 1 to 2 hours for moderate cases. Effects last less than 2 hours and symptoms can reappear 1 to 3 hours after a treatment. Previously feared rebound edema and tachycardia appear to be uncommon.[93]

Corticosteroids

Systemic corticosteroids are used to treat croup symptoms because the primary underlying pathophysiology involves inflammation with swelling and narrowing of the airways. Routine use of corticosteroids has been controversial because their effectiveness in the treatment of croup had not been clearly established.[94,95] In one meta-analysis, dexamethasone doses >3 mg/kg resulted in significant clinical improvement 12 to 24 hours after IM administration. More recently, a single dose of dexamethasone (0.6 mg/kg) intramuscularly was shown to reduce hospitalizations significantly more than placebo and provided benefit comparable to nebulized budesonide (2 mg) and considerably greater benefit than budesonide five hours after treatment.[99C] Both PO and IM doses of dexamethasone are believed to provide comparable resolution of symptoms.[96–98] Budesonide is a corticosteroid with strong topical anti-inflammatory properties and low systemic toxicity.[99] Generally, multiple doses of corticosteroids are not necessary because croup usually is short-term in duration. Although the risks of short-term corticosteroids are few, the potential for GI bleeding and immunosuppression need to be considered on an individual patient basis. R.G. should receive a single dose of dexamethasone 5 mg PO, as soon as possible after his initial assessment.

Antibiotics

Antibiotics should be used only if a bacterial superinfection is suspected. Although rare, S. aureus (most common), H. influenzae, S. pneumoniae, and M. catarrhalis can cause bacterial tracheitis.[100] If bacterial croup is presumed, antibiotics directed against the most common pathogens should be initiated. Second- and third-generation cephalosporins (e.g., cefuroxime, cefotaxime, ceftriaxone) are active against all of these organisms. Because of the potential for rapid deterioration in patients with bacterial croup, parenteral antibiotics are recommended until the patient has adequately responded to therapy. Once the patient is stable and culture and sensitivity results are available, oral antibiotics should be considered for the remaining 10-day course of antibiotic therapy (see Table 96-3).

EPIGLOTTITIS
Clinical Presentation

25. How does the management of R.G. differ from that of a child with epiglottitis (supraglottitis)?

R.G. has a classic presentation of nonbacterial croup. If he had bacterial epiglottitis, his symptoms would have been markedly different, and his condition would have been considered a medical emergency. Epiglottitis occurs primarily in older infants and young children and is associated with more severe symptoms, including a "toxic" appearance. The classic presentation is a child who develops fever and a sore throat; within a few hours, the child begins to drool and develops signs of upper airway obstruction and systemic illness (e.g., pallor, hypotension, tachycardia, tachypnea, dehydration, and lethargy or irritability).[100] These symptoms are precursors to acute respiratory failure and require immediate evaluation for intubation. Historically, epiglottitis was most commonly caused by H. influenzae type B. Introduction of universal HIB vaccination (see Chapter 95, Immunizations) has decreased the incidence of epiglottitis dramatically, although other pathogens (e.g., group A, B, and C streptococci, S. pneumoniae, K. pneumoniae, Candida albicans, S. aureus, N. meningitides, and varicella zoster) can still cause the disease. If epiglottitis is diagnosed, empiric antibiotic therapy should be initiated as soon as the airway has been secured.

PERTUSSIS
Clinical Presentation

26. L.D., a 6 week old, 5-kg girl, has been diagnosed with pertussis. What organism causes pertussis and what are the clinical stages of presentation?

Pertussis is a relatively rare respiratory infection caused by Bordetella pertussis and can afflict young infants or unimmunized children; it is associated with high morbidity in children under 1 year of age. Vaccination with whole cell and acellular pertussis (as DTP or DTaP) has drastically reduced the incidence of pertussis infection in infants. However, the vaccine is not administered after age 7 years, and protective titers decrease with increasing age. As a result, adolescents and adults serve as a source of infection for unimmunized infants (see also Chapter 95, Pediatric Immunizations).[101–103] L.D., who at age 6 weeks may not yet have been immunized with DTaP, is an example of a child at risk for pertussis infection.

Treatment

27. What is the treatment of choice for L.D.?

Erythromycin is considered the antibiotic of choice for the treatment of pertussis.[103] It eradicates the organism from the respiratory secretions and, if initiated early enough (during the catarrhal phase), may shorten the duration of symptoms. Unfortunately, most patients are diagnosed after the time period when antibiotics are most effective. Azithromycin (a 5-day course) and clarithromycin (a 10-day course) are as effective and better tolerated than erythromycin for the treatment of pertussis in children.[104,105] Cough suppressants do not relieve the coughing spells and should not be prescribed.

Prophylaxis

28. **What are the benefits and risks of pertussis prophylaxis for L.D.'s siblings?**

Prophylaxis should be administered, regardless of age and vaccination status, when there is a documented case of pertussis. Household members and other close contacts should receive a 14-day course of erythromycin or TMP-SMX, or a 10-day course of clarithromycin, or a 5-day course of azithromycin.[105] Early prophylaxis reduces the *B. pertussis* carrier state and subsequently reduces secondary transmission, which can cause epidemic outbreaks of pertussis. Close contacts <7 years of age who have not competed the four-dose primary immunization series should complete the series with the minimal intervals. Children <7 years of age who have completed the series, but have not received a DTaP dose within 3 years, should be given a booster dose. Although members of L.D.'s family may have been vaccinated against pertussis, antibiotic prophylaxis is still recommended because the pertussis vaccine is not completely effective and the immunity from the vaccine decreases over time. Because little risk is associated with a short course of antibiotics, it is clearly beneficial to initiate erythromycin prophylaxis in L.D.'s family. Clarithromycin and azithromycin have fewer side effects (less GI upset) than erythromycin and may be considered for prophylaxis in patients who cannot tolerate the gastrointestinal effects of erythromycin.

MEASLES

29. **Measles is a highly contagious infection that can be complicated by involvement of the central nervous system and the respiratory tract. What is the role of empiric prophylactic antibiotics or adjunctive therapies in the treatment of measles?**

Mild cases of measles generally are without complications; however secondary bacterial infections such as otitis media and pneumonia occur in 5% to 15% of patients. The occurrence of bacterial complications does not warrant routine antimicrobial prophylaxis, but very young children (<1 year), those who have a history of recurrent bacterial respiratory tract infections (otitis media, pharyngitis, bronchitis), or those who require hospitalization may benefit from empiric antibiotic therapy against the common respiratory tract pathogens (see Table 96-2 and Chapter 95, Pediatric Immunizations).

Vitamin A is an important cofactor in the immune response, particularly to acute viral infections such as measles. Measles infection has the propensity to induce a vitamin A–deficient state during the acute infection and children with decreased vitamin A stores (i.e., malnourished, short-bowel syndrome, cystic fibrosis) have increased morbidity and mortality from measles infection. Children with severe measles

have been found to benefit from vitamin A therapy.[107–109] Administration of vitamin A 400,000 units within 5 days of the onset of the rash, reduced pulmonary complications, reduced fever, decreased hospital stay, and decreased mortality compared with a placebo group.[107,108] The World Health Organization recommends vitamin A supplementation in patients with measles if there is a high incidence of vitamin A deficiency in the region or if the mortality rate of measles is >1% (mortality in the United States is <1%). The AAP also recommends the use of vitamin A in children with measles.[110] For Infants <6 months of age, the recommended dose is 100,000 units as a single dose. Patients >6 months of age should receive a single dose of 200,000 units. A repeat dose in 24 hours and again 4 weeks later is recommended if the infected patient has evidence of significant vitamin A deficiency or malnutrition.

KAWASAKI'S DISEASE
Clinical Presentation and Diagnosis

30. **B.C., a 2-year-old, 12-kg boy, has had a fever for the last 6 days. He was started on amoxicillin 40 mg/kg per day 4 days ago without improvement. B.C. has become increasingly irritable and has developed a macular papular rash over his trunk, legs, and arms. B.C. is an otherwise healthy boy, his immunizations are current, and he has not had any contact with animals. On physical examination, B.C. has a temperature of 104°F (oral), a red swollen tongue with a "strawberry" appearance, cracked fissures on the lips, and enlarged cervical lymph nodes. He also has bilateral infection of the conjunctiva without discharge or pain. His heart examination is normal. Laboratory tests indicate a WBC count of 22,000 cell/mm³, an ESR of 96 mm/hr, and a platelet count of 540,000 cells/mm³. What signs and symptoms would suggest the diagnosis of Kawasaki's disease in B.C.? What are the prognosis and progression of this disease?**

Kawasaki's disease is a mucocutaneous lymph node syndrome that primarily occurs in children 6 months to 5 years of age.[111] The diagnosis of Kawasaki's disease is based on the presence of a constellation of symptoms, including fever for >5 days with at least four of the following findings: (1) mucous membrane changes (e.g., swollen lips, "strawberry" tongue, perioral fissures); (2) cervical lymphadenopathy; (3) bilateral conjunctivitis; (4) rash; and (5) swollen hands or feet with desquamation.[111,112] Several nondiagnostic characteristics such as arthritis, irritability, lack of response to antibiotic therapy, and urethritis occur frequently and suggest the diagnosis of Kawasaki's disease. Infants <1 year of age often present with atypical symptoms and may not meet the diagnostic criteria. B.C. fulfills the CDC criteria for diagnosis of Kawasaki's disease (listed above) and also has several laboratory findings suggestive of Kawasaki's disease such as elevated ESR and platelet count. After all other possible causes have been ruled out (e.g., scarlet fever, juvenile rheumatoid arthritis, toxic shock syndrome), Kawasaki's disease should be considered a diagnosis of exclusion. Although numerous infectious etiologies have been proposed, the cause of Kawasaki disease remains unknown and no specific test can confirm the diagnosis. B.C. is in the acute phase of Kawasaki's disease, which starts with fever and lasts 1 to 2 weeks without treatment.

Characteristic symptoms develop during the first week, but diagnosis can be difficult because one symptom appears as another resolves. The acute phase is followed by a subacute phase in which periungual desquamation (peeling of the skin of the palms and soles) and joint inflammation occur, and coronary aneurysms begin to form. In the final phase, called the *convalescent phase,* the patient begins to feel better and laboratory findings return to normal. However, coronary aneurisms continue to develop, reaching their largest size 4 to 6 weeks from the onset of fever.[113]

Kawasaki's disease has been the leading cause of acquired heart disease in children. It is associated with high morbidity and mortality, which can be significantly reduced with rapid and appropriate therapeutic management. Up to 25% of untreated Kawasaki's disease patients develop coronary aneurysms secondary to the disease process and approximately 5% persist beyond the convalescent phase.[114] These patients are at increased risk for serious cardiac events, such as myocardial infarction and/or death.[111]

Aspirin

31. **Why should B.C. be treated with aspirin?**

During the initial acute phase of the disease, high dose aspirin is prescribed to reduce fever, inflammation and clot formation. Although aspirin has not been found to reduce the risk of coronary aneurysm development,[115] dosages of 80 to 100 mg/kg per day are used to control fever and inflammation.[116] Once the child is afebrile and the ESR is <20 mm/hour, the aspirin dose is decreased to an "antiplatelet" dose of 3 to 5 mg/kg per day.[117] Low-dose aspirin is continued throughout the convalescent phase and then discontinued unless the patient has coronary damage. Risk factors that have been identified for the development of coronary aneurysms include the following: (1) Asian descent; (2) age younger than 5 years; (3) fever for >14 days; (4) platelet count >900,000/mm³; and (5) ESR >100 mm/hour.[115,119] Warfarin and dipyridamole may also be recommended for additional antithrombotic therapy in patients that have documented persistent coronary aneurysms >8 mm in size or ocular involvement.[120]

Because aspirin therapy is associated with Reye's syndrome, it should be temporarily discontinued in children who develop chickenpox or influenza. Aspirin should not be taken for 6 weeks after administration of the varicella vaccine. Children with large aneurysms should receive therapy with other antiplatelet agents until aspirin can be restarted.

DOSE AND MONITORING

32. **What dose of aspirin should be prescribed for B.C., and how should this therapy be monitored?**

B.C. should be given aspirin, 300 mg every 6 hours (100 mg/kg per day). Serum salicylate concentrations should be monitored to improve efficacy and reduce potential toxicity. Target trough salicylate concentrations of 200 to 300 mg/L (20 to 30 mg/dL) have been recommended, and steady state generally is achieved after 48 hours.[121] Oral absorption of aspirin can be decreased by as much as 50% in Kawasaki's disease patients; thus, higher doses may be needed to achieve desired therapeutic . concentrations.[121] Close monitoring of salicylate concentrations is recommended during high-dose therapy because bioavailability may change during the natural course of the disease and increase the risk of salicylate toxicity. Salicylates may cause GI bleeding and tinnitus, which also should be monitored. The aspirin dose can be decreased to an antiplatelet dose of 40 mg (3.3 mg/kg perday) after about 14 days and then discontinued after 6 to 8 weeks if coronary abnormalities are not present.

Intravenous Immunoglobulin

33. **Could B.C. benefit from intravenous immunoglobulin (IVIG) therapy? What would be an appropriate regimen and monitoring plan for this therapy?**

IVIG therapy is currently the standard of care in the treatment of Kawasaki's disease. Studies have found that IVIG can significantly decrease the incidence of coronary aneurysms if it is administered within 10 days of fever onset.[119] Therefore, based on his diagnosis of Kawasaki disease, B.C. should receive IVIG therapy as soon as possible. Several different treatment regimens have been investigated including 400 mg/kg per day for 4 days and 2 g/kg as a single dose over 8 to 12 hours.[122,123] Both regimens have proved to be beneficial effects in Kawasaki's disease, with limited data suggesting that the single-dose regimens may be more effective. The economic advantages of the single-dose therapy have made this regimen favorable, although adverse effects with high-dose regimens have been reported including isolated reports of congestive failure and hemorrhage.[123–125] IVIG generally is well tolerated by most patients. B.C. should receive a single dose of 24 g IVIG over 12 hours. He should be monitored closely for changes in vital signs (hypotension, hypertension, tachycardia, tachypnea) during the infusion. IVIG should be infused slowly, and rates should be increased incrementally to avoid these unwanted effects. Most patients rapidly respond to IVIG with resolution of fever, rash, and decreased ESR within 72 hours. A repeated course of IVIG may be considered if the fever has not resolved within 2 days after the dose of IVIG.[125]

RICKETTSIAL DISEASES

Rickettsial diseases are unique in that they infect mammals and are transmitted to humans via arthropods (ticks, lice, mites, fleas). The diseases are divided into three groups: spotted fever (Rocky Mountain spotted fever, rickettsialpox and boutonneuse fever), typhus (louse-bourne typhus, Brill-Zinsser disease, murine typhus) and "other" (Q fever, tsutsugamushi disease). The geographic and seasonal distribution of rickettsial infections mimic the presence of the vector.[127] Rickettsial infections vary in severity, ranging from a self-limited, mild illness to a life-threatening infection. The most severe and most frequently reported rickettsial disease in the United States is *Rickettsia rickettsii,* the tick-borne pathogen responsible for Rocky Mountain spotted fever (RMSF). Although initially thought to be limited to the Rocky Mountain region of the United States, RMSF is now reported in all geographic areas of the United States, southern Canada, Central America, Mexico, and parts of South America. RMSF causes an infectious vasculitis by invading and multiplying intracellularly in endothelial cells. The epidemiology, treatment, and prevention of RMSF is presented is presented in Chapter 75, Tick-Borne Diseases.

REFERENCES

1. Rowe PC. The Harriett Lane Handbook. Chicago: Year Book Medical Publishers, 2003.
2. Ballow M et al. Development of the immune system in very low birth weight (less than 1500 g) premature infants: concentrations of plasma immunoglobulins and patterns of infections. Pediatr Res 1986;20:899.
3. Byington CL. The diagnosis and management of otitis media with effusion. Pediatr Ann 1998; 27:96.
4. Paap CM, Nahata MC. Infectious diseases IV: viral and bacterial respiratory tract infections. In: Kuhn R, ed. Pediatric Pharmacotherapy. Lexington: University of Kentucky Press, 2003;11.
5. Robinson RR, Nahata MC. Respiratory syncytial virus (RSV) immune globulin and palivizumab for prevention of RSV infection. Am J Health-System Pharm 2000;57:259.
6. Mascitelli, L Pezzetta F. Recurrent otitis media in children. JAMA 2003;289:1382.
6B Hendley JO. Otitis Media. N Engl J Med 2002; 347:1169.
6C Little P et al. Pragmatic randomized controlled trial of two prescribing strategies for childhood acute otitis media. Br Med J 2001;322:336.
7. Korzyrskyj AL et al. Treatment of acute otitis media with a shortened course of antibiotics. JAMA 1998;279:1736.
8. Daley KA, Giebink GS. Clinical epidemiology of otitis media. Pediatr Dis J 2000;19:31.
9. Ruuskanen O et al. Viruses in acute otitis media: increasing evidence of clinical significance. Pediatr Infect Dis J 1991;10:425.
10. Bluestone CD et al. Ten-year review of otitis media pathogens. Pediatr Infect Dis J 1992;11:S7.
11. Ruuskanen O, Heikkinen T. Otitis media: etiology and diagnosis. Pediatr Infect Dis J 1994;13:S23.
12. Fliss DM et al. Medical sequelae and complications of acute otitis media. Pediatr Infect Dis J 1994; 13:S34.
13. Rovers MM et al. Day care and otitis media in young children. A critical overview. Eur J Pediatr 1999;158;1.
14. DiFranza JR, Lew RA. Morbidity and mortality in children associated with the use of tobacco products in other people. Pediatr 1996;97:560.
15. Niemela M et al. Pacifier as a risk factor for acute otitis media: a randomized, controlled trial of parental counseling. Pediatrics 2000;106(3):483.
16. Uhari M et al. A meta-analytic review of the risk factors of acute otitis media. Clinc Infect Dis 1996;22;1079
17. Fireman MA et al. Impact of the Pneumococcal Conjugate Vaccine on otitis media. Pediatr Infect Dis J 2003: 22(1):10.
18. Clements D et al. Influenza A vaccine decreases the incidence of otitis media in 6 to 30 month old children in day care. Arch Pediatr Adolesc Med 1995;149(10):1113.
19. Gunger AD, Bluestone CD. Antibiotic Therapy in otitis media. Curr Allergy Asthma Rep 2002:4:364.
20. Gaskins JD et al. Chemoprophylaxis of recurrent otitis media using trimethoprim/sulfamethoxazole. Drug Intell Clin Pharm 1982;16:387.
21. Barnett ED, Klein JO. The problem of resistant bacteria for the management of acute otitis media. Pediatr Clin North Am 1995;42:509.
22. Baquero F, Loza E. Antibiotic resistance of microorganisms involved in ear, nose and throat infections. Pediatr Infect Dis J 1994;13:S9.
23. Takata GS, et al. Evidence assessment of management of acute otitis media: the role of antibiotics in treatment of uncomplicated acute otitis media. Pediatrics 2001;108(2):239.
24. Dowell SF et al. Acute otitis media: management and surveillance in an era of pneumococcal resistance—a report from the drug-resistant *Streptococcus pneumoniae* therapeutic working group. Pediatr Infect Dis J 1999;18:1.
25. Bottenfield et al. Safety and tolerability of a new formulation of amoxicillin/clavulanate in the empiric treatment of pediatric acute otitis media caused by drug-resistant *Streptococcus pneumoniae*. Pediatr Infect Dis J 1998;17:963.
26. The Medical Letter. 2003;45(1148);5.
27. Cohen R et al. One dose ceftriaxone versus ten days of amoxicillin-clavulanate therapy for acute otitis media: clinical efficacy and change in nasopharyngeal flora. Pediatr Infect Dis J 1999:18:403.
28. Pichichero ME. Acute otitis media: Part II. Treatment in an era of increasing antibiotic resistance. Am Fam Physician 2000;61;2410.
29. Angelilli ML et al. Palatability of oral antibiotics among children in an urban primary care center. Arch Pediatr Adolesc Med 2000:154:267.
30. Chaput de Saintonge D et al. Trial of three-day and ten-day course of amoxicillin in otitis media. Br Med J 1982;284:1078.
31. Hendricks WA et al. Five vs ten days of therapy for acute otitis media. Pediatr Infect Dis J 1988;7:14.
32. Williams R, et al. Use of antibiotics in preventing recurrent otitis media and in treating otitis media with effusion. JAMA 1993;270(11):1344.
33. Rosenfeld RM et al. Systemic steroids for otitis media with effusion in children. Arch Otolaryngol Head Neck Surg 1991;117(9):984.
34. Berman S et al. Theoretical cost effectiveness of management options for children with persisting middle ear effusions. Pediatrics 1994;93:353.
35. Subcommittee on Management of Sinusitis and Committee on Quality Improvement. American Academy of Pediatrics: Clinical Practice Guideline: Management of Sinusitis. Pediatrics 2001;108(3):798.
36. Giebink GS. Childhood sinusitis: pathophysiology, diagnosis and treatment. Pediatr Infect Dis J 1994;13:S55.
37. Tinkelman DG, Silk HJ. Clinical and bacteriologic features of chronic sinusitis in children. Am J Dis Child 1989;143(8):938.
38. Barlan IB et al. Intranasal budesonide spray as an adjunct to oral antibiotic therapy for acute sinusitis in children. Ann Allergy Asthma Immunol 1997;78:598.
39. Meltzer EO et al. Intranasal flunisolide spray as an adjunct to oral antibiotic therapy for sinusitis. J Allergy Clin Immunol 1993;92:812.
40. McCormick DP et al. A double-blind, placebo-controlled trial of decongestant-antihistamine for the treatment of sinusitis in children. Clin Pediatr 1996;35:457.
41. Muntz HR. Allergic fungal sinusitis in children. Otolaryngol Clin North Am 1996;29(1)1.
42. Augmentin stability. Product Package Insert. GlaxoSmithKline, 2003.
43. Johnson CE et al. Cefixime compared with amoxicillin for the treatment of acute otitis media. J Pediatr 1991;119:117
44. Gieseker KE et al. Evaluating the American Academy of Pediatrics diagnostic standard for *Streptococcus pyogenes* pharyngitis: backup cultures verses repeat rapid antigen testing. Pediatrics 2003;11(1):666.
45. Giesker KE et al. Comparison of two rapid *Streptococcus pyogenes* diagnostic tests with a rigorous culture standard. Pediatr Inf Dis J 2002;10:922.
46. Van Cauwenberge PB, Vander Mijnsbrugge A. Pharyngitis: a survey of the microbiologic etiology. Pediatr Inf Dis J 1991;10(10):S39.
47. Pichichero ME et al. Incidence of streptococcal carriers in a private pediatric practice. Arch Pediatr Adolec Med 1999;153(6)624.
48. Shulman ST. Complications of streptococcal pharyngitis. Pediatr Infect Dis J 1994;13:S70.
49. Johnson DR et al. Epidemiologic analysis of Group A streptococci serotypes associated with severe systemic infections, rheumatic fever, or uncomplicated pharyngitis. J Infect Dis 1992;166:374.
50. Working group on severe streptococcal infections: defining the Group A streptococcal toxic shock syndrome. JAMA 1993;269:390.
51. Taubert KA et al. Nationwide survey of Kawasaki's disease and acute rheumatic fever. J Pediatr 1991;119:279.
52. Bronze MS, Dale JB. The reemergence of serious group A streptococcal infections and acute rheumatic fever. Am J Med Sci 1996;311(1):41.
53. Catanzaro F et al. The role of the streptococcus in the pathogenesis of rheumatic fever. Am J Med 1954;17:749.
54. Gerber MA et al. New approaches to the treatment of group A streptococcal pharyngitis. Curr Opin Pediatr 2001;13:51.
55. Pichichero ME. Cephalosporins are superior to penicillin for treatment of streptococcal tonsillopharyngitis: is the difference worth it? Pediatr Infect Dis J 1993;12:268.
56. Gerber MA et al. Once daily penicillin V therapy for pharyngitis. Pediatr Infect Dis J 1993;12.
57. Holm SE. Reasons for failures in penicillin treatment of streptococcal tonsillitis and possible alternatives. Pediatr Infect Dis J 1994;13;S66.
58. Hooten TM. A comparison of azithromycin and penicillin V for the treatment of streptococcal pharyngitis. Am J Med 1991;91:23S.
58B. Martin JM et al. Erythromycin-resistant group A streptococci in schoolchildren in Pittsburgh. N Engl J Med 2002;346:1200.
58C. Huovinen P. Macrolide-resistant group A streptococcus - Now in the United States. N Engl J Med 2002;346:1243.
59. Bisno AL et al. Diagnosis and management of group A streptococcal pharyngitis. A practice guideline. Clin Infect Dis 1997;25:574.
60. Chaudhary S et al. Penicillin V and rifampin for the treatment of Groups A streptococcal pharyngitis: a randomized trial of 10 days penicillin vs 10 days penicillin with rifampin during the final four days of therapy. J Pediatr 1985;106:481.
61. Tanz RR et al. Penicillin plus rifampin eradicates pharyngeal carriage of Group A streptococci. J Pediatr 1985;106:876.
62. Anon. Guidelines for the diagnosis of rheumatic fever, Jones criteria 1992. JAMA 1992;268(15):2069.
63. Proceedings of Jones' Criteria workshop. Circulation. 2002;106:2521
64. Pickering LK. Rheumatic Fever. 2000 Red Book: Report of the Committee on Infectious Diseases, 25th Ed. American Academy of Pediatrics. Elk Grove, IL;2000
65. Combined Rheumatic Fever Study Group. A comparison of short-term, intensive prednisone and acetyl-salicylic acid therapy in the treatment of rheumatic fever. N Engl J Med 1965;272:63.
66. Dromgoole SH, Furst DE. Salicylates. In: Evans WE et al, eds. Applied Pharmacokinetics: Principles of Therapeutics Drug Monitoring. Vancouver: Applied Therapeutics, 1992:32.
67. Cilliers AM et al. Anti-inflammatory treatment for carditis in acute rheumatic fever (Cochrane Review). In: The Cochrane Library, issue 2, 2003. Oxford: Update Software.
68. American Heart Association. Treatment of acute streptococcal pharyngitis and prevention of rheumatic fever. Pediatrics 1995;96:758.
69. Peters G et al. Report of the Committee on Infectious Diseases. Elk Grove Village, IL: American Academy of Pediatrics, 1994:438.
70. International Rheumatic Fever Study Group. Allergic reactions to long-term benzathine prophylaxis for rheumatic fever. Lancet 1991;337(8753):1308.
71. Sly PD et al. Do wheezy infants recovering from bronchiolitis respond to inhaled salbutamol? Pediatr Pulmonol 1991;10:36.
72. Lenney W, Milner AD. At what age do bronchodilator drugs work? Arch Dis Child 1978;53:532.
73. Lugo RA, Nahata MC. Pathogenesis and treatment of bronchiolitis. Clin Pharm 1993;12:95.
74. Schuh S et al. Nebulized albuterol in acute bronchiolitis. J Pediatr 1990;117:633.
75. Klassen TP et al. Randomized trial of salbutamol in acute bronchiolitis. J Pediatr 1991;118:807.
76. Ho L et al. Effect of salbutamol on oxygen saturation in bronchiolitis. Arch Dis Child 1991;66:1061.

77. Prendiville A et al. Hypoxaemia in wheezy infants after bronchodilator treatment. Arch Dis Child 1987;62:997.

78. Seidenberg J et al. Hypoxemia after nebulized salbutamol in wheezy infants: importance of aerosol acidity. Arch Dis Child 1991;66:672.

79. O'Callaghan C, Milner AD. Paradoxical deterioration in lung function after nebulized salbutamol in wheezy infants. Lancet 1986;2:1424.

80. Balmes JR et al. Acidity potentiates bronchoconstriction induced by hyposmolar aerosols. Am Rev Respir Dis 1988;138:35.

81. Seidenberg J et al. Effect of ipratropium bromide on respiratory mechanics in infants with acute bronchiolitis. Aust Paediatr J 1987;23:169.

82. Henry RL et al. Ineffectiveness of ipratropium bromide in acute bronchiolitis. Arch Dis Child 1983;58:925.

83. Brooks LJ, Cropp GJA. Theophylline therapy in bronchiolitis. Am J Dis Child 1981;135:934.

84. Schena JA et al. The use of aminophylline in severe bronchiolitis [Abstract]. Crit Care Med 1984; 12:225.

85. Tal A et al. Dexamethasone and salbutamol in the treatment of acute wheezing in infants. Pediatrics 1983;71:13.

86. McGeorge M. Severe obstructive bronchiolitis in infancy: treatment with hydrocortisone. Clin Pediatr 1964;3:11.

87. Leer JA et al. Corticosteroid treatment in bronchiolitis. Am J Dis Child 1969;117:495.

88. Springer C et al. Corticosteroids do not affect the clinical or physiological status of infants with bronchiolitis. Pediatr Pulmonol 1990;9:181.

89. Klassen TP et al. Dexamethosone in salbutamol treated inpatients with acute bronchiolitis: a randomized controlled study. J Pediatr 1997; 130(2):191.

90. Kelly HW, Murphy S. Corticosteroids for acute, severe asthma. Ann Pharmacother 1991;25:72.

91. Ewig JM. Croup. Pediatr Ann 2002;31(2):125.

92. Kelley PB, Simon JE. Racemic epinephrine in croup and disposition. Am J Emerg Med 1992; 10:181.

93. Waisman Y et al. Prospective randomized double-blind study comparing L-epinephrine and racemic epinephrine aerosols in the treatment of laryngotracheitis (croup). Pediatrics 1992;89:302.

94. Kairys SW et al. Steroid treatment of laryngotracheitis: a meta-analysis of the evidence from randomized trials. Pediatrics 1989;83:683.

95. Ausejo M et al. The effectiveness of glucocorticoids in treatment of croup: meta-analysis. Br Med J 1999;319(7210):595.

96. Geelhoed GC, Macdonald WB. Oral dexamethasone in the treatment of croup: 0.15 mg/kg. 0.3 mg/kg verses 0.6 mg/kg. Pediatr Pulmonol 1995; 20(6):362.

97. Donaldson D et al. Intramuscular versus oral dexamethasone for the treatment of moderate to severe croup: a randomized, double blind trial. Acad Emerg Med 2003;10(1):16.

98. Rittichier KK, Ledwith CA. Outpatient treatment of moderate croup with dexamethasone: intramuscular versus oral dosing. Pediatrics 2000;106(6): 1344.

99. Johnson DW et al. A comparison of nebulized budesonide, intramuscular dexamethasone and placebo for moderately severe croup. N Engl J Med 1998;339:498.

99B Jaffe DM. The treatment of croup with glucocorticoids. N Engl J Med 1998;339:553

99C Johnson DW et al. A comparison of nebulized budesonide, intramuscular dexamethasone, and placebo for moderately severe croup. N Engl J Med 1998; 339:498

100. Cressman WR, Myer CM III. Diagnosis and management of croup and epiglottitis. Pediatric Clin N Am 1994;41(2)265.

101. Birkebaek NH et al. Bordetella pertussis and chronic cough in adults. Clin Infect Dis 1999; 29(5)1239.

102. Gardner P. Indications for acellular pertussis vaccines in adults: the case for selective rather than universal recommendations. Clin Infect Dis 1999;28(Suppl 2):S131.

103. Cherry JD et al. Report of the task force on pertussis and pertussis immunization—1988. Pediatrics 1988;81(suppl):939.

104. Bace A et al. Short-term treatment of pertussis with azithromycin in infants and young children. Eur J CLin Microbiol Infect Dis 1999;18(4)296.

105. Aoyama T et al. Efficacy of short term treatment of pertussis with clarithromycin and azithromycin. J Pediatr 1996;129(5):761.

106. Barclay AJG et al. Vitamin A supplements and mortality related to measles: a randomized clinical trial. Br Med J 1987;294:294.

107. Hussey GD, Klein M. A randomized controlled trial of vitamin A in children with severe measles. N Engl J Med 1990;323:160.

108. D'Souza RM, D'Souza R. Vitamin A for preventing secondary infections in children with measles—a systematic review. J Trop Pediatr 2002;48(2):72.

109. Report of the Committee of Infectious Diseases. American Academy of Pediatrics. Vitamin A supplementation for measles. Pediatrics 1993;92:501.

110. Peters G et al. Report of the Committee on Infectious Diseases. Elk Grove Village, IL: American Academy of Pediatrics, 1994:284.

111. CDC. Kawasaki disease. MMWR 1980;29:61.

112. Barron KS. Kawasaki disease in children. Curr Opin Rheumatol 1998;10(1):29.

113. Klassen TP et al. Economic evaluation of intravenous immune globulin therapy for Kawasaki syndrome. J Pediatr 1993;122:538.

114. Nakashima L, Edwards DL. Treatment of Kawasaki disease. Clin Pharm 1990;9:755.

115. Koren G et al. Probable efficacy of high dose salicylates in reducing coronary involvement in Kawasaki disease. JAMA 1985;254:767.

116. Akagi T et al. Salicylate treatment in Kawasaki disease: high dose or low dose? Eur J Pediatr 1991;150:642.

117. Laupland KB, Davies H. Epidemiology, etiology and management of Kawasaki disease: state of the art. Pediatr Cardiol 1999;20(3):177.

118. Third International Kawasaki Disease Symposium Participants. Management of Kawasaki syndrome: a consensus statement prepared by the North-American participants of the third international Kawasaki syndrome symposium. Pediatr Infect Dis 1989;8:663.

119. Smith LBII et al. Kawasaki syndrome and the eye. Pediatr Infect Dis J 1989;8:116.

120. Koren G, MacLeod SM. Difficulty in achieving therapeutic serum concentrations of salicylate in Kawasaki disease. J Pediatr 1984;105:991.

121. Newburger JW et al. The treatment of Kawasaki syndrome with intravenous gamma globulin. N Engl J Med 1986;315:341.

122. Engle MA et al. Clinical trial of single dose intravenous gamma globulin in acute Kawasaki disease. Am J Dis Child 1989;143:1300.

123. Mori M et al. Predictors of coronary artery lesions after intravenous gamma-globulin treatment in Kawasaki Disease. J Pediatr 2000;137:177.

124. Comenzo RL et al. Immune hemolysis, disseminated intravascular coagulation, and serum sickness after large doses of immune globulin given intravenously for Kawasaki disease. J Pediatr 1992;120:926.

125. Sundel RP et al. Gamma globulin re-treatment in Kawasaki disease. J Pediatr 1993;123:657.

126. Peters G et al. Report of the Committee on Infectious Diseases. Elk Grove Village, IL: American Academy of Pediatrics, 1994:399.

127. www.cdc.gov/ncidod/dvrd/rmsf/index.htm

CHAPTER 97

Pediatric Nutrition

Michael F. Chicella, Emily B. Hak

Adequate nutrition is an essential component of the health maintenance of children and, in part, has been responsible for the dramatic reduction of infant mortality seen in the United States during the 20th century. Clinical experience has confirmed the value of optimal nutrition in resisting the effects of disease and trauma and in improving the response to medical and surgical therapy. The metabolic demands of rapid growth and maturation, in addition to the low nutritional reserves present during infancy, make the potential benefit of good nutrition to critically ill pediatric patients even greater.

Breast-feeding is the ideal method of feeding an infant up to 1 year of age. When this is not feasible, a wide variety of infant formulas are available that provide appropriate nutrients for infants using the oral route. A pediatric patient who has a functioning intestinal tract but is unable to achieve adequate oral intake can be fed enterally using a tube inserted into the stomach or small intestine. Indications for providing specialized enteral nutrition include malnutrition, malabsorption, hypermetabolism, failure to thrive, prematurity, and disorders of absorption, digestion, excretion, or utilization of nutrients.

Despite the many formulas and feeding techniques available, several medical and gastrointestinal (GI) dilemmas arise in infants and children that limit the use of the GI tract for nutritional support. Premature infants with severe respiratory disease, congenital abnormalities of the GI tract, or necrotizing enterocolitis are typical candidates for support with parenteral nutrition (PN). Older children with short bowel syndrome, severe malnutrition, intractable diarrhea, or inflammatory bowel disease have been managed successfully with PN therapy. Pediatric patients receiving chemotherapy for the treatment of malignancies or bone marrow transplant, and children with severe cardiac failure, also have been successfully rehabilitated with PN.

Many disorders that adversely affect nutrient intake or absorption also have an adverse impact on fluid and electrolyte status. Consequently, fluid, electrolyte, and nutrient management should be approached in an integrated manner. This chapter reviews selected aspects of fluid and electrolyte management and nutrition therapy for the pediatric population.

FLUID AND ELECTROLYTE MAINTENANCE

Management of fluid and electrolyte disturbances involves providing normal daily maintenance requirements, replacing deficits, and replacing ongoing losses. To design rational fluid therapy, it is necessary to know the normal composition of body water, to understand the routes through which water and solutes are lost from the body, and to understand the effects of disease and medications on water and electrolytes. Sodium-containing fluids are often referred to as fractions of normal saline (NS) (0.9% NaCl). Normal saline contains 154 mEq/L of sodium chloride.

Requirements

The general recommendations for calculating maintenance fluid, electrolyte, and nutrient requirements on the basis of weight are provided in Table 97-1. These requirements may be

Table 97-1 Daily Parenteral Nutrient Requirements in Children[1-5]

Nutrient	Weight/Age	Requirement
Macronutrients		
Fluid[1]	<1.5kg	150 mL/kg
	1.5–2.5 kg	120 mL/kg
	2.5–10 kg	100 mL/kg
	10–20 kg	1,000 mL +50 mL/kg for each kg >10 kg
	>20 kg	1,500 mL +20 mL/kg for each kg >20 kg
Calories	Up to 10 kg	100 kcal/kg
	20 kg	1,000 kcal + 50 kcal/kg for each kg >10 kg
	>20 kg	1,500 kcal + 20 kcal/kg for each kg >20 kg
Protein[a]	Infants	2–3 g/kg
	Older children	1.5–2.0 g/kg
	Adolescents and older	1.0–1.5 g/kg
Fat[b]	Infants and children	Initially: 0.5–1 g/kg then increase by 0.5–1 g/kg (maximum of 3 g/kg in preterm neonates, 4 g/kg older infants and children) (≥4% of calories as linoleic acid)
	>50 kg	One 500 mL bottle (100 g fat)
Electrolytes and Minerals[c]		
Sodium	Infants and children	2–4 mEq/kg
Potassium	Infants and children	2–3 mEq/kg
Chloride	Infants and children	2–4 mEq/kg
Magnesium	Preterm and term infants	0.25–0.5 mEq/kg
	Children >1 yr (or >12 kg)	4–12 mEq
Calcium	Preterm and term infants	2–3 mEq/kg
	Children >1 yr (or >12 kg)	10–20 mEq
Phosphorus	Preterm and term infants	1.0–1.5 mmol/kg
	Children >1 yr (or >12 kg)	10–20 mmol
Trace Elements		
Zinc	Preterm Infants	400 μg/kg
	Term Infants	
	<3 mo	250 μg/kg
	>3 mo	100 μg/kg
	Children	50 μg/kg (up to 5 mg)
Copper	Infants and children	20 μg/kg (up to 300 μg)
Manganese	Infants and children	1 μg/kg (up to 50 μg)
Chromium	Infants and children	0.2 μg/kg (up to 5 μg)
Selenium	Infants and children	2 μg/kg (up to 80 μg)

Vitamins	Preterm Infants < 2.5 kg (2 mL/kg MVI Pediatric)	Term Infants/Children <11 yr (5 mL MVI Pediatric)	Children >11 yr (10 mL MVI-12)
Vitamin A	280 μg/kg	700 μg	1 mg
Vitamin D	160 IU/kg	400 IU	200 IU
Vitamin E	2.8 mg/kg	7 mg	10 mg
Vitamin K[d]	80 μg/kg	200 μg	None
Thiamine	0.48 mg/kg	1.2 mg	3 mg
Niacin	6.8 mg/kg	17 mg	40 mg
Riboflavin	0.56 mg/kg	1.4 mg	3.6 mg
Pyridoxine	0.4 mg/kg	1 mg	4 mg
Vitamin B$_{12}$	0.4 μg/kg	1 μg	5 μg
Biotin	8 μg/kg	20 μg	60 μg
Vitamin C	32 mg/kg	80 mg	100 mg
Folic acid	56 μg/kg	140 μg	400 μg

[a]"Infant" amino acids contain histidine, taurine, tyrosine, and cysteine, which are essential in infants but not older patients.
[b]Because linoleic acid represents 54% of the fatty acid in soy bean oil and 77% in safflower oil, 7–10% of calories must be provided as fat emulsion. This can be given daily over 24 hours (preferred in patients predisposed to sepsis and preterm infants) or 2–3 times weekly.
[c]These doses are guidelines and all patients should be evaluated individually for appropriateness of dosing. For example, patients with short bowel syndrome may require large doses of magnesium and patients with renal insufficiency may require none to low amounts of potassium, calcium, phosphorous, and magnesium.
[d]For patients receiving MVI-12, it may be desirable to add vitamin K.

Table 97-2 Situations That Alter Maintenance Fluid Requirements

Situation	Mechanism	Extent of Change
Extreme prematurity	↑ skin losses	Varies
Radiant warmer use	↑ insensible water loss	20–40%
Croup tent	↓ evaporative water loss	20–50%
Diarrhea or vomiting	↑ GI loss	Varies
Fever	↑ insensible water loss	10–15% per °C
Renal dysfunction	↑ or ↓ renal loss	Varies
Hyperventilation	↑ pulmonary evaporative loss	Varies
Phototherapy for hyperbilirubinemia	↑ insensible water loss	10–20%
GI tract suction or ostomy	↑ GI loss	Varies
Mechanical ventilation	↓ insensible water loss	20–30%

GI, gastrointestinal.

altered when fluid and electrolyte losses are increased or when excretion is impaired.

When abnormal fluid losses are present from any of the sources listed in Table 97-2, they must be added to the patient's daily fluid and electrolyte formula. Replacement fluid is generally replaced 1 mL for every 1 mL lost but may be replaced as 0.5 mL for every 1 mL lost. In general, a solution of one-half normal saline (NS) with 20 mEq of KCl per liter is used to replace upper GI tract losses; however, the electrolyte content of GI secretions varies widely. The composition of a replacement fluid can be estimated based on knowledge of the usual electrolyte distribution of the fluid type being lost. Estimates are listed in Table 97-3. If serum electrolyte concentrations are abnormal, indicating that the replacement fluid is not appropriate, a sample of the fluid lost from the patient may be analyzed for electrolyte content, and electrolyte replacement fluid can be individualized.

In patients with severe renal dysfunction and oliguria, a factor of 40 mL/kg or 300 to 500 mL/m² may be used to estimate all other routes of insensible fluid loss; the patient's actual urine output (mL/day) then is added to this amount to arrive at a daily fluid amount. In some cases, urine output is increased in renal failure, and fluid and electrolyte management in these patients can be very complicated.

The requirements for fluid and calories normalized to body weight are much greater in very small children than in older children and adults as can be seen in Table 97-1. This is because infants have a much larger body surface area relative to weight, lose more fluid through evaporation, and dissipate more heat per kilogram than their older counterparts. Furthermore, very low birth weight (VLBW) infants cannot concentrate urine and are at increased risk for dehydration if inadequate fluids are provided.

Calculation of Maintenance Fluid and Electrolyte Requirements

1. P.J., a 2-day-old, 3.5-kg term female infant has developed abdominal distention, and her oral feedings have been stopped. Calculate a maintenance fluid and electrolyte prescription for her. Her admission serum electrolytes include the following: sodium (Na), 137 mEq/L (normal, 135 to 145 mEq/L); potassium (K), 4.2 mEq/L (normal, 3.5 to 5 mEq/L); chloride (Cl), 105 mEq/L (normal, 102 to 109 mEq/L); and bicarbonate (HCO_3^-), 23 mEq/L (normal, 22 to 29 mEq/L). While P.J. receives nothing by mouth (NPO), her fluid and electrolyte needs must be met intravenously. Estimate her requirements.

[SI units: Na, 137 mmol/L (normal, 135 to 145); K, 4.2 mmol/L (normal, 3.5 to 5.0); Cl, 105 mmol/L (normal, 102 to 109); HCO_3^-, 23 mmol/L (normal, 22 to 29)]

Although a commercially available intravenous (IV) solution will be used, each component of the solution can be calculated separately. Using the guidelines in Table 97-1, P.J.'s maintenance requirements can be estimated as follows:

Fluid	100 mL/kg × 3.5 kg = 350 mL/day or 15 mL/hr
Sodium	2–4 mEq/kg/day × 3.5 kg = 7–14 mEq/day
Potassium	2–3 mEq/kg/day × 3.5 kg = 7–10.5 mEq/day

(97-A)

Fluid and electrolyte requirements can be met by infusing a solution of 5% dextrose with one-quarter NS (38 mEq/L) and 20 mEq/L of KCl at 15 mL/hr. This provides 12 mEq (3.4 mEq/kg per day) of NaCl and 7 mEq (2 mEq/kg per day) of KCl in 360 mL (103 mL/kg per day) of fluid per day.

Adjustment for Ultraviolet Light Therapy

2. On the third day of life, P.J.'s indirect bilirubin is 15.2 mg/dL (normal, 0.6 to 10.5 mg/dL). It is decided to use phototherapy lights to treat her hyperbilirubinemia. How will this modify her maintenance fluid needs?

[SI unit: bilirubin, 259.92 μmol/L (normal, 10.3 to 179.5)]

Table 97-2 details situations that alter maintenance fluid needs. Phototherapy lights will increase P.J.'s insensible losses and will increase her maintenance fluid needs by 10% to 20%. This can be met by increasing her IV fluid rate to 17 mL/hr (116 mL/kg per day). Although her increased fluid loss will be free from solutes and the solution she is receiving contains

Table 97-3 Body Fluid Volumes and Electrolyte Content

Source	Volume (L/day)	Na⁺ (mEq/L)	K⁺ (mEq/L)	Cl⁻ mEq/L	HCO₃⁻ mEq/L
Salivary glands	1.5 (0.5–2)	10 (2–10)	26 (20–30)	10 (8–18)	30
Stomach	1.5 (0.1–4)	60 (9–116)	10 (0–32)	130 (8–154)	—
Duodenum	(0.1–2)	140	5	80	—
Ileum	3 (0.1–9)	140 (80–150)	5 (2–8)	104 (43–137)	30
Colon	—	60	30	40	—
Pancreas	(0.1–0.8)	140 (113–185)	5 (3–7)	75 (54–95)	115
Bile	(0.05–0.8)	145 (131–164)	5 (3–12)	100 (89–180)	35

sodium and potassium, the electrolytes she receives still will be within the range of normal, and her kidneys should be able to compensate for the small increase.

Dehydration
Clinical Presentation: Vomiting
ACUTE MANAGEMENT

3. H.S., a 2-year-old lethargic girl, is seen in her pediatrician's office with a 2-day history of vomiting and minimal oral intake. Yesterday, she required only three diaper changes instead of her usual eight and has needed only one change today. Her vital signs are as follows: temperature, 39°C; pulse, 140 beats/min (normal, 80 to 130 beats/min); respiratory rate, 30 breaths/ min (normal, 30 to 35 breaths/min); and blood pressure (BP), 80/45 mm Hg (normal, 80 to 115/50 to 80 mm Hg). On physical examination, her eyes appear sunken, her mucous membranes are dry, and her skin is dry and cool to touch. Although she is crying, there are no tears and the skin over her sternum tents when pinched. Her weight today is 11.4 kg; 3 weeks ago, it was 12.9 kg. What do these findings represent? What immediate treatment should be provided?

H.S.'s lethargy, decreased urine output, tearless crying, dry mucous membranes, dry skin with fever, sunken eyes, mild tachycardia with low normal blood pressure, and poor skin turgor are all signs of dehydration. This is consistent with her 2-day history of vomiting and poor intake. Her weight loss of 1.5 kg gives a further clue to the extent of dehydration. Dehydration or fluid loss is determined most accurately by weight loss. Because 1 g of body weight is approximately equal to 1 mL, her fluid deficit is estimated to be 1,500 mL. The percentage dehydration is estimated using the following formula:

$$\% \text{ dehydration} = \frac{\text{Normal body weight} - \text{Actual body weight}}{\text{Normal body weight}} \times 100 \quad (97\text{--}1)$$

If recent weights are unavailable, the extent of dehydration can be approximated from physical findings as described in Table 97-4. Tachycardia and marginal blood pressure dictate the need for immediate intravenous rehydration. Normal serum sodium concentration ranges from 135 to 145 mEq/L of sodium; thus, normal saline approximates the sodium concentration of plasma and is often used as a volume expander. In this patient, 10 to 20 ml/kg of normal saline (12.9 kg ×10 to 20 mL/kg = 129 to 258 mL) should be infused as rapidly as possible to establish normal blood pressure. For symptomatic patients, including those with seizures, the serum sodium concentration should be increased acutely only to the degree necessary to abate symptoms.

CALCULATION OF REQUIREMENTS

4. Calculate H.S.'s fluid and electrolyte needs. Her serum electrolyte results were as follows: Na, 128 mEq/L (normal, 135 to 145 mEq/L); K, 3.1 mEq/L (normal, 3.5 to 5 mEq/L); Cl, 88 mEq/L (normal, 102 to 109 mEq/L); and HCO$_3^-$, 30 mEq/L(normal, 22 to 29 mEq/L).

[SI units: Na, 128 mmol/L (normal, 135 to 145); K, 3.1 mmol/L (normal, 3.5 to 5); Cl, 88 mmol/L (normal, 102 to 109); HCO$_3^-$, 30 mmol/L (normal, 22 to 29)]

In addition to normal maintenance fluids, H.S. must be provided with fluids and electrolytes to replace her deficit secondary to dehydration and compensate for increased insensible water loss because of fever. Each component of the fluid can be calculated separately, using Equations 97-2 to 97-4.

$$\text{Fluid deficit} = \text{Weight loss (kg)} \times 1,000 \text{ mL/kg} \quad (97\text{--}2)$$

$$\text{Fever adjustment} = 10\% \times \text{Maintenance for each } °C > 37°C \quad (97\text{--}3)$$

$$(CD - CO) \times F_d \times \text{Weight} = \text{mEq required} \quad (97\text{--}4)$$

where CD is the concentration of sodium desired (mEq/L), CO is the concentration observed (mEq/L), F_d is the apparent distribution factor as a fraction of body weight (Table 97-5), and weight is the baseline weight before illness (kg). In consideration of both maintenance needs and current deficits, fluid and electrolyte requirements for H.S. would be estimated as follows.

Fluid

Maintenance	1,000 mL + (50 × 2.9) = 1,145 mL	
Fever	2°C × 0.1 (1,145) = 229 mL	**(97-B)**
Deficit	1.5 kg × 1,000 mL/kg = <u>1,500 mL</u>	
	Total fluid = 2,874 mL	

Sodium

Maintenance	3 mEq/kg × 12.9 kg = 38.7	
Deficit	(135 − 128 mEq/L) ×	**(97-C)**
	0.6 L/kg × 12.9 kg = 54.2	
	Total sodium ~ 93 mEq	

Chloride

H.S. has a mild metabolic alkalosis as evidenced by her serum chloride of 88 mEq/L and her serum bicarbonate of 30 mEq/L. This is most likely because of the loss of hydrogen and chloride in her vomitus. Thus, both the sodium and potassium replacements should be administered as chloride salts.

Table 97-4 Clinical Signs of Dehydration

Severity	% Dehydration	Psyche	Thirst	Mucous Membranes	Tears	Anterior Fontanel	Skin	Urine-Specific Gravity
Mild	<5	Normal	Slight	Normal to dry	Present	Flat	Normal	Slight change
Moderate	6–10	Irritable	Moderate	Dry	±	±	±	↑
Severe	10–15	Hyperirritable to lethargic	Intense	Parched	Absent	Sunken	Tenting	Greatly ↑

Table 97-5 Electrolytes and Apparent Distribution

Electrolyte	F_d (L/kg)
Sodium	0.6–0.7
Bicarbonate	0.4–0.5
Chloride	0.2–0.3

F_d, apparent distribution factor as a fraction of body weight.

Potassium

Potassium is primarily an intracellular ion. It moves in and out of cells in exchange for hydrogen ions to maintain a normal blood pH. Therefore, in metabolic alkalosis, the intracellular shift of potassium will make the serum potassium concentration decrease. When the pH normalizes, as will occur with rehydration, the hydrogen ions will move intracellularly and the potassium will move extracellularly, thus causing the serum potassium concentration to increase. Additionally, potassium is also excreted by the kidney in exchange for hydrogen ion conservation. These factors make the serum potassium concentration difficult to interpret. Intravascular volume depletion causes hypoperfusion of the kidney and may result in acute renal failure; therefore, the prudent approach is to give no potassium until urine output is clearly established. Then, only maintenance doses of potassium should be administered until a normal acid base and fluid status are established and the serum potassium can be assessed more accurately. Hence, H.S. should receive approximately 26 to 39 mEq of potassium (2 to 3 mEq/kg 12.9 kg) once urine flow is established.

ADMINISTRATION OF FLUID REQUIREMENTS

5. How should these calculated needs be given?

Requirements for the first 24 hours of parenteral fluid therapy should provide approximately 2,875 mL of fluid (maintenance fluid, fever replacement, and deficit replacement). In addition to fluid, at least 93 mEq of sodium (maintenance needs and deficit replacement) should be provided in the first 24 hours. It is important to provide sufficient amounts of sodium and water; therefore, the appropriate fluid should be $^{1}/_{4}$ NS or greater. Potassium is usually withheld until urine flow is established; as a result, initial fluids should not contain potassium. After urine flow begins, potassium should be added to meet the estimated daily requirement.

Rehydration fluids are usually dispensed in volumes less than the 24-hour requirement. This is to prevent wasting IV fluids due to changes in electrolyte needs during replacement therapy. Because this patient requires approximately 3 L of fluid, only 1 L would be prepared initially, and this would likely consist of dextrose 5% and 0.2% NS (or greater). Approximately 15 mEq/L of potassium would be added to the next liter of IV solution if the patient had a reasonable urine output.

The infusion rate should be calculated to provide one-third of the daily maintenance fluid plus one half of the deficit replacement during the first 8 hours. The remainder of the maintenance fluid (adjusted for fever) and deficit replacement should be administered over the next 16 hours. Usually, serum electrolytes are monitored every 6 to 8 hours during rehydra-

tion therapy to ensure that appropriate electrolytes are being provided. Usually, the concentration of serum electrolytes are monitored frequently during fluid replacement therapy of deficits. In general, the serum sodium concentration should not be increased >10 to 12 mEq/L per day. After the initial fluid deficits are replaced, the infusion rate of the IV fluid would be decreased to 48 mL/hr (1,152 mL or approximately maintenance fluid rate).

Clinical Presentation: Diarrhea

6. S.B., a 4-month-old, 5.9-kg boy, is seen in his pediatrician's office because of a 4-day history of diarrhea (five to eight large, liquid stools each day). On a well-child visit 4 weeks ago, his weight was 6 kg. Since the onset of diarrhea, he has only been receiving oral rehydration fluids. Physical examination reveals the following: temperature, 39.8°C; pulse, 110 beats/min (normal, 80 to 160 beats/min); respirations, 45 breaths/min (normal, 20 to 40 breaths/min); and BP, 100/58 mm Hg (normal, 75 to 105/40 to 65 mm Hg). His skin is pale, warm, and dry. He is very irritable, and his mucous membranes are dry. S.B.'s serum electrolytes are as follows: Na, 159 mEq/L (normal, 135 to 145 mEq/L); K, 3.3 mEq/L (normal, 3.5 to 5.0 mEq/L); Cl, 114 mEq/L (normal, 102 to 109 mEq/L); and HCO_3^-, 12 mEq/L (normal, 22 to 29 mEq/L). Correlate S.B.'s history and physical findings with the reported laboratory values.

[SI units: Na, 159 mmol/L (normal, 135 to 145); K, 3.3 mmol/L (normal, 3.5 to 5.0); Cl, 114 mmol/L (normal, 102 to 109); HCO_3^-, 12 mmol/L (normal, 22 to 29)]

Diarrheal fluid losses commonly contain high concentrations of bicarbonate, accounting for S.B.'s metabolic acidosis. This, in turn, has resulted in a rapid respiratory rate as the body attempts to compensate for the acidosis by eliminating carbon dioxide. The increased insensible water losses of fever and tachypnea have resulted in the loss of water in excess of sodium, producing hypernatremia.

ACUTE MANAGEMENT

7. How will S.B.'s management differ from that of H.S. (see Questions 3 to 5)?

Unlike H.S., S.B. has relatively normal vital signs and will not require rapid fluid replacement to correct hypotension. Hypernatremia in S.B. indicates fluid losses in excess of sodium and this should be corrected. With hypernatremia, the central nervous system (CNS) increases intracellular osmolarity load to prevent intracellular dehydration of cells in the CNS. Rapid correction of hypernatremia can cause excessive movement of water into the cells of the CNS and has been associated with seizures. Therefore, S.B.'s fluid and electrolyte deficits should be corrected over 2 to 3 days at a consistent rate rather than rapidly. In general, serum sodium should not be decreased >2 mEq/hr (maximum, 15 mEq/L per day).

CALCULATION OF REQUIREMENTS

8. Estimate S.B.'s fluid and electrolyte requirements to correct his deficits.

S.B.'s requirements are estimated using the same methods described in Question 4. First, the approximate extent of dehydration must be estimated. S.B.'s weight of 6 kg at the time of his well-child visit at 3 months of age was at the 50th percentile. If his growth has continued at this rate, his current pre-illness weight should be approximately 6.5 kg. This weight should be used to calculate his maintenance requirements. Thus, his water deficit is approximately 0.6 L, or 9%. Using this approximation, his fluid and electrolyte requirements can be estimated as follows.

Fluid

Maintenance	6.5×100 mL/kg = 650 mL/24 hr	
Fever	$2.8°C \times 0.1$ (650 mL) = 182 mL/24 hr	
Deficit	600 mL/3 days = 200 mL/24 hr	**(97-D)**
	Total daily needs = 1,032 mL or 43 mL/hr	

Sodium

Maintenance	3 mEq/kg $\times$ 6.5 kg = 19.5 mEq/24 hr	
Deficit	This is calculated at total body deficit (normal − actual)	
Norma:	145 mEq/L $\times$ 0.6 L/kg $\times$ 6.5 kg = 566 mEq	**(97-E)**
Actual	159 mEq/L $\times$ 0.6 L/kg $\times$ 5.9 kg = 563 mEq	
Deficit	= 3 mEq	
	or 1 mEq/day	

Potassium

As noted in Question 4, the serum potassium value of 3.3 mEq/L may not be indicative of S.B.'s total body potassium status. A metabolic acidosis in S.B. should have facilitated the movement of hydrogen ions into the cells and the movement of potassium from the intracellular to the extracellular space. Thus, the serum potassium of 3.3 mEq/L probably indicates a total body deficit. Nevertheless, potassium should not be administered until urine output is established. Thereafter, a maintenance potassium dosage of 13 to 20 mEq/day (approximately 2 to 3 mEq/kg) of potassium should be given. Serum electrolytes should be measured every 8 to 12 hours and the intake of all electrolytes should be readjusted based on the results.

Bicarbonate

With metabolic acidosis, bicarbonate should be administered as well. No maintenance amount is customarily given, but deficit replacement is calculated in a manner similar to that used for sodium (see Table 97-5). The volume of distribution of bicarbonate is 0.5 L/kg. For S.B. the bicarbonate deficit is as follows:

$$(23 − 12) \text{ mEq/L} \times 0.5 \text{ L/kg} \times 6.5 \text{ kg} = 36 \text{ mEq} \quad \textbf{(97-F)}$$

Initially, about half this amount should be replaced over the first 8 to 12 hours. His serum electrolytes then should be reassessed, and the dosages adjusted accordingly. The entire bicarbonate deficit need not be replaced at once because other compensatory mechanisms will contribute to endogenous bicarbonate sparing.

REPLACEMENT FLUID COMPOSITION

9. **Recommend an appropriate replacement fluid for S.B.'s therapy.**

S.B.'s fluid and electrolyte maintenance requirements and deficits should be corrected with dextrose 5% and approximately 0.2% NS with half as the chloride salt and half as

$NaHCO_3$. An infusion of this solution at 43 mL/hr should correct approximately half the calculated fluid and bicarbonate deficits within 24 hours in addition to his normal daily doses. After he urinates, 15 mEq/L KCl may be added to the next liter of solution to provide approximately 2.6 mEq/kg per day to this patient. The concentration of serum electrolytes should be measured often and the concentration of electrolytes in the replacement fluid should be adjusted every 8 to 12 hours based on laboratory results. The amount of fluid replacement should be modified based on whether this patient's diarrhea has resolved and fever has subsided.

ADMINISTRATION OF REQUIREMENTS

10. **By what route should the fluid calculated above be administered?**

Rehydration of the dehydrated patient may be achieved by either the oral or intravenous route. In some patients, vomiting may preclude effective oral rehydration. If the losses are diarrheal and there is no problem with vomiting, the oral route may be a cost-effective alternative to the parenteral route. Various solutions have been used to rehydrate children orally. In an asymptomatic dehydrated child, the sodium concentration of an oral rehydration fluid should contain at least 70 mEq/L of sodium.[6-8]

The composition of several products is shown in Table 97-6. A glucose concentration of 2% optimizes water and electrolyte absorption from the GI tract[9]; more concentrated glucose solutions may worsen rather than ameliorate diarrhea. Use of the oral route and the more concentrated sodium solutions may allow safe rehydration of hypernatremic dehydration in a shorter time frame than the 2 to 3 days previously noted.[9,10]

S.B.'s output must be measured to account for ongoing fluid loss. This often is accomplished by weighing the baby's diapers when they are dry and again when they are full. Composition of additional replacement fluids can be determined by using the average composition of the patient's losses (see Table 97-3). As an alternative, the composition of the losses may be determined by actual laboratory measurement. If prolonged therapy is necessary, specific analyses are recommended because of the wide range of normal values for diarrheal stool and other GI tract fluids. Because frequent adjustments may be necessary, replacement fluid should be administered separately if PN is being used as a maintenance solution.

Table 97-6   Composition of Oral Rehydration Products

Product	Na⁺ (mEq/L)	K⁺ (mEq/L)	Cl (mEq/L)	Bicarbonate Source (mEq/L)	Carbohydrate (%)
Gastrolyte	90	20	80	30 citrate	2
Rehydrate	75	20	65	30 citrate	2.5
Lytren	50	25	45	30 citrate	2
Pedialyte	45	20	35	30 citrate	2.5
WHO salts	90	20	80	30 bicarbonate	2

WHO, World Health Organization.

INFANT NUTRITION

Growth assessment is an important focus of pediatric health care during the first year of life. With the exception of the intrauterine period, the most rapid growth occurs during the first year. On average, a normally growing infant gains approximately 30 g/day. Typically, healthy infants weigh approximately three times their birth weight by their first birthday. Caloric requirements can be estimated using the formula provided in Table 97-1.

The American Academy of Pediatrics (AAP) has suggested that infant feeding be divided into three stages.[11] In the nursing period, only liquids are provided. During the transitional period, solid foods are introduced, but human milk, or commercially prepared infant formula, still provides the major source of the infant's caloric and nutrient supply. In the modified adult period, most nutrition is derived from the solid foods consumed by other household members.

At birth, the human GI tract is adapted for the consumption of a human milk–based diet. Intestinal lactase is present from 36 weeks' gestation and exhibits its maximum activity during infancy. Pancreatic amylase secretion is low, and the bile salt pool is decreased relative to older persons, resulting in decreased fat absorption.[12] Human milk provides nutrients in their most usable form for the developing GI tract.

Human Milk Feeding

11. M.E.'s mother will breast-feed her infant. What are the nutritional implications of this decision for M.E.?

Human milk is the ideal food for a human infant. There are three phases to human milk production. During the first 5 days of lactation, a viscous, yellow liquid known as colostrum is produced. Colostrum is rich in protein, minerals, and other substances (e.g., immunoglobulins). During the next 5 days, transitional milk is produced; in the last phase, mature human milk is produced. The exact nutritional content of human milk varies from mother to mother; however, mature human milk provides sufficient protein, minerals, and calories regardless of the mother's nutritional status.[13] Mature human milk generally provides 70 kcal/100 mL and fat accounts for >50% of the caloric content.[14] The fat in human milk is highly digestible and absorbable.[15] Forty percent of calories are provided as carbohydrates, primarily in the form of lactose, and the remaining 10% of calories are provided as protein. Whey and casein are the two primary proteins in mature human milk, with whey being the major protein component (whey:casein ratio of 55:45).[12] Human milk is of such biologic quality and bioavailability that adequate growth can be attained with a lower overall intake of protein than is provided by commercially prepared infant formulas, which contain lower whey:casein ratios.[15,13]

The iron content of human milk is inadequate for term infants; however, supplementation generally is unnecessary in the breast-fed infant.[16] Regardless of maternal status, the vitamin D and fluoride contents of human milk are inadequate. Thus, M.E. will require 400 IU of vitamin D and 0.25 mg/day of fluoride while she is exclusively breast-fed.[13,17]

12. Aside from nutrients, what other benefits are associated with human milk and breast-feeding?

Human milk provides the infant with protection against a wide variety of infectious diseases including otitis media, diarrhea, pneumonia, and bronchiolitis. Evidence further suggests that human milk provides protection against noninfectious disorders such as allergies, inflammatory bowel disease, insulin-dependent diabetes mellitus, and sudden infant death syndrome.[18] Human milk contains immunologically active cellular components and antibodies. These include secretory IgA, both T and B lymphocytes, macrophages, and neutrophils.[13,15] The lipases and amylase present in human milk may facilitate digestion of fat and carbohydrates in the still developing GI tract. Proteins present in human milk serve as carriers for trace minerals and facilitate their absorption.[13] Oligosaccharides and glycopeptides may promote the colonization of the GI tract by *Lactobacilli* and decrease colonization by *Bacteroides, Clostridia,* enterococci, and Gram-negative rods, all of which may be pathogenic.[15]

13. What potential complications are associated with breast-feeding. What instructions should be given to M.E.'s mother?

Complications associated with breast-feeding are few; however, there are some potential problems. "Breast milk jaundice" associated with an indirect (unconjugated) hyperbilirubinemia can occur in the breast-fed infant during the first week of life, and generally resolves by the fourth week of life. Although the infant's skin, sclera, and palate become yellow, this is generally not a dangerous condition. Nevertheless, if the bilirubin level becomes too high, the infant could develop an encephalopathy known as kernicterus. Therefore, the mother should temporarily stop breast-feeding and feed the infant formula until the jaundice starts to resolve.

Some maternal infections have the potential to be transmitted to the infant during breast-feeding. HIV and human T-lymphotropic virus 1 (HTLV-1) can be transmitted via breast milk and therefore maternal infections with these viruses are contraindications to breast-feeding.[19] Other viruses like herpes simplex virus can be transmitted if contact with active lesions occurs during breastfeeding. Similarly, some medications taken by the mother are detectable in her breast milk. Fortunately, only a few agents (e.g., antineoplastics, radiopharmaceuticals, ergot alkaloids, iodides, atropine, lithium, cyclosporine, chloramphenicol, bromocriptine) are absolute contraindications to breast-feeding.[19] (See Chapter 47, Teratogenicity and Drugs in Breast Milk, for additional information concerning the transfer of medications and chemicals into breast milk.)

Infant Formula

14. E.R.'s mother decides not to breast-feed her infant. She received a sample package of infant formula at the time of her discharge from the hospital. How are these products prepared and how do they differ from human milk?

Examples of infant formulas and their individual components are provided in Table 97-7. According to AAP guidelines for commercially prepared infant formula composition, formula should provide 20 kcal/oz; osmolality should be between 300 and 400 mOsm/L; protein quantity should be a minimum of 1.8 g/100 kcal and should not exceed 4.5 g/100

Table 97-7 Infant Formulas and Their Individual Components

Product	Calories per 100 mL	Carbohydrate (g/100 mL)	Carbohydrate Source	Protein (g/100 mL)	Protein Source	Fat (g/100 mL)
Human milk	70	7.2	Lactose	1	Whey 55%, casein 45%	4
Cow's Milk-Based Formulas						
Enfamil with iron[a]	67	7.5	Lactose	1.4	Whey 50%, casein 50%	3.6
Similac with iron[a,b]	68	7.2	Lactose	1.5	Nonfat milk, whey	3.6
Carnation Good Start	67	7.5	Lactose	1.5	Whey 100%	3.4
Soy-Based, Lactose-free Formulas						
Isomil	67	6.8	Corn syrup, sucrose	1.7	Soy, L-methionine	3.7
Nursoy	68	6.9	Sucrose	2.1	Soy, L-methionine	3.6
ProSoBee	67	7.2	Corn syrup	1.8	Soy, L-methionine	3.7
Alsoy	67	7.5	Maltodextrin, sucrose	1.9	Soy, L-methionine	3.3
Carnation Follow Up	67	8.8	Corn syrup	1.7	Nonfat milk	2.8
Similac Lactose Free	68	7.2	Maltodextrin, sucrose	1.5	Milk protein isolates	3.6
Enfamil LactoFree	67	7.3	Corn syrup	1.4	Milk protein isolates	3.5
Elemental, Premature Infant Formulas						
Alimentum	68	6.7	Sucrose, modified tapioca starch	1.9	Hydrolyzed casein	3.7
Nutramigen	67	9.1	Corn syrup, modified corn starch	1.9	Hydrolyzed casein	2.6
Pregestimil[b]	67	9.1	Corn syrup, modified corn starch	2.4	Hydrolyzed casein	2.7
NeoCate	67	7.1	Corn syrup	1.9	Free amino acids	2.8
Neosure Advance	75	7.7	Maltodextrin, lactose	1.9	Nonfat milk, whey	4.1
Enfamil Premature with Lipil[b]	67	7.3	Corn syrup, lactose	2	Nonfat milk, whey	3.4
Similac Special Care[a,b]	68	7.2	Corn syrup, lactose	1.8	Nonfat milk, whey	3.7

[a]Also available as a low iron formula.
[b]Also available as a 24 kcal/oz formula.
MCT, medium-chain triglyceride.

kcal; and fat quantity should be between 3.3 and 6 g/100 kcal, supplying between 30% and 54% of calories. Infant formulas generally begin with a cow's milk base; however, intolerance to pure cow's milk has resulted in several modifications. The predominant protein in cow's milk is casein, which is more difficult for infants to digest than the human milk protein, whey. Consequently, infant formulas generally have less casein than cow's milk, although not to the level of human milk. Casein:whey ratios of infant formulas and human milk are compared in Table 97-7. The casein present in cow's milk formulas also may be heat denatured to improve its digestibility. In addition, the fat source in cow's milk is replaced by one of several vegetable oils allowing for easier digestion. Last, the carbohydrate source in cow's milk–based formula is supplemented with lactose or sucrose because the lactose content of cow's milk is only 50% to 70% of that in human milk. Soy-based and protein hydrolysate formulas are available for infants who are intolerant of cow's milk–based formulas.

Soy-based formulas use soybean as the protein source. The soy is heat treated to enhance protein digestibility and improve the bioavailability of some nutrients. Although nutrients such as methionine, zinc, and carnitine are still present, their concentrations are relatively low. Therefore, methionine is routinely added to all soy-based formulas by the manufacturer. Zinc and carnitine may not be added and exogenous supplementation may be necessary. Soy-based formulas substitute sucrose, corn syrup, or a combination of the two for lactose as the carbohydrate source. Additionally, soy protein formulas are more expensive than cow's milk–based formulas. The AAP recommends that the use of soy-based formula be limited to patients with primary lactase deficiency (galactosemia); patients with secondary lactose intolerance from enteric infections or other causes; vegetarian families in which animal protein formulas are not desired; and infants who are potentially cow milk protein allergic, but who have not demonstrated clinical manifestations of allergy. Long term use of soy-based formulas in premature and low birth weight infants should not be recommended. Soy-based formulas have aluminum contamination, and have been associated with the development of rickets. Soy-based formulas are also not recommended for infants with documented allergic reactions to cow's milk protein because of the potential for cross-antigenicity between the two proteins. Soy protein formulas are not recommended for the routine management of colic.[20]

Protein hydrolysate formulas are another option for infants who are intolerant of cow's milk–based formulas. The milk proteins (i.e., casein and whey) are heat treated and enzymatically hydrolyzed to enhance digestibility of protein hydrolysate formulas, which are fortified with additional amino acids that are lost during processing. Like soy protein formulas, protein hydrolysates substitute sucrose, tapioca, or corn syrup for lactose as the carbohydrate source. Protein hydrolysate formulas often include significant amounts of medium-chain triglycerides (MCTs) because they are easily absorbed. Because the proteins are extensively hydrolyzed, these formulas probably are the least allergenic of the infant formulas and therefore may be appropriate for infants with

Table 97-7   Infant Formulas and Their Individual Components

Fat Source	Osmolality (mOsm/L)	Sodium (mEq/100 mL)	Potassium (mEq/100 mL)	Chloride (mEq/100 mL)	Calcium (mg/100 mL)	Phosphorus (mg/100 mL)	Iron (mg/100 mL)
Human milk fat	300	0.7	1.3	1.2	32	14	0.03
Palm, soy, coconut, safflower oil	300	0.8	1.9	1.2	53	36	1.3
Soy, coconut oil	290	1	2.1	1.5	57	37	1.2
Palm, soy, safflower	265	0.3	0.9	1.1	43	24	1
Soy, coconut, safflower oil	180	1.3	1.9	1.1	71	51	1.2
Soy, coconut, safflower oil	296	0.9	1.8	1.1	60	42	1.2
Palm, soy, coconut, safflower oil	200	1	2.1	1.5	71	56	1.2
Palm, soy, coconut, safflower oil	200	0.9	2	1.3	71	41	1.2
Palm, soy, coconut, safflower oil	326	0.4	1.2	1.6	80	54	1.2
Soy, coconut oil	180	0.9	1.8	1.2	57	38	1.2
Palm, soy, coconut, sunflower oil	200	0.3	1	1.9	54	37	1.2
MCT, safflower, soy oil	333	1.3	2	1.6	71	50	1.2
Corn oil	320	1.4	1.9	1.6	62	42	1.2
MCT, corn, soy oil	350	1.4	1.9	1.6	62	50	1.2
Soy, safflower, coconut oil	342	0.9	2.4	1.4	83	62	1.2
MCT, soy, coconut oil	250	1	2.7	1.6	78	46	1.2
MCT, soy, sunflower, safflower, crypthecodinium, mortierella alpina oil	260	0.6	0.9	1.7	110	55	1.8
MCT, soy, coconut, crypthecodinium, mortierella alpina oil	211	1.3	2.2	1.6	122	68	1.8

true allergy to cow's milk protein. Nevertheless, prospective studies on the safety of such a substitution in human infants have not been undertaken because it would be unethical to intentionally expose infants with documented allergies to a potential allergen. Protein hydrolysate formulas are the least palatable of the available pediatric formulas, and are more costly than other formulas.[21]

Infant formula is available from the manufacturer in three forms: ready-to-feed form, reconstitutable powder, and concentrated liquid. The ready-to-feed form is the most convenient but also the most expensive. The powder and the concentrated liquid are less expensive; however, both require that predetermined amounts of boiled water be added before use. To save money, some parents will dilute infant formula to a greater extent than is recommended to make the formula last longer. This practice should be discouraged since excessive free water intake by infants <1 year of age may result in hyponatremia and, ultimately, seizures. Similarly, supplementing an infant's diet with free water, for whatever reason, may also result in hyponatremia and seizures and should be discouraged. Recently, use of dry powder formula in the neonatal intensive care unit has been associated with severe bacterial infection. Because of this, dry powder formula in neonatal intensive care patients should be used cautiously.[22]

Introduction of Pure Cow's Milk

15. At her 2-month-old, well-child checkup, E.R. is found to have a hematocrit (Hct) of 33% (normal, 35% to 45%). After questioning her mother, the pediatrician learns that E.R. was taken off infant formula 1 month ago and changed to whole cow's milk to decrease food costs. How are these two findings related? What should be added to E.R.'s diet?

[SI unit: hematocrit, 0.35 (normal, 0.35 to 0.45)]

Pure cow's milk, straight from the dairy counter in the grocery store, is not recommended for infants younger than 1 year of age. Unlike human milk, the iron in cow's milk is present in inadequate concentrations and absorbed poorly from the human GI tract. For this reason, most infant formulas are fortified with iron. Cow's milk has been associated with GI blood loss in infants younger than 140 days of age.[23] When the milk is heated to a higher temperature than the usual pasteurization temperature, as it is in formula preparation, the association of cow's milk with GI bleeding is no longer present; therefore, the component responsible for the blood loss appears to be a heat-labile protein. Furthermore, cow's milk contains excessive amounts of solute that cannot be eliminated by the immature kidney. Also, cow's milk does not contain taurine, an amino acid that is important in retinal development.

To treat E.R.'s anemia, iron should be added to her diet. This can be done by changing back to an iron-fortified infant formula, feeding her an iron-fortified cereal, or giving a therapeutic ferrous sulfate liquid medication. The appropriate iron replacement dose for severe anemia is 4 to 6 mg/kg per day of elemental iron in divided doses with follow-up of the infant's hemoglobin and hematocrit.

Introduction of Solid Foods

16. At her 4-month-old, well-child checkup, M.E.'s mother asks her pediatrician about the introduction of "baby foods" into M.E.'s diet. When and how should solids be introduced?

Human milk or commercially prepared infant formula provides adequate nutrition for an infant for the first 12 months of life. Introduction of solid foods before the age of 4 months, while common in the past, is discouraged because the younger infant is unprepared to swallow foods other than liquids. Solids (first cereals, then fruits and vegetables) should be introduced when the child has good control of the head and neck movements (i.e., usually at the age of 4 to 6 months).[11] Preferably, one new food should be introduced at a time, at 1-week intervals, to allow assessment of food allergy.

Therapeutic Formulas
Phenylketonuria

17. L.B. is a 2-week-old infant whose newborn screen is positive for phenylketonuria (PKU). Discuss the concepts behind the production of therapeutic formulas and the dietary management of patients with inborn errors of metabolism. How must L.B.'s diet be modified?

Inborn errors of metabolism are disorders in which an enzyme or its cofactor is absent or insufficient to meet metabolic demands. As a result, one or more precursor compounds in a metabolic pathway can accumulate before the defective step. Correspondingly, one or more metabolic products that normally would have been generated after the defective step in the metabolic pathway are not sufficiently available.

The dietary management of metabolic errors is based on the following strategies:

- Reduce the intake of a precursor compound that cannot be metabolized.
- Supplement the deficient compounds that would have been produced if the normal metabolic pathway had not been blocked.
- Add a substrate that provides an alternative pathway for elimination of an accumulated toxin.

Therapeutic formulas are designed to reduce the intake of precursor compounds or to provide the deficient metabolic end-product.

When hydroxylation of phenylalanine to tyrosine does not take place, phenylalanine accumulates in the blood and results in mental retardation. Because PKU has been diagnosed in L.B., his diet should be modified using a formula containing little or no phenylalanine (e.g., Lofenalac, Phenex-1, Phenyl-Free). The tyrosine deficiency of PKU also can be managed by the addition of tyrosine to the phenylalanine-free therapeutic formulas that are available for patients with PKU. When L.B. progresses to solid foods, protein must be provided from predominately phenylalanine-free sources; therefore, patients with PKU should take in only minimal protein from table foods.[24]

Other Metabolic Errors

18. What other metabolic errors present in infancy require a specialized diet?

Other metabolic errors present in infancy include galactosemia (galactose cannot be metabolized to glucose), homocystinuria (methionine is not converted to cysteine), urea cycle disorders (ammonia detoxification is impaired), and maple syrup urine disease (metabolism of the branched chain amino acids, leucine, isoleucine, and valine is blocked).

These metabolic errors are managed by manipulating the diet.[25] In galactosemia, the carbohydrate source should not contain galactose or lactose. In homocystinuria, methionine should be present only in quantities sufficient to meet basic requirements, and cysteine should be supplemented. In the urea cycle disorders, protein often is provided only as essential amino acids, and a high-energy diet is provided to maximize the formation of nonessential amino acids from nitrogen and to minimize ammonia production. In maple syrup urine disease, natural protein is fed in small quantities to provide the minimal requirement of branched chain amino acids, and a branched chain–free supplement is added to provide adequate protein intake.

Route of Administration

Nutritional support using the GI tract is the preferred approach when possible. Enteral nutrition provides several advantages. First, interposition of the GI mucosa between the nutrient supply and the circulation allows absorptive function to provide a homeostatic control. Second, the flow of nutrients from the GI tract to the liver via the portal circulation before reaching the systemic circulation also assists homeostatic control. Third, the lack of enteral nutrition allows normal GI tract flora to overgrow and translocate into the blood, ultimately resulting in bacteremia. Finally, the intestinal mucosa depends on intraluminal absorption for much of its energy supply. Hence, provision of at least a small amount of enteral feeding, referred to as trophic feeds, helps to insure a healthy GI tract and may facilitate advancement to full enteral feedings at the appropriate time.[26,27]

Normal oral feeding is the most basic method for patients who are willing and able to eat or drink. Patients whose GI motility, structure, and function are normal but whose oral feeding is prevented by an altered state of consciousness, incoordination of sucking and swallowing, or other conditions that prevent adequate oral ingestion can be fed by a GI tube in intermittent boluses or by continuous infusion.

Bolus tube feedings more closely mimic the normal state. They periodically distend the stomach, which aids in gastric secretion and emptying. When bolus tube feeding is undertaken, the volume of formula required to provide sufficient calories for a 24-hour period is administered through the tube in equal aliquots every 2, 3, 4, or 6 hours. The frequency of administration depends on the patient's age, gastric capacity and their ability to maintain a normal serum glucose concentration between feedings. In general, younger and more premature infants require more frequent feedings. Intolerance to bolus tube feedings may be manifested as diarrhea, gastroesophageal reflux with emesis, or poor motility. Poor motility usually is apparent when large volumes of feeding, referred to as residuals, remain in the stomach when the next feeding is due.

Continuous tube feedings may be given at a constant rate of infusion by pump into the stomach or duodenum when bolus feedings have failed. This approach may be better tolerated by premature infants and children with diarrhea.[28]

Patients with intrinsic GI disease (Table 97-8) or malabsorption may require total or supplemental PN. Concurrent administration of low-volume, trophic enteral feedings may provide important nutrients to the gut mucosa even when the parenteral route supplies all of the necessary systemic nutrients.[26,27] Administration of PN into a peripheral vein is limited to those patients expected to require parenteral feeding only for a short time (i.e., 2 weeks) because the amount of nutrients that can be safely infused peripherally is limited. In patients who require long-term PN, the IV solution is more concentrated and must be administered into a central vein.

Nutritional Assessment

The patient's nutritional status should be assessed before beginning a nutritional support regimen and reassessed at regular intervals during the course of treatment. If the patient previously was well nourished, the goal is to maintain that status until a normal diet can be resumed. In a child who was previously malnourished, an effort should be made to promote "catch-up" growth and to normalize the biochemical nutritional measures. About one-third of children admitted to hospital are malnourished at the time of their admission.[29] Malnutrition in children is a risk factor for decreased social skills and impaired intellectual development.[30–32]

Table 97-8   Indications for Parenteral Nutrition Support
Extreme prematurity
Respiratory distress
Congenital GI anomalies
Duodenal atresia
Jejunal atresia
Esophageal atresia
Tracheoesophageal fistula
Pyloric stenosis
Congenital webs
Hirschsprung's disease
Malrotation
Volvulus
Abdominal wall defects
Omphalocele (herniation of viscera into the umbilical cord base)
Gastroschisis (defect of abdominal wall, any location except umbilical cord)
Congenital diaphragmatic hernia
Necrotizing enterocolitis
Chronic diarrhea
Inflammatory bowel disease
Chylothorax
Pseudoobstruction
Megacystic microcolon
Abdominal trauma involving viscera
Adverse effects of treating neoplastic disease
Radiation enteritis
Nausea and vomiting
Stomatitis, glossitis, and esophagitis
Anorexia nervosa
Cystic fibrosis
Chronic renal failure
Hepatic failure
Metabolic errors

GI, gastrointestinal.

Factors used to determine nutritional status in children include dietary history, weight, height, and visceral protein measurements (e.g., albumin, prealbumin, retinol binding protein, transferrin). Other measurements used in adults—such as 24-hour creatinine excretion, 24-hour nitrogen excretion, and nitrogen balance—are reserved for older children because complete collections of urine are difficult to obtain and because the percentage of non-urea nitrogen present in urine is variable in infants.

Anthropometric Measurements

Height, weight, and head circumference are used to determine nutritional status in infants and children. Standards for these measurements have been derived from pediatric patients in the United States and compiled into graphs referred to as growth curves. These were recently revised and are available at www.cdc.gov/growthcharts.[33] An individual patient's measurements are compared with the graph of normal values for their age group. As prematurely born infants age, a standard growth curve adjusted for prematurity can be used. Using these measurements, comparisons to standards are possible: weight for age, height for age, and weight for height.[33] A weight that is below the 5th percentile for the patient's height is considered an indication of acute malnutrition. Similarly, a height and weight that are below the 5th percentile for the patient's age indicates chronic malnutrition. It is important to consider the height and weight of the child's parents because genetics are important determinants of the height and weight that a child may ultimately achieve. Additionally, the revised growth charts include the body mass index (BMI) for age for children older than 2 years. The BMI helps identify children at risk for obesity and type 2 diabetes, two problems that have recently become a concern in children.[33]

Biochemical Measurements

Numerous biochemical indices are used in the assessment of nutritional status. Several, such as the quantitative excretion of compounds like 3-methyl-histidine and creatinine, are difficult to use in children because they require cumbersome 24-hour urine collections. Also, reliable standards for very young children are unavailable.

Of the biochemical markers of nutritional status, the most readily available and widely used is the serum albumin concentration. Although a low serum albumin can be a specific indicator of protein-calorie malnutrition, albumin's long half-life (20 days)[34] makes it an insensitive indicator for developing and resolving malnutrition.

Prealbumin, fibronectin, transferrin, and retinol-binding protein are plasma transport proteins that also can function as biochemical markers of nutritional status.[34–37] They have the advantage of being more sensitive than albumin to acute nutritional changes because their half-lives are shorter, and they are useful when exogenous albumin infusions are given.[38] Nevertheless, transferrin, fibronectin, and retinol-binding protein are influenced by factors other than nutrition (e.g., stress), and are less specific indicators of nutritional status.[39,40]

Laboratory and Clinical Assessments

The nutritional status of a patient receiving PN should be evaluated at regular intervals (e.g., weekly). The adverse effects of enteral and PN should include evaluations of the patient for signs and symptoms of fluid overload, GI losses (e.g., stool, emesis, ostomy output), and metabolic imbalances. The patient should be weighed and the fluid intake, urine output, and GI losses assessed daily.

Blood and urine glucose concentrations should be performed daily initially until the patient is stable on a formulation; subsequently, the frequency of monitoring can be reduced. Several laboratory tests also should be monitored routinely in those receiving PN (Table 97-9). The frequency of monitoring the subjective and objective data of a patient should be modified based on the clinical condition of the patient.

Clinical Presentation: Nutritional Assessment

19. T.C., a 4-month-old, lethargic boy, is seen in his pediatrician's office for routine well-baby care. At examination, he has a moderately distended abdomen and dry mucous membranes. No other remarkable abnormalities are noted. His weight is 6.5 kg (50th to 75th percentile for age). At a previous well-baby visit when he was 2 months old, T.C. weighed 5.6 kg (75th percentile for age), and his length was 57 cm (50th percentile for age). His mother reports that for the past 5 to 7 days, he has had five to eight large, liquid stools per day. His diet has not been changed and consists of 5 to 6 oz of a commercial, infant formula every 4 hours around the clock. He is to be hospitalized for evaluation of his diarrhea and weight loss and for fluid and nutritional management.

After correction of his initial fluid and electrolyte deficits, an assessment of his nutritional status shows the following: weight, 6.5 kg (50th to 75th percentile); length, 62 cm (50th percentile); albumin, 3.8 g/dL (normal, 4 to 5.3 g/dL); and prealbumin, 7 mg/dL (normal, 20 to 50 mg/dL). What do these data suggest about the nature of T.C.'s malnutrition?

[SI units: albumin, 38 g/L (normal, 40 to 53); prealbumin, 70 mg/L (normal, 200 to 500 mg/L)]

If T.C. had continued to gain weight at his previous rate, his weight, extrapolated from the appropriate growth chart,

Table 97-9 Routine Laboratory Monitoring of Pediatric and Neonatal Parenteral Nutrition[a]

Test	Frequency
Electrolytes, glucose, BUN, SrCr	Daily until stable, then 2–3 times/wk
Calcium	1–2 times/wk
Phosphorus	1–2 times/wk
Magnesium	1–2 times/wk
Triglycerides	QOD until stable on maximum fat dose, then weekly
PA or RBP	Weekly
Total protein, albumin	Weekly if PA, RBP not available
Alkaline phosphatase	Weekly
Bilirubin (total, direct)[a]	Weekly
Hgb, WBC count	Weekly
AST, ALT	Monthly

[a]Bilirubin (indirect) daily in the newborn, until normal.
ALT, alanine aminotransferase; AST, aspartate aminotransferase; BUN, blood urea nitrogen; Hgb, hemoglobin; PA, prealbumin; RBP, retinol binding protein; SrCr, serum creatinine; WBC, white blood cell.

should be approximately 7.2 kg. His growth in length has continued to progress at the same rate. Thus, the decrease in weight for age with a normal progression in length for age indicates malnutrition of a relatively short duration. This is further validated by a near-normal serum concentration of albumin with a decrease in prealbumin.

Role of Enteral Nutrition in Chronic Diarrhea

20. After initial IV rehydration and receiving nothing by mouth (NPO) for 48 hours, T.C.'s stool output has decreased dramatically. Is this characteristic of infants with chronic diarrhea? Should enteral intake be initiated?

A prompt decrease in stool output when enteral intake is stopped is typical of infants with chronic diarrhea. Nonetheless, evaluation of bowel function and adaptation has shown that enteral nutrition is superior to PN with regard to histologic recovery, improvement of D-xylose absorption,[41] protein absorption, and disaccharidase activity.[42–44] In fact, improvement in histology or absorptive function might not occur until enteral nutrients are given.[42,43] Thus, for T.C., every effort should be made to provide some nutrition enterally, whether this route is used exclusively[42] or in combination with supplemental PN.[44]

Choice of Formula

21. What type of enteral formula should be chosen for T.C.?

The enteral regimen should be initiated with a lactose free formula, such as an elemental formula or a soy-based formula. While any soy-based formula would be appropriate, Isomil DF is a soy-based formula with added fiber that is indicated for infants with diarrhea. Infants with chronic diarrhea can have small bowel mucosal damage and decreased disaccharidase activity.[43,44] Carbohydrate absorption depends on digestion of disaccharides and polysaccharides to monosaccharides through disaccharidase activity in the intestinal lumen. Substitution of free glucose orally may overcome the problem of carbohydrate digestion and absorption. However, the administration of large amounts of oral glucose should be limited because of its osmotic effect and potential to worsen diarrhea. Furthermore, incompletely absorbed carbohydrate is available to colonic bacteria for fermentation, the end-products of which may produce diarrhea through colonic irritation.

Unlike carbohydrate, protein rarely causes diarrhea,[45] but the mucosal damage present in patients with chronic diarrhea, such as T.C., may reduce the absorptive surface area so that protein malabsorption may occur. This can be minimized through the administration of a formula containing protein in the form of dipeptides and tripeptides, which are absorbed more efficiently than free amino acids.[3]

Dilution of hypertonic formulas to half strength may improve formula tolerance.[42] The concentration is increased in a step-wise fashion to full strength if there is no carbohydrate malabsorption and if stool output is not excessive (defined by Orenstein as ≥40% of enteral intake).[42] Tolerance may be improved by continuous infusion of the enteral product.[28] If enteral refeeding results in the return of diarrhea, fluid and electrolytes must be replaced with an equal volume of an IV solution of similar electrolyte composition to the stool loss.[42]

Monitoring

22. How can T.C.'s tolerance to the formula and his recovery of intestinal function be assessed?

Malabsorption or formula intolerance can be assessed by stool studies that would include assessing for the presence of reducing substances and stool pH. Lactose is a reducing sugar and its presence in stool is an assessment of carbohydrate absorption. The bacterial fermentation products of malabsorbed carbohydrates may result in a decreased stool pH which suggests malabsorption. To further evaluate carbohydrate absorption d-xylose may be given orally; a blood sample is drawn 4 to 5 hours later to determine the amount absorbed. This test may be of initial prognostic value in predicting which patients will require prolonged courses of treatment.[41] More than 5% of ingested fat in a stool collection (usually 3 days) is indicative of fat malabsorption. All these tests may be followed serially during treatment to help guide the refeeding process.

Reinstitution of Standard Formula

23. Once the diarrhea has resolved and the enteral diet is well tolerated, how should standard infant formula be reinstituted in T.C.?

Standard formula feedings are restarted somewhat arbitrarily in patients such as T.C., although the D-xylose absorption test may be a useful guide.[41,42] The diarrhea should have resolved completely, and full maintenance fluid and caloric intake should be established using an enteral elemental or soy-based formula. Regardless of the time chosen, a gradual step-wise conversion is suggested. A small volume of standard formula is substituted for an equal volume of elemental or soy-based formula and the substitution volume is increased daily until the elemental or soy-based formula is eliminated completely from the regimen.

If a specific nutrient intolerance has been identified, a standard formula that does not contain that nutrient must be selected. For example, a patient with cow's milk protein intolerance may require a soy protein formula.

Pediatric Parenteral Nutrition

Nutrient Requirements

The basic requirements for a parenteral nutrient regimen are listed in Table 97-1. These guidelines for the initiation of a nutrient regimen should be individualized to specific patient needs because requirements may vary from patient to patient. The correct regimen for any specific patient is that which supplies sufficient nutrients to promote a normal rate of growth without toxicity. In particular, patients with ongoing, abnormal nutrient losses may require much larger doses of certain nutrients. Individualization of the nutrient prescription cannot be overemphasized.

Although the vitamin doses recommended in Table 97-1 correspond to the guidelines of the American Medical Association—Nutrition Advisory Group clinical evaluation, the administration of these doses has revealed several problems. VLBW infants given higher doses of vitamin A than those listed in the table can still develop signs and symptoms of vitamin A deficiency.[4,46] This may be caused by binding of parenteral vitamin A to the plastic IV infusion bag or tubing. Vitamins D and E appeared to be adequately supplied by this dose (65% of the maximum shown in Table 97-1 for preterm infants, the full maximum dose for term infants and older children). In contrast to vitamin A, most water-soluble vitamin serum concentrations were adequate with the higher dose. Niacin, pantothenate, biotin, and vitamin C levels were above normal in premature infants. Vitamin B_{12} and folate levels were elevated in premature infants as well as older infants and children.[47] Thus, a completely appropriate parenteral vitamin product is not available yet. Additionally, parenteral vitamin products are contaminated with aluminum, which may accumulate in preterm neonates whose renal function is not fully developed. Currently available parenteral vitamin products are listed in Table 97-10.

Many of the requirements listed in Table 97-1 apply to nutrients administered by the enteral route as well. In some instances, the absorption of a particular nutrient from the GI mucosa is incomplete and enteral requirements are substantially higher. This is particularly true of the major minerals (calcium, magnesium, and iron) and trace elements.[48] In some cases, parenteral doses may be greater than enteral doses to achieve the same blood concentration.[3]

Indications

PN is indicated for any patient unable to take in sufficient nourishment to maintain normal growth. Some specific indications are listed in Table 97-8.

Very Low Birth Weight Infants

Extremely premature infants require specialized nutritional support for two distinct reasons. First, the third trimester in utero is a time of rapid growth and accumulation of protein, glycogen, fat, and minerals.[50] The infant born in the very early stages of the third trimester does not accumulate these stores and therefore must receive nutrients earlier than a more mature infant. Second, extreme prematurity is associated with poor coordination of the suck and swallow reflex, poor GI motility, and incomplete absorption.[51] Therefore, enteral nutrients may need to be administered via an orogastric or nasogastric tube, and PN supplementation probably will be needed.

Respiratory Distress

Respiratory distress may preclude the ability to consume sufficient nutrients enterally because high respiratory rates prevent coordinated breathing and swallowing. In infants who are hypoxic, or at high risk for hypoxia, aggressive enteral feedings during the acute phase of their illness may increase the likelihood of bowel ischemia. Often, these situations are resolved in 3 to 5 days, but this can rarely be predicted at the outset. Trophic feedings (1 to 5 mL/hr) are often implemented to maintain GI tract integrity. Nutritional support in such cases is initiated by giving parenteral fluids, which provide dextrose as a caloric source. This allows the infant to conserve endogenous energy substrates, an important consideration for the VLBW infant whose entire body composition may contain a 3- to 4-day energy supply.[50] PN should be initiated as soon as it becomes clear the enteral feeding will be impossible for 3 to 5 days or when several days have elapsed and no clear time frame can be determined for the establishment of enteral feeding. Although a short course (5 days) of PN may be used,

Table 97-10 Parenteral Multivitamin Products

Vitamin	MVI-Pediatric 5 mL Powder (Astra)	MVI-12 10 mL (Astra)	MULTI-12 5 mL (Sabex)	MULTI-12 PED 5 mL (4+1) Solution (Sabex)	Cernevit 5 mL Powder (Baxter)	Influvite-12 10 mL (Baxter)	Influvite Pediatric 5 mL (Baxter)
A (IU)	2,300	3,300	3,300	2,300	3,500	3,300	2,300
D (IU)	400	200	200	400	220	200	400
E (IU)	7	10	10	7	11.2	200	400
K (μg)	200	0	0	0	0	150	7
C (mg)	80	100	100	80	125	200	200
B1 (mg)	1.2	3	3	1.2	3.51	6	1.2
B2 (mg)	1.4	3.6	3.6	1.4	4.14	3.6	1.4
B6 (mg)	1	4	4	1	4.53	6	1
B3 (mg)	17	40	40	17	48	40	17
B5 (mg)	5	15	15	5	17.25	15	5
Biotin (μg)	20	60	60	20	69	60	20
Folic acid (μg)	140	400	400	140	414	600	140
B12 (μg)	1	5	5	1	6	5	1
	Polysorbate 80 50 mg Polysorbate 20 0.8 mg Mannitol 375 mg BHT 58 μg BHA 14 μg	Propylene glycol Sodium citrate Citric acid NaOH Polysorbate 20 BHA BHT Ethanolamide		Polysorbate 80 50 mg Mannitol 75 mg NaOH or HCl Sodium citrate or citric acid	Glycine 250 mg Glycocholic acid 140 mg Soybean Phosphatides 112.5 mg	Propylene glycol Polysorbate 80 50 mg	Polysorbate 80 50 mg Mannitol 7 mg

the quantity of nutrients supplied during the process of initiation and gradual increase to full requirements is so low that extremely short courses may be difficult to justify. However, peripheral PN using fat emulsion as a significant source of calories can provide up to 70 kcal/kg and, with appropriate types and amounts of protein, can result in modest weight gain and nitrogen equilibrium.

Gastrointestinal Anomalies

Infants with GI anomalies often require PN because the implementation of enteral feedings may be delayed. For example, GI tract atresias or stenosis may obstruct, or partially obstruct, the lumen of the GI tract. This prevents or slows the passage of fluids and nutrients and may result in vomiting, depending on the location of the obstruction. Similarly, infants with necrotizing enterocolitis have zones of ischemic bowel and are at risk for bowel perforation if fed enterally.[52] Infants with these disorders need PN until viability of the entire GI tract can be assured.

Chronic Renal Failure and Hepatic Disease

Chronic renal or hepatic disease requires modification of a normal diet to account for the impaired elimination of nitrogenous waste or impaired protein metabolism. Careful caloric supplementation with a reduced amount of protein may permit normal growth while minimizing excess urea production in an infant with renal failure.

24. Approximately 48 hours after discharge from the hospital, T.C. returns to the emergency department with abdominal distention and bloody diarrhea. He is diagnosed with postgastroenteritis syndrome. T.C. cannot receive nutrients enterally, and PN is to be initiated because he is nutritionally depleted. Describe how a regimen of PN should be instituted in T.C. What aspects of his disease may alter specific nutrient needs?

When initiating PN, the protein (amino acids), glucose (dextrose), fat (lipids or fat emulsion), fluid and electrolyte, mineral, and vitamin components of the regimen are managed as separate entities. In addition, the route of PN delivery is important to consider because the amount of glucose, potassium, and calcium must be limited if the infusion is given peripherally. In general, 12.5% dextrose, 40 mEq potassium per liter, and 10 mEq calcium per liter are the maximum amounts that should be provided by infusion into a peripheral vein. These nutrients can be increased if a central venous line is placed. The fluids, electrolytes, minerals, and vitamins are initiated at full daily maintenance doses after correction of any pre-existing abnormalities. Protein should be initiated at full daily doses in term infants and children with normal renal and hepatic function. Glucose and fat are started at lower doses and increased daily until requirements are reached. Forgetting to increase doses in T.C. will lead to underfeeding.

Protein should be started in T.C. at full daily requirements of 2 to 3 g/kg per day. Azotemia and acidosis have occurred in infants receiving >4 g/kg per day of protein; however, these complications are rare at the recommended dosage.

Parenteral glucose administration is initiated at 5 to 8 mg/kg per minute (7.2 to 11.5 g/kg per day). This closely approximates normal endogenous glucose production[53] and should be tolerated. At normal maintenance fluid rates, 10% glucose represents a generally well-tolerated starting solution for patients of virtually any age or size, except the VLBW infant. In T.C.'s case, the glucose concentration will begin and continue at 10% because of the peripheral line limitations. This concentration of glucose will provide 7.3 mg/kg per minute. If a central line later becomes necessary, the concentration of glucose can be increased by 5% each day until the caloric requirement is met. This glucose increment should be accompanied by blood and urine glucose monitoring. If the blood glucose is ≥150 mg/dL or if the urine glucose exceeds "trace" amounts, the PN infusion rate should be decreased by at least 25% and a second IV solution should be added to provide needed fluids and electrolytes. Alternatively, the dextrose concentration can be decreased or insulin can be infused concomitantly and titrated to a desired serum glucose concentration of 120 to 140 mg/dL.

Fat should be initiated at 1 g/kg per day and increased daily by 0.5 to 1 g/kg per day until the maximum dosage of 3 g/kg per day is reached. The daily fat dose should be infused at a constant rate because fats are better tolerated when infused over 24 hours.[54] Serum triglycerides should be monitored every other day while the dose of fat is being increased. Patients with a fasting triglyceride concentration of 150 mg/dL or less may have their fat dose increased. In patients who are receiving inadequate calories, triglycerides may be elevated because endogenous fats are being mobilized. If the triglyceride concentration is >150 mg/dL, the serum sample must be examined visually. A clear sample with a mildly elevated triglyceride concentration probably indicates the use of endogenous fat stores for energy. Conversely, a turbid or lipemic sample indicates the patient's inability to use the amount of intravenous fat administered. In this case, further increases in the fat dose should be delayed until triglyceride concentrations decrease.[55]

25. **T.C., has a single peripheral IV line. Can the glucose–amino acid solution and the IV fat emulsion be infused through the same IV line?**

Not only can they be infused through the same peripheral IV line, but doing so may prolong the patency of the IV site and reduce the likelihood of local complications, such as phlebitis.[56,57] Lipids dilute the hypertonic glucose–amino acid solution. However, the fat has two more important effects. It acts as a mechanical barrier to the vascular endothelium and has a local modulating effect on prostaglandin and leukotriene mediators of inflammation.[57]

Special Considerations and Complications

26. **J.H., a 4-day-old boy, was born at 31 weeks' gestation. His birth weight was 1,950 g, and he now weighs 2,000 g. On the first day of life, he was given a commercial preterm infant formula by orogastric tube in gradually increasing quantity with supplemental IV fluids. Now, on the fourth day of life, he has developed a distended abdomen and his stools contain bright red blood. An abdominal radiograph shows pneumatosis intestinalis (gas within the intestinal wall). All enteral feedings are stopped (NPO). What do these findings represent? What are the implications for J.H.'s nutritional management?**

Abdominal distention, bloody stools, and pneumatosis intestinalis are characteristic of necrotizing enterocolitis.[52] The causes of this disorder are unclear, but it occurs more often in premature than in term infants, may occur in clusters of cases, rarely is seen before enteral feeding is instituted, and may be associated with rapid increases in enteral intake.[58] Because J.H. will receive antibiotics for 10 to 14 days and remain NPO, he requires PN. The planned duration of the regimen makes central venous access a necessity.

Parenteral Nutrition
Goals of Long-Term Support

27. **The following day, intestinal perforation requires the resection of two-thirds of J.H.'s distal jejunum and one-third of his ileum, with creation of a jejunostomy. The ileocecal valve and the entire colon are left intact. During the operation, a central venous catheter is placed. What is the goal of PN for J.H.?**

J.H. will be NPO for a prolonged time. Therefore, the goals of his PN must be to promote normal growth as well as healing of his diseased gut and surgical wounds.

Because J.H. is a premature infant, it will be difficult to predict how well he will tolerate PN. VLBW infants tolerate normal doses of pediatric amino acids without difficulty; however, some clinicians initiate protein at a lower daily dose such as 1.0 g/kg per day and advance by 0.5 g/kg per day each day until a goal of 2 to 3 g/kg per day is achieved. The problem with this approach is that it is easy to forget to advance the protein, which leads to underfeeding. Fat should be started at 0.5 to 1 g/kg per day and increased by 0.5 g/kg per day up to 3 g/kg per day. Glucose should be initiated at 5 to 10 g/kg per day and increased by 2 to 3 g/kg until the desired caloric intake is achieved. Appropriate doses of electrolytes and minerals may be started immediately using the guidelines listed in Table 97-1.

Fat Emulsions: Complications

28. **What must be considered in making decisions regarding fat administration in J.H.?**

Although J.H. can receive adequate calories using only glucose and crystalline amino acids, he will require fat to provide a more physiologic diet and to prevent essential fatty acid deficiency (EFAD), which develops quickly in low birth weight infants who have little fat reserve.[59] J.H. should receive a minimum of 5% of his total caloric requirement as fat emulsion to minimize the risk of EFAD.[55] Ideally his nutrition regimen will provide approximately 40% of calories from fat, which is similar to what is provided by human milk.

Infusions of fat emulsions have been associated with impaired oxygen transport and pulmonary ventilation-perfusion mismatch. This adverse effect generally occurred when the dose of fat was ≥4 g/kg and infused over a relatively short (4 hours) period. Current practice is to gradually increase the doses of fat from 0.5 to 1 g/kg per day up to a maximum of 4 g/kg per day and to infuse the fat emulsion over 24 hours to minimize the likelihood of pulmonary problems and to promote clearance.

It is unclear if IV fat administration is detrimental to patients with sepsis. Rapid IV infusion of fat, and in vitro incubation of leukocytes with fat emulsion has resulted in impaired leukocyte chemotaxis and phagocytosis.[60] On the other hand, the linoleic acid in IV fat is the precursor to arachidonic acid, prostaglandins, thromboxane, interleukins, and immune-mediating cells. Theoretically, this may minimize bacteremia. Necrotizing enterocolitis, intestinal perforation, and surgery predispose J.H. to sepsis. Therefore, he should have his IV fat infused at an appropriate dose over 24 hours. Because fat clearance can be impaired during infection, it is also prudent to monitor his triglyceride concentrations.

Free fatty acids can displace bilirubin from its albumin binding sites thereby placing the infant at risk for kernicterus.[61] Therefore, before advancing the fat dose, the total bilirubin and direct bilirubin should be measured. Patients with an indirect bilirubin (total bilirubin − direct bilirubin) ≤10 mg/dL whose albumin levels are normal are at low risk for kernicterus. Indirect bilirubin usually peaks before 1 week of age. After the risk for indirect hyperbilirubinemia has passed, the fat dose may be increased as recommended in Table 97-1. The infusion of 1 g/kg over 24 hours is associated with minimal risk for decreased bilirubin binding[61]; however, rapid infusion of this same dose can displace bilirubin from albumin binding sites. Given the low level of indirect bilirubin found on routine monitoring (see Question 36) and the planned fat infusion rate, J.H. should not be at risk for kernicterus.

Egg phospholipids are used to emulsify fats; therefore, patients with a known allergy to eggs (e.g., fever, chills, urticaria, dyspnea, bronchospasm, chest pain) should not receive fat emulsion.[55]

Glucose Intolerance

29. **Because J.H is a premature infant, PN should be initiated using 5% glucose, 2.5 g/kg per day of amino acids, and 0.5 g/kg per day of fat emulsion. The volume of PN should be 240 ml based on a maintenance fluid requirement of 120 ml/kg (see Table 97-1). On the second day, he receives 10% glucose and 2.5 g/kg per day of amino acids and 1 g/kg per day of fat. On the third day, glucose is increased to 15%, amino acids remain at 2.5 g/kg, and fat emulsion is increased to 1.5 g/kg per day. On the fourth day, glucose is increased to 20%, amino acids remain at 2.5 g/kg, and fats are increased to 2 g/kg per day. After this solution has infused for 8 hours, his urine has 1% for glucose (normal, no glucose) and his blood glucose level is 210 mg/dL (normal, 120 mg/dL). Explain this new finding and the problems it may cause. How should hyperglycemia be managed?**

[SI unit: blood glucose, 11.7 mmol/L (normal, 6.66)]

Maximum glucose oxidation rates in milligrams per kilograms per minute are inversely related to age, and decrease from 15 to 18 mg/kg per minute in neonates and young infants to 4 to 5 mg/kg per minute in adults. In full term neonates and infants receiving maintenance fluids (100 mL/kg), glucose concentrations can be started at 10 g/kg per day (equivalent to dextrose 10%) and advanced by 5 g/kg (equivalent to dextrose 5%) every 24 hours up to approximately 25 g/kg per day (equivalent to dextrose 25%).

In preterm neonates, like J.H., dextrose is started at a lower dose and advanced at smaller increments, usually 2 to 3 g/kg per day. Glucose tolerance varies significantly, so each patient should be considered individually.

At J.H.'s prescribed fluid rate of 10 mL/hr, 20% glucose represents 16.7 mg/kg per minute of glucose. The hyperglycemia and glycosuria probably have occurred because the increases in the infusion rate have exceeded J.H.'s ability to adapt to the glucose dose. However, patients who have been euglycemic on their glucose dose and then become glucose intolerant should be evaluated for other causes, such as infection.[62]

Hyperglycemia and glycosuria may result in serum hyperosmolarity, osmotic diuresis, and dehydration. Regardless of the cause, the hyperglycemia should be treated by reducing the glucose administration rate. Therefore, the first step in managing the hyperglycemia would be to decrease J.H.'s PN rate. If needed, a second IV solution, without dextrose, may be added to meet his fluid requirements. For example, the PN solution could be decreased to 8 mL/hr to provide 13.3 mg/kg per minute of glucose. The sodium and potassium content of the second fluid should be identical to the concentration in the PN solution to avoid electrolyte imbalance. After this new fluid combination is initiated, the blood and urine glucose should again be monitored at frequent intervals. The rate of the PN infusion can be decreased further if hyperglycemia continues or increased if the hyperglycemia resolves. The second fluid and electrolyte infusion rate should be adjusted accordingly.

When the PN order is written for the subsequent days, the glucose increases should be made in smaller amounts up to the maintenance calorie requirements per day. Frequent blood and urine glucose monitoring must be continued. Severe glucose intolerance in patients who require PN can be managed with insulin to normalize serum glucose. Although insulin is compatible with PN solutions, it does adsorb to glass, polyvinyl chloride, and filters, resulting in decreased delivery of insulin.[63] The addition of albumin may decrease the binding of insulin to solution containers.[64] Frequently, pediatric patients have changing insulin requirements that prevent the addition of insulin to PN solutions. A separate continuous infusion of regular insulin (initial dose: 0.05 to 0.1 units/kg per hour) titrated to control serum glucose concentrations offers a practical solution to minimize waste of the PN solution.[65] It is essential to discontinue the insulin infusion if the PN solution is discontinued to avoid hypoglycemia.

Effects of Bronchopulmonary Dysplasia and Mechanical Ventilation

30. **J.H. remains dependent on a ventilator because of his immature lungs. How could J.H.'s respiratory disease influence his nutritional regimen?**

At older than 28 days of age, ventilator dependence defines J.H. as having bronchopulmonary dysplasia (BPD), a chronic lung disease of infancy. BPD is characterized by an increase in resting energy expenditure, increased work of breathing, and growth failure.[66,67] Therefore, J.H.'s caloric requirement may be higher than expected. Additionally, J.H.'s ventilator may also alter the approach to his caloric supply. Very high carbohydrate loads have been associated with an increase in carbon dioxide production.[68] This, in turn, may make it difficult to wean J.H. from the mechanical ventilator. As previously discussed, rapid infusions of fat emulsion also may also have a detrimental effect on pulmonary function. Fat emulsion should not be omitted from J.H.'s PN regimen; rather, a slower infusion rate, with gradual dose increases, while monitoring pulmonary function is appropriate.

Pediatric Amino Acid Formulations

31. **Why would a specialized pediatric amino acid solution be preferable to a standard adult formulation for J.H.?**

Patients 1 year of age or older tolerate standard adult amino acid preparations (e.g., Aminosyn [Abbott Laboratories] and Travasol [Baxter Healthcare]) well. For infants younger than 1 year of age, two specifically designed amino acid solutions—TrophAmine (B. Braun) and Aminosyn PF (Abbott Laboratories)—are available. TrophAmine is available as a 6% solution and a 10% solution and has a pH of 5.5. Aminosyn-PF is available as a 7% and 10% solution and has a pH of 5.4. The pH of these formulations decreases further when 40 mg of L-cysteine per gram of protein is added. Pediatric amino acid formulations (PAAFs) were developed in response to the abnormal plasma amino acid patterns noted in infants receiving adult amino acid formulations. The products were designed with the goal of producing plasma amino acid patterns closely matching those of 2-hour postprandial, human-milk–fed infants. Theoretically, normal plasma amino acid patterns will promote normal protein synthesis in growing infants.

PAAFS differ from conventional amino acid formulations in several ways. First, they contain a higher content of branch chain amino acids (leucine, isoleucine, and valine); and a lower content of glycine, methionine, and phenylalanine (Table 97-11). In addition, PAAFs have a higher percentage of essential amino acids with a wider distribution of the nonessential amino acids. Finally, PAAFs are unique in that they contain three essential amino acids for neonates: taurine, tyrosine (as N-acetyl-L-tyrosine), and cysteine (added as L-cysteine HCl). Adult solutions contain little if any of these amino acids. Neonates have immature liver functions. This results in decreased levels of both hepatic cystathionase and phenylalanine hydroxylase enzymes. Without these enzymes,

neonates cannot adequately convert methionine to cysteine or phenylalanine to tyrosine or synthesize taurine from cysteine. Deficiencies in these amino acids can have significant impact on the health of the neonate. For example, taurine has a role in retinal development, protection and stabilization of cell membranes, neurotransmission, regulation of cell volume, and bile acid conjugation. Taurine also may be important in decreasing or preventing cholestasis associated with long-term PN.

Several investigators have studied the clinical, nutritional, and biochemical effects of TrophAmine in term and preterm infants.[69,70] The use of TrophAmine was found to result in nearly normal amino acid patterns. In addition, patients receiving TrophAmine had greater weight gain and significantly better nitrogen utilization than similar groups using the adult formulations. TrophAmine and Aminosyn-PF over a 7-day period produce comparable weight gain and nitrogen retention.[71] In one study, some of the VLBW infants experienced metabolic acidosis.[69] L-cysteine, a HCl salt, provides an additional 5.7 mEq Cl/100 mg and may have contributed to the acidosis. While the manufacturer's recommended dose of 40 mg L-cysteine per gram of amino acid may be too much for the VLBW infant; the most appropriate dose of L-cysteine for the VLBW infant has not been determined.

To date, PAAFs have been effective in producing a positive weight gain, positive nitrogen balance, and normalizing amino acid patterns in preterm neonates. They also allow for the provision of larger doses of calcium and phosphorus because PAAFs lower the pH of the final PN solution. Providing larger amounts of calcium and phosphorus, in appropriate ratios, should minimize metabolic bone disease. Further evaluation of these products is needed to determine the magnitude of the proposed benefits (i.e., improved nitrogen retention, better weight gain, enhanced bone growth, and decreased cholestasis) and the most appropriate L-cysteine dose to use in VLBW infants. In any event, these potential benefits, and clinical experience with these products, have resulted in the use of PAAFs as the standard of care in infants requiring PN.

Carnitine

32. **Why would carnitine supplementation be warranted in J.II.?**

Carnitine has many functions within the body, but it primarily serves to transport long-chain fatty acids (LCFA) across the mitochondrial membrane where they undergo β-oxidation to produce energy. Deficiency in carnitine lessens LCFA availability for oxidation, resulting in the accumulation of LCFA and a decrease in ketone and adenosine triphosphate (ATP) production. This can adversely affect the CNS and skeletal and cardiac muscles. Carnitine deficiency in premature infants also has been linked to disorders such as GI reflux, apnea, and bradycardia.[72]

Whereas carnitine is a nonessential nutrient in adults and is readily available from a diet that includes meat and dairy products, it appears to be an essential nutrient in neonates and infants. This population has low body stores of carnitine and a decreased ability to synthesize it on their own. The premature infant has even lower stores of carnitine because carnitine accumulation occurs during the third trimester. Human milk and most cow's milk–based infant formulas contain carnitine.

Table 97-11 Pediatric Amino Acid Solutions

	TrophAmine 6%	Aminosyn-PF 7%
Essential Amino Acids (EAA) (mg/1 g Total Amino Acids)		
Isoleucine	81.7	76.3
Leucine	140.0	118.7
Lysine	81.7	67.9
Methionine	33.3	17.9
Phenylalanine	48.3	42.9
Threonine	41.7	51.4
Tryptophan	20.0	17.9
Valine	78.3	64.6
Cysteine HCl[a]	3.3	0
Histidine	48.3	31.4
Tyrosine	23.3	6.3
Taurine	2.5	7.1
Nonessential Amino Acids (mg/1 g Total Amino Acids)		
Alanine	53.3	70.0
Arginine	121.7	123.0
Proline	68.3	81.4
Serine	38.3	49.6
Glycine	36.7	38.6
L-aspartic acid	31.7	52.9
L-glutamic acid	50.0	82.3
Sodium (mEq/L)	5.0	3.4
Acetate (mEq/L)	56.0	32.5
Chloride (mEq/L)	<3	0
% essential amino acid	60.1	50.2
% branched chain amino acid (g amino acid/1 g nitrogen)	30.0	26.0

[a] 40 g of cysteine syringe available.

Some soy-based formulas have additional carnitine added during manufacturing. However, PN is not routinely supplemented with carnitine. Therefore, infants who are exclusively fed by PN are at risk for developing complications associated with carnitine deficiency.[72]

Because J.H. has two risk factors for the development of carnitine deficiency (prematurity and exclusive use of PN), and because carnitine has little or no adverse effects associated with its use, it is appropriate to provide J.H. with a carnitine supplement. Carnitine is available as both an oral and intravenous formulation. The recommended dose in J.H. is 10 to 20 mg/kg per day. The addition of carnitine directly to PN improves carnitine plasma concentrations and nutritional status.

Septicemia

33. J.H. was diagnosed with necrotizing enterocolitis and received 14 days of antibiotics. On his sixth day off antibiotics, he begins having 15 to 20 episodes of bradycardia per day. His physical examination is remarkable for cold extremities and slow capillary refill, but his chest radiographs show no acute change. Laboratory evaluation at this time includes electrolytes, blood glucose, complete blood count, and blood cultures, which are reported as follows: Na, 139 mEq/L (normal, 135 to 145 mEq/L); K, 4.7 mEq/L (normal, 3.5 to 5.0 mEq/L); Cl, 112 mEq/L (normal, 102 to 109 mEq/L); HCO_3^-, 17 mEq/L (normal, 22 to 29 mEq/L); glucose, 164 mg/dL (normal, 70 to 105 mg/dL); platelet count, 36,000/mm³ (normal, 150,000 to 450,000/mm³); and white blood cell (WBC) count, 24,300/mm³ (normal, 5,500 to 18,000). WBC differential includes 52% segmented neutrophils (normal, 20% to 50%) and 27% immature neutrophils (normal, 3% to 5%). Blood cultures are drawn; results will be unavailable for at least 24 hours. What is the likely cause of these findings? How might J.H.'s nutrition regimen affect the diagnostic evaluation and treatment selected?

[SI units: Na, 139 mmol/L (normal, 135 to 145); K, 4.7 mmol/L (normal, 3.5 to 5.0); Cl, 112 mmol/L (normal, 102 to 109); HCO_3^-, 17 mmol/L (normal, 22 to 29); glucose, 9.1 mmol/L (normal, 3.9 to 5.8); platelet count, 36 × 10⁹/L (normal, 150 to 450); WBC count, 24.3 × 10⁶ cells/L (normal, 5.5 to 18.0)]

This constellation of findings (metabolic acidosis, hyperglycemia, thrombocytopenia, leukocytosis, bradycardia, and poor perfusion) is nonspecific but could represent septicemia.

The presence of a central venous catheter predisposes J.H. to infection with Gram-negative bacteria and bacteria normally found on the skin (e.g., coagulase-negative staphylococci).[73] Cultures growing coagulase-negative staphylococci must not be presumed to be the result of contamination in symptomatic patients. The typical antimicrobial sensitivities of this organism dictate that vancomycin be among the empiric antibiotics. A third-generation cephalosporin to cover Gram-negative organisms should be added empirically as well.[74]

The central venous catheter, and the use of broad-spectrum antibiotics also predisposes J.H. to fungal infection.[75] Candidal infection may occur, and when fat emulsions are used, as in J.H., systemic infection with *Malassezia furfur* must be considered. *M. furfur* is a normal skin fungus that requires an exogenous source of fatty acids. The empiric use of antifungal drugs is not indicated in patients with *M. furfur*; however, the clinician should screen specifically for this fungus by culture.

Metabolic Bone Disease (Rickets)

34. On the chest radiograph taken to evaluate the septic episode just described, the radiologist notes that J.H. has two rib fractures and that the bones appear undermineralized. The most recent laboratory values show a serum calcium (Ca) of 9.3 mg/dL (normal, 8.5 to 10.5 mg/dL), a serum phosphorus of 3.6 mg/dL (normal, 4.0 to 8.5 mg/dL), and an alkaline phosphatase of 674 U/L (normal, 350 U/L). What diagnosis is suggested by these findings? How and why has J.H.'s nutrition regimen placed him at risk for this disease?

[SI units: Ca, 2.3 mmol/L (normal, 2.1 to 2.6); phosphorus, 1.16 mmol/L (normal, 1.3 to 2.7); phosphatase, 674 U/L (normal, 350)]

During the last trimester of pregnancy, bone accretion is accelerated reaching its peak at about 36 weeks. Premature infants, therefore, require larger calcium and phosphorous doses. However, limitations to venous access may preclude the infusion of concentrated calcium solutions peripherally, and their end-organs may be resistant to vitamin D. Thus, metabolic bone disease is not unexpected in a premature infant such as J.H.

Aluminum, a contaminant in some parenteral salt products (particularly calcium), also may play a role in impaired bone mineraliziation.[76] Low serum phosphorus with high alkaline phosphatase, undermineralized bones, and fractures resulting from routine handling are consistent with a diagnosis of rickets.

PN solutions provide calcium and phosphorus in much smaller amounts than the infant would accumulate in utero.[77] Solution pH, temperature, calcium salt, and final calcium and phosphorus concentrations influence their solubility in PN solutions. An acidic PN solution favors the solubility of these salts. The pH of commercially available amino acid preparations ranges from 5.4 (in the PAAFs) to 7 (in adult amino acid formulations). The addition of l-cysteine, with a pH of 1.5, also makes the solution more acidic. Since dextrose also is acidic, solutions with higher dextrose concentrations are more acidic. Of note, colder storage temperatures promotes calcium and phosphorus solubility. Therefore, refrigerated PN solutions may appear to be free of precipitate on visual inspection. However, calcium and phosphate may precipitate when warmed to room temperature, or when infused into patients with fever or in incubators. Calcium salt selection is another important consideration because the chloride salt dissociates rapidly and favors precipitation while the gluconate and gluceptate salts dissociate less quickly.

CALCIUM AND PHOSPHORUS SUPPLEMENTATION

35. How should the supply of these nutrients be altered to address J.H.'s rickets?

It is important to provide sufficient amounts of calcium and phosphorus. The provision of calcium and phosphorus either as a 1 to 1.3:1 molar ratio (or 1.3 to 1.7:1 weight ratio) will allow for adequate bone mineralization.[78] Providing alternating solutions containing either calcium or phosphorus alone results in wide fluctuations in plasma concentrations of these minerals and should be avoided.[79]

Although oral treatment of rickets would require supplemental vitamin D to enhance absorption of calcium and phosphorus, when these minerals are supplied parenterally, vitamin D doses similar to those in Table 97-1 are adequate.[80]

Parenteral pediatric multivitamin preparations provide an appropriate dose of vitamin D. Serum phosphorus concentrations should be monitored several times per week and phosphorus intake adjusted to prevent symptomatic hypophosphatemia. Serum calcium is not useful as an indicator of disease activity because it will remain normal at the expense of bone mineralization. This is demonstrated by J.H.'s serum calcium at the time of diagnosis (see Question 33).

Liver Disease Associated With Parenteral Nutrition

36. On the 56th day of life, J.H. is noted to be mildly jaundiced. A review of his laboratory tests reveal the following:

Test	Age (days)				
	22	29	36	43	50
AST (U/L) (normal, <40)	14	17	15	20	25
ALT (U/L) (normal, <28)	6	7	10	10	11
Alkaline phosphatase (IU/L) (normal, <350)	103	158	345	506	695
Bilirubin					
Indirect (normal, <1 mg/dL)	0.9	0.9	0.8	0.8	0.9
Direct (normal, <0.2)	0.1	0.1	0.8	1.6	3

Could this be related to his PN?

In past decades, hepatic damage has been reported in up to one-third of infants receiving PN,[81] with a higher prevalence (up to 50%) in VLBW infants such as J.H.[82] Although it is still a concern today, hepatic damage is less prevalent because there is better understanding of how to manage infants requiring long-term PN. The laboratory abnormalities reported in J.H. are typical of this complication. The first change observed is usually an elevated direct (conjugated) bilirubin, which can occur as early as 2 weeks after beginning PN.[83] Increases in the serum concentrations of the hepatic enzymes, AST and ALT, lag 2 weeks or more behind the rise in direct bilirubin.[83] Alkaline phosphatase also may rise, but it is a nonspecific indicator of liver disease. Alkaline phosphatase is produced by the liver, GI tract, and bones.[83] Although the laboratory results observed in J.H. are consistent with the pattern associated with liver disease induced by PN, PN-associated cholestasis is a diagnosis of exclusion; therefore, other causes, such as viral hepatitis, must be ruled out.

RISK FACTORS

37. What clinical factors placed J.H. at high risk for developing cholestatic liver disease secondary to PN?

Although components of PN solutions are commonly blamed for the development of cholestasis, there are many potential causes.[84] J.H. has several other risk factors for developing cholestasis, and prolonged enteral fasting may be the most significant.[85] Stimulation of bile flow and gallbladder contraction depend on GI hormones, which depend on enteral feeding for their release.[86] Absence of these secretogogues, therefore, can promote cholestasis.[87-89] Immature hepatic function secondary to prematurity also places J.H. at risk, as does the duration of PN therapy. As the duration of PN use increases, so does the prevalence of hepatic disease in premature infants; 25% of infants nourished in this manner for ≥30 days show evidence of cholestasis.[82] Surgical patients have a greater likelihood of developing hyperbilirubinemia than medical patients, especially those requiring GI surgery.[90,91] A large number of surgical procedures is associated with a higher risk of jaundice.[85] Finally, J.H.'s infection increases his risk for cholestasis.[92]

The use of adult amino acid preparations in infants increases the risk of cholestasis. In one study, the incidence of cholestasis in VLBW infants receiving TrophAmine was reduced to 23% relative to historical controls of 30% to 50%.[93] In another study comparing the two PAAFs, no difference in the incidence of cholestasis was found in infants 1 year old, and the overall incidence of cholestasis was 27%.[5] These investigators did not assess whether or not the patients were provided with l-cysteine, which may be important because l-cysteine is a precursor for taurine and taurine forms the water-soluble nontoxic bile acid, taurocholate.

Additional risk factors for cholestasis not present in J.H. are the administration of large amounts of protein or dextrose. Since amino acids are actively transported in hepatocytes, it is important to provide appropriate types and amounts of amino acids to minimize the development of cholestasis. In one study, a high-protein regimen (3.6 g/kg per day) was associated with an earlier onset and greater degree of cholestasis than a low-protein regimen (2.3 g/kg per day).[94] Similarly, dextrose overload is a known cause of hepatic steatosis and has been shown to decrease bile flow.[95] Therefore, overly aggressive feeding of J.H. with PN should be avoided.

In addition to the hepatic damage, gallstones have been reported in infants and children receiving PN.[96,97] The ileal resection performed during the acute phase of his necrotizing enterocolitis may put J.H. at increased risk for this hepatobiliary complication as well.[96]

38. What modifications can be made in J.H.'s regimen in the presence of cholestasis?

First, the institution of enteral feeding needs to be considered. Even low-volume trophic feeding may help alleviate the condition and should be attempted in cholestatic patients. Next, the protein and glucose dose provided by the PN should be evaluated. During cholestasis, calories should be provided using an appropriate mix of protein, carbohydrate, and fat.

Although the effect of cycling a patient off PN has not been evaluated in clinical trials, this should be considered. Cycling PN, when the infusion rate is gradually decreased to off for a period and then restarted and gradually increased to the desired rate, will decrease the length of time the liver is exposed to PN. Unfortunately, VLBW infants may become hypoglycemic even with very gradual decreases in infusion rate, so this option should be used with care. In any event, a short time off PN (e.g., 2 hours) should be attempted.

The trace elements provided by the formulation should be examined. Both copper and manganese are enterohepatically recycled and may accumulate in liver disease. Manganese may also contribute to hepatotoxicity and should be removed from J.H.'s PN solutions. Studies have not established when removal of copper and manganese is warranted. The inappropriate removal of copper could lead to anemia, osteopenia, and neutropenia.[49] Therefore, decreasing the copper dose and monitoring serum concentrations of both copper and manganese should guide therapy.

Pharmacologic interventions have had limited success in the management of PN-associated cholestasis. Neither phenobarbital nor bile acid binding agents, such as cholestyramine, are effective in reducing or reversing PN-associated cholestasis.[98,99] Ursodiol 10 to 20 mg/kg per day has been used successfully in the treatment of other cholestatic liver diseases, and preliminary reports indicate that it may also improve PN-associated cholestasis in children.[100] Ursodiol, a naturally occurring nontoxic bile acid, presumably works by displacing and replacing the endogenously produced, potentially toxic bile salts that accumulate with cholestasis.

The antibiotic, metronidazole, also appears promising in the prevention of PN-associated cholestasis in adults. Metronidazole inhibits the bacterial overgrowth in the GI tract that occurs with intestinal stasis. The bacteria are responsible for increased formation of hepatotoxic bile acids such as lithocholate; 15 mg/kg per day of metronidazole has been shown to prevent lithocholate accumulation.[101]

PROGNOSIS

39. **Project the course of J.H.'s liver disease if PN is discontinued and enteral feedings are instituted within 2 weeks. What may occur if enteral feedings cannot be instituted?**

If PN can be discontinued soon after the onset of cholestasis, the prospects for J.H. to recover normal hepatic function are good. Jaundice usually resolves within 2 weeks after PN is discontinued, and the biochemical abnormalities normalize soon thereafter.[102] The pathologic changes observed on biopsy resolve even more slowly. Biopsy evidence of cholestasis has been observed for up to 40 weeks after resolution of clinical and serologic evidence of hepatic disease.[102,103]

If enteral feedings cannot be instituted successfully, the prognosis for J.H.'s liver function is not as good. Studies have demonstrated that infants receiving PN for ≥90 days had biopsy evidence of irreversible liver damage.[88] Thus, it clearly is advantageous to convert J.H.'s nutrition to the enteral route as soon as he tolerates such a change.

TOLERANCE OF CONVERSION TO ENTERAL FEEDING

40. **On day 60 of life, J.H.'s intestinal remnants are reanastomosed. Given the desirability of feeding J.H. enterally as soon as possible, what aspects of his disease and surgery will influence his ability to tolerate such a regimen?**

J.H.'s surgery involved the resection of two-thirds of his jejunum and one-third of his ileum. Having his terminal ileum and ileocecal valve intact should have a positive impact on his ability to be successfully fed enterally. The terminal ileum is the site of absorption for vitamin B_{12}[104] and bile salts.[105] Absence of the ileocecal valve permits the overgrowth of colonic bacteria in the small intestine and may result in a malabsorption state by various mechanisms.[104] Because J.H. has his ileocecal valve, this should not be a concern.

Even infants with necrotizing enterocolitis without perforation may form strictures in areas of diseased intestine upon resolution of the acute illness.[52] Thus, feeding difficulties, surgery to correct strictures, and consequent periods of NPO may become necessary for J.H. again in the future.

Not all infants with necrotizing enterocolitis develop long-term nutritional difficulties. Without major intestinal resection, nutritional status and GI function can be normalized by 1 year of age or earlier.[106]

ENTERAL REFEEDING

41. **Plan a regimen for refeeding J.H. enterally.**

The re-initiation of enteral feedings in a patient such as J.H. who has undergone resection of a large part of his small intestine can be viewed as an attempt to provide four separate nutrient components: protein, fat, carbohydrate, and micronutrients. Each is subject to its own regulatory mechanisms and may independently lead to the success or failure of the entire regimen. An important problem underlying the absorption of all nutrients is the decrease in surface area available for absorption which resulted from J.H.'s resection. Absorptive adaptation of the surgically shortened intestine is more efficient with enteral nutrient administration, even if it is carried out only in small amounts as a supplement of PN.[45] Thus, trophic feeds should be initiated as early as possible.

A knowledge of the physiology of the small intestine underlies determination of the enteral prescription. It is important that the healthy sections of J.H.'s intestine have been reconnected because this procedure provides a larger total absorptive surface area.

Protein is unlikely to create diarrhea[45] but may be malabsorbed if the absorptive surface area is diminished. The malabsorption can be minimized by the administration of a formula containing protein in the form of short chain peptides that are absorbed more efficiently and are less osmotically active than free amino acids.[3]

Carbohydrate absorption has already been discussed (see Question 24). The same principles apply to the patient with a surgical short gut.

J.H. has a terminal ileum, thus, he is not at significant risk for excessive loss of bile acids and attendant fat malabsorption.[105] In patients without a terminal ileum, administration of part or most of the fat intake as MCTs will bypass the problem of fat absorption because these do not require bile for micelle formation, do not need to be re-esterified in the intestinal cell, and can be absorbed directly into the portal circulation bound to albumin.[107,108] EFAD will not be prevented by use of MCTs, however, and a source of long-chain fatty acids should be used in a quantity similar to that provided parenterally to satisfy this need (4 to 5% of total caloric intake as linoleic acid).

In addition to choosing an infant formula, it will be necessary to specify how it is to be given. In an infant who can coordinate the sucking and swallowing actions, oral feedings may be attempted; the infant who is incapable of such coordination will need to be fed through an orogastric or nasogastric tube. The tube feedings may be delivered by either continuous infusion or intermittent bolus administration. If patients receiving bolus feedings either orally or by tube develop diarrhea, substantial stool fluid and nutrient loss can occur. This can be minimized by changing the infant to a continuous feeding regimen.[30] Monitoring for carbohydrate and fat malabsorption can be achieved by measuring stool pH and reducing substances as well as quantitative fat excretion as outlined in Question 25.

REFERENCES

1. Holliday MA, Segar WE. The maintenance need for water in parenteral fluid therapy. Pediatrics 1957;19:823.
2. Al-Jurf AS et al. Effect of nutritional method on adaptation of the intestinal remnant after massive bowel resection. J Pediatr Gastroenterol Nutr 1985;4:245.
3. Greene HL et al. Guidelines for the use of vitamins, trace elements, calcium, magnesium, and phosphorus in infants and children receiving total parenteral nutrition: report of the subcommittee on pediatric parenteral nutrient requirements from the committee on clinical practice issues of the American Society for Clinical Nutrition. Am J Clin Nutr 1988;48:1324.
4. Greene HL et al. Persistently low blood retinol levels during and after parenteral feeding of very low-birth-weight infants: examination of losses into intravenous administration sets and a method of prevention by addition to a lipid emulsion. Pediatrics 1987;79:84.
5. Gura K, Forchielli M. Incidence of cholestasis in infants receiving parenteral nutrition: comparison of Aminosyn-PF and TrophAmine. J Patenter Enteral Nutr 1992;16(Suppl):28S.
6. Santosham M et al. Oral rehydration therapy of infantile diarrhea: a controlled study of well-nourished children hospitalized in the United States and Panama. N Engl J Med 1983;306:1070.
7. Santosham M et al. Oral rehydration therapy for acute diarrhea in ambulatory children in the United States: a double-blind comparison of four different solutions. Pediatrics 1985;76:159.
8. Pizzaro D et al. Oral rehydration in hypernatremic and hyponatremic diarrheal dehydration. Am J Dis Child 1983;137:730.
9. Meeuwisse GW. High sugar worse than high sodium in oral rehydration solutions. Acta Paediatr Scand 1983;72:161.
10. Guzman C et al. Hypernatremic diarrheal dehydration treated with oral glucose—electrolyte solution containing 90 or 75 mEq/L of sodium. J Gastroenterol Nutr 1988;7:694.
11. American Academy of Pediatrics, Committee on Nutrition. On the feeding of supplemental foods to infants. Pediatrics 1980;65:1178.
12. Bucuvalas JC et al. The neonatal gastrointestinal tract. In: Fanaroff AA et al, eds. Neonatal-Perinatal Medicine: Disease of the Fetus and Infant. St Louis: Mosby, 1987:894.
13. Anderson GH. Human milk feeding. Pediatr Clin North Am 1985;32:335.
14. Yom HC, Bremel RD. Genetic engineering of milk composition: modification of milk components in lactating transgenic animals. Am J Clin Nutr 1993;58(Suppl):299.
15. Garza C et al. Special properties of human milk. Clin Perinatol 1987;14:11.
16. Oski FA. Iron deficiency—facts and fallacies. Pediatr Clin North Am 1985;32:493.
17. American Academy of Pediatrics, Committee on Nutrition. Fluoride supplementation. Pediatrics 1986;77:758.
18. Dewey KG et al. Differences in morbidity between breast-fed and formula-fed infants. J Pediatr 1995;126.
19. Churchill RB, Pickering LK. The pros (many) and cons (a few) of breastfeeding. Contemp Pediatr 1998;15:18.
20. Committee on Nutrition. Soy-protein formulas: recommendations for use in infant feeding. Pediatrics 1983;72:359.
21. Committee on Nutrition. Hypoallergenic infant formulas. Pediatrics 1989;83:1068.
22. Anonymous. Enterobacter sakazakii infections associated with the use of powdered infant formula-Tennessee 2001. MMWR 2002;51:298.
23. Fomon SJ et al. Cow milk feeding in infancy: gastrointestinal blood loss and iron nutritional status. J Pediatr 1981;98:540.
24. Crump IM. Selected inborn errors of metabolism. In: Kelts DG, Jones EG, eds. Manual of Pediatric Nutrition. Boston: Little, Brown, 1984:211.
25. Collins JE et al. The dietary management of inborn errors of metabolism. Hum Nutr Appl Nutr 1985;39:255.
26. Dunn L et al. Beneficial effects of early hypocaloric enteral feeding on neonatal gastrointestinal function: preliminary report of a randomized trial. J Pediatr 1988;112:622.
27. Slagle TA, Gross SJ. Effect of early low-volume enteral substrate on subsequent feeding tolerance in very low-birth-weight infants. J Pediatr 1988;113:526.
28. Parker P et al. A controlled comparison of continuous versus intermittent feeding in the treatment of infants with intestinal disease. J Pediatr 1981;99:360.
29. Leleiko NS et al. Nutritional assessment of pediatric patients admitted to an acute-care pediatric service utilizing anthropometric measurements. J Parenter Enteral Nutr 1986;10:166.
30. Georgieff MK et al. Effect of neonatal caloric deprivation on head growth and 1-year developmental status in preterm infants. J Pediatr 1985;107:581.
31. Galler JR et al. Long-term effects of early kwashiorkor compared with marasmus. II. Intellectual performance. J Pediatr Gastroenterol Nutr 1987;6:847.
32. Galler JR et al. Long-term effects of early kwashiorkor compared with marasmus. III. Fine motor skills. J Pediatr Gastroenterol Nutr 1987;6:855.
33. 2000 CDC growth charts: United States. Retrieved April 1, 2003 from the World Wide Web: http://www.cdc.gov/growthcharts.
34. Thomas MR et al. Evaluation of transthyretin as a monitor of protein-energy intake in preterm and sick neonatal infants. J Parenter Enteral Nutr 1988;12:162.
35. Yoder MC et al. Comparison of serum fibronectin, prealbumin and albumin concentrations during nutritional repletion in protein calorie malnourished infants. J Pediatr Gastroenterol Nutr 1987;6:84.
36. Georgieff MK et al. Serum transthyretin levels and protein intake as predictors of weight gain velocity in premature infants. J Pediatr Gastroenterol Nutr 1987;6:775.
37. Moskowitz SR et al. Prealbumin as a biochemical marker of nutritional adequacy in premature infants J Pediatr 1983,102:749.
38. Vanlandingham S et al. Prealbumin: a parameter of visceral protein levels during albumin infusion. J Parenter Enteral Nutr 1982;6:230.
39. Ramsden DB et al. The interrelationship of thyroid hormones, vitamin A and the binding proteins following acute stress. Clin Endocrinol 1978;8:109.
40. Sandstedt S et al. Influence of total parenteral nutrition on plasma fibronectin in malnourished subjects with or without inflammatory response. J Parenter Enteral Nutr 1984;8:493.
41. Hill R et al. An evaluation of D-xylose absorption measurements in children suspected of having small intestinal disease. J Pediatr 1981; 99:245.
42. Orenstein SR. Enteral versus parenteral therapy for intractable diarrhea of infancy: a prospective, randomized trial. J Pediatr 1986;109:277.
43. Rossi TM et al. Extent and duration of small intestinal mucosal injury in tractable diarrhea of infancy. Pediatrics 1980;66:730.
44. Green HL et al. Protracted diarrhea and malnutrition in infancy: changes in intestinal morphology and disaccharidase activities during treatment with total intravenous nutrition or oral elemental diets. J Pediatr 1975;87:695.
45. Klish WJ, Putman TC. The short gut. Am J Dis Child 1981;135:1056.
46. Greene HL et al. Evaluation of a pediatric multiple vitamin preparation for total parenteral nutrition. II. Blood levels of vitamins A, D, and E. Pediatrics 1987;77:539.
47. Moore MC et al. Evaluation of a pediatric multiple vitamin preparation for total parenteral nutrition in infants and children. I. Blood levels of water soluble vitamins. Pediatrics 1987;77:530.
48. Hambridge M. Trace element deficiencies in childhood. In: Suskind RM, ed. Textbook of Pediatric Nutrition. New York: Raven, 1981:163.
49. Knight P et al. Calcium and phosphate requirements of preterm infants who require prolonged hyperalimentation. JAMA 1980;2432:1244
50. Heird WC et al. Intravenous alimentation in pediatric patients. J Pediatr 1972;80:351.
51. Topper WH. Enteral feeding methods for compromised neonates and infants. In: Lebenthal E, ed. Textbook of Gastroenterology and Nutrition in Infancy. New York: Raven, 1981:645.
52. Kleigman RJ, Fanaroff A. Necrotizing enterocolitis. N Engl J Med 1984;310:1093.
53. Pildres RS, Lilien LD. Carbohydrate metabolism in the fetus and neonate. In: Fanaroff AA, Martin RJ, eds. Behrman's Neonatal-Perinatal Medicine. St. Louis: Mosby, 1983;845.
54. Kao LC et al. Triglycerides, free fatty acids, free fatty acids/albumin molar ratio and cholesterol levels in serum of neonates receiving long-term lipid infusions: controlled trial of continuous and intermittent regimens. J Pediatr 1984;104:429.
55. Cochran EB, Phelps SJ, Helms RA. Parenteral nutrition in pediatric patients. Clin Pharm 1988;7:351.
56. Phelps SJ et al. Effect of the continuous administration of fat emulsion on the infiltration of intravenous lines in infants receiving peripheral nutrition solutions. J Parenter Enteral Nutr 1989;13:628.
57. Pineault M et al. Beneficial effect of coinfusing a lipid emulsion on venous patency. J Parenter Enteral Nutr 1989;13:637.
58. Zabielski PB et al. Necrotizing enterocolitis: feeding in endemic and epidemic periods. J Parenter Enteral Nutr 1989;13:520.
59. Friedman Z et al. Rapid onset of essential fatty acid deficiency in the newborn. Pediatrics 1976;58:640.
60. Herson VC et al. Effect of intravenous fat infusion on neonatal neutrophil and platelet function. J Parenter Enteral Nutr 1989;13:620.
61. Andrew G et al. Lipid metabolism in the neonate: II. The effect of Intralipid in bilirubin binding in vitro and in vivo. J Pediatr 1976;88:279.
62. Beisel WR. Metabolic response of the host to infections. In: Feigin RD, Cherry JD, eds. Textbook of Pediatric Infectious Disease. Philadelphia: WB Saunders, 1981:1.
63. Weber SS et al. Availability of insulin from parenteral nutrient solutions. Am J Hosp Pharm 1977;34:353.
64. Niemiec PW, Vanderveen TW. Compatibility considerations in parenteral nutrient solutions. Am J Hosp Pharm 1984;41:893.
65. Sajbel TA et al. Use of separate insulin infusions with total parenteral nutrition. J Parenter Enteral Nutr 1987;11:97.
66. Yeh TF et al. Metabolic rate and energy balance in infants with bronchopulmonary dysplasia. J Pediatr 1989; 114:448.
67. Kurzner SI et al. Growth failure in infants with bronchopulmonary dysplasia: nutrition and elevated resting metabolic expenditure. Pediatrics 1988; 81:379.
68. Covelli HD et al. Respiratory failure precipitated by high carbohydrate loads. Ann Intern Med 1981; 95:579.
69. Heird WC et al. Pediatric parenteral amino acid mixture in low birth weight infants. Pediatrics 1988;81:41.
70. Helms RA et al. Comparison of a pediatric versus standard amino acid formulation in preterm neonates requiring parenteral nutrition. J Pediatr 1987;110:466.
71. Adamkin D, McClead R. Comparison of two neonatal intravenous amino acid formulations in preterm infants: a multicenter study. J Perinatol 1991;11:375.

72. Crill CM et al. Carnitine: a conditionally essential nutrient in the neonatal population? J Pediatr Pharm Pract 1999;4:127.

73. Baumgart S et al. Sepsis with coagulase-negative staphylococci in critically-ill newborns. Am J Dis Child 1983;137:461.

74. Lowy FD, Hammer SM. Staphylococcus epidermidis infection. Ann Intern Med 1983;99:834.

75. Johnson DE. Systemic candidiasis in very low-birth-weight infants (1500 grams). Pediatrics 1984;73:138.

76. Koo WWK et al. Response of preterm infants to aluminum in parenteral nutrition. J Parenter Enteral Nutr 1989;13:516.

77. Ziegler EE et al. Body composition of the reference fetus. Growth 1976;40:329.

78. Koo WWK. Parenteral nutrition-related bone disease. J Parenter Enteral Nutr 1992;16:386.

79. Hoehn GJ et al. Alternate day infusion of calcium and phosphate in very low-birth-weight infants: wasting of the infused mineral. J Pediatr Gastroenterol Nutr 1987;6:752.

80. Koo WWK et al. Vitamin D requirements in infants receiving parenteral nutrition. J Parenter Enteral Nutr 1987;11:172.

81. Postuma R, Trevenen CL. Liver disease in infants receiving total parenteral nutrition. Pediatrics 1979;63:110.

82. Pereira GR et al. Hyperalimentation-induced cholestasis: increased incidence and severity in premature infants. Am J Dis Child 1981;135:842.

83. Vileisis RA et al. Laboratory monitoring of parenteral nutrition-associated hepatic dysfunction in infants. J Parenter Enteral Nutr 1981;5:67.

84. Merritt RJ. Cholestasis associated with total parenteral nutrition. J Pediatr Gastroenterol Nutr 1986;5:22.

85. Drongowski RA et al. An analysis of factors contributing to the development of total parenteral nu-trition-induced cholestasis. J Parenter Enteral Nutr 1989;13:586.

86. Lucas A et al. Metabolic and endocrine consequences of depriving preterm infants of enteral nutrition. Acta Paediatr Scand 1983;72:245.

87. Enzenauer RW et al. Total parenteral nutrition cholestasis: a cause of mechanical biliary obstruction. Pediatrics 1985;76:905.

88. Cohen C, Olsen MM. Pediatric total parenteral nutrition: liver histopathology. Arch Pathol Lab Med 1981;105:152.

89. Benjamin DR. Hepatobiliary dysfunction in infants and children associated with long-term total parenteral nutrition: a clinicopathologic study. Am J Clin Pathol 1981;76:276.

90. Kattwinkel J et al. The effects of age on alkaline phosphatase and other serologic liver function tests in normal subjects and patients with cystic fibrosis. J Pediatr 1973;82:234.

91. Bell RL et al. Total parenteral nutrition-related cholestasis in infants. J Parenter Enteral Nutr 1986;10:356.

92. Kubota A et al. Hyperbilirubinemia in neonates associated with total parenteral nutrition. J Parenter Enteral Nutr 1988;12:602.

93. Mauer E. Incidence of cholestasis in low birth weight neonates on TrophAmine. J Parenter Enteral Nutr 1991;15(Suppl):25S.

94. Vileisis RA et al. Prospective controlled study of parenteral nutrition-associated cholestatic jaundice: effects of protein intake. J Pediatr 1980; 96:893.

95. Hira Y et al. High caloric infusion induced hepatic impairment in infants. J Parenter Enteral Nutr 1979;3:146.

96. Roslyn JJ et al. Increased risk of gallstones in children receiving total parenteral nutrition. Pediatrics 1983;71:784.

97. Suita S et al. Cholelithiasis in infants: association with parenteral nutrition. J Parenter Enteral Nutr 1984;8:568.

98. Gleghorn EE et al. Phenobarbital does not prevent total parenteral nutrition-associated cholestasis in non-infected neonates. J Parenter Enteral Nutr 1986;10:282.

99. Levy JS et al. Prolonged neonatal cholestasis: bile acid patterns and response to cholestyramine [Abstract]. Mount Sinai J Med 1979;46:169.

100. Sandler RH et al. Use of ursodeoxycholic acid (UDCA) for children with severe liver disease from total parenteral nutrition (TPN); report of three cases [Abstract]. Pediatr Res 1989;25:124.

101. Lambert JR, Thomas SM. Metronidazole prevention of serum liver enzyme abnormalities during total parenteral nutrition. J Parenter Enteral Nutr 1985; 9:501.

102. Dahms BB, Halpin TC. Serial liver biopsies in parenteral nutrition-associated cholestasis of early infancy. Gastroenterology 1981;81:136.

103. Suita S et al. Follow-up studies of children treated with long-term intravenous nutrition (IVN) during the neonatal period. J Pediatr Surg 1982; 17:37.

104. Demetriou AA, Jones LK. Vitamins. In: Rombeau JL, Caldwell MD, eds. Clinical Nutrition Parenteral Nutrition. 2nd Ed. Philadelphia: WB Saunders, 1993.

105. Tyor MP et al. Metabolism and transport of bile salts in the intestine. Am J Med 1971;51:614.

106. Abbasi S et al. Long-term assessment of growth, nutritional status and gastrointestinal function in survivors of necrotizing enterocolitis. J Pediatr 1984; 104:550.

107. Record KE et al. Long-chain versus medium-chain length triglycerides: a review of metabolism and clinical use. Nutr Clin Pract 1986;1:129.

108. Sucher KP. Medium-chain triglycerides: a review of their enteral use in clinical nutrition. Nutr Clin Pract 1986;1:146.

Cystic Fibrosis

Sandra B. Earle

Cystic fibrosis (CF) affects 1 of every 3,200 live births, or approximately 30,000 children and adults in the United States One in 31 Americans carry the autosomal recessive gene for CF, which arises from a mutation in coding for the cystic fibrosis transmembrane regulator protein (CFTR) This genetic mutational error results in the complex, multi-system disease of cystic fibrosis, which is characterized by malabsorption and a state of chronic lung inflammation and infection.

The course and severity of cystic fibrosis are variable and unpredictable. The median life expectancy for a child born with CF in 1990 (i.e., about 40 years) was about double what would have been expected for a child diagnosed 20 years earlier because of advances in the management of this disorder. Although therapy continues to rely on treatment of symptoms rather than the underlying pathologic causes, continuing improved understanding of CF is likely to result in even better control and perhaps a cure. CF is still a lethal disease, but aggressive therapy can decrease the morbidity of this disease and increase the life expectancy of the patient.

HISTORY

In early history (~3,000 BC), the forehead of a newborn was licked crosswise for cleaning, and if a salty taste was perceived, the baby was considered "bewitched" and expected to soon die.[1] This early observation is consistent with the later discovery that patients with CF lose excess salt in their sweat and with the subsequent establishment of the "sweat chloride test" for the diagnosis CF.[2] The term "cystic fibrosis" was first used in 1938 to describe "cystic fibrosis of the pancreas" from postmortem pancreatic lesions.[3] Cystic fibrosis, therefore, is a relatively newly described disease; as a result, most patients cannot relate a long family history of this disease.[4]

GENETIC BASIS

Cystic fibrosis is caused by mutations in the CFTR, which is a member of the ATP Binding Cassette (ABC) family. CFTR is dependent upon cyclic adenosine monophosphate (cAMP) for chloride transport, and defective coding for CFTR inhibits the normal regulation of ion transport in and out of the cell on the apical surface of secretory epithelial cells.[5] CFTR also regulates the transport of bicarbonate and sodium ions, mucus rheology, pulmonary inflammation, and bacterial adherence.[6–10]

Approximately 5% of Whites are asymptomatic carriers of the CF mutation. The high frequency of this mutation has been attributed to a heterozygote-selective advantage that presumably protected the carrier against dehydration from cholera and other secretory diarrheal disease.[15–23]

More than a decade has passed since the identification and cloning of the gene responsible for cystic fibrosis, and more than 1,000 new CFTR mutations have been discovered.[12–14] These mutations have been grouped into five major classes according to the functional consequence of the defect (Fig. 98-1).[41,42] The most common variant is δF508, representing 66% of all mutations. Approximately 85% of all patients with CF have at least one copy of this mutation.[24] Interestingly, even among individuals with identical genotypes, there is a

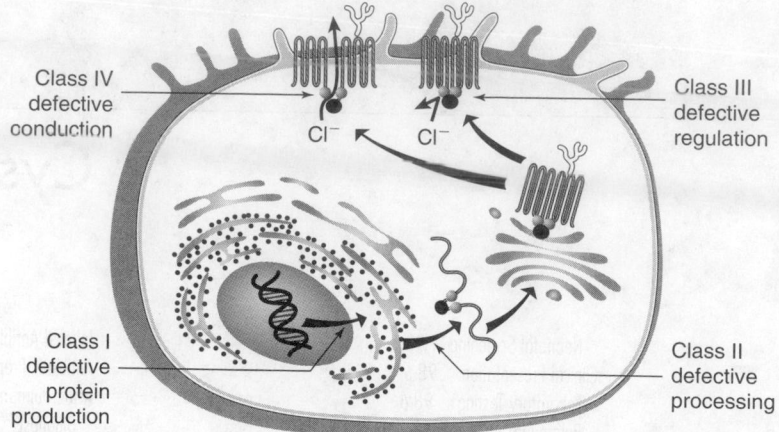

FIGURE 98-1 Classification of mutations: Class I mutations include those in which the production of the cystic fibrosis transmembrane regulator (CFTR) protein is blocked. These are called *stop mutations.* Defective protein processing is responsible for the Class II mutations. In this class, the protein is made, but it is unable to make its way from the point of origin on the endoplasmic reticulum to the apical membrane, where it is needed for proper operation. This includes the most common, δF508, mutation, which is due to improper folding of the protein. Class III mutations cause the disruption of the channel to open properly. Class IV mutations are unable to achieve proper ion conduction. Class V is a milder form of Class I mutations and includes mutations that cause reduced production of functional cystic fibrosis transmembrane regulator (CFTR).[41]

broad spectrum of disease severity.[25,26] Environmental and socioeconomic differences can influence disease severity, however, these factors alone cannot account for the wide variability in the severity of this disease.[27–31] Modifier genes and the contribution of genetic factors other than CFTR may have greater influences on disease severity.[32–39] As investigators better understand these genetic mutations and genetic modifiers, more effective therapies hopefully can be developed.[40]

CLINICAL MANIFESTATIONS

Genotype, environmental factors, and modifier gene status all contribute to the highly variable clinical course of CF. The linking of the loss of CFTR function to clinical manifestations of the disease, however, has been central to gaining an understanding of the disease and in the discovery of new therapies. Normally, CFTR is highly expressed on the membranes of epithelial cells of sweat glands, salivary glands, and male genital ducts as well as the pancreas, lung, kidney tubules, and digestive tract. The CFTR performs different functions in specific tissues; therefore, a dysfunctional or absent CFTR has different effects on different organs resulting in the multiorgan clinical manifestations of cystic fibrosis (Table 98-1).

Sweat Glands

The fluid secreted by the sweat glands in CF patients is normal, but a defect in the reabsorption of electrolytes leads to sweat with a high salt content. CFTR, in the apical membrane of the resorptive area of the sweat gland, functions as an ion channel for chloride transport and also activates an associated epithelial sodium channel (ENaC).[44] Normally, these channels efficiently reabsorb sodium chloride from sweat. In patients with CF, loss of these functioning channels blocks the ability of the sweat ducts to reabsorb salt, leading to sweat sodium chloride (NaCl) concentrations of >100 mM. (Fig. 98-2). The loss of these sodium and chloride ion channels serves as the

basis for the diagnostic sweat chloride test and as the scientific basis for the "infant who tastes of salt" in folklore.

Sinus Involvement

Nasal polyps, which are outgrowths of normal sinus epidermis, can be found in up to 20% of older CF patients and may become large enough to block nasal passages. The pathogenesis of these polyps is unknown, but the obstruction of nasal passages can lead to infection. The faulty ionic transport of chloride across the apical membrane of epithelial cells lining exocrine glands leads to dehydration of extracellular fluids and the development of thickened inspissated mucus in nasal and sinus passages. Most CF patients develop sinus disease with panpacification of the sinuses in 90% to 100% of patients older than 8 months of age; on radiographic examination, >90% of adult-age CF patients have pansinusitis, which can contribute to pulmonary exacerbations.[45,46] The impact of sinusitis on the CF population is significant.

Pancreatic Involvement

The exocrine and ultimately the endocrine function of the pancreas are affected in CF. Pancreatic enzymes normally are secreted into bicarbonate-rich fluid from the pancreatic duct, and CFTR is needed to secrete the bicarbonate into the lumen. The loss of CFTR function inhibits secretion of digestive enzymes and bicarbonate into the duodenum, and the enzymes are trapped in the pancreas by ductal obstruction. Over time, these enzymes (lipase, protease, amylase) accumulate and eventually begin to digest the pancreatic tissue.[10,47] The term *cystic fibrosis* arises from the fibrotic scar tissue that replaces the destroyed pancreas. Without these enzymes, there is poor digestion of fats and, to a lesser extent, proteins and carbohydrates are absorbed poorly. As a result, 85% of CF patients experience pancreatic insufficiency characterized by steatorrhea (fatty stools), decreased absorption of the fat-soluble vitamins

Table 98-1   **Clinical Manifestations of Cystic Fibrosis**[192]

Approximate Incidence (%)

Manifestation	Infants	Children	Adults
Pancreatic			
Insufficiency	80–85	85	90
Pancreatitis	—	1–2	2–4
Abnormal glucose tolerance	—	5/yr[a]	30
Diabetes mellitus	—	2–4	8–15
Hepatobiliary			
Biliary cirrhosis	—	10–20	>20
Cholelithiasis	—	5	5–10
Biliary obstruction	—	1–2	5
Intestinal			
Meconium ileus	10–15	—	—
Meconium ileus equivalent	—	1–5	10–20
Rectal prolapse	—	10–15	1–2
Intussusception	—	1–5	1–2
Gastroesophageal reflux	—	1–5	>10
Appendiceal abscess	—	0–1	1–2
Respiratory			
Upper			
Nasal polyps	<1	4–10	15–20
Pansinusitis	—	—	90–100
Lower			
Bronchiectasis	—	30–50	>90
Pneumothorax	—	1–2	10–15
Hemoptysis[b]	—	5–15	50–60
Genitourinary			
Delayed puberty	—	—	85
Infertility			
Males	—	—	98
Females	—	—	70–80

[a] ↑ in glucose intolerance of approximately 5% per year.
[b] Percentage includes both major and minor hemoptysis.

(A, D, E, and K), malnutrition, and failure to thrive. Early in life, serum concentrations of amylase and lipase are increased secondary to pancreatic autodigestion. This destructive process can result in either painful or asymptomatic chronic pancreatitis.

Eventually, the progressive destruction of the pancreas affects its endocrine function, leading to glucose intolerance in about 17% of children and 75% of adults.[48,49] Diabetes mellitus occurs in approximately 40% of adult patients with CF.[50] The additional diagnosis of diabetes in CF is associated with significantly increased morbidity and mortality,[51,52] and a decrease in insulin sensitivity is associated with pulmonary exacerbations.[53]

Intestinal Involvement

Meconium ileus occurs in approximately 10% to 15% of newborns with CF and is manifested by failure to pass meconium (the first stool) within the first 48 hours of life, abdominal distention, and bilious vomiting. Outside the neonatal period, distal intestinal obstruction syndrome (DIOS, also called *meconium ileus equivalent*) can occur at any age and results from the complete or partial obstruction of the intestine. Intestinal obstruction occurs in 10% to 20% of patients and results from the inspissation of intestinal secretions and incompletely digested intestinal contents. A right lower quadrant mass, abdominal distention, failure to pass stools, and vomiting may accompany DIOS.

Gastrointestinal reflux disease (GERD) is common in both children and adults with CF.[54–56] Children with CF should be screened for GERD and treated, if diagnosed. Other intestinal complications include rectal prolapse, intussusception, and appendiceal abscesses.

Hepatic Involvement

Liver disease has become more important in CF as life expectancy improves. CFTR, located on the apical surfaces of the cells lining the intrahepatic and extrahepatic bile ducts and the gallbladder, functions to facilitate ion transport.[57] In CF patients, the abnormal chloride efflux across the cells results in the reduction in water and sodium movement into the bile. The resulting decrease in the volume and flow of bile leads to stasis and obstruction of the biliary tree. With chronic obstruction there is inflammation, giving rise to the characteristic lesion of focal biliary cirrhosis.[58]

About 13% to 17% of children with CF suffer from clinically relevant liver disease, and about 2% progress to multilobular cirrhosis.[59,60] However, since sensitive, diagnostic markers of hepatobiliary disease are not available, prevalence rates are probably underestimated. Progressive cirrhosis is associated with portal hypertension, hypersplenism, esophageal varices, ascites, and in a small number of patients, complete hepatic failure requiring transplantation. Approximately 30% of CF patients have abnormal gallbladder function and size (absent or small gallbladder) with 5% to 10% of patients developing gallstones.[61]

Genitourinary Involvement

Approximately 98% of males with CF are infertile secondary to in utero obstruction of the vas deferens or related structures. Hormonal secretion and secondary sexual characteristics are normal. In a small number of patients, infertility may be the

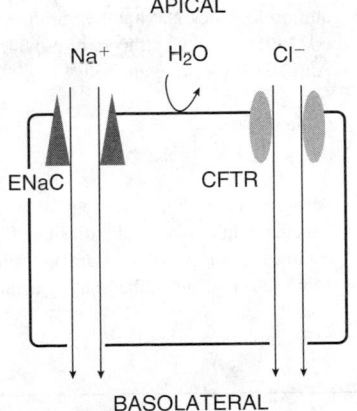

FIGURE 98-2 Normal salt (NaCl) absorption in the sweat duct with working epithelial sodium channel (ENaC) and cystic fibrosis transmembrane regulator (CFTR).

only manifestation of disease, and CF may go undiagnosed until fertility testing is performed. The prevalence of infertility is higher in women with CF and hypothesized to be related to the production of thick and tenacious cervical mucus. Hundreds of pregnancies have been carried successfully to term, but they are not without risk, especially for patients with moderate to severe pulmonary disease.[62]

Bone and Joint Involvement

CF patients have low bone mineral density, slower rate of bone formation, high rate of bone loss, accelerated rate of bone loss, and arthritis.[63,64] Although the severity of bone loss may correlate with the severity of pulmonary disease, insufficient intake or absorption of vitamin D can account for some of the morbidity.[64–66]

CF patients often suffer from intermittent arthritis symptoms, but only about 2% of CF patients have persistent symptoms. There are three types of intermittent CF arthritis: (1) hypertrophic osteoarthropathy, (2) immunoreactive, and (3) CF arthropathy. The first two types are associated with pulmonary disease flare-up. The third type, CF arthropathy, affects large joints and may be accompanied by fever and erythema nodosum.[67–71]

Pulmonary Involvement

The relationship of ion channel disruption resulting from CFTR dysfunction to the lung tissue destruction has yet to be firmly established. Presently, the CF gene mutation is believed to cause CFTR dysfunction, which in turn causes ion transporter defects, and subsequent changes in the airway secretions (Fig. 98-3). The changes in airway secretions promote the infection-inflammation-tissue damage cycle.

Chronic infection combined with inflammation has been the hallmark of lung disease in cystic fibrosis. The cycle of

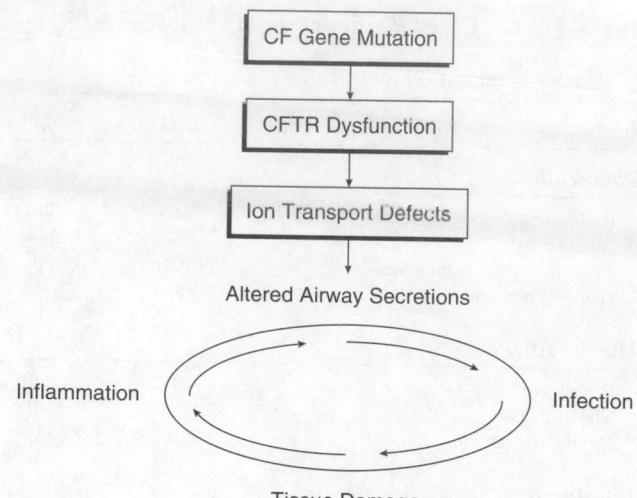

FIGURE 98-3 Pathologic cycle in lung disease. CFTR, cystic fibrosis transmembrane regulator.[193]

unchecked inflammation and infection has been the focus of much investigation and ongoing debate as to "Which came first—infection or inflammation."[72] Although the inflammatory response appears to set up bacterial colonization in the airways, infection also can stimulate an inflammatory response. In either case, the cycle of inflammation and infection eventually leads to lung tissue damage and bronchiectasis.[73]

This pattern of inflammation and infection has not been observed in any other tissue where CFTR is expressed. Differences in the CF patient's airway surface liquid, mucus, and other protective mechanisms in the lung are being studied, and some of these differences may help explain the inflammation-infection cycle (Table 98-2)

Table 98-2 Host Abnormalities That Predispose to Chronic Lung Infection

Abnormality	Proposed impact	Proposed intervention(s)
Abnormal cystic fibrosis transmembrane regulator (CFTR)	Altered secretions (low volume of airway surface fluid and hypertonicity) leads to thick dehydrated mucus, impairment of mucociliary escalator, and impaired defensin-mediated antimicrobial activity	• Chest physiotherapy • Inhaled DNase • Gene therapy[a] • Alter electrolyte and water balance by aerosolized amiloride (block Na+ uptake)[a] uridine triphosphate (UTP) (increase Cl efflux)[a], or provide novel peptides[b]
Increased expression of asialoganglioside (aGMI)	Increased *P. aeruginosa* and *S. aureus* binding to respiratory epithelial cells	• Anti-aGMI blocking antibody[b]
Defective CFTR-mediated uptake of *P. aeruginosa* by respiratory epithelial cells	Decreased clearance of internalized *P. aeruginosa* with sloughed epithelial cells	• Gene therapy[a]
Abnormal regulation of pro-inflammatory cytokines	• Hyperexuberant neutrophil recruitment and release of neutrophil oxidants	• Anti-inflammatory therapy, e.g., steroids or ibuprofen beneficial, but associated with side effects such as cataracts, poor growth, or gastrointestinal bleeding
Increased IL-8 expression and TNF-alpha	• Upregulation of human mucin genes	• More selective anti-inflammatory agents[b]
Variant mannose-binding lectin (MBL)	Polymorphisms may differentially bind bacterial surface carbohydrates	• MBL replacement[b]

[a]Investigational intervention.
[b]Theoretic intervention.
From Saiman L, Siegel J. Infection control recommendations for patients with cystic fibrosis: microbiology, important pathogens and infection control practices to prevent patient-to-patient transmission. Am J Infect Control 2003;31(3 Suppl):S1.

Infection

Despite repeated courses of aggressive antibiotic therapy, patients with CF eventually develop endobronchial bacterial colonization and infection. Understanding why bacteria seldom are eradicated is important to treating this disease.

The lower airways of a normal lung are always maintained free of pathogens through various lung defense mechanisms. For example, a thin film of liquid on the airway surfaces called the airway surface layer (ASL) contains antibiotics, antioxidants, proteases and other substances that work to eliminate pathogens. The ASL also signals molecules to turn on the cellular immune system by recruiting neutrophils and macrophages to the site of microbe invasion. In addition, the ASL can remove invading microbes from the lung by moving a mucus gel toward the mouth through ciliary motion. Mucociliary clearance of microbes and debris is aided by the cough reflex to keep the airways clean. Since coughing is an important defense mechanism necessary for CF patients, cough suppressants should not be prescribed or taken by a patient with CF.

Local antibacterial peptides (lysozyme, β-defensins) in the ASL are inactivated by high concentrations of salt like that found in CF ASL.[74,75] The ion channel dysfunction associated with CF can dehydrate and thicken mucus as well as deplete periciliary fluid and collapse cilia".[76,77] Thick mucus, which is not easily cleared, serves as a nidus for bacterial growth and when combined with impaired mucociliary clearance, promotes chronic bacterial infection.[78]

CF epithelial tracheal cells express high numbers of surface receptors for *Pseudomonas aeruginosa* and *Staphylococcus aureus*.[79] *S. aureus* is frequently responsible for the initial bacterial colonization, whereas *P. aeruginosa* is the most common pathogen isolated in chronically colonized patients.

The oxygen radicals produced by the inflammatory response in infected CF airways induce bacterial mutations of *P. aeruginosa* that lead to production of alginate, a biofilm that allows the organism to become more resistant to antibiotics. Mucoid *P. aeruginosa* bacteria also produce exotoxin A, protease, and elastase, which damage lung tissue and decrease the effectiveness of the neutrophils (PMNs) and macrophages.[83,84] *Burkholderia cepacia*, another opportunistic pathogen found in CF patients, is highly resistant to virtually all antibiotics. Patients may be asymptomatic or may have a fulminant infection leading to death. CF patients infected with mucoid strains of *P. aeruginosa* and *B. cepacia* experience increased morbidity and mortality.[80–82]

Viruses, fungi, and mycobacteria are also potential pathogens. Viruses may predispose patients to subsequent bacterial infection and may be responsible for activating the inflammation cycle. *Aspergillus fumigatus*, a fungus, has been associated with allergic bronchopulmonary aspergillosis (ABPA) in 5% to 25% of CF patients. ABPA is an immunologic reaction to *Aspergillus*, which can lead to progressive pulmonary fibrosis if left undiagnosed and untreated. Nontuberculous mycobacteria have emerged as pathogens in the CF population.[85,86] The clinical course associated with nontuberculous mycobacteria infection is variable and complicate the diagnosis and treatment of the CF patient.

Inflammation

Inflammation is the lung's response to chronic infection.[79,87] Neutrophils (PMNs) are "called" to the site of an infection by interleukin-1 (IL-1), interleukin-8 (IL-8), leukotriene (LTB$_4$), endotoxin, and tumor necrosis factor (TNF-α). When neutrophils arrive at the site, they release proteases, oxidants, elastases, and cytokines. Antiproteases and interleukin-10 (IL-10), an anti-inflammatory cytokine, subsequently are released in an effort to counterbalance the inflammatory system. The number of anti-inflammatory compounds are relatively low in CF patients, and levels of neutrophils, proteases, elastases, oxidants, and cytokines all are increased.[88–90] These abnormalities lead to a sustained and destructive cycle of unchecked inflammation that begins at a very early age.[87]

Arachidonic acid (AA), an agonist in the inflammation pathway, is increased, and docosahexaenoic acid (DHA), a downregulator of AA, is decreased in the bronchial lavage fluid in CF patients. This imbalance of fatty acids favors the inflammatory and mucus-producing AA and therefore provides an explanation for the role of CFTR in causing inflammation and increased mucus production in the airways.[91]

DIAGNOSIS

Diagnostic Criteria

Most children with CF are diagnosed in the first year of life (median age at diagnosis, 6 months), but 8% are not diagnosed until later (>18 years of age).[92] A positive diagnosis of CF is contingent on having one or more of the characteristics listed in Table 98-3, a history of CF in a sibling, or a positive newborn screening test result. These must then be accompanied by two positive sweat chloride tests, two positive nasal potential differences (NPD) tests, or identification of two CF mutations.[93] The classic triad of clinical signs and symptoms

---

Table 98-3 Phenotypic Features Consistent With Diagnosis of CF

1. Chronic sinopulmonary disease manifested by:
   - Persistent colonization/infection with typical CF pathogens (e.g., S. aureus, nontypeable *H. influenzae,* mucoid and nonmucoid *P. aeruginosa,* and *B. cepacia*
   - Chronic cough and sputum production
   - Persistent chest radiograph abnormalities (e.g., bronchiectasis, atelectasis, infiltrates, hyperinflation)
   - Airway obstruction manifested by wheezing and air trapping
   - Nasal polyps; radiographic or computed tomographic abnormalities of paranasal sinuses
   - Digital clubbing
2. Gastrointestinal and nutritional abnormalities including:
   - *Intestinal:* meconium ileus, distal intestinal obstruction syndrome, rectal prolapse
   - *Pancreatic:* pancreatic insufficiency, recurrent pancreatitis
   - *Hepatic:* chronic hepatic disease manifested by clinical or histologic evidence of focal biliary cirrhosis or multilobular cirrhosis
   - *Nutritional:* failure to thrive (protein–calorie malnutrition), hypoproteinemia and edema, complications secondary to fat-soluble vitamin deficiency
3. Salt loss syndromes: acute salt depletion, chronic metabolic alkalosis
4. Male urogenital abnormalities resulting in obstructive azoospermia (CBAVD)

CF, cystic fibrosis; CBAVD, congenital bilateral absence of the vas deferens. From Rosenstein BJ, Cutting GR. The diagnosis of cystic fibrosis: a consensus statement. Cystic Fibrosis Foundation Consensus Panel. J Pediatr 1998; 132(4):589.

for the diagnosis of CF are a positive sweat chloride test, gastrointestinal malabsorption, and chronic pulmonary disease. With the discovery of the CF gene, DNA typing is now available for 95% of the CF mutations.

When the pilocarpine iontophoresis test (i.e., sweat chloride test) is conducted at a certified CF center and is positive (>60 mEq/L) on two different days, the diagnosis of CF can be applied.[94] This test may be unreliable in infants less than 2 months of age because it is difficult to obtain a sufficient sample volume. A false-positive sweat chloride test for CF can result from glucose-6-phosphate dehydrogenase deficiency, hypothyroidism, glycogen storage disease, untreated adrenal insufficiency, and malnutrition.

A second diagnostic test for CF evaluates the pattern of increased NPDs. Abnormalities of ion transport in respiratory epithelia, results in patients with CF having a higher basal NPD, which reflects enhanced Na^+ transport across a relatively Cl^- impermeable barrier. This test can be effective in diagnosing CF in infants in the first few hours of life. Older children may need mild sedation before initiating the test for NPD. Inflamed mucosa or nasal polyps can generate a false-negative NPD. The NPD test should be repeated on a separate day at a reputable CF center if the first test is positive for CF.[95]

Genetic Testing
Prenatal Screening
If both parents are known to be carriers of CF, the American College of Medical Genetics (ACMG) and the American College of Obstetrics and Gynecology (ACOG) recommend prenatal screening.[105] Amniocentesis, chorionic villus sampling (CVS) and pancreatitis associated protein (PAP) all have been used to diagnose CF in utero. Genetic testing for CF should be conducted at a center that has knowledgeable genetic counselors who understand the validity and reliability of the tests as well as the sociomedical implications for a child diagnosed with CF.

Neonatal Screening
CF is one of many disorders that infants can be screened for shortly after birth. Whereas some experts support routine CF screening because it is not "harmful," others feel that the evidence is inadequate to show that early diagnosis is medically beneficial.[97–100] At birth, neonates with CF have increased serum concentrations of immunoreactive trypsinogen (IRT), which result from obstruction of the pancreatic ducts. This test has a low prevalence of false positives (5 of 1000). An elevated IRT, however, is not diagnostic of CF on its own. If a second screening still shows increased serum concentrations of IRT 4 to 6 weeks later, a follow-up sweat chloride test is indicated to confirm a diagnosis of CF, and blood samples also should be genotyped. Newborns who present with meconium ileus are always suspected of having CF; however, in this subset of patients, for reasons not understood, IRT has a high prevalence of false-negative results.[96] There is a growing consensus that early aggressive therapy improves the quality of life and extends the life-span of CF patients.[101–103] It is possible, therefore, that early screening of infants for CF will gain advocates and become widely accepted. If neonatal screening is to be effective, an infrastructure must be in place to provide education and counseling for families.[104]

Clinical Presentation

1. L.T., a 9-month-old boy whose well-baby visits have been sporadic, is brought to the pediatric primary care clinic. His mother states, "He can't seem to eat enough food and cries constantly." She says that he has 8 to 10 stools per day, but she thought this was because he ate so much. On further questioning she says that the stools are large, greasy, and foul smelling. He has never been hospitalized, but has had three ear infections and three chest colds, which were treated with antibiotics. When plotted on a standard growth curve, L.T. is found to be in the fifth percentile for both weight and height (7.5 kg and 68 cm). The pregnancy and delivery were uncomplicated, and L.T.'s medical history is otherwise unremarkable. Physical examination shows a poorly nourished, small-for-age infant in no apparent distress. Family history is unremarkable. Review of systems reveals diffuse crackles in the lower lung fields; all other systems are within normal limits. A sweat chloride test is ordered and results in a chloride concentration of 110 mEq/L (normal, <60 mEq/L). L.T.'s chest x-ray shows mild peribronchial thickening of both upper lobes. What subjective and objective data for L.T. are suggestive of the diagnosis of CF?

L.T. fulfills the classic triad for the diagnosis of CF: elevated sweat chloride, chronic recurrent pulmonary infections, and apparent pancreatic insufficiency. Although not showing symptoms of pulmonary infection at present, the baby has had several chest colds, and chest x-ray indicates chronic inflammation. As illustrated by L.T., the earliest chest x-ray shows peribronchial thickening in the upper lung fields. As the lung disease progresses, hyperinflation, as evidenced by increased anteroposterior diameter of the chest (barrel chest), and flattening of the diaphragm, is evident. Eventually, areas of collapse, consolidation, and abscess formation and bronchiectasis develop, indicating severe pulmonary tissue destruction. L.T.'s pancreatic insufficiency is suggested by his multiple daily fatty stools and failure to thrive despite a voracious appetite. In summary, a positive sweat test, evidence of GI malabsorption, and pulmonary involvement support the probable diagnosis of CF in L.T.

Laboratory Testing

2. What further testing can be done to confirm the diagnosis of CF in L.T.?

The sweat chloride test should be repeated on another day to affirm laboratory testing reliability and to rule out other conditions that can cause an elevated sweat chloride level (see Diagnostic Criteria above). Genetic testing can be done to identify CFTR mutations. Since genetic testing cannot identify all the possible mutations that can cause CF, genetic testing is not the diagnostic test of choice. A diagnosis of CF is likely if the second sweat chloride test is positive, especially in light of his clinical presentation.

Pulmonary Testing

3. What testing and follow-up should be completed to define L.T.'s pulmonary involvement?

Baseline pulmonary function tests, chest x-rays, oxygen saturation, and sputum cultures are a part of the normal workup. Spirometry should be performed every 6 months, and complete pulmonary function tests should be performed once a year. Arterial blood gases or pulse oximetry need to be completed on patients whose forced expiratory volume in 1 second (FEV$_1$) is <40% predicted. Unfortunately, children such as L.T., who are younger than 5 years of age, are unable to adequately perform the tasks associated with pulmonary function testing. Chest x-rays should be obtained annually, whenever the patient has a pulmonary-related hospital admission, and before any surgery. Respiratory tract cultures and sensitivities should be completed annually and before initiation of antibiotic therapy. Because obtaining a voluntary sputum sample from an infant is difficult, an oropharyngeal swab can be used to initiate a gag reflex and cough, and then a sputum sample is collected. The sputum sample obtained actually may contain only normal upper airway flora rather than bacteria colonizing the lower airway; therefore, it is important to interpret persistently normal flora from a sputum culture of an infant with caution.[156]

Gastrointestinal Testing

4. What testing and follow-up should be completed in L.T. to define GI and nutritional involvement?

L.T.'s head circumference, height, and weight should be plotted on standard growth charts every 3 months for the first year. An experienced, knowledgeable registered dietician should meet with the family to help them understand the importance of appropriate nutrition and help develop a plan for L.T. Nutritional assessments should be completed annually, or more often if L.T. shows evidence of weight loss or poor weight gain. Serum lipase and amylase, fasting blood glucose, liver function tests, albumin, pre-albumin, serum electrolytes, iron, and vitamins A, D, and E levels should be determined at least annually. An abdominal examination should be done to determine liver and spleen size and consistency at each office visit. Although quantification of fecal fat content may assist in the titration of pancreatic enzyme doses, an accurate dietary fat intake history is needed for accurate quantification. Many CF centers undertake this assessment only in patients who have demonstrated excessive pancreatic enzyme dose requirements.

THERAPY

The management of a patient with CF is costly and complex. The costs to care for a CF patient in 1995 were estimated to be $40,000 per year, and these costs have continued to escalate. In addition, the emotional, physical, and social effects of caring for a chronically ill child can be overwhelming. Family socioeconomic status also seems to be a predictor of a CF child's health. The risk of death in the lowest income group (<$20,000/year) increased by 44%, and patients in this group had consistently lower pulmonary functions and body weights than those with higher income.[31]

In a review of more than 18,000 CF patients (6 to 18 years of age), those who were monitored frequently and treated aggressively had better lung health as measured by FEV$_1$.[106] Aggressive preventive therapies, therefore, apparently result in better outcomes than treating problems as they arise.[101–103] Although a cure for CF is still the ultimate goal, new therapies to target malabsorption and the infection-inflammation cycle are being vigorously studied.

Control of Malabsorption

Patients with untreated CF have pancreatic insufficiency and are malnourished. Early diagnosis and treatment of malabsorption (i.e., meeting caloric needs, providing vitamin, mineral, and digestive enzymes) are beneficial to the patient.

Caloric Needs

Poor nutrition correlates with negative prognosis; therefore, maximizing the nutritional status of the CF patient is important. CF patients are hypermetabolic and do not absorb fats and proteins normally. Therefore, the CF diet must be high in calories, fat, and protein. An infant at diagnosis may need a total daily caloric goal of 120 to 150 kcal/kg to make up for lost time. Weight gain, fat stores, and growth then drive the daily caloric goal. When a patient has a significant weight loss or falls below the tenth percentile for weight or height for age, it is indicative of nutritional failure, which requires therapeutic intervention.[107] Some patients at nutritional risk benefit from nighttime enteral feedings.[108,109]

Vitamin and Mineral Supplementation

The malabsorption of fats in CF patients with pancreatic insufficiency also results in decreased GI absorption of the fat-soluble vitamins (A, D, E, and K). Approximately 45% of the CF population is deficient in one of these vitamins, even when pancreatic enzymes are being used appropriately.[110] The current recommendations for replacement therapy are listed in Table 98-4.[107] Vitamin K deficiency is a relatively uncommon finding in CF patients; however, a more sensitive measurement of vitamin K (e.g., PIVKA-II test) might uncover more widespread deficiency of this vitamin.[111–113] Zinc, calcium, sodium, and iron may also need to be given as supplements.

Enzyme Supplementation

The mainstay of treatment for pancreatic insufficiency is exogenous replacement of pancreatic digestive enzymes. The goals of pancreatic enzyme supplementation are to (1) improve weight gain, (2) minimize steatorrhea, and (3) eliminate abdominal cramping and bloating. Supplementation with currently available therapies does not fully restore fat absorption and the absorption of sufficient fat-soluble vitamins continues to be problematic.[114]

Table 98-4 Daily Recommended Doses of Fat-Soluble Vitamins for CF Patients and Vitamin Content in ADEK Formulations

Age	Vitamin A (IU)	Vitamin E (IU)	Vitamin D (IU)	Vitamin K (mg)
0–12 months	1,500	40–50	400	0.3–0.5
1–3 years	5,000	80–150	400–800	0.3–0.5
4–8 years	5,000–10,000	100–200	400–800	0.3–0.5
>8 years	10,000	200–400	400–800	0.3–0.5
Vitamin Content				
ADEK Chew Tab	9,000	150	400	0.15
ADEK drops	3,170	40	400	0.1

Adapted from Borowitz D et al. Consensus report on nutrition for pediatric patients with cystic fibrosis. J Pediatr Gastroenterol Nutr 2002;35(3):246.

The digestive enzymes (lipase, protease, and amylase in a mixture of approximately one part amylase to three parts protease and three parts amylase) are available in capsules (Table 98-5) that contain enteric-coated microspheres of these enzymes. The enteric coating protects these enzymes from gastric acid. Since the breakdown of fat is the most important function of these enzymes, dosing is based on the lipase content, and the dose varies according to weight, age, dietary fat intake, and severity of symptoms. The initial dose for infants is 2,000 to 2,500 units of lipase/kg per breast-feeding or per 120 mL of bottle-feeding: the dose is decreased to 1,000 units/kg per meal when infants begin to eat solid food. For children older than 4 years of age, 500 units of lipase/kg per meal is the empiric dose for enzyme supplementation.[115] A full dose is taken with meals, and half the prescribed dose is taken with snacks. Subsequent dosing adjustments are titrated to response.

The patient and family need to be aware that lack of weight gain, smelly, greasy stools, and abdominal pain or bloating may be signs of insufficient enzyme dosing. Generic substitutions of pancreatic enzymes have resulted in therapeutic failure and are not recommended.[122] Selected available products are listed in Table 98-5.

High-strength pancreatic enzymes have been associated with colonic strictures, which are accompanied by symptoms similar to that of distal intestinal obstruction syndrome (DIOS) and which must be differentiated from DIOS by ultrasound or x-ray.[116] Although cause and effect have not been firmly established, doses ≥6,500 units lipase/kg per meal have been associated with stricture formation. As a result, most recommend that the daily dose of lipase not exceed 10,000 units of lipase/kg.[117]

When patients require unusually high doses of enzyme supplements, it may be because of high gastric acidity. The enteric coating on the pancreatic enzyme microspheres dissolves at a pH of 5.8, and the enzymes are destroyed at a pH of 4.0. CF patients have longer postprandial periods of time when the pH is less than 4.0 in the bowel and also have significantly less time when the pH is >5.8. Since enzymes may

be less effective when the bowel pH is very low,[118] adding an H_2 antagonist or a proton pump inhibitor to increase the pH may help lower the enzyme dosing requirement.[119–121]

5. Significant laboratory findings for L.T. include the following: serum vitamin E, 2.5 mg/L (normal, 3 to 15.8 mg/L); vitamin A, 26 μg/dL (normal, 30 to 90 μg/dL); lipase, 47 U/L (normal, 0.1 to 208 U/L); amylase, <30 U/L (normal, 0 to 110); albumin, 2.7 g/dL (normal, 3.4 to 5.1 g/dL); all other laboratory values are within normal limits. Pancreatic enzymes are to be started in L.T. Develop a dosing and monitoring plan for his pancreatic enzyme therapy.

Dosing is empirically started at 1,000 U/kg of the lipase component. The initial dose for L.T., who weighs 7.5 kg, would be 7,500 units, with a full dose for meals and a half-dose for snacks. To simplify drug therapy, it is best to select a single capsule strength that can be used for both meals and snacks. Therefore, a product with close to the desired amount (e.g., Creon 10) should be selected and dosed as 1 capsule with meals, and half a capsule with light meals or snacks. For the best result, the supplements should be given at the beginning of the meal or snack.[157] This is challenging, especially for an infant. Capsules can be opened and the microspheres put on the nipple of a mother nursing her CF infant or on the nipple of a bottle. Alternatively, the capsules can be opened and added to a spoonful of cereal or applesauce and given just before nursing or giving a bottle. The microspheres should not be chewed or put on hot food or liquid because the coating can be destroyed. The dose of the pancreatic enzymes should be adjusted to minimize steatorrhea, and the dose increased as needed. L.T.'s family should also be taught the signs of constipation or stomach pain in an infant.

L.T.'s weight gain and growth should be assessed every 3 months for the first year. As L.T. grows, his enzyme requirements will change and eventually he will need to become responsible for taking them on his own before eating. Neighbors, friends, and teachers should store a few supplements for L.T. to accommodate spontaneous playing or eating of snacks.

6. In addition to enzyme replacement, what fat-soluble vitamin supplementation is appropriate for L.T.?

L.T.'s laboratory evaluation reveals vitamin A and E deficiencies, which are relatively common in patients with malabsorption. The long-term effects of inadequate fat-soluble vitamin intake are unclear. Vitamins A, D, E, and K, however, should be prescribed for L.T. because of the theoretical benefits, low cost, and low risk. L.T. should be started on 1 mL of ADEK drops daily (see Table 98-4). The L.T.'s levels for vitamins A, D, and E should be monitored yearly: his vitamin K need not be monitored unless risk factors are present or clotting difficulties are suspected.[107]

Control of Infection
Mobilization of Secretions
Sputum in CF patients is difficult to mobilize because pulmonary secretions are thick as a result of both the CFTR defect and the large amounts of viscous DNA from the breakdown of white blood cells and bacterial debris left over from chronic infections. Mechanical clearance methods and inhaled mucolytics can be helpful in mobilizing pulmonary secretions.

Table 98-5　Selected Pancreatic Enzymes

| Product[a] | Microencapsulated Enzymes | | |
	Lipase	Protease	Amylase
Creon 5	5,000	18,750	16,600
Creon 10	10,000	37,500	33,200
Creon 20	20,000	75,000	66,400
Pancrease	4,500	25,000	20,000
Pancrease MT 4	4,000	12,000	12,000
Pancrease MT 10	10,000	30,000	30,000
Pancrease MT 16	16,000	48,000	48,000
Pancrease MT 20	20,000	44,000	56,000
Ultrase	4,500	25,000	20,000
Ultrase MT 12	12,000	39,000	39,000
Ultrase MT 18	18,000	58,500	58,500
Ultrase MT 20	20,000	65,000	65,000

[a]Dosing and comparison of products based on lipase content.
Adapted from Drug Facts and Comparisons, Inc, 2003.

MECHANICAL METHODS

Methods used to mechanically break up and mobilize mucus in the pulmonary tree include traditional hand percussion and postural drainage (P&PD); oscillating positive end pressure (OPEP) with the flutter valve; high-frequency chest wall oscillation (HFCWO) with the ThAIRapy vest; intrapulmonary percussive ventilation (IPV); and autogenic drainage (a technique of deep breathing exercises). These mechanical approaches for mobilizing mucus are about equal in efficacy, and the selection of the most appropriate for a patient depends on the ability, motivation, preference, and resources of the patient.[139] When the traditional P&PD was compared with HFCWO and OPEP, clinical efficacy and safety were comparable, but 50% of patients preferred the HFCWO, 37% preferred OPEP, and 13% preferred P&PD.[140]

DORNASE ALFA

Dornase alfa (Pulmozyme), an inhaled recombinant form of human deoxyribonuclease I, selectively breaks up the DNA formed by the PMNs that block airways in the CF patient. It reduces exacerbation frequency in patients with advanced, moderate, and mild lung disease and is safe for use in infants.[141–144] This drug does not seem to benefit the patient experiencing an acute exacerbation.[145] Dornase alfa is very expensive, with costs averaging about $1,200/month; and the cost-benefit ratio for the use of dornase alfa continues to be debated.[146,147] More than 50% of CF patients are using dornase alfa.[92] Although inhaled hypertonic saline also improves mucociliary clearance in CF airways, it is less effective than dornase alfa and is not recommended.[148]

7. What mucus clearance methods would be appropriate for L.T.'s therapy?

Methods of mechanical assistance to remove pulmonary secretions are all equally effective, but hand P&PD would be the method of choice for L.T. because he is only 9 months old. His parents should be taught the method of using a cupped hand or a vibrator device to shake loose the secretions accumulated in L.T.'s lungs. The other methods of chest physiotherapy can be used when L.T. is older and better able to participate in these therapeutic approaches.

Dornase alfa improves sputum viscosity in CF patients, and patients are able to benefit from this drug early in the course of their lung disease.[141] In the Pulmozyme Early Intervention Trial (PEIT), the risk of pulmonary exacerbations was reduced by 34% in young patients with mild lung function abnormalities, and pulmonary function tests also were improved in patients with close to normal pulmonary function. The addition of dornase alfa is a viable consideration if the cost and scheduling of regular treatments are not issues for L.T.

Patient counseling is important if dornase alfa is prescribed for L.T. Because it is an enzyme that can be denatured, dornase alfa should not be mixed with other drugs. Only approved nebulizers can be used because of the variability of delivery of aerosolized medications from different nebulizers. Baseline pulmonary function tests should be obtained, and L.T. should be re-evaluated in 6 weeks. Evidence of improvement should include the following: diminished dyspnea and cough, increase in sputum production, increased appetite, improved subjective measures (e.g., perception of energy, ability

to sleep), and improvement in pulmonary function tests. Dornase alfa should be discontinued if the patient does not appear to be benefiting from therapy.[147]

Immunizations

8. Gram's stain of L.T.'s sputum reveals normal respiratory flora, and the throat culture is pending. What immunizations should be considered for L.T. at this time?

L.T. has no evidence of a pulmonary infection at this time. He should receive all childhood immunizations at the usual recommended times (see Chapter 95, Immunizations) and an annual flu vaccine as well. Prevention of influenza may help avoid the onset of a bacterial infection.

Antibiotic Therapy

Antibiotics are commonly used for the CF patient to improve or delay the decline of pulmonary function. The indications for antimicrobial use include (1) treatment for an exacerbation, (2) prevention of colonization with *P. aeruginosa,* and (3) maintenance therapy for chronic *P. aeruginosa.* Because pathogens often are not eradicated from the CF patients' airways, bacterial resistance to antibiotics commonly develops. As a result, CF patients may need to receive broad-spectrum antibiotics more often than might be indicated in other populations.[123–126]

DIFFERENCES IN KINETICS

The physiologic changes in the CF patient affects how the body absorbs, distributes, and clears drugs. Lack of bicarbonate secretion in the GI tract and prolonged GI transit times affect the rate and extent of absorption of some drugs (e.g., oral ciprofloxacin). CF patients have alterations in their body water to mass ratio, changing the apparent volume of distribution of drugs that are distributed to total body water.[127] For example, the volume of distribution is typically increased for aminoglycosides and β-lactams.

Both hepatic and renal clearances are increased for many drugs in CF patients. N acetyltransferase activity is increased,[128] but the P450 system does not seem to be greatly affected and remains isoenzyme dependent (i.e., CYP1A2, CYP2A6, CYP2C9, and CYP3A4 enzyme activity is not changed in CF patients).[129–131] CYP2C8 activity and biliary secretion, however, may be enhanced.[127] The malfunctioning CFTR is hypothesized to increase the renal tubular clearance of organic anion drugs in CF patients (e.g., penicillins and trimethoprim).[128,132–134]

These differences in renal tubular clearance and volumes of distributions make it necessary to adjust doses of some antibiotics in CF patients. Theoretically, increased clearance alone would necessitate shorter dosing intervals, and when coupled with a larger volume of distribution, larger daily doses may be needed as well. Table 98-6 contains an abbreviated list of suggested dosage regimens.

MONITORING AND ADVERSE EFFECTS

The prolonged, repeated use of aminoglycosides in patients with CF increases the risk for drug-related toxicity. It is interesting that nephrotoxicity, ototoxicity, and vestibular damage associated with aminoglycosides seem to be less common in CF patients than in the rest of the population.[135] Nevertheless,

Table 98-6 Antibiotic Doses For Cystic Fibrosis[194]

	Systemic Antibiotics		
Drug	Daily Dosage (mg/kg)	Frequency	Maximum Individual Dose (mg)
Amikacin	30	Divided Q 8–12 hr	TDM
Ceftazidime	150–225	Divided Q 8 hr	2,000
Cefuroxime	150–225	Divided Q 8 hr	1,500
Ciprofloxacin IV	30	Divided Q 8 hr	400
Ciprofloxacin PO	40	Divided Q 12 hr	1,000
Gentamicin	10–12	Divided Q 8–12 hr	TDM
Imipenem	40–80	Divided Q 6 hr	1,000
Oxacillin	200	Divided Q 6 hr	2,000
Piperacillin	200–400	Divided Q 6 hr	4,000
Ticarcillin/clavulanate	200–400	Divided Q 6 hr	3,100
Tobramycin	10–12 (8–10 adults)	Divided Q 8 hr	TDM
	Inhaled Antibiotics		
Drug	Dosage	Interval	
Amikacin	7.5 mg/kg/dose	BID–TID	
Gentamicin	2.5 mg/kg/dose	BID–TID	
TOBI	300 mg	BID	30 days on, 30 days off
Colistin	37.5–75 mg	BID–QID	

TDM, therapeutic drug monitoring (gentamicin/tobramycin desired C_{max} 12–15 mg/L); TOBI, tobramycin for inhalation.
Adapted from reference 194.

diligence in monitoring for these adverse effects are essential. The Cystic Fibrosis Center recommends urinalysis and blood urea nitrogen (BUN) and serum creatinine testing after each course of aminoglycosides. Some clinicians suggest audiometric assessments for patients who have had 10 or more courses of IV aminoglycosides.[135] The adverse effects most often seen with β-lactams are elevated liver enzymes, diarrhea, hypersensitivity reactions, and fungal overgrowth.

Broad-spectrum antibiotics may cause overgrowth of *Clostridium difficile* in the gut lumen or fungus in the oropharyngeal cavity. Patients should be asked to report any diarrhea, difficulty in swallowing, or white plaques in their mouth.

INHALED ANTIBIOTICS

CF patients frequently receive large doses of systemic antibiotics to treat lung infections. However, the site of infection in CF is the airway lumen, not the lung parenchyma. Aerosolized delivery of antibiotic administers the drug directly to the site of infection, theoretically improving drug delivery and decreasing systemic toxicity risk. Aerosolized tobramycin and colistin are the most studied in CF, but other antibiotics are also given via this route.[136,137] Inhaled tobramycin might have some advantage over inhaled colistin in patients with *Pseudomonas*.[138] More than 40% of all CF patients in the United States are currently using inhaled tobramycin.[92]

ANTIBIOTIC PROPHYLAXIS

9. When is it appropriate to give L.T. antibiotics to prevent lung infection and colonization?

Some clinicians prescribe prophylactic antibiotics in an effort to prevent *S. aureus* infections in young children and subsequent *Pseudomonas* infections. However, the most recent randomized study of cephalexin prophylaxis demonstrated a significant decrease in colonization with *S. aureus,* but a significant increase in *P. aeruginosa* infections.[158] Thus, routine antistaphylococcal prophylaxis is not recommended for young children with CF and would not be recommended for L.T.

ACUTE PULMONARY EXACERBATION
Diagnosis

10. B.W., a 19-year-old woman, was diagnosed with CF at 3 years of age after a history of chronic pneumonias. She now presents to the pulmonary clinic with increasing cough and sputum production over the past 2 weeks with a change in sputum color from white to green. She currently weighs 45.2 kg and states she has lost 4 pounds. B.W. is a slightly thin adult woman whose breathing is labored. Pulmonary function tests reveal an FEV_1 of 65% of predicted normal and a forced vital capacity (FVC) of 60% (her usual baselines are FEV_1, 85%, and FVC, 80%). *P. aeruginosa* grew out of her sputum sample taken at the clinic 4 weeks ago for the first time. Other pertinent laboratory findings are as follows: WBC count, 17,000/mm³ (normal, 4,500 to 11,000/mm³) with 4% bands (normal, 0% to 11%), 35% segmented neutrophils (normal, 36% to 66%), 50% lymphocytes (normal, 24% to 44%), 11% eosinophils (normal, 1% to 4%); BUN, 7 mg/dL (normal, 5 to 18 mg/dL); and creatinine, 0.5 mg/dL (normal, 0.6 to 1.3 mg/dL). All other blood work, liver function tests, and electrolytes are within normal limits. Heart rate and blood pressure are normal. Temperature is 99.2°F, respiratory rate is 25 breaths/min (normal, 12 to 16) with an oxygen saturation of 95% (normal, 97% to 100%). A number of new pulmonary infiltrates are seen on chest radiograph. Her current medications include the following: 1 multiple vitamin QD, 2 microencapsulated pancreatic enzyme capsules (16,000 U lipase/capsule) with meals, and 1 or 2 additional capsules with snacks as needed.

What subjective and objective findings does B.W. exhibit that would lead to the diagnosis of a pulmonary exacerbation?

The onset of a pulmonary exacerbation of CF usually is marked by an increase in symptoms such as an increase in sputum production (usually purulent), increased cough, dyspnea, weight loss, and a 15% to 20% decline in pulmonary function tests over baseline. All these findings are present in B.W. An increase in WBC count, fever, or appearance of a new infiltrate on chest radiograph may or may not be present. Traditional management for an acute CF exacerbation includes nutritional repletion, antibiotics, and chest physiotherapy.[125]

Early Treatment of Pseudomonas aeruginosa

11. **B.W. is admitted to the hospital for a "cleanout," consisting of aggressive chest physiotherapy, aggressive nutritional repletion, and antipseudomonal antibiotics. Since *P. aeruginosa* was found in her sputum 4 weeks ago, the following sensitivities to antibiotics were tested and noted as follows: *P. aeruginosa* strain resistant to all antibiotics except tobramycin and ceftazidime. What is the value in giving antibiotics at this time?**

If given in the early phase of colonization, antibiotics can prevent the switch to a chronic mucoid infection. A combination of inhaled colistin or tobramycin with oral ciprofloxacin (see Question 14 on restricted use of quinolones) or inhaled antibiotics alone have been used to treat early pseudomonas infection.[159,160] In 14 of 15 patients treated with inhaled tobramycin for 1 year, colonization was not only prevented, but *Pseudomonas* was eradicated.[161] Since pulmonary tissue damage probably is related to bacterial load because of the infection-inflammation cycle, decreasing bacterial burden may slow the progression of lung disease. Therefore, it would be beneficial to treat B.W. aggressively with antipseudomonal therapy.

Aminoglycoside Dosing

12. **Because of B.W.'s clinical presentation, her physician has decided to admit her to the hospital and treat her with antibiotics. Her physician inquires about the use of extended-interval dosing for B.W.'s aminoglycoside therapy. Based on available laboratory data, develop a medication regimen and monitoring plan.**

In patients with CF, *P. aeruginosa* infection must be treated with a combination of two antibiotics to avoid resistance. An aminoglycoside combined with a β-lactam is the most common approach. Given the aforementioned sensitivities for patient B.W., ceftazidime plus tobramycin would be a good initial choice of antibiotics for this exacerbation. Because her renal and liver functions are normal, standard CF dosing can be used.

Ceftazidime 2 g IV every 8 hours could be administered to B.W. by continuous infusion because the β-lactams are time-dependent bactericidal antibiotics and the administration of ceftazidime, as a constant infusion in a CF patient is thought to be safe and effective.[162]

Extended-interval dosing of aminoglycosides (i.e., Q 12 hr or Q 24 hr compared with Q 8 hr) is being used to treat infections to enhance ease and cost of administration and to,

theoretically, improve efficacy and limit toxicity. The efficacy of extended-interval dosing of aminoglycosides, however, needs further study in the CF population because of the altered pharmacokinetics in CF. Nevertheless, several studies with small sample sizes appear to indicate that the use of extended-interval dosing of aminoglycosides is safe and effective for both children and adults with CF.[163–166] A large, multicenter trial investigating this issue more fully is currently underway. Although the early studies look promising, extended-interval dosing should not be used until completion of this or other large clinical trials.[167]

In B.W., the initial dosing regimen of IV tobramycin would be 225 mg (5 mg/kg) every 12 hours. Target peak concentrations of 12 to 15 mg/L should be verified on the third dose. Target trough concentrations should be less than 2 mg/L. A serum trough tobramycin level should be measured at least every 7 days while B.W. is on therapy, along with serum concentrations of BUN and creatinine.

The course of therapy will be 2 weeks with an additional 7 days if B.W. fails to reach specified endpoints at day 14. Endpoints of therapy are based on clinical response. Ideally, pulmonary function tests of FEV_1 should improve by 10% to 20% and should be evaluated weekly. The purulent nature and volume of the sputum should decrease and a gradual overall improvement in subjective feeling should be noted. Improved appetite and increased weight gain should be assessed daily with the goal of reaching baseline weight.

Inhaled Tobramycin

13. **B.W.'s physician wants to start TOBI. Why should (or should not) inhaled aminoglycosides be added to the parenteral regimen?**

TOBI is a special formulation of tobramycin for inhalation. Aerosolized antibiotics have been used in combination with IV antibiotics for treatment of acute exacerbations. Although eradication of *P. aeruginosa* from the sputum may be increased with these combined routes of therapy, the response may be only temporary.[168] The evidence for the addition of inhaled antibiotics to parenteral therapy is not strong, but the evidence for using inhaled tobramycin prophylactically to reduce bacterial load and avoid future exacerbations is getting stronger. Improved pulmonary function, along with a decrease in exacerbations or hospitalizations has been demonstrated with TOBI prophylactic regimens.[124,168–171] TOBI can be prescribed as twice-daily inhalations (300 mg) administered as a 30-day on and 30-day off schedule. Although this is a time-consuming and expensive therapy, it has been deemed to be cost-effective.[172] B.W. should be discharged on TOBI 300 mg BID prophylactic cycle schedule.

ORAL ANTIBIOTICS

14. **B.W. reaches her clinical endpoints and is sent home on TOBI therapy. Six months later, she calls the clinic from her college dorm. She has signs of an exacerbation, but refuses IV antibiotics or hospitalization, because she is in the middle of final exams. What alternative to IV therapy is available to treat B.W.? She now weighs 53 kg.**

The quinolone family of antibiotics is currently the only option for oral coverage of *P. aeruginosa*. Emergence of resistant strains of staphylococcal and *Pseudomonas* species have led the CF medical community to restrict the use of quinolones to the treatment of acute CF exacerbations.[175,176] Oral ciprofloxacin has become widely used in CF patients, because it is less expensive, easy to administer, and as effective as IV therapy in an acute exacerbation.[173,174]

Quinolones are not approved for use in patients less than 18 years old because of the risk of arthropathy. Fortunately, one study of 634 children failed to demonstrate any arthropathy in the patients, although reversible arthralgias were noted.[177] This risk is further complicated by the underlying problems with bone metabolism seen in CF. Although this issue has not been fully resolved, quinolones are used with caution in certain pediatric populations. In addition, B.W. is of childbearing age and quinolones are relatively contraindicated because of possible effects on cartilage development in the fetus. If a quinolone is used, B.W. should be counseled to use appropriate birth control techniques.

Because of the past sensitivities of B.W.'s organisms and her refusal to be admitted to the hospital, ciprofloxacin 1,000 mg orally twice daily for 1 week can be initiated in addition to the aerosolized tobramycin.[178] After 1 week of the combined aerosol and oral therapies, B.W. should be re-evaluated for hospital admission if her condition worsens, or her therapy can be continued if her condition improves.

Control of Inflammation

The inflammatory response in CF airways can be treated with drugs that block PMN chemotaxis, proinflammatory cytokines, or any other step in the inflammatory cascade. Corticosteroids, nonsteroidal anti-inflammatory agents (NSAIDs), and macrolides all have been used to control the inflammation seen in CF lung disease.

Corticosteroids

15. **J.J., an 18-year-old young man with CF, returns to the clinic for a routine 6-month visit. He now has severe pulmonary disease as reflected by his pulmonary function tests (FEV$_1$ is 39% of predicted normal and FVC is 37%) and marked chest radiographic changes that include areas of bronchiectasis and hyperinflation. He is chronically colonized with a resistant strain of *P. aeruginosa* and has a chronic productive cough, which currently is at baseline. Because the lung damage in CF is from inflammation secondary to the bacterial infection, what anti-inflammatory therapies might be considered for use in J.J.?**

Oral corticosteroids are not recommended in the treatment of CF. Although prednisone 1 to 2 mg/kg every other day, can reduce the decline of lung function and decrease pulmonary exacerbations in patients with *Pseudomonas* infections, it also can result in cataracts, glucose intolerance and persistent growth retardation.[179–181] Inhaled steroids do not show an improvement in pulmonary function in CF patients when used alone.[182] However, many CF patients with concurrent reactive airway disease or asthma in addition to CF respond to corticosteroids.

Nonsteroidal Anti-Inflammatory Agents

NSAIDs have been used to slow lung function decline. High-dose ibuprofen (20 to 30 mg/kg BID with doses titrated to a therapeutic range of 50 to 100 mg/L) can significantly slow the annual rate of FEV$_1$ decline in children between 6 and 13 years of age.[149] Ibuprofen serum concentrations must be measured and monitored closely to stay in the therapeutic window because lower concentrations can increase PMN infiltration. Since these doses are much higher than the recommended doses to treat pain or fever, concerns about long-term side effects including GI bleeding and renal toxicity together with the need for frequent blood draws have not made this method of treatment common. Less than 5% of the CF population is using ibuprofen.[92,150]

16. **Is J.J. a candidate for high-dose ibuprofen? He has refused routine blood draws in the past and worries about the side effects of medication.**

For maximal benefit, ibuprofen therapy must be started early, before the disease is as advanced as J.J.'s. Since J.J. does not like the idea of having to come in for blood draws or the possible side effects of GI distress or renal impairment, high-dose ibuprofen should not be recommended.

Macrolide Antibiotics

17. **When and why would azithromycin be indicated for J.J.?**

Macrolide antibiotics have immunomodulatory properties in addition to antimicrobial activity and have been shown to improve pulmonary function tests, reduce exacerbations, and improve quality of life in children and adults with end-stage disease.[151–154] In a 3-month prospective, randomized, double-blind, placebo-controlled study of azithromycin (250 mg/day) in 60 adults with CF, FEV$_1$ improved, C-reactive protein decreased, and fewer IV antibiotics were needed in the azithromycin group.[153] In a 15-month, randomized, double-blind, placebo-controlled, crossover trial, 41 children with CF received azithromycin. FEV$_1$ improved by 5.4% in the treatment group, and most patients required fewer courses of antibiotics while on azithromycin. No change in sputum bacterial density, inflammation markers, exercise tolerance, or quality of life were detected.[152] The development of bacterial resistance with long-term use of azithromycin is of genuine concern, and patients should be followed up closely if azithromycin is initiated on this basis.[155]

Although there is no definitive place in CF therapy for azithromycin, a 6-month trial may be indicated for patients who do not respond to conventional therapy.[152] J.J.'s lung function should be monitored to see whether he is improving, and therapy should be continued for an additional 6 months.

Other Strategies

Some types of bone pain and insulin resistance can be related to the severity of CF. Insulin therapy can improve weight and lung function, in addition to glucose control. Clinical lung deterioration is seen in patients several years before the development of cystic fibrosis related diabetes (CFRD). A case report noted improvements in weight and lung function in four patients treated with low doses of insulin.[183]

18. **What other approaches may be tried to modify the course of CF in B.W. and J.J.?**

J.J. and B.W. are both colonized with *Pseudomonas* in their lungs. J.J. should be started on a trial of TOBI, and both patients may be candidates for dornase alfa inhalation therapy. Re-evaluation of the type of mechanical clearance method, nutritional status, and enzyme dose should be considered. J.J. and B.W. should also be tested for liver disease, bone disease, and insulin resistance. J.J. and B.W.'s disease course and weight history should be carefully evaluated along with a fasting blood glucose, HbA$_{1c}$, and oral glucose tolerance test.

FUTURE THERAPIES

20. **What kind of treatments might be available to help patients with CF in the future?**

Many drugs are being evaluated to intercede at various levels of the vicious pathologic cascade (see Fig. 98-3) seen in CF lung disease. Fixing the inactive or malfunctioning CFTR by repairing the mutant gene would be a cure for CF. Until that is possible, researchers must work their way through the various steps in the cycle: CFTR dysfunction can be restored; ion transport defects re-established; altered airway secretions repaired; inflammation stopped; infection cured; and tissue damage averted.

Correcting the Gene

Gene therapy to correct the CFTR in the lungs is being actively pursued. CFTR is expressed in low levels in the lungs so that only 6% to 10% of the cells need active CFTR to correct the chloride channel deficiency. Several vectors are being developed to deliver the good gene and allow it to be incorporated into these cells, including adenovirus (Ad), adeno-associated virus (AAV), liposomes, retroviral vectors, and a new compacted DNA. Ad vectors were selected because of their tropism toward pulmonary cells; however, problems with the humoral response of the host prompted efforts to make this a safer vector. AAV is encouraging because it does not cause clinical disease in humans; however, the ability to carry the correct genetic code is hampered by its small size. Phase II trial results for tgAAVCF, a product using an AAV vector, demonstrated good gene transfer, no side effects, improvement in lung function, and a decrease in IL-8.[184,185] Cationic liposomes lack immunogenicity and toxicity, but the expression of CFTR has been low and inconsistent.[186] Retroviral vectors are efficient, but safety issues arise when using a virus that can integrate randomly in cells.

Lastly, nanotechnology has been used to "compact" or tightly bind strands of DNA, making it tiny enough to pass through a cell membrane and into the nucleus. Phase I trials have been completed; compact DNA was put into a solution and dripped into the noses of 12 patients. The treatment was well tolerated and without side effects in all patients. The investigators feel encouraged in that "gene transfer may have occurred."[187]

CFTR Dysfunction

Several therapies are directed at restoring CFTR function. The most common mutation, δF508, is due to a misfolding of the responsible protein. There are several "chemical chaperones," such as cellular osmolytes and low-molecular-weight compounds, which, when added to cells, rescue the folding of mutated proteins like δF508 CFTR.[188] Gentamicin has been shown to restore a class I mutation in vitro, and 8-cyclopentyl-1,3 dipropylxanthine (CPX) and sodium 4-phenylbutyrate (4PBA) have restored the CFTR to the surface of the apical membrane.[189]

Ion Channel Modifiers

Amiloride, a sodium channel blocker, has been given by nebulization on an investigational basis to inhibit the reabsorption of sodium (and water) into the lung epithelium in an attempt to prevent dehydration of pulmonary secretions. Unfortunately in a multicenter study, amiloride was of no benefit.[190] Adenosine triphosphate (ATP) and uridine triphosphate (UTP) can modify chloride channels by stimulating chloride secretion through increasing intracellular calcium. ATP is degraded to adenosine, which is a bronchoconstrictor; therefore, this would not be beneficial in CF patients with reactive airway disease or asthma. Duramycin and isobutylmethylxanthine are two other compounds in early clinical trials that also act as chloride secretagogues. CPX, omeprazole, and lansoprazole have also been observed to restore channel function.[121,191]

Decreasing the Inflammation-Infection Cycle

Drugs that modulate the host immune and inflammatory response are also being investigated. Pentoxifylline inhibits neutrophil chemotaxis and degranulation; aerosolized α$_1$-antitrypsin and secretory leukoprotease inhibitor inactivate the elastase in the ASL (airway surface layer); colchicine has been shown to have an anti-inflammatory effect; and high doses of DHA (docosahexaenoic acid) have been proposed to rebalance the arachidonic acid imbalance.[91]

Providing a complete list of all the potentially helpful compounds to treat this complex disease is beyond the scope of this chapter. However, a tremendous amount of research is focused on developing new therapies for CF, and there is reason to have hope for more effective treatment of this disease, and some day a cure.

REFERENCES

1. Busch R. On the history of cystic fibrosis. Acta Univ Carol [Med] (Praha) 1990;36(1-4):13.
2. di Sant'Agnese PA et al. Abnormal electrolyte composition of sweat in cystic fibrosis of the pancreas. Pediatrics 1953;12:549.
3. Andersen DH. Cystic fibrosis of the pancreas and its relation to celiac disease, a clinical and pathological study. Am J Dis Child 1938;56:344.
4. Kubba AK, Young M. The long suffering of Frederic Chopin. Chest 1998;113(1):210.

5. Welsh MJ. Abnormal regulation of ion channels in cystic fibrosis epithelia. Faseb J 1990;4(10):2718.
6. Boucher RC et al. Na+ transport in cystic fibrosis respiratory epithelia. Abnormal basal rate and response to adenylate cyclase activation. J Clin Invest 1986;78(5):1245.
7. Smith JJ, M.J Welch. cAMP stimulates bicarbonate secretion across normal, but not cystic fibrosis airway epithelia. J Clin Invest 1992;89:1148.

8. Ballard ST et al. CFTR involvement in chloride, bicarbonate, and liquid secretion by airway submucosal glands. Am J Physiol 1999;277(4 Pt 1):L694.
9. Schwiebert EM et al. CFTR is a conductance regulator as well as a chloride channel. Physiol Rev 1999;79(1 Suppl):S145.
10. Lee MG et al. Cystic fibrosis transmembrane conductance regulator regulates luminal Cl-/HCO3-exchange in mouse submandibular and pancreatic ducts. J Biol Chem 1999;274(21):14670.

11. Andersen DH, Hodges RG. Celiac syndrome. V. Genetics of cystic fibrosis of the pancreas with a consideration of the etiology. Am J Dis Child 1946;72:62.

12. Rommens JM et al. Identification of the cystic fibrosis gene: chromosome walking and jumping. Science 1989;245(4922):1059.

13. Kerem B et al. Identification of the cystic fibrosis gene: genetic analysis. Science 1989;245(4922):1073.

14. Riordan J.R. Identification of the cystic fibrosis gene: cloning and characterization of complementary DNA. Science 1989;245(4922):1066.

15. Rodman DM, Zamudio S. The cystic fibrosis heterozygote—advantage in surviving cholera? Med Hypotheses 1991;36(3):253.

16. Romeo G et al. Why is the cystic fibrosis gene so frequent? Hum Genet 1989;84(1):1.

17. Gabriel SE et al. Cystic fibrosis heterozygote resistance to cholera toxin in the cystic fibrosis mouse model. Science 1994;266(5182):107.

18. Padua RA et al. The cystic fibrosis delta F508 gene mutation and cancer. Hum Mutat 1997;10(1):45.

19. Warren N et al. Frequency of carriers of cystic fibrosis gene among patients with myeloid malignancy and melanoma. Br Med J 1991;302(6779):760.

20. Neglia JP et al. The risk of cancer among patients with cystic fibrosis. Cystic Fibrosis and Cancer Study Group. N Engl J Med 1995;332(8):494.

21. Abraham EH et al. Cystic fibrosis hetero- and homozygosity is associated with inhibition of breast cancer growth. Nat Med 1996;2(5):593.

22. Laniado ME et al. Expression and functional analysis of voltage-activated Na+ channels in human prostate cancer cell lines and their contribution to invasion in vitro. Am J Pathol 1997;150(4):1213.

23. Southey MC et al. CFTR deltaF508 carrier status, risk of breast cancer before the age of 40 and histological grading in a population-based case-control study. Int J Cancer 1998;79(5):487.

24. Consortium, T.C.F.G.A., Cystic Fibrosis Mutation Data Base, in http://www.genet.sickkids.on.ca/cftr. 1998, The Cystic Fibrosis Genetic Analysis Consortium.

25. Kerem E et al. The relation between genotype and phenotype in cystic fibrosis: analysis of the most common mutation (delta F508). N Engl J Med 1990;323(22):1517.

26. Zielenski J. Genotype and phenotype in cystic fibrosis. Respiration 2000;67(2):117.

27. Corey M. Modelling survival in cystic fibrosis. Thorax 2001;56(10):743.

28. Nixon GM et al. Clinical outcome after early Pseudomonas aeruginosa infection in cystic fibrosis. J Pediatr 2001;138(5):699.

29. Schechter MS et al. The association of socioeconomic status with outcomes in cystic fibrosis patients in he United States. Am J Respir Crit Care Med 2001;163(6):1331.

30. Kovesi T et al. Passive smoking and lung function in cystic fibrosis. Am Rev Respir Dis 1993;148(5):1266.

31. O'Connor GT et al. Median household income and mortality rate in cystic fibrosis. Pediatrics 2003;111(4 Pt 1):e333.

32. Grasemann H et al. Endothelial nitric oxide synthase variants in cystic fibrosis lung disease. Am J Respir Crit Care Med 2003;167(3):390.

33. Merlo CA, Boyle MP. Modifier genes in cystic fibrosis lung disease. J Lab Clin Med 2003;141(4):237.

34. Bronsveld I et al. Chloride conductance and genetic background modulate the cystic fibrosis phenotype of Delta F508 homozygous twins and siblings. J Clin Invest 2001;108(11):1705.

35. Hull J, Thomson AH. Contribution of genetic factors other than CFTR to disease severity in cystic fibrosis. Thorax 1998;53(12):1018.

36. Drumm ML. Modifier genes and variation in cystic fibrosis. Respir Res 2001;2(3):125.

37. Arkwright PD et al. End-organ dysfunction in cystic fibrosis: association with angiotensin I converting enzyme and cytokine gene polymorphisms. Am J Respir Crit Care Med 2003;167(3):384.

38. Henrion-Caude A et al. Liver disease in pediatric patients with cystic fibrosis is associated with glu-

tathione S-transferase P1 polymorphism. Hepatology 2002;36(4 Pt 1):913.

39. Garred P et al. Association of mannose-binding lectin gene heterogeneity with severity of lung disease and survival in cystic fibrosis. J Clin Invest 1999;104(4):431.

40. Garred P et al. Mannose-binding lectin (MBL) therapy in an MBL-deficient patient with severe cystic fibrosis lung disease. Pediatr Pulmonol 2002; 33(3):201.

41. Welsh MJ, Ramsey BW. Research on cystic fibrosis: a journey from the Heart House. Am J Respir Crit Care Med 1998;157(4 Pt 2):S148.

42. Zielenski J, Tsui LC. Cystic fibrosis: genotypic and phenotypic variations. Annu Rev Genet 1995;29:777.

43. Hamilton JW. Gentamicin in pharmacogenetic approach to treatment of cystic fibrosis. Lancet 2001;358(9298):201.

44. Reddy MM et al. Activation of the epithelial Na+ channel (ENaC) requires CFTR Cl–channel function. Nature 1999;402(6759):301.

45. Ramsey B, Richardson MA. Impact of sinusitis in cystic fibrosis. J Allergy Clin Immunol 1992;90(3 Pt 2):547.

46. Umetsu DT et al. Sinus disease in patients with severe cystic fibrosis: relation to pulmonary exacerbation. Lancet 1990;335(8697):1077.

47. Sohma Y et al. HCO₃-transport in a mathematical model of the pancreatic ductal epithelium. J Membr Biol 2000;176(1):77.

48. Hardin DS, Moran A. Diabetes mellitus in cystic fibrosis. Endocrinol Metab Clin North Am 1999; 28(4):787, ix.

49. Solomon MP et al. Glucose intolerance in children with cystic fibrosis. J Pediatr 2003;142(2):128.

50. Moran A et al. Abnormal glucose metabolism in cystic fibrosis. J Pediatr 1998;133(1):10.

51. Finkelstein SM et al. Diabetes mellitus associated with cystic fibrosis. J Pediatr 1988. 112(3):373.

52. Lanng S et al. Influence of the development of diabetes mellitus on clinical status in patients with cystic fibrosis. Eur J Pediatr 1992;151(9):684.

53. Hardin DS et al. Insulin resistance is associated with decreased clinical status in cystic fibrosis. J Pediatr 1997;130(6):948.

54. Brodzicki J et al. Frequency, consequences and pharmacological treatment of gastroesophageal reflux in children with cystic fibrosis. Med Sci Monit 2002;8(7):CR529.

55. Ledson MJ et al. Prevalence and mechanisms of gastro-oesophageal reflux in adult cystic fibrosis patients. J R Soc Med 1998;91(1):7.

56. Heine RG et al. Gastro-oesophageal reflux in infants under 6 moths with cystic fibrosis. Arch Dis Child 1998;78(1):44.

57. Cohn JA et al. Localization of the cystic fibrosis transmembrane conductance regulator in human bile duct epithelial cells. Gastroenterology 1993; 105(6):1857.

58. Kopelman H. Cystic fibrosis. 6. Gastrointestinal and nutritional aspects. Thorax 1991;46(4):261.

59. Gaskin KJ et al. Liver disease and common-bile-duct stenosis in cystic fibrosis. N Engl J Med 1988. 318(6):340.

60. Colombo C et al. Analysis of risk factors for the development of liver disease associated with cystic fibrosis. J Pediatr 1994;124(3):393.

61. Sokol RJ, Durie PR. Recommendations for management of liver and biliary tract disease in cystic fibrosis. Cystic Fibrosis Foundation Hepatobiliary Disease Consensus Group. J Pediatr Gastroenterol Nutr 1999;28(Suppl 1):S1.

62. Geddes DM. Cystic fibrosis and pregnancy. J R Soc Med 1992;85(Suppl 1):36.

63. Elkin SL et al. Histomorphometric analysis of bone biopsies from the iliac crest of adults with cystic fibrosis. Am J Respir Crit Care Med 2002;166(11):1470.

64. Haworth CS et al. A prospective study of change in bone mineral density over one year in adults with cystic fibrosis. Thorax 2002;57(8):719.

65. Haworth CS et al. Low bone mineral density in adults with cystic fibrosis. Thorax 1999;54(11):961.

66. Sood M et al. Bone status in cystic fibrosis. Arch Dis Child 2001;84(6):516.

67. Dixey J et al. The arthropathy of cystic fibrosis. Ann Rheum Dis 1988;47(3):218.

68. Rush, P.J. et al. The musculoskeletal manifestations of cystic fibrosis. Semin Arthritis Rheum 1986; 15(3):213.

69. Newman AJ, Ansell BM. Episodic arthritis in children with cystic fibrosis. J Pediatr 1979;94(4):594.

70. Phillips BM, David TJ. Pathogenesis and management of arthropathy in cystic fibrosis. J R Soc Med 1986;79(Suppl 12):44.

71. Pertuiset E et al. Cystic fibrosis arthritis. A report of five cases. Br J Rheumatol 1992;31(8):535.

72. Hoiby N. Inflammation and infection in cystic fibrosis—hen or egg? Eur Respir J 2001;17(1):4.

73. Elborn JS et al. Host inflammatory responses to first isolation of Pseudomonas aeruginosa from sputum in cystic fibrosis. Pediatr Pulmonol 1993;15(5):287.

74. Smith JJ et al. Cystic fibrosis airway epithelia fail to kill bacteria because of abnormal airway surface fluid. Cell 1996;85(2):229.

75. Travis SM et al. Activity of abundant antimicrobials of the human airway. Am J Respir Cell Mol Biol 1999;20(5):872.

76. Matsui H. et al. Evidence for periciliary liquid layer depletion, not abnormal ion composition, in the pathogenesis of cystic fibrosis airways disease. Cell 1998;95(7):1005.

77. Trout L et al. Disruptive effects of anion secretion inhibitors on airway mucus morphology in isolated perfused pig lung. J Physiol (Lond) 2003;549:845.

78. Ballard ST et al. Liquid secretion inhibitors reduce mucociliary transport in glandular airways. Am J Physiol Lung Cell Mol Physiol 2002;283(2):L329.

79. Scheid P et al. Inflammation in cystic fibrosis airways: relationship to increased bacterial adherence. Eur Respir J 2001;17(1):27.

80. Henry RL et al. Mucoid Pseudomonas aeruginosa is a marker of poor survival in cystic fibrosis. Pediatr Pulmonol 1992;12(3):158.

81. Soni R et al. Effect of Burkholderia cepacia infection in the clinical course of patients with cystic fibrosis: a pilot study in a Sydney clinic. Respirology 2002;7(3):241.

82. Konstan MW, Berger M. Current understanding of the inflammatory process in cystic fibrosis: onset and etiology. Pediatr Pulmonol 1997;24(2):137; discussion 159.

83. Mahadeva R et al. Anti-neutrophil cytoplasmic antibodies (ANCA) against bactericidal/permeability-increasing protein (BPI) and cystic fibrosis lung disease. Clin Exp Immunol 1999;117(3):561.

84. Tager AM et al. The effect of chloride concentration on human neutrophil functions: potential relevance to cystic fibrosis. Am J Respir Cell Mol Biol 1998; 19(4):643.

85. Olivier KN et al. Nontuberculous mycobacteria. II: nested-cohort study of impact on cystic fibrosis lung disease. Am J Respir Crit Care Med 2003; 167(6):835.

86. Olivier KN et al. Nontuberculous mycobacteria. I: multicenter prevalence study in cystic fibrosis. Am J Respir Crit Care Med 2003;167(6):828.

87. Armstrong DS et al. Lower airway inflammation in infants and young children with cystic fibrosis. Am J Respir Crit Care Med 1997;156(4 Pt 1):1197.

88. Bonfield TL et al. Inflammatory cytokines in cystic fibrosis lungs. Am J Respir Crit Care Med 1995;152(6 Pt 1):2111.

89. Bonfield TL et al. Normal bronchial epithelial cells constitutively produce the anti-inflammatory cytokine interleukin-10, which is downregulated in cystic fibrosis. Am J Respir Cell Mol Biol 1995;13(3):257.

90. Bonfield TL et al. Altered respiratory epithelial cell cytokine production in cystic fibrosis. J Allergy Clin Immunol 1999;104(1):72.

91. Freedman SD et al. A membrane lipid imbalance plays a role in the phenotypic expression of cystic fibrosis in cftr(-/-) mice. Proc Natl Acad Sci USA 1999;96(24):13995.

92. Foundation CF. Patient Registry 2001 Annual Data Report, in epidemiology. 2002: Bethesda, MD.

93. Rosenstein BJ, Cutting GR. The diagnosis of cystic fibrosis: a consensus statement. Cystic Fibrosis Foundation Consensus Panel. J Pediatr 1998; 132(4):589.

94. Gibson L, Cooke R. A test for concentration of electorlytes in sweat in cystic fibrosis of the pancreas utilizing pilocarpine iontophoresis. Pediatrics 1959;23:545.

95. Knowles MR et al. Boucher, In vivo nasal potential difference: techniques and protocols for assessing efficacy of gene transfer in cystic fibrosis. Hum Gene Ther 1995;6(4):445.

96. Hammond KB et al. Efficacy of statewide neonatal screening for cystic fibrosis by assay of trypsinogen concentrations. N Engl J Med 1991; 325(11):769.

97. Merelle ME et al. Newborn screening for cystic fibrosis. Cochrane Database Syst Rev 2001(3): CD001402.

98. Farrell PM et al. Nutritional benefits of neonatal screening for cystic fibrosis. Wisconsin Cystic Fibrosis Neonatal Screening Study Group. N Engl J Med 1997;337(14):963.

99. Wagener JS. et al. A debate on why my state (province) should or should not conduct newborn screening for cystic fibrosis (14th Annual North American Cystic Fibrosis Conference). Pediatr Pulmonol 2001;32(5):385.

100. Farrell PM et al. Early diagnosis of cystic fibrosis through neonatal screening prevents severe malnutrition and improves long-term growth. Wisconsin Cystic Fibrosis Neonatal Screening Study Group. Pediatrics 2001;107(1):1.

101. Conway SP. Evidence-based medicine in cystic fibrosis: how should practice cahnge? Pediatr Pulmonol 2002;34(3):242.

102. Fiel SB. Early aggressive intervention in cystic fibrosis: is it time to redefine our "best practice" strategies? Chest 2003;123(1):1.

103. Koch C. Early infection and progression of cystic fibrosis lung disease. Pediatr Pulmonol 2002; 34(3):232.

104. Farrell M et al. Genetic counseling and risk communication services of newborn screening programs. Arch Pediatr Adolesc Med 2001;155(2):120.

105. Farrell PM, Fost N. Prenatal screening for cystic fibrosis: where are we now? J Pediatr 2002; 141(6):758.

106. Johnson C et al. Factors influencing outcomes in cystic fibrosis: a center-based analysis. Chest 2003;123(1):20.

107. Borowitz D et al. Consensus report on nutrition for pediatric patients with cystic fibrosis. J Pediatr Gastroenterol Nutr 2002;35(3):246.

108. Rosenfeld M et al. Nutritional effects of long-term gastrostomy feedings in children with cystic fibrosis. J Am Diet Assoc 1999;99(2):191.

109. Steinkamp G, von der Hardt H. Improvement of nutritional status and lung function after long-term nocturnal gastrostomy feedings in cystic fibrosis. J Pediatr 1994;124(2):244.

110. Feranchak AP et al. Prospective, long-term study of fat-soluble vitamin status in children with cystic fibrosis identified by newborn screen. J Pediatr 1999;135(5):601.

111. Rashid M et al. Prevalence of vitamin K deficiency in cystic fibrosis. Am J Clin Nutr 1999;70(3):378.

112. Wilson DC et al. Treatment of vitamin K deficiency in cystic fibrosis: effectiveness of a daily fat-soluble vitamin combination. J Pediatr 2001;138(6):851.

113. Beker LT et al. Effect of vitamin K1 supplementation on vitamin K status in cystic fibrosis patients. J Pediatr Gastroenterol Nutr 1997;24(5):512.

114. Guarner L et al. Fate of oral enzymes in pancreatic insufficiency. Gut 1993;34(5):708.

115. Borowitz DS et al. Use of pancreatic enzyme supplements for patients with cystic fibrosis in the context of fibrosing colonopathy. Consensus Committee. J Pediatr 1995;127(5):681.

116. Smyth RL et al. Strictures of ascending colon in cystic fibrosis and high-strength pancreatic enzymes. Lancet 1994;343(8889):85.

117. FitzSimmons SC et al. High-dose pancreatic enzyme supplements and fibrosing colonopathy in children with cystic fibrosis. N Engl J Med 1997;336(18):1283.

118. Robinson PJ et al Duodenal pH in cystic fibrosis and its relationship to fat malabsorption. Dig Dis Sci 1990;35(10):1299.

119. Heijerman HG. Ranitidine compared with dimethylprostaglandin E2 analogue enprostil as adjunct to pancreatic enzyme replacement in adult cystic fibrosis. Scand J Gastroenterol Suppl 1990;178:26.

120. Heijerman HG et al. Omeprazole enhances the efficacy of pancreatin (Pancrease) in cystic fibrosis. Ann Intern Med 1991;114:200.

121. Hendriks JJE et al. Changes in pulmonary hyperinflation and bronchial hyperresponsiveness following treatment with lansoprazole in children with cystic fibrosis. Pediatr Pulmonol 2001;31:59.

122. Hendeles L et al. Treatment failure after substitution of generic pancrelipase capsules. Correlation with in vitro lipase activity. JAMA 1990;263(18):2459.

123. Saiman L, Siegel J. Infection control recommendations for patients with cystic fibrosis: microbiology, important pathogens, and infection control practices to prevent patient-to-patient transmission. Am J Infect Control 2003.S1.

124. Ramsey BW et al. Intermittent administration of inhaled tobramycin in patients with cystic fibrosis. Cystic Fibrosis Inhaled Tobramycin Study Group. N Engl J Med 1999;340(1):23.

125. Ramsey BW. Management of pulmonary disease in patients with cystic fibrosis. N Engl J Med 1996;335(3):179.

126. Frederiksen B et al. Changing epidemiology of *Pseudomonas aeruginosa* infection in Danish cystic fibrosis patients (1974-1995). Pediatr Pulmonol 1999;28(3):159.

127. Kearns GL et al. Hepatic drug clearance in patients with mild cystic fibrosis. Clin Pharmacol Ther 1996;59(5):529.

128. Hutabarat RM et al. Disposition of drugs in cystic fibrosis. I. Sulfamethoxazole and trimethoprim. Clin Pharmacol Ther 1991;49(4):402.

129. Wang JP et al. Disposition of drugs in cystic fibrosis. VI. In vivo activity of cytochrome P450 isoforms involved in the metabolism of (R)-warfarin (including P450 3A4) is not enhanced in cystic fibrosis. Clin Pharmacol Ther 1994;55(5):528.

130. O'Sullivan TA et al. Disposition of drugs in cystic fibrosis. V. In vivo CYP2C9 activity as probed by (S)-warfarin is not enhanced in cystic fibrosis. Clin Pharmacol Ther 1993;54(3):323.

131. Hamelin BA et al. Caffeine metabolism in cystic fibrosis: enhanced xanthine oxidase activity. Clin Pharmacol Ther 1994;56(5):521.

132. Woodland C et al. Hypothetical framework for enhanced renal tubular secretion of drugs in cystic fibrosis. Med Hypotheses 1998;51(6):489.

133. Wang JP et al. Disposition of drugs in cystic fibrosis. IV. Mechanisms for enhanced renal clearance of ticarcillin. Clin Pharmacol Ther 1993; 54(3):293.

134. Weber A et al. Probenecid pharmacokinetics in cystic fibrosis. Dev Pharmacol Ther 1991;16(1):7.

135. Tan KH et al. Aminoglycoside prescribing and surveillance in cystic fibrosis. Am J Respir Crit Care Med 2003;167(6):819.

136. Kuhn RJ. Pharmaceutical considerations in aerosol drug delivery. Pharmacotherapy 2002; 22(3 Pt 2):80S.

137. Kuhn RJ. Formulation of aerosolized therapeutics. Chest 2001;120(3 Suppl):94S.

138. Hodson ME et al. A randomised clinical trial of nebulised tobramycin or colistin in cystic fibrosis. Eur Respir J 2002;20(3):658.

139. Varekojis SM et al. A comparison of the therapeutic effectiveness of and preference for postural drainage and percussion, intrapulmonary percussive ventilation, and high-frequency chest wall compression in hospitalized cystic fibrosis patients. Respir Care 2003;48(1):24.

140. Oermann CM et al. Comparison of high-frequency chest wall oscillation and oscillating positive expiratory pressure in the home management of cystic fibrosis: a pilot study. Pediatr Pulmonol 2001;32(5):372.

141. Quan JM et al. A two-year randomized, placebo-controlled trial of dornase alfa in young patients with cystic fibrosis with mild lung function abnormalities. J Pediatr 2001;139(6):813.

142. Fuchs HJ et al. Effect of aerosolized recombinant human DNase on exacerbations of respiratory symptoms and on pulmonary function in patients with cystic fibrosis. The Pulmozyme Study Group. N Engl J Med 1994;331(10):637.

143. Harms HK et al. Multicenter, open-label study of recombinant human DNase in cystic fibrosis patients with moderate lung disease. DNase International Study Group. Pediatr Pulmonol 1998; 26(3):155.

144. McCoy K et al. Effects of 12-week administration of dornase alfa in patients with advanced cystic fibrosis lung disease. Pulmozyme Study Group. Chest 1996;110(4):889.

145. Wilmott RW et al. Aerosolized recombinant human DNase in hospitalized cystic fibrosis patients with acute pulmonary exacerbations. Am J Respir Crit Care Med 1996;153(6 Pt 1):1914.

146. Grieve R et al. A cost-effectiveness analysis of rhDNase in children with cystic fibrosis. Int J Technol Assess Health Care 2003;19(1):71.

147. Cramer GW, Bosso JA. The role of dornase alfa in the treatment of cystic fibrosis. Ann Pharmacother 1996;30(6):656.

148. Wark PA, McDonald V. Nebulised hypertonic saline for cystic fibrosis. Cochrane Database Syst Rev 2003(1):CD001506.

149. Konstan MW et al. Effect of high-dose ibuprofen in patients with cystic fibrosis. N Engl J Med 1995;332(13):848.

150. Dezateux C, Crighton A. Oral non-steroidal anti-inflammatory drug therapy for cystic fibrosis. Cochrane Database Syst Rev 2000(2):CD001505.

151. Jaffe A et al. Long-term azithromycin may improve lung function in children with cystic fibrosis. Lancet 1998;351(9100):420.

152. Equi A et al. Long term azithromycin in children with cystic fibrosis: a randomised, placebo-controlled crossover trial. Lancet 2002;360(9338):978.

153. Wolter J et al. Effect of long term treatment with azithromycin on disease parameters in cystic fibrosis: a randomised trial. Thorax 2002;57(3):212.

154. Gaylor AS, Reilly JC. Therapy with macrolides in patients with cystic fibrosis. Pharmacotherapy 2002;22(2):227.

155. Prunier AL et al. Clinical isolates of *Staphylococcus aureus* with ribosomal mutations conferring resistance to macrolides. Antimicrob Agents Chemother 2002;46(9):3054.

156. Ramsey BW et al. Predictive value of oropharyngeal cultures for identifying lower airway bacteria in cystic fibrosis patients. Am Rev Respir Dis 1991;144(2):331.

157. Brady MS et al. Effectiveness of enteric coated pancreatic enzymes given before meals in reducing steatorrhea in children with cystic fibrosis. J Am Diet Assoc 1992;92(7):813.

158. Stutman HR et al. Antibiotic prophylaxis in infants and young children with cystic fibrosis: a randomized controlled trial. J Pediatr 2002;140(3):299.

159. Valerius NH et al. Prevention of chronic *Pseudomonas aeruginosa* colonisation in cystic fibrosis by early treatment. Lancet 1991;338(8769): 725.

160. Wiesemann HG et al. Placebo-controlled, double-blind, randomized study of aerosolized tobramycin for early treatment of *Pseudomonas aeruginosa* colonization in cystic fibrosis. Pediatr Pulmonol 1998;25(2):88.

161. Ratjen F et al. Effect of inhaled tobramycin on early *Pseudomonas aeruginosa* colonisation in patients with cystic fibrosis. Lancet 2001; 358(9286):983.

162. Bosso JA et al. A pilot study of the efficacy of constant-infusion ceftazidime in the treatment of endobronchial infections in adults with cystic fibrosis. Pharmacotherapy 1999;19(5):620.

163. Master V et al. Efficacy of once-daily tobramycin monotherapy for acute pulmonary exacerbations of cystic fibrosis: a preliminary study. Pediatr Pulmonol 2001;31(5):367.

164. Vic P et al. Efficacy, tolerance, and pharmacokinetics of once daily tobramycin for pseudomonas exacerbations in cystic fibrosis. Arch Dis Child 1998;78(6):536.

165. Whitehead A et al. Once-daily tobramycin in the treatment of adult patients with cystic fibrosis. Eur Respir J 2002;19(2):303.

166. Bragonier R, Brown NM. The pharmacokinetics and toxicity of once-daily tobramycin therapy in children with cystic fibrosis. J Antimicrob Chemother 1998;42(1):103.

167. Tan K, Bunn H. Once daily versus multiple daily dosing with intravenous aminoglycosides for cystic fibrosis. Cochrane Database Syst Rev 2000(4):CD002009.

168. Ramsey BW et al. Efficacy of aerosolized tobramycin in patients with cystic fibrosis. N Engl J Med 1993;328(24):1740.

169. Gibson RL et al. Significant microbiological effect of inhaled tobramycin in young children with cystic fibrosis. Am J Respir Crit Care Med 2003;167(6):841.

170. Steinkamp G et al. Long-term tobramycin aerosol therapy in cystic fibrosis. Pediatr Pulmonol 1989;6(2):91.

171. Moss RB. Long-term benefits of inhaled tobramycin in adolescent patients with cystic fibrosis. Chest 2002;121(1):55.

172. Heinzl B et al. Effects of inhaled gentamicin prophylaxis on acquisition of *Pseudomonas aeruginosa* in children with cystic fibrosis: a pilot study. Pediatr Pulmonol 2002;33(1):32.

173. Bosso JA et al. Ciprofloxacin versus tobramycin plus azlocillin in pulmonary exacerbations in adult patients with cystic fibrosis. Am J Med 1987;82(4A):180.

174. Hodson ME et al. Oral ciprofloxacin compared with conventional intravenous treatment for *Pseudomonas aeruginosa* infection in adults with cystic fibrosis. Lancet 1987;1(8527):235.

175. Blumberg HM et al. Rapid development of ciprofloxacin resistance in methicillin-susceptible and -resistant *Staphylococcus aureus*. J Infect Dis 1991;163(6):1279.

176. Radberg G et al. Development of quinolone-imipenem cross resistance in *Pseudomonas aeruginosa* during exposure to ciprofloxacin. Antimicrob Agents Chemother 1990;34(11):2142.

177. Chysky V et al. Safety of ciprofloxacin in children: worldwide clinical experience based on compassionate use. Emphasis on joint evaluation. Infection 1991;19(4):289.

178. Rubio TT et al. Pharmacokinetic disposition of sequential intravenous/oral ciprofloxacin in pediatric cystic fibrosis patients with acute pulmonary exacerbation. Pediatr Infect Dis J 1997;16(1):112; discussion 123.

179. Eigen H et al. A multicenter study of alternate-day prednisone therapy in patients with cystic fibrosis. Cystic Fibrosis Foundation Prednisone Trial Group. J Pediatr 1995;126(4):515.

180. Auerbach HS et al. Alternate-day prednisone reduces morbidity and improves pulmonary function in cystic fibrosis. Lancet 1985;2(8457):686.

181. Lai, HC et al. Risk of persistent growth impairment after alternate-day prednisone treatment in children with cystic fibrosis. N Engl J Med 2000;342(12):851.

182. Dezateux C et al. Inhaled corticosteroids for cystic fibrosis. Cochrane Database Syst Rev 2000(2):CD001915.

183. Dobson L et al. Clinical improvement in cystic fibrosis with early insulin treatment. Arch Dis Child 2002;87(5):430.

184. Aitken ML et al. A phase I study of aerosolized administration of tgAAVCF to cystic fibrosis subjects with mild lung disease. Hum Gene Ther 2001;12(15):1907.

185. Moss R. Respiratory Tract: planning and executing a gene therapy trial for the respiratory tract. In 6th Annual American Society of Gene Therapy Meeting. 2003; Washington, DC.

186. Alton EW et al. Cationic lipid-mediated CFTR gene transfer to the lungs and nose of patients with cystic fibrosis: a double-blind placebo-controlled trial. Lancet 1999;353(9157):947.

187. Konstan MW. Gene transfer using novel compacted DNA. In 6th Annual American Society of Gene Therapy Meeting. 2003; Washington, DC.

188. Jiang C et al. Partial restoration of cAMP-stimulated CFTR chloride channel activity in DeltaF508 cells by deoxyspergualin. Am J Physiol, 1998;275(1 Pt 1):C171.

189. Zeitlin PL et al. Evidence of CFTR function in cystic fibrosis after systemic administration of 4-phenylbutyrate. Mol Ther 2002;6(1):119.

190. Pons G et al. French multicenter randomized double-blind placebo-controlled trial on nebulized amiloride in cystic fibrosis patients. The Amiloride-AFLM Collaborative Study Group. Pediatr Pulmonol 2000;30(1):25.

191. McCarty NA et al. A phase I randomized, multicenter trial of CPX in adult subjects with mild cystic fibrosis. Pediatr Pulmonol 2002;33(2):90.

192. MacLusky L. Spectrum of clinical manifestations of cystic fibrosis. Pediatr Ann 1993;22:544.

193. Gardiner-Caldwell. Cystic fibrosis: Pathogenesis and therapies. In major pathogenic events in cystic fibrosis lung disease. Synermed Communications, NJ, 1994.

194. Scott CS, Milavetz G. Cystic Fibrosis. In Carter BL et al (eds). Pharmacotherapy Self-Assessment Module. Kansas City, MO. ACCP 1999;109.

CHAPTER 99

Geriatric Drug Use

Jiwon Kim, Andrea Cooper

Demographic and Economic Considerations

Demographic changes and U.S. medical progress in the last half of the 20th century have created imperatives to improve our knowledge about the health care and drug therapy of older adults. The Federal Interagency Forum on Aging-Related Statistics recently published its first chartbook, which provides information on the health and well-being of older Americans in the United States (Table 99-1).[1]

The oldest-old category or frail elderly (i.e., those older than 85 years of age) is going to have the greatest impact on the health care system because the numbers of people in this group have increased faster than any other age category. This group will triple its size by 2040, which is more than double the growth rate of the next fastest-growing category.[2] By 2050, at least half of Americans will live to age 85; they will number 19 million and comprise 5% of the total U.S. population.[3] Because the frail elderly are often dependent and in ill health, they require the highest level of health services. They have the highest health care expenditures, hospitalization rates, and home health visits.[1]

Approximately 4% of the 35 million U.S. residents 65 years of age or older in 1999 resided in long-term care facilities (LTCFs).[4] Elderly LTCF residents are predominantly women, 75 years and older, white non-Hispanic, and widowed. Although the prevalence of functional disability in the elderly is expected to be reduced,[5] the national expenditure for long-term care services for the elderly is expected to grow through year 2040.[4] Of older adults who live at home, about 10% in the 65- to 74-year-old age group and up to 50% in the over-85-year-old age group require assistance with everyday activities.[2] Up to 64% of those who receive care rely on informal care from children and other relatives.[1] Thus, it is important to include the caregiver in the counseling and monitoring of activities when feasible.

Health care for the elderly is increasingly based on a prospective reimbursement system in institutional settings. Managed care practices aim to minimize high-cost hospitalizations by shifting care to lower-cost alternatives, such as home health care, assisted living, and hospice care. The escalating costs and affordability of medications is a national concern, especially in the Medicare population. As reforms are put in place to enhance access to drugs, it is especially important to keep in mind that this population is particularly vulnerable to drug-related morbidity and mortality, which costs the U.S. health care system at least $30.1 billion annually.[6]

Table 99-1	**Profile of Older Americans**[1]

Current Status of the Older Population

- The older population, persons ≥65 years of age, numbered 35 million in 2000, representing 13% of the U.S. population. This means since 1900, the percentage of Americans aged ≥65 tripled (4.1% in 1900 to 13% in 2000), and their numbers have increased 10-fold (from 3.1 million to 35 million in 2000)
- There are more women than men among the older population. Among persons ≥65 years old in 2000, 58% were women. In the oldest old group, 70% of persons ≥85 years were women
- The older population is getting older. In 2000 the ≥85 age group (4 million) was 31 times larger than in 1900
- The expected number of years of life increased by approximately 60% since 1900. In 1997, life expectancy was 79.4 years for women and 73.6 years for men
- In 1995, among noninstitutionalized elderly ≥70 years of age, 79% had at least one of the seven chronic conditions common among the elderly (arthritis, hypertension, respiratory illnesses, heart disease, diabetes, stroke, and cancer)
- Among all persons ≥65 years of age, the five leading causes of death are heart disease, cancer, stroke, chronic obstructive pulmonary diseases, pneumonia and influenza, and diabetes

Future Growth of the Older Population

- Although the rate of growth slowed during the 1990s because of the relatively small number of births during the Great Depression of the 1930s, the most rapid increase is expected between the years 2010 and 2030, when the baby boom generation reaches age 65
- By 2030, there will be about 70 million older persons, 2.7 times their number in 1980. If current fertility and immigration levels remain stable, the only age groups to grow significantly will be those >55 years of age
- By 2030, persons aged ≥65 are expected to represent 20% of the population; the population ≥85 years of age will more than double to approximately 8.5 million persons

Table 99-2	**Factors That May Influence Functional Age**

Poor versus good or adequate nutrition
Smoking versus quit smoking versus never a smoker
Acute or chronic diseases versus good health
Acute or chronic drug therapy versus no drug use
"Couch potato" versus lifelong habit of exercise
Institutionalized versus living independently at home

denced by the scarcity of information on aging and pharmacologic effects. Resnick and Marcantonio have summarized six geriatric clinical care principles (Table 99-3).[7]

Absorption

Changes in the gastrointestinal (GI) tract with age may influence drug absorption. Gastric pH increases, intestinal blood flow diminishes, and some impairment of both active and passive transport mechanisms occurs.[8] However, the significance of these changes is not clear. One study found nearly 90% of healthy, independently living elders were able to acidify gastric contents (pH 3.5), even in the basal unstimulated state (ages, 65 to 96 years).[9] However, these volunteers were "functionally" young (see Table 99-2), with an average of only 2.1 self-reported disease states and 1.6 over-the-counter (OTC) and prescription medications. Assessment of age-associated changes in absorption requires careful attention to methodology. For example, samples must be collected for 4 to 6 half-lives in older subjects to obtain a complete area under the time-concentration curve (AUC). Also, intravenous (IV) and oral (PO) data must be compared in the same subject to validate the assumption that clearance is constant.

$$AUC = \frac{(S)(F)(Dose)}{Cl} \qquad (99\text{-}1)$$

where *(S)(F)* is the fraction of dose administered that will reach systemic circulation and *Cl* is clearance.

The following generalizations can be concluded: the extent of absorption is similar in older patients and in young adults, the rate of absorption is reduced or unaltered in older patients, and drugs that undergo first-pass metabolism are absorbed more completely in the older patient.

Age-Related Physiologic, Pharmacokinetic, and Pharmacodynamic Changes

An important determinant of drug-related problems in the aged is an increased physiologic vulnerability to medication adverse effects and an impaired ability to recover from drug-induced insults. The progressive decrease in the ability of each organ system to maintain homeostasis in the face of challenge is a definition of physiologic aging.[7] Disruption of homeostatic "balance" predisposes an older adult to disease or medication side effects. Homeostatic mechanisms in the cardiovascular and nervous systems are less efficient; drug metabolism and excretion decrease; body tissue composition and drug volume of distribution change; and drug receptor sensitivity may be altered. Age-associated changes are progressive, occurring gradually over a lifetime, rather than abruptly at any given age (e.g., 65 years of age). The physiologic processes of aging often result in an increased susceptibility to many diseases. However, older people remain a heterogeneous group, with chronologic age not always reflecting "functional age" (Table 99-2). Distinct separation of these interrelated factors is difficult because all may contribute to variability in drug response. In particular, pharmacodynamic changes in the aging population is a research topic fraught with many methodological and logistic constraints, as evi-

1. I.W., a 75-year-old woman, 5'4", 120 pounds, serum creatinine (SrCr) of 1.9 mg/dL, has an acute exacerbation of heart failure (HF). She is given furosemide 40 mg orally, but this produces little increase in urine output or resolution of her symptoms. What might be an explanation for I.W.'s lack of response to furosemide? How might the desired response to furosemide be achieved?

The extent of furosemide (Lasix) absorption is not changed in older patients, but the rate of absorption is slowed. This results in a diminished efficacy of the drug because active secretion into the urine (rate of entry) must reach the steep portion of the sigmoid dose-response curve for maximal effect of the drug.[10] I.W. should be given a 40 mg dose of furosemide intravenously to bypass the problem of decreased rate of absorption. High sodium intake or concurrent use of nonsteroidal anti-inflammatory drugs (NSAIDs) can also decrease the effectiveness of furosemide. Further increases in

Table 99-3 Geriatric Clinical Care Principles

Care Principle	Outcome/Example
Because of impaired physiologic reserve in older patients, disease often presents at an earlier stage	• Mild disease may tip the "balance" • Drug side effects may occur with agents and doses unlikely to be toxic in younger people • Stoic elderly may be less likely to seek help for dysfunction until symptoms are advanced
Presentation of a new disease depends on the organ system made most vulnerable by previous changes, and this "weak link" often differs from the organ newly diseased	• Presentation is often atypical, with the "weakest link" being the brain (confusion), lower urinary tract (incontinence), musculoskeletal system (falling), or cardiovascular system (fainting)
Clinical findings abnormal in younger patients are common in older people and may not be responsible for a particular symptom	• An elderly patient with syncope due to medications and dehydration, but with ventricular ectopy on a cardiac monitor, may be harmed by misdirected antiarrhythmic therapy
Because comorbid disease and drug use are common, symptoms are often due to multiple causes	• Incontinence may involve a combination of fecal impaction, drugs inducing confusion, and impaired mobility due to arthritis
Because many homeostatic mechanisms may be compromised concurrently, multiple abnormalities can be amenable to treatment and small improvements in several areas may yield dramatic benefits to overall function	• Falls associated with diabetic polyneuropathy are exacerbated by concomitant drug use, arthritis, and orthostatic hypotension, which are more easily treated than the underlying disease
Because older patients are more likely to suffer adverse consequences of disease, treatment and prevention may be equally or more effective	• Thrombolytics for AMI • β-Blockers after MI • Hypertension treatment • Immunization (influenza, pneumococcal pneumonia) • Fall prevention (modify drugs that induce orthostasis or confusion, remove environmental hazards, address balance, peripheral edema, nocturia)

AMI, acute myocardial infarction; MI, myocardial infarction.

the dose of furosemide may be necessary, with consideration of a continuous infusion in patients with severe chronic renal insufficiency (see Chapter 19, Heart Failure).[10]

Distribution

A number of changes that can affect the distribution of drugs in the body may occur with aging. Cardiac output decreases about 1% per year from ages 19 to 86.[11] In many older patients, this decline in cardiac output is accompanied by an increase in peripheral vascular resistance and a proportional decrease in hepatic and renal blood flow. However, noninstitutionalized older adults who are free of coronary artery disease or other debilitating health problems exhibit little age-related declines in cardiac output (functionally young).[12] Body composition undergoes changes during normal aging. Total body water and lean body mass both decline with age, and total fat content increases between ages 18 and 85 years from 18% to 36% in men and from 33% to 48% in women.[13,14] Thus, the volume of distribution (Vd) of drugs that are distributed primarily in body water or lean body mass (e.g., lithium, digoxin) is decreased in older adults; unadjusted dosing can result in higher blood levels. Conversely, the Vd of highly lipid-soluble drugs, such as long-acting benzodiazepines (e.g., diazepam), may be increased, thereby delaying maximal effects or resulting in accumulation with continued use.[15] Factors that may affect binding—with special applicability in older patients—include protein concentration, disease states, co-administration of other drugs, and nutritional status. Serum albumin concentrations fall progressively for each decade beyond 40 years of age, reaching a mean of 3.58 g/dL (normal, 4 g/dL) in those older than 80 years of age.[16]

Decreased albumin concentrations are important because albumin is a major site of drug binding. Increases in α_1-acid glycoprotein in older patients[17] affect the binding of weak bases such as lidocaine and propranolol. Data are lacking concerning age-related changes in tissue protein binding of drugs. However, the Vd of digoxin does decrease in subjects with impaired renal function, as does the myocardial-to-serum concentration ratio.[18] Finally, an important factor in determining the significance of changes in protein binding status is whether a drug is restrictively or nonrestrictively cleared.[19]

Altered Protein Binding

2. O.T., a 90-year-old woman, 5′8″, 132 pounds, is brought to the emergency department (ED) for evaluation of a "shaking spell." In the ED, another "spell" is observed, starting with shaking of the left arm and progressing into a generalized tonic-clonic seizure. A loading dose of phenytoin (Dilantin) 1,000 mg is given IV over 30 minutes. O.T. is admitted to the neurology unit for further evaluation and given phenytoin 300 mg QHS. What is your assessment of O.T.'s phenytoin therapy given her age? What laboratory tests should be ordered, and how often should these be monitored?

O.T. received an average phenytoin loading dose of 17 mg/kg (normal, 15 to 20 mg/kg) and is receiving the average daily maintenance dose. A sodium serum concentration should be obtained to rule out hyponatremia-induced seizure, and an albumin serum concentration should be obtained because of phenytoin's high (90%) protein binding. A phenytoin serum concentration should be measured before O.T. is discharged from the hospital to document that the desired therapeutic serum concentration has been achieved. The serum phenytoin concentration should be obtained whenever an adverse drug reaction or seizure occurs. A follow-up steady-state phenytoin serum concentration should be obtained in 10 to 14 days to determine if the current dose is appropriate.

3. The serum albumin concentration is 2.2 g/dL (normal, 3.2 to 5.2 g/dL), Na is 140 mEq/L (normal, 138 to 145 mEq/L), and the phenytoin serum concentration is 15 μg/mL (normal, 10 to 20 μg/mL). O.T. complains of drowsiness and has a wide-based, unsteady gait. What is the likely cause of her symptoms?

[SI units: albumin, 22 g/L (normal, 32 to 52); phenytoin, 59.5 mmol/L (normal, 40 to 80)]

O.T. could have a phenytoin free-fraction percentage of up to 18%, compared with the normal value of 10%, because of her low albumin serum concentration.[19] This would produce a free phenytoin concentration of 27 μg/mL (normal, 10 to 20 μg/mL), explaining O.T.'s symptoms (assuming O.T.'s serum phenytoin concentration is at steady state). In O.T.'s case, free phenytoin concentration monitoring would be appropriate, if available, and her dosage should be adjusted accordingly. A dietary consultation to examine the reason for her low albumin may contribute to her overall health.

Metabolism

O.T.'s phenytoin metabolism may be affected due to factors shown to influence hepatic drug metabolism, which include disease states, concurrent drug use, nutritional status, environmental compounds, genetic differences, gender, liver mass, and blood flow. Hepatic microsomal enzyme activity is reduced with increasing age in animals, but the clinical significance of this is controversial in humans. Large interindividual variation in liver metabolism exists for any given drug and in most cases may be more important than the changes associated with aging.[8,20–23] Also, liver mass declines and hepatic blood flow decreases 45% between the ages of 25 and 65.[24] Unfortunately, clinical tools for the assessment of hepatic metabolism are not readily available. Age-related changes in the liver metabolism of warfarin and long-acting benzodiazepines have been reported in humans.[25–27] Compounds undergoing phase I metabolism (reduction, oxidation, hydroxylation, demethylation) have a decreased or unchanged clearance, whereas compounds metabolized by phase II processes (conjugation, acetylation, sulfonation, glucuronidation) have no change in clearance with age. Drugs with high hepatic-extraction ratios, such as the nitrates, barbiturates, lidocaine, and propranolol, may have reduced hepatic metabolism in older adults.[28]

Reduction in Hepatic Reserve

4. D.A., an independently living 65-year-old man, 70″ tall and weighing 260 pounds, has a chief complaint of severe shortness of breath (SOB; respirations, 26 breaths/min), palpitations (heart rate [HR], 120 beats/min), and nausea. He has a history of chronic obstructive pulmonary disease (COPD) and heart failure (HF). D.A.'s current medications are theophylline-SR (Theo-Dur) 450 mg Q 8 hr, captopril (Capoten) 12.5 mg TID, and furosemide (Lasix) 20 mg QD. At his last visit to his physician 2 months ago, his theophylline serum concentration was 15

mg/mL (therapeutic range, 8 to 12 mg/mL). After a long history of heavy smoking, D.A. finally took his physician's advice and abruptly quit. The diagnosis of acute HF is made on the basis of the chest radiograph, 2% pitting edema, and "junky" sounding lungs. Based on the information given, what potential problems should be added to the list of differential diagnoses to be considered?

Theophylline toxicity should be suspected for two reasons: (1) lack of hepatic microsome/enzyme stimulation from his recent smoking cessation and (2) the known reduction of theophylline hepatic metabolism secondary to acute HF.[19] The theophylline dose should be held until the serum theophylline concentration is within the desired therapeutic range. In patients who are at high risk of developing theophylline toxicity, other treatment options such as a β-agonist and/or ipratropium by inhalation should be considered in place of theophylline (see Chapter 23, Asthma).

Although the potential for theophylline toxicity can be predicted reasonably in D.A., the sudden onset of clinical deterioration or an adverse effect often arises unexpectedly in many older patients. Patients often do well while medically stable only to abruptly experience a "cascade of disasters" when hospitalized or when they begin taking additional medications. As presented in the answer to Question 3, the process of aging can be associated with declining liver mass, decreased hepatic blood flow, altered nutritional status, and a host of other physiologic changes. These alterations result in a loss of "hepatic reserve," making the patient susceptible to adverse effects because new drugs compete for the same metabolic enzymes. The concept of a lost "reserve" in the elderly applies to other organ systems as well. Therefore, D.A.'s response to renally excreted drugs (e.g., captopril, furosemide) should also be considered during this episode of acute heart failure.

Excretion

Age-related changes in renal function result in more adverse drug events than any other age-related physiologic alterations. Compounding these changes in the kidney are the arteriosclerotic changes and a declining cardiac output that decrease renal perfusion by 40% to 50% between the ages of 25 and 65. This is accompanied by a corresponding decrease in glomerular filtration and urea clearance.[29] Urine concentrating ability declines with age, as does renal sodium conservation.[30,31] Tubular secretory capacity and creatinine clearance (Cl_{Cr}) also may be reduced.[32,33] The kidney loses functioning cells with age, and histologic studies reveal a decline in the absolute number of nephrons.[34] All these measures of kidney function decline uniformly, leading to the concept of the "intact nephron." Significant variability can occur in the rate of decline in renal function in a minority of elderly patients[35] (see Table 99-2).

The plasma half-life is prolonged for a number of renally excreted drugs in "healthy" older adults. The highest-risk drugs are those that depend entirely on the kidney for elimination. Examples of these are listed in Table 99-4.

Age-related changes in renal function are evaluated using the creatinine clearance, an estimate of glomerular filtration rate. The Cockcroft-Gault equation is used most commonly to estimate creatinine clearance.[36] Many controversies exist with regard to the use of this equation. One relates to whether one

Table 99-4 Drugs Highly Dependent on Renal Function for Elimination[a]

Acetazolamide	Diflunisal	Metoclopramide
Acyclovir	Digoxin	Nadolol
Allopurinol	Enalapril	Nitrosourea
Amantadine	Ethambutol	Penicillamine
Amiloride	Fluconazole	Pentamidine
Aminoglycosides	Flucytosine	Phenazopyridine
Amphotericin B	Fluoroquinolones	Plicamycin
Atenolol	(most)	Probenecid
Aztreonam	Furosemide	Procainamide
Bleomycin	Gallamine	Pyridostigmine
Bretylium	Gold sodium thioma-	Spironolactone
Captopril	late	Sulfamethoxazole
Cephalosporins	H₂ blockers (most)	Sulfinpyrazone
(most)	Imipenem	Thiazides
Chlorpropamide	Lisinopril	Ticarcillin
Cisplatin	Lithium	Trimethoprim
Clonidine	Methenamine	Vancomycin
Colistimethate	Methotrexate	

This list is not comprehensive; see references 159 and 160 for additional details.

should use the actual or lean body weight (LBW).[37,38] The use of LBW may reflect serum creatinine production more accurately because creatinine is produced in muscle mass, which is decreased in older patients. There is also a question of whether one should use the actual creatinine value when it is <1.0 or whether it should be rounded to 1.0. Finally, for certain subpopulations of older patients (i.e., ambulatory and healthy versus hospitalized, malnourished and/or critically ill) other methods may produce more accurate estimates of renal function.

Table 99-5 provides a composite picture of the age-related physiologic changes, disease states, and pharmacologic factors that affect pharmacokinetic processes in older adults.

Pharmacodynamic Changes

Homeostasis and Postural Hypotension

D.A. is susceptible not only to decreased clearance (i.e., hepatic metabolism, renal elimination) but also to pharmacodynamic changes. Pharmacodynamic changes are defined loosely in this chapter as alterations in concentration-response relationships or receptor sensitivity. Drug side effects that are mild or nonexistent in younger patients may be significant in older adults due to inefficient homeostatic adjustments. For example, the higher rate of orthostatic hypotension observed in older patients is often the result of impaired baroreceptor function and a failure of cerebral blood flow autoregulation. Orthostatic hypotension occurs in 20% of ambulatory patients older than 65 years of age and in 30% among those older than 75,[39] and it often is aggravated by drugs with sympatholytic activity (e.g., α-adrenergic blocking agents, phenothiazines, and tricyclic antidepressants [TCAs]), volume-depleting drugs (e.g., diuretics), and vasodilating agents (e.g., nitrates and alcohol).[40] In one study of 100 geriatric psychiatric outpatients, almost 40% complained of dizziness and falling, which were attributed to psychiatric medications.[41] Patients with impaired cardiac output and patients taking concurrent diuretic therapy (e.g., patient D.A.) are especially vulnerable. Also, aging impairs balance and posture maintenance, and drug effects on posture control may contribute to drug-induced falls in older adults.[42] Table 99-6 reviews the therapeutic agents commonly associated with adverse drug reactions that may affect the mobility of older patients.

Receptor Sensitivity

An exaggerated response to some drugs (e.g., nitrazepam, heparin [in females], and warfarin) may reflect an intrinsic, age-related change in receptor sensitivity.[43,44] The aging central nervous system (CNS) is particularly vulnerable to qualitative as well as quantitative alterations in drug response. The

Table 99-5 Changes Affecting Pharmacokinetic Parameters

Parameter	Physiologic Changes	Disease States	Pharmacologic Factors
Absorption (bioavailability, first-pass metabolism)	↑ Gastric pH ↓ Absorptive surface ↓ Splanchnic blood flow ↓ GI motility ↓ Gastric emptying rate	Achlorhydria, diarrhea, gastrectomy, malabsorptive syndromes, pancreatitis	Drug interactions, antacids, anticholinergics, cholestyramine, food
Distribution	↓ Cardiac output ↓ TBW ↓ Lean body mass ↓ Serum albumin ↑ α₁-Acid glycoprotein ↑ Body fat ↓ Altered relative tissue perfusion	CHF; dehydration; edema, ascites; hepatic failure; malnutrition; renal failure	Drug interactions, protein binding displacement
Metabolism	↓ Hepatic mass ↓ Enzyme activity ↓ Hepatic blood flow	CHF, fever, hepatic failure, malignancy, malnutrition, thyroid disease, viral infection, or immunization	Dietary makeup, drug interactions, insecticides, alcohol, smoking, induction of metabolism, inhibition of metabolism
Excretion	↓ Renal blood flow ↓ GFR ↓ Tubular secretion ↓ Renal mass	Hypovolemia, renal insufficiency	Drug interactions

CHF, congestive heart failure; GFR, glomerular filtration rate; GI, gastrointestinal; TBW, total body water.

Table 99-6 Adverse Drug Reactions That May Affect Mobility of the Older Patient

Medication Class	Adverse Drug Reaction
TCAs	Orthostatic hypotension, tremor, cardiac arrhythmias, sedation
Benzodiazepines and sedative hypnotics	Sedation, weakness, ↓ coordination, confusion
Narcotic analgesics	Sedation, ↓ coordination, confusion
Antipsychotics	Orthostatic hypotension, sedation, extrapyramidal effects
Antihypertensives	Orthostatic hypotension
β-Adrenergic blockers	↓ Ability to respond to work load

TCAs, tricyclic antidepressants.

aging brain, like the aging kidney, loses a significant number of active cells during later life, and some brain atrophy is a common, although not necessarily pathologic, finding in older adults. Normal aging also involves a reduction in cerebral blood flow and oxygen consumption, and increased cerebrovascular resistance.[45] Older adults often have cerebral blood flow rates that are as much as 20% lower than those of younger persons.[11] In addition, inhibitory and excitatory pathways in the CNS are delicately balanced to modulate cognitive functions and behavior. With aging, there is a selective decline in some pathways and the preservation of others. For example, cholinergic neurons in the neocortex and hippocampal areas of the brain normally decrease with age. Pathologic cholinergic deficits are associated with memory loss, confusion, and other cognitive impairments.[46] Drugs with anticholinergic properties are particularly notorious for inducing mental fuzziness and confusion in older patients. Several examples of therapeutic classes with anticholinergic properties are listed in Table 99-7.

Both central and peripheral responsiveness of adrenergic receptors decline with aging.[47] Monoamine-oxidase activity

Table 99-7 Categories of Anticholinergic Drugs That Can Induce Confusion in Older Patients

Therapeutic Class	Examples (Brand Name)
Antispasmodic	Belladonna (Generic)
	Dicyclomine (Bentyl)
	Propantheline (Probanthine)
Antiparkinson	Benztropine (Cogentin)
	Trihexyphenidyl (Artane)
Antihistamine	Diphenhydramine (Benadryl)
	Chlorpheniramine (Chlor-Trimeton)
Antidepressant	Amitriptyline (Elavil)
	Imipramine (Tofranil)
Antiarrhythmic	Quinidine
	Disopyramide (Norpace)
Neuroleptic	Thioridazine (Mellaril)
	Chlorpromazine (Thorazine)
Hypnotic	Hydroxyzine (Vistaril)
OTC agents	Antidiarrheals
	Doxylamine
	Cold remedies

OTC, over-the-counter.

increases with normal aging, and this is reflected by a decline in norepinephrine and dopamine levels in aging brains.[48] The decline in CNS dopamine synthesis is associated with increased sensitivity to dopamine blocking agents (e.g., neuroleptics, metoclopramide). On the other hand, β-receptor sensitivity to both β-agonists and β-antagonists decreases, even if the number of β-receptors does not decrease in older patients.[49–51] Because these neurologic and biochemical reserves are reduced as a normal consequence of aging, iatrogenic behavioral disorders are relatively common in older adults, and drugs are one of the most common causes of sudden, unexplained mental impairment in the older adult. For example, in one study, 11% of 300 patients older than 65 years of age experienced cognitive impairment as a result of an adverse drug reaction, and the risk increased nine-fold when patients were taking four or more prescription drugs.[52]

In conclusion, D.A. is susceptible to significant variations in response to his medications and needs to be monitored carefully because of both pharmacokinetic and pharmacodynamic alterations attributable to aging. His theophylline therapy in particular should be evaluated.

Problems Associated With Drug Use in Older Adults
Polymedicine
Multiple medication use is the primary cause of drug-related adverse events in the older population according to the Centers for Disease Control and Prevention (CDC).[53] Polydrug therapy thrives under conditions in which multiple chronic diseases exist in patients with communication problems, especially when the physician is under pressure to be time-efficient. These factors can lead to misdiagnoses and unclear drug indications. For these reasons, monitoring drug therapy in these patients is not only challenging but imperative. Busy health care providers often assign a low priority to nursing home patients in terms of individual attention, and much of the prescribing of medications and follow-up is done by telephone. Duplicative prescribing within the same drug class often occurs, and unrecognized drug side effects are treated with more drugs. With minimal actual patient contact, prescribers may continue drugs in patients long after the original problem has resolved to avoid the inconvenience of meticulous dosage adjustments and follow-up monitoring. Careful drug regimen review is essential to identify potentially unnecessary or inappropriate medications and to systematically taper and discontinue these agents, with attentive monitoring of the older person.[54–56]

Adverse Drug Events
An adverse drug event (ADE) includes preventable and nonpreventable events and accounts for errors related to prescribing and administration. The combining of several medications can also increase the risk of clinically significant drug interactions and subsequent ADEs in the elderly. Age per se is not an independent risk factor for ADEs, but rather, increased risk is derived from age-related factors (e.g., physiologic changes), chronic disease states, use of different health care providers, and inappropriate prescribing.[57]

Twenty-eight percent of hospitalization of older persons are a result of ADEs and poor medication adherence.[58] Adverse drug reactions in older patients cared for in the community may be as high as 35%.[59] An estimated 32,000 hip fractures, 163,000 cases of drug-induced cognitive impairment, and 61,000 cases of neuroleptic-induced Parkinsonism occur annually.[58]

ADEs can be difficult to detect in older patients because they often present atypically and with nonspecific symptoms, such as lethargy, confusion, light-headedness, or falls. Nevertheless, most adverse reactions represent extensions of a drug's pharmacologic effect, have identifiable predictors, and are preventable (Table 99-8).[60–62] Adverse drug reactions remain a significant problem, with some experts placing the health care costs for adverse drug reactions at $3.4 billion annually.[63]

ADVERSE DRUG REACTIONS IN OLDER PATIENTS

5. S.E., an 85-year-old woman, 5′2″ and 102 pounds, with a SrCr of 1.6 mg/dL, is admitted for chest pain, SOB, and to rule out myocardial infarction (MI). Her physician is concerned about oversedation with narcotics and prescribes ketorolac (Toradol) 30 mg Q 6 hr IV. She has a history of severe HF and angina for which she takes lisinopril 10 mg QD, furosemide 40 mg QD, aspirin 81 mg QD, and nitroglycerin SR 6 mg BID. The lisinopril dosage is increased to 20 mg QD and the furosemide dosage is also increased to 40 mg BID. Her BP is 110/66 mm Hg, and her urine output has been 20 to 30 mL/hr for 4 hours since ketorolac was initiated. What risk factors are present in S.E. for drug-induced renal problems?

[SI unit: SrCr, 141.4 μmol/L]

S.E. has a number of risk factors for the development of drug-induced acute renal failure (ARF). Angiotensin-converting enzyme (ACE) inhibitors are indicated for heart failure management and improve renal function by increasing cardiac output. However, they can diminish efferent arteriole glomerular capillary filtration pressure and precipitate ARF in predisposed patients. A 13% incidence of azotemia has been reported in LTCF residents started on a short course of NSAID treatment.[64] A low serum sodium concentration, high-dose diuretics, diabetes, severe HF (i.e., NYHA class IV), use of a long-acting ACE inhibitor, and concurrent NSAID use are all risk factors for drug-induced ARF (see Chapter 31, Acute Renal Failure). Patients with these risk factors should be monitored closely when an ACE inhibitor is initiated and when the dosage of an ACE inhibitor is increased (see Chapter 19, Heart Failure). Renal prostaglandins (PGE$_2$, PGI$_2$) increase or help maintain renal blood flow when renal function is compromised by intrinsic renal disease, HF, liver disease

with ascites, or hypertension; therefore, the use of a prostaglandin inhibitor such as ketorolac places S.E. at an increased risk for ARF. Furthermore, the ketorolac dose is excessive for S.E. based on the recommended maximum dose of 15 mg every 6 hours for elderly patients.[65]

Disease-Specific Geriatric Drug Therapy
Cardiovascular Disease in the Ambulatory Older Patient

6. T.M. is a 78-year-old woman who presents to a "brown bag" session being sponsored by the local senior center and school of pharmacy. She reports that recently she has begun to feel "sluggish" and has had several episodes of fainting. She lives at home alone on a modest, fixed retirement income. She has a number of chronic medical problems, including coronary artery disease (CAD), HF, hypertension, diabetes, and hyperlipidemia. She visits different specialists on a sporadic basis for management of her various disease states and takes "a lot of medications," whose names she does not know. She admits to skipping her medications periodically. T.M. usually maintains a fairly active social life, hosting and visiting her elderly friends regularly and attending the local seniors' lunch social three times a week. She is highly interested in matters relating to her health, and she often self-medicates with nonprescription medications and herbal remedies she hears about through her peers. Review of her "brown bag" reveals the following items: glyburide 2.5 mg BID, HCTZ 25 mg QD, propranolol 20 mg QID, niacin 500 mg TID, ASA 325 mg PRN, digoxin 0.25 mg QD, isosorbide dinitrate (ISDN) 20 mg QID, NTG 0.4 mg SL PRN, captopril 25 mg TID, furosemide 40 mg BID, acetaminophen 500 mg PRN, verapamil 60 mg QID, multi-vitamins with minerals, chlorpropamide 250 mg QD, calcium carbonate 500 mg TID, hawthorn tincture 20 drops BID, ibuprofen 200 mg PRN, rosiglitazone 2 mg BID, and dandelion 10 mL BID. She also drinks a glass of red wine with dinner and several cups of licorice tea with breakfast and lunch. What initial steps are necessary for safe and effective management of T.M.'s drug therapy?

Like many ambulatory older patients who are being treated for multiple chronic medical conditions, T.M. is at high risk for drug-induced problems secondary to nonadherence, medication errors, and inappropriate prescribing. She is representative of more than 9 million older adults who live at home alone. The isolated community-dwelling older patient is typically female, 75 years of age or older, has multiple medical issues, and takes multiple medications.[66] Many of these individuals lack close support and a daily routine, and may not be fully aware of the time of day or the day of the week. Limited time awareness makes adherence to complex medication regimens more difficult in this population. In addition to older people like T.M., a second high-risk group of older persons consists of those individuals who were recently discharged from the hospital. The post-discharge period can be a time of confusion for these patients, who often must cope with new drugs or replacement drugs added to an already complex pre-hospitalization regimen. A summary of the various factors contributing to nonadherence in the older patient is presented in Table 99-9.[67]

T.M. needs a primary care provider to manage her medical care and to follow-up on her new onset "sluggishness and fainting." She also should be advised to establish a relationship

---

Table 99-8 Predictors of Adverse Drug Events[60–62]

- >4 prescription medications
- Length of stay in hospital >14 days
- >4 active medical problems
- Admission to a general medical unit versus a specialized geriatric ward
- History of alcohol use
- Lower mean Mini-Mental Status Examination score (confusion, dementia)
- 2–4 new medications added to medication regimen during hospitalization

Table 99-9 Factors Influencing the Inability to Comply with a Medication Regimen

>3 chronic conditions
>5 prescription medications
≥12 medication dosages per day
Medication regimen changed ≥4 times during the past 12 months
≥3 prescribers involved
Significant cognitive or physical impairments (e.g., memory, hearing, vision, color discrimination, child-resistant containers)
Living alone in the community
Recently discharged from the hospital
Reliance on a caregiver
Low literacy
Medication cost
Demonstrated poor compliance history

Adapted from reference 67.

at one pharmacy that can monitor all her medications. Finally, T.M. should be counseled to discontinue alcohol, which can interact with several of her current medications.

7. **T.M. presents to the multi-disciplinary geriatric care team upon the advice of pharmacists and students at the "brown bag" session. During the pharmacy intake interview, she admits to selective adherence with many medications based on how they make her feel and their cost. Her "glass" of wine with dinner is 32 ounces four times a week. She also reveals that she has not been taking her furosemide and potassium supplement because she feels that they were contributing to her "sluggishness" and fainting. She is using hawthorne and dandelion instead. The geriatrician's summary of T.M.'s history and physical examination reads as follows: 78 year-old white female, 5′6″, 189 pounds. Vital signs: BP, 140/75 mm Hg; HR, 50 beats/min; temperature, 98.7°F; and respiratory rate, 18 breaths/min. Pertinent laboratory values: SrCr, 1.5 mg/dL (normal, 0.6 to 1.2 mg/dL); BUN, 35 mg/dL (normal, 8 to 18 mg/dL); Na, 153 mEq/L (normal, 138 to 145 mEq/L); K, 3.1 mEq/L (normal, 3.5 to 5 mEq/L); Mg, 1.5 mEq/L (normal, 1.6 to 2.4 mEq/L); glucose, 250 mg/dL (normal, 70 to 110 mg/dL); A1c, 9.5%, cholesterol, 259 mg/dL; LDL, 140 mg/dL; HDL, 40 mg/dL; triglycerides, 200 mg/dL; proteinuria; and digoxin level, 1.5 ng/mL. ECG showed sinus bradycardia with an old anterior MI. Echo: EF 25%. Problem list: new onset sluggishness and fainting, chest pain/SOB on exertion, 3(+) pitting edema bilaterally, NYHA class II–III HF, hypertension, type 2 diabetes, obesity, excessive alcohol intake, CAD, and hyperlipidemia. What factors may be contributing to T.M.'s feeling of sluggishness and fainting?**

[SI units: SrCr 114.39 μmol/L; BUN 12.5 mmol/L; Na 153 mmol/L; K 3.1 mmol/L; Mg 0.77 mmol/L; glucose 13.88 mmol/L]

HEART FAILURE

Heart failure is a common cause of morbidity and mortality in older patients. The standard therapy for heart failure alone commonly consists of 3 or more medications (diuretics, β-blockers, and ACE inhibitors, with or without digoxin and spironolactone) (see Chapter 19, Heart Failure). Standard use of multiple medications in the treatment of heart failure makes close monitoring of drug therapy essential. T.M. is currently taking verapamil, a powerful negative inotrope, which is contraindicated in patients with heart failure. Verapamil should be discontinued because it probably is contributing to her low heart rate and worsening of heart failure symptoms.

DIGOXIN

Age-related declines in renal function put older patients at increased risk for digoxin toxicity. T.M. is at even greater risk for digoxin toxicity because she is female, has reduced renal function secondary to her diabetes and heart failure, and is hypokalemic. Her heart rate of 50 beats/min is a clinical sign of iatrogenic bradycardia. This may be contributing to her sluggishness as well. At first glance, it may appear that T.M's digoxin level of 1.5 ng/mL does not support a diagnosis of digoxin toxicity. However, the suggested therapeutic range in HF patients with normal sinus rhythm is 0.5 to 0.9 ng/mL.[68] This range provides a safety margin in older patients like T.M. in whom other risk factors for digoxin toxicity are likely to be present. These include, for example, decreased lean muscle mass, interacting drugs, and renal insufficiency. The appropriate starting dose for digoxin in patients like T.M. should be no more than 0.125 mg QD.[69] The digoxin dose should be reduced to 0.125 mg QD at this time.

ANGIOTENSIN-CONVERTING ENZYME INHIBITORS

8. **T.M. has been taking captopril 25 mg TID. Why is this an inappropriate choice of ACE inhibitor for T.M.?**

ACE inhibitors, unless contraindicated, are a required part of all heart failure therapy, with proven benefits in reducing morbidity and mortality.[70–72] Although these benefits are considered a class effect, some ACE inhibitors may be more desirable than others in older patients. Multiple daily dosing of captopril in T.M. further complicates an already complex medication regimen. An ACE inhibitor that can be dosed once daily is more appropriate. Also, captopril relies heavily on renal clearance. An agent with a dual mechanism of clearance is more desirable to minimize the risk of toxicity. Fosinopril is a once-a-day ACE inhibitor that undergoes 50% renal and 50% hepatic clearance.[73] T.M.'s captopril should be discontinued and replaced with fosinopril. Other alternatives include enalapril or lisinopril. In light of her heart failure and reduced renal function, fosinopril should be initiated at 5 mg QD.[74]

β-BLOCKERS

9. **T.M. is being treated with propranolol 20 mg QID. Why is this an inappropriate choice of β-blocker for T.M.?**

The β-blockers carvedilol and metoprolol have been proven to reduce morbidity and mortality in patients with heart failure.[75–77] One of these agents should be prescribed in patients with heart failure, unless contraindicated. Other β-blockers should be considered contraindicated in heart failure. In T.M.'s case, propranolol should be discontinued for several reasons. It is probably contributing to her feeling of sluggishness because it is a nonselective β-blocker. Even if T.M. did not have a diagnosis of heart failure, propranolol is considered inappropriate for elderly patients, except to control violent behavior.[78] Also, selective β-blockers are preferred in patients with concomitant diabetes. In light of her diabetes and need for simplification of her medication regimen, metoprolol 12.5 mg QD is the most appropriate β-blocker for

T.M. and should be started when her current exacerbation of heart failure symptoms has resolved.

DIURETICS

T.M. has HCTZ and furosemide in her medication supplies. She continues to take the HCTZ even though she was told to discontinue it and start on furosemide. Situations like this are common; approximately 25% of older patients may be taking drugs that are not currently prescribed.[79] Patients often hoard medications because they are expensive and because they never know if they might have to take them again in the future. Some continue to take medications that have been discontinued because they do not realize they are duplicative and because instructions are misunderstood or inadequate. Loop diuretics are more effective than thiazides in the management of heart failure. HCTZ should be stopped and furosemide should be restarted to resolve T.M.'s current heart failure exacerbation. She should also be advised to limit or discontinue alcohol since the diuretic effect of alcohol can interfere with optimal furosemide therapy. T.M. is hypokalemic and should also be restarted on the potassium supplement.

ALTERNATIVE THERAPIES

10. **Is it safe and appropriate for T.M. to continue to use hawthorne and dandelion to treat her heart failure?**

Use of alternative therapies, including herbal preparations, continues to grow in the United States (see Chapter 3, Herbs and Nutritional Supplements). Unfortunately, consumers often look upon these agents as safe and without the potential risks and side effects associated with prescription drugs. This perception is especially dangerous in older patients, because some of these agents have the potential to interact with other drugs and exacerbate pre-existing conditions. T.M.'s herbal information network is well informed. Hawthorne may have beneficial roles in cardiovascular disease and has been approved for use by the German Commission E in NYHA class II-IIF.[80–82] However, hawthorne may interact with digoxin, increasing its toxicity, so the two agents should not be used concurrently. Dandelion root and leaves produce a mild diuretic action, but may interact with hypoglycemic agents because the herb also has a hypoglycemic effect.[81,83] T.M. should be counseled to discontinue use of both these herbal products. She also should be informed about the potential dangers of self-medication and the substitution of herbs for prescription medications.

CORONARY HEART DISEASE/HYPERLIPIDEMIA

11. **T.M. does not take her niacin because she experienced unbearable facial flushing. Despite her history of MI, she does not believe that cholesterol and "heart disease" are a major health concern for her because she is a woman. Is it important to manage cholesterol in an elderly woman with coronary heart disease (CHD)? Are women older than age 65 at greater, lower, or equal risk of death due to CHD compared with their male counterparts?**

Elevated cholesterol levels have been shown to increase the risk for CHD in older adults.[84–87] This increased risk is statistically significant even after adjusting for indicators of frailty and poor health.[84] Furthermore, CHD is the number one cause of death in women older than age 65.[88] Serum total cholesterol levels greater than 240 mg/dL are present in 42% of women older than 65 years of age compared with just 25% of men older than 65 years of age.[89] After age 65, the mortality from CHD is equal in men and women.[90]

12. **What is an optimal therapeutic plan for management of T.M.'s hyperlipidemia?**

T.M.'s treatment plan should begin with lifestyle and dietary modifications. However, her history of MI places her at extremely high risk, so she should also be started on lipid lowering therapy. Based on current cholesterol guidelines, the initial target for lipid lowering therapy is to lower LDL to an individualized goal based on patient risk factors (see Chapter 13, Dyslipidemias).[91] Statins are the drugs of choice for lowering LDL and should also be considered the drug of choice for lipid lowering in the elderly population as they are well tolerated.[92,93] Aggressive dosing of a statin is indicated in T.M. with a goal of lowering her LDL to less than 100 mg/dL because of her pre-existing history of CHD. T.M.'s triglycerides are not high enough to warrant the addition of a second agent. Discontinuation of alcohol would be beneficial since it can increase triglycerides as much as 50%.

13. **What other interventions should be implemented to optimize management of T.M.'s coronary artery disease?**

T.M. is experiencing anginal pain on her current regimen (see Chapter 17, Ischemic Heart Disease: Anginal Syndromes). Nonadherence with her complex medication regimen is most likely contributing to poor pain control. T.M. is taking ISDN four times a day; she should be taking once daily medications whenever possible to simplify her medication regimen. The ISDN could be replaced with a long-acting once daily nitrate and supplemented with NTG SL tablets as needed. She also may benefit from the addition of amlodipine for long term management in place of verapamil. As mentioned previously, the change from propranolol 20 mg QID to metoprolol 12.5 mg QD should increase her ability to take the medications as prescribed, thereby enhancing control of her angina. ASA in the dose range of 81 to 325 mg should be taken once daily to reduce her risk of death due to MI (see Chapter 18, Myocardial Infarction).

HYPERTENSION

14. **T.M. has isolated systolic hypertension. How should this be managed in light of her advanced age?**

T.M.'s blood pressure is well above the goal of less than 130/80 mm Hg for diabetic patients as set forth by the American Diabetes Association (ADA) and the Seventh Report of the Joint National Committee on Prevention, Detection, Evaluation, and Treatment of High Blood Pressure (JNC VII).[94,95] Hypertension is present in more than two-thirds of individuals >65 years of age.[96] Despite having the highest prevalence of hypertension, this population is the least likely to have their blood pressures adequately controlled.[97] Treatment of elderly patients, such as T.M., should be based on the same guidelines published for the general care of hypertension (see Chapter 14, Essential Hypertension). Standard doses of anti-hypertensive drugs and multiple drug therapy are needed in the majority of older patients. However, in many of these patients, lower initial doses are needed to minimize the risk of adverse effects such as postural hypotension. T.M. is taking furosemide, propranolol, isosorbide dinitrate, captopril, and verapamil, all of which have hypotensive effects. Since she has isolated systolic hypertension, she would likely benefit from a long-acting dihydropyridine calcium channel blocker at a low initial dose in place of verapamil. Amlodipine 2.5 mg QD is an appropriate initial dose for T.M's hypertension.[98]

Diabetes in the Elderly

15. T.M. reports that she has not taken chlorpropamide for years because she would get flushed when drinking wine with dinner. Also, she frequently felt light-headed and shaky when she took this drug. Because glyburide also causes symptoms of hypoglycemia, she takes it only sporadically. What is an optimal therapeutic plan for the management of T.M.'s diabetes?

Comprehensive diabetes education needs to be initiated, stressing the importance of weight loss, regular monitoring of blood glucose, and medication adherence. A 10% weight loss will improve her glucose control and have beneficial effects on her cardiovascular risk factors. T.M.'s alcohol consumption and self-reported erratic meal schedule may be contributing to the hypoglycemia. In addition to providing empty calories that can contribute to weight gain, alcohol also has inherent hypoglycemic effect that can exacerbate this side effect of her diabetes medication. Patients who are resistant to stopping alcohol altogether should be strongly encouraged to limit daily intake to one ounce of ethanol for men and one-half ounce for women. In T.M.'s case this would be one small glass of wine (3 to 4 ounces).[99] Chlorpropamide is an inappropriate choice in an older person because of its long half-life and side effect profile: protracted hypoglycemia and syndrome of inappropriate antidiuretic hormone (SIADH).[78] Glyburide also is long acting and causes severe hypoglycemia more commonly than other sulfonylureas. The elderly are more susceptible, even at low doses. Among the second generation sulfonylureas, glipizide or glimepiride are better choices. Alternatively, T.M. could be treated with a meglitinide, such as repaglinide, which does not require dose adjustment in elderly patients. Use of a meglitinide also allows for a more flexible meal pattern, since it is taken with each meal and is skipped if a meal is skipped.[100] Any new diabetes medication should be initiated in low doses and gradually titrated upward to avoid hypoglycemic episodes and to achieve glycemic goals in accordance with American Diabetes Association (ADA) guidelines.[94] Since the use of thiazolidinediones, such as rosiglitazone, is contraindicated in patients with heart failure, it should be discontinued in T.M. (see Chapter 50, Diabetes Mellitus).

Depression and the Older Patient

Significant depression is the most common mental illness among older adults, occurring in about 15%; it is a source of significant morbidity and mortality in this population.[101] Unfortunately, depression remains underrecognized and undertreated even though it is a major risk factor for suicide in the elderly, who have a suicide rate that is 5.5 times greater than the national average.[103,104] Older patients may be at increased risk of depression due to the high prevalence of comorbid medical conditions (i.e., stroke, cancer, MI, rheumatoid arthritis, dementia, Parkinson's disease, and diabetes mellitus).[105] Refer to Chapter 79, Mood Disorders I: Major Depressive Disorders, for further discussion of risk factors for depression and potential drug-induced causes. Most patients are treated in the primary care setting.[102]

16. J.W. is a married, 5'8", 110-pound, 79-year-old woman who comes in for a psychiatric evaluation. Her husband says she just has not been herself lately. The changes in J.W. began on a family vacation 6 months earlier when she got lost on the cruise ship. Since that incident she has become increasingly anxious and has developed insomnia. Although she does not feel sad or "depressed," she generally does not feel well. J.W.'s normally positive attitude toward life has become pessimistic. Her husband confirms that she has become more forgetful and no longer enjoys eating. In fact, she has lost 18 pounds over the past 2 months. J.W. no longer does her volunteer work at the local children's center. She says she wants to die because she is no longer the person she used to be, but she denies having any specific suicidal thoughts. Her medical history is significant for diabetes and hypertension, which are both well controlled on glipizide 5 mg QAM and HCTZ 25 mg QD. Her medical evaluation and physical examination are unremarkable. Laboratory results and head CT scan are within normal limits. J.W. is diagnosed as having a major depressive episode. What symptoms of depression are present in J.W.?

J.W.'s presenting symptoms are quite typical of major depression in an older patient, which is commonly quite different than that of younger depressed patients. Criteria set forth in the DSM IV for diagnosing depression were developed using younger subjects and may not be applicable to the older depressed patient.[106–108] Older patients are less likely to report suicidal thoughts, but are more likely to experience weight loss as a symptom of depression. Anxiety, irritability, somatic complains, or a change in functional ability may be more significant features in late life depression than depressed mood. Memory problems, such as J.W.'s forgetfulness, may be due to a lack of concentration or effort stemming from her depression. This is distinct from dementia, which manifests itself prominently with impairment in short-term and long-term memory (see Chapter 100, Geriatric Dementias). Therefore, depressed mood cannot be relied on for determining whether an older patient has a depressive disorder.[103] Table 99-10 lists

Table 99-10 Atypical Depressive Symptoms in the Older Adult

Agitation/anxiety/worrying
Reduced initiative and problem-solving capacities
Alcohol or substance abuse
Paranoia
Obsessions and compulsions
Irritability
Somatic complaints
Excessive guilt
Marital discord
Social withdrawal
Cognitive impairment
Deterioration in self care

Adapted from reference 103.

atypical depressive symptoms that may be found in older adults. The presence of any one of these symptoms should be considered a red flag and should prompt further evaluation for major depression.[104]

17. J.W.'s physician decides to prescribe anti-depressive medication. Which antidepressants are preferred for use in older adults?

Selection of an antidepressant drug for elderly patients must take into consideration age-related changes in pharmacokinetic, pharmacodynamic, and physiologic parameters that make this population more vulnerable to adverse effects. Although the available antidepressants are about equally effective, selective serotonin reuptake inhibitors (SSRIs) are better tolerated. Therefore, low-dose SSRIs should be considered first-line therapy for most older patients. Of course, this does not preclude the use of sound clinical judgment that incorporates the patient's history of response, comorbidities, and the drug's side effect profile. J.W. should start taking a low-dose SSRI with gradual dose titration to achieve control of her depressive symptoms. Table 99-11 lists recommended starting doses for SSRIs in older patients. Full antidepressant response may take twice as long in older patients compared with younger patients; it may take 8 to 12 weeks before assessment of J.W.'s full response can be made.[109]

Asthma and Chronic Obstructive Pulmonary Disease in the Elderly

Epidemiologic studies estimate the prevalence of asthma in the elderly to be between 6.5% and 17% and even higher for chronic obstructive pulmonary disease (COPD).[110,111] Although many patients have a history of childhood asthma that persists into adulthood, a significant proportion (up to 48%) are diagnosed with asthma after age 65.[112] Rates of hospitalization for asthma are highest in the older population, and asthma-related mortality for adults aged 65 to 74 years is higher compared with younger adults, possibly due to underdiagnosis and undertreatment of the disease.[113] Symptoms of asthma—including wheezing, cough, chest tightness, and dyspnea—are similar in both older and younger patients (see Chapter 23, Asthma). However, because the elderly are more likely to have coexisting medical conditions (e.g., heart failure, angina, COPD and gastroesophageal reflux disease [GERD]) with symptoms that mimic asthma, accurate diagnosis and assessment of severity is often more difficult.[114]

COPD is a major cause of morbidity and mortality in the older population[115,116] but is often undiagnosed because patients tend to accept worsening pulmonary function as part of the "normal" aging process or may be less aware of the symptoms of airflow obstruction.[117,118] Drug therapy for COPD in the elderly does not differ significantly from standard management regimens (see Chapter 24, Chronic Obstructive Pulmonary Disease). However, older patients with pulmonary disease and coexisting medical problems may be more sensitive to the adverse effects of pharmacologic agents.

18. J.C., a 67-year-old woman, 5'6", 145 pounds, presents to the ED with complaints of SOB for the past 2 days. She was in her usual state of health until 4 days ago when she developed flu-like symptoms consisting of fever, cough, and mild wheezing. J.C. has a history of asthma, diabetes, hypertension, headache, and GERD. Her current medications include glipizide 5 mg QD, lisinopril 10 mg QD, metoprolol 50 mg BID, lansoprazole 30 mg QD, ibuprofen 200 mg Q 6 hr PRN for headache, albuterol metered-dose inhaler (MDI) 2 puffs QID PRN for SOB, and fluticasone (44 µg) MDI 2 puffs BID. Her drug regimen has been unchanged for the past 2 years and she reports taking all medications as prescribed. The only recent change has been the need for albuterol every 3 to 4 hours for coughing and wheezing over the past few days. What factors (including medications) may have contributed to her acute asthma exacerbation?

Management of acute asthma exacerbations in previously stable elderly asthmatics should begin with a review of the medication history for asthma-inducing agents. Aspirin and other NSAIDs are known to induce acute bronchoconstriction in approximately 3% to 5% of adult asthmatics.[119] J.C. should be queried about her previous (especially recent) use of ibuprofen in relation to her asthma symptoms. If she reports worsening of her asthma following ingestion of ibuprofen, further use of aspirin and NSAIDs should be avoided. Alternative agents for pain control include acetaminophen or selective COX-2 inhibitors (e.g., celecoxib, rofecoxib). Nonselective β-blockers, including topical ophthalmic formulations, can precipitate acute bronchoconstriction and should be avoided in patients with reactive airway disease. While cardioselective β-blockers are generally considered safe for use in patients with asthma, it is important to recognize that cardioselectivity may be lost with higher dosages. Because J.C. has been taking low-dose metoprolol (a cardioselective agent) for years without problem, this medication is unlikely to be contributing to her current asthma exacerbation. One of the most important triggers for asthma exacerbations is respiratory infection (particularly viral). J.C. reports the recent onset of symptoms consistent with influenza and this is likely precipitating her current pulmonary symptoms. As a future prophylactic measure, J.C. should be counseled to receive the influenza vaccine annually. Additionally, because she is older than 65 years of age, she should receive a one-time pneumococcal vaccine to reduce the risk of developing pneumococcal pneumonia.

19. Are the medication regimens used to treat asthma in elderly patients different from those used in children and younger adults? Should J.C.'s asthma regimen be changed?

Medications used in the management of persistent form of asthma in the elderly are similar to those used in younger patients and consist of bronchodilators in combination with anti-inflammatory agents (see Chapter 23, Asthma). The primary difference relates to drug selection and monitoring which may be more complicated in the elderly because of the greater likelihood of co-existing medical conditions and increased potential for drug–disease and drug–drug interactions.

Table 99-11 SSRI Dosing in Older Adults

Drug	Initial Dosage	Maximum Dosage
Citalopram HBr	10 mg QD	40 mg QD
Escitalopram Oxalate	5 mg QD	20 mg QD
Fluoxetine HCL	5 mg QD	40 mg QD
Fluvoxamine	25 mg QHS	200 mg QHS
Paroxetine HCL	10 mg QD	40 mg QD
Sertraline HCL	25 mg QD	150 mg QD

Inhaled β_2-agonists are an important class of drugs used to treat asthma in all age groups. The low incidence of drug interactions and reduced side effect profile make inhaled β_2-agonists ideal for use in the older asthmatics. However, both inhaled and oral β_2-agonists can cause dose-dependent systemic side effects, such as tremor, tachycardia, hypokalemia, and arrhythmias which are of particular concern in patients with cardiac conditions.[114] Inhaled corticosteroids are the preferred treatment for all forms of persistent asthma and, in general, are well tolerated by older patients. However, elderly patients receiving high dose therapy are at an increased risk for osteoporosis, cataracts, skin thinning and bruising.[120] In addition to the well-known complications associated with systemic corticosteroid use (see Chapter 44, Connective Tissue Disorders: The Clinical Use of Corticosteroids), these agents can acutely cause confusion, agitation, and hyperglycemia. Theophylline should be used with caution in the elderly because of the potential for CNS stimulation, nausea, vomiting, and in higher doses arrhythmias and seizures.

J.C. is currently maintained on low doses of an inhaled corticosteroid (fluticasone) in combination with a short-acting β_2-agonist (albuterol), and this is an appropriate regimen for a patient with mild-persistent asthma. J.C.'s asthma control should be re-evaluated within the next 3 months. If her asthma symptoms are not well controlled, she may benefit from an increase in her fluticasone dose or the addition of a long-acting inhaled β_2-agonist (salmeterol or formoterol). Because J.C. is postmenopausal, she is at risk for osteoporosis; calcium and vitamin D supplementation should be initiated.

20. **J.C. was admitted to the hospital and given intravenous methylprednisolone for 4 days. She is discharged home with glipizide 5 mg QD, lisinopril 20 mg QD, fluticasone (44 μg) 2 puffs BID, albuterol 2 to 4 puffs Q 4 hr PRN, and prednisone 40 mg QD × 7 days. What are some of the important counseling points for J.C. regarding her discharge medications?**

Appropriate use of MDIs is difficult for most patients, but may be particularly problematic in the elderly population because of decreased hand strength or arthritis. The use of spacer/holding chamber devices can alleviate this problem by minimizing the coordination necessary for proper use of a MDI, resulting in improved pulmonary drug delivery. Additionally, spacers may reduce the incidence of systemic and local (cough, hoarseness, thrush) side effects associated with inhaled corticosteroids. J.C. should be discharged with a spacer device to use with her albuterol and fluticasone MDIs. Even though J.C. previously used a MDI, she should be asked to demonstrate her MDI technique and re-instructed, if necessary, to ensure she is using the inhaler and spacer correctly. If J.C. is unable to correctly use her MDIs with a spacer, use of breath-activated or dry-powder inhalers should be considered. Although J.C. is prescribed prednisone for a short course, counseling for J.C. should also include more frequent monitoring of blood glucose while she is taking systemic corticosteroid therapy because she also has diabetes.

Infectious Diseases in the Elderly

Infections are among the most common problems in the elderly and are a significant cause of morbidity and mortality. Infections are also one of the most frequent reasons for hospitalization of older ambulatory persons.[121] Antibiotic therapy for an infection in the elderly is often delayed because they present with atypical signs and symptoms. The older population also is more likely to have polymicrobial infections than younger people, and treatment duration is usually longer because of other comorbidities present in this population.[122]

PNEUMONIA

21. **Three days after J.C. is discharged from the hospital, she presents again to the ED. This time, she is accompanied by a neighbor who noted that J.C. suddenly became forgetful and confused and continued to have difficulty breathing. Her neighbor reports that J.C. has been staying in bed the past 2 days and has not eaten much. J.C. has a low-grade fever, and chest examination reveals faint breath sounds with light crackling rales over her right lung base. A chest radiograph confirms the diagnosis of pneumonia. How is J.C.'s clinical presentation consistent with community-acquired pneumonia in the elderly? How should she be treated for her respiratory infection?**

Pneumonia is the leading infectious cause of mortality in the elderly, who have a 5- to 10-fold increased risk of developing pneumonia compared with younger adults.[123] Most patients admitted to hospital for the treatment of community-acquired pneumonia (CAP) are elderly.[124] Risk factors for CAP in the elderly include alcoholism and asthma, but other medical conditions common in older population, such as dementia, congestive heart failure, cerebrovascular disease, and chronic obstructive lung disease, can also increase the risk of pneumonia in this population.[125] *Streptococcus pneumoniae,* the most common cause of CAP in the elderly, is responsible for up to 50% of cases.[126–128] Viral pneumonia is the second most common cause of lower respiratory infection in older ambulatory patients. Respiratory symptoms and fever are often subtle or absent in older patients with pneumonia; instead, like J.C. they may present only with altered mental status (delirium, acute confusion, memory problems) or a decline in functional status. Delirium or acute confusion is a common presentation in elderly patients who may have new-onset lower respiratory infection. Management of pneumonia in the elderly requires hospitalization in many cases because they are at greater risk for mortality and complications. Early empiric antibacterial therapy is particularly important for older patients with pneumonia (see Chapter 60, Respiratory Tract Infections). J.C. should be hospitalized again and treated aggressively for pneumonia with broad-spectrum IV antibiotics.

PREVENTION

22. **After 7 days of hospitalization, J.C. is discharged home with an oral antibiotic to finish the 14-day course of therapy. What preventive measures are available to J.C. after she is discharged?**

Both influenza and pneumococcal vaccinations are beneficial in the prevention of pneumonia in the older population.[129,130] Among the elderly residents of nursing homes, influenza vaccine was found to be up to 60% effective in preventing pneumonia and hospitalization, and it was up to 70% effective in preventing hospitalization of ambulatory older adults. Among the respiratory viruses, influenza virus causes the greatest morbidity and mortality.[131] Influenza virus damages respiratory epithelial cells, decreases cell-mediated immunity, and exacerbates or worsens many chronic underlying medical conditions common to the older population. A yearly influenza vaccine is therefore recommended for all persons aged 65 years and older. Amantadine, rimantadine or oseltamivir are effective for the early treatment of influenza and for prophylaxis against influenza. Unlike oseltamivir, which is active versus both influenza A and B, amantadine and rimantadine are only active versus influenza A. If amantadine or rimantadine are selected, they should be given at a reduced dose of 100 mg orally per day in older patients; the dose of amantadine should be further reduced in patients with renal impairment to avoid central nervous system side effects. Although the above agents are effective in the prevention of influenza, vaccination should be the primary prophylactic intervention. The pneumococcal vaccine has been shown to be up to 80% effective in preventing pneumococcal bacteremia in those older than 65 years of age,[132] although the reduction in the risk of pneumonia with pneumococcal vaccine is questionable.[133] Pneumococcal vaccine is nonetheless recommended in all adults aged 65 and older to prevent bacteremia. Pneumococcal vaccination is generally given one time, although a case can be made for repeating the dose every 5 to 7 years in the elderly because of their somewhat compromised immune status. J.C. should be offered both influenza and pneumococcal vaccines after she is discharged from the hospital.

URINARY TRACT INFECTION

23. **A.H. is a 72-year-old Hispanic woman who is currently wheelchair-bound because of pain in her right hip. Her granddaughter brings A.H. to the geriatric clinic because she has recently developed urinary incontinence. Her granddaughter reports that A.H. has been feeling weak the past 2 days and fell while getting out of the wheelchair. A urinalysis indicates the presence of a urinary tract infection (UTI), and A.H. is prescribed a 7-day course of ciprofloxacin 500 mg PO BID. Is this therapy appropriate?**

UTI is the most common bacterial infection in the elderly.[134] The frequency of bacteriuria in ambulatory older adults is 10% to 30% in women and 5% to 10% in men. These figures are even higher in elderly people residing in LTCFs. Impaired voiding with residual urine in older women and obstructive uropathy from prostatic disease in older men predispose them to bacteriuria. The severity of UTI in the older population ranges from mild cystitis to life-threatening urosepsis; both are more difficult to treat because of resistant organisms and age-related decreases in host defenses. The majority of UTIs in the older population do not present typically, but there are often nonspecific manifestations such as decline in functional status, cognitive impairment, weakness, falls, and urinary incontinence.[135] A.H.'s presentation (weakness, urinary incontinence, and a recent fall) is consistent with this pattern. As with most urinary tract infections, those in the elderly are caused primarily by *Escherichia coli*. However, other species of bacteria such as *Klebsiella* sp., *Proteus* sp., and *Enterococcus* sp. are also frequently involved (see Chapter 64, Urinary Tract Infections).[136]

Oral antibiotics are appropriate for most elderly patients with symptomatic UTI.[137] One study suggests that fluoroquinolones are significantly better tolerated than trimethoprim-sulfamethoxazole for the treatment of UTI in elderly women.[138] There was better clinical resolution at the end of the therapy and the incidence of drug-related adverse events was significantly lower in women treated with a fluoroquinolone. This study suggests that a fluoroquinolone may be the preferred agent for a broad range of UTIs in the elderly and should be considered as initial therapy in the majority of the older population. Ciprofloxacin is a reasonable choice for A.H. because *E. coli* is the most likely causative agent and fluoroquinolones are well tolerated in the elderly.

The most important effect of age on antibiotic therapy for UTI is impaired renal function. Many older patients have limited renal function reserve due to prostatic disease or chronic UTIs.[139] Nitrofurantoin should not be used in those patients with significantly impaired renal function. For those patients requiring IV therapy for UTI, aminoglycosides pose a distinct disadvantage in older patients due to their drug-related nephrotoxicity and the need for serum drug level monitoring.[139]

Osteoarthritis Pain

Arthritis is the most common cause of disability in people older than 75 years of age, with prevalence rates up to 30%.[140] It is also the most common cause of immobility in the older population, resulting in confinement in bed or to the house. Osteoarthritis, also called degenerative joint disease, is the most common type of joint disease in the older population. Its prevalence increases with age. Nonpharmacologic management of osteoarthritis, such as physical therapy and occupational therapy, have been shown to decrease pain and improve function in patients with osteoarthritis, both alone or in combination with appropriate analgesics.[141]

24. **C.W., a 71-year-old retired school teacher, has been suffering from osteoarthritis of his hands for 5 years. He is an active older adult who enjoys volunteer work at the local hospital. He presents to the geriatric clinic with increased arthritis pain, which is uncontrolled by his current pain medication. He also complains of increased heartburn and gastric reflux symptoms. He also takes several other medications for his diabetes, hypertension, hypercholesterolemia, and GERD. C.W.'s current medications include glipizide 10 mg QD, verapamil sustained-released 240 mg QD, atorvastatin 10 mg QD, famotidine 20 mg BID, docusate sodium 100 mg BID, and ibuprofen 200 mg QID PRN. What modifications can be made to his drug regimen to better control his arthritis pain and minimize side effects from his pain medication?**

Acetaminophen is the drug of choice for mild to moderate arthritis pain (see Chapter 43, Rheumatic Disorders). For elderly patients with reduced hepatic function or for those who drink more than two alcoholic beverages a day, the recommended maximum daily dose is 2.5 g/day.[142] Acetaminophen is preferred over NSAIDs in the elderly because of its low renal and GI toxicity. C.W.'s past medication history should be reviewed. If he has not tried acetaminophen in the past for his arthritis pain, acetaminophen 1 gm QID should be initiated. Older patients suffering from osteoarthritis pain often find relief from NSAIDs, which should be used with caution because of their potential GI side effects and renal toxicity. A meta-analysis reported a relative risk of 5.5 for serious GI complications with NSAIDs in older adults.[64] NSAID-associated renal toxicity is not as common as GI toxicity, but advanced age is one of the major risk factors.[142] Renal toxicities of NSAIDs in the elderly include sodium and water retention and increased risk for hypertension.[143] Thus, ibuprofen may be contributing to C.W.'s increased GERD symptoms and to his hypertension. Non-acetylated salicylates, such as salsalate, can be used if acetaminophen does not provide adequate pain relief. Compared to NSAIDs, non-acetylated salicytes have fewer renal and GI side effects. Currently available highly selective cyclooxygenase (COX)-2 inhibitors, such as rofecoxib and celecoxib, are preferred in older patients because they are less likely to cause GI side effects than non-selective agents; however, the risk of adverse renal events is equivalent.[142] A COX-2 inhibitor is also an option for C.W., who may experience reduced GI symptoms with equally effective pain relief compared to ibuprofen.

25. **C.W. reveals that he has tried acetaminophen without much relief of his pain. He is prescribed rofecoxib and tries it for several months, but his pain continues and he is still experiencing GI distress. What other pain medication options does C.W. have?**

For moderate to severe chronic pain due to osteoarthritis, the topical analgesic, capsaicin, has been shown to provide temporary pain relief. However, capsaicin requires multiple daily applications for effective management of pain, and optimal efficacy takes 4 to 6 weeks of continued use. Glucosamine and chondroitin have also been shown to decrease osteoarthritis pain and delay progression of the disease.[144] Glucosamine 1,500 mg combined with 1,200 mg chondroitin daily is recommended and is well tolerated in most elderly patients. However, glucosamine might increase the insulin resistance in diabetic patients, and C.W. should be counseled to monitor his blood glucose more closely when initiating this agent.

Another option for C.W. is long-acting opioid medications combined with acetaminophen, which can provide relief from pain with minimal side effects (see Chapter 9, Pain). Codeine and tramadol are "weak" opioids that have ceiling effects and generally do not provide adequate analgesia. The use of propoxyphene should be avoided in the elderly because of their limited efficacy and the risk for neural and cardiac toxicity.[145] Meperidine should be avoided as well in older adults because of its high potential for central nervous system side effects, especially in those with reduced renal function. C.W. is a candidate for opioid therapy. He should be started on the lowest dose of a short-acting formulation on a scheduled regimen and counseled on the side effects. Constipation may be a particular problem because he is also taking verapamil, which can also cause significant constipation. The elderly are also at increased risk for constipation due to age-related reduced bowel motility. To prevent opioid-associated constipation in C.W., prophylactic laxatives and stool softeners should be started at the initiation of opioid therapy. Bulk laxatives are ineffective and should be avoided. He should be counseled to drink adequate fluids as well.[145]

Rehabilitative Geriatric Medicine

The geriatric population forms a major part of rehabilitative medicine. Relative to persons younger than 65 years of age, people 65 and older have more than twice as much disability, four times the activity limitation, and about twice as many hospital stays lasting about 50% longer.[146] The goal of all rehabilitation programs is to develop a person to the fullest physical, psychological, social, vocational, avocational, and educational potential consistent with his or her physiologic, anatomic, and environmental limitations. Realistic goals based on functional activities that are essential to the independence and well-being of the individual should be established. The patient, family, and interdisciplinary rehabilitation team should work together to establish these goals. In the older person, rehabilitation often means working to obtain optimal function despite residual disability caused by an irreversible medical condition. Rehabilitation can take place in the home, hospital, or nursing home setting.

Functional Assessment

Meticulous clinical evaluation of the patient's medical and functional status is the first step in a rehabilitation program.[147] The functional status evaluation should include an assessment of age, gender, and environment-appropriate activities of daily living (ADLs). According to the National Center for Health Statistics, nearly 9% of non-institutionalized persons at least 70 years of age are unable to perform one or more ADLs.[148] ADLs include dressing, eating, bathing, grooming, using the toilet, and moving around within the home. Instrumental activities of daily living (IADLs) are other activities that determine an individual's functional independence. IADLs include food preparation, laundry, housekeeping, shopping, the ability to use the telephone, use of transportation, medication use, financial management, and child care if appropriate. Leisure and recreational activities important to a person's physical and psychological well-being can also be considered IADLs. A disability or dysfunction is defined as any deviation from the normal or characteristic ability of a person to perform tasks of living. Impairments are defined as abnormalities in organs or body systems that can lead to dysfunction. When the inability to perform tasks results in social disadvantage, the condition is viewed as a handicap.[149]

Pharmacists' Role in Geriatric Rehabilitation

26. **B.L., a 5'10", 180 pound, 78 year-old man, experienced an embolic stroke 7 days before transfer to the rehabilitation unit. His medical history is significant for atrial fibrillation and GERD. Medications at the time of transfer are digoxin 0.25 mg QD, warfarin 5 mg QD except 2.5 mg on Monday/Thursday, ranitidine 150 mg BID, metoclopramide 10 mg QID, metoprolol 50 mg BID, and milk of magnesia PRN for constipation. His laboratory values are as follows: Na, 135 mEq/L; K, 4.2 mEq/L; SCr, 1.5 mg/dL; BUN, 23 mg/dL, and digoxin level, 1.2 ng/mL. His vital signs are BP, 110/70 mmHg; HR, 60 beats/min; and temperature, 98.4°F. What is the pharmacist's role in the initial evaluation of B.L.?**

[SI units: Na 135 mmol/L; K 4.2 mmol/L; SrCr 132.6 mmol/L; BUN 8.2 mmol/L]

An interdisciplinary "geriatric assessment" team is essential to accomplishing a comprehensive functional evaluation of the rehabilitation patient. These teams, including a pharmacist member as the pharmacotherapy specialist, significantly reduce length of stay, readmissions, drug costs, and patient mortality.[150–152] A physician trained and certified in rehabilitation medicine (i.e., a physiatrist) usually leads the team. Other disciplines represented on the team are physical therapy, occupational therapy, speech therapy, recreational therapy, behavioral medicine (psychologist, social worker), and nursing. The pharmacist's role in the initial assessment is to obtain a complete medication history so that an accurate assessment of drug therapy can be made. Adverse reactions to medications can be detrimental to the functional capacity of the geriatric patient by worsening cognition, psychological state, vascular reflexes, balance, bowel and bladder control, muscle tone, and coordination, any of which may already be impaired by the present illness or injury. It is the responsibility of the team pharmacist to alert the rest of the team to drug-induced problems, facilitate medication adherence, provide medication education, advocate to discontinue unnecessary medications, screen for drug interactions, and recommend appropriate changes in therapy based on the physiologic effects of aging. The team pharmacist should also make some assessment of the individual's ability to self-medicate. Table 99-12 lists conditions and skills that have been identified as possible indicators of an older person's ability to self-medicate.

Table 99-12 Indicators of the Inability to Self-Medicate[161,162]

Cognitive impairments
>5 prescription medications
Inability to read prescription and auxiliary labels
Difficulty opening nonchildproof containers
Problems removing small tablets from containers
Inability to discriminate between medication colors and shapes

Drug Effects on Functional Ability

27. During the initial team meeting to discuss B.L., the physical therapist mentions that the patient walks with a stooped posture, has a shuffling gait, and poor balance. The speech therapist reports that B.L. has difficulty in swallowing, noting that the problem is out of proportion for the location of his stroke. A flat affect, crying episodes, fatigue, and drowsiness are reported by the occupational therapist. The psychologist notes confusion and possible dementia on neuropsychologic testing. Can any of B.L.'s problems be attributed to his current medication regimen?

Functional impairments in older adults can be medication induced.[153] Table 99-13 lists several examples of drugs that can interfere with the functional, physical, social, and psychologic assessment of the older patient. Dopamine depleting drugs may produce extrapyramidal side effects and interfere with physical and occupational therapy goals. Neuroleptics, tricyclic antidepressants, and excessive doses of antihypertensives can increase the risk of falls by causing orthostatic hypotension. Problems with balance and/or tinnitus may be precipitated by drugs that affect the vestibular system and cause damage to the eighth cranial nerve (e.g., aminoglycosides, loop diuretics, and high serum concentrations of aspirin). Long-term corticosteroid use may lead to proximal muscle wasting and slow the recovery of strength even when patients are undergoing aggressive rehabilitative therapy.

CNS medications may lead to oversedation and decrease the capability to learn, ambulate, eat, or use the toilet as well as increase the risk of falls. Drugs such as benzodiazepines, antihypertensives, neuroleptics, H₂ blockers, and analgesics have been reported to cause reversible cognitive impairment. Digoxin toxicity in the elderly may initially manifest as confusion, delirium, nightmares, or hallucinations. Medications

Table 99-13 Drug Effects on Other Assessments

Assessments	Drug Effects	Drug Examples
Functional	Movement disorders (extrapyramidal, tardive dyskinesia)	Neuroleptics, metoclopramide, amoxapine, methyldopa
	Balance (neuritis, neuropathies, tinnitus, dizziness; hypotension)	Metronidazole, phenytoin, aspirin, aminoglycosides, furosemide, ethacrynic acid, β-blockers, calcium channel blockers, neuroleptics, antidepressants, diuretics, vasodilators, benzodiazepines, levodopa, metoclopramide
Physical	Supporting structures (arthralgias, myopathies, osteoporosis, osteomalacia)	Corticosteroids, lithium, phenytoin, heparin
	Incontinence (urinary retention; secondary oversedation)	Anticholinergic agents, TCAs, neuroleptics, antihistamines, smooth muscle relaxants, nifedipine, phenylpropanolamine, prazosin; benzodiazepines, sedatives, hypnotics
	Sexual dysfunction	Hypotensive agents, CNS depressants, SSRI antidepressants
Social	Malnutrition	Drugs affecting appetite
	Poor dental health	Anticholinergic agents, glucose-containing oral liquid/chewable dosage forms
Psychologic	Cognitive impairment (metabolic alterations; memory loss, dementia)	β-Blockers, corticosteroids, diuretics, sulfonylureas, methyldopa, propranolol, hydrochlorothiazide, reserpine, neuroleptics, opiates, cimetidine, amantadine, benzodiazepines, anticonvulsants
	Behavioral toxicity (insomnia, nightmares, sedation, agitation, delirium, psychosis, hallucinations)	Anticholinergics, cimetidine, ranitidine, famotidine, digoxin, bromocriptine, amantadine, baclofen, levodopa, opiates, sympathomimetics, corticosteroids
	Depression	Reserpine, methyldopa, β-blockers, metoclopramide, corticosteroids, CNS depressants

Adapted from reference 153.
CNS, central nervous system; SSRI, selective serotonin reuptake inhibitors; TCA, tricyclic antidepressant.

that cause a relative dominance of dopamine over acetylcholine in the brain may produce psychosis, hallucinations, or delirium.

Depression is an important adverse reaction to look for in patients undergoing rehabilitation because it may mimic dementia on neuropsychologic testing. Depression may be worsened or induced by some antihypertensives (e.g., central agonists, highly lipophilic β-blockers). Metoclopramide is an important yet often overlooked potential contributor to depression.

B.L. is receiving several medications that may be contributing to the functional impairments found during the initial assessment. Metoclopramide has dopamine-blocking activity and can produce pseudo-Parkinson symptoms like those reported by the physical therapist. Dopamine blockers can also cause swallowing difficulties. Metoclopramide has also been known to produce mental depression in some patients that may or may not recur when the drug is re-instituted at lower dosages. B.L. is at even greater risk for these adverse effects from metoclopramide since it is primarily renally excreted and B.L. has reduced renal function, with an estimated creatinine clearance of 42 mL/min. H_2 blockers, such as ranitidine, can cause confusion and agitation in older patients with decreased renal function. Metoclopramide and ranitidine should be discontinued at this time. B.L.'s GERD should be reassessed and if chronic therapy is needed, a proton pump inhibitor (e.g., rabeprazole, others) is an appropriate choice since there is a low likelihood that it will cause functional impairment.

B.L.'s problem of depressive symptoms reported by the occupational therapist and potential dementia reported by his psychologist are compatible with CNS effects of metoprolol, a highly lipophilic β-blocker. Metoclopramide may also be a contributor to these findings. If B.L. must continue taking a β-blocker for additional rate control, he should be switched to an agent with low-lipid solubility, such as atenolol, which has a lower likelihood of producing CNS side effects. Otherwise, the dose of metoprolol should be reduced immediately and then tapered.

B.L.'s digoxin level is currently within normal limits, and he does not have any clinical signs of digoxin toxicity. However, the pharmacist team member should monitor B.L. for signs and symptoms of digoxin toxicity and make appropriate dose adjustments as necessary. Finally, B.L. should have an INR drawn to ensure that the dose of warfarin is correct.

The contribution of medication to functional deficits must not be overlooked when assessing patients undergoing rehabilitation. Beers has published defined criteria for determining medications that are potentially inappropriate in the elderly.[78] When using these criteria, it is important to keep in mind that these are "potentially" inappropriate medications. The pharmacotherapy specialist trained in geriatric care is responsible for applying patient-specific criteria, such as history of use and response, when evaluating the appropriateness of a drug in a particular patient.

Long-Term Care Facility (LTCF)

The LTCF environment is governed in part by the Omnibus Budget Reconciliation Act (OBRA) as well as by numerous other laws and regulations. Table 99-14 summarizes the man-

Table 99-14	**Basic Requirements of OBRA 1990 Legislation[163]**

Prospective DUR
Retrospective DUR
Education and intervention programs
Patient counseling and provision of information to patients/caregivers
Documentation of DUR and educational activities

DUR, drug utilization review; OBRA, Omnibus Budget Reconciliation Act.

dated responsibilities of the "supervising pharmacist" in a LTCF. The completion of these responsibilities must include monthly review of each resident's medication profile to determine the following:

1. Is each drug clearly indicated?
2. If indicated, is it being dosed and administered appropriately?
3. Are the laboratory results and vital signs being done appropriately and are they available for adequate evaluation of therapy?
4. Are any real or potential problems with drug side effects or interactions present?
5. What specific recommendations can be made to optimize this resident's drug therapy?
6. If neuroleptic agents are being prescribed, has their use been justified and is the therapy being monitored?
7. Have therapeutic goals been established for chronic drug therapies?
8. Are any unnecessary drugs present?

OBRA regulations require inclusion of a pharmacist on the pharmaceutical and infection control committees. The pharmacist is also required to participate in drug use evaluations. All medication errors and adverse drug reactions must be reported to the patient's physician and documented by the pharmacist or the nurse. The American Society of Consultant Pharmacists publishes detailed information concerning standards of practice in the LTCF environment.[154]

28. **As a new consulting pharmacist to a 60-bed skilled-nursing facility, several multiple drug use problems become apparent during initial chart reviews. A typical case is D.M., an 82-year-old man who has resided there for the past month. D.M.'s past medical history is significant for hypertension, depression, constipation, long-standing mild cognitive impairment that is now worsening, and dizziness. In the nurses' notes, it is documented that D.M. had a fall when getting out of bed last week.**

At admission, D.M.'s weight was 165 pounds; BP, 100/60 mmHg; pulse, 85 beats/min; and temperature, 98.6°F. Subsequent vital signs are not recorded systematically into his medical record. Sporadic documentation in the nurses' notes indicate little change from admission values. No laboratory information is available at this time. D.M. has no known allergies.

Current medications include felodipine 10 mg QD, diltiazem CD 240 mg QD, HCTZ 25 mg QD, nortriptyline 150 mg QHS, thioridazine 25 mg TID, haloperidol 0.5 mg BID, benztropine 1 mg BID, docusate sodium 100 mg BID, milk of magnesia 30 mL QD, flurazepam 15 mg QHS, and acetaminophen one to two 325 mg tablets Q 4 to 6 hr PRN pain. D.M. follows a 2-g sodium diet.

D.M. is ambulatory and takes his meals in the facility's cafeteria. He is not in any acute distress, but the nurses' notes indicate that D.M. is often confused and complains of dizziness when ambulating. His weight has decreased 4 pounds since being admitted. What should be expected of this LTCF with respect to medication monitoring, and what OBRA deficiencies can be found in the review of D.M.'s case?

Under OBRA, the establishment of goals of antihypertensive therapy and monitoring for these goals are required. D.M.'s blood pressure should be measured and documented in his medical record with a signature and date on a regular basis. D.M.'s dizziness, a symptom of orthostatic hypotension, may be due to overtreatment of his hypertension as evidenced by his low admission blood pressure. Orthostatic hypotension occurs in more than half of frail, elderly LTCF residents and is most common when patients first arise, indicating that this may have been the cause of D.M.'s recent fall. D.M. is currently being inappropriately treated with two calcium channel blockers. Discontinuation of one of them should reduce this patient's dizziness and help prevent future falls. Preferably, felodipine should be discontinued because dihydropyridine calcium channel blockers are known to cause orthostasis. The use of antipsychotic and anti-Parkinson agents also have been associated with orthostatic hypotension. Since D.M. is being treated with a diuretic, he should have a chemistry panel drawn to check for electrolyte abnormalities.

In the admission workup D.M. was described as having a longstanding history of mild cognitive impairment, but subsequent nursing notes suggest that his symptoms of disorientation and confusion worsened quickly after admission. Chronic dementia is not normally characterized by rapid deterioration of mental acuity (see Chapter 100, Geriatric Dementias). This should raise the suspicion that a reversible factor could be responsible for D.M.'s mental decline. Overprescribing of psychotropic drugs in institutionalized elderly patients is well documented.[155-157] The cognitive impairment of chronic degenerative dementia can be greatly exaggerated by D.M.'s treatment with flurazepam, nortriptyline, thioridazine, haloperidol, and benztropine.

Neuroleptics are some of the most commonly prescribed drugs in nursing home residents. It is only appropriate to use these drugs in elderly patients with documented psychotic behavioral disturbances or those with impulsivity and agitation associated with functional or organic disorders, such as degenerative dementia. Unfortunately, neuroleptics are often unnecessarily prescribed for anxiety, insomnia, confusion, "senility," and failure to conform to the institution's standards for behavior. OBRA regulations require that these drugs be used for a specified condition, at the lowest possible dosage, and for the shortest possible time. The regulations also mandate tapering of the dose and careful documentation of all clinical assessments that justify the ongoing need for neuroleptics. Even when a neuroleptic agent is indicated, the use of two or more, as in D.M., is irrational. Unless extrapyramidal symptoms have been clearly documented, D.M.'s treatment with benztropine is not indicated.

Antidepressant treatment may not be indicated for D.M., but if it is, nortriptyline is a poor choice because it has significant anticholinergic and sedating side effects (see prior discussion of depression in this chapter). D.M. is being treated with several sedating medications (flurazepam, haloperidol, and thioridazine). These agents may induce pseudodepression, which should resolve by reducing the number of sedating drugs. Flurazepam, a long-acting benzodiazepine, may increase the risk of falls and bone fractures in the geriatric population. Continuous nightly use of long-acting benzodiazepines increases the relative risk of hip fractures by 50% compared with shorter-acting benzodiazepines.[158] Elderly patients naturally sleep for shorter periods with a shallower sleep that is subject to frequent awakenings. Thus, the need for scheduled bedtime sleep agents must always be evaluated critically (see Chapter 77, Sleep Disorders).

In light of the atypical deterioration of D.M.'s cognitive function, the doses of all psychotropic medications should be gradually tapered down and then discontinued. A baseline assessment of D.M.'s cognitive function and psychiatric status should be performed by a geriatrician, psychiatrist, or clinical psychologist to establish the presence or absence of psychotic behavioral disturbances or depression. If any of these disorders are present, then each should be managed with a single drug, titrated to the appropriate therapeutic dose. In accordance with established immunization practices, D.M., other LTCF residents, and staff members should receive an annual influenza vaccine. A pneumococcal vaccination should also be administered to D.M. if he has not previously received one.

REFERENCES

1. Federal Interagency Forum on Aging-Related Statistics. Older Americans 2000: key indicators of well-being. Federal Interagency Forum on Aging-Related Statistics, Washington, DC: U.S. Government Printing Office, August 2000.
2. Congressional Budget Office. Projections of expenditure for long-term care services for the elderly. 1999.
3. U.S. Bureau of the Census. Current population reports, special studies. P23-190. 65+ in the United States. Washington, DC: U.S. Government Printing Office, 1996.
4. Jones A. The National Nursing Home Survey: 1999 summary. National Center for Health Statistics. Vital Health Stat 2002;13(152).
5. Singer BH. Manton KG. The effects of health changes on projections of health service needs for the elderly population of the United States. Proc Natl Acad Sci USA 1998;95(26):15618.
6. Johnson JA, Bootman JL. Drug-related morbidity and mortality; a cost of illness model. Arch Inern Med 1995;155:1949.
7. Resnick NM, Marcantonio DR. How should clinical care of the aged differ? Lancet 1997;350:1157.
8. Swift CG. Clinical pharmacology in the older patients. Scott Med J 1979;24:221.
9. Hurwitz A et al. Gastric acidity in older adults. JAMA 1997;278:659.
10. Rudy DW et al. Loop diuretics for chronic renal insufficiency. Ann Intern Med 1991;115:360.
11. Bender AD. The effect of increasing age on the distribution of peripheral blood flow in man. J Am Geriatr Soc 1965;13:192.
12. Riesenberg DE. Studies reshape some views of the aging heart. JAMA 1986;255:871.
13. Shock NW et al. Age differences in the water content of the body as related to basal oxygen consumption in males. J Gerontol 1963;18:1.
14. Novak IP. Aging, total body potassium, fat-free mass, and cell mass in males and females between ages 18 and 85 years. J Gerontol 1972;27:438.
15. Greenblatt DJ et al. Toxicity of high-dose flurazepam in the elderly. Clin Pharmacol Ther 1977;21:355.
16. Greenblatt DJ. Reduced serum albumin concentration in the older patients: a report from the Boston Collaborative Drug Surveillance Program. J Am Geriatr Soc 1979;27:20.
17. Israili ZH, Dayton PG. Human alpha-1 glycoprotein and its interactions with drugs. Drug Metab Rev 2001;33:161.
18. Jusko WJ, Weintraub M. Myocardial distribution of digoxin and renal function. Clin Pharmacol Ther 1974;16:449.
19. Mayersohn MB. Special pharmacokinetic considerations in the elderly. In: Evans WE et al, eds. Applied Pharmacokinetics: Principles of Therapeutic

Drug Monitoring. 3rd Ed. Vancouver: Applied Therapeutics, 1992.

20. Farah F et al. Hepatic drug acetylation and oxidation: effects of aging in man. Br Med J 1977;2:255.

21. O'Malley K et al. Effect of age and sex on human drug metabolism. Br Med J 1971;3:607.

22. Thompson EN et al. Effect of age on liver function with particular reference to bromsulphalein excretion. Gut 1965;6:266.

23. Triggs EJ et al. Pharmacokinetics in the older patients. Eur J Clin Pharmacol 1975;8:55.

24. Geokas MC et al. The aging gastrointestinal tract. Am J Surg 1969;117:881.

25. Hewick DS et al. The effect of age on sensitivity to warfarin sodium. Br J Pharmacol 1975;2:189P.

26. Shader RI et al. Absorption and disposition of chlordiazepoxide in young and older patients male volunteers. J Clin Pharmacol 1977;17:709.

27. Klotz U et al. Effects of age and liver disease on disposition and elimination of diazepam in adult man. J Clin Invest 1975;55:347.

28. Nies AS et al. Altered hepatic blood flow and drug disposition. Clin Pharmacokinet 1976;1:125.

29. Rowe JW et al. The effect of age on creatinine clearance in man: a cross sectional and longitudinal study. J Gerontol 1976;31:155.

30. Rowe JW et al. The influence of age on renal response to water deprivation in man. Nephron 1976;17:270.

31. Epstein M et al. Age as a determinant of renal sodium conservation. J Lab Clin Med 1976;87:411.

32. Baylis EM et al. Effects of renal function on plasma digoxin levels in elder ambulant patients in domiciliary practice. Br Med J 1972;1:338.

33. Leikola E et al. On oral penicillin levels in young and geriatric patients. J Gerontol 1957;12:48.

34. Palmer BF, Moshe L. Effect of aging on renal function and disease. In: Brenner BM, Rector FC, eds. Brenner and Rector's The Kidney. 5th Ed. Philadelphia: WB Saunders, 1996:2274.

35. Lindeman RD et al. Longitudinal studies on the rate of decline in renal function with age. J Am Geriatr Soc 1985;33:278.

36. Cockcroft DW, Gault MH. Prediction of creatinine clearance from serum creatinine. Nephron 1976;16:31.

37. O'Connell MB et al. Predictive performance of equations to estimate creatinine clearance in hospitalized elderly patients. Ann Pharmacother 1992;26:627.

38. Smythe M et al. Estimating creatinine clearance in elderly patients with low serum creatinine concentrations. Am J Hosp Pharm 1994;51:198.

39. Lipsitz LA. Orthostatic hypotension in the older patients. N Engl J Med 1989;321:952.

40. Davis TA et al. Orthostatic hypotension: therapeutic alternatives for geriatric patients. DICP Ann Pharmacother 1989;23:750.

41. Blumenthal MD et al. Dizziness and falling in elderly outpatients. Am J Psychiatry 1980;137:203.

42. Overstall PW et al. Falls in the older patients related to postural imbalance. Br Med J 1977;1:261.

43. Anonymous. Drugs in the older patients. Med Lett Drugs Ther 1979;21:43.

44. Castleden CM et al. Increased sensitivity to nitrazepam in old age. Br Med J 1977;1:10.

45. Smith BH et al. Aging and the nervous system. Geriatrics 1975;30:109.

46. Roth M. Senile dementia and its borderlands. Proc Annu Meet Am Psychopathol Assoc 1980;69:205.

47. Heinsimer JA et al. The impact of aging on adrenergic receptor function: clinical and biochemical aspects. J Am Geriatr Soc 1985;33:184.

48. Samorajski T. Age-related changes in brain biogenic amines. In: Schneider EL, ed. Aging. Clinical, Morphologic and Neurochemical Aspects in the Aging Central Nervous System. New York: Raven Press, 1975;1:199.

49. Fleg JL et al. Age-related augmentation of plasma catecholamines during dynamic exercise in healthy males. J Appl Physiol 1985;59:1033.

50. Scarpace PJ et al. Beta-adrenergic function in aging: basic mechanisms and clinical implications. Drugs Aging 1991;1:116.

51. Vestal RE et al. Reduced beta-adrenergic sensitivity in the elderly. Clin Pharmacol Ther 1979;26:181.

52. Larson EB et al. Adverse drug reactions associated with global cognitive impairment in older patients persons. Ann Intern Med 1987;107:169.

53. Anonymous. Surgeon General's workshop on health promotion and aging: summary recommendations of the medication working group. JAMA 1989;262:1755.

54. American Society of Consultant Pharmacists. Practice standards for long-term care pharmacy, 1998.

55. Zermansky AG et al. Randomized controlled trial of clinical medication review by a pharmacist of elderly patients receiving repeat prescriptions in general practice. Br Med J 2001;323:1.

56. Zhan C et al. Potentially inappropriate medication use in the community-dwelling elderly. JAMA 2001;286(22):2823.

57. Yoshikawa TT et al. Practical Ambulatory Geriatrics. St. Louis, MO: Mosby, 1998:23.

58. American Society of Consultant Pharmacists. Senior care pharmacy: the statistics. Consul Pharm 2000;15:310.

59. Hanlon JT et al. A randomized, controlled trial of a clinical pharmacist intervention to improve inappropriate prescribing in elderly outpatients with polypharmacy. Am J Med 1996;100:428.

60. Riedinger JL, Robbins LJ. Prevention of iatrogenic illness: adverse drug reactions and nosocomial infections in hospitalized older adults. Clin Geriatr Med 1998;14(4):681.

61. Gray SL et al. Adverse drug events in hospitalized elderly. J Gerontol 1998;53A(1):M59.

62. Gurwitz JH et al. Incidence and preventability of adverse drug events among older persons in the ambulatory setting. JAMA 2003;289(9):1107.

63. Johnson JA, Bootman JL. Drug-related morbidity and mortality; a cost of illness model. Arch Intern Med 1995;155:1949.

64. Beyth RJ, Shorr RI. Epidemiology of adverse drug reactions in the elderly by drug class. Drugs Aging 1999;14(3):231.

65. Roche Laboratories. Toradol package insert. Nutley, NJ: September 2002.

66. Lamy PP. The elderly, communications, and compliance. Pharm Times 1992;58:33.

67. Bero LA et al. Characterization of geriatric drug-related hospital readmissions. Med Care 1991;29:989.

68. Terra SG et al. Therapeutic range of digoxin's efficacy in heart failure: what is the evidence? Pharmacotherapy 1999;19(10):1123.

69. AHA/ACC Guidelines for the Evaluation and Management of Chronic Heart Failure in the Adult. A report of the American College of Cardiology/American Heart Association Task Force on Practice Guidelines. AHA/ACC Practice Guidelines 2001.

70. Heart Outcomes Prevention Evaluation (HOPE) study investigators. Effects of ramipril on cardiovascular and microvascular outcomes in people with diabetes mellitus: results of the HOPE study and MICRO-HOPE sub-study. Lancet 2000;355:253.

71. The Cooperative North Scandinavian Enalapril Survival Study (CONSENSUS) Group. Effects of enalapril on mortality in severe CHF. N Engl J Med 1987;316:1429.

72. The Studies of Left Ventricular Dysfunction (SOLVD) Investigators. Effect of enalapril on survival in patients with reduced ventricular ejection fraction and congestive heart failure. N Engl J Med 1991;325:293.

73. Williams BR, Kim J. Cardiovascular drug therapy in the elderly: theoretical and practical considerations. Drugs Aging 2003;20(6):445.

74. Bristol-Myers Squibb Company. Monopril package insert. Princeton, NJ: May 2003.

75. Packer M et al. U.S. Carvedilol Heart Failure Study Group. The effect of carvedilol on mortality in patients with chronic heart failure. N Engl J Med 1996;334:1349.

76. MERIT-HF Study Group. Effect of metoprolol CR/XL in chronic heart failure: metoprolol CR/XL randomized intervention trial in congestive heart failure (MERIT-HF). Lancet 1999;353:2001.

77. Krum H et al. Carvedilol Prospective Randomized Cumulative Survival (COPERNICUS) Study Group. Effects of initiating carvedilol in patients with severe chronic heart failure: results from the COPERNICUS Study. JAMA 2003;289(6):712.

78. Beers MH. Explicit criteria for determining potentially inappropriate medication use by elderly: an update. Arch Intern Med 1997;157:1531.

79. Green LW et al. Programs to reduce drug errors in the elderly: direct and indirect evidence from patient education. In: Improving Medication Compliance. Reston: National Pharmaceutical Council, 1985.

80. Hawthorn monograph. Natural Medicines Comprehensive Database 1999:427.

81. Dandelion, hawthorn, and herbal diuretics monographs. Review of Natural Products, Facts and Comparisons, 1998.

82. Valli G, Giardina E-GV. Benefits, adverse effects, and drug interactions of herbal therapies with cardiovascular effects. J Am Coll Cardiol 2002;39:1083.

83. Dandelion monograph. Natural Medicines Comprehensive Database 1999:283.

84. Corti MC et al. Clarifying the direct relation between total cholesterol levels and death from coronary heart disease in older persons. Ann Intern Med 1997;126:753.

85. Benfante R, Reed D. Is elevated serum cholesterol level a risk factor for coronary heart disease in the elderly? JAMA 1990;263:393.

86. Howard G et al. Does the association of risk factors and atherosclerosis change with age? Stroke 1997;28:1693.

87. Frost PH et al. Serum lipids and incidence of coronary heart disease, findings from the Systolic Hypertension in the Elderly Program (SHEP). Circulation 1996;94:2381.

88. Grundy SM et al. Cholesterol lowering in the elderly population. Arch Intern Med 1999;159:1670.

89. National Lipid Education Council. Treating dyslipidemia in the elderly: are we doing enough? Lipid Manage Newslett 1999;4:1.

90. Dalal D, Robbins JA. Management of hyperlipidemia in the elderly population: an evidence-based approach. South Med J 2002;95(11):1255.

91. Expert Panel on Detection, Evaluation, and Treatment of High Blood Cholesterol in Adults. Executive Summary of The Third Report of The National Cholesterol Education Program (NCEP) Expert Panel on Detection, Evaluation, And Treatment of High Blood Cholesterol In Adults (Adult Treatment Panel III). JAMA 2001;285(19):2486.

92. Grundy SM. The role of cholesterol management in coronary heart disease risk reduction in elderly patients. Endocrinol Metab Clin North Am 1998;27:655.

93. Illingworth DR. Management of hypercholesterolemia. Med Clin North Am 2000;84:23.

94. American Diabetes Association. Treatment of hypertension in adults with diabetes. Diabet Care 2003;26(Suppl 1):S80.

95. National High Blood Pressure Education Program. The seventh report of the Joint National Committee on Prevention, Detection, Evaluation, and Treatment of High Blood Pressure. NIH Publication No 03-5233. May 2003.

96. National High Blood Pressure Education Program. The sixth report of the Joint National Committee on Prevention, Detection, Evaluation, and Treatment of High Blood Pressure. Arch Intern Med 1997;157;2413.

97. Hyman DJ, Pavlik VN. Characteristics of patients with uncontrolled hypertension in the United States. N Engl J Med 2001;345:479.

98. Pfizer Laboratories. Norvasc package insert. New York, NY: December 2001.

99. Criqui MH, Golomb BA. Should patients with diabetes drink to their health? JAMA 1999;282(3):279.

100. Novo Nordisk Pharmaceuticals Inc. Prandin package insert. Princeton, NJ: October 2002.

101. Jeste DV et al. Consensus statement, The upcoming crisis in geriatric mental health: challenges and opportunities. Arch Gen Psychiatry 1999; 56:848.

102. Lebowitz BD. Diagnosis and treatment of depression in late life: an overview of the NIH consensus statement. Am J Ger Psych 1996;4:S3.

103. Sable JA et al. Late-life depression: how to identify its symptoms and provide effective treatment. Geriatrics 2002;57(2):18.

104. Pollack B. Clinical update: how to recognize and treat depression in older patients. Geriatrics 2000;55(1):67.

105. Reynolds CF, Kupfer DJ. Depression and aging: a look to the future. Psychiatr Serv 1999;50:1167.

106. American Psychiatric Association. Diagnostic and statistical manual of mental disorders. 4th Ed. Washington, DC: American Psychiatric Association, 1994.

107. Koenig HG, Blazer DG. Epidemiology of geriatric affective disorders. Clin Geriatr Med 1992; 8:235.

108. Blazer DG. Depression in the elderly: Myths and misconceptions. Psychiatr Clin North Am 1997; 20:111.

109. Georgotas A, McRue RE. The additional benefit of extending an antidepressant trial past seven weeks in the depressed elderly patient. Int J Geriatr Psychiatry 1989;4:191.

110. Renwick DS, Connolly MJ. Prevalence and treatment of chronic airflow obstruction in adults over the age of 45. Thorax 1996;51:164.

111. Parameswaran K et al. Asthma in the elderly: underperceived, underdiagnosed and undertreated: a community survey. Respir Med 1998;92:573.

112. Burr ML et al. Asthma in the elderly: an epidemiological survey. Br Med J 1979;1:1041.

113. Enright PL et al. Underdiagnosis and undertreatment of asthma in the elderly: Cardiovascular Health Study Research Group. Chest 1999; 116:603.

114. National Asthma Education and Prevention Program. Considerations for Diagnosing and Managing Asthma in the Elderly, 1997. NIH publication No. 97-4051.

115. Claessens MT et al. Dying with lung cancer or chronic obstructive pulmonary disease: insights from SUPPORT. J Am Geriatr Soc 2000;48:S146.

116. Renwick DS, Connolly MJ. Impact of obstructive airways disease on quality of life in older adults. Thorax 1996;51:520.

117. Pethcram IS et al. Assessment and management of acute asthma in the elderly: a comparison with younger asthmatics. Postgrad Med J 1982;58:149.

118. Connolly MJ et al. reduced subjective awareness of bronchoconstriction provoked by methacholine in elderly asthmatic and normal subjects as measured on a simple awareness scale. Thorax 1992;47:410.

119. Szczezeklik A, Stevenson DD. Aspirin-induced asthma: advances in pathogenesis and management. J Allergy Clin Immunol 2003;111:913.

120. National Institutes of Health. Expert Panel Report 2. Guidelines for the Diagnosis and Management of Asthma, 1997; NIH publication No. 97-4051.

121. Ruben FL et al. Clinical infections in the non-institutionalized geriatric age group: methods utilized and incidence of infections. The Pittsburgh Good Health Study. Am J Epidemiol 1995; 141:145.

122. Miller RA. The aging immune system: primer and prospectus. Science 1996;273:70.

123. Jokinen C et al. Incidence of community-acquired pneumonia in the population of four municipalities in Eastern Finland. Am J Epidemiol 1993; 137:977.

124. Marrie TJ. Community-acquired pneumonia in the elderly. Clin Infect Dis 2000;31:1066.

125. Lipsky BA et al. Risk factors for acquiring pneumococcal infections. Arch Intern Med 1986;146: 2179.

126. Porth A et al. The epidemiology of community-acquired pneumonia among hospitalized patients. J Infect 1997;34:41.

127. Burman et al. Diagnosis of pneumonia by cultures, bacterial and viral antigen detection tests, and serology with special references to antibodies against pneumococcal antigen. J Infect Dis 1991; 163:1087.

128. Kauppienen MT et al. the etiology of community-acquired pneumonia among hospitalized patients during a *Chlamydia pneumoniae* epidemic in Finland. J Infect Dis 1995;172:1330.

129. Gross PA et al. The efficacy of influenza vaccine in elderly persons: a meta-analysis and review of the literature. Ann Intern Med 1995;123:518.

130. Ortqvist A et al. Swedish pneumococcal vaccination study group. Randomized trial of 23-valent pneumococcal capsular polysaccharide vaccine in prevention of pneumonia in middle-aged and elderly people. Lancet 1998;351:399.

131. Couch RB et al. Influenza: its control in persons and populations. J Infect Dis 1986;153(3):431.

132. Shapiro ED et al. The protective efficacy of polyvalent pneumococcal polysaccharide vaccine. N Engl J Med 1991;325:1453.

133. Jackson LA et al. Effectiveness of pneumococcal polysaccharide vaccine in older adults. N Engl J Med 2003;348(18):1747.

134. Nicolle LE. Urinary tract infections in the elderly. J Antimicrob Chemother 1994;33(S):99.

135. Raz P. Urinary tract infection in the elderly women. Int J Antimicrob Agents 1998;10:177.

136. Ackermann RJ, Monroe PW. Bacteremic urinary tract infection in older people. J Am Geriatr Soc 1996;44:927.

137. Eykyn SJ. Urinary tract infections in the elderly. Br J Urol 1998,82(S):79.

138. Gomolin IH et al. Efficacy and safety of ciprofloxacin oral suspension versus trimethoprim:sulfamethoxazole oral suspension for treatment of older women with acute urinary tract infection. J Am Geriatr Soc 2001;49:1606.

139. McEvoy GK et al. eds. AHFS Drug Information. Bethesda: American Society of Health-System Pharmacists, Inc., 2002:838.

140. Felson DT. The course of osteoarthritis and factors that affect it. Rheum Dis Clin North Am 1993;19:607.

141. American Geriatrics Society Panel on Pain in Older Persons. The management of persistent pain in older persons. J Am Geriatr Soc 2002;50:S205.

142. Gloth FM. Pain management in older adults: prevention and treatment. J Am Geriatr Soc 2001;49(2):188.

143. Roche RJ, Forman WB. Pain management for the geriatric patients. Clin Podiatr Med Surg 1994;11(1):41.

144. Richy F et al. Structural and symptomatic efficacy of glucosamine and chondroitin in knee osteoarthritis: a comprehensive meta-analysis. Arch Intern Med 2003;163(13):1514.

145. Davis MP, Srivastava M. Demographics, assessment and management of pain the elderly. Drugs Aging 2003;20(1):23.

146. Brotman HB. Every ninth American: an analysis for the chairman of the select committee on aging, House of Representatives. Comm publication no. 1-97-332. Washington, DC: U.S. Government Printing Office, 1982.

147. DeLisa JA et al. Rehabilitation medicine, past, present, and future. In: DeLisa JA, ed. Rehabilitation Medicine: Principles and Practice. Philadelphia: Lippincott, 1988:3.

148. National Center for Health Statistics. Health, United States, 1999 with Health and Aging Chartbook. Hyattsville, MD: 1999.

149. World Health Organization. International classification of impairments, disabilities, and handicaps: a manual of classification relating to the consequences of disease. Geneva: WHO, 1980.

150. Karki SD et al. Impact of a team approach on reducing polypharmacy. Consult Pharm 1991;6:133.

151. Thomas DR et al. Inpatient community-based geriatric assessment reduces subsequent mortality. J Am Geriatr Soc 1993;41:101.

152. Bjornson DC, Hiner WO Jr. Evaluation of the effects of clinical pharmacists on inpatient healthcare outcomes. Presented at AJHP Midyear Clinical Meeting. Orlando, Florida, December 1992.

153. Owens NJ et al. The relationship between comprehensive functional assessment and optimal pharmacotherapy in the older patient. DICP Ann Pharmacother 1989;23:847.

154. American Society of Consultant Pharmacists. ASCP Policies, Standards, and Guidelines 2002.

155. Aparasu RR, Mort JR. Inappropriate prescribing for the elderly: Beers criteria-based review. Ann Pharmacother 2000;34:338.

156. Hanlon JT et al. Recent advances in geriatrics: drug-related problems in the elderly. Ann Pharmacother 2000;34:360.

157. Liu GG, Christensen DB. The continuing challenge of inappropriate prescribing in the elderly: an update of the evidence. J Am Pharm Assoc 2002;42(6):847.

158. Ray WA et al. Benzodiazepines of long and short elimination half-life and the risk of hip fracture. JAMA 1989;262:3303.

159. Arnoff GR et al. Drug prescribing in renal failure: Dosing guidelines for adults. 4th Ed. Philadelphia: American College of Physicians, 1999:18.

160. Swan SK, Bennett WM. Drug dosing guidelines in patients with renal failure. West J Med 1992; 156:633.

161. Murray MD et al. Factors contributing to medication noncompliance in older patients public housing tenants. Drug Intell Clin Pharm 1986;20:146.

162. Meyer ME et al. Assessment of geriatric patients' functional ability to take medication. Drug Intell Clin Pharm 1989;23:717.

163. Canaday BR. OBRA '90: A Practical Guide to Effecting Pharmaceutical Care. Washington, DC: American Pharmaceutical Association, 1994.

Geriatric Dementias

Bradley R. Williams

With the continuing growth in the elderly population, the incidence and prevalence of cognitive disorders continues to rise.[1,2] Alzheimer's disease (AD) is the most common cause of dementia, accounting for approximately half of all diagnosed cases.[3] Vascular dementias (VaD) and dementia with Lewy bodies (DLB) are the next most common dementias, with frontotemporal dementia, pseudodementia, and other forms occurring less often.[3,4] Almost 600,000 people each year die with dementia in the United States.[5]

Incidence and Prevalence

The exact incidence and prevalence of dementia are difficult to determine for several reasons, including a lack of universally accepted diagnostic criteria, demographic variables, and well-designed epidemiologic studies.[6–9] Prevalence estimates have ranged from 2.5% in Great Britain to 24.6% in the former Soviet Union.[7] Studies in the United States have estimated the prevalence of dementias to be from 3.5% to 16.1% for the population aged 65 and older.[10,11] The worldwide prevalence of AD appears to be about 1% of the elderly population, with an exponential age-related increase.[9,12] AD currently affects approximately 2.3 million Americans.[2] The prevalence in the United States may be more than 10% of those aged 65 and older, increasing sharply with age, from 3% among those 65 to 74 years to as much as 47.2% of those older than 85 years of age.[13,14] The incidence of dementia for people age 50 and older in the United States has been estimated at 527 new cases/100,000 population per year, with 437/100,000 diagnosed as AD.[15] The incidence increases with age, and women may be at a slightly higher risk than men.[1,16]

Life expectancy following a diagnosis of AD is reduced by as much as 69% for those diagnosed before age 70 and by 39% for those diagnosed after age 90.[17]

The cost of dementia is staggering. The annual direct and total costs of treating a dementia patient is estimated to be almost $18,000 and $174,000, respectively.[18] Managed care organizations spend 1.5 times more on patients with dementia than on nondemented enrollees.[19] The cost to society in the United States of treating dementia is almost $100 billion annually.[20]

Clinical Diagnosis

Dementia is a syndrome that exhibits impaired short-term and long-term memory as its most prominent feature. Multiple cognitive deficits that compromise normal social or occupational function must be present before dementia can be diagnosed. (Table 100-1).[21] Commonly, forgetfulness is the primary complaint of patients or the first symptom noted by the family.[21] Family members or others may note several symptoms that should prompt a medical evaluation (Table 100-2).[22] Memory loss often accompanies several diseases or disorders in elderly individuals. Therefore, a medical history, physical examination, and medication history are essential in excluding systemic illness or medication toxicity as causes of the dementia (Table 100-3).[23] Laboratory and other tests to assist in differentiating dementia from other disorders are listed in Table 100-4. In patients with primary degenerative dementia, or AD, test results will generally be normal; evidence of cerebrovascular disease is present in patients with vascular dementias.

Table 100-1 Diagnostic Criteria for Alzheimer-Type Dementia

1. The presence of multiple cognitive deficits manifested by both:
   - Impaired memory (ability to learn new information or to retrieve information previously learned), and
   - At least one of the following:
     Aphasia (language difficulties)
     Apraxia (diminished ability to perform motor activities in the presence of intact motor function)
     Agnosia (inability to recognize or name objects despite intact sensory function)
     Disruption of executive function (diminished ability to plan, organize)
2. The deficits above significantly interfere with normal work or social activities and represent a decline from previous ability to function
3. The deficits above cannot be attributed to any of the following:
   - CNS conditions that cause progressive cognitive or memory impairment (e.g., cerebrovascular disease)
   - Systemic conditions known to cause dementia (e.g., hypothyroidism, neurosyphilis, HIV infection)
   - Substance-induced conditions (e.g., drug toxicity)
4. The deficits do not occur exclusively during the course of a delirium
5. The disturbance is not better accounted for by another Axis I disorder (schizophrenia, major depressive disorder)

CNS, central nervous system; HIV, human immunodeficiency virus.
Adapted with permission from reference 21.

Table 100-2 Symptoms Suggesting Dementia

Symptom	Evidence
Difficulty learning or retaining new information	Repeats questions; difficulty remembering recent conversations, events, etc.; loses items
Unable to handle complex tasks	Cannot complete tasks that require multiple steps (e.g., difficulty following a shopping list)
Impaired reasoning	Difficulty solving everyday problems; inappropriate social behavior
Impaired spatial orientation and abilities	Gets lost in familiar places; difficulty with driving
Language deficits	Problems finding appropriate words (e.g., difficulty with naming common objects)
Behavior changes	Changes in personality; suspiciousness

Adapted from reference 22.

Table 100-3 Causes of Dementia Symptoms

CNS Disorders	Systemic Illness	Medications
Adjustment disorder (e.g., inability to adjust to retirement)	Cardiovascular disease	Anticholinergic agents
	Arrhythmia	Anticonvulsants
	Heart failure	Antidepressants
Amnestic syndrome (e.g., isolated memory impairment)	Vascular occlusion	Antihistamines
	Deficiency states	Anti-infectives
	Vitamin B_{12}	Antineoplastic agents
	Folate	Antipsychotic agents
Delirium	Iron	Cardiovascular agents
Depression	Infections	Antiarrhythmics
Intracranial causes	Metabolic disorders	Antihypertensives
Brain abscess	Adrenal	Corticosteroids
Normal pressure	Glucose	H_2-receptor antagonists
Hydrocephalus	Renal failure	Immunosuppressants
Stroke	Thyroid	Narcotic analgesics
Subdural hematoma		Nonsteroidal anti-inflammatory agents
Tumor		Sedative hypnotics and Anxiolytics
		Skeletal muscle relaxants

Table 100-4 Dementia Screening Tests

Test	Rationale for Testing
CBC with sedimentation rate	Anemic anoxia, infection, neoplasms
Metabolic screen	
Serum electrolytes	Hypernatremia, hyponatremia; renal function
BUN, creatinine	Renal function
Bilirubin	Hepatic dysfunction (e.g., portal systemic encephalopathy, hepatocerebral degeneration)
Thyroid function	Hypothyroidism, apathetic hyperthyroidism
Iron, B_{12}, folate	Deficiency states (B_{12}, folate neuropathies), anemias
Stool occult blood	Blood loss, anemia
Syphilis serology	Neurosyphilis
UA	Infection, proteinuria
Chest roentgenogram	Neoplasms, infection, airway disease (anoxia)
ECG	Cardiac disease (stagnant anoxia)
Brain scan	Cerebral tumors, cerebrovascular disease
Mental status testing	General cognitive screen
Depression testing	Depression, pseudodementia

BUN, blood urea nitrogen; CBC, complete blood cell count; ECG, electrocardiogram; UA, urinalysis.

Brain imaging, such as a computed tomography (CT) scan or magnetic resonance imaging (MRI), can be useful in establishing the presence of a dementia, but neither is diagnostic. A CT scan is useful when a space-occupying lesion, such as a tumor, is suspected as a possible cause. An MRI scan is capable of identifying small infarcts, such as those found in some vascular dementias, and atrophy of subcortical structures such as the brainstem.[23]

The initial test in mental status screening is generally the Folstein Mini-Mental Status Exam.[24] This test rapidly assesses orientation, registration, attention and calculation, recall, and language. Patients with dementia exhibit deficits in multiple areas. Those who score below the normal range on the Mini-Mental Status Exam or who exhibit symptoms characteristic of dementia receive further testing (see Tables 100-1 and 100-2). The Blessed Dementia Scale evaluates daily functional capacity (e.g., shopping, performing household tasks), activities of daily living (e.g., eating, dressing, toileting), and personality. The Blessed Information-Memory-Concentration Test evaluates orientation, memory, and concentration.[25] All screening tests are subject to limitations. Therefore, additional psychometric testing often is ordered to further establish the presence and type of dementia.[22]

Dementias may be classified as cortical or subcortical, according to the areas of the brain preferentially affected by the disorder. AD, a typical cortical dementia, disrupts the cerebral cortex. Patients with cortical dementias display impaired language rather than impaired speech, a learning deficit (amnesia), reduced higher cortical functions (e.g., inability to perform calculations, poor judgment), and an unconcerned or disinhibited affect. Subcortical dementias such as multiinfarct dementia primarily affect the basal ganglia, thalamus, and brainstem. Deficits include abnormal motor function, disrupted speech patterns rather than language difficulties, forgetfulness (impaired recall), slowed cognitive function, and an apathetic or depressed affect.[3]

ALZHEIMER'S DISEASE
Etiology

Although a number of etiologies have been advanced for AD, a definitive cause has yet to be determined. Aluminum toxicity, immunologic abnormalities, hereditary predisposition, viral infection, and cellular dysfunction are among the more commonly proposed causes.[3] Although elevated aluminum concentration has been noted in patients with Alzheimer-type dementia, this finding has not been consistent.[26-28] For example, patients with aluminum toxicity, as seen in dialysis dementia, do not exhibit AD-type lesions.[29] Increased concentrations of cerebral aluminum may be a secondary process resulting from an underlying pathologic condition.[30] Other reported risk factors for AD include young (15 to 19 years) or old (≥40 years) maternal age,[31-33] head trauma,[33,34] small head circumference and brain size,[35,36] and low intelligence.[37]

Genetics play a significant role in the development of Alzheimer-type dementia. The high familial occurrence of Alzheimer's dementia has been linked to autosomal-dominant traits on chromosomes 21, 14, and 1.[38] The risk to first-degree relatives of patients with AD is 24% to 48% and may be as high as 64% for offspring.[39-42] Familial dementia of the Alzheimer type is associated with an early onset, faster progression, family history of psychiatric problems, and more prominent language difficulties.[39,43-45] However, there is some association between changes on chromosome 14 and late-onset AD.[46,47]

In families with a history of Down syndrome or other defects on chromosome 21, the prevalence of Alzheimer-type dementia is increased significantly. AD affects virtually all Down syndrome patients who survive into old age.[44,48,49] Mutations on chromosome 14 are responsible for most cases of familial early-onset AD, whereas chromosome 1–associated mutations account for cases in only a small cohort of families.[50,51] However, differences in risk based on age at onset and discordance for the disease among monozygotic twins indicate some heterogeneity in the genetic etiology.[42,44,52] Clinically, patients with familial dementia of the Alzheimer type are indistinguishable from those with nonfamilial, or sporadic, forms of the disease, suggesting a combination of genetic and environmental causes.[31,45] Despite the familial patterns, these mutations account for only approximately 5% of all cases of AD.[53]

Abnormalities in serum protein and alterations in immune function often are found among patients with AD. Amyloid precursor protein (APP), a normal protein found throughout the body (e.g., platelets and peripheral lymphocytes),[54] maps on chromosome 21 and is produced in excess in patients with Down syndrome.[48] Because of overproduction or transcription errors, an abnormal subunit (i.e., β-amyloid) is produced.[48,55] This finding is consistent in families with a high incidence of Alzheimer-type dementia, especially those with early-onset (before age 65) forms.[44,48,55]

Mutations on chromosome 14 occur in the presenilin-1 gene, and mutations on chromosome 1 occur in the presenilin-2 gene.[50,51,56] These mutations also code for alterations in the processing of APP. The abnormal cleavage of APP produces a 42–amino acid form of β-amyloid that demonstrates a higher toxicity than other amyloid forms.[38]

Apolipoprotein E (ApoE), a protein that is involved in cholesterol and phospholipid metabolism, plays a role in the development of sporadic, late-onset AD.[57] The ApoE gene resides on chromosome 19 and possesses three alleles: $\epsilon 2$, $\epsilon 3$, and $\epsilon 4$. The $\epsilon 3$ allele is most common, the $\epsilon 2$ allele appears to be protective against AD, and the $\epsilon 4$ allele increases the risk for AD.[58,59] The presence of ApoE-4, the protein coded for by the $\epsilon 4$ allele, appears to increase the deposition of β-amyloid and promote its change to a more pathologic configuration.[38] Measurable memory decline in people with either one or two copies of the $\epsilon 4$ allele occurs much earlier than in those with no copies, and well in advance of the first clinical symptoms of AD.[60,61] The risk for developing AD by age 80 has been estimated at 47% for people with one copy of ApoE-$\epsilon 4$ and at 91% for those who carry two copies. In contrast, the risk is approximately 20% for those with no ApoE-$\epsilon 4$ copies.[58]

Amyloid protein can commonly be found in the neuritic plaques, which occur in Alzheimer-type dementia, and cerebral amyloid angiopathy occurs in 50% to 90% of patients with progressive dementia and neurofibrillary degeneration.[62,63] Amyloid protein also is noted in blood vessel walls of patients with AD.[54] β-Amyloid protein deposits occur early in the course of Alzheimer's dementia and are distinct from the amyloid proteins found in other amyloid disorders, such as primary amyloidosis or multiple myeloma.[30,54]

Neuropathology

Although brain atrophy is the most obvious finding among patients with Alzheimer-type dementia, it is not diagnostic for Alzheimer's or other dementias because some degree of atrophy accompanies normal aging.[64] Atrophic changes induced by AD are found primarily in the temporal, parietal, and frontal areas of the brain; the occipital region, primary motor cortex, and somatosensory areas generally are unaffected (Fig. 100-1).[3]

Neuronal changes in the cerebral cortex associated with AD include neurofibrillary tangles, neuritic plaques, amyloid angiopathy, and granulovacuolar degeneration. These changes lead to loss of neurons and synapses (Fig. 100-2).[38] Neurofibrillary tangles (NFTs) are found primarily in the pyramidal regions of the neocortex, hippocampus, and amygdala, but they also are noted in areas of the brainstem and locus ceruleus.[38,65] Tangles are a prominent feature of Alzheimer-type dementia but can be found in several other brain disorders (e.g., Down syndrome, postencephalitic Parkinson's disease) and even in normally aging brains, although they are generally less numerous and histologically different.[38,66] Conversely,

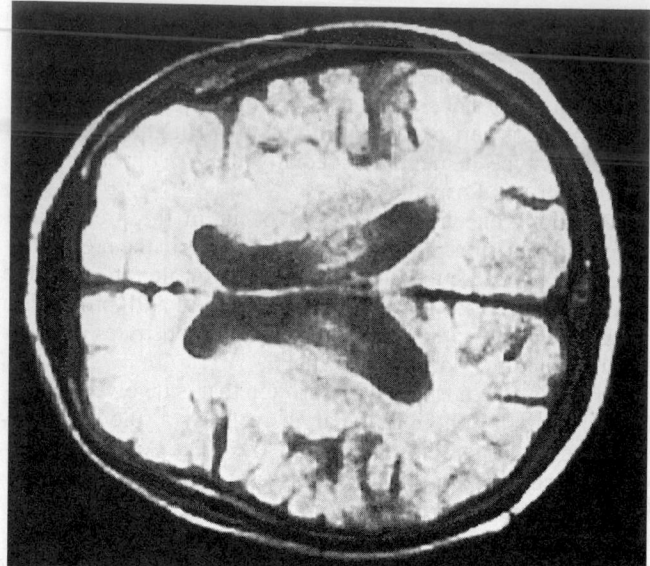

FIGURE 100-1 Alzheimer's disease: MRI scan. Ventricles are enlarged, and there is generalized atrophy, with greater atrophy present near the temporal areas.

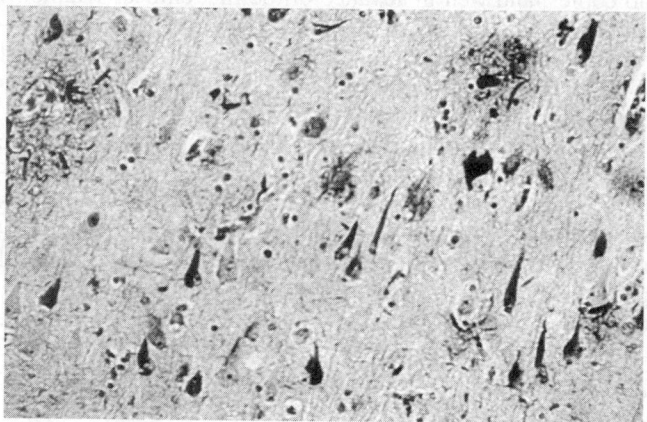

FIGURE 100-2 Numerous plaques (large, round bodies) and tangles (tear-shaped bodies) are found throughout the cortex in Alzheimer-type dementia.

Alzheimer-type dementia also may occur in the absence of neurofibrillary tangles.[66]

Tangles are composed of paired helical filaments, combinations of fibrils with a characteristic width and contour, containing a tau protein with an abnormal pattern of phosphate deposition.[38,67,68] Tangles are highly immunoreactive and are most likely to form in large pyramidal neurons. They typically begin in the transentorhinal cortex and spread to the limbic cortex and the neocortex.[38] Although the nerve structures (axons, dendrites, and nerve terminals) found within neurofibrillary tangles contain amyloid deposits, abnormal axons may occur independently of amyloid deposition. Thus, the presence of amyloid protein is not required for the development of tangles.[69] The presence of neurofibrillary tangles in the neocortical areas is associated with the presence of Alzheimer-type dementia, and their number in the nucleus basalis is correlated with the severity and duration of the disease.[70,71]

Neuritic plaques are spherical bodies of tissue composed of granular deposits and remnants of neuronal processes.[3] Diffuse plaques, considered to represent the early stage of plaque formation, contain no amyloid core. They have been found in areas in the cerebellum and throughout cerebral hemispheres that are not related to AD symptoms.[38] The typical neuritic plaques of AD may develop from preamyloid deposits with subsequent deposition of amyloid protein and accumulation of oligosaccharide, aggregation of amyloid subunits, and β-pleating of the protein.[72,73] They are spherical structures between 50 and 200 μm wide and exhibit a three-tiered structure: a central amyloid core, a middle region of swollen axons and dendrites, and an outer zone containing degenerating neuritic processes.[38] The plaques are concentrated in the cerebral cortex and hippocampus, but they also are found in the corpus striatum, amygdala, and hypothalamus.[3,74] Rare plaques also have been found in nondemented elderly patients.[70]

Plaques contain APP, which can be cleaved by a defective metabolic process to form β-amyloid.[75-77] In addition to β-amyloid, plaques also contain protein, apolipoprotein E, and acute-phase inflammatory proteins such as α_1-chymotrypsin and α_2-macroglobulin.[38,78] Although β-amyloid is found in normal as well as AD subjects, neurofibrillary tangles occurring in the plaques of nondemented subjects do not contain the abnormal protein seen in individuals with dementia.[70] The deposition of amyloid in neuritic plaques correlates with the severity of AD, and the density of cortical plaques is associated with decreased choline acetyltransferase and the severity of cognitive impairment.[75,79] β-Amyloid has been identified in plaques associated with Down syndrome and in both familial and sporadic forms of dementia of the Alzheimer type.[75,80] The process of development from the time of amyloid deposition to plaque formation may take as long as 30 years.[75,81]

In addition to neuritic plaques, APP and β-amyloid produce an amyloid angiopathy outside brain tissue. APP has been located in the adenohypophysis, adrenal gland, cardiac muscle, and peripheral nervous system.[76] Amyloid deposits, identical to those found in neuritic plaques, have been found in cerebral blood vessels as well as in the vasculature of skin, subcutaneous tissue, and intestine.[38,75,82]

A granulovacuolar degeneration is the other major histologic finding in AD. It consists of clusters of intracytoplasmic vacuoles that contain tiny granules. The vacuoles appear to be specifically located in the pyramidal neurons of the hippocampus. Granulovacuolar degeneration also can occur, albeit rarely, in individuals without dementia.[38]

The loss of cortical neurons that originate in the nucleus basalis and project into the cerebral cortex is the most significant histopathologic consequence of AD.[38,79,83,84] Cell loss, granulovacuolar degeneration, and neurons with neurofibrillary tangles are concentrated in this area.[38]

Accompanying these changes are decreased concentrations of several neurotransmitters and enzymes. Choline acetyltransferase levels are reduced 60% to 90% in the cortical and hippocampal regions.[38,79] Acetylcholine and acetylcholinesterase also are decreased, whereas muscarinic receptors in the cortex and hippocampus remain at normal levels or are moderately decreased.[3,79,85] Nicotinic receptor proteins also are reduced in patients with Alzheimer-type dementia when compared with age-matched controls.[86,87] Decreased choline acetyltransferase activity has been correlated with plaque density and disease severity.[79] Cortical synapse loss, especially in the midfrontal region, is associated with disease severity.[88]

Changes affecting acetylcholinesterase have significant implications for the management of AD symptoms. Many isoforms of AChE have been identified; they possess identical amino acid sequences, but display different postranslational modifications, predominate at diverse anatomic and microanatomic locations, and function in different ways.[89] The predominant form of AChE in the cortical and hippocampal regions of humans is G4, a tetrameric form that is membrane-bound. The monomeric form, G1, is found in a much lower concentration. There is a selective loss of the G4 form in patients with AD, allowing the G1 form to assume greater importance.

Although cholinergic activity is the most significantly affected by Alzheimer-type dementia, other neurochemical systems also are altered. Norepinephrine, serotonin, and γ-aminobutyric acid levels may be normal or moderately decreased.[38] Somatostatin and corticotropin-releasing factor also are reduced in patients with Alzheimer-type dementia.[79,90]

Clinical Presentation and Diagnosis

1. C.L., a 63-year-old woman, complains of increasing memory problems over the past 2 years. She states that she began writing reminder notes to herself but she often forgot to look at them. Eventually, she began to lose items around her house, forget appointments, and fail to pay some important bills. During the past 2 to 3 months, she has had difficulty following a shopping list and has become disoriented in the store. One week ago, she became agitated when she heard the low-battery alarm in her smoke alarm. C.L. admits to becoming increasingly depressed over her memory problems but denies appetite or sleep changes or suicidal ideation. She also denies hallucinations, delusional thoughts, or symptoms of anxiety. C.L.'s medical history is significant for non–insulin-dependent diabetes mellitus, which is diet controlled, and bilateral open-angle glaucoma, treated with dipivefrin 0.1%, 1 drop BID. Her family history is negative for stroke and positive for diabetes mellitus and hypertension. She reports that two or three of her maternal relatives had "memory problems" and that one aunt was diagnosed with AD 5 years ago.

Physical examination reveals a moderately obese woman who is well dressed and groomed. Her blood pressure (BP) is 140/86 mm Hg supine and 132/82 mm Hg standing, with pulse rates of 74 beats/min and 78 beats/min, respectively. She is awake and oriented to place and person. During the interview, she is reserved but becomes easily irritated with the physician.

The Folstein Mini-Mental score was 24/30, with errors in orientation, attention, and calculation (inability to spell "world" backward), recall, and language (difficulty with word finding). Her score on the Blessed Dementia Scale was 25/33, with deficits in personality, memory, concentration, and habits. Neurologic examination revealed no deficits. The rest of the physical examination was within normal limits.

Laboratory tests performed include renal and liver chemistries, thyroid function tests, glycosylated hemoglobin, vitamin B_{12} and folate levels, syphilis and HIV tests, complete blood count (CBC) with sedimentation rate, and urinalysis. All results were normal with the exception of a fasting glucose level of 150 mg/dL (normal, <126 mg/dL) and a glycosylated hemoglobin of 8.4% (normal, 4% to 6%). Chest radiograph and electrocardiogram (ECG) were normal. Depression testing revealed a sad, mildly anxious individual who was not depressed. What is the most probable diagnosis for C.L.?

[SI units: fasting glucose, 8.3 mmol/L; glycosylated hemoglobin, 0.084%]

C.L. is in the early stages of AD. She displays several trigger symptoms associated with dementia, including problems learning new information, difficulty with complex tasks (shopping), impaired reasoning (recognizing the smoke alarm battery warning), and increased irritability.[22] Her score of 24/30 on the Folstein Mini-Mental state indicates mild cognitive impairment as evidenced by errors in orientation, calculation, recall, and language.[24] Personality and habit changes and deficits in memory and concentration are revealed in C.L.'s score on the Blessed Dementia Scale.[25] Secondary medical causes of cognitive impairment can be eliminated by C.L.'s generally normal physical examination and laboratory test results. C.L.'s fasting glucose and glycosylated hemoglobin levels are mildly elevated but cannot account for her significant cognitive decline. MRI or CT scanning may be useful in many cases to help eliminate brain pathology, such as stroke, but the lack of any abnormal neurologic findings renders imaging in C.L. unnecessary.

Secondary psychiatric causes for C.L.'s decline also can be discounted. Although she is sad and anxious, the absence of alterations in appetite or sleep patterns, absence of suicidal thoughts, and the results of psychologic testing indicate C.L. is not depressed. She is fully conscious, alert, and oriented to place and person. She exhibits no psychotic behavior and no evidence of delirium.

C.L.'s slowly progressive decline, its impact on her social and occupational function (forgetting appointments, failing to pay bills), normal physical examination and laboratory findings, and family history meet the DSM-IV criteria for AD (see Table 100-1). Because she is younger than 65 years, she also may be classified as early-onset type.[21] Her history and course to date satisfy the criteria for Alzheimer-type dementia and do not indicate a likely alternative explanation for her condition. Thus, C.L. can be classified as probable AD according to the criteria established by the National Institute of Neurological and Communicative Disorders-Alzheimer's Disease and Related Disorders Association (NINCDS-ADRDA) Task Force (Table 100-5).[91]

2. C.L.'s children are very concerned about the family history for dementia. They ask if there are any tests they should receive at this time to determine their risk. What should they be told?

Although there is a strong genetic association with AD, such instances account for a small minority of cases.[53] There is no apparent family history of Down syndrome. Mutations in the presenilin-1 and presenilin-2 genes have been documented in only a few families worldwide.[92] The test that would most likely be performed is APOE-4 genotyping, but this is not recommended because the sensitivity and specificity of the test is not yet known.[92,93]

Prognosis

3. What is the likely prognosis for C.L.?

AD follows a predictable course that may progress over 10 years or more.[17,94] Two common rating scales for dementia are the Global Deterioration Scale and the Clinical Dementia

Table 100-5　NINCDS-ADRDA Criteria for Dementia of the Alzheimer Type[91]

Definite DAT
　Clinical criteria for probable DAT
　Histopathologic evidence for DAT (autopsy or biopsy confirmed)
Probable DAT
　Dementia established by clinical examination and documented by mental status testing (e.g., history and physical examination, Folstein Mini-Mental)
　Confirmation of dementia by neuropsychologic tests (e.g., Blessed Dementia Screen and other tests)
　Deficits in at least 2 areas of cognitive function (e.g., language and memory)
　Progressive deterioration of memory and other cognitive function
　Undisturbed consciousness
　Onset between the ages of 40 and 90
　Absence of systemic or other brain disease capable of producing dementia
Possible DAT
　Atypical onset, presentation, or progression of dementia with an unknown etiology
　Presence of a systemic or other brain disease capable of producing dementia, but not thought to be the cause of the dementia
　Gradually progressive decline in one intellectual function in the absence of another identifiable cause
Unlikely DAT
　Sudden onset
　Focal neurologic findings (e.g., ↑ DTRs, hemiparesis)

DAT, dementia of the Alzheimer type; DTRs, deep tendon reflexes; NINCDS-ADRDA, National Institute of Neurological and Communicative Disorders-Alzheimer's Disease and Related Disorders Association.

Rating Scale. According to the Global Deterioration Scale (Table 100-6), C.L.'s impaired social functioning, anxiety, and objective cognitive decline as well as her continued ability to concentrate and perform some complex skills, combined with her preserved affect and social interaction, are consistent with the features of stage three dementia of the Alzheimer type. This stage AD generally is associated with a period of mild cognitive decline.[95] The more general Clinical Dementia Rating Scale also places C.L. in the category of mild dementia.[96] Clinical diagnoses of AD using clinical criteria for probable AD have a sensitivity of approximately 85% when compared with autopsy-confirmed cases.[92,97]

Because of technologic advances, it is possible to diagnose dementia earlier and to keep patients alive into the final stages of the disease. The early diagnosis of AD in C.L. will allow her condition to be followed closely. Although it is less expensive to maintain a patient at home, caregiver burden can become a significant consideration.[98,99] Eventually, C.L. should be moved into a sheltered environment (e.g., a relative's home, residential care facility, or nursing home) before suffering an injury caused by her poor judgment (e.g., failing to dress properly for the weather, falling). In the later stages, interventions ranging from tube feedings to life support can prolong life. Death in the late stage of AD commonly is associated with the development of infections such as pneumonia, urinary tract infections, or decubitus ulcers.

Treatment

4.　What is an appropriate initial treatment strategy for C.L.?

Maintaining independence as long as possible is an important goal in treating a patient with dementia. Keeping patients in familiar surroundings allows them to function without the added burden of having to attempt to adapt to a strange environment. C.L. appears to be functioning reasonably well at home, although her forgetfulness is causing some problems for her. She is still eating well (her laboratory testing indicated no deficiencies in total protein or albumin, vitamin B_{12}, or folic acid) and performing normal daily activities such as dressing, grooming, bathing, and toileting. Some regular supervision from family members, neighbors, or household help will ensure that C.L. remains safe in her own home.

C.L.'s diabetes mellitus and general medical condition also should be monitored closely. Because both hyperglycemia and hypoglycemia can impair cognitive processes, either of these complications can exacerbate her memory problems. Concurrent diseases and many medications can reduce function and increase cognitive impairment in demented patients, so any new findings in C.L. must be evaluated carefully to distinguish new problems from a worsening of her dementia.

C.L.'s family needs to be educated about what to expect as her dementia progresses. They should be referred to the Alzheimer's Disease and Related Disorders Association (360 N. Michigan Avenue, Chicago, IL 60601; http://www.alz.org). This association has local affiliates in most major cities that often sponsor support groups and inform families of other resources available in the community.

5.　What pharmacotherapeutic options are available for C.L.? Which is most appropriate for C.L. and why?

To date, no drugs are available that can halt or reverse the progression of AD. Four agents have been approved by the Food and Drug Administration (FDA) for the treatment of memory deficits associated with AD. Before initiating pharmacologic treatment, it is important to evaluate the potential risks and benefits in C.L. Because of her declining cognitive capacity, she will be at higher risk for poor adherence to therapy and she may be unable to recognize or report possible adverse effects. Family supervision may be required to monitor therapy.

Table 100-6　Stages of Dementia of the Alzheimer Type

Stage of Cognitive Decline	Features
No cognitive decline	Normal cognitive state
Very mild cognitive decline	Forgetfulness, subjective complaints only; no objective decline
Mild cognitive decline	Objective decline through psychiatric testing; work and social impairment; mild anxiety and denial
Moderate cognitive decline	Concentration, complex skills decline; flat affect and withdrawal
Moderately severe cognitive decline	Early dementia; difficulty in interactions; unable to recall or recognize people or places
Severe cognitive decline	Requires assistance with bathing, toileting; behavioral symptoms present (agitation, delusions, aggressive behavior)
Very severe cognitive decline	Loss of psychomotor skills and verbal abilities; incontinence; total dependence

Adapted from reference 95.

Cholinesterase Inhibitors

Because acetylcholine is significantly reduced in AD, several efforts have been directed toward increasing its cerebral concentrations. This can be done by supplying choline as a precursor for synthesis, providing an agonist, or preventing acetylcholine degradation with a cholinesterase inhibitor (Fig. 100-3). Results of trials investigating precursor loading and agonists have been disappointing. Moderate success has been demonstrated with cholinesterase inhibitors.[100] However, the long-term value of this strategy is limited by the fact that the disease process is unaltered and neuronal degeneration continues.[101]

TACRINE

Tacrine, the first agent approved for the symptomatic treatment of mild to moderate AD, is an aminoacridine derivative that reversibly inhibits both acetylcholinesterase and butyrylcholinesterase (BuCHE).[102] It has a relatively low bioavailability, which is further decreased when the drug is taken with meals. Multiple daily doses are required because tacrine's half-life is short (Table 100-7).[103]

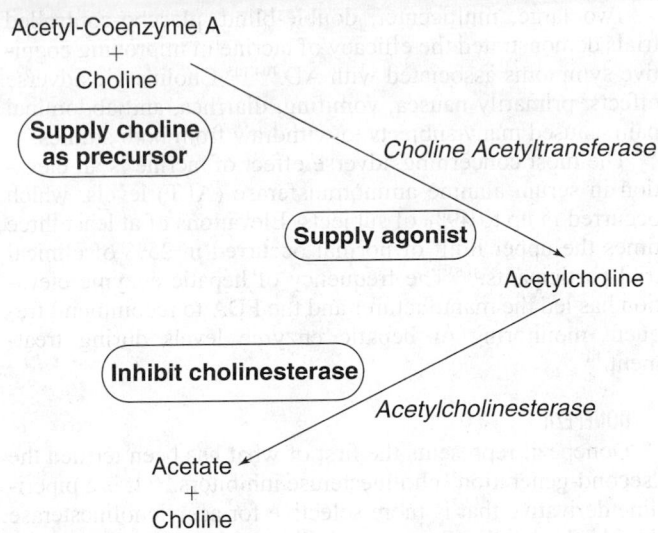

FIGURE 100-3 Potential strategies for cholinergic manipulation.

Table 100-7 FDA-Approved Drugs for Alzheimer's Disease

Generic Drug (Brand Name) and Mechanism	Dosage Form and Dosage	Indication and Effect	Adverse Effects	Other
Donepezil HCl (Aricept) Reversibly inhibits acetylcholinesterase, primarily in CNS	5, 10 mg tablets 5 mg daily, usually at bedtime Dose may be increased to 10 mg after 4–6 weeks	Symptomatic treatment of mild to moderate AD Small improvements in cognition and function occur within 12–24 weeks; benefits may last for at least 2 years	Cholinergic effects, particularly affecting the GI tract (nausea, anorexia, diarrhea); headache; bradycardia may occur	Completely bioavailable and may be given as a single daily dose due to long half-life (70 hr) Metabolized by CYP3A4 isoenzymes
Galantamine HBr (Reminyl) Reversibly inhibits acetylcholinesterase, primarily in CNS; also stimulates nicotinic receptors at a site distinct from that of acetylcholine	4, 8, 12 mg tablets 4 mg twice daily, with food Dose may be increased every 4–6 weeks in 4 mg BID increments, to a maximum dose of 12 mg BID	Symptomatic treatment of mild to moderate AD. Small improvements in cognition and function occur within 12–24 weeks. Benefits may last for more than 1 year.	Cholinergic effects, particularly affecting the GI tract (nausea, anorexia, diarrhea); headache; bradycardia may occur	Highly bioavailable. Initial dose is not therapeutic; slow titration increases tolerability. Metabolized by CYP2D6 and CYP3A4 isoenzymes.
Rivastigmine tartrate (Exelon) Reversibly inhibits acetylcholinesterase and butyrylcholinesterase, primarily in CNS	1.5, 3, 4.5, 6 mg tablets 1.5 mg twice daily, with food. Dose may be increased every 4–6 weeks in 1.5 mg BID increments, to a maximum dose of 6 mg BID	Symptomatic treatment of mild to moderate AD. Small improvements in cognition and function occur within 12–24 weeks. Benefits may last for more than 1 year	Cholinergic effects, particularly affecting the GI tract (nausea, anorexia, vomiting, diarrhea); headache; bradycardia may occur	Highly bioavailable. Therapeutic effect greatly exceeds biologic half-life (1 hr), allowing for twice daily dosing. Metabolized by hydrolysis. Initial dose is not therapeutic; administration with food and slow titration are necessary to increase tolerability.
Tacrine (Cognex) Reversibly inhibits acetylcholinesterase and butyrylcholinesterase, in CNS and periphery.	10, 20, 30, 40 mg tablets Initially 10 mg QID, with increases of 10 mg QID every 4 weeks; maximum dose is 40 mg QID	Symptomatic treatment of mild to moderate AD Small improvements in cognition and function occur within 12–24 weeks	Cholinergic effects, particularly affecting the GI tract (nausea, anorexia, vomiting, diarrhea); abdominal pain; headache; bradycardia may occur. Increases in ALT levels require frequent monitoring	Poor bioavailability, further reduced by giving with food Adverse effects limit patient tolerability Multiple daily doses require frequent dosing Metabolized by CYP1A2, CYP2D6 Initial dose is not therapeutic

AD, Alzheimer's disease; CNS, central nervous system; GI, gastrointestinal.
Adapted from references 102, 104, 105, 107, 108, 110, 114–116, 120–123, and 127.

Two large, multicenter, double-blind, placebo-controlled trials demonstrated the efficacy of tacrine in improving cognitive symptoms associated with AD.[104,105] Cholinergic adverse effects, primarily nausea, vomiting, diarrhea, and abdominal pain, caused many subjects to withdraw from both studies.

The most concerning adverse effect of tacrine is an elevation in serum alanine aminotransferase (ALT) levels, which occurred in up to 49% of subjects. Elevations of at least three times the upper limit of normal occurred in 25% of clinical trial participants.[106] The frequency of hepatic enzyme elevation has led the manufacturer and the FDA to recommend frequent monitoring of hepatic enzyme levels during treatment.[107]

DONEPEZIL

Donepezil represents the first of what has been termed the "second-generation" cholinesterase inhibitors.[100] It is a piperidine derivative that is more selective for acetylcholinesterase than butyrylcholinesterase and, like tacrine, it reversibly inhibits cholinesterase activity. Donepezil is completely bioavailable and exhibits a long half-life, allowing it to be given as a single daily dose.[108] It is highly protein bound, primarily to albumin (see Table 100-7).[109]

Donepezil improves cognition and global function in people with AD. In a multicenter, double-blind, placebo-controlled trial, subjects with mild to moderately severe AD improved over a 12-week treatment period.[110] Subjects taking 10 mg of donepezil at bedtime improved their cognitive function as measured by the Alzheimer's Disease Assessment Scale-Cognitive Subscale (ADAS-Cog), and their overall function as measured by the Clinician's Interview-Based Impression of Change with caregiver input (CIBIC-Plus).[111,112] A 24-week multicenter, placebo-controlled trial using dosages of 5 mg/day and 10 mg/day demonstrated similar results. Both 5- and 10-mg doses were superior to placebo; adverse effects were less common with the 5-mg dose.[113] A long-term, open-label follow-up study to these trials demonstrated that donepezil effects may persist for almost 3 years.[114] Interruption or discontinuation of donepezil treatment was followed by a return of cognition and function to baseline or below.

The most common adverse effects of donepezil are associated with cholinergic activity. They tend to be mild to moderate in nature and resolve with stabilization of the dose.[110,113] In a 144-week extension trial of donepezil, the most frequently encountered adverse effects were nausea, diarrhea, and headache.[114]

RIVASTIGMINE

Rivastigmine is a carbamate derivative that inhibits both acetylcholinesterase and butyrylcholinesterase activity. Butyrylcholinesterase provides an alternate pathway for acetylcholine metabolism. Rivastigmine inhibits the activity of both cholinesterases, primarily in the central nervous system.[115] Its acetylcholinesterase inhibition is greater for the G1 as compared to the G4 form.[116] The drug binds to the esteratic site of the AChE and BuChE molecule and slowly dissociates. Because of this, it is often referred to as a "pseudo-irreversible" inhibitor.[117] Rivastigmine's biologic half-life is approximately 1 hour, but because its slow dissociation extends its activity for at least 10 hours, it can be dosed twice daily. Rivastigmine is bound approximately 40% to serum proteins and is metab-

olized via hydrolysis to renally excreted inactive compounds.[116] Rivastigmine absorption is nearly complete, but because it undergoes a significant first-pass effect, the resultant bioavailability is approximately 36% (Table 100-7).

In two large clinical trials conducted in patients with mild to moderately severe AD, rivastigmine improved cognition, the ability to perform daily activities, and global function over 24 weeks.[118,119] In each multi-center, double-blind, placebo-controlled trial, subjects were randomized to receive placebo, low-dose (1 to 4 mg/day) or high-dose (6 to 12 mg/day) rivastigmine in two divided doses during a 26-week period. In one study, subjects in both dosage groups demonstrated statistically significant improvement after 26 weeks on the ADAS-cog and CIBIC-Plus scales.[118] In the other trial, only those subjects taking 6 to 12 mg/day improved on the same scales.[119] An open-label extension study that included subjects from both of the previous studies found that subjects taking 6 to 12 mg/day of rivastigmine had significantly better cognitive function after one year than did subjects who had originally received placebo.[120]

Adverse effects typically included nausea, vomiting, diarrhea and other cholinergically-mediated gastrointestinal effects.[121] They are most common when rivastigmine is taken on an empty stomach or when the dose escalation is too rapid. Headache, dizziness, and fatigue also are common adverse effects. Increasing the dose by 1.5 mg BID at 4-week intervals increases drug tolerability and reduces the frequency and severity of gastrointestinal side effects.

GALANTAMINE

Like other agents used to treat AD, galantamine enhances cholinergic activity by inhibiting acetylcholinesterase. However, it also stimulates nicotinic receptors at a site distinct from that stimulated by acetylcholine, an action that does not rely on the presence of acetylcholine.[122] This action is referred to as allosteric modulation. Galantamine is rapidly and completely absorbed, reaches peak serum levels in less than 2 hours, and has a half-life of approximately 5 hours. It exhibits low protein binding and has a large volume of distribution. Galantamine is metabolized primarily by CYP2D6 and CYP3A4 and is eliminated in the urine (Table 100-7).[123,124]

Clinical trials have shown galantamine to be effective for the symptomatic treatment of mild to moderate AD. Doses of 16 and 24 mg/day produced clinically meaningful improvement in ADAS-cog and CIBIC-Plus scores during a 5-month, randomized, placebo-controlled trial.[125] A similar trial conducted in Europe and Canada that evaluated patients over 6 months used doses of 24 and 32 mg/day. Both doses were more effective than placebo, but patients in the 32 mg/day group exhibited more adverse effects.[126] A 6-month, open label extension trial showed that patients treated with galantamine 24 mg/day maintained ADAS-cog scores throughout the entire 12 months of the study.[127]

As with the other cholinesterase inhibitors, cholinergic effects in the gastrointestinal tract are the most commonly encountered adverse effects. Nausea, diarrhea, vomiting, and anorexia were the most frequent events encountered during clinical trials.[124] They were typically present during the dose-escalation phases of the studies. A dose titration interval of 4 weeks reduces the severity of adverse effects and increases tolerability.

It is unlikely that a cholinesterase inhibitor will produce a dramatic or long-lasting improvement in C.L.'s cognitive abilities. Treatment, however, may slow her cognitive decline and help maintain her ability to care for herself for 1 year or more. The choice of drug is based on the agent most likely to produce a positive response with the fewest adverse effects. Ease of adherence must also be considered. Tacrine is the least useful choice because of its adverse effect profile and the need for 4 daily doses. All other cholinesterase inhibitors exhibit similar adverse effect profiles. Rivastigmine may be less prone to drug interactions because of its metabolic pathway. Donepezil can be given as a single daily dose. It is typically given at bedtime, which may make cholinergic side effects less troublesome. Therefore, C.L. should receive donepezil.

6. **How should treatment with donepezil be instituted in C.L., and how should therapy be monitored?**

C.L. should receive donepezil 5 mg at bedtime. She should be monitored for cholinergic side effects (particularly nausea and diarrhea), insomnia, headache, and dizziness, the adverse effects most commonly reported in clinical trials.[110,113] Her family and physician should look for improvements in her memory, orientation, and her ability to concentrate on complex tasks, such as shopping. She should also become less irritable. If she has not improved noticeably after 4 to 6 weeks, the dose of donepezil may be increased to 10 mg at bedtime.

If her condition does not respond to donepezil after a trial of 3 months, it is reasonable to switch C.L to another cholinesterase inhibitor. Both rivastigmine and galantamine have additional mechanisms of action that might prove beneficial. Rivastigmine is started at a dose of 1.5 mg twice daily (BID) with meals to slow absorption and improve tolerability. The dose may be increased at 4-week intervals by 1.5 mg BID, up to the maximum dose of 6 mg BID. Galantamine is started at 4 mg BID, and increased every 4 weeks by 4 mg BID, up to a maximum dose of 12 mg BID. Taking galantamine with meals may improve tolerability of gastrointestinal effects.

Investigational Agents

7. **C.L. tolerated donepezil well, with the exception of some mild nausea and occasional loose stools. She was once again able to engage in normal activities with the help of reminder notes, and she became much less irritable, according to her family.**

One year later, C.L. is exhibiting some decline in her cognition and is becoming more disoriented, particularly in the afternoon and evening. What other drug therapy strategies are being investigated for Alzheimer-type dementia, and which would be appropriate for C.L.?

Several other treatments are being studied. Some are medications already approved for other uses and others are new and investigational agents. Many protocols are aimed at treatments that modify the disease process rather than the associated behavioral problems. The Alzheimer's Association and many of its local chapters can provide information regarding the studies and their eligibility requirements.

MEMANTINE

Evidence that release of glutamate in the CNS can lead to excitotoxic reactions and cell death has led to research into the use of N-methyl-D-aspartate (NMDA) antagonists to treat AD and other neurodegenerative disorders.[128] Memantine is an uncompetitive NMDA receptor antagonist with moderate affinity and voltage-dependent binding. It is completely absorbed after oral administration, reaches peak serum concentrations in 3 to 8 hours, and is moderately protein bound (Table 100-7).[129]

Two large clinical trials have evaluated memantine in subjects with moderate to severe AD. A dose of 10 mg/day for 12 weeks increased functional ability (e.g., dressing, toileting, participating in group activities) and reduced care dependence compared with placebo.[130] A 28-week trial using a dose of 20 mg/day improved CIBIC-Plus scores, activities of daily living, and global function compared with placebo.[131] Common adverse effects include diarrhea, insomnia, dizziness, headache, and hallucinations.[129] Preliminary evidence suggests that the combined use of memantine and a cholinesterase inhibitor may be superior to a cholinesterase inhibitor alone.[132]

ESTROGENS

Estrogen has several beneficial effects on the brain, including improved cerebral blood flow, increased glucose transport and metabolism, and facilitated repair of damaged neurons.[133] Retrospective studies have demonstrated a link between postmenopausal estrogen replacement and improved performance on memory testing in older women.[134] A reduced risk for dementia has been found among postmenopausal estrogen users in some studies but not in others.[135] A secondary analysis of a 30-week clinical trial of tacrine revealed that estrogen use was a strong predictor of improvement among subjects who received tacrine.[136] In contrast, the Women's Health Initiative Study recently found that women taking combined estrogen and progestin were more likely to develop dementia than those who had not taken these hormones. The hazard ratio for developing dementia was 2.05.[137]

NONSTEROIDAL ANTI-INFLAMMATORY DRUGS

The recognition that acute-phase inflammatory proteins are present in neuritic plaques has led to the investigation of nonsteroidal anti-inflammatory drugs (NSAIDs) for the treatment or prevention of AD.[78] In retrospective studies, people who take NSAIDs have a lower prevalence of AD when compared with nonusers.[138–141] The reduced risk appears to be greatest for those who have used these agents for at least 2 years; acetaminophen does not appear to have any protective effects.[141] Prospective pilot studies using indomethacin and diclofenac/misoprostol in patients with mild to moderate AD have produced promising but inconclusive results.[142,143] Although a recent epidemiologic study demonstrated reduced risk for AD with NSAID use,[144] a 1-year clinical trial of both naproxen and rofecoxib showed no effect on cognition when compared with placebo.[145]

MONOAMINE OXIDASE INHIBITORS

Findings of decreased central norepinephrine and increased monoamine oxidase type B (MAO-B) among patients with Alzheimer-type dementia has led to the investigation of the MAO-B inhibitor, selegiline (Eldepryl), as a potential treatment.[65,146] Improvement in memory, attention, and social interaction, as well as reductions in anxiety, depression, and tension, have been demonstrated in some clinical trials, although others have found no significant benefit.[146-149] Mild improvement on dementia screening tests has been shown in a pilot study using selegiline in combination with tacrine or physostigmine.[150] An investigation that evaluated selegiline and α-tocopherol, alone and in combination, found that each agent independently delayed the progression of AD longer than did the combination.[151]

ALTERNATIVE MEDICINES

Extract of ginkgo biloba has been used for many years in Europe to improve memory performance. Although its mechanism is not well understood, it may function as an antioxidant and may increase cholinergic activity.[152-154] Increasing interest in alternative medicines in the United States has led many people to use the crude extract. Three published trials have evaluated EGb 761, a specific combination of constituents, as a treatment for AD. Two trials found modest improvement in memory without significant adverse effects,[153,154] whereas the third found no benefit after 24 weeks of treatment (see Chapter 3, Herbs and Nutritional Supplements).[155]

Two factors must be considered when referring C.L. for investigational treatments. The first is the appropriateness of individual therapies for her, and the second is the likelihood that she will be able to comply with a research protocol. C.L. was able to tolerate the cholinergic adverse effects of donepezil and thus would probably not experience difficulty with other cholinergic drugs. However, it is unlikely that a different cholinergic agent would provide superior results. The most recent evidence regarding hormone replacement therapy suggests that the benefits may not outweigh the potential risks. Likewise, NSAID therapy poses significant gastrointestinal, renal, and cardiovascular risks; therefore, they should not be used solely for the treatment of AD (see Chapter 43, Rheumatic Disorders).

Selegiline is currently available commercially as a treatment for Parkinson's disease, but research results for AD have not been overly promising (see Chapter 53, Parkinson's Disease). Because gingko biloba acts in a similar manner to cholinesterase inhibitors, its use is not likely to provide additional benefit.

Memantine has shown promise as an individual treatment and in combination with cholinesterase inhibitor therapy. This would be a reasonable strategy for C.L. if she could be enrolled in a clinical trial. Although C.L. will require significant supervision by her family to ensure that she can adhere to a protocol, she should be referred to a local investigator to be evaluated for inclusion in a clinical trial.

DEMENTIA WITH LEWY BODIES
Etiology

Lewy bodies are hyaline-containing inclusion bodies typically found in people with Parkinson's disease. Up to 25% of patients with dementia have Lewy bodies in the brainstem and cortex.[156] Many of these patients display extrapyramidal signs without the classic presentation of Parkinson's disease.[157] Evidence of AD, including β-amyloid deposits and neuritic plaques, is common.[156]

Clinical Presentation

8. J.F. is a 72-year-old woman who was diagnosed with mild cognitive impairment 6 months ago. She had been increasingly forgetful and confused for about 1 year before the diagnosis. Approximately 3 months ago, J.F. and her family decided that J.F. should move in with them so that she would not be left alone. Since moving in with the family, her son has noted that she seems "spaced out" at times. Some days, she appears to be very clear and not confused; other days she is very forgetful and requires assistance with daily tasks. Her daughter-in-law reported that J.F. has been unsteady on her feet at times and has fallen twice. Recently, J.F. reported seeing people coming out of the painting on the wall (a European street scene). "They were walking all through the house trying to steal anything that can be hidden in a coat pocket."

At the physician visit, J.F. was found to be medically stable. Vital signs, serum chemistries, and the CBC were within normal limits. Her MMSE score was 21/30. During the review of systems, J.F.'s daughter-in-law had to answer some questions because J.F. appeared to not hear or to ignore them. On physical examination she demonstrated mild cog-wheeling rigidity, bradykinesia, and masked facies; she did not display a resting tremor. What is the most likely explanation for J.F.'s presentation?

Given her physical health, inability to live by herself because of impaired cognition, and her MMSE score, J.F. meets the criteria for dementia. Her rigidity, bradykinesia, and masked facies are consistent with early Parkinson's disease (see Chapter 53, Parkinson's Disease). Although there are no specific diagnostic criteria for dementia with Lewy bodies (DLB), guidelines have been proposed. The guidelines include core features of dementia, fluctuating cognition, recurrent visual hallucinations, and motor signs of Parkinsonism. Supporting features include repeated falls, syncope, transient loss of consciousness, severe exacerbations of extrapyramidal symptoms with neuroleptic use, and delusions.[156] J.F. exhibits all the core features and has had some falls. Dementia with Lewy bodies is a likely explanation for her condition.

Treatment

9. **What is an appropriate treatment for J.F.?**

There are no specific treatments for DLB. Levodopa/carbidopa therapy should be started to help the symptoms of Parkinsonism. Because the use of older antipsychotic agents, such as haloperidol, may worsen her extrapyramidal symptoms, they should be avoided. Newer agents, such as olanzapine or quetiapine, may be less likely to exacerbate these symptoms but should be instituted with great caution.[157] Although a small, open-label trial of rivastigmine demonstrated benefit, it is too early to recommend cholinesterase inhibitors to treat DLB.[158]

VASCULAR DEMENTIAS
Etiology

Vascular dementia is a broad classification of cognitive disorders caused by vascular disease. The most common cause of vascular dementia is occlusion of cerebral blood vessels by a thrombus or embolus, leading to ischemic brain injury.[3,159] The term multi-infarct dementia (MID) refers specifically to the cognitive decline that follows multiple small or large cerebrovascular occlusions.[160] A number of diseases, including atherosclerosis, arteriosclerosis, and vasculitis, lead to the production of emboli and thrombi that potentially occlude brain vessels.[3] Hemorrhagic phenomena and disorders such as hypertension or cardiac disease can produce episodes of cerebral ischemia or hypoxia and are responsible for some cases of vascular dementia.[23,159] Specific risk factors for vascular dementias include advancing age, diabetes mellitus, small vessel cerebrovascular disease, hypertension, heart disease, hyperlipidemia, cigarette smoking, and alcohol use.[161–164]

Neuropathology

Vascular dementias typically are subcortical. Most patients with MID have blockage of multiple blood vessels and infarction of the cerebral tissue supplied by those vessels. When the distribution of a large artery or medium-sized arteriole is blocked, focal neurologic deficits can result (see Chapter 55, Cerebrovascular Disorders). Depending on the area affected, there may be significant cognitive impairment. More often, however, a patient may have suffered transient ischemic attacks (TIAs) or multiple microinfarcts that have remained unrecognized.[165,166] Patients with subcortical vascular dementias often exhibit small, deep ischemic infarcts in arterioles of the basal ganglia, thalamus, and internal capsule.[6,167] A history of atherosclerosis, diabetes mellitus, or hypertension often is present without a history of stroke.[165,168,169] MRI scans can be very useful in diagnosing vascular dementias because areas of cerebral infarction are easier to visualize than they are with CT scanning (Fig. 100-4). Lesions in white matter may occur in as many as 85% of patients with vascular dementia.[170] Deep white matter lesions known as leukoariosis often include demyelination and may represent early changes in dementia.[169,171,172] Although patients with Alzheimer-type dementia also may exhibit leukoariosis, it is much more prevalent in those with MIDs.[6,173] Blood flow in patients with leukoariosis

is reduced in all brain regions except parietal white matter, especially in the putamen and thalamus.[174] Patients with long-standing uncontrolled hypertension often develop multiple leukoariosis lesions leading to ischemic periventricular encephalopathy.[169] The lesions are too small to be visualized grossly but are evident on MRI scans.[159] Known as Binswanger's disease, this disorder is characterized by focal neurologic deficits, emotional lability, gait disturbances, and urinary incontinence.[169,175] Patients with Binswanger's disease exhibit activation of the coagulation-fibrinolysis pathway, which may lead to microthrombi and microcirculatory disturbances.[176]

Vascular dementias typically have an earlier onset than dementia of the Alzheimer type.[94] Unlike AD, males are affected more often than females, and survival is shorter for vascular dementia patients.[94,177]

Clinical Presentation

10. D.V., a 73-year-old man, is accompanied by his daughter for evaluation of "fuzzy thinking." Although his chief complaint is impaired memory, he denies significant impact on his daily routine. D.V. states his memory problem began 2 years ago after a dizzy spell and subsequent fall. However, his daughter states that the impairment began approximately 1 year before that episode. The memory loss has been slowly progressive. D.V. states that he feels useless because of his memory problems and his "boring" daily routine. Although D.V. is generally independent, he relies on his daughter for assistance with most financial matters. He has voluntarily quit driving because of a lack of confidence in his abilities. D.V.'s daughter reports that according to her mother, D.V. is sometimes disoriented at night when he awakens to urinate. He has no history of urinary incontinence. D.V. has a questionable history of TIAs but no focal neurologic deficits. He has a long history of mild hypertension, which is treated with a diuretic. He drinks alcohol occasionally and smokes about half a pack of cigarettes per day. His medical history is unremarkable except for the possible TIAs, hypertension, and a mildly enlarged prostate. His family history is positive for diabetes and heart disease.

On physical examination, D.V. is found to be a mildly obese man who is well dressed and groomed, alert, and oriented to person. His BP is 160/92 mm Hg sitting and 168/95 mm Hg standing. Cardiac examination is normal. Neurologic findings include somewhat diminished extraocular movements laterally and slightly asymmetric reflexes, with right greater than left. Muscle tone is normal in the lower extremities. He has a mild shuffling gait. Vibratory sensation is diminished but within normal limits for his age. His score on the Folstein Mini-Mental Status Exam was 22/30, including errors in orientation and recall. His score on the Blessed Dementia Scale was 16/33, with errors in memory and orientation. Psychologic evaluation found him to be mildly depressed.

A full laboratory analysis was generally within normal limits. D.V.'s serum potassium (3.8 mEq/dL) and sodium (138 mEq/dL) were in the low normal range, and his blood urea nitrogen (BUN) (18 mg/dL) was in the upper normal range. Serum total cholesterol was 246 mg/dL and fasting triglycerides were 230 mg/dL. A chest radiograph revealed a mildly enlarged heart; his

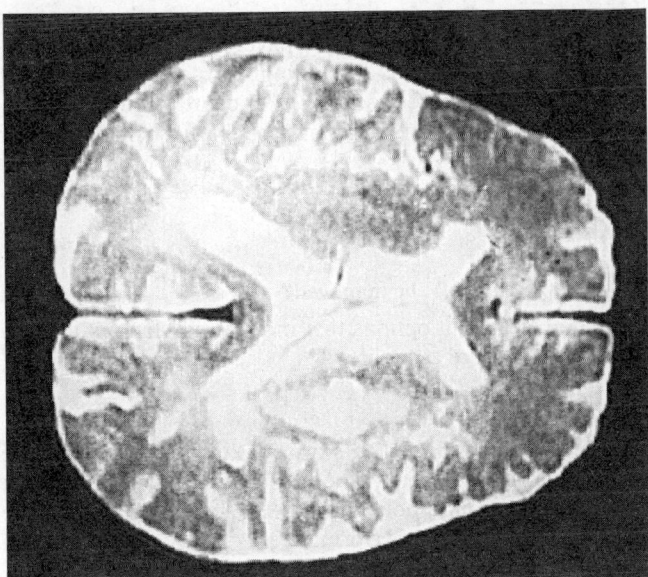

FIGURE 100-4 A large stoke is visible to the right of the ventricles. There is evidence of atrophy in the right temporal area.

ECG was normal. An MRI scan indicated generalized atrophy with enlarged ventricles, periventricular white matter ischemic changes, bilateral basal ganglion lacunar infarcts, and small cortical infarcts in the right parietal lobe. What subjective and objective evidence exists for a diagnosis of dementia in D.V.?

[SI units: BUN, 6.4 mmol/L of urea; total cholesterol, 6.36 mmol/L; triglycerides, 2.60 mmol/L]

D.V.'s major complaint is "fuzzy thinking" and impaired memory that he attributes to his dizzy spell and fall. However, his family began to note problems a full year before that episode, with progression over time. Although D.V. denies that his impairment significantly affects his daily routine, he has voluntarily stopped driving and relies on his daughter for assistance with financial matters. His memory difficulties appear to have affected his mood and made him feel useless. D.V. is disoriented at night when he awakens to urinate. These factors satisfy the DSM-IV criteria for interference with normal activities.[21]

Multiple deficits are present on both the Folstein Mini-Mental Status Exam[24] (orientation, recall) and on the Blessed Dementia Scale[25] (memory, orientation), indicating impaired short-term and long-term memory. D.V.'s inability to drive reflects poor judgment behind the wheel of a car; a disturbance of higher cortical function is indicated by his need for assistance with financial matters. There is no evidence of a delirium being present. Evidence of an organic cause is provided by the MRI scan.

Diagnosis

11. **What type of dementia does D.V. have?**

There is sufficient evidence to indicate that D.V. suffers from a vascular dementia. Although DSM-IV provides diagnostic criteria for vascular dementia (Table 100-8), it is not clear that D.V. satisfies the requirements.[21] Vascular dementias commonly present suddenly after a cerebrovascular insult. This is followed by a period of stability and further declines

Table 100-8   DSM-IV Criteria for Vascular Dementia

1. The presence of multiple cognitive deficits manifested by both:
   - Impaired memory ($\downarrow$ ability to learn new information or to retrieve information previously learned)
   - At least one of the following:
     Aphasia (language difficulties)
     Apraxia (diminished ability to perform motor activities in the presence of intact motor function)
     Agnosia (inability to recognize or name objects despite intact sensory function)
     Disruption of executive function (diminished ability to plan, organize)
2. The deficits above significantly interfere with normal work or social activities and represent a decline from previous ability to function
3. Focal neurologic deficits (e.g., hyperactive DTRs, gait disturbances, weak extremities) or laboratory evidence indicating cerebrovascular disease (e.g., multiple infarctions of the cortex or white matter) judged to be etiologically linked to the disorder
4. The deficits do not occur exclusively during the course of a delirium

DSM-IV, Diagnostic and Statistical Manual of Mental Disorders, 4th Ed; DTRs, deep tendon reflexes.
Adapted from reference 21.

after additional episodes, in a stepwise pattern. Cognitive impairments are variable and depend on the area of the brain affected by the insult.[21]

With the exception of the dizzy spell and fall, D.V.'s deterioration has had a pattern that resembles a downhill slide rather than stepwise decline. Although his cognitive deficits are "patchy" (e.g., he appears to have no language difficulty), they are not particularly prominent. D.V. displays some neurologic signs and symptoms, including diminished extraocular movements, asymmetric reflexes, and a mild shuffling gait, but they are subtle and might be easily missed by an untrained observer as being related to a dementia. Reliance solely on the clear presence of diagnostic criteria often may lead to a missed diagnosis.[178] The Hachinski Ischemic Scale ranks signs and symptoms associated with cognitive impairment of cerebrovascular origin and is used to help differentiate between AD and MID.[179] According to this scale, D.V.'s nocturnal confusion, depression, hypertension history, and focal neurologic signs and symptoms are sufficient to indicate vascular dementia.

D.V.'s history and clinical presentation do not suggest dementia caused by a single large or several small strokes. Large strokes produce significant motor damage, typically on one side of the body (the side contralateral to the stroke). Multiple smaller strokes cause prominent motor deficits in discrete areas controlled by the affected areas. Neither of these patterns describes D.V.'s condition. However, he clearly is exhibiting signs of dementia and has significant cerebrovascular disease. He possesses several risk factors for a vascular dementia, including hypertension, smoking, and hyperlipidemia. His MRI indicates a lacunar state, with multiple small infarcts in the deep penetrating arterioles at the base of the brain, particularly in the basal ganglia, internal capsule, thalamus, and pons (see Chapter 55, Cerebrovascular Disorders). These MRI findings are consistent with D.V.'s longstanding hypertension and neurologic presentation. The absence of a significant gait disturbance and urinary incontinence argues against Binswanger's disease.

Because diagnostic criteria for vascular dementias are vague, arriving at a specific diagnosis is difficult. Therefore, diagnostic criteria (Table 100-9) have been proposed for ischemic vascular dementia, providing a structure for the most common type of these disorders.[159] According to this diagnostic scheme, D.V. suffers from probable ischemic vascular dementia.

Treatment

12. **How should D.V. be managed?**

Several treatment options that modify risk factors for vascular dementias are available.

Smoking Cessation

D.V. should be counseled to stop smoking because cigarette smoking reduces cerebral blood flow and increases the risk for stroke.[180] Among smokers with MID, cessation of cigarette use improves cognitive performance.[181]

Antihypertensive Therapy

Hypertension and hyperlipidemia, both present in D.V., are additional risk factors for stroke and MID. Control of systolic hy-

Table 100-9 Proposed Diagnostic Criteria for Ischemic Vascular Dementia

Definite IVD (Requires Histopathologic Examination of the Brain)
  Clinical evidence of dementia
  Pathologic confirmation of multiple infarcts, some extracerebellar

Probable IVD
  Dementia
  Evidence of at least two ischemic strokes by history, neurologic signs, or neuroimaging, or a single stroke with clearly documented temporal relationship to the dementia onset
  Supporting evidence of multiple infarcts in regions affecting cognition, history of TIAs or vascular risk factors, elevated Hachinski score

Possible IVD
  Dementia, plus one or more of the following:
  • History or evidence of a single stroke (but not multiple strokes) without clearly documented temporal relationship to dementia onset
  • Binswanger's disease (without multiple strokes), including all of the following:
    Early-onset urinary incontinence unexplained by urologic disease, or gait disturbance not explained by peripheral cause
    Vascular risk factors
    Extensive white matter change on neuroimaging

IVD, ischemic vascular dementia; TIAs, transient ischemic attacks.
Adapted from reference 159.

pertension reduces the risk of stroke by 36% in elderly patients,[182] and maintaining the systolic BP between 135 and 150 mm Hg is associated with improved cognition among MID patients. A systolic BP that exceeds 150 mm Hg indicates inadequate control, whereas a systolic BP below 135 mm Hg may lead to inadequate cerebral perfusion.[181] As in nondemented individuals, nonpharmacologic treatment (e.g., diet, weight loss, exercise) is an essential component. The antihypertensive agent must be chosen carefully in this population to maximize compliance and minimize adverse reactions.[183] Both thiazide diuretics and β-adrenergic blockers may increase lipid levels, a potential complication in D.V. β-Adrenergic blockers and sympatholytic agents may cause depression or impair cognitive activity. Calcium channel blockers or angiotensin-converting enzyme (ACE) inhibitors are acceptable because they are well tolerated by elderly patients and may help preserve renal function in patients with diabetes mellitus (see Chapter 14, Essential Hypertension). Dihydropyridine calcium channel blockers have been shown to improve cognition in patients with dementia[184] and reduce the risk of dementia in elderly patients with isolated systolic hypertension.[185] Because D.V. has benign prostatic hyperplasia, he may benefit from the use of an α-adrenergic blocking agent, such as doxazosin (Cardura) 1 mg at bedtime, or terazosin (Hytrin) 1 mg at bedtime (see Chapter 101, Geriatric Urological Disorders). Evidence indicating an increased risk for negative cardiac outcomes, however, makes the α-adrenergic blocking agents less attractive choices.[186] The use of a vasodilating calcium channel blocker, such as amlodipine 5 mg/day, is an appropriate first choice. An ACE inhibitor such as benazepril (Lotensin) 10 mg/day is an appropriate alternative. Both these agents exhibit the advantage of once-daily dosing over some other agents within their respective classes. This feature is important for maximizing adherence in patients with declining memory.

Antiplatelet Therapy

Prophylaxis against future cerebrovascular events is indicated in MID, but few studies that have looked specifically at individuals with dementia are available. Cerebral perfusion and cognitive performance were improved in MID patients receiving aspirin 325 mg/day for 1 year when compared with a control population.[187] Aspirin dosages as low as 30 mg/day reduce the incidence of transient ischemic attacks and are associated with fewer adverse effects than higher dosages.[188]

Other agents that affect the coagulation process include clopidogrel (Plavix), ticlopidine (Ticlid), aspirin/dipyridamole (Aggrenox), and warfarin (Coumadin). None of these agents has been evaluated specifically in people with vascular dementias. Guidelines from the American College of Chest Physicians recommend the use of antiplatelet therapy in patients with a history of TIA or atherothrombotic stroke that is not of cardiogenic origin. Warfarin is recommended after cardioembolic cerebral ischemic events. According to those guidelines, aspirin 25 mg/dipyridamole extended-release 200 mg BID is recommended as the first line agent..[189]

Cholinesterase Inhibitors

Deficits in cholinergic transmission and nicotinic receptor binding abnormalities have been noted in vascular dementia.[190] Early clinical trials with donepezil,[191] galantamine,[192] and rivastigmine[193] have demonstrated improvement in cognition and daily function among patients with vascular dementia. As of yet, however, the use of these agents remains investigational.

BEHAVIORAL DISTURBANCES IN DEMENTIA

Several types of behavioral disturbances may develop during the course of a dementia, particularly during the later stages (Table 100-10).[95] The disturbances can be classified into two broad categories: psychologic behavior and nonpsychologic behavior. Psychologic behavior includes anxiety, depression, withdrawal, psychotic behaviors, and aggression; these respond reasonably well to both nonpharmacologic and pharmacologic intervention. Nonpsychologic behaviors such as wandering, inappropriate motor activity, shouting, and incontinence respond better to environmental modification than to drug therapy.[194,195] The first step in evaluating altered behavior in patients with dementia is to ensure that the problem is not the result of an unrecognized medical problem or to an adverse effect of a medication (see Chapter 99, Geriatric Drug Use).

Anxiety

13. T.G., an otherwise healthy 62-year-old man, has recently been diagnosed with AD. Recently, he has refused to go on his daily walks around the neighborhood because he is afraid he will get lost. He also expresses worry about the burden he will place on his family as his condition worsens. His concerns keep him awake at night, making him quite tired during the day. How should T.G.'s anxiety be managed?

Anxiety is a common problem in the early stages of dementia. Patients are aware of their progressive cognitive decline and have sufficient insight to understand the consequences. Anxiety and apprehension are common reactions.

Table 100-10 Behavior Disturbances in Dementia

Behavior	Typical Presentation	Treatment
Anxiety	Excessive worrying, sleep disturbances, rumination	Trazodone Buspirone (if no insomnia) Short-acting benzodiazepine SSRI antidepressant
Depression	Withdrawal, loss of appetite, irritability, restlessness, sleep disturbances	Trazodone SSRI antidepressant
General agitation	Repeated questions, wandering, pacing	Often unresponsive to medications; redirecting activity may be effective; safety-proofing the residence reduces wandering
Psychotic behaviors	Delusions (often of theft), hallucinations, misperceptions	Atypical antipsychotic, if associated with paranoid features SSRI antidepressant, if associated with withdrawal, tearfulness, themes of loss
Aggressive behaviors	Physical or verbal aggressiveness toward others, excessive yelling and screaming, manic features	Anticonvulsant, such as divalproex or carbamazepine, possibly in combination with an atypical antipsychotic

Adapted from references 194, 195, 197, 200, and 207.

T.G. exhibits a generalized anxiety disorder superimposed on his dementia that is interfering with his functional capacity more than his cognitive decline. Therefore, pharmacologic therapy would be appropriate.

In addition to their affects on cognition, galantamine and donepezil improve behavior and the ability of patients to care for themselves.[196,197] Therefore, a trial of a cholinesterase inhibitor is an appropriate initial treatment. If his anxiety continues, additional treatment should be considered.

Benzodiazepines are the most commonly used anxiolytics and will address T.G.'s insomnia as well as his anxiety. However, they are associated with several negative outcomes in the elderly, including confusion, amnestic syndromes, ataxia, and falls.[197] Long-acting benzodiazepines are generally considered inappropriate for geriatric patients because age-associated accumulation increases the risk of acute toxicity.[198] Benzodiazepines with short half-lives, such as alprazolam (Xanax), lorazepam (Ativan), or oxazepam (Serax), are preferable. Lorazepam 0.5 mg may be used on an as-needed basis, up to 4 times daily.

Trazodone is a sedative antidepressant that is effective for insomnia and agitated behaviors in patients with AD.[197,199] Treatment is started at 25 mg at bedtime (HS) and may be increased to a dose of 250 mg/day in divided doses. Another alternative treatment is buspirone, which does not cause the cognitive impairments associated with the benzodiazepines. Dosage begins at 5 mg three times daily and may be increased up to 15 mg three times daily. However, buspirone requires 3 to 4 weeks to become fully effective and will not concurrently manage T.G.'s insomnia because it has no sedative effect.[200]

Trazodone should be initiated at a dose of 25 mg at bedtime for T.G. if a cholinesterase inhibitor does not improve his sleep and anxiety. It may be increased by 25 mg/day at 5 to 7 day intervals, up to 100 mg. Doses above 100 mg/day should be split into two daily doses.

Psychosis

14. **T.G.'s mental status continues to decline to the point that he requires help with bathing and dressing. During a physician visit, he accuses his wife and children of stealing from him. He also cannot locate his coin collection, which he placed in a "safe"** location when his memory began to decline; during the night he rummages through the house looking for it. He believes his family has been plotting to steal all of his assets and then turn him out onto the street. T.G.'s son reports that T.G. has been verbally abusive and has threatened several members of the family recently. How should T.G.'s psychotic behavior be managed?

Delusions and hallucinations are common among demented individuals. Paranoid ideation or delusions have been reported in up to half of dementia patients.[201–203] Delusions typically involve suspicion of theft by family members, which may be secondary to the patient's inability to remember where valuable items were placed and incorrectly concluding that they were stolen.[202] Another common delusion is the misidentification of people or objects. Capgras syndrome, the belief that a person has been "replaced" by an identical-looking impostor, or the belief that photographs or television pictures are real individuals, may occur in almost half of demented individuals.[202,204,205]

Psychotic symptoms respond best to neuroleptic agents, although these are not highly effective, and no single antipsychotic is more effective than any other. Delusions, hallucinations, aggression, and uncooperativeness symptoms respond best, but overall improvement occurs in only about 18% of patients.[205,206]

The choice of a neuroleptic agent is determined by the symptoms displayed by the patient as well as the potential for adverse effects. First, it is important to evaluate the target symptoms to determine whether they will respond to pharmacotherapy. Then, an appropriate agent that has a relatively low risk for adverse effects can be chosen.[207] The atypical antipsychotic agents are better tolerated by older adults than are the conventional neuroleptics (see Chapter 78, Schizophrenia).[197,207,208]

T.G. is experiencing a delusion of theft, suspiciousness, and aggressive behavior. It is possible that the verbal abuse and threats are consequences of fear brought on by the false belief that his family is stealing from him and plans to abandon him. The delusions and suspiciousness may respond to the use of an antipsychotic agent, which may then diminish his aggression as well.

T.G. has no major contraindications to the use of any neuroleptic agent, and his target symptoms will probably respond to any of the available agents. Therefore, the choice can be made according to which antipsychotic agent is least likely to cause intolerable adverse effects. Risperidone has been evaluated in a case series and in a large double-blind, placebo-controlled trial.[209,210] In the case study series, symptoms improved in half of the patients taking dosages ranging from 0.5 mg every other day to 3 mg two times a day. However, 50% also experienced extrapyramidal symptoms (EPS), even at the lowest dosage used.[209] Subjects in the double-blind trial received either placebo or risperidone at dosages of 0.5 mg/day, 1 mg/day, or 2 mg/day for 12 weeks. Daily doses of 1 or 2 mg reduced psychosis and improved behavior, but EPS and somnolence were common adverse effects.[210] A recent report noted that cerebrovascular events occurred in 4% of patients treated with risperidone during clinical trials, compared to 2% of those taking placebo.[211] Low doses of olanzapine, 5 to 15 mg/day, were superior to placebo for reducing agitation, aggression, and psychosis during a 6-week study among nursing facility residents.[212] Somnolence and gait disturbances were the most common adverse effects. Quetiapine has not been well-studied, and clozapine poses significant toxicity risks and requires careful monitoring.[207] Because T.G. does not have cardiovascular or cerebrovascular risk factors and does not have gait or balance problems, either risperidone 0.25 mg HS or olanzapine 5 mg HS can be initiated. Doses of risperidone may be increased by 0.25 mg/day in weekly intervals, up to 1 mg/day; olanzapine doses can be increased by 5 mg/day, up to 15 mg/day. Once his behavior has stabilized, the medication should be continued for about 3 months. At that time, the dose should be decreased in weekly intervals to determine whether the medication is still required. T.G. should be monitored closely for adverse effects, including EPS, which can occur with the atypical antipsychotics.[207,213]

Aggressive Behaviors

15. After 3 months, T.G.'s delusions have subsided, but he continues to be verbally abusive and often displays angry, emotional outbursts, especially when he requires help with bathing or toileting. At other times, he is withdrawn and apathetic. He also has been found wandering in the neighborhood on three occasions. These behaviors persist despite treatment with olanzapine 5 mg BID. What alternative treatments can be attempted?

Although psychotic symptoms respond to neuroleptic agents, many other behaviors do not. More than 80% of patients with dementia exhibit at least one disruptive behavior such as angry outbursts, screaming, and abusive language, and more than 50% display multiple aggressive behaviors.[201,214,215] About 21% display assaultive or violent behavior.[201] Such behaviors typically are directed at caregivers, precipitated by receipt of assistance with activities of daily living such as bathing and toileting, and increase in frequency with dementia severity.[201,214,216] Several of these behaviors may be merely defensive responses to perceived threats in cognitively impaired individuals.[216] Behavioral disturbances must be addressed because they can have a negative effect on the patient's ability to perform activities of daily living.[217]

Some behaviors exhibited by T.G. are not likely to respond to medications. Wandering is typically unaltered by the use of medications unless the patient is oversedated. Nonpharmacologic treatments, such as periods of physical exercise and rest, or environmental modification are much more effective.[195,218]

T.G.'s reactions to assistance with bathing and toileting may be caused by confusion and fear. Breaking the tasks down to step-by-step procedures, accomplished individually, often helps to modify aggressive behaviors.[218]

Verbal abuse and aggressiveness place both the patient and caregiver at risk for injury. Anticonvulsant agents have been shown to reduce rage and aggressive behaviors in patients resistant to treatment with neuroleptics.[219] Carbamazepine and valproic acid (including divalproex) are the most well-studied agents.[220,221] Carbamazepine (Tegretol) 200 to 1,000 mg/day, titrated to a serum level of 5 to 8 μg/mL, reduces severe agitation in dementia patients.[220–222] Significant adverse effects include dizziness, drowsiness, ataxia, and agranulocytosis. Patients should be monitored for central nervous system (CNS) effects (e.g., increased confusion, daytime drowsiness) and require baseline and periodic CBCs with differentials. Carbamazepine also induces hepatic microsomal enzymes, causing more rapid metabolism of several drugs.

Valproic acid and divalproex, alone and in combination with a neuroleptic, also are effective in managing acute aggressive behaviors.[223–225] Common adverse effects are nausea, vomiting, and dizziness. They do not produce blood dyscrasias and are subject to fewer drug interactions than carbamazepine.[195] This makes these agents a better choice for the treatment of T.G.'s symptoms, and they may be added to his risperidone treatment unless his symptoms are determined to be caused by depression (see the following). The initial dosage of divalproex should be 125 mg/day; it may be increased by 125 mg/day every 3 to 6 days until the behavior improves or until a serum level of 82 μg/mL is reached.[219] When his behavior has stabilized, the risperidone dose should be reduced, and if T.G.'s psychotic symptoms do not recur, the drug may be discontinued. Likewise, divalproex treatment should be re-evaluated after 2 to 3 months.

Depression

16. How should T.G.'s social withdrawal and apathy be treated?

Depression often accompanies dementia and may significantly impair a patient's functional capacity, cognitive abilities, and communication.[226,227] T.G. is withdrawn and apathetic, symptoms suggestive of depression. Screaming also is thought to be a symptom of depression in individuals with dementia, perhaps reflecting feelings of loneliness, boredom, or the need for attention.[214,228] Because a definite diagnosis of depression relies heavily on a patient interview and response to questions, a formal diagnosis in patients with dementia is difficult, if not impossible. Therefore, one must rely on patient observation to make a clinical evaluation.

The selective serotonin reuptake inhibitors (SSRI) have not been well studied in patients with dementia, but are effective antidepressants with adverse effects that are better tolerated than those of the tricyclic antidepressants. Sertraline, in doses of 50 mg to 150 mg/day, was superior to placebo in reducing depression in AD patients during a 12-week trial.[229] Citalopram also has demonstrated effectiveness in small trials; in contrast, fluoxetine and fluvoxamine have not demonstrated benefit.[197]

Trazodone (Desyrel) reduces disruptive and aggressive behaviors in cognitively impaired patients and thus is a reasonable choice for treatment of depression in T.G.[195,230,231] This drug is sedating and may help with sleep disorders and is free of anticholinergic effects. It does, however, possess α-adrenergic blocking activity, which may cause orthostasis. If it is determined that T.G. is depressed, trazodone may be initiated at 50 mg at bedtime and increased to 100 mg at bedtime after several days. If necessary, dosages for T.G. can be increased by 50 mg/day every 5 to 7 days. If further dosage increases are needed, the total daily dose should be divided into two or three doses up to a maximum daily dose of 300 mg.[195] The trazodone should induce a restful sleep at night, increase T.G.'s sociability, and decrease his abusive behaviors. If he does not respond to trazodone, either sertraline 50 mg/day or citalopram 10 mg/day may be tried. Dosages may be increased weekly up to a maximum of 150 mg/day or 40 mg/day, respectively.

Social Support

17. T.G.'s family indicates that caring for him at home has become so burdensome that they are considering placing him in an institution. What social support services are available to families facing this decision?

Institutionalization is a typical outcome for patients in the late stages of dementia. The total care required to manage a dementia patient usually becomes unmanageable for most families as the disease progresses. Caregiver stress often is exacerbated by the patient's declining memory, inability to communicate, physical decline, incontinence, and the caregiver's loss of freedom and depression.[232] Caregivers commonly experience anger, helplessness, guilt, and worry and suffer from physical stressors such as fatigue and illness.[218]

Outside assistance is essential to families caring for a patient with dementia. Families should be referred to the Alzheimer's Disease and Related Disorders Association (360 N. Michigan Avenue, Chicago, IL 60601) as soon as a diagnosis of dementia is received. The association has local affiliates in most major cities. The book *The 36-Hour Day* is a valuable resource for families as well.[218] It describes the symptoms, behaviors, and problems that can be encountered when caring for a patient with dementia.

Support groups, individual and family counseling, and other sources of support are useful and may help families cope for a longer period.[233] However, the key intervention to reduce caregiver stress is respite care, which allows a family time away from the responsibilities of taking care of a frail individual.[234] Respite care brings a person into the home or allows the patient to go to a day-care center or similar environment on a regular schedule. Such programs may delay the need to institutionalize a patient.

PSEUDODEMENTIA
Clinical Presentation and Diagnosis

18. G.Y., an 86-year-old woman, lives alone in a low-income housing unit. Over the past 6 weeks, she has become disoriented and confused. A neighbor brought her to the hospital after finding her wandering through the neighborhood in her nightclothes. She eats only one meal a day—a frozen pot pie—because she generally forgets to eat her other meals. Several bills remain unpaid. She has difficulty sleeping and expresses little desire to live because "all my friends are gone." Her score on the Folstein Mini-Mental Status Exam is 18/30 with multiple deficits. Most errors are attributable to answers of "I don't know" or "I can't." She currently takes propranolol 40 mg TID for high BP, cimetidine 400 mg BID for gastroesophageal reflux disease, and temazepam 15 mg HS PRN for insomnia. What subjective and objective data support a diagnosis of pseudodementia in G.Y.?

Depression

G.Y. clearly exhibits cognitive impairment as evidenced by her symptoms of confusion and disorientation, forgetting to eat, wandering, and a low score on the Folstein Mini-Mental Status Exam.[24] However, the rapid course of her decline, her lack of effort on mental status testing, and the medications she is taking suggest that her impairment might be secondary to causes other than true dementia.[235]

Depression is the most common cause of pseudodementia, accounting for at least 50% of cases.[3] Depressive symptoms in G.Y. include self-neglect, insomnia, loss of desire to live, and lack of effort on mental status testing. When given a mental status screening test, depressed patients tend to give "I don't know" answers, which reflect dysphoria or an inability to cooperate, whereas demented patients typically provide incorrect answers.[3,235]

Medications

Medications often are responsible for cognitive impairment in older adults, accounting for dementia symptoms in approximately 12% of patients with cognitive impairment. Psychotropic medications, analgesics, antihypertensives, corticosteroids, and cimetidine often are implicated (see Chapter 79, Mood Disorders I: Major Depressive Disorders).[23,198,236]

Treatment

19. What is the proper treatment for G.Y.'s pseudodementia?

Initial therapy should consist of the discontinuation of her medications, all of which may be contributing to her cognitive decline. Because all the medications are relatively short acting, her mental status should improve significantly within 48 hours. At that time, her hypertension and gastroesophageal reflux disease can be re-evaluated and more appropriate therapy instituted, if warranted.

G.Y. should be evaluated for depression, and psychotherapy should be initiated if she is in fact depressed. She also should be referred to a social services agency or senior center to provide her with assistance and to offer her opportunities for social interaction.

REFERENCES

1. Jorm AF, Jolley D. The incidence of dementia: a meta-analysis. Neruology 1998;51:728.
2. Brookmeyer R et al. Projections of Alzheimer's disease in the United States and the public health impact of delaying onset. Am J Public Health 1998;88:1337.
3. Cummings J, Benson DF. Dementia: A Clinical Approach. 2nd Ed. Boston: Butterworth-Heinemann, 1992:45.
4. Knopman DS. An overview of common non-Alzheimer dementias. Clin Geriatr Med 2001; 17:281.
5. Lanska DJ. Dementia mortality in the United States: results of the 1986 National Mortality Followback Survey. Neurology 1998;50:362.
6. Cummings J et al. Reversible dementia: illustrative cases, definition, and review. JAMA 1980;243:2434.
7. Ineichen B. Measuring the rising tide: how many dementia cases will there be by 2001? Br J Psychiatry 1987;150:193.
8. Larson EB. Alzheimer's disease in the community [Editorial]. JAMA 1989;262:2591.
9. Henderson AS. The epidemiology of Alzheimer's disease. Br Med Bull 1986;42:3.
10. Kokmen E et al. Prevalence of medically diagnosed dementia in a defined United States population: Rochester, Minnesota, January 1, 1975. Neurology 1989;39:773.
11. Weissman MM et al. Psychiatric disorders (DSM-III) and cognitive impairment among the elderly in a US urban community. Acta Psychiatr Scand 1985;77:366.
12. Rocca WA et al. Frequency and distribution of Alzheimer's disease in Europe: a collaborative study of 1980–1990 prevalence findings. Ann Neurol 1991;30:381.
13. Evans DA et al. Prevalence of Alzheimer's disease in a community of older persons: higher than previously reported. JAMA 1989;262:2551.
14. Wernicke TF, Reischies FM. Prevalence of dementia in old age: clinical diagnoses in subjects aged 95 years and older. Neurology 1994;44:250.
15. Rocca WA et al. Incidence of dementia and Alzheimer's disease. Am J Epidemiol 1998;148:51.
16. Gao S et al. The relationship between age, sex and the incidence of dementia and Alzheimer's disease. Arch Gen Psychiatry 1998;55:809
17. Brookmeyer R et al. Survival following a diagnosis of Alzheimer's disease. Arch Neurol 2002;59:1764.
18. Ernst RL, Hay JW. The US economic and social costs of Alzheimer's disease revisited. Am J Public Health 1994;84:1261.
19. Gutterman EM et al. Cost of Alzheimer's disease and related dementia in managed-Medicare. J Am Geriatr Soc 1999;47:1065.
20. Meek PD et al. Economic considerations in Alzheimer's disease. Pharmacotherapy 1998;18:68S.
21. American Psychiatric Association, Diagnostic and Statistical Manual of Mental Disorders. 4th Ed. Washington, DC: American Psychiatric Association, 1994.
22. Costa PT Jr. et al. Recognition and initial assessment of Alzheimer's disease and related dementias. Clinical Practice Guideline No. 19. AHCPR publication no. 97-0702. Rockville, MD: US DHHS, PHS, AHCPR, November 1996.
23. Small GW et al. Diagnosis and treatment of Alzheimer disease and related disorders. JAMA 1997;278:1363.
24. Folstein MF et al. "Mini-mental state": a practical method for grading the mental state of patients for the clinician. J Psychiatr Res 1975;12:189.
25. Blessed G et al. The association between quantitative measures of dementia and of senile change in the cerebral grey matter of elderly subjects. Br J Psychiatry 1968;114:797.
26. Shore D et al. Serum aluminum in primary degenerative dementia. Biol Psychiatry 1980;15:971.
27. Markesbery WR et al. Instrumental neutron activation analysis of brain aluminum in Alzheimer disease and aging. Ann Neurol 1981;10:511.
28. Good PF et al. Selective accumulation of aluminum and iron in the neurofibrillary tangles of Alzheimer's disease: a laser microprobe (LAMMA) study. Ann Neurol 1992;31:286.
29. Glenner GG. The pathobiology of Alzheimer's disease. Ann Rev Med 1989;40:45.
30. Selkoe DJ. Alzheimer's disease: insights into an emerging epidemic. J Geriatr Psychiatry 1992;25:211.
31. Edwards JK et al. Are there clinical and epidemiological differences between familial and non-familial Alzheimer's disease? J Am Geriatr Soc 1991;39:477.
32. Rocca WA et al. Maternal age and Alzheimer's disease: a collaborative re-analysis of case-control studies. Int J Epidemiol 1991;20:S21.
33. Chandra V et al. Head trauma with loss of consciousness as a risk factor for Alzheimer's disease. Neurology 1989;39:1576.
34. Mortimer JA et al. Head trauma as a risk factor for Alzheimer's disease: a collaborative re-analysis of case-control studies. Int J Epidemiol 1991;20:S28.
35. Graves AB et al. Head circumference as a measure of cognitive reserve: association with severity of impairment in Alzheimer's disease. Br J Psychiatry 1996;169:86.
36. Mori E et al. Premorbid brain size as a determinant of reserve capacity against intellectual decline in Alzheimer's disease. Am J Psychiatry 1997;154:18.
37. Snowden DA et al. Linguistic ability in early life and cognitive function and Alzheimer's disease in late life. JAMA 1996;275:528.
38. Cummings JL et al. Alzheimer's disease: etiologies, pathophysiology, cognitive reserve, and treatment opportunities. Neurology 1998;51(Suppl 1):S2.
39. Huff FJ et al. Risk of dementia in relatives of patients with Alzheimer's disease. Neurology 1988;38:786.
40. Farrer LA et al. Assessment of genetic risk for Alzheimer's disease among first-degree relatives. Ann Neurol 1989;25:485.
41. Hoffman A et al. History of dementia and Parkinson's disease in 1st-degree relatives of patients with Alzheimer's disease. Neurology 1989;39:1589.
42. Farrer LA et al. Transmission and age-at-onset patterns in familial Alzheimer's disease: evidence for heterogeneity. Neurology 1990;40:395.
43. Chui HC et al. Clinical subtypes of dementia of the Alzheimer type. Neurology 1985;35:1544.
44. Van Duijn CM et al. Familial aggregation of Alzheimer's disease and related disorders: a collaborative re-analysis of case-control studies. Int J Epidemiol 1991;20:S13.
45. Luchins DJ et al. Are there clinical differences between familial and nonfamilial Alzheimer's disease? Am J Psychiatry 1992;149:1023.
46. Devi G et al. Validity of family history for the diagnosis of dementia among siblings of patients with late-onset Alzheimer's disease. Gen Epidemiol 1998;15:215.
47. Hayashi Y et al. Evidence for presenilin-1 involvement in amyloid angiopathy in the Alzheimer's disease-affected brain. Brain Res 1998;789:307.
48. St. George-Hyslop PH et al. The genetic defect causing familial Alzheimer's disease maps on chromosome 21. Science 1987;235:885.
49. Lai F, Williams RS. A prospective study of Alzheimer disease in Down syndrome. Arch Neurol 1989;46:849.
50. Mann DMA et al. Amyloid β protein (Aβ) deposition in chromosome 14-linked Alzheimer's disease: predominance of Aβ42(43). Ann Neurol 1996;40:149.
51. Levy-Lahad E et al. Candidate gene for the chromosome 1 familial Alzheimer's disease locus. Science 1995;269:973.
52. Creasey H et al. Monozygotic twins discordant for Alzheimer's disease. Neurology 1989;39:1474.
53. Whitehouse PJ. Genesis of Alzheimer's disease. Neurology 1997;48(Suppl 7):S2.
54. Joachim CL, Selkoe DJ. The seminal role of β-amyloid in the pathogenesis of Alzheimer's disease. Alzheimer Dis Assoc Disord 1992;6:7.
55. Murrell J et al. A mutation in the amyloid precursor protein associated with hereditary Alzheimer's disease. Science 1991;254:97.
56. Gustafson L et al. A 50-year perspective of a family with chromosome-14-linked Alzheimer's disease. Hum Genet 1998;102:253.
57. Poirier J et al. Apolipoprotein E4 allele as a predictor of cholinergic deficits and treatment outcome in Alzheimer disease. Proc Natl Acad Sci USA 1995;92:12260.
58. Corder EH et al. Gene dose of apolipoprotein E type 4 allele and the risk of Alzheimer's disease in late onset families. Science 1993;261:921.
59. Farrer LA et al. Effects of age, sex, and ethnicity on the association between apolipoprotein E genotype and Alzheimer's disease. JAMA 1997;278:1349.
60. O'Hara R et al. The APOE e4 allele is associated with decline on delayed recall performance in community-dwelling older adults. J Am Geriatr Soc 1998;46:1493.
61. Caselli RJ et al. Preclinical memory decline in cognitively normal apolipoprotein E-e4 homozygotes. Neurology 1999;53:201.
62. Glenner GG. Current knowledge of amyloid deposits as applied to senile plaques and congophilic angiopathy. In: Katzman R et al., eds. Alzheimer's Disease, Senile Dementia and Related Disorders. New York: Raven, 1978:493.
63. Chui HC. The significance of clinically defined subgroups of Alzheimer's disease. J Neural Transm 1987;24(Suppl):57.
64. Poirier J, Finch CE. Neurochemistry of the aging human brain. In: Hazzard WR et al., eds. Principles of Geriatric Medicine and Gerontology. New York: McGraw-Hill, 1990:905.
65. Bondareff W et al. Loss of neurons of origin of the adrenergic projection to cerebral cortex (nucleus locus ceruleus) in senile dementia. Neurology 1982;32:164.
66. Khachaturian ZS. Diagnosis of Alzheimer's disease. Arch Neurol 1985;42:1097.
67. Grundke-Iqbal I et al. Abnormal phosphorylation of the microtubule-associated protein tau in Alzheimer cytoskeletal pathology. Proc Natl Acad Sci USA 1986;83:4913.
68. Lee VMY et al. A68: a major subunit of paired helical filaments and derivatized forms of normal tau. Nature 1991;251:675.
69. Tabaton M et al. The widespread alteration of neurites in Alzheimer's disease may be unrelated to amyloid deposition. Ann Neurol 1989;26:771.
70. McKee AC et al. Neuritic pathology and dementia in Alzheimer's disease. Ann Neurol 1991;30:156.
71. Samuel WA et al. Severity of dementia in Alzheimer disease and neurofibrillary tangles in multiple brain regions. Alzheimer Dis Assoc Disord 1991;5:1.
72. Bugiani O et al. Preamyloid deposits, amyloid deposits, and senile plaques in Alzheimer's disease, Down syndrome, and aging. Ann NY Acad Sci 1991;640:122.
73. Mann DM. Neuropathology of Alzheimer's disease: towards an understanding of the pathogenesis. Biochem Soc Trans 1989;17:73.
74. Lassman H et al. Synaptic pathology of Alzheimer's disease. Ann NY Acad Sci 1993;695:59.
75. Beyreuther K et al. Mechanisms of amyloid deposition in Alzheimer's disease. Ann NY Acad Sci 1991;640:129.
76. Arai H et al. Expression patterns of β-amyloid precursor protein (β-APP) in neural and nonneural

human tissues from Alzheimer's disease and control subjects. Ann Neurol 1991;30:686.

77. Haass C et al. Normal cellular processing of the β-amyloid precursor protein results in the secretion of the amyloid β peptide and related molecules. Ann NY Acad Sci 1993;695:109

78. Aisen PS. Inflammation and Alzheimer's disease: mechanisms and therapeutic strategies. Gerontology 1997;43:143.

79. Coyle JT et al. Alzheimer's disease: a disorder of cortical cholinergic innervation. Science 1983; 219:1184.

80. Rumble BR et al. Amyloid A4 protein and its precursor in Down's syndrome and Alzheimer's disease. N Engl J Med 1989;320:1446.

81. Davies LB et al. A4 amyloid protein deposition and the diagnosis of Alzheimer's disease: prevalence in aged brains determined by immunocytochemistry compared with conventional neuropathologic techniques. Neurology 1988;38:1688.

82. Joachim CL et al. Amyloid β-protein deposition in tissues other than brain in Alzheimer's disease. Nature 1989;341:226.

83. Whitehouse PJ et al. Alzheimer's disease and senile dementia: loss of neurons in the basal forebrain. Science 1982;215:1237.

84. Whitehouse PJ et al. Alzheimer disease: evidence for selective loss of cholinergic neurons in the nucleus basalis. Ann Neurol 1981;10:122.

85. Weinberger DR et al. The distribution of cerebral muscarinic acetylcholine receptors in vivo in patients with dementia. Arch Neurol 1991;48:169.

86. Schroder H et al. Cellular distribution and expression of cortical acetylcholine receptors in aging and Alzheimer's disease. Ann NY Acad Sci 1991; 640:189.

87. Ladner CJ, Lee JM. Pharmacological drug treatment of Alzheimer disease: the cholinergic hypothesis revisited. J Neuropathol Exp Neurol 1998;57:719.

88. Terry RD et al. Physical basis of cognitive alterations in Alzheimer's disease: synapse loss is the major correlate of cognitive impairment. Ann Neurol 1991;30:572.

89. Krall WJ et al. Cholinesterase inhibitors: a therapeutic strategy for Alzheimer's disease. Ann Pharmacother 1999;33:441.

90. Nemeroff CB et al. Recent advances in the neurochemical pathology of Alzheimer's disease. Ann NY Acad Sci 1991;640:193.

91. McKhann G et al. Clinical diagnosis of Alzheimer's disease: report of the NINCDS-ADRDA Work Group, Department of Health and Human Services Task Force on Alzheimer's Disease. Neurology 1984;34:939.

92. Ronald and Nancy Reagan Institute. Consensus report of the Working Group on "Molecular and biochemical markers of Alzheimer's disease." Neurobiol Aging 1998;19:109.

93. Farlow MR. Alzheimer's disease: clinical implications of the apolipoprotein E genotype. Neurology 1997;48(Suppl 6):S30.

94. Barclay LL et al. Survival in Alzheimer's disease and vascular dementias. Neurology 1985;35:834.

95. Riesberg B et al. The global deterioration scale for assessment of primary degenerative dementia. Am J Psychiatry 1982;139:1136.

96. Hughes CP et al. A new clinical scale for the staging of dementia. Br J Psychiatry 1982;140:566.

97. Morris JC. Clinical and neuropathological findings from CERAD. In: Becker R, Giacobini E, eds. Alzheimer Disease: From Molecular Biology to Therapy. Boston: Birkhauser, 1996:7.

98. Ernst RL et al. Cognitive function and the cost of Alzheimer's disease. Arch Neurol 1997;54:687.

99. Gwyther LP. Social issues of the Alzheimer's disease patient and family. Am J Med 1998; 104(4A):17S.

100. Schneider LS. Treatment of Alzheimer's disease with cholinesterase inhibitors. Clin Geriatr Med 2001;17:337.

101. Brinton RD, Yamazaki RS. Advances and challenges in the prevention and treatment of Alzheimer's disease. Pharmaceut Res 1998; 15:386.

102. Crismon ML. Pharmacokinetics and drug interactions of cholinesterase inhibitors administered in Alzheimer's disease. Pharmacotherapy 1998; 18:47S.

103. Parnetti L. Clinical pharmacokinetics of drugs for Alzheimer's disease. Clin Pharmacokinet 1995; 29:110.

104. Farlow M et al. A controlled trial of tacrine in Alzheimer's disease. JAMA 1992;268:2523.

105. Knapp MJ et al. A 30-week randomized controlled trial of high-dose tacrine in patients with Alzheimer's disease. JAMA 1994;271:985.

106. Watkins PB et al. Hepatotoxic effects of tacrine administration in patients with Alzheimer's disease. JAMA 1994;271:992.

107. Parke-Davis. Cognex package insert. Morris Plains, NJ: November 1993.

108. Mihara M et al. Pharmacokinetics of E2020, a new compound for Alzheimer's disease, in healthy male volunteers. Int J Clin Pharmacol Ther Toxicol 1993;31:223.

109. Rho JP, Lipson LG. Focus on donepezil. Formulary 1997;32:677.

110. Rogers SL et al. Donepezil improves cognition and global function in Alzheimer's disease. Arch Intern Med 1998;158:1021.

111. Rosen WG et al. A new rating scale for Alzheimer's disease. Am J Psychiatry 1984;141:1356.

112. Knopman DS et al. The clinician interview-based impression (CIBI): a clinician's global change rating scale in Alzheimer's disease. Neurology 1994;44:2315.

113. Rogers SL et al. A 24-week, double-blind, placebo-controlled trial of donepezil in patients with Alzheimer's disease. Neurology 1998;50:136.

114. Doody RS et al. Open-label, multicenter, phase 3 extension study of the safety and efficacy of donepezil in patients with Alzheimer disease. Arch Neurol 2001;58:427.

115. Cutler NR et al. Dose-dependent CSF acetylcholinesterase inhibition by SDZ ENA 713 in Alzheimer's disease. Acta Neurol Scand 1998; 97:244.

116. Polinsky RJ. Clinical pharmacology of rivastigmine: a new-generation acetylcholinesterase inhibitor for the treatment of Alzheimer's disease. Clin Ther 1998;20:634.

117. Anand R et al. Clinical development of Exelon (ENA-713): the ADENA programme. J Drug Dev Clin Pract 1996;8:117.

118. Corey-Bloom J et al. A randomized trial evaluating the efficacy and safety of ENA 713 (rivastigmine tartrate), a new acetylcholinesterase inhibitor, in patients with mild to moderately severe Alzheimer's disease. Int J Geriatr Psychopharmacol 1998;1:55.

119. Rösler M et al. Efficacy and safety of rivastigmine in patients with Alzheimer's disease: international randomized controlled trial. BMJ 1999;318:633.

120. Farlow M et al. A 52-week study of the efficacy of rivastigmine in patients with mild to moderately severe Alzheimer's disease. Eur Neurol 2000; 44:236.

121. Williams BR et al. A review of rivastigmine. Clin Ther 2003;25:1634.

122. Maelicke A et al. Allosteric sensitization of nicotinic receptors by galantamine, a new treatment strategy for Alzheimer's disease. Biol Psychiatry 2001;49:279.

123. Mihailova D et al. Pharmacokinetics of galanthamine hydrobromide after single subcutaneous and oral dosage in humans. Pharmacology 1989;39:50.

124. Scott LJ, Goa KL. Galantamine: a review of its use in Alzheimer's disease. Drugs 2000;60:1095.

125. Tariot PN et al. A 5-month, randomized, placebo-controlled trial of galantamine in AD. Neurology 2000;54:2269.

126. Wilcock GK et al. Efficacy and safety of galantamine in patients with mild to moderate Alzheimer's disease: multicentre randomized controlled trial. BMJ 2000;321:1.

127. Raskind MA et al. Galantamine in AD: a 6-month randomized, placebo-controlled trial with a 6-month extension. Neurology 2000;54:2261.

128. Cacabelos R et al. The glutamatergic system and neurodegeneration in dementia: preventive strategies in Alzheimer's disease. Int J Geriatr Psychiatry 1999;14:3.

129. Jarvis B, Figgitt DP. Memantine. Drugs Aging 2003;20:406.

130. Winblad B et al. Memantine in severe dementia: results of the ⁹M-BEST study (benefit and efficacy in severely demented patients during treatment with memantine). Int J Geriatr Psychiatry 1999; 14:135.

131. Reisberg B et al. Memantine in moderate-to-severe Alzheimer's disease. N Engl J Med 2003; 348:1333.

132. Farlow MR et al. Memantine/donepezil dual therapy is superior to placebo/donepezil for treatment of moderate to severe Alzheimer's disease [Abstract]. Neurology 2003;60(Suppl 1):A412.

133. Birge SJ. The role of estrogen in the treatment of Alzheimer's disease. Neurology 1997;48(Suppl 7):S36.

134. Robinson D et al. Estrogen replacement therapy and memory in older women. J Am Geriatr Soc 1994;42:919.

135. Yaffe K et al. Estrogen therapy in postmenopausal women: effects on cognitive function and dementia. JAMA 1998;279:688.

136. Schneider LS et al. Effects of estrogen replacement therapy on response to tacrine in patients with Alzheimer's disease. Neurology 1996;46:1580.

137. Shumaker SA et al. Estrogen plus progestin and the incidence of dementia and mild cognitive impairment in postmenopausal women: the Women's Health Initiative Memory Study: a randomized controlled trial. JAMA 2003;289:2651.

138. Breitner JCS et al. Inverse association of anti-inflammatory treatments and Alzheimer's disease: initial results of a co-twin control study. Neurology 1994;44:227.

139. Anderson K et al. Do nonsteroidal anti-inflammatory drugs decrease the risk for Alzheimer's disease? Neurology 1995;45:1441.

140. Rich JB et al. Nonsteroidal anti-inflammatory drugs in Alzheimer's disease. Neurology 1995; 45:51.

141. Stewart WF et al. Risk of Alzheimer's disease and duration of NSAID use. Neurology 1997;48:626.

142. Rogers J et al. Clinical trial of indomethacin in Alzheimer's disease. Neurology 1993;43:1609.

143. Scharf S et al. A double-blind, placebo-controlled trial of diclofenac/misoprostol in Alzheimer's disease. Neurology 1999;53:197.

144. in t'Veld BA et al. Non-steroidal anti-inflammatory drugs and the risk of Alzheimer's disease. N Engl J Med 2001;345:1515.

145. Aisen PS et al. Effects of rofecoxib or naproxen vs. placebo in Alzheimer disease progression. JAMA 2003;289:2819.

146. Tariot PN et al. L-deprenyl in Alzheimer's disease. Arch Gen Psychiatry 1987;44:427.

147. Piccinin GL et al. Neuropsychological effects of L-deprenyl in Alzheimer's type dementia. Clin Neuropharmacol 1990;13:147.

148. Burke WJ et al. L-deprenyl in the treatment of mild dementia of the Alzheimer type: results of a 15-month trial. J Am Geriatr Soc 1993;41:1219.

149. Freedman M et al. L-deprenyl in Alzheimer's disease. Neurology 1998;50:660.

150. Schneider LS et al. A double-blind crossover pilot study of L-deprenyl (selegiline) combined with cholinesterase inhibitor in Alzheimer's disease. Am J Psychiatry 1993;150:321.

151. Sano M et al. A controlled trial of selegiline, alpha-tocopherol, or both as treatment for Alzheimer's disease. N Engl J Med 1997;336:1216.

152. Tyler V. Herbs of Choice: The Therapeutic Use of Phytomedicinals. New York: Pharmaceutical Products Press, 1994:108.

153. Le Bars PL et al. A placebo-controlled, double-blind, randomized trial of an extract of ginkgo biloba for dementia. JAMA 1997;278:1327.

154. Maurer K et al. Clinical efficacy of ginkgo biloba special extract EGb 761 in dementia of the Alzheimer type. J Psychiatric Res 1997;31:645.

155. van Dongen MCJM et al. The efficacy of ginkgo for elderly people with dementia and age-associated memory impairment: new results of a randomized clinical trial. J Am Geriatric Soc 2000;48:1183.

156. McKeith IG et al. Consensus guidelines for the clinical and pathological diagnosis of dementia with Lewy bodies (DLB): report of the consortium on DLB international workshop. Neurology 1996;47:1113.

157. Knopman DS. An overview of common non-Alzheimer dementias. Clin Geriatr Med 2001; 17:281.

158. McKeith IG et al. Rivastigmine in the treatment of dementia with Lewy bodies: preliminary findings from an open trial. Int J Geriatr Psychiatry 2000; 15:387.

159. Chui HC et al. Criteria for the diagnosis of ischemic vascular dementia proposed by the State of California Alzheimer's Disease Diagnostic and Treatment Centers. Neurology 1992;42:473.

160. Hachinski VC et al. Multi-infarct dementia: a cause of mental deterioration in the elderly. Lancet 1974; 2:207.

161. Tresch DD et al. Prevalence and significance of cardiovascular disease and hypertension in elderly patients with dementia. J Am Geriatr Soc 1985;33:530.

162. Meyer JS et al. Aetiological considerations and risk factors for multi-infarct dementia. J Neurol Neurosurg Psychiatry 1988;51:1489.

163. Zimetbaum P et al. Lipids, vascular disease, and dementia with advancing age. Arch Intern Med 1991;151:240.

164. Ross GW et al. Characterization of risk factors for vascular dementia. Neurology 1999;53:337.

165. Pullicino P et al. Small deep infarcts diagnosed on computed tomography. Neurology 1980;30:1090.

166. Goto K et al. Diffuse white-matter disease in the geriatric population. Radiology 1981;141:687.

167. Ishii N et al. Why do frontal lobe symptoms predominate in vascular dementia with lacunes? Neurology 1986;36:340.

168. Donnan GA et al. A prospective study of lacunar infarction using computerized tomography. Neurology 1982;32:49.

169. Roman GC. Senile dementia of the Binswanger type: a form of vascular dementia in the elderly. JAMA 1987;258:1782.

170. Wallin A, Blennow K. Pathogenetic basis of vascular dementia. Alzheimer Dis Assoc Disord 1991;5:91.

171. Hachinski VC et al. Leuko-araiosis. Arch Neurol 1987;44:21.

172. Munoz DG. The pathological basis of multi-infarct dementia. Alzheimer Dis Assoc Disord 1991;5:77.

173. Inzitari D et al. Vascular risk factors and leuko-araiosis. Arch Neurol 1987;44:42.

174. Kawamura J et al. Leukoariosis correlates with cerebral hypoperfusion in vascular dementia. Stroke 1991;22:609.

175. Babikian V, Ropper AH. Binswanger's disease: a review. Stroke 1987;18:2.

176. Tomimoto H et al. Coagulation activation in patients with Binswanger disease. Arch Neurol 1999; 56:1104.

177. Rocca WA et al. Prevalence of clinically diagnosed Alzheimer's disease and other dementing disorders: a door-to-door survey in Appignano, Macerata Province, Italy. Neurology 1990;40:626.

178. Nussbaum M et al. DSM-III criteria for primary degenerative dementia and multi-infarct dementia. Alzheimer Dis Assoc Disord 1992;6:111.

179. Hachinski VC et al. Cerebral blood flow in dementia. Arch Neurol 1975;32:632.

180. Rogers RL et al. Cigarette smoking decreases cerebral blood flow suggesting increased risk for stroke. JAMA 1983;250:2796.

181. Meyer JS et al. Improved cognition after control of risk factors for multi-infarct dementia. JAMA 1986; 256:2203.

182. SHEP Cooperative Research Group. Prevention of stroke by antihypertensive drug treatment in older persons with isolated systolic hypertension. JAMA 1991;265:3255.

183. Williams BR, Kim J. Cardiovascular drug therapy in the elderly: theoretical and practical considerations. Drugs Aging 2003;20:445.

184. Tollefson GD. Short-term effects of the calcium channel blocker nimodipine in the management of primary degenerative dementia. Biol Psychiatry 1990;27:1133.

185. Forette F et al. The prevention of dementia with antihypertensive treatment: new evidence from the Systolic Hypertension in Europe (Sys-Eur) study. Arch Intern Med 2002;162:2046.

186. The ALLHAT Officers and Coordinators for the ALLHAT Collaborative Research Group. Major cardiovascular events in hypertensive patients randomized to doxazosin vs. chlorthalidone: the Antihypertensive and Lipid-Lowering Treatment to Prevent Heart Attack Trial (ALLHAT). JAMA 2000;283:1967.

187. Meyer JS et al. Randomized clinical trial of daily aspirin therapy in multi-infarct dementia: a pilot study. J Am Geriatr Soc 1989;37:549.

188. Dutch TIA Trial Study Group. A comparison of two doses of aspirin (30 mg vs. 283 mg a day) in patients after a transient ischemic attack or minor ischemic stroke. N Engl J Med 1991;325:1261.

189. Albers GW et al. Antithrombotic and thrombolytic therapy for ischemic stroke. Chest 2001; 119:300S.

190. Erkinjuntti T. Cognitive decline and treatment options for patients with vascular dementia. Acta Neurol Scand 2002;106(Suppl 178):15.

191. Meyer JS et al. Donepezil treatment of vascular dementia. Ann N Y Acad Sci 2002;977:482.

192. Erkinjuntti T et al. Efficacy of galantamine in probable vascular dementia and Alzheimer's disease combined with cerebrovascular disease: a randomized trial. Lancet 2002;359:1283.

193. Moretti R et al. Rivastigmine in subcortical vascular dementia: an open 22-month study. J Neurol Sci 2002;203-204:141.

194. Maletta GJ. Management of behavior in elderly patients with dementias. Clin Geriatr Med 1988; 4:719.

195. Tariot PN. Treatment of agitation in dementia. J Clin Psychiatry 1999;60(Suppl 8):11.

196. Cummings JL et al. The relationship between donepezil and behavioral disturbances in patients with Alzheimer's disease. Am J Geriatr Psychiatry 2000;8:134.

197. Tariot PN et al. Pharmacologic therapy for behavioral symptoms of Alzheimer's disease. Clin Geriatr Med 2001;17:359.

198. Beers MH et al. Explicit criteria for determining potentially inappropriate medication use by the elderly. Arch Intern Med 1997;157:1531.

199. Aultzer DL et al. A double-blind comparison of trazodone and haloperidol for treatment of agitation in patients with dementia. Am J Geriatr Psychiatry 1997;5:60.

200. Burke WJ et al. Effective use of anxiolytics in older adults. Clin Geriatr Med 1998;14:47.

201. Swearer JM et al. Troublesome and disruptive behaviors in dementia. J Am Geriatr Soc 1988; 36:784.

202. Binetti G et al. Delusions in Alzheimer's disease and multi-infarct dementia. Acta Neurol Scand 1993;88:5.

203. Hirono N et al. Factors associated with psychotic symptoms in Alzheimer's disease. J Neurol Neurosurg Psychiatry 1998;64:648.

204. Neitch SM, Zarraga A. A misidentification delusion in two Alzheimer's patients. J Am Geriatr Soc 1991;39:513.

205. Rapp MS et al. Behavioural disturbances in the demented elderly: phenomenology, pharmacotherapy and behaviour management. Can J Psychiatry 1992;37:651.

206. Schneider LS et al. A meta-analysis of controlled trials of neuroleptic treatment in dementia. J Am Geriatr Soc 1990;38:553.

207. Schneider LS. Pharmacologic management of psychosis in dementia. J Clin Psychiatry 1999; 60(Suppl 8):54.

208. Kumar V et al. Pharmacologic management of Alzheimer's disease. Clin Geriatr Med 1998; 14:129.

209. Herrmann N et al. Risperidone for the treatment of behavioral disturbances in dementia: a case series. J Neuropsychiatry Clin Neurosci 1998;10:220.

210. Katz I et al. Comparison of risperidone and placebo for psychosis and behavioral disturbances in dementia: a randomized, double-blind trial. J Clin Psychiatry 1999;60:107.

211. Wooltorton E. Risperidone (Risperdal): increased rate of cerebrovascular events in dementia trials. Can Med Assoc J 2002;167:1269.

212. Street JS et al. Olanzapine treatment of psychotic and behavioral symptoms in patients with Alzheimer disease in nursing care facilities. Arch Gen Psychiatry 2000;57:968.

213. Maixner SM et al. The efficacy, safety, and tolerability of antipsychotics in the elderly. J Clin Psychiatry 1999;60(Suppl 8):29.

214. Cohen-Mansfield J et al. Screaming in nursing home residents. J Am Geriatr Soc 1990;38:785.

215. Cariaga J et al. A controlled study of disruptive vocalizations among geriatric residents in nursing homes. J Am Geriatr Soc 1991;39:501.

216. Bridges-Parlet S et al. A descriptive study of physically aggressive behavior in dementia by direct observation. J Am Geriatr Soc 1994;42:192.

217. Freels S et al. Functional status and clinical findings with Alzheimer's disease. J Gerontol 1992;47:M177.

218. Mace NL, Rabins PV. The 36 Hour Day. Baltimore: Johns Hopkins University Press, 1981:16.

219. Grossman E. A review of anticonvulsants in treating agitated demented elderly patients. Pharmacotherapy 1998;18:600.

220. Gleason RP, Schneider LS. Carbamazepine treatment of agitation in Alzheimer's outpatients refractory to neuroleptics. J Clin Psychiatry 1990;51:115.

221. Tariot PN et al. Efficacy and tolerability of carbamazepine for agitation and aggression in dementia. J Clin Psychiatry 1998;155:54.

222. Essa M. Carbamazepine in dementia. J Clin Psychopharmacol 1986;6:234.

223. Hass S et al. Divalproex: a possible treatment alternative for demented, elderly aggressive patients. Ann Clin Psychiatry 1997;9:145.

224. Porsteinsson AP et al. Placebo-controlled study of divalproex sodium for agitation in dementia. Am J Geriatr Psychiatry 2001;9:1.

225. Narayan M, Nelson JC. Treatment of dementia with behavioral disturbance using divalproex or a combination of divalproex and a neuroleptic. J Clin Psychiatry 1997;58:351.

226. Salzman C. Treatment of agitation, anxiety, and depression in dementia. Psychopharmacol Bull 1988;24:39.

227. Fitz AG, Teri L. Depression, cognition, and functional ability in patients with Alzheimer's disease. J Am Geriatr Soc 1994;42:186.

228. Carlyle W et al. ECT: an effective treatment in the screaming demented patient [Letter]. J Am Geriatr Soc 1991;39:637.

229. Lyketsos CG et al. Randomized, placebo-controlled, double-blind clinical trial of sertraline

in the treatment of depression complicating Alzheimer's disease: initial results from the Depression in Alzheimer's Disease Study. Am J Psychiatry 2000;157:1686.

230. Simpson DM, Foster D. Improvement in organically disturbed behavior with trazodone treatment. J Clin Psychiatry 1986;47:191.

231. Pinner E, Rich C. Effects of trazodone on aggressive behavior in seven patients with organic mental disorders. Am J Psychiatry 1988;145:1295.

232. Williamson GM, Schulz R. Coping with specific stressors in Alzheimer's disease caregiving. Gerontologist 1993;33:747.

233. Mittelman MS et al. An intervention that delays institutionalization of Alzheimer's disease patients: treatment of spouse-caregivers. Gerontologist 1993;33:730.

234. Knight BG et al. A meta-analytic review of interventions for caregiver distress: recommendations for future research. Gerontologist 1993;33:240.

235. Cole JO et al. Tricyclic use in the cognitively impaired elderly. J Clin Psychiatry 1983;44:14.

236. Larson EB et al. Adverse drug reactions associated with cognitive impairment in elderly persons. Ann Intern Med 1987;107:169.

CHAPTER 101

Geriatric Urologic Disorders

John F. Thompson

SEXUAL DYSFUNCTION

Sexual dysfunction has been described as a public health concern by a National Institutes of Health Consensus panel.[1,2] Sexual dysfunctions are highly prevalent in both sexes, ranging from 10% to 52% in men and from 25% to 63% in women.[3,4] In addition, advancing age is accompanied by a decrease in sexual function. Intercourse decreases from an average of once a week at the age of 65 to once every 10 weeks at the age of 80.[5] The frequency of sexual intercourse among the elderly actually has increased over the past 40 years, but still is substantially less than in younger individuals.[5–8] Although individual variations in frequency are large, most studies show that sexual activity among the elderly depends on the life pattern and past experiences of good or poor sexual func-

tion in each patient. Elderly patients may experience physiologic changes and encounter additional interference with sexual activity because of disability, disease, and medications. Furthermore, there is a decline in sexual interest with aging.[9]

Poor health often is cited by elderly women as a reason for not participating in sexual activity, and among men, erectile dysfunction is the leading cause of decline in activity.[5,10] The major factors that correlate with reduced sexual activity include an older spouse, poor mental or physical health, marital difficulties, previous negative sexual experiences, and negative attitudes toward sexuality in the aged.[11] During the postmenopausal years, women undergo substantial physiologic change. The major physiologic event of natural menopause is a decrease in estrogen production. There is little doubt that a decline in estrogen production is associated with many of the physiologic changes causing elderly women to report a low interest in sexual activity. The medical literature is replete with research and data on elderly male sexual dysfunction, but there are little, if any, data on female sexual dysfunction.

Male Sexual Dysfunction

Aging men may experience andropause, a syndrome consisting of weakness, fatigue, reduced muscle and bone mass, impaired hematopoiesis, oligospermia, sexual dysfunction, and psychiatric symptoms.[12] The relation between declining testosterone and andropause is not firmly established. Free testosterone levels begin to decline at the rate of 1% per year after age 40 years. By the age of 60 years, 20% of men have levels below the lower limit of normal.[14] The physiologic and psychological effects of declining hormone levels in men are less dramatic than those experienced by women.

Sexual function is considered an interaction among motivation, drive, desires, thoughts, fantasies, pleasures, experiences (referred to as the *libido*), penile vasocongestion, erection, orgasmic contractions, and ejaculations (referred to as *potency*).[15,16] Testosterone plays an important role in male libido and sexual behavior, and may play some role in penile erection. Elderly men show a strong correlation between advancing age and diminishing bioavailable serum testosterone levels.[17,18] Testosterone progressively declines after the seventh decade, partly because of testicular and hypothalamic-pituitary dysfunction.[19]

Male sexual dysfunction, denoting the inability to achieve a satisfactory sexual relationship, may involve inadequacy of erection or problems with emission, ejaculation, or orgasm. *Erectile dysfunction* is the inability to achieve and maintain a firm erection sufficient for satisfactory sexual performance.[20] *Premature ejaculation* refers to uncontrolled ejaculation before or shortly after entering the vagina. *Retarded ejaculation* usually is synonymous with delayed ejaculation. *Retrograde ejaculation* denotes backflow of semen into the bladder during ejaculation due to an incompetent bladder neck mechanism.

The neurologic structures in the brain most closely associated with sexual function and arousal are the limbic system and the hypothalamus. The psychogenic sexual arousal mechanism involving sensory organs (e.g., vision, auditory, olfactory, tactile) and imaginative stimuli participate in sexual function through the hypothalamus and limbic systems. Subsequent nerve transmission down the spinal cord to the autonomic nervous system and sacral and thoracolumbar centers mediates the penile erection. Furthermore, the reflexogenic mechanism of penile erection (stimulation of the genital area) also involves nerve transmission by the pudendal nerve to the sacral erection center. Neurotransmission in the peripheral nervous system is mediated by adrenergic and cholinergic stimulation and may be diminished in advanced age.[21] Neurochemical mediators also are involved with sexual function. For example, dopamine is associated with sexual arousal (stimulation), whereas serotonin has an inhibitory effect.[22,23] In the elderly, reduced onset of sexual arousal may be attributed to global cerebrovascular disease and diminished sensory input to the central nervous system (CNS). Peripheral mechanisms of sexual arousal also may be affected by aging.

Erectile dysfunction was once regarded as a psychosocial disorder. The cause of erectile dysfunction today is regarded as a variety of medical, psychological, and lifestyle factors. According to data from the Massachusetts Male Aging Study (MMAS), the combined prevalence of minimal, moderate, and complete erectile dysfunction among all elderly men is 52%.[24,24A] According to the Baltimore Longitudinal Study of Aging, erectile dysfunction was a problem in 8% of all healthy men by age 55, and the prevalence of erectile dysfunction increased to 25%, 55%, and 75% for men 65, 75, and 80 years of age, respectively.[25] Erectile dysfunction is estimated to affect as many as 30 million men in the United States. Five percent of males aged 45 years or older in the United States seek prescription drug therapy for erectile dysfunction, on an annual basis.[24B] By the year 2005, it is estimated that moderate to severe erectile dysfunction will to affect >50 million men.[15]

Approximately 80% of all cases of erectile dysfunction now are thought to be related to organic disease and subject to numerous influences.[15,26–28] In one study,[18] neurologic and vascular disorders were the primary causes of erectile dysfunction among elderly men, and psychogenic factors were the cause in <10%. The single most common etiology for erectile failure in the elderly is severe atherosclerosis (e.g., vascular disease and diabetes mellitus).[18] Cardiovascular disease, hypertension, diabetes mellitus, elevated low-density lipoprotein cholesterol, and cigarette smoking are associated with a greater probability of complete erectile dysfunction in men.[24] Therefore, prevention of cardiovascular disorders by interventions such as low-fat and low-cholesterol diets and abstinence from tobacco should minimize the development of geriatric sexual erectile dysfunction.

Different physiologic mechanisms are involved in erection, emission, ejaculation, and orgasm. Except for nocturnal emissions, ejaculation requires stimulation of the external genitalia. Ejaculation occurs in three phases. The first phase is termed emission. Efferent signals traveling in the hypogastric nerve activate secretions and transport sperm from the distal epididymis, vas deferens, seminal vesicles, and prostate to the prostatic urethra (Fig. 101-1). The second phase is the coordinated closing of the internal urethral sphincter and the relaxation of the external sphincter to direct the semen into the bulbous urethra. The coordinated closing of the internal sphincter and relaxation of the external sphincter is mediated by α- and β-adrenergic stimulation. The third phase, external ejaculation, involves the somatomotor efferent segment of the pudendal nerve to contract the bulbocavernosus muscle, which forces the semen through a pressurized conduit, the much-narrowed urethral lumen compressed by the engorged corpora cavernosa and corpus spongiosum (Fig. 101-2), to produce 2 to 5 mL of ejaculate.[27] In the elderly male, ejaculation is less vigorous and the total ejaculate is likely to be reduced.[29]

The hemodynamics of penile erection involve the pudendal artery (the major blood supply to the penis), of which the terminal portion divides into three branches: (1) the bulbourethral artery, (2) the dorsal artery, and (3) the cavernous artery. The cavernous artery supplies the corpora cavernosa; the dorsal artery, the glans penis; and the bulbourethral artery, the corpus spongiosum. The corpora cavernosa and the corpus spongiosum (also referred to as *corporal smooth muscle*) are the erectile muscle tissues and appear to be under β-

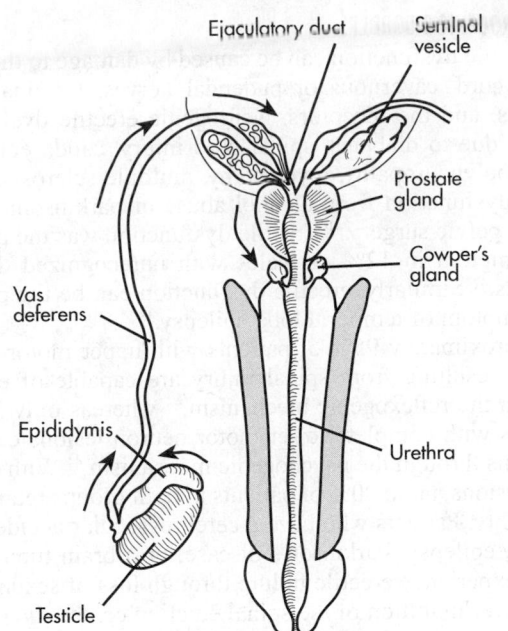

FIGURE 101-1 A diagram showing the sources and direction of seminal flow. (Reproduced with permission from reference 301.)

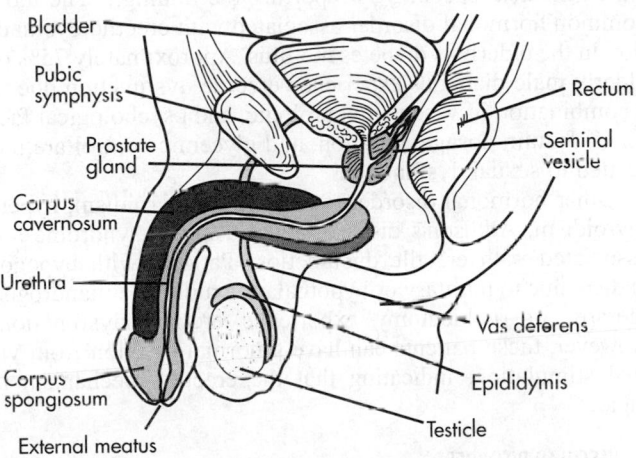

FIGURE 101-2 A diagram showing the relations of the bladder, prostate, seminal vesicles, penis, urethra, and scrotal contents. (Reproduced with permission from reference 301.)

adrenergic control.[15,27] Thoracolumbar or sacral erection-center stimulation shunts the blood to these structures and an erection ensues. The sympathetic nervous system also is involved in the constriction of veins in the erectile tissue that diminishes venous outflow. The resultant high intracavernous (IC) pressure converts a soft, flaccid organ to a blood-distended erect penis. Distention of the erectile tissue further results in compression of the venules, reducing the venous capacity to minimum, which allows full erection of the penis. These actions maintain erection in the corpora cavernosa without diverting too much cardiac output for penile erection.[30]

The biochemical basis of erection is simply an extension of the neuronal physiologic mechanisms. The erectile system involves neural initiation, cellular translation, and vascular transduction. Central initiation of an erection involves erectogenic stimuli (tactile) and/or erotic imagery at the cerebral cortex. The nuclei that integrate erectile signaling are highly specific.[31] The medial preoptic area (MPOA) of the hypothalamus may be the integration for the central control of erection. It receives sensory impulses from the amygdala that have inputs from cortical association areas.[31A] The signals generated follow the spinal pathways and create an erection through receptor interaction and cellular mechanisms in the vasculature in the periphery. As a result of erectogenic or erotic activity, dopamine, acting via the D_2-receptor, is the initiating neurotransmitter. Inhibitory stimuli such as anxiety can dampen the response or the dopaminergic system.

The cellular mechanisms that control the vascular response necessary for penile erection are similar to equivalent mechanisms elsewhere in the vasculature. Cellular mechanisms are designed to induce vascular relaxation and thus cause an erection. There are essentially two cellular factors that are believed to induce vascular relaxation. The first factor, prostaglandin E_1, which is released at the local level as a result of the spinal pathway message, causes adenyl cyclase to accelerate the production of cyclic adenosine monophosphate (cAMP) and results in intracellular release of potassium, a known vasodilator. A second factor involves the release of nitric oxide from local neuronal tissue. Nitric oxide is the main neurotransmitter mediating erection. Once called endothelium–derived relaxing factor, nitric oxide has been shown to induce relaxation of vascular smooth muscle.[6] Nitric oxide induces the formation of cyclic guanosine monophosphate (cGMP) in the vascular system; cGMP is postulated to activate protein G, leading to the phosphorylation of proteins regulating corporal smooth muscle through ion channel changes.[32] This results in the opening of potassium channels and hyperpolarization of the muscle cell membrane, sequestration of intracellular calcium by the endoplasmic reticulum, and blocking of calcium influx by calcium channel inhibition.[32A] Nitric oxide is released by endothelial cells and efferent neuronal cells in response to erectogenic stimuli.

The major arteries needed for an erection are the feeder pelvic vessels and the penile vessels themselves. In all of these components, there are multiple competing systems in a state of balance. The final vascular consequence of these actions depends on the intracellular response and the interaction of the vascular wall complex (smooth muscle, endothelium, nerves plus the effects of stromal and luminal blood pressure). The vascular wall complex is the interplay of vasodilators (prostaglandin E_1, nitric oxide, potassium), the inhibition of the vasoconstrictor mechanisms, and the resultant relaxation of the vascular wall.[33]

The process of orgasm is the least understood sexual process. Simultaneous with emission and ejaculation are involuntary rhythmic contractions of the anal sphincter, hyperventilation, tachycardia, and elevation of blood pressure. Because erectile dysfunction is more likely in male patients with coronary artery disease, the understanding of the cardiovascular stresses involved with sexual intercourse can aid in patient management. Cardiac and metabolic expenditures during sexual intercourse vary depending on the type of sexual activity. Healthy males with their usual female partners generally achieve a peak heart rate of 110 beats/minute with woman-on-top coitus and an average peak heart rate of 127 beats/minute with man-on-top coitus.[34] There is significant individual variation in cardiovascular response, when measured as oxygen uptake and metabolic expenditures, for male-on-top coitus.

In a study of medication-free patients with coronary artery disease who were in the New York Heart Association functional class I or II, sexual activity was compared with near-maximal exercise treadmill test.[35] Electrocardiographic changes representing ischemia during intercourse were found in one-third of the patients; however, two-thirds of these patients remained asymptomatic. All patients with ischemia during coitus also demonstrated ischemia during exercise treadmill testing. The average heart rate during coitus was 118 beats/minute, with some patients attaining a heart rate of 185 beats/minute at orgasm. Intercourse in patients with coronary artery disease may provoke increased ventricular ectopic activity that is not necessarily elicited by other stimuli.[36] These electrocardiographic changes and associated symptoms can be abolished with the use of β-blockers.[37] Sexual activity is a likely contributor to the onset of myocardial infarction only 0.9% of the time.[38] Coital death is rare, accounting for 0.6% of sudden death cases.[39] The hemodynamic changes associated with sexual activity may be far greater with an unfamiliar partner, in unfamiliar settings, and after excessive eating and alcohol consumption.

Erectile Dysfunction
Pathogenesis
Erection involves the neurologic, psychological, hormonal, arterial, and venous systems. In a study of 1,500 elderly men over a period of 10 years, organic erectile dysfunction was diagnosed in >1,050 subjects.[40] As a result of research in vascular physiology, neurophysiology, and neuropharmacology of the penis, most urologists today believe that up to 80% of elderly erectile dysfunction cases are organic in origin and that the remainder are due to psychological factors[41] (Table 101-1). In most elderly male sexual dysfunction studies, 50% involve vascular problems, and 30% relate to diabetes mellitus.[41A]

Table 101-1 Causes of Impotence

Vascular	Iatrogenic
Atherosclerosis	Pelvic radiation
Penile Raynaud's phenomenon	Lumbar sympathectomy
Neurologic	Prostatectomy
	Renal transplantation
Cerebrovascular accident	Spinal cord resection
Spinal cord damage	**Psychogenic**
Autonomic neuropathy	
Peripheral neuropathy	Performance anxiety
Endocrine	Depression
	Widower's syndrome
Diabetes mellitus	
Hypogonadism	
Prolactinomas	
Hyperthyroidism	
Hypothyroidism	

Adapted with permission from reference 74.

NEUROGENIC DISORDERS
Erectile dysfunction can be caused by damage to the brain, spinal cord, cavernous or pudendal nerves, terminal nerve endings, and the receptors. Neurogenic erectile dysfunction can be due to diabetes, spinal cord injury, cauda equina lesions, polyneuropathy, myelopathy, multiple sclerosis, dorsal nerve dysfunction from alcohol abuse or parkinsonism, and radical pelvic surgery.[41] Erectile dysfunction was the presenting symptom in 12% of males with unrecognized diabetes mellitus.[42] Similarly, erectile dysfunction can be the presenting symptom of temporal lobe epilepsy.[43]

Approximately 95% of patients with upper motor neuron lesions resulting from spinal injury are capable of erection through the reflexogenic mechanism,[44] whereas only 25% of patients with complete lower motor neuron lesions can have erections through the psychogenic mechanism.[44] With incomplete lesions, up to 90% of patients in both groups retain erectile ability. Patients who have a cerebrovascular accident, dementia, epilepsy, Parkinson's disease, or a brain tumor most likely experience erectile failure through loss of sexual interest or overinhibition of the spinal erection centers.[41]

HORMONAL DISORDERS
The incidence of erectile dysfunction with a hormonal cause has been estimated to be 5% to 35%, depending on which medical specialty is reporting the finding.[45] The most common hormonal disorder associated with erectile dysfunction in the elderly is diabetes mellitus. Approximately 75% of elderly male diabetics experience erectile dysfunction due to a combination of vascular, neurologic, and psychological factors.[46] Insulin dosage, duration, and glycemic control are unrelated to sexual dysfunction.

Other hormonal disorders such as hypothyroidism, hyperthyroidism, Addison's disease, and Cushing's syndrome are associated with erectile dysfunction. Patients with hypogonadism due to pituitary or hypothalamic tumors, antiandrogen therapy, or orchiectomy experience erectile dysfunction. However, these patients can have a normal erection from visual stimulation, indicating that the erectile mechanism is intact.[47]

VASCULAR DISORDERS
Atherosclerosis is the leading vascular disease associated with male erectile dysfunction. The age of onset of coronary artery disease parallels the onset of erectile dysfunction, indicating a generalized atherosclerotic etiology for the erectile dysfunction.[48] However, the degree of arteriolar narrowing and clinical presentation differs from patient to patient. Some patients can have severe coronary artery disease but retain the capability of a full erection. As long as the arterial flow into the penis exceeds the venous outflow, the patient can be potent. Narrowing of the arterial lumen lowers pressure in the cavernous arteries, and poor arterial flow can only partially fill the sinusoidal system. Overall, the partial filling of the sinusoidal system causes inadequate expansion of the sinusoidal wall, resulting in partial compression of the venules. The net effect is a partial erection, difficulty in maintaining an erection, or the most common complaint, early detumescence. Intrapenile arterial disease resulting from diabetes mellitus, atherosclerosis, or aging does not respond to present surgical techniques.

Signs and Symptoms

1. F.M., a 66-year-old man, was referred to a urologist because he was experiencing a loss of interest in sexual activity. He describes the inability to maintain a firm erection for the past 6 months in >75% of sexual attempts with his sexual partner. Physical examination was unremarkable except for an enlarged prostate gland and evidence of pubic and axillary hair loss. Vital signs were as follows: blood pressure (BP), 160/95 mm Hg; pulse, 88 beats/min; respirations, 14 breaths/min; and temperature, 98.7°F. Current medications include ramipril 5 mg/day and glyburide 5 mg/day. F.M.'s medical history is positive for cigarette smoking, hypertension, and diabetes mellitus. Significant laboratory results include the following: random blood sugar, 200 mg/dL (normal, 70 to 110); serum creatinine (SrCr), 1.5 mg/dL (normal, 0.6 to 1.2); blood urea nitrogen (BUN), 22 mg/dL (normal, 8 to 18); free testosterone level, 30 pg/mL (normal, 52 to 280); luteinizing hormone (LH), 4 MU/mL (normal, 1 to 8); follicle-stimulating hormone (FSH) level, 40 mIU/mL (normal, 4 to 25); and serum prolactin level, 28 ng/mL (normal, <20). What signs and symptoms does F.M. have that would suggest the need for a complete medical workup for erectile dysfunction?

[SI units: glucose, 11.1 mmol/L (normal, 3.9 to 6.1); SrCr, 132.6 μmol/L (normal, 50 to 110); BUN, 7.9 mmol/L urea (normal, 3.0 to 6.5); LH, 4 IU/L (normal, 1 to 8); FSH, 40 IU/L (normal, 4 to 25); serum prolactin, 28 μg/L (normal, <20)]

F.M. presents with the complaint of loss of interest in sexual activity and the inability to maintain a full erection during >75% of sexual encounters with his partner. On physical examination, F.M. is found to have a noticeable loss of pubic and axillary body hair. With longstanding androgen deficiency, there may be loss of hair in the androgen-dependent areas of the body, fine wrinkling of the skin around the mouth and eyes, noticeable loss of muscle mass and strength, altered body-fat distribution, and osteoporosis. In contrast, overt hypogonadism results in a change in the pattern of pubic hair from the male diamond shape to the female inverted triangle appearance. At this point it appears that F.M.'s loss of pubic and axillary hair is the result of androgen deficiency, with the cause yet to be determined. The laboratory results for gonadal function coincide with what is expected in an elderly male with erectile dysfunction (see Question 4).

Urologic Workup

2. What clinical evaluations and laboratory tests should be included in the medical workup of F.M. to determine the cause of his erectile dysfunction?

A detailed medical and sexual history and thorough physical examination are essential in the evaluation of sexual dysfunction. General medical history and physical examination should consider drug-induced erectile dysfunction (Table 101-2); cigarette smoking (cigar and pipe tobacco have not been associated with sexual dysfunction); prior surgery (e.g., transurethral resection of prostate [TURP], aortoiliac bypass, prostatectomy); prior physical trauma (e.g., herniated disc,

Table 101-2 Common Drug-Induced Alterations in Sexual Response

Drug Categories	Clinical Considerations
Antihypertensives	
Diuretic	
Thiazides	Temporal association with sexual dysfunction. Reported incidence varies between 0 and 32%[283-287]; however, impotence generally is not considered common. Mechanism believed to be a "steal syndrome" whereby blood is routed from erectile tissues to skeletal muscle.[84]
Spironolactone	Associated with ↓ libido, impotence, and gynecomastia. Mechanism may be hormone related. Incidence is dose related and reported to be 5–67%[84,288,289] and much more commonly encountered than with the thiazides. May be due to antiandrogen effects of drug.
Sympatholytics	
Methyldopa	Central action mediated causing vasodilation resulting in erectile dysfunction. Reported incidence: 10%.[84,88] Also ↓ libido.
Clonidine	Induces erectile dysfunction. Mechanism similar to methyldopa and other central α₂-agonists. Incidence reported to be 4–70% and dose related.[290-292] Also ↓ libido.
Guanabenz, guanfacine	Incidence and mechanism believed to be similar to other central α₂-agonists.
Nonselective β-Blockers	
Propranolol	Associated with erectile dysfunction and ↓ libido. Mechanism believed to be due to ↓ vascular resistance and central effects. Erectile dysfunction reported to begin at doses of 120 mg/day. Incidence may be as high as 100% at higher dosages.[81,88,293]
Selective β-Blockers	
Atenolol, metoprolol, pindolol, timolol (drops)	Incidence of erectile dysfunction is significantly less than nonselective β-blockers.[294]
α-Blockers	
Doxazosin, prazosin, terazosin	Associated with erectile dysfunction and priapism.[60,295] Reported incidence: 0.6–4%.[296] Mechanism is local α₁-blockade resulting in vasodilation. Erectile dysfunction and priapism appears to be unique to the nonspecific α₁-antagonists.
Phenoxybenzamine	Associated with priapism, retrograde ejaculation, and inhibited emissions during erection. Effects are dose related.[297,298]

Continued

Table 101-2   Common Drug-Induced Alterations in Sexual Response—cont'd

Drug Categories	Clinical Considerations
Direct Vasodilators	
Hydralazine	Associated with erectile dysfunction. Mechanism is vascular smooth muscle relaxation. Incidence not reported.[297]
Calcium Channel Blockers	
Nifedipine	Associated with erectile dysfunction. Mechanism believed to be vasodilation and possibly muscle relaxation. Reported incidence: <2%.[74]
Diltiazem, verapamil	Similar to nifedipine. Reported incidence: <1%.
Antiarrhythmics	
Class 1A	
Disopyramide	Associated with erectile dysfunction in patients treated for ventricular arrhythmias. Incidence not reported. Mechanism believed to be due to strong anticholinergic effect.[84,297]
Anticonvulsants	
Carbamazepine, phenytoin	May be associated with sexual dysfunction through decreasing DHEA, which is a precursor to testosterone, estrogen, and pheromones.[248]
Antidepressants	
Selective serotonin reuptake inhibitors	Drugs with prominent serotonin agonist effects commonly cause delayed ejaculation and anorgasmia. The reported incidence for delayed ejaculation among men is 2–12%; for anorgasmia among women users, the incidence appears to be <3%. This adverse effect is directly dose related.[248]
Tricyclic antidepressants (TCAs), monoamine oxidase inhibitors	Associated with impairment of sexual performance in both male and female: ↓ libido, anorgasmia, retrograde ejaculation, erectile dysfunction. Mechanism believed to be due to anticholinergic and serotonergic effects. Incidence not reported; several case studies in the literature.[21]
Trazodone	Associated with priapism in men and ↑ libido in women. Mechanism similar to TCAs. Incidence not reported but believed to be dose related.[21] (Note: The literature reports that overall there is less sexual dysfunction with desipramine than with other antidepressants.)
Antipsychotics	
Phenothiazines	Frequently associated with sexual dysfunction. Commonly, ↓ libido is reported. Mechanism is due to hyperprolactinemia secondary to central dopamine antagonism. Thioridazine is the most often reported offender. Erectile and ejaculatory pain are very common with this drug class; the α-antagonism and anticholinergic effects are responsible. Priapism is common with this drug group, owing to the peripheral α-blockade property. Incidence for all sexual dysfunction with this drug class: approximately 50% of users.[21]
Anxiolytics	
Short-acting barbiturates	Biphasic effect. At low doses, libido ↑, similar to ethanol, and at higher doses, CNS depression causes ↓ libido and performance.[21]
Benzodiazepines	Biphasic effect. At low doses, ↑ libido, whereas at higher dosages, CNS depression causes performance failure. Some reports of anorgasmia (men and women) and ejaculatory failure.[21]
Substances of Abuse	
Alcohol	Alcohol is thought to impair sexual function through its chronic effects on the nervous system. Short-term use of alcohol can induce erectile dysfunction through its sedative effects. More than 600 mL alcohol per week increases the probability of erectile dysfunction.[212]
Cocaine	Biphasic effect. At low doses, there is enhanced sexual desire (similar to amphetamines) and possibly performance. At higher dosages, there may be arousal dysfunction, ejaculatory dysfunction, anorgasmia. Freebasing has been associated with spontaneous orgasm. Continued use ("on a run") causes significant loss of sexual interest and performance ability. Chronic use associated with hyperprolactinemia resulting in ↓ libido.[21]
Ethanol	At low doses actually may enhance libido. Sexual dysfunction is dose related and due to CNS depressant effects.[84,88,295]
Hallucinogens	Biphasic effect for most drugs in this category. At low doses, libido is enhanced; at higher doses, libido is severely ↓. No reports on chronic use.[21]
Marijuana	Biphasic effect similar to ethanol. With chronic use there is a ↓ in libido. Mechanism may be due to ↓ testosterone. Incidence not reported.[21]
Opioids	Associated with sexual dysfunction: erection lubrication, orgasm, and ejaculation. Chronic use associated with ↓ libido. Mechanism may be due to α-antagonism, alterations in testosterone, and the intoxicating effects. Incidence not reported.[83,88,295,299]
Miscellaneous	
Amyl nitrate	Associated with intense and prolonged orgasms in both male and female. Impotence has been reported in some cases due to vasodilation.[21]
Cimetidine, ranitidine	Associated with ↓ libido and erectile dysfunction. Mechanism due to antiandrogen qualities and drug-induced elevation of prolactin. May be dose related.[88,300]
Metoclopramide	Associated with ↓ libido and erectile dysfunction. Mechanism is through CNS dopamine antagonism, resulting in hyperprolactinemia. Incidence not reported.[88]

CNS, central nervous system; DHEA, dehydroepiandrosterone; SSRIs, selective serotonin reuptake inhibitors; TCAs, tricyclic antidepressants.

testicular trauma); voiding dysfunction; visual field defects (visual field changes may be one of the first presenting symptoms of diabetes mellitus, the most common endocrine abnormality associated with male sexual dysfunction and may be associated with pituitary tumor pressure on the optic nerve); femoral artery bruits; testicular atrophy; Peyronie's plaques (a fibrous palpable plaque along the shaft of the penis, causing penile curvature and poor erection distal to the plaque, thought to be caused by atherosclerosis or severe vasculitis); pedal pulses; and neurologic examination. Hormonal and metabolic screening should be included with the history and physical examination.

Although laboratory-based diagnostic procedures are available, it is proposed that sexual function is best assessed in a naturalistic setting with patient self-report techniques. One such self-reporting tool, the International Index of Erectile Function (IIEF), has been demonstrated to address the relevant domains of male sexual function (erectile function, orgasmic function, sexual desire, intercourse satisfaction, and overall satisfaction), is psychometrically sound, and has been linguistically validated in 10 languages.[49]

F.M.'s endocrine status should include assessment of his diabetes, thyroid function tests, and a serum lipid profile. Neuropathy (as well as atherosclerosis) are common findings among male patients with diabetes mellitus, and both are potential causes of erectile dysfunction. Patients experiencing hypothyroidism may have decreased libido, and hypothyroidism is associated with hyperprolactinemia, which can result in an inhibition in the release of testosterone. Elevated serum lipids (e.g., total cholesterol, triglycerides) may be associated with significant vascular damage that could contribute to erectile dysfunction. Diabetes mellitus is best evaluated with a hemoglobin-A1$_c$ as well as a fasting blood sugar.[49A]

The serum concentrations of free testosterone, prolactin, and LH should be evaluated. Testosterone, like all other hormones secreted into the plasma, is available to tissues only in the free form (i.e., unbound to serum proteins, particularly the sex hormone–binding globulin). Only 1% to 2% of testosterone is free and physiologically active; therefore, measurement of the unbound serum testosterone provides the best estimate of biologically available testosterone. Low testosterone serum concentrations are associated with primary and secondary hypogonadism. Primary hypogonadism is associated with testicular disease (e.g., Leydig cell tumors), whereas secondary hypogonadism is the result of pituitary or hypothalamic disease.

The serum prolactin concentration should be determined, because a high serum concentration of prolactin inhibits release of testosterone from the testes. Therefore, a low serum testosterone concentration may be caused by hyperprolactinemia. Hyperprolactinemia may be due to prolactin adenomas, diabetes mellitus, or drug therapy (e.g., neuroleptics, metoclopramide).

LH stimulates testicular steroidogenesis and secretion of testosterone. LH increases the conversion of cholesterol to pregnenolone, a precursor of testosterone. FSH is required for spermatogenesis in early puberty, but is not a required gonadotropin for the maintenance of spermatogenesis in adult men. Normal testicular function depends on stimulation by the gonadotropin LH, which is secreted by the anterior pituitary gland. Consequently, a low normal serum concentration of LH is associated with secondary hypogonadism.

In patients with symptoms of prostatic disease, expressed prostatic secretions (EPS) should be examined because prostate inflammation has been associated with ejaculatory dysfunction. During prostatic inflammation, the EPS contains leukocytes and macrophages, and microscopic examination of the EPS can determine the degree of prostate inflammation. The presence of >20 white blood cells (WBCs) per high-powered field (HPF) in the EPS is abnormal, and indicative of prostatitis. Only about 5% of prostatitis can be attributed to a bacterial infection; the remaining 95% is due to unknown etiologies.

Ideally, assessment of erectile dysfunction should include urologic, endocrinologic, psychiatric, and neurologic evaluations as close together as possible. The chief complaint of erectile dysfunction must be identified carefully and described, because medical intervention is indicated if it occurs over a 6-month period and in >50% of attempts.[27] A detailed history should determine whether erectile dysfunction varies with partners, sexual settings, position, and masturbation, and if morning and nocturnal erections are impaired.

Clinicians should ask the patient to estimate the degree of penile rigidity, especially with regard to the ability for vaginal penetration, and ask about nocturnal penile tumescence to differentiate psychogenic from organic causes of erectile dysfunction. The examiner should ascertain the presence of associated problems (e.g., atherosclerosis, diabetes mellitus) and attempt to correlate these problems to identified concerns with libido, orgasm, and ejaculation. Ideally, the sexual partner should be present during history taking. A pattern of progressive erectile dysfunction often indicates organic cause, whereas a pattern of intermittent episodes of erectile dysfunction with an abrupt onset suggests a psychogenic cause.

Relationship of Medical History and Erectile Dysfunction

3. What is the relationship among hypertension, cigarette smoking, diabetes mellitus, and F.M.'s erectile dysfunction?

HYPERTENSION

Among elderly men, erectile dysfunction most often is due to neurovascular diseases.[18] The high degree of arteriosclerosis among elderly American men is the leading cause of erectile dysfunction.[18,50,51] In the MMAS, heart disease with hypertension and low serum high-density lipoprotein correlated with erectile dysfunction.[15] The hemodynamics of erection can be impaired in patients with myocardial infarction, coronary bypass surgery, cerebrovascular accidents, and peripheral vascular disease.[52–55] In several studies of impotent men, the number of abnormal penile vascular findings significantly increased when the history included hypertension and cigarette smoking.[56–58] In one report, 8% to 10% of all untreated hypertensive elderly males were impotent at the time of diagnosis of hypertension.[59] Control of blood pressure among hypertensive male patients does not necessarily improve erectile function, and antihypertensive medications can have a significant effect on erectile dysfunction and sexual performances (see Table 101-2).[60–62]

CIGARETTE SMOKING

The prevalence of cigarette smoking among men with erectile dysfunction is higher than in the general population.[57,63,64] When the relation between cigarette smoking and erectile physiology was studied in 314 men with erectile dysfunction,[65] smoking was noted to further compromise penile physiology in men experiencing difficulty maintaining erections long enough for satisfactory intercourse. Several investigators report lower penile blood pressure indices, penile arterial insufficiency, and abnormal blood perfusion associated with cigarette smoking.[57,66] Clearly, cigarette smoking is counterproductive in men with existing erectile dysfunction.

DIABETES MELLITUS

Diabetes mellitus clearly has been associated with erectile dysfunction. In the MMAS, male patients with diabetes mellitus were three times more likely to have erectile dysfunction than patients without diabetes.[15] Other investigators using exclusively diabetic populations have found a prevalence of erectile dysfunction as high as 75% among subjects.[67,68] The onset of erectile dysfunction in the diabetic patient occurs at an earlier age when compared with the general population. In a few cases, erectile dysfunction may be the presenting symptom of diabetes mellitus, and in most cases erectile dysfunction follows within 10 years of the diagnosis, regardless of insulin-dependence status.[69,70] Researchers disagree as to the exact contribution of diabetes mellitus to erectile dysfunction, but most of the literature supports an atherosclerotic etiology.[71,72] Other possible causes also include autonomic neuropathy and gonadal dysfunction.[69]

Gonadal Function in Erectile Dysfunction

4. What is the significance of the gonadal function results for F.M.?

GONADOTROPINS

Abnormalities of primary or secondary hypogonadism must be ruled out, particularly in patients with a decreased libido with or without erectile dysfunction. The results of F.M.'s gonadal function tests are relatively normal for an aged male. Testosterone serum levels decline with aging as a result of hypothalamic-pituitary changes or Leydig cell dysfunction. The understanding of changes that take place in the hypothalamic-pituitary level with advancing age is in a state of flux. For some time, most investigators focused on the increased serum concentration of male gonadotropins (LH, FSH), believing that all elderly males had some degree of primary hypogonadism.[73] However, other studies have shown that LH levels in elderly males are lower than the median of that in younger patients.[74] These findings show that LH levels do not increase in response to the decrease in testosterone serum concentrations in the aged male, indicating a defect in the hypothalamic-pituitary axis, leading to secondary hypogonadism.[75] Secondary hypogonadism results when there is a dysregulation of pituitary LH release, resulting in low serum testosterone levels.[41]

TESTICULAR SIZE AND AGING

Testicular size decreases with age; however, the testicular degeneration is sporadic, thereby allowing most elderly men to maintain a normal or slightly decreased sperm output.[73] Overall, spermatogenesis decreases and is accompanied by an increase in serum concentration of FSH. FSH elevation correlates well with a decline in the number of Sertoli cells that secrete inhibin. Inhibin normally decreases FSH.[76]

TESTOSTERONE

As a result of primary or secondary hypogonadism in the elderly male, there is a decline in available testosterone. Approximately 60% to 75% of circulating serum testosterone is bound to a β-globulin known as sex hormone–binding globulin or testosterone-binding globulin. Approximately 20% to 40% of testosterone is bound to serum albumin, and 1% to 2% is unbound, or free. The unbound portion of testosterone is the only active portion of the total serum testosterone concentration. Testosterone serum concentrations are 20% higher in the morning than in the evening, and this should be taken into consideration when evaluating laboratory results. In virtually all cases of male erectile dysfunction, the serum concentration of testosterone should be measured in the morning.

The production of testosterone is regulated by feedback with the hypothalamus and pituitary. The hypothalamus produces gonadotropin-releasing hormone (Gn-RH) in response to low testosterone levels. Gn-RH induces the pituitary to secrete LH and FSH, which in turn stimulate the Leydig cells of the testes to secrete testosterone. Less than 10% of cases of erectile dysfunction studied are due strictly to hypogonadism.[18,77] The role of testosterone in male erectile dysfunction is complex. After testosterone production decreases, libido eventually declines and precedes the decrease in frequency of erections.[78] Men given antiandrogens maintain their erectile capacity but have a decreased libido.[79] On the other hand, high dosages of androgens given to hypogonadal males clearly increase both the frequency of erections and libido.[80] It would seem reasonable to postulate that at physiologic levels, testosterone modulates the cognitive processes associated with sexual arousal more than it contributes to erectile capability.

ENDOCRINE DISORDERS

Many endocrine disorders can result in erectile dysfunction. Patients with prolactinomas commonly have erectile dysfunction, but prolactinomas account for <1% of erectile dysfunction cases.[81] Prolactin inhibits the release of testosterone, resulting in secondary hypogonadism. Hyperprolactinemia may be more prevalent in diabetic patients.[82] However, in the elderly, hyperprolactinemia often is secondary to the use of medications. F.M.'s serum prolactin level is elevated, most likely due to his diabetes mellitus.

In summary, aged males have a decrease in testosterone due to defects at the testicular and hypothalamic-pituitary function. Secondary hypogonadism in elderly males is quite common, and the point at which this becomes pathologic has not yet been established. Correspondingly, the use of hormonal therapy to treat physiologic secondary hypogonadism is extremely controversial. Therefore, the gonadal function tests for F.M. are normal for his age and do not provide an explanation for his erectile dysfunction.

Medications That Cause Erectile Dysfunction

5. What medications are known to contribute to male erectile dysfunction? Is it likely that a medication is causing F.M.'s erectile dysfunction?

Several general statements can be made regarding sexual function and medications. Drugs that affect libido generally have a central mode of action. For example, medication that blocks central dopamine transmission can decrease libido, and opiates have an antiandrogen effect.[83] Drugs that alter hemodynamics may interfere with erection. Excessive sympathetic tone is thought to cause the "steal syndrome," which increases blood flow to muscles, drawing blood away from the erectile tissue.[84] Drugs that block the peripheral sympathetic system may cause retrograde ejaculation, or no ejaculation at all. There are numerous drugs that have been associated with altering sexual function[85] (see Table 101-2).

Few studies exist in the literature that are solely devoted to drug-induced erectile dysfunction or sexual dysfunction.[61,62] However, a few studies and review articles list medications as one of many potential causes for male erectile dysfunction.[15,22,25,41,86] Most studies documenting drug-induced erectile dysfunction have been subjective and based on case reports, uncontrolled studies, and clinical impressions. Nevertheless, 16 of the most common 200 drugs prescribed in the United States have been reported to cause erectile dysfunction.[87]

In a study (MMAS) from the New England Research Institute at Boston University Medical Center, complete erectile dysfunction was most significant for smokers being treated with cardiac drugs.[15A] In this study, erectile dysfunction was statistically correlated with antihypertensive, vasodilator, cardiac, and hypoglycemic drugs. The probability of moderate as well as complete erectile dysfunction was particularly high for vasodilator drugs.[15] Although the MMAS is one of the most well-designed studies to date, the medications reported are not considered to be the universe of all medications associated with erectile dysfunction. Diagnosis of drug-induced sexual dysfunction should be restricted to a reproducible dose-related effect that disappears on discontinuation of the drug.[88] A much larger survey of a controlled study in a clinical population would be required to establish any suspect medication as causative, rather than temporal.

F.M.'s sexual dysfunction (e.g., loss of interest in sexual activity and erectile dysfunction) is not due to his current drug regimen, ramipril and glyburide. Even though the MMAS[15] reported a correlation between the use of antihypertensives and hypoglycemic drugs with erectile dysfunction, clinicians must look at the individual drugs themselves and the conditions for which they are prescribed. Sexual dysfunction has not been reported for ramipril, or any of the other angiotensin-converting enzyme (ACE) inhibitors, or for the hypoglycemic agent, glyburide. Although ramipril is an antihypertensive, its pharmacologic effects do not contribute to a decline in libido or cause erectile dysfunction (an advantage that ACE inhibitors have over other antihypertensive medications). Similarly, the pharmacologic action of glyburide does not contribute to F.M.'s decreased libido or erectile dysfunction. In most sexual dysfunction cases, it is less likely that the medication is the direct cause of the problem; rather, it is the medical condition for which the drugs were prescribed. The ability of a drug to induce sexual dysfunction simply is an extension of its pharmacologic actions. As a general rule, drugs that manipulate the sympathetic or the parasympathetic system, both centrally and peripherally, are associated with sexual dysfunction.

F.M. is a hypertensive diabetic patient who smokes cigarettes. These three factors (hypertension, diabetes, cigarettes) are more likely to be the cause of F.M.'s sexual dysfunction than are his medications. Again, in the MMAS[15] study, cigarette smoking combined with hypertension was determined to be the most significant cause of male erectile dysfunction. Diabetes mellitus is the most common hormonal disorder associated with erectile dysfunction in the elderly population.[46] The continued loss of interest in sexual activity experienced by F.M. most likely is the result of having experienced erectile dysfunction during past and present sexual events.

F.M.'s subjective and objective findings are quite common among elderly men. His sexual dysfunction is due to atherosclerosis and possible neuropathy secondary to diabetes mellitus. Since cigarette smoking is no doubt contributing to F.M.'s erectile dysfunction, cessation should be recommended; some improvement can be expected.[21] There is no need to alter F.M.'s drug regimen.

Management

Essentially, there are three levels to the management of erectile dysfunction. Level I mandates lifestyle and drug therapy modifications. Specifically, the patient should be instructed to modify smoking and alcohol use. The patient's drug regimen should be checked periodically to assure that drugs associated with ED are not being prescribed. If necessary, psychosocial counseling should be provided. After careful consideration, oral medications for management of ED should be instituted. If Level I therapies have failed or are not acceptable to the patient, then Level II therapy is instituted. These interventions include a vacuum construction device to elicit an erection, intracavernosal injections, or transurethral inserts. Level III management involves placement of a penile prothesis.

Pharmacotherapy

Any therapy directed at male sexual dysfunction must include the elimination of drugs causing adverse sexual effects. Drug therapy is directed primarily toward treatment of erectile dysfunction and includes hormonal therapy, bromocriptine, yohimbine, prostaglandin E$_1$, sildenafil, tadalafil, vardenafil, and apomorphine.

TESTOSTERONE

6. **Should F.M. be treated with testosterone?**

Primary hypogonadism with severely deficient serum levels of bioavailable testosterone is the only appropriate indication for the use of androgen hormone therapy.[89] The goal of androgen replacement therapy is to restore potency and libido by maintaining normal serum levels of testosterone.[90] Testosterone has no benefit in the treatment of eugonadal or mildly hypogonadal elderly men and actually may enhance the growth of undiagnosed adenocarcinoma of the prostate or cause further erectile dysfunction.[26] In eugonadal men, testosterone enhances the rigidity of the erection, but does not change the penile circumference.[90A] F.M. would not be a candidate for testosterone therapy.

7. **Which type of patient would benefit from testosterone therapy?**

Unless testosterone deficiency is severe, for example, if free testosterone serum levels are less than 7 to 8 pg/mL, testosterone replacement therapy will not improve the success rate of intercourse.[90B] Testosterone replacement in patients with primary hypogonadism generally restores libido and potency. In some patients with secondary hypogonadism caused by disorders of the hypothalamus or pituitary, Gn-RH analogs can be administered to differentiate between hypothalamic and pituitary abnormalities and to correct testosterone deficiency.[90] Libido and potency then are restored.

8. How should testosterone be used as a treatment for erectile dysfunction?

Testosterone replacement therapy is available in several formulations, including gels, topical body or scrotal patches, and intramuscular injection. In a study by Monga and colleagues,[90C] transdermal testosterone system (Testoderm-TTS) nonscrotal application was determined to provide improved erections and intercourse when compared with Testoderm scrotal patches. In this study, intramuscular testosterone or transdermal testosterone was favorably accepted by the study patients.

Because of poor drug bioavailability, oral testosterone replacement therapy is less effective than parenteral testosterone in achieving normal serum testosterone levels. Oral administration also is associated with a higher incidence of hepatotoxicity and adverse serum lipid effects.[26,91] A long-acting testosterone intramuscular formulation such as the enanthate or the cypionate ester is still considered the regimen of choice for the treatment of primary hypogonadism. A dose of 50 to 400 mg should be administered intramuscularly every 2 to 4 weeks. Side effects of testosterone therapy include early gynecomastia, increases in hematocrit (sometimes to the point of polycythemia), and fluid retention that may worsen hypertension or congestive heart failure (CHF).

Results of several studies have demonstrated that serum testosterone levels are normalized while using transdermal testosterone applications.[92–95] The system normalizes dihydrotestosterone:testosterone ratios and reduces LH levels toward the normal range. The testosterone transdermal (TTD) system is well tolerated, with application site reactions such as pruritus, burnlike blisters, and erythema being the most commonly reported events. Nightly applications of TTD system in men with hypogonadism results in a 24-hour serum testosterone concentration profile that mimics the circadian pattern observed in healthy young men.[78] The adhesive side of the TTD system should be applied to a clean, dry area of the skin on the back, abdomen, upper arms, or thighs. The patient should be instructed to avoid application over bony prominences or on a part of the body that may be subject to prolonged pressure during sleep or sitting (e.g., the deltoid region of the upper arm, the greater trochanter of the femur, and the ischial tuberosity); do not apply to the scrotum. The sites of application should be rotated, with an interval of 7 days between applications to the same site. The area selected should not be oily, damaged, or irritated.

Topical testosterone gel should be applied once daily in the morning to clean, dry skin on the upper arms, shoulders, or abdomen. Topical testosterone gel is available as a 1% gel in unit-dose packets containing a 25-mg or 50-mg dose. The dose can be as high as 100 mg per 24 hours. After the gel has dried on the site of application, it should be protected with clothing to prevent transfer to a nonuser. The patient's hands should be washed.

Commonly reported adverse effects in chronic users include acne, edema, gynecomastia, and dermatologic reactions to injections or transdermal applications of testosterone. The most serious risk of prolonged testosterone use is prostate carcinoma, although the association between high concentrations of testosterone and the risk of prostate carcinoma is controversial.[96,97] Three studies suggest that testosterone replacement therapy is relatively safe in hypogonadism.[98–100] Baseline assessment of the prostate should be done before starting testosterone replacement therapy. This should consist of a transrectal ultrasound, digital palpation of the prostate gland, and analysis of the total and free prostate-specific antigen (PSA) levels. Fine-needle biopsy of the prostate gland may be necessary in some hypogonadal men, because the PSA may not be completely reliable.[101]

BROMOCRIPTINE AND PERGOLIDE

9. Because F.M.'s prolactin serum concentration is 28 ng/mL, should bromocriptine (Parlodel) or pergolide (Permax) be prescribed to decrease his hyperprolactinemia and treat his erectile dysfunction?

[SI unit: prolactin, 28 μg/L]

Hyperprolactinemia may be treated with the ergot alkaloid, bromocriptine, or other dopamine agonists such as pergolide mesylate. Normalization of the serum prolactin level is mandatory if restoration of potency is to be achieved. However, even with normalization of prolactin levels, approximately 50% of elderly male patients are unable to achieve erectile function and desire.[90,91] Bromocriptine therapy may be initiated with twice-daily 1.25-mg doses taken with meals to minimize gastrointestinal upset. Thereafter, doses may be increased weekly, at a rate of no more than 2.5 mg/day. Because bromocriptine is associated with dizziness, drowsiness, hypotension, and cerebrovascular accidents, the patient should be forewarned.[26,90]

Pergolide mesylate, although not approved by the Food and Drug Administration (FDA) for sexual dysfunction, is useful for erectile dysfunction associated with hypogonadism and hyperprolactinemia. Pergolide is many times more potent than bromocriptine. The initial dose is 0.05 mg/day for 2 days; then on the third day, the dose may be increased by 0.1 to 0.15 mg, and every third day thereafter for 12 days. From the twelfth day on, the dose may be increased by 0.25 mg every third day until therapeutic effectiveness is noted. The average dose for pergolide is 1.0 mg three times a day. Maintenance doses of pergolide are administered three times a day to decrease the common side effect, nausea. As with bromocriptine, the patient should be forewarned about hypotension.[90D]

F.M. is not a candidate for treatment with either bromocriptine or pergolide because he does not have secondary hypogonadism, and his erectile dysfunction probably is secondary to atherosclerosis associated with his hypertension, diabetes, and cigarette smoking. Normalizing the prolactin serum level in F.M. would not correct his problem. Furthermore, the elevation of F.M.'s serum prolactin concentration is not significant enough to warrant drug therapy. With only a 50% (or less) response rate to bromocriptine or pergolide in elderly men, the risk of adverse reactions (e.g., dyskinesia, dizziness, hallucinations, dystonia, confusion, cerebrovascular accidents) does not outweigh the benefit of this drug therapy.

SILDENAFIL

10. Would sildenafil citrate (Viagra) be appropriate for F.M.? What are its side effects and contraindications? Does it interact with other drugs?

F.M. has diabetes mellitus and atherosclerosis and therefore is a candidate for sildenafil. In a multicenter, randomized, double-blind, placebo-controlled, flexible dose-escalation study, sildenafil was shown to be effective and well tolerated for erectile dysfunction in men with diabetes.[102] Sildenafil citrate is an orally active and selective inhibitor of cGMP-specific phosphodiesterase type 5, the predominant phosphodiesterase isoenzyme metabolizing cGMP in the corpus cavernosum. Sildenafil facilitates an erection in response to sexual stimulation by enhancing the nitric oxide–induced relaxation of corpus cavernosal smooth muscle. The results of double-blind, placebo-controlled clinical trials in men with erectile dysfunction of various causes have demonstrated that sildenafil significantly improves erectile function and the rate of successful sexual intercourse, with therapeutic outcomes approaching those of normal men of the same age.[103]

The typical dose of sildenafil is 50 mg orally, taken 1 hour before sexual activity. However, sildenafil citrate may be taken anywhere from 4 hours to 0.5 hour before sexual activity. The maximum recommended dosing frequency is once per day. The following factors are associated with increased plasma levels of sildenafil: age over 65 years (40% increase in area under the curve [AUC]), hepatic impairment (e.g., cirrhosis, 80% increase), severe renal impairment (creatinine clearance <30 mL/minute, 100% increase), and concomitant use of potent cytochrome P450 (CYP) 3A4 inhibitors (erythromycin, ketoconazole, itraconazole, 200% increase). Because higher plasma levels may increase both the efficacy and the incidence of adverse events, a starting dose of 25 mg should be considered in these patients. The dose may be increased to 100 mg or reduced to 25 mg. F.M. should be started on 25-mg tablets of sildenafil, and the dose may be increased under strict supervision.

F.M. should be counseled on the adverse effects of sildenafil. The vasodilating action of sildenafil affects both the arteries and the veins, so the most common side effects are headache and facial flushing.[104] Sildenafil causes small decreases in both systolic and diastolic blood pressures, but clinically significant hypotension is rare. Studies of sildenafil and nitrates taken together show much greater drops in blood pressure. For that reason, sildenafil is contraindicated in patients taking long-acting nitrates or short-acting, nitrate-containing medications.[26] In phase II/III studies before FDA approval, >3,700 patients received sildenafil and almost 2,000 received placebo in double-blind and open-label studies. Approximately 25% of patients had hypertension and were taking antihypertensive medications, and 17% were diabetic. In these studies, the incidence of serious cardiovascular adverse effects was similar to the double-blind sildenafil group, the double-blind placebo group, and the open-label group. Twenty-eight patients had experienced a myocardial infarction. When adjusted for patient-years of exposure, there were no significant differences in the myocardial infarction

rates between the sildenafil and the placebo group, and no deaths were attributed to sildenafil.[105,106] Nevertheless, several deaths due to myocardial infarction or arrhythmia have been associated with the use of sildenafil.[106A] Deaths associated with sildenafil (and presumably other PDE5 inhibitors) are most likely due to increased cardiac workload in patients with unstable angina.[106B]

Transient visual anomalies (mostly blue-green color-tinged objects, increased perception of light, and blurred vision) have been reported in patients taking sildenafil, especially at higher dosages (>100 mg). These visual effects appear to be related to the weaker inhibiting action of sildenafil on the enzyme, phosphodiesterase-6 (PDE-6), which regulates signal transduction pathways in the retinal photoreceptors. Sildenafil is 10-fold selective for PDE-5 over PDE-6. In patients with inherited disorders of retinal PDE-6, such as retinitis pigmentosa, sildenafil should be administered with extreme caution.

The vasodilator actions of nitrates are profoundly amplified with concomitant use of sildenafil. This interaction likely applies to all nitrates and nitric oxide donors, regardless of their predominant hemodynamic site of action. Sildenafil also may potentiate the inhaled form of nitrate, such as amyl nitrite, and therefore is contraindicated in patients using this product. Dietary sources of nitrates, nitrites, and L-arginine (the substrate from which nitric oxide is synthesized) do not contribute to the circulating levels of nitric oxide in humans and therefore are unlikely to interact with sildenafil. The anesthetic agent, nitrous oxide, is eliminated unchanged from the body, mostly via the lungs, within minutes of inhalation. It does not form nitric oxide in the human body and does not itself activate guanylate cyclase. As such, there is no contraindication to its use after administration of sildenafil.

It is unknown how much time must elapse from the time a patient takes sildenafil before a nitrate-containing medication might be given without the marked hypotensive effect being produced. On the basis of the pharmacokinetic profile of sildenafil, it can be assumed that the coadministration of a nitrate within 24 hours is likely to produce an exaggerated hypotensive response and therefore is contraindicated. After 24 hours, the administration of nitrates can once again be considered. In patients who may have a prolonged sildenafil half-life, the nitrate-free period must be extended. All patients taking nitrates must be warned of the contraindications and the potential consequences of taking sildenafil in the 24-hour interval after taking a nitrate preparation, including sublingual nitroglycerin. Although sublingual nitroglycerin is short-acting, its use within a 24-hour time period before sexual relations does suggest that it may be needed again after sildenafil-enhanced sexual activity.

Sildenafil is metabolized by both the CYP 2C9 pathway and the CYP 3A4 pathway. Thus, inhibitors of the CYP 3A4 isoenzyme, such as erythromycin or cimetidine, may lead to competitive inhibition of its metabolism; however, CYP 3A4 is a high-capacity pathway. The effects of erythromycin or cimetidine on the half-life and physiologic effects of sildenafil are not known, but clinicians should be warned about the potential interaction.

Inadequate physical sexual stimulation while using any of the PDE5 inhibitors may lead to treatment failure. Adequate sexual stimulation is needed to trigger the events leading to erection.[106C] PDE5-inhibitors cannot initiate an erection, they can only assist in the process. Some patients may need several attempts at sexual stimulation before they are successful with intercourse.

11. Is F.M. a candidate for tadalafil or vardenafil?

TADALAFIL

Similar to sildenafil, tadalafil (Cialis) is a selective inhibitor of phosphodiesterase 5 (PDE5). Tadalafil has several times more affinity for PDE5 than sildenafil.[106D] The clinical significance of this increased affinity for PDE5 is unknown because comparative clinical trials between the PDE5-inhibitors (sildenafil, tadalafil and vardenafil) have not been conducted. However, tadalfil and vardenafil have minimal or no effect on visual disturbance (impairment of blue/green color discrimination), which is well recognized side effect of sildenafil.[106E] Tadalafil's extended half-life of 17.5 hours relative to sildenafil most likely precludes its use in patients with angina or hypertension. Tadalafil is metabolized by the hepatic CYP 3A4 isozyme. Food has no effect on the oral absorption of tadalafil in contrast to sildenafil (bioavailability decreased by 29%). Tadalafil may be advantageous in a subset of patients, based on its shorter onset of action (16 minutes) and 24-hour duration of action.[106F] Specifically, patients with psychogenic or neurogenic ED and those with stable cardiovascular systems may prefer tadalafil because it offers the potential for multiple sessions of intercourse encounters with a single daily dose. F.M. has hypertension that most likely would be affected by tadalafil; therefore, extreme caution is advised. Perhaps the shorter-acting sildenafil would be the PDE5-inhibitor drug of choice for F.M. The warnings regarding the use of nitrates while taking tadalafil are similar to the warnings for sildenafil.

VARDENAFIL

Vardenafil (Levitra) is the third FDA-approved oral PDE5 inhibitor for treatment of erectile dysfunction. Vardenafil, like the other PDE5-inhibitors has an affinity for PDE6 and will therefore cause ocular adverse effects. The warnings regarding the use of nitrates while taking vardenafil are similar to the warnings for sildenafil. Patients using vardenafil may experience headache, flushing, or rhinitis; the incidence of these side effects are dose related.[106G] Vardenafil is metabolized by the hepatic CYP 3A4 isozyme and has a reported half-life of 5 hours.[106H] Thus, drugs known to inhibit the CYP 3A4 isozyme have the potential to prolong its half-life. Vardenafil 10 mg does not impair the ability of patients with stable coronary artery disease to exercise at levels equivalent to or greater than that attained during sexual intercourse.[106I]

12. What other drug therapy is available for F.M.?

YOHIMBINE

Yohimbine is an indole alkaloid derived from the bark of the West African yohimbine tree and has been classified as an aphrodisiac in many pharmacopoeias. Yohimbine hydrochloride is an α_2-adrenergic antagonist that decreases the outward blood flow from the penile corporal tissue. The effectiveness of yohimbine relies on an adequate penile blood supply. It has been used in treating erectile dysfunction among diabetics with some degree of success.[107] In a trial of men with psychogenic erectile dysfunction, yohimbine produced a 47% response rate versus 28% among placebo users.[108] This finding was affirmed in a subsequent study.[109] Men with psychogenic or neurogenic ED impotent men have some response.[107–109] In spite of its modest efficacy, yohimbine is used in patients who do not accept more invasive methods because it is safe, available, and easy to use. Because F.M. is experiencing vasculogenic, neurogenic, and psychogenic erectile dysfunction, his response to yohimbine may be none to slight, at best, owing to his atherosclerosis and resultant low penile blood supply. Again, the risk of side effects compared with the slight benefit that F.M. may experience suggests that other therapies be considered.

In some patients, yohimbine has been associated with nausea, tachycardia, a slight elevation in blood pressure, anxiety, and panic attacks.[91] The drug regimen used in clinical trials is 6 mg orally three times a day, and beneficial effects usually become apparent within 2 to 3 weeks.[22,107,108] In some of the trials, the point was made that the dose of 18 mg/day may be too low; however, dose-response trials would be necessary before higher doses could be recommended.

INTRACAVERNOUS INJECTIONS

In 1982, inadvertent injection of papaverine into the penis was found to produce an erection.[114] This landmark observation ushered in a new methodology for the diagnosis and therapy of erectile dysfunction. By 1986, papaverine injection into the penis had gained worldwide popularity for the treatment of erectile dysfunction.[115] In 1983, the α-blocker, phenoxybenzamine, also was noted to be effective.[116] Shortly thereafter, the combination of papaverine with another vasodilator, phentolamine, reportedly enhanced and prolonged the duration of erection.[117] These vasoactive drugs, when injected into the cavernosa, cause prolonged penile arterial vasodilation and venous compression, thus allowing the patient to achieve and maintain an erection. Erectile dysfunction responds favorably to the self-injection of vasoactive drugs into the penis.[115,118,119] Originally, the intracavernous (IC) regimen of papaverine with phentolamine was prescribed as a short-term measure taken while patients were awaiting the results of counseling or a penile implant. Currently, self-injection of vasoactive drugs has become accepted as a nonsurgical method of treating erectile dysfunction (Table 101-3).

Papaverine–Phentolamine Combination

Papaverine, a nonspecific phosphodiesterase inhibitor, increases the serum concentration of cAMP, resulting in penile arteriolar and corporal sinusoidal smooth muscle relaxation. In laboratory studies, papaverine blocks voltage-operated cal-

Table 101-3	Agents Used to Treat Vasculogenic Male Impotence		
Drugs	*Route*	*Mechanism*	
Papaverine	ICI	Phosphodiesterase inhibitor; penile arteriolar vasodilator	
Phentolamine	ICI	α-Adrenergic blockade; direct vasodilator	
Prostaglandin E₁	ICI	α-Blockade; vasodilator	
Atropine	ICI	Antimuscarinic; smooth muscle relaxant	

ICI, intracavernous injection.

cium channels, inhibits the release and storage of intracellular calcium, increases calcium efflux, and inhibits calcium-activated chloride and potassium currents in vascular smooth muscle.[120–122] Papaverine also may relax an elastic venous valve mechanism that is kept open by an α-adrenergically mediated smooth muscle contraction.[123–125]

Phentolamine exerts its relaxant effects by α-adrenergic receptor blockade of both α_1- and α_2-adrenoceptors. In addition, phentolamine also may have a direct, nonspecific relaxant effect on vessels.[126] The combined use of papaverine with phentolamine exerts a greater effect than would be experienced with either drug alone.[127] The use of alprostadil (prostaglandin E_1) by intracavernous injection is addressed in Question 18.

Candidates for Intracavernous Injection Therapy

13. **What objective data must be obtained to ensure that F.M. can receive IC injections safely?**

Patients who have failed to obtain a satisfactory erection while on oral drug therapy, such as sildenafil, tadalafil, yohimbine, or sublingual apomorphine (available in Europe), are candidates for the IC injections of vasoactive drugs. The patient must have a complete medical workup to include assessment of the penile arterial system. Doppler sonography of the penis identifies penile architecture, defines the thickness of any plaques, measures the diameter of cavernous arteries (before and after vasodilation), and allows visualization of the penile arteries. This noninvasive assessment of the individual penile arteries is much more accurate than the penile brachial pressure index (PBI). The PBI is the ratio of the penile systolic blood pressure (measured by continuous wave Doppler analysis) to the brachial artery systolic pressure. This method of assessment measures all the penile arteries rather than signals from a single penile artery. PBI ratios that are normal (i.e., >0.6) do not always indicate normal penile blood flow, because the PBI is obtained while the penis is flaccid. F.M. should have sonography combined with Doppler analysis to assess the adequacy of his penile arterial blood flow.

In some urologic practices, the functional evaluation of penile arteries is obtained by IC injection of vasoactive drugs at the office. If the patient develops a fully rigid erection within 12 minutes of injection of papaverine hydrochloride 30 to 60 mg or prostaglandin E_1 10 to 20 mg and maintains a rigid erection for 30 minutes, adequate arterial flow and an intact venous mechanism can be assumed.[27] The patient then is a candidate for at-home IC injection of vasoactive drugs.

14. **The Doppler sonography analysis of F.M.'s penile arteries showed severe atherosclerosis, indicating a vasculogenic etiology for his erectile dysfunction. Is F.M. still a candidate for IC injection therapy?**

Patients with psychogenic and/or neurogenic erectile dysfunction who respond to test doses of IC injections of a vasoactive drug are optimal candidates for IC injection therapy.[110] Patients with vasculogenic erectile dysfunction are less responsive to the IC injections of vasoactive drugs, and corporeal veno-occlusive dysfunction is the primary potential obstacle to this treatment.[128,129]

An abnormal veno-occlusive mechanism can result in penile venous incompetence, causing rapid detumescence or partial erection (referred to as venogenic erectile dysfunc-

tion). The veno-occlusive mechanism of the corpora cavernosa can be assessed through an elaborate and quite painful invasive process, using angiocatheters and iodinated contrast media. In a study to determine the effectiveness and safety of IC therapy in vasculogenic impotent men, 40% of the participants had arteriovenogenic erectile dysfunction, and 32% had venogenic erectile dysfunction (i.e., they had a dysfunctional veno-occlusive mechanism), with only 28% of participants having pure arteriogenic erectile dysfunction.[130] However, only 4% of the participants failed to achieve a sustained rigid erection; massive veno-occlusive mechanism dysfunction was cited as the reason. At a mean follow-up of 20 months, the remaining 96% of patients (including those with some degree of veno-occlusive mechanism dysfunction) still were using the IC injection therapy. Given these findings, F.M. has a good chance of responding to IC injection therapy, even if it is determined that he has some veno-occlusive disease. Absolute contraindications to IC injection therapy are anticoagulant therapy, Peyronie's disease, and idiopathic priapism.

Dosing

15. **What is the protocol for starting a patient on an IC injection therapy program for home use?**

The initial dose of the papaverine–phentolamine combination should take into consideration the underlying etiology for the erectile dysfunction, the findings of the Doppler sonography, and the patient's response to a test dose of the IC injection. Generally, patients with neurogenic erectile dysfunction are started on the lowest doses (usually 0.5 mL), whereas patients with severely compromised penile arterial blood flow would receive larger doses (e.g., 1.0 mL). It should be kept in mind that there may be excessive sympathetic stimulation in an anxious patient while at the physician's office, and more drug may be required to overcome the vasoconstriction,[131] This implies that at-home use may require a lower dose. The standard mixture for the most common vasoactive IC injection solution is 30 mg/mL of papaverine and 1 mg/mL of phentolamine, for a total volume of 10 mL. The initial test dose administered in the physician's office generally is 0.5 mL (but may be as low as 0.25 mL) of the 30:1 mixture, using a tuberculin syringe with a 26-gauge needle. The patient is observed for not only therapeutic effects, but also for adverse effects such as bradycardia, hypertension, dizziness, or flushing. If any of these adverse effects are observed, atropine should be injected intracavernously.[132] In the event that the patient's erection becomes prolonged beyond 30 to 60 minutes, the subsequent dose of papaverine–phentolamine should be reduced. Prolonged erection, which may progress to a pulsatile priapism, is the most significant complication of IC injections of vasoactive drugs. Treatment should be instituted immediately with epinephrine 1 mg/mL, 10 to 20 mL injected intracorporeally as an irrigant, and then aspirated.[110] Prolonged erections can lead to intracorporeal hypoxia, resulting in corporeal fibrosis.[132] In some cases, the physician may choose single-drug IC injection with papaverine 25 to 60 mg, or prostaglandin E_1 10 or 20 mg/dose.

Extemporaneous Compounding

16. **What procedures should be taken when extemporaneously compounding a papaverine–phentolamine injectable solution, and what expiration date is acceptable?**

The method used to extemporaneously compound the papaverine–phentolamine mixture was developed in the early 1980s without consideration of pharmaceutic product stability. Nevertheless, the compounding of the papaverine–phentolamine solution has not changed much from those early days. The final product usually consists of a 10-mL vial of papaverine and phentolamine in a ratio of 30:1 mg/mL. Papaverine hydrochloride is available in a 30-mg/mL, 10-mL multidose vial that also contains 0.5% chlorbutanol as a preservative. Phentolamine mesylate (Regitine) is available in vials containing 5 mg of active drug and 25 mg of mannitol, in a sterile lyophilized form. Extemporaneous compounding of this product requires sterile technique. One vial of papaverine and two vials of phentolamine are needed to make the final product. Using a small-gauge needle and 3-mL syringe, remove 2 mL (i.e., 60 mg) from the papaverine vial and use 1 mL to reconstitute the first vial of phentolamine. With the remaining 1 mL of papaverine solution in the syringe, reconstitute the second vial of phentolamine. Using the empty syringe, remove the solution from both phentolamine vials and instill this volume into the 10-mL papaverine multidose vial. Each milliliter of the final concentration in the papaverine vial should contain 30 mg of papaverine hydrochloride with 1 mg of phentolamine mesylate (plus 0.5% chlorbutanol and 5 mg of mannitol).

Currently, the FDA has not approved either papaverine or phentolamine alone or in combination as a treatment modality for erectile dysfunction. The addition of phentolamine mesylate to a multidose vial of papaverine hydrochloride for at-home patient use is not mentioned in the respective manufacturers' package inserts.[133,134] In a product-stability study, the combination of papaverine and phentolamine was stable for at least 40 days when stored at room temperature.[135] In this study, the concentration of papaverine hydrochloride was 25 mg/mL and phentolamine mesylate was 0.83 mg/mL. Thus, the common practice of using a 30-day expiration date on extemporaneously prepared papaverine–phentolamine multidose preparations is justified.

Patient Instructions

17. **What instructions should be provided to the patient for IC injection therapy?**

Once the dose of IC injection vasoactive drug is determined for the patient at the physician's office, the patient then is taught self-injection using a 26-gauge needle, 1-mL syringe.

Patients should be instructed to inject into the right side of the penis (lateral aspect), approximately 4 cm from the glans after the area has been cleaned with an alcohol swab. The tip of the needle should be placed into the center of the right corpus cavernosum with a quick jab. The injection is administered within a 1- to 2-minute period. If pain is felt in the glans penis, the rate of injection should be slowed (next time) to perhaps 3 or 4 minutes. Upon withdrawal of the needle, the puncture site is compressed and the penis should be massaged gently by squeezing intermittently for approximately 3 minutes to distribute the drug throughout the shaft. A tourniquet at the base of the penis is not necessary. Sterile technique should be stressed when discussing this procedure with patients.

The number of injections per month is limited by a 10-mL supply to prevent long-term complications. The 10-mL volume allows patients to have intercourse 10 to 20 times per month if doses of 0.5 to 1 mL are used.

Adverse Effects

18. **F.M. has been using papaverine–phentolamine 30:1 mixture at a dose of 1.0 mL per sexual episode over the past 6 months. He has injected himself 32 times. For the past month, he has noticed a lateral deviation of his penis when rigid, and now he feels a "hard spot" (induration) below the surface of the skin on the shaft. What are the adverse effects associated with repeated use of papaverine–phentolamine IC injections?**

Penile induration and corporeal fibrosis are complications of IC injections, particularly when papaverine hydrochloride is used. The appearance of induration and/or fibrosis significantly correlates to the number of injections administered.[136] Men with penile induration and/or fibrosis injected the papaverine–phentolamine mixture two and one-half times more often than those who did not suffer this side effect. Similarly, men who administered higher doses also were more likely to develop penile induration and/or fibrosis ($P < .01$). Hence, a 10-mL solution of the papaverine–phentolamine combination should be dispensed on a monthly basis to manage not only the frequency of use but the total dose used. The patient should be educated about the complications and side effects of penile injection with vasoactive drugs (Table 101-4).

Corporeal fibrosis, which may result in Peyronie's disease, is the limiting factor with any combination of papaverine, because the relative acidity of the drug (pH, 3 to 4) is associated with sclerosis.[137–140] The frequency of IC papaverine injections should be limited. At least 94% of patients using IC self-injection experience at least one complication, with 70% of users reporting at least two to three complications.[141] Pain at the site of injection is related more to the injection of the drugs than to the insertion of the needle.[142] The pain is described as a burning sensation in the glans penis occurring 30 seconds after the injection begins and lasting for 1 to 2 minutes after the injection is stopped. The most devastating complication, priapism, is experienced by approximately 4% of patients and requires treatment. Of interest, none of the patients who experienced priapism had vasculogenic impotence. Self-administration side effects such as pain, bruising, and swelling usually do not occur when physicians inject the vasoactive drugs into the penis.[136]

Systemic effects of papaverine–phentolamine initially were believed to be insignificant. However, the use of this mixture has been associated with abnormal liver function tests (LFTs) in 40% of recipients, mostly involving mild to moderate elevations of serum alkaline phosphatase and serum

Table 101-4 Side Effects of Papaverine-Phentolamine ICI for Vasculogenic Impotence

Prolonged erection	Penile induration
Priapism	Pain at injection site
Painless penile nodules	Bruising/bleeding at injection site
Peyronie's disease	Abnormal LFTs

ICI, intracavernous injection; LFTs, liver function tests.

lactic dehydrogenase.[136] Hepatotoxicity, which may have an immune mechanism, has been associated with papaverine injection infrequently. A patient may be advised to discontinue the use of this medication if the LFTs are indicative of hepatocellular injury.

The adverse effects from the use of papaverine–phentolamine generally do not prevent continued use of this therapy. However, after an episode of priapism, patients are instructed not to use the injection for at least 1 month.[141] Most patients who have experienced one or more adverse effects (e.g., bruising, pain, fibrosis, priapism) from the papaverine–phentolamine injections generally still resist penile implantation for as long as possible and continue the injection therapy.[141]

Several studies have reported various degrees of satisfaction among users of IC self-injection.[118,119,141] Eventually, most users discontinue the use of IC injection and consider a penile implant. Fortunately, complications resulting from IC injection of vasoactive drugs do not prevent successful prosthetic implantation.[141]

Alprostadil

19. **What other drugs can be used by IC injection in patients who are unresponsive to the papaverine–phentolamine mixture? How is alprostadil used to treat erectile dysfunction?**

Patients with vasculogenic erectile dysfunction are less likely to respond to papaverine–phentolamine by IC injection. These patients generally require larger doses of papaverine–phentolamine and thus are more likely to develop penile induration. However, 96% of patients with vasculogenic erectile dysfunction responded to a four-drug vasoactive mixture of papaverine hydrochloride 12.1 mg/mL, prostaglandin E_1 10.1 mg/mL, phentolamine mesylate 1.01 mg/mL, and atropine sulfate 0.15 mg/mL. The solution was obtained by mixing 250 mg papaverine hydrochloride (14.4 mL), 200 mg of prostaglandin E_1 (0.4 mL), 20 mg of phentolamine mesylate (2 mL), and 3 mg of atropine sulfate (3 mL), for a total of 19.8 mL.[130] Doses administered were from 0.1 to 1.0 mL via a 27-gauge self-injection device.

Prostaglandin E_1 (alprostadil) is available for IC injection, as a urethral insert (referred to as *medicated urethral system for erection* [MUSE]) and as a topical cream. All of these pharmaceutical preparations have been shown to be efficacious for men with erectile dysfunction,[20,144,144A] with users reporting successful intercourse 65% of the time. The efficacy of alprostadil was similar, regardless of the patient's age or the cause of erectile dysfunction, which included vascular disease, diabetes, surgery, and trauma. Prostaglandin E_1 has α-blocking properties mediated through a membrane receptor. It relaxes the cavernous and arteriolar smooth muscle while restricting venous outflow.[110] The addition of an oral α-blocker may have a beneficial effect in patients with erectile dysfunction for whom IC injection therapy alone fails. The synergistic effects of vascular dilation and blockade of sympathetic inhibition may explain this response.[145] Prostaglandin E_1 is an acceptable alternative to papaverine and patients experience few side effects.[146,147] However, the use of intracorporeal papaverine with prostaglandin E_1 has proved to be superior to prostaglandin E_1 alone.[143] Prostaglandin is metabolized in the local tissue and is unlikely to cause any systemic effects.[148] The most common side effects of urethral alprostadil inserts

are penile pain, which occurs in 29% to 49%[148A] of users, and hypotension within 1 hour of use, which occurs in 3.3% of users. Urethral bleeding has been reported in 5% or users. Patients should be advised about hypotension, particularly if they also are using nitrates or antihypertensive medications. Less than 2% of users have reported swelling of leg veins, leg pain, perineal pain, and rapid pulse. Penile induration has not yet been reported with use of prostaglandin E_1.

BENIGN PROSTATIC HYPERPLASIA

Benign prostatic hyperplasia (BPH), a common cause of urinary dysfunctional symptoms in elderly men, results from proliferation of the stromal and epithelial cells of the prostate gland.[149,150] There is both a static and a dynamic component to prostate enlargement. The static component increases the prostate size by smooth muscle cell proliferation in the prostate stroma, whereas the dynamic component contributes to an enlarged prostate through an increase in smooth muscle tone in the prostate and bladder neck. The term *benign prostatic hypertrophy* often is used inappropriately because the prostate gland pathology results from hyperplasia rather than hypertrophy. BPH rarely is detected in males less than 40 years of age. After age 40, the prevalence of BPH is age dependent.[151] Approximately 75% of men who live to the age of 70 develop clinical symptoms of BPH that are sufficiently severe to necessitate medical attention, and approximately 90% of octogenarians have evidence of BPH. Essentially, all men will develop BPH if they live long enough. The microscopic incidence of BPH is fairly constant among several Western and developing countries,[152] suggesting that the initiation of BPH may not be environmentally or genetically influenced. Although BPH and prostatic cancer often coexist, there is no compelling evidence that BPH predisposes patients to the development of prostate cancer.[153] However, the appearance of atypical prostatic hyperplasia correlates with the presence of latent prostatic carcinoma.[154]

The cause of BPH is unclear; however, most hypotheses are based on hormonal and aging processes. This is because intact, normally functioning testes are essential for BPH to develop,[155] and castration before puberty prevents the development of BPH. The prostate is dependent on androgens both for embryologic development and maintenance of size and function in the mature male.[156] Testosterone, the major circulating androgen, is metabolized to dihydrotestosterone (DHT) by 5α-reductase. There are two isoenzymes of 5α-reductase, designated type 1 and type 2. Type 2 is found predominantly in the prostate and other genital tissues, whereas type 1 is found throughout the body, as well as in the prostate.[156A] For testosterone to be active in the prostate, it must be converted to DHT; therefore, DHT is the obligate androgen responsible for normal and hyperplastic prostate growth. Within the prostate, DHT initiates RNA synthesis, protein synthesis, and cell replication. The exact role of testosterone may be only to initiate fibroadenomatous hyperplasia, eventually resulting in glandular enlargement.

Stromal hyperplasia in the prostate periurethral glands is one of the earliest microscopic findings in men with BPH.[152] As males increase in age, testosterone serum concentrations decrease and the peripheral conversion of testosterone to estrogen increases. At one time, estrogens were thought to initiate stromal hyperplasia, which in turn induces epithelial hyperplasia. However, it is now known that estrogens do not have a direct effect on the development of BPH and prostatic carcinoma, but progesterone does play a role in their pathogenesis. Progesterone receptors have been shown to exist in prostate stromal cells, whereas estrogen receptors were essentially nonexistent.[157]

Pathophysiology and Clinical Presentation

20. G.M., a 72-year-old man, presents to the emergency department with severe lower abdominal discomfort of 4 days' duration. He gives a history of having increasing difficulty initiating urination, a significant decrease in the force of his urinary stream, occasional midstream stoppage, and postvoid dribbling. Physical examination is unremarkable except for the abdominal and rectal examination. Abdominal examination reveals distention, tenderness, and increased dullness in the hypogastrium with a large mass, believed to be the bladder. Upon rectal examination, the prostate is found to be severely enlarged, firm, and rubbery without nodules or undue hardness. G.M. gives a history of nocturia (approximately four to five times a night) and daytime urinary frequency (eight to ten times a day). G.M. indicates that when he is able to urinate he does not feel relieved. Laboratory findings are as follows: BUN, 45 mg/dL (normal, 8 to 18); SrCr, 3.2 mg/dL (normal, 0.6 to 1.2); and serum PSA, 7.1 ng/mL (normal, 0.1 to 4.0). A urethral catheter was inserted, and 900 mL of urine was obtained. G.M. subsequently was scheduled for a urologic workup. What is the pathophysiologic basis for G.M.'s symptoms?

[SI units: BUN, 16.1 mmol/L urea; SrCr, 282.9 μmol/L; serum prostatic acid phosphatase, 3 units/L (normal, 2.5 to 11)]

Symptoms of BPH can be both obstructive and irritative, and descriptions of the symptoms need a frame of reference for standardization. The Boyarsky index, a questionnaire consisting of nine questions to quantify the severity of BPH,[158] has been developed. Five questions are designed to assess obstructive symptoms and four to assess irritative symptoms. Although there may be some limitations to the use of this questionnaire (Table 101-5), it is one of the most common measures used to quantify symptoms in BPH studies[152] and it correlates well with the pathophysiology of BPH. The format of the Boyarsky index is designed to help the clinician educate the patient about the obstructive and irritative symptoms of BPH. The Boyarsky index was the first of three patient questionnaires developed to quantitatively assess BPH and the effectiveness of individual treatment.[156] As such, this questionnaire has been used in numerous clinical trials to measure the outcome of interventions. The Boyarsky index is not useful in comparing different treatment therapies among BPH patients, because it has not been sufficiently validated for this purpose; rather, it is useful in evaluating an individual's response to therapy.

The Multidisciplinary Measurements Committee of the American Urologic Association (AUA) also has published a Urinary Symptom Index for Prostatism[159] (Table 101-6). The AUA recognized the importance of a validated symptom index for assessing the baseline severity of prostatism, disease progression, and the effectiveness of different therapies. The

Table 101-5   BPH Symptom Scoring System (Boyarsky Index)[a]

Nocturia

0	Absence of symptoms
1	Urinates 1 time/night
2	Urinates 2–3 times/night
3	Urinates ≥4 times/night

Daytime Frequency

0	Urinates 1–4 times/day
1	Urinates 5–7 times/day
2	Urinates 8–12 times/day
3	Urinates ≥13 times/day

Hesitance (Lasts ≥1 min)

0	Occasional (≤20% of the time)
1	Moderate (20–50% of the time)
2	Frequent (≥50% of the time)
3	Always present

Intermittency (Lasts ≥min)

0	Occasional (≤20% of the time)
1	Moderate (20–50% of the time)
2	Frequent (≥50% of the time)
3	Always present

Terminal Dribbling (At end of voiding)

0	Occasional (≤20% of the time)
1	Moderate (20–50% of the time)
2	Frequent (≥50% of the time)
3	Always present (may wet clothes)

Urgency

0	Absence
1	Occasionally difficult to postpone urination
2	Frequently difficult to postpone urination
3	Always difficult to postpone urination

Impairment of Size and Force of Urinary Stream

0	Absence
1	Impaired trajectory
2	Most of the time size and force are restricted
3	Urinates with great effort and stream is interrupted

Dysuria

0	Absence
1	Occasional burning sensation during urination
2	Frequent (>50% of the time) burning sensation
3	Frequent and painful burning sensation during urination

Sensation of Incomplete Voiding

0	Absence
1	Occasional sensation
2	Frequent (>50% of the time) sensation
3	Constant and urgent sensation, no relief on voiding

[a]Symptom scoring provides the clinician with a tool to measure the relative need for, and efficacy of, different interventions. No specific score is associated with the need for a specific intervention. A low symptom score in the absence of significant urine retention generally indicates that medical management can be attempted before considering surgical intervention.[158]
BPH, benign prostatic hyperplasia.

Table 101-6 **American Urological Association (AUA) Urinary Symptom Index for Prostatism**

	Score					
Symptom	Not at All	<1 In 5 Times	<1/2 the Time	=1/2 the Time	>1/2 the Time	Almost Always
1. Over the past month or so, how often have you had a sensation of not emptying your bladder completely after you finished urinating?	0	1	2	3	4	5
2. Over the past month or so, how often have you had to urinate again <2 hr after you finished urinating?	0	1	2	3	4	5
3. Over the past month or so, how often have you found you stopped and started several times when you urinated?	0	1	2	3	4	5
4. Over the past month or so, how often have you found it difficult to postpone urination?	0	1	2	3	4	5
5. Over the past month or so, how often have you had a weak urinary stream?	0	1	2	3	4	5
6. Over the past month or so, how often have you had to push or strain to begin urination?	0	1	2	3	4	5
7. Over the past month or so, how many times did you most typically get up to urinate from the time you went to bed at night until the time you got up in the morning?	0 times	1 time	2 times	3 times	4 times	5 times

Interpretation of AUA Symptom Index

AUA Symptom Score = Sum of questions 1–7 = _____

Mild prostatism ≤7
Moderate prostatism 8–18
Severe prostatism >18
Highest possible score 35

Reprinted with permission from reference 301.

AUA symptom index allows comparison between therapies and is the preferred questionnaire for BPH research. It has been validated through internal consistency reliability, constructive reliability, test-retest reliability, and criterion reliability.[156] However, the AUA index may not be BPH specific.[160] When 101 men and 96 women between the ages of 55 and 79 used the AUA index, urinary symptoms and severity of urinary symptoms were similar in both groups. Therefore, symptoms associated with prostatism can be associated with aging as well as BPH. The National Institutes of Health (NIH) convened a chronic prostatitis workshop to come to consensus on a new classification system for the diagnosis and management of prostatitis.[161] This group developed a symptom index that provides a valid outcome measure for men with prostatitis. This index attempts to quantify the pain and discomfort associated with prostatism, and should help differentiate prostatism from prostatic hyperplasia. The symptom index is self-administered.

G.M. presents with obstructive symptoms consistent with benign prostatic hyperplasia as follows: (1) a history of difficulty in initiating urination (hesitancy), (2) a decrease in urinary force, (3) occasional midstream stoppage, (4) postvoiding dribbling, and (5) a feeling of incomplete bladder emptying. The common obstructive symptom of decreased force and size of urine stream is due to urethral compression from prostate gland hyperplasia. Hesitancy, another obstructive symptom, is the result of the bladder detrusor muscle taking a longer time to generate the initial increased pressure to overcome urethral resistance. Urinary stream intermittency is due to the inability of the bladder detrusor muscle to sustain the increased pressure until the end of voiding. Terminal dribbling and incomplete emptying occur for the same reason, but also may be due to obstructive prostatic tissue at the bladder neck, causing a "ball valve" effect.

G.M. also has a history of classic irritative symptoms that are consistent with BPH as follows: (1) nocturia approximately four to five times a night and (2) daytime urinary frequency of 8 to 10 times a day. Incomplete emptying of the bladder results in shorter intervals between voiding, explaining the complaint of frequency. Also, a large prostate gland provokes the bladder to trigger a voiding response more frequently. This response is more pronounced if the prostate is growing intravesically and compromising the bladder volume. Bladder detrusor muscle becomes hypertrophied as a result of the greater bladder residual urine volume, which can result in increased detrusor muscle excitability. Clinically, this excitability may result in bladder instability. The symptoms of urinary frequency are more pronounced at night because cortical inhibitions are lessened and bladder sphincter tone is more relaxed during sleep. Obstructive symptoms are associated more with an enlarged prostate, and the predominance of irritative symptoms could suggest voiding dysfunctions in addition to those of BPH.

Urinary incontinence is not a common symptom of BPH. With advanced BPH, a large residual volume of urine in the bladder weakens the bladder sphincter and allows the escape of small amounts of urine, when the bladder is full. As the residual bladder volume increases, the ureters will dilate, resulting in stasis of urine in the ureters. The end result may be ascending hydronephrosis caused by the transmission of high pressure to nephrons, which produces renal damage (Fig. 101-3). This can account for abdominal discomfort and flank pain during voiding and ascending urinary tract infections.

Acute urinary retention in BPH may occur as a result of increasing size of the prostate gland. However, independent of gland size, drugs may precipitate acute urinary retention. Drugs such as alcohol, anticholinergic agents, α-adrenergic agents, and neuroleptics all have been associated with acute urinary retention in men with BPH. Commonly, when advanced BPH is present, acute urinary retention is exacerbated if the patient does not void at the first sign of urgency. G.M. is not taking any drugs commonly associated with urinary retention.

Clinical Findings

21. **What objective findings in G.M. are associated with BPH?**

G.M. presents with classic symptoms of BPH. The increasingly severe symptoms culminated in an episode of acute urinary retention as evidenced by inability to void and lower abdominal discomfort. Objective symptoms associated with

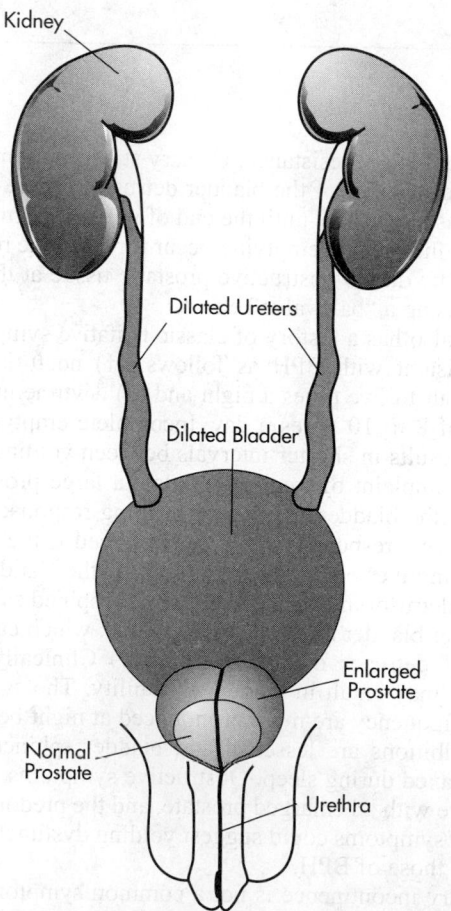

FIGURE 101-3 Flow of urine (color) is interrupted by compression from a prostate that has enlarged from normal size. In this diagram, the ureters and bladder are dilated by backed-up urine.

G.M.'s BPH are as follows: (1) abdominal tenderness with increased dullness in the hypogastrium; (2) the finding of an enlarged bladder; (3) an enlarged, firm, and rubbery prostate gland; and (4) a return of 900 mL of urine via urinary catheter. The normal serum acid phosphatase, normal PSA, and digital rectal examination of the prostate suggest that G.M. does not have prostatic carcinoma at this time (see following section). The elevated BUN and serum creatinine may suggest hydronephrosis as a result of his BPH.

Urinalysis

Because BPH patients also may have a urinary tract infection, a urinalysis with microscopic examination is essential. It is mandatory that G.M. give a urine specimen for urinalysis before the digital rectal examination of the prostate gland, because examination of the prostate causes prostatic secretions to be expelled into the urethra, which may contaminate the urine specimen and make it difficult to determine the source of an infection. The presence of WBCs and bacteria in the urine necessitates a workup for infection. Similarly, hematuria requires a workup for urinary tract pathology other than BPH. Because BPH also may cause hydronephrosis, renal function and serum electrolytes should be evaluated.

Digital Rectal Examination

A serum PSA followed by a digital rectal examination of the prostate remains a fundamental part of evaluating a man with prostatism. The prostate examination should determine the size, shape, consistency, and nodularity of this gland. Prostatic hyperplasia results in a large, palpable prostate with a smooth mucosal surface rectally. The discernment of the right and left prostate lobes is lost in BPH. The digital rectal examination of a patient with BPH commonly finds asymmetry of the prostate, with one side being larger than the other. Prostatic enlargement can be both in an anteroposterior and in a superoinferior direction. As a result, on digital rectal examination, the upper extent of prostate hyperplasia is not palpable. Occasionally, the degree of enlargement felt by digital rectal examination may be misleading, because a substantial portion of enlargement may be intravesical. The consistency of the gland may be soft or firm, depending on the predominance of glandular or fibromuscular elements.[162] The presence of firm-to-hard nodules; irregularities; induration; or a stony, hard prostate suggest possible prostate cancer. In those cases in which the prostate gland size or shape may be questioned, the patient should have a transrectal ultrasound (TRUS) to determine the gland volume.

Prostate-Specific Antigen

Prostate-specific antigen (PSA) is a glycoprotein enzyme (molecular weight, 33,000) that is secreted in the cytoplasm of the prostatic cells; it aids in the liquefaction of semen. There are claims that this enzyme is specific for prostate origin, although a few isolated instances of elevation in nonprostate tumors have been reported. PSA correlates reasonably well, on average, with prostate weight due to benign prostate glandular hyperplasia.[163] However, prostate cancer produces approximately 10 times the amount of PSA on a tissue volume basis than does BPH.[164] For the past decade, men 50 years of age or older have been encouraged to have an annual measurement of serum PSA and a digital rectal examination, as a basic screen for prostate cancer and to monitor the growth of the prostate gland. Several investigators have proposed age-adjusted PSA reference ranges, which reflect the size of the prostate gland[165-167] (see Table 101-7). Studies have resulted in several formulas that try to adjust the PSA for the effect of BPH. The best-known formula for predicting the PSA level (PSA serum density) is as follows[168]:

$$PSA \text{ in ng/mL or } \mu g/L = 0.12 \times \text{gland volume (in cubic centimeters [c3] by transrectal ultrasound [TRUS])}$$
$$TRUS \text{ gland volume} = \text{prostate height} \times \text{width} \times \text{length} \times 0.523$$

The PSA result for G.M. is slightly above the upper limit for his age. As such, he should have a TRUS to determine the prostate gland volume and hence, the PSA density. Once the prostate gland volume is determined, the significance of his PSA level of 7.1 can be determined.

Radiologic and Imaging Studies

22. **Why should G.M. have his urinary tract evaluated with radiologic and imaging studies?**

Visualization of the kidneys, ureters, and bladder (KUB) with intravenous pyelography (IVP) is commonly used to evaluate BPH in some institutions. However, the routine use of IVP is being questioned because this procedure does not visualize the bladder outlet during voiding and therefore cannot be used to detect obstruction directly. As noted, G.M. is suspected of having hydronephrosis because his BUN and serum creatinine are elevated. Thus, the nephrotoxic risk of IVP may outweigh its potential benefit.[169-171] Furthermore, when hydronephrosis is a concern, ultrasound is the preferred diagnostic maneuver, because it spares the patient exposure to radiation and possible adverse reactions to the contrast agent.[172] Presently, the consensus is that IVP is warranted only if hematuria is present.[162] Computed tomographic (CT) scanning and magnetic resonance imaging (MRI) have little value in BPH assessment.

Urodynamic Evaluation and Cystoscopy

23. **Why should G.M. have urodynamic evaluation and cystoscopy for his BPH?**

Because G.M. has been scheduled for a TURP, it is important to determine the extent of urinary flow obstruction and the urinary flow rate. An accurate determination of the urinary peak flow rate and the voided volume correlated with G.M.'s history will be useful in determining the degree of his urinary obstruction. Urodynamic evaluation involves assessing the urinary flow rate, bladder volume, detrusor pressure, and visualization of voiding. Peak *urinary flow rate* to assess prostatism is a useful method because it is noninvasive and requires only simple and inexpensive equipment.

The urinary flow rate depends on bladder volume,[173] and a nomogram that corrects for age has been developed.[174,175] Flow rate represents the contributions of bladder contraction and outlet opening during voiding. A low flow rate may reflect diminished bladder contractility (e.g., due to aging, disease, medications) or outlet obstruction. Thus, a low flow rate is not specific and cannot differentiate bladder outlet obstruction from an underactive detrusor muscle, nor does it discriminate well between those who will and those who will not benefit from TURP.[174-176] The use of urinary flow rates as predictors of TURP outcomes is controversial. Kadow and colleagues[177] found no significant difference in symptomatic outcomes from TURP when comparing pre-TURP urinary flow rates. In addition, although flow rates tend to improve after TURP, there is wide individual variation, and an increased postoperative peak flow does not always correlate with symptom relief.[178]

Voiding cystourethrography involves retrograde filling of the bladder with a contrast agent, followed by visualization of the bladder and urethra during the resting, voiding, and postvoiding phases. Although this procedure has the same problems as the IVP, it does have the advantage of providing a dynamic evaluation of the urethral outlet during micturition.[162] Voiding cystourethrography often is performed by technicians and read by radiologists who might not be well trained in lower urinary tract physiology and who therefore do not provide sensitive analyses.

In spite of its utility, pressure/flow analysis is not widely used in the evaluation of prostatism because the patient must be able to forestall voiding during bladder filling, and then void on command. As a result, interpretable data are obtained in only 60% to 86% of cases analyzed in optimal laboratory settings.[179]

Cystoscopy is used in prostatism to rule out intravesical pathology such as tumors or stones that also cause voiding symptoms and to evaluate bladder trabeculation, prostatic length and size, the presence of an enlarged median lobe, and the degree of obstruction. Like an IVP, cystoscopy is required if hematuria is present and also should be considered whenever there is pelvic pain with voiding.

In making treatment decisions, the roles of intravenous urography, the visual appearance of the prostate via cystoscopy, urodynamic studies, urine flow measurements, and the degree of obstructive and irritative voiding symptoms, collectively, remain controversial and do not provide data sufficient to dictate the best treatment for the patient.[180,181] Therefore, these tests are not necessary for G.M.

Nonpharmacologic Treatment
Transurethral Resection of the Prostate

24. **What nonpharmacologic treatment is best for G.M.? When should prostate surgery be undertaken in general?**

G.M.'s subjective and objective findings, particularly the acute urinary retention and hydronephrosis, collectively indicate the need for a transurethral resection of the prostate gland. G.M. has been advised by his urologist that a TURP is

Table 101-7	Age-Adjusted PSA Values	
Age Range (yr)	PSA Upper Limit (ng/mL)	PSA Density
40–49	2.5	0.08
50–59	3.5	0.10
60–69	4.5	0.11
70–79	6.5	0.13

PSA, prostate-specific antigen.

the treatment of choice given the severity of his presentation (e.g., large prostate gland with acute urinary retention) and that the procedure will relieve his symptoms, allow him to lead a relatively normal life, and avoid sequelae of prolonged obstruction.

TURP provides significant relief of BPH symptoms in 86%, 83%, 75%, and 75% of patients at 3 months, 1 year, 3 years, and 7 years, respectively.[181] Of patients with severe BPH, 93% report reduced symptoms 1 year after a TURP.[180] The TURP is considered the "gold standard" for the treatment of BPH and is used in 90% of patients with symptoms of residual urine or acute urinary retention.[152] As a result, surgical alternatives are always compared with the outcome studies of TURP.

The need for a TURP in G.M.'s situation is fairly clear. However, in most cases, the need for a TURP is less clear because the symptoms do not inevitably progress and men often are willing to live with their symptoms. Therefore, clinicians need to be able to talk to patients and help them answer the question of whether the discomfort, risk, and problems during the postsurgical recovery period are outweighed by the high probability that surgery will relieve symptoms. After conditions that clearly require surgery have been ruled out, the severity of a patient's symptoms and the degree to which they interfere with living a normal life are the dominant factors in any decision to proceed with prostate surgery. Because surgery for prostate enlargement most often is performed to improve the patient's quality of life, clinicians must counsel patients and help them make the decision.

ADVERSE EFFECTS

25. **What are the adverse effects that G.M. may experience after the TURP?**

The adverse effects that G.M. may experience can be divided into those that are immediate in onset and those that are late in onset. The immediate adverse effects are determined by the size of G.M.'s prostate gland, the time necessary to complete the TURP, and the surgical technique. One of the most devastating and potentially life-threatening adverse effects of the procedure is the postsurgical TURP syndrome.[152] Irrigating fluid (e.g., dextrose 5%) is forced through the urethra during the TURP procedure, and a certain amount of absorption occurs via the venous sinuses. Most TURP procedures last 45 minutes (or less), therefore approximately 1 to 2 L of fluid can be absorbed. If the procedure is prolonged, the patient may become hypervolemic and hyponatremic, resulting in cerebral edema and seizures. Preventive measures require frequent monitoring of the patient's serum sodium concentration during the procedure and correction of hyponatremia using 3% hypertonic saline and mannitol diuresis. The incidence of the postsurgical TURP syndrome is 2%. Other immediate complications of TURP include failure to void, hemorrhage, and urinary tract infections.

Late complications of the TURP include erectile dysfunction, urinary incontinence, and bladder neck contractures. Erectile dysfunction is the most devastating long-term adverse effect of the TURP procedure[152] and afflicts as many as 30%; however, the incidence generally is lower. The etiologic mechanism may be arterial damage that causes arterial insufficiency. Similarly, electrocautery during the TURP may cause thermal damage to the arterial supply and the nerves of the corpora cavernosa, resulting in fibrosis or venous leakage. In most cases, the patient has other risk factors for erectile dysfunction, such as atherosclerosis, peripheral vascular disease, and hypertension.

Retrograde ejaculation (i.e., the ejaculation of semen into the urinary bladder) is a common outcome of the TURP, particularly after a "complete" TURP. This is caused by damage within the urethra at the location of the prostate gland. Retrograde ejaculation is not harmful; however, it causes a strange sensation to which patients can become gradually accustomed.

Transurethral Incision of the Prostate

26. **Is TURP the only procedure available for G.M.?**

A reasonable alternative to TURP is the transurethral incision of the prostate (TUIP). TUIP is a reasonable procedure for men with small prostates, which nevertheless cause bladder outlet obstruction. The TUIP uses shallow incisions in the prostatic urethra area to relieve bladder outflow obstruction and preserve antegrade ejaculation[152] (retrograde ejaculation is a complication of TURP). The TUIP is advantageous in high-risk patients such as the elderly[182] because it can be performed under local anesthesia. However, the procedure does not provide a tissue specimen for pathology review, and the potential for missing an occult carcinoma is a real concern. In contrast, prostate tissue can be retrieved from a TURP and sent for pathology studies. However, men should not undergo a TURP purely to find out whether microscopic cancer is present, because a TURP does not reduce the risk of prostate cancer, which often develops in the outer shell of prostate tissue left behind at surgery. In terms of patient satisfaction, 88% of the TUIP group and 66% of the TURP group report good improvement in symptoms. Mean peak urinary flow improved by 67% in the TUIP group.[183] TUIP patients may undergo a TURP at a later time if the TUIP outcome is unacceptable.

Transurethral Dilation of the Prostate

Transurethral dilation of the prostate (TUDP) by balloon catheter is another alternative for high-risk patients who are not candidates for TURP (Table 101-8). After satisfactory anesthesia has been achieved, the balloon catheter is positioned in the prostatic urethra. If performed improperly, balloon inflation can damage the external sphincter and cause incontinence. The balloon is inflated for 15 minutes to dilate the tissue. Postoperatively, the patient is left with an indwelling urinary catheter, usually overnight. Balloon dilation is appropriate for patients with smaller prostates who wish to avoid potential side effects (i.e., retrograde ejaculation that is associated with TURP). The success rate of TUDP in comparison

---

Table 101-8 **Surgical Options for BPH**

Transurethral resection of the prostate (TURP)
Transurethral incision of the prostate (TUIP)
Transurethral (balloon) dilation of the prostate (TUDP)
Visual laser ablation of the prostate (VLAP)[a]

[a]Experimental.
BPH, benign prostatic hyperplasia.

with TURP is uncertain,[184] but hospital stays are shorter and there is less blood loss.

The most recent innovation (which still is experimental) for an alternative to the TURP is the visual laser ablation of the prostate gland (VLAP) via the urethra. The VLAP has been shown to result in spontaneous urination in all patients treated without operative complications.[185] Patients who respond successfully to the VLAP generally have small prostate glands (i.e., 40 g). As a minimally invasive method to partially remove an obstructing prostate, laser treatment warrants further study.

G.M. was determined to have a large prostate gland (i.e., most likely >40 g) and is not a candidate for any of the alternative procedures (i.e., TUIP, TUDP, or VLAP). Currently, patients with prostate glands >80 g are not candidates for TURP, but must undergo open surgical removal of the prostate adenoma. TURP for large glands necessitates >45 minutes of procedure time, which exposes the patient to a much higher risk for the postsurgical TURP syndrome.

Transurethral Microwave Hyperthermia

Local microwave hyperthermia, delivered transurethrally or transrectally, is a relatively new modality for treating BPH. In most cases, a catheter is inserted through the urethra all the way to the prostate. The tip of the catheter acts as an antenna that emits microwaves to heat the tissue. Water circulates through the catheter applicator to cool the system and protect adjacent tissue. Transurethral microwave hyperthermia does not correct all problems (e.g., incomplete emptying of the bladder). Nevertheless, it is an effective and convenient alternative to drug therapy. The procedure requires 1 hour and can be performed in an outpatient setting.[186]

Transurethral Enzyme Injection

The use of enzyme solubilization and ablation of prostatic tissue to alleviate urinary outlet obstruction has proved effective in dogs. Transurethral enzyme injection has potential as a minimally invasive, safe treatment modality for BPH that has limited requirements for anesthesia.[187]

Drug Therapy
α₁-Adrenergic Receptor Antagonists

27. **What drug therapy should be prescribed to treat G.M.'s prostatic hyperplasia?**

G.M. most likely will be scheduled for a TURP, because he presents with acute urinary retention and hydronephrosis due to a moderately enlarged prostate gland (i.e., >40 g and <80 g). However, he should be started and maintained on an α_1-adrenergic receptor antagonist to reduce the tension of the bladder neck, the prostate adenoma, and the prostatic capsule. Similarly, he should receive finasteride to induce atrophy of the prostate gland and halt progression of the disease (Table 101-9).

The prostatic capsule and BPH adenoma have plentiful α_{1A}-adrenergic receptors. There are three known subtypes of the α_1-adrenergic receptor: α_{1A}, α_{1B}, and α_{1D}. Inhibiting the α_{1A}-adrenergic receptors can reduce the smooth muscle tone of the prostatic urethra, thereby reducing the functional component of urethral constriction and obstruction.

Table 101-9   Causes of Incontinence

Resnick's Mnemonic: DIAPPERS

D	Delirium and dementia
I	Infections
A	Atrophic vaginitis, atrophic urethritis, atonic bladder
P	Psychological causes, depression
P	Pharmacologic agents
E	Endocrine (diabetes, hypercalcemia, hypothyroidism)
R	Restricted mobility
S	Stool impaction

Adapted from reference 243.

Phenoxybenzamine (Dibenzyline), a nonselective α-antagonist, has been 80% effective in increasing urinary flow rates, but its use is hampered by a 30% incidence of side effects (fatigue, dizziness, hypotension), which are exacerbated by its long half-life.[188,189] The dose of phenoxybenzamine is 5 to 20 mg/day orally. Prazosin (Minipress) 2 to 4 mg/day is more α_{1A}-selective and is less likely to cause side effects compared with phenoxybenzamine. The clinical efficacy of prazosin in improving urinary flow rates is somewhat less impressive.[188–190]

TERAZOSIN

Terazosin (Hytrin), a long-acting α_{1A}-adrenergic receptor antagonist, has significantly improved obstructive symptoms and urinary flow rates at doses of 1 to 5 mg/day.[156,191] The α_{1A} blockade alone does not account for the long-term clinical responses exerted by this drug in the treatment of benign prostatic hyperplasia. Terazosin has been shown to induce prostate smooth muscle cell apoptosis resulting in improvement of urinary symptoms. Terazosin (and doxazosin) has a quinazoline nucleus, which may account for this effect. Tamulosin, which is not a quinazoline, does not induce prostate smooth muscle cell apoptosis.[191A]

In most patients, the dose of terazosin will need to be increased to 5 to 10 mg/day to obtain desired results. However, orthostatic hypotension may occur in the beginning days of therapy or during dosage adjustment periods. In patients who, for whatever reason, stop their terazosin therapy for 2 or more days, therapy should be reinstituted cautiously to avoid the "first-dose" adverse effect of syncope.

Terazosin maintained the level of improvement in BPH symptom scores over a 30-month period. Only 10% of the patients experienced treatment failure.[156] In this long-term study, the systolic blood pressure in normotensive and hypertensive patients was decreased by 4 and 18 mm Hg, respectively. Apparently, terazosin typically only lowered the blood pressure significantly in the hypertensive patients.

Terazosin commonly is prescribed with finasteride to control the progression and symptoms of BPH despite the lack of adequate clinical studies.[192] The mechanisms of action for both of these drugs are different, and the combined use of both produces a synergistic effect. When combined with finasteride, a smaller terazosin maintenance dose (1 to 5 mg/day) can be used, resulting in fewer dose-related side effects (e.g., orthostatic hypotension and dizziness).

DOXAZOSIN

Doxazosin (Cardura), a quinazoline derivative, is a long-acting selective α_{1A}-adrenergic receptor antagonist structurally related to prazosin and terazosin. Doxazosin is prescribed primarily for hypertension, but also is useful in the treatment of BPH. Hypertension and BPH are linked by the sympathetic nervous system. Like terazosin, doxazosin improves urinary flow rates and symptoms in patients with BPH. These effects have been demonstrated in controlled clinical studies, within weeks, and over the long term. Doxazosin should be started at 1 mg/day. After 1 to 2 weeks, the dose can be increased over several weeks to 8 mg/day. As with other long-acting α_1-adrenergic receptor antagonists, the first dose should be taken at bedtime to minimize lightheadedness and syncope (the first-dose effect), and the blood pressure of the patient should be monitored periodically during therapy. Most patients require between 4 and 8 mg/day to effectively control the urinary symptoms of BPH. Dosages >4 mg/day are associated with a greater frequency of dizziness, orthostatic hypotension, and syncope.[193,194]

TAMSULOSIN

Tamsulosin, a nonquinazoline, is a long-acting α_{1A}-adrenergic receptor antagonist similar to doxazosin, terazosin, and prazosin. Tamsulosin and its metabolites are more specific for the prostatic α_{1A}-adrenergic receptors than any of the other α_{1A}-adrenergic receptor antagonists.[195] Apparently, tamsulosin and its metabolites are less specific for the vascular α_{1A}-adrenergic receptors, and therefore cause less orthostatic hypotension than the other α_{1A}-adrenergic receptor antagonists. Consequently, there is no need to titrate tamsulosin to the recommended daily dose range of 0.4 to 0.8 mg. Coadministration of tamsulosin with antihypertensives does not require dosage adjustment of the antihypertensives. Tamsulosin is very effective in treating bladder outlet obstruction associated with BPH.[196,197]

More than 90% of tamsulosin is absorbed following oral administration of a 0.4-mg dose under fasting conditions. Administration with food decreases the bioavailability by 30% and increases time to peak plasma concentration. Tamsulosin is hepatically metabolized by CYP isozymes, CYP 3A4 and CYP 2D6.[198] Impaired renal function increases total tamsulosin plasma concentration by approximately 100% during steady-state administration. However, because active, unbound drug levels are not affected, no dose modification is required in renally impaired patients with symptomatic BPH.[199] As with all α_{1A}-adrenergic receptor antagonists, tamsulosin does not affect the PSA and must be taken indefinitely to maintain its therapeutic effect.[200]

Androgen Suppression

Considerable information has accrued concerning the endocrine basis for control of BPH (Fig. 101-4), the effect of age on hormone dynamics in men, and the hormonal changes in the hypertrophic human prostate. Maintenance of morphology and functional activity of the adult human prostate is controlled by, and dependent on, androgens. Prostatic regression after androgen deprivation is an active process that requires the synthesis of macromolecules.[201] As a result of androgen deprivation,[202] the loss of stromal and epithelial prostate cells

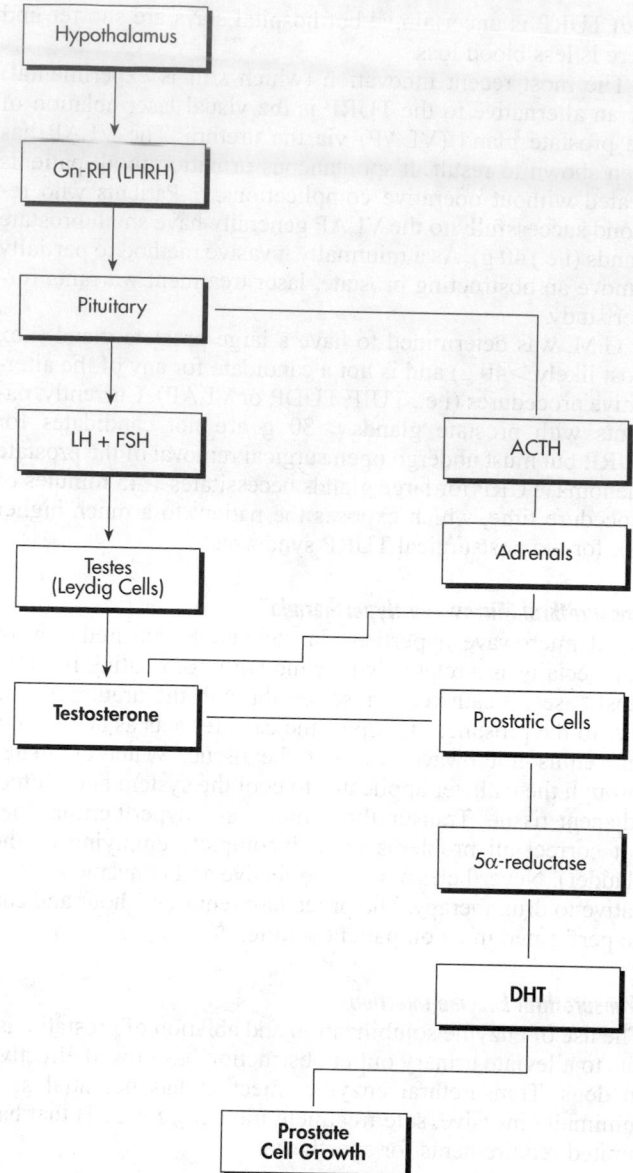

FIGURE 101-4 Pituitary-gonadal axis: endocrine basis for control of benign prostatic hyperplasia (BPH). The pituitary-gonadal axis plays an important role in prostatic growth. Neurons in the preoptic area of the hypothalamus secrete gonadotropin-releasing hormone (Gn-RH), also known as luteinizing hormone-releasing hormone (LHRH). LHRH is a small peptide that interacts with surface receptor sites on the plasma membrane of the pituitary cells. LHRH stimulates the pituitary to release both luteinizing hormone (LH) and follicle-stimulating hormone (FSH). LH secretion causes the Leydig cells of the testicle to produce testosterone. Testosterone appears to inhibit LHRH at the hypothalamic level and LH at the pituitary level. The adrenals only contribute approximately 1% of circulating testosterone. Testosterone diffuses into the prostatic cells, where it is converted to dihydrotestosterone (DHT) by 5α-reductase. DHT binds to steroid receptor complexes in the nucleus of the prostate, which causes cell growth. ACTH, corticotropin; DHT, dihydrotestosterone; FSH, follicle-stimulating hormone; Gn-RH, gonadotropin-releasing hormone; LH, luteinizing hormone. (Reproduced with permission from reference 151.)

is disproportionate, with four times greater loss of epithelial cells. Testosterone serves as the pro-hormone for the two active metabolites, DHT and 17-β-estradiol. Testosterone is metabolized to DHT by the enzyme 5α-reductase (type 1 and type 2). Thus, conversion of testosterone to DHT precludes its conversion to estrogen by the enzyme, aromatase, and the relative activity of these two enzymes is of paramount importance in prostate homeostasis.[203]

Although the mean plasma testosterone level in men falls after the age of 60, the level of testosterone in subjects with BPH and age-matched controls is not different.[204] Moreover, the onset of BPH starts some 10 to 20 years before the plasma testosterone levels decrease. However, the serum concentration of DHT is increased in men with BPH.[201,205,206] The mechanism responsible for accumulation of DHT has not been established, but there is a significant increase in 5α-reductase activity, which is known to produce DHT.[207,208]

One other major hormonal change associated with aging is the increased formation of estrogen from circulating androgens—in both the testes and the peripheral adipose tissue. Androgen conversion to estrogen via aromatase begins in males at approximately the third decade of life and increases with age,[209] but the plasma estrogen concentration is the same in men with BPH and age-matched controls without BPH.[205] Estrogen receptors are abundant in stroma cells,[210,211] more so in patients with prostatic carcinoma than in patients with BPH.[212] Estrogen stimulation of stromal tissue was once believed to explain the prostatic growth that continued with age despite the decline in testosterone secretion by the testes. However, progesterone receptors appear to be more abundant than estrogen receptors in the stromal and epithelial cells of prostate tissue of BPH patients. Thus, progesterone may play a more important role in the pathogenesis of BPH than estrogen. However, the known effect of DHT in initiating the BPH process is believed to be augmented by estrogen.[213] The number of prostate androgen receptors can be increased by estrogens and can be reversed by the administration of antiestrogens.[204] The increase in androgen receptors induced by estrogens may allow for continued androgen-mediated growth in spite of the declining amount of testosterone produced with old age.

α-Reductase Inhibitors
FINASTERIDE

Finasteride (Proscar), a competitive inhibitor of 5α-reductase (type 2), decreases the conversion of testosterone to DHT, the principal androgen responsible for stimulation of prostatic growth. After 7 days of treatment with all doses of finasteride, prostatic tissue DHT declined to ≤15% of control levels, and the testosterone concentration increased in a reciprocal manner.[214] When finasteride was administered in 1- and 5-mg doses to men with BPH for a total of 12 months, the symptom score and urinary flow improved significantly. Finasteride 5 mg daily decreased the median prostate volume by 24% and improved the maximal urinary flow rate by 2.9 mL/s.[214A] Adverse effects in the finasteride groups occurred in <5%, and side effects, such as decreased libido and ejaculatory dysfunction, were dose related.[215] The effectiveness of daily finasteride 5 mg was evaluated in 298 men over 24 months.[216] A slight improvement over the results reported at end of the 12-month period was noted. The median DHT levels had declined by 74.5% compared with 69.3% at 12 months, and prostate volume declined by 25.2% compared with 21.2% at 12 months. Patient symptom scores indicated slightly more improvement at 24 months, compared with 12 months. Obstructive symptom scores were responsible for the majority of improved symptoms reported. The prevalence of sexual adverse experiences at 24 months was similar to that at 12 months. In those men who experience finasteride induced sexual dysfunction, 50% will experience resolution after discontinuing the medication.[216A] Inhibition of DHT by 5α-reductase inhibitors does not affect testosterone-mediated functions on muscle mass, libido, or spermatogenesis. Thus, finasteride has an acceptable safety profile, halts disease progression, and improves the quality of life in patients with moderate BPH disease (i.e., enlarged prostate with symptoms of urinary obstruction, but not acute urinary retention). Finasteride improves objective pressure flow parameters after 1 year of therapy, and efficacy appears to be greatest in patients with large prostates (>40 g).[217] For those who do respond, the drug must be continued indefinitely because DHT serum concentrations return to pretreatment levels within 14 days of discontinuing finasteride, and prostate size returns to pretreatment levels within 4 months.[218,219]

Unlike leuprolide, finasteride does not affect the histologic features of BPH and prostate cancer.[220] Morphologic evaluation of finasteride-treated patients with symptomatic BPH undergoing adenectomy showed a reduction in the size of the prostate and an increase in the stroma:epithilial and stroma:lumen ratio.[221]

DUTASTERIDE

Dutasteride (Avodart) is a competitive and specific inhibitor of both type 1 and type 2 5α-reductase isoenzymes. A clear advantage of dutasteride over finasteride is the additional inhibition of 5α-reductase (type 1) in the peripheral tissues, which produces a further decline in serum DHT. In a prospective study of 2,951 men with moderate to severe BPH, dutasteride 0.5 mg per day decreased DHT serum levels by 90% at 1 month in 58% of patients. At 24 months, 85% of dutasteride-treated patients were noted to have a 90% reduction of serum DHT.[221A] Correspondingly, the patients noted improvement in urinary symptoms as early as 3 months after treatment and a significant ($P < 0.001$) improvement by the sixth month when compared with placebo-treated patients. Dutasteride reduces total serum PSA by approximately 40% after 3 months of treatment and by approximately 50% after 24 months.[221A] Common side effects of dutasteride are similar to those of finasteride: impotence (4.7%), decreased libido (3.0%), ejaculation disorder (1.4%) and gynecomastia (1.0%).

Antiandrogens: Flutamide

Flutamide (Eulexin) is an orally administered nonsteroidal antiandrogen that inhibits the binding of androgen to its receptor. The safety and effectiveness of flutamide were evaluated in a double-blind, placebo-controlled study of 31 males with symptomatic BPH.[222] Patients received a daily dose of 375 mg of flutamide for 12 weeks. There were no significant differences in the treatment and placebo groups with regard to any symptoms of prostatism (force of stream, frequency, nocturia). Based on the digital rectal examination, patients receiving flutamide had a significant reduction of prostate size. In 7 of 15 patients treated with flutamide developed nipple tenderness and decreased libido. In another study, there was no significant difference between flutamide and placebo.[223] In this same study, which used flutamide 250 mg three times daily, 53% of the patients experienced breast tenderness and 11% experienced diarrhea. Because flutamide is a potent hepatotoxin in certain patients, serial blood aminotransferase levels should be monitored during the first few months of therapy.[224] Flutamide also is associated with a 50% reduction in the serum concentration of PSA.[192,223] In summary, flutamide results in toxicity with limited effectiveness. However, its use may be justified in patients who are unable to tolerate finasteride with or without terazosin.

Gonadotropin-Releasing Hormone: Leuprolide

Analogs of Gn-RH can cause regression of BPH. Leuprolide acetate (Lupron) is a synthetic nonpeptide analog of natural-occurring Gn-RH. It desensitizes LH-releasing hormone receptors (when given continuously and in therapeutic doses), thereby preventing the release of gonadotropin. Chronic leuprolide acetate therapy will suppress testicular testosterone production, causing a "chemical-like" castration. Because it reversibly binds to Gn-RH receptors, testosterone production resumes when it is discontinued. In a double-blind, placebo-controlled study, patients with BPH received leuprolide 3.75 mg intramuscularly monthly for 24 weeks.[225] There were no statistically or clinically significant differences in the percentage change in total, obstructive, or irritative symptoms at 24 weeks between the placebo and leuprolide groups. Detrusor muscle pressure at maximum urine flow was improved at 24 weeks, and prostate volume was reduced. However, of those patients receiving leuprolide acetate, 92% developed hot flashes, and of the sexually active patients, 95% experienced a loss of potency.

Leuprolide should be reserved for patients with prostate cancer. Its high cost, questionable effectiveness, and castration-like adverse effects make it an undesirable choice for treatment of BPH.

Effect of Androgen Suppression on Prostate-Specific Antigen

28. What effect does androgen suppression have on PSA?

The FDA has approved Hybritech's PSA test for the screening of prostate cancer. The possibility that antiandrogen treatment of BPH could adversely affect the interpretation of the PSA screening test for prostate cancer is of concern. For example, androgen suppression with leuprolide acetate reduces prostate volume primarily by inducing involution of the epithelial elements of the prostate.[226] Because PSA primarily is produced by the epithelial cells of the prostate, these drugs can alter serum and prostate concentrations of PSA.[227] Finasteride 5 mg/day also can reduce the serum PSA level by 50%.[228] However, the serum PSA level reduction is predictable, and serum PSA levels can be recalculated during hormonal treatment for BPH. Nevertheless, patients receiving finasteride should have a digital rectal examination of their prostate periodically, have a PSA level measured, and have any suspicious findings investigated immediately.[216] Andro-

gen suppression therapy is not contraindicated in BPH solely on the basis of its effect on serum PSA levels.[229]

29. What over-the-counter medications are available for prostate disorders?

Saw Palmetto

Saw palmetto is an herbal product obtained from the fruit of the *Serenoa repens* tree. The active ingredients are phytosterols; β-sitosterol and β-sitosterol-3-O-glucosides are the most abundant. Saw palmetto has antiandrogen activity. Several trials have shown that it significantly improves benign prostatic hyperplasia symptoms,[229A,229B,229C,229D] to a degree similar to finasteride.[229E]

URINARY INCONTINENCE

Urinary incontinence, both acute and chronic, is a common disorder among elderly individuals, affecting approximately 50% of the institutionalized elderly and 20% of the community-dwelling elderly.[230,231] Neurologic impairment, immobility, female gender, and history of hysterectomy are independent risk factors for incontinence, but neither advanced age nor chronic bacteriuria seem to be. Incontinence has economic costs, medical (e.g., cystitis, urosepsis, pressure sores, perineal rashes, falls) and psychosocial (e.g., embarrassment, isolation, depression, predisposition to institutionalization) consequences. Nevertheless, incontinence often is a neglected condition. Only a minority of patients whose lives are seriously disrupted seek medical attention; when they do, their incontinence often is attributed to aging and not evaluated further.[230,232] Incontinence is not an inevitable consequence of aging. It is a pathologic condition that, when rationally approached, usually can be ameliorated or cured, often without invasive tests or surgery and almost invariably without an indwelling catheter (see Table 101-9).[233,234]

Neurophysiologic Considerations

The bladder can be thought of as a "balloon" with a narrow outlet, wrapped with a muscular layer, the detrusor muscle. The detrusor and the bladder outlet functions are coordinated neurologically to allow for storage and expulsion of urine.[235] The detrusor muscle is innervated by the parasympathetic nervous system, and the bladder neck is innervated by the sympathetic nervous system (α-adrenergic) (Fig. 101-5). The proximal smooth muscle (internal) sphincter in the bladder neck also is innervated through the sympathetic nervous system (α-adrenergic). The distal striated muscle (external) sphincter of the urethra is supplied by the somatic nervous system.

Urine storage is the result of detrusor muscle relaxation and closure of both the internal and external sphincters. Detrusor relaxation is accomplished by CNS inhibition of the parasympathetic tone; sphincter closure is mediated by a reflex increase in α-adrenergic and somatic activity. Voiding occurs when detrusor contraction is coordinated with sphincter relaxation. Detrusor contraction is mediated by the parasympathetic nervous system, and relaxation requires inhibition of somatic and sympathetic nerve impulses to the outlet. The bladder capacity is approximately 300 mL in the elderly and

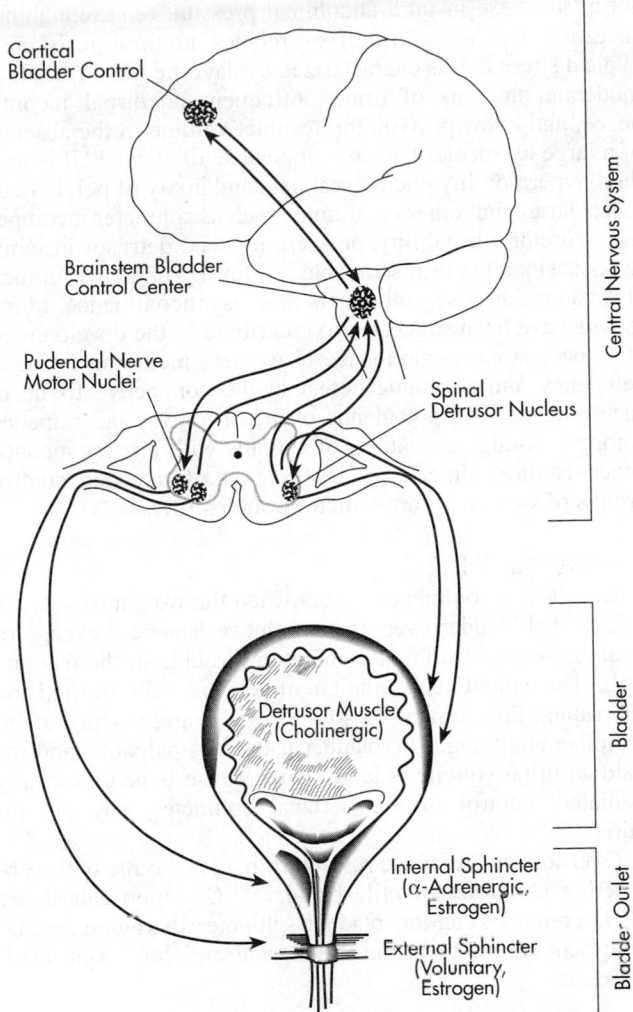

FIGURE 101-5 Neurologic bladder control. Three major components are involved in urine storage and release. (1) Central nervous system: Inhibition from the frontal lobe (cortical) micturition center permits bladder relaxation and filling, and sphincter closure to prevent leakage of urine. When cortical inhibition ceases (i.e., the patient wants to urinate), the brainstem (pontine) micturition center sends impulses down the spinal cord to the detrusor muscle, resulting in muscle contraction. (2) Bladder: Increase in bladder volume stimulates proprioception receptors in the bladder wall and sensory impulses are transmitted through the sacral nerves (S_2–S_4 roots) to trigger bladder contraction. This stimulus for bladder contraction is under inhibitory control by the central nervous system frontal lobe as described previously. Cholinergic stimulation results in bladder contraction. (3) Bladder outlet: The two major factors in maintaining urethral pressure are the internal and external sphincters. Internal sphincter: α-Adrenergic stimulation causes muscle contraction, preventing flow of urine. External sphincter: It consists of striated muscle under voluntary control. Contraction prevents flow of urine. Estrogen deficiency in women can result in decreased competence of the internal and external sphincters. (Reproduced with permission from reference 302.)

approximately 400 mL in young adults. The relationship between the detrusor and the outlet is coordinated by a micturition center located in the CNS, perhaps the pons.[236] The cortex and diencephalon also permit inhibition of what would otherwise be a reflex contraction of the detrusor muscle in response to bladder distention.

Age-Related Changes

Aging affects the lower urinary tract in several ways (Table 101-10). Structural and functional changes have been observed. Bladder capacity, the ability to postpone voiding, urethral and bladder compliance, maximal urethral closure pressure, and urinary flow rate all are reduced with normal aging.[236,237] For women, these changes are correlated with the decline of estrogen production. Estrogen has trophic effects on the epithelium and on tissues lining and surrounding the urethra, bladder outlet, and vagina. Atrophy of these tissues can result in friability, inflammation, susceptibility to infection, diminished periurethral blood flow, and prolapse of pelvic structures. All of these effects can precipitate symptoms of urinary incontinence. For men, the age-related changes in the prostate gland are responsible for many of the changes in urination. The most common age-related change, in both women and men, is involuntary bladder contractions (detrusor motor instability). These involuntary bladder contractions occur in up to 20% of asymptomatic, neurologically normal, continent elderly patients.[238–241]

In many elderly persons, nocturia is a common complaint and may stem from age-related increases in nocturnal urine production.[242] Each of these changes predisposes people to incontinence, but none alone precipitates it. This predisposition to incontinence, together with the increased likelihood that an older person will be subjected to additional pathologic, physiologic, or pharmacologic insults, underlies the higher incidence of incontinence in the elderly. The onset or exacerbation of incontinence in an older person is likely to be due to a precipitating factor outside the lower urinary tract.[243] Correspondingly, reversal of the precipitating factor may be sufficient to restore continence without correction of the underlying urologic abnormality.

Drug-Induced Urinary Incontinence

Occasionally, reports of female stress incontinence from α_1-adrenergic receptor antagonists, which have a relaxant effect on urethral smooth muscle, have appeared in the medical literature.[244–246] In one study, the incidence of genuine stress incontinence was significantly higher in women taking prazosin (86.2%) than in the nonprazosin group (65.7%) ($P <0.01$). In 55% of the women contacted in the prazosin group, urinary incontinence was improved or cured by prazosin withdrawal.[247] There was a significant increase in functional urethral length, maximum urethral closure pressure, and abdominal pressure transmission to the urethra after prazosin withdrawal. In one case report, switching from doxazosin to enalapril briefly improved the female patient's stress incontinence; however, she developed a persistent dry cough (from

Table 101-10	Age-Related Changes in Urologic Function

↓ bladder capacity
↑ residual urine
↑ uninhibited bladder contractions
↑ nocturnal sodium and fluid excretion
↓ urethral resistance in women
↑ urethral resistance in men
Weakness of pelvic floor muscles in women

the enalapril) that continued to cause episodic stress incontinence. Her cough and stress incontinence resolved when she was switched to amlodipine.[248]

Classification

Urinary incontinence can be classified several different ways. The two most basic types of urinary incontinence are (1) acute (or transient) and reversible or (2) chronic and persistent. Persistent urinary incontinence (PUI), which refers to incontinence that is not acute and occurs over a long period of time, can be classified further into four subgroups: (a) urge, (b) stress, (c) overflow, and (d) functional.

Acute Incontinence

Urinary incontinence that is of relatively recent onset or associated with an acute medical problem should prompt a review for reversible factors. These include the following: (1) cystitis, atrophic vaginitis, and urethritis; (2) CHF; (3) polyuria from diabetes; (4) delirium and acute confusional states; (5) immobility; and (6) medication side effects. The following medications are associated with acute onset urinary incontinence: (1) diuretics; (2) α-adrenergic agonists (e.g., pseudoephedrine); (3) α-adrenergic antagonists (e.g., terazosin); (4) anticholinergics; and (5) neuroleptics. The management of acute forms of urinary incontinence depends on the identification and elimination of the reversible factor.

For women with urethritis and atrophic vaginitis with irritative voiding symptoms, estrogen replacement can be very helpful. An intravaginal estrogen cream administered nightly for 7 days and followed by at least once-a-week application thereafter or oral conjugated estrogen 0.625 mg/day can be prescribed.[249] For women with an intact uterus, the conjugated estrogen should be given in a cyclic manner with a progestational agent. However, in keeping with the Women's Health Initiative Trial, serious risks including breast cancer and cardiovascular disease, appear to outweigh long-term benefits of this combination of hormone therapy.[249A]

Persistent Urinary Incontinence
URGE INCONTINENCE

Urge incontinence is the most common form of incontinence affecting the elderly and occurs when involuntary voiding is preceded by a warning of a few seconds to a few minutes. Urge PUI is characterized by precipitous urine leakage, most often after the urge to void is perceived. Urge PUI can be caused by a variety of genitourinary and neurologic disorders. It most often, but not always, is associated with detrusor motor instability (involuntary contraction of the bladder) or detrusor hyperreflexia (detrusor motor instability caused by a neurologic disorder). The most common causes are local genitourinary conditions such as cystitis, urethritis, tumors, stones, bladder diverticula, and outflow obstruction. Neurologic disorders such as stroke, dementia, parkinsonism, and spinal cord injury can be associated with urge PUI.[250]

STRESS INCONTINENCE

Stress incontinence, the involuntary leakage that occurs only during stress, is common in elderly women but uncommon in men (unless the sphincter has been damaged during a TURP or prostatectomy). Stress incontinence occurs when an abrupt increase in intra-abdominal pressure (e.g., coughing, sneezing, laughing, lifting) overcomes urethral resistance. Typical stress PUI is characterized by daytime loss of small to moderate amounts of urine, infrequent nocturnal incontinence, and a low postvoiding residual volume in the absence of a large cystocele. The common cause of stress PUI is urethral hypermobility due to weakness and laxity of pelvic floor musculature, but other conditions, such as sphincter incompetence, urethral instability, or stress-induced detrusor instability, occasionally are responsible.[236] Obesity or TURP in men also can predispose individuals to stress incontinence. Many factors have been suggested to contribute to the development of urinary stress incontinence in women, including estrogen deficiency and a genetic defect in the connective tissue in such patients. The prevalence of urinary stress incontinence among first-degree relatives of patients with urinary incontinence is three times ($P < 0.005$) that of matched control groups of women without micturition disorders.[251]

OVERFLOW INCONTINENCE

Overflow incontinence occurs when the weight of urine in a distended bladder overcomes outlet resistance. Leakage of small amounts of urine are common throughout the day and night. The patient may complain of hesitancy, diminished and interrupted flow, a need to strain to void, and a sense of incomplete emptying. The bladder usually is palpable, and the residual urine volume is large. If the cause is neurologically mediated, control of the perianal sphincter may be impaired.[252]

Overflow incontinence results from an anatomic outlet obstruction or an acontractile bladder.[250] Common causes are BPH, urethral stricture, bladder-sphincter dyssynergia, diabetic neuropathy, fecal impaction, and anticholinergic medication use.

FUNCTIONAL INCONTINENCE

Functional incontinence occurs when a continent individual is unable or unwilling to reach the toilet to urinate. Common causes are musculoskeletal disorders, muscle weakness, impaired mental status, use of physical restraints, psychological impairment, environmental barriers, and medications (e.g., sedatives, neuroleptics).

Clinical Presentation and Evaluation

30. H.K., an 83-year-old female resident of a nursing facility, developed urinary incontinence 3 years before admission. She has been managed with adult diapers and bladder training. What objective and subjective data are needed to determine the pathophysiology (and hence the classification) of H.K.'s urinary incontinence?

The rationale for the clinical evaluation of H.K. is to classify the imbalance between bladder pressure and bladder sphincter resistance and, as a result, institute appropriate medical or surgical management of her urinary incontinence.

Documentation of H.K.'s urinary incontinence is accomplished most easily by having her or one of her nurses keep an incontinence record. Observations should be recorded every 2 hours regarding whether the patient is wet or dry, as well as associated symptoms or circumstances. A record maintained over 3 to 4 days will facilitate assessment of the voiding pattern. Knowledge of the voiding pattern can be used to design bladder training programs and to detect iatrogenic causes (e.g., diuretic ingestion, use of restraints). Successful bladder training relies on estimating when the bladder is full.

Physical examination of H.K. is paramount in determining the cause and classification of her urinary incontinence. A complete neurologic examination is mandatory. Clinical findings may identify specific pathophysiologic abnormalities. H.K. should have a thorough pelvic examination to determine the contribution of atrophic vaginitis, uterine prolapse, and bladder anatomy. Funneling of the bladder neck suggests stress incontinence, and palpation of the bladder suggests overflow incontinence. The presence of physical restraints or musculoskeletal disability would suggest functional incontinence.

H.K.'s bladder should be catheterized immediately after urination to determine residual urine volume. Volumes >50 mL are abnormal and may indicate obstruction or an adynamic detrusor muscle. Although urodynamic studies are widely recommended and used, there is little evidence that these produce clinically useful data for institutionalized geriatric patients. A urinalysis, blood chemistries, renal function, and glucose tolerance test should be performed. An abnormal urinalysis may suggest pathology (e.g., infection) that can be managed medically. Urinary tract infection is common in the incontinent patient.

A number of treatment options exists for each type of urinary incontinence (Table 101-11). Proper evaluation should guide the clinician in choosing the optimal course of drug therapy. Drug therapy should be based on sound principles of neurophysiology, urology, and pharmacology. Basically, drug therapy is directed at decreasing bladder contractility (detrusor instability) and increasing outlet obstruction (bladder neck and proximal urethra).

31. The incontinence record maintained by the nursing staff indicates that H.K. has urinary urges quite frequently, resulting in urine leakage. Throughout the day and night, H.K. urinates four to five times. Physical examination reveals atrophic vaginitis, no funneling of the bladder neck, and no bladder distention.

Table 101-11	Drug Therapy of Persistent Urinary Incontinence
Type	Treatment With Initial Doses
Urge	Oxybutynin 2.5 mg QD–TID
	Flavoxate 100 mg TID–QID
	Imipramine 25 mg QD–TID
	Propantheline 15–30 mg TID
	Dicyclomine 10–20 mg TID
Stress	Pseudoephedrine 15–30 mg BID–TID
	Imipramine 25 mg QD
	Conjugated estrogens 0.625 mg QD[a]
	Vaginal estrogen cream 0.5–1.0 g two times/week
Overflow	Prazosin 0.5–1.0 mg QD (usually at HS)
	Bethanechol 10 mg TID
Functional	None

[a]If patient has uterus, consider cyclic therapy with a progestational agent to reduce risk for cervical cancer.

H.K. does have a history of stroke. The urinalysis is normal, as are the blood chemistries. Postvoiding bladder catheterization produced a residual urine volume of 30 mL. What is the pathophysiology and classification of H.K.'s incontinence?

Most neuropathic disease processes can change bladder function. As illustrated by H.K., a cerebrovascular accident is commonly associated with bladder dysfunction and incontinence in the elderly. Neurologic injury above the level of the micturition center in the spinal cord, in most cases, results in bladder spasticity. Sacral reflexes are intact, but loss of inhibition from higher CNS centers results in spastic bladder and inappropriate sphincter behavior. The degree of spasticity varies between the bladder and sphincter, as well as from patient to patient with the same CNS lesions. H.K. is suffering from a detrusor muscle that is spastic resulting from an unchecked sacral reflex. H.K.'s bladder dysfunction is classified as urge urinary incontinence of the persistent type.

Drug Therapy
Anticholinergic Agents

32. What drug therapy should be prescribed for H.K.?

H.K. is suffering from detrusor instability and requires anticholinergic drug therapy. Detrusor muscle stabilization through pharmacologic intervention and behavioral modification is the treatment of choice for urge PUI. The major neurohormonal stimulus for physiologic bladder muscle contraction is acetylcholine-induced stimulation of postganglionic parasympathetic cholinergic receptor sites on bladder smooth muscle.[253] Atropine and atropine-like substances depress true involuntary bladder contractions of any etiology.[254]

OXYBUTYNIN CHLORIDE
Oxybutynin (Ditropan, Generics) is available as an oral immediate-release tablet, an extended-release tablet, or a transdermal system. Oxybutynin is commonly used to produce an anticholinergic effect in the lower urinary tract. The transdermal system contains 36 mg of active drug and delivers 3.9 mg of oxybutynin per day when dosed twice a week.[254A] The transdermal system should be protected from moisture and humidity. Common side effects from the transdermal system at the application site are pruritus (14%) and site redness (8.3%). A comparison study of immediate-release oxybutynin and the transdermal system indicated that patients using the transdermal system experienced fewer side effects. Dry mouth was reported in 38% of the oxybutynin transdermal system users in contrast to 94% of those who used immediate-release tablets.[254B]

Oxybutynin has been described as a strong independent smooth muscle relaxant with local anesthetic activity that has minor anticholinergic effects.[255,256] This agent has been used successfully to depress uninhibited detrusor contractions in patients with and without neurogenic bladder dysfunction. Oxybutynin improves total bladder capacity, neuropathic voiding dysfunction, and bladder filling pressure.[257,258] The dosage of oxybutynin chloride suggested for the elderly is 2.5 mg up to three times a day; in some cases, the dosage may need to be increased to 5 mg three times a day. Because oxybutynin is a tertiary-amine anticholinergic compound, the potential for CNS toxicity increases as the dose is increased.

Compared with oral propantheline bromide 15 mg three times a day, a full dose of oral oxybutynin (5 mg three time a day) in one study produced a good response more frequently.[259] Once-daily controlled-release oxybutynin at doses of 5 to 30 mg reduced the number of incontinence episodes.[17,260] Maximum benefit was demonstrated by maintenance week 4 and was sustained as long as the patient continued therapy.[261]

TOLTERODINE TARTRATE

Tolterodine (Detrol, Detrol LA, Generic) is a competitive muscarinic receptor antagonist (anticholinergic) indicated for the treatment of overactive bladder symptoms of urinary frequency or urge incontinence. At doses of 1 to 2 mg twice a day, compared with a placebo, the number of urinary voids per 24 hours decreased ($P = 0.0045$), the volume of urine per void increased ($P < 0.001$), and the mean number of incontinence episodes decreased by 50% ($P < 0.19$).[262] There was no clinical or electrocardiographic evidence of significant cardiac adverse events in the group studied. Tolterodine has greater selectivity for the bladder than the salivary glands in vivo, which is not attributable to muscarinic receptor subtype selectivity.[263] Thus, tolterodine is much less potent in inhibiting salivation, suggesting that it may have less propensity to cause dry mouth in clinical use. The onset of pharmacologic action of tolterodine is <1 hour, and therapeutic efficacy is maintained during long-term treatment. In comparative trials, tolterodine and oxybutynin are equivalent in terms of efficacy. However, tolterodine is better tolerated.

Despite short terminal half-lives of 2 to 3 and 3 to 4 hours for tolterodine and its active 5-hydroxy metabolite, respectively, twice-daily dosing is effective because of the drug's long pharmacodynamic effects.[264] Dosage adjustment is recommended in the presence of hepatic impairment and during concurrent therapy with drugs that inhibit CYP 2D6 and CYP 3A4 isozymes.

Until pharmacoeconomic analyses are conducted that clearly justify use of this more expensive agent, tolterodine is perhaps best reserved for patients who are intolerant of or fail oxybutynin.

PROPANTHELINE BROMIDE

Propantheline bromide (Pro-Banthine, Generics) is an oral agent prescribed to produce an anticholinergic effect in the lower urinary tract. The adult dose is 15 to 30 mg every 4 to 6 hours. Higher doses sometimes are necessary and are well tolerated. Propantheline bromide is a quaternary ammonium anticholinergic compound that does not cross the blood–brain barrier.[255] As such, CNS side effects are insignificant. Oral administration of propantheline in the fasting state is preferred to improve bioavailability. The anticholinergic effects of propantheline on the detrusor muscle when compared with other anticholinergic agents are similar.[256] These anticholinergic agents differ primarily in their frequency of dosing and their side effect profiles. However, no other oral drug is available whose direct anticholinergic binding potential approximates that of atropine.[265]

Antispasmodics

Other drugs with anticholinergic properties also have local anesthetic and smooth muscle relaxant effects. These include tolterodine, flavoxate, oxybutynin, and dicyclomine. These drugs act directly on smooth muscle at a site that is metabolically distal to the cholinergic receptor. Because their effectiveness in treating urge incontinence is due to muscle relaxant property, rather than their anticholinergic effects, they are classified as antispasmodics.[255] All agents in this group should be prescribed for a 2-week trial period. If no improvement has been observed with one drug, trial with another may be appropriate.

DICYCLOMINE HYDROCHLORIDE

Dicyclomine hydrochloride (Bentyl) is a tertiary-amine and has dose-related CNS effects.[255] An oral dose of 20 mg three times a day will increase bladder capacity in patients with detrusor hyperreflexia. The dose for elderly patients is listed as 10 to 20 mg three times a day, but it may need to be increased to 30 mg three times a day.[256,266] As the dose is increased, anticholinergic side effects become prominent.

FLAVOXATE HYDROCHLORIDE

Evidence for the efficacy of flavoxate hydrochloride (Urispas) is weak. The recommended adult dose is 100 to 200 mg three to four times a day.

β-Adrenergic Agents: Terbutaline

Terbutaline (Brethine) 5 mg orally three times a day reportedly benefits select patients with urge PUI and does not have significant effects on the bladders of normal humans.[267] The human bladder muscle has β-adrenergic receptors that, when stimulated, will increase the capacity of the bladder. However, the effects of β-adrenergic stimulation in patients with detrusor hyperactivity is inadequately studied.

Although any of the aforementioned drugs would be useful for H.K., oxybutynin is considered the drug of choice for the elderly. Oxybutynin has fewer anticholinergic effects and a more prominent detrusor relaxation effect than any of the other drugs except tolterodine. However, tolterodine is a much more expensive agent when compared with oxybutynin and is best reserved for patients who are intolerant of or fail oxybutynin. Oxybutynin can be dosed once a day in some cases and in most cases, twice a day. Flavoxate, dicyclomine, and propantheline require at least three doses a day. The systemic anticholinergic side effects from oxybutynin, tolterodine, flavoxate, and dicyclomine are relatively mild compared with propantheline. A beginning dose of oxybutynin for H.K. would be 2.5 mg/day; the dose can be increased by increments of 2.5 mg/day, not to exceed 5 mg three times a day.

Monitoring H.K. necessitates evaluating her urinary frequency through patient (and where possible, nurse or caregiver) interviews. Specifically, a reduction in the urinary urgency sensation is the desired outcome. Too much anticholinergic therapy may result in urinary hesitancy and possibly urinary retention. If the patient has to concentrate on the act of micturition, the anticholinergic drug dose should be reduced. CNS and systemic side effects should be assessed as often as possible. As with all urge incontinent patients, urinary tract infection is quite common. If symptoms of dysuria appear, or if urinary urgency reappears, a urinalysis should be obtained.

Increasing Bladder Outlet Resistance

33. M.K., a 68-year-old woman, has been diagnosed with urinary stress incontinence. What drug therapy would be appropriate for this classification of PUI?

IMIPRAMINE HYDROCHLORIDE

Imipramine hydrochloride (Tofranil, Generics) is useful for increasing bladder capacity and increasing bladder outlet resistance.[268] The pharmacologic mechanism of tricyclic antidepressants (TCAs) in treating PUI has been studied extensively.[269] The results and conclusions of the data reported demonstrate that, at best, the mechanism of action on the lower urinary tract is speculative. All the TCAs have some degree of anticholinergic effect, both centrally and peripherally, but not at all sites. These drugs block the active transport system in the presynaptic nerve ending and prevent the uptake of norepinephrine and serotonin; they produce varying degrees of CNS sedation. All the TCAs antagonize histamine receptors, both H_1 and H_2, to some degree, and they desensitize some α_2-adrenergic receptors.[269,270] Imipramine has significant systemic anticholinergic effects, but it has weak anticholinergic effects at the detrusor muscle.[271] However, imipramine has a significant inhibitory effect on the detrusor muscle, which is neither anticholinergically nor adrenergically mediated. Its detrusor inhibitory effect may be the result of peripheral blockade of norepinephrine reuptake. The ability of imipramine to increase bladder outlet resistance is believed to be due to enhanced α-adrenergic effects in the smooth muscle of the bladder base and proximal urethra, where α-receptors outnumber β-receptors. Imipramine 75 mg/day produced continence in 68% of women with stress PUI within 4 weeks.[272]

The initial dose for imipramine is 25 mg orally at bedtime. The dose can be increased every third day by 25 mg until the patient is continent, side effects occur, or a dose of 150 mg/day is reached.[268] Most patients become continent within 7 to 10 days, and some patients may become continent in as few as 3 to 5 days. The usual adult dose for voiding dysfunction is 25 mg four times a day, and for geriatric patients the dose is 25 mg twice a day, because the serum half-life is prolonged in the elderly.[273] Weakness, fatigue, and postural hypotension are significant problems associated with imipramine. There has been a threefold increase in hip fractures reported among elderly patients taking imipramine.[274]

α-Adrenergic receptor stimulation at the detrusor muscle and proximal urethra will increase the maximum urethral pressure (MUP) and the maximum urethral closure pressure (MUCP).[275] Several oral α-adrenergic agonist agents are available. All of them should be used cautiously in the elderly because of side effects, which include anxiety, insomnia, blood pressure elevation, headache, tremor, weakness, palpitations, cardiac arrhythmias, and respiratory difficulties.[276]

ESTROGENS

Estrogens affect many aspects of uterine smooth muscle, including excitability, receptor density, and transmitter metabolism, especially adrenergic nerves.[281] The detrusor and urethra are embryologically related to the uterus, and significant work has been done on estrogenic hormone effects on the lower urinary tract. α-Adrenergic stimulation of the urethra is estrogen dependent,[256] and several studies have demonstrated the relationship of estrogen to α-adrenergic receptor density in the lower urinary tract.[282] Estrogen therapy, in the form of vaginal suppositories (1 mg/day), facilitates urinary storage in some postmenopausal female patients by increasing urethral outlet resistance and has an additive effect with α-adrenergic therapy (phenylpropanolamine 50 mg twice a day).[243] The use of estrogen in the treatment of stress PUI requires further study. The use of long-term estrogen treatment must be considered carefully in light of the controversy over whether estrogen therapy predisposes to the development of endometrial carcinoma. If estrogen is combined with α-adrenergic agonist therapy, the lowest effective maintenance dose should be prescribed.

Decreasing Bladder Outlet Resistance

Overflow incontinence in females resulting from outlet obstruction or weak detrusor muscle is now being treated with α_{1A}-blockers by many urologists. Traditional treatments include cholinergic agents (e.g., bethanechol), Foley catheter, surgical procedures or urethral caps. α_{1A}-Blockers such as prazosin, terazosin or doxazosin are certainly not the drugs of choice, but they can decrease outflow resistance by decreasing sphincter tone.[282A] The majority of α_{1A}-receptors are found in prostate tissue; however, these same receptors are also located in the spinal cord, bladder neck, urethra and periurethral tissue in women.[282B] The symptoms of urinary symptoms suggestive of prostatism are not gender specific. Well-controlled randomized cross-over studies are needed to determine the efficacy of α_{1A}-blockers in overflow incontinence.

REFERENCES

1. Lauman EO et al. Sexual dysfunction in the United States. JAMA 1999;281:537.
2. NIH Consensus Conference. Impotence. National Institutes of Health Consensus Development Panel on Impotence. JAMA 1993;270:83.
3. Rosen RC et al. Prevalence of sexual dysfunction in women: results of a survey study of 329 women in an outpatient gynecological clinic. J Sex Marital Ther 1993;19:171.
4. Spector IP, Casey MP. Incidence and prevalence of the sexual dysfunctions: a critical review of the empirical literature. Arch Sex Behav 1990;19:389.
5. Kinsey A et al, eds. Sexual Behavior in the Human Male. Philadelphia: WB Saunders, 1984.
6. Pfieffer E et al. Sexual behavior in aged men and women. Arch Gen Psychiatry 1986;19:735.
7. Bretschneider JG, McCoy NL. Sexual interest and behavior in healthy 80 to 102 year olds. Arch Sex Behav 1988;17:109.
8. Diokno AC et al. Correlates of sexual dysfunction in the elderly. J Urol 1988;139:496A.
9. Tordarello O, Boscia FM. Sexuality in aging: a study of a group of 300 elderly men and women. J Endocrinol Invest 1985;8(Suppl 2):123.
10. Starr BD, Weiner MD. The Starr-Weiner Report on Sex and Sexuality in the Mature Years. New York: Stein and Day, 1981.
11. Persson G. Sexuality in a 70-year-old urban population. J Psychosom Res 1980;24:137.
12. Sternbach H. Age-associated testosterone decline in men: clinical issues for psychiatry. Am J Psychiatry 1998;155:1310.
13. Lund BC et al. Testosterone and andropause: the feasibility of testosterone replacement therapy in elderly men. Pharmacotherapy 1999;19:951.
14. Vermeulen A, Kaufman JM. Ageing of the hypothalamopituitary-testicular axis in men. Horm Res 1995;43:25.
15. Feldman HA et al. Impotence and its medical and psychosocial correlates: results of the Massachusetts Male Aging Study. J Urol 1994;151:54.
16. Melman A. Evaluation of the first 70 patients in the center for male sexual dysfunction of Beth Israel Medical Center. J Urol 1984;131:53.
17. Shrom SH et al. Clinical profile of experience with 130 consecutive cases of impotent men. Urology 1980;13:511.
18. Mulligan T, Katz G. Why aged men become impotent. Arch Intern Med 1989;149:1365.
19. Hsueh WA. Sexual dysfunction with aging and systemic hypertension. Am J Cardiol 1988;61(Suppl):18H.
20. Padam-Nathan H et al. Treatment of men with erectile dysfunction with transurethral alprostadil. N Engl J Med 1997;336:1.
21. McWaine DE, Procci WR. Drug-induced sexual dysfunction. Med Toxicol 1988;3:289.

22. Deamer RL, Thompson JF. The role of medications in geriatric sexual function. Clin Geriatr Med 1991;7:95.

23. Mooradian AD et al. Endocrinology in aging. Dis Mon 1988;34:398.

24. Wein AJ, Van Arsdalen KN. Drug-induced male sexual dysfunction. Urol Clin North Am 1988;15:23.

24A. Johannes CB et al. Incidence of erectile dysfunction in men 40 to 69 years old: longitudinal results from the Massachusetts Male Aging Study. J Urol 2000;163:460.

24B. Hatzichristou DG. Sildenafil citrate: lessons learned from 3 years of clinical experience. Int J Impot Res 2002;14(Suppl 1):43.

25. Morley JE. Impotence. Am J Med 1986;80:897.

26. Krane RJ et al. Impotence. N Engl J Med 1989;321:1648.

27. Lue TF. Male sexual dysfunction. In: Tanagho EA, McAinich JW, eds. Smith's General Urology. Norwalk: Appleton & Lange, 1992:696.

28. Deslypere JP, Vermeulen A. Leydig cell function in normal men: effect of age, life-style, residence, diet, and activity. J Clin Endocrinol Metab 1984; 59:955.

29. Tesitouras PD. Effects of age on testicular function. Endocrinol Metab Clin North Am 1987;16:1045.

30. Lue TF, Tanagho EA. Physiology of erection and pharmacological management of impotence. J Urol 1987;137:829.

31. Heaton JPW et al. Recovery of erectile function by the oral administration of apomorphine. Urology 1995;45:200.

31A. Shabsigh R, Anastadiadis AG. Erectile dysfunction. Annu Rev Med 2003;54:153.

32. Lincoln TM, Cornell TL. Towards an understanding of the mechanism of action of cyclic AMP and cyclic GMP in smooth muscle relaxation. Blood Vessels 28;128:1991.

32A. Lue TF. Erectile dysfunction. N Engl J Med 2000;342:1802.

33. Burnett AL. Nitric oxide in the penis: physiology and pathology. J Urol 1997;157:320.

34. Bohlen JG et al. Heart rate, rate-pressure product, and oxygen uptake during four sexual activities. Arch Intern Med 1984;144:1745.

35. Drory Y et al. Myocardial ischemia during sexual activity in patients with coronary artery disease. Am J Cardiol 1995;75:835.

36. Johnson BL, Fletcher GF. Dynamic electrocardiographic recording during sexual activity in recent post-myocardial infarction and revascularization patients. Am Heart J 1979;98:736.

37. Jackson G. Sexual intercourse and angina pectoris. Int Rehabil Med 1981;3:35.

38. Muller JE et al. Triggering myocardial infarction by sexual activity: low absolute risk and prevention by regular physical exertion. Determinants of Myocardial Infarction Onset Study. JAMA 1996;275:1405.

39. Ueno M. The so-called coital death. Jpn J Leg Med 1963;17:330.

40. Padam-Nathan H et al. Evaluation of the impotent patient. Semin Urol 1986;4:225.

41. Whitehead ED et al. Diagnostic evaluation of impotence. Postgrad Med 1990;88:123.

41A. Goldstein I and The Working Group for the Study of Central Mechanisms in ED. Male sexual circuitry. Sci Am 2000;283:70.

42. Deutsch S et al. Previously unrecognized diabetes mellitus in sexually impotent men. JAMA 1980; 244:2430.

43. Spark RF et al. Hypogonadism, hyperprolactinaemia, and temporal lobe epilepsy in hyposexual men. Lancet 1984;1:413.

44. Gerstenberg TC, Bradly WE. Nerve conduction velocity measurement of dorsal nerve of the penis in normal and impotent men. J Urol 1985;21:90.

45. Spark RF et al. Impotence is not always psychogenic: newer insights into hypothalamic-pituitary-gonadal dysfunction. JAMA 1980;243:750.

46. Rubin A, Babbott D. Impotence and diabetes mellitus. JAMA 1958;168:498.

47. Bancroft J, Wu FCW. Changes in erectile responsiveness during androgen therapy. Arch Sex Behav 1983;12:59.

48. Michal V et al. Arterial lesions in impotence: phalloarteriography. Int Angiol 1984;3:247.

49. Rosen RC et al. The international index of erectile function (IIEF): a multidimensional scale for assessment of erectile dysfunction. Urology 1997; 49:822.

49A. Jardin A et al. Recommendations of the First International Consultation on Erectile Dysfunction. In: Jardin A et al, eds. Erectile Dysfunction. Plymouth: Plymbridge Distributors, 2000:711.

50. Spina M et al. Age-related changes in the composition of and mechanical properties of the tunica media of the upper thoracic human aorta. Arteriosclerosis 1983;3:64.

51. Smulyan H et al. Effect of age on arterial distensibility in asymptomatic humans. Arteriosclerosis 1983;3:199.

52. Wabrek AJ, Burchell RC. Male sexual dysfunction associated with coronary heart disease. Arch Sex Behav 1980;9:69.

53. Gundle MJ et al. Psychological outcome after aortocoronary artery surgery. Am J Psych 1980;137:1591.

54. Agarwal A, Jain DC. Male sexual dysfunction after stroke. J Assoc Physicians India 1989;37:505.

55. Ruzbarsky V, Michal V. Morphologic changes in the arterial bed of the penis with aging. Relationship to the pathogenesis of impotence. Invest Urol 1977;15:194.

56. Morley JE et al. Relationship of penile brachial pressure index to myocardial infarction and cerebrovascular accidents in older men. Am J Med 1988;84:445.

57. Virag R et al. Is impotence an arterial disorder? Lancet 1985;1:181.

58. Shabsigh R et al. Cigarette smoking and other vascular risk factors in vasculogenic impotence. Urology 1991;38:227.

59. Oaks WW, Moyer JH. Sex and hypertension. Med Aspects Hum Sex 1972;6:128.

60. Bulpitt CJ et al. Changes in symptoms of hypertensive patients after referral to hospital clinic. Br Heart J 1976;38:121.

61. Report of Medical Research Council Working Party on Mild to Moderate Hypertension. Adverse reaction to bendroflumethiazide and propranolol for the treatment of mild hypertension. Lancet 1981;2:539.

62. Veterans Administrative Cooperative Study Group on antihypertensive agents. Comparison of prazosin with hydralazine in patients receiving hydrochlorothiazide: a randomized double blind clinical trial. Circulation 1981;64:722.

63. Wabrek AJ et al. Noninvasive penile arterial evaluation in 120 males with erectile dysfunction. Urology 1983;22:230.

64. Condra M et al. Prevalence and significance of tobacco smoking in impotence. Urology 1986;27:495.

65. Hirshkowitz M et al. Nocturnal penile tumescence in cigarette smokers with erectile dysfunction. Urology 1992;34:101.

66. DePalma RG et al. A screening sequence for vasculogenic impotence. J Vasc Surg 1987;5:228.

67. Zemel P. Sexual dysfunction in the diabetic patient with hypertension. Am J Cardiol 1988;61:27H.

68. Rubin A, Babbott D. Impotence and diabetes mellitus. JAMA 1958;168:498.

69. Whitehead ED, Klyde BJ. Diabetes-related impotence in the elderly. Clin Geriatr Med 1990;6:771.

70. McCulloch DK et al. The prevalence of diabetic impotence. Diabetologia 1980;18:279.

71. Kannel W et al. The role of diabetes in congestive heart failure: the Framingham study. Am J Cardiol 1974;34:29.

72. Lehman TP, Jacobs JA. Etiology of diabetic impotence. Urology 1983;129:291.

73. Morley JE, Kaiser FE. Testicular function in the aging male. In: Armbrecht HJ, ed. Endocrine Function and Aging. New York: Springer-Verlag, 1989:456.

74. Morely JE et al. Sexual function with advancing age. Med Clin North Am 1989;73:1483.

75. Snyder PJ et al. Serum LH and FSH response to synthetic gonadotropins in normal men. J Clin Endocrinol Metab 1975;41:938.

76. Tenover JS et al. Decreased serum inhibin levels in normal elderly men: evidence for a decline in Ser-

toli cell function with aging. J Clin Endocrinol Metab 1988;67:455.

77. Kaiser FE et al. Impotence and aging: clinical and hormonal factors. J Am Geriatr Soc 1988;36:511.

78. Skakkeback N et al. Androgen replacement with oral testosterone in hypogonadal men: a double-blind controlled study. Clin Endocrinol (Oxf) 1981;14:49.

79. Bancroft J. Endocrinology of sexual function. Clin Endocrinol Metab 1980;4:253.

80. Davidson JM et al. Hormonal changes and sexual function in aging men. J Clin Endocrinol Metab 1983;57:71.

81. Morley JE. Impotence. Am J Med 1986;80:897.

82. Mooradian AD et al. Hyperprolactinemia in male diabetics. Postgrad Med J 1985;61:11.

83. Mirin SM et al. Opiate use and sexual function. Am J Psychiatry 1980;137:909.

84. McWaine DE, Procci WR. Drug-induced sexual dysfunction. Med Toxicol 1988;3:289.

85. Bissada NK, Finkbbeiner AE. Urologic manifestations of drug therapy. Urol Clin North Am 1988; 15:725.

86. Crenshaw TL, Goldberg JP. Sexual Pharmacology: Drugs That Affect Sexual Function. New York: WW Norton, 1996.

87. Morley JE. Impotence in older men. Hosp Pract 1988;23:139.

88. Wein AJ, Van Arsdalen KN. Drug-induced male dysfunction. Urol Clin North Am 1988;15:23.

89. Morley JE. Impotence. Am J Med 1986;80:897.

90. Whitehead ED et al. Treatment alternatives for impotence. Postgrad Med 1990;88:139.

90A. Scruti A et al. The effects of testosterone administration and visual erotic stimuli on nocturnal penile tumescence in normal men. Horm Behav 1990;24:435.

90B. Guay AT et al. Efficacy and safety of sildenafil for treatment of erectile dysfunction in a population with associated organic risk factors. J Androl 2001;22:793.

90C. Monga M et al. Patient satisfaction with testosterone supplementation for the treatment of erectile dysfunction. Arch Androl 2002;48(6):433.

90D. Lamberts SW, Quik RF. A comparison of the efficacy and safety of pergolide and bromocriptine in the treatment of hyperprolactinemia. J Clin Endocrinol Metab 1991;72:635.

91. Morley JE, Kaiser FE. Sexual function with advancing age. Med Clin North Am 1989;73:1483.

92. Yu Z et al. Transdermal testosterone administration in hypogonadal men: comparison of pharmacokinetics at different sites of application and at the first and fifth days of application. J Clin Pharmacol 1997;37:1129.

93. McCellan KJ, Goa KL. Transdermal testosterone. Drugs 1998;55:253.

94. Winters SJ. Current status of testosterone replacement therapy in men. Arch Fam Med 1999;8:257.

95. Parker S, Armitage M. Experience with transdermal testosterone replacement therapy for hypogonadal men. Clin Endocrinol (Oxf) 1999;50:57.

96. Gann PH et al. Prospective study of sex hormone levels and risk of prostate cancer. J Natl Cancer Inst 1996;88:1118.

97. Nomura A et al. Serum androgens and prostate cancer. Cancer Epidemiol Biomarkers Prev 1996;5:621.

98. Sih R et al. Testosterone replacement in older hypogonadal men: a 12 month randomized controlled trial. J Clin Endocrinol Metab 1997;82: 1661.

99. Hajjar R et al. Outcomes of long-term testosterone analysis. J Clin Endocrinol Metab 1997;82:3793.

100. Zgliczynski S et al. Effect of testosterone replacement therapy on lipids and lipoproteins in hypogonadal and elderly men. Atherosclerosis 1996; 121:35.

101. Morgentaler A et al. Occult prostate cancer in men with low serum testosterone levels. JAMA 1996;276:1904.

102. Rendell MS et al. Sildenafil for treatment of erectile dysfunction in men with diabetes: a randomized controlled trial. JAMA 1999;281:421.

103. Cheitlin MD et al. ACC/AHA Expert Consensus Document: use of sildenafil in patients with cardiovascular disease. J Am Cardiol 1999;33:273.

104. Goldstein I et al. Oral sildenafil in the treatment of erectile dysfunction. N Engl J Med 1998;538:1397.

105. Morales A et al. Clinical safety of oral sildenafil citrate (Viagra) in the treatment of erectile dysfunction. Int J Impot Res 1998;10:69.

106. Mitka M. Viagra leads as rivals are moving up. JAMA 1998;280:119.

106A. Cohen JS. Comparison of FDA reports of patient deaths associated with sildenafil and with injectable alprostadil. Ann Pharmacother 2001;35:285.

106B. Arruda-Olson AM. Mahoney DW. Nehra A. et al. Cardiovascular effects of sildenafil during exercise in men with known or probable coronary artery disease. A randomized crossover trial. JAMA 2002;287:719.

106C. Sadovsky R et al. Three-year update of sildenafil citrate efficacy and safety. Int J Clin Pract 2001; 3:196.

106D. Angulo J et al. Tadalafil enhances NO-mediated relaxation of human arterial and trabecular penile smooth muscle. Annual Meeting of the European Association for the Study of Diabetes; 2001;Glascow, Scotland [Abstract].

106E. Vickers MA, Satyanarayana R. Phosphodiesterase type 5 inhibitors for the treatment of erectile duysfunction in patients with diabetes mellitus. In J Impot Res 2002;14:466.

106F. Padma-Nathan H. Cialis™ (tadalafil) provides prompt response and extended period of responsiveness for the treatment of men with erectile dysfunction (ED). J Urol 2001;(Suppl):165:224.

106G. Porst H et al. The efficacy and tolerability of vardenafil, a new, oral, selective phosphodiesterase type 5 inhibitor, in patiens with erectile dysfunction: the first at home clinical trial. Int J Impot Res 2001;13:192.

106H. Steidle CP et al. Pharmacokientics of vardenafil in the elderly and subgroup data on efficacy and safety in elderly patients with erectile dysfunction [Abstract]. J Am Geriatr Soc 2001;49(4) S103.

106I. Thandani U et al. The effect of vardenafil, a potent and highly selective phosphodiesterase-5 inhibitor for the treatment or eretile dysfunction, on the cardiovascular response to exercise in patients with coronary disease. J Am Coll Cardiol 2002; 40(11):2006.

107. Morales A et al. Is yohimbine effective in the treatment of organic impotence? Results of a controlled trial. J Urol 1987;137:1168.

108. Morales A et al. Oral and transcutaneous pharmacological agents in the treatment of impotence. Urol Clin North Am 1988;15:87.

109. Reid K et al. Double blind trial of yohimbine in treatment of psychogenic impotence. Lancet 1987;2:421.

110. Lue T et al. Physiology of erection and pharmacological management of impotence. J Urol 1987; 137:829.

111. Carson CC, Mino RD. Priapism associated with trazodone therapy. J Urol 1988;139:369.

112. Nelson RP. Nonoperative management of impotence. J Urol 1988;139:2.

113. Sacerdote A et al. Recovery from diabetic impotence during improved diabetic control and inositol supplementation unassociated with improvement in bulbocavernous reflex latency. Diabetes 1985;34:204A.

114. Virag R. Intracavernous injection of papaverine for erectile failure. Lancet 1982;2:328.

115. Sidi AA et al. Intracavernous drug-induced erections in the management of male erectile dysfunction: experience with 100 patients. J Urol 1986; 135:704.

116. Brindley GS. Cavernosal alpha-blockade: a new technique for investigating and treating erectile impotence. Br J Psychiatry 1983;143:332.

117. Zorgniotti AW, Lefleur RS. Auto-injection of the corpus cavernosum with a vasoactive drug combination for vasculogenic impotence. J Urol 1985;133:39.

118. Nelson RP. Injections of papaverine and Regitine into the corpora cavernosa for erectile dysfunction: clinical results in 60 patients. South Med J 1989;82:26.

119. Watters GR et al. Experience in the management of erectile dysfunction using the intracavernosal self-injection of vasoactive drugs. J Urol 1988;140:1417.

120. Brading AF et al. The effects of papaverine on the electrical and mechanical activity of the guinea pig ureter. J Physiol 1983;334:79.

121. Huddart H et al. Inhibition by papaverine of calcium movements and tension in the smooth muscle of rats vas deferens and urinary bladder. J Physiol 1984;349:183.

122. Wang Q, Large WA. Modulation of noradrenaline-induced membrane currents by papaverine in rabbit vascular smooth muscle cells. J Physiol 1991;439:501.

123. Brindley GS. Neurophysiology of erection. In: Proceedings of the First World Meeting on Impotence. Paris, France: 1984:39.

124. Brindley GS. New treatment for priapism. Lancet 1984;2:220.

125. Juenemann KP et al. Hemodynamics of papaverine and phentolamine induced penile erection. J Urol 1986;136:158.

126. Juenemann KP et al. Further evidence of venous outflow restriction during erection. Br J Urol 1986;58:320.

127. Keogh E et al. Treatment of impotence by intrapenile injections: a comparison of papaverine versus papaverine and phentolamine: a double-blind crossover study. J Urol 1989;142:726.

128. Lue T et al. Functional evaluation of penile veins by cavernosography in papaverine induced erections. J Urol 1986;135:479.

129. Wespes E, Schulman C. Systemic complications of intracavernous papaverine injections in patients with venous leakage. Urology 1988;31:114.

130. Montorsi F et al. Effectiveness and safety of multidrug intra-cavernous therapy for vasculogenic impotence. Urology 1993;42:554.

131. Katlowitz N et al. Effect of multidose intracorporeal injection and audiovisual sexual stimulation in vasculogenic impotence. Urology 1993;42:695.

132. Nelson RP. Injections of papaverine and Regitine into the corpora cavernosa for erectile dysfunction: clinical results in 60 patients. South Med J 1989;82:26.

133. Eli Lilly and Company. Papaverine Hydrochloride USP Injection, package insert. Indianapolis, IN: 1994 April.

134. Ciba Pharmaceuticals. Phentolamine Mesylate USP package insert. Woodbridge, NJ: 1994 April.

135. Benson G, Seifert W. Is phentolamine stable in solution with papaverine? J Urol 1988;140:970.

136. Levine SB et al. Side-effects of self-administration of intracavernous papaverine and phentolamine for the treatment of impotence. J Urol 1989;141:54.

137. Larsen EH et al. Fibrosis of corpus cavernosum after intra-cavernous injection of phentolamine/ papaverine. J Urol 1987;137:292.

138. Malloy TR, Malkowicz B. Pharmacologic treatment of impotence. Urol Clin North Am 1987;14:297.

139. Abozeid M et al. Chronic papaverine treatment: the effect of repeated injections on the simian erectile and penile tissue. J Urol 1987;138:1263.

140. Fuchs M, Brawer M. Papaverine-induced fibrosis of the corpus cavernosum. J Urol 1989;141:125.

141. Girdley FM et al. Intracavernous self-injection for impotence: a long-term therapeutic option? Experience in 78 patients. J Urol 1988;140:972.

142. Keogh EJ et al. Treatment of impotence by intrapenile injections. A comparison of papaverine versus papaverine and phentolamine: a double-blind, crossover trial. J Urol 1989;142:726.

143. Zaher TF. Papaverine plus prostaglandin E₁ versus prostaglandin alone for intracorporeal injection therapy. Int Urol Nephrol 1998;30:193.

144. Kunelius P, Lukkarinen O. Intracavernous self-injection of prostaglandin E₁ in the treatment of erectile dysfunction. Int J Impot Res 1999;11:21.

144A. Steidle C et al. Topical alprostadil cream for the treatment of erectile dysfunction: a combined analysis of the phase II program. Urology 2002;60(6):1077.

145. Kaplan SA et al. Combination therapy using oral alpha-blockers and intracavernosal injection in men with erectile dysfunction. Urology 1998; 52:739.

146. Ishii N et al. Therapeutic trial with prostaglandin E₁ for organic impotence. Abstract presented at Second World Meeting on Impotence. Prague, Czechoslovakia, 1986.

147. Sarsody M et al. A prospective double-blind trial of intra-corporeal papaverine versus prostaglandin E₁ in the treatment of impotence. J Urol 1989;141:551.

148. Hedlund H, Andersson K. Contraction and relaxation induced by some prostanoids in isolated human penile erectile tissue and cavernous artery. J Urol 1985;134:1245.

148A. Hellstrom WJ. A double-blind placebo controlled evaluation of the erectile response to transurethral alprostadil. Urology 1996;48:851.

149. Walsh PC. Benign prostatic hyperplasia. In: Walsch PC et al, eds. Campbell's Urology, 5th Ed. Philadelphia: WB Saunders, 1986:1248.

150. Standberg JD. Comparative pathology of benign prostatic hypertrophy. In: Lepor H, Lawson RK, eds. Prostatic Diseases. Philadelphia: WB Saunders, 1993:212.

151. Berry SJ et al. The development of human benign prostatic hyperplasia with age. J Urol 1984;132:474.

152. Narayan P. Neoplasms of the prostate. In: Tanago EA, McAninch JW, eds. Smith's General Urology. Norwalk: Appleton & Lange, 1992:378.

153. Greenwald P et al. Cancer of the prostate among men with benign prostatic hyperplasia. J Natl Cancer Inst 1970;53:335.

154. Takahashi S et al. Latent prostatic carcinomas found at autopsy in men over 90 years old. Jap J Clin Oncol 1992;22(2):117.

155. Issacs JT, Coffey DS. Etiology and disease process of benign prostatic hyperplasia. Prostate Suppl 1989;2:34.

156. Lepor H. Medical therapy for benign prostatic hyperplasia. Urology 1993;42:483.

156A. Bartsch G et al. Dihydrotestosterone and the concept of 5-alpha reductase inhibition in human benign hyperplasia. Eur Urol 2000;37:367.

157. Hiramatsu M et al. Immunolocalization of oestrogen and progesterone receptors in prostatic hyperplasia and carcinoma. Histopathology 1996;28:163.

158. Boyarsky S et al. A new look at bladder neck obstruction by the Food and Drug Administration regulators: guidelines for the investigation of benign prostatic hypertrophy. Trans Am Assoc Genitourin Surg 1977;68:29.

159. Barry MJ et al. The American Urological Association symptom index for benign prostatic hyperplasia. J Urol 1992;148:1549.

160. Lepro H, Machi G. Comparison of AUA Symptom Index in unselected males and females between fifty-five and seventy nine years of age. Urology 1993;42:36.

161. Litwin M et al. The National Institutes of Health chronic prostatitis symptom index: development and validation of a new outcome measure. J Urol 1999;162:369.

162. DuBeau CE, Resnick NM. Controversies in the diagnosis and management of benign prostatic hypertrophy. Adv Intern Med 1991;37:55.

163. Dalkin BL et al. Prostate specific antigen levels in men older than 50 years without clinical evidence of prostatic carcinoma. J Urol 1993;150:1837.

164. Reissigl A et al. Comparison of different prostate-specific antigen cutpoints for early detection of prostate cancer: results of a large screening study. Urology 1995;46:662.

165. Borer JG et al. Age specific prostate-specific antigen reference ranges: population specific. J Urol 1998;159:444.

166. Slovacek KJ et al. Use of age-specific normal ranges for serum prostate-specific antigen. Arch Pathol Lab Med 1998;122:330.

167. Richardson TD, Osterling JE. Age-specific reference ranges for serum prostate-specific antigen. Urol Clin North Am 1997;24:339.

168. Ravel R. Laboratory aspects of cancer. In Ravel R, ed. Clinical Laboratory of Medicine, 6th Ed. St Louis: CV Mosby, 1995:566.

169. Talner LB. Specific causes of obstruction. In: Pollack HM, ed. Clinical Urology, 2nd Ed. Philadelphia: WB Saunders, 1990:1629.

170. Mushlin AI, Thornbury JR. Intravenous pyelography. The case against its routine. Ann Intern Med 1989;111:58.

171. Wasserman NF et al. Assessment of prostatism: role of intravenous urography. Radiology 1987;165:831.

172. Webb JAW. Ultrasonography in the diagnosis of renal obstruction. Sensitive but not very specific. Br J Med 1990;301:944.

173. Siroky MB et al. The flow rate nomogram: I. Development. J Urol 1979;122:665.

174. Haylen BT et al. Maximum and average urine flow rates in normal male and female populations. Br J Urol 1989;64:30.

175. Marshall VR et al. The use of urinary flow rates obtained from voided volumes less than 150 mL in the assessment of voiding ability. Br J Urol 1983;55:28.

176. Lepor H, Rigaud C. The efficacy of transurethral resection of the prostate in men with moderate symptoms of prostatism. J Urol 1990;143:533.

177. Kadow C et al. Prostatectomy or conservative management in the treatment of benign prostatic hypertrophy. Br J Urol 1988;61:432.

178. Bruskewitz RC et al. 3 year follow-up of urinary symptoms after transurethral resection of the prostate. J Urol 1989;142:1251.

179. Chancellor MB et al. Bladder outlet obstruction and impaired detrusor contractility: a blinded comparison of the video-urodynamic diagnosis versus the diagnosis based on a detrusor contractility parameter, a urethral resistant parameter, and a sustained/ fade index. Neurourol Urodyn 1990;9:209.

180. Fowler FJ et al. Symptom status and quality of life following prostatectomy. JAMA 1988;259:3018.

181. Bruskewitz RC, Christensen MM. Critical evaluation of transurethral resection and incision of the prostate. Prostate 1990;3:27.

182. Loughlin KR et al. Transurethral incisions and resection of the prostate under local anesthesia. Br J Urol 1987;60:105.

183. Orandi A. Transurethral incision of the prostate compared with transurethral resection of the prostate in 132 matching cases. J Urol 1987;138:810.

184. Keane PF et al. Balloon dilation of the prostate: technique and early results. Br J Urol 1990;65:354.

185. Marks LS. Serial endoscopy following visual laser ablation prostatectomy. Urology 1993;42:66.

186. Baert L et al. Transurethral microwave hyperthermia for benign prostatic hyperplasia: the Leuven clinical experience. J Endourol 1993;7:61.

187. Darson MF, Barret DM. Transurethral enzyme injection—future management of benign prostatic hyperplasia. Mayo Clin Proc 1998;73:908.

188. Lepor H. The role of alpha-adrenergic blockers in the treatment of benign prostatic hypertrophy. Prostate Suppl 1990;3:75.

189. Caine M. The present role of alpha-adrenergic blockers in the treatment of benign prostatic hypertrophy. J Urol 1986;136:1.

190. Lepor H. Nonoperative management of benign prostatic hypertrophy. J Urol 1989;141:1283.

191. Dunzendorfer U. Clinical experience: symptomatic management of BPH with terazosin. Urology 1988;32(Suppl):27.

191A. Kyprianou N. Doxazosin and terazosin suppress prostate growth by inducing apoptosis: clinical significance. J Urol 2003;169(4):1520.

192. Lepor H, Machi G. The relative efficacy of terazosin versus terazosin and flutamide for the treatment of symptomatic BPH. Prostate 1992;20:89.

193. Fulton B et al. Doxazosin: an update of its clinical pharmacology and therapeutic applications in hypertension and benign hyperplasia. Drugs 1995;49(2):295.

194. Pool JL. Doxazosin: a new approach to hypertension and benign prostatic hyperplasia. Br J Clin Pract 1996;50:154.

195. Taguchi K et al. Effects of tamsulosin metabolites at alpha-1 adrenoceptor subtypes. J Pharmacol Exp Ther 1997;280:1.

196. Chapple CR et al. Tamsulosin, the first prostate selective alpha-1a-adenoceptor antagonist—a meta analysis of two randomized, placebo controlled, multicenter studies in patients with benign prostatic obstruction. Eur Urol 1996;29:145.

197. Murayama K et al. Clinical evaluation of tamsulosin hydrochloride on bladder outlet obstruction associated with benign prostatic hyperplasia; effect on urethral pressure profile and cystometrogram. Hinyokika Kiyo 1997;43:799.

198. Kamimura H et al. Identification of cytochrome P450 involved in metabolism of the alpha-1 adrenoceptor blocker tamsulosin in human liver microsomes. Xenobiotica 1998;28:909.

199. Wolzt M et al. Pharmacokinetics of tamsulosin in subjects with normal and varying degrees of impaired renal function: an open-label single-dose and multiple-dose study. Eur J Clin Pharmacol 1998;54:367.

200. Narayan P. Tamsulosin: the United States trials. Geriatrics 1998;53:S29.

201. Isaacs JT et al. Changes in the metabolism of dihydrotestosterone in the hyperplastic human prostate. J Clin Endocrinol 1983;56:139.

202. DeKlerk DP, Coffey DS. Quantitative determination of prostatic epithelial and stromal hyperplasia by a new technique: biomorphometrics. Invest Urol 1978;16:240.

203. Matzkin H, Braf Z. Endocrine treatment of benign prostatic hypertrophy: current concepts. Urology 1991;37:1.

204. Wilson JP. The pathogenesis of benign prostatic hyperplasia. Am J Med 1980;68:745.

205. Bartsh W et al. Hormone blood levels and their interrelationships in normal men and men with benign prostatic hypertrophy. Acta Endocrinol 1979;90:727.

206. Ghanadian et al. Serum dihydrotestosterone in patients with benign prostatic hypertrophy. Br J Urol 1977;49:541.

207. Siiteri PK, Wilson JD. Dihydrotestosterone in prostatic hypertrophy, the formation and content of DHT in the hypertrophic prostate of man. J Clin Invest 1970;49:1737.

208. Bruchovsky N, Lieskovsky G. Increased ration of 5-alpha reductase: 3-alpha (Beta)-hydroxysteroid dehydrogenase activities in the hyperplastic human prostate. J Endocrinol 1979;80:289.

209. Habenicht UF et al. Development of a model for the induction of estrogen-related prostatic hyperplasia. Prostate 1986;6:181.

210. Geller J, Albert JD. BPH and prostate cancer: results of hormonal manipulation. In: Bruchovsky N et al, eds. Regulation of Androgen Action. Berlin: Conrgessdruck R. Bruckner, 1985:51.

211. Charisiri N, Pierrepoint CG. Examination of the distribution of estrogen receptor between the stromal and epithelial compartments of the prostate. Prostate 1980;1:357.

212. Feldman HA et al. Impotence and its psychological correlates: results of the Massachusetts male aging study. J Urol 1994;151:54.

213. DeKlerk DP et al. Comparison of spontaneous and experimentally induced canine prostatic hypertrophy. J. Clin Endocrinol Metab 1979;64:842.

214. McConnell JD et al. Finasteride, an inhibitor of 5 alpha-reductase, suppresses prostatic dihydrotestosterone in men with benign prostatic hyperplasia. J Clin Endocrinol Metab 1992;74:504.

214A. Lowe FC et al. Long-term 6-year experience with finasteride in patients with benign prostatic hyperplasia. Urology 2003;61(4):791.

215. Gormley GJ et al. The effect of finasteride in men with benign prostatic hyperplasia. The finasteride study group. N Engl J Med 1992;327:1185.

216. Stoner E et al. Maintenance of clinical efficacy with finasteride therapy for 24 months in patients with benign prostatic hyperplasia. Arch Intern Med 1994;83:154.

216A. Weeslls H. et al. Incidence and severity of sexual adverse prostatic hyperplasia. Urol 2003;61(3):579.

217. Abrams P et al. Improvement of pressure flow parameters with finasteride is greater in men with large prostates. Urology 1999;161:1513.

218. Anon. Finasteride for benign prostatic hypertrophy. Med Lett Drugs Ther 1992;34:83.

219. MK-906C Finasteride Study Group. One year experience in the treatment of benign prostatic hyperplasia with finasteride. J Androl 1991;12:372.

220. Yang XJ et al. Does long-term finasteride therapy affect the histological features of benign prostatic tissue and prostate cancer on needle biopsy? PLESS Study Group (Proscar Long-Term Efficacy and Safety Study). Urology 1999;53:696.

221. Montironi R et al. Treatment of benign prostatic hyperplasia with 5-alpha-reductase inhibitor: morphological changes in patients who fail to respond. J Clin Pathol 1996;49:324.

221A. Roehrborn C et al. Efficacy and safety of a dual inhibitor of 5-alpha-reductase types 1 and 2 (dutasteride) in men with benign prostatic hyperplasia. Urology 2002;60:434.

222. Caine M et al. The treatment of benign prostatic hypertrophy with flutamide (SCH 13521): a placebo-controlled study. J Urol 1975;114:564.

223. Stone NN. Flutamide in treatment of benign prostatic hypertrophy. Urology 1989;34(Suppl):64.

224. Wysowski DK, Fourcroy JL. Flutamide hepatotoxicity. J Urol 1996;155:209.

225. Eri LM, Tveter KJ. A prospective placebo controlled study of the luteinizing hormone releasing hormone agonist leuprolide as a treatment for patients with benign prostatic hyperplasia. J Urol 1993;150:359.

226. Keane PF et al. Response of the benign hypertrophied prostate to treatment with an LHRH analogue. Br J Urol 1988;62:163.

227. Oesterling JE. Prostate specific antigen: a critical assessment of the most useful tumor marker for adenocarcinoma of the prostate. J Urol 1991;145:907.

228. Guess HA et al. The effect of finasteride on prostate specific antigen in men with benign prostatic hyperplasia. Prostate 1992;22:31.

229. Lepor H. Medical therapy for benign prostatic hyperplasia. Urology 1993;42:483.

229A. Descotes JL et al. Placebo-controlled evaluation of the efficacy and tolerabilty of permixon in benign prostatic hyperplasia. Clin Drug Invest 1995;9:291.

229B. Carbin BE et al. Treatment of benign prostatic hyperplasia with phytosterols. Br J Urol 1990;66:639.

229C. Bayne CW et al. Serenoa repens: a 5 alpha-reductase type I and II inhibitor—new evidence in a coculture model of BPH. Prostate 1999;40:232.

229D. Gordon AE, Shaughnessy AF. Saw palmetto for prostate disorders. Am Fam Physician 2003;67(6):1281.

229E. Carraro JC et al. Comparison of phytotherapy (Permixon) with finasteride in the treatment of benign prostate hyperplasia: a randomized international study of 1,098 patients. Prostate 1996;29:231.

230. Ouslander JG et al. Urinary incontinence in elderly nursing home patients. JAMA 1982;248:1194.

231. Mohide EA. The prevalence and scope of urinary incontinence. Clin Geriatr Med 1986;2:639.

232. Thomas TM et al. Prevalence of urinary incontinence. Br J Med 1980;281:1243.

233. Marron et al. The nonuse of urethral catheterization in the management of urinary incontinence in the teaching nursing home. J Am Geriatr Soc 1983;31:278.

234. Colling J et al. The effects of patterned urge-response toileting (PURT) on urinary incontinence among nursing home residents. J Am Geriatr Soc 1992;40:135.

235. Gosling JA, Chilton CP. The anatomy of the bladder, urethra, and pelvic floor. In: Mundy AR et al, eds. Urodynamics: Principles, Practice, and Application. New York: Churchill Livingstone, 1984:3.

236. Resnick NM, Yalla SV. Management of urinary incontinence in the elderly. N Engl J Med 1985; 313:800.

237. Rud T. Urethral pressure profile in continent women from childhood to old age. Acta Obstet Gynecol Scand 1980;59:331.

238. Jones KW, Schoenberg HW. Comparison of the incidence of bladder hyperreflexia in patients with benign prostatic hypertrophy and age-matched female controls. J Urol 1985;133:425.

239. Ouslander JG et al. Genitourinary dysfunction in a geriatric outpatient population. J Am Geriatr Soc 1986;34:507.

240. Castleden CM et al. Clinical and urodynamic studies in 100 elderly incontinent patients. Br J Med 1981;282:1103.

241. Overstall PW et al. Experience with an incontinence clinic. J Am Geriatr Soc 1980;28:535.

242. Ouslander JG, Bruskewitz R. Disorders of micturition in the aging patient. Adv Intern Med 1989;34:165.

243. Resnick NM. Voiding dysfunction in the elderly. In: Yalla SV et al, eds. Principles and Practice of Urodynamics and Neuro-Urology. New York: Macmillan, 1986:180.

244. Marshall HJ, Beevers DG. Alpha-adrenoceptor blocking drugs and female urinary incontinence: prevalence and reversibility. Br J Clin Pharmacol 1996;42:507.

245. Menefee SA et al. Stress urinary incontinence due to prescription medications: alpha-blockers and angiotensin converting enzyme inhibitors. Obstet Gynecol 1998;91:853.

246. Dwyer PL, Teele JS. Prazosin: a neglected cause of genuine stress incontinence. Obstet Gynecol 1992;79:117.

247. Montejo-Gonzales AL et al. SSRI-induced sexual dysfunction: fluoxetine, paroxetine, sertraline and fluvoxamine in a prospective, multicenter, and descriptive clinical study of 344 patients. J Sex Marital Ther 1997;23:176.

248. Crenshaw TL, Goldber JP. Sexual pharmacology: drugs that affect sexual function. New York: WW Norton, 1996.

249. Mandel FP et al. Biological effects of various doses of vaginally administered conjugated equine estrogens in postmenopausal women. J Clin Endocrinol Metab 1983;57:133.

249A. Writing Group for The Women's Health Initiative Investigators. Risks and benefits of estrogen plus progestin in healthy postmenopausal women: principal results from the Women's Health Initiative randomized controlled trial. JAMA 2002; 288:321.

250. Ouslander JG. Causes, assessment, and treatment of incontinence in the elderly. Urology 1990; 36(Suppl):25.

251. Mushkat Y et al. Female urinary stress incontinence—does it have familial prevalence? Am J Obstet Gynecol 1996;174:617.

252. Blaivas JG et al. The bulbocavernous reflex in urology: a prospective study of 299 patients. J Urol 1981;126:197.

253. Jensen D Jr. Pharmacological studies of the uninhibited neurogenic bladder. Acta Neurol Scand 1981;64:175.

254. Blaivas J et al. Cystometric response to propantheline in detrusor hyperreflexia: therapeutic implications. J Urol 1980;124:259.

254A. Product Information for Oxytrol. Watson Pharmaceuticals. Corona, CA 92880. February 14, 2003.

254B. Davila GW et al. A short-term, multicenter, randomized double-blind dose titration study of the efficacy and anticholinergic side effects of transdermal compared to immediate release oral oxybutynin treatment of patients with urge urinary incontinence. J Urol 2001;166:140.

255. Brown JH. Atropine, scopolamine and related antimuscarinic drugs. In: Gilman AG et al, eds. Goodman and Gilman's The Pharmacological Basis of Therapeutics. New York: Pergamon Press, 1990:150.

256. Wein AJ. Pharmacological treatment of incontinence. J Am Geriatr Soc 1990;38:317.

257. Moisey CU et al. The urodynamic and subjective results of the treatment of detrusor instability with oxybutynin chloride. Br J Urol 1980;52:472.

258. Hehir M, Fitzpatrick JM. Oxybutynin and the prevention of urinary incontinence in spina bifida. Eur Urol 1985;11:254.

259. Gajewski JB, Awad JA. Oxybutynin versus propantheline in patients with multiple sclerosis and detrusor hyperreflexia. Urology 1986;135: 966.

260. Goldenberg MM. An extended-release formulation of oxybutynin chloride for the treatment of overactive urinary bladder. Clin Ther 1999;21:634.

261. Gleason DM et al. Evaluation of a new once-daily formulation of oxybutynin for the treatment of urinary urge incontinence. Ditropan XL Study Group. Urology 1999;54:420.

262. Millard R et al. Clinical efficacy and safety of tolterodine compared to placebo in detrusor overactivity. J Urol 1999;161:1551.

263. Hills JC et al. Tolterodine. Drugs 1998;55:813.

264. Guay DR. Tolterodine, a new antimuscarinic drug for treatment of bladder overactivity. Pharmacotherapy 1999;19:267.

265. Levin RM et al. The muscarinic cholinergic binding kinetics of the human urinary bladder. Neurourol Urodyn 1982;1:122.

266. Marion Merrel Dow. Bentyl package insert. Kansas City, MO: 1994 April.

267. Norlen L et al. Beta-adrenoceptor stimulation of the human urinary bladder in vivo. Acta Pharmacol Toxicol 1981;43:5.

268. Castleden CM et al. Imipramine—a possible alternative to current therapy for urinary incontinence in the elderly. J Urol 1981;125:218.

269. Hollister LE. Current antidepressants. Ann Rev Pharmacol Toxicol 1986;26:23.

270. Baldessarini RJ. Drugs and the treatment of psychiatric disorders. In: Gilman AG et al, eds. Goodman and Gilman's The Pharmacological Basis of Therapeutics. New York: Pergamon Press, 1990:383.

271. Levin RM et al. Analysis of the anticholinergic and musculotropic effects of desmethylimipramine on the rabbit urinary bladder. Urol Res 1983;11:259.

272. Gilja I et al. Conservative treatment of female stress incontinence with imipramine. J Urol 1984;132:909.

273. Abernethy DR et al. Imipramine and desipramine disposition in the elderly. J Pharmacol Exp Ther 1985;232:183.

274. Ray WA et al. Psychotropic drug use and the risk of hip fracture. N Engl J Med 1987;316:363.

275. Wein AJ, Barrett DM. Voiding function and dysfunction: a logical and practical approach. Chicago: Year Book Medical Publishers, 1988:195.

276. Hoffman BB, Lefkowitz RJ. Catecholamines and sympathomimetic drugs. In: Gilman AG et al, eds. Goodman and Gilman's The Pharmacological Basis of Therapeutics. New York: Pergamon Press, 1990:187.

277. Awad S et al. Alpha-adrenergic agents in urinary disorders of the proximal urethra: 1. Stress incontinence. Br J Urol 1978;50:332.

278. SmithKline Beecham. Ornade Spansule, package insert. Philadelphia, PA: 1994.

279. Younglove RH et al. Medical management of unstable bladder. J Reprod Med 1980;24:215.

280. Lasagna L. Phenylpropanolamine—A Review. New York: John Wiley & Sons, 1988:191.

281. Gibson A. The influence of endocrine hormones on the autonomic nervous system. J Auton Pharmacol 1981;1:331.

282. Batra SC, Iosif CS. Female urethra: a target for estrogen action. J Urol 1983;129:418.

282A. Lepor H, Theune C. Randomized double-blind study comparing the efficacy of terazosin versus placebo in women with prostatism-like symptoms. J Urol 1995;154:116.

282B. Sivkov AV et al. Use of alpha 1-adrenergic blockers in voiding disorders in women. Urologiia 2002;5(Suppl):52(Abstract).

283. MRC Working Party on Mild to Moderate Hypertension. Adverse reactions to bendroflumethiazide and propranolol for the treatment of hypertension. Lancet 1981;2:539.

284. Bulbitt DJ, Fletcher AE. Drug treatment and quality of life in the elderly. Clin Geriatr Med 1990;6:309.

285. Bauer GE et al. Side-effects of antihypertensive treatment: a placebo-controlled study. Clin Sci Mol Med 1978;55:341s.

286. Bulpitt CJ, Dollery CT. Side-effects of hypotensive agents evaluated by self-administered questionnaire. Am J Cardiol 1973;3:485.

287. Hogan MJ et al. Antihypertensive therapy and male sexual dysfunction. Psychosomatics 1981; 21:234.

288. Mallett EC, Badlani GH. Sexuality in the elderly. Semin Urol 1987;5:141.

289. Zarren HS, Black PM. Unilateral gynecomastia and impotence during low dose spironolactone administration in men. Milit Med 1975;140:417.

290. Ebringer A et al. The use of clonidine in the treatment of hypertension. Lancet 1970,1:524.

291. Laver MC. Sexual behavior patterns in male hypertensives. Aust NZ J Med 1974;4:29.

292. Onesti G et al. Clonidine: a new antihypertensive agent. Am J Cardiol 1971;28:74.

293. Burnett WG, Chamine RA. Sexual dysfunction as a complication of propranolol therapy in men. Cardiovasc Med 1979;4:811.

294. Buffum J. Pharmacosexology: the effects of drugs on sexual function: a review. J Psychoactive Drugs 1982;14:5.

295. Troutman WG. Drug-induced sexual dysfunction. In: Knoben JE, Anderson PO, eds. Handbook of Clinical Drug Data, 6th Ed. Hamilton, IL: Drug Intelligence Publications, 1988:112.

296. Amery A et al. Double-blind crossover study with a new vasodilator—prazosin—in the treatment of mild hypertension. Excerpta Medica International Congress Series 1974;331:100.

297. Van Arsdalen KN, Wein AJ. Drug induced sexual dysfunction in older men. Geriatrics 1984;39:63.

298. Caine M et al. Phenoxybenzamine for benign prostatic obstruction. Urology 1981;17:542.

299. Buffum JC. Pharmacosexology update: heroin and sexual function. J Psychoactive Drugs 1983;15:317.

300. Beeley L. Drug-induced sexual dysfunction and infertility. Adverse Drug React Acute Poisoning Rev 1984;3:23.

301. Longe RL, Calvert JC. Physical Assessment: A Guide for Evaluating Drug Therapy. Vancouver, WA: Applied Therapeutics, 1994.

302. Ferri FF, Fretwell MD. Practical Guide to the Care of the Geriatric Patient. St. Louis: CVMosby, 1992.

Page numbers in *italics* denote figures; those followed by a t denote tables.

Dobutamine (continued)
for cardiogenic shock, 22-18, 22-20–22-21, 22-27
for echocardiographic stress imaging study, 17-9
effects on hemodynamics, 22-21
for heart failure, 19-16, 19-55, 19-56, 19-59, 19-60
receptor sensitivity and pharmacologic effect, 22-19t
for septic shock, 22-32–22-33

Docetaxel
adverse effects
emesis, 8-11, 8-11t
hypersensitivity reactions, 89-18t
neurotoxicity, 89-20t, 89-21
for breast cancer, 91-6
clinical pharmacology, 88-18t
for lung cancer, 88-25t, 91-14
for ovarian cancer, 91-15
for prostate cancer, 91-21

Docosanol, for herpes infection, 72-7
Docusate, in pregnancy, 46-10
Dofetilide
for atrial fibrillation, 20-11, 20-13
classification, antiarrhythmic, 20-6t
drug interactions, 20-11
heart failure caused by, 19-19

Dolasetron, for emesis, 10-25, 10-27t, 10-28
chemotherapy-induced, 8-12t
postoperative, 8-7t
radiation-induced, 8-8

Dolobid. (see Diflunisal)
Dolophine. (see Methadone)
Domperidone
for anorexia nervosa, 82-16
effect on TSH and TRH, 49-10
for gastroesophageal reflux in infants, 93-10

Donepezil HCl
for Alzheimer's disease, 100-7t, 100-8, 100-9
for anxiety, in dementia, 100-14
for vascular dementia, 100-13

Dopamine
for acute tubular necrosis, 31-12
for cardiogenic shock, 22-18–22-20, 22-27
effects on hemodynamics, 22-20
for heart failure, 19-16, 19-55, 19-59
receptor sensitivity and pharmacologic effect, 22-19t
for septic shock, 22-32
structure of, 53-7

Dopamine agonists
for Parkinson's disease, 53-2, 53-4, 53-5t, 53-6, 53-7–53-12
pharmacologic and pharmacokinetic properties of, 53-7t
structure of, 53-7

Doral. (see Quazepam)
Dornase alfa, for cystic fibrosis, 98-9
Dorzolamide
adverse effects, 51-11
for glaucoma, 51-5, 51-9t

Doxacurium
adverse effects, 10-14, 10-14t
classification, 10-14t
elimination, 10-16t, 10-17

pharmacokinetic/pharmacodynamic properties, 10-16t

Doxapram
adverse effects, 94-38
for apnea in neonates, 94-38

Doxazosin
for benign prostatic hyperplasia, 3-19, 101-22
for hypertension, 6-11t, 14-14, 14-15–14-16, 14-39–14-40, 14-40t
in renal disease, 32-20
in vascular dementia, 100-13
sexual dysfunction and, 101-5t

Doxepin
adverse effects, 79-13t
for headache, 52-24
for insomnia, 83-9
in lactation, 79-18
orthostatic hypotension and, 79-26
for pain
chronic, 9-25
neuropathic, 9-30
pharmacology of, 79-12t
for pruritus, 38-13
for sleep disorders, 77-14

Doxercalciferol, for secondary hyperparathyroidism, 32-25–32-26
Doxil. (see Doxorubicin)
Doxorubicin
for acute lymphoblastic leukemia, 90-33
adverse effects
cardiotoxicity, 89-22–89-24, 91-27
emesis, 8-10
extravasation, 89-15, 89-16t
hand-foot syndrome, 89-12
heart failure, 19-5
hypersensitivity reactions, 89-18t
infertility, 89-34
ocular, 51-15t
radiation reactions, 89-13
for bladder cancer, 91-16
for breast cancer, 88-24t, 91-4, 91-6
clinical pharmacology, 88-18t
for gastric cancer, 88-25t
for Hodgkin's lymphoma, 88-26t, 90-17
for Kaposi's sarcoma, 70-41
liposomal, 88-18t
for multiple myeloma, 88-26t, 90-18, 90-19t, 90-20
for neuroblastoma, 91-24–91-25, 91-24t, 91-25t
for non-Hodgkin's lymphoma, 70-42, 88-26t, 90-14–90-15
for osteosarcoma, 91-28
for ovarian cancer, 91-15
for rhabdomyosarcoma, 91-29
for Wilms' tumor, 91-27

Doxycycline
for acne, 39-7
bile concentration, 63-3t
for bite wounds, 67-9
for *Borrelia burgdorferi,* 56-13t
for bronchitis, 60-4
for *Chlamydia,* 56-13t
for chronic obstructive pulmonary disease (COPD), 24-12, 24-23

dosage for respiratory tract infections, 60-11t
for ehrlichiosis, 75-13
for endemic relapsing fever, 75-10
for enterococcal endocarditis, 59-19
for gonorrhea, 65-3, 65-5, 65-7, 65-9t
for *Legionella,* 56-12t
for Lyme disease, 75-5, 75-5t, 75-7
for lymphogranuloma venereum, 65-12
for malaria, 74-6, 74-7
for *Moraxella catarrhalis,* 56-12t
for *Mycoplasma,* 56-13t
for nongonococcal urethritis, 65-11
for pediatric infections, 96-7t
for pelvic inflammatory disease, 65-6t, 65-8, 65-9
phototoxicity, 75-7
for pneumonia, 60-9, 60-20t
for Rocky Mountain Spotted Fever, 75-15
for septic arthritis, 66-12
for *Streptococcus pneumoniae,* 56-11t
for syphilis, 65-15t, 65-16
for *Treponema pallidum,* 56-13t
for urinary tract infections, 64-5t, 64-11
for *Vibrio cholerae* diarrhea, 62-7
for *Vibrio parahaemolyticus* diarrhea, 62-7

Doxylamine, 76-6t
D-penicillamine. (see Penicillamine)
Dramamine. (see Dimenhydrinate)
Drixoral. (see Dexbrompheniramine)
Dronabinol, 83-17
for emesis, 8-3t, 8-15
for HIV wasting syndrome, 70-39, 70-39t

Droperidol
for emesis, 8-3, 9-34, 10-26t
chemotherapy-induced, 8-13t, 8-16
postoperative, 8-6–8-8, 8-7t
for opioid-induced nausea, 9-34

Drospirenone, 45-2, 45-5t
Drotrecogin α, for septic shock, 22-34–22-35
DTIC-Dome. (see Dacarbazine)
DTP vaccines, 95-2t, 95-3t, 95-4–95-5
Dulcolax. (see Bisacodyl)
Duloxetine, 79-21
DuoDERM, 41-18
Duramorph. (see Morphine)
Duramycin, for cystic fibrosis, 98-13
Duranest. (see Etidocaine)
Duricef. (see Cefadroxil)
Dutasteride, for benign prostatic hyperplasia, 101-23
Duteplase. (see Tissue plasminogen activator)
Dyazide. (see Triamterene-hydrochlorothiazide)
Dyclonine, for mucositis/stomatitis, 89-7t, 89-8
Dymelor. (see Acetohexamide)
DynaCirc. (see Isradipine)
Dynapen. (see Dicloxacillin)
Dyrenium. (see Triamterene)

EACA (epsilon aminocaproic acid), 55-17
Echinacea, 3-15–3-18
adverse effects, 3-17
for allergic rhinitis, 25-24
anti-infective effects, 3-18
for cold prevention, 3-17, 72-18
for cold treatment, 3-16
drug interactions, 35-37
for hematologic recovery after chemotherapy, 3-17–3-18
in immune deficiency, 3-17
indications and dosing, 3-2t
mechanism of action, 3-16–3-17
pharmacokinetics and dosing, 3-17
in pregnancy, 47-27
preparations, 3-15–3-16
for wound healing, 3-18

Echothiophate iodide, for glaucoma, 51-7, 51-10t
Edrophonium, for neuromuscular blockade reversal, 10-15
Efavirenz
adverse effects, 56-17t, *69-15*
characteristics, 69-8t
contraindications, 69-19t
drug interactions, 61-20–61-21, 61-21t, 69-19t, 69-21t, 70-29, 70-31t
for HIV, initial therapy, 69-18t
resistance mutations, *69-26*
site of activity, *69-3*

Effexor. (see Venlafaxine)
EGFR (epidermal growth factor receptor) inhibitors, adverse effects, 89-12–89-13
Elavil. (see Amitriptyline)
Eldepryl. (see Selegiline)
Electrolytes, in parenteral nutrition, 37-12, 37-12t
Eletriptan
drug interactions, 52-9–52-10
for headache, 52-4, 52-8t, 52-9–52-10

Elimite. (see Permethrin)
Elitek. (see Rasburicase)
Ellence. (see Epirubicin)
Eloxatin. (see Oxaliplatin)
Elspar. (see L-asparaginase)
Emadine. (see Emedastine)
Emcyt. (see Estramustine)
Emedastine, for allergic conjunctivitis, 25-17, 25-17t, 51-17
Emergency contraceptive pills, 45-23–45-24
Emetine for amebiasis, 74-9, 74-10
Emetrol. (see Phosphorated carbohydrate solution)
Eminase. (see Anistreplase)
EMLA topical anesthetic cream, 93-15–93-16
Emtricitabine
adverse effects, 56-17t
characteristics, 69-7t

Emtriva. (see Emtricitabine)
E-Mycin. (see Erythromycin)
Enalapril
drug interactions, 19-39
for heart failure, 19-27–19-30, 19-31t, 19-32, 19-33, 19-35, 76-8
for hypertension, 14-28, 14-31t
in intermittent claudication, 15-7

Page numbers in *italics* denote figures; those followed by a t denote tables.

LIVERPOOL
JOHN MOORES UNIVERSITY
AVRIL ROBARTS LRC
TITHEBARN STREET
LIVERPOOL L2 2ER
TEL 0151 231 4022